CANCER
Principles & Practice
of Oncology

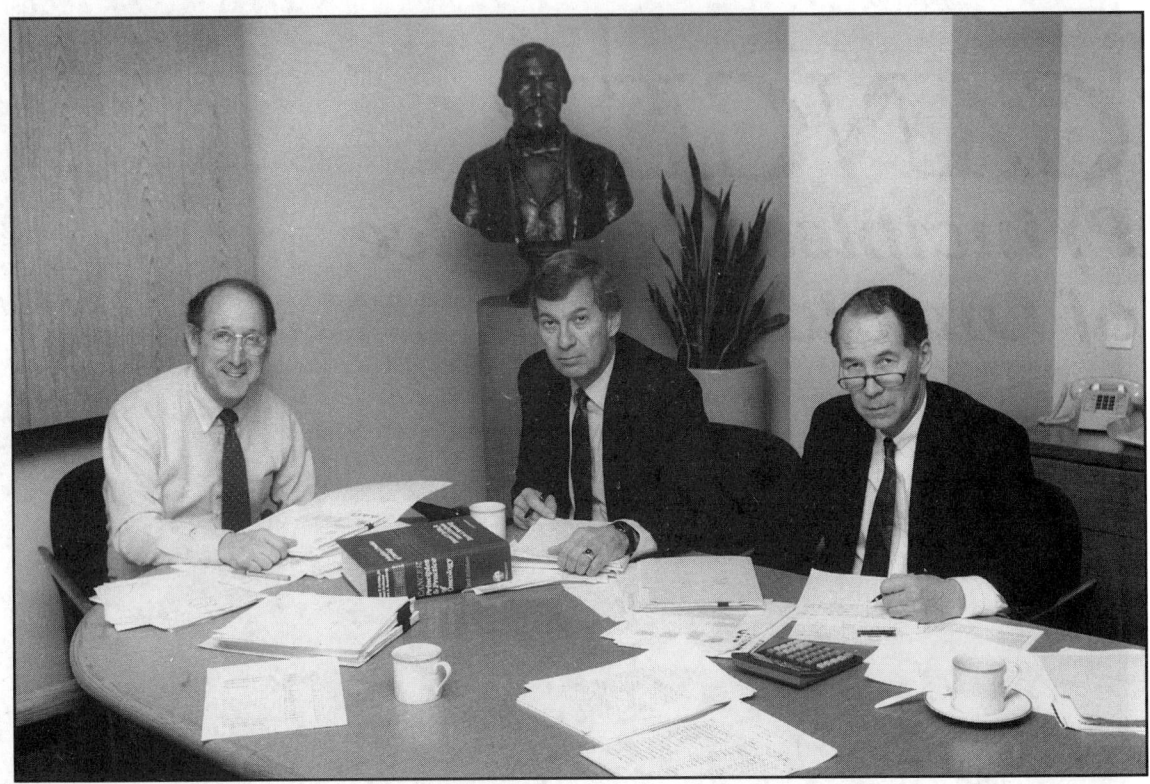

EDITED BY

Vincent T. DeVita, Jr., MD
Director, Yale Comprehensive Cancer Center, Professor of Medicine,
Yale University School of Medicine, New Haven, Connecticut

Samuel Hellman, MD
Dean, Division of the Biological Sciences and The Pritzker School of Medicine,
Vice President for the Medical Center, The University of Chicago,
Chicago, Illinois

Steven A. Rosenberg, MD, PhD
Chief of Surgery, National Cancer Institute, Professor of Surgery, Uniformed
Services University of the Health Sciences School of Medicine,
Bethesda, Maryland

214 Contributors

CANCER
Principles & Practice of Oncology

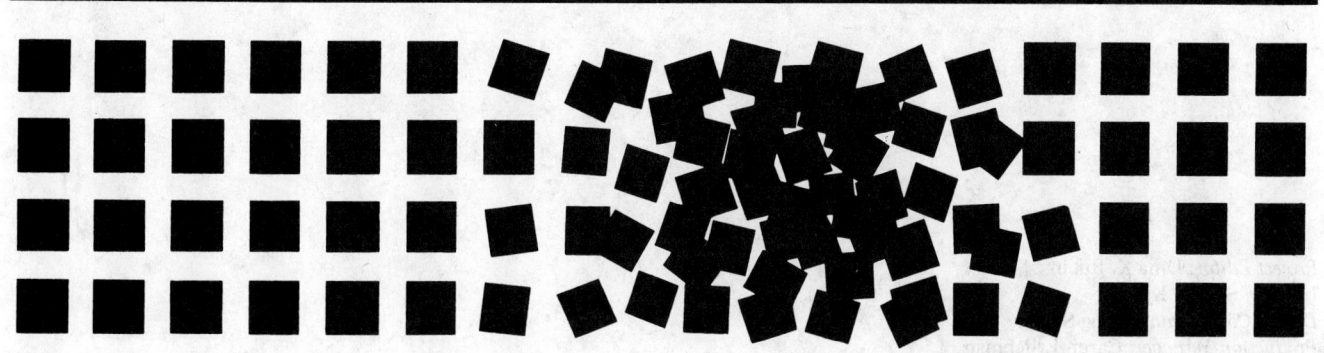

4th Edition

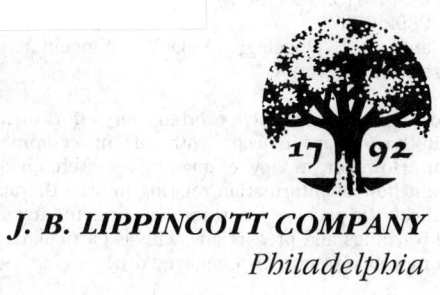

J. B. LIPPINCOTT COMPANY
Philadelphia

Project Editor: Dina K. Rubin
Indexer: Sandra King
Design Coordinator: Doug Smock
Production Manager: Caren Erlichman
Production Coordinator: Sharon McCarthy
Compositor: Tapsco Incorporated
Printer/Binder: Courier Book Company/Westford
Color Insert Printer: Village Craftsmen/Princeton Polychrome Press

4th Edition

6 5 4 3 2

Library of Congress Cataloging in Publications Data

Cancer: principles and practice of oncology/[edited by] Vincent T. DeVita, Jr., Samuel Hellman,
  Steven A. Rosenberg; 214 contributors.—4th ed.
    p.   cm.
  Includes bibliographical references.
  Includes index.
  ISBN 0-397-51214-7 (one-vol. ed.)
  ISBN 0-397-51321-6 (two-vol. set)
  ISBN 0-397-51322-4 (vol. 1)
  ISBN 0-397-51323-2 (vol. 2)
  ISSN 0892-0567
    1. Cancer. 2. Oncology. I. DeVita, Vincent T., Jr. II. Hellman, Samuel.
  III. Rosenberg, Steven A.

The authors and publisher have exerted every effort to ensure that drug selection and dosage
set forth in this text are in accord with current recommendations and practice at the time of
publication. However, in view of ongoing research, changes in government regulations, and
the constant flow of information relating to drug therapy and drug reactions, the reader is
urged to check the package insert for each drug for any change in indications and dosage and
for added warnings and precautions. This is particularly important when the recommended
agent is a new or infrequently employed drug.

Dedicated to

Mary Kay
Rusty
Alice

CONTRIBUTORS

Daniel M. Albert, MD
Frederick Davis Professor and Chairman, Department of Ophthalmology, University of Wisconsin Medical School, Madison, Wisconsin

H. Richard Alexander, MD
Clinical Assistant Professor of Surgery, Uniformed Services University of the Health Sciences, Senior Investigator, Surgery Branch, National Cancer Institute, National Institutes of Health, Bethesda, Maryland

Michael Andreeff, MD, PhD
Professor of Medicine, University of Texas Medical School, Chief, Section of Leukemia, Chief, Section of Experimental Hematology, The University of Texas M.D. Anderson Cancer Center, Houston, Texas

Karen H. Antman, MD
Associate Professor, Dana-Farber Cancer Institute, Harvard Medical School, Boston, Massachusetts

John G. Armstrong, MD, MRCPI
Assistant Professor of Radiation Oncology in Medicine, Cornell University Medical College, Assistant Attending, Memorial Sloan-Kettering Cancer Center, New York, New York

Mary Austin-Seymour, MD
Associate Professor, Department of Radiation Oncology, University of Washington, Seattle, Washington

Alan R. Baker, MD
Senior Investigator, Surgery Branch, National Cancer Institute, Bethesda, Maryland

Charles M. Balch, MD
Professor and Head, Division of Surgery, Professor of Immunology, Chairman, Department of General Surgery, Associate Chairman, Department of Surgery, University of Texas Medical School at Houston, Houston, Texas

Renato Baserga, MD
Professor of Microbiology and Immunology, Thomas Jefferson University, Deputy Director, Jefferson Cancer Center, Philadelphia, Pennsylvania

Clair J. Beard, MD
Instructor, Harvard Medical School, Attending, Joint Center for Radiation Therapy, Boston, Massachusetts

Colin B. Begg, MD
Chairman, Department of Epidemiology and Biostatistics, Memorial Sloan-Kettering Cancer Center, Professor of Biostatistics, Cornell University Medical College, New York, New York

Nathan A. Berger, MD
Professor of Medicine, Biochemistry and Oncology, Chief, Hematology and Oncology Division, Director, Ireland Cancer Center, University Hospitals of Cleveland, Case Western Reserve University, Cleveland, Ohio

Leslie Bernstein, PhD
Professor of Preventive Medicine, Norris Comprehensive Cancer Center, University of Southern California, Los Angeles, California

Georg A. Bjarnason, MD
Assistant Professor, Department of Medicine, Assistant Professor of Clinical Pharmacology, University of Toronto, Attending Physician, Toronto-Bayview Regional Cancer Centre, Toronto, Ontario, Canada

Alan Blum, MD, FAAFP
Associate Professor, Department of Family Medicine, Baylor College of Medicine, Houston, Texas

Gianni Bonadonna, MD
Professor of Hematology, University of Milan School of Medicine, Director, Department of Medicine, Istituto Nazionale Tumori, Milan, Italy

Murray F. Brennan, MD
Professor of Surgery, Cornell University, Chairman, Department of Surgery, Alfred P. Sloan Chair in Surgery, Memorial Sloan-Kettering Cancer Center, New York, New York

Frank J. Brescia, MD, MA

Clinical Assistant Professor, Department of Medicine, Clinical Assistant Professor, Department of Community and Preventive Medicine, New York Medical College, Visiting Assistant Professor of Medicine, Albert Einstein College of Medicine, Adjunct Professor, Department of Philosophy, Georgetown University, Medical Director, Calvary Hospital, Bronx, New York

Samuel Broder, MD

Director, National Cancer Institute, Bethesda, Maryland

Jan C. Buckner, MD

Associate Professor of Oncology, Mayo Graduate School of Medicine, Mayo Clinic, Rochester, Minnesota

Paul A. Bunn, Jr, MD

Professor of Medicine, Director, University of Colorado Cancer Center, Head, Division of Medical Oncology, University Hospital, Denver, Colorado

Julie E. Buring, ScD

Associate Professor, Department of Preventive Medicine, Harvard Medical School, Associate Epidemiologist, Brigham and Women's Hospital, Boston, Massachusetts

Brian I. Carr, MD, MRCP, PhD

Professor of Surgery and Medicine, University of Pittsburgh, Chief, Hepatobiliary Tumor Service, Presbyterian University Hospital of Pittsburgh, Pittsburgh, Pennsylvania

Ephraim S. Casper, MD

Associate Professor of Clinical Medicine, Cornell University Medical College, Associate Attending Physician, Gastrointestinal Oncology Service, Division of Solid Tumor Oncology, Department of Medicine, Memorial Sloan-Kettering Cancer Center, New York, New York

J. Robert Cassady, MD

Professor of Radiation Oncology, Head, Department of Radiation Oncology, The University of Arizona, Arizona Health Sciences Center, Tucson, Arizona

Ronald A. Castellino, MD

Chairman, Department of Radiology, Memorial Sloan-Kettering Cancer Center, New York, New York

Bruce A. Chabner, MD

Director, Division of Cancer Treatment, National Cancer Institute, Bethesda, Maryland

Richard E. Champlin, MD

Professor of Medicine, Chief, Section of Bone Marrow Transplantation, The University of Texas M.D. Anderson Cancer Center, Houston, Texas

Grace H. Christ, DSW

Assistant Professor, Columbia University School of Social Work, New York, New York

Edward Chu, MD

Senior Clinical Investigator, National Cancer Institute, NCI—Navy Medical Oncology Branch, Bethesda, Maryland

Carolyn K. Clifford, PhD

Chief, Diet and Cancer Branch, Division of Cancer Prevention and Control, National Cancer Institute, Bethesda, Maryland

Alfred M. Cohen, MD

Professor of Surgery, Cornell University Medical College, Chief, Colorectal Service, Department of Surgery, Memorial Sloan-Kettering Cancer Center, New York, New York

Daniel G. Coit, MD, FACS

Assistant Professor of Surgery, Cornell University Medical School, Assistant Attending Surgeon, Memorial Sloan-Kettering Cancer Center, New York, New York

C. Norman Coleman, MD

Alvan T. and Viola D. Fuller—American Cancer Society Professor, Chairman, Joint Center for Radiation Therapy, Harvard Medical School, Boston, Massachusetts

Joseph Corson, MD

Professor of Pathology, Chief of Surgical Pathology, Brigham and Women's Hospital, Harvard Medical School, Boston, Massachusetts

Kenneth H. Cowan, MD, PhD

Head, Medical Breast Cancer Section, Medicine Branch, National Cancer Institute, Bethesda, Maryland

Gregory A. Curt, MD

Clinical Director, National Cancer Institute, National Institutes of Health, Bethesda, Maryland

William S. Dalton, PhD, MD

Associate Professor of Medicine and Pharmacology/Toxicology, Director, Bone Marrow Transplant Program, University of Arizona, Tucson, Arizona

John M. Daly, MD

Jonathan E. Rhoads Professor of Surgery, University of Pennsylvania, Chief, Division of Surgical Oncology, Hospital of the University of Pennsylvania, Philadelphia, Pennsylvania

Albert B. Deisseroth, MD, PhD

Professor of Medicine, Internist, The University of Texas M.D. Anderson Cancer Center, Houston, Texas

Thomas F. DeLaney, MD

Boston University School of Medicine, Chairman, Department of Radiation Oncology, Boston University Medical Center, The University Hospital, Boston, Massachusetts

Robert L. DeLaPaz, MD

Associate Professor of Radiology, Cornell University Medical School, Memorial Sloan-Kettering Cancer Center, New York, New York

Susan S. Devesa, PhD

Biostatistics Branch, Epidemiology and Biostatistics Program, National Cancer Institute, Bethesda, Maryland

Sarah S. Donaldson, MD, FACR

Catharine and Howard Avery Professor of Radiation Oncology, Stanford University School of Medicine, Chief of Radiation Oncology Service, Lucille Salter Packard Children's Hospital at Stanford, Stanford, California

Ross C. Donehower, MD

Johns Hopkins Oncology Center, Johns Hopkins University School of Medicine, Baltimore, Maryland

John L. Doppman, MD

Professor of Radiology, Georgetown University School of Medicine, Washington, DC

Director, Diagnostic Radiology Department, Warren Grant Magnuson Clinical Center, National Institutes of Health, Bethesda, Maryland

John D. Earle, MD

William H. Donner Professor of Oncology, Mayo Medical School, Mayo Clinic, Rochester, Minnesota

Lawrence H. Einhorn, MD

Distinguished Professor of Medicine, Indiana University Medical Center, Indiana University Hospital, Indianapolis, Indiana

William D. Ensminger, MD, PhD

Professor, Internal Medicine and Pharmacology, University of Michigan, University of Michigan Medical Center, Ann Arbor, Michigan

Elihu H. Estey, MD

Associate Professor of Medicine, Department of Hematology, The University of Texas M.D. Anderson Cancer Center, Houston, Texas

William R. Fair, MD
Professor of Surgery (Urology), Cornell University Medical College, Chief, Urologic Surgery Service, Memorial Sloan-Kettering Cancer Center, New York, New York

John C. Flickinger, MD
Associate Professor of Radiation Oncology, University of Pittsburgh School of Medicine, Presbyterian University Hospital, Pittsburgh, Pennsylvania

Kathleen M. Foley, MD
Professor, Neurology, Neuroscience and Clinical Pharmacology, Cornell University Medical College, Chief, Pain Service, Department of Neurology, Memorial Sloan-Kettering Cancer Center, New York, New York

Arlene A. Forastiere, MD
Associate Professor of Oncology, Johns Hopkins University School of Medicine, Johns Hopkins Oncology Center, Baltimore, Maryland

Joseph F. Fraumeni, Jr, MD
Associate Director for Epidemiology and Biostatistics, National Cancer Institute, Bethesda, Maryland

Alison G. Freifeld, MD
Medical Officer, Infectious Diseases Section, Pediatric Branch, National Institutes of Health, Bethesda, Maryland

Michael A. Friedman, MD
Associate Director, Cancer Therapy Evaluation Program, National Cancer Institute, Bethesda, Maryland

Zvi Y. Fuks, MD
Professor of Radiation Oncology, Department of Medicine, Cornell University Medical College, Chairman and Attending Radiation Oncologist, Department of Radiation Oncology, Memorial Sloan-Kettering Cancer Center, New York, New York

Janice Lynn Gabrilove, MD
Assistant Professor of Medicine, Cornell University Medical College, Assistant Associate Physician, Memorial Sloan-Kettering Cancer Center, Associate Member, Sloan-Kettering Institute, New York, New York

Patrice M. Gallelli, PT
Staff Physical Therapist, Department of Rehabilitation Medicine, Clinical Center, National Institutes of Health, Bethesda, Maryland

Ellen J. Gallina, RN, BSN, OCN
Assistant Director, Research Nursing, Memorial Sloan-Kettering Cancer Center, New York, New York

Lynn H. Gerber, MD
Adjunct Associate Professor, George Washington University, Washington, DC

Chief, Department of Rehabilitation Medicine, Clinical Center, National Institutes of Health, Bethesda, Maryland

Robert J. Ginsberg, MD, FRCS(C)
Professor of Surgery, Cornell University Medical College, Chief, Thoracic Surgery, Memorial Sloan-Kettering Cancer Center, New York, New York

Eli J. Glatstein, MD
Professor and Chairman, Department of Radiation Oncology, The University of Texas Southwestern Medical Center at Dallas, Chairman, Department of Radiation Oncology, Zale Lipshy University Hospital, Parkland Memorial Hospital, St. Paul Medical Center, Dallas, Texas

David W. Golde, MD
Enid A. Haupt Professor of Hematologic Oncology, Head, Division of Hematologic Oncology, Memorial Sloan-Kettering Cancer Center, New York, New York

Richard J. Gralla, MD
Director, Ochsner Cancer Institute, Alton Ochsner Medical Foundation, New Orleans, Louisiana

F. Anthony Greco, MD
Professor of Medicine, Vanderbilt University Medical Center, Nashville, Tennessee

Peter Greenwald, MD, DrPH
Director, Division of Cancer Prevention and Control, National Cancer Institute, National Institutes of Health, Bethesda, Maryland

Michael R. Grever, MD
Associate Director, Developmental Therapeutics Program, Division of Cancer Treatment, National Cancer Institute, Bethesda, Maryland

Thomas W. Griffin, MD
Professor and Chairman, Department of Radiation Oncology, University of Washington, Director, University Cancer Center, University Hospital Medical Center, Seattle, Washington

Jerome E. Groopman, MD
Dina and Raphael Recanati Chair in Immunology, Associate Professor of Medicine, Harvard Medical School, Chief, Division of Hematology/Oncology, Department of Medicine, New England Deaconess Hospital, Boston, Massachusetts

Philip H. Gutin, MD
Professor of Neurological Surgery and Radiation Oncology, School of Medicine, University of California, San Francisco, California

John D. Hainsworth, MD
Associate Professor of Medicine, Vanderbilt University, Nashville, Tennessee

Eric J. Hall, DPhil, DSc
Professor of Radiology and Radiation Oncology, Director, Center for Radiological Research, Columbia University, New York, New York

Gerald E. Hanks, MD
Professor and Chairman, Department of Radiation Oncology, Fox Chase Cancer Center, Philadelphia, Pennsylvania

Curtis C. Harris, MD
Chief, Laboratory of Human Carcinogenesis, National Cancer Institute, Bethesda, Maryland

Jay R. Harris, MD
Professor of Radiation Oncology, Department of Radiation Oncology, Harvard Medical School, Departments of Radiation Oncology, Beth Israel Hospital and Dana-Farber Cancer Institute, Joint Center for Radiation Therapy, Boston, Massachusetts

Louis B. Harrison, MD
Associate Professor of Radiation Oncology, Cornell University Medical College, Chief, Brachytherapy Service, Department of Radiation Oncology, Memorial Sloan-Kettering Cancer Center, New York, New York

Michael J. Hawkins, MD
Department of Medicine, Division of Medical Oncology, Georgetown University Medical Center, Vincent T. Lombardi Cancer Research Center, Washington, DC

Daniel M. Hays, MD
Professor of Surgery and Pediatrics, University of Southern California School of Medicine, Director, Oncology Follow-up Clinic, Childrens Hospital, Los Angeles, California

Brian E. Henderson, MD
Professor of Preventive Medicine, Director, Norris Comprehensive Cancer Center, University of Southern California, Los Angeles, California

Charles H. Hennekens, MD, DrPH
Professor of Medicine and Preventive Medicine, Harvard Medical School, Senior Physician, Brigham and Women's Hospital, Boston, Massachusetts

Jeanne E. Hicks, MD
Adjunct Associate Professor of Rehabilitation Medicine, Department of Orthopedic Surgery, Georgetown University, Assistant Professor of Medicine, George Washington School of Medicine, Assistant Professor of Medicine, Uniformed Armed Services Institute, Washington, DC

Deputy Chief, Department of Rehabilitation Medicine, Clinical Center, National Institutes of Health, Bethesda, Maryland

Waun Ki Hong, MD
Professor of Medicine, Chief, Section of Head, Neck and Thoracic Medical Oncology, Charles A. LeMaistre Chair in Thoracic Oncology, The University of Texas M.D. Anderson Cancer Center, Houston, Texas

Robert N. Hoover, MD
Chief, Environmental Epidemiology Branch, Epidemiology and Biostatistics Program, National Cancer Institute, Bethesda, Maryland

Richard T. Hoppe, MD
Professor, Department of Radiation Oncology, Stanford University, Stanford, California

William J. Hoskins, MD
Chief, Gynecology Service, Memorial Sloan-Kettering Cancer Center, New York, New York

Alan N. Houghton, Jr, MD
Associate Professor, Cornell University Medical College, Member and Chief, Clinical Imunology Service, Memorial Sloan-Kettering Cancer Center, Attending Physician, Memorial Hospital, New York, New York

Peter M. Howley, MD
Chief, Laboratory of Tumor Virus Biology, National Cancer Institute, Bethesda, Maryland

William J.M. Hrushesky, MD
Professor of Medicine and Microbiology/Immunobiology, Albany Medical College, Adjunct Professor, Clinical Engineering, Rensselaer Polytechnic Institute, Adjunct Professor, Pharmaceutics, Albany College of Pharmacy, Senior Attending Oncologist, Stratton Veterans Administration Medical Center, Albany, New York

Susan Molloy Hubbard, RN, BSN
Director, International Cancer Information Center, Associate Director, National Cancer Institute, Bethesda, Maryland

Daniel C. Ihde, MD
Professor of Medicine, Uniformed Services University of the Health Sciences, Deputy Director, National Cancer Institute, Bethesda, Maryland

Elaine S. Jaffe, MD
Chief, Hematopathology Section, Deputy Chief, Laboratory of Pathology, National Cancer Institute, National Institutes of Health, Bethesda, Maryland

Robert T. Jensen, MD
Chief, Digestive Diseases Branch, National Institute of Diabetes, Digestive and Kidney Diseases, National Institutes of Health, Bethesda, Maryland

Hagop Kantarjian, MD
Associate Professor, Associate Internist, The University of Texas M.D. Anderson Cancer Center, Houston, Texas

Judith E. Karp, MD
Associate Professor of Oncology and Medicine, The Johns Hopkins Oncology Center, The Johns Hopkins University School of Medicine, Baltimore, Maryland

Special Assistant to the Director, National Cancer Institute, Bethesda, Maryland

Michael J. Keating, MD
Professor of Medicine, Internist, University of Melbourne, Australia

Associate Vice President for Clinical Investigations, The University of Texas M.D. Anderson Cancer Center, Houston, Texas

David P. Kelsen, MD
Professor of Medicine, Cornell University Medical College, Attending Physician, Chief, Gastrointestinal Oncology Service, Memorial Sloan-Kettering Cancer Center, New York, New York

Issa F. Khouri, MD
Junior Faculty Associate, Section of Bone Marrow Transplantation and the Department of Hematology, The University of Texas M.D. Anderson Cancer Center, Houston, Texas

Leo J. Kinlen, MB, BS, FRCP, DPhil
Director, Cancer Research Campaign Cancer Epidemiology Group, Department of Public Health and Primary Care, University of Oxford, Radcliffe Infirmary, Oxford, England

Timothy J. Kinsella, MS, MD
Chair, Department of Human Oncology, University of Wisconsin Medical School, Madison, Wisconsin

Mark G. Kris, MD
Associate Member, Memorial Sloan-Kettering Cancer Center, Associate Professor of Medicine, Cornell University Medical College, Associate Attending Physician, Memorial Hospital, New York, New York

Larry E. Kun, MD
Professor, Departments of Radiology and Pediatrics, University of Tennessee College of Medicine, Chairman, Department of Radiation Oncology, St. Jude Children's Research Hospital, Memphis, Tennessee

Robert C. Kurtz, MD
Member, Memorial Hospital, Director, Gastrointestinal Endoscopy Unit and Attending Physician, Gastroenterology and Nutrition Service, Department of Medicine, Memorial Sloan-Kettering Cancer Center, New York, New York

Steven M. Larson, MD
Professor of Radiology, Cornell University Medical College, Chief and Attending Physician, Nuclear Medicine Service, Department of Radiology, Memorial Hospital, New York, New York

Marguerite S. Lederberg, MD
Associate Professor of Clinical Psychiatry, Cornell University Medical College, Attending Psychiatrist, Memorial Sloan-Kettering Cancer Center, New York, New York

Steven A. Leibel, MD
Member, Vice-Chairman and Clinical Director, Attending Radiation Oncologist, Department of Radiation Oncology, Memorial Sloan-Kettering Cancer Center, New York, New York

Bernard Levin, MD
Professor of Medicine, Vice-President for Cancer Prevention (ad interim), Chief, Section of Gastrointestinal Oncology and Digestive Diseases, The University of Texas M.D. Anderson Cancer Center, Houston, Texas

Victor A. Levin, MD
Chairman and Professor, Department of Neuro-Oncology, Clinic Chief, The University of Texas M.D. Anderson Cancer Center, Houston, Texas

Stephen F. Levinson, MD, PhD
Assistant Professor, University of Rochester, School of Medicine and Dentistry, Senior Staff Physiatrist, Department of Rehabilitation Medicine, Clinical Center, National Institutes of Health, Bethesda, Maryland

Frederick P. Li, MD
Professor of Medicine, Dana-Farber Cancer Institute, Harvard Medical School, Boston, Massachusetts

Allen S. Lichter, MD
Professor of Radiation Oncology, Chairman, Department of Radiation Oncology, The University of Michigan Medical Center, Ann Arbor, Michigan

Charles J. Lightdale, MD
Professor of Medicine, Cornell University Medical College, Attending Physician, Gastroenterology Service, Memorial Sloan-Kettering Cancer Center, New York, New York

W. Marston Linehan, MD

Assistant Professor of Surgery, Uniformed Services University of the Health Sciences, Head, Urologic Oncology Section, Surgery Branch, National Cancer Institute, Bethesda, Maryland

Michael P. Link, MD

Professor of Pediatrics, Division of Hematology/Oncology, Stanford University School of Medicine, Lucille Salter Packard Children's Hospital at Stanford, Stanford, California

Lance A. Liotta, MD, PhD

Pathologist, Case Western Reserve University, Chief, Laboratory of Pathology, National Cancer Institute, Deputy Director of Intramural Research, National Institutes of Health, Bethesda, Maryland

Marc E. Lippman, MD

Professor of Medicine and Pharmacology, Georgetown University Medical School, Director, Vincent T. Lombardi Cancer Research Center, Georgetown University Medical Center, Washington, DC

Dan L. Longo, MD, FACP

Director, Biological Response Modifiers Program, Division of Cancer Treatment, National Cancer Institute-Frederick Cancer Research and Development Center, Frederick, Maryland

Matthew Loscalzo, ACSW

Assistant Director, Department of Social Work, Memorial Sloan-Kettering Cancer Center, New York, New York

Michael T. Lotze, MD

Professor of Surgery, Molecular Genetics and Biochemistry, Department of Surgery, University of Pittsburgh, Chief, Section of Surgical Oncology, University of Pittsburgh Medical Center, Pittsburgh, Pennsylvania

Ian T. Magrath, MB, FRCP, FRCPath

Head, Lymphoma Biology Section of the Pediatric Branch of the National Cancer Institute, Bethesda, Maryland

Martin M. Malawer, MD, FACS

Director, Orthopedic Oncology, The Cancer Institute, Washington Hospital Center, Professor of Orthopedic Surgery, The George Washington University School of Medicine and Health Sciences, and Children's National Medical Center, Washington, DC

Consultant, Surgery Branch, National Cancer Institute, National Institutes of Health, Bethesda, Maryland

Mary Jane Massie, MD

Associate Professor of Clinical Psychiatry, Cornell University Medical College, Attending Psychiatrist, Memorial Sloan-Kettering Cancer Center, New York, New York

Peter Mauch, MD

Associate Professor, Department of Radiation Oncology, Harvard Medical School, Boston, Massachusetts

John Mendelsohn, MD

Professor of Medicine, Cornell University Medical College, Chairman, Department of Medicine, Winthrop Rockefeller Chair in Medical Oncology, Memorial Sloan-Kettering Cancer Center, New York, New York

Joel D. Meyers, MD*

Professor of Medicine, University of Washington School of Medicine, Head, Program in Infectious Diseases, Fred Hutchinson Cancer Research Center, Seattle, Washington

Anthony B. Miller, MB, FRCP

Professor and Chairman, Department of Preventive Medicine and Biostatistics, University of Toronto, Toronto, Ontario, Canada

---

* Deceased.

Donald L. Miller, MD

Professor of Radiology, Georgetown University School of Medicine, Washington, DC

Director, Vascular/Interventional Radiology, Diagnostic Radiology Department, Warren Grant Magneson Clinical Center, National Institutes of Health, Bethesda, Maryland

Bruce D. Minsky, MD

Associate Professor of Radiation Oncology, Cornell University Medical College, Associate Attending Physician, Department of Radiation Oncology, Memorial Sloan-Kettering Cancer Center, New York, New York

Felix Mitelman, MD

Professor and Chairman, Department of Clinical Genetics, University of Lund, Director, Department of Clinical Genetics, University Hospital, Lund, Sweden

Drogo K. Montague, MD

Staff Urologist, The Cleveland Clinic Foundation, Cleveland, Ohio

Charles S. Morrow, MD, PhD

Medicine Branch, National Cancer Institute, Bethesda, Maryland

Monica Morrow, MD

Associate Professor of Surgery, University of Chicago, Director, Multidisciplinary Breast Program, University of Chicago Hospitals, Chicago, Illinois

Rosemary T. Moynihan, CSW

Coordinator, Mental Health Program, Comprehensive Care Center for HIV, St. Joseph's Hospital and Medical Center, Paterson, New Jersey

John J. Mulvihill, MD

Chair and Professor of Human Genetics, University of Pittsburgh, Acting Director, Department of Medical Genetics, Children's Hospital of Pittsburgh, Pittsburgh, Pennsylvania

Charles E. Myers, MD

Chief, Clinical Pharmacology Branch, National Cancer Institute, National Institutes of Health, Bethesda, Maryland

John E. Niederhuber, MD

Emile Holman Professor of Surgery, Professor of Microbiology, Chairman of Surgery, Stanford Hospital, Stanford, California

Jeffrey A. Norton, MD

Professor of Surgery, Chief of Endocrine and Cancer Surgery, Washington University School of Medicine, Barnes Hospital, St. Louis, Missouri

Edward H. Oldfield, Jr, MD

Chief, Surgical Neurology Branch, National Institute of Neurological Disease and Stroke, The Clinical Center, National Institutes of Health, Bethesda, Maryland

James R. Oleson, MD, PhD

Professor, Department of Radiation Oncology, Duke University Medical Center, Durham, North Carolina

Takis S. Papas, PhD

Chief, Laboratory of Molecular Oncology, National Cancer Institute, Bethesda, Maryland

David R. Parkinson, MD

Chief, Investigational Drug Branch, Cancer Therapy Evaluation Program, Senior Staff, Immunotherapy Service, Surgery Branch, Clinical Oncology Program, Division of Cancer Treatment, National Cancer Institute, Bethesda, Maryland

Harvey I. Pass, MD

Head, Thoracic Oncology Section, Senior Investigator, Surgery Branch, National Cancer Institute, Bethesda, Maryland

Carlos A. Perez, MD

Director, Radiation Oncology Center, Mallinckrodt Institute of Radiology, Washington University Medical Center, St. Louis, Missouri

Archibald S. Perkins, MD, PhD
Assistant Professor, Department of Pathology, Yale University School of Medicine, New Haven, Connecticut

Lester J. Peters, MD
Professor and Head, Division of Radiotherapy, The University of Texas M.D. Anderson Cancer Center, Houston, Texas

Philip A. Pizzo, MD
Professor of Pediatrics, Uniformed Services University for the Health Sciences, Chief of Pediatrics, Head, Infectious Diseases, National Cancer Institute, Bethesda, Maryland

David G. Poplack, MD
Head, Pharmacology and Experimental Therapeutics Section, Pediatric Branch, National Cancer Institute, Bethesda, Maryland

Joe B. Putnam, Jr, MD
Assistant Surgeon and Assistant Professor of Surgery, The University of Texas M.D. Anderson Cancer Center, Department of Thoracic Surgery, Active Staff, Division of Thoracic and Cardiovascular Surgery, Department of Surgery, Hermann Hospital, Houston, Texas

Eddie Reed, MD
Chief, Medical Ovarian Cancer Section, Medical Branch, National Cancer Institute, Bethesda, Maryland

Jerome P. Richie, MD
Elliott C. Cutler Professor of Surgery, Harvard Medical School, Chairman, Harvard Program in Urology, Chief of Urology, Brigham and Women's Hospital, Boston, Massachusetts

E. Chester Ridgway, MD
Professor of Medicine, University of Colorado Health Sciences Center, Head, Division of Endocrinology, Program Director, General Clinical Research Center, Denver, Colorado

Juan Rosai, MD
James Ewing Alumni Professor and Chairman, Department of Pathology, Member, Memorial Sloan-Kettering Cancer Center, Professor of Pathology, Cornell University School of Medicine, New York, New York

J.C. Rosenberg, MD, PhD
Professor of Surgery, Wayne State University, Chief of Surgery, Hutzel Hospital, Detroit, Michigan

Ronald K. Ross, MD
Professor of Preventive Medicine, Norris Comprehensive Cancer Center, University of Southern California, Los Angeles, California

Jack A. Roth, MD
Professor and Chairman, Department of Thoracic Surgery, Bud S. Johnson Chair, Professor of Tumor Biology, The University of Texas M.D. Anderson Cancer Center, Houston, Texas

Eric K. Rowinsky, MD, FACP
Associate Professor of Oncology, Division of Pharmacology and Experimental Therapeutics, The Johns Hopkins Oncology Center, Baltimore, Maryland

Janet D. Rowley, MD
Blum-Riese Distinguished Service Professor, Departments of Medicine and of Molecular Genetics and Cell Biology, University of Chicago, Chicago, Illinois

Paul Russo, MD
Assistant Professor of Surgery, Cornell Medical College, Assistant Attending Surgeon, Urology Service, Memorial Sloan-Kettering Cancer Center, New York, New York

Bijan Safai, MD, DSc
Professor of Medicine, Cornell University Medical College, Chief, Dermatology Service, Memorial Sloan-Kettering Cancer Center, New York, New York

Jose A. Sahel, MD
Professor des Universites, Universite Louis Pasteur, Praticien Hospitalier, Clinique Ophtalmologique, Hopitaux Universitaires de Strasbourg, Strasbourg, France

Sydney E. Salmon, MD
Regents Professor of Internal Medicine, The University of Arizona, College of Medicine, Director, Arizona Cancer Center, Tucson, Arizona

Donna Sammarino, BSN, MA
Nurse Manager, Memorial Sloan-Kettering Cancer Center, New York, New York

Peter T. Scardino, MD
Professor and Chairman, Scott Department of Urology, Baylor College of Medicine, Chief of Service, The Methodist Hospital, Houston, Texas

Wendy S. Schain, EdD
Medical Care Consultant, National Cancer Institute, Bethesda, Maryland

Consultant, Long Beach Memorial Hospital, Long Beach, California

Stimson P. Schantz, MD
Associate Professor of Surgery, Cornell University Medical Center, Associate Attending Surgeon, Head and Neck Service, Department of Surgery, Memorial Sloan-Kettering Cancer Center, New York, New York

Donna S. Scheib, MS, CCC/Speech-Language-Pathology
Clinical Coordinator, Speech-Language-Pathology Section, Department of Rehabilitation Medicine, Clinical Center, National Institutes of Health, Bethesda, Maryland

Howard I. Scher, MD, FACP
Associate Professor of Medicine, Cornell University Medical College, Chief, Genitourinary Oncology Service, Associate Attending Physician, Division of Solid Tumor Oncology, Department of Medicine, Memorial Sloan-Kettering Cancer Center, New York, New York

Richard L. Schilsky, MD
Professor of Medicine, Director, Cancer Research Center, University of Chicago, Attending Physician, University of Chicago Hospitals and Clinics, Chicago, Illinois

Leslie R. Schover, PhD
Staff Psychologist, The Center for Sexual Function, The Cleveland Clinic Foundation, Cleveland, Ohio

Morton K. Schwartz, MD
Professor of Molecular Pharmacology and Therapeutics, Sloan-Kettering Division, Cornell University, Graduate School of Medical Sciences, Attending Clinical Chemist, Chairman, Department of Clinical Chemistry, Memorial Sloan-Kettering Cancer Center, New York, New York

Claudia A. Seipp, RN, CCN
Oncology Nurse Clinician, Surgery Branch, National Cancer Institute, Bethesda, Maryland

Roy B. Sessions, MD, FACS
Professor and Chairman, Georgetown University Medical School, Chief of Otolaryngology–Head and Neck Surgery, Member, Vincent Lombardi Cancer Center, Georgetown University Medical Center, Washington, DC

Arun Seth, MD
Scientist, Laboratory of Molecular Oncology, National Cancer Institute, Bethesda, Maryland

Brenda Shank, MD, PhD
Chairman and Professor, Radiation Oncology Department, Mount Sinai School of Medicine, Director and Attending, Radiation Oncology Department, Mount Sinai Hospital, New York, New York

Richard J. Sherins, MD
Medical Staff, Department of Medicine, Fairfax Hospital, Fairfax, Virginia

Peter G. Shields, MD
Senior Clinical Investigator, Laboratory of Human Carcinogenesis, Division of Cancer Etiology, National Cancer Institute, Bethesda, Maryland

William U. Shipley, MD, FACR
Professor of Radiation Oncology, Harvard Medical School, Head, Genitourinary Oncology, Department of Radiation Oncology, Massachusetts General Hospital, Boston, Massachusetts

Richard M. Simon, PhD
Chief, Biometric Research Branch, Division of Cancer Treatment, National Cancer Institute, Bethesda, Maryland

Jeffrey Sklar, MD, PhD
Professor of Pathology, Harvard Medical School, Director, Divisions of Molecular Oncology and Diagnostic Molecular Biology, Department of Pathology, Brigham and Women's Hospital, Boston, Massachusetts

Barbara C. Sonies, PhD
Adjunct Teaching Faculty, University of Maryland, George Washington University, Chief, Speech-Language-Pathology Section, Department of Rehabilitation Medicine, Clinical Center, National Institutes of Health, Bethesda, Maryland

Stephen T. Sonis, DMD, DMSc
Professor of Oral Medicine, Harvard School of Dental Medicine, Chief, Division of Dentistry, Brigham and Women's Hospital, Boston, Massachusetts

C.A. Stein, MD, PhD
Assistant Professor of Medicine and Pharmacology, Columbia University, New York, New York

Laurel Judith Steinherz, MD, FAAP, FACC
Associate Professor, Department of Pediatrics, Cornell University Medical College, Associate Attending Pediatrician, Cardiology, Director of Pediatric Cardiology, Memorial Sloan-Kettering Cancer Center, Associate Attending Pediatrician, The New York Hospital-Cornell Medical Center, New York, New York

William G. Stetler-Stevenson, MD, PhD
Medical Officer, Laboratory of Pathology, National Cancer Institute, Bethesda, Maryland

Diane E. Stover, MD, FACCP
Associate Professor of Clinical Medicine, Cornell University Medical College, Chief, Pulmonary Service, Head, Division of General Medicine, Memorial Sloan-Kettering Cancer Center, New York, New York

Chris H. Takimoto, MD, PhD
Senior Staff Fellow, National Cancer Institute, NCI—Navy Medical Oncology Branch, Bethesda, Maryland

Moshe Talpaz, MD
Professor of Medicine, Chief, Section of Biologic Studies, The University of Texas M.D. Anderson Cancer Center, Houston, Texas

Joel E. Tepper, MD
Professor and Chair, Department of Radiation Oncology, University of North Carolina School of Medicine, Chair, Department of Radiation Oncology, University of North Carolina Hospitals, Chapel Hill, North Carolina

Philip E. Thorpe, PhD
Professor, Department of Pharmacology, Serena S. Simmons Distinguished Chair in Immunopharmacology, University of Texas Southwestern Medical Center, Dallas, Texas

Michael H. Torosian, MD
Assistant Professor of Surgery, University of Pennsylvania School of Medicine, Attending Surgeon, The Hospital of the University of Pennsylvania, Philadelphia, Pennsylvania

Margaret A. Tucker, MD
Chief, Genetic Epidemiology Branch, Division of Cancer Etiology, National Cancer Institute, Bethesda, Maryland

Jonathan W. Uhr, MD
Professor of Internal Medicine, Professor and Chairman of Microbiology, University of Texas Southwestern Medical Center, Dallas, Texas

Walter J. Urba, MD, PhD, FACP
Director, Clinical Services Program, Program Resources, Inc./DynCorp, National Cancer Institute-Frederick Cancer Research and Development Center, Frederick, Maryland

George F. Vande Woude, PhD
Director, ABL-Basic Research Program, National Cancer Institute-Frederick Cancer Research and Development Center, Frederick, Maryland

Susan Vande Woude, DVM
Staff Veterinarian, Assistant Professor, Department of Pathology, Colorado State University, Fort Collins, Colorado

Ellen S. Vitetta, PhD
Sheryle Simmons-Patigian Distinguished Chair in Cancer Immunobiology, Director, Cancer Immunobiology Center, Professor of Microbiology, University of Texas Southwestern Medical School, Dallas, Texas

Nicholas J. Vogelzang, MD
Associate Professor of Medicine, Pritzker School of Medicine, University of Chicago, Section of Hematology/Oncology, University of Chicago Medical Center, Chicago, Illinois

Ralph O. Wallerstein, MD, FACP
Kaiser Permanente, Denver, Colorado

Thomas J. Walsh, MD
Senior Investigator, Section of Infectious Diseases, Pediatric Branch, National Cancer Institute, Bethesda, Maryland

McClellan M. Walther, MD
Senior Investigator, Urologic Oncology Section, Surgery Branch, Division of Cancer Treatment, National Cancer Institute, Bethesda, Maryland

Raymond P. Warrell, Jr, MD
Associate Professor of Medicine, Cornell University Medical College, Associate Member, Memorial Sloan-Kettering Cancer Center, New York, New York

Jeffrey S. Weber, MD, PhD
Senior Investigator, Surgery Branch, National Cancer Institute, Bethesda, Maryland

Lois L. Weinstein, CSW
Director, Department of Social Work, Memorial Sloan-Kettering Cancer Center, New York, New York

Raymond B. Weiss, MD
Professor of Medicine, Uniformed Services University of the Health Sciences, Bethesda, Maryland

Chief of Medical Oncology, Walter Reed Army Medical Center, Washington, DC

Jessie Whitehurst, PT
Staff Physical Therapist, Department of Rehabilitation Medicine, Clinical Center, National Institutes of Health, Bethesda, Maryland

Donald C. Wright, MD
Associate Professor, University of Pittsburgh School of Medicine, Department of Neurosurgery, Presbyterian University Hospital, Pittsburgh, Pennsylvania

Joachim Yahalom, MD
Associate Professor of Radiation Oncology, Cornell University Medical College, Associate Member, Memorial Sloan-Kettering Cancer Center, New York, New York

James C. Yang, MD
Senior Investigator, Surgery Branch, National Cancer Institute, Bethesda, Maryland

Charles W. Young, MD
Professor of Medicine, Cornell University Medical College, Member, Memorial Sloan-Kettering Cancer Center, New York, New York

Robert C. Young, MD
President, Fox Chase Cancer Center, Philadelphia, Pennsylvania

PUBLISHER'S FOREWORD

The physicians and surgeons who edit textbooks all have the same objective—the writing and publication of a textbook which, although edited by several and written by many, will nonetheless seem to reflect the knowledge and clinical wisdom of one mind. As every student and practitioner knows, the realization usually falls short of intention. What was to have been a divisible whole turns out to be a confusing, perplexing mosaic of contradiction, with some of the pieces missing. Such are the characteristics of most multiauthored textbooks in medicine and in surgery. There are few exceptions.

Cancer: Principles and Practice of Oncology is an exception, as thousands of oncologists, surgeons, and internists throughout the world have recognized since the publication of the first edition in January 1982. That the book *seems* to reflect one mind is no accident. As described in the Publisher's Foreword to the first edition, before the text was written the editors had exhaustive sessions with their contributors, sessions which, in many cases, lasted far into the night. Chapters were drafted and redrafted. The three editors and I (representing the publisher) met together for 1 week, and all editors re-viewed all chapters—together. The chapters were then returned to the contributors with suggestions for amplification or clarification, or the deletion or addition of illustrations, drawings, and tables. The revised chapters were once again reviewed before being delivered to the publisher.

As with the first edition, so with the second, the third, and now the fourth. After the initial changes were decided on, the chapters were assigned, written, reviewed collectively, revised, and then reviewed again. The result of such effort you hold in your hands, and I am convinced that this is now the most rigorously edited and the most comprehensive textbook to have been written in oncology.

There are many rewards in medical publishing, but the most gratifying reward is to be associated with a textbook that is the best, that really works, and that has made a positive difference in the lives of cancer patients throughout the world, including me.

J. Stuart Freeman, Jr

PREFACE

Two basic ideas guided the preparation of the original edition of *Cancer: Principles and Practice of Oncology.* The first was that the text should present a dynamic, well-balanced consideration of the current practice of oncology without overemphasis on one or another subspecialty or treatment modality. The second was that this balance should be maintained on the leading edge of the changing fields that interface with all of oncology by expeditious publication of future editions of the text. Over the years we have had no reason to change these precepts. Hence, the fourth edition of *Cancer: Principles and Practice of Oncology,* appearing 11 years after the first, preserves the balance although the content has changed.

The first third of the text, emphasizing the principles of oncology, reflects the extent to which the revolution in molecular biology has permeated cancer medicine. There are new chapters on the use of molecular methods in diagnosis, in assessing prognosis, and in estimating minute amounts of residual disease, which hold promise for overcoming the limitations of current cancer treatment; there is an expanded chapter on the pharmacology of cancer chemotherapy. This part of the text continues to serve as a primer on the science of cancer.

Much of the second section also is new. Different perspectives and new information on diagnosis and treatment have been integrated with the appropriate stage of the cancers in question, including the assimilation of the use of biologics as supportive and treatment measures.

A striking change over the past 11 years has been the emergence of effective and less morbid therapy, including effective systemic therapy for some of the most stubborn of visceral malignancies, such as colorectal and breast cancer. The last part of the text emphasizes the management and treatment of complications of cancer and emerging new approaches.

The management of complications has been the quiet revolution in the practice of oncology. New, more effective antiemetics and marrow protective agents have made standard treatments more tolerable, and also have opened the door to methods to enhance treatment. Since the last edition, the era of gene therapy has begun to reach the oncology clinics, in a preliminary way, and this is described in the new edition.

As we have emphasized in prior prefaces, the chance a cancer patient has of surviving is maximized by early diagnosis and the prompt administration of the most effective treatment. Increasingly, this treatment is multimodal and tailored so that each aspect of the separate therapies interdigitate with the others like the pieces of a crossword puzzle. We have attempted to collect all of this information in one text to best serve the physician and the patient.

Vincent T. DeVita, Jr, MD
Samuel Hellman, MD
Steven A. Rosenberg, MD, PhD

ACKNOWLEDGMENTS

The editors are especially grateful to those persons whose excellent help and unflagging enthusiasm contributed to this book.

Alice Rosenberg assumed responsibility for the overall compilation of the contributions to this book and for many of the organizational details involved in its assembly.

Dona D'Maggio and Nola Roth contributed to the preparation and compilation of many of the manuscripts.

Stuart Freeman, Editor, Oncology Program, J. B. Lippincott Company, has worked closely with the editors from the book's inception in 1978 through the completion of all four editions. His valuable advice and continuing encouragement have contributed greatly to the preparation of all four.

CONTENTS

2

Principles of Molecular Cell Biology of Cancer: General Aspects of Gene Regulation **23**

ARUN SETH
TAKIS S. PAPAS

Transcription   23
Regulation of the Regulators   30
Transcription Factors in Muscle Cell Development   31
Transcription Factors in Oncogenesis   32

3

Principles of Molecular Cell Biology of Cancer: Oncogenes **35**

ARCHIBALD S. PERKINS
GEORGE F. VANDE WOUDE

Identification of Oncogenes and Tumor Suppressor Genes   36
Tumor Suppressor Genes or Recessive Oncogenes   41
Dominant Oncogenes Involved in Signal Transduction   47
Transformed Cell Phenotype, Antineoplastic Drugs, and the Cell Cycle   54

4

Principles of Molecular Cell Biology of Cancer: The Cell Cycle **60**

RENATO BASERGA

The Cell Cycle   60
Tumor Growth   60
Gene Expression and Cell Proliferation   61
Molecular Biology of the Cell Cycle   62

5

Principles of Molecular Cell Biology of Cancer: Chromosome Abnormalities in Human Cancer and Leukemia **67**

JANET D. ROWLEY
FELIX MITELMAN

Chromosome Nomenclature   67
Myeloid Disorders   68
Malignant Lymphoid Disorders   73
Solid Tumors   78
Conclusions   87
Glossary of Cytogenetic Terminology   87

6

Principles of Molecular Cell Biology of Cancer: Molecular Approaches to Cancer Diagnosis **92**

JEFFREY SKLAR

General Considerations   92
Purposes of Molecular Tests in Cancer Diagnosis   93

7

Principles of Molecular Cell Biology of Cancer: Growth Factors **114**

JOHN MENDELSOHN
MARC E. LIPPMAN

8

Principles of Molecular Cell Biology of Cancer: Cancer Metastasis **134**

LANCE A. LIOTTA
WILLIAM G. STETLER-STEVENSON

9

Epidemiology of Cancer **150**

JOSEPH F. FRAUMENI, JR   SUSAN S. DEVESA
ROBERT N. HOOVER   LEO J. KINLEN

10

Principles of Carcinogenesis: Viral **182**

PETER M. HOWLEY

11

Principles of Carcinogenesis: Chemical **200**

PETER G. SHIELDS
CURTIS C. HARRIS

12

Principles of Carcinogenesis: Physical **213**

ERIC J. HALL

13

Principles of Oncologic Pathology **228**

JUAN ROSAI

14
Principles of Surgical Oncology **238**
STEVEN A. ROSENBERG

Historical Perspective   *238*
The Operation   *239*
Roles for Surgery   *242*

15
Principles of Radiation Therapy **248**
SAMUEL HELLMAN

Physical Considerations   *248*
Biologic Considerations   *255*
Tumor Radiobiology   *264*
Clinical Considerations   *268*

16
Principles of Chemotherapy **276**
VINCENT T. DEVITA, JR

History   *276*
Chemotherapy As Part of the Initial Treatment of Cancer   *276*
Clinical Endpoints in Evaluating Response to Chemotherapy   *277*
Principles Governing the Use of Combination Chemotherapy   *278*
**Impact of the Goldie-Coldman Hypothesis on Design of Clinical Trials
Using Combination Chemotherapy**   *279*
Response to Chemotherapy Is Affected by the Biology of Tumor Growth   *280*
**Biochemical Resistance to Chemotherapy Is the Major Impediment
to Successful Treatment**   *281*
Concept of Dose Intensity   *283*
In Vitro Tests to Select Chemotherapeutic Agents for Individualized Treatment   *286*
Cancer Drug Development   *286*
Early Clinical Trials of Antitumor Agents   *288*
Overcoming the Limitations of Cancer Treatment   *289*

17
Principles and Applications of Biologic Therapy **293**
STEVEN A. ROSENBERG

Basic Principles of Tumor Immunology   *293*
Immunotherapy   *305*

27

Cancer of the Pancreas **849**

MURRAY F. BRENNAN
TIMOTHY J. KINSELLA
EPHRAIM S. CASPER

28

Hepatobiliary Neoplasms **883**

MICHAEL T. LOTZE
JOHN C. FLICKINGER
BRIAN I. CARR

29

Cancer of the Small Intestine **915**

DANIEL G. COIT

36

Cancer of the Urethra and Penis 1114

WILLIAM R. FAIR
ZVI Y. FUKS
HOWARD I. SCHER

37

Cancer of the Testis 1126

LAWRENCE H. EINHORN
JEROME P. RICHIE
WILLIAM U. SHIPLEY

38

Gynecologic Tumors **1152**

WILLIAM J. HOSKINS
CARLOS A. PEREZ
ROBERT C. YOUNG

39

Cancer of the Ovary **1226**

ROBERT C. YOUNG
CARLOS A. PEREZ
WILLIAM J. HOSKINS

40

Cancer of the Breast **1264**

JAY R. HARRIS
MONICA MORROW
GIANNI BONADONNA

41

Cancer of the Endocrine System **1333**

JEFFREY A. NORTON
BERNARD LEVIN
ROBERT T. JENSEN

42

Sarcomas of Soft Tissues **1436**

JAMES C. YANG   ELI J. GLATSTEIN
STEVEN A. ROSENBERG   KAREN H. ANTMAN

46

CHARLES M. BALCH
ALAN N. HOUGHTON
LESTER J. PETERS

47

JOSE A. SAHEL
JOHN D. EARLE
DANIEL M. ALBERT

48

Neoplasms of the Central Nervous System **1679**

VICTOR A. LEVIN
PHILIP H. GUTIN
STEVEN LEIBEL

49

Solid Tumors of Childhood **1738**

PHILIP A. PIZZO   DANIEL M. HAYS
MARC E. HOROWITZ   LARRY E. KUN
DAVID G. POPLACK

50
Leukemias and Lymphomas of Childhood **1792**

DAVID G. POPLACK   IAN T. MAGRATH
LARRY E. KUN   PHILIP A. PIZZO

51
Hodgkin's Disease **1819**

VINCENT T. DEVITA, JR
SAMUEL HELLMAN
ELAINE S. JAFFE

52
Lymphocytic Lymphomas **1859**

DAN L. LONGO   PETER MAUCH
VINCENT T. DEVITA, JR   WALTER J. URBA
ELAINE S. JAFFE

53

Cutaneous Lymphomas **1928**

PAUL A. BUNN, JR
RICHARD T. HOPPE

54

Acute Leukemia **1938**

MICHAEL J. KEATING
ELIHU ESTEY
HAGOP KANTARJIAN

55

Chronic Leukemias **1965**

ALBERT B. DEISSEROTH   HAGOP KANTARJIAN
MICHAEL ANDREEFF   ISSA F. KHOURI
RICHARD CHAMPLIN   MOSHE TALPAZ
MICHAEL J. KEATING

56

Plasma Cell Neoplasms **1984**

SYDNEY E. SALMON
J. ROBERT CASSADY

60
Oncologic Emergencies **2111**

* *Deceased.*

65

Genetic Counseling of the Cancer Patient **2529**

JOHN J. MULVIHILL

66

Evaluation and Management of Disability: Rehabilitation Aspects of Cancer **2538**

LYNN H. GERBER   JESSIE WHITEHURST
STEPHEN LEVINSON   DONNA SCHEIB
JEANNE E. HICKS   BARBARA C. SONIES
PATRICE GALLELLI

67

*Practical Guide to Chemotherapy Administration for Physicians
and Oncology Nurses* **2570**

ELLEN J. GALLINA

68

Information Systems in Oncology **2581**

CANCER
Principles & Practice
of Oncology

PRINCIPLES OF ONCOLOGY

Cancer: Principles & Practice of Oncology, Fourth Edition,
edited by Vincent T. DeVita, Jr., Samuel Hellman, Steven A. Rosenberg.
J.B. Lippincott Co., Philadelphia © 1993.

Susan Vande Woude
George F. Vande Woude

CHAPTER **1**

Principles of Molecular Cell Biology of Cancer: Introduction to Methods in Molecular Biology

One of the most significant achievements of the 1980s was the discovery that a human gene could functionally replace a defective gene in yeast called p34[cdc2] and allow the yeast cell to grow and divide.[1] There have been 1 billion years of evolution since man diverged from yeast, but the function of specific genetic information has been preserved. The product of this gene is responsible for regulating progression through the cell cycle and determining when to duplicate DNA and when to partition the DNA into daughter cells at mitosis.[2] An earlier edition of this series stated that oncogenes reside in the hierarchy of genes that regulate the cell cycle.[3] Oncogenes and tumor suppressor genes have recently been shown to influence or be influenced by p34[cdc2]. This connection depicts the molecular basis for the transformed phenotype of the tumor cell.

Absolute measurements in molecular biology and genetic engineering have provided the first descriptions of the molecular elements responsible for triggering the events that lead to cancer. Terms like DNA sequence, molecular cloning, polymerase chain reaction, gene therapy, transgenic animals, and germline transmission describe a new armamentarium of techniques used in molecular biology research. These methods have been used to identify, isolate, and characterize the molecular elements that have been implicated in normal and abnormal biologic processes in human and animal cells (see the glossary at the end of this chapter).

Recent technologic achievements promise important applications of this new information for clinical diagnosis and treatment of human cancer. Specific cellular genes are associated with specific tumor types, such as c-*MYC* in Burkitt lymphoma or c-*ABL* in chronic myelogenous leukemia, and mutations in the p53 tumor suppressor gene are found in most human tumors.[4-9] In these instances, the tools of molecular biology have become unambiguous diagnostic reagents. In other cancers, certain molecular alterations lead to proliferation, and correlations of genetic changes with tumor progression from benign to neoplastic have also been made. Perhaps the best model of this is human colorectal cancer, in which a series of chromosomal deletions and mutations in oncogenes and tumor suppressor genes are associated with progression from normal colonic epithelial morphology to metastatic colonic adenocarcinoma.[10]

The rapidly emerging biotechnology requires familiarity with the specialized terminology it brings with it. This chapter introduces the names of molecular structures and techniques used in molecular biology, molecular genetics, and genetic engineering.

STRUCTURE OF DNA

All of the genetic information of an organism is encoded in the DNA genome in each living cell.[11] In the nucleus, DNA is condensed into chromatin along a chromosome. In mammals, if each DNA molecule were unwound and laid end to end, the DNA from just one cell would be 1 m long. Every

3

somatic cell possesses two copies of the genome, one received from each parent, and each copy has an estimated complexity of 50,000 to 100,000 genes. It is the differential expression of these genes that determines all genetic characteristics from animal speciation and embryologic development to cellular and tissue functions. This information is encoded in DNA by

the precise ordering of four chemically distinct monomeric units called nucleotides. There are two types of nucleotides: purine bases (deoxyadenylic acid [A] and deoxyguanylic acid [G]) and pyrimidine bases (deoxythymidylic acid [T] and deoxycytidylic acid [C]). These nucleotides or bases are linked in chains and can number several billion per mammalian ge-

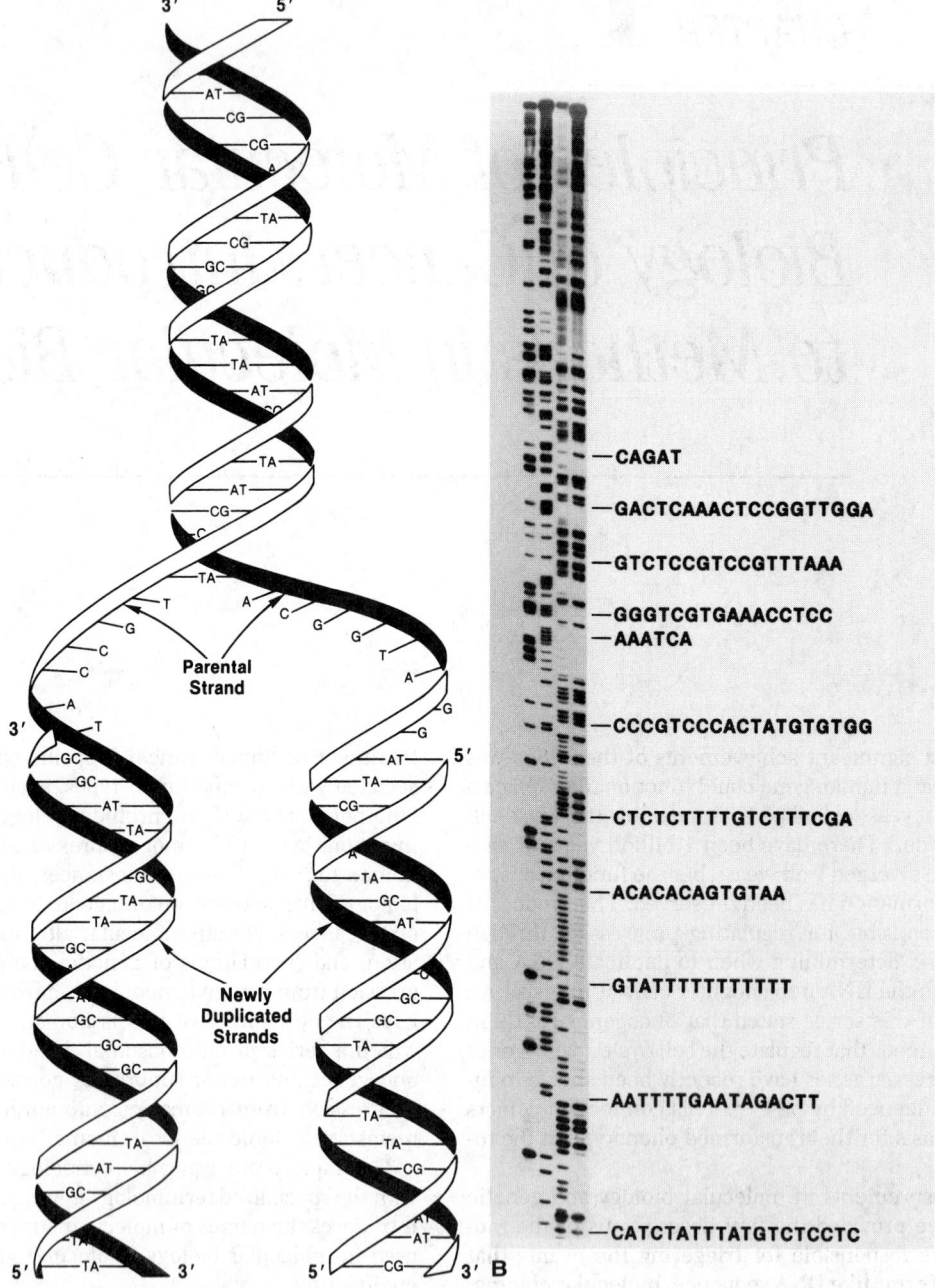

FIGURE 1–1.   Structure of DNA. **(A)** The precise order of monomeric deoxyribonucleic acids (adenylic [A], thymidylic [T], guanylic [G], and cytodylic [C] acids) in the DNA molecule encodes all the genetic information for each organism. The DNA molecule consists of two strands in opposite polarity as determined by the orientation of the monomer nucleotide bases and indicated by a 5' to 3' notation. The two strands of opposite polarity are held together by weak bonds between pairs of nucleotide bases. Notice that A always pairs with T, and G pairs with C. When DNA is duplicated by DNA polymerase, the newly synthesized strand is formed by linking the appropriate base pairs as directed by the template of the parental strand. **(B)** DNA sequence. The precise order of the nucleotide bases in á DNA strand can be determined by DNA sequencing. In this Maxam-Gilbert sequencing reaction, four reactions that cleave at different sites in the DNA strand have been performed and are electrophoresed in a polyacrylamide gel matrix. The banding patterns of the resulting DNA strands are then compared to determine the DNA sequence.

nome (Fig. 1–1A). The precise order of nucleotides, called the DNA sequence, confers the specificity of the genetic code. Sequence analysis can be determined by several methods and is the ultimate characterization of the genetic information within an individual (Fig. 1–1B). It is this principle that underlies the effort to sequence the genomes of a variety of organisms, from prokaryotes to humans.

GENE EXPRESSION

The flow of information in eukaryotic cells is from DNA into RNA in a process called transcription; RNA is then used as a blueprint for protein in a process called translation (Fig. 1–2). RNA polymerase is the enzyme that transcribes genes into RNA, which is formed from monomeric nucleotides called RNA bases.[12,13] The RNA copy of the DNA that is destined to form protein molecules is called messenger RNA (mRNA). Synthesis of the message is initiated from a promoter region in the DNA (Fig. 1–2), and the primary RNA transcript consists of a series of coding and noncoding regions (called exons and introns, respectively). The mRNAs are processed before leaving the nucleus for translation. Splicing removes the introns from the transcript and, usually in the nucleus, a series of adenylic acid nucleotides is added to the terminal end of the mRNA molecule; this molecule is said to be polyadenylated. The mRNA is then transported to the cytoplasm and translated into protein.

Translation occurs on the ribosomes within the cell. The first portion of the molecule, the untranslated leader, is not a protein coding sequence. The amino acid sequence of a protein is determined by the ribonucleotide sequence of the mRNA, which was derived from the DNA sequence.[14] For mRNA to be translated into the specific protein for which it encodes, interactions among translation-initiation enzymes, cofactors, amino acid-charged transfer RNAs (tRNAs), and ribosomes must take place. The coding region of the mRNA is dictated by series of triplets of nucleotides, called codons, which specify a particular amino acid. The relation of triplet codons to their respective amino acids is known as the genetic code (Table 1–1). A series of codons that can be transcribed into protein is known as an open reading frame. The order of the amino acids in a protein chain is responsible for the three-dimensional structure of the protein and its biologic and biochemical activity. More detailed information on the regulation of transcription and translation is found in Chapter 2.

DNA STRUCTURAL ANALYSIS

The properties associated with DNA structure provide the basis for modern genetic engineering technology. Each DNA molecule consists of two strands paired together in a double helix (Fig. 1–1A). Each nucleotide has polarity, and each strand of DNA has a direction. The notation 5′ to 3′ describing this direction indicates the sites of the ribose sugar backbone where the nucleotides are joined. Complementary strands run in opposite directions, and combined, they form the double helix. The strands are held together by hydrogen bonds between nucleotides on opposing strands. An A nucleotide always pairs

FIGURE 1–2. Gene transcription and translation. Messenger RNA synthesis by polymerase II is initiated from a site in the gene called a promoter, and RNA is transcribed from the complementary (antisense) DNA strand of the structural (protein-coding) gene. Thus, the 5′ (upstream) end of the RNA is transcribed from a DNA sequence in the 3′ to 5′ orientation (*line 1*). The first portion usually lacks structural (protein-coding) information and is referred to as an untranslated (ut) leader. The newly transcribed structural information is interrupted by intervening sequences (introns, I_1 to I_3), which are processed (spliced) from the transcript to leave only structural coding exons (E_1 and E_2) (*lines 2 and 3*). The transcribed messenger RNA (mRNA) is terminated by the addition of approximately 200 adenine nucleotide bases. The process is called polyadenylation, and the sequence is referred to as the poly A tail. The mRNA is transported to the cytoplasm, where it is translated, or decoded, into protein in cytoplasmic structures called polyribosomes. The decoding is performed by transfer RNA (tRNA) molecules that recognize the specific nucleotide codon information and provide the appropriate amino acid for linking to the growing polypeptide chain.

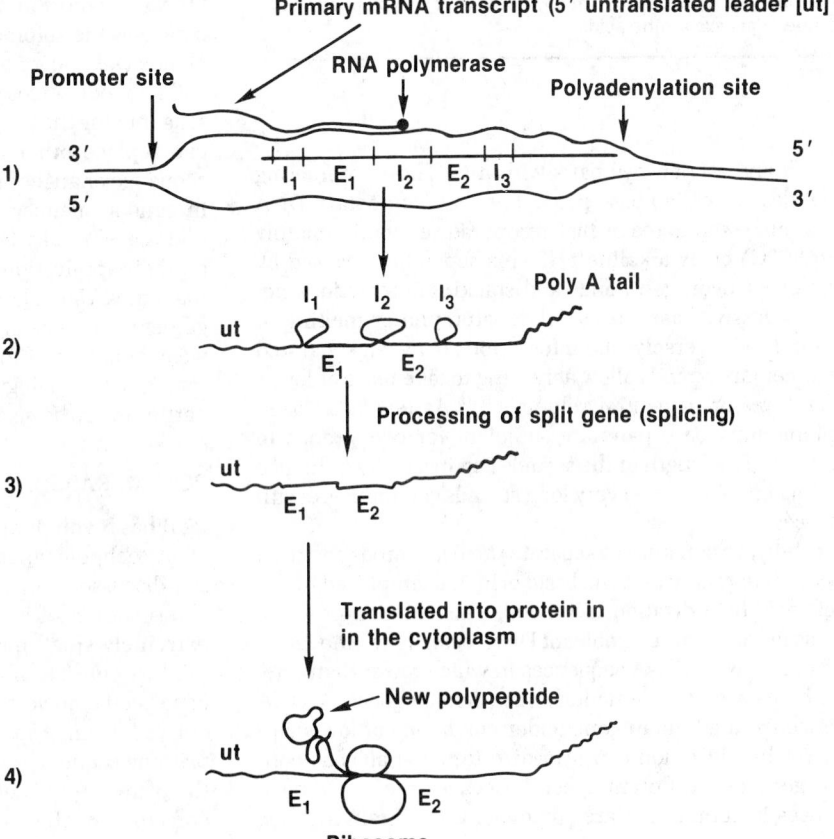

TABLE 1–1. The Genetic Code

First Position in Codon*	Second Position in Codon				Third Position in Codon (3' End)
	U	C	A	G	
U	Phe	Ser	Tyr	Cys	U
	Phe	Ser	Tyr	Cys	C
	Leu	Ser	Ter	Ter	A
	Leu	Ser	Ter	Trp	G
C	Leu	Pro	His	Arg	U
	Leu	Pro	His	Arg	C
	Leu	Pro	Gln	Arg	A
	Leu	Pro	Gln	Arg	G
A	Ile	Thr	Asn	Ser	U
	Ile	Thr	Asn	Ser	C
	Ile	Thr	Lys	Arg	A
	Met	Thr	Lys	Arg	G
G	Val	Ala	Asp	Gly	U
	Val	Ala	Asp	Gly	C
	Val	Ala	Glu	Gly	A
	Val	Ala	Glu	Gly	G

* The three RNA nucleotide bases coding the amino acid codons are given in first, second, and third positions in the 5' to 3' notation. For example, the codon 5' AUG 3' in mRNA specifies methionine, and CUC specifies leucine. UAA, UAG, and UGA are translational termination signals (Ter). AUG codes for methionine and is the first amino acid or initiation signal of every protein, but it also codes for internal methionines. Uridine (U), cytidine (C), adenine (A), and guanine (G) are nucleotide bases. Alanine (Ala), arginine (Arg), asparagine (Asn), aspartic (Asp), cysteine (Cys), glutamic (Glu), glutamine (Gln), glycine (Gly), histidine (His), isoleucine (Ile), leucine (Leu), lysine (Lys), methionine (Met), phylalanine (Phe), proline (Pro), serine (Ser), threonine (Thr), tyrosine (Tyr), tryptophan (Trp), and valine (Val) are amino acids.

with a T, and a G always pairs with a C. These interacting nucleotides are called base pairs. The complementary DNA strands can be separated by high temperature (approximately 70° to 80°C) or by alkaline pH. This separation, caused by disruption of hydrogen bonds and stacking interactions between successive bases, is called denaturation or melting of the strands. Conversely, the interactions between separated complementary strands allow annealing to take place at lower temperatures or in neutral solutions.[5–18] As few as a dozen complementary base pairs are sufficient for two strands to anneal.[19–21] The length of the strands can markedly influence annealing efficiency, and very long strands can interfere with the process.

The ability to denature or separate the two strands and then allow them to reanneal is the basic principle employed in the nucleic acid hybridization technique. This reaction provides the basis for much of recombinant DNA technology. Annealing can occur between DNA sequences in which fewer than 75% of the bases are complementary (i.e., homologous). A DNA sequence from a human gene under conditions of low stringency for hybridization can hybridize to the analogous conserved gene of a different species, because the genes have sequences in common or are homologous in certain regions.

DNA DUPLICATION AND NICK TRANSLATION

DNA is duplicated in vivo by DNA polymerase.[22–23] The parental strand is used as a template by this enzyme; nucleotides are covalently joined as they base pair with the parent strand (Fig. 1–1A). The new DNA molecules, each consisting of a parent strand and a newly synthesized strand, are partitioned to each new daughter cell during mitosis and cell division.

DNA polymerase is used extensively in vitro to copy a DNA sequence. The polymerase begins at a nick within the DNA and replaces the nucleotides in the damaged strand. When isotopically labeled nucleotides (usually isotopes of ^{32}P or ^{3}H) are included in the reaction, the DNA becomes uniformly labeled.[24,25] This reaction is referred to as nick translation. The isotopically labeled DNA sequence can then be denatured, mixed with other DNA fragments in solution or on a solid matrix, and allowed to reanneal. In this manner, a labeled DNA sequence hybridizes only to the unique copy among the more than 50,000 genes in the DNA molecule of a mammalian cell and serves as the molecular biologist's tool for finding the proverbial needle in a haystack.

A variation of the nick translation technique is called random priming. Six base pair fragments of DNA with random sequences are combined with denatured DNA strands. The mixture is allowed to hybridize (anneal) and the short fragments serve as "primers" for DNA polymerase. Because more radiolabeled nucleotides are incorporated using this method, the probe that is generated can be very high in specific radiolabeling activity and is therefore more sensitive.[26]

OLIGONUCLEOTIDE PRIMERS

One of the most important technologic advances in molecular biology is the automated synthesis of oligodeoxyribonucleotide chains (i.e., oligonucleotides).

Oligonucleotides can be used as primers, short probes, and reagents for the polymerase chain reaction (PCR). Their use can replace other recombinant DNA techniques if specific sequence changes are to be incorporated (often as mutations) in gene sequences. These single strands of deoxyribonucleotides are usually between 6 and 100 bases long, depending on their application. They are synthesized on programmable machines that chemically bond successive nucleotides together to produce the desired nucleic acid.[27–29] Within 10 years we expect that, if for no other reason than their requirement for PCR technology, oligonucleotide synthesizers will be a part of every basic and clinical research laboratory.

POLYMERASE CHAIN REACTION

PCR has revolutionized molecular diagnosis and recombinant DNA technology; applications of this technique in oncology are discussed in other chapters. PCR allows detection and identification of a segment of DNA or RNA that occurs in extremely small quantities within a sample.[30] The reaction mixture consists of the sample to be assayed for the presence of a specific nucleic acid, a thermostable bacterial polymerase derived from *Thermus aquaticus* (*Taq* polymerase), short priming sequences (i.e., oligonucleotides) complementary to the 3' and 5' ends of the DNA sequence to be analyzed, and cofactors for the enzymatic reaction.

These reagents are combined and placed in a programmable heat block that varies the temperature conditions for the sequential steps in the amplification reaction (Fig. 1–3). The DNA within the sample is denatured by heating to temperatures of 91° to 94°C. Rapid cooling allows annealing of oligonucleotide primers to the appropriate segment of DNA within the unknown sample. The temperature is then raised to 75° to 80°C, the optimal temperature for *TAQ* polymerase, to synthesize the target sequence between the oligonucleotide primers. This cycle is repeated approximately 30 times. During each cycle, the target sequence is doubled, and at the end of 30 reactions, one copy of DNA is amplified 2^{30} times. After the first cycle, newly synthesized fragments are used as the template, and the amplified fragment becomes the sequence between the two primers. This fragment can be detected by gel electrophoresis, Southern analysis, or sequencing. If RNA is to be assayed, it is first converted to DNA using the retroviral enzyme reverse transcriptase, and the DNA is assayed as described.

Some of the more important implications of this technology for oncology are in diagnosis and genetic screening and in the detection of residual disease in patients after cancer treatment.[31-33] This simple but powerful technology has also modified the conventional methods used in molecular biology.

DNA RESTRICTION ANALYSIS

One of the most important contributions to the study of DNA was the identification of restriction enzymes. These enzymes recognize specific short DNA sequences (usually 4- to 8-bp palindromes) and cleave the DNA strands at that site.[34] These enzymes are produced by bacteria as part of the restriction-

POLYMERASE CHAIN REACTION

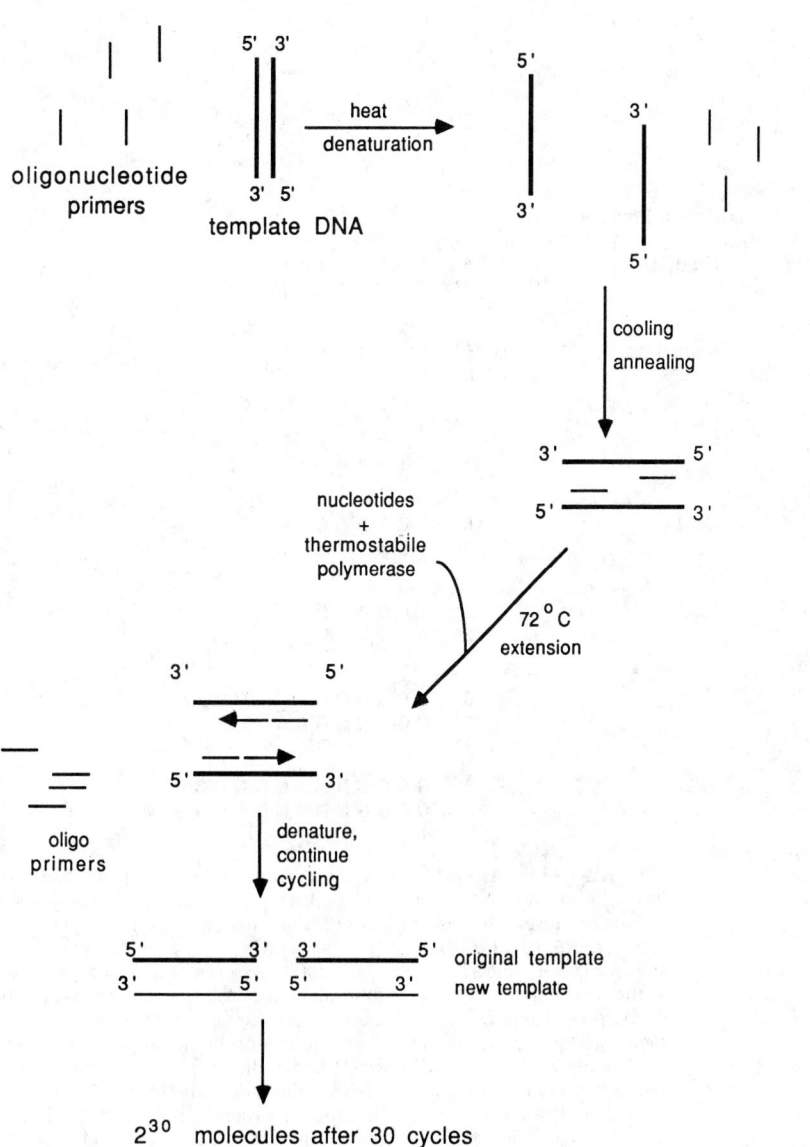

FIGURE 1–3. Steps in the polymerase chain reaction amplification reaction. Template DNA and oligonucleotide primers homologous to 3' and 5' regions of the target sequence are combined with *Taq* polymerase, nucleotides, and cofactors. Heat is applied to denature the DNA strands, and then the reaction is cooled to allow annealing of the primers to the template. The reaction is heated to 72°C to allow extension by the polymerase. The cycle is continued, using the newly synthesized strands as new templates. Theoretically, the target sequence is amplified 2^{30} times after 30 cycles.

modification system that protects the bacteria from invasion by foreign DNA.[34-38] Restriction sites, as these recognition sequences are called, are protected from cleavage by a modification enzyme that adds a methyl group to one base in the site and renders it resistant to change by the restriction enzyme.[38] Several hundred restriction enzymes that recognize more than 150 specific nucleotide sequences in double-stranded DNA have been identified. The recognition sites of several restriction enzymes are shown in Figure 1–4A. Foreign DNA entering the cell is not modified by methylation enzymes and is subject to digestion by the restriction enzyme. In the laboratory, these enzymes are powerful tools for dissecting DNA genetic information and are fundamental to recombinant DNA technology.

In a DNA molecule of random nucleotide sequences, a 6-base recognition sequence would be expected to occur once in every 4096 bp (*i.e.*, 1 in 4^6 bases). In human DNA, which is approximately 3×10^9 bp long, a 6-base recognition restriction enzyme cuts the DNA into several million fragments, but the DNA genome of a small DNA tumor virus may lack or have only a few cleavage sites for the same enzyme.[27] It is possible to fractionate the digested DNA fragments according to size in an agarose gel matrix by electrophoresis. The mobilities of the DNA fragments in this matrix are approximately proportional to the $\log_{10}$ of their length in base pairs.[39] The DNA fragments can be visualized with ultraviolet light after staining the gel with ethidium bromide. This compound intercalates between DNA base pairs and fluoresces under ultraviolet light. The genomic DNA from human cells is cut several million times by the same enzyme and appears as a smear when resolved by gel electrophoresis and visualized by ethidium bromide staining (Fig. 1–4B).

PCR can be used to generate restriction sites that flank a given length of DNA. Oligonucleotide primers are synthesized that are homologous to the 3' and 5' ends of the sequence to be amplified and that have an artificial restriction site distal to the homologous annealing sequence. During the amplification process, the target DNA sequence is produced with

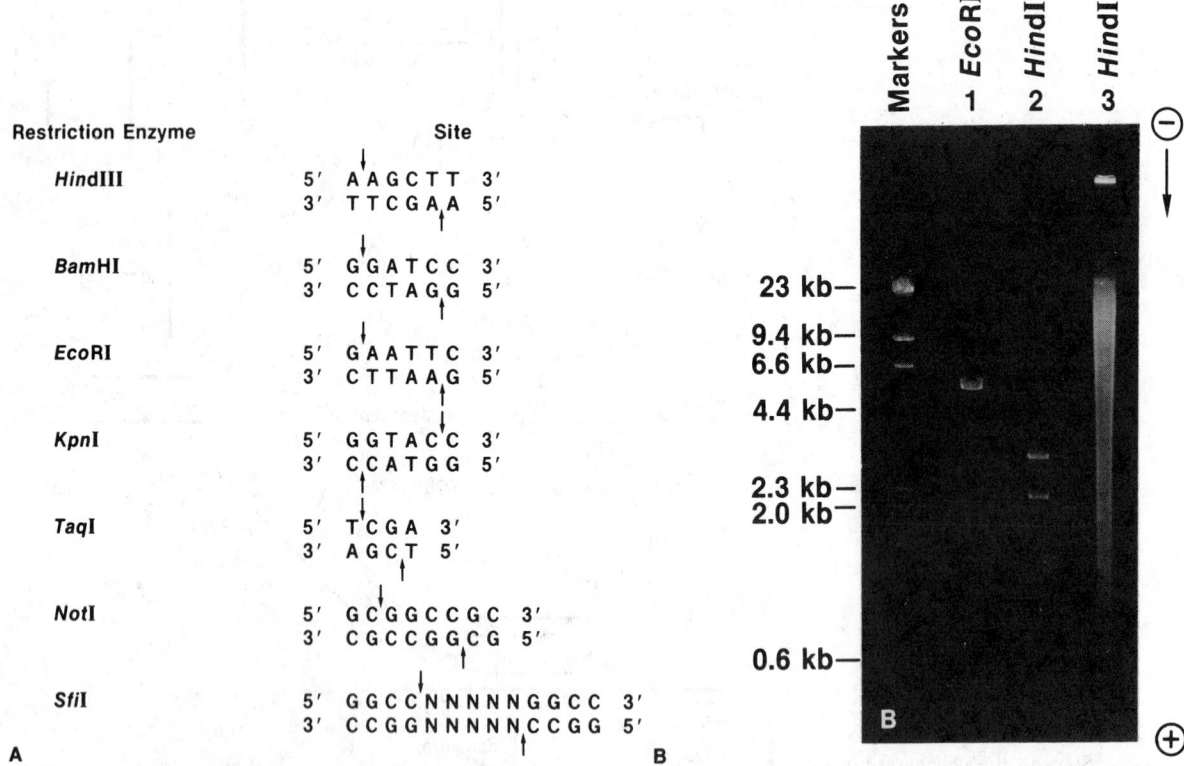

FIGURE 1–4. **(A)** Restriction enzyme recognition sites. The 6-base nucleotide sequence recognition sites in double-strand DNA for *Hind*III, *Bam*HI, *Eco*RI, and *Kpn*I are underlined. The orientation 5' to 3' is important because with these enzymes the double-strand enzyme cleavage is staggered, leaving a 4-base 5' single-strand overhang (*Hind*III, *Bam*HI, and *Eco*RI) or a 4-base 3' overhang (*Kpn*I). Three additional recognition sites for the enzymes *Taq*I, *Not*I, and *Sfi*I are shown. These enzymes cleave double-strand DNA everywhere in the molecule that the recognition sequence appears. The overhang allows recombinant DNA gene splicing in the presence of DNA ligase to occur between a heterogenous population of similarly digested DNA fragments. **(B)** Fractionation of restriction fragments by electrophoresis. One microgram of purified polyomavirus DNA is digested with *Eco*RI (*lane 1*) or *Hind*III (*lane 2*) and subjected to agarose gel electrophoresis. Ten micrograms of human placental DNA is digested with *Hind*III (*lane 3*) and likewise subjected to electrophoresis. After the gel is stained with ethidium bromide, the resolved DNA fragments can be visualized by long-wave UV light. The extreme left lane shows DNA fragments of known size, in kilobase pairs (kb).

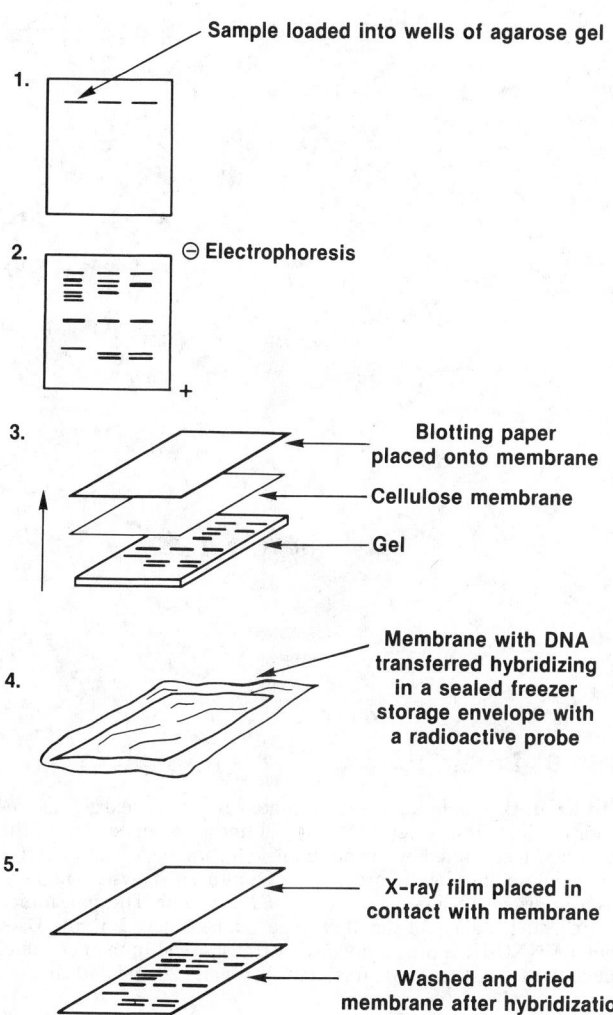

1. Sample loaded into wells of agarose gel

2. ⊖ Electrophoresis

   +

3. Blotting paper placed onto membrane

   Cellulose membrane

   Gel

4. Membrane with DNA transferred hybridizing in a sealed freezer storage envelope with a radioactive probe

5. X-ray film placed in contact with membrane

   Washed and dried membrane after hybridization

Schematic of Steps in the Southern Transfer Analysis

A

flanking restriction sites. The fragment is isolated, cut with a restriction enzyme, and cloned into a vector as described later.[40]

DETECTION OF GENES AND GENE PRODUCTS

SOUTHERN ANALYSIS

Any one of the 50,000 or more genes in the mammalian genome can be detected by a technique called Southern transfer analysis.[41] Restriction enzyme-cleaved DNA is resolved in one dimension by agarose gel electrophoresis as described earlier (Fig. 1–4B). After electrophoresis, the gel is exposed to an alkaline solution, which denatures the DNA strands within it. The DNA is then transferred to a membrane that traps the single-strand, size-sorted DNA fragments (Fig. 1–5A). The DNA is immobilized on the membrane by drying in a vacuum oven. This filter, or blot, containing the transferred DNA can then be placed in a hybridization solution with a radioactive probe. Isotopic labeling of one strand of DNA followed by hybridization with the complementary strand results in a radioactive hybrid product. After hybridization and washing to remove nonspecific sticking of the probe to the filter, the blot is exposed to x-ray film. The position of the gene that is homologous to the probe can be visualized.

This technique has identified related genes, such as oncogenes, within cells of different species. It has also allowed correlation between regions of cellular oncogenes (c-*ONC*) with viral oncogenic sequences (v-*ONC*). Figure 1–5B illustrates an autoradiograph. Mouse, human, and quail DNAs were digested with a restriction enzyme and subjected to agarose gel electrophoresis. The gel was blotted and hybridized with a mouse *MOS* oncogene probe.[42] The mouse probe detects the

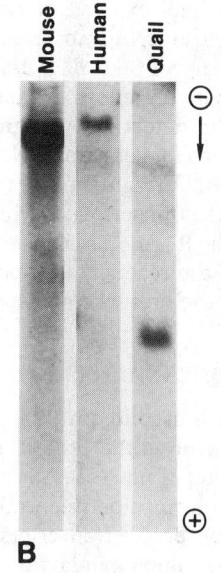

Mouse   Human   Quail

⊖

⊕

B

FIGURE 1–5. **(A)** Schematic of the steps in Southern analysis. **1.** A 20 × 20 cm 0.5% to 1.0% agarose gel, 3 or 4 mm thick, is formed in a conventional gel electrophoresis apparatus. **2.** Restriction enzyme-digested DNA samples are loaded into preformed wells, and the gel is subjected to an electrophoretic field to fractionate the restricted DNA fragments. **3.** For blotting, the gel is placed in a tray on top of absorbent paper wetted with buffer, and a cut-to-size wetted membrane is placed atop the gel and is sandwiched with dry absorbent paper to draw (blot) the resolved DNA fragments onto the DNA-trapping membrane. **4.** After the DNA is fixed to the membrane and nonspecific binding sites are blocked with a special medium, the membrane is sealed in a plastic envelope with a suitable isotopically labeled probe and placed under hybridization conditions, usually overnight. **5.** The excess isotopic label is washed off, and the membrane is exposed to x-ray film for 12 hours or more. The film is developed to reveal hybridizing fragments. **(B)** Southern transfer analysis detection of the *MOS* oncogene in mouse, quail, and human cellular genomic DNA. Twenty micrograms each of mouse BALB/c DNA digested with *Eco*RI, human placental DNA digested with *Hin*dIII, and quail QT6 cell line DNA digested with *Bam*HI were subjected to electrophoresis in an agarose gel. The electrophoretically resolved DNA in the gel was then transferred to a nitrocellulose membrane by the procedure of Southern analysis, and a mouse *MOS*-specific isotopically labeled probe was hybridized to the DNA blotted onto the membrane. After hybridization, the membrane was exposed to x-ray film for 12 hours to detect the radioactive fragments containing nucleotide sequences homologous to *MOS*.

homologous sequences in mouse DNA and detects homologous cellular genes in human and quail DNAs. This result shows that the *MOS* gene sequences are conserved in the three animal species. Thousands of probes have been used to detect genomic sequences in the DNA of viruses and living organisms.

PCR can also be used to detect and isolate homologous genes. For example, degenerate oligonucleotide primers are synthesized in the codons of conserved segments of open reading frames. During PCR, the only primers corresponding to the correct sequence in the target gene are selected and amplified. The fragments produced can be analyzed by electrophoresis, Southern analysis, direct DNA sequencing, or molecular cloning.

PULSED-FIELD GEL ELECTROPHORESIS

The traditional Southern blot technique has many applications in the analysis of DNA but suffers from the limitation that fragments larger than 20 kb are poorly resolved on conventional agarose gels. Variations of this technique have been described that use alterations in the electrical field applied to the DNA and result in increased resolution of large DNA fragments. Although there are several variations of this method, they all use pulses of current instead of a constant field to increase resolution.[43] The pulsed-field gel electrophoresis (PFGE) causes the DNA molecules to align in a linear fashion within the field. Variations of this method involve applying current at different angles to the gel and are referred to as orthogonal field agarose gel electrophoresis (OFAGE).[44] In field-inversion gel electrophoresis (FIGE), the polarity of the field is biased to favor DNA mobility in one direction as pulses of current are applied.[45]

During conventional electrophoresis, large DNA fragments run together in the gel. The size range in which fragments resolve using FIGE depends on the electrode placement and the duration of the pulses. Fragments as large as 7 million base pairs have been separated in this way.[46] Large-fragment DNA analysis uses restriction enzymes that recognize larger recognition sites (*e.g.*, 8-bp sequence) and theoretically cleaves a random DNA strand once every 65,536 bp. If digestion by the enzyme does not go to completion, a partial digestion can be compared with a complete digestion to determine fragment relations.[47]

The power to resolve large fragments allows construction of physical maps of small genomes or chromosomes. The genome of *Escherichia coli,* which is approximately 10 million base pairs, has been mapped.[48] The maps of other bacterial chromosomes, yeast chromosomes, and mammalian chromosomes are being constructed in this manner.[49]

DNA from a human cell line containing a *MET* protooncogene rearrangement was digested with *Sfi*I (restriction site: 5' GGCC↓NNNNNGGCC 3') and subjected to FIGE (Fig. 1–6). The DNA was transferred to a filter using a modified Southern technique and probed with an isotopically labeled *MET* oncogene probe. The rearrangement of the gene is indicated by the appearance of the larger fragment size in the human tumor cell line.[50]

NORTHERN ANALYSIS

Northern analysis, a variation of the Southern technique, detects RNA molecules and transcripts (mRNA) instead of

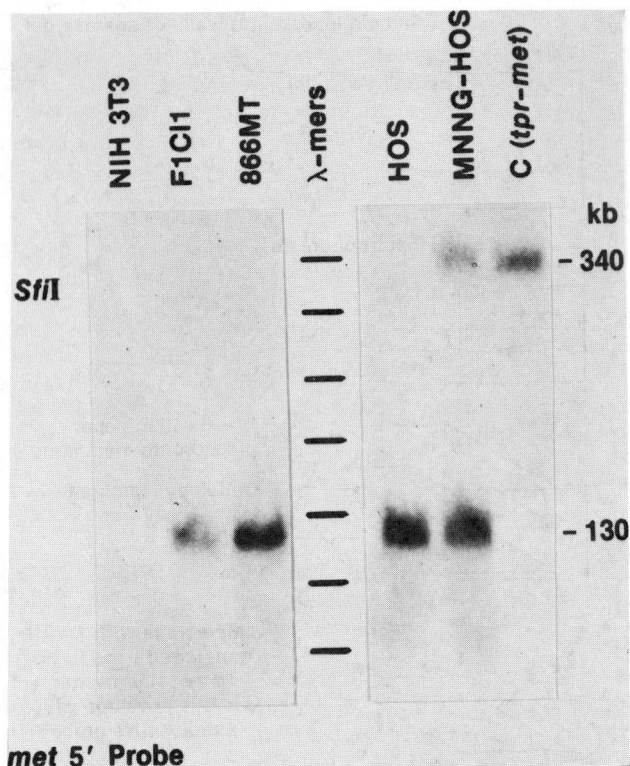

FIGURE 1–6.   DNA fragments separated by pulsed-field gel electrophoresis. DNA from several human cell lines was digested with the enzyme *Sfi*I, separated by the pulsed-field technique, transferred to a nitrocellulose filter by the procedure of Southern analysis. The filter was hybridized with a probe from the *MET* oncogene. The appearance of a rearranged allele of the *MET* gene can be observed in the DNA from a MNNG-HOS line, a chemically transformed human cell line. Notice the separation of the fragments between 120 and 340 kb.

cleaved DNA fragments. Extracted RNA is run on a denaturing agarose gel, blotted to membranes, and probed in a hybridization reaction similar to the one described for Southern analysis.[27,51] Northern analyses can reveal quantitative and qualitative information on steady-state mRNA transcripts and can identify amplified gene expression (*e.g.*, c-*MYC* or m-*MYC* in tumor cells) or hybrid RNA transcripts in rearranged genomic loci (*e.g.*, the novel 8-kb *BCR-ABL* hybrid transcript expressed in chronic myelogenous leukemia).[52,53]

PCR can be used to detect RNA fragments by a method similar to that described for detecting DNA fragments. Before the PCR reaction, mRNA fragments are treated with the retroviral enzyme reverse transcriptase, which makes a single-strand DNA copy of the RNA. This DNA serves as the template for the remainder of the reaction. The product is assayed as described earlier for the presence of a specific sequence.[54]

RNASE PROTECTION ANALYSIS

Several techniques are used to quantitate mRNA levels; the basic methodology involves the protection of double-strand hybrids from the action of nucleases. S1 nuclease protection analysis uses hybrids formed between mRNA and a specific DNA probe to identify specific transcripts. An isotopically labeled DNA fragment, complementary to the specific RNA in question, is denatured and mixed with total or poly A-enriched

RNA. Conditions are provided that favor RNA-DNA hybridization. The enzyme S1 nuclease is used to digest all single-stranded DNA and RNA molecules; hybrid molecules are left intact. These complexes are analyzed by polyacrylamide gel electrophoresis (Fig. 1–7).[54,55] Because RNA-DNA annealing conditions are selective, S1 nuclease protection analysis is very sensitive and can be used to detect one mRNA molecule in 100 cells if large amounts of RNA are available. This method is useful for the examination of low-abundance transcripts. A variation of this method uses RNA-RNA hybridization conditions.[27]

PCR, although not yet strictly quantitative, is the most sensitive detection method available for RNA or DNA. Theoretically, one RNA molecule can be amplified to quantities sufficient to sequence.[56]

WESTERN ANALYSIS

Southern analysis and Northern analysis are used to detect DNA and RNA, respectively, and the name Western analysis has been used to describe an equivalent technique to detect proteins. Protein isolated from tissues or cells is subjected to electrophoresis on polyacrylamide gels, often with the detergent sodium dodecylsulfate, to separate the molecules by molecular weight. The protein is then transferred to a filter using high-voltage electrophoresis (transfer of RNA or DNA to a filter is done by capillary action and compressive forces). The filter with transferred protein is exposed to specific antibodies; enzyme-linked or isotopically labeled antispecies antibodies or proteins that bind specifically to antibodies are applied to the filter. The protein bands recognized by the antibodies are visualized calorimetrically or by autoradiographic methods.[27,57,58]

ISOLATION AND CHARACTERIZATION OF GENES

DNA SEQUENCING

The precise order of the nucleotide bases in a DNA strand can be determined by DNA sequencing. Historically, two methods have been used. The Maxam-Gilbert technique end-labels DNA strands isotopically.[27,59] Single-strand DNA is subjected to four different reactions. These reactions cleave randomly at one of four sites: C, T and C, A and G, or G. After the reactions have occurred, the samples are subjected to polyacrylamide gel electrophoresis. The strands are separated by size; comparison of the banding patterns from the four reactions allows sequence analysis of the parental strand (Fig. 1–1B).

The second procedure for sequence analysis incorporates a DNA polymerization step. The DNA to be sequenced is again divided into four different polymerization reactions. A small quantity of one nucleotide (a different one in each reaction) is replaced by dideoxynucleotides. Isotopically labeled nucleotides are also incorporated into the reaction mixture for autoradiographic analysis of the synthetic products. The reaction proceeds using the parental strand as a template; incorporation of a dideoxynucleotide results in chain termination. (This same strategy makes AZT [3-azido-3′-thymidine] a successful drug for treating acquired immunodeficiency syndrome.) Size resolution by polyacrylamide electrophoresis of all four reactions allows sequence determination. This sequencing method, known as the Sanger or dideoxy technique, is more widely used today.[27,60]

Automated sequencing is being developed to aid the human genome project (*e.g.,* Applied Biosystems automated sequencing system). The technology helps to standardize se-

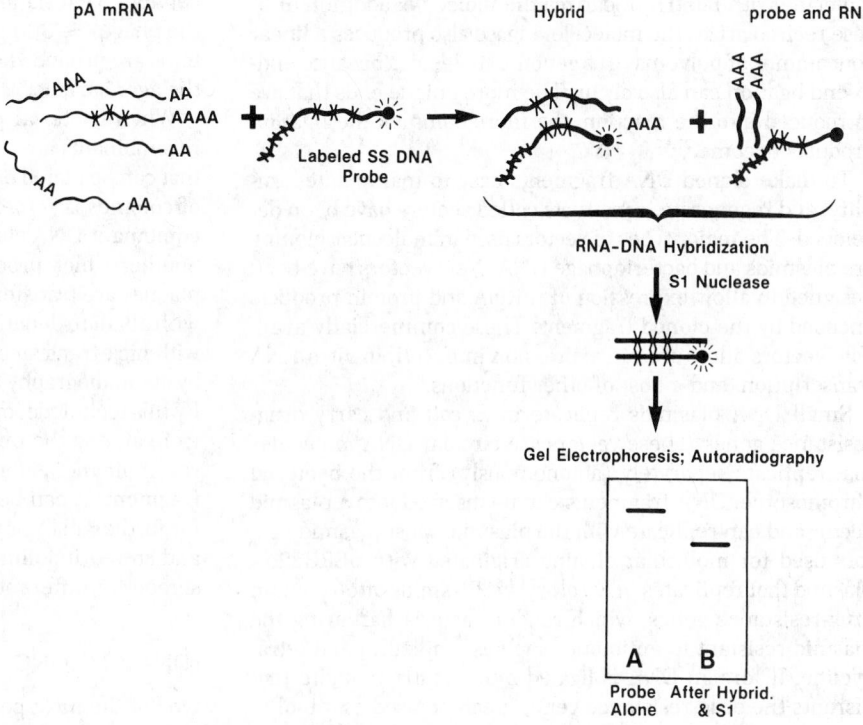

FIGURE 1–7. S1 nuclease analysis. S1 nuclease is used to demonstrate that a specific transcript is present in a population of mRNAs. An isotopically labeled single-strand DNA probe is denatured and mixed with mRNAs. Buffer and temperature conditions favoring RNA-DNA annealing are provided. S1 nuclease is added, which degrades all single-strand DNA and RNA in the mixture; only the double-strand RNA-DNA product is resistant to digestion. The product is analyzed by gel electrophoresis and autoradiography for size and abundance.

quencing results, reduce human error, and decrease the labor involved in the sequencing process.[61]

After sequences are compiled, they are entered into one of several computer databases (*e.g.*, GenBank, European Molecular Biology Laboratory, and National Biomedical Research Foundation) and processed by several programs (*e.g.*, PC/Gene [IntelliGenetics, Inc.], Sequence Analysis Software Package [University of Wisconsin], or Genepro [Riverside Scientific Enterprises]). This allows homology comparisons to be performed among the thousands of proteins and nucleic acids already entered, provides others with access to the data, and screens for interesting regions of the molecule, such as specific types of helices, metal-binding regions, or kinase homology regions. The latter capability is expanding dramatically, and it will eventually replace the need for three-dimensional crystallographic analyses.

MOLECULAR CLONING

Modern molecular biology depends on the technology of molecular cloning, which can be defined as the isolation and amplification of defined DNA fragments. Molecular cloning is a straightforward process involving the manipulation of DNA with enzymes followed by screening with probes to isolate the desired nucleic acid sequence. PCR technology has significantly simplified this process, because it enables DNA amplification from a sample that can be visualized as a band on a gel and then molecularly cloned or sequenced.

The initial step in molecular cloning involves the use of restriction enzymes to cleave the DNA (usually genomic) into a series of fragments. Another critical enzyme used in molecular cloning is DNA ligase. This enzyme reseals the cohesive ends of two DNA fragments.[62] The genome of polyomavirus is a circular double-stranded DNA molecule (Fig. 1–4B). Its genome is 5292 bp long, and it contains a single *Bam*HI recognition site (Fig. 1–4A).[63] Cutting the circular molecule with *Bam*HI linearizes the molecule; addition of ligase recircularizes the molecule. Ligase also produces a linear concatamer of polyomavirus genome molecules because end-to-end ligation can also occur. The more unique ends that are introduced into the reaction, the more complex the ligation products become.[27,62]

To make cloned DNA fragments easy to manipulate, amplify, and regenerate, constructs called vectors have been developed. The major types of vectors used in molecular cloning are plasmids and bacteriophage DNA. New vectors have been designed to allow expression of mRNA and protein products encoded by the cloned fragment. These commercially available vectors allow protein expression in *E. coli*, in vitro RNA transcription, and a host of other functions.[27]

Small DNA plasmids replicate in *E. coli* and carry drug-resistance genes. These vectors are circular DNA molecules that replicate separately (autonomously) from the bacterial chromosome. DNA fragments can be inserted into a plasmid vector and can replicate with the plasmid. Most plasmid vectors used for molecular cloning originated with pBR322, a plasmid that replicates in *E. coli*.[27,64,65] Plasmids often contain drug-resistance genes, which render bacteria harboring the plasmid resistant to antibiotics such as ampicillin and tetracycline. If foreign DNA is ligated into a restriction site that disrupts the drug resistance gene, it can be used as a tool to screen for recombinants (*i.e.*, bacterial plasmids with foreign DNA inserts), because only plasmids with disrupted drug resistance genes are sensitive to the antibiotic. Commercially available plasmids also use the *LACZ* gene as a marker for inserts. When grown on X-gal (5-bromo-4-chloro-3-indolyl-β-D-galactopyranoside), an artificial substrate for the *LACZ*-encoded enzyme, in the presence of an *LACZ* gene promotor, isopropylthio-β-D-galactopyranoside, bacteria with intact plasmids produce blue colonies. Plasmids that have incorporated inserts are white. A combination of drug resistance and *LACZ* expression can be used to select for bacteria that have incorporated a plasmid and have an insert (Fig. 1–8).[27,66]

Although well suited for the cloning of small DNA fragments, plasmids do not accommodate larger DNA fragments. To molecularly clone larger fragments, bacteriophage vectors have been developed. Bacteriophages are bacterial viruses; they have been modified to function as vectors by removing sections of their genome that are not essential for autonomous replication. Foreign DNA fragments of up to 20 kb can be cloned into these vectors. Bacteriophage λ is the prototypic bacteriophage vector, but commercially available forms provide a wide variety of capabilities, including in vivo and in vitro expression.[27]

A genomic library is a collection of recombinant molecules that theoretically represents every DNA sequence within the genome of the organism being studied. One million recombinant clones of random genomic fragments with an average length of 15 kb should contain 15 billion base pairs of genomic sequence and would presumably be representative of the 3 billion base pair mammalian or human genome. To construct such a library, genomic DNA is digested with a restriction enzyme to yield fragments of the appropriate size. The fragments are mixed with a vector (usually λ phage, because they accommodate large fragments) that has been cut with the same restriction enzyme. Ligase is added to join the vector with the inserts. After packaging in vitro with phage coat proteins, the infectious recombinant phages are mixed with susceptible bacteria and plated on agar. Bacteria infected with the phage ($\approx$ 300 phages per cell) are lysed after phage proteins are produced and clear areas known as plaques form on the agar surface.[27,67]

When bacterial plasmids are used as vectors, the ligated recombinants are transformed into a competent bacterial host that can be plated on agar. In this case, an appropriate number of colonies is screened with a probe to detect the desired recombinant DNA clone. Screening is performed similar to the Southern blot procedure described previously; colonies or plaques are transferred to membranes, the filters are treated with alkali to denature the DNA, and the filters are hybridized with nick-translated probe.[68,69] Positive colonies are identified by autoradiography and matched to colonies on the agar plates. By this technique, one recombinant molecule can be identified from among the millions of host genomic fragments. After a recombinant is identified as one containing the desired DNA fragment, it can be grown in microgram or gram quantities for further analysis (Fig. 1–8). DNA libraries can be amplified and stored indefinitely, and they can be used repeatedly to screen for different recombinants.[27]

cDNA CLONING

One of the most powerful techniques in molecular biology is cDNA cloning, because it allows the study of cell-specific gene

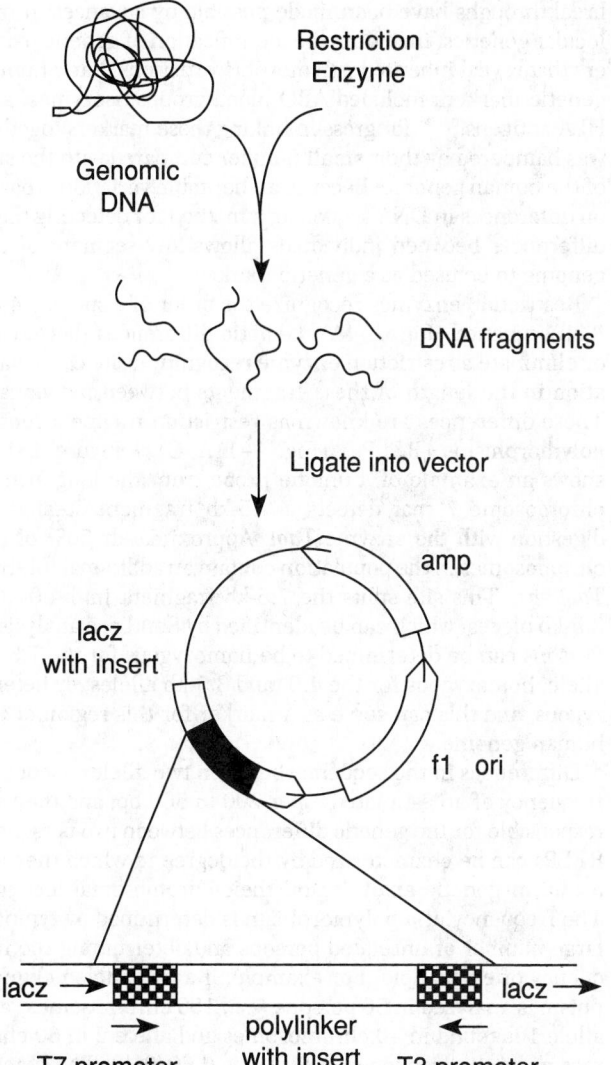

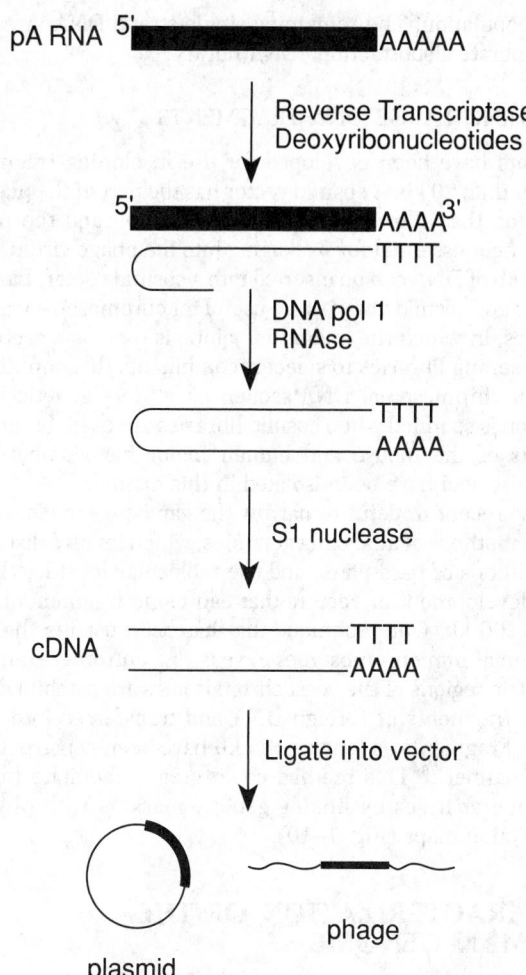

FIGURE 1–8. Genomic cloning. To isolate specific genomic sequences, DNA is extracted from tissues or cells and digested into small (5–25 kb) fragments with a restriction enzyme. DNA fragments can be sorted by size by using column fractionation or elution from agarose gels. The fragments are then ligated into appropriate vectors (usually λ phage for this size fragment) that have also been cut with restriction enzymes. The vectors with inserts are amplified in DNA and screened using probes as described in the text. The plasmid vector shown illustrates a drug-resistance gene (*AMP*), a replication origin that allows autonomous replication (f1 ori), and a β-galactosidase gene cloning site (*lacZ*). When the *lacZ* gene is interrupted by a genomic insert, induced bacteria that incorporate the plasmid are unable to cleave the gene promotor isoprophylthio-β-D-glactopyranose, and resultant colonies are white. Colonies with uninterrupted plasmids are blue. Also shown as part of the insertion site is a polylinker that is a manufactured stretch of DNA containing many tandem restriction sites. The polylinker provides a variety of convenient ligation sites for the insert. T7 and T3 promoters allow for RNA synthesis of the insert in both directions. This provides the ability to synthesize highly specific single-strand probes from the insert or allows for in vitro transcription of the insert.

FIGURE 1–9. cDNA cloning. Polyadenylated messenger RNA (mRNA) is incubated with free deoxynucleotides and the enzyme reverse transcriptase (usually isolated from avian myeloblastosis virus). This enzyme synthesizes a DNA copy of the mRNA template. A "hairpin loop" is formed at the 5' end. DNA polymerase (DNA POL1) is added for the synthesis of the second strand; RNAse digests the RNA template. S1 nuclease cleaves the hairpin loop, and a double-strand copy of the mRNA remains. The fragments are ligated into vectors (usually plasmids as the DNAs are relatively short, 0.5–5 kb). The collection of cDNA clones is then amplified in bacteria and screened using probes as described in the text.

expression. In this technique, mRNA isolated from specific cells or tissues is reverse transcribed to generate single-strand DNA copies of the transcripts. DNA polymerase is then used to generate double-strand DNA fragments, which can be cloned into vectors (Fig. 1–9).[27,70] cDNA libraries differ from genomic libraries by being limited to only the transcribed

portion of genes and, therefore, are greatly reduced in complexity. These libraries are useful in providing amplified copies of specific sequences; for example, a cDNA library from reticulocytes will contain many copies of globin cDNA, whereas this gene occurs only twice in a genomic library.

cDNA libraries prepared in a similar manner have been useful for identifying transcripts that are differentially regulated in related cell types in the so-called subtraction cloning technique. For example, to identify novel transcripts that are expressed in mitogenically stimulated cells but not in resting cells, single-strand cDNA prepared from the former is annealed with an excess of RNA prepared from the latter. RNA-DNA hybrids representing sequences common to both cell types are removed by several separation techniques.[71–74] After repeating the cycle several times, the sequences common to both cell types are markedly reduced. This enhances the concentration of novel sequences for the mitogenically stimulated cell population. The remaining single-strand DNAs are used to generate a subtraction cDNA library.

CLONING LARGE DNA FRAGMENTS

Vectors have been developed for use in cloning fragments larger than 20 kb. A cosmid vector has the part of the plasmid genome that allows autonomous replication and the phage sequences essential for packaging into the phage virion.[75] Up to 50 kb of DNA can be inserted into a cosmid vector. Lambda phage and cosmid libraries are useful for chromosome walking studies, in which the end of one clone is used as a probe for rescreening libraries to select recombinants that contain adjacent chromosomal DNA sequences.[76] More genetic information is spanned when cosmid libraries are used. Large segments of the mouse and human major histocompatibility complex loci have been isolated in this manner.[77]

The recent impetus to narrow the gap between classic genetic methods of analyzing genomes, which involve distances in millions of base pairs, and the molecular level has led to the development of vectors that can clone fragments larger than 100 kb. One technique that has been used is the generation of minichromosomes in yeast.[78] Centromeric and telocentric regions of the yeast chromosomes are combined with large fragments of foreign DNA and transferred into yeast cells. Fragments as long as 125 kb have been constructed in this manner.[78] This method could greatly facilitate human genome analyses by linking genetic markers with physical restriction maps (Fig. 1–10).

CHARACTERIZATION OF THE HUMAN GENOME

RESTRICTION FRAGMENT LENGTH POLYMORPHISMS

Dramatic advances have occurred recently in identifying and understanding numerous genetic disorders, including muscular dystrophy, cystic fibrosis, retinoblastoma, colon cancer, small cell lung cancer, and familial polyposis coli.[10,79–93] These breakthroughs have been made possible by advances in molecular genetics, including the identification of genetic markers that reveal inherited polymorphic variations. Early human genetic markers included ABO blood groups, isozymes, and HLA antigens.[94–96] Progress in linking these markers together was hampered by their small number compared with the size of the human genome. Because all heritable variation is based on differences in DNA sequence, a method for detecting these differences between individuals allows any segment of the genome to be used as a genetic marker.

Restriction enzymes recognize the order of a specific 4- to 8-bp sequence (Fig. 1–4A). Genetic differences that create or eliminate a restriction enzyme recognition site cause variation in the length of these fragments between individuals. These differences are known as restriction fragment length polymorphisms (RFLPs) (Fig. 1–11A–C).[97] Figure 1–11A shows an example of a unique probe from the long arm of chromosome 7 that detects a 7.5-kb fragment created by digestion with the enzyme *Taq*I. Approximately 50% of the chromosomes in the population contain an additional internal *Taq*I site. This site splits the 7.5-kb fragment into 4.0- and 3.5-kb pieces, which can be identified by Southern analysis.[98] Persons can be determined to be homozygous for the 7.5-kb allele, homozygous for the 4.0- and 3.5-kb alleles, or heterozygous, and this can serve as a marker for this region of the human genome.

Differences in the sequence between two alleles occur at a frequency of an estimated 1 per 200 to 500 bp, and they are responsible for the genetic differences between two persons.[99] RFLPs can be characterized by the degree to which they are useful in genetic analysis and their chromosomal location. The frequency of a polymorphism is determined by typing a large number of unrelated persons and determining the frequency of each allele. For example, if a two-allele polymorphism is analyzed in 50 persons (*i.e.*, 100 chromosomes) and allele 1 is found in 40 chromosomes and allele 2 in 60 chromosomes, the frequency of 2 to 1 is 0.60/0.40. The heterozygosity of an RFLP is related to the frequency and is a measure of the percentage of persons who are heterozygotes. The

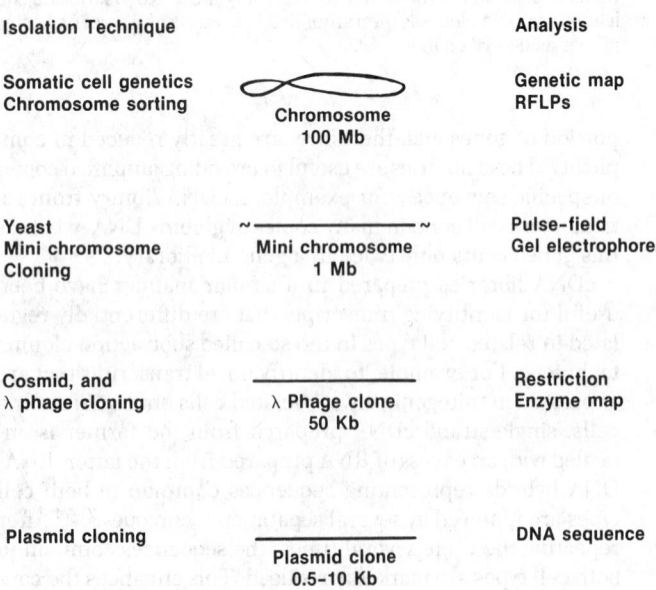

FIGURE 1–10. Cloning and analyzing the human genome. Techniques for capturing portions of genetic information and the types of analyses that they make possible are compared. Somatic cell hybrids and fluorescence-activated cell sorting allow whole chromosomes (50–200 Mb) to be isolated. These techniques assist in the construction of genetic linkage maps of chromosomes. Chromosomes can be broken down into 0.1- to 1.0-Mb fragments by cloning into yeast minichromosomes. These fragments can be used to generate a physical map using pulsed-field gel electrophoresis. Minichromosomes can be subdivided by cloning into cosmid and phage vectors, and these subclones can be characterized by conventional restriction mapping. Fragments for the phage clones can be inserted into plasmid vectors, and the nucleotide sequence can be determined.

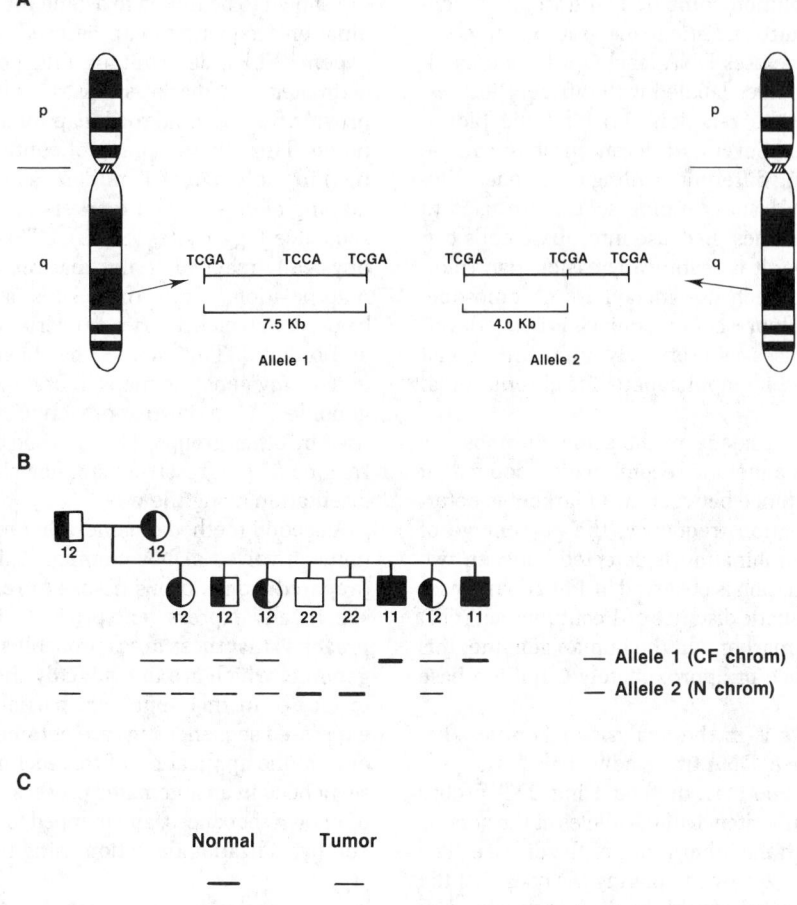

FIGURE 1-11. Use of a DNA-based genetic marker. **(A)** An example of a restriction fragment-length polymorphism (RFLP). A diagram of human chromosome 7 shows the position of the *MET* protooncogene at 7q31. The sequence TCGA is the recognition sequence of the *Taq*I restriction enzyme, which generates a 7.5-kb fragment. **(B)** Use of an RFLP in genetic diagnosis. The *MET* gene is tightly linked to the cystic fibrosis (CF) gene, and they are almost always inherited together. In this family, allele 1 is on the CF chromosome and the affected children (*filled symbols*) have a 1,1 genotype. Those with a 1,2 genotype are unaffected carriers and 2,2 children are unaffected noncarriers. **(C)** RFLP detection of DNA deletion in a tumor. This hypothetical example shows how the deletion of all or part of a chromosome can be detected by comparing tumor and normal DNA from the same patient. **(D)** (See color insert between pages 72 and 73.) Fluorescent in situ hybridization of a nonisotopically labeled *HUD*5 probe to human chromosomes. The photograph on the left depicts fluorescent signals on chromosomes counterstained with propidium iodide, and the photograph on the right illustrates *DAPI*-banding of the same metaphase spread. The signals in this and other cells examined are located at band 15q21. (Courtesy of J. Testa, Fox Chase Cancer Center, Philadelphia, PA)

polymorphism information content is a measure of the percentage of families in which both parents are heterozygous for a given polymorphism.[97]

GENETIC MAPPING AND LINKAGE ANALYSIS

Probes that detect RFLPs can be mapped to chromosomes by physical and genetic methods. The physical methods include somatic cell hybridization and in situ hybridization.[100,101] Somatic cell hybridization assigns a gene to a given chromosome according to its segregation in a panel of interspecies hybrid cell lines. For example, a series of human/hamster hybrids contain different cell lines with predominantly hamster chromosomes. Human chromosomal assignments are made by mapping which cell lines contain the given human gene or

its marker and correlating this information with the human chromosome content of the cell line. This technique can be aided by PCR; oligonucleotide primers from the ends of the gene or marker sequence are added to DNA extracted from each hybrid cell line. The gene is easily determined by sequence amplification.[102]

In situ hybridization is a more precise localization technique. An isotopically labeled probe is applied to the chromosomes, which are then covered with photographic emulsion. After the emulsion is developed, the number of grains over the chromosome is quantitated. A newer technique uses a fluorescent-labeled probe applied directly to interphase chromosomes (see Color Fig. 1–11D after p. 72) and is referred to as fluorescent in situ hybridization (FISH).[103]

The use of fluorescent probes enhances the speed of the

reaction and spatial resolution compared with isotopic techniques, which often require statistical analysis to map sites. The fluorescent technique uses DNA labeled with photoactivated biotin; avidin molecules labeled with different fluorescent tags are added to the reaction and bind the biotin-hybridized DNA probes. Several different probes can be examined at once by using different labeling techniques. Fluorescent microscopes or laser-scanning scopes are used to identify labeled chromosomes. Because interphase cells can be used in this technique, it is technically easier than traditional in situ methods, which use metaphase chromosome preparations.[103,104] This fluorescent technique is being developed to detect genetic diseases prenatally on a commercial basis, and it has far-reaching applications for chromosomal mapping.

Two markers that are resident on the same chromosome are inherited together in a meiotic recombination-dependent fashion. The genetic distance between two markers is determined by the recombination frequency, the percentage of meioses in which a recombination is detected between two markers. If the recombination is observed in 1 of 100 meioses (a frequency of 1%), a genetic distance of 1 centimorgan (cM) occurs between the two markers. In the human genome, this is equivalent to a distance of approximately 1 million base pairs.[105]

A major use of RFLPs is in the analysis of families that segregate a human disease. DNA from individuals in the pedigree is analyzed by the Southern method using DNA probes that detect RFLPs. The inheritance of the alleles of the genetic marker is correlated with the inheritance of the disease. The data are statistically analyzed by calculating the odds that the association between the marker and the disease occurred by chance. This information is used to calculate an LOD score (the log of the odds). An LOD score of 3 (odds of 1000 to 1) is taken as formal proof of linkage.[106] An example of that linkage is displayed in Figure 1–11B. RFLP markers discovered in the *MET* protooncogene on human chromosome 7 were used to analyze pedigrees segregating the recessive genetic disease cystic fibrosis. In the first families analyzed, there was a perfect correlation between the marker and the disease, resulting in an LOD score of 8 (100,000,000 to 1).[98] This finding mapped the cystic fibrosis defect to chromosome 7q31.1-31.3. The cystic fibrosis gene has been subsequently cloned using chromosomal walking and jumping techniques to scan this region of the human genome.[80] Other genes that have been identified using chromosomal localization data include those for neurofibromatosis type I, multiple polyposis coli, and Li-Fraumeni syndrome.[90–93,107,108]

These examples illustrate the applications of RFLP linkage analysis. Carrier detection and prenatal diagnosis of diseases and traits can be identified using these markers. RFLP analysis has been used in analysis of human cancers to determine loss of heterozygosity in somatic cell tumors. This technology has been essential for the discovery and isolation of tumor suppressor genes.

HUMAN GENETIC LINKAGE MAP

The first step toward sequencing the human genome is to generate a map of spaced genetic markers for each chromosome by developing a genetic linkage map.[78] Just as RFLPs

are shown to be linked to a gene for a genetic disease, recombination frequencies can be used to determine the link between RFLPs, determining linkage on a chromosome. It is estimated that markers must be placed at 2-cM intervals to provide the essential road map for sequencing the human genome. This allows cloning of continuous units of DNA (contigs) in the range of 1 million base pairs by analysis of overlapping clones.[109] The markers used for mapping are called sequence-tagged sites (STSs); STSs are short sequences from physically mapped clones that represent uniquely identified map positions. From these sites, a bottom-up approach can be used, in which a series of overlapping clones are sequenced and ordered. This method has been partially successful for generating genomic maps in organisms with relatively small genomes. A top-down approach to genomic mapping is being used by other groups. This method breaks chromosomes into regions of progressively smaller size, determining the map orientation along the way.[109]

A second method of generating mapped sites along the genome involves cDNA cloning. This approach maps cDNA prepared from various tissues to regions of the genome that specifically express gene products. One advantage to this approach is that these areas probably represent only 10% of the genome, which are undoubtedly the most important regions to locate. In this approach, partial cDNA sequences called expressed sequence tags are obtained as chromosomal markers. In one application of this technique, clones are partially sequenced in an automated process, compared with a database of known sequences, and mapped to a chromosome by somatic cell hybridization detection using the PCR.[102]

MOLECULAR CLONING OF THE HUMAN GENOME

The isolation of the entire human genome as a set of ordered, overlapping molecular clones represents a major undertaking for researchers. This is minimally equivalent to 150,000 λ phage clones, 60,000 cosmid clones, or 3000 yeast minichromosomes (Fig. 1–10). An ordered set of 1 million base pair fragments would be extremely useful as a source for identifying a gene responsible for a genetic disease or a chromosomal aberration in a specific neoplasm. Available clones from that region would obviate the need to screen for markers and greatly speed the process of reverse genetics.[110]

MODELS USING RECOMBINANT DNA TECHNOLOGY

TRANSGENIC ANIMALS

The term transgenic was coined to define organisms that carry genetic material that has been introduced into the germline. The inserted genetic information or transgene can be a segment of genomic DNA from a homologous or heterologous species or even from prokaryotes or viruses. Most often, genes are introduced into the germline of these animals by using regulatory sequences that direct expression to specific cells or tissue types. There are three mechanisms for the introduction of genes into the germline. Most often, DNA is directly injected into the pronucleus of a mouse embryo. This is accomplished by the use of a modified microscope that allows manipulation of the embryo with a suction pipette and injection of the pronucleus with an injection pipette.[111,112] A second method of gene introduction into embryos has been accomplished using retroviral vectors.[113] A third method is embryonic stem cell transfection.

After microinjection, embryos are transplanted into pseudopregnant foster mothers and carried to term. At birth, DNA is extracted from each offspring and assayed for the introduced gene by PCR or Southern analysis. Test breeding is conducted with positive animals, and approximately 25% carry the gene in the germline. Most often, the newly acquired trait is transmitted in a mendelian fashion.[112,114,115]

Despite the microinjected recombinant DNA being arbitrarily localized in the genome, it is usually subjected to normal gene regulation.[112] Many new mouse strains have been developed with novel phenotypes that can be traced to the newly inserted genetic information and its expression in specific cells or organs. Ectopic or increased expression of oncogenes in transgenic animals frequently generates phenotypes that can aid in understanding gene function.

Transgenic mice have been helpful in understanding how oncogenes may generate tumors. Stable lineages of transgenic mice have been developed that express oncogenes and reproducibly experience preneoplastic lesions that progress to various cancers. For example, c-*MYC* transgenics develop mammary adenocarcinomas if the oncogene is driven by a mouse mammary tumor virus promoter. If instead an immunoglobulin regulatory region is attached to the c-*MYC* oncogene, pre-B and B-cell lymphomas result. Similarly, c-*FOS* transgenics develop osteosarcomas, and *MOS* introduced into a mouse germline produces multiple endocrine neoplasia. These are only a few examples of how oncogene function can be studied in this in vivo system. Expression of these genes, how they alter differentiation, and how neoplastic transformation occurs can be studied using transgenic animals.[114,116–118]

The use of transgenic mice provides an exceptional system for studying protocols for gene therapy, and several different genetic defects have been corrected using this procedure. A strain of dwarf mice that is defective in growth hormone production was partially cured by the introduction of a rat growth hormone into the germline.[119] Another strain of mouse with a mutation in the β-globin gene was "cured" by microinjection with a normal mouse β-globin construct.[114]

EMBRYONIC STEM CELL TRANSFER

An alternative method to the introduction of foreign genes into the germline involves the manipulation of cultured embryonic stem cells. These cells are pluripotent cells that can be altered in vitro, and then reunited with blastocyst cells to form chimeric animals. Genes are introduced into these cells by means of electrical or chemical methods. Cells can be selected that have incorporated the desired genome. In the most sophisticated application of this technique, genes are introduced that undergo homologous recombination with a target gene. The usual goals of this application are to disrupt the normal function of a gene and to develop animal models. The important application of this technology will be to mimic the mutations found in human genes, such as cystic fibrosis, in the homologous mouse gene, providing an animal model for studying the human genetic disorder.[120]

IMPLICATIONS FOR ONCOLOGY

GENE THERAPY

The goals of gene therapy are to introduce a gene into a patient's body to target and repair malfunctioning cells with minimal side effects. This process has the clearest applications in the patient with a single gene defect that renders the affected gene nonfunctional. One of the first human applications of this technique was in oncology; gene therapy trials are underway for patients with advanced melanoma. Gene therapy holds great promise for the treatment of many diseases that now lack specific therapies.[121–124]

Depending on the type of disease being treated, three strategies for gene therapy can be adopted. Dysfunctional genes can be replaced, altered to become functional, or augmented with healthy genes working at different loci within the cell. Of these options, gene augmentation therapy is currently the most plausible. An example of gene augmentation is the addition of a functional adenosine deaminase gene to patients with severe combined immunodeficiency.[121–124]

Prerequisites for gene therapy are understanding the defect of the disease and having a normal functional gene cloned and characterized. Genes are introduced by several methods. Naked DNA can be inserted into the patient's somatic cells, which are transplanted back into the patient, but this has not been found to be very efficient. Virus vectors have also been exploited as delivery vehicles for the normal genes. Retroviruses, and to a lesser extent papovaviruses and adenoviruses, have been designed for these techniques. The viral genomes are altered to render them nonvirulent but capable of infecting certain cell types. Retroviral vectors are most suitable because they efficiently integrate into the host chromosome. The functional replacement gene is inserted in a position within the viral genome to render it capable of being expressed after it has entered the appropriate tissue. The virus is then administered to the patient or the target cells to allow transformation to the desired functional phenotype. Bone marrow is a suitable target site for gene therapy, because it is readily accessible and manipulable in vitro and contains stem cells to perpetuate the altered genotype. Liver and the central nervous system are also potential targets for gene therapy.[121]

Human cancer is often associated with aberrant gene expression or mutations in specific genes, and it is possible that neoplastic processes can be altered by gene therapy. Alternatively, tumor cells altered by gene therapy may be destroyed by the insertion of toxic genes or genes rendering them sensitive to chemotherapeutic agents. Another approach to inactivating neoplastic cells is to insert an antisense oncogene into the tumor cells. These genes are transcribed in the reverse orientation to the oncogene. Because the sequences are complementary, the mRNAs hybridize; the oncogene activity is depleted because the gene cannot be translated.[121]

The first application of gene therapy to the treatment of cancer differs from all of the aforementioned strategies and has been called "adoptive immunotherapy." Tumor-infiltrating lymphocytes (TILs) are removed from the surgical specimens obtained from patients with advanced lymphoma. These cells are treated with interleukin-2 to cause cell proliferation. These cells are transfused back into patients, and some advanced melanomas respond successfully to this treatment.[125] The next step in this process is to infect the TILs with a retroviral vector and marker gene to monitor the fate of the infused cells, determine the safety of the retroviral vector, and assay the activity of the marker gene within the tumor tissue.[126] The third phase, which is underway, uses a second retroviral vector that contains a gene for tumor necrosis factor (TNF). It is hoped that the TILs will target the metastatic melanoma, infiltrate the tumor, and release TNF to aid the destruction of the tumor tissue. Depending on the outcome of this clinical trial, it is likely that methods incorporating several facets of the biologic basis of neoplasia will be used in future gene therapy protocols.[127]

DIAGNOSIS, RISK, PROGNOSIS, AND THERAPY

As the molecular alterations of neoplasia are defined, cancers can be better categorized by the tools of molecular biology. RFLP and Southern analysis of tumor tissue may pinpoint specific subtypes of neoplasias that have a similar biologic behavior, and the DNA analysis of tumors may aid diagnosis and prognosis.[128] Similarly, as the genetic predisposition to certain tumors is defined, DNA screening tests may be conducted for at-risk patients to predict tumor occurrence with more certainty.[93] These persons can then be screened by more invasive conventional methods to arrive at earlier diagnoses of neoplasia.

These technologies also have therapeutic applications. One example is the use of gene therapy. Future therapeutic advances will hinge on understanding the molecular basis for cell transformation in different tissues. After the molecular mechanisms are understood, drugs can be designed to interrupt the abnormal cellular events that lead to malignant transformation. As we progress in characterizing the molecular basis for cancer pathogenesis, the tide will be turned and the assault on cancer will be won.

GLOSSARY OF TERMS USED IN MOLECULAR BIOLOGY AND ONCOGENE RESEARCH

Acute transforming retroviruses
Viruses that have acquired sequences from the host genome that confer the property of causing rapid tumor formation in animals or morphologic transformation in cells in culture. The acquired sequences are called viral oncogenes.

Anneal
To form hydrogen bonded base pairs between complementary strands of nucleic acids.

Antisense
The noncoding strand of the DNA within the RNA-coding region of the gene. It is complementary to the "sense" strand and is used as a template for RNA synthesis.

Bacteriophage
Bacterial viruses, which have been extensively modified for use as molecular cloning vehicles.

cDNA library
A collection of clones representative of the mRNA of a given cell type. The cDNA, or complementary DNA, is formed using mRNA and the enzyme reverse transcriptase.

Centimorgan (cM)
A unit of genetic distance. A centimorgan is equivalent to a meiotic recombination frequency of 1%. In the human genome with approximately 3×10^6 base pairs and 3000 cM, 1 cM is roughly equal to 1 million base pairs.

Chloramphenicol acetyl transferase (CAT)
A prokaryotic enzyme that is used in a reporter gene assay to measure protein synthesis in vitro.

Chromosome walking
Molecular walking, jumping, and other techniques have been developed to aid in identifying a locus (*e.g.*, gene responsible for a genetic disorder) from a genetically linked marker DNA sequence.

***cis*-acting DNA elements**
DNA segments that serve as binding sites for transcriptional activators or repressors.

Coding sequence
That part of the genome or mRNA that is translated into protein.

Concatamer
A series of fragments ligated together in head-to-tail fashion.

Conditional expression
Gene expression that occurs only in response to certain stimuli or specific conditions.

Consensus sequence
A characteristic nucleotide sequence that is identified with a gene regulation function.

Constitutive expression
A gene that is expressed at the same level for most of the cell cycle.

Cosmid
A cloning vector designed to carry large fragments of DNA. The vector contains sequences of λ bacteriophage that allow the DNA to be packaged as a phage particle. Inside the bacterium, the cosmid replicates as a plasmid. Cosmid vectors can be used to clone fragments as large as 50 kb.

DNA sequence
The precise order of the four nucleotides, adenine (A), guanine (G), cytosine (C), thymidine (T), as they are linked together to form the DNA chain. This DNA sequence encodes the genetic information of an organism.

DNA transfection
The transfer of DNA into cells in culture. The foreign DNA can integrate with the host chromosome and be expressed as an identifiable phenotype.

DNase footprinting
A technique that allows the determination of the specific DNA sequences in the binding sites of a DNA-binding protein or protein complex.

Embryonic stem cell
A pluripotent cell derived from embryonal tissue. These cells can be modified with foreign genetic information, transferred back to the embryo, and generate chimeric offspring.

Enhancers
DNA elements of various lengths that can be located upstream or downstream from a gene in polarity and enhance gene transcription.

Exon
A gene sequence that is retained in fully mature mRNA. An exon usually contains protein-coding information.

Gene therapy

Techniques that introduce foreign genetic material into a patient to correct an underlying disease.

Gene transcription

Synthesis of an RNA molecule by polymerization of nucleotides complementary to a DNA template. This RNA molecule is a precursor of mRNA and represents a faithful complementary copy of the DNA sequence from which it was transcribed. A specific sequence (promoter) in front of the gene identifies the initiation site for transcription. In RNA, uridine (U) occupies positions that thymidine (T) occupies in DNA.

Genetic code

The 3-bp code (codon) of a nucleic acid that translates into an amino acid sequence.

Genomic library

A collection of clones containing genomic DNA fragments. The library should contain enough clones so that every region of the genome is represented at least once.

Heteroduplex

A double-stranded DNA molecule formed by hybridization of complementary single strands derived from two different sources. Only stretches of homologous or complementary DNA sequences can form double-stranded regions, and noncomplementary DNA stretches remain as single strands and are visible as such by electron microscopy.

Hybridization

The annealing or base pairing of two single-stranded DNA or RNA molecules that are homologous or complementary.

Inducible

Capable of being "turned on" in a specific situation; the β-lactamase gene of *E. coli* is "induced" under conditions of low glucose and high galactose concentrations.

Initiation codon

The ribonucleotides AUG that translate into the amino acid methionine; this is always the first amino acid codon of every mRNA.

Insertional mutagenesis

The process of interrupting the structure—regulatory elements or protein-coding information—of a gene by insertion of foreign genetic information.

In situ hybridization

Application of a labeled probe directly on a tissue, cell, or chromosome preparation. Areas of homology can be identified directly using this technique.

Intron

A noncoding DNA sequence that interrupts the coding portions of a gene (exons); it is excised to create the fully processed mRNA.

Linkage map

A set of closely spaced genetic markers, usually RFLPs, that have been mapped to the same chromosome. If the linkage map covers the entire chromosome, any gene responsible for an inherited disease can in theory be located.

Linker scanning

A method of in vitro mutagenesis wherein restriction enzyme cleavage sites are inserted at different positions along the gene so that sequences 5' and 3' to the insertions are not altered. Gene function is then assayed to identify functional domains.

Long terminal repeat

A repetitive element of the integrated provirus that is generated during viral DNA synthesis and contains the transcription control elements that regulate virus expression.

Messenger RNA (mRNA)

An RNA molecule that represents a faithful copy of the amino acid-coding sequences of a gene. Noncoding sequences (introns) have been removed. With few exceptions, mRNA possesses a stretch of about 300 adenine bases (poly A tail) attached to its 3' end; this tail is not encoded by DNA.

Minichromosome

A large fragment of DNA that can replicate in yeast cells. Minichromosomes are constructed by adding yeast centromere and telomere sequences to foreign DNA fragments. Human DNA fragments as large as 125 kb have been cloned in yeast, and it may be possible to clone segments of 1 million or more base pairs.

Mobility shift

An assay that allows identification of extracts that contain specific DNA-binding proteins.

Molecular cloning

The insertion of a foreign DNA segment of finite length into a vector that replicates in a specific host. The host-vector systems are defined by the NIH Guidelines for Research Involving Recombinant DNA Molecules.[129]

Nick translation

A method that replaces nucleotides in double-stranded DNA with the same but isotopically labeled nucleotides after treatment with DNase I and repair with DNA polymerase. Both strands are labeled by this technique.

Northern analysis

Detection of specific RNA transcripts using electrophoresis, transfer to nitrocellulose membranes, and hybridization with molecular probes.

Null mutation

A mutation that eliminates or inactivates a gene from the genome of an organism.

Oligonucleotide

A short strand of nucleotides, usually DNA (deoxyribonucleotide) 6 to 100 bp long. These molecules are used as probes or primers in polymerization reactions.

Oncogene

An "activated" form of a cellular protooncogene, normally positive regulators of signal transduction events and the cell cycle. When activated, they represent a gain of function to the cell.

Oncoprotein

Protein encoded by an oncogene that is capable of inducing neoplastic transformation. These can be mutated forms of normal cellular proteins or the normal products expressed at an inappropriate time or amount (protooncoproteins).

Plasmid

An autonomously replicating circular DNA found in some bacteria. Plasmids have been modified to make convenient vectors for molecular cloning.

Polyadenylation

The addition of a stretch of approximately 200 riboadenylic acid residues to the end of an RNA polymerase II transcript.

Polymerase chain reaction (PCR)

A technique that uses a thermostable polymerase in a series

of annealing and polymerization reactions to amplify nucleic acid sequences in an exponential fashion.

Primer extension

An assay that uses mRNA and a complementary oligonucleotide (primer) to synthesize a DNA antisense copy of the mRNA. It is used to determine mRNA 5′ structure.

Promoter

A DNA sequence that signals RNA polymerase to initiate transcription.

Pulsed-field gel electrophoresis (PFGE)

A modification of agarose gel electrophoresis of DNA in which fragments of several megabases can be resolved. The technique uses pulses of current in the reverse direction or at angles to the gel to accomplish the increased resolution. Orthogonal field gel electrophoresis (OFAGE) and field inversion gel electrophoresis (FIGE) are variations of this technique.

Recombinant DNA

A DNA molecule constructed by joining a fragment of DNA from a different source to a vector, such as a circular bacterial plasmid. The vector is opened at a specific site, a given DNA fragment from another source is inserted, and the circle is closed again. The recombinant DNA is amplified in a host cell that can replicate the vector.

Reporter gene

A gene whose activity can be easily assayed; it is used as a marker of gene expression in transcription or translation systems, or both.

Restriction enzymes

Enzymes made by certain strains of bacteria to protect themselves against invading foreign DNA (*e.g.*, bacteriophage DNA). These enzymes cut DNA at specific recognition sites.

Restriction fragment length polymorphism (RFLP)

A variation between individuals in the size of fragments produced by restriction enzyme digestion. The variation is inherited and can be used as a genetic marker in linkage analysis.

Retrovirus

A plus-stranded RNA genome virus that is reverse transcribed into DNA during infection and replication. The DNA copy integrates into the host chromosomal DNA. This DNA template, called a provirus, is transcribed into virion RNA and produces translatable mRNA that codes for virion or oncogene protein products.

Reverse genetics

The use of information on the chromosomal location of a genetic disease gene to clone the gene itself. In some instances, chromosomal abnormalities have provided the essential clues, and in other cases, genetic linkage data have been used to localize the gene.

Reverse transcriptase

An enzyme encoded by all retroviruses that copies the viral RNA genome into a DNA copy which subsequently integrates into the host genome. This enzyme is widely used in the laboratory for cloning purposes to copy RNA into DNA.

RNAse protection

Detection of small quantities of RNA using nucleic acid hybridization with specific probes, followed by digestion of any single-stranded species that remain.

S1 nuclease protection analysis

An assay designed to elucidate mRNA structure; it uses RNA-DNA hybridization conditions and single-strand-specific S1 nuclease enzyme to digest nonannealed RNA or DNA species.

Site-directed mutagenesis

A technique used to introduce a specific mutation at a specific site in a DNA sequence.

Somatic cell hybridization

Combinations of chromosomes from different species to make viable cells in vitro. These linkages can be used for chromosomal mapping studies.

Southern analysis

A technique for detecting specific sequences in DNA. A DNA sample is digested with restriction enzymes. The restriction fragments are fractionated by size on agarose gels, transferred to a nitrocellulose membrane, and subjected to hybridization using an isotopically labeled nucleic acid probe.

Subtraction cloning

Use of serial RNA-DNA hybridization reactions with removal of annealed species to enrich for transcripts unique to a particular cell type.

Trans-acting factors

Gene products that regulate transcription at specific sites along the DNA strand.

Transgenic mouse

A mouse generated by the introduction of a recombinant DNA molecule at the one-cell embryo stage. The founder mouse is shown to contain the recombinant DNA molecule by, for example, examining DNA extracted from a segment of the tail. New strains are developed if the founder mouse is able to transmit the acquired gene in a mendelian fashion.

Tumor suppressor gene

A cellular gene whose loss of function leads to cell transformation and tumor development.

Tyrosine kinases

Protein enzymes that have specificity for phosphorylating tyrosine residues on target proteins.

Upstream elements

DNA sequences located 5′ to the RNA start site of a gene that are involved in regulating its expression.

Western analysis

A technique used to identify a unique protein within a sample; the methodology is similar to Southern and Northern analyses.

Acknowledgments

Research done in Dr. G. Vande Woude's laboratory was supported by the National Cancer Institute, Department of Health and Human Services, under contract No. NO1-CO-74101 with ABL. The contents of this publication do not necessarily reflect the views or policies of the Department of Health and Human Services, nor does mention of trade names, commercial products, or organizations imply endorsement by the U.S. Government.

REFERENCES

1. Lee MG, Nurse P. Complementation used to clone a human homologue of the fission yeast cycle control gene *CDC2*. Nature 1987;327:31.

2. Nurse P, Bisset Y. Gene required in G_1 for commitment to cell cycle and in G_2 for control of mitosis in fission yeast. Nature 1981;292:558.

3. Park M, Vande Woude G. Principles of molecular cell biology of cancer: Oncogenes. In: DeVita VT Jr, Hellman S, Rosenberg SA, eds. Cancer: Principles and practice of oncology. 3rd ed. Philadelphia: JB Lippincott, 1989:45–66.

4. Leder P, Battey J, Lenoir G, et al. Translocations among antibody genes in human cancer. Science 1983;222:765.

5. Groffee J, Stephenson JR, Heisterkamp N, et al. Philadelphia chromosomal breakpoints are clustered within a limited region, BCR, on chromosome 22. Cell 1984;36:93.

6. Canaani E, Steiner-Saltz D, Aghai E, et al. Altered transcription of an oncogene in chronic myeloid leukaemia. Lancet 1984;1:593.

7. Collins SJ, Kubonishi I, Miyoshi I, et al. Altered transcription of the c-ABL oncogene in K-562 and other chronic myelogenous leukemia cells. Science 1984;225:72.

8. Hollstein M, Sidransky D, Vogelstein B, et al. P53 mutations in human cancers. Science 1991;253:49.

9. Stephens T. Closing in on p53's normal function. J Natl Inst Health Res 1991;3:34.

10. Fearon ER, Vogelstein, B. A genetic model for colorectal tumorigenesis. Cell 1990;61: 759.

11. Lewin B. Genes. 3rd ed. New York: John Wiley & Sons.

12. Roeder R. Eukaryotic nuclear RNA polymerases. In: Losick R, Chamberlin M, eds. RNA polymerases. Cold Spring Harbor, NY: Cold Spring Harbor Laboratory, 1986: 285–329.

13. Corden J, Wasylyk B, Buchwalder A, et al. Promoter sequences of eukaryotic protein-coding genes. Science 1980;209:1406.

14. Watson JD. Molecular biology of the gene. 3rd ed. Menlo Park, NJ: Benjamin Cummings, 1976.

15. Bonner TI, Brenner DJ, Beufeld BR, et al. Reduction in the rate of DNA reassociation by sequence divergence. J Mol Biol 1973;81:123.

16. Casey J, Davidson N. Rates of formation and thermal stabilities of RNA:DNA and DNA:DNA duplexes at high concentrations of formamide. Nucleic Acids Res 1977;4: 1539.

17. Hutton JR. Renaturation kinetics and thermal stability of DNA in aqueous solutions of formamide and urea. Nucleic Acids Res 1977;4:3537.

18. McConaughy BL, Laird CD, McCarthy BJ. Nucleic acid reassociation in formamide. Biochemistry 1969;8:3289.

19. Suggs SV, Wallace RB, Hirose T, et al. Use of synthetic oligonucleotides as hybridization probes: Isolation of cloned cDNA sequences for human B_2-microglobulin. Proc Natl Acad Sci USA 1981;78:6613.

20. Wallace RB, Shaffer J, Murphy RF, et al. Hybridization of synthetic oligodeoxyribonucleotides to ζX174 DNA: The effect of single base pair mismatch. Nucleic Acids Res 1979;6:3543.

21. Wallace RB, Johnson MJ, Hirose T, et al. The use of synthetic oligonucleotides as hybridization probes: II. Hybridization of oligonucleotides of mixed sequence to rabbit β-globin DNA. Nucleic Acids Res 1981;9:879.

22. Richardson CC. Enzymes in DNA metabolism. Annu Rev Biochem 1969;38:795.

23. Kornberg A. Aspects of DNA replication. Cold Spring Harb Symp Quant Biol 1980; 43:1.

24. Rigby PWJ, Dieckmann M, Rhodes C, et al. Labeling deoxyribonucleic acid to high specific activity in vitro by nick translation with DNA polymerase I. J Mol Biol 1977;113: 237.

25. Maniatis T, Jeffrey A, Kleid DG. Nucleotide sequence of the rightward operator of phage lambda. Proc Natl Acad Sci USA 1975;72:1184.

26. Feinberg AP, Vogelstein B. A technique for radiolabeling DNA restriction endonuclease fragments to high specific activity. Anal Biochem 1983;132:6.

27. Sambrook J, Fritsch EF, Maniatis T. Molecular cloning: A laboratory manual. 2nd ed. Cold Spring Harbor, NY: Cold Spring Harbor Laboratory, 1989.

28. Narang SA. DNA synthesis. Tetrahedron 1983;39:3.

29. Itakura K, Rossi JJ, Wallace RB. Synthesis and use of synthetic oligonucleotides. Annu Rev Biochem 1984;53:323.

30. Saiki RK, Gelfand DH, Stoffel S, et al. Primer-directed enzymatic amplification of DNA with a thermostabile DNA polymerase. Science 1988;239:487, 1988.

31. Saiki RK, Scharf S, Faloona KB, et al. Enzymatic amplification of β-globin genomic sequences and restriction site analysis for diagnosis of sickle cell anemia. Science 1985;230:1350.

32. Lee M-S, Chang K-S, Cabanillas F, et al. Detection of minimal residual cells carrying the t(14;18) by DNA sequence amplification. Science 1987;237:175.

33. Crescenzi M, Seta M, Herzig GP, et al. Thermophilic polymerase chain amplification of t(14;18) chromosome breakpoints and the detection of minimal residual disease. Proc Natl Acad Sci USA 1988;85:4869.

34. Roberts R. Restriction and modification enzymes and their recognition sequences. Nucleic Acid Res 1982;10:117.

35. Linn S, Arber W. Host specificity of DNA produced by Escherichia coli. X. In vitro restriction of phase fd replicative form. Proc Natl Acad Sci USA 1968;59:1300.

36. Smith HO, Wilcox KW. A restriction enzyme from Hemophilus influenzae. I. Purification and general properties. J Mol Biol 1970;51:379.

37. Kelly TJ Jr, Smith HO. A restriction enzyme from Hemophilus influenzae. II. Base sequence of the recognition site. J Mol Biol 1970;51:393.

38. Roberts RJ. Restriction and modification enzymes and their recognition sequences. Nucleic Acids Res 1981;9:75.

39. Helling RB, Goodman HM, Boyer HW. Analysis of endonuclease R-EcoRI fragments of DNA from lamdoid bacteriophages and other viruses by agarose-gel electrophoresis. J Virol 1974;14:1235.

40. Scharf SJ. Cloning with PCR. In: Innis MA, Gelfand DH, Sninsky JJ, White TJ, eds. PCR protocols: A guide to methods and applications. San Diego: Academic Press, 1990: 84–92.

41. Southern EM. Detection of specific sequences among DNA fragments separated by gel electrophoresis. J Mol Biol 1975;98:503.

42. Blair DG, Oskarsson M, Wood TG, et al. Activation of the transforming potential of a normal cell sequence: A molecular model for oncogenesis. Science 1981;212:941.

43. Schwartz DC, Cantor CR. Separation of yeast chromosome-sized DNAs by pulsed field gradient gel electrophoresis. Cell 1984;37:67.

44. Carle GF, Olson MV. Separation of chromosomal DNA molecules from yeast by orthogonal field-alternation gel electrophoresis. Nucleic Acids Res 1984;12:5647.

45. Chu G, Vollrath D, Davis RW. Separation of large DNA molecules by contour-clamped homogeneous electric fields. Science 1986;234:1582.

46. Vollrath D, Davis RW. Resolution of DNA molecules greater than 5 megabases by contour-clamped homogeneous electric fields. Nucleic Acids Res 1987;15:7865.

47. Lawrance SK, Smith CL, Srivastava R, et al. Megabase-scale mapping of the HLA gene complex by pulsed field gel electrophoresis. Science 1987;235:1387.

48. Smith CL, Econome JG, Schutt A, et al. A physical map of the Escherichia coli K12 genome. Science 1987;236:1448.

49. O'Brien SJ. Genetic Maps 1987: A compilation of linkage and restriction maps of genetically studied organisms, vol 4. Cold Spring Harbor, NY: Cold Spring Harbor Laboratory, 1987.

50. Dean M, Park M, Vande Woude GF. Characterization of the rearranged TRP-MET oncogene breakpoint. Mol Cell Biol 1987;7:921.

51. Alwine JC, Kemp DJ, Stark GR. Method for detection of specific RNAs in agarose gels by transfer to diazobenzyloxymethyl-paper and hybridization with DNA probes. Proc Natl Acad Sci USA 1977;74:5350.

52. Shtivelman E, Lifshitz B, Gale RP, et al. Fused transcript of ABL and BCR genes in chronic myelogenous leukemia. Nature 1986;315:550.

53. Grosveld G, Verwoerd T, Van Agthoven T, et al. The chronic myelocytic cell line K562 contains a breakpoint in BCR and produces a chimeric BCR/c-ABL transcript. Mol Cell Biol 1986;6:607.

54. Favaloro J, Treisman R, Kamen R. Transcriptional maps of polyoma virus specific RNA: Analysis by two-dimensional nuclease S1 gel mapping. Methods Enzymol 1980;65: 718.

55. Berk AJ, Sharp PA. Sizing and mapping of early adenovirus mRNAs by gel electrophoresis of S1 endonuclease-digested hybrids. Cell 1977;12:721.

56. Powell LM, Wallis SC, Pease RJ, et al. A novel form of tissue-specific RNA processing produces apolipoprotein-B48 in intestine. Cell 1987;50:831.

57. Towbin H, Staehelin T, Gordon J. Electrophoretic transfer of proteins from polyacrylamide gels to nitrocellulose sheets: Procedure and some applications. Proc Natl Acad Sci USA 1979;76:4350.

58. Burnette WN. "Western blotting": Electrophoretic transfer of proteins from sodium dodecylsulfate polyacrylamide gels to unmodified nitrocellulose and radiographic detection with antibody and radioiodinated protein A. Anal Biochem 1981;112:195.

59. Maxam AM, Gilbert W. A new method for sequencing DNA. Proc Natl Acad Sci USA 1977;74:560.

60. Sanger F, Nicklen S, Coulson AR. DNA sequencing with chain-terminating inhibitors. Proc Natl Acad Sci USA 1977;74:5463.

61. Labouze E. Automatic DNA sequencing and the human genome project. Impact Sci Soc 1988;149:75.

62. Bugaiczyk A, Boyer HW, Goodman HM. Ligation of EcoRI endonuclease-generated DNA fragments into linear and circular structures. J Mol Biol 1975;96:171.

63. Soeda E, Arrand JR, Smolar N, et al. Coding potential and regulatory signals of the polyoma virus genome. Nature 1980;283:445.

64. Bolivar F, Backman K. Plasmids of Escherichia coli as cloning vectors. Methods Enzymol 1979;68:245.

65. Bernard HU, Helinski DR. Bacterial plasmid cloning vehicles. In: Setlow JK, Hollaender A, eds. Genetic engineering, vol 2. New York: Plenum Press, 1980:113.

66. Yanisch-Perron C, Vieira J, Messing J. Improved M13 phage cloning vectors and host strains: Nucleotide sequences of the M13mp18 and pUC19 vectors. Gene 1985;33: 103.

67. Maniatis T, Hardison RC, Lacy E, et al. The isolation of structural genes from libraries of eukaryotic DNA. Cell 1987;15:687.

68. Grunstein M, Hogness D. Colony hybridization: A method for the isolation of cloned DNAs that contain a specific gene. Proc Natl Acad Sci USA 1975;72:3961.

69. Benton WD, Davis RW. Screen λgt recombinant clones by hybridization to single plaques in situ. Science 1977;1986:180.

70. Okayama H, Berg P. High-efficiency cloning of full-length cDNA. Mol Cell Biol 1982;2: 161.

71. Alt FW, Enea V, Bothwell ALM, et al. Probes for specific mRNAs by subtractive hybridization: Anomalous expression of immunoglobulin genes. In: Axel R, Maniatis T, Fox CF, eds. Eukaryotic gene regulation. New York: Academic Press, 1979:407–419.

72. Duguid JR, Rohwer RG, Seed B. Isolation of cDNAs of scrapie-modulated RNAs by subtractive hybridization of a cDNA library. Proc Natl Acad Sci USA 1988;85: 5738.

73. Sive HL, St. John T. A simple subtractive hybridization technique employing photoactivatable biotin and phenol extraction. Nucleic Acids Res 1988;16:10937.

74. Travis GH, Sutcliffe JG. Phenol emulsion-enhanced DNA-driven subtractive cDNA cloning: Isolation of low-abundance monkey cortex specific mRNAs. Proc Natl Acad Sci USA 1988;85:1696.

75. Saito I, Stark GR. Charomids: Cosmid vectors for efficient cloning and mapping of large or small restriction fragments. Proc Natl Acad Sci USA 1986;83:8664.

76. Watson JD, Tooze J, Kurtz DT. Recombinant DNA: A short course. New York: Scientific American Books, 1983.

77. Steinmetz M, Moor KW, Frelinger JA, et al. A pseudogene homologous to mouse transplantation antigens: Transplantation antigens are encoded by light exons that correlate with protein domains. Cell 1981;25:683.

78. Burke DT, Carle GF, Olson MV. Cloning of large segments of exogenous DNA into yeast by means of artificial chromosome vectors. Science 1987;236:806.

79. Kunkel LM, Beggs, AH, Hoffman EP. Molecular genetics of Duchenne and Becker muscular dystrophy: Emphasis on improved diagnosis. Clin Chem 1989;35:21.

80. Rommens JM, Iannuzzi MC, Kerem B-S, et al. Identification of the cystic fibrosis gene: Chromosome walking and jumping. Science 1989;245:1059.

81. Riordan JR, Rommens JM, Kerem B-S, et al. Identification of the cystic fibrosis gene: Cloning and characterization of complementary DNA. Science 1989;245:1066.

82. Kerem B-S, Rommens JM, Bucharan JA. Identification of the cystic fibrosis gene: Genetic analysis. Science 1989;245:1073.

83. Friend SH, Bernards R, Rogelj S, et al. A human DNA segment with properties of the gene that predispose to retinoblastoma and osteosarcoma. Nature 1986;323:643.

84. Lee W, Bookstein R, Hong F, et al. Human retinoblastoma, susceptibility gene: Cloning, identification, and sequence. Science 1987;235:1394.

85. Knudson, AG. Hereditary cancers: Clues to mechanisms of carcinogenesis. Br J Cancer 1989;59:661.

86. Fearon ER, Cho R, Nigro JM, et al. Identification of a chromosome 18q gene that is altered in colorectal cancers. Science 1990;247:49.

87. Vogelstein B, Fearon ER, Hamilton SR, et al. Genetic alterations during colorectal-tumor development. N Engl J Med 1988;319:525.

88. Baker SJ, Fearon ER, Nigro JM. Chromosome 17 deletions and p53 gene mutations in colorectal carcinoma. Science 1989;244:217.

89. Yokota J, Wada M, Shimosato Y, et al. Loss of heterozygosity on chromosomes 3, 13, and 17 in small-cell carcinoma and on chromosomes 3 in adenocarcinoma of the lung. Proc Natl Acad Sci USA 1987;84:9252.

90. Dunlop MG, Wyllie AH, Nakamura Y, et al. Genetic linkage map of six polymorphic DNA markers around the gene for familial polyposis on chromosome 5. Am J Hum Genet 1990;47:482.

91. Groden J, Thliveris HA, Samowitz W, et al. Identification and characterization of the familial adenomatous polyposis coli gene. Cell 1991;66:589.

92. Joslyn G, Carlson M, Thliveris HA, et al. Identification of deletion mutations and three new genes at the familial polyposis coli locus. Cell 1991;66:601.

93. Dunlop MG, Wyllie AH, Steel CM, et al. Linked DNA markers for presymptomatic diagnosis of familial adenomatous polyposis. Lancet 1991;337:313.

94. Race R, Sadnger R. Blood groups in man. 6th ed. Oxford: Blackwell, 1975:610.

95. Thomas G, Bodmer W, Bodmer J. The HLA system as a model for studying the interaction between selection, migration and linkage. In: Karlin S, Nevo E, eds. Population genetics and ecology. New York: Academic Press, 1976:465.

96. Ploegh HL, Orr HT, Strominger JL. Major histocompatibility antigens: The human (HLA-A, -B, -C) and murine (H-LK, -D) class I molecules. Cell 1981;24:287.

97. Botstein D, White R, Skolnick M, et al. Construction of a genetic linkage map in man using restriction fragment length polymorphisms. Am J Hum Genet 1980;32:314.

98. White R, Woodward S, Leppert M, et al. A closely linked genetic marker for cystic fibrosis. Nature 1985;318:45.

99. White RL, Barker D, Holm T, et al. Approaches to linkage analysis in the human. In: Caskey CT, White RL, eds. Banbury report 14: Recombinant DNA applications to human disease. Cold Spring Harbor, NY: Cold Spring Harbor Laboratory, 1983.

100. O'Brien SJ, Nash WG. Genetic mapping in mammals. Chromosome map of domestic cat. Science 1982;216:257.

101. Harper ME, Saunders GF. Localization of single copy DNA sequences on G-banded human chromosomes by in situ hybridization. Chromosoma 1981;83:431.

102. Adams MD, Kelley JM, Gocayne JD, et al. Complementary DNA sequencing: Expressed sequence tags and the human genome project. Science 1991;252:1651.

103. Pinkel D, Straume T, Gray JW. Cytogenetic analysis using quantitative, high-sensitivity, fluorescence hybridization. Proc Natl Acad Sci USA 1986;83:2934.

104. Lichter P, Tang, CC, Call K, et al. High-resolution mapping of human chromosome 11 by in situ hybridization with cosmid clones. Science 1990;247:64.

105. Donis-Keller H, Green P, Helms C, et al. A genetic linkage map of the human genome. Cell 1987;51:319.

106. Morton NE. Sequential tests for the detection of linkage. Am J Hum Genet 1955;7:277.

107. Wallace MR, Marchuk DA, Andersen LB, et al. Type 1 neurofibromatosis gene: Identification of a large transcript disrupted in three NF1 patients. Science 1990;249:181.

108. Malkin D, Li FP, Strong LC, et al. Germ line p53 mutations in a familial syndrome of breast cancer, sarcomas, and other neoplasms. Science 1990;250:1233.

109. Watson JD. The human genome project: Past, present, future. Science 1990;248:44.

110. Orkin SH. Reverse genetics and human disease. Cell 1986;47:845.

111. Gordon JW, Scangos GA, Plotkin DJ, et al. Genetic transformation of mouse embryos by microinjection of purified DNA. Proc Natl Acad Sci USA 1980;77:7380.

112. Palmiter RD, Brinster RL. Germ-line transformation of mice. Annu Rev Genet 1986;20:465.

113. Hughes SH. Will retroviral vectors be used to make transgenic livestock? Ag Biotech News Info 1991;3:25.

114. DeTolla L. Transgenic animal models. Comp Pathol Bull 1990;22:1.

115. Hogan B, Constantini F, Lacy E. Manipulating the mouse embryo. Cold Spring Harbor, NY: Cold Spring Harbor Laboratory Press, 1986.

116. Schulz N, Propst F, Rosenberg MP, et al. Pheochromocytomas and C-cell thyroid neoplasms in transgenic c-*MOS* mice: A model for the human multiple endocrine neoplasia type 2 syndrome. Cancer Res 1992;52:450.

117. Hanahan, D. Transgenic mice as probes into complex systems. Science 1989;246:1265.

118. Khillan JS, Oskarsson MK, Propst F, et al. Defects in lens fiber differentiation are linked to c-*MOS* overexpression in transgenic mice. Genes Dev 1987;1:1327.

119. Hammer RE, Palmiter RD, Brinster RL. Partial correction of murine hereditary disorder by germ-line incorporation of a new gene. Nature 1987;311:65.

120. Capecchi MR. Altering the genome by homologous recombination. Science 1989;244:1288.

121. Friedmann T. Progress toward human gene therapy. Science 1989;244:1275.

122. Verma IM. Gene therapy. Sci Am 1990;263:68.

123. Miller AD. Progress toward human gene therapy. Blood 1990;76:271.

124. Karson EM. Prospects for gene therapy. Biol Reprod 1990;42:39.

125. Rosenberg SA, Packard BS, Aebersold PM, et al. Use of tumor-infiltrating lymphocytes and interleukin-2 in the immunotherapy of patients with metastatic melanoma: A preliminary report. N Engl J Med 1988;319:1676.

126. Rosenberg SA, Aebersold PM, Cornetta K. Gene transfer into humans: Immunotherapy of patients with advanced melanoma, using tumor-infiltrating lymphocytes modified by retroviral gene transduction. N Engl J Med 1990;323:570.

127. Culliton BJ. Gene therapy: Into the home stretch. Science 1990;249:974.

128. Sato T, Tanigama A, Yamakawa K, et al. Allelotype of breast cancer: Cumulative allele losses promote tumor progression in primary breast cancer. Cancer Res 1990;50:1784.

129. National Institutes of Health: Guidelines for Research Involving Recombinant DNA Molecules. Federal Register 1982;47:38050–38068.

Cancer: Principles & Practice of Oncology, Fourth Edition,
edited by Vincent T. DeVita, Jr., Samuel Hellman, Steven A. Rosenberg.
J.B. Lippincott Co., Philadelphia © 1993.

Arun Seth

Takis S. Papas

CHAPTER **2**

Principles of Molecular Cell Biology of Cancer: General Aspects of Gene Regulation

The human genome contains 50,000 to 100,000 genes. Each gene codes for a specific product, an RNA or a protein, which has a unique function in cellular metabolism. Whether the cell is a neuron or hepatocyte, its genetic information is essentially the same. How each cell determines its phenotype and maintains its cellular function throughout its life is an elegant, complex achievement.

Genomic DNA is contained in chromosomes. In the cell nucleus, genomic DNA is highly coiled in an exquisitely ordered structure to facilitate regulated expression. Myriad protein-nucleotide interactions occur during gene expression that eventually result in translation. The events that occur during these processes are discussed in this chapter. Gene expression, the molecular basis for cell division, specialization, and differentiation, is a vast topic. Current molecular biologic techniques have just begun to reveal the mechanisms of the detailed cellular processes leading to phenotypic expression. The elucidation of these processes can clarify normal cell function and unravel the mechanisms in cell dysfunction.

TRANSCRIPTION

Transcription in eukaryotic cells is a cooperative process that is mediated by specific DNA-dependent RNA polymerases and a multiplicity of regulatory factors.[1] There are at least three RNA polymerases in the cell nucleus, and each has a unique function. In the nucleolus, RNA polymerase I transcribes ri-

bosomal RNA (rRNA), which is the major nucleic acid constituent of the protein-synthesizing ribosomes. In the nucleoplasm, RNA polymerase II transcribes messenger RNA (mRNA), the protein-encoding transcript, and RNA polymerase III transcribes transfer RNA (tRNA), which locates the appropriate amino acid into the correct codon position of mRNA to initiate peptide synthesis and adds amino acids to the growing peptide chain.[2] All RNAs are transcribed from a DNA template using four ribonucleotides (*i.e.*, ATP, GTP, CTP, UTP), which are similar to the deoxyribonucleotides in DNA but which possess a 2' hydroxyl (OH) in the phosphate backbone. Eukaryotic RNA polymerases contain two large subunits and several small subunits that range in size from 500 to 600 kd. These polymerases are highly conserved among eukaryotes.[2,3] Most studies have been directed toward understanding RNA polymerase II because of its importance in gene regulation and understanding how the interaction of RNA polymerase II with different nuclear factors regulates the transcription processes.[4]

Gene regulation involves *cis*-acting elements, which are defined DNA sequences called promoters, enhancers, or silencers. These sequences are recognition sites for a variety of protein factors that specifically regulate transcription.[5] For minimal mRNA transcription by RNA polymerase II, two classes of promoters have been described.[6] The first class contains a "TATA box" sequence that is located approximately 30 bp upstream (5') from the start site (Fig. 2–1). In vitro studies have shown that the TATA box is sufficient for basal

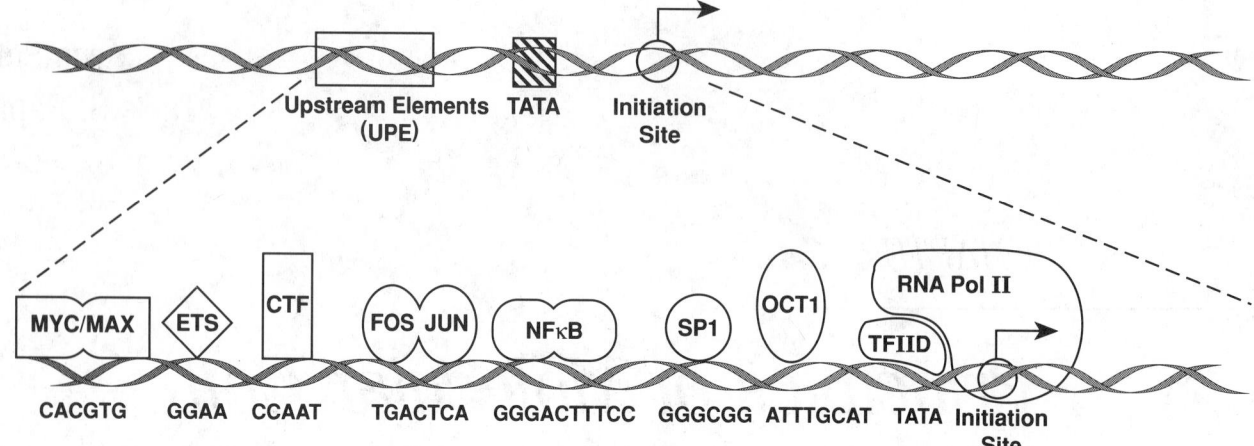

FIGURE 2–1. In the schematic of the transcriptional control region of a eukaryotic gene transcribed by RNA polymerase II, initiation sites (*arrows*), TATA sequences (*hatched boxes*), and upstream elements (*open boxes*) are shown. The transactivating factors that bind to particular DNA sequences are indicated symbolically. The upstream elements that are essential for transcriptional activation may contain binding sites for various factors, some of which are depicted. The diagram is somewhat speculative, and all of the binding sites shown here may not be present within the transcriptional control region of a single gene. During the transactivation process, factors may shift their positions to interact with other factors or with RNA POLII.

transcription by RNA polymerase and requires only the TATA sequence binding factor (TFIID), transcription factor for RNA polymerase II, for accurate selection of the initiation site.[7] The level of transcription from this core promoter is minimal unless there is interaction with the other DNA-binding proteins that complex with *cis*-acting upstream elements or enhancers. The second class of promoters lack a TATA box sequence, and transcription initiation generally occurs at multiple sites. In vitro studies indicate that even these promoters require the TATA binding protein TFIID, but the exact differences between the TATA box-dependent and TATA box-independent modes of transcription initiation have not been determined.[8]

UPSTREAM ELEMENTS AND ENHANCERS

Upstream elements are specific sequences located 5' from the start sites and occur in most eukaryotic promoters.[9] A variety of upstream elements and enhancers have been molecularly characterized (*i.e.*, essential sequences have been determined)

and are known to modify the rate of transcription from specific promoters. Enhancers act on promoters in an orientation-independent manner and can be located at great distances 5' or 3' from the responsive promoter sequence. Upstream elements and enhancer sequences can positively or negatively mediate the regulation of transcription, thereby regulating the expression of essential genes during embryologic development and cellular differentiation processes.[10]

Upstream Elements

The core sequences of upstream elements range from 4 to 8 bases (Table 2–1) and are part of a large number of cellular and viral promoters. They are always proximal to the transcriptional initiation start site of their target promoters (Fig. 2–1). The DNA sequences CCAAT and GGGCGG are frequently used in transcription regulation of a large number of genes. Other sequences, such as metal ion-, heat-, or hormone-responsive elements are found only in a limited number of promoters.[9] Specific proteins bind to upstream elements and

TABLE 2–1. DNA-Binding and Transactivation Domains of Transcription Factors

Transcription Factor	DNA-Binding Domain	Core Sequence	Transactivation Domain	Reference
AP1 (JUN/FOS)	Leucine zipper	TGACTCA		25
MYOD	Helix-loop-helix	CANNTG		30
λ-434 repressor	Helix-turn-helix	ACAANNNNTTGT		18
MYB	Tryptophan repeat	PyAACt/gG		41
ETS	Tryptophan repeat	GGAA		42
SP1	Zinc finger	GGGCGG	Glutamine-rich	48
OCT1/OCT2	Homeo/POU	ATTTGCAT	Acidic domain	47
CTF		CCAAT	Proline-rich	49

N is A, G, C or Tbase, Py is Pyrimidine.

stimulate transcription by directly interacting with the RNA polymerase II or by binding to RNA polymerase II by at least one other factor.[6] The upstream elements can act in an orientation-independent manner relative to the start site. The strength and tissue specificity of a promoter are determined by the number and type of upstream elements, but distance between a particular upstream element and the start site also affects the rate of transcription.

Enhancers

Enhancers are DNA elements that activate gene transcription.[11] Unlike the upstream elements, enhancers can be located at great distances upstream or downstream from the start site. They also act in an orientation-independent manner.[11] The first evidence for enhancers came from the discovery of elements that "enhanced" transcription in viral promoters.[12] The first cellular enhancer was identified in the immunoglobulin (Ig) heavy chain gene locus.[13] The enhancer in the SV40 DNA tumor virus promoter is able to stimulate the transcription of a linked β-globin gene by as much as 20-fold when placed in a recombinant construct in either orientation. The Ig enhancer is located downstream (3') from the start site in the first intron of the Ig gene (Fig. 2–2) and induces transcription in specific cell types.[13] In vitro studies suggest that different transcription factors bind to the same SV40 enhancer region in different cell types, indicating that this specific sequence motif is able to regulate gene expression in different cell types by interacting with unique tissue or cellular factors, enabling the virus to grow in a variety of host cells and tissues.

Viral Enhancers

All viruses possess sequences that allow expression from their genome in the host cells. DNA enhancer sequences have been identified in papovaviruses (*e.g.*, SV40, polyoma), herpesviruses (*e.g.*, HSV-1, HSV-2, CMV), adenoviruses, hepatitis B virus, and retroviruses. The enhancers play a critical role in tissue tropism and in the development of site-specific cancers of infected animals by provirus insertion next a proto-oncogene. SV40 and polyoma enhancers have been studied in great detail.[11] SV40 contains two transcription units for regulating early and late viral events. The early events involve DNA duplication by expression of SV40 large T antigen, and the late gene products are capsid proteins. The early and late genes are transcribed from opposite strands. The early transcription unit is expressed during the initial phase of the SV40 viral infection cycle and contains a 72-bp repeat enhancer element that stimulates the transcription of linked genes in many tissue and cell types. Unlike the SV40 enhancer, the polyoma enhancer is restrictive and shows greater activity in murine than primate cells.[14]

The retroviral enhancers are located within the long terminal repeat regions that flank the viral genome and influence tissue tropism of the virus and cellular targets for tumorigenesis.

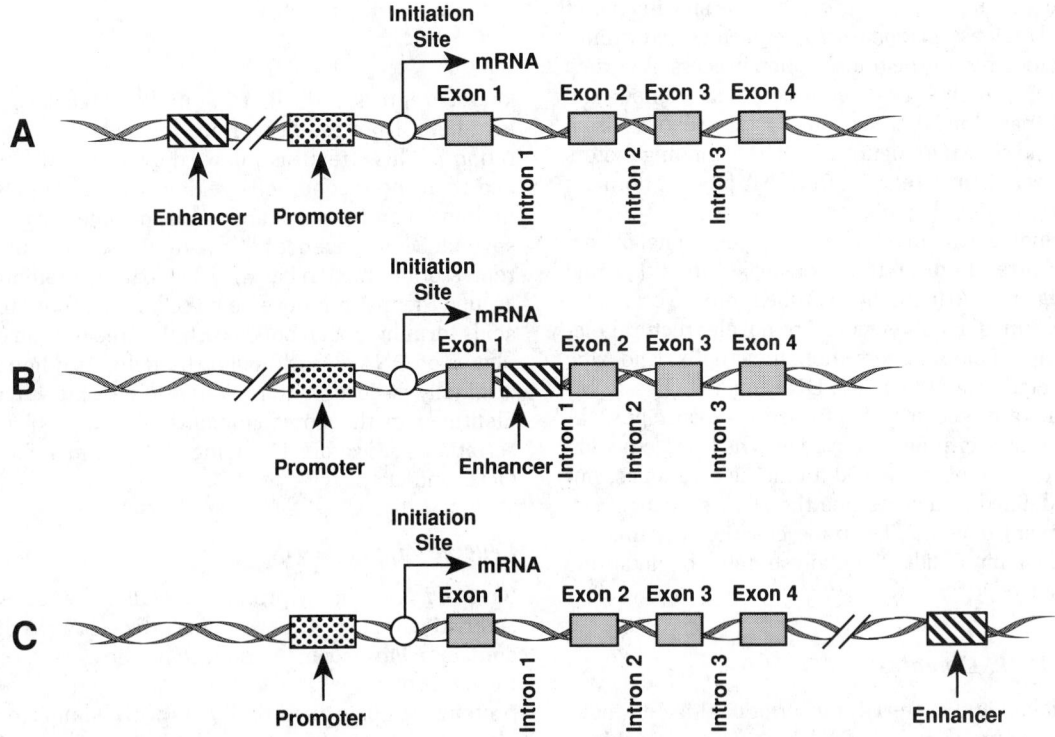

FIGURE 2–2. Locations of enhancer sequences in different genes. The enhancers may be located at great distances from the promoter and also upstream or downstream from the promoter or within the intervening sequences of a gene. **(A)** In the albumin gene, the enhancer is located at the 5' end, upstream from the promoter region. **(B)** The immunoglobulin enhancer is located within the first intron of the gene. **(C)** The enhancer of the T-cell receptor is located in the 3' noncoding region.

Cellular Enhancers

Cellular enhancers are most often found upstream from the mRNA start site, but they are also located within the first intron or at the 3′ end of the target gene (Fig. 2–2).[13,15] The cellular enhancers for the Ig heavy chain and κ light chain gene locus are located within the first intron.[11] The Ig heavy chain enhancer regulates the temporal and tissue-specific expression of Ig genes in B cells or during lymphoid cell differentiation.[11,13] This enhancer is 140 bp long and contains binding sites for several transcriptional factors, which cooperate to effect maximal levels of Ig mRNA expression.[11,13] The Ig heavy chain enhancer and the promoter act synergistically.[11,13] Both contain an octamer motif (Table 2–1) that can be recognized by two transcription factors called OCT1 and OCT2 (also called OTF1 and OTF2) (Fig. 2–1).

DNA-BINDING DOMAINS OF TRANSCRIPTION FACTORS

Many DNA-binding sites called *cis*-regulatory regions have been identified in promoters and enhancers by DNA footprinting and gel electrophoretic mobility shift assays.[6,16] When a protein binds to a specific DNA sequence, it protects this sequence from DNAase and DNA sequencing reagents; as a result, the lack of bands in a DNA sequence ladder, called the footprint, can be easily read. If a protein binds to a radioactively labeled DNA oligonucleotide, its electrophoretic mobility is retarded (shifts) compared with the unbound DNA, and the DNA-protein binding can be measured.[9,16] Specific regulatory proteins are known to bind to these sequences and regulate gene transcription in a positive or negative fashion. The stability of binding of these proteins to the specific target sequences, and their association with other factors, determines the ultimate efficiency of the transcription process. A variety of DNA-binding proteins have been identified, cloned, and characterized; many bind to the specific DNA sequences listed in Table 2–1 and shown in Figure 2–1. These binding factors have at least two distinct regions: the DNA-binding domain, and the transactivation domain.[4,6,9]

The DNA-binding domains of nuclear transcriptional factors have been localized to discrete regions of 60 to 100 amino acids and have been structurally classified into several categories.[4,9] These modular subregions are novel structural elements, such as leucine zippers, helix-turn-helix, and zinc fingers, that regulate and facilitate DNA binding. The DNA-binding domains are necessary only for sequence-specific DNA binding, not for transcriptional activation. The transactivation domains are regions of 50 to 100 amino acid residues, but they are not defined structures like the DNA sequence recognition or binding domains. The transactivation domains can be rich in acidic amino acids or contain stretches of glutamine or proline residues.[4,6,9,17]

Helix-Turn-Helix Domains

Many mammalian and bacterial transcriptional factors have a helix-turn-helix motif in their DNA-binding domain that is responsible for recognizing and binding to specific DNA sequences.[18] Although the region required for binding is much larger, the specificity is determined by the helix-turn-helix motif, which is 20 amino acids long (Fig. 2–3). In the pro-

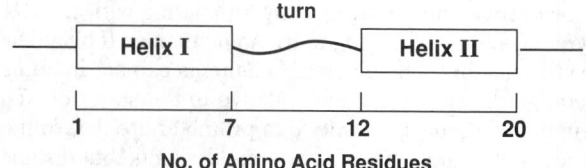

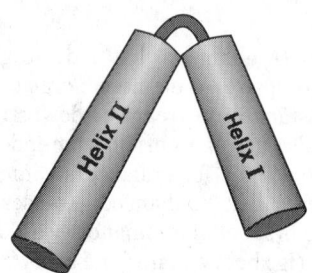

FIGURE 2–3. Structure of the helix-turn-helix DNA-binding domain. The helix-turn-helix structure is a common feature of several bacterial DNA-binding proteins, such as λ and *E. coli* repressors. A similar helix-turn-helix structure has also been found in various homeo and POU domains containing eukaryotic transcription factors. The helix-turn-helix structure was determined by x-ray crystallographic analysis of the phage λ repressor protein bound to the synthetic DNA fragment. The first helix is composed of 7 amino acids, and the second helix contains 9 amino acids. A glycine residue at position nine within the turn is common to all DNA-binding proteins containing helix-turn-helix domain. Some of the hydrophobic amino acids within helix I and helix II are also shared among different transcription factors. The helix-turn-helix structure makes contact with the major groove in DNA.

karyote repressor, the first 7 amino acid residues of the helix-turn-helix from the helix I are involved in sequence recognition.[18] This stretch is followed by a turn of 4 amino acids and then the second helix region, which consists of the remaining 9 amino acids and is responsible for binding to the specific DNA sequences.[19,20] X-ray crystallography of DNA-λ repressor interaction has revealed that the protein winds itself around the major groove, and the amino groups of the amino acids form hydrogen bonds with the free oxygen of the phosphates of DNA.[19,20] Although the helix-turn-helix motif was originally discovered in prokaryotic systems, it has also been identified in the homeodomains of many eukaryotic transcriptional activators, including such common factors as Pit1, Oct1, and Oct2.[21,22]

Leucine Zippers

Several DNA-binding proteins contain leucine residues characteristically spaced at every seventh position in their binding domain.[23] This leucine periodicity in the α-helix configuration forms a region with a hydrophobic "face" by which these proteins can pair or form dimers with homologous or heterologous partners, thereby modulating or facilitating binding to DNA at specific sites by adjacent basic amino acid residues (Fig. 2–4).[23] These structures are called leucine zippers (Fig. 2–4), and even though the leucine residues in these proteins do not make contact with DNA, they are required for holding

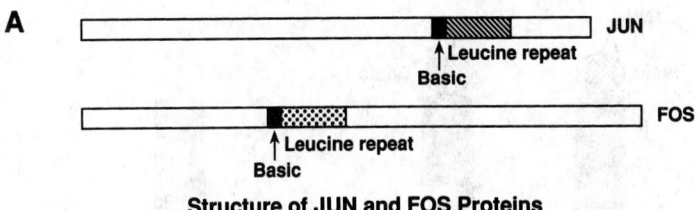

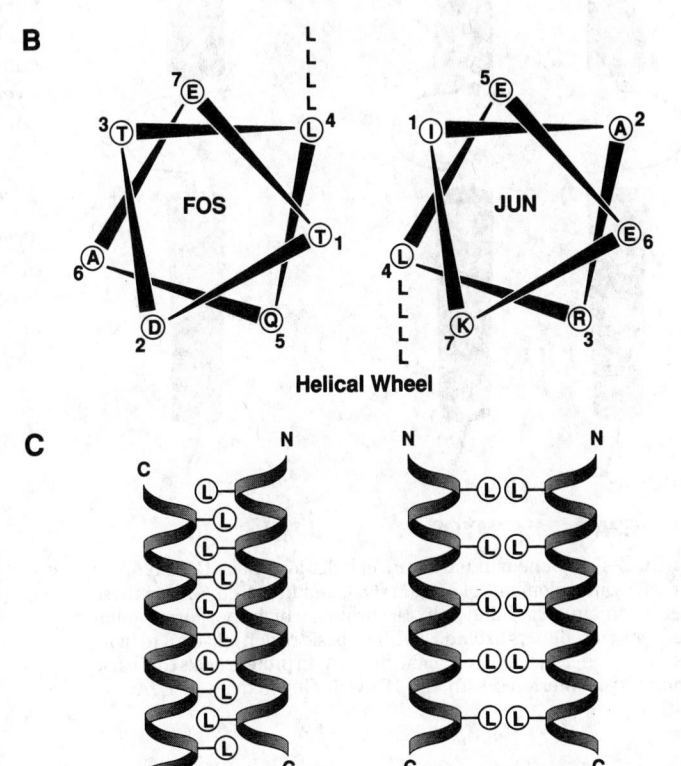

FIGURE 2–4. Schematic structure of JUN and FOS proteins and the DNA-binding domains. **(A)** The bars indicate JUN and FOS proteins; the solid box identifies the basic region located upstream of the leucine repeat region, depicted by the hatched box (JUN) or the stippled box (FOS). **(B)** An α-helical representation of the DNA-binding domain sequence of FOS and JUN proteins is displayed according to previously described reports. The first leucine residue of the leucine repeat region (zipper) is included at position 4 of the helical wheel, and every seventh residue at this position is a leucine. **(C)** α-Helices of the FOS and JUN leucine repeat regions in which every seventh amino acid is a leucine residue. Both the configurations (parallel and antiparallel) are depicted. Previously, an antiparallel configuration was thought to be the correct model, but x-ray crystallographic data indicate that the correct arrangement of leucine is in a parallel configuration.

homodimers or heterodimers in a particular configuration needed for DNA binding.[24] The region that makes contact with DNA is adjacent to the conserved leucines and is highly enriched in basic and hydrophobic amino acid residues.

A variety of proteins, identified in species from yeast to human, belong to this family of transcription factors.[25] The most extensively studied members of this family are the yeast transcriptional activator GCN4 and the protooncogene products of *FOS* and *JUN*.[26,27] The leucine zipper regions between the proteins JUN and GCN4 can be interchanged without any loss of transcriptional activity.[27,28] There are several members of the JUN and FOS family of gene products, all of which are able to form heterodimers that are collectively referred to as the AP1 transcriptional factors.[27] AP1 is required for the transcriptional activation of most mammalian genes. The leucine zipper region is found in many types of transcription factors, such as C/EBP.[25] It is also conserved in the *MYC* oncogene family of proteins. In fact, the MYC proteins contain the leucine zipper and a helix-loop-helix motif that provides another level of sophistication by which interaction with even a larger number of regulatory proteins can be effected.[27]

Helix-Loop-Helix Domains

The helix-loop-helix family of transcription factors include genes that are involved in cell proliferation and transformation (*MYC* family) and those that are found at breakpoints in chromosomal translocations associated with malignancies (*e.g.*, *MYC, SCL, LYL1*).[28] Members of this family of transcription factors (*e.g.*, MYOD, MYF, myogenin) can regulate differentiation, such as myogenesis. The DNA-binding domain of these proteins consists of 50 to 60 amino acid residues that can form two amphipathic helices separated by a loop (Fig. 2–5).[29] This domain is involved in protein-protein interactions to form homodimers or heterodimers, which bind DNA in a sequence-specific manner. The helix-loop-helix family of proteins have been classified in three groups. Group A proteins are ubiquitously expressed and include E2A and the product of *DAUGHTERLESS*.[29] Group B proteins are expressed in a tissue-specific manner and include achaete-scute, MYOD, and myogenin.[29] Group C proteins consist primarily of *MYC*-family members.[29] It has been suggested that the tissue-specific group B proteins can complex with ubiquitously expressed group A

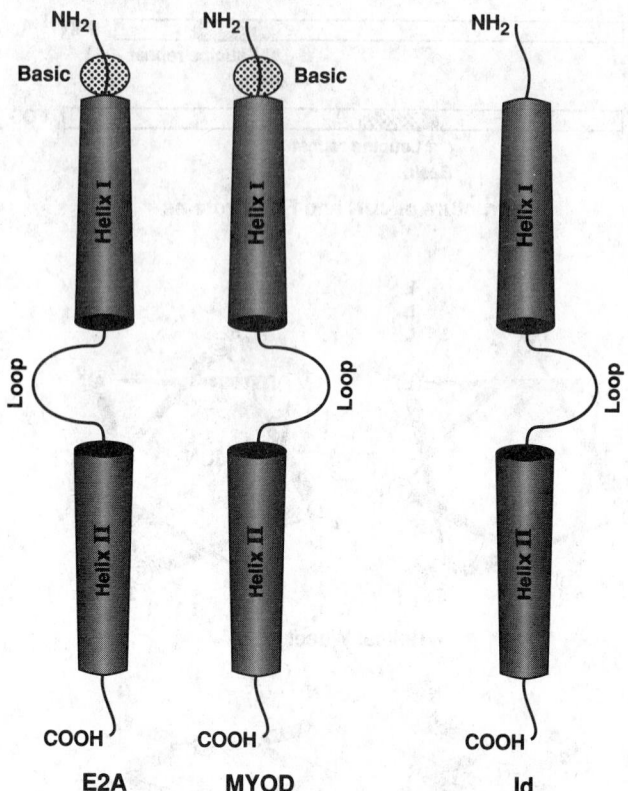

FIGURE 2–5. Schematic structure of helix-loop-helix DNA-binding and dimerization domains of E2A, MYOD, and Id proteins. All of these proteins contain helix I and helix II, through which they form homodimers or heterodimers to bind DNA. The basic region adjacent to helix I makes sequence-specific contact with DNA. Id protein lacks this basic region, and it interferes with the DNA-binding activity of E2A and *MYOD*.

proteins to form stable heterodimers that interact with κE2 sequences in different tissues. For example, the E2A and MYOD heterodimers form more stable complexes with enhancer sequences than do E2A or MYOD homodimers.[30]

A basic motif similar to that found in the leucine zipper-containing proteins is also located at the N-terminal side of helix I in helix-loop-helix proteins (Fig. 2–5) and is involved in DNA binding.[30] A subclass of helix-loop-helix family proteins (*e.g.*, ID, EMC) has been identified that lacks the adjacent basic region and functions as negative regulators of transcription in a heterodimeric form with MYOD or E2A and is referred to as a dominant-negative regulator.[31,32]

Zinc Fingers

So-called metal finger proteins (*e.g.*, zinc fingers) were originally identified in the transcriptional factor III (TFIIIA) of *Xenopus laevis*, which is involved in the regulation of 5S RNA expression.[33] This class of DNA-binding domain possesses cysteine and histidine residues that interact with metal ions such as zinc, forming the unique conformational structure of zinc fingers (Fig. 2–6). This widely conserved region that interacts with metal ions is a common feature of many DNA-binding proteins from yeast to mammals.[33,34] In *Drosophila*, the zinc finger protein Kruppel plays a crucial role in gap-segmentation development (*i.e.*, generating the embryo's ini-

tial seven segments), and the glucocorticoid receptors are all zinc finger-containing DNA-binding proteins (Fig. 2–6).[35–37]

Two types of zinc finger motifs have been described: Cys-Cys–His-His (*i.e.*, Cys-His or C_2H_2) and the cysteine cluster Cys-Cys–Cys-Cys (*i.e.*, Cys-Cys or C_x).[38] C_2H_2 is the prototype finger domain, in which the cysteine and histidine residues are usually repeated tandemly.[38] In the glucocorticoid receptors, *TAT* of HIV is nonrepetitive and the "x" residue may vary, representing 4, 5, or 6 amino acids. Some of the amino acids located between the cysteines and histidines are highly conserved in the C_2H_2-type fingers, but the amino acids between cysteines in the C_x type fingers are not apparently conserved.[35–38]

Tryptophan Repeats

Tryptophan repeat domains have, thus far, been identified only in the *MYB* and *ETS* protooncogene families of protein products.[39] In each repeat, three tryptophan residues are separated by 17 or 18 amino acids.[40] MYB contains three tryp-

A

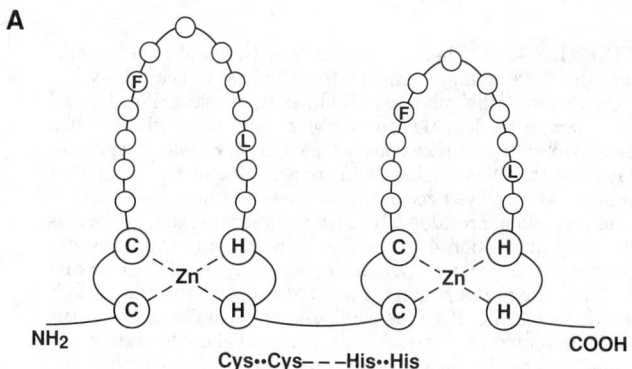

B

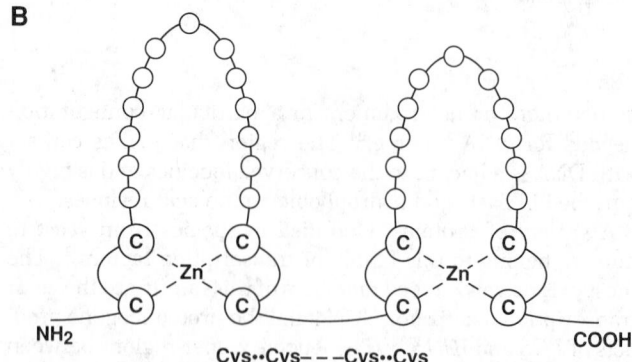

FIGURE 2–6. **(A)** Structure of the Cys-His (Cys··Cys---His··His) and **(B)** Cys-Cys (Cys··Cys---Cys··Cys) zinc fingers. The zinc finger structure of the transcription factor IIIA and glucocorticoid receptor was determined by two-dimensional nuclear magnetic resonance of the proteins bound to the zinc atoms. The nonconserved amino acids are indicated by open circles and the conserved amino acids are indicated by one-letter codes. Cys-His fingers are always present in tandem repeats and contain conserved phenylalenine and leucine residues in the finger structure. These types of fingers were originally discovered in the transcription factor IIIA of *Xenopus laevis*. The Cys-Cys finger does not contain any conserved amino acid in the finger portion and is present in the glucocorticoid receptor and other members of the steroid hormone receptor family. The probable role of zinc fingers is to bind DNA and RNA in a sequence-specific manner.

tophan repeat domains, and more than one repeat is necessary for specific DNA binding.[40] The tryptophan residues form a hydrophobic core, which enables neighboring basic amino acids to form a configuration that facilitates DNA binding.[41]

The ETS proteins also contain tryptophan repeats in their sequence-specific DNA-binding domains, but these proteins contain only one tryptophan repeat. Like MYB, the ETS proteins contain hydrophobic and basic amino acids located in this region, which may be involved in contacting DNA.[42]

Homeodomains

Homeodomains, or homeoboxes, were originally discovered in *Drosophila* genes that control embryogenesis. Mutations in these domains lead to homeotic transformations, such as legs growing in the place of antennae.[43] The homeodomains are 60 amino acids long and were found in a large number of transcription factors.[21,22,44] These domains bind to AT-rich DNA sequences (Table 2–1).[43] Physical studies of one of the *Drosophila* homeodomain proteins complexed with DNA revealed that a part of the homeodomains forms a helix-turn-helix structure similar to that observed in the bacterial repressor protein-DNA complexes. The homeodomain-containing transcription factors bind to DNA as monomers, unlike the λ repressor, which binds as a dimer.[18,19] Two human transcriptional factors, OCT1 and OCT2, contain homeodomains that share only a 35% sequence homology with a *Drosophila* homeodomain factor called antennapedia (ANTP). However, the helix-turn-helix structure is maintained in the *Drosophila* ANTP and in the OCT1 and OCT2 homeodomains.

POU Domains

OCT1 and OCT2 DNA-binding domains that bind to octamer core sequences (Table 2–1 and Fig. 2–1) and the pituitary-specific transcription factor PIT1 and a number of genes involved in the development of *Cainorhabditis elegans* include the homeodomains as part of a larger binding domain referred to as the POU domain.[21,22] These domains are approximately 150 amino acids long and can be divided into two subdomains: POU-specific domains and classic POU homeodomain.[21] The entire POU region is required for specific DNA binding, because mutations in either domain alter DNA binding efficiency. Although the mammalian OCT1 and OCT2 proteins bind to the same octamer DNA sequence, their expression in a cell-type-specific fashion regulates different sets of genes. OCT1 is expressed ubiquitously, but OCT2 is expressed in B cells and regulates immunoglobulin gene expression.[44,45]

Other Binding Domains

Several transcription factors bind DNA in a sequence-specific manner but lack any of the aforementioned DNA-binding domains. NFκB was originally identified in B cells and is responsible for regulating transcription of immunoglobulin κ genes by binding to the enhancer element.[46] The NFκB has two subunits of 50 and 65 kd and is restricted to the cytoplasm by complexing with a 48-kd IκB, which prevents NFκB movement to the nucleus and therefore prevents it from regulating gene expression.[46,47] Both subunits of NFκB (50 and 65 kd) possess homology to the proteins coded by the c-*REL* pro-

tooncogene family and the *Drosophila* gene *dorsal*.[46,47] The DNA-binding and dimerization domains of NFκB/REL are located at the N terminus, but the transactivation domain is at the C terminus.[47]

TRANSACTIVATOR OR TRANSCRIPTIONAL DOMAINS

Transactivation domains lack DNA-binding activity but provide specificity for protein-protein interaction and are directly or indirectly involved in promoting gene transcription by helping to assemble active transcription complexes.[6,9,42] Some transcriptional activators completely lack DNA-binding domains, such as HSV/VP16, but others, such as GAL4, CTF, OCT1 or OCT2, and SP1, possess a transactivating domain separate from their specific DNA-binding domain (Table 2–1).[47–50]

There are several types of transactivation domains that possess short stretches of 40 to 100 amino acids that are rich in acidic amino acids (*e.g.*, aspartic or glutamic residues) or in glutamine or proline residues.[47–49] Transactivator proteins lacking a DNA-binding domain function by interacting with another protein(s) with DNA-binding specificity.[50] A classic example of the latter interaction is the herpesvirus transactivator VP16 with the OCT1 transcription factor.[50] In this complex, the DNA-binding domain of OCT1 binds to a specific DNA sequence, while the acidic transactivating domain of VP16 is responsible for regulating transcription.[50]

Acidic Transactivating Domains

Acidic transactivating domains were first identified and characterized in the yeast transcription factor GAL4.[17] This transactivating domain is rich in acidic amino acid residues that can form an amphipathic α-helix, which is thought to be the structure responsible for interacting with other transcription regulatory proteins.[47] If the GAL4 acidic domain is deleted, the resulting protein binds DNA but fails to activate transcription.

Because transcriptional activating regions are interchangeable, chimeras with the GAL4 DNA-binding domain have been used to screen and identify transactivating regions of other proteins by assaying for stimulation of GAL4 promoter transcription.[17,47] The herpesvirus protein VP16 contains an acidic activating domain but lacks a DNA-binding domain.[50] This protein activates transcription by interacting with OCT1 DNA-binding protein.[50] Thus, VP16 transactivates expression in a manner that is dependent on the OCT1 DNA-binding site. The direct target of the VP16 acidic activator is TFIIB, a subunit of the general RNA polymerase II transcription factor.[6,9]

Glutamine-Rich Transcriptional Activator Domains

The transactivator domain of the mammalian transcription factor SP1 is glutamine rich.[48] Another transcriptional factor with a glutamine-rich domain is the *Drosophila* protein, ANTP.[48] The SP1 glutamine-rich domain is one of the most potent activators, and if interchanged with the glutamine-rich domain of *Drosophila* ANTP, it demonstrates that the transcriptional activation is primarily due to this domain, because there is not significant homology between the glutamine regions of SP1 and ANTP.[48] SP1 protein contains additional activating domains that are adjacent to the glutamine-rich domain and contribute to the glutamine-rich stimulation of transcription.[48] Other transcriptional factors, such as mammalian OCT2, JUN, AP2, and SRF and yeast GAL11, HAP1, and HAP2, have been shown to contain putative glutamine-rich transactivator domains and may transactivate transcription through this domain.[9]

Proline-Rich Transcriptional Activator Domains

A third type of transcriptional activator domain is rich in proline residues. Proline-rich regions have been identified by deletion mutagenesis in a mammalian transcription factor, such as CTF or SRF.[9,49] This region also stimulates gene expression when linked to heterologous DNA-binding domains, such as GAL4.

The different transactivating domains of transcription factors function by different mechanisms. Acidic domains may interact with proteins having positively charged domains, the glutamine-rich domains form hydrogen bonds with their partners, and proline-rich domains may form unique structures that preferentially interact with specific transcription regulatory factors.[17,47–49] The possible number of combinations of activator domains with DNA-binding factors to couple with transcriptional complexes (*e.g.*, RNA polymerase II) are staggering, and their consequences can be quite diverse at the level of gene transcription. In this way, the systems have evolved to deliver a stoichiometric amount of a gene product to the cell.

REGULATION OF THE REGULATORS

Through controlled gene expression, an organism regulates its development. We have discussed how protein-protein interactions and protein-DNA binding regulate gene transcription, but the stoichiometric amount of a factor in the cell is regulated by synthesis at mRNA and protein levels. Cell-specific or tissue-specific gene expression is regulated at the level of RNA transcription or protein translation. Transcriptional regulation can occur at the level of initiation and elongation (*e.g.*, c-*MYC*-related mRNA), transport of mRNA into cytoplasm through the action of SNRP complexes, or alternate splicing mechanisms to yield alternate mRNA forms with a different cytoplasmic stability or unique coding information.[42] Stability is most affected through capping at the 5′ end and polyadenylation at the 3′ end of the mRNA. Gene regulation at the translational level can be affected by factors that influence the rate of protein synthesis or protein stability or by posttranslational modification, such as phosphorylation at specific sites to influence interprotein or intraprotein interactions.[51] The interactions have been observed with growth factors or cell cycle control proteins in response to external stimuli. Transcription is also regulated in a positive and negative fashion by interaction of transcription factors with specific proteins.[52]

TRANSCRIPTIONAL REGULATION

The presence of a transcription factor in a cell is regulated by the level of its mRNA expression and its stability. The levels of mRNA can be affected by external factors, such as growth factors, or intracellularly by second messengers, such as cAMP. TPA (12-O-tetradecanoylphorbol-13-acetate) and serum growth factors induce the transcription of *FOS, JUN,* and *ETS* through the protein kinase C signal transduction pathway.[53–55] Similarly, an intracellular second messenger, such as cAMP, stimulates the pituitary-specific factor PIT1 through the activation of the cAMP response element, binding CREB protein.[56] The transcription factors can also be auto-regulated positively or negatively by their own products or by gene products of their own family members. Transcription factors such as JUN, ETS1, and a muscle differentiation factor (MYOD) are positively autoregulated, but the MYC and FOS transcription factors are negatively autoregulated.[57–61]

Alternate splicing is another mechanism for controlling the expression of transcription factors.[62] For example, the alternately spliced *MYB* mRNA results in a truncated product that lacks the transactivation domain, but it retains the DNA-binding domain.[62] This truncated product interferes with the binding of the normal MYB protein to its target site. Alternate splicing is a widely used mechanism in transcription regulation and has been observed with various other genes, such as the E2 gene product of bovine papillomavirus, as well as the FOS, ID, and *MYOD* gene products in an interaction referred to as dominant-negative.[63,64]

TRANSLATIONAL REGULATION

Although the translational controls of transcription factors are less well characterized than the transcriptional controls, posttranslational modifications are essential for function. Phosphorylation, perhaps the most important posttranslational modification, plays a key role in regulating the activity of many proteins.[65] Most transcription factors are phosphoproteins, and their activity can be directly regulated by phosphorylation or dephosphorylation. Sites of protein phosphorylation are on serine or threonine residues, and the phosphorylation is carried out by protein kinases, such as protein kinase C, cyclic AMP-dependent kinases, casein kinase II, calmodulin-dependent protein kinase, or the major cell cycle regulator p34^{cdc2} kinase.[65,66] An example of phosphorylation regulation is that of the phosphorylated form of the MYB protein that does not bind to the *MYB*-specific DNA sequences.[67] Phosphorylation of the heat-shock transcription factor results in an increased level of transcription of the target genes. In this case, the negatively charged phosphate residues in the transactivation domain of the heat-shock factor mimic the acidic transactivation domains.[17]

An example of how phosphorylation affects transcriptional activity is the CREB. This protein binds to DNA only in a dimeric form, and the phosphorylation of monomers by cAMP-dependent protein kinase favors dimer formation.

Other posttranslational modifications are less frequently used to regulate transcription activity, such as glycosylation. Glycosylation of SP1 does not affect the DNA-binding activity, but it reduces transcriptional activation activity.

The stability or half-life of a transcriptional factor plays an important role in its transcriptional activation. Most factors are present in low concentrations and have short half-lives.[67] TPA increases the half-life of the ETS2 transcription factor from 20 minutes to 2.5 hours.[67] This induction is ETS2 specific, because MYC and ETS1 do not appear to be affected by such treatment.[67] In this case, the increased half-life of ETS2 could lead to sustained activation of its relevant target genes.

PROTEIN-PROTEIN INTERACTIONS: POSITIVE AND NEGATIVE REGULATION

Protein-protein interaction, especially in transactivation domains, plays an important role in the regulation of transcriptional factors.[6,9,42] Many transcription factors form homodimers, heterodimers, or protein oligomers that are essential in the transactivation process.[29] The dimerization domains discussed previously have been identified in these factors by their influence on DNA binding (Figs. 2–4 and 2–5); these domains include the leucine zipper and helix-loop-helix motifs.

Leucine zipper domains present in the gene products of c-*JUN* and c-*FOS* are important motifs for the formation of homodimers or heterodimers (*e.g.*, JUN-JUN, FOS-FOS, JUN-FOS).[53] The JUN-FOS heterodimer binds DNA with high affinity to the specific TGACTCA DNA sequence (*i.e.*, AP1 site) (Table 2–1), and the homodimer JUN-JUN binds with low affinity and can be displaced by JUN-FOS.[25] The FOS-FOS homodimer (but none of the monomer proteins) binds to this sequence, illustrating how protein-protein interactions greatly alter binding affinity.[25,27,53]

Another dimerization domain, the helix-loop-helix motif (Fig. 2-5), is associated with many transcription factors.[29,68] For example, MYOD forms heterodimers with a ubiquitously expressed transcription factor, E2A, and this complex binds specifically to muscle creatine kinase enhancer, promoting muscle-specific expression.[29] Some transcription factors, such as the MYC family, contain helix-loop-helix and leucine zipper dimerization motifs.[68] An MYC dimerization protein (Max) also contains the helix-loop-helix and LZ domains, and in this heterodimeric form, the complex binds specifically to the CAGCTG core sequence.[68] The interaction between MYC and Max proteins is highly specific, and no other helix-loop-helix or leucine zipper protein has yet been found that binds to the MYC or Max proteins.[68]

The heterodimerization of different transcriptional factors provides the enormous potential for unique interaction with a greater variety of target gene promoters.

NEGATIVE REGULATION

FOS and JUN heterodimers bind to a specific DNA sequence to activate transcription. However, FOSB2 protein, a product of differentially spliced FOSB2 mRNA, inhibits the formation of the active FOS-JUN complex by dominant interaction with JUN protein.[69] This FOSB2-JUN complex binds to the AP1 site, but does not activate transcription and therefore serves as a dominant-negative transcription regulator.[69]

Another protein that interferes with the FOS-JUN complex is inhibition protein-1 (IP1).[70] This protein complexes with the FOS-JUN dimers and prevents transcriptional activation.[70] However, the phosphorylation of IP1 by the cAMP-dependent protein kinase dissociates this protein from the FOS-JUN complex and, through cAMP, restores FOS-JUN activity.

Another interesting dominant-negative protein inhibitor, ID, is expressed in all except fully differentiated cells.[31] This protein contains the helix-loop-helix region, but it lacks the adjacent basic domain required for DNA-binding activity (Fig. 2–5).[31] ID complexes with MYOD, E2A, and other transcriptional activators of the helix-loop-helix family and prevents their binding to DNA, thereby interfering with the transcriptional activation and differentiation.[31,32] This inhibitor plays an important role in differentiation by downregulating the activity of helix-loop-helix proteins required for this process.[31]

NFκB is very important in regulating the expression of immunoglobulin κ chain during B-cell development.[46] In the active complex, this factor is composed of two subunits, a 50-kd and a 65-kd protein.[47a] A dominant-negative inhibitory factor, IκB, forms a complex with the active form of NFκB, and this interaction makes the complex inactive by preventing its migration from the cytoplasm into the nucleus.[46,47A] As with IP1, phosphorylation of the IκB results in the dissociation of the inhibitor from the NFκB complex, allowing it to move into the nucleus and transactivate relevant target genes.[47A,70] The formation of the NFκB-IκB complex is through ankyrin repeat sequences that are present in the 50-kd NFκB subunit and the IκB protein. The ankyrin repeat was originally discovered in ankyrin, a red blood cell cytoskeleton protein, and is composed of 33 amino acid residues that are often located in tandem arrays that have been implicated in protein-protein interactions.[71]

TRANSCRIPTION FACTORS IN MUSCLE CELL DEVELOPMENT

Gene regulation is responsible for the processes of cell proliferation and differentiation. During the last decade, there has been an explosion in the duplication and characterization of the products involved in these processes. Many genes code transcription factors, which control the expression of downstream effector genes that promote differentiation or development. A good example is the system of development and differentiation of skeletal muscle because the role of transcription factors in this process is fairly well understood.[71]

TRANSCRIPTION FACTORS THAT ACTIVATE MUSCLE DEVELOPMENT

Muscle development in mouse and humans is induced by a family of transcriptional factors that include MYOD, myogenin, MYF3, MYF4, MYF5, and MYF6.[72-74] MYOD was the first myogenic factor discovered.[74] Its gene, molecularly cloned from a myoblast cell line, encodes a 318 amino acid nuclear phosphoprotein that transactivates the expression of several genes to regulate muscle development.[74] Cell lines derived from diverse cell types such as hepatomas, neuroblastomas, melanomas, and 10T1/2 fibroblasts can be converted into myoblasts by the expression of MYOD.[74] This indicates that MYOD can directly activate muscle-specific development in fibroblast cells and in a variety of other cell types. Moreover, it indicates that MYOD interacts with factors that are expressed in a wide variety of cell types to effect muscle-specific expression.[74] Several cell lines, such as HeLa and monkey CV-1 cells, are refractory to myogenic conversion by MYOD expression, suggesting that these cells express negative factors like ID or that positive-acting factors are absent.[74]

MYOD activates muscle-specific gene expression during muscle development by specifically binding to a CANNTG (N = A, G, C, or Tbase) DNA core sequence.[30] Such core sequences have been identified in the *MYOD* promoter and other gene family members; MYOD regulates itself and its family members.[29,30] MYOD has been shown to form an active complex with the E2A gene product, and this complex activates transcription of the muscle creatine kinase gene.[29,30] The human muscle regulatory factors MYF3 and MYF4 are the human homologs of MYOD and myogenin and are also capable of inducing muscle cell differentiation in 10T1/2 cells.[73] Although these family members bind to the same core DNA sequence, they require distinct cooperating factors for muscle development.[72,73] The *MYF* genes are differentially expressed during muscle development. Different muscle cell subtypes express different factors.[73] However, for complete myogenic development, expression of all three factors—MYF3, MYF4, and MYF5—are required.[73] Myogenin is expressed in all muscle cell lines and types, suggesting that this factor is absolutely required for muscle development.

Expression of other genes, such as *MYD* and *SKI,* can convert fibroblasts to myoblasts.[75,76] These genes are not related to the *MYOD* family and appear to mediate muscle development through pathways different from those used by *MYOD.* The *SKI* gene was originally identified as a transduced viral oncogene, and when expressed in the skeletal muscles of trans-genic mice under the control of a long terminal repeat, it causes profound hypertrophy of fast muscle fibers.[76,77]

TRANSCRIPTION FACTORS IN ONCOGENESIS

Spontaneous human cancers arise from a series of somatic cellular changes caused by chromosome deletions, rearrangements, or point mutations. The oncogenes are damaged versions of normal cellular protooncogenes that perform important cellular functions such as cell growth and differentiation. A number of protooncogene products (*e.g.,* FOS, JUN, MYC, ETS, REL, MYB) are localized in the nucleus and function as transcription factors.[29,42,46,64,68] A limited number of genes called tumor suppressor genes play a major role in neoplasia. The most celebrated of these tumor suppressor genes are *RB* and p53, which are normally involved in controlling cell growth.[78] In the case of *RB,* mutation or deletion of both the alleles results in the loss of normal function, leading to uncontrolled cancer growth. On the other hand, p53 can, in the heterozygous state, contribute to tumorigenesis. Mutations of the p53 gene are the most common genetic lesions in human cancer and have also been frequently reported as part of the Li-Fraumeni syndrome. The p53 gene, which is located on

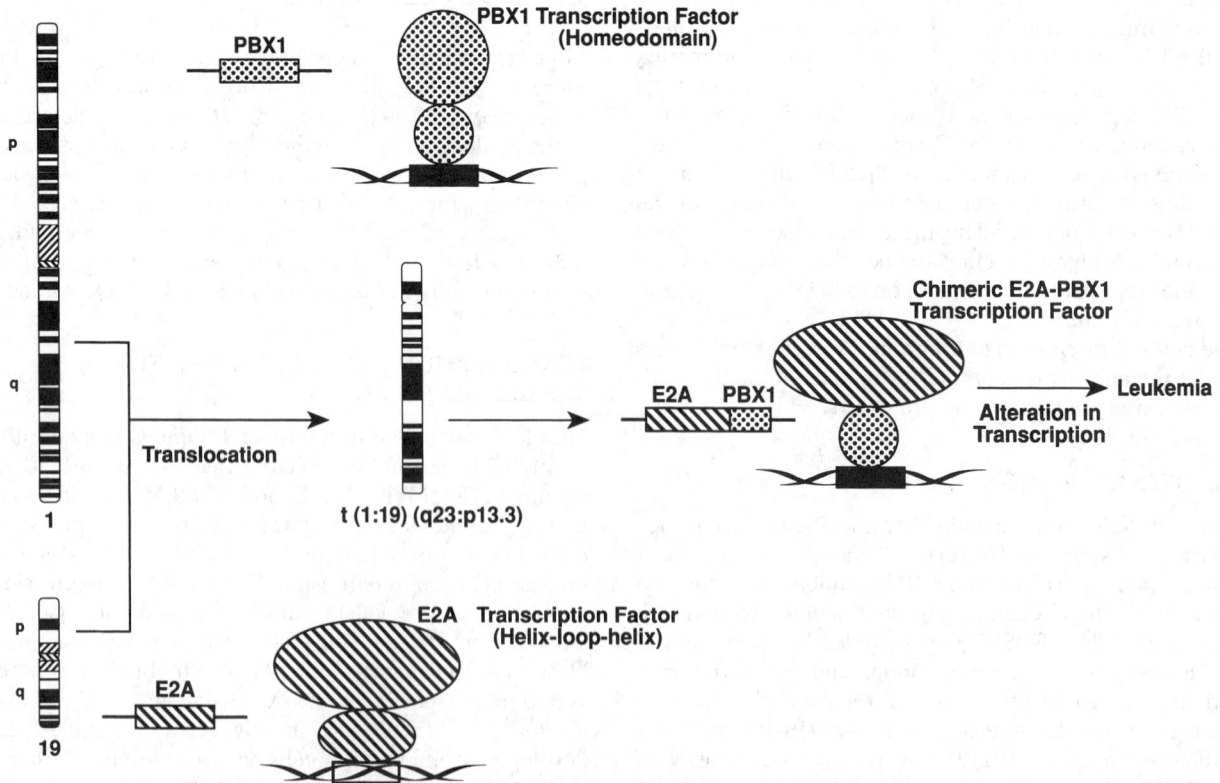

FIGURE 2–7.   Generation of a chimeric transcription factor (E2A-PBX1) as a result of chromosomal translocation and its role in pre-B ALL. In the t(1;19)(q23;p13.3) translocation, a ubiquitously expressed helix-loop-helix–containing transcription factor E2A is fused to a homeodomain-containing transcription factor (PBX1), generating a chimeric transcription factor with oncogenic activity. This chimeric transcription factor (E2A-PBX1) binds to the promoter-enhancer region of those genes that are normally bound by PBX1; however, it regulates gene expression through E2A target proteins. PBX1 was formerly called PRL.

chromosome 17p, is a transcriptional factor and controls various growth-related genes.[78]

Several transcription factors that contain the helix-loop-helix and homeodomains have been found in nonrandom chromosomal translocation breakpoints and are believed to be directly involved with a variety of leukemias.[28,79,80] The *MYC* protooncogene was the first oncogene discovered at a nonrandom chromosomal translocation breakpoint in Burkitt lymphoma. The MYC product is a member of the helix-loop-helix family of transcriptional factors. A growing number of other helix-loop-helix-containing transcriptional factors (*e.g.*, products encoded by *LYL1*, *TAL1*, *SCL*) have been found to be structurally disrupted after chromosomal translocations.[28,79,80] Given that these helix-loop-helix proteins complex with other transcription factors, it is not surprising that inappropriate expression or damage to these transcription regulator genes alters hematopoietic differentiation or activated cell proliferation.[80]

A homeobox-containing gene, *HOX11*, which is normally expressed in liver cells, was found to be inappropriately expressed in T cells after t(10;14) translocation.[79] The inappropriate expression of this gene in nonliver cells may activate a battery of genes as part of the liver differentiation program that are normally silent in these cells.[79] Alternatively, oncogenesis may result from repression by Hox11 of genes that are required for normal T-cell differentiation.

Two novel nonrandom chromosomal translocations (t[15;17] and t[1;19]) are involved in acute promyelocytic leukemia (APL) and pre-B-cell leukemia.[79,80] Both translocations generate chimeric transcription factors (Fig. 2–7).

Molecular characterization of the t(15;17) breakpoint has shown that most chromosome 17 breakpoints involve the first intron of the retinoic acid receptor gene[81] (*i.e.*, *RARα*, a gene related to the superfamily of steroid and thyroid hormone receptors). This genetic rearrangement produces a chimeric protein that contains the DNA-binding and hormone-responsive domains from RARα fused to another gene product, PML (a new transcription factor).[79,80] The fusion product (PML-RARα) appears to interfere with promyelocyte differentiation. This is important in explaining why retinoic acid and its analogs cause remission of APL disease and potential restoration of normal hematopoietic differentiation.[79,80] The truncated RARα fusion product is easily detected by molecular techniques. The fusion product has been sequenced, and a sensitive polymerase chain reaction assay has been developed to monitor patients with APL for response to retinoid therapy and for residual disease after treatment with chemotherapeutic agents.[79,80]

Pre-B-cell acute lymphoblastic leukemia (ALL) involves a frequent chromosomal translocation t(1;19) whose breakpoint results in the fusion of two different genes, yielding a novel chimeric transcription regulator.[79,80] The 5′ portion of the chimeric protein contains a truncated form of the transactivator regulator E2A, and the 3′ portion contains a DNA-binding-specific homeodomain from the transcriptional factor called PBX1 (previously called PRL).[81] The chimeric protein (E2A-PBX1) is a consistent feature in cells containing the t(1;19) translocation (Fig. 2–7). The contribution of the chimeric protein (containing two distinctive regions, the helix-loop-helix protein-protein interaction activator domain and the DNA-binding-specific homeodomain) in the pathogenesis

of this pre-B-cell malignancy may result from inappropriate target activation during B-cell differentiation that results in the arrest of maturation.

Novel oncogene products arise from nonrandom chromosomal translocations. Molecular cloning and characterization of these nonrandom chromosomal translocation breakpoints continues to provide new insights into the molecular basis of specific neoplasias. Future research in these areas will provide innovative diagnostic probes and perhaps lead to the development of therapies directed at inhibiting the disruptive chimeric products.

Acknowledgment

The contents of this publication do not necessarily reflect the views or policies of the Department of Health and Human Services, nor does mention of trade names, commercial products, or organizations imply endorsement by the U.S. Government.

REFERENCES

1. Lewin B. Building the transcription complex. In: RNA polymerase-promoter interactions. Genes, vol 4. New York: John Wiley & Sons, 1989.
2. Shenk T. Transcriptional control regions: Nucleotide sequences requirements for initiation by RNA polymerase II and III. Curr Top Microbiol Immunol 1981;93:25–40.
3. Saltzman AG, Weinmann R. Promoter specificity and modulation of RNA polymerase II transcription. FASEB J 1989;3:1723–1733.
4. Johnson PF, McKnight SL. Eukaryotic transcriptional regulatory proteins. Annu Rev Biochem 1989;58:799–838.
5. Murphy S, Moorefield B, Pieler T. Common mechanisms of promoter recognition by RNA polymerases II and III. Trends Genet 1989;5:122–126.
6. Dynan WS, Tjian R. Control of eukaryotic messenger RNA synthesis by sequence-specific DNA-binding proteins. Nature 1985;316:774–777.
7. Buratowski S, Hahn S, Guarente L, et al. Five intermediate complexes in transcription initiation by RNA polymerase II. Cell 1989;56:549–561.
8. Garrity PA, Wold BJ. Tissue specific expression from a compound TATA-dependent and TATA-independent promoter. Mol Cell Biol 1990;10:5646–5654.
9. Maniatis T, Goodbourn S, Fisher JA. Regulation of inducible and tissue specific gene expression. Science 1987;236:1237–1244.
10. Klausner RD, Harford JB. *Cis-trans* models for post-transcriptional gene regulation. Science 1989;246:870–872.
11. Serfling E, Jasin M, Schaffner W. Enhancers and eukaryotic gene transcription. Trends Genet 1985;1:224–230.
12. Levinson B, Khoury G, Vande Woude GF, Gruss B. Activation of the SV40 genome by the 72 base-pair tandem repeats of Moloney sarcoma virus. Nature 1982;259:568–572.
13. Gillies SD, Morrison SL, Oi VT, Tonegawa S. A tissue-specific transcription enhancer element is located in the major intron of a rearranged immunoglobulin heavy chain gene. Cell 1983;33:717–728.
14. Herbomel P, Bourachot B, Yaniv, M. Two distinct enhancers with different cell specificities co-exist in the regulatory region of polyoma. Cell 1984;39:653–662, 1984.
15. Karpinski BA, Yang L-H, Cacheris P, et al. The first intron of the 4F2 heavy-chain gene contains a transcriptional enhancer element that binds multiple nuclear proteins. Mol Cell Biol 1989;9:2588–2597.
16. Maniatis T, Fritsch EF, Sambrook J. Molecular cloning: A laboratory manual. Cold Spring Harbor, NY: Cold Spring Harbor Laboratory, 1989.
17. Ptashne M. How gene activators work. Sci Am 1989;260:24–31.
18. Harrison SC, Aggarwal AK. DNA recognition by proteins with the helix-turn-helix motif. Ann Rev Biochem 1990;59:933–969.
19. Dodd IB, Egan JB. Improved detection of helix-turn-helix DNA-binding motifs in protein sequences. Nucleic Acids Res 1990;18:5019–5024.
20. Clarke ND, Beamer LJ, Goldberg HR, et al. The DNA binding arm of λ repressor: Critical contacts from a flexible region. Science 1991;254:267–270.
21. Rosenfeld MG. POU-domain transcription factors: Pou-er-ful developmental regulators. Genes Dev 1991;5:897–907.
22. Ruvkun G, Finney M. Regulation of transcription and cell identity by POU domain proteins. Cell 1991;64:475–478.
23. Landschulz WH, Johnson PF, McKnight SL. The leucine zipper: A hypothetical structure common to a new class of DNA-binding proteins. Science 1988;240:1759–1764.
24. O'Shea EK, Rutkowski R, Kim PS. Evidence that the leucine zipper is a coiled coil. Science 1991;243:538–542.
25. Busch SJ, Sassone-Coysi P. Dimers, leucine zippers and DNA binding domains. Trends Genet 1990;6:36–40.
26. Hope IA, Struhl K. Functional dissection of a eukaryotic transcriptional activator protein GCN4 of yeast. Cell 1986;46:885–894.

27. Stouhl K. The DNA binding domains of the JUN oncoprotein and the yeast GCN4 transcriptional activator are functionally homologous. Cell 1987;50:841–846.
28. Mellentin JD, Smith SD, Cleary ML. *LYL-1*, a novel gene altered by chromosomal translocation in T cell leukemia, codes for a protein with a helix-loop-helix DNA binding motif. Cell 1989;58:77–83.
29. Murre C, McCaw PS, Baltimore D. A new DNA binding and dimerization motif in immunoglobulin enhancer binding, daughterless, MyoD, and myc proteins. Cell 1989;56:777–783.
30. Lassar AB, Buskin JN, Lockshon D, et al. MYOD is a sequence-specific DNA binding protein requiring a region of *MYC* homology to bind to the muscle creatine kinase enhancer. Cell 1989;58:823–831.
31. Benezra R, Davis RL, Lockshon D, et al. The protein ID: A negative regulator of helix-loop-helix DNA binding proteins. Cell 1990;61:49–59.
32. Christy BA, Sanders LK, Lau LF, et al. An ID-related helix-loop-helix protein encoded by a growth factor-inducible gene. Proc Natl Acad Sci USA 1991;88:1815–1819.
33. Koster M, Pieler T, Poting A, et al. The finger motif defines a multigene family represented in the maternal mRNA of *Xenopus laevis* oocytes. EMBO J 1988;7:1735–1741.
34. Klug A, Rhodes D. "Zinc fingers": A novel protein motif for nucleic acid recognition. Trends Biochem Sci 1987;12:464.
35. Green S, Chambon P. Oestradiol induction of a glucocorticoid-responsive gene by a chimaeric receptor. Nature 1987;325:75–78.
36. Schule R, Muller M, Kaltschmidt C, et al. Many transcription factors interact synergistically with steroid receptors. Science 1988;242:1418–1420.
37. Frankel AD, Bredt DS, Pabo CO. Tat protein from human immunodeficiency virus forms a metal-linked dimer. Science 1988;240:70–73.
38. Evans RM, Hollenberg SM. Zinc fingers: Gilt by association. Cell 1988;52:1–3.
39. Anton IA, Frampton J. Tryptophans in MYB proteins. Nature 1988;336:719.
40. Saikumar P, Murali R, Reddy EP. Role of tryptophan repeats and flanking amino acids in MYB-DNA interactions. Proc Natl Acad Sci USA 1990;87:8452–8456.
41. Biedenkapp H, Borgmeyer U, Sippel AE, et al. Viral *MYB* oncogene encodes a sequence-specific DNA-binding activity. Nature 1988;335:835–837.
42. Seth A, Ascione R, Fisher B, et al. The *ETS* gene family. Cell Growth Differentiation 1992;3:327–334.
43. Kemler I, Bucher E, Seipel K, et al. Promoters with the octamer DNA motif (ATGCAAAT) can be ubiquitous or cell type-specific depending on binding affinity of the octamer site and OCT-factor concentration. Nucleic Acids Res 1991;19:237–242.
44. Scholer HR, Hatzopoulos AK, Balling R, et al. A family of octamer-specific proteins present during mouse embryogenesis: Evidence for germline-specific expression of an OCT factor. EMBO J 1989;8:2543–2550.
45. Dressler GR. An update on the vertebrate homeobox. Trends Genet 1989;5:129–130.
46. Lenardo MJ, Baltimore D. NF-κB. A pleiotropic mediator of inducible and tissue-specific gene control. Cell 1989;58:227–229.
47. Lin Y-S, Green MR. Mechanism of action of an acidic transcriptional activator in vitro. Cell 1991;64:971–981.
47a.Nolan GP, Ghosh S, Liou H-C, et al. DNA binding and IκB inhibition of the cloned p65 subunit of NF-κB, a *rel*-related polypeptide. Cell 1991;64:961–969.
48. Courey AJ, Holtzman DA, Jackson SP, et al. Synergistic activation by the glutamine-rich domains of human transcription factor Spl. Cell 1989;59:827–836.
49. Mermod N, O'Neill EA, Kelly TJ, et al. The proline-rich transcriptional activator of CTF/NF-I is distinct from the replication and DNA binding domain. Cell 1989;58:741–753.
50. Stern S, Tanaka M, Herr W. The OCT-1 homoeodomain directs formation of a multi-protein-DNA complex with the HSV transactivator VP16. Nature 1989;341:624–628.
51. Eisenman RN, Thompson CB. Oncogenes with potential nuclear function: *MYC, MYB*, and *FOS*. Cancer Surv 1986;5:309–327.
52. Jones NC, Rigby PWJ, Ziff EB. Trans-acting protein factors and the regulation of eukaryotic transcription: Lessons from studies on DNA tumor viruses. Genes Dev 1988;2:267–281.
53. Curran T. The *FOS* oncogene. In: Reddy EP, Skalka AM, Curran T, eds. The oncogene. Amsterdam: Elsevier, 1988:307–325.
54. Lamph WW, Wamsley P, Sassone-Corsi P. Induction of protooncogene *JUN/AP1* by serum and TPA. Nature 1988;334:629–631.
55. Koizumi S, Fisher RJ, Fujiwana S, et al. Isoforms of the human ETS-1 protein: Generation by alternative splicing and differential phosphorylation. Oncogene 1990;5:675–681.
56. Pei D, Shih C. Transcriptional activation and repression by cellular DNA-binding protein C/EBP. J Virol 1990;64:1517–1522.
57. Angel P, Hattori K, Smeal T, et al. The *JUN* proto-oncogene. Cell 1988;5:875–885.
58. Seth A, Papas TS. The c-*ETS*1 protooncogene has oncogenic activity and is positively autoregulated. Oncogene 1990;5:1761–1767.
59. Davis RL, Cheng PF, Lassar AB, Weintraub H. The MYOD DNA binding domain containing a recognition code for muscle-specific gene activation. Cell 1990;60:733–746.
60. Leder P, Battey J, Lenoir G, Moulding G, Murphy W, Potter H, Stewart T, Taub R. Translocations among antibody genes in human cancer. Science 1983;222:765–771.
61. Sassone-Corsi P, Sisson JC, Verma IM. Transcriptional autoregulation of the protooncogene *FOS*. Nature 1988;334:314–319.
62. Weber BL, Westin EH, Clarke MF. Differentiation of mouse erythroleukemia cells enhanced by alternatively spliced c-*MYB* mRNA. Science 1990;249:1291–1293.
63. McBride AA, Byrne JC, Howley PM. E2 polypeptides encoded by bovine papillomavirus type 1 form dimers through the common carboxyl-terminal domain: Transactivation is mediated by the conserved amino-terminal domain. Proc Natl Acad Sci USA 1989;86:510–514.
64. Nakabeppu Y, Nathans D. A naturally occurring truncated form of FOSB that inhibits *FOS/JUN* transcriptional activity. Cell 1991;64:751–759.
65. Kemp BE, Pearson RB. Protein kinase recognition sequence motifs. Trends Biochem Sci 1990;15:342–346.
66. Featherstone C. The complexities of the cell cycle. Trends Biochem Sci 1989;14:85–87.
67. Fujiwara S, Fisher RJ, Bhat NK, Diaz de La Espina, SM, Papas TS. A short lived nuclear phosphoprotein encoded by the human *ETS*2 protooncogene is stabilized by activation of protein kinase C. Mol Cell Biol 1988;8:4700–4706.
68. Blackwood EM, Eisenman RN. Max: A helix-loop-helix zipper protein that forms a sequence-specific DNA-binding complex with *MYC*. Science 1991;251:1211–1217.
69. Yen J, Wisdom R, Tratner I, et al. An alternative spliced form of FOSB is a negative regulator of transcriptional activation and transformation by FOS proteins. Proc Natl Acad Sci USA 1991;88:5077–5081.
70. Auwerx J, Sassone-Corsi P. IP-1: A dominant inhibitor of *FOS/JUN* whose activity is modulated by phosphorylation. Cell 1991;64:983–993.
71. Lamarco K, Thompson C, Brien B, et al. Identification of ETS and Notch related subunits in GA binding proteins. Science 1991;253:789–792.
72. Olson EN. *MYOD* family: A paradigm for development? Genes Dev 1990;4:1454–1461.
73. Braun T, Bober E, Winter B, et al. MYF-6, a new member of the human gene family of myogenic determination factors: Evidence for a gene cluster on chromosome 12. EMBO J 1990;9:821–831.
74. Weintraub H, Davis R, Tapscott S, et al. The *MYOD* gene family: Nodal point during specification of the muscle cell lineage. Science 1991;251:761–766.
75. Pinney DF, Pearson-White SH, Konieczny SF, Latham KE, Emerson CP Jr. Myogenic lineage determination and differentiation: Evidence for a regulatory gene pathway. Cell 1988;53:781–793.
76. Colmenames C, Stavnezer E. The *SKI* oncogene induces muscle differentiation in quail embryo cells. Cell 1989;59:293–303.
77. Sutrave P, Kelly AM, Hughes SH. *SKI* can cause selective growth of skeletal muscle in transgenic mice. Genes Dev 1990;4:1462–1472.
78. Levine A, Momand J, Finlay C. The p53 tumor suppressor gene. Nature 1991;351:453–456.
79. Chen Q, Cheng J-T, Tsai L-H, et al. The *TAL* gene undergoes chromosome translocation in T-cell leukemia and potentially encodes a helix-loop-helix protein. EMBO J 1990;9:415–424.
80. Kamps MP, Murre C, Sun X, et al. A new homeobox gene contributes the DNA binding domain of the t(1;19) translocation protein in pre-B ALL. Cell 1990;60:547–555.
81. Ezzell C. Spliced and diced receptor gene explains rare leukemia. J Natl Inst Health Res 1991;3:55–60.

Cancer: Principles & Practice of Oncology, Fourth Edition,
edited by Vincent T. DeVita, Jr., Samuel Hellman, Steven A. Rosenberg.
J.B. Lippincott Co., Philadelphia © 1993.

Archibald S. Perkins
George F. Vande Woude

CHAPTER **3**

Principles of Molecular Cell Biology of Cancer: Oncogenes

Oncologists are confronted daily with the unrelenting nature and lethal consequences of abnormal cell proliferation. Armed with the best pharmacologic and radiologic armamentarium, they try to turn the tide in favor of restoring health. Advanced forms of treatment require elucidation of the molecular mechanisms of neoplastic transformation and proliferation. For instance, potential anticancer drugs are being developed that block the farnesylation of the *RAS* oncoprotein. The clinician should have an understanding of the rationale for the actions of these drugs and an understanding of molecular oncogenesis.

Such pragmatism aside, the field of cancer research is fascinating in its own right and becomes more so as our understanding progresses. Cancer is a multistep process in which multiple genetic alterations must occur, usually over the span of years, to have a cumulative effect on the control of cell differentiation, cell division, and growth control.[1] As in cancer-predisposing syndromes, these genetic alterations are sometimes carried in the germline. Among human tumors, heritable mutations are by far the exception. Most alterations are acquired in the form of chromosomal translocations, deletions, inversions, amplifications, or point mutations. Certain oncogenic viruses play important roles in a few human tumors, such as human papillomavirus in cervical cancer and certain skin tumors, Epstein-Barr virus in nasopharyngeal carcinoma and Burkitt's lymphoma, and human T-cell leukemia viruses (*e.g.*, HTLV-I, HTLV-II) in T-cell leukemia. Transforming retroviruses play an important role in the development of experimental tumors in animals, and these viruses have yielded a wealth of information about the mechanisms of oncogenesis.

During the past decade, we have witnessed extraordinary advances in understanding the mechanisms of oncogenesis, primarily through a synthesis of what were once separate cancer research disciplines. The application of the techniques of molecular biology in the field of tumor virology, cytogenetics, and cell biology led to the discovery of the transforming genes of tumor viruses, the genes activated at the breakpoints of nonrandom chromosomal translocations of lymphomas and leukemias, the correlation between growth factors or growth factor receptors and certain transforming genes, and the existence of transforming genes that are activated in vivo and in vitro by direct-acting chemical carcinogens.[2-4]

The transforming genes are collectively called *oncogenes*, and their study has elucidated the process of cellular transformation and may ultimately reveal the intricate processes by which cells communicate, grow, divide, and differentiate. Oncogene products are positive effectors of transformation. They superimpose their activity on the cell to elicit the transformed phenotype and can be considered positive regulators of growth. To the transformed cell, they represent a gain in function. Tumor suppressor gene products are negative growth regulators and their loss of function results in expression of a transformed phenotype.[5]

The preceding two chapters described the technologic advances that researchers are using to unravel the mysteries of genome order and gene regulation. They provide a useful introduction, because the genes and their products described in this chapter appear to regulate the biologic processes of cell division and differentiation.

In this chapter, we describe oncogenes and their normally functioning cellular counterparts, called *protooncogenes*. Protooncogenes are important regulators of biologic processes. The term protooncogene is misleading, because it wrongly implies that these genes latently reside in the genome for the sole purpose of expressing the neoplastic phenotype, although they are essential to the normal biologic processes, such as cell division. They are localized in different cell compartments (Fig. 3–1A), are expressed at different stages of the cell cycle, and appear to be involved in the cascade of events that maintain the ordered procession through the cell cycle (Fig. 3–1B).

The cell cycle is regulated by external mitogens (*e.g.*, growth factors, peptide and steroid hormones, lymphokines), which activate a process called signal transduction whereby specific signals are transmitted throughout the cell to the nucleus. The process is also mediated by nonintegral membrane-associated proteins belonging to the tyrosine kinase and *RAS* gene families (Fig. 3–1A). Signals generated by mitogenic stimulation can lead to the expression of specific genes coding for proteins localized to the nucleus (Fig. 3–1A). Certain members of the nuclear oncogene protein family have been shown to be transactivators of specific RNA transcripts.

IDENTIFICATION OF ONCOGENES AND TUMOR SUPPRESSOR GENES

A revolution is taking place in the field of cancer research. The primary avenues for studying neoplasia were made traditionally in animal tumor systems. Starting with the discovery of the Rous sarcoma virus in 1911 and continuing with the identification of transforming genes within retroviruses, the chicken, mouse, rat, and cat have dominated the research scene.[6] The current study of the genes involved in human tumors has gained important ground, because advances have been made in our understanding of heritable cancer-predisposing syndromes such as familial adenomatous pol-

yposis, retinoblastoma, Wilms' tumor, Von Recklinghausen's neurofibromatosis (VRNF), and the Li-Fraumeni syndrome. These findings have elucidated the mechanisms of oncogenesis and reinforced the validity of studying animal tumors, because certain genes altered in these syndromes were first discovered in an animal tumor system.[7]

Oncogenes have been discovered by the study of acutely transforming retroviruses and common sites of retroviral insertion, study of the transforming genes in DNA tumor viruses, DNA-mediated gene transfer in cell culture, identifying genes at translocation breakpoints in human tumors, and isolation of tumor suppressor genes by analyzing chromosomal deletions. One remarkable feature of this research is that identical or closely related genes have been identified as oncogenes by using different approaches and experimental systems.

RETROVIRUSES AND ONCOGENES

The first oncogenes were identified in studies of cancer-causing retroviruses. An important step in the retrovirus infection cycle is the stable yet random integration of the provirus into the host chromosome, which can alter expression of the region of the host chromosome into which it inserts; if the locus is a protooncogene, the provirus insertion can contribute significantly to tumorigenesis.[8-10] This insertional activation of protooncogenes occurs frequently in animal tumors, but has not yet been found to play a role in human tumors. The tumors are typically leukemias or lymphomas, and the viruses are named leukemia or leukosis viruses. The long latent period of disease caused by these retroviruses is partially the result of the low probability that proviruses will integrate into or adjacent to a host cellular protooncogene. Many novel oncogenes have been discovered on the basis of the knowledge that provirus insertion causes leukemias and lymphomas after long latent periods by inserting adjacent to protooncogene loci (Table 3–1).

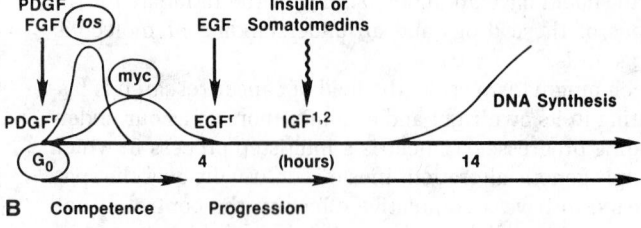

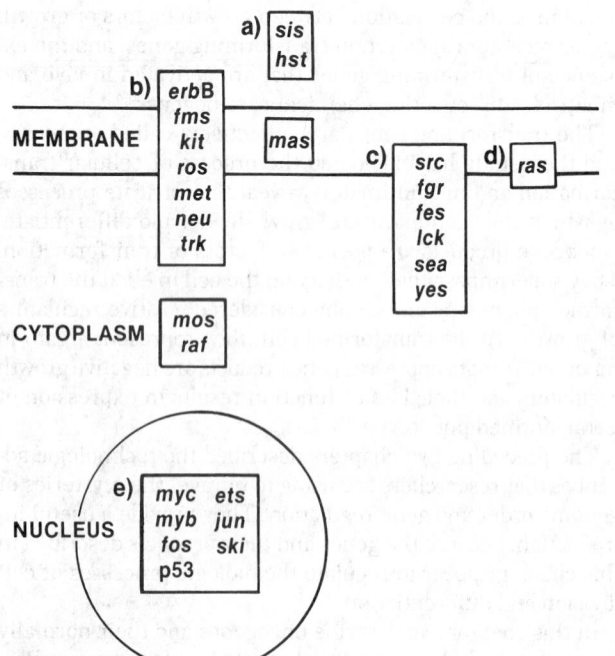

FIGURE 3–1. **(A)** Schematic presentation of the cellular compartments in which oncogene or protooncogene products are localized. The cell cycle is regulated by growth factors (external mitogenic signals), transmembrane tyrosine kinase growth factor receptor membranes, nonintegral membrane-associated proteins of the *SRC* gene family and *RAS* gene family, and oncogenes localized in the nucleus. **(B)** Stimulation of quiescent murine fibroblasts to enter the G_1 phase of growth by addition of platelet-derived growth factor (PDGF) or fibroblast growth factor (FGF). A transient increase in the expression of both C-*FOS* and C-*MYC* follows PDGF or FGF stimulation or treatment of cells with phorbol ester TPA plus a calcium ionophore. Cells rendered competent require epidermal growth factor and insulin-like growth factors to progress through DNA synthesis and the cell cycle.

TABLE 3–1. Oncogenes Source and Properties

RNA Tumor Virus	Oncogene	Alternative Method of Identification	Species of Origin	Source	Properties	Reference
Integral Membrane Tyrosine Kinases						
Susan McDonough feline sarcoma virus	v-*FMS*		Cat	Sarcoma	From CSF 1 receptor	206
Avian erythroblastosis virus	v-*ERBB*		Chicken	Sarcoma/ erythroblastosis	From EGF receptor	206
HZ4 feline sarcoma virus	v-*KIT*		Cat	Sarcoma		207
UR2 avian sarcoma virus	v-*ROS*		Chicken	Sarcoma		208
	NEU	DNA transfection	Rat	Neuroblastoma		26
	MET	DNA transfection	Human	MNNG-treated human osteosarcoma cell line	From HGF/SF receptor	27
	TRK	DNA transfection	Human	Colon carcinoma	From NGF receptor	28
Membrane-Associated Tyrosine Kinases						
Rous sarcoma virus	v-*SRC*		Chicken	Sarcoma		206
Yamaguchi-79 sarcoma virus	v-*YES*		Chicken	Sarcoma		206
Gardner-Rasheed feline sarcoma virus	v-*FGR*		Cat	Sarcoma		206
Fujinami sarcoma virus	v-*FPS*		Chicken	Sarcoma		206
Snyder-Theilen virus	v-*FES*		Cat	Sarcoma		206
Abelson murine leukemia virus	v-*ABL*		Mouse	Leukemia		206
Hardy Zuckerman 2 feline sarcoma virus	v-*ABL*		Cat	Sarcoma		206
Serine-Threonine Kinases						
Moloney murine sarcoma virus	v-*MOS*		Mouse	Sarcoma		206
3611 murine	*RAF*		Mouse	Sarcoma		206
Growth Factor Families						
Simian sarcoma virus	v-*SIS*		Woolly monkey	Glioma/ fibrosarcoma	B chain PDGF	206
	INT-2	Proviral insertion	Mouse	Mammary carcinoma	Member of FGF family	209
	KS3	DNA transfection	Human	Kaposi sarcoma	Member of FGF family	31
	HST	DNA transfection	Human	Stomach carcinoma	Member of FGF family	30
RAS Family						
Harvey murine sarcoma virus	v-H-*RAS*		Rat	Erythroleukemia	GTP binding/ GTPase	206
Kirsten murine sarcoma virus	v-K-*RAS*		Rat	Sarcoma	GTP binding/ GTPase	206
	N-*RAS*	DNA transfection	Human DNA	Various	GTP binding/ GTPase	213
Nuclear Protein Family						
Myelocytomatosis-29 virus	v-*MYC*		Chicken	Carcinoma myelocytomatosis	Binds DNA	206
	N-*MYC*	Gene amplification	Human	Neuroblastoma		44
	L-*MYC*	Gene amplification	Human	Small cell lung carcinoma		210

(continued)

TABLE 3–1. *(Continued)*

RNA Tumor Virus	Oncogene	Alternative Method of Identification	Species of Origin	Source	Properties	Reference
Avian myeloblastosis virus	v-*MYB*		Chicken	Myeloblastosis	Binds DNA	206
FBJ murine sarcoma	v-*FOS*		Mouse	Osteosarcoma	Binds DNA	206
Sloan-Kettering avian sarcoma virus	v-*SKI*		Chicken	Carcinoma		206
	v-*JUN*		Chicken		Binds DNA	211
	p53		Mouse/human	Expressed at high levels in transformed cells	Binds SV40 large T/and adenovirus E1B	77
Others						
Reticuloendotheliosis virus, strain T	v-*REL*		Turkey	Lymphatic leukemia		206
E26 avian leukemia virus	v-*ETS*		Chicken			206
Avian erythroblastosis virus	v-*ERBA*		Chicken	Erythroblastosis	Derived from steroid receptor for triiodothyronine	206
	MAS	DNA transfection	Human	Mammary carcinoma	Transmembrane protein	29
	INT1	Proviral insertion	Mouse	Mammary carcinoma		212

In contrast to the leukemia or leukosis retroviruses, acute transforming retroviruses can produce tumors in newborn animals in less than 2 weeks. The difference between the latent periods for disease caused by these two viral classes can be traced to differences in their genetic content. The acute transforming retroviruses possess nucleic acid sequences acquired (transduced) from the genetic information of the host cell, and these gene sequences are responsible for the rapid transforming activity. These host-derived genes are called viral oncogenes (v-*ONC*), and many have been identified in acute transforming retroviruses (Table 3–2).

The acute transforming retroviruses are laboratory curiosities, but identification of their v-*ONC* sequences and comparison with the protooncogenes from which they were derived have provided a unique source of genes with transforming potential and a fundamental knowledge of se-

TABLE 3–2. Cellular Genes Activated by Insertional Mutagenesis

Gene	Virus	Disease	Animal	Reference
c-*MYC*	ALV, CSF, REV	Bursal lymphoma	Chicken	9
	MLV	T-cell lymphoma	Mouse	213
	FeLV	T-cell lymphoma	Cat	213
c-*ERBB*	ALV	Erythroleukemia	Chicken	213
c-*MYB*	MLV	Lymphosarcoma	Mouse	213
c-H-*RAS*	MAV	Nephroblastoma	Chicken	213
c-*MOS*	IAP	Plasmacytoma (cell line)	Mouse	213
IL2	GaLV	T-cell lymphoma (cell line)	Ape	213
IL3	IAP	Myelomonocytic leukemia	Mouse	213
INT1	MMTV	Mammary carcinoma	Mouse	212
INT2	MMTV	Mammary carcinoma	Mouse	209
PIM1	M-MLV	T-cell lymphoma	Mouse	213
TCK (1SKT)	M-MLV	Thymoma (cell line)	Mouse	213
PVT (MIS1)	M-MLV	T- or B-cell lymphoma	Mouse/rat	213
MLVI1	M-MLV	T-cell lymphoma	Rat	213
MLVI2	M-MLV	T-cell lymphoma	Rat	213
MLVI3	M-MLV	T-cell lymphoma	Rat	213
EVI1	MCF-MLV	Myeloid lymphoma	Mouse	213
EVI2	MCF-MLV	Myeloid lymphoma	Mouse	213

quences necessary for their activation. Because acute transforming retroviruses are replicated like viruses, they are subject to a very high mutation rate. This, coupled with investigator-mediated selection for increased tumorigenic potential, can result in viruses with numerous changes in v-*ONC* sequences, compared with the protooncogene sequence, and mutations can be identified that increase tumorigenic potential. These mutations include multiple point mutations, deleted upstream or downstream exons, and changes in transcriptional and posttranscriptional regulatory elements. For example, deletion of a 3′ noncoding region sequence that normally inhibits c-*FOS* expression posttranscriptionally allows v-*FOS* to be produced at high levels.[11] Many v-*ONC* genes are expressed as fusion gene products with viral genes (*i.e.*, *GAG* and *ENV*) and at high levels under the constitutive control of the retroviral long terminal repeat.[2] The *GAG-* or *ENV-ONC* fusion products may contribute to transforming potential by misdirecting an oncogene product to an improper cellular location. Moreover, the target cell specificity of the retrovirus can result in the expression of the oncogene in an inappropriate cell type. For instance, *GAG* sequences are required for v-*ABL* transformation of lymphoid cells.[12] The v-*RAS* genes contain point mutations in the same position as in activated c-*RAS* genes in human tumors, and the v-*SRC* gene in the Rous sarcoma virus contains both point mutations and a carboxy-terminal deletion, which is essential for activating the *SRC* protooncogene.[13,14]

DNA TUMOR VIRUS TRANSFORMING GENES

The discovery that the middle T antigen of polyomavirus associates with pp60[src] and forms an active tyrosine kinase complex sets the stage for the extraordinary discoveries of the mechanisms by which other DNA tumor virus oncogenes cause cellular transformation. The viral oncogenes of adenovirus E1A and SV40 (T antigen) and human papillomaviruses (E6 and E7), although totally unrelated in structure, replication mechanisms, or target host cell, were all found to associate with the tumor suppressor gene products of RB1 and p53.

HUMAN ONCOGENES DETECTED BY DNA TRANSFECTION

DNA transfection, or gene transfer, analysis was first used to study and identify the transforming genes of RNA and DNA tumor viruses.[15,16] NIH/3T3 cells, which are maintained as a contact-inhibited nontumorigenic cell line, are frequently used for the assay. Transformation by transfection is monitored by morphologic changes.[17] Genomic DNA from mouse and human chemically induced or naturally occurring tumor cell lines give rise to foci or morphologically altered cells when transfected onto nontransformed mouse cell monolayers.[18] The transforming foreign DNA from the newly transformed mouse cells can be molecularly cloned.[19]

Many of the transfectable human transforming genes are related to the *RAS* family of oncogenes (Table 3–1). These oncogenes were first identified in acute transforming retroviruses of the Harvey and Kirsten sarcoma viruses and were designated c-H-*RAS* and c-K-*RAS*.[20,21] A *RAS* gene family member identified in a human neuroblastoma cell line and a

human promyelocytic leukemia cell line were designated N-*RAS* (Table 3–1).[22,23] Approximately 15% of human tumor cell lines and fresh tumor biopsies have activated *RAS* oncogenes as detected by this assay, and this number may be much higher in certain specific human tumors like colorectal cancers.[24,25]

Several novel transforming genes that are not members of the *RAS* gene family nor related to the viral oncogenes of the acute transforming retroviruses have been identified by DNA transfection assays. These include the *NEU*, *MET*, *TRK*, *MAS*, *HST*, and *KS3* oncogenes.[26–31] With the exception of the *MAS* oncogene, which appears to be a unique integral membrane protein, the other oncogenes are members of the tyrosine kinase growth factor receptor family (*NEU*, *MET*, or *TRK*) or the fibroblast growth factor (FGF) family (*HST*, *KS3*).

ONCOGENES IDENTIFIED BY CHROMOSOME ABNORMALITIES

Nonrandom chromosomal abnormalities have been invaluable for identifying genes involved in oncogenesis and for providing diagnostic clues for certain tumors. A curious and significant correlation exists between the type of chromosomal abnormality and the histopathologic type of tumor in which it is found, suggesting that certain lineages are susceptible to the transforming effects caused by deregulation of the particular gene at that translocation. Most of the abnormalities characterized are in hematologic malignancies, due to the relative ease with which these tumors can be grown in culture. Nonrandom abnormalities in chromosomes from solid tumors continue to be described and have already yielded important information.

Table 3–3 lists the translocations, inversions, and deletions for which the resident genes have been identified and cloned. Many of these involve T-cell receptor (TCR) or immunoglobulin (Ig) loci, which occur in T- and B-cell malignancies, respectively. Sequence analysis of the joint between these loci and the foreign loci reveal canonical heptamer-nonamer sequences. These are used by the recombinase system during somatic rearrangement of the TCR and Ig genes, indicating that the translocation most likely arose by a recombination error. By juxtaposing the protooncogene with the TCR or Ig loci, it becomes transcriptionally deregulated, structurally altered, or both. Such alterations are thought to be responsible for the oncogenic effects of these translocations.

One common feature in several of the genes that are deregulated by translocation in hematopoietic malignancies is that they encode proteins with significant homology to known transcriptional regulatory proteins (Table 3–3). For example, MYC, LYL1, and TAL-SCL proteins contain helix-loop-helix domains, which have been identified in a number of transcription factors.[32] This motif is thought to be involved in facilitating homo- or heterodimerization, which is required for high-affinity, site-specific binding to DNA. The t(15;17) translocation characteristic of acute promyelocytic leukemia results in the deregulated production of a chimeric protein containing much of the retinoic acid receptor α, which normally functions as a transcription factor in the presence of its ligand.[33,34] The deregulated expression of these factors may disrupt normal control of cellular events such as differentiation

TABLE 3–3. Chromosomal Genes Located at Translocation Breakpoints in Human Tumors

Tumor	Chromosomal Abnormality	Gene(s) Involved	Gene Features or Function	References
Chronic myelogenous leukemia	t(9;22)(q34;q11)	BCR-ABL, p210 gene product	Fusion gene involving nonreceptor tyrosine kinase (ABL)	36
T-cell acute lymphoblastic leukemia (T ALL)	t(9;22)(q34;q11)	BCR-ABL	p180 gene product	214
Follicular center cell lymphoma	t(14:18)(q32;q21)	BCL2 activation	Prevents apoptosis	214
Burkitt lymphoma	t(8:14)(q24;q32)	c-MYC IG locus	Transcription factor (?)	214
Acute promyelocytic leukemia	t(15;17)	APL-RARA fusion	Fusion gene involving the retinoic acid receptor X; deregulates gene expression	33, 34
T ALL	t(11,14)(p15;q11)	TCR locus, TTG1, rhombotin	Zinc finger gene, nuclear homology to CRIP	32
T ALL	t(7;19)(q34;p13)	LYL1 (βTCR)	Nuclear, helix-loop-helix	32
Pre-B ALL	t(1;19)(q23;p13.3)	E2A-PR1 fusion	Fusion gene containing homeobox from PRL	32
T ALL	t(1;14)(p32;q11)	SCL(tal;TCL5)	Helix-loop-helix gene	32
T ALL	del(1) p33	SCL/SIL (SCL interrupter locus)	SIL-SCL fusion gene	32
T ALL	t(10;14)	HOX11 or TCL3	Homeobox gene	32
T ALL	t(7;9)	TAN1	Homolog of Drosophila notch gene	215
B-cell lymphoma	t(11;14)(q13;132)	PRAD1, BCL1	Cyclin D	216
Amplifications in breast and squamous cell carcinomas	inv(11)	G₁ cyclin gene		218
Parathyroid adenoma	inv(11)	PRAD1	Cyclin D	217

or cell division, presumably through the altered expression of subordinate genes.

At least 95% of patients with chronic myelocytic leukemia (CML) possess a typical Philadelphia chromosome resulting from the q34;q11 translocation between chromosomes 9 and 22. In this translocation, the c-*ABL* protooncogene (Tables 3–1 and 3–3) is translocated from chromosome 9 band q34 to chromosome 22 band q11. The breakpoints that occur in chromosome 22q11 are clustered within a 5-kilobase (kb) genomic region, and this region has been referred to as the breakpoint cluster region (*BCR*). In contrast, the breakpoints in the c-*ABL* locus on chromosome 9q34 differ considerably from patient to patient, with estimated differences of greater than 100 kb. Despite this, a transcription unit in the *BCR* locus provides the promoter and 5′ end sequences that result in a fused 8.5-kb *BCR-ABL*-encoded hybrid mRNA encoding a novel fusion protein of 210 kilodaltons (kd).[35,36] In this disease, DNA rearrangements in the *BCR* locus, the expression of the novel 8.5-kb *BCR-ABL*-encoded mRNA, and the detection of the novel 210-kd BCR-ABL protein are all diagnostic for Philadelphia-positive (Ph¹) CML.[37] A second type of Philadelphia chromosome is seen in a small percentage of patients with CML and most Ph¹-positive acute lymphocytic leukemia (ALL). This involves the intron region of *BCR*, rather than the main breakpoint cluster region. This variant Ph¹ confers a worse prognosis and, at the molecular level, results in a 7.0-kb fusion mRNA that encodes a p185$^{bcr-abl}$ chimeric protein.

It is not understood how this rearrangement contributes to CML, but after the p210$^{bcr-abl}$ gene is reintroduced into the bone marrow cells of mice, the mice develop a CML-like disease.[38] Transgenic mice made with the p185$^{bcr-abl}$ gene succumb to acute myeloid or lymphoid leukemias.[39] The normal c-*ABL* product is a member of the tyrosine kinase family and may be involved in signal transduction. To attain transforming ability, the *ABL* tyrosine kinase must be activated, and it appears that *BCR*-encoded sequences in the chimeric protein are essential for this activation.[40] This is most likely achieved by direct physical binding of kinase regulatory domain of ABL (an SH2 domain) to an SH2-binding region in BCR.[41]

Several cellular oncogenes are amplified in human tumors (Table 3–4). The c-*MYC* protooncogene locus is amplified in a promyelocytic leukemia both in the primary tumor and in the cell line HL-60, which was derived from the tumor.[42,43] Other oncogenes like c-*ERBB* (*EGFR*), *NEU* (*HER-2*), and c-*MYC* family members are amplified in specific tumor types (Table 3–4), and multiple copies of these genes have been associated with poor prognosis. Multiple copies of N-*MYC* (first identified as an amplified gene in human neuroblastoma) have been correlated with advanced stages of the disease.[44] The amplification of *MYC* family members in small cell lung carcinoma is also associated with a more malignant progression of the disease.[45] The *MYC* family members appear to be associated with the progression of neuroblastomas and small cell lung carcinomas, and the c-*ERBB* or *EGFR* gene has been found amplified in glioblastomas and squamous carcinomas.

Chromosomal abnormalities also involve deletions of various lengths in portions of chromosomes in different patients, but analysis of the chromosomes often reveals common de-

TABLE 3–4. Cellular Oncogenes Amplified in Human Tumors

Tumor	Oncogene	Amplification
Small cell lung cancers	c-*MYC*	up to 80×
	N-*MYC*	up to 50×
	L-*MYC*	up to 20×
Neuroblastomas	N-*MYC*	up to 250×
Glioblastomas	c-*ERBB* (EGFR)	up to 50×
Mammary carcinoma	c-*ERBB2* (HER2)	up to 30×

(Park M, Vande Woude GF. Principles of molecular cell biology of cancer: Oncogenes. In: DeVita VT Jr, Hellman S, Rosenberg SA, eds. Cancer: Principles and practice of oncology. 3rd ed. Philadelphia: JB Lippincott, 1989)

leted regions. The loss of DNA from certain regions of chromosomes, thought to unmask recessive mutations in the remaining allele and often referred to as recessive oncogenes or tumor suppressor genes, has been associated with several tumors, especially childhood tumors such as retinoblastoma and Wilms tumor.[46–48] Patients with retinoblastoma have deletions in chromosome 13 band q14, and patients with Wilms tumor have deletions in chromosome 11 band p13 and p15.[47,49] The genes located within these regions that are implicated in oncogenesis have been molecularly cloned.

TUMOR SUPPRESSOR GENES OR RECESSIVE ONCOGENES

In 1970, DeMars postulated that cancer-prone persons are heterozygous for the cancer-predisposing gene and that cancer develops due to a somatic mutation at the remaining normal allele.[50] Knudson developed a mathematical model based on his observations of the incidence and age of onset of unilateral and bilateral cases of familial retinoblastoma.[46] This model predicted that one additional mutation was the rate-limiting step in the development of tumors in familial cases, such as the loss of heterozygosity, but two events were needed in nonfamilial cases. This hypothesis fit with the high incidence of bilateral tumors in familial cases and the earlier age of onset in familial cases than in nonfamilial cases.

The list of the heritable types of cancer in which Knudson's model of mutation applies continues to grow.[51] Several types of tumors contain chromosome deletions or loss of heterozygosity, which strongly suggests that the tumors arise, at least in part, after the loss of a tumor suppressor gene (Table 3–5). These tumors include retinoblastoma, Wilms' tumor, VRNF, familial adenomatous polyposis, and Li-Fraumeni syndrome. Nonfamilial cancers also arise through this mechanism, but both alleles must be mutated or lost, one allele is mutated and the other is lost, or mutation of one allele can act as a dominant-negative mutation to incapacitate the function of the normal allele.[5,51]

TABLE 3–5. Allele Losses in Human Tumors Defined by DNA Studies

Tumor Predisposition	Site of Allele Loss	Corresponding Loci*
Retinoblastoma	13q	13q D, L
Osteosarcoma	13q	
Wilms	11p	?11p D (not yet confirmed by linkage)
Rhabdomyosarcoma	11p	
Hepatoblastoma	11p	
Hepatocellular carcinoma	11p	
Bladder	11p	
Renal carcinoma	3p	Family with t(3,8) Von Hippel-Lindau 3p L
Lung, small-cell	3p,13q,17p	
Lung, other types	3p (13q,17p, less frequent)	
Breast	11p,13q	
Stomach	13q	
Colon	5q,17p,18q,22, others	Polyposis 5q D, L
Insulinoma	11	MEN 1 11qL
Pheochromocytoma	1p,22	MEN2 10L NF-1 17L
Medullary thyroid carcinoma	1p	MEN-2 10L
Meningioma	22	NF-2 22L
Acoustic neuroma	22	
Melanoma	Various	

* D, chromosomal deletion; L, chromosomal loss.
(Ponder B. Gene losses in human tumours. Nature 1988;335:400)

RETINOBLASTOMA

Retinoblastoma accounts for 1% of all cancer deaths among children and is the most common malignant eye tumor. It can be multifocal and bilateral, and 40% of the cases are familial.

The model of gene loss as the basis for the genesis of retinoblastoma gained support from cytogenetic studies. Karyotypic analysis of tumor tissue and nontumor tissue revealed deletions in the region of chromosome 13q14, lending support to the loss-of-function mutation theory.[49] Unambiguous support came with the demonstration that DNA probes to the chromosome 13q14 failed to detect this DNA in tumors, but nontumor DNA from the same patient exhibited the expected two somatic cell copies.[48] These investigations further showed that there was reduction to homozygosity (or loss of heterozygosity) in the tumor DNA for genes in the vicinity of chromosome 13q14, due to nondisjunction, mitotic recombination, or gene conversion. Cavenee and coworkers later showed that it was the normal allele that was lost in somatic tissue during tumor development, consistent with the loss of a tumor suppressor gene.[52]

Cloning of the RB Gene

Equipped with DNA probes for the region of chromosome 13 and RNA extracted from retinoblastomas, Friend, Dryja, and coworkers were able to isolate the gene that confers susceptibility to retinoblastoma.[53] The gene (*RB1*) encodes a 928-residue protein designated p105-RB, reflecting its apparent molecular weight. By RNA analysis, the gene was found to be expressed in most tissues, which was surprising, because in familial retinoblastoma only two types of tumors develop: retinoblastomas and, after long latent periods, osteosarcomas.[54] One possibility is that p105-RB performs different functions in different tissues, or perhaps due to compensatory mechanisms, some tissues are resistant to the effects of *RB1* mutation. Critical to the recessive oncogene theory was the demonstration that by reintroducing a normal *RB1* gene into tumor cells, it was possible to restore a nontransformed phenotype, a finding that may ultimately have implications for cancer treatment.[55]

Other human tumors display mutations in *RB1* (Table 3–6): osteosarcomas, a high percentage of small cell lung carcinomas, soft tissue sarcomas, a small proportion of breast carcinomas, and genitourinary carcinomas.[53,56–63]

TABLE 3–6.   Tumors With Alterations at *RB1*

Tumor Type	References
Osteosarcoma	53
Small cell lung carcinomas	56
	57
Soft tissue sarcomas	58
	59
Breast carcinomas	60
	61
Genitourinary carcinomas	62
	57
	63

The RB1 Gene Product p105-RB: A Nuclear Phosphoprotein Involved in Cell Cycle Regulation

The nuclear protein p105-RB is found in phosphorylated and unphosphorylated forms.[60] In resting primary human peripheral blood lymphocytes, only underphosphorylated forms of p105-RB are present. Stimulation with mitogens leads to the appearance of phosphorylated p105-RB and to DNA synthesis.[64] Similarly, phosphorylation of p105-RB is highest at the start of S phase, and lowest after mitosis and entry into G_1.[65] When cells in culture are induced to differentiate, p105-RB becomes hypophosphorylated, suggesting that only the hypophosphorylated form can suppress cell proliferation.[64,65]

A dramatic breakthrough in the understanding of p105-RB function was obtained by Harlow and coworkers, who were studying the cellular proteins that interact with the adenovirus E1A oncoprotein. The viral oncoprotein contains a conserved region called transforming domain 2 (residues 121–139), which is essential for E1A transforming ability. Likewise, the large T antigen of SV40 contains a short domain (residues 105–114), also required for transformation, that bears structural homology to domain 2 of E1A. These domains act as binding sites for cellular proteins that play a role in E1A- or large T antigen-mediated transformation.[66] Harlow and coworkers, studying proteins that interact with transforming domain 2 of E1A, identified one as p105-RB.[67] Similar studies were then performed with SV40 large T antigen and subsequently with the human papillomavirus E7 oncoprotein.[65,68] All of these viral oncoproteins bind to the same region of p105-RB with high affinity. Although binding to p105-RB is linked to their transforming ability, it is likely that adenovirus and SV40, which normally do not participate in cell transformation, capture control of the cell cycle by binding to p105-RB to facilitate viral replication.[69]

SV40 T antigen binds preferentially to p105-RB in its unphosphorylated form, which indicated that the phosphorylated form of p105-RB is the inactive form, and only in the unphosphorylated form can p105-RB exert its growth suppressing effects.[70] By complexing with unphosphorylated p105-RB, the viral oncoproteins inactivate p105-RB and prevent it from interacting with its cellular targets and suppressing growth. The net effect is the same as that observed with the inactivating mutations found in tumors that bear point mutations that prevent phosphorylation.[71] With no active form of p105-RB, the cell proceeds uncontrolled through the cell cycle. The most likely point at which p105-RB exerts its effect is the G_1 to S transition, although in most cell lineages, it probably does not act alone in controlling this transition. In certain cell lineages, p105RB may act alone, which would explain the restricted appearance of familial tumors. In the absence of viral oncoproteins, p105-RB activity is regulated by phosphorylation and dephosphorylation, which implies that certain cellular kinases and phosphatases play key roles in cell cycle regulation. The growth inhibitor transforming growth factor-β (TGF-β) blocks the phosphorylation of p105-RB and may keep it in its active, growth-suppressing form.[72]

What are the normal cellular targets that bind to p105-RB? Studies on the p105-RB structure-function relations have found that a large central "pocket" exists on the protein, to which the three aforementioned viral oncoproteins bind, and it is a region for the growth-suppressing activity of p105-RB.

With this pocket serving as a ligand, seven different cellular proteins that bind it were identified.[73] One of these proteins is a cellular transcription factor, E2F, which was first identified because of its role in the regulation of the adenovirus E2 promoter. E2F binds to the hypophosphorylated form of p105-RB and is released by phosphorylation.[74] Similarly, it is postulated that E1A, large T antigen, or phosphorylation of p105-RB cause the release of the transcription factor.[74] Release of E2F from p105-RB by either mechanism would allow it to become active. E2F binds in a sequence-specific manner to DNA to promote RNA transcription, and in addition to regulating adenovirus E2 transcription, it probably regulates a number of cellular genes involved in cell cycle regulation. By binding E2F, the hypophosphorylated form of p105-RB may retard or prevent movement into S phase.

In addition to E2F regulation, p105-RB may also block serum stimulation of c-*FOS* expression and abrogate a key cellular response to this growth stimulus.[75] The repression of c-*MYC* transcription by TGF-β appears to be mediated by p105-RB, which suggests that p105-RB may be an important mediator of TGF-β-induced growth suppression.[76] The identification of *RB* and the characterization of its function are important advances in our understanding of the mechanism of oncogenesis.

TUMOR SUPPRESSION AND P53

First identified as a tumor antigen in SV40-transformed cells and later as a cellular protein involved in SV40 transformation, p53 has emerged in recent years as a central player in many human tumors. Alterations at the p53 locus on chromosome 17p have been found in a large percentage and wide variety of human tumors and are the most common alterations in human cancers (Table 3–5).[77,78] Indeed, 75% to 80% of colon tumors show abnormalities at both p53 alleles: one allele is often deleted, and the other has point mutations, which are usually missense mutations that yield an altered protein product. Analysis of mutations in p53 may provide a powerful marker of prognosis and may emerge as part of a routine patient workup.

In SV40-transformed cells, p53 was found to form a tight complex with the SV40-encoded large T antigen. This suggested a possible role for p53 in transformation, and evidence that has mounted over the ensuing years supports this notion.

The p53 gene was shown to cooperate with activated p21[ras] to transform primary rat embryo fibroblasts, acting in the same group as c-*MYC* or E1A in this assay, and to rescue cells from senescence (Table 3–7). It was later realized that the "normal" gene used in these experiments bore a point mutation that rendered it oncogenic; the normal allele does not transform cells, but it can, as a tumor suppressor gene, reverse the transformed phenotype of tumor cells and is thus similar to *RB*.[79,80] Persons with the cancer-predisposing Li-Fraumeni syndrome are born with mutations in one allele of the p53 gene and develop tumors that bear mutations at both alleles, as predicted by Knudson's hypothesis.[81]

In the absence of normal p53, the mutant allele, depending on the mutation, can act to alter cell growth. In other tumors, both alleles are deleted, and there is no p53.[82] The lack of a normal p53 allele in naturally occurring tumors argues that p53 functions as a true tumor suppressor gene to control cell growth and division. However, malignant transformation can also occur when certain mutants of p53 are expressed in a cell containing at least one normal p53 allele. These mutations, referred to as dominant negative, probably act by binding to and inhibiting the function of the normal p53 protein in the cell, which is analogous to the role that SV40 T antigen plays in altering p53. These dominant negative mutations are quite similar to having alterations at both alleles.

The point mutations found in the p53 gene are highly clustered (Fig. 3–2), probably indicating features of the protein that contribute to its transforming activity.[77] Most alterations occur in one of three amino acids: 175, 248, and 273. Other mutations are clustered within four short regions. Certain mutations are more common in certain tumor types, which may reflect the types of mutagens that different organs are exposed to or may indicate that different cell types are sensitive only to certain p53 mutations.[78] The different mutations can be expected to have different effects on the protein's structure and function. For instance, mutations at amino acid 175 are more efficient than those at 273 in cooperation with *RAS*. Patients with Li-Fraumeni syndrome have mutations only in one p53 allele in amino acids 245 to 258. These mutations are predictably not dominant, and in the heterozygous state, the carriers of this mutant allele are normal. Mice with p53 germline deletion develop normally but display a high tumor incidence that occurs months earlier in the homozygous state than in the heterozygous state.[83] As more is learned about the

TABLE 3–7. Oncogene Complementation Groups in Rat Embryo Fibroblast Transformation Assay

Group I Rescue From Senescence (S Phase)	Group II Morphologic Transformation (M Phase)
E1A	E1B
SV40 large T	Polyoma middle T
Polyoma large T	H-*RAS*
c-*MYC*	K-*RAS*
N-*MYC*	N-*RAS*
p53	

(Hunter T. Cooperation between oncogenes. Cell 1991;64:249)

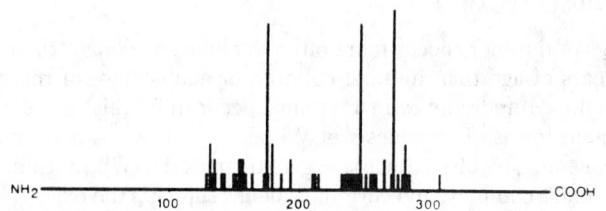

FIGURE 3–2. The human p53 gene with the distribution of p53 mutations. The 393 codons of the human p53 gene are represented by a horizontal bar. The percentage of mutations that occur at each codon of the p53 gene are represented by the vertical bar. Data obtained from a sequence of 94 different primary tumors, xenografts, or cell lines derived from tumors (*e.g.*, brain, breast, colon, esophageal, lung, neurofibrosarcomas, osteosarcomas, rhabdomyosarcomas, T-cell lymphomas).

different domains of p53 and what roles they play, the significance of this mutational clustering will undoubtedly become clear.

Although certain genetic mutations cause p53 protein to accumulate in the cytoplasm, the protein is usually localized to the nucleus, is phosphorylated, and may exist in large oligomeric forms.[77,84] The amino acid sequence of p53 does not appear to have any recognizable motifs, but it does contain an acidic, proline-rich amino-terminal domain, hydrophobic internal segments, and basic portions at the carboxy-terminus. Cotransfection studies have shown that certain mutant forms cooperate with *RAS*, and the normal gene can suppress transformation by *RAS, MYC*, or the adenovirus E1A gene, suggesting that normal p53 is dominant and can downregulate the product of these oncogenes.[85,86] The protein product of p53 has been implicated in two different, but perhaps compatible, nuclear processes: DNA replication and RNA transcription. It has been shown to bind DNA in a nonspecific and a specific manner, but mutant p53 proteins fail to bind or bind abnormally.[87,88] One site that p53 appears to bind is adjacent to the origin of replication of SV40, and wild-type, but not mutant, p53 proteins can block SV40 T antigen replication functions.[89] The protein product of p53 may interfere with the virus life cycle, necessitating its inactivation by a viable virus. It is conceivable that p53 may bind to cellular origins to block replication, but its mode of action is unknown. It has been suggested that p53 may be a regulator of RNA transcription. Regions of the p53 protein, when linked to a sequence-specific DNA-binding protein, can activate transcription from promoters that contain binding sites for the chimeric protein.

Unlike *RB*, it is not clear how or where p53 regulates cell growth and cell cycling. By introducing a normal p53 gene, it is possible to severely lengthen cell doubling time or stop growth of transformed cells that lack a normal p53 gene.[90] When a temperature-sensitive mutant of p53 is used, growth arrest and apoptosis can be induced by shifting to the temperature permissive for wild-type p53 function.[91] With this shift, the p53 localizes to the nucleus and has a shortened half-life.[92] Inactivation of normal p53 can also occur through the action of several virally encoded proteins, including SV40 T antigen, adenovirus E1B, and oncogenic human papillomavirus E6 protein.[93–95] The ability of these proteins to inactivate p53 has evolved to ensure that the host cells undergo uncontrolled division, which would allow efficient viral replication.

WILMS' TUMOR

Several tumors occur more often in children younger than 5 years of age than in older children or adults. Two of these, Wilms' tumor and retinoblastoma, occur in familial and sporadic forms. The genesis of Wilms' tumor, as with retinoblastoma, involves the loss of genetic material. Wilms' tumor is more complex, and current evidence supports the existence of three distinct loci for Wilms' tumor: two on 11p and one not yet localized.

Interesting associations have been noticed between the occurrence of Wilms' tumor and certain congenital anomalies. Aniridia and urogenital anomalies are found in 2% of patients with Wilms' tumor, and a certain percentage are associated with mental retardation. Associations also exist between Wilms' tumor and gonadoblastoma and ambiguous genitalia, hence the eponym WAGR (*W*ilms', *a*niridia, *g*enitourinary anomalies [or *g*onadoblastoma or ambiguous *g*enitalia], and *r*etardation) syndrome.[96,97] The WAGR syndrome is associated with deletions involving 11p13, a finding that provided the first hint of the location of the Wilms'' tumor locus.[97] The gene for aniridia is clearly distinct from the Wilms' tumor locus, because two families with aniridia were found to have a translocation at 11p13, yet did not suffer from Wilms' tumor.[98] However, the loci for genitourinary anomalies and Wilms' tumor are more closely linked.[47] By DNA hybridization studies, loss of heterozygosity was found for markers on 11p, and in 15% to 20% of tumors, this appears to involve band 13. These tumors include sporadic and familial cases of Wilms' tumor.[47]

Beckwith-Wiedemann syndrome (*i.e.*, exophthalmos, macroglossia, and gigantism) is associated with several embryonal cancers (*i.e.*, Wilms' tumor, hepatoblastoma, adrenocortical carcinoma, and rhabdomyosarcoma) and often involves deletions in chromosome band 11p15 instead of 11p13.[99] DNA from these tumors shows loss of heterozygosity for markers on 11p, and linkage analyses of families with this syndrome place the locus at band p15.[100,101] Hemihypertrophy is yet another syndrome that has been associated with an increased incidence of Wilms' tumor.[102] The similarities between Beckwith-Wiedemann syndrome and the organomegaly found in gestational diabetes led to the consideration that overexpression of IGF II, which maps to 11p15, may play an etiologic role.[103] Although this is supported by certain findings, it is unlikely that overexpression of IGF II plays a role in Wilms' tumors, because there is no evidence that the IGF II gene is specifically mutated in Wilms' tumors, and genetic analysis implicates gene loss rather than overexpression in Wilms' tumor.[47]

Comparison of diseases associated with 11p13 or 11p15 indicate that they represent loci with some similar and some different effects on tumorigenesis. The histopathology of Wilms' tumor associated with 11p13 is different from that associated with 11p15.[104] The syndromes with which the two are associated are distinct: 11p13 with genitourinary anomalies and 11p15 with Beckwith-Wiedemann syndrome. Although both loci are associated with Wilms' tumor, the 11p15 locus is also associated with adrenocortical carcinomas and hepatoblastomas.

Familial cases of Wilms' tumor are rare and are typically not associated with the 11p13 locus, although one case has been clearly linked to mutations at 11p13.[105] Analysis of three large Wilms' tumor pedigrees failed to find linkage to either of the 11p loci, indicating the existence of a third locus, which remains unmapped in the human genome.

A candidate gene (*WT1*) for the Wilms' tumor locus on 11p13 was cloned and found to encode a zinc finger protein.[106,107] Mutations in this gene appear to be responsible for at least some cases of sporadic and familial Wilms' tumor.[105,108] In one sporadic tumor, a 25-bp deletion is present in *WT1* that deletes one of the four zinc fingers, and the other *WT1* allele is apparently normal.[108] Thus, the mutant protein may have a dominant-negative effect. Alternatively, if the normal allele is subject to abnormal feedback inhibition by the mutant protein or is silenced by imprinting, a significant gene-dosage effect may be at play. The *WT1* alterations have been associated with two pedigrees of familial Wilms' tumor, and in both cases, there were associated genital defects (*e.g.*, hypospadias and cryptorchidism). In both cases, patients carried one normal and one mutant allele in the germline, but only the mutant allele (encoding a truncated protein product) was detected in the tumor DNA.

The presence of four zinc finger motifs in the *WT1* gene product suggests that it is a sequence-specific DNA-binding protein involved in the regulation of RNA transcription. A high-affinity binding site for the protein has been identified and bears similarity to the binding site for another zinc finger protein, EGR-1 (named for early growth response).[109] EGR-1 is induced by a number of mitogenic stimuli and positively regulates a number of target genes involved in differentiation and cell growth.[110] The *WT1* gene product can act to repress EGR-1-mediated gene transcription, and in vivo, *WT1* may slow cell proliferation so that cell differentiation may occur.[111] Mutation or deletion of the *WT1* coding region could prevent tissue-specific differentiation pathways from proceeding normally.

An important corollary to the supposition that Wilms' tumor occurs by the loss of a tumor suppressor gene is that by replacing the normal allele, it is possible to reverse the transformed phenotype of Wilms' tumor cells. Weissman and coworkers[112] showed that the tumor phenotype of cells from a Wilms' tumor can be partially suppressed by transfer of chromosome 11, and additional work has localized this region to genetic material from 11p15, rather than 11p13.[113] Although attempts to reverse the transformed phenotype by introducing a normal *WT1* gene have been unsuccessful, this may be due to the unavailability of a Wilms' tumor cell line that bears a mutation at *WT1* rather than at the other implicated loci.

Although much has been learned about the cause of Wilms' tumor, two of the three (or more) Wilms' tumor loci have yet to be cloned, leaving much of the story to be told.

VON RECKLINGHAUSEN'S NEUROFIBROMATOSIS

Of the several forms of neurofibromatosis, VRNF is the most common, occurring with a frequency of 1 in 3000. Fifty percent of the cases represent new mutations, making *VRNF* the most commonly mutated allele that has been followed in the general population. Although the expressivity of the disease varies in familial cases, the penetrance is 100%, and it is transmitted as an autosomal dominant trait that maps to human chromosome 17q. Myriad lesions may present in VRNF, the most common of which are the subcutaneous neurofibromas that are composed of proliferating neurites, Schwann cells, and fibroblasts. In 3% of patients, these tumors undergo malignant transformation. Other features of the disease include café au lait spots; pigmented iris hamartomas (Lisch's nodules); a propensity to develop other tumors, such as meningiomas, optic gliomas, pheochromocytomas, Wilms' tumor, rhabdomyosarcoma, or acute nonlymphocytic leukemia; and bone lesions, such as erosive defects, scoliosis, intraosseous cystic lesions, subperiosteal bone cysts, and pseudarthrosis of the tibia.

Genetic linkage analysis led to the mapping of the gene for VRNF to chromosome 17 in the region of 17q11 to 17q22, and further localization was provided by a translocation in-

volving 17q11.2.[114,115] Two separate cloning efforts led to the identification of a candidate *NF1* gene.[7,116] One approach took advantage of two VRNF alleles that contained translocation involving chromosome 17 with breakpoints 60 kb apart. Molecular access to the region was provided by a DNA probe, called *EVI2A*, that mapped between the two translocation breakpoints. *EVI2A* (for ecotropic viral integration site-2) was identified as a common site of retroviral insertion in virally induced myeloid leukemias that arose in the inbred mouse strain, BXH-2.[117] Starting from *EVI2A*, two adjacent genes were identified, called *EVI2B* and *OMGP*, but extensive analysis of these three genes failed to uncover any mutations in VRNF patients. However, further chromosome walking and cloning led to the isolation of *NF1*, a much larger gene (270–390 kb) that is transcribed in the opposite orientation relative to *EVI2A*, *EVI2B*, and *OMGP*, and whose exons flank the three smaller genes (Fig. 3–3).[7] *NF1* is transcribed to an 11- to 13-kb mRNA, which is translated to a 250- to 280-kd protein.

Through several techniques, mutations have been found so far in 10% of VRNF patients; the large size of the gene may underlie the difficulties of finding mutations in all cases. These mutations include translocations, deletions, an *Alu* sequence insertion into an intron, and several point mutations.[118] These studies leave little doubt that *NF1* is the gene for VRNF, although several puzzles remain. It is unclear whether both alleles must be lost or mutated for tumorigenesis. Certain aspects of the VRNF phenotype, such as the benign neurofibromas, may require loss of only one allele, but the development of neurofibrosarcomas may require mutations at both alleles.

Analysis of the coding region for NF1 has revealed significant homology to the catalytic domains of the mammalian GAP (*RAS* p21 GTPase-activating protein) and the yeast IRA1 and IRA2 (inhibitory regulators of the *RAS*-cAMP pathway genes).[119,120] The homology to IRA1 and IRA2 extends well beyond the catalytic domain, suggesting that NF1 may function more like IRA1 and IRA2 than GAP. GAP catalyzes the conversion of active GTP-containing *RAS* p21 to the inactive GDP-bound form and has been considered to be an important regulator or effector of *RAS* p21 function.[121–124] Transforming mutants of *RAS* p21 are resistant to the GTPase-activating effect of GAP. Overexpression of GAP in NIH/3T3 cells can suppress transformation by normal *RAS*, but not by activated *RAS*. It was of great interest to determine whether NF1 could play a similar role in regulating the GTP/GDP status of p21^{ras} and the activity of p21^{ras} in transformation. It appears that this is indeed the case. A fragment of the NF1 that contains the region with homology to the GAP and IRA1 catalytic domain can stimulate the GTPase activity of *RAS* p21 and can complement *IRA* mutants in yeast.[125,126] The *NF1* gene product may play an important role in the regulation of *RAS* p21 or *RAS* p21-related proteins, and the alterations of *NF1* in VRNF may play an important role in deregulating this pathway.

Two models are proposed to explain NF1 involvement in the *RAS* pathway and in tumorigenesis. One possibility is that it inhibits *RAS* function by maintaining p21^{ras} in the GDP-bound form. Loss of both *NF1* alleles in neurofibromas would allow GTP-bound p21^{ras} levels to increase, stimulating the *RAS* pathway. Alternatively, *NF1* encodes an effector of differentiation for neuronal cells and acts downstream of p21^{ras}. Knocking out both alleles would disrupt proper differentiation.

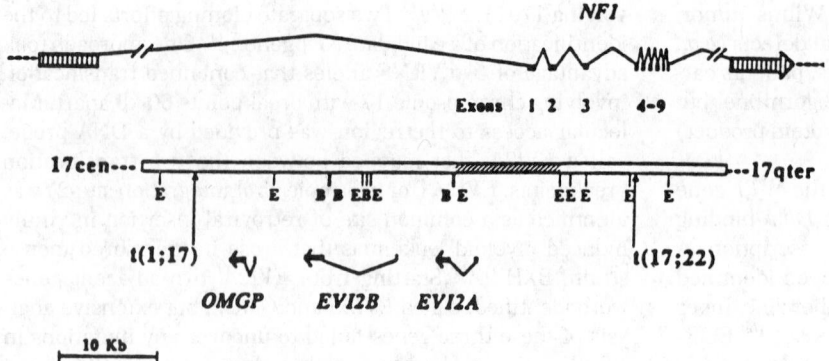

FIGURE 3–3. Partial genomic structure of *NF1*. The *NF1* gene (*above map*) spans two translocation breaks, t(1;17) and t(17;22), in an orientation opposite from three other genes in this region (*below map*). Solid bars in the top line represent the nine *NF1* exons already identified, and the striped boxes represent the regions of the *NF1* gene where intron-exon boundaries are still unknown. Arrowheads indicate the orientation of transcription. (Adapted from Viskochil D, Buchberg AM, Xu G, et al. Deletions and a translocation interrupt a cloned gene at the neurofibromatosis type 1 locus. Cell 1990;62:187)

The *NF1* gene is expressed in many normal tissues. It is unclear why only particular cell types are susceptible to the effects of its mutation, but it may be that certain tissue-specific pathways that involve NF1 are more sensitive to *NF1* mutations than other pathways.

The progression to malignant neurofibrosarcomas occurs in 3% of patients with VRNF, a frequency that suggests that VRNF patients are predisposed to the development of malignancy compared with the general population and that additional mutations are required for the development of malignant tumors. Analysis of DNA from neurofibrosarcomas has revealed deletions on 17p that often involves the locus for p53, which is located on 17p.[127]

FAMILIAL ADENOMATOUS POLYPOSIS

Familial adenomatous polyposis (FAP) is an autosomal dominant condition in which patients develop innumerable neoplastic polyps that carpet the entire colon. The onset is usually in the second or third decade, and 100% of the patients eventually develop colorectal carcinoma. Gardner's syndrome is a related disorder, which consists of polyposis coli, osteomas, and desmoid tumors. FAP and Gardner's syndrome are probably caused by the same gene, with differences created by other loci or environmental effects. Both genes are linked to the same region of 5q21.[128]

Localization of FAP to 5q was first established by Herrera and coworkers.[129] Linkage analysis confirmed this mapping.[128] Vogelstein and colleagues[130] reported that sporadic (nonfamilial) cases are also linked to 5q. Nakamura and associates[128] and Kinzler and coworkers[131] isolated cosmid clones of human DNA from this region that flanked the gene for FAP. Two mammoth DNA cloning efforts then led to the identification and molecular cloning of the responsible gene at the FAP locus.[131,132] A number of genes were identified in this region: *FER, APC, TB2,* and *MCC.* The *FER* gene mapped very close to where the FAP locus was expected to be and exhibited homology to tyrosine kinase oncogenes. Probes for these genes were used to analyze FAP tumor DNA and RNA for alterations. RNA from tumors derived from two FAP patients was analyzed for changes in the *FER* gene, without success, making it unlikely that this was the FAP gene. The *APC, TB2,* and *MCC* genes were all clustered within 200 kb and located at the center of a region that was shown to have allelic deletions in sporadic tumors.

Initial studies with *MCC* revealed the disruption of the gene in one tumor and somatically acquired point mutations in six other sporadic colorectal tumors.[133] None of these mutations was a "silent" mutation, but all resulted in nonconservative amino acid changes. These data suggested that *MCC* (*i.e.,* mutated in colorectal carcinoma) was the FAP gene. However, extensive analysis of the *MCC* gene in affected individuals from 90 FAP kindreds failed to reveal any germline mutations.

The *APC* gene appeared promising, because an 800-bp insertion into the gene was found in 1 of 200 sporadic tumors analyzed. Alterations were detected in *APC* DNA from 5 of 103 kindreds susceptible to FAP or Gardner's syndrome. These included missense mutations and nonsense mutations, which, in the case of the latter, cosegregated perfectly with the disease in one family. Four additional mutations of *APC* have been reported.[132] Analysis of sporadic tumors uncovered four somatically acquired mutations (two nonsense mutations, one frame-shift insertion, and a splice donor mutation), suggesting that alterations at *APC* are responsible for both FAP and Gardner's syndrome. Among 10 of the sporadic tumors, 8 exhibited a normal *APC* allele, and the other two exhibited allelic deletions of chromosome 5q. These data suggest dominant-negative or gene-dosage effects. The natural history of colorectal disease in patients with FAP and Gardner's syndrome suggests that both alleles need not be mutated for the development of adenomatous polyps; hundreds to thousands of polyps develop, making it unlikely that mutation at the normal 5q allele is required. Analyses of DNA from these polyps have failed to reveal loss of 5q DNA. The formation of carcinomas may require the loss of the normal allele, because loss of heterozygosity has been found in FAP carcinomas.[130] Further analyses of mutations in *APC* and *MCC* are necessary to resolve the relation between different mutations and disease phenotype.

What can be said of the protein products of *MCC* and *APC*? By DNA sequence analysis, *APC* is predicted to encode a 2843-amino acid polypeptide. The NH$_2$-terminal 25% of the protein shows similarities to myosins, intermediate filaments, and plakoglobin (a protein that is a cytoplasmic component of gap junctions and is allelic with the *Drosophila armadillo* locus).[134] The carboxy-terminal 75% of APC shows short regions of homology to the *RAL2* gene in yeast, which may play a role in *RAS* regulation.[135] The *MCC* gene is predicted to encode an 829-amino acid polypeptide with a 19-residue stretch of the G protein-coupled m3 muscarinic acetylcholine receptor. This segment has been found to include sequences that specify the particular G protein with which the receptor interacts. These findings suggest that MCC may be involved in the regulation of a signalling pathway, most likely the Ca^{++}/phosphoinositide pathway, perhaps as a negative regulator.

Further analysis of MCC and APC revealed the presence of potential α-helical structures with heptad repeats (apolar-X-X-apolar-X-X-X) that might allow homo- or heterodimerization in a coiled-coil arrangement, in which two extended filamentous helical regions wrap around each other to form bimolecular or oligomeric complexes.[131,136] Such structures can be formed with a number of other proteins, including the nuclear lamins, vimentin, myosins, and keratins. These macromolecular complexes create a diverse array of intracellular structures that regulate cell shape, motility, and compartmentalization. Dominant-acting structural mutations could be envisaged in MCC or APC, in which the mutant protein would dimerize with and incapacitate the gene product of the normal allele. Precedent for such mutations exists for a number of genes encoding structural proteins.[136] Additional work is needed to establish the roles that *APC* and *MCC* play in the development of colorectal carcinoma.

CHROMOSOME 18Q DELETIONS IN COLORECTAL CARCINOMAS

Deletions involving chromosomes 17p and 18q occur in more than 70% of the colorectal tumors, which suggests that important tumor suppressor genes are located in these regions and that loss or mutation of one or both alleles at these loci constitute key steps in carcinogenesis.[130] The tumor suppressor gene on 17p is most likely p53, although other genes may be involved.[137,138] Vogelstein and coworkers localized the common region of deletion on chromosome 18 to 18q21-qter, and molecular access to the region was provided by an anonymous DNA probe that was found to be deleted in one or both alleles in tumor DNA but not in surrounding normal tissue.[130,139] Among 120 tumor DNAs analyzed, 71% showed deletion of this anonymous probe, and one showed acquisition of a different-sized band when compared with normal DNA from the same patient, suggesting that the anonymous probe was within the tumor suppressor locus, which proved to be the case.

A candidate gene named *DCC* for *d*eleted in *c*olorectal *c*arcinomas was successfully cloned using a novel cloning strategy, and the gene was found to be expressed at low levels in most tissues tested.[140] Expression was very low or absent in 88% of the colorectal carcinomas, consistent with its role as a tumor suppressor gene. In support of this notion, 13% of the colorectal carcinomas contained somatically acquired mutations in *DCC*, including deletions, point mutations, and insertions.

The predicted protein product of *DCC* is a 750-amino acid polypeptide with a 25-bp hydrophobic leader sequence typical of membrane-bound proteins. The sequence exhibits a high degree of homology to neural cell adhesion molecules.[141] There are four immunoglobulin-like domains of the C2 class, and potential N-linked glycosylation sites and fibronectin type III-related domains, all of which are features found on cell adhesion molecule family members.

The prediction that *DCC* encodes a cell adhesion molecule and that disruption of one or both alleles serves to further the transformed phenotype fits well with accepted notions in tumor cell biology. Cellular differentiation is directly influenced by intercellular adhesion mediated by cellular adhesion molecules, which establish and maintain cell-cell and cell-matrix or cell-basement membrane contacts that are essential features of a properly oriented, normal epithelium.[141]

DOMINANT ONCOGENES INVOLVED IN SIGNAL TRANSDUCTION

The products of oncogenes presumably display at least a subset of the activities of the protooncogene product. Therefore, the functional properties of the protooncogene product must be characterized to understand the role of an oncogene in tumorigenesis. Because these genes have been conserved during evolution, they have closely related counterparts in multicellular organisms, and these genes can be studied in animal model systems and in genetically well-characterized organisms. The conservation of protooncogenes in different animal species can be studied with the use of nucleic acid hybridization techniques (see Chap. 1).

The DNA sequences of certain protooncogenes are highly conserved between species, a measure that must be related to their function.[142] Of special interest are the protooncogene homologs found in organisms that are well suited for classic genetic studies, such as yeast or *Drosophila*. In these organisms, the phenotypic influence of mutated protooncogene homologs on cell division or differentiation and embryologic development can be tested, and genes can be identified that suppress the mutant phenotype, thereby identifying other members of the biochemical pathway. The nucleotide sequences of most of the oncogenes listed in Table 3–1 have been determined, and many of their RNA and protein products have been characterized. They have also been compared with the nucleotide or predicted amino acid sequences of the host protooncogene from which they were derived and with the homologous protooncogenes in other species, especially in humans. For instance, the *WNT1* oncogene (formerly called *INT1*), first identified as a common proviral integration site in mammary tumors induced by mouse mammary tumor virus (MMTV) was shown to be a developmentally regulated gene (*wingless*) of *Drosophila* and responsible for the formation of the dorsal axis during development in *Xenopus* embryos.[143,144] In the mouse, however, animals homozygous for the deletion of *WNT1* fail to develop a normal midbrain or cerebellum and die soon after birth.[145] Studies of *RAS* genes in yeast, *Drosophila*, and *Caenorhabditis elegans* are increasing our understanding of what is apparently a conserved biochemical pathway of signal transduction.[121,146,147]

The roles of dominantly acting oncogenes in malignant transformation can be addressed by asking what function they play in normal cells, as protooncogenes, and how that is altered in tumors. Many of the genes whose alteration or deregulation lead to cancer are involved in cell division and the control of cell division by means of signal transduction.

Experiments on virally induced tumors in animals, growth control in cell culture, and genes involved in human neoplasia have led to the discovery of a plethora of genes and their encoded gene products that are involved in signal transduction. The coordinated growth, differentiation, and adaptation that are essential for multicellular organisms are mediated through complex pathways. The pathways propagate and amplify signals from outside the cell to specific targets within the cell (*e.g.*, the cytoskeleton and the nucleus). Because growth is not a common event in many organs of mature multicellular organisms, these pathways must be highly regulated. They start at the extracellular membrane, where cell surface receptors interact with ligands (*e.g.*, growth factors) that are soluble or present on other cells or in their extracellular matrix.

Growth factors initiate the signal, which is mediated through respective receptors and leads to cell proliferation or differentiation.[148] Growth factors, cytokines, or antigens must be supplied to cells in culture to stimulate cell proliferation and growth.[148] Transformed cells show partial or complete relaxation of the requirements for growth factors (Table 3–8), and factor dependence can be abrogated by infecting cells with acute transforming retroviruses containing specific oncogenes.[148] The viral oncogene products can override factor dependency by perhaps mimicking the action of ligands, their receptors, or some downstream signal in the ordered procession of events that follows mitogenic stimulation.[149] Ligand binding to the cell surface receptor induces a conformational change in the cytoplasmic domain of the receptor, and in the case of tyrosine kinase growth factor receptors, this results in receptor clustering and activation of receptor function.[150] Through autophosphorylation, receptor clustering, or both, the activated receptor serves as a nidus for the assembly of complex, multiprotein signal transducers (Fig. 3–4).

The proteins involved in these complexes and the means by which they are recruited and activated are only now being elucidated, but many proteins implicated in oncogenesis appear to be involved. These include the protein products of *YES, FYN, RAS,* c-*SRC,* c-*RAF,* and *LCK* and other proteins, such as phosphatidylinositol-3 (PI-3) kinase, *RAS*-GAP, protein kinase C (PKC), and phospholipase Cγ (PLCγ).[150] Considering the complexity and diversity of the responses mediated by these signalling systems (*e.g.*, fibroblast migration and proliferation in wounds, T-cell activation by binding of antigen, and differentiation of neuroblasts into neurites), it is clear that specificity must emerge out of a set of pathways and responses that overlap considerably from one system to another.

Although much progress has been made in elucidating the signal transduction pathway, significant gaps exist in our un-

TABLE 3–8. Altered Properties of Tumor Cells

Characteristic	G_1/S	G_2/M
Cellular morphology		+
Nuclear structure		+
Cytoskeleton		+
Growth characteristics and cell metabolism	+	+
Anchorage independence and loss of contact inhibition		+
Changes in extracellular matrix		+
Genetic instability		+

(Vande Woude GF, Schulz N, Zhou R, et al. Cell cycle regulation, oncogenes, and antineoplastic drugs. In: Fortner JG, Rhoads JE, eds. Views of cancer research: General Motors Cancer Research Foundation. Philadelphia: JB Lippincott, 1990:128)

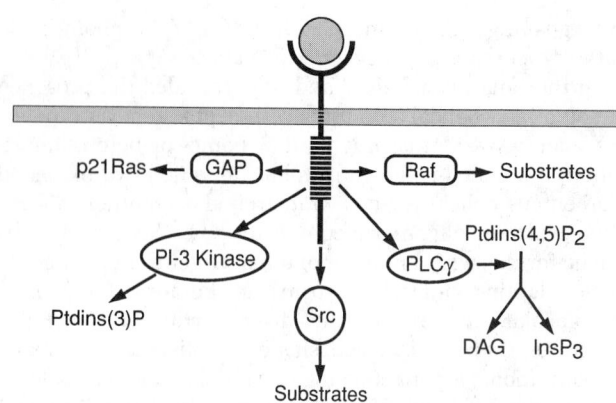

FIGURE 3–4. Substrates of receptor tyrosine kinases. A prototype receptor tyrosine kinase and known intracellular substrates are shown. The dashed line to Raf indicates that its activation may be by mechanisms other than direct tyrosine phosphorylation. (Adapted from Aaronsen, SA. Growth factors and cancer. Science 1991;254:1146)

derstanding, particularly in bridging the events at the cell membrane with events in the nucleus. It appears that oncoproteins, like their nontransforming counterparts, play important roles in these signalling pathways. Each control point along the pathway can be the target of deregulation by oncoproteins, either overexpressed or ectopically expressed proteins that bear no alteration in their normal structure, or mutated versions of their normal counterparts, bearing point mutations or truncations. By causing deregulation of the signalling, oncoproteins can force a cell into uncontrolled cell division or invasive growth. The nature of these mutations has contributed to our understanding of functional domains within these proteins and how the proteins are regulated.

EXTRACELLULAR GROWTH FACTORS

Of the many growth factors identified, those most likely to play a role in human cancers are Sis and TGF-α, CSF1, HST, and HGF-SF (hepatocyte growth factor-scatter factor).[151–155] The *SIS* oncogene, first identified in the simian sarcoma virus, encodes a protein highly related to the β chain of platelet-derived growth factor (PDGF) and is implicated in certain astrocytomas, sarcomas, and gliomas.[149,153,156] PDGF is an important serum mitogen required for the growth of mesenchymal cells in culture. TGF-α is related to epidermal growth factor (EGF), binds to the EGF receptor (EGFR), and induces the same spectrum of responses as EGF, which includes premature eyelid opening and incisor eruption in neonatal mice.[157] IGF II has also been implicated in oncogenesis, because it maps in the human genome within a region of chromosome 11p15, where alterations have been found in the cancer-predisposing disorder, Beckwith-Wiedemann syndrome.[47]

Several other oncogenes are related or identical to polypeptide growth factors. The *KS3* oncogene identified in gene transfer experiments with genomic DNA from a Kaposi's sarcoma, INT2, activated by MMTV proviral insertion in mouse mammary carcinomas and *HST,* a transforming gene identified by DNA transfection, are all members of the basic and acidic fibroblast growth factor (FGF) family.[30,31,148,158] The human *KS3* and *HST* oncogenes are identical, but distinct from the closely related mouse *INT2* gene. The expression of *INT2* is most abundant in primitive mouse endodermal cells. The low level of *INT2* expression activated by proviral insertion in mouse mammary tumors may stimulate in an autocrine fashion inappropriate cell proliferation. The fibroblast growth factors exhibit angiogenic properties and are related to polypeptide mitogens that apparently recognize different cell-type receptors.[148]

The growth factor ligands for two tyrosine kinase receptor protooncogenes have recently been identified. The receptors, *TRK* and *MET*, were originally identified as transforming genes, but their natural ligands were unknown. Nerve growth factor (NGF) is now known to be the extracellular ligand for the *TRK*-encoded receptor, and HGF-SF is the ligand for the *MET*-encoded receptor.[27,28,159,160] It is unclear whether NGF plays a role in human tumors. HGF was originally identified as a mitogenic factor for hepatocytes and was recently shown to be identical to SF, which causes epithelial cells to change in shape and become motile and invasive in in vitro assays.[161]

TYROSINE KINASE RECEPTORS

Many tyrosine kinase receptors have emerged from the myriad approaches to finding oncogenes. To this sizable number can be added other tyrosine kinase receptors cloned on the basis of homology or of their role in *Drosophila* or *Caenorhabditis elegans* development.[162] These receptors fall into six classes, each of which is named for the prototype of its class (Fig. 3–5). There is also a miscellaneous class that includes additional oncogenes, such as *LTK*, c-*ROS*, *MET*, *SEA*, and *RET*.[162] These receptors contain common structural features that are important to their function.[150,162] All have large, glycosylated, extracellular ligand-binding domains. Many, such as the PDGF receptor (PDGFR), function as homodimers or as heterodimers of α and β chains. The heterodimer may mediate different types of signals than the homodimer.

The cytoplasmic portion of these cell surface receptors contain tyrosine kinase domains that are required for signal transduction. Certain receptors, such as those in the PDGFR family, have a split kinase domain, with an autophosphorylation site in the middle.[162] The EGFR family also contains several autophosphorylation sites, which are located at the carboxy-terminal (cytoplasmic) tail of the protein. These sites modulate receptor activity and provide recognition sites for receptor targets. After the binding of ligand to the extracellular domain, these receptors undergo dimerization and activation of tyrosine kinase. This leads to autophosphorylation (in the case of EGFR) and binding and phosphorylation of other intracellular target proteins. Both N-terminal and C-terminal rearrangements appear to activate the transforming potential of these transmembrane receptor tyrosine kinase family members. The alterations may remove downmodulating domains of the protein and result in the constitutive activation of what is normally a conditionally regulated enzyme activity.

SIGNALLING COMPLEXES AND SECOND MESSENGERS

Several mechanisms come into play in the transduction process. The lipid bilayer of the plasma membrane allows lateral movement of receptors, dimerization or patching of receptors, and close interaction between the cytoplasmic tails of adjacent receptors (for cross-phosphorylation) and between the receptors and a number of proteins localized to the inner surface of the plasma membrane. This movement of receptors may be mediated by p21^{ras}, because in B lymphocytes, p21^{ras} patches together with surface immunoglobulin at the plasma membrane.[163] Some of the proteins that are part of the signalling process are localized at the plasma membrane by a number of structural motifs, such as basic motifs (*e.g.*, p21^{K-ras}) and posttranslational modifications, including myristylation (*e.g.*, pp60^{src} and related gene products), farnesylation (*e.g.*, p21^{ras}), and palmitylation (*e.g.*, p21^{H-ras}).[150] Other proteins are recruited to the plasma membrane within seconds to minutes after receptor activation. Key proteins in this group include RAS-GAP, PI-3 kinase, PKC, and PLCγ (Fig. 3–4).[150,164] Depending on the cell type and the receptor, some of these proteins congregate at specific sites of the activated receptor on the inner surface of the plasma membrane to form the signal transduction complex. The path diverges at this point to follow the transduction process into the cell along several disparate routes to end at common points: the cytoskeleton, which is the key effector of changes in cell shape and motility; the nucleus, where regulation of cell cycle and transcription takes place; and perhaps other points, such as back to the plasma membrane to affect ion channels and cell-cell interactions.

The plasma membrane appears to be involved in the generation of molecules that propagate the signal by serving as a pool of substrates for several key enzymes within the complex. These enzymes include PLCγ, which catalyzes the breakdown of phosphatidylinositol phosphates to generate diacylglycerol (DAG); phospholipase D, which converts phosphatidylcholine to a precursor of DAG; and PI-3 kinase, which causes the generation of phosphatidylinositol derivatives with a phosphate group on the D3 position.[150] These seemingly simple signalling molecules have diverse effects on the cell, including activation of PKC by DAG, release of calcium from intracellular stores by inositol triphosphates, translocation of certain enzymes to the plasma membrane, and regulation of cytoskeletal proteins by polyphosphoinositides.[150,165]

In addition to the phospholipid second messengers, there are several proteins that are key messengers in the signalling process, including PLCγ, p120$^{ras-GAP}$, and pp74^{raf}.

An important advance in our understanding of the interactions of receptor tyrosine kinases with other molecules was the identification of a domain within several key proteins that appears to be responsible for the binding to phosphotyrosine. This domain, called SH2 (for SRC homology region 2), is present in a number of other proteins, including pp60^{src}, PLCγ, PI-3 kinase, RAS-GAP, CRK, ABL, and VAV, and SRC-related proteins, like FPS.[150] The number of proteins with an SH2 domain continues to grow. This domain is thought to have the structure of a pocket, where the binding to the negatively charged phosphotyrosines is stabilized by three consistently placed arginines. The SH2 domain allows the interaction of these regulatory proteins with the phosphotyrosines on the cytoplasmic domain of activated receptors, thereby initiating the subsequent signalling events. It appears that the SH2 domain of SRC can interact with a phosphotyrosine of SRC itself, located at the carboxy-terminus (P-Tyr-527), and that this interaction keeps the tyrosine kinase activity inhibited

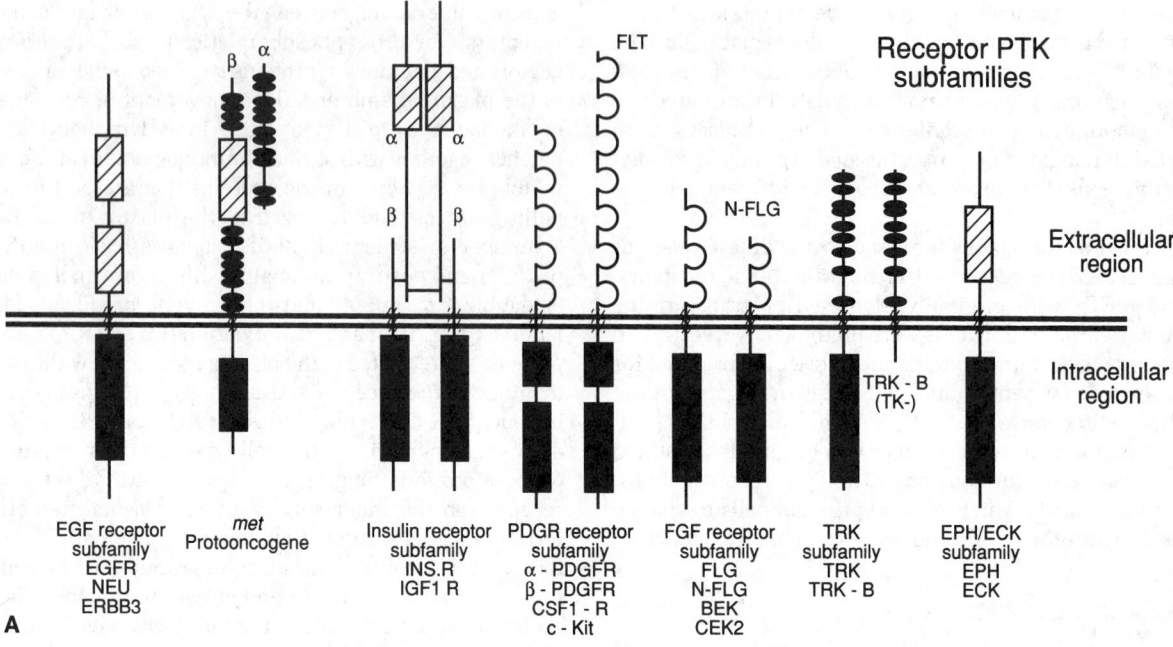

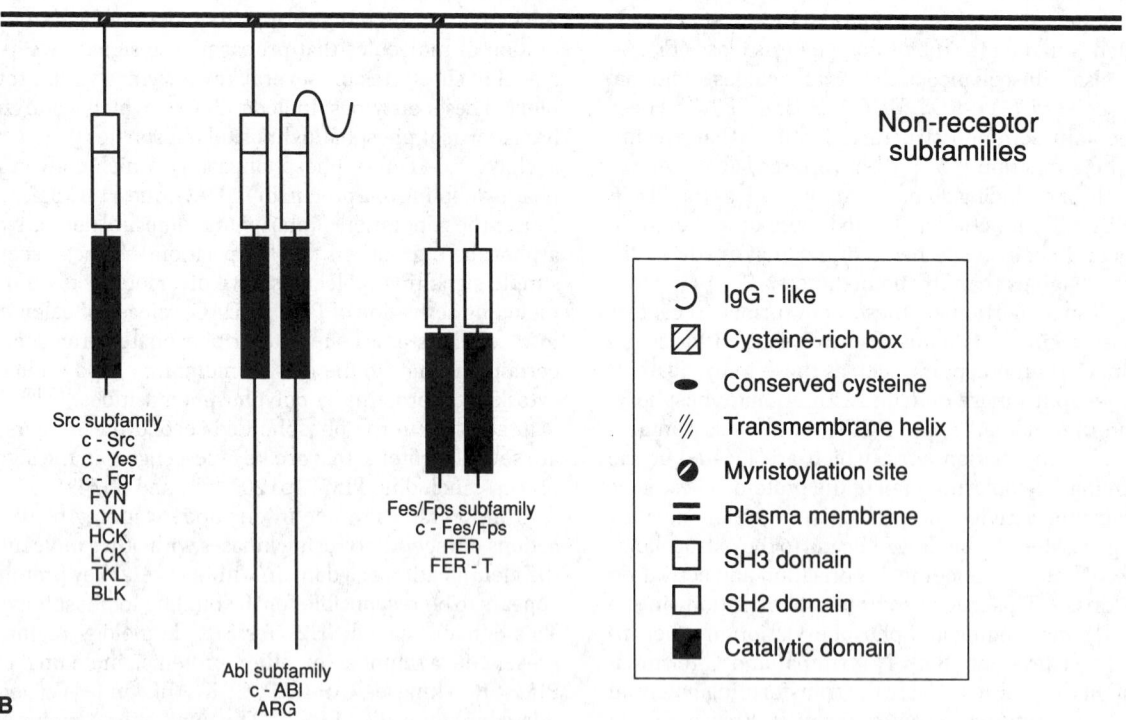

FIGURE 3–5. Depiction of the six different classes of tyrosine kinase receptors, and comparison of **(A)** the *MET* receptor and **(B)** nonreceptor tyrosine kinases. The plasma membrane is depicted as the horizontal double line, with the extracellular portion above and the cytoplasmic portion below. Inset is a key to the structural domains.

and the SRC SH2 domain occupied.[150] This repression of SRC activity can be alleviated by dephosphorylating P-Tyr-527 or by presenting SRC with another SH2-containing protein, such as CRK, to occupy P-Tyr-527.[150] Consistent with this, oncogenic forms of SRC lack P-Tyr-527 and have constitutive tyrosine kinase activity. It appears to be through SH2 domain–P-Tyr interactions that SRC and PDGFR can recruit other signalling molecules to the membrane to form an active complex. Raf protein, which has been shown to be an important molecule in the signalling process, does not possess an SH2 domain nor a lipophilic posttranslational modification, and its recruitment into the signalling complex must be mediated by as yet unidentified proteins.

Phospholipase Cγ is a major enzyme regulating the generation of phosphatidyl inositol-derived second messengers, including diacylglycerol (the physiologic activator of protein kinase C) and inositol triphosphates. The latter three molecules control the level of Ca^{2+} in growth factor-treated cells, which may be an important mediator of cell growth control, perhaps by the regulation of calmodulin-dependent kinases.[165] Within seconds of receptor tyrosine kinase activation, PLCγ becomes physically associated with and phosphorylated by the receptor, which leads to the accumulation of the described second messengers. Tumor promoters, such as phorbol esters, can activate this pathway through stimulation of protein kinase C.

Key regulatory proteins in the signal transduction cascade are p120$^{ras-GAP}$ and the related protein, the *NF1* gene product. These proteins are intimately involved in negatively regulating and possibly mediating the function of p21^{ras}.[123] They accomplish this by catalyzing the conversion of active, GTP-bound p21^{ras} to inactive, GDP-bound p21^{ras}. These proteins only regulate normal p21^{ras}; they cannot regulate mutant, oncogenic forms of p21^{ras}. Normal p21^{ras} can transform cells in culture by overexpression, but less efficiently than activated p21^{ras}. Overexpression of GAP in cells transformed by normal p21^{ras} reverts their phenotype, but overexpression has no effect on activated p21^{ras}-transformed cells.[166] This argues strongly that p120$^{ras-GAP}$ regulates normal p21^{ras} and that the amino acids that are mutated in p21^{ras} to render it oncogenic appear to be essential for the action of p120$^{ras-GAP}$.[167]

T-cell activation by antigen binding was shown to involve an increase in the ratio of GTP- to GDP-bound p21.^{ras} T-cell activation (and the increase in active p21^{ras}) can also be mediated by phorbol esters, which activate PKC. The effect of PKC on active p21^{ras} levels occurs through a decrease in p120$^{ras-GAP}$ (or a GAP-like protein) activity, which indicates that PKC caused an increase in the GTP to GDP p21^{ras} ratio by preventing interaction with p120$^{ras-GAP}$.[168] Although these studies indicate that p120$^{ras-GAP}$ acts upstream of p21^{ras} to prevent GTP hydrolysis, other studies have shown that it can act downstream and function to transmit the mitogenic signals of p21^{ras} to cellular targets.[122,124,169] These findings appear to be contradictory, but it is possible that p120$^{ras-GAP}$ may function upstream and downstream of p21^{ras} in the signal transduction pathway.

After p21^{ras} is in its GTP-bound, active form, what does it do? It is a key mediator of several complex cellular events. It may play an important role in T-cell activation and transformation. RAS also appears to play a role in differentiation.[170]

The downstream players in these phenomena have not been identified, but some progress has been made. The regulation of the transcription factor Jun occurs by an inhibitor that binds to and inactivates this factor. Jun is an important transcription factor, because it responds to growth factors by stimulating cellular gene transcription and can be oncogenic.[171]

The *RAF* gene product, pp74^{raf}, is a serine-threonine kinase, activated by phosphorylation on tyrosine or serine and presumably involved in transmitting mitogenic signals to the nucleus.[172] Constitutively activated forms of *RAF* are tumorigenic.[173] Activation by phosphorylation occurs in response to a variety of stimuli, including treatment with phorbol esters and the binding of growth factors to receptors. When activated, pp74^{raf} is found in a complex with ligand-activated receptor tyrosine kinases and signal transduction protein mediators, such as PLCγ, p120$^{ras-GAP}$, and p13 kinase.[174] In vitro, receptor tyrosine kinases can directly activate pp74^{raf} through phosphorylation on tyrosine.[174] With in vivo stimulation of pp74^{raf}, serine or threonine kinase activity can be mediated by multiple signal transduction pathways, involving serine-threonine or tyrosine kinase.[175] The activation of pp74^{raf} also appears to depend on p21^{ras}, because dominant-negative mutants of *RAS* can block the serum-induced phosphorylation and activation of pp74^{raf}.[176] The *RAS*-induced activation of transcription of certain target genes appears to occur exclusively through pp74^{raf}.[177] Activation of pp74^{raf} results in the transcription of several "early growth response" genes, including c-*FOS* and *EGR*, the genes for two transcription factors that control the transcription of subordinate genes expressed during cell proliferative responses.

PKC is a serine-threonine kinase that is activated by tumor-promoting phorbol esters or the phosphatidyinositol-derived second messenger, DAG, and is an important mediator of the nuclear effects of growth factor signalling.[178] PKC can directly affect gene transcription by inactivating an inhibitor of the transcription factor NFκB. The inhibitor, IκB, is phosphorylated by PKC to cause dissociation from NFκB, allowing the latter to move to the nucleus where it can activate the transcription of target genes.[179]

RAS FUNCTION

New insight into the regulation of p21^{ras} and its normal role in the cell have emerged from studies of a variety of systems. The importance of the four terminal residues of p21^{ras} for transformation led to the finding that it was the site of prenylation by a thioether linkage to a cysteine residue.[24,180] In the case of the p21^{ras} proteins encoded by K-*RAS*B and H-*RAS*, this prenyl group is all-*trans*-farnesol, a 15-carbon modification. Another prenyl modification, geranylgeranylation (20 carbons), is much more common, and both modifications appear to mediate the attachment of proteins to membranes.[181] The necessity of farnesylation for proper p21^{ras} function indicates that the protein must attach to membranes to perform its role in signal transduction. Because only a small fraction of cellular proteins are farnesylated and this modification is necessary for p21^{ras}-mediated transformation, the enzyme(s) that catalyze this modification are the focus of intense research, to understand p21^{ras} function and to identify a potential target of inhibition of *RAS*-induced transformation.

One of these enzymes, farnesyltransferase is a heterodimeric enzyme consisting of α and β subunits, each having an apparent molecular mass of 50 kd. The β subunit has been molecularly cloned and is homologous to its yeast counterpart (*DPR1-RAM1*).[121,182] Mutations in these yeast genes are defective for mating and cell division, demonstrating that farnesylation is an important cell process.[183] The α subunit appears to be common to farnesyltransferase and geranyl-geranyltransferase, but their β subunits are distinct.[184] The substrate for the farnesyltransferase holoenzyme is the tetrapeptide, cysteine-aliphatic-aliphatic-X, where X is any amino acid, and the enzyme can be inhibited from farnesylating p21^{ras} by such tetrapeptides, suggesting the possibility of therapeutic intervention in tumors that have activated p21^{ras}.[185]

Over 30 small GTP-binding proteins that are related to RAS have been identified.[121] These include well-characterized proteins, such as the *E. coli* elongation factor EF-TU and the mammalian G proteins that are involved in the coupling of receptors to second messenger-generating enzyme complexes. In yeast, the RAS homologs RAS1 and RAS2 couple nutrition-sensing cell surface molecules to the cAMP-generating systems and inhibit starvation-induced responses, such as exit from the cell cycle and sporulation, when nutrients are available. Transforming or oncogenic mutants of RAS fail to downregulate during starvation. The correlation with mammalian RAS function is still unclear, because RAS in higher eukaryotes does not appear to regulate cAMP.

Three classes of RAS-related proteins are emerging.[121] *RAP1* was first identified as a gene that could cause phenotypic reversion of *RAS*-transformed cells, and it has been postulated that RAP1 competes with RAS for downstream targets that block its action. A GTPase-accelerating protein (another GAP family member) specific for RAP1 has been identified and molecularly cloned and bears no sequence homology to other GAPs.[186] Because RAP1 is found in a complex of proteins with cytochrome b in neutrophils, it has also been postulated to play a role in inflammatory responses.

The RHO family represents a second class of RAS-related proteins.[121] These proteins exhibit 30% homology with RAS, also have a CAAX motif for prenylation, and possess GTPase activity. An RHO-specific GAP protein has been identified.[187] RHO appears to be involved in the regulation of the cytoskeleton, because microinjection of RHO into cells causes a dramatic change in shape. Such a role is also the case for a yeast homolog, CDC42, which is involved in the control of cell polarity and budding, two processes in which the cytoskeleton plays a major role.[188]

The third family of RAS-related proteins may play a part in facilitating vesicular transport and secretion. In this class are two yeast genes, *SEC4* and *YPT1*. In *SEC4* mutants, vesicles accumulate at the plasma membrane and are unable to fuse with it. The *YPT1* mutants are blocked in an earlier step in the secretion pathway.[121] Mammalian proteins of this class (*e.g.*, RAB) can complement the yeast mutations, and also appear to be associated with vesicles.

What does the study of these RAS-related proteins tell us about the function of RAS and its role in malignant transformation? These proteins are involved with cell shape and vesicular transport. Because the function of RAS proteins depends on their isoprenylation, it is likely that they must attach to membrane structures. Perhaps in the process of vesicular transport, RAS-related proteins tag the organelle and catalyze its movement by mediating attachment to the cytoskeleton. The p21^{ras} patches together with immunoglobulin at the cytoplasmic membrane, and this process depends on actin polymerization.[163] More work is needed to substantiate a role for p21^{ras} in signal transduction by the cytoskeleton or membrane structures.

NUCLEAR ONCOGENE AND PROTOONCOGENE PROTEINS

Several of the nuclear proteins encoded by protooncogenes and oncogenes are directly involved in the regulation of gene expression that leads to cell proliferation, division, and differentiation (see Chap. 2). Many of these nuclear proteins bind DNA in a site-specific manner and can activate or repress transcription from adjacent transcription units. Interesting homologies exist between several nuclear oncogene products and transcriptional regulatory proteins identified through work on gene regulation. For instance, c-JUN is the mammalian homolog of the yeast transcription factor GCN4; c-REL is homologous to NF-κB, which is involved in the regulation of immunoglobulin genes, interleukin-2 (IL-2), IL-2 receptor, and interferon-β, and to *DORSAL*, a *Drosophila* gene involved in the control of ventral-dorsal polarity; and c-*ERBA* codes for a thyroid hormone receptor.[171]

Several other nuclear oncoproteins contain structural motifs indicative of a role in DNA binding and transcriptional regulation or DNA replication. The proteins encoded by the *MYC* family of genes (*i.e.*, c-*MYC*, N-*MYC*, and L-*MYC*) have a helix-loop-helix domain, a motif present in several developmentally important transcription factors that mediates dimerization. These proteins also contain a leucine zipper region, which is also involved in dimerization. A group of newly identified proteins has been identified by virtue of T-cell-specific translocations of their respective genes that result in their activation.[32] This group includes LYL and SCL, which contain helix-loop-helix motifs, and PBX, which, as the product of a chimeric translocation gene, contains a helix-loop-helix and a homeobox motif (another DNA-binding motif). The t(15;17) translocation characteristic of acute promyelocytic leukemia results in the production of a novel fusion protein comprised of APL joined to the retinoic acid receptor α (Table 3-3).

Several nuclear oncogenes participate in the same complementation group of the cooperative oncogene assay (Table 3-7) or are transcriptionally activated by mitogenic stimulation (*e.g.*, MYC, FOS).[189] If quiescent serum-starved (growth-arrested) murine fibroblasts are stimulated with serum or growth factors, the cells immediately enter G$_1$, and there is a transient increase in the level of c-*MYC* and c-*FOS*. The induction varies from a peak at 30 minutes for c-*FOS* (Fig. 3-1B) to a much later time for the stimulation of p53 RNA expression, which peaks 18 to 24 hours poststimulation in late G$_2$, before M phase.[190] The induction of the expression of these nuclear protein-encoding protooncogenes is observed with PDGF or fetal calf serum, but the cells only become competent for DNA replication.[191] If PDGF is removed, the cells remain competent, and apparently the expression of a family of genes referred to as competence genes (*e.g.*, FOS and MYC) has already occurred.[191] EGF and insulin-like growth factors are required for cells to progress through G$_1$ and enter

S phase (Fig. 3–1B). Collectively, these studies suggest that the transient expression of nuclear protein-encoding oncogenes is required for cells to traverse specific points in the cell cycle. The expression of FOS and MYC in this system greatly precedes the onset of DNA synthesis and probably is not directly involved in DNA replication.

Expression of c-MYB and c-MYC decreases dramatically during terminal differentiation, and evidence indicates that they play a role in cell proliferation.[192] It is also postulated that constitutive expression of c-MYC prevents differentiation and promotes cell division.[193] Because the expression of these genes appears to occur at specific points in the cell cycle, their expression may promote proliferation or promote differentiation by being specifically expressed, as shown for c-FOS for which expression is observed during promonocyte differentiation and macrophage proliferation.[194]

There is a growing body of evidence indicating that products of the nuclear protein-encoding oncogenes can regulate gene expression. Many of the nuclear oncoproteins specifically bind nucleic acids (e.g., MYC, MYB, ETS, FOS, p53, JUN, and ERBA).[88,171] Moreover, the products of MYB, ETS, MYC, FOS, JUN, and ERBA and E1A directly or indirectly alter the expression of specific cellular genes.[171]

The c-FOS and c-JUN gene products are components of the transcription complex AP1, and both contain a leucine zipper dimerization motif.[171] Although JUN can homodimerize to yield a functional complex, Fos can only heterodimerize with JUN, or perhaps other leucine zipper proteins, to be functional. These complexes bind to the AP1 recognition sequence, TGACTCA, and can influence expression of adjacent target genes. AP1 is the nuclear transcription factor that mediates transcription regulation by phorbol ester tumor promoters and numerous growth factor stimuli.[171] The c-FOS product has been directly implicated in the downregulation of transcription of an adipocyte-specific differentiation gene, and gene regulation can be positive or negative.[195] The C-terminal 48 amino acids of c-FOS are deleted in transforming FOS, but the difference in transforming ability of the two is not evident and may result from deregulated expression of either gene. In the case of the murine osteosarcoma virus (FBJ-MuSV), transformation may be due to the strong viral long terminal repeat promoters.

Perhaps the most dramatic evidence demonstrating the role of nuclear protein-encoding oncogenes as *trans*-acting factors comes from the studies of the c-JUN oncogene.[171] DNA sequence analysis revealed that the C terminus of the c-JUN protein was homologous to the C terminus of the transcriptional activator protein GCN4 from yeast *Saccharomyces cerevisiae*. Furthermore, a chimeric GCN4 gene sequence containing the DNA-binding domain of c-JUN rescued yeast strains that lacked the GCN4 gene (*i.e.*, null mutations). The consensus DNA-binding sequence for the yeast GCN4 gene is the same as that of the mammalian transcription factor AP1. This discovery led to the demonstration that the c-JUN oncoprotein is the transforming homolog of a component of the normal AP1 transcription factor.[171] The AP1 product interacts with phorbol ester-inducible promoter elements and with the enhancer elements found in many viral and cellular transcription control sequences. This finding suggests that the unregulated or ectopic expression of a normal transcription regulator protein contributes to tumor development. Of interest now is the

identification of genes regulated by AP1 or c-JUN that directly affect growth and expression of a neoplastic phenotype.

The c-JUN and v-JUN products differ in that the latter lacks a 27-amino acid segment called the delta (Δ) region. This domain and an adjacent A1 domain mediate the interaction between c-JUN and tissue-specific inhibitory c-JUN binding proteins. This provides a theoretical basis for the transforming ability of v-JUN. Transformation by v-SRC or mutant p21^{ras} can alleviate the Δ-A1 region-mediated repression of c-JUN activity, but the exact pathway by which this occurs is unclear.[196]

A different role has been proposed for the nuclear oncoprotein v-ERBA, which is a nuclear receptor for the thyroid hormones triiodothyronine and thyroxine.[197] v-ERBA by itself does not appear to express transforming potential, but its presence potentiates the transforming potential of v-ERBA by specifically interrupting the differentiation of erythroblasts.[198] The thyroid hormone receptor is known to positively and negatively regulate the expression of many genes. In the absence of ligand, the receptor can bind DNA in a sequence-specific manner, but cannot activate transcription. In such a way, it can act as a transcriptional repressor. In the presence of ligand, it can activate transcription. The v-ERBA product arrests the expression of genes that play an important role in erythroid differentiation.[199] Because of mutations in the v-ERBA gene, it does not bind T_3 or T_4 and is therefore ligand independent.[171] As with other nuclear protein-encoding oncogenes, the v-ERBA product probably acts constitutively to upregulate or downregulate expression of target genes, apparently interrupting the regulation of genes that are essential for erythroblast differentiation. Compared with native thyroid hormone receptor, the v-ERBA product is truncated at both ends.

The protooncogene c-MYB plays an important role in the control of early myeloid and erythroid differentiation, probably by controlling the expression of differentiation-specific genes. A DNA-binding site for MYB has been identified, and MYB activates transcription from synthetic and native promoters that contain the sequence.[171] By using a temperature-sensitive MYB gene, it has been shown that in certain myeloid cell lines a decrease in active MYB in the cell allows differentiation along the myeloid lineage to proceed.[200] Oncogenic versions of MYB are deleted on their 5' end, in a region that encodes a phosphorylation site that may be important in the regulation of the MYB protein, and loss of these sequences may lead to unregulated activity.[201] Alternatively, point mutations within the DNA-binding domain may yield a protein with altered specificity, allowing it to activate inappropriate genes.

The v-REL oncogene is a truncated version of c-REL, and its product is homologous to the transcription factor NF-κB and *dorsal*.[171] The v-REL gene was first identified in the turkey reticuloendotheliosis virus, which causes B-cell lymphomas in chickens. The *dorsal* product is required for establishing the dorsal-ventral axis in *Drosophila* and shares 80% homology with REL over a 250-amino acid region.[171] NF-κB is a heterodimer with subunits of 50 and 65 kd, of which the 50-kd subunit is 60% homologous to c-REL. Both dorsal and NF-κB proteins are regulated by movement from the cytoplasm, where they are inactive by virtue of being bound to inhibitor proteins, to the nucleus, where they are active. The inhibitor of NF-κB, called IκB, also binds REL and releases the transcription factors after phosphorylation by PKC. REL proteins can bind to the same DNA sequence as NF-κB and can act as a repressor of transcription on promoters containing this sequence.[171] How the truncation leads to transformation remains unclear.

TRANSFORMED CELL PHENOTYPE, ANTINEOPLASTIC DRUGS, AND THE CELL CYCLE

With the wealth of information describing the molecular pathology of cancer, we can begin to explain how oncogenes and tumor suppressor genes contribute to the transformed phenotype (Table 3–8). Although antineoplastic drugs are discovered through empiric testing, it is possible that oncogene activation or loss of tumor suppressor genes render tumor cells more sensitive to these drugs. A general mechanism explaining how and why existing antineoplastic drugs work can lead to improvements in their use and can revolutionize how new drugs are identified and used.

How do so many different oncogenes cause similar phenotypes in cells they transform? Oncogenes and tumor suppressor genes participate in common signal transduction pathways, and it is likely that the transformed phenotype must be derived from a common cellular process that is aberrantly modified when these genes are activated or deleted. Signal transduction regulates cell cycle progression, DNA synthesis, and cell division. It has recently been proposed that many of the phenotypes of transformed cells are due to aberrant expression of M phase of the cell cycle during interphase.[202]

Dramatic discoveries have been made during the past several years in identifying the genes responsible for the regulation of progression through the cell cycle. The major cell cycle oscillator, $p34^{cdc2}$, governs entry into S phase, during which DNA is synthesized (Fig. 3–6), and M phase (mitosis

or meiosis) is presumably regulated through phosphorylation of specific targets or substrates. This protein kinase is conserved from yeast to man in structure (65% homology) and in function.[203] $P34^{cdc2}$ kinase is believed to be directed toward its targets by associating with different members of a family of proteins (*i.e.*, cyclins) that appear and disappear at specific stages of the cell cycle (Fig. 3–6A). Thus, G_1 cyclins appear before S phase and are believed to initiate entry into S phase when they associate with a p34 kinase product. A direct link has been established between oncogenes and cyclins. The G_1 cyclins have been directly implicated in several human cancers (Tables 3–3 and 3–9). Cyclin A appears early in S phase and has recently been shown to be necessary for DNA synthesis.[204] Many oncogenes and tumor suppressor genes are believed to be targets of phosphorylation by the cyclin A–$p34^{cdc2}$ complex. This could facilitate their association or dissociation with substrates as positive or negative growth regulators.

The B cyclins function primarily during M phase, and their association with $p34^{cdc2}$ gives rise to M-phase promoting factor (MPF).[202] MPF is extremely active as a kinase and maximal activity occurs at metaphase of meiosis or mitosis. M-phase metaphase is considered to be the second major cell cycle control point (entry into S is the first) and the final step of the cell cycle.[202] Anaphase represents entry into interphase of the next cycle. MPF has been known for many years as the universal regulator of M phase (from yeast to man), no doubt due to the conservation of $p34^{cdc2}$. MPF is believed to be responsible during M phase for nuclear envelope breakdown, chromosome condensation, and spindle formation.

Several oncogenes (*e.g.*, MOS, SRC, RAS) that are considered paradigm transforming genes have M-phase activity.[202] The MOS protooncogene functions only during meiosis. It specifically initiates meiosis I by activating MPF and stabilizes MPF at metaphase II of meiosis, the stage corresponding to an un-

A

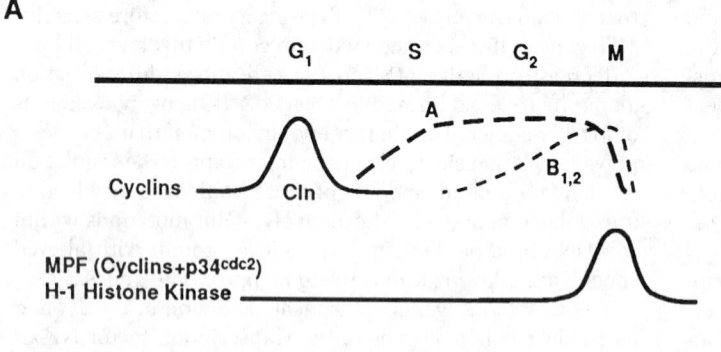

B

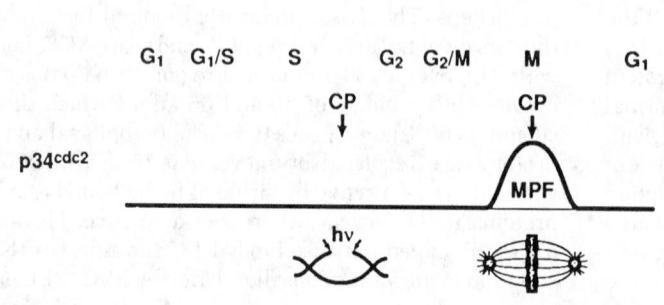

FIGURE 3–6. Cell cycle regulation and checkpoint function. **(A)** The major cell cycle oscillator, $p34^{cdc2}$, associates with different cyclins that appear and disappear during specific stages of the cell cycle. The kinase p24 is directed toward its targets by association with the specific cyclins. G_1 cyclins appear to regulate entry into S phase, and the cyclin A–$p34^{cdc2}$ complex functions during S phase. The highest p34 kinase levels are displayed in metaphase of mitosis and called MPF for M-phase promoting factor. MPF consists of a complex between B cyclins and $p34^{cdc2}$. **(B)** Checkpoint functions were first identified in yeast. They are manifested by pauses in the cell cycle where the fidelity of the process is checked. Numerous checkpoint genes have been identified; only two are indicated. One is involved in sensing repair of radiation damage. The other is part of many checkpoint functions associated with the spindle. This is an important part of the cycle to check for errors, just before cytokinesis.

TABLE 3–9. Cyclin Genes Associated
With Human Tumors

Gene	Tumor	References
Cyclin A	Hepatocellular carcinoma (HBV insertion)	219
D11S287E	Benign parathyroid adenoma (11q13)	217
or *PRAD1*	B-cell malignancies (11q13)	216
or *BCL1*? (*CYL1* or cyclin D1)*	B-cell malignancies and breast cancer (amplified)	220 218, 221

* Also characterized as G_1 cyclins.

TABLE 3–10. Selected Antineoplastic Agents

G_1 + S Phase (Upstream)	M Phase (Downstream)
Tamoxifen (antiestrogen)	Vincristine (tubulin binding)
Prednisone (corticosteroid)	Vinblastine (tubulin binding)
Dacarbazine (DNA alkylation)	Taxol (tubulin binding)
Mechlorethamine (DNA alkylation)	Doxorubicin (topoisomerase II inhibitor)
Cisplatin (DNA crosslinking)	Daunorubicin (topoisomerase II inhibitor)
Methotrexate (DNA synthesis)	Etoposide (topoisomerase II inhibitor)
5-fluorouracil (DNA synthesis)	Bleomycin (DNA crosslinking)
Cytosine arabinoside (DNA synthesis)	

(Vande Woude GF, Schulz N, Zhou R, et al. Cell cycle regulation, oncogenes, and antineoplastic drugs. In: Fortner JG, Rhoads JE, eds. Views of cancer research: General Motors Cancer Research Foundation. Philadelphia: JB Lippincott, 1990:128)

fertilized egg. The major function of this protooncogene product is to stabilize MPF at the last major control point in the cell cycle. As an oncogene, *MOS* is expressed constitutively, during interphase. This leads to the hypothesis that many phenotypes of transformed cells may represent M-phase activities (Table 3–8).[202] The altered morphology of tumor cells could be due to expression of some of the cytoskeletal changes of M phase (related to *MOS, RAS,* or *SRC* function) during interphase.[202] This model can also explain how oncogenes cooperate. The rat embryo fibroblast cooperating oncogene assay (Table 3–7) previously described is believed to mimic tumor progression.[189] One class of oncogenes rescue cells from senescence, and the second class are responsible for morphologic transformation. Oncogenes that rescue cells from senescence promote entry in S phase (Table 3–9); G_1 cyclins also fit in this class. The oncogenes in the second class responsible for morphologic transformation may do so by promoting expression of M-phase events during interphase.[202]

It is possible that many oncogenes and tumor suppressor genes discovered may only affect the two major compartments of the cell cycle: entry into S phase or M phase. Tumor progression may be a combination of events that lead to increased loss of control over entry into S phase plus an increase in the number and extent of M-phase activities expressed during interphase. Tumor progression is due to the genetic instability (Table 3–8), and this property is central to the cancer process.

We have proposed that genetic instability of transformed cell is also due to the oncogene alteration of an important cell cycle function called checkpoints (Fig. 3–6B).[202] Checkpoints, first described by Hartwell and Weinert, are pauses in the cell cycle where the fidelity of the process is checked.[205] Presumably, they work by signalling the cell directly or indirectly to proceed through the cycle. Checkpoints should be downstream of repair genes and upstream of $p34^{cdc2}$. Oncogenes with downstream M-phase activity could compromise checkpoint functions when expressed during interphase. It is possible that oncogenes or tumor suppressor genes serve as checkpoint genes.

Compromise of checkpoint function can explain how, in the same tumor lineage, point mutations, deletions, amplifications, and translocations can occur. Moreover, if oncogenes and tumor suppressor genes are responsible for malignant transformation and their activation or deletion leads to checkpoint compromise, tumor cells should be more vulnerable to antineoplastic drugs than normal cells. This model

can provide a unifying hypothesis for the genetic instability of tumor cells, tumor progression, and the sensitivity of tumor cells to antineoplastic agents.

The vulnerability of tumor cells to drugs that target S phase (*e.g.*, DNA alkylating agents) or M phase (*e.g.*, tubulin-binding vinca alkaloids or taxol and topoisomerase II inhibitors) may be due to the cancer cell continuing through the cell cycle with too many errors, while the normal cell stops at the appropriate checkpoints until the necessary repairs are made. This implies that antineoplastic drug damage to normal cells must be repairable. Recognizing that drugs may function at different stages of the cell cycle and on multiple targets, it is rather striking that many antineoplastic drugs can be assigned as acting preferentially chiefly on S-phase or M-phase activ-

TABLE 3–11. Selected Chemotherapeutic Regimens

Malignancy	G_1 or S Phase (Upstream)	M Phase (Downstream)
Acute lymphocytic leukemia	Prednisone	Vincristine
	L-Asparaginase	Daunorubicin
	Cytosine arabinoside	Etoposide
Acute nonlymphocytic leukemia	Cytosine arabinoside	Daunorubicin
Testicular cancer	Cisplatin	Bleomycin
		Vinblastine or etoposide
	Mechlorethamine	
Hodgkin lymphoma	Procarbazine	Vincristine
	Prednisone	
		Doxorubicin
	Dacarbazine	Vincristone
		Bleomycin

(Vande Woude GF, Schulz N, Zhou R, et al. Cell cycle regulation, oncogenes, and antineoplastic drugs. In: Fortner JG, Rhoads JE, eds. Views of cancer research: General Motors Cancer Research Foundation. Philadelphia: JB Lippincott, 1990:128)

ities (upstream or downstream) (Table 3–10).[202] Many of the drugs damage DNA or function during M phase to affect chromosome partitioning. If oncogenes allow progression through the cell cycle with the damage caused by these agents, drugs acting at different stages or targets of the cell cycle would be expected to act in synergy. Remarkably, certain empirically established protocols are combinations of S-phase and M-phase agents (Table 3–11). Regimens for acute lymphocytic leukemia, acute nonlymphocytic leukemia, testicular cancer, and Hodgkin lymphoma use a combination of drugs that act upstream and downstream, and the preponderance of S-phase or M-phase agents in the MOPP or ABVD regimens for Hodgkin lymphoma may explain their relative efficacies.

Although new approaches to identify and design antineoplastic drugs will certainly target the biochemical activities of oncogene and altered tumor suppressor gene products, knowing how oncogenes function in the cell cycle may also elucidate the mechanisms of action of existing antineoplastic drugs. This could provide new ways to use these drugs and aid in designing new and better strategies.

Acknowledgments

Research performed in Dr. G. Vande Woude's laboratory was supported by the National Cancer Institute, DHHS, under contract No. N01-C0-74101 with ABL. The contents of this publication do not necessarily reflect the views or policies of the Department of Health and Human Services, nor does mention of trade names, commercial products, or organizations imply endorsement by the U.S. Government.

REFERENCES

1. Foulds L. The natural history of cancer. J Chron Dis 1958;8:2.
2. Bishop JM. Cellular oncogenes and retroviruses. Annu Rev Biochem 1983;52:301.
3. Klein G, Klein E. Evolution of tumours and the impact of molecular oncology. Nature 1985;315:190.
4. Hunter T, Cooper JA. Viral oncogenes and tyrosine phosphorylation. In: Boyer PD, Krebs EG, eds. Enzyme control by protein phosphorylation. New York: Academic Press, 1986:191.
5. Marshall CJ. Tumor suppressor genes. Cell 1991;64:313.
6. Rous P. A sarcoma of fowl transmissible by an agent separable from the tumor cells. J Exp Med 1911;13:397.
7. Viskochil D, Buchberg AM, Xu G, et al. Deletions and a translocation interrupt a cloned gene at the neurofibromatosis type 1 locus. Cell 1990;62:187.
8. Weiss R, Teich N, Varmus H, et al. RNA tumor viruses. Cold Spring Harbor, NY: Cold Spring Harbor Laboratory, 1982.
9. Hayward WS, Neel BG, Astrin SM. Activation of a cellular ONC gene by promoter insertion in ALV-induced lymphoid leukosis. Nature 1982;290:475.
10. Blair DG, Oskarsson M, Wood TG, et al. Activation of the transforming potential of a normal cell sequence: A molecular model for oncogenesis. Science 1981;212:941.
11. Curran T, Miller AD, Zokas L, et al. Viral and cellular FOS proteins: A comparative analysis. Cell 1984;36:259.
12. Prywes R, Foulkes JG, Rosenberg N, et al. Sequences of the A-MuLV protein needed for fibroblast and lymphoid cell transformation. Cell 1983;34:569.
13. Levinson AD. Normal and activated RAS oncogenes and their encoded products. Trends Genet 1986;2:81.
14. Takeya T, Hanafusa H. Structure and sequence of the cellular gene homologous to the RSV SRC gene and the mechanism for generating the transforming virus. Cell 1983;32:881.
15. Hill M, Hillova J. Virus recovery in chicken cells tested with Rous sarcoma cell DNA. Nature 1972;237:35.
16. Graham FL, Van Der Eb AJ. A new technique for the assay of infectivity of human adenovirus 5 DNA. Virology 1973;52:456.
17. Blair DG, Cooper CS, Oskarsson MK, et al. New method for detecting cellular transforming genes. Science 1982;218:1122.
18. Shih C, Shilo BZ, Goldfarb MP, et al. Passage of phenotypes of chemically transformed cells via transfection of DNA and chromatin. Proc Natl Acad Sci USA 1979;76:5714.
19. Goldfarb M, Shimizu K, Perucho M, et al. Isolation and preliminary characterization of a human transforming gene from T24 bladder carcinoma cells. Nature 1982;296:404.
20. Der CJ, Krontiris TG, Cooper GM. Transforming genes of human bladder and lung carcinoma cell lines are homologous to the RAS genes of Harvey and Kirsten sarcoma viruses. Proc Natl Acad Sci USA 1982;79:3637.
21. Parada LF, Tabin CJ, Shih C, et al. Human EJ bladder carcinoma oncogene is homologue of Harvey sarcoma virus RAS gene. Nature 1982;297:474.
22. Perucho M, Goldfarb M, Shimizu K, et al. Human tumor-derived cell lines contain common and different transforming genes. Cell 1981;27:467.
23. Murray MJ, Shilo B-Z, Shih C, et al. Three different human tumor cell lines contain different oncogenes. Cell 1981;25:355.
24. Barbacid M. RAS genes. Annu Rev Biochem 1987;56:779.
25. Bos JL, Fearon ER, Hamilton SR, et al. Prevalence of RAS gene mutations in human colorectal cancers. Nature 1987;327:293.
26. Coussens L, Yang-Feng TL, Liao Y, et al. Tyrosine kinase receptor with extensive homology to EGF receptor shares chromosomal location with NEU oncogene. Science 1985;230:1132.
27. Cooper CS, Park M, Blair DG, et al. Molecular cloning of a new transforming gene from a chemically transformed human cell line. Nature 1984;311:29.
28. Martin-Zanca D, Hughes SH, Barbacid M. A human oncogene formed by the fusion of truncated tropomyosin and protein tyrosine kinase sequences. Nature 1986;319:743.
29. Fasano O, Birnbaum D, Edlund L, et al. New human transforming genes detected by a tumorigenicity assay. Mol Cell Biol 1984;4:1695.
30. Yoshida T, Miyagawa K, Odagiri H, et al. Genomic sequence of HST, a transforming gene encoding a protein homologous to fibroblast growth factors and the INT-2-encoded protein. Proc Natl Acad Sci USA 1987;84:7305.
31. Bovi PD, Curatola AM, Kern FG. An oncogene isolated by transfection of Kaposi's sarcoma DNA encodes a growth factor that is a member of the FGF family. Cell 1987;50:729.
32. Cleary ML. Oncogenic conversion of transcription factors by chromosomal translocation. Cell 1991;66:619.
33. DeThé M, Lavau C, Marchio A, et al. The PML-PARX fusion mRNA generated by the t(15;17) translocation in acute promyelocytic leukemia encodes a functionally altered RAR. Cell 1991;66:675.
34. DeThé M, Chomrene C, Lanotte M, et al. The t(15;17) translocation of acute promyelocytic leukaemia fuses the retinoic acid receptor α gene to a nove transcribed locus. Nature 1990;347:558.
35. Collins SJ, Kubonishi I, Miyoshi I, et al. Altered transcription of the c-ABL oncogene in K-562 and other chronic myelogenous leukemia cells. Science 1984;225:72.
36. Konopka, JB, Watanabe SM, Witte ON. An alteration of the human c-ABL protein in K562 leukemia cells unmasks associated tyrosine kinase activity. Cell 1984;37:1035.
37. Witte ON. Functions of the ABL oncogene. Cancer Surv 1986;5:183.
38. Daley GQ, Van Etten RA, Baltimore D. Induction of chronic myelogenous leukemia in mice by the P210[MD30]BCR/ABL gene of the Philadelphia chromosome. Science 1990;247:824–830.
39. Heisterkamp N, Jenster G, ten Hoeve J. Acute leukaemia in BCR/abl transgenic mice. Nature 1990;344:251.
40. Lugo TG, Pendergast AM, Muller AJ, et al. Tyrosine kinase activity and transformation potency of BCR/abl oncogene products. Science 1990;247:1079.
41. Pendergast AM, Muller AJ, Havlik MH, et al. BCR sequences essential for transformation by the BCR/ABL oncogene bind to ABL SH2 regulatory domain in a nonphosphotyrosine-dependent manner. Cell 1991;66:161.
42. Collins S, Groudine M. Amplification of endogenous MYC-related DNA sequences in a human myeloid leukaemia cell line. Nature 1982;298:679.
43. Dalla Favera R, Wong-Staal F, Gallo RC. Onc gene amplification in promyelocytic leukaemia cell line HL-60 and primary leukaemic cells of the same patient. Nature 1982;299:61.
44. Schwab M, Varmus HE, Bishop JM. Chromosome localization in normal cells and neuroblastomas of a gene related to c-MYC. Nature 1984;308:288.
45. Little CD, Nau MM, Carney DN, et al. Amplification and expression of the c-MYC oncogene in human lung cell lines. Nature 1983;306:194.
46. Knudson AG. Mutation and cancer: Statistical study of retinoblastoma. Proc Natl Acad Sci USA 1971;68:820.
47. Haber DA, Housman DE. The genetics of Wilms' tumor. Adv Cancer Res 1992;59:41.
48. Cavenee WK, Dryja TP, Phillips RA, et al. Expression of recessive alleles by chromosomal mechanisms in retinoblastoma. Nature 1983;305:779.
49. Francke U. Retinoblastoma and chromosome 13. Birth Defects 1978;12:131.
50. DeMars R. Fundamental cancer research: 23rd annual symposium. Baltimore: Williams & Wilkins, 1970:105.
51. Ponder B. Gene losses in human tumours. Nature 1988;335:400.
52. Cavenee WK, Hansen MF, Nordenskjold M, et al. Genetic origin of mutations predisposing to retinoblastoma. Nature 1985;305:779.
53. Friend SH, Bernards R, Rogelj S, et al. A human DNA segment with properties of the gene that predisposes to retinoblastoma and osteosarcoma. Nature 1986;323:643.
54. Lee W-H, Bookstein R, Hong F, et al. Human retinoblastoma susceptibility gene: Cloning, identification, and sequence. Science 1987;235:1394.
55. Bookstein R, Rio P, Madreperla SA, et al. Promoter deletion and loss of retinoblastoma gene expression in human prostate carcinoma. Proc Natl Acad Sci USA 1990;87:7762.
56. Harbour JW, Lai S-L, Whang-Peng J, et al. Abnormalities in structure and expression of the human retinoblastoma gene in SCLC. Science 1988;241:353.
57. Horowitz JM, Park S-H, Bogenmann E, et al. Frequent inactivation of the retinoblastoma anti-oncogene is restricted to a subset of human tumor cells. Proc Natl Acad Sci USA 1990;87:2775.

58. Friend SH, Horowitz JM, Gerber MR. Deletions of a DNA sequence in retinoblastomas and mesenchymal tumors: Organization of the sequence and its encoded protein. Proc Natl Acad Sci USA 1987;84:9059.

59. Reissmann PT, Simon MA, Lee W, et al. Studies of the retinoblastoma gene in human sarcomas. Oncogene 1989;4:839.

60. Lee EY-HP, To H, Shew J-H, et al. Inactivation of the retinoblastoma susceptibility gene in human breast cancers. Science 1988;241:218.

61. T'Ang A, Varley JM, Chakraborty S, et al. Structural rearrangement of the retinoblastoma gene in human breast carcinoma. Science 1988;242:263.

62. Bookstein R, Shew J-Y, Chen P-L, et al. Suppression of tumorigenicity of human prostate carcinoma cells by replacing a mutated *RB* gene. Science 1990;247:712.

63. Strohmeyer T, Reissmann P, Cordon-Cardo, C, et al. Correlation between retinoblastoma gene expression and differentiation in human testicular tumors. Proc Natl Acad Sci USA 1991;88:6662.

64. Chen P-L, Scully P, Shew J-Y, et al. Phosphorylation of the retinoblastoma gene product is modulated during the cell cycle and cellular differentiation. Cell 1989;58:1193.

65. DeCaprio JA, Ludlow JW, Lynch D, et al. The product of the retinoblastoma susceptibility gene has properties of a cell cycle regulatory element. Cell 1989;58:1085.

66. Figge J, Webster T, Smith, TF, et al. Prediction of similar transforming regions in simian virus 40 large T, adenovirus E1A, and *MYC* oncoproteins. J Virol 1988;62:1814.

67. Whyte P, Buchkovich KJ, Horowitz JM, et al. Association between an oncogene and an antioncogene: The adenovirus E1A proteins bind to the retinoblastoma gene product. Nature 1988;334:124.

68. Dyson N, Howley PM, Munger K, et al. The human papilloma virus-16 E7 oncoprotein is able to bind to the retinoblastoma gene product. Science 1989;243:934.

69. Green MR. When the products of oncogenes and anti-oncogenes meet. Cell 1989;56:1.

70. Ludlow JW, DeCaprio JA, Huang C-M, et al. SV40 large T antigen binds preferentially to an underphosphorylated member of the retinoblastoma susceptibility gene product family. Cell 1989;56:57.

71. Kaye FJ, Kratzke RA, Gerster JL, et al. A single amino acid substitution results in a retinoblastoma protein defective in phosphorylation and oncoprotein binding. Proc Natl Acad Sci USA 1990;87:6922.

72. Laiho M, DeCaprio JA, Ludlow JW, et al. Growth inhibition by TGF-β linked to suppression of retinoblastoma protein phosphorylation. Cell 1990;62:175.

73. Kaelin WG Jr, Palas DC, DeCaprio JA, et al. Identification of cellular proteins that can interact specifically with the T/E1A-binding region of the retinoblastoma gene product. Cell 1991;64:521.

74. Chellappan SP, Hiebert S, Mudryi M, et al. The E2F transcription factor is a cellular target for the RB protein. Cell 1991;65:1053.

75. Robbins PD, Horowitz JM, Mulligan RC. Negative regulation of human c-*FOS* expression by the retinoblastoma gene product. Nature 1990;346:668.

76. Pietenpol JA, Stein RW, Moran E, et al. TGF-β1 inhibition of c-*MYC* transcription and growth in keratinocytes is abrogated by viral transforming proteins with pRB binding domains. Cell 1990;61:777.

77. Levine AJ, Momand J, Finlay CA. The p53 tumour suppressor gene. Nature 1991;351:453.

78. Hollstein M, Sidransky D, Vogelstein B, et al. P53 mutations in human cancers. Science 1991;253:49.

79. Finlay CA, Hinds PW, Tan T-H, et al. Activating mutations for transformation by p53 produce a gene product that forms an hsc70-p53 complex with an altered half-life. Mol Cell Biol 1988;8:531.

80. Chen P-L, Chen Y, Bookstein R, et al. Genetic mechanisms of tumor suppression by the human p53 gene. Science 1990;250:1576–1580.

81. Malkin D, Li FP, Strong LC, et al. Germ line p53 mutations in a familial syndrome of breast cancer, sarcomas, and other neoplasms. Science 1990;250:1233.

82. Mulligan LM, Matlashewski GJ, Scrable HJ, et al. Mechanisms of p53 loss in human sarcomas. Proc Natl Acad Sci USA 1990;87:5863.

83. Donehower LA, Harvey M, Slagle BL, et al. Mice deficient for p53 are developmentally normal but susceptible to spontaneous tumors. Nature 1992;356:215.

84. Sturzbecher H, Brain R, Miamets T, et al. Mouse p53 blocks SV40 DNA replication in vitro and downregulates T antigen DNA helicase activity. Oncogene 1988;3:405.

85. Finlay CA, Hinds PW, Levine AJ. The p53 proto-oncogene can act as a suppressor of transformation. Cell 1989;57:1083.

86. Eliyahu D, Michalovitz D, Eliyahu S, et al. Wild-type p53 can inhibit oncogene-mediated focus formation. Proc Natl Acad Sci USA 1989;86:8763.

87. Steinmeyer K, Deppert W. DNA binding properties of muring p53. Oncogene 1988;3:501.

88. Kern SE, Kinzler KW, Bruskin A, et al. Sequence-specific binding of p53 to DNA. Science 1991;252:1708.

89. Friedman PN, Kern SE, Vogelstein B, et al. Wild-type, but not mutant, human p53 proteins inhibit the replication activities of simian virus 40 large tumor antigen. Proc Natl Acad Sci USA 1990;87:9275.

90. Baker SJ, Markowitz S, Fearon ER, et al. Suppression of human colorectal carcinoma cell growth by wild-type p53. Science 1990;249:912.

91. Yonish-Rouach E, Resnitsky D, Lotem J, et al. Wild-type p53 induces apoptosis of myeloid leukaemic cells that is inhibited by interleukin-6. Nature 1991;352:345.

92. Ginsberg D, Michael-Michalovitz D, Ginsberg D, et al. Induction of growth arrest by a temperature-sensitive p53 mutant is correlated with increased nuclear localization and decreased stability of the protein. Mol Cell Biol 1991;11:582.

93. Lane DP, Crawford LV. T-antigen is bound to host protein in SV40-transformed cells. Nature 1979;278:261.

94. Sarnow P, Ho YS, Williams J, et al. Adenovirus E1b—58-kd tumor antigen and SV40 large tumor antigen are physically associated with the same 54-kd cellular protein in transformed cells. Cell 1982;28:387.

95. Werness BA, Levine AJ, Howley PM. Association of human papillomavirus types 16 and 18 E6 proteins with p53. Science 1990;248:76.

96. Anderson SR, Geertinger P, Larsen H-W, et al. Aniridia, cataract and gonadoblastoma in a mentally retarded girl with deletion of chromosome 11: A clinicopathological case report. Ophthalmologica 1978;176:171.

97. Riccardi VM, Sujansky E, Smith AC, et al. Chromosomal imbalance in the aniridia-Wilms' tumor association: 11p interstitial deletion. Pediatrics 1978;61:604.

98. Moore JW, Hyman S, Antonarakis SE, et al. Familial isolated aniridia associated with a translocation involving chromosomes 11 and 22 [t(11;22) p13;q12.2)]. Hum Genet 1986;72:297.

99. Waziri M, Patil SR, Hanson JW, et al. Abnormality of chromosome 11 in patients with features of Beckwith-Wiedemann syndrome. J Pediatr 1983;102:873.

100. Koufos A, Hansen MF, Copeland NG, et al. Loss of heterozygosity in three embryonal tumours suggests a common pathogenetic mechanism. Nature 1985;316:330.

101. Koufos A, Grundy P, Morgan K, et al. Familial Wiedemann-Beckwith syndrome and a second Wilms tumor locus both map to 11p15.5. Am J Hum Genet 1989;44:711.

102. Meadows AT, Lichtenfeld JL, Koop CE. Wilms' tumor in three children of a woman with congenital hemihypertrophy. N Engl J Med 1974;291:23.

103. Gardner LI. Pseudo-Beckwith-Wiedemann syndrome: Interaction with maternal diabetes. Lancet [Letter] 1973;2:911.

104. Beckwith JB, Kiviat NB, Bonadio JF. Nephrogenic rests, nephroblastomatosis, and the pathogenesis of Wilms' tumor. Pediatr Pathol 1990;10:1.

105. Pelletier J, Bruening W, Li FP, et al. *WT1* mutations contribute to abnormal genital system development and hereditary Wilms' tumour. Nature 1991;353:431.

106. Rose EA, Glaser T, Jones C, et al. Complete physical map of the WAGR region of 11p13 localizes a candidate Wilms' tumor gene. Cell 1990;60:495.

107. Call KM, Glaser T, Ito CY, et al. Isolation and characterization of a zinc finger polypeptide gene in the human chromosome 11 Wilms' tumor locus. Cell 1990;60:509.

108. Haber DA, Buckler AJ, Glaser T, et al. An internal deletion within an 11p13 zinc finger gene contributes to the development of Wilms' tumor. Cell 1990;61:1257.

109. Rauscher FJ III, Morris JF, Tournay, OE, et al. Binding of the Wilms' tumor locus zinc finger protein to the EGR-1 consensus sequence. Science 1990;250:1259.

110. Lemaire P, Vesque C, Schmitt J, et al. The serum-inducible mouse gene *Krox*-24 encodes a sequence-specific transcriptional activator. Mol Cell Biol 1990;10:3456.

111. Madden SL, Cook DM, Morris JF, et al. Transcriptional repression mediated by the WT1 Wilms tumor gene product. Science 1991;253:1550.

112. Weissman BE, Saxon PJ, Pasquale SR, et al. Introduction of a normal human chromosome 11 into a Wilms' tumor cell line controls its tumorigenic expression. Science 1987;236:175.

113. Dowdy SF, Fasching CL, Araujo D, et al. Suppression of tumorigenicity in Wilms' tumor by the p15.5-p14 region of chromosome 11. Science 1991;254:293.

114. Goldgar DE, Green P, Parry DM, et al. Multipoint linkage analysis in neurofibromatosis type 1: An international collaboration. Am J Hum Genet 1989;44:6.

115. Ledbetter DH, Rich DC, O'Connell P, et al. Precise localization of NF1 to 17q11.2 by balanced translocation. Am J Hum Genet 1989;44:20.

116. Wallace, MR, Marchuk DA, Andersen LB. Type 1 neurofibromatosis gene: Identification of a large transcript disrupted in three NF1 patients. Science 1990;249:181.

117. Buchberg AM, Bedigian HG, Jenkins NA, et al. EVI-2, a common integration site involved in murine myeloid leukemogenesis. Mol Cell Biol 1990;10:465B.

118. Korf B. Launching the gene for neurofibromatosis 1. Neurofibromatosis Res Newslett 1990;7:1.

119. Tanaka K, Nakafuku M, Satoh T, et al. *S. cerevisiae* genes *IRA1* and *IRA2* encode proteins that may be functionally equivalent to mammalian *RAS* GTPase activating protein. Cell 1990;60:803.

120. Buchberg AM, Cleveland LS, Jenkins NA, et al. Sequence homology shared by neurofibromatosis type-1 gene and IRA-1 and IRA-2 negative regulators of the RAS cyclic AMP pathway. Nature 1990;347:291.

121. Hall A. The cellular functions of small GTP-binding proteins. Science 1990;249:635.

122. Wigler M. GAPs in understanding RAS. Nature 1990;346:696.

123. Lowy DR, Zhang K, Declue JE. Regulation of p21[MD30]RAS activity. Trends Genet 1991;7:346.

124. McCormick F. *RAS* GTPase activating protein: signal transmitter and signal terminator. Cell 1989;56:5.

125. Xu G, Lin B, Tanaka K, et al. The catalytic domain of the neurofibromatosis type 1 gene product stimulates *RAS* GTPase and complements *IRA* mutants of *S. cerevisiae.* Cell 1990;63:835.

126. Ballester R, Marchuk D, Boguski M, et al. The NF1 locus encodes a protein functionally related to mammalian GAP and yeast IRA proteins. Cell 1990;63:851.

127. Menon AG, Anderson KM, Riccardi VM, et al. Chromosome 17p deletions and p53 gene mutations associated with the formation of malignant neurofibrosarcomas in von Recklinghausen neurofibromatosis. Proc Natl Acad Sci USA 1990;87:5435.

128. Nakamura Y, Lathrop M, Leppert M, et al. Localization of the genetic defect in familial adenomatous polyposis within a small region of chromosome 5. Am J Hum Genet 1988;43:638.

129. Herrera L, Kakati S, Gibas L, et al. Gardner syndrome in a man with an interstitial deletion of 5q. Am J Med Genet 1986;25:473.

130. Vogelstein B, Fearon ER, Hamilton SR, et al. Genetic alterations during colorectal tumor development. N Engl J Med 1988;319:525.

131. Kinzler KW, Nilbert MC, Su LK, et al. Identification of FAP locus genes from chromosome 5q21. Science 1991;253:661.

132. Groden J, Thliveris A, Samowitz W, et al. Identification and characterization of the familial adenomatous polyposis coli gene. Cell 1991;66:589.

133. Kinzler KW, Nilbert MC, Vogelstein B, et al. Identification of a gene located at chromosome 5q21 that is mutated in colorectal cancers. Science 1991;251:1366.

134. Peifer M, Weischaus E. The segment polarity gene *armadillo* encodes a functionally modular protein that is the *Drosphila* homolog of human plakoglobin. Cell 1990;63:1167.

135. Fukui Y, Miyake S, Satoh M, et al. Characterization of the *Schizosaccharomyces pombe* *RA12* gene implicated in activation of the RAS1 gene product. Mol Cell Biol 1989;9:5617.

136. Bourne HR. Colon cancer. Consider the coiled coil. Nature 1991;351:188.

137. Baker SJ, Fearon ER, Nigro JM, et al. Chromosome 17 deletions and p53 gene mutations in colorectal carcinomas. Science 1989;244:217.

138. Chen L-C, Neubauer A, Kurisu W, et al. Loss of heterozygosity on the short arm of chromosome 17 is associated with high proliferative capacity and DNA aneuploidy in primary human breast cancer. Proc Natl Acad Sci USA 1991;88:3847.

139. Fearon ER, Vogelstein B. A genetic model for colorectal tumorigenesis. Cell 1990;61:759.

140. Fearon ER, Cho KR, Nigro JM, et al. Identification of a chromosome 18q gene that is altered in colorectal cancers. Science 1990;247:49.

141. Edelman GM. Morphoregulatory molecules. Biochemistry 1988;27:3533.

142. Shilo B-Z, Weinberg RA. DNA sequences homologous to vertebrate oncogenes are conserved in *Drosophila melanogaster*. Proc Natl Acad Sci USA 1981;78:6789.

143. Rijsewijk F, Schuermann M, Wagenaar E, et al. The *Drosophila* homolog of the mouse mammary oncogene *INT-1* is identical to the segment polarity gene *wingless*. Cell 1987;50:649.

144. Sokol S, Christian JL, Moon RT, et al. Injected *WNT* RNA induces a complete body axis in *Xenopus* embryos. Cell 1991;67:741.

145. McMahon AP, Bradley A. The *WNT-1* (*int-1*) proto-oncogene is required for development of a large region of the mouse brain. Cell 1990;62:1073.

146. Simon MA, Bowtell DDL, Dodson GS, et al. RAS1 and putative guanine nucleotide exchange factor perform crucial steps in signalling by the sevenless protein tyrosine kinase. Cell 1991;67:701.

147. Greenwald I, Broach JR. Cell fates in *C. elegans*: In medias *RAS*. Cell 1990;63:1113.

148. Cross M, Dexter TM. Growth factors in development, transformation, and tumorigenesis. Cell 1991;64:271.

149. Doolittle RF, Hunkapiller MW, Hood LE, et al. Simian sarcoma virus *ONC* gene, v-*SIS*, is derived from the gene (or genes) encoding a platelet-derived growth factor. Science 1983;221:275.

150. Cantley, LC, Auger K, Carpenter C. Oncogenes and signal transduction. Cell 1991;64:281.

151. Bishop JM. The molecular genetics of cancer. Science 1987;235:305.

152. Bishop JM. Oncogenes and clinical cancer. In: Weinberg RA, ed. Oncogenes and the molecular origins of cancer. Cold Spring Harbor, NY: Cold Spring Harbor Laboratory Press, 1989;327.

153. Bishop JM. Molecular themes in carcinogenesis. Cell 1991;64:235.

154. Rosen EM, Meromsky L, Setter E. Smooth muscle-derived factor stimulates mobility of human tumor cells. Invasion Metastasis 1990;10:49.

155. Weidner KM, Behrens J, Vandekerckhove J. Scatter factor: Molecular characteristics and effect on the invasiveness of epithelial cells. J Cell Biol 1990;111:2097.

156. Eva A, Robbins KC, Andersen PR, et al. Cellular genes analogous to retroviral *ONC* genes are transcribed in human tumour cells. Nature 1982;295:116.

157. Carpenter G, Cohen S. Epidermal growth factor. Ann Rev Biochem 1979;48:193.

158. Dickson C, Peters G. Potential oncogene product related to growth factors. Nature 1987;326:833.

159. Kaplan DR, Hempstead B, Martin-Zanace D, et al. The *TRK* proto-oncogene product: A signal transducing receptor for nerve growth factor. Science 1991;252:554.

160. Bottaro DP, Rubin JS, Faletto DL, et al. Identification of the hepatocyte growth factor receptor as the c-*MET* proto-oncogene product. Science 1991;251:802.

161. Weidner, KM, Arakaki N, Hartmann G. Evidence for the identity of human scatter factor and human hepatocyte growth factor. Proc Natl Acad Sci USA 1991;88:7001.

162. Hanks SK. Eukaryotic protein kinases. Curr Opin Struc Biol 1991;1:369.

163. Graziadei L, Riabowol K, Bar-Sagi D. Co-capping of *RAS* proteins with surface immunoglobins in B lymphocytes. Nature 1990;347:396.

164. Aaronson SA. Growth factors and cancer. Science 1991;254:1146.

165. Majeras PW, Ross TS, Cunningham TW, et al. Recent insights in phosphatidylinositol signaling. Cell 1990;63:459.

166. Zhang K, DeClue JE, Vass WC. Suppression of c-*RAS* transformation by GTPase-activating protein. Nature 1990;346:754.

167. Maruta H, Holden J, Sizeland A, et al. The residues of RAS and RAP proteins that determine their GAP specificities. J Biol Chem 1991;266:11661.

168. Downward J, Graves JD, Warne PH. Stimulation of p21[MD30]RAS upon T-cell activation. Nature 1990;346:719.

169. Yatani A, Okabe K, Polakis P. RAS p21 and GAP inhibit coupling of muscarinic receptors to atrial K⁺ channels. Cell 1990;61:769.

170. Bar-Sagi D, Feramisco JR. Microinjection of the *RAS* oncogene protein into PC12 cells induces morphological differentiation. Cell 1985;42:841.

171. Lewin B. Oncogenic conversion by regulatory changes in transcription factors. Cell 1991;64:303.

172. Morrison DK. The Raf-1 kinase as a transducer of mitogenic signals. Cancer Cells 1990;2:377.

173. Rapp UR, Goldsborough MD, Mark, GE. Structure and biological activity of v-*RAF*, a unique oncogene transduced by a retrovirus. Proc Natl Acad Sci USA 1983;80:4218.

174. Morrison DK, Kaplan DR, Escobedo JA. Direct activation of the serine/threonine kinase activity of Raf-1 through tyrosine phosphorylation by the PDGF β-receptor. Cell 1989;58:649.

175. Lee R-M, Rapp UR, Blackshear PJ. Evidence for one or more Raf-1 kinase(s) activated by insulin and polypeptide growth factors. J Biol Chem 1991;266:10351.

176. Troppmair J, Bruder JT, App H, et al. RAS controls coupling of growth factor receptors and protein kinase C in the membrane to Raf1 and B-Raf protein serine kinases in the cytosol. Oncogene (in press).

177. Bruder JT, Heideker G, Rapp UR. Serum, TPA, and RAS-induced expression from AP-1/ETS-driven promoters requires c-Raf-1 kinase. Genes Dev 1992;6:545.

178. Nishizuka Y. Studies and perspectives on protein kinase C. Science 1986;233:305.

179. Ghosh S, Baltimore D. Activation in vitro of NF-κB by phosphorylation of its inhibitor 1κB. Nature 1990;344:678.

180. Casey PJ, Solski PA, Der CJ, et al. p21[MD30]RAS is modified by a farnesyl isoprenoid. Proc Natl Acad Sci USA 1989;86:8323.

181. Glomset JA, Gelb MH, Farnsworth CC. Prenyl proteins in eukaryotic cells: A new type of membrane anchor. Trends Biochem Sci 1990;15:139.

182. Chen WJ, Andres DA, Goldstein JL. cDNA cloning and expression of the peptide-binding β subunit of rat p21[MD30]RAS farnesyltransferase, the counterpart of yeast DPR1/RAM1. Cell 1991;66:327.

183. Schafer WR, Trueblood CE, Yang CC, et al. Enzymatic coupling of cholesterol intermediates to a mating pheromone precursor and to the RAS protein. Science 1990;249:1133.

184. Reiss Y, Goldstein, JL, Seabra MC. Inhibition of purified p21[MD30]RAS farnesyl: Protein transferase by Cys-AAX tetrapeptides. Cell 1990;62:81.

185. Seabra MC, Reiss Y, Casey PJ, et al. Protein farnesyltransferase and geranylgeranyltransferase share a common α subunit. Cell 1991;65:429.

186. Rubinfeld B, Munemitsu S, Clark R, et al. Molecular cloning of a GTPase activating protein specific for the K*REV*-1 protein p21[MD30]RAP1. Cell 1991;65:1033.

187. Garrett MD, Self AJ, vanOers C, et al. Identification of distinct cytoplasmic targets for RAS/R-RAS and RHO regulatory proteins. J Biol Chem 1989;264:10.

188. Bender A, Pringle JR. Multicopy suppression of the *CDC24* budding defect in yeast by CDC24 and three newly identified genes including the *RAS*-related gene *RSR1*. Proc Natl Acad Sci USA 1989;86:9976.

189. Hunter T. Cooperation between oncogenes. Cell 1991;64:249.

190. Greenberg ME, Ziff EB. Stimulation of mouse 3T3 cells induces transcription of the c-*FOS* oncogene. Nature 1984;311:433.

191. Pardee AB. G₁ events and regulation of cell proliferation. Science 1989;246:603.

192. Eisenman RN, Thompson CB. Oncogenes with potential nuclear function: *MYC*, *MYB*, and *FOS*. Cancer Surv 1986;5:309.

193. Prochowkni EV, Kukowska J. Deregulated expression of c-*MYC* by murine erythroleukemia cells prevents differentiation. Nature 1986;32:848.

194. Mitchell RL, Zokas L, Schreiber RD, et al. Rapid induction of the expression of proto-oncogene *FOS* during human monocytic differentiation. Cell 1985;40:209.

195. Distel RJ, Ro H-S, Rosen BS, et al. Nucleoprotein complexes that regulate gene expression in adipocyte differentiation: Direct participation of c-*FOS*. Cell 1987;49:835.

196. Baichwal VR, Tijan R. Control of c-*JUN* activity by interaction of a cell-specific inhibitor with regulatory domain δ: Differences between v- and c-*JUN*. Cell 1990;63:815.

197. Sap J, Munoz A, Damm K, et al. The v-*ERB*-A protein is a high affinity receptor for thyroid hormone. Nature 1986;324:635.

198. Frykberg L, Palmieri S, Beug H, et al. Transforming capacities of avian erythroblastosis virus mutants deleted in the v-*ERB*-A or *ERBB* oncogenes. Cell 1983;32:227.

199. Zenke M, Kahn P, Disela C, et al. v-*ERBA* specifically suppresses transcription of the avian erythrocyte anion transporter (band 3) gene. Cell 1988;52:107.

200. Beug H, Blundell P, Graf T. Reversibility of differentiation and proliferative capacity in avian myelomonocytic cells transformed by tsE26 leukemia virus. Genes Dev 1987;1:277.

201. Luscher B, Christenson E, Lichtfield DW, et al. *MYB* binding inhibited by phosphorylation at a site deleted during oncogenic activation. Nature 1989;344:517.

202. Vande Woude GF, Schulz N, Zhou R, et al. Cell cycle regulation, oncogenes, and antineoplastic drugs. In: JG Fortner, Rhoads JE, eds. Views of cancer research: General Motors Cancer Research Foundation. Philadelphia: JB Lippincott, 1990:128.

203. Lee M, Nurse P. Cell cycle control genes in fission yeast and mammalian cells. Trends Genet 1988;4:287.

204. Maller J. Personal communication.

205. Hartwell LH, Weinert TA. Checkpoints: Controls that ensure the order of cell cycle events. Science 1989;246:629.

206. Vande Woude GF, Gilden RV. Principles of cancer biology: The molecular biology of cancer. In: DeVita VT Jr, Hellman S, Rosenberg SA, eds. Cancer: Principles and practice of oncology, vol 2. Philadelphia: JB Lippincott, 1985:23–47.

207. Besmer P, Murphy JE, George PC, et al. A new acute transforming feline retrovirus and relationship of its oncogene v-*KIT* with the protein kinase gene family. Nature 1986;320:415.

208. Bargmann CI, Hung M-C, Weinberg RA. Multiple independent activations of the *NEU* oncogene by a point mutation altering the transmembrane domain of p185. Cell 1986;45:649.

209. Peters G, Brookes S, Smith R, et al. Tumorigenesis by mouse mammary tumor virus: Evidence for a common region for provirus integration in mammary tumors. Cell 1983;33:369.

210. Nau MM, Brooks BJ, Battey J, et al. L-*MYC*, a new *MYC*-related gene amplified and expressed in human small lung cancer. Nature 1985;318:69.

211. Maki Y, Bos TJ, Davis C, et al. Avian sarcoma virus 17 carries the *JUN* oncogene. Proc Natl Acad Sci USA 1987;84:2848.

212. Nusse R, Varmus HE. Many tumors induced by the mouse mammary tumor virus contain a provirus integrated in the same region of the host genome. Cell 1982;31:99.

213. Park M, Vande Woude GF. Principles of molecular cell biology of cancer: Oncogenes. In: DeVita VT Jr, Hellman S, Rosenberg SA, eds. Cancer: Principles and practice of oncology. 3rd ed. Philadelphia: JB Lippincott, 1989.

214. Solomon E, Borrow J, Goddard AD. Chromosome aberrations and cancer. Science 1991;254:1153.

215. Ellisen LW, Bird J, West DC. *TAN-1*, the human homolog of the *Drosphila Notch* gene is broken by chromosomal translocations in T lymphoblastic neoplasms. Cell 1991;66:649.

216. Tsujimoto Y, Ynis J, Onorato-Showe L, et al. Molecular cloning of the chromosomal breakpoint of B-cell lymphomas and leukemias with the t(11;14) chromosome translocation. Science 1984;224:1403.

217. Motokara T, Bloom T, Kim HG, et al. A novel cyclin encoded by a *BCL1*-linked candidate oncogene. Nature 1991;350:512.

218. Matsushime H, Roussel MF, Ashmun RA, et al. Colony-stimulating factor 1 regulates novel cyclins during the G_1 phase of the cell cycle. Cell 1991;65:701.

219. Wang J, Chenivesse X, Henglein B, et al. Hepatitis B virus integration in a cyclin A gene in a hepatocellular carcinoma. Nature 1990;343:555.

220. Lammie GA, Fantl V, Smith R, et al. D11S287, a putative oncogene on chromosome 11q13, is amplified and expressed in squamous cell and mammary carcinomas and linked to *BCL-1*. Oncogene 1991;6:439.

221. Xiong Y, Connolly T, Futcher B, et al. Human D-type cyclin. Cell 1991;65:691.

Cancer: Principles & Practice of Oncology, Fourth Edition,
edited by Vincent T. DeVita, Jr., Samuel Hellman, Steven A. Rosenberg.
J.B. Lippincott Co., Philadelphia © 1993.

Renato Baserga

CHAPTER 4

Principles of Molecular Cell Biology of Cancer: The Cell Cycle

Tissues and organs consist of populations of cells held together by intercellular substance that is secreted (*e.g.*, collagen). The growth of tissues and organs may occur by an increase in the number of cells, an increase in the size of cells, or both.[1] In animals, growth in number usually predominates over growth in size, although some growth in size also occurs during normal and abnormal growth. In *Homo sapiens*, growth in cell number is by far the most important component in development. An adult grows to an average of 10^{15} cells from a single fertilized egg. Although there is a threefold to fourfold increase in the size of cells from newborn to adult humans, most growth is due to an increase in cell number. After humans reach maturity, the number of cells remains essentially constant. However, even in adults, cell division continues at a brisk rate. Approximately 10^{12} cells die each day and must be replaced. Most of the cells that die come from tissues and organs like the gastrointestinal tract, skin, and bone marrow.

In the adult animal, the number of cells that are produced equals the number of cells that die. This simple equation is fundamental to our understanding of normal and abnormal growth. If the number of cells that are produced exceeds the number of cells that die in a given period of time, there is growth. If fewer cells are produced than die, the organ or tissue shrinks, producing atrophy, a negative form of growth that often occurs with disuse or old age.

THE CELL CYCLE

In every population of cells, there are three subpopulations (Fig. 4–1). The first group is cycling cells that continuously proliferate, going from one mitosis to the next one. The second is composed of terminally differentiated cells that irrevocably

leave the growth cycle and are destined to die without dividing again. A third subpopulation of nondividing cells are not cycling and do not divide but can reenter the cell cycle if an appropriate stimulus is applied (G_0 cells).[1] Fig. 4–1 also shows that cycling cells go through four different phases that are defined as G_1, S phase, G_2, and mitosis.

G_0 or quiescent cells are normally present in the living animal. In the adult liver, most of the cells are in G_0. However, if two thirds of the liver are surgically removed, the remaining liver cells quickly resume the cell cycle, proliferate, and restore the liver roughly to its original size. There are several other types of G_0 cells in the body. One that is of particular interest to medical oncologists is the stem cell of the bone marrow. These stem cells are capable of reproducing themselves and of producing all the different lineages of hemopoietic cells from lymphocytes to erythrocytes to megakaryocytes. Most of the bone marrow stem cells are in G_0, a fortunate occurrence because these cells are often protected from chemotherapeutic agents used to treat leukemia or metastatic cancer. The bone marrow depletion caused by chemotherapeutic agents stimulates the protected stem cells to reenter the cell cycle and eventually repopulate the bone marrow. The G_0 cells in cell populations help to optimize our therapeutic approaches. In tissue cultures, the G_0 state is achieved by restricting the availability of certain growth factors.

TUMOR GROWTH

Figure 4–1 reveals that any population of cells can grow in number by any one of three mechanisms: shortening the length of the cell cycle, resulting in more cells being produced

60

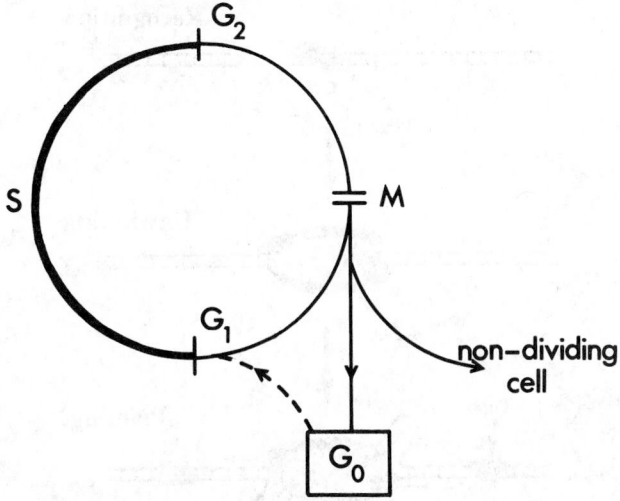

FIGURE 4–1. In the cell cycle, continuously dividing cells go from one mitosis (M) to the next, passing through G_1, S (DNA synthesis phase), and G_2. Some cells leave the cycle temporarily, entering a G_0 state from which they can be rescued by appropriate mitogenic stimuli. Other cells leave the cycle permanently, entering terminal differentiation.

per unit time; decreasing the rate of cell death; and moving G_0 cells into the cell cycle, again resulting in more cells produced per unit time. All three mechanisms operate in normal and abnormal growth. In tumors, there is sometimes a shortening of the cell cycle compared with normal cells, or there is an increase in the growth fraction (*i.e.*, fraction of proliferating cells) or a decrease in the rate of cell loss.[1]

In most tumors, all three mechanisms are important in determining the aggressiveness of the tumor, which is best characterized by its doubling time.[2] Steel summarized data from various sources on the doubling time of human tumors and their metastases.[3] They range from as little as 17 days for Ewing sarcoma to more than 600 days for certain adenocarcinomas of the colon and rectum. However, the fastest growing tumor is probably Burkitt's lymphoma, for which the clinical doubling time is 38 to 116 hours, with a mean of 66 hours, or less than 3 days. The doubling time is the real measure of aggressiveness of a tumor, providing a better index of aggressiveness than the mitotic index or the degree of anaplasia that are so dear to traditional pathologists.

GENE EXPRESSION AND CELL PROLIFERATION

Many genes are growth regulated, which means that there are genes whose steady-state mRNA levels increase when quiescent fibroblasts, lymphocytes, or other types of cells are stimulated to proliferate by growth factors or by any other mechanism. Several protooncogenes, including c-*MYC*, c-*FOS*, and c-*MYB*, are growth regulated, and because protooncogenes are in some way involved in the regulation of cellular proliferation, it has been assumed that growth-regulated genes are also growth regulatory and that they control cell proliferation. This is not true for three reasons. First, the expression of some growth-regulated genes and protooncogenes (*e.g.*, c-

FOS) is also induced in situations in which cell proliferation does not occur or is inhibited. Second, some exquisitely growth-regulated genes do not have any growth regulatory function. The best example is the thymidine kinase gene, which is growth regulated and yet is a dispensable gene that can be eliminated without affecting the growth of cells in culture or of certain animals, like the squirrel.

The third reason is somewhat more complicated. Cellular proliferation and the cell cycle are complex processes that require the correct expression of several genes and the appropriate modifications of many gene products. The function of gene products can be inhibited by the use of appropriate antibodies, or antisense RNA, or by exposing the cells to antisense oligodeoxynucleotides. Targeting these inhibitors to a variety of cellular RNAs or proteins like those of c-*RAS*, c-*MYC*, c-*FOS*, *CDC2*, c-*MYB*, and *PCNA* results in inhibition of cellular proliferation. This is not surprising. The *CDC2* and *PCNA* gene products, for instance, are both proteins necessary for DNA replication. If the production of these proteins is inhibited, DNA synthesis is inhibited, and cell proliferation will grind to a halt. Does that make *PCNA* and *CDC2* growth regulatory? The answer is yes or maybe, depending on the definition of growth regulatory. The products of the *PCNA* and *CDC2* genes are necessary for cellular proliferation, and in this context, they are growth regulatory. However, under this broad definition, many other gene products and cellular components are growth regulatory, including ATP and essential amino acids. There is nothing wrong in calling so many genes and molecules growth regulatory, except that by doing so the heuristic content of the word becomes almost trivial.

If an antibody or an antisense RNA or an antisense oligodeoxynucleotide targeted to an appropriate gene product blocks cell cycle progression, the targeted gene is said to be required for cellular proliferation. The term *growth regulatory* should be reserved only for those genes that actually regulate the extent of cellular proliferation, such as the ability to induce cellular proliferation in quiescent cells. Unfortunately, if we use this much stricter definition, cellular growth regulatory genes have not yet been identified. There are some viral gene products, such as the SV40 T antigen or the adenovirus E1A protein, that can cause quiescent mammalian cells to enter DNA synthesis and divide without addition of growth factors, but there is no single cellular gene that microinjected or transfected into quiescent cells causes them to divide.

There is substantial evidence that the molecular biology and the biochemistry of chromosomal replication and mitosis are essentially similar in all animal cells, but the expression of some genes important in cell proliferation is specific to cell types, and in the case of common genes required for cellular proliferation, the regulation of expression may differ from one cell type to another. For instance, the expression of c-*MYB* is necessary for the entry of hemopoietic cells into S phase, but c-*MYB* is not expressed in most fibroblasts and epithelial cells, in which its function is probably taken over by similar but different genes. Hemopoietic cells use some growth factor receptors that are different from the growth factor receptors used by fibroblasts or epithelial cells. In other cases, the genes are the same but the way in which they are regulated differs. Differences among different cell types should not be underestimated, because they are probably the basis of some differential responses to chemotherapeutic agents.

MOLECULAR BIOLOGY OF THE CELL CYCLE

The three fundamental components of the cell cycle are chromosomal replication (*i.e.*, S phase), doubling of the other cellular components (*i.e.*, doubling in size), and mitosis. Growth in size occurs throughout the cell cycle at a steady pace, but S phase and mitosis occur in discrete periods.[1] The all-or-none characteristic of S phase and mitosis and the fact that cellular proliferation is triggered by subtle changes in the environment (*e.g.*, small variations in the concentration of certain growth factors) define the cell cycle as a perfect example of a nonlinear chemical clock.

THE S PHASE

The replication of chromosomal DNA in mammalian cells is not completely understood, but considerable progress has been made by studying the replication of SV40 DNA, which, being a simple system, is more amenable to analysis. Several investigators have established in vitro systems capable of supporting the complete replication of plasmid DNA containing the SV40 origin of replication. Except for the requirement for the SV40 large T antigen, all other proteins involved in the replication reaction are of cellular origin. It is reasonable, therefore, to assume that the mechanism of SV40 DNA replication is fundamentally similar to that of cellular DNA replication.[5]

Several cellular proteins are necessary for SV40 DNA replication in vitro: DNA polymerase α-primase complex, topoisomerases I and II, replication protein A (RP-A), protein phosphatase 2A, PCNA, replication factor C (RF-C), and DNA polymerase δ. The model proposed for SV40 DNA replication by Kelly and coworkers is illustrated in Figure 4–2.[5] RP-A (also known as replication factor-A or RF-A) is a multisubunit cellular protein, which is required in step 2 and also functions as an auxiliary protein for DNA polymerases α and δ. It is phosphorylated at the G_1-S boundary and dephosphorylated at mitosis, providing a link between DNA replication and cell cycle-regulated protein phosphorylation.[6]

Cellular extracts from G_1 cells cannot support DNA replication in vitro, but extracts from S phase cells can. Roberts and coworkers have shown that the activation of DNA replication in S-phase extracts reflects the appearance at the G_1-S boundary of an essential cellular replication factor, called RF-S.[7] The human RF-S contains the homolog of *Schizosaccharomyces pombe* $p34^{cdc2}$ kinase, which is also required for mitosis and whose mechanism of action is described in that section. D'Urso and colleagues ". . . suggest that accumulation of a cyclin during G_1 leads to the activation of the p34 kinase at the start of S phase. DNA synthesis would begin when phosphorylation of specific replication proteins by the $p34^{cdc2}$ kinase promoted the formation of functional initiation complexes at chromosomal replication origins."[7]

The DNA building blocks, the deoxynucleotides, are also necessary for DNA replication, and the cell must synthesize them. All enzymes necessary for the synthesis of deoxynucleotides (*e.g.*, dihydrofolate reductase, thymidylate synthase, and so forth) are also necessary for entry into S and cellular proliferation. Chromosomal proteins (*e.g.*, histones and nonhistones) must also be synthesized to protect the integrity of

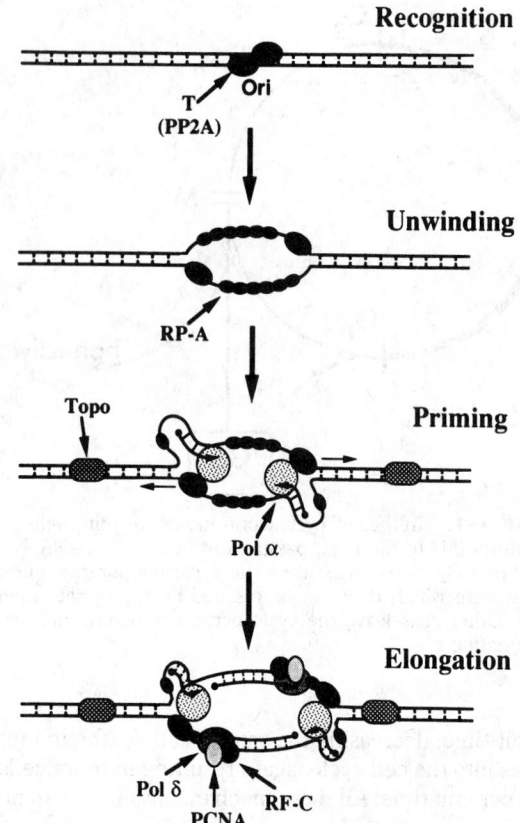

FIGURE 4–2.   In DNA replication, the first step is binding of T antigen to the origin of replication, which is facilitated by ATP. In the second step, T antigen catalyzes the unwinding of the duplex in a reaction that requires ATP and replication factor-A (RP-A) and is stimulated by phosphatase 2A. In the third step, short DNA chains are synthesized by the DNA polymerase α-primase complex, which is the only activity capable of starting de novo DNA synthesis. Elongation of DNA chains requires the topoisomerases, DNA polymerase δ, RF-C, and PCNA. (Weinberg DH, Collins KL, Simancek. Reconstitution of simian virus 40 DNA replication with purified proteins. Proc Natl Acad Sci USA 1990;87:6769–6771)

chromosomal structure and function. Not surprisingly, the inhibition of the synthesis of these proteins leads to a complete cessation of DNA replication.[1] The DNA synthesis genes and genes coding for enzymes required for the synthesis of the DNA building blocks are extremely sensitive to low concentrations of cycloheximide (an inhibitor for protein synthesis), indicating that their transcriptional activation depends on prior de novo protein synthesis.

MITOSIS

In eukaryotic cells, mitosis is initiated by the activation of the $p34^{cdc2}$ protein kinase, which in mammalian cells is the homolog of the yeast *START* gene, designated as *CDC2* in *S. pombe* and *CDC28* in *S. cerevisiae*. Given its central role, it is important to know how the $p34^{cdc2}$ is activated and how the $p34^{cdc2}$ kinase induces the biochemical and morphologic changes of mitosis. Two excellent reviews of this subject were written by Moreno and Nurse[8] and by Lewin.[9]

M phase is characterized by the activation of a kinase, known under various names (*e.g.*, maturation-promoting factor, histone H1 kinase), whose catalytic subunit is the *CDC2* gene product of *S. pombe* or its homolog in mammalian cells. The catalytic subunit is the CDC2 protein or its equivalent, and the regulatory subunits belong to the category of cyclins, which are a heterogenous group of proteins involved also in the G_1 to S transition. The activation of p34^{cdc2} for mitosis is a complex process, diagrammed in Figure 4–3.

After the p34^{cdc2} kinase is active, it phosphorylates substrates. The embarrassingly heterogenous list of possible targets includes histone H1, lamins, nucleolin, myosin light chain, pp60^{src}, SW 15 and T antigen, and probably others.[9] To these, Moreno and Nurse add RNA polymerase II, cyclin B, EF1β, and EF1γ, from which they deduce an amino acid consensus sequence for phosphorylation by p34: S/T-P-X-Z, where X is a polar amino acid and Z is usually a basic amino acid.[8] Notice that the phosphorylated residue can be serine or threonine. Moreno and Nurse give an attractive explanation for the presence of so many substrates; they implicated the many structural and functional changes that occur during mitosis.[8] Thus, phosphorylation of lamins (a component of the nuclear envelope) may alter coiled-coil interactions in lamin dimers and promote the dissolution of the nuclear membrane that characterizes mitosis. Histone H1 phosphorylation may change nucleosome packing leading to chromosome condensation, a feature that can be observed at the microscope. Phosphorylation of pp60^{src} may account for the cytoskeletal reorganization occurring at mitosis, and phosphorylation of

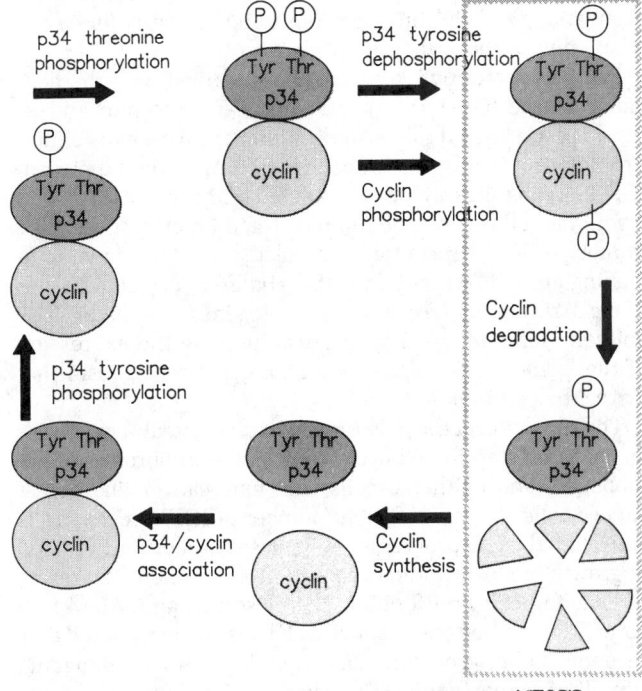

FIGURE 4–3. Mitotic activation of p34^{cdc2}. Activation of p34^{cdc2} involves threonine 167 phosphorylation and tyrosine 15 dephosphorylation of p34 and its association with a phosphorylated cyclin, which is proteolytically degraded, leaving the activated p34 kinase. After mitosis, cyclins are synthesized de novo, and the cyclin-p34 association leads to an inactive complex, in which the p34 subunit is phosphorylated on tyrosine 15, and the cycle repeats itself. (Lewin B. Driving the cell cycle: M phase kinase, its partners, and substrates. Cell 1990;61:549–551)

nucleolar proteins may provide the basis of nucleolus disassembly. Phosphorylation of RNA polymerase II and other DNA-binding proteins may be responsible for the inhibition of transcription during mitosis.

Although some of these explanations are still speculative, a picture of mitosis is clearly emerging, with the p34^{cdc2} kinase solidly in the center. On one side of it are the changes necessary for its activation, and on the other side, the structural and functional changes that p34^{cdc2} can cause by the phosphorylation of appropriate substrates. For a pathologist who started his scientific career looking at mitotic figures, it is thrilling to know that the complicated morphologic changes of mitosis are written in the language of molecular biology.

At least two protooncogenes, c-*MOS* and c-*RAS*, play an important role in the control of mitosis.[10] The mechanism of action of these two protooncogenes in mitosis is not yet known, but they seem to activate the p34-cyclin complex.

CONTROL OF CELLULAR PROLIFERATION: G_0 AND G_1

Some of the molecules involved in chromosomal replication and mitosis have been identified. They provide targets for inhibiting cellular proliferation. Antisense strategies or antibodies to these targets consistently arrest the cell cycle. However, if we adopt the strict definition of control of cell proliferation, these are not the genes or the gene products that decide whether the cell should divide. In the case of chromosomal replication, many of the genes coding for the proteins of the DNA-synthesizing apparatus are almost synchronously activated at the G_1-S boundary. Something regulates their expression, and it is this something that decides whether the cell should enter S phase, because without the products of these genes, there is no DNA synthesis. What is the delicate balance of positive and negative stimuli that results in the activation of the G_1-S boundary genes? Is there a candidate gene (or genes) that could be considered the activator of all these other genes?

There is a very promising candidate in budding yeast. DNA synthesis genes are periodically expressed in the yeast cell cycle. The upstream promoter sequences of all these genes have in common a palindromic hexamer element, ACGCGT, which Lowndes and associates[11] and Gordon and Campbell have shown capable of conferring cell cycle regulation of expression to heterologous genes.[12] Lowndes and colleagues also showed that a protein (which they called DSCI) binds to this hexamer, and that this protein is cell cycle regulated.[11] These are the same genes (*e.g.*, DNA polymerase genes, primase genes, *PCNA*, *CDC2*) that are induced at the G_1-S boundary in mammalian cells. In the immediate 5′ flanking sequences of the *PCNA* and DNA polymerase α genes of mammals, there are two repeats of a ACGCGG hexamer, whose homology to the yeast hexamer is striking.

The next step is to identify candidate genes for the DSCI protein and for those proteins that may cooperate with or regulate the expression of the mammalian counterpart of DSCI. Looking for candidates among growth-regulated genes is like looking for a needle in a haystack. The number of genes whose mRNA levels are growth regulated is very large.[13–15] Even allowing some overlap, it is clear that many genes may be required for cell proliferation but do not necessarily control it. Some of them (*e.g.*, c-*FOS*) are induced even in conditions that have nothing to do with cellular proliferation. However, we can make a distinction between early growth-regulated genes and late growth-regulated genes. As a rule, early growth-regulated genes (*e.g.*, c-*FOS*, c-*MYC*, c-*JUN*) are insensitive to cycloheximide even at high concentrations, indicating that de novo protein synthesis is not required for their activation. The expression of late growth-regulated genes (*e.g.*, thymidine kinase gene, DNA polymerase α gene, *PCNA*) is extremely sensitive to cycloheximide, even at concentrations that decrease cellular protein synthesis by only 30% to 40%.[15]

Because of the large number of genes whose expression increases in cells stimulated to proliferate, only a few genes, whose role in the control of cell proliferation is supported by substantial evidence are considered here. C-*MYC* is one of these genes.[16] Circumstantial evidence includes the fact that it is the cellular equivalent of a retroviral transforming gene, that it is induced by platelet-derived growth factor (PDGF) and other growth factors (*i.e.*, it is growth regulated), and that antisense oligodeoxynucleotides to c-*MYC* RNA inhibit cell proliferation. It is often rearranged or amplified in certain tumors, and if overexpressed in fibroblasts, it can abrogate the requirement for PDGF.[17,18] C-*MYC* can mimic all the sets of events that are induced by PDGF, one of two growth factors that are necessary and sufficient for the growth of fibroblasts. Another crucial gene is that for IGF-I; the IGF-I requirement can be abrogated by a constitutively expressed c-*MYB*, which suggested that c-*MYC* and c-*MYB* are the two genes required for the activation of the DNA synthesis genes.[19] It turns out, however, that c-*MYB* activates the genes for IGF-I and the IGF-I receptor, providing an example of autocrine stimulation. But this also raises again the question: how does the activation of the IGF-I receptor regulate the expression of the DNA synthesis genes?

THE ROLE OF CYCLINS
AND OF THE IGF-1 RECEPTOR

C-*MYC* and c-*MYB* certainly play a role in cell cycle progression, but it is obvious that several other oncogene products are involved in or can modify growth regulation. Hunter lists 51 protooncogene products.[20]

That oncogene products that are growth factors or growth factor receptors can modify the control of cellular proliferation makes sense. For instance, *ERBB*, in its truncated form as v-*ERB*, encodes a permanently activated epidermal growth factor (EGF) receptor, constantly transmitting a mitogenic signal. With transcription factors, the explanation is not so simple, but it still is reasonable. Transcription factors may activate cell cycle genes or genes whose products can neutralize the products of antiproliferative genes. A good example is c-*MYB*. It can activate transcription from the IGF-I and the IGF-I receptor genes, leading to autocrine stimulation and back to growth factors and their receptors.[19,21] Other oncogenes are involved in signal transduction, which is only a step removed from activated receptors. C-*MOS* is involved in the phosphorylation of cyclin B, which is required for mitosis and meiosis, and pp60[c-src] may also be involved in mitosis.

It is still not clear how some of the protooncogenes alter growth regulation. That they are required is acceptable, but

why would they stimulate cell division when overexpressed, amplified, or mutated? And why are there so many of them? The problem of too many oncogenes is the same as that of too many antioncogenes. If there is a single controlling event, how can so many different gene products bypass it? If multiple events are required, why are c-*MYB* and c-*MYC* enough to stimulate cell proliferation?

There are cyclins involved in the G₂ to M transition. In humans, two mitosis-associated cyclins have been cloned and sequenced: cyclin A and cyclin B. Cyclin A is identical to p60, a protein that associates with p34[cdc2] in interphase cells and with adenovirus E1A in transformed cells.[22] G₁ cyclins have limited but significant sequence similarities to mitotic cyclins. G₁ cyclins have been well characterized in yeast. Wittenberg and Reed said ". . . the most notable property of G₁ cyclins is that their accumulation or activation appears to be rate limiting for the execution of START."[23] START is the *CDC2*-*CDC28* regulated step. These proteins are encoded by three genes, *CLN1*, *CLN2*, and *CLN3*, which are redundant. Any two of the genes can be deleted without affecting cell growth, but the function of the remaining gene is essential. A human cDNA related to CLN-type cyclins was isolated by Xiong and colleagues and called cyclin D1.[24] It is overexpressed in glioblastoma cell lines and is identical to *PRAD1*, a gene overexpressed in parathyroid tumors and possibly related to the *BCL1* oncogene.[25] Two mouse cyclin-like genes, regulated by CSF-1 during the G₁ phase of the macrophage cell cycle have also been identified and cloned.[26] The role of cyclins in the control of the G₁-S transition is a key question in future investigation, and the first problem to be solved is finding at what point of the cell cycle they act.

Pardee's restriction point can be identified with the activation of the IGF-1 receptor.[27] The IGF-1 receptor and its ligand play a crucial role in determining the extent of cellular proliferation in a variety of cell types.[28] After the number of IGF-1 binding sites on the cellular membrane reaches a certain level, the cell can respond to IGF-1 and enter S phase. The number of IGF-1 receptors is regulated by many agents, including growth factors like PDGF and EGF, protooncogenes like c-*MYC* and c-*MYB*, and DNA oncogenes like the SV40 T antigen. Some of these agents also increase the expression of the ligand, IGF-1, creating an autocrine mechanism that drives the cell into S phase.

The activation of the IGF-1 receptor undoubtedly constitutes an essential step in cell cycle progression in fibroblasts, hemopoietic and epithelial cells, and lung cancer and breast cancer cells. After a sufficient number of IGF-1 receptors is activated, the cell progresses to S phase without further need of growth factors or unique copy gene expression.[27] In terms of enabling cell proliferation, the closest thing to the SV40 large T antigen or the adenovirus E1A is the activated IGF-1 receptor. Other growth factors (*e.g.*, PDGF, EGF, mitogenic stimuli of hemopoietic cells) require a functional IGF-1 receptor to stimulate cell proliferation, but an activated, overexpressed IGF-1 receptor does not need the activation of other receptors, such as the PDGF or EGF receptors.[28,29] The IGF-1 receptor is upstream of the onset of S phase and precedes and regulates the increase in mRNA levels of the DNA synthesis genes like the DNA polymerase α gene, thymidine kinase gene, *PCNA*, and *CDC2*.[30] It is downstream from c-*MYC*, other early growth-regulated genes, and c-*MYB*.

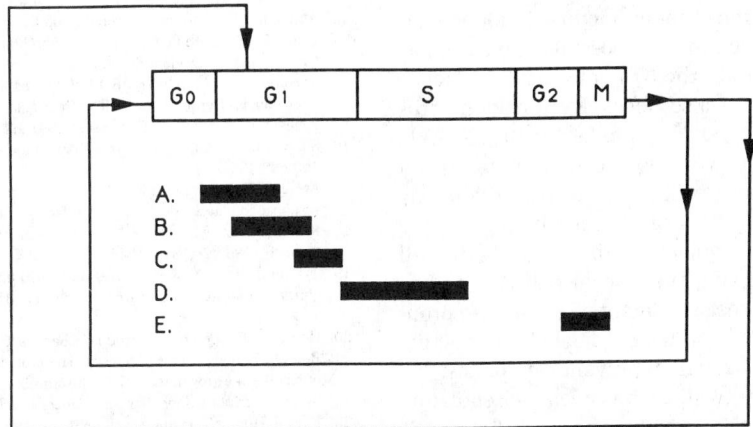

FIGURE 4–4. Cell cycle regulation of gene expression. The time of gene expression during the cell cycle (including G_0) is represented by the heavy lines. **(A)** Early growth-regulated genes (*i.e.*, a set of transcripts necessary for the G_0 to G_1 transition). Prototypes are c-*MYC* and c-*FOS*, but many others are known. **(B)** G_1 genes provide a set of transcripts necessary for cell cycle progression during G_1. Prototypes are ornithine decarboxylase, C-*MYB* and the mostly unknown genes complementing G_1-specific temperature-sensitive mutants of the cell cycle. **(C)** Genes at the restriction point (*i.e.*, genes necessary to pass through the restriction point). Prototypes are IGF1 and IGF1 receptor and the genes immediately controlled by the activation of the IGF1 receptor. It is not clear yet where G_1 cyclins fit, whether before or after the IGF1 receptor. **(D)** DNA synthesis genes provide all the genes required for chromosomal replication. Prototypes are DNA polymerases α and δ, CDC2, and PCNA. Antioncogenes, like the products of the p53 and *Rb* genes, could act at this point or between the activation of the IGF1 receptor and the transcription of the DNA synthesis genes. **(E)** Genes required for the S to M transition. Prototypes are p34^{cdc2} and associated cyclins A and B, and C-*MOS*.

The uncertain role of G_1 cyclins is emphasized in Figure 4–4, a schematic representation of gene expression during cell cycle progression in animal cells. Only a few representative key genes are given. Each of those areas is a target for therapeutic manipulations.

TUMOR SUPPRESSOR GENES

One way to slow cellular proliferation is to reduce the expression of genes whose products stimulate cell division. Another alternative is to increase the expression of genes or to increase the activity of gene products that suppress cellular proliferation. The latter alternative has gained ascendancy with the discovery of antioncogenes or tumor suppressor genes. These have been reviewed by Bishop[31] and by Marshall.[32]

The concept of tumor suppressor genes stems from a 30-year-old observation that hybrid cells generated by the fusion of tumorigenic and nontumorigenic cells are nontumorigenic, unless certain chromosomes are lost from the hybrids, which generate tumorigenic variants. The identification of tumor suppressor genes has depended on the study of certain human tumors, especially retinoblastoma and Wilms' tumor. Chromosomal deletions in these conditions have allowed isolation of genes that have an antiproliferative effect; the number of such genes have been rapidly expanding, and Table 4–1 gives a list of tumor suppressor genes and other factors that may exert an inhibitory effect on cellular proliferation.

We are concerned here only with how these genes may regulate cell cycle progression. The products of the *RB1* and p53 genes bind to viral oncogene proteins, such as the E1A transforming protein of adenovirus or the SV40 large T antigen.[33,34] These oncogenes may act by neutralizing the inhibitory effect of RB1 or p53 proteins. In cell cycle terms, researchers are looking for a cellular equivalent of E1A or T,

and the search is on for cellular proteins that bind to the p105-RB protein or to the p53 protein. Cyclin A has been shown to bind to E1A, and it seems that the *CDC2* kinase is part of the E1A-cyclin A complex.[35] The *NF1* antioncogene may exercise negative control over the RAS proteins.

There is ambiguity about how these genes may inhibit cellular proliferation. Bishop[31] and Marshall[32] point out that the RB1 and p53 gene products could be directly involved in DNA

TABLE 4–1. Genes With Antiproliferative Action

Inhibitory Gene or Factor	*Remarks*
RB1	Retinoblastoma gene; also deleted in osteosarcomas and other tumors
p53	P53 protein; binds oncogene products; deleted in some tumors
WT1	Wilms tumor
DCC	Carcinoma of the colon
NF1	Neurofibromatosis type I
FAP	Carcinoma of the colon
MEN1	Multiple endocrine neoplasias
Prohibitin	A cDNA clone capable of inhibiting cell proliferation
GAS genes	Growth-arrested genes, overexpressed in G_0 cells
C/EBP	CAAT-binding protein; inhibits cell proliferation
Statin	Overexpressed in growth-arrested and senescent cells

(Modified from Bishop JM. Molecular themes in oncogenesis. Cell 1991;64:235–248)

synthesis or indirectly as transcription factors. Evidence has been presented for both functions; it is possible that they may have a dual function. After all, the *NF1* transcription factor, a CCAAT binding protein, is also necessary for adenovirus DNA replication.[36] Another transcription factor, the CCAAT-enhancer binding protein (C/EBP), is also an inhibitor of cell proliferation, indicating that regulation of transcription may play both a positive and negative role in cell division.[37]

Growth in cell number is regulated by the length of the cell cycle, the growth fraction, and the rate of cell death. The wild-type p53 induces apoptosis; a mutant p53 loses the property of regulating cell death.[38] Another candidate for regulating the rate of cell death is *BCL2*, which prevents apoptosis.[39]

There are other attractive candidates as negative regulators of cell proliferation, like the growth-arrest-specific (GAS) genes, whose mRNAs are maximally expressed in G_0 cells, and prohibitin, whose mRNA inhibits entry into S phase.[40,41]

It is difficult to determine the extent of the role of antioncogenes in the cell cycle. Marshall, in his review, limited himself to comment on the peculiar fact that there are already multiple suppressor genes.[32] An unbiased perspective must await the discovery and definition of other antioncogenes and their products.

REFERENCES

1. Baserga R. The biology of cell reproduction. Cambridge, MA: Harvard University Press, 1985.
2. Bresciani F, Paoluzi R, Benassi M. Cell kinetics and growth of squamous cell carcinomas in man. Cancer Res. 1974;34:2405–2415.
3. Steel GG. Growth kinetics of tumors. Oxford: Clarendon Press, 1977.
4. Baserga R. The cell cycle: Myths and realities. Cancer Res 1990;50:6769–6771.
5. Weinberg DH, Collins KL, Simancek P. Reconstitution of simian virus 40 DNA replication with purified proteins. Proc Natl Acad Sci USA 1990;87:8692–8696.
6. Din S, Brill SJ, Fairman MSP, et al. Cell cycle-regulated phosphorylation of DNA replication factor A from human and yeast cells. Genes Dev 1990;4:968–977.
7. D'Urso G, Marraccino RL, Marshak DR, et al. Cell cycle control of DNA replication by a homologue from human cells of the p34^{cdc2} protein kinase. Science 1990;250:786–791.
8. Moreno S, Nurse P. Substrates for p34^{cdc2}: In vivo veritas? Cell 1990;61:549–551.
9. Lewin B. Driving the cell cycle: M phase kinase, its partners, and substrates. Cell 1990;61:743–752.
10. Daar I, Nebreda AR, Yew N, Sass P, Paules R, Santos E, Wigler M, Vande Woude GF. The *RAS* oncoprotein and M-phase activity. Science 1991;253:74–76.
11. Lowndes NF, Johnson AL, Johnston LH. Coordination of expression of DNA synthesis genes in budding yeast by a cell cycle regulated transcription factor. Nature 1991;350:247–250.
12. Gordon CB, Campbell JL. A cell cycle-responsive transcriptional control element and a negative control element in the gene encoding DNA polymerase α in *Saccharomyces cerevisiae*. Proc Natl Acad Sci USA 1991;88:6058–6062.
13. Almendral JM, Sommer D, MacDonald-Bravo H, et al. Complexity of the early genetic response to growth factors in mouse fibroblasts. Mol Cell Biol 1988;8:2140–2148.
14. Lau LF, Nathans D. Identification of a set of genes expressed during the G_0—G_1 transition of cultured mouse cells. EMBO J 1985;4:3145–3151.
15. Hofbauer R, Denhardt D. Cell cycle-regulated and proliferation stimulus-responsive genes. Eukaryotic Gene Expression 1991;1:247–300.
16. Studzinski GP. Oncogenes, growth and the cell cycle: An overview. Cell Tissue Kinet 1989;22:405–424.
17. Armelin HAM, Armelin MCS, Kelly K, et al. Functional role for c-*MYC* in mitogenic response to platelet-derived growth factor. Nature 1984;310:655–660.
18. Kaczmarek L, Hyland JK, Watt R, et al. Micro-injected c-*MYC* as a competence factor. Science 1985;228:1313–1315.
19. Travali S, Reiss K, Ferber A, et al. Constitutively expressed c-*MYB* abrogates the requirement for insulin-like growth factor I in 3T3 fibroblasts. Mol Cell Biol 1991;2:731–736.
20. Hunter T. Cooperation between oncogenes. Cell 1991;64:249–270.
21. Reiss K, Ferber A, Travali S, et al. The protooncogene c-*MYB* increases the expression of insulin-like growth factor I and insulin-like growth factor I receptor messenger RNAs by a transcriptional mechanism. Cancer Res 1991;51:5997–6000.
22. Pines J, Hunter T. Human cyclin A is adenovirus E1A associated protein 60 and behaves differently from cyclin B. Nature 1990;346:760–763.
23. Wittenberg C, Reed SL. Control of gene expression and the yeast cell cycle. Crit Rev Eukaryotic Gene Expression 1991;1:189–205.
24. Xiong X, Connolly T, Futcher B, et al. Human D-type cyclin. Cell 1991;65:691–699.
25. Motokura T, Bloom T, Kim HG, et al. A novel cyclin encoded by a *BLC-1*-linked candidate oncogene. Nature 1991;350:512–515.
26. Matsushime H, Roussel MF, Ashmun RA et al. Colony-stimulating factor 1 regulates novel cyclins during the G_1 phase of the cell cycle. Cell 1991;65:701–713.
27. Pardee AB. G_1 events and regulation of cell proliferation. Science 1989;246:603–608.
28. Baserga R. The IGF-1 receptor as the restriction point of the cell cycle. Ann NY Acad Sci (in press).
29. Pietrzkowski Z, Lammers R, Carpenter G, et al. Constitutive expression of IGF-1 and IGF-1 receptor abrogates all requirements for exogenous growth factors. Cell Growth Diff 1992;3:199–205.
30. Surmacz E, Nugent P, Pietrzkowksi Z, Baserga R. The role of the IGF-1 receptor in the regulation of *CDC2* mRNA in fibroblasts. Exp Cell Res 1992;199:275–278.
31. Bishop JM. Molecular themes in oncogenesis. Cell 1991;64:235–248.
32. Marshall CJ. Tumor suppressor genes. Cell 1991;64:313–326.
33. Whyte P, Buchkovich K, Horowitz JM, et al. Association between an oncogene and an antioncogene: The adenovirus E1A proteins bind to the retinoblastoma gene product. Nature 1988;334:124–129.
34. De Caprio JA, Ludlow JW, Figge J, et al. SV40 large tumor antigen forms a specific complex with the product of the retinoblastoma susceptibility gene. Cell 1988;54:275–283.
35. Pines J, Hunter T. Human cyclin A is adenovirus E1A-associated protein p60 and behaves differently from cyclin B. Nature 1990;346:760–763.
36. Jones KA, Kadonaga JT, Rosenfeld PJ, et al. A cellular DNA-binding protein that activates eukaryotic transcription and DNA replication. Cell 1987;48:79–89.
37. Umek RM, Friedman AD, McKnight SL. CCAAT-enhancer binding protein: A component of a differentiation switch. Science 1991;251:288–292.
38. Yonish-Rouach E, Resnitzky D, Loten J, et al. Wild-type p53 induces apoptosis of myeloid leukaemic cells that is inhibited by interleukin-6. Nature 1991;352:345–347.
39. Williams GT. Programmed cell death: Apoptosis and oncogenesis. Cell 1991;65:1097–1098.
40. Ciccarelli C, Philipson L, Sorrentino V. Regulation of expression of growth arrest-specific genes in mouse fibroblasts. Mol Cell Biol 1990;10:1525–1529.
41. Nuell MJ, Stewart DA, Walker L, et al. Prohibitin, an evolutionarily conserved intracellular protein that blocks DNA synthesis in normal fibroblasts and HeLa cells. Mol Cell Biol 1991;2:1372–1381.

Cancer: Principles & Practice of Oncology, Fourth Edition,
edited by Vincent T. DeVita, Jr., Samuel Hellman, Steven A. Rosenberg.
J.B. Lippincott Co., Philadelphia © 1993.

Janet D. Rowley
Felix Mitelman

CHAPTER **5**

Principles of Molecular Cell Biology of Cancer: Chromosome Abnormalities in Human Cancer and Leukemia

The association of specific chromosome abnormalities with particular types of human cancer has been established by investigators during the past decade. Many of the genes involved in consistent chromosome rearrangements, notably translocations but also deletions, have already been identified. For several of the rearrangements, some of the changes in gene structure and function have been defined, and several principles that may be applicable to all chromosome rearrangements in human malignant disease are beginning to emerge. It has been established that multiple genetic changes are usually required to transform a normal cell into a fully malignant cell (*e.g.*, colon cancer).

Detailed information about the relevant chromosome rearrangements is contained in several recent reviews, and only a summary is presented here.[1-7] The fourth edition of the Catalog of Chromosome Aberrations in Cancer has just been published.[8] A comparison of the number of abnormal karyotypes in the different editions of the catalogs according to the type of neoplasia is summarized in Figure 5–1. Although carcinomas account for the greatest proportion of malignant disease, they represent only about 20% of the karyotypic data; most information is available for leukemia and lymphoma.

Virtually all malignant tumors have an abnormal karyotype. Although studies of leukemia in the 1960s and early 1970s detected an abnormal karyotype in only about 50% of patients,

the use of improved techniques led to the identification of clonal abnormalities in at least 80% to 90% of patients.[9] Some malignant diseases, such as Hodgkin's disease or chronic lymphocytic leukemia, continue to show a high frequency of normal karyotypes or inadequate samples. These diseases are characterized by malignant cells with a low mitotic index, and it is likely that the dividing cells studied often do not represent the malignant cells. The use of fluorescence in situ hybridization techniques with appropriate probes in the analysis of interphase cells provides a new and powerful tool to overcome this impediment.

This discussion is restricted to clonal abnormalities, which are defined as at least two cells with the same extra chromosome or structural rearrangement or three cells with the same missing chromosome.[10]

CHROMOSOME NOMENCLATURE

The simplest change is a gain or loss of a whole chromosome. Common structural alterations are *translocations*, which involve the exchange of material between two or more chromosomes, *deletions*, which involve loss of DNA from a chromosome, and *inversions*, in which a single chromosome is broken in two places, and the central portion is inverted (Fig.

67

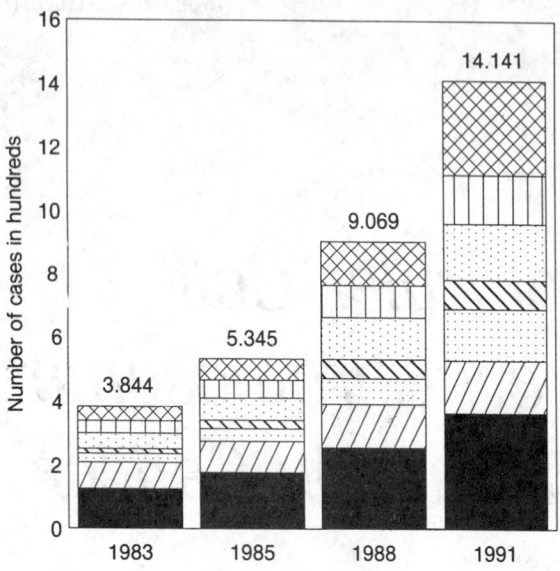

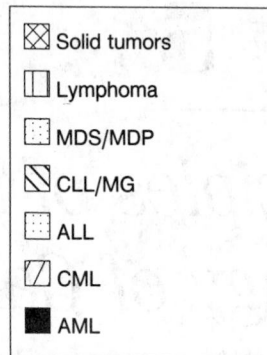

NUMBER OF ABNORMAL KARYOTYPES
MITELMAN'S CATALOG

FIGURE 5–1. Graph showing the proportion of abnormal karyotypes in the four catalogs by disease type. The number above the bar is the total number of abnormal karyotypes in each edition. Chronic myeloid leukemia patients with only a t(9;22) are not included.

5–2). International meetings during the last 30 years have established a universally accepted system for chromosome nomenclature.[10] The total chromosome number is followed by the sex chromosomes, and gains and losses of whole chromosomes are identified by a + or − before the chromosome number. A gain or loss of part of a chromosome is identified by a + or − after the chromosome number; p and q represent the short and long arm, respectively. Each chromosome band is numbered sequentially from the centromere. Translocations are indicated by t; the chromosomes involved are given in the first set of brackets and the breakpoints are given in the second set of brackets. Other abnormalities will be defined as they are described.

To be relevant to the malignant disease, chromosomes for analysis must be obtained from the tumor cells. For leukemia, bone marrow cells processed directly or after 1 to 3 days of culture are used; lymph nodes or solid tumors are minced to yield a cell suspension that can be harvested immediately or cultured for a short period of time.[11,12] The cells are exposed to a hypotonic solution, fixed, and stained according to a variety of protocols.

MYELOID DISORDERS

CHRONIC MYELOID LEUKEMIA

Chronic Phase

The first consistent chromosome abnormality in any malignant disease was identified in chronic myeloid leukemia (CML), and the analysis of CML has provided unique insights into leukemogenesis for the last 30 years. The Philadelphia or Ph chromosome was shown with banding to involve chromosome 22 (22q−).[13] The correct chromosome defect was shown to be a translocation involving chromosomes 9 and 22;

this was the first consistent translocation specifically associated with any human or animal disease (Fig. 5–3A).[14] Its reciprocal nature was established when the Abelson protooncogene, *ABL*, normally on chromosome 9, was identified on the Ph chromosome.[15] About 92% of Ph-positive patients with CML have the standard 9;22 translocation; the remainder have a complex translocation involving three or more different chromosomes, two of which are chromosomes 9 and 22.[16,17] Virtually all chromosomes have been involved in these variant translocations, but chromosome 17 is affected more often than are other chromosomes. The genetic consequences of the standard t(9;22) or the complex translocations involving at least three chromosomes is to move the *ABL* protooncogene on chromosome 9 next to a gene on chromosome 22, called *BCR*. The molecular analysis of the translocation has provided important information about the specific interactions of the two genes involved in the translocation.

Acute Phase

When patients with CML enter the terminal acute phase, most patients show additional chromosome abnormalities, resulting in cells with modal chromosome numbers of 47 to 50.[16] Different abnormal chromosomes occur singly or in combination in a distinctly nonrandom pattern, most commonly a second Ph, an isochromosome for the long arm of chromosome 17 [i(17q)], or a +8. Chromosome loss occurs only rarely; that most often seen is −7, which occurs in 3% of patients.[16]

Patients who have no prior history of CML are classified as having Ph-positive acute leukemia. Some Ph-positive ALL patients have a different breakpoint in *BCR*. In CML patients, the Ph chromosome is present in granulocytic, erythroid, and megakaryocytic cells, in some B cells, and probably in a few T cells.[17] In blast crisis, some blasts have intracytoplasmic

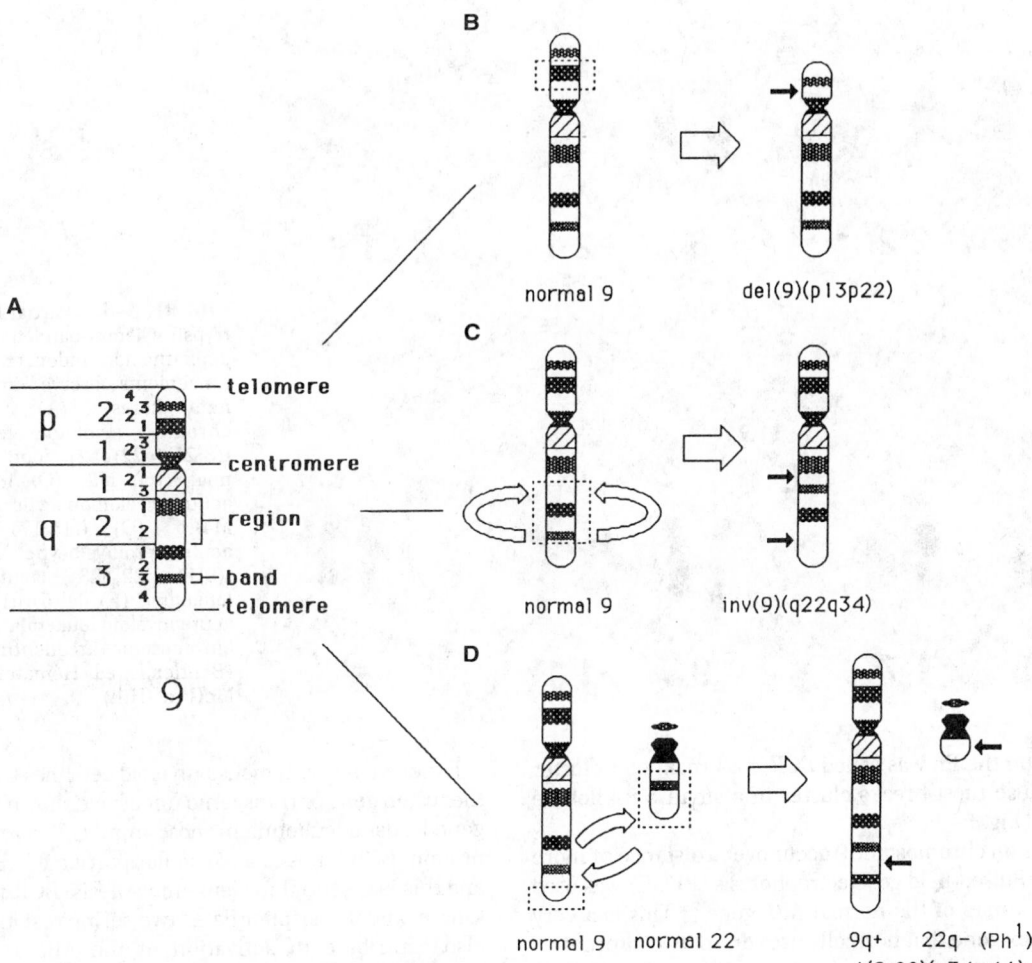

FIGURE 5–2. A normal chromosome and three chromosome abnormalities observed in human neoplasms. **(A)** Diagram of the banding pattern of a normal chromosome 9. The chromosome arms (p, short arm; q, long arm), regions, and band numbers are indicated on the left of the chromosome; specific chromosome structures are indicated on the right of the chromosome. **(B)** Diagram of the mechanism of an interstitial deletion of the short arm of chromosome 9, a common abnormality in acute lymphoblastic leukemia. Chromosome breaks occur in bands 9p13 and 9p22, and the intervening chromosome segment (band 9p21 and parts of bands 9p13 and 9p22) is lost [del(9)(p13p22)]. **(C)** Diagram of the mechanism of a paracentric inversion. Chromosome breaks occur in two bands within a single chromosome arm (in this case, in 9p22 and 9p34); the intervening segment is inverted, and the chromosome breaks are repaired [inv(9)(q22q34)]. **(D)** The mechanism of the reciprocal translocation involving chromosomes 9 and 22, t(9;22)(q34;q11), which gives rise to the Philadelphia (Ph) chromosome in the malignant cells of patients with chronic myeloid leukemia. Breaks occur in bands q34 and q11 of chromosomes 9 and 22, respectively, followed by a reciprocal exchange of chromosome material. This rearrangement results in the translation of the *ABL* oncogene, normally located at 9p34, adjacent to the *BCR* gene on chromosome 22, giving rise to a chimeric *BCR-ABL* gene, whose protein product plays a role in the transformation of hematopoietic cells. (Beutler E, ed. Hematology, New York: McGraw-Hill, 1990:79)

IgM, which is characteristic of pre-B cells, and these cells have an immunoglobulin gene rearrangement.[18]

Ph-negative Leukemia

Marrow cells from some patients thought to have CML appear to lack a Ph chromosome and usually have a normal karyotype. Somewhat surprisingly, the survival of these patients is substantially shorter than that of those whose cells are Ph-positive.[19] A review of the histology of 50 Ph-negative patients showed that most of them did not have CML, but they instead had some type of myelodysplasia, most commonly chronic myelomonocytic leukemia or refractory anemia with excess

blasts.[20,21] However, some patients with clinically typical CML who lack a Ph chromosome cytogenetically have evidence of the insertion of *ABL* sequences into the *BCR* gene, often as a consequence of complex cytogenetic rearrangements.[22,23] The proportion of all CML patients who fall into this category is not confirmed, but it may be 3% to 7%. It appears that the sine qua non of CML is the juxtaposition of *BCR* and *ABL*.

Molecular Analysis of the 9;22 Translocation

The *ABL* gene was first identified because of its homology to the viral oncogene that had been isolated from a mouse pre-B-cell leukemia. The breakpoint junction in CML was cloned,

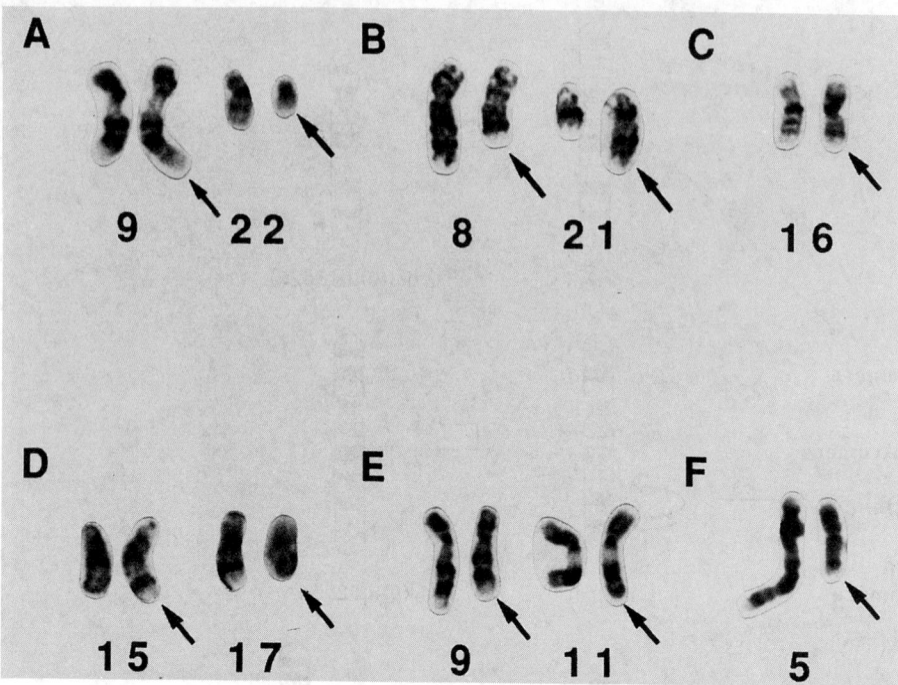

FIGURE 5–3. Partial karyotypes from trypsin-Giemsa-banded metaphase cells, depicting nonrandom chromosome rearrangements observed in myeloid malignant diseases. **(A)** t(9;22)(q34;q11), chronic myeloid leukemia. **(B)** t(8;21)(q22;q22), acute myeloid leukemia, type M2. **(C)** inv(16)(p13q22), acute myelomonocytic leukemia, type M4Eo. **(D)** t(15;17) (q22;q11–12), acute promyelocytic leukemia. **(E)** t(9;11)(p22;q23), acute monoblastic leukemia. **(F)** del(5)(q13q33) in T-cell acute myeloid leukemia. The rearranged chromosomes are identified with arrows. (Beutler E, ed. Hematology, New York: McGraw-Hill)

and the site on the Ph was called *BCR*, for breakpoint cluster region, because most breaks cluster in a small 5.8-kilobase (kb) region (Fig. 5–4).[24]

The breaks on chromosome 9 occur over a distance of more than 200 kb. Pulsed-field gel electrophoresis (PFGE) was used to construct a map of the normal *ABL* gene.[25] This is a very large, complex gene that normally uses one of two alternative beginnings, exon Ia or Ib. During transcription, either of these can be spliced at the same point on the remainder of the gene, which is called the common splice acceptor site or exon II. The breakpoints in the *ABL* gene of various CML patients and cell lines occur in many locations upstream (5′) of exon II. However, the same size (8.5 kb) mRNA is found in all CML patients; this occurs because the *BCR* exons are spliced to *ABL* exon II, resulting in a chimeric mRNA that is translated into a chimeric protein (p210 BCR-ABL).[26,27]

Experiments with mouse myeloid cell lines transfected with the fusion gene or transgenic mice have shown that the fusion gene leads to leukemia in most animals.[28,29] In the BCR-ABL protein, BCR binds to a particular portion of ABL called SH2, and this is essential for leukemogenesis. BCR is also a serine kinase, and it phosphorylates two serine residues in ABL that also contribute to activation of the ABL tyrosine kinase activity.[30]

The cloning of the translocation breakpoint has major implications for the diagnosis of CML and Ph-positive ALL and for monitoring patients during the course of their disease. The *BCR-ALL* fusion gene can be detected with standard Southern blot analysis or PFGE or with the polymerase chain reaction using appropriate primers.[31] In addition, fluorescence in situ hybridization can be used to detect the Ph chromosome in metaphase chromosomes and in interphase cells.[32,33]

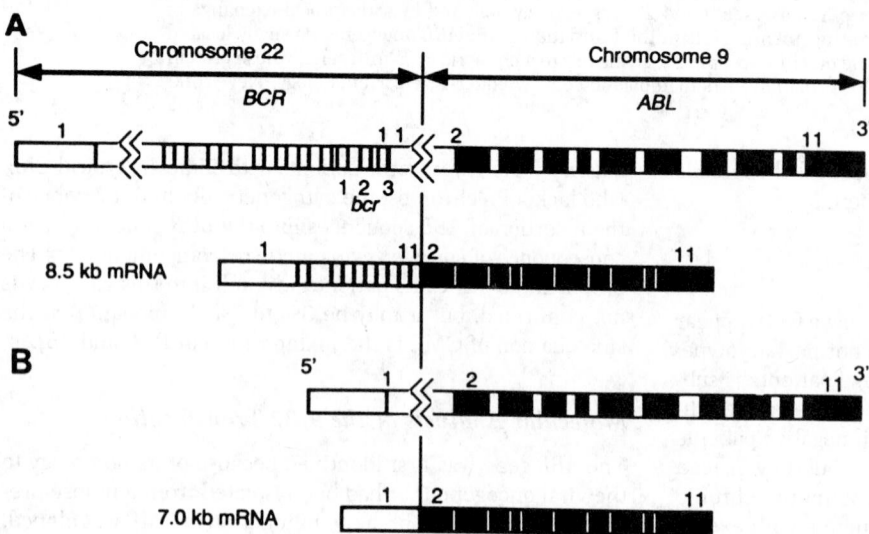

FIGURE 5–4. **(A)** Map of the *BCR-ABL* fusion gene in chronic myeloid leukemia (CML) and in some adult acute lymphoblastic leukemia (ALL) patients. In this example, the breakpoint has occurred between the third and fourth exons included in the BCR region, which are equivalent to exons 11 and 121 in the *BCR* gene. The chimeric mRNA is diagramed below the gene. **(B)** Map of the fusion gene in some ALL patients showing the breakpoint in the first intron of *BCR*. The breakpoint in *ABL* is identical to that in CML in this example. Because only one *BCR* exon is included, the mRNA is much smaller than in CML.

DE NOVO ACUTE MYELOID LEUKEMIA

Although it was possible by the late 1970s to show a close association between specific chromosome rearrangements and a particular subtype of acute myeloid leukemia (AML) as defined by the French-American-British Cooperative Group (FAB classification), the genes involved in these rearrangements are just now being identified.[34] The chromosome abnormalities associated with each subtype are listed in Table 5–1. The most frequent abnormalities are a gain of chromosome 8 and a loss of chromosome 7, which are seen in most subtypes of AML; the most characteristic structural aberrations are presented in the next sections.

The 8;21 Translocation

A translocation between chromosomes 8 and 21 (t[8;21] [q22;q22]) was first identified in 1973 (Fig. 5–3B).[35] It occurs in about 10% to 12% of adult AML patients.[16,36] The t(8;21), the most frequent abnormality in children with AML, is reported in 17% to 19% of karyotypically abnormal cases.[11,37]

The abnormality is usually restricted to patients with a diagnosis of AML-M2 (*i.e.*, acute myeloblastic leukemia with maturation), but a few patients are classified as having AML-M4.[36]

Chromosomes 8 and 21 can participate in three-way rearrangements similar to those involving chromosomes 9 and 22 in CML, and the t(8;21) is often accompanied by the loss of a sex chromosome. Among the cases reviewed at the Fourth International Workshop on Chromosomes in Leukemia and Lymphoma, 28 (85%) of 33 male patients had −Y, and 8 (67%) of 12 female patients had −X.[36] Although the significance is unclear, the *CSF2R* gene (formerly *GM-CSF*) for the receptor is located in the pseudoautosomal region of the X and Y chromosomes, which is the segment of the two chromosomes that is homologous and that pairs during meiosis.[38]

The translocation breakpoint has recently been cloned by two groups.[39,40] Little is known about the function of the genes on chromosome 8 or 21, but the translocation results in a fusion gene. Probes from the junction on chromosome 21 are already in use for fluorescence in situ hybridization.

TABLE 5–1. Nonrandom Chromosomal Abnormalities in Malignant Myeloid Diseases

Disease	Chromosomal Abnormality	Percent of Patients
CML	t(9;22)(q34;q11)	100
CML blast phase	t(9;22)(q34;q11) with +8, +Ph¹, +19, or i(17q)	70
AML-M2	t(8;21)(q22;q22)	18
APL-M3, M3V	t(15;17)(q22;q11–12)	60–100
AMMoL-M4Eo	inv(16)(p13q22) or t(16;16)(p13;q22)	100 (25% of M4)
AMoL-M4 or M5	t(1;11)(q21;q23)	
	t(2;11)(q21;q23)	
	t(6;11)(q27;q23)	
	t(10;11)(p11–p15;q23)	35
	ins(10;11)(p11;q23q24)	
	t(11;17)(q23;q25)	
	t(11;19)(q23;p13)	
	t(11q13 or q23), del(11)(q23)	
AMoL-M5	t(9;11)(q22;q23), t(11q13 or q23)	30
AML	+8	13
	−7 or del(7q)	9
	−5 or del(5q)	6
	t(6;9)(p23;q34)	2
	t(3;3)(q21;q26) or inv(3)(q21q26)	2
	del(20q)	5
	t(12p) or del(12p)	2
Therapy-related ANLL	−7 or del(7q) and/or −5 or del(5q)	90
	der(1)t(1;7)(p11;p11)	2
	t(3;21)(q26;q22)	1
	der(5)t(5;7)(q11;p11)	<1
	t(9;11)(p22;q23)	<1

* CML, chronic myelogenous leukemia; AML, acute myeloblastic leukemia; AML-M2, AML with maturation; AMMoL, acute myelomonocytic leukemia; AMMoL-M4Eo, acute myelomonocytic leukemia with abnormal eosinophils; AMoL, acute monoblastic leukemia; APL-M3, acute promyelocytic leukemia, hypergranular (M3) and microgranular (M3V); Ph¹, Philadelphia chromosome; ANLL, acute nonlymphocytic leukemia.

The 15;17 Translocation

A structural rearrangement involving chromosomes 15 and 17 in acute promyelocytic leukemia (APL) was first recognized in 1977 (Fig. 5–3D).[41] All of the 66 APL patients at the University of Chicago had the t(15;17); about 80% of APL patients with aberrations reported in the literature had t(15;17).[8] This rearrangement is unique to APL. Patients with an acute promyelocytic transformation of CML have a t(15;17) in addition to the t(9;22).

This translocation breakpoint has been cloned by four groups.[42,43] The affected gene on chromosome 17 is the retinoic acid receptor α (*RARA*), and the gene on chromosome 15 is called *PML*. The critical genetic rearrangement is on the derivative chromosome 15. The fusion gene formed consists of the 5′ portion of the *PML* gene and exon 3 and the remaining 3′ portions of the *RARA* gene, including its DNA binding and retinoic acid response elements. The *PML* gene also has segments that appear to be homologous to zinc fingers.[44]

Biondi and colleagues were able to detect rearrangements using probes from chromosomes 15 and 17 in all 26 APL patients, two of whom were cytogenetically "normal."[45] Because a fusion gene is formed, the polymerase chain reaction can also be used for diagnosis and monitoring of patients. Fluorescence in situ hybridization can be used to detect the rearrangement in metaphase and interphase cells (Color Fig. 5–5). The fact that *RARA* is involved in the translocation is especially interesting in view of the unique response of APL patients to retinoic acid derivatives.

The 6;9 Translocation

A translocation involving chromosomes 6 and 9 [t(6;9)(p23;q34)] was first described in two patients in 1976, but no common features were detected.[9] It occurs in about 2% of all AML patients. Review of slides from 9 patients with the t(6;9)

revealed that 8 of them had an increase in morphologically normal basophils in the bone marrow ranging from 1.5% to 12% (the normal value is 0.2%). Of the 9 patients, 5 were classified as M2, 3 as M4, and 1 as M1.[46] The same proportions were found in 16 patients analyzed in Rotterdam.[47]

Molecular Analysis of the t(6;9)

This breakpoint was cloned by Grosveld's laboratory and a fusion gene is formed. The gene on chromosome 9, named *CAN*, is about 300 kb telomeric from *ABL*; it is a large gene, greater than 230 kb, and codes for a 220-kd protein.[47] The breaks all occur in one intron between exons 3 and 4. The gene on chromosome 6, named *DEK*, is about 40 kb and codes for a 43-kd protein. The breaks also all occur within the same intron in *DEK*. Neither protein shows substantial homology to known protein sequences. The critical junction is on the derivative chromosome 6 with the formation of a *DEK-CAN* fusion gene and protein. The fusion gene appears to be invariant and therefore the polymerase chain reaction can be used to detect the translocation.

Aberrations of 11q23

The close association of translocations, or less often deletions, of the long arm of chromosome 11 (especially 11q23) and acute monoblastic leukemia (M5) was first observed by Berger et al (Fig. 5–3E).[48] Abnormalities of 11q occurred most frequently in monoblastic leukemia in children (75%) and less often in adults (30%). About 22% of patients with M5 leukemia had an aberration involving 11q; 25% of these patients were younger than 1 year of age, and another 25% were younger than 20 years of age.[36] Although the other chromosome involved in the translocation varies, a t(9;11)(p22;q23) is common.[49]

The breakpoint has been identified in four translocations involving 11q23: t(9;11), t(6;11), t(11;19), and t(4;11) in

COLOR FIGURE 5–5. In situ hybridization of DNA probes to metaphase chromosomes and interphase cells from normal and leukemic samples. Panels A through I illustrate the use of DNA probes labeled with biotin or digoxygenin and detected with FITC-conjugated avidin (green-yellow signal) or rhodamine-conjugated antidigoxygenin (red signal). The left photographs in A and in C through I illustrate material stained with DAPI to visualize the same cells or chromosomes on the right that have been labeled with various DNA probes detected with various fluorochromes. **(A)** Normal cells hybridized with α satellite probes to the centromere of chromosomes 7 (FITC) and 8 (rhodamine). There are two green signals and two red signals in each cell. **(B)** Interphase cell from a patient with chronic lymphoblastic leukemia probed with an α satellite probe for the centromere of chromosome 12. The trisomy 12 is easily detected; the cell has been counterstained with ethidium bromide. **(C)** Metaphase chromosomes and **(D)** interphase cell from an acute myeloid leukemia patient with trisomy 11. The α satellite probes for the centromeres of 8, 9, or 11 are detected with rhodamine (*arrow*), mixture of rhodamine and FITC (*long arrow*), or FITC (*arrowhead*), respectively. **(E–H)** Metaphase cells from leukemic samples probed with chromosome-specific DNA libraries to detect a variety of structural abnormalities. **(E)** Chromosome 1 library detects the two normal chromosomes and the long arm of chromosome 1 translocated to chromosome 6 [dic(1;6)(p13;p22)] at 9 o'clock. **(F)** Use of a chromosome 4 library can identify structurally rearranged chromosomes in a metaphase cell with very poor morphology. The probe identifies the normal 4 (*center*), deleted 4q (*top*), and t(4;13)(q25;p13) (*bottom*). **(G)** The use of a chromosome 8 probe clarified the abnormality in this sample (initially −8,+mar). The normal 8 (*left*) and an isochromosome 8q (*right*) leading to trisomy for 8q were identified. **(H)** The use of a chromosome 7 library identified an unknown marker (*left*) as a del(7q) in a patient initially karyotyped as −7,+mar. The normal 7 is at the bottom. **(I)** Interphase cell from a patient with acute promyelocytic leukemia and the t(15;17). Cosmid probes from chromosomes 15 distal to the breakpoint (detected with FITC) and 17 proximal to the breakpoint (detected with rhodamine and Texas red) identify the normal chromosomes 15 (*upper center left*) and 17 (*lower*) and the orange fusion signal of the der(17) chromosome (*center*). **(J)** Use of chromogenic detection and light microscopy. (*Left*) A normal metaphase cell hybridized with a chromosome 17 centromere probe that was biotinylated and finally detected with horseradish peroxidase. (*Right*) A cosmid probe on 15q also detected with horseradish peroxidase.

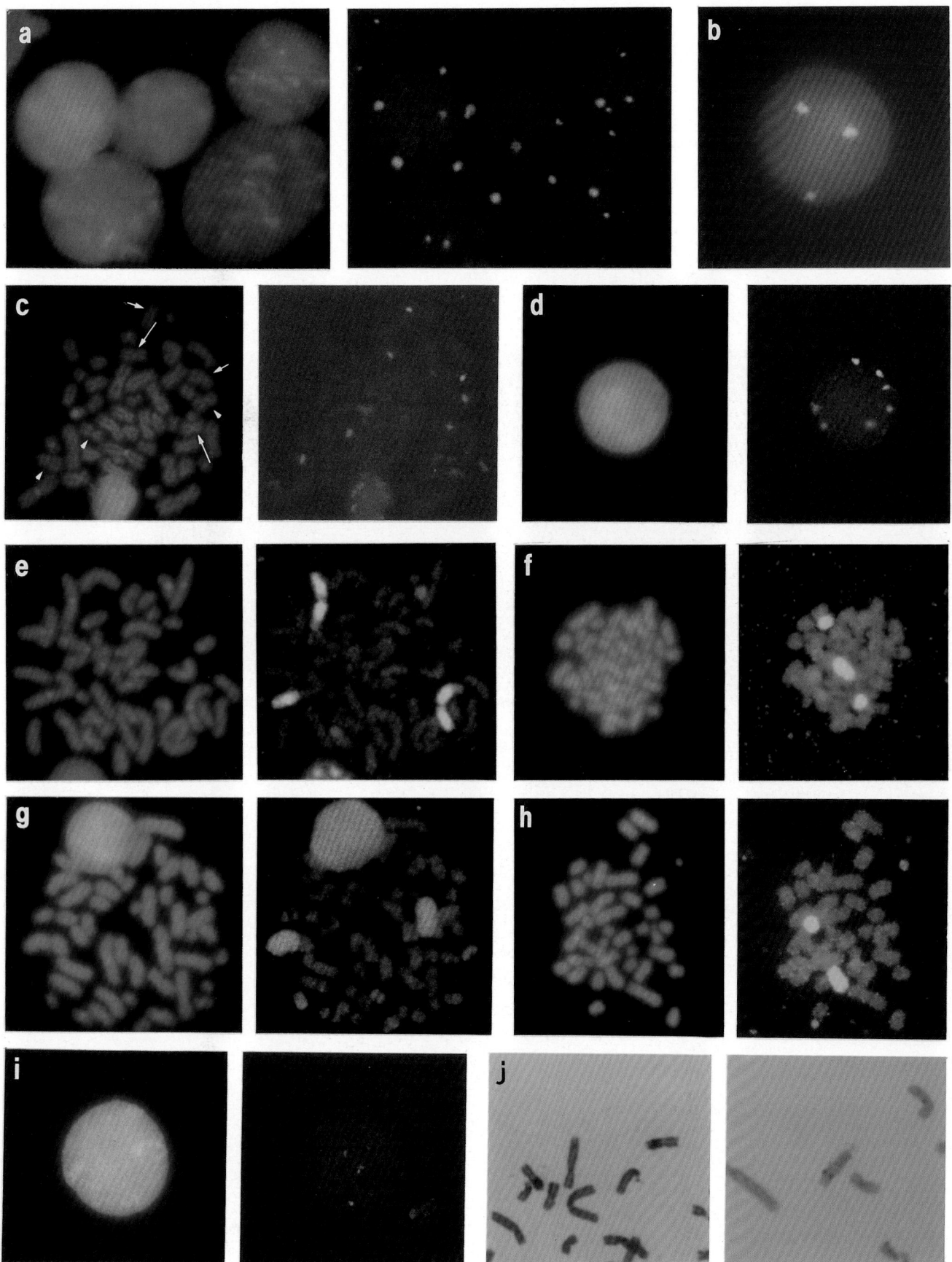

COLOR FIGURE 5–5.

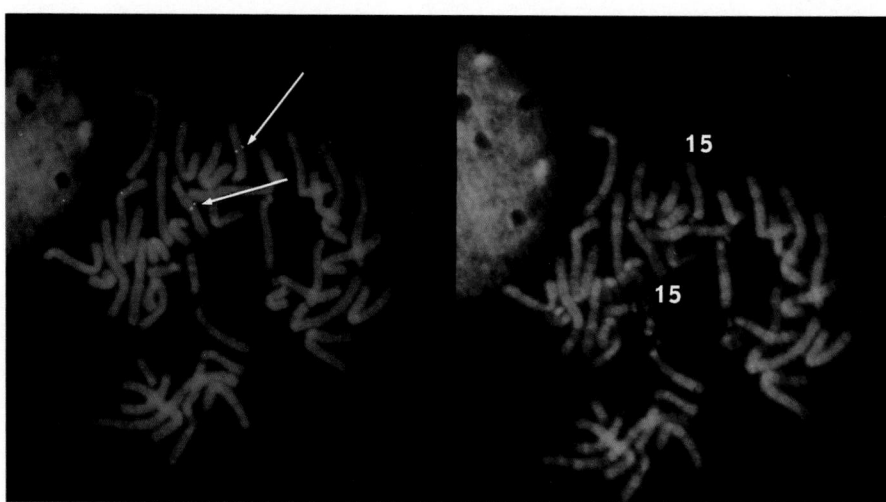

COLOR FIGURE 1–11D. Fluorescent in situ hybridization of a nonisotopically labeled *HUD*5 probe to human chromosomes. The photograph on the left depicts fluorescent signals on chromosomes counterstained with propidium iodide, and the photograph on the right illustrates *DAPI*-banding of the same metaphase spread. The signals in this and other cells examined are located at band 15q21. (Courtesy of J. Testa, Fox Chase Cancer Center, Philadelphia, PA)

acute lymphoblastic leukemia.[50,51] It is located about 100 kb telomeric to the *CD3* γ and δ gene cluster. The cDNA of the gene, called *MLL*, is large (11.5 kb) and appears to have alternative exon splicing; several smaller transcripts (*i.e.*, 11.0, 5.5, and 1.5 kb) have also been detected. The consequences of the translocation are unknown, but all of the translocations in myeloid leukemias identified have resulted in fusion genes that code for chimeric proteins.

Aberrations of Chromosome 16

Another clinicocytogenetic association involves myelomonocytic (M4) leukemia with abnormal eosinophils. Arthur and Bloomfield described 5 patients with a deleted chromosome 16 [del(16)(q22)] who had AML M2 or M4 in which the bone marrow contained an excess of eosinophils (8–54%).[52] A related entity was described for 33 patients from the University of Chicago.[53] Most of these patients had M4 leukemia with eosinophils (M4Eo) that showed large irregular basophilic granules; one third lacked increased eosinophils because the marrow had fewer than 5% eosinophils. Twenty-seven patients had an inversion of chromosome 16, inv(16)(p13q22), and 6 had a t(16;16)(p13;q22) (Fig. 5–3C). The morphologic features of the eosinophils are so specific that pathologists can accurately predict which patients will have an inv(16) or a t(16;16) by examining the bone marrow aspirate.

This chromosome abnormality has clinical implications as well. Among 32 treated patients, 78% achieved a complete remission, compared with 36% of 58 other acute myelomonocytic leukemia patients. The median survival time was more than 65 weeks for patients with abnormal chromosome 16 compared with 29 weeks for those with a normal 16.[53] These data confirm an observation reported by Keating and coworkers that increased marrow eosinophils were a good prognostic sign.[54] The projected median survival for all Fourth International Workshop on Chromosomes in Leukemia and Lymphoma patients was 8 months; those with a t(8;21) had the longest median survival (13 months), and those with abnormalities of chromosomes 5 and 7, t(15;17), or hyperdiploidy had the shortest survivals (3–4 months) The data on survival were updated in 1988, and the prognostic importance of the karyotype was reaffirmed.[55]

TREATMENT-ASSOCIATED ACUTE MYELOID LEUKEMIA AND MYELODYSPLASTIC SYNDROMES

A distinctive disorder of bone marrow morphology and function that terminates in a myelodysplastic syndrome (MDS) or in AML has been recognized as a late complication of cytotoxic therapy used in the treatment of malignant and nonmalignant diseases.[56] Characteristic nonrandom chromosome abnormalities are commonly observed in bone marrow cells of patients with treatment-associated MDS or AML. These abnormalities differ in their type and frequency from those seen in de novo AML. Sixty-one of 63 treatment-associated MDS or AML patients had an abnormal karyotype, and 55 of these had an abnormality of one or both chromosomes 5 and 7.[57] These observations have been confirmed by others.[58,59] In a series of 29 patients with del(5q), band 5q31 was consistently missing in every patient (Fig. 5–3F). In contrast, only about 16% of patients with de novo AML have a similar

abnormality of chromosome 5, 7, or both.[60] These patients frequently had significant occupational exposure to potential environmental carcinogens, such as chemicals, solvents, or pesticides.[61,62] A number of growth factors or growth factor receptors have been mapped to region 5q23–32; whether any of them play a role in mutagen-associated leukemia is unknown.[63]

With the increasing use of topoisomerase II inhibitors in high doses, especially etoposide and teniposide, a new subtype of treatment-associated AML has appeared. The leukemia occurs earlier than that induced by alkylating agents (at about 3 years rather than 5 years after treatment), lacks a preleukemic phase, and often has balanced translocations involving 11q23 and 21q22.[64–67]

POLYCYTHEMIA VERA

An abnormal chromosome clone occurs in 14% of untreated patients with polycythemia vera, in 30% of treated patients, and in 85% of patients who transform to AML.[5,16] Marrow cells frequently contain additional chromosomes (+8 or +9); these also occur together, which is otherwise rare. Structural rearrangements most often involve a deletion of the long arm of chromosome 20 (30% of patients) or a duplication of the long arm of chromosome 1, especially bands 1q25–1q32 (20% of patients). Different abnormalities have been observed in the leukemic phase of polycythemia vera: −7 (20%) and del(5q) (40%). These changes may be related to prior treatment.

MYELODYSPLASTIC SYNDROMES

MDS are a heterogenous group of disorders.[68] Clonal chromosome abnormalities can be detected at diagnosis in marrow cells of 40% to 70% of patients with MDS.[69–71] The proportion varies with the risk that a subtype will transform to AML, which is highest for refractory anemia with excess blasts and refractory anemia with excess blasts in transformation. The common chromosome changes, +8, −5/del(5q), −7/del(7q), and del(20q), are similar to those seen in de novo AML. The absence of the common recurring translocations such as t(8;21) or t(15;17) seen in de novo AML is probably significant. In general, the chromosome changes do not correlate with the specific subtypes of myelodysplastic syndrome. A subset of older patients have a similar interstitial deletion of the long arm of chromosome 5, which has led to the designation "5q syndrome."[72] These patients can have a relatively benign course that extends over several years.

MALIGNANT LYMPHOID DISORDERS

The chromosome abnormalities in lymphoid disorders, especially in the non-Hodgkin's lymphomas (NHL), have been reviewed in considerable detail.[2,73–75] This section considers the consistent translocations seen in Burkitt's lymphoma and some cases of B-cell ALL, aberrations in ALL and some T-cell disorders, and the recurring cytogenetic features of NHL and CLL.

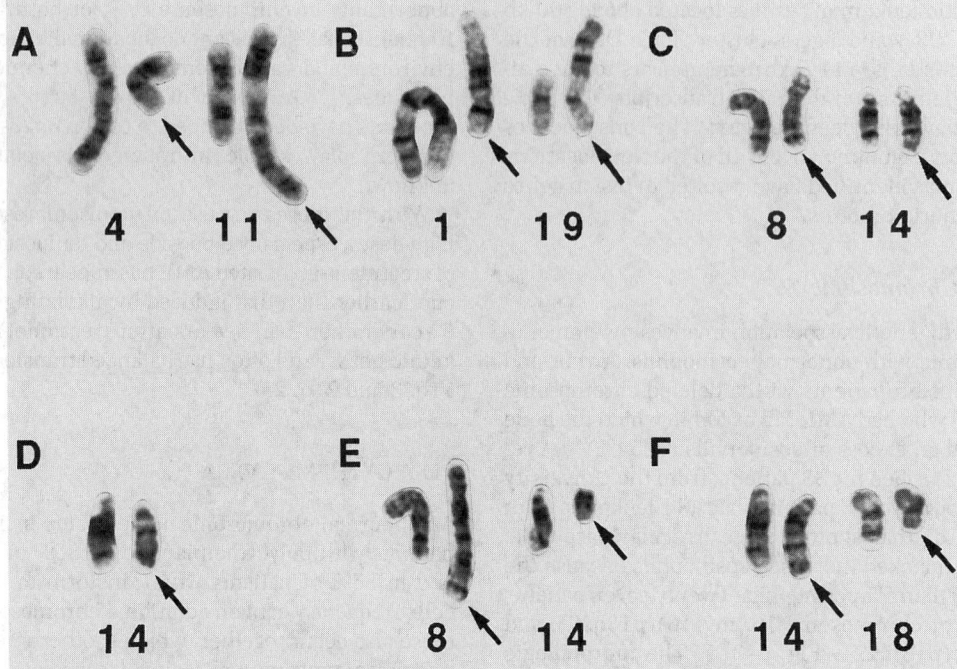

FIGURE 5–6. Partial karyotypes of trypsin-Giemsa-banded metaphase cells depicting nonrandom chromosome rearrangements observed in lymphoid malignant diseases. **(A)** t(4;11)(q21;q23) in acute lymphoblastic leukemia (ALL). **(B)** t(1;19)(q21;p13) in pre-B cell ALL. **(C)** t(8;14)(q24;q32) in B-cell ALL and Burkitt's lymphoma. **(D)** inv(14)(q11q32) in T-cell leukemia/lymphoma. **(E)** t(8;14)(q24;q11) in T-cell leukemia/lymphoma. **(F)** t(14;18)(q32;q21) in B-cell non-Hodgkin's lymphoma. The rearranged chromosomes are identified with arrows. (Beutler E, ed. Hematology, New York: McGraw-Hill)

LYMPHOMA

The 8;14 Translocation

In 1972, Manolov and Manolova discovered that cells of Burkitt's lymphomas had an additional band at the end of the long arm of one chromosome 14 (14q+).[76] In 1976, Zech and co-workers first observed that the end of one chromosome 8 was consistently absent, and they suggested that the missing part of chromosome 8 was translocated to chromosome 14 (t[8;14][q24;q32]) (Fig. 5–6C).[77] The t(8;14) has also been observed in nonendemic Burkitt's tumors from America, Europe, and Japan that are Epstein-Barr virus negative, con-

TABLE 5–2. Cytogenetic-Immunophenotypic Correlations: Malignant T-Lymphoid Diseases

Phenotype	Rearrangement	Involved Genes	
Acute lymphoblastic leukemia			
Early-B precursor	t(4;11)(q21;q23)	?	MLL
Common	t(9;22)(q34;q11)	BCR	ABL
	t(1;19)(q23;p13)	PBX1	E2A
Pre-B	t(5;14)(q31;q32)	IGH	IL3
B(SIg⁺)	t(8;14)(q24;q32)	IGH	MYC
(Also BL and NHL)	t(2;8)(p11–12;q24)	IGK	MYC/PVT1
	t(8;22)(q24;q11)	IGL	MYC/PVT1
Chronic lymphocytic leukemia			
	t(11;14)(q13;q32)	IGH	BCL1
	t(14;19)(q32;q13)	IGH	BCL3
	t(2;14)(p13;q32)		
	t(18;22)(q21;q11)	IGL	BCL2
	+12		
	del(13q)		
Non-Hodgkin's lymphoma			
Follicular	t(14;18)(q32;q21)	IGH	BCL2
	t(11;14)(q13;q32)	IGH	BCL1
	t(10;14)(q24;q32)	IGH	LYT10

firming that it is a highly characteristic chromosome anomaly in Burkitt's tumors (Table 5–2). This translocation has also been observed in other lymphomas, particularly those of the diffuse large cell type. Two related translocations involve a break in 8q24. One variant translocation involves chromosome 2 with a break in the short arm [t(2;8)(p12;q24)], and the other involves chromosome 22 with a break in band 22q11. All three translocations have also been identified in patients with B-cell ALL.

The protooncogene *MYC* (*i.e.*, cellular homolog of the avian myelocytomatosis virus) is located in 8q24. The immunoglobulin genes (heavy chain and κ and λ light chain genes) are located at the breakpoints 14q23, 2p12, and 22q11, respectively. These translocations result in the juxtaposition of *MYC* and one of the immunoglobulin genes, leading to abnormal regulation of *MYC* expression.[78,79]

The 14;18 Translocation

Considering karyotypic aberrations in lymphoid diseases as a whole, a break in chromosome 14 at band q32, with translocation of material from elsewhere to the broken chromosome 14, is the single most common change. The only other major recurring translocation, the t(14;18)(q32;q21), is the most common translocation in lymphoma (Fig. 5–6F). This was first identified by Fukuhara and coworkers in 6 of 9 patients with poorly differentiated lymphocytic lymphoma, now called "malignant lymphoma, follicular, predominantly small cleaved cell" (FSC) in the Working Formulation Classification System.[80,81] This finding was confirmed by many others.[73–75] The correlation between karyotype and histology in 260 patients reviewed at the Fifth International Workshop on Chromosomes in Leukemia and Lymphoma is summarized in Figure 5–7.[75] The t(14;18) is common in follicular lymphomas, and the t(8;14) is common in small noncleaved cell lymphoma. Tumors with a t(14;18) and large cell morphology may have a gain of chromosome 7 or a deletion of the long arm of chromosome 6 ([del]6q) that appears to correlate with a more malignant phenotype.[73,74,80]

The translocation junction has been cloned, and a gene on chromosome 18 called *BCL2* has been identified.[82] In the lymphoma cells, the expression of the normal gene is suppressed and an abnormal chimeric *BCL2-IGH* mRNA is expressed that appears to block programmed cell death.[83] Transgenic mice bearing a *BCL2-IGH* minigene have expansion of resting B cells with a prolonged life span.[84]

CHRONIC LYMPHOCYTIC LEUKEMIA

Chronic lymphocytic leukemia (CLL) is the most common leukemia in the United States and Europe, accounting for about 30% of all leukemias. It is considered to be a monoclonal neoplastic proliferation mainly of small B lymphocytes. Clonal abnormalities have been detected in approximately one third of the patients. These include trisomy for chromosome 12 (31%), translocations involving 14q32 (19%), and structural abnormalities of chromosome 13 (23%) (Table 5–2).[85–86] The use of fluorescence in situ hybridization techniques has already had a major impact on the analysis of CLL.[87,88] Centromere probes for chromosome 12 have been used to show that 30% of the CLL patients at the University of Chicago have trisomy 12 (Color Fig. 5–5). Reanalysis of standard cytogenetic preparations revealed an extra chromosome 12 in patients with samples previously designated normal or inadequate. There are somewhat conflicting reports about the prognostic significance of these abnormalities.[85–86] A more accurate assessment, at least for trisomy 12, will be possible with the use of fluorescence in situ hybridization.

The 14q32 Translocations

Two translocations in CLL have been cloned. One of these is the t(11;14)(q13;q32), which involves the *IGH* locus on 14q32 and *BCL1*.[89] No gene was identified as *BCL1*, but recent data suggest that another gene, *PRAD1*, identified in parathyroid adenomas may be *BCL1*.[90] *BCL1* rearrangements have been found in CLL and in 30% to 50% of centrocytic lymphomas and intermediate lymphocytic lymphomas.[91] The second translocation is the t(14;19)(q32;q13), which involves *IGH* and *BCL3*.[86,92] It has recently been shown that *BCL3* is a member of the *IFKB* gene family, which act as inhibitors to the *NFKB* gene family, which code for transcription factors activating a number of genes in hematopoietic cells, especially *IGK* in B cells.[93]

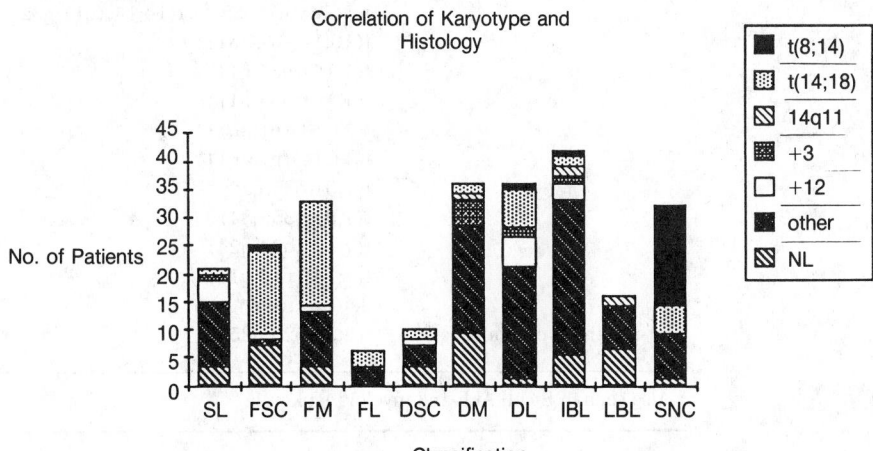

Correlation of Karyotype and Histology

No. of Patients

Classification: SL FSC FM FL DSC DM DL IBL LBL SNC

Legend: ■ t(8;14) ▨ t(14;18) ◩ 14q11 ▦ +3 □ +12 ■ other ◿ NL

FIGURE 5–7. Histogram showing the most common chromosome changes that were identified in 260 lymphomas studied before treatment and reviewed at the Fifth International Workshop on Chromosomes in Leukemia/Lymphoma; each tumor was classified according to the Working Formulation.

ACUTE LYMPHOCYTIC LEUKEMIA

Although the correlation of cytogenetic changes with morphology in AML led to the identification of the specific associations described in a previous section, this correlation was not useful in ALL, except for the t(8;14) and its variants in L3 B-cell ALL. However, with the widespread use of precise immunophenotyping, the correlation of certain chromosome rearrangements with specific immunologic subsets of ALL has been established (Tables 5–2 and 5–3). The poor morphology of metaphase chromosomes from ALL patients impeded an accurate karyotypic analysis until recently.

ALL is the most frequent leukemia in children. It was rigorously demonstrated for the first time at the Third International Workshop on Chromosomes in Leukemia that the karyotype is an important independent prognostic factor in ALL.[94] Of 330 patients reviewed at the Third Workshop, 112 appeared to have a normal karyotype; the largest group (39 patients) with a well-defined abnormality had a Ph chromosome.

Ph-Positive Acute Lymphocytic Leukemia

The Ph chromosome is the most frequent rearrangement, comprising 17.3% of adult ALL. In the Workshop material, the children with a Ph chromosome had the second highest median leukocyte count (75,000/mm³), all were classified as non-B, non-T ALL, and they had a poor median survival of only 15 months. By identifying this chromosomal abnormality, it is possible to detect patients who have a poor prognosis.

The breakpoints appear identical to those in CML; recent molecular analysis indicates that the breakpoint in the *BCR* gene on chromosome 22 is more proximal in some patients with Ph-positive ALL. Ph-positive ALL patients have an abnormal-size chimeric *BCR-ABL*-encoded mRNA (7.0–7.4 kb) and ABL protein (p185[bcr-abl]) (Fig. 5–4).[95,96] It is possible to use several DNA probes from the *BCR* gene and PFGE to differentiate the CML from the ALL breakpoint; this can also be done with the polymerase chain reaction using the appropriate primers. A preliminary analysis of samples from adult ALL patients with probes for *BCR* and *ABL* has detected the presence of the Ph translocation in about 30% of patients.[97]

The 4;11 Translocation

Of 216 Workshop patients with chromosomal abnormalities, 18 (8.3%) had a t(4;11)(q21;q23) (Fig. 5–6A). Half of the patients were children, and the median age was 1 year. The association of the t(4;11) with neonatal or early childhood ALL is particularly interesting in view of the low incidence of ALL in this age group; acute leukemias in this age group are usually of the myeloid type, and they involve a break in 11q23. Children with t(4;11) had very high leukocyte counts (median, 214,000/mm³), which is a poor prognostic factor. Children and adults had a short median survival of 9 and 7 months, respectively. Only patients with abnormalities involving 8q24 or 14q32 had shorter survivals. Although the morphology of some cells often appears lymphoid, other features suggest a monocytic leukemia. A t(4;11) cell line showed rearranged heavy and light chain (κ) genes, although the cells lacked cytoplasmic immunoglobulin and were probably in a very early stage of B-cell differentiation.[98] However, when cultured with the phorbol ester, TPA, a monocytic-like phenotype was induced. The *MLL* gene at 11q23 is involved in this translocation in AML and in monoblastic leukemia.[51] By using PFGE and a probe for *CD3D*, the breakpoints in 8 patients could be identified.[99]

The 1;19 Translocation

A t(1;19)(q21;p13) has been identified in about 25% of patients with a pre-B phenotype; they have cytoplasmic immunoglobulin and are CALLA positive (Fig. 5–6B).[94,100–102] The translocation breakpoints have recently been cloned. It is the first translocation in lymphoid leukemias that does not

TABLE 5–3. Cytogenetic-Immunophenotypic Correlations: Malignant T-Lymphoid Diseases

Phenotype	Rearrangement	Involved Genes	
Acute lymphoblastic leukemia	t(8;14)(q24;q11)	*TCRA*	*MYC*
	inv(14)(q11q32.3)	*TCRA*	*IGH*
	inv(14)(q11q32.1)/t(14;14)(q11;q32)	*TCRA*	*(TCL1)*
	t(10;14)(q24;q11)	*TCRD*	*HOX11*
	t(1;14)(p34;q11)	*TCRD*	*TAL1(SCL)*
	t(1;14)(p34;q11)	*TCRD*	*LCK*
	t(11;14)(p15;q11)	*TCRD*	*RBTN1(TTG)*
	t(11;14)(p13;q11)	*TCRD*	*RBTN2*
	t(7;9)(q35;q32)	*TCRB*	*TAL2*
	t(7;9)(q35;q34)	*TCRB*	*TAN1*
	t(7;10)(q34;q24)	*TCRB*	*HOX11*
	t(7;14)(p15;q11)		
	del(9p),t(9p)*	*IFNA/B?*	
KI-1-positive lymphoma	t(2;5)(p23;q35)		

* Also seen in B-cell ALL and myeloid leukemia.

involve an immunoglobulin or T-cell receptor gene.[103,104] The gene on chromosome 19 is *E2A*, which functions as a transcription factor; the gene on chromosome 1, called *PBX1*, is a homeobox gene. The breakpoints in *E2A* are clustered within one small intron, but they are spread within a large intron of at least 50 kb in *PBX1*. The translocation results in a chimeric gene with the 5' region derived from *E2A* and the 3' region from *PBX1*. The DNA binding portion of *E2A* is replaced by that of the *PBX1*. The aberrant mRNA from this fusion gene is highly conserved and can be detected with the polymerase chain reaction.[105]

Hyperdiploid Acute Lymphocytic Leukemia

The leukemic cells of a substantial number of patients with ALL are characterized by a gain of many chromosomes and fewer structural abnormalities.[94,106,107] Chromosome numbers usually range from 50 to 60. Although identical karyotypes are unusual, certain additional chromosomes are commonly seen. Among 31 hyperdiploid Third Workshop patients (14% of patients with abnormalities), +21, +6, +18, +14, +4, and +10, in decreasing frequency, were seen in 10% to 33% of patients.[94] Some of these chromosomes, particularly chromosomes 10, 18, and 21, are also seen as additional chromosomes in patients with near-haploid ALL, with chromosome numbers of 26 to 36 (median, 28). The median age of the 22 children with this abnormality was 3 years, and that of all 31 patients was 5 years, which was less than that of patients with other abnormalities. The leukocyte count was low (median, 6000/mm^3). These patients have all of the previously recognized factors, including age between 3 and 7 years, low leukocyte count, and non-T, non-B markers, that indicate a good prognosis. In the Sixth International Workshop on Chromosomes in Leukemia and Lymphoma follow-up study of the Third Workshop patients, the complete remission rate for children was 95%, with a median remission duration longer than 95 months. The median survival of the children with hyperdiploidy is longer than that of those with a normal karyotype; for adults, the median survival for the two groups is comparable.[55]

Chromosome losses were less frequent and involved chromosomes 9, 7, 13, 20, or 8, in that order. With regard to karyotype and age, patients with a deletion of 6q and a modal chromosome number greater than 50 were younger, and those with a Ph chromosome or a 14q+ were older than patients with other abnormalities. The highest remission rates were for patients with a normal karyotype and a modal number greater than 50; the lowest were seen in patients with a Ph chromosome, a 14q+ chromosome, a t(8;14), and a t(4;11).[55]

T-CELL DISORDERS

Although fewer leukemias of T-cell origin have been studied, a distinct pattern of nonrandom karyotypic abnormalities is emerging (Table 5-3). Rearrangements involving chromosome 14 (14q11) and chromosome 7 (7q35--q36 and 7p15) occur in T-cell malignancies, but have been observed in ataxia-telangiectasia as well; breaks involving these regions are very rare in other malignant diseases.[101,108-112] One recurring rearrangement in T-cell neoplasia, particularly CLL, is a paracentric inversion of chromosome 14 with a proximal break-

point at q11 and a distal breakpoint at q32 (Fig. 5-6D).[108,113] A closely related rearrangement, t(14;14)(q11;q32), is seen in T-cell neoplasia and in phytohemagglutinin-stimulated T lymphocytes from patients with ataxia-telangiectasia and in the leukemic cells of ataxia-telangiectasia patients in whom this disease evolved.[111,112] Breaks in 14q11 occur relatively frequently in adult T-cell leukemia-lymphoma patients in Japan; 14q11 breaks are much less common in patients in other countries.[75,109,114,115] Williams and her associates described a t(11;14)(p13;q13) in the leukemic cells of 4 of 16 patients with T-cell ALL.[101] The breaks may occur in 14q11 or 14q32 or in both bands in the same patient; in B-cell disorders, breaks usually occur only in 14q32, and they rarely involve 14q11.[108] The data confirm the importance of 14q11 in T-cell neoplasia.[111]

The molecular analysis of translocation junctions in malignant T cells led to the discovery of many new genes, only a few of which can be described here. A complete list of these genes is included in Table 5-3. The first cloned translocations at 14q11 involved the α chain of the T-cell receptor (*TCRA*) and the δ chain for the receptor (*TCRD*). The t(8;14)(q24;q11) is analogous to the t(8;14)(q24;q32) in Burkitt lymphoma in that the involved gene on chromosome 8 is *MYC* but is *TCRA* on chromosome 14 (Fig. 5-6E). The break in *MYC* was 3' of the third exon (similar to those affecting the *IG* light chain genes) and in *TCRA* was just 5' of one of the J segments.[116,117]

Another gene, *TAL1*, is involved in a translocation and a deletion.[118,119] *TAL1* is expressed in hematopoietic progenitor cells, and its product is a member of the helix-loop-helix family of transcription factors that also includes products of *LYL1* and *TAL2*. The t(1;14)(p34;q11) involving *TAL1* and *TCRD* is seen in 5% of T-cell ALL patients. A precise 92-kb deletion of sequences just 5' of *TAL1* is seen in about 25% of T-cell ALL patients. The consequence of both aberrations is the removal of the 5' regulatory sequences for the *TAL1* gene and its aberrant expression in T cells. The β chain of the T-cell receptor (*TCRB*) at 7q34-35 is also involved in translocations.

MOLECULAR ANALYSIS OF CONSISTENT CHROMOSOME ABNORMALITIES IN HEMATOPOIETIC NEOPLASMS

How and When Consistent Translocations Occur

We do not know how consistent structural rearrangements occur. They may be random, with selection eliminating the majority that do not provide a proliferative advantage. Alternatively, certain changes may occur preferentially; some tantalizing data that need to be explored show an association of chromosome rearrangements in tumor cells from patients with fragile sites affecting one of the chromosome bands broken in the tumor cells.[120-122] Croce[123] proposed that many of the chromosome rearrangements in B- and T-cell tumors involve the heptamer and nonamer sequences used in the normal recombination of the V-D-J segments of the immunoglobulin and T-cell receptor genes, because these sequences may be found in the nonantigen receptor gene at the site of the translocation (*e.g., MYC, BCL2, TAL1*).[119,123-125]

An equally important issue is when the translocations or other chromosome aberrations occur in the multistage process of malignant transformation of a particular cell. Some chromosome changes occur as part of the further evolution of the malignant phenotype (*e.g.*, blast crisis of CML), and they are relatively late events. Fialkow and his colleagues presented evidence supporting the proposal that there is expansion of an altered clone with the translocation as an added event.[126] Transgenic mice whose cells have a vector containing the *MYC-IGH* junction from a murine plasmacytoma develop B-cell tumors that are clonal, indicating that one or more additional changes occur in one cell, resulting in clonality.[127]

Specificity of Chromosome Rearrangements

There is a remarkable specificity of certain chromosome rearrangements for particular subtypes of leukemia, lymphoma, and sarcoma. The location of the breakpoints and critical protooncogenes is illustrated in Figure 5–8. The mechanisms by which this specificity is achieved are unknown, but certain proteins required for promotion of gene expression are synthesized in a cell-type and developmental-stage-specific manner.[128] These proteins are only present in the appropriate cell type, and the particular gene is activated in a developmentally regulated manner only in that cell type. The chromosome rearrangements affecting *MYC* in B-cell and T-cell tumors indicate that the specificity resides in the gene that is uniquely active in a particular cell type. The immunoglobulin genes in B cells and *TCRA* in T cells are activators for *MYC* in B cells or T cells, respectively.

Some of the genetic consequences of the translocations and some differences in the various leukemias can now be identified (Table 5–4). All of the breakpoints cloned in myeloid leukemias have resulted in fusion genes with relatively limited variability (Table 5–5).

Most lymphoid leukemias involve one of the immune receptor genes and another gene whose protein-coding region is normal; the malignant phenotype appears to be a consequence of the inappropriate expression of the affected gene. As shown in Table 5–4, most other genes affected are transcription activators, and the translocation often results in an increased level of expression of these genes. In some cases (*e.g.*, *RBTN1* and *RBTN2*), these genes are normally expressed in brain tissue but are inappropriately expressed in hematopoietic cells. Fusion genes also result from translocations in lymphoblastic leukemia, notably the *BCR-ABL* fusion in Ph-positive ALL and the *E2A-PBX1* fusion in the t(1;19).

All of the translocations that involve transcription factors (excluding *BCL3* and *LYT10* because they both function as inhibitors and bind to the NFKB p50 transcription factor) are present in acute leukemias. This suggests that inappropriate or excessive expression of these factors leads to a much more aggressive phenotype. It should be emphasized that cloning translocation breakpoints is a very powerful tool for identifying new genes. Of those listed in Table 5–4, only *MYC*, *E2A*, and *RARA* had been previously identified.

We have made relatively little progress in identifying the genes involved in the most common chromosome deletions in hematopoietic neoplasms. Although many laboratories are mapping the deletion in 5q, 6q, 9p, and 20q, only the genes first identified in deletions in solid tumors have been shown to play any role in the leukemias. This includes *TP53* on 17p in CML in blast crisis and *RB1* on 13q in CLL.[85]

SOLID TUMORS

Despite recent technical improvements in cancer cytogenetics, solid tumors still comprise only 20% of the 15,000 neoplasms studied with banding techniques.[8] The acquisition of reliable knowledge about the essential genomic rearrangements in solid tumors has also been hampered by other problems. Most investigations have been made on highly advanced tumors, often metastatic lesions or effusions, with many additional abnormalities acquired during tumor progression. However, the chromosomal anomalies are often highly complex even when the analysis is performed on biopsies taken at diagnosis from primary tumors. Differentiating primary, pathogenetically essential changes and secondary aberrations is usually more difficult in solid tumors than in leukemias. Nonetheless, a growing number of consistent cytogenetic abnormalities are now being revealed in benign and malignant solid tumors.[3–7] Some of the associations are as specific as the various cytogenetic-morphologic correlations known from hematologic malignancies; others are still tentative. The most characteristic recurrent rearrangements are summarized in Table 5–6. Only a few of the chromosome rearrangements have been characterized at the molecular level.

BENIGN TUMORS

Epithelial Neoplasms

The only benign epithelial neoplasm studied in sufficient number to permit reasonably well-founded conclusions is the mixed tumor of the salivary gland (*i.e.*, pleomorphic adenoma).[129,130] More than 75% of the abnormal stem lines have abnormalities that affect only one or two of chromosomes 3, 8, and 12. Three cytogenetic subgroups of tumors can be determined: aberrations of 3p21, 8q12, or 12q13–15. The first two breakpoints often are involved in a t(3;8)(p21;q12), shown schematically in Figure 5–9. This may be considered a standard rearrangement, with the other 3p21 and 8q12 changes representing variant translocations. Aberrations affecting 12q occur independently of the 3p or 8q abnormalities. A comparison of the breakpoint regions of the three cytogenetic subgroups of salivary gland adenomas with recurring breakpoints in other neoplasms reveals some interesting features. The 3p21 breakpoint may be close to the breakpoints in small cell lung cancer and kidney cancer, and the 12q13–15 cluster region overlaps with the breakpoint sites found in uterine leiomyomas and benign and malignant lipogenic tumors.

Mesenchymal Neoplasms

Most lipomas are karyotypically abnormal.[131,132] Three major cytogenetic subgroups can be identified: reciprocal, apparently balanced translocations between 12q13–15 and various other chromosomes, including the specific rearrangement t(3;12)(q27–28;q13–15); one or more supernumerary ring chromosomes in addition to an otherwise apparently normal karyotype; and other aberrations. Both the 12q13–15 abnormalities and the ring chromosomes have been found as sole anomalies and probably represent primary changes.

Clonal chromosome abnormalities may be detected in ap-

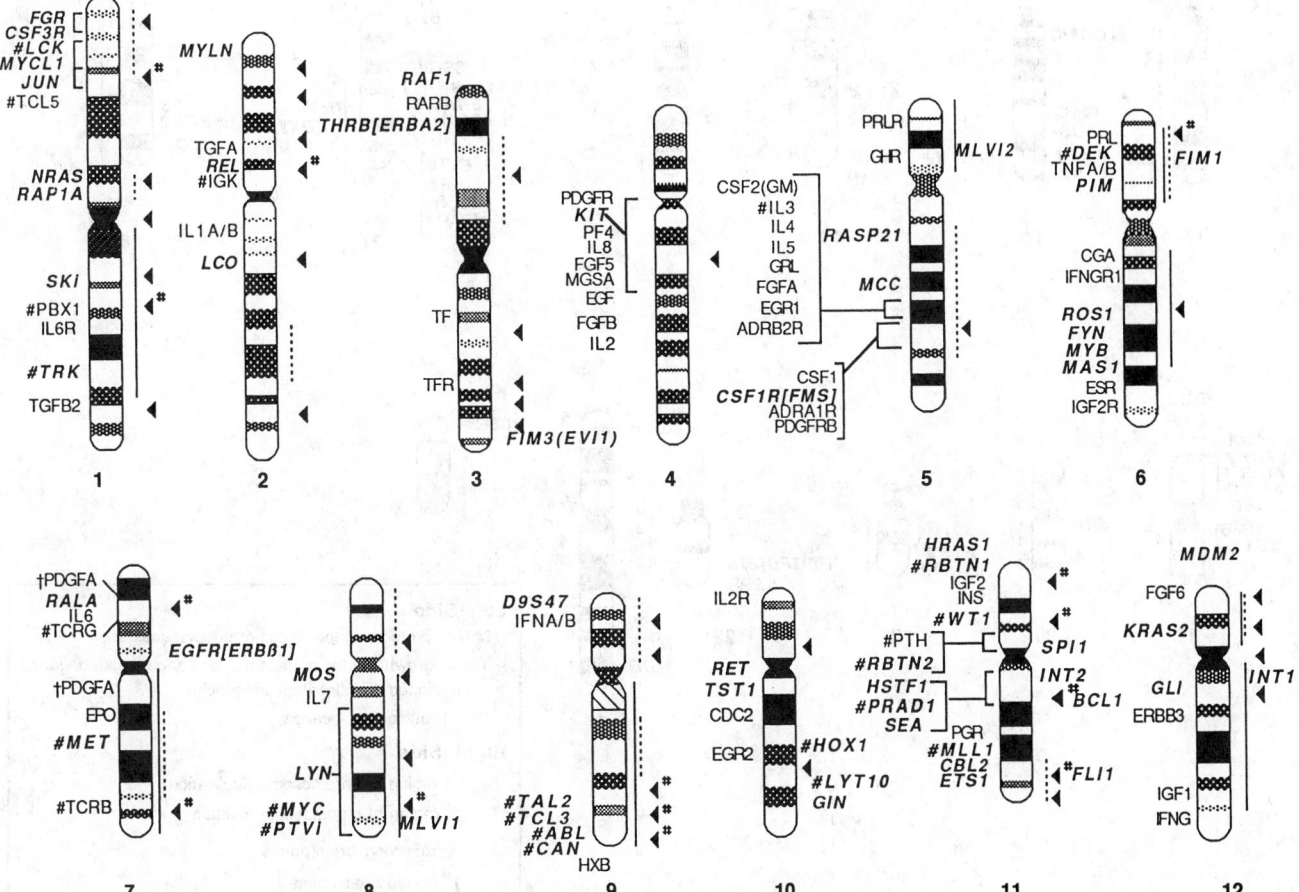

FIGURE 5–8. Chromosome locations of protooncogenes or of genes that appear to be important in malignant transformation and the breakpoints observed in recurring chromosome abnormalities in human leukemia, lymphoma, and solid tumors. Known protooncogenes are indicated in bold italics, and other cancer-related genes are listed in standard type. The protooncogenes and their locations are placed to the left of the appropriate chromosome band (*arrow*) or region (*bracket*). The breakpoints in recurring translocations, inversions, and other rearrangements are indicated with an arrowhead to the right of the affected chromosome band. The solid vertical lines on the right indicate regions frequently present in triplicate; the dashed lines indicate recurring deletions. Recurring viral integration sites and cloned translocation breakpoints with no identified transcripts are indicated to the right of the appropriate band. Genes or recurring breakpoints that have been cloned are identified by #. The locations of the cancer-specific breakpoints are based on the Report of the Committee on Structural Chromosome Changes in Neoplasia, Human Gene Mapping 11. (Author's note: Any map of this sort involves selection as to the genes that should or should not be included; I have been relatively conservative. Also for recurring breakpoints and deletions, I have included only those listed as Status I or II in HGM11.) (Prepared by Michelle S. Rebelsky, modified from Rowley JD. Molecular cytogenetics: Rosetta stone for understanding cancer. Cancer Res 1990;50:3816–3825)

proximately 20% of histologically benign uterine leiomyomas. These include t(12;14)(q14–15;q23–24), del(7)(q21q31), trisomy 12, and rearrangements of 6p.[133–135] Clonal evolution may occur, often as chromosome 1 aberrations or the formation of ring chromosomes. When multiple aberrations are found, the leiomyomas tend to be of the cellular type and to have mitotic activity or even to have histologic features justifying a diagnosis of bizarre or atypical myoma.[136]

Neurogenic Neoplasms

Meningiomas are the only benign neurogenic tumors that have been extensively investigated.[137,138] Most cases are characterized by the loss of one chromosome 22 or occasionally by a del(22q). Both observations are compatible with the hypothesis that tumor suppressor gene loss is the essential outcome of the cytogenetic aberration. Analyses of loss of polymorphic loci along the long arm of chromosome 22 have narrowed the likely position of this putative tumor suppressor locus to 22q12–qter.[139]

MALIGNANT TUMORS

Sufficient data to allow a meaningful discussion of the characteristic karyology of malignant neoplasms are available for at least some tumors of the respiratory and digestive systems, breast, reproductive organs, urinary tract, skin, bone, connective tissues, and the nervous system.

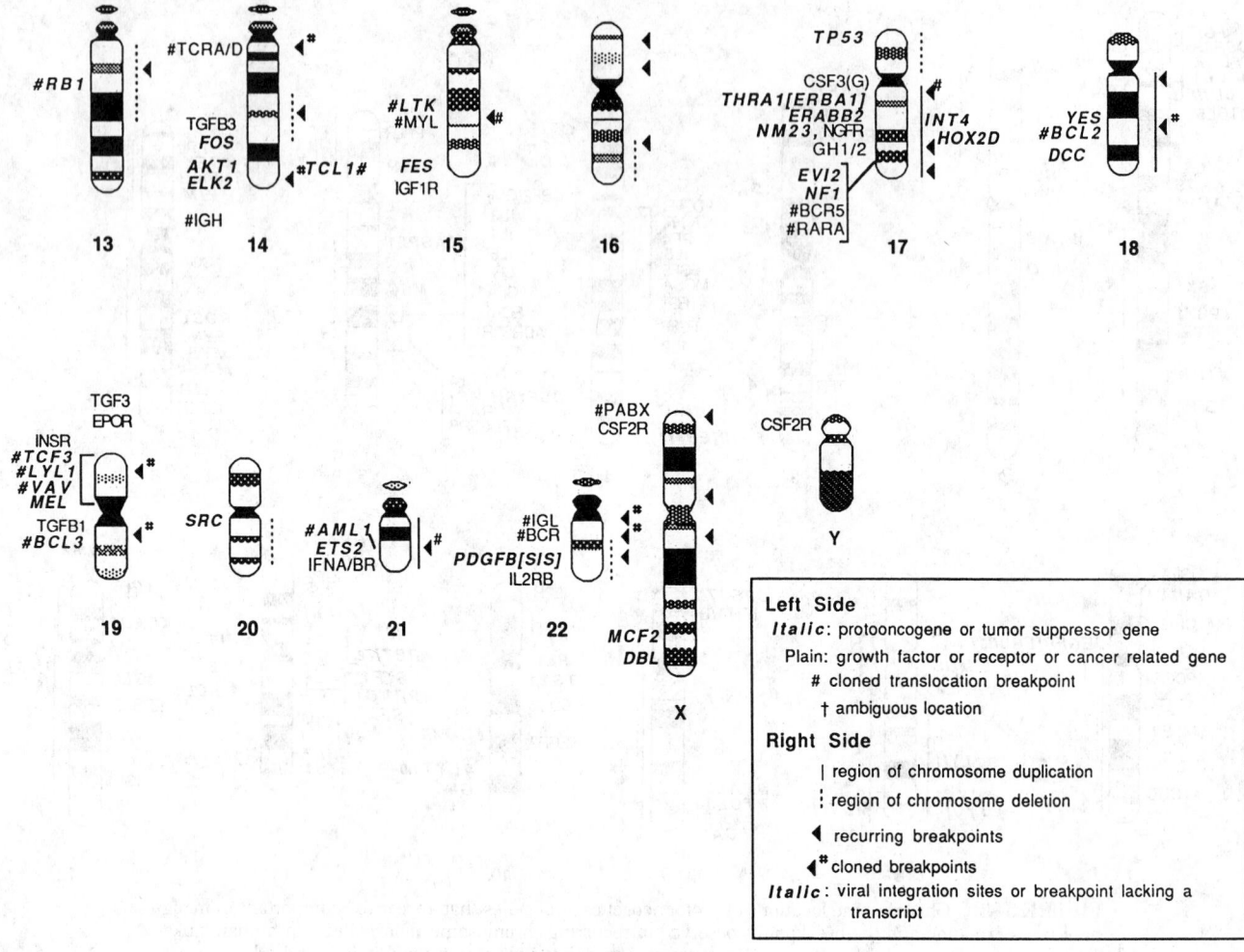

FIGURE 5–8.   *(Continued)*

Upper Airways

Few karyotypically abnormal squamous cell carcinomas of the head and neck region (*i.e.*, mouth, pharynx, larynx) have been published.[140–142] Cytogenetically unrelated clones are a recurring feature. This could mean that the primary genetic alteration is submicroscopic and that the visible aberrations are only secondary, or the finding could indicate multiclonal carcinogenesis within a cancer-prone epithelial field. However, equally possible is the interpretation that the clonal aberrations, which are mostly balanced translocations, are not representative of the tumor parenchyma at all but are instead in stromal fibroblasts or other subepithelial cells.

The distribution of breakpoints in the chromosomal rearrangements in head and neck squamous cell carcinomas seems to be nonrandom; bands 1p22 and 11q13 are preferentially involved.[142] Cytogenetic signs of gene amplification, such as double minute chromosomes and homogenously staining regions, are also detected.

Lung

Of the four major histologic subtypes of bronchogenic carcinomas, only small cell lung carcinomas have been investi-

gated cytogenetically in any number.[143–146] More than 90% of these tumors have a deletion of the short arm of chromosome 3, with loss of 3p14–23 as the minimal region of deletion (Fig. 5–10). The 3p− markers are not confined to the small cell subtype, because they have also been found in other bronchogenic carcinomas, including adenocarcinoma. More data are needed before the prevalence of 3p− in lung cancers of various histologies can be established.[147] The consistent loss of chromosome material, often with variable deletion breakpoints, is compatible with loss of tumor suppression activity as the essential mechanism.

Pleura

The karyotypes of the mesotheliomas so far studied have been complex, and no specific aberrations are known.[148,149] Common numeric changes include −1, −3, +7, −9, +11, −14, and −22, and the most common structural rearrangements are deletions and translocations of 1p, 3p, 9p, and 22q.

Breast

Because of the extreme numeric and structural complexity encountered, the number of breast carcinomas studied is in-

TABLE 5–4. Functional Classification of Transforming Genes at Translocation Junctions

Genes	Site Affected	Rearrangement	Disease
SRC family (TYR protein kinases)			
ABL	9q34	t(9;22)	CML/ALL
LCK	1p34	t(1;7)	T ALL
Serine protein kinase			
BCR	22q11	t(9;22)	CML/ALL
Cell surface receptor			
TAN1	9q34	t(7;9)	T ALL
Growth factor			
IL3	5q31	t(5;14)	Pre-B ALL
Inner mitochondrial membrane protein			
BCL2	18q21	t(14;18)	NHL
Transcriptional regulating factors			
BCL3	19q13	t(14;19)	B CLL
LYT10	10q24	t(10;14)	B NHL
PBX	1q23	t(1;19)	Pre-B ALL
E2A	19p13	t(1;19)	Pre-B ALL
CAN	9q34	t(6;9)	AML
HOX11	10q24	t(10;14)/t(7;10)	T ALL
LYL1	19p13	t(7;19)	T ALL
MYC	8q24	t(8;14)	B ALL/T ALL
PML	15q22	t(15;17)	APL
RARA	17q12	t(15;17)	APL
TAL1(SCL)	1p34	t(1;14)	T ALL
TAL2	9q32	t(7;9)	T ALL
RBTN1(TTG1)	11p15	t(11;14)	T ALL
RBTN2	11p13	t(11;14)	T ALL

TABLE 5–5. Alterations of Transcription Factors in Translocations

Deregulated Expression	Gene (Band)	Fusion Protein	Translocation
TCRA/D (14q11)	RBTN1* (11p15)	E2A/PBX1*	t(1;19)
	RBTN2* (11p13)		
	HOX11* (10q24)		
	TAL1* (1p34)	PML*/RARA	t(15;17)
	MYC (8q24)		
TCRB (7q34)	TAL2* (9q32)	DEK/CAN*	t(6;9)
	LYL1* (19p13)		
	RBTN2* (11p13)		
	HOX11* (10q24)		
IGH/K/L (14q32) (2p12) (22q11)	MYC (8q24)		

* Gene(s) identified by cloning breakpoint.

TABLE 5–6. Characteristic Karyotypic Abnormalities in Solid Tumors

Tumor Type	Type of Rearrangement
Epithelial Tumors	
Pleomorphic adenoma	Translocations of 12q13–15
	t(3;8)(p21;q12)
Lung carcinoma	del(3)(p14–23)
Kidney carcinoma	del(3)(p14–23)
	t(3;5)(p13;q22)
Bladder carcinoma	i(5p)
	Trisomy 7
	Monosomy 9
Wilms tumor	del(11)(p13)
Ovarian carcinoma	t(19;?)(p13;?)
Prostate carcinoma	del(7)(q22)
	del(10)(q24)
Mesenchymal Tumors	
Lipoma	Translocations of 12q13–15
	Ring chromosomes
Leiomyoma	Structural changes of 12q13–15
	del(7)(q21q31)
	Trisomy 12
Liposarcoma (myxoid)	t(12;16)(q13.3;p11.2)
Synovial sarcoma	t(X;18)(p11;q11)
Rhabdomyosarcoma	t(2;13)(q35–37;q14)
Malignant fibrous histiocytoma	t(19;?)(p13;?)
Neurogenic, Neuroectodermal, and Germ Cell Tumors	
Meningioma	Monosomy 22
	del(22)(q12–13)
Astrocytoma	del(9)(p13–24)
	dmin
Neuroblastoma	del(1)(p32–36)
	hsr/dmin
Retinoblastoma	del(13)(q14)
	i(6p)
Malignant melanoma	Deletions of 6q
	i(6p)
Ewing's sarcoma	t(11;22)(q24;q12)
Askin's tumor	
Peripheral neuroepithelioma	
Germ cell tumors	i(12p)

sufficient for any reliable evaluation of the pathogenetic significance of the various changes. Some information about nonrandom structural rearrangements can nevertheless be gained from the confusing picture.[150–153] Chromosome 1 is undoubtedly preferentially involved; almost 80% of all cytogenetically abnormal cases have recognizable structural changes of this chromosome. Most are various translocations affecting 1p, most commonly the region 1p11–21 and particularly band 1p13. Other genomic regions that are frequently rearranged, often leading to loss of genetic material, are 3p, 6q, 11p, 11q, 16q, and 17p.

Uterus

Most cytogenetically characterized uterine carcinomas have been squamous cell carcinomas of the cervix; only about 20% are endometrial adenocarcinomas.[154–156] The chromosomal picture in both tumor types has been extremely variable and complex, allowing complete karyotyping in only a minority of cases. No single cytogenetic abnormality has been consistently associated with either tumor type. Chromosome 1 is involved in a nonrandom manner and has been affected in 80% of all cytogenetically abnormal cases. The aberrations of chromosome 1 comprise numeric and structural rearrangements, without obvious breakpoint clustering to specific bands or regions.

Ovary

Chromosome 1 abnormalities are the most common cytogenetic change in ovarian carcinomas of various histologic types and have been found in more than 80% of cases successfully studied with banding techniques.[157–159] The aberrations include deletions, duplications, translocations, and inversions of the short and the long arms and formation of 1q isochromosomes. The breakpoints have mostly been mapped to 1p36 and the distal half of the long arm. Other recurrent chromosome arrangements include structural abnormalities of 6q and 11p, mostly leading to loss of genetic material, and 19p+ markers, in which the material added to 19p13 is unknown. Highly differentiated carcinomas are usually less karyotypically complex than their poorly differentiated counterparts.

Prostate

Most prostatic adenocarcinomas that have been cytogenetically analyzed have had normal karyotypes; only a few tumors with clonal chromosome aberrations have been reported.[160,161] No consistent abnormalities are known, but structural rearrangements of chromosome arms 2p, 7q, and 10q are the most common changes, especially deletions of 7q and 10q with breakpoints in 7q22 and 10q24.

Testis

A specific chromosome anomaly, an isochromosome for the short arm of chromosome 12, i(12p), has consistently been found in various histologic types of germ cell tumors of the testis, including seminomas, teratomas, embryonal cell carcinomas, and tumors of mixed histology.[162–165] Data are limited, but the i(12p) seems to be much more common in testicular tumors than in corresponding ovarian germ cell tumors.

Large Bowel

Adenocarcinomas of the colon and rectum are the most extensively studied malignant epithelial neoplasms in man. Despite the large number of cases studied, the cytogenetic results have been extremely hard to interpret because of the often low technical quality of the preparations and the complexity of the changes. Half of all tumors have stem line karyotypes in the hypotriploid-hypotetraploid region, and most have a

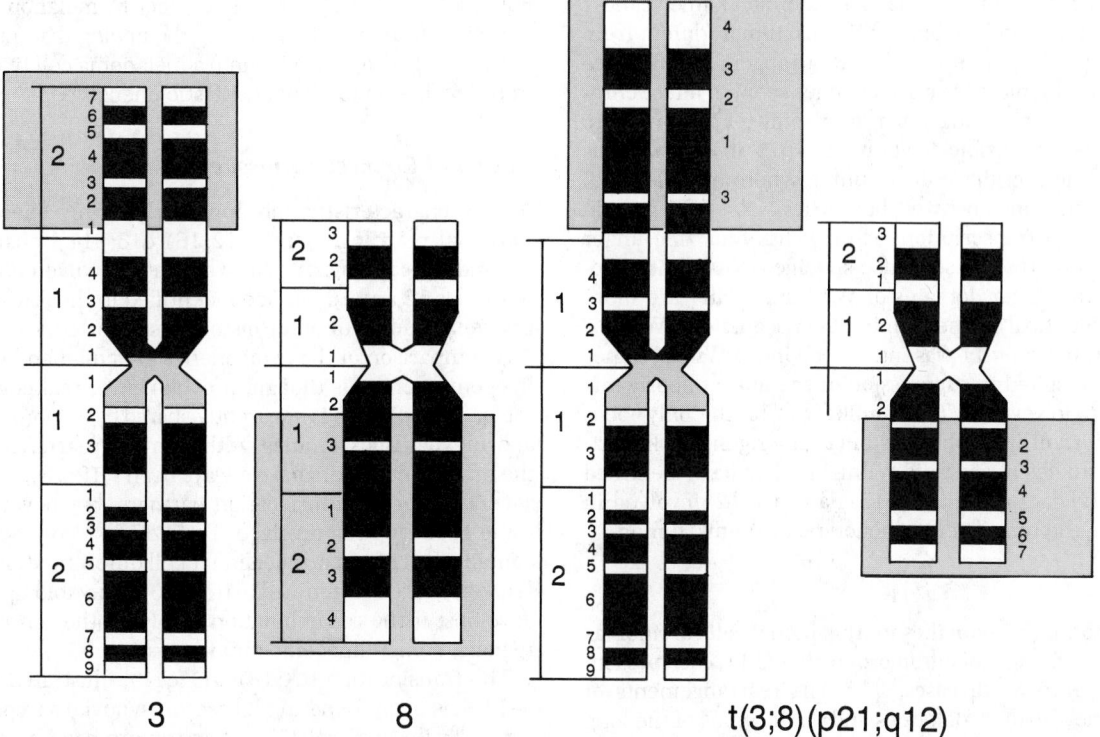

3   8   t(3;8)(p21;q12)

FIGURE 5–9. The reciprocal translocation t(3;8)(p21;q12) characterizes a subgroup of salivary gland adenomas.

number of unidentified marker chromosomes. At least four nonrandom cytogenetic abnormalities can be differentiated: structural changes of chromosome 1, trisomy 7, rearrangements of 17p usually leading to loss of the short arm, and loss of one chromosome 18.[166,167]

Molecular genetic studies have added significantly to our knowledge of the genetic changes that characterize colorectal tumorigenesis and have emphasized the fact that multiple genetic changes are required to change a normal cell into a fully malignant cell. Vogelstein and coworkers pinpointed five critical genes—*MCC* and *APC* on chromosome 5, *KRAS* on chromosome 11, *TP53* on chromosome 17, and *DCC* on chromosome 18—that are important in the development of colorectal tumors.[168,169] Except for *KRAS*, cytogenetic studies have been crucial in identifying the chromosomal regions harboring all of these genes, and further studies may reveal chromosomal sites of other genes that, if deregulated, rearranged, or lost, may be of pathogenetic significance.

Kidney

Structural rearrangements of the short arm of chromosome 3, with breakpoints mapping to 3p11–21, are the changes most consistently seen in renal cell carcinomas. The one feature common to these 3p aberrations appears to be the net loss of chromosomal material. The changes have commonly been interstitial or terminal deletions, and in other cases, reciprocal translocations between 3p and other chromosomes have occurred with concomitant loss of variable 3p segments.[170–172]

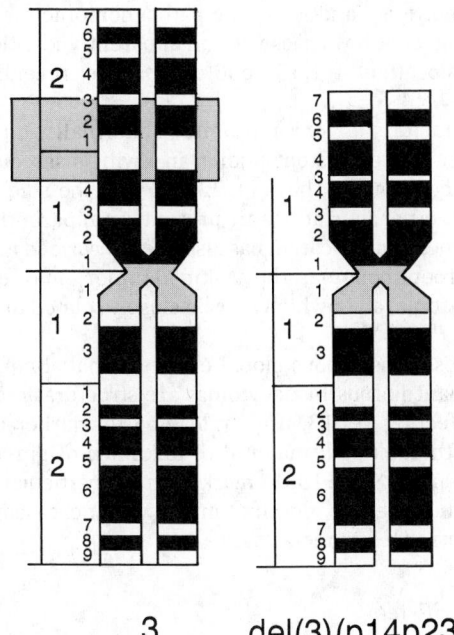

3   del(3)(p14p23)

FIGURE 5–10. A deletion of the short arm of chromosome 3, illustrated as a del(3)(p14p23), is the most consistent cytogenetic rearrangement in lung carcinomas. In other carcinomas, especially of the kidney, 3p– is also common.

The karyotypic profile of the most common kidney cancer of childhood, nephroblastoma or Wilms' tumor, differs from that of renal cell carcinomas.[173-176] Rearrangements of 3p are uncommon. The most frequent changes seem to affect chromosome 1, often resulting in partial trisomy for the long arm. Some tumors have visible deletions of 11p13, in which a locus (*WT1*) for the aniridia-Wilms' tumor syndrome is located. *WT1* has been cloned by two laboratories.[177,178] WT1 protein appears to be a transcription factor; it has four zinc finger domains, hallmarks of a sequence-specific DNA-binding protein. The zinc finger domains of WT1 and EGR1 are more than 60% identical in their amino acid sequences. When a normal chromosome 11 was introduced into a Wilms' tumor cell line, it resulted in suppression of the line's tumorigenic capacity.[179] However, *WT1* is unlikely to be the only locus that is important in nephroblastoma tumorigenesis. In fact, molecular studies of sporadic Wilms' tumors have identified another candidate gene in 11p15, named *WT2*, involved in suppressing the tumorigenic phenotype of Wilms' tumor.[180]

Bladder

The most common anomalies in transitional cell carcinomas are structural changes of chromosomes 1 and 11, each present in about a third of all cases.[181,182] The rearrangements of chromosome 1 include deletions and duplications of the long and short arms and a variety of translocations with breakpoints usually localized to the central segments of the long arm. The chromosome 11 abnormalities include isochromosome formation for 11p and 11q, translocations with a diversity of breakpoints on both arms, and deletions, usually del(11p). The abnormalities affecting both chromosomes are highly variable and possibly represent secondary, nonspecific changes. In contrast, three frequently recurring abnormalities—an isochromosome for the short arm of chromosome 5, trisomy 7, and monosomy 9—have been described as sole anomalies and are therefore credible candidates for a primary role in transitional cell carcinogenesis.

Skin

Although very few skin cancers have been cytogenetically investigated, recent studies of preinvasive and infiltrating squamous cell carcinomas and basal cell carcinomas have produced interesting and unexpected results.[183-185] Several abnormal clones, which often are unrelated, have been found. The number of cases studied is small, but the remarkably diverse karyotypic pictures hint that the tumors may be multiclonal rather than monoclonal. Additional cytogenetic evidence indicating similar polyclonality was also reported for squamous cell carcinomas of the aerodigestive tract. The combined data seem to indicate a fundamental pathogenetic difference between these epithelial tumors and most hematologic and mesenchymal neoplasms, for which karyotypic findings strongly support a monoclonal origin.

Chromosomes 1, 6, and 7 are nonrandomly involved in malignant melanomas.[186-188] The most common abnormalities of chromosome 1 are various deletions of the short arm, with breakpoints mostly in the region 1p11–22. The chromosome 7 involvement is mostly in the form of trisomy. The nonrandom involvement of chromosome 6 is due to numerous translocations and deletions of the long arm, with clustering to 6q12–25. The importance of 6q loci in melanoma tumorigenesis is further underscored by the finding that introduction of a normal chromosome 6 into a melanoma cell line resulted in the reversion to a nonneoplastic phenotype.[189]

Bone and Connective Tissue

A very characteristic and apparently highly specific chromosomal rearrangement, t(12;16)(q13;p11), characterizes myxoid liposarcomas.[190] No systematic involvement of chromosomes 12 and 16 has been identified in the few malignant lipogenic tumors of other histologies reported.

A comparison of the cytogenetics of benign and malignant lipogenic tumors is thought-provoking. A breakpoint cluster region in 12q13–15 is apparently shared by a lipoma subgroup and myxoid liposarcomas. Although the rearrangements in the malignant tumors have always been t(12;16), in lipomas, several different translocation partners, but never chromosome 16, have been involved. The 12q13–15 region probably contains loci of importance in fat cell differentiation. If these sequences are recombined in t(12;16), a myxoid liposarcoma develops; if the recombination involves other chromosomal regions, benign lipogenic tumors result.

The translocation t(X;18)(p11;q11), illustrated in Figure 5–11, has been found in all cases of synovial sarcomas studied.[191,192] Because relatively few tumors have been investigated, it is too early to know how frequent and how specific this rearrangement is. The t(X;18) is the first cancer-associated structural rearrangement that involves one of the sex chromosomes.

The reciprocal translocation t(2;13)(q35–37;q14) has been described in a large proportion of rhabdomyosarcomas, usually of the alveolar type, but also in the undifferentiated and embryonal forms.[193,194] The t(2;13) has not been reported in any other tumor type, and it may be pathognomonic for rhabdomyosarcomas. A few cases with an apparently identical variant translocation, t(1;13)(p36;q14), have recently been reported.[195,196]

A characteristic chromosomal abnormality, t(11;22)(q24;q12), is a consistent finding in Ewing's sarcoma (Fig. 5–12). Occasionally, the t(11;22) may be the sole change, but usually other aberrations are present. An apparently identical reciprocal translocation has also been described in peripheral neuroepithelioma, the Askin's tumor, and esthesioneuroblastoma, all of which may be closely related to Ewing's sarcomas.[197-199]

The most conspicuous clonal chromosomal abnormalities in malignant fibrous histiocytomas are structural rearrangements affecting 19p13, usually leading to marker chromosomes with additional material of unknown origin attached to band 19p13.[200] The 19p13 markers are of particular interest because they seem to identify tumors with increased risk for local recurrences or metastases.

Nervous System

No specific karyotypic abnormalities have been detected in malignant gliomas. The most frequent findings, occurring in half of these tumors, have been double minute chromosomes. Deletions and translocations involving 9p, trisomy 7, and loss of chromosomes 10, 22, and the sex chromosomes are also

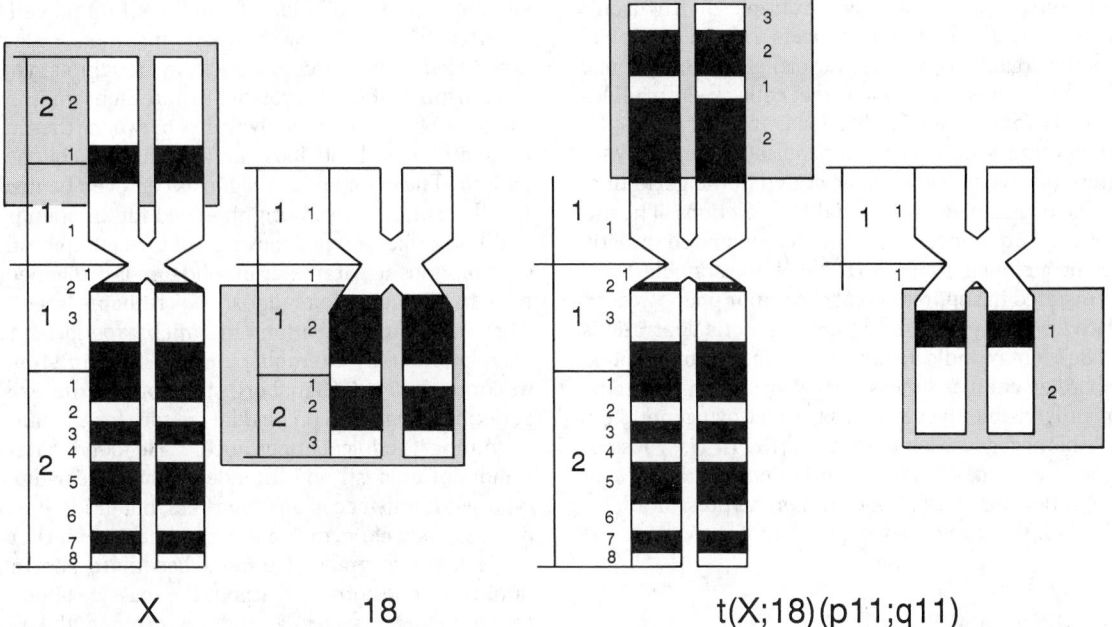

X 18 t(X;18)(p11;q11)

FIGURE 5–11. The reciprocal translocation t(X;18)(p11;q11) is specific for synovial sarcoma.

found.[201-203] It has recently been shown that a homozygous or heterozygous deletion of the interferon-α gene cluster, located on 9p, is present in more than 25% of glioma samples or cell lines derived from these tumors. These deletions are present only in patients with stage III and IV disease.[204]

The predominant abnormalities in neuroblastomas are deletions and other rearrangements of the terminal portion of 1p.[205-208] Although the breakpoints are variable, the segment from 1p31 to 1pter is usually deleted with a consensus deletion of band 1p36.[207] As many as 67% of all investigated tumors also display homogenously staining regions or double minute chromosomes. The homogenously staining regions and double minute chromosomes are more frequent in advanced tumors and especially in established cell lines. These phenomena appear to be linked to amplification of the *MYC* oncogene.

The most consistent acquired cytogenetic abnormality in retinoblastoma, found in about 33% of all cases, is an isochromosome for the short arm of chromosome 6.[209,210] Less consistent but even more frequent (50%) are various structural rearrangements of chromosome 1, mostly leading to a net increase of 1q material. Monosomy 13 or 13q deletions are discernible in fewer than 20% of all tumors. Apparently, visible chromosome deletions are a relatively minor mechanism for the production of hemi- or homozygosity at the retinoblastoma locus (*RB1*) in 13q14.

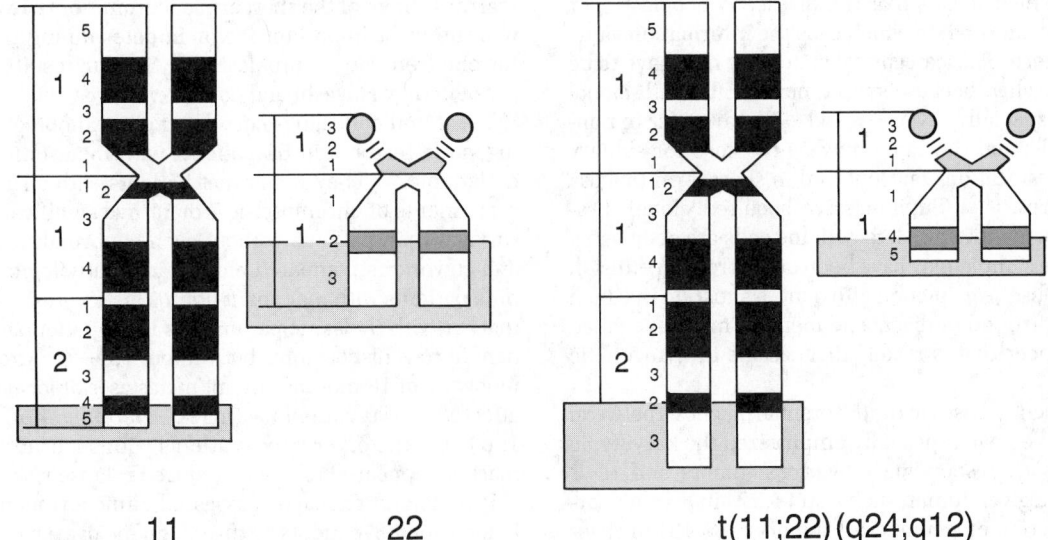

11 22 t(11;22)(q24;q12)

FIGURE 5–12. The reciprocal translocation t(11;22)(q24;q12) characterizes Ewing's sarcoma and the rarer variants of peripheral neuroepithelioma, Askin's tumor, and esthesioneuroblastoma.

Retinoblastoma is a paradigmatic example of Knudson's two-hit model, which explains how cancers that are autosomal dominant at the organism level may nevertheless be autosomal recessive at the level of individual target cells.[211] Both alleles of the retinoblastoma susceptibility locus in 13q14 must be inactivated before the cell becomes neoplastic. Patients with bilateral tumors have one allele inactivated in the germ line; some even have visible, constitutional 13q deletions. The importance of the 13q14 locus has been demonstrated directly by introducing a cloned, intact *RB1* gene into retinoblastoma cells. This resulted in suppression of the tumor phenotype.[212]

The relative scarcity of detectable cytogenetic aberrations affecting 13q14 may indicate that deletions in and around 13q14 jeopardize cellular fitness if they are so large as to be microscopically visible. Nevertheless, direct cytogenetic evidence of a homozygous deletion in 13q13–14 (*i.e.*, loss of the *RB1* locus in 13q14) was recently demonstrated, supporting the notion that loss of both tumor suppressor alleles is necessary before a tumor develops.[213]

CLINICAL IMPORTANCE
OF SOLID TUMOR CYTOGENETICS

For hematologic neoplasms, cytogenetic analysis now plays an integral part in the diagnostic workup of patients. The karyotypic findings in peripheral blood, bone marrow, or lymph node cells may unequivocally establish that the disease process is neoplastic, determine the type of neoplasm, and provide information of prognostic value. In practice, cytogenetics and other diagnostic modalities complement each other to achieve a picture in any given case that is as accurate and detailed as possible. Close cooperation between clinician, pathologist, and geneticist is of the essence.

The technical difficulties and the still limited data base have precluded the introduction of cytogenetics into routine diagnostic practices for solid tumors, although this situation may now be changing. As is the case in hematology, the major clinical usefulness of a chromosome analysis often lies in the digital nature of the result. Clonal chromosome aberrations are present, which means that the disease is neoplastic, or the karyotype is normal, in which case the information value is practically zero. This categorical statement may have to be modified somewhat, because simple numeric but still clonal aberrations (especially −X or −Y and +7) may occur in non-neoplastic cells, and the same may be the case for solitary reciprocal translocations encountered in short-term mucosa and skin cultures.[214–217] But if massive, acquired, clonal chromosomal abnormalities are detected, the cells are neoplastic. In practice, the sample may have been taken from an effusion of unknown cause (*e.g.*, pleural effusion), a situation in which classic cytologic or other diagnostic methods may have failed to detect a cancer that is readily diagnosable by cytogenetic methods.

Another difficulty arises in the differential diagnosis between tumor types. We have repeatedly emphasized the karyotypic characteristics corresponding to various tumors and their specificity for a given tumor, such as t(11;22) in Ewing's sarcoma (and the related neural crest tumors), t(2;13) in rhabdomyosarcoma, t(X;18) in synovial sarcoma, and t(12;16) in myxoid liposarcoma. Cytogenetics has already provided significant help in one of the most difficult differential diagnostic situations, the evaluation of small cell, round cell tumors in children.[218] Because Ewing's sarcoma, metastatic neuroblastoma, rhabdomyosarcoma, and non-Hodgkin's lymphoma all have distinguishing karyotypic features, chromosome analysis may differentiate unequivocally between these diagnostic possibilities with obvious therapeutic consequences for the patient. The cytogenetic diagnosis can even be made on fine-needle aspirates, obviating the need for an open biopsy.[219]

Whether karyotype features will turn out to be an independent prognostic parameter in solid tumor cytogenetics, as they have in hematologic malignancies, remains largely untested. There are some situations in which prognostic-cytogenetic correlations may exemplify the direction of similar reports to come. In 1986, Sandberg summarized the existing cytogenetic information on bladder tumors for the purpose of determining its clinical importance.[181] He found that noninvasive tumors of grades I and II tended to have near-diploid karyotypes with only occasional markers, but grade II tumors were often grossly abnormal and had numerous markers. Superficially invasive grade II tumors had more aberrations than noninvasive lesions but without the massive abnormalities of the more aggressive carcinomas. Among the noninvasive papillary tumors, the presence of cytogenetic markers appeared to have predictive value: tumors recurred in 90% of the patients with markers compared with fewer than 5% in whom no abnormal chromosomes were found.

The karyotype seems to be prognostically important in neuroblastoma. Kaneko and colleagues reported that a near-triploid chromosome number was associated with excellent prognosis and that the prognosis for patients with near-diploid or pseudodiploid tumors was dismal.[208] Hypotetraploid tumors seemed to have karyotypic and clinical features in common with the near-diploid or pseudodiploid tumors. The conclusion was that, at least from a clinical point of view, the near-triploid tumors constitute a distinct entity. Christiansen and Lampert analyzed patients with neuroblastoma of different stages and showed a 90% probability of surviving among patients lacking a 1p rearrangement, compared with a survival rate of less than 10% among patients with an abnormal 1p.[220] They concluded that the tumor karyotype, particularly whether a visible rearrangement of the short arm of chromosome 1 was present, was the most important factor in determining the outcome for children with neuroblastoma. Similar results have been presented by Hayashi and coworkers.[206]

Trent and colleagues correlated clinical outcome with cytogenetic features in 62 patients with metastatic malignant melanoma.[221] They found that patients with structural rearrangements of chromosome 7 or 11 had significantly shorter survival than patients without such abnormalities. Rydholm and coworkers compared clinical and pathologic features in nine patients with malignant fibrous histiocytoma and a 19p+ marker with the same parameters in 13 patients with malignant fibrous histiocytoma but without 19p+.[222] After a median follow-up of 18 months, distant metastases or local recurrence affected 8 of 9 patients with 19p+ but only 4 of 13 without 19p+. On the other hand, patients with supernumerary ring markers appeared to have a reduced relapse risk.

Pejovic and colleagues assessed clinicocytogenetic correlations for 88 patients with malignant ovarian tumors and found that chromosome abnormalities were present more often among seropapillary tumors and that cases with abnormal karyotypes on average were of higher stage with more frequent residual tumor mass after initial surgery.[223] Patients with clonal abnormalities had significantly shorter survival than those with a normal karyotype, and a multivariate analysis identified abnormal karyotype as being independently associated with short survival in advanced clinical stages of ovarian carcinoma.

Many of these correlations are preliminary, but they all illustrate the important point that chromosomal abnormalities may serve as disease markers. When these are statistically compared with other parameters, the associations that emerge may help improve diagnostic and prognostic precision. This development has already taken place in hematologic cytogenetics, and solid tumor cytogenetics is now quickly headed in the same direction.

CONCLUSIONS

One of the most surprising revelations has been the observation that many protooncogenes are located in the bands that are involved in consistent translocations (Fig. 5–8).[1,6,224,225] The evidence in Burkitt's lymphoma and in CML provided the impetus for investigation of other translocations. The successful cloning of several critical genes from solid tumors, based on their location within recurring chromosome deletions, contributed dramatically to our understanding of the genetic basis of malignant transformation.[226]

The analysis of various tumors for alterations in protooncogenes has revealed that many are abnormal as a result of translocations, amplification, or mutations. The relation of the change in the protooncogene to the multistage process of malignant transformation may be unclear. This ambiguity is not a problem with chromosome translocations; the evidence is overwhelming that the t(8;14) in Burkitt's lymphoma and the t(9;22) in CML are an integral component of the cascade of events leading to the transformation of a normal to a malignant cell. The ever-increasing number of recurring translocations reviewed in this chapter provides a potential gold mine for identifying new genes that are unequivocally related to the malignant phenotype of the affected cell.

The detection of recurring chromosome deletions provided the clues to the location of genes whose loss of function was a critical component leading to the malignant phenotype of many cells in solid tumors. Some of these genes have already been cloned: *RB1* (13q14), *TP53* (17p), *WT1* (11p13), *MCC* and *APC* (5q21), and *DCC* (18q21). The genes on 1p, 3p, 5q, 6q, 9p, 20q, and 22q that are important in carcinomas and leukemias have not yet been identified, but they will be cloned within the foreseeable future.

The ultimate measure of success will be the application of the insights into the critical genetic changes in malignant cells to the development of innovative, more effective treatments for cancer. Perhaps in the future, each subtype of tumor will be diagnosed and treated in a way that is most appropriate for its specific genetic defect. This should lead to a new era of cancer therapy that is more effective and less toxic.

GLOSSARY OF CYTOGENETIC TERMINOLOGY

Centromere
The constriction along the length of the chromosome that is the site of the spindle fiber attachment. The position of the centromere determines whether chromosomes are metacentric (X-shaped, such as chromosomes 1, 3, 16, 19, and 20) or acrocentric (inverted V-shaped, such as chromosomes 13 through 15, 21, 22, and Y). During mitosis, the two exact copies of the DNA in each chromosome are separated by shortening of the spindle fibers attached to opposite sides of the dividing cell.

Clone
In the cytogenetic sense, clone is defined as two cells with the same additional or structurally rearranged chromosome or three cells with loss of the same chromosome.

Deletion
A segment of a chromosome is missing as the result of two breaks and loss of the intervening piece.

Diploid
Normal chromosome number and composition of chromosomes.

Haploid
Only one half the normal complement (*i.e.*, 23 chromosomes in humans).

Hyperdiploid
Additional chromosomes; the modal number is 47 or greater in humans.

Hypodiploid
Loss of chromosomes with modal number 45 or less in humans.

Inversion
Two breaks occur in the same chromosome with rotation of the intervening segment. If both the breaks are on the same side of the centromere, it is called a *paracentric* inversion. If they are on opposite sides, it is called a *pericentric* inversion.

Isochromosome
A chromosome that consists of identical copies of one chromosome arm with loss of the other arm. An isochromosome for the long arm of chromosome 17 [i(17q)] contains two copies of the long arm (separated by the centromere) with loss of the short arm of the chromosome.

Karyotype
Arrangement of chromosomes from a particular cell according to a well-established system such that the largest chromosomes are first and the smallest ones are last. The normal female karyotype is 46,XX; the normal male karyotype is 46,XY.

Translocation
A break in at least two chromosomes with exchange of material; in a reciprocal translocation, there is no obvious loss of chromosomal material.

REFERENCES

1. Rowley JD. Molecular cytogenetics: Rosetta stone for understanding cancer: Clowes award lecture. Cancer Res 1990;50:3816–3825.
2. Rowley JD. Recurring chromosome abnormalities in leukemia and lymphoma. Semin Hematol 1990;27:122–136.
3. Heim S, Mitelman F. Primary chromosome abnormalities in human neoplasia. Adv Cancer Res 1989;52:1–43, 1989.
4. Heim S, Mitelman F. Cytogenetics of solid tumors. Adv Histopathol 1992;15:37–66.
5. Sandberg AA. The chromosomes in human cancer and leukemia. 2nd ed. New York: Elsevier, 1990.
6. Mitelman F, Kaneko Y, Trent JM. Report of the committee on chromosome changes in neoplasia. Cytogenet Cell Genet 1991;58:1051–1075.
7. Solomon E, Borrow J, Goddard AD. Chromosome aberrations and cancer. Science 1991;254:1153–1160.

8. Mitelman F. Catalog of chromosome aberrations in cancer. 4th ed. New York: Wiley-Liss, 1991.

9. Rowley JD, Potter D. Chromosomal banding patterns in acute nonlymphocytic leukemia. Blood 1976;47:705–721.

10. Mitelman F, ed. ISCN (1991) guidelines for cancer cytogenetics, supplement to an international system for human cytogenetic nomenclature. Basel: S. Karger, 1991.

11. Testa JR, Rowley JD. Chromosomes in leukemia and lymphoma with special emphasis on methodology. In: Catovsky D, ed. The leukemic cell. Edinburgh: Churchill-Livingstone, 1981:184–202.

12. Mandahl N. Methods in solid tumor cytogenetics. In: Rooney DE, Czepulkowski BH, eds. Human cytogenetics: A practical approach, vol 2. Malignancy and acquired chromosome abnormalities. : IRL Press, 1991.

13. Nowell PC, Hungerford DA. A minute chromosome in human granulocytic leukemia. Science 1960;132:1497.

14. Rowley JD. A new consistent chromosomal abnormality in chronic myelogenous leukemia. Nature 1973;243:290–293.

15. de Klein A, van Kessel AG, Grosveld G, et al. A cellular oncogene is translocated to the Philadelphia chromosome in chronic myelocytic leukemia. Nature 1982;300:765–767.

16. Rowley JD, Testa JR. Chromosome abnormalities in malignant hematologic diseases. In: Klein G, Weinhouse S, eds. Advances in Cancer Research. New York: Academic Press, 1983:103–148.

17. de Klein A, Hagemeijer A. Cytogenetic and molecular analysis of the Ph^1 translocation in chronic myeloid leukemia. Cancer Surv 1984;3:515–529.

18. Bakhshi A, Minowada J, Arnold A, et al. Lymphoid blast crises of chronic myelogenous leukemia represent stages in the development of B-cell precursors. N Engl J Med 1983;309:826–831.

19. Whang-Peng J, Canellos GP, Carbone PP, et al. Clinical implications of cytogenetic variants in chronic myelocytic leukemia (CML). Blood 1968;32:755–766.

20. Pugh WC, Pearson M, Vardiman JW, et al. Philadelphia chromosome-negative chronic myelogenous leukaemia: A morphologic reassessment. Br J Haematol 1985;60:457–467.

21. Travis LB, Pierre RV, DeWald GW. Ph^1-negative chronic granulocytic leukemia: A nonentity. Am J Clin Pathol 1986;85:186–193.

22. Morris CM, Reeve AE, Fitzgerald PH, et al. Genomic diversity correlates with clinical variation in Ph^1-negative chronic myeloid leukemia. Nature 1986;320:281–283.

23. Weinstein ME, Grossman A, Perle MA, et al. The karyotype of Philadelphia chromosome negative, *BCR* rearrangement-positive chronic myeloid leukemia. Cancer Genet Cytogenet 1988;35:223–229.

24. Groffen J, Stevenson JR, Heisterkamp N, et al. Philadelphia chromosomal breakpoints are clustered within a limited region, *BCR*, on chromosome 22. Cell 1984;36:93–99.

25. Westbrook CA, Rubin CM, Carrino JJ, et al. Long-range mapping of the Philadelphia chromosome by pulsed-field gel electrophoresis. Blood 1988;79:697–702.

26. Konopka JB, Watanabe SM, Witte ON. An alteration of the human c-ABL protein in K562 leukemia cells unmasks associate tyrosine kinase activity. Cell 1984;37:1035–1042.

27. Shtivelman E, Lifshitz B, Robert P, et al. Fused transcript of *ABL* and *BCR* genes in chronic myelogenous leukaemia. Nature 1985;315:550–554.

28. Daley GQ, Van Etten RA, Baltimore D. Induction of chronic myelogenous leukemia in mice by the p210$^{bcr/abl}$ gene of the Philadelphia chromosome. Science 1990;247:824–830.

29. Heisterkamp NN, Jenster G, ten Hoeve J, et al. Acute leukemia in BCR/ABL transgenic mice. Nature 1990;344:251–253.

30. Maru Y, Witte ON. The *BCR* gene encodes a novel serine/threonine kinase activity within a single exon. Cell 1991;67:459–468.

31. Kawasaki ES, Clark SS, Coyne MY, et al. Diagnosis of chronic myeloid and acute lymphocytic leukemias by detection of leukemia-specific mRNA sequences amplified in vitro. Proc Natl Acad Sci USA 1988;85:5698–5702.

32. Tkachuk DC, Westbrook CA, Andreeff M, et al. Detection of BCR-ABL fusion in chronic myelogenous leukemia by in situ hybridization. Science 1990;250:559–562.

33. Arnoldus EPJ, Wiegant J, Noordermeer IA, et al. Detection of the Philadelphia chromosome in interphase nuclei. Cytogenet Cell Genet 1990;54:108–111.

34. Bennett JM, Catovsky D, Daniel M-T, et al. Proposals for the classification of the acute leukemias: French-American-British (FAB) Co-operative Group. Br J Haematol 1976;33:451–458.

35. Rowley JD. Identification of a translocation with quinacrine fluorescence in a patient with acute leukemia. Ann Genet 1973;16:109–112.

36. Fourth International Workshop on Chromosomes in Leukemia. Cancer Genet Cytogenet 1984;11:249–360.

37. Leverger G, Bernheim A, Daniel M-T, et al. Cytogenetic study of 130 childhood acute nonlymphocytic leukemias. Med Pediatr Oncol 1988;16:227–232.

38. Gough NM, Gearing DP, Nicola NA, et al. Localization of the human GM-CSF receptor gene to the X-Y pseudoautosomal region. Nature 1990;345:734–736.

39. Gao J, Erickson P, Gardiner K, et al. Isolation of a yeast artificial chromosome spanning the 8;21 translocation breakpoint, t(8;21)(q22;q22.3), in acute myelogenous leukemia. Proc Natl Acad Sci USA 1991;88:4882–4886.

40. Miyoshi H, Shimizu K, Kozu T, et al. The t(8;21) breakpoints on chromosome 21 in acute myeloid leukemia clustered within a limited region of a novel gene, *AML1*. Proc Natl Acad Sci USA 1991;88:10431–10434.

41. Rowley JD, Golomb HM, Vardiman J, et al. Further evidence for a non-random chromosomal abnormality in acute promyelocytic leukemia. Int J Cancer 1977;20:869–872.

42. Borrow J, Goddard AD, Sheer D, et al. Molecular analysis of acute promyelocytic leukemia breakpoint cluster region on chromosome 17. Science 1990;249:1577–1580.

43. de Thé H, Chomienne C, Lanotte M, et al. The t(15;17) translocation of acute promyelocytic leukaemia fuses the retinoic acid receptor α gene to a novel transcribed locus. Nature 1990;347:558–562.

44. Kakezuka A, Miller WH, Umesona K, et al. Chromosomal translocation t(15;17) in human acute promyelocytic leukemia fuses RARα with a novel putative transcription factor, PML. Cell 1991;66:663–674.

45. Biondi A, Rambaldi A, Alcalay M, et al. *Rar-α* gene rearrangements as a genetic marker for diagnosis and monitoring in acute promyelocytic leukaemia. Blood 1991;77:1418–1422.

46. Pearson MG, Vardiman JW, Le Beau MM, et al. A new cytogenetic subset of acute non-lymphocytic leukemia: t(6;9) associated with bone marrow basophilia. Am J Hematol 1985;18:393–403.

47. von Lindern M, Poustka A, Lerach H, et al. The (6;9) chromosome translocation, associated with a specific subtype of acute nonlymphocytic leukemia, leads to aberrant transcription of a target gene on 9p34. Mol Cell Biol 1990;10:4016–4026.

48. Berger R, Bernheim A, Sigaux F, et al. Acute monocytic leukemia chromosome studies. Leuk Res 1982;6:17–26.

49. Hagemeijer A, Hahlen K, Sizoo W, et al. Translocation (9;11)(p21;q23) in three cases of acute monoblastic leukemia. Cancer Genet Cytogenet 1982;5:95–105.

50. Rowley JD, Diaz MO, Espinosa R, et al. Mapping chromosome band 11q23 in human acute leukemia with biotinylated probes: Identification of 11q23 translocation breakpoints with a yeast artificial chromosome. Proc Natl Acad Sci USA 1990;87:9358–9362.

51. Ziemin-van der Poel S, McCabe N, Gill HJ, et al. Identification of a gene (*MLL*) which spans the breakpoint in 11q23 translocations associated with human leukemias. Proc Natl Acad Sci USA 1991;88:10735–10739.

52. Arthur DC, Bloomfield CD. Partial deletion of the long arm of chromosome 16 and bone marrow eosinophilia in acute nonlymphocytic leukemia: A new association. Blood 1983;61:994–998.

53. Larson RA, Williams SF, Le Beau MM, et al. Acute myelomonocytic leukemia with abnormal eosinophils and inv(16) or t(16;16) has a favorable prognosis. Blood 1986;68:1242–1249.

54. Keating MJ, Smith TL, Kantarjian H, et al. Cytogenetic patterns in acute myelogenous leukemia: A major reproducible determinant of outcome. Leukemia 1988;2:403–412.

55. Sixth Workshop on Chromosomes in Leukemia. Cancer Genet Cytogenet 1989;40:141–132.

56. Tucker MA, Coleman CN, Cox RS, et al. Risk of second cancers after treatment for Hodgkin's disease. N Engl J Med 1988;318:76–81.

57. Le Beau MM, Albain KS, Larson RA, et al. Clinical and cytogenetic correlations in 63 patients with therapy-related myelodysplastic syndromes and acute nonlymphocytic leukemia: Further evidence for characteristic abnormalities of chromosomes No. 5 and 7. J Clin Oncol 1986;4:325–345.

58. Arthur DC, Bloomfield CD. Banded chromosome analysis in patients with treatment-associated acute non-lymphocytic leukemia. Cancer Genet Cytogenet 1984;12:189–199.

59. Pedersen-Bjergaard J, Philip P, Larsen SO, et al. Chromosome aberrations and prognostic factors in therapy-related myelodysplasia and acute nonlymphocytic leukemia. Blood 1990;76:1083–1091.

60. Larson RA, Le Beau MM, Vardiman JW, et al. The predictive value of initial cytogenetic studies in 148 adults with acute nonlymphocytic leukemia. Cancer Genet Cytogenet 1983;10:219–236.

61. Mitelman F, Nilsson PG, Brandt C, et al. Chromosome pattern, occupation and clinical features in patients with acute nonlymphocytic leukemia. Cancer Cytogenet 1981;4:187–214.

62. Golomb HM, Alimena G, Rowley JD, et al. Correlation of occupation and karyotype in adults with acute nonlymphocytic leukemia. Blood 1982;60:404–411.

63. Rowley JD, Le Beau MM. Cytogenetic and molecular analysis of therapy-related leukemia. In: Diamond L, Wolman S, eds. Viral oncogenesis and cell differentiation: Memorial symposium volume for Dr. Charlotte Friend. NY Acad Sci 1989;567:130–140.

64. Ratain MJ, Kaminer LS, Bitran JD, et al. Acute nonlymphocytic leukemia following etoposide and cisplatin combination chemotherapy for advanced non-small cell carcinoma of the lung. Blood 1987;70:1412–1417.

65. Piu C-H, Behm FG, Raimondi S, et al. Secondary acute myeloid leukemia in children treated for acute lymphoid leukemia. N Engl J Med 1989;321:136–142.

66. Pedersen-Bjergaard J, Philip P. Balanced translocations involving chromosome bands 11q23 and 21q22 are highly characteristic of myelodysplasia and leukemia following therapy with cytostatic agents targeting at DNA–topoisomerase II. Blood [Letter] 1991;78:1147–1148.

67. Larson RA, Le Beau MM, Ratain MJ, et al. Balanced translocations involving chromosome bands 11q23 and 21q22 in therapy-related leukemia. Blood 1992;79:1892–1893.

68. Bennett JM, Catovsky D, Daniel MT, et al. Proposals for the classification of the myelodysplastic syndromes. Br J Haematol 1982;51:189.

69. Third MIC Cooperative Study Group (1987). Morphologic, immunologic, and cytogenetics (MIC) working classification of the primary myelodysplastic syndromes and therapy-related myelodysplasias and leukemias. Cancer Genet Cytogenet 1988;32:1–10.

70. Jacobs RH, Cornbleet MA, Vardiman JW, et al. Prognostic implications of morphology and karyotype in primary myelodysplastic syndromes. Blood 1986;67:1765–1772.

71. Yunis JJ, Lohell M, Arnesen MA, et al. Refined chromosome study helps define prognostic subgroups in most patients with primary myelodysplastic syndrome and acute myelogenous leukemia. Br J Haematol 1988;68:189–194.

72. Van Den Berghe H, Cassiman JJ, David G, et al. Distinct hematological disorder with deletion of long arm of No. 5 chromosome. Nature 1974;251:437–438.

73. Yunis JJ, Frizzera G, Oken MM, et al. Multiple recurrent genomic defects in follicular lymphoma; a possible model for cancer. N Engl J Med 1987;316:79–84.

74. Offit K, Jhanwar SC, Ladanyi M, et al. Cytogenetic analysis of 434 consecutively ascertained specimens of non-Hodgkin's lymphoma: Correlations between recurrent aberrations, histology, and exposure to cytotoxic treatment. Genes Chrom Cancer 1991;3:189–201.

75. Fifth International Workshop on Chromosomes in Leukemia-Lymphoma. Correlation of chromosome abnormalities with histologic and immunologic characteristics in non-Hodgkin's lymphoma and adult T-cell leukemia-lymphoma. Blood 1987;70:1554–1564.

76. Manolov G, Manolova Y. Marker band in one chromosome 14 from Burkitt lymphomas. Nature 1972;237:33–34.

77. Zech L, Haglund U, Nilsson K, et al. Characteristic chromosomal abnormalities in biopsies and lymphoid-cell lines from patients with Burkitt and non-Burkitt lymphomas. Int J Cancer 1976;17:47–56.

78. Leder P, Battey J, Lenoir G, et al. Translocations among antibody genes in human cancer. Science 1983;222:765–771.

79. Cesarman E, Dalla-Favera R, Bently D, et al. Mutations in the first exon are associated with altered transcription of c-MYC in Burkitt lymphoma. Science 1987;238:1272–1275.

80. Fukuhara S, Rowley JD, Variakojis D, et al. Chromosome abnormalities in poorly differentiated lymphocytic lymphoma. Cancer Res 1979;39:3119–3128.

81. Working formulation for clinical usage: National Cancer Institute sponsored study of classification of non-Hodgkin's lymphomas. Cancer 1982;49:2112–2135.

82. Tsujimoto Y, Finger LR, Yunis JJ, et al. Cloning of the chromosome breakpoint of neoplastic B cells with the t(14;18) chromosome translocation. Science 1984;226:1098–1099.

83. Cleary ML, Sklar J. Cloning and structural analysis of cDNA's for BCL-2 and a hybrid BCL-2/immunoglobulin transcript resulting from the t(14;18) translocation. Cell 1986;47:19–28.

84. Hockenberry D, Zutter M, Hickey W, et al. BCL-2 protein is topographically restricted in tissues characterized by apoptotic cell death. Proc Natl Acad Sci USA 1991;88:6961–6965.

85. Juliusson G, Oscher DG, Fitchett M, et al. Prognostic subgroups in B-cell chronic lymphocytic leukemia defined by specfic chromosomal abnormalities. N Engl J Med 1990;323:720–724.

86. Bird ML, Ueshima Y, Rowley JD, et al. Chromosome abnormalities in B-cell chronic lymphocytic leukemia and their clinical correlations. Leukemia 1989;3:182–191.

87. Perez Losada A, Wessman M, Tianinen M, et al. Trisomy 12 in chronic lymphocytic leukemia: An interphase cytogenetic study. Blood 1991;78:775–779.

88. Anastasi J, Le Beau MM, Vardiman JW. Detection of trisomy 12 in chronic lymphocytic leukemia by fluorescence in situ hybridization to interphase cells: A simple and sensitive method. Blood 1992;79:1796–1801.

89. Tsujimoto Y, Yunis J, Onorato-Showe L, et al. Molecular cloning of the chromosomal breakpoint of B-cell lymphomas and leukemias with the t(11;14) chromosome translocation. Science 1984;224:1403–1406.

90. Rosenberg CL, Wong E, Petty EM, et al. PRAD1, a candidate BCL1 oncogene: Mapping and expression in centrocytic lymphoma. Proc Natl Acad Sci USA 1991;88:9638–9642.

91. Williams ME, Meeker TC, Swerdlow SH. Rearrangement of the chromosome 11 BCL-1 locus in centrocytic lymphoma: Analysis with multiple breakpoint probes. Blood 1991;78:493–498.

92. Ohno H, Takimoto G, McKeithan TW. The candidate proto-oncogene BCL-3 is related to genes implicated in cell lineage determination and cell cycle control. Cell 1990;60:991–997.

93. Nucifora G, Zhang Q, Dickstein J, et al. BCL3: A putative new member of the IkB family of transcriptional factor inhibitors. Abstract presented at 1992 AACR meeting (in press).

94. The Third International Workshop on Chromosomes in Leukemia. Cancer Genet Cytogenet 1981;4:95–142.

95. Clark SS, McLaughlin J, Crist WM, et al. Unique forms of the abl tyrosine kinase distinguish Ph¹-positive CML from Ph¹-positive ALL. Science 1987;235:85–88.

96. Chan LC, Karhi KK, Rayter SI, et al. A novel ABL protein expressed in Philadelphia chromosome positive acute lymphoblastic leukaemia. Nature 1987;325:635–637.

97. Hooberman AL, Westbrook CA, Davey F, et al. Molecular detection of the Philadelphia (Ph¹) chromosome in acute lymphoblastic leukemia (ALL): Clinical, cytogenetic, and immunophenotypic correlations in a CALGB study. Blood 1989;72:52a.

98. Stong RC, Korsmeyer SJ, Parkin JL, et al. Human acute leukemia cell line with the t(4;11) chromosomal rearrangement exhibits B-lineage and monocytic characteristics. Blood 1986;67:391–397.

99. Chen C-S, Medberry PS, Arthur DC, et al. Breakpoint clustering in t(4;11)(q21;q23) acute leukemia. Blood 1991;78:2498–2504.

100. Michael PM, Levin MD, Garson OM, et al. Translocation 1;19—a new cytogenetic abnormality in acute lymphocytic leukemia. Cancer Genet Cytogenet 1984;12:333–341.

101. Williams DL, Look AT, Melvin SL, et al. New chromosomal translocations correlate with specific immunophenotypes of childhood acute lymphoblastic leukemia. Cell 1984;36:101–109.

102. Crist WM, Shuster JJ, Behm FG, et al. Poor prognosis of children with pre-B acute leukemia is associated with t(1;19)(q23;p13): A Pediatric Oncology Group study. Blood 1990;76:117–122.

103. Mellentin JD, Murri C, Donlon TA, et al. The gene for enhancer binding proteins E12/E47 lies at the t(1;19) breakpoint in acute leukemias. Science 1989;246:379–382.

104. Kamps MP, Murre C, Sun X-H, et al. A new homeobox gene contributes the DNA binding domain of the t(1;19) translocation protein in pre-B ALL. Cell 1990;60:547–556.

105. Hunger SP, Galili N, Carroll AJ, et al. The t(1;19)(q23;p13) results in consistent fusion of E2A and PBX1 coding sequences in acute lymphoblastic leukemia. Blood 1991;77:687–693.

106. Williams DL, Look AT, Harber J, et al. Chromosomal translocations play a unique role in influencing prognosis in childhood acute lymphoblastic leukemia. Blood 1986;68:205–212.

107. Rubin CM, Le Beau MM, Mick R, et al. Impact of chromosomal translocations on prognosis in childhood acute lymphoblastic leukemia. J Clin Oncol 1991;9:2183–2192.

108. Ueshima Y, Rowley JD, Variakojis D, et al. Cytogenetic studies on patients with chronic T cell leukemia/lymphoma. Blood 1984;63:1028–1038.

109. Miyamoto K, Tomita N, Ishii A, et al. Chromosome abnormalities of leukemia cells in adult patients with T-cell leukemia. JNCI 1984;73:353–362.

110. Raimondi SC, Pui C-H, Behm FG, et al. 7q32-q36 translocations in childhood T cell leukemia: Cytogenetic evidence for involvement of the T cell receptor B-chain gene. Blood 1987;69:131–134.

111. Kaiser-McCaw B, Hecht F, Harnden DG, et al. Somatic rearrangement of chromosome 14 in human lymphocytes. Proc Natl Acad Sci USA 1974;72:2071–2075.

112. Aurias A. Analyse cytogenetique de 21 cas d'ataxie-telangiectasie. J Genet Hum 1981;29:235–247.

113. Zech L, Gahrton G, Hammarstrom L, et al. Inversion of chromosome 14 marks human T-cell chronic lymphocytic leukemia. Nature 1985;309:858–860.

114. Sadamori N, Nishino K, Kusano M, et al. Significance of chromosome 14 anomaly at band q11 in Japanese patients with adult T-cell leukemia. Cancer 1986;58:2244–2250.

115. Rowley JD, Haren JM, Wong-Staal F, et al. Chromosome pattern in cells from patients positive for human T-cell leukemia virus. In: Gallo RC, Essex ME, Gross L, eds. Human T-cell leukemia-lymphoma viruses. Cold Spring Harbor, NY: Cold Spring Harbor Press, 1984:85–89.

116. Shima EA, Le Beau MM, McKeithan TW, et al. Gene encoding the alpha chain of the T-cell receptor is moved immediately downstream of c-MYC in a chromosomal 8;14 translocation in a cell line from a human T-cell leukemia. Proc Natl Acad Sci USA 1986;83:3439–3443.

117. Mathieu-Mahul D, Caubet JF, Bernheim A. Molecular cloning of a DNA fragment from human chromosome 14(14q11) involved in T cell malignancies. EMBO J 1985;4:3427–3433.

118. Brown L, Cheng J-T, Chen Q, et al. Site-specific recombination of the TAL-1 gene is a common occurrence in human T cell leukemia. EMBO J 1990;9:3343–3351.

119. Aplan PD, Lombardi DP, Ginsberg AM, et al. Disruption of the human SCL locus by "illegitimate" V-(D)-J recombinase activity. Science 1990;250:1426–1429.

120. Sutherland GR, Hecht F. Fragile sites on human chromosomes. New York: Oxford University Press, 1985.

121. Yunis JJ, Soreng AL. Constitutive fragile sites and cancer. Science 1984;226:1199–1204.

122. Le Beau MM. Chromosomal fragile sites and cancer-specific rearrangements. Blood 1986;67:849–858.

123. ar-Rushdi A, Nishikura K, Erickson J, et al. Differential expression of the translocated and the untranslocated c-MYC oncogene in Burkitt lymphoma. Science 1983;222:390–393.

124. Rabbitts TH, Boehm T, Mengle-Gaw L, et al. Chromosomal abnormalities in lymphoid tumours: Mechanism and role in tumour pathogenesis. Trends Genet 1988;4:300–304.

125. Tycko B, Sklar J. Chromosomal translocations in lymphoid neoplasia: A reappraisal of the recombinase model. Cancer Cells 1990;2:1–8.

126. Fialkow PJ, Singer JW. Tracing development and cell lineages in human hemopoietic neoplasia. In: Weissman IL, ed. Leukemia. Dahlem Konferenzen. Berlin: Springer-Verlag, 1985:203–222.

127. Adams JM, Cory S. Transgenic models of tumor development. Science 1991;254:1161–1167.

128. Nomiyama H, Fromental C, Xiao JH, et al. Cell-specific activity of the constituent elements of the simian virus 40 enhancer. Proc Natl Acad Sci USA 1987;84:7881–7885.

129. Bullerdiek J, Chilla R, Haubrich J. A causal relationship between chromosomal rearrangements and the genesis of salivary gland pleomorphic adenomas. Arch Otorhinolaryngol 1988;245:244–249.

130. Sandros J, Stenman G, Mark J. Cytogenetic and molecular observations in human and experimental salivary gland tumors. Cancer Genet Cytogenet 1990;44:153–167.

131. Mandahl N, Heim S, Arheden K, et al. Three major cytogenetic subgroups can be identified among chromosomally abnormal solitary lipomas. Hum Genet 1988;79:203–208.

132. Sreekantaiah C, Leong SPL, Karakousis C, et al. Cytogenetic profile of 109 lipomas. Cancer Res 1991;51:422–433.

133. Nilbert M, Heim S. Uterine leiomyoma cytogenetics. Genes Chrom Cancer 1990;2:3–13.

134. Mark J, Havel G, Grepp C, et al. Chromosomal patterns in human benign uterine leiomyomas. Cancer Genet Cytogenet 1990;44:1–13.

135. Pandis N, Heim S, Bardi G, et al. Chromosome analysis of 96 uterine leiomyomas. Cancer Genet Cytogenet 1991;55:11–18.

136. Pandis N, Heim S, Willén H, et al. Histologic-cytogenetic correlations in uterine leiomyomas. Int J Gynecol Cancer 1991;1:163–168.

137. Mark J. Chromosomal abnormalities and their specificity in human neoplasms: An assessment of recent observations by banding techniques. Adv Cancer Res 1977;24:165–222.

138. Zang K. Cytological and cytogenetical studies on human meningioma. Cancer Genet Cytogenet 1982;6:249–274.

139. Dumanski JP, Rouleau GA, Nordenskjöld M, et al. Molecular genetic analysis of chromosome 22 in 81 cases of meningioma. Cancer Res 1990;50:5863–5867.

140. Jin Y, Heim S, Mandahl N, et al. Multiple clonal chromosome aberrations in squamous cell carcinomas of the larynx. Cancer Genet Cytogenet 1990;44:209–216.

141. Jin Y, Heim S, Mandahl N, et al. Unrelated clonal chromosomal aberrations in carcinomas of the oral cavity. Genes Chrom Cancer 1990;1:209–215.

142. Jin Y, Higashi K, Mandahl N, et al. Frequent rearrangement of chromosomal bands 1p22 and 11q13 in squamous cell carcinomas of the head and neck. Genes Chrom Cancer 1990;2:198–204.

143. Whang-Peng J, Lee EC. Cytogenetics of human small cell lung cancer. Recent Results Cancer Res 1985;97:37–46.

144. Campbell L, Brown J, Garson OM, et al. Cytogenetic abnormalities in lung cancer. In: Hansen HH, ed. Basic and clinical concepts of lung cancer. Boston: Kluwer Academic, 1989:123–136.

145. Lukeis R, Irving L, Garson M, et al. Cytogenetics of non-small cell lung cancer: Analysis of consistent non-random abnormalities. Genes Chrom Cancer 1990;2:116–124.

146. Miura I, Siegfried JM, Resau J, et al. Chromosome alterations in 21 non-small cell lung carcinomas. Genes Chrom Cancer 1990;2:328–338.

147. Birrer MJ, Minna JD. Genetic changes in the pathogenesis of lung cancer. Annu Rev Med 1989;40:305–317.

148. Tiainen M, Tammilehto L, Rautonen J, et al. Chromosomal abnormalities and their correlations with asbestos exposure and survival in patients with mesothelioma. Br J Cancer 1989;60:618–626.

149. Hagemeijer A, Versnel MA, Van Drunen E, et al. Cytogenetic analysis of malignant mesothelioma. Cancer Genet Cytogenet 1990;47:1–28.

150. Dutrillaux B, Gerbault-Seureau M, Zafrani B. Characterization of chromosomal anomalies in human breast cancer. A comparison of 30 paradiploid cases with few chromosome changes. Cancer Genet Cytogenet 1990;49:203–217.

151. Geleick D, Müller H, Matter A, et al. Cytogenetics of breast cancer. Cancer Genet Cytogenet 1990;46:217–229.

152. Mitchell ELD, Santibanez-Koref MF. 1p13 is the most frequently involved band in structural chromosomal rearrangements in human breast cancer. Genes Chrom Cancer 1990;2:279–289.

153. Pandis N, Heim S, Bardi G, et al. Improved technique for cytogenetic analysis of human breast cancer. Genes Chrom Cancer 1992;5:14–20.

154. Couturier J, Vielh P, Salmon RJ, et al. Chromosome imbalance in endometrial adenocarcinoma. Cancer Genet Cytogenet 1988;33:67–76.

155. Atkin NB, Baker MC, Fox MF. Chromosome changes in 43 carcinomas of the cervix uteri. Cancer Genet Cytogenet 1990;44:229–241.

156. Milatovich A, Heerema NA, Palmer CG. Cytogenetic studies of endometrial malignancies. Cancer Genet Cytogenet 1990;46:41–54.

157. Pejovic T, Heim S, Mandahl N, et al. Consistent occurrence of a 19p+ marker chromosome and loss of 11p material in ovarian seropapillary cystadenocarcinomas. Genes Chrom Cancer 1989;1:167–171.

158. Bello MJ, Rey JA. Chromosome aberrations in metastatic ovarian cancer: relationship with abnormalities in primary tumors. Int J Cancer 1990;45:50–54.

159. Pejovic T, Heim S, Mandahl N, et al. Chromosome aberrations in 35 primary ovarian carcinomas. Genes Chrom Cancer 1992;4:58–68.

160. Brothman AR, Peehl DM, Patel AM, et al. Frequency and pattern of karyotypic abnormalities in human prostate cancer. Cancer Res 1990;50:3795–3803.

161. Lundgren R, Mandahl N, Heim S, et al. Cytogenetic analysis of 57 primary prostatic adenocarcinomas. Genes Chrom Cancer 1992;4:16–24.

162. Delozier-Blanchet CD, Walt H, Engel E, et al. Cytogenetic studies of human testicular germ cell tumours. Int J Androl 1987;10:69–77.

163. Bosl GJ, Dmitrovsky E, Reuter VE, et al. Isochromosome of chromosome 12: Clinical useful marker for male germ cell tumors. JNCI 1989;81:1874–1878.

164. Castedo SMMJ, de Jong B, Oosterhuis JW, et al. Chromosomal changes in human primary testicular nonseminomatous germ cell tumors. Cancer Res 1989;49:5696–5701.

165. Castedo SMMJ, de Jong B, Oosterhuis JW, et al. Cytogenetic analysis of ten human seminomas. Cancer Res 1989;49:439–443.

166. Muleris M, Salmon R-J, Dutrillaux B. Cytogenetics of colorectal adenocarcinomas. Cancer Genet Cytogenet 1990;46:143–156.

167. Bardi G, Johansson B, Pandis N, et al. Cytogenetic aberrations in colorectal adenocarcinomas and their correlation to clinicopathologic features. (submitted).

168. Fearon ER, Vogelstein B. A genetic model for colorectal tumorigenesis. Cell 1990;61:759–767.

169. Kinzler KW, Nilbert MC, Su L-K, et al. Identification of FAP locus genes from chromosome 5q21. Science 1991;253:661–665.

170. Dal Cin P, Li FP, Prout Jr GR, et al. Involvement of chromosomes 3 and 5 in renal cell carcinoma. Cancer Genet Cytogenet 1988;35:41–46.

171. Kovacs G, Frisch S. Clonal chromosome abnormalities in tumor cells from patients with sporadic renal cell carcinomas. Cancer Res 1989;49:651–659.

172. Walter TA, Berger CS, Sandberg AA. The cytogenetics of renal tumors. Where do we stand, where do we go? Cancer Genet Cytogenet 1989;43:15–34.

173. Kondo K, Chilcote RR, Maurer HS, et al. Chromosome abnormalities in tumor cells from patients with sporadic Wilms' tumor. Cancer Res 1984;44:5376–5381.

174. Douglass EC, Wilimas JA, Green AA, et al. Abnormalities of chromosomes 1 and 11 in Wilms' tumor. Cancer Genet Cytogenet 1985;14:331–338.

175. Slater RM, de Kraker J, Voûte PA, et al. A cytogenetic study of Wilms' tumor. Cancer Genet Cytogenet 1985;14:95–109.

176. Solis V, Pritchard J, Cowell JK. Cytogenetic changes in Wilms' tumor. Cancer Genet Cytogenet 1988;34:223–234.

177. Call KM, Glaser T, Ito CY, et al. Isolation and characterization of a zinc finger polypeptide gene at the human chromosome 11 Wilms' tumor locus. Cell 1990;60:509–520.

178. Gessler M, Poustka A, Cavenee W, et al. Homozygous deletion in Wilms' tumours of a zinc-finger gene identified by chromosome jumping. Nature 1990;343:774–778.

179. Weissman BE, Saxon PJ, Pasquale SR, et al. Introduction of a normal human chromosome 11 into a Wilms' tumor cell line controls its tumorigenic expression. Science 1987;236:175–180.

180. Dowdy SF, Fasching CL, Araujo D, et al. Suppression of tumorigenicity in Wilms tumor by the p15.5-p14 region of chromosome 11. Science 1991;254:293–295.

181. Sandberg AA. Chromosome changes in bladder cancer: Clinical and other correlations. Cancer Genet Cytogenet 1986;19:163–175.

182. Perucca D, Szepetowski P, Simon M-P, et al. Molecular genetics of human bladder carcinomas. Cancer Genet Cytogenet 1990;49:143–156.

183. Aledo R, Dutrillaux B, Lombard M, et al. Cytogenetic study on eleven cutaneous neoplasms and two pre-tumoral lesions from xeroderma pigmentosum patients. Int J Cancer 1989;44:79–83.

184. Heim S, Mertens F, Jin Y, et al. Diverse chromosome abnormalities in squamous cell carcinomas of the skin. Cancer Genet Cytogenet 1989;39:69–76.

185. Mertens F, Heim S, Mandahl N, et al. Cytogenetic analysis of 33 basal cell carcinomas. Cancer Res 1991;51:954–957.

186. Parmiter AH, Nowell PC. The cytogenetics of human malignant melanoma and premalignant lesions. In: Nathanson L, ed. Malignant melanoma: Biology, diagnosis, and therapy. Boston: Kluwer Academic, 1988:47–61.

187. Trent JM, Thompson FH, Meyskens Jr FL. Identification of a recurring site involving chromosome 6 in human malignant melanoma. Cancer Res 1989;49:420–423.

188. Cowan JM, Francke U. Cytogenetic analysis in melanoma and nevi. In: Nathanson L, ed. Melanoma research: Genetics, growth factors, metastases and antigenes. Boston: Kluwer Academic, 1991:3–16.

189. Trent JM, Stanbridge EJ, McBride HL, et al. Tumorigenicity in human melanoma cell lines controlled by introduction of human chromosome 6. Science 1990;247:568–571.

190. Turc-Carel C, Limon J, Dal Cin P, et al. Cytogenetic studies of adipose tissue tumors. II. Recurrent translocation t(12;16)(q13;p11) in myxoid liposarcomas. Cancer Genet Cytogenet 1986;23:291–299.

191. Turc-Carel C, Dal Cin P, Limon J, et al. Involvement of chromosome X in primary cytogenetic change in human neoplasia: Nonrandom translocation in synovial sarcoma. Proc Natl Acad Sci USA 1987;84:1981–1985.

192. Limon J, Mrozek K, Mandahl N, et al. Cytogenetics of synovial sarcoma: Presentation of ten new cases and review of the literature. Genes Chrom Cancer 1991;3:338–345.

193. Douglass EC, Valentine M, Etcubanas E, et al. A specific chromosomal abnormality in rhabdomyosarcoma. Cytogenet Cell Genet 1987;45:148–155.

194. Wang-Wuu S, Soukup S, Ballard E, et al. Chromosomal analysis of sixteen human rhabdomyosarcomas. Cancer Res 1988;48:983–987.

195. Biegel JA, Meek RS, Parmiter AH, et al. Chromosomal translocation t(1;13)(p36;q14) in a case of rhabdomyosarcoma. Genes Chrom Cancer 1991;3:483–484.

196. Douglass ED, Rowe ST, Valentine M, et al. Variant translocations of chromosome 13 in alveolar rhabdomyosarcoma. Genes Chrom Cancer 1991;3:480–482.

197. Turc-Carel C, Aurias A, Mugneret F, et al. Chromosomes in Ewing's sarcoma. I. An evaluation of 85 cases and remarkable consistency of t(11;22)(q24;q12). Cancer Genet Cytogenet 1988;32:229–238.

198. Mugneret F, Lizard S, Aurias A, et al. Chromosomes in Ewing's sarcoma. II. Nonrandom additional changes, trisomy 8 and der(16)t(1;16). Cancer Genet Cytogenet 1988;32:239–241.

199. Douglass EC, Rowe ST, Valentine M, et al. A second nonrandom translocation, der(16)t(1;16)(q21;q13), in Ewing sarcoma and peripheral neuroectodermal tumor. Cytogenet Cell Genet 1990;53:87–90.

200. Mandahl N, Heim S, Willén H, et al. Characteristic karyotypic anomalies identify subtypes of malignant fibrous histiocytoma. Genes Chrom Cancer 1989;1:9–14.

201. Bigner SH, Mark J, Burger PC, et al. Specific chromosomal abnormalities in malignant human gliomas. Cancer Res 1988;88:405–411.

202. Jenkins RB, Kimmel DW, Moertel CA, et al. A cytogenetic study of 53 human gliomas. Cancer Genet Cytogenet 1989;39:253–279.

203. Bigner SH, Mark J, Bigner DD. Cytogenetics of human brain tumors. Cancer Genet Cytogenet 1990;47:141–154.

204. Olopade OI, Jenkins RB, Ransom DT, et al. Molecular analysis of deletion of the short arm of chromosome 9 in human gliomas. Cancer Res 1992;52:2523–2529.

205. Brodeur GM, Fong C. Molecular biology and genetics of human neuroblastoma. Cancer Genet Cytogenet 1989;41:153–174.

206. Hayashi Y, Kanda N, Inaba T, et al. Cytogenetic findings and prognosis in neuroblastoma with emphasis on marker chromosome 1. Cancer 1989;63:126–132.

207. Weith A, Martinsson T, Cziepluch C, et al. Neuroblastoma consensus deletion maps to 1p36.1–2. Genes Chrom Cancer 1989;1:159–166.

208. Kaneko Y, Kanda N, Maseki N, et al. Different karyotypic patterns in early and advanced stage neuroblastomas. Cancer Res 1987;47:311–318.

209. Kusnetsova LE, Prigogina EL, Pogosianz HE, et al. Similar chromosomal abnormalities in several retinoblastomas. Hum Genet 1982;61:201–204.

210. Squire J, Gallie BL, Phillips RA. A detailed analysis of chromosomal changes in heritable and non-heritable retinoblastoma. Hum Genet 1985;70:291–301.

211. Knudson AG. Hereditary cancers disclose a class of cancer genes. Cancer 1989;63:1888–1891.

212. Huang H-JS, Yee J-K, Shew JY, et al. Suppression of the neoplastic phenotype of the RB gene in human cancer cells. Science 1988;242:1563–1566.

213. Lemieux N, Milot J, Barsoum-Homsy M, et al. First cytogenetic evidence of homozygosity for the retinoblastoma deletion in chromosome 13. Cancer Genet Cytogenet 1989;43:73–78.

214. Kovacs G, Brusa P. Clonal chromosome aberrations in normal kidney tissue from patients with renal cell carcinoma. Cancer Genet Cytogenet 1989;37:289–290.

215. Heim S, Mandahl N, Jin Y, et al. Trisomy 7 and sex chromosome loss in human brain tissue. Cytogenet Cell Genet 1989;52:136–138.

216. Elfving P, Cigudosa JC, Lundgren R, et al. Trisomy 7, trisomy 10, and loss of the Y chromosome in short-term cultures of normal kidney tissue. Cytogenet Cell Genet 1990;53:123–125.

217. Lindström E, Salford LG, Heim S, et al. Trisomy 7 and sex chromosome loss are not representative of tumor parenchyma cells in malignant glioma. Genes Chrom Cancer 1991;3:474–479.

218. Fletcher JA, Kozakewich HP, Hoffer FA, et al. Diagnostic relevance of clonal cytogenetic aberrations in malignant soft-tissue tumors. N Engl J Med 1991;324:436–442.

219. Åkerman M, Alvegård T, Eliasson J, et al. A case of Ewing's sarcoma diagnosed by fine needle aspiration, light microscopy, electron microscopy and chromosomal analysis. Acta Orthop Scand 1988;59:589–592.

220. Christiansen H, Lampert F. Tumour karyotype discriminates between good and bad prognostic outcomes in neuroblastoma. Br J Cancer 1988;57:121–126.

221. Trent JM, Meyskens FL, Salmon SE, et al. Relation of cytogenetic abnormalities and clinical outcome in metastatic melanoma. N Engl J Med 1990;322:1508–1511.

222. Rydholm A, Mandahl N, Heim S, et al. Malignant fibrous histiocytomas with a 19p+ marker chromosome have increased relapse rate. Genes Chrom Cancer 1990;2:296–299.

223. Pejovic T, Himmelmann A, Heim S, et al. Prognostic impact of chromosome aberrations in ovarian cancer. Br J Cancer 1992;65:65–78.

224. Mitelman F, Heim S. Consistent involvement of only 71 of the 329 chromosomal bands of the human genome in primary neoplasia-associated rearrangements. Cancer Res 1988;48:7115–7119.

225. Bishop JM. The molecular genetics of cancer. Science 1987;235:305–311.

226. Weinberg RA. Tumor suppressor genes. Science 1991;254:1138–1146.

Cancer: Principles & Practice of Oncology, Fourth Edition,
edited by Vincent T. DeVita, Jr., Samuel Hellman, Steven A. Rosenberg.
J.B. Lippincott Co., Philadelphia © 1993.

Jeffrey Sklar

CHAPTER **6**

Principles of Molecular Cell Biology of Cancer: Molecular Approaches to Cancer Diagnosis

The last 15 years have yielded many important advances in understanding the biology of human cancer. This period has also witnessed the introduction of powerful techniques for the detection of molecular alterations in cells and tissues. During the last decade, these two areas of research have combined to foster the development of a growing field in contemporary medicine—the molecular diagnostics of cancer.

Although this field has emerged only recently, some molecular tests for cancer have already gained an accepted role in the diagnosis of certain cancers. Other tests now under investigation are showing promise. This chapter discusses both tests in current use and those with potential for future application. Emphasis is placed on tests that focus on nucleic acids, principally on DNA, as diagnostic markers; however, tests directed at antigenic markers also deserve mention, particularly as alternatives for detecting the same genetic or physiologic changes identified by study of nucleic acids.

GENERAL CONSIDERATIONS

Interest in molecular diagnostics stems from major advantages that this approach offers in sensitivity and objectivity compared with conventional methods for diagnosing cancer. Conventional cancer diagnosis has depended for many years primarily on histopathologic evaluation of tissue biopsy specimens. Histopathologic diagnosis uses microscopy to identify anatomic abnormalities in the cytologic features of cells, in the cellular architecture of tissues, and in the frequency of certain cell types in biopsy specimens. Histopathologic diagnoses are based fundamentally on morphologic criteria, and the judgment of what is abnormal may be heavily influenced by the training and experience of the observer. In contrast, molecular diagnosis is based on more objective criteria, such as the presence, absence, or prevalence of a signal obtained from analysis of a tissue sample. Interpretation of the results tends to be less subject to observer variability. Futhermore, under many conditions, histopathologic methods can probably detect no more than about 1% to 10% neoplastic cells relative to the total cells in a biopsy sample. Molecular diagnostic methods are usually significantly more sensitive, and some tests are capable of routinely detecting as few as one neoplastic cell among 10^5 to 10^6 total cells.

Molecular approaches to cancer diagnosis can be considered from several different perspectives, for example, from the standpoint of the particular diagnostic purposes for which the tests can be applied (Table 6–1). Molecular tests can also be discussed in terms of the variety of molecular markers that can be assessed for diagnostic purposes, and in terms of the different techniques used for detecting these markers. In addition, molecular diagnosis of cancer can be discussed on a disease-by-disease basis. The first part of this chapter overviews the molecular diagnostics of cancer from each of these four general perspectives. Within the framework of these

TABLE 6–1.   Multiple Perspectives in the Molecular Diagnosis of Cancer

Purposes	*Molecular Markers*	*Techniques*	*Disease Examples*
Primary diagnosis	Cytogenetic abnormalities	In situ hybridization for DNA or RNA	Hematopoietic cancers Myeloid leukemia (chronic myelocytic, acute promyelocytic)
Staging dissemination	DNA rearrangements	Flow cytometry and image analysis microscopy	Lymphocytic cancers (non-Hodgkin lymphoma, lymphocytic leukemias)

Determining prognosis	Point mutation, deletion, and amplifications of or around oncogenes and tumor suppressor genes	Southern blot hybridization	Solid cancers
			  Neuroblastoma
			  Breast cancer
			  Bladder cancer

Detecting residual disease after therapy	Total DNA content	Polymerase chain reaction combined with:	Melanoma
Diagnosing inherited predisposition	Viral nucleotide sequences RNA sequences	Standard gel electrophoresis Southern blot hybridization Sequence analysis Oligonucleotide hybridization Chemical modification of heteroduplexes RNase protection Oligonucleotide ligation Single-strand conformation polymorphism gel electrophoresis Gradient denaturing gel electrophoresis	Retinoblastoma
	Antigens	Immunohistochemistry	

perspectives, the second part of this chapter illustrates how molecular approaches have been used to address diagnostic problems in certain types of cancer.

PURPOSES OF MOLECULAR TESTS IN CANCER DIAGNOSIS

There are at least five purposes for which molecular tests can be applied in the diagnosis of cancer. The first application is for the primary diagnosis of cancer, to determine whether or not tissue within a biopsy specimen contains a malignant neoplasm and what type of neoplasm it might be. Second, molecular tests offer opportunities for sensitive staging of cancers to determine the extent to which dissemination has occurred once a neoplasm has been diagnosed. Third, molecular tests sometimes provide information about the prognosis of a case or the biologic behavior expected for a particular tumor. Fourth, molecular tests can monitor residual disease after therapy to adjust treatment more effectively. Fifth, molecular tests are beginning to make possible the analysis of the genetic predisposition for developing certain cancers.

Conventional histopathology can also be used for the first four applications above, but molecular approaches usually provide greater sensitivity. The last application—the detection of cancer predisposition—is an aspect of cancer diagnosis that is not possible with conventional methods beyond a few isolated situations and is unique to molecular diagnostics.

MOLECULAR MARKERS IN CANCER DIAGNOSIS

Many molecular structures can serve as markers for molecular diagnosis of cancers. Most of these markers are closely related to the basic biology of cancer. In simple terms, cancer can be regarded as a genetic disease, in that the malignant progenitors from which tumors arise seem to have acquired a critical number of mutations within genes affecting cell growth or differentiation.[1] Some of these mutations may be in oncogenes—a class of genes that produce proteins with functions affecting cell proliferation and embryologic development of tissues.[2,3] Other mutations may occur in so-called *tumor suppressor genes*, the products of which appear to inhibit proliferation, sometimes by binding to and inactivating products of oncogenes.[4,5] After the threshold of sufficient mutations has been reached, the malignant cell proliferates in an uncontrolled fashion.[6] Each of the critical mutations required for the malignant character of the original transformed cell is transmitted to the progeny of that cell. The progeny constitute a clone with all members genetically similar if not identical to the progenitor cell. Additional mutations, in oncogenes, tumor suppressor genes, or elsewhere, may also accumulate in subclones of this progeny, and these mutations may further modify the growth or behavior of the subclone in a wide variety of ways. In principle, any mutation or mutant gene product that contributes to the malignant phenotype is a reasonable target for the molecular diagnosis of cancer. Additionally, markers that reflect the clonality of the proliferation can be useful for the cancer diagnosis.

An important example of such markers are the various cytogenetic abnormalities associated with different forms of human cancer.[7-10] In one sense, these cytogenetic abnormalities are not molecular markers but morphologic markers, because they have traditionally been detected microscopically by changes in the appearance of metaphase chromosomes. However, new molecular techniques can identify these abnormalities in interphase cells, and the data provided are more quantitative than morphologic. Cytogenetic abnormalities found in cancer include the following:

chromosomal translocations, involving the exchange of chromosomal material between chromosomes;

interstitial deletions, in which a segment within a chromosome is inverted;

chromosomal deletions, in which a whole chromosome or portion of a chromosome is lost from the cell;

chromosomal duplication, consisting of the duplication usually of whole chromosomes but sometimes of subchromosomal segments;

homogenously staining regions (HSRs) caused by numerous tandem iterations within chromosomes of small chromosomal segments containing some critical gene; and

double minute chromosomes, due to the extrachromosomal amplification of small chromosomal segments akin to the intrachromosomal amplifications that lead to formation of HSRs.

Some cytogenetic abnormalities are specific; that is, a particular chromosomal aberration is consistently detected in a given form of cancer. Other cytogenetic abnormalities are nonspecific and are found in different kinds of cancers. However, cytogenetic abnormalities or combinations of two or more cytogenetic abnormalities that are not specific themselves may be characteristic of certain cancers. Cytogenetic abnormalities are not always easy to detect by standard techniques, but recent developments may enhance the value of cytogenetic markers in cancer diagnosis in the near future.

An important type of molecular marker closely related to cytogenetic abnormalities is provided by DNA rearrangements found in cancer cells. In theory, any cytogenetic abnormality may be detected as a rearrangement in DNA. Submicroscopic aberrations in chromosomes may also produce DNA rearrangements potentially useful in cancer diagnosis. The result of DNA rearrangements is the juxtaposition of nucleotide sequences generally not found in normal tissues. The juxtapositions of sequences at the breakpoints of chromosomes are among the most widely applied molecular markers for cancer diagnosis because there are convenient, sensitive methods for their detection. DNA sequences at the breakpoints of chromosomal translocations have been particularly useful.

Deletions of chromosome segments or specific genes may be potentially valuable markers for cancer diagnosis, especially because the loss of such tumor suppressor genes as *RB1* and *TP53* appears to be a common event in oncogenesis. Some of these deletions may be detectable as cytogenetic abnormalities. However, unlike novel juxtapositions of DNA sequences created at the breakpoints of chromosomal abnormalities, deletions of DNA have had limited value as diagnostic

markers. This is because deletions represent the loss of a marker—a situation that poses a number of practical problems for diagnostic application. One such problem is due to the heterogeneity of most biopsy tissues; often the neoplastic component represents only a fraction of the cells in the specimen, making loss of a specific gene or nucleotide sequence from bulk tissue DNA difficult to discern.

On the other hand, DNA amplification has a number of advantages as a diagnostic marker. In general, amplifications, including those due to HSRs or double minutes, are easily detectable and quantifiable. Increased amplification of certain genes seems to be correlated with prognosis in certain forms of cancer.

A type of marker that cannot be detected by cytogenetic methods is point mutation in DNA. The mutations that have been most extensively studied can be divided into two categories: mutations that alter or increase the activity of oncogenes, and mutations that inactivate tumor suppressor genes.

Total DNA content within tissues can also be useful as a marker for cancer.[11-12] Deviations in DNA content within cells relative to normal cells (the DNA index) may indicate duplications or losses of individual chromosomes (aneuploidy) or extra haploid sets of chromosomes (polyploidy). In addition, the profile of DNA content among the cells of a tissue reflects the fraction of cells in the S and G_2 phases of the cell cycle. Higher numbers of cells in these fractions have been correlated with poorer prognosis in many forms of cancer.

In the few cancers known to be associated with viruses, viral nucleic acids or proteins can be used as markers for cancer diagnosis.[13] The most significant viruses in this context are human T-cell leukemia virus type 1 (associated with adult T-cell leukemia/lymphoma), Epstein-Barr virus (associated with Burkitt's lymphoma, non-Hodgkin's lymphomas in immunosuppressed individuals, and nasopharyngeal carcinoma), and human papilloma virus types 16 and 18 (associated with cervical carcinoma).[14-17] Each of these viruses appears to be involved in the transformation process, possibly as one of the factors in the multistep progression to malignancy. However, infection of the virus precedes development of the cancer in each of these neoplasms. Therefore, when viral material or evidence of viral infection (*e.g.*, antiviral antibody) is used as a diagnostic marker, the amount of viral material present within a tissue must be considered along with other clinical and pathologic data.

In some cases, the RNA and protein products of genes associated with tissue-specific patterns of expression may constitute worthwhile markers for diagnosis. Most commonly, these markers are used to obtain information about the tissue origin of a tumor and its expected behavior and prognosis. Cellular immunoglobulins may be used as markers of clonality in B-lineage lymphocytic neoplasms by determining that the population of cells within a biopsy sample express predominantly κ or λ light-chain protein rather than the 2:1 κ to λ ratio usually found in reactive lymphocytic processes.[18] It may also be possible to detect occult metastasis by analysis of tissue-specific gene products, especially by using highly sensitive molecular biologic methods.

A last type of marker, which is fundamentally different in several ways from most other diagnostic markers, is relevant to the detection of clonality. Like products of tissue-specific genes but unlike markers associated with cancer per se (*e.g.*, cytogenetic abnormalities or oncogene mutations), markers of clonality are acquired by cells before neoplastic transformation. Furthermore, in contrast to products of tissue-specific genes, markers of clonality vary from cell to cell within a tissue.

The use of these markers of clonality in the diagnosis of cancer is based on the clonal nature of neoplasia. Cells of virtually all neoplasms, whether benign or malignant, are clonal, whereas cells in reactive or hyperplastic processes tend to be polyclonal. Cells of neoplasms therefore share uniform clonal markers, whereas the cells in reactive tissues are diverse. In essence, assays of clonal markers measure the fraction of cells within a tissue sample that carry the same form of the marker and are thus presumed to be clonal. Some clonal markers can be used to monitor residual malignant disease after therapy by demonstrating the persistence of cells bearing the distinctive marker indicative of the original malignant clone. Prime examples of diagnostically useful clonal markers are antigen receptor gene rearrangements in lymphocytic tumors. Inactivation of X chromosomes in females heterozygous for some X-linked gene have been widely used to confirm the clonality of tumors by examination of isotypes of proteins or by analysis of methylation in X chromosome DNA.[19–22] As diagnostic procedures, studies of X chromosome inactivation suffer from the fact that they apply only to women and, furthermore, only to women who are heterozygous for assayable genes.

TECHNIQUES FOR DETECTION OF MOLECULAR MARKERS IN CANCER DIAGNOSIS

The value of molecular markers for cancer diagnosis depends on their accessibility to detection by various analytic strategies. For the most part, these strategies have been developed from a small set of basic techniques that frequently are modified or combined to assist in marker detection. Often several strategies are available for detection of the same marker, and these strategies differ in convenience, specificity, sensitivity, speed, expense, and appropriateness for particular clinical situations. This discussion is limited to those core techniques having general applicability to molecular testing in cancer diagnosis. A number of specific strategies for marker detection with special significance for the diagnosis of certain cancers are discussed later in this chapter.

IN SITU HYBRIDIZATION TECHNIQUES

Until recently, cytogenetic markers were studied exclusively by karyotyping of metaphase cells. Because of the technical difficulty in obtaining high-quality preparations of condensed, metaphase chromosomes from cancer cells and the skill required for proper identifications of abnormalities in these chromosomes using standard banding techniques, this approach to cytogenetics has largely been limited to centers with special expertise in this field. This has been particularly true for most solid tumors because tissue culture methods for karyotyping cells of solid tumors have not produced metaphase cells as reliably as have methods applied to leukemias and lymphomas.

In the last few years, an alternative approach has been developed for obtaining cytogenetic information from cells and tissues. This approach involves in situ hybridization of DNA probes to metaphase chromosomes deposited on microscope slides or to chromatin within intact interphase cells in smears or tissue sections. In situ hybridization to chromosomes is usually monitored by fluorescence, as discussed below, and is therefore referred to as *fluorescence in situ hybridization* (FISH).[23–25] The DNA probes used for in situ hybridization to chromosomes may consist of mixtures of DNA fragments covering whole chromosomes, fragments containing chromosome-specific repeated sequences (*e.g.*, the pericentromeric α satellite sequences), or fragments containing unique, nonrepetitive sequences. The lower limit of fragment size for unique sequence fragments is about 4 or 5 kb, but fragments of more than 25 kb, such as those propagated in bacterial cosmid cloning vectors or in yeast artificial chromosomes, give better results. An exciting prospect is the rapid production of probes for virtually any region of the genome by dissecting chromosomal bands from metaphase chromosomes with fine glass needles directed by micromanipulators. DNA within a small collection of bands dissected from a particular region may be amplified into a pool of probe fragments using the polymerase chain reaction (see below).

In situ hybridization of probes to complementary sequences in the chromosomes is detected by attaching molecular tags such as biotin or digoxigenin to the probe, usually by incorporating modified nucleotides into the probe DNA. The hybridized preparation is then incubated with antibody that is specific for the tag and has been conjugated to a fluorochrome (*e.g.*, fluorescein isothiocyanate or Texas red). The results are examined with a fluorescent microscope. Antibodies conjugated to peroxidase or alkaline phosphatase—enzymes that generate a colored reaction product when supplied with appropriate substrates—can also be used to localize the hybridized probe, thereby eliminating the need for a microscope equipped with fluorescence optics. By either detection system, chromosomes appear as blobs within interphase nuclei, whereas subchromosomal probes give a much more finely circumscribed signal or dot, as in the case of unique sequence probes. Applied to metaphase chromosomes, the signal is confined precisely to a band or subband.

In situ hybridization as a method for detecting cytogenetic abnormalities in cells has many advantages. For one, it is fast when performed on interphase cells; information can be obtained within a few hours. It is more sensitive than conventional karyotyping in that changes too small to be identified by standard chromosome banding techniques are detectable with in situ probes. The method can also be carried out on formalin-fixed, paraffin-embedded tissues—the way that tissues are prepared and stored for standard histopathologic examination. In situ hybridization to smears or sections of tissues permits at least some correlation with morphology, a feature not shared by conventional karyotypic analysis and a major advantage when dealing with heterogenous biopsy tissues.

In situ hybridization is probably best suited for detecting numerical changes in chromosomes or regions of chromosomes, including interstitial deletions.[26] However, chromosomal translocations can be detected by the simultaneous use of two probes containing DNA sequence known to lie on either side of a translocation breakpoint in one of the two reciprocal translocation products.[27] Presence of the translocation is indicated by the apposition of two of four dots normally produced in diploid cells. Identification of this result may be facilitated by labeling the two probes with different tags recognized with antibodies conjugated to different fluorochromes.

The chief disadvantage of using in situ hybridization to obtain cytogenetic information is that it provides data only on those regions of the genome complementary to the probe. In contrast, conventional karyotypic analysis scans the whole genome for abnormalities. In addition, in situ hybridization is susceptible to a number of artefacts, for instance, superimposition of signals from two chromosomes, high background staining of nonspecific sites within nuclei, or simply inadequate hybridization to DNA in some chromosomes.

Because of the many positive attributes of in situ hybridization, it is likely that in coming years cytogenetic analysis of biopsy tissues will be applied for all the diagnostic purposes discussed above and will have a major role in primary diagnosis. It will probably also be applied increasingly for detecting a predisposition to cancer by revealing constitutive deletions of tumor suppressor genes, such as deletions of the *RB1* gene associated with the predisposition to retinoblastoma and other cancers. The principal limitation of cytogenetic analysis is sensitivity, which is defined by how many cells or metaphase chromosome spreads can conveniently be screened for abnormalities and the reliability of the results obtained on a single cell. Because of this limitation, cytogenetics will not be a definitive method for monitoring disease after therapy.

In situ hybridization can also be performed to detect RNA within cells deposited on microscope slides or in tissue sections.[28–31] The cells are subjected to mild proteolytic enzyme digestion to expose the nucleotide sequences in the RNA and then hybridized with a radiolabeled probe or a probe linked to a molecular tag such as biotin. After hybridization with radioactive probes, the whole slide is coated with a thin layer of photographic emulsion and set aside in the dark for autoradiography to proceed. Days to weeks later, the slide is developed and the position of exposed emulsion over the cells or tissues is viewed under the microscope. Radioactive probes are usually labeled with ^{35}S, which gives better localization than ^{32}P and more intense signal than ^{3}H. The position of hybridized, chemically labeled probe is detected with antibody conjugated to an enzyme that generates an insoluble, colored product from a soluble substrate at the site of hybridization.

The chief diagnostic application of in situ hybridization to RNA is for the characterization of the tissue origin of a neoplasm. Its major advantage is its applicability to formalin-fixed, paraffin-embedded tissues. However, even in expert hands in situ hybridization gives variable results, sometimes even from region to region in the same tissue section. In addition, immunohistochemistry (see below) offers a more reliable alternative technique. It yields similar information in most situations, with the possible exception of a cell or tissue that secretes a protein so rapidly that insufficient amounts of intracellular protein may be present for detection.

TECHNIQUES FOR THE MEASUREMENT OF DNA CONTENT

Total DNA within cells for evaluation of ploidy or S phase fraction can be analyzed by flow cytometry or image analysis microscopy. Flow cytometry is performed on disaggregated cells or nuclei in suspension; image analysis microscopy is performed on cells in smears or in tissue sections. Flow cytometry, like image analysis microscopy, can be carried out with fixed and paraffin-embedded tissues. For either method, the cells are first stained with dyes that bind quantitatively to DNA. Fluorescent dyes are used for flow cytometry. The stained cells are then analyzed in a flow cytometer, which excites the dye with a laser beam and measures the fluorescence emitted by individual cells as they pass before a photomultiplier tube one cell at a time. The fluorescence data is compiled in a histogram indicating the distribution of DNA content among the cells in the tissue. For image analysis microscopy, nonfluorescent dyes are used, and the amount of dye bound is measured by special instrumentation in cells selected for analysis under the microscope. Information provided on DNA content by flow cytometry and image analysis microscopy has been correlated with prognosis in studies of a variety of cancers, including carcinoma of the colon and breast.[32–35]

SOUTHERN BLOT HYBRIDIZATION

A mainstay technique for the molecular diagnosis of cancer is Southern blot hybridization analysis.[36] Southern blot analysis provides a method for detecting changes or differences in DNA nucleotide sequence, particularly when these changes involve rearrangements of sizable stretches of DNA, including deletions and amplifications rather than point mutations or small deletions. The technique is also useful for detection of viral genomes in tumor tissues. The Southern blot procedure is performed on total cellular DNA extracted from a tissue specimen. The purified DNA is digested in vitro with one or occasionally two bacterial restriction enzymes. Each of these enzymes cleaves DNA at sites consisting of 4 to 8 base pairs of DNA sequence specifically recognized by a given enzyme. The DNA fragments resulting from enzyme digestion are separated according to size by electrophoresis in an agarose gel, where fragments of equal size form a large series of invisible bands. After electrophoresis, the DNA in the gel is denatured by soaking the gel in base. It is then transferred to a nylon or nitrocellulose membrane by applying the membrane to the gel and drawing a buffered solution through the gel and membrane by capillary action into some absorbent material or under suction. The DNA sticks on encountering the membrane, forming a replica of the bands in the gel. After transfer is complete, the membrane is dried and incubated with a denatured hybridization probe radiolabeled with ^{32}P. During this step, the probe anneals with the appropriate band or bands containing DNA complementary to the probe. After hybridization has taken place (about 24 hours), the membrane is washed to remove unhybridized or weakly hybridized probe. It is dried and autoradiographed against x-ray film to produce an image of the bands containing the DNA of interest.

The conditions of hybridization and washing (*e.g.*, the temperature and ionic strength of the solutions in either step) affect the extent of complementarity required between the probe and target for a band to be detected. By raising the stringency of conditions, for example, higher temperature and lower ionic strength, only bands containing perfect or near-perfect matches to sequences within the probe appear in the autoradiogram. Detection of DNA amplifications by Southern blot hybridization with probes containing sequence within the amplified unit is a straightforward matter of assessing the intensity of the amplified band compared with the band obtained with normal control tissue lacking the amplification. Even simpler is Southern blot analysis for viral genomes, in which the result is the presence or absence of a band in the Southern blot autoradiogram. Other markers for which Southern blot analysis has served as an invaluable method for detection are antigen receptor gene rearrangements and many chromosomal translocations; however, the principles underlying detection for these markers is more complex than for amplifications or viral genomes. Antigen receptor gene rearrangements and chromosomal translocations result in the novel juxtaposition of DNA sequences about a site of DNA breakage and joining. The relative positions of restriction sites flanking these positions define a restriction fragment that is not produced by digestion of DNA inherited through the germline. These fragments (along with unrearranged germline fragments) can be detected by hybridization probe containing sequence on one side of the break.

Southern blot hybridization has also been used to detect deletions of DNA by revealing the loss of DNA sequence polymorphisms within the deleted DNA segment. These normal variations in DNA affect the size of some restriction fragments, for instance, by a single base pair that creates or destroys a restriction site, or by the variable number of reduplications of so-called *mini-* and *micro-satellite sequences* between two restriction sites.[37–40] Such polymorphisms are widely distributed throughout human populations, and not infrequently two different allelic fragments of DNA can be detected from normal tissues with a single hybridization probe. Differences in allelic fragments detected in this manner are referred to as *restriction fragment length polymorphism* (RFLP). Loss of one of these allelic fragments indicates the presence of deletions in one chromosomal homolog.[41,42]

Southern blot hybridization can be applied for all the major diagnostic purposes. Its most important limitation is its restricted sensitivity (no more than about 1%; that is, one neoplastic cell in 100 total cells), meaning that its use in staging or in detection of residual disease is suboptimal. Another limitation is that the method works reliably on DNA extracted only from frozen or ethanol-fixed tissue. Also, breakpoints in some chromosomal translocations occur over such large distances in DNA that it is difficult to find probe/restriction enzyme combinations that can reliably detect all translocations identifiable by cytogenetics.

PULSED-FIELD GEL ELECTROPHORESIS IN SOUTHERN BLOT ANALYSIS

Because of the latter problem, Southern blot analysis has sometimes been combined with pulsed-field gel electrophoresis to detect chromosomal translocations.[43] This type of gel system is capable of separating megabase fragments of DNA, unlike standard agarose gels, which do not resolve fragments over about 25 kb in length.[44–46] Pulsed-field gels and standard gels use an agarose matrix to separate the fragments. The basic difference is that in the simplest form of pulsed-field gel electrophoresis, two electrical fields are applied to the fragments migrating in the gel, each at an angle to the overall direction of fragment migration. The two fields are applied in an alternating manner, so that the very long fragments of DNA must continually realign themselves in an electric field before moving along the vector of that field. The time required for realignment is presumably a function of fragment length. Once fragments over about 25 kb long are aligned, they apparently migrate at the same speed (the property that accounts for the poor resolution of larger DNA fragments in standard gel electrophoresis). To generate large fragments for pulsed-field gels, the DNA is extracted from cells and digested while embedded in agarose plugs so that the long, fragile strands of DNA are not sheared by the currents that occur in free solution. Restriction enzymes that cut at eight nucleotide recognition sequences are most often used. After separation of fragments by pulsed-field electrophoresis, the DNA within the gel can be treated just as DNA in a routine Southern blot.

The advantage of pulsed-field gel electrophoresis combined with Southern blot analysis is that it permits scanning of large stretches of DNA with a single hybridization probe. However, reproducible digestion of DNA in agarose plugs is often difficult. Consistently high-quality results require considerable experience with the technique. Furthermore, the method can only be applied to fresh cells. Consequently, pulsed-field gel electrophoresis has not been widely used for diagnostic purposes.

THE POLYMERASE CHAIN REACTION

The most important recent innovation in the molecular diagnosis of cancer has been the introduction of the polymerase chain reaction (PCR).[47–49] PCR is a procedure in which regions of DNA in a complex genome can be enormously amplified in vitro by bacterial enzyme DNA polymerase, provided the nucleotide sequences immediately flanking these regions are known. The essential principle behind this procedure is that under the proper conditions, DNA polymerase copies each strand of a double-stranded DNA template. But DNA polymerase cannot begin DNA synthesis de novo at any point in the template. Rather, DNA polymerase can only copy the DNA of the template by adding nucleotides to the 3′ end of a preexisting strand of DNA annealed to the template DNA.

In PCR, 3′ ends for extension by DNA polymerase are provided by a pair of single-stranded oligonucleotides, referred to as *primers*, each about 15 to 40 nucleotides in length. These primers are constructed in automated instruments, called *DNA synthesizers*, to be complementary to specific sequences in opposite strands of the template on either side of the region to be amplified. Once annealed to the two strands of the template, the 3′ ends of the two primers face each other. During the amplification procedure, double-stranded DNA template (*e.g.*, total cellular DNA) is denatured at high temperature, after which the temperature is lowered to allow annealing of the primers to both strands of the template and then brought to a third temperature for copying of the DNA between the two primers.

The region of template to be copied is determined by choosing two primers with sequences complementary to template DNA flanking that region. Using the same pair of primers, DNA can be amplified by copying the DNA template over and over again in repetitive cycles of heating and cooling of the reaction. Shifting between the temperatures necessary for denaturation, annealing, and primer extension is facilitated by the availability of heat-resistant DNA polymerase purified from the bacterium *Thermophilus aquaticus* and of programmable thermal cycling incubators. In each cycle of primer extension, the DNA synthesized during the previous cycle becomes the template for the current cycle, so that in theory, newly synthesized single-stranded fragments of DNA accumulate at a rate of 2^n, where n equals the number of cycles completed for each copy of starting template. After completion of the amplification reaction, complementary single-stranded fragments anneal to one another at low temperature, producing a collection of double-stranded fragments, the size of which is precisely determined by the positions of the two sequences complementary to the primers in the genomic template DNA. Because DNA polymerase is usually capable of synthesizing strands only up to several kilobases in length before falling off the template, the PCR technique is limited to amplifying regions of DNA no larger than this.

The products of PCR reactions are assayed by gel electrophoresis. Successful amplification results in a band at a position corresponding to the size predicted from the locations of the two oligonucleotide sites in the template. So much fragment product is generated when the target sequence is abundant in the DNA that a band can often be seen directly by viewing the gel under an ultraviolet lamp after it has been stained with ethidium bromide, a fluorescent dye molecule that binds between the base pairs of double-stranded DNA. More sensitive detection of a reaction product can be carried out by performing Southern blot hybridization analysis of the reaction products using a probe consisting of a conventional radiolabeled DNA fragment, a radiolabeled oligonucleotide complementary to sequences internal to the two priming oligonucleotides, or radiolabeled PCR product itself. Southern blot analysis with an internal probe also confirms the specificity of the products. A nonradioactive method sometimes used to confirm or increase the specificity of PCR uses so-called *nested primers*—after a series of cycles with one pair of primer, a portion of the reaction mixture is reamplified with a second pair of primers complementary to DNA internal to the first primer pair. PCR combined with Southern blot analysis of the products is capable of routinely detecting a unique target sequence within the total DNA of 10^5 human genomes in one amplification reaction. These numbers are only limited by the maximal amount of human genomic DNA (about 2 μg, the equivalent of about 2×10^5 cells) that can be tested in a single amplification reaction.

Indeed, the extreme sensitivity of PCR is the cause of its principal drawback. Because only a single template can give rise to a positive result, contamination of the reaction by exogenous amplifiable sequences can be an occasional problem even in laboratories that exercise great care to guard against such occurrences. The source of contamination in most instances is probably the inadvertent transfer of small amounts of product from one reaction to the ingredients of another reaction that uses the same primers. Measures usually taken to prevent artefactual results due to contamination include ultra-clean set-up rooms for preparation of the reactions, pipettes containing aerosol barriers, and ultraviolet irradiation of the reaction mixture before addition of polymerase and template DNA. Additionally, control reactions from which

template DNA has been omitted should always be performed and analyzed in parallel with any PCR test to ensure that reagents other than the template are not contaminated. Products can also be precisely sized on gels, analyzed by Southern blot hybridization, or subjected to nucleotide sequence analysis to distinguish bona fide product expected for a specific amplification reaction from artefactual product that may have been amplified during reactions.

A less significant problem with PCR is that the results are not directly quantifiable because in practice the amplification signal does not continue to grow indefinitely with increasing numbers of cycles. Instead, a plateau is reached so that virtually the same signal can be obtained from a few templates as from many. A partial solution to this problem is to perform PCR on serial dilutions of the template with normal DNA until an amplification product is no longer obtained. Assuming a single target sequence can generate a product, the inverse of the dilution at which product no longer appears is roughly equal to the number of targets in the undiluted template DNA.

The advantages of PCR far outweigh its disadvantages. The amplification capabilities of the procedure mean that very small numbers of total cells are sufficient for analysis. The small size of the amplification target (which may be made as small as 40 or 50 base pairs by selecting appropriate primers) makes PCR possible on partially degraded DNA or on the highly fragmented DNA normally obtained by extraction from formalin-fixed, paraffin-embedded tissue. PCR is also fast, because an amplification of 25 to 30 cycles, which is about standard, can be completed in a few hours. Furthermore, if maximal sensitivity is not an overriding concern, analysis can be carried out without having to use radioactive probes.

PCR has been applied directly or indirectly for detection of all kinds of nucleic acid markers and in detection strategies designed for each of the major diagnostic purposes relevant to cancer. The ability to amplify a product from one cell in 10^5 makes PCR the technique of choice for any strategy directed at sensitive staging of cancer or monitoring of residual disease after therapy. For example, if breakpoints are known to cluster within the span of DNA over which PCR is efficient (*i.e.*, less than about 1 or 2 kilobases), some chromosomal translocations can be detected by the amplification of DNA using primers complementary to sequence on either side of the breakpoint (Fig. 6–1). Additionally, PCR can aid in the diagnosis of those cancers associated with viral infections by demonstrating viral DNA sequences in the cells of the tumor. Similarly, PCR can be used to detect with sensitivity transcripts of RNA from specific cellular genes by performing amplifications on cDNA synthesized in vitro from RNA by reverse transcriptase.

PCR COMBINED WITH TECHNIQUES FOR DETECTION OF POINT MUTATIONS

Another important application of PCR is the amplification and isolation of regions of DNA to identify point mutations. In this regard, PCR is far more powerful than Southern blot analysis, which can only detect point mutations that alter restriction sites in the vicinity of DNA complementary to the sequences in hybridization probes. To detect point mutations, PCR must be combined with some other technique for analysis of sequence within the amplification product. Direct sequence

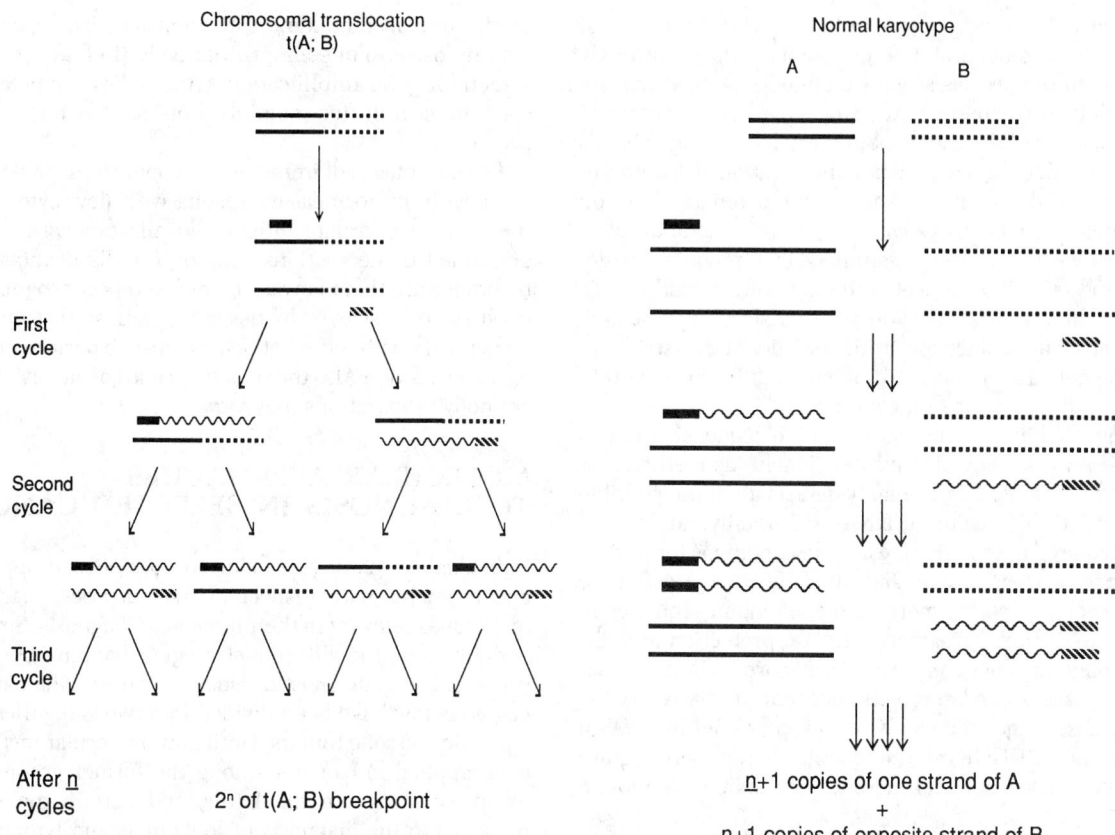

FIGURE 6–1. The polymerase chain reaction (PCR) for amplification of DNA. Successful amplification of DNA across a chromosomal translocation breakpoint (*left*) is compared with attempted amplification of DNA from cells lacking the translocation (*right*). The double helical DNA of one of the two involved chromosomes, chromosome A, is represented by solid lines, and the DNA of the other chromosome, B, by dashed lines. The two oligonucleotide primers are shown as solid and cross-hatched small rectangles where they anneal to the denatured strands of the DNA. DNA synthesized during primer extension steps is indicated by wavy lines. The lengths of the newly synthesized strands are heterogenous after the first cycle of synthesis. In subsequent cycles, the primer extensions occur off of previously synthesized DNA strands, and the strands are homogenous and correspond to the distance between the 5' ends of the two primers.

analysis is the most definitive technique for achieving this objective but is also the most laborious.[51,52] Consequently, a number of alternative techniques have been applied for screening PCR products for sequence variations. One of these techniques is hybridization of radiolabeled oligonucleotide probes to PCR products immobilized on membranes under sufficiently stringent conditions to distinguish single base mismatches between the probe and the target sequence.[52,53] Several chemical methods have also been adapted for detection of point mutations. For example, a DNA heteroduplex of PCR target and radiolabeled probe can be treated with osmium tetroxide or hydroxylamine to modify unhybridized cytidine or thymidine nucleotides, followed by cleavage at the modified nucleotide with piperidine.[54,55] The resulting fragments can be assayed by gel electrophoresis and autoradiography. Mismatched guanosine and thymidine nucleotides can also be modified by carbodiimide. Primer extension from the ends of the heteroduplexes containing the modified nucleotides is blocked at the position of the modifications, producing two small fragments.[56]

Enzyme-mediated techniques for detecting point mutations include RNase protection, a method that makes use of radio-labeled RNA probes, often called *riboprobes*, which may be generated by transcription of mutant PCR fragments.[57] After hybridization of the riboprobe to the target PCR fragments in solution, RNase A or T_1 is used to digest the riboprobe at unhybridized nucleotides. Intact riboprobe demonstrated by gel electrophoresis indicates complete complementarity between target and probe. Point mutations can also be detected by using *E. coli* DNA polymerase in vitro to selectively add a single nucleotide complementary to the mutant base of a DNA template at the 3' end of an annealed oligonucleotide primer.[58] A last enzymatic technique is based on the ability of bacteriophage T4 DNA ligase to join the 3' and 5' ends of two adjacent oligonucleotides hybridized to a single strand of DNA only if the 3' and 5' nucleotides in the respective oligonucleotides are both complementary to the single strand DNA.[59] Therefore, an oligonucleotide complementary to the mutation at its 3' or 5' end participates in a ligation reaction, whereas one that differs at this position does not.

Two purely electrophoretic techniques have been introduced for detecting point mutations. Denaturing gradient gel electrophoresis (DGGE), discussed in greater detail below, makes use of the fact that a gradient of chemical denaturants added to a polyacrylamide gel induces local separation of strands in PCR products at different points in the gel strongly dependent on the precise sequence of nucleotides in that region of the PCR fragment.[57] Any single-strandedness greatly reduces mobility of the fragment in the gel, resulting in bands at the position in the gel where the concentration of denaturant has opened the double helix. The second technique relies on the principle referred to as *single-strand conformational polymorphism* (SSCP).[60,61] Double-stranded PCR products are denatured and quickly reannealed to allow intrastrand bonds. The three-dimensional structures assumed by each strand, and the consequent electrophoretic mobility of that structure in agarose gels, can be affected by small differences within the nucleotide sequence of the strand.

Although each of the alternatives to full-sequence analysis may be less work, they all have deficiencies as methods for detecting mutations. None reliably detects all of the possible mutations within a region of DNA, and usually experimentation is required to establish the correct conditions for finding a difference between mutant and wild type DNA. Most of the techniques can detect no more than one mutant sequence in about 10^2 to 10^3 total fragments. RNase protection and differential oligonucleotide protection are more sensitive, but at least in the case of the latter technique, only a very restricted region of DNA sequence can be checked at one time. With the exception of DGGE, all the techniques routinely require radioactivity. The chemical methods use toxic or explosive reagents.

IMMUNOHISTOCHEMISTRY

The last basic technique pertinent to the molecular diagnosis of cancer is immunohistochemistry.[62,63] Unlike the other techniques discussed above, the marker assessed by this technique rarely involves nucleic acids, but consists primarily of antigenic proteins and polysaccharides. For this reason and because it has been applied for years before nucleic acids were used in cancer diagnosis, immunohistochemistry is sometimes not considered a molecular technique. However, it seems inappropriate to exclude immunohistochemistry from a discussion of molecular diagnosis of cancer because it often presents a clear and convenient alternative to techniques that detect nucleic acid markers.

The essential feature of immunohistochemistry is the use of antibodies directed against antigenic markers. The antibodies may be polyclonal, derived from the sera of immunized animals, or monoclonal, derived from mouse hybridomas. Antibodies can be used to stain cells in suspensions or cells disaggregated from solid tissues, and in smears or tissue sections on microscope slides. Binding of antibodies to cells on slides is analyzed by light microscopy, whereas binding to cells in suspensions or disaggregated from solid tissues is analyzed by flow cytometry. The signal detected in flow cytometry, and less often in microscopy, is fluorescence by way of antibodies conjugated to fluorescent tags or indirectly by using anti-antibodies (*e.g.,* rabbit antimouse IgG antibody) conjugated to fluorescent tags. Antibodies conjugated to such enzymes as peroxidase and alkaline phosphatase are frequently employed for immunohistochemistry on slides.

Immunohistochemistry is mostly used to detect expression of tissue-specific genes, for instance, to identify the tissue of origin for a specific tumor. It can also be used quantitatively (in microscopy) or semiquantitatively (in flow cytometry) to screen for gene amplifications. Antibodies can potentially be used to search for mutant proteins (such as oncogene products).

The advantages of immunohistochemistry include its speed, the possibility to measure results with flow cytometry, and the ability to correlate antigenic localization with microscopy of stained tissue sections. Among the disadvantages of the technique are that many antigenic epitopes recognized by antibodies are destroyed by tissue fixation, so that immunohistochemistry with these antibodies must be performed on fresh or frozen tissues. Also the sensitivity and specificity of different antibody preparations may vary.

MOLECULAR APPROACHES TO DIAGNOSIS IN SELECTED CANCERS

Individual forms of cancer often pose special opportunities and problems with respect to the purposes, markers, and techniques relevant to their molecular diagnosis. Several cancers illustrate the different strategies that have been applied successfully to diagnostic issues in cancer. The cancers discussed below have been divided into two categories—hematopoietic and solid tumors. Until now, molecular methods have been applied to cancers among the former group far more extensively than to the latter, and certain molecular approaches to the diagnosis of leukemias and lymphomas are almost routine. The reasons for this difference are several, including the availability of definitive markers for several hematopoietic cancers, primarily in the form of specific, consistent chromosomal translocations. Fewer consistent markers have been characterized at a molecular level for solid tumors. Furthermore, the special problems of primary diagnosis of hematopoietic cancers, particularly concerning non-Hodgkin lymphoma, the importance of accurate subtyping of these leukemias and lymphomas, and concern about residual disease in the setting of chemotherapy and bone marrow transplantation have also spurred progress in molecular diagnosis of these tumors. Although work has been slower for solid tumors, a number of molecular strategies have been presented for the diagnosis of these cancers, and these methods represent valuable paradigms for future developments in this field.

HEMATOPOIETIC TUMORS

Myeloid Leukemias

Among those cancers on which molecular diagnosis has had the greatest impact is chronic myelocytic leukemia (CML). The marker in this disease has been the Philadelphia chromosome (Ph[1]), t(9;22) (q34;q11), demonstrable in about 95% of CMLs.[64,65] This translocation is apparently an important factor, although not by itself a sufficient factor, in the malignant transformation of the pluripotential stem cell that is the primary transformed progenitor in this cancer. The translocation is amenable to detection by conventional cytogenetics, FISH, Southern blot hybridization,[66–68] and PCR. Application of the first three techniques closely follows the general strategies presented earlier in this chapter. On the other hand, application of PCR to the Ph[1] chromosome requires modification of the usual strategy for detecting chromosomal translocation breakpoints.

At the level of molecular genetic level, the Ph¹ chromosome joins the 5′ portion of the *BCR* gene located on chromosome 22 with the 3′ portion of the *ABL* gene on chromosome 9[69–71] (Fig. 6–2). The chimeric *BCR-ABL* gene is transcribed into a novel 8.5-kb mRNA, which in turn is translated into a 210-kd protein not found in normal cells. The 210-kd protein has greatly increased tyrosine kinase activity (a common property of many oncogene products) compared with that associated with the normal *ABL* protein.[72] The function of the *BCR* protein in nontransformed cells is unknown, although it may bind to the *ABL* protein (consequently, the translocation may be conceptualized as resulting in the ultimate enhancement of this interaction).

Although the structures of the *BCR-ABL* mRNA and the 210-kd protein are conserved between different cases of CML, the precise position of the breakpoints within DNA varies considerably. This is because the breaks occur within introns, the sequence of which is excised from the initial forms of the *BCR* and *ABL* transcripts to produce the mature 8.5-kb mRNA and which therefore are not expressed as protein. Breaks in *BCR* range over several kilobases and in *ABL* over much greater distances. The actual number of *BCR* and *ABL* introns included in the *BCR-ABL*-encoded mRNA and protein may differ slightly from case to case, but these optional introns are small and do not change the overall size of the products to an appreciable degree.[73] The variability in the positions of the breaks in DNA preclude the use of a single pair of PCR primers to amplify DNA across the breakpoint. To circumvent

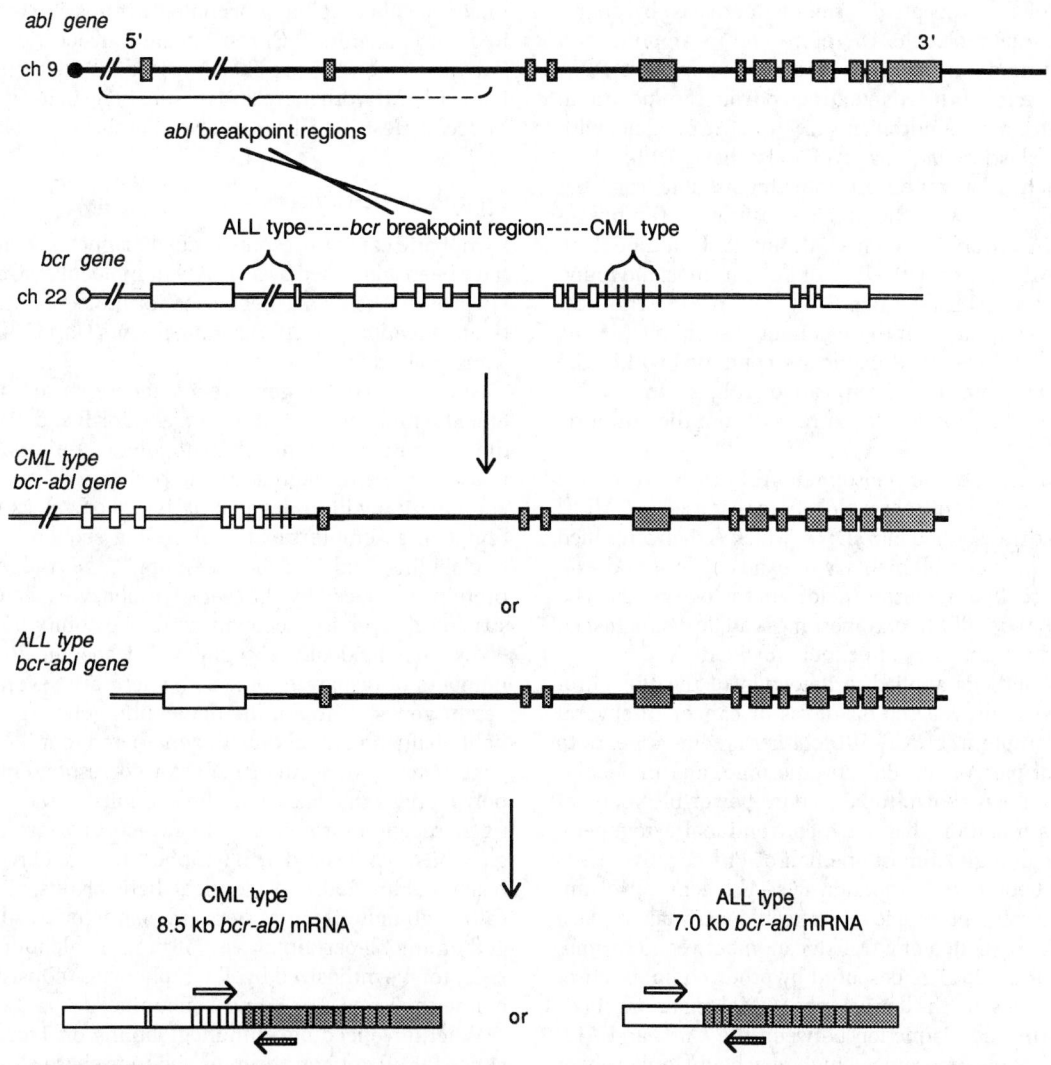

FIGURE 6–2. Structure of *BCR*, *ABL*, and *BCR-ABL* genes involved in the Philadelphia chromosomes found in chronic myelocytic and acute lymphoblastic leukemias. Boxes represent exons. The normal *BCR* and *ABL* genes span about 115 and 245 kb of DNA, respectively. The exon structure of the two types of RNA transcribed from the chimeric *BCR-ABL* genes is shown at the bottom of the figure. The relative positions of *BCR* and *ABL* oligonucleotide primers (*horizontal arrows*) that can be used in PCR to distinguish the two types of translocations are illustrated with respect to the structure of the RNAs. Detection of *BCR-ABL* RNA by PCR requires an initial round of reverse transcription using a primer complementary to *ABL* RNA sequence, followed by DNA amplification of the cDNA using primers complementary to sequence on either side of the fusion point between the genes. ALL, acute lymphoblastic leukemia; CML, chronic myelocytic leukemia.

this problem, investigators have performed so-called *reverse* PCR on RNA from blood or bone marrow cells with primers complementary to nucleotide sequence in the exons of *BCR* and *ABL*, which flank the introns containing the break-points.[74–77] In the first step of the procedure, the *BCR-ABL* mRNA is transcribed into single-strand cDNA by reverse transcriptase with an *ABL* primer. Nucleotide sequences in the cDNA are then amplified with primers for the *BCR* and *ABL* exons.

The threshold of detection for CML cells by PCR is about one in 10^5 to 10^6. This number is necessarily vague because it depends on how many *BCR-ABL* mRNA molecules are present in CML cells. Levels of *BCR-ABL* mRNA may vary from case to case, between stages of the disease, among cell types (*e.g.*, megakaryocyte, lymphocyte, and granulocyte), and even from cell to cell. The major disadvantage of this strategy for disease detection is that RNA is much less stable than DNA and the risk of false negative results is increased by degradation of the target molecule. Therefore, control amplification must be performed using primers for some omnipresent RNA to test the integrity of the RNA extracted from the specimen.

About 3% to 6% of children and 15% to 20% of adults with acute lymphoblastic leukemia (ALL) also have a Ph^1 chromosome, which is cytogenetically indistinguishable from that found in CML. However, the precise position of the break-points in DNA differs between CML and ALL, although in rare cases, CML may have the type of Ph^1 chromosome found predominantly in ALL (see Fig. 6–2).[73–78] In ALL, the *BCR* breakpoints cluster far 5' of those generally seen in CML. As a result, 8 to 12 fewer *BCR* exons are contained within the *BCR-ABL* gene product of Ph^1-positive ALL, so that a 7.0 mRNA and 190-kd protein are expressed from the chimeric gene.

Detection of the Ph^1 chromosome in ALL has been carried out by a PCR strategy entirely analogous to that used in CML.[74] RNA is reverse transcribed into cDNA, which is then amplified with PCR primers complementary to exons of *BCR* and *ABL* flanking the breakpoint cluster regions in the two genes. The CML and ALL types of Ph^1 chromosomes can be distinguished by choosing different pairs of primers for PCR.

Molecular methods applied to detection of the Ph^1 chromosome have improved the diagnosis of cancer in several ways. For example, the *BCR-ABL* chimeric gene appears to be the critical part of the Ph^1 chromosome, and molecular methods have been shown to be a more powerful means of detecting this mutation than have conventional cytogenetic methods. Accordingly, almost one half of Ph^1-negative cases of CML have been found to contain *BCR-ABL* genes, presumably because a submicroscopic rearrangement has taken place or because the presence of a translocation between chromosomes 9q34 and 22q11 is obscured by other complex chromosomal changes in the karyotypes.[67] Molecular methods have also permitted distinction between the CML and ALL forms of the Ph^1 chromosome, which may be the only way of separating lymphoid blast crisis of CML from de novo ALL. Identification of the Ph^1 chromosome in ALL, in turn, seems to signify a poorer than average prognosis for ALL. This finding is, however, subject to modification as new therapeutic protocols come into usage. In addition, the position of breakpoints in the *BCR* gene may affect the prognosis in CML, although this issue is controversial.[79–82] PCR detection of *BCR-ABL*

mRNA can be used to monitor patients for residual disease after therapy, for instance, after bone marrow transplantation.[77]

Although CML has led the way for molecular diagnosis among myelocytic leukemias, other forms of myelocytic leukemias are likely to be diagnosed by molecular methods in the near future. The breakpoint of the chromosomal translocation t(15;17)(q22;q11–12), associated with virtually all cases of acute promyelocytic (M3) leukemia (APL),[83] has been molecularly characterized and shown to result in formation a chimeric gene joining a newly discovered gene *PML* to the gene for the retinoic acid receptor $\alpha(RARA)$.[84] This gene fusion has been demonstrated to be a reliable marker detectable by Southern blot hybridization and PCR.[85] FISH should also be of value. The importance of applying these techniques for the diagnosis has been underscored by the observation that treatment of patients with all trans-retinoic acid results in a high incidence of complete morphologic remission in APL but not in other leukemias.[84] Chromosomal translocation breakpoints have also recently been characterized for the t(6;9)(p23;q34) found in AML with increased mature bone marrow basophils.[86] Molecular tests for this marker will probably be available soon.

Lymphocytic Cancers

Lymphatic cancer presents special diagnostic challenges that have been addressed by a variety of molecular strategies. Two types of markers have been used for molecular diagnosis: antigen receptor gene rearrangements, and chromosomal translocation breakpoints.

Antigen receptor gene rearrangements are markers for clonal lymphocyte proliferation and for B and T lymphocytic differentiation among hematopoietic tumors.[87–97] These markers arise through a unique process of somatic DNA recombination within developing lymphocytes as the cells attempt to assemble functional coding sequences for immunoglobulins and T-cell receptors.[98–102] Antigen receptor proteins produced by different lymphocytes show enormous structural diversity, accounting for the ability of these molecules to individually recognize and specifically bind large numbers of disparate antigens. There are seven antigen receptor genes—three immunoglobulin genes (heavy chain, κ light chain, and λ light chain genes) and four T-cell receptor genes (*i.e.*, β, α, γ, and δ genes)—corresponding to types of polypeptides that make up the subunits of the complete antigen receptor proteins. Cell-surface or secreted immunoglobulins, synthesized by B lymphocytes, contain two identical heavy chains and two identical light chains of κ or λ type (although multiple tetramers are characteristically linked together among certain classes of immunoglobulins).[103] T-cell receptors, synthesized by T lymphocytes, consist of a heterodimer of α and β or γ and δ subunits.[104]

Whether encoding immunoglobulins or T-cell receptors, genes for all antigen receptor subunits share a common general structure (Fig. 6–3A). The form of these genes transmitted through the germline consists of several sets of multimember gene segments (V, J, C, and in some genes, D segment sets, with the D segments lying between the V and J segment sets) distributed over the long stretches of DNA making up each gene. As lymphocytes differentiate, one member from each of the V, D, and J sets (and sometimes

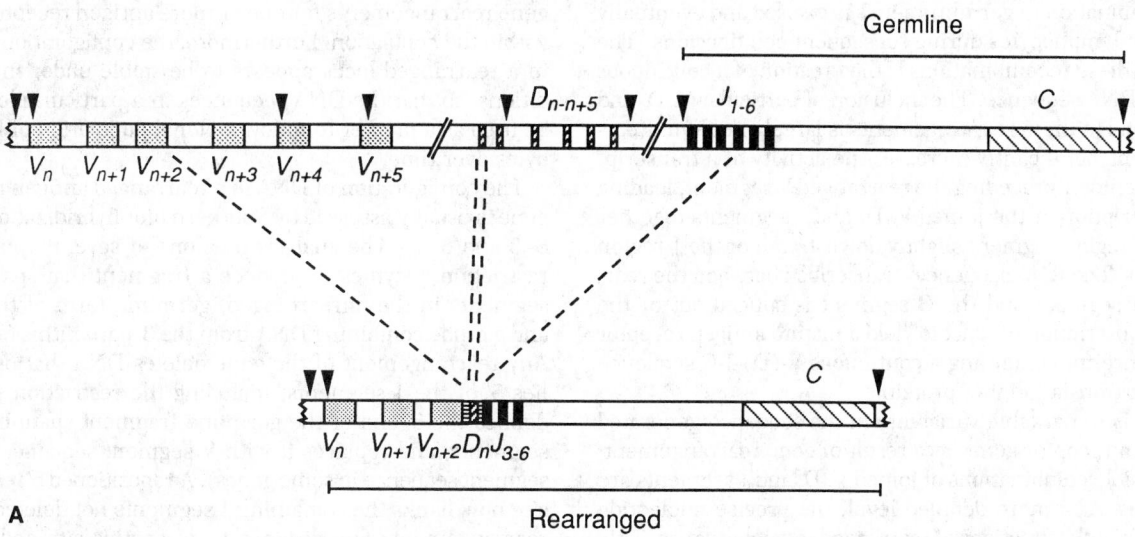

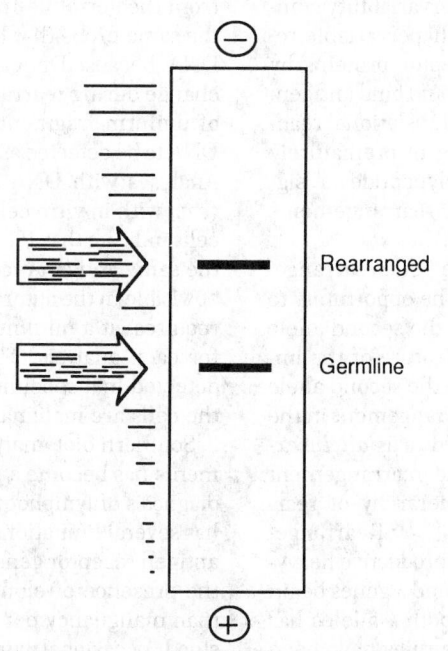

FIGURE 6–3. Principles of Southern blot hybridization analysis of antigen receptor gene rearrangement. **(A)** A hypothetical rearrangement in the immunoglobulin heavy-chain gene. The germline positions of V, D, J, and C gene segments in chromosomal DNA is shown on the top line of the figure; the configuration of segments after rearrangement is shown below. Downward arrowheads show the positions of restriction enzyme cleavage sites in the cDNA. The bracketed lines above and below the chromosomal DNA indicate the size of the germline and the rearranged DNA fragments that span the J segment region and are released from DNA after cleavage by the restriction enzyme. **(B)** Autoradiogram from analysis of a tissue specimen in which at least 1% of the lymphocytes contain the rearrangement illustrated in A. The positions where polyclonal rearranged fragments, clonal rearranged fragments (*upper arrow*), and germline fragments (*lower arrow*) would array themselves in the gel are shown to the left of the autoradiogram. After hybridization with a radiolabeled hybridization probe containing DNA of the J segments and 3' of them, only the clonal rearranged fragment and the germline fragment are detected as discrete bands in the autoradiogram. The polyclonal rearranged fragments are not sufficiently abundant to be detected.

two members of the D region set in the case of the δ T cell receptor gene) become joined together through a series of recombination events. The DNA that lies between these sites of recombination in germline genes is excised and eventually lost from lymphocytes during subsequent cell divisions. The result of these recombinations is the creation of a continuous V-(D)-J DNA sequence. The inclusion of particular V, D, and J segments in these rearrangements is largely random. Rearrangement significantly increases the activity of a transcriptional promoter preceding the rearranged V segment, leading to transcription of the joined V, D, and J segments together with a C-region segment slightly downstream of the J-region segments. The RNA sequences transcribed between the rearranged J segment and the C segment is spliced out of the initial transcription product to yield a mature antigen receptor gene transcript containing a continuous V-(D)-J-C sequence ready for translation into protein.

There is remarkable variability in the sequence generated in antigen receptor genes as a result of gene rearrangement. The possible combinations of joined V, D, and J segments are numerous. At a more detailed level, the precise nucleotide sequences at the junctions of rearranged segments vary greatly due to small deletions and insertions (except in immunoglobulin light-chain genes) of nucleotides between the segments.[105-106] Consequently, the amino acid sequences at the junctions of V, D, and J segments show hypervariability compared with the rest of the molecule. These hypervariable regions encode portions of the antigen receptor proteins by which the antigen receptor proteins contact and bind antigen. However, some of these junctions shift the translational reading frame of codons out of phase, resulting in prematurely terminated or missense antigen receptor polypeptides. A significant fraction of all antigen receptor gene rearrangements end up being nonproductive for this reason.

The high degree of waste inherent in the gene rearrangement process is partly compensated for by the opportunity to attempt productive gene rearrangement in the second allele for each gene. A striking but unexplained feature of the immune system is that lymphocytes rearrange the second allele for an antigen receptor gene only if the rearrangement in the first allele is defective—a principle referred to as *allelic exclusion*.[107] Additional economy in the gene rearrangement process is achieved through an ordered hierarchy of rearrangements among immunoglobulin genes.[108-110] Rearrangements in κ genes generally occur only after a productive heavy-chain gene rearrangement has taken place, and λ genes begin to rearrange only after rearrangement in both κ alleles has failed, although certain exceptions to these rules have been found.

The order of rearrangement events among T-cell receptor genes is less clear.[111-113] Most T lymphocytes bear heterodimers of α and β T-cell receptor subunits on their cell surfaces, but a small minority bear γ/δ dimers. Apparently, γ and δ genes rearrange earlier in T-lymphocyte ontogeny than do α and β genes. The prevailing view is that α/β cells and γ/δ cells represent separate lineages and that cells that rearrange α genes do not rearrange δ genes (which are actually embedded within the α locus) and vice versa.[114]

Most pertinent to the diagnosis of lymphocytic cancers is that the configuration of rearranged gene segments in an antigen receptor locus is specific for the lymphocyte in which that rearrangement occurred and any clonal progeny of that lymphocyte. Therefore, a population of lymphocytes can be identified as clonal by demonstrating uniform antigen receptor gene rearrangements for one or more antigen receptor genes within the population. Furthermore, the configuration of DNA in a rearranged locus appears to be stable under most conditions, so that the DNA sequences in a particular locus can be used as a marker to follow a clonal population of lymphocytes over time.

The configuration of DNA in a rearranged antigen receptor gene is usually assessed by Southern blot hybridization (Figs. 6–3 and 6–4). The analysis uses one of several appropriate restriction enzymes to produce a fragment that spans the J segments in the unrearranged, germline form of the gene, and a probe containing DNA from the 3′ part of this region.[115] Any rearrangement of the gene deletes DNA that originally lies 5′ of the J segments, including the restriction site that defines the 5′ end of the germline fragment spanning the J segments, and replaces it with V segment sequence (and D segment sequence in some genes). A repositioned 5′ restriction site now flanks the remaining J segments not deleted during rearrangement. The distance between this site and the retained restriction site on the 3′ side of the J segments is almost always different than that in germline DNA. The size of the fragment produced from this region is consequently distinct from the germline fragment. This fragment is detected with the same probe that hybridizes to the unrearranged germline DNA, because DNA at the 3′ portion of the fragment does not change during rearrangement. However, a sufficient number of uniform fragments must be present in a digest of tissue DNA to be detected as a band in a Southern blot autoradiogram. Analyses with DNA from pure populations of lymphocytes (*e.g.*, with in vitro cell lines) mixed with DNA from germline cells indicate that 1% to 5% of cells in a specimen must contain the same antigen receptor gene rearrangement for a band to be visible in the autoradiogram.[88] The Southern blot procedure requires, at a minimum, DNA from about 5×10^5 total cells for each analysis. Therefore, a lymphocytic cancer can be detected in a specimen of this size if about 5000 or more of the cells are malignant.

Southern blot analysis of antigen receptor gene rearrangements has become a widely accepted adjunct to morphologic diagnosis of lymphocytic cancers. Nevertheless, this approach has several limitations. From a biologic point of view, uniform antigen receptor gene rearrangements in biopsy tissue reflect the presence of clonal lymphocytes in the specimen rather than malignancy per se. For reasons that are not well understood, occasional lymphocytic cancers lack detectable gene rearrangements.[116] Furthermore, some rare clinically benign disorders are apparently clonal, although many of these disorders are associated with a high incidence of lymphoma or lymphocytic leukemia.[117-124] Consequently, it may be that these disorders represent premalignant processes that contain some of the genetic alterations necessary for full-blown malignancy. In any event, clonality is not the equivalent of malignancy, and the detection of clonal antigen receptor gene rearrangements must be interpreted circumspectly and in light of other diagnostic information.

In addition, antigen receptor gene rearrangements must be used cautiously to infer the lymphocytic lineage of a given tumor. Some lymphocytic neoplasms that are B-lineage by

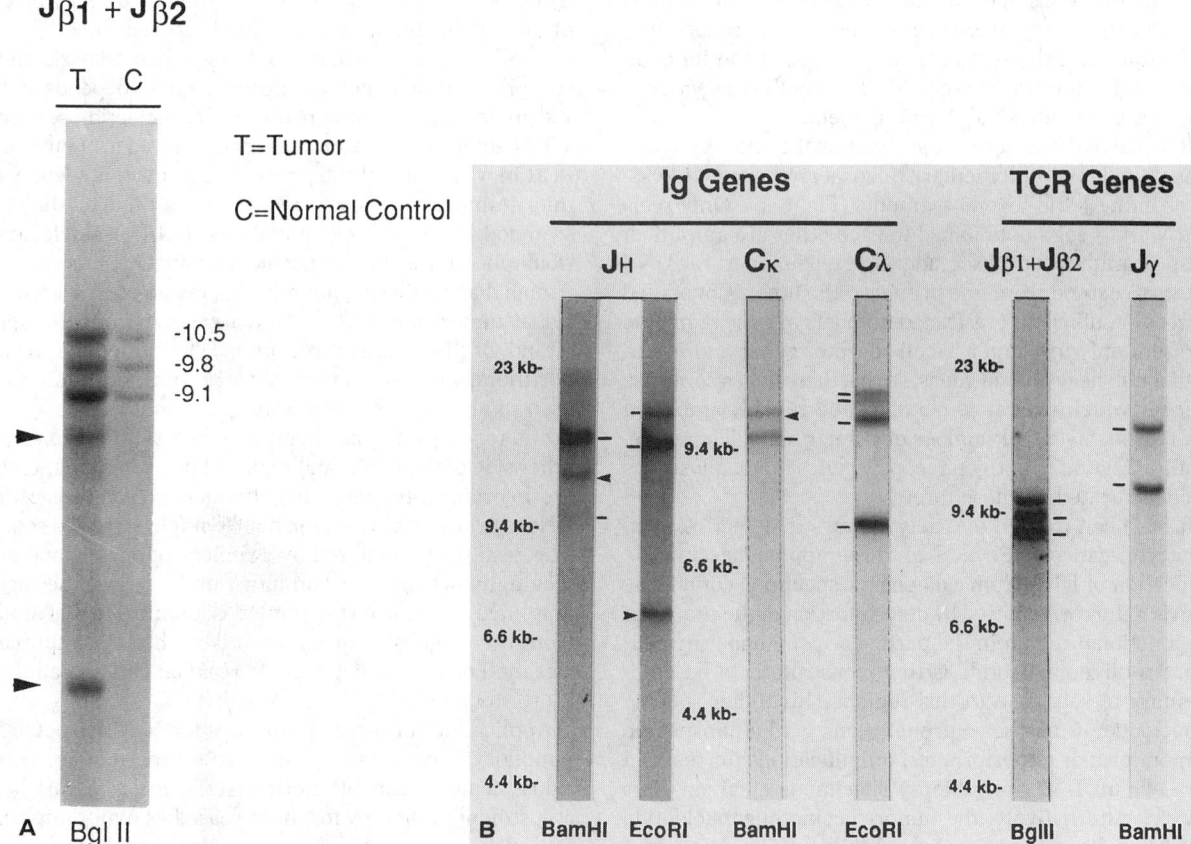

FIGURE 6–4. Southern blot autoradiograms from analysis of antigen receptor genes in non-Hodgkin lymphomas. **(A)** Analysis of beta T-cell receptor genes in a T-cell lymphoma. DNA from the tumor (T) was analyzed alongside DNA from the same patient's peripheral blood (C), which was histologically free of tumor cells. Both DNAs were digested with the BglII restriction enzyme before electrophoresis. Hybridization was performed with a mixture of probes for the two J-segment clusters in the gene. The arrows indicate the two clonal rearranged bands (apparently both β T-cell receptor alleles had been rearranged in the tumor). The sizes of the fragments in kilobases is shown for the three germline bands. Three germline bands are present due to hybridization for each of the two J-segment clusters and a common polymorphism in the DNA sequence affecting a BglII site flanking the second J-segment cluster. **(B)** An expanded panel of analyses in a case of B-cell lymphoma. All three immunoglobulin genes and two T-cell receptor genes (β and γ) were analyzed. The probe used for each analysis is shown above the autoradiograms; the restriction enzymes are shown below. Results for the immunoglobulin heavy-chain gene were confirmed by performing analyses with two separate restriction enzymes (BamHI and EcoRI). The germline fragments are indicated by dashes; clonal rearranged fragments by arrows. Multiple germline bands arise from the presence of several J-segment clusters in the gene or certain cross-hybridizing sequences having partial homology to that of the probe. The positions of size marker fragments run in parallel with the test samples are shown to the left of the autoradiograms. The results are consistent with a B-lineage tumor because only immunoglobulin genes and no T-cell receptor genes show clonal rearrangement. A tumor exhibiting this pattern of rearrangements would be expected to express immunoglobulin containing κ rather than λ light chains.

antigenic markers and contain clonal immunoglobulin gene rearrangements also contain clonal T-cell receptor gene rearrangements.[125,126] The inverse is sometimes true for T-lineage neoplasms. This situation especially pertains to immature lymphocytic cancers, such as pre–B-cell acute lymphoblastic leukemias. Moreover, clonal antigen receptor genes are sometimes found in certain myeloid leukemias.[127,128] However, a consistent pattern of rearrangement in several genes (*e.g.*, rearrangements of heavy- and light-chain immunoglobulin genes and germline T-cell receptor genes) can help confirm the lymphocytic lineage indicated by antigenic data.

From a technical point of view, Southern blot analysis of

antigen receptor gene rearrangements suffers from limited sensitivity, in terms of the fraction of clonal cells within a specimen that are detectable and the total number of cells required for analysis. Efforts have been made to overcome these disadvantages by applying PCR to antigen receptor gene rearrangements. The marker in these approaches to diagnosis of lymphocytic cancers is the unique, clonotypic sequences at the junctions between rearranged gene segments. These sequences are created at the time of V(D)J joining by the combined effects of different gene segments participating in the rearrangement, exonucleolytic deletions that remove variable numbers of base pairs from the ends of these segments, and the addition of random G:C-rich sequence called *N sequence* to the segment ends before they are joined together. The deletions and the N sequences inserted at the junction range from 0 to about 30 base pairs. The result is a sequence specific for each individual rearrangement.

PCR is carried out across the junctional region by using oligonucleotides complementary to conserved nucleotide sequences in the J and V gene segments (Fig. 6–5). Only rearranged V and J segments joined to each other are amplified, because germline V and J segments are too far apart for DNA synthesis to extend from one primer to the other. Conserved sequences or sufficiently restricted numbers of gene segments are present only in γ and δ T-cell receptor genes and in immunoglobulin heavy-chain genes, so that these genes comprise the set for which rearrangements can be reliably amplified with a reasonably small number of primer pairs. Therefore, PCR amplification of antigen receptor genes for diagnosis has been concentrated on these three genes.

PCR has been used in a variety of ways to detect residual lymphocytic cancers. Several of these approaches involve amplification of DNA from a diagnostic specimen containing unequivocal tumor, followed by determination of the sequence at the junctional region in the particular gene under investigation. An olignonucleotide is then constructed to be complementary to sequence in this region. This tumor-specific oligonucleotide is used as a primer along with a nonspecific V segment primer to perform test amplifications for residual tumor cells on DNA from biopsy specimens obtained after therapy.[129] Alternatively, the tumor-specific oligonucleotide is radiolabeled and used as a hybridization probe on antigen receptor DNA amplified from the posttherapy specimen.[130,131] For δ T-cell receptor genes, a modified procedure takes advantage of a convenient, conserved V-segment restriction site to cleave a fragment off of the PCR product amplified

from the diagnostic specimen and thereby directly produce a probe for the tumor-specific junctional sequence.[132]

Another approach that avoids sequence analysis and construction of tumor-specific oligonucleotides depends on V- and J-segment primers designed to have nucleotide sequence of a T7 bacteriophage promoter incorporated at their 5′ end.[133] PCR in which one of the primers contains this sequence permits immediate transcription of one strand of the double-stranded DNA product into labeled RNA. A single-stranded riboprobe for the tumor-specific rearrangement is synthesized from a diagnostic specimen in this fashion. To search for residual tumor, target RNA is synthesized from the opposite strand of the antigen receptor DNA amplified from the posttherapy specimen using a pair of primers similar to that used to amplify DNA of the original tumor, except that the promoter sequence has been attached to the primer on the other side of the junctional region. The probe and target RNA are hybridized together and then subjected to digestion by RNase A, which cleaves mismatch single-stranded sequence. The results are analyzed by gel electrophoresis and autoradiography, which reveal an intact probe only if the sequence amplified from the test specimen is identical to that amplified from the diagnostic specimen. Like other PCR approaches, this method can detect a single residual cancer cell in about 2×10^5 total cells.

Applications of these approaches for sensitive detection of lymphocytic cancers have focused on the monitoring of residual acute lymphoblastic leukemia, in large part because adjustment in therapy for this disease has major implications for balancing the chances of cure against the risks of short- and long-term side effects from overtherapy. Early results suggest that this approach can predict relapse long before conventional methods, but large-scale prospective studies now in progress will ultimately prove how often residual tumor

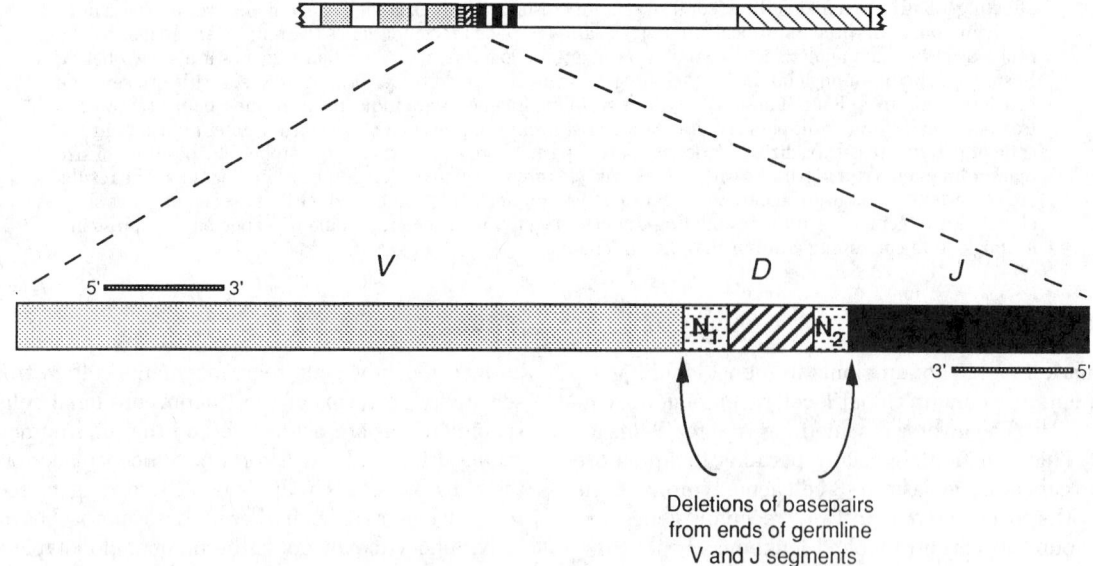

Deletions of basepairs
from ends of germline
V and J segments

FIGURE 6–5.   A rearranged antigen receptor gene highlighting the components of the junctional region with two N sequences flanking a D segment. Oligonucleotide primers complementary to conserved sequences within the V and J segments are shown at positions where they might anneal to the DNA for polymerase chain reaction amplification of the junctional region.

present at the 10^{-5} level actually has practical clinical consequences.[134]

PCR has also been adapted for diagnosing lymphocytic cancer when the total number of lymphocytes in the specimen is low. Such situations include early stages of cutaneous T-cell lymphoma (CTCL) and non-Hodgkin lymphoma involving the central nervous system. Skin lesions in early CTCL are often difficult to distinguish clinically and histologically from chronic dermatitis. Sections of the skin may show only a sparse infiltrate of various mononuclear cells lacking significant atypia and other clearcut morphologic features of malignancy. Not infrequently, there are too few lymphocytes in the tissues for analysis of clonality by Southern blot hybridization with antigen receptor gene probes. Similarly, cerebrospinal fluid from patients with lymphoma in the brain may show a small number of neoplastic lymphocytes that cannot be separated histologically from reactive lymphocytes due to infection or inflammatory conditions.

To address these diagnostic issues, rearranged antigen receptor genes in DNA extracted from biopsy specimens have been amplified by PCR to assess the clonality of the lymphocytes in the sample. The amplification procedure is essentially the same as that used to determine the clonotypic junctional sequences of rearranged antigen receptor genes for monitoring residual lymphocytic cancer: PCR is performed using oligonucleotide primers complementary to conserved sequences in the V and J segments of the gene under examination. The fraction of PCR products containing identical sequences across the junctional region is then evaluated by gel electrophoresis. The simplest strategy is to analyze the products in standard agarose gels, which separate the products by size. Detection of a discrete band in the gel indicates that in at least 1% of the rearrangements the net number of base pairs lost by exonucleolytic deletions plus those added as N sequences is the same.[135,136] Polyclonal lymphocytic populations yield only a smear of many bands within the gel and no discrete bands.

Standard agarose gels demonstrate only that the PCR products amplified from the antigen receptor gene rearrangements of a specimen are or are not of equivalent size. A more specific method for rapidly analyzing PCR products is denaturing gradient gel electrophoresis (DGGE).[137] This method is based on the fact that single-stranded regions within partially denatured double-stranded DNA fragments greatly reduce the electrophoretic mobility of the fragment in a gel. Stepwise regional denaturation of DNA can be induced by gradually raising the temperature or by increasing the concentration of such chemical denaturants as urea and formamide. The temperature or denaturant concentration at which the strands of DNA begin to unravel is highly sensitive to the nucleotide sequence in that region of DNA, so that even a single base pair change can significantly change the conditions that produce denaturation. In DGGE, the PCR fragments are analyzed in a polyacrylamide gel that has incorporated into it an increasing gradient of urea and formamide. Driven through the gel by an electric field, the fragments migrate until a level of denaturants is encountered at which the strands of DNA in the fragment begin to come apart. The fragments undergoing denaturation essentially stop at this point, and if sufficient numbers of fragments stop in the same place (*i.e.*, if the fragments have identical sequences) a discrete band appears in the gel (Fig. 6–6). The diverse PCR products generated from the DNA of polyclonal tissues denature at different positions within the gel and therefore produce only a diffuse smear. Controlled studies performed by amplifying rearranged antigen receptor genes from mixtures of cell line DNA and polyclonal lymphocyte DNA indicate that the method is sensitive enough to detect 0.1% clonal fraction among lymphocytic cell populations.

Analysis of PCR products amplified from antigen receptor gene rearrangements by standard electrophoresis or by DGGE has the added virtue of permitting direct visualization of the results in the gel under ultraviolet light after staining with ethidium bromide. This means that autoradiography is not necessary, and compared with Southern blot analysis, results can be obtained in 1 or 2 days rather than 1 week. The major limitation of this approach is that its use is restricted to those genes listed above because of problems in finding consensus PCR primers for other genes. Analysis of CTCL, for example, must be based on amplification of γ T-cell receptor genes instead of β T-cell receptor genes, which would be expected to be rearranged in a higher percentage of cases. Nevertheless, DGGE analysis of CTCL specimens suggests that about 85% of cases contain clonal γ T-cell receptor rearrangements detectable by this technique.[138]

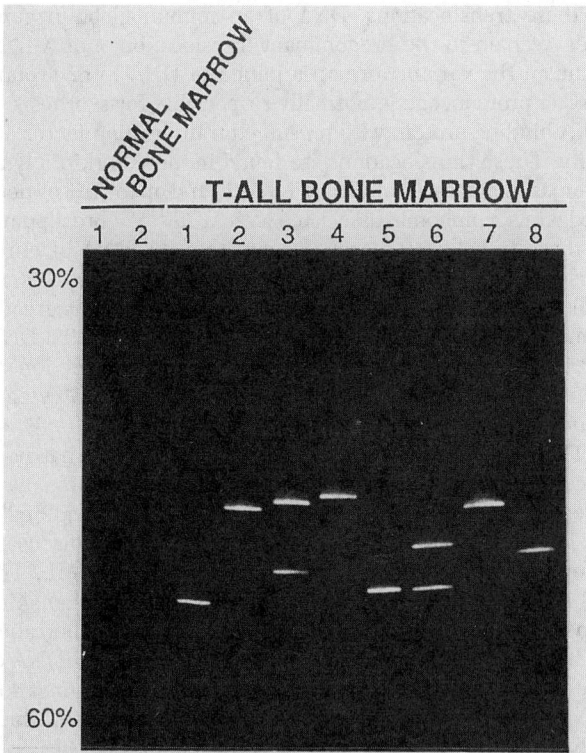

FIGURE 6–6. Antigen receptor gene rearrangements analyzed by the polymerase chain reaction and gradient denaturing gel electrophoresis. A polyacrylamide gel containing γ T-cell receptor gene DNA was amplified from a series of normal bone marrow specimens or bone marrow specimens containing T-lineage acute lymphoblastic leukemia. The relative concentration of chemical denaturants (urea and formamide) is indicated at the top and bottom of the gel. The gel has been stained with ethidium bromide and photographed under ultraviolet light.

In addition to antigen receptor gene rearrangements, chromosomal translocations have been used as diagnostic markers for lymphocytic cancers, but to a much lesser extent. A large number of recurrent chromosomal translocations have been identified in lymphocytic cancers, and DNA surrounding the breakpoints have been molecularly cloned from a growing subset of these chromosomal aberrations.[139] Many of these translocations have had limited diagnostic use because they are rare, although it remains to be determined whether or not any of the rarer translocations may correlate with subtle clinical characteristics that would be diagnostically useful in delineating new subtypes of lymphocytic cancer. For example, the t(11;14)(q13;q32), which was identified several years ago in infrequent cases of chronic lymphocytic leukemia and small lymphocytic leukemia, has recently been shown to be present in over 50% of lymphocytic lymphomas of intermediate differentiation (also referred to as *centrocytic lymphoma* or *mantle zone lymphoma*), a rare form of chronic B-lineage non-Hodgkin's lymphoma.[140,141]

Another practical problem associated with the use of translocations as diagnostic markers is that the positions of breakpoints within the chromosomal DNA are too heterogenous to permit detection of the translocation with a reasonable number of hybridization probes or PCR primers. This situation pertains most clearly to the t(8;14)(q24;q32) and its variant forms t(2;8)(p11;q24) and t(8;22)(q24;q11).[139–142] In each of these translocations, DNA of an immunoglobulin gene (heavy chain in the predominant translocation; κ or λ light chain in the variant forms) is joined to DNA in or around *MYC*, a protooncogene normally responsible for synthesis of DNA-binding protein with presumed transcription factor activity. These translocations are found in most Burkitt's lymphomas, many cases of L2 and L3 ALL, and up to 75% of non-Hodgkin's lymphomas associated with AIDS.[143,144] Breakpoints in these translocations can occur within the DNA of chromosome 8 over a distance of several hundred kilobases on either side of *MYC*. Although the scatter of breakpoints greatly complicates routine detection of rearrangements of *MYC* DNA for diagnostic purposes, it does not preclude detection of translocations involving *MYC* by means of standard cytogenetics or potentially by FISH.

The two translocations in lymphocytic cancers that have received the most attention for diagnostic applications have been the t(9;22)(q34;q11) in ALL and the t(14;18)(q32;q21) in follicular B-cell lymphoma. The t(9;22) was discussed above in the context of the Ph¹ chromosome in CML. The t(14;18) is found in over 90% of follicular lymphomas, making it perhaps the most common specific chromosomal aberration in hematopoietic cancers.[145] The translocation joins DNA of the immunoglobulin heavy-chain gene on chromosome 14 to DNA of the protooncogene *BCL2*, the protein product of which is found at the inner membrane of mitochondria and has been experimentally implicated in the delay of programmed cell death (apoptosis) of B cells in follicular centers of activated lymph nodes.[140–148] Among (14;18) translocations, the breaks in *BCL2* occur predominantly within two cluster regions 3' of the coding sequence: a major breakpoint cluster region (MBR, in about 60% to 70% of cases) and a minor cluster region (MCR, in about 20% to 25% cases).[149,150] Within each cluster region, most breaks are distributed over several hundred base pairs. In virtually all cases, DNA at the sites is joined to J segments in the immunoglobulin heavy-chain locus.

The concentration of breakpoints in (14;18) translocations within defined regions of DNA permits reliable detection of this marker by Southern blot hybridization with probes for *BCL2* or PCR with primers for J segment sequence and MBR or MCR.[151–153] In practice, neither Southern blot analysis nor PCR of the t(14;18) have been widely applied for diagnosis. Problems in the primary diagnosis of a specimen as lymphoma are usually resolved by analysis of immunoglobulin gene rearrangements and assignment to the follicular subtype is usually based on morphology. In addition, application of PCR for detection of residual disease has been restricted because chemotherapy does not affect long-term survival and the goal of therapy has largely been tumor control rather than cure. The recent discovery that (14;18) translocations can be detected by PCR in about 50% of lymph nodes showing reactive hyperplasia also suggests that this marker may not be as specific as earlier thought.[154] Nevertheless, these considerations do not pertain to assessment of bone marrow for residual follicular lymphoma in the treatment of patients by autologous bone marrow transplantation. Studies indicate that marrow grafts found to be free of disease by PCR for the t(14;18) show a far better prognosis.[155]

SOLID TUMORS

Neuroblastoma

Neuroblastoma is perhaps the one example of a solid tumor in which one type of molecular diagnosis is routine. The diagnostic marker analyzed in this disease is amplification of N-*MYC*, a protooncogene homologous to *MYC*.[156] The purpose of analyzing N-*MYC* amplification in neuroblastoma is the determination of prognosis. Increased numbers of N-*MYC* correlate with poorer prognosis independent of stage.[157] For example, in one large study, patients whose tumors have had 1, 3 to 10, or more than 10 copies of N-*MYC* per cell showed a progression-free survival after 18 months of 70%, 30%, and 5%, respectively.[158] The standard method for evaluating N-*MYC* amplification is Southern blot hybridization with a N-*MYC* probe. Amplification is indicated by increased intensity of the N-*MYC* band in the Southern blot autoradiogram.

Amplification of N-*MYC* is not the only useful molecular marker in neuroblastoma. DNA content, assessed by flow cytometry, and deletions in the short arm of chromosome 1, assessed by cytogenetics or perhaps in the future by FISH, also have predictive value.[159] Combined with N-*MYC* amplification, these two other variables define three distinct prognostic groups. Patients in the first group have tumors with a hyperdiploid or triploid modal chromosome number and lack 1p deletions or N-*MYC* amplifications. These patients are generally under 1 year of age and have a good prognosis for survival. In the second group are patients with tumors having near-diploid or near-tetraploid chromosome numbers without 1p deletions or N-*MYC* amplifications. These patients tend to be older than patients in the first group and more often follow a slowly progressive, fatal course. The last group of patients have tumors with near-diploid or near-tetraploid chromosome numbers and 1p deletions or N-*MYC* amplifications. Patients in this group are older on average than those in the other groups, present in a more advanced stage, and die more quickly. These three groups appear to be stable, with no conversion or progression between groups. In this respect, neuroblastoma epitomizes the power of a multiparameter molecular approach to cancer prognosis.

Breast Cancer

Molecular diagnosis in breast cancer has largely focused on the issue of predicting relapse in women without histopathologic evidence of spread to axillary lymph nodes. With local therapy alone (surgery with or without radiation), up to 30% of these women relapse within 5 years of diagnosis. Some patients among this group should receive chemotherapy, but treatment of all node-negative patients would subject many patients who may not benefit to the risks and discomfort of systemic therapy. To aid in this dilemma, attempts have been made to correlate a number of molecular markers with increased likelihood of relapse. Among the genes and gene products studied in this regard have been the epidermal growth factor receptor (EGFR), cathepsin D, and *NM23*, a gene for an NDP-kinase originally identified by its differential levels of activity in murine melanoma cell lines which show differing potential for metastasis after inoculation into animals.[160-164] Tumors expressing elevated levels of the first two genes and reduced levels of the last gene appear to be more likely to relapse.

The gene that has been studied more than any other for evaluating prognosis in breast cancer is *ERBB2* (or *HER2/NEU*).[165] The oncogene *ERBB2* encodes a surface membrane protein with homology to EGFR. About 25% to 30% of breast cancers show amplification of the gene, which also correlates closely with increased levels of *ERBB2* RNA and protein. Numerous studies of the gene have revealed an association between *ERBB2* amplification and earlier relapse and decreased survival, independent of node status. In fact, after the number of involved lymph nodes, *ERBB2* amplification is the most reliable known predictor of disease-free and overall survival.[166-171] More recently, *ERBB2* amplification has been detected in about 30% of ovarian cancers and overexpression has been correlated with poorer prognosis.[172]

Analysis of the *ERBB2* gene in breast and ovarian cancer illustrates the range of methods for detection that may be applicable to many genetic markers in human cancers. Amplification of the gene has been studied by Southern blotting, Northern blotting, Western blotting, and immunohistochemistry. Each method has certain virtues, but in terms of convenience, immunohistochemistry is easiest and permits simultaneous assessment of morphology, an important advantage because most tumors show significant admixture of malignant and normal tissues. However, immunohistochemistry is less directly quantifiable than other methods and the antibodies available for staining the tissues work only on frozen specimens.

Bladder Cancer

Recent work in bladder cancer presents a potentially valuable model for the molecular monitoring of early relapse in many cancers that can be followed by examination of exfoliated cells. Relapse is a particular problem in bladder cancer because of the propensity for development of recurrent tumors throughout the urinary epithelium in patients who have had a single tumor fulgurated or excised. The marker used to monitor recurrence is mutation in the *TP53* tumor suppressor gene. *TP53* encodes a protein that binds viral oncoproteins, such as the E7 protein of human papillomavirus, and may normally help to negatively regulate key events in the cell cycle by binding cellular proteins or by interacting directly with DNA.[173,174] *TP53* is probably the most commonly mutated gene known in human cancer, and about 50% of bladder carcinomas contain mutations in this gene. Because recurrent tumors appear to represent metastases rather than independent primary cancers, these recurrences can be expected to have the same *TP53* mutations as the original tumor.[175] Therefore, once the specific mutation has been identified in the original tumor, patients can be followed for recurrences by screening for the tumor-specific mutation in cells present in urine sediments.[176]

The strategy used to monitor recurrences involves initial PCR amplification of p53 gene DNA from the original tumor. Nucleotide sequence of the amplification product is analyzed to determine the precise mutation in the *TP53* gene. Based on this information, short, radiolabeled oligonucleotides complementary to the region of *TP53* containing the mutation are prepared for use as hybridization probes to screen cells in subsequent urine specimens. Such oligonucleotides anneal selectively to mutant *TP53* DNA rather than normal DNA by performing the hybridization at suitable stringency, despite the fact that the mutant and normal sequences differ by only a single base pair.

To screen for recurrences, *TP53* DNA is amplified from the cells of these urine specimens, and the amplification products are ligated into the DNA of M13 bacteriophage genomes. These recombinant genomes are transfected into *E. coli*, which are then grown in a lawn of bacteria on agar plates. The infected cells produce plaques containing recombinant phages and their DNA, which can be transferred directly to membranes similar to those used for Southern blotting by simply laying the membrane over the surface of the plate. After removing the membrane and drying it to bind the DNA, the entire membrane is incubated with the tumor-specific oligonucleotide under properly stringent conditions. Plaques containing mutant *TP53* DNA are identified as dark spots on autoradiograms of the hybridized membranes. In this manner, one tumor cell among about 5000 to 10,000 total exfoliated cells can be detected in urine specimens.

Strategies like the one described for monitoring recurrence in bladder cancer may be applicable to colon, lung, and other cancers using mutations in *TP53* or other genes. Practical shortcomings inherent in this strategy also highlight some of the areas in which molecular monitoring of residual disease could be substantially improved. One such area is the efficient detection of point mutations in oncogenes. In many instances, as in *TP53*, mutations in these genes tend to be clustered in particular regions of the genes. This fact makes finding of a tumor-specific mutation easier than it would be otherwise by making it possible to focus sequence analysis on those regions likely to contain mutations. Nevertheless, sequence analysis is still required to determine the exact mutation, and a method that could quickly identify the mutations in critical genes without employing full-scale sequence analysis would greatly simplify any molecular approach to cancer involving detection of point mutations. The procedure for screening follow-up specimens by analysis of phage plaques is also too cumbersome to anticipate that it will gain widespread and routine use. Furthermore, the sensitivity of the screening procedure may be too low to detect the earliest stages of relapse. Development of new methods to test specimens directly and more sensitively for specific point mutations could change these situations.

Melanoma

An example of a molecular approach designed for sensitive detection of metastasis and with implications for many cancers has recently been described in melanoma. In a small study involving only positive and negative control patients, circulating melanoma cells were detected in the blood of 4 of 7 patients with metastatic melanoma.[177] The method involved synthesizing cDNA from the RNA of peripheral blood cells, followed by PCR amplification of tyrosinase DNA using oligonucleotide primers specific for this gene. Blood from healthy volunteers or patients with other forms of cancer failed to produce an amplification product with these primers. Reconstitution experiments with melanoma cell lines and normal blood showed a sensitivity for detecting tumor cells down to about one tumor cell in 10^6 total cells.

The capability and clinical relevance of detecting circulating tumor cells by the above approach in melanoma patients without known metastases remains to be determined. In principle, a similar approach could be used for detecting metastases in virtually any cancer for which RNA of an appropriate gene could serve as a tumor marker. An appropriate gene would be any gene expressed in the cancer but not expressed in cells normally resident at the site of possible metastasis (*e.g.*, lymph node or bone marrow). The approach is not unlike using immunohistochemistry or flow cytometry to screen for metastatic cells with antibodies against differentiation antigens. The advantage of a molecular approach using PCR is that it is probably more sensitive and not limited to markers expressed on the cell surface (or for that matter, to genes expressed as protein at all, as long as the RNA for the gene is present). A potential pitfall of this approach is the phenomenon *illegitimate transcription* where in many normal tissues small amounts of RNA are expressed by genes that have no real physiologic role in the cell.[178] This would give rise to a normal low level background signal which would have to be distinguished from the signal generated from the metastatic cells. In some cases, normal cells containing small amounts of marker RNA may yield results resembling those obtained from few cells containing high levels of marker RNA. Indeed, after many cycles of PCR, faint signals were obtained for tyrosinase RNA in the blood of normal controls for the study of metastatic melanoma.[178]

Retinoblastoma

Retinoblastoma is the outstanding example of a cancer with a well-known incidence of familial predisposition,[179] and efforts have been mounted in recent years to use molecular methods for identifying those patients at risk. The key to this diagnosis is the *RB1* gene, a tumor suppressor gene that encodes a 105-kd product and shares with the *TP53* product the ability to bind certain viral oncoproteins.[180–183] In normal cells of many tissues, *RB1*-encoded product also binds to a number of nuclear proteins. The capacity of RB1 product to bind other proteins seems to be controlled by phosphorylation of the RB1 product, which in turn may be regulated by $p34^{cdc2}$ kinase, an enzyme involved in the progression of the cell from the G_0 to G_1 phases of the cell cycle. In retinoblastoma cells, both *RB1* alleles are inactivated by mutation or deletion.[184–188]

Detection of an inherited defect in *RB1* to assess risk in individuals with a family history of retinoblastoma can be performed in several ways. About 0.5% to 3% of patients have a cytogenetic deletion centered about chromosome 13 band q14, the site of the *RB1* gene. Because the deletion is transmitted through the germline, karyotyping can be carried out for this deletion on leukocytes or fibroblasts. In those patients without cytogenetic deletions, inheritance of the defective copy of *RB1* can be followed by RFLP analysis, when nontumor tissues from affected and unaffected family members are available and study of these tissues reveals an RFLP linked to the defective allele.[188] With the molecular cloning of the *RB1* gene itself, it is also possible to screen blood or other tissues directly for the critical mutation. If point mutations are involved, diagnosing increased risk is complicated by the usual difficulties of finding single base changes in large genes.

CONSIDERATIONS FOR THE FUTURE

Diagnostic molecular analysis of cancer is only beginning to affect the practice of oncology. The extent to which molecular approaches to diagnosis will change cancer medicine will depend on how well these new approaches meet particular needs. Some molecular approaches to diagnosis simply seem to improve the accuracy of diagnosis by conventional methods, whereas other approaches provide information that cannot be obtained in other ways. Examples of this kind of information include the presence of minimal disease and findings suggesting poor prognosis. Whether or not this information is of clinical value will require large prospective studies that involve therapeutic protocols modified in accordance with the results of molecular tests.

Another need is the development of more convenient techniques. By and large, molecular tests for cancer diagnosis are labor-intensive, time-consuming, and expensive relative to other laboratory tests. Introduction of simplified procedures will undoubtedly increase the use of molecular diagnoses. Part of the simplification process might involve the automation of steps, little of which has been accomplished in this field. In any event, until tests become fully automated, increased numbers of laboratory personnel will have to be trained in the existing methods before molecular diagnostic tests become more widely available than they are now.

Conventional practices by which patient specimens are stored must also be altered for patients to benefit maximally from the application of molecular diagnostic tests. As in the past, standard methods for the storage of specimens include fixation in formaldehyde, embedding in paraffin, or preservation as air-dried smears on glass microscope slides. Some molecular techniques (for instance, PCR) will work on specimens stored in these ways, but most of molecular techniques, including PCR, function much better with frozen or ethanol-fixed tissues. Surgeons, oncologists, and pathologists should be mindful of this difference if there is any chance that molecular tests may be used in a case. Additionally, lack of tissues preserved in the proper manner will inhibit retrospective studies, which often provide preliminary evidence for the value of a new diagnostic strategy.

Finally, physicians must make themselves aware of the capabilities and limitations of molecular approaches to cancer diagnosis. Education in the appropriate uses of these tests should probably begin in medical school and continue through fellowship training and beyond. Only by expanded awareness among physicians of the potential of these techniques will the opportunities offered by these tests for improved patient care be fully realized.

REFERENCES

1. Bishop JM. Molecular themes in oncogenesis. Cell 1991;64:235–248.
2. Hunter T. Cooperation between oncogenes. Cell 1991;64:249–270.
3. Cantley LC, Auger KR, Carpenter C, et al. Oncogenes and signal transduction. Cell 1991;64:281–302.
4. Marshall CJ. Tumor suppressor genes. Cell 1991;64:313–326.
5. Weinberg RA. Tumor suppressor genes. Science 1991;254:1138–1146.
6. Fearon ER, Vogelstein B. A genetic model for colorectal tumorigenesis. Cell 1990;61:759–767.
7. Heim S, Mitelman F. Cancer cytogenetics. New York, Alan R. Liss, 1987.
8. Mitelman F. Catalogue of chromosomal aberrations in cancer. New York: Wiley-Liss, 1991.
9. Sandberg AA. The chromosomes in human cancer and leukemia. New York: Elsevier, 1990.
10. Solomon E, Borrow J, Goddard AD. Chromosome aberrations and cancer. Science 1991;254:1153–1160.
11. Friedlander ML, Hedley DW, Taylor IW, Clinical and biological significance of aneuploidy in human tumours. J Clin Pathol 1984;37:961–974.
12. Barlogie B, Raber MN, Schumann J, et al. Flow cytometry in clinical cancer research. Cancer research 1983;43:3982–3997.
13. Zur Hausen H. Viruses in human cancers. Science 1991;254:1167–1173.
14. Reitz MSJ, Kalyanarraman VS, Robert-Gurnoff M, et al. Human T cell leukemia lymphoma virus: the retrovirus of adult T cell leukemia/lymphoma. J Inf Dis 1983;147:399–405.
15. Henle W, Henle G. The Epstein-Barr virus in Burkitt's lymphoma and nasopharyngeal carcinoma. Ann Clin Lab Sci 1974;4:109–114.
16. Hanto DW, Frizzera G, Purtilo DT, et al. Clinical spectrum of lymphoproliferative disorders in renal transplant recipients and evidence for the role of Epstein-Barr virus. Cancer Res 1981;41:4253–4261.
17. Boshart M, Gissman L, Ikenberg H, et al. A new type of human papilloma virus, its presence in genital cancer biopsies and in cell lines derived from cervical cancer. EMBO J 1984;3:1151–1157.
18. Levy R, Warnke R, Dorfman RF, et al. The monoclonality of human B-cell lymphomas. J Exp Med 1972;145:1014–1028.
19. Fialkow PJ. Clonal and stem cell origins in blood neoplasms. In: Lobue J, Gordon AR, Silber R, Muggia FM, eds. Contemporary hematology/oncology. New York: Plenum Press, 1980:11.
20. Migeon BR. Glucose-6-phosphate dehydrogenase as a probe for the study of X-chromosome inactivation in human females. Isozymes Curr Top Biol Med Res 1983;9:189–200.
21. Vogelstein B, Fearon ER, Hamilton SR, et al. Use of restriction fragment length polymorphisms to determine the clonal origin of human tumors. Science 1985;227:642–645.
22. Vogelstein B, Fearon ER, Hamilton SR, et al. Clonal analysis using recombinant DNA probes from the X-chromosome. Cancer research 1987;47:4806–4813.
23. Langer-Safer P, Levine M, Ward D. Immunological method for mapping genes on Drosophila polytene chromosomes. Proc Natl Acad Sci USA 1982;79:4381–4385.
24. Lichter P, Cremer T, Tang CJ, et al. Rapid detection of human chromosome 21 aberrations by in situ hybridization. Proc Natl Acad Sci USA 1988;85:9664–9668.
25. Pinkel D, Landegent J, Collins C, et al. Fluorescent in situ hybridization with human chromosome-specific libraries: Detection of trisomy 21 and translocations of chromosome 4. Proc Natl Acad Sci USA 1988;87:9138–9142.
26. Anastasi JA, Le Beau MM, Vardiman JW, et al. Detection of trisomy 12 in chronic lymphocytic leukemia by fluorescence in situ hybridization to interphase cells: A simple and sensitive method. Blood 1992;79:1796–1801.
27. Tkachuk D, Westbrook C, Andreeff M, et al. Detection of BCR-ABL fusion in chronic myelogenous leukemia by in situ hybridization. Science 1990;250:559–562.
28. Huten E, Kuroiwa A, Gehring WJ. Spatial distribution of transcripts from the segmentation gene *fushi tarazu* during *Drosophila* embryologic development. Cell 1984;37:833–841.
29. Grody WW, Cheng L, Lewin KJ. Application of in situ DNA hybridization technology to diagnostic surgical pathology. Path Annu 1987;22(2):151–175.
30. DeLellis RA, Wolfe HJ. New techniques in gene product analysis. Arch Pathol Lab Med 1987;111:620–627.
31. Angerer LM, Angerer RC. Localization of mRNAs by in situ hybridization. Methods Cell Biol 1991;35:37–71.
32. Hood DL, Petras RE, Edinger M, et al: DNA ploidy and cell cycle analysis of colorectal carcinoma by flow cytometry: A prospective study of 137 cases using fresh whole cell suspensions. Am J Clin Pathol 1990;93:615–620.
33. Meling GI, Rognum TO, Clausen OP, et al: Association between DNA ploidy pattern and cellular atypia in colorectal cancers: A new clinical application of DNA flow cytometric study? Cancer 1991;67:1642–1649.
34. Kallioniemi OP, Blanco G, Alarackko M, et al. Improving the prognostic value of DNA flow cytometry in breast cancer by combining DNA index and S-phase fraction: A proposed classification of DNA histograms in breast cancer. Cancer 1988;62:2183–2190.
35. Dressler LG, Seamer MT, Owens MA, et al. DNA flow cytometry and prognostic factors in 1331 frozen breast cancer specimens. Cancer 1988;61:420–427.
36. Southern E. Detection of specific sequences among DNA fragments separated by gel electrophoresis. J Mol Biol 1975;98:503–517.
37. Kan YW, Dozy AM. Antenatal diagnosis of sickle-cell anaemia by DNA analysis of amniotic-fluid cells. Lancet 1978;2:910–912.
38. Botstein D, White RL, Skolnick M, et al. Construction of a genetic linkage map in man using restriction fragment length polymorphisms. Am J Hum Genet 1980;32:314–331.
39. Jeffreys AJ, Wilson V, Thein SL. Hypervariable minisatellite regions in human DNA. Nature 1985;314:67–73.
40. Nakamura Y, Leppert M, O'Connell P, et al. Variable number of tandem repeats (VNTR) markers for human gene mapping. Science 1987;235:1616–1622.
41. Koufos A, Hansen M, Copeland N. Loss of heterozygosity in three embryonal tumors suggests a common pathogenetic mechanism. Nature 1985;316:330–334.
42. Cavenee W, Hansen M, Nordenskjold M, et al. Genetic origin of mutations predisposing to retinoblastoma. Science 1985;228:501–503.
43. Westbrook CA, Rubin CM, Carrino JJ, et al. Long range mapping of the Philadelphia chromosome by pulse field gel electrophoresis. Blood 1988;71:697–702.
44. Schwartz DC, Cantor CR. Separation of yeast chromosome-sized DNAs by pulsed field gradient gel electrophoresis. Cell 1984;37:67–75.
45. Carle GF, Olson MV. Separation of chromosomal DNA molecules from yeast by orthogonalized alternation gel electrophoresis. Nucleic Acids Res 1984;12:5647–5664.
46. Chu G, Vollrath D, Davis RW. Separation of large DNA molecules by contour-clamped homogeneous electric fields. Science 1986;234:1582–1585.
47. Saiki R, Bugawan T, Horn G, et al. Analysis of enzymatically amplified βave-globin and HLA-DQ DNA with allele-specific oligonucleotide probes. Nature 1986;324:163–166.
48. Mullis KB, Faloona FAS. Specific synthesis of DNA in vitro via a polymerase-catalyzed chain reaction. Methods Enzymol 1987;155:335–350.
49. Saiki RK, Gelfand DH, Stoffel S, et al. Primer-directed enzymatic amplification of DNA with a thermostable DNA polymerase. Science 1988;239:487–491.
50. Wong C, Dowling CE, Saiki RK, et al. Characterization of beta-thalassaemia mutations using direct genomic sequencing of amplified single copy DNA. Nature 1987;330:384–386.
51. Gyllensten UB, Erlich HA. Generation of single-stranded DNA by the polymerase chain reaction and its application to direct sequencing of the HLA-DQA locus. Proc Natl Acad Sci USA 1988;85:7652–7656.
52. Bos JL, Verlaan de Vries M, Janssen AM, et al. Three different mutations in codon 61 of the human N-ras gene detected by synthetic oligonucleotide hybridization. Nucleic Acids Res 1984;12:9155–9163.
53. Bos JL, Fearon ER, Hamilton SR, et al. Prevalence of ras gene mutations in human colorectal cancers. Nature 1987;327:293–297.
54. Cotton RGH, Rodrigues NR, Campbell RD. Reactivity of cytosine and thymine in single-base-pair mismatches with hydroxylamine and oxmium tetroxide and its application to the study of mutations. Proc Natl Acad Sci USA 1988;86:4397–4401.
55. Dahl H-HM, Lamande SR, Cotton RGH. Detection and localization of base changes in RNA using a chemical cleavage method. Anal Biochem 1989;183:263–268.
56. Ganguly A, Prockop DJ. Detection of single-base mutations by reaction of DNA heteroduplexes with a water-soluble carbodiimide followed by primer extension: Application to products from the polymerase chain reaction. Nucleic Acids Res 1990;18:3933–3939.
57. Myers RM, Lumelsky N, Lerman LS, et al. Detection of single base substitutions in total genomic DNA. Nature 1985;313:495–498.
58. Kuppuswamy MN, Hoffmann JW, Kasper CK, et al. Single nucleotide primer extension to detect genetic diseases: Experimental application to hemophilia B (factor IX) and cystic fibrosis genes. Proc Natl Acad Sci USA 1991;88:1143–1147.
59. Landegren U, Kaiser R, Sanders J, et al. A ligase-mediated gene detection technique. Science 1988;241:1077–1080.
60. Orita M, Iwahana H, Kanazawa H, et al. Detection of polymorphisms of human DNA by gel electrophoresis as single-strand conformation polymorphisms. Proc Natl Acad Sci USA 1989;86:2766–2770.
61. Orita M, Suzuki Y, Sekiya T, et al. Rapid and sensitive detection of point mutations and DNA polymorphisms using the polymerase chain reaction. Genomics 1989;5:874–879.
62. DeLellis RA, ed. Diagnostic immunohistochemistry. New York: Masson, 1981.
63. Gatter KC, Alcock C, Heryet A, et al. Clinical importance of analyzing malignant tumors of uncertain origin with immunohistological techniques. Lancet 1985;1:1302–1305.
64. Nowell P, Hungerford D. A minute chromosome in human granulocytic leukemia. Science 1960;132:1497.

65. Rowley JD. A new consistent chromosomal abnormality in chronic myelogenous leukemia identified by quinicrine fluoroescence and Giemsa staining. Nature 1973;243:290–293.

66. de Klein A, Hagemerger A. Cytogenetic and molecular analysis of the Philadelphia translocation in chronic myelogenous leukemia. Cancer Surv 1984;3:515–529.

67. Ganessan TS, Rassool F, Gino A-P, et al. Rearrangement of the BCR gene in Ph chromosome-negative chronic myelogenous leukemia. Blood 1986;68:957–960.

68. Blennerhassett GT, Furth ME, Anderson P, et al. Clinical evaluation of DNA probe assay for Philadelphia translocation in chronic myelogenous leukemia. Leukemia 1988;2:648–657.

69. Hagemeyer A, Bottsma D, Spurr N, et al. A cellular oncogene is translocated to the Philadelphia chromosome in chronic myelocytic leukemia. Nature 1982;300:765–767.

70. Groffen J, Stevenson J, Heisterkamp N, et al. Philadelphia chromosome breakpoints are clustered within a limited region, BCR, on chromosome 22. Cell 1984;36:93–99.

71. Kurzrock R, Gutterman JU, Talpaz M. The molecular genetics of Philadelphia chromosome-positive leukemias. N Engl J Med 1988;319:990–998.

72. Konopka J, Watahabe S, Witte O. An alteration of the human c-ABL protein K562 leukemia cells unmasks associated tyrosine kinase activity. Cell 1984;37:1035–1042.

73. Selleri L, von Lindern M, Hermans A, et al. Chronic myeloid leukemia may be associated with several BCR-ABL transcripts including the acute lymphoid leukemia-type 7 kb transcript. Blood 1990;75:1146–1153.

74. Kawasaki ES, Clark SS, Coyne MY, et al. Diagnosis of chronic myelogenous leukemia and acute leukemia by detection of leukemia-specific mRNA sequences amplified in vitro. Proc Natl Acad Sci USA 1988;85:5689–5694.

75. Rothe MS, Antin JH, Bingham EL, et al. Detection of Philadelphia chromosome-positive cells by polymerase chain reaction following bone marrow transplant for chronic myelogenous leukemia. Blood 1989;74:882–885.

76. Lee M-S, LeMaistre A, Kantarjian HM, et al. Detection of two alternative BCR/ABL mRNA junctions and minimal residual disease in Philadelphia chromosome positive chronic myelogenous leukemia by polymerase chain reaction. Blood 1989;73:2165–2170.

77. Gabert J, Thuret I, Lafage M, et al. Detection of residual BCR/ABL translocation by polymerase chain reaction in chronic myelogenous leukemia patients after bone marrow transplant. Lancet 1989;2:1125–1128.

78. Hermans A, Heisterkamp N, von Lindern M, et al. Unique fusion of BCR and c-ABL genes in Philadelphia chromosome-positive acute lymphoblastic leukemia. Cell 1987;51:31–40.

79. Mills KI, MacKenzie ED, Birnie GD. The site of the breakpoint within the BCR is a prognostic factor in Philadelphia in positive CML patients. Blood 1988;72:1237–1241.

80. Johansson B, Mertens F, Fiorentos T, et al. Remarkably long survival of a patient with Ph 1-positive chronic myeloid leukemia and 5' BCR rearrangement. Leukemia 1990;4:448–449.

81. Jaubert J, Martiat P, Dowding C, et al. The position of the M-BCR breakpoint does not predict the duration of chronic phase or survival in chronic myeloid leukemia. Br J Haematol 1990;74:30–35.

82. Ogawa H, Sugiyama H, Soma T, et al. No correlation between locations of BCR breakpoints and clinical states in Ph1-positive CML patients. Leukemia 1989;3:492–496.

83. Rowley JD, Golomb HM, Vardiman J, et al. Further evidence for a non-random chromosomal abnormality in acute promyelocytic leukemia. Int J Cancer 1977;20:869–872.

84. Borrow J, Goddard AD, Sheer D, et al. Molecular analysis of acute promyelocytic leukemia breakpoint cluster region on chromosome 17. Science 1990;249:1577–1580.

85. Chang KS, Lu JF, Wang G, et al. The t(15;17) breakpoint in acute promyelocytic leukemia cluster. Blood 1992;79:554–558.

86. von Lindern M, Poustka A, Lerach H, et al. The (6;9) chromosomal translocation, associated with a specific subtype of acute non-lymphocytic leukemia, leads to aberrant transcription of a target gene on 9q34. Mol Cell Biol 1990;10:4016–4026.

87. Arnold A, Cossman J, Bakhshi A, et al. Immunoglobulin gene rearrangement was unique clonal markers in human lymphoid neoplasms. N Engl J Med 1983;309:1593–1598.

88. Cleary ML, Chao J, Warnke R, et al. Immunoglobulin gene rearrangement as a diagnostic criterion of B cell lymphoma. Proc Natl Acad Sci USA 1984;81:593–597.

89. Aisenberg AC, Krontiris TG, Mak TW, et al. Rearrangement of the gene for the beta chain of the T-cell receptor in T-cell chronic lymphocytic leukemia and related disorders. N Engl J Med 1985;313:529–533.

90. Bertness V, Kirsch I, Hollis G, et al. T-cell receptor gene rearrangements as clinical markers of human T-cell lymphomas. N Engl J Med 1985;313:534–538.

91. Weiss LM, Hu E, Wood GS, et al. Clonal rearrangements of T-cell receptor genes in mycosis fungoides and dermatopathic lymphadenopathy. N Engl J Med 1985;313:539–544.

92. Flug F, Pelicci PG, Bonetti R, et al. T-cell receptor gene rearrangements as markers of lineage and clonality in T-cell neoplasms. Proc Natl Acad Sci USA 1985;82:3460–3464.

93. O'Connor NTJ, Wainscoat JS, Weatherall DJ, et al. Rearrangement of the T-cell-receptor β-chain gene in the diagnosis of lymphoproliferative disorders. Lancet 1985;1:1295–1297.

94. Sklar J, Weiss L, Cleary ML. Diagnostic molecular biology of non-Hodgkin's lymphomas. In: Berard CW, Dorfman RF, ed. Malignant lymphoma. Baltimore: Williams & Wilkins, 1987:204–224.

95. Korsmeyer SJ. Antigen receptor genes as molecular markers of lymphoid neoplasms. J Clin Invest 1987;79:1291.

96. Sklar J, Weiss LM. Applications of antigen receptor gene rearrangements to the diagnosis and characterization of lymphoid neoplasms. Ann Rev Med 1988;39:315–334.

97. Cossman J, Uppendamp M, Sundeen J, et al. Molecular genetics and the diagnosis of lymphoma. Arch Pathol Lab Med 1988;112:117–127.

98. Hozumi N, Tonegawa S. Evidence for somatic rearrangement of immunoglobulin genes coding for variable and constant regions. Proc Natl Acad Sci USA 1976;73:3628–3632.

99. Seidman J, Leder P. The arrangement and rearrangement of antibody genes. Nature 1978;276:790–795.

100. Tonegawa S. Somatic generation of antibody diversity. Nature 1983;302:575–581.

101. Alt F, Blackwell TK, DePinko RA, et al. Regulation of genome rearrangement events during lymphocyte differentiation. Immunol Rev 1986;89:5–30.

102. Alt FW, Blackwell TK, Yancopoulos GD. Development of the primary antibody repertoire. Science 1987;238:1079–1987.

103. Abbas AK, Lichtman AH, Pober JS. Cellular and molecular immunology. Philadelphia: WB Saunders, 1991:38–50.

104. Abbas AK, Lichtman AH, Pober JS. Cellular and molecular immunology. Philadelphia: WB Saunders, 1991:139–167.

105. Alt FW, Baltimore D. Joining of immunoglobulin heavy chain gene segments: Implications from a chromosome with evidence of three D-J$_H$ fusion. Proc Natl Acad Sci USA 1982;167:4118–4122.

106. Desiderio SV, Yancopoulos GD, Paskind M, et al. Insertion of N regions into heavy-chain genes in correlated with expression of terminal deoxytransferase in B cells. Nature 1984;311:752–755.

107. Alt FW, Yancopoulos GD, Blackwell TK, et al. Ordered rearrangement of immunoglobulin heavy chain variable region segments. EMBO J 1984;3:1209–1219.

108. Korsmeyer SJ, Hieter PA, Ravetch JV, et al. Developmental hierarchy of immunoglobulin gene rearrangements in human leukemic pre–B-cells. Proc Natl Acad Sci USA 1981;78:7096–7100.

109. Hieter PA, Korsmeyer SJ, Waldmann TA, et al. Human immunoglobulin light-chain genes are deleted or rearranged in lambda-producing B cells. Nature 1981;290:368–372.

110. Korsmeyer SJ, Hieter PA, Sharrow SO, et al. Normal human B cells display ordered light chain gene rearrangements and deletions. J Exp Med 1982;156:975–985.

111. Raulet DH, Garman RD, Saito H, et al. Developmental regulation of T-cell receptor gene expression. Nature 1985;314:103–107.

112. Snodgrass HR, Dembic Z, Steinmetz M, et al. Expression of T-cell antigen receptor genes during fetal development in the thymus. Nature 1985;315:232–233.

113. Pardoll DM, Fowlkes BJ, Bluestone JA, et al. Differential expression of two distinct T-cell receptors during thymocyte development. Nature 1987;326:79–81.

114. Winoto A, Baltimore D. Separate lineages of T cells expression the alpha beta and delta gamma receptors. Nature 1989;338:430–432.

115. Sklar J. Antigen receptor genes. structure, function, and techniques for analysis of their rearrangements. In: Knowles D, ed. Neoplastic hematology. Baltimore: Williams & Wilkins, 1992.

116. Weiss LM, Picker LJ, Grogan TM, et al. Absence of clonal beta and gamma T-cell receptor gene rearrangements in a subset of peripheral T-cell lymphomas. Am J Pathol 1988;130:436–442.

117. Weiss LE, Wood GS, Trela M, et al. Clonal T cell populations in lymphomatoid papulosis: Evidence for a lymphoproliferative origin for a clinically benign disease. N Engl J Med 1986;315:475–479.

118. Kadin ME, Vonderheid EC, Sako D, et al. Clonal composition of T cells in lymphomatoid papulosis. Am J Pathol 1987;126:13–17.

119. Fishleder A, Tubbs R, Hesse B, et al. Uniform detection of immunoglobulin gene rearrangements in benign lymphoepithelial lesions. N Engl J Med 1987;316:1118–1121.

120. Weiss LM, Wood GS, Reynolds TC, et al. Clonal T cell populations in pityriasis lichenoides et varioloiformis acuta (Mucha-Habermann disease). Am J Pathol 1987;126:417–422.

121. Neri A, Jakobiec FA, Pelicci PG, et al. Immunoglobulin and T cell receptor beta chain gene rearrangement analysis of ocular adnexal lymphoid neoplasms: Clinical and biologic implications. Blood 1987;70:1519–1529.

122. Foa R, Pelicci PG, Migone M, et al. Analysis of T-cell receptor beta chain (T beta) gene rearrangements demonstrates the monoclonal nature of T-cell chronic lymphoproliferative disorders. Blood 1986;67:247–250.

123. Hanson CA, Frizzera G, Patton DF, et al. Clonal rearrangement for immunoglobulin and T-cell receptor genes in systemic Castleman's disease: Association with Epstein-Barr virus. Am J Pathol 1988;131:84–91.

124. Sigal SH, Saul SH, Auerbach HE, et al. Gastric small lymphocytic proliferation with immunoglobulin gene rearrangement in pseudolymphoma versus lymphoma. Gastroenterology 1989;97:195–201.

125. Kitchingman GR, Rovigatti U, Maauer AM, et al. Rearrangement of immunoglobulin heavy chain genes in T cell acute lymphoblastic leukemia. Blood 1985;654:725–729.

126. Greaves MF, Chan LC, Furley SM, et al. Lineage promiscuity in hemopoietic differentiation and leukemia. Blood 1986;67:1–11.

127. Ha K, Minden M, Hozumi N, et al. Immunoglobulin gene rearrangement in acute myelogenous leukemia. Cancer Res 1984;44:4658–4660.

128. Cheng G, Minden M, Toyonaga B, et al. T cell receptor and immunoglobulin gene rearrangements in acute myeloblastic leukemia. J Exp Med 1986;163:414–424.

129. Tycko B, Palmer JD, Link MP, et al. Polymerase chain reaction amplification of rearranged antigen receptor genes using junction-specific oligonucleotides: Possible application for detection of minimal residual disease in ALL. Cancer Cells 1989;7:47–52.

130. D'Auriol L, Macintyre E, Galibert F, et al. In vitro amplification of T cell gene rearrangements: A new tool for the assessment of minimal residual disease in acute lymphoblastic leukemias. Leukemia 1989;3:155–158.

131. Yamada M, Wasserman R, Lange B, et al. Minimal residual disease in childhood B-

lineage lymphoblastic leukemia. Persistence of leukemic cells during the first months of treatment. N Engl J Med 1990;323:448–455.

132. Hansen-Hagge TE, Yokota S, Bartram CR. Detection of minimal residual disease in acute lymphoblastic leukemia by in vitro amplification of rearranged T-cell receptor beta sequences. Blood 1989;74:1762–1767.

133. Veelken H, Tycko B, Sklar J. Sensitive detection of clonal antigen receptor gene rearrangements for the diagnosis and monitoring of lymphoid neoplasia by a PCR-mediated ribonuclease protection assay. Blood 1991;78:1318–1326.

134. Tycko B, Ritz J, Sallan S, et al. Unpublished data.

135. McCarthy KP, Sloane JP, Wiedemann LM. Rapid method for distinguishing clonal from polyclonal B cell populations in surgical biopsy specimens. J Clin Pathol 1990;43:429–432.

136. Trainor KJ, Brisco MJ, Story CJ, et al. Monoclonality in B-lymphoproliferative disorders detected at the DNA level. Blood 1990;75:2220–2222.

137. Bourguin A, Tung RM, Galili N, et al. Rapid, non-radioact detection of clonal T cell receptor gene rearrangements in lymphoid neoplasms. Proc Natl Acad Sci USA 1990;87:8536–8540.

138. Sklar J, Tung R, Kadin M. Unpublished data.

139. Showe LC, Croce CM. The role of chromosomal translocation in B- and T-cell neoplasia. Annu Rev Immunol 1987;5:253–277.

140. Tsujimoto Y, Finger LR, Yunis J, et al. Cloning of the chromosomal breakpoints of neoplastic B cells with the t(14;18) chromosomal translocation. Science 1984;226:1097–1099.

141. Williams ME, Meeker TC, Swerdlow SH. Rearrangement of the chromosome 11 BCL-1 locus in centrocytic lymphoma: Analysis with multiple breakpoint probes. Blood 1991;78:493–498.

142. Croce CM, Nowell PC. Molecular basis of B cell neoplasia. Blood 1985;65:1–7.

143. Pelicci P-G, Knowles DMI, McGrath I, et al. Chromosomal breakpoints and structural alterations of the c-MYC locus differ in endemic and sporadic forms of Burkitt lymphoma. Proc Natl Acad Sci USA 1986;83:2984–2988.

144. Hulaska FG, Russo G, Kaut J, et al. Molecular resemblance of an AIDS-associated lymphoma and endemic Burkitt's lymphoma: Implications for their pathogenesis. Proc Natl Acad Sci USA 1989;86:8907–8911.

145. Offit K, Jhanwar SC, Ladanyi M, et al. Cytogenetic analysis of 434 consecutively ascertained specimens of non-Hodgkin's lymphoma: Correlations between recurrent aberrations, histology, and exposure to cytotoxic treatment. Genes Chromosome Cancer 1991;3:189–201.

146. Cleary ML, Sklar J. Nucleotide sequence of a t(14;18) chromosomal bp in follicular lymphoma and demonstration of a breakpoint cluster region near a transcriptionally active locus on chromosome 18. Proc Natl Acad Sci USA 1985;82:7439–7443.

147. Bakhshi A, Jensen JP, Goldman P, et al. Cloning the chromosome bp of t(14;18) in human lymphomas: clustering around JH on chromosome 14 and near a transcriptional unit on chromosome 18. Cell 1985;41:899–906.

148. Hockenberry D, Nuuez G, Milliman C, et al. Bcl-2 is an inner mitochondrial membrane protein that blocks programmed cell death. Nature 1990;348:334–336.

149. Cleary ML, Galili N, Sklar J. Detection of a second t(14;18) breakpoint cluster region in follicular lymphoma. J Exp Med 1986;164:305–310.

150. Weiss LM, Warnke R, Sklar J, et al. Molecular analysis of the t(14;18) chromosomal translocation in malignant lymphoma. N Engl J Med 1987;317:1185–1189.

151. Lee M-S, Chang K-S, Cabanillas F, et al. Detection of minimal residual cell carrying the t(14;18) by DNA sequence amplification. Science 1987;237:175–178.

152. Crescenzi M, Seto M, Herzig GP, et al. Thermostable DNA polymerase chain amplification of t(14;18) chromosome breakpoints and detection of minimal residual disease. Proc Natl Acad Sci USA 1988;85:4869–4873.

153. Ngan BY, Nourse J, Cleary ML. Detection of chromosomal translocation t(14;18) within the minor cluster region of BCL2 by polymerase chain reaction and direct genomic sequencing of the enzymatically amplified DNA in follicular lymphomas. Blood 1989;73:1759–1762.

154. Limpens J, de JD, van KJH, et al. BCL-2/JH rearrangements in benign lymphoid tissues with follicular hyperplasia. Oncogene 1991;6:2271–2276.

155. Gribben J, Freedman A, Neuberg D, et al. Immunologic purging of marrow assessed by PCR before autologous bone marrow transplantation for B-cell lymphoma. N Engl J Med 1991;325:1525–1533.

156. Schwab M, Alitalo K, Klempnauer KH, et al. Amplified DNA with limited homology to MYC cellular oncogene is shared by human neuroblastoma cell lines and a neuroblastoma tumor. Nature 1983;305:245–248.

157. Brodeur GM, Seeger RC, Schwab M, et al. Amplification of N-MYC in untreated human neuroblastomas correlates with advanced disease stage. Science 1984;224:1121–1124.

158. Seeger RC, Brodeur GM, Sather H, et al. Association multiple copies of the N-MYC oncogene with rapid progression of neuroblastomas. N Engl J Med 1985;313:1111–1116.

159. Brodeur GM. Neuroblastoma-clinical applications of molecular parameters. Brain Pathol 1990;1:47–54.

160. Sainsbury JR, Farndon JR, Needham GK, et al. Epidermal-growth-factor receptor status as predictor of early recurrence of and death from breast cancer. Lancet 1987;1:1398–1402.

161. Tandon AK, Clark GM, Chamness GC, et al. Cathepsin D and prognosis in breast cancer. N Engl J Med 1990;322:297–302.

162. Steeg PS, Bevilacqua G, Kopper L, et al. Evidence for a novel gene associated with low tumor metastatic potential. JNCI 1988;80:200–204.

163. Bevilacqua G, Sobel ME, Liotta LA, et al. Association of low nm23 RNA levels in human primary infiltrating ductal breast carcinomas with lymph node involvement and other histopathological indicators of high metastatic potential. Cancer Res 1989;49:5185–5190.

164. Hennessey C, Henry JA, May FEB, et al. Expression of the anti-metastatic gene NM23 in human breast cancer: Association with good prognosis. JNCI 1991;83:281–285.

165. Slamon DJ, Clark GM, Wong SG, et al. Human breast cancer: Correlation of relapse and survival with amplification of the HER-2/neu oncogene. Science 1987;235:177–182.

166. Wright C, Angus B, Nicholson S, et al. Expression of c-ERBB-2 oncoprotein: A prognostic indicator in human breast cancer. Cancer Res 1989;49:2087–2090.

167. Paik S, Hazan R, Fisher ER, et al. Pathologic findings from the national surgical adjuvant breast and bowel project: Prognostic significance of ERBB-2 protein overexpression in primary breast cancer. 1990;8:103–112.

168. Ro J, El-Naggar A, Ro JY, et al. c-ERBB-2 amplification in node-negative human breast cancer. Cancer Res 1989;49:6941–6944.

169. Paterson MC, Dietrich KD, Danyluk J, et al. Correlation between c-ERBB-2 amplification and risk of recurrent disease in node-negative breast cancer. Cancer Res 1991;51:556–567.

170. Gullick WJ, Love SB, Wright C, et al. c-ERBB-2 protein overexpression in breast cancer is a risk factor in patients with involved and uninvolved lymph nodes. Br J Cancer 1991;63:434–438.

171. Winstanley J, Cooke T, Murray GD, et al. The long term prognostic significance of c-ERBB-2 in primary breast cancer. Br J Cancer 1991;63:447–450.

172. Slamon DJ, Godolphin W, Jones LA, et al. Studies of the HER-2/NEU proto-oncogene in human breast and ovarian cancer. Science 1989;244:707–712.

173. Scheffner M, Werness BA, Huibregtse JM, et al. The E6 oncoprotein encoded by human papillomavirus types 16 and 18 promotes the degradation of p53. Cell 1990;63:1129–1136.

174. Levine AJ, Momand J, Finlay CA. The p53 tumour suppressor gene. Nature 1991;351:453–456.

175. Sidransky D, Frost P, Von Eschenbach A, et al. Clonal origin bladder cancer. N Engl J Med 1992;326:737–740.

176. Sidransky D, von Eschenbach A, Tsai YC, et al. Identification of p53 gene mutations in bladder cancers and urine samples. Science 1991;252:706–709.

177. Smith B, Selby P, Southgate J, et al. Detection of melanoma cells in peripheral blood by means of reverse transcriptase and polymerase chain reaction. Lancet 1991;338:1227–1229.

178. Chelly J, Concordet J-P, Kaplan J-C, et al. Illegitimate transcription: Transcription of any gene in any cell type. Proc Natl Acad Sci USA 1989;86:2617–2621.

179. Knudson AG. A statistical study of retinoblastoma. Proc Natl Acad Sci USA 1971;68:820–825.

180. Lee WH, Bookstein R, Hong F, et al. Human retinoblastoma susceptibility gene: Cloning, identification, and sequence. Science 1987;235:1394–1399.

181. Bookstein R, Lee EY, To H, et al. Human retinoblastoma susceptibility gene: genomic organization and analysis of heterozygous intragenic deletion mutants. Proc Natl Acad Sci USA 1988;85:2210–2214.

182. Dyson N, Howley PM, Munger K, et al. The human papilloma virus-16 E7 oncoprotein is able to bind to the retinoblastoma gene product. Science 1989;243:934–937.

183. Wagner S, Green MR. Retinoblastoma: A transcriptional tryst. Nature 1991;352:189–190.

184. Benedict WF, Murphree AL, Banerjee A, et al. Patient with 13 chromosome deletion: Evidence that the retinoblastoma gene is a recessive cancer gene. Science 1983;219:973–975.

185. Dryja TP. Homozygosity of chromosome 13 in retinoblastoma. N Engl J Med 1984;310:550–553.

186. Friend SH, Bernards R, Rogel S, et al. A human DNA segment with properties of the gene that predisposes to retinoblastoma and osteosarcoma. Nature 1986;323:643–646.

187. Lee EY, Huang S, Shew JY, et al. Diverse mutations lead to inactivation of the retinoblastoma gene. Prog Clin Biol Res 1991;362:221–240.

188. Cowell JK, Hungerford J, Rutland P, et al. Genetic and cytogenetic analysis of patients showing reduced esterase-D levels and mental retardation from a survey of 500 individuals with retinoblastoma. Ophthalmic Paediatr Genet 1989;10:117–127.

189. Wiggs J, Nordenskjold M, Yandell D, et al. Prediction of the risk of hereditary retinoblastoma, using DNA polymorphisms within the retinoblastoma gene. N Engl J Med 1990;318:151–157.

Cancer: Principles & Practice of Oncology, Fourth Edition,
edited by Vincent T. DeVita, Jr., Samuel Hellman, Steven A. Rosenberg.
J.B. Lippincott Co., Philadelphia © 1993.

John Mendelsohn
Marc E. Lippman

CHAPTER **7**

Principles of Molecular Cell Biology of Cancer: Growth Factors

Growth factors are polypeptide molecules that regulate cell growth and function by binding with high affinity to specific receptor molecules in the plasma membrane and stimulating receptor-mediated activation of intracellular signal transduction pathways. This provides a mechanism by which molecules in the extracellular environment can modulate the key intracellular biochemical regulatory pathways that are active in both normal and malignant cells. Although the initial focus of research on growth factors was on stimulatory ligands and their receptors, it has become clear that there are inhibitory ligands and receptors with equally important regulatory effects on cell proliferation. Table 7–1 lists the main nonhematopoietic growth factors and receptors that are found in normal and malignant human cells. It is taken from one of a number of excellent review articles recommended for more information on this interesting subject.[1-5] The recent volumes edited by Sporn and Roberts provide detailed monographs on each of the growth factors.[6]

AUTOCRINE STIMULATION

Growth factors are found in all tissues of the body. The concept that simultaneous production of a growth factor and expression of its specific receptor by the same cell could result in self-stimulation was based on the landmark description by DeLarco and Todaro of the autostimulatory pathway of EGF receptor activation in cultured tumor cells.[7] These and other obser-

vations were expanded into a hypothesis of autocrine growth regulation by Sporn and Todaro.[8,9] They postulated that autoproduction of growth factors essential for proliferation could provide a mechanism by which a cell could escape from the requirement for those particular growth factors in its environment, resulting in unregulated cell growth (Fig. 7–1). This escape from growth regulation is one of the primary characteristics of malignant cell transformation.

Receptors and their growth factors are frequently coexpressed in primary tumor tissues and human cancer cell lines. Evidence for the existence of autostimulatory growth factor pathways comes from many studies with tumor cell lines cultured in the absence of an exogenous supply of growth factors and studies of comparable cultures grown in the presence of monoclonal antibodies that bind to receptors or growth factors.[10] By blocking the capacity of the growth factor to activate the receptor, these antibodies can prevent receptor activation and thereby inhibit cell proliferation.

Blood levels of most growth factors are low, although platelets are a repository of growth factors such as transforming growth factor-α (TGF-α), platelet-derived growth factor (PDGF), and transforming growth factor-β (TGF-β), which are released after platelet activation at a wound or inflammatory site.[11] In physiologic conditions, the growth factors that act on a particular cell are thought to be produced primarily in the immediate vicinity by the cell itself or by adjacent cells.[12] The latter form of stimulation has been called paracrine, and it has been shown that this type of interaction can

114

TABLE 7–1. Properties of a Selection of Polypeptide Growth Factors

Growth Factors	Description	Known Localization/ Sources	Known Targets	Receptors
PDGF AA, AB, and BB	Dimers of A (17 kd) and B (16 kd) chains. B chain is product of c-*SIS* protooncogene.	Platelets, placenta, preimplantation embryos, endothelial cells	Mesenchymal cells, glial cells, smooth muscle, placental trophoblasts	Two species of glycoprotein. Both tyrosine kinases. Type α (170 kd) binds all PDGF dimers. Type β (180 kd) binds PDGF BB and AB weakly.
EGF and TGF-α	Major forms are 6 kd, with some larger species detected. EGF and TGF-α proteins are 40% identical. Both are released by proteolysis of membrane-bound precursors.	EGF: submaxillary gland, Brunner's gland, mRNA (but not 6 kd protein) in variety of newborn mouse tissues. TGF-α: Preimplantation mouse embryos, later embryos, placenta. Common in transformed cells.	Epithelial, mesenchymal, and glial cells	Protein tyrosine kinase (175 kd). Product of the c-*ERBB* protooncogene. Receptor for EGF, TGF-α, and vaccinia virus growth factor.
TGF-β1, TGF-β2, and TGF-β3	25 kd homodimers. Secreted as latent complexes.	Preimplantation mouse embryos, later embryos. Widespread throughout adult tissues and cultured cells.	Wide variety of cell types	Type 1, 50 kd; type 2, 70 kd; type 3, 280–330 kd. Each type binds TGF-β1, -β2, and -β3. Type 1 and 2 may be main mediators of responses.
IGF1 and IGF2	7 kd. Related to each other and to proinsulin.	IGF1 mainly produced in liver. IGF2 mRNA in variety of cells, including some tumor cells, but protein sometimes undetectable. Both present in plasma, in association with specific binding proteins.	Wide variety of cell types	IGF1 receptor (130 kd + 90 kd)$_2$ protein tyrosine kinase binds IGF1 and -2. IGF2 receptor (250 kd) binds IGF2, identical to mannose-6-phosphate receptor.
FGF1 and FGF2	Acidic and basic FGF, respectively. 16–17 kd. Occasionally larger forms. No consensus signal peptide. 55% identical. Also related to other FGFs and interleukin-1 family.	Low mRNA levels in wide range of normal and transformed cells. Proteins widely distributed, associated with extracellular matrix.	Variety of endothelial, epithelial, mesenchyme, and neuronal cell types	(150 kd) FGF1 and (130 kd) FGF2 receptors both protein tyrosine kinases. High cross-reactivity of FGF1 and -2 binding.
FGF3	27–32 kd alternative translation products of *INT*2 protooncogene.	mRNA in mouse embryonic tissues, brain, testes, mouse mammary tumor, and teratocarcinoma cells.	Unknown	Unknown
FGF4	19 kd glycoprotein product of *HST* (human) or *KS3* (mouse) protooncogenes.	Unknown	Vascular endothelial cells, fibroblasts	Unknown
FGF5	26 kd glycoprotein.	Unknown	Fibroblasts	Unknown

(Cross M, Dexter TM. Growth factors in development, transformation, and tumorigenesis. Cell 1991;64:271–280)

occur between cells of the same or different histologic type.[8] For example, breast cancer cell lines can be stimulated by insulin-like growth factor-2 (IGF2), which is produced by fibroblasts in malignant lesions but not by fibroblasts in normal tissues.[13] PDGF produced by breast cancer cells can activate the fibroblasts, which bear PDGF receptors, but not breast cancer cells, because they do not express PDGF receptors.[14]

Many growth factors are synthesized as portions of larger precursor molecules that contain hydrophobic sequences that anchor them in the plasma membrane.[15] After synthesis and transport in the endoplasmic reticulum and Golgi, these molecules are expressed on the cell surface. The soluble growth factor polypeptide is then released by proteolytic cleavage from the precursor molecule into the extracellular environment, where it can activate receptors on the cell that produced it (autocrine) or on adjacent cells (paracrine) (see Fig. 7–1).

The membrane-bound form of a growth factor, TGF-α, can also activate receptors.[16,17] Using a mutated form of TGF-α,

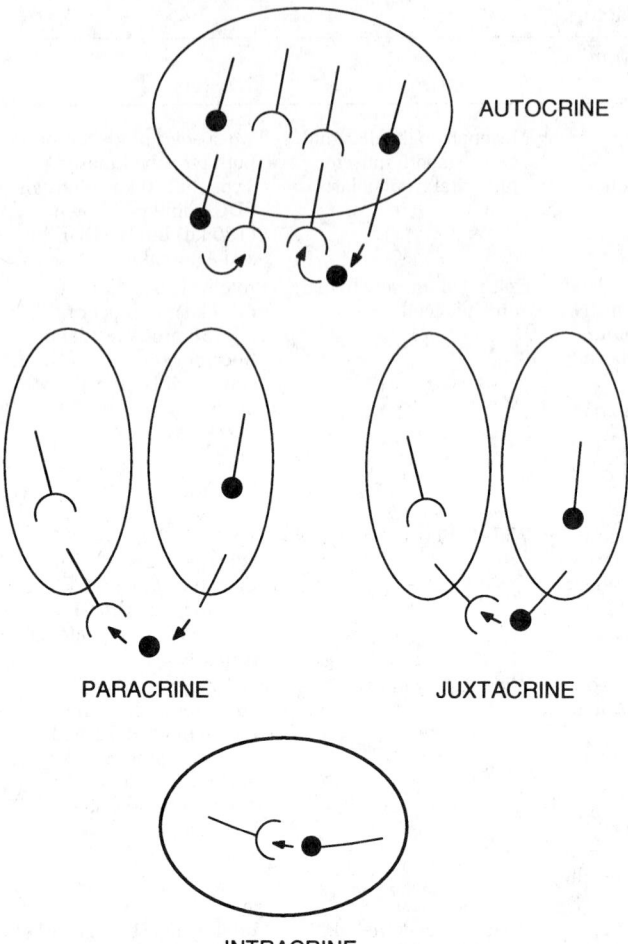

FIGURE 7–1. Interactions between cells producing growth factors and receptors. ●—, precursor for growth factor; ●, soluble growth factor released into extracellular space; ——(, receptor.

which encodes a noncleavable form of the precursor molecule, pro–TGF-α variants can be made to accumulate on the cell surface. These can bind to receptors on adjacent cells and activate tyrosine phosphorylation.[18] It is possible that receptor activation might commonly occur through cell-to-cell contact mediated by membrane-bound factor acting on a receptor on an adjacent cell, a process called juxtacrine stimulation (see Fig. 7–1).[18]

Because the receptor and its growth factor may be produced by the same cell, it is possible that the union of growth factor and receptor could occur intracellularly before expression of either of the molecules on the cell surface (intracrine, see Fig. 7–1). This occurs in a cell line transformed with the v-*SIS* oncogene, but whether this is a generalized physiologic mechanism mediating responses to PDGF is unknown.[19,20] Evidence from other studies suggests that the receptor for PDGF must be expressed on the cell surface to mediate signal transduction through its activated tyrosine kinase.[21] Exploration of the autocrine pathway for epidermal growth factor (EGF) or TGF-α in A431 cells, which express the EGF receptor and TGF-α, suggests that the major pathway of autocrine activation occurs extracellularly, mediated by binding

of growth factor to receptors that are expressed on the cell surface.[22]

Serum is a source of growth factors, many of which are released by platelets during the clotting process. The requirement for serum in synthetic cell culture media is thought to be primarily attributable to its content of growth factors and hormones.[23] Many cells can be cultured in chemically defined medium without serum if they produce the growth factors required for proliferation or if these agents are provided in the culture medium. Characteristically, tumor cells in serum-free cultures have reduced requirements for growth factors, indicating that they produce the factors or have bypassed the need for them.[12] Although the receptor for a particular growth factor is not known to differ from one cell type to another, the group or constellation of receptors expressed does vary between cells from different tissues. Cells from different tissues require tailored "cocktails" of growth factor supplements, typically between three and five, to grow optimally in serum-free cultures. Cells deprived of these essential growth-promoting agents proliferate at reduced rates or are prevented from dividing.[24] The differences in growth factor requirements provide some potential for selectivity and specificity in the application of antireceptor agents to cancer therapy.

GROWTH FACTORS AND THEIR RECEPTORS

More than 40 growth factors have been described. They are remarkably consistent across phyla, suggesting that they control regulatory pathways that are fundamental to the living process. The main group of nonhematopoietic growth factors mediates its effects by means of receptors containing an intrinsic protein tyrosine kinase (Fig. 7–2).[25,26] These receptors are transmembrane glycoproteins that have an extracellular ligand-binding domain and an intracellular tyrosine kinase domain that mediates signal transduction into growth-regulatory pathways. The binding of ligand (growth factor) to monomeric receptors activates formation of homodimers or oligomers (Fig. 7–3).[27] This stimulates the tyrosine kinase domains to carry out transphosphorylation on selected tyrosine residues of their paired partner. The dimeric receptor, with phosphorylated tyrosine residues, is now ready to bind with high affinity to the substrates for its activated intrinsic tyrosine kinase.

The primary amino acid sequences of the extracellular domains of growth factor receptors are known in many cases. The spacing of cysteine residues in these domains allows predictions of tertiary structure into one of two major categories: immunoglobulin-like domains, in which a series of looped structures is created by the formation of disulfide bonds between cysteines, and cysteine-rich domains, in which complex tertiary folding results from the formation of disulfide bonds, creating pockets to which ligands can bind with high affinity (see Fig. 7–2).[25] There is intensive effort to resolve the molecular details of growth factor binding sites, because this would allow the design of specific pharmacologic agonists and antagonists.

When growth factors bind to and activate their specific receptors, the event causes activation of a cascade of biochemical reactions collectively referred to as signal transduction path-

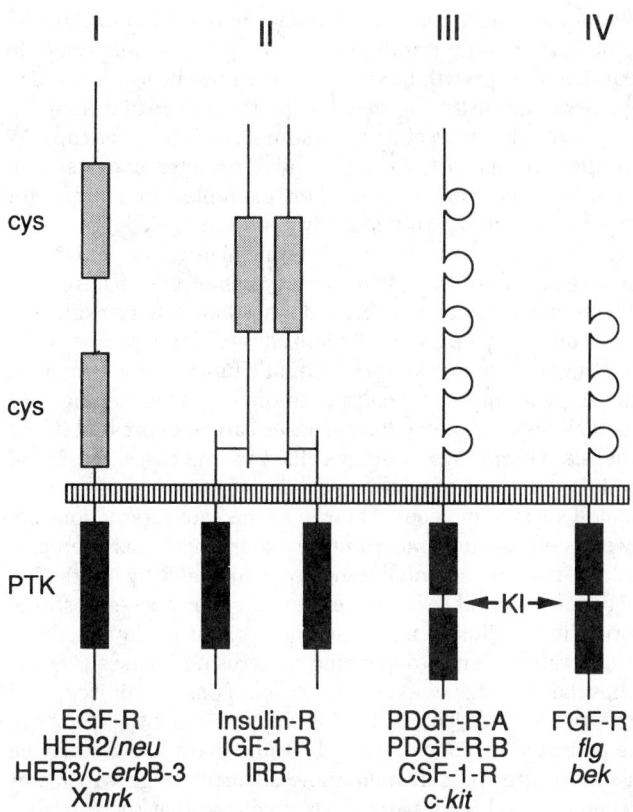

FIGURE 7–2. Growth factor receptor subclasses. Cys, cysteine rich region; PTK, protein tyrosine kinase; KI, kinase insert region. (Ullrich A, Schlessinger J. Signal transduction by receptors with tyrosine kinase activity. Cell 1990;61:203–212)

of forms of PI phosphorylated in the 3, 4, and 5 positions, confirming that PI3K is regulated by tyrosine kinases in vivo.[37]

GAP interacts with the p21 protein product of the *RAS* oncogene, which is activated in many types of cancer. RAS belongs to the family of G proteins that bind GTP (guanosine triphosphate) and have intrinsic GTPase activity. GAP regulates the capacity of RAS to hydrolyse GTP to GDP.[38] Intracellular injection of RAS-neutralizing antibodies can block the mitogenic effects of PDGF and transiently revert the malignant phenotype of cells transformed with the *SRC* oncogene.[39] This confirms the connection between activation of a receptor tyrosine kinase and RAS.

The serine-threonine kinase, RAF, also complexes with the PDGF receptor after stimulation by PDGF, but this may be through mechanisms different from the other substrates.[33] Other molecules that bind to activated receptor kinases have yet to be characterized.

The signal transduction pathway initially involves molecules that bind to cell surface membrane proteins, but it progresses to stimulate molecules with the capacity to regulate cell function. Within an hour of receptor activation, there is expression

ways.[2,25] These pathways initiate cell cycle traversal and differentiation. After binding of EGF or PDGF, several proteins become physically associated with and are phosphorylated by the activated receptors. These candidate substrates for the activated intrinsic tyrosine kinase activity of receptors for growth factors include phospholipase C-γ (PLCγ), phosphotidylinositol 3′-kinase (PI3K), RAS guanosine triphosphatase activating protein (GAP), and the RAF protein product of the cellular oncogene c-*RAF*, which is a serine-threonine kinase.[28–33]

One of the best characterized substrates is PLCγ, which hydrolyses phosphotidylinositol 4,5-bisphosphate to produce two second messengers: inositol trisphosphate, which acts to release calcium from intracellular storage compartments into the cytosol, and diacylglycerol, which is a specific activator of the versatile serine-threonine kinase, protein kinase C (PKC).[34,35] The latter can stimulate uptake of calcium from the extracellular environment. A rise in cytoplasmic calcium concentrations is a rapid event after activation of receptor tyrosine kinases, occurring within less than a minute. Within minutes after receptor activation, there is phosphorylation of multiple substrates on serine and threonine residues by PKC, S6 kinase, or other related kinases.

PI3K phosphorylates the inositol ring of phosphotidylinositol in the D3 position in response to activation by a variety of tyrosine kinases.[36] PDGF stimulation induces accumulation

Subclass I

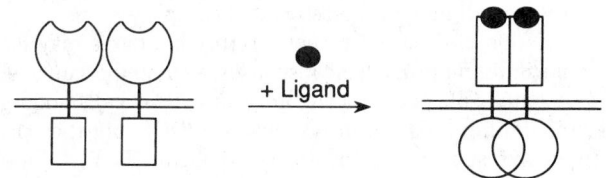

Subclass II

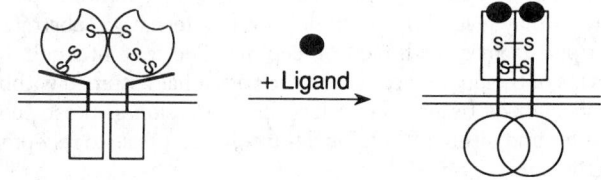

Subclass III

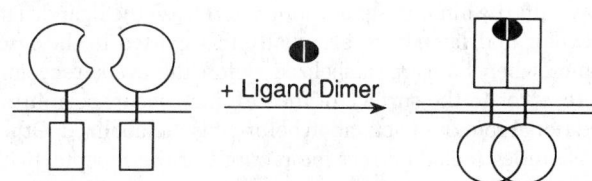

FIGURE 7–3. Models of receptor subclass-specific variations of the mechanism of activation by dimerization. Receptor activation may occur by binding of monomeric ligands resulting in a conformational change of the extracellular domain and dimer formation (subclass I), by interaction of the ligand with a disulfide-stabilized receptor dimer and subsequent intracomplex conformational change (subclass II), or by mediation of dimer formation through a dimeric ligand (subclass III). (Ullrich A, Schlessinger J. Signal transduction by receptors with tyrosine kinase activity. Cell 1990;61:203–212)

of genes whose products have the capacity to regulate transcription of RNA. These include *FOS*, the mRNA for which typically rises within 15 minutes and declines within an hour, and *MYC*, which follows expression of *FOS* and remains elevated for a longer period of time.[40]

Although the substrates for activated receptor kinases differ widely in their enzymatic activities, each (with the exception of RAF) shares a conserved domain containing SH2 (SRC *homology*) domains that bind with high affinity to tyrosine-phosphorylated proteins.[37] SH2 domains apparently regulate protein-protein interactions by recognizing peptide sequences that contain phosphotyrosine. The adjacent amino acids may be important in providing specificity by restricting binding to phosphotyrosines on certain protein molecules. The diversity of cellular responses to growth factors could be regulated by the affinities with which different SH2 domains on substrates interact with receptors. One result of EGF receptor or PDGF receptor autophosphorylation on tyrosine residues is high-affinity binding to substrates such as PLCγ, PI3K, and GAP.[37]

These substrates for the EGF receptor also share SH3 domains, which are analagous to a region in SRC and may mediate binding to cellular membranes or to cytoskeletal proteins.[37] Taken together, the SH2 and SH3 domains may serve as chemical links that bind enzymes and substrates together in the growth factor-mediated signal transduction pathway and create cell membrane-associated complexes.

Activation of different receptor tyrosine kinases may lead to quite different physiologic responses, even in the same cell. For example, oligodendrocyte progenitor OA-2 cells undergo terminal differentiation in response to PDGF, but they proliferate in response to fibroblast growth factor (FGF).[41,42] P12 neuronal cells differentiate in response to NGF, but they proliferate after stimulation with EGF.[2] The same growth factor, TGF-β, may inhibit proliferation of a particular fibroblast cell line in the presence of EGF but stimulate proliferation in the presence of PDGF.[43] These data suggest that future experiments may lead to the identification of alternative substrates for particular growth factor receptors. The state of a cell, in terms of the phenotypic characteristics it has assumed within a specialized tissue, may select for expression of these substrates and ultimately channel the cell's response to receptor activation.

The binding of a growth factor to its receptor does not permanently activate a signal transduction pathway. The receptor and its bound ligand are efficiently internalized, typically within less than an hour.[44] In the endosomes, the reduced pH may shift the binding equilibrium and release the ligand. The receptor and ligand are eventually transported to the lysosomes, where both are catabolized. Before this event, recycling of receptor to the surface of the cell may occur, permitting additional rounds of activation before it is metabolized. Other possibilities include direct interactions of the receptor with nuclear components.

Although activation of particular substrates occurs within minutes after binding of growth factors to receptors, the stimulation of receptor tyrosine kinase activity must be maintained for 5 to 6 hours to activate movement into the active phases of the cell cycle that lead to cell division.[45,46] The half-life of a receptor after exposure to growth factor is typically in the range of 4 hours. To maintain an active receptor-mediated

signal for longer than a few hours, new receptors must be synthesized and put into place in the plasma membrane. In parallel, new growth factor molecules must be synthesized to make contact with the new receptors and activate them. In response to a variety of external stimuli, cells have the capacity to alter the quantity of a particular receptor expressed on their surface membranes. For example, EGF receptor expression can be stimulated by exposure to EGF.[47]

An important mechanism for modulating the activity of growth factor receptors involves tyrosine phosphatases.[48,49] These enzymes can efficiently dephosphorylate tyrosine residues on the cytoplasmic portions of receptors, thereby deactivating the tyrosine kinase enzymatic function and removing the high-affinity phosphotyrosine binding sites for the SH2 regions on substrates. Phosphatases can be expressed in the surface membranes of many cells. In some cases, the extracellular portions of tyrosine kinases are structurally similar to cell surface molecules known to mediate interactions between cells during embryonic development. It has been postulated that contact inhibition may be mediated by interaction between external segments of tyrosine phosphatases, stimulating intracellular enzymatic activity that could deactivate proliferation signals depending on tyrosine kinases.[50] Some phosphatases have extracellular domains reminiscent of growth factor receptors, raising the possibility that they can be activated by polypeptides. Tyrosine phosphatases may be inserted into the cell membrane adjacent to growth factor receptors, and Schlessinger has predicted that there is a tyrosine phosphatase for every tyrosine kinase.[48] The contribution of tyrosine phosphatases to the regulation of receptor function is not yet determined.

Activation of signal transduction pathways can also be accomplished by binding of growth factors to receptors with biochemical characteristics entirely different from tyrosine kinases. Bombesin activates a receptor that belongs to the class of neurotransmitters.[2] These receptors are anchored into the plasma membrane by seven helical transmembrane domains and lack an intrinsic tyrosine kinase. The *MAS* oncogene encodes an oncoprotein with seven membrane-spanning regions that is a receptor for angiotensin.[51] Activation of this super family of receptors by specific ligands such as bombesin, angiotensin, adrenergic agents, or serotonin activates guanine nucleotide binding proteins (G proteins), which interact with adenylate cyclase, PLC, and other biochemical mediators of signal transduction.[52]

A third mechanism for signal transduction by receptors is characteristic of many of the hematopoietic growth factors and the interleukins.[2] The receptors for these growth factors and cytokines contain specific extracellular binding sites but have no known internal biochemical activity. However, the intracellular portions of these receptors are able to couple with and activate members of the SRC family of intracytoplasmic tyrosine kinases, creating the capacity to use signalling pathways similar to the growth factor receptors of epithelial and connective tissue cells. The *SRC* family of intracytoplasmic tyrosine kinases includes seven closely related genes (i.e., v-*SRC*, v-*YES*, v-*FGR*, *HCK*, *LYN*, *FYN*, *LCK*) and two more distantly related genes (i.e., v-*ALT*, v-*FPS*/v-*FES*).[3] Five of these were discovered as mammalian and avian transforming retroviruses. *HCK*, *LYN*, *FYN*, and *LCK* were identified on the basis of similarities to known tyrosine kinases at the nucleic acid level or the protein level, and their roles in signal transduction may be related to their capacity to bind to transmembrane receptors.

Recent evidence indicates the existence of yet another class of growth factor receptors. These are the receptors for members of the TGF-β/activin family.[53] The receptors are transmembrane molecules with intracellular portions that are serine-threonine kinases.[54-56] These findings provide new insight into the nature of the negative growth regulating signals that counterbalance the growth prompting effects of tyrosine kinase activators.

GROWTH FACTORS AND MALIGNANCY

Many converging lines of evidence strongly suggest that growth factors play a central role in malignancy.

The original observation of autostimulation of proliferation in cells expressing a growth factor and its receptor has been followed by studies showing that many primary human tumors and human tumor cell lines express high levels of growth factor receptors and are capable of producing the relevant growth factors, establishing conditions conducive to autocrine or paracrine stimulation.

In the early 1980s, several laboratories established that protein tyrosine kinase activity was a property of the EGF receptor and the oncogenic pp60[src] protein and that the two molecules were antigenically related.[57-59] In 1983 and 1984, the discovery was made that three viral oncogenes shared extensive amino acid sequence homology with growth factors and receptors: v-SIS with the B chain of PDGF, v-ERBB with the EGF receptor, and v-FMS with the receptor for macrophage colony stimulating factor.[60-65] It had been shown previously that viral oncogenes were derived from cellular genes (*i.e.*, protooncogenes), and the new information pinpointed

growth factor and receptor pathways as sources in the cellular genome for the virally transmitted oncogenic activity. Because expression of viral oncogenes is alone sufficient to induce malignant transformation of some cells, the conclusion was drawn that unregulated growth factor activity could mediate malignant transformation.

Many oncogenes are analogs of cellular protooncogenes that code for growth factors, their receptors, soluble tyrosine protein kinases, or biochemical pathways mediated by tyrosine kinase activation.[1-5] A partial list of oncogenes that are related to protooncogenes for growth factors and receptors is presented in Table 7-2.

The mechanisms by which these oncogenes mediate malignant transformation vary. The v-SIS oncogene encodes a polypeptide that shares 90% homology with its protooncogene (B chain of PDGF).[13,60,61] The product of v-SIS can form a homodimer that activates PDGF receptors, and the unregulated activation of proliferation mediated by this receptor can produce malignant behavior in cells that are suspectable (presumably due to biochemical changes or to their particular stage of differentiation). The oncogene v-ERBB is a defective version of its protooncogene, which encodes the EGF receptor, and two modifications in its structure have been characterized that explain its malignant potential.[62-64] The oncogene encodes a receptor that lacks the extracellular domain that is the binding site for EGF, and it also lacks the carboxyl terminal residues, which are presumed to have a regulatory function. Another example is provided by the *NEU* oncogene, originally isolated from a carcinogen-induced neuroblastoma in rats. In this case, conversion of the protooncogene to an oncogene involves a single nucleotide change, altering one amino acid in the transmembrane region.[66] However, the search for mutated receptors and growth factors in primary human tumor specimens has revealed only a few examples.

Experiments using recombinant molecular technology have demonstrated that constitutive overexpression of cellular on-

TABLE 7-2. Oncogenes Related To Protooncogenes That Encode Growth Factors or Receptors

Oncogene	Protooncogene	Origin
v-SIS	PDGF (B chain)	Simian retrovirus
v-ERBB	EGF receptor*	Avian retrovirus
NEU/HER2L	Receptor*	Rat neuroblastoma
v-ERBB2	Receptor*	
v-FMS	CSF1 receptor	Feline retrovirus
v-ROS	Insulin receptor, β chain	Avian retrovirus
MET	Hepatocyte growth factor receptor*	Human osteosarcoma
K-FGF/HST	FGF4*	Human stomach cancer, Kaposi sarcoma
INT2	Related to FGF3	Murine mammary tumors
TRK family	NGF receptor family*	Human colon carcinoma
v-KIT	KIT ligand receptor	Feline retrovirus
v-SEA	Related to insulin receptor	Avian erythroblastosis, sarcoma virus
v-ERBA	T3 receptor	Avian retrovirus

* Indicates evidence for involvement in human cancer.
(Adapted from Leutz A, Graf T. Relationships between oncogenes and growth control. In: Sporn MB, Roberts AB, eds. Peptide growth factors and their receptors, vol II. Berlin: Springer-Verlag, 1990: 655-703)

cogenes encoding growth factors or their receptors can cause nonmalignant cells to display a malignant phenotype. Typically, this is measured by anchorage independent growth in soft agar culture and by the capacity to form successful xenografts in nude mice. For example, malignant properties can be conferred merely by overexpression of protooncogene *HER2*, *TGF-β*, or *PDGF*. Unregulated expression *TGF-α* can result in mammary carcinogenesis in transgenic mice, indicating that this protooncogene can be oncogenic without modification but only in certain tissues.[67-69] In these animals, the only other malignant tumor observed was hepatocellular carcinoma.

In several reports, expression of high levels of growth factor receptors in primary human tumor specimens was correlated with a poor clinical prognosis for these patients. Increased expression of *NEU*/*HER2*/c-*ERBB2* is associated with a worse prognosis in adenocarcinoma of the breast and ovary.[70-74] High EGF receptor levels are prognostically adverse in adenocarcinoma of the breast, transitional bladder cancer, and squamous lung carcinoma.[75-79]

From this accumulation of observations, it is reasonable to postulate that expression of high levels of growth factor receptors or the relevant growth factors form autocrine or paracrine activation pathways that give a selective advantage to malignant human cells. This could result in enhancement of tumor cell growth rate. These tumor cells would be better able to withstand an environment in which exogenous essential growth factors are scarce. The capacity to subvert growth regulation by bypassing the requirement that certain essential growth factors be provided in the extracellular environment may in itself be sufficient for oncogenesis. In other situations, enhanced activation of growth factor and receptor pathways can play an important supporting role in a series of oncogenic events that may include other regulatory pathways in human cells.

SPECIFIC GROWTH FACTORS

TGFA/EGF FAMILY

EGF was first described by Stanley Cohen, who purified it using accelerated eyelid opening and tooth eruption in newborn mice as an assay.[80] EGF stimulates proliferation of cultured cells and activates a specific high-affinity membrane receptor with protein tyrosine kinase activity, which mediates its proliferative effects on cells.[44,45,81]

The EGF receptor is activated by a family of growth factors. For mammalian cells, in addition to EGF, these include TGF-α, amphiregulin, and a newly described heparin-binding EGF.[15,45,82,83] The precursors of these molecules are transmembrane glycoproteins. The extracellular domain of the TGF-α precursor contains a 50-amino acid portion that is cleaved from the precursor molecule by the activity of elastase-like proteolytic enzymes to form mature, soluble TGF-α.[15] The precursor for amphiregulin contains a similar polypeptide in a region of the extracellular portion, and the precursor for EGF itself contains eight redundant EGF-like structural units in addition to the portion that includes the latent EGF molecule. The spacing of six cysteine residues within the soluble EGF family of growth factors is rigidly conserved, and these

dictate the tertiary structure of the molecule through disulfide bonding. The intracytoplasmic portion of these molecules is not known to have a function. TGF-α and EGF have only 35% homology, but they bind with indistinguishable affinity to the EGF receptors in most tissues that have been examined.[15,44] Each activates receptor downregulation, although release of TGF-α from the receptor is more rapid in the mildly acidic endosomes, which may allow more efficient recycling of the receptor than when it is bound to EGF. TGF-α is more potent than EGF in activating angiogenesis.[84]

TGF-α is produced by many tumor cell lines and by cells transformed by retroviruses and oncogenes. It was first discovered when conditioned medium from cultures of transformed cells was found to stimulate growth of fibroblasts in soft agar.[7] It was found that this particular stimulatory property required concurrent exposure to a pair of ligands, TGF-α and TGF-β, both of which were present in the conditioned medium.[85]

Introduction of TGF-α cDNA into cells is transforming, but weaker than some other cellular protooncogenes in that these cells have less capacity to form xenografts in athymic mice.[86] Expression of vectors with EGF receptors can transform cells, but this usually depends on addition of exogenous ligand.[87-89] Expression of TGF-α in transgenic mice produces breast and liver malignancies and generates epithelial and pancreatic hyperplasia.[67-69] Many normal adult and embryonic tissues express the messenger RNA for TGF-α and the growth factor protein.[81]

Although TGF-α and EGF act primarily by stimulating cell proliferation, they also can have inhibitory effects. For example, they can inhibit the growth of hair follicle cells.[90] This property has been used to cause de-epilation of wool from sheep. These two growth factors in high concentrations also inhibit the growth of cultured tumor cell lines that express extraordinarily high levels of EGF receptors. Activation of EGF receptors by amphiregulin can stimulate proliferation in some types of cells and inhibit others.[82] The mechanisms that determine these two opposed pathways are not yet determined.

The receptor for EGF and TGF-α is a transmembrane 170-kd glycoprotein.[44,45,81] The external portion is the binding site for ligands. This is connected by a transmembrane hydrophobic region to the intracellular portion of the molecule, which contains a tyrosine kinase with binding sites for ATP and substrate and a C-terminal tail with three tyrosine residues that are substrates for the intrinsic kinase. Binding of ligand causes dimerization (or oligomerization) with activation of tyrosine kinase activity that mediates transphosphorylation of both of the receptors.[25] Substrates for the receptor were described earlier.

Many types of epithelial malignancies display increased EGF receptors on their cell-surface membranes. Examples include cancer of the lung, glioblastoma, breast cancer, head and neck cancer, and cancer of the bladder.[75-77,91-95] Gene amplification is not a commonly reported finding in these tumors, with the exception of the glioblastomas.[94] Only in the case of high-grade glioblastomas have mutant EGF receptors been described.[96] Increased receptor expression is often associated with increased production of TGF-α by the same tumor cells.[97] This establishes conditions conducive to receptor activation by an autocrine stimulatory pathway.

The role of the EGF receptor in breast cancer has been under study for more than a decade. After a report that EGF stimulated the proliferation of MCF-7 cells in chemically defined medium, it was discovered that each of 13 breast cancer cell lines that grow attached to the surface of culture dishes express high-affinity EGF receptors in varying amounts and that some of these lines are stimulated by addition of EGF to serum-free medium.[98,99] The same investigators found that EGF binding to specimens of primary human breast tumors was independent of estrogen binding, and 20% of tumors were positive for EGF receptors and negative for estrogen receptor.[100] Subsequent reports found a significant inverse correlation between the expression of EGF receptors and estrogen receptors in primary breast tumors and more frequent expression of EGF receptors on metastases than on primary tumors.[101-104] Breast cancer cell lines that exhibit high levels of EGF receptor expression were found to have low estrogen receptors.[105] Except for one cell line, MDA 468, the gene for the EGF receptor is not amplified, and increased transcription may explain the high levels of receptors observed in some mammary cell lines.[105]

Messenger RNA for TGF-α was expressed in more than half of primary breast adenocarcinoma specimens examined, and immunoreactive and biologically active TGF-α was significantly higher in malignant effusions from breast cancer patients than in effusions from noncancer patients.[106,107] As with the receptor, the expression of the TGF-α ligand is higher in lymph node metastases than in primary malignant breast tissue. Studies with breast cell lines also have demonstrated TGF-α production.[108] The level of TGF-α may be regulated by estrogen, which can induce increased TGF-α production in several breast cancer lines.[106,109]

TGF-α and EGF have a role in normal breast growth and development. They stimulate the lobular-alveolar development of the mouse mammary gland in explant cultures and in vivo.[110] Normal breast tissues express EGF receptors and nonmalignant human mammary cell lines express the EGF receptor and express and secrete TGF-α.[99,103,111] Furthermore, TGF-α is a growth-promoting factor for nontransformed breast cell lines in serum-free culture.[111]

Clinical studies of primary breast cancer specimens have revealed important correlations between the levels of EGF receptors and the prognosis and response to therapy. Relapse-free survival and total survival are significantly shorter for EGF receptor-positive than EGF receptor-negative tumors.[75,76] There also is evidence for lack of response to endocrine therapy in patients with EGF receptor-positive tumors.[112] The absence of EGF receptors is as good as the presence of estrogen receptors for predicting an objective response to estrogen therapy. It is clear that EGF receptors play a regulatory role in a significant subpopulation (approximately half) of breast cancer patients.

Additional data in support of this conclusion are derived from using anti-EGF receptor monoclonal antibodies (MoAbs) as reagents to explore for the presence of autocrine stimulating pathways in cultured human cells. Studies have been performed with nonmalignant and malignant breast cell lines using anti-EGF receptor MoAbs that block activation of signal transduction mediated by the receptor. The data from these experiments are best presented by considering three types of response to MoAb 225 or other anti-EGF receptor monoclonal antibodies. Some cell lines, which can proliferate without exogenous TGF-α and are strongly inhibited by MoAb 225, presumably have an active and obligatory autocrine pathway. Other cell lines proliferate in response to exogenous TGF-α, and this is inhibited by MoAb 225. Some cells that express EGF receptors do not respond to TGF-α and ignore the presence of MoAb 225, suggesting they do not require receptor activation for growth.[106,113,114] Treatment of cultures with an MoAb against TGF-α can also inhibit growth of EGF/TGF-α dependent mammary epithelial cells.[115]

EGF receptors are expressed on normal bowel epithelium. Anti-EGF receptor MoAbs can inhibit the proliferation of a cultured nonmalignant colon cell line derived from an adenomatous polyp.[116] Several colon carcinoma lines coexpress EGF receptors and TGF-α. As with the breast cell line, anti-receptor MoAb has the capacity to block proliferation of some of these colon carcinoma cell lines.[117]

Examination of primary specimens of human lung cancer tissue using immunohistochemical techniques have demonstrated that high levels of EGF receptors are displayed on most squamous carcinomas, most adenocarcinomas, and none of the small cell lung cancers.[91-93] There was a high expression of TGF-α in almost all squamous cancers and adenocarcinomas of the lung.[118] As with breast cancer, high levels of EGF receptor expression in lung cancer tissue are associated with a poor survival.[78,79] High expression of TGF-α correlated with reduced 5-year survival. The proliferation of cultured lung cancer cell lines of the squamous carcinoma and adenocarcinoma types can be inhibited by additional of anti-EGF receptor monoclonal antibody.[119,120] In parallel, antibody against TGF-α inhibit proliferation of adenocarcinoma cell lines known to produce TGF-α and express EGF receptors.[121]

Could interruptions in the activation of EGF receptors lead to clinically useful antitumor effects? Until receptor structure is solved and small peptides can be designed to block ligand binding sites, monoclonal antibodies selected for their capacity to block binding provide the best model system for exploring antireceptor therapy. Receptor blockade with antibody could take advantage of the large number of tumors in which the EGF receptor level is markedly elevated, making it a relatively tumor-specific antigen. In addition, malignant cells may have a greater propensity than normal cells to respond to deprivation of an essential growth promoting factor by continuing imbalanced growth leading to cell death, rather than arresting in G_1 phase of the cell cycle.[122-124]

A number of laboratories have produced anti-EGF receptor MoAbs that block EGF/TGF-α binding and prevent activation of tyrosine kinase. These include MoAbs 225, 528, 425, and 108.[125-129] Preclinical studies exploring the antiproliferative effects of anti-EGF receptor MoAbs in cell culture have been mentioned. Studies of nude mouse xenografts of breast, bowel, and lung cancer cell lines expressing high levels of EGF receptors also have demonstrated the antitumor effects of anti-EGF receptor MoAbs in vivo when administered for a 3-week period.[120,130,131] The cell lines studied were dependent on TGF-α for optimal growth in culture, and it is likely that they require TGF-α for optimal growth in vivo. The results of these series of studies involving the three most common human malignancies, and others, provide convincing evidence that the EGF receptor blockade is worthy of clinical trials.

Pilot clinical trials with anti-EGF receptor MoAb therapy

have explored targeted radiotherapy, using labeled antibody 425 and antibody R1, which does not block EGF binding.[132,133] A recent phase I dose escalation trial was carried out with a single dose of MoAb 225 in patients with advanced squamous lung carcinoma, which invariably express high levels of EGF receptors. The antibody was labeled with indium 111 for visualization by nuclear scanning. There were two important conclusions: doses of 120 mg produced concentrations of antibody in the blood that were saturating for EGF receptors for more than 3 days without any toxicity, and primary lung tumors and metastases greater than or equal to 1 cm in diameter were visualized with doses of 40 mg or more.[134] Studies with repeated injections of 225 MoAb in a chimerized or humanized form are the next step in testing EGF receptor blockade therapy.

C-ERBB2

The nomenclature for this growth factor receptor is currently unsettled. The term "NEU" derives from its original description in a series of ethylnitrosourea induced rat neuroblastomas.[135] HER2 reflects its homology to the human epidermal growth factor receptor.[136] ERBB2 reflects its homology to the product of *ERBB*, the acutely transforming avian erythroblastosis viral gene, which is a truncated form of the human epidermal growth factor receptor. We shall refer to it as ERBB2.

The c-*ERBB2* gene is located on chromosome 17 at q21 and specifies a transmembrane receptor-like phosphoglycoprotein that is closely related in structure but is still biologically distinct from the epidermal growth factor receptor, c-ERBB.[137–141] This gene was first discovered as a transforming oncogene in a series of ethylnitrosourea-induced rat neuroblastomas, in which it was called *NEU*.[135] The transforming potential of the human *ERBB2* gene is fully achieved by single point mutation in transgenic mice or by overexpression in NIH-3T3 cells.[136,142–144] ERBB2 is amplified in many adenocarcinomas and is overexpressed in almost 30% of human breast cancer patients.[73,145,146] That the overexpression rather than genetic aberration of the gene may be transforming, coupled with the fact that this gene has been found to be overexpressed in breast carcinomas, supported the view that increased expression of this gene could have significance for the pathogenesis of breast disease.[104] In addition, p185^{erbB2} is necessary for the maintenance of the malignant phenotype of cells transformed by *ERBB2*.[71,146] Amplification or overexpression of the *ERBB2* protooncogene correlates with poor prognosis in breast, ovarian, and non-small cell lung carcinomas.[70,71,73,145,146] In addition to these clinical studies, in vitro studies strongly suggest that overexpression of p185^{erbB2} may have an important role in malignant progression.[147–149] Moreover, p185^{erbB2} overexpression has been associated with tumor cell resistance to several cytotoxic mechanisms, including the actions of platinum, tumor necrosis factor on breast cancer cells, and the action of natural killer cells or tamoxifen on breast cancer cells.[136,150–153]

Data from transfection studies and transgenic mice suggest a role for *ERBB2* in the pathogenesis of breast cancer, which agrees with prognostic studies.[142,143] Immunostaining of primary tumors revealed that if a tumor is positive, it usually shows a very homogenous staining of all tumor cells, including the preinvasive and metastatic components. Several groups reported a higher incidence of *ERBB2* overexpression in ductal carcinoma in situ than in infiltrating ductal carcinoma.[154] *ERBB2* is usually observed in all stages of breast cancer in metastatic sites and the primary tumor.[73] This suggests that overexpression may be an early event in progression. Overexpression alone cannot account for an increased invasive potential, because a very high proportion of comedo-type intraductal carcinomas overexpress the protein.[73] These findings indicate that *ERBB2* overexpression in itself is not a sufficient condition for invasiveness and point to the importance of determining what are the necessary cofactors in the acquisition of this phenotype by some *ERBB2*-overexpressing cells.

Colony formation of NIH-3T3 cells transformed by *ERBB2* overexpression could be inhibited by an anti-ERBB2 antibody.[155] An anti-p185NEU monoclonal antibody generated against mutated rat NEU protein inhibited growth of NIH-3T3/NEU cells in soft agar and in nude mice.[156] Treatment of SK-Br-3 cells with 4D5 (anti-ERBB2) inhibited their colony formation in soft agar and reduced the activity of receptor tyrosine kinase.[155,157–159]

In addition to its prognostic significance in breast cancer, *ERBB2* is overexpressed in a variable proportion of tumors of ovary, stomach, and adenocarcinoma of the lung. In each of these cases, preliminary data suggested that overexpression or gene amplification is associated with a decreased disease-free and overall survival.

It is not yet clear how the ERBB2 protein alters cell growth in normal or cancer cells. There is a close sequence similarity between ERBB2 and EGF receptor.[137,139] This similarity strongly suggests analogous functions: the extracellular domain of the ERBB2 protein binds extracellular ligands and transduces a signal to the cell by tyrosine kinase activity of its intracellular domain. A four-domain model for the organization of the EGF receptor has been proposed where subdomain III contributes most of the determinants involved in ligand binding and signal transduction, and a similar structure has been proposed for the ERBB2 protein.[139,160] Interference of ERBB2 association with its ligand could provide a significant tool for therapeutic applications and differentiate biologic pathways.

To understand the function of p185^{erbB2} and to evaluate its potential as a therapeutic target for neoplasia, it is necessary to identify specific p185^{erbB2} ligands. The identification and purification of a 30-kd (gp30) growth factor secreted by MDA-MB-231 human breast cancer cell has been described.[157,161] A monoclonal antibody against the extracellular domain of p185^{erbB2} (4D5) was able to compete with gp30 for binding to p185^{erbB2}.[157] In addition, a polypeptide with an apparent molecular weight of 75 kd (p75) has been identified.[158] Purified gp30 stimulated phosphorylation of p185^{erbB2} in cells that overexpress ERBB2, gp30 also binds to EGF receptor, but p75 interacts exclusively with p185^{erbB2} and shows no binding or activation of EGF receptor.[157,158,161] Gp30 and p75 have biphasic growth effects. Low concentrations induced cell proliferation in ERBB2-overexpressing cells, but relatively high concentrations inhibited growth in cells that overexpressed ERBB2.[157,158] Gp30 and p75 are able to induce phosphorylation of p185^{erbB2} in a dose-dependent manner. These two polypeptides are candidate ligands for the ERBB2 oncogene product and may play a role in eventual therapeutic strategies.

PLATELET-DERIVED GROWTH FACTOR

Platelet-derived growth factor was first described as a constituent of α granules in platelets that had the capacity to stimulate proliferation of smooth muscle cells and fibroblasts.[4,13,162] The active growth factor is a 30-kilodalton homodimer or heterodimer formed by A and B chains, which have 60% homology and show strict conservation of eight cysteine residues.[163] These molecules are synthesized as higher-molecular-weight precursors and are subjected to proteolytic processing. All three combinations occur: AA, AB, and BB.

There are two 170- to 180-kd receptors for PDGF that have similar structures.[164] The extracellular portions contain five immunoglobulin-like domains, created by the formation of sulfhydryl bonds, and these have 30% similarity in their amino acid sequences. The intracellular portions each contain tyrosine kinase domains into which are inserted an interrupting sequence of approximately 100 amino acids. Similar inserts are found in the tyrosine kinase portion of the CSF1 receptor and the c-*KIT* product, and they are felt to be the sites for binding of the SH2 domains on substrates for these receptors.[37,165] Mutations in the kinase insert can block the mitogenic signal by altering binding of substrates. Because the PDGF ligand is a covalently bound dimer (unlike EGF/TGF-α), there is no difficulty explaining the observation that the bivalent growth factor binds to dimeric PDGF receptors (see Fig. 7–3).[25] The α receptor can bind A and B forms of PDGF, but the β receptor chain prefers the B isoform. On binding of ligand to the extracellular portions of the two receptor chains, a receptor homodimer or heterodimer is formed, and autophosphorylation of receptor tyrosine residues is stimulated.

The substrates that are involved in signal transduction by the activated receptor include PLCγ, phosphotidylinositol 3′-kinase, GAP and RAF1. Each of these molecules can be coprecipitated with the PDGF receptor. The stimulation of PDGF receptors results in induction of a larger number of genes within a few hours. These include transcription factors such as c-*FOS*, c-*JUN*, c-*MYC*, and c-*MYB* and a variety of other proteins that may be only indirectly involved with cell proliferation.[166,167]

Receptors for PDGF are prominent on mesenchymal cells, including fibroblasts and smooth muscle cells.[11] The release of PDGF from platelets during the conversion of plasma to serum suggests a role for this growth factor in the connective tissue proliferation associated with inflammation and tissue repair. PDGF has also been implicated in the proliferation of periendothelial smooth muscle cells, which is a prominent feature of the pathology of atherogenesis.[168]

The observation that the v-*SIS* oncogene product shares close homology with the B chain of PDGF stimulated gene transfer experiments which demonstrated that constitutive expression of the B chain or A chain of PDGF protooncogene can cause cell transformation, although the A chain is less efficient.[60,61,169–171] PDGF is produced by some tumor cell lines that lack receptors for the growth factor (*e.g.,* mammary carcinoma cell lines).[172] In the case of breast cancer, it has been suggested that the tumor cells may stimulate adjacent non-malignant fibroblast, resulting in the fibrosis that is commonly an accompanying feature of breast malignancy.[13]

PDGF alone cannot stimulate cell division in cultured BALB/c 3T3 cells, but it can do so only if an additional growth factor such as EGF or IGF1 is added. A model was developed to explain this sequence by postulating that PDGF confers "competence" for cell cycle traversal, and the other growth factors produce "progression" through the cell cycle.[173,174] This division of functions has not been documented in all cells, but it provides a very useful way to dissect the interactions of multiple growth factors in the stimulation of cell growth. Studies of cell cycle progression in serum deprived cultures suggest that competence factors act early in G_0/G_1 phase, and progression factors act later in G_1 phase.

INSULIN-LIKE GROWTH FACTORS

The insulin-like growth factors, IGF-I and IGF-II, are part of a family of ligands, receptors, and binding proteins that have a significant role in normal development and growth. As their names imply, IGF-I and IGF-II show considerable homology to insulin, or more directly, pro-insulin.[175–177] The primary structures of IGF-I and IGF-II were first described in the late 1970s by Rinderknecht and Humbel.[178,179] Numerous studies have shown that IGF-I and IGF-II can be potent mitogens for a wide variety of human cell lines, including lines derived from malignant tumors. It was this potent growth-promoting activity in cell culture models that sparked the interest of laboratories in the possible role of IGF-I and IGF-II as tumor growth regulators.

IGF-I is also known as somatomedin-C, the mediator of the effects of human growth hormone. The mature form of IGF-I is a 70-amino acid polypeptide, which is secreted in response to pituitary growth hormone in normal humans.[180] The protein is thought to be primarily produced in the liver, but mRNA for the peptide has been identified in the tissues throughout the body.[181] IGF-I appears to be one of the most important mediators of growth in normal humans.

In contrast to the defined role of IGF-I in normal growth physiology, the function of IGF-II is much less clear. IGF-II is a 67-residue peptide and is found in considerable quantity in fetal tissue, leading to the hypothesis that it serves as a fetal growth promoter.[182] In animals, primarily focusing on rodents, IGF-II levels are high in the fetus, but drop precipitously at the time of birth. The function of IGF-II in adults is not understood.[182]

The cell surface receptors for IGF-I and IGF-II have been characterized and cloned. The biologic functions of the IGF-I and IGF-II receptors, also called the type I and type II IGF receptors, respectively, appear to be quite distinct. The IGF-I or type I IGF receptor is very similar structurally to the human insulin receptor. It is a single gene product that is posttranslationally modified to form a transmembrane heterotetramer comprised of two α and two β chains. Each α chain has a molecular weight of 130,000, and the chains comprise the extracellular ligand binding domain. The β chains include a small extracellular domain that is linked to the α chain and the transmembrane and intracellular portions of the receptor, the latter of which possesses tyrosine kinase activity.[183,184] In contrast, the IGF-II or type II IGF receptor is a single transmembrane polypeptide that does not possess tyrosine kinase activity.[185] Although some efforts to quantify IGF-I receptors in human malignancy have been carried out, these have been largely uninterpretable because of the existence of these receptors in large quantities on normal cellular components contaminating tumor biopsies.

Considerable cross-reactivity exists between the various ligands and receptors in the insulin and IGF family.[186] IGF-I binds with high affinity to the type I receptor and with reduced affinity to the insulin receptor. Neither IGF-I nor insulin appear to bind with high affinity to the type II IGF receptor.[187,188] It is possible that the type II IGF receptor, like the IGF-binding proteins discussed later, binds free IGF-II, modifying the interaction of the ligand with the type I and type II receptors. Circulating forms of the type II IGF receptor have been identified in the serum of rats, monkeys, and humans.[189-191]

The family of IGF ligands and receptors is complemented by a group of IGF-binding proteins. The aggregate function of these binding proteins in IGF physiology is not understood. Multiple binding proteins have been described in human serum.[192] The binding protein appears to stabilize IGF-I and IGF-II in the serum, preventing their degradation. The serum half-life of the IGFs in the presence of binding protein is on the order of hours, but unbound IGF is degraded in minutes.[193]

IGF-I and IGF-II are potent mitogens for breast cancer epithelial cells.[194,195] IGF overexpression has also been reported in sarcomas that are of purely mesenchymal origin with no significant epithelial component.[196,197] Similarly, IGF overexpression has been found in Wilms tumor, a pediatric tumor of mesenchymal origin.[198,199] In situ hybridization studies with IGF-I demonstrated that IGF-I mRNA could be detected in the stroma of normal tissue surrounding the breast tumor but not in the stromal or epithelial elements of the tumor itself.[200] In cell culture, virtually all cancer cell lines are stimulated by insulin and IGF-I.

In breast cancer, αIR3, a MoAb that blocks binding to the type I IGF receptor, blocked the mitogenic effects of IGF-I and IGF-II but not insulin. αIR3 also was able to block more than 80% of radiolabelled IGF-I binding to MCF-7 human breast cancer cells but did not block radiolabelled IGF-II binding. This suggests that, although type I and type II receptors are expressed in breast cancer cells, the mitogenic response to IGF-I and IGF-II is mediated by the type I receptor.[201] Others have reported similar findings.[202] The major issue in terms of eventual therapeutic efforts is whether it will be safe to inhibit pathways modulated by the IGFs given their important role in normal cellular function.

HEPARIN-BINDING GROWTH FACTORS

Before considering the heparin-binding growth factors as a group, it is worthwhile to summarize information on angiogenesis in tumors.

Angiogenesis is required for growth of normal and neoplastic tissue.[203] The generation of new capillaries in response to an angiogenic stimulus involves several steps.[204] Initially, angiogenic stimuli induce increased levels of proteases in endothelial cells,[205] allowing localized degradation of the venular basement membrane. Endothelial cells then migrate toward the angiogenic stimulus and proliferate to form a nascent capillary, with ultimate appearance of a lumen.[206-212]

It is becoming increasingly evident that "tumor growth is angiogenesis-dependent."[203] Tumor growth in animals is limited by the extent of vascularization, and inhibitors of angiogenesis that are not cytotoxic or cytostatic in vitro can inhibit tumor growth in vivo.[213-217] Neovascularization may be a critical determinant of the metastatic potential of a tumor. Tumor cells may not gain entry into the systemic circulation in significant numbers until tumor neovascularization has occurred, and larger, more vascular tumors may shed more tumor cells into the bloodstream.[218,219] Newly formed vessels in tumors are hyperpermeable to plasma proteins, possibly due to gaps in the endothelial lining; this vascular abnormality could facilitate entry of tumor cells into the circulation.[220]

Cancers often demonstrate an initial prevascular or in situ phase and a more advanced vascular phase.[221-223] The appearance of angiogenic activity in a histologically benign or in situ malignant lesion may be an important indicator that neovascularization and transition to a more malignant, invasive cancer will occur.[224-228] Neovascularization is associated with a propensity for bleeding, more rapid tumor growth, and greater likelihood of metastasis. In a clinical-histopathologic study of tumor neovascularization in patients with breast cancer, the degree of neovascularization in the patient's primary lesion (as assessed by microscopic quantitation of microvessels) was found to be a significant, independent predictor of the likelihood of metastatic spread of breast cancer.[229] Similarly, tumor neovascularization is common in human melanomas that have a Breslow's thickness of greater than 0.75 mm.[223,230] Melanomas thicker than 0.75 mm at diagnosis are much more likely to have metastasized before surgical excision.[231] In a quantitative, histologic study of patients with intermediate-thickness melanomas (0.75–4.0 mm), the degree of vascularization at the tumor base is an important, independent predictor of the likelihood of recurrence-free survival.[230]

The formation of new blood vessels involves the migration, proliferation, and differentiation of vascular endothelial cells. These processes are physiologically controlled by growth factors and growth factor modulators. Heparin-binding growth factors and transforming growth factors (TGFs), heparin and related compounds, and other substances have been shown to modulate angiogenesis.[204] The heparin-binding growth factors are particularly potent in stimulating motility and proliferation of endothelial cells and inducing several known members, which are now denoted as HBGF1 through HBGF7 (Table 7–3).[232,233]

TABLE 7–3. Unifying Nomenclature for the Fibroblast Growth Factor (FGF) Family of Peptides

Protein Name	Historical Name
FGF1	Acidic FGF, ECGF, HBGF1
FGF2	Basic FGF, HBGF2
FGF3	INT2
FGF4	K-FGF, HST1
FGF5	FGF5
FGF6	FGF6, HST2
FGF7	KGF

ECGF, endothelial cell growth factor; HBGF, heparin-binding growth factor; HST, HST oncogene product; KGF, keratinocyte growth factor.

A new family of non-FGF-related heparin-binding growth factors, the pleiotrophins, also has intense angiogenic activity.[234-236] This activity stimulates endothelial cell growth and is expressed commonly and at high levels by breast cancer, prostate cancer, and melanoma tumor samples. In this terminology, acidic fibroblast growth factor (aFGF) is HBGF1, and basic fibroblast growth factor (bFGF) is HBGF2. HBGFs have been isolated from a wide variety of normal and neoplastic tissues and in vitro cultured cells. In addition to their effects in stimulating endothelial cells and angiogenesis, HBGFs have demonstrated mitogenic and differentiation-inducing effects on several other types of normal cells.[204,232,237,238]

Steroid-induced proliferation of some hormonally responsive cell lines may be mediated by production of an autocrine-stimulatory HBGF. A high level of overexpression of HBGF2 or expression of a secreted form of HBGF2 (after cellular transfection with various HBGF2 constructs) have produced a transformed phenotype in NIH-3T3, BALB/c 3T3, or BHK21 cells.[232,233,238,240] An expression vector coding for the Kaposi *FGF* (K-*FGF*) oncogene was transfected into a human adrenal cortex cell line (SW-13 cells). In contrast to the parent cell line, K-*FGF* transfected SW-13 cells were clonogenic in soft agar and tumorigenic in athymic nude mice.[241]

The immunohistochemical localization of HBGF2 has been evaluated in paraffin blocks of human astrocytomas, a type of tumor that often demonstrates prominent vascular hyperplasia or angiogenesis.[242] Expression of HBGF2 was most prominent in the highest-grade astrocytomas (glioblastomas), which microscopically demonstrate the most cellular atypia, hypercellularity, and vascular hyperplasia (and which carry the poorest prognosis). These results are consistent with a role for HBGF2 in tumor growth and angiogenesis. Recent studies provide evidence of the role of HBGFs in the pathogenesis of human glioblastomas.[243,244]

Heparin has variable effects on the activities of HBGFs in vitro and in animals. In general, heparin potentiates HBGF1 activities, apparently by stabilization of HBGF1, but heparin has little effect on HBGF2 activities.[232,245] For example, heparin can potentiate the mitogenic effect of HBGF1 on human umbilical vein endothelial cells in vitro, but it has no effect on HBGF2 stimulation of growth of these cells.[246] In vivo, heparin was found to enhance HBGF1-induced angiogenesis or tumor-induced angiogenesis in the chick embryo chorioallantoic membrane model.[247-249]

The effects of several other sulfated polysaccharides on HBGF activities and angiogenesis have been examined in recent years. Pentosan polysulfate (PPS), a semisynthetic product manufactured from birch shavings, can effectively block HBGF activities in several in vitro and in vivo systems. PPS effectively inhibits HBGF-dependent growth of a human adrenal carcinoma cell line (SW-13), but heparin at more than 100-fold higher concentrations has no effect.[250] PPS has been found to be more effective than heparin in inhibiting the growth of a vascular smooth muscle cell line.[251] PPS is more effective than heparin in inhibiting formation of pulmonary metastases after intravenous injection of tumorigenic hepatoma cells in rats.[252]

Several other modulators of HBGF activities and angiogenesis have been described. Suramin, a polycyclic polysulfated antiparasitic drug, can block the binding of HBGF1 or HBGF2 to HBGF receptors and is showing promise as an anticancer drug in early clinical trials in prostate cancer.[253,254] However, suramin has protean effects on biologic activities of many other growth factors, including PDGF, EGF, and TGF-β, as well as inhibiting several key enzymes and metabolic pathways in mammals.[254-257] The clinical anticancer utility of suramin may be limited by the significant adverse effects of this drug, among which are induction of adrenal insufficiency and neuropathies. It is possible that a more selective inhibitor of angiogenesis would have comparable or greater anticancer activity with less clinical toxicity.

Other agents that inhibit HBGF activities or angiogenesis include protamine, sulfated polysaccharide-peptidoglycan complexes, platelet factor 4, and fumagillin and fumagillin analogs.[258-265] Marked elevations of plasma levels of platelet factor 4 occur in patients treated with PPS or other sulfated polysaccharides.[266] Protamine has been evaluated in clinical trials in cancer patients and may have some activity in retarding clinical tumor progression.[267] However, interest in protamine has been limited because it lacks potency as an antiangiogenic agent; administration of therapeutic doses is inconvenient; and there is significant potential for adverse effects (unrelated to antiangiogenic effects) when high antiangiogenic doses of this drug are administered.[217] Certain synthetic fumagillin analogs, notably AGM-1470, demonstrate potent antiangiogenic activity and little toxicity in animals and promising activity in inhibiting growth of transplantable tumors in mouse modes.[264,265] These new agents will be of great interest for future clinical studies.

The fibroblast growth factors act through a homologous series of cell surface receptors whose intracellular domains encode a tyrosine kinase activity. Four species have been described, although even more diversity exists through potential for multiple splicing. No receptor for the pleiotrophins has been described.

NERVE GROWTH FACTOR

Nerve growth factor (NGF), the first growth factor to be identified, was discovered by Levi-Montalcini and Hamburger.[268] Sympathetic neurons and a subtype of sensory neurons are dependent on NGF for growth and survival in culture.[269] The growth factor occurs in high concentrations in the salivary gland, as does EGF. Although NGF is not known to be oncogenic, its potential role is suggested by the discovery that the *TRK* oncogene encodes the receptor for NGF and that NGF stimulation of cells expressing *TRK* induces mitogenesis.[270] The *TRK* oncogene, found in DNA extracts from a human colon carcinoma, was discovered as a transforming factor for NIH-3T3 cells.[271] It has membrane-spanning and tyrosine kinase domains in addition to the binding site for NGF. Several new forms of NGF-related growth factors and TRK-related receptors have been described.

BOMBESIN

Bombesin is 14 amino acids long, was isolated from frog skin, and is a homolog of the mammalian gastrin-releasing peptide.[272] Administration of either of these peptides intravenously stimulates gastric acid secretion by means of gastrin secretion. Some small-cell carcinoma cell lines produce bombesin and are stimulated by it.[273,274] Bombesin can enhance the growth of normal human bronchial epithelial cells in serum-free cultures. The peptide is also mitogenic for Swiss 3T3 murine embryonal fibroblasts, and this effect is potentiated by insulin, PDGF or EGF.[275] A MoAb that binds to bombesin has been shown to inhibit proliferation of non-small cell carcinoma cells in culture and in nude mouse xenografts.[274] A trial of antibombesin MoAb therapy for small cell carcinoma has been initiated.

GROWTH INHIBITORY CYTOKINES

TRANSFORMING GROWTH FACTOR-β

Transforming growth factor-β is the prototypic member of a family of polypeptide regulatory molecules, which includes activins, inhibins, bone morphogenic proteins, and the müllerian inhibitory substance in mammals.[53,276,277] It was originally identified as a transforming component (with TGF-α) of the factors in conditioned medium of certain tumor cell line cultures that had the capacity to stimulate the growth of fibroblasts in soft agar.[7,85] Although its name is based on the transforming properties that were initially identified, this growth factor has an array of functions that regulate many normal cellular processes involved in morphogenesis, differentiation, and wound healing.

TGF-β1, the best characterized molecule of this group of growth factors, is synthesized as the C-terminal domain of a precursor molecule that is a secretory polypeptide.[278] After secretion, the pro-region remains attached to the TGF-β1 domain, and two such precursor molecules form a dimer that has only latent biologic activity. This latent complex was originally found in platelets, but it may be released directly into the environment, where it is bound to the extracellular matrix and to specific binding proteins.[279] Cleavage by proteolytic digestion or by alterations in pH can release an active 25-kilodalton TGF-β dimer from the latent complex.[280] Most cells synthesize TGF-β in one of its molecular forms.

In the TGF-β family, there are four additional molecular forms that are closely related to TGF-β1, each of which forms dimers that express biologic activity. The multiplicity of TGF-β forms and the sequence conservation within each form through a number of species suggest important specific roles for each form of TGF-β.[53,276,277]

The effects of TGF-β, activins, and probably all members of this family are mediated by a pair of membrane-spanning receptors: type I with a mass of 53 kilodalton and type II with a mass of 70 kilodalton.[53] Each can bind ligand with high affinity, and it is not known whether activation involves dimerization of receptors. Although the type I receptor remains to be characterized, type II activin and TGF-β receptors have been cloned and have the sequence of a serine-threonine kinase in their intracytoplasmic portions.[54-56] This equips the receptor to enter signal transduction pathways on activation by its ligand. The capacity of these receptors to discriminate between different TGF-β forms may create the opportunity for selectivity in responses by different cells and tissues. However, both receptor types are expressed on most cells, and there is no apparent pattern to the relative expression of receptors on particular cell lines and tissues.

Another protein with the capacity to bind TGF-β is β-glycan, previously designated as the type III receptor.[53] β-Glycan can exist as a transmembrane protein or be released into the extracellular space in a soluble form. It is speculated that these abundant molecules could function as a reservoir or a clearance system for bioactive TGF-β.[53]

The capacity of TGF-β to inhibit proliferation of a variety of malignant epithelial tumor cell lines has attracted attention to its possible use as an anticancer agent. However, it also inhibits the proliferation of normal epithelial cells in the breast, liver, bronchus, kidney, skin, and intestine.[276] It has been postulated that TGF-β may be the major biologic regulator of normal cells that have the capacity to repopulate tissues.[276] In this model, tumorigenesis involves escape from cellular regulation by TGF-β. For example, although retinal cells bear receptors for TGF-β, retinoblastoma cells lack these receptors, and this may permit the cell to escape regulation by TGF-β in the retina.[281] Although loss of receptors is an unusual event, other mechanisms, such as alteration in intracellular signal transduction pathways or suppressor genes, may deactivate the regulatory capacity of the TGF-β receptor.

The inhibitory effects of TGF-β on cell proliferation extend beyond the epithelium. Remarkable growth-inhibiting activity has been observed in endothelial, fibroblast, neuronal, lymphoid, and hematopoietic cell types. The degree of inhibition varies. The responding cells display delayed progression through or arrest in the late G_1 phase of the cell cycle.[282,283]

These observations have led to the hypothesis that TGF-β may have utility in inhibiting the immune system or in temporarily arresting the production of bone marrow stem cells to protect them from chemotherapy.[276] T-lymphocyte activation can increase the production of TGF-β, and TGF-β can inhibit the IL-2 induced upregulation of IL-2 receptors. These events may physiologically dampen the IL-2 mediated proliferative response of these immune cells.[284]

Analysis of the effects of TGF-β is complicated by its capacity to activate opposite responses (*e.g.*, growth stimulation and suppression), sometimes in the same target cells. This may depend on the particular growth conditions. In the case of ARK-LB mouse fibroblasts, growth in serum (a source of mitogens) is slowed by TGF-β, but in serum-free culture, growth may be enhanced. The mechanism of growth enhancement is thought to be indirect, through induction of expression of PDGF, which can activate the growth of the fibroblasts by autocrine stimulation.[282,285] Osteoblasts are also stimulated to proliferate in culture by TGF-β.

Exposure of cells to TGF-β alters the phenotype, which may play a major role in differentiation and embryologic morphogenesis.[53,276] For example, the differentiation of preadipocytes and myoblasts is regulated by TGF-β1. Sites of intense development and morphogenesis in the connective tissues of the embryo express high levels of TGF-β, suggesting a role in function and remodeling of embryonic structures.

TGF-β may play a role in inflammation and repair in several ways.[53,276] It is a potent chemotactic factor and activator of macrophages. It stimulates the production of components of extracellular matrix, such as collagen and fibronectin. It inhibits expression of proteolytic enzyme activity that could destroy newly formed connective tissue by reducing the production of enzymes like collagenase and stromalysin and by upregulating the production of protease inhibitors. TGF-β also upregulates expression of integrin receptors for molecules like collagen and fibronectin, thereby increasing the adhesion of cells to matrix proteins.[53] The regulation of integrin expression may modulate the capacity of cells to interact with other cells, by altering cell-to-cell adhesion.

The mechanism of growth inhibition at the molecular level is not fully understood. One line of evidence suggests a role for TGF-β in inhibiting the expression of c-*MYC*, which could reduce the transcription of genes key to proliferation.[286] An alternative mechanism involves the demonstrated capacity of TGF-β stimulation to reduce phosphorylation of the RB protein.[283] Because RB phosphorylation is required to release bound nuclear transcription regulators and allow entry into S phase, this observation could provide an explanation for the arrest of cells in late G$_1$ phase after exposure to TGF-β.

Activins and inhibins are growth factors consisting of heterodimeric and homodimeric molecules related to the TGF-β family.[287] These growth factors were originally recognized as gonadal protein hormones that modulated follicle-stimulating hormone production by the anterior pituitary. The activin and inhibin molecules share a common β chain and differ in the second chain, which can be an α chain (inhibins) or another β chain (activins).[287,288] In addition to regulating pituitary function, activins and inhibins regulate hormone production in gonadal tissues and differentiation of erythroid and neural cells.

Müllerian-inhibiting substance (MIS) is structurally and biochemically related to TGF-β.[289] It is expressed in the testes, and this causes regression of the müllerian duct during fetal development. It also is expressed transiently and at low levels in the ovary. MIS inhibited the colony growth of a number of primary ovarian and endometrial cancers from patients and the cell lines derived from these sources.[290,291]

MAMMASTATIN

A regulatory peptide produced by normal human mammary epithelial cells has been described.[292] This peptide has relative tissue specificity for normal mammary cells and mammary cancer cells and can inhibit their proliferation. Its production and secretion are increased by pharmacologic concentrations of estrogens (but not by tamoxifen). Preliminary sequence information has suggested some sequence homology to the inhibin family. The identification of this molecule raises the possibility that, in some cases, progression of mammary neoplasia may represent inadequate production of or failure to respond to tissue-specific inhibitors. For the former case, administration of the growth inhibitor can be envisioned as an anticancer therapy.

THE INTERFERONS

The interferons (IFNs) are secreted proteins that were discovered as biologic agents interfering with virus replication.[293] They have numerous functions, including modulation of the immune system and regulation of cell proliferation and differentiation. Recent reviews of the IFNs offer more detailed discussions of the complex actions of these cytokines.[294,295]

One superfamily of IFNs consists of at least 18 IFN-α genes and 6 IFN-α2 genes expressed in leukocytes, plus a single IFN-β gene expressed in fibroblasts.[294,295] These bind to a class of receptors that are not yet well characterized. IFN-α, produced by activated T lymphocytes and natural killer cells, binds to a different receptor.

Binding of IFN to receptors activates a number of the signal transduction pathways described previously but does not appear to involve tyrosine kinase. Several IFN-responsive tran-

scription factors have been identified. These activate transcription of specific mRNAs by binding to IFN-responsive DNA sequences that activate target genes.[295] Exposure of cells to IFN activates production of more than 30 proteins, which vary widely in their functions. Among the best characterized is the (2',5') oligo A synthetase family of enzymes, which convert ATP into 2',5'(A)n, where n ranges from 2 to 15.[296] This enzyme, which is stimulated by double-stranded RNA, activates RNase L, which cleaves single-stranded RNA and may interfere with virus replication. Other IFN-induced proteins include the major histocompatibility complex class I and class II antigens, which are involved in cell recognition and the processing of antigens.

IFNs can inhibit the proliferation of a wide variety of cells. Their action is generally cytostatic rather than cytotoxic, and inhibition of progression through cell cycle phases has been demonstrated. However, stimulation of cell proliferation has also been observed in some experimental situations.

By activating immune and inflammatory cells and regulating immunoglobulin secretion, IFNs influence the physiologic processes involved in host defense mechanisms. They may also play a role in the pathogenesis of chonic inflammatory and autoimmune diseases.

Therapeutic utility of IFN administration has been demonstrated for hairy cell leukemia, chonic leukemias, and Kaposi's sarcoma. These and other potential clinical applications are described elsewhere in this volume.

TUMOR NECROSIS FACTOR

Tumor necrosis factor (TNF) is a protein containing 157 amino acids that is produced by activated macrophages and other cells.[297-299] It binds to specific 55-kd and 75-kd receptors. Activation of a G protein may be an important pathway of signal transduction. TNF released at the site of inflammation acts on receptors on endothelial cells, T and B lymphocytes, and granulocytes to stimulate immune and inflammatory responses. In these processes, there is overlap with the functions of interleukin-1 and the interferons. It is believed that many of the physiologic changes associated with endotoxemia are activated by TNF and related cytokines.

TNF and a related molecule, lymphotoxin, are now known as TNF-α and TNF-β. They have cytotoxic effects on a variety of tumor cells in experimental systems, but TNF can stimulate the proliferation of certain fibroblast lines. The mechanisms of these effects require clarification. More detailed descriptions of potential clinical applications of TNF are found elsewhere in this volume.

GROWTH FACTORS AND THEIR RECEPTORS AS TARGETS FOR ANTICANCER THERAPY

Growth factor pathways, mediated by specific growth factors and their receptors, appear to play critical roles in progression of human neoplasia. A critical test of this idea will be the application of this approach to the design of anticancer therapy. Toxic effects can render these approaches ineffective, and clinical trials will be required. Successful therapies against growth factors and their receptors have been explored in vitro and in a variety of experimental systems (Fig. 7–4):

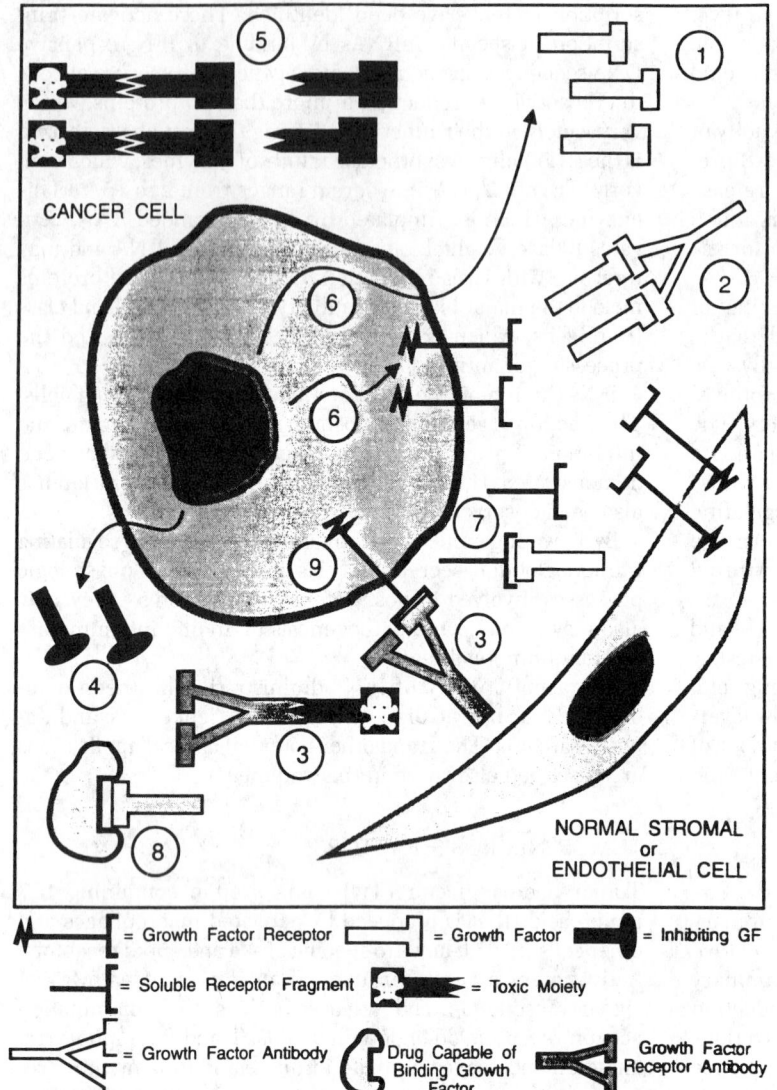

CANCER CELL

NORMAL STROMAL
or
ENDOTHELIAL CELL

⊢⊦⟍ = Growth Factor Receptor   ▭— = Growth Factor   ◼—• = Inhibiting GF

⊢— = Soluble Receptor Fragment   ☠◼— = Toxic Moiety

Y = Growth Factor Antibody   ⊃ Drug Capable of Binding Growth Factor   Growth Factor Receptor Antibody

FIGURE 7–4. Potential sites for therapeutic intervention in growth factor receptor pathways. (For explanation of numbers, refer to the text.)

1. High concentrations of growth factors may themselves be growth inhibitory in cells that overexpress the cognate growth factor receptor.
2. Antibodies directed against individual growth factors could inhibit the growth of tumor cells dependent on those growth factors. An example is the efficiency of monoclonal antibodies against bombesin.[274] These antibodies have blocked the growth of some human small cell carcinomas of the lung when inoculated into athymic nude mice. Limited clinical trials with this antibody have been undertaken.
3. Growth factor receptor antibodies alone or as conjugates or chimeric molecules with a variety of toxins, radionuclides, and drugs can inhibit or destroy tumor cells.[10,300,301] Significant activity against HTLV-I leukemia has been reported with antibody against the IL-2 receptor.[302] Monoclonal antibodies against the receptors for EGF,[132–134] HER2/ERBB2, and transferrin are being studied. Because of the ability to block the physiologic activity of specific receptors, this approach has great appeal.
4. The use of ligands that inhibit cancer growth is a direct approach. For example, the peptide mammastatin from

human breast epithelial cells directly inhibits the growth of breast cancer.[292] The eventual usefulness of this approach will be determined by the specificity of the effect. For example, although TGF-β can inhibit many epithelial tumor cell lines, its effect on the host are likely to be overwhelmingly debilitating.[303]
5. Growth factor fragments capable of blocking their cognate receptor sites may be growth inhibitory. These fragments (or the entire growth factor or peptide analogs) can be conjugated to or recombinantly expressed with a series of noxious substances, allowing targeting directly to cancer sites. This topic is reviewed elsewhere.[304]
6. Antisense oligodeoxynucleotides may be employed to downregulate the production of any translated product of interest, including growth factors or growth factor receptors or at least potentially mutated genetic elements putatively responsible for various tumors.[305]
7. Extracellular domains of membrane-spanning cell surface receptors may function as highly specific but inert binding sites for stimulatory ligands. These could be given systemically.
8. There are agents capable of interacting with growth

factors or other cell products contributing to malignant behavior and inactivating them or blocking their access to growth factor receptors. For example, suramin and pentosan polysulfate have the ability to interact with growth factors and block their binding to growth factor receptors.[306,307]

9. Interference with a signal transduction cascade after the binding of the growth factor to its receptor could deactivate the effect of a growth factor. The development of a series of tyrosine kinase inhibitors may eventually lead to drugs capable of blocking the effects of individual growth factors.[308]

10. Neovascularization, or tumor-induced angiogenesis, is a mandatory component of tumor progression beyond 1 or 2 mm.[221] Many of the described therapeutic approaches have been suggested as inhibitors of angiogenesis, and new agents derived from naturally occurring inhibitors of angiogenesis are entering clinical trials.

Many of these approaches are not mutually exclusive and combinations of biologic therapy (*e.g.*, blocking a specific growth factor receptor while simultaneously attempting to lower biologically available concentrations of that growth factor) make intuitive sense. All of these therapeutic approaches have developed from our expansion of fundamental cellular and molecular biologic studies of cancer rather than empiric observations.

REFERENCES

1. Cross M, Dexter TM. Growth factors in development, transformation, and tumorigenesis. Cell 1991;64:271–280.
2. Aaronson SA. Growth factors and cancer. Science 1991;254:1146–1153.
3. Leutz A, Graf T. Relationships between oncogenes and growth control. In: Sporn MB, Roberts AB, eds. Peptide growth factors and their receptors, vol II. Berlin: Springer-Verlag, 1990:655–703.
4. Heldin C-H, Westermark B. Growth factors as transforming proteins. Eur J Biochem 1989;184:487–496.
5. Varmus H. An historical overview of oncogenes. In: Weinberg RA, ed. Oncogenes and the molecular origins of cancer. Cold Spring Harbor, NY: Cold Spring Harbor Laboratory Press, 1989:3–44.
6. Sporn MB, Roberts AB, eds. Peptide growth factors and their receptors, vols I and II. Berlin: Springer-Verlag, 1990.
7. De Larco JE, Todaro GJ. Growth factors from murine sarcoma virus-transformed cells. Proc Natl Acad Sci USA 1978;75:4001–4005.
8. Sporn MB, Todaro GJ. Autocrine secretion and malignant transformation of cells. N Engl J Med 1980;308:878–880.
9. Sporn MB, Todaro GJ. Autocrine growth factors and cancer. Nature 1985;313:747–751.
10. Mendelsohn J. Antibodies to growth factors and receptors. In: DeVita VT Jr, Hellman S, Rosenberg SA, eds. Biologic therapy of cancer. Philadelphia: JB Lippincott, 1991:601–612.
11. Deuel TF. Polypeptide growth factors: Roles in normal and abnormal cell growth. Annu Rev Cell Biol 1987;3:443–492.
12. Goustin AS, Leof EB, Shipley GD, Moses HL. Growth factors and cancer. Cancer Res 1986;46:1015–1029.
13. Cullen KJ, Smith HS, Hill S, Rosen N, Lippman ME. Growth factor mRNA expression by human breast fibroblasts from benign and malignant lesions. Cancer Res 1991;51:4978–4985.
14. Heldin C-H, Westermark B. Platelet-derived growth factor: Mechanism of action and possible in vivo function. Cell Reg 1990;1:555–566.
15. Massagué J. Transforming growth factor-α. J Biol Chem 1990;265:21393–21396.
16. Brachmann R, Lindquist PB, Nagashima M, et al. Transmembrane TGF-α precursors activate EGF/TGF-α receptors. Cell 1989;56:691–700.
17. Wong ST, Winchell LF, McCune BK, et al. The TGF-α precursor expressed on the cell surface binds to the EGF receptor on adjacent cells, leading to signal transduction. Cell 1989;56:495–506.
18. Anklesaria P, Teixido J, Laiho M, Pierce JH, Greenberger JS, Massagué J. Cell–cell adhesion mediated by binding of membrane-anchored transforming growth factor-alpha to epidermal growth factor receptors promotes cell proliferation. Proc Natl Acad Sci USA 1990;87:3289–3293.
19. Huang JS, Huang SS, Deuel TF. Transforming protein of simian sarcoma virus stimulates autocrine cell growth of SSV-transformed cells through platelet-derived growth factor cell surface receptors. Cell 1984;39:79–87.
20. Keating MT, Williams LT. Autocrine stimulation of intracellular PDGF receptors in v-*SIS*–transformed cells. Science 1988;239:914–916.
21. Hannink M, Donoghue DJ. Autocrine stimulation by the v-*SIS* gene product requires a ligand-receptor interaction at the cell surface. J Cell Biol 1988;107:287–298.
22. Van de Vijver M, Kumar R, Mendelsohn J. Ligand-induced activation of A431 cell EGF receptors occurs primarily by an autocrine pathway that acts upon receptors on the surface rather than intracellularly. J Biol Chem 1991;266:7503–7508.
23. Barbes D, Sat G. Serum-free cell culture: A unifying approach. Cell 1980;22:649–655.
24. Sato G, Pardee AB, Sirbasku D. Growth of cells in hormonally defined media. Cold Spring Harbor Conferences on Cell Proliferation, vol 9. Cold Spring Harbor, NY: Cold Spring Harbor Laboratory Press, 1982.
25. Ullrich A, Schlessinger J. Signal transduction by receptors with tyrosine kinase activity. Cell 1990;61:203–212.
26. Hunter T. A thousand and one protein kinases. Cell 1987;50:823–829.
27. Honegger AM, Kris RM, Ullrich A, Schlessinger J. Evidence that autophosphorylation of solubilized EGF-receptors is mediated by intermolecular cross phosphorylation. Proc Natl Acad Sci USA 1989;86:925–929.
28. Wahl M, Nishibi S, Suh P-G, Rhee SG, Carpenter G. Epidermal growth factor stimulates tyrosine phosphorylation of phospholipase C-II independently of receptor internalization and extracellular calcium. Proc Natl Acad Sci USA 1989;86:1568–1572.
29. Margolis B, Rhee SG, Felder S, et al. EGF induces phosphorylation of phospholipase C-II: A potential mechanism for EGF receptor signaling. Cell 1989B;57:1101–1107.
30. Meisenhelder J, Suh P-G, Rhee SG, Hunter T. Phospholipase C-gamma is a substrate for the PDGF and EGF receptor protein-tyrosine kinases in vivo and in vitro. Cell 1989;57:1109–1122.
31. Varticovski L, Druker B, Morrison D, Cantley L, Robert T. The colony stimulating factor-1 receptor associates with an activated phosphatidylinositol-3 kinase. Nature 1989;342:699–702.
32. Molloy CJ, Bottaro DP, Fleming TP, Marshall MS, Gibbs JB, Aaronson SA. PDGF induction of tyrosine phosphorylation of GTPase activating protein. Nature 1989;342:711–714.
33. Morrison DK, Kaplan DR, Escobedo JA, Rapp UR, Roberts TM, Williams LT. Direct activation of the serine/threonine kinase activity of RAF1 through tyrosine phosphorylation by the PDGF-β receptor. Cell 1989;58:649–657.
34. Rhee SG, Suh P-G, Ryu S-H, Lee SY. Studies of inositol phospholipid-specific phospholipase C. Science 1989;244:546.
35. Kikkawa U, Kishimoto A, Nishizuka Y. The protein kinase C family: Heterogeneity and its implications. Annu Rev Biochem 1989;58:31.
36. Whitman M, Downes CP, Keeler M, Keller T, Cantley L. Type I phosphatidylinositol kinase makes a novel inositol phospholipid, phosphatidylinositol-3-phosphate. Nature 1988;332:644.
37. Koch CA, Anderson D, Moran MF, Ellis C, Pawson T. SH2 and SH3 domains: Elements that control interactions of cytoplasmic signaling proteins. Science 1991;252:668–674.
38. Trahey M, McCormick F. A cytoplasmic protein stimulates normal N-RAS p21 GTPase, but does not affect oncogenic mutants. Science 1987;238:542.
39. Mulcahy LS, Smith MR, Stacey DW. Requirement for *RAS* proto-oncogene function during serum-stimulated growth of NIH 3T3 cells. Nature 1985;313:241–243.
40. Eisenman RN. Nuclear oncogenes. In: Weinberg RA, ed. Oncogenes and the molecular origins of cancer. Cold Spring Harbor, NY: Cold Spring Harbor Laboratory Press, 1989:175–221,
41. Raff MC, Lillien LE, Richardson WD, Burne JF, Noble MD. Platelet-derived growth factor from astrocytes drives the clock that times oligodendrocyte development in culture. Nature 1988;333:562.
42. McKinnon RD, Matsui T, Dubois-Dalcq M, Aaronson SA. FGF modulates the PDGF-driven pathway of oligodendrocyte development. Neuron 1990;5:603.
43. Roberts AB, Anzano MA, Wakefield LM, Roche NS, Stern DF, Sporn MB. Type β transforming growth factor: A bifunctional regulator of cellular growth. Proc Natl Acad Sci USA 1985;82:119–123.
44. Carpenter G. Receptors for epidermal growth factor and other polypeptide mitogens. Annu Rev Biochem 1987;56:881–914.
45. Carpenter G. Epidermal growth factor. Annu Rev Biochem 1979;48:193–216.
46. Fox CF, Das M. Internalization and processing of the EGF receptor in the induction of DNA synthesis in cultured fibroblasts: The endocyte activation hypothesis. J Supramol Struct 1979;10:199–214.
47. Clark AJL, Ishii S, Richert N, Merlino GT, Pastan I. Epidermal growth factor regulates the expression of its own receptor. Proc Natl Acad Sci USA 1985;82:8374–8378.
48. Marx J. Biologists turn on to "off-enzymes." Science 1991;251:744–746.
49. Hunter T. Protein-tyrosine phosphatases: The other side of the coin. Cell 1989;58:1013–1016.
50. Kreuger NX, Streuli M, Saito H. Structural diversity and evolution of human receptor-like tyrosine phosphatases. EMBO J 1990;9:3241.
51. Jackson TR, Blair LAC, Marshall J, Goedert M, Hanley MR. The *MAS* oncogene encodes an angiotensin receptor. Nature 1988;335:437–440.
52. Lebacq-Verheyden A-M, Trepel J, Sausville EA, Battey JF. Bombesin and gastrin-releasing peptide: Neuropeptides, secretogogues, and growth factors. In: Sporn MB, Roberts AB, eds. Peptide growth factors and their receptors, vol II. Berlin: Springer-Verlag, 1990:71–124.
53. Massagué J. The transforming growth factor-β family. Annu Rev Cell Biol 1990;6:597–641.
54. Mathews LS, Vale WW. Expression cloning of an activin receptor, a predicted transmembrane serine kinase. Cell 1991;65:973–982.

55. Attisano L, Wrana JL, Cheifetz S, Massagué J. Novel activin receptors: Distinct genes and alternative mRNA splicing generate a repertoire of serine/threonine kinase receptors. Cell 1992;68:97–108.

56. Lin HY, Wang X-F, Ng-Eaton E, Weinberg RA, Lodish HF. Expression cloning of the TGF-β type II receptor, a functional transmembrane serine/threonine kinase. Cell 1992;68:775–785.

57. Chinkers M, Cohen S. Purified EGF receptor-kinase interacts specifically with antibodies to Rous sarcoma virus transforming protein. Nature 1981;290:516–519.

58. Erikson E, Shealy DJ, Erikson RL. Evidence that viral transforming gene products and epidermal growth factor stimulate phosphorylation of the same cellular protein with similar specificity. J Biol Chem 1981;256:11381–11384.

59. Cooper JA, Hunter T. Similarities and differences between the effects of epidermal growth factor and Rous sarcoma virus. J Cell Biol 1981;91:878–883.

60. Doolittle RF, Hunkapiller MW, Hood LE, et al. Simian sarcoma virus oncogene, v-sis, is derived from the gene (or genes) encoding a platelet-derived growth factor. Science 1983;221:275–277.

61. Waterfield MD, Scrace GT, Whittle N, et al. Platelet-derived growth factor is structurally related to the putative transforming protein p28sis of simian sarcoma virus. Nature 1983;304:35–39.

62. Downward J, Yarden Y, Mayes E, et al. Close similarity of epidermal growth factor receptor and v-ERB-B oncogene protein sequences. Nature 1984;307:521–528.

63. Young-Hua X, Ishii S, Clark AJL, et al. Human epidermal growth factor receptor cDNA is homologous to a variety of RNAs overproduced in A431 carcinoma cells. Nature 1984;309:806–810.

64. Lin CR, Chen WS, Kruiger W, et al. Expression cloning of human EGF receptor complementary DNA: Gene amplification and three related messenger RNA products in A431 cells. Science 1984;224:843–845.

65. Sherr CJ, Rettenmeier CW, Sacca R, Roussel MF, Look AT, Stanley ER. The c-fms proto-oncogene product is related to the receptor for the mononuclear phagocyte growth factor, CSF-1. Cell 1985;41:665–676.

66. Stern DF, Heffernan PA, Weinberg RA. p185^HER2, a product of the NEU proto-oncogene, is a receptor-like protein associated with tyrosine kinase activity. Mol Cell Biol 1986;6:1729–1740.

67. Sandgren EP, Luetteke NC, Palmiter RD, Brinster RL, Lee DC. Overexpression of TGF α in transgenic mice: Induction of epithelial hyperplasia, pancreatic metaplasia, and carcinoma of the breast. Cell 1990;61:1121–1135.

68. Jhappan C, Stahle C, Harkins RN, Fausto N, Smith GH, Merlino GT. TGF α overexpression in transgenic mice induces liver neoplasia and abnormal development of the mammary gland and pancreas. Cell 1990;61:1147–1155.

69. Matsui Y, Halter SA, Holt JT, Hogan BL, Coffey RJ. Development of mammary hyperplasia and neoplasia in MMTV-TGF α transgenic mice. Cell 1990;61:1147–1155.

70. Slamon DJ, Godolphin W, Jones LA, et al. Studies of the HER-2/NEU proto-oncogene in human breast and ovarian cancer. Science 1989;244:707–712.

71. Wright C, Angus B, Nicholson S, et al. Expression of c-ERBB-2 oncoprotein: A prognostic indicator in human breast cancer. Cancer Res 1989;49:2087–2090.

72. King CR, Swain SM, Porter L, Steinberg SM, Lippman ME, Gelmann EP. Heterogeneous expression of ERBB-2 messenger RNA in human breast cancer. Cancer Res 1989;49:4185–4191.

73. Van de Vijver MJ, Peterse JL, Mooi WJ, et al. Neu-protein overexpression in breast cancer: Association with comedo-type ductal carcinoma in situ and limited prognostic value in stage II breast cancer. N Engl J Medicine 1988;319:1239–1245.

74. Gullick WJ. The role of the epidermal growth factor receptor and the c-ERBB-2 protein in breast cancer. Int J Cancer 1990;5S:55–61.

75. Harris AL, Nicholson S, Sainsbury JRC, et al. Epidermal growth factor receptor: A marker of early relapse in breast cancer and tumor stage progression in bladder cancer—interactions with NEU. In: Furth M, Greaves M, eds. The molecular diagnostics of human cancer, vol 7. Cold Spring Harbor, NY: Cold Spring Harbor Laboratory Press, 1989:353–357.

76. Sainsbury JRC, Malcolm AJ, Appleton DR, Farndon JR, Harris AL. Presence of epidermal growth factor receptor as an indicator of poor prognosis in patients with breast cancer. J Clin Pathol 1985;38:1225–1228.

77. Neal DE, Bennett MK, Hall RR, et al. Epidermal growth factor receptors in human bladder cancer: Comparison of invasive and superficial tumors. Lancet 1985;1:366–368.

78. Hendler F, Shum-Siu A, Nanu L, Yuan D, Ozanne B. Increased EGF receptors and the absence of an alveolar differentiation marker predict a poor survival in lung cancer. Proc Am Clin Onc [Abstract] 1989;8:223.

79. Veale D, Ashcroft T, Marsh C, Gibson GJ, Harris AL. Epidermal growth factor receptors in non-small cell lung cancer. Br J Cancer 1987;55:513–516.

80. Cohen S. Isolation of a mouse submaxillary gland protein accelerating incisor eruption and eyelid opening in the new born animal. J Biol Chem 1962;237:1555–1562.

81. Carpenter G, Wahl MI. The epidermal growth factor family. In: Sporn MB, Roberts AB, eds. Peptide growth factors and their receptors, vol I. Berlin: Springer-Verlag, 1990:69–171.

82. Shoyab M, Plowman GD, McDonald VL, Bradley JG, Todaro GJ. Structure and function of human amphiregulin: A member of the epidermal growth factor family. Science 1989;243:1074–1076.

83. Higashiyama S, Abraham JA, Miller J, Fiddes JC, Klagsbrun M. A heparin-binding growth factor secreted by macrophage-like cells that is related to EGF. Science 1991;251:936–939.

84. Schreiber AB, Winkler ME, Derynck R. Transforming growth factor alpha: A more potent angiogenic mediator than epidermal growth factor. Science 1986;232:1250–1253.

85. Anzano M, Roberts AB, Meyers CA, et al. Sarcoma growth factor from conditioned medium of virally transformed cells is composed of both type alpha and type beta transforming growth factors. Proc Natl Acad Sci USA 1983;80:6264–6268.

86. Rosenthal A, Lindquist PB, Bringman TS, Goeddel DV, Derynck R. Expression in rat fibroblasts of a human transforming growth factor-alpha cDNA results in transformation. Cell 1986;46:301–309.

87. Riedel H, Massoglia S, Schlessinger J, Ullrich A. Ligand activation of overexpressed epidermal growth factor receptors transforms NIH 3T3 mouse fibroblasts. Proc Natl Acad Sci USA 1988;85:1477–1481.

88. Di Fiore PP, Pierce JH, Fleming TP, et al. Overexpression of the human EGF receptor confers an EGF-dependent transformed phenotype to NIH 3T3 cells. Cell 1987;51:1063–1070.

89. Velu TJ, Beguinot L, Vass WC, et al. Epidermal growth factor-dependent transformation by a human EGF receptor proto-oncogene. Science 1987;238:1408–1410.

90. Thorburn GD, Waters MJ, Dolling M, Young IR. Fetal maturation and epidermal growth factor. Proc Aust Phys Pharmacol Soc 1981;12:11–15.

91. Ozanne B, Richards CS, Hendler F, Burns D, Gusterson B. Over-expression of the EGF receptor is a hallmark of squamous cell carcinomas. J Pathology 1986;149:9–14.

92. Sobol RE, Astarita RW, Hofeditz C, et al. EGF receptor expression in human lung carcinomas defined by a monoclonal antibody. JNCI 1987;79:403–407.

93. Veale D, Kerr N, Gibson GH, Harris AL. Characterization of epidermal growth factor receptor in primary human non-small cell lung cancer. Cancer Res 1989;49:1313–1317.

94. Libermann TA, Razon N, Bartal AD, Yarden Y, Schlessinger J, Soreq H. Expression of epidermal growth factor receptors in human brain tumors. Cancer Res 1984;44:753–760.

95. Eisbruch A, Blick M, Lee JS, Sacks PG, Gutterman J. Analysis of the epidermal growth factor receptor gene in fresh human head and neck tumors. Cancer Res 1984;47:3603–3605.

96. Humphrey PA, Wong AJ, Vogelstein B, et al. Anti-synthetic peptide antibody reacting at the fusion junction of deletion-mutant epidermal growth factor receptors in human glioblastoma. Proc Natl Acad Sci USA 1990;87:4207–4211.

97. Derynck R, Goeddel DV, Ullrich A, et al. Synthesis of messenger RNAs for transforming growth factors α and β and the epidermal growth factor receptor by human tumors. Cancer Res 1987;47:707–712.

98. Osborne CK, Hamilton B, Titus G, Livingston RB. Epidermal growth factor stimulation of human breast cancer cells in culture. Cancer Res 1980;40:2361–2366.

99. Fitzpatrick SL, LaChance MP, Schultz GS. Characterization of epidermal growth factor receptor and action on human breast cancer cells in culture. Cancer Res 1984;44:3442–3447.

100. Fitzpatrick SL, Brightwell JB, Wittliff JL, Barrows GH, Schultz GS. Epidermal growth factor binding by breast tumor biopsies and relationship to estrogen receptor and progestin receptor levels. Cancer Res 1984;44:3448–3453.

101. Perez R, Pascual M, Macias A, Lage A. Epidermal growth factor receptors in human breast cancer. Breast Cancer Res Treat 1984;4:189–193.

102. Sainsbury JRC, Sherbet GV, Farndon JR, Harris AL. Epidermal growth factor receptors and oestrogen receptors in human breast cancer. Lancet 1985;1:364–366.

103. Travers MT, Barrett-Lee PJ, Berger U, et al. Growth factor expression in normal, benign, and malignant breast tissue. Br Med J 1988;296:1621–1624.

104. Koenders PG, Beex LKVAM, Geurtz-Moespot A, Heuvel JJTM, Kienhuis CBM, Benraad TJ. Epidermal growth factor receptor-negative tumors are predominantly confined to the subgroup of estradiol receptor-positive human primary breast cancers. Cancer Res 1991;51:4544–4548.

105. Davidson NE, Gelmann EP, Lippman ME, Dickson RB. Epidermal growth factor receptor gene expression in estrogen receptor-positive and negative human breast cancer cell lines. Mol Endocrinol 1987;1:216–223.

106. Bates SE, Davidson NE, Valverius EM, et al. Expression of transforming growth factor-α and its messenger ribonucleic acid in human breast cancer: Its regulation by estrogen and its possible functional significance. Mol Endocrinol 1988;2:543–555.

107. Ciardiello F, Kim N, Liscia DS, et al. mRNA expression of transforming growth factor-α in human breast carcinomas and its activity in effusions of breast cancer patients. JNCI 1989;81:1165–1171.

108. Dickson RB, Bates SE, McManaway ME, Lippman ME. Characterization of estrogen responsive transforming activity in human breast cancer cell lines. Cancer Res 1986;46:1707.

109. Dickson RB, Huff KK, Spencer EM, Lippman ME. Induction of epidermal growth factor-related polypeptides by 17β-estradiol in MCF-7 human breast cancer cells. Endocrinology 1985;118:138.

110. Vonderhaar BK. Local effects of EGF, α-GF and EGF-like growth factors on lobuloalveolar development of the mouse mammary gland in vivo. J Cell Physiol 1987;132:581–584.

111. Valverius EM, Bates SE, Stampfer ME, Clark R, McCormick F, Salomon DS, Lippman ME, Dickson RB. Transforming growth factor-α production and epidermal growth factor receptor expression in normal and oncogene transformed human mammary epithelial cells. Mol Endocrinol 1989;3:203–214.

112. Nicholson S, Halcrow P, Farndon JR, Sainsbury JRC, Chambers P, Harris AL. Expression of epidermal growth factor receptors associated with lack of response to endocrine therapy in recurrent breast cancer. Lancet 1989;1:182–185.

113. Ennis BW, Valverius EM, Lippman ME, Bellot F, Kris R, Schlessinger J, Masui H, Goldenberg A, Mendelsohn J, Dickson RB. Monoclonal anti-EGF receptor antibodies inhibit the growth of malignant and non-malignant human mammary epithelial cells. Mol Endocrinol 1989;3:1830–1838.

114. Bates SE, Valverius EM, Ennis BW, et al. Expression of TGF-α/EGF receptor pathway in normal human breast epithelial cells. Endocrinol 1990;126:596–607.

115. Ciardiello F, McGeady ML, Kim N, et al. TGF-α expression is enhanced in human mammary epithelial cells transformed by an activated c-Ha-*RAS* proto-oncogene but not by the c-*NEU* proto-oncogene, and overexpression of the TGF-α cDNA leads to transformation. Cell Growth Differ 1990;1:407–420.

116. Markowitz SD, Molkentin K, Gerbic C, Jackson J, Stellato T, Willson JKV. Growth stimulation by coexpression of transforming growth factor α and epidermal growth factor-receptor in normal and adenomatous human colon epithelium. J Clin Invest 1990;86:356–362.

117. Karnes WE Jr, Walsh JH, Wu SV, et al. Autocrine stimulation of EGF receptors by TGF-α regulates autonomous proliferation of human colon cancer cells. Gastroenterology 1992;102(2):474–485.

118. Baselga J, Mendelsohn J, Cordon-Cardo C. Unpublished data.

119. Reiss M, Stash EB, Vellucci VF, Zhou Z. Activation of the autocrine transforming growth factor alpha pathway in human squamous carcinoma cells. Cancer Res 1991;51:6254–6262.

120. Lee M, Kris RM, Bellot F, et al. EGF receptor monoclonal antibodies inhibit the growth on non-small cell lung cancer in vitro and in vivo. Proc Am Assoc Cancer Res [Abstract 243] 1990;31:41.

121. Imanish K, Yamaguchi K, Kuranami M, Kyo E, Hozumi T, Abe K. Inhibition of growth of human lung adenocarcinoma cell lines by anti-transforming growth factor-α monoclonal antibody. JNCI 1989;81:220–223.

122. Holley RW. Control of growth of mammalian cells in cell culture. Nature 1975;258:487–492.

123. Pardee AB, Dubrow R, Hamlin JL, Kletzien RF. Animal cell cycle. Annu Rev Biochem 1978;47:715.

124. Vande Woude GF, Schulz N, Zhou R, et al. Cell cycle regulation, oncogenes, and antineoplastic drugs. In: Fortner J, Rhoads JE, eds. Accomplishments in cancer research. Philadelphia: JB Lippincott, 1990;129–143.

125. Kawamoto T, Sato JD, Le A, Polikoff J, Sato GH, Mendelsohn J. Growth stimulation of A431 cells by EGF: Identification of high affinity receptors for epidermal growth factor by an anti-receptor monoclonal antibody. Proc Natl Acad Sci USA 1983;80:1337–1341.

126. Sato JD, Kawamoto T, Le AD, Mendelsohn J, Polikoff J, Sato GH. Biological effect in vitro of monoclonal antibodies to human EGF receptors. Mol Biol Med 1983;1:511–529.

127. Rodeck U, Herlyn M, Herlyn D, et al. Tumor growth modulation by a monoclonal antibody to the epidermal growth factor receptor: Immunologically mediated and effector cell-independent effects. Cancer Res 1987;47:3692–3696.

128. Rodeck U, Williams N, Murthy U, Herlyn M. Monoclonal antibody 425 inhibits growth stimulation of carcinoma cells by exogenous EGF and tumor-derived EGF/TGF-α. J Cell Biochem 1990;44:69–79.

129. Aboud-Pirak E, Hurwitz E, Pirak ME, Bellot F, Schlessinger J, Sela M. Efficacy of antibodies to epidermal growth factor receptor against KB carcinoma in vitro and in nude mice. JNCI 1988;80:1605–1611.

130. Mendelsohn J. Potential clinical applications of anti-EGF receptor monoclonal antibodies. In: Furth M, Greaves M, eds. The molecular diagnostics of human cancer, vol 7. Cold Spring Harbor, NY: Cold Spring Harbor Laboratory Press, 1989:359–362.

131. Masui H, Boman B, Hyman J, Castro L, Mendelsohn J: Treatment with anti-EGF receptor monoclonal antibody causes regression of DiFi human colorectal carcinoma xenografts. Proc Am Assoc Cancer Res [Abstract 2340] 1991;32:394.

132. Brady LW, Woo DV, Marko A, et al. Treatment of malignant gliomas with ^{125}I-labeled monoclonal antibody against epidermal growth factor receptor. Antibody Immunoconj Radiopharmaceut 1990;3:169–179.

133. Kalofonos HP, Pawlikowska TR, Hemingway A, et al. Antibody guided diagnosis and therapy of brain gliomas using radiolabeled monoclonal antibodies against epidermal growth factor receptor and placental alkaline phosphatase. J Nucl Med 1989;30:1636–1645.

134. Divgi CR, Welt C, Kris M, et al. Phase I and imaging trial of indium-111 labeled anti-EGF receptor monoclonal antibody 225 in patients with squamous cell lung carcinoma. JNCI 1991;83:97–104.

135. Schecter AL, Stern DF, Vaidyanathan L, Decker SJ. The NEU oncogene: An *ERBB*-related gene encoding a 185,000 Mr tumour antigen. Nature 1984;312:513–516.

136. Huziak RM, Schlessinger J, Ullrich A. Increased expression of the putative growth factor receptor p 185 (HER2) causes transformation and tumorigenesis of NIH3T3 cells. Proc Natl Acad Sci USA 1987;84:7159–7163.

137. Coussens L, Yang-Feng TL, Liao YC, et al. Tyrosine kinase receptor with extensive homology to EGF receptor shares chromosomal location with the NEU oncogene. Science 1985;230:1130–1139.

138. Fukushige SI, Matsubaru K, Yoshida M. Localization of a novel v-*ERBB*-related gene, c-*ERBB*-2 on chromosome-17 and its amplification in a gastric cell line. Mol Cell Biol 1986;6:955–958.

139. Yamamoto T, Ikawa S, Akiyama T, et al. Similarity of protein encoded by the human c-*ERBB*-2 gene to epidermal growth factor receptor. Nature 1986;319:230–234.

140. Schechter AL, Stern DF, Vaidyanathan L. An *ERBB* related gene encoding a 185,000-Mr tumor antigen. Nature 1984;312:513–516.

141. Semba K, Kamata N, Toyoshima K, Yamamoto T. V-*ERBB* related protooncogenes, c-*ERBB*-2, is distinct from the c-*ERBB*-1/epidermal growth factor-receptor gene and is amplified in human salivary gland adenocarcinoma. Proc Natl Acad Sci USA 1985;82:6497–6501.

142. Muller W, Sinn E, Patengale P, Wallace R, Leder P. Single-step induction of mammary adenocarcinoma in transgenic mice bearing the activated c-*NEU* oncogene. Cell 1988;54:105–115.

143. Bouchard L, Lamarre L, Tremblay P, Jolicoeur P. Stochastic appearance of mammary tumors in transgenic mice carrying the *MMTV/c-NEU* oncogene. Cell 1989;57:931–936.

144. DiFiore PP, Pierce JH, Kraus MH, Segatto O, King CR, Aaronson SA. *ErbB-2* is a potent oncogene when overexpressed in NIH/3T3 cells. Science 1986;237:178–182.

145. Slamon DJ, Clark GM, Wong SG, Levin WJ, Ullrich A, McGuire WL. Human breast cancer correlation of relapse and survival with amplification of the *HER-2/NEU* oncogene. Science 1987;235:177–182.

146. Paik S, Fisher ER, Fisher B, et al. Pathological findings from National Surgical Adjuvant Breast Project (protocol B-06), prognosis significance of ERBB-2 protein overexpression in primary breast cancer. J Clin Oncol 1990;8:103–112.

147. Shih C, Padhy L, Murray M, Weinberg RA. Transforming genes of carcinoma and neuroblastomas introduced into mouse fibroblasts. Nature 1981;290:261–264.

148. Bargamann CI, Hung MC, Weinberg RA. Transforming genes of carcinoma and neuroblastomas introduced into mouse fibroblasts. Nature 1986;319:226–230.

149. Segatto O, King CR, Pierce JH, DiFiore PP, Aaronson SA. Different structural alterations upregulate in vitro tyrosine kinase activity and transforming potency of the *ERBB-2* gene. Mol Cell Biol 1988;8:5570–5574.

150. Hancock MC, Langton BC, Chan T, et al. A monoclonal antibody against c-ERB 132 protein enhances the cytotoxicity of *cis*-diaminine dichoroplatinum against human breast and Oranian tumor cell lines. Cancer Res 1991;51:4575–4580.

151. Wiltschke C, Tyl E, Steininger A, et al. Increased NK-cell activity correlates with low or negative expression of the *HER-2/NEU* oncogene in breast cancer patients. Proc Am Assoc Cancer Res 1991;32:203.

152. Borg A, Baldetorp B, Ferno M, Killander D, Olsson H, Sigurdsson H. *ERBB2* amplification in breast cancer with a high rate of proliferation. Oncogene 1991;6:137–143.

153. Nicholson S, Wright C, Sainsbury RC, et al. Epidermal growth factor receptor (EGFr) as a marker for poor prognosis in node-negative breast cancer patients: *Neu* and tamoxifen failure. J Steroid Biochem Mol Biol 1990;37:811–814.

154. Yokota J, Yamamoto T, Toyoshima K, et al. Amplification of c-*ERBB* oncogene in human adenocarcinoma in vivo. Lancet 1986;1:765–767.

155. Hudziak R, Lewis G, Winget M, Fendly B, Shepard H, Ullrich A. P185HER2 monoclonal antibody has antiproliferative effects in vitro and sensitizes human breast tumor cells to tumor necrosis factor. Mol Cell Biol 1989;9:1165–1172.

156. Drebin J, Link V, Stern D, Weinberg R, Greene M. Down-modulation of an oncogene protein product and reversion of the transformed phenotype by monoclonal antibodies. Cell 1985;41:695–706.

157. Lupu R, Colomer R, Zugmaier G, Shepard M, Slamon D, Lippman ME. Direct interaction of a ligand for the ERBB2 oncogene product with the EGF receptor and p185ERBB2. Science 1990;249:1552–1555.

158. Lupu R, Colomer R, Kannan B, Lippman ME. Characterization of a growth factor that binds exclusively to the ERBB2 receptor and induces cellular responses. Proc Natl Acad Sci USA 1992;89:2287–2291.

159. Kumar R, Shephard HM, Mendelsohn J: Regulation of phosphorylation of the c-*ERBB2/HER2* gene product by a monoclonal antibody and serum growth factor(s) in human mammary carcinoma cells. Mol Cell Biol 1991;11:979–986.

160. Lax I, Bellot F, How K, Ullrich A, Givol D, Schlessinger J. Functional analysis of the ligand binding site of EGF-receptor utilizing chimeric receptor. EMBO J 1989;8:167–173.

161. Lupu R, Wellstein A, Sheridan J, et al. A novel biologically active polypeptide structurally and functionally related to TGFα: Purification and characterization. Biochem 1992 (in press).

162. Raines EW, Bowen-Pope DF, Ross R. Platelet-derived growth factor. In: Sporn MB, Roberts AB, eds. Peptide growth factors and their receptors, vol I. Berlin: Springer-Verlag, 1990:174–262.

163. Betsholtz C, Johnsson A, Heldin C-H, et al. cDNA sequence and chromosomal localization of human platelet-derived growth factor A-chain and its expression in tumour cell lines. Nature 1986;320:695–699.

164. Heldin C-H, Backstrom G, Ostman A, et al. Binding of different dimeric forms of PDGF to human fibroblasts: Evidence for two separate receptor types. EMBO J 1988;7:1387–1394.

165. Yarden Y, Escobedo JA, Kuang W-J, et al. Structure of the receptor for platelet-derived growth factor helps define a family of closely related growth factor receptors. Nature 1986;323:226–232.

166. Cochran BH, Reffel AC, Stiles CD. Molecular cloning of gene sequences regulated by platelet-derived growth factor. Cell 1983;33:939–947.

167. Almendral JM, Sommer D, MacDonal-Bravo H, et al. Complexity of the early genetic response to growth factors in mouse fibroblasts. Mol Cell Biol 1988;8:2140–2148.

168. Ross R. The pathogenesis of atherosclerosis: An update. N Engl J Med 1986;314:488–500.

169. Clarke MF, Westin E, Schmidt D, et al. Transformation of NIH 3T3 cells by a human c-*sis* cDNA clone. Nature 1984;308:464–467.

170. Gazit A, Igarashi H, Chiu I-M, et al. Expression of the normal human *sis/PDGF* coding sequence induces cellular transformation. Cell 1984;39:80–97.

171. Beckmann MP, Betsholtz C, Heldin C-H, et al. Human PDGF-A and -B chains differ in their biological properties and transforming potential. Science 1988;241:1346–1349.

172. Rozengurt E, Sinnett-Smith J, Taylor-Papadimitriou J. Production of PDGF-like growth factor by breast cancer cell lines. Int J Cancer 1985;36:247–252.

173. Pledger WJ, Stiles CD, Antoniades HN, Scher CD. Induction of DNA synthesis in BALB/c 3T3 cells by serum complements: Reevaluation of the commitment process. Proc Natl Acad Sci USA 1977;74:4481–4485.

174. Pledger WJ, Stiles CD, Antoniades HN, Scher CD. An ordered sequence of events is required before BALB/c 3T3 cells become committed to DNA synthesis. Proc Natl Acad Sci USA 1978;75:2839–2843.

175. Blundell TL, Humbel RE. Hormone families: Pancreatic hormones and homologous growth factors. Nature 1980;287:781–787.

176. Baxter TL. The somatomedins: Insulin-like growth factors. Adv Clin Chem 1986;25: 49–115.

177. Nissley SP, Rechler MM. Insulin-like growth factors: Biosynthesis, receptors, and carrier proteins. Horm Proteins Peptides 1986;12:127–203.

178. Rinderknecht E, Humbel RE. The amino acid sequence of human insulin-like growth factor I and its structural homology with proinsulin. J Biol Chem 1978;253:2769–2776.

179. Rinderknecht E, Humbel RE. Primary structure of human insulin-like growth factor II. FEBS Lett 1978;89:283–286.

180. Mathews LS, Norstedt G, Palmiter RD. Regulation of insulin-like growth factor I gene expression by growth hormone. Proc Natl Acad Sci USA 1988;83:9343–9347.

181. Han VKM, Lund PK, Lee DC, D'Ercole AJ. Expression of somatomedin/insulin-like growth factor messenger ribonucleic acids in the human fetus: Identification, characterization, and tissue distribution. J Clin Endocrinol Metab 1988;66:422–429.

182. Zapf J, Froesch VR. Insulin-like growth factors/somatomedins: Structure, secretion, biological actions and physiological roles. Horm Res 1986;24:121–130.

183. Ullrich A, Gray A, Tam AW, et al. Insulin-like growth factor I receptor primary structure: Comparison with insulin receptor suggests structural determinants that define hormonal specificity. EMBO J 1986;5:2503–2512.

184. Massagué J, Czech MP. The subunit structures of two distinct receptors for insulin-like growth factors I and II and their relationship to the insulin receptor. J Biol Chem 1982;257:5038–5045.

185. Morgan DO, Edman JC, Standring DN, et al. Insulin-like growth factor II receptor as a multifunctional binding protein. Nature 1987;329:301–307.

186. Fraddin JE, Eastman RC, Lesniak MA, Roth J. Specificity spillover at the hormone receptor—exploring its role in human disease. N Engl J Med 1989;320:640–645.

187. Ewton DZ, Falen SL, Florini JR. The type II insulin-like growth factor (IGF) receptor has low affinity for IGF analogs: Pleiotypic action of IGFs on myoblast are apparently mediated by the type I receptor. Endocrinology 1987;120:115–123.

188. Rosenfeld RG, Conover CA, Hodges D, et al. Heterogeneity of insulin-like growth factor-I affinity for the insulin-like growth factor-II receptor: Comparison of natural, synthetic and recombinant DNA-derived insulin-like growth factor-I. Biochem Biophys Res Comm 1987;143:199–205.

189. MacDonald RG, Tepper MA, Clairmont KB, Perreaux SB, Czech MP. Serum form of the rat insulin-like growth factor II/mannose 6-phosphate receptor is truncated in the carboxyl-terminal domain. J Biol Chem 1989;264:3256–3261.

190. Gelato MC, Kiess W, Lee L. The insulin-like growth factor II/mannose-6-phosphate receptor is present in monkey serum. J Clin Endocrinol Metab 1988;67:669–675.

191. Causin C, Waheed A, Braulke T, et al. Mannose 6-phosphate/ insulin-like growth factor II-binding proteins in human serum and urine—their relation to the mannose 6-phosphate/insulin-like growth factor II receptor. Biochem J 1988;252:795–799.

192. Baxter RC, Martin JL. Binding proteins for the insulin-like growth factors: Structure, regulation and function. Prog Growth Factor Res 1989;1:49–68.

193. Cohen KL, Nissley SP. The serum half-life of somatomedin activity: Evidence for growth hormone dependence. Acta Endocrinol 1976;83:243–258.

194. Yee D, Cullen KJ, Paik S, et al. Insulin-like growth factor II mRNA expression in human breast cancer. Cancer Res 1988;48:6691–6696.

195. Karey KP, Sirbasku DA. Differential responsiveness of human breast cancer cell lines MDF-7 and t47D to growth factors and 17β estradiol. Cancer Res 1988;48:4083–4092.

196. Hoopener JWM, Mosselman S, Roholl PJM. Expression of insulin-like growth I and II genes in human smooth muscle tumours. EMBO J 1988;7:1379–1385.

197. Tricoli JV, Rall LB, Karakousis CP. Enhanced levels of insulin-like growth factor messenger RNA in human colon carcinomas and liposarcomas. Cancer Res 1986;46:6169–6173.

198. Reeve AE, Eccles MR, Wilkins RJ, Bell GI, Millow LJ. Expression of insulin-like growth factor II transcripts in Wilms' tumor. Nature 1985;317:258–260.

199. Scott J, Cowell J, Robertson ME, et al. Insulin-like growth factor II gene expression in Wilms' tumour and embryonic tissues. Nature 1985;317:260–262.

200. Yee D, Paik S, Lebovic G, et al. Analysis of IGF-I gene expression in malignancy—evidence for a paracrine role in human breast cancer. Mol Endocrinol 1989;3:509–517.

201. Cullen KJ, Yee D, Sly WS, Perdue J, Hampton B, Lippman ME, Rosen N. Insulin-like growth factor receptor expression and function in human breast cancer. Cancer Res 1990;50:48–53.

202. Osborne CK, Coronado EB, Kitten LJ, et al. Insulin-like growth factor-II (IGF-II): A potential autocrine/paracrine growth factor for human breast cancer acting via the IGF-I receptor. Mol Endocrinol 1989;3:1701–1709.

203. Folkman J. What is the evidence that tumors are angiogenesis dependent? JNCI 1990;82: 4–6.

204. Folkman J, Klagsbrun M. Angiogenic factors. Science 1987;235:442–447.

205. Gross J, Moscatell D, Rifkin D. Increased capillary endothelial cell protease activity in response to angiogenic stimuli in vitro. Proc Natl Acad Sci USA 1983;80:2623–2627.

206. Ausprunk D, Folkman J. Migration and proliferation of endothelial cells in preformed and newly formed blood vessels during tumor angiogenesis. Microvasc Res 1977;14: 53–65.

207. Zetter B. Migration of capillary endothelial cells is stimulated by tumour-derived factors. Nature 1980;285:41–43.

208. Azizkhan R, Azizkhan J, Zetter B, Folkman J. Mast cell heparin stimulates migration of capillary endothelial cells in vitro. J Exper Med 1980;152:931–944.

209. Birdwell C, Gospodarowicz D, Nicolson G. Factors from 3T3 cells stimulate proliferation of cultured vascular endothelial cells. Nature 1977;268:528–531.

210. Gospodarowicz D, Moran J, Braun D, Birdwell C. Clonal growth of bovine vascular endothelial cells: Fibroblast growth factor as a survival agent. Proc Natl Acad Sci USA 1976;73:4120–4124.

211. Folkman J, Haudenschild C, Zetter B. Long-term culture of capillary endothelial cells. Proc Natl Acad Sci USA 1979;76:5217–5221.

212. Folkman J, Haudenschild C. Angiogenesis in vitro. Nature 1980;288:551–556.

213. Algire G, Chalkley H, Legallais F, Park H. Vascular reaction of normal and malignant tumors in vivo. I. Vascular reactions of mice to wounds and to normal and neoplastic transplants. JNCI 1945;6:73–85.

214. Gimbrone M, Leapman S, Coran R, Folkman J. Tumor dormancy in vivo by prevention of neovascularization. J Exp Med 1972;136:261–276.

215. Knighton D, Ausprunk D, Tapper D, Folkman J. Avascular and vascular phases of tumour growth in the chick embryo. Br J Cancer 1977;35:347–356.

216. Nicosia R, Tchao R, Leighton J. Angiogenesis-dependent tumor spread in reinforced fibrin clot culture. Cancer Res 1983;43:2159–2166.

217. Folkman J. Angiogenesis and its inhibitors. In: DeVita V, Hellman S, Rosenberg S, eds. Important advances in oncology 1985. Philadelphia: JB Lippincott, 1985: 42–62.

218. Liotta L, Kleinerman J, Saidel G. The significance of hematogenous tumor cell clumps in the metastatic process. Cancer Res 1976;36:889–894.

219. Liotta L, Kleinerman J, Saidel G. Quantitative relationships of intravascular tumor cells, tumor vessels, and pulmonary metastases following tumor implantation. Cancer Res 1974;34:997–1004.

220. Nagy J, Brown L, Senger D, et al. Pathogenesis of tumor stroma generation: A critical role for leaky blood vessels and fibrin deposition. Biochem Biophys Acta 1988;948: 305–326.

221. Folkman J, Watson K, Ingber D, Hanahan D. Induction of angiogenesis during the transition from hyperplasia to neoplasia. Nature 1989;339:58–61.

222. Silman F, Boyce J, Fruchter R. The significance of atypical vessels and neovascularization in cervical neoplasia. Am J Obstet Gynecol 1981;139:154–159.

223. Srivastava A, Laidler P, Hughes L, Woodcock J, Shedden E. Neovascularization in human cutaneous melanoma: A quantitative morphological and Doppler ultrasound study. Eur J Cancer Clin Oncol 1986;22:1205–1209.

224. Chodak G, Haudenschild C, Gittes R, Folkman J. Angiogenic activity as a marker of neoplastic and preneoplastic lesions of the human bladder. Ann Surg 1980;192: 762–771.

225. Jensen H, Chen I, DeVault M, Lewis A. Angiogenesis induced by "normal" human breast tissue: A probable marker for precancer. Science 1982;218:293–295.

226. Brem S, Jenson H, Gullino P. Angiogenesis as a marker for preneoplastic lesions of the human breast. Cancer 1978;41:239–244.

227. Brem S, Gullino P, Medina D. Angiogenesis: A marker for neoplastic transformation of mammary papillary hyperplasia. Science 1977;195:880–882.

228. Jensen H. Angiogenesis induced by normal human breast tissue. In: Rifkin D, Klagsbrun M, eds. Angiogenesis—mechanisms and pathology. Current communications in molecular biology. Cold Spring Harbor, NY: Cold Spring Harbor Laboratory, 1987:155–157.

229. Weidner N, Semple J, Welch W, Folkman J. Tumor angiogenesis and metastasis-correlation in invasive breast carcinoma. N Engl J Med 1991;324:1–8.

230. Srivastava A, Laidler P, Davies R, Horgan K, Hughes L. The prognostic significance of tumor vascularity in intermediate-thickness (0.76–1.0 mm thick) skin melanoma. Am J Pathol 1988;133:419–423.

231. Breslow A. Thickness cross sectional areas and depth of invasion in the prognosis of cutaneous melanoma. Ann Surg 1970;172:902–908.

232. Burgess W, Maciag T. The heparin-binding (fibroblast) growth factor family of proteins. Annu Rev Biochem 1989;58:575–606.

233. Baird A, Klagsbrun M. The fibroblast growth factor family. Cancer Cells 1991;3:239–243.

234. Li YS, Milner PG, Chauhan AK, et al. Cloning and expression of a developmentally regulated protein that induces mitogenic and neurite outgrowth activity. Science 1990;250:1690–1694.

235. Merenmies J, Rauvala H. Molecular cloning of the 18-kDa growth-associated protein of developing brain. J Biol Chem 1990;265:16721–16724.

236. Wellstein A, Fang WJ, Khatri A, et al. A heparin-binding growth factor secreted from breast cancer cells homologous to a developmentally regulated cytokine. J Biol Chem 1992;269(4):2582–2587.

237. Sato Y, Rifkin D. Autocrine activities of basic fibroblast growth factor: Regulation of endothelial cell movement, plasminogen activator synthesis and DNA synthesis. J Cell Biol 1988;107:1199–1205.

238. Rifkin D, Moscatelli D. Recent developments in the cell biology of basic fibroblast growth factor. J Cell Biol 1989;109:1–6.

239. Thompson J, Haudenschild C, Anderson K, DiPietro J, Anderson WF, Maciag T. Heparin-binding growth factor 1 induces the formation of organoid neovascular structures in vivo. Proc Natl Acad Sci USA 1989;86:7928–7932.

240. Yamanishi H, Nonomura N, Tanaka A, et al. Proliferation of Shionogi carcinoma 115 cells by glucocorticoid-induced autocrine heparin-binding growth factors in serum-free medium. Cancer Res 1991;51:3006–3010.

241. Blam S, Mitchell R, Tischer E, Rubin J, Siva M, Silver S, Fiddes J, Abraham J, Aaronson S. Addition of growth hormone secretion signal to basic fibroblast growth factor results in cell transformation and secretion of aberrant forms of the protein. Oncogene 1988;3: 129–136.

242. Neufeld G, Mitchell R, Ponte R, Gospodarowicz D. Expression of human basic fibroblast growth factor cDNA in baby hamster kidney-derived cells results in autonomous cell growth. J Cell Biol 1988;106:1385–1394.

243. Wellstein A, Lupu R, Zugmaier G, et al. Autocrine growth stimulation by secreted Kaposi fibroblast growth factor but not by endogenous basic fibroblast growth factor. Cell Growth Differ 1990;1:63–71.

244. Hanneken A, Lutty G, McLeod D, Robey F, Harvey A, Hjelmeland L. Localization of basic fibroblast growth factor to the developing capillaries of the bovine retina. J Cell Physiol 1989;138:115–120.

245. Lobb R, Harper J, Fett J. Purification of heparin-binding growth factors. Anal Biochem 1986;154:1–14.

246. Herbert J, Cottineau M, Driot F, Pereillo J, Maffrand J. Activity of pentosan polysulfate and derived compounds on vascular endothelial cell proliferation and migration induced by acidic and basic FGF in vitro. Biochem Pharmacol 1988;37:4281–4288.

247. Thomas K, Rios-Candelore M, Gimenez-Gallego G, DiSalvo J, Bennett C, Rodkey J, Fitzpatrick S. Pure brain-derived acidic fibroblast growth factor is a potent angiogenic vascular endothelial cell mitogen with sequence homology to interleukin 1. Proc Natl Acad Sci USA 1985;82:6409–6413.

248. Lobb R, Alderman E, Fett J. Induction of angiogenesis by bovine brain-derived class 1 heparin-binding growth factor. Biochemistry 1985;24:4969–4973.

249. Taylor S, Folkman J. Protamine is an inhibitor of angiogenesis. Nature 1982;297: 307–312.

250. Wellstein A, Zugmaier G, Califano J, Broder S, Lippman M. Xylanpolyhydro-gensulfate inhibits fibroblast growth factor dependent growth of human tumor cells. Proc Am Assoc Cancer Res [Abstract 2320] 1989;30:583.

251. Paul R, Herbert J, Maffrand J, et al. Inhibition of vascular smooth muscle cell proliferation in culture by pentosan polysulfate and related compound. Thromb Res 1987;46: 793–801.

252. Kobayashi M, Yamashita T, Tsubura E. Inhibition of blood-borne pulmonary metastasis by sulfated polysaccharides. Tokushima J Exp Med 1979;26:41–51.

253. Huang J, Huang S, Kuo M. Bovine brain-derived growth factor: Purification and characterization of its interaction with responsive cells. J Biol Chem 1986;261:11600–11607.

254. Coffey R, Leci E, Shipley G, Moses H. Suramin inhibition of growth factor receptor binding and mitogenicity in AKR-2B cells. J Cell Physiol 1987;132:143–148.

255. Garrett J, Coughlin S, Niman H, Tremble P, Gleis G, Williams L. Blockade of autocrine stimulation in simian sarcoma virus-transformed cells reverses down-regulation of platelet-derived growth factor receptors. Proc Natl Acad Sci USA 1984;81:7466–7470.

256. Betsholtz C, Johnsson A, Heldin C, Westermark B. Efficient reversion of simian sarcoma virus-transformation and inhibition of growth factor-induced mitogenesis by suramin. Proc Natl Acad Sci USA 1986;83:6440–6444.

257. Calcaterra N, Vicario L, Roveri O. Inhibition by suramin of mitochondrial ATP synthesis. Biochem Pharmacol 1988;37:2521–2527.

258. Taylor S, Folkman J. Protamine is an inhibitor of angiogenesis. Nature 1982;297: 307–312.

259. Neufeld G, Gospodarowicz D. Protamine sulfate inhibits mitogenic activities of the extracellular matrix and fibroblast growth factor, but potentiates that of epidermal growth factor. J Cell Physiol 1987;132:287–294.

260. Inoue K, Korenaga H, Tanaka N, Sakamoto N, Kadoya S. The sulfated polysaccharide-peptidoglycan complex potently inhibits embryonic angiogenesis and tumor growth in the presence of cortisone acetate. Carbohydrate Res 1988;181:135–142.

261. Tanaka N, Sakamoto N, Inoue K, et al. Antitumor effects of an antiangiogenic polysaccharide form an *Arthrobacter* species with or without a steroid. Cancer Res 1989;49: 6727–6730.

262. Maione T, Gray G, Petro J, et al. Inhibition of angiogenesis by recombinant human platelet-factor-4 and related peptides. Science 1990;247:77–79.

263. Sharpe R, Byers H, Scott C, Bauer S, Maione T. Growth inhibition of murine melanoma and human colon carcinoma by recombinant human platelet-4. JNCI 1990;82:848–853.

264. Ingber D, Fujita T, Kishimoto S, et al. Synthetic analogs of fumagillin that inhibit angiogenesis and suppress tumor growth. Nature 1990;348:555–557.

265. Kusaka M, Sudo K, Fujita T, et al. Potent anti-angiogenic action of AGM-1470: Comparison to the fumagillin parent. Biochem Biophys Res Commun 1991;174:1070–1076.

266. MacGregor I, Dawes J, Pepper D, Prowse C, Stocks J. Metabolism of sodium pentosan polysulphate in man measured by a new competitive binding assay for sulphated polysaccharides comparison with effects upon anticoagulant activity, lipolysis, and platelet alpha-granule proteins. Thromb Haemost 1985;53:411–414.

267. Hughes L. Treatment of malignant disease with protamine sulfate. Lancet 1964;1: 408–409.

268. Levi-Montalcini R, Hamburger V. Selective growth stimulating effects of mouse sarcoma on the sensory and sympathetic nervous system of the chick embryo. J Exp Zool 1951;123:233–287.

269. Levi-Montalcini R. The nerve growth factor 35 years later. Science 1987;237:1154–1162.

270. Cordon-Cardo C, Tapley P, Jing S, et al. The *TRK* tyrosine protein kinase mediates the mitogenic properties of nerve growth factor and neurotrophin-3. Cell 1991;66: 173–183.

271. Martin-Zanca D, Hughes SH, Barbacid M. A human oncogene formed by the fusion of truncated tropomyosin and protein tyrosine kinase sequences. Nature 1986;319:743–748.

272. Lebacq-Verheyden A-M, Trepel J, Sausville EA, Battey JF. Bombesin and gastrin-releasing peptide: Neuropeptides, secretogogues, and growth factors. In: Sporn MB, Roberts AB, eds. Peptide growth factors and their receptors, vol II. Berlin: Springer-Verlag, 1990;71–124.

273. Carney DN, Bunn PA, Gazdar AF, et al. Selective growth in serum-free hormone-supplemented medium of tumor cells obtained by biopsy from patients with small cell carcinoma of the lung. Proc Natl Acad Sci USA 1981;78:3186–3189.

274. Cuttitta F, Carney DN, Mulshine J, et al. Bombesin-like peptides can function as autocrine growth factors in human small-cell lung cancer. Nature 1985;316:823–826.

275. Rozengurt E, Sinnett-Smith J. Bombesin stimulation of DNA synthesis and cell division in cultures of Swiss 3T3 cells. Proc Natl Acad Sci USA 1983;80:2936–2940.

276. Sporn MB, Roberts AB. Transforming growth factor-β: Multiple actions and potential clinical applications. JAMA 1989;262:938–941.

277. Lyons RM, Moses HL. Transforming growth factors and the regulation of cell proliferation. Eur J Biochem 1990;187:467–473.

278. Derynck R, Jarrett JA, Chen EY, et al. Human transforming growth factor—β complementary DNA sequence and expression in normal and transformed cells. Nature 1985;316:701–705.

279. Assoian RK, Komoriya A, Meyers CA, Miller DM, Sporn MB. Transforming growth factor-β in human platelets. J Biol Chem 1983;258:7155–7160.

280. Gentry LE, Lioubin MN, Purchio AP, Marquardt H. Molecular events in the processing of recombinant type 1 pre-pro-transforming growth factor beta to the mature polypeptide. Mol Cell Biol 1988;8:4162–4168.

281. Kimchi, A, Wang X-F, Weinberg RA, Cheifetz S, Massagué J. Absence of TGF-β receptors and growth inhibitory responses in retinoblastoma cells. Science 1988;240:196–198.

282. Shipley GD, Tucker RF, Moses HL. Type β-transforming growth factor/ growth inhibitor stimulates entry of monolayer cultures of AKR-2B cells into S-phase after prolonged prereplicative interval. Proc Natl Acad Sci USA 1985;82:4147–4151.

283. Laiho M, DeCaprio JA, Ludlow JW, Livingston DM, Massagué J. Growth inhibition by TGF-β linked to suppression of retinoblastoma protein phosphorylation. Cell 1990;62: 175–185.

284. Kehrl JH, Wakefield LM, Roberts AB, et al. Production of transforming growth factor beta by human T lymphocytes and its potential role in the regulation of T cell growth. J Exp Med 1986;163:1037–1050.

285. Leof EB, Proper JA, Goustin AS, Shipley GD, DiCorleto, PE, Moses HL. Induction of c-*SIS* mRNA and activity similar to platelet-derived growth factor β: A proposed model for indirect mitogenesis involving autocrine activity. Proc Natl Acad Sci USA 1986;83: 2453–2457.

286. Pietenpol JA, Stein RW, Moran E, et al. TGF-β1 inhibition of c-*MYC* transcription and growth in keratinocytes is abrogated by viral transforming proteins with pRB binding domains. Cell 1990;61:777–785.

287. Vale W, Hsueh A, Rivier C, Yu J. The inhibin/activin family of hormones and growth factors. In: Sporn MB, Roberts AB, eds. Peptide growth factors and their receptors, vol II. Berlin: Springer-Verlag, 1990;211–248.

288. Burger HG, Igarashi M. Inhibin: Definition and nomenclature, including related substances. J Clin Endocrinol Metab [Letter] 1988;66:885–886.

289. Cate RL, Donahoe PK, MacLaughlin DT. Müllerian-inhibiting substance. In: Sporn MB, Roberts AB, eds. Peptide growth factors and their receptors, vol II. Berlin: Springer-Verlag, 1990;179–210.

290. Donohoe PK, Fuller AF Jr, Scully RE, Guy Sr, Budzik GP. Müllerian inhibiting substance inhibits growth of a human ovarian cancer in nude mice. Ann Surg 1981;194:472–480.

291. Fuller AF Jr, Guy Sr, Budzik GP, Donohoe PK. Müllerian-inhibiting substance inhibits colony growth of a human ovarian carcinoma cell line. J Clin Endocrinol Metab 1982;54: 1051–1055.

292. Ervin PR, Kaminski MS, Cody RL, Wicha MS. Production of mammastatin, a tissue-specific growth inhibitor, by normal human mammary cells. Science 1989;244:1585–1587.

293. Isaacs A, Lindenmann J. Virus interference. I. The interferon. Proc R Soc Lond [Biol] 1957;147:258–267.

294. Vilček J. Interferons. In: Sporn MB, Roberts AB, eds. Peptide growth factors and their receptors, vol II. Berlin: Springer-Verlag, 1990:3–38.

295. Sen GC, Lengyel P. The interferon system. J Biol Chem. 1992;267:5017–5020.

296. Chebath J, Benech P, Hovanessian A, Galabru J, Revel M. Four different forms of interferon-induced 2′,5′-oligo(a) synthetase identified by immunoblotting in human cells. J Biol Chem 1987; 262:3852–3857.

297. Old LJ. Tumor necrosis factor. Sci Am 1988;258:59–75.

298. Beutler B. Cachetin/tumor necrosis factor and lymphotoxin. In: Sporn MB, Roberts AB, eds. Peptide growth factors and their receptors, vol II. Berlin: Springer-Verlag, 1990:39–70.

299. Spriggs DR. Tumor necrosis factor: Basic principles and preclinical studies. In: DeVita VT Jr, Hellman S, Rosenberg SA, eds. Biologic therapy of cancer. Philadelphia: JB Lippincott, 1991.

300. Mendelsohn J. Growth factor receptors as targets for antitumor therapy with monoclonal antibodies. In: Waldmann H, ed. Monoclonal antibody therapy, vol 45. Prog Allergy. Basel: Karger, 1988:147–160.

301. Siegall CB, Epstein S, Speir E, Hla T, Forough R, Maciag T, Fitsgerald DJ, Pastan I. Cytotoxic activity of chimeric proteins composed of acidic fibroblast growth factor and *Pseudomonas* exotoxin on a variety of cell types. FASEB J 1991;5:2843–2849.

302. Waldmann TA, Grant A, Tendler C, et al. Lymphokine receptor-directed therapy: A model of immune intervention. J Clin Immun 1990;10:19S–29S.

303. Zugmaier G, Lippman ME. Effects of TGFβ on normal and malignant mammary epithelium. In: Diez KA, Sporn MB, eds. Transforming growth factor βs. Ann NY Acad Sci 1990;593:272–275.

304. Pastan I, Fitzgerald D. Recombinant toxins for cancer treatment. Science 1991;254: 1173–1177.

305. Castle V, Varani J, Fligiel S, Prochownik EV, Dixit V. Antisense-mediated reduction in thrombospondin reverses the malignant phenotype of a human squamous carcinoma. J Clin Invest 1991;87:1883–1888.

306. Stein CA, LaRocca RV, Thomas R, McAtee N, Myers CE. Suramin: An anticancer drug with a unique mechanism of action. J Clin Oncol 1989;7:499–508.

307. Tanaka NG, Sakamoto N, Korenaga H, Inoue K, Ogawa H, Osada Y. The combination of a bacterial polysaccharide and tamoxifen inhibits angiogenesis and tumour growth. Int J Radiat Biol 1991;60:79–83.

308. Dvir A, Milner Y, Chomsky O, Gilon C, Gazit A, Levitzki A. The inhibition of EGF-dependent proliferation of keratinocytes by tyrphostin tyrosine kinase blockers. J Cell Biol 1991;113:857–865.

Cancer: Principles & Practice of Oncology, Fourth Edition,
edited by Vincent T. DeVita, Jr., Samuel Hellman, Steven A. Rosenberg.
J.B. Lippincott Co., Philadelphia © 1993.

Lance A. Liotta
William G. Stetler-Stevenson

CHAPTER **8**

Principles of Molecular Cell Biology of Cancer: Cancer Metastasis

THE CLINICAL SIGNIFICANCE OF INVASION AND METASTASIS

Tumor invasion and metastasis is the major cause of treatment failure for cancer patients. About 30% of patients with newly diagnosed solid tumors (excluding skin cancers other than melanoma) already have clinically detectable metastases. Of those 70% of cancer patients who are clinically free of metastasis, about half can be cured by local tumor therapy alone.[1] The remaining patients have clinically occult micrometastases that ultimately become manifest. Thus, 60% of patients have microscopic or clinically evident metastases at the time of primary tumor treatment. Most patients suffer from multiple metastases. The formation of metastatic colonies is a continuous process commencing early in the growth of the primary tumor and increasing with time.[2–9] A few large identifiable metastases in a given organ frequently are accompanied by a greater number of micrometastases that were seeded more recently. The size and age variation in metastases, their dispersed anatomic location, and their heterogenous composition hinder surgical removal and limit the effective concentration of anticancer drugs that can be delivered to the metastatic colonies.[1–4] The patient with metastatic disease succumbs to the direct anatomic compromise caused by the metastasis or to complications associated with antimetastatic therapy.

Tumors of comparable size can have widely divergent metastatic potential depending on their intrinsic aggressiveness and histologic type.[3–5] For many common epithelial tumors,

the onset of tumor-cell dissemination occurs soon after primary tumor vascularization. It has been calculated that most metastases from breast carcinomas are initiated when the primary tumor is less than 0.125 cm^3, and this is in accord with experimental studies.[6–9] Fidler has shown that the subpopulation of highly metastatic tumor cells preexists at a very early stage in the development of the heterogenous primary tumor.[4] These highly aggressive cells may be selected out because they have a higher probability of successfully producing a metastatic colony compared with other subpopulations of primary tumor cells.

Although the clinical significance of the most insidious expression of the malignant phenotype has been well appreciated, advances in understanding the molecular mechanisms involved in metastasis formation have lagged behind other developments in the cancer field. Progress has been hindered by the sheer complexity of this multistep tumor-host interaction, which also includes angiogenesis and immunologic mechanisms. To tackle the problem, investigators have separated invasion and metastasis into a series of defined sequential steps and focused on one step at a time. For each step, new experimental models had to be developed, and a combined effort using the disciplines of cell biology, protein biochemistry, and molecular genetics has resulted in an explosion of new information. General themes are emerging that yield new strategies for prognosis and therapy of human metastatic cancer.

A group of coordinated cellular processes, not just one gene product, is responsible for metastasis. Furthermore, negative factors may be as important as positive elements (Fig. 8–1). Some genetic changes result in an imbalance of growth regulation, leading to uncontrolled proliferation. Unrestrained growth does not, by itself, result in invasion and metastasis. The latter phenotype may require additional genetic changes. Tumorigenicity and metastatic potential have overlapping and separate features. Invasion and metastasis can be facilitated by proteins that stimulate tumor-cell attachment to host cellular or extracellular matrix determinants, tumor-cell proteolysis of host barriers such as the basement membrane, tumor-cell locomotion, and tumor-cell colony formation in the target organ for metastasis. Facilitory proteins may act at many levels intracellularly or extracellularly but are counterbalanced by factors that can block their production, regulation, or action. A common theme has emerged: in addition to loss of growth control, an imbalanced regulation of motility and proteolysis appears to be required for invasion and metastasis. Moreover, these same functions are also necessary for angiogenesis. Angiogenesis by normal endothelial cells and metastasis by tumor cells are functionally linked but differ in terms of regulation.

HETEROGENEITY OF THE METASTATIC PHENOTYPE

During the last 10 years, neoplasms have become widely recognized as biologically heterogenous. At the time of diagnosis, most neoplasms consist of different populations of cells with diverse biologic characteristics. Subpopulations differ in immunogenicity, growth rates, karyotype, pigment production, hormone production, receptor content, and susceptibility to cytotoxic drugs. Fidler and Hart have emphasized that neoplasms can be heterogenous for the propensity to invade and metastasize and that the aggressive subpopulation may be selected out in the formation of metastasis.[4] The first experimental proof of metastatic heterogeneity was provided by Fidler and Kripke in 1977.[10] Working with the murine B16 melanoma, the investigators used a modified fluctuation assay

of Luria and Delbruck.[11] They discovered that preexisting subpopulations growing in the same tumor exhibit heterogenous metastatic potential.

The process of metastasis is not random. Instead, it is a cascade of linked sequential steps that must be traversed by tumor cells if a metastasis is to develop (Fig. 8–2, Table 8–1). Each step involves multiple tumor-host interactions. To be successful, a metastatic tumor cell must leave the primary tumor and invade local host tissue. It must then enter the circulation, survive in the circulation, arrest at the distant vascular bed, extravasate into the organ interstitium and parenchyma, and multiply to initiate a metastatic colony. Interruption of the metastatic cascade at any of these steps can prevent the production of clinically symptomatic metastasis. A large foundation of experimental work suggests that during each stage of metastasis the rules of "survival of the fittest" apply. Metastasis is thus the result of a highly selective competition favoring the survival of a minor subpopulation of metastatic cells that preexist within the primary neoplasm.

Fidler's subpopulation concept is well accepted, but the size of this subpopulation has remained a significant unknown. Estimating the size of the metastatic subpopulation is of clinical significance because a prognostic assay based on a sample of the primary tumor would be highly inaccurate if the aggressive subpopulation were only a very small proportion of the total number of the tumor cell sample. Many investigators were discouraged about studying metastasis when the metastatic subpopulation of the primary tumor appeared to be very low in abundance and fleeting in animal models.[12] However, those who questioned this dogma did not find significant evidence of a difference between the average metastatic propensity of cells in the primary tumor compared with its established metastasis. Recently, Kerbel has addressed the subpopulation question experimentally using genetic markers.[12] He determined that the metastatic subpopulation dominates the primary tumor mass early in its growth. The dominance may be due to selective growth of the metastatic subpopulation in response to local cytokines. Measurement of the average level of a molecular marker in a primary tumor

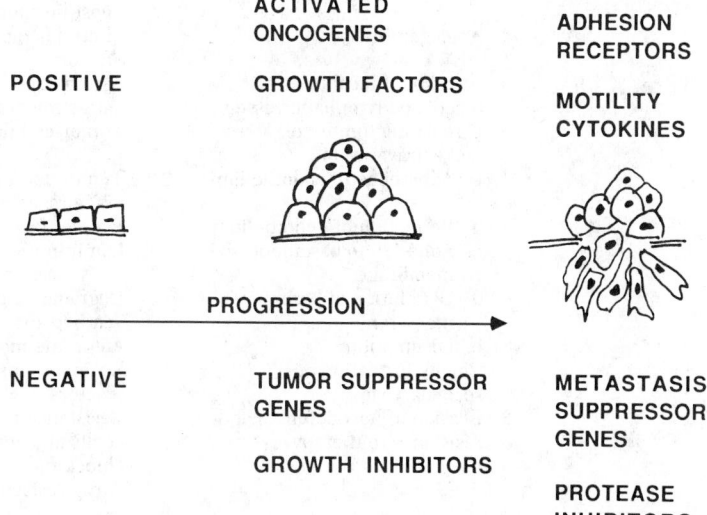

FIGURE 8–1. Positive and negative elements that regulate tumor progression from noninvasive to invasive carcinoma. Uncontrolled proliferation may result from the increase in growth factors or activated oncogenes or from the loss of growth inhibitors or suppressor oncogenes such as p53 or *RB*. Further progression to the invasive phenotype may involve the augmentation of gene products that facilitate invasion or the loss of proteins that suppress invasion.

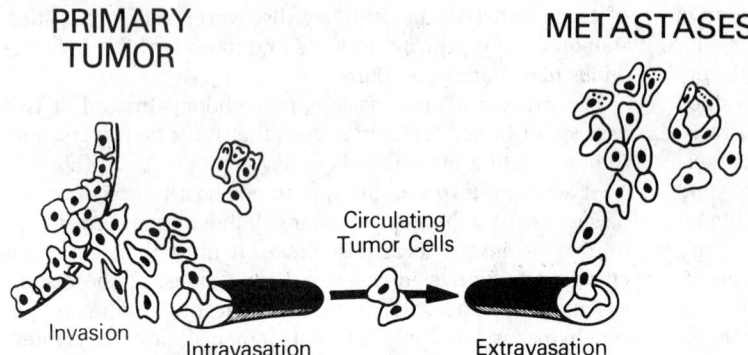

PRIMARY TUMOR

METASTASES

Circulating Tumor Cells

Invasion   Intravasation   Extravasation

FIGURE 8–2. Overview of the metastatic cascade. Tumor cells invade at the primary tumor site and enter the interstitial stroma, thereby gaining access to blood vessels for further dissemination. Tumor cells then invade the vascular wall and are dislodged into the circulation both as single cells and in tumor-cell clusters. Circulating tumor cells arrest in the precapillary venules of the target organ by adherence or mechanical trapping. They must then exit the circulation by disrupting the endothelial basement membrane to initiate a metastatic colony.

sample is likely to reflect the general metastatic propensity of the entire tumor. This has been borne out by a number of clinical studies indicating that the average level of specific protein markers or amplified oncogenes measured in the primary tumor can be correlated with clinical parameters of metastasis and recurrence.[13–16]

MULTIPLE GENE PRODUCTS ARE INVOLVED IN THE COMPLEX METASTATIC CASCADE

A metastatic colony is the result of a complicated series of tumor-host interactions (see Table 8–1). Primary tumor initiation and progression are followed by the transition from in situ to locally invasive cancer that is accompanied by angiogenesis.[3,4,17] Newly formed tumor vessels are often defective

and easily invaded by tumor cells within the primary mass.[9,17] Tumor cells also invade preestablished host blood vessels at the invasion front. Tumor cells are discharged into the venous drainage in single-cell form and in clumps. For rapidly growing 1-cm tumors, millions of tumor cells can be shed into the circulation every day.[9] Fortunately for the patient, only a very small percentage (less than 0.01%) of circulating tumor cells initiate metastatic colonies.[3] Tumors generally lack a well-formed lymphatic network.[18] Therefore, communication of tumor cells with lymphatic channels occurs only at the tumor periphery and not within the tumor mass. Tumor cells entering the lymphatic drainage are carried to regional lymph nodes where they arrest in the large lymphatics of the subcapsular sinus. Within 10 to 60 minutes after initial arrest in the lymph node, a significant fraction of the tumor cells detach and enter the afferent lymphatics. These tumor cells eventually end up in the regional or systemic venous drainage due to the nu-

TABLE 8–1. Tumor–Host Interactions During the Metastatic Cascade

Metastatic Cascade Event	Potential Mechanisms
1. Tumor initiation	Carcinogenic insult, oncogene activation or derepression, chromosome rearrangement
2. Promotion and progression	Karyotypic, genetic, and epigenetic instability; gene amplification; promotion of associated genes and hormones
3. Uncontrolled proliferation	Autocrine growth factors or their receptors; receptors for host hormones such as estrogen
4. Angiogenesis	Multiple angiogenesis factors including known growth factors
5. Invasion of local tissues, blood, and lymphatic vessels	Serum chemoattractants, autocrine motility factors, attachment receptors, degradative enzymes
6. Circulating tumor-cell arrest and extravasation	Tumor-cell homotypic or heterotypic aggregation
a. Adherence to endothelium	Tumor-cell interaction with fibrin, platelets, and clotting factors; adhesion to RGD-type receptors
b. Retraction of endothelium	Platelet factors, tumor-cell factors
c. Adhesion to basement membrane	Laminin receptor, thrombospondin receptor
d. Dissolution of basement membrane	Degradative proteases, type IV collagenase, heparanase, cathepsins
e. Locomotion	Autocrine motility factors; chemotaxis factors
7. Colony formation at secondary site	Receptors for local tissue growth factors; angiogenesis factors
8. Evasion of host defenses and resistance to therapy	Resistance to killing by host macrophages, natural killer cells and activated T cells; failure to express or blocking of tumor specific antigens; amplification of drug resistance genes

merous lymphatic hematogenous communications. The regional lymph node does not function as a true mechanical barrier to tumor dissemination. Lymphatic and hematogenous dissemination occurs in parallel.

CIRCULATING TUMOR CELL ARREST AND EXTRAVASATION

Circulating tumor cells use a variety of means to arrest in the vessels of the target organ where they initiate metastatic colonies. About 80% of the circulating tumor cells are in single-cell form and directly attach to the intact endothelial surface or to preexisting regions of exposed subendothelial basement membrane. Clumps of circulating tumor cells or tumor cells aggregated with host leukocytes, fibrin, or platelets can directly embolize in the precapillary venules by mechanical impaction. Tumor cells in single-cell or clump form adhere to the endothelial luminal surface of arterioles. The fate and time course of the arrested tumor cells differs depending on the mechanism and location of lodgement. Tumor cells that adhere to the surface of venule or capillary endothelium rapidly (1 to 4 hr) induce the active retraction of the endothelial cells.[3,19–21] The tumor cell then attaches avidly to the exposed basement membrane. After the tumor cells have attached, the adjacent endothelial cells extend over the tumor cell and separate it from the bloodstream. Tumor cells located between the endothelium and the basement membrane are held up in this location for 8 to 24 hr. Local dissolution of the basement membrane is then observed in association with a tumor-cell pseudopodia traversing the basement membrane. This step is soon followed by complete extravasation of the tumor cell and quite often by reestablishment of blood flow in the breached vessel.[19] Tumor cells arrested in the arterial tree can remain in this location for 2 to 3 weeks. Endothelial retraction does not occur after arterial arrest. Intraarterial tumor cells can actually proliferate and expand as colonies. As the tumor colonies enlarge, they become covered by a host endothelial surface that lacks a basement membrane. After the tumor colony fills the arteriole, mechanical damage to the endothelium occurs, and this exposes the basement membrane. Tumor cells at the periphery of the interarterial colony then invade through the basement membrane and the elastic lamina of the arteriole wall to gain an extravascular position.[19]

At all stages of the metastatic cascade, tumor cells must overcome host defenses.[3–5,22–24] Although tumor-specific antigens have been identified in animal models, it remains unclear whether similar antigens play a role in human tumors and whether the recognition of these antigens can be boosted by adjuvant immunotherapy.[22,24] Limited effectiveness of adjuvant immunotherapy of metastases may be due to tumor antigen heterogeneity, tumor antigen shedding, or absence of tumor-cell immunogenicity. Nonspecific host defenses such as macrophages and natural killer cells may be more effective against heterogenous tumor-cell population.[24] In animal models, these effector cells play an important role in the elimination of circulating tumor cells and destruction of micrometastasis.[24]

Extravasated tumor cells proliferate as colonies but require a new vascular supply to grow larger than 0.5 mm.[25–27] Recent studies have demonstrated a close correlation between neo-

vascularization of the primary tumor and the frequency of metastasis formation in human breast cancer.[28] Angiogenesis is necessary at the beginning and at the end of the metastatic cascade. A metastasis can itself metastasize, further amplifying the level of tumor dissemination. Numerous clinical reports provide circumstantial evidence for the existence of dormant metastases.[1,3] Up to one third of the mortality from breast cancer, for instance, occurs more than 5 years after removal of the primary tumor. Three potential mechanisms of tumor dormancy have been distinguished in animals: immunologic restraint such that the tumor population death rate equals its growth rate; constitutive dependency of tumor cells on host growth factors; and avascularity causing the metastasis to be limited in size due to deficiency in nutrient diffusion.[3]

METASTASIS ORGAN DISTRIBUTION

The distribution of metastases varies widely depending on the histologic type and anatomic location of the primary tumor. The most frequent organ location of distant metastasis in many types of cancer appears to be the first capillary bed encountered by the circulating cells. These include sarcomas metastasizing to lung, lung cancer to brain, and colorectal tumor dissemination to liver. Many metastatic sites cannot be predicted based on anatomic considerations alone and can be considered as examples of organ tropism. For example, clear cell carcinoma of the kidney often metastasizes to bone and thyroid, breast carcinoma to ovaries, and ocular melanoma to the liver.

There is an increasing list of animal tumor models that show preference of metastasis to one or more distant sites.

TABLE 8–2. Organ Preference of Metastatic Colonization Using Animal Tumors That Have Not Undergone Purposeful Selection

Animal Species	Designation and Type of Tumor	Common Colonization Site(s)
Mouse	X5563 plasmacytoma	Spleen
Mouse	Kobayashi's plasmacytoma	Bone
Mouse	C198 reticuloendothelioma	Liver → lung, spleen
Mouse	Type A reticulum cell sarcoma	Liver → spleen
Mouse	RAW117 large-cell lymphoma	Liver → other sites
Mouse	B16 melanoma	Lung → other sites
Mouse	K-1735 melanoma	Lung
Mouse	M-5076 monocytic sarcoma	Liver → ovary → other sites
Rat	R39 sarcoma	Kidney, adrenal
Rat	Flexner-Jobling carcinoma	Kidney, adrenal
Guinea pig	Line 10 hepatocarcinoma	Liver, lymph node
Chicken	HV-transformed lymphoma	Liver
Rabbit	VX₂ carcinoma	Liver, lung

(Modified from Nicolson GL. Organ specificity of tumor metastasis: Role of preferential adhesion, invasion, and growth of malignant cells at specific secondary sites. Cancer Metastasis Rev 1988;7:143–188)

In many cases, organ preference for metastasis in these models cannot simply be explained based on anatomic considerations. Organ preference of metastatic colonization can be observed in some animal tumors that have not undergone purposeful selection (Table 8–2). In other models, organ selectivity has been experimentally amplified by sequential in vivo passage through the target organ (Table 8–3).

Many investigators have implanted organ grafts into ectopic sites. The transplanted organ grafts were used as target sites for tumor-cell hematogenous colonization. Hart and Fidler observed that intravenously injected B16-F10 melanoma cells colonized the native lung and subcutaneous lung grafts.[4] To colonize the ectopic site, the tumor cells must have clearly left the first capillary arrest site in the lungs and traveled to the ectopic site. In control mice, ectopic kidney grafts were not colonized by circulating B16-F10 tumor cells, indicating a clear organ selectivity for lung, but not for kidney.

Theoretic mechanisms for organ tropism include the following:

Tumor cells disseminate equally in all organs, but preferentially grow only in specific organs. Preferential growth may be induced by local growth factors or hormones present in the target organ for metastasis.

Circulating tumor cells may adhere preferentially to the endothelial luminal surface only in the target organ for metastasis. This hypothesis predicts organ-specific endothelial determinants.

Circulating tumor cells may respond to soluble factors diffusing locally out of the target organ. Such factors could act in a chemotactic fashion to attract the tumor cells to extravasate. They could also cause the circulating tumor cells to aggregate and therefore embolize in the target organ.

Research with animal models indicates that all of these mechanisms play roles to varying degrees, depending on the tumor model system.[3,21]

TABLE 8–3.   Organ Preference of Metastasis in Some Selected Human and Animal Tumor Models

Tumor System Subline	Lung	Liver	Brain	Ovary	Spleen	Lymph Node
Murine B16 Melanoma (I.V. or IC)						
B16-F10	++++	±	–	+	±	±
B16-B15b	+++	–	+++	–	–	±
B16-O13	++	–	–	+++	–	±
Murine RAW117 Large-Cell Lymphoma (I.V. or IC)						
RAW117-L17	+++	++++	–	–	++	–
Murine Lewis Lung Carcinoma (IM, IC, or IS)						
HL	++++	–	–	–	–	+
HH	±	++++	±	±	–	+
Chicken MD Lymphoma (I.V.)						
AL-2	–	++++	–	±	–	–
AL-3	–	+	–	+++	–	–
Human A375 Melanoma (I.V. in Nude Mice)						
A375-SM	++	–	–	–	–	+
A375-L	+	++	–	–	–	–
Human PC-3 Prostatic Carcinoma (I.V. in Athymic Mice)						
PC-3-125-IN	++++	–	–	–	–	–
PC-3-1-LN	++++	+	–	+	±	+++
Human KM12 Colon Carcinoma (IS or IC in Nude Mice)						
KM20C	+	+++	–	–	–	+
KM23C	+	+++	–	–	–	++
Human MeWo Melanoma (I.V. in Nude Mice)						
MeWo	+	–	–	–	–	–
MeWo-70-W	++	–	++	+	–	–

Metastases: –, none; ±, sometimes; +, few; ++, moderate; +++, many; ++++, large numbers and heavy tumor burden; I.V., intravenous; IC, intracecum; IM, intramuscular; IS, intrasplenic.
(Modified from Nicolson GL. Organ specificity of tumor metastasis: Role of preferential adhesion, invasion and growth of malignant cells at specific secondary sites. Cancer Metastasis Rev 1988;7: 143–188)

BASEMENT MEMBRANE DISRUPTION DURING TRANSITION FROM IN SITU TO INVASIVE TUMORS

The mammalian organism is composed of a series of tissue compartments separated from each other by two types of extracellular matrix: basement membranes and interstitial stroma.[5] The matrix determines tissue architecture, has important biologic functions, and serves as a mechanical barrier to invasion. During the transition from in situ to invasive carcinoma, tumor cells penetrate the epithelial basement membrane and enter the underlying interstitial stroma (see Fig. 8–1). After the tumor cells enter the stroma, they gain access to lymphatics and blood vessels for further dissemination (see Fig. 8–2). Fibrosarcomas and angiosarcomas, developing from stromal cells, invade surrounding muscle basement membrane and destroy myocytes. Tumor cells must cross basement membranes to invade peripheral nerves and most types of organ parenchyma. During intravasation or extravasation, the tumor cells of any histologic origin must penetrate the subendothelial basement membrane.[3,5] In the distant organ where metastatic colonies are initiated, extravasated tumor cells must migrate through the perivascular interstitial stroma before tumor colony growth occurs in the organ parenchyma. Therefore, tumor-cell interaction with the extracellular matrix occurs at multiple stages in the metastatic cascade.

General and widespread changes occur in the organization, distribution, and quantity of the epithelial basement membrane during the transition from benign to invasive carcinoma.[29,30] For example, benign proliferative disorders of the breast such as fibrocystic disease, sclerosing adenosis, intraductal hyperplasia, fibroadenoma, and intraductal papilloma are all characterized by disorganization of the normal epithelial stromal architecture. Extreme forms can mimic the appearance of invasive carcinoma. However, no matter how extensive the architectural disorganization, these benign disorders are always characterized by a continuous basement membrane separating the epithelium from the stroma.[29] In contrast, invasive ductal carcinoma, invasive lobular carcinoma, and tubular carcinoma consistently possess a defective extracellular basement membrane with zones of basement membrane loss around the invading tumor cells in the stroma.[29] The basement membrane is also markedly defective adjacent to tumor cells in lymph node and organ metastases. In some focal regions of well-differentiated carcinoma, partial basement membrane formation can be identified. These findings can be applied directly to diagnostic problems in surgical pathology such as the differentiation of tangential sections of in situ lesions from true invasion or differentiation of severe adenosis from invasive carcinoma. Loss of basement membranes in human rectal carcinomas significantly correlates with increased incidence of metastasis and poor 5-year survival.[30]

THREE-STEP THEORY OF INVASION

A three-step hypothesis has been proposed to describe the sequence of biochemical events during tumor-cell invasion of the extracellular matrix (Fig. 8–3).[5] The first step is tumor-cell attachment to the matrix. This attachment may be me-

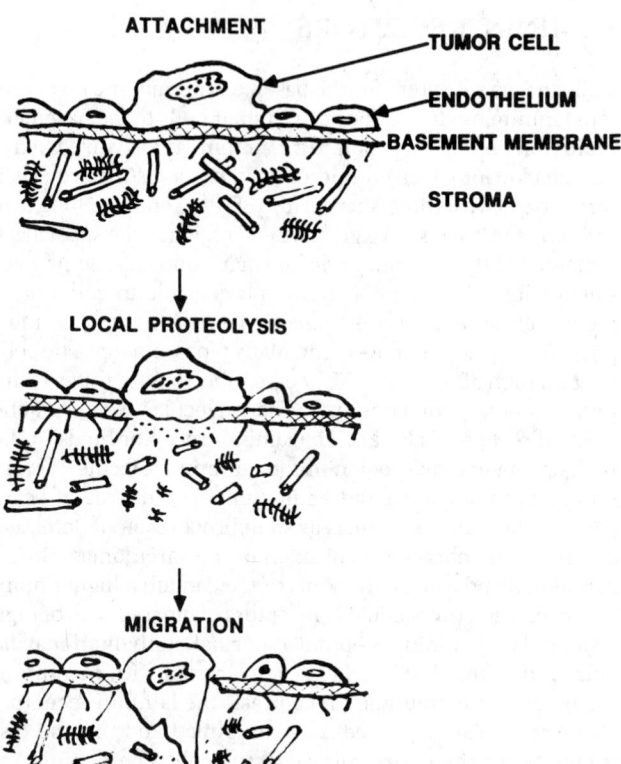

FIGURE 8–3. Three-step hypothesis of tumor-cell invasion of extracellular matrix. **(A)** The first step is tumor-cell attachment to the matrix. This process may be mediated by specific attachment factors such as laminin (in the case of the basement membrane) and fibronectin. **(B)** The second step is local degradation of the matrix by tumor-cell–associated proteases. Such proteases may degrade both the attachment proteins and the structural collagenous proteins of the matrix. Proteolysis may be localized at the tumor-cell surface, where the amount of active enzyme outbalances the natural protease inhibitors present in the matrix. **(C)** The third step is tumor-cell locomotion into the region of the matrix modified by proteolysis. The direction of locomotion may be influenced by chemotactic factors. Invasion of the extracellular matrix may continue by cyclic repetition of these three steps.

diated through specific glycoproteins such as laminin and fibronectin and through tumor-cell plasma membrane receptors. After attachment, the tumor cell secretes hydrolytic enzymes (or induces host cells to secrete enzymes) that can locally degrade the matrix (including degradation of the attachment glycoproteins). Matrix lysis most likely takes place in a highly localized region close to the tumor-cell surface where the amount of active enzyme outbalances the natural protease inhibitors present in the serum and in the matrix itself. In contrast to the invasive tumor cell, when a normal cell or benign tumor cell attaches to the matrix it may respond by shifting into a resting or differentiated state. The third step is tumor-cell locomotion into the region of the matrix modified by proteolysis. The direction of the locomotion may be influenced by host-derived chemotactic factors and tumor-cell–derived motility factors. The chemotactic factors derived from serum, organ parenchyma, or the matrix itself may influence the organ specificity of metastasis.[3,21] Continued invasion of the matrix may take place by cyclic repetition of these three steps.

LAMININ RECEPTORS

Cell-surface receptors for the basement membrane glycoprotein laminin mediate adhesion of tumor cells to the basement membrane before invasion.[31,32] Laminin, as visualized by rotary shadowing electron microscopy, has a distinctive cruciform shape with three short arms (35 nm) and one long arm (75 nm).[33] All arms have globular end regions. The specialized structure of the laminin molecule may contribute to its multiple biologic functions. Laminin plays a role in cell attachment, cell spreading, mitogenesis, neurite outgrowth, morphogenesis, and cell movement. Many types of neoplastic cells contain high affinity (nM Kd) cell-surface binding sites (laminin receptors) for laminin.[31] The molecular weight of the isolated receptor is 65 kd. The laminin receptor binds to the B-chain (short-arm) region of the laminin molecule.[34] Laminin receptors may be altered in number or degree of occupancy in human carcinomas as an indirect result of defective basement membrane organization in the carcinomas. Breast carcinoma and colon carcinoma tissue contain a higher number of exposed (unoccupied) receptors compared with benign lesions. The laminin receptors of normal epithelium may be polarized at the basal surface and occupied with laminin in the basement membrane. In contrast, the laminin receptors on invading carcinoma cells are amplified and may be distributed over the entire surface of the cell. The laminin receptor has been shown experimentally to play a role in hematogenous metastasis.[35] Treating tumor cells with the receptor-binding fragment of laminin at low concentrations markedly inhibits or abolishes lung metastasis from hematogenously introduced tumor cells. The mechanism of action involves blocking the adhesion of circulating tumor cells to the subendothelial basement membrane.

RGD RECOGNITION RECEPTORS
(INTEGRINS)

A family of cell-surface glycoproteins called *integrins* bind with low affinity to a variety of adhesion proteins including fibronectin, von Willebrand's factor, fibrin, vitronectin, type I collagen, and thrombospondin.[36] The integrins are a complex of α (140 kd) and β (95 kd) subunit proteins. The functions of several of the integrins are inhibited by peptides related to the Arg-Gly-Asp (RGD) sequence of fibronectin. The RGD sequences present on a wide variety of proteins may serve as recognition sites for binding of integrins. It is likely that specific ligand sequences adjacent to the RGD site confers preferential recognition of one type of adhesion protein by certain members of the integrin family.[37] Integrin proteins are believed to align adhesion proteins such as fibronectin on the cell surface with cytoskeletal components such as talin and actin, thus altering cell shape.[38,39] Integrin-type proteins may play an adhesive role in platelet–tumor-cell interactions, binding of lymphoid cells to endothelium, and the interaction of circulating tumor cells with endothelial surfaces, fibrin, von Willebrand's factor, or thrombospondin. In keeping with this concept, coinjection of tumor cells with large quantities of RGD peptides has been reported to inhibit metastasis formation in animal models.[40] The RGD peptides may interfere with the adhesion of tumor cells to the endothelial surface, which may directly or indirectly be mediated through integrin proteins.

CADHERINS: ROLE OF CELL-CELL ADHESION IN TUMOR-CELL INVASION

A number of cell-surface glycoproteins have been described that mediate intercellular adhesion. The possible role of one class of these molecules, the integrins, in tumor-cell invasion has already been discussed. Another class of cell adhesion molecules, the cadherins, are essential for the Ca^{2+}-dependent process of cell-cell adhesion.[41] This family is divided into subclasses with varying tissue distribution, and three types of cadherins have been identified in mammals. These molecules are designated *E-*, *N-* and *P-cadherins*.

The potential role of E-cadherin (homologous to uvomorulin) in preventing tumor-cell invasion has recently been highlighted by several studies. Investigators have shown that epithelial Madin-Darby canine kidney (MDCK) cells acquired in vitro invasive capacity when treated with monoclonal anti–E-cadherin antibodies.[42] These studies have been extended through genetic manipulation of E-cadherin levels in MDCK cells and murine mammary gland epithelial cells.[43] Transfection of plasmids encoding sense (overexpression) or antisense (downregulation) E-cadherin-specific RNA enabled the overexpression of E-cadherin in highly invasive clones and partial downregulation in noninvasive clones. High expression of E-cadherin showed reproducible loss of the invasive phenotype in two types of in vitro invasion assays. On the other hand, partial downregulation of E-cadherin levels rendered cells invasive. Decreased adhesion of tumor cells to neighboring tumor or host cells would favor their emigration from the local site and their penetration of extracellular matrix, consistent with the three-step hypothesis. These studies provide direct evidence that E-cadherin acts as an invasion suppressor molecule.

TUMOR-CELL MOTILITY FACTORS

Cell motility is necessary for tumor cells to traverse many stages in the complex cascade of invasion. Such stages may include the detachment and subsequent infiltration of cells from the primary tumor into adjacent tissue, the migration of the cells through the vascular wall into the circulation (intravasation), and the extravasation of the cells to a secondary site. The movement of cells through biologic barriers, such as the endothelial basement membranes of the vasculature, may occur by means of chemotactic mechanisms. Studies on in vitro chemotaxis of some tumor cells indicate that compounds such as complement-derived materials, collagen peptides, formyl peptides, and certain connective tissue components can act as chemoattractants.[17,44,45] Although these agents may contribute to the directional aspects of a motile response, they are not sufficient to initiate the intrinsic locomotion of tumor cells. The availability of soluble attractants to the tumor cell depends greatly on the host, even in those cases in which the production of attractants is the result of interaction between the tumor cell and host tissue. At best, the cell would have access to such motility stimuli at sporadic and irregular intervals. Such conditions are unfavorable to a sustained migration of highly invasive cells. With these considerations in mind and stimulated by the studies of Anzano and coworkers[46] (in which they demonstrated autocrine growth factors for transformed cells), we investigated the possibility that such cells elaborate autocrine motility factors. The action of these substances could explain in part the markedly invasive character and the metastatic property of malignant neoplastic cells. Under the influence of such an autocrine material, a tumor cell might move out into the surrounding host tissue and also exert a recruiting effect on adjacent tumor cells in the presence of a gradient of attractant. Conceivably, such factors might also attract fibroblastic cells of the host, resulting in the phenomenon of desmoplasia, characteristic of invasive tumors.

We have found that the human melanoma cell line A2058 and human breast carcinoma cells produce in culture a material that markedly stimulates their own motility.[47-49] These cells respond in a dose-dependent manner to concentrations of conditioned medium obtained by incubating confluent cells in serum-free medium, an indication that the motility factor is derived from the cell. Motility was measured by the modified Boyden's chamber procedure. Using this assay and the so-called *checkerboard analysis,* we have also found that the conditioned medium factor has chemotactic (directional) and chemokinetic (randomly motile) properties.[48] The transducer system activated by autocrine motility factor (AMF) involves phospholipase C and phospholipase A_2.[48] Early events in migration may involve pseudopodia protrusion.[49] During the course of invasion, the same tumor cell must interact with a variety of extracellular matrix proteins as it traverses each tissue barrier. For example, the tumor cell encounters laminin and type IV collagen when it penetrates the basement membrane, and type I collagen and fibronectin when it crosses the interstitial stroma. Cells express specific cell-surface receptors that recognize extracellular matrix proteins. The first example of such a receptor is the laminin receptor, which binds to laminin with a nanomolar affinity. Laminin receptors are augmented in actively invading tumor cells and may play an important role in tumor-cell interaction with the basement membrane. RGD recognition receptors are another class of cell-surface proteins that bind extracellular matrix proteins, which in turn contain the protein sequence Arg-Gly-Asp.[36] Such proteins include fibronectin, collagen type I, and vitronectin. The process of cell migration undoubtedly requires a series of adhesion and detachment steps resulting in traction and propulsion.

Studies using the AMF-stimulated motility as a model system have revealed an important function of pseudopodia protrusion in this process. AMF stimulates motility on different substrata; therefore, its action is independent of the mechanism of attachment. Furthermore, AMF induces the rapid protrusion of pseudopodia in a time- and dose-dependent manner.[49] Isolation of the induced pseudopodia reveals that they are highly enriched in their content of laminin and fibronectin matrix receptors. Because cell pseudopodia formation is a prominent feature of actively motile cells, we can set forth a working hypothesis to explain the early events in cell motility. Cytokines such as AMF that stimulate intrinsic motility may induce exploratory pseudopodia before cell translocation. Such pseudopodia may express augmented levels of matrix receptors

(and possibly proteinases). The protruding pseudopodia may serve multiple functions including acting as sense organs to interact with the extracellular matrix proteins and thereby locate directional cues, providing propulsive traction for locomotion, and inducing local matrix proteolysis to assist in the penetration of the matrix.[50,51]

PROTEINASES AND TUMOR-CELL INVASION: FROM CORRELATION TO CAUSALITY

Proteolysis occurs in normal tissue but is limited in duration and subject to strict regulation at many levels. A general aspect of malignant neoplasms may be an imbalance of proteolysis, which favors invasion. Proteolysis of tissue barriers is not a property unique to tumor cells. It is used, for example, during trophoblast implantation, embryo morphogenesis, tissue remodeling, parasitic and bacterial invasion, and angiogenesis. Furthermore, the defect in the tumor cell cannot be simply unbridled production of degradative enzymes, because cell migration during invasion requires attachment and deattachment of the cell as it moves forward. Lysis of all matrix components around the tumor cell would remove the substratum necessary for proper cell traction. The invading tumor cell probably uses proteolysis in a highly organized manner spatially and temporally, which does not differ functionally from the operating mode of normal cells that migrate through tissue barriers. The difference is that tumor cells couple proteolysis with motility to achieve invasion at times and places that would be inappropriate for normal cells.

The metastasis field has progressed from establishing a correlation between proteolysis and malignant progression to the finding that the actual blockade of certain proteinases prevents invasion and metastasis. A positive association with tumor aggressiveness has been noted for various classes of degradative enzymes including heparanases,[52,53] serine,[54] thiol,[55,56] and metal-dependent enzymes.[57-60] A cascade including all these enzymes is probably involved in the invasive process, and more than one enzyme is necessary but not sufficient. This conclusion is justified by the many findings that inhibitors for metalloproteinases or inhibitors of serine proteinases can each block tumor-cell invasion of native or reconstituted connective tissue barriers in vitro.[61-64] The enzymes involved in tumor invasion and metastasis may well resemble the proteolytic cascades involved in blood coagulation.

Plasminogen activator, specifically urokinase-type plasminogen activator (uPA), has been closely linked to the metastatic phenotype.[65,66] Anti-uPA antibodies block human HEP-3 cell invasion in the chick chorioallantoic membrane assay and murine B16-F10 melanoma cell metastasis after tail vein injection.[67,68] Overexpression of uPA in H-*RAS*-transformed 3T3 cells enhanced lung invasion and experimental metastasis formation.[69] Serine-proteinase inhibitors also block tumor-cell invasion through human amniotic membranes.[63]

Among the list of enzymes involved in cancer, a large body of information has been accumulated concerning the matrix metalloproteinase gene family (Fig. 8–4). These enzymes have been grouped into three broad categories based on substrate preference: interstitial collagenases, type IV collagen-

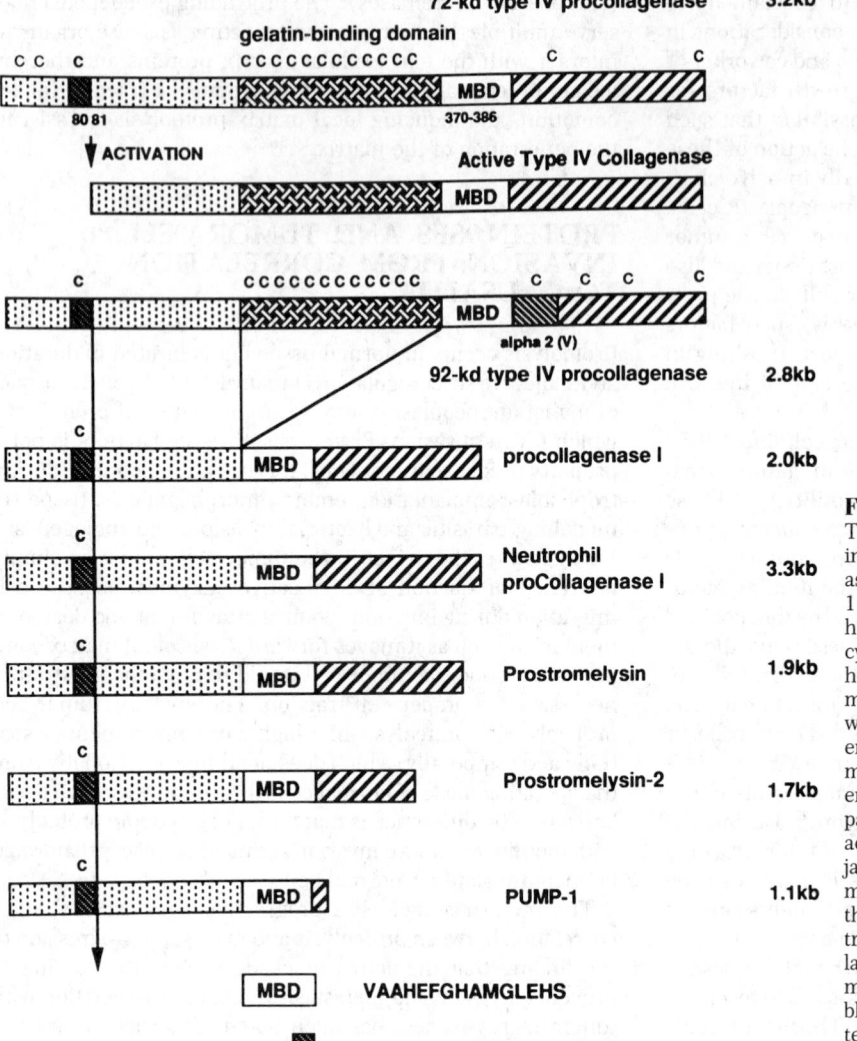

FIGURE 8–4. Matrix metalloproteinase family. Type IV procollagenase (72-kd and 92-kd forms), interstitial procollagenase, neutrophil procollagenase, prostromelysin, prostromelysin-2, and PUMP-1 are aligned to show regions of protein sequence homology. Type IV procollagenases contain a cysteine-rich, substrate-binding domain that shows homology to fibronectin but is absent from the other matrix metalloproteinase enzymes. On treatment with organomercurial compounds in vitro, all seven enzymes are activated with the concomitant removal of an aminoterminal segment of the latent enzyme. The removed segment contains an unpaired cysteine residue within the conserved amino acid sequence PRCGVPDV located immediately adjacent to the proenzyme cleavage site. Site-directed mutagenesis studies have shown that alterations in this sequence result in spontaneous activation of transin, the rat homologue of stromelysin. In the latent proenzyme, this sequence interacts with the metal ion through the unpaired cysteinyl residue to block activity (see Fig. 8–2). Pertubation of this interaction affects activation. MBD, active site metal ion binding domain.

ases (gelatinases), and stromelysins.[70] The interstitial collagenase is the best characterized and specifically degrades type I collagen.[60] Neutrophil collagenase, which has recently been cloned, appears very similar in substrate specificity.[71] The stromelysins are three related gene products, stromelysin, stromelysin-2, and PUMP1, which degrade a variety of matrix components including proteoglycans and noncollagenous glycoproteins such as laminin and fibronectin, and the noncollagenous domains of type IV collagen. The role of stromelysin in tumor progression has recently been reviewed.[72] The type IV collagenases are named for their selective ability to cleave type IV collagen in a pepsin-resistant triple-helical domain, generating characteristic ¼ aminoterminal and ¾ carboxyl terminal fragments.[73] Both 72-kd and 92-kd type IV collagenases exist, and cDNA cloning has demonstrated that each is a unique gene product.[74,75]

All classes of matrix metalloproteinases are secreted as inactive zymogens, and enzyme activation is an important control step in proteolysis. Recent observations have detailed a model for matrix metalloproteinase proenzyme activation.[76–79] The essential feature of this model is that the latent form of the matrix metalloproteinase enzymes all have a metal atom sulfhydryl side-chain interaction that results in a catalytically inert active center. The sulfhydryl group in this interaction is donated by the CYS-73 residue, which is contained in a highly conserved peptide present in all known members of this metalloproteinase family. The metal atom is presumably the zinc atom of the active site. Disruption of this interaction results in conformational rearrangement and rapid attainment of protease activity (Fig. 8–5). The implication of this model is that mutations in the CYS-73 residue result in intrinsic enzyme activation, which may play a role in tumor progression. The in vivo mechanism of normal metalloproteinase activation is unknown but may involve the action of other proteinases in solution or by a cell-surface-dependent mechanism.[80–82] The latter would allow for precise cellular control at the point of matrix interaction. Among the matrix metalloproteinase family members, an accumulating body of evidence supports a positive correlation between type IV collagenase activity and tumor-cell invasion.[52,59,83,84] Augmented type IV collagenase activity is associated with the genetic induction of a metastatic phenotype.[85–88] Furthermore, use of

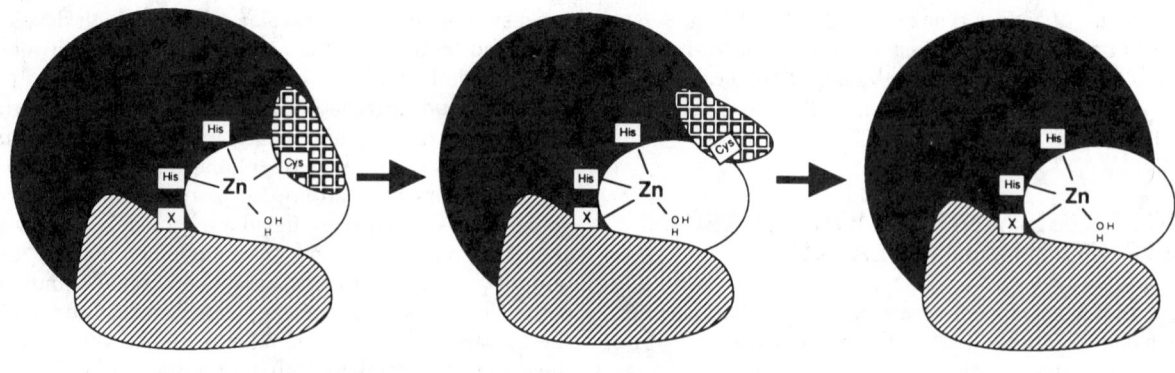

Latent Proenzyme   Active Proenzyme   Active Enzyme

FIGURE 8–5.   Model of matrix metalloproteinases latent state and enzyme activation. Latency of the proenzyme is maintained by an interaction between the unpaired cysteinyl residue (CYS-73) of the profragment and the zinc atom at the active site. Disruption of the zinc atom–sulfhydryl group interaction results in full collagenolytic activity after conformational rearrangement. The zinc atom coordination site contains two histidyl residues (His) and shows homology with thermolysin. The third coordination position of the active enzyme is an unidentified amino acid residue (X). After conformational rearrangement and attainment of proteolytic activity, the active enzyme undergoes autoproteolytic removal of the aminoterminal profragment to generate a stable active enzyme species.

agents that specifically inhibit type IV collagenase activity or block collagenase secretion prevent tumor-cell invasion in vitro.[54,89] Immunohistochemical studies using affinity purified, anti-72kd type IV collagenase antibodies demonstrate that low levels of this enzyme are produced by normal, nontumorigenic, nonmetastatic cells such as the myoepithelial cells of the human breast.[76,90] Benign proliferative lesions of the breast, benign polyps of the colon, and normal colorectal and gastric mucosa all show negligible immunoreactivity for 72-kd type IV collagenase. In contrast, almost all invasive colonic and gastric adenocarcinomas are positive for this antigen.[91,92] Downregulation of type IV collagenolytic activity by retinoic acid treatment of human melanoma cells has been correlated with a loss of the invasive phenotype.[83] Studies of the mechanism of this effect reveal that retinoic acid treatment of these human melanoma cells results in a reduction of the steady-state level of the 72-kd type IV collagenase mRNA and loss of the invasive capacity.[93] These results suggest that the 72-kd type IV collagenase enzyme is a normal cell component that is dramatically overexpressed in many invasive and metastatic human cancers.

NATURAL PROTEINASE INHIBITORS ARE INVASION SUPPRESSORS

The secretion and the activation of metalloproteinases are not enough to ensure that they degrade the target matrix substrate.[94,95] This is because natural inhibitor proteins, produced by the host or by the tumor cell itself, can block the latent or the active metalloproteinases.[95] Natural proteinase inhibitor proteins, such as tissue inhibitor of metalloproteinases (TIMPs)[96] or plasminogen activator inhibitors (PAIs), may therefore function as metastasis suppressor proteins, which act to inhibit tumor-cell invasion of the extracellular matrix. TIMP-1, the original member of the TIMP family,[97] is a glycoprotein with an apparent molecular size of 28.5 kd that forms a complex of 1:1 stoichiometry with activated interstitial

collagenase, activated stromelysin, and the 92-kd type IV collagenase. Transfection of antisense RNA, which blocks TIMP-1 expression, enhances the malignant phenotype.[98] One explanation for this result is that the antisense RNA blocked the production of TIMP-1, which normally prevented the malignant phenotype. In animal models, administration of recombinant TIMP-1 blocks metastasis.[99,100]

Recently, Stetler-Stevenson and coworkers have isolated, purified, determined the complete primary structure, and cloned a second member of the TIMP family, TIMP-2.[101,102] An identical inhibitor was isolated from endothelial cells by DeClerck.[103,104] TIMP-1 and TIMP-2 are regulated independently and oppositely by TPA, TGFβ, and other cytokines. TIMP-2 is a 21-kd protein that selectively forms a complex with the latent proenzyme form of the 72-kd type IV collagenase. The secreted protein has 194 amino acid residues and is not glycosylated. TIMP-2 shows 37% identity and overall 65.6% homology to TIMP-1 at the deduced amino acid sequence level. The position of the 12 cysteine residues in TIMP-2 are conserved with respect to those present in TIMP-1, as are 3 of the 4 tryptophan residues; yet the 2 proteins are immunologically distinct. TIMP-2 inhibits at a 1:1 ratio the type IV collagenolytic activity and the gelatinolytic activity associated with the 72-kd enzyme. Unlike TIMP-1, TIMP-2 is capable of binding to the latent and activated forms of the 72-kd type IV collagenase and abolishing the hydrolytic activity of all members of the metalloproteinase family.[102,105] The 92-kd type IV procollagenase can be found as a complex with TIMP-1.[75] Activation of the latent 72-kd or 92-kd type IV collagenase TIMP complex can be reversed by binding of a second mole of TIMP-1 or TIMP-2. This suggests that on these enzymes there are two separate TIMP binding sites and that binding of TIMP-1 or TIMP-2 to the latent proenzymes serves a different function than the inactivation that occurs after binding to the active species. The areas of the two proteins that differ in homology may contain the regions responsible for the functional differences.[102] The net 72-kd type IV collagenase activity consequently depends on the balance between the levels of activated enzyme and TIMP-2 (Fig. 8–6). TIMP-2 is a potent inhibitor of cancer cell invasion through reconstituted extracellular matrix.[106] TIMP-2 produced by the same tumor cells that make collagenase, therefore, exists as a natural suppressor of invasion.

ANGIOGENESIS AND TUMOR INVASION ARE FUNCTIONALLY RELATED

The formation of new blood vessels, or angiogenesis, permits the expansion of a tumor mass in three dimensions.[25,27] Prevascular tumors may persist as thin asymptomatic lesions, restricted by the limits of oxygen and nutrient diffusion. In contrast, vascularized tumors expand locally and by metastasis. Local shedding of cancer cells into the tumor venous drainage is commenced at the onset of tumor angiogenesis, is quantitatively related to the surface area of new tumor vessels, and may be facilitated by the immature nature of the newly formed vessels.[9]

Tumors can induce angiogenesis through a variety of soluble factors.[26,107] Angiogenesis is not one event, but a cascade of processes emanating from microvascular endothelial cells. Endothelial cells resting in the parent vessel are stimulated to degrade the endothelial basement membrane, migrate into the perivascular stroma, and initiate a capillary sprout.[108] The direction of the migration is pointed toward the source of the angiogenesis stimulus. The sprout subsequently expands and assumes a tubular structure. Endothelial proliferation permits

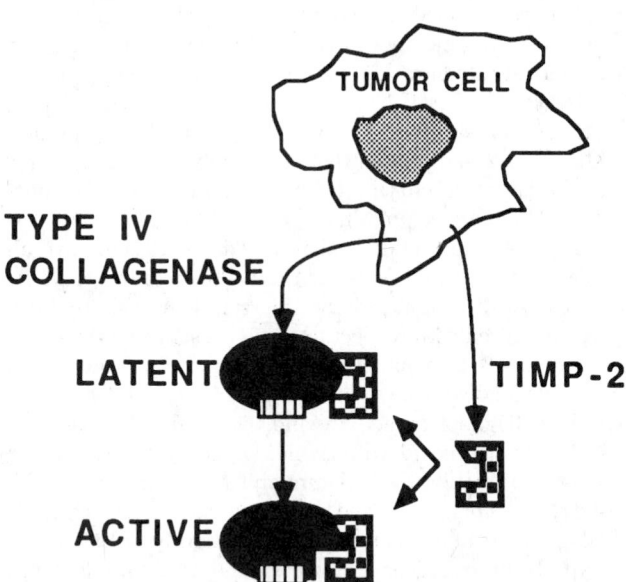

FIGURE 8–6. Suppressor role for TIMP-2. Tumor cells can produce both metalloproteinases and TIMPs. TIMP-2 binds with 1:1 stoichiometry to latent 72-kd type IV collagenase and may block physiologic activation. It also binds to the activated form of the enzyme and to the activated form of other members of the matrix metalloproteinase family. Type IV collagenolysis by the 72-kd type IV collagenase enzyme occurs only if the local levels of the activated enzyme exceed the local levels of TIMPs. Therapeutic administration of TIMP-2 could prevent 72-kd type IV collagenase enzyme activation and abolish the activity of activated enzyme.

extension of the microvascular tubules, which develop into loops and then into a functioning circulatory network. The exit of endothelial cells from the parent vessel involves cell migration and degradation of the extracellular matrix in a manner that may be functionally indistinguishable from cancer cell invasion of the extracellular matrix.[109,110]

Investigators have attempted to recapitulate early angiogenic events in vitro by developing models of endothelial growth, migration, and extracellular matrix interactions.[64,107,110] These in vitro assays reveal that stimulated endothelial cells can produce degradative proteinases and invade the extracellular matrix similar to tumor cells. Moreover, these model systems indicate that a finely tuned balance between proteinase and proteinase inhibitor regulates vascular morphogenesis and invasion.[81,111] Migrating endothelial cells produce type IV collagenase and other members of the matrix metalloproteinase family and serine proteinases. Specific inhibitors of type IV collagenase, general metalloproteinase inhibitors, and serine-proteinase inhibitors block endothelial cell invasion of the extracellular matrix.[64,112] These inhibitors block tumor-cell invasion in the same assay.[61,63,113]

Mignatti and coworkers reported that TIMP-1 inhibited in vitro endothelial-cell invasion of human amniotic membranes.[64] Moses and colleagues reported that cartilage-derived inhibitor (CDI), a TIMP-related protein isolated from bovine articular cartilage, could block angiogenesis and also inhibit endothelial proliferation.[112] Pepper and coworkers have shown that agents that induce angiogenesis in vivo, such as basic fibroblast growth factor (bFGF), induce urokinase type PA and plasminogen activator inhibitor-1 (PAI-1).[94,107] However, the kinetics of the amplitude of the uPA and PAI-1 mRNA induction by angiogenic agents showed a ratio tilted towards enhanced proteolysis. TGFβ1 could tip the balance to antiproteolysis, which results in the formation of solid endothelial cords rather than tubes in three-dimensional matrix culture. This finding is in accord with the results of Montesano and coworkers, who studied the formation of endothelial angiomas in a fibrin gel culture.[111] All endothelioma cell lines produced uPA but not PAI and formed hemangioma-like cystic structures in culture. When the excess proteolytic activity was blocked by the exogenous serine-proteinase inhibitor aprotinin (Trasylol), the endothelioma cells formed cords instead of sacular structures (Fig. 8–7). The balance between serine-proteinase and inhibitor can influence the morphology of the capillary tubule. The mechanism may involve the mechanical restraints of the three-dimensional matrix. Some level of proteinase activity at the surface of an endothelial cord may be required to lyse the adjacent matrix, causing an expansion of the cord diameter and permitting lumen formation in the longitudinal center of the cord. If such proteolysis is increased, then the surrounding destruction of the matrix may be excessive and create a cavity lined by endothelial cells. This would be the configuration of the cyst-like hemangioma structures generated by the endothelioma cells in the study of Montesano and coworkers.[111]

The common feature of many agents that induce angiogenesis, such as bFGF, has been a specific triad of multifunctional stimulation of capillary endothelial cells. This triad of functions is motility, proteolysis, and growth. Motility is necessary for endothelial cell chemotaxis toward the angiogenesis stim-

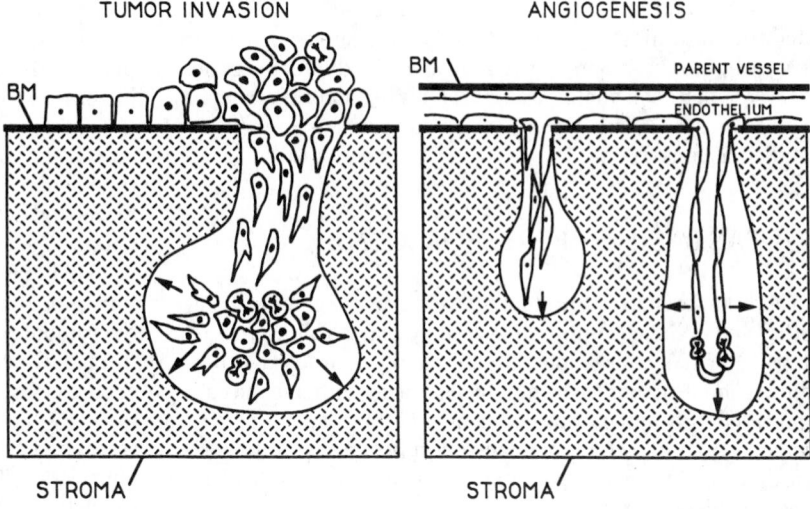

FIGURE 8–7. Functional similarity of tumor invasion and angiogenesis. (*Left*) Transition from in situ to invasive carcinoma is associated with dissolution of the basement membrane and migration into the interstitial stroma (containing stromal cells and matrix molecules). Proliferation of tumor cells expands the secondary colony. (*Right*) Early phases of angiogenesis involve dissolution of the parent-vessel basement membrane and endothelial migration into the stroma, forming a sprout toward the angiogenic stimulus. Lateral proteolysis of the stroma (that is not excessive) permits expansion of the sprout diameter and lumen formation. Proliferation of endothelial cells is required for elongation of the vascular tree. Angiogenic factors such as basic fibroblast growth factor induce endothelial migration, proteolysis, and proliferation.

ulus and lining up of the endothelial cells to form a sprout. Proteolysis is required for capillary sprout penetration into, and lateral expansion within, the extracellular matrix. Lateral expansion that is not excessive is associated with lumen formation. Finally, proliferation of the endothelial cells is needed to populate the expanding vascular network. This same triad of properties also defines an invasive tumor cell and provides aspects of equivalence between angiogenesis and tumor invasion. The major difference between the tumor cell and the endothelial cell may be that the tumor cell is unregulated or autoregulated in these three properties. The endothelial cell, on the other hand, can revert to a nonangiogenic state when the angiogenic stimulus is removed. The implication of this model is that antiinvasion compounds should be antiangiogenic. An antiinvasion compound should also block metastasis growth by blocking angiogenesis.

METASTASIS AND TUMORIGENICITY CAN BE UNDER SEPARATE GENETIC CONTROL

Five years ago, investigators in the metastasis field were sure that the new developments in oncogenes were relevant only to tumorigenicity and that separate genes would be found that evoke the metastatic process. At the time, biologic assays of oncogenes were restricted to scoring tumorigenicity. Little attention had been paid to metastasis formation. Nevertheless, when the proper studies were done, it was found that transfection of certain oncogenes in the correct recipient cell could induce the complete phenotype of invasion and metastasis. Although the search for specific metastasis-inducing genes goes on, oncogene transfection has provided a model to switch on the effector processes that are required for the cell to carry out invasion and metastasis. These models have revealed that some metastasis effector genes can be regulated independently from those that confer tumorigenicity. The incidence of aberrant gene expression and genetic alterations of the *RAS* and *MYC* gene families have been shown to be important in progression of human cancers and may be useful as prognostic indicators.[114] Thorgeirsson and coworkers were the first to report that the activated (mutated) *RAS* oncogene sequences, when transfected into mouse embryo-derived fibroblasts (NIH-3T3 cells), produced numerous metastases.[115] The resultant highly metastatic cells were not more resistant to host immune-cell lysis (macrophage or NK cells) compared with control cells, indicating that the *RAS* oncogene had augmented the intrinsic aggressiveness of the NIH-3T3 cells. Transfection of H-*RAS*-family oncogenes has been shown to induce metastasis in fibroblasts and epithelial cells of rodent and human origin.[85,86,88,116–119] H-*RAS* is not the only oncogene that can induce metastatic potential. At much lower efficiency, the serine-threonine kinases v-*MOS*, v-*RAF*, and A-*RAF*;[117,120] the tyrosine kinases v-*SRC*, v-*FES*, and v-*FMS*;[117] and the phosphoprotein p53[121] have been demonstrated to induce the metastatic phenotype in the appropriate recipient cell.

Two observations indicate that the downstream pathways used in *RAS* induction of tumorigenicity and metastasis have dissimilar features. First, the adenovirus 2E1A gene has been demonstrated to suppress *RAS* induction of metastatic potential with no inhibition of soft agar colony formation or tumorigenicity.[122] Second, cells are capable of being transformed by *RAS* but do not metastasize.[85,123] These results are best explained by assuming that invasion and metastasis require activation of a set of effector genes over and above those required for unrestrained growth alone. The failure of *RAS* to induce metastasis in certain experimental systems probably reflects a deficiency in, or a suppression of, some of these effector proteins. Several candidate effector proteins have been associated with metastasis in *RAS* transfection models, including proteinases (*e.g.*, type IV collagenase), cathepsin L, and motility-associated cytokines.[47,74,86,88,124] In these *RAS* transfection models, certain effector genes are activated or suppressed, possibly in a coordinated manner, to induce metastasis formation. Oncogenes such as v-*SRC* and *RAS*, tumor-promoting phorbol esters and growth factors such as EGF and PDGF induce transin (rat homolog of human stromelysin) mRNA transcript levels. The observation that these agents all induce a rapid stimulation of c-*FOS* that precedes the induction of transin mRNA and the knowledge that protein synthesis is required for this induction suggest that c-*FOS* may act as a third messenger and directly modulate transin gene transcription.[72,125] Some oncogene-associated effector genes may regulate cell motility and proteolysis, and this forms a common thread with separate work on proteinases, motility, and angiogenesis.

METASTASIS SUPPRESSOR GENES

In addition to motility, proteolysis, and growth, genetic instability and cellular communication may play a role in metastasis. Normal cells cooperate to form an ordered three-dimensional tissue. Metastatic cells, on the other hand, act independently and may be deficient in certain aspects of cell-to-cell signaling, which regulates morphogenesis. In this regard, the *NM23* gene, a potential metastasis suppressor gene, has provided a fresh new set of hypotheses.

The *NM23* gene was identified on the basis of its reduced expression at the RNA level in a series of seven cell lines, all derived from a single K-1735 murine melanoma.[126] *NM23* RNA levels were reduced 10-fold in five high metastatic potential K-1735 melanoma lines compared with two related, low metastatic potential K-1735 melanoma lines. Quantitative reductions in *NM23* RNA levels were observed in multiple cell lines and tumors in four rodent metastasis model systems. The identification of a potential metastasis suppressor gene was in keeping with the results of cell fusion experiments, in which fusion of normal cells with metastatic cells resulted in tumorigenic nonmetastatic cells.[84,127] *NM23* RNA and protein levels were also examined in a prospective series of human infiltrating ductal breast carcinomas using in situ hybridization and immunoperoxidase staining.[128,129] Tumors from breast cancer patients with evidence of metastasis to the lymph nodes at surgery contained low *NM23* RNA levels, which correlates with markedly reduced survival in patients with node-negative or well-differentiated breast cancer.[130]

The first clue to *NM23* function came from its virtual identity with the *Drosophila* gene product AWD.[131–133] Mutations that result in reduced *AWD* expression or the production of a mutated protein do not significantly alter embryonic development but do alter the development of multiple tissues postmetamorphosis, when presumptive adult tissue in the imaginal discs begins to divide and differentiate. These abnormalities include altered morphology of the wing discs, larval brain and proventriculus, aberrant differentiation of the wing, leg and eye-antennae imaginal discs and ovaries, and cell necrosis, predominately in the wing discs. *NM23/AWD* may contribute to the normal development of tissues, which may include signal transduction of cell-to-cell communication. Loss of *NM23/AWD* expression may lead to a disordered state, favoring aberrant development or tumor progression to the metastatic state. The second clue to *NM23* function came from study of *Dictyostelium*,[134] rat,[135] and *Myxococcus*,[136] in which cDNA clones for nucleoside diphosphate (NDP) kinases were isolated and were highly similar in amino acid sequence to *NM23/AWD*. This strong amino acid homology was confirmed by the identification of *AWD* as a nucleoside 5'-phosphate (NDP) kinase.[137] NDP kinases comprise a ubiquitous class of enzymes that catalyze the transfer of the terminal phosphate group of

5'-triphosphate nucleotides to 5'-diphosphate nucleotides through the formation of enzyme-bound high-energy phosphate intermediates.[138,139] The cellular NDP kinase is an oligomer of individual NDP kinase subunits, ranging from 3 to 6 subunits depending on the cell type. Each subunit has a size of 17 to 18 kd. NDP kinases exhibit heterogeneity in their subunit number and amino acid sequences, and in membrane and cytoplasmic localization, which implies functional heterogeneity.

NDP kinases are known to participate in at least two major functions that could play a role in cancer and development: microtubule assembly or disassembly and signal transduction through G proteins.[140–144] Microtubule assembly requires the exchange or transphosphorylation without exchange of GDP to GTP. Nickerson and Wells have isolated a microtubule-associated NDP kinase, which may catalyze such transphosphorylation.[140] In this fashion, NM23-like NDP kinases could regulate cellular functions using microtubule machinery, including mitotic spindle formation and cell locomotion.[137] NDP kinases have also been shown to form a complex with a variety of G proteins involved in cyclic AMP pathways.[135,142–144] It is likely that NDP kinases form a complex with other classes of G proteins regulating a diversity of second messenger pathways.[139] This could serve to channel GTP onto the G protein during activation or to transphosphorylate the GDP to GTP without exchange. Aberrant G proteins have been demonstrated to contribute to oncogenesis.[145] Based on these functional roles, members of the NDP kinase family could be expected to have suppressor or inducer functions in the developmental and cancer processes, depending on whether they were normal or mutated and on which signal response pathways were involved.

NEW STRATEGIES FOR METASTASIS DIAGNOSIS AND THERAPY

The elucidation of biochemical and genetic mechanisms that play a role in cancer metastases (see Table 8–1) has led to new strategies for cancer diagnosis and therapy. Because normal host parenchymal cells do not invade and metastasize, the biochemical changes expressed in the malignant phenotype may be a target for strategies that are more selective for tumor cells than conventional cytotoxic agents.

The most immediate application of these basic research findings is in the area of tumor diagnosis and prognosis. The clinical aggressiveness of a patient's individual tumor could be more accurately predicted by the measurement of genes or gene products functionally associated with the phenotype of invasion and metastases. These include oncogenes such as *RAS*, *MYC*, and *NEU*, newly discovered genes such as *NM23*, which may be associated with suppression of the metastatic phenotype,[126,146] and genes that encode receptors, proteinases, and motility factors associated with invasion. The average levels of such metastasis markers may be measured in a sample of the patient's tumor tissue. On the other hand, antibodies or genetic probes for the markers could be applied to a histologic section of the tumor to study the tumor-cell population distribution of the marker. In this manner, the proportion of tumor cells reacting with the marker could be used as an index of the aggressive tumor subpopulation. Application of antibodies to metastases-associated antigens by the surgical pathologist may increase the accuracy of identifying micrometastases in lymph nodes. Furthermore, immunohistochemical applications are not limited to tumor-associated antigens. Host antigens may also be altered in the vicinity of the tumor. This is the case for host basement membranes, which are locally fragmented or lost in the area of tumor cell invasion. Loss of basement membrane antigens has already proven useful in detecting breast cancer microinvasion and in the grading and staging of colorectal tumors.[29,30]

Some of the proteins associated with invasion and metastases are secreted by the tumor cell. Examples are degradative enzymes such as type IV collagenase and heparanase, or hormone-like proteins such as tumor autocrine motility factors and growth factors. After secretion by the tumor cell, the proteins (whole or as fragments) may accumulate in the blood or urine of the patient. Measurement of the level of the proteins by sensitive immunoassay procedures may be a means to detect occult metastases, estimate the body burden of metastatic disease, and detect local tumor recurrence. Furthermore, in the case of bladder cancer, the level of the marker in the urine may reflect the invasive stage of the transitional cell carcinoma.

Tumor-cell proteins functionally associated with the metastatic phenotype may be quantitatively augmented in tumor cells composing the metastatic foci. Systematically administered antibodies or synthetic ligands that bind to tumor-cell proteins may preferentially accumulate in the metastatic foci compared with other body sites. This could be useful in the radioscintigraphic detection of clinically occult metastases. Furthermore, if the antibody or ligand is coupled to a toxic agent, it may selectively kill the tumor cells in the metastatic foci.

An increased understanding of the mechanisms of tumor cell invasion may lead to the development of pharmacologic agents or strategies that block tumor-cell invasion. In theory, blocking any of the necessary steps for invasion listed in Table 8–1 could prevent tumor-cell invasion. Tumor angiogenesis may depend on mechanisms similar to cancer invasion, including proteolysis. Consequently, an antiinvasion agent may also block tumor angiogenesis. Chronic systemic treatment or local administration with an antiinvasion agent may be clinically useful in preventing the transition from in situ to invasive cancer in high-risk patients, reducing local tumor recurrence and invasion after surgical removal of primary tumors, and inhibiting metastasis formation by circulating tumor cells disseminated by inoperable primary tumors, metastases, or released during surgical manipulation of the primary tumor.

The goal of metastasis research is to develop strategies to selectively eradicate established metastasis. This could be based on the targeting of toxic agents to the metastatic foci. Actual killing of the tumor cells in the metastatic foci may not be necessary to prevent the usual clinical outcome of metastatic disease. Inhibition of metastasis growth by chronic treatment regimens may achieve the same end. This is a hopeful area for therapy strategies, because it has been found that common cellular pathways may be dearranged by genetic events, such as increased *RAS* expression, in such a way as to increase the growth and invasion of tumor cells. An example of a common pathway is the inositol phosphate cascade operating through phospholipase C and protein kinase C. This pathway may be altered by a number of oncogenes. Agents that normalize this pathway in tumor cells may act to suppress growth and invasion.

REFERENCES

1. Sugarbaker EV. Patterns of metastasis in human malignancies. Cancer Biol Rev 1981;2:235.
2. Weiss L, Gilbert HA. Bone Metastasis. Boston: G. K. Hall, 1981.
3. Schirrmacher V. Experimental approaches, theoretical concepts, and impacts for treatment strategies. Adv Cancer Res 1985;43:1–32.
4. Fidler IJ, Hart IR. Biologic diversity in metastatic neoplasms—origins and implications. Science 1982;217:998–1001.
5. Liotta LA. Tumor invasion and metastasis—role of the extracellular matrix: Rhoads Memorial Award Lecture. Cancer Res 1986;46:1.
6. Tubiana M, Chauvel P, Renaud A, Malaise EP. Vitresse de croissance et histoire naturelle du cancer du sein. Bull Cancer 1975;62:341.
7. Koscielny S, Tubiana M, Valleron A-J. A simulation model of the natural history of breast cancer. Br J Cancer 1985;52:515.
8. Bauer W, Igot J-P, Le Gal Y. Chronologie du cancer mammaire utilisant un modele de croissance de Fompertx. Ann Anat Pathol (Paris) 1980;25:39.
9. Liotta L, Kleinerman J, Saidel G. Quantitative relationships of intravascular tumor cells, tumor vessels and pulmonary metastases following tumor implantation. Cancer Res 1974;34:1001–1004.
10. Fidler IJ, Kripke ML. Metastasis results from pre-existing variant cells within a malignant tumor. Science 1977;197:893.
11. Luria SE, Delbruck M. Mutations of bacteria from virus sensitivity to virus resistance. Genetics 1945;28:491.
12. Kerbel RS. Growth dominance of the metastatic cancer cell: Cellular and molecular aspects. Adv Cancer Res 1990;55:87–131.
13. McGuire WL, Tandon AK, Allred DC, et al. How to use prognostic factors in axillary node negative breast cancer patients. JNCI 1990;92:1006–1015.
14. Slamon DJ, Godolphin W, Jones LA, et al. Studies of the HER-2/neu proto-oncogene in human breast and ovarian cancer. Science 1989;244:707–712.
15. Lidereau R, Callahan R, Dickson C, et al. Amplification of the int-2 gene in primary human breast tumors. Oncogene Res 1988;2:285–291.
16. Tandon AK, Clark GM, Chamness GC, et al. Cathepsin D and prognosis in breast cancer. N Engl J Med 1990;322:297.
17. Furcht LT. Critical factors controlling angiogenesis: Cell products, cell matrix, and growth factors. Lab Invest [Editorial] 1986;55:505.
18. Guillino PM, Grantham F. The vascular space of growing tumors. Cancer Res 1964;24:1727.
19. Lapis K, Paku S, Liotta LA. Endothelialization of embolized tumor cells during metastasis formation. Clin Exp Metastasis 1988;6:73.
20. Wallace AC, Chew E, Jones DS. The arrest and extravasation of cancer cells in the lung. In: Weiss L, Gilbert HA, eds. Pulmonary metastasis. Boston: G.K. Hall, 1978:26.
21. Nicolson GL, Dilski K, Basson C, Welch DR. Preferential organ attachment and invasion in vitro by B16 melanoma cells selected for differing metastatic colonization and invasive potential. Invasion Metastasis 1985;5:144.
22. Frost P, Kerbel RS. Immunology of metastasis. Can the immune response cope with disseminated tumor? Metastasis Rev 1983;2:239.
23. Old LJ. Cancer immunology—The search for specificity. Cancer Res 1981;41:361.
24. Hanna N, Fidler IJ. Relationship between metastatic potential and resistance to natural killer cell mediated cytotoxicity in three murine tumor systems. JNCI 1981;66:1183.
25. Folkman J. Tumor angiogenesis: Therapeutic implications. N Engl J Med 1971;285:1182–1186.
26. Folkman J, Klagsbrun M. Angiogenic factors. Science 1987;235:442–447.
27. Folkman J, Watson K, Ingber D, Hanahan D. Induction of angiogenesis during the transition from hyperplasia to neoplasia. Nature 1989;339:58–61.
28. Weidner N, Semple JP, Welch WR, Folkman J. Tumor angiogenesis and metastasis—correlation in invasive breast carcinoma. N Engl J Med 1991;324:1–8.
29. Barsky SH, Siegal GP, Jannotta F, et al. Loss of basement membrane components by invasive tumors but not by their benign counterparts. Lab Invest 1983;49:140.
30. Forrester SJ, Talbot IC, Critshley DR. Laminin and fibronectin in rectal adenocarcinoma: Relationship to tumor grade, stage and metastasis. Br J Cancer 1984;50:51.
31. Wewer UM, Liotta LA, Jaye M, et al. Altered levels of laminin receptor mRNA in various human carcinoma cells that have different abilities to bind laminin. Proc Natl Acad Sci USA 1986;83:7137.
32. Rao CN, Margulies I, Tralka S, et al. Isolation of a subunit of laminin and its role in molecular structure and tumor cell attachment. J Biol Chem 1982;257:9740.
33. Engel J, Odermatt E, Engel A, et al. Shapes, domain organization and flexibility of laminin and fibronectin—two multifunctional proteins of the extracellular matrix. Mol Biol 1981;150:97.
34. Wewer UM, Taraboletti G, Sobel ME, et al. Laminin receptor: Role in tumor cell migration. Cancer Res 1987;47:5691.

35. Barsky SH, Rao CN, Williams JE, Liotta LA. Laminin molecular domains which alter metastasis in a murine model. J Clin Invest 1984;74:843.
36. Hynes RO. Integrins: A family of cell surface receptors. Cell 1987;48:549.
37. Ruoslathi E, Pierschbacher MD. Arg-Gly-Asp: A versatile cell recognition signal. Cell 1986;44:517.
38. Yamada KM, Kennedy DW. Dualistic nature of adhesive protein function: Fibronectin and its biologically active peptide fragments can autoinhibit fibronectin function. J Cell Biol 1984;99:29.
39. Horwitz A, Duggan C, et al. Binding of fibronectin receptors to talin. Nature 1986;320: 531.
40. Humphries MJ, Olden K, Yamada KM. A synthetic peptide from fibronectin inhibits experimental metastasis of murine melanoma cells. Science 1986;233:467.
41. Takeichi M. Cadherins: A molecular family important in selective cell–cell adhesion. Annu Rev Biochem 1990;59:237–252.
42. Behrens J, Mareel MM, Van Roy FM, Birchmacher W. Dissecting tumor cell invasion: Epithelial cells acquire invasive properties after the loss of uvomorulin-mediated cell-cell adhesion. J Cell Biol 1989;108:2435–2447.
43. Uleminckx K, Vakaet L, Mareel M, Fiers W, Van Roy F. Genetic manipulation of E-cadherin expression by epithelial tumor cells reveals an invasion suppressor role. Cell 1991;66:107–119.
44. Lam WC, Delikatny JE, Orr FW, et al. The chemotactic response of tumor cells: A model for cancer metastasis. Am J Pathol 1981;104:69.
45. McCarthy JB, Basara ML, Palm SL, et al. Stimulation of haptotaxis and migration of tumor cells by serum spreading factor. Cancer Metastasis Rev 1985;4:125.
46. Anzano MA, Roberts AB, Smith JM, et al. Sarcoma growth factors from conditioned media of virally transformed cells composed of both type alpha and beta growth factors. Proc Natl Acad Sci USA 1983;80:6264.
47. Liotta LA, Mandler R, Murano G, et al. Tumor cell autocrine motility factor. Proc Natl Acad Sci USA 1986;83:3302–3306.
48. Stracke ML, Guirguis R, Liotta LA, et al. Pertussis toxin inhibits stimulated motility independently of the adenylate cyclase pathway in human melanoma cells. Biochem Biophys Res Commun 1987;146:339.
49. Guirguis R, Margulies IMK, Taraboletti G, et al. Cytokine-induced pseudopodial protrusion is coupled to tumor cell migration. Nature 1987;329:261.
50. Bokoch GM, Gilman AG. Inhibition of receptor-mediated release of arachidonic acid by pertussis toxin. Cell 1984;39:301.
51. Smith CD, Cox CC, Snyderman R. Receptor-coupled activation of phosphoinositide-specific phospholipase C by an N protein. Science 1986;232:97.
52. Nakajima M, Welch D, Belloni PN, Nicolson GL. Degradation of basement membrane type IV collagen and lung subendothelial matrix by rat mammary adenocarcinoma cell clones of differing metastatic potentials. Cancer Res 1987;47:4869–4876.
53. Nakajima M, Morikawa K, Fabra A, Bucana CD, Fidler IJ. Influence of organ environment on extracellular matrix degradative activity and metastasis of human colon carcinoma cells. JNCI 1990;82:1890–1898.
54. Reich R, Thompson E, Iwamoto Y, et al. Effects of inhibitors of plasminogen activator, serine proteinases, and collagenase IV on the invasion of basement membranes by metastatic cells. Cancer Res 1988;48:3307–3312.
55. Recklies AD, Poole AR, Mort JS. A cysteine proteinase secreted from human breast tumours is immunologically related to cathepsin B. Biochem J 1982;207:633.
56. Sloane BR, Honn KV. Cysteine proteinases and metastasis. Cancer Metastasis Rev 1984;3:249.
57. Ostrowski LE, Rinch J, Kreig P, Matrisian L. Expression pattern of a gene for a secreted metalloproteinase during late stages of tumor progression. Mol Carcing 1988;1:13–19.
58. Liotta LA, Abe S, Robey P, Martin G. Preferential digestion of basement membrane collagen by an enzyme derived from a metastatic murine tumor. Proc Natl Acad Sci USA 1979;76:2268–2272.
59. Liotta LA, Tryggvason K, Garbisa S, et al. Metastatic potential correlates with enzymatic degradation of basement membrane collagen. Nature 1980;284:67–68.
60. Templeton NS, Brown PD, Levy AT, Margulies IMK, Liotta LA, Stetler-Stevenson WG. Cloning and characterization of human tumor cell interstitial collagenase. Cancer Res 1990;50:5431–5437.
61. Thorgeirsson UP, Liotta LA, Kalebic T, et al. Effect of natural protease inhibitors and a chemoattractant on tumor cell invasion in vitro. JNCI 1982;69:1049.
62. Wang M, Stearns ME. Blocking of collagenase secretion by estamustine during in vitro tumor cell invasion. Cancer Res 1988;48:6262–6271.
63. Mignatti P, Robbins E, Rifkin D. Tumor invasion through the human amniotic membrane: Requirement for a proteinase cascade. Cell 1986;47:487–498.
64. Mignatti P, Tsuboi R, Robbins E, Rifkin D. In vitro angiogenesis on the human amniotic membrane: Requirement for basic fibroblast growth factor-induced proteinases. J Cell Biol 1989;108:671–682.
65. Dano K, Andreasen PA, Grondahl-Hansen J, et al. Plasminogen activators, tissue degradation and cancer. Adv Cancer Res 1985;44:139.
66. Sappino A-P, Busso N, Belin D, Vassalli J-D. Increase of urokinase type plasminogen activator gene expression in human lung and breast carcinomas. Cancer Res 1987;47: 4043.
67. Ossowski L, Reich E. Antibodies to plasminogen activator inhibit human tumor metastasis. Cell 1983;35:611–619.
68. Esheicher A, Wohlwend A, Belin D, Vassalli JD. Characterization of the cellular binding site for the urokinase type plasminogen activator. J Biol Chem 1989;264:1180–1189.
69. Axelrod JH, Reich R, Mishkin R. Expression of human recombinant plasminogen activators enhance invasion and experimental metastasis of Ha-RAS-transformed NIH 3T3 cells. Mol Cell Biol 1989;9:2133–2141.
70. Wilhelm, S, Collier I, Kronberg A, et al. Human skin fibroblast stromelysin: Structure, glycosylation, substrate specificity, and differential expression in normal and tumorigenic cells. Proc Natl Acad Sci USA 1987;84:6725–6729.
71. Hasty KA, Pourmotabbed TF, Goldberg GI, et al. Human neutrophil collagenase. J Biol Chem 1990;265:11421–11424.
72. Matrisian L, Bowden T. Stromelysin/transin and tumor progression. Semin Cancer Biol 1990;1:107–115.
73. Fessler L, Duncan K, Tryggvason K. Identification of the procollagen IV cleavage products produced by a specific tumor collagenase. J Biol Chem 1984;259:9783–9789.
74. Collier IE, Wilhelm SM, Eisen AZ, et al. H-RAS oncogene transformed human bronchial epithelial cells (TBE-1) secrete a single metalloproteinase capable of degrading basement membrane collagen. J Biol Chem 1989;263:6579–6587.
75. Wilhelm SM, Collier IE, Marmer BL, Eisen AZ, Grant GA, Goldberg GI. SV40-transformed human lung fibroblasts secrete a 92-kDa type-IV collagenase which is identical to that secreted by normal human macrophages. J Biol Chem 1989;264:17213–17221.
76. Stetler-Stevenson WG, Krutzsch HC, Wacher MP, Margulies IMK, Liotta LA. The activation of human type IV collagenase proenzyme. J Biol Chem 1989;264:1353–1356.
77. Stetler-Stevenson WG, Talano J, Gallagher M, Krutzsch HC, Liotta LA. Inhibition of human type IV collagenase by a highly conserved peptide sequence derived for its prosegment. Am J Med Sci 1991;302:163–170.
78. Vallee BL, Auld DS. Zinc coordination function and structure of zinc enzymes and other proteins. Biochemistry 1990;29:5647–5659.
79. Van Wart HE, Birkedal-Hansen H. The cysteine switch: A principle of regulation of metalloproteinase activity with potential applicability to the entire matrix metalloproteinase gene family. Proc Natl Acad Sci USA 1990;87:5578–5582.
80. Brown PD, Levy AT, Margulies I, Liotta L, Stetler-Stevenson WG. Independent expression and cellular processing of the 72-kDa type IV collagenase and interstitial collagenase in human tumorigenic cell lines. Cancer Res 1990;50:6184–6191.
81. Herron GS, Banda MJ, Clark EJ, Gavrilovic J, Werb Z. Secretion of metalloproteinases by stimulated capillary endothelial cells. II. Expression of collagenase and stromelysin activities is regulated by endogenous inhibitors. J Biol Chem 1986;261:2814–2818.
82. He C, Wilhelm SM, Pentland AP, et al. Tissue cooperation in a proteolytic cascade activating human interstitial collagenase. Proc Natl Acad Sci USA 1989;86:2632–2636.
83. Nakajima M, Lotan D, Baig MM, et al. Inhibition of retinoic acid of type IV collagenolysis and invasion through reconstituted basement membrane by metastatic rat mammary adenocarcinoma cells. Cancer Res 1989;49:1698–1706.
84. Turpeenniemi-Hujanen T, Thorgeirsson UP, Hart IR, et al. Expression of collagenase IV (basement membrane collagenase) activity in murine tumor cell hybrids that differ in metastatic potential. JNCI 1985;75:99–108.
85. Muschel RJ, Williams JE, Lowy DR, Liotta LA. Harvey RAS induction of metastatic potential depends upon oncogene activation and the type of recipient cell. Am J Pathol 1985;121:1–8.
86. Garbisa S, Pozzatti R, Muschel R, et al. Secretion of type IV collagenolytic protease and metastatic phenotype: Induction by transfection with c-Ha-RAS but not c-Ha-RAS plus Ad2-Ela. Cancer Res 1987;47:1523–1528.
87. Bonfil DR, Reddel RR, Ura H, et al. Invasive and metastatic potential of a v-Ha-RAS-transformed human bronchial epithelial cell line. JNCI 1989;81:587–594.
88. Ura H, Bonfil RD, Reich R, et al. Expression of type IV collagenase and procollagen genes and its correlation with the tumorigenic, invasive, and metastatic abilities of oncogene-transformed human bronchial epithelial cells. Cancer Res 1989;49:4615–4621.
89. Wang BS, McLouglin GA, Richie JP, Mannick JA. Correlation of the production of plasminogen activator with tumor metastasis in B16 mouse melanoma cell lines. Cancer Res 1980;40:288.
90. Monteagudo C, Merino M, San-Juan J, Liotta L, Stetler-Stevenson W. Immunohistologic distribution of type IV collagenase in normal, benign and malignant breast tissue. Am J Pathol 1990;136:585–592.
91. D'Errico A, Garbisa S, Liotta LA, Castronovo V, Stetler-Stevenson WG, Griogioni WG. Augmentation of type IV collagenase, laminin receptor, and Ki67 proliferation antigen associated with human colon, gastric and breast carcinoma progression. Mod Pathol 1991;4:239–246.
92. Levy A, Cioce V, Sobel ME, et al. Increased expression of the 72 kDa type IV collagenase in human colonic adenocarcinoma. Cancer Res 1991;51:439–444.
93. Hendrix M, Wood R, Seftor E, et al. Retinoic acid inhibition of human melanoma cell invasion through a reconstituted basement membrane and its relation to decreases in the expression of proteolytic enzymes and motility factor receptor. Cancer Res 1990;50: 4121–4130.
94. Levin EG, Santell L. Association of a plasminogen activator inhibitor (PAI-1) with the growth substratum and membrane of human endothelial cells. J Cell Biol 1987;105: 2543–2649.
95. Gottesman M. The role of proteases in cancer. Semin Cancer Biol 1990;1:97–160.
96. Carmichael DF, Sommer A, Thomson R, et al. Primary structure and cDNA cloning of human fibroblast collagenase inhibitor. Proc Natl Acad Sci USA 1986;83:2407–2411.
97. Murphy G, Cawston T, Reynolds J. An inhibitor of collagenase from human amniotic fluid: Purification, characterization and action on metalloproteinases. Biochem J 1981;195:167–170.
98. Khokha R, Waterhouse P, Yagel S, et al. Antisense RNA-induced reduction in metal-

loproteinase inhibitor causes mouse 3T3 cells to become tumorigenic. Science 1989;243: 947–950.

99. Schultz, RM, Silberman S, Persky B, Bajowski AS, Carmichael DF. Inhibition by recombinant tissue inhibitor of metalloproteinases of human amnion invasion and lung colonization by murine B16-F10 melanoma cells. Cancer Res 1988;48:5539–5545.

100. Alvarez OA, Carmichael DF, DeClerck YA. Inhibition of collagenolytic activity and metastasis of tumor cells by a recombinant human tissue inhibitor of metalloproteinases. JNCI 1990;82:589–595.

101. Stetler-Stevenson WG, Krutzsch HC, Liotta LA. TIMP-2, a new member of the metalloproteinase inhibitor family. J Biol Chem 1989;264:17374–17378.

102. Stetler-Stevenson WG, Brown P, Onisto M, Levy A, Liotta L. Tissue inhibitor of metalloproteinases-2 (TIMP-2) mRNA expression in tumor cell lines and human tumor tissues. J Biol Chem 1990;265:13933–13938.

103. DeClerck Y, Yean T, Ratzkin B, Lu H, Langley K. Purification and characterization of two related but distinct metalloproteinase inhibitors secreted by bovine aortic endothelial cells. J Biol Chem 1989;264:17445–17453.

104. Boone T, Johnson M, DeClerck Y, Langley K. cDNA cloning and expression of a metalloproteinase inhibitor related to tissue inhibitor of metalloproteinases. Proc Natl Acad Sci USA 1990;87:2800–2804.

105. Goldberg GI, Marmer BL, Grant GA, Eisen AZ, Wilhelm S, He C. Human 72-kDa type IV collagenase forms a complex with a tissue inhibitor of metalloproteinase inhibitor. Proc Natl Acad Sci USA 1989;86:8207–8211.

106. Albini A, Melchiori A, Parodi A, Liotta LA, Brown PD, Stetler-Stevenson WG. TIMP-2 inhibits tumor cell invasion. JNCI 1991;83:775–779.

107. Pepper MS, Belin D, Montesano R, Orci L, Vassalli JD. Transforming growth factor beta 1 modulates basic fibroblast growth factor-induced proteolytic and angiogenic properties of endothelial cells in vitro. J Cell Biol 1990;111:743–755.

108. Ausprunk DH, Folkman J. Migration and proliferation of endothelial cells in preformed and newly formed blood vessels during angiogenesis. Microvasc Res 1977;14:53–65.

109. Cliff WJ. Observations on healing tissues: A combined light and electron microscopic investigation. Philos Trans R Soc Lond (Biol) 1963;246:305–325.

110. Kalebic T, Garbisa S, Glaser B, Liotta LA. Basement membrane collagen: Degradation by migrating endothelial cells. Science 1983;221:281–283.

111. Montesano R, Pepper MS, Mohle-Steinlein U, Risau W, Wagner EF, Orci L. Increased proteolytic activity is responsible for aberrant morphogenetic behavior of endothelial cells expressing the middle T oncogene. Cell 1990;62:435–445.

112. Moses MA, Sudhalter J, Langer R. Identification of an inhibitor of neovascularization from cartilage. Science 1990;248:1408–1410.

113. Thorgeirsson UP, Turpeenniemi-Hujanen T, Neckers LM, et al. Protein synthesis but not DNA synthesis is required for tumor cell invasion in vitro. Invasion Metastasis 1984;4:73.

114. Field JK, Spandidos, DA. The role of RAS and MYC oncogenes in human solid tumours and their relevance in diagnosis and prognosis. Anticancer Res [Review] 1990;10:1–22.

115. Thorgeirsson UP, Turpeenniemi-Hujanen T, Williams JE, et al. NIH 3T3 cells transfected with human tumor DNA containing activated RAS oncogenes express the metastatic phenotype in nude mice. Mol Cell Biol 1985;5:259–262.

116. Hill SA, Wilson A, Chambers AF. Clonal heterogeneity, experimental metastatic ability, and p21 expression in H-RAS-transformed NIH 3T3 cells. JNCI 1988;80:484–490.

117. Greenberg AH, Eagen SE, Wright JA. Oncogenes and metastatic progression. Invasion Metastasis 1989;9:360–378.

118. Theodorescu D, Cornil I, Fernandez B, Kerbel RS. Overexpression of normal and mutated forms of c-Ha-RAS induce orthotopic bladder invasion in a human transitional cell carcinoma. Proc Natl Acad Sci USA. 1990;87:9047–9051.

119. Nicolson GL. Tumor cell instability, diversification and progression to the metastatic phenotype: From oncogene to oncofetal expression. Cancer Res 1987;47:1473.

120. Egan SE, Wright JA, Jarolim L, Yanagihara K, Bassim RH, Greenberg AH. Transformation by oncogenes encoding protein kinases induces the metastatic phenotype. Science 1987;238:202.

121. Pohl J, Goldfinger N, Rader-Pohl A, Rolter V, Schirrmacher V. P53 increases experimental metastatic capacity of murine carcinoma cells. Mol Cell Biol 1988;8:2078.

122. Pozzatti RP, Muschel RJ, Williams JR, Howard B, Liotta LA, Khoury G. Primary rat embryo cells transformed by one or two oncogenes show different metastatic potentials. Science 1986;232:223–227.

123. Tuck AB, Wilson SM, Chambers AF. Ras transfection and expression does not induce progression from tumorigenicity to metastatic ability in mouse LTA cells. Clin Exp Metastasis 1990;8:417–431.

124. Mason RW, Gal S, Gottesman MM. The identification of the major excreted protein (MEP) from a transformed mouse fibroblast cell line as a catalytically active precursor form of cathepsin L. Biochem J 1987;248:449.

125. Kerr LD, Holt JT, Matrisian LM. Growth factors regulate transin gene expression by c-FOS-dependent and c-FOS-independent pathways. Science 1988;242:1424–1427.

126. Steeg PS, Bevilacqua G, Kopper L, et al. Evidence for a novel gene associated with low tumor metastatic potential. JNCI 1988;80:200.

127. Sidebottom E, Clark SR. Cell fusion segregates progressive growth from metastasis. Br J Cancer 1983;47:399.

128. Bevilacqua G, Sobel ME, Liotta LA, Steeg PS. Association of low nm23 RNA levels in human primary infiltrating ductal breast carcinomas with lymph node involvement and other histopathological indicators of high metastatic potential. Cancer Res 1989;49: 5185.

129. Barnes R, Masood S, Barker E, et al. Low nm23 protein expression in infiltrating ductal breast carcinomas correlates with reduced patient survival. Am J Pathol 1991;139: 2245–2250.

130. Hennessy C, Henry JA, May FEB, Westley BR, Angus B, Lennard TWJ. Expression of the anti-metastatic gene nm23 in human breast cancer: Association with good prognosis. JNCI 1991;83:281–285.

131. Dearolf C, Hersperger E, Shearn A. Development consequences of AWD, a cell-autonomous lethal mutation of *Drosophila* induced by hybrid dysgenesis. Dev Biol 1988;129:159–168.

132. Dearolf C, Tripoulas N, Biggs J, Shearn A. Molecular consequences of AWD, a cell-autonomous lethal mutation of *Drosophila* induced by hybrid dysgenesis. Dev Biol 1988;129:169–178.

133. Rosengard AM, Krutzsch HC, Shearn A, et al. Reduced nm23/AWD protein in tumor metastasis and aberrant *Drosophila* development. Nature 1989;342:177.

134. Wallet V, Mutzel R, Troll H, et al. *Dictyostelium* nucleoside diphosphate kinase highly homologous to nm23 and AWD proteins involved in mammalian tumor metastasis and *Drosophila* development. JNCI 1990;18:1199–1202.

135. Kimura N, Shimada N, Nomura K, Watanabe K. Isolation and characterization of a cDNA clone encoding rat nucleoside diphosphate kinase. J Biol Chem 1990;265:15744–15749.

136. Munoz-Dorado J, Inouye M, Inouye S. Nucleoside diphosphate kinase from *Myxococcus xanthus*. I. Cloning and sequencing of the gene. J Biol Chem 1990;265:2702–2706.

137. Biggs J, Hersperger E, Steeg PS, Liotta LA, Shearn A. A *Drosophila* gene which is homologous to a mammalian metastasis associated gene codes for a nucleoside diphosphate kinase. Cell 1990;63:933–940.

138. Parks R, Agarwal R. Nucleoside diphosphokinases. In: Boyer P, ed. The enzymes. New York: Academic Press, 1973:307–334.

139. Liotta LA, Steeg PS. Clues to the function of Nm23 and Awd proteins in development signal transduction, and tumor metastasis provided by studies of *Dictyostelium discoideum*. JNCI 1990;82:1170–1172.

140. Nickerson J, Wells W. The microtubule-associated nucleoside diphosphate kinase. J Biol Chem 1988;259:11297–11304.

141. Kikkawa S, Takahashi K, Takahashi K-I, Shimada N, Ui M, Kimura N, Katada T. Conversion of GDP to GTP by nucleoside diphosphate kinase on the GTP-binding proteins. J Biol Chem 1990;265:21536–21540.

142. Kimura N, Johnson G. Increased membrane-associated nucleotide diphosphate kinase activity as a possible basis for enhanced guanine nucleotide dependent adenylate cyclase activity induced by picolinic acid treatment of simian virus 40-transformed normal rat kidney cells. J Biol Chem 1983;258:12609–12617.

143. Kimura N, Shimada N. Membrane-associated nucleoside diphosphate kinase from rat liver. J Biol Chem 1988;263:4647–4653.

144. Kimura N, Shimada N. Evidence for complex formation between GTP binding protein (Gs) and membrane-associated nucleoside diphosphate kinase. Biochem Biophys Res Commun 1990;168:99–106.

145. McCormick F. Gasp: Not just another oncogene. Nature 1989;340:678–679.

146. Leone A, Flatow U, King CR, et al. Reduced tumor incidence, metastatic potential and cytokine responsiveness of nm23 transfected melanoma cells. Cell 1991;65:25–35.

147. Nicolson GL. Organ specificity of tumor metastasis: Role of preferential adhesion, invasion, and growth of malignant cells at specific secondary sites. Cancer Metastasis Rev 1988;7:143–188.

Cancer: Principles & Practice of Oncology, Fourth Edition, edited by Vincent T. DeVita, Jr., Samuel Hellman, Steven A. Rosenberg. J.B. Lippincott Co., Philadelphia © 1993.

Joseph F. Fraumeni, Jr   Susan S. Devesa

Robert N. Hoover   Leo J. Kinlen

CHAPTER **9**

Epidemiology of Cancer

Epidemiology is the study of variations in disease frequency among population groups and the factors that influence these variations. Its principal objective is the finding of causes so that, ideally, preventive measures may be applied. By focusing on events that necessarily precede the onset of disease, epidemiology contrasts to clinical medicine, in which the primary concern is the diagnosis and treatment of individual patients. In epidemiology, the perennial reference point for individual patients is the population from which they come. This approach encompasses not only unaffected members of the group in question, which may be useful for comparison purposes, but also all affected persons in that population, avoiding the selection factors that can determine the experience of individual clinicians.

After dramatic improvements in the control of infectious disease during this century, the attention of epidemiologists has increasingly turned toward the study of chronic illnesses. The resulting advances include some of the most important discoveries in the cause and prevention of cancer. The impact of epidemiology on cancer touches the clinician, experimentalist, policy maker, and even the lay public, whose attention is often drawn to epidemiologic observations and environmental issues by the news media, sometimes in an unbalanced way.

Practicing physicians must often interpret epidemiologic findings for their patients. They have opportunities to use epidemiologic data that will protect high-risk individuals, to collaborate in epidemiologic studies, and to make clinical observations relevant to etiology. The large volume of research into the origins of cancer and its prevention makes it increasingly important for the clinical oncologist to understand the principles and methods of epidemiology.

HISTORICAL PERSPECTIVE

Epidemiologic observations in cancer have a long and fascinating history.[1] In 1700, the Italian occupational physician Bernardino Ramazzini observed that breast cancer was more common in nuns than other women, and he suggested the influence of celibacy. In 1775, the British surgeon Percivall Pott reported the first description of occupational carcinogenesis in the form of scrotal cancer among chimney sweeps. In the 18th century there were also reports of cancer risks associated with tobacco, namely snuff taking and nasal cancer by Hill in 1761 and pipe smoking and lip cancer by von Soemmering in 1795. Perhaps the first modern epidemiologic study of cancer was in 1842 by Rigoni-Stern, who attempted to quantify the risks of uterine cancer in the city of Verona among nuns and other women and showed that the disease was significantly less common in the former group. Important occupational cancers were also observed in the 19th century: lung cancer (first described as "mediastinal lymphoma") among the metal miners of Schneeberg and Joachimsthal by Harting and Hesse in 1879 and bladder cancer among aniline dye workers by Rehn in 1895. In 1888, Hutchinson reported the first suggestion of drug-induced cancer with an account of skin cancers in patients treated with an arsenic-containing solution.

These historical observations and many others that followed illustrate the importance of clinical observations as a source of new discoveries in cancer etiology.[2,3] They also include an early indication of the long latent interval in human carcinogenesis, because Pott observed that some of the men with scrotal cancer had not worked as chimney sweeps since boyhood. Furthermore, they show how some causes can be detected (and diseases prevented) before specific agents and mechanisms are elucidated by laboratory investigators. Many decades elapsed before evidence was available to indicate that polycyclic hydrocarbons, radioactive substances, and aromatic amines explained some of the early findings described previously.

AIMS OF EPIDEMIOLOGY

Several words are key to the definition of the term *epidemiology,* which is the study of the distribution and determinants of disease frequency in human populations.[4] The word *humans* differentiates the approach from laboratory disciplines in cancer research that use animals and other test systems in their experiments. The study of *populations* stands in contrast to clinical research, which usually involves investigations at the individual patient or case series level. The term *frequency* indicates the orientation of epidemiology towards quantifying the occurrence of disease and the risks attributable to various causes. The phrase *distribution and determinants* points to the two major approaches of epidemiology. In general, descriptive studies examine the distribution of disease frequency in populations that can be useful in generating etiologic hypotheses, whereas analytic studies test hypotheses by pursuing differences in the personal characteristics or exposures among individuals.

The main contribution of cancer epidemiology is the detection and quantification of the risks associated with specific environmental exposures and host factors. These associations may lead to causal inferences, providing the basis for instituting preventive measures. Epidemiologic data support the concept that carcinogenesis is a lengthy multistage process that is affected by a wide variety of factors.[5-7] Some factors appear to act early as initiators, others later as promoters, and still others at both early and late stages. Certain agents act together to accelerate the carcinogenic process, such as the way smoking combines synergistically with asbestos to produce lung cancer or with alcohol to produce oral and esophageal cancers. Furthermore, the process may be retarded by dietary factors, such as certain micronutrients that appear to diminish the risk of various cancer sites including smoking-related lung cancer.

The aims of epidemiology are to uncover new etiologic leads through peculiarities in the distribution of cancer, quantify the risks associated with different exposures (some of which may be protective), promote insights into the mechanisms of carcinogenesis, and assess the efficacy of preventive measures. Although the usual observational methods of epidemiology have succeeded in identifying many causes of cancer, future progress may depend to a considerable degree on innovative strategies that employ laboratory techniques in epidemiologic investigations.

DESCRIPTIVE STUDIES

There is perhaps no disorder that shows a uniform incidence in all human groups. Cancers are striking in the variations they show according to such factors as age, sex, race, time, socioeconomic class, marital status, and geographic location. Descriptive (or demographic) studies, by revealing the patterns of disease in populations, have provided many clues to cancer causes. Variations by age, area, and time are often remarkable, even allowing for the fluctuations that might be expected as a result of chance and differences in diagnostic and reporting practices.[6] The descriptive patterns are useful also in monitoring variations and trends that might point to new environmental hazards, in evaluating the effects of cancer prevention, screening, and treatment activities and in predicting future trends that may help set priorities in various aspects of oncology.[8]

MEASURES OF CANCER FREQUENCY

Descriptive studies measure rates, which are based on three items of information: the number of persons affected by the disease (numerator), the length of the period covered (time), and the population from which they are derived (denominator). The expression of disease in this manner allows the rates in one population to be compared with the rates in another. Often these rates must be adjusted for such factors as age, race, and social class, which might otherwise spuriously influence the comparison.[9] The rates most often used in cancer epidemiology concern incidence, mortality, and prevalence, with each having its particular uses and limitations. When measures of occurrence are not based on populations at risk, they usually represent proportions, even though sometimes labeled as rates (*e.g.,* case-fatality rates). Sample calculations of these measures are derived from numbers given in Table 9–1.

The incidence rate provides a direct measure of the probability of developing cancer, and it is defined as the

$$\frac{\text{Number of persons developing cancer in a unit of time}}{\text{Total population living at that time}}$$

Most often the unit of time is 1 year, with the midyear population serving as the denominator. The rates are usually expressed per 100,000 or per million persons. For example, from the data in Table 9–1 the annual occurrence of Hodgkin disease per 100,000 residents in Connecticut is calculated as follows:

$$\text{Incidence rate} = \frac{120}{3,126,488} \times 100,000$$

$$= 3.8 \text{ per } 100,000 \text{ per year}$$

Incidence rates may be crude (all ages), as in this example, or age-specific. Because of the great dependence of cancer incidence on age, age-specific rates are more informative. However, when summary figures are necessary to compare rates between population groups with different age distributions, they should be age-adjusted; this is done by multiplying each age-specific rate by the percent of individuals in a standard population (*e.g.,* the 1970 U.S. population) with the same ages, and then summing to produce a single value. For etiologic studies, incidence rates tend to be more informative than mortality rates, because they cover all diagnosed cases (not merely the fatal ones) at a time which is closer to the point of causation. The information on incident cancers is usually

TABLE 9–1. Patients With Hodgkin's Disease and Pancreatic Cancer, Connecticut, 1982

Type of Cancer	Patients Alive at Start of Year*	New Cases in Year†	Deaths in Year‡
Hodgkin's disease	1151	120	26
Pancreatic cancer	220	326	297

* Prevalence data estimated from data of Feldman AR, et al. The prevalence of cancer. N Engl J Med 1986;315:1394.
† Incidence data from Connecticut Tumor Registry.
‡ Mortality data from National Center for Health Statistics.
Estimated populations were 3,112,469 on January 1, 1982, for prevalence and 3,126,488 on July 1, 1982, for incidence and mortality.

more extensive and reliable, with details often available on histologic type and stage.

The mortality or death rate is defined as the

$$\frac{\text{Number of persons dying of cancer in a unit of time}}{\text{Total population living at that time}}$$

From data in Table 9–1, the mortality rate for Hodgkin disease is computed as follows:

$$\text{Mortality rate} = \frac{26}{3,126,488} \times 100,000$$

$$= 0.8 \text{ per } 100,000 \text{ per year}$$

For etiologic research, mortality rates most clearly reflect the occurrence of those cancer sites with the worst prognosis, and are vulnerable to well-known inaccuracies and variations in death-certificate reporting of diagnoses. However, mortality data are often the only statistics available in certain locations and periods, and they have been especially useful for evaluation of long-term trends and geographic variations on a national or international scale. For several cancers with poor survival, mortality rates nearly equal incidence rates. Even with improvements in survival of many cancers, mortality rates help in clarifying incidence trends for certain cancers (*e.g.*, breast and prostate) that may be distorted by heightened efforts at case finding.[6,8] Mortality rates are also useful in evaluating the impact of advances in cancer prevention and treatment on the general population. The combined analyses of incidence, mortality, and survival statistics that comprise the Surveillance, Epidemiology, and End Results (SEER) Program of the National Cancer Institute (NCI) provide valuable data on the patterns of cancer in the United States.[10] When comparing cancer incidence or mortality rates in different countries, investigators sometimes use truncated age groups (*e.g.*, 35–64 years) to exclude the elderly whose rates are most subject to variations in medical care and reporting.

The case-fatality rate is a measure of the severity or lethality of disease. A proportion rather than a true rate, it is usually expressed as a percentage and defined as the

$$\frac{\text{Number of deaths from cancer}}{\text{Number of persons developing cancer}} \times 100\%$$

From data in Table 9–1, case-fatality rates are estimated as follows:

$$\text{Case fatality (Hodgkin's disease)} = \frac{26}{120} \times 100\% = 21.7\%$$

$$\text{Case fatality (pancreatic cancer)} = \frac{297}{326} \times 100\% = 91.1\%$$

Because the cases and deaths usually refer to the same period of time, this concept is less meaningful in chronic than in acute diseases and is generally replaced by survival rates that are discussed later.

The prevalence rate is seldom used in etiologic studies of cancer, but provides a useful measure for planning health services by estimating the burden of disease in the population.[11] Also called *point prevalence*, it is defined as the

$$\frac{\text{Number of persons with cancer at a given point in time}}{\text{Total population living at that time}}$$

From the data in Table 9–1, the prevalence of Hodgkin's disease on January 1, 1982 is calculated as follows:

$$\text{Prevalence} = \frac{1,115}{3,112,469} \times 100,000$$

$$= 37.0 \text{ per } 100,000$$

Table 9–2 summarizes the various kinds of rates for Hodgkin's disease and pancreatic cancer. Hodgkin's disease displays lower incidence and mortality rates than pancreatic cancer, but a higher prevalence rate due to its much lower case-fatality rate (or conversely, higher survival rate).

Proportional rates or relative frequencies are used when details of the population that produce a series of cancer cases

TABLE 9–2. Measures of Frequency for Hodgkin's Disease and Pancreatic Cancer, Connecticut, 1982

Rate	Hodgkin's Disease	Pancreatic Cancer
Mortality	0.8	9.5
Incidence	3.8	10.4
Prevalence	37.0	7.1

Crude rates per 100,000 population per year are calculated from data in Table 9–1.

or deaths are unknown. This may occur in surveys of hospital patients or death certificates, in which the proportions of different cancers may be compared with those in the general population for each sex and age group. Proportional mortality ratios are sometimes used in studies of occupational groups.[12] Because the denominator refers to total deaths rather than the population at risk, the magnitude of the ratio for a particular cancer may be misleading, because it also fluctuates according to the number of deaths from other causes. Positive findings emerging from this type of survey should be interpreted cautiously and pursued by more definitive investigation.

CORRELATIONAL STUDIES

Descriptive studies may use the correlational (or ecologic) approach, in which the rates of disease in populations are compared with the geographic or temporal distribution of suspected risk factors.[13] The association is often expressed in terms of correlation or regression coefficients. Although a correlational study may be helpful in formulating hypotheses about carcinogenic risks, it falls short of establishing causal relations. Correlational studies have the advantage of being inexpensive and quick because they often use statistics assembled for other purposes.[13]

The primary weakness of such studies for etiologic research, as with descriptive studies generally, is that the exposures concern populations rather than individuals. Moreover, the exposure measures are usually crude and subject to confounding factors. For example, in early surveys of lung cancer, the temporal increases among men were consistent with the effects of an increasing prevalence of cigarette smoking, but this correlation by itself provided only weak evidence of causation, because other factors such as air pollution and improvements in diagnosis showed a similar pattern. It required analytic studies that pursued these leads to establish the cause-and-effect relation between smoking and lung cancer. Correlational studies also may provide supporting evidence in evaluating relations detected by analytic or laboratory studies. This is illustrated by the more recent temporal increases in lung cancer among women, who have lagged about 25 years behind men in their adoption of smoking habits. Another example is the geographic correlation in developing countries between primary liver cancer and intake of foodstuffs contaminated by aflatoxin, a potent hepatocarcinogen in laboratory animals.[6] Although correlational data may provide clues to the causes, an investigator must be careful not to draw a premature or inappropriate conclusion, sometimes referred to as an *ecologic fallacy*.[13]

SOURCES OF DATA

Descriptive studies employ mainly population-based statistics on mortality, incidence, and survival to calculate rates, although clinical series from hospital-based registries or other sources may also provide clues to the cause and natural history of cancer.

Death Certificates

In many countries, a death certificate is prepared for legal purposes for each person who dies.[14] In addition to demographic variables, the certificate usually includes the underlying and secondary causes of death. Although in 1900 only 11 states in the United States contributed to the national registration system, by 1933 all 48 states were included. Alaska and Hawaii were added in 1959 and 1960 with their entry into the Union. The National Center for Health Statistics tabulates the deaths annually and calculates rates using population estimates provided by the Census Bureau. The data are also made available on computer magnetic tape for research purposes. A national death registry for the United States was established in 1979. This National Death Index is frequently used to identify persons in epidemiologic studies who have died.

The NCI has examined the national cancer mortality data in several periods. An early tabulation by age, race, sex, and form of cancer included deaths starting in 1930 and continuing through 1955.[15] Geographic variations in cancer mortality at the state level were evaluated for the years 1950 to 1967.[16] Analyses at the county level for 1950 to 1969[17] formed the basis for computer-generated color atlases portraying geographic patterns on a small-area scale for whites and nonwhites.[18,19] More recently, cancer mortality was tabulated at the county level by decade from 1950 through 1979.[20] Using data through 1980, maps of cancer mortality were prepared according to state economic area to examine trends in the geographic patterns.[21,22] Computer graphics have also been used to display national trends by age, race, and sex for 1950 to 1977.[23] Long-term trends in U.S. cancer mortality and incidence were examined for 1935 to 1974[24] and more recently for 1947 to 1984.[25] The geographic and temporal variations of cancer mortality have also been analyzed on an international scale.[26]

Despite the value of mortality data for epidemiologic study, reservations are often expressed about the quality of diagnoses reported on death certificates, even though most cancers diagnosed before death are properly recorded on the certificates.[27] Changes in diagnostic and certification practices and in coding rules may produce spurious trends, and it is prudent to consider each observation on its merits. Death certificates are also of great value to epidemiologists in comparing the mortality of a specific group under study with that of the general population. However, the death certificates of the study group must be coded according to the same rules as for the standard or reference population.

Population-Based Registries

The complete ascertainment of all newly diagnosed cases of cancer in a defined population is a difficult and expensive task. There is no system for gathering incidence data for the entire United States, but such data have been collected for specific areas in different time periods. The longest ongoing population-based resource is the Connecticut Tumor Registry, which has incidence data available from 1935.[28] Several other registries covering states or cities have been in existence for varying periods.

The NCI has coordinated several periodic surveys of cancer incidence in selected areas of the country. The first survey was in 1937 to 1939 and the second in 1947 to 1948,[29] with both covering the same 10 metropolitan areas and referred to as the Ten-Cities Surveys. Information was gathered on cases diagnosed during 1 calendar year in each of the areas, although the specific year varied among the areas. A special survey of cases diagnosed during 1950 was conducted in Iowa to compare cancer incidence patterns among rural and urban residents.[30] The Third National Cancer Survey included cases diagnosed during 1969 to 1971 in two states and seven cities.[31] Since 1973, the SEER program has included several population-based cancer registries that continuously gather information on cancer incidence, mortality, and survival.[10,32,33] The SEER registries cover more than 10% of the U.S. population. Although not a probability sample of the entire population, considerable geographic and ethnic variations are represented. It has been possible to evaluate the long-term trends in cancer incidence by focusing on the geographic areas common to the various surveys.[24,25] In other countries, cancer reporting systems have been in existence for varying periods, starting with the Danish Cancer Registry in 1942. The International Agency for Research on Cancer has compiled data from many of the registries in five successive volumes of *Cancer Incidence in Five Continents*, the most recent providing data generally for 1978 to 1982.[34] This resource has been immensely valuable for proposing etiologic hypotheses.

In conjunction with the operation of a cancer registry, patients may be followed to ascertain their medical condition and vital status. Such survival data are useful in understanding incidence and mortality trends, and in measuring the dissemination and effect of treatment improvements in the general population. Although not population-based, the End Results Group of the NCI compiled survival data starting in 1950.[35,36] Since the advent of the SEER program in 1973, it has been possible to continuously monitor population-based survival

Hospital-Based Registries

Although hospital-based cancer registries are valuable for clinical, administrative, and educational purposes, the data have limited use for epidemiologic studies.[39] However, such a registry may be an important component of a population-based cancer reporting system, and provides a means of identifying patients for case-control studies. In addition, a hospital registry may be useful in investigating the natural history of cancer and the risk of developing second primary cancers, and in assembling a clinical series that may provide clues to environmental or genetic factors in carcinogenesis.

PATTERNS OF CANCER OCCURRENCE

MAGNITUDE OF THE PROBLEM

In the United States, cancer is second only to heart disease as a cause of death and accounts for 22% of all deaths.[40] Among women aged 35 to 74, it is the leading cause of death. More than 1 million newly diagnosed cases of cancer and 500,000 deaths due to cancer are predicted for the United States during 1992 (Table 9–3). Lung cancer is the most common form, accounting for 15% of the cases and 28% of the deaths. Almost as many cases of colorectal cancer occur as lung cancer, but there are more than twice as many deaths from lung cancer. The next most common are cancers of the breast and prostate, so that these four cancers account for 56% and 55% of the

TABLE 9–3. Estimated New Cases and Deaths in the United States for Major Forms of Cancer—1992

Type of Cancer	Number of Cases	Number of Deaths
All sites	1,130,000	520,000
Lung	168,000	146,000
Colon and rectum	156,000	58,300
Breast	181,000*	46,300
Prostate	132,000	34,000
Urinary tract	78,100	20,200
Uterus	45,500*	10,000
Oral cavity and pharynx	30,300	7,950
Skin	32,000†	8,800‡
Pancreas	28,300	25,000
Leukemia	28,200	18,200
Ovary	21,000	13,000
All other sites	229,600	132,250

* Invasive cancers only; more than 20,000 carcinomas in situ of the breast and 55,000 carcinomas in situ of the cervix are estimated.
† Melanoma only; more than 600,000 nonmelanoma skin cancers are estimated.
‡ Melanoma 6700; other skin cancers 2100.
(Boring CC, Squires TS, Tong T. Cancer statistics, 1992. CA 1992; 42:19. Based on incidence data from National Cancer Institute SEER program 1986–1988 and mortality data from the National Center for Health Statistics. All figures are rounded.)

total cancer cases and deaths, respectively. The 11 sites shown in Table 9–3 comprise 80% of all cancer cases and 75% of cancer deaths.

Table 9–4 presents the age-adjusted incidence and mortality rates for 44 specific forms of cancer among white males and females in the United States for the period 1984 to 1988. Among males the mortality rate is highest for lung cancer, followed by colorectal and prostate cancers, whereas among females the rates are highest for lung and breast cancers, followed by colorectal cancer. However, the highest incidence rates are for prostate and breast cancers among males and females, respectively, survival rates for which are both considerably better than for lung cancer. All cancers show higher rates among men except for those of the breast, gallbladder, and thyroid.

INTERNATIONAL VARIATION

It has been estimated that about 75% to 80% of all cancer in the United States is due to environmental factors.[6] To obtain this estimate, rates for the lowest-risk countries were subtracted from rates prevailing in the United States. The lowest risk is considered the baseline level for so-called *spontaneous tumors* that in theory cannot be prevented.

Table 9–5 shows in rank form the international variation for a number of cancers based on recent statistics from volume 5 of *Cancer Incidence in Five Continents*.[34] The variation ranges from 155-fold for melanoma to fivefold for leukemia and is not believed to be greatly affected by differences in diagnostic and reporting practices between countries.[3,6] Although genetic

TABLE 9–4. Average Annual Age-Adjusted Incidence and Mortality Rates Per 100,000 Among U.S. Whites by Primary Cancer Site, 1984–1988

Type of Cancer	Incidence (SEER)		Mortality (U.S.)	
	Males	Females	Males	Females
All sites	433.1	339.8	212.7	138.3
Lip	2.8	0.3	0.1	0.0
Salivary gland	1.3	0.8	0.3	0.1
Nasopharynx	0.6	0.3	0.3	0.1
Other oral cavity and pharynx	11.6	5.0	3.7	1.5
Esophagus	5.2	1.6	4.9	1.2
Stomach	10.6	4.5	6.6	3.0
Small intestine	1.3	0.9	0.4	0.2
Colon	42.3	31.4	20.9	14.8
Rectum	19.3	11.3	3.6	2.1
Liver	2.9	1.2	2.9	1.3
Gallbladder	0.8	1.4	0.5	1.0
Other biliary	1.4	1.0	0.8	0.6
Pancreas	10.7	7.9	9.8	6.9
Larynx	8.3	1.6	2.3	0.4
Lung and bronchus	82.5	37.8	72.5	27.6
Pleura	1.4	0.2	0.3	0.1
Nasal cavity and sinuses	0.8	0.5	0.2	0.1
Bones and joints	1.0	0.7	0.5	0.3
Soft tissue	2.5	1.8	1.2	1.0
Melanoma of skin	12.6	9.7	3.2	1.7
Other nonepithelial skin	5.2	0.8	1.3	0.3
Breast	0.8	108.8	0.2	27.3
Cervix uteri	—	7.8	—	2.7
Uterus excluding cervix	—	22.7	—	3.4
Ovary	—	14.6	—	7.9
Vagina	—	0.6	—	4.2
Vulva	—	0.6	—	0.3
Prostate	92.2	—	22.2	—
Testis	4.7	—	0.3	—
Penis	0.8	—	0.2	—
Bladder	32.1	7.8	6.0	1.7
Kidney	11.6	5.6	4.8	2.2
Ureter	0.9	0.3	0.1	0.1
Eye and orbit	0.8	0.6	0.1	0.1
Brain and other nervous system	7.6	5.5	5.2	3.5
Thyroid	2.5	6.0	0.3	0.4
Hodgkin's disease	3.5	2.7	0.9	0.5
Non-Hodgkin's lymphoma	16.6	11.2	7.3	5.0
Multiple myeloma	4.7	3.2	3.2	2.2
Acute lymphocytic leukemia	1.8	1.2	0.8	0.5
Chronic lymphocytic leukemia	4.2	2.0	1.7	0.7
Acute myeloid leukemia	2.8	1.9	2.2	1.5
Chronic myeloid leukemia	1.7	1.0	1.0	0.6
Other leukemias	2.8	1.7	2.8	1.7
All other sites	15.9	12.2	17.0	11.5

Rates are age-adjusted based on the 1970 U.S. standard population. Incidence data are from the National Cancer Institute SEER program, and national mortality data are from the National Center for Health Statistics.

factors may play some role (*e.g.*, in melanoma, which tends to affect fair-skinned populations), evidence suggests that the international differences are mainly due to environmental factors. The patterns observed in Table 9–5 are in fact likely to underestimate the true global variation, because some regions with exceptionally high rates of certain cancers are not covered by registries (*e.g.*, esophageal cancer in parts of China and Iran, liver cancer in parts of Africa and Asia, and urinary tract cancer in areas endemic with schistosomiasis or Balkan nephropathy).[3] Furthermore, the differences would be more pronounced if data were available for certain subtypes of cancer such as Burkitt's lymphoma and Kaposi's sarcoma, or subsites such as the gingival-buccal mucosa which comes in contact with smokeless tobacco and related products.

MIGRANT PATTERNS

Further evidence for environmental factors can be found in studies of migrant populations, such as the Japanese who moved to Hawaii and California. After migration, with the adoption of new habits, the risk of various cancers has moved away from the rate prevailing in the country of origin toward that of the new country.[41] Among Japanese migrants, increases in the risk of large bowel cancer were evident within a few decades of migration, whereas changes in breast cancer rates continue for generations. In contrast to general environmental exposures, lifestyle practices may change slowly among migrants, depending on the speed and extent of acculturation.

Migrant patterns have been studied by comparing the cancer mortality rates in the U.S. white population by country of birth with the corresponding rates in the country of origin.[42] Figure 9–1 shows the age-adjusted mortality rates for colorectal and stomach cancers.[43] Stomach cancer rates among migrants are generally lower than in the country of origin, but higher than among whites born in the United States. In contrast, colorectal cancer mortality in most countries is lower than in the United States, but the rates among migrants not only approach those of the U.S.-born whites but even exceed them in some instances. Those born in Mexico, however, have retained rates that are about 50% those of native-born white Americans. In addition, colorectal cancer mortality among the foreign-born has not reached U.S. rates as frequently for women as for men. When mortality from other cancers among the U.S. foreign-born is compared with statistics in the countries of origin, the rates for breast, corpus uteri, and prostate cancers are generally more closely aligned with those of U.S. native-born whites. Analytic studies among migrants should provide insights into lifestyle factors in cancer causation.

CANCER MAPS

Although variations within countries are not as great as those seen internationally, the computer-generated mapping of cancer death rates in the United States at the county level for the period 1950 to 1969 revealed several high-risk areas that have led to the investigation of environmental exposures.[18,19] For example, the elevated rates for lung cancer among men along the eastern seaboard drew attention to the unexpected scale and impact of asbestos exposures in shipyards during World War II (Fig. 9–2).[44] Similarly, a clustering of high-risk

TABLE 9–5. International Variation in Cancer Incidence*

Type of Cancer	Ratio (H/L)	High (H) Incidence Area	Rate†	Low (L) Incidence Area	Rate†
Melanoma	155	Australia (Queensland)	30.9	Japan (Osaka)	0.2
Lip	151	Canada (Newfoundland)	15.1	Japan (Osaka)	0.1
Nasopharynx	100	Hong Kong	30.0	U.K. (South Western)	0.3
Prostate	70	U.S. (Atlanta, black)	91.2	China (Tianjin)	1.3
Liver	49	China (Shanghai)	34.4	Canada (Nova Scotia)	0.7
Penis	42	Brazil (Recife)	8.3	Israel (Born Eur. and Am.)	0.2
Oral cavity	34	France (Bas-Rhin)	13.5	India (Poona)	0.4
Cervix uteri (F)	28	Brazil (Recife)	83.2	Israel (non-Jews)	3.0
Esophagus	27	France (Calvados)	29.9	Romania (Urban Cluj)	1.1
Stomach	22	Japan (Nagasaki)	82.0	Kuwait (Kuwaitis)	3.7
Thyroid	22	Hawaii (Chinese)	8.8	Poland (Warsaw City)	0.4
Multiple myeloma	22	U.S. (Alameda, black)	8.8	Phillipines (Rural)	0.4
Kidney	21	Canada (NWT and Yukon)	15.0	India (Poona)	0.7
Corpus uteri (F)	21	U.S. (Bay Area, white)	25.7	India (Nagpur)	1.2
Lung	19	U.S. (New Orleans, black)	110.0	India (Madras)	5.8
Colon	19	U.S. (Connecticut, white)	34.1	India (Madras)	1.8
Testis	17	Switzerland (Urban Vaud)	10.0	China (Tianjin)	0.6
Bladder	16	Switzerland (Basel)	27.8	India (Nagpur)	1.7
Lymphosarcoma	12	Switzerland (Basel)	9.2	Japan (Rural Miyagi)	0.8
Pancreas	11	U.S. (Los Angeles, Korean)	16.4	India (Poona)	1.5
Hodgkin's disease	10	Canada (Quebec)	4.8	Japan (Miyagi)	0.5
Brain	9	N.Z. (Polynesian Islanders)	9.7	India (Nagpur)	1.1
Larynx	8	Brazil (Sao Paulo)	17.8	Japan (Rural Miyagi)	2.1
Ovary (F)	8	N.Z. (Polynesian Islanders)	25.8	Kuwait (Kuwaitis)	3.3
Rectum	8	Israel (Born Eur. and Am.)	22.6	Kuwait (Kuwaitis)	3.0
Breast (F)	7	Hawaii (Hawaiian)	93.9	Israel (non-Jews)	14.1
Leukemia	5	Canada (Ontario)	11.6	India (Nagpur)	2.2

* Among males unless specified as females (F); rates based on less than 10 cases are excluded.
† Average annual rate per 100,000, age-adjusted based on the world standard population; rates generally are for the period 1978–1982.
(Muir C, Parkin M. International Agency for Research on Cancer, based on data abstracted from Muir C, Waterhouse J, Mack T. et al. eds. Cancer incidence in five continents, vol 5. Lyon: International Agency for Research on Cancer, 1987)

areas in Louisiana was traced in part to heavy smoking by the Cajun population.[45] Furthermore, studies of the elevated rates for oral cancer among women in the rural south have pointed to the hazards associated with the practice of snuff dipping (Fig. 9–3).[46] A recent update of the cancer maps through the period 1970 to 1980 has revealed patterns resembling those in the earlier atlas, but with a tendency toward greater uniformity of rates around the country.[21,22] Yet some new clustering emerged, including elevated rates of lung and oral cancers among women in Florida and along the Pacific coast that seem related to smoking habits, and high rates of non-Hodgkin's lymphoma in central regions that may be associated with agricultural exposure to herbicides.[47] The U.S. cancer maps were soon followed by similar atlases from other countries, the total reaching 22 at last count.[48] Most remarkable are the maps from China that have disclosed dramatic variations in mortality and have stimulated analytic studies in areas with exceptionally high rates.[49] In Scandinavian countries that have national cancer registries, atlases based on incidence data have been useful in identifying high-risk communities, particularly for less lethal tumors (*e.g.*, endometrium) that are not measured well by mortality statistics.

TIME TRENDS

A major indication of the importance of environmental factors lies in the variation in the mortality and incidence of certain cancers over time. Mortality rates for some forms of cancer in the United States have changed greatly over the last 57 years, whereas rates for several other cancers have remained relatively stable (Fig. 9–4).[50] Most striking has been the tenfold increase in lung cancer mortality. The upward trend started earlier among males than among females, for whom the rate of increase accelerated during the 1960s. However, the rates among males have not been rising as rapidly during the 1980s as in previous years. These trends reflect the changing prevalence of smoking habits in the male and female populations.[51] Lung cancer mortality among females has sur-

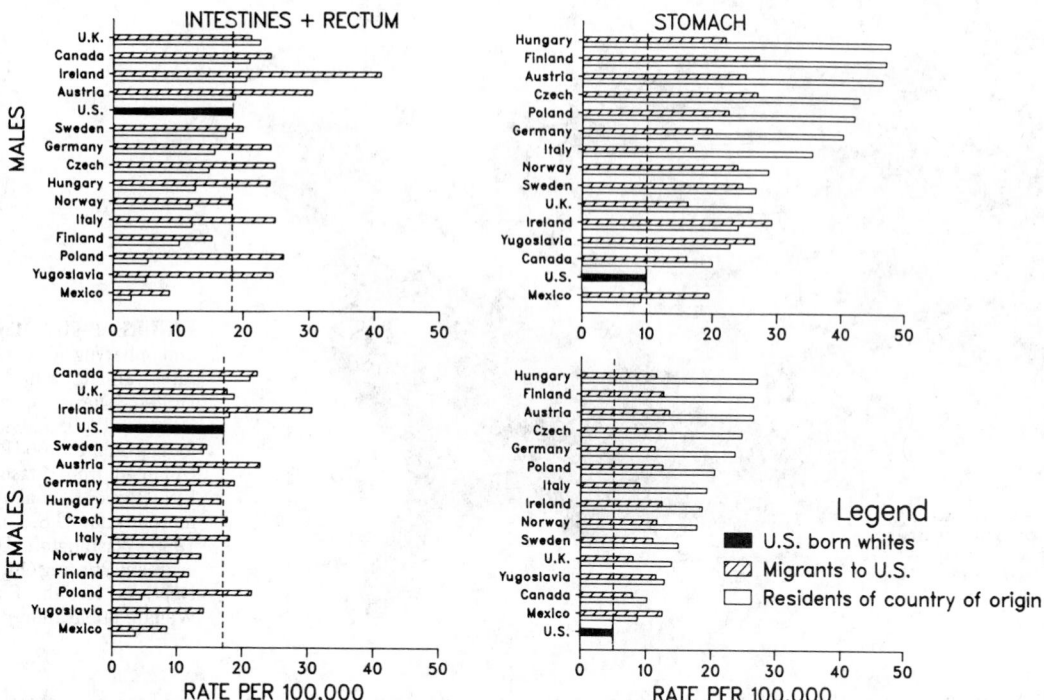

FIGURE 9–1. Average annual mortality rates for intestinal and stomach cancers among U.S.-born whites, migrants from selected countries from 1959 to 1961, and residents of the countries of origin, 1960. Rates standardized for age on the 1950 U.S. population. (Data from Lilienfeld AM, Levin ML, Kessler II. Cancer in the United States. Cambridge, MA: Harvard University Press, 1972)

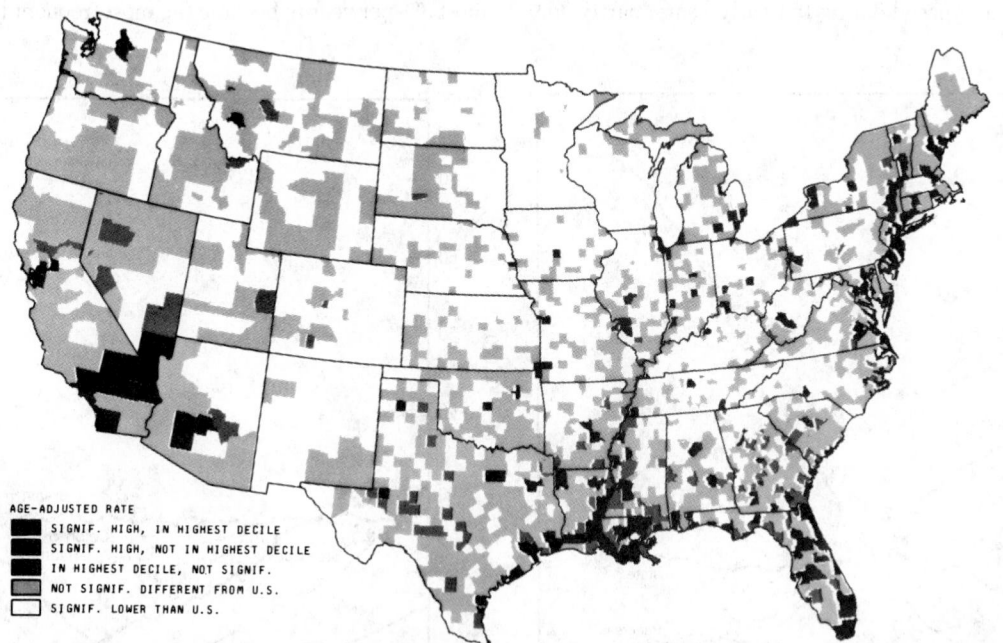

FIGURE 9–2. Mapping of lung cancer mortality rates among white men for United States state economic areas, 1950 to 1969. Rates standardized for age on the 1960 U.S. population. (Adapted from Mason TJ, McKay FW, Hoover R, et al. Atlas of cancer mortality for U.S. counties: 1950–1969. Washington, DC, U.S. Government Printing Office; 1975. U.S. Dept. of Health, Education, and Welfare publication [NIH] 75-780)

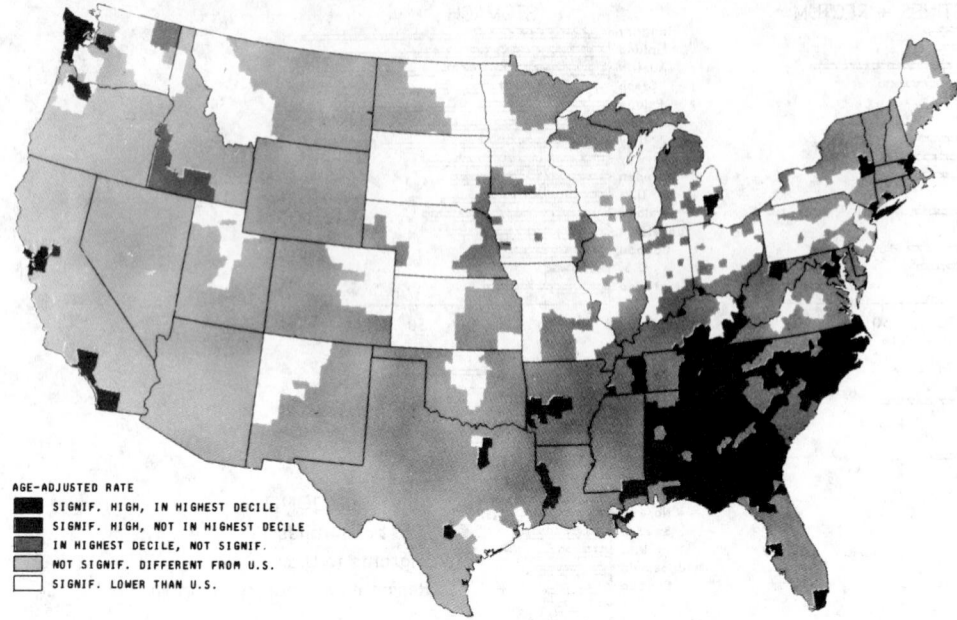

FIGURE 9–3. Mapping of oral and pharyngeal cancer mortality rates among white females for United States state economic areas, 1950 to 1969. Rates standardized for age on the 1960 U.S. population. (Adapted from Mason TJ, McKay FW, Hoover R, et al. Atlas of cancer mortality for U.S. counties: 1950–1969. Washington, DC, U.S. Government Printing Office; 1975. U.S. Dept. of Health, Education, and Welfare publication [NIH] 75-780)

passed that for breast cancer, the rate for which has not changed substantially over the past 50 years. Notable declines are apparent for stomach cancer and uterine cancer (reflecting downward mortality trends for cancers of the cervix and corpus uteri). Colorectal cancer rates increased until the late 1940s in both sexes and have leveled off among males and declined among females. Rates for several forms of cancer (*e.g.*, pancreas) increased during the early years, partly due to improvements in diagnosis and the accuracy of death certificates. The decreases noted for liver cancer are likely to reflect greater precision in the diagnosis and certification of primary cancer at this site.

Incidence data spanning about 40 years are shown in Figure 9–5 for the white population in five geographic areas of the country.[25] Among males, lung cancer incidence increased almost 3% per year to become the most frequent form of cancer

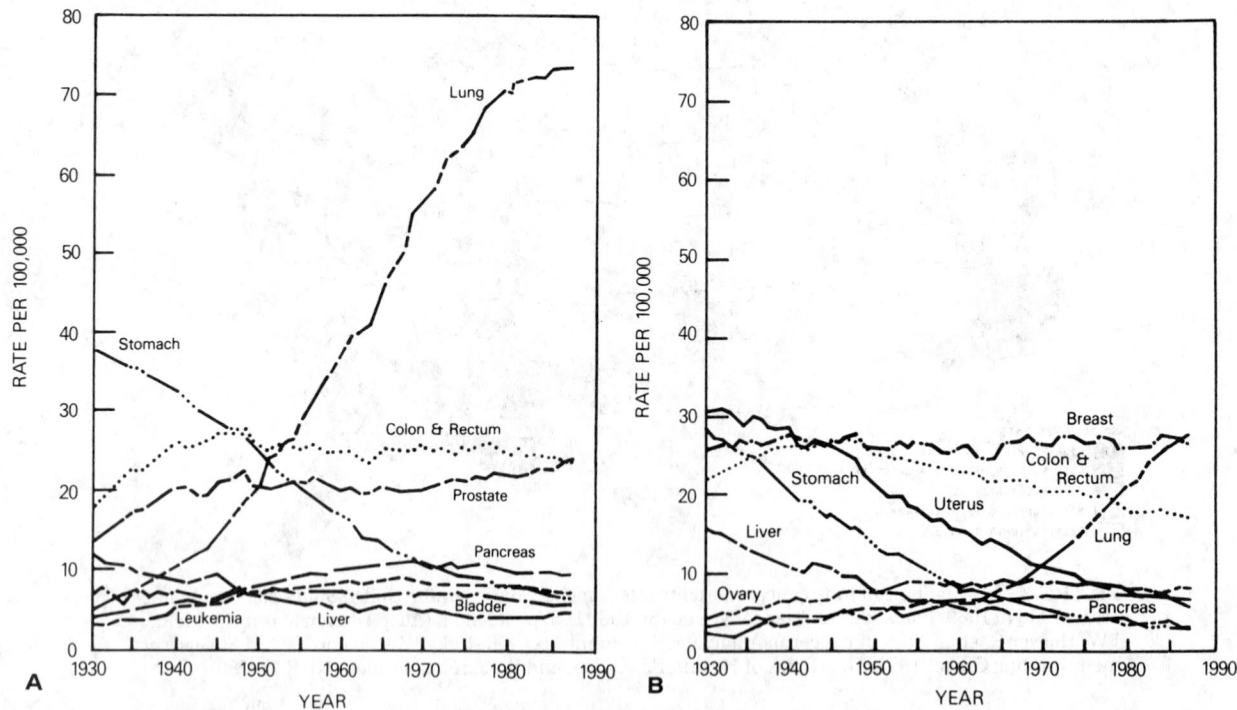

FIGURE 9–4. Cancer mortality trends for selected sites in the U.S. population, 1930 to 1987, among **(A)** males and **(B)** females. Rates standardized for age on the 1970 U.S. population. (Data from the National Center for Health Statistics; and Bureau of the Census; and Boring CC, Squires TS, Tong T. Cancer statistics, 1991. CA 1991;41:19)

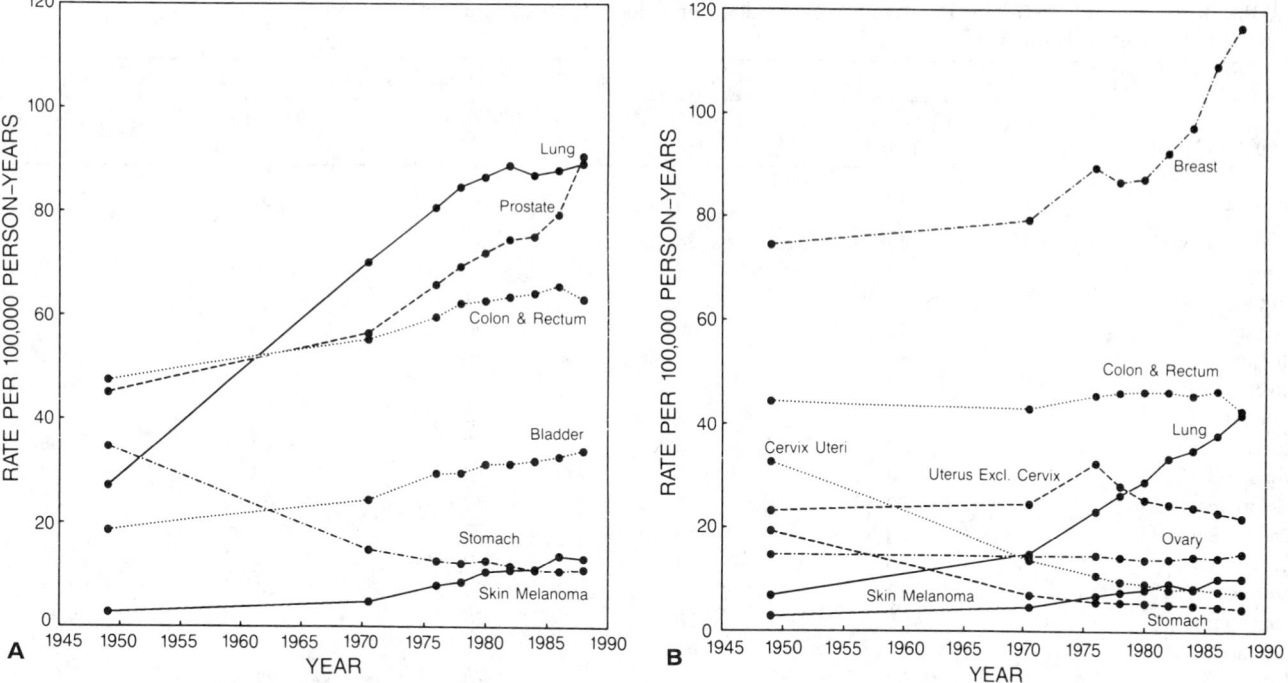

FIGURE 9–5. Cancer incidence trends for selected sites in five geographic areas of the United States, 1947 to 1988, among **(A)** white males and **(B)** white females. Rates standardized for age on the 1970 U.S. population. (Data from Devesa SS, Silverman DT, Young JL Jr, et al. Cancer incidence and mortality trends among whites in the United States, 1947–84. J Natl Cancer Inst 1987;79:701 and Surveillance, Epidemiology, and End Results program)

until recently; the leveling off in recent years may reflect a decrease in smoking prevalence. Prostatic cancer incidence rose to become the most common cancer among white males, due at least partly to the improved detection of early-stage or latent carcinomas.[52] Some of the increases in bladder cancer among males may be due to changing criteria by cancer registries, notably for papillomas, but trends in smoking must also play a role. Increases of 33% in colorectal cancer and declines of 68% in stomach cancer among males are consistent with a number of dietary hypotheses under active investigation.[53] Melanoma incidence rose nearly fourfold among males, probably due in part to the changing patterns of exposure to sunlight.[54]

Among females, breast cancer incidence rose 56% from the late 1940s to the late 1980s, with most of the increases occurring during the last decade. The striking rise during the early 1970s has been attributed to increased public awareness of breast cancer that precipitated earlier diagnoses, but reasons for the continuing increases, especially among women aged 55 and older, are unclear. Incidence rates have risen most sharply for localized tumors of the breast, and increases in early detection appear to be contributing to the trend.[33,55] In contrast to the prominent upward trend among males, colorectal cancer rates among females have remained relatively stable. Although lung cancer incidence rates are considerably lower among females than males, the proportional increases of almost 6% per year have been greater. The rates for cancer of the body of the uterus appeared stable until the 1970s, when a substantial increase of more than 30% occurred and was followed by decreases of similar magnitude. This pattern follows the upturn and subsequent downturn in the use of

menopausal estrogens that have been implicated in the development of endometrial cancer.[56] Incidence rates for invasive cancer of the cervix uteri declined more than 75% over the 40-year period, or about 4% per year, one of the largest observed for any cancer site in either sex. The decrease is due partly to the increased use of cervical cytology to detect precursor lesions,[57] but the increasing prevalence of women with a hysterectomy has contributed to the trend.[58] Declines of 77% in stomach cancer incidence and increases of almost threefold in melanoma are apparent among females, resembling the trends among males.

SURVIVAL TRENDS

Five-year relative survival rates among whites for all cancers combined rose from 39% in the early 1960s to 52% during the 1980s (Table 9–6). Interpretation of the trends should consider that the data come from two sources: the End Results Group for the earliest two periods and the SEER program for the subsequent intervals.[33] The relative survival rate is adjusted to take into account the expected mortality prevailing in the general population. The trend for all sites combined reflects not only improvements in survival for a number of specific cancers but also changes in their relative frequency. Large increases in survival rates have occurred for Hodgkin's disease, skin melanoma, and cancers of the testis, prostate, and bladder. Increases are seen also for leukemia, non-Hodgkin's lymphoma, and several other forms of cancer, due to better methods of treatment and perhaps earlier diagnosis. Melanoma and cancers of the thyroid, testis, and corpus uteri have shown 5-year survival rates of 80% or more in recent

TABLE 9–6. Trends in 5-Year Relative Survival Rates for Selected Sites of Cancer Among U.S. Whites, 1960–1987

Type of Cancer	Year of Diagnosis				
	1960–1963* (%)	1970–1973* (%)	1974–1976† (%)	1977–1980† (%)	1981–1987† (%)
All sites	39	43	50	50	52
Oral cavity and pharynx	45	43	55	54	54
Esophagus	4	4	5	6	9
Stomach	11	13	14	16	16
Colon	43	49	50	53	58
Rectum	38	45	48	51	55
Liver	2	3	4	3	5
Pancreas	1	2	3	2	3
Larynx	53	62	66	67	68
Lung and bronchus	8	10	12	13	13
Melanoma of skin	60	68	80	82	82
Breast (females)	63	68	75	75	78
Cervix uteri	58	64	69	68	68
Corpus uteri	73	81	89	86	84
Ovary	32	36	36	38	38
Prostate	50	63	67	72	76
Testis	63	72	78	88	93
Bladder	53	61	74	76	79
Kidney	37	46	52	51	53
Brain and nervous system	18	20	22	24	24
Thyroid	83	86	92	92	94
Hodgkin's disease	40	67	71	73	77
Non-Hodgkin's lymphoma	31	41	47	48	51
Multiple myeloma	12	19	24	25	26
Leukemia	14	22	34	36	36

* Rates based on data from the End Results Group using a series of hospital registries and one population-based registry.
† Rates based on data from the SEER program with follow-up of patients through 1988.
(National Cancer Institute: Cancer Statistics Review 1973–1988, Bethesda, MD, 1991)

years. Survival rates for those with esophageal, stomach, liver, pancreatic, and lung cancers remain poor.

The stage at diagnosis varies substantially by cancer site (Table 9–7). More than 75% of lip and corpus uteri cancers are localized when first detected, as are skin melanomas. At the other extreme are pancreatic and ovarian cancers, more than 50% of which have spread to distant sites. Survival figures for most cancers are greatly affected by the extent of disease at the time of detection. Patients with colon, rectum, bladder, or kidney cancers diagnosed at a localized stage experience 5-year survival rates exceeding 80%, whereas rates are lower than 10% if the cancer has spread to one or more distant sites. The impact of stage at diagnosis is only slightly less striking for melanoma and cancers of the breast and cervix. This suggests that major improvements in overall cancer survival and in mortality rates may be achieved through development and implementation of techniques enabling earlier detection and treatment. Generally less favorable survival rates among blacks than whites are at least partly due to more advanced stages of cancer at the time of diagnosis.[33]

The impact of improved treatment has been remarkable for childhood cancer (Table 9–8).[33] Five-year relative survival rates for all types combined improved from 28% during the early 1960s to 67% in the 1980s. Acute lymphocytic leukemia has been transformed from a virtually fatal cancer with a 4% survival rate to one with a 73% probability of 5-year survival. Children diagnosed with Hodgkin's disease during the early 1960s experienced a 52% survival rate, whereas those diagnosed during the 1980s achieved rates approaching 90%. For Wilms' tumor, survival rates increased from 33% to 84% over the same period. Improvements in therapy and survival have resulted in dramatic declines in childhood cancer mortality in recent years.[59]

AGE CURVES

Because of the marked rise in cancer incidence with advancing age, it was suggested that some aspect of the aging process increases susceptibility to cancer, perhaps by impairing immune function. It is now believed that the relation of many

TABLE 9–7. Stage Distribution and 5-Year Relative Survival Rates According to Stage at Diagnosis for Selected Sites of Cancer Among U.S. Whites, 1981–1987*

Type of Cancer	Stage Distribution (%)†			Relative Survival Rates (%)		
	Localized	Regional	Distant	Localized	Regional	Distant
Lip	78	13	1	93	82	‡
Salivary gland	49	34	9	91	52	30
Nasopharynx	19	46	19	75	43	25
Other oral and pharynx	32	47	12	66	40	17
Esophagus	25	21	27	21	6	0
Stomach	16	35	36	57	16	2
Colon	33	41	20	91	60	6
Rectum	41	36	16	83	50	5
Liver	22	21	26	13	5	2
Pancreas	10	21	51	7	4	1
Larynx	51	37	6	84	54	31
Lung and bronchus	18	31	39	41	14	2
Melanoma of skin	81	8	4	90	50	14
Breast (females)	52	38	7	92	72	19
Cervix uteri	48	32	10	89	54	14
Corpus uteri	76	11	9	93	72	29
Ovary	22	21	52	87	39	19
Prostate	61	14	18	89	80	29
Testis	62	23	13	97	96	67
Bladder	74	19	3	91	46	9
Kidney	42	25	28	84	56	8
Brain and nervous system	72	18	1	24	26	26
Thyroid	55	36	6	99	93	50

* Rates based on data from the SEER program with follow-up of patients through 1988.
† Percentages do not add to 100 due to some cases with unknown stage.
‡ Inadequate numbers to calculate.
(National Cancer Institute: Cancer Statistics Review 1973–1988, Bethesda, MD, 1991, and unpublished SEER data)

TABLE 9–8. Trends in 5-Year Relative Survival Rates for Selected Forms of Cancer Among U.S. White Children Under 15 Years of Age, 1960–1987

Type of Cancer	Year of Diagnosis				
	1960–1963* (%)	1970–1973* (%)	1974–1976† (%)	1977–1980† (%)	1981–1987† (%)
All forms	28	45	55	62	67
Acute lymphocytic leukemia	4	34	53	68	73
Acute myeloid leukemia	3	5	16	25	25
Wilms's tumor	33	70	74	80	84
Brain and nervous system	35	45	54	56	58
Neuroblastoma	25	40	49	52	55
Bone	20	30	52	47	56
Hodgkin's disease	52	90	80	88	87
Non-Hodgkin's lymphoma	18	26	43	50	68

* Rates based on the End Results Group using a series of hospital registries and one population-based registry.
† Rates based on the SEER program with follow-up of patients through 1988.
(National Cancer Institute: Cancer Statistics Review 1973–1988, Bethesda, MD, 1991)

cancers to increasing age mainly reflects the importance of duration of exposure to carcinogens and of long induction periods.[5]

Figure 9–6 shows the age distribution for selected cancers in the white population, with incidence plotted on a semilog scale. Most epithelial cancers are rare under age 30 but then rise progressively with age (*e.g.*, cancers of the colon and rectum, prostate, and bladder), although at the oldest ages a slight downturn in the curve is probably related to underdiagnosis. For cancers of female reproductive sites, the rates appear to reach a plateau or decline at postmenopausal ages, consistent with an influence of endogenous hormones. Only a few nonepithelial cancers rise sharply with age, notably multiple myeloma and chronic lymphocytic leukemia.[5] Deviations from the usual age trends are illustrated by the cancers plotted in Figure 9–6C. Peaks for leukemia and nervous system cancer occur not only at older ages but also in early childhood, suggesting the influence of prenatal factors. The bimodal age curve for Hodgkin's disease has received much attention, and some evidence suggests that the young adult peak may result from an infectious agent.[60] Also intriguing is the pattern of testis cancer, with a peak occurrence among young adult men and a rising incidence over time that remains unexplained.[61] The rates for invasive cervical cancer increase sharply with age among young women, but then level off after age 35.

Table 9–9 shows the incidence rates for the major cancers among white children by age group and sex for the period 1984 to 1988. Except for lymphomas and bone tumors, the highest incidence occurs in children under 5 years. In general, boys have somewhat higher rates than girls in all three age groups, especially for the lymphomas.

ETHNIC VARIATION

The SEER program provides data indicating striking racial and ethnic variations in cancer incidence in the United States (Tables 9–10 and 9–11). For males, the rates for all cancers combined are highest in blacks, followed by whites and Hawaiian Americans, whereas for females the rates are highest for Hawaiian Americans, followed by whites and blacks. The lowest rates in both sexes are in Native Americans. Compared with other groups, whites have especially high rates for melanoma, Hodgkin's disease, non-Hodgkin's lymphoma, leukemia, and cancers of the lip, breast, corpus uteri, ovary, testis, bladder, brain, colon, and rectum. Blacks have elevated rates for multiple myeloma and cancers of the oral cavity, esophagus, colon, pancreas, larynx, lung (males), cervix uteri, and prostate. Hispanic Americans have especially high rates for cervix cancer, and to some extent for cancers of the stomach and biliary tract (especially females), whereas Native Amer-

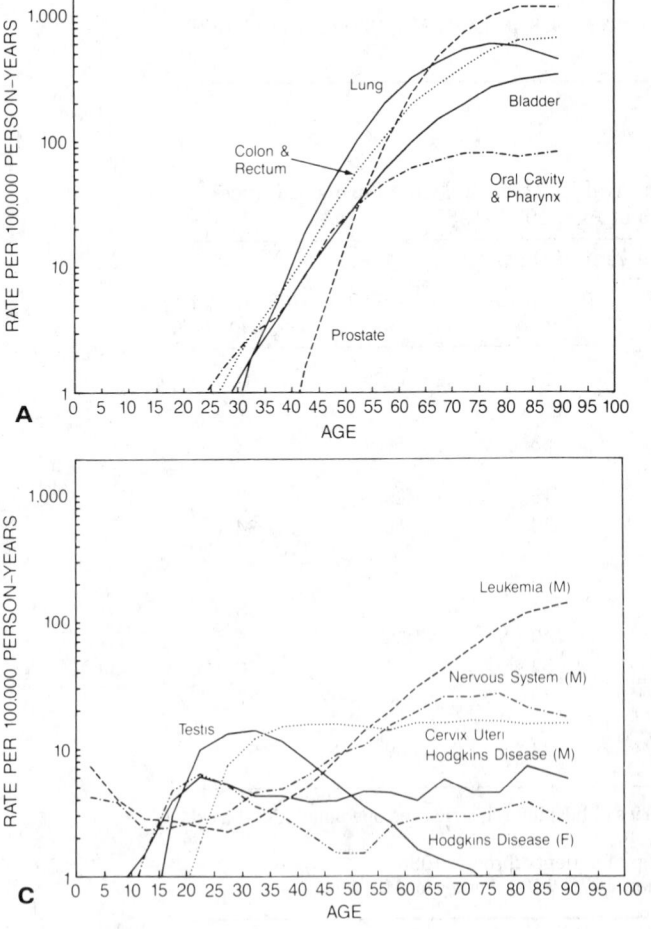

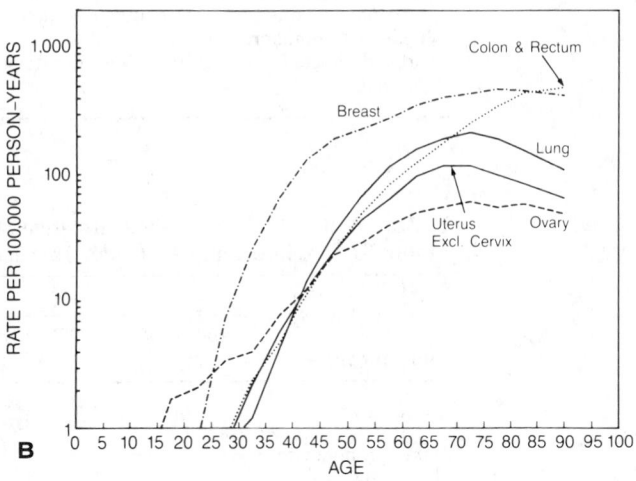

FIGURE 9–6. Age-specific incidence patterns in the U.S. white population, Surveillance, Epidemiology, and End Results program, 1984 to 1988, for selected epithelial cancers among **(A)** males and **(B)** females, and **(C)** for selected nonepithelial cancers and cancer of the cervix.

TABLE 9–9. Age-Specific Incidence Rates for Selected Forms of Cancer Among U.S. White Children, 1984–1988*

Type of Cancer	Boys			Girls		
	0–4†	5–9	10–14	0–4	5–9	10–14
All forms	21.5	13.0	12.8	18.8	9.8	11.9
Leukemia	7.5	4.0	2.8	6.8	2.6	2.6
Brain and central nervous system	4.2	3.8	2.3	3.6	3.2	2.3
Lymphoma	0.8	2.2	3.4	0.4	1.1	2.2
Neuroblastoma	3.6	0.4	0.0	2.8	0.4	0.1
Soft tissue	0.6	0.4	0.5	0.7	0.3	0.7
Wilm tumor	1.6	0.6	0.1	1.9	0.6	0.1
Bone	0.1	0.5	1.6	0.1	0.6	1.4
Retinoblastoma	1.0	0.1	0.0	1.2	0.1	0.0
All others	2.1	1.0	2.1	1.3	0.9	2.5

* Average annual rates per 100,000 population.
† Age given in years.
(National Cancer Institute: Cancer Statistics Review 1973–1988, Bethesda, MD, 1991, and unpublished SEER data)

TABLE 9–10. Average Annual Age-Adjusted Incidence Rates per 100,000 for Selected Cancer Sites by Racial and Ethnic Group, 1975–1985, U.S. Males

Type of Cancer	Whites	Blacks	Hispanics	American Indians	Chinese	Japanese	Filipinos	Hawaiians
All sites	404.1	490.2	265.5	184.5	292.7	303.6	242.0	398.9
Lip	3.7	0.2	3.3	0.0	0.1	0.1	0.0	0.0
Nasopharynx	0.6	1.0	0.9	0.5	13.9	1.4	2.9	1.5
Other oral cavity and pharynx	11.8	20.5	5.2	1.7	6.2	6.0	6.8	10.1
Esophagus	4.9	18.4	2.9	1.9	6.1	5.6	4.9	15.1
Stomach	11.5	20.5	20.8	26.1	14.5	38.6	9.6	40.4
Colon	40.3	40.7	17.9	8.4	33.6	42.1	24.0	25.8
Rectum	20.0	14.9	11.5	5.0	19.3	23.4	16.9	18.7
Liver	2.7	5.2	4.3	4.5	19.5	7.1	10.2	9.8
Gallbladder	0.8	0.8	1.5	8.9	1.2	1.5	1.2	1.4
Other biliary	1.6	1.2	2.2	2.8	2.2	3.9	2.1	2.5
Pancreas	11.2	16.9	12.4	9.0	8.7	9.9	7.9	10.6
Larynx	8.6	12.3	4.2	1.1	2.9	3.9	2.8	6.5
Lung and bronchus	82.1	119.6	32.2	14.2	61.2	48.4	39.9	108.2
Melanoma of skin	9.8	0.8	1.6	2.2	0.4	1.5	1.2	1.6
Prostate	77.3	122.8	71.5	45.5	32.5	45.7	47.4	59.6
Testis	4.2	0.8	3.0	1.8	1.9	1.3	0.5	2.6
Bladder	30.2	15.1	10.9	3.6	13.9	12.5	6.0	10.6
Kidney	10.3	9.6	8.7	9.2	4.9	6.1	4.6	6.9
Brain and other nervous system	7.3	4.3	4.9	3.1	3.0	3.1	3.4	3.1
Thyroid	2.3	1.4	2.9	2.3	4.5	6.2	6.8	7.4
Hodgkin's disease	3.5	2.7	3.3	0.7	0.8	0.8	1.7	1.4
Non-Hodgkin's lymphoma	13.0	8.5	6.9	4.7	10.2	9.2	9.8	10.9
Multiple myeloma	4.6	10.3	2.8	2.7	2.2	1.7	4.6	5.9
Leukemia	13.8	11.1	7.8	5.5	7.7	6.9	8.8	9.5
All others	27.8	30.7	21.8	18.7	21.3	16.6	18.0	28.6

Based on data from the SEER program. Data for Hispanics and American Indians are from New Mexico, whereas those for Chinese, Japanese, and Filipinos are from San Francisco and Hawaii. Rates are age-adjusted based on the 1970 U.S. standard population.

TABLE 9–11. Average Annual Age-Adjusted Incidence Rates per 100,000 for Selected Cancer Sites by Racial and Ethnic Group, 1975–1985, U.S. Females

Type of Cancer	Whites	Blacks	Hispanics	American Indians	Chinese	Japanese	Filipinos	Hawaiians
All sites	316.1	296.6	220.4	168.8	242.2	214.0	202.6	344.1
Lip	0.3	0.1	0.4	0.0	0.0	0.1	0.0	0.0
Nasopharynx	0.3	0.5	0.2	0.0	6.7	0.3	1.6	1.1
Other oral cavity and pharynx	5.2	6.2	1.7	0.6	1.3	2.1	5.3	5.3
Esophagus	1.6	5.0	0.8	0.3	1.2	0.8	1.9	2.2
Stomach	5.1	8.5	10.0	12.3	8.7	19.0	7.2	17.9
Colon	32.3	35.0	16.7	8.1	23.7	25.7	14.9	16.3
Rectum	12.8	10.8	7.6	3.2	10.9	10.9	8.1	8.1
Liver	1.1	1.7	1.9	2.6	4.7	2.4	3.2	2.7
Gallbladder	1.6	1.1	7.1	17.1	1.0	1.7	1.8	1.3
Other biliary	1.1	0.8	1.3	4.4	1.9	2.4	0.7	2.6
Pancreas	7.7	11.5	10.8	4.3	7.8	6.0	4.8	9.2
Larynx	1.5	2.2	0.9	0.0	0.2	0.2	0.7	1.6
Lung and bronchus	29.7	31.2	15.6	4.6	27.6	13.2	17.9	45.8
Melanoma of skin	8.2	0.7	2.2	0.7	0.7	1.0	0.9	1.0
Breast	91.5	76.4	50.9	25.6	58.7	57.1	45.6	104.6
Cervix uteri	8.8	19.7	17.1	20.0	10.5	5.8	10.8	14.5
Uterus excluding cervix	27.1	14.8	11.2	5.2	18.2	17.6	11.0	28.0
Ovary	14.1	9.8	11.3	8.9	10.3	8.5	9.7	13.2
Bladder	7.7	5.5	3.3	0.4	4.0	4.4	3.1	6.0
Kidney	4.7	4.6	4.2	6.2	2.5	2.2	2.2	2.8
Brain and other nervous system	5.1	2.9	2.4	1.8	2.7	2.2	1.3	4.2
Thyroid	5.5	3.5	7.9	6.1	6.9	6.6	17.3	13.7
Hodgkin's disease	2.6	1.2	1.3	0.5	0.8	0.3	1.3	0.9
Non-Hodgkin's lymphoma	9.6	5.7	5.5	4.8	6.5	5.9	7.1	6.6
Multiple myeloma	3.1	6.8	2.8	2.2	1.7	1.3	2.6	5.6
Leukemia	8.0	7.0	6.3	4.5	4.7	5.1	6.4	7.0
All others	20.2	23.6	18.8	24.4	18.1	11.1	15.3	22.2

Based on data from the SEER program. Data for Hispanics and American Indians are from New Mexico, whereas those for Chinese, Japanese, and Filipinos are from San Francisco and Hawaii. Rates are age-adjusted based on the 1970 U.S. standard population.

icans have remarkably high rates for cancers of the stomach, biliary tract, cervix, and kidney (females). Chinese Americans experience elevated rates for cancers of the nasopharynx and liver, whereas Japanese Americans have high rates for stomach cancer and (in males) for cancers of the colon, rectum, and thyroid. Filipino Americans have high rates for cancers of the thyroid, whereas Hawaiian Americans show elevated rates for cancers of the lung (notably in females), breast, corpus uteri, stomach, and thyroid. Like migrant populations, the racial and ethnic variations in cancer occurrence within the United States offer special opportunities for studies aimed at clarifying the environmental and host determinants of cancer.

SOCIOECONOMIC PATTERNS

Although racial and ethnic variations in rates may reflect genetic influences, many are influenced strongly by environmental factors, some of which may be associated with socioeconomic status. Data from the Third National Cancer Survey[31] were used to estimate the associations of cancer incidence with median family income and educational achievement as indicated by census tract of residence and to evaluate the impact of adjustment for socioeconomic disparities on the observed black-to-white relative risks.[62] Overall, cancer incidence rates among whites were 20% greater in the lowest income group than in the highest, with a continuous gradient in risk (Table 9–12). This pattern varied by primary site. Cervix cancer was almost four times as frequent among women in the lowest relative to the highest category, for reasons that are not clear. Rates for esophageal cancer among men varied more than twofold, in line with socioeconomic differences in the use of alcohol and tobacco and nutritional status. Striking inverse gradients were also apparent for lung and stomach cancers among males, reflecting smoking and perhaps nutritional patterns. In contrast, positive gradients with income level were apparent for both breast and corpus uteri cancers, which may parallel the distribution of reproductive and menstrual risk factors.

An important question is the extent to which socioeconomic

TABLE 9–12. Relative Risks for All Cancers and Selected Sites by Socioeconomic Status (SES) and Race, 1969–1971*

Site of Cancer	Income Level Among Whites					Black/White Relative Risks	
	Low	2	3	4	High	SES Unadjusted	SES Adjusted†
All sites (males)	1.20	1.09	1.07	1.02	1.00	1.10	1.0
Esophagus (males)	2.13	1.69	1.34	1.20	1.00	3.05	2.3
Stomach (males)	1.39	1.26	1.16	1.02	1.00	1.48	1.2
Lung (males)	1.65	1.44	1.33	1.18	1.00	1.10	0.9
Breast (females)	0.70	0.73	0.80	0.83	1.00	0.85	0.8
Cervix uteri	3.82	2.69	1.95	1.39	1.00	1.74	1.2
Corpus uteri	0.75	0.83	0.88	0.89	1.00	0.70	0.6

* Data derived from the Third National Cancer Survey, 1969–1971. All relative risks adjusted for age and geographic area.
† Also adjusted for income and education.

factors account for the black-to-white differentials in cancer incidence. When adjusted for racial variations in socioeconomic status, the excess risk among blacks is diminished for cancers of the esophagus, stomach, lung, and cervix. These patterns generally were still apparent in recent years.[63,64] Socioeconomic status may also influence cancer survival and mortality patterns by affecting access to diagnosis and treatment.

ANALYTIC STUDIES

The major contribution of epidemiology has been to test etiologic hypotheses through analytic studies, usually involving cohort or case-control designs. These studies obtain data on suspected risk factors and disease occurrence at the individual instead of at the aggregate (population) level. By using specific methods to select and compare groups of subjects while controlling for other relevant variables, the risk of disease associated with exposure can be estimated.[4,13,14] In designing these studies, the groups should be sufficiently large and the time intervals between initial exposure and tumor onset sufficiently long to identify the lowest excess risk considered important to detect. Reliable and valid estimates of exposure should be sought, with quantitative measurements to permit dose-response evaluations. Studies must be designed to minimize potential sources of bias (*i.e.*, systematic error) and to permit the detection and control of confounding (*i.e.*, the distortion of exposure-disease associations by extraneous variables).

COHORT STUDIES

Cohort studies, also referred to as *follow-up studies* or *prospective studies*, identify groups of individuals with and without a particular exposure, follow them over time to determine subsequent health outcomes, and compare their mortality or incidence rates of disease.[4,65] An association is suggested when the rates of disease are different in the exposed than in the unexposed group. These investigations may be based on current exposures and future health outcomes, referred to as *prospective cohort studies*. More often, they use information on exposures collected in the past and are termed *retrospective*

cohort studies. Instead of an unexposed comparison group, general population mortality or incidence rates (specific for age, sex, race, geographic area, and calendar time) are often used to estimate an expected number of events. This method assumes that in the absence of the specific exposure of interest the study group would have the same probability of developing the disease as the general population. The cohort approach is used mainly when it is possible to evaluate high exposures in clearly defined subgroups of the population. It has been especially helpful, for example, in assessing the carcinogenic risk from occupational hazards, smoking, or medical exposures such as radiation and certain drugs.

CASE-CONTROL STUDIES

Case-control studies, also called *case-referent studies* or *retrospective studies*, identify persons with a particular disease (cases) and a group of similar persons without the disease (controls), and then collect information on past exposures by interview or other methods.[4,65] If the proportion of cases with a certain exposure is greater than that of the controls, an association may be indicated. The case-control approach is especially suited for studying uncommon diseases. Although used primarily to test hypotheses, the approach occasionally has taken the form of an exploratory study when a disease is so poorly understood that hypotheses need to be formulated for subsequent investigation. In general, both cases and controls should be selected from the same source, which may be either population-based or hospital-based. Because factors associated with hospitalization may be over-represented among hospital controls, careful consideration should be given to the diagnostic composition of this group. Bias is minimized by selecting hospital controls with a variety of disorders and excluding conditions related to the exposure in question.[66]

COMPARISON OF METHODS

The case-control and cohort methods have different strengths and weaknesses. Case-control studies provide a more efficient means of studying rare diseases, with fewer individuals needed, a shorter study period, and generally lower costs compared with the cohort approach. In addition, there are greater opportunities to evaluate more than one risk factor and interactions between them.[67] On the other hand, the case-control approach cannot directly estimate the actual rate associated with a particular exposure and is subject to recall and other biases that affect the comparability of cases and controls and the precision of past exposure measures.[4] Such studies also are usually limited to evaluating one disease at a time.

The advantages of cohort studies are their capacity to measure directly incidence or mortality rates associated with a particular exposure; to reduce subjective biases by obtaining information before the disease develops; to detect associations between a particular exposure and multiple outcomes; and to evaluate temporal relations such as latency period and the duration of an effect. Cohort studies are usually expensive and complex undertakings. They require large numbers of exposed individuals, particularly when uncommon diseases are being investigated, and care in dealing with such problems as persons lost to follow-up or biased estimates of risk, as produced by the healthy worker effect of occupational studies.[4] Moreover, they may not permit as ready an ascertainment of potential confounding factors. To remedy this particular deficiency, case-control studies within defined cohorts, or nested case-control studies, are often initiated.

MEASURES OF ASSOCIATION

For cohort studies, the chief measures of association are based on rates of disease (Table 9–13). The relative risk (RR) is the disease rate in the exposed population, I_e, divided by the

TABLE 9–13. Measures of Association From a Cohort Study

	Affected Persons (Cases)	Total Persons (or Person-Time)
Exposed	a	n_e
Not exposed	c	n_0
Total	a + c	N

Relative risk (RR) = $\dfrac{a/n_e}{c/n_0}$

Attributable risk in the exposed (A_e) = $\dfrac{a}{n_e} - \dfrac{c}{n_0}$

Attributable risk percent in the exposed ($A_e\%$) = $\dfrac{(a/n_e) - (c/n_0)}{a/n_e}$

$\qquad\qquad = \dfrac{RR - 1}{RR} \times 100\%$

Population attributable risk (A_p) = $\dfrac{a + c}{N} - \dfrac{c}{n_0}$

Population attributable risk percent ($A_p\%$)

$\qquad = \dfrac{(a + c)N - (c/n_0)}{(a + c)N}$

$\qquad = \dfrac{RR - 1}{RR + 1/P - 1} \times 100\%$

where P is the proportion of the population that is exposed, or n_e/N

disease rate in the referent population (usually nonexposed, I_0).[4] The relative risk from a cohort study is defined as

$$RR = \frac{I_e}{I_0} = \frac{a/n_e}{c/n_0}$$

This measure gives the relative disease risk between two populations. An RR of 2.0 would indicate that the exposed group has twice the risk of the unexposed group (*i.e.*, a 100% increase in risk). An important aspect of the calculation is the concept of person-time. Usually individuals are followed for different periods owing to variable times of entry to and exit from observation because of either death or loss to follow-up. To accommodate the variable follow-up periods and still preserve the concept of a rate, each person is counted in the denominator only for the interval of time under observation, resulting in measures of person-years or person-months.[4]

An association may also be measured by the risk difference, often referred to as the *attributable risk* (A_e). This estimate results from the subtraction of the rate among the unexposed from that among the exposed. The attributable risk is defined as

$$A_e = I_e - I_0 = \frac{a}{n_e} - \frac{c}{n_0}$$

The attributable risk means that if the relation observed is causal, the difference between the rates of exposed and unexposed groups is the amount of disease attributable to that exposure.[4] When expressed as a percentage of the total disease rate in an exposed group, the attributable risk percent ($A_e\%$) is the proportion of the exposed group's total risk that is due to the exposure.[68]

The measures of relative risk and attributable risk have somewhat different uses. The magnitude of the RR indicates the strength of a relation between exposure and disease and the likelihood of causality. The A_e is influenced not only by the magnitude of the difference between the exposed and unexposed but also by the rate of disease in the absence of exposure.

The amount of disease attributable to a particular exposure can be estimated not only among the exposed but also in the population as a whole.[68] This measure reflects the amount of disease that would be eliminated in a definable population if the exposure were removed and is referred to as the *population attributable risk* (A_p). It is calculated by subtracting the rate among the unexposed from the rate that exists in the total population. The population attributable risk is defined as

$$A_p = I_t - I_0 = \frac{a + c}{N} - \frac{c}{n_0}$$

The magnitude of this estimate is influenced by the size of the relative difference in risk between the exposed and unexposed, by the level of the disease among the unexposed, and by the prevalence of the exposure in the population. When this risk is expressed as a proportion of the total disease rate in the population, it is called the *population attributable risk percent* ($A_p\%$) or the etiologic fraction.[69]

These measures are illustrated by a recent cohort study involving 1-year survivors of ovarian cancer from five randomized trials.[70] The incidence rates for acute nonlymphocytic leukemia and preleukemia were evaluated among women treated with no chemotherapy, with cyclophosphamide, and with melphalan. The corresponding rates were 0.18, 3.21, and 11.46 cases per 1000 women per year. Compared with those receiving no chemotherapy, the RR of leukemic conditions was 18 (3.21/0.18) for women given cyclophosphamide and 64 (11.46/0.18) for those given melphalan. The magnitude of these risks suggests that the drugs are causally related to leukemia. However, the risk differences obtained by subtracting rates among the exposed from the unexposed groups were not great. The A_e associated with cyclophosphamide is about 3 per 1000 per year, and with melphalan, about 11 per 1000 per year. Given the life-threatening problems posed by ovarian cancer, these risks should not deter physicians from using a therapy whose proven benefit outweighs these risks. Also, when the A_e is not large, it is possible to see how difficult it is for a clinician or even a large group practice to suspect a leukemia risk related to treatment.

If exposure to all alkylating agents were removed, it would have little impact on the total leukemia rate in the general population because relatively few persons are exposed to these drugs. However, in the clinical populations under study, the overall rate of leukemic conditions was 2.29 per 1000 patients per year. As shown in Table 9–14, subtracting the rate among those not treated with chemotherapy (0.18 per 1000 per year) from the rate for all patients combined yields a population attributable risk of 2.11 cases per 1000 women per year, or an etiologic fraction of 92% in the clinical populations.

For case-control studies, the enumeration of exposed and unexposed populations is not available, as it is in cohort studies, to directly measure rates (or risks). Fortunately, data from

TABLE 9–14. Risks of Leukemia and Preleukemia Associated With Chemotherapy

	Cases	Person-Years at Risk	Rate per 1000
Any Chemotherapy	33	4295	7.68
No Chemotherapy	2	10,983	0.18
Total	35	15,278	2.29

Relative risk (RR) $= \dfrac{33/4275}{2/10,983} = \dfrac{7.68}{0.18} = 42.4$

Attributable risk in the exposed (A_e) $= 33/4275 - 2/10,983$

$\qquad\qquad = 7.50$ per 1000

Attributable risk percent in the exposed (A_e%) $= \dfrac{42.4 - 1}{42.4} \times 100\%$

$\qquad\qquad = 98\%$

Population attributable risk (A_p) $= \dfrac{35}{15,278} - \dfrac{2}{10,983}$

$\qquad\qquad = 2.11$ per 1000

Population attributable risk percent (A_p%)

$\qquad = \dfrac{35/15,278 - 2/10,983}{35/15,278} \times 100\%$

$\qquad = 92\%$

(Adapted from Greene MH, Harris EL, Gershenson DM, et al. Melphalan may be a more potent leukemogen than cyclophosphamide. Ann Intern Med 1986;105:360)

TABLE 9–15. Measures of Association From a Case-Control Study

	Cases	Controls
Exposed	a	b
Not exposed	c	d
Total	a + c	b + d

Relative odds (R) $= \dfrac{ad}{bc}$

Attributable risk percent in the exposed (A_e%) $= \dfrac{R - 1}{R} \times 100\%$

Population attributable risk percent (A_p%) or etiologic fraction

$$= \dfrac{P_0(R - 1)}{1 + P_0(R - 1)} \times 100\%$$

$$= \dfrac{(R - 1)P_e}{R} \times 100\%$$

where P_0 is the exposure rate in the controls, or $\dfrac{b}{b + d}$ and

P_e is the exposure rate in the cases, or $\dfrac{a}{a + c}$

cross-classification tables in a case-control study can be used to calculate reasonable estimates of relative and attributable risks. If the sampling fractions for the cases and the controls are known (*i.e.*, the proportion of all the cases in a defined population that is present in the case series and the proportion of the same population present in the control series), they can be used to estimate the rates among the exposed and unexposed groups and to calculate relative and attributable risks. For most case-control studies, however, sampling fractions are unknown. In this circumstance, the calculation of relative odds, also termed an *odds ratio*, usually gives a good approximation of the relative risk (Table 9–15).[4] The absolute measures of attributable risk cannot be estimated directly, but algebraic properties of cross-classification tables allow estimations of the attributable risk percent and the etiologic fraction (see Table 9–15).[68]

Calculation of these measures is illustrated in Table 9–16, based on a national case-control study of bladder cancer that evaluated the risks associated with smoking.[71] The study estimated a relative risk of 2.2 for cigarette smoking, with 55% of bladder cancer among smokers attributable to their smoking and 43% of bladder cancer in the U.S. population due to smoking. These figures are consistent with the direct estimates of risk from cohort studies.

INTERVENTION STUDIES

Also referred to as *experimental studies*,[65] controlled intervention trials represent a third strategy of analytic epidemiology. Intervention studies are especially useful for confirming causal relations suggested by cohort or case-control studies and for directly evaluating the effect of possible preventive measures. This method permits control over extraneous variables and biases that may influence results by the random allocation of subjects to study and control groups.

TABLE 9-16. Risks of Bladder Cancer Associated With Cigarette Smoking

	Cases	Controls
Smokers	2324	3581
Nonsmokers	657	2198
Total	2981	5779

Relative odds (R) $= \dfrac{(2324)(2198)}{(657)(3581)} = 2.2$

Attributable risk percent in the exposed $(A_e\%) = \dfrac{2.2 - 1}{2.2} \times 100\%$

$$= 55\%$$

Population attributable risk percent $(A_p\%)$ or etiologic fraction

$$= \dfrac{\dfrac{3581}{5779}(2.2 - 1)}{1 + \dfrac{3581}{5579}(2.2 - 1)} \times 100\%$$

$$= 43\%$$

Alternatively, $\dfrac{(2.2 - 1)}{2.2} \times \dfrac{2324}{2981} \times 100\% = 43\%$

(Adapted from Hartge P, Silverman D, Hoover R, et al. Changing cigarette habits and bladder cancer risk: A case-control study. JNCI 1987;78:1119)

There are no clear guidelines as to when evidence is sufficient to conduct intervention trials, yet when there is a reasonable likelihood of benefit resulting from intervention (and any potential for harm), ethical questions may arise. In the field of cancer cause and prevention, opportunities for intervention have been limited for various reasons, including the long latency periods that may be involved before an effect is seen. However, intervention studies are gaining emphasis in the evaluation of diet and nutrition, especially the use of various micronutrient supplements that may inhibit late stages of the carcinogenic process. Also underway are hepatitis B vaccine trials in endemic areas for liver cancer. After intervention, the follow-up and analytic procedures to evaluate outcomes resemble those employed for cohort studies.

STRENGTHS AND LIMITS OF EPIDEMIOLOGY

STRENGTHS

In contrast to laboratory studies, epidemiology directly evaluates the experience of human populations and their response to various environmental exposures and host factors (the risk of disease). The consequences of an exposure can be measured as it actually occurs in the population. Questionable extrapolations from other species are also avoided. Although positive findings from animal studies may indicate a potential human risk, epidemiology offers the only means of quantifying the risk. Furthermore, even when the specific causal agent cannot be clearly identified (*e.g.*, the precise carcinogens in cigarette smoke), sufficient information can be obtained for the disease to be prevented.

LIMITATIONS

Cancer epidemiology has certain limitations. First, epidemiologic studies are mainly observational, relying on natural occurrences in human populations, and the opportunities for experiment are rare and limited to efforts at prevention. Second, epidemiology can seldom indicate a cause with great specificity, particularly when the exposures are multiple or when surrogate measures of exposure are used (*e.g.*, occupation or area of residence), although laboratory techniques may be helpful in such circumstances. Third, study groups chosen on the basis of one characteristic may be distinctive in another, and it may be difficult to disentangle them even with refined analytic methods. Fourth, it is hard to incriminate an agent when there is relative uniformity of exposure in a given population, which may be the case with some dietary factors (*e.g.*, high fat intake). Finally, evidence of an environmental hazard is usually obtained from high or intermediate levels of exposure. As in animal studies, it is difficult to detect causal relations when the exposure level is low or the excess risk is small compared with the baseline incidence rate. In such situations, the numbers of subjects needed to provide definite results may be virtually impossible to assemble for the purposes of a single study.

BIOCHEMICAL AND MOLECULAR EPIDEMIOLOGY

The power of certain studies may be increased by incorporating laboratory methods into analytic investigations, an approach termed *biochemical* or *molecular epidemiology*.[72,73] The analysis of biologic samples in the laboratory can permit the study of exposure to oncogenic viruses. It may also be possible to detect past exposures to chemical and physical agents and to clarify early preneoplastic events, various host factors, and mechanisms of action. The approach provides new opportunities to evaluate carcinogenic risks associated with dietary factors and with markers of genetic predisposition. In view of rapid experimental advances, biochemical and molecular epidemiology is a challenging multidisciplinary approach that should help to elucidate further the causes of cancer. Such studies are complex undertakings that require careful planning and teamwork, including the collaboration of clinicians.

SOURCES OF CLUES

Because an analytic study is designed to evaluate an association between a disease and an antecedent factor, there must be some previous indication or suspicion of such an association. The lead may come from descriptive or correlational studies or from another analytic study. The most fruitful source of etiologic clues has been the alert clinician who has uncovered some of the most striking examples of environmental cancer, starting with Pott's discovery of scrotal cancer among chimney sweeps. Usually the clinician recognizes an excessive number of patients with the same tumor and traces the cluster to a particular cultural, occupational, or iatrogenic exposure.[2] Clinical observations have linked asbestos with mesothelioma, vinyl chloride with hepatic angiosarcoma, furniture-making with nasal adenocarcinoma, radium-dial painting with osteosarcoma, and prenatal exposure to diethylstilbestrol with clear-cell adenocarcinoma of the vagina among offspring. Clinicians were able to detect these associations because the tumors are rare in the general population and involve exceptionally high risks. In most instances, the associations required epidemiologic study less to confirm them than to quantify them. Clinicians have also identified a wide variety of heritable conditions associated with susceptibility to cancer.[74] Opportunities for the practicing physician to make significant etiologic discoveries were highlighted recently at a symposium entitled "Unusual Occurrences as Clues to Cancer Etiology."[75] On the other hand, epidemiologists can identify causes of cancer that may seem less dramatic in relative risks but are important to public health, such as smoking and asbestos in lung cancer.

Another source of leads has been provided by experimental studies, especially those relating chemicals to tumors in laboratory animals. In the case of mustard gas and 4-aminobiphenyl, for example, carcinogenic risks were found in humans after the substances were shown to induce tumors in animal studies.[2] Whatever the sequence of observations, there is no question that clinical, epidemiologic, and experimental data greatly complement one another in determining the risks and mechanisms involved in carcinogenesis. When all approaches are brought to bear on a particular hypothesis, advances in understanding the carcinogenic process may be extraordinary.

INTERPRETATION OF EPIDEMIOLOGIC STUDIES

SAMPLE SIZE AND POWER

A fundamental aspect of planning or evaluating a study is the number of subjects needed to test an etiologic hypothesis.[13] The power of a study is the likelihood of detecting a postulated level of risk. The larger the sample size, the greater the power to detect a specified risk, and the smaller the sample size, the weaker the power.

Issues of sample size and power are of great concern when evaluating negative results of epidemiologic studies.[76] Only large studies may confidently exclude low to moderate levels of risk, whereas negative results of a small study should be viewed with caution because they usually lack adequate power.

NONCAUSAL ASSOCIATIONS

When interpreting the results of analytic studies, one must ask whether the associations observed between exposure and disease are the result of bias, confounding, chance, or cause-and-effect. Bias or systematic error is usually the result of imperfections in study design or conduct, and often cannot be corrected in the analysis. Many types of bias have been described,[73] but most can be grouped as biases of selection or information.[66] Selection bias involves systematic differences in exposure between those selected and not selected into the study. For example, a case-control study might include only cases referred to a particular institution or only survivors, so that differences observed might reflect factors influencing referral patterns or survival. A similar bias in a cohort study may result from differences in the loss to follow-up between exposed and unexposed groups. Information bias involves differences in measuring the factor in question between groups and is best illustrated by recall bias or interviewer bias, both

of which may affect the outcome of case-control studies. For example, in studies of childhood cancer, parents of cases might provide more reliable or thorough responses than parents of controls because of the soul-searching they have undergone. Also, interviewers might tend to probe more deeply into past events if a subject is known to be a case rather than a control.

Confounding refers to the effect of an extraneous variable that may account, entirely or partly, for an apparent association between exposure and disease, or may obscure a real association.[13,66] Confounding can usually be evaluated and accommodated during analysis by adjustment procedures, including the stratification of subjects on the suspected variable. To be a confounder, a variable must be related to the exposure and related causally to the disease. For example, cigarette smoking could contribute to an excess of lung cancer among industrial groups that smoke more heavily than the average. Conversely, a relation between oral contraceptives and invasive cervical cancer became apparent only after adjustment was made for the interval since last Pap smear, because in this study the frequency of screening was found to be related both to pill use and the development of cervical cancer.[78] Whereas analytic methods can control for known confounders, they cannot do this for unknown confounders, which are free to distort observed risk estimates. The advantage of experimental studies is that the randomization process tends to ensure that the prevalence of all potential confounders is similar among the randomized groups.

The role of chance is evaluated in epidemiologic studies by the use of significance testing and confidence limits. If a risk estimate is statistically significant at a specified level (*e.g.,* 0.05, or 1 in 20) or if the 95% confidence limits exclude 1.0, chance can be assumed to be an unlikely explanation. It does not exclude the operation of a chance event, but only indicates that chance would explain a risk estimate of the observed magnitude or greater only 1 out of 20 times. In studies involving multiple comparisons, some significant associations can be anticipated by the play of chance, and each finding should be considered on its own merits.

DETERMINING CAUSALITY

In interpreting associations found in epidemiologic studies, the investigator is influenced by the magnitude of the risk estimates, their statistical significance (likelihood of being due to chance), and especially the rigor of the study design to avoid methodologic pitfalls. If bias, confounding, and chance are excluded as likely explanations for an association, the issue of causality must be considered through a process of scientific judgment that extends beyond any statement of statistical probability.[13,14,66] During the controversy over cigarette smoking and lung cancer, a set of criteria was formulated to assist the epidemiologist in making causal inferences.[79,80] These criteria provide useful guidelines for determining causality and refer especially to the strength and specificity of an association, the presence of a dose-response gradient, the consistency and reproducibility of results, biologic plausibility and coherence, and an appropriate temporal sequence. It may not be possible to satisfy all the criteria in any particular instance, although evidence that the exposure preceded the disease is obviously crucial.[66] With smaller relative risks, especially when interactions between multiple exposures and susceptibility states seem important, the term *risk factor* is often used instead of *causal agent*. The finding of small relative risks should not be readily dismissed as due to chance or bias but explored further by examining possible interactions with other risk factors or susceptible subgroups of the population.

Causal inferences from epidemiology usually develop gradually after taking into account all relevant biologic information, including laboratory studies. Although epidemiologic observations can accumulate to the point at which causation is virtually inescapable, strictly speaking it is not possible to prove causality by these means alone. Nevertheless, causation can often be shown to be sufficiently probable to provide a compelling basis for preventive and public health action and certainly so in the case of cigarette smoking and lung cancer.

CAUSES OF CANCER

This section provides a brief overview of cancer risk factors, based mainly on evidence from analytic epidemiology, including recent observations relevant to the practicing oncologist. The contributions of epidemiology to cancer cause and prevention are presented elsewhere in greater detail.[6,7,81,82] Best known is the success of the epidemiologic approach in discovering or confirming lifestyle and other environmental exposures as causes of cancer (Table 9–17).

TOBACCO

Among the carcinogenic hazards identified so far, tobacco smoking is the most important in Western countries and increasingly so in developing countries. Smoking has been firmly linked to cancers not only of the lung but also of the larynx, mouth, pharynx, esophagus, bladder, and pancreas.[83] Recent evidence indicates that smokers are also prone to cancers of the kidney parenchyma[84] and pelvis,[85] cervix,[86] nasal passages,[87] stomach[88] and leukemia.[89] The wide variety of neoplasms related to smoking is hardly surprising in view of the large number of chemicals detected in cigarette smoke and delivered to a highly vascular and absorptive organ. In the United States it appears that smoking, especially of cigarettes, accounts for about 40% of all cancer deaths in men and about 20% in women, with lung cancers representing the largest proportion. For smokers of two or more packs per day, the risk of lung cancer is about 20 times that of nonsmokers, and is much greater for squamous and small cell carcinomas than for adenocarcinomas.

Epidemiologic studies have demonstrated the benefits of stopping smoking, with lower risks relative to those of continuing smokers appearing within a few years of quitting.[6,83] This is consistent with evidence that smoking exerts an effect at late and early stages of carcinogenesis. The introduction of lower tar levels in cigarettes and of filter tips has also reduced the risk of lung cancer, although not nearly to the extent seen with cessation of smoking.[90] The risks of cigar and pipe smokers resemble those of cigarette smokers for cancers of the oral cavity, larynx, and esophagus, but are lower for lung cancer.

Smokeless tobacco is also of concern, because oral cancer has been linked with snuff dipping, a common practice in rural southern parts of the United States.[46] Under suspicion are the high levels of tobacco-specific nitrosamines that have been detected in snuff and in the saliva of snuff users. In parts of Asia, oral cancer is common in people who use tobacco quids often mixed with betel, lime, and other agents.[91] Overall, these findings have prompted recent public health and legislative measures in the United States aimed at discouraging the use of smokeless tobacco, especially among young people.

Passive smoking has been hotly debated as a risk factor for lung cancer. Evidence suggests that nonsmoking women married to smokers have experienced an excess risk on the order of 30%.[92,93] Passive or involuntary smoking is a real concern, because tobacco smoke constituents and metabolites can be detected in the body fluids of exposed nonsmokers. Moreover, a cause-and-effect relation with lung cancer is suggested by the replication of findings in different populations, by a dose-response effect with excess risks of about 70% among heavily exposed nonsmokers, by cell-type patterns resembling those associated with active smoking, and by the similarity in risk estimates between heavy passive smokers and light active smokers.

ALCOHOL

Consumption of alcoholic beverages has been shown to potentiate the effects of tobacco smoking on cancers of the mouth, pharynx, esophagus, and larynx and has been estimated to account for about 3% of all cancer deaths.[94,95] It has been difficult to study the effects of alcohol alone and the nature of its interaction with smoking because of small numbers in certain categories of exposure (especially drinkers who abstain from smoking). In a large-scale case-control study of oral cancer, the risks shown in Table 9–18 increased with intake of alcohol among nonsmokers, but in combination with smoking the risks multiplied to 35-fold among heavy consumers of both products.[96] Combined exposures were found to account for about 75% of all oral and pharyngeal cancers. The risks were higher with hard liquor or beer than with wine. For esophageal cancer, the highest recorded risks from alcohol are those associated with the consumption of home-brewed apple brandies in the northwest part of France. For larynx cancer, the alcohol effect is more prominent for tumors in the supraglottic segments than for tumors in the intrinsic segments. Because ethanol is not carcinogenic in laboratory animals, the mechanism by which alcohol acts is not clear. It may involve nutritional deficiencies that accompany prolonged heavy drinking, contaminants such as nitrosamines and hydrocarbons, or increased permeability of mucous membranes to other carcinogens. Further evidence for a topical effect comes from a recent analysis suggesting an excess risk of oral cancer associated with the use of mouthwash high in alcohol content.[97]

Alcohol is an important cause of hepatic cirrhosis, which is sometimes complicated by hepatocellular carcinoma, although alcohol may also have an independent effect on the risk of this cancer. The role of alcohol in other cancers remains uncertain. Rectal cancer in men has shown positive geographic correlations with beer consumption, but the findings from analytic studies have been inconsistent. For example, cohort studies of brewery workers (who receive a free

TABLE 9–17. Environmental Causes of Human Cancer

Agent	Type of Exposure	Site of Cancer
Aflatoxin	Contaminated foodstuffs	Liver
Alcoholic beverages	Drinking	Mouth, pharynx, esophagus, larynx, liver
Alkylating agents (melphalan, cyclophosphamide, chlorambucil, semustine)	Medication	Leukemia
Androgen-anabolic steroids	Medication	Liver
Aromatic amines (benzidine, 2-naphthylamine, 4-aminobiphenyl)	Manufacturing of dyes and other chemicals	Bladder
Arsenic (inorganic)	Mining and smelting of certain ores, pesticide manufacturing and use, medication, drinking water	Lung, skin, liver (angiosarcoma)
Asbestos	Manufacturing and use	Lung, pleura, peritoneum
Benzene	Leather, petroleum, and other industries	Leukemia
Bis(chloromethyl)ether	Manufacturing	Lung (small cell)
Chlornaphazine	Medication	Bladder
Chromium compounds	Manufacturing	Lung
Estrogens	Medication	
Synthetic (diethylstilbestrol)		Vagina, cervix (adenocarcinoma)
Conjugated (Premarin)		Endometrium
Steroid contraceptives		Liver, cervix
Immunosuppressants (azathioprine, cyclosporine)	Medication	Non-Hodgkin's lymphoma, skin (squamous carcinoma and melanoma), soft-tissue tumors (including Kaposi's sarcoma)
Ionizing radiation	Atomic bomb explosions, treatment and diagnosis, radium dial painting, uranium and metal mining	Most sites
Isopropyl alcohol production	Manufacturing by strong acid process	Nasal sinuses
Leather industry	Manufacturing and repair (boot and shoe)	Nasal sinuses, bladder
Mustard gas	Manufacturing	Lung, larynx, nasal sinuses
Nickel dust	Refining	Lung, nasal sinuses
Parasites	Infection	
Schistosoma haematobium		Bladder (squamous carcinoma)
Clonorchis sinensis		Liver (cholangiocarcinoma)
Pesticides	Application	Non-Hodgkin's lymphoma, lung
Phenacetin-containing analgesics	Medication	Renal pelvis
Polycyclic hydrocarbons	Coal carbonization products and some mineral oils	Lung, skin (squamous carcinoma)
Tobacco chews, including betel nut	Snuff dipping and chewing of tobacco, betel, lime	Mouth
Tobacco smoke	Smoking, especially cigarettes	Lung, larynx, mouth, pharynx, esophagus, bladder, pancreas, kidney
Ultraviolet radiation	Sunlight	Skin (including melanoma), lip
Viruses	Infection	
Epstein-Barr virus		Burkitt's lymphoma, nasopharyngeal carcinoma
Hepatitis B and C virus		Hepatocellular carcinoma
Human immunodeficiency virus		Kaposi's sarcoma, non-Hodgkin's lymphoma
Human papillomavirus		Cervix, other anogenital tumors
Human T-lymphotropic virus type I		T-cell leukemia/lymphoma
Vinyl chloride	Manufacturing of polyvinyl chloride	Liver (angiosarcoma)
Wood dusts	Furniture manufacturing (hardwood)	Nasal sinuses (adenocarcinoma)

TABLE 9–18. Relative Risks For Oral and Pharyngeal Cancer Associated With Smoking and Drinking

Smoking Status*	Number of Alcoholic Drinks Per Week				
	<1	1–4	5–14	15–29	30+
Nonsmoker	1.0	1.3	1.6	1.4	5.8
Former smoker	0.7	2.2	1.4	3.2	6.4
Light smoker	1.7	1.5	2.7	5.4	7.9
Moderate smoker	1.9	2.4	4.4	7.2	23.8
Heavy smoker	7.4	0.7	4.4	20.2	37.7

* Light, moderate, and heavy smokers. 1–19, 20–39, and 40+ cigarettes per day for 20+ years, respectively.
(Adapted from Blot WJ, McLaughlin JK, Winn DM, et al. Smoking and drinking in relation to oral and pharyngeal cancer. Cancer Res 1988;48:3282)

beer allocation) have revealed an excess risk of rectal cancer in Dublin but not in Copenhagen.[98] Recent interest has centered on the possible relation of alcohol with breast cancer, with a series of prospective studies showing an excess risk and dose-response gradient.[99,100] Further investigation is needed to determine if this relation is causal, or if indirect, how it is mediated, especially because the elevated risk in some studies is associated with consumption levels as low as 1 to 2 drinks per day.

OCCUPATIONAL HAZARDS

The study of occupational groups has identified more carcinogens than any other branch of cancer epidemiology and has led to cancer prevention by reducing or eliminating hazardous exposures in the workplace.[101,102] Occupational exposures appear to account for about 5% of all cancer deaths, although the proportion is higher in certain areas for particular cancers, such as those of the bladder and lung. Most carcinogenic exposures in the workplace were first detected by clinicians, whereas others were noticed initially by epidemiologists as in the case of asbestos (lung cancer), inorganic arsenic (lung cancer), and the leather industry (nasal cancer) or by experimentalists, as in the case of 4-aminobiphenyl.[2] All compounds shown to be carcinogenic in humans have been positive in long-term animal testing, except for arsenic and alcohol. This argues for the importance of bioassay programs, but the exceptions remind us that it is not prudent to rely solely on laboratory work.

Asbestos represents the major occupational carcinogen in many countries due to its induction of lung cancers rather than mesotheliomas. This is true even though the relative risk for lung cancer is little more than twofold and that for mesothelioma is well over 100-fold, because lung cancer is much more common than mesothelioma in people unexposed to asbestos. A multiplicative relation exists between asbestos exposure and smoking in the development of lung cancer.[103] American shipyard workers (whose exposure to asbestos was heavy during World War II) have experienced a high incidence, but the far greater excess among smokers than nonsmokers indicates a synergism between the risk factors (Fig. 9–7).[44] The risks also vary according to the type of asbestos

fiber and are highest for crocidolite, which is banned in many countries. Much research is in progress on man-made mineral fibers, but there is no clear evidence of a carcinogenic risk to humans.[102]

Many of the occupational cancers listed in Table 9–17 are characterized by high relative risks and rarity in the general population. A challenge facing epidemiologists is to detect hazards with smaller relative risks that may have a greater impact on the public health when the exposure is widespread and the tumor in question is common. This problem is particularly acute for lung cancer because variations in the prevalence and duration of smoking may inhibit the detection of occupational risks. Recent studies have implicated various occupational exposures including phenoxyacetic acid herbicides with non-Hodgkin's lymphoma,[47] motor exhausts with lung and bladder cancers,[104,105] and formaldehyde with nasal and nasopharyngeal cancers.[106] Such findings illustrate that the discovery of occupational hazards may have implications beyond the workplace, because they point to potential risks experienced at a lower level by the general public.

ENVIRONMENTAL POLLUTION

Pollutants in the urban air have long been suspected in the cause of lung cancer. Fossil fuel combustion products, especially polycyclic hydrocarbons, are of special concern. The subject has been difficult to study, primarily due to the overpowering effects of smoking, which first became popular in urban areas. Nevertheless, there is suggestive evidence that atmospheric pollution plays a limited role in the causation of lung cancer.[6]

Asbestos bodies and calcified pleural plaques are common in urban populations, but the risks of cancer after nonoccupational exposures are uncertain. There are many case reports suggesting that mesotheliomas may result from neighborhood

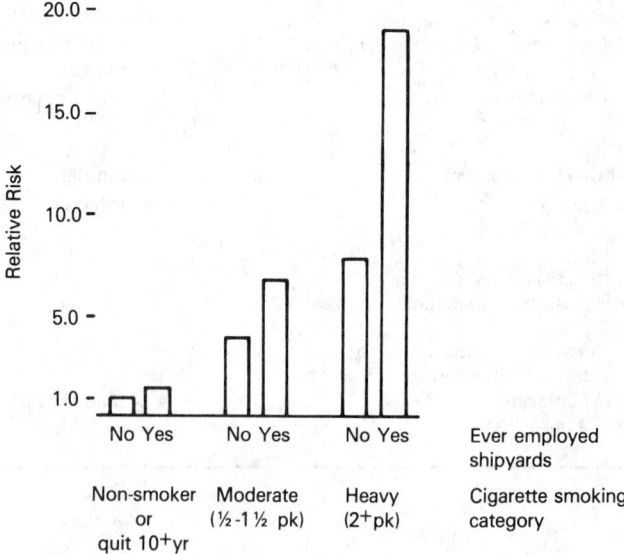

FIGURE 9–7. Relative risk of lung cancer according to usual cigarette-smoking category and employment in shipyards during World War II. (Blot WJ, Harrington JM, Toledo A, et al. Lung cancer after employment in shipyards during World War II. N Engl J Med 1978;299:620)

exposures to asbestos industries and from household contact with asbestos dust, perhaps through the laundering of work clothing.[107] A striking example of an environmental carcinogen is the naturally occurring zeolite fiber in parts of Turkey that causes a high mortality from pleural mesothelioma.[108] Another hazard may result from airborne arsenic, because increased mortality rates for lung cancer have been reported in both sexes in the neighborhood of arsenic-emitting smelters and cannot be explained by smoking and occupational exposures.[109]

There is much interest in the role of indoor air pollution by radon gas and tobacco smoke in the cause of lung cancer. In China, the high rates of lung cancer among nonsmoking women have been related to cooking oil vapors generated by wok cooking[110] and to effluents from coal-heating stoves.[111] Also under investigation are contaminants in drinking water, especially because several halogenated organic compounds produced during chlorination are carcinogenic and mutagenic in laboratory tests. A large case-control study of bladder cancer has found a modest excess risk associated with prolonged use of chlorinated surface water,[112] and studies are underway to see if this risk can be confirmed and whether it extends to other cancers. In Taiwan, high levels of inorganic arsenic in drinking water have been linked to skin cancer and possibly other cancers.[113] It has been estimated that only about 2% of cancer deaths are due to environmental pollution,[6] but this estimate is based on limited data and may be modified by the results of future research.

IONIZING RADIATION

Along with tobacco smoking, more is known about the carcinogenic effects of ionizing radiation than about any other human carcinogen.[114–116] This dates from early observations on radiologists to the comprehensive studies among survivors of the atomic bombs in Japan and among patients receiving radiotherapy for cervical cancer and ankylosing spondylitis. It is difficult to measure directly the effects of low doses of ionizing radiation such as x-rays or γ rays, and extrapolations have to be made from populations exposed to high and moderate doses for medical, occupational, or military reasons. Although much has been learned about the carcinogenic risks of radiation therapy for different conditions, there are little firm data about risks from the lower doses of diagnostic radiation, except for a 50% increase in leukemia and other childhood cancers associated with prenatal exposures.

About 5% of all cancer deaths may be attributed to radiation,[116] but the upper limit might be somewhat higher if certain estimates are confirmed about the risk of lung cancer associated with indoor levels of radon emanating mainly from soils containing uranium deposits. Studies of underground miners exposed to relatively high doses of α-radiation have shown excess lung cancer risks, even at levels that might be attained through long-term residential exposure in some parts of the United States.[117] More reliable data should come from ongoing case-control studies of lung cancer that involve careful measurements of indoor radon.

Nearly all sites of the body appear vulnerable to the carcinogenic effects of radiation, with the most radiosensitive tissues being the bone marrow, breast, and thyroid.[118] The patterns of risk provide insights into mechanisms of carcinogenesis and guidelines for radiation protection. For example, radiogenic leukemia shows a distinctive wave-like pattern with the excess risk starting 2 to 4 years after exposure, peaking at 6 to 8 years, and declining to normal within 25 years. In contrast, radiogenic carcinomas have a minimal latent period of 5 to 10 years and a temporal distribution that resembles the natural age-specific incidence curve, suggesting the influence of other factors acting at a later stage of carcinogenesis. The advent of large-scale mammography has renewed interest in the breast cancer experience of atomic bomb survivors and women exposed to medical x-rays. Despite a reasonably linear dose-response curve for breast cancer, the radiation effect is most pronounced among young women and is not evident among those who were exposed after age 40. This finding is reassuring for women in midlife who are most likely to undergo periodic screening with mammography.

Recent reports of increases in childhood leukemia among families living near nuclear facilities in the United Kingdom were not confirmed in France or the United States.[119] Persons living in areas of high natural background radiation in China,[120] and patients given radioactive iodine in Sweden[121] were not found to be at increased cancer risk. These data suggest that radiation given gradually over time may cause less cancers overall than if the same radiation dose were given over a brief interval.

SOLAR RADIATION

Ultraviolet (UV) radiation from sunlight is the major risk factor for skin cancer, both squamous and basal cell carcinomas and melanoma.[122] The evidence includes the tendency of tumors to arise on sun-exposed sites, the high incidence associated with outdoor activities, and the predisposition of fair-complexioned people who sunburn easily. Exceptionally high risks of skin cancer occur among persons with genetic diseases exacerbated by sunlight (xeroderma pigmentosum and albinism). Furthermore, in experimental animals, repeated doses of UV radiation, particularly in the UV-B spectral range (290 to 320 nm), can induce skin cancer. In addition, about one half of the melanomas appear to arise from dysplastic nevi, a precursor state that should greatly expand opportunities for early detection and treatment.[123]

Because incidence data for nonmelanoma skin cancer are not collected routinely by most population-based cancer registries, special surveys in the United States were conducted in the 1970s as an adjunct to the SEER program together with measures of UV-B radiation at ground level.[124] The gradient with UV-B levels was steepest for squamous cell carcinoma followed by basal cell carcinoma, and was least apparent for melanoma (Fig. 9–8). These differences are consistent with analytic studies suggesting that intermittent (recreational) exposures associated with sunburning are important in melanoma,[54] whereas cumulative (occupational) exposures appear more closely related to nonmelanoma skin cancer. The steady rise in the incidence and mortality rates for melanoma may be related to short-term intense sun exposures that have accompanied changes in leisure-time activities and clothing habits. Increases in squamous cell carcinoma of the skin have also been documented.[125] There is no evidence so far that ground-level measures of UV-B have increased,[126] but recent reports of stratospheric ozone depletion have prompted con-

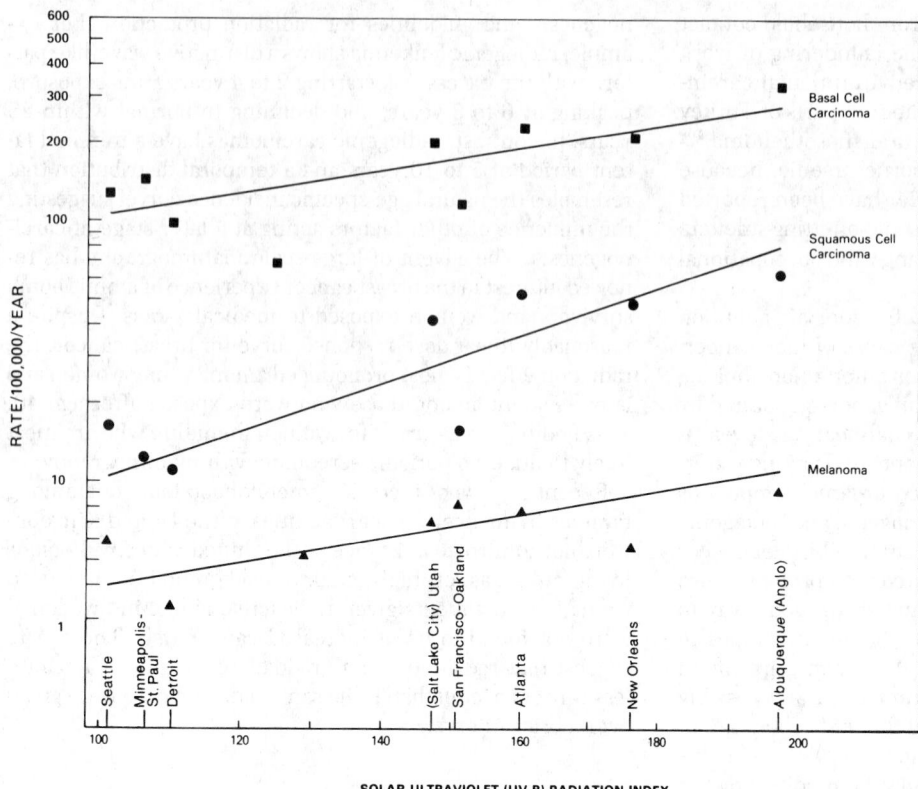

FIGURE 9–8. Annual age-adjusted incidence rates for basal and squamous cell carcinomas and melanoma among white females, according to annual UV-B measurements at selected areas of the United States. (Scotto J, Fraumeni JF Jr. Skin [other than melanoma]. In: Schottenfeld D, Fraumeni JF Jr, eds. Cancer epidemiology and prevention. Philadelphia; WB Saunders, 1982:996. Melanoma data are from the Surveillance, Epidemiology, and End Results program [1973–1976] and nonmelanoma data from a special survey [1977–1978]. Regression lines are based on exponential model.)

cerns about future trends in skin cancer that would presumably result from increases in UV-B reaching the earth's surface. International efforts are under way to phase out chlorofluorocarbons (used in aerosol propellants and air conditioners) that may reduce the protective ozone layer.

MEDICATIONS

Several of the carcinogens listed in Table 9–17 have been detected by studies of patients exposed to medicinal agents that may account for as much as 2% of all cancers. Some drugs have been withdrawn from clinical practice, whereas others are retained because their benefits are judged to outweigh their side effects. A major discovery was that synthetic estrogens given during pregnancy produced adenocarcinomas of the vagina and cervix several years later in daughters exposed in utero.[127] This was the first demonstration of transplacental carcinogenesis in humans. Endometrial cancer can result from conjugated estrogens taken for menopausal symptoms, and some studies have suggested an excess of breast cancer in long-term users.[128] Oral contraceptives are still under evaluation, with some studies suggesting an elevated risk of breast cancer when there is early and prolonged use or when there exist predisposing conditions such as familial occurrence or benign breast disease.[129] Also, a relation of pill use to invasive cervical cancer is suggested by recent studies that have made careful attempts to control for confounding variables such as sexual activity and screening history.[78] A reduced risk of endometrial and ovarian cancers has been reported with the combined oral contraceptives, especially after long-term use. The effects of exogenous hormones, along with the relation of female cancers to reproductive and menstrual variables, indicate the importance of investigating endogenous hormones as risk factors.[130]

An excess risk of acute nonlymphocytic leukemia has been noted among patients receiving alkylating agents, especially melphalan, cyclophosphamide, and chlorambucil.[70] The monitoring of carcinogenic risks should be part of randomized therapy trials. For example, when semustine (methylcyclohexylchloroethyl nitrosurea [MeCCNU]) was evaluated as adjuvant therapy for gastrointestinal cancer, the risks of leukemia and preleukemia were found to be elevated, with a clear dose-response relation (Table 9–19).[131,132] This finding demonstrates the importance of carefully weighing risks and benefits in designing treatment regimens that involve alkylating agents, especially for those cancer patients with a low risk of relapse or for patients with nonmalignant diseases.

Immunosuppressive agents, particularly azathioprine, have been assessed mainly by studies of renal transplant recipients. The risk of non-Hodgkin's lymphoma is high within a few months of transplantation and remains at about the same level.[133,134] This rapid onset is in marked contrast to the usual behavior of chemical carcinogens and suggests activation of a latent oncogenic virus by immunologic mechanisms. Contrary to the prediction of the so-called *immunosurveillance hypothesis* as first proposed, the increase of other cancers is not generalized but is confined to particular types such as squamous carcinoma of the skin, melanoma, Kaposi's sarcoma, liver cancer, and cervical cancer (Table 9–20). Although the risk of posttransplant lymphoma might be influenced by antigenic stimulation by the graft, patients treated with azathioprine for other conditions have shown a tenfold

TABLE 9–19. Risk of Leukemic Disorders According to Dose of Semustine

	Cumulative Dosage (mg/m²)				
	0	1–	500–	750–	1000+
Number of leukemic disorders	1	3	3	7	5
Number of patients	1,566	714	442	633	278
Relative risk*	1.0	8.7	10.5	18.7	36.9
5-year cumulative risk (%)†	0.1	0.8	1.2	1.1	2.5

* The referent category was those who did not receive semustine. Maximum likelihood estimates of relative risk were adjusted for survival times.
† Cumulative probabilities were estimated by the Kaplan-Meier technique (Kaplan EL, Meier P. Nonparametric estimation from incomplete observations. J Am Stat Assoc 1958;53:457)
(Boice JD Jr, Greene MH, Killen JY Jr, et al. Leukemia after adjuvant chemotherapy with semustine [methyl-CCNU]—Evidence of a dose-response effect. N Engl J Med 1986;314:119)

excess of lymphoma.[134] A predominance of lymphomas has been seen with primary immunodeficiency disorders such as ataxia-telangiectasia, Wiskott-Aldrich syndrome, and the X-linked lymphoproliferative syndrome.[135] For lymphomas in the latter group and in transplant patients, there is evidence of causation by the Epstein-Barr virus.[136] This finding is consistent with animal experiments, indicating that immunosurveillance primarily operates against viral-induced neoplasms.

Recent studies have suggested that nonsteroidal antiinflammatory drugs such as aspirin may protect against large bowel cancer, perhaps through its effect on prostaglandin metabolism.[137]

VIRUSES

The laboratory discovery of many different oncogenic viruses in animals has long suggested that some human cancers have similar causes, but convincing evidence in humans was slow to emerge until recently.[138] The proportion of viral-related cancer in the United States has been roughly estimated at 5%,[6] but one can only speculate about upper bounds as rapid advances in molecular virology are made. However, the estimate must surpass 5% in certain developing countries. Furthermore, other infectious agents are receiving increasing attention, notably the relation between *Helicobacter pylori* infection and the risk of gastric cancer.[139]

The Epstein-Barr virus (EBV) is widely considered the necessary cause of endemic Burkitt lymphoma and probably also of nasopharyngeal cancer.[140] In Burkitt's lymphoma, holoendemic malaria appears to enhance the oncogenic effect of EBV and produce uneven distribution and occasional clustering of the lymphoma in Africa. EBV appears involved also in the lymphomas that occur in certain immunodeficiency disorders, perhaps by interacting with immunologic and genetic mechanisms. The relation of EBV to nasopharyngeal cancer has been suggested by the higher antibody levels seen in patients than in controls and the presence of viral genome in epithelial cells from the tumor. The high rates of this cancer in southern China cannot be attributed to EBV infection alone, and other risk factors such as consumption of salted fish or histocompatibility antigens appear to be involved.

Hepatitis B virus (HBV) infection is an important cause of hepatocellular carcinoma, especially in endemic regions of Asia and Africa. The most convincing evidence comes from a cohort study of 22,707 men in Taiwan in which the risk of liver carcinoma was more than 200 times greater among carriers of hepatitis B surface antigen than among noncarriers

TABLE 9–20. Relative Risk of Certain Cancers in Renal Transplant Recipients in Two Major Studies (With Observed Cancers in Parentheses)

Types of Cancer	United Kingdom–Australasian Study	American College of Surgeons Study*
All types†	2.8 (86)	2.8 (136)
Non-Hodgkin's lymphoma	45.9 (42)	26.9 (53)
Primary liver cancer	37.5 (3)	20.0 (4)
Skin melanoma	8.7 (2)	2.5 (5)
Other cancer‡	1.3 (39)	1.7 (74)

* Based on unpublished data from Hoover RN and Fraumeni JF Jr, 1989.
† Excludes cervix cancer in situ and nonmelanoma skin cancer, although increases in squamous carcinoma of skin have been reported.
‡ Includes excesses of mesenchymal tumors, notably Kaposi's sarcoma.
(Adapted from Kinlen LJ. Immunosuppressive therapy and cancer. Cancer Surv 1, 1982;1:565)

(Table 9–21).[141] The oncogenic effects of hepatitis B may be enhanced by early-life infection and dietary exposures to aflatoxin. Infection with hepatitis C virus may also increase the risk of liver cancer.[142]

The high incidence of adult T-cell leukemia in some areas of Japan and the Caribbean has been linked to infection with the human T-lymphotropic virus type I (HTLV-I), the first retrovirus to be detected in humans.[143] In endemic areas, the virus appears to be transmitted early in life and may also be spread by sexual activity, parenteral drug use, and blood transfusions.

Another human retrovirus, the human immunodeficiency virus (HIV), has been shown to cause the acquired immunodeficiency syndrome (AIDS).[144] Recognized since 1981, AIDS in the United States affects mainly homosexual men, hemophiliacs, and intravenous drug users and predisposes patients to Kaposi's sarcoma and non-Hodgkin's lymphoma. The much higher incidence of Kaposi's sarcoma among male homosexuals than other high-risk groups with AIDS suggests that an oncogenic agent is superimposed on HIV infection and is also sexually transmitted. The classic or endemic form of Kaposi's sarcoma in Africa and Mediterranean areas has been associated with cytomegalovirus infection in some studies, but the findings in AIDS patients suggest that it is a passenger virus.

The relation of cervical cancer to multiple sexual partners has long suggested the venereal transmission of an infectious agent. Although herpes simplex virus type 2 was a candidate agent for some time, the chief suspect is the human papillomavirus (HPV). DNA sequences from certain HPV types, notably HPV-16 and HPV-18, have been found in a high percentage of biopsies from invasive cervical cancer.[145] HPV has been isolated also from many vulvar, penile, and anal cancers and from squamous cell skin cancers associated with the genetic syndrome of epidermodysplasia verruciformis.

Investigations of clusters of leukemia or lymphoma in the community have provided no solid clues to cause, and particularly for childhood leukemia, statistical studies have not detected any general tendency for space-time clustering of these malignancies. However, space-time clustering would not be expected if a disease is a rare response to some underlying infective agent. The mixing of previously separated groups of people, especially in rural areas, has been associated with increases in childhood leukemia consistent with an infective

basis.[146] A viral origin for Hodgkin's disease in young adults has been suggested by its association with certain childhood environments, such as small family size, that would tend to reduce or delay early-life exposures to infections, such as in paralytic poliomyelitis.[60] EBV has been suspected, because an increased risk of Hodgkin's disease has been reported among persons with infectious mononucleosis and among those with elevated levels of antibodies to EBV antigens.[147] Recent molecular viral studies have suggested that in some cases the relation between EBV and Hodgkin's disease may be causal.[148] Despite mounting evidence of oncogenic viruses in humans, there is little indication that any form of cancer is contagious.

DIET AND NUTRITION

When viewed in the light of experimental work showing how dietary manipulation can influence the yield of tumors in laboratory animals, the recent growth of interest in dietary causes of human cancer seems not merely logical but overdue. International correlations and migrant studies also suggest that certain aspects of the affluent Western diet contribute to a sizable but uncertain proportion of all cancers. Various hypotheses about causative and protective factors are under intensive study, but the specific dietary components are elusive and the mechanisms of action appear complex. Problems stem from the inherent limitations of nutritional methods such as dietary recall, but progress may come from cohort studies in which specimens have been stored for subsequent biochemical assay, from molecular markers of intermediate endpoints, and from intervention studies to determine whether certain dietary modifications and nutrient supplements exert a protective effect against cancer.

Dietary fat has been suggested as a risk factor for certain cancers, especially of the breast and large bowel, by the strongly positive correlations that exist between age-adjusted rates in different countries and per capita consumption of fat.[149] Although the results of case-control and cohort studies have not provided strong support for the fat hypothesis in breast cancer,[53,150] recent studies have suggested a relation of colon cancer to dietary sources of animal fat.[151,152] It is not known whether this association operates through fat or one of its correlates (*e.g.,* protein, cooking-derived carcinogens). Furthermore, no positive relation has been found between the levels of serum cholesterol, which are influenced by fat intake, and subsequent risk of breast or large bowel cancers. The issue is complicated by methodologic difficulties in estimating or measuring intake of fat and different types of fat, the limited variation in fat consumption within many countries, problems in evaluating dietary habits in early life (which may be especially important for breast cancer), and difficulties in differentiating fat per se from calories (because fat is more calorigenic than other macronutrients). Calories may influence the risk of breast and other reproductive cancers by increasing body weight or size, for obesity is an established risk factor for certain cancers in women, especially cancer of the endometrium.[56] It is possible that obesity elevates the risk of endometrial and breast cancers by increasing the serum levels of circulating estrogens through a conversion from androstenedione in adipose tissue and perhaps also by a lowering of the sex-hormone binding globulin.[130] Caloric intake is also related to physical activity, which lowers the risk of colon cancer[151] and perhaps other tumors.

TABLE 9–21. Deaths From Liver Disease According to Hepatitis B Surface Antigen (HBsAg) Status on Recruitment Into Study

HBsAg Status	Cause of Death		Population at Risk	Mortality From Liver Cancer*
	Liver Cancer	Cirrhosis		
Positive	40	17	3,454	1,158
Negative	1	2	19,253	5
Total	41	19	22,707	181

* Mortality from primary hepatocellular carcinoma per 100,000 during study period.
(Adapted from Beasley RP, Hwang L-Y, Lin C-C, et al. Hepatocellular carcinoma and hepatitis-B virus. Lancet, 1981;2:1129)

A low intake of certain food groups may predispose persons to cancer, and a lower consumption of vegetables and fruit has been one of the more consistent findings in dietary studies of cancer.[153] A protective action for fiber was proposed by Burkitt, who was impressed by the low rates of colon cancer in parts of Africa where fiber intake and stool bulk were high. Correlational studies have indicated that fiber intake, especially when measured as nonstarch polysaccharides, tends to be lower in high-incidence regions.[154] Although the results are less consistent, there is some support from case-control studies that fiber protects against colon cancer.[155] The subject is complicated by the relatively crude characterization of fiber and by difficulty in separating the effects of micronutrients found in fiber sources such as fruits and vegetables.

Micronutrients may be responsible for the inverse gradients in risk associated with the intake of fruits and vegetables. Several epithelial cancers, especially of the lung, show this negative relation both in case-control studies and some cohort studies employing serologic tests; the effect has been attributed by some workers to beta-carotene,[53,156] although other carotenoids deserve attention.[153] More limited evidence suggests that vitamin C may protect against gastric and certain other cancers, perhaps by blocking the endogenous formation of nitrosamines. However, other components of fruits and vegetables have been suggested as protective factors in experimental and epidemiologic studies. For example, indole compounds in cruciferous vegetables may decrease the risk of colon cancer,[157] and allyl sulfide in garlic and onions may lower the risk of gastric cancer.[88] Vitamin D and calcium have been suggested as protective factors for colon and breast cancers.[158,159] The effects of vitamin E, selenium, and folic acid are also under study. Mixed or multiple deficiencies in the diet may be involved in some tumors, especially among populations with high risks of esophageal cancer.[160] Intervention studies are ideally suited to test the micronutrient hypotheses after sufficient information is obtained from analytic studies and laboratory animals, and the results of several ongoing trials are awaited with interest.

Other dietary factors, including additives and contaminants, have attracted attention. The consumption of aflatoxin, a carcinogenic metabolite of the fungus *Aspergillus flavus*, has been linked to liver cancer by correlation studies, followed by a case-control study,[161] and recently by characteristic p53 mu-

tations in tumors associated with high aflatoxin intake.[162] A relation between salted foods and stomach cancer has been claimed in some studies,[88] but this has not been consistently observed. The consumption of salted fish containing high concentrations of nitrosamines has been linked to the high rates of nasopharyngeal cancer in Hong Kong and southern China.[163] Coffee intake has been associated with bladder and pancreatic cancers, but this has not been confirmed in many other studies and there is no evidence for a causal relation. The artificial sweeteners saccharin and cyclamate cause bladder cancer in laboratory animals, but a large case-control study of bladder cancer indicated that the risk in humans at past levels of consumption is small if present at all.[164] Cooking practices may generate polycyclic hydrocarbons, heterocyclic aromatic amines, or other carcinogens in the food at high temperatures, but relevant epidemiologic data are scarce.[165]

GENETIC SUSCEPTIBILITY

Although the geographic and ethnic differentials for most cancers appear largely determined by environmental influences, genetic factors may contribute to some high rates (*e.g.*, nasopharyngeal cancer among Chinese and gallbladder cancer among Native Americans) and some low rates (*e.g.*, testicular cancer and Ewing's sarcoma among blacks in Africa and the United States). Genetic susceptibility is most evident for skin cancer, with geographic and ethnic variations corresponding to the degree of protective skin pigmentation. The apparently limited evidence for genetic factors based on these patterns does not exclude even large variations in individual susceptibility. Furthermore, the relatively small differences in risk between close relatives of patients with various cancers and other people are in fact consistent with large differences in genetic predisposition. The truth of this perhaps surprising statement can be demonstrated mathematically.[166] Only with advances in biochemical and molecular methods will it be possible to further define the impact of genetic factors or genetic-environmental interactions in causing cancer. For example, the phenotype associated with the rapid metabolic oxidation of certain drugs appears to influence the risk of smoking-related lung cancer,[167] supporting the long-held suspicion that certain persons have a higher risk of smoking-induced lung cancer than others because of genetic consti-

TABLE 9–22. Hereditary Neoplasms

	Inheritance	Features
Retinoblastoma	AD	Susceptibility to second primary tumors, including osteosarcoma of leg and radiogenic sarcoma of orbit; chromosome deletion (13q14) in some cases
Nevoid basal cell carcinoma	AD	Basal cell cancers of skin increased by UV and ionizing radiation; medulloblastoma, ovarian fibromas, and developmental defects in some cases
Multiple endocrine neoplasia I	AD	Adenomas of anterior pituitary, parathyroid, pancreatic islet cells, thyroid, and adrenal cortex; carcinoid tumors of intestine and bronchus in some cases
Multiple endocrine neoplasia II	AD	Pheochromocytoma and medullary thyroid carcinoma; parathyroid tumors and neurofibromas in some cases
Polyposis coli	AD	Multiple adenomatous polyps and adenocarcinomas of large bowel; some families exhibit osteomas, fibromas, lipomas, and epidermal cysts (Gardner's syndrome)
Dysplastic nevus syndrome	AD	Hereditary melanomas derived from nevi, especially after sun exposure

AD, autosomal dominant.

tution. The claim is sometimes made that the proportion of people who are susceptible to cancer is limited, with variations only in the specific sites affected (Cramer's hypothesis). This notion has been shown to be false[5] and has given way to mutation models and genetic hypotheses[168] that are stimulating further research into the nature of cancer susceptibility genes.

Although only a small fraction of cancer is inherited in a mendelian fashion, over 200 single-gene disorders have been linked to neoplasia.[169] This does not include several constitutional cytogenetic disorders that predispose persons to cancer, such as Down's syndrome with leukemia, Klinefelter's syndrome with mediastinal teratoma, gonadal dysgenesis with gonadoblastoma, and aniridia with Wilms' tumor.[74,166] Table 9–22 lists some cancers that occur as an inherited trait (hereditary neoplasms) and Table 9–23 presents those arising as a complication of inherited precursor lesions (preneoplastic states). In several of the listed syndromes, sunlight contributes to multiple skin cancers, including the dysplastic nevus syndrome predisposing to melanoma, and xeroderma pigmentosum predisposing to various skin cancers. Genetically de-

termined neoplasms tend to occur earlier in life than other cancers of the same anatomic type and often have a multifocal origin. In a growing number of syndromes, alterations in tumor suppressor genes and oncogenes are being recognized. In some conditions, such as familial adenomatous polyposis, the cascade of mutations are defining key events involved in the multistage mechanisms of carcinogenesis.[170] In addition, common neoplasms such as breast and colon cancers show small familial risks on the order of twofold to threefold, but among subgroups on patients with onset at young ages and bilateral or multifocal origin, the risks may be as high as 20- to 30-fold.[171] Some families show remarkable aggregations of site-specific cancer that appear consistent with autosomal dominant inheritance. Recent linkage analysis of families prone to early-onset breast cancer has pointed to a susceptibility gene located on chromosome 17q21.[172]

Because cancer is so common, it is sometimes difficult to know whether familial clusters are simply due to chance, especially if different types of cancer are involved.[173] In this circumstance, it can be useful to consider the possibility of a

TABLE 9–23. Hereditary Preneoplastic Syndromes

	Inheritance	Neoplasms
Phacomatoses		
Neurofibromatosis	AD	Sarcomatous change in the neurofibromas of 10% of cases; gliomas of brain and optic nerve, acoustic neuromas, meningiomas, and acute leukemia
Tuberous sclerosis	AD	Hamartomatous growths in several organs; brain tumors, chiefly giant-cell astrocytoma, in 1–3% of patients
von Hippel-Lindau syndrome	AD	Angiomatosis of retina and cerebellum; renal adenocarcinoma, pheochromocytoma, and ependymoma in some cases
Peutz-Jeghers syndrome	AD	Rare malignant change in hamartomatous polyps of gastrointestinal tract; ovarian neoplasms in 5% of female patients
Cowden's multiple hamartoma syndrome	AD	Oral papillomas, cystic mastopathy and breast cancer, thyroid and colonic neoplasms
Genodermatoses		
Xeroderma pigmentosum	AR	Various skin cancers in all patients exposed to sunlight
Albinism	AR	Skin cancers, chiefly squamous, in sun-exposed areas
Epidermodysplasia verruciformis	AR	Skin cancers, chiefly squamous, in multiple warts induced by papillomavirus
Werner's syndrome (adult progeria)	AR	Soft tissue sarcoma, other tumors
Chromosome Instability		
Bloom's syndrome	AR	Acute leukemia, non-Hodgkin's lymphoma, other cancers
Fanconi's anemia	AR	Acute myelomonocytic leukemia and squamous carcinoma of mucous membranes; hepatoma reported after androgen-anabolic steroids
Immunodeficiency		
Ataxia-telangiectasia	AR	Non-Hodgkin's lymphoma, acute lymphocytic leukemia, stomach cancer, other tumors; heterozygous carriers prone to cancer, especially of the breast
Common variable immunodeficiency	?AR	Non-Hodgkin's lymphoma, stomach cancer
Wiskott-Aldrich syndrome	XR	Non-Hodgkin's lymphoma, acute leukemia
X-linked (Bruton's) agammaglobulinemia	XR	Non-Hodgkin's lymphoma, acute leukemia
X-linked lymphoproliferative syndrome	XR	Non-Hodgkin's lymphoma, plasmacytoma

AD, autosomal dominant; AR, autosomal recessive; XR, X-linked recessive.

familial multiple-cancer syndrome. A distinct pattern is seen, for example, with a familial aggregation involving several childhood and adult cancers, including soft-tissue and bone sarcomas, breast carcinoma, brain tumors, leukemia, and adrenocortical neoplasms (Li-Fraumeni syndrome).[174,175] Family members with this syndrome are prone to multiple primary cancers, including radiogenic sarcomas. Recently, molecular studies of these cancer-prone families have identified germline mutations of p53, a tumor suppressor gene on chromosome 17p13 that often occurs as somatic mutations in a number of human cancers.[176] By delineating genetic and familial syndromes of cancer, clinicians have been instrumental not only in helping to identify and protect high-risk individuals but also in pointing experimentalists to new research opportunities. A multidisciplinary approach to genetic susceptibility ranging from clinical observations and epidemiology to molecular biology shows promise in identifying carcinogenic mechanisms and may have consequences in cancer prevention that are at least as important as the detection of environmental carcinogens.

REFERENCES

1. Shimkin MB. Contrary to nature. National Institutes of Health (NIH) report 76-720. Washington, DC: US Government Printing Office, 1977.
2. Doll R. Pott and the prospects for prevention. Br J Cancer 1975;32:263.
3. Doll R. The epidemiology of cancer. Cancer 1980;45:2475.
4. MacMahon B, Pugh TF. Epidemiology: Principles and methods. Boston: Little, Brown, 1970.
5. Doll R. An epidemiologic perspective of the biology of cancer. Cancer Res 1978;38:3573.
6. Doll R, Peto R. The causes of cancer. JNCI 1981;66:1191.
7. Schottenfeld D, Fraumeni JF Jr, eds. Cancer epidemiology and prevention. Philadelphia: WB Saunders, 1982.
8. Muir CS, Malhotra A. Changing patterns of cancer incidence in five continents. Gann Monogr Cancer Res 1987;33:3.
9. Hill AB. Principles of medical statistics. New York: Oxford University Press, 1966.
10. Young JL Jr, Percy CL, Asire AJ, eds. Surveillance, Epidemiology, and End Results Program: Incidence and mortality data, 1973—1977. NCI Monogr 1981;57.
11. Feldman AR, Kessler L, Myers MH, et al. The prevalence of cancer: Estimates based on the Connecticut Tumor Registry. N Engl J Med 1986;315:1394.
12. Decoufle P, Thomas TL, Pickle LW. Comparison of the proportionate mortality ratio and standardized mortality ratio risk measures. Am J Epidemiol 1980;111:263.
13. Kelsey JL, Thompson WD, Evans AS. Methods in observational epidemiology. New York: Oxford University Press, 1986.
14. Lilienfeld A, Pederson E, Dowd JE. Cancer epidemiology: Methods of study. Baltimore: Johns Hopkins Press, 1967.
15. Gordon T, Crittenden M, Haenszel W. Cancer mortality trends in the United States, 1930–1955. NCI Monogr 1961;6:133.
16. Burbank F. Patterns in cancer mortality in the United States: 1950–1967. NCI Monogr 1971;33.
17. Mason TJ, McKay FW. US cancer mortality by county: 1950–1969. US Dept. of Health, Education, and Welfare publication (NIH) 74-615. Washington, DC: US Government Printing Office, 1974.
18. Mason TJ, McKay FW, Hoover R, et al. Atlas of cancer mortality for US counties: 1950–1969. US Dept. of Health, Education, and Welfare publication (NIH) 75-780. Washington, DC: US Government Printing Office, 1975.
19. Mason TJ, McKay FW, Hoover R, et al. Atlas of cancer mortality among US nonwhites: 1950–1969. US Dept. of Health, Education, and Welfare publication (NIH) 76-1204. Washington, DC: US Government Printing Office, 1976.
20. Riggan WB, Van Bruggen J, Acquavella JF, et al. US cancer mortality rates and trends, 1950–1979, vols 1–3. EPA publication 600/1-83-015a. Washington, DC: US Government Printing Office, 1983.
21. Pickle LW, Mason TJ, Howard N, et al. Atlas of US cancer mortality among whites, 1950–1980. Dept. of Health and Human Services publication (NIH) 87-2900. Washington, DC: US Government Printing Office, 1987.
22. Pickle LW, Mason TJ, Howard N, et al. Atlas of US cancer mortality among nonwhites, 1950–1980. National Institutes of Health publication 90-1582. Washington, DC: US Government Printing Office, 1990.
23. McKay FW, Hanson MR, Miller RW. Cancer mortality in the United States: 1950–1977. NCI Monogr 1982;59.
24. Devesa SS, Silverman DT. Cancer incidence and mortality trends in the United States: 1935–1974. JNCI 1978;60:545.
25. Devesa SS, Silverman DT, Young JL Jr, et al. Cancer incidence and mortality trends among whites in the United States, 1947–1984. JNCI 1987;79:701.
26. Segi M, Aoki K, Kurihara M. World cancer mortality. Gann Monogr Cancer Res 1981;26:121.
27. Percy C, Miller BA, Ries LAG. Effect of changes in cancer classification and the accuracy of cancer death certificates on trends in cancer mortality. Ann NY Acad Sci 1990;609:87.
28. Heston JF, Kelly JB, Meigs JW, et al, eds. Forty-five years of cancer incidence in Connecticut: 1935–1979. NCI Monogr 1986;70.
29. Dorn HF, Cutler SJ. Morbidity from cancer in the United States. I and II. Public Health Monogr 1959;56.
30. Haenszel W, Marcus SC, Zimmerer EG. Cancer morbidity in urban and rural Iowa. Public Health Monogr 1956;37.
31. Cutler SJ, Young JL Jr (eds). Third National Cancer Survey: Incidence data. NCI Monogr 1975;41.
32. Horm JW, Asire AJ, Young JL Jr, et al, eds. SEER Program: Cancer incidence and mortality in the United States, 1973–1981. Dept. of Health and Human Services publication (NIH) 85-1837. Bethesda, MD: National Institutes of Health, 1984.
33. National Cancer Institute. Cancer statistics review 1973–1988. NIH publication 91-2789. Bethesda, MD: National Institutes of Health, 1991.
34. Muir C, Waterhouse J, Mack T, et al. Cancer incidence in five continents, vol V. Lyon: International Agency for Research on Cancer, 1987.
35. Axtell LM, Asire AJ, Myers MH. Cancer patient survival report number 5. US Dept. of Health, Education, and Welfare publication (NIH) 77-992. Bethesda, MD: National Institutes of Health, 1976.
36. Myers MH, Hankey BF. Cancer patient survival experience. NIH publication 80-2148. Bethesda, MD: National Institutes of Health, 1980.
37. Ries LG, Pollack ES, Young JL Jr. Cancer patient survival: Surveillance, Epidemiology, and End Results Program, 1973–1979. JNCI 1983;70:693.
38. Young JL Jr, Ries LG, Pollack ES. Cancer patient survival among ethnic groups in the United States. JNCI 1984;73:341.
39. Newell GR. Hospital- and population-based tumor registries. Cancer Bull 1983;35:283.
40. Boring CC, Squire TS, Tong T. Cancer statistics 1992. CA 1992;42:19.
41. Haenszel W. Migrant studies. In: Schottenfeld D, Fraumeni JF Jr, eds. Cancer epidemiology and prevention. Philadelphia: WB Saunders, 1982:194.
42. Lilienfeld AM, Levin ML, Kessler II. Cancer in the United States. Cambridge, MA: Harvard University Press, 1972.
43. Ziegler RG, Devesa SS, Fraumeni JF Jr. Epidemiologic patterns of colorectal cancer. In: DeVita VT Jr, Hellman S, Rosenberg SA, eds. Important advances in oncology 1986. Philadelphia: JB Lippincott, 1986:209.
44. Blot WJ, Harrington JM, Toledo A, et al. Lung cancer after employment in shipyards during World War II. N Engl J Med 1978;299:620.
45. Pickle LW, Correa P, Fontham E. Recent case-control studies of lung cancer in the United States. In: Mizell M, Correa P, eds. Lung cancer: Causes and prevention. Deerfield Beach, FL: Verlag-Chemie International, 1984:101.
46. Winn D, Blot WJ, Shy CM, et al. Snuff dipping and oral cancer among women in the southern United States. N Engl J Med 1981;304:745.
47. Hoar SK, Blair A, Holmes FF, et al. Agricultural herbicide use and risk of lymphoma and soft-tissue sarcoma. JAMA 1986;256:1141.
48. Boyle P, Muir CS, Grundmann E, eds. Cancer mapping: Recent results in cancer research, vol 114. Berlin: Springer-Verlag, 1989.
49. Liu JY, Liu BQ, Li GY, et al. Atlas of cancer mortality in the People's Republic of China: An aid for cancer control and research. Int J Epidemiol 1981;10:127.
50. Boring CC, Squire TS, Tong T. Cancer statistics 1991. CA 1991;41:19.
51. National Center for Health Statistics. Health: United States 1990. US Dept. of Health and Human Services publication (PHS) 91-1232. Washington, DC: US Government Printing Office, 1991.
52. Potosky AL, Kessler L, Gridley G, et al. Rise in prostatic cancer incidence associated with increased use of transurethral resection. JNCI 1990;82:1624.
53. Willett WC. Diet and human cancer. In: Brugge J, Curran T, Harlow E, et al, eds. Origins of human cancer: A comprehensive review. Cold Spring Harbor, NY: Cold Spring Harbor Laboratory Press, 1991:191.
54. Elwood JM, Hislop TG. Solar radiation in the etiology of cutaneous malignant melanoma in Caucasians. NCI Monogr 1982;62:167.
55. Miller BA, Feuer EJ, Hankey BF. The increasing incidence of breast cancer since 1982: Relevance of early detection. Cancer Causes and Control 1991;2:67.
56. Weiss NS. Epidemiology of carcinoma of the endometrium. In: Lilienfeld AM, ed. Reviews in cancer epidemiology, vol 2. New York: Elsevier, 1983:46.
57. Cramer DW. Uterine cervix. In: Schottenfeld D, Fraumeni JF Jr, eds. Cancer epidemiology and prevention. Philadelphia: WB Saunders, 1982:881.
58. Pokras R, Hufnagel VG. Hysterectomies in the United States, 1965–1984. Vital and health statistics, series 13, vol 92. US Dept. of Health and Human Services publication (PHS) 88-1753. Washington, DC: US Government Printing Office, 1987.
59. Miller RW, McKay FW. Decline in US childhood cancer mortality. JAMA 1984;251:1567.
60. Gutensohn N, Cole P. Epidemiology of Hodgkin's disease. Semin Oncol 1980;7:92.
61. Brown LM, Pottern LM, Hoover RN, et al. Testicular cancer in the United States: Trends in incidence and mortality. Int J Epidemiol 1986;15:164.
62. Devesa SS, Diamond EL. Association of breast cancer and cervical cancer incidences with income and education among whites and blacks. JNCI 1980;65:515.
63. McWhorter WP, Schatzkin AG, Horm JW, et al. Contribution of socioeconomic status to black/white differences in cancer incidence. Cancer 1989;63:982.
64. Baquet CR, Horm JW, Gibbs T, et al. Socioeconomic factors and cancer incidence among blacks and whites. JNCI 1991;83:551.

65. Hutchison GB. The epidemiologic method. In: Schottenfeld D, Fraumeni JF Jr, eds. Cancer epidemiology and prevention. Philadelphia: WB Saunders, 1982:3.

66. Rothman KJ. Modern epidemiology. Boston: Little, Brown, 1986.

67. Cole P. The evolving case-control study. J Chronic Dis 1979;32:15.

68. Cole P, MacMahon B. Attributable risk percent in case-control studies. Br J Prev Soc Med 1971;25:242.

69. Miettinen OS. Proportion of disease caused or prevented by a given exposure, trait or intervention. Am J Epidemiol 1974;99:325.

70. Greene MH, Harris EL, Gershenson DM, et al. Melphalan may be a more potent leukemogen than cyclophosphamide. Ann Intern Med 1986;105:360.

71. Hartge P, Silverman D, Hoover R, et al. Changing cigarette habits and bladder cancer risk: A case-control study. JNCI 1987;78:1119.

72. Shields PG, Harris CC. Molecular epidemiology and the genetics of environmental cancer. JAMA 1991;266:681.

73. Perera FP, Weinstein IB. Molecular epidemiology and carcinogen-DNA adduct detection: New approaches to studies of human cancer causation. J Chronic Dis 1982;35:581.

74. Miller RW. Genes, syndromes, and cancer. Pediatr Rev 1986;8:153.

75. Miller RW, Watenabe S, Fraumeni JF Jr, et al. eds. Unusual occurrences as clues to cancer etiology. Proceedings of the 18th International Symposium of the Princess Takamatsu Cancer Research Fund, 1987. Tokyo: Japan Scientific Societies Press, 1988.

76. Wald NJ, Doll R, eds. Interpretation of negative epidemiological evidence for carcinogenicity. IARC Scientific publication 65. Lyon: International Agency for Research on Cancer, 1985.

77. Sackett DL. Bias in analytic research. J Chronic Dis 1979;32:51.

78. Brinton LA, Huggins GR, Lehman HF, et al. Long-term use of oral contraceptives and risk of invasive cervical cancer. Int J Cancer 1986;38:339.

79. Hill AB. The environment and disease: Association or causation? Proc R Soc Med 1965;58:295.

80. Report of the Advisory Committee to the Surgeon General. Smoking and health. Public Health Service publication 1103. Washington, DC: US Government Printing Office, 1964.

81. Vessey MP, Gray M, eds. Cancer risks and prevention. Oxford: Oxford University Press, 1985.

82. Tomatis L, ed. Cancer: Causes, occurrence and control. IARC scientific publication 100. Lyon: International Agency for Research on Cancer, 1990.

83. International Agency for Research on Cancer. Tobacco smoking. IARC Monographs on the Evaluation of the Carcinogenic Risk of Chemicals to Humans, vol 38. Lyon: International Agency for Research on Cancer, 1986.

84. McLaughlin JK, Mandel JS, Blot WJ, et al. A population-based case-control study of renal cell carcinoma. JNCI 1984;72:275.

85. McLaughlin JK, Blot WJ, Mandel JS, et al. Etiology of cancer of the renal pelvis. JNCI 1983;71:287.

86. Brinton LA, Schairer C, Haenszel W, et al. Cigarette smoking and invasive cervical cancer. JAMA 1986;255:3265.

87. Brinton LA, Blot WJ, Becker JA, et al. A case-control study of cancers of the nasal cavity and paranasal sinuses. Am J Epidemiol 1984;119:896.

88. You WC, Blot WJ, Chang YS, et al. Diet and the high risk of stomach cancer in Shandong, China. Cancer Res 1988;48:3518.

89. Kinlen LJ, Rogot E. Leukemia and smoking habits among United States veterans. Br Med J 1988;297:657.

90. Lubin JH, Blot WJ, Berino F, et al. Patterns of lung cancer risk according to type of cigarette smoked. Int J Cancer 1984;33:569.

91. International Agency for Research on Cancer. Tobacco habits other than smoking: Betel-quid and areca-nut chewing and some related nitrosamines. IARC Monographs on the Evaluation of the Carcinogenic Risk of Chemicals to Humans, vol 37. Lyon: International Agency for Research on Cancer, 1985.

92. Blot WJ, Fraumeni JF Jr. Passive smoking and lung cancer. JNCI 1986;77:993.

93. Wald NJ, Nanchahal K, Thompson SG, et al. Does breathing other people's tobacco smoke cause lung cancer? Br Med J 1986;293:1217.

94. Tuyns AJ. Alcohol. In: Schottenfeld D, Fraumeni JF Jr, eds. Cancer epidemiology and prevention. Philadelphia: WB Saunders, 1982:293.

95. Rothman KJ. The proportion of cancer attributable to alcohol consumption. Prev Med 1980;9:174.

96. Blot WJ, McLaughlin JK, Winn DM, et al. Smoking and drinking in relation to oral and pharyngeal cancer. Cancer Res 1988;48:3282.

97. Winn DM, Blot WJ, McLaughlin JK, et al. Mouthwash use and oral conditions in the risk of oral and pharyngeal cancer. Cancer Res 1991;51:3044.

98. Jensen OM. Cancer morbidity and causes of death among Danish brewery workers. Int J Cancer 1979;23:454.

99. Schatzkin A, Jones DY, Hoover RN. Alcohol consumption and breast cancer in the epidemiologic follow-up study of the first National Health and Nutrition Examination Survey. N Engl J Med 1987;316:1169.

100. Willett WC, Stampfer MJ, Colditz GA, et al. Moderate alcohol consumption and the risk of breast cancer. N Engl J Med 1987;316:1174.

101. Decoufle P. Occupation. In: Schottenfeld D, Fraumeni JF Jr, eds. Cancer epidemiology and prevention. Philadelphia: WB Saunders, 1982:318.

102. Saracci R. Occupation. In: Vessey MP, Gray M, eds. Cancer risks and prevention. Oxford: Oxford University Press, 1985:99.

103. Saracci R. Asbestosis and lung cancer: An analysis of the epidemiological evidence on the asbestos-smoking interaction. Int J Cancer 1977;20:323.

104. Silverman DT, Hoover RN, Mason TJ, et al. Motor exhaust-related occupations and bladder cancer. Cancer Res 1986;46:2113.

105. Hayes RB, Thomas T, Silverman DT, et al. Lung cancer in motor exhaust-related occupations. Am J Ind Med 1989;16:685.

106. Blair A, Saracci R, Stewart PA, et al. Epidemiologic evidence on the relationship between formaldehyde exposure and cancer. Scand J Work Environ Health 1990;16:381.

107. Tagnon I, Blot WJ, Stroube RB, et al. Mesothelioma associated with the shipbuilding industry in coastal Virginia. Cancer Res 1980;40:3875.

108. Artvinll M, Baris YI. Malignant mesotheliomas in a small village in the Anatolian region of Turkey: An epidemiologic study. JNCI 1979;63:17.

109. Brown LM, Pottern LM, Blot WJ. Lung cancer in relation to environmental pollutants emitted from industrial sources. Environ Res 1984;34:250.

110. Gao YT, Blot WJ, Zheng W, et al. Lung cancer among Chinese women. Int J Cancer 1987;40:604.

111. Mumford JL, He XZ, Chapman RS, et al. Lung cancer and indoor air pollution in Xuan Wei, China. Science 1987;235:217.

112. Cantor KP, Hoover R, Hartge P, et al. Bladder cancer, drinking water source, and tap water consumption: A case-control study. JNCI 1987;79:1269.

113. Chen CJ, Chuang YC, You SL, et al. A retrospective study on malignant neoplasms of bladder, lung and liver in blackfoot disease in endemic area of Taiwan. Br J Cancer 1986;53:399.

114. Boice JD Jr, Fraumeni JF Jr, eds. Radiation carcinogenesis: Epidemiology and biological significance. Progress in cancer research and therapy, vol 26. New York: Raven Press, 1984.

115. United Nations Scientific Committee on the Effects of Atomic Radiation. Sources, effects and risks of ionizing radiation. New York: United Nations, 1988.

116. National Research Council, Committee on the Biological Effects of Ionizing Radiations (BEIR V): Health effects of exposure to low levels of ionizing radiation. Washington, DC: National Academy Press, 1990.

117. National Research Council, Committee on the Biological Effects of Ionizing Radiations (BEIR IV). Health risks of radon and other internally deposited alpha-emitters. Washington, DC: National Academy Press, 1988.

118. Boice JD Jr, Land CE. Ionizing radiation. In: Schottenfeld D, Fraumeni JF Jr, eds. Cancer epidemiology and prevention. Philadelphia: WB Saunders, 1982:231.

119. Jablon S, Hrubec Z, Boice JD Jr. Cancer in populations living near nuclear facilities. JAMA 1991;265:1403.

120. Wang Z, Boice JD Jr., Wei L, et al. Thyroid nodularity and chromosome aberrations among women in areas of high background radiation in China. JNCI 1990;82:478.

121. Holm LE, Hall P, Wiklund K, et al. Cancer risks after I-131 therapy for hyperthyroidism. JNCI 1991;83:1072.

122. Scotto J, Fears TR, Fraumeni JF Jr. Solar radiation. In: Schottenfeld D, Fraumeni JF Jr, eds. Cancer epidemiology and prevention. Philadelphia: WB Saunders, 1982:254.

123. Greene MH, Clark WH, Tucker MA, et al. Acquired precursors of cutaneous malignant melanoma: The familial dysplastic nevus syndrome. N Engl J Med 1985;312:91.

124. Scotto J, Fraumeni JF Jr. Skin (other than melanoma). In: Schottenfeld D, Fraumeni JF Jr, eds. Cancer epidemiology and prevention. Philadelphia: WB Saunders, 1982:996.

125. Glass AG, Hoover RN. The emerging epidemic of melanoma and squamous cell skin cancer. JAMA 1989;262:2097.

126. Scotto J, Cotton G, Urback F, et al. Biologically effective ultraviolet radiation: Surface measurements in the United States, 1974–1985. Science 1988;239:762.

127. Herbst AL, Cole P, Colton T, et al. Age incidence and risk of diethylstilbestrol-related clear cell carcinoma of the vagina and cervix. Am J Obstet Gynecol 1977;128:43.

128. Steinberg KK, Thacker SB, Smith J, et al. A meta-analysis of the effect of estrogen replacement therapy on the risk of breast cancer. JAMA 1991;265:1985.

129. UK National Case-Control Study Group. Oral contraceptive use and breast cancer risk in young women. Lancet 1989;1:973.

130. Henderson B, Ross RK, Pike MC. Toward the primary prevention of cancer. Science 1991;254:1131.

131. Boice JD Jr, Greene MH, Killen JY Jr, et al. Leukemia and preleukemia after adjuvant treatment of gastrointestinal cancer with semustine (methyl-CCNU). N Engl J Med 1983;309:1079.

132. Boice JD Jr, Greene MH, Killen JY Jr, et al. Leukemia after adjuvant chemotherapy with semustine (methyl-CCNU)—Evidence of a dose-response effect. N Engl J Med 1986;314:119.

133. Hoover R, Fraumeni JF Jr. Risk of cancer in renal-transplant recipients. Lancet 1973;2:55.

134. Kinlen LJ. Immunosuppressive therapy and cancer. Cancer Surv 1982;1:565.

135. Filopovich AH, Spector BD, Kersey J. Immunodeficiency in humans as a risk factor in the development of malignancy. Prev Med 1980;9:252.

136. List AF, Greco FA, Vogler LB. Lymphoproliferative diseases in immunocompromised hosts: The role of the Epstein-Barr virus. J Clin Oncol 1987;5:1673.

137. Thun MJ, Namboodiri MM, Heath CW Jr. Aspirin use and reduced risk of fatal colon cancer. N Engl J Med 1991;325:1593.

138. Evans AS. Viruses. In: Schottenfeld D, Fraumeni JF Jr, eds. Cancer epidemiology and prevention. Philadelphia: WB Saunders, 1982:364.

139. Correa P. Is gastric carcinoma an infectious disease? N Engl J Med 1991;325:1170.

140. Levine PH, Ablashi DV, Nonoyama M, et al. eds. Epstein-Barr virus and human disease. Clifton, NJ: Humana Press, 1987.

141. Beasley RP, Hwang LY, Lin CC, et al. Hepatocellular carcinoma and hepatitis B virus: A prospective study of 22,707 men in Taiwan. Lancet 1981;2:1129.

142. Simonetti RG, Camma C, Fiorello F, et al. Hepatitis C virus infection as a risk factor for hepatocellular carcinoma in patients with cirrhosis: A case-control study. Ann Int Med 1992;116:97.

143. Blattner WA. Human retroviruses. In: Feigin RD, Cherry JD, eds. Textbook of pediatric infectious diseases. 2nd ed. Philadelphia: WB Saunders, 1987:1795.

144. Goedert JJ, Blattner WA. The epidemiology and natural history of human immunodeficiency virus. In: DeVita VT Jr, Hellman S, Rosenberg SA, eds. AIDS: Etiology, diagnosis, treatment and prevention. 2nd ed. Philadelphia: JB Lippincott, 1988.

145. Zur Hausen H. Papillomaviruses in human cancer. Cancer 1987;59:1692.

146. Kinlen LJ, Clarke K, Hudson C. Evidence from population mixing in British New Towns 1946–1985 of an infective basis of childhood leukemia. Lancet 1990;2:577.

147. Mueller N, Evans A, Harris NL. Hodgkin's disease and Epstein-Barr virus: Altered antibody pattern before diagnosis. N Engl J Med 1989;320:689.

148. Pallesen G, Hamilton-Dutoit SJ, Rowe M, et al. Expression of Epstein-Barr virus latent gene products in tumour cells of Hodgkin's disease. Lancet 1991;337:320.

149. Armstrong BK, McMichael AJ, MacLennan R. Diet. In: Schottenfeld D, Fraumeni JF Jr, eds. Cancer epidemiology and prevention. Philadelphia: WB Saunders, 1982:419.

150. Kinlen LJ. Fat and breast cancer. Cancer Surv 1987;6:585.

151. Whittemore AS, Wu-Williams AS, Lee M, et al. Diet, physical activity, and colorectal cancer among Chinese in North America and China. JNCI 1990;82:915.

152. Willett WC, Stampfer MJ, Colditz GA, et al. Relation of meat, fat, and fiber intake to the risk of colon cancer in a prospective study among women. N Engl J Med 1990;323:1664.

153. Ziegler RG. Vegetables, fruits, and carotenoids and the risk of cancer. Am J Clin Nutr 1991;53S:251.

154. Bingham SA, Williams DRR, Cummings JH. Dietary fibre consumption in Britain: New estimates and their relation to large bowel cancer mortality. Br J Cancer 1985;52:399.

155. Greenwald P, Lanza E. Role of dietary fiber in the prevention of cancer. In: DeVita VT Jr, Hellman S, Rosenberg SA, eds. Important advances in oncology 1986. Philadelphia: JB Lippincott, 1986:37.

156. Ziegler RG, Mason TJ, Stemhagen A, et al. Carotene intake, vegetables, and the risk of lung cancer among white men in New Jersey. Am J Epidemiol 1986;123:1080.

157. Graham S, Dayal H, Swanson M, et al. Diet in the epidemiology of cancer of the colon and rectum. JNCI 1978;61:709.

158. Garland CF, Comstock GW, Garland FC, et al. Serum 25-hydroxyvitamin D and colon cancer: Eight-year prospective study. Lancet 1989;2:1176.

159. Garland FC, Garland CE, Gorham ED, et al. Geographic variation in breast cancer mortality in the United States: A hypothesis involving exposure to solar radiation. Prev Med 1990;19:614.

160. Kinlen LJ. Meat and fat consumption and cancer mortality: A study of strict religious orders in Britain. Lancet 1982;1:946

161. Bulatao-Jayme J, Almero EM, Castro MCA, et al. A case-control dietary study of primary liver cancer risk from aflatoxin exposure. Int J Epidemiol 1982;11:112.

162. Hsu IC, Metcalf RA, Sun T, et al. Mutational hotspot in the p53 gene in human hepatocellular carcinoma. Nature 1991;350:427.

163. Yu MC, Ho JHC, Lai SH, et al. Cantonese-style salted fish as a cause of nasopharyngeal carcinoma: Report of a case-control study in Hong Kong. Cancer Res 1986;46:956.

164. Hoover RN, Strasser PH. Artificial sweeteners and human bladder cancer. Lancet 1980;1:837.

165. Adamson RH. Mutagens and carcinogens formed during cooking of foods and methods to minimize their formation. In: DeVita VT Jr, Hellman S, Rosenberg SA, eds. Cancer prevention. Philadelphia: JB Lippincott, 1990:1.

166. Easton D, Peto J. The contribution of inherited predisposition to cancer incidence. Cancer Surv 1990;9:395.

167. Ayesh R, Idle JR, Ritchie JC, et al. Metabolic oxidation phenotypes as markers for susceptibility to lung cancer. Nature 1984;312:169.

168. Knudson AG. Hereditary cancer, oncogenes, and antioncogenes. Cancer Res 1985;45:1437.

169. Mulvihill JJ. Clinical genetics of pediatric cancer. In: Pizzo P, Poplack DP, eds. Principles and practice of pediatric oncology. Philadelphia: JB Lippincott, 1989:19–38.

170. Kinzler KW, Nilbert MC, Su LK, et al. Identification of FAP locus genes from chromosome 5q21. Science 1991;253:661.

171. Anderson DE. Familial predisposition. In: Schottenfeld D, Fraumeni JF Jr, eds. Cancer epidemiology and prevention. Philadelphia: WB Saunders, 1982:483.

172. Hall JM, Lee MK, Newman B, et al. Linkage of early-onset familial breast cancer to chromosome 17q21. Science 1990;250:1684.

173. Mulvihill JJ. Clinical ecogenetics: Cancer in families. N Engl J Med 1985;312:1569.

174. Li FP, Fraumeni JF Jr. Soft-tissue sarcomas, breast cancer, and other neoplasms: A familial syndrome? Ann Intern Med 1969;71:747.

175. Garber JE, Goldstein AM, Kantor AG, et al. Follow-up study of twenty-four families with Li-Fraumeni syndrome. Cancer Res 1991;51:6094.

176. Malkin D, Li FP, Strong LC, et al. Germ line p53 mutations in a familial syndrome of breast cancer, sarcomas, and other neoplasms. Science 1990;250:1233.

Cancer: Principles & Practice of Oncology, Fourth Edition,
edited by Vincent T. DeVita, Jr., Samuel Hellman, Steven A. Rosenberg.
J.B. Lippincott Co., Philadelphia © 1993.

Peter M. Howley

CHAPTER **10**

Principles of Carcinogenesis: Viral

Viral oncology has its foundations in scientific observations made at the turn of the century defining the transmissibility of avian leukemia in Denmark in 1908 and of an avian sarcoma in chickens in 1911.[1,2] These important discoveries were not appreciated at the time and their impact on virology and medicine was not recognized for decades. The importance of the work of Peyton Rous, who showed that cell-free extracts from a sarcoma in chickens could induce tumors in injected chickens within a few weeks, even when passed through filters that retained bacteria, was recognized by a Nobel prize in 1968.[2] Rous's original work pointed out that this infectious agent was not only capable of inducing tumors, but also imprinted the phenotypic characteristics of the original tumor on the recipient cell. This early work was relegated to the rank of avian curiosities, however, and its importance was not recognized for several decades.

In the 1930s, Richard Shope published a series of papers demonstrating cell-free transmission of tumors in rabbits. The first studies involved fibromatous tumors found in the footpads of wild cottontail rabbits, which could be transmitted by injecting cell-free extracts in either wild or domestic rabbits.[3] Subsequent studies have shown that this virus, referred to as the *Shope fibroma virus*, is a pox virus. Additional studies by Shope demonstrated that cutaneous papillomatosis in wild cottontail rabbits could also be transmitted by cell-free extracts. In some cases, these benign papillomas progress spontaneously into squamous cell carcinomas in infected domestic rabbits or in the infected cottontail rabbits.[4,5] In general, the field of viral oncology lay dormant until the discovery in the early 1950s of the murine leukemia viruses by Ludwig Gross[6] and of the mouse polyoma virus by Gross, Stewart, and Eddy.[7,8] These findings of tumor viruses in mice led many cancer researchers and virologists to the field of viral oncology in the hope that these initial observations could be extended to hu-

mans and that a fair proportion of human tumors might have a viral origin. The Special Viral Cancer Program at the National Cancer Institute grew from this intense interest in viral oncology and in identifying human tumor viruses.

Many of the most important developments in modern molecular biology derive from studies in viral oncology from the 1960s and 1970s. The discovery of reverse transcriptase, the development of recombinant DNA technology, the discovery of mRNA splicing, the discovery of oncogenes, and tumor suppressor genes are all developments that derive directly from studies in viral oncology. Oncogenes were first recognized as cellular genes that had been acquired by retroviruses through recombinational processes to convert them into acute-transforming RNA tumor viruses (see Chap. 3). The recognition that oncogenes participate in many different types of tumors and can be involved at different stages of tumorigenesis and viral oncology has contributed to our understanding of nonviral carcinogenesis. It is likely that the direct-transforming, oncogene-transducing retroviruses do not play a major causative role in naturally occurring cancers in animals or in humans, but rather represent laboratory generated recombinants. Human viruses with oncogenic properties are listed in Table 10–1. This list includes viruses such as the transforming adenoviruses, which are capable of transforming normal cells into malignant cells in the laboratory but which have not been associated with any known human tumors. The list also includes the papillomaviruses, which have been associated etiologically with specific human cancers and have been shown to encode transforming viral oncogenes. Finally, it includes viruses that have been closely linked with a specific human tumor, such as the hepatitis B virus and hepatocellular carcinoma, for which the evidence of a viral oncogene is still unclear. This chapter focuses on those viruses associated with specific human cancers and discusses the biology and perti-

TABLE 10–1. Human Viruses With Oncogenic Properties

Virus Family	Type	Human Tumor	Cofactors
Adenovirus	Types 2, 5, 12	None	—
Hepadnavirus	Hepatitis B (HBV)	Hepatocellular carcinoma	Aflatoxin, alcohol, smoking
Herpesvirus	Epstein-Barr (EBV)	Burkitt's lymphoma	Malaria
		Immunoblastic lymphoma	Immunodeficiency
		Nasopharyngeal carcinoma	Nitrosamines, HLA genotype
Papillomaviruses	HPV-16, -18, -33, -39	Anogenital cancers and some upper airway cancers	Smoking?, other factors
	HPV-5, -8, -17	Skin cancer	Genetic disorders, sunlight
Polyomavirus	BK, JC	?Neural tumors	—
		?Insulinomas	
Retroviruses	HTLV-I	Adult T-cell leukemia/lymphoma	Uncertain
	HTLV-II	Hairy cell leukemia	Unknown

nent molecular biology of these viruses. Evidence of the association of each of these viruses with specific types of human neoplasia is presented, and the mechanisms by which these viruses may contribute to malignant transformation are discussed.

Table 10–1 also lists cofactors believed to be important in the carcinogenic processes associated with each of these viruses. None of these viruses is sufficient alone to induce the specific neoplasia with which it is associated. Each of the viruses associated with these human cancers is thought to be involved at an early step in carcinogenesis. Subsequent cellular genetic events such as somatic mutations are thought to be important at each step in the multistep process of malignant progression.

HUMAN RETROVIRUSES

The first two tumor viruses described were both retroviruses. These were the avian leukemia virus described by Ellermann and Bang[1] and the avian sarcoma virus described by Peyton Rous at the turn of the century.[2] Among the tumor viruses, the retroviruses have been a primary subject of research by virologists, oncologists, and molecular biologists. During the past 25 years, retroviruses have provided us with reverse transcriptase and oncogenes and have been engineered into vectors for the effective delivery of DNA to cells for gene therapy. Interest in viruses as infectious tumor agents was spurred by the findings of Ludwig Gross, who in the 1950s described retroviruses that could cause tumors in mice.[6,7] In the early 1960s, William Jarrett discovered the feline leukemia virus (FeLV), which was found to induce leukemia and aplasia in cats.[9] Studies with FeLV were important because subsequent studies established that the leukemia associated with FeLV could be communicated in the natural setting and was not limited to the laboratory. This provided a major impetus to look for retroviruses as possible tumor viruses, possibly related to leukemia in humans. With the retroviruses associated with leukemia in animals such as chickens, mice, and cats, there is extensive viral replication and the virus

particles can often be easily seen by electron microscopy.[10] The studies of the late 1960s and through the 1970s that looked for a human retrovirus in human blood disorders relied heavily on the electron microscope.

The Nobel Prize–winning experiments of Howard Temin and David Baltimore showed that these viruses contained enzymes called *reverse transcriptase* that were involved in transcribing the single-stranded RNA copy of the input viral RNA into DNA.[11,12] This enzymatic activity is associated with retrovirus particles and can be readily assayed from infected cells. Assays for reverse transcriptase activities unique to retroviruses provided an alternative and sensitive assay for these viruses. Nonetheless, almost 70 years passed between Peyton Rous's initial description of the avian sarcoma virus and the first unequivocal evidence of a human retrovirus.

HUMAN T-CELL LEUKEMIA VIRUS TYPE I

The first substantiated reports of a human retrovirus were published in 1980 and 1981 by Gallo and colleagues[13,14] and soon after by Yoshida and colleagues in Japan.[15] These isolates were from human T-cell leukemia cell lines. The human T-cell leukemia virus type I (HTLV-I) is the virus etiologic agent of adult T-cell leukemia (ATL). This leukemia is endemic in Kyushu and Shikoku, the southernmost islands of Japan. A causal relation between HTLV-I and ATL was initially suggested by epidemiologic studies showing geographic clustering of ATL implicating an infectious agent.

ATL was first described by Takatsuki and colleagues in 1977 and is a malignancy of mature CD4 positive lymphocytes.[16,17] It is endemic in parts of Japan and in the Caribbean and in parts of Africa.[18–20] The tumor resembles mycosis fungoides and Sézary syndrome but is more aggressive; the median survival from the time of diagnosis is only 3 to 4 months. It affects visceral organs and the skin and often induces hypercalcemia. In the Gallo laboratory, the isolation of HTLV-I from a leukemia cell line of a patient was a consequence and extension of the basic research in that laboratory identifying a T-cell growth factor referred to as *interleukin*-2 (IL-2).[14,21] This growth factor is released by T cells after stimulation with phytohemagglutinin (PHA), which causes T-cells to proliferate. PHA activates T cells not only to secrete IL-2 but also to develop receptor molecules on their surface for the growth factor molecules. With IL-2 bound to its receptor, the cells begin to divide.

After the isolation of HTLV-I from initial American and Japanese patients, immunologic assays were developed to detect antibodies specific for the viral antigens. Such serologic assays became the basis of subsequent epidemiologic and transmission studies. Studies revealed that virus infection was more widespread in the endemic areas than was the prevalence of malignancies.[18] A person infected with HTLV-I has about a 1% lifetime risk of developing ATL. A preleukemic disease in the form of a chronic lymphocytosis is often seen before the development of acute leukemia or lymphoma.[22] ATL generally occurs in early adulthood, about 20 to 30 years after initial infection.

Although retroviruses are often referred to as *leukemia viruses,* the spectrum of diseases with which they are associated is not limited to leukemia. For instance, the avian leukemia viruses are also associated with an autoimmune wasting disease and osteoporosis. The FeLVs can also be associated with anemia, aplasia, and immunodeficiency. Certain mouse leukemia viruses can also induce paralysis and neuropathies. Similarly, HTLV-I infection has been associated with other diseases in humans. HTLV-I has been associated with an increased susceptibility to opportunistic infections and a degenerative neurologic disease. In West Indian patients, this disease is referred to as *tropical spastic paraparesis* (TSP)[23,24] and a similar disease in Japan is known as *HTLV-I-associated myelopathy* (HAM).[25] The specific risk factors important in determining the development of leukemia, immunodeficiency, or TSP in the HTLV-I infected individual are not known.

HUMAN T-CELL LEUKEMIA VIRUS TYPE II

The second human retrovirus, HTLV-II, was first described in a cell line established from a patient with an unusual form of hairy cell leukemia.[26] Morphologically, the cells resemble those of a hairy cell leukemia; however, they contain markers of a T-cell lineage, whereas most hairy cell leukemias contain B-cell markers. Unlike HTLV-I, HTLV-II has not been found to be endemic in any specific population of humans. Its association with specific leukemias is not established, because not enough cases have been available for clear epidemiologic studies. HTLV-II is distinct from HTLV-I but shares considerable nucleic acid homology.[27,28]

HUMAN IMMUNODEFICIENCY VIRUS

A discussion of the human immunodeficiency viruses (HIV-1 and HIV-2) is beyond the scope of this chapter. The HIVs, also human retroviruses, were initially referred to as *HTLVs* but are now recognized to be distinct members of the retrovirus subclass called *lentiviruses.*[29] Like HTLV-I and HTLV-II, the HIVs also infect CD4-positive cells, but beyond that the viruses are not closely related. HIV-1 and HIV-2 are associated with acquired immunodeficiency syndrome (AIDS) and do not appear to be directly associated with any specific human tumors, although there is a high incidence of specific tumors in patients with AIDS.[30] One of the earliest diagnostic features of AIDS in young homosexual men can be Kaposi's sarcoma, which was regarded as an extremely rare tumor before the AIDS epidemic. Other tumors often observed in AIDS patients include non-Hodgkin's lymphomas and papillomavirus-associated perianal squamous cell carcinomas. Some of the tumors seen in AIDS patients may have a viral origin. The lymphomas may be accounted for in part by the emergence of cells transformed by the Epstein-Barr virus progressing to malignancy. It is also possible that HTLV-I accounts for some lymphomas in patients with AIDS. The genital warts and perianal squamous cell carcinomas seen in these patients have been shown to harbor specific human papillomavirus DNA types and are discussed later in this chapter.

THE MECHANISM OF TRANSFORMATION

Only a subset of individuals seropositive for HTLV-I develops ATL. The virus is not casually transmitted but is transmitted through sexual contact or through contaminated blood. Recent evidence suggests that the virus can be transmitted from mother to infant through mother's milk.[31,32] There is a latency period between the time of infection and the development of ATL in those patients who go on to develop the malignancy, which can vary from a few years to as long as 40 years.

How is this virus involved in leukemogenesis? Several lines of evidence suggest a direct role. The first is epidemiologic. Infants born in an endemic area who have been infected have the same likelihood of developing ATL whether they remain in the endemic area or move to another part of the world. The virus alone appears sufficient to initiate the chain of events leading to malignancy independent of subsequent environmental factors.

Additional evidence for a role of HTLV-I as an etiologic agent in ATL comes from the molecular biology of the virus. In retrovirus-infected cells, the provirus (*i.e.,* the double-stranded DNA copy of the viral RNA genome) is integrated into the cellular genome at random positions as part of the life cycle of the virus. Within HTLV-I–infected cells, the provirus is also randomly integrated into the host chromosome.[33] In the leukemic cells of an ATL patient, the viral sequences are found integrated in the same place in each cell, and the site of integration varies from leukemia to leukemia.[34,35] This indicates that ATL is clonal and is derived from a single cell. It also indicates that the viral infection necessarily precedes the origin of the tumor.

HTLV-I is able to transform human umbilical cord blood lymphocytes (T-cells) in vitro, turning them from normal cells into immortalized precancerous cells. The mechanism by which HTLV-I induces leukemogenesis is different from that of the other chronic leukemia retroviruses such as the avian leukosis virus. The combination of the clonality of the tumor cells and the random nature of the integration sites of the provirus from tumor to tumor indicates that HTLV-I transforms by a novel mechanism for retroviruses. Before the detailed studies of HTLV-I, two mechanisms were known by which a retrovirus could induce malignancy. One mechanism involved the transduction of an oncogene directly by the retrovirus. Oncogenes are cellular genes often involved in the regulation of cellular growth. In fact, the avian sarcoma virus is capable of inducing tumors in chickens because it has acquired extra nucleic acids from the cellular oncogene *SRC*. Retroviruses containing an oncogene are themselves defective for viral replication but give rise to a rapidly developing cancer after infection of the appropriate cell. The tumors that result from infection with a retrovirus containing an oncogene are not necessarily monoclonal. The genetic events leading to the recombinational events between the cellular and viral nucleic acids are rare. These viruses are important to the molecular virologist but are of little consequence to the cause of naturally occurring cancers in humans or in animals.

The slow-acting leukemogenic retroviruses, such as FeLV and the mouse leukemia virus (MuLV), do not contain oncogenes and therefore induce leukemia in a manner similar to the HTLV-I-associated human malignancies in that only a minority of the infected animals develop leukemia. There is a long latency between the time of infection and the time of tumor formation. In addition, the tumors are clonal. The difference between the mechanisms of leukemogenesis of these slow-acting leukemogenic retroviruses and of HTLV-I is that although the provirus integrates randomly into the cellular chromosomes in infected cells, it is found preferentially in the vicinity of protooncogenes in the tumors that develop. For these viruses to induce malignancy, the provirus must integrate in a region of the host genome in a manner that enables the regulatory sequences of the provirus to interact with the nearby oncogene to promote cellular proliferation. The mechanism by which this occurs is referred to as *promoter insertion* if the proviral LTR (long terminal repeat) acts as a promoter to initiate transcription of the protooncogene, or *enhancer insertion* if it acts as an enhancer to activate the expression of protooncogene. In the avian leukosis virus, the integration of the retrovirus occurs in the vicinity of the c-*MYC* oncogene, resulting in the deregulation of its expression.[36]

The HTLV-I provirus can therefore act at a distance. This suggests that the viral genome encodes a factor that is critical in the early stages of leukemogenesis. HTLV-I and its relative HTLV-II belong to a distinct group of retroviruses that has been referred to as *trans-regulating retroviruses*. This group for retroviruses includes the bovine leukemia virus, the biology of which is somewhat similar to that of HTLV-I and HTLV-

II.[37] These viruses differ from the chronic leukemia viruses and the acute leukemia viruses in that they contain additional genomic sequences at the 3' end of the genome, called the *X region* by Yoshida, who first described it (Fig. 10–1).[38] Subsequent studies have indicated that this region encodes transregulatory factors.[39-42] Two unique regulatory genes, *TAX* and *REX*, are encoded by this region.[43] The *TAX* gene serves as a master key for activating transcription from the viral LTR, and the *REX* gene is involved in regulating viral mRNA levels. The *TAX* gene product acts to increase the transcriptional activity of the viral promoter in the LTR.[41,44,45]

In addition, the *TAX* gene product has been shown to activate transcription of some nonviral genes, including the IL-2 gene and IL-2 receptor.[46] One mechanism by which HTLV-I could induce cellular proliferation and immortalization may involve an autocrine loop through the stimulation of both IL-2 and its receptor. TAX-mediated activation of cellular genes may also involve paracrine mechanisms. Among the cellular genes that TAX has been shown to activate is the granulocyte-macrophage colony-stimulating factor (GM-CSF).[47] TAX-stimulated GM-CSF secreted by T cells could affect T-cell growth by activating or increasing the number of macrophages that could then activate T cells through the release of additional cytokines such as IL-1. A final mechanism by which HTLV could mediate transformation is direct stimulation of T cells by the virus itself or some viral structural component through interaction with cellular receptors.

HEPATITIS B VIRUS

Hepatitis B virus (HBV) is the cause of hepatitis B, a major worldwide public health problem. In endemic parts of the world such as Far East Asia and tropical Africa, about 10% of the population are chronic carriers of the HBV. In these areas, chronic active hepatitis and liver cirrhosis associated with HBV infection are the major causes of mortality. Furthermore, HBV has been shown by epidemiologic studies to be of great importance in the cause of hepatocellular carcinoma (HCC).[48] In China alone, there are between 500,000 and 1,000,000 cases of HCC annually.

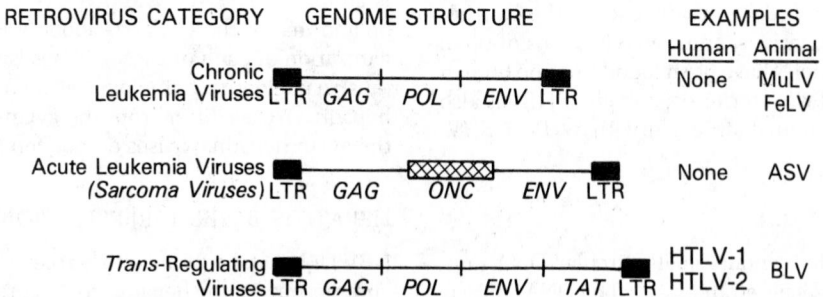

FIGURE 10–1. The genomic organization of different types of retroviruses. The prototype retrovirus is represented in the figure by the chronic leukemia viruses. It contains regulatory sequences at each end derived from the long terminal repeat (LTR) elements of the virus as well as the viral proteins coded for by *GAG*, *POL*, and *ENV*. The acute transforming retroviruses are defective viruses. In addition to losing viral gene segments, they have acquired onc sequences from the cellular genome. The transregulatory retroviruses contain sequences, 3* to the env gene, that encode regulatory factors. This region has been referred to as the *X region* and encodes the *TAX* and *REX* genes. ASV, avian sarcoma virus; BLV, bovine leukemia virus; FeLV, feline leukemia virus; MLV, murine leukemia virus.

HBV is a member of a group of animal viruses referred to as the *hepadnaviruses* (for hepatotropic DNA viruses). HBV is the only human member of this group of viruses.[49] Other members of this group include the woodchuck hepatitis virus (WHV), the Beechey ground squirrel hepatitis virus (GSHV), and the Peking duck hepatitis B virus (DHBV).[50–52] Each of these viruses has a similar structure and each is hepatotropic, leading to persistent viral infections of the liver. The animal hepatitis viruses have been important contributors to our understanding of the molecular biology of these viruses. Of the hepadnaviruses, only HBV and WHV have been associated with chronic active hepatitis and HCC.

DISCOVERY

The hepatitis B surface antigen (HBsAg) was discovered in 1963 by Baruch Blumberg while studying human serum protein polymorphisms.[53,54] Studies that associated this antigen with acute hepatitis B infection gave it the name *hepatitis-associated antigen* (HAA); it is now known as *hepatitis B surface antigen*.[55,56] This antigen is the surface or envelope protein of the hepatitis B virus particle, and its presence in the serum of infected patients remains the most useful marker of an active HBV infection.[57] Until recently, HBV had not been successfully grown in tissue culture and the serum from infected patients became the principal source of viral material for the characterization of the virus.

During an HBV infection, virus particles are present at high titer in the serum with up to 10^5 to 10^9 virions per ml visible by electron microscopy.[58] In addition to the complete virion particles, the serum also contains empty viral envelopes consisting of spheric or filamentous particles 22 nm in diameter.[59] The virion of 42 nm in diameter consists of an envelope and a nucleocapsid containing the double-stranded circular DNA molecule and the DNA polymerase. This virion particle was first described by Dane and is sometimes referred to as the *Dane particle*.[57] The outer envelope contains the HBsAg and consists of protein, carbohydrate, and lipid. The capsid carries the hepatitis B core antigen (HBcAg). The outer envelope of the virion with the HBsAg can be removed with treatment with nonionic detergents such as Nonidet P-40, releasing the free core particles (Fig. 10–2). Treatment of the virion core with a strong detergent such as SDS releases the double-stranded viral DNA. The concentrations of the incomplete viral forms in the serum usually greatly exceed the concentrations of the complete virions, and concentrations of up to 10^{13} 22-nm spheric particles have been found in some human sera.[59] This spectrum of virus forms described for HBV is also found in the serum of animals infected with WHV, GSHV, and DHBV.[50–52]

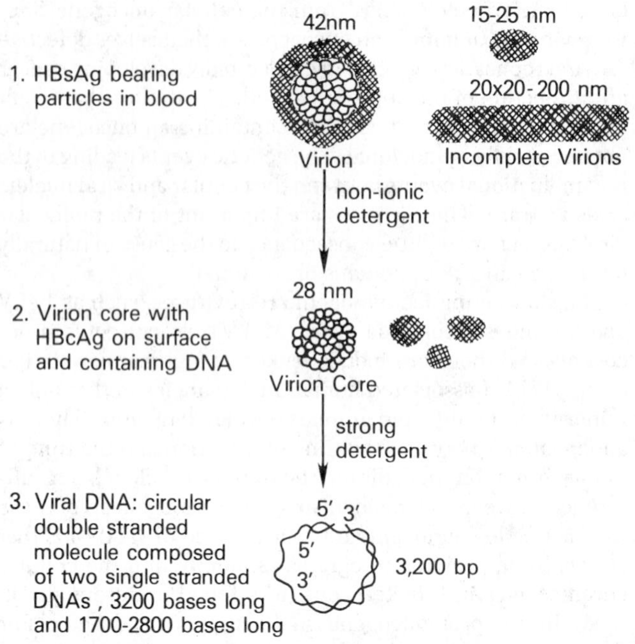

HEPATITIS B VIRAL DNA

Hepatitis B viral particles contain small, circular DNA molecules that are partially double stranded.[60,61] The DNA consists of a long strand with a constant length of 3220 bases and a shorter strand that varies in length from 1700 to 2800 bases in different molecules (Fig. 10–3).[61] The virion particles contain a DNA polymerase activity capable of repairing the single-stranded DNA region to make two fully double-stranded molecules, each about 3220 bases in length.[62] For this reaction, DNA synthesis initiates at the 3' end of the short strand which,

FIGURE 10–2. Hepatitis B virus forms in the blood of infected humans. The virion core is released by nonionic detergent. The viral genome consists of a long strand (3200 bases) and a shorter strand (1700–2800 bases). (Redrawn from Robinson WS. Hepatitis B virus. In: Fields BN, ed. Virology. New York: Raven Press, 1984:1384)

as noted above, is heterogenous among different DNA molecules. DNA synthesis terminates at the uniquely located 5' end of the short strand when it is reached. The long strand is not a closed molecule but contains a nick at a unique site about 300 bp from the 5' end of the short strand.

The HBV genome has four open reading frames (ORFs). These ORFs are designated as *S* and *pre-S, C, P,* and *X*.[61,63] S and pre-S represent two contiguous reading frames and code for the viral surface glycoproteins. Region C contains the coding sequences for the structural protein of the nucleocapsid. The P gene encodes the viral polymerase, which contains reverse transcriptase activity. The X ORF encodes a basic polypeptide that is a transcriptional transactivator and can upregulate the activity of hepadnaviral promoters.[64,65] The overall structure of the genomes of all of the animal hepadnaviruses is similar.[63] The WHV and GSHV genomes are about 3300 bp and that of the DHBV is about 3000 bp. The genomic organization of each of these viruses is similar and there is extensive nucleotide homology between them. The mammalian hepadnaviruses differ from the avian hepadnaviruses in that the avian hepadnaviruses do not contain the X region.[63]

HEPATITIS B VIRAL REPLICATION

HBV DNA can be found either free or integrated into the host chromosome of the hepatocyte.[66,67] Free HBV DNA represents intermediate forms of replication for the viral genome and can be detected during acute and some chronic stages of HPV infection. Integrated sequences are usually found during chronic virus infection and in HCC. The replication mechanism for the hepadnaviruses, first discovered by Summers and Mason for DHBV and later confirmed for HBV, is different from that of other DNA viruses.[68,69] The replication cycle in-

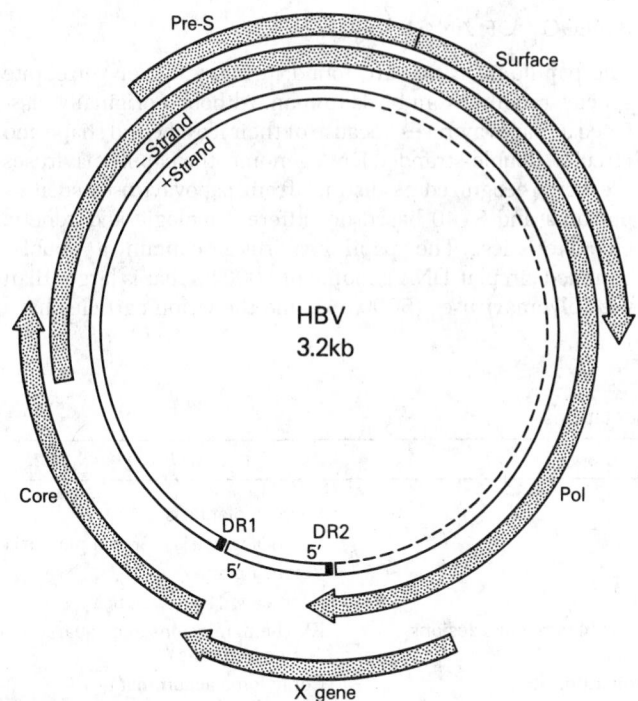

FIGURE 10–3. Physical and genetic map of HBV DNA. The arrows surrounding the genome represent the four large open reading frames of the L(−) strand with the genes they encode. The broken line is the S(+) DNA strand. The positions of the 5' ends of the DNA strands are indicated. The locations of the direct repeats (DR1 and DR2) involved in the initiation of DNA replication are also indicated.[63,69]

volves a reverse transcription step resembling that of the retroviruses in that a central feature is the use of an RNA copy of the genome as an intermediate in replication. The hepadnaviruses differ from the retroviruses in that the retrovirus virions contain RNA and the intermediate form of replication is integrated DNA. The virions of the hepadnaviruses contain DNA and the intermediate replication form is RNA. Integration of the hepadnaviral genome is not a necessary intermediate step for viral genome replication. The similarity between the retroviruses and the hepadnaviruses is also reflected in the genomic organization in that all of the genes are necessarily encoded on only one strand. The order of the genes within the retroviruses (*i.e.*, GAG, POL, and ENV) is similar to that of their counterparts for the hepadnaviruses (core, polymerase, and surface antigen). There are other subtle differences in the transcriptional programs used to generate the mRNAs for these different viruses. A further similarity between these viruses is the finding that a subset of these viruses encode transcriptional regulatory factors. For HTLV-I, the X region encodes TAX, a transcriptional activator. Evidence from several laboratories indicates that the X gene of the mammalian hepadnaviruses similarly encodes transcriptional transactivator.

HBV AND HEPATOCELLULAR CARCINOMA

Considerable evidence indicates an etiologic involvement of HBV with human HCC. This evidence stems primarily from epidemiologic studies. There is a striking correlation between the worldwide geographic incidence of HCC and the prevalence of HBsAg chronic carriers.[70] Compelling evidence for

the role of HBV in HCC comes from the prospective epidemiologic studies performed by Palmer Beasley in Taiwan.[48] His studies revealed a relative risk for HBsAg-positive males to be 217 compared with noncarriers. Furthermore, 51% of the deaths from these carriers were caused by cirrhosis of the liver or HCC, compared with only 2% among the control population. Among the noncarriers, 90% had evidence of a previous Sézary's syndrome HBV infection but did not have evidence of the HBsAg chronic carrier state. This indicated that the high incidence of HCC was clearly related to the carrier state and not to a previous HBV infection. The age distribution of HBV infections, which occurs at early ages in this population of the Taiwanese, indicated that the tumors appear after a mean duration of 35 years of HBV infection. Between 60% and 90% of the HCC patients also had cirrhosis.

These epidemiologic data do not preclude a role for other factors in the HCC. In fact, factors such as aflatoxin have been recognized as having a role in some cases of liver cancer. Also, chronic hepatitis due to hepatitis C virus (HCV), an RNA virus with similarities to flaviviruses, has been strongly implicated in some cases of HBV negative HCC.

What is the functional role of HBV in HCC? In general, the only HBV DNA sequences in HCC are integrated into the host cellular DNA. Different tumors display different patterns of integration, indicating that the insertion of the viral DNA into the host chromosome is not site specific. In a given tumor, all cells have the same pattern of HBV DNA integration, indicating that the integration event necessarily precedes the clonal expansion of the tumor supporting an etiologic role of HBV in HCC. The integrated viral genomes of HBV are usually highly rearranged within tumors with a variety of deletions, inversions, and point mutations. Although occasional integrated genomes do retain one or more viral genes intact, no gene is consistently preserved intact.

What is the role of HBV DNA in HCC? There is no compelling evidence that HBV encodes a transforming protein. The viral X protein is a transcriptional activator and it is possible that alteration of its structure or regulation contributes directly to growth deregulation. Transgenic mice, which overexpress the HBV X protein, develop liver tumors.[71] The role of the HBV gene product in tumorigenesis in these mice may be indirect, however, because it may also be HBV-transgenic mice that overexpress the large surface antigen of HBV that develop liver tumors.[72] In this case, it seems that the role of HBV is indirect by provoking an immune-mediated liver injury and triggering hepatocellular regeneration. Such regeneration expands the pool of cells at risk for additional genetic lesions. Those cells with the appropriate genetic mutations could then undergo clonal expansion and ultimately progression to HCC. Mechanisms by which HBV DNA integration could directly contribute to tumorigenesis would be protooncogene activation by insertion of the viral DNA or the inactivation of tumor suppressor alleles by such integration. There is evidence for insertional activation in WHV-induced hepatomas, in which about 20% of the tumors show WHV DNA inserted into an N-MYC locus. An extensive search for comparable events in HBV-associated human HCC has turned up only rare examples.[73,74] Direct and indirect roles of HBV in hepatocellular carcinogenesis, as discussed here, could contribute. HCC is probably the result of multiple steps in carcinogenesis.

PAPILLOMAVIRUSES

The viral nature of human warts was first demonstrated at the turn of the century by transmission using a cell-free filtrate.[75] This important group of viruses has remained refractory to standard virologic studies, however, because none of the papillomavirus has been successfully propagated in the laboratory in tissue culture. There has been a virtual explosion in our knowledge of the papillomaviruses during the past decade as a result of advances in basic research.

BIOLOGY OF AN HPV INFECTION

The papillomaviruses are found in many higher vertebrate species ranging from birds to man. Although originally classified as papovaviruses because of their icosahedral shape and circular, double-stranded DNA genome, the papillomaviruses are now recognized as distinct from papovaviruses such as polyoma and SV40 based on different biologic and genetic characteristics. The papillomaviruses contain a double-stranded circular DNA genome of 8000 bp that is larger than the polyomaviruses (5000 bp), and the virion particles have

TABLE 10–2. Human Papillomaviruses and Their Clinical Associations

HPV Type	Location	Isolated From	Associated With
1	Cutaneous	Verruca plantaris	Verruca plantaris
2	Cutaneous	Verruca vulgaris	Verruca vulgaris; verruca plantaris
3	Cutaneous	Verruca plana	Verruca plana
4	Cutaneous	Verruca vulgaris	Verruca vulgaris; verruca
5	Cutaneous	Pityriasis versicolor-like macular lesions of EV	EV (benign lesions and squamous cell carcinoma)
6	Genital mucosa	Condyloma acuminatum	Condyloma acuminata Laryngeal papilloma Buschke-Löwenstein tumor
7	Cutaneous	Butchers' wart	Butchers' wart
8	Cutaneous	Macular lesions (EV, cell carcinomas)	EV (benign and squamous)
9	Cutaneous	EV lesions	EV (benign)
10	Cutaneous	Verruca plana	Verruca plana
11	Genital mucosa	Laryngeal papilloma	Condyloma acuminata Laryngeal papilloma
12	Cutaneous	Macular lesions (EV)	EV (benign)
13	Oral mucosa	FEH	Focal epithelial hyperplasia
14	Cutaneous	Flat warts (EV)	EV (Benign) EV (squamous cell carcinoma)
15	Cutaneous	Flat warts (EV)	EV (benign)
16	Genital mucosa	Cervical carcinoma	CIN; cervical cancer
17	Cutaneous	Macular lesions (EV)	EV (benign lesions and squamous cell carcinoma)
18	Genital mucosa	Cervical carcinoma	CIN Cervical carcinoma
19	Cutaneous	Macular lesions (EV)	EV (benign)
20	Cutaneous	Flat warts (EV)	EV (benign) EV (squamous cell carcinoma)
21	Cutaneous	Flat warts (EV)	EV (benign)
22	Cutaneous	Macular lesions (EV)	EV (benign)
23	Cutaneous	Macular lesions (EV)	EV (benign)
24	Cutaneous	Macular lesions (EV)	EV (benign)
25	Cutaneous	Macular lesions (EV)	EV (benign)
26	Cutaneous	Verruca vulgaris (immunosuppressed patient)	
27	Cutaneous	Verruca (immunosuppressed patient)	
28	Cutaneous	Verruca plana	
29	Cutaneous	Verruca vulgaris	
30	Genital and oral mucosa	Laryngeal carcinoma	CIN
31	Genital mucosa	CIN	CIN Cervical carcinoma
32	Oral mucosa	FEH	FEH Oral papilloma

(continued)

TABLE 10–2. *(Continued)*

HPV Type	Location	Isolated From	Associated With
33	Genital mucosa	Cervical carcinoma	CIN
			Cervical carcinoma
34	Genital mucosa (cutaneous)	Bowen's disease (cutaneous)	CIN (genital)
35	Genital mucosa	Cervical adenocarcinoma	CIN
			Cervical carcinoma
36	Cutaneous	Actinic keratosis	EV (benign)
37	Cutaneous	Keratoacanthoma	
38	Cutaneous	Malignant melanoma	
39	Genital mucosa	PIN	CIN
			Cervical carcinoma
40	Genital mucosa	PIN	CIN
41	Cutaneous	Disseminated warts	Cutaneous squamous cell carcinoma
42	Genital mucosa	Vulvar papilloma	CIN
43	Genital mucosa	Vulvar hyperplasia	CIN (normal cervical mucosa)
44	Genital mucosa	Vulvar condyloma	CIN (normal cervical mucosa)
45	Genital mucosa	CIN	CIN
			Cervical carcinoma
46	Cutaneous	Macular lesions (Hodgkin's disease patient)	EV (benign)
47	Cutaneous	Macular and verrucae lesions (EV)	EV (benign)
48	Cutaneous	Squmous cell carcinoma (transplant patient)	
49	Cutaneous	Verruca plana (immunosuppressed patient)	
50	Cutaneous	EV (benign)	
51	Genital mucosa	CIN	CIN
			Cervical carcinoma
52	Genital mucosa	CIN	CIN
			Cervical carcinoma
53	Genital mucosa	Normal cervical mucosa	
54	Genital mucosa	Condyloma acuminatum	
55	Genital mucosa	Bowenoid papulosis	
56	Genital mucosa (malignant and potential)	CIN	CIN
		Cervical carcinoma	
57	Oral and genital mucosa (cutaneous)	Inverted papilloma of the maxillary sinus	CIN
			Verruca vulgaris
58	Genital mucosa	CIN	
59	Genital mucosa	Vulvar intraepithelial neoplasia	
60	Cutaneous	Epidermoid cyst	

CIN, cervical intraepithelial neoplasia; EV, epidermodysplasia verruciformis; FEH, focal epithelial hyperplasia; PIN, penile intraepithelial neoplasia.
(Modified from DeVilliers E-M. Heterogeneity of the human papillomavirus group. J Virol 1989;63: 4898–4903)

a correspondingly larger capsid diameter (55 nm versus 40 nm). The papillomaviruses have not been propagated in tissue culture under standard conditions. The development of a permissive cell culture system for papillomavirus replication would be a major advance in the study of the biology of this virus.

More than 65 types of HPVs have been characterized, and new types are being recognized on a regular basis.[76] Unlike some human viruses such as adenoviruses, it has not been possible to type the papillomaviruses by serologic methods because antisera that can distinguish between the different HPV types are not available. As a consequence, the viruses have been typed by DNA hybridization under controlled conditions of stringency. Viruses differing by more than 50% DNA homology when assayed under stringent conditions are considered as different types.[76] Some of the HPVs and the clinical syndromes with which they are associated are presented in Table 10–2.

The productive functions of the papillomavirus, including vegetative viral DNA synthesis and the expression of late viral genes, occur only in the fully differentiated squamous epithelial cells of a papilloma. Vegetative viral DNA synthesis has been detected by in situ hybridization techniques only in the squamous epithelial cells of the stratum spinosum and of the granular layer of the epidermis, but not in the basal layer nor in the underlying dermal fibroblasts. Viral capsid protein production and virus assembly occur in the upper stratum spinosum and in the granular layer in which the epithelial cells are terminally differentiated. It is generally believed that the viral genome is present in the epithelial cells of the basal layer and that the expression of specific viral genes in the basal layer and in the lower layers of the epidermis is responsible for the cellular proliferation that is one characteristic of a wart. As the cells of the epidermis migrate upward through the stratum spinosum into the granular layer, they undergo a program of differentiation. The control of papillomavirus late gene expression is tightly linked to the differentiation state of the squamous epithelial cells.[77] The basis for this transcriptional control is not known.

Papillomaviruses have a specific tropism for squamous epithelial cells and HPV types have specificity for different anatomic sites. HPV-1, which is associated with plantar warts, has only been observed to replicate in heavily keratinized epithelium such as the palm or the sole, whereas HPV-16 has a preference for mucosal squamous epithelium. HPV-1 does not replicate in cervical epithelium and HPV-16 is generally not observed in the skin of the hand or foot. Specialized keratinocytes from different anatomic sites may have distinct differentiation patterns, evident from the types of keratin proteins they synthesize and from the pattern of synthesis of other epithelial specific proteins such as involucrin. The ability of HPVs to proliferate at a particular anatomic site may therefore reflect a specific interaction between viral and cellular gene regulatory factors involved in transcription.

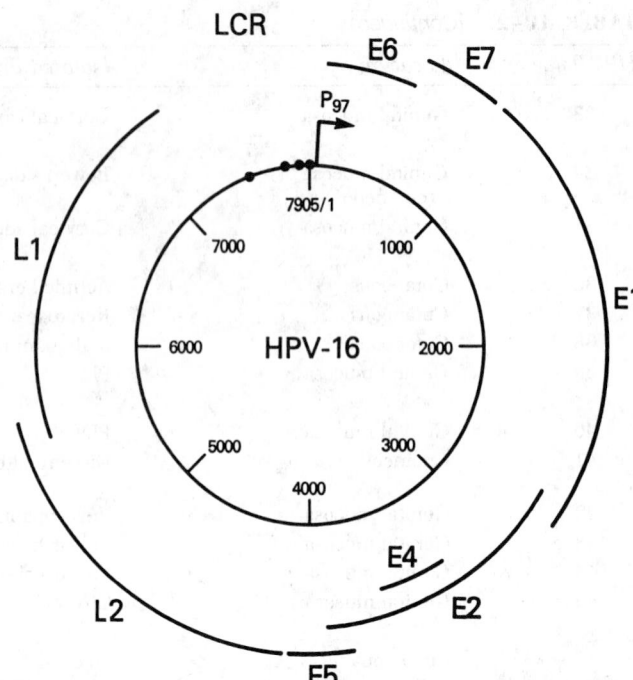

FIGURE 10–4.   The genomic map of human papillomavirus type 16 (HPV-16) deduced from the DNA sequence. The nucleotide numbers are noted within the circular maps. Transcription proceeds clockwise, and the major open reading frames are E1 to E7, L1, and L2. The only transcriptional promoter mapped to data for HPV-16 is designated P_{97}. A_E and A_L represent the putative polyadenylation signals for the early and late transcripts, respectively. The viral long control region (LCR) contains the putative viral transcriptional and replication regulatory elements. The closed circles on the genome represent the four E2 binding sites noted in the LCR. (Romanczuk H, Howley PM. Disruption of either the E1 or the E2 regulatory gene of human papillomavirus type 16 increases viral immortalization capacity. Proc Natl Acad Sci USA 1992;81:3160)

HPV GENOMIC ORGANIZATION

All HPV types examined to date have a similar genomic organization. The DNA genomes of each of the HPVs sequenced and the other animal papillomaviruses contain about 8000 bp of genetic information. All of the open reading frames (ORFs) that could serve to encode proteins for these viruses are located on only one of the two viral DNA strands. RNA studies have indicated that only one strand is transcribed.

The HPV genome can be divided into two distinct regions: an *early region* that encodes the viral proteins involved in viral DNA replication, transcriptional regulation, and cellular transformation, and a *late region* that encodes the viral capsid proteins. This functional division is largely based on genetic studies done with the bovine papillomavirus.[78] The organization of a typical HPV-16 is shown in Figure 10–4. The genes in the early region are designated *E1, E2,* and so forth, whereas the genes in the late region are designated *L1* and *L2.* From studies with the HPVs, it is likely that E4 encodes a so-called *late gene* that is expressed only in productively infected keratinocytes.[79] Although this ORF is located with the early ORFs, its function may be important only in the vegetative replication of the virus.

In productively infected tissue (*i.e.,* tissues in which viral particles are made such as warts), mRNA is transcribed from both the early and late regions of the genome.[80,81] Nonpro-

ductive infection of host cells (as seen in the lower cells of the epithelium in a wart) is accompanied by mRNA being transcribed from only the early region of the genome.[82] The restricted expression of the genome to only the early region involves regulation of transcription at the levels of the initiation of RNA synthesis, RNA stability, and transcriptional termination.[77]

The functional analysis of the molecular biology of papillomaviruses has been most extensively studied for the bovine papillomavirus (BPV-1), which is capable of transforming a variety of rodent fibroblast cell lines in tissue culture.[83–85] In these transformed cells, the DNA remains as a stable extrachromosomal plasmid and this system has served as an excellent model for studying latent infection by papillomavirus.[86] This virus has served as the prototype for unraveling aspects of the biology of the papillomaviruses over the past decade. Two independent transforming activities have been mapped in BPV-1 to the *E5* gene and to the *E6* gene.[87] The *E2* gene of BPV-1 encodes factors that are involved in the regulation of a conditional transcriptional enhancer located in the virally control region, LCR.[88,89] Mutations in the *E2* gene result in a decreased transformation efficiency of the BPV-1 and affect DNA replication.[90–92] The effect on transformation is indirect through the requirement for transcriptional activity of the viral genes that are directly required for transformation (*E5* and *E6*).

E2 has a direct role in viral DNA replication.[93] The *E2* genes of other papillomaviruses have also been shown to encode transcriptional regulatory functions.[94,95] In the bovine papillomavirus, the *E1* gene encodes a protein necessary for extrachromosomal replication in transformed cells.[96,97] In the BPV system, the *E7* gene has been reported to have a role in maintaining the high copy of plasmid DNA in transformed cells.[98] No function has been found for the *E3* ORF of BPV-1. The *E8* ORF may also be involved in plasmid replication. The *L1* ORF of the papillomaviruses encodes the major caption protein and the *L2* ORF encodes a minor caption protein.[99,100] The *L1* and *L2* ORFs are only expressed in the terminally differentiated keratinocytes.[77,80]

Although initial studies with the papillomaviruses on transformation focused on the BPV-1 because it was so effective at transforming rodent cells in tissue culture, recent studies have focused more on HPV-16 and HPV-18, which are associated with human cervical cancer. Although the genomic organization of the human papillomaviruses is similar to that of BPV-1, there appear to be important differences in the mechanisms by which they transform cells. The principal transforming genes for the cancer-associated HPVs have been mapped to *E6* and *E7*. *E7* is by itself sufficient for the transformation of primary rodent cells.[101-103] *E7* is also capable of cooperating with an activated *RAS* oncogene to transform primary rodent cells.[102] Expression of *E6* and *E7* together is sufficient for the efficient immortalization of primary human cells, most notably primary human keratinocytes, which are the normal host cells for the human papillomaviruses.[104,105]

PAPILLOMAVIRUSES IN CANCER

Only a subgroup of the papillomaviruses are associated with lesions that may progress to cancer (Table 10–3). The Shope papillomavirus (abbreviated as CRPV because it infects cottontail rabbits) was first identified by Shope as the etiologic agent of cutaneous papillomatosis in rabbits.[4] CRPV has been extensively studied as a model for papillomavirus-induced carcinogenesis.[5,106] One of the features of carcinogenic progression with the papillomaviruses is the synergy between the virus and carcinogenic external factors (see Table 10–3). In

CRPV, carcinomas develop at an increased frequency in virus-induced papillomas that are painted with cool tar or methylcholanthrene.[107,108] These CRPV-associated carcinomas contain copies of the viral DNA that are transcriptionally active, which supports the hypothesis that these viruses play an active role in the cancers that develop.[109,110]

In cattle, BPV-4 has been associated with esophageal papillomatosis and squamous cell carcinomas of the upper alimentary tract.[111,112] Interestingly, only those cattle from the highlands of Scotland that are infected with BPV-4 and feed on bracken fern (which contains a radiomimetic substance) have a high incidence of squamous cell carcinomas of the esophagus and foregut.[111] In contrast to the CRPV-associated carcinomas in which the viral DNA can invariably be found, extensive analysis of the squamous cell carcinomas of the upper alimentary tract in these cattle infected with BPV-4 has failed to reveal a consistent pattern of viral DNA sequences within the malignant tumors.[113] In these alimentary tract tumors, the continued presence of BPV-4 DNA sequences may not be required for the maintenance of the cancer.

EPIDERMODYSPLASIA VERRUCIFORMIS

Epidermodysplasia verruciformis (EV) is a rare lifelong disease in humans that usually begins in infancy or childhood. The disease is characterized by disseminated polymorphic cutaneous lesions that resemble flat warts and also as reddish macules sometimes referred to as *pityriasis-like lesions*.[114] About one third of patients with EV develop multiple skin cancers usually during the third or fourth decade of their lives. Papillomavirus particles have been detected within the benign lesions and not in the carcinomas. It has been proposed that EV is linked to a rare, recessive, abnormal allele of an X-linked gene. Patients with EV often have impaired cell-mediated immunity, which is believed to play a role in the lifelong infection by papillomaviruses. Of interest is that the carcinomas that develop in these patients arise in sun-exposed areas, and ultraviolet radiation may play a cocarcinogenic role with papillomaviruses in the cause of these cancers. EV is a rare disease, yet it has been under intense study by dermatologists and virologists. Over 15 different HPV types have been isolated from individual lesions in a small number of patients with this rare disease (see Table 10–2). The cuta-

TABLE 10–3. Papillomaviruses Associated With Lesions That May Progress To Cancer

Investigations	Papillomaviruses	Cancers	Other Factors
Rous et al[5,106]	CRPV (Shope)	Skin cancer	Methylcholanthrene
Jarrett et al[111]	Bovine (BPV-4)	Tongue, esophageal, foregut cancers	Bracken
Ford et al[225]	Bovine (not typed)	Ocular cancers	Ultraviolet light
Vanselow et al[226]	Ovine	Skin cancer	Ultraviolet light
Orth[115]	Human (HPV-5, -8 and others)	Skin cancer in patients with epidermodysplasia verruciformis	Ulraviolet light
Durst et al[147] Boshart et al[148] Beaudenon et al[150]	Human (HPV-16, -18, -31; high-risk HPVs)	Anogenital cancers, cancers	Smoking? herpes factors

neous carcinomas in patients with EV can be bowenoid carcinomas, in situ carcinomas, or invasive squamous cell carcinomas. Of the HPV types found in patients with EV only a subset of them is associated with a risk of malignant progression, most notably HPV-5 and HPV-8.

Extensive studies have been done by Gerard Orth from the Pasteur Institute in Paris and Stephonia Jablonska in Warsaw in analyzing the HPVs in cancers from patients with EV. They have investigated a total of 28 tumors from 14 patients. HPV genomes have been found in 27 of the 28 samples. Twenty-one of these contained HPV-5 DNA, five contained HPV-8 DNA, and one contained HPV-14 DNA.[115] HPV-5 has been found in metastatic squamous cell carcinoma lesions in some patients with EV.[116,117] Still other investigators have found additional HPVs in carcinomas in EV patients. HPV-3 has been found in an in situ vulvar carcinoma of an EV patient[118] and HPV-17 has been found in a cutaneous EV carcinoma by a group of Japanese investigators.[119] The specific association of carcinomas in patients with EV is not strictly limited to HPV-5 and HPV-8. Although metastasis is uncommon in the cancers in these patients, the presence of HPV-5 in the two metastatic lymph node lesions examined strengthens the argument for an etiologic role for HPV in these carcinomas.[115,116] Further studies have established that the viral genomes are transcriptionally active within these carcinomas[120] and that HPV-5 and HPV-8 encode transforming proteins.[121]

GENITIAL CARCINOMAS

The epidemiology of genital warts follows a pattern characteristic of a venereal-transmitted disease with a high prevalence in populations of women of high promiscuity.[122,123] There are two general types of genital wart virus infections that can be differentiated by their clinical appearance: condyloma acuminata and flat genital warts. Condyloma acuminata can be localized to the penis, the vulva, the perineum, the anus, and rarely the uterine cervix, and they are caused by papillomaviruses. Particles have been demonstrated by the electron microscope, and papillomavirus-specific antigens have been detected using antisera to a common papillomavirus antigen.[124–126] HPV-6 was directly cloned from a condyloma acuminata, and using its DNA and that of the closely related HPV-11, Harald zur Hausen and colleagues in Germany were able to demonstrate HPV DNA in over 90% of the lesions of condyloma acuminata examined.[127,128] Less frequently, other HPV types can be found in condyloma acuminata. Malignant conversion of condyloma acuminata into squamous cell carcinoma is uncommon. A lesion described by Buschke and Löwenstein as a *giant condyloma* has characteristics similar to that of a locally invasive squamous cell carcinoma.[129] These tumors have been associated with HPV-6 and HPV-11.[127,130] However, most cervical carcinomas and other genital tract carcinomas have been negative when examined for HPV-6 and HPV-11.

Compelling evidence linking an HPV infection with cervical carcinoma came from the recognition that the morphologic changes previously interpreted on pap smears and tissue sections of the cervix as cervical dysplasia were due to a papillomavirus infection.[131–133] The characteristic cell that is diagnostic for a cervical papillomavirus infection is the koilocyte.[134] Electron microscopy has demonstrated papillomavirus particles in koilocytotic cells, supporting the papillomavirus etiology.[135,136] Numerous studies have found papillomavirus specific capsid antigens and HPV DNA within cervical dysplastic cells, confirming the viral cause of cervical dysplasia.

Epidemiologic studies have implicated an infectious agent in the cause of human cervical carcinoma.[137,138] Venereal transmission of a carcinogenic factor with a long latency has been suggested by such studies. Sexual promiscuity, an early age of onset of sexual activity, and poor sexual hygienic conditions are known risk factors for cervical carcinoma. There is a correlation between the incidence rates of cervical cancer and penile carcinoma in different geographic areas, although the incidence rates for penile carcinoma are 20-fold lower when compared with those of cervical carcinoma. The similar ratio of incidence between cervical carcinoma and penile carcinoma is maintained in areas of high, medium, or low prevalence, suggesting that the etiologic factors for penile and cervical carcinoma may be the same. The male factor also appears to implicate a venereal transmitted agent. Women who are monogamous are at a higher risk for cervical carcinoma if their spouses have multiple sexual partners.

The possible involvement of an infectious agent in the cause of cervical carcinoma has prompted many studies evaluating genital pathogens as potential causative agents. Infections by *Trichomonas*, *Chlamydia*, and such bacteria as syphilis and gonorrhea have not been linked to cervical carcinoma. In the late 1960s and early 1970s, genital infection by herpes simplex virus (HSV) type 2 was considered as an etiologic candidate.[139,140] Support for the notion that HSV might be a cancer-associated virus came from studies demonstrating the ability of HSV to transform certain rodent cells in the laboratory in vitro and from serologic studies suggesting a higher frequency of antibodies to HSV-2 in patients with cervical carcinoma. Subsequent molecular studies attempting to demonstrate HSV RNA or HSV DNA in cervical cancer tissues could not provide convincing evidence for a role for HSV in cervical cancer.[141] A large prospective epidemiologic study by Vonka failed to support the involvement of HSV-1 of HSV-2 infections in cervical cancer.[142,143]

The association of an HPV with cervical dysplasia (also referred to as *cervical intraepithelial neoplasia* [CIN]) provided impetus for a close examination of cervical cancer for HPV sequences. The natural history linking CIN to carcinoma in situ and to invasive squamous cell carcinoma of the cervix had already been well established.[144–146] Initial experiments revealed HPV sequences in occasional cases of cervical carcinoma and of anogenital carcinoma, but no consistent pattern of positivity emerged. Using radioactively labeled HPV-11 DNA under conditions of hybridization of low stringency, zur Hausen and colleagues examined human cervical carcinoma DNAs related to HPV DNAs and identified two new papillomavirus DNAs: HPV-16 and HPV-18.[147,148] Using HPV-16 and HPV-18 DNAs as probes, these DNAs were demonstrated in about 70% of cervical carcinomas.[149] Low-stringency hybridization has led to the identification of about 20 different HPVs associated with genital tract lesions. HPV-31, HPV-33, HPV-39, HPV-42, and other HPVs are each associated with a small percentage of cervical carcinomas.[150,151] Specific HPVs are regularly found in human cervical carcinoma tissues and in other human genital carcinomas including penile, vulvar, and perianal carcinomas. The availability of HPV DNA probes has permitted the extensive analysis of specific clinical lesions. For instance, bowenoid papulosis of the penis is associated with HPV-16 and is the male counterpart of CIN in the female.[152,153] The human papillomaviruses associated with anogenital lesions can be classified as either high-risk or low-risk, based on whether the genital tract lesions with which these HPVs are associated are at significant risk for malignant progression. The low-risk viruses such as HPV-6 and HPV-11 are associated with venereal warts, and the high-risk viruses such as HPV-16 and HPV-18 are associated with CIN and cervical cancer. Other high-risk viruses are HPV-31, HPV-33, HPV-35, HPV-39, HPV-45, HPV-51, HPV-52, and HPV-56. It appears that about 80% to 90% of cervical carcinomas contain the DNA of a high-risk HPV.

Studies of cervical cancers and derived cell lines that are HPV positive indicate that the DNA is usually integrated, although there are cases in which DNA is apparently also extrachromosomal. If the DNA is integrated, the pattern of integration is clonal, indicating that the association of the HPV preceded the clonal outgrowth of the tumor. Integration of the viral DNA is not at specific sites in the host chromosome, although in some cell lines the integration event has occurred in the vicinity of known oncogenes. For instance, in the HeLa cells (an HPV-18-positive cervical carcinoma cell line), the integration of the viral genome has occurred within about 50 kb of the c-*MYC* locus on human chromosome 8.[154] It is not known whether such an integration event provides a selective advantage to the progression of a preneoplastic lesion to a cancer. It does seem plausible that in some cancers the integration of the viral DNA could result in genetic changes that might contribute to carcinogenic progression.

In HPV-positive cancers, there appears to be a selection for the integrity of the *E6–E7* coding region and the upstream regulatory region. Furthermore, the *E6* and *E7* genes are regularly expressed in HPV-positive cervical cancers.[154-156] Interestingly, integration of the viral genome into the host chromosome in the cancers is often associated with disruption of the viral *E1* or *E2* genes.[154,155] Like the bovine papillomavirus, the HPV *E2* gene encodes transcriptional regulatory factors.[94,95] Integration in a manner to disrupt expression of the *E2* ORF, therefore, could result in the derepression of the promoter upstream of *E6* and *E7* and lead to deregulated expression of the viral *E6* and *E7* genes. A recent study has confirmed that disruption of either the *E1* or the *E2* regulatory gene of HPV-16 increases the immortalization capacity of the viral genome.[157]

An emerging theme among DNA tumor viruses (including the HPVs) is that the transformation properties of the proteins encoded by these viruses may be due in part to their interaction with critical cellular regulatory proteins (Fig. 10–5). The *E7* proteins encoded by the high-risk HPVs share sequence similarity to adenovirus E1A. This sequence similarity can also be extended to SV40 large T antigen and involves regions in all three proteins that are critical for the transformation properties of these oncoproteins. The regions of amino acid sequence similarity between *E7* and adenovirus E1A that are shared with SV40 large T antigen are regions that have been shown to participate in the binding of important cellular regulatory proteins, including the product of the retinoblastoma tumor suppressor gene, p*RB*.[158-161]

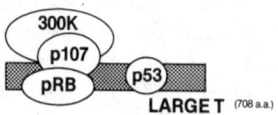

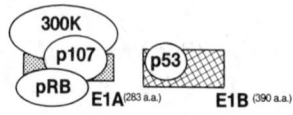

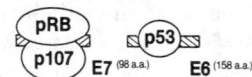

FIGURE 10–5. The transforming proteins encoded by three distinct groups of DNA tumor viruses target similar cellular proteins. The tumor suppressor gene products pRB and p53 are described in the text. The 300K and p107 proteins are cellular proteins that have also been shown to interact with the indicated viral oncoproteins. The binding of HPV E6 oncoproteins to p53 is mediated by the cellular protein E6-AP.[224] (Modified from Werness BA, Levine AJ, Howley PM: Association of human papillomavirus types 16 and 18 E6 proteins with p53. Science 1990;248:76)

The transforming properties of the *E6* protein were first revealed by studies using primary human cells, most importantly, primary human squamous epithelial cells.[104,105] The efficient immortalization of primary human cells requires both the *E6* and *E7* genes of the high-risk HPVs.[104,105,162] The ability of the *E6* and *E7* proteins together to efficiently immortalize primary human keratinocytes is a characteristic of the high-risk HPVs, but not of the low-risk HPVs.[163,164] Like SV40 large T antigen and the 55-kd protein encoded by adenovirus E1B, the *E6* proteins of the high-risk HPVs can enter into a complex with p53, a cellular protein with tumor suppressor activity, and can promote the degradation of p53 in vitro.[165,166] The functional inactivation of p53 and pRB through their interactions with *E6* and *E7*, respectively, appear to be important events in cervical carcinogenesis. Analysis of human cervical carcinoma cell lines has revealed that the p53 and pRB genes are intact and expressed in those cervical carcinoma cell lines that are HPV positive. In contrast, mutations were identified in both the p53 and pRB genes in two HPV-negative cervical carcinoma cell lines. These results support the notion that inactivation of the normal functions of the tumor suppressor proteins, pRB and p53, is an important step in human cervical carcinogenesis, either by mutation (as in HPV-negative cancers) or from complex formation with the HPV oncoproteins in HPV-positive cell lines.[167]

HPV infections by themselves are not sufficient for carcinogenic progression. Only a small fraction of those individuals who are infected by a specific HPV eventually develop cervical carcinoma. The genetic information carried by the virus is not sufficient for malignant progression and other factors must be involved in the progression of viral-associated lesions to genital tract cancers. Papillomavirus infections may work synergistically with these other factors. Epidemiologic studies have suggested that smoking is a risk factor for developing cervical carcinoma.[168-170] It has been suggested that the tobacco condensate in women who smoke accumulates in the vaginal fluids, bathing the cervix and acting as a cofactor with the papillomavirus infection.[171] It also has been postulated that herpes virus infection acts synergistically with specific papillomaviruses to induce human cervical carcinoma.[172]

OTHER HUMAN CANCERS ASSOCIATED WITH PAPILLOMAVIRUSES

The availability of specific HPV DNA probes has provided investigators with the opportunity to carry out extensive screenings of various human cancers for HPV sequences. Based on animal models, it seemed that carcinomas of any squamous epithelium or of an epithelium that can undergo squamous metaplasia could be associated with an HPV. Studies examining oral carcinomas and upper airway carcinomas have revealed some HPV-positive carcinomas.[173-175] HPV DNA has been found in benign oral papillomas,[176-179] and oral focal epithelial hyperplasia has been firmly established as having a papillomavirus cause.[180,181] In addition, papillomavirus DNA sequences have been found to be associated with some cases of oral leukoplakia.[177,182] HPV-16 sequences have been described in a verrucous carcinoma of the larynx. HPV-11 has been found in a squamous cell carcinoma of the lung arising in a young adult with a history of laryngotracheobronchial papillomatosis.[183] In this patient, HPV-11 DNA was also found within metastatic lesions in the liver and lymph nodes. The viral genome was transcriptionally active, suggesting that expression of the virus played an active role in the carcinogenic progression. Esophageal carcinomas in humans have not been convincingly shown to be associated with an HPV. The esophagus is lined by a squamous epithelium, and squamous cell papillomas of the esophagus have been described in humans.[184,185] Additional studies are warranted to investigate a possible role of HPV in human esophageal cancers.

EPSTEIN-BARR VIRUS

The Epstein-Barr virus (EBV) was the first human tumor virus to be recognized as such. It was discovered during studies of lymphoma in young children in certain parts of East Africa and was first described by Dennis Burkitt in 1958.[186] Although this childhood lymphoma had been previously recognized, it had not been defined as a unique entity with characteristic clinical, pathologic, and epidemiologic features until the studies of Burkitt.[186,187] In these early descriptive studies, Burkitt suggested that the lymphoma could be due to a virus because its geographic distribution was similar to that of yellow fever in a belt across equatorial Africa. In 1964, Epstein and Barr described virus particles of the herpesvirus family in lymphoblastoid lines cultured from explants of Burkitt's lymphoma (BL).[188,189] The finding of such virus particles in lymphoid lines was not limited to explants of BL tissue, however. They could also be seen in cell lines established from patients with other malignancies, from patients with infectious mononucleosis and, occasionally, from normal individuals.

EBV is a double-stranded DNA virus belonging to the herpesvirus family. Other members of the human herpesvirus family include herpes simplex viruses types 1 and 2, varicella zoster virus, the cytomegalovirus, and the more recently described human herpes virus type 6. Morphologically, the mature virus is essentially indistinguishable from the other members of the herpes family. These are large viruses of 150 to 180 nm in diameter with a large double-stranded DNA genome of about 170,000 bp. In addition to its central core of genetic material, the virus particle is also composed of a capsid layer made up of capsomeres in an icosahedral shape and an outer lipoprotein envelope. Because of its tropism for lymphoid cells in vivo and in vitro, EBV is considered a member of the γ herpesviruses. Individual members of this group are specific for either B or T lymphocytes and include Marek's disease virus of chickens and two viruses that infect New World monkeys: herpes ateles and herpes saimiri.

EBV VIRAL GENOME

As noted above, the genome is a double-stranded DNA molecule of about 170,000 bp.[190] The organization is complex with regions of repeated DNA sequences and multiple tandem copies (6 to 12) of a 500 base pair terminal repeat unit at the end of the linear genome. If the cell nucleus is in the latent state, the genome exists in a circular form. Its ability to circularize may involve homologous recombination through these terminal repeated DNA sequences. The EBV genome has been sequenced in its entirety, and the availability of this DNA sequence information has permitted the identification of ORFs and genes for subsequent genetic and molecular studies.[191]

EBV ANTIGENS

Many antigens have been identified in EBV-infected and EBV-transformed cells using immunologic means. The viral capsid antigens (VCA) are detected in cells producing EBV particles, as are the membrane antigens (MA).[192] These are late antigens because their expression occurs after the onset of vegetative viral DNA synthesis in the life cycle of the virus. The MA antigens are responsible for eliciting virus-neutralizing antibody.[193] The EBV-induced early antigens (EA) are synthesized early, before the onset of DNA replication in the virus replication cycle. This group of antigens can be subdivided into the diffuse (D) and restricted (R) components based on the distribution of the antigens and the sensitivity of the patterns to fixation.[194]

All cells that harbor and express the EBV genome in a latent state express a viral antigen complex in the nucleus, which is referred to as the EBV-induced nuclear antigen (EBNA).[195] This antigen serves as an excellent immunologic marker for the presence of the viral DNA and is expressed in virtually every cell containing the viral genome. EBNA consists of a group of at least 6 different EBV encoded proteins. The individual EBNA gene products and the genes that encode them have been identified using different methods including the generation of antisera to specific proteins encoded by specific genes. Two of these genes, *EBNA2* and *LMP,* have proven to be particularly important with regard to viral latency and the immortalization of human lymphocytes by EBV. *EBNA1* is a DNA-binding protein that binds to a specific portion of the

EBV genome called *ORIP* to permit latent replication of the viral DNA.[196] *EBNA2* is an acidic protein that can serve as a transcriptional transactivator of both viral and cellular genes. Viral proteins whose expression can be increased by *EBNA2* include the latent membrane protein (LMP)[197,198] and terminal protein, which is expressed in latently infected cells.[199] Cellular proteins that can be activated by *EBNA2* include the B-cell activation antigens, CD21, CD23, and the protooncogene c-*FGR*.[200–202]

Other EBV proteins expressed in latently infected cells include the *EBNA3-A*, *EBNA3-B*, and *EBNA3-C* proteins. These proteins are found in the nuclear matrix, chromatin, and nucleoplasmic fractions, but their functions are unknown. The *EBNA-LP* is encoded in a leader segment for each of the *EBNA* mRNAs and is translated from some of these mRNAs; it is referred to as the *leader protein*. The function of this protein is not known. Several latent membrane proteins (LMPs) are encoded by the virus. The expression of LMP is itself activated by *EBNA2*. Along with *EBNA2*, *LMP* (previously referred to as *BNLF1*) is required for immortalization of B lymphocytes. LMP has been shown to alter the effect of the growth properties of rodent cells, epithelial cells, and B lymphocytes. *LMP* is a membrane protein that is predicted based on its amino acid structure to span the plasma membrane six times with both the amino terminus and carboxy terminus located in the cytoplasm. The function of *LMP* is not known, although, based on its amino acid sequence, it has transport properties that resemble those of the multiple drug resistance gene.

The role of specific EBV genes in EBV-associated malignancies is not clear. Immortalization genes have been mapped to *EBNA2* and *LMP*, and these two genes are presumed to play a direct role in inducing cellular immortalization in B lymphocytes as an early event in leukemogenesis. The role of other genes in this process cannot be ruled out because genetic studies on the immortalizing and transforming functions of EBV have been limited.

BURKITT'S LYMPHOMA

Burkitt's lymphoma occurs several years after the primary infection with EBV. Burkitt's lymphoma is a monoclonal lymphoma, as opposed to infectious mononucleosis, which is a polyclonal disease.[203] African Burkitt's lymphoma is characterized by rapid growth of the tumor at nonlymphoid sites such as the jaw or the retroperitoneum. The tumor is of B-cell origin and is closely related to the small noncleaved cells of normal lymphoid follicles.[204] The biopsy specimens from African Burkitt's lymphoma invariably contain the EBV genome and are positive for EBNA.[205] This contrasts with the non-African Burkitt's lymphoma, in which only 15% to 20% of the tumors contain the EBV genome. EBV has a worldwide distribution and infects most (more than 90%) individuals before adulthood. The clustering of Burkitt's lymphoma in the equatorial belt of East Africa remains unexplained. It has been hypothesized that alterations of the immune system, possibly due to hyperstimulation by endemic malaria, may play an important role in the outcome of an EBV infection to individuals in this region.[206,207] Individuals from this region show impairment of virus-specific cytotoxic T-cell activity. Normally, it is the T-cell response to EBV infection that limits

B-cell proliferation and is directly stimulated by EBV.[208] It has been postulated that the failure of the T-cell immune response to control this proliferation could lead to excessive B-cell proliferation and, as such, provide a suitable background for further mutation, oncogenic transformation, and lymphomagenesis. Burkitt's lymphomas regularly contain abnormalities of those chromosomes that contain the immunoglobulin genes, most notably chromosomes 2, 14, and 22. The most common abnormality observed in more than 90% of Burkitt's lymphoma is a translocation of the long arm of chromosome 14 containing the heavy-chain immunoglobulin genes to chromosome 8, which in turn contains the c-*MYC* oncogene.[209] Less frequent translocations involve chromosome 2 (κ light chain) and chromosome 22 (λ light chain).[210] These translocations generally involve reciprocal translocations to the distal arm of chromosome 8 (band 884), containing the c-*MYC* protooncogene.[211] Burkitt's lymphomas are believed to have abnormal expression of the c-*MYC* oncogene after this translocation, and it is believed that this abnormal expression is a result of the proximity of the c-*MYC* oncogene to the transcriptional control elements of the immunoglobulin genes.[211,212]

The chromosomal abnormalities noted above are not detected in the peripheral blood lymphocytes of Burkitt's lymphoma patients nor are they found in nonmalignant lymphoblastoid cell lines that can be derived from such patients. The translocation appears to be specific for Burkitt's lymphoma and would appear to occur at a step after the immortalization by EBV. In 1979, George Klein suggested a scenario for the involvement of EBV in the cause of African Burkitt's lymphoma.[213] The first step involves the EBV-induced immortalization of B lymphocytes in a primary infection. The second step involves the stimulated proliferation of EBV-positive B cells. This step is facilitated in the geographic areas where Burkitt's lymphoma is endemic (presumably because of the presence of malaria), through B-cell triggering and the suppression of T cells involved in the control of the proliferation of EBV-infected cells. This pool of cells becomes increased in size as a target cell population for random chromosomal rearrangements. The third and final step is the reciprocal translocation involving a chromosomal locus with an immunoglobulin gene and the c-*MYC* gene on chromosome 8. This leads to the deregulation of the c-*MYC* gene, to the development of the malignant clone, and to the appearance of a tumor mass.[214] Alternative scenarios have been proposed in which the order of the steps are rearranged such that the B-cell activation by malaria precedes the chromosomal translocation and is followed by EBV infection.[215] Regardless, the components of these two scenarios each account for the geographic distribution of Burkitt's lymphoma, the critical involvement of EBV in lymphomagenesis, and the eventual selection and clonal outgrowth of a population of cells with the critical translocation involving the deregulation of the c-*MYC* gene on chromosome 8.

NASOPHARYNGEAL CARCINOMA

Nasopharyngeal carcinoma (NPC) has also been linked to EBV.[216] NPC occurs in adults from ages 20 to 50, although in certain parts of Africa the age distribution extends to children as well. In general, males outnumber females 2 to 1. Although worldwide the annual incidence rates are low, there are areas in China (especially the southern province) in which there is a high rate of about 10 cases per 100,000 persons per year. Because the incidence among individuals of Chinese descent remains high, irrespective of where they live, a genetic susceptibility has been proposed. For the Cantonese in Singapore, the annual rates of 29 per 100,000 are higher than for other racial groups living in the same locale. A correlation of certain HLA haplotypes has been noted among the Chinese, but these associations do not hold true for evaluation of NPC in Tunisia. Environmental factors have been implicated as risk factors for NPC, including fumes, chemicals, smoke, and ingestion of salt-cured fish.

EBV genomes are found in nearly all biopsies of undifferentiated NPC specimens from all over the world.[217,218] The genome exists in the epithelial cells of the tumors.[219] The EBV genome is transcriptionally active within these tumors, and the regions transcribed in the NPC biopsies are the same as those expressed in latently infected lymphocytes.[220] These molecular observations are consistent with an active role for EBV in the neoplastic processes involved in NPC. Patients with NPC have elevated levels of IgG antibodies to EBV capsid and early antigens. Furthermore, they have serum IgA antibodies to capsid and early antigen, most likely reflecting the local production of such antibodies in the nasopharynx. No characteristic chromosomal translocations have been found in NPCs. Attempts to identify mutated or activated cellular oncogenes in NPC also have not been successful.

The presence of immunoglobulin markers for EBV (IgA/VCA and IgA/EA) has provided the opportunity for early serologic identification of patients with NPC. The frequency of IgA antibody to the EBV capsid antigen of 150,000 Chinese studied was found to be 1%. About 20% of the patients with elevated IgA antibodies to VCA had NPC when biopsied. Early detection using serologic tests can be applied in areas where NPC is prevalent, possibly leading to early therapeutic intervention.[221]

LYMPHOMA IN IMMUNODEFICIENT INDIVIDUALS

EBV is associated with lymphomas in patients with acquired or congenital immunodeficiencies. These lymphomas can be distinguished from the classical Burkitt's lymphomas in that the tumors are often polyclonal. The tumors also do not demonstrate the characteristic chromosomal abnormalities of Burkitt's lymphoma described earlier. The pathogenesis of these lymphomas involves a deficiency in the affector mechanisms needed to control EBV-transformed cells. The prototypic model for this disease has been the X-linked lymphoproliferative (XLP) syndrome.[222] Patients with XLP who develop acute infectious mononucleosis exhibit the usual atypical lymphocytosis and polyclonal elevation of serum immunoglobulins and increases in specific antibody to VCA and to EA. During these infections, patients with XLP fail to mount and sustain an anti-EBNA response after acute infection. The unique vulnerability of males with XLP to EBV infection is most likely due to an inherited immune regulatory defect that results in the failure to govern the cytotoxic T cells and NK cells required to cope with EBV.

Patients with iatrogenic immunodeficiencies, such as organ transplant recipients, are at an increased risk for lymphomas, and these lymphomas often contain EBV DNA and EBNA. Also, patients with AIDS are at a higher risk for developing polyclonal lymphomas associated with EBV.

REFERENCES

1. Ellermann V, Bang O. Experimentelle leukamie bei huhnern. Zentralbl Bakteriol Abt I 1908;46:595–609.
2. Rous P. A sarcoma of the fowl transmissible by an agent separable from the tumor cells. J Exp Med 1911;13:397–411.
3. Shope RE. A filtrable virus causing a tumor-like condition in rabbits and its relationship to virus myxomatosum. J Exp Med 1932;56:803–822.
4. Shope RE. Infectious papillomatosis of rabbits. J Exp Med 1933;58:607–629.
5. Rous P, Beard JW. The progression to carcinoma of virus-induced rabbit papillomas (Shope). J Exp Med 1935;62:523–548.
6. Gross L. Pathogenic properties, and "vertical" transmission of the mouse leukemia agent. Proc Soc Exp Biol Med 1951;62:523–548.
7. Gross L. A filtrable agent, recovered from Akr leukemia extracts, causing salivary gland carcinomas in C3H mice. Proc Soc Exp Biol Med 1953;83:414–421.
8. Steward SE. Leukemia in mice produced by a filterable agent present in AKR leukemic tissues with notes on a sarcoma produced by the same agent. Anat Rev 1953;117:532.
9. Jarrett WFH, Martin WB, Crighton GW, et al. Transmission experiments with leukemia (lymphosarcoma). Nature 1964;202:566–567.
10. Bernard W. The detection and study of tumor viruses with electron microscopy. Cancer Res 1960;20:712–727.
11. Temin HM, Mizutani S. RNA-dependent DNA polymerase in virions of Rous sarcoma virus. Nature 1970;226:1211–1212.
12. Baltimore D. RNA-dependent DNA polymerase in virions of RNA tumor viruses. Nature 1970;276:1209–1211.
13. Poiesz BJ, Ruscetti FW, Gazdar AF, et al. Detection and isolation of type C retrovirus particles from fresh and cultured lymphocytes of a patient with cutaneous T-cell lymphoma. Proc Natl Acad Sci USA 1980;77:7415–7419.
14. Poiesz BJ, Ruscetti FW, Reitz MS, et al. Isolation of a new type C retrovirus (HTLV) in primary uncultured cells of a patient with Sézary T-cell leukemia. Nature 1981;294:268–271.
15. Yoshida M, Miyoshi I, Hinuma Y. Isolation and characterization of retrovirus from cell lines of human adult T-cell leukemia and its implication in disease. Anat Rev 1953;117:532.
16. Uchiyama T, Yodoi J, Sagawa K, et al. Adult T-cell leukemia-clinical and hematological features of 16 cases. Blood 1977;50:481–492.
17. Hattori T, Uchiyama T, Tibana K, et al. Surface phenotype of Japanese adult T-cell leukemia cells characterized by monoclonal antibodies. Blood 1981;58:645–647.
18. Hinuma Y, Nagata K, Misoka M, et al. Adult T cell leukemia: Antigen in an ATL cell line and detection of antibodies to the antigen in human sera. Proc Natl Acad Sci USA 1981;78:6476–7480.
19. Blattner WA, Kalyanaraman VS, Robert-Guroff M, et al. The human type C retrovirus, in HTLV, in blacks from the Caribbean region, and relationship to adult T cell leukemia/lymphoma. Int J Cancer 1982;30:257–265.
20. Hunsman G, Schneider J, Schmitt J, et al. Detection of serum antibodies to adult T-cell leukemia virus in non-human primates and in people form Africa. Int J Cancer 1983;32:329–332.
21. Morgan DA, Ruscetti FW, Gallo RC. Selective in vitro growth of T-lymphocytes from normal human bone marrows. Science 1991;193:1007.
22. Yamaguchi K, Nishimura H, Kawano K, et al. A proposal for smoldering adult T-cell leukemia: Diversity in clinical pictures of adult T-cell leukemia. Jpn J Clin Oncol 1983;13:189–200.
23. Gessain A, Barin F, Vernant JC, et al. Antibodies to human lymphotropic virus type-I in patients with tropical spastic paraparesis. Lancet 1985;2:407–410.
24. Bartholomew C, Cleghorn F, Charles W, et al. HTLV-I and tropical spastic paraparesis. Lancet 1986;2:99–100.
25. Osame M, Usuku K, Izumo S, et al. HTLV-I associated myelopathy: A new clinical entity. Lancet 1986;1:1031–1032.
26. Kalyanaraman VS, Sarngadharan MG, Robert-Guroff M, et al. A new subtype of human T-cell leukaemia virus (HTLV-11) associated with a T-cell variant of hairy cell leukaemia. Science 1982;218:571–573.
27. Gelmann EP, Franchini G, Manzari V, et al. Molecular cloning of a unique human T-cell leukemia virus (HTLV-II). Proc Natl Acad Sci USA 1984;81:993–997.
28. Shaw GM, Gonda MA, Flickinger GH, et al. Genomes of evolutionary divergent members of human T-cell leukemia virus family (HTLV-I and HTLV-II) are highly conserved, especially in pX. Proc Natl Acad Sci USA 1984;81:4544–4548.
29. McClure MO, Weiss RA. Human immunodeficiency virus and related viruses. Curr Top AIDS 1987;1:95–117.
30. Pinching A, Weiss RA: AIDS and the spectrum of HTLV-III/LAV infection. Int Rev Exp Pathol 1986;28:1–44.
31. Tajima K, Tominaga S, Suchi T, et al. Epidemiological analysis of the distribution of antibody to adult T-cell leukemia virus. Gann 1982;73:893–901.
32. Okochi K, Sato H, Hinuma Y. A retrospective study on transmission of adult T-cell leukemia virus by blood transfusion: Sero-conversion in recipients. Vox Sang 1983;46:245–253.
33. Seika M, Eddy R, Shows TR, et al. Non-specific integration of the HTLV provirus genome into adult T-cell leukemia cells. Nature 1984;309:640–642.

34. Yoshida M, Seiki M, Yamaguchi K, et al. Monoclonal integration of human T-cell leukemia provirus in all primary tumors of adult T-cell leukemia suggest causative role of human T-cell leukemia virus in the disease. Proc Natl Acad Sci USA 1984;81: 2534–2537.

35. Wong-Staal F, Hahn B, Manzari V, et al. A survey of human leukemias for sequences of a human retrovirus, HTLV. Nature 1983;302:626–628.

36. Hayward WS, Neel BG, Astrin SM. Activation of a cellular onc gene by promoter insertion in ALV-induced lymphoid leukosis. Nature 981;290:475–480.

37. Burny A, Buck C, Chantrenne H, et al. Bovine leukemia virus: Molecular biology and epidemiology. In: Klein G, ed. Viral Oncology. New York: Raven Press, 1980:231–280.

38. Seiki M, Hattori S, Hirayama Y, et al. Human adult T-cell leukemia virus: Complete nucleotide sequence of provirus genome integrated in leukemia cell DNA. Proc Natl Acad Sci USA 1983;80:3618–3622.

39. Sodroski JG, Rosen CA, Haseltine WA. Trans-acting transcriptional activation of the long terminal repeat of human T lymphotropic viruses in infected cells. Science 1984;225:381–385.

40. Fujisawa J, Seiki M, Kiyokawa T, et al. Functional activation of long terminal repeat of human T-cell leukemia virus type 1 by transacting factor. Proc Natl Acad Sci USA 1985;82:2277–2281.

41. Febler BK, Paskalis H, Klienman-Eqing C, et al. The pX protein of HTLV-I is a transcriptional activator of its long terminal repeats. Science 1985;229:675–679.

42. Chen ISY, Slamon DJ, Rosenblatt JD, et al. The x gene is essential for HTLV replication. Science 1985;229:54–58.

43. Kiyokawa T, Seiki M, Iwashita S, et al. p27x-III and p21x-III, proteins encoded by the pX sequence of human T-cell leukemia virus type I. Proc Natl Acad Sci USA 1985;82: 8359–8363.

44. Fujisawa J, Seika M, Sato M, et al. A transcriptional enhancer sequence of HTLV-I is responsible for trans-activation mediated by p40 or HTLV-I. EMBO J 1986;5:713–718.

45. Rosen CA, Sodroski JG, Haseltine WA. Location of cis-acting regulatory sequences in the human T-cell leukemia virus type 1 long terminal repeat. Proc Natl Acad Sci USA 1985;82:6502–6506.

46. Greene WC, Leonard WJ, Wano Y, et al. Trans-activator gene of HTLV-11 induces IL-2 cellular gene expression. Science 1986;232:877–880.

47. Wano Y, Feinberg M, Hosking JB, et al. Stable expression of the tax gene of type I human T-cell leukemia virus in human T cells activates specific cellular genes involved in growth. Proc Natl Acad Sci USA 1988;85:9733–9737.

48. Beasley RP, Lin CC, Hwang L, et al. Hepatocellular carcinoma and hepatitis B virus: A prospective study of 22,707 men in Taiwan. Lancet 1981;2:1129–1133.

49. Robinson WS, Marion PL, Feitelson M, et al. The hepadnavirus group: hepatitis B and related viruses. In: Szmuness W, Alter HJ, Maynard JW, eds. Viral hepatitis—1981 International Symposium. Philadelphia: Franklin Institute Press, 1982:57–68.

50. Summers J, Smolec JM, Snyder R. A virus similar to human hepatitis B virus associated with hepatitis and hepatoma in woodchucks. Proc Natl Acad Sci USA 1978;74:4533–4537.

51. Marion PL, Oshiro L, Regnery DC, et al. A virus in Beechey ground squirrels that is related to hepatitis B virus of man. Proc Natl Acad Sci USA 1980;77:2941–2945.

52. Mason WS, Seal G, Summers J. Virus of Peking ducks with structural and biological relatedness to human hepatitis B virus. J Virol 1980;36:829–836.

53. Blumberg BS, Alter HJ, Visnich S. A "new" antigen in leukemia sera. JAMA 1965;191: 541–546.

54. Alter HJ, Blumberg BS. Further studies on a "new" human isoprecipitin system (Australia antigen). Blood 1966;27:297–309.

55. Blumberg BS, Gerstley BJS, Hungerford DA, et al. A serum antigen (Australia antigen) in Down's syndrome leukemia and hepatitis. Ann Intern Med 1967;66:924–931.

56. Prince AM. An antigen detected in the blood during the incubation period of serum hepatitis. Proc Natl Acad Sci USA 1968;60:814–821.

57. Dane DS, Cameron CH, Briggs M. Virus-like particles in serum of patients with Australia antigen associated hepatitis. Lancet 1970;2:695–698.

58. Almeida JD. Individual morphological variatin seen in Australia antigen positive sera. Am J Dis Child 1972;123:303–309.

59. Kim CY, Tilles JG. Purification and biophysical characterization of hepatitis B antigen. J Clin Invest 1970;52:1176–1186.

60. Summers JA, O'Connell A, Millman I. Genome of hepatitis B virus: Restriction enzyme cleavage and structure of DNA extracted from Dane particles. Proc Natl Acad Sci USA 1975;72:4597–4601.

61. Tiollais P, Pourcel C, Dejean A. The hepatitis B virus. Nature 1985;317:489–495.

62. Landers TA, Greenberg HB, Robinson WS. Structure of hepatitis B Dane particle DNA and nature of the endogenous DNA polymerase reaction. J Virol 1977;23:368–376.

63. Ganem D, Varmus HE. The molecular biology of hepatitis B virus. Annu Rev Biochem 1987;56:651–693.

64. Spandau D, Lee C. Trans-activation of viral enhancers by the hepatitis B virus X protein. J Virol 1988;62:427–434.

65. Colgrove R, Simon G, Ganem D. Transcriptional activation of homologous and heterologous genes by the hepatitis B virus X gene product in cells permissive for viral replication. J Virol 1992;63:4019–4026.

66. Shafritz DA, Shouval D, Sherman H, et al. Integration of hepatitis B virus DNA into the genome of liver cells in chronic liver disease and hepatocellular carcinoma. N Engl J Med 1981;305:1067–1073.

67. Brechot C, Pourcel C, Hadchouel M, et al. State of hepatitis B virus DNA in liver diseases. Hematology 1982;2:27–34.

68. Summers J, Mason WS. Replication of the genome of a hepatitis B-like virus by reverse transcription of an RNA intermediate. Cell 1982;29:403–415.

69. Seeger C, Ganem D, Varmus HE. Biochemical and genetic evidence for the hepatitis B virus replication strategy. Science 1986;232:477–484.

70. Szmuness W. Hepatocellular carcinoma and the hepatitis B virus: Evidence for a causal association. Prog Med Virol 1978;24:40–69.

71. Kim C-Y, Koike K, Saito I, et al. HBx gene of hepatitis B virus induces liver cancer in transgenic mice. Nature 1991;351:317–320.

72. Chisari FV, Klopchin K, Moriyama T, et al. Molecular pathogenesis of hepatocellular carcinoma in hepatitis B virus transgenic mice. Cell 1989;59:1145–1156.

73. Dejean A, Bougueleret K, Grzeschik K, et al. Hepatitis B virus DNA integration in a sequence homologous to v-erbA and steroid receptor genes in a hepatocellular carcinoma. Nature 1986;322:70–72.

74. Wang J, Chenivesse X, Henglein B, et al. Hepatitis B virus integration in a cyclin A gene in a hepatocellular carcinoma. Nature 1990;343:555–557.

75. Ciuffo G. Imnfesto positivo con filtrato di verruca volgare. Giorn Ital Mal Venereol 1907;48:12–17.

76. DeVilliers E-M. Heterogeneity of the human papillomavirus group. J Virol 1989;63: 4898–4903.

77. Baker CC, Howley PM. Differential promoter utilization by the bovine papillomavirus in transformed cells and productively infected wart tissues. EMBO J 1987;6:1027–1035.

78. Lowy DR, Dvoretzky I, Shober R, et al. In vitro tumorigenic transformation by a defined sub-genomic fragment of bovine papilloma virus DNA. Nature 1980;287:72–74.

79. Doorbar J, Campbell D, Grand RJ, et al. Identification of the human papilloma virus-1a E4 gene products. EMBO J 1986;5:355–362.

80. Engel LW, Heilman CA, Howley PM. Transcriptional organization of bovine papillomavirus type 1. J Virol 1983;47:516–528.

81. Amtmann E, Sauer G. Bovine papilloma virus transcription: Polyadenylated RNA species and assessment of the direction of transcription. J Virol 1982;43:59–66.

82. Heilman CA, Engel L, Lowy DR, et al. Virus-specific transcription in bovine papillomavirus-transformed mouse cells. Virology 1982;119:22–34.

83. Black PH, Hartley JW, Rowe WP, et al. Transformation of bovine tissue culture cells by bovine papilloma virus. Nature 1963;199:1016–1018.

84. Thomas M, Boiron M, Tanzer J, et al. In vitro transformation of mice by bovine papillomavirus. Nature 1964;202:709–710.

85. Dvoretzky I, Shober R, Lowy DR. Focus assay in mouse cells for bovine papillomavirus. Virology 1980;103:369–375.

86. Law MF, Lowy DR, Dvoretzky I, et al. Mouse cells transformed by bovine papillomavirus contain only extrachromosomal viral DNA sequences. Proc Natl Acad Sci USA 1981;78: 2727–2731.

87. Spalholz BA, Howley PM. Papillomavirus-host cell interactions. In: Klein G, ed. Advances in viral oncology, vol 8. New York: Raven Press, 1989:27–53.

88. Spalholz BA, Yang YC, Howley PM. Transactivation of a bovine papilloma virus transcriptional regulatory element by the E2 gene product. Cell 1985;42:183–191.

89. Lambert PF, Spalholz BA, Howley PM. A transcriptional repressor encoded by BPV-1 shares a common carboxy-terminal domain with the E2 transactivator. Cell 1987;50: 69–78.

90. Groff DE, Lancaster WD. Genetic analysis of the 3′ early region transformation and replication functions of bovine papillomavirus type 1. Virology 1986;150:221–230.

91. Rabson MS, Yee C, Yang YC, et al. Bovine papillomavirus type 1 3′ early region transformation and plasmid maintenance functions. J Virol 1986;60:626–634.

92. DiMaio D. Nonsense mutation in open reading frame E2 of bovine papillomavirus DNA. J Virol 1986;57:475–480.

93. Ustav M, Stenlund A. Transient replication of BPV-1 requires two viral polypeptides encoded by the E1 and E2 open reading frames. EMBO J 1991;10:449–457.

94. Phelps WC, Howley PM. Transcriptional trans-activation by the human papillomavirus type 16 E2 gene product. J Virol 1987;61:1630–1638.

95. Hirochika H, Broker TR, Chow LT. Enhancers and trans-acting E2 transcriptional factors of papillomaviruses. J Virol 1987;61:2599–2606.

96. Sarver N, Rabson MS, Yang YC, et al. Localization and analysis of bovine papillomavirus type 1 transforming functions. J Virol 1984;52:377–388.

97. Lusky M, Botchan MR. Genetic analysis of bovine papillomavirus type 1 trans-acting replication factors. J Virol 1985;53:955–965.

98. Berg LJ, Singh K, Botchan M. Complementation of a bovine papilloma virus low-copy-number mutant: Evidence for a temporal requirement of the complementing gene. Mol Cell Biol 1986;6:859–869.

99. Pilacinski WP, Glassman DL, Krzyzek RA, et al. Cloning and expression in Escherichia coli of the bovine papillomavirus L1 and L2 open reading frames. Biotechnology 1984;1: 356–360.

100. Komly CA, Breitburd F, Croissant O, et al. The L2 open reading frame of human papillomavirus type 1a encodes a minor structural protein carrying type-specific antigens. J Virol 1986;60:813–816.

101. Bedell MA, Jones KH, Laimins LA. The E6-E7 region of human papillomavirus type 18 is sufficient for transformation of NIH 3T3 and rat-1 cells. J Virol 1987;61:3635–3640.

102. Phelps WC, Yee CL, Münger K, et al. The human papillomavirus type 16 E7 gene encodes transactivation and transformation functions similar to those of adenovirus E1A. Cell 1988;53:539–547.

103. Matlashewski G, Schneider J, Banks L, et al. Human papillomavirus type 16 DNA cooperates with activated ras in transforming primary cells. EMBO J 1987;6:1741–1746.

104. Münger K, Phelps WC, Bubb V, et al. The E6 and E7 genes of the human papillomavirus type 16 together are necessary and sufficient for transformation of primary human keratinocytes. J Virol 1989;63:4417–4421.

105. Hawley-Nelson P, Vousden KH, Hubbert NL, et al. HPV16 E6 and E7 proteins cooperate to immortalize human foreskin keratinocytes. EMBO J 1989;8:3905–3910.

106. Rous P, Kidd JG, Smith WE. Experiments on the cause of the rabbit carcinomas derived from virus-induced papillomas. J Exp Med 1953;96:159–174.

107. Rous P, Kidd JG. The carcinogenic effect of a virus upon tarred skin. Science 1936;83: 468–469.

108. Kidd JG, Rous P. Effect of the papillomavirus (Shope) upon tar warts of rabbits. Proc Soc Exp Biol Med 1937;37:518–520.

109. Wettstein FO, Stevens JG. Variable-sized free episomes of Shope papilloma virus DNA are present in all non-virus-producing neoplasms and integrated episomes are detected in some. Proc Natl Acad Sci USA 1982;79:790–794.

110. Nasseri M, Wettstein FO. Differences exist between viral transcripts in cottontail rabbit papillomavirus-induced benign and malignant tumors as well as non-virus-producing and virus-producing tumors. J Virol 1984;51:706–712.

111. Jarrett WFH, McNeil PE, Grimshaw WIR, et al. High incidence area of cattle cancer with a possible interaction between an environmental carcinogen and a papillomavirus. Nature 1978;274:215–217.

112. Jarrett WFH, Murphy J, O'Neill BW, et al. Virus-induced papillomas of the alimentary tract of cattle. Int J Cancer 1978;22:323–328.

113. Campo MS, Moar MH, Sartirana ML, et al. The presence of bovine papillomavirus type 4 DNA is not required for the progression to, or the maintenance of, the malignant state in cancers of the alimentary canal in cattle. EMBO J 1985;4:1819–1825.

114. Lutzner M. An autosomal recessive disease characterized by viral warts and skin cancer: A model for viral oncogenesis. Bull Cancer 1978;65:169–182.

115. Orth G. Epidermodysplasia verruciformis: A model for understanding the oncogenicity of human papillomaviruses. Ciba Found Symp 1986;120:157–174.

116. Ostrow RS, Bender M, Niimura M, et al. Human papillomavirus DNA in cutaneous primary and metastasized squamous cell carcinomas from patients with epidermodysplasia verruciformis. Proc Natl Acad Sci USA 1982;79:1634–1638.

117. Pfister H, Gassenmaier A, Nurnberger F, et al. Human papilloma virus 5-DNA in a carcinoma of an epidermodysplasia verruciformis patient infected with various human papillomavirus types. Cancer Res 1983;43:1436–1441.

118. Green M, Brackmann KH, Sanders PR, et al. Isolation of a human papillomavirus from a patient with epidermodysplasia verruciformis: Presence of related viral DNA genomes in human urogenital tumors. Proc Natl Acad Sci USA 1982;79:4437–4441.

119. Yutsudo M, Shimakage T, Hakura A. Human papillomavirus type 17 DNA in skin carcinoma tissue of a patient with epidermodysplasia verruciformis. Virology 1985;144: 295–298.

120. Yutsudo M, Hakura A. Human papillomavirus type 17 transcripts expressed in skin carcinoma tissue of a patient with epidermodysplasia verruciformis. Int J Cancer 1987;39:586–589.

121. Iftner T, Bierfelder S, Csapo Z, et al. Involvement of human papillomavirus type 8 genes E6 and E7 in transformation and replication. J Virol 1988;62:3655–3661.

122. Underwood PB, Hester L. Diagnosis and treatment of premalignant lesions of the vulva. Am J Obstet Gynecol 1971;110:849–857.

123. Waugh M. Condylomata acuminata. Br Med J 1972;2:527–528.

124. Dunn AE, Ogilvie MM. Intranuclear virus particles in human genital wart tissue: Observation on the ultrastructure of epidermal layer. J Ultrastruct Res 1968;22:282–295.

125. Oriel JD, Almeida JD. Demonstration of virus particles in human genital warts. Br J Vener Dis 1970;46:37–42.

126. Woodruff JD, Braun L, Cavalieri R, et al. Immunologic identification of papillomavirus antigen in condyloma tissues from the female genital tract. Obstet Gynecol 1980;56: 727–732.

127. Gissmann L, de Villiers EM, zur Hausen H. Analysis of human genital warts (condylomata acuminata) and other genital tumors for human papillomavirus type 6 DNA. Int J Cancer 1982;29:143–146.

128. Gissmann L, Wolnik L, Ikenberg H, et al. Human papillomavirus types 6 and 11 DNA sequences in genital and laryngeal papillomas and in some cervical cancers. Proc Natl Acad Sci USA 1983;80:560–563.

129. Buschke A, Löwenstein L. Uber carcinomahnliche condylomata acumina des penis. Arch Dermatol Syph 1931;163:30–46.

130. Boshart M, zur Hausen H. Human papillomaviruses in Buschke-Löwenstein tumors: Physical state of the DNA and identification of a tandem duplication in the noncoding region of a human papillomavirus 6 subtype. J Virol 1986;58:963–966.

131. Meisels A, Fortin R. Condylomatous lesions of the cervix and vagina. I. Cytologic patterns. Acta Cytol 1976;20:505–509.

132. Purola E, Savia E. Cytology of gynecologic condyloma acuminatum. Acta Cytol 1977;21: 26–31.

133. Laverty CR, Russell P, Hills E, et al. The significance of noncondylomatous wart virus infection of the cervical transformation zone. Acta Cytol 1978;22:195–201.

134. Koss LG, Durfee GR. Unusual patterns of squamous epithelium of the uterine cervix: Cytologic and pathologic study of koilocytotic atypia. Ann N Y Acad Sci 1956;63:1245–1261.

135. Della Torre G, Pilotti S, De Palo G, et al. Viral particles in cervical condylomatous lesions. Tumori 1978;64:549–553.

136. Hills E, Laverty CR. Electron microscopic detection of papilloma virus particles in selected koilocytotic cells in a routine cervical smear. Acta Cytol 1979;23:53–56.

137. Kessler IL. Human cervical cancer as a venereal disease. Cancer Res 1976;36:783–791.

138. Zur Hausen H. Human papillomaviruses and their possible role in squamous cell carcinomas. Curr Top Microbiol Immunol 1977;78:1–30.

139. Rawls WE, Tompkins WAF, Figueroa ME, et al. Herpes simplex virus type 2: Association with carcinoma of the cervix. Science 1968;161:1255–1256.

140. Nahmias AJ, Josey WE, Naib ZM, et al. Antibodies to herpes virus hominus types 1 and 2 in humans. II. Women with cervical cancer. Am J Epidemiol 1970;91:547–552.

141. zur Hausen H. Herpes simplex virus in human genital cancer. Int Rev Exp Pathol 1983;25:307–326.

142. Vonka V, Kanda J, Hirsch I, et al. Prospective study on the relationship between cervical neoplasia and herpes simplex type-2 virus. II. Herpes simplex type-2 antibody presence in sera taken at enrollment. Int J Cancer 1984;33:61–66.

143. Vonka V, Kanda J, Jelinek J, et al. Prospective study on the relationship between cervical neoplasia and herpes simplex type-2 virus. I. Epidemiological characteristics. Int J Cancer 1984;33:49–60.

144. Peterson O. Spontaneous course of cervical precancerous conditions. Am J Obstet Gynecol 1956;72:1063–1071.

145. Kinlen LJ, Spriggs AI. Women with positive cervical smears but without surgical intervention: A follow up study. Lancet 1978;2:463–465.

146. Richart RM, Barrow BA. A follow-up study of patients with cervical dysplasia. Am J Obstet Gynecol 1969;105:386–393.

147. Durst M, Gissmann L, Idenburg H, et al. A papillomavirus DNA from a cervical carcinoma and its prevalence in cancer biopsy samples from different geographic regions. Proc Natl Acad Sci USA 1983;80:3812–3815.

148. Boshart M, Gissmann L, Ikenberg H, et al. A new type of papillomavirus DNA, its presence in genital cancer biopsies and in cell lines derived from cervical cancer. EMBO J 1984;3:1151–1157.

149. Gissmann L, Schwarz E. Persistence and expression of human papillomavirus DNA in genital cancer. In: Evered D, Clark S, eds. Papillomaviruses. CIBA Symposium 120. Chichester: John Wiley & Sons, 1986:190–197.

150. Beaudenon S, Kremsdorf D, Croissant O, et al. A novel type of human papillomavirus associated with genital neoplasias. Nature 1986;321:246–249.

151. Beaudenon S, Kremsdorf D, Obalek S, et al. Plurality of genital human papillomaviruses: Characterization of two new types with distinct biological properties. Virology 1987;161: 374–384.

152. Ikenberg H, Gissmann L, Gross G, et al. Human papillomavirus type-16-related DNA in genital Bowen's disease and in Bowenoid papulosis. Int J Cancer 1983;32:563–565.

153. Gross G, Hagedorn M, Ikenberg H, et al. Bowenoid papulosis. Presence of human papillomavirus (HPV) structural antigens and of HPV 16-related DNA sequences. Arch Dermatol 1985;121:858–863.

154. Durst M, Croce C, Gissmann L, et al. Papillomavirus sequences integrate near cellular oncogenes in some cervical carcinomas. Proc Natl Acad Sci USA 1987;84:1070–1074.

155. Schwarz E, Freese UK, Gissmann L, et al. Structure and transcription of human papillomavirus sequences in cervical carcinoma cells. Nature 1985;314:111–114.

156. Yee C, Krishnan-Hewlett I, Baker CC, et al. Presence and expression of human papillomavirus sequences in human cervical carcinoma cell lines. Am J Pathol 1985;119: 361–366.

157. Romanczuk H, Howley PM. Disruption of either the E1 or the E2 regulatory gene of human papillomavirus type 16 increases viral immortalization capacity. Proc Natl Acad Sci USA 1992;89:3159–3163.

158. DeCaprio JA, Ludlow JW, Figge J, et al. SV40 large tumor antigen forms a specific complex with the product of the retinoblastoma susceptibility gene. Cell 1988;54:275–283.

159. Whyte P, Williamson NM, Harlow E. Cellular targets for transformation by the adenovirus E1A proteins. Cell 1989;56:67–75.

160. Ewen MB, Ludlow JW, Marsilio E, et al. An N-terminal transformation-governing sequence of SV40 large T antigen contributes to the binding of both p110 RB and a second cellular protein, p120. Cell 1989;58:257–267.

161. Münger K, Werness BA, Dyson N, et al. Complex formation of human papillomavirus E7 proteins with the retinoblastoma tumor suppressor gene product. EMBO J 1989;8: 4099–4105.

162. Hudson JB, Bedell MA, McCance DJ, et al. Immortalization and altered differentiation of human keratinocytes in vitro by the E6 and E7 open reading frames of human papillomavirus type 18. J Virol 1990;64:519–526.

163. Barbosa MS, Vass WC, Lowy DR, et al. In vitro biological activities of the E6 and E7 genes vary among HPVs of different oncogenic potential. J Virol 1991;65:292–298.

164. Schlegel R, Phelps WC, Zhang Y-L, et al. Quantitative keratinocyte assay detects two biological activities of human papillomavirus DNA and identifies viral types associated with cervical carcinoma. EMBO J 1988;7:3181–3187.

165. Werness BA, Levine AJ, Howley PM. Association of human papillomavirus types 16 and 18 E6 proteins with p53. Science 1990;248:76–79.

166. Scheffner M, Werness BA, Huibregtse JM, et al. The E6 oncoprotein encoded by human papillomavirus types 16 and 18 promotes the degradation of p53. Cell 1990;63:1129–1136.

167. Münger K, Yee CL, Phelps WC, et al. Biochemical and biological differences between E7 oncoproteins of the high- and low-risk human papillomavirus types are determined by amino-terminal sequences. J Virol 1991;65:3943–3948.

168. Clarke EA, Morgan RW, Newman AM. Smoking as a risk factor in cancer of the cervix: Additional evidence from a case control study. Am J Epidemiol 1982;115:59–66.

169. Wigle DT. Smoking and cancer of the cervix: Hypothesis. Am J Epidemiol 1980;111: 125–127.

170. Winkelstein W Jr. Smoking and cancer of the uterine cervix. Am J Epidemiol 1977;106: 257–259.

171. Hoffman D, Hecht SS, Haley NJ, et al. Tumorigenic agents in tobacco products and their uptake by chewers, smokers and nonsmokers. J Cell Biochem 1985;9C:33.

172. Zur Hausen H. Human genital cancer: Synergism between two virus infections or synergism between a virus infection and initiating events. Lancet 1982;2:1370–1372.

173. Kahn T, Schwarz E, zur Hausen H. Molecular cloning and characterization of the DNA

of a new human papillomavirus from a laryngeal carcinoma. Int J Cancer 1986;37: 61–65.

174. Loning T, Ikenberg H, Becker J, et al. Analysis of oral papillomas, leukoplakias, and invasive carcinomas for human papillomavirus type related DNA. J Invest Dermatol 1985;84:417–420.

175. Brandsma JL, Steinberg BM, Abramson AL, et al. Presence of human papillomavirus type 16 related sequences in verrucous carcinoma of the larynx. Cancer Res 1986;46: 2185–2188.

176. Jenson AB, Lancaster WD, Hartman DP, et al. Frequency and distribution of papillomavirus structural antigens in verrucae, multiple papillomas, and condylomata of the oral cavity. Am J Pathol 1982;107:212–218.

177. Lind P, Syrjanen K, Koppang HS, et al. Immunoreactivity and human papillomavirus (HPV) on oral precancer and cancer lesions. Scand J Dent Res 19;94:419–426.

178. De Villiers EM, Neumann C, Le JY, et al. Infection of the oral mucosa with defined types of human papillomaviruses. Med Microbiol Immunol (Berl) 1986;174:287–294.

179. Naghasfar Z, Sawada E, Kutcher MK, et al. Identification of genital tract papillomaviruses HPV-6 and HPV-16 in warts of the oral cavity. J Virol 1985;62:660–667.

180. Pfister H, Hettich I, Runne U, et al. Characterization of human papillomavirus type 13 from focal epithelial hyperplasia Heck lesions. J Virol 1983;47:363–366.

181. Beaudenon S, Praetorius F, Kremsdorf D, et al. A new type of human papillomavirus associated with oral focal epithelial hyperplasia. J Invest Dermatol 1987;88:130–135.

182. Syrjanen S, Syrjanen K, Lambert MA. Detection of human papillomavirus DNA in oral mucosal lesions using in situ DNA hybridization applied on paraffin sections. Oral Surg Oral Med Oral Pathol 1986;62:660–667.

183. Byrne JC, Tsao MS, Fraser RS, et al. Human papillomavirus-11 DNA in a patient with chronic laryngotracheobronchial papillomatosis and metastatic squamous-cell carcinoma of the lung. N Engl J Med 1987;317:873–878.

184. Syrjanen K, Pyrhonen S, Aukee S, et al. A tumor probably caused by human papillomavirus (HPV). Diagn Histopathol 1982;5:291–296.

185. Winkler B, Capo V, Reumann W, et al. Human papillomavirus infection of the esophagus. Cancer 1985;55:149–155.

186. Burkitt D. A sarcoma involving the jaws in African children. Br J Surg 1958;46:218–223.

187. Burkitt D. Determining the climatic limitations of a children's cancer common in Africa. Br Med J 1962;2:1019–1023.

188. Epstein MA, Barr YM. Cultivation in vitro of human lymphoblasts from Burkitt's malignant lymphoma. Lancet 1964;1:252–253.

189. Epstein MA, Achong BG, Barr YM. Virus particles in cultured lymphoblasts from Burkitt's lymphoma. Lancet 1964;1:702–703.

190. Kieff E, Dambaugh T, Heller M, et al. The biology and chemistry of Epstein-Barr virus. J Infect Dis 1982;146:506–517.

191. Baer R, Bankier AT, Biggin MD, et al. DNA sequence and expression of B95-8 Epstein Barr virus genome. Proc Natl Acad Sci USA 1984;310:207–211.

192. Hummel M, Kieff E. Mapping of polypeptides encoded by the Epstein-Barr virus genome in productive infection. Proc Natl Acad Sci 1982;79:5698–5698.

193. de Schryver A, Klein G, Henle W, et al. Comparison of EBV neutralization tests based on abortive infection or transformation of lymphoid cells and their relation to membrane reactive antibodies (anti-MA). Int J Cancer 1974;13:353–362.

194. Henle G, Henle W, Klein G. Demonstration of two distinct components in the early antigen complex of Epstein-Barr virus-infected cells. Int J Cancer 1971;8:272–282.

195. Reedman BM, Klein G. Cellular localization of an Epstein-Barr virus (EBV) associated complement-fixing antigen in producer and non-producer lymphoblastoid cell lines. Int J Cancer 1973;11:499–520.

196. Yates J, Warren N, Reisman D, et al. A cis-acting element from the Epstein-Barr viral genome that permits stable replication of recombinant plasmids in latently infected cells. Proc Natl Acad Sci USA 1984;81:3806–3810.

197. Abbot SD, Rowe M, Cadwallader K, et al. Epstein-Barr virus nuclear antigen 2 induces expression of the virus-encoded latent membrane protein. J Virol 1990;64:2126–2134.

198. Wang F, Tsang S, Kurilla MG, et al. Epstein-Barr virus nuclear antigen 2 transactivates latent membrane protein LMP 1. J Virol 1990;64:3407–3416.

199. Zimber-Strobl U, Suentzenich KO, Laux G, et al. Epstein-Barr virus nuclear antigen-2 activates transcription of the terminal protein gene. J Virol 1991;65:415–423.

200. Cordier M, Calender A, Billaud M, et al. Stable transfection of Epstein-Barr virus nuclear antigen 2 in lymphoma cells containing the EBV P3HR1 genome induces

expression of B-cell activation molecules CD21 and CD23. J Virol 1990;64:1002–1013.

201. Wang F, Gregory C, Sample C, et al. Epstein-Barr virus latent membrane protein (LMP 1) and nuclear proteins 2 and 3C are effectors of phenotypic changes in B-lymphocytes: EBNA 2 and LMP 1 cooperatively induce CD23. J Virol 1990;64:2309–2318.

202. Knutson JC. The level of c-fgr RNA is increased by EBNA-2, Epstein-Barr virus gene required for B-cell immortalization. J Virol 1990;64:2530–2536.

203. Fialkow PJ, Klein E, Klein G, et al. Immunoglobulin and glucose-6-phosphate dehydrogenase as markers of cellular origin in Burkitt lymphoma. J Exp Med 1973;138:89–101.

204. Mann RB, Bernard CW. Burkitt's tumor: Lessons from mice, monkeys, and man. Lancet 1979;2:84.

205. Magrath I. Clinical and pathobiological features of Burkitt's lymphoma and their resistance to treatment. In: Levine PH, Ablashi DV, Pearson GR, et al, eds. Epstein-Barr virus and associated diseases. Boston: M. Nijhoff Publishing, 1986:631–643.

206. Kafuko GW, Burkitt DP. Burkitt's lymphoma and malaria. Int J Cancer 1970;6:1–9.

207. Morrow RH Jr. Epidemiological evidence for the role of falciparum malaria in the pathogenesis of Burkitt's lymphoma. In: Lenoir GM, O'Connor G, Olweny CLM, eds. A human cancer model. IARC Scientific Publication, 1985:177–186.

208. Moss DJ, Burrows SR, Catelino DJ, et al. A comparison of Epstein-Barr virus-specific T-cell immunity in malaria-endemic and nonendemic regions of Papua New Guinea. Int J Cancer 1983;31:727–732.

209. Manolov G, Manolova Y. Marker band in one chromosome 14 from Burkitt lymphomas. Nature 1972;237:33–34.

210. Lenoir GM, Taub R. Chromosomal translocations and oncogenes in Burkitt's lymphoma. In: Goldman JM, ed. Leukaemia and lymphoma research: Genetic rearrangements in leukaemia and lymphoma. London: DG Harnden, 1986:152–172.

211. Leder P, Battey J, Lenoir G, et al. Translocations among antibody genes in human cancer. Science 1983;222:765–771.

212. Erikson J, Finan J, Nowell PC, et al. Translocation of immunoglobulin V H genes in Burkitt's lymphoma. Proc Natl Acad Sci USA 1982;79:5611–5615.

213. Klein G. Lymphoma development in mice and human: Diversity of initiation is followed by convergent cytogenetic evolution. Proc Natl Acad Sci USA 1979;76:2442–2446.

214. Klein G, Klein E. Evolution of tumors and the impact of molecular oncology. Nature 1985;315:190.

215. Lenoir GM, Bornkamm GW. Burkitt's lymphoma, a human cancer model for the study of multistep development of cancer: Proposal for a new scenario. Adv Viral Oncol 1987;7:173–206.

216. Henle W, Henle G. Epstein-Barr virus and human malignancies. Adv Viral Oncol 1985;5:201–238.

217. zur Hausen H, Schulte-Holthausen H, Klein G, et al. EBV DNA in biopsies of Burkitt tumors and anaplastic carcinomas of the nasopharynx. Nature 1970;228:1056–1058.

218. Andersson-Anvret M, Forsby N, Klein G, et al. Relationship between the Epstein-Barr virus and undifferentiated nasopharyngeal carcinoma: Correlated nucleic acid hybridization and histopathological examination. Int J Cancer 1977;20:486–494.

219. Raab-Traub N, Flynn K, Pearson G, et al. The differentiated form of nasopharyngeal carcinoma contains Epstein-Barr virus DNA. Int J Cancer 1987;39:25–29.

220. Pagano JS. Epstein-Barr virus transcription in nasopharyngeal carcinoma. J Virol 1983;48:580–590.

221. De the G, Zeng Y. Population screening for EBV markers: Toward improvement of nasopharyngeal carcinoma control. In: Epstein MA, Achog BG, eds. The Epstein-Barr virus. New York: John Wiley & Sons, 1986:237–248.

222. Purtilo DT, Sakamoto K, Barnabai V, et al. Epstein-Barr virus-induced diseases in boys with the X-linked lymphoproliferative syndrome (XLP): Updates on studies of the registry. Am J Med 1982;73:49–56.

223. Robinson WS. Hepatitis B virus. In: Fields BN, ed. Virology. New York: Raven Press, 1985:1384–1406.

224. Huibregtse JM, Scheffner M, Howley PM: A cellular protein mediates association of p53 with the E6 oncoprotein of human papillomavirus types 16 or 18. EMBO J 1991;10:4129–4135.

225. Ford JN, Jennings PA, Spradbrow PB, et al. Evidence for papillomaviruses in ocular lesions in cattle. Res Vet Sci 1982;32:257–259.

226. Vanselow BA, Spradbrow PB, Jackson AR. Papillomaviruses, papillomas and squamous cell carcinomas in sheep. Vet Rec 1982;110:561–562.

Cancer: Principles & Practice of Oncology, Fourth Edition,
edited by Vincent T. DeVita, Jr., Samuel Hellman, Steven A. Rosenberg.
J.B. Lippincott Co., Philadelphia © 1993.

Peter G. Shields

Curtis C. Harris

CHAPTER **11**

Principles of Carcinogenesis: Chemical

Chemical carcinogenesis has its roots in the epidemiology of cancer.[1] In 1759, John Hill reported that tobacco snuff caused oral cavity cancers.[2] Soon after, Percival Pott published his findings that working as a chimney sweep, exposure to soot, and poor hygiene led to scrotal cancer.[3] Other associations followed, such as bladder cancer with aromatic amines,[4] benzene with leukemia,[5] and lung cancer with tobacco smoke.[6,7] Epidemiologic relations were also explored in the laboratory. As early as 1918 and in reaction to Pott's findings, Yamigawa and Ichikawa reported that coal tar could cause skin cancer in laboratory animals,[8] which was followed by similar findings for individual chemicals. This chapter presents some of the basic principles of chemical carcinogenesis, focusing on topics that are especially relevant to the understanding of human carcinogenesis. The molecular epidemiology of human cancer, an emerging field in cancer research, is explored. Reviews of the research accomplishments in the field of chemical carcinogenesis are available and contain more extensive bibliographies.[1,9,10]

MULTISTAGE CARCINOGENESIS

Carcinogenesis is a multistage process driven by genetic damage and epigenetic changes (Fig. 11–1). The traditional view of carcinogenesis is derived primarily from studies of animal models, but more recent studies rely on the molecular analysis of cancer-related genes in human cells.[1] Tumor initiation begins in cells through mutations from exposure to carcinogens. These mutated cells may have an altered responsiveness to their microenvironment and a selective growth advantage when compared with the surrounding normal cells. The tumor-initiated cells also may have a decreased responsiveness to the intercellular and intracellular signals that maintain their architecture and regulate homeostatic growth. For example, initiated cells may be less responsive to negative growth factors, terminal cell differentiation, or programmed cell death. Selective clonal expansion of the initiated cells may also occur by physical perturbation of the normal microenvironment (*e.g.,* wounding of mouse skin or partial hepatectomy in rodents), chemical agents (*e.g.,* phorbol esters on mouse skin or rat liver and phenobarbital), microbial agents (*e.g.,* influenza virus enhancement of rodent lung carcinogenesis or hepatitis virus in human liver carcinogenesis), or other inflammatory processes. Tumor promotion results in further selective clonal expansion and proliferation of the initiated cells, thereby enhancing the probability of additional genetic damage through endogenous mutations or DNA-damaging agents. During tumor progression, malignant cells continue to exhibit progressive phenotypic changes[11] and genomic instability, including gene amplification, chromosomal aberrations, and altered gene expression.[12,13]

The classic view of two-stage carcinogenesis, in which tumor initiation (mutation) is followed by tumor promotion (epigenetic changes), has been conceptually important but is too simplistic. There may be six or more independent mutational events.[14,15] Furthermore, chemical carcinogens may be genotoxic, nongenotoxic, or cause epigenetic effects.[16,17] Dose-response relations may be linear or nonlinear.[18,19] Endogenous mutagenic mechanisms, such as DNA oxy-radical damage, depurination, polymerase infidelity, and deamination of 5-methylcytosine also contribute to carcinogenesis.[20–23] None-

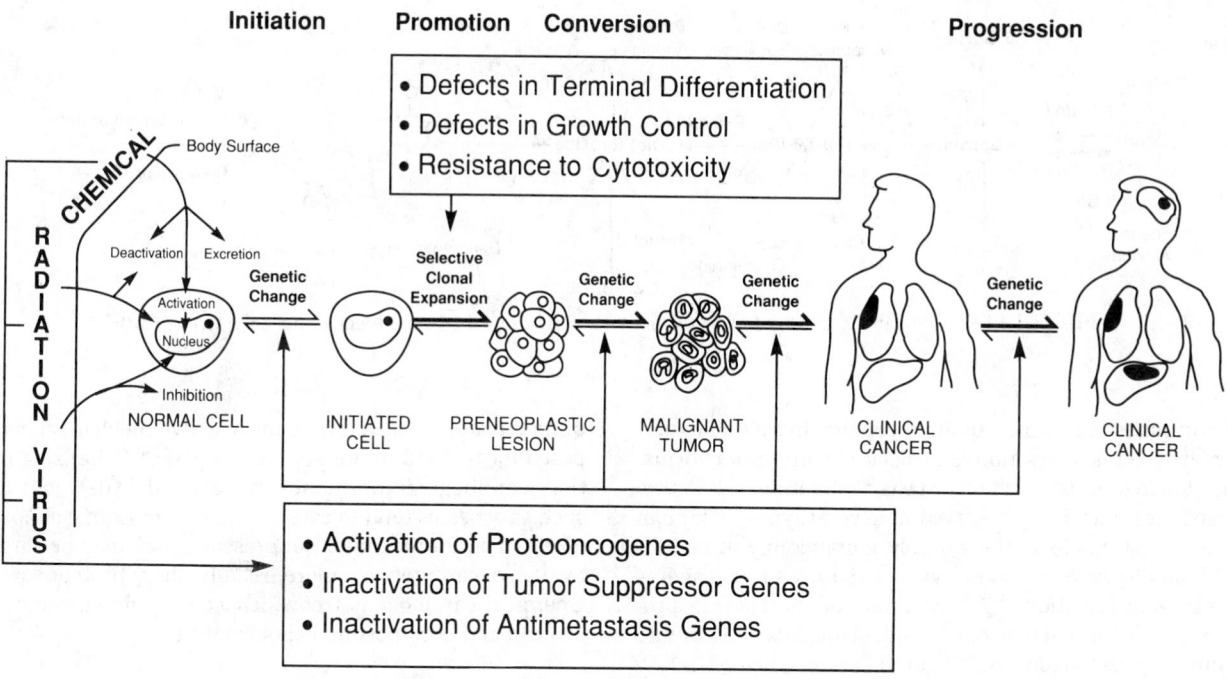

FIGURE 11–1. Multistage model of carcinogenesis.

theless, a debate continues regarding the relative importance of endogenous versus exogenous mutagenic events and the value of animal bioassays or short-term mutagenic assays for the assessment of human cancer risk.[23–26] Societal and regulatory decisions crucial to public health are at issue in this debate.

CARCINOGEN METABOLISM AND DNA DAMAGE

Most chemical carcinogens require metabolic activation through the generation of highly reactive electrophiles. These form DNA adducts by covalently binding to nucleic acids, exerting a promutagenic effect. Metabolic activation is generally catalyzed by cytochrome P450 enzymes through oxidation. Cytochrome P450 genes are continually being identified; organisms can have over 200 distinct P450 enzymes.[27] A proposed nomenclature for individual genes uses the prefix *CYP* followed by an arabic numeral, letter, and numeral that indicate the family, subfamily, and gene number, respectively.[28] The families designated *CYP1, CYP2, CYP3,* and *CYP4* are primarily responsible for metabolism of foreign chemicals.[29] Family and subfamilies are determined by the percentage of gene sequence homology. The ability to isolate and clone human cDNA has allowed the determination of substrate specificity for individual P450 enzymes, in many cases confirming earlier work using purified rodent proteins.[27]

The ability to metabolize carcinogens varies widely among animal species.[27] Cytochrome P450 enzymes also vary among different tissues within and among species.[30,31] Although interspecies differences have long been known to be quantitative, the metabolic activation pathways are qualitatively similar.[31] These observations support the qualitative extrapolation of carcinogenesis data from laboratory animals to humans,

whereas quantitative differences are partly responsible for interspecies, interindividual, and intertissue responses to carcinogens.[32]

The metabolism of any individual carcinogen can be complex because it can be a substrate for several enzymes. For example, significant progress has been achieved in elucidating the metabolic activation and detoxification pathways for polycyclic aromatic hydrocarbons (PAH), such as benzo[*a*]pyrene (BP).[33] These compounds are composed of fused benzene rings that are essentially water insoluble but are readily absorbed through the lungs and gastrointestinal tract. They are commonly found as combustion products of fossil fuels (*e.g.,* coal, wood, diesel exhaust) and vegetable matter. Consequently, PAHs are common environmental pollutants. BP is metabolically activated by phase 1 enzymes forming a reactive diolepoxide (Fig. 11–2). Initially, CYP1A1 and epoxide hydroxylase catalyze the conversion of BP to a dihydrodiol. Then, cytochrome CYP3A4 converts this product to the diolepoxide (BP-7,8-diol 9,10-epoxide). Along this pathway, intermediates may be detoxified by conjugation, oxidation, or reduction and then excreted in urine or feces.

CRITICAL DNA TARGETS: PROTOONCOGENES AND TUMOR SUPPRESSOR GENES

Protooncogenes are normal cellular genes that can be inappropriately *activated* to cause dysregulation of cell growth and differentiation, which increases the *probability* of neoplastic transformation. They can be activated by carcinogens through nucleotide base substitutions, chromosomal translocations, and gene amplification. Among the best-studied protooncogenes is the *RAS* family. *RAS* protein products are involved in signal transduction pathways initiated by growth factors

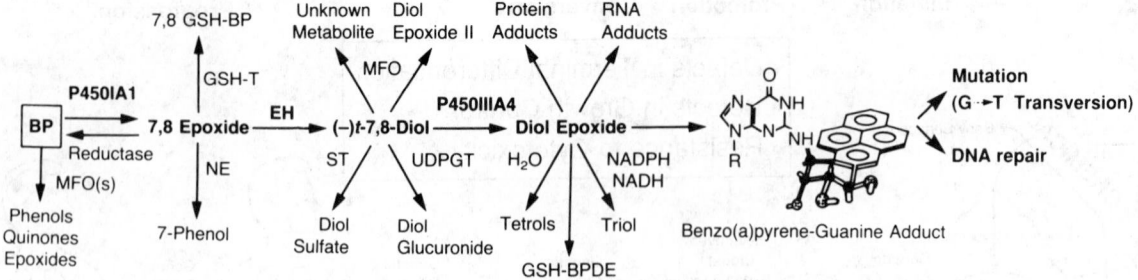

FIGURE 11–2.   Metabolic activation, deactivation, and formation of DNA adducts for benzo[a]pyrene (BP).

and hormones at cell membrane receptors. In several experimental systems, activation is associated with tumor formation,[34] angiogenesis,[35] and metastasis.[36] Mutation of *RAS* protooncogenes have been observed in several types of human cancers.[37] Base substitutions occur nonrandomly at codons 12, 13, and 61 in vitro and in vivo on exposure to such agents as PAHs and radiation.[34,38–40] Mutation of the Ha-*RAS* protooncogene is an early event in rodent models of skin and mammary carcinogenesis.[38,41] In addition, the v-Ha-*RAS* transgene can substitute for the initiation step in mouse skin carcinogenesis in transgenic mice.[42,43]

In contrast to protooncogenes, tumor suppressor genes are normal cellular genes that can be inappropriately *inactivated* to cause dysregulation of growth and differentiation pathways. This also increases the *probability* of neoplastic transformation. Tumor suppressor genes perform different functions (Table 11–1). Although the loss of suppressor gene function is dominant in carcinogenesis, the inheritable trait is recessive; loss of function for both alleles is the basis of the two-hit hypothesis for carcinogenesis.[44,45] Alternatively, suppressor genes can be inactivated by genomic imprinting,[46] increased proteolytic digestion of gene products,[47] or other dominant negative mechanisms.[48] Based on target size theory, the inactivation of a single allele of a tumor suppressor gene (in which mutations at multiple sites may cause inactivation) should have an intrinsically higher probability than activation of a protooncogene (in which only a few mutations at specific codons can cause activation). The requirement for inactivation of both alleles of a tumor suppressor gene counterbalances this probability except in those cases in which an inactivated allele is inherited (*e.g.*, familial polyposis coli, Li-Fraumeni syndrome, Wilms' tumor, or retinoblastoma) or the process

TABLE 11–1. Examples of Functions of Putative Tumor Suppressor Genes

- Induce terminal differentiation
- Maintain genomic stability
- Trigger senescence
- Regulate cell growth
    Signal transducers of negative growth factors
    Regulators, *e.g.*, PTPase-γ, of tyrosine kinases
- Induce proteases
- Induce programmed cell death
- Alter DNA methylase activity
- Modulate histocompatibility antigens
- Regulate angiogenesis
- Facilitate cell–cell communication

of inactivation is by a dominant negative mechanism as proposed for the p53 tumor suppressor gene.[48,49] Ionizing radiation, carcinogenic hormones, metals, aldehydes, and fibers such as asbestos tend to cause gross chromosomal abnormalities.[50] Therefore, tumor suppressor genes may be targeted by these carcinogens more readily than protooncogenes. Chemical carcinogens frequently cause promutagenic DNA adducts and chromosomal abnormalities.

MUTATIONAL SPECTRUM

The mutational spectra of endogenous and exogenous carcinogens are largely responsible for activating protooncogenes and inactivating tumor suppressor genes. Studies using prokaryotic, simple eukaryotic, and site-specific mutagenesis assays have suggested that carcinogenic agents produce a fingerprint of DNA adducts and mutations. Similar evidence exists in eukaryotic studies such as exogenous gene insertion by shuttle vector[51,52] or endogenous gene analysis.[53] These can become mutated at specific loci to produce detectable phenotypic changes (adenine phosphoribosyl transferase [APRT], dihydrofolate reductase [DHFR], and hypoxanthine-guanine phosphoribosyl transferase [HPRT]). However, these assays may underestimate mutational frequency because gene deletions, chromosomal nondisjunction, and frameshift mutations cause loss of other genes essential for cell survival. In addition, certain mutations may cause clonal expansion or inhibition of the mutant cell, further complicating the interpretation of the mutational spectrum.

A comparison of the spontaneously occurring mutational spectrum at the *APRT* locus in Chinese hamster ovary (CHO) cells with spectra induced by ionizing radiation, ultraviolet radiation, or benzo[a]pyrene diolepoxide is shown in Table 11–2. The mutational spectrum of ultraviolet light is consistent with mutagenesis models of promutagenic cyclobutane and pyrimidine-pyrimidone photoproducts. Ionizing radiation, in contrast, most frequently causes deletions, although specific point mutations are also observed. Benzo[a]pyrene diolepoxide, which binds to the 2-amino group of deoxyguanosine, produces predominantly G:C→T:A transversions; a similar mutational spectrum for benzo[a]pyrene diolepoxide has been observed in human cell assays.[54] The *HPRT* locus is of particular interest because of the potential to compare mutational spectra in cultured cells with those in human lymphocytes of persons exposed in vivo to environmental carcinogens.[55]

The molecular analysis of mutationally activated *RAS* protooncogenes in animal models suggests that mutational spectra

TABLE 11–2. Percent Distribution of Mutations in the Endogenous Adenine Phosphoribosyl Transferase Locus in Chinese Hamster Ovary Cells

Mutagen	Transitions		Transversions				Deletions	Insertions
	G:C → A:T	A:T → G:C	G:C → T:A	G:C → C:G	A:T → C:G	A:T → T:A		
Spontaneous	71	0	13	3	0	7	6	0
Ultraviolet radiation	61	2	5	10	5	12	2	2
Ionizing radiation	19	6	6	6	19	13	31	0
Benzo[a]pyrene diolepoxide	5	0	62	14	0	9	5	5

reflect DNA-adduct formation.[1] For example, mutations found in activated *RAS* protooncogenes of rodent tumors after *N*-nitroso compound exposure are predominantly G:C→A:T base substitutions; these are likely due to methylation of deoxyguanosine at the O^6 position followed by mispairing with thymine during DNA synthesis.[56] Although there are several guanine residues in *RAS* codons that would generate a transforming protein if substituted with adenine, the animal experiments have revealed that the mutations occur overwhelmingly at only certain mutation sites (codons 12, 13, and 61). Unexplained mutational specificities have been observed in other experimental systems and may reflect the differences in the spectrum of promutagenic carcinogen-DNA adducts, specificity of DNA repair enzymes, or resultant amino acid changes that are silent or nonlethal.[57–59] The mutational spectra of activated *RAS* protooncogenes in tumors and preneoplastic lesions of laboratory animals may be instructive in the interpretation of mutations in human cancers. The spectra of Ki-*RAS* protooncogene mutations in human adenocarcinomas vary according to tissue site, although the base substitution is not always specific. For example, G:C→T:A transversions occur in lung tumors, which can be caused by PAH exposure, endogenous mutagens (8-OH-deoxyguanosine caused by oxy-radical damage), DNA depurination, or polymerase infidelity.[60,61]

The p53 tumor suppressor gene is ideally suited for analysis of mutational spectra. First, p53 is well conserved in evolution and the DNA sequence of 5 domains are more than 90% homologous among humans and rodents.[62] Second, p53 is mutated in diverse types of human cancer.[63] Third, a wide spectrum of mutational types and codon sites has been observed that presumably define regions of the p53 protein likely to be essential for tumor suppression, cell-cycle control, and interactions with cellular and viral proteins. Most mutations in human tumors occur in the evolutionarily highly conserved domains in exons 5 to 8 of the p53 gene.[63] Moreover, the missense mutations are predominantly transitions at G:C base pairs, and 95% of the amino acids are entirely conserved in mouse, rat, monkey, and human. Mutational spectra also vary among cancer types (Table 11–3). The G:C→A:T transitions are most frequent in colon tumors and 68% occur at CpG dinucleotides. These findings are consistent with endogenous mutational mechanisms due to deamination of 5-methylcytosine residues. More than half of the p53 mutations in colon tumors are at hotspot codons 175, 248, 273, or 282, each of which is a CpG dinucleotide. In contrast to colon tumors, CpG dinucleotides are less frequently found at mutation sites of other human cancers. For example, G:C→T:A transversions are seen commonly in breast and lung cancers but not in colon tumors. CpG→TpG mutations occur with intermediate frequency in esophageal cancers, but 36% of these mutations are at A:T pairs, which may be due in part to DNA depurination or exposure to chemical carcinogens such as urethane (a contaminant of certain alcoholic beverages) or acetyladehyde (a metabolite of ethanol).

The most striking p53 mutational spectrum is found in hepatocellular carcinomas from Qidong, People's Republic of China[64] and southern Africa.[65] Eleven out of 12 base substitution mutations in 26 tumors were at the third base position of codon 249, and all but one were G:C→T:A transversions. One additional mutation at codon 157 was also a G:C→T:A transversion. These tumors were from patients who live in geographic areas where aflatoxin B_1 and hepatitis B virus are major risk factors for liver cancer. Aflatoxin B_1, a product of mold that grows in crops, forms promutagenic adducts on deoxyguanosine and induces primarily G:C→T:A transversions and G:C→A:T transitions in experimental systems.[66] Analysis of liver tumors from geographical areas where aflatoxin B_1 is considered not to be a significant risk factor will help determine whether exposure to this carcinogen or another coincident carcinogen may be responsible for these p53 mutations.

CHEMICAL-VIRAL INTERACTIVE EFFECTS

Interactive effects of chemicals, viruses, physical agents, and host factors have been observed (Table 11–4). One example is the relation of aflatoxin B_1 and hepatitis virus to the development of hepatocellular carcinoma. Hepatitis B virus (HBV) and more recently hepatitis C virus have been linked to primary hepatocellular carcinoma.[67] Geographic location of HBV carriers indicates that factors such as aflatoxin B_1 and alcoholic beverages are also important. Another example is in uranium miners, in whom the coexposure of tobacco smoke and radon significantly acts to increase risk of lung cancer.[68] Occupational asbestos exposure and tobacco consumption also act synergistically to increase the incidence of bronchogenic carcinoma.[69] In the laboratory, in vitro DNA strand breaks increase with the combined exposure.[70] Moreover, tobacco smoke and asbestos, through their ability to induce inflammation and lipid peroxidation, cause oxidative DNA damage.[71,72] Another consideration for the interactive effect is the ability of asbestos to adsorb PAHs and act as a carrier for the carcinogen.[73]

TABLE 11–3. Examples of Human Cancers With Base Substitution Mutations in the p53 Gene

Worldwide Cancer Burden (Rank)[182]	Cancer	Number of Mutations Detected in Tumor Cell Lines and Tumors*	Mutational Hotspots (Codon)	Mutations					
				A:T	G:C	CpG → TpG	G:C → A:T	G:C → T:A	G:C → C:G
1	Stomach	6		2	4	2	3	1	0
2	Lung	70	273	7	63	14	22	32	9
3	Breast	63		15	48	14	27	12	9
4	Colon	48	175, 248, 272, 282	10	38	30	36	0	2
7	Esophagus	38		12	26	7	16	10	0
8	Liver	22	249	2	20	0	3	16	1
11	Bladder	15		3	12	5	7	2	3
9, 12	Leukemia and lymphomas	84	175, 213, 248, 272, 282	26	58	35	45	6	7
—	Skin	16		0	16	1	11†	4	1
—	Sarcomas	12		0	12	7	8	2	2
—	Brain	24	273	4	20	9	17	2	1
—	Ovary	14		3	11	1	6	1	4

* Mutation screening by an RFLP analysis of one site is not included.
† Includes tandem double mutations.

ASSESSMENT OF CANCER RISK IN HUMANS

Our understanding of carcinogenesis and risk to human health comes from experimental models and methods including mutagenesis assays, mammalian cell-culture experiments, animal studies, classic epidemiology, and molecular epidemiology. The usefulness of each method can be contrasted with its limitations (Table 11–5). The evaluation of an individual patient must rely on an accurate history, physical examination, and research data. The latter is often beyond the scope of the practitioner, but methods of individual cancer risk assessment have been proposed and resources are available.[74] Some known or potential human carcinogens are indicated in Table 11–6.

Short-term assays for mutagenesis provide quick and inexpensive screens for potential carcinogens.[75,76] Among the most widely used and sensitive is the Ames' assay, in which frameshift mutations or base-pair substitutions are measured in *Salmonella typhimurium* bacteria.[77] The Ames' assay also

TABLE 11–4. Interactive Effects of Carcinogens, Viruses, and Host Factors

Type	Example	Associated Tumor
Chemical-chemical	Tobacco smoke and alcoholic beverages	Otolaryngeal, esophageal
Viral-chemical	HPV and tobacco smoke	Cervical
	EBV and N-nitrosamine	Nasopharyngeal
	HBV and aflatoxin B₁	Liver
Physical-chemical	Asbestos and tobacco smoke	Lung
	Radon and tobacco smoke	Lung
Chemical-host	PAH and CYP2D6	Lung
	Tobacco smoke and CYP2D6	Lung
Physical-host	Asbestos and CYP2D6	Lung
	Sunlight and xeroderma pigmentosum	Skin
	Radiation and *RB*-deficient genotype	Osteosarcoma
Viral-host	EBV and X-linked immunodeficiency syndrome	Lymphoma

HPV, human papilloma virus; EBV, Epstein-Barr virus; HBV, hepatitis B virus; CYP2D6, ctytochrome P-450 CYP2D6 metabolic phenotype determined by debrisoquine sulfate administration and measurement of urinary metabolites; PAH, polycyclic aromatic hydrocarbon; *RB*, retinoblastoma susceptibility gene.

TABLE 11–5.　Testing for Carcinogenicity

Method	Advantages	Disadvantages
In vitro testing	Economical Rapid results Human cells can be used	Uncertain in vitro to in vivo extrapolations Frequent false-positives and false-negatives Mutagenicity is not carcinogenicity Substantial interlaboratory variation
Animal bioassay	More predictive of human experience than short term tests Elucidates species differences	Expensive Doses are higher than those experienced by humans Uncertain animal to human extrapolation
Classic epidermiology	Direct measurement of human experience Covariables examined Dose-response data	Insensitive Does not prove causation Unknown confounding variables
Molecular epidemiology	Measures internal dosimeter of exposure and genetic predisposition Identifies risk in an individual	Early stage of development and validation

TABLE 11–6.　Selected Known or Potential Human Carcinogens[183]

Known or Potential Carcinogen*	Target Organs	Known or Potential Carcinogen*	Target Organs
Chemical		**Industry†**	
Aflatoxin	Liver	Aluminum production	Lung, bladder
4-Aminobiphenyl	Bladder	Auramine manufacture	Bladder
Arsenic	Skin, lung	Boot and shoe manufacture	Bone marrow, nasal sinus
Asbestos	Lung, pleura	Coal gasification	Skin, lung, bladder
Benzene	Bone marrow	Coke production	Skin, lung, kidney
Benzidine	Bladder	Furniture and cabinet manufacture	Nasal
Benzo[a]pyrene	Skin, lung	Iron and steel founding	Lung
Beryllium	Lung	Hematite mining (radon)	Lung
bis(chloromethyl)ether	Lung	Isopropyl alcohol manufacture	Nasal sinus
Cadmium	Prostate, lung	Magenta manufacture	Bladder
Chromium	Lung	Paints	Lung
Coal tar and pitch	Skin, lung, bladder	Rubber industry	Bone marrow, bladder
Nickel compounds	Lung, nasal cavity	**Viral**	
Vinyl chloride	Liver, lung, brain	Epstein-Barr virus	Nasopharynx
Mineral oils	Skin	Hepatitis B	Liver
Mustard gas	Lung	Hepatitis C	Liver
2-Napthylamine	Bladder	Human immunodeficiency	Lymphatic
Shale oils	Skin	Human T-lymphocyte	Lymphatic, bone marrow
Soots	Skin, lung	Human papilloma	Cervical
Lifestyle and Diet			
Betel quid with tobacco	Oral		
Tobacco smoke	Multiple sites		
Alcoholic beverage	Oral, esophageal, pancreas, liver		
Smoked, salted, pickled foods	Gastrointestinal		
High fat diet	Colon, mammary		

* Carcinogenic agents or activities in this table are classified by the International Agency For Research on Cancer as recognized human carcinogens. The list is not all inclusive.
† Refers to only some occupations within an industry.
(Tomatis L, Aitio A, Wilbourn J, Shuker L., Human carcinogens so far identified. Jpn J Cancer Res 1989;80:795–807)

has been used as a biomonitor in humans. Urine from cigarette smokers, for example, is mutagenic.[78] Other short-term assays use Chinese hamster ovary cells, mouse lymphoma cells, V79 cells, or rat hepatocytes to measure forward mutations, sister chromatid exchanges, and unscheduled DNA synthesis.[79] Although short-term assays are useful in identifying potentially carcinogenic compounds in the respective cell system, the same sensitivity makes the results difficult to extrapolate to humans; positive results might be unique to the strain. Factors such as metabolism, repair, and exposure cannot be assessed.

Laboratory animal studies provide an important source for the identification of potential carcinogens in humans, mostly because few better alternatives exist. These animal bioassays are also expensive and time-consuming, preventing the testing of a large number of chemicals.[76,80] As recommended by the National Toxicology Program, carcinogenicity bioassay studies should use lifetime exposures in rats and mice with maximally tolerated doses (MTD), that is, those not producing clinically evident toxic effects. To infer that a carcinogenic effect is present in laboratory animals, dose-response relations, overall mortality rates, and consistency with data from other species must be examined. The limitations in these experiments include the routine use of the MTD that potentially increases cell replication and endogenous mutations; interspecies and interstrain differences; use of rodents known to have high spontaneous rates of cancer; an inability to account for metabolic differences between high- and low-dose exposure; and difficulty in interpreting data from doses that commonly exceed those experienced by humans.[81-83]

Human investigations provide the most relevant data regarding human risk. Classic epidemiology measures the incidence or prevalence of disease in human populations. Epidemiologic studies have identified previously unknown risks such as asbestos-related pleural mesothelioma, benzene-induced leukemia, and bladder cancer in dye workers. Epidemiologic methods by themselves do not demonstrate causation. The assessment of causation can be aided by Sir Austin Bradford-Hill's proposed criteria, which consider the strengths of an association, consistency, specificity, temporality, biologic gradients, biologic plausibility, coherence, and analogies.[84] Study design and controlling for confounding variables are important determinants of a true association. For example, assessing cancer mortality rates from death certificates can be unreliable because the certificate diagnosis frequently is not accurate. Loss of persons in follow-up, inappropriate choice of control populations, ascertainment bias secondary to an unrelated cancer cluster, and "healthy worker effects" may also influence outcomes. The latter effect can be important if an occupation impacts on risk factors, for example, by not allowing tobacco consumption at the workplace. It is also important to examine existing exposure data and dose-response relations. Finally, statistical methods, beyond the scope of this chapter, must be carefully chosen to determine whether a finding is attributable to chance.

The concordance between different methods for inferring human cancer risk is variable. In such cases as aflatoxin B$_1$, mustard gas, radon, and vinyl chloride, animal testing revealed a carcinogenic risk before human epidemiologic evidence was available.[83] Comparing DNA reactivity based on chemical structure, mutagenicity, carcinogenicity in laboratory animals and epidemiology, most chemicals that have positive results in one method are generally positive with other methods, although 100% concordance does not exist. Sensitivity for short-term assays is high but specificity is low.[83,85] For example, chemicals that are predictive of reactivity by chemical structure are commonly mutagenic, but 84% of tested carcinogens and 66% of noncarcinogens are mutagenic.[83,86] Chemicals that are not predictive of reactivity and are nonmutagenic are carcinogenic less than 5% of the time. The concordance from animal to human experience is wide ranging (5% to 70%), although carcinogens that are more potent in one species tend to be more potent in others.[85,87]

The physician can look to various regulatory, governmental, or review organizations for extensive evaluation of the scientific literature. Some organizations generate documents reporting the findings of a panel of experts who critically review the scientific literature, whereas others simply summarize data from other organizations. Several lists of carcinogens have also been published, but the evaluations of the literature and the definitions can vary greatly among organizations.[74] The physician should be aware of the purposes and goals of an organization when requesting its information. Quantitative risk assessment methods are used by regulatory agencies to estimate the risk to a population exposed to a particular carcinogen at a specific dose. Risk assessments serve public health interests as they attempt to predict the frequency of cancer in a population before epidemiologic investigations can be performed and adverse outcomes occur. Several mathematical models rank relative risks and suggest regulatory exposures limits. Risk assessments include four general steps.[88]

1. Hazard assessment, which qualitatively reviews scientific literature to determine whether a hazard might exist
2. Dose-response assessment, which evaluates the doses used in scientific studies and relates them to human exposures
3. Exposure assessment, which examines a population thought to be at risk with regard to the quantity, duration, and routes of exposure. Necessary information includes quantitative measurements of relevant media such as soil, water, air, or body fluids.
4. Risk characterization, which incorporates the above information and evaluates the assumptions and the uncertainties to estimate risk. At the conclusion, an incidence of cancer will be predicted, such as 1 additional person in 1 million persons.

Each of these steps requires assumptions that are open to debate, such as subjective evaluations of the literature, extrapolations from laboratory animals to humans, and mathematical methods. It is tempting to extrapolate conclusions of a formal risk assessment to risk for a given individual, especially if that person is a cancer patient. Such an exercise is inherently flawed because risk assessments calculate risk in a group of people and do not assess coexposures or inheritable variables that may increase or decrease an individual's risk of cancer. Separately, risk assessments must be reevaluated when experimental or epidemiologic data become available. One example is dioxin exposure, whose laboratory animal carcinogenicity data led to strict regulation in humans and with considerable cost. However, recent data have led the Environmental Protection Agency to review its policy.[89]

MOLECULAR EPIDEMIOLOGY OF HUMAN CANCER

Molecular epidemiology is a multidisciplinary field that seeks to explore cancer risk through molecular genetics and biochemical methods.[90] In contrast to classic epidemiology, which identifies cancer risk in populations, molecular epidemiology explores cancer risk in individuals. This strategy includes exposure assessments by measuring biologically effective doses of carcinogens in target tissues (or surrogate tissues) and an analysis of host susceptibility factors, within the framework of well-designed epidemiologic studies.

EXPOSURE ASSESSMENT

Carcinogen-DNA adducts, somatic gene mutations, and cytogenetic changes can be measured in the DNA of target cells or in surrogate blood cells.[90–94] The observation that carcinogen-DNA adducts formed in cultured human tissues are generally the same as those found in experimental animal cancer models has encouraged investigators to search for DNA adducts in humans. Carcinogen-DNA adducts are the result of exposure, absorption, metabolism, and DNA repair. The amount of a carcinogen that reaches the target DNA reflects the biologically effective dose and can be distinguished from the relevance of ambient air or other environmental measurement of exposure. A variety of assays are available to identify carcinogen-DNA adducts in human tissues.[90,91] Studies using laboratory animals generally demonstrate a relation between dose, adduct level, and carcinogenicity.[91,95] It is expected that human epidemiologic studies will bear a similar relation.

The most important lifestyle risk factor in carcinogenesis is tobacco smoke exposure.[96] Due to aggressive advertising and the addictive nature of cigarettes, tobacco smoke has become the major cause of cancer. Of growing concern is the documentation that passive exposure to tobacco smoke also increases the risk of lung cancer.[97,98] Putative adducts have been correlated with consumption by the ^{32}P-postlabeling assay in human lung,[99–101] alveolar lavage cells,[102] and placenta,[103] but not in lymphocytes[104] or oral mucosa.[105] Tobacco-specific N-nitrosamines are potent carcinogens in laboratory animals.[96] Levels are higher in secondary rather than mainstream smoke, highlighting the role of passive smoke exposure. Hemoglobin adducts are increased in smokers over nonsmokers, whereas even higher levels are reported in snuff dippers.[106] Nitrosamine-related adducts have also been found in the human lung.[107,108] Urine also can be used as a biomarker for tobacco smoke exposure because it is mutagenic in smokers. However, this cannot be solely attributed to tobacco because dietary heterocyclic amines also are found in the urine.[109]

PAHs, associated with an increased risk of lung and skin cancer, can cause adducts found in the white blood cells of persons exposed to coke oven emissions, tobacco smoke, and urban areas (*e.g.*, from industrial pollution).[110–116] Dietary exposure resulting from the overcooking of meats and fish also results in elevated adduct levels.[117] Adducts also have been found in human lung and placental samples.[118] Wide interindividual variations in levels have been noted, presumably reflecting variable cancer risk in individuals.

Among the best-studied dietary carcinogens are the aflatoxins produced by *Aspergillus flavus* and *Aspergillus parasiticus*. These molds are contaminants of corn, peanuts, sorghum, and rice. The risk of hepatocellular carcinoma correlates with the degree of contamination by geographic region.[119] Adduct levels also correlate with regional exposure and are inversely correlated with residence in industrialized countries.[119,120] N-nitrosamines also are dietary (and tobacco smoke) carcinogens whose adducts can be measured in DNA.[121–126] In this case, adduct levels are elevated in Chinese persons with esophageal cancer[121] and in Japanese persons with liver cancer,[121] confirming the risk associated with these adducts and their parent N-nitroso compounds.

INTERINDIVIDUAL VARIATION AND HOST SUSCEPTIBILITY FACTORS

> No one supposes that all the individuals of the same species are cast in the very same mould. These individual differences are highly important for us. . . .
> Charles Darwin, *The Origin of Species*, 1859

Metabolic Activation and Deactivation

Physicians and scientists have repeatedly recognized person-to-person differences in behavior, morphology, and risk of disease. Such interindividual differences reflect inherited and acquired factors. For example, inherited differences in susceptibility to physical or chemical carcinogens have been observed, including an increased risk of sunlight-induced skin cancer in people with xeroderma pigmentosum,[127] bladder cancer in dye stuff workers with a poor acetylator phenotype,[128] and bronchogenic carcinoma in tobacco smokers who have an extensive debrisoquine hydroxylator phenotype.[129,130] Because most chemical carcinogens require metabolic activation to exert their oncogenic effects, interindividual variation in metabolism is considered to be an important determinant of cancer susceptibility.[32]

PAH metabolism is probably the best example of the effects of interindividual variation and cancer risk. Several thousand-fold interindividual variation has been observed in lung.[32] Placental aryl hydrocarbon hydroxylase (AHH) activity, which is under direct genetic control, can be induced by maternal exposure to environmental carcinogens (*e.g.*, tobacco smoke or dietary factors).[131,132] Higher AHH activity is generally correlated with higher adduct level.[101] The induction process itself may have a genetic component,[133] and inducible activity is higher in cultured lymphocytes from lung cancer cases compared with controls.[134] The ability to form benzo[a]pyrene diolepoxide–DNA adducts was higher in lung cancer patients than in controls.[135,136] A highly inducible allelic variant of CYP1A1 has been identified in humans.[137,138] A restriction fragment length polymorphism for CYP1A1 has also been described that is associated with increased risk of tobacco smoking associated lung cancer in a Japanese study.[139]

CYP2D6 activity, another P450 cytochrome, is polymorphic and has also been linked to lung cancer risk.[129,130] CYP2D6 hydroxylates xenobiotic antihypertensives (including debrisoquine), antidepressives, and a carcinogenic tobacco-specific N-nitrosamine.[140] An individual's polymorphic phenotype is inherited in an autosomal recessive manner. The rate of 4-hydroxylation of debrisoquine varies several thousand-fold among people. Lung, liver, and advanced bladder cancer patients are more likely to have the extensive hydroxylator phenotype when compared with noncancer controls.[129,141,142] The increased risk in lung cancer is found primarily for histologic types other than adenocarcinoma of the lung and increases in persons who are occupationally exposed to high amounts of asbestos or PAHs.[130,143]

Acetylation of carcinogenic aromatic amines has been proposed as a cancer risk factor.[144] The N-acetylation polymorphism is controlled by two autosomal alleles at a single locus in which rapid acetylation is the dominant trait and slow acetylation is recessive. The slow acetylator phenotype has been linked to occupationally induced bladder cancer in dye workers exposed to large amounts of N-substituted aryl compounds.[128] In contrast, the rapid acetylator phenotype is more commonly found in cases from two studies of colon cancer[145,146] but not in another.[147] Whether this association is due to metabolism of a carcinogenic aromatic amine in the colonic epithelium is not known.

Glutathione S-transferases (GST) are multifunctional proteins that catalyze the conjugation of glutathione and electrophiles, including the ultimate carcinogenic metabolite of benzo[a]pyrene.[148,149] The three isoenzymes of GST (α, μ, and π) vary in their substrate specificity, tissue distribution, and activities among individuals.[150] Expression of GST-μ is inherited as an autosomal dominant trait[151] and individuals with low GST-μ activity may be at a greater risk for lung cancer caused by cigarette smoking.[152,153]

Protooncogenes and Tumor Suppressor Genes

Genetic differences in protooncogenes and tumor suppressor genes can also be predictive of cancer risk. Inheritance of a germline mutation in the tumor suppressor gene p53[154,155] and perhaps *RB*[156] predisposes to the development of cancer. It has been found that inheritance of rare alleles for H-*RAS*, detected by a restriction enzyme digest and Southern blot analysis, is found more frequently in lung cancer cases than controls.[157,158] These alleles may provide an unstable site where recombination or amplification occurs. The relation of this polymorphism to lung and other cancers has been extensively reviewed.[159] Analysis of the L-*MYC* protooncogene also demonstrates a polymorphic restriction enzyme site. The site present allele has been detected more frequently in persons with soft tissue sarcomas and gastric and lung cancer, although not consistently in lung cancer.[160–162] The association also suggests a worse prognosis at the time of diagnosis in renal cell cancer patients.

DNA Repair Rates

DNA repair enzymes modify carcinogenic damage by the removal of DNA adducts. Studies of cells from donors with xeroderma pigmentosum have been particularly important in expanding our understanding of DNA excision repair and its possible relation to risk of cancer.[127] DNA repair rates, but not fidelity, can be determined by measuring unscheduled DNA synthesis and removal of DNA adducts. Substantial interindividual variations in DNA repair rates have been observed.[163] The fidelity of DNA repair also may vary among individuals, and recent advances in the identification of mammalian DNA repair genes and their molecular mechanisms provide an opportunity for investigation.[164,165] In addition to finding severely depressed excision repair rates in xeroderma pigmentosum cells (*e.g.*, complementation group A), a fivefold variation among individuals in unscheduled DNA synthesis induced by UV exposure of lymphocytes in vitro has been found in the general population.[163] A significant reduction in unscheduled DNA synthesis induced in vitro by N-acetoxy-2-acetylaminofluorene has been observed in mononuclear leukocytes from individuals with a history of cancer in first-degree relatives compared with those without a family history.[166,167]

Interindividual variation has been noted in the activity of O^6-alkyldeoxyguanine-DNA alkyltransferase; this enzyme removes the adduct O^6-deoxyguanine caused by N-nitrosamine exposure. It is a suicide protein that transfers adducted alkyl groups to itself and becomes irreversibly inactivated. Cell cytotoxicity and tumor-cell resistance are negatively correlated with levels of this enzyme.[168] Wide variations in DNA repair activity have been observed in different types of tissues,[169,170] and cells may have lower repair rates after terminal differentiation.[171] The activity of this DNA repair enzyme is inhibited by certain aldehydes[169] and alkylating cancer chemotherapeutic agents.[172] A decrease in this DNA repair activity has been observed in fibroblasts from patients with lung cancer compared with donors with melanoma or noncancer controls.[173] Therefore, acquired or inherited deficiency in O^6-alkylguanine-DNA-alkyltransferase may be a cancer risk factor in tobacco smokers.

CARCINOGENICITY OF CHEMOTHERAPY

The carcinogenic effect of some chemotherapeutic agents in humans has been well documented and supported by laboratory animal studies (almost an 85% concordance), and reviews with extensive bibliographies are available.[174–176] The International Agency For Research on Cancer, through working groups of scientists and physicians, has identified about 20 single agents or combination chemotherapy regimens for which there is sufficient evidence of a carcinogenic effect in humans, and about 50 others in which a carcinogenic effect is suspected (Table 11–7).[174,177] The identification of a carcinogenic effect does not preclude its use for treatment in patients. The decision process depends on the specific risks and benefits, considering the prognosis and life expectancy of the patient with and without treatment.

Carcinogenic chemotherapeutic agents generally exhibit target organ specificity. The bone marrow, lymphatic system, and urinary bladder are most commonly affected. As with other carcinogens, genotoxic agents generally act by forming promutagenic DNA adducts and crosslinking,[174] although chromosomal aberration also occurs.[178] P450 metabolic activation is not necessarily required. Nitrogen mustard–type compounds (including nitrogen mustard, chlorambucil, melphalan, and chloronaphazine) have highly reactive electrophilic centers that react with DNA to form adducts without metabolic activation. Cyclophosphamide, in contrast, is a nitrogen mustard that undergoes cytochrome P450 metabolism in the liver, where it is converted to acrolein and 4-hydroxycyclophosphamide. This latter compound breaks down spontaneously to phosphoramide mustard, which then reacts with DNA.

TABLE 11–7. Selected Pharmaceutical Agents That Are Known or Potential Human Carcinogens*

Agent	Animal Target Organ	Human Target Organ
Phenacetin	Urinary tract, nasal	Kidney
Chloramphenicol	—†	Bone marrow
Doxorubicin	Mammary, skin	—
Azacitidine	Bone marrow, lymph, lung, skin	—
Chloronaphazine	Skin, lung	Bladder
Bischloroethylnitrosourea	Lung, neurologic, peritoneum	Bone marrow
Busulphan	Thymus, ovary	Bone marrow
Chlorambucil	Lung, bone marrow, ovary	Bone marrow
Chlorzotocin	Peritoneum	Bone marrow
Cisplatin	Lung, bone marrow	—
Cyclophosphamide	Mammary, bone marrow, bladder, liver, testis, neurologic	—
Melphalan	Lymphatic, lung	Bladder, bone marrow
Nitrogen mustard	Skin, lung, lymphatic	Bone marrow
Procarbazine	Lung, bone marrow, kidney	Skin
Streptozocin	Liver, pancreas	—
Thiotepa	Lung, lymphatic, bone marrow, uterus, mammary	—
Arsenic salts	Lung, stomach	Bone marrow
Coal tars	Skin	Skin
8-Methoxypsoralen & UVA	Skin	Skin
Testosterone	Cervix, uterus, prostate	Skin
Nonsteroid estrogen	Vagina, cervix, uterus, ovary, mammary	Liver Vagina, cervix
Estrogen replacement	Kidney	Endometrium
Azathioprine	Lymphatic	Lymphatic
Cyclosporine	Lymphatic	Lymphatic

* Classified by the Agency for Research on Cancer as known or possible human carcinogens. This list is not all inclusive.
† Cancer not observed.

Chemotherapy combinations can significantly raise the risk of secondary tumors, especially nonlymphocytic leukemias. The combination of lomustine, cyclophosphamide, and vincristine led to a leukemia incidence of 14% over 4 years after treatment.[179] Nitrogen mustard, vincristine, prednisone, and procarbazine for the treatment of Hodgkin's disease yield leukemia rates up to 17%.[180] More than six cycles increased the relative risk from 9 to 14. Radiation further increases the risk of leukemia.[181]

REFERENCES

1. Harris CC. Chemical and physical carcinogenesis: Advances and perspectives. Cancer Res 1991;51:5023S–5044S.
2. Hill J. Cautions against the immoderate use of snuff. London: R. Baldwin and J. Jacobson, 1761.
3. Pott P. Chirurgical observations relative to the cancer of the scrotum. London: L. Hawes, W. Clark, and R. Collins, 1775.
4. Rehn L. Blasengeschwulste bei fuchsin-arbeiten. Arch Klin Chir 1895;50:588–600.
5. Delore P, Borgomano C. Leucemie alignee au cours de l'intoxication benzenique: Sur l'origine toxique de certaines leucemies aigues et leur relations avec les anemies graves. J Med Lyon 1928;9:227.
6. Doll R, Hill AB. Smoking and carcinoma of the lung: Preliminary report. Br Med J 1950;2:739–748.
7. Wynder EL, Graham EA. Tobacco smoking as a possible etiologic factor in bronchogenic carcinoma. JAMA 1950;143:329–336.
8. Yamagiwa K, Ichikawa K. Experimental study of the pathogenesis of carcinoma. J Cancer Res 1918;3:1–21.
9. Brugge J, Curran T, Harlow E, McCormick F. Origins of human cancer. Cold Spring Harbor, NY: Cold Spring Harbor Laboratory Press, 1991.
10. Cooper C, Grover P, eds. Chemical carcinogenesis and mutagenesis I and II. Berlin: Springer-Verlag, 1990.
11. Foulds L. The experimental study of tumor progression: A review. Cancer Res 1954;14:317–339.
12. Rowley JD. Molecular cytogenetics: Rosetta stone for understanding cancer—The 29th G. H. A. Clowes memorial award lecture. Cancer Res 1990;50:3816–3825.
13. Schimke RT. The search for early genetic events in tumorigenesis: An amplification paradigm. Cancer Cells 1990;2:149–151.
14. Peto R, Roe FJ, Lee PN, Levy L, Clack J. Cancer and ageing in mice and men. Br J Cancer 1975;32:411–426.
15. Fearon ER, Vogelstein B. A genetic model for colorectal tumorigenesis. Cell 1990;61:759–767.
16. Butterworth BE, Slaga TJ. Nongenotoxic mechanisms in carcinogenesis: Banbury Report, vol 25. Cold Spring Harbor, NY: Cold Spring Harbor Laboratory Press, 1987.
17. Wilson VL, Smith RA, Longoria J, Liotta MA, Harper CM, Harris CC. Chemical carcinogen-induced decreases in genomic 5-methyldeoxycytidine content of normal human bronchial epithelial cells. Proc Natl Acad Sci USA 1987;84:3298–3301.
18. Lutz WK. Dose-response relationship and low dose extrapolation in chemical carcinogenesis. Carcinogenesis 1990;11:1243–1247.
19. Swenberg JA, Richardson FC, Boucheron JA, et al. High- to low-dose extrapolation: Critical determinants involved in the dose response of carcinogenic substances. Environ Health Perspect 1987;76:57–63.
20. Loeb LA. Mutator phenotype may be required for multistage carcinogenesis. Cancer Res 1991;51:3075–3079.

21. Lutz WK. Endogenous genotoxic agents and processes as a basis of spontaneous carcinogenesis. Mutat Res 1990;238:287–295.
22. Breimer LH. Molecular mechanisms of oxygen radical carcinogenesis and mutagenesis: The role of DNA base damage. Mol Carcinogen 1990;3:188–197.
23. Weinstein IB. Mitogenesis is only one factor in carcinogenesis. Science 1991;251: 387–388.
24. Ames BN, Gold LS. Too many rodent carcinogens: Mitogenesis increases mutagenesis. Science 1990;249:970–971.
25. Infante PF. Prevention versus chemophobia: A defense of rodent carcinogenicity tests [comments]. Lancet 1991;337:538–540.
26. Hay A. Carcinogenesis: Testing times for the tests [news]. Nature 1991;350:555–556.
27. Gonzalez FJ, Crespi CL, Gelboin HV. DNA-expressed human cytochrome P450s: A new age of molecular toxicology and human risk assessment. Mutat Res 1991;247: 113–127.
28. Nebert DW, Nelson DR, Coon MJ, et al. The P450 superfamily: Update on new sequences, gene mapping and recommended nomenclature. DNA Cell Biol 1991;10:1–20.
29. Gonzalez FJ. Molecular genetics of the P-450 superfamily. Pharmacol Ther 1990;45: 1–38.
30. Autrup H, Harris CC. Metabolism of chemical carcinogens by human tissues. In: Harris CC, Autrup H, eds. Human carcinogenesis. New York: Academic Press, 1983:169–194.
31. Harris CC. Human tissues and cells in carcinogenesis research. Cancer Res 1987;47: 1–10.
32. Harris CC. Interindividual variation among humans in carcinogen metabolism, DNA adduct formation and DNA repair. Carcinogenesis 1989;10:1563–1566.
33. Hall M, Grover PL. Polycyclic aromatic hydrocarbons: Metabolism, activation, and tumour initiation. In: Cooper CS, Grover PL, eds. Chemical carcinogenesis and mutagenesis I. Berlin: Springer-Verlag, 1990:327–372.
34. Barbacid M. *RAS* genes. Annu Rev Biochem 1987;56:779–827.
35. Bouck N. Tumor angiogenesis: The role of oncogenes and tumor suppressor genes. Cancer Cells 1990;2:179–185.
36. Liotta LA, Steeg PS, Stetler-Stevenson WG: Cancer metastasis and angiogenesis: An imbalance of positive and negative regulation. Cell 1991;64:327–336.
37. Bishop JM: Molecular themes in oncogenesis. Cell 1991;64:235–248.
38. Brown K, Buchmann A, Balmain A. Carcinogen-induced mutations in the mouse c-Ha-*RAS* gene provide evidence of multiple pathways for tumor progression. Proc Natl Acad Sci USA 1990;87:538–542.
39. Newcomb EW, Diamond LE, Sloan SR, Corominas M, Guerrero I, Pellicer A. Radiation and chemical activation of *RAS* oncogenes in different mouse strains. Environ Health Perspect 1989;81:33–37.
40. Marshall CJ, Vousden KH, Phillips DH. Activation of c-Ha-*RAS*-1 proto-oncogene by in vitro modification with a chemical carcinogen, benzo(a)pyrene diol-epoxide. Nature 1984;310:586–589.
41. Sukumar S. An experimental analysis of cancer: Role of *RAS* oncogenes in multistep carcinogenesis. Cancer Cells 1990;2:199–204.
42. Bailleul B, Surani MA, White S, et al. Skin hyperkeratosis and papilloma formation in transgenic mice expressing a *RAS* oncogene from a suprabasal keratin promoter. Cell 1990;62:697–708.
43. Leder A, Kuo A, Cardiff RD, Sinn E, Leder P. v-Ha-*RAS* transgene abrogates the initiation step in mouse skin tumorigenesis: Effects of phorbol esters and retinoic acid. Proc Natl Acad Sci USA 1990;87:9178–9182.
44. Knudson AG Jr. Mutation and cancer: Statistical study of retinoblastoma. Proc Natl Acad Sci USA 1971;68:820–823.
45. Cavenee WK, Dryja TP, Phillips RA, et al. Expression of recessive alleles by chromosomal mechanisms in retinoblastoma. Nature 1983;305:779–784.
46. Sapienza C. Genome imprinting, cellular mosaicism and carcinogenesis. Mol Carcinogen 1990;3:118–121.
47. Scheffner M, Werness BA, Huibregtse JM, Levine AJ, Howley PM. The E6 oncoprotein encoded by human papillomavirus types 16 and 18 promotes the degradation of p53. Cell 1990;63:1129–1136.
48. Herskowitz I. Functional inactivation of genes by dominant negative mutations. Nature 1987;329:219–222.
49. Green MR. When the products of oncogenes and anti-oncogenes meet. Cell 1989;56: 1–3.
50. Barrett JC. The relationship between mutagenesis and carcinogenesis. In: Brugge J, Curren T, Harlow E, McCormick F, eds. Origins of human cancer. Cold Spring Harbor, NY: Cold Spring Harbor Laboratory Press, 1991:101–112.
51. Sarasin A. Shuttle vectors for studying mutagenesis in mammalian cells. J Photochem Photobiol [B] 1989;3:143–155.
52. Basu AK, Essigmann JM. Site specifically modified oligodeoxynucleotides as probes for the structural and biological effects of DNA-damaging agents. Chem Res Toxicol 1988;1:1–18.
53. Skandalis A, Glickman BW. Endogenous gene systems for the study of mutational specificity in mammalian cells. Cancer Cells 1990;2:79–83.
54. Yang JL, Chen RH, Maher VM, McCormick JJ. Kinds and location of mutations induced by (+)-7β,8-dihydroxy-9,10-epoxy-7,8,9,10-tetrahydrobenzo[a]pyrene in the coding region of the hypoxanthine (guanine) phosphoribosyltransferase gene in diploid human fibroblasts. Carcinogenesis 1991;12:71–75.
55. Albertini RJ, Sullivan LM, Berman JK, et al. Mutagenicity monitoring in humans by autoradiographic assay for mutant T lymphocytes. Mutat Res 1988;204:481–492.
56. Loechler EL, Green CL, Essigmann JM. In vivo mutagenesis by O^6-methylguanine built into a unique site in a viral genome. Proc Natl Acad Sci USA 1984;81:6271–6275.
57. Doniger J, Notario V, DiPaolo JA. Carcinogens with diverse mutagenic activities initiate neoplastic guinea pig cells that acquire the same N-RAS point mutation. J Biol Chem 1987;262:3813–3819.
58. Brookes P. Chemical carcinogens and *RAS* gene activation. Mol Carcinogen 1989;2: 305–307.
59. Topal MD. DNA repair, oncogenes and carcinogenesis. Carcinogenesis 1988;9:691–696.
60. Wood ML, Dizdaroglu M, Gajewski E, Essigmann JM. Mechanistic studies of ionizing radiation and oxidative mutagenesis: Genetic effects of a single 8-hydroxyguanine (7-hydro-8-oxyguanine) residue inserted at a unique site in a viral genome. Biochemistry 1990;349:7024–7032.
61. Lindahl T, Nyberg B. Rate of depurination of native deoxyribonucleic acid. Biochemistry 1972;11:3610–3618.
62. Soussi T, Caron de Fromentel C, May P. Structural aspects of the p53 protein in relation to gene evolution. Oncogene 1990;5:945–952.
63. Hollstein M, Sidransky D, Vogelstein B, Harris CC. P53 mutations in human cancers. Science 1991;253:49–53.
64. Hsu IC, Metcalf RA, Sun T, Welsh J, Wang NJ, Harris CC. P53 gene mutational hotspot in human hepatocellular carcinomas from Qidong, China. Nature 1991;350: 427–428.
65. Bressac B, Kew M, Wands J, Ozturk M. Selective G to T mutations of p53 gene in hepatocellular carcinoma from southern Africa. Nature 1991;350:429–431.
66. McMahon G, Davis EF, Huber LJ, Kim Y, Wogan GN. Characterization of c-Ki-*RAS* and N-*RAS* oncogenes in aflatoxin B$_1$-induced rat liver tumors. Proc Natl Acad Sci USA 1990;87:1104–1108.
67. Harris CC. Hepatocellular carcinogenesis: Recent advances and speculations. Cancer Cells 1990;2:146–148.
68. Committee on the Biological Effects of Ionizing Radiation National Research Council (BEIR IV): Health risks of radon. Washington, DC: National Academy Press, 1988:1.
69. Saracci R. The interactions of tobacco smoking and other agents in cancer etiology. Epidemiol Rev 1987;9:175–193.
70. Jackson JH, Schraufstatter IU, Hyslop PA, et al. Role of oxidants in DNA damage: Hydroxyl radical mediates the synergistic DNA damaging effects of asbestos and cigarette smoke. J Clin Invest 1987;80:1090–1095.
71. Mossman BT, Marsh JP. Evidence supporting a role for active oxygen species in asbestos-induced toxicity and lung disease. Environ Health Perspect 1989;81:91–94.
72. Kamp DW, Dunne M, Weitzman SA, Dunn MM. The interaction of asbestos and neutrophils injures cultured human pulmonary epithelial cells: Role of hydrogen peroxide. J Lab Clin Med 1989;114:604–612.
73. Mossman BT, Eastman A, Landesman JM, Bresnick E. Effects of crocidolite and chrysotile asbestos on cellular uptake and metabolism of benzo(a)pyrene in hamster tracheal epithelial cells. Environ Health Perspect 1983;51:331–335.
74. Shields PG, Harris CC. Environmental causes of cancer. Med Clin North Am 1990;74: 263–277.
75. Lave LB, Omenn GS. Cost-effectiveness of short-term tests for carcinogenicity. Nature 1986;324:29–34.
76. Ashby J, Morrod RS. Detection of human carcinogens. Nature 1991;352:185–186.
77. Ames BN, McCann J, Yamasaki E. Methods for detecting carcinogens and mutagens with the *Salmonella*/mammalian-microsome mutagenicity test. Mutat Res 1975;31: 347–364.
78. Yamasaki E, Ames BN. Concentration of mutagens from urine by absorption with the nonpolar resin XAD-2: Cigarette smokers have mutagenic urine. Proc Natl Acad Sci USA 1977;74:3555–3559.
79. Santella RM. In vitro testing for carcinogens and mutagens. In: Brandt-Rauf PW, ed. Occupational medicine—state of the art reviews. Philadelphia: Hanley & Belfus, 1987: 39–46.
80. Lave LB, Ennever FK, Rosenkranz HS, Omenn GS. Information value of the rodent bioassay. Nature 1988;336:631–633.
81. Ames BN, Magaw R, Gold LS. Ranking possible carcinogenic hazards. Science 1987;236: 271–280.
82. Lijinsky W. In vivo testing for carcinogenicity. In: Cooper CS, Grover PL, eds. Chemical carcinogenesis and mutagenesis I. Berlin: Springer-Verlag, 1990:179–209.
83. Tomatis L, Bartsch H. The contribution of experimental studies to risk assessment of carcinogenic agents in humans. Exp Pathol 1990;40:251–266.
84. Hill AB. The environment and disease: Association or causation. Proc Royal Soc Med 1965;58:295–300.
85. Tennant RW, Margolin BH, Shelby MD, et al. Prediction of chemical carcinogenicity in rodents from in vitro genetic toxicity assays. Science 1987;236:933–941.
86. Ashby J, Tennant RW. Definitive relationships among chemical structure: Carcinogenicity and mutagenicity for 301 chemicals tested by the U.S. NTP. Mutat Res 1991;257:229–306.
87. Purchase IF. Range of experimental evidence in assessing potential human carcinogenicity. Arch Toxicol Suppl 1980;3:283–293.
88. Russell M, Gruber M. Risk assessment in environmental policy-making. Science 1987;236:286–290.
89. Culliton BJ. US government orders new look at dioxin. Nature 1991;352:753.
90. Shields PG, Harris CC. Molecular epidemiology and the genetics of environmental cancer. JAMA 1991;266:681–687.
91. Wogan GN. Markers of exposure to carcinogens. Environ Health Perspect 1989;81: 9–17.
92. Menichini P, Abbondandolo A. Somatic gene mutations in humans. In: Gledhill BL, Mauro F, eds. Trends in biological dosimetry. New York: Wiley-Liss, 1991:267–279.
93. Albertini RJ, Robison SH. Human population monitoring. In: Li AP, Heflich RH, eds. Genetic toxicology: A treatise. Caldwell, NJ: Telford Press, 1991:375–420.

94. Wolff S. Biological dosimetry with cytogenetic endpoints. In: Gledhill BL, Mauro F, eds. Trends in biological dosimetry. New York: Wiley-Liss, 1991:351–362.

95. Lutz WK. Quantitative evaluation of DNA binding data for risk estimation and for classification of direct and indirect carcinogens. J Cancer Res Clin Oncol 1986;112: 85–91.

96. Hoffmann D, Hecht SS. Advances in tobacco carcinogenesis. In: Cooper CS, Grover PL, eds. Chemical carcinogenesis and mutagenesis I. Berlin: Springer-Verlag, 1990: 63–102.

97. Fielding JE, Phenow KJ. Health effects of involuntary smoking. N Engl J Med 1988;319: 1452–1460.

98. Wu-Williams AH, Samet JM. Environmental tobacco smoke: Exposure-response relationships in epidemiologic studies. Risk Anal 1990;10:39–48.

99. Dunn BP, Vedal S, San RH, et al. DNA adducts in bronchial biopsies. Int J Cancer 1991;48:485–492.

100. Phillips DH, Hewer A, Martin CN, Garner RC, King MM. Correlation of DNA adduct levels in human lung with cigarette smoking. Nature 1988;336:790–792.

101. Geneste O, Camus AM, Castegnaro M, et al. Comparison of pulmonary DNA adduct levels, measured by ^{32}P-postlabelling and aryl hydrocarbon hydroxylase activity in lung parenchyma of smokers and ex-smokers. Carcinogenesis 1991;12:1301–1305.

102. Izzotti A, Rossi GA, Bagnasco M, De Flora S. Benzo[a]pyrene diolepoxide-DNA adducts in alveolar macrophages of smokers. Carcinogenesis 1991;12:1281–1285.

103. Everson RB, Randerath E, Santella RM, Cefalo RC, Avitts TA, Randerath K. Detection of smoking-related covalent DNA adducts in human placenta. Science 1986;231:54–57.

104. Phillips DH, Schoket B, Hewer A, Bailey E, Kostic S, Vincze I. Influence of cigarette smoking on the levels of DNA adducts in human bronchial epithelium and white blood cells. Int J Cancer 1990;46:569–575.

105. Chacko M, Gupta RC. Evaluation of DNA damage in the oral mucosa of tobacco users and non-users by ^{32}P-postlabeling assay. Carcinogenesis 1988;9:2309–2313.

106. Carmella SG, Kagan SS, Kagan M, et al. Mass spectrometric analysis of tobacco-specific nitrosamine hemoglobin adducts in snuff dippers, smokers, and nonsmokers. Cancer Res 1990;50:5438–5445.

107. Wilson VL, Basu AK, Essigmann JM, Smith RA, Harris CC. O^6-alkyldeoxyguanosine detection by ^{32}P-postlabeling and nucleotide chromatographic analysis. Cancer Res 1988;48:2156–2161.

108. Shields PG, Povey AC, Wilson VL, Weston A, Harris CC. Combined high performance liquid chromatography/^{32}P-postlabeling assay of N7-methyldeoxyguanosine. Cancer Res 1990;50:6580–6584.

109. Peluso M, Castegnaro M, Malaveille C, et al. ^{32}Postlabelling analysis of urinary mutagens from smokers of black tobacco implicates 2-amino-1-methyl-6-phenylimidazo[4,5-b]pyridine (PhIP) as a major DNA-damaging agent. Carcinogenesis 1991;12:713–717.

110. Harris CC, Vahakangas K, Newman MJ, et al. Detection of benzo[a]pyrene diolepoxide-DNA adducts in peripheral blood lymphocytes and antibodies to the adducts in serum from coke oven workers. Proc Natl Acad Sci USA 1985;82:6672–6676.

111. Van Schooten FJ, Van Leeuwen FE, Hillebrand MJ, et al. Determination of benzo[a]pyrene diol epoxide-DNA adducts in white blood cell DNA from coke-oven workers: The impact of smoking. JNCI 1990;82:927–933.

112. Perera FP, Hemminki K, Young TL, Brenner D, Kelly G, Santella RM. Detection of polycyclic aromatic hydrocarbon-DNA adducts in white blood cells of foundry workers. Cancer Res 1988;48:2288–2291.

113. Bryant MS, Vineis P, Skipper PL, Tannenbaum SR. Hemoglobin adducts of aromatic amines: Associations with smoking status and type of tobacco. Proc Natl Acad Sci USA 1988;85:9788–9791.

114. Hemminki K, Grzybowska E, Chorazy M, et al. DNA adducts in humans environmentally exposed to aromatic compounds in an industrial area of Poland. Carcinogenesis 1990;11: 1229–1231.

115. Phillips DH, Hemminki K, Alhonen A, Hewer A, Grover PL. Monitoring occupational exposure to carcinogens: Detection by ^{32}P-postlabelling of aromatic DNA adducts in white blood cells from iron foundry workers. Mutat Res 1988;204:531–541.

116. Foiles PG, Miglietta LM, Quart AM, Quart E, Kabat GC, Hecht SS. Evaluation of ^{32}P-postlabeling analysis of DNA from exfoliated oral mucosa cells as a means of monitoring exposure of the oral cavity to genotoxic agents. Carcinogenesis 1989;10:1429–1434.

117. Rothman N, Poirier MC, Baser ME, et al. Formation of polycyclic aromatic hydrocarbon-DNA adducts in peripheral white blood cells during consumption of charcoal-broiled beef. Carcinogenesis 1990;11:1241–1243.

118. Manchester DK, Weston A, Choi JS, et al. Detection of benzo[a]pyrene diol epoxide-DNA adducts in human placenta. Proc Natl Acad Sci USA 1988;85:9243–9247.

119. Groopman JD, Cain LG, Kensler TW. Aflatoxin exposure in human populations: Measurements and relationship to cancer. CRC Crit Rev Toxicol 1988;19:113–145.

120. Wild CP, Jiang YZ, Sabbioni G, Chapot B, Montesano R. Evaluation of methods for quantitation of aflatoxin-albumin adducts and their application to human exposure assessment. Cancer Res 1990;50:245–251.

121. Huh NH, Satoh MS, Shiga J, Rajewsky MF, Kuroki T. Immunoanalytical detection of O4-ethylthymine in liver DNA of individuals with or without malignant tumors. Cancer Res 1989;49:93–97.

122. Wilson VL, Weston A, Manchester DK, et al. Alkyl and aryl carcinogen adducts detected in human peripheral lung. Carcinogenesis 1989;10:2149–2153.

123. Herron DC, Shank RC. Methylated purines in human liver DNA after probable dimethylnitrosamine poisoning. Cancer Res 1980;40:3116–3117.

124. Foiles PG, Miglietta LM, Akerkar SA, Everson RB, Hecht SS. Detection of O^6-methyldeoxyguanosine in human placental DNA. Cancer Res 1988;48:4184–4188.

125. Umbenhauer D, Wild CP, Montesano R, et al. O^6-methyldeoxyguanosine in oesophageal DNA among individuals at high risk of oesophageal cancer. Int J Cancer 1985;36: 661–665.

126. Wild CP, Montesano R. Immunological quantitation of human exposure to aflatoxins and N-nitrosamines. In: Vanderlaan M, Stanker LH, Watkins BE, Roberts DW, eds. Immunoassays for trace chemical analysis: Monitoring toxic chemicals in humans, food, and the environment. Washington, DC: American Chemical Society, 1991:215–228.

127. Cleaver JE. Do we know the cause of xeroderma pigmentosum? Carcinogenesis 1990;11: 875–882.

128. Cartwright RA, Glashan RW, Rogers HJ, et al. Role of N-acetyltransferase phenotypes in bladder carcinogenesis: A pharmacogenetic epidemiological approach to bladder cancer. Lancet 1982;2:842–845.

129. Ayesh R, Idle JR, Ritchie JC, Crothers MJ, Hetzel MR. Metabolic oxidation phenotypes as markers for susceptibility to lung cancer. Nature 1984;312:169–170.

130. Caporaso NE, Tucker MA, Hoover R, et al. Lung cancer and the debrisoquine metabolic phenotype. JNCI 1990;85:1264–1272.

131. Conney AH. Induction of microsomal enzymes by foreign chemicals and carcinogenesis by polycyclic aromatic hydrocarbons: The G. H. A Clowes Memorial Lecture. Cancer Res 1982;42:4875–4917.

132. Manchester DK, Jacoby EH. Sensitivity of human placental monooxygenase activity to maternal smoking. Clin Pharmacol Ther 1981;30:687–692.

133. Nowak D, Schmidt-Preuss U, Jorres R, Liebke F, Rudiger HW. Formation of DNA adducts and water-soluble metabolites of benzo[a]pyrene in human monocytes is genetically controlled. Int J Cancer 1988;41:169–173.

134. Kouri RE, McKinney CE, Slomiany DJ, Snodgrass DR, Wray NP, McLemore TL. Positive correlation between high aryl hydrocarbon hydroxylase activity and primary lung cancer as analyzed in cryopreserved lymphocytes. Cancer Res 1982;42:5030–5037.

135. Farmer PB, Bailey E, Gorf SM, et al. Monitoring human exposure to ethylene oxide by the determination of haemoglobin adducts using gas chromatography-mass spectrometry. Carcinogenesis 1986;7:637–640.

136. Hawke LJ, Farrell GC. Increased binding of benzo[a]pyrene metabolites to lymphocytes from patients with lung cancer. Cancer Lett 1986;30:289–297.

137. Peterson DD, McKinney CE, Ikeya K, et al. Human CYPIA1 gene: Co-segregation of the enzyme inducible phenotype and a restriction fragment length polymorphism. Am J Hum Genet 1991;48:720–725.

138. McLemore TL, Adelberg S, Liu MC, McMahon NA. Expression of cytochrome P450IA1 gene in lung cancer patients: Evidence for cigarette smoke-induced expression in normal lung and altered gene regulation in primary pulmonary carcinomas. JNCI 1990;82:1333–1339.

139. Kawajiri K, Nakachi K, Imai K, Yoshii A, Shinoda N, Watanabe J. Identification of genetically high risk individuals to lung cancer by DNA polymorphisms of the cytochrome P450IA1 gene. FEBS Lett 1990;263:131–133.

140. Crespi CL, Penman BW, Gelboin HV, Gonzalez FJ. A tobacco smoke-derived nitrosamine, 4-(methylnitrosamino)-1-(3-pyridyl)-1-butanone, is activated by multiple human cytochrome P450s including the polymorphic human cytochrome P4502D6. Carcinogenesis 1991;12:1197–1201.

141. Idle JR, Mahgoub A, Sloan TP, Smith RL, Mbanefo CO, Bababunmi EA. Some observations on the oxidation phenotype status of Nigerian patients presenting with cancer. Cancer Lett 1981;11:331–338.

142. Kaisary A, Smith P, Jaczq E, et al. Genetic predisposition to bladder cancer: Ability to hydroxylate debrisoquine and mephenytoin as risk factors. Cancer Res 1987;47:5488–5493.

143. Caporaso N, Hayes RB, Dosemeci M, et al. Lung cancer risk, occupational exposure, and the debrisoquine metabolic phenotype. Cancer Res 1989;49:3675–3679.

144. Beland FA, Kadlubar FF. Metabolic activation and DNA adducts of aromatic amines and nitroaromatic hydrocarbons. In: Cooper CS, Grover PL, eds. Chemical carcinogenesis and mutagenesis I. Berlin: Springer-Verlag, 1990:268–325.

145. Lang NP, Chu DZ, Hunter CF, Kendall DC, Flammang TJ, Kadlubar FF. Role of aromatic amine acetyltransferase in human colorectal cancer. Arch Surg 1986;121: 1259–1261.

146. Ilett KF, David BM, Detchon P, Castleden WM, Kwa R. Acetylation phenotype in colorectal carcinoma. Cancer Res 1987;47:1466–1469.

147. Ladero JM, Gonzalez JF, Benitez J, et al. Acetylator polymorphism in human colorectal carcinoma. Cancer Res 1991;51:2098–2100.

148. Jerina DM, Bend JA. Glutathione S-transferases. In: Jollow D, Kocsis JJ, Synder R, Vaino H, eds. Biological reactive metabolites. New York: Plenum Press, 1977:207–236.

149. Robertson IGC, Guthenberg C, Mannervik B, Jernstrom B. The glutathione conjugation of benzo(a)pyrene diol-epoxide by human glutathione transferases. In: Cooke M, Dennis AJ, eds. Polynuclear aromatic hydrocarbons: A decade of progress. Columbus, OH: Battelle Press, 1988:799–808.

150. Mannervik B. The isoenzymes of glutathione transferase. Adv Enzymol 1985;57:357–417.

151. Seidegard J, Pero RW. The hereditary transmission of high glutathione transferase activity towards trans-stilbene oxide in human mononuclear leukocytes. Hum Genet 1985;69:66–68.

152. Seidegard J, Pero RW, Miller DG, Beattie EJ. A glutathione transferase in human leukocytes as a marker for the susceptibility to lung cancer. Carcinogenesis 1986;7: 751–753.

153. Seidegard J, Pero RW, Markowitz MM, Roush G, Miller DG, Beattie EJ. Isoenzyme(s) of glutathione transferase (class Mu) as a marker for the susceptibility to lung cancer: A follow up study. Carcinogenesis 1990;11:33–36.

154. Malkin D, Li FP, Strong LC, et al. Germ line p53 mutations in a familial syndrome of breast cancer, sarcomas, and other neoplasms. Science 1990;250:1233–1238.

155. Srivastava S, Zou ZQ, Pirollo K, Blattner WA, Chang EH. Germline transmission of a mutated p53 in a cancer-prone family with Li-Fraumeni syndrome. Nature 1990;348: 747–749.

156. Sanders BM, Jay M, Draper GJ, Roberts EM. Non-ocular cancer in relatives of retinoblastoma patients. Br J Cancer 1989;60:358–365.

157. Krontiris TG, DiMartino NA, Colb M, Parkinson DR. Unique allelic restriction fragments of the human Ha-RAS locus in leukocyte and tumour DNAs of cancer patients. Nature 1985;313:369–374.

158. Sugimura H, Caporaso NE, Hoover RN, et al. Association of rare alleles of the Harvey *RAS* protooncogene locus with lung cancer. Cancer Res 1990;50:1857–1862.

159. Vineis P, Caporaso N. The analysis of restriction fragment length polymorphism in human cancer: A review from an epidemiological perspective. Int J Cancer 1991;47:26–30.

160. Kawashima K, Shikama H, Imoto K, et al. Close correlation between restriction fragment length polymorphism of the L-MYC gene and metastasis of human lung cancer to the lymph nodes and other organs. Proc Natl Acad Sci USA 1988;85:2353–2356.

161. Ishizaki K, Kato M, Ikenaga M, Honda K, Ozawa K, Toguchida J. Correlation of L-*MYC* genotypes to metastasis of gastric cancer and breast cancer. JNCI 1990;82:238–239.

162. Tamai S, Sugimura H, Caporaso NE, et al. Restriction fragment length polymorphism analysis of the L-*MYC* gene locus in a case-control study of lung cancer. Int J Cancer 1990;46:411–415.

163. Setlow RB. Variations in DNA repair among humans. In: Harris CC, Autrup H, eds. Human carcinogenesis. New York: Academic Press, 1983:231–254.

164. Hoeijmakers JHJ, Bootsma D. Molecular genetics of eukaryotic DNA excision repair. Cancer Cells 1990;2:311–320.

165. Lindahl T, Wood RD, Karran P. Molecular deficiencies in human cancer-prone syndromes associated with hypersensitivity to DNA damaging agents. In: Brugge J, Curren T, Harlow E, McCormick F, eds: Origins of human cancer. Cold Spring Harbor, NY: Cold Spring Harbor Laboratory Press, 1991:163–170.

166. Pero RW, Bryngelsson C, Bryngelsson T, Norden A. A genetic component of the variance of N-acetoxy-2-acetylaminofluorene-induced DNA damage in mononuclear leukocytes determined by a twin study. Hum Genet 1983;65:181–184.

167. Pero RW, Johnson DB, Markowitz M, et al. DNA repair synthesis in individuals with and without a family history of cancer. Carcinogenesis 1989;10:693–697.

168. Scudiero DA, Meyer SA, Clatterbuck BE, Mattern MR, Ziolkowski CH, Day RS. Sensitivity of human cell strains having different abilities to repair O^6-methylguanine in DNA to inactivation by alkylating agents including chloroethylnitrosoureas. Cancer Res 1984;44:2467–2474.

169. Grafstrom RC, Pegg AE, Trump BF, Harris CC. O^6-alkylguanine-DNA alkyltransferase activity in normal human tissues and cells. Cancer Res 1984;44:2855–2857.

170. Yarosh DB. The role of O^6-methylguanine-DNA methyltransferase in cell survival, mutagenesis and carcinogenesis. Mutat Res 1985;145:1–16.

171. Grafstrom RC, Fornace AJ Jr, Autrup H, Lechner JF, Harris CC. Formaldehyde damage to DNA and inhibition of DNA repair in human bronchial cells. Science 1983;220:216–218.

172. Sagher D, Karrison T, Schwartz JL, Larson R, Meier P, Strauss B. Low O^6-alkylguanine DNA alkyltransferase activity in the peripheral blood lymphocytes of patients with therapy-related acute nonlymphocytic leukemia. Cancer Res 1988;48:3084–3089.

173. Rudiger HW, Schwartz U, Serrand E, et al. Reduced O^6-methylguanine repair in fibroblast cultures from patients with lung cancer. Cancer Res 1989;49:5623–5626.

174. Ludlum DB. Therapeutic agents as potential carcinogens. In: Cooper CS, Grover PL, eds. Chemical carcinogenesis and mutagenesis I. Berlin: Springer-Verlag, 1990:153–175.

175. Casciato DA, Scott JL. Acute leukemia following prolonged cytotoxic agent therapy. Medicine (Baltimore) 1979;58:32–47.

176. Marselos M, Vainio H. Carcinogenic properties of pharmaceutical agents evaluated in the IARC monographs programme. Carcinogenesis 1991;12:1751–1766.

177. International Agency for Research on Cancer. Monographs on the evaluation of carcinogenic risks to humans: Overall evaluations of carcinogenicity—an updating of IARC monographs volumes 1 to 42. Lyon: International Agency for Research on Cancer, 1987.

178. Vyas RC, Adhvaryu SG, Shah VC. Effects of CCNU therapy on human chromosomes. Mutat Res 1988;206:163–166.

179. Pedersen-Bjergaard J, Osterlind K, Hansen M, Philip P, Pedersen AG, Hansen HH. Acute nonlymphocytic leukemia, preleukemia, and solid tumors following intensive chemotherapy of small cell carcinoma of the lung. Blood 1985;66:1393–1397.

180. Kaldor JM, Day NE, Clarke EA, et al. Leukemia following Hodgkin's disease [comments]. N Engl J Med 1990;322:7–13.

181. Valagussa P, Santoro A, Fossati-Bellani F, Banfi A, Bonadonna G. Second acute leukemia and other malignancies following treatment for Hodgkin's disease. J Clin Oncol 1986;4:830–837.

182. Parkin DM, Laara E, Muir CS. Estimates of the worldwide frequency of sixteen major cancers in 1980. Int J Cancer 1988;41:184–197.

183. Tomatis L, Aitio A, Wilbourn J, Shuker L. Human carcinogens so far identified. Jpn J Cancer Res 1989;80:795–807.

Cancer: Principles & Practice of Oncology, Fourth Edition,
edited by Vincent T. DeVita, Jr., Samuel Hellman, Steven A. Rosenberg.
J.B. Lippincott Co., Philadelphia © 1993.

Eric J. Hall

CHAPTER **12**

Principles of Carcinogenesis: Physical

This chapter discusses the induction of cancer by three physical agents: ionizing radiation, ultraviolet radiation, and mineral fibers. On one hand, these agents occur naturally in the environment, but on the other hand they are also man-made or man-enhanced. Low frequency electric and magnetic fields, as well as hyperthermia, are also discussed because it has been suggested (but not proved) that they may also be associated with an increased incidence of malignancies. Life on earth has always been exposed to ionizing radiations in the form of cosmic rays or radioactivity in the earth. To this must be added man-made radiations from medical radiology and nuclear power and man-enhanced sources, such as naturally occurring radon. Radon is enhanced because humans live in houses sealed against the heat or cold, where radon concentrates and decays. Ultraviolet radiation (UVR) from sunlight is natural, although the migration of fair-skinned people to warmer and sunnier climes greatly increases the incidence of UVR-induced cancer in humans. Asbestos also is a naturally occurring fiber. However, as a carcinogen it must be classified as man-enhanced, because it is hazardous only when it is mined and used in commercial products.

Studies of cancer induction by these physical agents have two distinct aims: first, to estimate the risk of cancer to the human population after exposure, and second, to elucidate mechanisms of cancer induction.

IONIZING RADIATIONS

HISTORIC PERSPECTIVE

Within 6 years of the discovery of x-rays, a causal relation was suspected between skin cancer and exposure to radiation.[1]

An association between leukemia and radiation exposure was suspected a few years later.[2] Martland first suspected the induction of cancer in humans by ingested radionuclides from a study of the radium dial painters in 1931.[3] There are many examples of an excess cancer incidence in human populations exposed to radiation, and there are excellent accounts of the experiences of early radiation workers.[4,5] Radiation protection standards in pioneering days were based largely on early effects, such as skin reaction, but the risk of cancer induction is currently the dominant factor in determining occupational exposure limits.

CHARACTERISTICS OF IONIZING RADIATION

A radiation is said to be ionizing if it has sufficient energy to eject one or more orbital electrons from an atom or molecule. The important characteristic of ionizing radiations is the local release of large amounts of energy, sufficient to break strong chemical bonds that are biologically important.

Ionizing radiations are classified as *electromagnetic* or *particulate*. Charged particles, such as electrons, protons, α particles, or heavy ions may ionize directly. Uncharged particles, notably neutrons, interact with the nuclei of atoms through which they pass and give up their energy to produce recoil protons, α particles, and heavier nuclear fragments, which go on to produce ionizations. X-rays and γ-rays are electromagnetic radiations at the short wavelength end of the spectrum. They give up part or all of their energy to orbital electrons of the atoms through which they pass, producing fast recoil electrons that have sufficient energy to be ionizing.

The dose, or quantity, of radiation is expressed in terms of the energy absorbed per unit mass of tissue. The unit is the

Gray, defined as 1 joule per kilogram. In the case of densely ionizing radiations, the track structure becomes important; energy absorption on a macroscopic scale (*i.e.,* dose) is then not an adequate description, and it is necessary to consider energy absorption in small volumes comparable to the dimensions of cellular components. The reader is referred to reviews of concepts of microdosimetry and nanodosimetry.[6-9]

The quality of a radiation is expressed in terms of the average density of ionization along the tracks of the charged particles. X-rays give rise to secondary electrons that are sparsely ionizing; they are referred to as *low linear energy transfer (low LET) radiation*. By contrast, α particles, with greater mass and slower velocity, are densely ionizing and are described as *high LET radiation*. Exposure to equal absorbed doses of high and low LET radiations do not result in the same biologic effect. The relative biologic effectiveness (RBE) of high LET radiations, such as neutrons and α particles, is greater than that of low LET radiations, such as x-rays or γ-rays. (RBE is the ratio of absorbed dose of a reference radiation, conventionally x-rays, to the absorbed dose of a test radiation to result in the same level of biologic effect). This is true for chromosomal aberrations, cell lethality, oncogenic transformation in vitro, or cancer induction in vivo. RBE values as high as 50 or more have been measured for some biologic endpoints at low doses.[10] The maximally effective radiation has a LET of about 100 keV/μm and results in a track in which the ionizations are separated, on average, by about 2 nm; this corresponds closely with the diameter of the DNA double helix as illustrated in Figure 12–1. This suggests that double-strand breaks may be the most important radiation-induced lesions, and other evidence suggests that the interaction of two double-strand breaks may be responsible for many radiation-induced biologic effects.

RADIATION DOSES TO WHICH THE HUMAN POPULATION IS EXPOSED

Life on earth has evolved against a background of ionizing radiations arising from cosmic rays and from radioactivity in the earth. The human population also is exposed to various synthetic or human-enhanced sources. The best estimate of the average annual effective dose equivalent from all sources to the U.S. population is 3.6 millisievert (mSv).[11] The composition of this dose is illustrated in Figure 12–2. Only in recent years has the importance of radon as the principal source of radiation to the U.S. general population been recognized. The home is the source of this exposure to radon, a naturally occurring radioactive gas that emanates from the ground and from building materials. Inside the home, it decays to short-lived radioactive daughters that attach to aerosol particles and are deposited in the tracheobronchial tree. The concern is the risk of lung cancer from the high LET α particles emitted during the decay of the daughter products, polonium 218 and polonium 214.[12-14] The potential exposure to radon varies widely in different parts of the country, depending on the uranium content of rock and soil; an even more uncertain factor is exposure to thoron, another radioactive gas that could contribute to lung dose.

Estimates of the number of lung cancers in the United States that result from radon vary from 4000 to 50,000 per year. Estimates are based on measured radon levels in homes and cancer risks extrapolated from epidemiologic studies of uranium miners and other underground miners, who are exposed to much higher levels of radon. The estimates vary according to the models and assumptions made.[12,13,15,16] The Environmental Protection Agency recommends an annual average radon level of 4 pCi/L of air as the level in homes at which remedial measures should be considered. This could affect as many as 8% to 12% of homes across the nation. The radiation dose associated with this radon level is much larger than that allowed for the general public from other radiation sources, which underlines the present equivocal view of radon; no one knows how seriously to take it.

Medical radiography results in about 15% of the total annual effective dose equivalent. The number of medical radiologic procedures exceeds the U.S. population (*i.e.,* the number of x-ray examinations averages more than one per person for every man, woman, and child in the United States). The av-

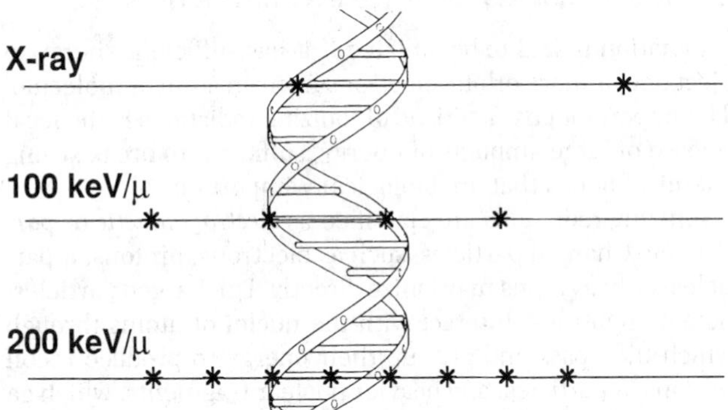

FIGURE 12–1. The radiation that is most effective biologically has a linear energy transfer of about 100 keV/μm. For this radiation the average separation between ionizing events coincides approximately with the diameter of the DNA double helix (20A or 2 nm), so that double strand breaks are produced most efficiently.

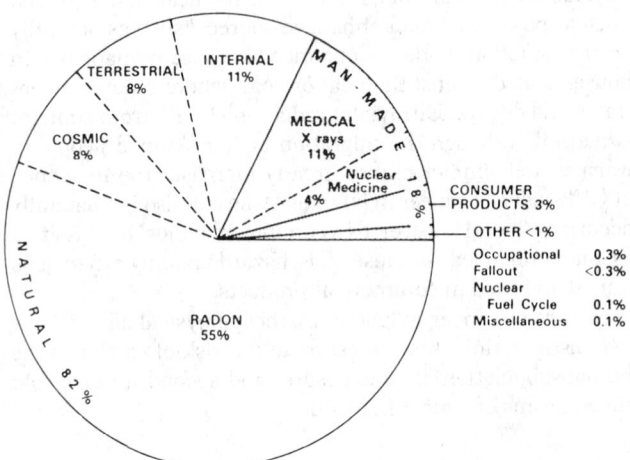

FIGURE 12–2. Estimated contribution of various radiation sources to the total average effective dose equivalent in the U.S. population. The estimates of some of the contributing sources, for example, radon, have uncertainties on the order of a factor of two or three. (NCRP Report 93: Ionizing Radiation Exposure of the Population of the United States. Bethesda, MD, NCRP, 1987)

erage bone marrow dose is estimated to be about 1 mSv, but individual doses vary widely. There are two balancing trends. Individual doses from a given procedure have been falling for the past two decades as faster films are developed and equipment is improved. On the other hand, computed tomography (CT) scans are ordered with increasing frequency, and these involve doses of several cGy, which tends to push the average dose up.

RADIATION-INDUCED CANCERS

There is a wealth of experience concerning cancer and leukemia induced in human populations by radiation.

1. Skin cancer was common in early x-ray workers, who worked around accelerators before radiation safety standards were introduced.
2. Lung cancer occurred in pitchblender miners and in uranium miners. Breathing radon gas led to the deposit of radon daughter products in the lungs, which emit intense α rays.[13,14]
3. Bone tumors were observed in radium dial painters, persons who painted luminous dials on clocks and watches with paint containing radium, which they ingested by licking the brush into a point.[3]
4. An excess incidence of liver cancer was reported in patients in whom the contrast material thorotrast was used; this contained thorium, an α emitter.[17]
5. The survivors of the atomic bomb attacks on Hiroshima and Nagasaki represent the most important single group. Leukemia and a whole spectrum of solid tumors have been observed.[18,19]
6. A small excess incidence of leukemia has been observed in patients suffering from ankylosing spondylitis who received radiotherapy for the relief of pain.[20-22]
7. Thyroid cancer has been reported in children irradiated for what was perceived to be an enlarged thymus, or epilated with x-rays for the treatment of ringworm of the scalp.[23-27]
8. There is an excess incidence of breast cancer in patients receiving radiotherapy for postpartum mastitis and also in patients with tuberculosis who were fluoroscoped many times during the management of artificial pneumothorax.[28-30]

Some of these instances are of little more than historical interest, because the radiation doses involved are not known with any certainty, but others are sufficiently quantitative to allow estimates to be made of the risk of cancer as a function of dose.

SENSITIVITY OF DIFFERENT TISSUES

Animal experiments, as well as the human experience, show that exposure to ionizing radiations in sufficient doses may induce cancer. The susceptibility of tissues varies widely, but all appear to be at risk.[31,32] There is no obvious relation between natural susceptibility and sensitivity to radiation-induced cancer. For example, thyroid cancer has a *low* natural and *high* radiation incidence. Breast cancer has a *high* incidence of natural and radiation-induced cancer. Colon cancer has a *high* natural and *low* radiation-induced incidence.

STOCHASTIC NATURE OF RADIATION-INDUCED CANCER

Radiation-induced cancer and the genetic effects of radiation are considered to be *stochastic late effects*. A stochastic effect has two characteristics. First, it has no threshold. Second, the severity of the effect is independent of the dose, although the probability of it occurring increases with dose. The far-reaching implication of this is that any dose, however small, carries with it some risk of inducing cancer. There are two justifications for this assumption. First, experimental evidence suggests no threshold, although it is not practical for dose-response curves to be taken down to very low doses. Second, the suggested mechanisms of cancer include processes such as a point mutation or a chromosome deletion that could be the consequence of the passage of a single charged particle track.

THE LATENT PERIOD

There is always a latent interval between irradiation and the appearance of an induced malignancy. Leukemia has the shortest latent period; excess cases appeared in the survivors of Hiroshima and Nagasaki by 5 to 7 years postirradiation.[18,19] By contrast, solid tumors have a longer latency and continue to appear in excess incidence for over 40 years.[18,19] Some of the latent interval may be due to the time required for the tumor to reach a sufficient size to be detectable; on the other hand, the processes of initiation, promotion, and progression also take time. Ideas concerning the latent period have changed in recent years, largely as a consequence of the continuing study of the Japanese survivors. Latency is no longer considered as a fixed time interval, because solid cancers induced by radiation tend to appear at the age at which the naturally occurring cancers of the same type are seen.[19] The latent period, therefore, is longer when exposure is early in life. This suggests that age-dependent host factors are important, and that the expression of cells initiated in the young are suppressed until the necessary host milieu is present.

DOSE-RESPONSE RELATIONS

Dose-response curves for the incidence of cancer as a function of dose are extremely complex (Fig. 12–3). For low LET radiations, excess incidence is proportional to dose at low doses; as the dose increases, the curve is concave upwards, indicating a linear-quadratic dependence on dose for acute exposures. At some point, the curve bends over as cell killing dominates over the initiation of more cells to a transformed state. A curve of this general form has been observed for many malignancies in experimental animals, notably for leukemia in mice and for oncogenic transformation in vitro.[34-38] For low LET radiations at low dose-rate, the dose-response curve remains linear over a wider range of doses and appears to be a continuation of the low-dose region of the acute dose-response curve.

This pattern of response, observed experimentally, is predicted by models of carcinogenesis that involve interaction of lesions and that allow for repair. The linear-quadratic form of the acute dose-response curve reflects the contributions of a single track (αD) and multiple tracks (αD^2), respectively. At low dose-rate, the number of tracks of ionizing events for

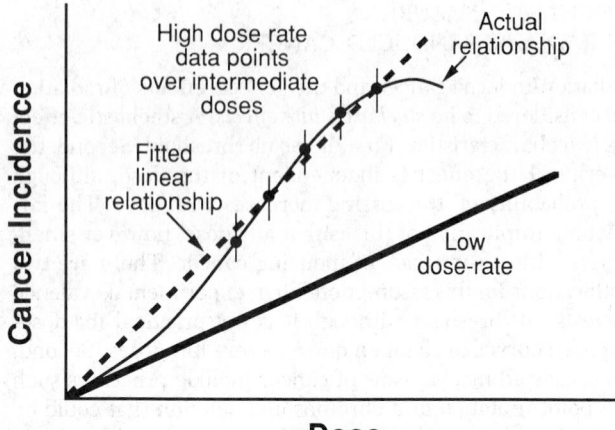

FIGURE 12–3. The data points for excess solid cancers in a human population exposed to an acute dose of low dose of low linear energy transfer (LET) radiation are frequently fitted by a linear function of dose. The data available are usually poor and cover a limited dose range. There are biophysical reasons to believe that the actual relation is more complex; excess cancer incidence rises as a linear-quadratic function of dose, but bends over at higher doses as cell killing becomes important. For low-dose-rate exposures of low LET radiation, excess cancer incidence approximates a linear function of dose, which is a continuation of the linear low-dose component of the high-dose-rate relation.

a given total dose is unchanged, but the probability of interactions between tracks is greatly diminished when the radiation is spread out over a long time. Time is biologically important because of repair.

For high LET radiations, dose-response relations tend to be steep and a linear function of dose. Consequently, RBE values are high, particularly at low doses. In contrast to the situation for low LET radiations, the biologic effect of a given dose of high LET radiation is not reduced by protraction of the dose by continuous low dose-rate or by fractionation. In the case of oncogenic transformation in vitro, induction of mammary tumors in mice and even the induction of lung tumors in humans by radon inhalation in low doses appear to be more effective than high doses.[39–41] Biophysical models have been invoked to account for this so-called *inverse dose-rate effect*.[43]

RISK ESTIMATES

Risk estimates for radiation-induced cancer by low LET radiation are based on the human experience. The most recent reassessments by the Committee on the Biological Effects of Ionizing Radiation (BEIR-V) of the National Academy of Sciences, and by the United Nations Scientific Committee on the Effects of Atomic Radiation (UNSCEAR) depend almost entirely on the atomic bomb survivors, but estimates are commensurate with those derived from other exposed human populations.[19,44]

Models used in the past were based on absolute or relative risk. An absolute risk model assumes that radiation produces a crop of malignancies over and above the natural incidence and unrelated to it. A relative risk model assumes that radiation increases the natural risk by a multiplicative factor. The choice of a projection model is crucial, because the major source of data for risk estimates is the atomic bomb survivors of whom

about one half are still alive. To estimate lifetime risks for the U.S. population from these data, therefore, involves projections in time and across populations. The favored model is a time-dependent relative risk model. The excess cancer incidence is assumed to be a function of dose, $(dose)^2$, age at exposure, time since exposure, and in some cases, sex. In fact, the best fit dose-response relation for most cases turned out to be a linear function of dose; only leukemia showed a significant dose squared term. The probable explanation for this finding is illustrated in Figure 12–4.

Table 12–1 summarizes risk estimates from the BEIR-V and UNSCEAR reports, comparing similar categories of cancers for which calculations were made. These estimates relate to an acute exposure of low LET radiation. It is not known whether lowering the dose-rate reduces the carcinogenic effect in humans, but data from animal experiments suggest a dose-rate effectiveness factor in the range of 2 to 10. The International Commission on Radiological Protection (ICRP) suggests an overall risk estimate of 4% per Sv for a working population and 5% for the general population.[4,5]

GENETIC FACTORS

There is no clear-cut proof of the influence of genetic factors on radiation-induced cancer, but some evidence is suggestive. The fact that in mice there are strain differences in radiation-induced (and natural) incidences of cancer attests to the importance of inherited factors, although susceptibility may be related to host factors that influence expression rather than initiation. When subjected to ionizing radiations in vitro, the cells of individuals with severe genetic diseases have been shown to produce chromatid abberations and to be sensitive to killing.[46–50] Perhaps more to the point, an elevated risk of cancer is associated with some genetic conditions, notably ataxia-telangiectasia,[51] but an increased susceptibility to radiation-induced cancer has not been shown. An important question, often posed but not answered, is whether the heterozygous state of any of the genetic disorders carries an increased risk. Second cancers in patients treated for cancer in

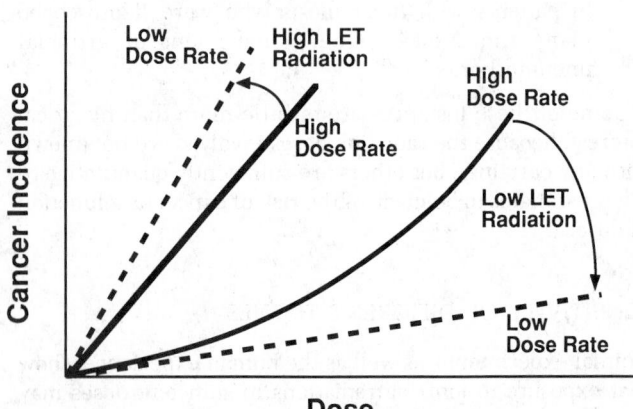

FIGURE 12–4. For low LET radiations, such as x-rays and γ-rays, excess cancer incidence increases as a linear-quadratic function of dose if the radiation is delivered in an acute exposure at high dose-rate. At low dose-rate, cancer incidence increases as a linear function of dose; the dose-response relation is an extrapolation of the initial slope of the high-dose-rate curve.

TABLE 12–1. Excess Cancer Mortality for Lifetime Risk of 100,000, 0.1 Sv

	BEIR V* (U.S. Population)		UNSCEAR 88† (Japanese Population)	
	Males	Females		
Breast	—	70	Breast	60
Respiratory	190	150	Lung	151
Digestive system	170	290	Stomach	126
Other solid	300	220	Colon	79
Leukemia	110	80	Other solid	194
			Leukemia	100
Total	770	810	Total	710

* (Data from National Research Council. Health effects of exposure to low levels of ionizing radiation. [BEIR V]. Washington, DC: National Academy Press, 1990)
† (Data from United Nations Scientific Committee on the Effects of Anatomic Radiation [UNSCEAR]. Genetic and somatic effects of ionizing radiation: Report E88 IX7. New York: United Nations, 1988)

childhood have a distinct pattern that reflects genetic susceptibility, but again it is not clear whether this susceptibility extends to radiation-induced cancer.

AGE AND SEX

Although the natural incidence of cancer generally increases with age, the risk of radiation-induced cancer is often greater when exposure occurs at younger ages. This is true of cancers of the breast,[18,19] lung,[18,52] stomach,[18,52] thyroid,[23,24] and connective tissue.[53] The recent reanalysis of the atomic bomb survivors shows that the change of susceptibility with age is particularly dramatic for breast cancer in women. Survivors who were less than 10 years old at the time of exposure are most susceptible, with risk decreasing steadily thereafter, becoming very small by late middle age.[19] In the case of leukemias in humans, the age dependency of susceptibility is more complex. The risk of leukemia was greater in 50-year-old spondylitic patients treated with x-rays than in patients under 25 years.[21] In the recent reevaluation of the atomic bomb survivors by the BEIR-V committee, a greater sensitivity was noted for radiation-induced leukemia before than after the age of 20 years.

The overall risk of radiation-induced cancer is estimated to be slightly higher in women than in men by about 10% (see Table 12–1). The difference can be largely accounted for by sex-specific tumors, principally those in the breast, which appears to be a susceptible tissue. Thyroid cancer after external radiation may also occur with higher frequency in women than in men.[23] On the other hand, male atomic bomb survivors appear to have been at greater risk than females for leukemia and cancers of the respiratory system.

RISKS OF CARCINOGENESIS AFTER RADIOTHERAPY

The risk of second malignancies after radiation therapy is a subject not without controversy. Some investigators report that doses between 40 and 60 Gy to limited areas do not significantly increase the incidence of second cancers.[54–56] In contrast, others report excess carcinogenesis when substantial doses are given to healthy organs.[57] Chemotherapy for Hodgkin's disease is reported to substantially elevate the risk of second malignancies, especially leukemia and bladder cancer.[60–62] Now that the combination of chemotherapy and radiation therapy is so commonly used, it is increasingly difficult to dissect out the risk of radiation alone. For this reason, two large studies reported recently are important. Both involve large numbers of patients with carcinoma of the uterine cervix. These form an ideal study group because survival is good, accurate dosimetry is possible, chemotherapy is rarely given, and surgically treated patients are available for comparison. Boice and colleagues reported a study of 150,000 patients treated for carcinoma of the uterine cervix.[63] Doses on the order of several hundred Gray were found to increase the risk of cancer of the bladder, rectum, vagina and possibly bone, uterine corpus, cecum, and non-Hodgkin's lymphoma. For all female genital cancer taken together, a sharp dose-response gradient was observed, reaching a fivefold increase for doses more than 150 Gy. Several Gray increased the risk of stomach cancer and leukemia. Cancer of the kidney was significantly increased among 15-year survivors. The situation concerning breast cancer was complex. For most cancers commonly associated with radiation, risks were highest among long-term survivors and appeared to be concentrated among women irradiated at younger ages.

Arai and his colleagues surveyed over 11,000 patients in Japan treated for cancer of the uterine cervix with radiotherapy alone, surgery alone, or postoperative radiation therapy.[64] They concluded that organs in the irradiated field, such as the rectum and bladder, showed an evident increase in the incidence of second cancers. The incidence of leukemia was also increased after radiation therapy.

It would appear, therefore, that when a sufficiently large number of patients are studied with adequate controls, radiation therapy does induce a small but significant incidence of second malignancies in heavily irradiated tissues and in organs more remote from the target area that receive a few Gray. Radiation is a known carcinogen and it should come as no surprise that elevated risks are seen after radiotherapy. Despite the large number of patients studied, at most about 5% of all second cancers could be convincingly linked to the radiation treatment.[63]

RISKS OF CANCER AFTER DIAGNOSTIC RADIOLOGY

The most recent estimate of the annual number of diagnostic radiographic examinations in the United States puts the figure at about 281 million.[65] Because the induction of leukemia has long been associated with radiation, the mean annual bone marrow dose from diagnostic procedures is clearly important. This is variously estimated as 0.75 to 1.14 mGy for adults. The collective effective dose equivalent from all diagnostic procedures performed in hospitals and doctors offices in the U.S. was estimated in 1980 to be 92,000 person-sievert.[65] This estimate may be low for the 1990s because of the increased use of CT scans. The population receiving diagnostic x-rays is substantially skewed with regard to age and sex distribution, so that a more realistic weighted collective effective dose equivalent may be smaller by about 36%.[65]

This widespread use of radiation for diagnostic purposes has led to the estimate that the practice of radiology in hospitals and doctors' offices for 1 year could induce about 1740 fatal and 580 nonfatal malignancies, about half of which may be leukemia.[66] A more pertinent figure, perhaps, is the risk to the individual of dying of cancer as a result of the radiation received in a given procedure. The risks for a barium enema and a radiograph of the extremities (representing procedures with the highest and lowest effective dose equivalent) are, respectively, 1 in 17,000 and 1 in 2.5 million. Compared with other risks of life, these are small and must be balanced against the medical benefit. For example, 1 in 17,000 is about the annual risk of accidental death for a worker in the manufacturing industries, whereas 1 in 2.5 million is about the annual risk of being hit by lightning.

Screening procedures, especially mammography, are a special case. To result in a benefit, a screening procedure should not induce more cancers than it detects. Studies designed to prove the benefit of screening by mammography in terms of a reduction in breast cancer mortality have produced results that are equivocal and contradictory. Both the prognosis for breast cancer and the susceptibility to radiation-induced cancer vary with age. Consequently, it is agreed that screening leads to a reduction in breast cancer mortality in older but not in younger patients. For the radiation doses associated with mammography (about 0.20 cGy), the risk–benefit ratio is favorable after about 45 years of age.[67]

RISKS FROM NUCLEAR POWER

The contribution of the nuclear industry to the radiation exposure of the general population (see Fig. 12–2) is small and well within the variation in natural background radiation that occurs from one area to another around the country. The health of workers in the nuclear industry has been carefully monitored for over 50 years. The most recent comprehensive report of a study of over 95,000 workers in the British nuclear industry shows strong evidence of the familiar "healthy worker effect," because mortality is lower in radiation workers than in the general population, both overall and for most specific causes including cancer.[68] This healthy worker effect is attributed to the selection of fit individuals to work in the industry and the benefits of relatively high socioeconomic status.[69] There is less strong evidence for a dose-related mortality from leukemia.[68]

A recent report has made a statistical association between preconceptual radiation exposure and the subsequent development of leukemia or lymphoma in the children of Sellafield workers.[70] Sellafield is the site of a nuclear reprocessing plant in Great Britain. There is an apparent cluster of leukemias in children living near the plant and it has been suggested that the cause is a germline mutation induced by preconceptual irradiation of the fathers, who received large doses of radiation while working at the plant. However, the report is based on a handful of cases, has geneticists puzzled as to the mechanism of transmission, and is not supported by data from the children of individuals irradiated at Hiroshima and Nagasaki[71] or by evidence from other nuclear sites in the United Kingdom.[72]

It is not the routine discharge of radioactivity by the nuclear industry that is the source of the fear in which many people hold nuclear power. Rather, it is the risk of a catastrophic incident causing large numbers of deaths and economic disruption. Two names come to mind—Three Mile Island and Chernobyl. Although they are often linked, in fact they differ by a factor of more than a million in the amount of radioactivity released.

In the case of Three Mile Island, radioactive noble gases were released, but the inventory of solid decay products in the reactor core remained contained. By the worst estimate, there would be only 1 radiation-induced cancer death in the 2 million people around the reactor.[73] By contrast, much of the radioactive inventory of the reactor core at Chernobyl was released, and many excess cancer deaths may be expected.[74]

Table 12–2 is perhaps the best summary of collective doses—that is, the sum of the product of dose × the number of people who received that dose—and their health impact in terms of cancer, genetic effects, and deleterious consequences to children exposed in utero.[75] There are many difficulties in making such estimates, and various attempts differ by a factor of two or three.

There are three groups of exposed people to consider:

1. The 135,000 people who were evacuated from the immediate area around Chernobyl will receive in their lifetime a collective dose of about 16,000 person Gy—that is, an average exposure of about 0.12 Gy. Using the cancer risk estimates from the UNSCEAR and BEIR committees, which are based on the Japanese survivors, there could be about 410 excess cancer cases in this group, over and above the 17,000 cancer cases from natural cases. This 2% to 3% increase might be detectable in a careful study comparable to that undertaken at Hiroshima and Nagasaki.
2. The 75 million people in European USSR received a collective lifetime dose of 470,000 person Gy—an average of about 7 mGy and about a tenth of the lifetime exposure from natural background radiation. This is estimated to result in 11,000 radiation-induced fatal cancers, compared with the 9.4 million that occur naturally in this population. No study could detect this approximately 0.1% excess.
3. The rest of the Northern Hemisphere, including Europe, Asia, and the United States, received doses to the individual that are a tiny fraction of the natural background. Extrapolating risk estimates derived from atomic bomb survivors who received a large acute dose down to doses

TABLE 12–2. Projected Chernobyl Health Impacts in the Northern Hemisphere: Comparison of Spontaneous and Estimated Radiation-Induced Effects*

	Population (10^6)	Collective Lifetime Dose (10^6 Person-Gy)	Fetal Cancer Natural (10^3)	Fetal Cancer Rad-Induced (10^3)	Severe Mental Retardation Natural (10^3)	Severe Mental Retardation Rad-Induced (10^3)	Genetic Disorders Natural (10^3)	Genetic Disorders Rad-Induced (10^3)
USSR Evacuees	0.135†	16	17	0.41	0.013	0.018‡	6.9	0.06
European USSR	75	470	9400	11	7.2	0.27	3900	0.75
Asian USSR	225	110	28,000	2.5	22	0.06	12,000	0.18
Europe (other)	400	580	72,000	13	38	0.33	21,000	0.93
Asia (other)	2600	27	450,000	0.6	240	—	130,000	0.04
USA	226	1.1	41,000	0.02	22	—	12,000	—
Northern hemisphere	3500	1200	600,000	28	340	0.7	180,000	1.9

* The possibility of zero health effects at very low doses and dose rates cannot be excluded.
† Recently revised by the Soviets to 0.116.
‡ This value may be an overestimate; recent Soviet discussions indicate that pregnant women were evacuated early and received average individual doses on the order of 0.5 rad.
(National Technical Information Service, U.S. Department of Commerce. Report to the U.S. Dept of Energy: Health and environmental consequences of the Chernobyl nuclear power plant accident, 22161. Report DOE/ER 0332, 1987)

that are a fraction of natural background and spread out over many years involves many uncertainties.

The total estimate for all three population groups referred to above is 28,000 cancer deaths and 1900 genetic disorders in a population of over 1 billion. This number represents an extremely small percentage (0.1%) increase over background that could never be detected. These estimates may easily be wrong by a factor of two or three, but they spell a disaster by any standards. The Chernobyl disaster is the single greatest in the history of nuclear power, but it ranks alongside other man-made disasters and such natural disasters as earthquakes and floods. The death toll is probably comparable to the *annual* death rate caused by the effects of domestic radon—a natural radiation hazard. Over a lifetime, radon would be a much higher source of risk, even for the Chernobyl evacuees.

In judging nuclear power, the most relevant figure is the risk of loss of life per unit of energy produced, compared with other methods that can be used to generate electricity. Table 12–3, adapted from Fremlin,[76] compares the risk of loss of

TABLE 12–3. Risk of Loss of Human Life (Per Giga Watt–Year of Energy Produced)

	Accidents Workers	Accidents Public	Operation Workers	Operation Public
Hydroelectric	0.01–0.1	5	0.01–0.1	—
Coal-electric	1.0	0.01–0.1	0.6	5
Oil-electric	0.25	0.1–0.2	0.05	5
Nuclear-electric	0.01	0.01	0.03	0.01

(Adapted from Fremlin JH. Power production: What are the risks? 2nd ed. Bristol: Adam Hilger, 1989)

life per giga watt—year of energy produced by hydroelectric, coal, oil, nuclear, and other sources; routine operation and the results of accidents are included in this survey. According to these figures, nuclear power is by far the safest form of power production.

Studies such as this do little to convince the person in the street, however. The risk from nuclear power is considered more frightening because the cancer risk occurs in the general public. For coal-produced power (for example), the risks are incurred by those who dig and transport the coal, and accidents in coal mines and railways are accepted as normal. Hydroelectric power poses a high risk of accidents from burst dams, which in this century have resulted in several of the biggest disasters involving loss of life from man-made sources.

MECHANISMS OF RADIATION CARCINOGENESIS

There is much evidence that human cancers frequently result from the activation of a dominant acting oncogene or the deletion of a suppressor gene. These ideas are particularly attractive because they provide a paradigm for explaining common pathways for carcinogenesis by different agents. Oncogenes are known to be activated by a point mutation, a chromosomal translocation, or by gene amplification.[77-80] The removal of a suppressor gene is likely to involve a small or a large deletion. Radiation is known to be highly effective at producing deletions and chromosome translocations, and rather less efficient at point mutations. These mechanisms are attractive possibilities for radiation-induced cancer, but they have not been demonstrated in any specific human malignancy induced by radiation. A dominant-acting transforming gene has been demonstrated in radiation-induced oncogenic transformation in vitro, but the gene has not been sequenced.[81] Activated K-*RAS* and N-*RAS* were reported in a proportion of murine thymic lymphoma induced by x-rays or neutrons, but are probably not the causative step.[82,83]

ULTRAVIOLET RADIATION CARCINOGENESIS

Skin cancers are the most common type of human cancers, with about 500,000 new cases diagnosed annually in the United States.[84] Basal cell carcinomas occur four times more frequently than squamous cell carcinoma in men, and six times more frequently in women.[85] Both types of cancer occur more frequently in men than in women and about 70 times more frequently in whites than in blacks.[85] The cancers usually occur on areas exposed to sunlight, and occur at higher rates in southern latitudes of the United States. The incidence, particularly of basal cell carcinoma, is increasing but fortunately the cure rate exceeds 95%. In humans and in experimental animals, protracted or multiple exposures with high total fluences of UVR usually are required to produce carcinomas of the skin.

The evidence for a causal relation between UVR and melanoma is compelling, but is not as strong as that for nonmelanoma skin cancer.[86,87] Indeed, the possible involvement of UVR in the cause and pathogenesis of cutaneous melanoma is controversial.[88] Because there is little evidence to suggest that UVR is directly involved in melanoma carcinogenesis by causing neoplastic transformation of melanocytes, it has been postulated that the effects of UVR on the immune system may play a role in the pathogenesis of this type of skin cancer.[88–90] The marked increase in the incidence of melanoma in developed nations is a cause of considerable concern because of the high mortality rate associated with this form of cancer.[91] An important question is whether the incidence of melanoma would increase with a depletion of the ozone layer. The answer to this question depends on the validity of the causal relation between melanoma and UVR, which is controversial and in doubt.

VARIATION IN SUSCEPTIBILITY TO UVR-INDUCED NONMELANOTIC SKIN CANCER

Skin cancer incidence rates vary markedly among different populations. Although skin cancer is by far the most common form of cancer among white populations, it is infrequent among darkly pigmented ethnic groups because of the protection to UV-B afforded by melanin. The range of variation is about 50-fold. Those of Celtic ancestry have a particularly high susceptibility to skin cancer. For example, it was found in Philadelphia that those of Irish origin had about 5 times as much skin cancer as Italians.[92] In Hawaii, it was found that whites had more than 40 times the skin cancer incidence of Asians,[93] and in New Mexico and the United States in general, the Anglo Americans had a skin cancer incidence about six times that of Hispanic Americans.[94]

HISTORICAL PERSPECTIVE

The importance of sunlight in the cause of human skin cancer was recognized as early as 1894, but experiments with rats and mice showed that the UVR in sunlight was responsible for carcinogenesis.[95–97] Studies with animals also showed that UV-B (280–320 nm) was responsible for the induction of skin cancer.[98–101] UV-A (320–400 nm) also causes skin cancer in animals when given at high doses over a long period.[102–105]

OZONE DEPLETION AND SKIN CANCER

The ozone layer in the stratosphere acts as a highly effective absorbing layer that prevents the most biologically effective wavelengths of UVR, especially UV-B (280–320 nm) from reaching the earth and exposing the human population. Any increase in the fluence of UV-B resulting from a depletion of the ozone layer might be expected to increase the probability of skin cancer, especially basal cell and squamous cell carcinoma.[106] In the early 1970s, concern about ozone depletion arose for the first time, especially in regard to skin cancer and damage to the eye. Early on, it was feared that supersonic airplanes would inject nitrogen oxides into the stratosphere, resulting in ozone depletion.[107–109] More recently, chlorofluorocarbons are suspected as a cause of ozone depletion in the stratosphere.[110,111] There is evidence of a global reduction in ozone, which causes concern that an increase in skin cancer may result.

Estimates of effective UVR doses in the past were based on the spectral dependence of sunburn or mutations in DNA.[112] These data contained little information on long-wave UVR (UV-A, 315–380 nm). Recently, experiments with hairless mice have provided data on the carcinogenic effectiveness of UVR including UV-A.[113–115]

Although depletion of the ozone layer leads to an increase in UV-B, it has little effect on UV-A. Using these new data for the complete UV spectrum, and dose-response curves for carcinogenesis in mice, it is estimated that a 1% decrease in ozone yields a 1.56% increase in carcinogenic UV, which may lead to a 2.7% increase in nonmelanoma skin cancer.[106]

MECHANISMS OF UVR-INDUCED CANCER

UVR is a potent DNA-damaging agent and a known inducer of skin cancer in experimental animals. There is good evidence to believe that most nonmelanoma human skin cancers result from repeated exposures to sunlight and that this is a result of UVR-induced DNA damage. UVR primarily produces pyrimidine dimers, a form of DNA damage that differs from the lesions induced by any other carcinogen. Furthermore, enzymatic photoreactivation of UVR-induced pyrimidine dimers suppresses the induction of oncogenic transformation in human fibroblasts in vitro.[116] The prevalence of skin cancer on sun-exposed body sites in individuals with the inherited disorder xeroderma pigmentosum suggests that defective repair of UVR-induced DNA damage can lead to cancer.

By observing the rate of appearance of skin tumors in mice after daily UV irradiations were discontinued, UV carcinogenesis was divided into two main processes, one UV driven and one purely time dependent. This latter component could be a simple growth stage, but histopathology suggests that it may also entail a transition from active keratosis to squamous cell carcinoma.[117]

Activated *RAS* oncogenes have been identified in human skin cancer cells. In most cases, the mutations in the *RAS* oncogenes have been localized to pyrimidine-rich sequences, implying that these sites are probably the targets for UVR-induced DNA damage and subsequent mutation and transformation.[118] The presence of activated *RAS* oncogenes in benign and self-regressing keratoacanthomas in both humans and in animals indicates that they play a role in the early stages of carcinogenesis.[119,120]

Perhaps the most compelling evidence of a mechanism comes from a recent report by Brash and colleagues, who found that 14 of 24 invasive squamous cell carcinomas of the skin (58%) in a series of New England and Swedish patients contained mutations in the p53 tumor suppressor gene, each altering the amino acid sequence.[121] Involvement of UVR in these mutations is indicated by the presence in three of the tumors of a CC → TT double-base change, which is only known to be induced by UV. Additional evidence of UVR involvement comes from the occurrence of mutations exclusively at dipyrimidine sites, including a high frequency of C → T substitutions. The p53 mutations in internal malignancies do not show these UV-specific mutations.

ULTRAVIOLET RADIATION AND IMMUNOLOGY

The surprising conclusion that exposure to UVR could have systemic immunologic consequences evolved mainly from animal experiments. It was shown that during the course of chronic exposure to UVR mice lost their ability to reject transplants of highly antigenic UVR-induced skin cancers. This occurred long before there was evidence of development of primary skin cancer, even if they were transplanted into unirradiated areas.[122] Later studies led to the conclusion that repeated exposure of mouse suppressor T lymphocytes to UVR, specifically UV-B radiation, inhibited the immune response against UVR-induced tumors.

Photocarcinogenesis appears to involve at least three separate activities of UVR:

1. Transformation of normal cells into neoplastic cells.
2. The production of antigenic changes in the skin.
3. The induction of suppressor T lymphocytes directed against these antigens.

It is not clear how exposure of the skin to UVR brings about systemic changes in immune function, but it appears to be a real phenomenon.[123,124]

There is growing evidence to suggest that UVR can also alter immunologic processes in humans. Exposure of human skin to UVR led to suppressor-cell induction, and there is evidence that suppressor cells are present in patients with sunlight-induced skin cancers but not in patients with skin cancers induced by x-rays.[125-127] The most compelling evidence comes from the demonstration that exposure of human skin to low doses of UVR results in a markedly decreased contact hypersensitivity response in patients with sunlight-induced skin cancer.[127] These studies suggest that the ability of UVR to induce suppressor cell formation may be a predisposing factor in skin cancer development and may also have a role in human infectious diseases.

Exposure to UVR over a long period after an initial exposure to x-rays increases the carcinogenic effect of the ionizing radiation.[128] The interaction between UVR and x-rays appears to be synergistic, but the enhancing effect of the UVR is probably not specific. It is likely that the UVR acts to suppress the immune system as previously described.

XERODERMA PIGMENTOSUM

Xeroderma pigmentosum is an autosomal recessive disease which occurs with a frequency of about one in a quarter of a million people in the United States and Europe, but reportedly higher in Egypt and Japan.[129-131] The disease was first reported more than a century ago, at which time the genetic aspects and the possible role of sunlight were noted.[132] As early as 1929, it was suggested that the xeroderma pigmentosum trait might be an essential characteristic of persons who develop skin cancer.[133] About half of the patients with xeroderma pigmentosum also have neurologic abnormalities, but few have all the lesions characteristic of the De Sanctis-Cacchione syndrome.[130] Various ocular lesions such as cloudiness of the cornea, pigmentation, and telangiectasia of the conjunctiva have been recognized from the outset to be part of the syndrome.[129,130]

The parents of patients with xeroderma pigmentosum are heterozygotes and clinically normal,[130] although it has been suggested that they are at a higher risk for skin cancer.[134] By 1968 it was demonstrated that fibroblasts cultured from the skin of xeroderma pigmentosum patients were defective in the excision repair of UVR-induced DNA damage.[135] The picture is complicated, however, and the causal relation between defective DNA repair and cancer is far from clear-cut. Seven complementation groups have been identified that are deficient in excision repair, implying the involvement of many different genes.[136-138] An eighth group shows no LNS abnormalities or the characteristic sensitivity to sunlight, but the cells are more susceptible to UVR-induced mutations.[136-139] The area of photoimmunology has been reviewed extensively.[140,141]

ASBESTOS

CLASSIFICATION OF FIBERS

Asbestos is a broad commercial term for a group of naturally occurring hydrated mineral silicates that crystallize in a fibrous habit. The family of asbestos minerals can be classified as *serpentine*, meaning that the fibers are curly and pliable, or *amphibole*, meaning needle-like fibers (Fig. 12–5). Chrysotile, which accounts for 90% of the world's production of asbestos, is the most common fibrous serpentine. Crocidolite and amosite are the most common amphibole fibers.

HISTORIC PERSPECTIVE

The widespread use of asbestos and attempts to control its use are recent, but the mineral itself has been with us a long time. The Romans wove asbestos into tablecloths that could be tossed into the fire for cleaning. In one of Genghis Khan's northern provinces, Marco Polo saw inhabitants weaving an indestructible cloth from fibers dug from the earth.

At the turn of the century, asbestos was being used on an industrial scale as a fire retardant and thermal insulator, and it was soon shown to cause asbestosis.[142] Its association with the causation of lung cancer and mesothelioma in asbestos miners was demonstrated in the 1950s, and in asbestos textile weavers, pipe insulators, and shipyard workers in the 1960s.[143-146] The danger of developing asbestos-related diseases appears to extend beyond that of a simple occupational hazard because it has been documented in family members of asbestos workers[147] and in individuals living in the neighborhood of industrial sources of asbestos.[148]

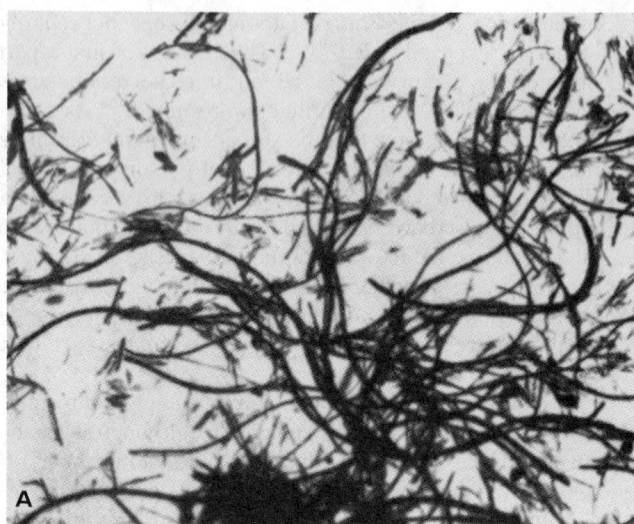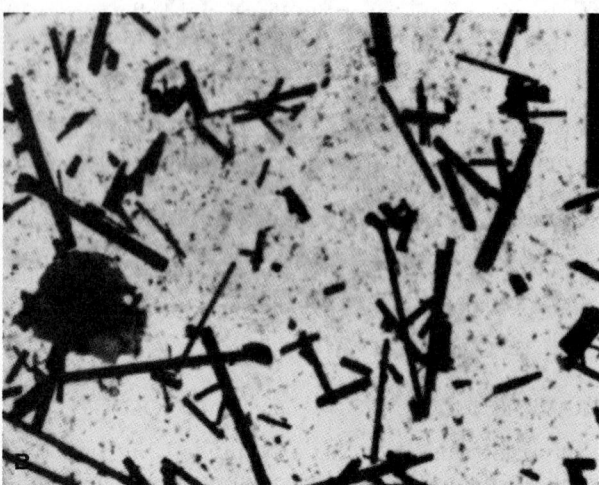

FIGURE 12–5. **(A)** Chrysotile fibers represent the group of curly fibers known as *serpentine*. **(B)** Amosite fibers represent the group of needle-like fibers known as *amphibole*. (Courtesy of Dr. Robert Nolan, The City University of New York, Brooklyn, NY)

By the 1970s and 1980s, the Government took action through the Occupational Safety and Health Administration and the Environmental Protection Agency. The new regulations were not a problem—industry bore the cost and they were regarded as humane and probably overdue. The seeds of the debate concerning the public policy and risk assessment of asbestos date from the advice of scientists at the Mount Sinai Medical Center in New York, who decided that evidence warranted the removal of asbestos already in place in buildings. Testimony was given to Congress that in-place asbestos posed a serious threat to the general population, including millions of school children. Other scientists claim that removing asbestos may, in effect, result in greater risks than leaving it in place, and in any case argue that the asbestos in most buildings in the United States is chrysotile, which they believe does not pose a threat at low doses, based on human epidemiologic data obtained from chrysotile miners.[149]

Although the debate over asbestos continues, it is not known whether the widespread contamination by small amounts of fibers poses a hazard. Meanwhile, vast sums of money and a whole industry have grown up around asbestos abatement.

MINERALS: DISEASE AND SIZE

Fibers that are long and thin are more carcinogenic than those that are short and thick. Studies have indicated that fibers that are carcinogenic tend to be longer than about 8 μm and less than 1.5 μm in diameter with a length to diameter ratio greater than 3:1.[150] Indications of the importance of size and shape of particles in the production of disease were obtained by the use of fine glass fibers in intrapleural inoculation experiments in rats.[151,152] Because fine glass fibers also produced mesothelioma, these data suggested that the crystal structure and chemical composition of the various fibrous materials used were not as important as the physical shape and configuration. Further evidence comes from the fact that leaching of asbestos fibers to remove any surface contamination does not reduce their carcinogenic potential.[153,154]

HEALTH RISK OF ASBESTOS

Epidemiologic investigations of the association of mesothelioma with asbestos exposure indicate that mesothelioma is much more likely to result from exposure to amphibole than chrysotile fibers.[155-159] However, an increased incidence of lung cancer has been demonstrated from exposure to all types of asbestos, an incidence that is synergistically increased by cigarette smoking.[160]

Among exposed workers, lung cancer is the number one malignant disease associated with asbestos, followed by mesothelioma. There is also a modest increase in gastrointestinal cancers and suggestion of an increase in cancers of the kidney, pancreas, esophagus, and colon. Mesothelioma is pathognomonic of fiber carcinogenesis, particularly asbestos.[161,162] About 20% of mesothelioma cases occur among those in whom occupational exposure has not been documented. These tumors arise from the mesothelial surfaces of the pleura and peritoneum and have a pleomorphic histologic appearance. The tumors spread over the pleural and peritoneal surfaces and do not invade the underlying tissues deeply, but they do metastasize. Mesothelioma is difficult to treat and the prognosis is, in general, poor.

The risks posed by environmental exposure to mineral fibers is thought to be mainly the induction of mesothelioma. It appears to have affected significant numbers of people who may have had only low-level exposures to asbestos in the workplace. Asbestosis, on the other hand, requires intensive exposures that are rare these days even in industry. Lung cancer is by far the most common cancer among asbestos workers, and is still a concern despite modern conditions, although most workers smoke. But most experts believe that for the general public, smokers and nonsmokers alike, lung cancer induction as a result of fiber exposure is less important than mesothelioma. City dwellers, for example, breathe in thousands of fibers from shedding car brakes. In about one third of known cases of mesothelioma, the patients could recall no industrial exposure to asbestos. In 1960, mesothelioma was killing an estimated two dozen Americans every year; by the 1980s, the figure was 1000 to 3000 deaths. Some experts were predicting that it would overtake lung cancer as a cause of death by the end of the century, but rates have flattened and there is no sign of that happening. Among women, whose asbestos exposure has primarily been environmental, the mesothelioma rate has remained flat for the last 20 years and the cancer remains rare.

Mossman and her colleagues argue that the reason is that chrysotile is not effective at producing mesothelioma—even at the highest industrial concentrations. The lungs wash the fibers out before they can cause serious harm. Only the amphiboles, according to Mossman and colleagues, have been shown to be highly carcinogenic and pose a risk at low levels in the environment.[163] With the exception of the United States and South Africa, the industrialized nations have accepted this so-called *amphibole hypothesis* and regulate chrysotile fibers less stringently. In the United States, no distinction between fiber types is made in formulating asbestos regulations.

LATENCY AND MODELS FOR RISK ESTIMATES

Tumors appear in asbestos workers anywhere from 15 to 40 years after exposure. The latency period appears to correlate with the type of cancer, the level of exposure, and the age at first exposure. The latency shortens as exposure levels increase and lengthens for older workers.[164] Among the asbestos-related diseases, mesothelioma appears to have the longest latency period. In general, tumor incidence peaks around 35 to 40 years after onset of exposure. There is abundant evidence to suggest that a threshold exposure level exists for fiber-induced pulmonary fibrosis. In addition, there is strong evidence to indicate a link between fibrosis and lung cancer.[164]

Risk estimation based on extrapolation from high- to low-dose exposure has been proposed, but there is uncertainty about the appropriate models to be used. It has been assumed that the dose-response relations for mesothelioma and lung cancer are linear, with the assumption that there is no threshold for disease, a hypothesis that is still open to debate. Credible quantitative estimates of risk are much more scarce for asbestos than for ionizing radiations. The fact that radiation, cigarette smoke, and asbestos—three important environmental carcinogens to which the general public are exposed—can interact in a synergistic or supraadditive way in cancer induction highlights the complexity of risk assessment. Historic perspectives on fiber-induced toxicity have recently been reviewed.[163,165]

MECHANISMS OF ASBESTOS CARCINOGENESIS

The mechanisms of cancer induction by fibers are not fully understood, but some progress has been made. Asbestos and glass fibers are phagocytosed by cells in culture, accumulating in the perinuclear region of the cytoplasm. Cells appear to selectively phatocytose the longer fibers, with the shorter fibers accumulating on the cell surface.[166,167] In Syrian hamster embryo cells in culture, asbestos fibers induce a dose-dependent increase in micronuclei and chromosome aberrations, as well as in oncogenic transformation.[167–170]

Aneuploidy is a consistent finding, as it is in the early stages of other types of tumors.[168] In C_3H 10T1/2 cells cultured in vitro, asbestos fibers were found to be cytotoxic in a dose-dependent manner; at concentrations that alone produced a barely detectable level of oncogenic transformations, asbestos interacted strongly with γ-rays and particularly with alpha particles in a synergistic way.[153,154,171]

Until recently, most reports on the mutagenicity of asbestos have largely been negative. However, studies using assay systems with large nonessential genomic targets, such as the human-hamster hybrid (A_L) cells, suggest that asbestos fibers are mutagenic and produce large multilocus deletions.[172] This explains why several earlier studies failed to detect fiber mutagenicity in other mutation assays, because large deletions are not compatible with the survival of the mutants.[173]

Several investigators have examined chromosomal aberrations in human mesotheliomas, but changes appeared inconsistent from tumor to tumor. The most common abnormalities involved inversions, translocations, and deletions of chromosomes 1, 3, 7, 9, 17, and 22.[174–176] Constitutively enhanced expression of the *PDGFB* gene, the protooncogene c-*SIS*, was observed in human mesothelioma cell lines when compared with normal human mesothelial cells.[177,178] The identification of activated transforming genes in human mesothelioma and the loss of specific chromosomal regions as a result of fiber-induced chromosomal deletions suggest a possible role for tumor protooncogenes on suppressor genes in fiber-related tumors. Although suggestive, no molecular studies have identified a causative step.

ELECTRIC AND MAGNETIC FIELDS

The role of electric and magnetic fields in cancer induction is a topic of much public interest, but adequate scientific evidence to make judgments is simply not available. There are two situations that are of concern: low-frequency electric and magnetic fields around electric power transmission lines and high static magnetic fields connected with magnetic resonance imaging (MRI) systems, both clinical and experimental.

LOW-FREQUENCY ELECTRIC AND MAGNETIC FIELDS

Electric and magnetic fields produced, for example, by electric power transmission lines have recently been added to the list of environmental agents that some believe to pose a threat to public health by causing or promoting cancer.

Conventional wisdom holds that the fields associated with power systems could not be a threat to human health because the physical interactions of such fields with the body are too weak to have a significant effect on biology at the level of the cell, in as much as they are small compared with thermal noise;[179] unlike x-rays, power frequency fields do not break chemical bonds; and unlike microwaves, power frequency fields cannot cause significant tissue heating.

Despite these indisputable facts, it is well established that some animals, including eels, sharks, and pigeons are able to detect extremely weak magnetic fields and use them for homing or finding prey. This demonstrates that at least some specialized cells, presumably in the brain, are exquisitely sensitive to such fields. A number of laboratory experiments have demonstrated that cell membranes can be sensitive to even weak low-frequency electromagnetic fields. An Office of

Technology Assessment report places the experiments in four categories:[180]

1. Modulation of ion flows
2. Interference with DNA synthesis and RNA transcription
3. Interaction with the response of normal cells to various agents and biochemicals such as hormones, neurotransmitters, and growth factors
4. Interaction with the biokinetics of cancer cells.

Despite the wealth of published data there is no consensus among those who work in the field as to which effects are valid; none have been replicated, whereas many have been contradicted.

Low-frequency electromagnetic fields have not been shown to cause chromosomal damage, but some experiments do indicate that the cell membrane is the site of the interaction between electromagnetic low frequency fields and the cell. This has led to the hypothesis that electromagnetic fields may play a role in tumor promotion rather than initiation.

The question of an association between cancer and low-frequency electromagnetic fields arose because of epidemiologic studies on childhood cancer in Denver.[181] This study reported a positive association between childhood cancer and homes they classified as near high-current configuration distribution lines, those likely to produce stronger than average magnetic fields. The study has been criticized on a number of grounds, and studies since then have yielded mixed results. Two studies found no association, but two others reported positive results, including that of Savitz, which is the latest and most thorough study.[181-186] Three studies were designed to examine the association between adult cancer and residential exposure to electromagnetic fields, but there are so many confounding problems that they do not provide enough evidence to draw any meaningful conclusions.[187-189]

Occupational exposure is another matter. More than 20 studies from several countries have looked for an association between malignancies, particularly leukemia and brain cancer, and workers exposed to electromagnetic radiations in electrical industries. The data have been reviewed by Tenforde[190] and Savitz.[191] There is an indication that occupational exposure is associated with an enhanced leukemia risk. This does not necessarily imply a causative link, because industrial jobs often involve exposure to other hazardous agents, particularly chemical solvents.

As recently as a few years ago, scientists were making categorical statements that on the basis of all available evidence there were no health risks to the human population from low-frequency electromagnetic fields. The emerging evidence no longer allows such categorical assertions; at the same time, the evidence does not provide convincing proof that such risks are an important consideration.

MAGNETIC RESONANCE IMAGING

The proliferation of magnetic resonance imaging (MRI) for clinical diagnostic use and for research purposes has led to a rapid increase in the number of individuals exposed to magnetic fields that are much higher than those found in nature. Operators and patients are exposed to enormously high fields of several tesla. A larger number of individuals in buildings above or below the floor on which such facilities are housed are exposed (often unwittingly) to magnetic fields that are ten times that of the earth's field.

The potential health hazards from medical MRI studies may result from the concurrent exposure to a high static magnetic field, time varying pulsed magnetic gradient fields, and a radiofrequency electromagnetic field. There are some well-understood effects on the orientation of bacteria and insects to magnetic fields and the generation of visual flickers and radiofrequency hearing.[192] However, there are no known hazards in humans except for the magnetic force on such metallic implants as surgical clips and pacemakers.[192,193]

The only federal regulation requires that areas be posted if the magnetic field strength exceeds 5 gauss, the intent being to avoid possible effects on pacemakers. Experiments seeking to determine the effects of MRI on cell lethality in bacteria or mammalian cells, chromosomal aberrations, mutations, and oncogenic transformations have all shown no effect.[194-198] Experiments with mice also indicate that prolonged exposure to MRI examination conditions does not lead to teratogenic effects either.[199] There is no evidence of a carcinogenic potential for the magnetic fields associated with MRI. As for low-frequency electric and magnetic fields associated with power transmission, the possibility that magnetic fields are promoters cannot be ruled out.

HYPERTHERMIA AND ERYTHEMA AB IGNE

Erythema ab igne is a macular reticulated skin discoloration seen after heat exposure, conductive or radiative. It is a common finding on the anterior aspects of the legs of old people who sit close to fires (ab igne) over a long period,[200] and also after chronic direct conductive heating with hot water bottles on heating pads for pain relief in pancreatic and cancer patients.[201-203]

The documentation of premalignant changes in the skin where erythema ab igne has developed has come from many parts of the world: old people in the United Kingdom;[200] women exposed to peat fires in Ireland;[204] the use of warming pans called *kangri* applied to the skin under clothes during the winter in Kashmir;[205] and the use of hot brick beds *(kang)* in Northwest China.[206] This represents an example of normal tissue damage caused by chronic hyperthermia, which is clearly carcinogenic. In contrast, experimental studies with in vitro assays for oncogenic transformation have shown that heat alone does not produce transformed foci.[207,208] Heat treatments that resulted in little or much cell killing did not produce transformants, but x-ray treatments resulting in similar levels of cell killing produce a substantial incidence of dose-dependent transformation. An extensive study with laboratory animals reached a similar conclusion, namely that heat alone did not induce tumors.[209] On the other hand, later studies by the same group showed that hyperthermia could potentiate the carcinogenic effect of x-rays as judged by tumors appearing in the back legs of mice.[210,211] It has been suggested that the appearance of malignancies after erythema ab igne may be due not to a direct carcinogenic effect of the heat itself but to the continued stimulation of cell division in skin cells by the chronic application of heat.[212] This suggestion is consistent with all of the available information from in vivo and in vitro studies.

REFERENCES

1. Frieben A. Demonstration lines cancroids des rechten Handruckens, das sich nach langdauernder Einwirkung von Rontgenstrahlen entwichelt hatte. Fortschr Geb Röntgenstr 1902;6:106.

2. Von Jagic N, Schwarz G, von Siebenrock L. Blutbefunde bei Röntgenologon. Berl Klin Wochenschr 1911;48:1220–1222.

3. Martland HS. The occurrence of malignancy in radioactive persons: A general review of data gathered in the study of the radium dial painters with special reference to the occurrence of osteogenic sarcoma and the interrelationship of certain blood diseases. Am J Cancer 1931;15;2435–2516.

4. Grigg ERN. The trail of the invisible light. Springfield, IL: Charles C Thomas, 1965.

5. Upton AC. Physical carcinogenesis: Radiation—history and sources. In: Becker FF, ed. Cancer: A comprehensive treatise. 2nd ed. New York: Plenum Press, 1982:551–567.

6. Kellerer AM, Rossi HH. A generalized formulation of dual radiation action. Radiat Res 1978;75:471–488.

7. Kellerer AM, Rossi HH. Biophysical aspects of radiation carcinogenesis. In Becker FF (ed). Cancer: A Comprehensive Treatise. 2nd ed. New York: Plenum Press, 1982: 569–616.

8. Goodhead DT. An assessment of the role of microdosimetry in radiobiology. Radiat Res 1982;91:45–76.

9. Zaider M, Rossi HH. Microdosimetry and its application to biological processes. In: Onton CG, ed. Radiation dosimetry. New York: Plenum Press, 1986:171–242.

10. International Commission on Radiation Units and Measurements (ICRU). The quality factor in radiation protection: ICRU Report 40. Bethesda, MD: International Commission on Radiation Units and Measurements, 1986.

11. National Council on Radiation Protection and Measurements (NCRP). Ionizing radiation exposure of the population of the United States: NCRP report 93. Bethesda, MD: NCRP, 1987.

12. National Council on Radiation Protection and Measurements (NCRP). Exposures from the uranium series with emphasis on radon and its daughters: NCRP report 77. Bethesda, MD: NCRP, 1984.

13. National Research Council, Committee on the Biological Effects of Ionizing Radiation (BEIR). Health risks of radon and other internally deposited alpha emitters. Washington, DC: National Academy Press, 1987.

14. Harley N, Samet JM, Cross FT, et al. Contribution of radon and radon daughters to respiratory cancer. Environ Health Perspect 1986;70:17–21.

15. United Nations Scientific Committee on Effects of Atomic Radiation (UNSCEAR). Ionizing radiation: Sources and biological effects—report to the general assembly with annexes. New York: United Nations, 1988.

16. National Research Council, Committee on the Biological Effects of Ionizing Radiation (BEIR). The effects on populations of exposure to low levels of ionizing radiation. Washington, DC: National Academy Press, 1980.

17. Blomberg R, Larsson LE, Lindell B, Lindren E. Late effects of Thorotrast in cerebral angiography. Acta Radiol [Diag] (Stockh) 1963;1:995–1006.

18. Preston DL, Kato H, Kopecky KJ, et al. Studies of the mortality of A-bomb survivors. 8. Cancer mortality, 1950–1982. Radiat Res 1987;111:151–178.

19. National Research Council. Health effects of exposure to low levels of ionizing radiation (BEIR V). Washington, DC: National Academy Press, 1990.

20. Darby SC, Doll R, Gill SK et al. Long-term mortality after a single treatment course with x-rays in patients treated for ankylosing spondylitis. Br J Cancer 1987;55:179–190.

21. Smith PG, Doll R. Mortality among patients with ankylosing spondylitis after a single treatment course with x-rays. Br Med J 1982;284:449–460.

22. Court-Brown WM, Doll R. Mortality from cancer and other causes after radiotherapy for ankylosing spondylitis. Br Med J 1965;2:1327–1332.

23. Shore RE, Woodard ED, Hempelmann LH. Radiation-induced thyroid cancer. In: Boice JD Jr, Fraumeni JF Jr, eds. Radiation carcinogenesis: Epidemiology and biological significance. New York: Raven Press, 1984:131–138.

24. Ron E, Modan B. Thyroid and other neoplasms following childhood scalp irradiation. In: Boice JD Jr, Fraumeni JF Jr, eds. Radiation carcinogenesis: Epidemiology and biological significance. New York: Raven Press, 1984:139–151.

25. Ron E, Modan B, Boice JD. Mortality following radiotherapy for ringworm of the scalp. Am J Epidemiol 1988;127:713–725.

26. Shore RE, Woodard E, Hildreth N, et al. Thyroid tumors following thymus irradiation. JNCI 1985;74:1177–1184.

27. Schneider AB, Shore RE, Freedman E, et al. Radiation-induced thyroid and other head and neck tumors: Occurrence of multiple tumors and analysis of risk factors. J Clin Endocrinol Metab 1986;63:107–112.

28. Shore RE, Woodard E, Dvoretsky P, et al. Breast cancer among women given x-ray therapy for acute post partum mastitis. JNCI 1986;77:689–696.

29. Boice JD, Monson RR. X-ray exposure and breast cancer. Am J Epidemiol 1976;104: 349–350.

30. Boice JD Jr, Land CE, Shore RE, Norman JE, Tokunaga M. Risk of breast cancer following low-dose exposure. Radiology 1979;131:589–597.

31. Storer JB. Radiation carcinogenesis. In: Becker FF, ed. Cancer: A comprehensive treatise, vol 1. 2nd ed. New York: Plenum Press, 1982:629–659.

32. Beebe GW. Assessment of health risks from exposure to ionizing radiation. In: Prentice RL, Whittemore AS, eds. Environmental epidemiology: Risk assessment. Philadelphia: SIAM, 1982:3–11.

33. Upton AC. The dose response relation in radiation induced cancer. Cancer Res 1961;21: 717–729.

34. Upton AC, Randolph ML, Conklin JW. Late effects of fast neutrons and gamma-rays in mice influenced by the dose rate of irradiation: Induction of neoplasia. Radiat Res 1970;41:467–491.

35. Ullrich RL, Storer JB. Influence of gamma radiation on the development of neoplastic disease in mice. III. Dose-rate effects. Radiat Res 1979;80:325–342.

36. Han A, Hill CK, Elkind MM. Repair of cell killing and neoplastic transformation at reduced dose rates of ^{60}Co gamma rays. Cancer Res 1980;40:3328–3332.

37. National Council on Radiation Protection and Measurements (NCRP). Influence of dose and its distribution in time and dose-response relationships for low-LET radiations: NCRP report 64. Washington, DC: NCRP, 1980.

38. Hall EJ, Hei TK. Oncogenic transformation of cells in culture: Pragmatic comparisons of oncogenicity, cellular and molecular mechanisms. Int J Radiat Oncol Biol Phys 1986;12:1909–1921.

39. Hill CK, Buonaguro FM, Myers CP, et al. Fission-spectrum neutrons at reduced dose rates enhance neoplastic transformation. Nature 1982;298:67–69.

40. Miller RC, Brenner DJ, Geard CR, Komatsu K, Marino SA, Hall EJ. Oncogenic transformation by fractionated doses of neutrons. Radiat Res 1988;114:589–598.

41. Ullrich RL. Tumor induction in BALB/c mice after fractionated or protracted exposures to fission-spectrum neutrons. Radiat Res 1984;97:587–597.

42. Darby SC, Doll R. Radiation and exposure rate. Nature 1990;344:824.

43. Brenner DJ, Hall EJ. The inverse dose-rate effect for oncogenic transformation by neutrons and charged particles: A plausible interpretation consistent with published data. Int J Radiat Biol 1990;58(5):745–758.

44. United Nations Scientific Committee on the Effects of Atomic Radiation (UNSCEAR). Genetic and somatic effects of ionizing radiation: Report E88 IX7. New York: United Nations, 1986.

45. International Commission on Radiological Protection (ICRP). Recommendations, report 60. Ann ICRP 1991;21(1–3):1–201.

46. Taylor AMR, Harnden DG, Arlett, CF, et al. Ataxia telangiectasia: A human mutation with abnormal radiation sensitivity. Nature 1975;258:427–429.

47. Arlett CF, Lehmann AR. Human disorders showing increased sensitivity to the induction of genetic damage. Annu Rev Genet 1978;12:95–115.

48. Lewis PD, Carr JB, Arlett CF, et al. Increased sensitivity to gamma irradiation of skin fibroblasts in Friedrich's ataxia. Lancet 1979;2:474–475.

49. Smith PJ, Paterson MC, Kraemer KH. In vitro radiosensitivity in a patient with dermatomysitis and cancer. Lancet 1981;2:1216–217.

50. Sandford KK, Parshad R, Green MH, et al. Hypersensitivity to G_2 chromatid radiation damage in familial dysplastic naevus syndrome. Lancet 1987;2:1111–1116.

51. Kersey JH, Spector BD. Immune deficiency disease. In: Fraumeni JF Jr, ed. Persons at high risk of cancer: An approach to cancer etiology and control. New York: Academy Press, 1975:55–67.

52. Wakabayashi T, Kato H, Ikeda T, et al. Studies of the mortality of A-bomb survivors, part III: Incidence of cancer in 1959–78 based on the tumor registry, Nagasaki. Radiat Res 1983;93:112–146.

53. Kim JH, Chu FC, Woodard MR, et al. Radiation-induced soft-tissue and bone sarcoma. Radiology 1978;129:501–508.

54. Boice JD, Hutchison GB. Leukemia in women following radiotherapy for cervical cancer: Ten-year follow-up of an international study. JNCI 1980;65:115–129.

55. Kapp DS, Fisher D, Grady KJ, Schwartz PE. Subsequent malignancies associated with carcinoma of uterine cervix, including an analysis of the effects of patient and treatment parameters on incidence and sites of metachronous malignancies. Int J Radiat Oncol Biol Phys 1982;8:197–205.

56. Lee JY, Perez CA, Ettinger N, et al. The risk of second primaries subsequent to irradiation for cervix cancer. Int J Radiat Oncol Biol Phys 1982;8:207–211.

57. Czesnin K, Wronkowski Z. Second malignancies of the irradiated area in patients treated for uterine cervix cancer. Gynecol Oncol 1978;6:309–315.

58. Sadove AM, Block M, Rossof AH, et al. Radiation carcinogenesis in man: New primary neoplasms in field of prior therapeutic radiation. Cancer 1981;48:1139–1143.

59. Messerschmidt GL, Hoover R, Young RC. Gynecologic cancer treatment: Risk factors for therapeutically induced neoplasia. Cancer 1981;48:442–450.

60. Coleman CN. Second malignancy after treatment of Hodgkin's disease: An evolving picture. J Clin Oncol 1986;4:821–824.

61. Pederson BJ, Larson SD. Incidence of acute nonlymphocytic leukemia, preleukemia and acute myeloproliferative syndrome up to 10 years after treatment of Hodgkin's disease. N Engl J Med 1982;307:965–975.

62. Wall PL, Clausen KP. Carcinoma of urinary bladder in patients receiving cyclophosphamide. N Engl J Med 1975;293:271–273.

63. Boice J Jr, Engholm G, Kleinman RA, et al. Radiation dose and second cancer risk in patients treated for cancer of the cervix. Radiat Res 1988;116:3–55.

64. Arai T, Nakano T, Fukuhisa K, et al. Second cancer after radiation therapy for cancer of the uterine cervix. Cancer 1991;67:398–405.

65. National Council on Radiation Protection and Measurements (NCRP). Exposure of the US population from diagnostic medical radiation, report 100. Bethesda, MD: NCRP, 1989.

66. Hall EJ. Risk of cancer causation by diagnostic x-rays. Cancer Prev (March) 1990; 1–9.

67. National Council on Radiation Protection and Measurements (NCRP). Mammography: A user's guide, NCRP report 85. Bethesda, MD: NCRP, 1986.

68. Kendall GM, Muirhead CR, MacGibbon BH, et al. Mortality and occupational exposure to radiation: First analysis of the National Registry for Radiation Workers. Br Med J 1992;304:220–225.

69. Beral V, Inskip H, Frazer P, Booth M, Coleman D, Rose G. Mortality of employees of the United Kingdom Atomic Energy Authority, 1946–1979. Br Med J 1985;291:440–447.

70. Gardner, MJ, Snee MP, Hall AJ, Powell CA, Downes S, Terrell JD. Results of a case-control study of leukaemia and lymphoma among young people near Sellafield nuclear plant in West Cumbria. Br Med J 1990;300:845–854.
71. Yoshimoto Y, Schull WJ, Kato H, Neel JV. Mortality among the offspring (F) of atomic bomb survivors 1946–1985. Technical Report 1–91. Hiroshima: Radiation Effects Research Foundation, 1991.
72. Urquhart JD, Black RJ, Muirhead MJ, et al. Case-control study of leukemia and non-Hodgkin's lymphoma in children in Caithness near the Dounreay nuclear installation. Br Med J 1991;302:687–692.
73. The Ad Hoc Population Dose Assessment Group. Population dose and health impact of the accident at the Three Mile Island nuclear station: A preliminary assessment for the period March 28 through April 7, 1979. Washington, DC: US Government Printing Office, 1979.
74. Nenot JC. Overview of the radiological accidents in the world, updated to December 1989. Int J Radiat Biol 1990;57:1073–1085.
75. National Technical Information Service, US Department of Commerce. Report to the US Department of Energy: Health and environmental consequences of the Chernobyl nuclear power plant accident. Report DOE/ER 0332. Springfield, VA: US Department of Energy, 1987.
76. Fremlin JH. Power production: What are the risks? 2nd ed. Bristol: Adam Hilger, 1989.
77. Watson JD, Hopkins NH, Roberts JW, Steitz JA, Weiner AM. Molecular biology of the gene. 4th ed. Menlo Park, CA: Benjamin Cummings, 1987.
78. Bos JL. The RAS gene family and human carcinogenesis. Mutat Res 1988;195:255–271.
79. Brodeur GM, Seeger RC, Schwab M, Varmus HE, Bishop JM. Amplification of N-myc in untreated human neuroblastomas correlates with advanced disease stage. Science 1984;224:1121–1124.
80. Dalla-Favera RS, Martinotti S, Gallo R, Erikson J, Croce C. Translocation and rearrangement of the c-myc oncogene locus in human undifferentiated B-cell lymphomas. Science 1983;219:963–967.
81. Freyer GA, Gurvits I. Isolation and identification of an oncogene induced by gamma radiation in C₃H 10T1/2 cells. In: Chapman JD, Dewey WC, Whitmore GF, eds. Radiation research: A twentieth century perspective. San Diego: Academic Press, 199:146.
82. Guerrero J, Villasonte A, Corces V, Pellicer A. Activation of a c-K-RAS oncogene by somatic mutation in mouse lymphomas induced by gamma radiation. Science 1984;225:1159–1162.
83. Sloan R, Newcomb EW, Pellicer A. Ionizing radiation and RAS oncogene activation. J Cancer Res Clin Oncol 1990;116(Suppl):808.
84. Scotto J, Fears TR, Fraumeni JF. Incidence of non-melanoma skin cancers in the United States. NIH publication 83-2433. Washington, DC: National Institutes of Health, 1983.
85. Scotto J, Fraumeni JF Jr. Skin (other than melanoma). In: Schottenfeld D, Fraumeni JF Jr, eds. Cancer epidemiology and prevention. Philadelphia: WB Saunders, 1982:996–1011.
86. Fitzpatrick TB, Sober AJ. Sunlight and skin cancer. N Engl J Med 1985;313:818–819.
87. Scotto J, Fears TR. The association of solar ultraviolet and skin melanoma incidence among Caucasians in the United States. Cancer Invest 1987;5:275–283.
88. Kopf AW, Kripke ML, Stern RS. Sunlight and malignant melanoma. J Am Acad Dermatol 1984;11:674–684.
89. Romerdahl CA, Donawho C, Fidler IJ, et al. Effect of ultraviolet-B radiation on the in vivo growth of murine melanoma cells. Cancer Res 1988;48:4007–4010.
90. Donawho CK, Kripke ML. Evidence that the local effect of ultraviolet radiation on the growth of murine melanomas is immunologically mediated. Cancer Res 1991;51:4176–4181.
91. Magnus K. Incidence of malignant melanoma of the skin in the five Nordic countries: Significance of solar radiation. Int J Cancer 1977;20:477–485.
92. Urbach F. Geographic distribution of skin cancer. J Surg Oncol 1971;3:219–234.
93. Quisenberry W. Ethnic differences in skin cancer in Hawaii. NCI Monogr 1963;10:181–189.
94. Fears T, Scotto J. Changes in skin cancer morbidity between 1971–72 and 1977–78. JNCI 1982;69:365–370.
95. Unna PG. Die Histopathologic der Hautkrankheiten. Berlin: Hirschwald, 1894.
96. Findlay GM. Ultraviolet light and skin cancer. Lancet 1928;215:1070–1073.
97. Rotto AH. Cancer et soleil: Carcinomes et sarcomes provoquees par l'action de soleil in toto. Bull Cancer (Paris) 1934;23:590–616.
98. Blum HF. Carcinogenesis by ultraviolet light. Princeton, NJ: Princeton University Press, 1959.
99. Urbach F. The biologic effects of ultraviolet radiation. New York: Pergamon Press, 1969.
100. Epstein JH. Photocarcinogenesis: A review. NCI Monogr 1978;50:13–25.
101. Forbes PD. Experimental photocarcinogenesis: An overview. J Invest Dermatol 1981;77:139–143.
102. Zigman S, Fowler J, Kraus AL. Black light induction of skin tumors in mice. J Invest Dermatol 1976;67:723–725.
103. Forbes PD, Davies RE. Quantity, quality and mode of UV administration as denominators of photocarcinogenesis. Curr Probl Dermatol 1986;15:290–302.
104. Van Weelden H, de Gruijl FR, Van der Leun JC. Tumors induced by UV-A in mice. Photochem Photobiol [Abstract] 1983;37:S79.
105. Strickland P. Photocarcinogenesis by near-ultraviolet (UVA) radiation in Sencar mice. J Invest Dermatol 1986;87:272–275.
106. Kelfkens G, de Gruijl FR, Van der Leun JC. Ozone depletion and increase in annual carcinogenic ultraviolet dose. Photochem Photobiol 1990;52:819–823.
107. Carter LJ. The global environment: MIT study looks for danger signals. Science 1970;169:660–662.
108. Johnston H. Reduction of stratospheric ozone by nitrogen oxide catalysts from supersonic transport exhaust. Science 1971;173:517–522.
109. Cutchis P. Stratospheric ozone depletion and solar ultraviolet radiation on earth. Science 1974;184:13.
110. National Research Council. Causes and effects of changes in stratospheric ozone: Update 1983. Washington, DC: National Academy Press, 1984.
111. Prather MJ, McElroy MB, Wofsy SC. Reductions in ozone at high concentrations of stratospheric halogens. Nature 1984;312:227–231.
112. Green AES, Hedinger RA. Models relating ultraviolet light and non-melanoma skin cancer incidence. Photochem Photobiol 1978;28:283–291.
113. Cole CA, Forbes PD, Davies RE. An action spectrum for photocarcinogenesis. Photochem Photobiol 1986;43:275–284.
114. Sterenborg HJCM, Van der Leun JC; Passchier WF, Bosnjakovic BFM, eds. Human exposure to ultraviolet radiation risks and regulations. Amsterdam: Elsevier, 1987:173–190.
115. Slaper H. Skin cancer and UV exposure: Investigations on the estimation of risks. Utrecht, The Netherlands: University of Utrecht; 1987:147–154. Thesis.
116. Sutherland BM, Cimino JS, Delihas N, et al. Ultraviolet light-induced transformation of human cells to anchorage-independent growth. Cancer Res 1980;40:1934–1939.
117. de Gruijl FR, van der Leun JC. Development of skin tumors in hairless mice after discontinuation of ultraviolet irradiation. Cancer Res 1991;51:979–984.
118. Ananthaswamy HN, Pierceall WE. Molecular mechanisms of ultraviolet radiation carcinogenesis. Photochem Photobiol 1990;52:1119–1136.
119. Corominas M, Kamino H, Leon J, Pellicer A. Oncogene activation in human benign tumors of the skin (keratoacanthomas): Is HRAS involved in differentiation as well as proliferation? Proc Natl Acad Sci USA 1989;86:6372–6376.
120. Kumar R, Sukumar S, Barbacid M. Activation of RAS oncogenes preceding the onset of neoplasia. Science 1990;248:1101–1104.
121. Brash DE, Rudolph JA, Simon JA, et al. A role for sunlight in skin cancer: UV-induced p53 mutations in squamous cell carcinoma. Proc Natl Acad Sci USA 1991;88:10124–10128.
122. Kripke ML, Fisher MS. Immunologic parameters of ultraviolet carcinogenesis. JNCI 1976;57:211–215.
123. Kripke ML. Immunologic mechanisms in UV radiation carcinogenesis. Adv Cancer Res 1981;34:69–106.
124. Hostetler LW, Kripke ML. Origin and significance of transplantation antigens induced on cells transformed by UV radiation. In: Greene MI, Hamaoka T, eds. Development and recognition of the transformed cell. New York: Plenum Press, 1987:307–329.
125. Cooper KD, Fox P, Neises G, et al. Effects of ultraviolet radiation on human epidermal cell alloantigen presentation: Initial depression of Langerhans cell-dependent function is followed by the appearance of T6⁻Dr⁺ cells that enhanced epidermal alloantigen presentation. J Immunol 1985;134:129–137.
126. Baadsgaard O, Fox D, Cooper KD. Human epidermal cells from ultraviolet light-exposed skin preferentially activate autoreactive CD4⁺2H4⁺ suppressor-inducer lymphocytes and CD8⁺ suppressor/cytotoxic lymphocytes. J Immunol 1988;140:1738–1744.
127. Frentz G, de Cunha Bang F, Munch-Petersen B, et al. Increased number of circulating suppressor T lymphocytes in sun-induced multiple skin cancers. Cancer 1988;61:291–297.
128. Fry RJM. Radiation protection guidelines for the skin. Int J Radiat Biol 1990;57:829–839.
129. Robbins JH, Kraemer KH, Lutzner MA, et al. Xeroderma pigmentosum: An inherited disease with sun sensitivity, multiple cutaneous neoplasms and abnormal repair. Ann Intern Med 1974;80:221–248.
130. Kraemer K, Lee MM, Scotto J. Xeroderma pigmentosum: Cutaneous, ocular and neurological abnormalities in 830 published cases. Arch Dermatol 1987;123:241–250.
131. Hashem N, Bootsma D, Keijzer W, et al. Clinical characteristics, DNA repair, and complementation groups in xeroderma pigmentosum patients from Egypt. Cancer Res 1980;40:13–18.
132. Hebra F, Kaposi M; Tay W, trans. On diseases of the skin including the exanthemata, vol 3. London: New Sydenham Society, 1974:252–258.
133. Haxthausen H, Hausmann N. Die Lichterkrankugen der Haut. Vienna: Urban und Schwartzenberg, 1929.
134. Swift M, Chase C. Cancer in families with xeroderma pigmentosum. JNCI 1979;62:1415–1421.
135. Cleaver JE. Defective repair replication of DNA in xeroderma pigmentosum. Nature 1968;218:652–656.
136. Jung EG. New form of molecular defect in xeroderma pigmentosum. Nature 1970;228:361–362.
137. Burk PG, Lutzner MA, Clarke DD, et al. Ultraviolet-stimulated thymidine incorporation in xeroderma pigmentosum lymphocytes. J Lab Clin Med 1971;77:759–767.
138. Cleaver JE. Xeroderma pigmentosum: Variants with normal DNA repair and normal sensitivity to ultraviolet light. J Invest Dermatol 1972;58:124–128.
139. Maher VM, Ouelette LM, Curren RD, et al. Frequency of ultraviolet light-induced mutations is higher in xeroderma pigmentosum variant cells. Nature 1976;261:593–595.
140. Kripke M. Review: Effects of UV radiation on tumor immunity. JNCI 1990;82:1392–1396.
141. Kripke M. Photoimmunology. Photochem Photobiol 1990;52:919–924.
142. Murray HM. Report of Departmental Committee on Compensation for Industrial Diseases: Minutes of evidence, CD3946. London: Her Majesty's Stationery Office, 1907:127–128.

143. Mossman BT, Gee JBL. Asbestos related diseases. N Engl J Med 1989;320:1721.
144. Selikoff IJ, Churg J, Hammond EC. Asbestos exposure and neoplasia. JAMA 1964;188: 22–26.
145. Selikoff IJ, Hammond EC, Churg J. Asbestos exposure, smoking and neoplasm. JAMA 1968;204:106–112.
146. Selikoff IJ, Hammond EG, Seidman H. Mortality experience of asbestos insulation workers in the United States and Canada. Ann NY Acad Sci 1979;330:91–116.
147. Anderson HA, Lilis R, Daum SM, Fischbein AS, Selikoff IJ. Household contact asbestos neoplastic risk. Ann NY Acad Sci 1976;271:311–323.
148. Hammond EC, Garfinkel L, Selikoff IJ, Nicholson WJ. Mortality experience of residents in the neighborhood of an asbestos factory. Ann NY Acad Sci 1979;330:417–422.
149. Warner JC, Pooley FD, Berry G, Seal RME, Munday DE, Morgan J, Clark NJ. A pathological and mineralogical study of asbestos-related deaths in the United Kingdom in 1977. Ann Occup Hyg 1982;26:423–431.
150. Stanton MF, Layara M, Tegeris A, et al. Relation of particle dimension to carcinogenicity in amphibole asbestosis and other fibrous minerals. JNCI 1981;67:965–975.
151. Stanton MF, Wrench C. Mechanisms of mesothelioma induction with asbestos and fibrous glass. JNCI 1972;48:797–821.
152. Ilgren EB, Wagner JC. Background incidence of mesotheliomas: Animal and human evidence. Regul Toxicol Pharmacol 1991;13:133–149.
153. Hei TK. Oncogenic transformation by asbestos fibers and alpha particles. In: Effects of mineral dusts on cells. NATO ASI series, vol 30. Heidelberg: Springer-Verlag, 1989; 389–397.
154. Hei TK, Kushner S. Radiation and asbestos fibers: Interaction and possible mechanism. In: Cerutti PA, Nygaard OF, Simic MG, eds. Anticarcinogenesis and radiation protection. New York: Plenum Press, 1987:345–348.
155. Dement J, Harris Jr RL, Symons MJ, Shy CM. Exposures and mortality among chrysotile asbestos workers. Part II. Mortality. Am J Ind Med 1983;4:421–433.
156. Finkelstein M. Mortality among employees of an Ontario asbestos-cement factory. Am Rev Respir Dis 1984;129:754–761.
157. Hughes JM, Weill H, Hammand YY. Mortality of workers employed in two asbestos cement manufacturing plants. Br J Ind Med 1987;44:161–174.
158. McDonald AD, Fry JS, Woolley AJ, McDonald JC. Dust exposure and mortality in an American factory using chrysotile, amosite and crocidolite in mainly textile manufacture. Br J Ind Med 1983;40:368–374.
159. Ohlson CG, Hogstedt C. Lung cancer among asbestos cement workers: A Swedish cohort study and a review. Br J Ind Med 1985;42:397–402.
160. Selikoff IJ, Hammond EC, Churg J. Asbestos exposure, smoking and neoplasia. JAMA 1968;204:106–112.
161. Nicholson WJ, Perbep G, Selikoff IJ. Occupational exposure to asbestos: Population at risk and projected mortality. Am J Ind Med 1987;3:259–311.
162. Omenn GS, Merchant J, Boatman E, et al. Contribution of environmental fibers to respiratory cancer. Environ Health Perspect 1986;70:51–56.
163. Mossman BT, Bignon J, Corn M, Seaton A, Gee JBL. Asbestos: Scientific developments and implications for public policy. Science 1990;247:294–301.
164. Newhouse M. Epidemiology of asbestos-related tumors. Semin Oncol 1981;8:250–257.
165. Selikoff IJ. Historical developments and perspectives in inorganic fiber toxicity in man. Environ Health Perspect 1990;88:269–276.
166. Hesterberg TW, Butterich CJ, Oshimura M, et al. Role of phagocytosis in Syrian hamster cell transformation and cytogenetic effects induced by asbestos and short and long glass fibers. Cancer Res 1986;46:5795–5802.
167. Hesterberg TW, Barrett JC. Dependence of asbestos and mineral dust-induced transformation of mammalian cells in culture on fiber dimension. Cancer Res 1984;44: 2170–2180.
168. Hesterberg TW, Barrett JC. Induction of asbestos fibers of anaphase abnormalities: Mechanism for aneuploidy induction and possibly carcinogenesis. Carcinogenesis 1985;6:473–475.
169. Oshimura M, Hesterberg TW, Tsutsui T, et al: Correlation of asbestos-induced cytogenetic effects with cell transformation of Syrian hamster embryo cells in culture. Cancer Res 1984;44:5017–5022.
170. Oshimura M, Hesterberg TW, Barrett JC. An early nonrandom karyotypic change in immortal Syrian hamster cell lines transformed by asbestos: Trisomy of chromosome 11. Cancer Genet Cytogenet 1986;22:225–237.
171. Hei TK, Geard CR, Osmak RS, et al. Correlation of in vitro genotoxicity and oncogenicity induced by radiation and asbestos fibres. Br J Cancer 1985;52:591–597.
172. Hei TK, Hall EJ, Osmak R. Asbestos, radiation and oncogenic transformation. Br J Cancer 1984;50:717.
173. Hei TK, He ZY, Piao CQ, and Waldren CA. The mutagenicity of mineral fibers. NATO ASI series A 1991 (in press).
174. Popescu NC, Chahinian AP, DiPaolo JA. Nonrandom chromosome alterations in human malignant mesothelioma. Cancer Res 1988;48:142–147.
175. Gibas Z, Li FP, Antman KH, Bernal S, Stahel R, Sandberg AA. Chromosome changes in malignant mesothelioma. Cancer Genet Cytogenet 1986;20:191–201.
176. Tiainen M, Tammilehto L, Mattson K, Knuutila S. Nonrandom chromosomal abnormalities in malignant pleural mesothelioma. Cancer Genet Cytogenet 1988;33:251.
177. Gerwin BI, Lechner JF, Reddel RR, et al. Comparison of production of transforming growth factor-β and platelet-derived growth factor by normal human mesothelial cells and mesothelioma cell lines. Cancer Res 1987;47:6180–6184.
178. Versnel MA, Hagemeijer A, Bouts MJ, Van der Kwast TH, Hoogsteden HC. Expression of c-sis (PDGF B-chain) and PDGF A-chain genes in ten human malignant mesothelioma cell lines derived from primary and metastatic tumors. Oncogene 1988;2: 601–605.
179. Adair RK. Biological effects on the cellular level of electric field pulses. Health Phys 1991;61:395–399.
180. Nair I, Morgan MG, Florig HK. US Congress, Office of Technological Assessment for the Office of Technological Assessment. Biological effects of powerline frequency electric and magnetic fields. Background Paper OTA-BP-E-53. Washington, DC: US Government Printing Office, 1989.
181. Wertheimer N, Leeper E. Electrical wiring configurations and childhood cancer. Am J Epidemiol 1979;109:273–284.
182. Fulton JP, Cobb S, Preble L, Leone L, Forman E. Electrical wiring configurations and childhood leukemia in Rhode Island. Am J Epidemiol 1980;111:292–296.
183. Myers A, Clayden AD, Cartwright RA, Cartwright SC. Childhood cancer and overhead power lines: A case-control study. Br J Cancer 1990;62:1008–1014.
184. Tomenius L. 50-Hz electromagnetic environments and the incidence of childhood tumors in Stockholm County. Bioelectromagnetics 1986;7:191–207.
185. Savitz DA, John EM, Kleckner RC. Magnetic field exposure from electric appliances and childhood cancer. Am J Epidemiol 1990;131:763–773.
186. Savitz Da, Wachtel HA, Barnes F, John EM, Tvrdik JG. Case-control study of childhood cancer and exposure to 60-hertz magnetic fields. Am J Epidemiol 1988;128(1):21–38.
187. Wertheimer N, Leeper E. Adult cancer related to electrical wires near the home. Int J Epidemiol 1982;11:345–355.
188. Stevens RG, Savitz DA. Is electromagnetic fields and cancer an issue worthy of study? Cancer 1992;69:603–607.
189. McDowall ME. Mortality of persons resident in the vicinity of electricity transmission facilities. Lancet 1983;77:246.
190. Cole P. An epidemiologic perspective on electromagnetic fields and cancer. Florida Department of Environmental Regulation, March 1987.
191. Savitz DA, Calle EE. Leukemia and occupational exposure to electromagnetic fields: Review of epidemiological surveys. J Occup Med 1987;29:47–51.
192. Budinger TE. Hazards of magnetic resonance imaging. In: Medical magnetic resonance. Budinger TE, Margulis AR, eds. Berkeley, CA: Society of Magnetic Resonance in Medicine, 1988:327–343.
193. Persson BRR, Stahlberg F. Health and safety of clinical NMR examinations. Boca Raton, FL: CRC Press, 1989.
194. White A, Handler PP, Smith EL: Principles of biochemistry. 5th ed. New York: McGraw-Hill, 1973.
195. Wolff S, Crooks LE, Brown P, Howard R, Painter RB. Test for DNA and chromosomal damage induced by nuclear magnetic resonance imaging. Radiology 1980;136:707.
196. Wolff S, James LT, Young GB, Margulis AR, Bodyyote J, Afzal V. Magnetic resonance imaging: Absence of in vitro cytogenetic damage. Radiology 1985;155:163.
197. Schwartz JL, Crooks LE. NMR imaging produces no observable mutations or cytotoxicity in mammalian cells. AJR 1982;139:583.
198. Geard CR, Osmak RS, Hall EJ, Simon HE, Maudsley AA, Hilal SK. Magnetic resonance and ionizing radiation: A comparative evaluation in vitro of oncogenic and genotoxic potential. Radiology 1984;152:199.
199. Heinrichs WL, Fong P, Moseley ME, et al. Analysis of teratogenesis and reproductive toxicity in Balb/C mice after midpregnancy MRI or MRS exposures. In: Proceedings of the Society of Magnetic Resonance in Medicine, 4th Annual Meeting. Berkeley, CA: Society of Magnetic Resonance in Medicine 1985:922.
200. Peterkin GAG. Malignant change in erythema ab igne. Br Med J 1955;2:1599–1602.
201. Butler ML. Erythema ab igne, a sign of pancreatic disease. Am J Gastroenterol 1977;67: 77–79.
202. Mok DWH, Blumgart LH. Erythema ab igne in chronic pancreatic pain: A diagnostic sign. J R Soc Med 1984;77:299–301.
203. Ashby MA. Erythema ab igne in cancer patients. J R Soc Med 1985;78:925–926.
204. Cross F. On a turf (peat) fire cancer: Malignant change superimposed on erythema ab igne. Proc R Soc Med 1967;60:1307–1308.
205. Neve EF. One cause of cancer as illustrated by epithelioma in Kashmir. Br Med J 1910;2:589.
206. Laycock HT. The 'kang cancer' of North-West China. Br Med J 1948;1:982.
207. Harisiadis L, Miller RC, Harisiadis A, Hall EJ. Oncogenic transformation and hyperthermia. Br J Radiol 1980;53:479–482.
208. Raaphorst GP, Azzam EI, Sargent MD, Einspenner M, Borsa J. The oncogenic potential of x-rays and/or hyperthermia in C3H 10T1/2 cells. Br J Radiol 1981;54:638–639.
209. Urano M. Long-term observation of mouse foot reaction after hyperthermia: Hyperthermia may or may not be carcinogenic? Br J Radiol 1981;54:534–536.
210. Urano M, Kenton LA, Kahn J. The effect of hyperthermia on the early- and late-appearing mouse foot reactions and on radiation carcinogenesis. Part II. Effect on radiation carcinogenesis (thermal enhancement and oxygen enhancement). Int J Radiat Oncol Biol Phys 1989;16:437–442.
211. Urano M, Kenton LA, Kahn J. The effect of hyperthermia on the early and late appearing mouse foot reactions and on the radiation carcinogenesis: Effect on the early and late appearing reactions. Int J Radiat Oncol Biol Phys 1988;15:159–166.
212. Hall EJ. Cell proliferation, not cancer, produced ab igne? Int J Hyperthermia 1985;1(4): 392–393.

Cancer: Principles & Practice of Oncology, Fourth Edition,
edited by Vincent T. DeVita, Jr., Samuel Hellman, Steven A. Rosenberg.
J.B. Lippincott Co., Philadelphia © 1993.

Juan Rosai

CHAPTER 13

Principles of Oncologic Pathology

Oncologic pathology is the branch of pathology that deals with the characterization of neoplasms on the basis of morphologic (shape-related) features, whether at the gross, microscopic, or ultrastructural level. It is a powerful tool for the evaluation of the common traits and differences among the innumerable types of neoplasms that can affect the human body, and it remains the basis for their identification and classification. Oncologic pathology provides clues to the genesis of these tumors and allows fairly accurate predictions about their natural history. The discipline is constantly being enriched by new technologies such as immunohistochemistry or in situ hybridization, which in most instances complement rather than replace conventional methods.

The morphologic study of human tumors in this century developed along two separate roads that eventually merged. The first emphasized the study of the nature (and, by inference, the histogenesis) of tumor cells and resulted in elaborate classifications based on analogies with the corresponding normal adult and embryonal counterparts; the second concerned itself with the expected behavior of tumors as judged from their appearance and therefore with the concepts of benignancy and malignancy. Current classifications of human neoplasms reflect, in an imperfect and sometimes imprecise manner, the attempt to name and arrange tumors according to a combination of histogenetic and behavioral traits.

CLASSIFICATION OF TUMORS

HISTOGENESIS

The traditional principle of tumor histogenesis, which has dominated the thinking in this field for more than a century,

is that neoplasms characterized by a certain phenotype arise from normal cells of similar phenotype. According to this scheme, rhabdomyosarcoma is viewed as a tumor originated from skeletal muscle cells, synovial sarcoma as a tumor originated from synovial cells, and so forth. As logical as this assumption appears, it is difficult to reconcile with the observations that some tumors show features of two or more distinct cell types and that some neoplasms occur where their presumed normal parent cells are absent (*e.g.,* synovial sarcoma arising at a distance from a synovial membrane, or osteosarcoma developing away from the skeletal system). Considerable evidence has accumulated in recent years to indicate that this histogenetic assumption is incorrect, and that most if not all neoplasms arise from immature cells, which in the course of neoplastic transformation acquire phenotypic features equivalent to those of one or more normal cell types. More often than not, this differentiation develops along lines analogous to those expected under normal conditions for that particular cell. For instance, primitive epithelial cells located at the base of the crypts of Lieberkühn in the intestinal mucosa differentiate under normal conditions along one or another of four specialized cell lines: absorptive cell, goblet cell, enterochromaffin cell, and Paneth cell. Correspondingly, neoplasms arising from these primitive cells do differentiate along one or another of these various pathways, sometimes singly and sometimes in combination (although in substantially different percentages).[1]

This change in interpretation does not mandate a change in terminology. The names assigned to the various tumors remain the same but have acquired a different significance. Therefore, rhabdomyosarcoma is no longer defined as a malignant tumor *arising* from striated muscle cells, but as a malignant tumor *differentiating* in the direction of striated muscle cells.

BEHAVIOR

The traditional classification of neoplasms by behavior is into benign and malignant types. These designations are determined by the expected behavior of the tumor rather than its microscopic appearance, although the two parameters are closely related. In the many cases in which there is a divergence, the behavioral aspects take precedence as far as terminology is concerned. For example, the better-differentiated chondrosarcomas have a microscopic appearance similar to that of normal cartilage, whereas some parathyroid adenomas are highly atypical and pleomorphic.

The division of tumors into benign and malignant represents a gross oversimplification of the wide behavioral range exhibited by these lesions, in terms of local aggressiveness and metastatic potential. Two interesting semantic changes have taken place recently in this regard. In the past, tumors were often designated malignant if they had the capacity to metastasize but also if they manifested an aggressive behavior locally. The tendency now is to restrict the term *malignant* to tumors with metastasizing properties. Several changes in terminology have occurred because of this policy, particularly in the field of soft tissue tumors. Tumors formerly diagnosed as well-differentiated liposarcomas in the superficial soft tissue are now commonly diagnosed as atypical lipomas.[2] The other development has been the creation of a new tumor category between the benign and malignant types, variously designated (depending on the site) as *borderline, intermediate,* or *undetermined.* Most tumors so named represent malignancies of such a low grade that a cure can be achieved in many cases by a conservative therapeutic approach. The best examples are in the field of gynecologic pathology and are represented by borderline serous tumors of the ovary and smooth muscle tumors of undetermined malignant potential of the uterine corpus.[3,4]

GRADING OF TUMORS

Determination of the microscopic type of a malignancy does not always provide all the information needed to predict the clinical course or to decide on the therapy. For instance, diagnoses such as prostatic adenocarcinoma or liposarcoma span an extremely wide range of lesions, from the slow growing, rarely metastasizing, and highly curable to the rapidly growing, often metastasizing, and rarely curable. Microscopic grading is an attempt to determine the degree of malignancy independently from cell type and is based on the evaluation of several parameters, which vary depending on the system being studied. They include cellularity, pleomorphism, mitotic activity, type of margins, amount of matrix formation, and presence of hemorrhage, necrosis, or inflammation. Not surprisingly, many of these parameters are closely interrelated. For soft tissue tumors, the number of mitotic figures, and extent of necrosis seem to be the most important parameters.[5,6]

The number of grades varies from system to system, but in general the three-grade system (well differentiated, moderately differentiated, and poorly differentiated, or undifferentiated; or grades I, II, and III, respectively) has proved to be the most reproducible and the best suited to predict survival.

The microscopic type or subtype of a tumor is related to its grade; for instance, embryonal rhabdomyosarcoma is by definition a high-grade neoplasm. The significance of a parameter depends greatly on the type of lesion. Marked variations may exist between various areas of the same tumor, and accurate grading requires representative, well-fixed, and well-stained histologic material. Tumors for which microscopic grading correlates with prognosis include soft tissue sarcomas,[7] squamous cell carcinomas of various organs, breast carcinoma,[8] and prostatic adenocarcinoma.[9]

PRECANCEROUS CONDITIONS AND CARCINOMA IN SITU

Probably no field in tumor pathology is more confusing and controversial yet as important clinically as that of the so-called *precancerous conditions.* The term embraces all the morphologically recognizable disorders thought to predispose a person to the development of malignancy. Because cancer is a multistep process in most instances, the concept can be expressed as the morphologic identification of the various steps that precede the development of a full-blown malignancy.[10] It is unfortunate that the terminology used for conceptually and often morphologically comparable processes differs so much depending on the organ systems in which they develop. It includes terms such as *dysplasia, atypical hyperplasia, atypical proliferation, intraepithelial neoplasia,* and *carcinoma in situ.* In some organs, such as the stomach, the terms *severe dysplasia* and *carcinoma in situ* are used synonymously; in others, such as the uterine cervix, a distinction has been made between them. Conceptually, hyperplasia and atypical hyperplasia are reversible processes, but carcinoma in situ is not.

Although the continuum from hyperplasia to neoplasia can be convincingly demonstrated, the precise boundaries between them cannot be determined with an acceptable degree of accuracy. Because of this difficulty, the alternative designation *intraepithelial neoplasia* has been advanced. The proponents of this terminology defend it on the grounds that the difference between the terms of *dysplasia* or *atypical hyperplasia* and *carcinoma in situ* (CIS) gives the morphologic spectrum a semantic dividing point that is far sharper in words than in the histologic images.[11] Instead, they maintain, a term such as *intraepithelial neoplasia* coupled with a grading system to indicate increasing degrees of severity can accomplish the following: emphasize the biologic and clinical unity of the two apparent conditions of dysplasia and CIS; remove from the pathologist the difficult and subjective task of distinguishing between severe dysplasia and CIS; indicate that although the grading of an intraepithelial lesion is of collective prognostic value, such grading offers no grounds for assuring a patient that this abnormality will or will not develop into an invasive carcinoma; allow for a unity of therapeutic approach and "prevent the state of affairs where a diagnosis of carcinoma in situ is regarded as a definite and often urgent indication for treatment whilst one of dysplasia, often differentiated from carcinoma in situ on relatively flimsy and uncertain pathologic grounds, is either not treated adequately or is ignored."[11]

The term *carcinoma in situ* (or the analogous term for melanocytic lesions, *melanoma in situ*) is being used with decreasing frequency in most sites. The statements that follow reflect in an eloquent fashion this increasingly popular point of view:

The best terminology for atypical intraepithelial lesions should accurately reflect the limitations of our knowledge about the process of carcinogenesis: 1) our inability to distinguish between atypical hyperplasia (reversible) from intraepithelial neoplasia (irreversible) and 2) our lack of criteria to recognize fully cancerized cells capable of invasion. The terminology should be simple and reproducible so that therapeutic protocols may be applied. It seems best to speak of atypical intraepithelial proliferation.[12]

The multi-step theory of neoplasia makes the definition of a malignancy in situ easy. Malignancy in situ is a state in which one or several cells and their progeny have acquired the potential to invade and to metastasize, but have not as yet exercised this option. The problem is that we cannot recognize these fully transformed cells until they actually invade the underlying tissue. In other words, a true malignancy in situ is not diagnosable at the present time by microscopy.[13]

The diagnosis of carcinoma in situ (melanoma in situ, malignancy in situ) is a contradiction in terms, the prototype of an oxymoron.[14]

METHODS IN ONCOLOGIC PATHOLOGY

The standard procedure for the pathologic evaluation of tissue specimens for tumors is (and is likely to remain for a long time) their examination under a light microscope after formalin fixation, paraffin embedding, and staining of the sections with hematoxylin-eosin. This technique has proved one of the most durable in the medical laboratory and has remained essentially unchanged—except for the automation of some of the steps—for more than half a century. Although it has some drawbacks, it offers considerable advantages over the many alternatives that have been proposed over the years: it is quick, inexpensive, suitable for most situations, and comparatively easy to master. Most important, it allows an accurate microscopic diagnosis in most cases. However, it cannot answer all of the questions that a given case may pose at the plain diagnostic level. It often proves insufficient when dealing with etiologic, histogenetic, or pathogenetic questions, or when trying to predict the responsiveness of a given tumor to one type of therapy or another. As a consequence, an increasingly sophisticated array of "special" techniques has evolved in an attempt to deal with these matters in a more effective fashion.

SPECIAL FIXATIVES

Buffered 10% formalin remains the standard fixative. A mercuric chloride-based fixative generally known by the abbreviation B5 currently is preferred over formalin for the study of hematolymphoid malignancies, mainly because of the superior cytologic details it provides. Zenker's solution is another mercuric chloride-based fixative and provides nearly identical results.

Several attempts have been made to introduce fixatives that are equally satisfactory for light microscopic and ultrastructural examination, but on the whole these have been unsuccessful.[15] Whether more recent attempts to devise fixatives compatible with routine use but providing better antigenic preservation than formalin (for the purposes of immunohistochemical evaluations) will be better accepted remains to be seen.

SPECIAL STAINS

Of the extensive battery of special stains listed in the manuals on histologic techniques, the tumor pathologist will find that only a few are of real diagnostic utility. This is particularly the case since the advent of immunohistochemistry, with its superior sensitivity and specificity.

The special stains most commonly used for human tumors are the following:

1. Periodic acid-Schiff (PAS) stain. This stain—one of the few in which the precise chemical nature of the reaction is known—demonstrates glycogen (in a specific fashion when used with a diastase-digested control) and is therefore routinely used for the study of Ewing sarcoma, which contains this polymer in large amounts. It also demonstrates various types of mucosubstances. Furthermore, it is the stain of choice for the demonstration of the intracytoplasmic granules that characterize the rare soft tissue neoplasm known as alveolar soft part sarcoma.

2. Silver (argentaffin and argyrophil) stains. The argentaffin reaction depends on the presence in the tissue of a substance that reduces silver salts. This substance is often of the phenolic group, which includes catecholamines or indolamines. Tumors that are typically argentaffin include carcinoid tumors and paragangliomas.

   In the argyrophilic reaction, an extraneous reducing agent is added to precipitate the silver. For all its pitfalls, it remains the best nonimmune light microscopic technique for the detection of neuroendocrine differentiation in tumors. Numerous technical variations have been proposed, of which we prefer the unmodified Grimelius' technique.[16]

3. Trichrome stains. The principal value of this family of stains consists in the evaluation of type and amount of extracellular material, particularly collagen. The three tissue structures demonstrated by the various dyes comprising this stain are nuclei, cytoplasm, and collagen, the latter being the only one having some degree of specificity. Despite assertions to the contrary, it is not useful to distinguish fibroblastic from smooth muscle or peripheral nerve tumors.

4. Phosphotungstic acid-hematoxylin (PTAH) stain. This stain traditionally has been used for the demonstration of intracytoplasmic filaments, but has been largely superseded by immunohistochemical techniques.

5. Stains for neutral lipids. Of these stains, oil red O is most commonly employed. In tumor pathology, the utility of fat stains is minimal. These stains are of no use in the differential diagnosis of liposarcoma; many liposarcomas contain little or no fat, whereas many nonadipose tissue neoplasms exhibit considerable amounts of fat, probably as a result of degenerative changes.

6. Mucin stains. The combination of Alcian blue and PAS is probably the most inclusive mucin stain, because it demonstrates mucosubstances of neutral, slightly acidic, and highly acidic types. These stains are useful as a sign of glandular differentiation in epithelial tumors. When combined with enzymatic digestion with hyaluronidase, they are of some utility in the differential diagnosis of soft tissue tumors, because cartilaginous neoplasms usu-

ally contain sulfated (hyaluronidase-resistant) mucins, in contrast to most other myxoid neoplasms.

ENZYME HISTOCHEMISTRY

Enzyme histochemistry is of little use in tumor diagnosis. The only techniques used with some frequency are those for chloroacetate esterase (Leder's stain, for cells of the myeloid series and mast cells),[17] acid phosphatase (for cells of the histiocytic series),[18] alkaline phosphatase (for endothelial cells and germ cells),[19] and the DOPA reaction (for melanocytes and related melanin-producing cells).

Because enzymes are proteins and therefore immunogenic, they can also be demonstrated with immunohistochemical techniques even when no longer active.[20]

TISSUE CULTURE

Pioneer work carried out in the Department of Pathology at Columbia-Presbyterian Hospital in New York City showed that histogenetic clues can sometimes be obtained from primary cultures of human tumors, taking advantage of the fact that tumor cells can express features of differentiation in vitro that are not easily appreciable in vivo.[21] The best known example is neuroblastoma, which grows neurites within 24 hours of having been placed in culture medium. Another is melanoma, which can make abundant melanin in vitro while being totally amelanotic in vivo. In some instances, the tumor differentiation has been induced in vitro by the addition of an exogenous agent such as cyclic AMP.[22] The most interesting recent example of this phenomenon is the neural differentiation that has been obtained in Ewing sarcoma of bone by the addition of AMP or TPA to the medium.[23] The most useful application of short-time tissue culture techniques is in the differential diagnosis of small round cell tumors of infancy. However, at a practical and strictly diagnostic level, the utility of tissue culture techniques remains limited.[24]

ELECTRON MICROSCOPY

The use of electron microscopy in tumor diagnosis has diminished considerably since the advent of immunohistochemistry. However, it remains a powerful tool when used selectively and intelligently after a differential diagnosis has been formulated at the light microscopic level.[25-30]

Electron microscopy can contribute to the differential diagnosis between carcinoma, melanoma, and sarcoma; adenocarcinoma and mesothelioma; anterior mediastinal tumors (*i.e.*, thymoma, thymic carcinoid, malignant lymphoma, seminoma); small round cell tumors (*i.e.*, Ewing's sarcoma, embryonal rhabdomyosarcoma, malignant lymphoma, neuroectodermal tumors); and spindle cell tumors of soft tissues (*i.e.*, muscular, pericytic, schwannian). It is also useful in detecting neuroendocrine differentiation in tumors (through the demonstration of dense core secretory granules), in identifying the cells of histiocytosis X (through the finding of Birbeck granules), and in confirming a diagnosis of alveolar soft part sarcoma (through the demonstration of membrane-bound intracytoplasmic crystals).

The main limitations of electron microscopy as a diagnostic tool relate to sampling (only a small portion of the tumor can be studied), paucity of truly specific ultrastructural features, and the ever-present danger of misinterpreting entrapped nonneoplastic elements as belonging to the tumor.

IMMUNOHISTOCHEMISTRY

The immunohistochemical method has contributed more than any other special technique to the histopathologic diagnosis of tumors. Basically, it consists of the application of immunologic principles and techniques—with their remarkable degree of specificity and sensitivity—to the study of cells and tissues.[31-33] It can be applied to routinely processed material (even if stored for long periods) and allows accurate correlations with the traditional morphologic parameters. It is compatible with most fixatives and is feasible even in material that has been decalcified.[34] It can also be applied to cytologic preparations and to electron microscopy, and can be used in conjunction with more conventional techniques (such as silver stains) in the same section.

For all its attributes, immunohistochemistry is fraught with numerous potential pitfalls. False-negative results can occur because of inappropriateness, denaturation, or wrong concentration of the antibody; loss of antigen through autolysis or diffusion; or presence of this antigen at a density below the level of detection. False-positive results can result from cross-reactivity with other antigens; nonspecific binding of the antibody to the tissue; entrapment of normal tissues by the tumor cells; and release of soluble proteins from the cytoplasm of normal cells invaded by the tumor, with permeation of the interstitium followed by nonspecific absorption or possibly phagocytosis by the tumor cells.[35,36] Other factors that have resulted in misinterpretations include the anomalous positive stains caused by ectopic antigen expression and hitherto unrecognized cross-reactions. Many markers thought to be specific for a certain cell, tissue, or tumor have proved to be shared by other tissues or tumors, and proper controls must therefore be used. An ingenious multitumor tissue block has been devised to test several tumor types in a quick and inexpensive fashion.[37]

The list of antigens that has been detected with immunohistochemistry is very large. Theoretically, any substance that is antigenic and whose antigenicity is at least partially retained in tissue sections can be demonstrated with this technique. The most important immunohistochemical markers in diagnostic tumor pathology are the following:

1. *Intermediate filaments.* Keratin serves as a marker of epithelial differentiation, vimentin as a generic marker of mesenchymal cells, desmin as a marker of muscle differentiation, neurofilaments as a marker of neural differentiation, and glial fibrillary acidic protein as a marker of glial differentiation.[38-43] Twenty or more antigenically distinct subclasses of keratin have been described having a tissue-related distribution in the various epithelia that is often recapitulated by the respective neoplasms.[44]

2. *Markers of muscle differentiation.* In addition to desmin, these markers include smooth muscle actin, skeletal muscle actin, myoglobin, and the product of *MYOD1* gene. All but the first are specific for striated muscle.[45-48]

3. *Lymphoid markers.* A huge number of monoclonal antibodies are available against the multitude of cell surface markers present in lymphocytes and related hematopoietic cells, sometimes as an expression of cell type or subtype and sometimes as a sign of a functional status, such as activation. Of those detectable in formalin-fixed, paraffin-embedded material, the most useful are leukocyte common antigen (LCA, a pan-lymphoid marker), L-26 (a pan-B-cell marker), UCHL1 (a pan-T-cell marker), Ber-H2 (analogous to Ki-1 and expressed by the Reed-Sternberg cells of Hodgkin's disease and the cells of so-called anaplastic large-cell lymphoma), and LeuM1 (expressed in Reed-Sternberg cells and in some T-cell lymphomas).[49]

4. *S-100 protein.* Although more ubiquitous than originally believed, the demonstration of this marker is of use in the diagnosis of melanocytic, schwannian, and cartilaginous neoplasms.[50,51]

5. *HMB-45.* This is a helpful although not entirely specific marker of activated melanocytes, particularly those of malignant melanoma.[52]

6. *Carcinoembryonic antigen (CEA).* This marker is mainly expressed by epithelial neoplasms, particularly those of glandular nature. Its main use is in the differential diagnosis between adenocarcinoma (usually positive) and malignant mesothelioma (nearly always negative).[53]

7. *Epithelial membrane antigen (EMA).* This is a general marker for epithelial differentiation.[54]

8. *Chromogranin, neuron-specific enolase,* and *synaptophysin.* These are markers of neural or neuroendocrine differentiation.[55-57]

9. Various peptide hormones (*e.g.,* gastrin, insulin, calcitonin, ACTH). These are markers of specific endocrine cell types.

10. Organ-related markers, such as thyroglobulin (for thyroid follicular cells),[58] prostatic specific antigen (for prostatic epithelium),[59] and *GCDFP-15* (for apocrine epithelium and breast carcinoma).[60]

11. *Human chorionic gonadotropin (HCG), α-fetoprotein,* and *human placental lactogen.* These are markers for various germ cell malignancies.

12. *Factor VIII-related antigen* and *Ulex europaeus I lectin.* These are markers of endothelial cells.[61,62]

13. *Type-IV collagen* and *laminin.* These are markers for basement membrane deposition.[63]

14. Markers for microorganisms, including viruses (*e.g.,* cytomegalovirus, human papillomavirus), bacteria, fungi, and parasites.

15. *Hormone receptors.* Reliable monoclonal antibodies are available for the detection of estrogen, progesterone, and androgen receptors in tissues (see Chap. 40).[64-67]

FLOW CYTOMETRY

Flow cytometry consists of the simultaneous measurement of several parameters while a suspension of cells flows through a beam of light past stationary detectors. It allows the analysis of 5000 to 10,000 cells per second for features such as cell size, cytoplasmic granularity, cell viability, cell cycle tissue, DNA content, surface marker phenotype, and enzyme content.

The main limitation of the technique is that cells must be in a single-cell suspension to be analyzed. This requirement is easily achieved in blood and other fluids, but obtaining satisfactory samples from nonhematopoietic solid tumors is more difficult. However, suitable techniques have been developed for most tumors, including a preparation of nuclear suspensions recovered from thick sections of routine formalin-fixed paraffin-embedded tissue blocks.[68,69] The main clinical uses of flow cytometry in solid tumors are as follows:[70-73]

To support a diagnosis of malignancy when the morphologic changes are equivocal, through the demonstration of an aneuploid cell population

To subclassify lesions of borderline malignancy

To provide prognostic information independent of stage and grade

To monitor response to therapy

To document the appearance of tumor relapse

To help determine whether two anatomically separate tumors of similar histology (whether synchronous or metachronous) are independent.

NUCLEIC ACID HYBRIDIZATION

Hybridization techniques are based on the application of recombinant DNA technology. The labeling of the probes can be done with radioactive or nonradioactive compounds (*e.g.,* bromodeoxyuridine).[74-79] Visualization of mRNA in tumor cells is being used increasingly to detect specific gene expressions, particularly those encoded by oncogenes and neuroendocrine-related genes.[80]

The two major techniques for hybridization of nucleic acids are the transfer or blotting methods (*i.e.,* Southern blotting for DNA, Northern blotting for RNA, and Western blotting for proteins) and in situ hybridization. The latter technique allows the visualization of cellular DNA or RNA in tissue sections, single cells, or chromosome preparations. The advantages of in situ hybridization over the transfer method are that it can be applied to small samples (in some instances even to paraffin-embedded material) and that it allows detection of the reaction product in specific cell types and subtypes or even subcellular sites. It allows a close correlation between the reaction and the morphologic appearance of the cells in which the reaction has occurred, a feature that represents the *desideratum* of any special technique in pathology.

Two important applications of nucleic acids hybridization in tumor pathology are in the evaluation of oncogenes and in the study of gene rearrangements in lymphoid diseases.

OTHER METHODS FOR ANALYSIS OF CELL PROLIFERATION

In addition to flow cytometry, several other methods exist for the evaluation of the degree of cellular proliferation.[81] These include mitotic count, thymidine labeling, microspectrophotometric analysis, and histochemical or immunohistochemical detection.

Mitotic Count

The older and most widely used method for evaluating cell proliferation is mitotic count. It is usually applied to routinely processed sections, the standard figure quoted being the number of mitoses in ten consecutive high-power fields (usually the combination of a 10× eyepiece and a 40× objective). Its most useful application is in the evaluation of mesenchymal neoplasms, particularly uterine smooth muscle tumors. Despite its apparent objectivity, results vary considerably depending on the thickness of the section, fields chosen, density of tumor cells (in absolute terms and in relation to nonneoplastic elements), type of microscope used, delay in fixation, and observer's variability in the identification of mitotic figures. Some of these handicaps can be eliminated by expressing the number of mitotic figures as percentages of tumor cells present.[82]

Thymidine Labeling

Thymidine labeling of fresh tumor tissue is followed by fixation, paraffin-embedding, and radioautography. The labeled nuclei are those that have incorporated the tritiated thymidine and are therefore in the S phase (DNA synthesis). An alternative (nonradioactive) marker is bromodeoxyuridine, a thymidine analog that is incorporated into nuclear DNA during the S phase and is detectable immunohistochemically.[83,84]

Microspectrophotometric Analysis

This analysis is performed by staining tissue sections with the Feulgen reaction (which is specific for DNA) and determining the DNA content (expressed in arbitrary units) in a microspectrophotometer.

Histochemical or Immunohistochemical Detection

Histochemical or immunohistochemical analysis can detect substances related to cell growth and division. These include the following: Ki-67, a monoclonal antibody that binds to nuclear antigens expressed by cells in the proliferative phases G_1, G_2, M, and S;[85-87] proliferating cell nuclear antigen (PCNA, cyclin), one of several cycle-related nuclear proteins that is maximally elevated in late G1 and S phases of proliferating cells;[88,89] and nucleolar organizing region-associated proteins (AgNor), a marker of cell activation demonstrable with a simple silver technique.[90-92]

IMAGE ANALYSIS

The quantitative analysis of images has been explored as a method to generate prognostic and perhaps diagnostic information on tumors and other lesions. It can objectively quantify individual cytologic criteria, such as nuclear size, variation in size and shape, and degree of roundness.[93-95] It can also be applied at the architectural level to measure the total surface (and, by inference, the volume) of tumor involving a given site. For instance, in a study of prostatic carcinoma diagnosed on transurethral resection, the area of tumor as measured by image analysis was a better predictive factor for survival than the conventional method of calculating the percentage of involved chips.[96] Image analysis can also be used to measure immunohistochemical stainings for hormone receptors or any other markers.[97]

DIAGNOSTIC CYTOLOGY

Diagnostic cytology (cytopathology) deals with the morphologic examination of individual cells (as opposed to tissues in histopathology). Specimens used for this purpose are obtained in one of three ways: by exfoliation or desquamation from an epithelial surface (such as cervical smears obtained with a spatula or brush); by fluid from a body cavity, whether obtained spontaneously (*i.e.*, urine) or by aspiration (*i.e.*, pleural or ascitic fluid); and by fine-needle aspiration of solid lesions. Whatever the source of the material, the cytologic preparation is then spread on a glass slide, fixed, and stained. The Papanicolaou's stain is the one most commonly used, because of the greater nuclear details it is supposed to provide.

The criteria for the evaluation of cytologic specimens vary from organ to organ, but the basic criteria are common and relate to specific features of the nucleus and cytoplasm. Abnormalities in nuclear structure are grouped under the term *dyskaryosis* and include coarse or dense granularity, hyperchromasia, abnormal (large, multiple, or irregularly shaped) nucleoli, and variations in the shape and size of the nuclei. Abnormal mitoses may also be present. Two other common features of malignant tumor are *pleomorphism* (a pronounced variation in shape) and *anisocytosis* (a pronounced variation in size). The nuclear-cytoplasmic ratio generally increases, largely because of the increased nuclear size but also (in many cases) because of the smaller amount of cytoplasm compared with the corresponding normal cells. The cell-to-cell relations are likely to be altered.

FINE-NEEDLE ASPIRATION BIOPSY

The cytologic procedure generally known as *fine-needle aspiration biopsy* had its inception more than 50 years ago at Memorial Hospital in New York City.[98,99] All the basic rules that still govern the performance of this method were carefully set down in articles published by Dr. Fred Stewart. For some reason, the popularity of the procedure declined at that institution, to be revived decades later in Europe (particularly in Scandinavian countries) by clinicians, until achieving popularity on a worldwide basis.[100-103]

Aspiration biopsy is most useful in tumor diagnosis. Experience is needed to obtain optimal results, which vary markedly depending on seemingly trivial items such as the needle size and design, the way the needle is inserted and withdrawn from the needle track, the direction of the smear preparation, the type of slide (plain or frosted), and the staining method. It has been stated that mastery of the interpretation of aspiration biopsy cytology lies in the ability to translate cytologic appearances into tissue patterns with diagnostic significance. Reliance on individual cell features to the exclusion of pattern, as practiced by cytopathologists having little background knowledge of tissue pathology, decreases diagnostic accuracy and reflects a lack of understanding of the method.

An important and much discussed issue is the reliability of the technique, usually measured in terms of false-negative and false-positive results. These are difficult figures to obtain and to evaluate for several reasons, including the standards against which they are compared (*i.e.*, histopathologic diagnosis versus clinical outcome), the impact of actually performing and interpreting the aspirate as opposed to receiving a specimen taken by others for processing and review, and the statistical methods employed.

The main sites in which fine-needle aspiration is used are the breast, lymph nodes, salivary glands, thyroid, lung, intraabdominal organs, prostate, bone, and soft tissue.

Breast

The breast has been one of the preferred sites for the use of the fine-needle aspiration technique from its inception. The reported series list 10% or fewer false-negative figures for breast carcinoma and a negligible number of false-positive diagnoses. In the past, most studies in this field were directed at clinically apparent breast masses. Recently, Swedish investigators have developed a stereotactic device for the sampling of subclinical, mammographically detected breast lesions. The technique has been adopted on a trial basis by several groups in the United States, but it is too early to make a statement about its effectiveness.

Lymph Nodes

The original use of the technique in lymph nodes was in the diagnosis of leukemia, malignant lymphoma, and infectious diseases. Its main use now is to confirm a clinical diagnosis of metastatic carcinoma and to determine the type and site of the primary tumor whenever indicated. The sensitivity for tumor diagnosis is more than 95%, and the specificity for the absence of malignant tumor is more than 97%.

Salivary Glands

Benign mixed tumor is the most common neoplasm of the major salivary glands and is also the one most easily recognized in specimens from fine-needle aspiration. Warthin's tumor is also readily identifiable. Adenoid cystic carcinoma gave rise to serious interpretive problems in the past, but with the establishment of better cytologic patterns, it is recognized with ease in most instances. Problems still arise in recognizing acinic cell carcinomas and mucoepidermoid carcinoma, because of their well-differentiated nature.

Most salivary gland swellings are inflammatory in nature. Cytologically, most can be recognized easily because of the admixture of normal-appearing ductal and acinar cells and inflammatory cells.

Thyroid

The most common application of the fine-needle aspiration technique is in the evaluation of the single cold nodule. In deciding whether the nodule represents a true neoplasm or part of a nodular hyperplasia (adenomatoid goiter), the sensitivity and specificity of the technique are more than 90% accurate. In determining the tumor type, cytology is accurate in the identification of papillary carcinoma (including most of its variants), poorly differentiated and undifferentiated carcinoma, and medullary carcinoma. The main difficulty rests in distinguishing between follicular adenoma and low-grade (*i.e.*, well-differentiated, minimally invasive) follicular carcinoma. This is because the distinction is largely based on capsular and vascular invasion, two criteria that cannot be

identified cytologically. However, because statistically follicular carcinomas are more likely to be more cellular and their nuclei more hyperchromatic than those of adenoma, a reasonably accurate "index of suspicion" for malignancy has been devised.

In practice, the three most common diagnoses made in thyroid fine-needle aspiration are nonneoplastic disorder (nodular goiter or thyroiditis), papillary carcinoma, and follicular neoplasm (not otherwise specified). The latter two diagnoses generally indicate the need for an operation.

Lung

Improvements in fluoroscopy have made the fine-needle aspiration procedure in the lung accurate and cost-effective, allowing the diagnosis of small lesions. In most series, false-positive results are fewer than 1%, but false-negative results occur in fewer than 10% of cases. For lung carcinoma, cytology allows typing just as accurately as histopathology, particularly in regard to the tumor for which typing carries the greatest practical importance (*i.e.*, small cell carcinoma).

Transthoracic fine-needle aspiration is perhaps the only aspiration procedure associated with occasional but significant complications. These include pneumothorax (about 10%), air embolism, and hemorrhage.

Intraabdominal Organs

More fine-needle aspirations are being performed in tumors in the abdominal cavity and retroperitoneum, including such sites as the liver, biliary tree, pancreas, adrenal, kidney, and retroperitoneal soft tissues. This has been related to the better localization of the lesion as a result of computed tomography, magnetic resonance imaging, and ultrasonography. For carcinomas of the ovary and uterus (usually recurrent in the pelvis), aspiration procedures can be carried out transvaginally or transrectally. The diagnosis of recurrent carcinoma involving the pelvis is easily made in most cases.

Prostate

Use of fine-needle aspiration in the prostate is controversial. Although the method is performed easily in an office setting, is relatively free of complications, is repeatable during the same visit or subsequent visits, and is cost-effective and reliable, urologists in the United States are reluctant to use the technique on a large scale. In the reported series, accuracy has ranged from 63% to 91%.

Bone and Soft Tissue

For bone lesions, the main use of aspiration cytology has been to identify metastatic tumors, with excellent results in terms of sensitivity and specificity. High-grade soft tissue sarcomas are identified with ease on cytologic preparations, because they usually lack the cell cohesiveness of metastatic carcinomas. The cell pattern may suggest a specific diagnosis, such as liposarcoma or leiomyosarcoma.

Cytologic material can be subjected to most of the special techniques that have been introduced over the years in histopathology. These include conventional special stains (*e.g.*,

PAS or mucicarmine), immunohistochemistry, electron microscopy, cytogenetics, molecular diagnostics, ploidy determination, and image analysis.[104-106] In image analysis, several efforts are being made to develop automated screening devices for the detection of abnormal cells in cytologic specimens from the female genital tract.[107] These devices use quantitative parameters to define limits of normality for the digital analysis of smears or monolayers. These instruments have the potential to serve as prescreening or rescreening devices for quality assurance, but large-scale prospective testing is required to decide how much of this potential can be realized.

INTRAOPERATIVE CONSULTATION

Intraoperative consultation (often referred to as *frozen section*) is one of the most important activities that the tumor pathologist performs. Introduced in this country by Welch in 1891 and developed for intraoperative pathologic diagnosis at the Mayo Clinic by Wilson and MacCarthy in 1905,[108] it is now used routinely in all pathology laboratories. It requires extensive experience, a good background in clinical medicine and anatomic pathology, sound judgment, and a keen awareness of the limitations of the method.

The reasons for doing a frozen section vary from organ to organ, but the basic indications remain the same. The three legitimate purposes of a frozen section are to establish the presence and nature of a lesion, to determine the adequacy of surgical margins, and to establish whether the sample obtained is adequate for the purpose for which it was taken (*i.e.,* for diagnosis or for special procedures such as hormone receptors or cell markers). If the result of the procedure will not influence in any way the subsequent course of the operation, the procedure is not indicated.

The overall accuracy of the procedure has been tested on numerous occasions and is consistently very high.[108-112] The Association of Directors of Anatomic and Surgical Pathology has estimated that an acceptable accuracy threshold is 3% (as measured by the number of cases in which a major disagreement existed between the frozen section and the permanent diagnosis).[113] Reasons for these discrepancies include mistaken interpretation of the slide, inadequate sampling of the gross specimen received, inadequate technical quality of the material, and lack of crucial clinical information. The first two together account for about 90% of the mistakes.

To carry out the procedure effectively, the pathologist should be thoroughly briefed on the patient's clinical history. Ideally, the surgeon and the pathologist should discuss the case beforehand, and the pathologist should review any previous slides on the case. The standard technique involves sampling of the tissue received, freezing, cutting of sections in a cryostat, staining of those sections with hematoxylin-eosin or an equivalent stain, and examination under the microscope. Ideally, this procedure takes about 5 minutes per specimen, although extra time must be allowed if multiple sections or specimens need to be examined on one case or if several cases are submitted at the same time.

Some groups have resurrected cytology to supplement and sometimes replace the frozen-section procedure as a way to provide an intraoperative diagnosis, a technique described as early as 1927. The proposal is attractive on several grounds,

one of them being the considerable amount of time saved (it takes 1 minute or less per slide and 5 to 10 minutes for a frozen section).[114,115] Although there are some specimens for which this technique is not feasible (*e.g.,* surgical margins or assessment of depth of invasion), there are many others in which it can provide as much information as the frozen section (or sometimes even more) and in a more expeditious fashion. Additional advantages are that the tissue is better conserved for subsequent permanent sections (a feature particularly important with small samples) and that it provides more thorough sampling of large, multiple, or highly necrotic specimens.

REFERENCES

1. Cox WF Jr, Pierce GB. The endodermal origin of the endocrine cells of an adenocarcinoma of the colon of the rat. Cancer 1982;50:1530–1538.
2. Azumi N, Curtis J, Kempson RL, et al. Atypical and malignant neoplasms showing lipomatous differentiation: A study of 111 cases. Am J Surg Pathol 1987;11:161–183.
3. Bostwick DG, Tazelaar HD, Ballon SC, et al. Ovarian epithelial tumors of borderline malignancy: A clinical and pathologic study of 109 cases. Cancer 1986;58:2052–2065.
4. Hart WR, Billman JK. A reassessment of uterine neoplasms originally diagnosed as leiomyosarcomas. Cancer 1978;41:1902–1910.
5. Collan Y. General principles of grading lesions in diagnostic histopathology. Pathol Res Pract 1989;185:539–543.
6. Donjuijsen K. Mitosis counts: Reproducibility and significance in grading of malignancy. Hum Pathol 1986;17:1122–1125.
7. Costa J, Wesley RA, Glatstein E, et al. The grading of soft tissue sarcomas. Cancer 1984;53:530–541.
8. Henson DE, Ries L, Freedman LS, et al. Relationship among outcome, stage of disease, and histologic grade for 22,616 cases of breast cancer: The basis for a prognostic index. Cancer 1991;68:2142–2149.
9. Gleason DF. Histologic grading and clinical staging of prostatic carcinoma. In: Tannenbaum M, ed. Urologic pathology: The Prostate. Philadelphia: Lea & Febiger, 1977: 171–198.
10. Medline A, Farber E. The multi-step theory of neoplasia. In: Anthony PP, MacSween RNM, eds. Recent advances in histopathology. New York: Churchill Livingston, 1981: 19.
11. Buckley CH, Butler EB, Fox H. Cervical intraepithelial neoplasia. J Clin Pathol 1982;35: 1–13.
12. Rywlin AM. Dysplasia: On the terminology of atypical intraepithelial proliferations. Am J Dermatopathol 1981;3:183–185.
13. Rywlin AM. Malignant melanoma in situ, precancerous melanosis, or atypical intradermal melanocytic proliferation. Am J Dermatopathol 1984;6:97–99.
14. Clark WH Jr. Malignant melanoma in situ. Hum Pathol 1990;21:1197–1199.
15. McDowell EM, Trump BF. Histologic fixatives suitable for diagnostic light and electron microscopy. Arch Pathol Lab Med 1976:100:405–414.
16. Smith DM Jr, Haggitt RC. A comparative study of generic stains for carcinoid secretory granules. Am J Surg Pathol 1983;7:61–68.
17. Leder L-D. The chloroacetate esterase reaction: A useful means of histological diagnosis of hematological disorders from paraffin sections of skin. Am J Dermatopathol 1979;1: 39–42.
18. Beckstead JH, Halveson PS, Ries CA, et al. Enzyme histochemistry and immunohistochemistry on biopsy specimens of pathologic human bone marrow. Blood 1981;57: 1088–1098.
19. Beckstead JH. Alkaline phosphatase histochemistry in human germ cell neoplasms. Am J Surg Pathol 1983;7:341–349.
20. Sheibani K, Tubbs RR. Enzyme immunohistochemistry: Technical aspects. Semin Diagn Pathol 1984;1:235–250.
21. Murray MR, Stout AP. The classification and diagnosis of human tumors by tissue culture methods. Tex Rep Biol Med 1954;12:898–915.
22. Giuffrè L, Schreyer M, Mach J-P, et al. Cyclic AMP induces differentiation in vitro of human melanoma cells. Cancer 1988;61:1132–1141.
23. Cavazzana AO, Miser JS, Jefferson J, et al. Experimental evidence for a neural origin of Ewing's sarcoma of bone. Am J Pathol 1987;127:507–518.
24. Ioachim HL. Tissue culture of human tumors: Its use and prospects. Pathol Annu 1970;5:217–256.
25. Bonikos DS, Bensch KG, Kempson RL. The contribution of electron microscopy to the differential diagnosis of tumors. Beitr Pathol 1976;158:417–444.
26. Erlandson RA. Application of transmission electron microscopy to human tumor diagnosis: An historical perspective. Cancer Invest 1987;5:487–505.
27. Fisher C. The value of electron microscopy and immunohistochemistry in the diagnosis of soft tissue sarcomas: A study of 200 cases. Histopathology 1990;16:441–454.
28. Ghadially FN. Diagnostic electron microscopy of tumours. 2nd ed. London: Butterworth, 1985.
29. Mackay B, Silva EG. Diagnostic electron microscopy in oncology. Pathol Annu 1980; 15 (part 2):241–270.

30. Williams MJ, Uzman BG. Uses and contributions of diagnostic electron microscopy in surgical pathology: A study of 20 Veterans Administration hospitals. Hum Pathol 1984;15:738–745.

31. Battifora H. Recent progress in the immunohistochemistry of solid tumors. Semin Diagn Pathol 1984;1:251–271.

32. DeLellis RA, Dayal Y. The role of immunohistochemistry in the diagnosis of poorly differentiated malignant neoplasms. Semin Oncol 1987;14:173–192.

33. Mukai K, Rosai J. Applications of immunoperoxidase techniques in surgical pathology. In: Fenoglio CM, Wolff M, eds. Progress in surgical pathology, vol 1. New York: Masson Publishing, 1980.

34. Mukai K, Yoshimura S, Anzai M. Effects of decalcification on immunoperoxidase staining. Am J Surg Pathol 1986;10:413–419.

35. Buffa R, Crivelli O, Fiocca R, et al. Complement–mediated unspecific binding of immunoglobulins to some endocrine cells. Histochemistry 1979;63:15–21.

36. Eusebi V, Bondi A, Rosai J. Immunohistochemical localization of myoglobin in non-muscular cells. Am J Surg Pathol 1984;8:51–55.

37. Battifora H. The multitumor (sausage) tissue block: Novel method for immunohistochemical antibody testing. Lab Invest 1986;55:244–248.

38. Azumi N, Battifora H. The distribution of vimentin and keratin in epithelial and non-epithelial neoplasms: A comprehensive immunohistochemical study on formalin- and alcohol-fixed tumors. Am J Clin Pathol 1987;88:286–296.

39. Battifora H. Clinical applications of the immunohistochemistry of filamentous proteins. Am J Surg Pathol 1988;12:24–42.

40. Denk H, Krepler R, Artlieb U, et al. Proteins of intermediate filaments: An immunohistochemical and biochemical approach to the classification of soft tissue tumors. Am J Pathol 1983;110:193–208.

41. De Armond SJ, Eng LF, Rubinstein LJ. The application of glial fibrillary acidic (GFA) protein immunohistochemistry in neurooncology. Pathol Res Pract 1980;168:374–394.

42. Leader M, Collins M, Patel J, et al. Vimentin: An evaluation of its role as a tumor marker. Histopathology 1987;11:63–72.

43. Osborne M, Weber K. Tumor diagnosis by intermediate filament typing. Lab Invest 1983;48:372–394.

44. Moll R, Franke WW, Schiller DL, et al. The catalog of human cytokeratins: Patterns of expression in normal epithelia, tumors and cultured cells. Cell 1982;31:11–24.

45. Mukai K, Rosai J, Hallaway BE. Localization of myoglobin in normal and neoplastic human skeletal muscle cells using an immunoperoxidase method. Am J Surg Pathol 1979;3:373–376.

46. Rosai J, Dias P, Parham DM, et al. MyoD1 protein expression in alveolar soft part sarcoma as confirmatory evidence of its skeletal muscle nature. Am J Surg Pathol 1991;15:974–981.

47. Schurch W, Skalli O, Seemayer TA. Intermediate filament proteins and actin isoforms as markers for soft tissue tumor differentiation and origin. 1. Smooth muscle tumors. Am J Pathol 1987;128:91–103.

48. Skalli O, Gabbiani G, Babai F, et al. Intermediate filament proteins and actin isoforms as markers for soft tissue tumor differentiation and origin. II. Rhabdomyosarcomas. Am J Pathol 1988;130:515–531.

49. Kurtin PJ, Pinkus GS. Leukocyte common antigen: A diagnostic discriminant between hematopoietic and nonhematopoietic neoplasms in paraffin sections using monoclonal antibodies. Correlation with immunologic studies and ultrastructural localization. Hum Pathol 1985;16:353–365.

50. Kahn HJ, Marks A, Thom H, et al. Role of antibody to S-100 protein in diagnostic pathology. Am J Clin Pathol 1983;79:341–347.

51. Nakajima T, Watanabe S, Sato Y, et al. An immunoperoxidase study of S-100 protein distribution in normal and neoplastic tissues. Am J Surg Pathol 1982;6:715–727.

52. Leong AS–Y, Milios J. An assessment of a melanoma–specific antibody (HMB-45) and other immunohistochemical markers of malignant melanoma in paraffin embedded tissues. Surg Pathol 1989;2:137–146.

53. Sheahan K, O'Brien MJ, Burke B, et al. Differential reactivities of carcinoembryonic antigen (CEA) and CEA-related monoclonal and polyclonal antibodies in common epithelial malignancies. Am J Clin Pathol 1990;94:157–164.

54. Pinkus GS, Kurtin PJ. Epithelial membrane antigen: A diagnostic discriminant in surgical pathology. Hum Pathol 1985;16:929–940.

55. Chejfec G, Falkmer S, Grimelius L, et al. Synaptophysin: A new marker for pancreatic neuroendocrine tumors. Am J Surg Pathol 1987;11:241–247.

56. Lloyd RV. Immunohistochemical localization of chromogranin in normal and neoplastic endocrine tissues. Pathol Annu 1987;22:69–90.

57. Seshi B, True L, Carter D, et al. Immunohistochemical characterization of a set of monoclonal antibodies to human neuron-specific enolase. Am J Pathol 1988;131:258–269.

58. Albores-Saavedra J, Nadji M, Civantos F, et al. Thyroglobulin in carcinoma of the thyroid. Hum Pathol 1983;14:62–66.

59. Nadji M, Tabei SZ, Castro A, et al. Prostatic-specific antigen: An immunohistologic marker for prostatic neoplasms. Cancer 1984;48:1229–1232.

60. Mazoujian G, Pinkus GS, Davis S, et al. Immunohistochemistry of a gross cystic disease fluid protein (GCDFP-15) of the breast: A marker of apocrine epithelium and breast carcinomas. Am J Pathol 1983;110:105–112.

61. Miettinen M, Holthofer H, Lehto V-P, et al. *Ulex europaeus* I lectin as a marker for tumors derived from endothelial cells. Am J Clin Pathol 1983;79:32–36.

62. Mukai K, Rosai J, Burgdorf WHC. Localization of factor VIII–related antigen in vascular endothelial cells using an immunoperoxidase method. Am J Surg Pathol 1980;4:273–276.

63. Miettinen M, Foidart J-M, Ekblom P. Immunohistochemical demonstration of laminin, the major glycoprotein of basement membranes, as an aid in the diagnosis of soft tissue tumors. Am J Clin Pathol 1983;79:306–311.

64. Carcangiu ML, Chambers JT, Voynick RM, et al. Immunohistochemical evaluation of estrogen and progesterone receptor content in 183 patients with endometrial carcinoma. Part I. Clinical and histologic correlations. Am J Clin Pathol 1990;94:247–252.

65. Chambers JT, Carcangiu ML, Voynick IM, et al. Immunohistochemical evaluation of estrogen and progesterone receptor content in 183 patients with endometrial carcinoma. Part II. Correlation between biochemical and immunohistochemical methods and survival. Am J Clin Pathol 1990;94:255–260.

66. McCarty KS Jr, McCarty KS Sr. Histochemical approaches to steroid receptor analyses. Semin Diagn Pathol 1984;2:297–308.

67. Pascal RR, Santeusanio G, Sarrell D, et al. Immunohistologic detection of estrogen receptors in paraffin-embedded breast cancers: Correlation with cytosol measurements. Hum Pathol 1986;17:370–375.

68. Frierson HF Jr. Flow cytometric analysis of ploidy in solid neoplasms: Comparison of fresh tissues with formalin-fixed paraffin-embedded specimens. Hum Pathol 1988;19:290–294.

69. Pelstring RJ, Hurtubise PE, Swerdlow SH. Flow-cytometric DNA analysis of hematopoietic and lymphoid proliferations: A comparison of fresh, formalin-fixed and B5-fixed tissues. Hum Pathol 1990;21:551–558.

70. Coon JS, Landay AL, Weinstein RS. Biology of disease: Advances in flow cytometry for diagnostic pathology. Lab Invest 1987;57:453–479.

71. Lovett EJ III, Schnitzer B, Keren DF, et al. Application of flow cytometry to diagnostic pathology. Lab Invest 1984;50:115–140.

72. Merke DE, McGuire WL. Ploidy, proliferative activity and prognosis: DNA flow cytometry of solid tumors. Cancer 1990;65:1194–1206.

73. Wersto RP, Liblit RL, Koss LG. Flow cytometric DNA analysis of human solid tumors: A review of the interpretation of DNA histograms. Hum Pathol 1991;22:1085–1098.

74. DeLellis RA, Wolfe HJ. The application of in situ hybridization techniques to endocrine pathology: An overview. Endocrinol Pathol Update 1990;1:293–310.

75. Grody WW, Cheng L, Lewin KJ. Application of in situ DNA hybridization technology to diagnostic surgical pathology. Pathol Annu 1987;22:151–175.

76. Polak JM, McGee JO'D, eds. In Situ Hybridization: Principles and practice. Oxford: Oxford University Press, 1990.

77. Sklar J. DNA hybridization in diagnostic pathology. Hum Pathol 1985;16:654–658.

78. Samoszuk M. Rapid detection of Epstein-Barr viral DNA by nonisotopic in situ hybridization: Correlation with the polymerase chain reaction. Am J Pathol 1991;96:448–453.

79. Schad CR, Kraker WJ, Jalal SM, et al. Use of fluorescent in situ hybridization for marker chromosome identification in congenital and neoplastic disorders. Cytogenetics 1991;96:203–210.

80. Bartow SA. Diagnostic and prognostic applications of oncogenes in surgical pathology. Am J Surg Pathol 1990;14:5–15.

81. Woosley JT. Measuring cell proliferation. Arch Pathol Lab Med 1991;115:555–557.

82. Ellis PSJ, Chir B, Whitehead R. Mitosis counting: A need for reappraisal. Hum Pathol 1981;12:3–4.

83. Lloveras B, Edgerton S, Thor AD. Evaluation of in vitro bromodeoxyuridine labeling of breast carcinomas with the use of a commercial kit. Am J Clin Pathol 1990;95:41–47.

84. Waldman FM, Chew K, Ljung B-M, et al. A comparison between bromodeoxyuridine and 3H thymidine labeling in human breast tumors. Mod Pathol 1991;4:718–722.

85. Deshmukh P, Ramsey L, Garewal HS. Ki-67 labeling index is a more reliable measure of solid tumor proliferative activity than tritiated thymidine labeling. Am J Clin Pathol 1990;94:192–195.

86. Brown DC, Gatter KC. Monoclonal antibody Ki-67: Its use in histopathology. Histopathology 1990;17:489–504.

87. Gerdes J, Li L, Schleuter C, et al. Immunobiochemical and molecular biologic characterization of the cell proliferation-associated nuclear antigen that is defined by monoclonal antibody Ki-67. Am J Pathol 1991;138:867–873.

88. Kamel OW, Lebrun DP, Davis RE, et al. Growth fraction estimation of malignant lymphomas in formalin-fixed paraffin-embedded tissue using anti-PCNA/cyclin 19A2. Am J Pathol 1991;138:1471–1477.

89. Van Dierendonch JH, Wijsman JH, Keijzer R, et al. Cell-cycle-related staining patterns of anti-proliferating cell nuclear antigen monoclonal antibodies: Comparison with BrdUrd labeling and Ki-67 staining. Am J Pathol 1991;138:1165–1172.

90. Derenzini M, Pession A, Trere D. Quantity of nucleolar silver-stained proteins is related to proliferating activity in cancer cells. Lab Invest 1990;63:137–140.

91. Smith R, Crocker J. Evaluation of nucleolar organizer region-associated proteins in breast malignancy. Histopathology 1988;12:113–115.

92. Ruschoff J, Plate K, Bittinger A, et al. Nucleolar organizer regions (NORS). Pathol Res Pract 1989;185:878–885.

93. Baak JPA, Kurver PHJ, Boon ME. Computer-aided application of quantitative microscopy in diagnostic pathology. Pathol Annu 1982;17(part 2):287–306.

94. Beck JS, Anderson JM. Quantitative methods as an aid to diagnosis in histopathology. Rec Adv Histopathol 1987;13:255–269.

95. Dawson AE, Austin RE, Weinberg DS. Nuclear grading of breast carcinoma by image analysis. Am J Clin Pathol 1991;95:S29–S37.

96. Foucar E, Haake G, Dalton L, et al. The area of cancer in transurethral resection specimens as a prognostic indicator in carcinoma of the prostate: A computer-assisted morphometric study. Hum Pathol 1990;21:586–592.

97. El-Badawy N, Cohen C, Derose PB, et al. Immunohistochemical progesterone receptor assay: Measurement by image analysis. Am J Clin Pathol 1991;96:704–710.

98. Martin HE, Ellis EB. Biopsy by needle puncture and aspiration. Ann Surg 1930;92:169–181.

99. Stewart F. The diagnosis of tumors by aspiration. Am J Pathol 1933;9:801–812.

100. Frable WJ. Fine–needle aspiration biopsy: A review. Hum Pathol 1983;14:9–28.

101. Frable WJ. Needle aspiration biopsy: Past, present, and future. Hum Pathol 1989;20:504–517.

102. Koss LG. Aspiration biopsy: A tool in surgical pathology. Am J Surg Pathol 1988;12:43–53.

103. Lever JV, Trott PA, Webb AJ. Fine needle aspiration cytology. J Clin Pathol 1985;38:1–11.

104. Dardick I, Yazdi HM, Brosko C, et al. A quantitative comparison of light and electron microscopic diagnoses in specimens obtained by fine–needle aspiration biopsy. Ultrastruct Pathol 1991;15:105–130.

105. Flens MJ, Van der Valk P, Tadema TM, et al. The contribution of immunocytochemistry in diagnostic cytology: Comparison and evaluation with immunohistology. Cancer 1990;65:2704–2711.

106. Weinraub J, Redard M, Wenger D, et al. The application of immunocytochemical techniques to routinely fixed and stained cytologic specimens. Pathol Res Pract 1990;186:658–665.

107. Hutchinson ML, Cassin CM, Ball HG. The efficacy of an automated preparation device for cervical cytology. Am J Clin Pathol 1991;96:300–305.

108. Zarbo RJ, Hoffman GG, Howanitz PJ. Interinstitutional comparison of frozen-section consultation: A college of American pathologist Q-probe study of 79647 consultation in 297 North American institutions. Arch Pathol Lab Med 1991;115:1187–1194.

109. Dankwa EK, Davies JD. Frozen section diagnosis: An audit. J Clin Pathol 1985;38:1235–1240.

110. Holaday WJ, Assor D. Ten thousand consecutive frozen sections: A retrospective study focusing on accuracy and quality control. Am J Clin Pathol 1974;61:769–777.

111. Howanitz PJ, Hoffman GG, Zarbo RJ. The accuracy of frozen section diagnoses in 34 hospitals. Arch Pathol Lab Med 1990;114:355–359.

112. Silva EG, Kraemer BB. Intraoperative pathologic diagnosis: Frozen section and other techniques. Baltimore: Williams & Wilkins, 1987.

113. Association of Directors of Anatomic and Surgical Pathology. Recommendations on quality control and quality assurance in anatomic pathology. Am J Surg Pathol 1991;15:1007–1009.

114. Abrams J, Silverberg SG. The role of intraoperative cytology in the evaluation of gynecologic disease. Pathol Annu 1989;24(part 2):167–187.

115. Mair S, Lash RH, Suskin D, et al. Intraoperative surgical specimen evaluation: Frozen section analysis, cytologic examination, or both? Am J Clin Pathol 1991;96:8–14.

Cancer: Principles & Practice of Oncology, Fourth Edition,
edited by Vincent T. DeVita, Jr., Samuel Hellman, Steven A. Rosenberg.
J.B. Lippincott Co., Philadelphia © 1993.

Steven A. Rosenberg

CHAPTER **14**

Principles of Surgical Oncology

Surgery is the oldest treatment for cancer and, until recently, was the only treatment that could cure patients with cancer. The surgical treatment of cancer has changed dramatically over the last several decades. Advances in surgical techniques and a better understanding of the patterns of spread of individual cancers have allowed surgeons to perform successful resections for an increased number of patients. The development of alternate treatment strategies that can control microscopic disease has prompted surgeons to reassess the magnitude of surgery necessary.

The surgeon who treats cancer must be familiar with the natural history of individual cancers and with the principles and potentialities of surgery, radiation therapy, chemotherapy, immunotherapy, and other new treatment modalities. The surgeon has a central role in the prevention, diagnosis, definitive treatment, palliation, and rehabilitation of the cancer patient. The principles underlying each of these roles of the surgical oncologist are discussed in this chapter.

HISTORICAL PERSPECTIVE

Although the earliest discussions of the surgical treatment of tumors are found in the Edwin Smith papyrus from the Egyptian Middle Kingdom (about 1600 B.C.), the modern era of elective surgery for visceral tumors began in frontier America in 1809.[1,2] Ephraim MacDowell removed a 22-pound ovarian tumor from a patient, Mrs. Jane Todd Crawford, who survived for 30 years after the operation. This procedure, the first of 13 ovarian resections performed by MacDowell, was the first elective abdominal operation and provided a great stimulus to the development of elective surgery.

The treatment of most tumors depended on two subsequent developments in surgery. The first of these was the introduc-

tion of general anesthesia by two dentists, Dr. William Morton and Dr. Crawford Long. The first major operation using general ether anesthesia was an excision of the submaxillary gland and part of the tongue, performed by Dr. John Collins Warren on October 16, 1846, at the Massachusetts General Hospital. The second major development stimulating the widespread application of surgery resulted from the introduction of the principles of antisepsis by Joseph Lister in 1867. Based on the concepts of Pasteur, Lister introduced carbolic acid in 1867 and described the principles of antisepsis in an article in *The Lancet* in that same year.

These developments freed surgery from pain and sepsis and greatly increased its use for the treatment of tumors. In the decade before the introduction of ether, only 385 operations were performed at the Massachusetts General Hospital. By the last decade of the 19th century, more than 20,000 operations per year were performed at that same hospital.[3]

Table 14–1 lists some selected milestones in the history of surgical oncology. Although this list does not include all of the important developments, it does provide the tempo of the application of surgery to cancer treatment.[4] Major figures in the evolution of surgical oncology included Albert Theodore Billroth who, in addition to developing meticulous surgical techniques, performed the first gastrectomy, laryngectomy, and esophagectomy. In the 1890s, William Stewart Halsted elucidated the principles of en bloc resections for cancer, as exemplified by the radical mastectomy. Examples of radical resections for cancers of individual organs include the radical prostatectomy by Hugh Young in 1904, the radical hysterectomy by Ernest Wertheim in 1906, the abdominoperineal resection for cancer of the rectum by W. Ernest Miles in 1908, and the first successful pneumonectomy performed for cancer by Evarts Graham in 1933. Modern technical innovations continue to extend the surgeon's capabilities. Recent examples

TABLE 14–1. Selected Historical Milestones in Surgical Oncology

Year	Surgeon	Event
1809	Ephraim McDowell	Elective abdominal surgery (excised ovarian tumor)
1846	John Collins Warren	Use of ether anesthesia (excised submaxillary gland)
1867	Joseph Lister	Introduction of antisepsis
1860–1890	Albert Theodore Billroth	First gastrectomy, laryngectomy, and esophagectomy
1878	Richard von Volkmann	Excision of cancerous rectum
1880s	Theodore Kocher	Development of thyroid surgery
1890	William Stewart Halsted	Radical mastectomy
1896	G. T. Beatson	Oophorectomy for breast cancer
1904	Hugh H. Young	Radical prostatectomy
1906	Ernest Wertheim	Radical hysterectomy
1908	W. Ernest Miles	Abdomenoperineal resection for rectal cancer
1912	E. Martin	Cordotomy for the treatment of pain
1910–1930	Harvey Cushing	Development of surgery for brain tumors
1913	Franz Torek	Successful resection of cancer of the thoracic esophagus
1927	G. Divis	Successful resection of pulmonary metastases
1933	Evarts Graham	Pneumonectomy
1935	A. O. Whipple	Pancreaticoduodenectomy
1945	Charles B. Huggins	Adrenalectomy for prostate cancer

include the development of microsurgical techniques that enable the performance of free grafts for reconstruction, automatic stapling devices, sophisticated endoscopic equipment that allows for a wide variety of "incisionless" surgery, and major improvements in postoperative management and critical care of patients that have extended the safety of major surgical therapy.

Critics who feel that the application of surgery has reached a plateau beyond which it will not progress should remember the words of famous British surgeon, Sir John Erichsen, who in his introductory address to the medical institutions at University College, said,

. . . there must be a final limit to the development of manipulative surgery, the knife cannot always have fresh fields for conquest and although methods of practice may be modified and varied and even improved to some extent, it must be within a certain limit. That this limit has nearly, if not quite, been reached will appear evident if we reflect on the great achievements of modern operative surgery. Very little remains for the boldest to devise or the most dextrous to perform.

These comments, published in *The Lancet* in 1873, preceded most important developments in modern surgical oncology.

THE OPERATION

ANESTHESIA

Modern anesthetic techniques have greatly increased the safety of major oncologic surgery. Regional and general anesthesia play important roles in a wide variety of diagnostic techniques, in local therapeutic maneuvers, and in major surgery. These techniques should be understood by all oncologists.

Anesthetic techniques may be divided into regional and general anesthesia. Regional anesthesia involves a reversible blockade of pain perception by the application of local anesthetic drugs. These agents generally work by preventing the activation of pain receptors or by blocking nerve conduction. Agents commonly used for regional anesthesia are shown in Table 14–2.[5] Topical anesthesia refers to the application of local anesthetics to the skin or mucous membranes. Good surface anesthesia of the conjunctiva and cornea, oropharynx and nasopharynx, esophagus, larynx, trachea, urethra, and anus can result from the application of these agents.

Local anesthesia involves injecting anesthetic agents directly into the operative field. *Field block* refers to injection of local anesthetic by circumscribing the operative field with a continuous wall of anesthetic agent. Lidocaine (Xylocaine) in concentrations from 0.5% to 1% is the most common anesthetic agent used for this purpose. Peripheral nerve block results from the deposition of a local anesthetic surrounding major nerve trunks. It can provide local anesthesia to entire anatomic areas.

Major surgical procedures in the lower portion of the body can be performed using epidural or spinal anesthesia. Epidural anesthesia results from the deposition of a local anesthetic agent into the extradural space within the vertebral canal. Catheters can be left in place in the epidural space, allowing the intermittent injection of local anesthetics for prolonged operations. The major advantage of epidural over spinal anesthesia is that it does not involve puncturing the dura, and the injection of foreign substances directly into the cerebrospinal fluid is avoided.

Spinal anesthesia involves the direct injection of a local anesthetic into the cerebrospinal fluid. Puncture of the dural sac generally is performed between the L2 and L4 vertebrae. Spinal anesthesia provides excellent anesthesia for intraabdominal operations, operations on the pelvis, or procedures involving the lower extremities. Because the patient is awake during spinal anesthesia and is breathing spontaneously, it often has been thought that spinal anesthesia is safer than

TABLE 14–2.   Regional Anesthetic Agents

Technique	Local Anesthetic	Concentration Range (%)	Duration of Action	Maximal Safe Dose (mg)
Topical anesthesia (mucous membranes)	Lidocaine	2–4	15 min	100
	Cocaine	4–10	30 min	100–200
	Tetracaine	1–2	45 min	40
	Benzocaine	2–10	Several hours	
Local infiltration	Procaine	0.5	¼–½ h	1000
	Lidocaine	0.5–1	½–1 h	500
	Mepivacaine	0.5–1	½–1 h	500
	Tetracaine	0.025–0.1	2–3 h	75
Major nerve block	Lidocaine	1–2	1–2 h	500
	Mepivacaine	1–2	1–2 h	500
	Tetracaine	0.1–0.25	2–3 h	75

(Adapted from Brunner EA, Eckenhoff JE. Anesthesia. In: Sabiston DC Jr, ed. Textbook of surgery. Philadelphia: WB Saunders, 1977)

general anesthesia. There is no difference in the incidence of intraoperative hypotension with spinal anesthesia compared with general anesthesia, and there is no clear benefit in using spinal anesthesia for patients with ischemic heart disease.[6] Because patients are awake during spinal anesthesia and can become agitated during the surgical procedure, spinal anesthesia actually can cause more myocardial stress than general anesthesia. The health status of patients with preoperative evidence of congestive heart failure is more likely to be worsened by general anesthesia than by spinal anesthesia. In one series, heart failure developed de novo in 4% of adults over the age of 40 years who were undergoing major surgery, and worsened in 22% of patients who had a history of heart failure.[6] Spinal anesthesia was not associated with any new or worsened heart failure. Because of local irritating effects of general anesthesia on the lung, it has been suggested that spinal anesthesia may be safer for patients with severe pulmonary disease.

General anesthesia refers to the reversible state of loss of consciousness produced by chemical agents that act directly on the brain. Most major oncologic procedures are performed under general anesthesia, which can be induced using intravenous or inhalational agents. The advantages of intravenous anesthesia are the extremely rapid onset of unconsciousness and improved patient comfort and acceptance. Ultrashort-acting barbiturates such as sodium thiopental, or tranquilizers such as the benzodiazepines or droperidol, are the most frequently used intravenous agents for general anesthesia or for sedation during regional anesthesia.

A variety of inhalational anesthetic agents are in clinical use. The most popular is nitrous oxide, usually in combination with narcotics and muscle relaxants. This technique provides a safe form of general anesthesia with the use of nonexplosive agents. Two other agents in widespread use are the fluorinated hydrocarbons, halothane (Fluothane) and enflurane (Ethrane). Although they are used frequently, the fluorinated hydrocarbons have a variety of side effects. Halothane depresses myocardial function, reduces cardiac output, causes significant vasodilation, and sensitizes the myocardium to endogenous and administered catecholamines, which can lead to life-threatening cardiac arrhythmias. In rare instances, halothane

can cause severe hepatotoxicity, which begins 2 to 5 days after surgery. Enflurane also depresses myocardial function but does not appear to sensitize the myocardium to catecholamines and has not been associated with hepatic toxicity. The newest of the halogenated hydrocarbons is isoflurane, which was introduced in 1980. Isoflurane depresses the myocardium less than halothane or enflurane, but it has more potent vasodilatory properties.

Virtually all general anesthetics affect biochemical mechanisms, including depression of bone marrow, alteration of the phagocytic activity of macrophages, and exhibition of immunosuppressive properties. General anesthetic agents, such as cyclopropane and diethyl ether, are rarely used because of their explosive potential.

Intravenous neuromuscular blocking agents, called *muscle relaxants*, are commonly used during general anesthesia. These agents are nondepolarizing (*e.g.,* curare), preventing access of acetylcholine to the receptor site of the myoneural junction, or depolarizing (*e.g.,* succinylcholine), acting in a manner similar to that of acetylcholine by depolarizing the motor end plate. These agents induce profound muscle relaxation during surgical procedures but have the disadvantage of inhibiting spontaneous respiration because of paralysis of respiratory muscles. Succinylcholine is short acting (3–5 minutes) with a rapid recovery phase. Curare-induced paralysis lasts for 30 to 40 minutes after usual clinical doses of 0.3 to 0.5 mg/kg. Pancuronium is a newer nondepolarizing agent that has fewer side effects than curare but can induce tachycardia by means of sympathetic stimulation.

DETERMINATION OF OPERATIVE RISK

As with any treatment, the potential benefits of surgical intervention in cancer patients must be weighed against the risks of surgery. The incidence of operative mortality is of major importance in formulating therapeutic decisions and varies greatly in different patient situations (Table 14–3). The incidence of operative mortality is a complex function of the basic disease process that involves surgery, anesthetic technique, operative complications, and, most importantly, the

TABLE 14–3. Determinants of Operative Risk

General health status
Severity of underlying illness
Degree to which surgery disrupts normal physiologic functions
Technical complexity of the procedure (related to incidence of complications)
Type of anesthesia required
Experience of personnel

general health status of patients and their ability to withstand operative trauma.

In an attempt to classify the physical status of patients and their surgical risks, the American Society of Anesthesiologists has formulated a General Classification of Physical Status that appears to correlate well with operative mortality.[7] Patients are classified into five groups depending on their general health status.

Class I. The patient has no organic, physiologic, biochemical, or psychiatric disturbance. The pathologic process for which the operation is to be performed is localized and does not entail a systemic disturbance. (Examples: a fit patient with a lipoma or an otherwise healthy woman with a fibroid uterus)

Class II. Mild to moderate systemic disturbances caused by the condition to be surgically treated or the pathophysiologic processes. The extremes of age are included here, the neonate or the octogenarian, even though no discernible systemic disease is present. Extreme obesity and chronic bronchitis also are included in this category. (Examples: nonlimiting or only slightly limiting organic heart disease, mild diabetes, essential hypertension, or anemia)

Class III. Severe systemic disturbance or disease from whatever cause, even though it may not be possible to define firmly the degree of disability. (Examples: severely limiting organic heart disease, severe diabetes with vascular complications, moderate to severe degrees of pulmonary insufficiency, angina pectoris, or healed myocardial infarction)

Class IV. Indicative of the patient with severe systemic disorders that already are life-threatening and not always correctable by an operation. (Examples: severely cachectic patients with metastatic cancer; patients with organic heart disease showing marked signs of cardiac insufficiency, persistent anginal syndrome, or active myocarditis; advanced degrees of pulmonary, hepatic, renal, or endocrine insufficiency; severe neutropenia or thrombocytopenia in cancer patients)

Class V. The moribund patient who has little chance of survival but who submitted to operation in desperation. Most of these patients require an operation as a resuscitative measure with little, if any, anesthesia. (Examples: burst abdominal aneurysm with profound shock, major cerebral trauma with rapidly increasing intracranial pressure, massive pulmonary embolus)

Emergency Operation (E). Any patient in classes I through V who is operated on as an emergency is considered to be in poor physical condition. The letter *E* is placed beside the numerical classification. (Examples: perforation of a viscus, major hemorrhage from a gastrointestinal mass, or hitherto uncomplicated hernia now incarcerated and associated with nausea and vomiting)

Operative mortality usually is defined as mortality that occurs within 30 days of a major operative procedure. In oncologic patients, the basic disease process is a major determinant of operative mortality. Patients undergoing palliative surgery for widely metastatic disease have a high operative mortality even if the surgical procedure can alleviate the symptomatic problem. Examples of these situations include surgery for intestinal obstruction in patients with widespread ovarian cancer and surgery for gastric outlet obstruction in patients with cancer of the head of the pancreas. These simple palliative procedures are associated with mortality rates of 20% to 30% in most series because of the debilitated state of the patient and the rapid progression of the basic disease.

Mortality caused by anesthetic administration alone is related directly to the physical status of the patient. In a review of 32,223 operations, Dripps and colleagues determined the mortality thought to be related to anesthetic administration alone (Table 14–4).[8] It is extremely difficult to differentiate the mortality caused by anesthesia from that resulting from other contributors to operative mortality. However, this analysis indicates that operative mortality due to anesthesia in physical status class 1 patients is extremely low, less than 1 in every 16,000 operations. The anesthetic mortality increased with worsened physical status. Most cancer patients undergoing elective cancer surgery fall somewhere between physical status 2 and 3. An anesthetic mortality rate of 0.1% to 0.2% is a realistic estimate for this group.

In an attempt to determine the operative mortality from anesthesia alone, similar estimates to that found by Dripps and colleagues have been obtained. For example, Moir found the fatality rate for women undergoing cesarean sections in Great Britain to be 1 in 1250 to 2000 deliveries.[9] The mortality thought to be caused by anesthesia alone was 1 patient in every 6000 to 7500 deliveries. A similar estimate was obtained by Collins and associates, who estimated that the mortality resulting from general anesthesia alone was about 1 in 3000 to 5000 in otherwise healthy patients.[10] Several health factors can increase the risks of the operative procedure. If the patient recently had a myocardial infarction, the risk of cardiac death associated with surgery increases significantly.[11] A recurrent myocardial infarction or cardiac death occurs in about 30% of patients who have surgery within 3 months after a myocardial infarction and in about 15% of patients who have surgery 3 to 6 months after an infarction. The risk of a recurrent infarction or cardiac death decreases to about 5% after 6 months and remains about constant regardless of how much longer the patient survives. Operative risks are similar after subendocardial and transmural infarctions.

Patients with a preoperative history of pulmonary edema

TABLE 14–4. Anesthetic Mortality Related to Physical Status

Physical Status	Number of Patients	Number of Deaths	Anesthetic Mortality (%)
Class I	16,192	0	<.006
Class II	12,154	7	0.058
Class III	4070	11	0.27
Class IV	720	17	2.4
Class V	87	4	4.6
Total	33,223	39	0.12

(Adapted from Dripps RD, Lamont A, Eckenhoff JE. The role of anesthesia in surgical mortality. JAMA 1961;178:261)

or with clinical evidence of congestive heart failure by pre-operative physical examination and chest x-ray films have a markedly increased risk for developing perioperative pulmonary edema. In a study of patients over the age of 40 undergoing major surgery, 23% of patients with a history of pulmonary edema developed cardiogenic pulmonary edema in the postoperative period, compared with 2% of patients with no history of congestive heart failure.[6,11] Because of the complexities of evaluating the general health status of a patient, multivariate analyses have been performed to determine which factors independently predict the development of complications. An example of one such multivariate analysis is presented in Table 14–5.[11] In this series of 1001 patients over the age of 40 who underwent major noncardiac surgical procedures, nine separate factors were used to group the patients into categories with substantially different risks of cardiac complications. Each factor listed in Table 14–5 was associated with a number of points, and the total number of points determined the risk class. For patients in class I (0 to 5 points), 0.7% of patients had cardiac complications from the surgical procedure, and 0.2% of patients died of cardiac causes. The risk of cardiac complications and death in class II patients (6 to 12 points) was 5% and 2%, respectively. In class III patients (13 to 25 points), the probability of nonfatal complications was 11%, but the risk of death remained at 2%. In class IV risk patients (26 or more points), 56% of patients died of cardiac causes, and an additional 22% had life-threatening, nonfatal complications.

The impact of general health status on operative mortality is seen when operative mortality as a function of age is analyzed. Palmberg and colleagues studied the postoperative mortality of 17,199 patients undergoing general surgical pro-

cedures.[12] The overall mortality rate of patients under 70 years was 0.25%, compared with 9.2% for patients over 70 years. In these elderly patients, the operative mortality rate for emergency operations was 36.8%, compared with 7.8% for elective surgical procedures. The four leading causes of operative mortality that accounted for about 75% of all postoperative deaths in this age group were pulmonary embolism, pneumonia, cardiovascular collapse, and the primary illness itself.

More recently, Hoskings and colleagues reviewed the outcome of surgery performed on 795 patients 90 years of age or older.[13] Surgery was generally well tolerated. As with younger patients, the American Society of Anesthesiology classification was an important predictor of outcome.

Reports of most surgical series include an account of operative mortality and operative complications. These results, combined with a consideration of the general health status of the patient, allow a reasonable estimate of the operative mortality for any given surgical intervention in the treatment of cancer.

ROLES FOR SURGERY

PREVENTION OF CANCER

Because surgeons are often the primary providers of medical care, they are responsible for educating patients about carcinogenic hazards and about direct surgical intervention for the prevention of cancer. All surgical oncologists should be aware of the high-risk situations that require surgery to prevent subsequent malignant disease.

TABLE 14–5. Correlation Between Signs and Symptoms of Preoperative Heart Failure and Risk of Perioperative Pulmonary Edema After Major Surgery in Patients Over Age 40

Signs and Symptoms	Total Patients (No.)	Patients Developing Cardiogenic Pulmonary Edema (%)
No history of congestive heart failure	853	2*
History of left heart failure but not evident on preoperative examination or chest roentgenogram	87	6*
Left heart failure by preoperative physical examination or chest roentgenogram	66	16*
Preoperative NYHA functional class for congestive heart failure		
I	935	
II	15	7
III	34	6
IV	17	25†
History of pulmonary edema	22	23‡
S3 gallop	17	35‡
Jugular venous distention and signs of left heart failure	23	30‡

* $p < 0.01$ for all pairs.
† $p < 0.001$ for class IV versus all others.
‡ $p < 0.01$ when comparing patients to those without these findings.
(Goldman L. Cardiac risks and complications of noncardiac surgery. Ann Surg 1983;198:780–791)

Underlying conditions or congenital or genetic traits are associated with an extremely high incidence of subsequent cancer. When these cancers are likely to occur in nonvital organs, it is necessary to remove the offending organ to prevent subsequent malignancy.[14] Examples of diseases associated with a high incidence of cancer that can be prevented by prophylactic surgery are presented in Table 14–6. An excellent example is presented by patients with the genetic trait for multiple polyposis of the colon. If colectomy is not performed in these patients, about half will develop colon cancer by the age of 40. By the age of 70, virtually all patients with multiple polyposis will develop colon cancer.[14] It is therefore advisable for all patients containing the mutant gene for multiple polyposis to undergo prophylactic colectomy before the age of 20 to prevent these cancers.

In this situation, as for many of the other familial conditions associated with a high incidence of cancer, the surgeon has a responsibility for alerting the family to the hereditary nature of the disorder and its possible occurrence in the other family members. Another disease associated with a high incidence of cancer of the colon is ulcerative colitis. About 40% of patients with total colonic involvement ultimately die of colon cancer if they survive the ulcerative colitis.[15] Three percent of children with ulcerative colitis develop cancer of the colon by the age of 10, and 20% develop cancer during each ensuing decade.[16] Colectomy is indicated for patients with ulcerative colitis if the chronicity of this disease is well established.

Other disorders that require early treatment to prevent subsequent cancers include cryptorchidism and multiple endocrine neoplasia. Cryptorchidism is associated with a high incidence of testicular cancer that probably can be prevented by early prophylactic surgery. Patients with multiple endocrine neoplasia (types II and III) should be screened for the presence of C-cell hyperplasia using pentagastrin-stimulation tests. If thyrocalcitonin levels are increased after this provocative test, thyroidectomy should be performed to prevent the subsequent clinical occurrence of medullary cancer of the thyroid gland.

A more complex example of the role of surgery in cancer prevention involves women at high risk for breast cancer. Because the risk of cancer in some women is increased substantially over the normal risk (but does not approach 100%),

TABLE 14–6. Surgery That Can Prevent Cancer

Underlying Condition	Associated Cancer	Prophylactic Surgery
Cryptorchidism	Testicular	Orchiopexy
Polyposis coli	Colon	Colectomy
Familial colon cancer	Colon	Colectomy
Ulcerative colitis	Colon	Colectomy
Multiple endocrine neoplasia, types II and III	Medullary cancer of the thyroid	Thyroidectomy
Familial breast cancer	Breast	Mastectomy
Familial ovarian cancer	Ovary	Oophorectomy

(Adapted from Mulvihill JJ. Cancer control through genetics. In: Arrighi FE, Rao PN, Stubblefield E, eds. Genes, chromosomes, and neoplasia. New York: Raven Press, 1980)

counseling is required. Women in this situation must carefully balance the benefits and risks of prophylactic mastectomy. A careful understanding of the factors involved in increased breast cancer incidence is essential for the surgical oncologist to provide sound advice in this area. Statistical techniques can provide approximations of the risk for patients depending on the frequency of disease in the family history, the age at the first pregnancy, and the presence of fibrocystic disease. For example, a woman with a family history of breast cancer in a sister or mother, who has fibrocystic disease, and is nulliparous or had a first pregnancy at a late age has an 18% probability of developing breast cancer over a 5-year period.[14] These estimates can be of value in advising women about prophylactic mastectomy.

DIAGNOSIS OF CANCER

The major role of surgery in the diagnosis of cancer lies in the acquisition of tissue for exact histologic diagnosis. The principles underlying the biopsy of malignant lesions vary depending on the natural history of the tumor under consideration. Various techniques exist for obtaining tissues suspected of malignancy, including aspiration biopsy, needle biopsy, incisional biopsy, and excisional biopsy.

Aspiration biopsy involves the aspiration of cells and tissue fragments through a needle that has been guided into the suspect tissue. Cytologic analysis of this material can provide a tentative diagnosis of the presence of malignant tissue. However, major surgical resections should not be undertaken solely on the basis of the evidence of aspiration biopsy. Even the most experienced cytologist can mistake inflammatory or benign reparative changes for malignant cells. This error is inherent in the uncertainties of an individual cell analysis and, even in the best of hands, provides an error rate substantially higher than that of standard histologic diagnosis.

Needle biopsy refers to obtaining a core of tissue through a specially designed needle introduced into the suspect tissue. The core of tissue provided by needle biopsies is sufficient for the diagnosis of most tumor types. Soft tissue and bony sarcomas often present major difficulties in differentiating benign and reparative lesions from malignancies and often cannot be diagnosed accurately. If these latter lesions are considered in the diagnosis, attempts should be made to obtain larger amounts of tissue than are possible from a needle biopsy.

Incisional biopsy refers to removal of a small wedge of tissue from a larger tumor mass. Incisional biopsies often are necessary for diagnosing large masses that require major surgical procedures for even local excision. Incisional biopsies are the preferred method of diagnosing soft tissue and bony sarcomas because of the magnitude of the surgical procedures necessary to extirpate these lesions definitively. The treatment of many visceral cancers cannot be undertaken without an incisional biopsy, but be aware of opening new tissue planes contaminated with tumor by performing excisional biopsies for large lesions. An inappropriately performed excisional biopsy can compromise subsequent surgical excision. When this is a possibility, incisional biopsies should be performed.

In excisional biopsy, an excision of the entire suspected tumor tissue with little or no margin of surrounding normal tissue is done. Excisional biopsies are the procedure of choice for most tumors if they can be performed without contaminating new tissue planes or further compromising the ultimate surgical procedure.

There is little evidence that differences exist between incisional and excisional biopsies with respect to tumor spread. Several studies comparing incisional and excisional biopsies of suspected melanoma lesions found no differences in ultimate outcome in these patients, but the surgeon should avoid cutting directly into suspected tumor if it is not necessary to do so.[17,18]

The following principles guide the performance of all surgical biopsies.

1. Needle tracts or scars should be placed carefully so that they can be conveniently removed as part of the subsequent definitive surgical procedure. Placement of biopsy incisions is extremely important, and misplacement often can compromise subsequent care. Incisions on the extremity generally should be placed longitudinally so as to make the removal of underlying tissue and subsequent closure easier.
2. Care should be taken not to contaminate new tissue planes during the biopsy. Large hematomas after biopsy can lead to tumor spread and must be scrupulously avoided by securing excellent hemostasis during the biopsy. For biopsies on extremities, the use of a tourniquet may help in controlling bleeding. Instruments used in a biopsy procedure are another potential source of contamination of new tissue planes. It is not uncommon to take biopsy samples from several suspected lesions at one time. Care should be taken not to use instruments that may have come in contact with tumor when obtaining tissue from a potentially uncontaminated area.
3. Choice of biopsy technique should be selected carefully to obtain an adequate tissue sample for the needs of the pathologist. For the diagnosis of selected tumors, electron microscopy, tissue culture or other techniques may be necessary. Sufficient tissue must be obtained for these purposes if diagnostic difficulties are anticipated.
4. Handling of the biopsy tissue by the pathologist is also important. When the orientation of the biopsy specimen is important for subsequent treatment, the surgeon should mark distinctive areas of the tumor carefully to facilitate subsequent orientation of the specimen by the pathologist. Different fixatives are best for different types or sizes of tissue. If all biopsy specimens are placed in formalin immediately, the opportunity to perform valuable diagnostic tests may be lost. The handling of excised tissue is the surgeon's responsibility. Biopsy tissue obtained from breast cancer lesions, for example, should be saved for estrogen receptor studies and placed in cold storage until ready for processing.

Surgery also has a role in diagnosing pathologic states in cancer patients that do not directly involve the diagnosis of cancer. Cancer patients often are immunosuppressed by their disease or their treatment and are subject to opportunistic infections not commonly seen in most general surgical patients. Open lung or liver biopsies are often important in diagnosing these lesions adequately and in planning suitable therapy.

Oncologists are becoming increasingly aware of the need for precise staging of patients when planning treatment. Lack of proper staging information can lead to poor treatment planning and compromise the ability to cure patients. Staging laparotomy can be important in determining the exact extent of spread of lymphomas (see Chap. 52).

In performing accurate surgical staging, the surgeon must be familiar with the natural history of the disease under consideration. The development of ovarian cancer treatment is an excellent example. The tendency of ovarian cancer to metastasize to the undersurface of the diaphragm is a good example of the need to biopsy an anatomic site that would not normally be biopsied by most surgeons. Extensive surgical staging may be required before undertaking other major surgical procedures with curative intent. For example, biopsy of the celiac and paraaortic lymph nodes in patients with cancer of the esophagus is often important so that unnecessary esophageal resections can be avoided.

Placement of radioopaque clips during biopsy and staging procedures is important to delineate areas of known tumor and as a guide to the subsequent delivery of radiation therapy to these areas.

TREATMENT OF CANCER

Surgery can be a simple, safe method to cure patients with solid tumors when the tumor is confined to the anatomic site of origin. Unfortunately, when patients with solid tumors present to the physician for the first time, about 70% already have micrometastases beyond the primary site. The extension of the surgical resection to include areas of regional spread can cure some of these patients, although regional spread often is an indication of undetectable distant micrometastases.

The emergence of effective nonsurgical therapies has had profound impact on the treatment of cancer patients and on the role and responsibilities of the surgeon treating the cancer patient. John Hunter, a brilliant 18th-century surgeon, characterized surgery as being "like an armed savage who attempts to get that by force which a civilized man would get by strategem."

Although surgery continues to be the most important aspect of the treatment of most patients presenting with solid tumors, modern clinical research in oncology has been devoted to applying other adjuvant "strategems" to improve the cure rates of those 70% who ultimately fail surgical therapy alone.

The role of surgery in the treatment of cancer patients can be divided into six separate areas. In each area, interactions with other treatment modalities can be essential for a successful outcome.

1. Definitive surgical treatment for primary cancer, selection of appropriate local therapy, and integration of surgery with other adjuvant modalities
2. Surgery to reduce the bulk of residual disease (Examples: Burkitt's lymphoma, ovarian cancer)
3. Surgical resection of metastatic disease with curative intent (Examples: pulmonary metastases in sarcoma patients, hepatic metastases from colorectal cancer)
4. Surgery for the treatment of oncologic emergencies
5. Surgery for palliation
6. Surgery for reconstruction and rehabilitation

Surgery for Primary Cancer

There are three major challenges confronting the surgical oncologist in the definitive treatment of solid tumors:

1. Accurate identification of patients who can be cured by local treatment alone
2. Development and selection of local treatments that provide the best balance between local cure and the impact of treatment morbidity on the quality of life
3. Development and application of adjuvant treatments that can improve the control of local and distant invasive and metastatic disease

The selection of the appropriate local therapy to be used in cancer treatment varies with the individual cancer type and the site of involvement. In many instances, definitive surgical therapy that encompasses a sufficient margin of normal tissue is sufficient local therapy. The treatment of many solid tumors falls into this category, including the wide excision of primary melanomas in the skin that can be cured locally by surgery alone in about 90% of cases. The resection of colon cancers with a 5-cm margin from the tumor results in anastomotic recurrences in less than 5% of cases.

In other instances, surgery is used to obtain histologic confirmation of diagnosis, but primary local therapy is achieved through the use of a nonsurgical modality such as radiation therapy. Examples include the treatment of Ewing sarcoma in long bones and the treatment of selected primary malignancies in the head and neck. In each instance, selection of the definitive local treatment involves careful consideration of the likelihood of cure balanced against the morbidity of the treatment modality.

The magnitude of surgical resection is modified in the treatment of many cancers by the use of adjuvant treatment modalities. Rationally integrating surgery with other treatments requires a careful consideration of all effective treatment options. The surgical oncologist must be thoroughly familiar with adjuncts and alternatives to surgical treatment. It is a knowledge of this rapidly changing field that separates the surgical oncologist from the general surgeon most distinctly.

In some instances, effective adjuvant modalities have led to a decrease in the magnitude of surgery. The evolution of childhood rhabdomyosarcoma treatment is a striking example of the successful integration of adjuvant therapies with surgery in the treatment of cancer.[19,20]

Childhood rhabdomyosarcoma is the most common soft tissue sarcoma in infants and children. Before 1970, surgery alone was used almost exclusively, and 5-year survivals of from 10% to 20% were commonly reported. Local surgery alone failed in patients with rhabdomyosarcomas of the prostate and extremities because of extensive invasion of surrounding tissues and the early development of metastatic disease. The failure of surgery alone to control local disease in patients with childhood rhabdomyosarcoma led to the introduction of adjuvant radiation therapy. This resulted in a marked improvement in local control rates that was further improved dramatically by the introduction of combination chemotherapy with vincristine, dactinomycin, and cyclophosphamide. Long-term cure rates are in the range of 80%. Many other examples of the integration of surgery with other treatment modalities appear throughout this book.

Surgery for Residual Disease

The concept of cytoreductive surgery has received much attention in recent years.[21,22] In some instances, the extensive local spread of cancer precludes the removal of all gross disease by surgery. The surgical resection of bulk disease in the treatment of selected cancers may well lead to improvements in the ability to control residual gross disease that has not been resected. Studies that suggest the merit of this approach are discussed in Chapters 50 and 39 (Burkitt's lymphoma and ovarian cancer, respectively).

Enthusiasm for cytoreductive surgery has led to the inappropriate use of surgery for reducing the bulk of tumor in some cases. Clearly, cytoreductive surgery is of benefit only when other effective treatments are available to control the residual disease that is unresectable. Except in rare palliative settings, there is no role for cytoreductive surgery in patients in whom little other effective therapy exists.

Surgery for Metastatic Disease

The value of surgery in the cure of patients with metastatic disease tends to be overlooked. As a general principle, patients with a single site of metastatic disease that can be resected without major morbidity should undergo resection of that metastatic cancer. Many patients with few metastases to lung or liver or brain can be cured by surgical resection (see Chap. 61, sections 1, 2, and 3). This approach is especially true for cancers that do not respond well to systemic chemotherapy. The resection of pulmonary metastases in patients with soft tissue and bony sarcomas can cure as many as 30% of patients. As effective systemic therapy is developed for the treatment of these diseases, cure rates may increase. Studies have shown that similar cure rates occur in patients with adenocarcinomas when resected metastatic disease to the lung is the sole clinical site of metastases. Small numbers of pulmonary metastases often are the only clinically apparent metastatic disease in patients with sarcomas. However, this is rare in the natural history of most adenocarcinomas. If solitary metastases to the lung do occur in patients with carcinoma of the colon or other adenocarcinomas, then surgical resection is indicated.

Similarly, there is increasing enthusiasm for the resection of hepatic metastases, especially from colorectal cancer, in patients in whom the liver is the only site of known metastatic disease. In patients with solitary hepatic metastases from colorectal cancer, resection can lead to long-term cure in about 25% of patients. This far exceeds the cure rates of any other available treatment.

The resection for cure of solitary brain metastases should also be considered when the brain is the only site of known metastatic disease. The exact location and functional sequelae of resection should be considered when making this treatment decision.

SURGERY FOR ONCOLOGIC EMERGENCIES

As in the treatment of all patients, emergencies arise for oncologic patients that require surgical intervention. These generally involve the treatment of exsanguinating hemorrhage, perforation, drainage of abscesses, or impending destruction of vital organs. Each category of surgical emergency is unique and requires an individual approach (see Chap. 60, section 4).

The oncologic patient often is neutropenic, thrombocytopenic, and has a high risk of hemorrhage or sepsis. Perforations of an abdominal viscus can result from direct tumor invasion or from tumor lysis resulting from effective systemic treatments. Perforation of the gastrointestinal tract after effective treatment for lymphoma involving the intestine is not uncommon. The ability to identify patients at high risk for perforation may lead to the use of surgery to prevent this problem. Surgery to decompress cancer invading the CNS represents another surgical emergency that can lead to preservation of function.

Surgery for Palliation

Surgical resection often is required for the relief of pain or functional abnormalities. The appropriate use of surgery in these settings can improve the quality of life for cancer patients. Palliative surgery may include the relief of mechanical problems such as intestinal obstruction or the removal of masses that are causing severe pain or disfigurement.

Surgery for Reconstruction and Rehabilitation

Surgical techniques are being refined that aid in the reconstruction and rehabilitation of cancer patients after definitive therapy. The ability to reconstruct anatomic defects can substantially improve function and cosmetic appearance. The development of free flaps using microvascular anastomotic techniques is having a profound impact on the ability to bring fresh tissue to resected or heavily irradiated areas. Loss of function (especially of extremities) often can be rehabilitated by surgical approaches. This includes lysis of contractures or muscle transposition to restore muscular function that has been damaged by previous surgery or radiation therapy.

THE SURGICAL ONCOLOGIST

Several factors have led to a recent increase in the development of surgical oncology and to the organization of separate sections of surgical oncology in large hospitals and departments of surgery within universities. This enthusiasm derives from the recognition that modern oncologic management requires levels of expertise in cancer surgery, chemotherapy, and radiation therapy that are not common to most general surgeons, and a desire to use effectively the resources being committed to cancer care and research by hospitals, private foundations, and the federal government. A sense of urgency has existed because some surgical leaders believe that the surgeon is experiencing a declining intellectual role in modern cancer treatment and research and that steps must be taken to reassert the surgeon's role in modern oncology.

Many surgeons have resisted the development of surgical oncology as a specialty area because of the fear of fragmenting the field of general surgery. A survey of 124 university surgery departments in the United States between January and July of 1985, revealed that 38% had formal divisions of surgical oncology compared with the divisions of medical oncology present in 95%, radiation oncology in 94%, pediatric oncology in 76%, and gynecologic oncology in 79%.[23] Of the 47 divisions of surgical oncology that did exist, only 13 (28%) had formal clinical training programs in surgical oncology.[21] This lack of emphasis on surgical oncology at universities may be a factor in the decreasing success of surgeons in obtaining grant support from the National Cancer Institute. From 1980 through 1985, an analysis of 6407 applications submitted from clinical departments of medical schools for peer-reviewed grants re-

vealed that 44% were submitted from departments of medicine and only 16% from departments of surgery.[22] Thirty-four percent of applications submitted from departments of medicine were awarded, compared with 25% from departments of surgery.[24]

The development of surgical oncology as a specialty area of surgery depends on a clear delineation of its role. There are six major areas in which the modern surgical oncologist can play a valuable role in the care of cancer patients at major treatment centers:[25]

1. Organize surgical oncology teaching programs for staff, residents, and students.
2. Provide expert consultation for unusual or difficult oncologic patient problems.
3. Provide unique surgical expertise in surgical cases unfamiliar to general surgeons (*e.g.*, major soft tissue resections, exenterations, head and neck resections, isolation-perfusions).
4. Organize clinical research protocols for surgical oncology patients.
5. Coordinate surgical oncology efforts with medical and radiation oncologists.
6. Conduct experimental research programs in oncology where possible.

The rapid development of new information in surgery, chemotherapy, and medical oncology, in addition to newer disciplines of immunotherapy, hyperthermia, and phototherapy, requires the continuing education of all surgical staff. Surgical oncologists maintain close contact with all of these areas and should be responsible for teaching programs for general surgical staff, residents, and students.

Because of the unique training and exposure to oncologic problems, the surgical oncologist has expertise in dealing with unusual or difficult oncologic patient problems and can provide expert consultation in these areas. The surgical oncologist is trained to perform many types of surgical procedures not commonly performed by general surgeons. Although most surgeons are able to perform many of the standard cancer resections, some operations are not performed frequently by general surgeons and can be performed better by a specialist in surgical oncology.

In most hospital settings, general surgeons operate on cancer patients. It is often essential, however, that patients receiving care for various cancers enter clinical protocols that help answer important questions related to the treatment of that cancer. The surgical oncologist can help organize clinical research protocols for surgical oncology patients treated by all surgeons at that institution. A large surgical group should have a surgical specialist capable of coordinating efforts with medical and radiation oncologists. Successful coordination with these nonsurgical specialists requires expertise in medical oncology and radiation therapy that is not common among most general surgeons.

The surgical oncologist can also be involved in administering and defining the need for adjuvant treatments. Adjuvant chemotherapy commonly is administered by surgeons when the chemotherapy regimens use well-known single or combination agents. The future development of immunotherapies and other new adjuvant treatments can be logically administered by surgical oncologists to their patients after recovery from the surgical procedure.

The surgical oncologist, when the situation allows, is in a position to perform experimental research in oncology that can lead to the introduction of new diagnostic and treatment regimens in clinical care. Laboratory research programs that contribute to basic knowledge of cancer biology also provide an important source of stimulation to residents and students.

The emergence of a subspecialty of surgical oncology within general surgery requires that special attention be given to the training of surgeons interested in pursuing this area of clinical care. Although it is generally agreed that all surgical oncologists should be well-trained general surgeons, attempts have been made to define additional areas of expertise that must be studied. In 1978, a group of surgical oncologists met under the sponsorship of the Society of Surgical Oncology and the Division of Cancer Research, Resources, and Centers of the National Cancer Institute to develop guidelines for the training of surgical oncologists.

The guidelines adopted by this meeting included suggestions for such training.[26,27]

1. Two-year training program on a surgical oncology service after completion of eligibility for general surgical certification by the American Board of Surgery or other surgical specialty board
2. Training at an institution whose cancer program is approved by the Commission on Cancer of the American College of Surgeons and whose clinical resources provide a sufficient variety and volume of clinical material to ensure exposure to a broad variety of clinical cancer problems
3. Training at a center with sufficient basic science resources to provide education in these areas, with exposure to basic and clinical research
4. Training at an institution that provides adequate operative experience, including standard curative and palliative procedures, with broad exposure to surgical procedures unique to the oncologic patient
5. A full-time assignment during the training period to radiation oncology and chemotherapy services to allow the trainee to gain confidence and knowledge in these nonsurgical disciplines

These training recommendations are designed to provide general surgeons with the expertise in oncology and nonsurgical disciplines necessary to bring the best aspects of all disciplines of modern oncology to the care of the cancer patient.

REFERENCES

1. Brested JH. The Edwin Smith surgical papyrus. Chicago: University of Chicago Press, 1930.
2. Thorwald J. Science and the secrets of early medicine. New York: Harcourt, Brace, and World, 1962.
3. Wangensteen OH. Has medical history importance for surgeons? Surg Gynecol Obstet 1975;140:434.
4. Hill GJ. Historic milestones in cancer surgery. Semin Oncol 1979;6:409–427.
5. Brunner EA, Eckenhoff JE. Anesthesia. In: Sabiston DC Jr, ed. Textbook of surgery. Philadelphia: WB Saunders, 1977.
6. Goldman L, Caldera DL, Nussbaum SR, et al. Multifactorial index of cardiac risk in noncardiac surgical procedures. N Engl J Med 1977;297:845–850.
7. Dripps RD, Eckenhoff JE, Vandam LD. Introduction to anesthesia. Philadelphia: WB Saunders, 1977.
8. Dripps RD, Lamont A, Eckenhoff JE. The role of anesthesia in surgical mortality. JAMA 1961;178:261.
9. Moir DD. Maternal mortality and anesthesia. Br J Anaesth 1980;52:1–3.
10. Collins VJ. Principles of anesthesiology. Philadelphia: Lea & Febiger, 1976.
11. Goldman L. Cardiac risks and complications of noncardiac surgery. Ann Surg 1983;198:780–791.
12. Palmberg S, Hirsjarvi E. Mortality in geriatric surgery. Gerontology 1979;25:103–112.
13. Hoskings MP, Warner MA, Lobdell EM, Offord KP, Melton LJ. Outcomes of surgery in patients 90 years of age and older. JAMA 1989;261:1909–1915.
14. Mulvihill JJ. Cancer control through genetics. In: Arrighi FE, Rao PN, Stubblefield E, eds. Genes, chromosomes, and neoplasia. New York: Raven Press, 1980.
15. MacDougall IPM. The cancer risk in ulcerative colitis. Lancet 1964;2:655.
16. Devroede GJ, Taylor WF, Sauer WG. Cancer risk and life expectancy of children with ulcerative colitis. N Engl J Med 1971;285:17.
17. Epstein E, Bragg K, Linden GJ. Biopsy and prognosis of malignant melanoma. JAMA 1969;208:1369.
18. Knutson CO, Hori JM, Spratt JS Jr. Melanoma. Curr Probl Surg 1971 Dec; 3–55.
19. Kilman JW, Clatworthy HW Jr, Newton WA, et al. Reasonable surgery for rhabdomyosarcoma: A study of 67 cases. Ann Surg 1973;3:346.
20. Heyn RM, Holland R, Newton WA, et al. The role of combined chemotherapy in the treatment of rhabdomyosarcoma in children. Cancer 1974;34:2128–2142.
21. Silberman AW. Surgical debulking of tumors. Surg Gynecol Obstet 1982;155:577–585.
22. Wong RJ, De Cosse JJ. Cytoreductive surgery. Surg Gynec Obstet 1990;170:276–281.
23. Lawrence W Jr, Wilson RE, Shingleton WW, et al. Surgical oncology in university departments of surgery in the United States. Arch Surg 1986;121:1088–1093.
24. Avis FP, Ellenberg S, Friedman MA. Surgical oncology research—a disappointing status report. Ann Surg 1988;207:262–266.
25. Rosenberg SA. The organization of surgical oncology in university departments of surgery. Surgery 1984;95:632–634.
26. Leffall LD Jr. Presidential address. Surgical oncology—expectations for the future. Cancer 1980;42:2925–2928.
27. Schweitzer RJ, Edwards MH, Lawrence W, et al. Training guidelines for surgical oncology. Cancer 1981;48:2336–2340.

Cancer: Principles & Practice of Oncology, Fourth Edition,
edited by Vincent T. DeVita, Jr., Samuel Hellman, Steven A. Rosenberg.
J.B. Lippincott Co., Philadelphia © 1993.

Samuel Hellman

CHAPTER **15**

Principles of Radiation Therapy

To understand the practice of radiation therapy, one must seek its roots in principles derived from three separate areas. The first is practical radiation physics. This must be understood much as the surgeon understands the use of the equipment available in the operating room and as the internist understands the pharmacologic basis of therapeutics. The basic concepts of physics necessary to consider radiation therapy in the disease-related chapters are introduced in this chapter.

The second important discipline to be understood is cell, tissue, and tumor biology. This chapter describes the fundamental principles of radiation biology and cell kinetics; cell kinetics in relation to chemotherapy and radiation therapy is discussed in Chapter 4. These two discussions provide the rudiments of cell biology necessary to understand the uses of radiation.

A large clinical experience in radiation use has resulted in certain principles of treatment. These are discussed separately and related to the physical and biologic concepts that may underlie their success.

PHYSICAL CONSIDERATIONS

Only the most important concepts of the physics of ionizing radiation can be discussed in this chapter. If more detailed information is needed, a standard textbook of radiation physics is a more appropriate source of information.[1]

Ionizing radiation is energy that, during absorption, causes the ejection of an orbital electron. A large amount of energy is associated with ionization. Ionizing radiation can be electromagnetic or particulate, and electromagnetic radiation can be considered as a wave and as a packet of energy (a photon). It is the particulate nature of electromagnetic radiation that explains much of its biologic activity. The packet of energy is large enough to cause ionizations, and these are distributed unevenly through tissue. Examples of particulate radiation are the subatomic particles: electrons, protons, α particles, neutrons, negative pimesons, and atomic nuclei. All of these have been experimentally considered or are being used in radiation therapy.

ELECTROMAGNETIC RADIATION

Electromagnetic radiation consists of roentgen and γ radiation. They differ only in the way in which they are produced: γ rays are produced intranuclearly, and roentgen rays are produced extranuclearly. In practice, this means that γ rays used in radiation therapy are produced by the decay of radioactive isotopes and that almost all of the roentgen rays used in radiation therapy are made by electrical machines. Exceptions are roentgen rays produced by orbital electron rearrangements, as in the decay of ^{125}I, which is a radioactive isotope but produces photons by extranuclear processes. Iodine 125 also emits a small number of γ rays from the nucleus.

The intensity of electromagnetic radiation dissipates as the inverse square of the distance from the source. The dose of radiation 2 cm from a point source is 25% of the dose at 1 cm.

The relative prevalence of the three dominant absorption mechanisms of electromagnetic radiation depends on the energy of the radiation. The first is photoelectric absorption, which predominates at lower energies. In this circumstance, the photon interaction results in the ejection of a tightly bound orbital electron. The vacancy left in the atomic shell is then filled by another electron falling from an outer shell of the same atom or from outside the atom. All or most of the photon energy of the transition is lost in this process. Photoelectric absorption varies with the cube of the atomic number (Z^3).

248

This has significant practical implications because it explains why materials with high atomic numbers, such as lead, are such effective shielding materials. It also means that bones absorb significantly more radiation than soft tissues at lower photon energies, the basis for conventional diagnostic radiology.

The second type of radiation absorption is the Compton type. In this process, the photon interaction is with a distant orbital electron that has a low binding energy. In this absorptive process, the photon does not give up all its energy to a single electron; an appreciable portion reappears as a secondary photon, which is created in the interaction. In contrast to the photoelectric effect, the probability of Compton absorption does not depend much on atomic number, but rather on electron density. This explains why films made at supervoltage energy do not show much difference between bone and soft tissue, but air cavities are clearly distinguished.

The third type of absorption is the pair production process. This type of absorption requires an incident photon energy greater than 1.02 MeV. In this process, positive and negative electrons are produced at the same time.

The fundamental quantity necessary to describe the interaction of radiation with matter is the amount of energy absorbed per unit mass. This quantity is called *absorbed dose*, and the *rad* was the most commonly used unit. Absorbed dose is measured in joules per kilogram; another name for 1 joule/kg is the Gray (1 Gray = 100 rad), which is now the recommended unit. The roentgen (R) is a unit of roentgen rays or γ rays based on the ability of radiation to ionize air. At the energies used in radiation therapy, 1 R of roentgen rays or γ rays results in a dose of somewhat less than 1 rad (0.01 Gy) in soft tissue.

The different ranges of electromagnetic radiations used in clinical practice are *superficial radiation* or roentgen rays from about 10 to 125 KeV; *orthovoltage* radiation or electromagnetic radiation between 125 and 400 KeV; and *supervoltage* or megavoltage radiation for energies above 400 KeV. There are important differences between these classes. As energy increases, the penetration of the roentgen rays increases (Fig. 15–1), and at supervoltage energies, absorption in bone is not higher than that in surrounding soft tissues, as is the case with lower energies. This is because at supervoltage energies, Compton absorption predominates. Compared with orthovoltage, supervoltage radiation is skin sparing, meaning that the maximum dose is not reached in the skin, but instead occurs below the surface. The electrons created in the interaction travel some distance and do not attain full intensity until they reach some depth, resulting in a reduced dose to the skin. With orthovoltage radiation, the skin frequently is the dose-limiting normal tissue.

RADIATION TECHNIQUES

Two general types of radiation techniques are used clinically—*brachytherapy* and *teletherapy*. In brachytherapy, the radiation device is placed within or close to the target volume. Examples of this are interstitial and intracavitary radiation used in the treatment of many gynecologic and oral tumors. Teletherapy uses a device located at a distance from the patient, as is the case in most orthovoltage or supervoltage machines.

Because the radiation source is close to or within the target volume with brachytherapy, the dose is determined largely by inverse-square considerations. This means that the geometry of the implant is important. Spatial arrangements have been determined for different types of applications based on the particular anatomic considerations of the tumor and important normal tissues. An example of isodose distribution around an intracavitary application for carcinoma of the cervix is shown in Figure 15–2. The dose decreases rapidly as the distance from the applicator increases. This emphasizes the importance of proper placement. The applicator pictured is used to treat the cervix, uterus, and important paracervical tissues, while limiting excessive irradiation of the bladder and rectum in front of and behind the tumor.

Historically, the removable interstitial and intracavitary sources used were radium and radon, the latter primarily for permanent implants. Marie Curie, the discoverer of radium, recognized its importance early and championed the medical use of these isotopes. They were important tools in early cancer therapy but now have been largely replaced by manmade isotopes, which overcome most of the disadvantages of the naturally occurring ones.

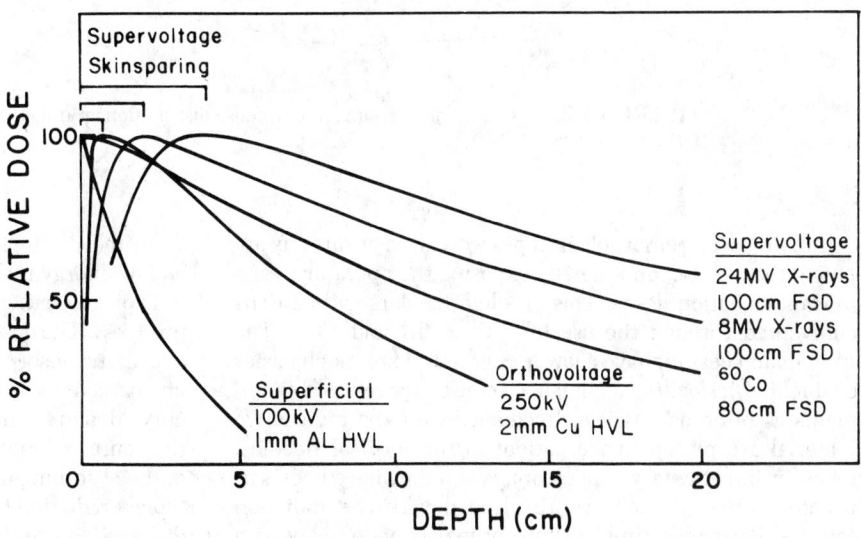

FIGURE 15–1. Relative dose at different depths for various types of ionizing radiation.

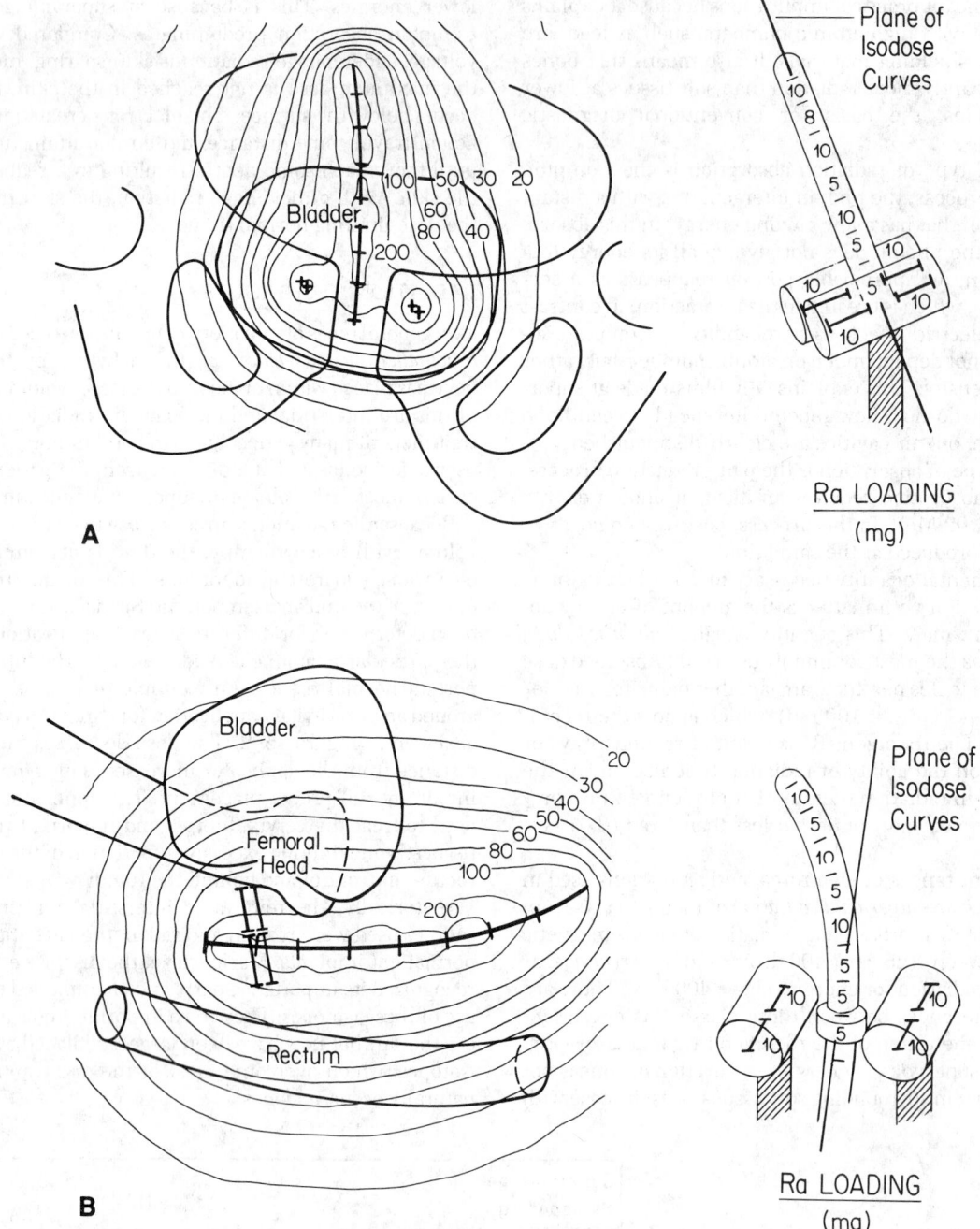

FIGURE 15–2. **(A)** Anteroposterior view of isodose distribution around an intrauterine radium applicator. **(B)** Lateral view.

Initially, even removable isotopes were used by directly applying the isotope, and thereby exposing the operator to significant radiation doses. This problem has largely been circumvented through the use of ^{137}Cs, ^{192}Ir, and ^{60}Co. The iridium and cesium have a lower energy and are much easier to shield. *Afterloading* techniques are used for removable implants as often as possible. Receptacles for the radioactive material are placed in the patient in the form of needles, tubes, or intracavitary applicators. When they have been satisfactorily placed they are afterloaded with the radiation sources. Permanent implants are primarily done today with

^{198}Au and ^{125}I. Iodine 125 is also used for removable implants. Its low energy makes shielding a simple matter.

Typical teletherapy isodose distributions are shown in Figure 15–3. The dose depends on inverse-square considerations and tissue absorption. The distribution of radiation depends on characteristics of the machine and the patient. The isodose curve depends on the energy of radiation, the distance from the source of radiation, and the density and atomic number of the absorbing material. The beam of radiation produced in typical radiation treatment may be modified to make isodose distributions conform to the specific target volume, and in-

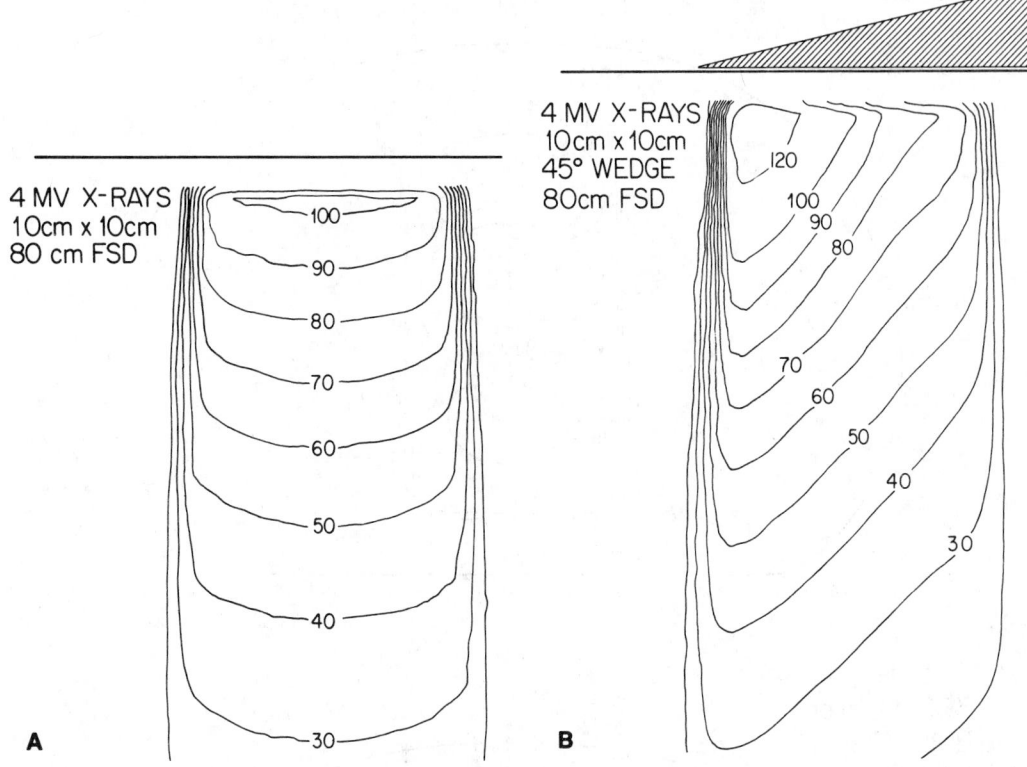

FIGURE 15–3. Isodose distributions for **(A)** 4 MeV without a wedge filter and **(B)** 4 MeV with a wedge filter.

dividually designed shields are used to protect vital normal tissues.

Figure 15–4 shows some radiation treatment plans in which the target volumes are depicted. This volume contains the tumor and the normal tissues intimately involved with the tumor. The diagram also contains the transited normal tissues or *transit volume*. The purpose of the treatment plan is to maximize the dose to the target volume and minimize the dose to the transit volume. *It is important that the tumor dose is relatively homogenous, because the maximum dose in the target volume is often the cause of complications, and the minimum dose in the target volume determines the likelihood of tumor recurrence.*

Beam-Modifying Devices

In modern radiation therapy, teletherapy is given almost exclusively with supervoltage equipment. These radiations are produced by the decay of radioactive cobalt or with the production of roentgen rays in the range of 2 to 35 MeV (the most common are 4–8 MeV). Higher-energy photons and electrons can be made by various electrical machines, of which the most common are linear accelerators.

Regardless of the radiation source, the beam must be modified for clinical use. With electrical machines, the beam tends to have a much greater intensity in the center than on the sides. Modification to give a uniform dose of radiation across the beam is done with a *flattening filter* (unnecessary in cobalt units). For the beam to be limited to the designated size, collimators are placed in the head of the machine. These usually

are made of materials that have a high Z value and can be varied to conform to the exact rectangular beam dimensions desired.

It is sometimes desirable for the beam to be more intense on one side than the other. This is especially important when fields at angles to each other are to be used. To modify the beam in this fashion, wedge filters are used (see Fig. 15–3B). These wedge-shaped pieces of metal absorb the beam differentially, depending on the thickness that produces the desired angled isodose curves. Depending on the anatomic volume being treated, it is often desirable to outline the beam differently from that which can be constructed by rectangular collimators. In these circumstances, certain areas within the beam should be shielded. To do this, individually fashioned blocks are made to conform to the individual distributions desired for each patient and each beam. They are made of material with a high Z, such as lead or the commercial product Libowitz metal, composed of bismuth, lead, tin, and cadmium.

The primary radiation beam is rectangular. This rectangle may be varied for individual patients, using the secondary collimators in the head of the machine. These can then be further modified by individually constructed blocks made to the contour of the normal tissue (Fig. 15–5). The newest equipment has multileaf collimators, which permit the collimator to follow closely the desired portal contour, rather than being restricted to a rectangular shape.

RADIATION TREATMENT

Once the decision has been made to treat a patient with radiation, pretreatment procedures must be performed. First,

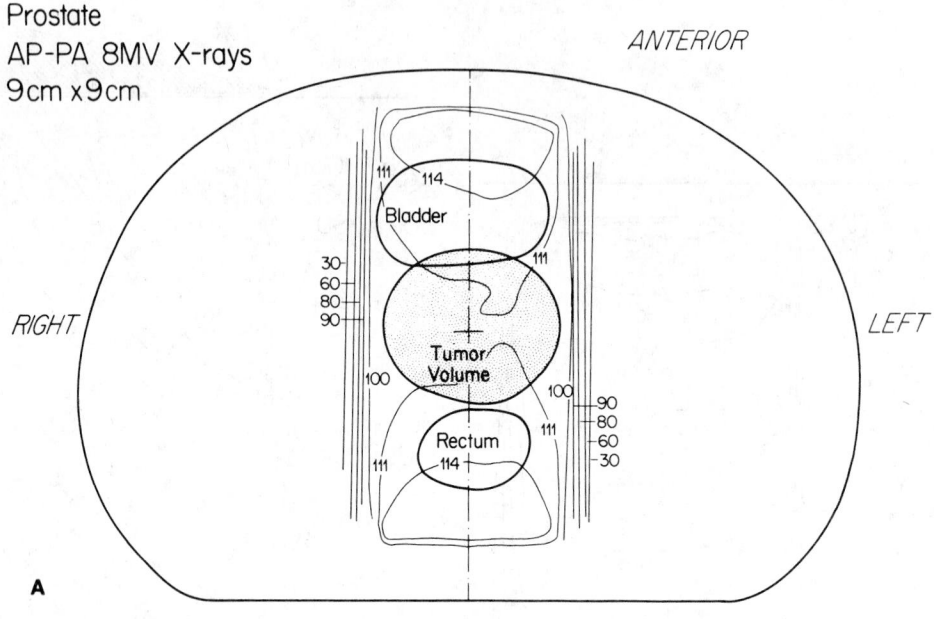

Prostate
AP-PA 8MV X-rays
9cm x9cm

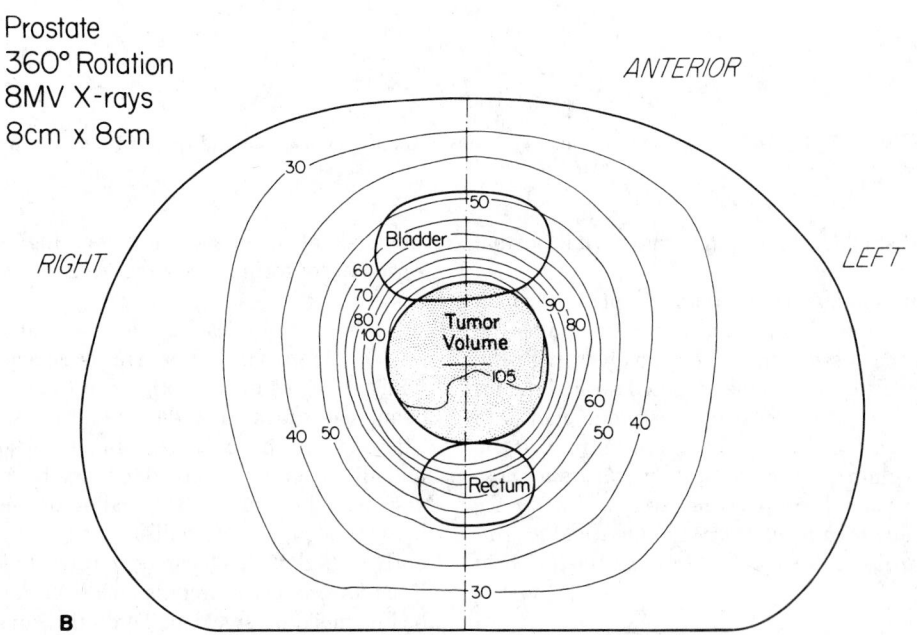

Prostate
360° Rotation
8MV X-rays
8cm x 8cm

FIGURE 15–4.   Typical supervoltage treatment plans for **(A)** opposing fields, **(B)** rotation, **(C)** three field, and **(D)** wedge rotation.

there must be accurate localization of the target volume and determination of the dose-limiting, transited normal tissues. This localization requires physical examination, radiography, ultrasonography, computed tomography (CT), and other diagnostic procedures. Before this, the clinician must understand the natural history of the disease and its patterns of spread. CT has greatly changed the process of tumor localization by allowing much greater accuracy in determining the location of normal tissues and tumor.

Once localization has been completed, the treatment-planning process begins, in which alternative techniques of treatment are considered. The selection of the appropriate

treatment plan is made by the clinician consulting with the radiologic physicist and dosimetrist. This team effort must consider the best beam distribution, homogeneity within the target volume, and appropriate minimizing of dose in the transit volume.

Once the appropriate treatment plan has been accepted, the technique is tested using a radiation simulator. This device mimics the treatment machine but produces superficial radiation that can be used for direct imaging with an image intensifier and for producing radiographs that delineate exactly the beam location. Treatment simulation often causes modifications to be made in the treatment plan, allowing fur-

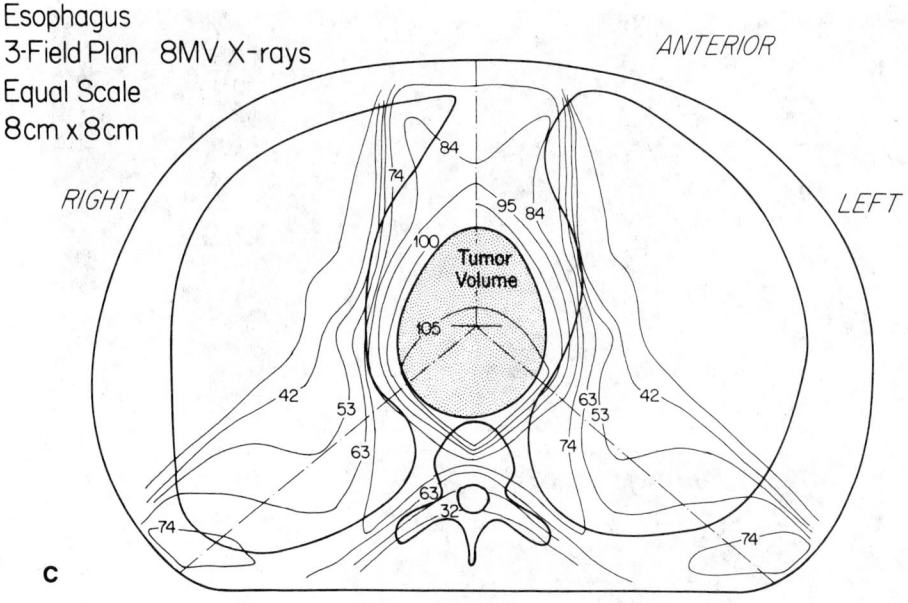

Esophagus
3-Field Plan   8MV X-rays
Equal Scale
8cm x 8cm

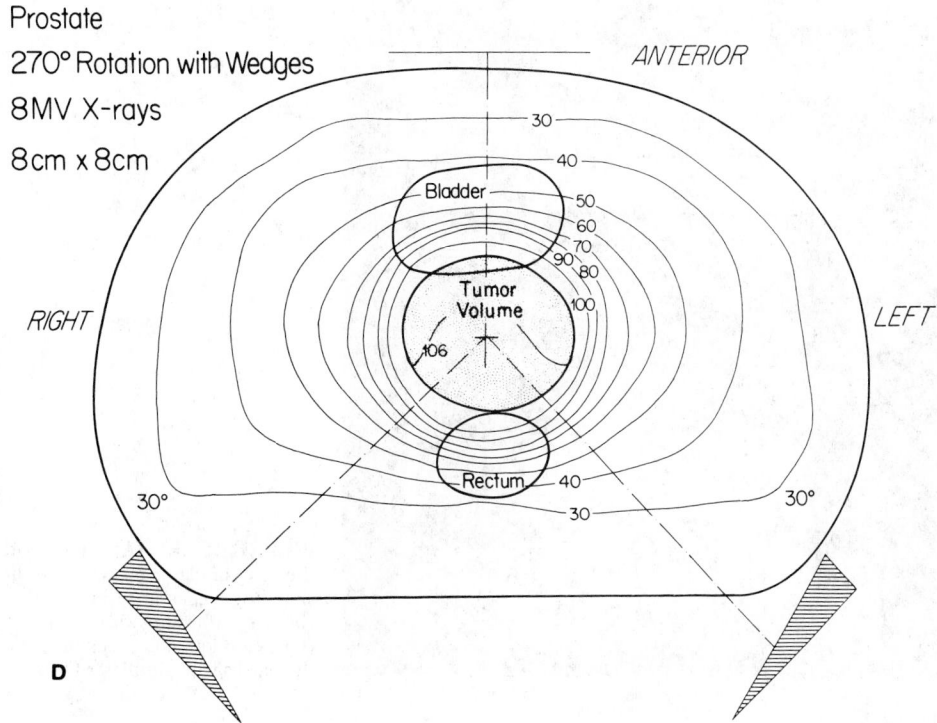

Prostate
270° Rotation with Wedges
8MV X-rays
8cm x 8cm

FIGURE 15–4.   *(Continued)*

ther sparing of normal tissues. Simulator films must be compared with the check or portal films made with the supervoltage machine, which confirm the treatment plan (see Fig. 15–5). Image quality is poor because they do not distinguish bone from soft tissue. This is because supervoltage radiation is absorbed primarily by the Compton process, which does not depend on Z. In contrast, the simulator films are made with radiations of 80 to 110 KeV, which are in the photoelectric range and therefore dependent on Z^3.

For the treatment to be applied as designed on the radiation

simulator, proper immobilization and marking techniques must be used. These also ensure that daily treatments are given to the same volume. Markings on the patient's skin may be temporary or permanent. Usually temporary marks are used to supplement the permanent small dots or "tattoos," ensuring that the treatment is given to the same volume each day. Should the patient require further therapy at a later date, these markings accurately indicate the location of previous treatment portals. Within the treatment room, light localizers describe the outline of the field, and small laser dots are used

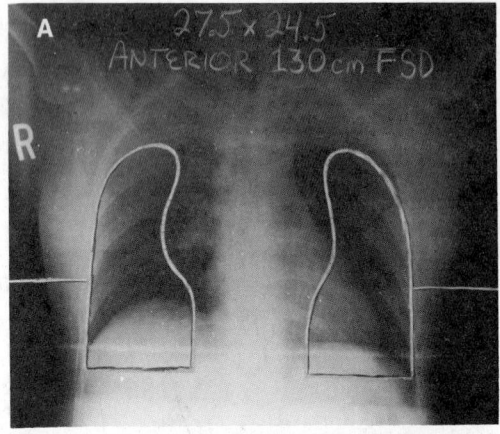
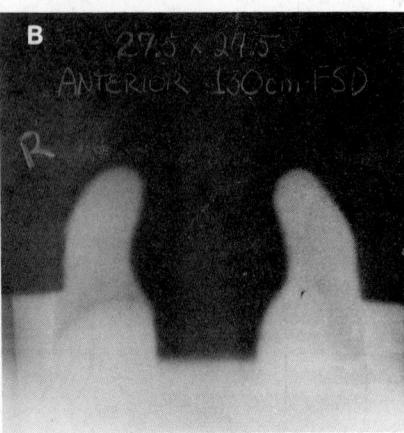
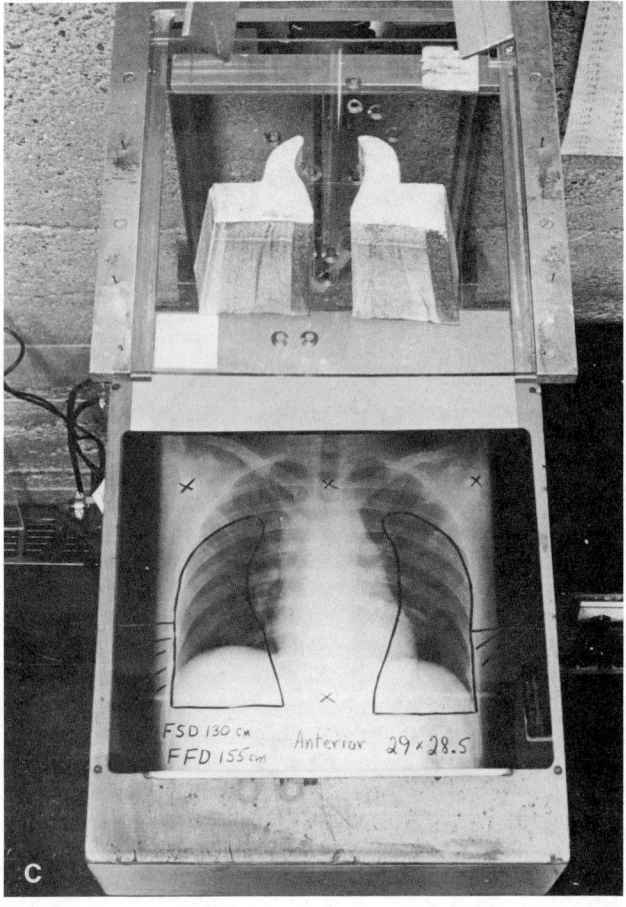

FIGURE 15–5. **(A)** A film made on a therapy simulator on which outlines for shielding blocks are drawn. **(B)** Supervoltage portal film with blocks in place. **(C)** Technique for checking accuracy of the blocks with simulator films.

to check whether the patient is in the correct position. Immobilization of the patient usually is achieved by devices made of foam, plastic, plaster, and other materials that can be made to conform to each patient's anatomy. It is most important that the patient be put in a position that is comfortable and easily reproduced from day to day.

Electron Therapy

With the development of betatrons and high-energy accelerators, electron beam therapy has become available for teletherapy. Electrons differ greatly in their characteristic depth-dose distributions (Fig. 15–6). The maximum dose is reached

and followed by a prompt fall. There is little skin sparing with electron beam therapy, but it is the most useful radiation in the treatment of superficial tumors because the deeper tissue is spared by the prompt fall in the radiation dose. With higher electron energy, the penetration is greater and the fall in depth dose is not as steep.

A major problem with electrons is that absorption can be modified greatly by bone or air-containing tissues. Bone greatly reduces the depth dose because it absorbs much more of the radiation; the contrary is true for air-containing spaces.

Electron beams are used primarily as a "boost" or supplementary treatment after photon therapy. Higher-energy electrons have had only limited use in radiation therapy, but new

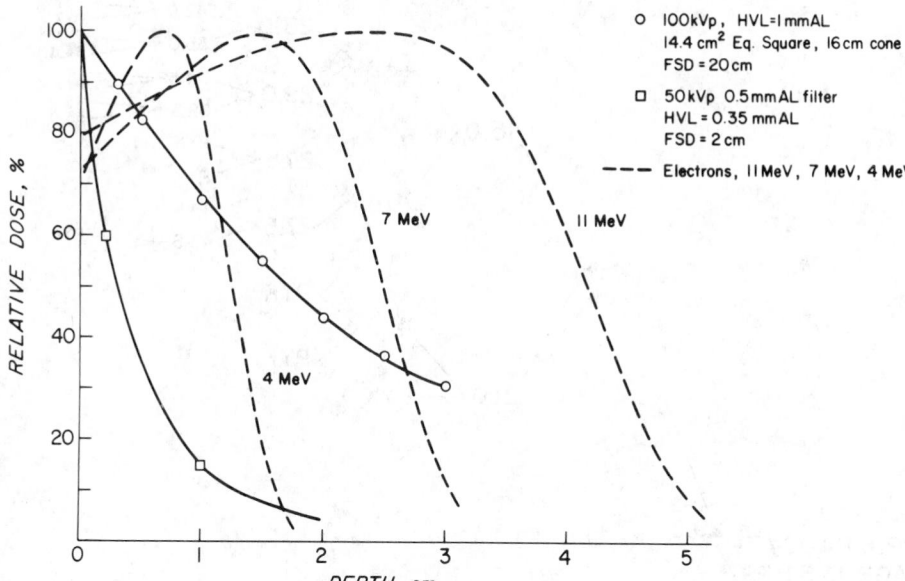

FIGURE 15–6. Electron and superficial roentgen ray depth–dose curves.

devices, such as the microtron, produce relatively pure high-energy electrons, whose characteristics are being explored for the definitive treatment of deep-seated and other tumors.

BIOLOGIC CONSIDERATIONS

RADIATION INTERACTION WITH BIOLOGIC MATERIALS

Because mammalian cells may be considered dilute aqueous solutions, there are two possible mechanisms of interaction with biologically important molecules—the direct effect of radiation on the important target molecule, and the indirect effect produced by intermediary radiation products. For most events, the important target molecule is thought to be the DNA, and when considering the maintenance of reproductive integrity, it is useful to assume that DNA is the target. Whatever the critical target, it can be affected directly by ionizing radiation that causes a change in the molecular structure of the biologically important molecule. This direct effect is most common for high linear energy transfer (LET) radiation. Alternatively, the photon may interact with water, the predominant molecule in these dilute solutions, to produce free radicals. All of these forms of radiation are short-lived; they can interact with biologically important material, causing a detrimental effect, or they can react innocently and revert to their former state. The likelihood of interaction or reversion can be modified by reaction with molecular oxygen, which favors prolonging the life of a reactive species, or by reaction with sulfhydryl compounds, which reduce the life span of the free radicals by combining with them to return to innocuous substances.

CELL SURVIVAL CONSIDERATIONS

Radiation effects, whether direct or indirect, are random, an important principle in the general nature of cell killing. The biologically important effects of radiation therapy are those concerned with reproductive integrity. It usually is assumed that DNA is the critical target for this radiation effect, although it has not been proved with certainty. Other biologically important effects of radiation (*e.g.*, edema) are far more likely to be caused by its action on membranes.

A cell that is damaged by radiation and loses its reproductive integrity may divide once or more often before all the progeny are rendered reproductively sterile. This is an important consequence of radiation; it means that an irradiated cell does not appear damaged until it faces at least the first division. At the time of reproduction, there are a number of possible paths for this cell:

1. It may die while trying to divide.
2. It may produce unusual forms as a result of aberrant attempts at division.
3. It may stay as it is, unable to divide, but physiologically functional for a long period of time. Such functional but sterile cells do not appear different from fertile cells.
4. It may divide, giving rise to one or more generations of daughter cells before some or all of the progeny become sterile. Those colonies in which some reproductively viable progeny emerge may then regrow.
5. The cell may suffer no alterations in the divisional process or only minor ones.

Usually some delay in division is produced, even in cells that are not damaged lethally. An example of cellular pedigrees photographed in vitro is shown in Figure 15–7.[2]

Survival Curves

Survival curves plot the fraction of cells surviving radiation against the dose given. Survival is determined by the ability to form a macroscopic colony. The simplest relation can be seen for bacteria in which survival is a constant exponential function of dose. The importance of this exponential relation is that for a given dose increment, a constant proportion, rather than a constant number, of cells is killed. Because of the randomness of radiation damage, if there is on average one lethal lesion per cell, some cells have one lesion, some more than one, and some less than one. Under such circum-

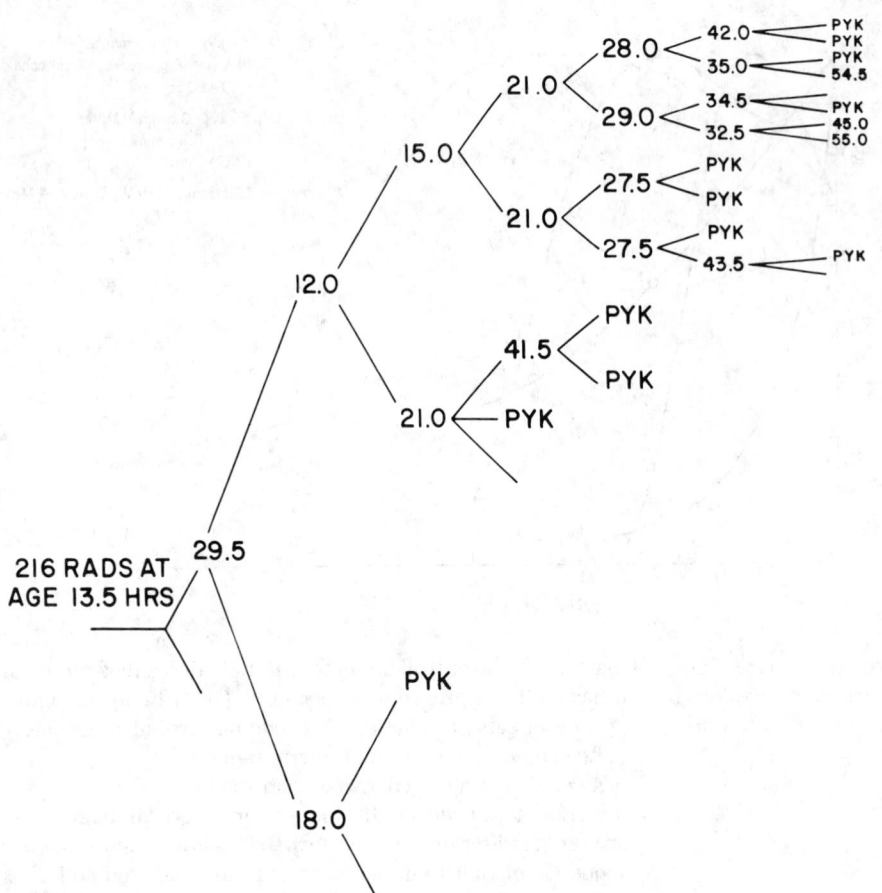

FIGURE 15–7. Two cell pedigrees indicating cell-cycle times and the outcome of cells irradiated in vitro. PYK-pyknosis. (Thompson LH, Suit HD. Proliferation kinetics of x-irradiated mouse L cells studied with time lapse photography II. Int J Radiat Biol 1969;15:347–362)

stances, the proportion of cells that have less than one, that is, no lethal events, is e^{-1}, or a survival fraction of 0.37. The dose required to reduce the survival fraction to 37% on the exponential curve is known as the D_o. This term is related to the slope of the exponential survival curve. If a smaller dose is required to reduce the survival fraction to 37%, the cells are more sensitive to radiation.

Survival curves of most mammalian cells differ from those of bacterial cells by having a "shoulder" in the low-dose region and the exponential relation at higher doses. This shoulder indicates a reduced efficiency of cell killing. Such an idealized curve is shown in Figure 15–8 with the important shorthand terminology used to describe survival curves. The terminal exponential portion is described by the D_o, whereas the initial shoulder region can be described by the extrapolation number n or the D_q, the quasi-threshold dose. The former is the number on the ordinate found when the exponential portion is extrapolated to O dose, whereas D_q is the dose at which the straight portion of the survival curve extrapolated backward intersects the line where the survival fraction is unity. If any two of these are known, the third can be calculated. The survival curve is described as follows: $\log e^n = D_q/D_o$. This curve is best described by a linear quadratic model with the following formula:[3]

$$S = e^{-(\alpha D + \beta D^2)}$$

Survival curves have been determined for benign or neoplastic mammalian cells in culture. There are no general characteristics of tumor cells that make them different from normal cells in culture. The survival curves for various human tumors thought to be sensitive and resistant to radiation were studied by Weichselbaum and colleagues, who failed to show any survival-curve characteristics that allow these two to be separated.[4] Therefore, the differences in clinical response cannot be explained by simple acute differences in survival curves.

Normal tissues also have been studied using clonogenic survival as an endpoint, with survival curves determined analogously to those for cells in tissue culture. The simplest clonal system, as originally described by Till and McCulloch, is that used for murine bone marrow stem cells.[5] When bone marrow cells are injected into lethally irradiated recipient animals, colonies are formed in the animals' spleens. These can be used to assess the reproductive integrity of the injected cells. The viability of the small intestinal clonogenic mucosal cells can be assessed by looking at sections of the small intestine at various times after irradiation and determining the appearance of colonies derived from cells surviving this radiation.[6] Using these and other techniques, the general properties of survival curves of normal and tumor cells are shown in Table 15–1. There are no characteristic differences in survival curves between normal tissues and tumors. Tumors generally resemble their normal tissue of origin in this respect.

Repair of Radiation Damage

When cells are irradiated, lethal damage can occur, or the damage may be modified and not lead irrevocably to cell death.

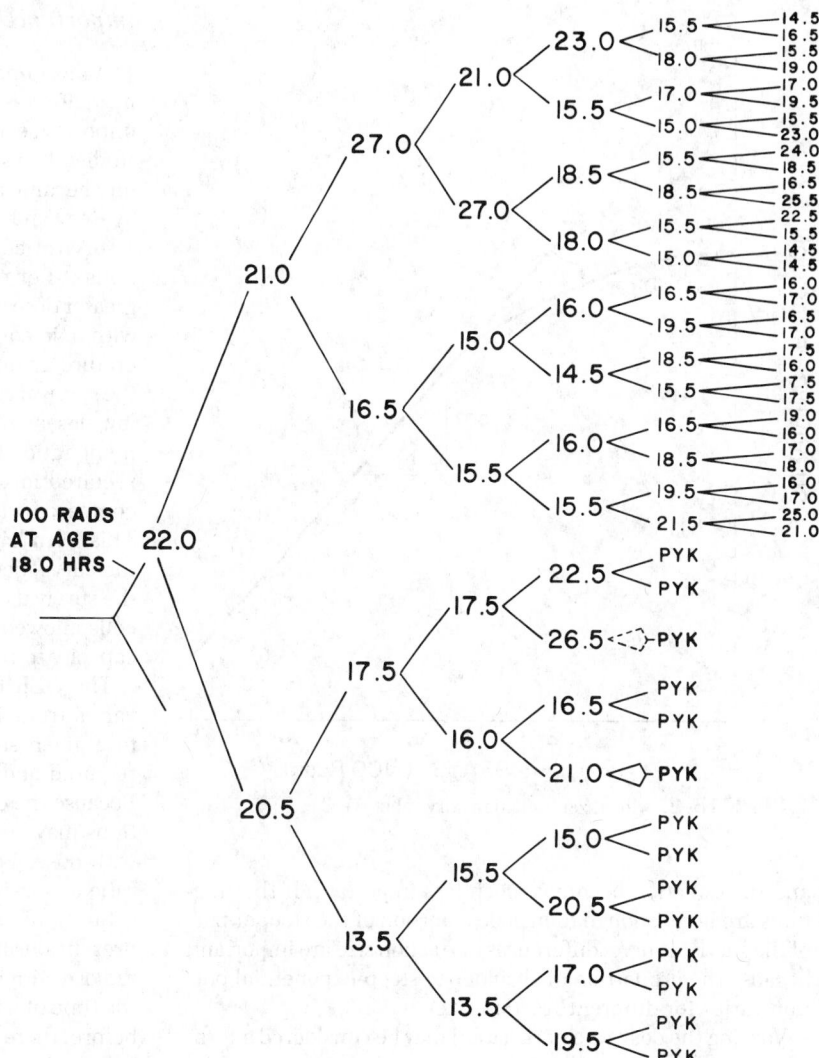

FIGURE 15–7.   *(Continued)*

Such amelioration of radiation damage is called *repair*. Repair can be divided into potentially lethal damage repair and sublethal damage repair.

Potentially lethal damage, under certain circumstances, leads to cell death. If postirradiation conditions are modified to allow repair, cells that would have died can be salvaged. In general, postirradiation conditions that suppress cell division are the ones most favorable to repair of potentially lethal damage. The simplest example of this was shown first in bacteria for ultraviolet and x-radiation.[7] A similar effect was seen in mammalian cells and persists into the first few postirradiation generations.[8–10] Potentially lethal damage repair may be most important in relating the cell culture studies of human tumors to their clinical response. Weichselbaum and colleagues have shown that osteogenic sarcoma, a tumor characteristically thought to be resistant to radiation, has a great capacity for potentially lethal damage repair compared with tumors that may be much more responsive to radiation.[11] After irradiation in the clinical circumstance, the tumor cell may not be faced with the necessity of rapid cell division, and it may have the opportunity for potentially lethal damage repair.

One explanation for the shoulder of the radiation survival curve is that the cell can repair some of the radiation damage, including a great proportion of the damage incurred with low doses of radiation. This is called *sublethal damage*. Elkind and colleagues have studied the shoulder and its return by using divided doses of radiation.[12] They have shown that if the dose of radiation is divided into two fractions and a few hours elapse between radiation doses, the shoulder will return. Therefore, two doses of radiation separated in time are less effective than the same total dose given as a single dose. The difference between a single dose and the divided dose that produce equivalent cell kills is the D_q if all the doses are sufficiently large to cause the loss in cell survival to extend to the exponential portion of the survival curve (Fig. 15–9).

The D_q is a measure of sublethal damage repair. Table 15–2 shows the D_q for bone marrow, skin, lung, and gastrointestinal mucosa. The contrast is striking. Bone marrow stem cells have a small D_q, whereas the others have considerable sublethal damage repair capacity. This suggests that multiple small fractions of radiation can preserve these tissues, but not bone marrow. Radiation fractionation schemes must account for whether the fraction size is sufficient to be off the shoulder. If all of the variations are on the shoulder, there will be little difference in cell kill. With such small fractions, essentially all the damage that can be repaired is being repaired already,

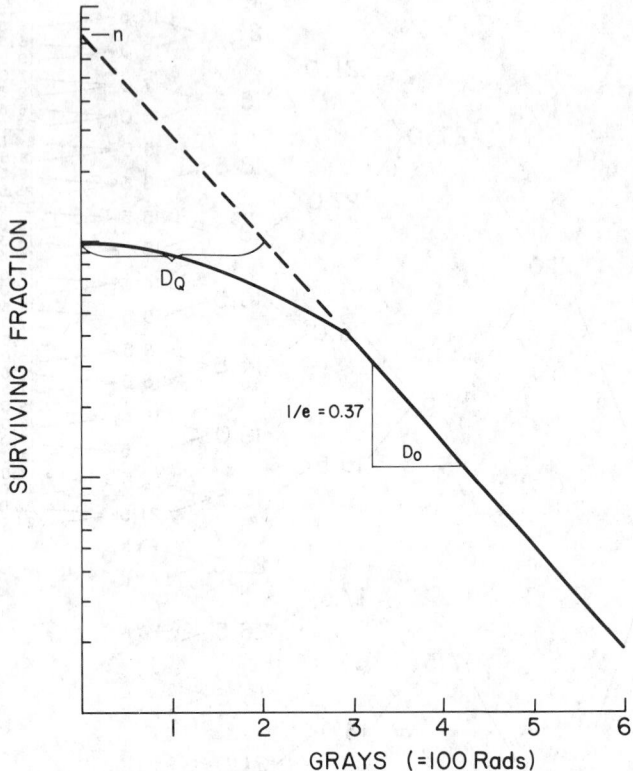

FIGURE 15–8. Idealized radiation survival curve.

Importance of Oxygen

The most important modifier of the biologic effect of ionizing irradiation is molecular oxygen. First noted in the 1920s, its importance was not realized until Mottram and colleagues studied it systematically.[14-16] The general scientific community became aware of this phenomenon with the publications by Read and Gray in the early 1950s.[15,16] Figure 15–11 shows a survival curve for cells under aerobic and hypoxic conditions.[17] For equivalent cell killing at every level of survival, greater doses are required under hypoxic conditions compared with oxic conditions. There is some disagreement in the literature as to whether the dose ratio is the same throughout the survival curve. Most data suggest a smaller difference when low doses are used. A shorthand term, the oxygen enhancement ratio (OER), often is used. OER is the ratio of dose required for equivalent cell killing in the absence of oxygen compared with the dose required in the presence of oxygen. This term has most relevance on the exponential portion of the curve, because there appears to be a reduced shoulder on the survival curve of cells under hypoxic conditions.[17] Tumor cells allowed to grow into physiologic hypoxia have reduced capacity to repair sublethal damage (Fig. 15–12).

The OER range for different cells that have been studied varies from about 2.5 to 3.5. This means that for reduction to a given survival level, three times as much radiation is required under hypoxic conditions as under oxic conditions. Because the curves are exponential, the ratio of survival fractions may be much greater at a given dose and will increase with dose. For example, in Figure 15–11, at 1000 rad the ratio of survival is 30.

Study of the phenomenon reveals that oxygen must be present during irradiation. Figure 15–13 shows the relative radiosensitivity of cells as a function of the oxygen tension at the time of irradiation. A low oxygen tension must be reached before there is a protective effect of hypoxia. The exact mechanism of the oxygen effect has not been determined definitively. It is believed that oxygen affects the initial chemical products of the interaction of radiation with biologic material. The important free radicals have short half-lives. A useful way to think about them is that they may return to an innocuous state or remain highly reactive molecules. Oxygen appears to favor the latter, whereas the presence of high levels of sulfhydryl compounds favors the former.

Thomlinson and Gray recognized the importance of the

and fractionation becomes much less important. If the fractions are large enough to include a portion of the steeper part of the survival curve, differences in fraction size are important, because the proportion of shoulder-to-steep-exponential portion varies for different fraction sizes.

Varying the dose rate of radiation may be considered a form of radiation fractionation. When the dose rate is low, such as during interstitial or intracavitary irradiation, it can be considered as a large number of small doses on the shoulder of the survival curve.[12] Therefore, differences between the dose-limiting normal tissues and the tumor in their shoulder characteristics and differences in the break point between shoulder and steep exponential will have great clinical implications for such continuous radiation. An example of this for cells in culture is shown in Figure 15–10.

TABLE 15–1. Survival Curve Parameters for Some Mammalian Cells In Vivo or In Vitro

Cell Type	How Determined	D_0 (Rad)	n	D_q (Rad)
Hamster V-79 fibroblast	In vitro	~160	~7	250–300
Chang liver	In vitro	150	2	150
HeLa	In vitro	130	4	180
P 388 leukemia	In vivo	130	8.5	280
Mouse bone marrow	In vivo	90–100	1.5–2.0	~60
Mouse small intestine	In vivo	100	50	390
Mouse chondroblast	In vivo	160	9	350
Rat endothelium	In vivo	170	7	340

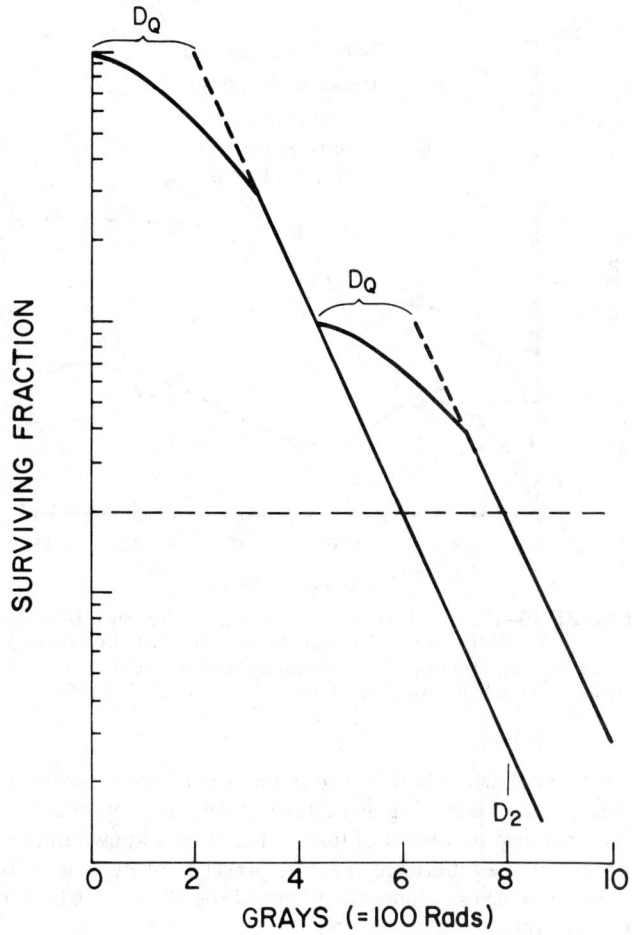

FIGURE 15–9. Two-dose radiation survival curves demonstrating return of the shoulder.

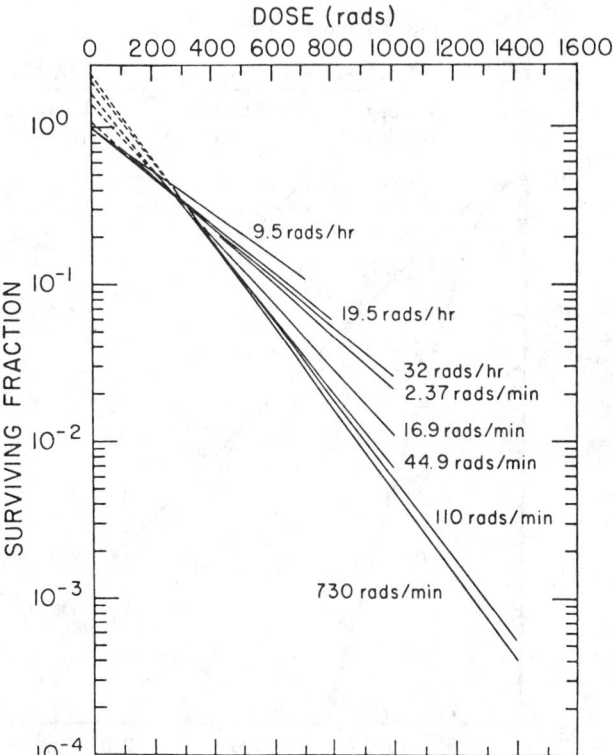

FIGURE 15–10. In vitro survival curves for cells irradiated at different dose rates. (Hall EJ. Radiation dose-rate: A factor of importance in radiobiology and radiotherapy. Br J Radiol 1972;45:81–97)

oxygen effect in a classic paper in which they showed that tumors from humans frequently had anoxic regions.[19] Calculations of oxygen diffusion from capillaries and metabolism predicted that the oxygen tension would decrease to zero at about 150 μm. They measured the width of tumor cords and showed that tumors can be modeled as shown in Figure 15–14. Those cells within about 100 μm of the capillary are well oxygenated; those beyond 150 μm are anoxic and necrotic; and those between 100 and 150 μm are hypoxic at an oxygen tension that might protect cells from radiation. This model has had a profound influence on radiobiologic and radiotherapeutic thinking. If all tumors look this way and such hypoxic

regions contain cells that ultimately could cause tumor regrowth, then no clinically apparent tumor would be cured by radiation therapy. Because this is not the case, this paradox must be explained.

Laboratory experiments have indicated that immediately after a single dose of radiation, the surviving tumor cells are mainly the original hypoxic cells. After a period of time, the proportion of hypoxic cells returns to the preradiation level. This has been called *reoxygenation*.[20] The term can be confusing because these are indirect experiments and do not record the fate of individual cells. The results of these experiments can be explained by suggesting that tumor cells do reoxygenate for several reasons:

1. Reduced total tumor cell population relative to the surface area of tumor blood vessels
2. Reduced separation of hypoxic cells from the blood vessels resulting from preferential cell kill of oxygenated cells
3. Increased oxygen diffusion
4. Decreased intratumoral pressure that opens blood vessels

Alternatively, a large number of these hypoxic cells might in fact be doomed because, with proliferation in the oxic regions, they will be pushed outward, ultimately forced to reside in the anoxic regions, and therefore die. They may have only a limited clinical importance in determining tumor curability. It is likely that different mechanisms occur under different circumstances in the laboratory and in the clinic.

TABLE 15–2. D_q Determination for Some Normal Tissues

Normal Tissue	D_q (Gy)*
Mouse skin	~4.00
Mouse intestine	3.50–4.00
Mouse lung	~3.75
Mouse bone marrow	0–0.60

* Average calculated from literature.

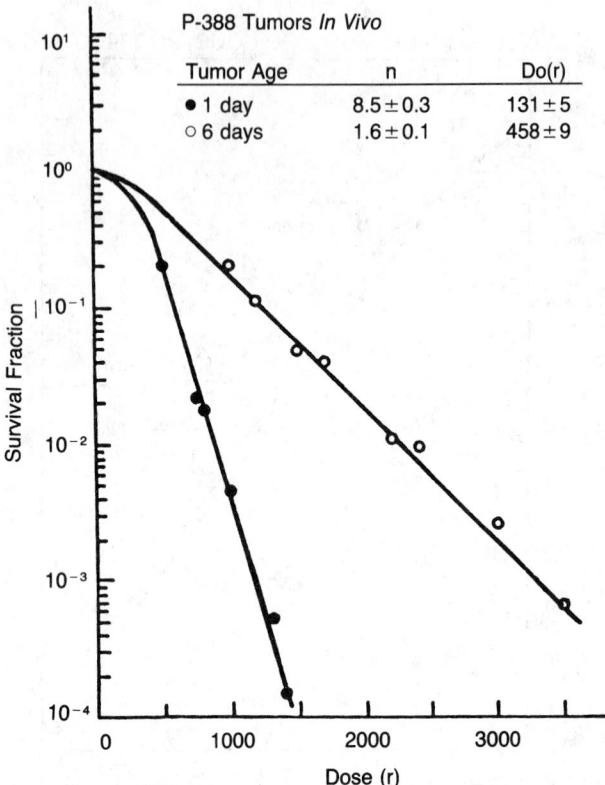

FIGURE 15–11. In vivo survival curves for oxic and hypoxic tumor cells. (Belli JA, Dicus GJ, Bonte FJ. Radiation response of mammalian tumor cells: 1. Repair of sublethal damage in vivo. J Natl Cancer Inst 1967;38:673–682)

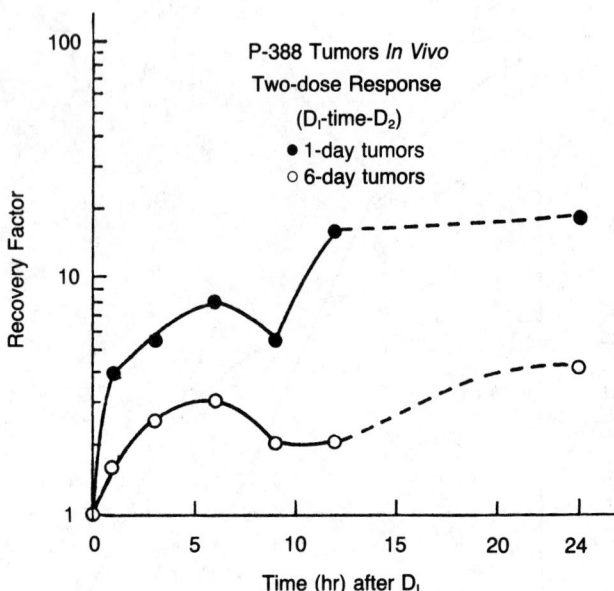

FIGURE 15–12. In vivo curves comparing two-dose survival to single-dose survival for oxic and hypoxic tumor cells. (Belli JA, Dicus GJ, Bonte FJ. Radiation response of mammalian tumor cells: 1. Repair of sublethal damage in vivo. J Natl Cancer Inst 1967;38:673–682)

The clinical importance of the oxygen effect has led to clinical and laboratory experiments, including the use of high-pressure oxygen with radiation therapy to improve results. These studies have indicated that with a small number of radiation fractions, hyperbaric oxygen increases curability. If normal fractionation schemes are used, hyperbaric oxygen often fails to show an advantage. There are, however, some reports of tumors of the head, neck, and uterine cervix that indicate that hyperbaric oxygen with 10 fractions of radiation results in greater cure than conventional daily fractionation.[21-23] Table 15–3 depicts the results with head and neck cancers. Despite these promising studies, the hyperbaric oxygen technique is cumbersome, difficult for the patient, and prohibits the use of the careful beam definition and beam modification so important in radiation therapy. The technique has been abandoned in most radiotherapy centers.

A more attractive alternative has been the development of *hypoxic cell sensitizers.* In the 1960s, Adams and colleagues began searching for compounds that would mimic oxygen in its effect.[24,25] They sought agents that would be metabolized slowly and reach all portions of the tumor. This is an important distinction, because high-pressure oxygen increases diffusion only slightly, whereas slowly metabolized sensitizers can reach all areas of the tumor. Although newer methods were based on replacing molecular oxygen, there are other effects of the nitroimidazoles, the most well-studied class of these agents. They appear to be cytotoxic to hypoxic cells and may sensitize cells to chemotherapeutic agents.[26,27] How important these

last two points are in their use remains to be seen. However, this general class of agents offers a whole new approach to the chemical treatment of tumors based on a known tumor-normal tissue difference (*i.e.,* the presence of hypoxic cells in tumors). These agents are discussed specifically in Chapter 69, section 10.

A practical clinical concern is whether the presence of anemia affects tumor response to radiation. Historic review and a prospective study from the Princess Margaret Hospital (Table 15–4) appear to indicate that anemia results in an adverse effect on tumor curability by radiation, presumably because it increases the hypoxic component of tumor cells.[28]

A recent review of intercapillary distance and tissue oxygen tension correlates local recurrence with evidence of hypoxia using these parameters in studying carcinoma of the cervix.[29]

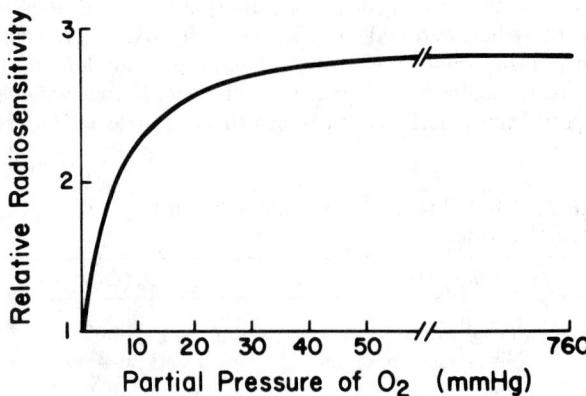

FIGURE 15–13. Radiation sensitivity as a function of ambient oxygen pressure. (Modified from Deschner EE, Gray LH. Influence of oxygen tension on x-ray induced chromosomal damage in Ehrlich ascites tumor cells irradiated in vitro and in vivo. Radiat Res 1959;11:115–146)

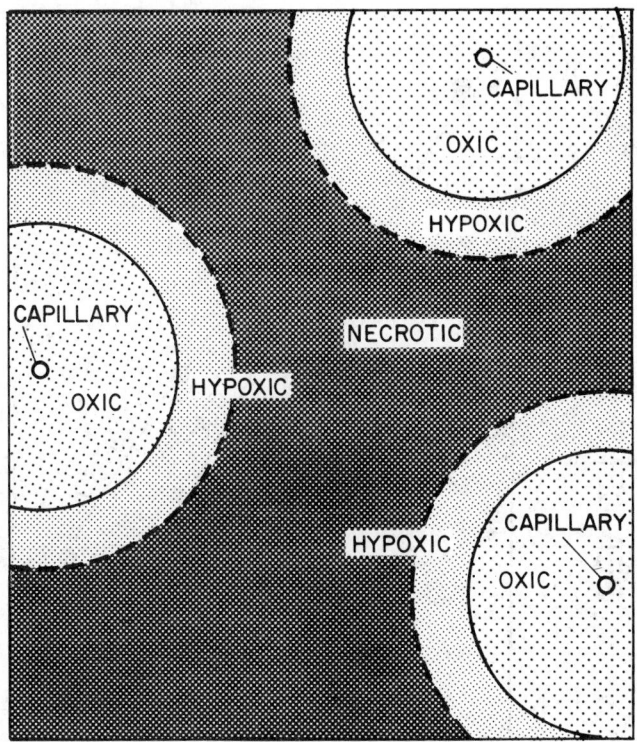

FIGURE 15–14.   Diagrammatic representation of a tumor.

These studies emphasize the promise of techniques that improve tissue oxygenation in the treatment of epithelial cancers. In vitro measurement of hypoxia using radioactively labeled hypoxic sensitizers may alter selection of appropriate tumors for such therapeutic manipulation.[30,31]

Variable Radiation Response During the Division Cycle

As described in Chapter 4, the cell cycle can be divided into four phases: G_1, S, G_2, and M. Terasima, Tolmach, and Sinclair studied synchronized populations to determine whether there is a difference in response to radiation as a function of the cell's position in the division cycle.[32,33] They found that generally the mitotic phase (M) is most sensitive and G_2 almost as sensitive. G_1 is relatively sensitive in cells with a short G_1. Cells gradually increase in resistance as they proceed through the late G_1 and S phases, reaching a maximum of resistance in the late S phase. In cells with a long G_1, there

TABLE 15–3.   Results of a Randomized Prospective Trial of Hyperbaric Oxygen in the Radiation Treatment of Head and Neck Cancer

	Local Control	Survival at 4 Years
HP O_2	61%	56%
Conventional treatment	40%	27%

(Henk JM, Kindler PB, Smith CW. Radiotherapy and head and neck cancer: Final report on the first clinical trial. Lancet 1977;2:101–103)

TABLE 15–4.   Effect of Anemia on Pelvic Recurrence in Stage IIB–III Cervical Cancer

	Control		Transfused
Hemoglobin (g/dl)	<12	>12	>12
Pelvic recurrence	50%	23%	16%
	(10/20)	(11/48)	(11/67)

(Bush RS, Jenkin RP, Allt WE, et al. Definitive evidence for hypoxic cells influencing cure in cancer therapy. Br J Cancer 1978;37:302–306)

appears to be a peak of resistance early in G_1. These findings in vitro seem to be true in vivo as well for normal and tumor cells.[34,35]

The changes in radiation response are reflected in changes in the shoulder of the survival curve and in the terminal slope. These differences can be large. The difference between the most resistant and the most sensitive can show slope ratios equal to that of the oxygen effect. The clinical consequence of a dose of 200 rad is shown in Table 15–5 for two different radiation fractionation schemes: one used in Hodgkin's disease (20 fractions) and one used in epithelial cancer (32 fractions).[36] Note how small differences in survival fractions after a single dose may change the final survival level achieved. All of these fractional survivals are within the range seen for cells in different parts of the cell cycle.

A second consequence of differential cell killing and the mitotic delay induced by radiation is a tendency to partially synchronize the cells. The timing of the second dose of a fractionated scheme may be critical. This synchronization is short-lived because cells desynchronize rapidly and redistribute themselves according to the original cell age distribution. This phenomenon, which could pose a clinical problem or a clinical advantage, does not seem to be important unless there is incomplete redistribution between fractions.

Cell Proliferation

During a course of fractionated radiation, the ultimate response of the tumor and normal tissue depends on whether there has been cell proliferation between the fractions, thereby

TABLE 15–5.   Calculated Cumulative Survival Fraction*

Survival Fraction	X^{32} $X =$	X^{20} $X =$
10^{-11}	0.45	0.28
10^{-10}	0.49	0.32
10^{-9}	0.52	0.35
10^{-8}	0.56	0.40
10^{-7}	0.60	0.45
10^{-6}	0.65	0.50
10^{-5}	0.70	0.56

* Calculated cumulative survival fraction for either 32 or 20 equal fractions when the fractional survival is varied.
(Hellman S. Cell kinetics, models, and cancer treatment: Some principles for the radiation oncologist. Radiology 1975;114:219–223)

increasing the number of cells exposed to radiation. This may be caused by cell proliferation within the irradiated volume (*i.e.*, within the tumor or normal cell renewal tissue) or by cells that immigrate from unirradiated adjacent areas. The latter situation is seen in the skin, oral gastrointestinal mucosa, or from great distances, as found with bone marrow and lymph node repopulation. The balance between radiation-induced cell killing and repopulation is responsible for most of the clinical findings seen during fractionated radiotherapy treatment.

In addition to spontaneous repopulation, there may be an induced cell proliferation or *recruitment* of cells.[37,38] Physiologically, many tissues of the body respond to trauma by being recruited into rapid proliferation (*e.g.*, after a wound in the skin, a break of the bone, or a partial hepatectomy). The reparative process requires proliferation of the undamaged cells. Similarly, when the oral mucosa is irradiated, there is strong evidence that the cell-cycle time is decreased and that net cell proliferation increases. This also may occur in some tumors but appears to be of less magnitude than that in normal tissues.[39] Part of the differential effect of fractionated radiation may lie in differential recruitment of normal versus tumor cells.

Transcriptional Activation, Gene Induction and Regulation After Ionizing Radiation

A new class of actions of ionizing radiation may explain a number of perplexing effects. Immediately after exposure to ionizing radiation, there appear to be expression of genes such as *FOS*, *JUN*, and *EGR1*.[39a,39b] This appears to occur in the presence of protein synthesis and is felt to be due to transcriptional activation and inhibition of protein degradation. Radiation also induces TNF-α.[39c,39d] This may produce additive, synergistic, and distant cytotoxic effects of radiation. PDGF-α and FGF are induced and released from vascular endothelium.[39e] It is suggested that this release stimulates proliferation of smooth muscle cells in the smaller arterioles and contributes to the undesirable long-term vascular events associated with radiation exposure.[39f]

Pharmacologic Modification of Radiation Effects

Pharmacologic agents can modify the basic parameters of radiation response. Figure 15–15 shows a radiation survival curve for cells that have semiconservatively incorporated the halogenated pyrimidine bromodeoxyuridine (BUDR) into their DNA. Under such circumstances, these cells are more sensitive to radiation, their survival curve having the slope and the shoulder modified.[40] This occurs only when the halogenated pyrimidines BUDR or iododeoxyuridine (IUDR) are incorporated into the DNA; their presence at the time of radiation is not sufficient (see Fig. 15–15). Sublethal damage repair also is markedly inhibited under these circumstances. Clinical experiments using these agents are discussed in Chapter 69, section 9.

A second class of agents includes those that primarily affect the shoulder and only slightly affect the slope. The two most important agents here are dactinomycin and doxorubicin. Sublethal damage apparently is inhibited by dactinomycin but not by doxorubicin.[41–47] The mechanisms by which these drugs

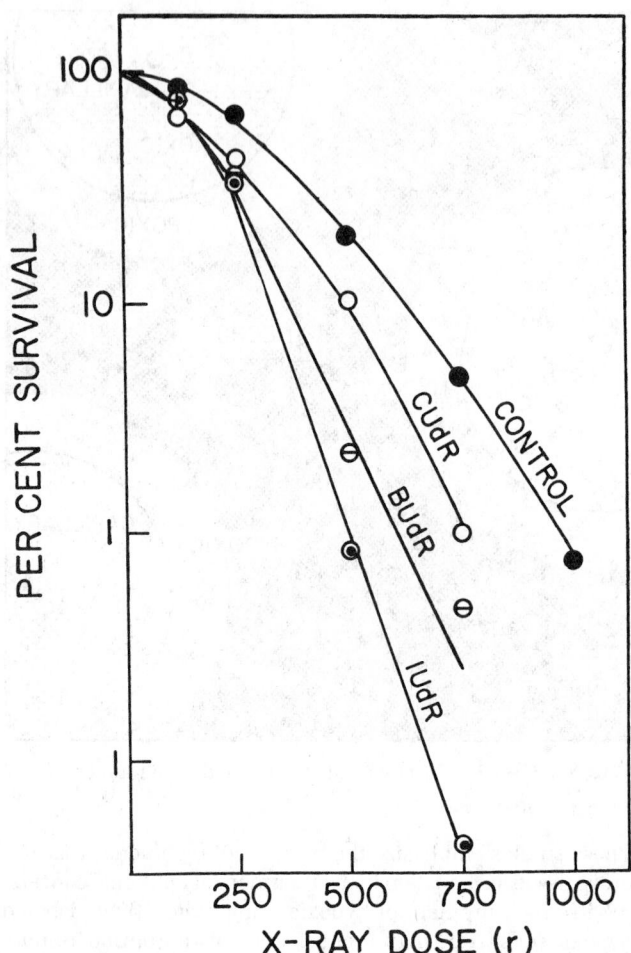

FIGURE 15–15. Radiation survival curve for cells incorporating halogenated pyrimidines. (Szybalski W. X-ray sensitization by halopyrimidines. Cancer Chemother Rep 1974;58:539–557)

affect radiation response are complicated. From a clinical standpoint, there appears to be strong evidence that these drugs can and do modify radiation effects when given simultaneously. Further, when given after radiation therapy, they can recall the irradiated volumes by erythema on the skin or by producing pulmonary reactions.[42,45,48,49] It is not known whether this is due to interaction between the damage done by radiation and that by drug or whether it represents only additivity of the effects.

Chemicals may also interact with radiation by preferentially killing cells that are more resistant to radiation. For example, agents that preferentially destroy cells in the most resistant phase of the cell cycle (S), along with radiation, will increase the cell kill; an example of this is hydroxyurea.[50] Hypoxic sensitizers also kill hypoxic cells and therefore act similarly in destroying a population of cells resistant to radiation. Radioprotective agents such as sulfhydryl-containing compounds act in the reverse fashion and tend to make cells more resistant.[51]

Agents with dose-limiting normal tissue toxicities different from radiation may be used effectively with radiation. This is one of the basic principles of multiple-drug chemotherapy— add agents with nonoverlapping toxicities. This also works well with radiation.

The combined effects of drugs and radiation, or of two drugs, can be divided into the following types:

1. Independent—the agents act independently, their mechanisms of action are independent, and their damage is independent.
2. Additivity—the agents act on the same loci, and therefore their sublethal damage and their lethal damage are additive. Because of additive sublethal damage, the lethality of the two together may be greater than the lethality of each alone added together.
3. Synergism—the two agents have a result that is more effective than pure additivity.
4. Antagonism—the cell killing is less than independent action.

The most important parameter for the clinician is the therapeutic index. The sigmoid curve of tumor cure and that of dose-limiting toxicity are portrayed in Figure 15–16. If both curves are moved but their relative place (one to the other) is not changed, then the proportion cured for a given level of toxicity is unchanged. Drug-roentgen-ray interaction is useful only when the curves are separated and not merely displaced. This is discussed further in Chapter 69, section 10, where halogenated pyrimidines in clinical trials are discussed.

HIGH LINEAR ENERGY TRANSFER RADIATION

Most of the previous discussion has been concerned with sparsely ionizing radiation, such as that produced by photons or high-energy electrons. More densely ionizing radiation is produced by larger atomic particles. The biologic actions of these two types of radiation are different and relate to the density of ionization. LET is the rate of energy loss along the path of the particle (de/dl). High LET radiations are densely ionizing, with de/dl being high. In general, the density of ionization depends on Z^2/v^2, where Z is the atomic number and v is the particle velocity. Photons and electrons are characterized by high energy and low mass. Therefore, the density

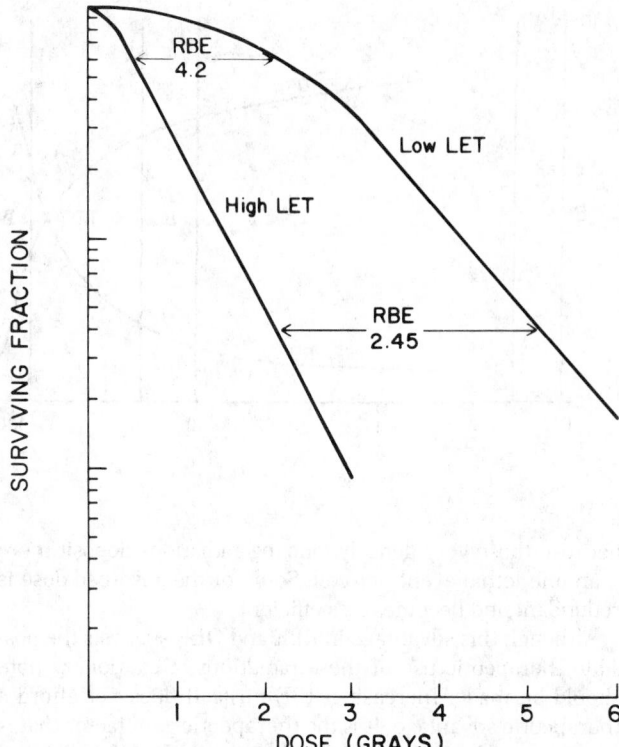

FIGURE 15–17. Survival fractions for high and low LET radiations.

of ionization is low until the secondary electrons come to rest at the end of their path. Particulate radiation ionizes directly. α particles and stripped nuclei have a high LET; neutrons have an intermediate LET due to recoil protons. The Z^2 is large for large particles, intermediate for protons, and low for photons.

RELATIVE BIOLOGIC EFFECTIVENESS

Relative biologic effectiveness (RBE) is a commonly used parameter in radiation biology. It is the dose ratio of different average LET beams required to produce the same biologic effect. This term generally is a descriptive one, but its numerical value is fraught with many difficulties because it varies with the biologic endpoint used. High LET radiation differs from low LET radiation in affecting the shoulder and the slope of the radiation survival curves (Fig. 15–17) If the biologic endpoint of interest is associated with a high survival fraction, then the RBE will be large because it considers shoulder differences and those of the terminal slope. If the biologic endpoint involves a low survival fraction, the RBE will be less because it primarily considers slope differences. In general, RBE increases as the dose decreases. Not only is the shoulder reduced, but other measures of sublethal damage repair or potentially lethal damage repair are markedly reduced with high LET radiation.

A general explanation is that the ionization is so dense that when a cell is hit, the damage is so great that it cannot be repaired. It is also true that the oxygen effect decreases as the LET increases. With very high LET radiation, there is no oxygen effect. Figure 15–18 plots RBE and OER as a function of LET.[52] With very high LET radiation, there is a fall in RBE

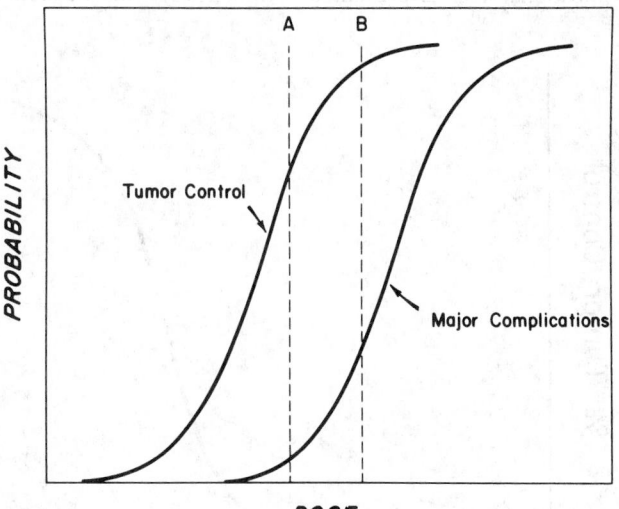

FIGURE 15–16. Sigmoid curves of tumor control and complications. **(A)** Dose for tumor control with minimum complications. **(B)** Maximum tumor dose with significant complications.

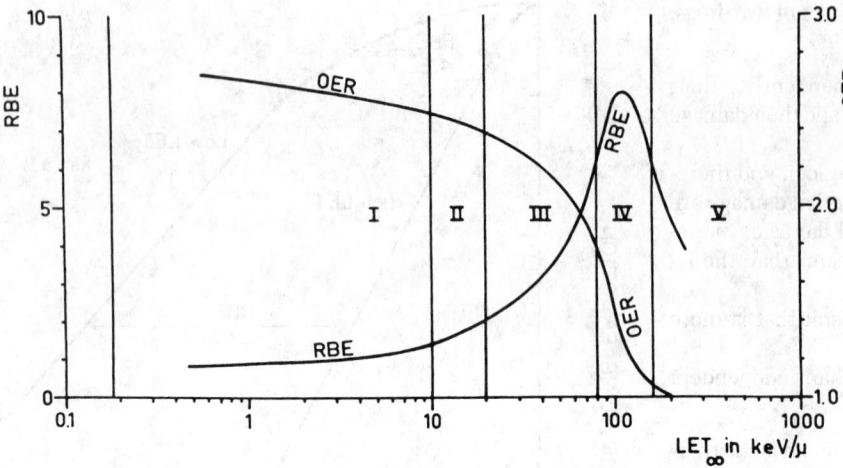

FIGURE 15–18. Oxygen enhancement ratio (OER) and relative biologic effectiveness as a function of linear energy transfer OER. Five regions of LET are suggested: I, corresponds to shouldered survival curves and is affected greatly by fraction size and dose rate; II, transition region; III, exponential survival curve, independent of fractionization and dose rate. RBE changes considerably with LET, as does OER; IV, transition region; V, LET in excess of 160 KeV/u independent of fractionization and dose rate. RBE decreases as LET increases, since any cell damaged is so extensively damaged by high density of interactions that some interactions are "wasted." (Barendsen GW. Response of cultured cells, tumors and normal tissues to radiations of different linear energy transfer. Curr Top Radiat Res 1968;4:293–356)

because these very densely ionizing radiations deposit more than one lethal event per cell. Some of the absorbed dose is redundant and becomes less efficient.

Although this advantage in RBE and OER suggests the possible therapeutic use of these radiations, a cautionary note should be made. Increasing RBE in itself does not afford a therapeutic advantage. It is the therapeutic gain factor that is important—the RBE of the tumor compared with the RBE of the normal tissue. This is complicated and greatly depends on the specific tumor and the dose-limiting normal tissue being considered (see Chap. 69, section 10).[53]

TUMOR RADIOBIOLOGY

Many experiments have been done using animal tumors. In general, these tumors are spontaneous tumors occurring with reasonably high frequency in certain strains of mice (*e.g.,* mammary carcinoma in C3H mice) or tumors induced by carcinogens. Such primary tumors of animals are difficult to use experimentally because their production is time consuming, and numbers of tumors of the same size and location are limited, restricting some experimental designs. A much more common technique is the use of transplanted tumors. These are tumors that may have occurred spontaneously or from the application of a carcinogen but have now been transplanted from animal to animal. They grow with predictable and known kinetics. Although this is a great advantage in experimental work, it does increase the likelihood that the application of the results may be somewhat limited. Because these tumors are selected for rapid growth and for the ability to transplant serially, they may not represent tumors that occur spontaneously in the host animal.

Tumors can be used in radiobiologic experiments and assayed in a number of ways. The simplest is to study the likelihood for cure. A researcher implants a tumor into animals, allows it to grow to palpable size, treats it with a specific regimen, and then determines how many tumors of this type in various host animals are cured. If the dose of radiation is plotted against the likelihood for cure, a sigmoid curve is generated (Fig. 15–19).[54] There is insufficient cell kill to cause tumor cure at very low doses. As the dose is raised (to about one lethal event per cell), the statistics of random cell kill become

important. Occasionally, tumors will have zero viable cells and are cured. The likelihood of cure rises rapidly with dose at this portion of the curve; it starts to plateau when the maximum effect of the particular technique is reached. The dose required to increase a 10% likelihood of tumor control to 90% is about three times the D_o dose. This sigmoid relation is important, because it is true not only for tumors in experimental animals but also for clinical situations.

The shape and steepness of the sigmoid dose-response relation for tumors can be affected by many factors. If the radiation survival curve is shallow for individual tumor cells (*i.e.,* the D_o is large), then the dose-response curve will also be shallow. It will also be affected by host defense mechanisms. This curve is steep with nonimmunogenic tumors or abrogated immune response, but it is significantly shallower in immunogenic tumors.[55] The shallowness means that there will be occasional cures at low doses and occasional failures at very high doses.

A similar sigmoid relation is seen when plotting the likelihood for complications against tumor control. Figure 15–16 shows the two sigmoid curves, one for cure and one for complications. This is presented optimistically—the important

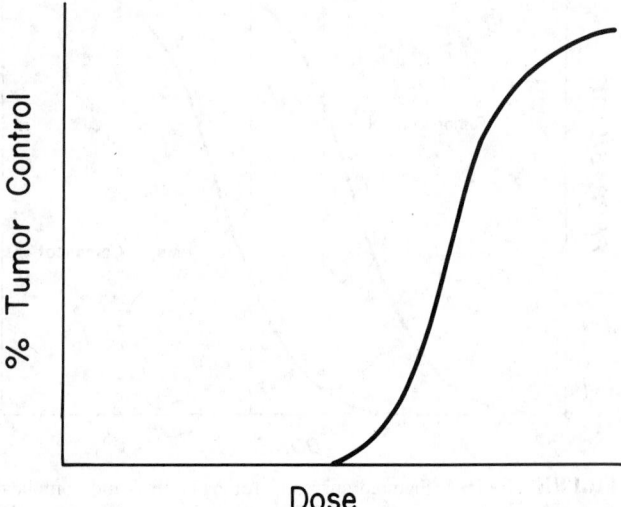

FIGURE 15–19. Sigmoid curve of tumor control.

complication curve is placed to the right of the tumor cure curve. The difference between these curves is a measure of therapeutic gain. Much of clinical medicine and research in cancer treatment is concerned with separating these curves.[53] After the curves are separated, for a given level of complications, the likelihood of cure can be increased. Or, for a high likelihood of cure, the likelihood of complications can be decreased.

Another method of measuring the response of tumors to treatment is to determine their growth delay after treatment. The longer the time for regrowth, the more effective the treatment. Assuming that tumors grow and regrow with the same kinetics when they are at similar sizes, the separation between the original curve and the regrowth curve is a direct measure of cell kill.[56] A direct measure of tumor cell kill is to remove the tumor after treatment, separate the cells, and score the surviving colony-forming cells in vivo or in vitro. Assay techniques include transplantation and measurement in recipient animals of death, tumor growth, or the number of colonies in the lung, liver, or brain. In vitro techniques require tumors to adapt to grow in vivo and in vitro.

Tumors, like normal tissues, have certain physiologic characteristics. We associate some of these with the definition of malignancy: continued growth and extension into surrounding tissues and the ability to metastasize. In addition, growing tumors must induce a blood supply to meet their increasing metabolic needs. The production of these blood vessels appears to result from the release of a substance described by Folkman and colleagues as "tumor angiogenesis factor" and may have important clinical implications. If tumors can be prevented from producing such substances, they cannot grow beyond a size supported by diffusion alone.[57-59] From the radiobiologic point of view it means that when irradiating a tumor, the radiobiology of the tumor and the vascular endothelial cells are important. Complete destruction of the ability of tumor blood vessels to proliferate will effectively limit tumor growth.

As tumors grow, they often exceed their blood supply and develop areas of necrosis and hypoxia (Fig. 15–14). The proportion of hypoxic cells in a tumor can be determined by studying the radiation survival curves. In Figure 15–20, curve A represents a well-oxygenated cell population, curve B describes hypoxic cells, and curve C represents a mixture of oxic and hypoxic cells (as in a tumor). Extrapolation of the curves to the ordinate gives the proportion of hypoxic cells within a tumor, first described by Powers and Tolmach.[60] In most experimental tumors studied, the percentage of hypoxic cells is 10% to 20%.

Calculation of the likelihood to cure tumors based on D_o, n, repopulation, repair, and hypoxia indicates that, because each fraction of radiation increases the proportion of hypoxic cells, the treatment regimens should not be effective. Because radiotherapy cures a large number of tumors that have hypoxic components and show necrosis on pathologic examination, this conclusion must be erroneous. After multiple fractions of radiation, a marked increase in the proportion of the more resistant hypoxic cells could be expected, but, in fact, the proportion remained constant when observed 72 hours after the last of five radiation fractions. Kallman has called this *reoxygenation*.[20] Hypoxic cells may not be important in tumors that are cured but may be important in some tumors that are

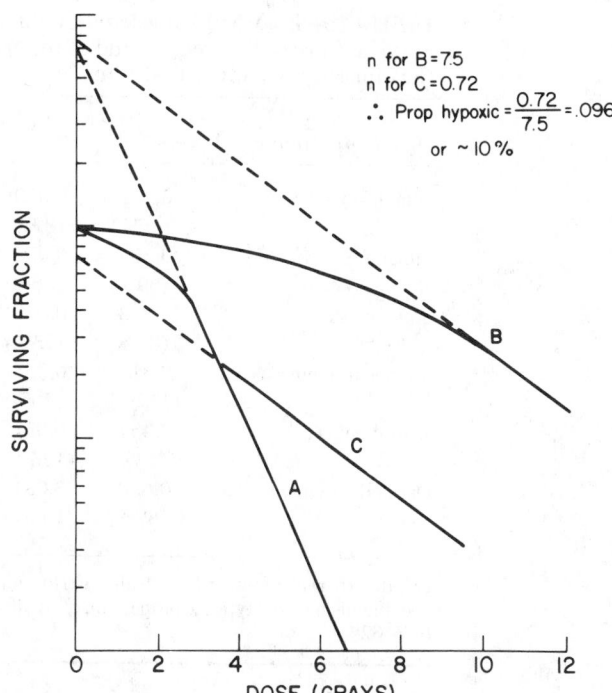

FIGURE 15–20. Idealized survival curves for (**A**) oxic tumor cells; (**B**) hypoxic tumor cells; and (**C**) a tumor containing both oxic and hypoxic tumor cells.

not cured. Clinical evidence that this is significant includes the benefits of correcting anemia, hyperbaric oxygen, and the hypoxic sensitizers. All appear to favorably influence tumor curability in certain clinical circumstances.

There has been a renaissance in trying to determine whether there are appropriate laboratory correlates for clinical radiation treatment.[61,62] Table 15–6 shows important parameters found by in vitro survival determinations for six histologic groups of human tumor cells.[63] The first four parameters have been described earlier. S_2 and S_8 are the survival fractions found with 2 Gy and 8 Gy, respectively. $\bar{D}$ is the mean inactivation dose, a mathematically determined characteristic of the initial portion of the survival curve. It appears that S_2 and $\bar{D}$ correlate directly with clinical radiocurability, whereas α is inversely related. All of these are measures of the initial portion of the radiation survival curve; S_2 is the most closely correlated with clinical practice, because doses between 1.5 and 2.5 Gy are used most often in patient care.

Because doses are repeated, small differences in S_2 can have significant consequences. Table 15–5 shows that, in a typical 32-fraction radiation treatment, the difference between survival fractions of 0.45 and 0.60 results in an ultimate survival fraction of 10^{-11} compared with 10^{-7}, respectively. Also, certain tumors that are known to be difficult to cure by radiation have been shown to have great capacity to repair radiation damage, as measured by allowing the cells time for repair before plating them for in vitro growth.[64] That these two simple laboratory determinations correlate with clinical results gives hope that in vitro techniques can be used to determine mechanisms of modifying clinical parameters. This does not mean that the other biologic parameters such as oxygenation, position in the cell cycle, and cell proliferation are not im-

TABLE 15–6. Mean Values and Coefficients of Variation (in Parentheses) of the Survival Curves' Parameters and of the Surviving Fractions at 2 Gy (S_2) and at 8 Gy (S_8) for Human Tumor Cell Lines

Histologic Groups	α	β	n	D_0 (Gy)	S_2 (%)	S_8 (%)	$\bar{D}$ (Gy)
Glioblastomas (5)	0.241 (86%)	0.029 (37%)	12 (71%)	1.44 (28%)	58 (34%)	4.98 (111%)	3.10 (38%)
Melanomas (19)	0.255 (69%)	0.053 (56%)	73 (265%)	1.04 (27%)	51 (28%)	1.11 (109%)	2.43 (25%)
Squamous cell carcinomas (6)	0.273 (39%)	0.045 (25%)	5 (38%)	1.28 (11%)	49 (18%)	0.88 (49%)	2.35 (25%)
Adenocarcinomas (6)	0.311 (117%)	0.055 (79%)	37 (166%)	1.04 (26%)	48 (37%)	0.39 (130%)	2.22 (28%)
Lymphomas (7)	0.451 (42%)	0.051 (126%)	1.8 (79%)	1.48 (34%)	34 (27%)	0.57 (121%)	1.77 (22%)
Oat cell carcinomas (6)	0.650 (37%)	0.081 (183%)	1.8 (104%)	1.51 (70%)	22 (42%)	0.14 (85%)	1.33 (21%)

(Modified from Malaise EP, et al. Distribution of radiation sensitivities for human tumor cells of specific histological types: Comparison of in vitro to in vivo data. Int J Radiat Oncol Biol Phys 1986;12: 617–624)

portant; no doubt all add to the complexity of correlating the clinical response with in vitro determinations.

NORMAL TISSUE RADIATION BIOLOGY

To understand normal tissue radiation biology, an appreciation of the cell kinetics of cell renewal tissues is vital (see Chap. 4). The effects on organ function depend on the reproductive requirements of the irradiated cells. Tissues whose functional activity does not require cell renewal (*e.g.,* muscle and neurologic tissue) are considered resistant to radiation. Both muscle and neurologic tissue also have important vasculo-connective tissue stroma that support them.[65] These stromal cells may be required to divide, and therefore determine the organ response to radiation. The radiation response of endothelial cells demonstrates a D_q = 340 rad, n = 7, and a D_o = 170 rad, values similar to those of epithelial cells.[66]

Many tissues of the body require continued cellular proliferation for their function, and they promptly demonstrate the effects of radiation. These cell renewal tissues include the skin and its appendages, the gastrointestinal mucosa, bone marrow, reproductive tissues, and many exocrine glands. Clonogenic survival curves for bone marrow stem cells, gastrointestinal epithelial cells, and skin are all available. In slowly proliferating tissues (*e.g.,* lung), the effects of radiation are seen much later, but the effects depend on radiation damage to proliferating cells.

Tissues such as the liver and bone require little or no proliferation during the steady state, and normal function can be maintained despite large doses of radiation. However, both of these respond to injury with rapid cell renewal. If trauma (fracture or partial hepatectomy) occurs, then the cells die when they attempt repair. Irradiation of the liver has few consequences in moderate doses, but if this is followed by a partial hepatectomy, hepatic failure can occur. This has been of clinical importance in the preoperative irradiation of right-sided

Wilms' tumors attached to the liver, in which a significant amount of liver must be removed.[67] Under such circumstances it is far better to operate, allow the liver to regenerate, and then irradiate.

Patients who have received large amounts of radiation to the bone do perfectly well unless the bone is fractured. The damaged bones will fail to be reconstituted or will heal slowly, causing a significant deformity and disability to the patient. These examples are included to stress that it is not the different cells that have such great differences in radiation response, but rather that the proliferative requirements of different tissues largely determine the radiation effects. If the proliferative requirements are low, the organ is considered resistant to radiation. If the proliferative requirements are high, it is considered radiosensitive. There may be some common limitations on all systems based on the radiosensitivity of the vascular connective tissue and endothelial cells.[65] Stem cells of the cell renewal tissues may have a limited proliferative capacity, and stem cell exhaustion appears to be a cause of late organ failure after irradiation.[68]

Many other effects of radiation that do not depend on reproductive viability may have clear clinical relevance. For example, radiation is damaging to the cell membrane and changes membrane transport. Subsequent radiation-induced edema is seen with moderate doses of radiation. These non-reproductive effects of radiation are far less well understood but may be important in understanding the effects of radiation on nondividing tissue—most importantly, the central nervous system.

Large doses of whole-body irradiation have obvious clinical consequences, which generally are not relevant to conventional radiation therapy. However, because whole-body irradiation has been used in low doses in treating the lymphomas and in high doses in treating metastatic carcinoma, this will be discussed briefly.

After large doses of radiation, the prodromal syndrome of

nausea, vomiting, diarrhea, cramps, fatigue, sweating, fever, and headache occurs. Three distinct modes of death may occur. The first, with very high doses of radiation (>10,000 rad), is seen within hours and appears to result from neurologic and cardiovascular damage. Because this occurs so quickly, it probably is not caused by failure of a proliferating cell system but rather by extranuclear events within these organs. At intermediate doses of radiation (500–1000 rad), death occurs within days. It is associated with extensive gastrointestinal mucosal damage, resulting in prolonged, severe, bloody diarrhea, dehydration, and secondary infection occurring as the gastrointestinal mucosa is denuded. At lower doses of radiation (around the LD_{50}), death is caused by hematopoietic failure. This has a latency period because the formed blood elements are nondividing and bone marrow failure does not occur until the progeny of the proliferating cells are required to maintain the patient. The lymphocyte level falls promptly as some of these cells die without dividing. The granulocyte level will fall on about day 5 or 6, and thrombocytopenia will occur later. Anemia does not occur as a direct result of a failure of red cell production because of the long life of the red cell, but it may be caused by hemorrhage.

Whole-body irradiation appears to have significant antitumor activity exceeding that seen when the same dose is given to the tumor alone.[69,70] Very low doses of whole-body radiation in humans (10 to 15 rad, 2 to 3 times per week for 6 to 10 fractions) may be effective treatment for lymphomas and may cause marked depression of the formed blood elements. The mechanism of action of this type of treatment is not understood. The effects on tumor and normal tissue are greater than can be explained by the typical survival curve. One possible explanation is the release of TNF-α after radiation.[39c,39d,39f] Perhaps the release of this and other factors may contribute to the general effects of low-dose whole-body radiation and the abscopal (distant) effects of regional irradiation.

ADVERSE EFFECTS OF RADIATION

Some biologic considerations of localized radiation may decrease the likelihood for tumor control. First and most discussed is the effect of radiation on the *immune response*. High-dose, whole-body irradiation has a well-known and profound effect on the immune response. However, this generalized treatment rarely is used in clinical therapy, except as preparation for bone marrow transplantation.

Shortly after the discovery of roentgen rays, whole-body irradiation before the administration of antigens was found to suppress the production of antibodies. After whole-body irradiation, there is a prompt fall in the lymphocyte count. The lymphocytes appear to have two types of radiation response: About 80% die a prompt, intermitotic death, but some lymphocytes survive the radiation. When assayed on the basis of reproductive capacity by exposure to mitogens after irradiation or other functional endpoints, their radiation survival curves looked similar to that of hematopoietic cells with a D_o of about 70 to 80 rad and an n of about 1.[71] Response depends on the classes of lymphocytes involved, the extent of cell proliferation required, cell traffic, and the balance between suppressor and helper systems. The following conclusions concerning the effect of radiation on the immune response can be made[71]:

1. B lymphocytes are radiosensitive and undergo interphase and mitotic death after irradiation.
2. All functional T-cell subpopulations have sensitive precursor cells. Suppressor T-cell precursors may undergo interphase death.
3. The homing potential of cells is affected by radiation.
4. Resting cells are more sensitive to interphase death than are the same cells when stimulated to divide before irradiation. (In the latter case they have an n and D_o similar to those of hematopoietic stem cells.)
5. The effects of whole-body irradiation are qualitatively and quantitatively different from those caused by localized or regional irradiation.

Whole-body irradiation is more effective in preventing response to new antigens than in modifying response to a previously encountered antigen. Survival of second-set skin grafts are affected much less than are initial grafts. Localized radiation, as used in radiation therapy, affects the immune response by decreasing the number of circulating lymphocytes, presumably by irradiating and destroying them as they pass through the irradiated volume. The consequences of this irradiation appear to be small if the tumor has been in place for a significant time before the irradiation and if the irradiated volume is small. If an animal is irradiated at the time the tumor is implanted, the immune response will be inhibited. However, this rarely is the clinical situation. There have been reports suggesting the deleterious effects of localized radiation on the immune response affecting survival in breast cancer, but this does not appear to be the case in the original series studied or in subsequent studies.[72–74]

Localized radiation, despite producing a chronic lymphopenia of T and B cells, does not affect the immune response to bacterial or viral agents because treated patients do not seem to be more susceptible. This is the case with the immune suppression produced by whole-body irradiation or systemic chemotherapy. Regional irradiation of the lymph nodes adjacent to tumors has been associated with increased curability in head and neck tumors in adults without adverse effects.[75]

There also may be adverse effects of radiation on the patient other than those on host-defense mechanisms. Radiation-induced *mutagenesis* is of concern for germline and somatic cells. If the gonads are irradiated, there is an increased likelihood of mutation with increasing doses, without any evidence of a threshold dose or of an ameliorating effect of fractionation. At higher doses, there is significant cell killing, and the dose-response curve is no longer linear, presumably because the cells that mutated received sufficient radiation to become sterile. Abnormal live births are uncommon after gonadal irradiation because most radiation-induced mutations are recessive. Further, dominant mutations, when they occur, usually are lethal. There is some evidence in the mouse that the risk of mutation decreases with time after ovarian irradiation. Whether this is true in humans and the mechanism by which it occurs in animals are not known. It does not appear to be true for irradiation of the testes.

The mutagenic effects of radiation depend on the type of irradiation. The RBE for high LET radiation can be extremely high for mutations. It is difficult to quantify the risk because experiments with mice indicate a large difference in the mutation rate for different loci, with as much as a 1000-fold variation in the mutation rate.[76] In general, the prudent figure used is that the mutation rate doubles with about every 50 rad.

Perhaps of even greater concern are somatic mutations, especially those that may lead to tumors. A great deal of evidence indicates that low doses of radiation increase the incidence of tumors after significant latent periods. This information comes largely from whole-body exposures to the atomic bomb and experience with patients irradiated for benign diseases.[77-79] In general, there appears to be a linear increase in tumor incidence with dose until high doses are reached, at which point the incidence reaches a plateau or even falls.[80-81] Presumably, this is true again because of cell killing. Figure 15–21 is an example of this biphasic dose-response curve. Such tumor induction is associated with a latent period of 3 to 5 years for leukemia but is much longer for solid tumors. There are different ages at which tumor induction is most likely. For example, the induction of breast cancer by radiation appears primarily with exposure in the first and second decades of life and decreases with radiation later in life.[82]

Except for irradiation of children, it is difficult to demonstrate a significantly increased incidence of tumors in patients receiving therapeutic radiation for malignant disease. This may be an example of the biphasic nature of the tumor induction curve. For example, long-term studies of patients with carcinoma of the cervix do not show increased incidence of pelvic cancer.[82,83] In contrast, when patients are irradiated to the same volume for benign diseases with much lower doses or radiation, an increased tumor incidence can be seen.[78] There appears to be a difference between the tumorigenicity of radiation doses used for benign disease (200 to 1000 rad) and that seen when therapeutic doses of radiation are used. Radiation is a teratogen when a woman is exposed during the rapidly proliferating period of embryogenesis, between weeks 2 and 16.

CLINICAL CONSIDERATIONS

It is often suggested that the goal of treatment is the greatest probability of uncomplicated cure. Although this is desirable, circumstances actually may dictate a different policy. Consider Figure 15–16, in which the curve for complications is to the right of the sigmoid curve for tumor control. The ideal dose would be that which gives as many cures as possible before the steep portion of the complication curve, as shown by line A. This may not be the optimal dose. It depends on the consequences of tumor failure and the nature of the complications. If tumor failure can be salvaged by subsequent surgery but complications are severe, long-lived, and difficult to manage, then line A is the optimal line.[53] An example of this would be the treatment of T2 and T3 glottic cancer. On the other hand, if complications are not severe or remediable, but cancer failure is fatal, then line B would be appropriate. This is the case in stage II and III carcinoma of the uterine cervix. There is no simple answer. Often the worst complication of treatment is tumor recurrence.

There are many clinical examples of sigmoid dose-response curves. An example for tumors of the head and neck is shown in Figure 15–22 and for Hodgkin's disease in Figure 15–23.[84,85] In Figure 15–22, the ordinate is arranged to convert a sigmoid curve to a straight line. These are simple because they do not consider time-dose relations or tumor volume. An instructive clinical experience is described by Stewart and Jackson in which a consistent ~10% change in dose was used.[86] Figure 15–24 shows the results in tumor control and

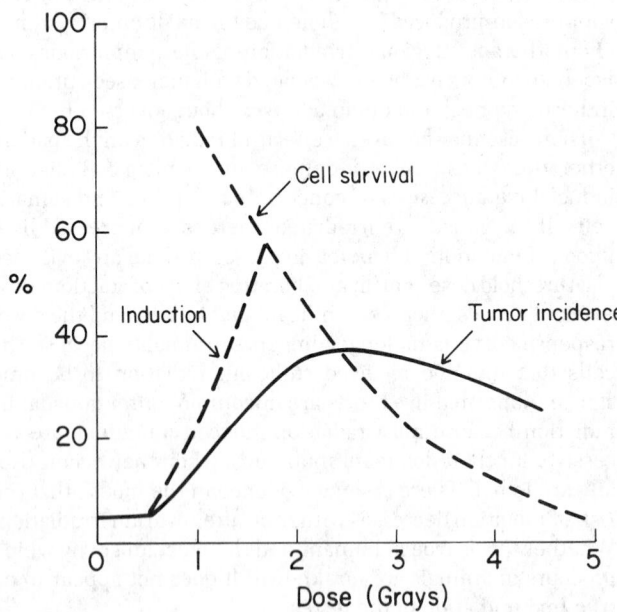

FIGURE 15–21. Biphase curve of tumor incidence. (Redrawn from Gray LH. Radiation biology and cancer. In: Cellular Radiation Biology, pp 7–25. M. D. Anderson Hospital and Tumor Institute 18th Symposium on Fundamental Cancer Research. Baltimore: Williams & Wilkins, 1965; and Upton AC, Randolph ML, Conklin JW. Late effects of fast neutrons and gamma rays in mice as influenced by the dose rate of irradiation: Induction of neoplasia. Radiat Res 1970;41:467–491)

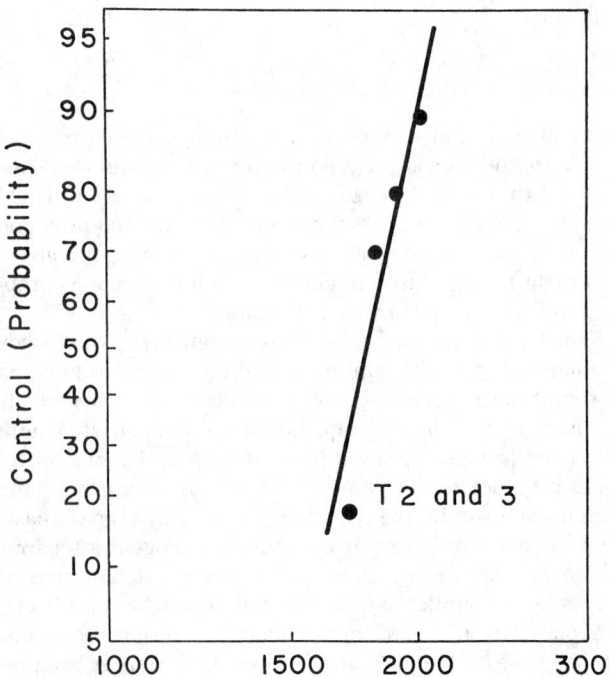

FIGURE 15–22. Tumor control versus dose for supraglottic carcinoma. (Shukovsky LJ. Dose, time, volume relationships in squamous cell carcinoma of the supraglottic larynx. Am J Roentgenol Rad Ther Nucl Med 1970;108:27–29)

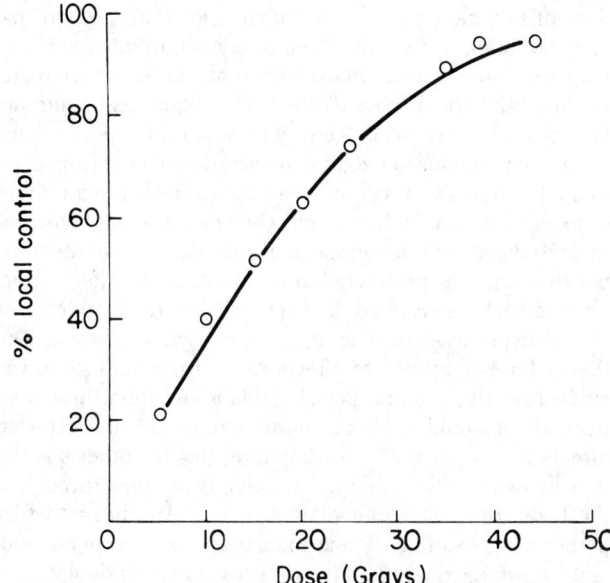

FIGURE 15–23. Tumor control versus dose. (Kaplan HS. Evidence for a tumoricidal dose level in the radiotherapy of Hodgkin's disease. Cancer Res 1966;26:1221–1224)

between tumor and normal tissues. It also shows displacement of the curve for cure as a function of tumor size.

Even though tumors have a very steep dose—response relations, significant intertumor heterogeneity may cause great flattening in the radiation dose—control curves.[87] There is considerable heterogeneity between tumors of the same histologic type and location, and this consideration explains the shallower nature of the clinical dose—response curves compared with those for experimental animals. These analyses further indicate that when the tumor control probability is low, the major reason is the high survival fraction associated with the initial fraction, that is, a high S_2. This emphasizes the importance of identifying prospectively tumors that have a high S_2.

FRACTIONATION

Early in this century, as the practice of radiation therapy evolved, the virtues of dividing the radiation into small fractions were noticed. The reasons given were often incorrect, but the clear observation was that fractionation of the dose allowed more effective tumor cure without excessive complications.

Fractionation considers the size and number of radiation increments. *Protraction* considers the time during which the radiation is given. Both factors affect all radiation therapy plans. The fashioning of a plan for fractionated radiation therapy for carcinoma of the larynx by Coutard, whose work was based on the principles of Regaud, laid the foundation for the development of radiation therapy.[88,89] The principles of such treatment were as follows:

1. Fractionation is important.
2. There is a relation between the acute reaction of the skin and oropharyngeal mucosa to cure and to late effects.

complications. The small increase in dose markedly improved the curability of the larger tumors, presumably because this dose is on the steep portion of the sigmoid dose-response curve. It did not change the cure rate for small tumors very much because, presumably, the dose already was large enough to be on the top of the dose-response curve, where changes in dose do not affect the cure appreciably. Similarly, complications were not increased very much. The point indicating complications was to the right, still on the shallow portion of the curve. This is a good example of separation of response

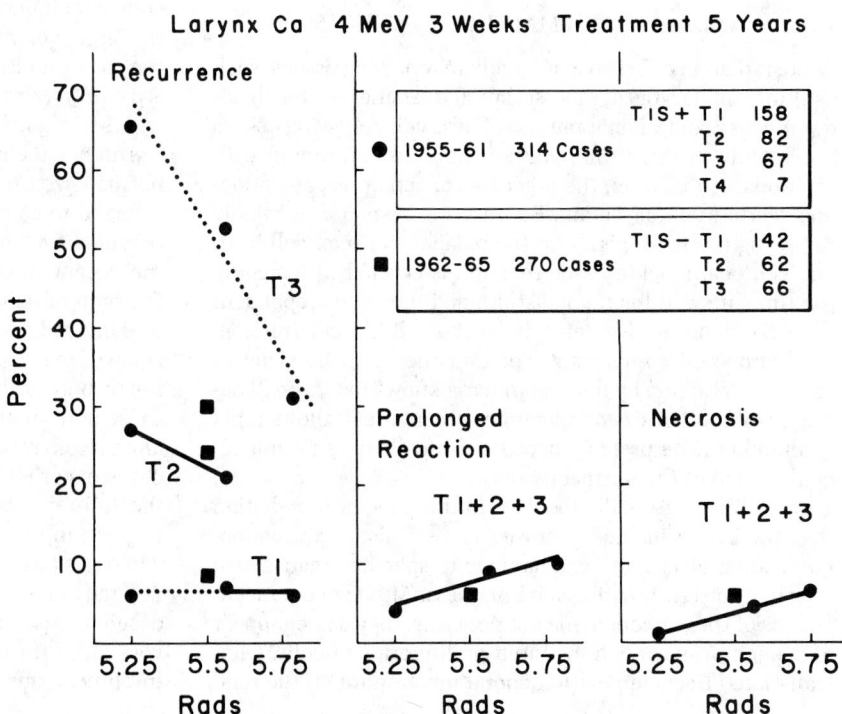

FIGURE 15–24. Tumor control versus dose for cancer of the larynx. (Stewart JG, Jackson AW. The steepness of the dose response curve both for tumor and normal tissue injury. Laryngoscope 1975;85:1107–1111)

It was believed that one had to have complete epidermititis and mucositis resulting in confluent reactions with primary healing from outside the treated area to have a dose sufficient to cure the tumor. The fractionation schemes recommended resulted in tolerable late effects.

The association between acute and late effects has sometimes led radiotherapists astray. This relation depends on the fractionation scheme, the energy of radiation used, and other factors. In general, acute effects are much more dependent on time than late effects. Late effects are influenced primarily by the total dose and fraction size.

CONTINUOUS RADIATION

Another important technique of radiation therapy that evolved in the early part of the century was the application of continuous radiation by interstitial or intracavitary application.[90] If the dose rate was too high or the volume too large, unacceptable complications occurred. Rules for treatment were developed that resulted in the cure of certain tumors without unacceptable complications. These required that the dose rate be kept moderate (less than 100 rad/hour) and an attempt at a good implant geometry be made to avoid unnecessary hot and cold spots.

The whole question of homogeneity of dose is much more difficult with intracavitary and interstitial irradiation than with external beam techniques. To a great extent, the clinical use of radioactive isotopes, especially by implantation techniques, developed separately from external beam radiation therapy. Some physicians only practiced one or the other of these techniques. More recently, external beam and interstitial treatment have been used together to take advantage of the virtues of both modalities. Good examples of this combined treatment are described in the chapters dealing with tumors of the head and neck and uterine cervix (see Chaps. 22 and 38).

ACUTE AND LATE NORMAL TISSUE EFFECTS

Acute radiation effects occur largely in renewing tissues, such as skin, oropharyngeal mucosa, small intestine, rectum, bladder mucosa, and vaginal mucosa. These cell-renewing tissues are rapidly proliferating, and as they are confronted with fractionated radiation, the processes of repair, repopulation, and recruitment all obtain. Because the response of rapidly renewing tissues depends on the balance between cell birth and cell death, acute tissue reaction is crucially affected by the time allowed for repopulation, and therefore dependent on protraction. It also depends on the cell kill per fraction, so fraction size is important. The radiotherapist observing an excessive reaction by the oral mucosa knows that a small decrease in fraction size or a small treatment break allows rapid resolution of the problem because these changes permit reconstitution of the normal tissue.

Late effects are really the dose-limiting factor in radiation therapy. These include necrosis, fibrosis, fistula formation, nonhealing ulceration, and damage to specific organs, such as spinal cord transection and blindness. Although the mechanisms of these phenomena are not clear, they do not appear to depend primarily on the rapid proliferation of cells. Clinically late effects appear to depend much more on the total dose of radiation and the size of the radiation fraction than on protraction. Only if the same fractionation scheme is used with the same normal tissue endpoint, the same irradiated volume, and the same treatment technique, can acute and late effects be correlated. If any of these parameters are varied, the acute reactions to radiation may be dissociated from eventual late effects and will be misleading. There are a number of examples in radiation therapy in which the total dose was increased and the fraction size was increased or kept the same, but the time was protracted to minimize acute effects. Such techniques have resulted in unacceptable late complications.

Two hypotheses for late effects are worth discussion. One theory holds that all late effects result from damage to vasculoconnective stroma. Because this is common throughout the body, it would suggest a common mechanism for the late effects in any organ.[65] A variation on this hypothesis is that it is damage to the endothelial cells, ubiquitous throughout the body, that determines late effects.[66] An alternative hypothesis suggests that the acute and the late effects of radiation and cytotoxic chemotherapy are caused by cell depletion of the targeted cell-renewal tissues. Acute effects depend on the balance between cell killing and compensatory replication of the stem and proliferative cells. The development of late effects requires that stem cells have only a limited proliferative capacity.[91,92] Compensation for extensive or repeated cell killing may exhaust this capacity, resulting in eventual tissue failure.[64,93]

ALTERING THE THERAPEUTIC INDEX

Goodman and Gilman define the therapeutic index as the relation between desired and undesired effects of therapy.[94] For the oncologist, separation of the sigmoid curve of complications from that of local control (see Fig. 15–16) is the graphic representation of manipulation of the therapeutic index. Some techniques of time-dose relations used by the radiotherapist to take advantage of this are fractionation, protraction, split-course technique, interstitial treatment, and manipulation of the target volume. Although fractionation has been discussed, the use of multiple small fractions two, three, or more times a day, *hyperfractionation,* is just beginning to be explored, with some good results.[95–97]

Another technique to reduce complications is the use of normal-sized fractions given more than once a day. This is referred to as multifraction, multiple daily fractions, or *accelerated fractionation.*[98] In the experiments that stimulated the recent interest, the investigators administered 2 daily fractions of radiation separated by 6 hours, and compared this to daily radiation given as a single fraction.[99] Six hours is believed to be long enough to allow complete sublethal damage repair but not long enough for significant proliferation. Because both methods are daily treatments, repair can be separated from repopulation and recruitment. The general results of the experiments were presented as the recovered radiation, the difference between the dose obtained when the radiation is given in two divided doses separated by 6 hours and that when it is given in one fraction. When the single fraction was 200 rad or less, there was little recovered dose. The recovered dose increased rapidly between 200 and 800 rad; then, with very large fractions, the recovered dose tended to level off. In clinical situations, when typical radiation doses of about

200 rad are divided into two smaller fractions, only a little more should be given because the recovered dose is small. This has been confirmed in a number of clinics.[100] The use of such hyperfractionation is being tried for several tumors, but it is too soon to determine whether it will be useful.

When tumor cells are proliferating rapidly, accelerated fractionation makes sense. Waiting 24 hours between each fraction may allow significant proliferation. Perhaps the best example of the changing therapeutic index obtained with accelerated fractionation is the enhanced success in treating Burkitt's lymphoma.[101]

In general, most radiotherapists administer conventional radiation in fractions between 180 and 250 rad each day. This allows tumor control without excessive acute or late effects. The fraction size that is tolerated in terms of acute effects depends on the volume irradiated (the larger the volume, the smaller the fraction size), the amount and type of dose-limiting normal tissue, the age of the patient, and other clinical factors.

Small changes in fraction size will make a big difference in tolerance. Patients often are given small breaks during the treatment. These rest periods usually are caused by weekend interruptions of daily fractionation. This protraction of the treatment allows for repopulation and recruitment. The days of rest also allow amelioration of many acute effects, and they may allow time for tumor regression, resulting in reoxygenation.

An attempt to formalize and extend treatment breaks is the so-called *split course technique.*[102-104] Two to 3 weeks are allowed in the middle of treatment for recovery from the acute effects and to permit tumor regression. When the dose of radiation is not increased, there is some evidence that this treatment (although better tolerated) may be associated with less tumor control.[105] When the split course is administered with an increase in total dose, the results seem to be comparable to conventional fractionation but perhaps with greater late effects.

Interstitial irradiation is administered in radium needle implants, gold and radon seed implants, iridium wire implants, and other techniques for permanently or temporarily placing radioactive material into tissues. It requires biologic and physical considerations. There is great inhomogeneity in even the most geometrically perfect implant. There is large inhomogeneity of dose and a similar variation in dose rate; the dose rate of radiation is greater in areas of high dose. With temporary implants, the radiologist attempts to administer a calculated dose of between 30 and 100 rad per hour to the minimum tumor location. This is impossible with permanent implants because isotopes decrease their radiation intensity as they decay. The most commonly used isotopes have been radon and ^{198}Au. More recently, ^{125}I has been used and has created unusual new considerations. The half-life of ^{125}I is long (60 days), resulting in a significant amount of the dose being given so slowly that there may be significant cell division occurring in the tumor and some normal cells. Therefore the important dose may not be the total dose, but rather the dose per cell cycle, which is different for each cell type and different as the isotope decays. Also, ^{125}I irradiates primarily by the emission of very low-energy photons, some of which are absorbed by the seeds themselves, leading to even further inhomogeneity.[106]

When implants can be used alone or in combination with external irradiation, the results tend to be better in terms of the therapeutic index than with external beam techniques alone. The high local dose, continuous radiation, and even inhomogeneity allowing normal tissue regrowth all contribute to better cosmetic and functional results and cure of the tumor. Examples are breast cancer and tumors of the tongue and other head and neck sites.[107]

Tumor volume also is important in clinical radiotherapy. Although the gross tumor extent can be determined, most clinicians recognize that a characteristic of tumors is to extend far beyond those macroscopically identifiable borders. Determination of the target volume must include this consideration, but if a larger volume must be irradiated, then a smaller dose is tolerated. Conversely, if the volume of the tumor is larger, then a larger dose is required. This dilemma limited the success of early radiotherapy of certain tumors by reducing the target volume, resulting in recurrences at the treatment margins, or by causing significant complications in the treatment of large target volumes. Today, distinctions are made between gross tumor and the subclinical extensions into apparently normal tissues. Subclinical disease means small numbers of cells, perhaps favorable to irradiation (well-oxygenated), which can be controlled with modest doses of radiation (Table 15–7). The large number of cells present in the clinically evidenced tumor requires higher doses (see curves in Figs. 15–22 and 15–23). This difference has led to the development of techniques for administering different doses to microscopic tumor extensions and to the gross tumor. These include shrinking field techniques, boost treatments, and certain strategies of combined surgery and radiotherapy.

Shrinking field technique means giving the largest potential tumor bed a moderate dose of radiation, then reducing the target volume to the tumor and its immediate confines, raising the dose. This can be done by reducing the fields, by changing the treatment technique and target volume, or by using a treatment technique that gives the desired moderate dose to the larger volume and a higher dose to the smaller volume. A modification of this is the *boost technique,* in which the maximum tolerated dose is given to a volume and then very localized radiation is used to raise the dose to the tumor bed. An implant or an electron boost can be used for this. Attempts have been made to consider fractionation, protraction, and even implantation used with external beam in some form of some mathematical formulae, all of which tend to simplify complex clinical circumstances and can be misleading.

The normal tissues that limit the dose of radiation given may be so close to the tumor that any target volume that in-

TABLE 15–7. Control (%) of Subclinical Disease

Dose (Gy)	Adenocarcinoma of the Breast	Carcinoma of Upper Aerodigestive Tract
30–35	60%–70%	60%–70%
40	80%–90%	>90%
50	>90%	>90%

(Fletcher GH. Clinical dose-response curves of human malignant epithelial tumours. Br J Radiol 1973; 46:1–12)

cludes a tumor must include these normal tissues. Dose-limiting normal tissues are distinguished from these normal tissues transited by the radiation but not in the target volume, although both may produce complications and be dose-limiting. Radiotherapy with detailed treatment planning, CT scanning, and techniques such as computer-controlled radiation therapy, may reduce the dose to the transit volume, possibly changing the therapeutic index.[109] However, it is unlikely that there will be significant physical techniques for reducing the dose to normal tissues in the target volume. This can be done only by some biologic mechanism that distinguishes tumor from normal tissues.

RADIOSENSITIVITY

The term *radiosensitivity* is used in different ways in the literature and can mean what we define as radiosensitivity, radioresponsiveness, or radiocurability. Each is a somewhat different concept. Radiosensitivity means the innate sensitivity of the cells to radiation. For cells that die a reproductive death, this is related to the slope of the survival curve or the D_o.

Radioresponsiveness means the clinical appearance of tumor regression promptly after moderate doses of radiation. This may be a function of the cell's radiosensitivity, but it also may be a function of the active cell kinetics of a tumor. Bergonie and Tribondeau first established an association between the rate of proliferation and the response of normal tissues, although they considered this to be radiosensitivity.[110] A similar relation was presumed to apply to tumors. Because cells will not die until they face mitosis, some tumors that proliferate rapidly will regress rapidly, but they also may regrow rapidly. This is often confused with radiosensitivity. An excellent example is the adenoidcystic tumor of the salivary gland or cylindroma. Such tumors are radioresponsive, but they require very large doses to be cured.

Radiocurability means that the tumor-normal tissue relations are such that curative doses of radiation can be applied regularly without excessive damage to normal tissues. Examples of such radiocurable tumors are carcinomas of the cervix, larynx, breast, and prostate, in addition to Hodgkin's disease and seminomas. Some of these are radioresponsive, some are radiosensitive, and some are neither.

RADIATION AND SURGERY

Radiation and surgery can be combined in many different ways. The general rationale for combining surgery and radiation is that the mechanism of failure for the two techniques is different. Radiation rarely fails at the periphery of tumors, where cells are small in number and well vascularized. When radiation fails, it usually does so in the center of the tumor where there are large volumes of tumor cells often under hypoxic conditions. Surgery, in contrast, is limited by the required preservation of vital normal tissues adjacent to the tumor. In resectable cancers, the gross tumor can be removed, but it is these vital normal tissues that limit the anatomic extent of the dissection. When surgery fails under these circumstances, it is usually due to microscopic tumor cells left behind. It seems logical, therefore, to consider combining the two techniques.

Radiation can be given before or after surgery. Preoperative radiation has the advantages of sterilizing cells at the edges of the resection, sterilizing cells that perhaps would be dislodged and seeded at the time of surgery, and in the special circumstance of unresectable tumors, reducing the tumor volume sufficiently to allow resection. It is not clear how often this really results in a cure, because it may only change gross tumor to microscopic tumor and still result in tumor recurrence. It does seem to benefit selected cases of large unresectable cancers.[111]

There are disadvantages in the use of preoperative irradiation. The pathology reports are not valuable because, if sufficient time is allowed between the radiation and the surgery, the destruction of tumor caused by preoperative radiation prevents ascertainment of the tumor's initial anatomic extent. In contrast, if the tumor is slow-growing or if the surgery is done shortly after the radiation, the consequences of the radiation will not be represented in the pathologic evaluation of the material because sufficient time was not allowed for tumor destruction and regression.

Another disadvantage is that the patient is irradiated before the careful staging available at surgical exploration, and some patients who would not benefit from preoperative radiation are given this treatment (*e.g.,* preoperative radiation to a colorectal carcinoma in a patient with occult liver metastases). Metastases may be found only at the time of surgery.

A disadvantage often mentioned is the delay before surgical resection. This may not be a disadvantage, because as long as the patient's tumor is being treated, the order of treatments should make no difference. The radiation dose usually is moderate (4000 to 5000 rad) and given in conventional 200-rad fractions 5 days a week or in smaller total doses given more quickly in larger fractions. If the total dose of radiation is kept small (less than or equal to 2000 rad), then the delay between radiation and surgery is small. When the dose reaches about 4000 rad, it is valuable to delay the surgery (usually 4 to 6 weeks) to allow the tissues to recover from the radiation. If the total dose is greater than 5000 rad, then the surgery often will be more difficult. However, with moderate doses of radiation and some time allowed between radiation and surgery, the resection can proceed without difficulty.

The use of smaller doses of radiation over short periods of time, without surgical delay, has many advantages and is becoming the preferred technique. With this technique the pathology is less distorted, tumor reduction does not occur significantly, and the surgeon is not lulled into doing too small an operation. If the major value of the preoperative radiation is to prevent seeding, then large doses of radiation are not necessary. For example, preoperative use of intrauterine radium before surgical treatment of carcinoma of the endometrium is an effective way of preventing seeding. This can be done immediately before surgery.

Postoperative radiation has a number of advantages as well. The subgroup of patients who may be helped by radiation can be defined accurately as a consequence of the surgical exploration and pathologic review. Unnecessary irradiation to patients who are not likely to benefit can be avoided, and the target volumes are tailored to meet what is found at surgery. Time can be allowed for wound healing so that the radiation will not interfere with this process. A disadvantage of such treatment is that it has no effect on seeding at the time of surgery. Surgery also may alter the physiology of the tumor left behind because of reduction of the vascular supply. Cells that were well-oxygenated may be rendered physiologically hypoxic and more resistant to radiation. Another disadvantage in the peritoneal cavity is that the surgery causes loops of bowel to be fixed in specific positions and increases the likelihood of small intestinal damage by radiation.

There is some uncertainty as to which technique is better for particular clinical circumstances. Both preoperative and postoperative radiation appear to be valuable and the choice of the method, the dose of radiation, and time between radiation and surgery should be considered in terms of the goals planned.

An additional technique for combining surgery with radiation is limited surgical removal of the gross tumor. Because the gross tumor limits the radiotherapeutic treatment, new interest has been raised in using surgery as the boost technique. Full courses of radiation combined with tumorectomy are given. This surgery can be done before or after the irradiation. An example of this is the "lumpectomy" used in the treatment of breast masses before definitive radiation (see Chap. 40).[112,113] In the latter there appears to be evidence that the removal of gross tumor displaces the sigmoid curve of cure to lower radiation doses and makes it change more steeply with dose (Fig. 15–25).

RADIATION AND CHEMOTHERAPY

The principles of combination radiation and chemotherapy were discussed earlier and emphasized that the purpose of such combined treatment is not to decrease the dose of radiation to gain the same effect, but rather to increase the therapeutic index. This may be achieved using techniques that take advantage of the different mechanisms of action of systemic chemotherapy and regional irradiation. Chemotherapeutic agents that directly modify the radiation survival curve may be used. A good example of this is the use of dactinomycin in the treatment of childhood rhabdomyosarcoma or Wilms tumor. A second way to increase the therapeutic index is to use drugs that specifically affect tumor response to radiation; the most exciting of these are the hypoxic sensitizers because they affect hypoxic cells that usually are restricted to tumors.

A third mechanism is the combination of drugs and roentgen rays with independent action or additivity. This is just beginning to be explored but appears to be of value in increased local control achieved in head and neck cancer when chemotherapy is given before radiation.[114] Also, enhanced local control is obtained when radiotherapy is followed by or administered concomitantly with adjuvant chemotherapy in locally advanced breast cancer.[115]

Because the major advantage of chemotherapy is its wide distribution throughout the body, the combination of radiation and chemotherapy may improve the therapeutic index because, like the combination of surgery and irradiation, the target volumes are different. Adjuvant chemotherapy with radiation for breast cancer, or with surgery and radiation for colon cancer, may improve survival because the chemotherapy is effective against occult micrometastases outside the radiation field. Similarly, radiation may be of value in the treatment of leukemia by chemotherapy because the radiation can be applied to specific sanctuary sites, such as the central nervous system. This is discussed further in Chapter 49.

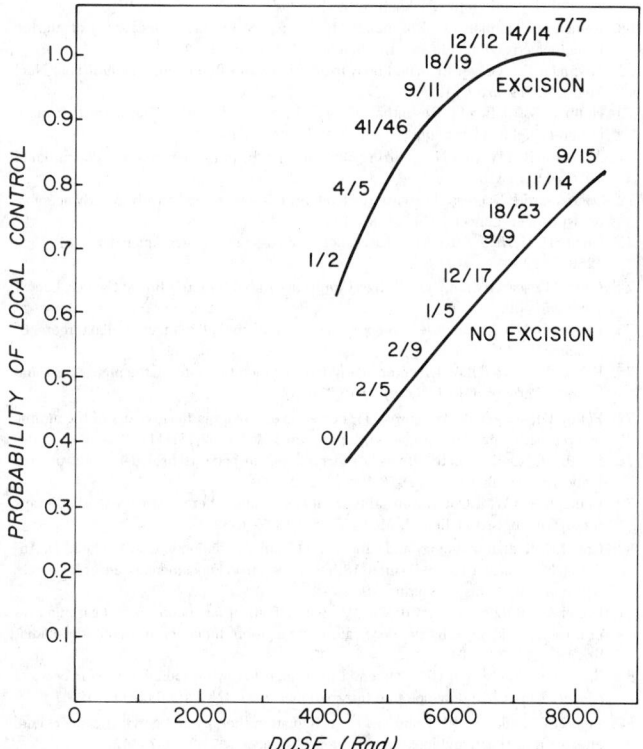

FIGURE 15–25. Tumor control versus dose for breast cancer stages II and III. (Hellman S. Improving the therapeutic index in breast cancer treatment. Cancer Res 1980;40:4335–4342)

REFERENCES

1. Johns HE, Cunningham JR. The physics of radiology. Springfield, IL: Charles C Thomas, 1977.
2. Thompson LH, Suit HD. Proliferation kinetics of x-irradiated mouse L cells studied with timelapse photography, part II. Int J Radiat Biol 1969;15:347–362.
3. Elkind MM. The initial part of the survival curve: Does it predict the outcome of fractionated radiotherapy? Radiat Res 1988;144(3):425–436.
4. Weichselbaum RR, Nove J, Little JB. X-ray sensitivity of human tumor cells in vitro. Int J Radiat Oncol Biol Phys 1980;6:437–440.
5. Till JE, McCulloch EA. A direct measurement of the radiation sensitivity of normal mouse bone marrow cells. Radiat Res 1961;14:213–222.
6. Withers HR, Elkind MM. Microcolony survival assay for cells of mouse intestinal mucosa exposed to radiation. Int J Radiat Biol 1970;17:261–267.
7. Alper T, Gillies NE. Restoration of *Escherichia coli* Strain B irradiation: Its dependence on suboptimal growth conditions. J Gen Microbiol 1958;18:461–472.
8. Phillips RA, Tolmach LJ. Repair of potentially lethal damage in x-irradiated HeLa cells. Radiat Res 1966;29:413–432.
9. Little JB, Hahn GM, Frindel E, et al. Repair of potentially lethal radiation damage in vitro and in vivo. Radiology 1973;106:689–694.
10. Belli JA, Shelton M. Potentially lethal radiation damage: Repair of mammalian cells in culture. Science 1969;165:490–492.
11. Weichselbaum R, Little JB, Nove J. Response of human osteosarcoma in vitro to irradiation: Evidence for unusual cellular repair activity. Int J Radiat Biol 1977;31:295–299.
12. Elkind MM, Sutton H. Radiation response of mammalian cells grown in culture: part 1. Repair of x-ray damage in surviving Chinese hamster cells. Radiat Res 1960;13:556–593.
13. Hall EJ. Radiation dose-rate: A factor of importance in radiobiology and radiotherapy. Br J Radiol 1972;45:81–97.
14. Mottram JC. Factors of importance in radiosensitivity of tumors. Br J Radiol 1936;9:606–614.
15. Read J. The effect of ionizing radiation on the broad beam root: The dependence of the x-ray sensitivity on dissolved oxygen. Br J Radiol 1952;25:89–99.
16. Gray LH, Coger AD, Ebert M, et al. The concentration of oxygen dissolved in tissues at the time of irradiation as a factor in radiotherapy. Br J Radiol 1953;26:638–648.
17. Belli JA, Dicus GJ, Bonte FJ. Radiation response of mammalian tumor cells: part 1. Repair of sublethal damage in vivo. JNCI 1967;38:673–682.

18. Deschner EE, Gray LH. Influence of oxygen tension on x-ray induced chromosomal damage in Ehrlich ascites tumor cells irradiated in vitro and in vivo. Radiat Res 1959;11:115–146.

19. Thomlinson RH, Gray LH. The histological structure of some human lung cancers and possible implications for radiotherapy. Br J Cancer 1955;9:539–549.

20. Kallman RF. The phenomenon of reoxygenation and its implications for fractionated radiotherapy. Radiology 1972;105:135–142.

21. Henk JM, Kindler PB, Smith CW. Radiotherapy and head and neck cancer: Final report of the first clinical trial. Lancet 1977;2:101–103.

22. Henk JM, Smith CW. Radiotherapy and head and neck cancer: Interim report of second clinical trial. Lancet 1977;2:104–105.

23. Watson ER, Halman KE, Dische S, et al. Hyperbaric oxygen and radiotherapy: A Medical Research Council trial in carcinoma of the cervix. Br J Radiol 1978;51:879–887.

24. Adams GE, Dewez DL. Hydrated electrons and radiobiological sensitization. Biochem Biophys Res Commun 1963;12:473–477.

25. Adams GE, Ahmed L, Fielden EM, et al. The development of some nitroimidazoles as hypoxic cell sensitizers. Cancer Clin Trials 1980;3:37–42.

26. Stratford LJ, Adams GE. Effect of hyperthermia on differential cytotoxicity of a hypoxic cell radiosensitizer RO-07-0582 on mammalian cells in vitro. Br J Cancer 1977;35:307–313.

27. Rose CM, Millar JL, Peacock JH, et al. Differential enhancement of toxicity in tumors and normal tissues by misonidazole. In: Proceedings of the Key Biscayne Conference on Hypoxic Cell Sensitizers and Radioprotectors. New York: Masson, 1980.

28. Bush RS, Jenkin RP, Allt WE, et al. Definitive evidence for hypoxic cells influencing cure in cancer therapy. Br J Cancer 1978;37:302–306.

29. Kolstad P. Intercapillary distance, oxygen tension, and local recurrence in cervix cancer. Scan J Clin Lab Invest 1968;106(Suppl):145–157.

30. Urtasun RC, Koch CJ, Franko AJ, et al. A novel technique for measuring human tissue PO_2 at the cellular level. Br J Cancer 1986;54:453–457.

31. Urtasun RC, Chapman JD, Raleigh JA, et al. Binding of ^{3}H-misonidazole to solid human tumors as a measure of tumor hypoxia. Int J Rad Oncol Biol Phys 1986;12:1263–1267.

32. Terasima R, Tolmach LJ. X-ray sensitivity and DNA synthesis in synchronous populations of HeLa cells. Science 1963;140:490–492.

33. Sinclair WK, Morton RA. X-ray sensitivity during the cell generation cycle of cultured Chinese hamster cells. Radiat Res 1966;29:450–474.

34. Chaffey JT, Hellman S. Differing responses to radiation of murine bone marrow stem cells in relation to the cell cycle. Cancer Res 1971;31:1613–1615.

35. Madoc-Jones H, Mauro F. Age response to x-rays vinca alkaloids and hydroxyurea of murine lymphoma cells synchronized in vivo. JNCI 1970;45:1131–1143.

36. Hellman S. Cell kinetics, models, and cancer treatment: Some principles for the radiation oncologist. Radiology 1975;114:219–223.

37. Chaffey JT, Hellman S. Radiation fractionation as applied to murine colony-forming units in differing proliferative states. Radiology 1969;93:1167–1172.

38. Chaffey JT, Hellman S. Studies on dose fractionation as measured by endogenous spleen colonies in the mouse. Radiology 1968;90:363–365.

39. Hermens AF, Barendson GW. Changes in cell proliferation characteristics in a rat rhabdomyosarcoma before and after x-irradiation. Eur J Cancer Clin Oncol 1969;5:173–189.

39a. Sherman ML, Datta R, Hallahan DE, et al. Ionizing radiation regulates expression of the *c-jun* proto-oncogene. Proc Natl Acad Sci USA 1990;87:5663–5666.

39b. Hallahan DE, Sukhatme VP, Sherman ML, et al. Protein kinase C mediates x-ray inducibility of nuclear signal transducers EGR1 and JUN. Proc Natl Acad Sci USA 1991;88:2156–2160.

39c. Hallahan DE, Spriggs DR, Beckett MA, et al. Increased tumor necrosis factor αmRNA after cellular exposure to ionizing radiation. Proc Natl Acad Sci USA 1989;86:10104–10107.

39d. Sherman ML, Datta R, Hallahan DE, et al. Tumor necrosis factor gene expression is transcriptionally and post-transcriptionally regulated by ionizing radiation in human myeloid leukemic cells and peripheral blood monocytes. J Clin Ivest 1991;87:1794–1797.

39e. Witte L, Fuks Z, Haimovitz-Friedman A, et al. Effects of radiation on the release of growth factors from cultured bovine, porcine and human endothelial cells. Cancer Res 1989;49:5066–5072.

39f. Weichselbaum RR, Hallahan DE, Sukhatme V, et al. Biological consequences of gene regulation after ionizing radiation exposure. JNCI 1991;83:480–484.

40. Szybalski W. X-ray sensitization by halopyrimidines. Cancer Chemother Rep 1974;58:539–557.

41. Piro AJ, Taylor CC, Belli JA. Interaction between radiation and drug damage in mammalian cells, part 1. Delayed expression of actinomycin D/x-ray effects in exponential and plateau phase cells. Radiat Res 1975;63:346–362.

42. D'Angio GJ, Farber S, Maddock CL. Potentiation of x-ray effects by actinomycin D. Radiology 1959;73:175–177.

43. Bases RE. Modification of the radiation response determined by single-cell techniques: Actinomycin D. Cancer Res 1959;19:1223–1229.

44. Elkind MM, Whitmore GF, Alescio T. Actinomycin D: Suppression of recovery in x-irradiated mammalian cells. Science 1964;143:1454–1456.

45. Pinkel D. Actinomycin D in childhood cancer: A preliminary report. Pediatrics 1959;23:342–347.

46. Hellman S, Hannon E. Effects of Adriamycin on the radiation response of murine hematopoietic stem cells. Radiat Res 1976;67:162–167.

47. Belli JA, Piro AJ. The interaction between radiation and adriamycin damage in mammalian cells. Cancer Res 1977;37:1624–1630.

48. Cassady JR, Richter MP, Piro AJ, et al. Radiation-adriamycin interactions: Preliminary clinical observations. Cancer 1975;36:946–949.

49. Donaldson SC, Glick JM, Wilbur JR: Adriamycin activating a recall phenomenon after radiation therapy. Ann Intern Med 1974;81:407–408.

50. Sinclair WK. Hydroxyurea: Effects on Chinese hamster cells grown in culture. Cancer Res 1967;27:297–308.

51. Yuhas JM, Yurconic M, Kligerman MM, et al. Combined use of radioprotective and radiosensitizing drugs in experimental radiotherapy. Radiat Res 1977;70:433–443.

52. Barendsen GW. Response of cultured cells, tumours, and normal tissues to radiations of different linear energy transfer. Curr Top Radiat Res 1968;4:293–356.

53. Bloomer WD, Hellman S. Normal tissue responses to radiation therapy. N Engl J Med 1975;293:80–83.

54. Holthusen H. Erfahrungen über die Vertaglichkeitsgrenze fur Röntgenstrahler und deren Nutzanwendung zur Verhutung von Schaden. Strahlentherapie 1936;57:254–269.

55. Suit HD, Goitein M. Rationale for use of charged-particle and fast-neutron beams in radiation therapy. In: Meyn RE, Withers HR, eds. Radiation biology in cancer research. New York: Raven Press, 1980.

56. Thomlinson RH. An experimental method for comparing treatments of intact tumors in animals and its application to the use of oxygen in radiotherapy. Br J Cancer 1960;14:555–576.

57. Folkman J, Tyler K. Tumor angiogenesis: Its possible role in metastasis and invasion. In: Day B, Myers WP, Stans Garattini S, et al, eds. Cancer invasion and metastasis: Mechanisms and therapy, vol 5. New York: Raven Press, 1977:95–103.

58. Folkman J. Tumor angiogenesis: A possible control point in tumor growth. Ann Intern Med 1975;82:96–100.

59. Folkman J, Langer R, Linhardt RJ, et al. Angiogenesis inhibition and tumor regression caused by heparin or a heparin fragment in the presence of cortisone. Science 1983;221:719–725.

60. Powers WE, Tolmach LV. A multicomponent x-ray survival curve for mouse lymphosarcoma cells irradiation in vitro. Nature 1963;197:710–711.

61. Fertil B, Malaise EP. Inherent cellular radiosensitivity as a basic concept for human tumor radiotherapy. Int J Radiat Oncol Biol Phys 1981;7:621–629.

62. Deacon J, Peckham MJ, Steel GG. The radioresponsiveness of human tumours and the initial slope of the cell survival curve. Radiother Oncol 1984;2:317–323.

63. Malaise EP, Fertil B, Chavaudra N, et al. Distribution of radiation sensitivities for human tumor cells of specific histological types: Comparison of in vitro to in vivo data. Int J Radiat Oncol Biol Phys 1986;12:617–624.

64. Weichselbaum RR, Dahlberg W, Little JB. Inherently radioresistant cells exist in some human tumors. Proc Natl Acad Sci USA 1985;82:4732–4735.

65. Rubin P, Casarett GW. Clinical radiation pathology. Philadelphia: WB Saunders, 1968.

66. Reinhold HS, Buisman GH. Radiosensitivity of capillary endothelium. Br J Radiol 1973;46:54–57.

67. Filler RM, Tefft M, Vawter GF, et al. Hepatic lobectomy in childhood: Effects of x-ray and chemotherapy. J Pediatr Surg 1969;4:31–41.

68. Reincke U, Hannon EC, Rosenblatt M, Hellman S. Proliferative capacity of murine hematopoietic stem cells in vitro. Science 1982;215:1619–1622.

69. Medinger FG, Craver LF. Total-body irradiation. Am J Roentgenol Radium Ther Nucl Med 1942;48:651–671.

70. Hellman S, Chaffey JT, Rosenthal DS, et al. Place of radiation therapy in the treatment of non-Hodgkin's lymphomas. Cancer 1977;39:843–851.

71. Anderson RE, Warner NL. Ionizing radiation and the immune response. Adv Immunol 1976;24:215–335.

72. Stjernsward J. Decreased survival related to irradiation postoperatively in early operable breast cancer. Lancet 1974;2:1285–1286.

73. Levitt SH, McHugh RB. Early breast cancer and postoperative irradiation. Lancet 1975;2:1258–1259.

74. Cancer Research Campaign (Kings/Cambridge) Trial for Early Breast Cancer. Lancet 1980;2:55–60.

75. Fletcher GH. Clinical dose-response curves of human malignant epithelial tumors. Br J Radiol 1973;46:1–12.

76. Kohn HI, Melvold RW. Divergent x-ray-induced mutation rates in the mouse for Hand "7 locus" groups of loci. Nature 1976;259:209–210.

77. Folley JH, Borges W, Yamawaki T. Incidence of leukemia in survivors of the atomic bomb in Hiroshima and Nagasaki, Japan. Am J Med 1952;13:311–321.

78. Smith PG, Doll R. Late effects of x-irradiation in patients healed for metropathia hemorrhagica. Br J Radiol 1976;49:224–232.

79. Court Brown WM, Doll R. Mortality from cancer and other causes after radiotherapy for ankylosing spondylitis. Br Med J 1965;2:1327–1332.

80. Gray LH. Radiation biology and cancer. In: Cellular radiation biology—The M.D. Anderson Hospital and Tumor Institute 18th Symposium on Fundamental Cancer Research. Baltimore: Williams & Wilkins, 1965:7–25.

81. Upton AC, Randolph ML, Conklin JW: Late effects of fast neutrons and gamma rays in mice as influenced by the dose rate of irradiation: Induction of neoplasia. Radiat Res 1970;41:467–491.

82. Boice JD, Hutchinson GB. Leukemia in women following radiotherapy for cervical cancer: Ten-year follow-up of an international study. JNCI 1980;65:115–129.

83. Zippen C, Bailar JC III, Kohn HI, et al. Radiation therapy and cervical cancer: Late effects on life span and leukemia incidence. Cancer 1971;28:937–942.

84. Shukovsky LJ. Dose, time, volume relationships in squamous cell carcinoma of the supraglottic larynx. Am J Roentgenol Rad Ther Nucl Med 1970;108:27–29.

85. Kaplan HS. Evidence for a tumoricidal dose level in the radiotherapy of Hodgkin's disease. Cancer Res 1966;26:1221–1224.

86. Stewart JG, Jackson AW. The steepness of the dose-response curve both for tumor and normal tissue injury. Laryngoscope 1975;85:1107–1111.

87. Zagars GK, Schultheiss TE, Peters LJ. Inter-tumor heterogeneity and radiation dose-control curves. Radiother Oncol 1987;8:353–362.

88. Coutard H. Roentgen therapy of epitheliomas of the tonsillar region, hypopharynx, and larynx from 1920 to 1926. AJR 1932;28:313–331.

89. Regaud C, Ferroux R. Discordance des effets des rayons X, d'une part dans la peau, d'autre part dans le testicule par le fractionement de la dose: Diminution de l'efficacite dans le peau, maintien de l'efficacite dans le testicule. Compt Rend Soc Biol 1927;97: 431–434.

90. Danlos H. Quelques considerations sur le traitement des dermatoses par le radium. J Physiotherapie (Paris) 1905;3:98–106.

91. Botnick L, Hannon EC, Hellman S. Multisystem stem cell failure after apparent recovery from alkylating agents. Cancer Res 1978;38:1942–1947.

92. Hellman S, Botnick LE. Stem cell depletion: An explanation of the late effects of cytotoxins. Int J Radiat Oncol Biol Phys 1977;2:181–184.

93. Harris JR, Recht A, Almaric R, et al. Time course and prognosis of local recurrence following primary radiation therapy for early breast cancer. J Clin Oncol 1984;2:37–41.

94. Goodman LS, Gilman A. The pharmacological basis of therapeutics. London: Macmillan, 1970:21.

95. Withers HR, Peters LJ, Thames HD, et al: Hyperfractionation. Int J Radiat Oncol Biol Phys 1982;8:1807–1809.

96. Withers HR, Thames HA, Peters LJ. Dose fractionation and volume effects in normal tissues and tumors. Cancer Treat Symp 1984;1:75–83.

97. Shank B, Chu FCH, Dinsmore R, et al. Hyperfractionated total body irradiation for bone marrow transplantation: Results in seventy leukemia patients with allogeneic transplants. Int J Radiat Oncol Biol Phys 1983;9:1607–1611.

98. Thames HD Jr, Peters LJ, Withers HR, et al. Accelerated fractionation vs hyperfractionation: Rationales for several treatments per day. Int J Radiat Oncol Biol Phys 1983;9:127–138.

99. Dutreix J, Wambersie A, Bounik C. Cellular recovery in human skin reactions: Application to dose, fraction number, overall time relationship in radiotherapy. Eur J Cancer Clin Oncol 1973;9:159–167.

100. Marks RD, Witherspoon BJ, Davis LW, et al. Hyperfractionation—where do we stand: A preliminary report. Int J Radiat Oncol Biol Phys 1978;4(Suppl):139–140.

101. Norin T, Onyango J. Radiotherapy in Burkitt's lymphoma: Conventional or superfractionated regime—early results. Int J Radiat Oncol Biol Phys 1977;2:399–406.

102. Scanlon P. Split-dose radiotherapy: The original premise. Int J Radiat Oncol Biol Phys 1980;6:527–528.

103. Sambrook DK. Split-course radiation therapy in malignant tumors. Am J Roentgenol 1964;91:37–45.

104. Parsons JT, Thar TL, Bova FJ, et al. An evaluation of split-course irradiation for pelvic malignancies. Int J Radiat Oncol Biol Phys 1980;6:175–181.

105. Parsons JT, Bova FJ, Million RR. A re-evaluation of the University of Florida split-course technique for squamous carcinoma of the head and neck. Int J Radiat Oncol Biol Phys 1980;6:1645–1652.

106. Ling CC, Anderson LL, Shipley WU: Dose inhomogeneity in interstitial implants using ^{125}I seeds. Int J Radiat Oncol Biol Phys 1979;5:419–425.

107. Pierquin B, Chassagne D, Baillet F, et al. Clinical observations on the time factor in interstitial radiotherapy using iridium-192. Clin Radiol 1973;24:506–509.

108. Beadle GF, Silver B, Botnick L, et al. Cosmetic results following primary radiation therapy for early breast cancer. Cancer 1984;54:2911–2918.

109. Levene MB, Kijewski PK, Chin LM, et al. Computer controlled radiation therapy. Radiology 1978;129:769–775.

110. Bergonie J, Tribondeau L. Interpretation of some results of radiotherapy and an attempt at determining a logical technique of treatment. Radiat Res 1959;11:587–588.

111. Kligerman MM. Radiotherapy and rectal cancer. Cancer 1977;39:896–900.

112. Harris JR, Beadle GF, Hellman S. Clinical studies on the use of radiation therapy as primary treatment of early breast cancer. Cancer 1984;53:705–711.

113. Hellman S. Improving the therapeutic index in breast cancer treatment. Cancer Res 1980;40:4335–4342.

114. Ervin TJ, Weichselbaum RR, Fabian RL, et al. Advanced squamous carcinoma of the head and neck: A preliminary report of neoadjuvant chemotherapy with cisplatin, bleomycin, and methotrexate. Arch Otolaryngol 1984;110:241–245.

115. Harris JR, Sawicka J, Gelman R, et al. Management of locally advanced carcinoma of the breast. Int J Radiat Oncol Biol Phys 1983;9:345–349.

Cancer: Principles & Practice of Oncology, Fourth Edition,
edited by Vincent T. DeVita, Jr., Samuel Hellman, Steven A. Rosenberg.
J.B. Lippincott Co., Philadelphia © 1993.

Vincent T. DeVita, Jr

CHAPTER **16**

Principles of Chemotherapy

HISTORY

Cancer chemotherapy had its roots in the work of Paul Ehrlich, who coined the word chemotherapy. Ehrlich's use of rodent models of infectious diseases to develop antibiotics led George Clowes, at Roswell Park Memorial Institute in Buffalo, New York, in the early 1900s, to develop inbred rodent lines that could carry transplanted tumors.[1] These types of models served as the testing ground for potential cancer chemotherapeutic agents and only recently have been effectively supplemented by human cells grown in culture. Alkylating agents, the first modern chemotherapeutic agents, were a product of the secret war gas program in both world wars. An explosion in Bari Harbor during World War II[2,3] and the exposure of seamen to mustard gas led to the observation that alkylating agents caused marrow and lymphoid hypoplasia, which led to their use in humans with hematopoietic neoplasms such as Hodgkin's disease and lymphocytic lymphomas, first attempted at Yale-New Haven Medical Center in 1943. Because of the secret nature of the gas warfare program, this work was not published until 1946.[1,4] The demonstration of dramatic regressions in advanced lymphomas with chemicals caused much excitement and later much disappointment, because the tumors invariably grew back. After Farber's observation on the effects of folic acid on leukemic cell growth in children with lymphoblastic leukemia and the development of the folic acid antagonists as cancer drugs, the chemotherapy of cancer began in earnest. The cure of childhood leukemias and Hodgkin's disease with combination chemotherapy in the 1960s proved that human cancers, even in their advanced stages, could be cured by drugs, and the application to the chemotherapy of solid tumors began.

CHEMOTHERAPY AS PART OF THE INITIAL TREATMENT OF CANCER

There are four ways chemotherapy is generally used[5]: as an induction treatment for advanced disease, as an adjunct to the local methods of treatment, as the primary treatment for patients who present with localized cancer, and by direct installation into sanctuaries or by site-directed perfusion of specific regions of the body most affected by the cancer.

The term *induction chemotherapy* has been used to describe the drug therapy given as the primary treatment for patients who present with advanced cancer for which no alternative treatment exists.[6] Development of new treatments is based on the effectiveness of the cancer drugs in rodent models. Combinations of drugs are fashioned based on the effectiveness, the level of cross-resistance, and the limiting toxicity of the available drugs when used alone in similar patient populations. Patients who fail after one drug treatment and require further chemotherapy pose a particularly difficult treatment problem because of the volume of tumor, their poor general health, and drug resistance. Induction chemotherapy in these patients is referred to as *salvage treatment*.

Adjuvant chemotherapy denotes the use of systemic treatment after the primary tumor has been controlled by an alternative method, such as surgery and radiotherapy. The selection of an adjuvant treatment program for a particular patient is based on response rates in separate groups of patients with advanced cancers of the same histologic type. The determination of a population of patients as suitable for adjuvant treatment is based on available data on their average risk of recurrence after local treatment alone and on disease variables known to influence prognosis adversely.

Primary chemotherapy denotes the use of chemotherapy as the initial treatment for patients who present with localized cancer for which there is an alternative, but less than completely effective, treatment. This approach also has been called *neoadjuvant chemotherapy,* but the term *primary chemotherapy* is more accurate.[7,8] For chemotherapy to be used as the primary treatment of a partially curable, localized cancer, there must be considerable evidence for the effectiveness of the drug program against advanced disease of the same type.

CLINICAL ENDPOINTS IN EVALUATING RESPONSE TO CHEMOTHERAPY

INDUCTION CHEMOTHERAPY

In induction chemotherapy for advanced cancer, it is possible to determine the response to drugs on a case-by-case basis. The partial response rate is usually defined as the fraction of patients that demonstrates at least a 50% reduction in measurable tumor mass; such responses usually are not of much value clinically, because they usually are brief and offset by the drug toxicity associated with continuous treatment. However, partial responses are useful in the evaluation of new drugs, or new drug programs, to determine whether the particular experimental approach is worth pursuing further. *The most important indicator of the effectiveness of chemotherapy is the complete response rate—it is the prerequisite for cure.* When new programs consistently produce more than an occasional complete remission, they have invariably later proved of practical value in medical practice. The qualitative and quantitative differences in the clinical value between a complete and a partial response are such that complete responses should always be reported separately. The most important indicator of the quality of a complete remission is the relapse-free survival from the time all treatment is discontinued. This criteria is the only clinical counterpart of the quantifiable cytoreductive effect of drugs in rodent systems. A current trend among many clinical investigators is the use of "freedom from progression" of patients who have attained complete and partial responses, measured as a combined group.[8] This method is said to be an indicator of the practical potential of a new treatment, but it obscures the value of a relapse-free survival of complete responders as the major determinant of the quality of remission and the potential for cure. Other endpoints, such as median response duration and median survival, are also of little practical value until treatment results have been refined so that the complete response rate is higher than 50%.

ADJUVANT CHEMOTHERAPY

There was great excitement concomitant with the use of chemotherapy as an adjunct to local treatments. The promise was great, because tumor volume is at a minimum when adjuvant therapy is initiated, and it was assumed that treatment with drugs at this stage would produce a much higher cure rate or that treatment intensity could be reduced and side effects thereby diminished, without loss of therapeutic effectiveness. Both assumptions have little scientific basis. Failure

to appreciate the problems surrounding the assessment of the response of a group of patients to adjuvant chemotherapy is the source of some of the current disillusionment with the positive, but less than dramatic, results achieved with adjuvant chemotherapy in common tumors, such as breast and colorectal cancers.[9,10]

It should be remembered that the major indicator of effectiveness of a chemotherapy program—the complete remission rate—is lost in the adjuvant setting, because the primary tumor has already been removed. In the clinic, treatment is selected for individual patients based on response rates in an entirely different population of patients with advanced disease with the same histologic type. Relapse-free survival remains the major endpoint, but the micrometastases in the population of adjuvant-treated patients consist of a mixture of tumor cells, some of which can be expected to be sensitive to chemotherapy, and others resistant. The relapse-free survival in the adjuvant setting, therefore, measures time to regrowth of cells unresponsive, partially responsive, or very sensitive to chemotherapy and is the equivalent of the duration of remission of complete and partial responders and the interval of regrowth in patients who would have been classified as nonresponders. In this sense, it is similar to the use of freedom from progression in patients with advanced disease. Attempts to use in vitro assays of drug sensitivity from the biopsy material of primary tumors to overcome the shortcomings of the absence of an indicator of individual response have not proved practical.

PRIMARY CHEMOTHERAPY

The unique feature of using chemotherapy in patients with localized tumor, before or instead of purely local treatments, is the preservation of the presenting tumor mass as a biologic marker of responsiveness to the drugs. As with induction chemotherapy for patients with advanced cancer, it is possible to determine, on a case-by-case basis, the potential effectiveness of a new treatment program. By definition, the presenting tumor mass is also the largest aggregate of tumor in the body and, historically, the oldest, and it is therefore the aggregate mass of tumor cells most likely to contain one or more resistant cell lines.[11] Being the largest mass of cells, it is also the mass with the least favorable cell kinetics. It is reasonable to assume, then, that whatever the effect of chemotherapy the physician sees on the primary tumor, a similar or greater effect is occurring fairly uniformly in micrometastatic deposits. A poor response of the primary tumor to chemotherapy indicates a group of patients for which alternative methods of treatment should be used quickly. Another feature of primary chemotherapy is the ability to delineate partial responders with varying degrees of prognosis, as determined by the state of the residual tumor mass after an initial good but partial response. Removal of residual tumor and histologic examination of the tissue allow determination of the viability of the remaining tumor mass. The response duration of complete and partial responders must be catalogued separately.

The most important issue facing investigators of primary chemotherapy is whether an effective primary chemotherapy treatment, pursued flexibly and intensively to complete remission, plus two or more additional cycles of treatment, will define a significant fraction of patients whose disease is cured by chemotherapy alone, without the addition of alternative treatments. In carefully selected patients with some stages of the commonest tumors for which there is less than satisfactory standard treatment, such studies are ethically and theoretically sound and are being pursued. Such an approach could result in briefer, less morbid, and more effective treatment programs.[5]

The use of chemotherapy as the primary treatment is reviewed, when appropriate, in each of the disease-oriented chapters. Table 16–1 lists tumors in which primary chemotherapy for localized forms of the cancer in question have already been incorporated in clinic protocols (first and second categories) and in which current clinical trials show considerable progress (third category).[12–17]

SPECIAL USES OF CHEMOTHERAPY

Special uses of chemotherapy include (1) the installation of drugs into the spinal fluid, directly through a lumbar puncture needle or into an implanted Ommaya reservoir, to treat meningeal leukemia and lymphoma, and into the pleural or the pericardial space to control effusions; (2) splenic infusion to control spleen size; (3) hepatic artery infusion to treat hepatic metastases selectively; (4) carotid artery infusion to treat head and neck cancers and brain tumors; and (5) intraperitoneal installation of drugs using dialysis techniques. These uses are discussed throughout this book in relation to specific cancers. In all instances, the rationale for directed chemotherapy is based on achieving a higher concentration over time ($C \times T$) against the target tumor tissue while sparing normal tissue. The usefulness of intracerebrospinal fluid and intrapleural administration of drugs is already established. Hepatic infusion

TABLE 16–1. Primary Chemotherapy

Neoplasms in Which Chemotherapy Is the Primary Therapeutic Modality

Localized diffuse large cell lymphoma
Burkitt's lymphoma
Childhood Hodgkin's disease
Wilms' tumor
Embryonal rhabdomyosarcoma
Small cell lung cancer

Neoplasms in Which Primary Chemotherapy Can Allow Less Mutilating Surgery

Anal carcinoma
Bladder carcinoma
Breast cancer
Laryngeal cancer
Osteogenic sarcoma
Soft tissue sarcomas

Neoplasms in Which Clinical Trials Indicate an Expanding Role for Primary Chemotherapy in the Future

Non-small-cell lung cancer
Breast cancer
Esophageal cancer
Nasopharyngeal cancer
Other cancers of the head and neck region

of chemotherapy has been simplified and improved enough by the development of technology for the infusion of drugs that a reevaluation of this approach is justified (see Chap. 61, section 3). It is now possible to measure the active principles of cancer drugs and their targets within the biologic range, and drugs can be infused in timing with the body's circadian rhythm (see Chap. 69, section 7).

The intraperitoneal administration of drugs to treat ovarian cancer, a disease that kills almost exclusively by local effects in the abdomen, is now being investigated, because it allows a wide distribution of antitumor drugs in the smallest interstices of the abdominal cavity, and because a higher $C \times T$ at the tumor is achieved (see Chaps. 18 and 39).[18,19] The concentration of drug available in the peritoneal cavity for some drugs with this "belly bath" technique far exceeds the plasma level achievable with systemic administration. The effects are particularly marked for drugs such as 5-fluorouracil, which is metabolized in the liver and excreted by the kidney, and doxorubicin and cisplatin, which, because of their molecular size, diffuse more slowly across the peritoneal membrane. A similar approach is being explored with abdominal installation of photoaffinity compounds, with subsequent exposure to laser light sources (see Chap. 69, section 7).

Drugs can also be encompassed in lipid bilayer droplets called *liposomes*.[20–22] The surface characteristics of liposomes can be altered to direct their delivery to specific organ sites or into resistant cell lines. Labile liposomes that dissolve at temperatures of 41°C can deposit drugs selectively in preheated areas.[21] A disadvantage of liposomes, however, is their failure to leave the vascular system except in the sinusoids of the liver and the spleen; liposome encapsulation of drugs for targeted delivery has been of limited value.[22]

PRINCIPLES GOVERNING THE USE OF COMBINATION CHEMOTHERAPY

With some exceptions (*e.g.*, choriocarcinoma and Burkitt's lymphoma), single drugs do not cure cancer. It became apparent in the 1960s that drug combinations are necessary to produce durable clinical responses. In the early years of chemotherapy, drug combinations were developed based on known biochemical actions of available anticancer drugs rather than on their clinical effectiveness. These programs were largely ineffective.[23–27] The era of effective combination chemotherapy began when an array of active drugs from different classes became available for use in combination in the treatment of leukemias and lymphomas. Combination chemotherapy has now been extended to the treatment of most other malignancies, as described throughout this text.

Combination chemotherapy accomplishes three important objectives not possible with single-agent treatment. It provides maximal cell kill within the range of toxicity tolerated by the host for each drug; it provides a broader range of coverage of resistant cell lines in a heterogenous tumor population; and it prevents or slows the development of new resistant lines.

The following principles have been useful in the selection of drugs in the most effective drug combinations, and they guide the development of new programs:

1. Only drugs known to be partially effective when used alone should be selected for use in combination. If avail-

able, drugs that produce some fraction of complete remission are preferred to those that produce only partial responses.

2. When several drugs of a class are available and are equally effective, a drug should be selected on the basis of toxicity that does not overlap with the toxicity of other drugs to be used in the combination. Although such selection leads to a wider range of side effects and more general discomfort for the patient, it minimizes the risk of a lethal effect caused by multiple insults to the same organ system by different drugs and allows dose intensity to be maximized.

3. Drugs should be used in their optimal dose and schedule.

4. Drug combinations should be given at consistent intervals. The treatment-free interval between cycles should be the shortest possible time necessary for recovery of the most sensitive normal target tissue, which is usually the bone marrow.

Omission of a drug from a combination may allow overgrowth by a cell line sensitive to that drug alone and resistant to other drugs in the combination. Also, arbitrarily reducing the dose of an effective drug to add other less effective drugs may reduce the dose of the most effective agent below the threshold of effectiveness and destroy the capacity of the combination to cure that particular patient.

Bone marrow has a storage compartment that can supply mature cells to the peripheral blood for 8 to 10 days after the stem cell pool has been damaged by cytotoxic drugs. Events measured in the peripheral blood are usually a week behind events occurring in the bone marrow. In previously untreated patients, leukopenia and thrombocytopenia are discernible on the ninth or tenth day after initial dosing. Nadir blood counts are noted between days 14 to 18, with recovery apparent by day 21 and usually complete by day 28. Prior treatment with drugs or x-radiation may alter this sequence by depleting the stem cell pool, shortening the time to the appearance of leukopenia and thrombocytopenia, and prolonging the recovery time. Curiously, when the second half of a combination given in the clinic on a day 1, day 8 schedule is omitted, leukopenia and thrombocytopenia comparable with that seen with the full combination usually occur, suggesting that the second set of doses does not cause an equal increment in bone marrow suppression, possibly because the stem cell compartment is still in a quiescent state. This result also suggests that, in most instances, the day-8 doses can be given safely, even if leukopenia and thrombocytopenia have already become evident. The interval of greatest importance in the clinic is the duration of the nadir level of leukocytes and platelets. The highest risk of infection or bleeding occurs with granulocyte counts lower than 500/dl and platelet counts lower than 20,000/dl. If this nadir lasts only 4 to 7 days, it is tolerated by most patients without supplemental support. Increasing doses of most anticancer drugs, within the range of the maximally tolerated dose, usually does not ablate the marrow or even prolong the time to recovery. Repeated dosing during the phase of early recovery of the marrow (days 16–21), however, may cause severer toxicity in the second treatment cycle in patients whose marrow is not the source of, or involved with, the tumor.

These types of data led to the familiar 2-week interval between cycles of the most effective drug combinations (new cycles begin on day 28 after the first dose) to accommodate the recovery time of human bone marrow. Although this treatment schedule is suitable for some tumors, the regrowth characteristics of others, such as diffuse large cell lymphomas, Burkitt's lymphoma, and leukemia, often permit the tumor volume to return to pretreatment levels in the interval required for bone marrow recovery, and other approaches to cycling drug combinations are now being explored. One such approach has been to use non-marrow-toxic chemotherapeutic agents, cycled with marrow-toxic agents, to permit the bone marrow to recover despite continuous treatment. This method has been useful in patients with rapidly growing diffuse large cell lymphomas. It is limited by the sensitivity of the tumor in question to the available non-marrow-toxic agents. The availability of colony-stimulating factors as supportive tools (see Chap. 62, section 2) is altering the design of clinical trials as well. Colony-stimulating factors have been coupled with cytotoxic combination chemotherapy, and the nadir leukopenia can usually be avoided or ameliorated.[28–32]

IMPACT OF THE GOLDIE-COLDMAN HYPOTHESIS ON DESIGN OF CLINICAL TRIALS USING COMBINATION CHEMOTHERAPY

In 1943, Luria and Delbruck described a principle in bacterial genetics important to our understanding of the development of spontaneous resistance to cancer chemotherapy that led to a reconsideration of how chemotherapy was used in clinical trials.[33] They observed that the bacterium *Escherichia coli* developed resistance to bacterial viruses (bacteriophage), not by surviving exposure, but by expanding clones of bacteria that had spontaneously mutated to a type inherently resistant to phage infection. In 1979, Goldie and Coldman applied this principle to the development of resistance by cancer cells to anticancer drugs without prior exposure to these drugs.[34] They proposed that the nonrandom cytogenic changes now known to be associated with most human cancers probably were tightly associated with the development of the capacity to resist the action of certain types of anticancer drugs.[35] They developed a mathematical model that predicted that tumor cells mutate to drug resistance at a rate intrinsic to the genetic instability of a particular tumor and that these events would begin to occur at population sizes between 10^3 and 10^6 tumor cells (1000–1 million cells), much lower than the mass of cells considered to be clinically detectable (10^9, or 1 billion cells). The probability that a given tumor will contain resistant clones when a patient is newly diagnosed would be a function of the mutation rate and the size of the tumor. If the mutation rate is as infrequent as 10^{-6}, a tumor composed of 10^9 cells (a 1-cm mass) would still be certain to have at least one drug-resistant clone; however, the *absolute number* of resistant cells in a tumor composed of 10^9 cells would be relatively small. Therefore, in the clinic, such tumors should initially respond to treatment with a complete or partial remission, but then recur as the resistance clone(s) expanded to repopulate the mass or masses. Such a pattern is seen with the use of chemotherapy in many drug-responsive cancers in the clinic.

The Goldie-Coldman hypothesis, therefore, predicts that

resistance should be a problem even with small tumor burdens, and the maximal chance for cure occurs when all available effective drugs are given simultaneously.[34] Because this would involve using 8 to 12 drugs simultaneously, this approach has not been tested in the clinic because of the fear that the use of more than five cytotoxic drugs, at full doses, would not be possible. The alternative approach, using two programs of equally effective, noncross-resistant drug combinations in alternating cycles, has been under evaluation for more than 10 years. Unfortunately, many studies purporting to test the Goldie-Coldman hypothesis have been poorly designed. In many instances, inadequate testing has been done to determine whether the alternate combination is truly noncross-resistant and as equally effective as the primary treatment (in most instances, it is not),[1] which it must be to fulfill the hypothesis as described by Goldie and Coldman. Second, dosing is rarely controlled, so that doses of essential drugs are modified downward, a priori, without testing the impact of such dose reductions on outcome. A more recent approach is the use of half of the drugs of each of the effective combination on days 1 and 8, respectively (so-called hybrid combinations). This approach is being tried in patients with Hodgkin's disease and diffuse large cell lymphomas. The use of alternating cycles of combination chemotherapy has not yet proved to be significantly more effective than are full doses of a single effective combination program.

In 1986, Day reanalyzed the Goldie-Coldman hypothesis and relaxed the requirement for symmetry in the model.[36,37] Although his model verified the basic tenets of the Goldie-Coldman hypothesis, it suggested a different approach to sequencing combinations: In many instances, the sequential use of combinations should out-perform alternating cycles, because no two combinations are likely to be strictly noncross-resistant or have equal cell killing capacity, the symmetry assumed by Goldie and Coldman. Day formulated "the worst-drug rule," which refers to any strategy using more or earlier doses of a treatment that is the least effective of two or more available options.[38] The worst-drug rule has interesting implications. First, it is a nonintuitive approach. If two treatments are available, treatments A and B, and B is known to be better, a physician is more likely to use B first. However, cells that are resistant to the best treatment, B, must be eliminated by the weaker program, A, and because it is the weaker program, one cannot wait too long to use it or the overgrowth of the population resistant to B will place the physician and patient in a situation difficult to overcome. The model predicts that, if six cycles of A and B are planned, using the weaker program—A—first performs better. There have been clinical examples in which sequential therapies have outperformed alternating cyclical use of the same programs if the dose intensity of the two regimens is carefully controlled.[39]

No rigid schedule can accommodate all the variables assumed to be important for maximum effectiveness of combination chemotherapy and the requirements of the patients in the practice of medical oncology. Physicians must often adjust doses at intervals to administer drugs safely. The certainty that the therapeutic effect of a drug or drug combination can be lost if the dose or schedule is altered should temper these judgments. Reductions in dose rates also often result in only minimal decreases in toxicity but major reductions in the capacity to attain a complete remission in patients with

drug-responsive tumors.[38] The physician and the patient must consider the risk of dying from cancer prematurely compared with the transient benefits of reducing the acute side effects of treatment. Adhering to the standard sliding scale for dose adjustments, usually published with most new treatments, is the most appropriate way to make the necessary adjustments without compromising long-term outcome. In addition to providing guidelines for dose reduction, these sliding scales provide consistency between patients, and between studies, by preserving the intervals between cycles and the integrity of each drug combination. These alternatives and their potential impact on the quality and quantity of life should be made clear to patients as part of the informed consent process if they are to share intelligently in decisions about dose modifications made by their physicians.[40]

RESPONSE TO CHEMOTHERAPY IS AFFECTED BY THE BIOLOGY OF TUMOR GROWTH

In the early 1960s Skipper and colleagues identified the guiding principles of present-day chemotherapy, using the rodent leukemia L1210 as a model.[41-43] Applying these principles to the drug treatment of human cancers required an understanding of the differences not only between the growth characteristics of this rodent leukemia and of human cancers but also in growth rates of normal target tissues in mice and humans. For example, L1210 leukemia is a rapidly growing tumor with a high percentage of cells synthesizing DNA, as measured by the uptake of tritiated thymidine (the labeling index). Because L1210 leukemia has a growth fraction of 100% (*i.e.*, all of its cells are actively progressing through the cell cycle), its life cycle is consistent and predictable.[44]

The relation between cell number and survival in L1210 leukemia is linear, as shown in Figure 16–1. The time to death of animals bearing L1210 leukemia is the interval required to achieve a population size of about 10^9 (1 billion) cells. With a growth fraction of 100% and a doubling time of 12 hours, 10^9 cells accumulate by 19 days after the injection of a single cell, by 10 days after the injection of 10^5 cells, and by 5 days after the administration of 10^8 cells. Skipper and associates postulated that the increase in host lifespan after cytotoxic chemotherapy of L1210 leukemia was largely due to the cytocidal effect of treatment on the tumor cell population. In these early elegant mouse experiments, they calculated the residual number of cells after treatment by extrapolating back from the duration of prolongation of life after a single treatment. An increase of 2 days in life would be equivalent to a 90% destruction of tumor cells (a 1-log kill), or a reduction in the cell number from 10^6 to 10^5. A 99.999% destruction of tumor cells, a number that seems enormous to most clinicians, represents only a 5-log kill and does not cure animals unless the initial inoculum is small, perhaps 10^4 cells or fewer. If multiple treatments are given, the net tumor cell kill per treatment is the sum of the surviving cells plus the regrowth of the tumor cell population before the next treatment.

The killing effects of cancer drugs in this model tumor follow log-kill kinetics, that is, if a particular dose of an individual drug kills three logs of cells and reduces tumor burden from

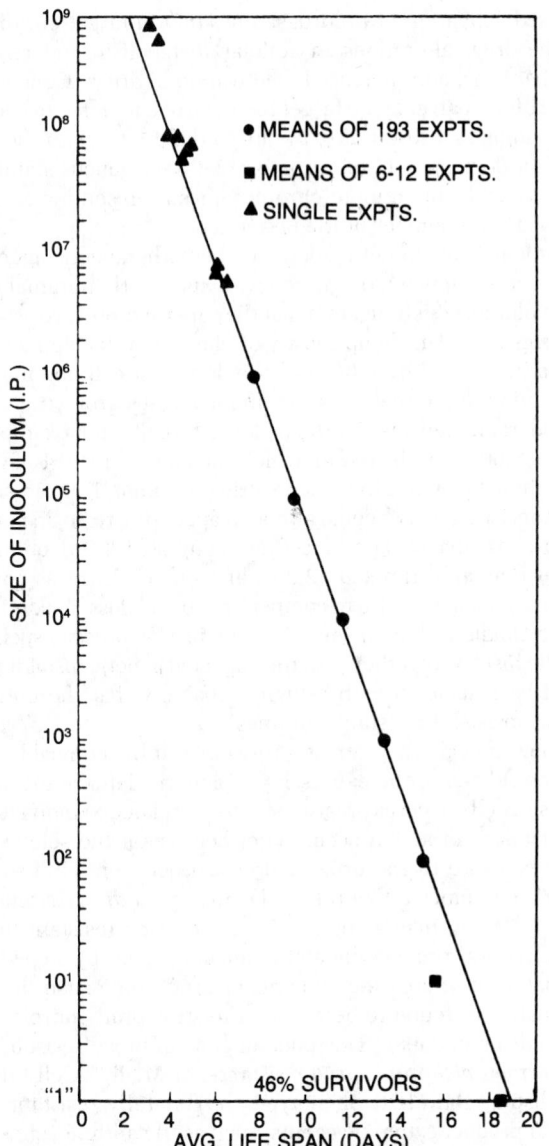

FIGURE 16–1. Relation between size of tumor cell inoculation and time to death of the host in L1210 leukemia in CDF₁ mice.

10^{10} to 10^7 cells, the same dose used at a tumor burden of 10^5 cells reduces the tumor mass to 10^2. The cell kill, therefore, is proportional, regardless of tumor burden. This model fits the response of L1210 murine leukemia to chemotherapy. When treatment failed in the experiments of Skipper and colleagues, it was because the initial tumor burden was too high to allow the delivery of curative doses of chemotherapy to eradicate the last leukemia cell. The cardinal rule of chemotherapy—the invariable inverse relation between cell number and curability—was established in this model and applies to all others. Skipper and colleagues proceeded to show that with an understanding of these basic facts, this rodent leukemia could be cured by specifically designed doses and schedules tied to tumor volume and growth characteristics.[41]

Although murine leukemias seemed to follow exponential kinetics, available data suggested that most human tumors did not appear to grow exponentially. For example, the concept of log kill would have predicted that some large tumors in the clinic should have been more sensitive to treatment than has been experienced. In toto, the available data in human cancers support a Gompertzian model of tumor growth and regression. The critical distinction between Gompertzian and exponential growth is that in Gompertzian kinetics, the growth fraction of the tumor is not constant but decreases exponentially with time (exponential growth is matched by exponential retardation of growth). The growth fraction peaks when the tumor is about 37% of its maximum size. In a Gompertzian model, when a patient with advanced cancer is treated, the tumor mass is larger, its growth fraction is low, and the fraction of cells killed is therefore small. An important feature of Gompertzian growth is that response to chemotherapy depends on where the tumor is in its growth curve. Gompertzian-growing tumors will respond to cytotoxic drugs in a Gompertzian fashion. Therefore, predictions can also be made about the behavior of small tumors, such as tumor burdens that might be present after primary surgical therapy. When the tumor is clinically undetectable, its growth fraction would be at its largest and, although the numerical reduction in cell number is small, the fractional cell kill from a "known to be effective" therapeutic dose of chemotherapy would be higher than it would be later in the tumor course. This observation initially was used to justify dose reductions at lower tumor volumes, which may account for some of the disappointment in the outcome of adjuvant studies in breast cancer, because there is no scientific justification for such dose reductions if residual cancer cells survive the treatment. The Gompertzian growth model is important for another reason: It impacts on the patterns of regrowth of residual tumor cells. In breast cancer, Norton has analyzed data from multiple adjuvant studies and also the only available studies of untreated patients who presented with localized cancers who were followed until death.[37,38,45,46] He found that in all instances a Gompertzian growth model precisely fitted the growth curves of these tumors. In adjuvant situations, the model showed that relapse-free survival and survival curves cannot discriminate between residual cell populations of 1 or 1 million cells, because the regrowth of residual cell populations will be faster at smaller residual volumes than it will be at larger residual volumes, producing identical endpoints sometimes at 5 years after diagnosis. Therefore, the effect of dose alterations cannot be differentiated using standard assay systems of effectiveness. Experimental observations imply that there are kinetic reasons for the failure of chemotherapy to cure large tumors and for the inadequate assessment of the effectiveness of drug adjuvant treatment. The data imply that short of total eradication of micrometastases (cure), varying residual volumes produce similar 5-year relapse-free survival and obscure the deleterious effect of dose reductions. This information has been useful in the design of new adjuvant treatment protocols in breast cancer.

BIOCHEMICAL RESISTANCE TO CHEMOTHERAPY IS THE MAJOR IMPEDIMENT TO SUCCESSFUL TREATMENT

The cancer cell presents a variable and moving target for anticancer drugs. The interrelation of pharmacokinetics and tumor and normal target cell kinetics is the fulcrum of clinical cancer chemotherapy. The therapeutic and toxic effects of chemotherapeutic agents are related to the time the active principle is exposed in an effective concentration to its target (Fig. 16–2). The same degree of cytotoxicity can be achieved, on different schedules, from the same concentration of drug multiplied by the time of exposure (C × T). This relation obtains across different species when the drugs are metabolized and excreted in a similar fashion. This principle has made it possible to translate doses of drugs devised in animals to humans for early clinical testing.[47,48] A given concentration of drug multiplied by the time of exposure to its target (C × T) generally is equally cytotoxic in populations of cells with equivalent growth characteristics and sensitivity to the agent(s) in question.

When the active principles of an anticancer drug reach their target, however, another obstacle to the capacity to kill the cancer cell appears: specific and permanent biochemical resistance to the drug. Resistance to drugs occurs de novo in cancer cells (intrinsic resistance) or is concomitant to exposure to drugs (acquired resistance).[48–57]

Many specific mechanisms of drug resistance have been revealed whereby cancer cells demonstrate the ability to circumvent a well-defined pathway of attack by an individual cytotoxic agent. These mechanisms are discussed in detail in Chapter 18 and are summarized in Figure 16–2.[49] Mechanisms of primary drug resistance include decreased uptake caused by changes in drug-specific transport mechanisms, de-

creased activation of prodrugs, alteration in target enzymes of the drug, alterations in cellular metabolism and repair mechanisms, and increased inactivation of drugs. Gene amplification of an enzyme target has been documented to occur in a tumor as a result of exposure to the drug,[57] with the attendant development of chromosomal homogenous staining regions or double-minute chromosomes representing an increased copy number of the target gene.

Some tumors do not respond to chemotherapeutic agents, however, even when diagnosed with apparently minimal tumor volume, which suggests that they are inherently resistant to drugs or are made up mostly of clones that have mutated to resistance and have become the dominant cell line in the population due to cell loss. As tumor masses grow, there is considerable cell loss from shedding of cells, for example, into the lumen of the bowel, which can amount to 90% of the total tumor volume. In such a setting, a tumor 1 cm in size and consisting of 10^9 cells, although appearing to be an early tumor, may have experienced as many as 1200 doublings rather than an estimated 32 doublings, if cell loss was not a factor, to reach that size to compensate for cell loss. According to the Goldie-Coldman somatic mutation hypothesis, such a kinetic history, together with the expected genetic instability, could be associated with a high probability that the entire mass consists of resistant cell lines.

It now appears that intrinsic resistance at the clinical level may be related to the expression of generic defense mechanisms in cells, whereas resistance that is related to individual mechanisms of action occurs later because of the selection after exposure to the drug or drugs in question. One such generic resistance is that referred to to as *multidrug resistance* (MDR). When malignant cell lines are made resistant to a single natural product chemotherapeutic agent, by stepwise incubation in increasing amounts of drug, some such lines, curiously, are found to be resistant to structurally unrelated cytotoxic compounds. This phenomenon of broad resistance was termed *pleiotropic drug resistance*, or MDR.[58] Cell lines that display the MDR phenotype are generally resistant to natural product cytotoxic agents, such as the anthracyclines, vinca alkaloids, epipodophyllotoxins, and actinomycin D. Because all these agents are believed to have different mechanisms of action, investigation of MDR has focused on the cell's basic defense mechanism against toxic agents that humans are exposed to naturally in the environment.

MDR has been shown to be associated with decreased intracellular drug accumulation and the presence of a 170-kd plasma membrane–associated glycoprotein (P-glycoprotein) that is not detectable in most parenteral drug-sensitive lines.[59,60] P-glycoprotein content has been directly correlated with the degree of the decrease in intracellular accumulation of the toxins and the drug resistance exhibited by the cell.[61,62] These observations suggest that the appearance of P-glycoprotein is associated with resistance perhaps by regulating the transport of toxins out of the cell. Most, but not all, cell lines with the MDR phenotype that have since been established show increased expression of the gene encoding P-glycoprotein, the *MDR* gene.[63–70] Recently, the gene for cystic fibrosis has been cloned and shown to produce a protein with marked homology to the P-glycoprotein, and additional data suggest that impaired drug influx may be a separate phenomenon. A great deal of evidence suggests that the P-

DNA Damage and Chemosensitivity

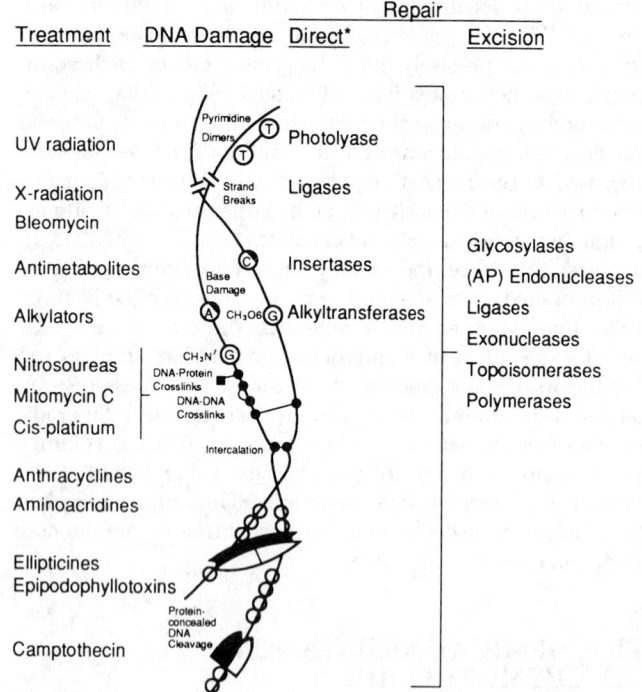

FIGURE 16–2. Schematic illustration of DNA damage and repair mechanisms in cells exposed to cytotoxic modalities. *Reversal/removal. AP, apurinic (apyrimidinic) site. (Epstein, RA. Drug-induced DNA damage and tumor chemosensitivity. J Clin Oncol 1990;8:2062–2084)

glycoprotein is an energy-dependent drug efflux pump, whose primary function is to extrude chloride ions. P-glycoprotein also binds photoaffinity analogs of the natural product vinblastine, a reaction that is competitively inhibited by unlabeled vinblastine and by anthracyclines.[68–72] Several agents, including the calcium channel blocker verapamil, quinidine, and nifedipine, can bind to the P-glycoprotein and compete with the vinblastine analogs for binding with the P-glycoprotein. Full-length cDNA sequences encoding the mouse and human P-glycoprotein gene have been isolated, and their nucleotide sequences determined. The deduced amino acid sequence of this protein shows structural similarities to a well-characterized bacterial membrane transport protein.[72–74] P-glycoprotein RNA expression has been found in high levels in normal adrenal gland and kidney tissue and in moderate levels in liver and colon tissue.[75] Recently, P-glycoprotein has been shown to be expressed on CD-34+ bone marrow stem cells, but not in more mature cells of the hematopoietic system, and in the endothelial lining of blood vessels. Both observations have important implications for the design of treatment protocols.[8,76,82] Because colon, kidney, and liver tissues are exposed to naturally occurring environmental toxins, the role of the P-glycoprotein in health may be one of protecting by facilitating efflux of these toxins or to serve as an alternative ion transport mechanism.

The range of expression of P-glycoprotein by human tumors is under intensive study.[77–79,82–84] In general, P-glycoprotein is highly expressed in tumors intrinsically resistant to chemotherapy and poorly expressed in drug-responsive tumors, unless they are sampled after relapse. These data provide avenues to pursue clinically. Protocols can be designed to use agents not affected by the pump in resistant tumors, or natural product anticancer drugs can be given early in the course of the disease, before MDR is expressed in most cells.[38] Agents that block the pump mechanism also can be used simultaneously with natural product anticancer drugs. These approaches are reviewed in reference 38 and in Chapter 69, section 6.

Another type of multidrug resistance often follows on the heels of that associated with the P-glycoprotein expression and is associated with the topoisomerase enzymes.[85–88] Topoisomerases are necessary for DNA replication, and they catalyze changes in the secondary and tertiary structures of DNA to relax DNA tension during transcription and cell division. Topoisomerase II appears to be the enzyme that is the target of antineoplastic drugs that act as DNA-intercalating agents, such as etoposide and the anthracyclines. The only known class of topoisomerase I-targeting drugs—the camptothecins—has shown unprecedented activity against human cancers in animal models and is currently undergoing clinical trials. Topoisomerases, therefore, may represent the final common pathway of cytotoxicity of several different classes of antineoplastic agents. Drugs that act through interaction with the topoisomerases do so by preventing the religation of DNA through the formation of cleavable complexes. Resistance may occur through alterations in production and function of the enzymes. For example, an etoposide-resistant Chinese hamster ovary cell line that was cross-resistant to the structurally dissimilar agents m-AMSA, mitoxantrone, and the anthracycline doxorubicin demonstrated altered topoisomerase II activity.[89] In addition, alteration in the topoisomerase

I-like activity was found in Chinese hamster cells selected for resistance to ellipticine and cross-resistance to m-AMSA and etoposide.[90]

As a result of these data, there is considerable excitement about the prospect of improving the effectiveness of chemotherapy by circumventing both types of MDR, by preventing the development of resistance or by interfering with the mechanisms themselves.

CONCEPT OF DOSE INTENSITY

For drug-sensitive cancers in favorable kinetic circumstances, the factor limiting the capacity to cure is proper dosing. The dose-response curve in biologic systems is usually sigmoidal in shape, with a threshold, a lag phase, a linear phase, and a plateau phase. For radiation therapy and chemotherapy, it is the difference between the dose-response curves of normal and tumor tissue that must be exploited during treatment. In experimental models, the dose-response curve is usually steep in the linear phase. Almost without exception in rodents bearing transplantable tumors, a reduction of doses in the linear phase of the dose-response curve results in a loss of the capacity to cure the tumor before there is a diminution in the response rate. That is, complete remissions will continue to be observed, but with dose reduction as small as 20%, the last few residual cells may not be eliminated, and relapse is inevitable. There is an extremely important lesson in these animal data for clinicians who, in their daily practice, judge the adequacy of their therapy by measuring the response rate of visible or palpable tumor masses and only much later are able to evaluate the treatment by survival results. This point is illustrated in Table 16–2, which summarizes data from numerous experiments conducted by Skipper and colleagues at the Southern Research Institute using the transplantable and palpable Ridgway osteosarcoma tumor model.[91,92] Reduction in the average dose intensity of the two-drug combination of L-phenylalanine mustard (L-PAM) and cyclophosphamide causes a marked decrease in the cure rate *before a significant reduction in the complete remission rate occurs.* On the average, a dose reduction of approximately 20% leads to a loss of 50% of the cure rate. The converse is also true. In high-growth-

TABLE 16–2. Ridgway Osteogenic Sarcoma: Response to Different Dose Intensity of Two-Drug Combination of Cyclophosphamide and L-PAM

| | RDI | | | |
CPA	L-PAM	Average	% CR	% Cures
0.38	0.82	0.60	100	60
0.75	0.18	0.47	100	44
0.25	0.55	0.44	100	10
0.50	0.12	0.31	10	0
0.17	0.36	0.27	0	0

RDI, relative dose intensity; CPA, cyclophosphamide; L-PAM, L-phenylalanine; CR, complete response. Tumors weighed 2–3 g.
(Modified from Skipper HE. Booklet No. 5. Birmingham: Southern Research Institute, 1986)

TABLE 16–3. Sample Calculations: Dose Intensity, Relative Dose Intensity, and Average Relative Dose Intensity

	Dose Intensity	Relative Dose Intensity
Calculation of Dose Intensity		
Test Schedule		
Cyclophosphamide 80 mg/m²/d (continuously)	560 mg/m²/wk	
Calculation of Relative Dose Intensity		
Standard		
Cyclophosphamide 80 mg/m²/d (continuously)	560 mg/m²/wk	
Test Schedule		
Cyclophosphamide 100 mg/m²/d (d 1–14, q 28 d)	350 mg/m²/wk	350/560 = 0.62
Calculation of Average Relative Dose Intensity		
Standard*		
Cyclophosphamide 2 mg/kg/d	560 mg/m²/wk	
Methotrexate 0.7 mg/kg/wk	28 mg/m²/wk	
5-Fluorouracil 12 mg/kg/wk	480 mg/m²/wk	
Test Regimen		
Cyclophosphamide 100 mg/m²/d (1–14)	350 mg/m²/wk	350/560 = 0.62
Methotrexate 40 mg/m²/d 1, 8	20 mg/m²/wk	20/28 = 0.71
5-Fluorouracil 600 mg/m²/d 1, 8	300 mg/m²/wk	300/480 = 0.62
Repeat cycles every 28 d		*Average* 0.65

* Assume standard regimen to be CMF. To convert mg/kg to mg/m², multiply by 40.
(Hryniuk WM: The importance of dose intensity in the outcome of chemotherapy. In: DeVita VT, Hellman S, Rosenberg SA, eds. Important advances in oncology. Philadelphia: JB Lippincott, 1988: 121–142)

fraction tumors, a twofold increase in dose often leads to a tenfold increase (1 log) in tumor cell kill. Although animal models are not the perfect analog for human cancers, the invariable nature of these data indicates that the general principle is transferable to the clinic and is ignored at great peril. Because anticancer drugs are toxic, it is often appealing to avoid acute, but not life-threatening, toxicity by diminishing the dose or increasing the intervals between cycles of treatment. This kind of ad hoc adjustment of dosing is probably the main reason for treatment failure in patients with *drug-sensitive human tumors* undergoing their first chemotherapy treatment.

It has been difficult to compare the impact of different dosing practices in treatment programs. Hryniuk and colleagues analyzed treatment outcome in a number of different tumors as a function of what they have termed *dose intensity*.[93–98] They defined dose intensity as the amount of drug delivered per unit of time, expressed as mg/m²/wk, regardless of the schedule or route of administration. Relative dose intensity (RDI) is the amount of drug delivered per unit of time relative to an arbitrarily chosen standard single drug, or, for a combination regimen, the decimal fraction of the ratio of the average dose intensity of all drugs of the test regimen compared with the standard regimen. A sample calculation of the RDI for a commonly used regimen, the cyclophosphamide, methotrexate, 5-fluorouracil (CMF) combination for breast cancer, is provided in Table 16–3.[94] To calculate the average RDI for a regimen containing fewer drugs than the standard regimen, a dose intensity of zero is assigned to the missing drug(s),

and the average RDI of the test regimen is divided by the total number of drugs in the standard.[94] The dose intensity of various programs is compared over whatever time frame the treatment programs are administered. Calculations can be made of intended dose intensity, the dose intensity as described in the treatment protocol, or actual or received dose intensity. Received dose intensity calculations are more useful data because they reflect the impact of dose reductions and necessary treatment delays imposed in actual practice.

Because calculations are made based on the amount of drugs given per week, regardless of schedule, treatment delays are given equal weight with dose reductions. Calculations of the dose intensity, therefore, require the assumption that differences in scheduling does not influence treatment outcome. Although this first appears to be heretical, close scrutiny of all available data in humans and rodents shows that scheduling influences outcome mostly by affecting toxicity, in this way allowing higher doses to be administered over the same time frame. An example can be found in the use of methotrexate in rodents and humans. Daily administration of low doses of methotrexate is extremely toxic and severely limits the dose and duration of therapy with this drug. A twice-weekly schedule, which is much more effective in rodents and humans, allows much higher doses to be delivered for longer durations, because this schedule is associated with less toxicity. The dose intensity of the twice-weekly schedule, therefore, is much greater than that of the daily oral schedule, if the calculation is based on mg/m²/wk of delivered drug. In practice, the impact of scheduling on the calculation of dose intensity can be neutralized by comparing programs in which drugs with toxicities affected by scheduling, such as the antimetabolites, are given on similar schedules.

Calculation of an average RDI of a drug combination also assumes that each drug has an equal efficacy against the tumor in question. However, the impact of any single drug or combinations of two or three drugs in a multidrug combination can be assessed separately. This measurement has been done by Hryniuk and colleagues to show the greater impact of cisplatin in a drug combination for ovarian cancer[94-98] and by others[99-102] to show the importance of adequate doses of alkylating agents and vinca alkaloids in lymphoma treatment. This kind of analysis can help identify the most effective drug in a combination and is important because such data can help avoid adjustments that radically alter the effectiveness of a program. Also, by identifying the most important drugs, protocols can be developed that emphasize the dose intensity of these agents compared with other less effective drugs.[36] Negative alterations in dose intensity of the most effective drug in a combination of drugs has great impact, as illustrated in Table 16–4, which displays the effects of the two-drug combination of L-PAM and the antimetabolite 6-mercaptopurine (6-MP) against the Ridgway osteogenic sarcoma model. In this instance, L-PAM is the more effective drug. The relation of average dose intensity of the two drugs to outcome is erratic, but the relation of the dose intensity of L-PAM to outcome is linear. Decreases in the dose intensity of L-PAM reduce the effect of the combination, even if the dose of 6-MP is increased to compensate for these reductions. In fact, any decrease in the dose intensity of L-PAM below 55% of the optimal single-dose schedule results in a loss of the capacity of this combination to cure animals, regardless of the dose of 6-MP.

TABLE 16–4. Ridgway Osteogenic Sarcoma: Effect of Varying Dose Intensity of More Effective Drug, L-PAM

Relative Dose Intensity				*Observed*	
		Ratio			
L-PAM	6-MP	*(L-PAM/6-MP)*	*Average*	*% CR*	*% Cures*
0.82	0.49	1.7	0.66	100	60
0.73	1.3	0.56	1.0	90	50
0.55	1.0	0.55	0.78	90	20
0.55	0.33	1.7	0.44	80	20
0.36	0.67	0.54	0.52	56	0
0.36	0.21	1.7	0.29	30	0
0.27	1.5	0.18	0.89	70	0
0.24	0.44	0.57	0.35	0	0
0.24	0.15	1.6	0.20	0	0
0.18	1.0	0.18	0.59	0	0
0.12	0.67	0.18	0.50	0	0
0.08	0.44	0.18	0.26	0	0

L-PAM, L-phenylalanine mustard; 6-MP, mercaptopurine. Tumors weighed 2–3 g. Varying the dose intensity of L-PAM has a greater impact on outcome than can be overcome by increasing the dose of 6-MP.
(Skipper HE. Booklet No. 4. Birmingham: Southern Research Institute, 1986)

To judge adequately the dosing of a particular protocol, data on total dose of each drug used and cumulative doses of each drug are necessary. Collection of such data is not part of routine practice, and reports are not generally available in the literature. To assess the impact of dosing schedules in practice and in clinical trials, such data should be required before papers are accepted for publication.

A positive relation between dose intensity and response rate has been demonstrated in advanced ovarian, breast, and colon cancers and in the lymphomas.[92,93,95,98,100-102]

Calculations of the impact of dose intensity on outcome are particularly important in estimating the value and exploring some of the pitfalls of adjuvant chemotherapy. The steep dose-response curve for anticancer drugs indicates that dose reductions in adjuvant drug treatment programs are likely to be associated with significantly less therapeutic effect. Dose reduction, however, has been the norm in the design of adjuvant trials. An example is the standard CMF regimen for breast cancer referred to in Table 16–3. The model for the regimen was published in 1974 by Canellos and associates.[100] It produced an impressive complete remission rate of approximately 30%, but its toxicity was considerable. As a result, when it was advanced for use in a cooperative group setting, first for advanced disease[99] and later for adjuvant trials by Bonadonna and colleagues,[101] its doses were arbitrarily reduced without pretesting the impact of such reductions on outcome. In addition, further reduction was made, a priori, for patients older than 60 years of age, with the assumption that such reductions would be required because of age. When the effect of these reductions is related to outcome, there is a strong suggestion of a negative impact.[99,102] In premenopausal women the differences in relapse-free survival at the high and low doses of CMF are statistically significant. The most important point, however, is that the average dose intensity of CMF as used in clinical trials and in the community is probably only half the dose intensity of the original program. These dose reductions exceed the levels that animal models predict would lead to a loss in the capacity to cure.

Another example of the potential impact dose intensity can have on the design of clinical trials has been provided by Hryniuk, as shown in Figure 16–3.[93] The dose intensity of 5-fluorouracil is plotted against the response rate for advanced colorectal cancer in panel A. Points indicated by the asterisks are from a single study in which response was reported for actual delivered doses at three different levels.[103] The steep nature of the dose-response curves should be noted. Panel B of Figure 16–3 plots the same three points from the single study but adds the doses used in four published adjuvant studies.[103-108] The doses in all of these studies are well below the level that most investigators would consider the threshold for producing useful responses in advanced colorectal cancer. The effect of dose intensity on the capacity to cure advanced Hodgkin's disease and diffuse large cell lymphomas is also striking and is described in detail in Chapters 51 and 52.

Increasing the dose intensity can be a useful way to improve the effect of certain drugs or combinations of drugs, but it is not useful in all clinical circumstances. Large tumor burdens tend to shift the dose-response curve to the right. At the low end of the curability curve (*i.e.,* in the presence of the highest tumor burdens), increasing the dose intensity often leads to unacceptable toxicity and may not produce more impressive

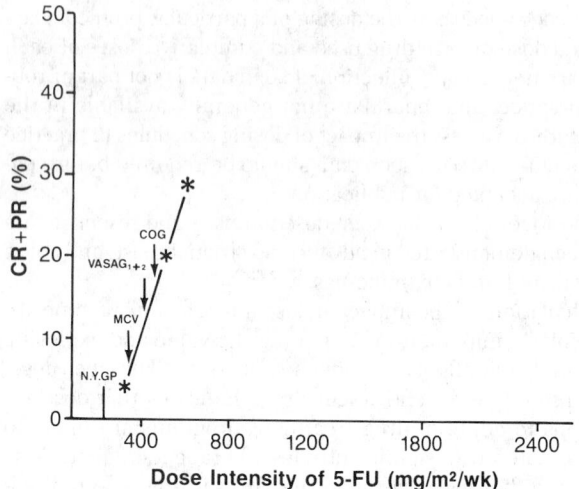

A

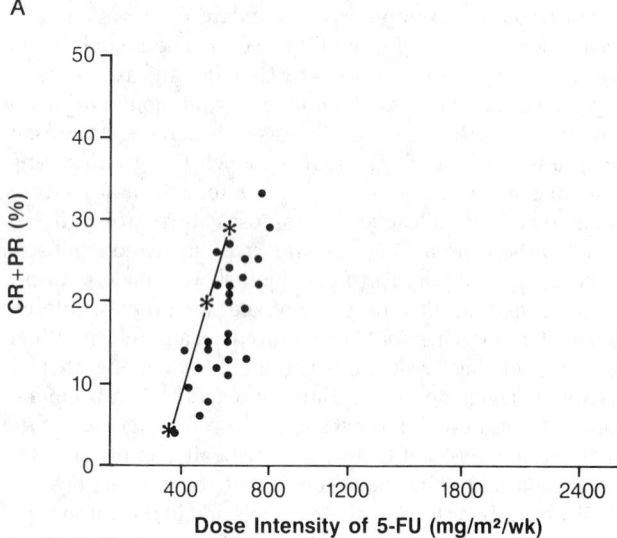

B

FIGURE 16–3. **(A)** Response rate at various intended dose intensity of 5-fluorouracil in advanced colorectal cancer. Each point represents results from one arm of a randomized trial. *Asterisks* indicate results of three doses from a single study, and *solid circles* indicate received dose intensity. **(B)** Dose intensities of 5-fluorouracil used in four adjuvant studies of colorectal cancer superimposed on the dose-response line for advanced disease shown in panel **A**. *Asterisks* represent received dose intensity from single study (see text). (Hryniuk WM. The importance of dose intensity in the outcome of chemotherapy. In: DeVita VT Jr, Hellman S, Rosenberg SA, eds. Important Advances in Oncology 1988. Philadelphia: JB Lippincott, 1988:125)

treatment outcomes, because the dose-response curve is flat. In addition, regimens that are already curing nearly 100% of a subset of patients, such as the combination of platinum, vinblastine, and bleomycin in low-burden testicular cancer and the nitrogen mustard, vincristine, procarbazine, prednisone (MOPP) chemotherapy program in stage IIIA Hodgkin's disease, cannot be expected to be improved on by augmenting dose intensity. However, for most drugs and most tumors, there appears to be a threshold dose that produces responses, and the remarkable success of high-dose chemotherapy programs with bone marrow transplantation support in refractory lymphomas, breast cancer, childhood sarcomas, and neuro-

blastomas suggests that maximizing dose intensity can improve the chances of cure in drug-responsive tumors.

IN VITRO TESTS TO SELECT CHEMOTHERAPEUTIC AGENTS FOR INDIVIDUALIZED TREATMENT

Short-term assays are not useful in determining the primary treatment for patients for whom a known and effective treatment exists. The assays are also of minimal value for the remainder of newly diagnosed patients and for those with drug-sensitive tumors who fail the first trial of chemotherapy. The basic problem is that the pool of available active drugs is too small for most cancers to make those assays useful beyond clinical judgment. They can, however, be of some use to avoid patient exposure to the toxicity of drugs that are unlikely to be effective, but the tests are too cumbersome and expensive for routine practice. No convincing reports in the literature have indicated that short-term assays provide additional benefit beyond what the clinician can provide by using good judgment and a knowledge of the effectiveness of the limited number of available single agents.

CANCER DRUG DEVELOPMENT

The steps in the development of anticancer drugs are shown in Figure 16–4. The most important step in the drug selection process is mass screening, the mechanism used to narrow the universe of chemicals potentially useful for the treatment of human cancers to a manageable number of high-priority drugs for clinical testing.[105-109] The mass screening effort is conducted by the National Cancer Institute (NCI) drug development program.

Many currently available anticancer drugs active against human leukemias and lymphomas were identified and developed as a result of the NCI system. The input to this type of screening program reached its maximum of 40,000 compounds screened per year in 1975. In 1975, a major change was made in the NCI screening program because of the avail-

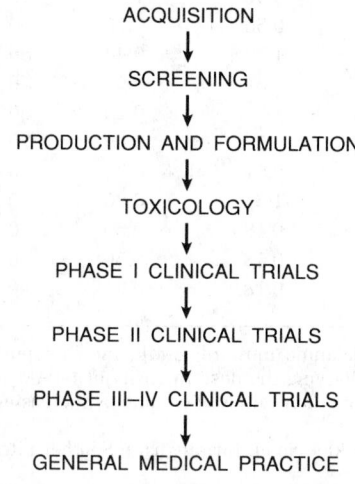

FIGURE 16–4.   Steps in cancer drug development.

ability of new rodent models. More rational selection of compounds was coupled with a panel of transplantable rodent tumor screens designed to match the histologic type of common visceral cancers. These rodent solid tumor screens were matched to human tumor cell lines of the same type grown in nude mice. This panel posed the question of the clinical specificity of the preclinical models. The panel of tumors was changed periodically to pose additional questions to the screening process.[110] Taxol, a new agent of considerable interest, was not active in traditional screens but was selected by the new screening panel. Later, human tumors grown in soft agar and under the renal capsule were also introduced into the screening program to further test the hypothesis that the use of human tissue in short-term assays could better select compounds more active in the clinic than could simpler rodent tumor models. Problems with the technical details of these in vitro systems led to their discontinuation.[110-113]

As it became possible to maintain human tumor cells in defined media, the screening program was again changed by developing disease-oriented panels of human tumor cell lines grown in defined media.[113,115] The initial selection of cell lines for this screening panel was based on several considerations, including the use of representatives of major histologic subtypes, the use of multiple cell lines for each tumor type, and the use of cell lines that retain appropriate features of the tumor of origin. The cell lines currently in use include lung, ovarian, and renal cancer; malignant melanoma; brain tumors; and leukemia. Because of the interest in the phenomenon of MDR and the likelihood that it is one of the factors limiting the effectiveness of chemotherapy, a human breast cancer line and an MDR variant of this line, selected for resistance to doxorubicin, are included, along with a murine leukemia and a comparable doxorubicin-induced MDR variant of this murine leukemia. These cell lines provide the potential for identifying new agents with particular activity against MDR cell populations.

A key element in screening strategy is to maintain the capacity for high-volume screening. The most commonly used approach is a colorimetric growth inhibition assay that is based on the metabolic reduction of the tetrazolium salt formazan inside viable cells. Under appropriate conditions, a linear relation is obtained between viable cell number and formazan optical density, measured using a standard enzyme immunosorbent assay plate reader.[116] Automation of this assay has made it possible to maintain an adequate volume of in vitro screening (10,000 compounds per year) at less expense. Preliminary analysis of screening results indicates that individual cell lines show characteristic degrees of in vitro chemosensitivity to individual test compounds with known patterns of clinical activity. Ease of automation of the colorimetric assay and the stability of the cell lines have largely overcome the technical problems associated with clonogenic or subrenal capsular assays.[113,117] The central goal of the in vitro-based, disease-oriented screening program is to identify new antitumor drug candidates that would not have been discovered by the previously available screening program. Clinical testing of these new leads, as with previous versions of preclinical screening, will ultimately be the only way to establish or disprove the validity of the new screen for identifying new drugs active against the common refractory human solid tumors.

In the early days of screening, the acquisition of agents was purely random. Random acquisition of chemicals for screening was associated with two major problems: repetitive screening of compounds already tested and screening of analogs of drugs already known to be active rather than the identification of new structures. Modern molecular biology techniques present an unusual opportunity to select materials, defined at the molecular level, that might prove useful in the inhibition of vital cell functions.

Inherent in all screening systems is the tenet that biologic activity in some preclinical system must be demonstrated before human testing is performed. No currently marketed, useful chemotherapeutic agent is devoid of such preclinical antitumor effect.

Toxicology testing has evolved during the last decade from complicated testing in rodents, dogs, and monkeys to a less expensive and simpler system that relies on toxicity testing primarily in mice. Large amounts of data accumulated since the beginning of anticancer drug development have allowed comparisons to be made across species with respect to common toxicity of chemicals. These data have shown that there is no safety advantage in using larger animal species instead of rodents. In the current system, implemented in 1980, the dose-response curve of a new drug is first developed in mice. The lethal dose (LD) in 10% of animals is determined, and the reproducible lethal dose in 10% of tested animals (LD_{10}) is used as the basis for establishing the initial dose in clinical trials. Usually, 10% of the LD_{10} dose in rodents is selected for the initial human dose; this dose is first tested for toxicity in dogs, before use in humans, to minimize the risks associated with administering an unknown compound to humans. Although the correlation of toxic effects on rapidly dividing normal tissue between rodents, dogs, monkeys, and humans is good, correlation of other toxic effects is not as consistent.[118] Therefore, routine pathologic examination of rodent tissue is not always performed before clinical testing.

All drugs should be given with reference to body weight or surface area. The preferable reference point is body surface area, because better cross-species comparisons can be made, and because calculations based on body surface area allow doses to be determined for adults and children without further

TABLE 16–5. Representative Surface Area to Weight Ratios (km) of Various Species*

Species	Body Weight (kg)	Surface Area	Surface Area to Weight Ratio (km)
Mouse	0.02	0.0066	3.0
Rat	0.15	0.025	5.9
Monkey	3	0.24	12
Dog	8	0.40	20
Human			
Child	20	0.80	25
Adult	60	1.6	37

* To express a mg/kg dose in any given species as the equivalent mg/m² dose, multiply the dose by the appropriate *km*. In the adult human, for example, 100 mg/kg is equivalent to 100 mg/kg × 37 kg/m² = 3700 mg/m².

TABLE 16–6. Equivalent Surface Area Dosage Conversion Factors*

	Mouse, 20 g	Rat, 150 g	Monkey, 3 kg	Dog, 8 kg	Human, 60 kg
Mouse	1	$\frac{1}{2}$	$\frac{1}{4}$	$\frac{1}{6}$	$\frac{1}{12}$
Rat	2	1	$\frac{1}{2}$	$\frac{1}{4}$	$\frac{1}{7}$
Monkey	4	2	1	$\frac{3}{5}$	$\frac{1}{3}$
Dog	6	4	$\frac{5}{3}$	1	$\frac{1}{2}$
Human	12	7	3	2	1

* This table shows approximate factors for converting doses expressed in terms of mg/kg from one species to an equivalent *surface area* dose expressed in the same terms mg/kg in the other species. For example, given a dose of 50 mg/kg in the mouse, what is the appropriate dose in the human, assuming equivalency on the basis of mg/m^2?

$$50 \text{ mg/kg} \times \tfrac{1}{12} = 4.1 \text{ mg/kg}$$

adjustment. The assumptions leading to the dose conversion factors have been described in detail by Freireich and coworkers[48] and are shown in Table 16–5, which is useful in converting doses in milligram per kilogram to the comparable milligram per square meter dose. Table 16–6 shows the procedure for conversion of a milligram per kilogram dose in rodents, monkeys, or dogs to the equivalent dose in humans.

EARLY CLINICAL TRIALS OF ANTITUMOR AGENTS

Antitumor agents pass through four phases of clinical testing before they are accepted for general medical practice, marketed, or discarded (see Fig. 16–4).[119-123] The average time from discovery of an effective antitumor agent to marketing of that agent is quite long, in the range of 10 to 12 years, and is expensive, costing $40 million to $80 million.

Although the main purpose of phase I trials is to identify a maximally tolerated dose (MTD) in one of several schedules suggested by the preclinical data, patients are entered into phase I trials with therapeutic intent. For most of the effective anticancer drugs, some therapeutic effect was often seen even in phase I trials. Because a limited number of patients with a variety of diseases are treated in phase I trials, and because doses may be less than the ultimate therapeutic range in a fraction of the patients, the absence of any positive effect in a phase I trial is not a sufficient reason to discontinue testing of a drug. The only reason not to proceed to a phase II study is prohibitive toxicity in phase I trials. Escalation of doses in phase I trials is usually done by a modified Fibonacci system: Doses are first doubled and then increased at decreasing increments of 66%, 50%, and 33% in succeeding groups of patients (usually three at a time) until limiting toxicity is observed.[119] Attempts have been made to rationalize and accelerate dose escalation by the systematic use of preclinical pharmacologic data.[124] This approach has relied on the assumption that the elimination rate of a drug determines its time concentration curve (C ×T), and it further assumes that for agents showing no major differences in target cell sensitivity, schedule dependence, or toxicity between mice and

humans, the C × T at the mouse LD_{10} and the human MTD should be similar. These assumptions lead naturally to a simple algorithm for escalating doses by targeting the human C × T in a phase I trial to the mouse C × T at LD_{10}.[121] The steps are as follows:

1. Determine the mouse LD_{10} (part of the routine preclinical toxicology testing discussed earlier).
2. Determine the mouse C × T at LD_{10}.
3. Begin human testing at a safe starting dose (currently one tenth of the mouse-equivalent LD_{10}).
4. Determine the human C × T at the starting dose in phase I.
5. Escalate doses in subsequent patients based on how close the C × T at the starting dose is to the target C × T.

Preliminary studies have suggested that applying this procedure may save 20% to 50% of the escalation steps for many agents. This approach is now being tested prospectively in the NCI phase I testing program.

The definition of a dose as maximally tolerated depends on how much toxicity the patient and physician are willing and able to tolerate. It has been amply demonstrated that for several drugs, such as cyclophosphamide, thiotepa, 1,3-bis(2-chlorethyl)-1-nitrosourea, and etoposide, the MTD, as determined from toxic effects other than bone marrow suppression, is three to ten times higher than the conventional MTD determined by granulocytopenia. The fact that the response rates are commonly a function of dose gives a strong impetus to further trials exploring the upper end of the dose-response curve. As a result, an alternative approach to phase I testing is under consideration, that is, to redefine the MTD as the dose at which unacceptable non-marrow-related toxicity supervenes, despite deployment of all the modern aspects of care. This approach should be greatly facilitated by the availability of colony-stimulating factors, if they succeed in eliminating bone marrow suppression as the rate-limiting step in early testing. It seems prudent to delay decisions on escalation of new agents past the conventionally determined MTD until more information about their clinical characteristics is available.

The purpose of phase II studies is to develop estimates of the response rate to a particular drug of patients with specified tumor types. Phase II studies determine activity rather than clinical usefulness and answer a biologic and clinical question. The outcome of the phase II trial is a decisive point in the development of a drug. These results determine whether a new treatment should be pursued.

When a drug enters phase II testing in individual diseases, it should be tested in a patient group with easily evaluated endpoints of responsiveness, provided it is ethically permissible to do so. This ambition is best fulfilled by enrolling patients with advanced cancer, but who have a maximal performance status, a minimal heterogeneity of metastatic sites, and a minimal amount of prior chemotherapy.[125] This means that for tumors sensitive to chemotherapy, patients who have failed no more than one prior regimen are ideal for study. For the less sensitive epithelial cancers, in many instances previously untreated patients can and should be entered into phase II studies. In view of the poor record of most single agents in heavily pretreated patients with advanced disease, such a strategy seems sensible, because for patients with advanced drug-resistant cancer, the likelihood of toxicity is much greater than is the likelihood of therapeutic benefit.

The number of patients accrued to phase II trials should be appropriate for the scientific goals of the study. In ideal circumstances, a drug that produces no antitumor effect in 14 patients with the same tumor type, particularly if the heterogeneity of the distribution of metastases is minimized, has a greater than 95% chance of being ineffective against that tumor and could reasonably be eliminated from further studies against that specific cancer. One or two responses, however, increase the chance of efficacy sufficiently to dictate an expansion of the trial to 30 or more patients, so as not to miss a drug with a response rate in the 20% range. In general, partial response rates higher than 20% place the agent in a category of potential clinical usefulness to be determined in further studies. Response rates in the range of 5% to 10% are consistent with observer variation in phase II trials. Response rates lower than than 20% can be meaningful, however, if the quality of the response is good. For example, a few complete remissions, even if the overall frequency of complete response is low, should lead to a decision to proceed with further testing in that disease, because complete disappearance of disease, however infrequent, is an important sign of a potentially effective new treatment. Because multiple doses and schedules may be tested, a phase II trial for each drug, schedule, and tumor type is required before a drug can be disqualified from further clinical use. Given all these confounding variables, a complete phase II trial often requires 600 or more patients.

At the completion of a phase II trial, a decision is made to proceed with or discard the agent. This decision is based on a lack of efficacy or an excessive or intolerable toxicity, against the background of the observed therapeutic effect. Because it is not possible to test each new agent against every tumor type, the potential for discarding agents that might be useful in rare tumors is significant. The early testing results of cisplatin are particularly instructive and illustrative of the problems faced by industry in cancer drug development. Cisplatin showed little activity against the common tumors in its early testing, because it was tested in heavily pretreated patients. Because its use was associated with considerable toxicity, it was almost discarded. Incidental testing in patients with testicular cancer, who are not generally part of major phase II studies, however, revealed interesting activity, and cisplatin was quickly advanced to use in combination with other drugs to treat advanced testicular cancer with curative intent. It was proposed for marketing on the basis of its usefulness in testicular cancer, but few data on its single-agent activity in this disease were available to the Food and Drug Administration in its appraisal of the new drug application, and marketing was delayed almost 3 years, despite nearly uniform enthusiasm for the drug in the oncology community. Only subsequent to widespread aftermarketing testing of cisplatin in other tumors did its broader effectiveness become apparent. This drug has now proved to be not only the mainstay of curative treatment of advanced testicular cancer but an important part of the therapy in lung and bladder cancer, head and neck cancer, ovarian cancer, and other common tumors. The U.S. Government recognized its role in delaying the marketing of this important drug by extending its patent life by 3 years.

If a drug is found effective in phase II trials, phases III and IV testing establishes its place in the therapeutic armamentarium. These clinical trials usually require large numbers of patients and are difficult to perform. The issue of randomized versus historical controls in phases III and IV trials is an important one and is discussed in detail in Chapter 19.

OVERCOMING THE LIMITATIONS OF CANCER TREATMENT

Since it has become apparent that chemotherapy could cure advanced cancers of some types, the question of why it could not cure more cancers, particularly those of the more common histologic types, has plagued investigators. In general, the limitations of cancer treatment have been difficult to overcome until the recent migration of molecular biology methodology to the clinic. The major limitations of cancer treatment are (1) the inability to determine precisely which cancers have metastasized at the time of diagnosis, (2) the inability to detect minimal residual disease after apparently successful treatment, (3) the inability to escalate doses of effective anticancer drugs to the high end of the dose-response curve, (4) the hurdle presented by the unexpected expression of MDR, and (5) the inability to measure the moment-to-moment impact of treatment on cancer cells.

The issue of determining which cancers have metastasized has been addressed indirectly by using panels of prognostic factors, which has proven too crude for practical use in most cancers. It is now being addressed on the molecular level by probing for expression of genes that normally control cell migration; this subject is reviewed in Chapter 8. Molecular diagnosis has advanced to the stage in which the ability to detect minimal residual disease has improved from crude morphologic methods and other tests that detect approximately 1 cancer cell in 20 or 100 normal cells to the ability to detect one malignant cell in 1 million normal cells, using tests such as the polymerase chain reaction. These approaches are reviewed in Chapter 6. We are now in the age in which the availability of colony-stimulating factors (see Chap. 62, section 2) and autologous bone marrow transplantation (see Chap. 62, section 1) are effectively allowing significant dose escalation, and the problems presented by the expression of MDR are in focus and attackable at the clinical level (see Chap. 69, section 6). Although scientists and practitioners are not yet able, at the clinical level, to monitor the impact of cancer treatment on cancer cells moment by moment, techniques such as magnetic resonance spectroscopy and positron emission tomography are available that offer promise. The capacity to measure instantaneously the impact of treatment should radically alter schedules of drug administration to whatever is required to kill cancer cells and no more.

Chemotherapy can cure about 15% of patients with advanced cancers, many of which occur in young patients. The impact of these successes, measured in person-years of life saved, is, however, disproportionately great because the younger average age at diagnosis results in a highly significant salvage of person-years of productive life. Systemic treatment also bears a special burden, because of fear of toxicity in the minds of physicians and patients, beyond that associated with surgery or radiation therapy, and because the effects of systemic therapy cannot be limited precisely to the region in-

TABLE 16–7.   Evolution of Cancer Treatment*

RSR (%)	Date	Surgery	Radiation Therapy	Systemic Therapy
(±0)	1894	Radical mastectomy	X-Rays discovered	
20	1920	Antibiotics	250 kv units	Transplantable rodent tumors
	1946	Supportive care		Nitrogen mustard in lymphomas
	1955	Radical surgery		Choriocarcinoma
33	1957	Micrometastases	Cobalt units	
	1961		Linear accelerator	Drug cures of leukemia and advanced Hodgkin's disease
36	1970	Resection of metastases	Radiosensitizers	Adjuvant therapy
				Immunotherapy
				Hybridoma technology
—			Particle therapy	MDR
41	1980	Conservative surgery	Neutron generators	Biologics
		Reconstructive surgery	Treatment planning with CT scans	MoABS
				Dose intensity
				ABMT
49	1985	Tailoring procedures to other treatments	Hyperthermia	Primary chemotherapy
				Overcoming drug resistance
—			Conformal RRx	Biochemotherapy
	1990	Detect capacity to metastasize		Attacking the signaling system
				Antisense compounds
				Monitor response to treatment
				Determine residual disease

* Illustrates the complexity of integrating advances in each field over a long time span. RSR, relative survival rates from NCI Surveillance, Epidemiology, and End Results (SEER) Program; MDR, multidrug resistance; CT, computed tomography; ABMT, autologous bone marrow transplant; RRx, radiation therapy; MoABS, monoclonal antibodies (also see chapters on principles of surgical oncology [14], radiation therapy [15], and biologic therapy [17]).

volved by tumor. Even though more sophisticated techniques of delivering systemic therapy to target organs have been developed, systemic toxicity is always a concomitant of systemic treatment. The same is true of biologicals. The promise of diminished side effects with the use of biological materials because they were natural products has not been fulfilled. A general principle is that all chemicals, natural or xenobiotic, when used in pharmacologic doses, produce significant side effects.

Patients cured of cancer by any modality generally find the toxicity associated with the treatment a justifiable experience. For those patients with advanced unresponsive cancers, however, who have the burden of progressive tumor and impending death, the risks and side effects of treatment should be carefully balanced against the potential benefits. Patients who are offered systemic therapy with a potential for cure should be treated aggressively; those for whom palliation is the only choice should not be overly burdened with extremely toxic treatments that may prolong life minimally and in an uncomfortable fashion. In practice, this means that patients with metastatic cancer for which no known effective systemic treatment exists often are best advised to avoid treatment with standard anticancer drugs or to take part in one of the many clinical trials testing new treatments.

To expand the benefits of chemotherapy, more use of anticancer drugs before and after surgery and radiotherapy is required when tumor burden is minimal, kinetic features of cell growth are favorable, and drug resistance is less likely to be present or easier to overcome. Because patients sometimes feel free of tumor after surgery, however, they may be less willing to accept the additional trauma of chemotherapy, unless the benefits are carefully explained and accurately and honestly balanced against the chances of recurrence.

Cancer treatment has progressed considerably, despite the frustrations. Nonetheless, the separation of the specialties remains a significant problem; it is often difficult to integrate newer approaches in each field into the practice of medicine. Each field has grown separately,[4] and yet the solutions to clinical problems require the careful integration of components of each specialty.[36] The evolution of the three approaches to cancer treatment are summarized in Table 16–7, which illustrates the complexity of integrating fields that have evolved slowly over eight decades, a time span that considerably exeeds the lifespan of clinical investigators, the change agents in cancer medicine.

REFERENCES

1. Marshall EK Jr. Historical perspectives in chemotherapy. In: Goldin A, Hawking IF, eds. Advances in chemotherapy. Vol 1. New York: Academic Press, 1964:1–8.
2. Hersh SM. Chemical and biological warfare: America's hidden arsenal. New York: Bobbs Merrill, 1968.

3. Alexander SF. Final report of Bari mustard casualties. Allied Force Headquarters, Office of the Surgeon, APO 512, June 20, 1944.

4. DeVita VT. The evolution of therapeutic research in cancer. N Engl J Med 1978;298: 907–910.

5. DeVita VT. On the value of response criteria in therapeutic research. Le Bulletin Du Cancer, Colloquim INSERM-John Libbey Series, Proceedings of the 2nd International Congress on Neo-Adjuvant Chemotherapy 1988;75(9):863–869.

6. Holland JF. Induction chemotherapy: An old term for an old concept. In: Neoadjuvant chemotherapy. Colloque INSERM 1986;137:45–47.

7. Frei A III, Clark JR, Miller D. The concept of neoadjuvant chemotherapy. In: Salmon SE, ed. Adjuvant therapy of cancer V. Orlando: Grune & Stratton, 1987:67.

8. Muggia FM. Primary chemotherapy: Concepts and issues. In: Primary chemotherapy in cancer medicine. New York: Alan R Liss, 1985:377–383.

9. DeVita VT. The relationship between tumor mass and resistance to treatment of cancer. Cancer 1983;51:1209–1220.

10. Skipper HE: Critical variables in the design of combination chemotherapy regimens to be used alone or in adjuvant setting. In: Neoadjuvant chemotherapy. Colloque INSERM 1986;137:11–12.

11. Goldie JH. Scientific basis for adjuvant and primary (neoadjuvant) chemotherapy. Semin Oncol 1987;14:1–7.

12. Bonadonna G. Veronesi U, Brambilla C, et al. Primary chemotherapy to avoid mastectomy in tumors with diameters of three centimeters or more. JNCI 1990;82:1539–1541.

13. Jacobs C. Adjuvant and neoadjuvant treatment of head and neck cancers. Semin Oncol 1991;18:504–514.

14. Kelsen DP, Bains M, Burt M. Neoadjuvant chemotherapy and surgery of cancer of the esophagus. Semin Surg Oncol 1990;6(5):268–273.

15. Herr HN, Whitmore NF, Morse MJ et al. Neoadjuvant chemotherapy in invasive bladder cancer: The evolving role of surgery. J Urol 1990;144:1083–1088.

16. Jacquillat C, Weil M, Baillet F, et al. Results of neoadjuvant chemotherapy and radiation therapy in the breast conserving treatment of 250 patients with all stages of infiltrative breast cancer. Cancer 1990;66:119–129.

17. DeVita VT. Primary chemotherapy can avoid mastectomy but there is more to it than that. JNCI [Editorial] 1990;82(19):1522–1523.

18. Dedrick RL, Myers CE, Bungay PM, et al. Pharmacokinetic rationale for peritoneal drug administration in treatment of ovarian cancer. Cancer Treat Rep 1978;62:1–11.

19. Jones RB, Myers CE, Guarino AM, et al. High volume intraperitoneal chemotherapy ("belly bath") for ovarian cancer: Pharmacologic basis and early results. Cancer Chemother Pharmacol 1978;1:161–166.

20. Papahadjopoulos D, Poste G, Vail WJ, et al. Use of lipid vesicles as carriers to introduce actinomycin D into resistant tumor cells. Cancer Res 1976;36:2988–3012.

21. Weinstein JM, Magin RL, Cysyk RL, et al. Treatment of solid L1210 murine tumors with local hyperthermia and temperature-sensitive liposomes containing methotrexate. Cancer Res 1980;40:1388–1396.

22. Weinstein JN. Liposomes as drug carriers in cancer therapy. Cancer Treat Rep 1984;68:127–135.

23. Nathanson L, Hall TC, Schilling AC, et al. Concurrent combination chemotherapy of human solid tumors: Experience with three-drug regimen and review of the literature. Cancer Res 1969;29:419–425.

24. Potter VR. Sequential blocking of metabolic pathways in vivo. Proc Soc Exp Biol Med 1951;76:41–46.

25. Elion GB, Singer S, Hitchings GH. Antagonists of nucleic acid derivatives: VIII. Synergism in combinations of biochemically related antimetabolites. J Biol Chem 1954;208:477–488.

26. Sartorelli AC. Approaches to the combination chemotherapy of transplantable neoplasms. Prog Ext Tumor Res 1965;6:228–288.

27. DeVita VT, Schein PS. The use of drugs in combination for the treatment of cancer: Rationale and results. N Engl J Med 1973;288:998–1006.

28. Morstyn, Campbell L, Souza LM, et al. Effect of granulocyte colony stimulating factor on neutropena induced by cytotoxin chemotherapy. Lancet 1988;1:667–672.

29. Antman KS, Griffin JD, Elias A, et al. Effect of recombinant human granulocyte-macrophage colony-stimulating factor on chemotherapy induced myelosuppression. N Engl J Med 1989;319:593–598.

30. Gabrilove J, Jakubowski A, Scher H, et al. Granulocyte colony-stimulating factor reduces neutropenia and associated morbidity of chemotherapy for transitional cell carcinoma of the urothelium. N Engl J Med 1988;318:1414–1422.

31. Ganser A, Volkers B, Ottman OG, et al. Recombinant human granulocyte-macrophage colony-stimulating factor in patients with myelodysplasia syndrome: Toxicity, pharmacokinetics and hematological effects. J Clin Oncol 1989;7:629–637.

32. Champlin RE, Nimer SD, Ireland P, et al. Treatment of refractory aplastic anemia with recombinant human granulocyte-macrophage-colony-stimulating factor. Blood 1989;73:694–699.

33. Luria SE, Delbruck M. Mutations of bacteria from virus sensitivity to virus resistance. Genetics 1943;28:491–511.

34. Goldie JH, Coldman AJ. A mathematic model for relating the drug sensitivity of tumors to the spontaneous mutation rate. Cancer Treat Rep 1979;63:1727–1733.

35. Yunis J. The chromosomal basis of human neoplasia. Science 1983;221:227–236.

36. Day RS. Treatment sequencing, asymmetry and uncertainty: Protocol strategies for combination chemotherapy. Cancer Res 1986;46:3876–3885.

37. Norton L, Day R. Potential innovations in scheduling in cancer chemotherapy. In: DeVita VT, Hellman S, Rosenberg SA, eds. Important advances in oncology 1991. Philadelphia: JB Lippincott, 1991:57–73.

38. DeVita VT. The influence of information on drug resistance on protocol design: The Harry Kaplan Memorial Lecture given at the Fourth International Conference on Malignant Lymphoma, June 6–9, 1990, Lugano, Switzerland. Ann Oncol 1991;2:93–106.

39. Buzzoni R, Bonadonna G, Valagussa P, et al. Adjuvant chemotherapy with doxorubicin plus cyclophosphamide, methotrexate, and flourouracil in the treatment of resectable breast cancer with more than three positive axillary nodes. J Clin Oncol 1991;9:2134–2140.

40. DeVita VT. Only if you believe in magic. In: Jones SE, Salmon SE, eds. Adjuvant therapy of cancer, 4th ed. Orlando: Grune & Stratton, 1984:3–16.

41. Skipper HE, Schabel FM Jr, Wilcox WS. Experimental evaluation of potential anticancer agents: XII. On the criteria and kinetics associated with "curability" of experimental leukemia. Cancer Chemother Rep 1964;35:1–111.

42. Skipper HE. Reasons for success and failure in treatment of murine leukemias with the drugs now employed in treating human leukemias. In: Cancer chemotherapy. Vol 1. Ann Arbor, MI: University Microfilms International, 1978:1–166.

43. Skipper HE, Schabel FM Jr, Mellet LB, et al. Implications of biochemical, cytokinetic, pharmacologic, and toxicologic relationships in the design of optimal therapeutic schedules. Cancer Chemother Rep 1950;54:431–450.

44. Yankee RA, DeVita VT, Perry S. The cell cycle of leukemia L1210 cells in vivo. Cancer Res 1968;27:2381–2385.

45. Norton LA. A Gompertzian model of human breast cancer growth. Cancer Res 1988;48:7067–7071.

46. Bloom H, Richardson M, Harris B. Natural history of untreated breast cancer (1804–1933): Comparison of treated and untreated cases according to histologic grade of malignancy. Med J 1962;2:213.

47. Schabel FM Jr, Simpson-Herren L. Some variables in experimental tumor systems which complicate interpretation of data from in vivo kinetic and pharmacologic studies with anticancer drugs. Antibiot Chemother 1978;23:113–127.

48. Freireich EJ, Gehan EA, Rall DP, et al. Quantitative comparison of toxicity of anticancer agents in mouse, rat, dog, monkey and man. Cancer Chemother Rep 1966;50:219–244.

49. Epstein RA. Drug-induced DNA damage and tumor chemosensitivity. J Clin Oncol 1990;8:2062–2084.

50. Brockman RW. Circumvention of resistance: Pharmacologic basis of cancer chemotherapy. In: Proceedings of the 27th Annual Symposium on Fundamental Research. Baltimore: Williams & Wilkins, 1975;691–711.

51. DeVita VT Jr, Young RC, Canellos GP. Combination versus single agent chemotherapy: Review of the basis of selection of drug treatment of cancer. Cancer 1975;35:98.

52. Hutchinson DJ, Schmid FA. Cross-resistance and collateral sensitivity. In: Mihich E, ed. Drug resistance and selectivity: Biochemical and cellular basis. New York: Academic Press, 1973:73–126.

53. Hutchinson DJ. Cross-resistance and collateral sensitivity studies in cancer chemotherapy. In: Haddow A, Weinhouse S, eds. Advances in cancer research. Vol 7. New York: Academic Press, 1963:235–350.

54. Klein M. A mechanism for the development of resistance to streptomycin and penicillin. J Bacteriol 1947;53:463–467.

55. Furth J, Kahn MC. The transmission of leukemia of mice with a single cell. Am J Cancer 1937;31:276–282.

56. Goldin A, Venditti JM, Humphries SR, et al. Influences of the concentration of leukemic inoculum on the effectiveness of treatment. Science 1956;123:840.

57. Ozols RJ, Cowan KH. New aspects of clinical drug resistance: The role of gene amplification and the reversal of drug refractory cancer. In: DeVita VT Jr, Hellman S, Rosenberg SA, eds. Important advances in oncology 1986. Philadelphia: JB Lippincott, 1986:129–157.

58. Biedler JL, Riehm H. Cellular resistance to actinomycin D in Chinese hamster cells in vitro: Cross-resistance, radioautographic and cytogenic studies. Cancer Res 1970;30:1174–1184.

59. Juliano RL, Ling V. A surface glycoprotein modulating drug permeability in Chinese hamster ovary cell mutants. Biochem Biophys Acta 1976;455:152–162.

60. Bech-Hanson NT, Till JE, Ling V. Pleiotropic phenotype of colchicine-resistant CHO cells: Cross-resistance and collateral sensitivity. J Cell Physiol 1976;88:23–32.

61. Ling V, Thompson LH. Reduced permeability in CHO cells as a mechanism of resistance to colchicine. J Cell Physiol 1973;83:103–116.

62. Kartner N, Riordan JR, Ling V. Cell surface P-glycoprotein as associated with multidrug resistance in mammalian cell lines. Science 1983;221:1285–1288.

63. Fojo AT, Whang-Peng J, Gottesman MM, et al. Amplification of DNA sequences in human multidrug resistant KB carcinoma cells. Proc Natl Acad Sci USA 1985;82:7661–7665.

64. Gros P, Croop J, Roninson I, et al. Isolation and characterization of DNA sequences amplified in multidrug-resistant hamster cells. Proc Natl Acad Sci USA 1986;83:337–341.

65. Fairchild CR, Ivy SP, Kao-Shan CS, et al. Isolation of amplified DNA sequences associated with pleiotropic drug resistance from human breast cancer cells. Cancer Res 1987;47:5141–5148.

66. Scotto KW, Biedler JL, Melera PW. Amplification and expression of genes associated with multidrug resistance in mammalian cells. Science 1986;232:751–755.

67. Roninson IB, Abelson HT, Housman DE, et al. Amplification of specific DNA sequences correlates with multidrug resistance in Chinese hamster cells. Nature 1984;309:2070–2076.

68. Corwell MM, Safa AR, Felsted RL, et al. Membrane vesicles from multidrug-resistant human cancer cells contain a specific 150 to 170-kDa protein detected by photoaffinity labelling. Proc Natl Acad Sci USA 1986;83:3847–3850.

69. Safa AR, Glover CI, Meyers CB, et al. Vinblastine photoaffinity labeling of a high molecular weight surface membrane glycoprotein specific for multidrug-resistant cells. J Biol Chem 1986;261:6137–6140.

70. Cornwell MM, Pastan I, Gottesman MM. Certain calcium channel blockers bind specifically to multidrug-resistant human KB carcinoma membrane vesicles and inhibit drug binding to P-glycoprotein. J Biol Chem 1987;262:2166–2170.

71. Gros P, Croop J, Housman D. Mammalian multidrug-resistance gene: Complete cDNA sequence indicates strong homology to bacterial transport proteins. Cell 1986;47:371–374.

72. Chen C-J, Chin JE, Ueda K, et al. Internal duplication and homology to bacterial transport proteins in the mdr1 (P-glycoprotein) gene from multidrug-resistant human cells. Cell 1986;47:381–389.

73. Gerlach JH, Endicott JA, Juranka PF, et al. Homology between P-glycoprotein and a bacterial haemolysin transport protein suggests a model for multidrug resistance. Nature 1986;324:485–489.

74. Pasten IH, Gottesman MM. Molecular biology of multidrug resistance in human cells. In: DeVita VT, Hellman S, Rosenberg SA, eds. Important advances in oncology 1988. Philadelphia: JB Lippincott, 1988:3–16.

75. Fojo AT, Ueda K, Slamon DJ, et al. Expression of a multidrug-resistant gene in human tumors and tissues. Proc Natl Acad Sci USA 1987;84:265–269.

76. Chaudhary PM, Roninson IB. Expressions and activity of P-glycoprotein, a multidrug efflux pump, in human hematopoietic stem cells. Cell 1991;66:85–94.

77. Endicott JA, Juranka PF, Sarangi F, et al. Simultaneous expression of two P-glycoprotein genes in drug sensitive Chinese hamster ovary cells. Mol Cell Biol 1987;7:4075–4081.

78. Gros P, Ben Neriah Y, Croop JM, et al. Isolation and expression of a complementary cDNA that confers multidrug resistance. Nature 1986;323:728–731.

79. Van Der Bliek AM, Baas F, Ten Houte de Lange T, et al. The human *MDR3* gene encodes a novel P-glycoprotein homologue and gives rise to alternatively spliced mRNAs in liver. EMBO J 1987;6:3325–3331.

80. Goldstein IJ, Glaskic H, Fojo A, et al. Expression of a multidrug resistant gene in human cancers. JNCI 1989;81:116–124.

81. Cordon-Cardo C, O'Brien JP, Boccin J, et al. Expression of the multidrug resistance gene product (P-glycoprotein) in human normal and tumor tissues. J Histochem Cytochem 1990;38:1277–1287.

82. Cordon-Cardo C, O'Brien JP, Casals D, et al. Multidrug-resistance gene (P-glycoprotein) is expressed by endothelial cells at blood-brain barrier sites. Proc Natl Acad Sci USA 1989;86:695–698.

83. Weinstein RS, Kusaac JR, Kluskons LF, et al. P-glycoprotein in pathology: The multidrug resistance gene family in humans. Human Pathol 1990;21:34–48.

84. Cordon-Cardo C, O'Brien JP. The multidrug resistance phenotype in human cancer. In: DeVita VT, Hellman S, Rosenberg SA, eds. Important advances in oncology 1991. Philadelphia: JB Lippincott, 1991:19–39.

85. Marsh W, Center MS. Adriamycin resistance in HL60 cells and accompanying modifications of a membrane protein contained in drug-sensitive cells. Cancer Res 1987;47:5080–5086.

86. Danks MK, Yalowich JC, Bech WT. Atypical multiple drug resistance in a human leukemic cell line selected for resistance to teniposide (VM-26). Cancer Res 1987;47:1297–1301.

87. Ross WE, Sullivan DM, Chow KC. Altered function of DNA topoisomerases as a basis for antineoplastic drug action. In: DeVita VT, Hellman S, Rosenberg S, eds. Important advances in oncology 1988. Philadelphia: JB Lippincott, 1988:65–81.

88. Liu LF, D'Arpa P. Topoisomerase-targeting antitumor drugs: Mechanisms of cytotoxicity and resistance. In: DeVita VT, Hellman S, Rosenberg SA, eds. Important advances in oncology 1992. Philadelphia: JB Lippincott, 1992:79–93.

89. Glisson B, Gupta R, Hodges P, et al. Cross resistance to intercalating agents in an epipodophyllotoxin-resistant Chinese hamster ovary cell line: Evidence for a common intracellular target. Cancer Res 1986;46:1939–1942.

90. Pommier Y, Kerrigan D, Schwartz RE, et al. Altered DNA topoisomerase II activity in Chinese hamster cells resistant to topoisomerase II inhibitors. Cancer Res 1986;46:3075–3081.

91. Skipper H. Data and analyses having to do with the influence of dose intensity and duration of treatment (single drugs and combinations) on lethal toxicity and the therapeutic response of experimental neoplasms. Birmingham: Southern Research Institute, Booklets 13, 1986, and 2–13, 1987.

92. DeVita VT, Hubbard SM, Longo DL. The chemotherapy of lymphomas: Looking back, moving forward—The Richard and Linda Rosenthal Foundation Award Lecture. Cancer Res 1987;47:5810–5824.

93. Hryniuk WM. The importance of dose intensity in the outcome of chemotherapy. In: DeVita VT, Hellman S, Rosenberg SA, eds. Important advances in oncology 1988. Philadelphia: JB Lippincott, 1988:121–142.

94. Hryniuk W, Levine MN. Analysis of dose intensity for adjuvant chemotherapy trials in stage II breast cancer. J Clin Oncol 1986;4:1162–1170.

95. Hryniuk WM. Average relative dose intensity and the impact on design on clinical trials. Semin Oncol 1987;14:65–74.

96. Levin L, Hryniuk W. Dose intensity analysis of chemotherapy regimens in ovarian carcinoma. J Clin Oncol 1987;5:756–767.

97. Hryniuk W, Bush H. The importance of dose intensity in chemotherapy of metastatic breast cancer. J Clin Oncol 1984;2:1281–1288.

98. Hryniuk W. Is more better? J Clin Oncol [Editorial] 1986;4:621–622.

99. Canellos GP, Pocock SJ, Taylor SG III, et al. Combination chemotherapy for metastatic breast cancer: Prospective comparison of multiple drug therapy with L-phenylalanine mustard. Cancer 1976;38:1882–1886.

100. Canellos GP, DeVita VT, Gold GL, et al. Cyclical combination chemotherapy for advanced breast cancer. Br Med J 1974;1:218–220.

101. Bonadonna G, Brusamalino MP, Valagussa R, et al. Combination chemotherapy as an adjuvant treatment in operable breast cancer. N Engl J Med 1976;298:405–410.

102. Bonadonna G, Valagussa R. Dose-response effect of adjuvant chemotherapy in breast cancer. N Engl J Med 1981;304:10–15.

103. Horton J, Olson KB, Sullivan J, et al: 5-Fluorouracil in cancer: An improved regimen. Ann Intern Med 1970;78:897–900.

104. Grage TB, Moss SE. Adjuvant chemotherapy in cancer of the colon and rectum: Demonstration of effectiveness of prolonged 5-FU chemotherapy in a prospectively controlled randomized trial. Surg Clin North Am 1981;61:1321–1329.

105. Higgins GA, Dwight RW, Smith JV, et al. Fluorouracil as an adjuvant to surgery in carcinoma of the colon. Arch Surg 1971;102:339–343.

106. Higgins GA Jr, Humphrey E, Juler GL, et al. Adjuvant chemotherapy in the surgical treatment of large bowel cancer. Cancer 1976;38:1461–1467.

107. Goldin A, Schepartz SA, Venditti JM, et al. Historical development and current strategy of the National Cancer Institute Drug Development Program. In: DeVita VT, Busch H, eds. Methods of cancer research. Vol XVI, Cancer drug development, part A. New York: Academic Press, 1979:165–247.

108. Zubrod CG, Schepartz S, Leiter J, et al. The chemotherapy program of the National Cancer Institute: History, analysis, and plans. Cancer Chemother Rep 1966;50:349–540.

109. Hirschberg E. Patterns of response of animal tumors to anticancer agents. Cancer Res 1963;23(suppl 5, part 2):521–980.

110. Driscoll JS. The preclinical new drug research program of the National Cancer Institute. Cancer Treat Rep 1984;68:63–76.

111. Shoemaker RH, Wolpert-DeFilippes MK, Venditti JM. Potentials and drawbacks of the human tumor stem cell assay. Behring Inst Mitt 1984;74:262–272.

112. Rockwell S. Effects of clumps and clusters on survival measurements with clonogenic assays. Cancer Res 1985;45:1601–1607.

113. Shoemaker RH, Wolpert-DeFilippes MK, Kern DH, et al. Application of a human tumor colony-forming assay to new drug screening. Cancer Res 1985;45:2145–2153.

114. Boyd M, Shoemaker R, Alley M, et al. New NCI disease-oriented drug screening program. In: Proceedings of the 5th NCI-EORTC Symposium on New Drugs in Cancer Therapy, Amsterdam, 1986.

115. Boyd MR, Shoemaker RH, McLemore TL, et al. New drug development. In: Roth JA, Ruckdescel JC, Weisenburger THE, eds. Thoracic oncology. Philadelphia: WB Saunders, 1987.

116. Mosmann T. Rapid colorimetric assay for cellular growth and survival: Application to proliferation and cytotoxicity assays. J Immunol Methods 1983;65:55–63.

117. Shoemaker RH. New approaches to antitumor drug screening: The human tumor colony forming assay. Cancer Treat Rep 1986;70:9–12.

118. Rozencweig M, Von Hoff DD, Staquet MJ, et al. Predictive value of animal toxicology with anticancer agents prior to early clinical trials. Clin Res [Abstract] 1979;27(2):391A.

119. DeVita VT, Oliverio VT, Muggia FM, et al. The drug development program and clinical trials programs of the Division of Cancer Treatment, National Cancer Institute. Cancer Clin Trials 1979;2:195–216.

120. Muggia FM, Rozencweig M, Chiuten DF, et al. Phase II trials: Use of a clinical tumor panel and overview of current resources and studies. Cancer Treat Rep 1980;64:1–9.

121. Wooley PV, Schein PS. Clinical pharmacology and phase I trial design. In: DeVita VT, Busch H, eds. Methods in cancer research. Vol XVII, Cancer drug development, part B. New York: Academic Press, 1979:177–199.

122. Muggia FM, McGuire WP, Rozencweig M. Rationale, design and methodology of phase II clinical trials. In: DeVita VT, Busch H, eds. Methods in cancer research. Vol XVII, Cancer drug development, part B. New York: Academic Press, 1979:199–215.

123. Collins JM, Zaharko DS, Dedrick RL, et al. Potential roles for preclinical pharmacology in phase I clinical trials. Cancer Treat Rep 1986;70:73.

124. Goldin A, Venditti JM. Progress report on the screening program at the Division of Cancer Treatment, National Cancer Institute. Cancer Treat Rev 1980;7:167.

125. Marsoni S, Hoth D, Simon R, et al. Clinical drug development: An analysis of phase II trials, 1970–1985. Cancer Treat Rep 1987;71:71.

Cancer: Principles & Practice of Oncology, Fourth Edition,
edited by Vincent T. DeVita, Jr., Samuel Hellman, Steven A. Rosenberg.
J.B. Lippincott Co., Philadelphia © 1993.

Steven A. Rosenberg

CHAPTER **17**

Principles and Applications of Biologic Therapy

Biologic therapy is cancer treatment that produces antitumor effects primarily through the action of natural host defense mechanisms or the administration of natural mammalian substances. Biologic therapy has emerged as an important fourth modality for the treatment of cancer (reviewed by DeVita and colleagues).[1] Its increased application is the result of a better understanding of the basic aspects of host defense mechanisms against cancer and rapid biotechnologic developments that made molecules available in quantities large enough for use in manipulating biologic processes in vivo. Although this field is still in its infancy, there are many examples of the successful application of biologic therapy to human cancers.

BASIC PRINCIPLES OF TUMOR IMMUNOLOGY

Most applications of biologic therapy for cancer have attempted to stimulate immune defense mechanisms. The immune system evolved as a means to detect and eliminate molecules or pathogens that are recognized as "nonself" but not react to host (self) tissues. Many immunotherapies attempted to cause the tumor to appear more "foreign" compared with normal tissues or tried to magnify relatively weak host immune reactions to growing tumors.

The immune system differs from most other organ systems because its cells are not in constant contact with each other. They circulate freely throughout the body in and out of the circulatory and lymphatic systems. Immune reactivity involves the integrated action of lymphocytes, monocytes, macrophages, basophils, eosinophils, dendritic cells, endothelial cells, and many other cells throughout the body. Although separate functions have been assigned to these cell types, it is now clear that they interact in many ways and can regulate each other's activities.

Immune cells secrete two major classes of soluble protein. The first of these lymphocyte products to be recognized was the antibody. Antibodies are a group of proteins composed of one or several units, each of which is composed of two pairs of different polypeptide chains (*i.e.*, heavy and light chains). Each unit possesses two recognition sites, which are capable of combining with the immunizing antigen. The unique bond between antigen and antibody is part of the basis for the exquisite specificity that is the hallmark of immunologic reactivity. The existence of circulating antibodies was first demonstrated in 1890, and until recently, scientific studies of antibodies monopolized the study of immune reactions.

During the past 20 years, it became clear that selected subpopulations of lymphoid cells can secrete a second (nonantibody) class of protein molecules. These molecules are not biochemically similar to antibodies, are produced in tiny amounts, and are not normally detectable in the circulation. Collectively called cytokines, they represent a new class of hormones with actions on many different target cells within and outside the immune system. Increasing knowledge of a wide variety of cytokines has dramatically altered our understanding of the functions of the immune system and created new possibilities for cancer immunotherapy.

CELLS OF THE IMMUNE SYSTEM

The central cell in immune function is the lymphocyte. Lymphocytes constitute approximately 20% of blood leukocytes and fall into three major classes—B cells, T cells, and null cells—on the basis of ontogeny and function. Analysis of cell-surface molecules, usually using monoclonal antibodies, revealed substantial heterogeneity in human leukocytes and lymphocytes. In 1982, the First International Workshop on Human Leukocyte Differentiation Antigens was held in Paris to attempt to codify the proliferating number of cell-surface determinants detected on leukocytes and the antibodies used to detect them. As a result of the testing of large numbers of antibodies on target cells of many different leukocyte types, cluster analysis permitted the definition of groups of antigens that are similar and those that are clearly different on each type of target cell. This workshop defined the clusters of differentiation (CD), which are now used to describe cell-surface components on leukocytes. A summary of selected CD classifications, the cells on which they are found, and the principal antibodies that are used to detect them as assigned by the Fourth International Workshop are shown in Table 17–1.

In birds, B cells develop in a special organ called the bursa of Fabricius. There is no anatomic counterpart of this bursa in humans, and it is thought that human B cells develop in the bone marrow and acquire surface immunoglobulin, which acts as their antigen receptors. B cells also develop receptors for lymphokines, enabling their regulation by T-cell products. B cells require the presence of antigen and help from antigen-specific T cells to produce and secrete antibodies.

The term "T cells" was derived from the role of the thymus in the differentiation of these lymphocytes. Lymphoid cells produced in the bone marrow traffic to the thymus late in fetal life, differentiate there, and then seed secondary lymphoid tissues. In the thymus, T cells are thought to express antigen-specific receptors and to differentiate into the various T-cell subpopulations. Many lymphocytes die in the thymus during ontogeny, which is thought to be part of the mechanism for the loss of self-reactive clones. T cells are involved in cellular immune reactions and recognize antigen by means of receptor molecules quite distinct from the immunoglobulin found on B cells. The T-cell receptor is generated from the recombination of germline genes to produce a wide diversity of receptors that can bind antigen together with major histocompatibility complex (MHC) molecules. The generation of diversity in T-cell receptors is similar to that of antibodies. The T-cell receptor for antigen is associated with a glycoprotein complex, CD3, present on all mature human T cells. B cells can recognize antigen alone, but T cells recognize antigen in association with MHC molecules.

Although T cells were initially subtyped by functions (*e.g.*, helper, suppressor, cytotoxic), it is now possible to identify two major T-cell subsets, each of which is restricted to recognizing one of the two major classes of MHC molecules. Class I molecules (serologically defined as HLA-A, B, or C) are involved with the presentation of processed antigen to T cells expressing the CD8 molecule. Similarly, MHC class II molecules (currently recognized as DP, DQ, and DR) present antigen to T cells expressing the CD4 molecule. This molecule is the cellular target for the human immunodeficiency virus, and the profound immunodepression observed in the acquired immunodeficiency syndrome (AIDS) is probably related to the destruction of this T-cell subset. Helper and cytotoxic functions can be ascribed to cells of each lineage, and other antigens have been useful to further delineate functional subsets within each of these T-cell populations.

A third population of lymphocytes, null cells, express neither T-cell nor B-cell surface markers. These cells appear to be a distinct lineage of lymphoid cells that bear some T-cell markers early in differentiation and later acquire markers also present on macrophages and neutrophils. Although the principal function of null cells is unknown, natural killer (NK) cells and lymphokine-activated killer (LAK) cells are derived from this subpopulation. NK cells can lyse a select group of cultured cell lines without a known prior exposure to an immunizing stimulus. LAK cells develop the ability to kill fresh tumor cells after exposure of these lymphoid precursors to the lymphokine interleukin-2 (IL-2). Cells mediating antibody-dependent cellular cytotoxicity also are found in the null cell population.

Other important cells in the immune system are the reticuloendothelial cells, predominantly monocytes and macrophages. Monocytes are long-lived circulating cells that develop into tissue macrophages. Macrophages are highly phagocytic cells that possess a variety of physiologic protective functions. They are also capable of presenting antigen to lymphocytes and may play a role in carrying antigen from the periphery to other immune sites. Other cell types derived from bone-marrow stem cells play a similar antigen-presenting role, including the Langerhans cells of the skin, follicular dendritic cells in lymph nodes, B cells, and endothelial cells.

IMMUNE EFFECTOR MECHANISMS RESULTING IN CELL DESTRUCTION

A variety of immune effector mechanisms can cause destruction of vascularized tissue or of circulating tumor cells (Table 17–2).

Antibodies can mediate cell destruction by the binding of complement or by action as an opsonin to facilitate phagocytosis by macrophages or by other phagocytic cells bearing Fc receptors.

The direct interaction of an immune cell with a target cell can also result in lysis, and a variety of immune cytotoxic cells have been described. The best-characterized lytic immune cell is the cytotoxic T lymphocyte (CTL). These T cells can interact with specific cell-surface antigens by an interaction with the T-cell receptor and a class I or II MHC molecule. This lysis appears to involve direct cell contact and can occur quickly, with the initial lytic events initiated within minutes of the adhesion of the target cell to the lymphocyte. Although binding of the CTL to the tumor target occurs by means of the T-cell receptor, other means for binding lytic cells to targets also produce lysis. One such mechanism is antibody-dependent cellular cytotoxicity. In this lysis, antibody bound to immune cells serves as a crosslink to a cytolytic cell bearing an Fc receptor. The Fc receptor on the immune effector binds to the free Fc portion of the antibody on the target cell; after this cross-linkage, lysis of the target cell occurs. Similarly, the phenomenon of lectin-dependent cellular

TABLE 17–1. Workshop Antigen Designation by the Nomenclature Committee of the Fourth International Workshop on Human Leukocyte Differentiation Antigens (to be Approved by IUIS/WHO)*

CD Designation	Selection of Assigned Monoclonal Antibodies	Main Cellular Reactivity	Recognized Membrane Component	Sequence/ CH-Structure Analyzed
CD1a	NA1/34; T6; VIT6; Leu-6	Thy, DC, B subset	gp49	Y
CD1b	WM-25; 4A76; NUT2	Thy, DC, B subset	gp45	Y
CD1c	L161; M241; 7C6; PHM3	Thy, DC, B subset	gp43	Y
CD2	9.6; T11; 35.1	T	CD58 (LFA-3) receptor, gp50	Y
CD2R	T11.3; VIT13; D66	Act. T	CD2 epitopes restr. to act. T	Y
CD3	T3; UCHT1; 38.1; Leu-4	T	CD3-complex (5 chains), gp/p26, 20, 16	Y
CD4	T4; Leu-3a; 91.D6	T subset	Class II/HIV receptor, gp59	Y
CD5	T1; UCHT2; T101; HH9; AMG4	T, B subset	gp67	Y
CD6	T12; T411	T, B subset	gp100	
CD7	3A1; 4A; CL1.3; G3–7	T	gp40	Y
CD8	α chain: T8; Leu-2a; M236; UCHT4; T811 β chain: T8/2T8-5H7	T subset	Class I receptor, gp32, αα or αβ dimer	Y
CD9	CLB-thromb/8; PHN200	Pre-B, M, Plt	p24	
CD10	J5, VILA1, BA-3	Lymph. Prog., cALL, Germ Ctr. B, G	Neutral endopeptidase, gp100, CALLA	Y
CD11a	MHM24; 2F12; CRIS-3	Leukocytes, broad	LFA-1, gp180/95	Y
CD11b	Mol; 5A4.C5; LPM19C	M, G, NK	C3bi receptor, gp155/95	
CD11c	B-LY6; L29; BL-4H4	M, G, NK, B sub	gp150/95	
CDw12	M67	M, G, Plt	(p90–120)	
CD13	MY7, MCS-2, TÜK1, MOU28	M, G	Aminopeptidase N, gp150	Y
CD14	Mo2, UCHM1, VIM13, MoP15	M, (G), LHC	gp55	Y
CD15	My1, VIM-D5	G, (M)	3-FAL, X-hapten	Y
CD16	BW209/2; HUNK2; VEP13; Leu-11c	NK, G, Mac.	FcRIII, gp50–65	Y
CDw17	GO35, Huly-m13	G, M, Plt	Lactosylceramide	
CD18	MHM23; M232; 11H6; CLB54	Leucocytes broad	β chain to CD11a,b,c	Y
CD19	B4; HD37	B	gp95	Y
CD20	B1; 1F5	B	p37/32, ion channel?	Y
CD21	B2; HB5	B subset	C3d/EBV rec. (CR2), p140	Y
CD22	HD39; S-HCL1; To15	Cytopl. B/surface B subset	gp135, homology to myelin assoc. gp (MAG)	Y
CD23	Blast-2, MHM6	B subset, act. M, Eo	FcεRII, gp45–50	Y
CD24	VIBE3; BA-1	B, G	gp41/38?	
CD25	TAC; 7G7/B6; 2A3	Activated T, B, M	IL-2R β chain, gp55	Y
CD26	134-2C2; TS145	Activated T	Dipeptidylpeptidase IV, gp120	Y
CD27	VIT14; S152; OKT18A; CLB-9F4	T subset	p55 (dimer)	
CD28	9.3; KOLT2	T subset	gp44	Y
CD29	K20; 4B4; A-1A5	Broad, T subset	VLA β-, integrin β1 chain, Plt GPIIa	Y
CD30	Ki-1; Ber-H2; HSR4	Activated T, B; Sternberg-Reed	gp120, Ki-1	
CD31	SG134; TM3	Plt, M, G, B, (T)	gp140, Plt GPIIa	
CDw32	CIKM5; 41H16; IV.3	M, G, B	FcRII, gp40	Y
CD33	My9; H153; L4F3	M, Prog., AML	gp67	Y
CD34	My10, B1-3C5, ICH-3	Prog	gp105–120	Y
CD35	TO5, CB04, J3D3	G, M, B	CR1	Y
CD36	5F1, CIMeg1	M, P, (B)	gp90, Plt GPIV	
CD37	HD28; HH1; G28-1	B, (T, M)	gp40–52	Y
CD38	HB7; T16	Lymph. Prog., PC, act. T	p45	Y
CD39	AC2; G28-2	B subset, (M)	gp70–100	
CD40	G28-5	B, carcinomas	gp50, homology to NGF receptor	Y
CD41	LO-PL3b; PBM 6.4; CLB-thromb/7	Plt	Plt GPIIb/IIIa complex	Y
CD42a	FMC25; BL-H6; GR-P	Plt	Plt GPIX, gp23	Y
CD42b	PHN89; PHN103; GN287	Plt	Plt GPIb, gp135/25	Y
CD43	OTH 71C5; G19-1; MEM-59	T, G, brain	Leukosialin, gp95	Y
CD44	GRHL1; F10-44-2; 33-383; BRIC35	T, G, brain, RBC	Pgp-1, gp80–95	Y
CD45	T29/33; BMAC 1; AB187	Leucocytes	LCA, T200	Y
CD45RA	G1-15; FB-11-13; 73.5	T subset, B, G, M	Restricted T200, gp220	Y

(continued)

TABLE 17–1. *(Continued)*

CD Designation	Selection of Assigned Monoclonal Antibodies	Main Cellular Reactivity	Recognized Membrane Component	Sequence/ CH-Structure Analyzed
CD45RB	PT17/26/16	T subset, B, G, M	Restricted T200	Y
CD45RO	UCHL1	T subset, B, G, M	Restricted T200, gp180	Y
CD46	HULYM5; 122-2; J4B	Leucocytes broad	Membrane cofactor protein (MCP), gp66/56	Y
CD47	BRIC 126; CIKM1; BRIC 125	Broad	gp47–52, N-linked glycan, Rh assoc.	
CD48	WM68; LO-MN25; J4-57	Leukocytes	gp41, PI-linked	
CDw49b	CLB-thromb/4; Gil4	Plt, act. T, Thy	VLA-α2 chain, Plt GP1a	Y
CDw49d	B5G10; HP2/1; HP1/3	M, T, B, LHC, Thy	VLA-α4 chain, gp150	
CDw49f	GoH3	Plt, (T)	VLA-α6 chain, gp140	
CDw50	101-1D2; 140-11	Leucocytes broad	gp180/108 PI-linked	
CD51	13C2; 23C6; NKI-M7; NKI-M9	Plt, (B)	VNR-α chain	Y
CDw52	097; YTH66.9; Campath-1	Leucocytes	Campath-1, gp21–28	
CD53	HI29; HI36; MEM-53; HD77	Leucocytes	gp32–40, PI-linked	
CD54	7F7; WEHI-CAMI	Broad, act.	ICAM-1	Y
CD55	143-30; BRIC 110; BRIC 128; F2B-7.2	Broad	Decay accelerating factor	Y
CD56	Leu-19; NKH1; FP2-11.14, L185	NK, act. lymphocytes	gp220/135, NKH1, isoform of N-CAM	Y
CD57	Leu-7; L183; L187	NK, T, B sub, brain	gp110, HNK1	
CD58	G26; BRIC 5; TS2/9	Leukocytes, epithel	LFA-3 gp40–65	Y
CD59	Y53.1; MEM-43	Broad	gp18–20	
CDw60	M-T32; M-T21; M-T41; UM4D4	T sub	NeuAc-NeuAc-Gal-	Y
CD61	Y2/51; CLB-thromb/1; VI-PL2; BL-E6	P, (B)	Integrin β3-, VNR-β chain, Plt GPIIIa	Y
CD62	CLB-thromb/6; CLB-thromb/5; RUU-SP1.18.1	Plt act.	GMP-140 (PADGEM), gp140	Y
CD63	RUU-SP2.28; CLB-gran/12	Plt act., M, G, T, B	gp53	
CD64	Mab32.2; Mab22	M	FcRI, gp75	Y
CDw65	VIM2; HE10; CF4; VIM8	G, M	Ceramide-dodecasaccharide 4c	Y
CD66	CLB gran/10; YTH71.3	G	Phosphoprotein pp 180–200	
CD67	B13.9; G10F5; JML-H16	G	p100, PI-linked	
CD68	EBM11; Y2//131; Y-1/82A; Ki-M7; Ki-M6	Macrophages	gp110	
CD69	MLR3; L78; BL-Ac/p26; FN50	Act. B, T	gp32/28, AIM	
CDw70	Ki-24; HNE 51; HNC 142	Act. B, -T, Sternberg-Reed cells	Ki-24	
CD71	138-18; 120-2A3; MEM-75; VIP-1; Nu-T1R2	Proliferating cells, Mac.	Transferrin receptor	Y
CD72	S-HCL2; J3-109; BU-40; BU-41	B	gp43/39	
CD73	1E9.28.1; 7G2.2.11; AD2	B subset, T subset	Ecto-5′-nucleotidase, p69	
CD74	LN2; BU-43; BU-45	B, M	Class II assoc. invariant chain, gp41/35/33	
CDw75	LN1; HH2; EBU-141	Mature B, (T subset)	p53?	
CD76	HD66; CRIS-4	Mature B, T subset	gp85/67	
CD77	38.13(BLA); 424/4A11; 424/3D9	Restr. B	Globotriaosylceramide (Gb3)	
CDw78	Anti-Ba; LO-panB-a; 1588	B, (M)	?	

Thy, thymocytes; DC, dendritic cells; B, B cells; T, T cells; M, monocytes; Plt, platelets; G, granulocytes; Prog, progenitor cells; Germ Ctr. B, germinal center B cells; NK, natural killer cells; Mac., macrophages; Cytopl., cytoplasmic; Sternberg-Reed, Reed-Sternberg cells; LHC, epidermal Langerhans cells; Epithel, epithelial cells; act., activated; NGF, nerve growth factor; Eo, eosinophil; PC, plasma cell.
* Members: Workshop Council: A. Bernard, P. Beverley, L. Boumsell, T. Kishimoto, W. Knapp, A. McMichael, C. Milstein, S. F. Schlossman, E. Reinherz, G. Riethmüller, T. A. Springer, R. Winchester. Workshop Organizers: T-Cell Section: P. Rieber, R. Kurrle, S. Meuer. B-Cell Section: B. Dörken, G. Moldenhauer, P. Möller, A. Pezzutto, R. Schwartz-Albiez. Myeloid Antigen Section: W. Knapp, P. Bettelheim, S. Gadd, U. Köller, O. Majdic, C. Peschel, T. Radaszkiewicz, H. Stockinger, P. A. T. Tetteroo, E. van der Schot. NK-/NL-Section: R. E. Schmidt. A. C. Feller, M. R. Hadam, J. Johnson, J. Schubert, R. Schwinzer, M. Stoll, P. Uciechowski, K. Wonigeit. Activation Antigen Section: H. Stein, R. Schwarting. Platelet Section: A. E. G. Kr.v.d. Borne, L. G. de Bruijne-Admiraal, P. W. Modderman, H. K. Niewenhuis, Statistics Section: W. R. Gilks, L. Oldfield, A. Rutherford.
(From J Immunol 1989;143:758–759)

TABLE 17–2. Immune Effector Mechanisms Resulting in Cell Destruction

Antibody-mediated lysis (plus complement or antibody as an opsonin for macrophages and other Fc-receptor-positive cells).
Direct cell-mediated lysis
    Cytotoxic T lymphocytes
    Antibody-dependent cellular cytotoxicity
    Lectin-dependent cellular cytotoxicity
    Natural killer cells
    Lymphokine-activated killer cells
    Macrophage lysis
Release of toxic mediators from lymphocytes and other immune cells

cytotoxicity involves the association of a lytic cell with a target using a lectin such as concanavalin A or phytohemagglutinin as the cross-linking agent.

The NK cells can lyse selected cultured target cells without a prior sensitizing stimulus. The most common target for NK cells is the K562 leukemia cell line. NK lymphocytes have little or no ability to kill fresh tumor cells, and their physiologic role as an antitumor effector mechanism is unclear.

LAK cells are lymphocytes that acquire the ability to lyse a broad array of tumor cells after incubation in IL-2. The precursor of LAK cells is a null lymphocyte, and most mature LAK cells do not bear T-cell or B-cell markers. However, one subpopulation of LAK cells has been shown to be CD3 positive, and precursor and effector LAK cells appear to bear the Leu-19 cell-surface marker. LAK cells can lyse a broad array of malignant, but not normal, fresh target cells in 4-hour chromium-release assays. LAK cells also can lyse normal and malignant cultured lines. LAK cells are capable of lysing most cells that have their membranes perturbed by malignant transformation, culture, or other activation processes.

Activated macrophages also recognize and lyse tumor cells. Although most lymphocyte-mediated lysis can easily be detected in 4 hours, the measurement of significant macrophage-mediated lysis often requires 48 to 72 hours.

Many of the cytokines secreted by immune cells can mediate toxicity of tissue directly or by the recruitment of other inflammatory processes. For example, tumor necrosis factor can interfere with the blood supply of tumors. Interferon-γ has an antiproliferative effect on some tumor cells. Many chemotactic and vascular permeability factors that are involved in inflammatory responses also can indirectly mediate tumor destruction and may play a role in tumor immune phenomena.

CYTOKINES

Cytokines are soluble proteins produced by mononuclear cells of the immune system (usually lymphocytes or monocytes) that have regulatory actions on other cells of the immune system or target cells involved in immune reactions. Cytokines produced by lymphocytes are referred to as lymphokines, and cytokines produced by monocytes are referred to as monokines. Cytokines are true hormones, acting on other cells at a distance from the secreting cells.

It has been known for 25 years that the soluble substances produced by immune cells are involved in immune function and regulation. These cytokines were first identified by the function they exhibit in in vitro assays. Lymphokines that inhibited the migration of macrophages were known as migration-inhibition factors, and other factors that activated macrophages were known as macrophage-activation factors. This identification of cytokines on the basis of function led to a confusing situation in which the same molecules were often described by various investigators using different assays for their detection.

Substantial progress in this field resulted from the use of molecular biologic techniques to clone the genes for these cytokines, express them in bacteria, purify them to homogeneity, and produce large amounts of homogenous cytokines for detailed study. A new nomenclature referring to cytokines as interleukins (meaning "between leukocytes") has been introduced that supplants the acronyms based on functional properties. In 1979, a meeting of the Second International Lymphokine Workshop in Ermatingen, Switzerland, reached a consensus that a variety of lymphokines that had been referred to as T-cell growth factor, thymocyte-stimulating factor, thymocyte mitogenic factor, killer-cell helper factor costimulator, and secondary CTL-inducing factor were all the same molecule and should be referred to as IL-2. The term "interleukin-1" was adopted to refer to a monocyte product previously called lymphocyte-activating factor. Since that time, many cytokines have been described, some of which are listed in Tables 17–3 and 17–4. This list is rapidly expanding as new hormones produced by cells of the immune system are described. Each of the cytokines has multiple names, as shown in Table 17–5. The principal cell sources of the individual cytokines are shown in Table 17–6.[2]

Cytokines are proteins or glycoproteins, mostly with molecular weights in the range of 15,000 to 40,000, and many are glycosylated, although it appears that the glycosylation is often not essential for function. In many cases, the cytokines described in mouse and man are structurally related. For example, IL-1α shows a 61% to 65% amino acid homology among human, rabbit, and mouse. Some lymphokines exhibit species specificity; for example, IL-1, IL-2, IL-5, and IL-6 derived from man are active on cells from mouse and man, but IL-3, IL-4, and interferon-γ (INF-γ) derived from man are active only on human cells and not on mouse cells.

Each cytokine presumably reacts with receptors specific for that cytokine on the cell surface. Little is known about most cytokine receptors, except the IL-2 receptor, which is present in low-, intermediate-, and high-affinity forms, depending on the specific aggregation of 55-kd and 75-kd polypeptide chain receptors.

Most research on cytokines has involved in vitro studies or animal studies. Many cytokines, such as INF-α, INF-β, INF-γ, IL-2, tumor necrosis factor, and the colony-stimulating factors, have reached clinical application in patients with cancer. The clinical uses of colony-stimulating factors are discussed in Chapter 62.

TUMOR ANTIGENS

Immune Response to Tumors in Rodents and Humans

Early attempts to identify tumor antigens in mouse models by immunizing mice with spontaneous or carcinogen-induced

(text continues on page 301)

TABLE 17–3. Interleukins and Their Biologic Activities

Interleukin	Molecular Weight (kd)*	Biologic Effects	References
IL-1α and β	14–17	Costimulates T cells; induces IL-2 production; increased IL-2 receptor number and binding; growth-factor activation; induction/release of other cytokines; augments IL-2-induced LAK activity; induces CSF production by accessory cells; hemopoietin 1 activity; activates endothelial cells and macrophages; induces acute-phase responses; mediates catabolic processes, inflammation, and nonspecific resistance to infection; enhances growth of virulent strains of *E. coli*; costimulates proliferation and differentiation of B cells; induces maturation of pre-B cells	5–10
IL-2	15	Costimulates T cells; activates cytotoxic responses in T cells; stimulates monocytes to become tumoricidal; chemotactic for T cells; cofactor for growth and differentiation of B cells; induction/release of cytokines; induces non-MHC-restricted CTL killing; costimulates proliferation and differentiation of B cells	3, 7–9, 11–15
IL-3	28	Initiates growth of mature inducer T cells (Thy-1$^+$, Lyt-1$^+$, 2$^-$) and of Thy-1$^+$, Lyt-1$^-$, 2$^-$, T3$^+$ non-MHC-restricted CTL (in mouse); supports mast cell growth; stimulates early progenitor cell growth (erythrocyte, monocyte, granulocyte, megakaryocyte); supports growth of pre-B-cell lines	7–9, 16–19
IL-4	15–20 (≥60 hyperglycos-ylated)	Costimulates (in proliferation of normal resting T cells); stimulates thymocyte proliferation and differentiation to CTLs (in presence of lectin or phorbol myristate acetate); helper factor for CTL generation in primary MLC and induces/amplifies in vitro primed MLC memory cells; promotes growth of TILs cytotoxic for autologous human melanoma; generates LAK activity and augments IL-2-Induced LAK activity (in mouse); supports mast cell growth; synergizes with other growth factors to promote colony growth; induces monocyte cytotoxicity (in mouse); induces MHC class II antigens on B cells and monocytes; growth factor for activated B cells; increases expression of Fc$_c$ receptors; increases IgG1 and IgE secretion by B cells; decreases IgG2a, IgG2b, IgM, and IgG3 secretion by B cells	7–9, 20–26
IL-5	12–18 (45–60, hyperglycos-ylated)	Cofactor for induction of CTL differentiation; induces IL-2 receptor expression on T and B cells; causes release of soluble IL-2 receptor; enhances IL-2-mediated LAK activity (in mouse); induces proliferation and differentiation of eosinophil precursors; increases proliferation of activated normal B cells; increases IgA and IgM secretion by B cells	7–9, 25–29
IL-6†	21–29	Costimulates T cells; induces IL-2 production; CTL differentiation factor; augments human NK and LAK cytotoxicity; augments human and mouse ADCC; enhances MHC class I expression; enhances tumor-associated antigen (CEA) expression on human colorectal adenocarcinoma cells; induces acute phase responses; synergizes with other growth factors to promote colony growth; enhances Ig secretion by B cells; induces B-cell differentiation	4, 7–9, 30–34
IL-7	25	Costimulates purified T cells (in presence of Con A or PMA); induces LAK activity; generates and expands allospecific CTL and antitumor CTL; induces cytokine secretion and tumoricidal activity by human monocytes; supports the growth of B-cell precursors	9, 35–38
PF4 Superfamily (IL-8, RANTES/ SIS)	8–16	Strongly chemotactic for neutrophils, T and B cells, and monocytes; enhnaces or inhibits growth of hematopoietic progenitors (depending on cofactor)	39–40
IL-9	32–39	Stimulates antigen-specific T helper cell clones; stimulates mast cell growth; supports erythroid colony formation; potentiates IL-4-induced IgE synthesis by B cells	41–47
IL-10	17–21	Cytokine synthesis inhibitory factor for T helper-1 cells; inhibits macrophage activity and monocyte-dependent stimulation of NK cell production of IFN-γ; costimulates with IL-2 or IL-4 the proliferation of activated but not resting T cells; increases the number of CTL precursors; augments CTL activity; stimulates B cell proliferation; increases MHC class II molecules on unstimulated B cells; increases viability of resting B cells; costimulates (with IL-3 or IL-4) enhanced growth of mast cell lines and progenitors	48–55
IL-11	24	No T-cell or NK/LAK activities defined; stimulates T-cell-dependent development of Ig-producing B cells; synergizes with IL-3 in supporting megakaryocyte colony formation; supports the proliferation of committed macrophage progenitors	56, 57

(continued)

TABLE 17–3. *(Continued)*

Interleukin	Molecular Weight (kd)*	Biologic Effects	References
Il-12	75 (heterodimer of 40 and 35 subunits)	Stimulates antigen-activated CD4$^+$ and CD8$^+$ T cells (independent of IL-2); synergizes with IL-2 in induction of CTL and additive with IL-2 and CTL proliferation; enhances NK activity; stimulates IFN-γ secretion by resting and activated human PBLs	58–61

IL, interleukin; CSF, colony stimulating factor; LAK, lymphokine-activated killer cell; CTL, cytotoxic T lymphocyte; MHC, major histocompatibility complex; MLC, mixed lymphocyte culture; TIL, tumor-infiltrating lymphocyte; ADCC, antibody dependent cellular cytotoxicity; CEA, carcinoembryonic antigen; NK, natural killer cell; Con A, concanavalin A; PMA, phorbol myristate acetate; kd, kilodalton; PF4, platelet factor-4; PBL, peripheral blood lymphocyte.
* Molecular weights vary with degree of glycosylation; all interleukins except IL-12, are single polypeptide chains. IL-10 shares extensive sequence homology and biologic activity to an open reading frame in the Epstein-Barr virus BCRF1; this suggests that BCRF1 may play an important role in EBV's interaction with the infected host's immune system.
† Originally termed IFN-β2; its antiviral activities are disputed.
(Mulé JJ, Rosenberg, SA. Catalogue of cytokines. Biol Ther Cancer Updates 1992;2:1–11)

TABLE 17–4. Interferons, Colony Stimulating Factors, and Tumor Necrosis Factor With Their Biologic Activities

Cytokine	Molecular Weight (kd)*	Biologic Effects	References
IFN-α or β1†	16–27	Antiproliferative to certain tumor cells; promotes partial reversal of the malignant phenotype; enhances the expression of surface molecules, including β2-microglobulin, Fc receptors, tumor-associated antigens, and MHC class I antigens; augments NK activity; modulates B-cell function; inhibits suppressor T-cell activity; activates monocytes/macrophages; exerts antiviral activity; interacts (enhance, inhibit) with growth factors, oncogenes and other cytokines; activates CTL	62
IFN-γ	15.5–25	Exerts antiviral activity; augments NK activity; induces expression of MHC class I and II molecules; activates macrophages; interacts (enhance, inhibit) with other cytokines; induces IL-2 receptors; mediates antimicrobial activity; regulates lipid metabolism; induces B-cell Ig production; suppresses IL-4 activities on B cells; activates CTL; enhances tumor-associated antigen expression; regulates differentiation	
TNF-α‡	17 (secretory), 26 (membrane form)	Stimulates T-cell proliferation; enhances NK activity; induces macrophage tumoricidal activity; directly cytotoxic to some tumor cells; induces systemic acute phase responses; activities PMNs; costimulates mitogen activated B cells; enhances expression of MHC class I and class II molecules; stimulates production of other cytokines, including colony stimulating factors; affects (reduces or increases) expression of oncogene products; induces cytokine receptor expression; activates endothelial cells (expression of adhesion molecules); mediates catabolic processes, septic shock and inflammation; induces myeloid differentiation	63–66
G-CSF	20–25	Stimulates growth of granulocyte colonies; activates mature granulocytes; increases antibody-dependent, neutrophil-mediated cytotoxicity; stimulates proliferation and differentiation of leukemic cells	19
GM-CSF	18–30	Stimulates growth of granulocyte, monocyte, and early erythrocyte progenitors; stimulates some megakaryocyte progenitors; enhances ADCC; activates mature granulocytes and monocytes; some stimulation of proliferation of leukemic progenitors; chemotactic for monocytes and PMNs; upregulates CR3 receptors on PMNs and monocytes; stimulates production of other cytokines (M-CSF and TNF) by monocytes	
M-CSF	45–70	Stimulates growth of monocyte colonies; supports survival of macrophages; activates mature monocytes; enhances ADCC by monocytes; stimulates	

(continued)

TABLE 17–4. *(Continued)*

Cytokine	Molecular Weight (kd)*	Biologic Effects	References
		production/secretion of cytokines, plasminogen activator, oxygen reduction products, acidic isoferritins by macrophages; enhances Fc receptor, CR3 receptor and MHC class II expression on macrophages; stimulates macrophage pinocytosis; chemotactic	

IFN, interferon; PMN, polymorphonuclear leukocyte; TNF, tumor necrosis factor; CR3, complement receptor-3; G, granulocyte; M, macrophage; also see Table 17–3 footnote.
* Molecular weights vary according to level of glycosylation; G- and GM-CSF are single polypeptide chains, M-CSF is a homodimer.
† There exist >20 closely related genes for IFN-α (subtypes: 80–85% amino acid homology to each other; 90% nuclear homology); only a single gene for IFN-γ, and possibly two genes for IFN-β.
‡ TNF-β lymphotoxin (LT). LT is produced by lymphocytes, is approximately 30% homologous with TNF-α, acts at the same receptor, and shares multiple biologic activities with TNF-α. There may exist other members of this cytokine family that have yet to be purified, sequenced, and cloned; these proteins have been implicated in monocyte- and lymphocyte-mediated tumor cell killing and are not neutralized by monoclonal antibodies to TNF-α or TNF-β.
(Mulé JJ, Rosenberg SA. Catalogue of cytokines. Biol Ther Cancer Updates 1992; 2:1–11)

TABLE 17–5. Alternative Names of Recombinant Cytokines

Cytokine	Alternative Names
IL-1α or β	B-cell activating factor (BAF); B-cell differentiation factor (BDF); catabolin; endogenous pyrogen (EP); hematopoietin-1 (HP1); lymphocyte-activating factor (LAF); leukocyte endogenous mediator (LEM); mitogenic protein (MP); mononuclear cell factor (MCF); proteolysis-inducing factor (PIF); serum amyloid A (SAA) inducer; T-cell replacing factor III (TRF-III)
IL-2	Killer helper factor (KHF); T-cell-derived growth factor (TCGF); T-cell maturation/stimulating factor (TMF/TSF); T-cell replacing factor (TRF)
IL-3	Burst promoting activity (BPA); eosinophil colony stimulating factor (Eo-CSF); erythroid colony stimulating factor (ECSF); hemopoietic cell growth factor (HPGF); hematopoietin-2 (HP2); mast cell growth factor (MCGF); megakaryocyte colony stimulating factor (MEG-CSF); multipotential colony stimulating factor (Multi-CSF); persisting cell stimulating factor (PSF)
IL-4	B-cell growth factor (BCGF); B-cell stimulating factor-1 (BSF1); B-cell stimulating factor p1 (BSFp1); macrophage fusion factor (MFF); mast cell growth factor II (MCGF-II); T-cell growth factor II (TCGF-II)
IL-5	B-cell growth factor II (BCGF-II); eosinophil colony stimulating factor (Eo-CSF); eosinophil differentiation factor (EDF); IgA-enhancing factor (IgA-EF); killer helper factor (KHF); T-cell replacing factor (TRF)
IL-6	B-cell differentiation factor (BCDF); B cell stimulatory factor 2 (BSF-2); B-cell stimulatory factor p2 (BSFp2); HP-1; cytotoxic T-cell differentiation factor (CDF); hepatocyte stimulating factor (HSF); hybridoma/plasmacytoma growth factor (HPGF); interferon-β2 (IFN-β2); 26-kd protein
IL-7	Pre-B-cell growth factor (pBCGF)
IL-8 (PF4 superfamily)	Monocyte-derived neutrophil chemotactic factor (MDNCF); neutrophil activating factor/protein (NAF/NAP); neutrophil chemotactic factor (NCF); T-cell chemotactic factor (TCF)
RANTES/SIS (PF4 superfamily)	Family members include the cytokines: Regulated on activation, normal T expressed and secreted (RANTES); I-309; macrophage inflammatory protein-1α or β (MIP-1α or β); monocyte chemotactic protein-1 (MCP1); HC14
IL-9	40-kd protein (P40)
IL-10	Cytokine synthesis inhibitory factor (CSIF); B-cell-derived T-cell growth factor (B-TCGF); mast cell growth factor III (MCGF-III)
IL-11	No alternative names associated
IL-12	Cytotoxic lymphocyte maturation factor (CLMF); natural killer cell stimulatory factor (NKSF)
IFN-α or β	No alternative names associated
IFN-γ	Macrophage activating factor (MAF); T-cell replacing factor (TRF)
TNF-α	Cachectin
TNF-β	Lymphotoxin (LT)
G-CSF	Colony-stimulating factor-β (CSFβ)
GM-CSF	Colony-stimulating factor-α (CSFα); neutrophil inhibition factor (NIF); pluripoietin
M-CSF	Colony-stimulating factor-1 (CSF1)

(Mulé JJ, Rosenberg SA. Catalogue of cytokines. Biol Ther Cancer Updates 1992; 2:1–11)

TABLE 17–6. Principal Cell Sources of Cytokines

Cytokine	Principal Cell Sources*
IL-1 α, β	Monocytes/ macrophages; dendritic cells; B, T, and NK cells; keratinocytes; fibroblasts; endothelial and epithelial cells
IL-2	T cells
IL-3	T cells; myelomonocytic cell lines
IL-4	T cells; mast cells
IL-5	T cells
IL-6	T cells; monocyte/macrophages; fibroblasts
IL-7	Stromal cells
PF4	IL-8: Monocytes/macrophages; RANTES/SIS: T cells, monocytes/macrophages, fibroblasts
IL-9	T helper cells
IL-10	T cells; Th_2 cells (in mouse); B cells
IL-11	Stromal cells
IL-12	B lymphoblastoid cell lines; PHA-stimulated peripheral blood lymphocytes or mixed lymphocyte culture cells
IFN-α	Leukocytes
IFN-β	Fibroblasts
IFN-γ	T cells; NK cells; monocytes/macrophages
TNF-α	Monocytes/macrophages; T cells
G-CSF	Stromal cells; endothelial cells; monocytes/ macrophages
GM-CSF	Fibroblasts; stromal cells; endothelial cells; T cells
M-CSF	Fibroblasts; stromal cells; monocytes/ macrophages

* Cells generally require activation for cytokine release.
(Mulé JJ, Rosenberg SA. Catalogue of cytokines. Biol Ther Cancer Updates 1992;2:1–11)

tumors were confused by the immune reactions that arose to normal transplantation antigens present on tumors. The development of inbred mouse strains made it possible to differentiate tumor antigens from normal histocompatibility antigens and led to the first demonstrations that tumors did contain unique tumor-associated antigens on their surface.

In 1943, Gross demonstrated that the intradermal immunization of inbred mice against a methylcholanthrene-induced sarcoma could result in immunization of that mouse against subsequent tumor challenge.[71] These findings encouraged studies of the nature of the immune response to transplantable tumors in inbred mice, which demonstrated that tumor-specific antigens did exist in a variety of murine tumors.[72–77] These tumor antigens could not be detected in the normal tissues of mice, as demonstrated by studies showing that immunization with tumor cells did not immunize mice against normal tissue grafts from the mouse donating the tumor.[74] Immunity to tumor antigens existed in the same mice in which the tumors had originated, demonstrating that the tumor antigens were not the result of minor allogeneic differences between the transplantable tumor and the host.[75] Tumor antigens were found on a variety of tumors induced with chemical or physical carcinogens and on spontaneous tumors.[78–82]

Tumors induced by chemical carcinogens appear to have limited cross-reactivity, as evidenced by immunization-challenge experiments; even two sarcomas induced in the same mouse do not crossreact.[73–76,83–85] The uniqueness of tumor antigens on chemically induced tumors contrasts with the shared antigens that are often found on virally induced

tumors.[86–88] The sharing of antigens on tumors induced by RNA and DNA viruses has facilitated the study of the biologic and molecular nature of these antigens. For example, studies performed with SV40-induced tumors identified the large T antigen, which is expressed primarily in the nucleus and is necessary to maintain the malignant phenotype of these tumor cells.[89,90] Similarly, the polyoma virus has a middle T antigen and small T antigen localized in the nucleus that can be detected by serologic tests. Boon and coworkers isolated the genes that code for murine tumor-associated antigens induced by chemical mutagenesis.[91] The isolated genes from several murine tumors bear little homology with one another or with other known genes.

In most animal studies of tumor immunity, tumor antigens are detected in experiments in which animals are immunized and then challenged with the same transplantable tumor. Lack of growth of a tumor challenge after immunization is taken as evidence for the existence of tumor antigens. In vitro assays involving reactivity of the tumor cell with antibodies or immune cells can also provide evidence for the existence of tumor antigens. Although tumors induced by high doses of chemical carcinogens or by viruses often exhibit high levels of immunogenicity in mice, it has been thought that spontaneous murine cancers are far less immunogenic.[92,93] The ability to detect tumor-associated antigens depends on the method used, and as more sensitive methods for detecting tumor antigens are developed, unsuspected antigens are likely to be observed.

There is a significant difference in the nature of the antigens recognized by humoral and cellular detection systems. Humoral antibodies detect specific epitopes on antigenic molecules, and it is the interaction of these molecules with the variable region of the antibody that produces recognition. In contrast, antigens recognized by T-cell receptors recognize processed peptides on the surface of the tumor cell or on an antigen-presenting cell in conjunction with MHC molecules. CD4-positive lymphocytes recognize small peptides bound to MHC class II molecules, and CD8-positive cells recognize peptides attached to class I molecules. Monoclonal antibodies are not capable of detecting the small processed peptides on MHC molecules on the cell surface, and the nature of the antigens recognized by humoral and cellular immune responses are therefore quite different.

Tumor-infiltrating lymphocytes (TIL) provide a valuable reagent for detecting cellular immune responses to tumor antigens, revealing unique tumor antigens on a variety of methylcholanthrene-induced sarcomas in inbred mice.[94–98] TIL can recognize tumor antigens based on direct lysis of tumor cells or by the specific release of cytokines such as INF-γ, granulocyte-macrophage colony-stimulating factor, or tumor necrosis factor-α when the TIL are co-cultured with the specific tumor. These TIL are derived from animals bearing established tumors and may differ from the cellular immune responses that are detected in animals that are highly immunized against the tumor as a result of artificial manipulations.

The detection of tumor antigens on human cancers presents unique problems because of the inability to use the immunization-challenge experiments, which have so effectively demonstrated tumor antigens on animal tumors. Attempts to detect human tumor antigens have relied almost exclusively on the availability of in vitro assays that could detect humoral or cellular immune responses.

TABLE 17–7. Characteristics of Human Lymphoid Cells Reactive With Cancer Antigens

Characteristics	Lymphokine-Activated Killer Cells	In Vitro Sensitized Cells	Tumor-Infiltrating Lymphocytes
Source	Peripheral blood lymphocytes or other lymphoid organs	Peripheral blood lymphocytes or draining lymph nodes	Tumor
Culture conditions			
Tumor stimulation	None	Repeated feeding with inactivated autologous tumor	Tumor present in initial culture, no restimulation
IL-2	High dose	Low dose	High dose
Feeder cells	None	B-cell lines	None
Duration	3–5 days	>4 weeks	>4 weeks
In vitro cytolytic activity			
Specificity	None	Restricted to autologous tumor (predominantly melanomas)	Restricted to autologous tumor (predominantly melanomas)
Effector phenotype	$CD11b^+$, $CD16^+$, $CD56^+$; $CD3^+$ or $CD3^-$	$CD3^+$, $CD8^+$, or $CD4^+$	$CD3^+$, $CD8^+$, or $CD4^+$

(Topalian SL, Rosenberg SA. Adoptive cellular therapy: Basic principles. In: DeVita VT, Hellman S, Rosenberg SA, eds. Biologic therapy of cancer. Philadelphia: JB Lippincott, 1991:178–196)

Cellular Immune Reactions for Detecting Human Tumor Antigens

Early studies to detect cellular immune reactivity to human tumor antigens depended on the isolation of lymphocytes from patients with growing tumors and tests of these lymphocytes against fresh or cultured tumor from the same patient. Assays depended on the ability of fresh lymphocytes to kill or prevent colony formation by tumor cells or measuring the ability of tumor cells to promote proliferation of reactive lymphocytes.[99–102] These studies demonstrated the cell-mediated recognition of antigens on fresh cancer cells, although difficulty with reproducibility of reagents and the relatively weak responses obtained prevented careful analysis of these phenomena.

The use of IL-2 enabled in vitro expansion of lymphoid cells reactive with the tumor.[103] In most studies, lymphocytes were co-cultivated with the tumor, and after expansion of the lymphocytes, tests for specific reactivity were conducted. Many MHC-restricted T-cell reactivities to specific tumor antigens were found (reviewed by Hellström and Hellström and by Schreiber).[104,105] IL-2 was also used to generate LAK cells capable of recognizing fresh tumors but not fresh normal cells in a non-MHC restricted fashion.[106–109] Comparison of the characteristics of human lymphoid cells that have been obtained from cancer-bearing patients that are capable of recognizing determinants on fresh tumors (Table 17–7) contrasts with the properties of LAK cells, in vitro sensitized cells, and TIL.[110]

TIL are lymphoid cells that infiltrate into solid tumors and can be grown in vitro in IL-2.[94,95,110–133] TIL have presumably been previously sensitized against autologous tumor antigens in vivo. The lymphocytes invading into the stroma of tumors have a higher proportion of tumor-reactive cells than can be found in the circulation or in lymph nodes. The isolation and expansion of TIL in IL-2 has confirmed specific MHC-restricted immune reactions to a variety of tumors, including melanomas, kidney cancers, colorectal cancers, and lymphomas.[110–136]

These techniques are still being developed. A summary of the in vitro properties of human TIL are shown in Table 17–8. The ability to identify specific reactive lymphocytes varies

TABLE 17–8. In Vitro Studies of Human Tumor-Infiltrating Lymphocytes

TIL can be grown in IL-2 from approximately 80% of human cancers of a variety of histologic types including melanoma, renal cell cancer, colon cancer, breast cancer, ovarian cancer, and others.

TIL with specific cytolytic activity for fresh cancer cells can be grown from approximately one third of patients with melanoma.

TIL are mainly CD3+ and can be CD8+, CD4+, or mixtures of both. Smaller numbers of CD56+ TIL may be present.

Specific lysis by TIL can be inhibited with antibodies to CD3 or to MHC class I molecules.

Growth of TIL from melanoma patients in IL-2 plus IL-4 results in increased in vitro lytic specificity for autologous melanoma.

Incubation of cultured tumors in interferon-γ increases their susceptibility to lysis by TIL.

TIL with lytic specificity for autologous tumor have not been obtained from patients with colorectal cancer, breast cancer, or sarcomas and only rarely from patients with renal cell cancer.

Direct positive panning techniques using antibody-coated flasks can be used to separate and grow highly purified subpopulations of CD4+ and CD8+ TIL.

Repeated immunoselection using TIL with specific lysis can be used to identify tumor lines resistant to lysis by autologous TIL. These immunoselected tumor lines can be used to identify multiple tumor antigens on a single tumor.

Shared tumor antigens on allogeneic melanomas that are recognized in an MHC-restricted fashion can be identified by testing lysis by specific TIL on panels of HLA-typed melanoma cultures. HLA-A2 is a common restriction element in the recognition of melanoma antigens.

MHC-restricted recognition of shared melanoma antigens on allogeneic melanomas was demonstrated by using HLA-A2-restricted specific TIL to lyse allogeneic melanomas transfected with the gene for HLA-A2.

Nonlytic TIL with specific immune recognition of human tumor antigens can be recognized by the specific release of cytokines (such as granulocyte-macrophage colony-stimulating factor, TNF, and interferon-γ) after incubation with autologous tumor. Specific reactivity has been identified in patients with melanoma and breast cancer.

In vitro lysis of autologous tumor by TIL exhibits mild but significant correlation with the clinical response.

significantly among tumor types and in different laboratories. TIL are capable of recognizing tumor-associated antigens by direct lysis in short-term chromium release assays or by the specific secretion of cytokines, such as INF-γ, granulocyte-macrophage colony-stimulating factor, or tumor necrosis factor-α, if the lymphocytes are co-cultivated with the tumor.[131] An example of the specific reactivity of TIL against melanomas is shown in Figure 17–1, which illustrates the lytic activity of TIL against tumor. An example of specific cytokine secretion by TIL used to identify tumor-specific antigens on breast cancers is shown in Figure 17–2. CTL and TIL have identified cross-reactive antigens on melanomas.[132,133,136] Melanomas commonly share tumor antigens that are restricted by different MHC class I determinants. HLA-A2 seems to be a very common restriction element used in the detection of melanoma antigens, although many other class I determinants can serve as restriction elements.

The availability of CTL and TIL to identify tumor antigens enabled early attempts to clone the genes that code for tumor antigens. The first of these genes was described by Boon and colleagues, who identified a class of tumor antigens on melanomas that they referred to as the MAGE family of antigens.[137] These genes exist in normal cells, but they appear to be expressed only on tumor cells.

Antibodies for Detecting Tumor Antigens

Immunoglobulins in all species have the same basic structure and consist of two polypeptide chains, the light chain with a molecular weight of approximately 23,000 and the heavy chain with a molecular weight of 55,000 to 70,000 (reviewed by Rudokoff).[138] The detailed primary and tertiary structure of antibodies is well known. The schematic representation of an IgG antibody molecule is shown in Figure 17–3.

Five different classes of immunoglobulins have been identified based on structural differences within the heavy chain constant regions. These classes are called IgM, IgG, IgA, IgD, and IgE. The characteristics of the immunoglobulin classes are summarized in Table 17–9. IgG constitutes the predominant immunoglobulin fraction in sera, and most antibody activity is associated with IgG antibodies. IgM constitutes about 5% to 10% of serum immunoglobulins and is the largest of the immunoglobulin molecules. IgA is the predominant immunoglobulin in exocrine secretions, and IgE immunoglobulins are involved in allergic reactions. The exact function of IgD immunoglobulins is unknown.

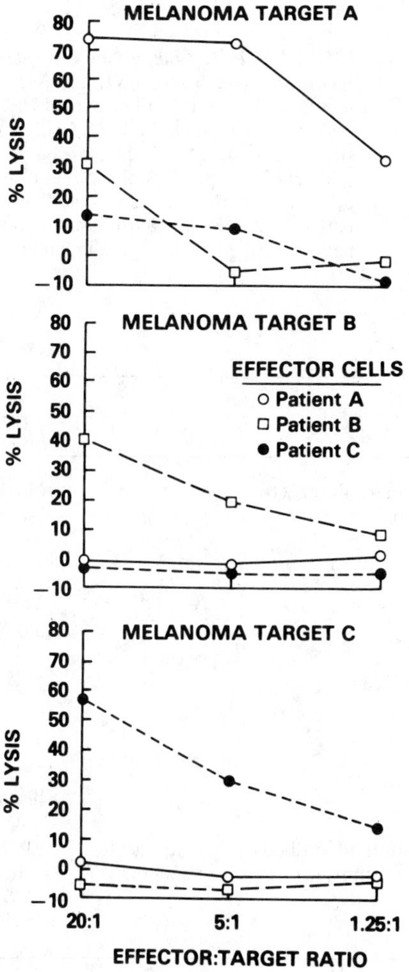

FIGURE 17–1. Specific tumor-infiltrating lymphocyte (TIL) lysis of autologous melanoma but not other allogeneic melanomas. TIL from three patients (○, patient A; □, patient B; ●, patient C) were tested simultaneously against melanoma from these patients. Only the autologous tumors exhibited significant lysis.

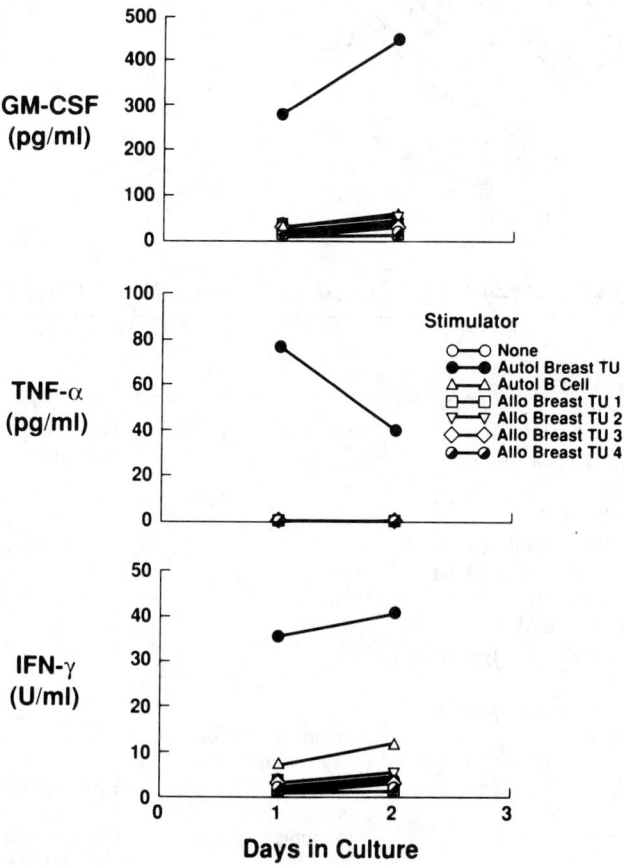

FIGURE 17–2. Demonstration of unique tumor antigens on breast cancer as evidenced by specific cytokine secretion by TIL. TIL from a patient with breast cancer secreted granulocyte-macrophage colony-stimulating factor, TNF-α, and interferon γ only when cocultured with the autologous breast cancer (●) and not with an autologous B-cell line (△) or with four other allogeneic breast cancers: □, ▽, ◇, and ◗.

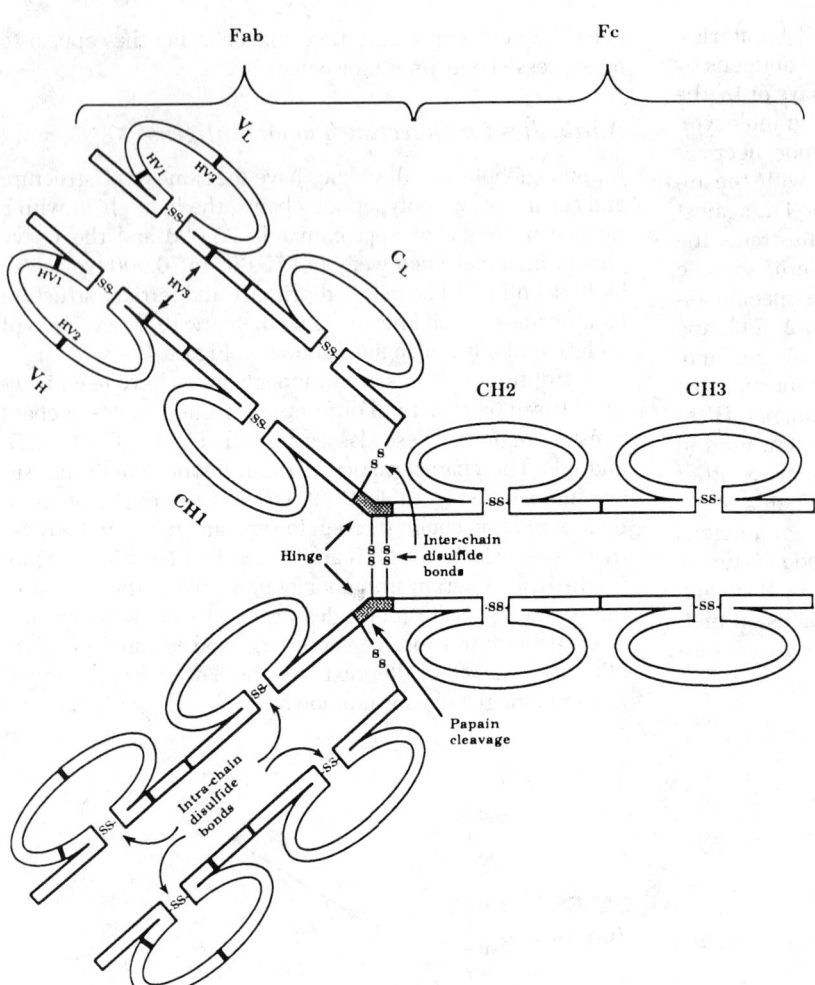

FIGURE 17–3. Schematic representation of an IgG antibody molecule. VL and VH, variable domains of the light and heavy chains; CL, constant region of the light chain; CH1, CH2, and CH3, constant domains of the heavy chain; HV1, HV2, and HV3, hypervariable or complementarity-determining regions; SS, disulfide bonds; Fab, papain-derived antigen-binding fragment; Fc, papain-derived crystallizable fragment.

TABLE 17–9. Characteristics of Immunoglobulin Classes

Property	Class				
	IgG	*IgM*	*IgA*	*IgD*	*IgE*
Common form	Monomer	Pentamer, monomer	Monomer, dimer, etc.	Monomer	Monomer
Molecular weight	150,000	950,000	160,000	175,000	190,000
Classic complement fixation	+	+	−	−	−
Carbohydrate (%)	3	~10	~9	10	12
Serum concentration (mg/ml)	~12	~1.5	~3	0.03	0.0003
Half-life (days)	23	5	6	3	2
Additional polypeptides	−	J chain	J chain, secretory piece	−	−
Placental transfer	+	−	−	−	−
Cell binding	Mononuclear cells and neutrophils	−	−	−	Basophils and mast cells
Other major functions	Predominant antibody in secondary immune response	Primary immune response; lymphocyte surface receptor	Predominant antibody in secretions	Lymphocyte receptor (?)	Effector of allergic and anaphylactic reactions

(Rudikoff S. Principles of tumor immunity: Biology of antibody-mediated responses. In: DeVita VT, Hellman S, Rosenberg SA, eds. Biologic therapy of cancer. Philadelphia: JB Lippincott, 1991:22–34)

Multiple attempts have been made to identify antibodies capable of recognizing tumor antigens in cancer patients. One unambiguous example of the ability of polyclonal antibodies to detect tumor antigens was provided by Klein and colleagues, who demonstrated that many patients with Burkitt's lymphoma have antibodies to antigens expressed on the surface of the lymphoma cells.[139] These cells express multiple tumor-associated antigens on the surface and in the nucleus that appear characteristic of virally induced antigens. It has been more difficult to use polyclonal antibodies to detect antigens in patients with solid tumors, although reports of antibodies reactive with antigens found on malignant melanomas and a variety of other tumors have appeared.[140-146] It has been possible to raise sera from other species that are capable of recognizing antigens that are preferentially expressed on tumors. The best examples of this are the use of heteroantibodies to recognize carcinoembryonic antigen or α-fetoprotein, which have played an important role in monitoring these tumors. The development of monoclonal antibodies greatly improved the ability to detect tumor antigens using humoral reactions.

Kohler and Milstein were the first to demonstrate that somatic cells could be fused with murine myelomas and that monoclonal antibodies with unique specificities could be produced.[147] A vast array of monoclonal antibodies have now been produced against a wide variety of human tumor-associated antigens (reviewed by Schlom).[148] Most hybridoma cell lines can produce between 1 and 10 μg of immunoglobulin per 1 ml in culture, and ascites fluids can produce between 1 and 10 mg of immunoglobulin per 1 ml. In the generation of most monoclonal antibodies, mice are immunized against a specific antigen, and their cells are fused with the mouse myeloma cell. It is, however, possible to use human lymph node or peripheral blood cells for fusion with human myelomas. These human monoclonal antibodies may be able to identify antigens that are not immunogenic in the mouse and are less immunogenic in humans than murine monoclonal antibodies. It is possible to make recombinant chimeric monoclonal antibodies that contain the variable region of murine origin and the constant region of human origin.

Examples of monoclonal antibodies to human tumor antigens are shown in Table 17–10. Many of the tumor antigens recognized by monoclonal antibodies are oncofetal antigens that recognize determinants shared by fetal tissue, differentiation antigens that preferentially react with cells in a given state of differentiation, or tissue-specific antigens that are unique to individual tissue types. Virtually all monoclonal antibodies have at least some reactivity with normal tissues, although the degree of cross-reactivity can be minimal. The potential clinical applications of monoclonal antibodies are summarized in Table 17–11.

IMMUNOTHERAPY

Strategies for the immunotherapy of cancer can be divided into active and passive approaches (Table 17–12). Active immunotherapy refers to the immunization of the tumor-bearing host with materials designed to elicit an immune reaction capable of eliminating or retarding tumor growth. Active immunotherapy can be subdivided into nonspecific or specific immunization. Most early attempts at the immunotherapy of

cancer used nonspecific active approaches to immune stimulation with adjuvants such as bacillus Calmette-Guérin (BCG), *Corynebacterium parvum*, and levamisole. Attempts at immunotherapy used immunization with tumor cells or tumor-cell extracts alone or in vaccines, often in conjunction with immune stimulators such as BCG. These early approaches were almost uniformly unsuccessful in humans and have largely been abandoned.

The advent of recombinant cytokines provided a more selective means for stimulating the immune system. Treatment with the interferons or with IL-2 is a form of nonspecific active immunotherapy, although the selective action of these purified lymphokines provides a greater ability to manipulate immune responses than was previously possible.

Many studies have demonstrated that the tumor-bearing host is immunosuppressed by growing tumor, and attempts at active immunotherapy may therefore have intrinsic disadvantages. Recent efforts have concentrated on passive approaches to immunotherapy, which involve the transfer to the tumor-bearing host of previously sensitized immunologic reagents (*e.g.*, cells or antibody) that have the ability to mediate antitumor responses directly or indirectly. The term "adoptive immunotherapy" usually denotes passive immunotherapy with cells (*e.g.*, lymphocytes, macrophages). Recent efforts have been devoted to developing adoptive immunotherapies using LAK cells, TIL, or other means for in vitro stimulation of cells with antitumor reactivity.

The development of techniques for generating monoclonal antibodies has greatly improved the ability to obtain preparations with specific reactivity to human tumor-associated antigens. These antibodies are being employed alone or conjugated with toxins or radiolabels in cancer treatment.

In addition to active and passive approaches, the immune system can be used in a variety of indirect ways to mediate antitumor responses, including removal of blocking factors from serum or inhibition of essential tumor growth factors.

ACTIVE NONSPECIFIC IMMUNOTHERAPY

In the absence of detailed information concerning the immune reaction to murine or human tumors, early attempts to perform immunotherapy involved nonspecific stimulation of the immune system with the hope that a nonspecific increase in immune reactivity would lead to a concomitant increase in the putative immune reaction to established tumors. Much of this early work was stimulated by the anecdotal observations of Coley, who at the turn of the 20th century observed that sarcomas in patients with advanced cancer could undergo significant regression after they experienced severe infections.[149] Mixed bacterial toxins were used to treat patients with a variety of cancers, and several instances of cancer regression were reported. This work has not been successfully repeated, but it spurred testing of many bacterial products for the immunotherapy of animal and human cancers.

Hersh extensively analyzed studies of the use of nonspecific immunotherapy in experimental and human cancers and divided these agents into nonspecific host defense stimulants or nonspecific immunomodulatory agents.[150] Some of these agents are listed in Tables 17–13 and 17–14. Most immune stimulants used intact bacteria or bacterial products or the purified active compounds in these materials. Agents that were

TABLE 17–10. Representative Monoclonal Antibodies to Human Tumor Antigens*

Tumor Type	Monoclonal Antibodies	Antigen†	Tumor Type	Monoclonal Antibodies	Antigen†
Carcinoma			Bladder	T43	87-kd gp
Pancarcinoma	17-1A	37–41-kd gp		T138	25-kd gp
	73.3	37–41-kd gp		HBA4	40-, 78-, 130-kd gp complex
	B72.3	TAG-72, HMW gp		J143	30-, 120-, 140-kd gp
	CC49, CC83	TAG-72, HMW gp		3G2-C6	90 kd
	L6	Ganglioside	Ovarian	OVB3	Unknown
	Mov-2	Glycoprotein		OC125	CA 125, HMW > 200 kd
	AR-3	CAR-3		OM-1	Unknown
Breast	HMFG-1, -2	HMW gp		NB12123	NB/70K
	111D5	HMW gp		MOv-1	Glycoprotein
	DF-3	HMW gp		MOv-18, -19	38–40-kd gp
	MAM-6	HMW gp		OC133	Unknown
	115D8	HMW gp, HMGF membrane		ID3, ID5	Unknown
	F36/22			OV-TL3	Unknown
	24-17.1	HMW gp	Melanoma	96.5	97-kd sialo gp
	323/A3	95 kd, transferrin receptor		48.7	Proteoglycan
	MBr1, 2, 3	43-kd gp		R24	GD₃, glycolipid
	SP-2	Unknown		14.18	GD₂ disialoganglioside
		90 kd		11C64	GD₃ disialoganglioside
Lung				140.240	87-kd gp
Small cell	Anti-Leu-7	110-kd gp		9.2.27	HMW, >440–500 kd
	TFS-4	Unknown	Central nervous system tumors	BF3, GE2	Unknown
	MO1-1	Unknown		CNT-2, -11, -8	130 kd, 70 kd, unknown
Non-small cell	KS 1/4, 1/7	40-kd gp		3F8	Ganglioside GD₂
	LuCA-1, -4	230-kd, 240-kd protein, 300-kd protein	Leukemias/ lymphomas	Anti-TAC	T-cell receptor
	E10/15	80-kd protein		T101	65-kd gp
	43-9F	50–200-kd gp complex		L17F12	T-cell differentiation antigen
	Po66	50 kd		Anti-T11, -T3	50 kd, 25 kd
Gastrointestinal	19-9	Sialyated Leᵃ		Anti-3A1	40 kd
	HAG-1, -2	115-kd gp, 20–230-kd gp complex		Anti-B1, -B4	35 kd, 95 kd
	ST-4-39	HMW mucin-like gp		CALLA	100 kd
	DuPAN-2	HMW mucin-like gp		Anti-MO2, -MY9	55 kd, 67 kd
	AR2-20, -28	190-kd protein		Antiidiotype	Idiotype of Ig
	VII 23	CEA, 180-kd gp		Anti-Lym-1, -2	Lym-1, -2
	T84.66	CEA, 180-kd gp	Sarcomas	791T/36	72-kd protein
	F33-37	CEA, 180-kd gp	Human monoclonal antibodies	MBE6	Unknown
	NP 1-4	CEA, 180-kd gp		MCA series	Unknown
	COL 1–15	CEA, 180-kd gp		Ri 37	Unknown
	791T/36	72-kd gp		3B7	Unknown
	7E6A5	40-kd protein		L72	GD₂
	Cora	75-kd, 95-kd gp complex		CA27, CF29, JD39	Unknown
	D612	48-kd gp		H1-C4	Forssman gp
	CAA	HMW-gp			
Prostate	F5	33–34-kd protein			
	IF3, 2G7, 1C5	34-kd protein			
	Anti-PAP	100-kd protein			
	P6.2	Unknown			
	Alpha-Pro3	54-kd protein			
	83.21	Unknown			

HMW, high molecular weight; gp, glycoprotein.
* This table represents only a partial listing of antihuman tumor monoclonal antibodies, and inclusion or exclusion from this table does not denote relative importance for cancer diagnosis or therapy. Some reactive antigens are listed as unknown as originally reported, but they since may have been identified.
(Schlom J. Antibodies in cancer therapy: Basic principles of monoclonal antibodies. In: DeVita VT, Hellman S, Rosenberg SA, eds. Biologic therapy of cancer. Philadelphia: JB Lippincott, 1991: 464–481)

TABLE 17–11. Clinical Applications of Monoclonal Antibodies

I. Diagnosis
  A. Screening of body fluids (serum, sputum, effusions, urine, cerebrospinal fluid) for the presence of circulating TAA
  B. Nuclear scanning with radiolabeled MoAb
    1. Detection of primary or metastatic lesions (I.V., subcutaneous, or IP administration of radiolabeled MoAb)
    2. Lymphoscintigraphy to detect lymph node involvement
  C. The use of radiolabeled MoAb and intraoperative γ detecting probe
  D. Immunopathology
    1. The diagnostic dilemma: malignant versus benign
    2. Differential diagnosis of tumor type
    3. Subclassification of tumor based on TAA expression
      a. Metastatic potential
      b. Specific favored sites of metastasis
      c. Predicted response (or lack thereof) to specific therapeutic regimens
      d. Prognosis

II. Monitoring of disease progression
  A. Screening of body fluids (see IA) for circulating TAA
  B. Nuclear scanning with radiolabeled MoAb to detect or quantitate tumor recurrence (see IB)
  C. Immunopathology for detection of occult metastases
    1. Aspiration cytology
    2. Lymph node or bone marrow biopsy
    3. Cytology of body fluids
III. Therapy
  A. Direct cytotoxicity of MoAb
    1. Complement mediated
    2. Cell mediated
  B. Drug conjugation of MoAb (*e.g.*, doxorubicin)
  C. Toxin conjugation of MoAB (*e.g.*, ricin)
  D. Radionuclide conjugation of MoAb (*e.g.*, α or β emitters)
  E. Ex vivo tumor removal from harvested bone marrow
  F. Inhibition of receptors for growth factors
  G. Administration of antiidiotype MoAbs to induce specific active immunity to tumor antigens

TAA, tumor-associated antigen; MoAb, monoclonal antibody.
(Schlom J. Antibodies in cancer therapy: Basic principles of monoclonal antibodies. In: DeVita VT, Hellman S, Rosenberg SA, eds. Biologic therapy of cancer. Philadelphia: JB Lippincott, 1991:464–481)

TABLE 17–12. Classification of Cancer Immunotherapies

Classification	Examples
Active immunotherapy	
Nonspecific	Immune adjuvants such as BCG, *C. parvum*, levamisole
	Interferon
	IL-2
Specific	Immunization with tumor-cell vaccines
Passive immunotherapy	
Antibodies	Monoclonal or polyclonal antibodies alone or conjugated with toxins or radiolabels
Cells	LAK cells, tumor-infiltrating lymphocytes
Indirect	Removal or blocking factors, inhibition of growth factors or angiogenic factors

TABLE 17–13. Nonspecific Host Defense Stimulants

Category	Examples	Category	Examples
Intact microorganisms	Viable: BCG	Purified or synthetic components	Peptidoglycans
	Viable inactivated: OK-432 (Picibanil)		Muramyl dipeptide (MDP)
	Nonviable: *C. parvum*		MDP derivatives
Microbial cell wall	BCG cell-wall skeleton		Trehalose dimycolate (P_3)
	Nocardia cell-wall skeleton		Endotoxins (lipopolysaccharide)
	Methanol extraction residue of BCG		Modified endotoxins (detoxified)
Glucans	Glucan (yeast)	Interferon inducers polynucleotides	Poly IC
	Lentinan (fungal)		Poly IC-LC
	Pachymaran (fungal)		Poly AU
	Scizophyllan (fungal)		Ampligen
		Pyan copolymers	MVE-2
Protein-bound polysaccharide	PSK (Krestin) (fungal)	Low-molecular-weight inducers	Pyrimidinones (ABPP, AIPP)
Microbial glycoproteins	*Klebsiella* glycoprotein (Biostim)	Delivery systems	Oil in water emulsions: CFA
			Water in oil emulsions: Ribi reagents
			Liposomes

BCG, bacillus Calmette-Guérin; *C. parvum*, *Corynebacterium parvum;* IC, inosinic-cytidylic acid; LC, poly L-leucine; AU, adenylic-uridylic acid: CFS, complete Freud's adjuvant; MVE-2, methyl vingl ether fraction 2.
(Hersh EM, Taylor CW. Immunotherapy by active immunization: Use of nonspecific stimulants and immunomodulators. In: DeVita VT, Hellman S, Rosenberg SA, eds. Biologic therapy of cancer. Philadelphia: JB Lippincott, 1991:613–626)

TABLE 17–14.   Nonspecific Immunomodulatory Agents

Category	Examples
Natural products and derivatives	
Thymic hormone extracts	Thymosin fraction 5, TPI, thymic humoral factor (THF)
Synthetic thymic hormones	Thymosin-α1, thymopoeitin, pentapeptide, THF-α2
Lymphocyte extracts	Transfer factor, immunogenic RNA
Tuftsin	Tuftsin
Enkephalins and endorphins	Methionine enkephalin
Chemical immunomodulators	
Sulfur-containing	Levamisole, diethyldithiocarbamates
Cyanoaziridines	Azimexon, ciamexon, imexon
Tellurium-based	AS101, tellurium chloride
Other	Isoprinosine
Vitamins	Retinoids, vitamin C
Regulators of physiologic mechanisms	PGE-2 synthesis inhibitors: indomethacin
	H-2 receptor antagonists: cimetidine
	Suppressor-cell modulation by cytoxic chemotherapy (cyclophosphamide)

(Hersh EM, Taylor CW. Immunotherapy by active immunization: Use of nonspecific stimulants and immunomodulators. In: DeVita VT, Hellman S, Rosenberg SA, eds. Biologic therapy of cancer. Philadelphia: JB Lippincott, 1991:613–626)

thought to modulate immune reactions also came from natural products, such as the thymus gland or lymphocyte extracts, or from synthetic chemicals.

Many early studies were performed using BCG, a modified form of the tubercle bacillus. BCG increased immune reactions in some murine models, including increased antibody formation and accelerated graft rejection.[150,151] Mathé and coworkers[152,153] showed that the administration of BCG could improve the survival of mice with transplantable leukemias, and positive results reported in early trials of BCG in patients with acute lymphocytic leukemia led to studies of BCG for of many human cancers in the adjuvant setting and in patients with advanced disease (reviewed by Hersh and Taylor).[150] Suggestions of a positive impact in nonrandomized studies led to tests of many immune stimulants in animal and human cancers.

Almost without exception, active nonspecific immunotherapy has been unsuccessful in the treatment of patients with advanced cancer. Early reports of the effectiveness of these nonspecific agents alone or in combination with other therapies in patients with melanoma, lung cancer, and other tumors in the adjuvant setting or in patients with advanced disease could not be confirmed in prospective randomized trials, and most of these approaches have been abandoned.[150]

The exploration of these approaches in the 1970s and early 1980s was preceded by a paucity of experimental information suggesting that nonspecific immune stimulatory approaches could impact established cancer in animals, hampering the

rational design of human trials. The reports of Mathé and coworkers of the effect of BCG in acute lymphoblastic leukemia were followed by studies at the M.D. Anderson Cancer Center demonstrating prolonged remission durations and survival using this approach.[153,154] The historically controlled investigations could not be confirmed in prospective randomized trials.[155–157]

Much impetus for the exploration of BCG and other nonspecific immune stimulants came from early studies demonstrating that BCG scarification could prolong remission duration in patients with stage II melanoma after lymph node dissection.[158] However, multiple randomized trials failed to confirm these results.[159–161] Some studies found that patients who had an empyema after surgery for lung cancer had a better survival than those without infection.[162] A randomized trial showed an improvement in survival for patients who received intrapleural BCG after surgery.[163] However, this result could not be confirmed by large randomized studies by the Lung Cancer Study Group.[164]

Perhaps the most compelling success of systemic nonspecific immunotherapy was provided by the addition of levamisole to chemotherapeutic agents in adjuvant therapy, which improved survival among patients with colon cancer (see Chap. 30).[165–167] The precise mechanism of action of levamisole is unknown.

Active nonspecific immunotherapy has twice been effective when administered by local injection or instillation for the treatment of localized cancer deposits. Direct BCG injection into cutaneous metastases in patients with melanoma resulted in the rejection of a high proportion of injected deposits (reviewed by Morton and colleagues).[168] The results of several studies of intralesional therapy are summarized in Table 17–15. Recommendations for treatment have been carefully delineated by Morton and coworkers.[168] Very little or no impact is seen in noninjected lesions, but good local control of injected lesions can be achieved by this approach. The use of live BCG organisms can result in disseminated BCG infection, and this has led to increased emphasis on the use of nonviable preparations for intralesional therapy. A prospective trial by Cohen and associates demonstrated that intralesional injection of dinitrochlorobenzene, an organic compound, was as effective as BCG in causing the regression of intracutaneous and subcutaneous melanoma deposits.[169]

Another successful application of BCG therapy involves the instillation of BCG into the bladder for the treatment of patients with superficial bladder cancers (reviewed by Herr).[170] In 1976, Morales and colleagues[171] reported that BCG could eliminate visible tumors and prevent tumor recurrences in patients with superficial bladder cancers, and several studies have confirmed this result. BCG is now accepted as one of several agents that can be used for instillational therapy for bladder cancer (see Chap. 34).

ACTIVE SPECIFIC IMMUNOTHERAPY

A primary feature of the immune system is its exquisite specificity of response. Successful immunization to prevent bacterial and viral diseases led to the hope that immunization against tumors could lead to potent immune responses capable of affecting the growth of established cancers. The many attempts to develop tumor "vaccines" included immunization

TABLE 17–15. Intralesional Therapy of Malignant Melanoma

Investigations	Therapy*	Patients	Local Response†	Toxicity‡
Morton	BCG	8	CR 5 (62%)	Fever, ulceration
Bornstein	BCG	15	CR 1 (7%), PR 4 (27%)	Fever, flu-like sx
Pinsky	BCG	25	CR 10 (40%), PR 5 (20%)	Flu-like sx, elevated LFTs
Grant	BCG, tumor cells + BCG, antibodies	10	CR 2 (20%), PR 3 (30%)	Flu-like sx, systemic infection, anaphylaxis
Mastrangelo	BCG	1	CR	Minimal
Morton	BCG	45	CR 90% (ID), CR 31% (SC-lesions)	Fever, systemic infection
Lieberman	BCG	6	CR 4 (66%)	Flu-like sx, elevated LFTs
Mastrangelo	BCG	1	CR (lesions), PR (pulm. met)	Flu-like sx
Richman	BCG, epilesional scarification	13	CR 3 (23%), PR 4 (31%)	Fever, elevated LFTs
Sieger	BCG/lymphocytes/vaccine	101	CR 61 (60%)	Flu-like sx
Yamamura	BCG-CWS, oil-attached	1	PR	Fever, flu-like sx
Sopkova	BCG	19	CR 4 (21%), PR 14 (74%)	Flu-like sx
Mastrangelo	BCG	15	CR 2 (13%), PR 3 (20%)	Flu-like sx, hepatic granulomas
Cohen	BCG	9	CR 6 (67%)	Flu-like sx, DIC
Krown	MER-BCG	18	CR 8 (44%), PR 4 (22%)	Flu-like sx, elev. LFTs, thrombocytopenia
Nathanson	BCG	28	CR 3 (11%), PR 9 (32%)	Flu-like sx, systemic infection
Storm	BCG	27	CR 10 (37%), PR 10 (37%)	Flu-like sx, elevated LFTs
Lokich	MER-BCG	6	CR 2 (33%), PR 2 (50%)	Flu-like sx
Plesnicar	BCG, XRT	19	CR 14 (74%), PR 1 (5%)	Flu-like sx, ulceration
Bauer	BCG	45	CR 30 (67%), PR 13 (29%)	Flu-like sx, systemic infection
Tisman	PPD	1	CR (2/2 lesions)	Local flare
Lokich	PPD	5	NR	Minimal inflammation
Cohen	DNCB	5	CR 61% (110/179 lesions)	Ulceration
Cohen	DNCB	9	CR 6 (67%)	Ulceration
Felix	Vitamin A	3	PR 50% (lesions)	Minimal
Adler	LAK cells	3	CR 33% (4/12 lesions)	Minimal
			PR 8% (1/12 lesions)	Minimal
von Wussow	IFN-α, r-IFN-α2b	51	CR 31% (16/51 lesions)	Flu-like sx, granulocytopenia
			PR 14% (7/51 lesions)	Flu-like sx, granulocytopenia
Irle	Human MoAb anti-GD2	8	CR 45% (10/22 lesions)	Erythema
			PR 23% (5/22 lesions)	Erythema
Irle	Human MoAb anti-GM2	2	CR 1 (50%)	Minimal

* BCG, bacillus Calmette-Guérin; CWS, cell wall skeleton; MER, methanol extracted residue; XRT, radiation therapy; PPD, purified protein derivative; DNCB, dinitrochlorobenzene; LAK, lymphokine-activated killer; IFN, interferon; MoAb, monoclonal antibody.
† CR, complete response; PR, partial response; ID, intradermal; SQ, subcutaneous; NR, no response.
‡ sx, symptoms; LFTs, liver function enzymes; DIC, disseminated intervascular coagulation.
(Morton DL, Hunt KK, Bauer RL, Lee JD. Clinical application using intralesional therapy. In: DeVita VT, Hellman S, Rosenberg SA, eds. Biologic therapy of cancer. Philadelphia: JB Lippincott, 1991: 627–642)

with autologous or allogeneic tumor cells using living cells, inactivated cells, or cell fragments alone or in conjunction with immune adjuvants such as BCG or with viruses.

It was possible to immunize mice against challenge with a variety of syngeneic tumors. Unfortunately, the ability to immunize a normal mouse against a subsequent tumor challenge did not translate into an ability to affect the growth of established tumor. The magnitude of an immune response necessary to prevent tumor implantation is probably far less than that required to diminish the growth of established tumor. The growing tumor probably can subvert immune effector mechanisms, which do not exist against a fresh tumor implant.

The local production of suppressor factors, the modulation of tumor antigens or MHC antigens on tumors, or the presence of circulating soluble suppressor factors all may interfere with the ability of the immune system to attack an established tumor. Virtually no models of active specific immunotherapy have been effective against established tumors in murine models. Although work with BCG tumor cell vaccines in guinea pig hepatoma models did showed some positive results, this information has not been easily transferable to other model systems.[172]

As in many areas of tumor immunology, the lack of suitable animal models did not inhibit conduction of clinical studies

TABLE 17–16. Characteristics of Interferons

Type of Interferon	No. of Species	No. of Amino Acids	Predominant Cellular Source	Molecular Mass (kd)	Glycosyl-ation	Chromosomal Location of Interferon	Chromosomal Location of Receptor	Inducers
α	>20	166	Leukocytes	16,000–27,000	≥3 species	9p21	21q21	Virus, double-stranded RNA
β	1*	166	Fibroblasts	20,000	Yes	9p21	21q21	Virus, double-stranded RNA
γ	1	146	T cells	15,500–25,000	Yes	12q24	6q	Mitogens, specific antigens

* IFN-β2 is identical to IL-6 and its antiviral properties have been disputed.
(Kurzrock R, Gutterman JU, Talpaz M. Interferons α, β, γ: Basic principles and preclinical studies. In: DeVita VT, Hellman S, Rosenberg SA, eds. Biologic therapy of cancer. Philadelphia: JB Lippincott, 1991:247–274)

of active specific immunotherapy for the treatment of human malignancy. Studies of this approach in patients with leukemia, melanoma, renal cell cancer, lung cancer, ovarian cancer, and sarcomas have been conducted using a variety of immunization schemes (reviewed by Hoover and Hanna).[173] Studies of patients with malignant melanoma have been particularly prominent, including the use of autologous unmodified melanoma cells, allogeneic unmodified melanoma cells, neuraminidase-treated melanoma cells, virally infected melanomas, and subcellular melanoma fractions. Although objective regressions of disease have been reported, the reproducibility and clinical significance of these results are uncertain.

A trial of BCG therapy for patients with colon cancer was conducted by Hoover and colleagues.[173–175] Patients with clinical stage B2 or C colorectal cancer underwent surgery to remove all gross disease and were then randomized to receive autologous tumor cells with BCG or to have no additional therapy. Patients with lesions below the peritoneal reflection also received 5040 cGy of pelvic irradiation after the immunotherapy was completed. Preliminary analysis of these results in patients with colon cancer suggested a decrease in the probability of recurrence in patients receiving immunotherapy, although no significant differences in survival rates were demonstrated. No differences in the probability of recurrence or probability of survival was observed among patients with rectal cancer.[173] Further follow-up and confirmatory studies are necessary before definitive conclusions can be drawn.

Attempts at active specific immunotherapy using gene-modified tumor cells have been conducted in animals.[176] Insertion of genes coding for cytokines into tumor cells can increase their immune recognition and lead to more potent cellular immune responses than were generated by unmodified tumor cells. This approach is considered in more detail in Chapter 69. Clinical tests of this phenomenon have recently begun in the Surgery Branch of the National Cancer Institute.

INTERFERONS

The interferons are a family of proteins that are produced by cells in response to viral infection or stimulation with double-stranded RNA, antigens, or mitogens (reviewed by Kurzrock and colleagues).[177] They were first described by Isaacs and Lindenmann in 1957.[178] The interferons can interfere with subsequent viral challenge, and they have many immunomodulatory and antiproliferative effects.

The characteristics of the three major groups—INF-α, INF-β, and INF-γ—are shown in Table 17–16. There are more than 20 closely related genes coding for INF-α with approximately 80% to 85% amino acid homology with one another. There appear to be two genes that code for IFN-β and only a single gene identified for IFN-γ. IFN-β is quite similar in many of its properties to IFN-α. The gene for IFN-γ has three introns, and there are no introns in the genes that code for IFN-α and IFN-β. IFN-α and IFN-β are stable to pH 2, although IFN-γ is labile at this pH. IFN-β and IFN-γ are glycosylated, but most IFN-α species are not.

TABLE 17–17. Biologic Properties of the Interferons

Properties Shared by IFN-α, β, and γ	Properties Exhibited Exclusively or Preferentially by IFN-γ

Immunomodulatory activities
  NK-cell activation
  Cytotoxic T-cell activation
  Induction of MHC class I antigens
Antiviral activity
  Induction of 2′,5′ A synthetase
  Induction of protein kinase
Antiproliferative activity
Inhibition of angiogenesis
Regulation of differentiation
Interaction with growth factors, oncogenes, and other cytokines
Enhancement of tumor-associated antigens
	Immunomodulatory activity
	  Activation of monocytes/macrophages
	  Stimulation of MHC class II antigens
	  Induction of B-cell immunoglobulin production
	  Induction of IL-2 receptors
	Antimicrobial activity (mediated by monocytes/macrophages)
	Regulation of lipid (triglyceride) metabolism

(Kurzrock R, Gutterman JU, Talpaz M. Interferons α, β, γ: Basic principles and preclinical studies. In: DeVita VT, Hellman S, Rosenberg SA, eds. Biologic therapy of cancer. Philadelphia: JB Lippincott, 1991:247–274)

IFN-α can be produced by a variety of cells including macrophages and lymphocytes. IFN-β is produced mainly by fibroblasts and epithelial cells. IFN-γ can be produced by a variety of lymphocyte subtypes, such as CD4- or CD8-positive cells, NK cells, and LAK cells. Secretion of IFN-γ occurs after stimulation by mitogens or antigens. Interferons have a variety of biologic properties as shown in Table 17–17. These properties include immunomodulatory activities, antiviral activities, the ability to interfere with cell proliferation, inhibition of angiogenesis, regulation of differentiation, and enhancement of the expression of a variety of cell-surface antigens.[177] Although the direct antiproliferative activity of the interferons is thought to play a major role in the antitumor effects of these compounds, other actions of the interferons may also be important.

The interferons have antitumor activity against a variety of tumor types, including hairy cell leukemia, chronic myelogenous leukemia, cutaneous T-cell lymphoma, and Kaposi's sarcoma (reviewed by DeVita and colleagues).[1] The response rates of various solid tumors and hematologic malignancies to treatment with IFN-α are summarized in Tables 17–18 and 17–19. IFN-α and-β, but not IFN-γ, demonstrate direct antitumor activity. The side effects associated with interferon therapy are shown in Table 17–20. The incidence and severity of side effects is highly dose and schedule dependent.

PASSIVE IMMUNOTHERAPY WITH ANTIBODIES

The development of monoclonal antibodies with relatively unique antitumor specificity led to multiple attempts to use them in cancer therapy (see Table 17–11). Unmodified antibodies can mediate complement-dependent cytotoxicity or antibody-dependent cellular cytotoxicity. Various materials

TABLE 17–18. Response of Various Solid Tumors to Interferon-α

Tumor Type	Response Rate (%)*
Cervical intraepithelial neoplasia	80–90
Basal cell cancer	90
Superficial bladder cancer	60–70
Malignant neuroendocrine tumors	30–80
Kaposi sarcoma (AIDS-related)	35
Ovarian cancer	
Parenteral	10–15
Intraperitoneal	40
Gliomas	30
Renal cell cancer	15–20
Nasopharyngeal cancer	20
Melanoma	10–15
Colorectal cancer	<10
Osteogenic sarcoma	<10
Lung (small and non-small cell)	<10
Breast cancer	<10

* Responses signify partial or complete tumor regression.
(Kurzrock R, Talpaz M, Gutterman JU. Interferons—clinical applications. In: DeVita VT, Hellman S, Rosenberg SA, eds. Biologic therapy of cancer. Philadelphia: JB Lippincott, 1991:334–345)

TABLE 17–19. Response of Various Hematologic Malignancies to Interferon-α

Tumor Type	Response Rate (%)*
Hairy cell leukemia	80–90
Chronic myelogenous leukemia	
Newly diagnosed	70–80
Advanced	10–25
Philadelphia-negative myeloproliferative disorders, essential thrombocythemia and polycythemia vera	75
Cutaneous T-cell lymphomas	
No prior therapy	80
Previously treated	55
Non-Hodgkin lymphomas (relapsed)	
Low grade	40–50
Intermediate and high grade	15
Hodgkin disease (relapsed)	20
Multiple myeloma	
No prior therapy	50
Previously treated	15–25
Chronic lymphocytic leukemia	10–15
Acute leukemia	10–20

* Responses signify partial or complete tumor regression.
(Kurzrock R, Talpaz M, Gutterman JU. Interferons—clinical applications. In: DeVita VT, Hellman S, Rosenberg SA, eds. Biologic therapy of cancer. Philadelphia: JB Lippincott, 1991:334–345)

including drugs, toxins, or radionuclides, are conjugated to monoclonal antibodies to aid in their antitumor effectiveness. Monoclonal antibodies can be used to clear tumor from bone marrow, or antiidiotypic monoclonal antibodies can induce specific active immunity to tumor antigens. Each of these approaches has been extensively explored in clinical trials, although each must still be considered experimental. The use of monoclonal antibodies with immunotoxins is considered separately in Chapter 69.

The advantages of monoclonal antibody therapies include their relative selectivity for tumor tissue and the relative lack of toxicity associated with their administration. Although

TABLE 17–20. Common Toxicities in Hairy Cell Leukemia Patients Receiving Interferon

Toxicity	Patients (%)
Flu-like symptoms	75–100
Rashes	40–50
Gastrointestinal complaints	15–40
Elevated hepatic enzymes	20–80
Neurologic complaints	5–20
Chronic fatigue	0–45

(Kurzrock R, Talpaz M, Gutterman JU. Interferons—clinical applications. In: DeVita VT, Hellman S, Rosenberg SA, eds. Biologic therapy of cancer. Philadelphia: JB Lippincott, 1991:344–345)

monoclonal antibodies can bind in vivo to tumors, their ability to destroy tissue is minimal unless aided by other mechanisms. Potential problems with use of monoclonal antibodies include the relatively low amount of the total antibody injected that actually arrives at the tumor and the poor diffusion of immunoglobulin molecules throughout large tumor masses. Monoclonal antibodies can be inhibited by soluble antigen, which can bind to their combining site and prevent attachment to antigens in tissues. A major problem with the use of murine monoclonal antibodies is the development of human anti-mouse antibodies (HAMA) that can inactivate the injected antibodies. Recombinant chimeric monoclonal antibodies that use the constant region of the human antibody and the variable combining region of the mouse antibody results in decreased production of HAMA.

One use of monoclonal antibodies under active investigation is the conjugation of these antibodies to radioisotopes. The radioisotopes in common use in these studies are shown in Table 17–21.

The use of antibodies in treating specific cancers is considered throughout this book. Particularly effective antitumor responses have been seen in the treatment of B-cell lymphomas using antiidiotypic antibodies (reviewed by Levi and Miller).[180] The use of anti-TAC antibodies for the treatment of T-cell leukemia or lymphomas has also provided promising results (reviewed by Waldmann).[181]

INTERLEUKIN-2 AND ADOPTIVE IMMUNOTHERAPY

Biologic Aspects of Interleukin-2

IL-2, a lymphokine produced by activated T cells, has a wide variety of actions and plays a central role in immune regulation (reviewed by Smith).[182] The binding of antigen in conjunction with IL-1 stimulates T cells to release IL-2, which is the second signal in lymphocyte mitogenesis. The primary action of IL-2 is its ability to stimulate the growth of activated T cells that bear IL-2 receptors, although IL-2 has a variety of other actions on T cells (see Table 17–3), B cells, macrophages, epidermal Langerhans' cells, and oligodendroglia.[183-192]

TABLE 17–21. Selected Radioisotopes for Radioimmunotherapy

Radionuclide	Decay Mode (MeV Energy)*	Half-life
[131]I	β minus (0.606)	8.0 d
[90]Y	β minus (2.27)	64 h
[124]I	EC, β plus (2.14)	4.2 d
[67]Ga	β minus (0.57)	58.5 h
[125]I	EC	60.2 d
[186]Re	β minus (1.07)	88.9 h
[212]Bi	α decay (2.25)	1 h
	β minus	
[211]At	α decay (5.868)	7.2 h

* For β decay, maximum energy is given.
(*Radiological Health Handbook.* Bureau of Radiological Health, Washington, DC: US Government Printing Office, 1970)

Human IL-2 was first isolated from supernatant fluids of cultured mitogen- or alloantigen-activated T cells.[183] The leukemic cell line Jurkat produces high concentrations of human IL-2, and using this cell line, the gene coding for human IL-2 was isolated and expressed in *E. coli*.[194-198]

Human cells contain a single copy of the IL-2 gene, which consists of four exons and three introns on chromosome 4. The cDNA consists of a single open reading frame coding for 153 amino acids. The first 20 N-terminal amino acids are hydrophobic and are cleaved to give the mature protein, which

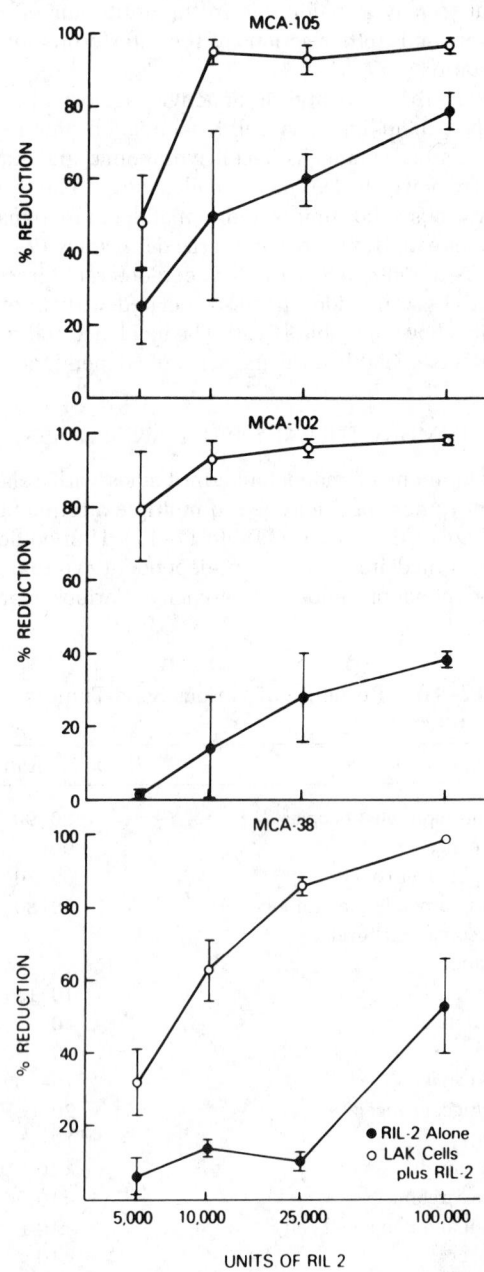

FIGURE 17–4. Therapy for established liver metastases in mice using recombinant IL-2 alone (●) or LAK cells plus recombinant IL-2 (○). Various doses of recombinant IL-2 were administered intraperitoneally every 8 hours for 5 days. At each dose of recombinant IL-2, more effective reduction in established 3-day liver metastases occurred if LAK cells were also administered.

consists of 133 amino acids and has a predicted molecular weight of 15,420. The residue at position 3 of the mature molecule is O-glycosylated, and size and charge heterogeneity are attributable to this posttranslational modification. The IL-2 molecule contains a single disulfide bond between residues 58 and 105 that appears to be essential for the full activity of the molecule. One form of IL-2 in clinical use contains a site-specific mutation with a serine-for-cysteine substitution that allows the production of a stable molecule containing the full biologic activity of native IL-2.[196,197]

IL-2 interacts with cells by binding to specific receptors on the cell surface. High-affinity receptors with a K_d of 10^{-11} M are the principal ones that mediate the physiologic response of T cells to IL-2 and comprise about 10% of the IL-2 receptors. A second group of receptors bind IL-2 with low affinity (K_d 10^{-8} M). It now appears that a 55-kd protein recognized by the anti-TAC monoclonal antibody mediates low-affinity IL-2 binding. A 75-kd IL-2 receptor protein of intermediate affinity has also been identified, and it appears that high-affinity receptors involve the interaction of IL-2 with a combination of the 55-kd and the 75-kd IL-2 receptor molecules.[198]

Many of the actions of IL-2 suggested that this molecule might be of value in cancer therapy.[199] IL-2 causes lymphoid proliferation and, in some cases, reverses immunodeficiency in vitro and in vivo. For example, in vivo administration of IL-2 restores depressed allogeneic responses in cyclophosphamide-treated mice, restores allograft responses in T-depleted rodents, and can restore the cytotoxic response of lymphoid cells from patients with AIDS to cultured NK-sensitive tumor cells.[200-202] IL-2 also causes proliferation of endogenous and adoptively transferred lymphoid cells in vivo.[203,204]

Lymphoid cells incubated with IL-2 develop a capacity to lyse fresh tumor cells.[205-209] This generation of LAK cells occurs in vitro and in vivo and has served as the basis for the development of adoptive immunotherapies for the treatment of cancer in humans. Moreover, the direct administration of IL-2 to tumor-bearing animals mediates the regression of established hepatic, pulmonary, and subdermal metastases in several murine tumor models.[210-214] Figure 17–4 and Table 17–22 present some of the characteristics of the effects of IL-2 in animals.

Other actions of IL-2 that suggest an ability to alter tumor growth include its augmentation of the therapeutic effect of the adoptive transfer of lymphoid cells and its effects on the emigration of lymphoid cells from the peripheral blood.[204,215-219] Administration of IL-2 causes the in vivo release of other lymphokines and hormones that mediate physiologic effects, often in concert with IL-2.[220]

Clinical Applications of IL-2 in Cancer Patients

The variety of physiologic effects of IL-2 encouraged exploration of its use in treating advanced cancers in humans. Initial clinical studies used IL-2 derived from the high-producer Jurkat cell line, although only small quantities of purified IL-2 could be obtained. Expression of the gene for IL-2 in *E. coli* led to the availability of virtually unlimited amounts of recombinant IL-2, and most clinical trials have used this material.

TABLE 17–22. Immunotherapy of Murine Tumors With Interleukin-2 Alone

Liver and lung micrometastases (3-day) from a variety of immunogenic and nonimmunogenic sarcomas, melanomas, and adenocarcinomas can be inhibited by IL-2 administration.

Lung macrometastases (10-day) from two immunogenic sarcomas, but not from two nonimmunogenic sarcomas, can be inhibited by IL-2 administration.

A direct relation exists between the dose of IL-2 and the therapeutic effect.

High-dose IL-2 administration leads to in vivo lymphoid proliferation in visceral organs, and these cells have LAK activity in vitro.

The immunotherapeutic effect of IL-2 on 3-day micrometastases is mediated by asialo-GM1-positive LAK cells. In immunogenic tumors, Lyt 2-positive cells also participate.

The immunotherapeutic effect of IL-2 on 10-day macrometastases is mediated by Lyt 2-positive cells.

Immunosuppression with radiation or cyclophosphamide can inhibit IL-2 activity against 3-day metastases but can enhance the effects of IL-2 on 10-day macrometastases.

The sensitivity of macrometastases to therapy with IL-2 appears to be directly related to the expression of MHC antigens (class I) on the tumor.

The administration of IL-2 can enhance the therapeutic effect of concomitantly administered LAK cells, TIL, and specifically sensitized T lymphocytes.

Several schedules of IL-2 administration have been explored in humans.[220-235] Most studies have used the bolus administration of IL-2 at doses between 72,000 and 720,000 IU/kg intravenously every 8 hours. IL-2 can also be administered by continuous infusion at doses from 6,000,000 to 42,000,000 IU/m²/day. Administration of IL-2 by bolus injection is less toxic than IL-2 administered by continuous infusion. Approximately three times more IL-2 can be tolerated by bolus than by continuous infusion. After the administration of IL-2, lymphopenia occurs, but the lymphocytes rebound substantially after IL-2 administration is discontinued. If small amounts of IL-2 are administered for more than 1 week, lymphocytosis may also occur. Serum levels of INF-γ and other hormones increase. After intravenous bolus injection, recombinant IL-2 is cleared from the circulation with an alpha distribution phase of 6.9 minutes and a beta clearance phase of approximately 70 minutes.[220]

In the treatment of patients with advanced cancer, IL-2 has been used alone or in conjunction with the adoptive transfer of LAK cells or TIL. Most experience with the clinical use of IL-2 has been in patients with melanoma and renal cell cancer, although a few patients with other histologic types of cancer have been treated. Approximately 5% to 10% of patients with renal cell cancer have complete regressions of metastatic cancer, and another 10% to 15% have objective partial regressions (see Chap. 33). The Surgery Branch, NCI experience with IL-2 therapy is shown in Table 17–23.[176]

On May 4, 1992, the Food and Drug Administration approved IL-2 for use in the United States for the treatment of patients with metastatic renal cell cancer. IL-2 became the first biologic response modifier to be approved for the treatment of patients with advanced cancer that acted solely

TABLE 17–23. Results of Immunotherapy in Patients With Advanced Cancer

	No. of Patients Treated With IL-2			CR + PR (%)
Cancer Diagnosis	Evaluable*	CR	PR	
Renal	60	5	6	18
Melanoma	41	1	9	24
Colorectal	12	0	0	
Non-Hodgkin's lymphoma	11	0	0	
Breast	3	0	0	
Other†	9	0	0	
Total	136	6	15	15

CR, complete response; PR, partial response.
* Includes all treated patients except four who died from therapy.
† Two patients, each with hepatoma and brain cancer; one each with sarcoma, lung, ovary, pancreas, and uterine cancer.

through immune mechanisms. Unlike interferon, IL-2 has no direct antiproliferative effect on cancer cells. FDA approval to administer IL-2 was restricted to the treatment of patients with advanced renal cell cancer at a dose of 720,000 IU/kg every 8 hours to tolerance. Two cycles are administered, separated by 7 to 10 days, and a second course of treatment is given to patients who are stable or are responding to treatment. The FDA review included 255 patients treated at a variety of institutions with this high-dose IL-2 regimen (Table 17–24).

The toxicity associated with IL-2 administration is considered in the next section.

Adoptive Immunotherapy

Adoptive immunotherapy—the transfer to the tumor-bearing host of cells with antitumor activity—has substantial therapeutic attractiveness as an approach to treating human cancer.[176,221–223,236,237] Early cell-transfer experiments in animals demonstrated that the cellular arm of the immune response is crucial in mediating the rejection of allogeneic grafts and syngeneic tumors. In most experimental systems, the transfer of immune cells, but not of antibody directed against cellular antigens, produces immunity to tissue transplants.

The major obstacle to the development of successful adoptive immunotherapies for the treatment of cancer in humans has been the inability to develop immune cells with specific

TABLE 17–24. FDA Review of Patients With Advanced Renal Cell Cancer Treated With High-Dose Interleukin-2

Investigations	No. of Patients	Complete Responses	Partial Responses
Surgery Branch, NCI	68	5	9
NCI Extramural phase II studies	124	3	11
Cetus phase II studies	63	1	8
Total	255	9	28

reactivity for human tumors that could be obtained in large enough numbers for transfer to tumor-bearing patients. However, several new approaches have been developed for generating human cells with reactivity to tumor, and the initial clinical experience with the adoptive transfer of these cells has been encouraging.[176,221–223]

Lymphokine-Activated Killer Cells and Interleukin-2

Beginning in 1980, Rosenberg and colleagues described a technique for generating lymphoid cells from mice and humans that were capable of lysing fresh tumor cells but not normal cells.[205–210] The incubation of resting murine splenocytes or human peripheral blood lymphocytes with IL-2 for 3 to 4 days generates LAK cells that can lyse fresh tumor cells.

The characteristics of LAK cells have been extensively studied.[205–210,238,239] These cells represent a lytic population quite distinct from NK cells or CTL, and their phenotypic surface markers are characteristic of non-MHC-restricted killer cells. LAK cells can be CD3 positive or negative, are nonadherent and E-rosette negative, and bear NK-like markers, such as CD16 and CD56. IL-2 is the sole signal required for the generation of LAK cells, as demonstrated by experiments using purified homogenous recombinant IL-2. The nature of the determinants recognized on fresh tumor targets by LAK cells is unknown, although the determinants appear to be broadly expressed on fresh and cultured tumor cells and

TABLE 17–25. Immunotherapy of Murine Tumors With Lymphokine-Activated Killer Cells Plus Interleukin-2

Liver and lung micrometastases (3-day) from a variety of immunogenic and nonimmunogenic sarcomas, melanomas, and adenocarcinomas can be inhibited by treatment with LAK cells plus IL-2.

A direct relation exists between therapeutic effect and the dosage of IL-2 and the dose of LAK cells.

The precursor of the LAK cell effective in vivo is Thy 1⁻, Ig⁻, ASGM1⁺.

Three-day incubation of splenocytes is optimal for the generation of LAK cells effective in vivo.

Immunotherapy of micrometastases with LAK cells and IL-2 is effective in hosts suppressed by total body irradiation or treatment with cyclophosamide. Therapy is also effective in B mice (thymectomized, lethally irradiated, reconstituted with T-cell-depleted bone marrow).

Immunotherapy of micrometastases with allogeneic LAK cells plus IL-2 is effective.

LAK cells effective in immunotherapy can be generated from the splenocytes of tumor-bearing mice.

Metastases that persist after in vivo therapy with LAK cells plus IL-2 are sensitive to LAK-cell lysis both in vitro and in subsequent in vivo experiments. We have been unable to generate LAK-resistant tumor cells.

Administration of IL-2 leads to in vivo proliferation of transferred LAK cells.

Diffuse intraperitoneal carcinomatosis can be successfully treated with intraperitoneal LAK cells plus IL-2.

LAK cells can mediate antibody-dependent cellular cytotoxicity, and thus administration of IL-2 alone or LAK cells plus IL-2 can enhance the in vivo therapeutic efficacy of monoclonal antibodies with antitumor reactivity.

on cultured normal cells. Fresh normal cells, with the possible exception of monocytes, do not appear to bear cell-surface determinants recognized by LAK cells.

After the description of the LAK cell phenomenon, animal studies evaluated the use of LAK cells in the adoptive immunotherapy of established tumors. These studies demonstrated that the adoptive transfer of LAK cells in conjunction with IL-2 can mediate the regression of established pulmonary, hepatic, and subdermal metastases from in a variety of animals.[240-244] IL-2 stimulated in vivo expansion of LAK cells with maintenance of cellular function.[203,204] The results are summarized in Table 17–25. In these systems, the significant antitumor effects of the administration of IL-2 alone are usually improved by the adoptive transfer of LAK cells.

Clinical trials using IL-2 and LAK cells plus IL-2 for the treatment of advanced cancer in humans were developed (Table 17–26). Early studies of the use of activated killer cells began with the use of phytohemagglutinin-activated killer

cells, because sufficient amounts of IL-2 were not available to generate LAK cells.[245,246] Similarly, clinical trials of IL-2 alone began with the use of natural Jurkat-derived IL-2.[247] After recombinant IL-2 became available, studies with LAK cells alone or with recombinant IL-2 alone were attempted.[220,246] No antitumor responses were seen in any of the early studies using activated killer cells alone. After these phase I studies, a combination of LAK cells and recombinant IL-2 was administered to patients with advanced cancer, and the tumors of some patients regressed.[221,222]

An outline of the protocol using IL-2 plus LAK cells is shown in Figure 17–5. In the Surgery Branch of the National Cancer Institute, 178 patients were treated with IL-2 and LAK cells. The results are shown in Table 17–27. Most experience with this treatment approach has been obtained in patients with renal cell cancer or melanoma. Approximately 10% of patients with these diseases obtain complete regressions of metastatic cancer, and about 20% have objective partial regres-

TABLE 17–26. Surgery Branch, National Cancer Institute Clinical Immunotherapy Studies

Year	Investigations	No. of Patients	Findings
1980	Adoptive transfer of long-term cultured peripheral blood lymphocytes	3	Small numbers (up to 5×10^8) of long-term cultured peripheral blood lymphocytes could be infused safely into humans
1981	Adoptive transfer of phytohemagglutinin-activated killer (PAK) cells	10	Large numbers (up to 1.7×10^{11}) of activated killer cells, obtained from up to 15 successive leukaphereses, could be safely infused into humans
1982	Adoptive transfer of PAK cells plus cyclophosphamide	6	Activated killer cells could be infused safely in conjunction with high-dose cyclophosphamide (50 mg/kg)
1983	Adoptive transfer of PAK cells plus activated macrophages	5	Activated killer cells plus activated macrophages could be infused safely
1983	Administration of natural (Jurkat-derived) IL-2	16	Natural (Jurkat-derived) IL-2 could be infused safely into humans at doses up to 2 mg
1984	Adoptive transfer of lymphokine-activated killer (LAK) cells	6	LAK cells (activated with recombinant IL-2) could be infused safely into humans
1984	Administration of recombinant IL-2	23	Recombinant IL-2 (from *E. coli*) could be administered safely though significant toxicity was seen at high doses
1985	Administration of LAK cells plus recombinant IL-2	25	Regression of metastatic cancers in some patients
1986	Administration of high-dose bolus IL-2 alone	10	Regression of metastatic cancer in 3 patients with melanoma
1987	Administration of high dose IL-2 alone or with LAK cells	156	Regression of metastatic cancers in some patients
1988	Adoptive transfer of tumor-infiltrating lymphocytes (TIL); pilot trial ± IL-2, ±cyclophosphamide	12	TIL could be infused safely with IL-2 and cyclophosphamide
1988	Adoptive transfer of TIL plus IL-2 and cyclophosphamide	25	Regression of metastatic cancer in 11 of 20 patients with melanoma
1989	Administration of IL-2 plus interferon-α	94	Established maximal doses in regression of metastatic renal cell cancer and melanoma
1989	Administration of IL-2 plus tumor necrosis factor	38	No additive antitumor effects of tumor necrosis factor
1990	Adoptive transfer of gene-modified TIL (bacterial neophosphotransferase)	5	First administration of foreign genes into humans; techniques found to be safe and feasible
1990	Adoptive transfer of TIL plus IL-2 and interferon-α	Ongoing	
1991	Adoptive transfer of TNF gene-modified TIL plus IL-2	Ongoing	

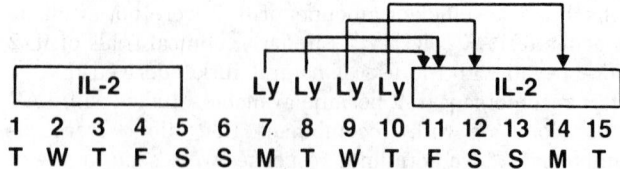

Ly: lymphocytapheresis
IL-2: intravenously every 8 hours
LAK: intravenous infusion of cells

FIGURE 17–5. Schematic representation of the clinical protocol for treatment of patients with advanced cancer using LAK cells and IL-2 in the Surgery Branch, National Cancer Institute.

sions.[176,221–223] About 15% of patients with metastatic colorectal cancer experience objective regression of their tumors. There has been little experience with other tumor types.

Regression of metastatic cancer has been observed in lung, liver, bone, skin, subcutaneous tissue, and circulating tumor cells. If tumor regression occurs at one site, it tends to occur at all sites; mixed responses are unusual.

Because meaningful clinical responses have been seen in patients given high-dose IL-2 and in patients receiving LAK cells and IL-2, Rosenberg and colleagues conducted a prospective randomized trial using patients with advanced cancer and comparing high-dose IL-2 alone or administered in conjunction with LAK cells. Preliminary results from this trial are shown in Table 17–28 and in Figures 17–6 and 17–7. Although no advantage was seen with the administration of LAK cells in patients with renal cell cancer, there is a strong trend toward improvement in survival with LAK cell administration in patients with advanced melanoma. Examples of patient responses to treatment with IL-2 alone or IL-2 plus LAK cells are shown in Figures 17–8 and 17–9.

Studies have also been conducted using LAK cells and IL-

TABLE 17–27. Results of Immunotherapy in Patients With Advanced Cancer

Cancer Diagnosis	No. of Patients Treated With LAK/IL-2			CR + PR (%)
	Evaluable*	CR	PR	
Renal	72	8	17	35
Melanoma	48	4	6	21
Colorectal	30	1	4	17
Non-Hodgkin's lymphoma	7	1	3	57
Sarcoma	6	0	0	
Lung	5	0	0	
Other†	10	0	0	
Total	178	14	30	25

* Includes all treated patients except one lost to follow-up and one who died from therapy.
† One patient each with cancer of breast, brain, esophagus, ovary, testes, thyroid, gastrinoma, unknown primary and two patients with Hodgkin's lymphoma.
CR, complete response; PR, partial response.

TABLE 17–28. Respose to Immunotherapy

Malignancy	Patient Group	No. of Patients Treated*	
		LAK/IL-2	IL-2
All cancers	Total	90	91
	Evaluable	85	79
	CR	10	4
	PR	14	12
Melanoma	Total	29	26
	Evaluable	27‡	22
	CR	3	0
	PR	3	6
Renal	Total	48	48
	Evaluable	46§	41
	CR	7	4
	PR	8	6
Colorectal	Total	8	10
	Evaluable	8‖	10
	CR	0	0
	PR	2	0
Non-Hodgkin's lymphoma	Total	4	5
	Evaluable	3¶	4
	CR	0	0
	PR	1	0
Other	Total†	1	2
	Evaluable	1	2
	CR	0	0
	PR	0	0

CR, complete response; PR, partial response.
* The only patients not evaluated were those who received no treatment with IL-2 (*i.e.*, dropped out before any therapy).
† LAK/IL-2, 1 thyroid; IL-2, 1 breast, 1 hepatoma.
‡ Two of these received no LAK cells (2 NR).
§ One of these received no LAK cells (NR). Another received no LAK cells in the first course (CR) but received LAK/IL-2 after a recurrence.
‖ Two of these received no LAK cells (2 NR).
¶ One of these received no LAK cells (1 NR).

2 locally for the treatment of intraperitoneal cancer or brain tumors (Table 17–29).[248–257]

Many questions remain concerning the use of IL-2 and LAK cells in cancer therapy. The dose-response and schedule-dependent characteristics of IL-2 have not been clearly established. Are higher response rates obtained with higher doses? What is the optimal administration schedule of IL-2 and cells? A need exists to test this immunotherapy approach for a variety of cancers at different sites. Are brain metastases affected? A need exists for simpler means of raising more potent cells for use in adoptive immunotherapy. Studies of the pathophysiology of IL-2 toxicities and means for decreasing these toxicities are needed.

Toxicity of Treatment

The adoptive transfer of activated killer cells alone causes little toxicity.[245,246] However, administration of high-dose recombinant IL-2 can be associated with substantial dose-limiting toxic side effects in several organ systems.[221,222,228] Many of the side effects of IL-2 are probably attributable to

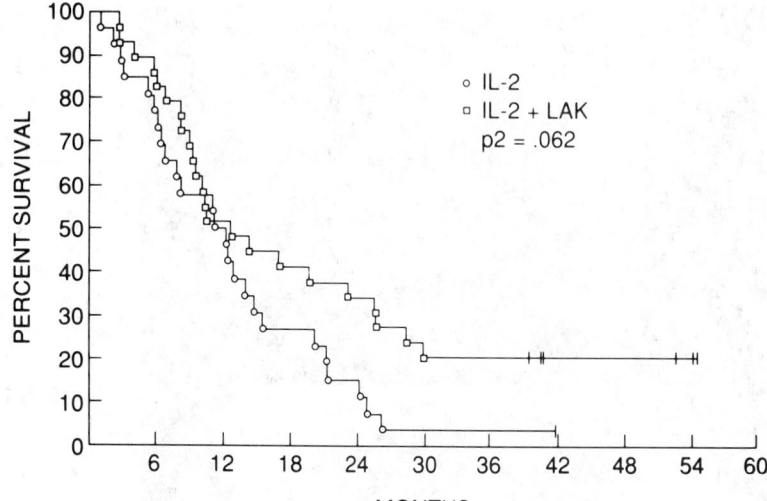

FIGURE 17–6. Results of a prospective randomized trial of patients with advanced melanoma who received either IL-2 alone (○) or IL-2 plus LAK cells (□). Patients receiving IL-2 plus LAK cells demonstrated a trend toward improved survival ($p_2 = 0.062$).

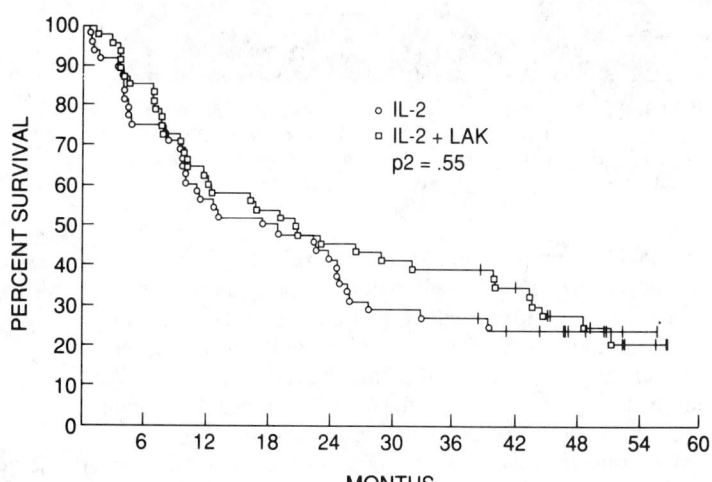

FIGURE 17–7. Results of a prospective randomized trial of patients with advanced renal cell cancer who received IL-2 alone (○) or LAK cells plus IL-2 (□). No difference in long-term survival was seen ($p_2 = 0.55$).

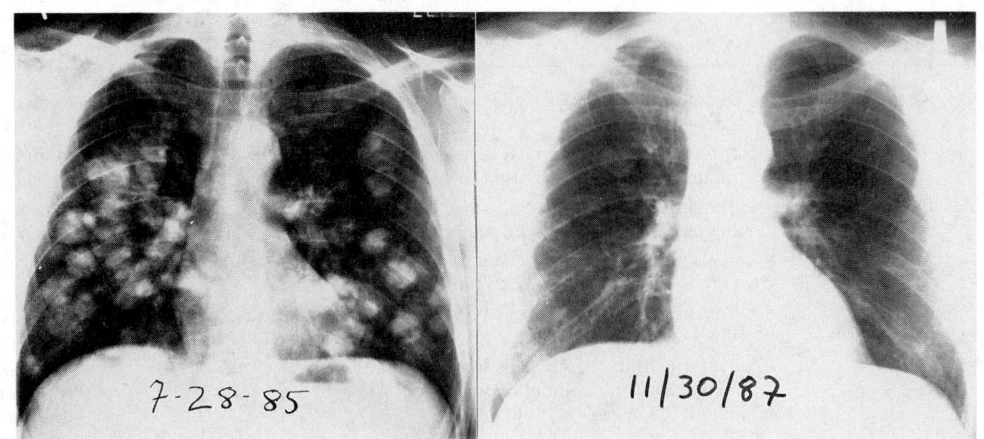

FIGURE 17–8. Regression of lung metastases in a patient with advanced malignant melanoma treated with recombinant IL-2 alone.

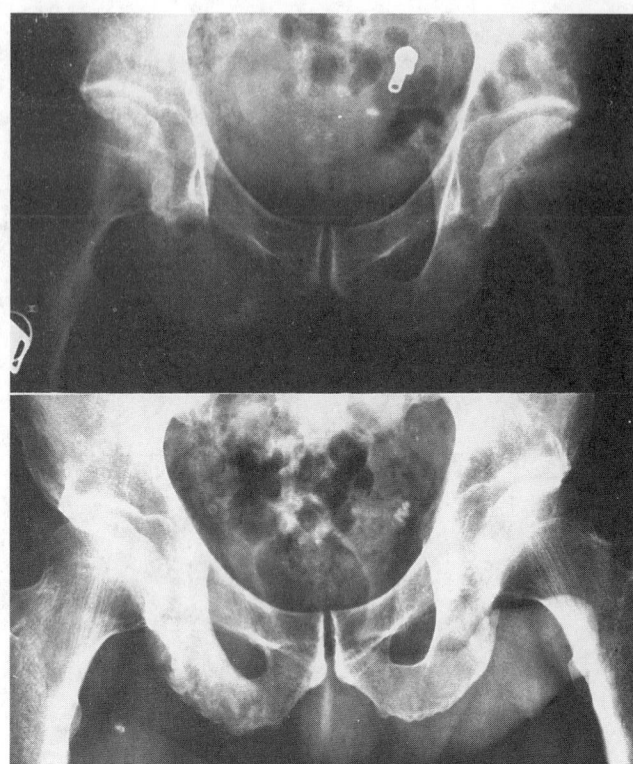

FIGURE 17–9. Complete regression of bony metastasis from renal cell cancer in the pubic ramus of a patient treated with LAK cells plus IL-2. This patient had complete regression of bony and lung metastases and remains free of disease more than 4 years after treatment.

lymphoid infiltrates in vital organs, to a vascular permeability leak induced by IL-2 that leads to fluid retention and interstitial edema that can compromise organ function, and to the ability of IL-2 to prompt secretion of other lymphokines such as INF-γ, which have a range of physiologic effects and toxicities of their own.[220,258,259] The side effects of IL-2 appear to be completely reversible after administration ceases.

The clinical course of a typical patient receiving IL-2 and LAK cells is summarized in Figure 17–10. Soon after admin-

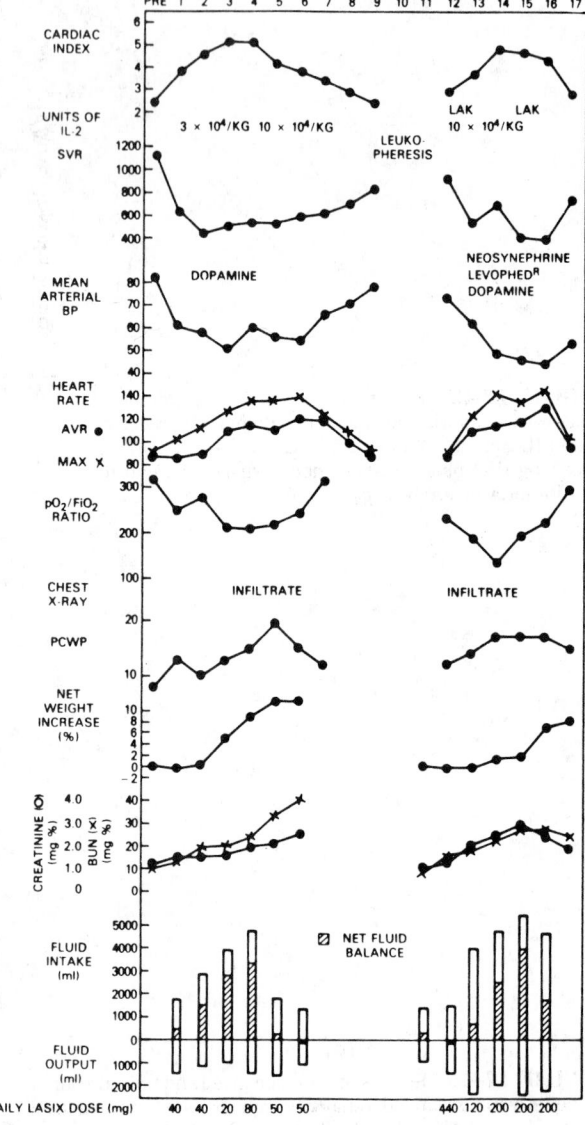

FIGURE 17–10. Sequential clinical measurements in a patient receiving treatment with LAK cells and IL-2.

TABLE 17–29. Regional Therapy for Malignant Brain Tumors With Lymphokine-Activated Killer Cells and Interleukin-2

Investigations	Treatment	No. of Patients	Comments
Jacobs, 1986[252]	Direct injection of LAK cells into tissue surrounding tumor cavity	15	No measurable tumor at time of treatment
Ingram, 1987[254]	Plasma clot containing LAK cells placed into resected tumor bed (PHA + IL-2 used in cell incubation)	55	No measurable tumor at time of treatment; survival data pending
Merchant, 1988[255]	Direct injection of LAK cells into tissue surrounding the tumor cavity during craniotomy	20	No measurable tumor at time of treatment; survival data pending
Yoshida, 1988[253]	Direct injection of LAK cells into recurrent cavity with 50 to 400 units of IL-2; multiple treatments	23	Tumor regression in 6 tumor patients
Barba, 1990[256]	Direct injection of LAK cells plus IL-2 into tumor or resected tumor cavity using an Ommaya reservoir	9	One partial response; neurologic side effects secondary to cerebral edema
Nitta, 1990[257]	Direct injection of LAK cells into tumor site after "debulking" in conjunction with anti-CD3-antiglioma bispecific antibody	10	"Regression" of tumor in 4 patients; no recurrence in any patient at 8 to 18 months follow-up

TABLE 17–30. Toxicity of Treatment With Interleukin-2

No. of patients	652
No. of courses	1039
Chills	399*
Pruritus	180
Necrosis	5
Anaphylaxis	1
Mucositis (requiring liquid diet)	30
Alimentation not possible	4
Nausea and vomiting	666
Diarrhea	596
Hyperbilirubinemia, maximum (mg/dl)	
2.1–6.0	547
6.1–10.0	179
10.1+	83
Oliguria	
<80 ml/8 h	347
<240 ml/24 h	42
Weight gain (% body weight)	
0.0–5.0	377
5.1–10.0	436
10.1–15.0	175
15.1–20.0	38
20.1+	13
Elevated creatinine, maximum (mg/dl)	
2.1–6.0	637
6.1–10.0	85
10.1+	10
Hematuria (gross)	2
Edema (symptomatic nerve or vessel compression)	17
Tissue ischemia	2
Respiratory distress	
Not intubated	67
Intubated	41
Bronchospasm	9
Pleural effusion (requiring thoracentesis)	17
Somnolence	114
Coma	33
Disorientation	215
Hypotension (requiring pressors)	508
Angina	22
Myocardial infarction	6
Arrhythmias	78
Anemia requiring transfusion (no. of units transfused)	
1–5	377
6–10	95
11–15	24
16+	14
Thrombocytopenia, minimum (/µl)	
<20,000	131
20,001–60,000	361
60,001–100,000	285
Central line sepsis	63
Death	10

* Unless otherwise stated, numbers refer to patients.
(Rosenberg SA, Lotze MT, Yang JC, Aebersold PM, Linehane WM, Seipp CA, White DE. Experience with the use of high-dose interleukin-2 in the treatment of 652 cancer patients. Ann Surg 1989;210:474–484)

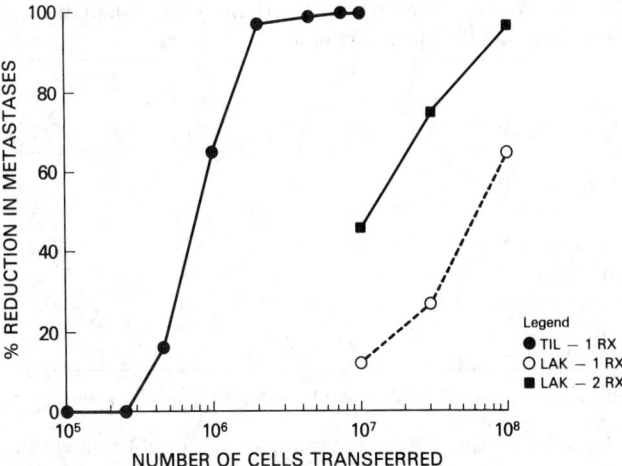

FIGURE 17–11. Titration of LAK cells and TIL administered with IL-2 in mice bearing 3-day lung metastases from a transplantable sarcoma. ●, TIL, one treatment; ○, LAK cells, one treatment; ■, LAK cells, two treatments. TIL appear to be 50 to 100 times more potent than LAK cells in reducing established lung metastases.

istration of IL-2, a drop in systemic vascular resistance occurs and is associated with tachycardia, decreased mean arterial blood pressure, and an increase in cardiac index.[260,261] As IL-2 administration continues, weight gain occurs secondary to the requisite replacement of fluid lost from the intravascular space by the capillary leak. Urine output drops, and serum creatinine rises, probably because of prerenal azotemia.[262–264] Vasopressors are often used early in treatment in an attempt to limit the need for fluid replacement, because exogenous fluid contributes to the interstitial edema, which can lead to

TABLE 17–31. Immunotherapy of Murine Tumors With Tumor-Infiltrating Lymphocytes and Interleukin-2

The administration of TIL plus IL-2 is 50 to 100 times more effective than LAK cells plus IL-2 in reducing established (day 3) lung micrometastases.

The administration of TIL plus IL-2 plus cyclophosphamide is effective in treating mice with advanced lung (day 14) or liver (day 8) metastases. All three agents are required for effective treatment.

The phenotype of TIL effective in vivo is CD3+, CD4−, CD8+.

TIL raised from tumors that express class I antigens only after transfection with genes coding for class I can mediate the regression of micrometastases from the parental tumor after treatment of the mouse with interferon-γ.

Local tumor irradiation synergizes with TIL and IL-2 administration in mediating the regression of established metastases. Local irradiation can substitute for cyclophosphamide.

TIL with improved antitumor activity in vivo can be generated from tumor suspensions by using immunomagnetic beads to isolate lymphocytes followed by incubation of lymphocytes in low-dose IL-2.

In mice cured of lung micrometastases by administration of TIL, live TIL can be identified in vivo 3 months after injection.

The specific secretion of interferon-γ by TIL when cultured with tumor is the best in vitro correlate of the in vivo antitumor effectiveness of TIL. Nonlytic TIL that specifically secrete interferon-γ can effectively treat established lung micrometastases.

TABLE 17–32. Treatment of Patients With Melanoma With Tumor-Infiltrating Lymphocytes

Patient Status*	NR	Objective Response (PR + CR)	PR + CR (all)	Percentage
No previous IL-2				
IL-2 + CY	17	11	11/28	39
IL-2 (no CY)	7	4	4/11	36
Previous IL-2				
IL-2 + CY†	3	3	3/6	50
IL-2 (no CY)	4	1	1/5	20

NR, no response; CY, cyclophosphamide; PR, partial response; CR, complete response.
* Excludes patients with brain metastases at start of treatment (all NR).
† Excludes two patients who received IL-2 at 186,000 IU/kg; both were NR.
(Rosenberg SA. The immunotherapy and gene therapy of cancer. J Clin Oncol 1992;10:180–199)

respiratory compromise and a decrease in arterial oxygenation. Weight gain, renal dysfunction, and hepatic dysfunction can occur. These toxicities and others seen in 65 patients treated by Rosenberg and associates are summarized in Table 17–30.[265-273] The treatment-related mortality rate in 273 patients given high-dose IL-2 was 1.5%.

Tumor-Infiltrating Lymphocytes and Interleukin-2

TIL are lymphocytes that infiltrate growing tumors and can be isolated by growing single-cell suspensions from the tumor in IL-2. The characteristics of TIL are presented in Tables 17–7 and 17–8.

In animals, the adoptive transfer of TIL can be from 50 to 100 times as potent as LAK cells in mediating the regression of established micrometastases (Fig. 17–11)[94] A summary of studies using TIL plus IL-2 for the immunotherapy of murine tumors is presented in Table 17–31.

TIL have been isolated from virtually all types of human tumors and can recognize tumor-associated antigens (see Figs. 17–1 and 17–2).[110-136] Based on these in vitro and in vivo studies, pilot trials of TIL for the treatment of advanced cancers in humans have begun.[274,275] The results of a pilot trial employing patients with metastatic melanoma treated with TIL in the Surgery Branch of the National Cancer Institute are presented in Table 17–32.

TIL traffic to and accumulate in tumor deposits.[276,277] This finding led to attempts to genetically alter TIL to increase their antitumor activity at the tumor site. In an initial phase of this effort, TIL transduced with the gene for neomycin phosphotransferase were infused into patients with advanced melanoma.[278] This study and additional efforts to develop gene therapies for patients with cancer are considered in Chapter 69.

REFERENCES

1. DeVita VT Jr, Hellman S, Rosenberg SA, eds. Biologic therapy of cancer. Philadelphia: JB Lippincott, 1991:1–800.

2. Mulé JJ, Rosenberg SA. Catalogue of cytokines. Biol Ther Cancer Updates 1992;2:1–11.
3. Rosenberg SA, Grimm EA, McGrogan M, Doyle M, Kawasaki E, Koths K, Mark DF. Biological activity of recombinant interleukin-2 produced in E. coli. Science 1984;223:1412–1415.
4. Koj A. The role of interleukin-6 as the hepatocyte stimulating factor in the network of inflammatory cytokines. In: Sehgal PB, Grieninger G, Tosato G, eds. Regulation of the acute phase and immune responses: Interleukin-6. Ann NY Acad Sci 1989;557:1–8.
5. Lomedico PT, Gubler U, Hellmann P, et al. Cloning and expression of murine interleukin-1 cDNA in Escherichia coli. Nature 1984;312:458–462.
6. Dinarello CA. Biology of interleukin-1. FASEB J 1988;2:108–115.
7. O'Garra A, Umland S, DeFrance T, Christiansen J. B cell factors are pleiotropic. Immunol Today 1990;9:45–54.
8. Oettgen HF, Old LJ. The history of cancer immunology. In: DeVita VT, Hellman S, Rosenberg SA, eds. Biologic therapy of cancer. Philadelphia: JB Lippincott, 1991:87–119.
9. Mulé JJ, Rosenberg SA. Combination cytokine therapy: Experimental and clinical trials. In: DeVita VT, Hellman S, Rosenberg SA, eds. Biologic therapy of cancer. Philadelphia: JB Lippincott, 1991:393–416.
10. Porat R, Clark BD, Wolff SM, Dinarello CA. Enhancement of growth of virulent strains of Escherichia coli by interleukin-1. Science 1991;254:430–432.
11. Morgan DA, Ruscetti FW, Gallo RC. Selective in vitro growth of T-lymphocytes from normal bone marrows. Science 1976;193:1007–1008.
12. Tanaguchi T, Matsui H, Fujita T, Takaoka C, Kashina N, Yoshimoto R, Hamuro J. Structure and expression of a cloned cDNA for human interleukin-2. Nature 1983;302:305–309.
13. Smith KA. Interleukin-2: Inception, impact, and implications. Science 1988;240:1169–1176.
14. Lotze MT. Interleukin-2: Basic principles. In: DeVita VT, Hellmann S, Rosenberg SA, eds. Biologic therapy of cancer. Philadelphia: JB Lippincott, 1991:123–141.
15. Mulé JJ, Rosenberg SA. Interleukin-2: Preclinical trials. In: DeVita VT, Hellmann S, Rosenberg SA, eds. Biologic therapy of cancer. Philadelphia: JB Lippincott, 1991:142–158.
16. Ihle JN, Keller J. Interleukin-3 regulation of hematopoietic stem cell differentiation. Prog Clin Biol Res 1985;184:85–94.
17. Ihle JN. Biochemical and biological properties of interleukin-3: A lymphokine mediating the differentiation of a lineage of cells that includes prothymocytes and mastlike cells. Contemp Top Mol Immunol 1985;10:93–119.
18. Ihle JN, Weinstein Y, Rapp UR, Cleveland JL, Reddy EP. Mechanisms in interleukin-3 regulated growth and differentiation. Adv Exp Med Biol 1987;213:149–162.
19. Metcalf D, Morstyn G. Colony-stimulating factors: General biology. In: DeVita VT, Hellmann S, Rosenberg SA, eds. Biologic therapy of cancer. Philadelphia: JB Lippincott, 1991:417–444.
20. Smith CA, Rennick DM. Characterization of a murine lymphokine distinct from interleukin-2 and interleukin-3 (IL-3) possessing a T-cell growth factor activity and a mast-cell growth factor activity that synergizes with IL-3. Proc Natl Acad Sci USA 1986;83:1857–1861.
21. Grabstein K, Eisenman J, Mochizuki D, et al. Purification to homogeneity of B cell stimulating factor: A molecule that stimulates proliferation of multiple lymphokine-dependent cell lines. J Exp Med 1986;163:1405–1414.
22. Yokota T, Otsuka T, Mosmann T, et al. Isolation and characterization of a human interleukin cDNA clone, homologous to mouse B cell stimulatory factor 1, that expresses B cell- and T cell-stimulating activities. Proc Natl Acad Sci USA 1986;83:5894–5898.
23. Noma Y, Sideras P, Naito T, Bergstedt-Lindquist S, et al. Cloning of cDNA encoding the murine IgG1 induction factor by a novel strategy using SP6 promoter. Nature 1986;319:640–646.
24. Paul WE. Interleukin-4/B-cell stimulatory factor 1: One lymphokine, many functions. FASEB J 1987;1:456–461.
25. Yokota T, Arai N, DeVries J, et al. Molecular biology of interleukin 4 and interleukin 5 genes and biology of their products that stimulate B cells, T cells and hemopoietic cells. Immunol Rev 1988;102:137–187.
26. Street NE, Mosmann TR. IL-4 and IL-5: The role of two multifunctional cytokines and their place in the network of cytokine interactions. Biotherapy 1990;2:347–362.
27. Azuma C, Tanabe T, Konishi M, et al. Cloning of cDNA for human T-cell replacing factor (interleukin-5) and comparison with the murine homologue. Nucleic Acids Res 1986;14:9149–9158.
28. Campbell HD, Tucker WQ, Hort Y, Martinson ME, et al. Molecular cloning, nucleotide sequence, and expression of the gene encoding human eosinophil differentiation factor (interleukin-5). Proc Natl Acad Sci USA 1987;84:6629–6633.
29. Aoki T, Kikuchi H, Miyatake S-I, et al. Interleukin-5 enhances interleukin-2-mediated lymphokine-activated killer activity. J Exp Med 1989;170:583–588.
30. Hirano T, Yasukawa K, Harada H, et al. Complementary DNA for a novel interleukin (BSF-2) that induces B lymphocytes to produce immunoglobulin. Nature 1986;324:73–76.
31. Chiu C-P, Moulds C, Coffman RL, Rennick D, Lee F. Multiple biological activities are expressed by a mouse interleukin-6 cDNA clone isolated from bone marrow stromal cells. Proc Natl Acad Sci USA 1988;85:7099–7103.
32. Wong GG, Clark SC. Multiple actions of interleukin-6 within a cytokine network. Immunol Today 1988;9:137–141.
33. Van Snick J. Interleukin-6: An overview. Annu Rev Immunol 1990;8:253–280.
34. Matsuda T, Hirano T. Interleukin-6 (IL-6). Biotherapy 1990;2:363–373.
35. Namen AE, Lupton S, Hjerrild K, et al. Stimulation of B cell progenitors by cloned murine interleukin-7. Nature 1988;333:571–574.
36. Goodwin RG, Lupton S, Schmierer A, et al. Human interleukin-7: Molecular cloning

and growth factor activity on human and murine B-lineage cells. Proc Natl Acad Sci USA 1989;86:302–308.

37. Jicha DL, Mulé JJ, Rosenberg SA. Interleukin-7 generates antitumor cytotoxic T lymphocytes against murine sarcomas with efficacy in cellular adoptive immunotherapy. J Exp Med 1991;174:1511–1515.

38. Alderson MR, Tough TW, Ziegler SF, Grabstein KH. Interleukin-7 induces cytokine secretion and tumoricidal activity by human peripheral blood monocytes. J Exp Med 1991;173:923–930.

39. Matsushima K, Oppenheim JJ. Interleukin 8 and MCAF. Novel inflammatory cytokines inducible by IL-1 and TNF. Cytokine 1989;1:2–13.

40. Schall TJ. Biology of the RANTES/SIS cytokine family. Cytokine 1991;3:165–183.

41. Uyttenhove C, Simpson R, Van Snick J. Functional and structural characterization of P40, a mouse glycoprotein with T cell growth factor activity. Proc Natl Acad Sci USA 1988;85:6934–6939.

42. Van Snick J, Goethals A, Renauld J-C, et al. Cloning and characterization of a cDNA for a new mouse T cell growth factor (P40). J Exp Med 1989;169:363–368.

43. Donahue RE, Yang YC, Clark SC. Human P40 T-cell growth factor (interleukin-9) supports erythroid colony formation. Blood 1990;75:2271–2275.

44. Renauld JC, Goethals A, Houssiau F, Merz H, Van Roost E, Van Snick J. Human P40/IL-9: Expression in activated CD4+ T cells, genomic organization, and comparison with the mouse gene. J Immunol 1990;144:4235–4241.

45. Hultner L, Moeller J. Mast cell growth-enhancing activity (MEA) stimulates interleukin-6 production in a mouse bone marrow-derived mast cell line and a malignant subline. Exp Hematol 1990;18:873–877.

46. Moeller J, Hultner L, Schmitt E, Breuer M, Dormer P. Purification of MEA, a mast cell growth-enhancing activity, to apparent homogeneity and its partial amino acid sequencing. J Immunol 1990;144:4231–4234.

47. Holbrook ST, Ohls RK, Schibler KR, Yang YC, Christensen RD. Effect of interleukin-9 on clonogenic maturation and cell-cycle status of fetal and adult hematopoietic progenitors. Blood 1991;77:2129–2134.

48. Vieira P, deWaal-Malefyt R, Dang M-N, et al. Isolation and expresson of human cytokine synthesis inhibitory factor cDNA clones: Homology to Epstein-Barr virus open reading frame BCRFI. Proc Natl Acad Sci USA 1991;88:1172–1176.

49. Hsu D-H, deWaal-Malefyt R, Fiorentino DF, et al. Expression of interleukin-10 activity by Epstein-Barr virus protein BCRFI. Science 1990;250:830–832.

50. Thompson-Snipes L, Dhar V, Bond MW, et al. Interleukin-10: A novel stimulatory factor for mast cells and their progenitors. J Exp Med 1991;173:507–510.

51. Go NF, Castle BE, Barrett R, et al. Interleukin-10, a novel B cell stimulatory factor: Unresponsiveness of X chromosome-linked immunodeficiency B cells. J Exp Med 1990;172:1625–1631.

52. MacNeil IA, Suda T, Moore KW, Mosmann TR, Zlotnik A. IL-10, a novel growth cofactor for mature and immature T cells. J Immunol 1990;145:4167–4173.

53. Mosmann TR, Moore KW. The role of IL-10 in crossregulation of TH1 and TH2 responses. Immunol Today 1991;12:A49–53.

54. Fiorentino DF, Zlotnik A, Vieira P, et al. IL-10 acts on the antigen-presenting cell to inhibit cytokine production by TH1 cells. J Immunol 1991;146:3444–3451.

55. Chen WF, Zlotnik A. IL-10: A novel cytotoxic T cell differentiation factor. J Immunol 1991;147:528–534.

56. Paul SR, Bennett F, Calvetti JA, et al. Molecular cloning of a cDNA encoding interleukin-11, a stromal cell-derived lymphopoietic and hematopoietic cytokine. Proc Natl Acad Sci USA 1990;87:7512–7516.

57. Kawashima I, Ohsumi J, Mita-Honjo K, et al. Molecular cloning of cDNA encoding adipogenesis inhibitory factor and identity with interleukin-11. FEBS Lett 1991;283:199–202.

58. Stern AS, Podlaski FJ, Hulmes JD, et al. Purification to homogeneity and partial characterization of cytotoxic lymphocyte maturation factor from human B-lymphoblastoid cells. Proc Natl Acad Sci USA 1990;87:6808–6812.

59. Gubler U, Chua A, Schoenhaut DS, et al. Coexpression of two distinct genes is required to generate secreted bioactive cytotoxic lymphocyte maturation factor. Proc Natl Acad Sci USA 1991;88:4143–4147.

60. Wolf SF, Temple PA, Kobayashi M, et al. Cloning of cDNA for natural killer cell stimulatory factor, a heterodimeric cytokine with multiple biologic effects on T and natural killer cells. J Immunol 1991;146:3074–3081.

61. Chan SH, Perussia B, Gupta JW, et al. Induction of interferon production by natural killer cell stimulatory factor: Characterization of the responder cells and synergy with other inducers. J Exp Med 1991;173:869–879.

62. Kurzrock R, Talpaz M, Gutterman J. Interferons-α, β, γ: Basic principles and preclinical studies. In: DeVita VT, Hellmann S, Rosenberg SA, eds. Biologic therapy of cancer. Philadelphia: JB Lippincott, 1991:247–274.

63. Carswell EA, Old LJ, Kassel RL, et al. An endotoxin-induced serum factor which causes necrosis of tumors. Proc Natl Acad Sci USA 1975;72:3666–3670.

64. Pennica D, Hayflick JS, Bringman TS, et al. Cloning and expression in *Escherichia coli* of the cDNA for murine tumor necrosis factor. Proc Natl Acad Sci USA 1985;82:6060–6064.

65. Wang AM, Creasey AA, Ladner MB, et al. Molecular cloning of the complementary DNA for human tumor necrosis factor. Science 1985;228:149–154.

66. Spriggs DR. Tumor necrosis factor: Basic principles and preclinical studies. In: DeVita VT, Hellmann S, Rosenberg SA, eds. Biologic therapy of cancer. Philadelphia: JB Lippincott, 1991:354–377.

67. Wong GG, Temple PA, Leary AC, et al. Human CSF-1: Molecular cloning and expression of 4-kb cDNA encoding human urinary protein. Science 1987;235:1504–1508.

68. Ralph P, Warren MK, Ladner MB, Kawasaki ES, Boosman A, White TJ. Molecular and biological properties of human macrophage growth factor, CSF-1. Cold Spring Harbor Symp Quant Biol 1986;51:679–683.

69. Bock SN, Cameron RB, Kragel P, Mulé JJ, Rosenberg SA. Biological and antitumor effects of recombinant human macrophage colony-stimulating factor in mice. Cancer Res 1991;51:2649–2654.

70. Sanda MG, Bolton E, Mulé JJ, Rosenberg SA. In vivo administration of recombinant macrophage colony-stimulating factor induces macrophage-mediated antibody-dependent cytotoxicity of tumor cells. J Immunother 1992;12:132–137.

71. Gross L. Intradermal immunization of C3H mice against a sarcoma that originated in an animal of the same line. Cancer Res 1943;3:326–333.

72. Foley EJ. Antigenic properties of methylcholanthrene-induced tumors in mice of the strain of origin. Cancer Res 1953;13:835–837.

73. Baldwin RW. Immunity to methylcholanthrene-induced tumors in inbred rats following atrophy and regression of implanted tumors. Br J Cancer 1955;9:652–665.

74. Prehn RT, Main JM. Immunity to methylcholanthrene-induced sarcomas. JNCI 1957;18:769–778.

75. Klein G, Sjögren HO, Klein E, Hellström KE. Demonstration of resistance against methylcholanthrene-induced sarcomas in the primary autochthonous host. Cancer Res 1960;20:1561–1572.

76. Old LJ, Boyse EA, Clarke DA, Carswell EA. Antigenic properties of chemically-induced tumors. Ann NY Acad Sci 1962;101:80–106.

77. Globerson A, Feldmann M. Antigenic specificity of benzo[a]pyrene-induced sarcomas. JNCI 1964;32:1229–1243.

78. Vaage J. Nonvirus-associated antigens in virus-induced mouse mammary tumors. Cancer Res 1968;28:2477–2483.

79. Morton DL, Miller GF, Wood DA. Demonstration of tumor-specific immunity against antigens unrelated to the mammary tumor virus in spontaneous mammary adenocarcinomas. JNCI 1969;42:289–301.

80. Carswell EA, Wanebo HJ, Old LJ, Boyse EA. Immunogenic properties of reticulum cell sarcomas of SJL/J mice. JNCI 1970;44:1281–1288.

81. Koch S, Zaleberg JR, McKenzie IFC. Description of a murine B lymphoma tumor-specific antigen. J Immunol 1984;133:1070–1077.

82. Baldwin RW. Tumor-specific immunity to spontaneous rat tumors. Int J Cancer 1966;1:257–264.

83. Basombrio MA. Search for common antigenicity among twenty-five sarcomas induced by methylcholanthrene. Cancer Res 1970;30:2458–2462.

84. Basombrio MA, Prehn RT. Studies on the basis of diversity and time of appearance of chemically-induced tumors. NCI Monogr 1972;35:117–124.

85. Baldwin RW, Price MR. Neoantigen expression in chemical carcinogenesis. In: Becker FF, ed. Cancer: A comprehensive treatise vol 1. 2nd ed. New York: Plenum, 1982:507–548.

86. Defendi V. Effects of SV40 virus immunization on growth of transplantable SV40 and polyoma virus tumors in hamsters. Proc Soc Exp Biol Med 1963;113:12–16.

87. Khera KS, Ashkenazi A, Rapp F, Melnick JL. Immunity in hamsters to cells transformed in vitro among the papovaviruses. J Immunol 1963;91:604–613.

88. Sjögren HO, Hellström I, Klein G. Resistance of polyoma virus-immunized mice to transplantation of established polyoma tumors. Exp Cell Res 1961;23:204–208.

89. Chang CR, Martin RG, Livingston DM, et al. Relationship between T-antigen and tumor-specific transplantation antigen in simian virus 40-transformed cells. J Virol 1979;29:69.

90. Livingston DM, Bradley MK. The simian virus 40 large T antigen. A lot packed into a little. Mol Biol Med 1987;4:63–80.

91. Boon T, Van Pel A, DePlaen E, et al. Genes coding for T-cell-defined tumor transplantation antigens: Point mutations, antigenic peptides, and subgenic expression. Cold Spring Harb Symp Quant Biol 1989;1:587–596.

92. Hewitt HB, Blake ER, Walder AS. A critique of the evidence for active host defense against cancer based on personal studies of 27 murine tumors of spontaneous origin. Br J Cancer 1976;33:241–259.

93. Middle JG, Embleton MJ. Naturally arising tumors of the inbred WAB/Not rat strain. II. Immunogenicity of transplanted tumors. JNCI 1981;67:637–643.

94. Rosenberg SA, Spiess P, Lafreniere R. A new approach to the adoptive immunotherapy of cancer with tumor-infiltrating lymphocytes. Science 1986;233:1318–1321.

95. Topalian SL, Rosenberg SA. Tumor infiltrating lymphocytes (TIL). Evidence for specific immune reactions against growing cancers in mice and humans. In: DeVita VT, Hellman S, Rosenberg SA, eds. Important advances in oncology. Philadelphia: JB Lippincott, 1990;19–41.

96. Barth RJ, Mulé JJ, Asher AL, Sanda MG, Rosenberg SA. Identification of unique murine tumor associated antigens by tumor infiltrating lymphocytes using tumor specific secretion of interferon-gamma and tumor necrosis factor. J Immunol Methods 1991;140:269–279.

97. Hellström I, Hellström KE, Sjögren HO, et al. Demonstration of cell-mediated immunity to human neoplasms of various histological types. Int J Cancer 1971;7:1–16.

98. Hellström I, Hellström KE, Shepard TH. Cell-mediated immunity against antigens common to human colonic carcinomas and fetal gut epithelium. Int J Cancer 1970;6:346–351.

99. Herberman RB, Oldham RK. Problems associated with study of cell-mediated immunity to human tumors by microcytotoxicity assays. JNCI 1975;55:749–753.

100. Hellström I, Hellström KE. Cell-mediated reactivity to human tumor-type associated antigens: Does it exist? J Biol Response Mod 1983;2:310–320.

101. Vanky F, Klein E. Specificity of auto-tumor cytotoxicity exerted by fresh, activated and propagated human T lymphocytes. Int J Cancer 1982;29:547–553.

102. Vanky F, Klein E, Willems J, et al. Lysis of autologous tumor cells by blood lymphocytes tested at the time of surgery. Correlation with the postsurgical clinical course. Cancer Immunol Immunother 1986;21:69–76.

103. Morgan DA, Ruscetti FW, Gallo RG. Selective in vitro growth of T-lymphocytes from normal bone marrow. Science 1976;193:1007–1008.

104. Hellstrom KE, Hellstrom I. Principles of tumor immunity: Tumor antigens. In: DeVita VT, Hellman S, Rosenberg SA, eds. Biologic therapy of cancer. Philadelphia: JB Lippincott, 1991:35–52.

105. Schreiber H. Tumor Immunology. In: Paul W, ed. Fundamental immunology. New York: Raven Press, 1989:923–956.

106. Lotze MT, Strausser JL, Line BR, Rosenberg SA. Tumor lysis by human T lymphocytes in long-term culture and their distribution in vivo: Implications for immunotherapy. Surg Forum 1980;30:404–406.

107. Grimm EA, Mazumder A, Zhang HZ, Rosenberg SA. The lymphokine activated killer cell phenomenon: Lysis of NK-resistant fresh solid tumor cells by IL-2 activated autologous human peripheral blood lymphocytes. J Exp Med 1982;155:1823–1841.

108. Grimm EA, Rosenberg SA. The human lymphokine-activated killer cell phenomenon. In: Pick E, Candy M, eds. Lymphokines. New York: Academic Press, 1983:279–311.

109. Rosenstein M, Yron I, Kaufmann Y, Rosenberg SA. Lymphokine activated killer cells: Lysis of fresh syngeneic NK-resistant murine tumor cells by lymphocytes cultured in interleukin-2. Cancer Res 1984;44:1946–1953.

110. Topalian SL, Rosenberg SA. Adoptive cellular therapy: Basic principles. In: DeVita VT, Hellman S, Rosenberg SA, eds. Biologic therapy of cancer. Philadelphia: JB Lippincott, 1991:178–196.

111. Galili U, Vanky F, Rodriquez L, et al. Activated T lymphocytes within human solid tumors. Cancer Immunol Immunother 1979;6:129–133.

112. Whiteside TL, Miescher S, Hurlimann J, et al. Separation, phenotyping, and limiting dilution analysis of T-lymphocytes infiltrating human solid tumors. Int J Cancer 1986;38:803–811.

113. Whiteside TL, Miescher S, Hurlimman J, et al. Clonal analysis and in situ characterization of lymphocytes infiltrating human breast carcinomas. Cancer Immunol Immunother 1986;23:169–178.

114. Paine J, Handa H, Yamasaki T, et al. Immunohistochemical analysis of infiltrating lymphocytes in central nervous system tumors. Neurosurgery 1986;18:766–772.

115. Itoh K, Tilden AB, Balch CM. Interleukin-2 activation of cytotoxic T-lymphocyte infiltrating into human metastatic melanomas. Cancer Res 1986;46:3011–3017.

116. Kurnick JT, Kradin RL, Blumberg R, et al. Functional characterization of T lymphocytes propagated from human lung carcinoma. Clin Immunol Immunopathol 1986;38:367–380.

117. Rabinowich H, Cohen R, Bruderman I, et al. Functional analysis of mononuclear cells infiltrating into tumors: Lysis of autologous human tumor cells by cultured infiltrating lymphocytes. Cancer Res 1987;47:173–177.

118. Muul LM, Spiess PJ, Director EP, et al. Identification of specific cytolytic immune responses against autologous tumor in humans bearing malignant melanoma. J Immunol 1987;138:989–995.

119. Heo DL, Whiteside TL, Johnson JT, et al. Long-term interleukin-2-dependent growth and cytotoxic activity of tumor-infiltrating lymphocytes from human squamous cell carcinomas of the head and neck. Cancer Res 1987;47:6353–6362.

120. Itoh K, Platsooucas CD, Balch CM. Autologous tumor-specific cytotoxic T lymphocytes in the infiltrate of human metastatic melanomas: Activation by interleukin-2 and autologous tumor cells and involvement of the T cell receptor. J Exp Med 1988;168:1419–1441.

121. Kuppner MC, Hamou MF, de Tribolet N. Immunohistological and functional analyses of lymphoid infiltrates in human glioblastomas. Cancer Res 1988;48:6926–6932.

122. Saito T, Tanaka R, Yoshida S, et al. Immunohistochemical analysis of tumor-infiltrating lymphocytes and major histocompatibility antigens in human gliomas and metastatic brain tumors. Surg Neurol 1988;29:435–442.

123. Heo DS, Whiteside TL, Kanbour A, et al. Lymphocytes infiltrating human ovarian tumors. I. Role of Leu-19 (NKH1)-positive recombinant IL-2 activated cultures of lymphocytes infiltrating human ovarian tumors. J Immunol 1988;140:4042–4049.

124. Belldegrun A, Muul LM, Rosenberg SA. Interleukin-2 expanded tumor-infiltrating lymphocytes in human renal cell cancer: Isolation, characterization, and anti-tumor activity. Cancer Res 1988;48:206–214.

125. Radrizzani M, Gambacorti-Passerini C, Parmiani G, et al. Lysis by interleukin-2 stimulated tumor-infiltrating lymphocytes of autologous and allogeneic tumor target cells. Cancer Immunol Immunother 1989;28:67–73.

126. Topalian SL, Solomon D, Rosenberg SA. Tumor-specific cytolysis by lymphocytes infiltrating human melanomas. J Immunol 1989;142:3714–3725.

127. Tagaki S, Chen K, Schwarz R, et al. Functional and phenotypic analysis of tumor-infiltrating lymphocytes isolated from human primary and metastatic liver tumors and cultured in recombinant interleukin-2. Cancer 1989;63:102–111.

128. Balch CM, Riley LB, Bae TJ, et al. Patterns of human tumor infiltrating lymphocytes in 120 human cancers. Arch Surg 1990;125:200–205.

129. Haas GP, Solomon D, Rosenberg SA. Tumor infiltrating lymphocytes from non renal urological malignancies. Cancer Immunol Immunother 1990;30:342–350.

130. Rivoltini L, Avienti F, Orazi A, et al. Phenotypic and functional analysis of lymphocytes infiltrating pediatric tumors, with a characterization of the tumor phenotype. Cancer Immunol Immunother 1992;34:241–251.

131. Schwartzentruber DJ, Topalian SL, Mancini MJ, et al. Specific release of granulocyte-macrophage colony-stimulating factor, tumor necrosis factor-a, and IFN-γ by human tumor-infiltrating lymphocytes after autologous tumor stimulation. J Immunol 1991;146:153–164.

132. Hom SS, Topalian SL, Simoni ST, et al. Common expression of melanoma tumor-associated antigens recognized by human tumor-infiltrating lymphocytes: Analysis by HLA restriction. J Immunother 1991;10:153–164.

133. Darrow TL, Slingluff CL, Seigler HF. The role of class I antigens in recognition of melanoma cells by tumor-specific cytotoxic T lymphocytes: Evidence for shared tumor antigens. J Immunol 1989;142:3329–3335.

134. Stotter H, Wiebke EA, Tomita S, et al. Cytokines alter target cell susceptibility to lysis: II. Evaluation of tumor infiltrating lymphocytes. J Immunol 1989;142:1767–1773.

135. Kawakami Y, Rosenberg SA, Lotze MT. Interleukin-4 promotes the growth of tumor-infiltrating lymphocytes cytotoxic for human autologous melanoma. J Exp Med 1988;168:2183–2191.

136. Kawakami Y, Zakut R, Topalian SL, et al. Shared human melanoma antigens: Recognition by tumor infiltrating lymphocytes in HLA-A2.1-transfected melanomas. J Immunol 1992;148:638–643.

137. Van der Bruggen P, Traversari C, Chomez P, et al. A gene encoding an antigen recognized by cytolytic T lymphocytes on a human melanoma. Science 1991;254:1643–1647.

138. Rudikoff S. Principles of tumor immunity: Biology of antibody-mediated responses. In: DeVita VT, Hellmann S, Rosenberg SA, eds. Biologic therapy of cancer. Philadelphia: JB Lippincott, 1991:22–34.

139. Klein G, Clifford P, Klein E, et al. Search for tumor-specific immune reactions in Burkitt's lymphoma patients by the membrane immunofluorescence reaction. Proc Natl Acad Sci USA 1966;55:1628–1635.

140. Lewis MG, Ikonopisov RL, Nairn RC, et al. Tumor-specific antibodies in human malignant melanoma and their relationship to extent of disease. Br Med J 1969;3:547–552.

141. Morton DL, Malmgren RA, Holmes EC, et al. Demonstration of antibodies against human malignant melanoma by immunofluorescence. Surgery 1968;64:233–240.

142. Morton DL, Malmgren RA. Human osteosarcomas: Immunologic evidence suggesting an associated infectious agent. Science 1968;162:1279–1281.

143. Sjögren HO, Hellström I, Bansal SC. Elution of "blocking factors" from human tumors capable of abrogating tumor cell destruction by specifically immune lymphocytes. Int J Cancer 1972;9:274–283.

144. Cornain S, deVries JE, Collard J, et al. Antibodies and antigen expression in human melanoma detected by the immune adherence test. Int J Cancer 1975;16:981–997.

145. Shiku H, Takahashi T, Oettgen HF, et al. Cell surface antigens of human malignant melanoma: II. Serological typing with immune adherence assays and definition of two new surface antigens. J Exp Med 1976;144:873–881.

146. Real FX, Mattes MJ, Houghton AN, et al. Class 1 (unique) tumor antigens of human melanoma. Identification of a 90,000 dalton cell surface glycoprotein by autologous antibody. J Exp Med 1984;160:1219–1233.

147. Kohler G, Milstein C. Continuous culture of fused cells secreting antibodies of predefined specificity. Nature 1975;256:495–497.

148. Schlom J. Antibodies in cancer therapy: Basic principles of monoclonal antibodies. In: DeVita VT, Hellmann S, Rosenberg SA, eds. Biologic therapy of cancer. Philadelphia: JB Lippincott, 1991:464–481.

149. Coley WB. A report of recent cases of inoperable sarcoma successfully treated with mixed toxins of erysipelas and *Bacillus prodigiosus*. Surg Gynecol Obstet 1911;13:174–190.

150. Hersh EM, Taylor CW. Immunotherapy by active immunization. In: DeVita VT, Hellmann S, Rosenberg SA, eds. Biologic therapy of cancer. Philadelphia: JB Lippincott, 1991:613–626.

151. Old LJ, Benacerraf B, Clarke D, et al. The role of the reticuloendothelial system in the host reaction to neoplasia. Cancer Res 1961;21:1281–1300.

152. Mathé G, Pouillart P, Lapeyraque F. Active immunotherapy of L1210 leukaemia applied after the graft of tumor cells. Br J Cancer 1989;23:814–824.

153. Mathé G, Amiel JL, Schwarzenberg L, et al. Active immunotherapy for acute lymphoblastic leukemia. Lancet 1969;2:697–699.

154. Gutterman JU, Hersh EM, Rodriguez V, et al. Chemoimmunotherapy of adult acute leukemia in prolongation of remission in myeloblastic leukemia with BCG. Lancet 1974;2:1405–1416.

155. Medical Research Council Leukaemia Committee and the Working Party on Leukaemia in Childhood: Treatment of acute lymphoblastic leukaemia. Comparison of immunotherapy (BCG), intermittent methotrexate, and no therapy after a five-month intensive cytotoxic regimen (Concord trial). Br Med J 1971;4:189–194.

156. Foon KA, Smalley RV, Riggs CW, et al. The role of immunotherapy in acute myelogenous leukemia. Arch Intern Med 1983;143:1726.

157. Volger WR. Results of randomized trials of immunotherapy for acute leukemia. Cancer Immunol Immunopharmacol 1980;9:15.

158. Gutterman JU, Mavligit GM, McBride CM, et al. Active immunotherapy with BCG for recurrent malignant melanoma. Lancet 1973;1:1208–1212.

159. Fisher RI, Terry WD, Hodes RJ, et al. Adjuvant immunotherapy or chemotherapy for malignant melanoma: Preliminary report of the National Cancer Institute randomized clinical trial. Surg Clin North Am 1981;61:1267–1277.

160. Veronesi U, Adamus J, Albert C, et al. A randomized trial of adjuvant chemotherapy and immunotherapy in cutaneous melanoma. N Engl J Med 1982;307:913–916.

161. Terry WT, Rosenberg SA. Immunotherapy of human cancer. New York: Elsevier-North Holland, 1982.

162. Ruckdeschel JC, Codish SD, Stranahan A, et al. Postoperative empyema improves survival in lung cancer: Documentation and analysis of a natural experiment. N Engl J Med 1972;287:1013–1017.

163. McKneally MF, Maver C, Kausel HW, et al. Regional immunotherapy of lung cancer with intrapleural BCG. Lancet 1976;1:377–379.

164. Holmes EC, Hill LD, Gail M, et al. A randomized comparison of the effects of adjuvant therapy on resected stages II and III non-small cell carcinoma of the lung. Ann Surg 1985;202:335–341.

165. Laurie JA, Moertel CG, Fleming TR, et al. Surgical adjuvant therapy of large-bowel carcinoma: An evaluation of levamisole and the combination of levamisole and fluorouracil. J Clin Oncol 1989;7:1447–1456.

166. Verhaegen H, DeCree J, DeCock W, et al. Levamisole therapy in patients with colorectal

cancer. In: Terry W, Rosenberg SA eds. Immunotherapy of human cancer. New York: Elsevier, 1982:225–229.

167. Moertel CG, Fleming TR, Macdonald JS, et al. Levamisole and fluorouracil for adjuvant therapy of resected colon carcinoma. N Engl J Med 1990;322:352–358.

168. Morton DL, Hunt KK, Bauer RL, Lee JD. Clinical application using intralesional therapy. In: DeVita VT, Hellmann S, Rosenberg SA, eds. Biologic therapy of cancer. Philadelphia: JB Lippincott, 1991:627–642.

169. Cohen MH, Jessup JM, Felix EL, et al. Intralesional treatment of recurrent metastatic cutaneous malignant melanoma: A randomized prospective study of intralesional bacillus Calmette-Guérin versus intralesional dinitrochlorobenzene. Cancer 1978;41:2456–2463.

170. Herr H. Instillation therapy for bladder cancer. In: DeVita VT, Hellmann S, Rosenberg SA, eds. Biologic therapy of cancer. Philadelphia: JB Lippincott, 1991:643–650.

171. Morales A, Eidinger D, Bruce AW. Intracavitary BCG in the treatment of superficial bladder tumors. J Urol 1976;116:180–184.

172. Hanna MG Jr, Pollack VA, Peters LC, et al. Active specific immunotherapy of established micrometastases with BCG plus tumor cell vaccines: Effective treatment of BCG side effects with isoniazid. Cancer 1982;49:659–664.

173. Hoover HC Jr, Hanna MG Jr: Immunotherapy by active specific immunization. In: DeVita VT, Hellmann S, Rosenberg SA, eds. Biologic therapy of cancer. Philadelphia: JB Lippincott, 1991:670–681.

174. Hoover HC Jr, Surdyke M, Dangel R, et al. Delayed cutaneous hypersensitivity to autologous tumor cells in colorectal cancer patients immunized with an autologous tumor cell: Bacillus Calmette-Guerin vaccine. Cancer Res 1984;44:1671–1676.

175. Hoover HC Jr, Surdyke MG, Dangel RB, et al. Prospectively randomized trial of adjuvant active-specific immunotherapy for human colorectal cancer. Cancer 1985;55:1236–1243.

176. Rosenberg SA. The immunotherapy and gene therapy of cancer. J Clin Oncol 1992;10:180–199.

177. Kurzrock R, Gutterman JU, Talpaz M. Interferons α, β, γ: Basic principles and preclinical studies. In: DeVita VT, Hellmann S, Rosenberg SA, eds. Biologic therapy of cancer. Philadelphia: JB Lippincott, 1991:247–274.

178. Isaacs A, Lindenmann J. Virus interference: I. The interferon. Proc R Soc Lond [Biol] 1957;147:258–267.

179. Kurzock R, Talpaz M, Gutterman JU. Interferons—clinical applications. In: DeVita VT, Hellmann S, Rosenberg SA, eds. Biologic therapy of cancer. Philadelphia: JB Lippincott, 1991:334–345.

180. Levy R, Miller RA. Antibodies in cancer therapy: B-cell lymphomas. In: DeVita VT, Hellmann S, Rosenberg SA, eds. Biologic therapy of cancer. Philadelphia: JB Lippincott, 1991:512–522.

181. Waldmann TA. Antibodies in cancer therapy: Clinical applications. T-cell leukemia/lymphomas. In: DeVita VT, Hellman S, Rosenberg SA, eds. Biologic therapy of cancer. Philadelphia: JB Lippincott, 1991:523–532.

182. Smith KA. Interleukin-2: Inception, impact and implications. Science 1988;240:1169–1175.

183. Morgan DA, Ruscetti FW, Gallo RG. Selective in vitro growth of T lymphocytes from normal human bone marrow. Science 1976;193:1007–1008.

184. Stern JB, Smith KA. Interleukin-2 induction of T-cell G1, progression and c-*MYB* expression. Science 1986;233:203–206.

185. Kornfeld H, Berman JS, Beer DJ, et al. Induction of human T lymphocyte motility by interleukin 2. J Immunol 1985;134:3887–3890.

186. Nedwin GE, Svederdky LP, Bringman TS, et al. Effect of interleukin 2, interferon-α, and mitogens on the production of tumor necrosis factors α and β. J Immunol 1985;135:2492–2497.

187. Waldmann TA, Goldman CK, Robb RJ, et al. Expression of interleukin-2 receptors on activated human B cells. J Exp Med 1984;160:1450–1466.

188. Jung LKL, Toshiro H, Fu SM. Detection and functional studies of p60–65 (Tac antigen) on activated human B cells. J Exp Med 1984;160:1597–1602.

189. Malkovsky M, Loveland B, North M, et al. Recombinant interleukin-2 directly augments the cytotoxicity of human monocytes. Nature 1987;325:262–264.

190. Hancock WW, Muller WA, Cotran RS. Interleukin 2 receptors are expressed by alveolar macrophages during pulmonary sarcoidosis and are inducible by lymphokine treatment of normal human lung macrophages, blood monocytes, and monocyte cell lines. J Immunol 1987;138:185–191.

191. Steiner G, Tschachler E, Tani M, et al. Interleukin 2 receptors on cultured murine epidermal Langerhans cells. J Immunol 1986;137:155–159.

192. Benveniste EN, Merrill JE. Stimulation of oligodendroglial proliferation and maturation by interleukin-2. Nature 1986;321:610–613.

193. Steiner G, Tschachler E, Tani M, et al. Interleukin-2 receptors on cultured murine epidermal Langerhans cells. J Immunol 1986;137:155–159.

194. Gillis S, Watson J. Biochemical and biological characterization of lymphocyte regulatory molecules: V. Identification of an interleukin-2 producing human leukemia T cell line. J Exp Med 1980;152:1709–1715.

195. Taniguchi T, Matsui H, Fujita T, et al. Structure and expression of a cloned cDNA for human interleukin-2. Nature 1983;302:305–307.

196. Rosenberg SA, Grimm EA, McGrogan M, et al. Biological activity of recombinant human interleukin-2 produced in E. coli. Science 1984;223:1412–1415.

197. Doyle MV, Lee MT, Fong S. Comparison of the biological activities of human recombinant interleukin-2$_{125}$ and native interleukin-2. J Biol Response Mod 1985;4:96–109.

198. Sharon M, Klausner RD, Cullen BR, et al. Novel interleukin-2 receptor subunit detected by cross-linking under high-affinity conditions. Science 1987;234:859–863.

199. Rosenberg SA, Lotze MT, Mulé JJ. New approaches to the immunotherapy of cancer. Ann Intern Med 1988;108:853–864.

200. Merluzzi VJ, Walker MM, Fananes RB. Inhibition of cytotoxic T-cell clonal expansion by cyclophosphamide and the recovery of cytotoxic T-lymphocyte precursors by supernatants from mixed lymphocyte cultures. Cancer Res 1981;41:850–853.

201. Clason AE, Duarte AJS, Kupiec-Weglinski JW, et al. Restoration of allograft responsiveness in B rats by interleukin-2 and/or adherent cells. J Immunol 1982;129:252–259.

202. Rook AH, Masur H, Lane HC, et al. Interleukin-2 enhances the depressed natural killer and cytomegalovirus-specific cytotoxic activities of lymphokines from patients with the acquired immune deficiency syndrome. J Clin Invest 1983;72:398–407.

203. Ettinghausen SE, Lipford EH III, Mulé JJ, et al. Systemic administration of recombinant interleukin-2 stimulates in vivo lymphoid cell proliferation in tissues. J Immunol 1985;135:1488–1497.

204. Ettinghausen SE, Lipford EH III, Mulé JJ, et al. Recombinant interleukin-2 stimulates in vivo proliferation of adoptively transferred lymphokine activated killer (LAK) cells. J Immunol 1985;135:3623–3635.

205. Yron I, Wood TA, Spiess P, et al. In vitro growth of murine T cells. V: The isolation and growth of lymphoid cells infiltrating syngeneic solid tumors. J Immunol 1980;125:238–245.

206. Lotze MT, Grimm E, Mazumder A, et al. In vitro growth of cytotoxic human lymphocytes. IV: Lysis of fresh and cultured autologous tumor by lymphocytes cultured in T cell growth factor (TCGF). Cancer Res 1981;41:4420–4425.

207. Grimm EA, Ramsey KM, Mazumder A, et al. Lymphokine-activated killer cell phenomenon. II: The precursor phenotype is serologically distinct from peripheral T lymphocytes, memory CTL, and NK cells. J Exp Med 1983;157:884–897.

208. Rosenstein M, Yron I, Kaufman Y, Rosenberg SA. Lymphokine activated killer cells: Lysis of fresh syngeneic NK-resistant murine tumor cells by lymphocytes cultured in interleukin-2. Cancer Res 1984;44:1946–1953.

209. Rayner AA, Grimm EA, Lotze MT, et al. Lymphokine-activated killer (LAK) cell phenomenon: Analysis of factors relevant to the immunotherapy of human cancer. Cancer 1985;55:1327–1333.

210. Rosenberg SA. Adoptive immunotherapy of cancer using lymphokine activated killer cells and recombinant interleukin-2. In: DeVita VT, Hellman S, Rosenberg SA, eds. Important advances in oncology. Philadelphia: JB Lippincott, 1986:55–91.

211. Rosenberg SA, Mulé JJ, Speiss PJ, et al. Regression of established pulmonary metastases and subcutaneous tumor mediated by the systemic administration of high dose recombinant IL-2. J Exp Med 1985;161:1169–1188.

212. Lafreniere R, Rosenberg SA. Successful immunotherapy of murine experimental hepatic metastases with lymphokine-activated killer cells and recombinant interleukin-2. Cancer Res 1985;45:3735–3741.

213. Mulé JJ, Yang JC, Lafreniere R, et al. Identification of cellular mechanisms operational in vivo during the regression of established pulmonary metastases by the systemic administration of high-dose recombinant interleukin-2. J Immunol 1987;139:285–294.

214. Papa MZ, Mulé JJ, Rosenberg SA. The anti-tumor efficacy of lymphokine-activated killer cells and recombinant interleukin-2 in vivo: Successful immunotherapy of established pulmonary metastases from weak and non-immunogenic murine tumors of three distinct histologic types. Cancer Res 1986;46:4973–4978.

215. Donohue JH, Rosenstein M, Chang AE, et al. The systemic administration of purified interleukin-2 enhances the ability of sensitized murine lymphocyte lines to cure a disseminated syngeneic lymphoma. J Immunol 1984;132:2123–2128.

216. Shu S, Chou T, Rosenberg SA. In vitro sensitization and expansion with viable tumor cells and interleukin-2 in the generation of specific therapeutic effector cells. J Immunol 1986;136:3891–3898.

217. Shu S, Chou T, Rosenberg SA. Generation from tumor-bearing mice of lymphocytes with in vivo therapeutic efficacy. J Immunol 1987;139:295–304.

218. Rosenberg SA, Spiess P, Lafreniere R. A new approach to the adoptive immunotherapy of cancer with tumor-infiltrating lymphocytes. Science 1986;223:1318–1321.

219. Spiess PJ, Yang JC, Rosenberg SA. The in vivo anti-tumor activity of tumor infiltrating lymphocytes expanded in recombinant interleukin-2. JNCI 1987;79:1067–1075.

220. Lotze MT, Matory YL, Ettinghausen SE, et al. In vivo administration of recombinant human interleukin-2 II: Half-life, immunologic effects and expansion of peripheral lymphoid cells in vivo with recombinant IL-2. J Immunol 1985;135:2865–2875.

221. Rosenberg SA, Lotze MT, Muul LM; Leitman S, et al. Observations on the systemic administration of autologous lymphokine-activated killer cells and recombinant interleukin-2 to patients with metastatic cancer. N Engl J Med 1985;313:1485–1492.

222. Rosenberg SA, Lotze MT, Muul LM, et al. A progress report on the treatment of 157 patients with advanced cancer using lymphokine activated killer cells and interleukin-2 or high-dose interleukin-2 alone. N Engl J Med 1987;316:889–897.

223. Rosenberg SA, Lotze MT, Yang JC, Aebersold PM, Linehan WM, Seipp CA, White DE. Experience with the use of high-dose interleukin-2 in the treatment of 652 cancer patients. Ann Surg 1989;210:474–484.

224. Lotze MT, Chang AE, Seipp CA, et al. High-dose recombinant interleukin-2 in the treatment of patients with disseminated cancer: Responses, treatment-related morbidity and histologic findings. JAMA 1986;256:3117–3124.

225. Gambacorti-Passerini C, Radrizzani M, Marolda R, et al. In vivo activation of lymphocytes in melanoma patients receiving escalating doses of recombinant interleukin-2. Int J Cancer 1988;41:700–706.

226. Richards JM, Barker E, Latta J, et al. Phase I study of weekly 24-hour infusions of recombinant human interleukin-2. JNCI 1988;80:1325–1328.

227. Sosman JA, Kohler PC, Hank JA, et al. Repetitive weekly cycles of interleukin-2. II. Clinical and immunologic effects of dose, schedule, and addition of indomethacin. JNCI 1988;80:1451–1461.

228. Thompson JA, Lee DJ, Lindgren CG, et al. Influence of dose and duration of infusion of interleukin-2 on toxicity and immunomodulation. J Clin Oncol 1988;6:669–678.

229. Sarna GP, Figlin RA, Pertcheck M, et al. Systemic administration of recombinant

methionyl human interleukin-2 (Ala 125) to cancer patients: Clinical results. J Biol Response Mod 1989;8:16–24.

230. Nasr S, McKolanis J, Pais R, et al. A phase I study of interleukin-2 in children with cancer and evaluation of clinical and immunologic status during therapy. A Pediatric Oncology Group study. Cancer 1989;64:783–788.

231. Allison MAK, Jones SE, McGuffey P. Phase II trial of outpatient interleukin-2 in malignant lymphoma, chronic lymphocytic leukemia, and selected solid tumors. J Clin Oncol 1989;7:75–80.

232. Hersh EM, Murray JL, Hong WK, et al. Phase I study of cancer therapy with recombinant interleukin-2 administered by intravenous bolus injection. Biotherapy 1989;1:215–226.

233. Goldstein D, Sosman JA, Hank JA, et al. Repetitive weekly cycles of interleukin-2: Effect of outpatient treatment with a lower dose of interleukin-2 on non-major histocompatibility complex-restricted killer activity. Cancer Res 1989;49:6832–6839.

234. Creekmore SP, Harris JE, Ellis TM, et al. A phase I clinical trial of recombinant interleukin-2 by periodic 24-hour intravenous infusions. J Clin Oncol 1989;7:276–284.

235. Bukowski RM, Goodman P, Crawford ED, et al. Phase II trial of high-dose intermittent interleukin-2 in metastatic renal cell carcinoma: A Southwest Oncology Group study. JNCI 1990;82:143–146.

236. Rosenberg SA, Terry W. Passive immunotherapy of cancer in animals and man. Adv Cancer Res 1977;25:323–388.

237. Rosenberg SA. The adoptive immunotherapy of cancer: Accomplishments and prospects. Cancer Treat Rep 1984;68:233–255.

238. Roberts K, Lotze MT, Rosenberg SA. Separation and functional studies of the human lymphokine-activated killer cell. Cancer Res 1987;47:4366–4371.

239. Phillips LL. Dissection of the LAK phenomenon. J Exp Med 1986;164:814–825.

240. Mulé JJ, Shu S, Schwarz SL, Rosenberg SA. Adoptive immunotherapy of established pulmonary metastases with LAK cells and recombinant interleukin-2. Science 1984;225:1487–1489.

241. Lafreniere R, Rosenberg SA. Adoptive immunotherapy of murine hepatic metastases with lymphokine activated killer (LAK) cells and recombinant interleukin-2 (RIL-2) can mediate the regression of both immunogenic and non-immunogenic sarcomas and an adenocarcinoma. J Immunol 1985;135:4273–4280.

242. Mulé JJ, Ettinghausen SE, Spiess PJ, et al. The anti-tumor efficacy of lymphokine-activated killer cells and recombinant interleukin-2 in vivo: An analysis of survival benefit and mechanisms of tumor escape in mice undergoing immunotherapy. Cancer Res 1986;46:676–683.

243. Mulé JJ, Yang J, Shu S, et al. The anti-tumor efficacy of lymphokine-activated killer cells and recombinant interleukin-2 in vivo: Direct correlation between reduction of established metastases and cytolytic activity of lymphokine-activated killer cells. J Immunol 1986;136:3899–3909.

244. Shiloni E, Lafreniere R, Mulé JJ, et al. Effect of immunotherapy with allogeneic lymphokine-activated killer cells and recombinant interleukin-2 on established pulmonary and hepatic metastases in mice. Cancer Res 1986;46:5633–5640.

245. Mazumder A, Eberlein TJ, Grimm EA. Phase I study of the adoptive immunotherapy of human cancer with lectin-activated autologous mononuclear cells. Cancer 1984;53:896–905.

246. Rosenberg SA. Immunotherapy of cancer by the systemic administration of lymphoid cells plus interleukin-2. J Biol Response Mod 1984;3:501–511.

247. Lotze MT, Frana LW, Sharrow SO, et al. In vivo administration of purified human interleukin-2 I: Half-life and immunologic effects of the Jurkat cell line-derived IL-2. J Immunol 1985;134:157–166.

248. Steis R, Bookman M, Clark J, et al. Intraperitoneal lymphokine activated killer (LAK) cell and interleukin-2 (IL-2) therapy for peritoneal carcinomatosis toxicity, efficacy, and laboratory results (abstract). Proc Annu Meet Am Soc Clin Oncol 1987;6:250.

249. Urba WJ, Clark JW, Steis RG, et al. Intraperitoneal lymphokine-activated killer cell/interleukin-2 therapy in patients with intraabdominal cancer: Immunologic considerations. JNCI 1989;81:602–611.

250. Yasumoto K, Miyazaki K, Nagashima A, et al. Induction of lymphokine activated killer cells by intrapleural instillations of recombinant interleukin-2 in patients with malignant pleurisy due to lung cancer. Cancer Res 1987;47:2184–2187.

251. Shimizu K, Okamoto Y, Miyao Y, et al. Adoptive immunotherapy of human meningeal gliomatosis and carcinomatosis with LAK cells and recombinant interleukin-2. J Neurosurg 1987;66:519–521.

252. Jacob SK, Wilson DJ, Kornblith PL, et al. Interleukin-2 or autologous lymphokine-activated killer cell treatment of malignant glioma: Phase I trial. Cancer Res 1986;46:2101–2104.

253. Yoshida S, Tanaka R, Takai N, et al. Local administration of autologous lymphokine-activated killer cells and recombinant interleukin-2 to patients with malignant brain tumors. Cancer Res 1988;48:5011–5016.

254. Ingram M, Jacques S, Freshwater DB, et al. Salvage immunotherapy of malignant glioma. Arch Surg 1987;122:1483–1486.

255. Merchant RE, Merchant LH, Cook SHS, et al. Intralesional infusion of lymphokine-activated killer (LAK) cells and recombinant interleukin-2 (rIL-2) for the treatment of patients with malignant brain tumor. Neurosurgery 1988;23:725–732.

256. Barba D, Saris SC, Holder C, et al. Immunotherapy of human glial tumors: Report of multiple dose intratumoral infusions of lymphokine-activated killer cells and interleukin-2. J Neurosurg 1988;70:175–182.

257. Nitta T, Sato K, Yagita H, et al. Preliminary trial of specific targeting therapy against malignant glioma. Lancet 1990;335:368–371.

258. Rosenstein M, Ettinghausen SE, Rosenberg SA. Extravasation of intravascular fluid mediated by the systemic administration of recombinant interleukin-2. J Immunol 1986;137:1735–1742.

259. Ettinghausen SE, Puri RK, Rosenberg SA. Increased vascular permeability in organs mediated by the systemic administration of lymphokine-activated killer cells and recombinant interleukin-2 in mice. JNCI 1988;80:177–188.

260. Ognibene FP, Rosenberg SA, Lotze M, et al. Interleukin-2 administration causes reversible hemodynamic changes and left ventricular dysfunction similar to those seen in septic shock. Chest 1988;94:750–754.

261. Lee RE, Lotze MT, Skibber JM, et al. Cardiorespiratory effects of immunotherapy with interleukin-2. J Clin Oncol 1989;7:7–20.

262. Belldegrun A, Webb DE, Austin HA, et al. Effects of interleukin-2 on renal function in patients receiving immunotherapy for advanced cancer. Ann Intern Med 1987;106:817–822.

263. Webb, DE, Austin HA, Belldegrun A, et al. Metabolic and renal effects of interleukin-2 immunotherapy for metastatic cancer. Clin Nephrol 1988;30:141–145.

264. Belldegrun A, Webb DE, Austin HA, et al. Renal toxicity of interleukin-2 administration in patients with metastatic renal cell cancers: Effect of pretherapy nephrectomy. J Urol 1989;141:499–503.

265. Denicoff KD, Rubinow DR, Papa MZ, et al. The neuropsychiatric effects of the treatment with interleukin-2 and lymphokine-activated killer cells. Ann Intern Med 1987;107:293–300.

266. Gaspari AA, Lotze MT, Rosenberg SA, et al. Dermatologic changes associated with interleukin-2 administration. JAMA 1987;258:1624–1629.

267. Schwartzentruber D, Lotze MT, Rosenberg SA. Colonic perforation: An unusual complication of therapy with high-dose interleukin-2. Cancer 1988;62:2350–2353.

268. Lee RE, Gaspari AA, Lotze MT, et al. Interleukin-2 and psoriasis. Arch Dermatol 1988;124:1811–1815.

269. Denicoff KD, Durkin TM, Lotze MT, et al. The neuroendocrine effects of interleukin-2 treatment. J Clin Endocrinol Metab 1989;69:402–410.

270. Kragel AH, Travis WD, Steis RG, et al. Myocarditis or acute myocardial infarction associated with interleukin-2 therapy for cancer. Cancer 1990;66:1513–1516.

271. Bock SN, Lee RE, Fisher B, et al. A prospective randomized trial evaluating prophylactic antibiotics to prevent triple-lumen catheter-related sepsis in patients treated with immunotherapy. J Clin Oncol 1990;8:161–169.

272. Atkins MB, Mier JW, Parkinson DR, et al. Hypothyroidism after treatment with interleukin-2 and lymphokine-activated killer cells. N Engl J Med 1988;318:1557–1563.

273. Schwartzentruber DJ, White DE, Zweig MH, et al. Thyroid dysfunction associated with immunotherapy for patients with cancer. Cancer 1991;68:2384–2390.

274. Kradin RL, Lazarus DS, Dubinett SM, et al. Tumor-infiltrating lymphocytes and interleukin-2 in treatment of advanced cancer. Lancet 1989;1:577–580.

275. Rosenberg SA, Packard BS, Aebersold PM, et al. Use of tumor-infiltrating lymphocytes and interleukin-2 in the immunotherapy of patients with metastatic melanoma: Special report. N Engl J Med 1988;319:1676–1680.

276. Fisher B, Packard BS, Read EJ, et al. Tumor localization of adoptively transferred indium-111 labeled tumor infiltrating lymphocytes in patients with metastatic melanoma. J Clin Oncol 1989;7:250–261.

277. Griffith KD, Read EJ, Carrasquillo CS, et al. In vivo distribution of adoptively transferred indium-111 labeled tumor infiltrating lymphocytes and peripheral blood lymphocytes in patients with metastatic melanoma. JNCI 1989;81:1709–1717.

278. Rosenberg SA, Aebersold P, Cornetta K, et al. Gene transfer into humans—Immunotherapy of patients with advanced melanoma, using tumor-infiltrating lymphocytes modified by retroviral gene transduction. N Engl J Med 1990;323:570–578.

Cancer: Principles & Practice of Oncology, Fourth Edition,
edited by Vincent T. DeVita, Jr., Samuel Hellman, Steven A. Rosenberg.
J.B. Lippincott Co., Philadelphia © 1993.

Bruce A. Chabner

CHAPTER **18**

Anticancer Drugs

The primary goal of clinical pharmacology is to develop a rational basis for the treatment of disease. Unfortunately, the required information is often not forthcoming for many years after the empiric discovery of active pharmacologic agents, and only then are important drug actions and interactions understood. In dealing with highly toxic agents that possess a narrow therapeutic index, such information is all the more important. The effective use of chemotherapeutic agents in oncology requires a higher level of pharmacologic understanding than any other subspecialty of internal medicine, because the margin for error is slim and the consequences of an error in dosage or dose adjustment may be lethal.

The objective of this chapter is to provide the fundamental information on drug action, metabolism, disposition, and toxicity in humans to allow optimal clinical use of anticancer drugs. This discussion assumes that the reader has a basic understanding of cell constituents; the general scheme of synthesis of DNA, RNA, and protein; and the fundamental principles of drug transport, metabolism, and excretion. For a review of these topics, refer to primary texts in biochemistry and pharmacology.[1,2] The synthesis of DNA and its precursors are summarized in Figure 18–1.

Safe drug use requires a choice of an appropriate route and schedule of administration, a determination of safe dosage range, an awareness of routes of drug elimination and an adjustment of dose to accommodate organ dysfunction, an awareness of the incidence and course of potentially life-threatening toxicity, and a knowledge of drug interactions as influenced by dose and schedule to maximize favorable in-

teractions and minimize toxicity. Each of these points should be considered in developing a new protocol or in using an unfamiliar protocol for the first time. Each patient brings unique disease-related or preexisting problems to the therapist, requiring careful consideration of the choice of drugs and dosage. Every effort should be made to employ the best protocol in full doses, but the oncologist must always be aware of the unique challenges presented by each patient.

A few tables are provided to allow rapid confirmation of the essential drug characteristics. Dose, toxicity, and pharmacokinetics of the most important agents are summarized in Table 18–1. Table 18–2 provides dose adjustment guidelines for agents affected by organ dysfunction. The indicated dose adjustments are only approximations, and subsequent doses should be calibrated against dose-limiting toxicity, such as myelosuppression.

Recently, with the development of techniques for bone marrow storage and reinfusion, and the availability of marrow colony-stimulating factors, it has been possible to employ cancer drugs in doses that would be uniformly fatal in the absence of these rescue measures. High-dose protocols have revealed new organ toxicities not appreciated at conventional doses. In general, these regimens should be used only in patients with normal renal, hepatic, and cardiac function. Examples of this type of therapy with typical regimens are given elsewhere in this text. The reader is referred to Chapter 68, section 1 for a practical guide to the administration of chemotherapy and its complications.

(text continues on page 328)

TABLE 18–1. Dose, Toxicity, and Pharmacokinetics of Major Antineoplastic Agents

Class	*Acute Toxicity* Route	Dose* (mg/m²)	Injection Vehicle	Infusion Duration	Dose Frequency
Plant Derivatives					
Taxol	I.V.	130–250	1:10 dilution in NS	24 h	q 3 wk
Vincristine	I.V.	1–1.4	10 ml NS	1–5 min	qwk
Vinblastine	I.V.	6	10 ml NS	1–5 min	qwk
	I.V.	2	NS	24 h × 5 d	q 3 wk
Vindesine	I.V.	2	10 ml NS	1–5 min	qwk
VP-16	I.V.	75–100	20 ml NS/ml reconstituted drug	1–5 min	qd × 5
	PO	200			2 d qwk
VM-26	I.V.	67	20 ml NS/ml	1–5 min	qwk
Antibiotics					
Dactinomycin	I.V.	0.6	500 µg/ml SW	1–5 min	qd × 5
Doxorubicin	I.V.	75	5 mg/ml SW	1–5 min	q 3 wk
	I.V.	20	5 mg/mL SW	1–5 min	qwk
Daunorubicin	I.V.	30	1 mg/ml SW	1–5 min	3 d, q 3 wk
Idarubicin	I.V.	13	1 mg/ml SW	1–5 min	qd × 3
Mithramycin	I.V.	1.75	500 µg/ml SW, then add to 100 ml D$_5$W	15–30 min	qod to toxicity
for high Ca^{2+}	I.V.	0.75	500 µg/ml SW	1–5 min bolus	qd × 3–4 d
Mitomycin C	I.V.	10	500 µg/ml SW	1–5 min bolus	qd × 3, q 3 wk
Bleomycin	I.V.	2–15	5 U/ml NS	1-min test dose, then I.V. bolus	qwk
	IM	2–15	15 U/ml NS		qwk
	SC	2–15	15 U/ml NS		qwk
Antimetabolites					
Methotrexate (high-dose)	I.V.	>500	100 ml D$_5$W or NS	10 min–1 h	q 3 wk
with leucovorin	I.V.	15	In vehicle	Bolus	q 6 h × 7 doses
Methotrexate	I.V.	25	10–25 ml D$_5$W or NS	Bolus	Twice weekly
	IM	25	2 ml NS		Twice weekly
	IT	12 (total dose)	10 ml Elliot B	1–5 min	q 4d
5-Fluorouracil	I.V.	500	Any convenient volume NS	Bolus	qwk or qd × 5 q 4w
	I.V.	800–1200	Any convenient volume NS	24 h × 5 d	q 3–4 wk
	IA	800–1200	Any convenient volume NS	24 h	qd × 14–21 d
5-Fluorouracil	I.V.	375–600	Any convenient volume NS	Bolus	qwk × 6
with leucovorin	I.V.	500	200 ml D$_5$W	2-h infusion begin 1 h before 5-FU	qwk × 6
5-Fluorodeoxyuridine	IA	5–20	Any convenient volume NS	24 h	qd × 14–21 d
6-Mercaptopurine	PO	100			qd × 5
6-Thioguanine	I.V.	100	15 mg/ml NS	Bolus	qd × 5
Cytarabine (cytosine arabinoside)	I.V.	100	20 mg/ml NS	Bolus or continuous infusion	q 12 h × 5–10 d
	I.V.	2000–3000	50 mg/ml SW then dilute in 150 ml D$_5$W	1 h	q 12 h × 6 d
5-Azacytidine	I.V.	200	Reconstitute vial in 20 ml SW, dilute in 150 ml D$_5$W	15–30 min	qd × 5
Hydroxyurea	I.V.	1000–1500	100 mg/ml SW	1–5 min	qd × 5
	PO	1000			qd

Acute Toxicity					
Leukocyte	*Platelet*	*Nausea/Vomiting*	*Other Toxicity*	*Elimination*	*Plasma Half-Life (h)†*
Moderate	Moderate	Mild	Anaphylactoid response, sensory neuropathy, alopecia	M	6–8
Mild	Mild	Mild	Distal neuropathy, inappropriate ADH	M	2.6
Marked	Marked	Mild	Mucositis	M	3.1
Marked	Marked	Mild	Mucositis	M	3.1
Moderate	Mild	Mild	Neurotoxicity	M	1.6
Moderate	Mild	Mild	Distal neuropathy	M, R	6
Moderate	Mild	Moderate			
Moderate	Mild	Mild	Distal neuropathy	M, R	3
Marked	Marked	Moderate	Alopecia, mucositis	M, R	?
Marked	Marked	Moderate	Alopecia, cardiomyopathy	M	3/25
Moderate	Moderate	Moderate	Alopecia, less cardiomyopathy	M	3/25
Marked	Marked	Moderate	Alopecia, cardiomyopathy	M	3/?
Marked	Marked	Moderate	Alopecia, mucositis, cardiomyopathy	M	34
Mild	Marked	Severe	Renal, hepatic, neurologic, fever, rash	M	?
Mild	Mild	Mild			
Marked	Marked	Moderate	Renal, pulmonary	M	?
Rare	Rare	Mild	Skin, pulmonary fibrosis, fever, allergic reactions	R	0.4/2
Mild	Mild	Moderate	Hepatic dysfunction, renal failure	R M	2/8
Moderate-marked	Moderate-marked	Mild	Stomatitis	R	2/8
Moderate-marked	Moderate-marked	Mild	Stomatitis	R	2/8
Mild	Mild	None	Fever, motor dysfunction	R	12 (CSF)
Moderate-marked	Moderate-marked	Mild	Cerebellar, conjunctivitis	M	0.3
Mild	Mild	Moderate	Mucositis, diarrhea	M	0.3
Mild	Mild	Moderate	Catheter-related	M	0.3
Marked	Marked	Mild	Diarrhea, stomatitis	M	0.3
Mild	Mild	Moderate	Catheter-related	M	0.3
Moderate-marked	Moderate-marked	Mild	Cholestasis	M	0.3–0.6
Moderate-marked	Moderate-marked	Mild	Cholestasis	M	1.5
Marked	Marked	Moderate	Cholestasis, mucositis	M	0.15
Marked	Marked	Marked	Cholestasis, mucositis, cerebral and cerebellar, conjunctivitis, pneumonitis	M, R	
Marked	Marked	Severe	Neurotoxicity, mucositis	M	Rapid
Marked	Moderate	Moderate	None	R, M	1.7
Marked	Marked	Mild		R, M	1.7

(continued)

TABLE 18–1. *(Continued)*

	Acute Toxicity				
Class	Route	Dose* (mg/m²)	Injection Vehicle	Infusion Duration	Dose Frequency
Deoxycoformycin	I.V.	4	Any volume NS	Bolus	q 2 wk
Fludarabine	I.V.	25		30 min	qd × 5
Alkylating Agents					
Cyclophosphamide	I.V.	400	20 mg/ml SW	Bolus	qd × 5
	PO	100			qd × 14
Ifosfamide	I.V.	1200–2400	Any volume D_5W or NS	24 h	qd × 5
and Mesna	I.V.	1800–2400	With ifosfamide	24 h	qd × 5.5
Melphalan	PO	4			qd
	I.V.	8	Reconstituted vial dilute in 100–200 ml D_5W	30–45 min	qd × 5
Busulfan	PO	2–6			qd
CCNU	PO	100–150			q 6 wk
MeCCNU	PO	150–200			q 6 wk
BCNU	I.V.	200–225	Reconstituted vial diluted to 100 mg/ml D_5W	30–45 min	q 6 wk
Streptozotocin	I.V.	500	Reconstituted vial diluted to 100 mg/ml D_5W	10–15 min	qd × 5 q 3–4 wk
Chlorambucil	PO	1–3			qd
cis-diamminedi-chloroplatinum	I.V.	50–100	200–500 ml NS	30–60 min	q 3–4 wk
		20	150 ml NS	1 h	qd × 5
	I.V.	40	250 ml 3% saline	1 h	qd × 5
CBDCA (carboplatin)	I.V.	300	Any volume D_5W	30–60 min	q 3–4 wk
Aziridinylbenzo-quinone (AZQ)	I.V.	18–20	150 ml NS	10–15 min	Days 1 and 8 of 28-d cycle
	I.V.	8	150 ml NS	10–15 min	qd × 5
Miscellaneous					
DTIC (Dacarbazine)	I.V.	200	10 mg/ml D_5W	10–15 min	qd × 5
mAMSA	I.V.	120	250 ml D_5W	2 h	qd × 5
Procarbazine	PO	100			qd × 10–14 d
Hexamethylmelamine	PO	150			qd × 14 d
Mitoxantrone	I.V.	14	10 ml NS	30 min	q 3 wk

I.V., intravenous; PO, oral; SC, subcutaneous; IM, intramuscular; IT, intrathecal; IA, intraarterial; NS, normal saline; D_5W, dextrose (5 g/dl) in water; SW, sterile water; R, renal; M, metabolic; F, fecal.
* Doses are typical of those used in combination regimens, but appropriate modification must be made depending on other drugs used, organ dysfunction, and other considerations.
† Slash indicates multiple half-lives.
‡ Prehydration and posthydration are indicated.

MICHAEL R. GREVER
BRUCE A. CHABNER

SECTION 1

Cancer Drug Discovery and Development

Despite the success of modern cancer chemotherapy in selected tumors, the continued commitment of government, academic, and industry laboratories to the arduous tasks involved with the discovery of new cancer therapeutic agents remains critically important.[3,4] Approximately 50 years of effort in cancer drug discovery and development have thus far resulted in 66 approved products for the treatment of malignancy in the United States. However, although major advances have been made in the chemotherapeutic management of some patients, particularly the hematologic malignancies, half of all cancer patients either fail to respond or will relapse from the initial response and ultimately die from their metastatic disease. The hope for improvement in treatment outcome for most patients with metastatic disease resides in continued research designed to optimize the administration of the currently available agents and to discover novel therapeutic products.

Beyond the intellectual challenge of drug discovery, formi-

| Acute Toxicity | | | | | Plasma |
Leukocyte	Platelet	Nausea/Vomiting	Other Toxicity	Elimination	Half-Life (h)†
Mild	Mild	Mild	None	R	1/10
Moderate	Mild	Mild	Pneumonitis, neurotoxicity	R, M	9.3
Marked	Mild	Moderate	Cystitis, water retention, alopecia	M	1–4
Moderate	Mild	Mild			
Moderate	Moderate	Mild	Neurotoxicity, urothelial toxicity	M	5–6
None	None	None	None	M	?
Moderate	Moderate	Mild	Leukemia	M	2
Marked	Marked	Moderate			
Marked	Marked	Mild	Pulmonary fibrosis	M	?
Marked	Marked	Moderate	Leukemia, pulmonary fibrosis, renal failure	M	?
Marked	Marked	Moderate	Leukemia, pulmonary fibrosis, renal failure	M	?
Marked	Marked	Marked	Leukemia, pulmonary fibrosis, renal failure	M	1.0
Mild	Mild	Moderate-marked	Renal failure, hyperglycemia, hepatic enzyme elevation	R	0.25
Moderate	Moderate	Mild	Leukemia	M	1.5
Moderate	Moderate	Severe	Renal failure, Mg^{2+} wasting, peripheral neuropathy	R, M	0.3
Mild	Mild	Moderate			
Moderate	Moderate	Marked	Neurotoxicity, ototoxicity	M	0.3
Marked	Marked	Mild		R	
Moderate	Moderate	Moderate	Cumulative myelosuppression	M	0.5
Moderate	Moderate	Moderate	Cumulative myelosuppression	M	0.5
Mild	Mild	Marked	Flulike syndrome, venoocclusive	M	0.65
Moderate	Moderate	Mild	Cardiac arrhythmias	M	7
Moderate	Moderate	Mild	Sensitivity to amines	M	?
Mild	Mild	Moderate	Neurotoxicity	M	5
Moderate	Moderate	Mild	Cholestasis, cardiac	M	0.25/37

dable effort, time, and expense are required for the complex developmental process that moves a new agent from discovery to its ultimate approval for use in the treatment of malignancy. Numerous pitfalls may threaten the progress of a promising agent (*e.g.*, excessive early toxicity, ineffective route or schedule of administration, inappropriate formulation, long-term unpredicted toxicities, and delays in the execution of clinical trials). Although the time to drug approval for the treatment of cancer during the past five decades has varied considerably, depending on the specific agent (*e.g.*, 6 to 12 years from the time of initiation of clinical trials), it is generally agreed that the entire process needs to be expedited, including both the preclinical and clinical components of investigation. In other areas of medicine, the time to develop specific drugs may be equally long and difficult, but the fatal consequence of unsuccessful treatment of malignancy continues to impart a sense of urgency in cancer medicine.

DRUG DISCOVERY

AN OVERVIEW: HOW DRUGS ARE DISCOVERED

This section considers strategies for identifying new chemical entities, either synthesized chemicals or compounds extracted or derived from plant, microbial, or marine animal sources.

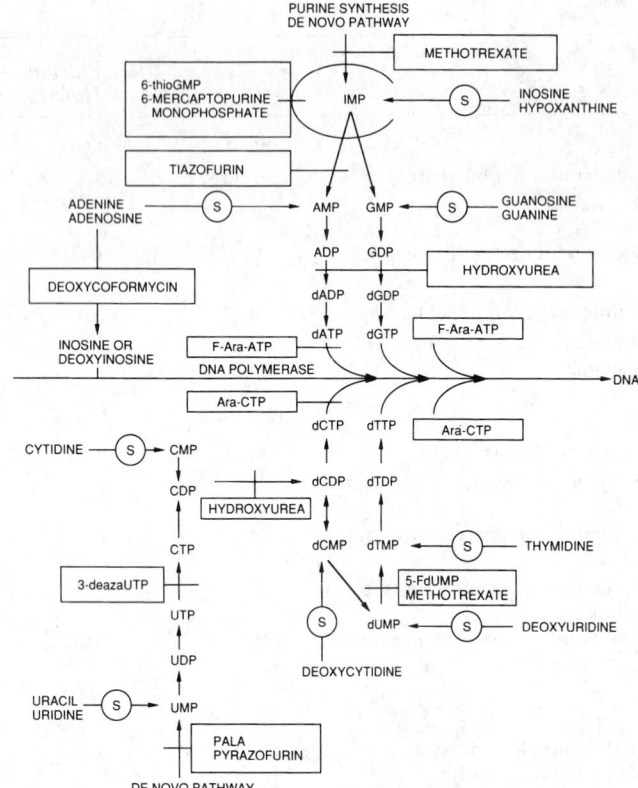

PYRIMIDINE SYNTHESIS

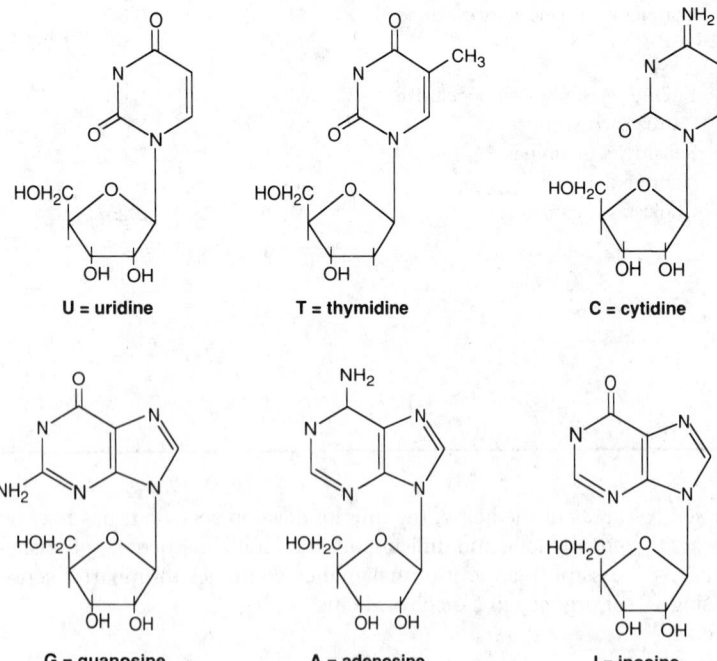

FIGURE 18–1. Pathways for synthesis of triphosphate precursors of DNA and site of action of antimetabolites. Salvage pathways of nucleotide biosynthesis are indicated by ─Ⓢ→ . Agents, or their metabolites, that inhibit specific synthetic reactions are enclosed in box, □. The inhibited pathway is indicated by ┿ ; d, deoxyribose; MP, monophosphate; DP, diphosphate; TP, triphosphate.

TABLE 18–2. Drugs Requiring Dose Modification for Organ Dysfunction

Agent	Organ Dysfunction	Suggested Dose Modification
Methotrexate	Renal failure or ↓ creatinine clearance	In proportion to ↓ creatinine clearance (normal 60 ml/min/m^2)
Cisplatin	Renal failure	In proportion to creatinine clearance
Cyclophosphamide	Renal failure (creatinine clearance < 25 ml/min)	50% decrease
Bleomycin	Renal failure (creatinine clearance < 25 ml/min)	50–75% decrease
Streptozotocin	Renal failure (creatinine clearance < 25 ml/min)	50–75% decrease
Carboplatin Hydroxyurea VP-16 Deoxycoformycin	Renal failure	In proportion to creatinine clearance
mAMSA Vincristine Vinblastine	Hepatic dysfunction	1. Only approximate guidelines can be offered and are probably inaccurate (see text). 2. For bilirubin of >1.5 mg/100 ml, reduce initial dose by 50%. 3. For bilirubin of >3 mg/100 ml, reduce initial dose by 75%.

The parallel process for discovery and development of biologic agents is discussed elsewhere in this text.

In establishing a program for drug discovery, cancer researchers must address two fundamental questions: What screening system will be used to detect a compound of interest? What compounds will be tested in this system? The answers to these two questions will determine whether the research effort is empiric, with few preconceived notions about where to search for compounds and what to use as the screen, or whether it focuses on a specific biologic target, such as an oncogene, and tests a specific set of materials, such as natural products and rationally synthesized inhibitors of a target enzyme. The history of cancer drug discovery basically reflects an evolution from highly empiric approaches, based on testing of randomly selected compounds against rapidly proliferating murine leukemias, to the current, more focused testing of natural products, rationally synthesized agents, and "biologic" products against well-characterized tumor cell lines or molecular targets. However, even in its earliest days, cancer drug discovery attracted scientists who had a theoretical basis for testing certain types of compounds. Perhaps the best examples are the fluoropyrimidines, synthesized by Heidelberger and colleagues (see related section elsewhere in this chapter), and the antifolates, tested by Farber and associates.

The story of the discovery of antifolates is particularly instructive in that it illustrates the important interplay between cancer biology and drug discovery. The earliest uses of an antifolate as a chemotherapeutic agent resulted from the astute observations of Farber, who observed an "acceleration" of the leukemic process in patients being treated with folic acid.[5]

A series of folic acid antagonists were provided to Farber and colleagues by the medicinal chemists at Lederle Laboratories.[5] Although structure-activity relations of antifolates, and the intracellular target of these compounds, were unknown at this time, it was clear from laboratory studies that modified folates could inhibit tumor cell growth. The initial clinical trial involved the administration of pteroylaspartic acid (an analog of folic acid or pteroylglutamate) to a moribund patient with progressive acute myelogenous leukemia and resulted in a markedly hypocellular bone marrow without actually producing clinical benefit. The investigators were sufficiently encouraged, however, to administer a "more powerful" folic acid antagonist, aminopterin (2,4-diaminopteroylglutamate), to children with advanced stages of acute leukemia. Substitution of an NH$_2$-group at the 4 position of the folate pteridine ring created a tight-binding inhibitor of dihydrofolate reductase and yielded drugs with the potential to induce remissions. Approximately 10 of the first 16 patients treated with aminopterin demonstrated evidence of hematologic and clinical improvement. These early clinical experiences provided the foundation for medicinal chemists to synthesize a number of agents that have structural similarities to naturally occurring folates, and they exposed an interesting array of antifolate actions in which specific substitutions lead to radically different enzymatic sites of action (Fig. 18–2).

From these primitive beginnings, rational design efforts have progressed to the use of computer modeling of drug-enzyme interactions as the basis for cancer drug discovery. Advances in crystallographic and nmr characterization of ligands and their target molecules have enhanced the potential for rational design, although as yet no effective cancer drugs

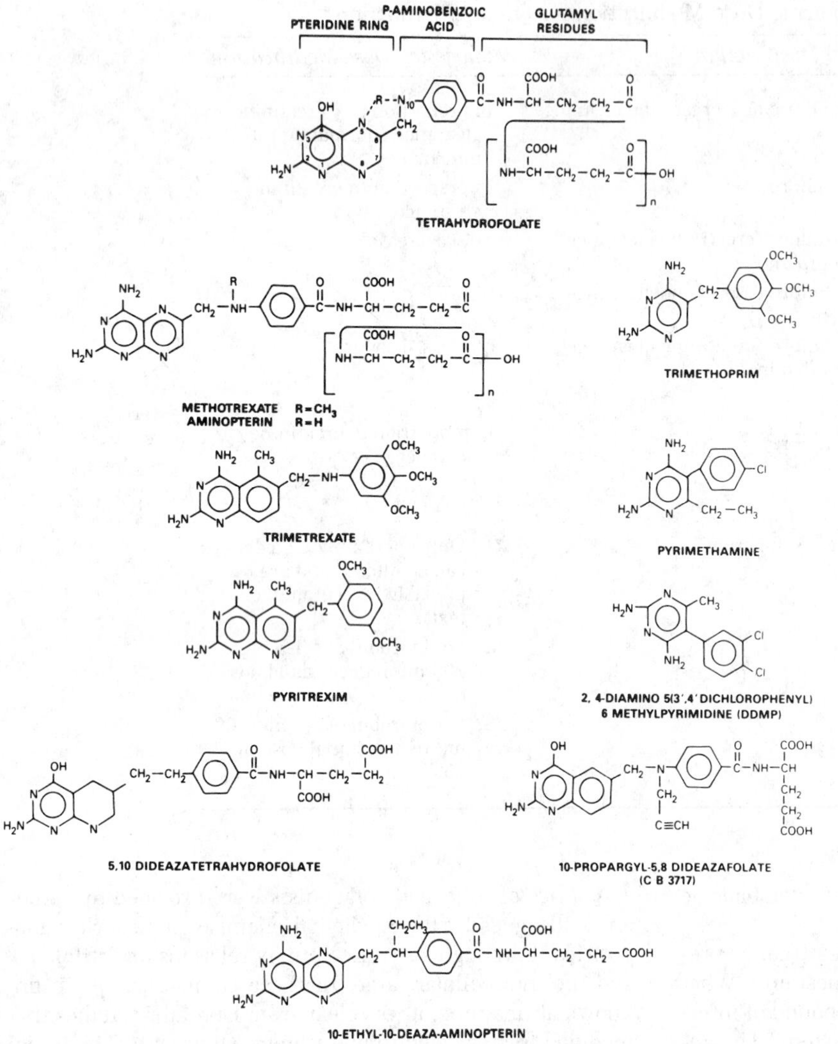

FIGURE 18–2. The structures illustrate the variety of analogs now in clinical use, all based on the structure of tetrahydrofolate. The 2,4-diaminopteroyl glutamates (methotrexate, aminopterin, and 10-ethyl-10-deazaaminopterin) as well as other lipid-soluble 2,4-diamino structures, such as trimetrexate, inhibit dihydrofolate reductase. 5,10-Dideazatetrahydrofolate inhibits an entirely different target (GAR transformylase, an early enzyme in purine synthesis), whereas 5,8-dideazafolates strongly inhibit thymidylate synthase, a third folate-dependent enzyme. (Chabner BA, Collins JM, eds. Cancer chemotherapy: Principles and practice. Philadelphia: JB Lippincott, 1990:113)

have actually resulted from these efforts. Symmetric inhibitors of the protease of human immunodeficiency virus type-1 (HIV-1) have been designed recently on the basis of the three-dimensional symmetry of the active enzyme site, thus demonstrating that this approach is feasible and has potential merit.[6]

In most current drug discovery efforts, the rational and empiric approaches are being combined. Lead compounds are identified as inhibitors for molecular targets through so-called molecular screening.[7] The lead compound can then be modified or enhanced by chemical analog synthesis based on a variety of considerations, including a detailed study of target-inhibitor interaction. The complete characterization of the target and its interaction with the lead agent provides the basis for enhancing drug-target interaction. A key decision in this approach is the selection of a suitable target (enzyme, growth factor receptor, or oncogene product).

Although early efforts in cancer drug discovery tested agents either from the broad universe of synthetic chemicals or from a more targeted rational effort, recent attention has turned increasingly to natural products as an important untapped source of promising lead compounds with unique sites of action as antineoplastic drugs.[8] The enormous diversity and complexity of chemical entities that have evolved as part of

nature's chemical warfare cannot be duplicated by compounds synthesized in the laboratory and available for screening. Approximately 30% of the currently effective antineoplastic agents are from natural sources or are derivatives of a natural product lead. Certain themes run through the efforts to discover and use natural products. Active compounds often have exceedingly complex structures that defy efforts at total synthesis. Problems of supply and dependence on a natural resource must be anticipated. Second, structure-activity relations are difficult to elucidate because of the basic problems presented by the unusual chemistry of these compounds and by the multiple chiral centers in these molecules (Fig. 18–3).

Among the natural products, microbial antibiotics have been the most important source of cytotoxic agents. As a result of the great advances in the field of microbiology during the 1940s, with the dawn of the era of effective antibiotic therapy, potent anticancer drugs were sought in fermentation broths obtained from soil microbes, including bacteria, fungi, and related organisms. The discoveries of the actinomycins, anthracyclines, bleomycins, deoxycoformycin, and other agents have contributed valuable new entities to the repository of effective antineoplastic agents. Natural product drug discovery, however, must be complemented by efforts to improve leads through chemical modification and analog synthesis.

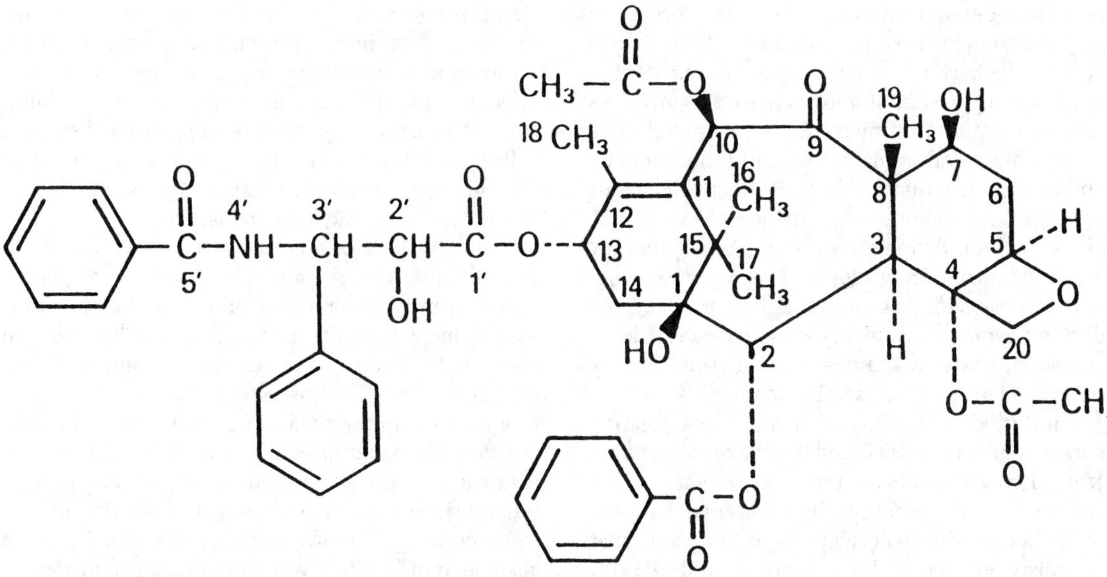

FIGURE 18–3. Structure of taxol, which contains 11 optimally active sites (indicated by *heavy triangular bond lines*). The requirement for stereospecific substitutions greatly complicates attempts at total synthesis. (Chabner BA. PPO Updates 1991;5[1])

The discovery and subsequent clinical development of anthracyclines revealed a pattern typical of the interplay of chemistry, biology, and clinical pharmacology in yielding improved chemotherapy.

Daunorubicin, isolated from a colony of *Streptomyces* in 1957, eventually was demonstrated to have substantial antileukemic activity in patients.[9] Additional research to induce mutant strains of the fungus *Streptomyces* resulted in the isolation of doxorubicin. Although the difference between these two anthracyclines is limited chemically to a single hydroxyl group, there is a substantial difference in their antitumor activity. Doxorubicin has been more effective than daunorubicin in the treatment of metastatic carcinomas and sarcomas. The cardiac toxicity associated with the chronic administration of both these agents, however, has provided an impetus to design numerous anthracycline analogs. None of these anthracycline analogs is devoid of cardiac toxicity, but closely related molecules may have significant advantages. For example, the anthraquinones (*e.g.*, mitoxantrone) demonstrate less cardiotoxicity and have remission-inducing activity in acute nonlymphocytic leukemia.[10] Anthrapyrazoles, because of their aminoquinone substitutions, also have less of a tendency to form semiquinone free radicals and, in early clinical study, have demonstrated significant antitumor activity in patients with metastatic breast cancer.[11,12] There may be cross-resistance between the anthracyclines, the anthraquinones, and the anthrapyrazoles with respect to their target, topoisomerase II, but the ultimate benefit may be a reduction in the cardiac toxicity and perhaps an extension of the antitumor spectrum.[11] Thus, the important role of the medicinal chemist in modifying the chemical structure of a natural product, and thereby enhancing its therapeutic index, can be appreciated.

Natural product research has yielded other effective antineoplastic drugs. Although most of these agents have been found in fermentation broths of microbial organisms, plants have also provided effective antineoplastic agents. One of the earliest plant-derived drugs resulted from a chance observation. More than 40 years ago, Noble and colleagues were investigating interesting plant extracts used by primitive peoples.[13] This attempt to take advantage of tribal medications, primarily natural products, represented an early entrée into the discipline known as *ethnopharmacology.*

The leaves of the Jamaican periwinkle plant, *Vinca rosea*, were used to make a tea that was reported to be of benefit in diabetes.[13] During the initial animal investigations, the extract of these leaves was administered orally to both rats and rabbits without any observed effect on the blood sugar levels. Subsequent administration of the aqueous extract of the periwinkle plant by injection to rats had a dramatic lethal effect within a week. The postmortem examination of the animals eventually demonstrated that the rats died of sepsis related to bone marrow suppression. Isolation and chemical characterization of the responsible chemical factors were accomplished using a bioassay-guided approach (*i.e.*, granulocytopenia in the treated animals) for identifying the effective component of this aqueous extract of the plant. The compound was determined to be an organic base, and subsequently was called *vincaleukoblastine.* This agent demonstrated carcinostatic activity against both a transplanted murine mammary adenocarcinoma and a rat-transplanted sarcoma.[13] Its mechanism of action—inhibition of microtubule formation—proved to be unique and provided the basis for an entirely new field for targeted drug development.

Rather than using the complicated biologic endpoint of the peripheral blood granulocyte count from an intact animal, simple and more rapid screens, such as in vitro cell cytotoxicity assays, are currently employed to guide fractionation of extracts for isolation and characterization of active principles. After the final chemical identification of the plant-derived chemical antineoplastic entity, validation of antitumor activity in an in vivo tumor model is still required. Sufficient supplies of the drugs isolated from natural product sources are needed to conduct adequate in vivo confirmatory studies. Adequate supply was a problem with the periwinkle extract in its early development, and it remains problematic for many natural product agents now being isolated.

Several new plant-derived natural products have proved to be of extreme interest in the treatment of cancer. Taxol, which was isolated from the bark of the Pacific yew tree in 1971,[14] has a unique mechanism of antitumor activity that involves promotion and stabilization of microtubule assembly.[15] The product has demonstrated remarkable antitumor activity against a number of human tumor xenografts, including breast cancer, ovarian cancer, and other malignancies.

The major obstacle to defining its role in cancer therapy relates to the difficulties in drug supply. The complex molecule, with its stereospecific substitutions, has not yet been synthesized. Semi-synthesis from 10-acetyl baccatin III has been accomplished, and new sources of taxol from nursery species have been identified (see section on taxol).

Another natural product that has been under investigation for many years, but only recently found to have broad activity, is derived from the bark of *Camptotheca accuminata*, a tree prized for its medicinal properties in traditional Chinese medicine.[16] The camptothecin derivatives are unique in that they inhibit topoisomerase I.[17,18] Both topotecan and CPT-11, which are derivatives of camptothecin, have significant activity in patients with advanced malignancies.[19-21] Because camptothecin is amenable to chemical synthesis, efforts are being directed at further defining the optimal structural analog. The most promising new analog, 9-aminocamptothecin, awaits initiation of clinical investigation.[22]

Marine organisms represent a largely unexplored and untapped source of unique toxic chemicals. These toxins are elaborated by sponges and other sessile saltwater organisms as defenses against their predators. Several highly potent agents demonstrating interesting antitumor activity against unique molecular targets in preclinical models include the bryostatins (a protein kinase C inhibitor) and the dolastatins and hali-chondrins (microtubule-binding agents).[8,23-25] Although the marine environment represents an untapped potential source for interesting new chemical entities, certain unique problems affect this biosphere. Scale-up procurement of bulk material from marine sources could present new challenges in biomass collection. The potency of many of these agents may ameliorate this supply problem, if selectivity against the tumor (and not the normal host) can be demonstrated.

Cancer drug discovery may result from a totally fortuitous experimental observation. The discovery of platinum complexes as antiproliferative agents with remarkable clinical activity demonstrates the importance of enlightened empiricism combined with dogged persistence in clinical testing and development. In 1965, Rosenberg observed that an electric current passing through platinum electrodes could inhibit *Escherichia coli* bacterial cell division.[26] This discovery was confirmed by the subsequent testing of platinum complexes into murine tumor model systems. Cisplatin inhibited the development of sarcomas, and other platinum complexes were also found to be effective in the preclinical models. The early clinical trials demonstrated antitumor activity in patients with advanced malignancies, but the excessive initial toxicity (nephrotoxicity) raised serious concern among the clinical investigators. The demonstration that adequate hydration and slow infusion reduce the degree of renal toxicity permitted further evaluation of the agent. The responses observed in testicular cancer and ovarian cancer led to approval of the drug approximately 6 years after the initial clinical trial. This excellent anticancer drug might have been discarded in error without the foresight of both preclinical and clinical investigators who were convinced of the drug's potential, were committed to the systematic testing of the drug, and were clever enough to find ways to deal with its toxicity.

TABLE 18–3. Comparison of Cancer Screening Devices

Screen	Advantages	Disadvantages
Tumor Cell Line-Based Assays		
Tumor Cell Line	High-volume assay	Mechanism of action not defined by this approach
	Has identified many current cancer drugs	
	Defines agent with effect on tumor cell and displays the pattern of cellular response	May define agents that are nonspecifically toxic to cells
	Defines agents that cross cell membrane and withstand the intracellular milieu	Does not elucidate the cellular target responsible for the observed effect
Mechanism/Molecular Targeted Assays		
Mechanistic or Molecular Targeted	High-volume assay	Despite scientific appeal, approach only recently implemented
	Has a rational basis for drug discovery	
	May provide agents specifically aimed at a critical point in the tumor cell	No guarantee that agents will enter the cell or withstand intracellular milieu
	Potential selective antitumor activity	
	May provide novel classes of antitumor agents	No guarantee that agents will be selective

CANCER DRUG SCREENING

Most of the antineoplastic agents have been discovered through empiric screening efforts or represent chemical modifications of lead compounds discovered in cancer screenings.

Screening methods can either be simple, such as a cell line or an enzymatic target, or complex, such as an animal tumor in vivo. In general, current efforts favor in vitro systems that accommodate high volumes of unknown compounds. The endpoint of the cancer screen may be a biologic target (*e.g.*, tumor cell cytotoxicity, growth inhibition, differentiation) or a biochemical-molecular target that is known to be important for the survival of malignant cells. Both approaches to screening are reasonable and have respective advantages and liabilities, as identified in Table 18–3. Both the cell line and molecular approach may be combined through the use of genetically engineered cell lines that express a particular molecular target. Cell lines have the advantage of a cell membrane and intracellular enzymatic machinery that activate or degrade candidate compounds.

The evolution of strategies at the National Cancer Institute (NCI) illustrates the changes in screening that have resulted from advances in cancer biology. The early NCI cancer screening efforts used murine leukemias (L1210 and P388) as the sentinel or index tumors in an in vivo screening effort.[27] The screen identified agents that had efficacy in humans in the treatment of leukemias and lymphoproliferative malignancies, such as hydroxyurea and the nitrosoureas. However, the failure of this screen to identify active drugs for the major solid tumors led to subsequent changes in the approach of the NCI in 1975 when animal solid tumors and human tumor xenografts were added as a secondary in vivo tumor panel.[27] In 1985, a second major change was made.[27,28] The availability of growing numbers of cell lines derived from human solid tumors and characterized with respect to drug response patterns, growth factor dependence, oncogene expression, and other features presented an opportunity to focus screening efforts on the unique biology of human solid tumors.

A number of human solid tumor cell lines were selected to provide a disease-oriented approach to drug discovery in contrast with the previous compound-oriented drug discovery methods. A total of 60 human tumor cell lines derived from seven cancer types (*e.g.*, lung, colon, melanoma, kidney, ovary, brain, leukemia) formed the original cell line panel. The initial concept proposed that leads demonstrating disease specificity would be identified, and activity could be subsequently examined further by in vivo testing in nude mice, using the most sensitive in vitro index tumor cell lines.

In the current NCI anticancer screen, each candidate agent is tested over a broad concentration range against every cell line in the panel.[27–29] Active compounds are selected for further testing based on several different criteria: disease-type specificity in the in vitro assay, unique structure, potency, and demonstration of a unique pattern of cellular cytotoxicity or cytostasis, indicating a unique mechanism of action or intracellular target. The agents selected for further investigation are then subjected to additional testing to assess their in vivo therapeutic index.[30] The current version of the cancer drug screening program of the NCI has been operational since 1990, and a number of novel chemical entities have been identified for further evaluation. This high-capacity screen can accommodate approximately 10,000 individual chemicals tested annually, with additional capacity for screening natural product extracts. Approximately 5% of the compounds tested in the initial screen show sufficient activity to warrant further evaluation in in vivo screens or biochemical-molecular assays.

The concept of cancer drug discovery that is based on high-volume screens, whether oriented toward a cell line-based or molecular target, relies on the acquisition of a large source of materials for examination. In the case of the NCI, an extensive program for acquiring both defined chemical entities and diverse natural products has been pursued.

The pharmaceutical industry is also actively engaged in the procurement of large numbers of interesting chemical structures and natural products for testing in their respective cancer screens, many of which focus on specific molecular targets. Decisions must be made to choose among the large number of unknown entities for initial testing and to aid in the prioritization of known active compounds for further development. Computerized programs have been developed to assist in this prioritization and to enhance the diversity of potential chemical entries and crude natural products introduced into the screening process.[31] For example, consider the problem of representing, analyzing, and storing the data generated by the substances tested in the in vitro screen of the NCI. As depicted in Figure 18–4, drug testing data are represented as a *mean graph* that displays growth inhibition in a standard bar graph presentation.[27] The mean graph is constructed by projecting bars to the right or left of the mean, depending on whether a cell line is more or less sensitive than the average line in the panel. Further, the length of each bar is proportional to the relative sensitivity of the cell lines. Thus, each drug can be represented by a characteristic "fingerprint" of cell line responsiveness, indicated by the bar graph presentation shown in Figure 18–4.

After an agent has been tested in the cancer screen, its unique response pattern can be compared with the results from all other agents within the database. A computer program called COMPARE uses a simple algorithm for aligning and contrasting the patterns for each compound with the patterns of other compounds in the database.[32] A compound is entered into the program as a "seed," and the computer database elicits a list of those agents that have similar patterns of tumor cellular responsiveness. In Table 18–4, an example is presented for the introduction of a seed compound and the resulting list of agents that had similar patterns of cellular cytotoxicity. A correlation coefficient is also expressed relating the closeness of the seed to those agents listed by the computer program. Close correlations between agents appear to have biologic and pharmacologic importance, implying a common intracellular target despite a dissimilarity in structure (*e.g.*, tubulin-binding agents, topoisomerase-interactive agents).[25] The COMPARE program has several important uses. It can identify the intracellular target or mechanism of action of a new compound through a comparison of its fingerprint with known agents, and it can search for compounds previously tested in the cancer screen that have a fingerprint similar to that of a lead compound known to inhibit a unique target. The comparison allows recognition that a new agent does not "match" with compounds that have known mechanisms of action, which may be the most interesting lead of all.

Computerized approaches to data analysis might also be used to search for agents interacting with specific molecular

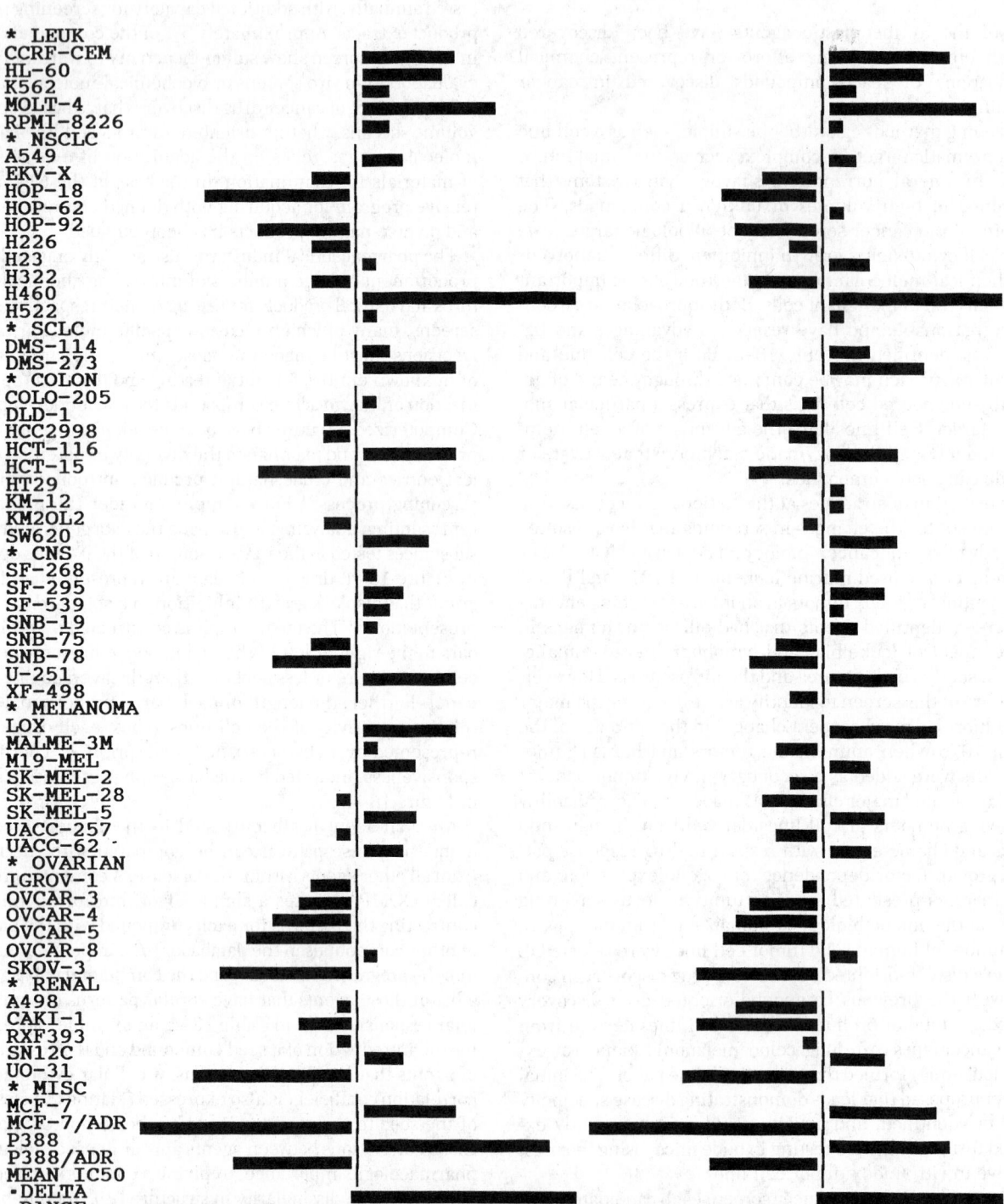

FIGURE 18–4.   Mean graph representation of antitumor effects in the cancer screen. The effects of a specific agent on the tumor cell lines in the NCI's cancer screen can be depicted by the construction of a mean graph presentation of the data. Screening results for two anthracyclines are presented. A mean concentration of the agent that produces the same level of response for all the cell lines in the screen forms an anchor point for this graphic presentation. The individual response of each cell line to the agent is then depicted by a bar graph extending either to the right or left of the mean, depending on whether the cell line was either more or less sensitive than the average response, respectively. The length of each bar is proportional to the relative sensitivity compared with the mean determination.

TABLE 18–4. The COMPARE Program

Parent = Taxol			
NSC Number	High Concentration	Correlation Coefficient	Chemical Name
153858	1.00E-09	0.812	Maytansine
49842	2.50E-06	0.767	Vinblastine sulfate
332598	5.00E-06	0.745	Rhizoxin
609395	1.00E-08	0.703	Halichondrin B
757	6.25E-04	0.691	Colchicine
67574	1.00E-03	0.628	Vincristine sulfate
376128	1.00E-08	0.628	Dolastatin

An extensive data base has been generated from the many agents tested in the NCI's Cancer Screen. The unique patterns of cellular response can be used to characterize an agent by its "fingerprint" of cytostasis or cytotoxicity. Agents that have common cellular targets can be identified by the use of the computerized data base. For example, introduction of a "seed" or "parent" compound into the COMPARE Program will elicit a list of those agents that exhibit similar patterns of tumor cell response. In the example in this table, the agents listed are known to be tubulin-interactive agents. The correlation coefficient for the relation of each agent to the seed or parent compound is provided. High concentration refers to the highest concentration of the agent used during the screening experiment. NSC Number refers to the individual identification number assigned to each agent submitted to the NCI.

targets. For example, because certain cell lines are known to contain an oncogene such as K-*RAS* or *HER2/NEU*, it is possible to search the database for agents active against only those cell lines.

MOLECULAR-TARGETED SCREENING

From a scientific perspective, a compelling argument can be made for focusing on a defined molecular target and using computer approaches to construct specific molecules that would interact with the target.

With the rapid advances being made in defining the molecular pathology of neoplastic cells, specific oncogenes and aberrant suppressor genes have been identified that are expressed uniquely in malignant tissue. The discovery of inappropriately expressed or mutated genes has provided an impetus for the establishment of numerous screens designed to detect specific inhibitors or modulators of the products of these abnormal genes. Intracellular signaling pathways that mediate the actions of growth factors and oncogenes on cell proliferation, such as protein kinases, G-proteins, and transcription activators, provide additional novel targets for anticancer drugs. Because there is considerable overlap of access to growth-factor signaling pathways (many signals use the same distal steps), signal transduction inhibitors may lack specificity for the neoplastic cells.[33]

Advocates for the use of the mechanistic approaches to new drug discovery have emphasized the potential for selectivity that may result from the use of molecular targeting.[7,34] The expression of identical molecular or biochemical targets in normal tissue must always be considered. Mutant oncogenes and their products appear to be most promising and include the chimeric protein that results from the *BCR-ABL* translocation in chronic myelogenous leukemia and the interference with tumor suppression resulting from the binding of papillomavirus proteins to the *RB* gene in cervical carcinoma.

In chronic myelogenous leukemia or a subpopulation of patients with acute lymphocytic leukemia, a characteristic reciprocal translocation between chromosomes 9 and 22 occurs.[35] The protooncogene (*ABL*) from chromosome 9 is translocated at the breakpoint cluster region (*BCR*) on chromosome 22. A fusion protein, BCR-ABL, with dysregulated tyrosine kinase function results and has been implicated in the neoplastic transformation of the hematopoietic stem cells.[35,36] Two forms of this activated BCR-ABL protein, p210 and p185, that differ in the *BCR*-derived base sequences have been identified. In general, the p185 form of this protein has been associated with a more aggressive neoplastic transformation process in either the animal models or the human form of the disease.

The aberrant tyrosine kinase resulting from these abnormal genetic rearrangements (*BCR-ABL*) within the hematopoietic stem cells does not exist in normal host cells. This abnormal gene provides an ideal molecular target for therapeutic intervention.

In vitro data suggest that expression of this genetic rearrangement is essential to maintaining the malignant phenotype.[37] In addition, transfection of the specific DNA for the *BCR-ABL*-encoded protein kinase into the hematopoietic stem cells of mice results in the induction of a malignant disorder in vivo with similarities to the clinical illness in humans.[38] These murine models provide an opportunity to test promising new therapeutic products in vivo.

Another potential target for therapeutic intervention has evolved from a better understanding of the impact of suppressor gene dysfunction in the malignant process. More than 80% of cervical carcinomas have evidence of integrated DNA sequences from papillomaviruses.[39] Human papillomavirus 16 has been implicated frequently in a causal role of this malignancy. Extensive molecular investigation of the association of human papillomavirus with cervical carcinoma has identified specific nuclear proteins that interact with the tumor-suppressor gene *RB*.[40] In fact, the complex protein-protein interaction between the E7 protein from HPV-16 and the retinoblastoma suppressor protein (pRB) is believed to be important in the cellular transformation that leads to cervical carcinoma. Expression of the E7 protein apparently occurs both within cells from patients with cervical carcinoma and from cell lines derived from this malignancy. The inactivation of the *RB* tumor-suppressor gene by this protein appears to be reversible. There is significant interest in searching for agents that could selectively interfere with this deleterious E7-RB interaction.

Although there are advantages and disadvantages involved with empiric cell line screening or highly targeted mechanistic-molecular targeted approaches, the function of a screen is to provide leads from a host of potential agents or extracts. Subsequent in vitro and in vivo secondary testing, coupled with lead optimization, is necessary to refine the initial promising leads and to identify the optimal drug candidate for introduction into the clinic.[41]

DRUG DEVELOPMENT

Although there is an urgent need to move promising new therapies into clinical trial, important and clinically relevant information may be lost by proceeding immediately from a primary in vitro screen to a clinical trial without defining the in vivo activity of an agent, its pharmacokinetics and schedule dependency in animals, and its profile of toxicity for normal and malignant cells and tissues.

Secondary in vitro studies to examine the effects of varying exposure time to an agent and to define its potential mechanism of action are useful for the investigators planning the in vivo studies. Examination of the dose-response data for several tumor cell lines should permit a selection of the optimal tumor system for subsequently evaluating in vivo efficacy. Further, preliminary pharmacologic studies in nontumor-bearing animals provide useful information about the plasma concentrations achievable and an estimate of the acute toxicity after systemic administration of a new agent. Success in identifying new therapies relies on the expeditious, yet careful, conduct of those studies pertinent to developing a promising in vitro observation (derived from the screen or the molecular model) into an actual drug.[42-45]

IN VIVO ANTITUMOR ASSAYS CURRENTLY IN USE

In the NCI development schema, the human tumor cell line most sensitive to an active candidate in vitro is selected for testing as a xenograft in a subcutaneous implant site in a nude mouse.

Failure to demonstrate in vivo efficacy for agents that display strong in vitro evidence of antitumor activity should prompt additional studies to determine whether there is a pharmacokinetic or metabolic explanation for the loss of activity. The initial lead, either discovered by an empiric screen or as a result of rational chemical design, is rarely the optimal chemical entity for clinical investigation. Lead optimization and an iterative process between chemists and tumor biologists may be required to enhance the in vivo therapeutic index. Factors such as poor solubility and rapid in vivo metabolism may be corrected by analog development. More potent and less toxic derivatives can often be developed, provided the molecule is amenable to modification.

PRECLINICAL PHARMACOLOGY

Preclinical studies in mice, rats, and dogs provide essential information about pharmacokinetics and provide a basis for rational schedule development for the new drugs in humans. Factors such as bioavailability (for agents administered by the oral route), metabolism, renal excretion, and penetration into the central nervous system contribute to the understanding of how best to test a new drug in humans. Although there is no guarantee that the human subject will handle a new drug in the same way as the animal species, in most instances the major pathways for drug metabolism and excretion are qualitatively, if not quantitatively, the same across species.

Pharmacokinetic information in animals can also provide a rational basis for dose escalation in humans. Collins and associates have hypothesized that dose-limiting toxicity in mice and humans is a function of drug exposure, as measured by the area under the drug concentration in plasma × time curve ($C \times T$).[46] They predict that animals and humans encounter dose-limiting toxicity at the same $C \times T$ for any given drug and that the experimentally determined dose-limiting $C \times T$ can be used as a target for dose escalation in humans. An

analysis of recent experience with phase I drug trials suggests that for most, but not all, drugs, the relationship of $C \times T$ to toxicity holds across species.[46] This work allows the clinical investigator to base initial dose escalation on measurements of $C \times T$. Dose escalation can proceed in a more rapid fashion than formerly possible using empiric schemes, and wasteful multiple steps in dose escalation can be avoided. This approach, although apparently valid in retrospective studies, has not been tested in a prospective manner.

Drugs that demonstrate substantial interspecies variation in patterns of target tissue activation are not good candidates for this approach. For example, drugs activated by deoxycytidine kinase, such as fludarabine phosphate, are much more toxic to human marrow cells than to mouse bone marrow, because the enzyme concentration is higher in human cells. In this instance, toxicity in humans is not accurately predicted by the $C \times T$ approach. Further, drug candidates that are excessively potent may have biologic effects at plasma concentrations lower than the level of reproducible detection and are not candidates for pharmacologically guided dose escalation.

FORMULATION STUDIES

Although the preliminary pharmacologic and toxicologic studies may begin before a decision on the final formulation of a product, the IND-directed toxicology should be performed with the final formulation. In addition, other critical studies may be influenced by the formulation (*e.g.*, bioavailability of an oral formulation, insolubility of an agent demonstrating interesting antitumor activity in the cancer screen). Three important factors that have an impact on formulation studies include solubility, stability, and dosage requirements.[47]

Because the route of drug administration for antineoplastic agents has primarily been through an intravenous approach, the solubility issue has provided a substantial challenge for a number of agents with limited aqueous solubility. Efforts to improve the solubility of an agent have primarily involved physical measures, including the use of various mixed solvent systems. Recently, novel approaches, including the use of micronization, liposomal encapsulation, and other unique delivery systems (*e.g.*, cyclodextrins and coacervate systems) have been investigated in an effort to improve methods of drug delivery to tissues. Major efforts are needed to expand the vehicles that are available for intravenous drug delivery of agents with limited aqueous solubility and stability.

The prodrug approach uses chemical modification to solve the difficulty associated with drug insolubility. The most recent example of a successful prodrug approach was the synthesis of the monophosphate of 2-fluoro-adenine arabinoside (fludarabine).[48] In essence, the halogenated nucleoside was poorly soluble in aqueous solution. In contrast, the monophosphate (fludarabine) was more soluble and readily cleaved enzymatically in vivo to the 2-fluoro-adenine arabinoside. The nucleoside is rapidly rephosphorylated after transport to the intracellular compartment, and thus can be effective as an anticancer agent.[48]

TOXICOLOGIC INVESTIGATION

Preclinical toxicologic testing is frequently the final step in the progression of a new chemotherapeutic drug from discovery to initial phase I testing in humans. The major objectives of the preclinical toxicologic studies include (1) definition of the qualitative and quantitative organ toxicities (including dose and schedule dependencies); (2) the reversibility of these effects; and (3) the initial safe starting dose proposed for humans. In general, the best approach is to ensure that the preclinical toxicologic studies reflect the intended clinical investigations in humans (*i.e.*, identical formulation, schedule(s), and route(s) of drug administration, and dose levels anticipated to reflect the likely experience in patients).

The actual protocols for performing the preclinical toxicology at the NCI have changed dramatically during the last two decades.[49,50] Numerous schedules of drug administration were examined in a variety of animal species in the era before 1980. The emphasis later focused on mouse lethality studies for the initial dose-range–finding studies (*i.e.*, LD_{10}, LD_{50}, and LD_{90}). The subsequent toxicologic studies were performed on fixed schedules to refine the doses associated with lethal and nonlethal toxicities. The preclinical toxicities reported correlated reasonably well with the subsequent clinical observations.[49,51–53] However, the extent of useless information relating to highly lethal murine doses (LD_{50} and LD_{90}) led to redesign of the toxicologic studies.

The current toxicologic investigations accepted by the Food and Drug Administration involve a simplified two-step approach. The initial step focuses on acute toxicity in small animals (*e.g.*, mice), and the major endpoint is a determination of the LD_{10}, the dose that produces lethality in approximately 10% of the mice.

The subsequent second phase of preclinical toxicologic investigation is more extensive. The emphasis is given to a careful qualitative and quantitative characterization of the organ-specific toxicities in rodents associated with the schedule and route of administration that is to be used in the initial clinical trial. Attention is given to defining accurately those toxicities that are likely to be observed at doses slightly higher than the highest nontoxic dose. Careful investigation of the doses in the animals that approximate the highest projected tolerable dose in that model should provide data that are more relevant to the anticipated clinical experience in patients.

In the past, most new antineoplastic agents were tested clinically on two relatively fixed schedules of drug administration (*i.e.*, single-bolus intravenous dose once every 3–4 weeks and 5 consecutive days of treatment repeated at 3- to 4-week intervals). The most frequently employed toxicologic protocols reflect each of these schedules. Some newer agents entering preclinical evaluation for cancer therapy are being proposed for continuous intravenous infusion or oral dosing. It is critically important that the preclinical toxicologic protocol simulates the planned therapeutic approach in patients.

Because there may be substantial variation between species in their tolerance to a drug, the safety of a projected starting dose in humans is confirmed by examining the preclinical toxicities in at least two species. Both the qualitative and the quantitative toxicities are usually well defined after investigation of a small animal model (*e.g.*, mouse) and a larger animal (*e.g.*, dog). Only occasionally is testing needed in an additional large animal (*e.g.*, monkey), although this species may be useful for defining central nervous system pharmacokinetics.

Certain organ-specific toxicities are reliably detected with the current toxicologic models (*e.g.*, myelosuppression and gastrointestinal toxicity). In contrast, hepatic and renal toxicities are often missed or falsely positive in animal testing. Toxicities involving the heart, lung, nervous system, pancreas, and integument are even less reliably appreciated. The preclinical evaluation can, at best, establish a safe starting dose for humans and predict acute organ toxicity. A complete definition of the toxicologic profile of a new agent usually emerges only after extensive clinical experimentation.

CONCLUSION

The processes of drug discovery and development of anticancer agents involve substantial time, effort, and resources. The approaches to identify the new therapies are constantly being evaluated and modified. The strategies employed for drug discovery range from empiric screening (the source of most of the current active drugs) to carefully designed proposals to exploit the major advances in cancer biology. However, the process of testing a new agent and bringing it to clinical trial only begins with the discovery of a new active principal. Efficient development of new discoveries demands the cooperation of a multidisciplinary team of investigators who understand and respond to the urgent need for new cancer agents.

REFERENCES

1. Chabner BA, Collins JM, eds. Cancer chemotherapy: Principles and practice. Philadelphia: JB Lippincott, 1990.
2. Pinedo HM, Longo DL, Chabner BA, eds. Cancer chemotherapy and biological modifiers, Annual 14. Amsterdam: Elsevier, 1992.
3. Driscoll J. The preclinical new drug research program of the National Cancer Institute. Cancer Treat Rep 1984;68:63–76.
4. Chabner BA, Shoemaker D. Drug development for cancer: Implications for chemical modifiers. Int J Radiat Oncol Biol Phys 1989;16:907–909.
5. Farber S, Diamond LK, Mercer RD, Sylvester RF, Wolff JA. Temporary remissions in acute leukemia in children produced by folic acid antagonist, 4-aminopteroyl-glutamic acid (aminopterin). N Engl J Med 1948;238:787–793.
6. Erickson J, Neidhart DJ, VanDrie J, et al. Design, activity, and 2.8 a crystal structure of a C2 symmetric inhibitor complexed to HIV-1 protease. Science 1990;249:527–250.
7. Johnson RK. Screening methods in antineoplastic drug discovery. JNCI 1990;82:1082–1083.
8. Suffness M, Newman DJ, Snader K. Discovery and development of antineoplastic agents from natural sources. Bioorg Marine Chem 1989;3:131–168.
9. Weiss RB, Sarosy G, Clagett-Carr K, Russo M, Leyland-Jones B. Anthracycline analogs: The past, present, and future. Cancer Chemother Pharmacol 1986;18:185–197.
10. Smith IE. Mitoxantrone (novantrone): A review of experimental and early clinical studies. Cancer Treat Rev 1983;10:103–115.
11. Werbel LM, Elslager EF, Fry DW, et al. 5-Aminoanthrapyrazoles (CI-937, CI-941, CI-942): A novel class of DNA binders with broad-spectrum anticancer activity. In: Harrap KR, Conners TA, eds. New avenues in developmental cancer chemotherapy. Orlando: Academic Press, 1987:355–365.
12. Smith IE, Talbot DC, Mansi JL, Judson IR, Calvert AH. Anthrapyrazole CI-941: A highly active new drug against advanced breast cancer. Proc Am Soc Clin Oncol [Abstract 94] 1991;10:55.
13. Noble RL, Beer CT, Cutts JH. Role of chance observations in chemotherapy: *Vinca rosea*. Ann NY Acad Sci 1958;76:882–894.
14. Wani MC, Taylor HL, Wall ME, Coggon P, McPhail AT. Plant antitumor agents: VI. The isolation and strucure of taxol, a novel antileukemic and antitumor agent from *Taxus brevifolia*. J Am Chem Soc 1971;93:2325–2327.
15. Schiff PB, Fant J, Horwitz SB. Promotion of microtubule assembly *in vitro* by taxol. Nature 1979;277:665–667.
16. Wall ME, Wani MC, Cook CE, et al. Plant antitumor agents: I. The isolation and structure of camptothecin, a novel alkaloidal leukemia and tumor inhibitor from *Camptotheca accuminata*. J Am Chem Soc 1966;88:3888–3890.
17. Hsiang Y-H, Hertzberg R, Hecht S, Liu LF. Camptothecin induces protein-linked DNA breaks via mammalian DNA topoisomerase I. J Biol Chem 1985;260:14873–14878.
18. Hsiang Y-H, Liu LF. Identification of mammmalian DNA topoisomerase I as an intracellular target of the anticancer drug camptothecin. Cancer Res 1988;48:1722–1726.
19. Rowinsky E, Grochow L, Hendricks C, et al. Phase I and pharmacologic study of topotecan

(SK & F 104864): A novel topoisomerase inhibitor. Proc Am Soc Clin Oncol [Abstract 240] 1991;10:93.

20. Sirott MN, Saltz L, Young C, et al. Phase I and clinical pharmacologic study of intravenous topotecan. Proc Am Soc Clin Oncol [Abstract 284] 1991;10:104.

21. Ohno R, Okada K, Masoaka T, et al. An early phase II study of CPT-11: A new derivative of camptothecin, for the treatment of leukemia and lymphoma. J Clin Oncol 1990;8: 1907–1912.

22. Giovanella BC, Stehlin JS, Wall ME, et al. DNA topoisomerase I-targeted chemotherapy of human colon cancer in xenografts. Science 1989;246:1046–1048.

23. Pettit GR, Herald CL, Doubek DL, et al. Isolation and structure of bryostatin 1. J Am Chem Soc 1982;104:6846–6848.

24. Bai R, Pettit GR, Hamel E. Dolastatin 10, a powerful cytostatic peptide derived from a marine animal: Inhibition of tubulin polymerization mediated through the vinca alkaloid binding domain. Biochem Pharmacol 1990;39:1941–1949.

25. Bai RL, Paull KD, Herald CL, et al. Halichondrin B and homohalichondrin B, marine natural products binding in the vinca domain of tubulin: Discovery of tubulin-based mechanism of action by analysis of differential cytotoxicity data. J Biol Chem 1991;266: 15882–15889.

26. Rosenberg B. Fundamental studies with cisplatin. Cancer 1985;55:2303–2316.

27. Boyd MR. Status of the NCI preclinical antitumor drug discovery screen. PPO Updates 1989;3:1–12.

28. Skehan P, Storeng R, Scudiero D, et al. New colorimetric cytotoxicity assay for anticancer-drug screening. JNCI 1990;82:1107–1112.

29. Chabner BA. In defense of cell-line screening. JNCI 1990;82:1083–1085.

30. Double JA, Bibby MC. Therapeutic index: A vital component in selection of anticancer agents for clinical trial. JNCI 1989;81:988–994.

31. Hodes L. Computer-aided selection of compounds for antitumor screening: Validation of a statistical-heuristic method. J Chem Inform Comput Sci 1981;21:123–190.

32. Paull KD, Shoemaker RH, Hodes L, et al. Display and analysis of patterns of differential activity of drugs against human tumor cell lines: Development of mean graph and COMPARE algorithm. JNCI 1989;81:1088–1092.

33. Powis G, Kozikowski A. Growth factor and oncogene signalling pathways as targets for rational anticancer drug development. Clin Biochem 1991;24:385–397.

34. Workman P. Philosophies of new anticancer drug development. J Drug Dev 1990;2: 193–197.

35. Kelliher M, Knott A, McLaughlin J, Wittee ON, Rosenberg N. Differences in oncogenic potency but not target cell specificity distinguish the two forms of the bcr/abl oncogene. Mol Cell Biol 1991;11:4710–4716.

36. Lugo TG, Pendergast AM, Muller AJ, Wittee ON. Tyrosine kinase activity and transformation potency of bcr-abl oncogene products. Science 1990;247:1079–1082.

37. Szczylik C, Skorski T, Nicholaides NC, et al. Selective inhibition of leukemia cell proliferation by BCR-ABL antisense oligodeoxynucleotides. Science 1991;253:562–565.

38. Kelliher MA, McLaughlin J, Wittee ON, Rosenberg N. Induction of a chronic myelogenous leukemia-like syndrome in mice with v-*ABL* and *BCR/ABL*. Proc Natl Acad Sci USA 1990;87:6649–6653.

39. Cooper GM. Viral oncogenes. In: Oncogenes. Boston: Jones and Bartlett, 1990:26.

40. Jones RE, Wegrzyn RJ, Patrick DR, et al. Identification of HPV-16 E7 peptides that are potent antagonists of E7 binding to the retinoblastoma suppressor protein. J Biol Chem 1990;265:12782–12785.

41. Staquet MJ, Byar DP, Green SB, Rozencweig M. Clinical predictivity of transplantable tumor systems in the selection of new drugs for solid tumors: Rationale for a three-stage strategy. Cancer Treat Rep 1983;67:753–766.

42. Corbett TH, Wozniak A, Gerpheide S, Hanka L. In vitro and in vivo models for detection of new antitumor drugs. In: Hanka LJ, Kondo T, White RJ, eds. Proceedings of a workshop at the 14th International Congress of Chemotherapy at Kyoto. Tokyo: University of Tokyo Press, 1985:5–14.

43. Grindey GB. Current status of cancer drug development: Failure or limited success? Cancer Cells 1990;2:163–171.

44. Bogden AE. The subrenal capsule assay and its use as a drug screening system. In: Hellman K, Carter SK, eds. Fundamentals of cancer chemotherapy. New York: McGraw-Hill, 1987:173–179.

45. Corbett TH, Valeriote FA, Baker LH. Is the P388 murine tumor no longer adequate as a drug discovery model? Invest New Drugs 1987;5:3–20.

46. Collins JM, Grieshaber CK, Chabner BA. Pharmacologically guided phase I clinical trials based upon preclinical drug development. JNCI 1990;82:1321–1326.

47. Davignon JP, Craddock JC. The formulation of anticancer drugs. In: Hellman K, Carter SK, eds. Fundamentals of cancer chemotherapy. New York, McGraw-Hill, 1987:212–227.

48. Brockman RW, Cheng YC, Schabel FM, Montgomery JA. Metabolism and chemotherapeutic activity of 9-B-D-arabinofuranosyl-2-fluoroadenine against murine leukemia L1210 and evidence for its phosphorylation by deoxycytidine kinase. Cancer Res 1980;40: 3610–3615.

49. Grieshaber CK, Marsoni S. Relation of preclinical toxicology to findings in early clinical trials. Cancer Treat Rep 1986;70:65.

50. Lowe MC, Davis RD. The current toxicology protocol of the National Cancer Institute. In: Hellman K, Carter SK, eds. Fundamentals of cancer chemotherapy. New York: McGraw-Hill, 1987:228–235.

51. Schein P, Anderson T. The efficacy of animal studies in predicting clinical toxicity of cancer chemotherapeutic drugs. Int J Clin Pharmacol 1973;8:228–238.

52. Lowe M. Large animal toxicological studies of anticancer drugs. In: Hellman K, Carter SK, eds. Fundamentals of cancer chemotherapy. New York: McGraw-Hill, 1987:228–235.

53. Schurig JE, Bradner WT. Small animal toxicology of cancer drugs. In: Hellman K, Carter SK, eds. Fundamentals of cancer chemotherapy. New York: McGraw-Hill, 1987: 248–261.

SECTION 2

CHARLES S. MORROW
KENNETH H. COWAN

Mechanisms of Antineoplastic Drug Resistance

Systemic chemotherapy is the principal means for treating advanced malignancy, and in the leukemias, lymphomas, and selected solid tumors, it is capable of cure. In the adjuvant setting, significant delays in recurrence of otherwise more resistant tumors may result from the early use of chemotherapy. However, in both settings, recurrences of tumor tend to be resistant to further treatment. In still other tumors, such as adenocarcinomas of the gastrointestinal tract and lung, drug resistance is present from the inception of treatment, and responses are infrequent. The biochemical and genetic processes that underlie the acquisition of the resistant phenotype have been the subject of intense study in the field of chemotherapy. This work has led to the identification of fundamental mechanisms of gene duplication, xenobiotic transport and inactivation, and DNA repair that mediate resistance. Various strategies for overcoming resistance have emerged from this research and are being tested in the clinic. An understanding of the principles of drug resistance and its circumvention is likely to become an increasingly important part of the practice of medical oncology.

Tissue culture models have been integral to the evolution of our understanding of drug resistance mechanisms. The selection of resistant cell lines through exposure to drugs in culture has allowed identification of resistance mechanisms at a molecular level. Murine tumor and xenograft models of tumor resistance to antineoplastic drugs, and analyses of patient tumor specimens, have confirmed the relevance of many of these cellular mechanisms. Additionally, animal studies have identified pharmacologic and anatomic factors unique to cancer-drug interactions in vivo. Although most of these mechanisms of antineoplastic drug resistance have been defined in experimental model systems, molecular analyses of human tumor specimens have indicated that similar mechanisms may underlie clinical drug resistance. These results suggest that the pharmacologic approaches to the reversal or the circumvention of drug resistance developed in vitro may be of value to selected patients.

In this section the authors discuss mechanisms of resistance to single agents or classes of drugs and to multiple structurally unrelated drugs. They consider the prevalence of these mechanisms in clinical practice and discuss strategies to overcome them.

GENERAL MECHANISMS OF RESISTANCE TO ANTINEOPLASTIC DRUGS

CELLULAR MECHANISMS

Selection of drug resistance by intermittent or continuous treatment of tumor cells with a single agent may result in cross-resistance to other structurally related drugs of the same class. This phenomenon of cross-resistance is expected on the basis of alterations in shared cytotoxic targets, drug transporters, and metabolic pathways. However, the resistant tumor cell line generally retains sensitivity to unrelated drugs.[1,2] In contrast, treatment of cells with one of several natural-product antineoplastic drugs frequently results in cross-resistance to multiple, structurally diverse cytotoxins with mechanisms of action that are often unrelated. When this pattern of multidrug resistance (MDR) is examined more closely, it is frequently found that although structurally dissimilar, the apparently unrelated cross-resistant drugs that comprise the phenotype actually have common cytotoxic targets, drug transporters, or metabolic pathways of activation or inactivation.

Decreased Drug Accumulation

Reduced intracellular accumulation of drug is one of the most common mechanisms of antineoplastic drug resistance. Resistance to the antifolate methotrexate (MTX) is frequently due to reduced drug influx secondary to alterations in the transport components, namely the folate-binding protein or the reduced folate transporter.[3] Similarly, a defective drug carrier has been implicated in resistance to nitrogen mustard.[4] Decreased drug accumulation may also be due to enhanced drug efflux. Perhaps the most important clinical example of this mechanism is the overexpression of the putative drug efflux pump associated with MDR, P-glycoprotein.[5]

Altered Drug Metabolism

In tumor cells that accumulate drug normally, resistance may be mediated by changes in drug activation, inactivation, or cofactors. Activation is required for the cytotoxic effect of many antimetabolites and some alkylating agents (*e.g.,* cyclophosphamide) that are administered as prodrugs. Natural or acquired resistance to the purine or pyrimidine analog antimetabolites may be mediated by reduced levels of the kinases and phosphoribosyl transferases necessary to convert these prodrugs to their cytotoxic nucleoside and nucleotide derivatives.[6] Additionally, inactivation of drugs, such as by increased deamination of pyrimidine and purine analogs, may also confer resistance to antimetabolites.[7,8] Alterations in cofactors involved in drug action may modulate cellular resistance to antineoplastic agents. For example, 5,10-methylene tetrahydrofolate enhances the inhibition of thymidylate synthase by 5-fluorodeoxyuridine monophosphate (FdUMP). Therefore, alterations in the level of this reduced folate may significantly influence the sensitivity of tumors cells to FdUMP and its prodrug, 5-fluorouracil (5-FU).

Altered Drug Targets

The drug resistance of tumor cells adapted to growth in the presence of antineoplastic agents may involve alterations in the intracellular drug target. Quantitative and qualitative alterations in dihydrofolate reductase, thymidylate synthase, and topoisomerase II have been associated with resistance to specific antineoplastic drug inhibitors of these enzymes.[9–11]

Enhanced DNA Repair Capacity

The final common pathway for cytotoxic effect of many of the cancer drugs, including the alkylating agents and topoisomerase-binding drugs, is DNA strand breakage. In addition, other classes of drugs, such as the antimetabolites, produce errors in base pairing, premature chain termination, or strand breaks. A poorly understood aspect of tumor resistance to chemotherapy is the process of repair of these lesions. With few exceptions, the specific enzymes responsible for the repair of various DNA lesions have not been identified. An example of such a repair system is the O^6-guanine alkyl transferase that removes adducts created by the nitrosoureas and diethyltriazinoimidazolecarboxamide (DTIC).[12] Enhanced repair capacity, which has been demonstrated best for cisplatin- and alkylating agent-resistant cells, could potentially confer resistance to multiple agents.[13]

RESISTANCE MECHANISMS APPARENT ONLY IN VIVO

Drug screening has identified a number of agents that show promising activity against tumor cells grown in culture yet show limited antitumor efficacy in vivo. Other drugs active against some tumor types are relatively ineffective against other tumors or tumors located in specific sites. Anatomic and pharmocologic sanctuaries may contribute to such resistance patterns. For example, the blood–brain and testicular barriers account for the high rate of local failure in these sites during otherwise effective systemic treatment of acute lymphocytic leukemia (ALL).[14] The relative resistance of some large solid tumors to chemotherapy is at least partially attributable to poor drug delivery to areas of poor vascularization and to areas of hypoxia and acidosis that may compromise the effectiveness of some chemotherapeutic agents. Therapeutic success is also influenced by idiosyncratic pharmacokinetic parameters such as variable absorption of an oral drug or altered metabolism and clearance of a drug.

Relative resistance to drugs may be conferred by factors present in the tissues and extracellular environment surrounding the tumor. For example, colon cancer cells were made MDR by culturing them in the presence of diacylglycerol, a protein kinase C activator present in the intestine.[15] Additionally, poorly defined host-tumor-drug interactions may play a role in the development of drug resistance in vivo. With the use of a tumor xenograft model, it was shown that tumor cells selected for resistance to cisplatin or cyclophosphamide in vivo became sensitive to the same drugs when grown in cell culture. Furthermore, when the cultured cells were reimplanted into animals, drug resistance was restored.[16] The authors suggest that novel host-dependent resistance mechanisms may exist that involve altered pharmacokinetics or tumor cell resistance mechanisms stimulated by host factors.

Agents that show significant cytotoxicity toward tumor cells grown in culture may fail clinically because of unexpected toxicity to normal host tissues.

RESISTANCE TO MULTIPLE DRUGS

Cells selected for resistance by treatment with one antineoplastic agent, although cross-resistant to drugs with similar mechanisms of cytoxicity from the same class, often retain sensitivity to unrelated drugs. Such resistance patterns are the rationale for treatment of cancer with regimens consisting of several chemotherapeutic agents. However, in many instances, tumor cells become refractory to multiple structurally unrelated drugs to which they have never been exposed either in the absence of prior treatment (de novo resistance) or in response to prior therapy (acquired resistance). These patterns are called MDR and are conveniently classified according to their association with the overexpression of the putative drug efflux pump P-glycoprotein, or with alterations in topoisomerase II or drug metabolizing pathways. Additionally, there are MDR patterns that resemble the P-glycoprotein-mediated MDR phenotype yet do not involve overexpression of P-glycoprotein and whose underlying resistance mechanisms are less well defined.

CLASSIC (P-GLYCOPROTEIN-MEDIATED) MULTIDRUG RESPONSE

The phenomenon of antineoplastic MDR was first described in cell lines selected for resistance to dactinomycin that simultaneously became resistant to vinca alkaloids, daunorubicin, and mitomycin C.[17] Subsequently, this MDR phenotype has been observed in many cell lines that share a pattern of cross-resistance to several lipophilic, natural-product drugs of disparate structure.

Classic MDR is conferred by an energy-dependent drug efflux pump, P-glycoprotein (p170) encoded by the *MDR1* gene.[5] MDR is associated with P-glycoprotein overexpression and with reduced drug accumulation secondary to enhanced drug efflux, a process sensitive to metabolic poisons. Gene transfer experiments have shown that P-glycoprotein overexpression is sufficient to confer MDR.[18,19,20]

Analyses of P-glycoprotein structure and tissue distribution further support its role as an energy-dependent transporter that has striking homology with some bacterial transport proteins.[21] Like the recently described cystic fibrosis gene, *MDR1* belongs to a family of genes that encode two pairs of 6 transmembrane regions and two putative nucleotide-binding domains.[5,22] Drug binding to P-glycoprotein has been demonstrated using photoaffinity analogs, and the multiple drug binding sites that have been identified may partially explain the remarkable ability of P-glycoprotein to process structurally diverse drugs.[23] In normal tissues, P-glycoprotein is localized on the luminal surfaces of renal tubules, colon, small intestine, bile canaliculi, and vascular epithelia of the brain and spinal cord.[24,25] The strategic location of P-glycoprotein on these luminal surfaces is consistent with its role as a transporter gene in normal and tumor tissues.

Classic MDR is associated with P-glycoprotein but is subject to significant phenotypic variability. For example, the relative cross-resistance to the drugs of the MDR phenotype varies depending on cell type and selecting drug. Multiple phenotypic changes in addition to overexpression of P-glycoprotein may occur with in vitro or in vivo selection, and such changes have been proposed to account for the variability in the magnitude of resistance and cross-resistance observed. However, one study showed an excellent correlation between the level of membrane P-glycoprotein and the degree of resistance to vinblastine in mouse cells infected with a human *MDR1* cDNA expression vector.[20] The linear correlation between resistance to vinblastine cytotoxicity and *MDR1* expression was preserved, regardless of whether the transfected clones had been selected by cytotoxic drug exposure or by immunofluorescence labeling and cell sorting. Although these results do not minimize the importance of other ancillary factors involved in some examples of MDR, they suggest that membrane P-glycoprotein density is sufficient to determine drug resistance level in carefully controlled situations using matched cell lines.

Mutations in the *MDR1* gene influence the MDR phenotype. A single amino acid substitution in position 185 of P-glycoprotein results in preferential resistance to colchicine compared with the wild-type gene. Expression of the mutant gene is associated with a relative decrease in colchicine accumulation by a mechanism that may involve altered release of drug into the extracellular space.[26] In addition to expression of alternative or mutant *MDR* genes, posttranslational modification of P-glycoprotein has been implicated in altered resistance. P-glycoprotein is phosphorylated by protein kinase C and by a novel membrane-associated kinase. The functional significance of these modifications is suggested by results that have shown an association between phorbol ester-induced P-glycoprotein phosphorylation by protein kinase C and decreased accumulation of vinblastine in MDR KB cells, and increased drug uptake when phosphorylation of P-glycoprotein was inhibited by Staurosporin.[27,28] Additionally, phenotypic heterogeneity in P-glycoprotein-associated MDR cells may be attributed to the coexistence of an entirely unrelated resistance mechanism.[29]

By understanding of the regulation of *MDR1* gene expression, it may be possible to consider strategies to block the evolution of P-glycoprotein overexpression in tumor cells or to reverse its overexpression once established. In vitro, the *MDR1* gene is frequently amplified or transcriptionally activated, or both, in cell lines selected for high levels of MDR. Additionally, it has been reported that increased P-glycoprotein mRNA may be induced by heat shock, heavy metals, cytotoxic drugs, toxic and ablative liver damage, ionizing radiation, and altered expression of the tumor suppressor gene, p53, or its mutant forms.[30–34] The latter observation, if confirmed, may provide a link between oncogenesis and the emergence of P-glycoprotein overexpression in some tumors.

The importance of P-glycoprotein in human cancer has been supported by numerous studies that have examined the levels of *MDR1*-encoded RNA or protein levels in tumor specimens. The *MDR1* gene product has been detected in a variety of tumors, including acute and chronic leukemias, ovarian cancer, multiple myeloma, breast cancer, neuroblastoma, soft tissue sarcomas, renal cell carcinoma, cervical cancer, and others.[35–50] Analyses of these results have tended to show an association between P-glycoprotein expression and a history of prior therapy or toxin exposure, presence of a tumor that is intrinsically or secondarily resistant to therapy, and poor treatment outcome. Elevated P-glycoprotein levels have been reported in acute nonlymphocytic leukemia (ANLL) patients during progressive disease or in association with poor prognostic groups.[35,36] There is some correlation in adult acute leukemias between increased P-glycoprotein and relapse, failure to achieve complete remission, or in vitro resistance to daunorubicin.[40] The *MDR1* gene is often expressed in treated and untreated neuroblastoma, but the gene tends to be more frequently and highly expressed in patients treated with doxorubicin-containing regimens than in untreated patients.[46] P-glycoprotein expression has been linked strongly to aggressive biologic behavior, poor treatment response, and poor outcome in patients with advanced neuroblastoma. Impressive correlations between aggressive, poorly responding disease and P-glycoprotein expression persisted when the presence of P-glycoprotein was corrected for confounding prognostic features. Elevated P-glycoprotein in childhood ALL and soft tissue sarcomas has been observed with greater frequency in patients who have been treated previously with an anthracycline-containing regimen, have failed remission induction, or have relapsed.[36,47] In a study of more than 400 patient tumor specimens, increased P-glycoprotein RNA was more prevalent in specimens derived from cancers that tended to be more resistant to therapy (*e.g.*, colon, kidney, adrenal gland, liver, pancreas) than in those derived from cancers that tend to be intrinsically sensitive to chemotherapy.[50] Additional prospective studies are required to confirm the clinical significance of P-glycoprotein in human cancer. However, results to date indicate that P-glycoprotein overexpression is associated with clinical evidence of drug resistance and treatment failure.[51] Determinations of P-glycoprotein levels in patients at diagnosis or relapse may have a major role in the design of future treatment protocols.

Similar phenotypes of resistance to multiple antineoplastic agents have been described that are associated with the expression of other membrane proteins. In many of these examples, resistance occurs independent of P-glycoprotein expression.[52-56] The mechanism of MDR in these cell lines and the role of these membrane proteins are currently unknown.

MULTIDRUG RESISTANCE ASSOCIATED WITH TOPOISOMERASE POISONS

Topoisomerases are nuclear enzymes that catalyze the formation of transient single- or double-strand DNA breaks, facilitate passage of DNA strands through these breaks, and promote rejoining of the DNA strands.[57] Additionally, an important site of the topoisomerase II action is the nuclear matrix, where it is believed to serve structural and enzymatic functions.[58] As a consequence of these activities, topoisomerases are thought to be critical for DNA replication, transcription, and recombination. The cytotoxicities of drugs that target topoisomerases (topiosomerase poisons or inhibitors) are thought to depend on the DNA cleavage activities of these enzymes. There are two classes of mammalian topoisomerases: Topoisomerase I catalyzes the formation of single-strand DNA breaks, whereas topoisomerase II catalyzes single- and double-strand breaks. During the cleavage reactions, reversible DNA-protein complexes (cleavable complexes) are formed that can be stabilized by interactions with drugs that act as topoisomerase poisons. Although the formation and stabilization of cleavable complexes can be dissociated from cytotoxicity under some circumstances, the formation of these complexes is believed to be the initiating event in topoisom-

TABLE 18–5.   Topoisomerase II Poisons

Nonintercalators	
	Etoposide (VP16)
Epipodophylotoxins	Teniposide (VM26)
Intercalators	
	Doxorubicin
Anthracyclines	Daunorubicin
Acridine	mAMSA (amsacrine)
Anthracenedione	Mitoxantrone
Antibiotic	Dactinomycin
Ellipticine	9-Hydroxyellipticine

erase poison-mediated cell death. Some of the topoisomerase II-acting drugs used clinically are listed in Table 18–5.

Several MDR cell lines have been described that display resistance to several or all of the drugs listed in Table 18–5.[59,60] Although many of these topoisomerase II poisons are also members of the classic MDR phenotype, the pattern of topoisomerase II-associated MDR differs significantly. Cells that display topoisomerase II-associated MDR retain sensitivity to the antimicrotubule drugs vincristine and vinblastine, which are associated with the P-glycoprotein-dependent MDR phenotype. Both quantitative and qualitative alterations in topoisomerase II activity may underlie topoisomerase-associated MDR. Decreased topoisomerase activity has been associated with reduced drug-induced DNA strand breaks in cells resistant to the cytotoxicity of topoisomerase II poisons.[61] Other studies have suggested that intrinsic changes in the enzyme properties, including point mutations in the topoisomerase II gene, may underlry some examples of topoisomerase-associated MDR.[11,62,63] The mutation in one of these topoisomerases is located in a putative ATP-binding domain and correlates with decreased catalytic activity and increased ATP requirement when compared with the wild-type topoisomerase.[64] A teniposide-resistant cell line has been characterized by a reduction in topoisomerase II activity associated with the nuclear matrix fraction.[65] The nature of the topoisomerase II alteration may influence the pattern of drug cross-resistance in topoisomerase-associated MDR. For example, cells that develop defective topoisomerase II activity on selection for resistance with m-AMSA may show cross-resistance to other intercalating agents but not to epipodophyllotoxins.[62] Collectively, these data indicate that reduced topoisomerase protein levels or specific alterations in enzyme activities may render cells more resistant to drugs by interfering with the formation of stable cleavable complexes and, hence, cytotoxic DNA strand breaks. The normal down-regulation of topoisomerase II in nondividing cells may explain the relative resistance to topoisomerase II poisons of some solid tumors that contain a large fraction of quiescent cells.[57]

The formation of stable cleavable complexes is believed to initiate the events leading to death in cells treated with topoisomerase poisons. However, it is possible partially to protect cells from topoisomerase-acting drug cytotoxicity by temporary inhibition of protein or nucleic acid synthesis, even though the drug-induced stabilization of cleavable complexes continues to occur.[58] These results indicate that cytotoxicity mediated by topoisomerase poisons is complex, involving processes distal to the formation of stable DNA-protein-drug ternary complexes. These processes may include the collision between DNA replication or transcriptional machinery with the cleavable complex, or they may involve the initiation of programmed cell death (apoptosis). Accordingly, alterations in these distal processes may confer resistance to topoisomerase poisons independently of changes in topoisomerase activity.

The drug camptothecin has been shown to mediate cytotoxicity by its interaction with topoisomerase I. As with topoisomerase II poisons, topoisomerase I-acting drugs can select cells that express a defective topoisomerase I with reduced ability to mediate camptothecin-induced DNA strand breaks.[66]

MULTIDRUG RESISTANCE ASSOCIATED WITH ALTERED DRUG-METABOLIZING ENZYMES

Acquired resistance to antineoplastic drugs in many respects parallels the response of normal tissues exposed to carcinogens. For example, in the Solt-Farber model of hepatic carcinogenesis, carcinogen exposure gives rise to preneoplastic liver nodules that show increased expression of the *MDR* gene, decreased activity of drug- and toxin-activating enzymes, and increased activity of enzymes that detoxify drugs and toxins.[32,67] A similar pattern of changes in drug-activating and -inactivating enzymes occurs when a breast cancer cell line is selected for MDR by chronic doxorubicin exposure.[68] Among the detoxifying enzymes increased in these models of drug resistance are the glutathione S-transferases (GSTs),[69] enzymes that catalyze the conjugation of electrophilic hydrophobic compounds to the thiol glutathione (GSH), and glutathione peroxidase, a second GSH-dependent enzyme that catalyzes the detoxification of hydroperoxides.

Antineoplastic agents and their metabolites that are reported to be substrates of GSTs are listed in Table 18–6. Whether GST levels in cancer cells are sufficient to confer clinically significant resistance is a matter of considerable debate. Gene transfer experiments using recombinant GST genes and tissue culture cells have suggested that some GST isozymes may confer a modest level of resistance to mephalan, chlorambucil, cisplatin, and doxorubicin.[70,71] Other experiments have failed to confirm any consistent resistance to doxorubicin, cisplatin, melphalan, chlorambucil, or BCNU in breast cancer cells transfected with any of the three major isozymes of soluble GSTs.[72] Additional studies may help clarify the role of GSTs in drug resistance.

APPROACHES FOR THE PREVENTION OR REVERSAL OF CLINICAL DRUG RESISTANCE

General approaches to overcome antineoplastic drug resistance include strategies to prevent the emergence of resistance, such as aggressive multiagent chemotherapy with noncross-resistant drugs, or attempts to avoid factors and drug schedules that tend to select for resistant tumors.

P-GLYCOPROTEIN-MEDIATED DRUG RESISTANCE

Since the original recognition that verapamil could partially restore drug sensitivity to cells made resistant to vincristine or doxorubicin, agents have been identified that can partially reverse the drug accumulation defects in classic MDR cells, including calcium channel blockers, cyclosporin A, calmodulin inhibitors such as phenothiazines, and other drugs.[73–75] Although the mechanism(s) by which these agents reverse MDR is incompletely understood, it is believed that direct interactions between these agents and P-glycoprotein interfere with antineoplastic drug efflux.

In the few trials done to date, responses have been observed in children with ALL refractory to standard therapy who were treated with vincristine and the calcium channel blocker diltiazem, in adults with doxorubicin-resistant solid tumors treated with that drug plus verapamil, and in children with refractory ALL treated with verapamil, vincristine, and etoposide.[76–78] However, these results were anecdotal, and no attempt was made to correlate response with P-glycoprotein expression. No responses and unacceptable cardiovascular toxicity were reported when 8 patients with refractory ovarian cancer were treated with doxorubicin and intravenously infused verapamil.[79] Trifluperazine, which also reverses MDR-type resistance in cell culture, was tested with doxorubicin and was found to produce responses in 7 of 21 patients with "acquired" resistance to chemotherapy.[80]

The correlation of P-glycoprotein level and response to the addition of a reversing agent has been addressed in studies of patients with malignant lymphoma and multiple myeloma.[81,82] Although responses have occurred in each of these studies, most of the patients had not been treated with an identical chemotherapy regimen before addition of verapamil and thus could not be labeled as refractory to therapy. Some of the responders had tumors that were positive for P-glycoprotein, and all had received some form of prior chemotherapy. Thus, it is likely, but not definitely established, that P-glycoprotein blockade with calcium channel blockers can enhance response in at least some patients with cancer. The optimal agent for reversal and the optimal regimen for its administration have not been established.

Cyclosporin A has shown great promise as an MDR-reversing agent in preclinical studies.[83–85] In one anecdotal report involving a patient with P-glycoprotein-expressing re-

TABLE 18–6. Substrates of GSTs Relevant to Anticancer Therapy

Antineoplastic Drugs

Alkylating Agents
  Chlorambucil
  Melphalan
  Cyclophosphamide
  1,3-bis(2-chloroethyl)-1-nitrosourea (BCNU)
Anthracenedione
  Mitoxantrone

Products of Membrane and DNA Oxidation

Fatty Acid Hydroperoxides
4-Hydroxyalkenals
?DNA Hydroperoxides

fractory acute myelocytic leukemia (AML), cyclosporin A treatment was able to reverse the defect of leukemic blasts in daunorubicin uptake in vitro and to restore transiently clinical responsiveness to chemotherapy in vivo.[86] The role of cyclosporin A in the reversal of MDR is the subject of more comprehensive clinical trials now in progress.

Collectively, these studies suggest that the use of MDR-reversing agents may benefit selected patients with P-glycoprotein-positive refractory tumors. What is needed before such reversing agents can be recommended are the results of additional clinical trials that correlate antitumor response with the presence of P-glycoprotein, as well as an identification of reversing agents with less toxicity and the determinations of optimal dosages and schedules. Additionally, preclinical studies have indicated that anti-P-glycoprotein antibodies, covalently linked to cellular toxins or used in conjunction with complement, can specifically reduce the burden of P-glycoprotein-positive tumor cells and restore sensitivity to vincristine.[87–90] The clinical usefulness of these immunologic agents is a matter for future investigations.

TOPOISOMERASE POISONS

Resistance to topoisomerase II drugs may occur as a consequence of P-glycoprotein overexpression or secondary to altered topoisomerase II activities. Resistance to anthracyclines or epipodophyllotoxins on the basis of P-glycoprotein overexpression does not usually result in resistance to the acridine known as amsacrine (mAMSA). Conversely, altered topoisomerase-mediated resistance to mAMSA and other intercalating agents is not necessarily associated with resistance to the nonintercalating epipodophyllotoxin class of topoisomerase II poisons.[62] Consequently, these results from in vitro studies suggest a rationale for the administration of alternative classes of topoisomerase II poisons in selected examples of clinical resistance to another class of topoisomerase II drug.[91]

RESISTANCE TO FREE RADICAL-ASSOCIATED DRUG TOXICITY

The generation of free radicals contributes to the cytotoxicities of some antineoplastic agents. Anthracyclines, such as doxorubicin, are important members of this class of antineoplastic agent. Although DNA-intercalating anthracyclines can confer cytotoxicity by several mechanisms, including stimulation of topoisomerase II-mediated DNA strand breaks, inhibition of nucleic acid synthesis, and perturbation of cell membranes, these compunds can also produce free radicals that contribute to cell death.[92,93] Therefore, cellular factors that limit hydrogen peroxide levels or that repair peroxidative damage to macromolecules may confer resistance to anthracyclines.

Although the relative importance of free radical production in tumor killing by anthracyclines has not been established, in experimental tumors measures that increase catalase or glutathione peroxidase activity inhibit response, whereas depletion of glutathione by buthionine sulfoximine (BSO) enhances cytotoxicity.[94,95] Others have not found evidence that glutathione levels or GSH-dependent enzyme activities influence response.[96,97] The possible role of GSTs in repairing oxidative damage to membranes and detoxifying lipid peroxides is suggested by biochemical studies in cell-free systems.[98]

Although the weight of experimental evidence suggests that anthracycline and anthracenedione toxicity is exerted through their interaction with topoisomerase II, the glutathione-dependent detoxification reactions may contribute to drug inactivation and may heighten drug resistance. Glutathione depletion by BSO and GST inactivation by ethacrynic acid are the subjects of ongoing clinical trials, with the aim of enhancing response to alkylating agents and anthracyclines.[99]

ALKYLATING AND PLATINUM DRUGS

Resistance to alkylating agents and platinum compounds may be mediated by decreased drug accumulation, increased drug inactivation, or increased repair of drug-induced damage. Preclinical studies have suggested that resistance mechanisms in the latter two categories may be circumvented by pharmacologic manipulations. Detoxification or inactivation of electrophilic alkylating agents and platinum compounds may occur as a consequence of their reactions with thiol-containing compounds, such as glutathione and metallothionein.[100] For example, glutathione conjugates form with a variety of alkylating agents in nonenzymatic and GST-catalyzed reactions. Associations have been reported between increased GST levels or specific GST isozymes and resistance to nitrosoureas, chlorambucil, and other nitrogen mustards.[71,101,102] Increased glutathione levels have also been reported with resistance to alkylating agents and cisplatin.[104] Although cisplatin can react spontaneously with glutathione, it is not known whether GSTs can catalyze this reaction. This issue is unresolved by conflicting reports that demonstrate elevation in pi class GST levels in some cisplatin resistant cells but not others.[105]

Although the clinical significance of GST and glutathione for alkylating agent resistance is controversial, preclinical data have prompted ongoing clinical trials using pharmacologic antagonists of GST or inhibitors of glutathione synthesis.[106]

Expression of the drug metabolizing enzyme aldehyde dehydrogenase (ALDH) has been associated with resistance to cyclophosphamide.[107] This enzyme converts aldophosphamide, a key metabolite of cyclophosphamide, mafosfamide, and other oxaphosphorines, to the inactive compound carboxyphosphamide. This reaction prevents the formation of the cytotoxic derivative of aldophosphamide, phosphoramide mustard. Increased expression has been associated with resistance to cyclophosphamide of tumor cells grown in vitro and of primative hematopoietic progenitor cells.[108] A number of substrates or inhibitors of ALDH-catalyzed reactions with aldophosphamide have been identified.[109] It remains to be determined whether any of these agents might offer therapeutic advantage to patients with refractory tumors or if these agents might contribute to toxicities.

Repair of DNA damage is a major cellular mechanism of circumventing alkylating agent toxicity. Alkylation of the O^6 position of guanine is believed to be an initiating event in the cytotoxicities of several agents, including the nitrosoureas BCNU, CCNU, and MeCCNU.[12] Repair of O^6-alkylguanine DNA intermediates by increased levels of O^6-alkylguanine DNA alkyltransferase has been associated with relative resistance to these drugs. Depletion of this alkyltranferase activity with O^6-benzylguanine or with O^6-methyl guanine enhances cytotoxicity to chloroethyl nitrosoureas in resistant cell lines in vitro, but in vivo treatment with O^6-methylguanine was limited by toxicity to the host.[12,110,111]

Cisplatin toxicity is also thought to be mediated by DNA damage—specifically, the formation of lethal intrastrand and interstrand DNA crosslinks. Increased DNA repair is associated with resistance to this compound.[112,113] DNA polymerase α is believed to be involved in DNA repair. The finding that coadministration of the DNA polymerase α inhibitor, aphidicolin, can potentiate cisplatin cytotoxicity in some resistant, but not sensitive, cells has prompted the consideration of clinical trials using this inhibitor with cisplatin.[106,112]

ANTIMETABOLITES

The cytotoxicities of most antimetabolite drugs for the treatment of cancer stem from their abilities to interfere with key steps in nucleic acid metabolism. Considered in this section are three clinically important compounds: the antifolate MTX and the pyrimidine analogs 5-FU and cytosine arabinoside (cytarabine). Resistance to antimetabolites may involve any of the steps in the complex pathway of drug transport, activation, and metabolism, interaction with its intracellular target, and elimination. Many mechanisms of resistance to these compounds have been described, and strategies to overcome them include dose escalation, pharmacologic manipulation of drug metabolism, and design of novel antimetabolites. The mechanism of action and clinical pharmacology of these drugs are discussed in greater detail elsewhere in this chapter.

MTX has clinically important activity against solid tumors and hematopoietic malignancies. Its mechanism of action and cellular pharmacology are described in the section on antifolates; with respect to resistance, each of the processes involved in its cellular action, including transport, polygluta-mation, and binding to dihydrofolate reductase, may be affected by changes in protein expression or gene amplification that affect these key steps.[3,114] Of considerable importance is the confirmation of amplification of the dihydrofolate reductase gene as a mechanism of clinical resistance to MTX.[115] Strategies designed to overcome resistance of MTX have been adopted and include the administration of high doses of MTX (with the rescue agent leucovorin), a regimen designed to overcome transport defects and increases in the target enzyme, dihydrofolate reductase.[14,116] The regimen may contribute to effective adjuvant therapy for osteogenic sarcoma and has more definite benefit in childhood ALL, for which entry of drug into the central nervous system helps to prevent meningeal leukemia.[14]

Lipid-soluble derivatives of MTX, such as trimetrexate and piritrexim, circumvent resistance due to deletion of the folate transporter(s) in tumor cells (Fig. 18–2) but have no advantage in cells that overexpress dihydrofolate reductase and, unfortunately, are subject to classic MDR-type resistance.[117,118] They have not proven to be effective in MTX-resistant tumors in the clinic.

5-FU, with its complex pathways for activation to FdUMP and FUTP, can be affected by deletion of any one of several steps in this sequence of activation.[9] In addition, increased expression or amplification of thymidylate synthase (TS; the target for FdUMP), or alteration in its affinity for FdUMP may lead to resistance in experimental models.[119,120] Although the specific enzymes may differ, MTX and 5-FU resistance share common mechanistic features.

To overcome 5-FU resistance, changes in drug schedule to continuous prolonged exposure, addition of an exogenous folate to increase binding to TS, and pretreatment with agents that enhance 5-FU activation (MTX and phosphonoacetyl-L-aspartate) have been employed.[121–124] Although these manipulations increase 5-FU effectiveness in animal models, only the addition of leucovorin has produced positive clinical results.

Like the antifolates and fluoropyrimidines, cytarabine progresses through a series of obligatory steps in its pathway to its final target, in this instance, incorporation into DNA. High doses of cytarabine have been employed clinically with definite benefit in relapsed patients with AML, perhaps related to the increased uptake of drug and increased activation. Specific mechanisms of resistance to this agent include decreased nucleoside transport, deletion of the initial activating enzyme (deoxycytidine kinase), increased inactivation by cytidine deaminase, and altered affinity of DNA polymerase for ara-CTP.[8,125] Clinical studies of resistance have not produced a clear picture of the reasons for development of resistance in patients with leukemia; perhaps the most convincing case can be made for deoxycytidine kinase deletion.

CONCLUSION

Most of the mechanisms of drug resistance described have been determined in cell culture and animal models. Evidence exists that many of these mechanisms operate in some cases of human cancer, but their relative importance in determining clinical drug resistance is only now emerging. No comprehensive evaluation of mechanisms of resistance has been undertaken in human disease. A thorough understanding of the targets of antineoplastic action and the precise mechanisms of resistance would allow the rational development of new drugs and treatment strategies. Additional studies are needed to identify as yet unrecognized resistance mechanisms and to develop specific resistance-reversing agents.

REFERENCES

1. Hill BT, Price LA, Goldie JH. The value of Adriamycin in overcoming resistance to methotrexate in cell culture. Eur J Cancer 1976;12:541.
2. Teicher BA, Cucchi CA, Lee JB, Flatow JL, Rosowsky A, Frei E III. Alkylating agents: In vitro studies of cross-resistance patterns in human cell lines. Cancer Res 1986;46:4379.
3. Sirotnak FM, Moccio DM, Kelleher LE, Goutsas LJ. Relative frequency and kinetic properties of transport defective phenotypes among methotrexate-resistant L1210 clonal cell lines derived in vivo. Cancer Res 1981;41:4447.
4. Goldenberg GJ, Vanstone CL, Israels LG, Isle D, Bihler D. Evidence for a transport carrier of nitrogen mustard in nitrogen mustard-sensitive, -resistance L5178Y lymphoblasts. Cancer Res 1970;30:2285.
5. Endicott JA, Ling V. The biochemistry of P-glycoprotein-mediated multidrug resistance. Annu Rev Biochem 1989;58:137.
6. Drahovsky D, Kreis W. Studies on drug resistance: II. Kinase patterns in P815 neoplasms sensitive and resistant to 1-β-D-arabinofuranosyl cytosine. Biochem Pharmacol 1970;19:940.
7. Hunt SW, Hoffee PA. Amplification of adenosine deaminase gene sequence in deoxy-coformycin-resistant rat hepatoma cells. J Biol Chem 1983;258:13185.
8. Stewart CD, Burke PJ. Cytidine deaminase and the development of resistance to cytosine arabinoside. Nature 1971;233:109.
9. Armstrong RA. Fluoropyrimidine activity and resistance at the cellular level. In: Kessel D, ed. Resistance to antineoplastic drugs. Boca Raton: CRC Press, 1989;317.
10. Haber DA, Beverly SM, Kiely ML, Schimke RT. Properties of altered dehydrofolate reductase encoded by amplified genes in cultured mouse fibroblasts. J Biol Chem 1981;256:9501.

11. Pommier Y, Kerrigan D, Schwartz RE, Swack JA, Swack AM. Altered DNA topoisomerase II activity in Chinese hamster cells resistant to topoisomerase II inhibitors. Cancer Res 1988;46:3075.
12. Erickson L. The role of O^6-methylguanine DNA methyltransferase (MGMT) in drug resistance and strategies for its inhibition. Semin Cancer Biol 1991;2:257.
13. Chao CCK, Lee YL, Cheng PW, Lin-Chao S. Enhanced host cell reactivation of damaged plasmid DNA in HeLa cells resistant to cis-diamminedichloroplatinum(II). Cancer Res 1991;51:601.
14. Poplack DG, Reaman G. Acute lymphoblastic leukemia in childhood. Pediatr Clin North Am 1988;35:903.
15. Dong Z, Ward NE, Fan D, Gupta KP, O'Brian CA. In vitro model for intrinsic drug resistance: Effects of protein kinase C activators on the chemosensitivity of cultured human colon cancer cells. Mol Pharmacol 1991;39:563.
16. Teicher BA, Herman TS, Holden SA, et al. Tumor resistance to alkylating agents conferred by mechanisms operative only in vivo. Science 1990;247:1457.
17. Biedler JL, Riehm H. Cellular resistance to actinomycin D in Chinese Hamster ovary cells in vitro: Cross resistance, radioautographic, and cytogenetic studies. Cancer Res 1970;30:1174.
18. Riordan JR, Ling V. Genetic and biochemical characterization of multidrug resistance. Pharmacol Ther 1985;28:51.
19. Ueda K, Cardarelli C, Gottesman MM, Pastan I. Expression of a full-length cDNA from the human *MDR1* gene confers resistance to colchicine, doxorubicin, and vinblastine. Proc Natl Acad Sci USA 1987;84:3004.
20. Choi K, Frommel TO, Stern RK, et al. Multidrug resistance after retroviral transfer of the human MDR1 gene correlates with P-glycoprotein density in the plasma membrane and is not affected by cytotoxic selection. Proc Natl Acad Sci USA 1991;88:7386.
21. Gros P, Croop J, Houseman D. Mammalian multidrug resistant gene: Complete cDNA sequence indicates strong homology to bacterial transport proteins. Cell 1986;47:371.
22. Riordan JR, Rommens JM, Kerem BS, et al. Indentification of the cystic fibrosis gene: Cloning and characterization of complementary DNA. Science 1989;245:1066.
23. Safa AR, Glover CJ, Meyers MB, Biedler JL, Felsted RL. Vinblastine photoaffinity labeling of a high molecular weight surface membrane glycoprotein specific for multidrug-resistant cells. J Biol Chem 1986;261:6137.
24. Gottesman MM, Pastan I. Resistance to multiple chemotherapeutic agents in human cancer cells. Trends Pharmacol Sci 1988;9:54.
25. Sugawara I, Hamada H, Tsuruo T, Mori S. Specialized localization of P-glycoprotein recognized by MRK 16 monoclonal antibody in endothelial cells of the brain and the spinal cord. Jpn J Cancer Res 1990;81:727.
26. Safa AR, Stern RK, Choi K, et al. Molecular basis of preferential resistance to colchicine in multidrug resistant human cells conferred by Gly-185—Val-185 substitution in P-glycoprotein Proc Natl Acad Sci USA 1990;87:7225.
27. Chambers TC, Chalikonda I, Elion G. Correlation of protein kinase C translocation, P-glycoprotein phosphorylation and reduced drug accumulation in multidrug resistant human KB cells. Biochem Biophys Res Commun 1990;169:253.
28. Ma LD, Marquardt D, Takemoto L, Center MS. Analysis of P-glycoprotein phosphorylation in HL60 cells isolated for resistance to vincristine. J Biol Chem 1991;266:5593–5599.
29. Friche E, Danks MK, Schmidt CA, Beck WT. Decreased DNA topoisomerase II in daunorubicin-resistant Ehrlich ascites tumor cells. Cancer Res 1991;51:4213.
30. Chin K-V, Chauhan SS, Pastan I, Gottesman MM. Regulation of mdr RNA levels in response to cytotoxic drugs in rodent cells. Cell Growth Differ 1990;1:361.
31. Chin KV, Ueda K, Pastan I, Gottesman MM. Modulation of activity of the promoter of the human MDR1 gene by Ras and p53. Science 1992;255:459.
32. Fairchild CR, Ivy SP, Rushmore T, et al. Carcinogen-induced mdr overexpression is associated with xenobiotic resistance in rat preneoplastic liver nodules and hepatocellular carcinomas. Proc Natl Acad Sci 1987;84:7701.
33. Hill BT, Deuchars K, Hosking LK, Ling V, Whelan RDH. Overexpression of P-glycoprotein in mammalian tumor cell lines after fractionated X irradiation in vitro. JNCI 1990;82:607.
34. Mickley LA, Bates SE, Richert ND, et al. Modulation of the expression of a multidrug resistance gene (mdr1/P-glycoprotein) by differentiating agents. J Biol Chem 1989;264:18031.
35. Ma DD, Scurr RD, Davey RA, Mackertich SM, Dowden G, Bell DR. Detection of a multidrug resistant phenotype in acute non-lymphoblastic leukaemia. Lancet 1987;1(8525):135.
36. Rothenberg ML, Mickley LA, Cole DE, et al. Expression of the mdr1 gene/P-170 gene in patients with acute lymphoblastic leukemia. Blood 1989;74:1388.
37. Sato H, Gottesman MM, Goldstein LJ, et al. Expression of the multidrug reistance gene in myeloid leukemias. Leuk Res 1990;14:11.
38. Holmes JA, Jacobs A, Carter G, Whittaker JA, Bentley DP, Padua RA. Is the mdr 1 gene relevant in chronic lymphocytic leukemia? Leukemia 1990;4:216.
39. Kuwazuru Y, Yoshimura A, Hanada S, et al. Expression of the multidrug transporter, P-glycoprotein, in chronic myelogenous leukemia in blast crisis. Br J Haematol 1990;74:24.
40. Marie J, Zittoun R, Sikic B. Multidrug resistance (*MDR1*) gene expression in adult acute leukemias: Correlations with treatment outcome and in vitro drug sensitivity. Blood 1991;78:586.
41. Bell DR, Gerlach JH, Kartner N, Buick RN, Ling V. Detection of P-glycoprotein in ovarian cancer: A molecular marker associated with multidrug resistance. J Clin Oncol 1985;3:311.
42. Schneider J, Efferth T, Kaufmann M, et al. Expression of the multidrug-resistance gene product P-glycoprotein in gynecological tumors. Cancer J 1990;3:202.
43. Dalton WS, Grogan TM, Rybski JA, et al. Immunohistochemical detection and quantitation of P-glycoprotein in multiple drug-resistant human myeloma cells: Association with level of drug resistance and drug accumulation. Blood 1989;73:747.
44. Keith WN, Stallard S, Brown R. Expression of mdr1 and GST π in human breast tumors: Comparison to in vitro sensitivity. Br J Cancer 1990;61:712.
45. Schneider J, Bak M, Efferth TH, Kaufmann M, Mattren J, Volm M. P-glycoprotein expression in treated and untreated breast cancer. Br J Cancer 1989;60:815.
46. Goldstein LJ, Fojo AT, Ueda K, et al. Expression of the multidrug resistant, MDR1, gene in neuroblastoma. J Clin Oncol 1990;8:128.
47. Chan HSL, Thorner PS, Haddad G, Ling V. Immunohistochemical detection of P-glycoprotein: Prognostic correlation in soft tissue sarcoma of childhood. J Clin Oncol 1990;8:689.
48. Mickisch G, Bier H, Bergler W, Bak M, Tschada R, Alken P. P-170 glycoprotein, glutathione and associated enzymes in relation to chemoresistance of primary human renal cell carcinomas. Urol Int 1990;45:170.
49. Riou GF, Zhou D, Ahomadegbe J, Gabillot M, Duvillard P, Lhomme C. Expression of multidrug resistance (MDR1) gene in normal epithelia and in invasive carcinomas of the uterine cervix. JNCI 1990;82:149.
50. Goldstein LJ, Galski H, Fojo A, et al. Expression of a multidrug resistance gene in human cancers. JNCI 1989;81:116.
51. Chan HSL, Haddad G, Thorner PS, et al. P-glycoprotein expression as a predictor of the outcome of therapy for neuroblastoma N Engl J Med 1991;325:1608.
52. Chen Y-N, Mickley LA, Schwartz AM, Acton EM, Hwang J, Fojo AT. Characterization of adriamycin-resistant human breast cancer cells which display overexpression of a novel resistance-related membrane protein. J Biol Chem 1990;265:10073.
53. Marquardt D, McCrone S, Center MS. Mechanisms of multidrug resistance in HL60 cells: Detection of resistance-associated proteins with antibodies against synthetic peptides that correspond to the deduced sequences of P-glycoprotein. Cancer Res 1990;50:1426.
54. Marsh W, Center M. Adriamycin resistance in HL60 cells and accompanying modification of a surface membrane protein contained in drug-sensitive cells. Cancer Res 1987;47:5080.
55. McGrath T, Latoud C, Arnold ST, Safa AR, Felsted RL, Center MS. Mechanisms of multidrug resistance in HL60 cells: Analysis of resistance associated membrane proteins and levels of mdr gene expression. Biochem Pharmacol 1989;38:3611.
56. Ohtsu T, Ishida Y, Tobinai K, et al. A novel multidrug resistance in cultured leukemia and lymphoma cells detected by a monoclonal antibody to 85kDa protein, MRK20. Jpn J Cancer Res 1989;80:1133.
57. Liu L. DNA topoisomerase poisons as antitumor drugs. Annu Rev Biochem 1989;58:351.
58. Fernandez DJ, Catapano CV. Nuclear matrix targets for anticancer agents. Cancer Cells 1991;3:134.
59. Glisson BS. Multidrug resistance mediated through alterations in topoisomerase II. Cancer Bull 1989;41:37.
60. Gupta RS. Genetic, biochemical, and cross-resistance studies with mutants of Chinese hamster ovary cells resistant to anticancer drugs, VM-26 and VP-16-213. Cancer Res 1983;43:1568.
61. Per S-R, Mattern MR, Mirabelli CK, Drake FH, Johnson RK, Crooke ST. Characterization of a subline of P388 leukemia resistant to amsacrine: Evidence of altered topoisomerase II function. Mol Pharmacol 1987;32:17.
62. Zwelling LA, Hinds M, Chan D, et al. Characterization of an amsacrine-resistant line of human leukemia cells: Evidence for a drug-resistant form of topoisomerase II. J Biol Chem 1989;264:16411.
63. Hinds M, Deisseroth K, Mayes J, et al. Identification of a point mutation in the topoisomerase II gene from a human leukemia cell line containing an amsacrine-resistant form of topoisomerase II. Cancer Res 1991;51:4729.
64. Buggs BY, Danks MK, Beck WT, Suttle DP. Expression of a mutant topoisomerase II in CCRF-CEM human leukemia cells selected for resistance to teniposide. Proc Natl Acad Sci USA 1991;7654.
65. Fernandez DJ, Danks MK, Beck WT. Decreased nuclear matrix DNA topoisomerase II in human leukemia cells resistant to VM-26 and m-AMSA. Biochemistry 1990;29:4235.
66. Tanizawa A, Pommier Y. Topoisomerase I alteration in a camptothecin-resistant cell line derived from Chinese hamster DC3F cells in culture. Cancer Res 1992;52:1848–1854.
67. Farber E. Cellular biochemistry of the stepwise development of cancer with chemicals. Cancer Res 1984;44:5463.
68. Fairchild CR, Ivy SP, Kao-Shaw C-S, et al. Isolation of amplified and overexpressed DNA sequences from adriamycin-resistant human breast cancer cells. Cancer Res 1987;47:5141.
69. Mannervik B, Danielson UH. Glutathione transferases-structure and catalytic activity. Crit Rev Biochem 1988;23:283.
70. Nakagawa K, Saijo N, Tsuchida S, et al. Glutathione S-transferase π as a determinant of drug resistance in transfectant cell lines. J Biol Chem 1990;265:4296.
71. Puchalski RB, Fahl WE. Expression of recombinant glutathione S-transferase π, Ya or Yb1 confers resistance to alkylating agents. Proc Natl Acad Sci USA 1990;87:2443.
72. Townsend AJ, Tu CP, Cowan KH. Expression of human mu or alpha class glutathione S-transferases in stably transfected human MCF-7 breast cancer cells: Effect on cellular sensitivity to cytotoxic agents. Mol Pharmacol 1992;41:230.
73. Tsuruo T, Iida H, Yamashiro M, Tsukagoshi S, Sakurai Y. Enhancement of vincristine- and adriamycin-induced cytoxicity by verapamil in P388 leukomia and its sublines resistant to vincristine and adriamycin. Biochem Pharmacol 1982;31:3138.
74. Akiyama S, Shiraishi N, Kuratomi Y, Nakagawa M, Kuwano M. Circumvention of multidrug resistance in P388 murine leukemia and its circumvention by calcium antagonists. Cancer Res 1985;45:1687.

75. Stewart DJ, Evans WK. Non-chemotherapeutic agents that potentiate chemotherapy efficacy. Cancer Treat Rev 1989;16:1.

76. Bessho F, Kinumaki H, Kobayashi M, et al. Treatment of children with refractory acute lymphocytic leukemia with vincristine and diltiazen. Med Pediatr Oncol 1985;13:199.

77. Presant CA, Kennedy PS, Wiseman C, et al. Verapamil reversal of clinical doxorubicin resistance in human cancer: A Wilshire Oncology Medical Group pilot phase I-II study. Am J Clin Oncol 1986;9:355.

78. Cairo MS, Siegel S, Arias N, Sender L. Clinical trial of continuous infusion verapamil, bolus vinblastine and continuous infusion VP-16 in drug-resistant pediatric tumors. Cancer Res 1989;49:1063.

79. Ozols RF, Cunnion RE, Klecker RW, et al. Verapamil and adriamycin in the treatment of drug-resistant ovarian cancer patients. J Clin Oncol 1987;5:641.

80. Miller RL, Bukowski RM, Budd GT, et al. Clinical modulation of deoxorubicine resistance by the caluodulin-inhibitor trifluperazine: A phase I/II trial. J Clin Oncol 1988;6:880.

81. Dalton WS, Grogan TM, Meltzer PS, et al. Drug resistance in multiple myloma and non-Hodgkin's lymphoma: Detection of P-glycoprotein and potential circumvention by addition of verapamil to chemotherapy. J Clin Oncol 1989;7:415.

82. Miller TP, Grogan TM, Dalton WS, et al. P-glycoprotein expression in malignant lymphoma and reversal of clinical drug resistance with chemotherapy plus high-dose verapamil. J Clin Oncol 1991;9:17–24.

83. Coley HM, Twentyman PR, Workman P. Improved cellular accumulation is characteristic of anthracyclines which retain high activity in multidrug resistant cell lines alone or in combination with verapamil or cyclosporin A. Biochem Pharmacol 1989;38:4467.

84. Hu XF, Martin TJ, Bell DR, Luise M, Zalcberg JR. Combined use of cyclosporin A and verapamil in modulating multidrug resistance in human leukemia cell lines. Cancer Res 1990;50:2953.

85. Nooter K, Sonneveld P, Oostrum R, Herweijer H, Hagenbeek T, Valerio D. Overexpression of the mdr1 gene in blast cells from patients with acute myelocytic leukemia is associated with decreased anthracycline accumulation that can be restored by cyclosporin-A. Int J Cancer 1990;45:263.

86. Sonneveld P, Nooter K. Reversal of drug-resistance by cyclosporin-A in a patient with acute myelocytic leukemia. Br J Haematol 1990;75:208.

87. Aihara M, Aihara Y, Schmidt-Wolf G, et al. A combined approach for purging multidrug-resistant leukemia cell lines in bone marrow using a monoclonal antibody and chemotherapy. Blood 1991;77:2079.

88. Fitzgerald DJ, Willingham MC, Cardarelli CO, et al. Monoclonal antibody-*Pseudomonas* toxin conjugate that specifically kills multidrug-resistant cells. Proc Natl Acad Sci USA 1987;84:4288.

89. Tong AW, Lee J Wang RM, Dalton WS, Tsuruo T Fay JW, Stone MJ. Elimination of chemoresistant multiple myloma clonogenic colony-forming cells by combined treatment with a plasma cell-reactive monoclonal antibody and a P-glycoprotein-reactive monoclonal antibody. Cancer Res 1989;49:4829.

90. Pearson JW, Fogler WE, Volker K, et al. Reversal of drug resistance in human colon cancer xenograft expressing *MDR1* complementary DNA by in vivo administration of MRK-11 monoclonal antibody. JNCI 1991;83:1386–1391.

91. Baguley BC, Holdaway KM, Fray LM. Design of DNA intercalators to overcome topoisomerase II-mediated multidrug resistance. JNCI 1990;82:398.

92. Myers CE, Mimnaugh E, Yeh G, Sinha BK. Biochemical mechanisms of tumor cell kill by the anthracyclines. In: Lown JW, ed. Anthracyclines and anthracenedione-based anticancer agents. Amsterdam: Elsevier, 1988:527–569.

93. Sinha BK. Free radicals in anticancer drug pharmacology. Chem Biol Interact 1989;69:293.

94. Sinha BK, Katki AG, Batist G, Cowan KH, Myers CE. Differential formation of hydroxy radicals by adriamycin in sensitive and resistant MCF-7 human breast cancer tumor cells: Implications for the mechanism of action. Biochemistry 1987;26:3776.

95. Dusre L, Mimnaugh EG, Myers CE, Sinha BK. Potentiation of doxorubicin cytoxicity by butathionine sulfoximine in multidrug-resistant human breast cancer cells. Cancer Res 1989;49:511.

96. Keizer HG, Rijn J, Pinedo HM, Joenje H. Effect of endogenous glutathione, superoxide dismutase, catalase, and glutathione peroxidase on adriamycin tolerance of Chinese hamster ovary cells. Cancer Res 1988;48:4493.

97. Townsend AJ, Morrow CS, Sinha BK, Cowan KH. Selenium-dependent glutathione peroxidase expression is inversely related to estrogen receptor content of human breast cancer cells. Cancer Comm 1991;3:265.

98. Alin P, Danielson UH, Mannervick B. 4-Hydroxyalk-2-enals are substrates for glutathione transferases. FEBS Lett 1985;179:267.

99. Tew KD, Bomber AW, Hoffman SJ. Ethracrynic acid and piriprost as enhancers of cytotoxicity in drug resistant cell lines. Cancer Res 1988;48:3622.

100. Lazo JS, Basu A. Metallothionein expression and transient resistance to electrophilic antineoplastic drugs. Cancer Biol 1991;2:267.

101. Buller AL, Clapper ML, Tew KD. Glutathione S-transferases in nitrogen mustard-resistant and -sensitive cell lines. Mol Pharmacol 1987;31:575.

102. Lewis AD, Hickson ID, Robson CN, et al. Amplication and increased expression of alpha class glutathione S-transferase-encoding genes associated with resistance to nitrogen mustards. Proc Natl Acad Sci USA 1988;85:8511.

103. Wolf CR, Hayward IP, Lawrie SS, et al. Cellular heterogeneity and drug resistance in two ovarian adenocarcinoma cell lines derived from a single patient. Int J Cancer 1987;39:695.

104. Hamilton TC, Ozols RF, Dabrow MB. Multidrug resistance to alkylating agents and platinum compounds: State of our knowledge. Oncology 1990;4:101.

105. Miyazaki M, Kohno K, Saburi Y, et al. Drug resistance to cisdiammine dichloroplatinum (II) in Chinese hamster ovary cell lines tranfected with glutathione S-transferase pi gene. Biochem Biophys Res Comm 1990;166:1358.

106. Ozols RF, O'Dwyer PJ, Hamilton TC, Young RC. The role of glutathione in drug resistance Cancer Treat Rev 1990;17(Suppl. A):45.

107. Colvin M, Russo JE, Hilton J, Dulik DM, Fenselau C. Enzymatic mechanisms of resistance to alkylating agents in tumor cells and normal tissues. Adv Enzyme Regul 1988;27:211.

108. Kastan MB, Schlaffer E, Russo JE, Colvin OM, Civin CI, Hilton J. Direct demonstration of elevated aldehyde dehydrogenase in human hematopoietic progenitor cells. Blood 1990;1947:1947.

109. Maki PA, Sladek NE. Potentiation of the cytotoxic action of mafosfamide by N-isopropyl-p-formylbenzamide, a metabolite of procarbazine. Cancer Res 1991;51:4170.

110. Dolan ME, Moschel RC, Pegg AE. Depletion of mammalian O6-alkylguanine-DNA alkyltransferase activity by O^6-benzylguanine provides a means to evaluate the role of this protein in protection against carcinogenic and therapeutic alkylating agents. Proc Natl Acad Sci USA 1990;87:5368.

111. D'Incalci M, Taverna P, Erba E, et al. O6-Methylguanine and temozolomide can reverse the resistance to chloroethylnitrosoureas of a mouse L1210 leukemia. Anticancer Res 1991;11:115.

112. Masuda H, Ozols RF, Gi-Ming L, Fojo A, Rothenberg M, Hamilton TC. Increased DNA repair as a mechanism of acquired resistance to *cis*-diamminedichloroplatinum (II) in human ovarian cancer cell lines. Cancer Res 1988;5313.

113. Sheibani N, Jennerwein MM, Eastman A. DNA repair in cells sensitive and resistant to *cis*-diamine dichloroplatinum (II): Host cell reactivation of damaged plasmid DNA. Biochemistry 1989;28:3120.

114. Curt GA, Allegra CJ. Methotrexate resistance: Mechanisms and implications. In: Kessel D, ed. Resistance to antineoplastic drugs. Boca Raton: CRC Press, 1989:369.

115. Curt GA, Carney DN, Cowan KH, et al. Unstable methotrexate resistance in human small cell carcinoma associated with double minute chromosomes. N Engl J Med 1983;308:199.

116. Ackland SP, Schilsky RL. High-dose methotrexate: A critical reappraisal. J Clin Oncol 1987;5:2017.

117. Lin JT, Bertino JR. Update on trimetrexate, a folate antagonist withantineoplastic and antiprotozoal properties. Cancer Invest 1991;9:159.

118. Assaraf YG, Molina A, Schinke RT. Cross-resistance to the lipid soluble antifolate trimetrexate in human carcinoma cells with the multidrug-resistant phenotype. JNCI 1989;81:290.

119. Bapat AR, Zarow C, Danenberg PV. Human leukemic cells resistant to FdUrd contain a thymidylate synthase with lower affinity for nucleotides. J Biol Chem 1983;258:4130.

120. Jenh CH, Geyer PK, Baskin F, Johnson LF. Thymidylate synthase gene amplification in fluorodeoxyuridine-resistant mouse cell lines. Mol Pharmacol 1985;28:80.

121. Calabro-Jones PM, Byfield JE, Ward JF, Sharp TR. Time-dose relationship for 5-fluorouracil toxicity against human epithelial cancer cells in vivo. Cancer Res 1982;42:4413.

122. Grem JL, Hoth OF, Hamilton JM, King SA, Leyland-Jones B. Overview of current status and future direction of clinical trials with 5-fluorouricil in combination with folinic acid. Cancer Treat Rep 1987;71:1249.

123. Cadman E, Heimer R, Davis L. The influence of methotrexate pretreatment on 5-fluorouicil metabolism in L1210 cells. J Biol Chem 1981;256:1695.

124. Grem JL, King SA, Leyland-Jones B. Biochemistry and clinical activity of N-(phosphonacetyl)-L-aspartate: A review. Cancer Res 1988;48:4441.

125. Montparler RL, Onetto-Pothier N. Drug resistance to cytosine arabinoside. In: Kessel D, ed. Resistance to antineoplastic drugs. Boca Raton: CRC Press, 1989:353.

MICHAEL J. HAWKINS

SECTION 3

Investigational Agents

Investigational agents play an integral role in the management of many cancer patients, especially in diseases that are resistant to standard agents. Extensive clinical research programs have been established worldwide, with most new agents emerging from the United States, Europe, and Japan. A comprehensive review of all the investigational agents currently being studied by pharmaceutical companies and governmental agencies in these countries is beyond the scope of this chapter. However, the agents currently in phases I and II clinical trials sponsored by the National Cancer Institute (NCI) serve as a representative sample and are summarized in Tables 18–7 and 18–8. Investigational agents for which clinical efficacy has been established are placed in a group C category pending commercial availability and may be obtained from the NCI for their respective indications (Table 18–9).) This section provides a more detailed discussion of agents that have shown promising clinical antitumor activity, because they may be more widely available in the future.

AMSACRINE

Amsacrine (*N*-[4-(9-acridinylamino)-3-methoxyphenyl]-methanesulfonamide, mAMSA), a 9-anilino derivative of the DNA binding dye acridine (Fig. 18–5), was synthesized by Bruce Cain and colleagues in New Zealand in 1974 and was found to have potent clinical activity against human acute nonlymphocytic leukemia.[1] It is particularly valuable because of its synergy with cytarabine, its activity in anthracycline-resistant patients, and its lower incidence of cardiotoxicity than with anthracyclines.[2] mAMSA was made available by the NCI under the group C guidelines in February 1982 for the treatment of ANLL (Table 18–9).

MECHANISM OF ACTION

Like other acridine dyes, mAMSA intercalates between strands of DNA and produces single- and double-strand breaks in DNA. Its cytotoxicity correlates closely with the formation of these breaks.[3] The DNA-cleaving enzyme topoisomerase II has been implicated in the action of the drug, in that the enzyme forms a tight complex with mAMSA and DNA. Although the normal action of topoisomerase II is to break and reseal DNA at points of torsion, resealing of breaks does not take place in the presence of mAMSA, and the protein remains bound to the free 5′ ends of the broken DNA strand.[4] mAMSA-induced strand breaks occur preferentially at specific base sequences in DNA; these sequences differ from the sites of preferential cleavage by etoposide and anthracyclines and may explain differences in tumor cell sensitivity to the various topoisomerase inhibitors.[5]

mAMSA-induced strand breakage and cytotoxicity are greatest during the S phase of the cell cycle, when topoisomerase levels within the cell increase to a maximum level.[6] Slowly dividing cells, such as fibroblasts and cells at confluence, are less sensitive to the drug. Cells selected for resistance to amsacrine have exhibited decreased levels of topoisomerase II and increased levels of glutathione S transferase, mutation

TABLE 18–7. Agents Currently in Phase I Clinical Trial

Agent	Mechanism of Action	Toxicities*
2-Chlorodeoxyadenosine	Antimetabolite	Renal and neurotoxicity, myelosuppression
Cyclopentenylcytosine	Antimetabolite	Myelosuppression
Chloroquinoxaline sulfonamide	Unknown	Rodents: neurotoxicity; Dogs: gastrointestinal; Humans: cardiotoxicity, hypoglycemia
ICI D1694	Inhibition of thymidilate synthetase	Myelosuppression, gastrointestinal
Fostriecin	Inhibition of DNA and RNA	Rodents: gastrointestinal and renal
		Dogs: gastrotintestinal and cardiovascular
Hepsulfam	Alkylator	Myelosuppression
Ipomeanol	Prodrug, metabolized to active form in the lung	Lung damage, particularly Clara cells
Mafosfamide	Alkylator	Animals: myelosuppression
		Humans: phlebitis, mucosal membrane irritation
Ormaplatin	DNA adduct formation	Gastrointestinal, myelosuppression
Pentosan	? Inhibition of growth factors	Anticoagulation, thrombocytopenia
Pyrazine diazohydroxide	DNA adduct formation	Myelosuppression, gastrointestinal
Pyrazoloacridine	Inhibition of DNA and RNA synthesis	Bolus I.V. administration: neurotoxicity
		Continuous I.V. administration: myelosuppression
Suramin	? Inhibition of growth factors	Coagulopathy, neurotoxicity, adrenal insufficiency, renal toxicity
Terephthalamidine	Unknown	Ocular toxicity, neurotoxicity
trans-Retinoic acid	Differentiator	Human: mucocutaneous and neurotoxicity

* Human unless otherwise noted.
I.V., intravenous.

TABLE 18–8. Agents Currently in Phase II Clinical Trial

Agent	Mechanism of Action	Received Phase II Dose (mg/m²)	Dose-Limiting Toxicities
Caracemide	Inhibition of DNA synthesis	550/d × 5, CIV	Neurotoxicity
Deoxyspergualin	Inhibition of polyamine synthesis	1800/d × 5, CIV	Hypotension
Didemnin-B	Inhibition of protein synthesis	6.3 q 4 wk	Myopathy, anaphylaxis
Echinomycin	DNA intercalation and inhibition of RNA synthesis	1.5 q 4 wk 1.2 q wk × 4	Nausea and vomiting (both schedules)
Edatrexate	Antifol	80 q wk	Oral mucositis
Fazarabine	Antimetabolite	48/d × 3, CIV 30/d × 5, bolus	Neutropenia (both schedules)
Hexamethylene bisacetamide	Differentiator	20 g/m²/d × 10, CIV 1–2 mmol Css, 5 d CIV	Thrombocytopenia, neurotoxicity
Homoharringtonine	Inhibition of protein synthesis	4/d × 5, CIV	Myelosuppression, hypotension (bolus administration)
Merbarone	Inhibition of topoisomerase II	1000/d × 5, CIV	Nephrotoxicity, phlebitis
Piroxantrone	Intercalator	150 q 3 wk	Leukopenia
Taxol	Tubulin active agent (stabilizer)	250/d, CIV	Leukopenia, neurotoxicity
Tiazofurin	Antimetabolite	800/d × 5, bolus	Neurotoxicity, myelosuppression
Topotecan	Inhibition of topoisomerase I	1.5–2/d × 5, bolus (solid tumors)	Neutropenia

CIV, continuous intravenous infusion; Css, concentration at steady state.

of the topoisomerase II gene, or alterations in the functional capacity of the topoisomerase II enzyme.[7,8] Other agents, such as etoposide and various anthracycline derivatives, that also cleave DNA through activation of topoisomerase II share cross-resistance with mAMSA in some mAMSA-resistant cell lines.[9] Although verapamil, a calcium channel blocker that reverses MDR, has been reported to enhance sensitivity to mAMSA in some cell lines, structural alterations of the topoisomerase II enzyme appear to represent the major mechanism of resistance to mAMSA.[10] Coincubation of cell lines with a topoisomerase I inhibitor, such as topotecan, antagonized the cytotoxicity of mAMSA and other topoisomerase II active agents.[11]

CLINICAL PHARMACOLOGY AND PHARMACOKINETICS

mAMSA is administered intravenously in doses of 100 to 150 mg/m² per day for 5 days. It is concentrated in the liver, where

TABLE 18–9. Agents Currently in the National Cancer Institute's Group C Category

Agent	Indication
5-Azacytidine	Refractory adult acute myelogenous leukemia (single-agent therapy)
Amsacrine (mAMSA)	Refractory adult acute myelogenous leukemia (single-agent therapy)
Erwinia asparaginase	Acute lymphocytic leukemia patients who are allergic to *Escherichia coli* L-asparaginase
Teniposide	First relapse or refractory acute lymphocytic leukemia Combination therapy with cytarabine

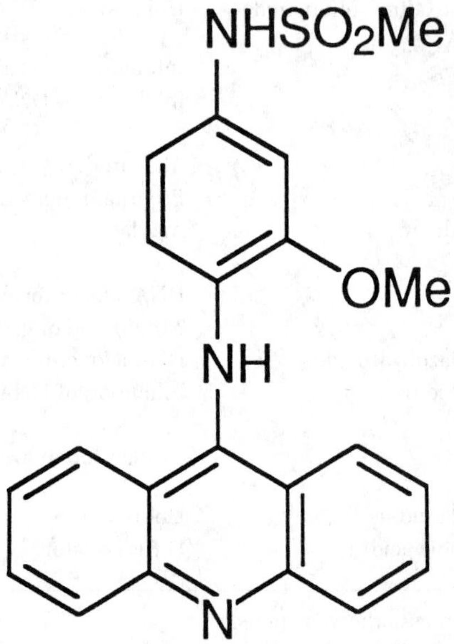

it undergoes conjugation to glutathione and excretion in bile.[12] Its primary plasma half-life is 7.4 hours, but the half-life is prolonged to 17 hours in patients with hepatic dysfunction, leading to recommendation of a 40% dose reduction in patients with serum bilirubin greater than 2 mg/100 ml. Less than 20% of drug is excreted unchanged in urine, and the need to reduce the dose in patients with renal failure is uncertain.[13] mAMSA is highly protein-bound in human plasma, with less than 5% of the drug in its free state in the therapeutic range of 1 to 100 μM.[14] Its ability to penetrate the blood–brain barrier is probably limited by this high degree of protein binding.

FIGURE 18–5. Amsacrine.

TOXICITY

The dose-limiting toxicities of mAMSA are pancytopenia, stomatitis, and mucositis.[15] Hepatotoxicity (which may delay excretion of mAMSA), nausea, vomiting, diarrhea, and alopecia are also common side effects.[16] Cardiotoxic events occur in 2% of patients receiving mAMSA, although many of these patients had previously received anthracyclines, and some were hypokalemic. Acute cardiac effects of mAMSA, occurring during or shortly after the infusion, may include prolongation in the QT interval, atrial and ventricular arrhythmias, and, rarely, acute heart failure. Toxicity may occur with the first dose of mAMSA and in the absence of prior cardiac disease or exposure to anthracyclines. Because of the frequent occurrence of QT prolongation with mAMSA therapy and the possibility that mAMSA may induce hypokalemia, treatment should not begin unless the serum potassium level is normal. With careful monitoring, mAMSA has been given safely to patients with preexisting heart disease.[17]

mAMSA is formulated in anhydrous *N,N*-dimethylacetamide, and contact of the undiluted solution with plastic should be avoided. Amsacrine is provided with a separate vial of L-lactic acid diluent. Although the combined orange-red solution is stable at room temperature and in ambient light for at least 48 hours, the reconstituted material is not bacteriostatic and should therefore be used within 8 hours of preparation. In preparing an intravenous injection of mAMSA, the drug should be diluted in dextrose and water rather than in saline, because the hydrochloride salt of mAMSA is poorly water soluble and may precipitate.[18]

TOPOISOMERASE I INHIBITORS

Camptothecin, a heterocyclic alkaloid, and its analogs are the only inhibitors of topoisomerase I possessing known antitumor activity (Fig. 18–6). Camptothecin was first isolated in 1966 from the stem wood of the *Camptotheca acuminata,* a tree native to northern China.[19] Based on the activity of the parent compound against the L1210 murine leukemia, the rat Walker's carcinosarcoma and tumors resistant to other chemotherapeutic agents, the sodium salt of camptothecin entered clinical trials in 1971.[19–21] It was later discovered that the sodium salt was inactive and all observed cytotoxicity resided in the intact lactone that formed slowly at neutral pH but at much higher rates in an acid environment. Although antitumor responses were observed in some patients, additional investigation of this agent ceased because of severe, unacceptable bladder toxicity that resulted from the formation of the cytotoxic lactone in acid urine.

Structure-activity relations for camptothecin have been elucidated subsequently.[22] Topoisomerase I inhibition and antitumor activity of the camptothecin molecule are lost when specific changes are made in the lactone ring (S to R stereoisomerization or other modifications of position 20; replacement of the 21-lactone by a lactam) or in the A-ring (addition of methoxy groups simultaneously to positions 10 and 11 or addition of an amino or nitro group to position 12). Topoisomerase I inhibition and antitumor potency increase with the addition of a methylenedioxy bridge at positions 10 and 11, an amino group at position 9, or a hydroxy group at position 10. Thus, the spatial region around position 12 is critical for activity, whereas selective substitutions at positions 9 or 10 can actually enhance potency.

Identification of these relations has led to the clinical development of a number of camptothecin analogs with greater solubility and improved therapeutic indices in preclinical models.[23] Topotecan (NSC 609699) incorporates a stable basic (dimethylamino)methyl side chain at the 9 position and a hydroxy group at the 10 position. CPT-11 (7-ethyl-10-[4-(1-piperidino)-1-piperidino] carbonyloxycamptothecin) was initially developed in Japan and has recently entered clinical trial in the United States. CPT-11 is converted in vivo to a major metabolite SN-38 (7-ethyl-10-hydroxycamptothecin),

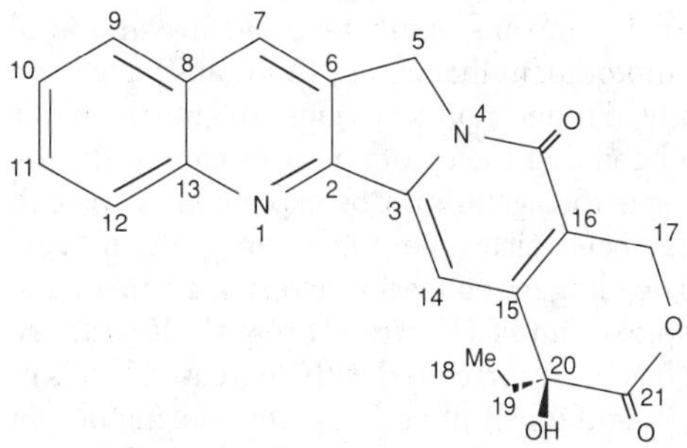

20(S) - camptothecin basic ring structure

Substitutions:

Compounds	Position		
	7	9	10
9-amino camptothecin	H	-NH$_2$	H
Topotecan	H	-CH$_2$-N(CH$_3$)(CH$_3$)	-OH
CPT-11	-CH$_2$-CH$_3$	H	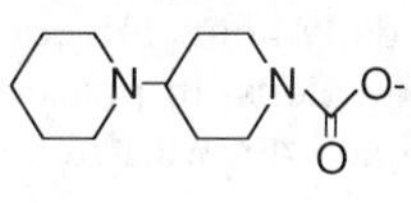 (piperidino-piperidino carbonyloxy)

FIGURE 18–6.   Camptothecin analogs.

which is approximately 100 times more potent than CPT-11 against tumor cell lines in vitro.[24-26] Based on data suggesting that less soluble analogs may be more active against cells expressing the MDR1 phenotype, two other camptothecin analogs (9-aminocamptothecin and 9-nitrocamptothecin) are in earlier stages of development. 9-Aminocamptothecin, 20(S)-camptothecin, and 10,11 methylenedioxy camptothecin have produced striking effects against human solid tumor xerografts in nude mice.[27]

MECHANISM OF ACTION

DNA topoisomerase I is the unique target for camptothecins.[28] Topoisomerase I transiently breaks a single strand of DNA, thereby reducing torsional strain and unwinding DNA ahead of the replication fork. Although eukaryotic cells lines lacking topoisomerase I may survive in culture, the enzyme has important roles in chromatin organization, in mitosis, and in DNA replication, recombination, and transcription. Human DNA topoisomerase I binds to its nucleic acid substrate noncovalently. The bound enzyme then creates a transient break in one DNA strand and concomitantly binds covalently to the 3'-phosphoryl end of the broken DNA strand. Topoisomerase I then allows passage of the unbroken DNA strand through the break site and religates the cleaved DNA. This reaction does not require an energy cofactor, because the binding of topoisomerase I with DNA occurs by way of a tyrosyl-phosphate bond that is released when the strand is religated. The intermediate, covalently bound enzyme-DNA complex is called a *cleavable complex,* because protein-linked single-strand DNA breaks can be detected when the reaction is aborted with a strong protein denaturant. The cleavable complex is in equilibrium with the noncovalently bound complex (*noncleavable complex*), which does not result in single-strand DNA breaks when exposed to denaturing conditions.

Although noncleavable complexes of topoisomerase I and DNA are the dominant form in normal circumstances, camptothecin shifts the equilibrium toward a cleavable ternary complex. The effect of camptothecin on the cleavable complex and the shift in equilibrium are rapidly reversed on withdrawal of the drug.[29] Camptothecin-induced DNA breaks have been detected frequently at replication forks close to growth points. It has been postulated that the cytotoxicity of camptothecin, a highly S-phase specific agent, may be explained by the collision of drug-stabilized cleavable complexes with moving replication forks, leading to replication arrest and conversion of cleavable complexes into DNA strand breaks.[30] Resistance to camptothecin has been correlated with decreased levels of topoisomerase I in some cell lines.[31] Camptothecins do not appear to be affected by classic P-170-mediated MDR.

CLINICAL PHARMACOLOGY AND PHARMACOKINETICS

A number of schedules of topotecan have been evaluated in phase I trials (Table 18–10). The maximum tolerated dose is highly schedule dependent. Patients tolerate less total drug when it is given in regimens that use continuous infusions or daily bolus injections compared with intermittent bolus injections. In phase I trials, responses have been observed in patients with non-small cell lung, ovarian, and esophageal

TABLE 18–10. Phase I Schedules Evaluated for Topotecan

Schedule	Recommended Cumulative Phase II Dose (mg/m^2 per Cycle)	Dose-Limiting Toxicities
30-min I.V. bolus × 1 q 28 d	17.5	Myelosuppression
30-min I.V. bolus × 5 q 21 d	7.5	Myelosuppression
24-h CIV q 21 d	12.5*	Myelosuppression
24-h CIV q 7 d × 3	6.0*	Myelosuppression
72-h CIV q 28 d	4.8*	Myelosuppression
120-h CIV q 28 d	3.4	Myelosuppression

* Highest dose achieved to date.
I.V., intravenous; CIV, continuous intravenous infusion.

cancer using daily administration of 0.5 to 1.5 mg/m^2 per day for 5 days, a regimen currently being tested in phase 2 (Table 18–8). Randomized trials will be conducted to compare the activity of other schedules of administration. Preliminary pharmacokinectic data for bolus administration have indicated median α and β half-lives of 9 and 103 minutes, respectively; total-body clearance of 2080 ml/min/m^2; and volume of distribution at steady state of 186 L/m^2.

Three regimens using bolus or short-duration infusions of CPT-11 have been studied extensively in clinical trials and do not differ markedly in the amount of drug that could be administered: 100 mg/m^2 weekly; 150 mg/m^2 every 2 weeks; and 200 mg/m^2 every 3 to 4 weeks. In contrast to the experience with topotecan, when CPT-11 is administered as a 120-hour continuous intravenous infusion, the maximum tolerated total dose is similar to that after bolus administration (150 mg/m^2).[32] In phase II trials, response rates in the range of 20% to 50% have been observed in ovarian cancer, colorectal carcinoma, small cell lung cancer, previously untreated non-small cell lung cancer, and non-Hodgkin's lymphoma.[33-36] CPT-11 pharmacokinetics are complex to interpret, because its major metabolite, SN-38, is more potent than the parent compound. After intravenous administration of 100 mg/m^2 over 30 minutes, the mean peak plasma levels of CPT-11 and SN-38 were 2566 and 43 ng/ml, respectively, and CPT-11 exhibited a triphasic plasma elimination pattern ($T_{1/2}$-α, -β, and -τ: 0.07, 2.2, and 18.2 hours, respectively).[37] When given by continuous infusion, the area under the plasma concentration versus time curve (AUC) for CPT-11 (but not SN-38) increased in a dose-dependent fashion, and there was less interpatient variation for the AUC of CPT-11 than for SN-38.[32] Preclinical models indicate that approximately 80% of CPT-11 and SN-38 are protein bound.[38] In preclinical models, approximately one third to one half of CPT-11 was excreted unchanged in the bile and urine, and SN-38 was found primarily in bile.[25]

As predicted by preclinical toxicology studies, reversible myelosuppression (predominantly neutropenia) has proved to be dose limiting for topotecan in phase I trials. Some patients develop elevation of serum hepatic transaminase and alkaline phosphatase levels. Alopecia and mild diarrhea have

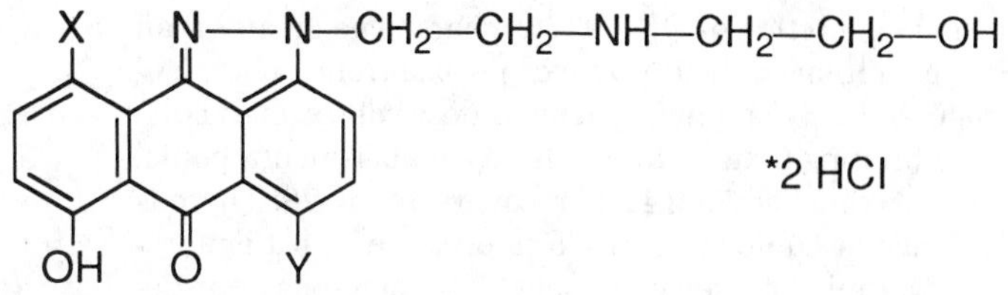

	X	Y
Piroxantrone	—OH	—NH—(CH$_2$)$_3$—NH$_2$
Biantrazole	—H	—NH—(CH$_2$)$_2$—NH (CH$_2$)$_2$OH
DUP 937	—OH	—NH—(CH$_2$)$_2$—NHCH$_3$

FIGURE 18–7. Structurally related anthrapyrazoles being studied in clinical trials.

also been reported. Leukopenia and diarrhea have been dose limiting for CPT-11 in essentially all trials reported to date.[32,33,35] In phase II trials of CPT-11 using bolus intravenous or short-duration infusions, leukopenia occurs more frequently than diarrhea,[32,33] whereas diarrhea becomes dose limiting when CPT-11 is given by continuous intravenous infusion for 5 days. Bladder toxicity, which was dose limiting for the sodium salt of camptothecin, has not been reported after administration of topotecan or CPT-11.

ANTHRAPYRAZOLES

The anthrapyrazoles are a series of 5-[(aminoalkyl)amino]-substituted anthra-[1,9-*cd*]pyrazol-6(2*H*)ones that were synthesized to develop DNA-binding agents with antitumor activity similar to that of the anthracyclines but with less cardiotoxicity.[39] In contrast with anthracenediones, such as mitoxantrone, the anthrapyrazoles incorporate a fourth ring into the chromophore nucleus (Fig. 18–7). Modifying the anthracenedione nucleus reduces the formation of semiquinone free radicals, a possible mechanism for anthracycline-induced cardiac toxicity. This series of agents is currently in early phase II clinical trials. One compound, biantrazole, has demonstrated considerable antitumor activity in doxorubicin-naive patients with breast cancer.

MECHANISM OF ACTION

The anthrapyrazoles intercalate DNA, cause protein-associated DNA single- and double-strand breaks, and relatively selectively inhibit DNA synthesis.[40] As a class, the anthrapyrazoles are highly effective in mice bearing P388 leukemia, L1210 leukemia, B16 melanoma, M5076 sarcoma, and MX-1 mammary xenograft.[41] However, 4 of 21 analogs tested were judged superior against mammary adenocarcinoma 16C, colon adenocarcinoma 11a, and the Ridgway osteogenic sarcoma, and three of these were then taken into clinical trial (Fig. 18–7). Although each agent produced at least six logs of net tumor cell kill against a parent P388 leukemia cell line, cell lines resistant to doxorubicin, mAMSA, and mitoxantrone were cross-resistant to the anthrapyrazoles, implicating topoisomerase II as their site of action. It is unclear whether the anthrapyrazoles are affected by MDR-type resistance.

CLINICAL PHARMACOLOGY, PHARMACOKINETICS, AND TOXICITY

The pharmacokinetics and recommended phase II doses for the three anthrapyrazole analogs studied in phase I trials are different (Table 18–11). Total body clearance and elimination half-life differ markedly for the three agents. In particular,

TABLE 18–11. Comparison of Pharmacokinetic Parameters of Three Anthrapyrazoles Currently in Clinical Trial

Drug	Elimination T$_{1/2}$	Total Body Clearance (ml/min/m^2)	Recommended Phase II Dose (mg/m^2)	Dose-Limiting Toxicity	Urinary Excretion (%)
Piroxantrone[42] NSC 349174 (DUP-942)	18±36 min	720±210	150 q 4 wk	Neutropenia	None detected
Piroxantrone[43]	30 min	1290	160 q 4 wk	Neutropenia	5
Biantrazole[44] NSC 357885 (DUP-941)	21±9 h	—	50 q 4 wk	Neutropenia	2–5
Biantrazole[45]	14±8 h	220	24 q wk	Neutropenia	12
NSC 374733[46] (DUP-937)	4.1 d	149±62	22 q 4 wk	Neutropenia	29

the urinary excretion of DUP-937 appears to be greater than urinary excretions of biantrazole or piroxantrone.

Although their maximum tolerated doses differ markedly, the dose-limiting toxicity for all three agents is neutropenia, which is maximal at day 14 and recovers by day 28. There is no evidence of cumulative myelosuppression in patients receiving multiple courses of therapy. The percentage of decrease in the leukocyte count correlates better with dose administered than with AUC. Other toxicities are mild and include nausea, vomiting, mucositis, diarrhea, lethargy, alopecia, and phlebitis (at the injection site). Transient elevations of the bilirubin have been reported after administration of DUP-937. There is no evidence of decreased cardiac ejection fraction after multiple courses of any anthrapyrazole, although the cumulative dose administered to most patients has been low. Cardiac arrhythmias have occurred in some patients receiving an anthrapyrazole, but the relation to treatment is not clear.

Biantrazole has demonstrated impressive antitumor activity in patients with breast cancer who had not previously received an anthracycline.[47] Of 30 patients treated, there were 18 partial and 1 complete responses (63% response rate), with a median response duration of 7 months. Studies with the other two agents in breast cancer are currently in progress.

RETINOIDS

The retinoids are a pharmacologic class of agents consisting of vitamin A (retinol) and its synthetic and naturally occurring analogs. Vitamin A has long been recognized as an essential fat-soluble substance necessary for normal growth, vision, and reproduction. In animals maintained on vitamin A-deficient diets, squamous epithelium undergoes metaplasia and neoplastic transformation. The retinoids appear to play a central role in the control of differentiation and proliferation,[48] perhaps through stimulation of a tumor growth factor-β autocrine loop. Excellent reviews summarize the extensive data on the role of retinoids as differentiating agents and their use in the treatment and the prevention of cancer.[49–51]

Despite promising results in animal models of tumor differentiation and inhibition of carcinogenesis, clinical trials using retinoids in the treatment of advanced malignant disease have generally yielded negative results.[51] However, recent results indicate significant clinical activity of retinoids in the treatment and the prevention of cancer. Patients with acute promyelocytic leukemia (APLL) achieve differentiation-induced complete remissions after treatment with all-*trans*-retinoic acid (tRA).[52,53] Patients with a history of successfully treated head and neck cancers have a reduced incidence of second malignancies when treated prophylatically with *cis*-retinoic acid (cRA).[54] A phase II trial of cRA and interferon-α in squamous cell carcinoma of the skin reported overall and complete response rates of 73% and 27%, respectively.[55] Similar results with this combination have been observed in cervical carcinoma.[56]

The basic structure of the retinoids consists of a cyclic endgroup, a polyene side chain, and a polar end group (Fig. 18–8). Because the initial attempts to administer pharmacologic doses of retinoids resulted in hepatotoxicity, modifications to the polar end group were pursued to create retinoids

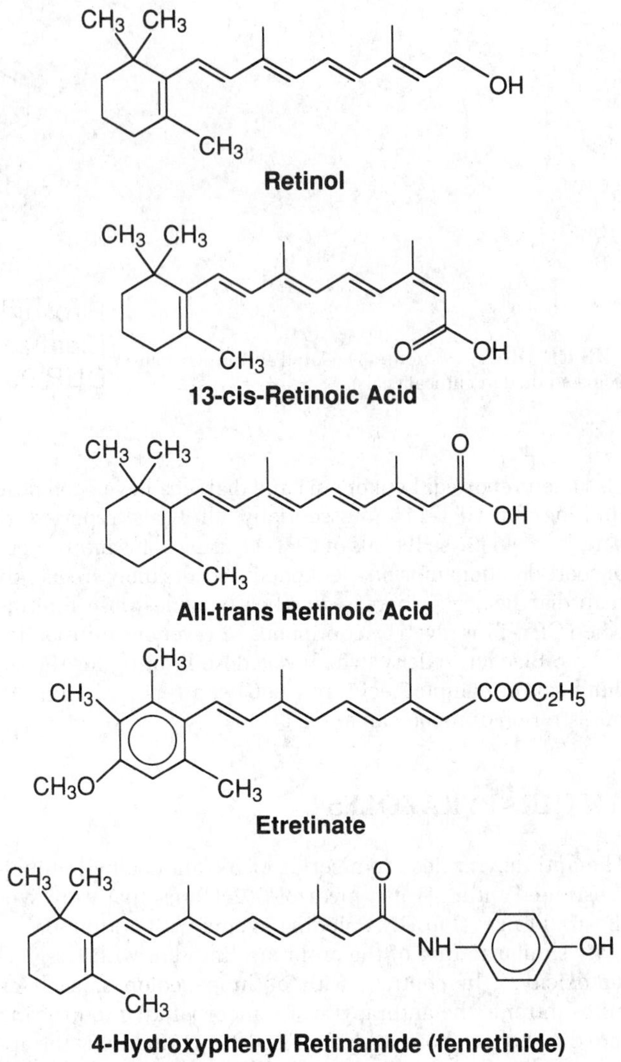

FIGURE 18–8. Commercially available and investigational retinoids.

that would not accumulate in the liver. Subsequent modifications of the retinol molecule have included aromatization of the cyclic end group (aromatic retinoids, *e.g.*, etretinate) and cyclization of the polyene side chain (arotinoids). The greatest clinical experience in the United States has been with cRA (Fig. 18–8), which is commercially available for the treatment of severe acne (Accutane). Because initial studies suggested a low therapeutic index for tRA, this agent has been administered primarily by the topical route. Etretinate (Tegison) is commercially available in the United States for the treatment of severe recalcitrant psoriasis. Fenretinide (N-[4-hydroxyphenyl]retinide), which concentrates in breast tissue, is being tested as a preventive agent for breast cancer.[57]

PHYSIOLOGY

The major dietary sources of vitamin A are carotenoids from plants and long-chain retinyl esters from animals.[58] Enzymatic conversion of beta-carotene to vitamin A occurs primarily in the intestinal mucosa, whereas retinyl esters are hydrolyzed in the intestinal lumen to retinol. Retinol is then esterified with long-chain fatty acids in the mucosal cell and transported in the lymphatics with chylomicrons to the plasma compartment. Chylomicron remnants containing retinyl ester are taken up by the hepatic parenchymal cells by endocytosis and vitamin A is stored in the liver primarily as retinyl palmitate. Although large amounts of vitamin A may be stored in the mammalian liver, under normal conditions plasma retinol levels tend to remain relatively constant.

tRA is formed naturally by intestinal cells from beta-carotene and from tissue anabolism of retinol and retinaldehyde and can perform the functions of vitamin A not related to vision or reproduction. In contrast with retinol, tRA is primarily absorbed through the venous portal system and is rapidly metabolized and eliminated. Although retinol binds to a specific protein (retinol-binding protein), tRA circulates in the plasma in tight association with albumin.

Distinct cytoplasmic-binding proteins (cellular retinoic acid-binding protein [CRABP] and cellular retinol-binding proteins) exist for tRA and retinol, although their function is not clear. These proteins may sequester retinoids in the cytoplasm and facilitate their metabolism to an inactive form. For example, overexpression of cellular proteins has been associated with decreased in vitro responses to retinoids, tissue content of the cellular proteins varies inversely with that of retinoic acid, and some tRA-sensitive leukemic cell lines have been documented to lack CRABP.[59]

The 50,000-kd nuclear retinoic acid receptors (RARs) α, β, and γ are members of the steroid-thyroid superfamily of nuclear receptors. RARs, normally present in human lung, mucosa, and skin, have been detected in human oral mucosa and in some squamous cell carcinoma and human leukemia cell lines.[60–62] In contrast to the cytoplasmic-binding proteins, presence of the nuclear RARs has correlated with sensitivity of malignant cells to retinoids, and transfection of the *RARA* gene into resistant cells restores sensitivity.[63] The human *RARA* gene is located at the breakpoint region for the 15:17 translocation associated with APL, a malignancy with striking sensitivity to tRA in the clinic.[64]

DIFFERENTIATING EFFECTS

Although changes in immunologic parameters follow administration of retinoids, their predominant therapeutic effect almost certainly results from differentiation of the malignant cell.[65] Retinoid-induced differentiation in vitro of myeloid leukemia, neuroblastoma, teratocarcinoma, and melanoma cell lines has been well documented, and a comprehensive list of retinoid-sensitive cell lines has been compiled recently.[66] However, the most compelling data to support a differentiating effect of the retinoids comes from the clinical trials using tRA in the treatment of APL.[67] After treatment with 20 to 45 mg/m² per day of tRA, malignant cells from patients with APL exhibit morphologic maturation, decreased proliferative capacity, and increased expression of maturation-associated cell-surface antigens. In addition, the 15:17 translocation can be identified in morphologically normal myeloid cells in the blood of APL patients after remission induction with tRA.

Retinoids may exert similar effects on epithelial-derived malignancies. Tracheal columnar ciliated epithelium and mucous cells grown in the absence of retinoids lose their normal morphology and undergo a proliferative squamous metaplasia.[68] Of the naturally occurring retinoids and their metabolites, tRA is the most active in reversing these changes. Based on these and other results, it is believed currently that differentiation and suppression of proliferation are intimately linked and that the retinoids effect these changes by regulating gene expression, possibly through stimulation of the autocrine inhibitory factor tumor growth factor-β.[48] Emerging clinical data suggest that retinoids have therapeutic activity in epithelial-derived malignancies.[54,55]

CLINICAL PHARMACOLOGY AND PHARMACOKINETICS

cRA has been studied more extensively in the clinic than any other retinoid, and its clinical pharmacology has been well characterized.[69] cRA is formulated in 10-, 20-, and 40-mg soft gelatin capsules, and the recommended starting dose for patients with acne is 0.5 to 1 mg/kg per day. After oral administration, cRA can be detected in the serum within 30 minutes and reaches maximal levels after approximately 3 hours. Plasma levels of the major metabolite of cRA, 4-oxo-cRA, exceed the level of the parent compound within 6 hours of administration, and the AUC for 4-oxo-cRA is typically fivefold greater than that of cRA. The elimination half-life for cRA generally is between 10 and 20 hours. Significant plasma levels of tRA have been reported in patients being treated with cRA, suggesting that significant in vivo isomerization occurs.[69] After oral weekly administration of high doses of cRA, peak plasma levels reach 3.8 ± 0.7 μg/ml after 400 mg/m² and do not increase higher than this level after doses as high as 1800 mg/m², suggesting saturable absorption mechanisms. Secondary peak plasma concentrations and highly variable terminal half-lives (3–101 hours) have been reported and may be the result of variable enterohepatic recirculation. For a given patient, chronic administration of cRA does not result in marked changes in the terminal half-life or steady-state plasma concentration.

Pharmacokinetic data from patients with APL treated with 45 mg/m²/day of tRA indicate a mean peak serum level of 309 ng/ml 3 hours after oral administration.[67] tRA is no longer detectable (<10 ng/ml) 8 hours after administration, and the elimination half-life is less than 1 hour. A marked decrease in plasma tRA concentrations occurs in most patients after 2 to 6 weeks of therapy, a factor that may contribute to retinoid resistance. Although the mechanism responsible for decreased circulating tRA levels is not known, tRA has been reported to increase levels of cytochrome P-450 and CRABPs, which could lead to respective increases in metabolism, tissue sequestration, or both.[70,71] The induction of accelerated clearance of tRA has been demonstrated in cynomolgus monkeys given equal doses of tRA or cRA; the AUC for tRA was approximately one half that for cRA, and although the AUC and C_{max} (maximum plasma concentration) for cRA did not change appreciably from day 1 to day 10, the corresponding values for tRA decreased by more than 60% during the same period.[72]

cRA and tRA are probably metabolized along similar pathways.[69,70,73,74] Each may be excreted in the bile as the glucuronide or may undergo P-450-mediated hydroxylation of the cyclohexenyl ring and subsequent oxidation to their respective

4-oxo-derivatives, the major metabolites found in the plasma and urine after administration of cRA or tRA.

Etretinate is supplied in 10- and 25-mg capsules, and the recommended starting dose for patients with severe psoriasis is 0.75 to 1 mg/kg per day. Bioavailability of oral etretinate is approximately 40%, and peak concentrations in the plasma are reached within 2 to 4 hours of administration.[74] Its major metabolite is the free aromatic acid (etretin), which can be detected in the plasma within 1 hour. Approximately 98% of etretinate and etretin circulate bound to plasma proteins. Elimination half-lives as long as 80 to 100 days have been reported for etretinate after long-term administration, and parent compound is still be detectable in the plasma 6 to 12 months after discontinuation of treatment. This observation may be related to the slow release of etretinate, a highly lipophilic compound, from storage sites in adipose tissue.

The mean ± SD elimination half-life and total body clearance of fenretinide were reported as 13.7 ± 1.9 hours and 57 ± 13 liter/h/m², respectively, in 3 patients receiving 300 mg/m².[75] The plasma half-life of the major biologically active metabolite of fenretinide, N-(4-methoxyphenyl) retinamide, was 23 hours. Within 2 weeks of starting fenretinide, mean plasma retinol and retinol-binding protein concentrations decreased by 60% and 47%, respectively.

TOXICITY

The side effects of the retinoids have been characterized extensively from reports of hypervitaminosis A and the extensive experience with cRA in nonmalignant conditions.[76] Within a few hours of ingesting toxic amounts of vitamin A, patients experience nausea, vomiting, anorexia, headache, dizziness, fatigue, and irritability, followed within a few days by generalized desquamation. Many of these symptoms are secondary to increased intracranial pressure (pseudotumor cerebri) caused by an increased production of cerebrospinal fluid. Physical findings may include cheilitis, hair loss, hepatosplenomegaly, bone tenderness, edema, and petechiae. Other toxicities associated with chronic hypervitaminosis A include fatty changes and sinusoidal fibrosis in the liver (which may not reverse completely in some patients); elevations of serum triglyceride and cholesterol levels accompanied by a decrease in high-density lipoproteins; increased muscle tone; and ocular abnormalities (conjunctivitis, xerophthalmia, diplopia, blurred vision, and corneal opacities). In some patients, neuropsychiatric manifestations (severe depression and psychosis) have predominated.

Fetal abnormalities are perhaps the most significant retinoid-related toxicity.[77] From 36 prospectively identified cRA-exposed pregnancies that were not electively terminated, there were eight (22%) spontaneous abortions and five infants (14%, one stillborn) with at least one major malformation. The relative risk compared with an unexposed pregnancy for the occurrence of a major malformation was estimated to be 26-fold (95% confidence interval, 11 to 58), comparable with that of thalidomide.

Although pseudotumor cerebri and hepatotoxicity are less common after therapy with cRA than with retinol, their side effects are otherwise similar. Hyperostosis is an additional, well-recognized side effect of cRA and is commoner after high doses and prolonged administration. Radiologic abnormalities

of bone have been found in as many as 75% of patients taking approximately 2 mg/kg per day for 1 year, and diffuse idiopathic skeletal hyperostosis has been reported in patients receiving chronic therapy for refractory ichthyosis.[78] Premature epiphyseal closure has been reported in younger patients treated with cRA.

The side effects of etretinate are similar to those of cRA, although skeletal abnormalities and alterations in lipid metabolism may be less common. Cutaneous toxicities of etretinate include increased skin fragility and a feeling of stickiness.[74] Hepatotoxicity may be more severe with etretinate and, due to its long plasma half-life, there are greater concerns regarding teratogenicity. In animal models, etretinate was teratogenic at doses as low as 2 to 4 mg/kg per day.

In the limited clinical experience with fenretinide, the drug has been tolerated well in women taking 200 mg daily for 1 year as adjuvant therapy for breast cancer.[57] Mucocutaneous and gastrointestinal toxicity was mild, and there was no evidence of hepatic damage or changes in lipid metabolism. Reversible, decreased night vision (nyctalopia) has been reported at higher doses and may be related to lower plasma retinol levels in patients receiving fenretinide.[79]

The side effects of systemic administration of tRA to patients with APL are similar to those of other retinoids.[67] Several patients receiving 45 mg/m² per day experienced increased intracranial pressure and required serial lumbar punctures, high-dose corticosteroids, and narcotic analgesia. Truncal or appendicular bone pain occurred in 10% to 20% of patients and, although generally self-limiting, at times required narcotic analgesia. Leukocytosis, due to differentiation of leukemic cells, may occur in patients with APL who are treated with tRA. Although an increasing leukocyte count usually indicates progression of an underlying leukemia, in tRA-treated patients with APL an initial leucocytosis probably indicates a response to therapy. Differentiated leukemic cells may obtain the functional characteristics of mature neutrophils, infiltrate into tissue, and cause organ dysfunction. Some patients with APL with respiratory syndrome, which sometimes occurred in the absence of peripheral leucocytosis, consisted of fever, pulmonary infiltrates, and plural and pericardial effusions, responded dramatically to high doses of dexamethasone.

REFERENCES

1. McCredie KB. Amsacrine: A new drug for hematological malignancies. Eur J Cancer 1985;21:1–3.
2. Minford J, Kerrigan D, Nichols M, et al. Enhancement of the DNA breakage and cytotoxic effects of intercalating agents by treatment with sublethal doses of 1-β-D-arabinofuranosylcytosine or hydroxyurea in L1210 cells. Cancer Res 1984;44:5583–5593.
3. Pommier Y, Zwelling LA, Kao-Shan C, et al. Correlations between intercalator-induced DNA strand breaks and sister chromatid exchanges, mutations, and cytotoxicity in Chinese hamster cells. Cancer Res 1985;45:3143–3149.
4. Rowe TC, Chen GL, Hsiang YH, et al. DNA damage by antitumor acridines mediated by mammalian DNA topoisomerase-II. Cancer Res 1986;46:2021–2026.
5. Pommier Y, Capranico G, Orr A, Kohn W. Local base sequence preferences for DNA cleavage by mammalian topoisomerase II in the presence of amsacrine or teniposide. Nucleic Acids Res 1991;19:5973–5980.
6. Markovits J, Pommier Y, Kerrigan D, et al. Topoisomerase-II-mediated DNA breaks and cytotoxicity in relation to cell proliferation and the cell cycle in NIH 3T3 fibroblasts and L1210 leukemia cells. Cancer Res 1987;47:2050–2055.
7. Lefevre D, Riou JF, Ahomadegbe JC, et al. Study of molecular markers of resistance to m-Amsa in a human breast cancer cell line: Decrease of topoisomerase II and increase of both topoisomerase I and acidic glutathione S transferase. Biochem Pharmacol 1991;41:1967–79.
8. Pommier Y, Kerrigan D, Schwartz RE, et al. Altered DNA topoisomerase-II activity in

Chinese hamster cells resistant to topoisomerase-II inhibitors. Cancer Res 1986;46: 3075–3081.

9. Pommier Y, Schwartz RE, Zwelling LA, et al. Reduced formation of protein-associated DNA strand breaks in Chinese hamster cells resistant to topoisomerase-II inhibitors. Cancer Res 1986;46:611–616.

10. Darken S, Ralph RK. Potentiation of 4'-(9 acridinylamino) methanesulphon-*m*-anisidine) action by verapamil. Cancer Lett 1986;30:25–33.

11. Kaufmann SH. Antagonism between camptothecin and topoisomerase II-directed chemotherapeutic agents in a human leukemia cell line. Cancer Res 1991;51:1129–36.

12. Shoemaker DD, Cysyk RL, Padmanabhan S, et al. Identification of the principal biliary metabolite of m-AMSA in rats. Drug Metab Dispos 1982;10:35–39.

13. Hall SW, Friedman J, Legha SS, et al. Human pharmacokinetics of a new acridine derivative 4'-(9-acridinylamino)methanesulfon-*m*-anisidide (NSC 249992). Cancer Res 1983;43:3422–3426.

14. Paxton JW, Jurlina JL, Foote SE. The binding of amsacrine to human plasma proteins. J Pharm Pharmacol 1986;38:432–438.

15. Cassileth PA, Gale RP. Amsacrine: A Review. Leuk Res 1986;10:1257–1265.

16. Weiss RB, Grillo-Lopez AJ, Marsoni S, et al. Amsacrine-associated cardiotoxicity: An analysis of 82 cases. J Clin Oncol 1986;4:918–928.

17. Arlin ZA, Feldman EJ, Mittelman A, et al. Amsacrine is safe and effective therapy for patients with myocardial dysfunction and acute leukemia. Cancer 1991;68:1198–1200.

18. Engelking C, Sullivan P, Agoliati G, et al. Amsacrine administration: A precautionary note. Cancer Chemother Pharmacol [Letter] 1984;13:150.

19. Wall ME, Wani MC, Cook CE, Palmer KH, McPhail AT, Sim GA. Plant antitumor agents: I. The isolation and structure of camptothecin, a novel alkaloidal leukemia and tumor inhibitor from *Camptotheca accuminata*. J Am Chem Soc 1966;88:3888–3890.

20. Dewys WD, Humphreys SR, Goldin A. Studies on therapeutic effectiveness of drugs with tumor weight and survival time indices of Walker 256 carcinosarcoma. Cancer Chemother Rep 1968;52:229–242.

21. Gallo RC, Whang-Peng J, Adamson RH. Studies on the antitumor activity, mechanism of action, and cell cycle effects of camptothecin. JNCI 1971;46:789–795.

22. Jaxel C, Kohn KW, Wani MC, et al. Structure-activity study of the actions of camptothecin derivatives on mammalian topoisomerase: I. Evidence for a specific receptor site and a relation to antitumor activity. Cancer Res 1989;49:1465–1469.

23. Johnson RK, McCabe FL, Faucette LF, et al. SK&F 104864, a water-soluble analog of camptothecin with a broad spectrum of activity in preclinical tumor models. Proc American Association for Cancer Research [Abstract] 1989;30:623.

24. Kunimoto T, Nitta K, Tanaka T, et al. Antitumor activity of 7-ethyl-10-[4-(1-piperidino)-1-piperidino]carbonyloxycamptothecin, a novel water-soluble derivative of camptothecin, against murine tumors. Cancer Res 1987;47:5944–5947.

25. Kaneda N, Yokokura T. Nonlinear pharmacokinetics of CPT-11 in rats. Cancer Res 1990;50:1721–1725.

26. Sasaki Y, Morita M, Tamura T, et al. In vitro and in vivo protein binding and in vitro and ex vivo antitumor activity of camptothecin derivative (CPT-11) and its metabolite (SN38). Proc Annu Meet Jpn Cancer Assoc [Abstract] 1990;49:397.

27. Giovanella BC, Stehlin JS, Wall ME, et al. DNA topoisomerase-I-targeted chemotherapy of human colon cancer in xenografts. Science 1989;246:1046–1048.

28. Schneider E, Hsiang Y-H, Liu LF. DNA topoisomerases as anticancer drug targets. Adv Pharmacol 1990;21:149–183.

29. Covey JM, Jaxel C, Kohn KW, et al. Protein-linked DNA strand breaks induced in mammalian cells by camptothecin, an inhibitor of topoisomerase I. Cancer Res 1989;49:5016–5022.

30. Hsiang Y-H, Lihou MG, Liu LF. Mechanism of cell killing by camptothecin: Arrest of replication forks by drug-stabilized topoisomerase I-DNA cleavable complexes. Cancer Res 1989;49:5077–5082.

31. Sugimoto Y, Tsukahara S, Oh-hara T. Decreased expression of DNA topoisomerase I in camptothecin-resistant tumor cell lines as determined by a monoclonal antibody. Cancer Res 1990;50:6925–6930.

32. Ohe Y, Sasaki Y, Shinkai T, et al. Pharmacokinetics with a 5-day continuous-infusion of a camptothecin derivative, CPT-11. Proc Am Soc Clin Oncol 1991;10:A336.

33. Takeuchi S, Takamizawa H, Takeda Y, et al. An early phase II study of CPT-11 in gynecologic cancers. Gan To Kagaku Ryoho 1991;18:579–584.

34. Shimada Y, Yoshino M, Wakui A, et al. Phase II study of CPT-11, new camptothecin derivative, in the patients with metastatic colorectal cancer. Proc Am Soc Clin Oncol 1991;10:A408.

35. Chabner BA. Camptothecins. J Clin Oncol [Editorial] 1992;10:3–4.

36. Ohno R, Okada K, Masoaka T, et al. An early phase II study of CPT-ll: A new derivative of camptothecin, for the treatment of leukemia and lymphoma. J Clin Oncol 1990;8:1907–1912.

37. Chabot GG, Barilero I, Armand JP, et al. Pharmacokinetics of the camptothecin analog CPT-11 and its active metabolite SN-38 in cancer patients. Proc American Association for Cancer Research [Abstract] 1991;32:175.

38. Sasaki Y, Morita M, Tamura T, et al. In vitro and in vivo protein binding and in vitro and ex vivo antitumor activity of camptothecin derivative (CPT-11) and its metabolite (SN38). Proc Annu Meet Jpn Cancer Assoc 1990;49:397.

39. Showalter HDH, Johnson JL, Werbel LM, et al. 5-[(Aminoalkyl)amino]-substituted anthra[1,9-*cd*] pyrazol-6(2*H*)-ones as novel anticancer agents: Synthesis and biological evaluation. J Med Chem 1984;27:253–255.

40. Frank SK, Mathiesen DA, Szurszewski M, et al. Preclinical pharmacology of the anthrapyrazole analog oxantrazole (NSC-349174, Piroxantrone). Cancer Chemother Pharmacol 1989;23:213–218.

41. Leopold WR, Nelson JM, Plowman J, et al. Anthrapyrazoles, a new class of intercalating agents with high-level, broad-spectrum activity against murine tumors. Cancer Res 1985;45:5532–5539.

42. Hantel A, Donehower RC, Rowinsky EK, et al. Phase I study and pharmacodynamics of piroxantrone (NSC 349174), a new anthrapyrazole. Cancer Res 1990;50:3284–3288.

43. Ames MM, Loprinzi CL, Collins JM, et al. Phase I and clinical pharmacological evaluation of piroxantrone hydrochloride (oxantrazole). Cancer Res 1990;50:3905–3909.

44. Foster BJ, Graham MA, Newell DR, et al. Phase I study of the anthrapyrazole CI-941 with pharmacokinetically guided dose escalation. Proc Am Soc Clin Oncol 1988;7:64.

45. Allan SG, Cummings J, Evans S, et al. Phase I study of the anthrapyrazole biantrazole: Clinical results and pharmacology. Cancer Chemother Pharmacol 1991;28:55–58.

46. Erlichman C, Moore M, Kerr I, et al. Phase I trial of the anthrapyrazole CI-937. Proc Am Soc Clin Oncol 1990;9:68.

47. Smith IE, Talbot DC, Mansi JL, et al. Anthrapyrazole CI-941: A highly active new drug against advanced breast cancer. Proc Am Soc Clin Oncol 1991;10:55.

48. Sporn MB, Roberts AB. Interactions of retinoids and transforming growth factor-β in regulation of cell differentiation and proliferation. Mol Endocrinol 1991;5:3–7.

49. Roberts AB, Sporn MB. Cellular biology and biochemistry of the retinoids. In: Sporn MB, Roberts AB, Goodman DS, eds. The retinoids. Vol 2. Orlando: Academic Press, 1984:209–286.

50. Lippman SM, Kessler JF, Meyskens FL Jr. Retinoids as preventive and therapeutic anticancer agents: I. Cancer Treat Rep 1987;71:391–405.

51. Lippman SM, Kessler JF, Meyskens FL Jr. Retinoids as preventive and therapeutic anticancer agents: II. Cancer Treat Rep 1987;71:493–515.

52. Huang ME, Ye YC, Chen SR, et al. Use of all-trans retinoic acid in the treatment of acute promyelocytic leukemia. Blood 1988;72:567–572.

53. Warrell RP Jr, Frankel SS, Miller WH Jr, et al. Differentiation therapy of acute promyelocytic leukemia with tretinoin (all-trans-retinoic acid). N Engl J Med 1991;324:1385–1393.

54. Hong WK, Lippman SM, Itri LM, et al. Prevention of second primary tumors with isotretinoin in squamous-cell carcinoma of the head and neck. N Engl J Med 1990;323:795–801.

55. Lippman SM, Parkinson DR, Weber RS, et al. Isotretinoin plus alpha-interferon: Effective therapy of advanced squamous cell carcinoma (scc) of the skin. Proc Am Soc Clin Oncol 1991;10:A650.

56. Lippman SM, Kavanagh JJ, Paredes-Espinoza, et al. 13-*cis*-Retinoic acid plus interferon α-2a: Highly active systemic therapy for squamous cell carcinoma of the cervix. JNCI 1992;84:241–245.

57. Costa A, Malone W, Perloff M, et al. Tolerability of the synthetic retinoid fenretinide* (HPR). Eur J Cancer Clin Oncol 1989;25:805–808.

58. Goodman DS. Vitamin A and retinoids in health and disease. N Engl J Med 1984;310:1023–1031.

59. Boylan JF, Gudas LJ. Overexpression of the cellular retinoic acid binding protein-I (CRABP-I) results in a reduction in differentiation-specific gene expression in F9 teratocarcinoma cells. J Cell Biol 1991;112:965–979.

60. Maden M, Ong DE, Summerbell D, et al. Spatial distribution of cellular protein binding to retinoic acid in the chick limb bud. Nature 1988;335:733–735.

61. Hu L, Crowe DL, Rheinwald JG, et al. Abnormal expression of retinoic acid receptors and keratin 19 by human oral and epidermal squamous cell carcinoma cell lines. Cancer Res 1991;51:3972–3981.

62. Gallagher R, Said F, Pua I, et al. Expression of retinoic acid receptor-α mRNA in human leukemia cells with variable responsiveness to retinoic acid. Leukemia 1989;3:789–795.

63. Collins S, Robertson K, Mueller L. Retinoic acid-induced granulocytic differentiation of HL-60 myeloid leukemia cells is mediated directly through the retinoic acid receptor (RAR-alpha). Mol Cell Biol 1990;10:2154–2163.

64. Mattei MG, Petkovich M, Mattei JF, et al. Mapping of the human retinoic acid receptor to the q21 band of chromosome 17. Hum Genet 1988;80:186–188.

65. Lotan R. Vitamin A analogs (retinoids) as biological response modifiers. Prog Clin Biol Res 1988;259:261–271.

66. Amos B, Lotan R. Retinoid-sensitive cells and cell lines. Methods Enzymol 1990;190:217–225.

67. Warrell RP. Retinoic acid and acute promyelocytic leukemia. Biol Ther Cancer Updates 1991;1:1–12.

68. Harris CC, Sporn MB, Kaufman DG, et al. Histogenesis of squamous metaplasia in the hamster tracheal epithelium caused by vitamin A deficiency or benzo(a)pyrene-ferric oxide. JNCI 1972;48:743–761.

69. Meyskens FL, Goodman GE, Alberts DS. 13-*cis*-retinoic acid: Pharmacology, toxicology, and clinical applications for the prevention and treatment of cancer. Crit Rev Oncol Hematol 1987;3:75–101.

70. Frolik CA, Roller PP, Roberts AB, et al. In vitro and in vivo metabolism of all-trans and 13-*cis*-retinoic acid in hamsters. J Biol Chem 1980;255:8057–8062.

71. Hirschel-Scholz S, Siegenthaler G, Saurat J-H. Ligand-specific and non-specific in vivo modulation of human epidermal cellular retinoic acid binding protein (CRABP). Eur J Clin Invest 1989;19:220–227.

72. Creech Kraft J, Slikker W, Bailey JR, et al. Plasma pharmacokinetics and metabolism of 13-*cis*- and all-*trans*-retinoic acid in the cynomolgus monkey and the identification of 13-*cis*- and all-*trans*-retinoyl-β-glucuronides. Drug Metab Dispos 1991;19:317–324.

73. Van Wauwe JP, Coene M-C, Goossens J, et al. Effects of cytochrome P-450 inhibitors on the in vivo metabolism of all-trans-retinoic acid in rats. J Pharmacol Exp Ther 1990;252:365–369.

74. Orfanos C, Ehlert R, Gollnick H. The retinoids: A review of their clinical pharmacology and therapeutic use. Drugs 1987;34:459–503.

75. Peng Y-M, Dalton WS, Alberts DS, et al. Pharmacokinetics of N-4-hydroxyphenyl-retinamide and the effect of its oral administration on plasma retinol concentrations in cancer patients. Int J Cancer 1989;43:22–26.

76. Strauss JS, Rapini RP, Shalita AR, et al. Isotretinoin therapy for acne: Results of a multicenter dose-response study. J Am Acad Dermatol 1984;10:490–496.
77. Lammer EJ, Chen DT, Hoar RM, et al. Retinoic acid embryopathy. N Engl J Med 1985;313:837–841.
78. Ellis CN, Madison KC, Pennes DR, et al. Isotretinoin therapy is associated with early skeletal radiographic changes. J Am Acad Dermatol 1984;10:1024–1029.
79. Modiano MR, Dalton WS, Lippman SM, et al. Phase II study of fenretinide (N-[4-hydroxyphenyl] retinamide) in advanced breast cancer and melanoma. Invest New Drugs 1990;8:317–319.

EDWARD CHU
CHRIS H. TAKIMOTO

SECTION 4
Antimetabolites

ANTIFOLATES

The era of antimetabolite chemotherapy began in 1948 with the demonstration that aminopterin, the 4-amino analog of folic acid, induced remissions in childhood leukemia.[1] Aminopterin has since been replaced by methotrexate (MTX), the 4-amino, 10-methyl analog of aminopterin (see Fig. 18–2). MTX remains the most widely used antifolate in cancer chemotherapy, with documented activity against leukemia, breast cancer, head and neck cancer, lymphoma, osteogenic sarcoma, and choriocarcinoma. Antifolates have been used in the treatment of psoriasis, rheumatoid arthritis, graft-versus-host disease, bacterial and plasmodial infections, and parasitic infections associated with the acquired immunodeficiency syndrome.[1a] This class of agents represents the best characterized and most versatile of all chemotherapeutic drugs in current clinical use.

MECHANISM OF ACTION

MTX is a tight-binding inhibitor of dihydrofolate reductase (DHFR), a critical enzyme in intracellular folate metabolism (Fig. 18–9). The importance of DHFR stems from its role in maintaining the intracellular folate pool in its fully reduced form as tetrahydrofolates. These compounds serve as 1-carbon carriers required for the de novo synthesis of pyrimidines and purines. 5,10-Methylenetetrahydrofolate provides a methyl group in the conversion of deoxyuridylate (dUMP) to thymidylate and is, itself, a reduced folate that is oxidized to dihydrofolate in a reaction catalyzed by thymidylate synthase (TS). 10-Formyltetrahydrofolate donates its 1-carbon group in the de novo purine synthesis reactions catalyzed by glycinamide ribonucleotide (GAR) transformylase and aminoimidazole carboxamide ribonucleotide (AICAR) transformylase. An intact DHFR pathway is therefore necessary for continued thymidylate and purine nucleotide biosynthesis.

The precise mechanism(s) by which MTX produces its cytotoxicity remains controversial. The classic proposal has been that MTX inhibits DHFR and depletes the intracellular reduced folate pool, resulting in the impaired synthesis of de novo purines and pyrimidines. However, after exposure of cells to concentrations of MTX that completely inhibit the synthesis of these DNA precursors, the level of intracellular reduced folates is only incompletely depleted (50–60%), a decrease insufficient to account for the observed inhibition of DNA synthesis.[2]

Additional cytotoxic actions of MTX result from its transformation to polyglutamate forms (see Fig. 18–9). MTX and physiologic folate polyglutamates are formed by the enzyme folylpolyglutamyl synthetase, which adds up to six glutamyl groups in a γ-peptide linkage. Polyglutamation occurs in tumor cells and, to a lesser extent, in normal tissues, reaching a maximum 12 to 24 hours after drug exposure.[3] As much as 80% of MTX found in malignant tissues is in the polyglutamated form.[4] The relative difference in polyglutamate formation in normal versus malignant cells may account for the selective activity of the drug. Polyglutamated derivatives are preferentially retained within cells. MTX polyglutamates bind to DHFR with similar affinity as the parent compound, but display slower rates of dissociation from the enzyme. They also directly inhibit other folate-dependent enzymes not inhibited by MTX, including TS and AICAR and GAR transfor-

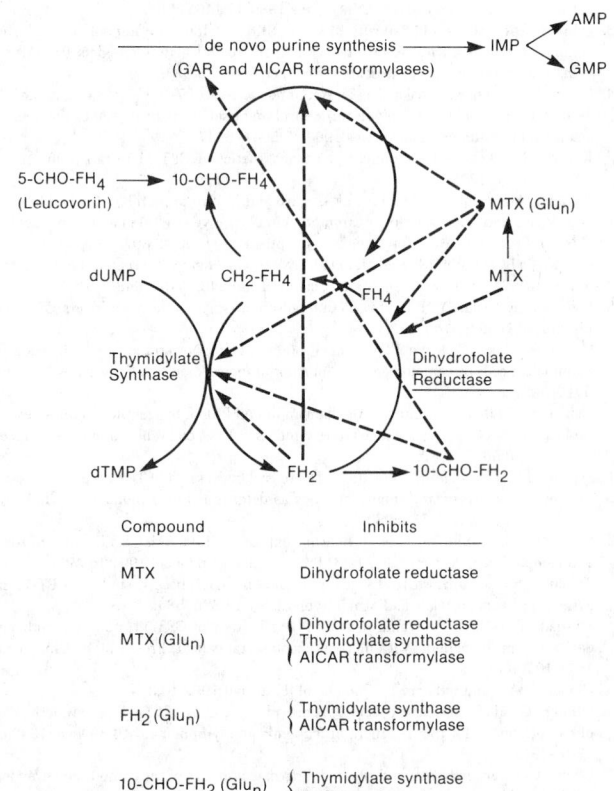

FIGURE 18–9. Sites of action of methotrexate (MTX), its polyglutamated metabolites [MTX(Glu_n)], and folate by-products of the inhibition of dihydrofolate reductase, including dihydrofolate (FH_2) and 10-formyl-dihydrofolate (10-CHO-FH_2). Also shown are 5-10-methylene tetrahydrofolic acid (CH_2-FH_4), the folate cofactor required for thymidylate synthesis, and 10-formyl-tetrahydrofolate (10-CHO-FH_4), the required intermediate in the synthesis of purine precursors. IMP, inosine monophosphate; AMP, adenosine monophosphate; GMP, guanine monophosphate; dUMP, deoxyuridylate; dTMP, thymidylate; GAR, glycinamide ribonucleotide transformylase; AICAR, aminoimidazole carboxamide ribonucleotide transformylase.

mylase.[2,5] In addition, the inhibition of DHFR leads to the accumulation of dihydrofolate polyglutamates, potent direct inhibitors of these same folate-dependent enzymes.[1a] The metabolic inhibition resulting from MTX exposure appears to be multifactorial, resulting from partial depletion of reduced folates and from direct inhibition of folate-dependent enzymes by MTX polyglutamates and dihydrofolate polyglutamates.

MTX cytotoxicity may also result from drug-induced single- and double-strand breakage of DNA.[6] These breaks appear to result from MTX-induced depletion of thymidylate and purine nucleotides, with impairment of the ability to repair sites of DNA damage. Moreover, an intracellular accumulation of dUMP results from the inhibitory effects of MTX on TS. Further metabolism of dUMP to the triphosphate nucleotide form (dUTP), which is then incorporated into DNA, results in inhibition of chain elongation and DNA synthesis. Excision repair of the DNA containing these incorporated dUTP moieties by the enzymes dUTP nucleotidohydrolase and uracil glycosylase may result in further DNA strand breaks and fragmentation.

MTX is most active against rapidly proliferating cells, because its cytotoxic effects occur primarily during the S phase of the cell cycle. During longer drug exposures, more cells are allowed to enter the DNA synthetic phase of the cell cycle, resulting in greater cell kill. In addition, MTX polyglutamate formation is substantially enhanced with longer periods of drug exposure, thereby increasing cytotoxicity. The cytotoxic effects of MTX are also greater with increasing drug concentrations. Therefore, MTX cytotoxicity is highly dependent on the absolute drug concentration and the duration of drug exposure.

MTX enters cells by the same active transport mechanisms used by physiologic folates. Intracellular drug concentrations reach steady state in less than 30 minutes. Folate transport is a complex process with at least two carrier-mediated, energy-dependent mechanisms existing in mammalian cells. The first is a relatively low-affinity, reduced folate carrier capable of transporting MTX and reduced folates, such as leucovorin, with affinity constants in the micromolar range.[1a] A second system uses a high-affinity, membrane-associated folate-binding protein with affinity constants for reduced folates and folic acid in the nanomolar range.[7] MTX is a relatively poor substrate for this folate-binding protein, with an affinity that is 10- to 30-fold lower than that of the reduced folates.[8] The relative function of each of these two distinct transport systems depends on the extracellular folate concentration and varies among different cell lines.[8a] Their role in MTX transport remains an active area of research. Nonglutamated antifolate compounds, such as trimetrexate, trimethoprim, and pyritrexim (see Fig. 18–2), do not rely on either of these folate carrier systems for cellular entry and are active against various cell lines resistant to MTX on the basis of decreased transport capacity.

In the presence of the cofactor, nicotinamide adenine nucleotide phosphate, MTX binds to the enzyme DHFR, resulting in a slow-forming, tight-binding inhibitory complex. Although this complex is tightly bound, its formation is reversible.[9] Because high levels of dihydrofolate can effectively compete with MTX for enzyme binding, excess free (unbound) drug is required to maintain complete DHFR enzyme inhibition.

Reduced folates, such as 5-formyltetrahydrofolate (leuco-

vorin), prevent the toxic effects of MTX. The predominant species of reduced folate in human plasma, 5-methyltetrahydrofolate, circulates with levels in the range of 5 to 50 nmol, a concentration inadequate to rescue cells. Administration of appropriate doses of leucovorin after high-dose MTX therapy can prevent toxicity to the bone marrow and gastrointestinal epithelium. The dose of leucovorin required to rescue normal tissues is dependent on the antifolate concentration at the time of antidote administration.[10] The competitive nature of this rescue suggests that leucovorin does more than simply replete intracellular reduced folate pools. Leucovorin is converted to intracellular folates that compete with MTX polyglutamates and dihydrofolate polyglutamates to overcome the inhibition of TS and AICAR transformylase.[11] In addition, MTX and reduced folates may also compete for transport into cells and for subsequent intracellular polyglutamation. The administration of exogenous thymidine also decreases MTX toxicity, but it is less practical and less effective than leucovorin. Although thymidine treatment bypasses the inhibition of de novo thymidylate synthesis, cells treated with MTX are still at risk from purine starvation. Administration of the bacterial enzyme carboxypeptidase G_2, which hydrolyzes MTX to inactive metabolites, currently is undergoing clinical testing as an alternative form of rescue from high-dose MTX therapy.[12]

MECHANISMS OF RESISTANCE

The development of cellular resistance to MTX remains a major obstacle to its effective clinical use. In experimental systems, resistance to antifolates may result from several mechanisms, including an alteration in antifolate transport, decreased capacity to polyglutamate MTX, and alterations in the target enzyme DHFR, including increased protein expression or decreased binding affinity for MTX.

Amplification of the *DHFR* gene is one of the most common forms of MTX resistance observed in experimental systems.[1a] The amplified gene may be stably integrated into chromosomal DNA in the form of a homogenously staining region (HSR), or it may exist in extrachromosomal pieces of DNA known as double-minute chromosomes.[13] HSR-mediated gene amplification is associated with the development of stable resistance to MTX. In contrast, double-minute chromosomes are unequally distributed during cell division, and, in the absence of continued selective pressure of MTX, cells eventually revert to a sensitive phenotype with wild-type levels of DHFR expression.

An alternative mechanism of resistance has been ascribed to mutations that result in a DHFR protein product with an altered binding affinity for MTX.[14] There is evidence that naturally occurring DHFR alleles with differing sensitivities to MTX may exist in cells and may provide a mechanism for the rapid emergence of MTX resistance.[15] Resistance to MTX may also arise from an acute increase in DHFR protein expression in response to MTX exposure. In experimental cell system, this acute elevation in DHFR expression results, in part, from an increase in the translational efficiency of DHFR mRNA.[16]

The exact clinical relevance of each of these various mechanisms of resistance to MTX and to other antifolates remains an active area of research. To date, *DHFR* gene amplification, defective transport, and decreased polyglutamate formation all have been observed in clinical specimens taken from MTX-resistant patients.[16a,17]

CLINICAL PHARMACOLOGY AND PHARMACOKINETICS

Accurate monitoring of MTX concentrations in plasma is essential for the safe and optimal use of this agent in cancer chemotherapy, particularly during high-dose use. At least four methods are presently available for the clinical monitoring of MTX drug levels, including the DHFR inhibition assay, the competitive protein-binding assay, a fluorescence-polarization radioimmunoassay technique, and an enzyme-linked immunoassay system.[1a] The immunoassay has similar sensitivity to the competitive binding assay, but crossreacts with the MTX metabolite 2,4-diamino-N^{10}-methylpteroic acid (DAMPA) and can give spuriously high results. High-performance liquid chromatography (HPLC) may be used to separate MTX and its various metabolites and, in particular, to measure MTX metabolites.

Oral MTX is well absorbed in doses less than 25 mg/m^2, but bioavailability is erratic at higher doses. Except in maintenance regimens, the drug is usually administered intravenously. The volume of distribution of MTX approaches that of total body water, and approximately 60% of the drug is bound to serum albumin at pharmacologic drug concentrations.[1a] Although plasma pharmacokinetics are variable, MTX generally follows a three-phase disappearance pattern. The initial distribution phase, which lasts for only a few minutes, is followed by a second phase lasting 12 to 24 hours, during which time the drug is eliminated with a half-life of 2 to 3 hours. The final phase of drug clearance has a half-life of 8 to 10 hours. The last two phases of drug elimination are considerably lengthened in patients with renal dysfunction. There is substantial evidence that a more rapid systemic clearance of drug is associated with a high risk of relapse in children receiving MTX for maintenance therapy of acute lymphocytic leukemia (ALL).[18]

The distribution of MTX into third-space fluid collections, such as pleural effusions and ascitic fluid, can substantially alter MTX pharmacokinetics. The slow release of accumulated MTX from these third spaces over time prolongs the terminal half-life of the drug, leading to potentially increased clinical toxicity.[19] Although no strict guidelines exist for the treatment of patients with ascites or pleural effusions, it is advisable to evacuate these fluid collections before treatment, monitor plasma drug concentrations closely, and reduce dosages in proportion to the terminal half-life of drug.

Elimination of MTX occurs primarily through renal excretion. MTX is filtered by the glomerulus and is actively secreted in the proximal tubule. Renal clearance usually equals or exceeds creatinine clearance. However, rates of drug clearance may vary widely and do not precisely parallel renal function. Renal excretion of MTX is inhibited by probenecid, penicillins, cephalosporins, aspirin, and nonsteroidal antiinflammatory drugs.[1a] The combination of MTX and nonsteroidal antiinflammatory drugs has been associated with severe MTX toxicity in patients receiving high-dose MTX.[20] Patients with impaired renal function (creatinine clearance less than 60 ml/min) should not be treated with high-dose MTX and should have standard MTX doses reduced in proportion to reductions in creatinine clearance.

The introduction of high-dose MTX regimens has led to the recognition of at least two MTX metabolites. 7-Hydroxy-methotrexate (7-OH-MTX) constitutes 20% to 46% of drug excreted in urine from 12 to 24 hours after the start of a high-dose infusion.[21] It is formed through the action of aldehyde oxidase in the liver and is a weak inhibitor of DHFR. 7-OH-MTX serves as a substrate for folylpolyglutamyl synthetase, and the resulting polyglutamates are inhibitors of the folate-dependent enzymes TS and AICAR transformylase, with a potency similar to that of MTX polyglutamates.[22] A second metabolite, DAMPA, a product of bacterial degradation of MTX in the gut lumen, is inactive and constitutes approximately 25% of the excreted drug at 24 to 48 hours after drug infusion.[23] The exact role of these metabolites in producing MTX toxicity or enhancing therapeutic activity is uncertain.

Biliary excretion of MTX represents approximately 10% of overall MTX drug clearance.[24] However, in the presence of renal dysfunction, enterohepatic circulation may represent an important determinant of drug elimination. Most of MTX excreted in bile is reabsorbed as intact drug, but an undefined fraction is converted by intestinal flora to DAMPA.[18] Intestinal binding of drug with oral charcoal or the anion-exchange resin cholestyramine enhances nonrenal drug excretion.[25] Given the relatively minor role of biliary excretion in drug elimination, no adjustments in MTX dose are necessary for patients with hepatic dysfunction.

SCHEDULES OF ADMINISTRATION

The safe use of high-dose MTX with leucovorin rescue requires a thorough understanding of MTX pharmacokinetics. High-dose MTX therapy has found application in the treatment of lymphomas, osteogenic sarcoma, and acute leukemia. These regimens employ otherwise lethal infusions of MTX given over 6 to 42 hours in doses of 500 mg/m^2 or higher. High-dose MTX can be safely administered to patients provided that careful attention is paid to intravenous fluid hydration, plasma drug level monitoring, and adequate administration of leucovorin. A typical high-dose MTX regimen is listed in Table 18–12.

During infusion of high-dose MTX, rapid renal excretion results in high urinary drug concentrations. Urinary MTX concentrations approaching 10 mmol/L exceed solubility, leading to intratubular precipitation and acute renal failure with potentially disastrous consequences. This complication can be avoided by vigorous hydration (3 liters of fluid/m^2/per 24 hours, beginning 12 hours before infusion and continuing for 36 hours), and urinary alkalinization to increase drug solubility (see Table 18–12). The MTX infusion should not begin until urine flow is 100 ml/hour and urine pH is 7 or greater, and these parameters need to be carefully monitored during the course of therapy. High-dose MTX therapy should not be used in patients with impaired renal function (creatinine clearance less than 60 ml/min).

Close monitoring of MTX plasma levels is essential for safe high-dose MTX therapy. The values presented in Table 18–12 are useful to guide the duration and the amount of leucovorin required to prevent severe MTX-associated toxicity.[26] Because of the competitive interaction between MTX and leucovorin, the dose of the rescue agent must be increased in proportion to the plasma concentration of MTX. Leucovorin therapy is continued until the plasma concentration decreases below 5×10^{-8} M. In patients with delayed MTX excretion,

TABLE 18–12. High-Dose Methotrexate Therapy

1. *Prehydration*
   In 12 h before treatment, establish diuresis with1.5 L/m^2 D$_5$W with 100 mEq HCO$_3^-$ and 20 mEq KCl per L. Test urine *p*H to assure neutrality (*p*H 7 or >7) at time of drug infusion.
2. *Drug Infusion*
   a. Jaffe regimen: 50–250 mg/kg MTX over 6-h infusion. Continue hydration (3 L/m^2) for 24 h. Begin leucovorin 2 h after end of drug infusion, 15 mg/m^2 1 M q 6h × 7 doses.
   b. Alternative: bolus administration of 50 mg/m^2 MTX intravenously followed by infusion of MTX over 36-h period at dose of 1.5 g/m^2. At 36 h, begin leucovorin infusion 200 mg/m^2 for 12 h. At 48 h, give leucovorin 25 mg/m^2 q 6h × 6 doses 1 M.
3. *Monitor Points*
   For Jaffe regimen and for 36-h infusion, drug levels 5 × 10^{-7} M at 48 h require additional leucovorin rescue.

Drug Level	*Dose Leucovorin*
5 × 10^{-7} M	15 mg/m^2 q 6h × 8 doses
1 × 10^{-6} M	100 mg/m^2 q 6h × 8 doses
2 × 10^{-6} M	200 mg/m^2 q 6h × 8 doses

Drug levels should be repeated every 48 h and leucovorin dose adjusted until drug concentration is less than 5 × 10^{-8} M.

MTX, methotrexate.

leucovorin is usually given intravenously, because its oral bioavailability is decreased at total doses higher than 40 mg.

Despite careful monitoring, persistent elevations of plasma MTX levels may sometimes occur. Plasma MTX levels higher than 10^{-5} M at 48 hours are poorly rescued even by high doses of leucovorin.[26] Hemodialysis and peritoneal dialysis are ineffective in removing MTX, with clearance rates of only 35 to 40 ml/min. Experimental approaches to the removal of toxic levels of MTX include hemoperfusion over a charcoal column, oral administration of activated charcoal or cholestyramine to increase enterohepatic drug loss, and infusions of the degradative enzyme carboxypeptidase G$_2$.[12]

MTX penetrates poorly into the cerebrospinal fluid (CSF). CSF levels are 30-fold lower than plasma levels at equilibrium.[27] However, after high-dose MTX therapy, peak CSF levels greater than the therapeutic threshold of 1 μM can be achieved. Systemic high-dose MTX therapy has been used to prevent meningeal leukemia and lymphoma. Intrathecal injection of MTX can also be used for prophylaxis. For treatment of meningeal carcinomatosis, injection of MTX through an indwelling Ommaya reservoir is recommended because drug administered into the CSF via the lumbar space poorly circulates into the ventricles. A total intrathecal dose of 12 mg is advised for all persons older than 3 years of age. In normal patients, the CSF half-life is approximately 12 hours, but it may be prolonged in patients with active meningeal disease. Delayed clearance from the CSF has been associated with an increased risk of MTX neurotoxicity.

TOXICITY

The primary toxic effects of MTX therapy are myelosuppression and gastrointestinal mucositis. The occurrence of these adverse effects and other toxicities depends on the dose, schedule, and route of drug administration. Mucositis usually

appears 3 to 7 days after MTX therapy and precedes the decrease in granulocyte and platelet count by several days. Myelosuppression and mucositis usually are completely reversed within 14 days, unless drug elimination mechanisms are impaired. In patients with compromised renal function, even small doses of MTX may result in serious bone marrow toxicity.

MTX-induced nephrotoxicity is thought to result from the intratubular precipitation of MTX and its metabolites, 7-OH-MTX and DAMPA, in acidic urine. Antifolates may also exert a direct toxic effect on the renal tubules. Vigorous hydration and urinary alkalinization reduce the incidence of renal failure to less than 1% in high-dose regimens.[1a]

MTX is associated with both acute and chronic hepatotoxicity. Acute elevations in hepatic enzyme levels, as well as hyperbilirubinemia, are often observed during high-dose therapy, but these usually return to normal within 10 days. Chronic administration of daily oral MTX, as used in the treatment of psoriasis, is associated with hepatic fibrosis in as many as 25% of patients.[28] On rare occasions, cirrhosis of the liver also may develop. Intermittent, weekly MTX therapy, rather than continuous daily treatment, is associated with a lower incidence of hepatotoxicity. Although the precise mechanism of MTX hepatotoxicity is not known, liver biopsies of patients with drug-induced liver disease demonstrate increased lipid deposition in the liver. In animal models, this pathologic picture can be reversed by administration of choline, suggesting that MTX hepatotoxicity may result from impaired choline synthesis.[29]

MTX causes a poorly defined, self-limited pneumonitis characterized by fever, cough, and interstitial pulmonary infiltrates.[30] Lung biopsies have not revealed consistent pathologic findings. Although a hypersensitivity reaction has been proposed as a possible explanation, rechallenge with MTX does not uniformly result in a return of symptoms. With the increasing use of chronic, low-dose MTX therapy for rheumatoid arthritis, there are now a number of cases of MTX-associated lung damage. No specific therapy for MTX pneumonitis is recommended other than withholding MTX therapy during the acute episode.

Three distinct neurotoxic syndromes are associated with intrathecal MTX therapy.[31] The most common syndrome is an acute chemical arachnoiditis that arises immediately after intrathecal drug administration. This syndrome is characterized by severe headaches, nuchal rigidity, vomiting, fever, and an inflammatory cell infiltrate in the CSF. These symptoms can be avoided by decreasing the dose of MTX. A subacute form of neurotoxicity is seen in approximately 10% of patients and occurs after the third or fourth course of intrathecal therapy. It is most common in adults with active meningeal leukemia and consists of motor paralysis, cranial nerve palsies, and seizures or coma, or both. A change in therapy is absolutely indicated, because continued intrathecal MTX therapy may result in death. The third syndrome is a chronic, demyelinating encephalopathy, typically occurring in children months to years after receiving intrathecal MTX. Patients present with dementia, limb spasticity and, in advanced cases, coma. Computed tomography (CT) scan reveals ventricular enlargement, cortical thinning, and diffuse intracerebral calcifications.[32]

High-dose systemic MTX therapy is occasionally associated

with an encephalopathy consisting of dementia and motor paresis developing in the second or third month after treatment.[33] Acute, transient cerebral dysfunction with symptoms of paresis, aphasia, behavioral abnormalities, and seizures occurs in 4% to 15% of patients.[34] Symptoms occur within 6 days of MTX treatment and usually completely resolve within 48 to 72 hours.

The underlying mechanism(s) of central nervous system (CNS) toxicity from MTX is unknown. Cranial irradiation decreases the blood–brain barrier to MTX and, because of the frequent combined use of these agents in patients, this interaction may represent an important mechanism of enhanced toxicity. There is no evidence to support the use of leucovorin in patients who develop neurotoxic symptoms.

True anaphylactic reactions to MTX are exceedingly rare. There have been a few reported cases of toxic skin erythema and desquamation of the hands after high-dose MTX therapy. In men treated with high-dose MTX, a reversible defect in spermatogenesis also may occur. However, no alterations in reproductive function have been reported in women treated with MTX.

NEW ANTIFOLATES

Several new antifolates have entered clinical trials (see Fig. 18–2). Lipophilic antifolates—such as trimetrexate and a related analog, pyritrexim—may be especially useful against human tumors resistant to MTX because of transport deficiency.[34a,35] In addition, several pteroyl glutamate analogs have shown superior preclinical activity, resulting from enhanced transport, more avid polyglutamation, or a unique site of action compared with MTX. 10-Ethyl-5-deaza-aminopterin, a potent inhibitor of DHFR with enhanced transport and more efficient polyglutamation relative to MTX, has activity against human lung cancer, mucositis being the dose-limiting toxicity.[36]

Two new antifolates, 10-propargyl-5,8-dideazafolate (CB3717) and *N*-(5-[*N*-(3,4-dihydro-2-methyl-4-oxoquinazolin-6-ylmethyl)-*N*-methylamino]-2-thenoyl)-L-glutamic acid (ICI D1694) are potent inhibitors of TS.[37] Both compounds are transported into cells by the reduced folate transport system and are metabolized intracellularly to their active polyglutamate forms. Unfortunately, in phase I clinical trials, CB3717 was associated with severe and erratic nephrotoxicity. D1694 is currently undergoing phase I testing. 5,10-Dideazatetrahydrofolate, a new antifolate that impairs de novo purine synthesis by virtue of its direct inhibitory effects on GAR transformylase, is presently undergoing phase II clinical investigation.[38]

FLUOROPYRIMIDINES

Most of the active antitumor agents presently in clinical use have been discovered by serendipitous observation or screening. 5-Fluorouracil (5-FU), synthesized by Dr. Charles Heidelberger and colleagues, represents a notable exception.[39] The rationale for the synthesis of fluorinated pyrimidines stemmed from the observation that rat hepatoma cells use uracil more efficiently than normal rat intestinal mucosa. This finding suggested that uracil might represent an exploitable target for cancer chemotherapy.

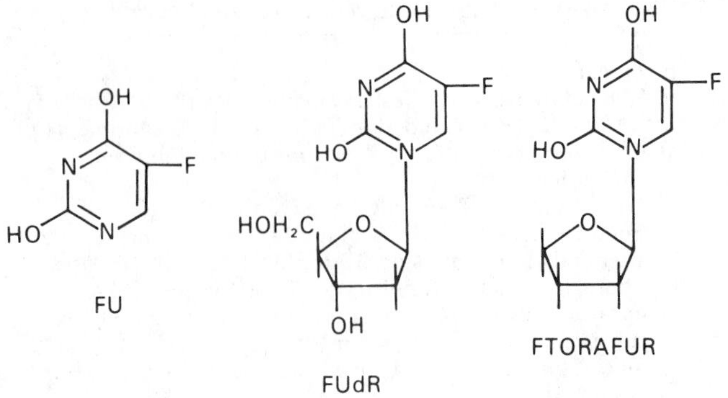

FIGURE 18–10. Structures of clinically useful 5-fluoropyrimidines.

The chemical structures of the fluoropyrimidines of clinical interest are shown in Figure 18–10. 5-FU has a fluorine atom substituted for hydrogen at the 5-carbon position of the pyrimidine ring. The deoxyribonucleoside derivative 5-fluoro-2'-deoxyuridine (FUDR) has been limited in its clinical use by rapid degradation in normal and tumor tissues. Currently, it is mainly used for intraarterial hepatic infusions. Activation to the nucleotide (ribose phosphate) form is essential for the antitumor activity of all the fluoropyrimidine compounds.

5-FU has antitumor activity (10–40% overall response rate) against many solid tumors, including breast, gastrointestinal, head and neck, and ovarian carcinomas. It has synergistic interactions with other antineoplastic agents, with irradiation, with physiologic nucleosides such as thymidine and uridine, and with the interferons. As a result, 5-FU is currently most often administered in the setting of combination therapy.

MECHANISM OF ACTION

The fluoropyrimidines require intracellular activation to exert their cytotoxic effects. These compounds are converted by multiple alternative biochemical pathways (Fig. 18–11) to one of several active cytotoxic forms. 5-FU is converted to FUDR by thymidine phosphorylase. Subsequent phosphorylation of FUDR by thymidine kinase results in formation of the active 5-FU metabolite, FdUMP. In the presence of the reduced folate, 5,10-methylenetetrahydrofolate, FdUMP forms a stable covalent complex with TS, inhibiting TS enzyme activity and leading to depletion of deoxythymidine triphosphate (dTTP), a necessary precursor for DNA synthesis.[40] Second, 5-FU may be anabolized to fluorouridine monophosphate (FUMP) through the sequential action of uridine phosphorylase and uridine kinase or through direct conversion by orotic acid phosphoribosyltransferase in the presence of 5'-phosphoribosyl-1-pyrophosphate (PRPP). FUMP may be further metabolized to fluorouridine triphosphate (FUTP), which may be incorporated into RNA or converted to the deoxyribonucleotide FdUMP.[41] Third, FdUMP may be subsequently phosphorylated to the triphosphate form, 5-fluoro-2'-deoxyuridine-5'-triphosphate, which may then be incorporated into DNA.[42]

Inhibition of TS by FdUMP is one of the principal mechanisms of 5-FU action. The TS-FdUMP-folate complex is slowly dissociable, with a half-life of 6 hours in intact cells. The presence of the reduced folate cofactor is critical for complex formation as well as for sustaining enzyme inhibition. Deple-

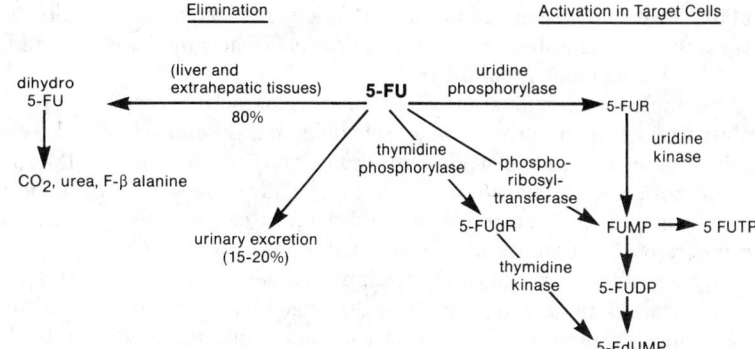

FIGURE 18–11. Pathways of 5-fluorouracil elimination and activation.

tion of intracellular reduced folates prevents ternary complex formation as demonstrated in various tissue culture systems.[43] Some tumors appear to be relatively deficient in reduced folates and are killed more effectively by 5-FU when it is given in combination with leucovorin (5-formyltetrahydrofolate, citrovorum factor). In the clinical setting, the combination of 5-FU and leucovorin has enhanced antitumor activity compared with 5-FU alone.[44,45]

5-FU is extensively incorporated into both nuclear and cytoplasmic RNA, and this incorporation alters RNA processing and function. However, the specific molecular locus for cytotoxicity by this RNA-mediated mechanism remains unclear. Incorporation of 5-FU into RNA inhibits the conversion of high-molecular-weight nuclear RNA species to lower-molecular-weight ribosomal RNA.[46] Relatively low concentrations of 5-FU inhibit polyadenylation of mRNA, thereby affecting the stability of this RNA species.[47] Incorporation of 5-FU into RNA affects both quantitative and qualitative aspects of protein synthesis; in the presence of RNA-containing 5-FU moieties, translational miscoding can occur.[48]

Incorporation of 5-FU into DNA, another mechanism of cytotoxicity, inhibits DNA elongation and alters DNA stability, with production of DNA single-strand breaks and DNA fragmentation.[49] The fluoropyrimidines may also induce DNA strand breaks without being directly incorporated into DNA, possibly through inhibition of DNA repair consequent to dTTP depletion.[50]

Uridine nucleotide sugars, such as uridine-5'-diphosphate (UDP)-glucose and UDP-N-acetylhexoseamines are substrates for glycosyltransferases, which catalyze the glycosylation of proteins and lipids. 5-FU also serves as a substrate for the synthesis of FUDP-sugars such as FUDP-hexoses and FUDP-N-acetylhexoseamines, which may alter cell membrane function.[51,52]

The relative contribution of each of these various mechanisms of action to the clinical activity of 5-FU remains unclear and may depend on the specific patterns of intracellular 5-FU metabolism that vary among different normal tissues and tumor types. The concentration of drug as well as the duration of exposure may also play a crucial role in determining the mechanism of cytotoxicity, with higher doses favoring an RNA-directed mechanism. However, the enhanced activity of 5-FU in combination with leucovorin suggests that the inhibition of TS is central to the clinical activity of 5-FU.

MECHANISMS OF RESISTANCE

Given the multiple sites of cytotoxic action of 5-FU and the multiple steps required for its activation, a number of different mechanisms of resistance have been identified in experimental and clinical settings. However, the relative frequency with which each of these mechanisms is responsible for resistance in humans is unknown.

In human and murine tumor cells, resistance to 5-FU can develop through deletion of one of the key enzymes (uridine kinase, uridine phosphorylase, or orotic acid phosphorylase) required for its activation. Increased activity of catabolic enzymes such as acid and alkaline phosphatases leading to decreased accumulation of 5-FU nucleotides has been implicated.[52] A relative deficiency of the reduced folate substrate 5,10-methylenetetrahydrofolate may also compromise the cytotoxic action of FdUMP on TS. Moreover, inability to convert 5,10-methylenetetrahydrofolate to a higher polyglutamate has also been correlated with resistance to 5-FU. Some resistant mutant cell lines have elevated intracellular cytidine triphosphate (CTP).[53] This increase in CTP pools results in feedback inhibition of uridine kinase and inhibits 5-FU conversion to the active nucleotide forms. Decreased incorporation of 5-FU into both RNA and DNA has also been found in various cell lines resistant to the fluoropyrimidines.[54]

Alterations in the target enzyme TS can lead to resistance to 5-FU. A decrease in binding affinity of the 5-FU metabolite FdUMP to the TS target, accompanied by 5-FU resistance, has resulted from mutations in the protein-coding region of the *TS* gene.[55,56] In cell lines made resistant to the fluoropyrimidines in vitro, increases in the levels of TS protein have been described, usually associated with amplification of the *TS* gene.[57] In cell lines made resistant to cisplatin or doxorubicin, simultaneous resistance to 5-FU develops on the basis of increased TS expression.[58] In this instance, the increase in *TS* results from increased transcription rather than from *TS* gene amplification. In many murine tumors and during clinical chemotherapy, the levels of TS protein acutely increase in malignant cells after exposure to 5-FU.[58,59] This process appears to be mediated through interference with FdUMP of the normal inhibitory effect of *TS* on translation of its own mRNA.[60] Although the precise mechanism by which TS enzyme induction remains an active area of investigation, it is known that this process allows the cells to resist rapidly the effects of 5-FU.

CLINICAL PHARMACOLOGY AND PHARMACOKINETICS

The most rapid and sensitive technique currently employed for measuring 5-FU is HPLC, using anion exchange or reverse-phase columns.[61] The sensitivity of these methods approaches 50 nM 5-FU in plasma and can be enhanced by derivatization of 5-FU with fluorescent conjugates. Magnetic resonance imaging with ^{19}F now allows monitoring of the pharmacokinetics and in vivo metabolism of 5-FU.[62]

A complete understanding of 5-FU pharmacokinetics is required to select the proper route, schedule, and dose of administration. Each route of administration—oral, intravenous, intraarterial, or intraperitoneal—has unique advantages and disadvantages that determine its usefulness in cancer chemotherapy. The clinical efficacy and pattern of toxicity seen with each of these routes can be explained, at least partially, by pharmacokinetic considerations. Prolonged exposures to low concentrations of 5-FU cause gastrointestinal toxicity and mucositis, and higher intermittent doses result in myelosuppression.

Oral bioavailability is erratic, as less than 75% of an oral dose reaches the systemic circulation. Plasma levels also vary as a result of variable first-pass metabolism in the liver.[63] Given these considerations, it is widely accepted that 5-FU should not be given by the oral route. After intravenous bolus or infusion, 5-FU penetrates well into the CSF and extracellular third-space fluids, such as ascites and pleural effusions. After conventional single doses of 400 to 600 mg/m^2 (10–15 mg/kg), peak plasma concentrations reach 0.2 to 1 mM, but rapid breakdown by dihydropyrimidine dehydrogenase to dihydrofluorouracil (DHFU) in the liver and other tissues leads to an abrupt fall in plasma concentrations. The primary plasma half-life of 5-FU is 6 to 20 minutes, but it may vary considerably between patients. Within a few hours of injection, plasma levels of 5-FU fall below 1 μM, the concentration thought to be the approximate threshold for exerting cytotoxic effects on normal tissue.

Because they are metabolized by the liver, 5-FU or FUDR can be infused directly into the hepatic artery or portal vein to maximize the exposure of hepatic metastases while limiting systemic toxicity. Intrahepatic arterial infusion at a rate of 30 mg/kg/day results in plasma levels in the range of 0.13 to 0.35 μM, thus explaining the relative lack of myelosuppression resulting from this form of therapy.[64] At this infusion rate, more than 50% of the infused drug is cleared in its first pass through the liver. Portal infusion of 5-FU in the adjuvant setting has been associated with a decreased incidence of hepatic metastases in patients with Dukes' stage B colon cancer after surgical resection of the primary tumor.[65] In the recent National Surgical Adjuvant Breast and Bowel Project, adjuvant portal vein infusion of 5-FU failed to reduce the incidence of hepatic metastases.[66] However, a significant increase in the disease-free survival was observed in treated patients, suggesting a systemic effect of the infused 5-FU.

5-FU may also be administered by the intraperitoneal route, particularly for the treatment of ovarian cancer, to take advantage of the high intraperitoneal concentration of drug (4 mM/L), the slow absorption of drug into the portal circulation, its rapid metabolism in the liver, and the relatively small amounts of drug that reach the systemic circulation.[67] Minimal systemic toxicity occurs when drug concentrations are maintained below 4 mM/L in the peritoneal cavity as a result of an approximately 300:1 gradient in drug concentration between the peritoneal fluid and the peripheral venous circulation. The efficacy of this therapy, however, remains uncertain.

More than 80% of administered 5-FU by an intravenous or intraarterial route is eliminated by metabolic conversion by dihydropyrimidine dehydrogenase to DHFU, and 20% is excreted intact in the urine. Rare persons deficient in this enzyme have greatly increased toxicity when treated with standard doses of 5-FU.[68] The primary metabolite, DHFU, is cleaved further to yield α-fluoroureidoproprionic acid, α-fluoro-β-alanine, and carbon dioxide. The liver, kidney, white blood cells, and gastrointestinal mucosa are the primary sites of 5-FU metabolism. Because metabolism occurs in extrahepatic tissues, doses of 5-FU do not need to be reduced in the presence of hepatic dysfunction.

Unlike the parent compound, the active 5-FU nucleotides, FdUMP and FUTP, have prolonged intracellular half-lives. Their decay rates vary among individual tissues, and their continued presence is a critical determinant of the duration and magnitude of drug effect.

CLINICAL TOXICITY

The primary effects of 5-FU are exerted on rapidly dividing tissues, specifically the gastrointestinal mucosa and the bone marrow. The spectrum of toxicities associated with 5-FU varies considerably according to the dose, schedule, and route of administration. After bolus intravenous therapy—using a 5-day course or single, weekly doses—myelosuppression is the dose-limiting toxicity observed, the nadir of leukopenia and thrombocytopenia generally occurring between the 9th and 14th day after the first injection of drug. Stomatitis and diarrhea are also frequent side effects, particularly in patients who receive a 5-day regimen. The diarrhea may be watery or bloody and life-threatening. Repeated episodes of watery diarrhea (more than three movements per day) for several days should alert the oncologist to the potential dangers of dehydration and sepsis, which represent a potentially fatal side effect. On complete recovery, subsequent courses of 5-FU therapy should be reinstituted at a reduced dose.

An alternative regimen using continuous intravenous infusion of 5-FU at doses of 30 mg/kg/day for 5 days gives equivalent therapeutic results but a different pattern of toxicity.[69] Gastrointestinal symptoms, such as stomatitis and diarrhea, are the principal dose-limiting toxicities, but myelosuppression is less intense. When 5-FU is given in combination with leucovorin in patients with metastatic colon cancer, enhanced gastrointestinal toxicity is observed irrespective of the 5-FU schedule.

Continuous intrahepatic infusion of 5-FU or FUDR is a useful alternative to intravenous therapy in patients with hepatic metastases. The response rates reported for the treatment of colon cancer patients with hepatic metastases approach 50%. Because at least 50% of 5-FU and more than 95% of FUDR are cleared in their first pass through the liver, systemic toxicity with this form of therapy is mild, consisting primarily of oral mucositis and gastrointestinal symptoms, such as nausea, vomiting, diarrhea and, less frequently, myelosuppression. Cholestatic jaundice associated with biliary sclerosis is a serious complication of intrahepatic infusion and is believed to result from perfusion of the blood supply to the gallbladder and upper bile duct with high local concentrations of drug. The median time to onset of biliary sclerosis is three treatment cycles and, although fluoropyrimidine therapy may be reinstituted at a lower dose after normalization of serum hepatic enzyme levels, most patients become progressively less tolerant. Catheter-related complications may also result from intrahepatic arterial infusion and include thrombosis of the extremity vessel used for percutaneous catheterization; hemorrhage or infection at the site of insertion; or slippage of the catheter into the gastroduodenal artery with resultant necrosis of the intestinal epithelium, hemorrage, and perforation. The physician must be alert to the sudden onset of epigastric pain or vomiting in the patient and understand the need to reassess catheter position promptly.

Less common adverse effects caused by 5-FU include dermatologic toxicity (hand-foot syndrome), which is often associated with continuous intravenous infusion therapy. Alopecia, dermatitis, increased pigmentation, and atrophy of the skin have been observed. 5-FU can enhance the cutaneous toxicity associated with radiation therapy, leading to onset of erythema and skin desquamation within 7 days of initiation of radiation. Acute neurologic symptoms, including somnolence, cerebellar ataxia, and upper motor signs, are primarily seen in patients receiving intracarotid infusions for head and neck tumors, but neurologic toxicity has been observed in patients given single-agent 5-FU in high doses. This syndrome is reproduced in animals by fluorocitrate, a neurotoxic 5-FU metabolite.[70] Several reports have detailed a syndrome of chest pain, serum enzyme elevations, and electrocardiographic changes consistent with myocardial ischemia in temporal association with 5-FU administration.[71] The underlying reason for this form of cardiac toxicity is unclear.

5-FU is also associated with significant ocular toxicity that includes blepharitis, epiphora, tear-duct stenosis, and acute and chronic conjunctivitis. The acute inflammatory response is reversible when the drug is discontinued early in the treatment course, but progression may require surgical correction of ectropion and tear-duct stenosis.

DRUG INTERACTIONS

Various antineoplastic compounds, including purine and pyrimidine analogs, and biochemical modulating agents have been used in combination with the fluoropyrimidines in an attempt to enhance both the cytotoxicity and therapeutic selectivity of fluoropyrimidine chemotherapy.

The interaction of 5-FU with MTX is of particular interest because of the frequent use of both drugs in combination chemotherapy. When given before 5-FU, MTX increases 5-FU nucleotide metabolite formation by increasing the intracellular content of phosphoribosylpyrophosphate (PRPP), a substrate required in the orotic acid phosphoribosyltransferase reaction.[72] Clinical studies provide supportive evidence for the importance of sequence in the interaction between 5-FU and MTX.[72]

In vitro studies have demonstrated that 5-FU cytotoxicity is increased with the addition of 5-formyltetrahydrofolate (leucovorin), a finding confirmed by randomized clinical trials.[44,73,74]

The interferons (IFNs) have been investigated extensively as biochemical modulators of fluoropyrimidine cytotoxicity. Synergistic cytotoxic interactions have been described for each of the IFNs (α, β, and γ) and 5-FU in various human cancer cell lines and in in vivo animal model systems.[75–77] Although the mechanism of interaction of the IFNs and 5-FU remains an active area of investigation, treatment with IFN-γ increases the formation of the 5-FU metabolite FdUMP in a human

leukemic cell line and inhibits the acute increase in TS in response to 5-FU exposure, thereby enhancing overall inhibition of this critical target enzyme.[78,79] In the treatment of advanced colorectal cancer, preliminary results of 5-FU with IFN-α suggest that IFN may enhance the antitumor activity of 5-FU.[80]

The interaction between 5-FU and inhibitors of the de novo pyrimidine synthetic pathway has potential clinical exploitation. N-(phosphonacetyl)-L-aspartate (PALA) inhibits aspartate transcarbamylase, the enzyme that catalyzes the second step in de novo pyrimidine synthesis. Pretreatment with PALA enhances 5-FU cytotoxicity by increasing incorporation of 5-FU nucleotide metabolites into RNA.[81] The combination of 5-FU and PALA has been tested in the clinic, and promising results have recently been reported with a low ("modulatory") dose of PALA (250 mg/m²) followed 24 hours later by a 24-hour infusion of high-dose 5-FU (2600 mg/m²).[82]

Thymidine and other nucleosides enhance 5-FU incorporation into RNA by various mechanisms. In addition, both thymidine and uridine inhibit 5-FU degradation by dihydropyrimidine dehydrogenase, thus prolonging the plasma half-life of 5-FU. In clinical trials, thymidine has enhanced 5-FU host toxicity due to altered pharmacokinetics, but does not improve clinical activity. Salvage of preformed thymidine may represent a potential mechanism by which malignant cells overcome the FdUMP-mediated inhibition of TS. The nucleoside transport inhibitor dipyridamole enhances 5-FU cytotoxicity by its ability to inhibit the uptake of thymidine, thereby decreasing the competing intracellular pools of dTTP for DNA synthesis, and by increasing the intracellular formation of FdUMP.[83] The combination of 5-FU with dipyridamole is currently under clinical investigation.

OTHER FLUOROPYRIMIDINES

Two analogs, ftorafur and 5'-deoxy-5-fluorouridine (dFUrd), have been tested clinically as depot forms of 5-FU, but neither has shown consistent activity. dFUrd is converted to the 5-FU base by uridine phosphorylase.[84] This enzyme is found in many normal tissues but seems to be in relatively higher levels in neoplastic cells. Myelosuppression and gastrointestinal toxicity are dose limiting, although a "hand-foot" dermatopathic syndrome and significant neurotoxicity that includes ataxia, altered mental status, diplopia, and a Wernicke-Korsakoff-like syndrome have also been observed.

CYTARABINE

Cytarabine (cytosine arabinoside; Ara-C) is one of several arabinose nucleosides isolated from the sponge *Cryptothethya crypta*.[85] It differs from its physiologic counterpart deoxycytidine by the presence of an OH group in the 2' position of the sugar (Fig. 18–12). Many arabinose nucleosides have been chemically synthesized or isolated from bacterial broths and tested for activity as antitumor agents. The most prominent of these are the cytidine analog arabinosyl-5-azacytidine and the purine analogs arabinosyl-adenine and fludarabine phosphate. Cytarabine has important clinical activity against human acute myelocytic leukemia (AML).

As a single agent, cytarabine induces remission in 50% of

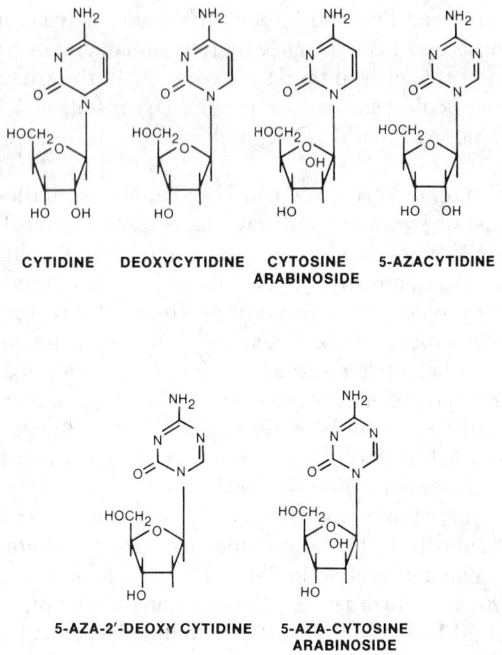

CYTIDINE   DEOXYCYTIDINE   CYTOSINE ARABINOSIDE   5-AZACYTIDINE

5-AZA-2'-DEOXY CYTIDINE   5-AZA-CYTOSINE ARABINOSIDE

FIGURE 18–12. Structure of physiologic cytidine nucleosides and related antimetabolites.

patients with AML, and it is the standard agent in combination with the anthracyclines for treatment of this disease. It is also used in combination therapy for the blast crisis of chronic granulocytic leukemia, for non-Hodgkin's lymphoma, and for childhood acute lymphocytic leukemia (ALL). It has minimal activity as a single agent against solid tumors, presumably because of its lack of metabolic activation in solid tumors and its selective action against rapidly dividing cells.

MECHANISM OF ACTION

In human cells, cytarabine is recognized as an analog of the physiologic nucleoside 2'-deoxycytidine and is metabolized by salvage pathway enzymes to its active cytotoxic form, ara-CTP. This nucleotide is a competitive inhibitor of DNA polymerase-α with respect to the normal substrate 2-deoxycytidine triphosphate (dCTP) ($K_i = 0.1\ \mu M$).[86] The inhibitory effects of cytarabine on DNA polymerase-α extend not only to semiconservative DNA replication but also to the repair of ultraviolet light damage to DNA.[87] A more important biochemical effect of cytarabine results from its incorporation into DNA, a process that correlates closely with cytotoxicity.[88] Incorporation of cytarabine into DNA leads to inhibition of template function, a marked slowing of chain elongation, and a defect in ligation of newly synthesized DNA fragments.[89] There is evidence indicating that cells exposed to cytarabine during the S phase of the cell cycle can reinitiate DNA synthesis, resulting in an abnormal duplication of limited portions of DNA.[90] These reduplicated segments increase the possibility of recombination, crossover, and gene amplification. In some cell lines cytarabine induces a pattern of internucleosomal DNA fragmentation reminiscent of apoptosis (*i.e.*, programmed cell death).[91]

Cytarabine has other biochemical effects, including inhibition of ribonucleotide reductase by the nucleotide ara-CTP

and inhibition of synthesis of membrane glycoproteins and glycolipids by the metabolite ara-CDP-choline, an analog of cytidine-5'-diphosphocholine.[92] In addition to its cytotoxic effects, cytarabine induces terminal differentiation of leukemic cells in tissue culture, an effect that is accompanied in some instances by decreased c-*MYC* oncogene expression.[93] These changes in both morphology and oncogene expression occur at concentrations above the threshold for cytotoxicity and may simply represent terminal injury of cells. However, molecular analysis of bone marrow specimens from some leukemic patients in remission has revealed persistence of leukemic markers, suggesting that differentiation may have occurred in response to cytarabine therapy.[94]

Cytarabine enters cells by an active nucleoside transport system that allows the rapid achievement of steady-state intracellular drug concentrations. There is a strong correlation between the number of transport sites and formation of the intracellular cytotoxic metabolite ara-CTP.[95] Transport into the cell is an important determinant of cytarabine sensitivity of human leukemic cells. At high drug concentrations (>10 μmol), cytarabine also enters cells by passive diffusion, a less efficient mechanism.

Cytarabine is converted intracellularly to its active form, aracytidine triphosphate (ara-CTP), through the sequential action of three enzymes: deoxycytidine kinase, deoxycytidylate (dCMP) kinase, and nucleoside diphosphate kinase. Two inactivating enzymes, cytidine deaminase and dCMP deaminase, may also act on cytarabine or ara-CMP, respectively, to form the inactive products ara-U or ara-UMP. Cytidine deaminase is widely distributed in mammalian tissues, including gastrointestinal epithelium, liver, and granulocytes.[96] The balance between intracellular activation and degradation is critical in determining the amount of drug that will ultimately be converted to the active nucleotide, ara-CTP. Because these deaminating enzymes are frequently found in high concentrations relative to activating enzymes, they may limit the intracellular accumulation of cytarabine-active nucleotides.

As an inhibitor of DNA synthesis, cytarabine kills cells selectively during the S phase of the cell cycle. Because longer exposures allow cytarabine to be incorporated into the DNA of a greater fraction of cells as they pass through S phase, the duration of exposure to cytarabine is directly correlated with cell kill. The cytotoxicity of cytarabine appears to be not only cycle specific but also dependent on the rate of DNA synthesis. Cytotoxic effects are greatest when cells are exposed to cytarabine during periods of rapid DNA synthesis. A second dose of cytarabine 8 to 10 days after the first dose may improve the therapeutic outcome.[96a]

MECHANISM OF RESISTANCE

The biochemical and molecular changes underlying the development of resistance to cytarabine were discussed in the section on drug resistance and include deoxycytidine (dCdr) kinase deficiency.[97] Recently, the potential clinical relevance of this mechanism of resistance has been confirmed in a study in which cell lines from a leukemic patient were established before and after high-dose cytarabine therapy.[98] The resistant cells had one fifth the pretreatment dCdr kinase activity found in sensitive cells, resulting in a significantly lower intracellular level of ara-CTP. A second mechanism of resistance, increased intracellular pools of dCTP, results from increased cytidine-5′-triphosphate (CTP) synthetase activity or through deficiency of dCMP deaminase.[99] Altered transport of cytarabine resulting from a decreased number of nucleoside transport sites has been described as another potential mechanism of resistance. In a clinical study, the cytarabine transport capacity of acute nonlymphocytic leukemic cells closely correlated with subsequent achievement of complete remission.[100]

A number of investigators have attempted to correlate resistance in the clinical setting with alterations in dCdr kinase, CdR deaminase, or cytarabine transport. Most studies have shown significant variation in enzyme levels among patients with AML or ALL with no clear pattern in resistant cells. Although the specific biochemical process(es) associated with resistance to cytarabine remains unclear, the current understanding of the cytotoxic action of cytarabine suggests that the uptake of cytarabine, formation of ara-CTP, and the half-life of ara-CTP in leukemic cells are the critical determinants of response.

CLINICAL PHARMACOLOGY AND PHARMACOKINETICS

A variety of assay methods have been used to measure cytarabine concentrations in plasma, including gas chromatography[100] and radioimmunoassay.[100a] The preferred method for cytarabine assay is HPLC. This technique cleanly separates cytarabine from its primary metabolite, ara-U, and it has the requisite specificity and sensitivity (0.1 μM).[101] A more rapid technique is the radioimmunoassay that uses a sheep antibody to a cytarabine conjugate with albumin.[102] This assay system is highly specific for cytarabine and probably more sensitive than HPLC. Because cytarabine is subject to deamination by cytidine deaminase in plasma, it is necessary to include tetrahydrouridine (THU), a cytidine deaminase inhibitor, in plasma samples immediately after blood samples are collected.

The presence of high concentrations of cytidine deaminase in the gastrointestinal epithelium and liver prevents the effective use of orally administered cytarabine. When administered by the intravenous route, cytarabine crosses into the CNS and reaches steady-state levels at 20% to 40% of those found simultaneously in plasma after 2 hours of continuous intravenous infusion.[103] Peak plasma concentrations approach 10 μmol after bolus doses of 100 mg/m^2 and are proportionately higher for doses up to 3 g/m^2 (above 100 μM) given over a 1- or 2-hour infusion. The plasma concentration of cytarabine declines rapidly, with a half-life of 7 to 20 minutes. A second half-life of 30 to 150 minutes has been detected by more sensitive methods, but is probably of little significance for standard-dose regimens. More than 70% of an administered dose is excreted in the urine in the form of the inactive metabolite ara-U. Within minutes of drug injection, ara-U becomes the predominant form of the drug in plasma. Its formation occurs in the plasma, liver, and granulocytes, and ara-U has a relatively longer half-life in plasma (3–6 hours) than does cytarabine.

Increases in plasma cytarabine concentrations are proportional for infusion rates of 0.1 to 2 g/m^2/day. At this highest dose, steady-state plasma levels reach 5 μM. At higher rates of infusion the deamination reaction is saturated and cytarabine plasma levels rise sharply, leading to serious toxicity. To allow rapid achievement of steady-state concentrations, a loading dose of three times the hourly infusion rate should be given.[104]

SCHEDULES OF ADMINISTRATION

Because of its rapid inactivation by cytidine deaminase and its maximal cytotoxic effects during the S phase of the cell cycle, cytarabine is usually administered in bolus doses of 100 mg/m^2 every 8 to 12 hours for 5 to 7 days or by continuous infusion. Other high- and low-dose schedules have been applied in treating leukemia. The more effective of these new regimens is a high-dose scheme, usually 2 to 3 g/m^2 given every 12 hours for 6 days.[105] Low-dose regimens of 3 to 20 mg/m^2/day for up to 3 weeks have been used mainly in the treatment of elderly patients with myelodysplastic syndromes.[106] The rationale for low-dose therapy is based on the presumption that low concentrations of cytarabine promote leukemic cell differentiation with less host toxicity. Unfortunately, low-dose regimens are still associated with the same myelosuppressive side effects as standard schedules.

In addition to conventional administration by intravenous bolus injection or infusion, cytarabine may be given by subcutaneous injection or infusion. Total drug exposure ($C \times T$) is twofold greater than that achieved by the same dose given by the intravenous bolus route.[107] Cytarabine may also be given intrathecally for the treatment of meningeal leukemia or meningeal carcinomatosis. Because deamination is minimal in the CSF, doses of 50 mg/m^2 result in peak levels of 1 mmol, which decline with a half-life of 2 hours. Cytotoxic concentrations of greater than 0.1 μM are maintained for up to 24 hours. Cytarabine is often used intrathecally as a substitute for MTX in patients experiencing MTX-associated neurotoxicity.

Cytarabine may also be administered by the intraperitoneal route, particularly for the treatment of ovarian cancer.[108] After instillation into the peritoneal cavity, cytarabine levels fall with a half-life of approximately 2 hours. Simultaneous plasma concentrations are 100- to 1000-fold lower, presumably because of cytarabine deamination in the liver.

TOXICITY

The main determinants of cytarabine toxicity are drug concentration and duration of drug exposure. In humans, single bolus doses of cytarabine, as high as 4 g/m^2, are fairly well tolerated because of the rapid inactivation of the parent compound and the brief period of exposure, but constant infusion of drug using total doses of 1 g/m^2 for 48 hours results in severe myelosuppression.[109]

The primary toxic side effects of cytarabine are myelosuppression and gastrointestinal epithelial injury. With standard doses of 200 mg/m^2/day for 5 to 7 days, leukopenia and thrombocytopenia reach their maximum in 7 to 14 days. Although the duration of myelosuppression usually lasts 14 to 21 days, it primarily depends on the dose of cytarabine, nature of concomitant therapy, and prior treatment experience.

Gastrointestinal toxicity is prominent in patients receiving cytarabine. The most frequent symptoms include nausea, vomiting, and diarrhea. A spectrum of pathologic changes is observed in the intestinal mucosa, ranging from superficial ulceration to intramural hematoma formation and perforation. Reversible intrahepatic cholestasis occurs frequently, but requires discontinuation of treatment in fewer than 25% of patients. In addition, cytarabine has been implicated as the cause of pancreatitis in a small number of patients.

High-dose cytarabine regimens, using 2 to 3 g/m^2 every 12 hours for 12 doses, cause severe but reversible myelosuppression and gastrointestinal toxicity. A more dangerous toxicity in 20% of patients receiving high-dose regimens involves cerebral and cerebellar dysfunction.[110] Patients older than 50 years of age are particularly susceptible to this toxicity and develop slurred speech, ataxia, confusion, and coma. CNS toxicity occurs more frequently in patients with abnormal serum creatinine levels, despite the fact that cytarabine is primarily eliminated by metabolism and not by urinary excretion. In most instances, the CNS toxicity is reversible, but occasionally has resulted in a fatal outcome. Pulmonary complications, which include noncardiogenic pulmonary edema and *Streptococcus viridans* pneumonia, are being reported with increasing frequency after high-dose cytarabine therapy.[111,112] Other side effects associated with high-dose cytarabine include conjunctivitis, a painful hand-foot syndrome, and, rarely, anaphylaxis. Neutrophilic eccrine hydradenitis, an unusual cutaneous reaction manifested as plaques or nodules, occurs during the second week after high-dose cytarabine administration.[113]

Cytarabine given intrathecally is infrequently associated with fever, seizures, and alterations in mental status occurring within 24 hours after administration. Intrathecal cytarabine should be given with caution in patients who have demonstrated evidence of MTX neurotoxicity.

Cytarabine is teratogenic in animals. Although cytarabine results in chromosomal breaks in cultured cells and in the bone marrow of patients, it is not an established carcinogen in humans.

DRUG INTERACTIONS

Synergistic activity between cytarabine and a number of antitumor agents, including alkylating agents, thiopurines, uridine analogs, and antifolates, has been observed in in vitro and animal tumor model systems. Specific biochemical and cellular kinetic mechanisms have been described for each of these interactions. Unfortunately, the direct application of these various combinations to the clinical setting has been difficult in view of the complex nature of biochemical and kinetic factors in humans. Cytarabine enhances cyclophosphamide, mAMSA, etoposide (VP-16), carmustine (BCNU), and cisplatin activity by inhibiting the repair of strand breaks associated with these agents. Although the precise mechanism of interaction remains unclear, pretreatment with MTX enhances ara-CTP formation in experimental tumors, resulting in greater cytarabine-associated cytotoxicity.[114] Inhibitors of ribonucleotide reductase, such as thymidine and hydroxyurea, also enhance cytarabine cytotoxicity in various cell lines by inhibiting formation of dCDP.[115] 3-Deazauridine and a new cytidine analog, cyclopentenyl cytosine, both inhibit CTP synthetase and lower the levels of dCTP. Both drugs enhance cytarabine cytotoxicity by increasing ara-CTP formation and its subsequent incorporation into DNA.[116]

Potent enhancement of cytarabine cytotoxicity is observed when patients are pretreated with THU, an inhibitor of cytidine deaminase. This compound significantly prolongs the plasma half-life of cytarabine, reduces the tolerable dose by 30-fold, and causes a marked increase in toxicity to the bone marrow.[117] Whether the combination of THU and cytarabine will alter the therapeutic efficacy of cytarabine awaits further investigation.

Biologic response modifiers that stimulate cell proliferation have also demonstrated a synergistic interaction with cytarabine. Treatment with interleukin-3 or GM-CSF before cytarabine results in greater kill of human leukemic cells than cytarabine alone, presumably through the ability of these biologics to increase entry of leukemic cells into the S phase of the cell cycle.[118]

OTHER CYTIDINE ANALOGS

Because of the rapid metabolism and short half-life of cytarabine, attempts have been made to develop new cytidine analogs or treatment strategies that preserve the inhibitory activity of cytarabine but are resistant to deamination. Cytarabine enclosed in liposomes has increased potency resulting from a prolonged half-life in plasma, but this enhanced activity has not translated into improved therapeutic efficacy. Various cytidine deaminase-resistant analogs have been developed, including N^4-acyl compounds, the anhydro analog cyclocytidine, and ara-CMP ester derivatives, but none have demonstrated enhanced therapeutic activity relative to cytarabine.[119–121]

Other cytidine nucleoside compounds with cytotoxic sites of action different from cytarabine have been developed. 5-Azacytidine (5-aza-C), 5-azacytosine arabinoside (ara-AC), and 3-deazauridine have entered clinical trials (see Fig. 18–12). 5-Aza-C has significant activity in the clinical treatment of leukemia. As with cytarabine, it is subject to deamination in plasma, liver, and tumor cells. In contrast with cytarabine, it is phosphorylated by uridine-cytidine kinase to 5-aza-CMP, which is then metabolized to its active, cytotoxic form, 5-aza-CTP, a substrate for RNA polymerase and a competitor with CTP for incorporation into RNA. This incorporation into RNA results in disassembly of polyribosomes, inhibition of RNA processing and function, and marked inhibition of protein synthesis. 5-Aza-C is also incorporated into DNA, resulting in inhibition of DNA methylation.[122] Reduction in cytosine methylation by 5-aza-C incorporation into DNA enhances the expression of a variety of genes, which may explain its ability to induce differentiation of both normal and malignant cells. Low-dose 5-aza-C has been used in clinical trials in an attempt to induce fetal hemoglobin synthesis in patients with sickle cell anemia and thalassemia, but concerns regarding its potential carcinogenicity have prevented routine clinical use.[123] Resistance to 5-aza-C develops mainly through deletion of the activating enzyme uridine-cytidine kinase.

5-Aza-C is rapidly removed from the plasma, through both metabolic clearance and chemical decomposition. Less than 2% of an administered dose remains in plasma as the parent drug 30 minutes after administration. This compound is a substrate for cytidine deaminase, but the metabolite 5-azauridine is chemically unstable and has not been identified in the plasma or urine of patients.

The primary toxicities observed with 5-aza-C are myelosuppression and severe, prolonged nausea and vomiting. When the drug is administered by prolonged or continuous infusion, symptoms of nausea and vomiting are more readily controlled. Other adverse effects include hepatotoxicity, particularly in patients with preexisting hepatic dysfunction, myalgias, transient fever, and pruritic skin rash. This drug has both mutagenic and teratogenic effects, although no second malignancies related to 5-aza-C treatment have been described.

Ara-AC is a synthetic pyrimidine nucleoside analog containing the structural features of both cytarabine and 5-aza-C (see Fig. 18–12). It readily undergoes decomposition in aqueous solution, and its stability is markedly enhanced when dissolved in dimethyl sulfoxide (DMSO). It enters cells through a nucleoside transport mechanism and is subsequently activated through phosphorylation by deoxycytidine kinase. This compound is a poor substrate for cytidine deaminase. Although its specific sites of cytotoxic action are not well defined, it is incorporated into DNA and thereby inhibits DNA synthesis and function.

Unlike cytarabine or 5-aza-C, ara-AC has demonstrated a broad spectrum of activity against a number of solid tumors in both in vitro and in vivo preclinical studies. The dose-limiting toxicity of ara-AC is myelosuppression, with leukopenia occurring more frequently than thrombocytopenia. Mild elevations in liver function tests predominantly manifested by increases in alkaline phosphatase have also been observed. Minor clinical responses have been reported in various tumor types, including AML and carcinomas of the testis and breast.[124] Further clinical trials are presently in progress to investigate the therapeutic activity of this agent against solid tumors.

PURINE ANALOGS

The development of purine analogs in antineoplastic chemotherapy began in 1951 with the initial reports on the 6-thiopurines by Hitchings and Elion.[125] 6-MP and 6-TG continue to be used principally in the management of acute leukemia. 6-MP has an important role in the maintenance therapy of ALL, and 6-TG is active in remission induction and in the maintenance therapy of acute myelogenous leukemia. Other purine analogs from the same research program include azathioprine, a potent immunosuppressive agent; allopurinol,

a xanthine oxidase inhibitor; and the antiviral agents acyclovir, gancyclovir, and arabinosyladenine (ara-A).[126] Two new purine analogs with promising clinical activity are deoxycoformycin, an adenosine deaminase inhibitor effective against hairy cell leukemia, and fludarabine phosphate, an agent useful in the treatment of chronic lymphocytic leukemia (CLL).

The 6-thiopurine analogs have a single substitution of a thiol group in place of the 6-hydroxyl group found in guanine or in the purine base (Fig. 18–13). 6-MP is a structural analog of hypoxanthine, and 6-TG is an analog of guanine. Azathioprine is a derivative of 6-MP and acts as a prodrug, providing for the sustained release of 6-MP.

MECHANISM OF ACTION

6-MP and 6-TG have similar effects on cellular biochemistry; they inhibit de novo purine synthesis and purine interconversion reactions and their nucleotide metabolites are incorporated into nucleic acids. The relative contribution of each of these actions to the mechanism of cytotoxicity of these agents is unclear.[127] Both 6-MP and 6-TG are converted to their respective monophosphates by hypoxanthine-guanine phosphoribosyl transferase (HGPRT; Fig. 18–14). These ribonucleotide monophosphates inhibit the first step of de novo purine synthesis at the level of the enzyme glutamine phosphoribosylpyrophosphate amidotransferase and block the conversion of inosinic acid to adenylic acid or to guanylic acid. This inhibition of purine nucleotide synthesis leads to the buildup of 5-phosphoribosylpyrophosphate (PRPP), which facilitates the activation of 6-MP and 6-TG to their active nucleotide forms by HGPRT. Inhibitors of de novo purine biosynthesis, such as MTX, are synergistic with 6-thiopurines because the MTX-induced block in purine synthesis expands the PRPP pool required for thiopurine activation. The triphosphate nucleotides of 6-TG and 6-MP incorporate into DNA, resulting in an increase in DNA strand breaks.[128] Incorporation of thiopurine nucleotides into DNA correlates with delayed cytotoxicity.[129]

Biochemical resistance to the 6-thiopurines results from a decreased ability to form active nucleotide metabolites. In experimental systems, resistant cells have a complete or partial deficiency of HGPRT.[130] Alterations in the affinity of HGPRT for the 6-thiopurines have also been described.[131] In

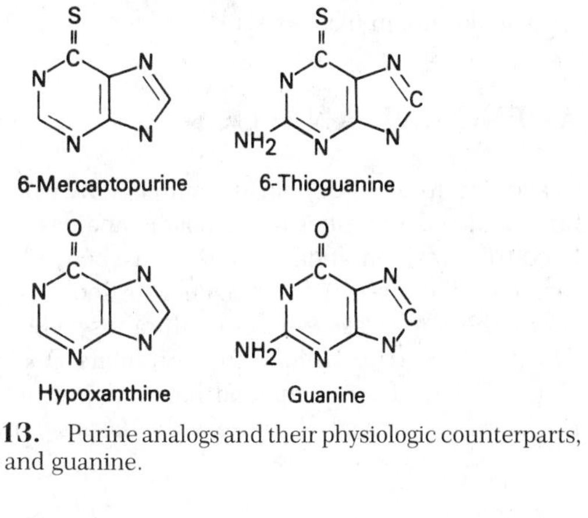

FIGURE 18–13. Purine analogs and their physiologic counterparts, hypoxanthine and guanine.

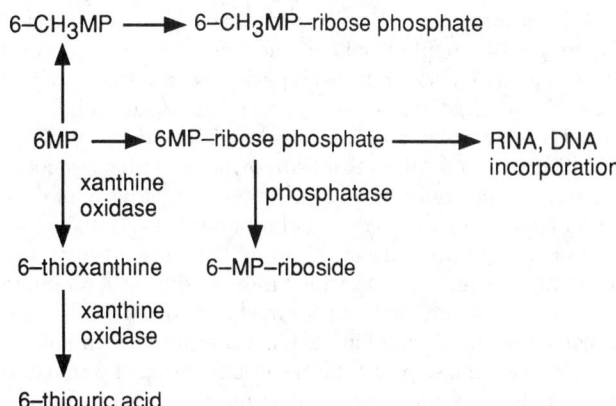

FIGURE 18–14. Pathways for activation and degradation of 6-mercaptopurine (6-MP).

clinical samples of human leukemia cells, resistance may result from increased concentrations of a membrane-bound alkaline phosphatase, or a conjugating enzyme, 6-thiopurine methyltransferase.[132,133]

CLINICAL PHARMACOLOGY AND PHARMACOKINETICS

HPLC analysis using the phenylmercury- or sulfonated-derivatives of the 6-TPs can now measure drug plasma levels as low as 0.1 μM.[134] Oral doses of 6-MP of 50 to 100 mg/m^2/day are commonly used in the maintenance therapy of ALL. Oral absorption is highly erratic with only 16% to 50% of an administered dose reaching the systemic circulation due to rapid first-pass metabolism in the liver.[135] Food intake and the antibiotic cotrimoxazole reduce drug absorption.[136,137] The variable bioavailability of oral 6-MP may be an important determinant of therapeutic outcome, because low plasma drug concentration-over-time measurements correlate with an increased risk of relapse in children with ALL.[138]

6-MP is well distributed into most body compartments, with the exception of the CSF. Approximately 30% of the drug binds weakly to plasma proteins. The plasma half-life is approximately 50 minutes after intravenous injection and 90 minutes after oral administration.[135] The major route of drug elimination is metabolic alteration by several pathways. 6-MP is oxidized to the inactive metabolite 6-thiouric acid by xanthine oxidase. Enhanced 6-MP toxicity may result from the concomitant administration of oral 6-MP and the xanthine oxidase inhibitor allopurinol. In patients receiving both 6-MP and allopurinol, the 6-MP dose should be reduced by 75%. 6-MP also undergoes S-methylation by the enzyme thiopurine methyltransferase to yield 6-methylmercaptopurine. After further phosphorylation, 6-methylmercaptopurine nucleotides also inhibit purine biosynthesis, but to a lesser extent than 6-MP nucleotides. The level of thiopurine methyltransferase varies considerably in patients and may correlate inversely with the 6-MP nucleotide content of erythrocytes and with drug toxicity.[133]

Renal excretion of 6-MP is minimal, but at high doses as much as 20% to 40% of the drug is removed by the kidneys.[139] Very high doses of 6-MP (>1000 mg/m^2) in children may cause renal precipitation of drug with hematuria and crystalluria.[140] In patients with renal dysfunction, dose reductions of 6-MP should be considered.

6-TG is administered orally in doses of 75 to 200 mg/m^2/day in the treatment of acute myelogenous leukemia. Its oral bioavailability is also erratic, with peak plasma levels occurring 2 to 4 hours after ingestion.[136] The median plasma half-life of 6-TG is approximately 90 minutes. The catabolism of 6-TG differs from 6-MP in that S-methylation with subsequent removal of the sulfur atom is an important pathway of drug elimination.[127] In a second catabolic pathway, 6-TG undergoes deamination by the enzyme guanine deaminase (guanase), resulting in 6-thioxanthine, which is then oxidized by xanthine oxidase to 6-thiouric acid. In contrast to 6-MP, 6-TG is not a direct substrate for xanthine oxidase. Because the inhibition of xanthine oxidase results in the accumulation of 6-thioxanthine, an inactive metabolite, adjustments in 6-TG dosage are not required for patients who also receive allopurinol.

TOXICITY

The major dose-related toxicities of 6-MP are myelosuppression and gastrointestinal toxicity. Leukopenia and thrombocytopenia are generally maximal 7 days after treatment, with full recovery occurring after 14 days. Gastrointestinal toxicities include nausea and vomiting, anorexia, diarrhea, and stomatitis. 6-MP hepatotoxicity occurs in as many as 30% of adult patients, with a clinical picture consisting primarily of cholestatic jaundice, although elevations of alkaline phosphatase and hepatic transaminases may also be seen.[141] Although hepatotoxicity is usually mild and reversible, frank hepatic necrosis can occur after high doses of 6-MP. Combinations of 6-MP with other known hepatotoxic agents should be avoided, and liver function tests should be closely monitored. The mechanism of liver toxicity is not known, but may relate to the P-450-dependent metabolism of 6-MP to a hepatotoxic metabolite.[127] 6-TG also causes dose-limiting bone marrow suppression but, in contrast with 6-MP, it causes fewer gastrointestinal side effects and less hepatotoxicity.

The 6-thiopurines and azathioprine, which release 6-MP through hepatic metabolism after oral administration, potently suppress cell-mediated immunity. These agents have been used to prevent rejection of transplanted organs and to treat autoimmune diseases, such as Crohn's disease, ulcerative colitis, and rheumatoid arthritis. Therapeutic immunosuppression occurs at 100 mg/day, a dose associated with only mild leukopenia. Long-term immunosuppressive therapy with azathioprine increases the risk of squamous carcinoma of the skin, histiocytic lymphoma, and Kaposi's sarcoma. These complications have not been reported after chronic 6-MP therapy. Other adverse effects associated with chronic 6-MP treatment include predispositions to bacterial and parasitic infections and teratogenic effects, particularly during the first trimester of pregnancy.

OTHER PURINE ANALOGS

Tiazofuran, a thiazole-4-carboxamide nucleoside analog, has modest clinical activity in refractory myeloid leukemia. Activation of tiazofuran results in formation of thiazole-4-carboxamide adenine dinucleotide, a structural analog of nicotinamide adenine dinucleotide (NAD) and a powerful inhibitor of inosine monophosphate dehydrogenase, a critical enzyme in de novo purine biosynthesis.[142] Although phase II studies of tiazofuran in patients with solid tumors have been disappointing, some activity has been reported in the treatment of acute myelogenous leukemia and chronic myelogenous leukemia in blast crisis.[143]

ADENOSINE ANALOGS

In addition to the 6-thiopurine compounds, which act as guanine analogs, a number of adenosine analogs have been isolated from fermentation broths or have been chemically synthesized. The first of these agents to find a role in clinical chemotherapy was 9-β-arabinofuranosyladenine (ara-A), which, in the triphosphate form, inhibits DNA polymerase (Fig. 18–15). This compound has antiviral activity against DNA viruses, particularly those of the herpes family. Although

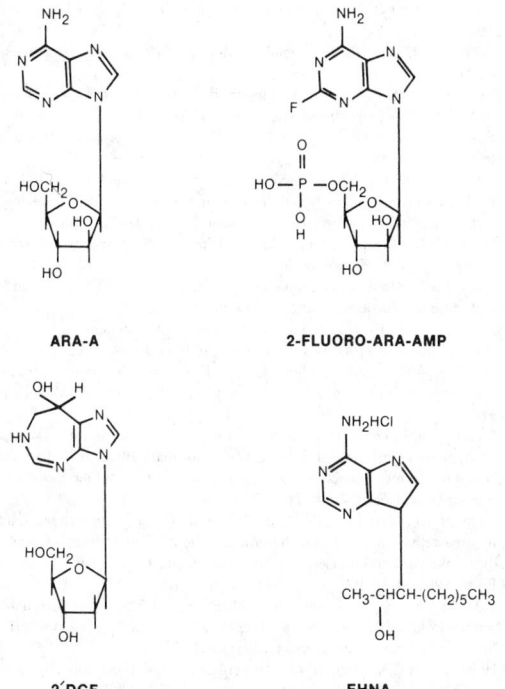

FIGURE 18–15. Adenosine antimetabolites (ara-A and 2-fluoro-ara-AMP) and inhibitors of adenosine deaminase [2'-deoxycoformycin (2'-DCF) and EHNA].

ara-A has demonstrated potent antitumor activity in animal tumor models, its clinical usefulness has been hindered by both its limited aqueous solubility and its rapid deamination by adenosine deaminase. The 2-fluoro derivative of ara-A is relatively resistant to adenosine deaminase but poorly soluble in water. Fludarabine (9-β-D-arabinofuranosyl-2-fluoroadeninemonophosphate; see Fig. 18–15), the monophosphate analog of 2-fluoro-ara-A, was subsequently synthesized. This compound is resistant to adenosine deaminase and has improved aqueous solubility.[144] It undergoes rapid dephosphorylation to 2-fluoro-ara-A in plasma and is subsequently phosphorylated intracellularly by deoxycytidine kinase and monophosphate and diphosphate kinase to the active cytotoxic triphosphate form. This metabolite inhibits DNA synthesis through its inhibitory effects on DNA polymerase and ribonucleotide reductase.[144] A number of clinical trials have shown that fludarabine is not active against solid tumors. However, it is an effective drug in the treatment of refractory or resistant CLL.[145] The major toxicities associated with fludarabine treatment are myelosuppression, infection, and peripheral sensorimotor neuropathy. At high doses (125 mg/m²/day for 5 days), significant delayed neurotoxicity may occur 21 to 43 days after initiation of therapy. Reported neurotoxic events include optic neuritis, cortical blindness, altered mental status, generalized seizures, and coma. The total body clearance of fludarabine correlates with creatinine clearance, suggesting the importance of renal excretion in its pharmacokinetics.[146]

An inborn genetic defect resulting in a deficiency of adenosine deaminase is associated with a significant impairment in T-cell-mediated immunity. This observation has stimulated interest in developing inhibitors of adenosine

deaminase for the treatment of human T-cell tumors and led to the identification of two inhibitors of this enzyme, 2'-deoxycoformycin (DCF) and erythro-9-(2-hydroxy-3-nanyl)-adenine (EHNA).[147,148] The tetrahedral configuration of DCF resembles the transition-state intermediate resulting from the adenosine deaminase-catalyzed hydrolysis of adenosine, and this structural resemblance is thought to be the principal factor in the high potency of DCF as an inhibitor of adenosine deaminase (K_i = 2.5 pmol). EHNA is less potent than DCF, but its lower affinity to tissue adenosine deaminase may result in more rapid elimination from tissues that are susceptible to the toxic effects of enzyme inhibition. Only DCF has been used in the clinical setting and, as a single agent, DCF is active against T-cell ALL, CLL, and mycosis fungoides. Currently, its most important clinical role is in the treatment of hairy cell leukemia, for which it is the most active single agent for remission induction.[149]

The precise mechanism(s) by which DCF exerts its cytotoxicity remains unclear. As a consequence of its inhibition of adenosine deaminase, DCF therapy results in a marked increase in the intracellular concentration of deoxyadenosine triphosphates (dATP) in lymphoid cells.[150] This increase in dATP pools leads to feedback inhibition of ribonucleotide reductase and a decrease in the levels of other deoxynucleotide precursors necessary for DNA synthesis.[151] A marked feedback inhibition of S-adenosylhomocysteine hydrolase also occurs, leading to inhibition of a host of transmethylation reactions. DCF is also phosphorylated in human T-lymphoblastoid cells to the monophosphate, diphosphate, and triphosphate forms, and incorporation of the triphosphate metabolite into DNA has been demonstrated.

DCF is highly toxic when given at dose levels of 10 mg/m²/day or higher. Disturbances in CNS function, such as somnolence, confusion and coma, significant impairment in renal function, hepatic enzyme elevation, conjunctivitis, immunosuppression, and nausea and vomiting are frequent side effects. At lower doses (4 mg/m² biweekly) the incidence of these side effects is low, and the drug is well tolerated. This schedule has proven to be effective in hairy cell leukemia, inducing a clinical and bone marrow remission in most treated patients. In the dose range of 2 to 10 mg/m², 80% to 100% of a dose of DCF is eliminated unchanged in the urine. A positive correlation exists between creatinine clearance and DCF clearance, and appropriate dose modification should be made in response to renal impairment.[152]

A third adenosine analog has shown early promise as an antileukemic agent. 2-Chlorodeoxyadenosine is resistant to adenosine deaminase and accumulates selectively as the 5'-triphosphate metabolite form in cells rich in deoxycytidine kinase, and its cytotoxic activity appears to be independent of cell division.[153] It is effective in the treatment of low-grade malignant disorders of the lymphoid tissue, including CLL, non-Hodgkin's lymphoma, and hairy cell leukemia. Although initial clinical studies demonstrated myelosuppression to be the dose-limiting toxicity, a single continuous 7-day infusion at 0.1 mg/kg/day, as has been employed effectively for treating hairy cell leukemia, causes minimal hematologic and nonhematologic toxicities.[154] Further studies are needed to define its pharmacologic properties and its spectrum of antitumor activity.

REFERENCES

1. Farber S, Diamond LK, Mercer RD, Sylvester RF, Wolff JA. Temporary remissions in acute leukemia in children produced by folic acid antagonist, 4-aminopteroylglutamic acid (aminopterin). N Engl J Med 1948;238:787–793.

1a. Allegra CJ. Antifolates. In: Chabner BA, Collins JM, eds. Cancer chemotherapy: Principles and practice. Philadelphia: JB Lippincott, 1990:110–153.

2. Chu E, Drake JC, Boarman D, et al. Mechanism of thymidylate synthase inhibition by methotrexate in human neoplastic cell lines and normal human myeloid progenitor cells. J Biol Chem 1990;256:8470–8478.

3. Jolivet J, Chabner BA. Intracellular pharmacokinetics of methotrexate polyglutamates in human breast cancer cells: Selective retention and less dissociable binding of 4-NH_2-10-CH_3-pteroylglutamate$_4$ and 4-NH_2-10-CH_3-pteroylglutamate$_5$ to dihydrofolate reductase. J Clin Invest 1983;72:773–778.

4. Winick NJ, Kamen BA, Balis FM, et al. Folate and methotrexate polyglutamate tissue levels in rhesus monkeys following chronic low-dose methotrexate. Cancer Drug Deliv 1987;4:25–29.

5. Allegra CJ, Hoang K, Yeh GC, et al. Evidence for direct inhibition of de novo purine synthesis in human MCF-7 breast cells as a principal mode of metabolic inhibition by methotrexate. J Biol Chem 1987;262:13520–13526.

6. Borchers AH, Kennedy DA, Straw JA. Inhibition of DNA excision repair by methotrexate in Chinese hamster ovary cells following exposure to ultra-violet irradiation or ethylmethanesulfonate. Cancer Res 1990;50:1786–1789.

7. Elwood PC. Molecular cloning and characterization of the human folate binding protein cDNA from placenta and malignant tissue culture (KB) cells. J Biol Chem 1989;264:14893–14901.

8. Jansen G, Westerhof GR, Jarmuszewski JA, et al. Methotrexate transport in variant human CCRF-CEM leukemia cells with elevated levels of the reduced folate carrier. J Biol Chem 1990;265:18272–18277.

8a. Sirotnak FM, Moccio DM, Kelleher LE, Goutsas LJ. Relative frequency and kinetic properties of transport defective phenotypes among methotrexate-resistant L1210 clonal cell lines derived in vivo. Cancer Res 1981;41:4447.

9. Cohen M, Bender RA, Donehower RC, et al. Reversibility of high affinity binding of methotrexate in L1210 murine leukemia cells. Cancer Res 1978;38:2866–2870.

10. Pinedo HM, Zaharko DS, Bull JM, et al. The reversal of methotrexate cytotoxicity to mouse bone marrow cells by leucovorin and nucleosides. Cancer Res 1976;36:4418–4424.

11. Allegra CJ, Boarman D. Interaction of methotrexate polyglutamates and dihydrofolate during leucovorin rescue in a human breast cancer cell line (MCF-7). Cancer Res 1990;50:3574–3578.

12. Adamson PC, Balis FM, McCully C, et al. Methotrexate pharmacokinetics following rescue with recombinant carboxypeptidase-G_2. Proc Am Soc Clin Oncol 1991;10:103.

13. Haber DA, Schimke RT. Unstable amplification of an altered dihydrofolate reductase gene associated with double-minute chromosomes. Cell 1981;26:355–359.

14. Dicker AP, Volkenandt M, Schweitzer BI, Banerjee D, Bertino JR. Identification and characterization of a mutation in the dihydrofolate reductase gene from the methotrexate-resistant Chinese hamster ovary cell line Pro^{-3} MTXRIII. J Biol Chem 1990;265:8317–8321.

15. Melera PW, Davide JP, Oen H. Antifolate-resistant Chinese hamster cells: Molecular basis for the biochemical and structural heterogeneity among DHFRs produced by drug-sensitive and drug-resistant cell lines. J Biol Chem 1987;262:1978–1990.

16. Cowan KH, Goldsmith ME, Ricciardone MD, et al. Regulation of dihydrofolate reductase in human breast cancer cells and in mutant hamster cells transfected with a human dihydrofolate reductase minigene. Mol Pharmacol 1986;30:69–73.

16a. Curt GA, Carney DN, Cowan KH, et al. Unstable methotrexate resistance in human small cell carcinoma associated with double minute chromosomes. N Engl J Med 1983;308:199.

17. Curt GA, Jolivet J, Carney DN, et al. Determinants of the sensitivity of human small-cell lung cancer cell lines to methotrexate. J Clin Invest 1985;76:1323–1329.

18. Evans WE, Crom WR, Abromowitch M, et al. Clinical pharmacodynamics of high-dose methotrexate in acute lymphocytic leukemia: Identification of a relation between concentration and effect. N Engl J Med 1986;314:471–474.

19. Chabner BA, Stoller RG, Hande KR, et al. Methotrexate disposition in humans: Case studies in ovarian cancer and following high-dose infusion. Drug Metab Rev 1978;8:107–117.

20. Thyss A, Milano G, Kubar J, et al. Clinical and pharmacokinetic evidence of a life-threatening interaction between methotrexate and ketoprofen. Lancet 1986;1:256.

21. Jacobs SA, Stoller RG, Chabner BA, et al. 7-Hydroxy methotrexate as a urinary metabolite in human subjects and rhesus monkeys receiving high-dose methotrexate. J Clin Invest 1976;57:534–538.

22. Sholar PW, Baram J, Seither R, et al. Inhibition of folate-dependent enzymes by 7-OH-methotrexate. Biochem Pharmacol 1988;37:3531–3534.

23. Donehower RC, Hande KR, Drake JC, et al. Presence of 2,4-diamino-N^{10}-methyl pteroic acid after high-dose methotrexate. Clin Pharmacol Ther 1979;26:63–72.

24. Calvert AH, Bondy PK, Harrap KR. Some observations on the human pharmacology of methotrexate. Cancer Treat Rep 1977;61:1647–1656.

25. Erttmann R, Landbeck G. Effect of oral cholestyramine on the elimination of high-dose methotrexate. J Cancer Res Clin Oncol 1985;110:48–51.

26. Stoller RG, Hande KR, Jacobs SA, et al. Use of plasma pharmacokinetics to predict and prevent methotrexate toxicity. N Engl J Med 1977;297:630–634.

27. Shapiro WR, Young D, Mehta BM. Methotrexate distribution in cerebrospinal fluid after intravenous ventricular and lumbar injections. N Engl J Med 1975;293:161–166.

28. Zachariae H, Kragballe K, Sogaard H. Methotrexate-induced cirrhosis. Br J Dermatol 1980;102:407–412.

29. Tuma DJ, Barak AJ, Sorrell MF. Interaction of methotrexate with lipotropic factors in rat liver. Biochem Pharmacol 1975;24:1327–1331.

30. Sostman HD, Matthay RA, Putman C, et al. Methotrexate-induced pneumonitis. Medicine (Baltimore) 1976;55:371–388.

31. Bleyer WA. The clinical pharmacology of methotrexate. Cancer 1978;41:36–51.

32. Peylan-Ramu N, Poplack DG, Blei CL, et al. Computer-assisted tomography in methotrexate encephalopathy. J Comput Assist Tomogr 1977;1:216–221.

33. Shapiro WR, Allen JC, Horten BC. Chronic methotrexate toxicity to the central nervous system. Clin Bull Memorial-Sloan Kettering 1980;10:49–52.

34. Walker RW, Allen JC, Rosen G, et al. Transient cerebral dysfunction secondary to high-dose methotrexate. Cancer 1984;53:1849–1851.

34a. Lin JT, Bertino JR. Update on trimetrexate, a folate antagonist with antineioplastic and antiprotozoal properties. Cancer Invest 1991;9:159.

35. Sigel CW, Macklin AW, Wolley TL, et al. Preclinical biochemical pharmacology and toxicology of piritrexim, a lipophilic inhibitor of DHFR. NCI Monogr 1987;5:111–120.

36. Sirotnak FM, DeGraw JI, Schmid FA, et al. New folate analogs of the 10-deaza-aminopterin series: Further evidence for markedly increased antitumor efficacy compared to methotrexate in ascites and solid murine tumor models. Cancer Chemother Pharmacol 1984;12:2630.

37. Jackman AL, Marsham PR, Moran RG, et al. Thymidylate synthase inhibitors: The in vitro activity of a series of heterocyclic benzoyl ring methyl-N$_{10}$-substituted-5,8-dideazafolates. In: Weber G, ed. Advances in enzyme regulation. Oxford: Pergamon Press, 1991:31;13–27.

38. Baldwin SW, Tse A, Gossett LS, et al. Structural features of 5,10-dideaza-5,6,7,8-tetrahydrofolate that determine inhibition of mammalian glycinamide ribonucleotide formyltransferase. Biochemistry 1991;30:1997–2006.

39. Heidelberger C, Chandhari NK, Dannenberg P, et al. Fluorinated pyrimidines: A new class of tumor inhibitory compounds. Nature 1957;179:663–666.

40. Sommer A, Santi DV. Purification and amino acid analysis of an active site peptide from thymidylate synthetase containing convalently bound 5'-fluoro-2'-deoxyuridylate and methylene tetrachloride. Biochem Biophys Res Commun 1974;57:689–696.

41. Mandel HG. Incorporation of 5-fluorouracil into RNA and its molecular consequences. Prog Mol Subcell Biol 1969;1:82–135.

42. Schuetz JD, Collins JM, Wallace HJ, et al. Alteration of the secondary structure of newly synthesized DNA from murine bone marrow cells by 5-fluorouracil. Cancer Res 1986;46:119–123.

43. Berger SH, Hakala MT. Relationship of dUMP and free FdUMP pools to inhibition of thymidylate synthase by 5-fluorouracil.

44. Petrelli N, Herrera L, Rustum Y, et al. A prospective randomized trial of 5-fluorouracil and methotrexate in previously untreated patients with advanced colorectal carcinoma. J Clin Oncol 1987;5:1559–1565.

45. Valone FH, Drakes R, Flam M, et al. Randomized trial of 5-FU vs leucovorin plus 5-FU vs sequential methotrexate, 5-FU, leucovorin in patients with advanced colorectal carcinoma: A Northern California Oncology Group Trial. Proc Am Soc Clin Oncol 1988;7:95.

46. Kanamaru R, Kakuta H, Sato T, et al. The inhibitory effects of 5-fluorouracil on the metabolism of preribosomal and ribosomal RNA in L-1210 cells in vitro. Cancer Chemother Pharmacol 1986;17:43–46.

47. Carrico CK, Glazer RI. The effect of 5-fluorouracil on the synthesis and translation of poly(A) RNA from regenerating liver. Cancer Res 1979;39:3694–3701.

48. Dolnick BJ, Pink JJ. Effects of 5-fluorouracil on dihydrofolate reductase mRNA from methotrexate-resistant KB cells. J Biol Chem 1985;260:3006–3014.

49. Cheng Y-C, Nakayama K. Effects of 5-fluoro-2'-deoxyuridine on DNA metabolism in HeLa cells. Mol Pharmacol 1983;23:171–174.

50. Yoshioka A, Tanaka S, Hiraoka O, et al. Deoxyribonucleoside triphosphate imbalance—fluorodeoxyuridine-induced DNA double strand breaks in mouse FM3A cells and the mechanism of cell death. J Biol Chem 1987;262:8235–8241.

51. Peters GJ, Laurensse E, Lankelma J, et al. Separation of several 5-fluorouracil metabolites in various melanoma cell lines: Evidence for the synthesis of 5-fluorouracil-nucleotide sugars. Eur J Clin Oncol 1984;20:1425–1431.

52. Fernandes DJ, Cranford SK. Resistance of CCRF-CEM cloned sublinnes to 5-fluorodeoxyuridine associated with enhanced phosphatase activities. Biochem Pharmacol 1985;34:125–132.

53. Aronow B, Watts T, Lassetter J, et al. Biochemical phenotype of 5-fluorouracil-resistant murine T-lymphoblasts with genetically altered CTP synthetase activity. J Biol Chem 1984;259:9035–9043.

54. Chu E, Lai G-M, Zinn S, Allegra CJ. Resistance of a human ovarian cancer line to 5-fluorouracil associated with decreased levels of 5-fluorouracil in DNA. Mol Pharmacol 1990;38:410–417.

55. Jastreboff MM, Kedzierska B, Rode W. Altered thymidylate synthase in 5-fluorodeoxyuridine-resistant cultured hepatoma cells. Biochem Pharmacol 1983;32:2259–2267.

56. Barbour KW, Berger SH, Berger FG. Single amino acid substitution defines a naturally occurring genetic variant of human thymidylate synthase. Mol Pharmacol 1990;37:515–518.

57. Berger SH, Jenh C-H, Johnson LF, et al. Thymidylate synthase overproduction and gene amplification in fluorodeoxyuridine-resistant human cells. Mol Pharmacol 1985;28:461–467.

58. Chu E, Drake JC, Koeller DM, et al. Induction of thymidylate synthase associated with multidrug resistance in human breast and colon cancer cell lines. Mol Pharmacol 1991;39:136–143.

59. Spears CP, Shahinian AH, Moran RG, et al. *In vivo* kinetics of thymidylate synthetase inhibition in 5-fluorouracil-sensitive and -resistant murine colon adenocarcinomas. Cancer Res 1982;42:450–456.

60. Chu E, Koeller DM, Casey JL, et al. Autoregulation of human thymidylate synthase messenger RNA translation by thymidylate synthase. Proc Natl Acad Sci USA 1991;88:8977–8981.

61. Peters GJ, Kraal I, Laurensse E, et al. Separation of 5-fluorouracil and uracil by ion pair reversed-phased high-performance liquid chromatography on a column with porous polymeric packing. J Chromatogr 1984;307:464–468.

62. Hull WE, Port RE, Herrmann R, et al. Metabolites of 5-fluorouracil in plasma and urine, as monitored by ^{17}F nuclear magnetic resonance spectroscopy, for patients receiving chemotherapy with or without methotrexate pretreatment. Cancer Res 1988;48:1680–1688.

63. Spicer DV, Ardalan B, Daniels JR, et al. Reevaluation of the maximum tolerated dose of continuous venous infusion of 5-fluorouracil with pharmacokinetics. Cancer Res 1988;48:459–461.

64. Christophidis N, Vajda FJE, Lucas I, et al. Fluorouracil therapy in patients with carcinoma of the large bowel: A pharmacokinetic comparison of various rates and routes of administration. Clin Pharmacokinetics 1978;3:330–336.

65. Taylor I, Machin D, Mullee M, et al. A randomized controlled trial of adjuvant portal vein cytotoxic perfusion in colorectal cancer. Br J Surg 1985;72:359–363.

66. Wolmark N, Rockette H, Wickerham DL, et al. Adjuvant therapy of Dukes' A, B, and C adenocarcinoma of the colon with portal-vein fluorouracil hepatic infusion: Preliminary results of National Surgical Adjuvant Breast and Bowel Project Protocol C-02. J Clin Oncol 1990;8:1466–1475.

67. Speyer JL, Collins JM, Dedrick RL, et al. Phase I and pharmacologic studies of 5-fluorouracil administered intraperitoneally. Cancer Res 1980;40:567–572.

68. Diasio RB, Schuetz JD, Wallace HJ, et al. Dihydrofluorouracil, a fluorouracil catabolite with antitumor activity in murine and human cells. Cancer Res 1985;45:4900–4903.

69. Lokich JJ, Bothe A, Fine N, et al. Phase I study of protracted venous infusion of 5-fluorouracil. Cancer 1981;48:2565–2568.

70. Keonig H, Patel A. Biochemical basis for fluoruracil neurotoxicity. Arch Neurol 1970;23:155–160.

71. Burger AJ, Mannino S. 5-Fluorouracil-induced coronary vasospasm. Am Heart J 1987;114:433–436.

72. Marsh JC, Bertino JR, Katz KH, et al. The influence of drug interval on the effect of methotrexate and fluorouracil in the treatment of advanced colorectal cancer. J Clin Oncol 1991;9:371–380.

73. Erlichman C, Fine S, Wong A, et al. A randomized trial of fluorouracil and folinic acid in patients with metastatic colorectal carcinoma. J Clin Oncol 1988;7:469–475.

74. Poon MA, O'Connell MJ, Moertel CG, et al. Biochemical modulation of fluorouracil: Evidence of significant improvement of survival and quality of life in patients with advanced colorectal carcinoma. J Clin Oncol 1989;7:1407–1418.

75. Miyoshi T, Ogawa S, Kanamori T, et al. Interferon potentiated cytotoxic effects of 5-fluorouracil on cell proliferation of established human cell lines originating from neoplastic tissues. Cancer Lett 1983;17:239–247.

76. Stolfi RL, Martin DS. Modulation of chemotherapeutic drug activity with polyribonucleotides or with interferon. J Biol Respon Modif 1985;4:634–639.

77. Wadler S, Wersto R, Weinberg V, et al. Interaction of fluorouracil and interferon in human colon cancer cell lines: Cytotoxic and cytokinetic effects. Cancer Res 1990;50:5735–5739.

78. Elias L, Sandoval JM. Interferon effects upon fluorouracil metabolism by HL-60 cells. Biochem Biophys Res Commun 1989;163:867–874.

79. Chu E, Zinn S, Boarman D, et al. Interaction of gamma interferon and 5-fluorouracil in the H630 human colon carcinoma cell line. Cancer Res 1990;50:5834–5840.

80. Wadler S, Lembersky B, Atkins M, Kirkwood J, Petrelli N. Phase II trial of fluorouracil and recombinant interferon alfa-2a in patients with advanced colorectal carcinoma: An Eastern Cooperative Oncology Group study. J Clin Oncol 1991;9:1806–1810.

81. Liang C-M, Donehower RC, Chabner BA. Biochemical interactions between N-(phosphonacetyl)-L-aspartate and 5-fluorouracil. Mol Pharmacol 1982;21:224–230.

82. Ardalan B, Singh G. A randomized phase I-II study of short-term infusion of high-dose 5-fluorouracil with or without N-(phosphonacetyl)-L-aspartic acid in patients with advanced pancreatic and colorectal cancer. J Clin Oncol 1988;6:1053–1058.

83. Grem JL, Fischer PH. Alteration of fluorouracil metabolism in human colon cancer cells by dipyridamole with a selective increase in fluorodeoxyuridine monophosphate levels. Cancer Res 1986;46:6191–6199.

84. Cook AF, Holman MJ, Kramer MJ, et al. Fluorinated pyrimidine nucleosides: III. Synthesis and antitumor activity of a series of 5'-deoxy-5-fluoropyrimidine nucleosides. J Med Chem 1979;22:1330–1335.

85. Bergmann W, Feeney R. Contributions to the study of marine products: XXXII. The nucleosides of sponges. J Org Chem 1951;16:981–987.

86. Chu MY, Fischer GA. A proposed mechanism of action of 1-β-D-arabinofuranosyl-cytosine as an inhibitor of the growth of leukemic cells. Biochem Pharmacol 1962;11:423–430.

87. Fram RJ, Kufe DW. Effect of 1-β-D-arabinofuranosyl cytosine and hydroxyurea on the repair of x-ray-induced DNA single-strand breaks in human leukemic blasts. Biochem Pharmacol 1985;34:2557–2560.

88. Fram RJ, Egan EM, Kufe DW. Accumulation of leukemic cell DNA strand breaks with Adriamycin and cytosine arabinoside. Leuk Res 1983;7:243–249.

89. Kufe DW, Munroe D, Herrick D, et al. Effects of 1-β-D-arabinosuranosyl-cytosine incorporation on eukaryotic DNA template function. Mol Pharmacol 1984;26:128–134.

90. Woodcock DM, Fox RM, Cooper IA. Evidence for a new mechanism of cytotoxicity of 1-β-D-arabinofuranosylcytosine. Cancer Res 1979;39:1418–1424.

91. Kharbanda SM, Sherman ML, Kufe DW. Transcriptional regulation of c-*jun* gene expression by arabinofuranosylcytosine in human myeloid leukemia cells. J Clin Invest 1990;86:1517–1523.

92. Hawtrey AO, Scott-Burden T, Robertson G. Inhibition of glycoprotein and glycolipid synthesis in hamster embryo cells by cytosine arabinoside and hydroxyurea. Nature 1974;252:58–60.

93. Bianchi Scarra GL, Romani M, Civiello DA, et al. Terminal erythroid differentiation in the K-562 cell line by 1-β-D-arabinofuranosylvytosine: Accompaniment by c-*myc* messenger RNA decrease. Cancer Res 1986;46:6327–6332.

94. Vogelstein ER, Burke PJ, Schiffer CA, et al. Differentiation of leukemia cells to polymorphonuclear leukocytes in patients with acute nonlymphocytic leukemia. N Engl J Med 1986;315:15–24.

95. Wiley JS, Taupin J, Jamieson GP, et al. Cytosine arabinoside transport and metabolism in acute leukemias and T-cell lymphoblastic lymphoma. J Clin Invest 1985;75:632–642.

96. Chabner BA, Hande KR, Drake JC, et al. Ara-C metabolism implications for drug resistance and drug interactions. Bull Cancer 1979;66:89–92.

96a. Vaughan WP, Karp JE, Burke PJ. Two cycle-timed sequential chemotherapy for adult acute nonlymphocytic leukemia. Blood 1984;67:975–980.

97. Tattersall MNH, Ganeshagura K, Hoffbrand AV. Mechanism of resistance of human acute leukaemia cells to cytosine arabinoside. Br J Haematol 1974;27:39–46.

98. Richel DJ, Colly LP, Arkesteijn GJA, et al. Substrate-specific deoxycytidine kinase deficiency in 1-β-D-arabinofuranosylcytosine-resistant leukemic cells. Cancer Res 1990;50:6515–6519.

99. de Saint Vincent BR, Buttin G. Studies on 1-β-D-arabinofuranosyl cytosine-resistant mutants of Chinese hamster cells: III. Joint resistance to arabinofuranosyl cytosine and to excess thymidine—a semidominant manifestation of deoxycytidine triphosphate pool expansion. Somatic Cell Genet 1979;5:67–82.

100. Boutagy J, Harvey DJ. Determination of cytosine arabinoside in human plasma by gas chromatography with a nitrogen-sensitive detector and by gas chromatography-mass spectrometry. J Chromatogr 1978;146:283–296.

100a. Piall EM, Aherne GW, Marks VM. A radioimmunoassay for cytosine arabinoside. Br J Cancer 1979;40:548–556.

101. Liversidge GG, Nishihata T, Higuchi T, et al. Simultaneous analysis of 1-β-D-arabinofuranosylcytosine, 1-β-D-arabinofuranosyluracil and sodium salicylate in biological samples by high-performance liquid chromatography. J Chromatogr 1983;276:375–383.

102. Shimada N, Ueda T, Yokoshima T, et al. A sensitive and specific radio-immunoassay for 1-β-D-arabinofuranosylcytosine. Cancer Lett 1984;24:173–178.

103. Ho DHW, Frei E III. Clinical pharmacology of 1-β-D-arabinofuranosylcytosine. Clin Pharmacol Ther 1971;12:944–954.

104. Wau SH, Huffman DH, Azarnoff DL, et al. Pharmacokinetics of 1-β-D-arabinofuranosylcytosine in humans. Cancer Res 1974;34:392–397.

105. Capizzi RL, Powell BL, Cooper MR, et al. Dose-related pharmacologic effects of high-dose ara-C and its use in combination with asparaginase for the treatment of patients with acute nonlymphocytic leukemia. Scand J Haematol 1986;34:17–23.

106. Wisch JS, Griffin JD, Kufe DW. Response of preleukemic syndromes to continuous infusion of low-dose cytarabine. N Engl J Med 1983;309:1599–1602.

107. Moloney WC, Rosenthal DS. Treatment of early acute nonlymphocytic leukemia with low-dose cytosine arabinoside. Haematol Blood Transfus 1961;26:59–62.

108. Markman M. The intracavitary administration of cytarabine to patients with non-hematopoietic malignancies: Pharmacologic rationale and results of clinical trials. Semin Oncol 1985;12:177–183.

109. Fre E III, Bickers JN, Hewlett JS, et al. Dose schedule and antitumor studies of arabinosyl cytosine (NSC 63878). Cancer Res 1969;29:1325–1332.

110. Herzig RH, Hines JD, Herzig GP, et al. Cerebellar toxicity with high-dose cytosine arabinoside. J Clin Oncol 1987;5:927–932.

111. Anderson BS, Luna MA, Yee C, et al. Fatal pulmonary failure complicating high-dose cytosine arabinoside therapy in acute leukemia. Cancer 1990;65:1079–1084.

112. Kern W, Kurrle E, Schmeiser T. Streptococcal bacteremia in adult patients with leukemia undergoing aggressive chemotherapy: A review of 55 cases. Infection 1990;18:138–145.

113. Flynn TC, Harris TJ, Murphy GF, et al. Neutrophilic eccrine hidradenitis: A distinctive rash associated with cytarabine therapy and acute leukemia. J Am Acad Dermatol 1984;11:584–590.

114. Cadman E, Eiferman F. Mechanism of synergistic cell killing when methotrexate precedes cytosine arabinoside: Study of L1210 and human leukemic cell. J Clin Invest 1979;64:788–797.

115. Harris AW, Reynolds EC, Finch LR. Effect of thymidine on the sensitivity of cultured mouse tumor cells to 1-β-D-arabinofuranosylcytosine. Cancer Res 1979;39:538–541.

116. Grem JL, Allegra CJ. Enhancement of the toxicity and DNA incorporation of arabinosyl-5-azacytosine and 1-β-D-arabinofuranosylcytosine by cyclopentenyl cytosine. Cancer Res 1990;50:7279–7284.

117. Kreis W, Wokcock TM, Gordon CS, et al. Tetrahydrouridine physiologic disposition and effect upon deamination of cytosine arabinoside in man. Cancer Treat Rep 1977;61:1347–1353.

118. Brach M, Klein H, Platzer E, et al. Effect of interleukin 3 on cytosine arabinoside-mediated cytotoxicity of leukemic myeloblasts. Exp Hematol 1990;18:748–753.

119. Ueda T, Nakamura T, Ando S, et al. Pharmacokinetics of N⁴-behenoyl-1-β-D-arabi-nofuranosylcytosine in patients with acute leukemia. Cancer Res 1983;43:3412–3416.

120. Ho DHW. Biochemical studies of a new antitumor agent, 0²,2'-cyclocytidine. Biochem Pharmacol 1974;23:1235–1244.

121. Kodama K, Morozumi M, Saitoh K, et al. Antitumor activity and pharmacology of 1-β-D-arabinofuranosylcytose-5'-stearyl-phosphate: An orally active derivative of 1-β-D-arabinofuranosylcytosine. Jpn J Cancer Res 1989;80:679–685.

122. Plagemann PGW, Behrens M, Abraham D. Metabolism and cytotoxicity of 5-azacytidine in cultured Novikoff rat hepatoma and P388 mouse leukemia cells and their enhancement by preincubation with pyrazofurin. Cancer Res 1978;38:2458–2466.

123. Ley TJ, DeSimone J, Anagnon NP, et al. 5-Azacytidine selectively increases gamma-globin synthesis in a patient with beta-thalassemia. N Engl J Med 1982;307:1469.

124. Sorbone A, Ford H Jr, Kelley JA, et al. Phase I and pharmacokinetic study of arabinofuranosyl-5-azacytosine (Fazarabine, NSC 281272). Cancer Res 1990;50:1220–1225.

125. Hitchings GH, Elion GB. The chemistry and biochemistry of purine analogs. Ann NY Acad Sci 1954;60:195–199.

126. Elion GB. Biochemistry and pharmacology of purine analogs. Fed Proc 1967;26:896–904.

127. McCormack JJ, Johns DG. Purine and purine nucleoside antimetabolites. In: Chabner BA, Collins JM, eds. Cancer chemotherapy: Principles and practice. Philadelphia: JB Lippincott, 1990:234–252.

128. Christie NT, Drake S, Meyn RE, et al. 6-Thiopurine-induced DNA damage as a determinant of cytotoxicity in cultured Chinese hamster ovary cells. Cancer Res 1984;44:3665–3672.

129. Tidd DM, Paterson ARP. Distinction between inhibition of purine nucleotide synthesis and the delayed cytotoxic reaction of 6-mercaptopurine. Cancer Res 1974;34:733–737.

130. Van Diggelen OP, Donahue TF, Shin SI. Basis for differential cellular sensitivity to 8-azaguanine and 6-thioguanine. J Cell Physiol 1979;98:59–71.

131. Calabresi P, Chabner BA. Chemotherapy of neoplastic diseases. In: Gilman AG, Rall TW, Nies AS, Taylor P, eds. The pharmacologic basis of therapeutics. New York: Pergamon Press, 1990:1202–1263.

132. Scholar EM, Calabresi P. Increased activity of alkaline phosphatases in leukemic cells from patients resistant to thiopurines. Biochem Pharmacol 1979;28:445–446.

133. Lennard L, Lillyman JS. Are children with lymphoblastic leukemia given enough 6-mercaptopurine? Lancet 1987;2:785.

134. Ding TL, Benet LZ. Determination of 6-mercaptopurine and azathioprine in plasma by high-performance liquid chromatography. J Chromatogr 1979;163:281–288.

135. Zimm S, Collins JM, Riccardi R, et al. Variable bioavailability of oral 6-mercaptopurine: Is maintenance chemotherapy in acute lymphoblastic leukemia being optimally delivered? N Engl J Med 1983;308:1005–1009.

136. Burton NK, Barnett MJ, Aherne GW, et al. The effect of food on the oral administration of 6-mercaptopurine. Cancer Chemother Pharmacol 1986;18:90–91.

137. Burton NK, Aherne GW. The effect of cotrimoxazole on the absorption of orally

138. Koren G, Ferrazini G, Sulh H, et al. Systemic exposure to mercaptopurine as a prognostic factor in acute lymphocytic leukemia in children. N Engl J Med 1990;323:17–21.

139. Coffey JJ, White CA, Lesk AB, et al. Effect of allopurinol on the pharmacokinetics of 6-mercaptopurine (NSC 755) in cancer patients. Cancer Res 1972;32:1283–1289.

140. Duttera MJ, Caralla RL, Gallelli JF, et al. Hematuria and crystalluria after high-dose 6-mercaptopurine administration. N Engl J Med 1972;287:292–294.

141. Einhorn, DI. Hepatotoxicity of 6-mercaptopurine. JAMA 1964;188:802–806.

142. Cooney DA, Jayaram HN, Gebeyehu G, et al. The conversion of 2-β-D-ribofuranosylthiazole-4-carboxamide to an analog of NAD with potent IMP dehydrogenase inhibitory properties. Biochem Pharmacol 1982;31:2133–2136.

143. Tricot GJ, Jayaram HN. Biochemically directed therapy of leukemia with tiazofurin, a selective blocker of inosine 5'-phosphate dehydrogenase activity. Cancer Res 1989;49:3696–3701.

144. Brockman RW, Cheng Y-C, Schabel FM Jr, et al. Metabolism and chemotherapeutic activity of 9-β-D-arabinofuranosyl-2-fluoroadenine against murine leukemia L1210 and evidence for its phosphorylation by deoxycytidine kinase. Cancer Res 1980;40:3610–3615.

145. Keating MJ, Kantarjian M, Talpaz J, et al. Fludarabine: A new agent with major activity against chronic lymphocytic leukemia. Blood 1989;74:19–25.

146. Desouza JV, Grever M, Neidhart JA, et al. Comparative pharmacokinetics and metabolism of fludarabine phosphate (NSC 312887) in man and dog. Proc Am Assoc Cancer Res 1984;25:361.

147. Agarwal RP, Spector T, Parks RE Jr. Tight-binding inhibitors: IV. Inhibition of adenosine deaminase by various inhibitors. Biochem Pharmacol 1977;26:359–367.

148. Lambe CU, Nelson DJ. Pharmacokinetics of inhibition of adenosine deaminase by erythro-9-(2-hydroxy-3-nonyl)-adenine in CBA mice. Biochem Pharmacol 1982;31:535–539.

149. Kraut EH, Bouroncle BA, Grever MR. Low-dose deoxycoformycin in the treatment of hairy cell leukemia. Blood 1986;68:1119–1122.

150. Mitchell BS, Edwards NL, Koller CA. Deoxyribonucleoside triphosphate accumulation by leukemic cells. Blood 1983;62:419–424.

151. Hershfield MS, Kredich NM, Koller CA, et al. S-Adenosylhomocysteine catabolism as a basis for acquired resistance during treatment of T-cell acute lymphoblastic leukemia with 1'-deoxycoformycin alone and in combination with 9-β-D-arabinofuranosyladenine. Cancer Res 1983;43:3451–3458.

152. Malspeis L, Weinrib AB, Staubus AE, et al. Clinical pharmacokinetics of 2'-deoxycoformycin. Cancer Treat Symp 1984;2:7–15.

153. Seto S, Carrera CJ, Kubota M, et al. Mechanism of deoxyadenosine and 2-chlorodeoxyadenosine toxicity to nondividing human lymphocytes. J Clin Invest 1985;75:377–383.

154. Piro LD, Carrera CJ, Carson DA, Beutler E. Lasting remissions in hairy-cell leukemia induced by a single infusion of 2-chlorodeoxyadenosine. N Engl J Med 1990;322:1117–1121.

BRUCE A. CHABNER
CHARLES E. MYERS

SECTION 5

Antitumor Antibiotics

BLEOMYCIN

One of the most unusual structures with antitumor activity is bleomycin, a mixture of low-molecular-weight (1500 daltons) peptides isolated from the fungus *Streptomyces verticullus*. Bleomycin is one of a family of antibiotic peptides that possess both antitumor and antimicrobial activity. It has found greatest usefulness in the treatment of germ cell tumors and lymphomas and is one of a few drugs that selectively kills tumor cells without affecting intestinal mucosa or bone marrow. The bleomycin mixture contains mostly the A_2 peptide, the unique pharmacologic properties of which have been characterized extensively.

The structure of the A_2 compound consists of a DNA-binding fragment and an iron-binding portion located at the opposite end of the molecule (Fig. 18–16). The primary action of bleomycin is to produce single-strand and double-strand breaks in DNA.[1] The sequence of events leading to DNA breakage begins with activation of the Fe^{2+}-bleomycin complex. Fe^{2+}, which is bound intimately to five nitrogen-containing groups in the bleomycin molecule, undergoes spontaneous or enzymatic activation, gaining an electron, and binding to O_2.[2] The activated complex of Fe^{2+}, oxygen, and bleomycin then binds to DNA as the result of intercalation by the bithiazole groups of the drug. Highly toxic oxygen intermediates, such as the superoxide or hydroxyl radicals, are then formed that attack the 4'-H of deoxyribose, leading to cleavage of the sugar and release of its attached base, usually thymine, cytosine, or their propenal adducts.[3] The action of bleomycin is specific for DNA and is exerted only weakly against RNA.

There is some base sequence specificity for the site of DNA cleavage. Bleomycin binds preferentially to the sequence GpT and cleaves the strand at the 3' side of G, releasing thymine as a thymine-propenal adduct.[4]

There appears to be some cytokinetic specificity to bleomycin cell kill.[5] Cells in synchronized culture systems are most susceptible during the premitotic or G2 phase, or in the mitotic phase of the cell cycle. However, cells exposed during G1 also are killed, and it is not known whether rapid cell division predisposes to cytotoxicity. The possibility of increasing cell kill by exposing cells during the G2 phase has

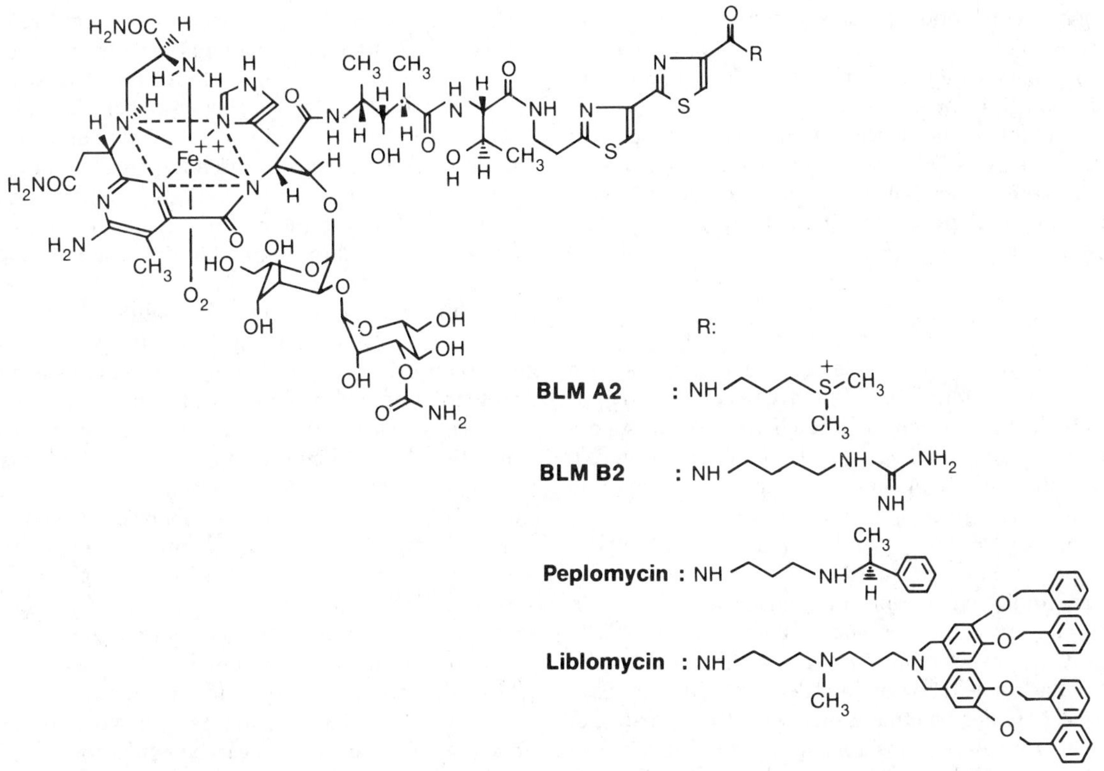

FIGURE 18–16. Structure of bleomycin-Fe(II) complex. The various substitutions on the amino-terminal end of the molecule are shown for bleomycin A$_2$ (BLM A2); for bleomycin B$_2$, also a component of the clinical preparation; and for two congeners, peplomycin and liblomycin.

prompted trials of bleomycin administration by continuous infusion.

The DNA lesions produced by bleomycin are visible as chromosomal breaks and deletions. Single-strand breaks predispose to the formation of double-strand breaks, which arise when the activated bleomycin-Fe^{2+}-O$_2$ complex is regenerated and attacks a GpT or GpC sequence on the opposing DNA strand.[6] It seems likely that repair processes play an important role in determining the lethality of these lesions, because repair of potentially lethal damage occurs in cultured cells exposed to this agent.[7] There is indirect evidence that the same processes required to repair ionizing radiation damage also are used in bleomycin repair and may be inhibited by calmodulin antagonists, such as trifluoperazine.[8] Glutathione enhances bleomycin cytotoxicity, as does misonidazole, and inhibitors of DNA repair, such as caffeine or 3-aminobenzamide, increase its lethality.[9,10] Several specific repair enzymes, including DNA polymerases, poly(ADP-ribose) polymerase, and ATP-dependent DNA ligase, have been implicated as important in repairing strand breaks induced by bleomycin.[11-13]

Little is known about the determinants of bleomycin resistance in tumor cells. A bleomycin-inactivating enzyme has been detected in both normal and malignant cells and is particularly prominent in the liver.[14] It has been purified and characterized as an aminopeptidase that hydrolyzes a broad spectrum of bleomycins and has homology to cathepsin H and other thiol proteinases.[15] The enzyme is found in low concentrations in lung and skin; its concentration in lung varies from one species to another and appears to determine the susceptibility to pulmonary injury.[16] Increased degradative activity has been found in resistant experimental tumors, as well as enhanced repair capacity and decreased drug uptake.[17-19]

CLINICAL PHARMACOLOGY AND PHARMACOKINETICS

The most sensitive and reliable technique for assay of bleomycin is radioimmunoassay; ^{125}I or ^{57}Co-bleomycin is used in this assay.[20]

Bleomycin is administered by parenteral injection subcutaneously, intramuscularly, or intravenously. There are no obvious differences in clinical response rates associated with the different routes, although continuous intravenous infusion has been used widely in the curative treatment of testicular cancer (see Chap. 35). Bleomycin has a two-phased plasma disappearance curve with half-lives of 24 minutes and 2 to 4 hours. Peak plasma concentrations reach 1 to 10 mU/ml after intravenous bolus doses of 15 U/m^2. The postinfusion half-life is approximately 3 hours, a value similar to the β-half-life after bolus administration. Most bleomycin is excreted unchanged in the urine in patients with normal renal function.[21]

Bleomycin pharmacokinetics are altered markedly in patients with abnormal renal function. A half-life of 21 hours has been observed in a patient with a creatinine clearance of 11 ml/min. It thus would be wise to decrease the dosage of bleomycin by 50% to 75% in patients with severely compromised renal function, who are at high risk for pulmonary toxicity, because of altered drug excretion rates.

In addition to conventional routes of administration, bleomycin may be injected into the pleural or peritoneal space to control malignant effusions.[22] Intracavitary doses of 60 U/m^2 provide effusion concentrations as high as 50 mU/ml, or approximately tenfold higher levels than in plasma. About 50% of an intracavitary dose enters the systemic circulation; the remaining fraction is metabolized in the pleural or peritoneal cavity or eliminated in its first pass through the portal circulation.

CLINICAL TOXICITY

In contrast with most antitumor agents, bleomycin has little myelosuppressive toxicity. Only at high doses (>25 U/m^2) or in patients with severely compromised bone marrow is a decrease in white blood cell count or platelet count observed. The primary toxicity of bleomycin is subacute or chronic pneumonitis that progresses to interstitial fibrosis.

The pathogenesis of bleomycin lung injury is not fully understood. The parent drug, as well as its terminal amine, can produce lung injury in experimental animals, and bleomycin stimulates collagen synthesis in isolated pulmonary fibroblasts in vitro.[23,24] Other experiments implicate a direct toxic effect on pulmonary arterioles and veins and demonstrate the release of fibrogenic peptides, such as tumor growth factor-β and interleukin-1, from alveolar macrophages.[25,26] Bleomycin also causes the release of nitric oxide.[27] Which of these effects is important in the evolution of clinical pulmonary injury has not been resolved.

The first signs of pulmonary toxicity are cough, dyspnea, pleuritic chest pain in some patients, and fever. Carbon monoxide diffusion capacity of the lung decreases progressively with increasing total doses of the drug, particularly above 250 mg, and the incidence of clinically significant pulmonary toxicity reaches 10% at total doses of 450 U or higher.[28] Carbon monoxide diffusion capacity does not appear to be a reliable predictor of impending pulmonary toxicity in asymptomatic patients, most of whom will experience a steady, dose-related decrease of 10% to 15% in this sign over the course of treatment.[29] Toxicity is most frequent in older patients (older than 70 years of age), in those with underlying lung disease such as emphysema, and in those previously treated with pulmonary or mediastinal irradiation. Bleomycin appears to predispose patients to respiratory failure after surgery, particularly if high concentrations of inspired O$_2$ are used during the procedure.[30] Although there appears to be a close relation between total dose and risk of pulmonary toxicity, well-documented cases have been observed at total doses lower than 100 U.

There are anecdotal cases, but no clear proof, to suggest that pulmonary fibrosis can be prevented or reversed with corticosteroid.

The clinical symptoms and radiograph findings of bleomycin-induced pulmonary toxicity are not distinguished easily from other syndromes commonly found in cancer patients, including progressive metastatic tumor (especially lymphangitic tumor), infectious processes such as *Pneumocystis carinii* or cytomegalovirus, and radiation injury. Radiologic abnormalities, including linear and nodular densities, which may become confluent, are detectable by CT scanning in approximately 40% of asymptomatic patients receiving

bleomycin, even though routine chest films are usually negative.[31,32] Symptomatic patients usually show bibasilar pulmonary infiltrates on chest film, although symptoms may precede the appearance of obvious radiologic findings. Gallium scans may detect drug-induced effects before routine chest films. Open lung biopsy is often required, and reveals an acute inflammatory infiltrate, interstitial and intraalveolar edema, pulmonary hyaline membrane formation, and intraalveolar and interstitial fibrosis. In addition, squamous metaplasia of the alveolar lining cells is often found. Radiologic evidence of pulmonary toxicity and abnormalities in carbon monoxide diffusion resolve in most asymptomatic patients after therapy is discontinued. Resolution of abnormalities is often incomplete in symptomatic patients. However, long-term follow-up of patients with testicular cancer treated with an average cumulative dose of bleomycin of 160 U/m^2 has demonstrated no significant reduction in pulmonary function (vital capacity or diffusion capacity of carbon monoxide) a median of 4 years after therapy.[33] The clinical management of patients with bleomycin lung injury requires drug discontinuation (although the lesion often becomes symptomatic after therapy has finished), attention to any element of pulmonary edema or infection, and the use of minimal levels of oxygen compatible with adequate respiration. Inflammatory changes tend to regress with time, but, in patients with extensive fibrosis, little reversal of these changes can be expected.

Bleomycin frequently produces an unusual cutaneous adverse reaction. Almost 50% of patients develop erythema, induration, thickening, and eventual peeling of the skin on the fingers, palms, and extremity joints. In addition, most patients develop hyperpigmentation of skin creases and a general darkening of the skin. Some patients also may develop Raynaud phenomenon during bleomycin therapy.

Less frequent side effects include acute hypertension, primarily in patients receiving doses greater than 25 U/day, and hyperbilirubinemia. Fever often is observed in the first 48 hours after drug administration, and occasional hypersensitivity reactions, with urticaria and bronchospasm, have been observed. These reactions usually do not necessitate withdrawal of the drug, but pretreatment with antihistamines and corticosteroids is recommended for patients who have a history of allergic reactions to bleomycin.

ANTHRACYCLINES

The first anthracyclines in clinical use, daunorubicin and doxorubicin, were produced from the *Streptomyces* species. These antibiotics are, in fact, part of a large group of highly colored bacterial products known as the *rhodomycins*. There are exhaustive reviews of the structure and properties of the rhodomycins.[34] These compounds, like daunorubicin and doxorubicin, have a planar anthraquinone nucleus attached to an amino sugar (Fig. 18–17). Within this group, or closely related to it, are compounds that have a wide range of antibacterial and antitumor activity.

As antitumor agents, anthracyclines are matched only by alkylating agents in terms of their clinical usefulness. Daunorubicin is one of the most effective agents in the treatment of ALL and AML. Doxorubicin, on the other hand, is used to treat solid tumors, such as carcinomas of the breast, lung,

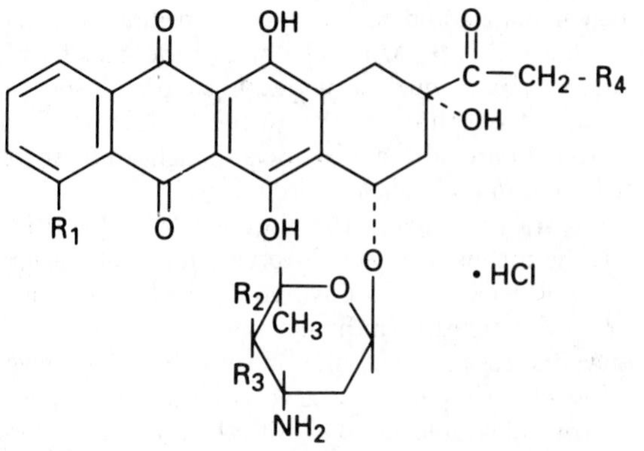

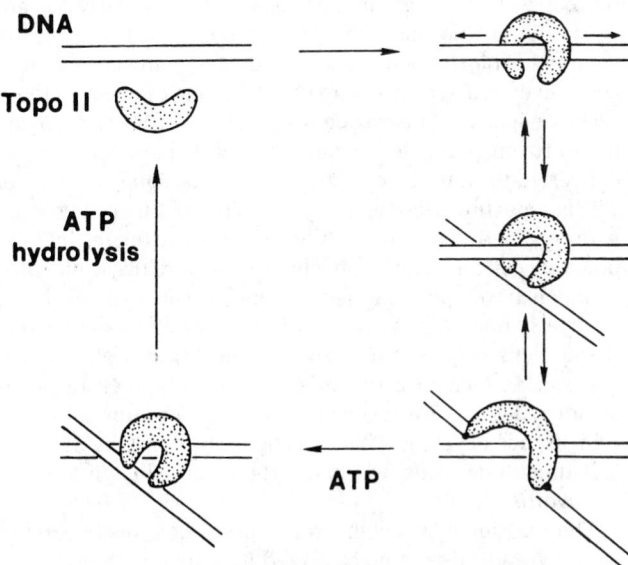

	Doxorubicin	Daunomycin	Epirubicin	Idarubicin
R_1 =	OCH_3	OCH_3	OCH_3	H
R_2 =	H	H	OH	H
R_3 =	OH	OH	H	OH
R_4 =	OH	H	OH	H

FIGURE 18–17. Structures of the four anthracyclines in current clinical use. Epirubicin differs from doxorubicin in the steric position of the 4'-OH group, whereas idarubicin differs from daunorubicin in lacking an A-ring methoxy substitution.

thyroid, and ovary, and soft tissue sarcomas. As a result of this clinical activity, more than 500 analogs have been synthesized or isolated from *Streptomyces*. It is likely these will provide the clinician with a number of new anthracyclines with different therapeutic spectra or altered toxicity. For this reason, emphasis in this section is placed on pertinent structure-activity relations.

MECHANISM OF ACTION

Although addition of doxorubicin or daunorubicin to tumor cells or lysed cell systems may result in a range of biochemical effects, the current view is that the antitumor activity and most toxicities are the result of free radical formation or triggering of topoisomerase II-dependent DNA fragmentation.

The organization of DNA in chromatin involves subjecting the DNA to variable degrees of supercoiled twisting.[35] Control of the degree of supercoiling of the DNA plays a critical role in DNA replication and gene function. As a result, there are several proteins whose function it is to control the degree of supercoiled twisting of the DNA. One of these is topoisomerase II (Fig. 18–18). This enzyme alters the degree of torsion in the DNA helix by creating a double-strand break that allows one portion of the DNA strand to pass through another. With each strand-passing event, the degree of supercoiled twist on the DNA double helix is increased or decreased. For topoisomerase II to create a double-strand break, it attaches to the phosphate backbone through formation of a tyrosine phosphate bridge. This results in a covalent attachment between the enzyme and the DNA helix. In addition, the enzyme acts to hold the DNA together so that the strands do not dissociate until the strand-passing process requires it to do so. Treatment of the DNA with strong alkali will denature the protein so that the double-strand breaks now become apparent, and at each break the denatured topoisomerase II may be found covalently linked to the DNA. This process gives rise to the characteristic protein-associated double-strand breaks diagnostic of topoisomerase II action. The anthracyclines appear to allow formation of the protein-associated double-strand breaks, but prevent the enzyme from finishing its cycle with religation of the broken strands. In addition, the alteration of

DNA helical structure that occurs on DNA intercalation by anthracyclines may trigger enhanced topoisomerase II activity. The net result is that addition of doxorubicin to tumor cells results in a dramatic increase in protein-associated breaks. Further, for most drugs that trigger topoisomerase II-associated DNA fragmentation, there is a consistent relation between break frequency and proportion of tumor cells killed. In addition, DNA intercalators that trigger topoisomerase II action generally exhibit a preference for specific DNA sequences.

Topoisomerase II is a major component of the nuclear matrix and the replication complex.[36] Because it is a portion of

FIGURE 18–18. Current concept of the strand-passing process catalyzed by topoisomerase II. The enzyme is thought to wrap itself around the DNA in a circular fashion and to move along the DNA until a site of topologic distortion is encountered. When a site of topologic distortion is encountered, the enzyme binds to a second segment of DNA, leading to covalent attachment and strand cleavage. In the process of ATP, the strand passage and regeneration of the free enzyme can proceed.

the nuclear matrix and can form covalent links with DNA, topoisomerase II is thought to be one of the sites by which DNA attaches to the nuclear matrix. In support of this, it can be shown that a high proportion of the DNA breaks caused by doxorubicin are adjacent to areas thought to be involved in attachment to the nuclear matrix.[37]

There is strong evidence that the topoisomerase II mechanism is the means by which doxorubicin and other anthracyclines kill leukemia and lymphoma cells, two disease groupings in which the anthracyclines play a major role.[38] Anthracycline-resistant cell lines in some instances have decreased levels of topoisomerase II or mutant enzymes that fail to form a cleavable complex with the drug. In addition, a similar mechanism of cytotoxicity appears to be involved in carcinoma of the lung, but there is less evidence for a role of topoisomerase II in the killing of breast, colon, or ovarian carcinoma cells by anthracyclines.[39,40]

The anthracyclines are able to form oxygen radicals by two independent mechanisms. The quinone functionality common to all clinically used anthracyclines may undergo a one-electron reduction to the corresponding semiquinone free radical. In the presence of oxygen, this semiquinone will rapidly donate its extra electron to molecular oxygen, resulting in regeneration of the parent anthracycline and superoxide. Superoxide is able to engage in a series of reactions that yield hydrogen peroxide and hydroxyl radical. The latter is one of the most reactive compounds known and rapidly attacks a wide range of important biologic targets, including DNA and cell membrane lipids. As a result, the most important of these reactions is the one in which hydrogen peroxide yields hydroxyl radical.

The enzymes that accomplish this reduction are all flavin-centered reductases and include microsomal cytochrome P450 reductase, mitochondrial NADH dehydrogenase, cytochrome b5 reductase, and xanthine oxidase.[41–44] These enzymes are found in most normal tissues and tumor cells. However, oxygen radical formation is also a product of many normal metabolic events, and pathways exist for the detoxification of these reactive species. Superoxide dismutase converts superoxide to hydrogen peroxide. In turn, hydrogen peroxide may be converted to water by catalase or by glutathione peroxidase. The latter action uses the tripeptide thiol glutathione to reduce hydrogen peroxide to water. Catalase tends to operate at high peroxide concentrations, but glutathione peroxidase operates at much lower peroxide levels. One reason that the heart muscle is unusually sensitive to anthracyclines is that this tissue lacks catalase, and doxorubicin destroys glutathione peroxidase.[45] This leaves cardiac tissue with no clear mechanism to detoxify hydrogen peroxide produced through doxorubicin redox cycling. This is particularly damaging in that it is hydrogen peroxide, which has the potential to give rise to the hydroxyl radical.

The reaction by which hydrogen peroxide gives rise to the hydroxyl radical may be catalyzed by transition metal ions, such as copper and iron. A second critical property of doxorubicin and other anthracyclines are that they effectively chelate Fe^{3+} and Cu^{2+}.[46,47] The resulting drug-metal complexes have a number of critical properties that render them destructive to mammalian cells.[48] First, they are effective catalysts of the reaction whereby hydrogen peroxide yields hydroxyl radical. Second, these drug-metal complexes bind to DNA and cell membranes. The combination of these two

properties results in efficient generation of hydroxyl radicals in the immediate vicinity of critical biologic targets. There is now a considerable body of evidence that these drug-iron complexes play a central role in the cardiac toxicity of the anthracyclines. ICRF-187, an edetate (EDTA) analog, effectively prevents clinical cardiac toxicity of doxorubicin by chelating iron and dramatically lessening hydroxyl radical formation.[49]

Although topoisomerase II has been shown to play a central role in the activity of the anthracyclines against leukemias and lymphomas, other evidence suggests a role for anthracycline-induced free radical formation in its killing of ovary, breast, and colon tumor cells.[50–54] Much of this evidence depends on the key roles that glutathione and glutathione peroxidase play in the detoxification of hydrogen peroxide and organic peroxides, a subject that is considered in detail in the section on drug resistance in this chapter.

One of the most unusual aspects of the anthracyclines is the ability of these agents to cause cardiomyopathy. Most of the existing evidence supports free radical formation as the basis for this toxicity. Other hypotheses have been put forward over the years, but none has survived experimental scrutiny for long. It is now clear that heart tissue is able to activate anthracyclines to a free radical at multiple sites, including the cytosol, mitochondria, and sarcoplasmic reticulum.[55] In addition, cardiac tissue has low levels of catalase, a key enzyme in the detoxification of hydrogen peroxide.[45] In addition, doxorubicin destroys glutathione peroxidase activity, a second major mechanism of peroxide removal. Doxorubicin stimulates oxygen-radical formation in the heart muscle while simultaneously abrogating the major mechanism by which the heart defends itself against oxygen radicals.

The major criticism of the free radical hypothesis was that free radical scavengers, such as tocopherol and N-acetylcysteine, have not been successful in preventing the cardiac toxicity in humans. However, at the time these studies were in progress, the unique involvement of iron in doxorubicin biochemistry was not appreciated. It is now known that in most experimental systems involving cells or subcellular organelles, iron must be present for doxorubicin free radical formation to result in significant damage. Doxorubicin is a remarkably active iron chelator, with measured binding affinities of 10^{28} to 10^{33}. The resulting iron—doxorubicin complex is extremely reactive in catalyzing a variety of free radical reactions, such as the conversion of hydrogen peroxide to hydroxyl radical. Neither tocopherol nor thiols such as N-acetylcysteine are effective in blocking this chemistry.

The logical conclusion of all of this work on doxorubicin chemistry is that the most critical step in the reactions leading up to free radical-induced cardiac injury is the reaction between doxorubicin, iron, and peroxide. Consistent with this hypothesis, the first clinically successful cardioprotective agent is an effective iron chelator, ICRF-187.[49]

CLINICAL PHARMACOLOGY AND PHARMACOKINETICS

Acquired resistance to the anthracyclines appears in most instances to be associated with the development of broad-spectrum drug resistance that typically extends to include the vinca alkaloids, etoposide, and taxol, but not the antimetabolites or alkylating agents. In most experimental systems, multidrug resistance is mediated by the *MDR* gene product—a cell surface glycoprotein that mediates ATP-dependent drug efflux.[56] It has become apparent that drug efflux pumps other than the *MDR* gene product exist.[57] The biology of the multidrug resistance efflux pump and its inhibition by various calcium channel blocking agents is more fully discussed in the section on mechanisms of antineoplastic drug resistance in this chapter.

Other mechanisms of multidrug resistance have been identified, including those that depend on a decreased activity or mutation in topoisomerase II or an increase in glutathione-dependent detoxification of peroxides, as discussed in the section on drug resistance in this chapter. However, the role of these drug efflux pumps in drug resistance in the clinical setting remains to be determined. Only within the past few years has adequate assay methodology become available for clinical monitoring of anthracyclines. Currently, the only valid assay methodology is with HPLC, which allows rapid resolution of doxorubicin and its metabolites.[58]

The major metabolites of anthracyclines are their side chain alcohols (e.g., doxorubicinol), which are the products of reduction by means of aldo-keto reductase. These compounds exhibit antitumor activity, although not as much as does the parent drug. The parent drug and these metabolites also predominate in bile and urine. The deoxyalglycones, other metabolites of interest, are one of the byproducts of semiquinone radical formation and, thus, are markers for this process in vivo. Other minor metabolites have been described, but their importance is not currently known.[59] Although the pharmacokinetics of doxorubicin are undoubtedly complex, its disappearance curves can be fit to a three-compartment model, with half-lives of 11 minutes, 3 hours, and 25 to 28 hours.[60] Clearance of doxorubicinol or daunorubicinol does not always parallel that of the parent drug. Epirubicin is unusual in that the major metabolite is the glucinomide.

The effects of renal and hepatic failure on doxorubicin and daunorubicin clearance are important to the clinician because this information may provide a basis for rational modification of drug dosage in cases of malfunction of these organs. Renal clearance of anthracyclines is minor in magnitude, and there is no need to modify drug dosages because of renal failure. All anthracyclines are metabolized significantly in the liver. As a result, drug doses often are modified because of abnormal liver function, especially elevated bilirubin. Precise guidelines based on sound pharmacokinetic information, however, are completely lacking, and this subject warrants further study. Nevertheless, existing information on the pharmacology of doxorubicin suggests that mild-to-moderate liver function abnormalities do not alter the pharmacokinetics of the drug. Further, administration of full doses of doxorubicin in the face of abnormal liver function has not been associated with increased drug toxicity.[61] Because the liver is the major site of doxorubicin clearance, these observations are somewhat surprising. It may be that the prolonged terminal phase of doxorubicin clearance (half-life of ~30 hours) is a function of the rate at which the drug dissociates from DNA rather than a function of liver metabolism.

TOXICITY

Anthracyclines cause bone marrow suppression and mucositis, which are dose limiting. Alopecia is a nearly universal adverse effect that, although not life-threatening, often causes significant patient distress. Extravasation of these agents leads to severe local reaction. Erythema and pain usually develop within 24 hours and can progress over weeks, resulting in deep ulceration that can reach tendon and bone. These lesions heal slowly and are difficult to skin graft. Multiple local measures used to manage this complication include ice packs and local injections of steroids, bicarbonate, or saline solution. The best approach is to take all possible precautions to avoid extravasation.

Perhaps the most perplexing reaction these agents cause is cardiac toxicity. Clinically, two aspects are involved: First is an acute syndrome that can be seen for hours to days after a dose of doxorubicin or daunorubicin; it is unrelated to cumulative dose and can manifest as disturbances in conduction and rhythm or pump failure. Electrocardiographic (ECG) studies have revealed supraventricular arrhythmias, heart block, and ventricular tachycardia. Second, ECG-gated pool scans have shown major drops in ejection fraction that reach a nadir within 24 to 48 hours after drug administration. In certain patients, this can cause acute congestive heart failure. Some of these patients develop pericardial effusions, and this whole complex has been called the *myocarditis-pericarditis syndrome*. Rarely, acute cardiac toxicity can cause the sudden demise of the patient.

The more common toxicity is a cumulative, dose-dependent cardiomyopathy that can lead to congestive heart failure in 1% to 10% of the patients who receive a total dose of 550 mg/m^2 of doxorubicin. The pathologic features of this lesion are unique and can be quantitated readily by endocardial biopsy. This technique is valuable in diagnosing the cause of congestive heart failure in patients who may have received doxorubicin and in detecting subclinical cardiac damage, which contraindicates further doxorubicin treatment. ECG-gated pool scan measurement of ejection fraction has proved valuable in detecting heart damage and is more practical than endocardial biopsy for widespread clinical use.

IMPORTANCE OF DOSE AND SCHEDULING

The traditional method of administering doxorubicin was as a bolus at a dosage of 45 to 75 mg/m^2 every 3 to 4 weeks. It is with this dosage that the risk of cardiac toxicity as a function of total dose was developed. It is now clear that this method of drug administration is not optimal. Repeated small doses (every week) or prolonged infusions (>96 hours) are associated with a much lower risk of cardiac toxicity without significantly compromising antitumor activity. On these schedules, gastrointestinal toxicity does, however, become a more significant problem.[62] Also, little has been done to work out how prolonged infusions of doxorubicin might be integrated into combination chemotherapy programs.

ANALOGS

Although enormous effort has been expended on anthracycline analog development, few agents that have seen clinical trial offer any advantage over daunorubicin or doxorubicin (Fig. 18–19). Epirubicin (4'-epidoxorubicin) has been claimed to be less cardiotoxic for equivalent therapeutic doses.[63] However, the advantage is not quantitatively impressive and may merely reflect differences in potency.

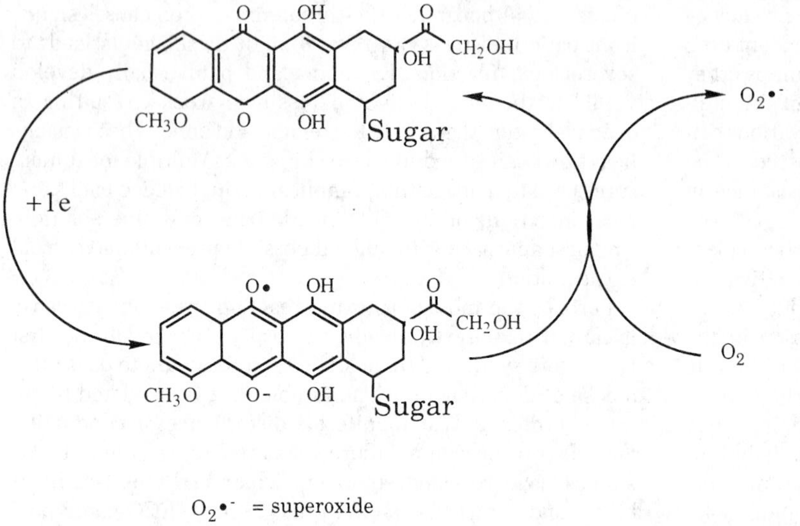

$O_2 \bullet^- $ = superoxide

FIGURE 18–19. One-electron reduction of doxorubicin. This reduction occurs at the quinone oxygens of the chromophore. The semiquinones react rapidly with oxygen, when it is available, to yield the one-electron reduction product of oxygen, superoxide.

Idarubicin (4-demethoxydaunorubicin) has proven superior to daunorubicin in the treatment of acute myelogenous leukemia and is also active in non-Hodgkin lymphoma and in breast cancer. This drug is rapidly converted to idarubicinol, and this metabolite has a longer half-life than the parent drug (50–60 hours compared with 10–15 hours).[64] As a result, circulating levels of idarubicinol are typically two or three times those of the parent drug. Idarubicin is unusual in that it is the only anthracycline in clinical use that retains its antitumor activity when administered orally. The bioavailability of the parent drug is approximately 20%. However, when idarubicinol is taken into account as an active metabolite, the bioavailability increases to 40%. Preclinical toxicology suggested that idarubicin might be devoid of cardiac toxicity. Unfortunately, clinical experience suggests that this drug is similar in its cardiac toxicity to that of all other currently used anthracyclines. Its primary metabolite, 4-demethoxy-13-hydroxydaunorubicin, is as cytotoxic as the parent and, because of slower elimination, exceeds the level of the parent in plamsa.[217] The drug is eliminated predominantly through the renal excretion of its 13-hydroxymetabolite.

5-Iminodaunomycin is inactive in all of the free radical chemistry described for doxorubicin and is not mutagenic or cardiotoxic.[65] It is, however, active in stimulating topoisomerase II cleavage of DNA. It is less potent than doxorubicin or daunorubicin. Nevertheless, it represents the first member of a structural class of anthracyclines in which topoisomerase activity can be clearly separated from free radical biochemistry and could signal a valuable direction for future development.

COMPOUNDS RELATED TO ANTHRACYCLINES

Mitoxantrone (Fig. 18–20) is a completely synthetic DNA intercalator based on the anthracenedione structure and may be viewed as an analog of the anthracyclines. As with most DNA intercalators, mitoxantrone has a chromophore composed of three planar aromatic rings. In this instance, the chromophore is an hydroxyquinone analogous to the anthracyclines. In place of the daunosamine sugar characteristic of the anthracyclines, mitoxantrone has two identical aminoalkyl side chains. As with the anthracyclines, mitoxantrone is able to undergo DNA intercalations and reduction to the corre-

sponding semiquinone.[66,67] However, because of the redox potential of this drug, the mitoxantrone semiquinone free radical is unreactive. As a result, mitoxantrone preserves the capacity of the anthracyclines to trigger topoisomerase-II-dependent DNA cleavage while exhibiting reduced cardiac toxicity.[68] Drug resistance is mediated by increased MDR protein, by reduced topoisomerase II activity, or by a unique drug efflux mechanism unrelated to the multidrug resistance system.[69] The pharmacokinetics of mitoxantrone are similar to those of doxorubicin and daunorubicin in that the initial distribution of the drug occurs with a half-life of 1 or 2 hours followed by a terminal half-life of 23 to 42 hours. Elimination of the parent drug into urine or stool accounts for less than 30% of the administered drug. Much of the fate of the drug remains to be determined, but extensive side chain oxidation to carboxylic acid groups appears to occur. Common schedules of administration are patterned after those used for the anthracyclines. Dose-limiting toxicity is granulocytopenia, with recovery complete by day 14 after usual doses of 10 to 14 mg/m². The drug also can cause thrombocytopenia, nausea and vomiting, and a bluish discoloration of the sclera, fingernails, and urine, but extravasation injury is uncommon. Mitoxantrone does cause cardiac toxicity, but this tends to be more of a problem in patients who have been pretreated with anthracyclines, and this drug is less cardiotoxic than the anthracyclines.[68] Perhaps as a consequence of the side chain oxidation discussed earlier, mitoxantrone has been reported to cause oxidative injury to the liver.[70] Although mitoxantrone does cause mucositis, it is much less emetogenic than the anthracyclines. In addition, alopecia is much less severe with mitoxantrone than with the anthracyclines. Although the therapeutic spectrum of mitoxantrone remains to be deter-

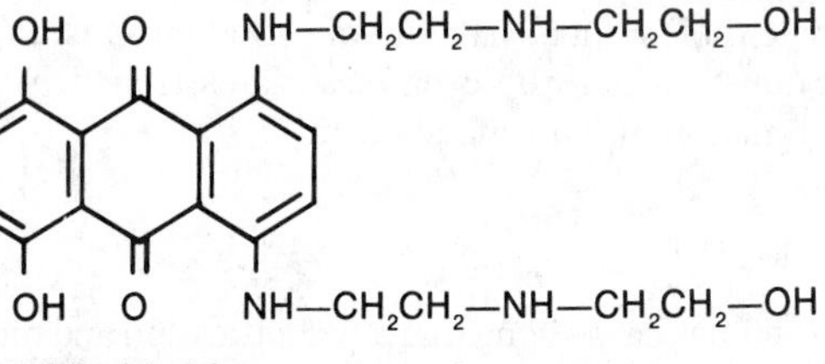

FIGURE 18–20. Structure of mitoxantrone.

mined, worthwhile antitumor activity has been seen in breast cancer, leukemias, and lymphomas.

The anthrapyrazoles, considered in the section on investigational agents elsewhere in this chapter, represent a related class of compounds with topoisomerase II-mediated activity and reduced cardiotoxicity in animals.

MITOMYCIN C

A number of considerations enter into the design of new anticancer drugs, including the identification of a tumor-selective target. Mitomycin C has evoked great interest because it is the only clinical agent that is known to undergo preferential activation in a hypoxic environment, such as found in human solid tumors. Its primary clinical use has been for gastrointestinal carcinoma and, more recently, non-small cell carcinoma of the lung. Several reviews offer more detail of the clinical activity and pharmacologic aspects of this agent.[71,72]

STRUCTURE AND MECHANISM OF ACTION

The structure of mitomycin C and its activation pathway are shown in Figure 18–21. Activation of the drug to an alkylating species can occur through enzymatic reduction, mediated by cytochrome b_5 reductase, DT-diaphorase, xanthine oxidase, or cytochrome P-450 reductase, or can occur in acid-catalyzed or base-catalyzed reactions in aqueous solution.[73,74] The role of enzymatic reduction in producing a clinically active species in vivo is uncertain and will depend on a number of factors, including the availability of oxygen, which tends to discourage the generation of a reactive semiquinone.[75] One-electron reduction generates the semiquinone species and creates electrophilic (and potentially alkylating) centers at carbons 1 and 10.[76] In an aerobic environment, reduction of mitomycin C initiates a chain of electron transfers that lead ultimately to formation of toxic hydroxyl and superoxide radicals.[77] Recent study indicates that bifunctional alkylation by mitomycin C occurs preferentially in a reducing environment, perhaps because O_2 tends to react with, and destroy, the activated one-electron reduction product through attack at the C-1 carbon.[78]

At least three reactive centers of the compound have been identified: the C-1 carbon of the mitosane ring (see Fig. 18–21); the quinone ring structure, which can undergo one or two electron reduction to form reactive species; and the urethane group, which can open to form an alkylating site at C-10. Once activated, mitomycin C alkylates and crosslinks DNA at the N^6 atom of adenine and the O^6, N^7, and N^2 atoms of guanine of DNA. Crosslinks result in inhibition of DNA synthesis and cell death.

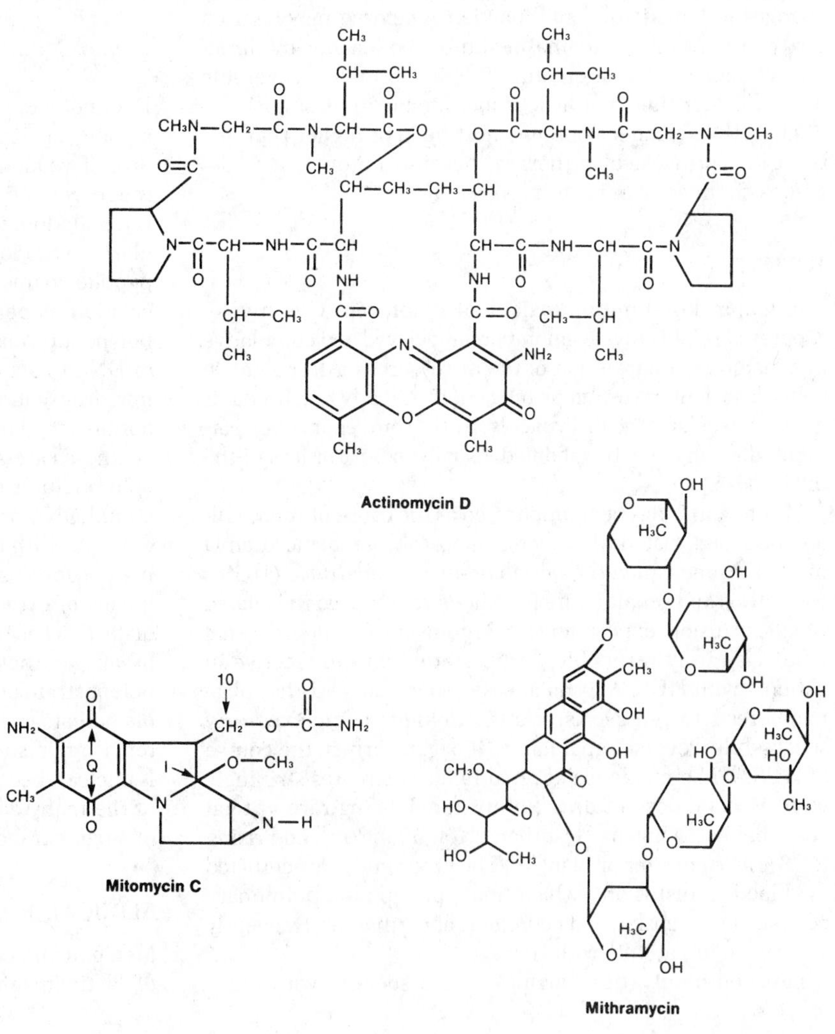

FIGURE 18–21. Antitumor antibiotics. Potential sites of activation of mitomycin C are indicated by *arrows* and include the carbon linked to a labile methoxy group (1), the C-10 carbon (10), and the quinone ring system (Q).

Although some investigators have found evidence for preferential "bioreductive" activation in hypoxic tumor cells in vitro, experiments in animals have not substantiated this preferential activity under hypoxic conditions.[79] Resistance to mitomycin C is poorly characterized. In some, but not all, cell lines that demonstrate broad-base multidrug resistance against natural-product drugs, mitomycin C resistance is associated with amplification of the P-170 glycoprotein.[80] In other resistant cells, decreased activation, in some instances associated with decreased DT-diaphorase activity, seems responsible for resistance.[81]

CLINICAL PHARMACOLOGY

The pharmacokinetics of mitomycin C have been reviewed by Dorr.[82] Usual doses of mitomycin C are 10 mg/m^2 in combination therapy protocols.

Metabolic activation by reduction occurs in all tissues and thus does not explain the selectivity of this agent for tumor tissue. As a result of this ubiquitous metabolism, clearance of the drug is rapid. As with the anthracyclines, renal clearance is minor, and the role of the liver is defined so poorly that no guidelines can be given for dose modification in the presence of liver or renal disease. The drug may be measured in biologic fluids by HPLC. The primary elimination half-life is 25 to 90 (mean 54) minutes. The plasma disappearance rate is uniform over the dose range of 15 to 60 mg/m^2 and is unaffected by changes in hepatic or renal function. The drug may be used for treatment of carcinoma in situ of the bladder by direct intravesicular installation; after 2 hours, 50% is recoverable in the bladder fluid, but little is measurable in plasma.[83]

The pH of bladder contents must be kept higher than pH 6 during intravesicular therapy, because mitomycin C degrades chemically at lower pHs.

TOXICITY

The major dose-limiting toxicity of mitomycin C is myelosuppression. This myelosuppression is delayed and cumulative in a fashion similar to that of the nitrosoureas. After a single bolus dose, leukocyte and platelet counts usually reach a nadir between weeks 4 and 6. Typically, by the third course of treatment, doses have to be modified, usually to 50% or less of the initial dose.

Mitomycin C has been implicated as the cause of renal failure, often associated with microangiopathic hemolytic anemia in a syndrome called the *hemolytic-uremic syndrome* (HUS). Hemolysis and renal failure have been reproduced in isolated renal perfusion experiments.[84] Mitomycin C-induced renal failure is rarely reversible; corticosteroids are ineffective in patients with HUS. Anecdotal case reports suggest that plasmapheresis to remove circulating immune complexes may successfully reverse renal failure if begun early in the course of HUS.[85] The incidence of renal failure increases strikingly with the total dose of drug administered, being rare at total doses below 30 mg/m^2, less than 2% at 50 mg/m^2, and rising to 28% at 70 mg/m^2 or higher.[86] The syndrome is exacerbated by blood transfusion, which may precipitate pulmonary edema. Hypertension and neurologic abnormalities frequently supervene in patients with HUS.[87]

Less commonly, this drug has been associated with interstitial pneumonitis and cardiomyopathy. The pneumonitis is uncommon, not dose-related, and exhibits pathologic characteristics similar to those of busulfan lung.[88] The incidence of pneumonitis is higher in patients receiving mitomycin C and a vinca alkaloid.[89] Pneumonitis is enhanced by raised oxygen tension and appears to be mediated by lipid peroxidation resulting from the generation of reactive oxygen species.[90] It may progress to extensive pulmonary fibrosis. The cardiomyopathy has been reported in patients receiving mitomycin C alone or in combination with doxorubicin. This phenomenon is not surprising, because doxorubicin and mitomycin C can be activated to radicals by reduction, and, in the former instance, this radical production has been proposed to be the cause of the cardiac toxicity. As in the HUS, the incidence of cardiotoxicity due to mitomycin C increases with total doses higher than 30 mg/m^2.[91]

DACTINOMYCIN

Dactinomycin is a member of a large class of similar drugs that were first isolated from *Streptomyces* species.[92] It is the only member of the class to achieve significant clinical use. Dactinomycin is effective in the treatment of Wilms' tumor, Ewing's sarcoma, embryonal rhabdomyosarcoma, and gestational choriocarcinoma. Responses also are seen in testicular cancer, Kaposi's sarcoma, and lymphoma.

STRUCTURE AND MECHANISM OF ACTION

Dactinomycin has an interesting structure. It is composed of a phenoxazone ring chromophore that gives a red color to the drug. Two identical cyclic polypeptides are bound to the chromophore (see Fig. 18–21). This antibiotic binds to DNA by intercalation, with the phenoxazone ring inserted perpendicularly to the long axis of the DNA double helix and the polypeptide chains extending along the minor groove. This intercalation depends on a specific interaction between the polypeptide chains and deoxyguanosine and blocks the ability of DNA to act as a template for RNA and DNA synthesis. At low drug concentrations, inhibition of RNA synthesis predominates, but at higher concentrations, RNA and DNA syntheses are affected.[93]

In addition to these effects, dactinomycin causes single-strand DNA breaks in a manner similar to that of doxorubicin.[94] As with doxorubicin, there are several possible explanations for this observation. Dactinomycin can be reduced by means of cytochrome P-450 reductase to a radical intermediate; this has been postulated as the cause of the single-strand breakage. Another hypothesis is that intercalation causes sufficient strain on the three-dimensional topography of the double helix to trigger enzymatic nicking and strand breakage by topoisomerase II. However, the role of single-strand breaks is unclear, because there is no correlation between the affinity of the many dactinomycin analogs for DNA, the occurrence of single-strand breaks, and cytotoxicity.

CLINICAL PHARMACOLOGY

Metabolism does not play a significant role in the clearance of dactinomycin, and most of the drug is excreted unchanged in bile and urine. Initial clearance of the drug from plasma is rapid and is dominated by tissue uptake and DNA binding. The slow phase (half-life of 36 hours) of the drug disappearance curve is determined by slow release of drug from tissue pools, with excretion into bile and urine.[95] Because human pharmacologic data are so fragmentary, no firm guidelines can be given for dose modification if there is liver or renal dysfunction.

TOXICITY

The most common dose-limiting toxicity of this agent is myelosuppression, but it occasionally may be gastrointestinal, manifested as ulceration of oral mucosa and gastrointestinal tract, accompanied by pain and diarrhea.

One of the most interesting and perplexing toxicities associated with dactinomycin is its interaction with x-irradiation. Combined treatment with these two modalities leads to accelerated skin and gastrointestinal toxicity. In addition, late radiation damage to lung and liver appears to be increased. It has been postulated that this effect results from the ability of dactinomycin to block repair of radiation-mediated DNA damage. This hypothesis does not explain the recall effect observed in patients treated with dactinomycin after x-irradiation. This recall reaction can be observed even after a period of several months between irradiation and drug treatment.

MITHRAMYCIN

Mithramycin (see Fig. 18–21), an antibiotic isolated from *Streptomyces plicatus,* not only has antitumor activity against testicular carcinoma but also has a specific hypocalcemic effect that is valuable in the treatment of malignant hypercalcemia.[96]

Mithramycin is an inhibitor of DNA-directed RNA synthesis. It is administered intravenously. Little is known about its pharmacokinetics and disposition in humans. Currently, there are no suitable assays for this drug. It is known to produce differentiation of human myeloid leukemia cells in culture and to produce remissions in the blastic phase of chronic myelogenous leukemia in humans, possibly through differentiation.[97] This agent has a number of unusual side effects in addition to its antitumor activity. It causes acute nausea and vomiting and, occasionally, diarrhea and stomatitis. More important, a hemorrhagic diathesis often is seen with daily treatment and is manifested as a decrease in platelet count, a lengthening of the prothrombin time, and a depression of clotting factors II, V, VII, and X. Deaths resulting from uncontrolled gastrointestinal hemorrhage have been reported with this schedule of administration. Mithramycin also has serious renal and hepatic toxicities, the mechanisms of which are unclear. An alternate-day regimen of 50 μg/kg/day appears to cause predictable and tolerable toxicity and is associated with a response rate of nearly 50% in testicular carcinoma. This schedule is maintained on an alternate-day basis until signs appear that signal hepatic (lactic dehydrogenase levels > 2000 U/100 ml), renal (azotemia), or clotting (prothrombin time > 15 seconds, platelet count < 100,000 cells/μl) dysfunction.

Other adverse reactions include fever, myalgias, headache, and, uncommonly, vascular thrombosis. Because of its many serious toxic side effects, mithramycin currently is indicated only for treatment of testicular neoplasms. However, in lower doses and for brief courses of treatment (15–25 μg/kg/day for 3 days), mithramycin effectively lowers serum calcium concentration in patients with hypercalcemia of malignant or nonmalignant origin. Its effects are mediated through decreased bone resorption and last for 7 to 21 days. In most instances, specific therapy directed against the neoplasm in question is required to produce permanent, effective control of the serum calcium level.

REFERENCES

1. Petering DH, Byrnes RW, Antholine WE. The role of redox-active metals in the mechanism of action of bleomycin. Chem Biol Interact 1990;73:133–182.
2. Ciriolo MR, Magliozzo RS, Peisach J. Microsome-stimulated activation of ferrous bleomycin in the presence of DNA. J Biol Chem 1987;262:6290–6295.
3. Kozarich JW, Worth L Jr, Frank BL, et al. Sequence-specific isotope effects on the cleavage of DNA by bleomycin. Science 1989;245:1396–1399.
4. Sugiyama H, Xu C, Murugesan N, et al. Chemistry of the alkali-labile lesion formed from Iron(II) bleomycin and d(CGCTTTAAAGCG). Biochemistry 1988;27:58–67.
5. Barraco SC, Humphrey RM. The effects of bleomycin on survival and cell progression in Chinese hamster cells in vitro. Cancer Res 1971;31:1218–1223.
6. Povrick LF, Han Y-H, Steighner RJ. Structure of bleomycin-induced DNA double-strand breaks: Predominance of blunt ends and single-base 5′ extensions. Biochemistry 1989;28:5808–5814.
7. Barranco SC, Novak JK, Humphrey RM. Studies on recovery from chemically induced damage in mammalian cells. Cancer Res 1975;35:1194–1204.
8. Chafouleas JG, Bolton WE, Means AR. Potentiation of bleomycin lethality by anticalmodulin drugs: A role for calmodulin in DNA repair. Science 1984;224:1346–1348.
9. Russo A, Mitchell JB, McPherson, et al. Alteration of bleomycin cytotoxicity by glutathione depletion or elevation. Int J Radiat Oncol Biol Phys 1984;10:1675–1678.
10. Nakatsugawa S, Dewey WC. The role in cancer therapy of inhibiting recovery from PLD induced by radiation or bleomycin. Int J Radiat Oncol Biol Phys 1984;10:1425–1430.
11. Sidik K, Smerdon MJ. Nucleosome rearrangement in human cells following short-patch repair of DNA damage. Biochemistry 1990;29:7501–7511.
12. Chatterjee S, Cheng MF, Berger NA. Hypersensitivity to clinically useful alkylating agents and radiation in poly(ADP-ribose)polymerase-deficient cell lines. Cancer Commun 1990;2:401–407.
13. Moore CW. Degradation of DNA and structure-activity relationship between bleomycins A$_2$ and B$_2$ in the absence of DNA repair. Biochemistry 1990;29:1342–1347.
14. Umezawa H, Hori S, Sawa T, et al. A bleomycin-activating enzyme in mouse liver. J Antibiot 1974;27:419–424.
15. Sebti SM, Mignano JE, Jani JP, et al. Bleomycin hydrolase: Molecular cloning, sequencing and biochemical studies reveal membership in the cysteine proteinase family. Biochemistry 1989;28:6544–6548.
16. Sehti SM, Lazo JS. Separation of the protective enzyme bleomycin hydrolase from rabbit pulmonary aminopeptidases. Biochemistry 1987;26:432–437.
17. Akiyama S, Kuwano M. Isolation and preliminary characterization of bleomycin-resistant mutants from Chinese hamster ovary cells. J Cell Physiol 1981;107:147.
18. Zuckerman JE, Raffin TA, Brown JM, et al. In vitro selection and characterization of a bleomycin-resistant subline of B16 melanoma. Cancer Res 1986;46:1748–1753.
19. Lazo JS, Braun ID, Labaree DC, et al. Characteristics of bleomycin-resistant phenotypes of human cell sublines and circumvention of bleomycin resistance by liblomycin. Cancer Res 1989;49:185–190.
20. Broughton A, Strong JE. Radioimmunoassay of bleomycin. Cancer Res 1976;36:1418–1421.
21. Alberts DS, Chen HSG, Liu R, et al. Bleomycin pharmacokinetics in man: I. Intravenous administration. Cancer Chemother Pharmacol 1978;1:177–181.
22. Alberts DS, Chen HSG, Mayersohn M, et al. Bleomycin pharmacokinetics in man: II. Intracavitary administration. Cancer Chemother Pharmacol 1979;2:127–132.
23. Raisfeld IH. Role of terminal substituents in the pulmonary toxicity of bleomycins. Toxicol Appl Pharmacol 1981;57:355–366.
24. Conley NS, Yarbro JW, Ferrari HA, et al. Bleomycin increases superoxide anion generation by pig peripheral alveolar macrophages. Mol Pharmacol 1986;30:48–52.
25. Adamson IY, Bowden DH. The pathogenesis of bleomycin-induced pulmonary fibrosis in mice. Am J Pathol 1974;77:185–189.
26. Suwabe A, Takahashi K, Yasui S, et al. Bleomycin-stimulated hamster alveolar macrophages release interleukin-1. Am J Pathol 1988;132:512–520.
27. Hout AE, Hacker MP. Role of reactive nitrogen intermediate production in alveolar macrophage-mediated cytostatic activity induced by bleomycin lung damage in rats. Cancer Res 1990;50:7863–7866.
28. Blum RH, Carter SK, Agre K. A clinical review of bleomycin—a new antineoplastic agent. Cancer 1973;31:903–914.

29. Comis RL. Detecting bleomycin pulmonary toxicity: A continued conundrum. J Clin Oncol 1990;8:765–767.

30. Goldiner PL, Carlon GC, Critkovic E, et al. Factors influencing post-operative morbidity and mortality in patients treated with bleomycin. Br Med J 1978;1:1664–1667.

31. Zucker PK, Khouri NF, Rosenshein NB. Bleomycin-induced pulmonary nodules: A variant of bleomycin pulmonary toxicity. Gynecol Oncol 1987;28:284–291.

32. Bellamy EA, Husband JE, Blaquiere RM, et al. Bleomycin-related lung damage: CT evidence. Radiology 1985;156:155–158.

33. Osanto S, Bukman A, Hoek F, et al. Long-term effects of chemotherapy in patients with testicular cancer. J Clin Oncol 1992;10:574–579.

34. DiMarco A, Galtani M, Orezzi PO. Daunomycin, a new antibiotic of the rhodomycin group. Nature 1964;201:706–707.

35. Zhang H, D'Arpe P, Liu LF. A model for tumor cell killing by topoisomerase poisons. Cancer Cells 1990;2:23–27.

36. Fernandes DJ, Catapano CV. Nuclear matrix targets for anticancer agents. Cancer Cells 1991;3:134–140.

37. Pommier Y, Capranico G, Orr A, Kohn KW. Local base sequence preferences for DNA cleavage by mammalian topoisomerase II in the presence of amsacrine or teniposide. Nucleic Acids Res 1991;19:5973–5980. [published erratum in Nucleic Acids Res 19:7003, 1991]

38. Zwelling LA. Topoisomerase II as a target of antileukemia drugs: A review of controversial areas. Hematol Pathol 1989;3:101–112.

39. Binaschi M, Capranico G, De IP, et al. Comparison of DNA cleavage induced by etoposide and doxorubicin in two human small-cell lung cancer lines with different sensitivities to topoisomerase II inhibitors. Int J Cancer 1990;45:347–352.

40. Kasahara K, Fujiwara Y, Sugimoto Y, et al. Determinants of response to the DNA topoisomerase II inhibitors doxorubicin and etoposide in human lung cancer cell lines. JNCI 1992;84:113–118.

41. Lown JW, Chen HH, Plambeck JA, Acton EM. Further studies on the generation of reactive oxygen species from activated anthracyclines and the relationship to cytotoxic action and cardiotoxic effects. Biochem Pharmacol 1982;31:575–581.

42. Myers CE, McGuire WP, Liss RH, et al. Adriamycin: The role of lipid peroxidation in cardiac toxicity and tumor response. Science 1977;197:165–167.

43. Sato S, Iwaizumi M, Handa K, Tamura Y. Electron spin resonance study on the mode of generation of free radicals of daunomycin, Adriamycin, and carboquone in NAD(P)H-microsome system. Gann 1977;68:603–608.

44. Doroshow JH. Anthracycline antibiotic-stimulated superoxide peroxide, and hydroxyl radical production by NADH dehydrogenase. Cancer Res 1983;43:4543–4551.

45. Doroshow JH, Locker GY, Myers CE. The enzymatic defenses of the mouse heart against reactive metabolites. J Clin Invest 1980;65:128–135.

46. Myers CE, Gianni L, Zweier J, et al. The role of iron in Adriamycin biochemistry. Fed Proc 1986;45:2792–2797.

47. Eliot H, Gianni L, Myers CE. Oxidative destruction of DNA by Adriamycin-iron complex. Biochemistry 1984;23:928–936.

48. Minotti G, Aust SD. The requirement of iron(III) in the initiation of lipid peroxidation. J Biol Chem 1987;262:1098–1104.

49. Speyer JL, Kramer GL, et al. Protective effect of the bispiperazinedione, ICRF-187, against doxorubicin-induced cardiac toxicity in women with advanced breast cancer. N Engl J Med 1988;319:745–752.

50. Dusre L. Mimnaugh EG, Myers CE, Sinha BK. Potentiation of doxorubicin cytoxicity by butathionine sulfoximine in multidrug-resistant human breast cancer cells. Cancer Res 1989;49:511.

51. Lai GM, Moscow JA, Alvarez MG, et al. Contribution of glutathione and glutathione-dependent enzymes in the reversal of Adriamycin resistance in colon carcinoma cell lines. Int J Cancer 1991;49:688–695.

52. Sinha BK, Katki AG, Batist G, et al. Adriamycin-simulated hydroxyl formation in human beast tumor cells. Biochem Pharmacol 1987;36:793–796.

53. Benchekroun MN, Catroux P, Montaudon D, Robert J. Development of mechanisms of protection against oxidative stress in doxorubicin-resistant rat tumoral cells in culture. Free Radic Res Commun 1990;11:137–144.

54. Chao CC, Huang YT, Ma CM, et al. Overexpression of glutathione-S-transferase and elevation of thiol pools in a multidrug-resistant human colon cancer cell line. Mol Pharmacol 1992;41:69–75.

55. Hacker MP, Lazo JS, Tritton TR, eds. Organ directed toxicities of anticancer drugs. The Hague: Martinus Nijhoff, 1988:31–40.

56. Juranka PF, Zastawny RL, Ling V. P-glycoprotein: Multidrug resistance and a superfamily of membrane-associated transport proteins. FASEB J 1989;3:2583–2592.

57. McGrath T, Latoud C, Arnold ST, et al. Mechanisms of multidrug resistance in HL60 cells: Analysis of resistance-associated membrane proteins and levels of *mdr* gene expression. Biochem Pharmacol 1989;38:3611–3619.

58. Israel M, Pegg WJ, Wilkinson PM, et al. Liquid chromatographic analysis of Adriamycin and metabolites in biological fluids. J Liquid Chromatogr 1978;1:795–809.

59. Takanashi S, Bachur NR. Adriamycin metabolism in man: Evidence from urinary metabolites. Drug Metab Disp 1976;4:79–87.

60. Benjamin RS. Pharmacokinetics of Adriamycin in patients with sarcomas. Cancer Chemother Rep 1974;58:271–273.

61. Sulkes A, Collins JM. Reappraisal of some dosage adjustment guidelines. Cancer Treat Rep 1987;71:229–233.

62. Benjamin RS, Chawla SP, Ewer MS, et al. Adriamycin cardiac toxicity—an assessment of approaches to cardiac monitoring and cardioprotection. In: Hacker MP, Lazo JS, Tritton TR, eds. Organ directed toxicities of anticancer drugs. The Hague: Martinus Nijhoff, 1988:41–55.

63. Myers CE. Anthracyclines. In: Pinedo HM, Longo DL, Chabner BA, eds. Cancer chemotherapy and biological response modifiers, Annual 9. Amsterdam: Elsevier, 1987:36–49.

64. Reid JM, Pendergrass TW, Krailo MD, et al. Plasma pharmacokinetics and cerebrospinal fluid concentrations of idarubicin and idarubicinol in pediatric leukemia patients: A Children's Cancer Study Group report. Cancer Res 1990;50:6525–6528.

65. Myers CE, Muindi JR, Zweier J, et al. 5-Iminodaunomycin: An anthracycline with unique properties. J Biol Chem 1987;262:11571–11577.

66. Ehninger G, Schuler U, Proksch B, et al. Pharmacokinetics and metabolism of mitoxantrone: A review. Clin Pharmacokinet 1990;18:365–380.

67. Novak RF, Kharasch ED. Mitoxantrone: Propensity for free radical formation and lipid peroxidation—implications for cardiotoxicity. Invest New Drugs 1985;3:95–99.

68. Henderson IC, Allegra JC, Woodcock T, et al. Randomized clinical trial comparing mitoxantrone with doxorubicin in previously treated patients with metastatic breast cancer. J Clin Oncol 1989;7:560–571.

69. Dalton WS, Cress AW, Alberats DS, et al. Cytogenetic and phenotypic analysis of a human colon carcinoma cell line resistant to mitoxantrone. Cancer Res 1988;48:1882–1888.

70. Llesuy SF, Arnaiz SL. Hepatoxicity of mitoxantrone and doxorubicin. Toxicology 1990;63:187–198.

71. Crooke ST, Bradner WT. Mitomycin C: A review. Cancer Treat Rev 1976;3:121–139.

72. Reich SD. Clinical pharmacology of mitomycin C. In: Carter SK, Crooke ST, eds. Mitomycin C: Current status and new developments. New York: Academic Press, 1979:243.

73. Keyes SR, Fracasso PM, Heimbrook DC, et al. Role of NADPH: Cytochrome C reductase and DT-diaphorase in the biotransformation of mitomycin C. Cancer Res 1984;44:5638–5643.

74. Iyengar BS, Remers WA. A comparison of mechanism proposed for the conversion of mitomycins into mitosenes. J Med Chem 1985;28:963–967.

75. den Hartigh J, Verweij J, Pinedo HM. Mitomycin C. In: Pinedo HM, Chabner BA, eds. Cancer chemotherapy, Annual 7. Amsterdam: Elsevier, 1985:83–90.

76. Tomasz M, Chowdary D, Lipman R, et al. Reaction of DNA with chemically or enzymatically activated DNA: Isolation and structure of the major covalent adduct. Proc Natl Acad Sci USA 1986;83:6702–6706.

77. Bachur NR, Gordon SL, Gee MV. A general mechanism for microsomal activation of quinone anticancer agents to free radicals. Cancer Res 1978;38:1745–1750.

78. Tomasz M, Chawla AK, Lipman R. Mechanism of monofunctional and bifunctional alkylation of DNA by mitomycin C. Biochemistry 1988;27:3182–3187.

79. Rockwell S. Effects of mitomycin C alone and in combination with x-rays on EMT-6 mouse mammary tumors in vivo. JNCI 1983;71:765–771.

80. Tsuruo T, Iida-Saito H, Kawabata H, et al. Characteristics of resistance to Adriamycin in human myelogenous leukemia K562 resistant to Adriamycin and in isolated clones. Jpn J Cancer Res 1986;77:682–692.

81. Dulhanty AM, Li M, Whitmore GF. Isolation of Chinese hamster ovary cell mutants deficient in excision repair and mitomycin C bioactivation. Cancer Res 1989;49:117–122.

82. Dorr RT. New findings in the pharmacokinetics, metabolic, and drug-resistance aspects of mitomycin C. Semin Oncol 1988;15(suppl 4):32–41.

83. van Helsdingen PJRO, Rikken CHM, Sleeboom HP. Mitomycin C resorption following repeated intravesical installations using different installation times. Urol Int 1988;43:42–46.

84. Cattell V. Mitomycin-induced hemolytic uremic kidney: An experimental model in the rat. Am J Pathol 1985;121:88–95.

85. Verweij J, Boven E, van der Meulen J, et al. Recovery from mitomycin C-induced haemolytic uraemic syndrome. Cancer 1984;54:2878–2881.

86. Valavaara R, Nordman E. Renal complications of mitomycin C therapy with special reference to the total dose. Cancer 1985;55:47–50.

87. Cantrell JE, Phillips TM, Schein PS. Carcinoma-associated hemolytic uremic syndrome: A complication of mitomycin C chemotherapy. J Clin Oncol 1985;3:723–734.

88. Oswoll ES, Kiessling PJ, Patterson JR. Interstitial pneumonia from mitomycin. Ann Intern Med 1978;89:352–355.

89. Kuedke D, McLaughlin TT, Daughaday C, et al. Mitomycin C and vindesine associated pulmonary toxicity with variable clinical expression. Cancer 1985;55:542–547.

90. Trush MA, Mimnaugh EG, Ginsburg E, et al. Studies on the in vitro interaction of mitomycin C, nitrofuantoin and paraquat with pulmonary microsomes: Stimulation of reactive oxygen-dependent lipid peroxidation. Biochem Pharmacol 1982;31:805.

91. Verweij J, Funke-Kuupper AJ, Teule GJJ, Pinedo HM. A prospective study on the dose dependency of cardiotoxicity induced by mitomycin C. Med Oncol Tumor Pharmacother 1988;5:159–163.

92. Selman Waksman Conference on Actinomycin: Their potential for cancer chemotherapy. Cancer Chemother Rep 1974;58:1–123.

93. Reich E, Franklin RM, Shatkin AJ, et al. Action of actinomycin D on animal cells and viruses. Proc Natl Acad Sci USA 1962;48:1238–1245.

94. Ross WE, Glaubiger DL, Kohn KW. Quantitative and qualitative aspects of intercalator-induced DNA damage. Biochim Biophys Acta 1979;562:41–50.

95. Tattersall NHM, Sodergren JE, Segupta SK, et al. Pharmacokinetics of actinomycin D in patients with malignant melanoma. Clin Pharmacol Ther 1975;17:701–708.

96. Kennedy BJ. Mithramycin therapy in testicular cancer. J Urol 1972;107:429–433.

97. Koller C, Miller DM. Preliminary observations on the therapy of the myeloid blast phase of chronic granulocytic leukemia with plicamycin and hydroxyurea. N Engl J Med 1986;315:1433–1437.

Miscellaneous Agents

HEXAMETHYLMELAMINE

Hexamethylmelamine (HMM) and its metabolite and experimental analog, pentamethylmelamine (PMM; Fig. 18–22), are structurally unique antitumor agents that have an uncertain mechanism of action but probably belong to the alkylator class of drugs. HMM has significant antineoplastic activity against ovarian cancer, breast cancer, the lymphomas, and small cell carcinoma of the lung. Despite partial elucidation of the complex metabolism of HMM, the active intermediate has not been identified with certainty. It likely acts as a DNA methylating agent, although clinically it does not display complete cross-resistance with cyclophosphamide, melphalan, other alkylators, or cisplatin. Its relatively mild myelosuppressive effects make this agent a candidate for combination therapy and encourage its use as second-line therapy for ovarian cancer.[1]

HMM consists of a symmetric 6-member triazene ring, with three attached dimethylamine groups. PMM, a more water-soluble analog that can be given intravenously, has one less methyl side group and is also present in plasma as a metabolite after oral administration of HMM. The methyl side groups of HMM and PMM are removed readily by a two-step process (microsomal oxidation to methylol groups, followed by *N*-demethylolation) to yield various possible methylmelamine derivatives and corresponding quantities of formaldehyde, a weakly cytotoxic compound.[2] HMM and its melamine metabolites are at best weakly cytotoxic in vitro in the absence of microsomes, but the methylol (R—CH_2OH) intermediates are highly cytotoxic in vitro. The actual site of HMM activation in humans is uncertain, and may be liver, intestinal mucosa, or tumor, or a combination thereof.[3]

Experimental studies with HMM labeled in the triazene ring or in the methyl groups have demonstrated covalent binding of both types of labeled compound to acid-insoluble material in tumor cells and normal tissues, indicating protein or nucleic acid alkylating action.[4] However, HMM is not consistently cross-resistant with classic alkylating agents in rodent tumors or in human cancer.

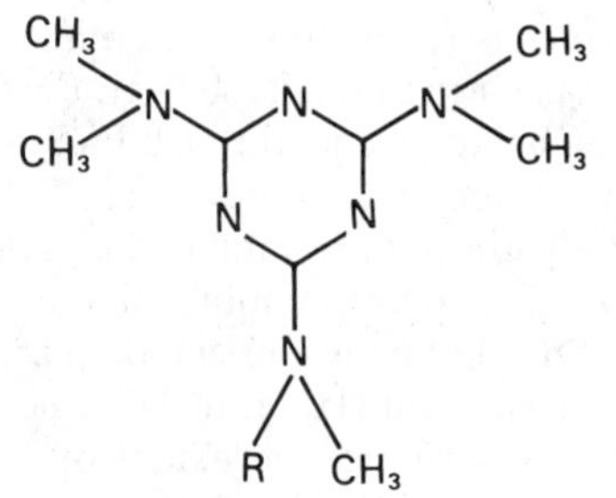

PMM and HMM are best measured by gas chromatography with a nitrogen detector or by gas chromatography-mass spectrometry.[5] Both of these methods can detect concentrations as little as 0.1 μM of either compound in plasma.

Because of its limited aqueous solubility, HMM is administered by the oral route. Usual doses of 4 to 12 mg/kg/day are given for courses of 14 to 21 days. The bioavailability of HMM by this route is variable, yielding peak blood levels of 0.2 to 20 μg/ml.[6] This erratic bioavailability likely results from variable first-pass metabolism in the liver and intestinal epithelium.[7] The parent compound has a half-life of 4.7 to 10.2 hours in plasma. PMM, given intravenously, has half-lives of 27 and 133 minutes, and therefore is eliminated somewhat faster than HMM.

HMM and PMM produce nausea and vomiting as their dose-limiting toxicity. These symptoms, produced by bolus administration of PMM, are particularly severe and have led to the use of more protracted infusion of PMM, which causes less emesis. Oral administration of HMM leads to a gradual increase in these symptoms over a period of days, limiting therapy to 2- to 3-week cycles. Higher daily doses of HMM (higher than 12 mg/kg/day) are tolerated for shorter periods.

PMM and HMM also produce neurotoxic symptoms. HMM treatment may lead to mood alterations, hallucinations, and peripheral neuropathy; these effects appear gradually during a protracted course of treatment and disappear when the drug is withdrawn. PMM has caused convulsive death in preclinical trials and acute coma after rapid intravenous injection in humans.

An intravenous formulation of HMM in intralipid has undergone initial clinical evaluation.[7] Its apparent advantage would be the avoidance of variable first-pass metabolism in the liver and intestinal mucosa. A single dose of 850 mg/m[2] or daily for five doses were well tolerated in phase I trials; however, no responses were observed, and there is no reason to believe that intravenous HMM will be more active than intravenous PMM, which has lesser antitumor activity and greater neurotoxicity than oral HMM. A trihydroxymethyl trimethylamine analog that does not require metabolic activation seems to have greater rationale for future development.[8]

Because HMM is a probable alkylating agent, it is not surprising that acute nonlymphocytic leukemia has been reported as a late complication of HMM treatment.[9]

DACARBAZINE

Dacarbazine (DTIC) [5-(3,3-dimethyl-1-triazeno)-imidazole-4-carboxamide] resulted from efforts to synthesize antimetabolite analogs of 5-amino-imidazole-4-carboxamide, an intermediate in purine biosynthesis. It was later learned that the imidazole nucleus is not essential to DTIC activity and that DTIC actually functions as an alkylating agent. It is active against a broad spectrum of murine solid and ascitic tumors, but its clinical effectiveness is limited to Hodgkin's disease, malignant melanoma, and soft tissue sarcomas.

The probable pathway of metabolic activation of this agent is shown in Figure 18–23 and consists of hepatic microsomal-mediated demethylation, followed by spontaneous rearrange-

R = CH_3 FOR HEXAMETHYLMELAMINE

R = H   FOR PENTAMETHYLMELAMINE

FIGURE 18–22. Structure of melamine derivatives.

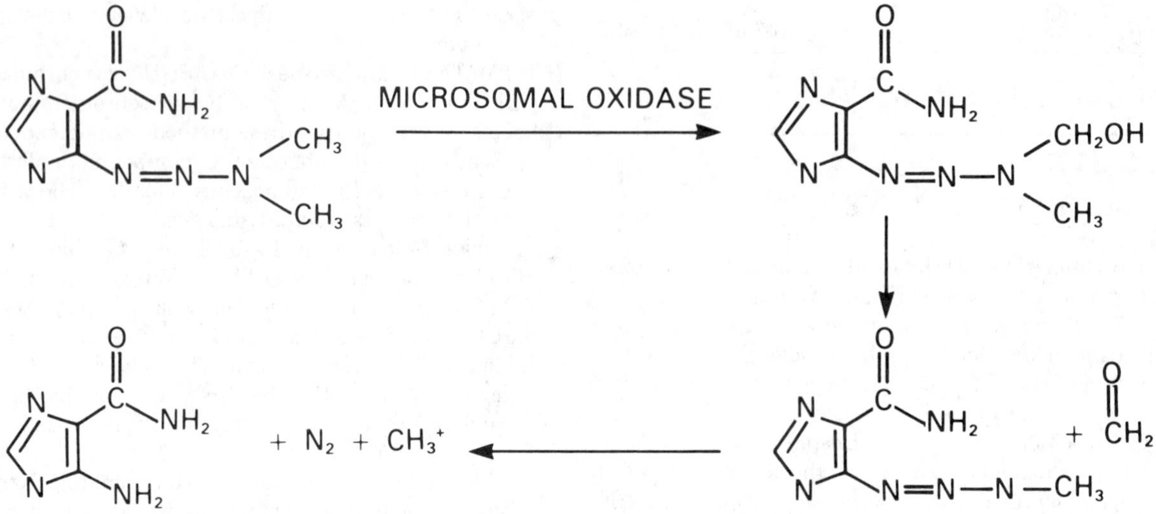

FIGURE 18–23. Metabolic activation of dacarbazine (DTIC). The initial step is enzymatically mediated, but the mechanism of subsequent reactions has not been clarified.

ment of the product, leading to elimination of a methyl diazonium cation (N ≡ $^{+}$NCH$_3$). This unstable cation further yields an active methyl cation (CH$_3$$^{1+}$) and N$_2$. Methylation of nucleic acids has been observed in experimental systems and in urinary nucleic acid excretion products in humans, but the active species of drug and the route of its generation are still not known.[10] In addition to the alkylating activity generated as described earlier, antimetabolite action has been ascribed to the side product methyltriazinoimidazole carboxamide, which inhibits purine nucleoside incorporation into DNA.[11]

When exposed to light, DTIC undergoes spontaneous decomposition, yielding diazoimidazole carboxamide and azahypoxanthine, an active antimetabolite in its own right. This light-activation pathway may account for the antitumor effects of DTIC in vitro in the absence of microsomes, but there is little evidence to support any relevance of this reaction sequence to in vivo toxicity.

DTIC appears to kill cells in all phases of the cell cycle and shows little schedule dependency in experimental studies. Triazine compounds, in addition to cytotoxicity, induce differentiation of malignant cells at sublethal concentrations.[12]

Preliminary information indicates that the drug is absorbed slowly and variably when given orally. A similar dose given intravenously yields fivefold higher peak blood levels. Its disappearance half-life from plasma is about 41 minutes. An ultimate metabolite, aminoimidazole carboxamide, has been detected in humans; as much as 50% of parent compound is excreted intact in the urine.[13] The drug penetrates poorly into the CNS in animals.

A variety of schedules of administration are used in humans. Intravenous doses vary from 150 to 300 mg/m^2/day for 5 to 10 days, depending on treatment history, concurrent therapy, and patient tolerance. The drug also has been given by intraarterial infusion, but this route lacks rationale because of the likely requirement for hepatic microsomal activation.

The most significant side effects are nausea and vomiting, which are severest during the first few days of treatment and which may be lessened by reducing the initial dose and gradually increasing the dose during the course of treatment.

Moderate myelosuppression may occur during the second or third week after treatment, but usually is not dose limiting. Other toxicities include a flu-like syndrome, photosensitivity, immunosuppression, and possible enhancement of doxorubicin cardiac toxicity.[14] Fulminant hepatic venoocclusive disease, associated with fever, eosinophilia, and acute hepatic necrosis, has been reported in patients receiving DTIC as adjuvant therapy for malignant melanoma. This reaction may be fatal.[15]

PROCARBAZINE

Procarbazine, N-isopropyl-α-(2-methylhydrazino)-p-toluamide hydrochloride, was discovered during a search for new monoamine oxidase inhibitors; it was found to have antitumor activity and has since become an important agent in the treatment of Hodgkin's disease and brain tumors.

The mechanism of action and metabolism of procarbazine are not understood completely. The drug undergoes microsomal activation, yielding as the end product an alkylating agent, probably a methyldiazonium ion.[16] However, metal catalyzed decomposition also occurs, yielding azoprocarbazine, a precursor of the alkylating azoxy metabolites.[17] The probable pathway for procarbazine activation in vivo is initiated when the methyl and benzyl azoxy metabolites are released into the bloodstream after absorption of procarbazine in the gut and its passage through the liver. Further activation of the azoxy metabolites occurs through P-450-mediated metabolism or by aldehyde or xanthine oxidase.[18] The latter non-P-450-activation pathways are inhibited by allopurinol. It is not known whether allopurinol-inhibitable activation is important to the clinical effectiveness of allopurinol.

Procarbazine-derived alkylation of DNA occurs at the O^6 and N^7 positions of guanine; the extent of O^6 methylation correlates with activity of the repair enzyme guanine O^6 alkyltransferase, the same enzyme linked to repair of alkylation by chloroethyl nitrosourea.[19]

The pharmacokinetics of procarbazine in humans have not been characterized completely. The parent drug disappears rapidly from plasma with a half-life of 7 minutes after intravenous administration. The primary excretion product is *N*-isopropylterephthalamic acid. Procarbazine-derived radioactivity in the CSF reaches equilibrium with plasma within 15 minutes after injection; the highly lipophilic azoxy metabolites also have been found in rat brains 10 to 30 minutes after intravenous administration.

The antitumor activity and the rate of microsomal metabolism of procarbazine are increased in rodents by pretreatment with phenobarbital, a microsomal enzyme inducer.[20] However, procarbazine itself inhibits microsomal biotransformation of pentobarbital and aminopyrene, indicating that it may have important interactions with antitumor drugs that undergo microsomal metabolism in humans, such as DTIC and cyclophosphamide.

Procarbazine usually is administered orally in daily doses of 100 mg/m^2 for 10 to 14 days. When given orally, procarbazine causes moderate nausea and a decrease in appetite, mild-to-moderate leukopenia and thrombocytopenia, and, less frequently, neurotoxicity, which is manifested by paresthesias of the extremities, drowsiness, or depression. These changes in mental status may be related to its inhibition of monoamine oxidase. Patients receiving procarbazine should be warned to avoid foods that contain significant quantities of tyramine, such as wine, bananas, yogurt, and ripe cheese, because these may provoke a hypertensive crisis. Other monoamine oxidase inhibitors, such as tricyclic antidepressants and sympathomimetic drugs, should not be used concomitantly with procarbazine. Potent hypnotics also should not be used, because procarbazine causes mild hypnotic effects and is known to depress the microsomal inactivation of other agents.

The neurotoxicity of procarbazine is the most prominent and disabling side effect when the drug is given intravenously.[21] Total doses of 2 g/m^2 by this route produce confusion or coma in patients but little myelosuppression. Clinical benefit of this schedule is uncertain.

Procarbazine has a disulfiram (Antabuse)-like action that may lead to sweating, flushing, and headache after ingestion of alcohol by patients receiving procarbazine. Hypersensitivity reactions also have been observed and frequently include a maculopapular rash and pulmonary infiltrates. In these authors' experience, the development of a rash is not cause for withdrawal of procarbazine. The rash usually abates with concurrent use of corticosteroids, and continued treatment with procarbazine plus corticosteroids does not lead to progressive cutaneous reaction or anaphylaxis.

Procarbazine is a potent immunosuppressant in rodents; it prolongs the survival of the first- or second-set skin grafts across major histocompatibility barriers.[22] Procarbazine is also highly teratogenic in rodents.[23] When exposed to the drug in utero, fetal rats acquire a variety of skeletal and nervous system abnormalities. However, clinical experience to date indicates that the drug can be used without teratogenic effect in women in all trimesters of pregnancy. Children born as a result of these pregnancies have not had birth defects.[24] The compound is highly mutagenic in the Ames assay and produces adenocarcinomas and acute nonlymphocytic leukemia in rodents and monkeys. An increased incidence of solid tumors and acute leukemias has been observed in patients receiving MOPP combination chemotherapy, particularly when chemotherapy is used with irradiation for Hodgkin's disease, and

it is believed that procarbazine is the leading carcinogen in these regimens. Its use in treating nonneoplastic diseases and in treating curable malignancies should be considered carefully because of these late toxicities. It also is highly toxic to the reproductive organs, producing azospermia and anovulation. These adverse effects on future reproductive capacity are greatest in adult men and in women in later reproductive years.[25]

L-ASPARAGINASE

The growth of malignant as well as normal cells depends on the availability of specific nutrients required for the synthesis of proteins, nucleic acids, and lipids. Some of these nutrients can be synthesized within the cell, but others are needed from external sources such as another organ (liver) or from food sources (essential amino acids). Nutritional therapy of cancer has been directed toward identifying the differences between the host and malignant cells that might be exploited in treatment; these attempts, for the most part, have been unsuccessful because of difficulties in producing a deficiency state by dietary means and because of a lack of clear differences between the rapidly proliferating host cells and the tumor. The only exception has been the use of L-asparaginase in the treatment of childhood acute leukemia.

In 1953, Kidd observed that the serum of guinea pigs had antileukemic effects when administered to mice.[26] Ten years later, Broome and coworkers demonstrated that the responsible factor copurified with the enzyme L-asparaginase.[27] Subsequently, highly purified preparations of enzyme from *Escherichia coli* and from *Erwinia carotovora* have shown significant activity against childhood ALL and have become standard components of induction regimens in this disease. Their antitumor effects result from the rapid and complete depletion of L-asparagine in the bloodstream and extracellular space, and resistance to this treatment is caused by an increase in L-asparagine synthetase activity in tumor cells. Resistance occurs through increased expression of a gene that is present but not transcribed in most tissues, leading to increased enzyme synthesis in response to the decrease in intracellular asparagine levels.[28]

The 133-kd, purified L-asparaginase enzyme, the gene for which has been cloned and sequenced, is composed of four subunits that each have one active catalytic site.[29-31] Preparations of enzyme from different bacterial strains and by different purification methods have differences in specific activity, isoelectric point, and substrate specificity and affinity. Of greater clinical importance, enzyme prepared from *Erwinia* does not cross-react immunologically with that from *E. coli*, despite their nearly 46% homology in amino acid sequence. Therefore, the *Erwinia* enzyme, which has equivalent therapeutic activity and nonimmunologic toxicity, may be used in patients who are hypersensitive to the *E. coli* L-asparagine.[32,33] The clinical preparations have an affinity constant for L-asparaginase of approximately 1×10^{-5} M, a figure tenfold higher than the minimum L-asparagine concentration at which the growth of sensitive tumors is inhibited in vitro.[34] An excess of enzyme is required to lower L-asparagine concentrations below the threshold for growth inhibition.

The cytotoxicity of L-asparaginase results from inhibition of protein synthesis and correlates well with the effects of the enzyme on the incorporation of an amino acid such as ^{3}H-valine into protein. Inhibition of nucleic acid synthesis also is observed in sensitive cells, but is believed to be secondary to the block in protein synthesis. Cells that are insensitive to asparagine depletion from growth medium in vitro are also insensitive to L-asparaginase and show little inhibition of RNA or protein synthesis in the presence of the enzyme. These resistant cells have high endogenous activity of asparagine synthetase.

Most bacterial L-asparaginase preparations contain significant L-glutaminase activity, which is 3% to 5% of the L-asparaginase activity. The enzyme from mammalian sources and from certain bacterial sources (*Vibrio succinogenes*) lacks L-glutaminase activity but has lesser affinity for L-asparagine.[35] Evidence suggests that the immunosuppressive properties of *E. coli* L-asparaginase may be caused by L-glutamine depletion[36] and that the cerebral dysfunction observed clinically may be the result of degradation of L-glutamine.

In an attempt to reduce immunogenicity, the *E. coli* enzyme has been conjugated to a variety of ligands, including DL-alanine, dextran, and polyethylene glycol (PEG).[37] Each of these manipulations increases the serum half-life of the enzyme, decreases immunogenicity, and has variable effects on enzyme activity. PEG-modified *E. coli* L-asparaginase has 50% of the enzymatic activity of the parent molecule, and in preliminary clinical trials retains activity in patients sensitized to the unmodified enzyme.[38] Because of its greatly prolonged plasma half-life, the PEG-modified enzyme is effective in doses of 2500 IU/m² once every 2 weeks, or about one tenth the dose of the native *E. coli* enzyme, in patients not previously sensitized to the *E. coli* enzyme. In hypersensitive patients, the dose of PEG-modified enzyme or its frequency of administration have not been established yet through clinical trials, but is likely to be at least 2500 IU/m²/week.

CLINICAL PHARMACOLOGY

L-Asparaginase levels are measured easily in biologic fluids by assays that detect ammonia release or by a coupled enzymic assay.[39,40] The drug is given intravenously, intramuscularly, or subcutaneously; the intramuscular route produces peak blood levels that are 50% lower than the intravenous route. The usual doses are 6000 (IU)/m² three days per week, although doses up to 25,000 IU/m² are used once per week as an alternative. Although blood levels of L-asparaginase are detectable for 1 to 3 weeks after these doses, widely spaced schedules of administration are not frequently used because of the increased risk of anaphylaxis.[41] Blood concentrations of L-asparagine decrease below 1 μmol within minutes of enzyme injection and cannot be measured for 7 to 10 days after completion of therapy.[42]

The concentration of L-asparaginase in plasma is proportional to the dose for doses up to 200,000 IU/m² and decreases with a primary half-life of 14 to 22 hours. In patients who are hypersensitive to the enzyme, plasma clearance is greatly accelerated and enzyme activity may be undetectable in plasma within 4 hours of administration.[43] The enzyme distributes primarily within the intravascular space. However, the concentration of asparagine in CSF falls rapidly, and an antileu-kemic effect is exerted here, despite the poor penetration of enzyme into the CSF. The drug can be given directly into the CSF but exits rapidly from this site, and there appears to be no clear therapeutic advantage for this route.

TOXICITY

The primary toxicities of L-asparaginase can be classified into two main groups: those related to immunologic sensitization to the foreign protein and those resulting from decreased protein synthesis. Positive skin tests to L-asparaginase rarely are observed before drug administration, but anaphylaxis may occur with the initial dose of drug. More commonly, hypersensitivity phenomena, such as urticaria, laryngeal edema, bronchospasm, or hypotension, occur after multiple courses of the enzyme. Passive hemagglutinating antibodies are observed in patients who subsequently develop anaphylaxis, and complement-fixing antibodies are found in serum after an anaphylactic episode.[43] In common protocols for treatment of childhood ALL, as many as 50% of children eventually exhibit hypersensitivity to *E. coli* L-asparaginase. The reason that all patients do not become sensitive to the bacterial protein may be the immunosuppressive properties of the drug itself (which inhibit delayed hypersensitivity) and its concomitant use with other immunosuppressive and neoplastic agents.

Hypersensitivity reactions are commoner in patients receiving the drug by the intravenous route, in those who have previously received the drug, and in those receiving more than 6000 IU/m²/day.

Other adverse effects are related to the inhibition of protein synthesis and include hypoalbuminemia; decrease in serum fibrinogen, prothrombin, antithrombin III, protein C and protein S, and other factors that lead to clotting and hemorrhagic complications; decreased serum insulin with hyperglycemia; decreased serum lipoproteins; and, in 25% of the patients, cerebral dysfunction with confusion, stupor, or frank coma.[292] The latter syndrome resembles ammonia toxicity, but is not correlated with serum ammonia levels and may be the result of low concentrations of L-asparagine or L-glutamine in the brain.

The most serious complication of inhibition of protein synthesis resulting from L-asparaginase therapy is thrombosis of a major vessel (artery or vein), usually occurring on the sixth to tenth day after the initiation of treatment and associated with the abrupt decrease in anticoagulant factors in the blood (*e.g.,* protein C, protein S, antithrombin III, plasminogen).[44,45] The decrease in anticoagulant factors during L-asparaginase therapy precedes the decrease in procoagulants, thus favoring thrombosis formation in the early phases of L-asparaginase treatment.[46] In addition, many patients with leukemia, including those with ALL, have evidence of increased coagulation before therapy, as indicated by the presence of elevated fibrinopeptides in blood, perhaps predisposing them to intravascular thrombosis.[47] L-Asparaginase should be discontinued immediately in patients with evidence of a vascular thrombosis. In the case of a documented thrombosis of a major vessel, anticoagulant therapy with heparin is indicated, although the danger of subsequent hemorrhage must be kept in mind, particularly in patients with dangerously low platelet counts or falling coagulant factors. Antithrombin III infusion has been demonstrated to reverse at least partially the evidence of a hypercoagulable state in patients receiving L-asparaginase and might be an appropriate intervention to prevent thrombosis in the first 10 days of treatment.[48]

Other toxicities are not as easily explained by the mode of action of the drug; the most important of these is acute pancreatitis, which occurs in fewer than 15% of patients, but which may progress to severe hemorrhagic pancreatitis. L-Asparaginase frequently causes abnormal liver function test findings, including increased serum bilirubin, serum glutamic oxalic transaminase, and alkaline phosphatase. Histologic examination of the liver reveals fatty metamorphosis.

Approximately two thirds of patients receiving L-asparaginase experience nausea, vomiting, and chills as an immediate reaction, but these side effects can be mitigated by antiemetics, antihistamines, or, in extreme cases, corticosteroids.

L-Asparaginase has no known effects on gastrointestinal mucosa or bone marrow and thus is a favorable agent for combination chemotherapy. The only well-established drug interaction is its ability to terminate MTX action,[49] probably by virtue of the inhibition of protein synthesis in tumor cells preventing their entry into S phase, the period of maximal vulnerability to MTX. When the enzyme is given after MTX administration, the action of the antifolate is abbreviated. Large doses of the antifolate are well tolerated if followed by L-asparaginase rescue, because of the limited time of exposure of the bone marrow and the gastrointestinal mucosa.

REFERENCES

1. Moore DH, Fowler WC Jr, Jones CP, Crumpler LS. Hexamethylmelamine chemotherapy for persistent or recurrent epithelial ovarian cancer. Am J Obstet Gynecol 1991;165:573–576.
2. Lake LM, Grunden EE, Johnson BM. Toxicity and antitumor activity of hexamethylmelamine and its N-demethylated metabolites in mice with transplantable tumors. Cancer Res 1975;35:2858–2863.
3. Ames MM. Hexamethylmelamine: Pharmacology and mechanism of action. Cancer Treat Rev 1991;18(suppl A):3–14.
4. Rutty CJ, Connors TA, Nguyen-Hoang-Nam, et al. In vivo studies with hexamethylmelamine. Eur J Cancer 1978;14:713–720.
5. Ames MM, Powis G. Determination of pentamethylmelamine and hexamethylmelamine in plasma and urine by nitrogen-phosphorous gas-liquid chromatography. J Chromatogr 1979;174:245–249.
6. D'Incalci M, Bolis G, Mangioni C, et al. Variable oral absorption of hexamethylmelamine in man. Cancer Treat Rep 1978;62:2117–2119.
7. Ames MM, Richardson RL, Kovach JS, et al. Phase I and clinical pharmacological evaluation of a parenteral hexamethylmelamine formulation. Cancer Res 1990;50:206–210.
8. Rutty CJ, Judson IR, Abel G, et al. Preclinical toxicology, pharmacokinetics and formulation of N^2, N^4, N^6-trihydroxymethyl-N^2, N^4, N^6-trimethylamine (Trimelamol), a water-soluble cytotoxic s-triazine which does not require metabolic activation. Cancer Chemother Pharmacol 1986;17:251–258.
9. Grubb BP, Thant M. Case report: Acute myelocytic leukemia in a patient treated with hexamethylmelamine. Am J Med Sci 1986;292:393–394.
10. Montgomery JA. Experimental studies at Southern Research Institute with DTIC (NSC-45388). Cancer Treat Rep 1976;60:125–134.
11. Hayward IP, Parson PG. Epigenetic effects of the methylating agent 5-(3-methyl-1-triazeno) imidazole-4-carboxamide in human melanoma cells. Aust J Exp Biol Med Sci 1984;62:597–606.
12. Tisdale MJ. Induction of haemoglobin synthesis in the human leukaemia cell line K562 by monomethyltriazenes and imidazotetrazinones. Biochem Pharmacol 1985;34:2077–2082.
13. Breithaupt H, Dammann A, Aigner K. Pharmacokinetics of decarbazine and its metabolite 5-aminoimidazole-4-carboxamide following different dose schedules. Cancer Chemother Pharmacol 1982;9:103.
14. Smith PJ, Ekert H, Waters KD, et al. High incidence of cardiomyopathy in children treated with Adriamycin and DTIC in combination chemotherapy. Cancer Treat Rep 1977;61:1736–1738.
15. Feaux de Lacroix W, Runne U, Hauk H, et al. Acute liver dystrophy with thrombosis of hepatic veins: A fatal complication of dacarbazine treatment. Cancer Treat Rep 1983;67:779–784.
16. Weinkam RJ, Shiba DA. Metabolic activation of procarbazine. Life Sci 1978;22:937–945.
17. Tweedie DJ, Fernandez D, Spearman ME, et al. Metabolism of azoxy derivatives of procarbazine by aldehyde dehydrogenase and xanthine oxidase. Drug Metab Dispos 1991;19:793–803.
18. Prough RA, Tweedie DJ. Procarbazine. In: Powis G, Prough RA, eds. Metabolism and action of anticancer drugs. London: Taylor & Francis, 1987:29–47.
19. Souliotis VL, Kaila S, Boussiotis VA, et al. Accumulation of O^6-methylguanine in human blood leukocyte DNA during exposure to procarbazine and its relationships with dose and repair. Cancer Res 1990;50:2759–2764.
20. Shiba DA, Weinkam RJ. Metabolic activation of procarbazine: Activity of the intermediates and the effects of pretreatment. Proc Am Assoc Cancer Res 1979;20:139.
21. Chabner BA, Sponzo R, Hubbard S, et al. High-dose intermittent intravenous infusion of procarbazine. Cancer Chemother Rep 1973;57:361–363.
22. Liske R. A comparative study of the activity of cyclophosphamide and procarbazine on the antibody production in mice. Clin Exp Immunol 1973;15:271–280.
23. Lee IP, Dixon RL. Mutagenicity, carcinogenicity, and teratogenicity of procarbazine. Mutat Res 1978;55:1–14.
24. Aviles A, Diaz-Maqueo JC, Talavera A, et al. Growth and development of children of mothers treated with chemotherapy during pregnancy: Current status of 43 children. Am J Hematol 1991;36:243–248.
25. Ortin TT, Shostak CA, Donaldson SS. Gonadal status and reproductive function following treatment for Hodgkin's disease in childhood: The Stanford experience. Int J Radiat Oncol Biol Phys 1990;19:873–880.
26. Kidd JG. Regression of transplanted lymphomas induced in vivo by means of normal guinea pig serum: I. Course of transplanted cancers of various kinds in mice and rats given guinea pig serum, horse serum, or rabbit serum. J Exp Med 1953;98:565–582.
27. Broome JD. Evidence that the L-asparaginase of guinea pig serum is responsible for its antilymphoma effects: I. Properties of the L-asparaginase of guinea pig serum in relation to those of the antilymphoma substance. J Exp Med 1963;118:99–120.
28. Worton KS, Kerbel RS, Andrulis IL. Hypomethylation and reactivation of the asparagine synthetase gene induced by L-asparaginase and ethyl methanesulfonate. Cancer Res 1991;51:985–989.
29. Bonthron DT. L-asparaginase II of *Escherichia coli* K-12: Cloning, mapping and sequencing of the ansB gene. Gene 1990;91:101–105.
30. Jennings MP, Beacham IR. Analysis of the *Escherichia coli* gene encoding L-asparaginase II, ansB, and its regulation by cyclic AMP receptor and FNR proteins. J Bacteriol 1990;172:1491–1498.
31. Jackson RC, Handschumacher RE. *Escherichia coli* L-asparaginase: Catalytic activity and subunit nature. Biochemistry 1970;9:3585–3590.
32. Eden OB, Shaw MP, Lilleyman JS, Richards S. Non-randomised study comparing toxicity of *Escherichia coli* and *Erwinia* asparaginase in children with leukaemia. Med Pediatr Oncol 1990;18:497–502.
33. Ohnama T, Holland JF, Meyer P. *Erwinia carotovora* asparaginase in patients with prior anaphylaxis to asparaginase from *E. coli*. Cancer 1972;30:376–381.
34. Haley EE, Fischer GA, Welch AD. The requirement for L-asparagine of mouse leukemia cells L5178T in culture. Cancer Res 1961;21:532–536.
35. Distasio JA, Neederman RA, Kafkewitz D, Goodman D. Purification and characterization of L-asparaginase with antilymphoma activity from *Vibrio succinogenes*. J Biol Chem 1976;251:6929–6933.
36. Haw T, Ohnuma T. L-Asparaginase: In vitro inhibition of blastogenesis by enzyme from *Erwinia carotovora*. Nature 1972;239:50–51.
37. Cao SG, Zhao QY, Ding ZT, et al. Chemical modification of enzyme molecules to improve their characteristics. Ann NY Acad Sci 1990;613:460–467.
38. Kawashima K, Takeshima H, Higashi Y, et al. High efficacy of monomethoxy-polyethylene glycol-conjugated L-asparaginase (PEG2-ASP) in two patients with hematological malignancies. Leuk Res 1991;15:525–530.
39. Tagami S, Matsuda K. An enzymatic method for the kinetic measurement of L-asparaginase activity and L-asparagine with an ammonia gas-sensing electrode. Chem Pharm Bull (Tokyo) 1990;38:153–155.
40. Cooney DA, Capizzi RL, Handschumacher RE. Evaluation of L-asparagine metabolism in animals and man. Cancer Res 1970;30:929–935.
41. Nesbit M, Chard R, Evans A, et al. Intermittent L-asparaginase therapy for acute childhood leukemia. Proceedings of the 10th International Cancer Congress, 1970:447.
42. Ohnuma T, Holland JF, Sinks LF. Biochemical and pharmacological studies with L-asparaginase in man. Cancer Res 1970;30:2297–2305.
43. Peterson RC, Handschumacher RF, Mitchell MS. Immunological responses to L-asparaginase. J Clin Invest 1971;50:1080–1090.
44. Castaman G, Rodeghiero F, Dini E. Thrombotic complications during L-asparaginase treatment for acute lymphocytic leukemia. Haematologica 1990;75:567–569.
45. Semeraro N, Montemurro P, Giordano P, et al. Unbalanced coagulation-fibrinolysis potential during L-asparaginase therapy in children with acute lymphoblastic leukemia. Thromb Haemost 1990;64:38–40.
46. Vigano-D'Angelo S, Gugliotta L, Mattioli-Belmonte M. L-Asparaginase treatment reduces the anticoagulant potential of the protein C system without affecting vitamin K-dependent carboxylation. Thromb Res 1990;59:985–994.
47. Rodeghiero F, Castaman G, Dini E. Fibrinopeptide A changes during remission induction treatment with L-asparaginase in acute lymphoblastic leukemia: Evidence for activation of blood coagulation. Thromb Res 1990;57:31–38.
48. Gugliotta L, D'Angelo A, Mattioli-Belmonte M, et al. Hypercoagulability during L-asparaginase treatment: The effect of antithrombin III supplementation in vivo. Br J Haematol 1990;74:465–470.
49. Capizzi R. Improvement in the therapeutic index of L-asparaginase by methotrexate. Cancer Chemother Rep 1975;6:37–41.

SECTION **7**

EDDIE REED

Platinum Analogs

The platinum coordination complexes represent the most important group of agents now in use for cancer treatment. They are curative in combination therapy for testicular cancer and ovarian cancer and play a central role in the treatment of lung, head and neck, and bladder cancers. Members of this group have highly unique and desirable pharmacologic actions, including synergy in combination with antimetabolites and radiation therapy, but they differ significantly in their patterns of toxicity and pharmacokinetics. The safe use of carboplatin and cisplatin, the two commonly used agents of the group, requires a thorough knowledge of these pharmacologic properties.

CHEMISTRY

COVALENT BOND CHARACTER

Platinum is in the third row of transition metals in the Periodic Table and has eight electrons in the outer d shell. Palladium and nickel, which occupy analogous positions in the second and first transition series, have similar configurations of outer electrons, but little or no antitumor activity. However, because the platinum atom has a much larger total number of electrons, the orbitals of its outer electrons are more polarizable, and bonds that are formed from these orbitals have more covalent character.

As a result of the covalent character of platinum, it possesses two essential properties: stereospecificity and energy barriers. Stereospecificity means that the bonds from the platinum atom have fixed bond angles and spacial configuration. The spacial configuration depends on whether the oxidation state of the platinum is +2 or +4; these oxidation states are usually designated as Pt(II) or Pt(IV), respectively. In Pt(II) complexes, the platinum atom has four bonds directed to the corners of a square at which the four ligand atoms are located. In Pt(IV) complexes, there are six bonds and six ligands: four in a planar square configuration as in Pt(II), plus one directly above and one directly below the platinum atom, an octahedral configuration. Because the bonds are fixed and not readily exchangeable, the complexes can have distinct isomers, such as *cis*- and *trans*-Pt(II) $(NH_3)_2Cl_2$. The *cis* isomer is the antitumor drug, cisplatin. The importance of stearic conformation is highlighted by the fact that the *trans* isomer has virtually no antitumor activity.

Like covalent bonds, the bonds to the platinum atom have energy barriers that limit the rate of bond formation or dissociation. Some platinum bonds, such as those to nitrogen, are essentially irreversible under physiologic conditions.

Reactions can occur in Pt(II) complexes in which one or both ligands is displaced by a competing nucleophile, in analogy to the reactions of alkylating agents. The Pt(II) complexes have significant chemical and biologic similarities to alkylating agents. Although both Pt(II) and Pt(IV) complexes can have potent antitumor activities, it is unclear whether Pt(IV) complexes may undergo ligand displacement reactions under physiologic conditions. The activity of Pt(IV) complexes may be the result of their reduction in vivo to the active Pt(II) state.[1]

REACTIONS IN WATER AND BIOLOGIC FLUIDS

The pharmacologic behavior of cisplatin is in part determined by its reactions in water, which are summarized in Figure 18–24. Although it is possible that a chloride ligand in cisplatin might, in some instances, be displaced directly in a reaction

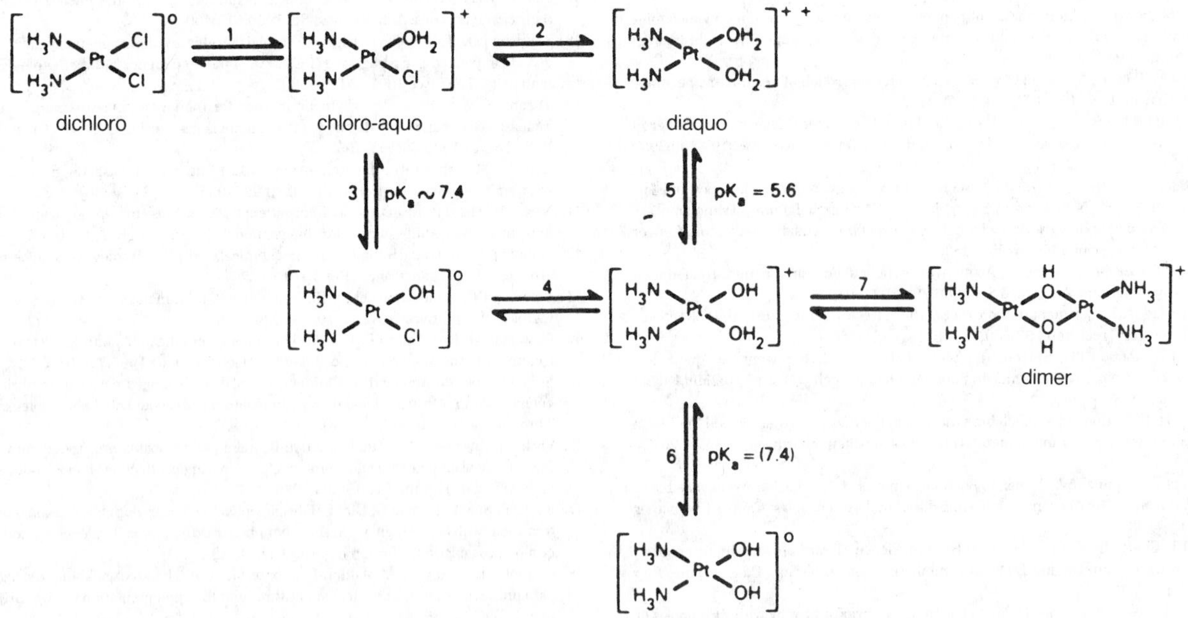

FIGURE 18–24. Aquation hydrolysis chemistry for cisplatin is shown. All reactions are theoretically possible under conditions of physiologic pH and saline concentration. Species that have a zero net charge are theoretically capable of crossing the cell membrane by passive diffusion.

with a macromolecule, it is generally agreed that the more usual path is by way of an initial aquation reaction in which a chloride is replaced by a water molecule. The aquation reaction is driven by the high concentration of water in the tissues. The aquated platinum complex can then react rapidly with a variety of strong binding sites.

In blood plasma, the high chloride concentration of approximately 100 mmol would keep cisplatin predominantly in the uncharged and relatively unreactive dichloro form. This form may react to some degree with sulfhydryl groups of plasma proteins. The free dichloro form could enter cells by passive diffusion. In the cytoplasm, the relatively low chloride concentration of approximately 4 mmol would favor the aquation reaction that would yield highly reactive species whose ionic charge may retard exit from the cell.

REACTIONS WITH DNA

Cisplatin can bind to all DNA bases, but in intact DNA, there appears to be preferential binding to the N7 positions of guanine and adenine.[2,3] This process may be because of the high nucleophilicity of the imidazole portion of the purine ring, particularly at the N7 position.[4] Cisplatin binds to RNA more extensively than does DNA, and to DNA more than protein, when binding is assessed as moles of drug per gram of macromolecule.[5]

In the reaction of cisplatin with DNA or other macromolecules, the two chloride ligands can (usually after aquation) react with two different sites so as to produce crosslinks (Fig. 18–25). The bond distance between the chloride-leaving groups of cisplatin is fixed at approximately 3 nm, and the corresponding bond distance for alkylating agents that can range between 7 and 10 nm.[3]

X-ray crystalographic techniques have disclosed the crystal and molecular structure of the intrastrand dGpG diammineplatinum adduct, which comprises approximately 60% of total platinum binding to DNA after in vitro or in vivo drug exposures. When cisplatin is covalently bound to the d(GpG) dinucleotide, the conformation of the dinucleotides largely depends on the stereochemical requirements for maintaining the planar platinum coordination relation. Further, it appears that the formation of an intramolecular hydrogen bond between a proton of the cisplatin amine ligand and an oxygen atom of the terminal 5′ phosphate of the purine nucleotide contributes to the stabilization of the platinum dinucleotide complex.[6] Gel electrophoretic methods allow determination of the effect of platinum DNA binding on the three-dimensional structure of the DNA double helix and have revealed that the platinum dGpG lesion causes bending of the DNA double helix by approximately 40° in the direction of the major groove.[7] These studies suggest that when platinum binds to DNA, the stereochemistry of the platinum(II) molecule is maintained and that DNA is modified in its three-dimensional conformation to accommodate the rigid structural conformation of the planar diammineplatinum(II) complex.

METHODS OF MEASUREMENT OF PLATINUM-DNA ADDUCTS

After the observation that cisplatin reacts with DNA, methods were developed to measure the binding of drug to DNA and the production of particular types of cisplatin-DNA lesions or

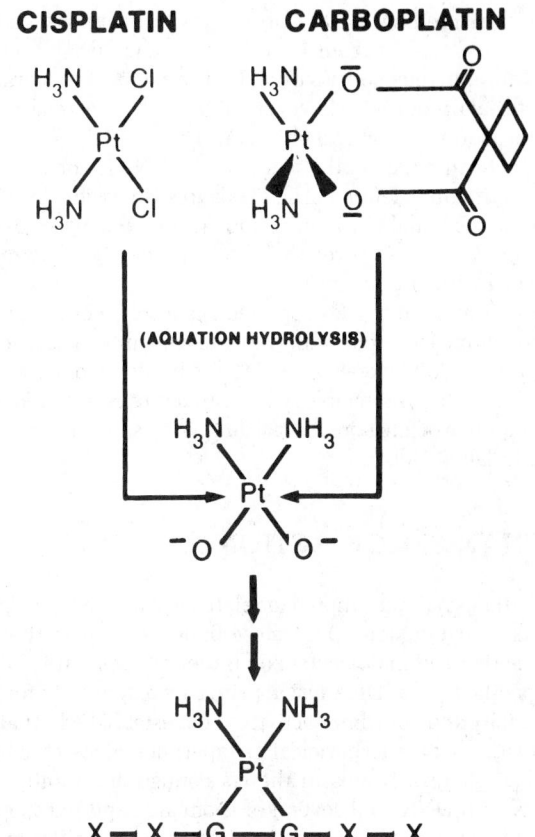

FIGURE 18–25. Cisplatin and carboplatin have leaving groups that generate identical reactive groups with DNA. Although the steps between intact drug and DNA-bound drug may differ substantially between cisplatin and carboplatin within the cell, both agents are capable of undergoing chemical aquation hydrolysis to form the platinum-based DNA reactive group.

adducts. There are now a number of methods available, which include two different methods of atomic absorption spectrometry (AAS), alkaline elution, enzyme-linked immunosorbent assays (ELISA), anion exchange/high-pressure liquid chromatography, microdensitometry of cellular nuclei, and several assays used in molecular biology studies.

The standard for the quantitation of elemental platinum is AAS, which uses high temperature to atomize molecules within a graphite chamber. The chamber is monitored by an optical system that reads the absorbance of the atomic cloud generated. With appropriate background or Zeeman correction, one can now obtain accurate measurements of platinum bound to DNA after therapeutic levels of drug exposure.[8]

The most commonly used method to assess cisplatin-induced DNA lesions in cells treated at pharmacologically relevant dosage is DNA alkaline elution.[9] In this method, cellular DNA is prelabeled with a radioisotope such as ^{3}H-thymidine. An alkaline solution is pumped slowly across a filter on which are deposited labeled cells and the rate of elution of the single-stranded DNA is determined. Using appropriate modifications of this technique, it is possible to quantify DNA interstrand crosslinks, DNA-protein crosslinks, and DNA strand breaks, all of which modulate the rate of DNA elution from the filter. The technique does not detect DNA intrastrand crosslinks or DNA-drug monoadducts.

A number of ELISA assays have been developed that can

assess drug binding to DNA in tissues from human cancer patients and tissues from experimental animals.[10,11] These assays differ in their sensitivity and in the extent of preparation of materials required. However their results correlate well with measurement of adduct by AAS.[12,13]

The determination of the nature of the DNA lesions formed by cisplatin after defined drug exposures is possible by high-performance liquid chromotography (HPLC) analyses of cisplatin-modified DNA after that DNA was degraded by enzymatic or hydrolytic means.[14]

Thomas and colleagues reported results of method development to measure platinum-DNA lesions in specific genes using the uvrABC excision nuclease complex from *Escherichia coli*.[15] This methodology has proved useful in addressing a number of questions regarding gene-specific repair of cisplatin-DNA adduct.[16]

MECHANISM OF ACTION

Many studies have attempted to relate cisplatin-induced DNA adducts to cytotoxicity, and most findings support the hypothesis that the major cytotoxic target of cisplatin is DNA. The specific type of DNA lesion primarily responsible for the cytotoxicity and antitumor activity is not established. Analogs of cisplatin that are tumoricidal in experimental systems have chemical leaving groups in the *cis* configuration and form adducts with DNA, and several of them are reported to have mechanisms of action that are in most respects similar to the parent compound.

The cytotoxicity of cisplatin against cells in culture has been found to be related directly to total platinum binding to DNA, to interstrand crosslinks, and to the formation of intrastrand bidentate N7 adducts at d(GpG) and d(ApG) (Fig. 18–26).[9,13,17–20] The relative percentages of these lesions have been studied after treatment of isolated DNA with cisplatin and after treatment of malignant and nonmalignant rodent

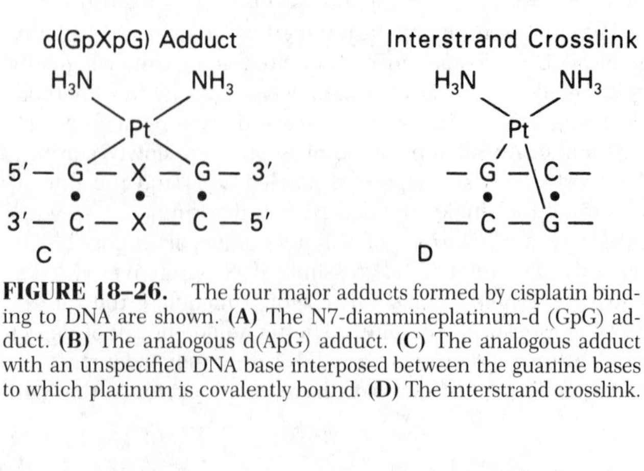

cells in human tumors and after treatment of cancer patients.[13,14,21,22] In each instance in which DNA adducts have been characterized, the d(GpG) lesion constitutes approximately 60% of total platinum binding to DNA, the d(ApG) lesion constitutes about 30% of total platinum binding, and the remaining 10% is a mixture of various intrastrand d(GpXpG) adducts, interstrand crosslinks (<1%), and monoadducts.

The mechanism by which DNA adducts lead to cell death is uncertain. Intrastrand guanine-guanine crosslinkage causes inhibition of DNA replication. Pinto and colleagues compared the ability of cisplatin and transplatinum to inhibit DNA systhesis using a single-strand DNA template and DNA polymerase I.[23] Cisplatin was much more effective than the *trans*-Pt(II) isomer at inhibiting DNA replication in this system. Cisplatin-induced inhibition occurred at sites of adjacent guanines on the template, suggesting that the intrastrand adducts between adjacent guanines were effective at inhibiting replication by DNA polymerase I in this system.[24] In this system as well, primary blocking lesions formed by cisplatin were at the sites of adjacent guanine bases. The effects of intrastrand adducts at d(ApG) or of interstrand crosslink on DNA replication have not yet been determined.

Because cisplatin can react avidly with many accessible sulfur and nitrogen sites on a variety of proteins, it is difficult to evaluate the possible importance of non-DNA targets in the mechanism of antitumor action or mechanism of toxicity. Platinum complexes bind extensively to sulfhydryl groups of plasma proteins, and it has been hypothesized that ligand exchange reactions with sulfhydryl groups of critical enzymes may be responsible for toxic effects on the kidney, gastrointestinal epithelium, and bone marrow.[25]

Although cytotoxicity correlates well with DNA adduct formation, selected cell lines may demonstrate rapid cell lysis when exposed to cisplatin, and they appear to have an impaired ability to tolerate the presence of cisplatin-DNA, cisplatin-protein lesions, or both.[26]

Consistent with these observations, Scanlon and coworkers reported alterations in the transmembrane transport of essential amino acids in cells sensitive to cisplatin.[27] Other researchers showed cisplatin suppression of Na^+-K^+-ATPase activity in kidney tissue[28] and have shown cisplatin-induced suppression of Ca^{2+} channel function.[29] Other intracellular effects reported include suppression of mitochondrial respiration and mitochondrial calcium accumulation,[30] inhibition of mitochondrial phosphate transport,[31] and inhibition of microtubule assembly.[32] Although DNA damage has been the intracellular effect most related to cisplatin-induced cell death, other effects may contribute to side effects or toxicity to specific tissues.

Diamminecyclobutane-dicarboxylatoplatinum (II), carboplatin, appears to have a subcellular mechanism of action similar to cisplatin, although its clinical spectrum of side effects differs somewhat from cisplatin. Against L1210 cells in vitro, carboplatin is 45 times less cytotoxic than cisplatin if compared on a molar basis.[33] In addition, peak levels of crosslinking occurred 6 to 12 hours later for carboplatin than with cisplatin. Additional studies by Knox and colleagues compared rates of DNA adduct formed during drug exposures, rates of dissociation of cisplatin and carboplatin from their *cis* leaving groups, and the relations of DNA binding to cell kill for both compounds.[34] The rate constant for the aquation of carboplatin

FIGURE 18–26. The four major adducts formed by cisplatin binding to DNA are shown. **(A)** The N7-diammineplatinum-d (GpG) adduct. **(B)** The analogous d(ApG) adduct. **(C)** The analogous adduct with an unspecified DNA base interposed between the guanine bases to which platinum is covalently bound. **(D)** The interstrand crosslink.

in phosphate buffer (pH 7) at 37°C was 7.2×10^{-7}/second and for cisplatin it was 8×10^{-5}/second, or 100-fold faster. Consistent with this finding, when plasmid DNA was treated with drug, a 100-fold larger concentration of carboplatin was needed to produce levels of DNA binding equivalent to that produced by cisplatin. When cells were treated, a 20- to 40-fold larger concentration of carboplatin was needed to produce levels of DNA binding equivalent to cisplatin. When cells were treated with the respective drugs and the same amount of DNA binding was obtained, cytotoxicity was the same for the two compounds, thus implicating DNA adduct formation as the common lesion formed by both drugs. Carboplatin and other cisplatin analogs that have shown preclinical tumoricidal activity form lesions with DNA that are recognized by the same antibodies that react with adducts formed by cisplatin, with the possible exception of tetraplatin, which has not been studied.[12]

Cis-diamminetetrachloroplatinum(IV), tetraplatin, has sparked interest by some investigators because of its apparent lack of cross-resistance with cisplatin in L1210 cells, human colon cancer cells, and human ovarian cancer cells.[35] There is evidence that platinum(IV) may actually be a prodrug of platinum(II) and that after a platinum(IV) complex enters the cell, it reacts with glutathione and is consequently reduced to a platinum(II) complex, which then reacts with DNA.[36,37]

DETERMINANTS OF SENSITIVITY AND RESISTANCE

Responsiveness to platinum complexes may depend on the presence of biochemical characteristics that may render certain types of cells unusually sensitive to this class of agents. Even within a given histologic type, different tumors may differ greatly in drug sensitivity.[38] Attempts to optimize chemotherapy have been directed at the mechanisms that determine drug sensitivity and the mechanisms of acquired resistance.

Cell lines established from fresh human tumors exhibit different levels of inherent sensitivity to cisplatin.[39,40] Resistant cell lines can be established by exposure of sensitive cells to cisplatin in vitro with continuous stepwise increases in drug concentration,[41,42] by exposure to other heavy metals such as cadmium and zinc,[43] or exposure of cells to compounds that augment intracellular sulfhydryl levels.[44] As a result of these studies, determinants of sensitivity and resistance to cisplatin can be grouped into three catagories: alterations in transmembrane transport of the drug, cytosolic quenching of the drug because of increased levels of sulfhydryl compounds, and enhanced DNA adduct repair capability.

Studies in cisplatin transmembrane transport as it relates to drug resistance have been conducted using paired wild-type (drug-sensitive) and mutant (resistant) cell lines.[45–48] Alterations in transmembrane transport of cisplatin are discussed here as a change in the ability to accumulate intracellular drug, relative to that of the parental cell line. Reduced intracellular accumulation of cisplatin after induced drug resistance in vitro has been described in human ovarian cancer cell lines,[46] human squamous carcinoma cell lines,[41] and murine leukemia cell lines.[45,47] Comparisons of a range of cell lines have shown correlations between intracellular accu-

mulation of drug and drug resistance in human prostate cancer cells and in HeLa cells, Chinese hamster ovary (CHO) cells, and Syrian hamster kidney cells.[48]

Two groups have reported the existence of membrane proteins that are reduced in cisplatin-resistant cells (suggesting the existence of a "pump" that actively takes up drug), and one group has reported a membrane protein that is increased in resistant cells (suggesting a pump that may actively efflux drug). Bernal and colleagues studied cell lines originating from tumors in the head and neck, lung, and cervix.[49] A membrane protein named SQM1 was reduced in cell lines made resistant to cisplatin or to methotrexate. Similarly, a 56-kd membrane protein has been identified in human ovarian cancer cells by Chen and associates; this protein is reduced in cisplatin-resistant cells.[50] Kawai's group has identified a 200-kd membrane glycoprotein that is overexpressed by cisplatin-resistant sublines of murine thymic lymphoma cells.[51]

Cisplatin in the unbound or the transient DNA-monoadduct state, or both, can be quenched in vitro by conjugation with thiourea, thus reducing the level of DNA interstrand crosslinks in L1210 leukemia cells and diminishing cytotoxicity. The use of sulfur compounds to quench cisplatin extracellularly and thereby to protect against excessive clinical toxicity has been reported by a number of investigators and is discussed later.

Evidence for cytosolic quenching by glutathione or by sulfhydryl-containing proteins has been obtained in malignant cell lines made resistant to cisplatin in vitro.[52–59] Some resistant cells have higher levels of intracellular glutathione.[52]

Several studies investigated the role of one or more such "inactivating" entities in different in vitro systems. Miyazaki and colleagues transfected the glutathione-S-transferase (GST) *PI* gene into CHO cells, which yielded cisplatin-resistant clones expressing high amounts of the GST mRNA.[54] In human small cell lung cancer cell lines, elevated glutathione level and glutathione synthesis rates were both correlated with increased resistance to cisplatin.[55] In these cell lines, pretreatment with D,L-buthionine-S,R-sulphoximine-depleted cells of glutathione increased the level of platinum-DNA damage and reduced DNA repair efficiency. The sulfhydryl-containing protein, metallothionein, is elevated in other cell lines made resistant to cisplatin by stepwise incubation with cisplatin or by exposures to cadmium or certain other heavy metals.[43,53] However, in L1210 and human ovarian carcinoma cell lines selected for cisplatin resistance, metallothionein levels were not increased.[56]

Augmented DNA repair capability plays a major role in cisplatin drug resistance in several mammalian cell lines, including human ovarian cancer cells, human bladder cancer cells, and resistant L1210 murine leukemia cells.[20,57,58] Preliminary data suggest that there may be specific DNA repair systems operative in cisplatin resistance as discussed later.[58–60]

The most well-defined system for repairing cisplatin-DNA damage is the uvrABC system of *E. coli*.[59] The uvrABC complex is composed of the enzyme products of three genes that are widely separated on the *E. coli* genetic map. The A, B, and C proteins form a complex that recognizes the damaged DNA and binds to the DNA damage site. The C protein cuts the damaged DNA strand at specific sites flanking the damaged DNA bases. After the adduct is removed with 10 to 12 adjacent DNA bases, a DNA polymerase can patch the site by copying the base sequence from the undamaged DNA strand. The uvrABC complex is not specific for cisplatin-induced DNA damage, however, and can repair ultraviolet (UV) dimers, psoralen-DNA crosslinks, and other bulky DNA lesions. In mammalian cells, the enzyme(s) responsible for repair of cisplatin adducts have not been identified conclusively.

Transfection of the human DNA repair gene *ERCC1*, which has homology with the *RAD10* DNA repair gene of yeast and with the uvrA gene in *E. coli* into UV-repair-deficient CHO cells of complementation group 1, increases cisplatin resistance fourfold to fivefold and reconstitutes the ability of the cells to remove cisplatin from cellular DNA.[58,60] *ERCC1* is expressed in every human malignant and nonmalignant tissue thus far examined.

Several groups have studied the potential role of DNA repair as a mechanism of resistance to cisplatin.[61,62] When the repair of intrastrand dGpG and dApG adducts was specifically examined, resistant sublines of L1210 removed as much as four times as many adducts as did the sensitive cell line during the rapid phase of adduct removal from cellular DNA. However, the extent of the repair capability did not closely correlate with the degree of resistance in the cell lines examined.[61] Repair capability can also be monitored as a function of the ability of cells to repair a cisplatin-modified plasmid, pRSVcat, after transfection of the plasmid into the cells. The plasmid contains platinated DNA sequences that code for the enzyme chloramphenicol acetyltransferase. Repair capability is assessed as the restoration of chloramphenicol acetyltransferase activity at defined time points after transfection.[62] This method for assessing repair of DNA adduct and assessment of drug accumulation and drug inactivation in the cytosol have implicated differences in repair as the primary factor accounting for different cisplatin sensitivity of two human ovarian cancer cell lines.[20]

Other studies support the contention that DNA repair is important in cisplatin drug resistance. Cisplatin-induced cell kill was potentiated by 3-aminobenzamide and by nicotinamide, both inhibitors of steps in the DNA repair process.[63] Although DNA repair appears to be an important component of cisplatin resistance in vitro, some cell lines appear to be inherently more sensitive to the presence of a given level of cisplatin-DNA lesions than other cells. These findings suggest that sensitivity to cisplatin may be a function not only of DNA repair but also of cellular tolerance for platinum-DNA lesions.[64]

Although the importance of DNA repair in cisplatin drug resistance is intuitively obvious, few studies have examined the repair of cisplatin-DNA lesions in human cell lines and the relation between such repair and cell survival. In one study, bladder cancer cell lines that were more resistant to cisplatin were also more efficient at removing platinum DNA adducts from cellular DNA than cisplatin-sensitive testis cancer cells. Inhibition of repair may augment cisplatin toxicity.[65] When cells are exposed to hydroxyurea or cytosine arabinoside, which inhibit excision repair, higher levels of interstrand crosslinks are found at late time points than after cisplatin alone.[66] In human ovarian cancer cells, in vitro acquired resistance to cisplatin may be associated with an increased capacity to remove cisplatin from cellular DNA as measured by AAS, and platinum-DNA adduct removal is delayed by aphidicolin, an inhibitor of DNA repair.[67]

Gene-specific repair may be a component of cisplatin drug resistance. CHO cells repair interstrand and intrastrand cisplatin-DNA lesions in the dihydrofolate reductase and c-*MYC* and c-*FOS* genes at an accelerated rate compared with repair of overall genomic DNA adducts.[16] Interstrand crosslinks and intrastrand adducts are more rapidly removed from actively transcribed portions of DNA than from nontranscribed DNA, and interstrand crosslinks are removed more rapidly than intrastrand adducts. Preliminary data from human ovarian cancer cells suggest that enhanced gene-specific repair may play a role in the development of resistance of these cells to cisplatin as well.[68]

Inhibition of repair of cisplatin-DNA damage in vivo appears to enhance response in athymic mice transplanted with human tumor xenographs, but results from the only clinical trial aimed at repair inhibition have not been encouraging.[69] Cantwell and colleagues treated 45 patients with non-small cell lung cancer with cisplatin at 50 mg/m^2, given during the eighth hour of a 24-hour high-dose hydroxyurea infusion.[70] The response rate observed was similar to that observed with cisplatin alone.

Acquired cellular resistance to cisplatin appears to be a multifactorial process that may encompass alterations in transmembrane transport of drug, intracellular levels of sulfhydryl-containing proteins, and the capacity to repair cisplatin-DNA lesions. Eastman and colleagues have attempted to quantitate the relative contribution of each factor to the observed levels of cisplatin resistance in L1210 sublines. They have constructed a conceptual model for the genetic transmission of those cellular properties that confer cisplatin drug resistance in L1210 cells with different patterns of cross-resistance to the agents cisplatin, DACH-platinum, melphalan, and cadmium.[57] In these studies, they show that reduced cellular accumulation of cisplatin may result in relatively low levels of cisplatin resistance (twofold to sixfold resistance) and that this trait is genetically recessive. It is not known whether this decreased cellular accumulation of drug results from reduced cellular uptake of cisplatin or from increased drug efflux. In these cell lines, augmented capacity to repair cisplatin-DNA adducts may result in relatively high levels of cisplatin resistance (up to 100-fold), and this trait is genetically dominant. Other studies in these cell lines showed that metallothionein played little or no role in cisplatin resistance and that intracellular glutathione levels were highly dependent on the culture medium and played a small role in cisplatin resistance.[57]

CLINICAL PHARMACOKINETICS AND DRUG ADMINISTRATION

The stability of cisplatin and several of its analogs is variable in solutions containing chloride ion.[71] In a solution containing 0.9% NaCl, cisplatin and tetraplatin are less than 90% stable for 6 hours. Lower NaCl concentrations result in greater rates of drug loss. Iproplatin is stable for 24 hours in intravenous glucose or saline solutions, but carboplatin stability is *decreased* in the presence of NaCl. Carboplatin should not be diluted with solutions containing chloride ions because of possible conversion of the compound to cisplatin.

CISPLATIN PHARMACOKINETICS

The clinical pharmacokinetics of cisplatin have been described by a number of investigators.[72-74] After an intravenous bolus infusion of drug in the dose range of 50 to 100 mg/m², the removal of cisplatin from the systemic circulation has a triphasic character. The half-life of the initial phase of removal, the $t_{1/2}$-α, is 20 to 30 minutes and represents removal of drug that is not protein bound. The half-life of the second phase of removal, the $t_{1/2}$-β, is 48 to 67 minutes in length and is also primarily a function of the removal of free drug from the circulation. These two phases are dependent on adequate renal function, because cisplatin that is excreted from the body is 90% removed by the kidneys as a combination of glomerular filtration and tubular secretion.[75] The third phase of drug removal from systemic circulation, the $t_{1/2}$-γ, is about 24 hours and represents removal of drug bound to blood proteins. This phase of removal is governed by a combination of factors, including protein catabolism, renal excretion, and biliary excretion of drug. Biliary excretion accounts for less than 10% of total drug removal from the systemic circulation.[76] The schedule of drug infusion can play a role in determining the duration of the initial phases of drug removal. Cisplatin given in the "high dose" (200 mg/m²/cycle) format has a $t_{1/2}$-α of 30 minutes.[74] The use of hypertonic saline has no effect on the pharmacokinetics of free or total platinum.[77]

Regional administration of cisplatin was originally developed by Myers[78] and explored in detail by Howell and others.[80] The studies of Howell and associates have shown that the clearances of cisplatin from the peritoneal and plasma compartments are independent of the cisplatin intraperitoneal dose.[80] Mean peritoneal clearance was 2.6 ± 1.4 L/m²/hour, and the mean plasma clearance after an intraperitoneal dose was 23.3 ± 15.2 L/m²/hour. The half-life of cisplatin in the intraperitoneal space is independent of dose, and peak intraperitoneal concentrations were as much as 21 times higher than the peak plasma concentrations.

CARBOPLATIN PHARMACOKINETICS

The clinical pharmacokinetics of carboplatin, the cisplatin analog with which the most clinical experience has been obtained, have been described by several investigators. In a phase I study of carboplatin administration as a 24-hour constant intravenous infusion, the half-life of ultrafilterable platinum, as measured by atomic absorption, was found to be 170 ± 34 minutes and was independent of dose.[81] When given in this manner, the maximal tolerated dose was 320 mg/m², and myelosuppression was the dose-limiting toxicity. Given as a 1-hour infusion at a dose of 100 mg/m², the half-life of unchanged drug, as measured by HPLC, was 105 ± 30.4 minutes.[82] In this 1-hour infusion study, the mean renal clearance of drug was comparable to the creatinine clearance but was only 61% of total body clearance, which may reflect drug elimination by degradation to aquation products that would not be measured in this HPLC assay. Oguri and colleagues investigated the pharmacokinetics of six different doses of carboplatin (ranging from 75 to 450 mg/m²) administered as a bolus intravenous infusion and found that the elimination of total platinum from the plasma was triphasic in nature and that the respective half-lives did not vary with dose.[83] The

initial half-life was 0.2 to 0.4 hours, the $t_{1/2}$-β was 1.3 to 1.7 hours, and the $t_{1/2}$-γ was 22 to 40 hours. Total body clearance of drug was also independent of dose.

Carboplatin clearance is dominated by renal excretion, with about 65% of an administered dose appearing in the urine during the first 24 hours. Renal excretion of cisplatin is about 25% over an equivalent time period. Therefore, based on the work of Van Echo and associates, carboplatin dose should be reduced in the setting of compromised renal function.[84] Recommended reductions include a starting standard dose of 360 mg/m² for a creatinine clearance greater than 60 ml/min; 250 mg/m² for 41 to 59 ml/min; and 200 mg/m² for 16 to 40 ml/min. Because carboplatin clearance correlates so closely with hematopoetic toxicity, complex formulas have been developed that can be used to predict bone marrow suppression.[84] Although these formulas predict well for carboplatin when it is used as a single agent, they may not be as useful when carboplatin is used in combination therapy.

Although the regional administration of cisplatin and carboplatin has been studied extensively, recent analyses suggest that intraperitoneal and other such approaches may not be as promising as once thought.[85]

CLINICAL MODULATION OF CISPLATIN TOXICITY

The interaction of cisplatin with thiols presents an opportunity to modulate the toxicity of the drug by coadministration of compounds such as diethyldithiocarbamate (DDTC) or WR-2721. These thiol-containing molecules react with and inactivate reactive intermediates derived from cisplatin. Although they are both capable of protecting animals from cisplatin and carboplatin toxicity, it is not clear that these protective effects are selective for normal tissue and that the intracellular pharmacokinetics of the platinum compounds are not altered unfavorably in the tumor. DDTC does not appear to alter the plasma pharmacokinetic profile of cisplatin,[86] and in at least one study, ameliorated nausea and vomiting.[87] However, when given with high-dose carboplatin (800 mg/m²),[88] DDTC caused autonomic toxicity and did not ameliorate the hematologic toxicity of the platinum compound.

In an attempt to allow escalation of cisplatin dose, WR-2721 has been used with cisplatin.[89] In a phase I trial of WR-2721 (450–910 mg/m²) and cisplatin (50–150 mg/m²), objective responses were observed in 25 of 53 patients with metastatic melanoma, 12 of 22 patients with locally recurrent or metastatic head and neck cancer, and 7 of 13 patients with metastatic breast cancer refractory to conventional chemotherapy. Most responses occurred at 120 to 150 mg/m² of cisplatin, apparently reflecting an amelioration of toxicity with preservation of the antineoplastic activity. Although WR-2721 was associated with transient hypotension during the intravenous infusion, this side effect did not add to the risk of nephrotoxicity from cisplatin. No patient developed febrile neutropenia or bleeding complications requiring platelet transfusions.

ORG2766 is an ACTH(4-9) analog, which in pharmacologic doses appears to mimic the endogenous signal involved in the in vivo repair of peripheral nerves after crush injury. In a randomized, double-blind, placebo-controlled study of 55 women with ovarian cancer, ORG2766 was given subcutaneously in a dose of 0.25 or 1 mg/m² before and after a regimen consisting of cisplatin and cyclophosphamide.[90] In the group receiving 1 mg/m^2, the threshold value for vibration perception was greatly decreased compared with the control group ($p < 0.005$), demonstrating objective amelioration of cisplatin-induced damage to peripheral nerves. This test result was also associated with fewer clinical neurologic signs and symptoms. The reduction in neurotoxicity was less prominent in the group receiving the 0.25 mg/m^2 ORG2766 dose. The disease response rate to chemotherapy was comparable in all treatment groups. In experimental studies of cisplatin neurotoxicity, although ORG2766 prevented cisplatin nerve damage as measured by sensory nerve conduction velocities, the ORG2766-treated rats and the control animals had similar cisplatin-DNA binding levels in ganglion cells.[91] However, adduct was not measured in Schwann cells of peripheral nerves, which may be the critical cells of question in any "stocking and glove" peripheral neuropathy. The mechanism of the protective effect of ORG2766 remains unclear.

CLINICAL PHARMACOLOGIC CORRELATES OF RESPONSE

An important objective of cancer pharmacology is to establish correlates of disease response. Correlates such as drug transport, target binding, or metabolism validate factors that are known to determine response in animal models, and if performed before therapy, may allow assignment of patients to optimal therapy. With respect to cisplatin response, the primary effort has focused on the measurement of platinum-DNA adduct in normal and malignant tissues. In particular, peripheral leukocytes provide a convenient and accessible tissue for monitoring adduct formation and repair and reflect interpatient variability in parameters that affect tumor response.

There is considerable evidence that formation of platinum-DNA adducts, as measured in peripheral leukocytes, correlates with response.[92-95] For example, in 25 patients with ovarian cancer treated with single-agent cisplatin, the correlation of adduct level and response yielded a two-sided p value of 0.0015. Of eight persons in this trial who failed to form measurable levels of adduct in their peripheral leukocytes in the 24 hours after treatment, none responded to therapy.[93] Similar positive correlations have been observed in patients with testicular cancer who received cisplatin as part of their combination chemotherapy.[94] In 24 patients with ovarian cancer, univariate analysis revealed that adduct level was the single strongest predictor of response ($p = 0.0058$) compared with Karnofsky status ($p = 0.125$), disease stage ($p = 0.189$), and other factors.[95] These findings imply that adduct levels in peripheral leukocytes parallel those in tumor and that the determinants of adduct formation or repair are common to both, a view supported by autopsy studies of adduct levels in bone marrow and tumor.[96] Additional studies, using various techniques for measuring levels of platinum-DNA adducts in normal tissues, have supported the hypothesis that adduct levels in normal and malignant tissues of an individual patient are closely correlated.[97] It is important to confirm this relation in larger prospective clinical trials.

These studies suggest that clinical resistance to cisplatin (and probably to other DNA damaging agents) may not be simply a function of tumor cell resistance, but may represent the relative ability of persons to protect cellular DNA in rapidly dividing tissues, an ability that may be governed by genetic factors, prior exposure to DNA damaging agents, or other factors.

TOXICITY

The clinical use of cisplatin can be limited by any of numerous drug-induced toxicities; their time course and frequency generally depend on the dose schedule of drug delivery. These toxicities may include renal dysfunction, nausea and vomiting, peripheral neuropathy, auditory impairment, myelosuppression, visual impairment, and in rare cases, seizures.[98-109] Of these dysfunctions, renal impairment, neurotoxicity, and ototoxicity are the most troublesome in that they are cumulative and are only partially reversible with discontinuation of therapy.[109a] Patients with testicular cancer treated with a mean cumulative dose of cisplatin of 483 mg/m^2 had an average decrease in creatinine clearance of 15% and a significant impairment in high-tone hearing 4 years after treatment.[109a] Other rarely reported ill effects have been attributed recently to cisplatin and include treatment-related leukemia, acute ischemic vascular events, cardiac arrhythmia, local neurotoxicity after intraarterial drug infusion, microscopic and biochemical damage to brain tissue, glucose intolerance, and pancreatitis.[110-119] However, these latter effects are relatively rare in clinical settings.

When used in the format of a single dose per cycle, the dose-limiting toxicity of cisplatin has consistently been nephrotoxicity and may be related to the peak plasma levels of drug.[101,120] Clinical predisposing factors may include hyperuricemia and hypoalbuminemia.[121] Acute renal failure may occur within 24 hours of drug administration, particularly in patients receiving inadequate pretreatment hydration, but in most patients receiving conventional doses of drug (≤ 100 mg/m^2/cycle) renal dysfunction is mild and reversible.[122] Patients have been retreated successfully with cisplatin after recovering from cisplatin-induced acute renal failure. In postmortem specimens taken from patients who have experienced renal toxicity, the areas of the kidney that histologically appear to be most damaged are the loops of Henle, the distal tubules, and the collecting ducts.[100] Substantial reductions in glomerular filtration rates occur acutely in the first 24 to 48 hours after drug administration, but in many patients renal function will return to normal after completion of therapy. Clinically, cisplatin-induced renal dysfunction may be manifested as a reduction in glomerular filtration rate, electrolyte imbalances (especially hypomagnesemia), or as frank renal failure. Renal toxicity may be worsened by the concomitant administration of other renal toxins, including aminoglycoside antibiotics and possibly amphotericin B. Renal toxicity may be lessened by vigorous intravenous hydration and the use of hypertonic saline, mannitol, or possibly organic phosphorothioates.

Cisplatin renal toxicity has been attributed to drug-protein interactions and the inactivation of specific renal brush border enzymes.[25,123] It is now clear that cisplatin renal toxicity can be divided into two phases: an acute phase and a chronic phase. The acute toxicity of the drug is characterized by hypomagnesemia, urinary enzyme excretion, acute reductions in glomerular filtration rate, and in some instances, a transient rise in blood urea nitrogen and serum creatinine, but the chronic phase of renal dysfunction is characterized by a stable, reduced creatinine clearance with or without elevations in serum creatinine.[99,101]

Studies of cisplatin-DNA adduct formation suggest that these two phases of cisplatin renal toxicity may have different pathophysiologic mechanisms.[96,124,125] In autopsy studies of two ovarian cancer patients who experienced cisplatin-related chronic renal toxicity, drug-DNA adduct levels could be measured in kidney tissues up to 9 months after their most recent dose of cisplatin, suggesting that persistence of these adducts in renal tissue DNA may play a role in the chronic phase of drug-related renal dysfunction. This finding raises the question that drug-DNA binding may have long-term functional sequelae.

Several rules should be kept in mind with respect to the administration of cisplatin or carboplatin, or both. Carboplatin dose should be reduced in the face of compromised renal function. Further, in patients who have received cisplatin in the past, serum creatinine is not a good indicator of the true level of renal function and a 24-hour creatinine clearance should be obtained. Hydration is extremely important for cisplatin regardless of dose, and hydration should be considered for carboplatin in "high-dose" regimens and in patients who have compromised renal function at the start of therapy.

Cisplatin is prepared for intravenous administration with the following incipient ingredients in the drug vial: the drug itself, mannitol, and NaCl. According to the package insert, when mixed with the appropriate volume of sterile water the solution contains 1 mg/ml of cisplatin, 10 mg/ml of mannitol, and 9 mg/ml of NaCl. This solution is then further diluted into saline-based solutions (preferably 100–150 mg of 0.95% NaCl or 3% NaCl) for intravenous administration. Before drug administration, the patient should be given intravenous hydration with 5% dextrose in normal saline or normal saline at a rate of 200 to 300 ml/hour for 2 to 4 hours before drug; and the same hydration regimen should be administered for 2 to 4 hours after cisplatin. Furosemide probably should not be used unless it is necessary to maintain urine flow. Cisplatin itself should be administered over 20 to 30 minutes in the 100- to 150-ml volume described earlier. Aluminum needles should not be used. Hypertonic saline may be used in conjunction with high-dose cisplatin.[126]

Neurotoxicity is a second general class of cisplatin-induced toxicity that may become chronic and disabling. When cisplatin is administered as five daily infusions rather than as a single bolus, neurotoxicity becomes dose limiting.[124] This general class of toxicity may include peripheral neuropathy, auditory impairment, and visual disturbances. Less commonly, cortical blindness, seizures, papilledema, and retrobulbar neuritis may also occur.

Cisplatin-induced peripheral neuropathy virtually always presents in "stocking and glove" distribution, and clinically resembles the neuropathy of vitamin B_{12} deficiency.[104,127] It has been suggested that this neuropathy may be caused by cisplatin disruption of normal cobalt metabolism, a necessary cofactor for vitamin B_{12}; however, effects on vitamin B_{12} metabolism have not been demonstrated in human tissues.[127,127a] Auditory impairment usually results in diminution of acuity at the high-frequency range of greater than 2000 Hz, but may affect the normal hearing range of 250 to 2000 Hz in 10% to

15% of cases.[105,128,129] Cisplatin-induced ototoxicity appears to be related to the loss of outer hair cells in the basal turns of the cochlear and is histologically similar to aminoglycoside-induced ototoxicity. It is postulated that this toxicity may be related to cisplatin-induced inhibition of Na^+-K^+-ATPase in the outer hairy cells of the cochlear. The incidence of clinically perceptible hearing impairment is directly related to total dose of cisplatin administered and to the peak serum levels of drug attained during drug administration. Unlike the case with nephrotoxicity, no clinical interventions are known to diminish this toxicity. However, the phosphonic acid antibiotic fosfomycin can significantly reduce cisplatin-induced ototoxicity in guinea pigs and could be considered for human use.[128]

Disturbances in color perception related to retinal cone dysfunction were observed in patients receiving "high-dose" cisplatin.[108] Other uncommon visual toxicities include cortical blindness, papilledema, and retrobulbar neuritis.[127] The neurophysiologic basis for this toxicity is unclear.

The most common immediate cisplatin-induced toxicity is nausea and vomiting, which can be dose limiting in some patients.[102,103,130] Currently it is unclear whether cisplatin primarily acts directly on the chemotactic trigger zone in the floor of the fourth ventricle or if cisplatin affects afferent nerves in the gastrointestinal tract and indirectly triggers the emetic center, which is in the body of the brain stem in close proximity to the chemotactic trigger zone.

Several antiemetics (*e.g.*, antihistamines, dopamine antagonists, cannabanoids, 5-hydroxytryptamine antagonists, corticosteroids) are useful in controlling this side effect. A reasonable antiemetic regimen may include one agent that has a direct antiemetic effect coadministered with dexamethasone. Corticosteroids appear to contribute to the efficacy of standard antiemetics in some patients. Care should be taken to continue antiemetic therapy at 2- to 4-hour intervals while the patient is awake throughout the first 24 hours after cisplatin administration. This precaution is extremely important, because a negative initial experience with cisplatin may result in future patient noncompliance. It is the experience of the author that it is better to overmedicate than undermedicate with antiemetics. Many patients experience delayed nausea and vomiting 24 to 120 hours after drug administration. This delayed nausea and vomiting may occasionally be refractory to antiemetics.

REFERENCES

1. Blatter EE, Vollano JF, Krishnan BS, Dabrowiak JC. Interaction of the antitumor agents *cis,cis,trans*-PtIV $(NH_3)_2Cl_2(OH)_2$ and *cis,cis,trans*-PtIV $[(CH_3)_2CHNH_2]_2Cl_2(OH)_2$ and their reduction products with PM2 DNA. Biochemistry 1984;23:4817–4820.
2. Pinto AL, Lippard SJ. Binding of the antitumor drug *cis*-diamminedichloroplatinum (II) (cisplatin) to DNA. Biochim Biophys Acta 1985;780:167–188.
3. Bau R, Gellert RW, Lehovec SM. Crystallographic studies on platinum-nucleoside and platinum nucleotide complexes. J Clin Hematol Oncol 1977;7:51–63.
4. Macquet JP, Jankowski K, Butour JL. Mass spectrometry study of DNA-cisplatin complexes: Perturbation of guanine-cytosine base pairs. Biochem Biophys Res Commun 1980;92:68–74.
5. Pascoe JM, Roberts JJ. Interaction between mammalian cell DNA and inorganic platinum compounds: I. DNA interstrand crosslinking and cytotoxic properties of platinum (II) compounds. Biochem Pharmacol 1974;23:1345–1357.
6. Sherman SE, Gibson D, Wang AHJ, Lippard SJ. Crystal and molecular structure of cis-[Pt(NH_3)_2{d(pGpG)}], the principal adduct formed by *cis*-diamminedichloroplatinum (II) with DNA. J Am Chem Soc 1988;110:7368–7381.
7. Rice JA, Crothers DM, Pinto AL, Lippard SJ. The major adduct of the antitumor drug *cis*-diamminedichloroplatinum (II) with DNA bends the duplex by ~40° toward the major grove. Proc Natl Acad Sci USA 1988;85:4158–4161.

8. Reed E, Sauerhoff S, Poirier MC. Quantitation of platinum-DNA binding in human tissues following therapeutic levels of drug exposure. Atom Spectrosc 1988;9:93–95.

9. Zwelling LA, Anderson T, Kohn KW. DNA-protein and DNA interstrand cross-linking by cis- and trans-platinum (II) diamminedichloride in L1210 mouse leukemia cells and its relation to cytotoxicity. Cancer Res 1979;39:365–369.

10. Poirier MC, Reed E, Zwelling LA, Ozols RJ, Litterst CL, Yuspa SH. The use of polyclonal antibodies to quantitate cis-diamminedichlorplatinum (II)-DNA adducts in cancer patients and animal models. Environ Health Perspect 1985;62:89–94.

11. Reed E, Litterst CL, Thill CC, Yuspa SH, Poirier MC. cis-Diamminedichloroplatinum (II)-DNA adduct formation in renal, gonadal, and tumor tissues of male and female rats. Cancer Res 1987;47:718–722.

12. Poirier MC, Egorin MJ, Fichtinger-Schepman AMJ, Yuspa SH, Reed E. DNA adducts of cisplatin and carboplatin in tissues of human cancer patients. In: Bartsch H, Hemminke K, O'Neill IK, eds. Damaging agents in humans: Applications in cancer epidemiology and prevention. Internation Agency for Research in Cancer Scientific Publications No. 89, July 1988:313–320.

13. Fichtinger-Schepman AMJ, van Oosterom AT, Lohman PHM, Berends R. cis-Diamminedichloroplatinum (II)-induced DNA adducts in peripheral leukocytes from seven cancer patients: Quantitative immunochemical detection of the adduct induction and removal after a single dose of cis-diamminedichloroplatinum (II). Cancer Res 1987;47:3000–3004.

14. Eastman A. Characterization of the adducts produced in DNA by cis-diamminedichloroplatinum (II) and cis-dichloro (ethylenediamine)-platinum (II). Biochemistry 1983;22:3927–3933.

15. Thomas DC, Okumoto DS, Sancar A, Bohr VA. Preferential DNA repair of (6-4) photoproducts in the dihydroxolate reductase gene of Chinese hamster ovary cells. J Biol Chem 1989;264:18005–18010.

16. Jones JC, Zhen W, Reed E, Parker RJ, Sancar A, Bohr VA. Gene-specific formation and repair of cisplatin intrastrand adducts and interstrand cross-links in Chinese hamster ovary cells. J Biol Chem 1991;266:7101–7107.

17. Roberts JJ, Knox RJ, Pera MF, Friedlos F, Lydall DA. The role of platinum-DNA interactions in the cellular toxicity and anti-tumor effects of platinum coordination compounds. In: Nicolini M, ed. Platinum and other metal coordination compounds in cancer chemotherapy. Boston: Martinus Nijhoff, 1988:16–31.

18. Zwelling LA, Michaels S, Szhwartz H, Dobson PP, Kohn KW. DNA cross-linking as an indicator of sensitivity and resistance of mouse L1210 leukemia to cis-diamminedichloroplatinum (II) and L-phenylalanine mustard. Cancer Res 1981;41:640–649.

19. Plooy ACM, van Dijk M, Lohman PHM. Induction and repair of DNA cross-links in Chinese hamster ovary cells treated with various platinum coordination compounds in relation to platinum binding to DNA, cytotoxicity, mutagenicity, and antitumor activity. Cancer Res 1984;44:2043–2051.

20. Parker RJ, Eastman A, Bostick-Bruton F, Reed E. Acquired cisplatin resistance in human ovarian cancer cells is associated with enhanced repair of cisplatin-DNA lesions and reduced drug accumulation. J Clin Invest 1991;87:772–777.

21. Eastman A. Reevaluation of interaction of cis-dischloro (ethylenediamine) platinum (II) with DNA. Biochemistry 1986;25:3912–3915.

22. Fichtinger-Schepman AMJ, Dijt FJ, De Jong WH, Van Oostorom AT, Brends F. In vivo cis-diamminedichloroplatinum (II)-DNA adduct formation and removal as measured with immunochemical techniques. In: Nicolini M, ed. Platinum and other metal coordination compounds in cancer chemotherapy. Boston: Martinum Nijhoff, 1988:32–46.

23. Pinto AL, Lippard SJ. Sequence-dependent termination of in vitro DNA synthesis by cis- and trans-diamminedichloroplatinum (II). Proc Natl Acad Sci USA 1985;82:4616–4619.

24. Gralla JD, Sasse-Dwight S, Poljak LG. Formation of blocking lesions at identical DNA sequences by the nitrosoruea and platinum classes of anticancer drugs. Cancer Res 1987;47:5092–5096.

25. Dedon PC, Borch RJ. Characterization of the reactions of platinum antitumor agents with biologic and nonbiologic sulfur-containing nucleophiles. Biochem Pharmacol 1987;36:1955–1964.

26. Ducore JM, Erickson LC, Zwelling LA, Laurent G, Kohn KW. Comparative studies of DNA cross-linking and cytotoxicity in Burkitt's lymphoma cell lines treated with cis-diamminedichloroplatinum (II) and L-phenylalanine mustard. Cancer Res 1982;42:897–902.

27. Scanlon KJ, Saferstein RL, Thies H, Gross RB, Waxman S, Guttenplan JB. Inhibition of amino acid transport by cis-diamminedichloroplatinum (II) derivatives in L1210 murine leukemia cells. Cancer Res 1983;43:4211–4215.

28. Uozumi J, Litterst CL. The effect of cisplatin on renal ATPase activity in vivo and in vitro. Cancer Chemother Pharmacol 1985;15:93–96.

29. Vassilev PM, Kanazirska MP, Charmamella LJ, Dimitrov NV, Tien HT. Changes in calcium channel activity in membranes from cis-diamminedichloroplatinum (II)-resistant and—sensitive L1210 cells. Cancer Res 1987;47:519–522.

30. Gordon JA, Gattone VH. Mitochondrial alterations in cisplatin-induced acute renal failure. Am J Physiol 1986;250:F991–F998.

31. Tkacova E, Kuzela S. Interaction of cis-diamminedichloroplatinum (II) with mitochondrial phosphate carrier. Neoplasma 1985;32:679–683.

32. Peyrot V, Briand C, Momburg R, Sari JC. In vitro mechanism study of microtubule assembly inhibition by cis-dichlorodiammine-platinum (II). Biochem Pharmacol 1986;35:371–375.

33. Micetich KC, Barnes D, Erickson LC. A comparative study of the cytotoxicity and DNA-damaging effects of cis-(diammino) (1,1-cyclobutanedicarboxylato)-platinum (II) and cis-diamminedichloroplatinum (II) on L1210 cells. Cancer Res 1985;45:4043–4047.

34. Knox RJ, Friedlos F, Lydall DA, Robberts JJ. Mechanism of cytotoxicity of anticancer platinum drugs: Evidence that cis-diamminedichloroplatinum (II) and cis-diammine-(1,1-cyclobutanedicarbosylato) platinum (II) differ only in the kinetics of their interaction with DNA. Cancer Res 1986;46:1972–1979.

35. Anderson WK, Quagliato DA, Haugwitz RD, Narayanan VL, Wolpert-DeFilippes MK. Syntheses, physical properties, and antitumor activity of tetrachloroplatinum (IV) stereoisomers of 1,2-diaminocyclohexane. Cancer Treat Rep 1986;70:997–1002.

36. Eastman A. Glutathione-mediated activation of anticancer platinum (IV) complexes. Biochem Pharmacol 1987;46:4177–4178.

37. Yung WKA, Siddik ZH, Newman RA, Steck PA. Cytotoxicity and intracellular platinum level of cisplatin, carboplatin and tetraplatin in cultured human glioma cells. Proc Am Assoc Cancer Res [Abstract] 1988;29:343.

38. Sariban E, Kohn KW, Zlotogorski C, et al. DNA cross linking responses of human malignant glioma cell strains to chloroethylnitrosoureas, cisplatin, and diaziquone. Cancer Res 1987;47:3988–3994.

39. Pera MF, Friedlos F, Mills J, Roberts JJ. Inherent sensitivity of cultured human embryonal carcinoma cells to adducts of cis-diamminedichloroplatinum (II) on DNA. Cancer Res 1987;47:6810–6813.

40. Roberts JJ, Friedlos F, Scott D, Ormerod MG, Rawlings CJ. The unique sensitivity of Walker rat tumour cells to difunctional agents is associated with a failure to recover from inhibition of DNA systhesis and increased chromosome damage. Mutat Res 1986;166:169–181.

41. Teicher BA, Holden SA, Kelley MJ, et al. Characterization of a human squamous carcinoma cell line resistant to cis-diamminedichloroplatinum (II). Cancer Res 1987;47:388–393.

42. Behrens BC, Hamilton TC, Masuda H, et al. Characterization of a cis-diamminedichloroplatinum (II) resistant human ovarian cancer cell line and its use in evaluation of platinum analogues. Cancer Res 1987;47:414–418.

43. Endresen L, Schjerven L, Rugstad HE. Tumours from a cell strain with a high content of metallothionein show enhanced resistance against cis-dichlorodiammineplatinum. Acta Pharmacol Toxicol (Copenh) 1984;55:183–187.

44. Zwelling LA, Filipski J, Kohn KW. Effects of thiourea on survival and DNA cross-link formation in cells treated with platinum (II) complexes, L-phenylalanine mustard and bis(2-chloroethyl) methylamine. Cancer Res 1979;39:4989–4995.

45. Hromas RA, North JA, Burns CP. Decreased cisplatin uptake by resistant L1210 leukemia cells. Cancer Lett 1987;36:197–201.

46. Andrews PA, Kim RW, Murphy MP, Howell SB. Altered cisplatin metabolism in cisplatin-resistant 2008 human ovarian carcinoma cells. Proc Am Assoc Cancer Res [Abstract] 1986;27:270.

47. Waud WR. Differential uptake of cis-diamminedichloroplatinum (II) by sensitive and resistant murine L1210 leukemia cells. Cancer Res 1987;47:6549–6555.

48. Eichholtz-Wirth H, Hietal B. The relationship between cisplatin sensitivity and drug uptake into mammalian cells in vitro. Br J Cancer 1986;54:239–243.

49. Bernal SD, Speak JA, Boeheim K, et al. Reduced membrane protein associated with resistance of human squamous carcinoma cells to methotrexate and cis-platinum. Mol Cell Biochem 1990;95:61–70.

50. Chen Y-N, Liu LC, Mickley LA, et al. Cisplatin (CP) resistance in human ovarian carcinoma cell lines. Proc Am Assoc Cancer Res [Abstract] 1990;31:335.

51. Kawai K, Kamatani N, Georges E, Ling V. Identification of a membrane glycoprotein overexpressed in muring lymphoma sublines resistant to cis-diamminedichloroplatinum (II). J Biol Chem 1990;265:13137–13142.

52. Hromas RA, Andrews PA, Murphy MP, Burns CP. Glutathione depletion reverses cisplatin resistance in murine L1210 leukemia cells. Cancer Lett 1987;34:9–13.

53. Andrews PA, Murphy MP, Howell SB. Metallothionein-mediated cisplatin resistance in human ovarian carcinoma cells. Cancer Chemother Pharmacol 1987;19:149–154.

54. Miyazaki M, Kohno K, Saburi Y, et al. Drug resistance to cis-diamminedichloroplatinum (II) in Chinese hamster ovary cell lines transfected with glutathione S-transferase PI gene. Biochem Biophys Res Commun 1990;166:1358–1364.

55. Meijer C, Mulder NH, Hospers GAP, Uges DRA, De Vries EGE. The role of glutathione in resistance to cisplatin in a human small cell lung cancer cell line. Br J Cancer 1990;62:72–77.

56. Schilder RJ, Hall L, Monks A, et al. Metallothionein gene expression and resistance to cisplatin in human ovarian cancer. Int J Cancer 1990;45:416–422.

57. Eastman A, Schulte N, Sheibani N, Sorenson CM. Mechanisms of resistance to platinum drugs. In: Nicolini M, ed. Platinum and other metal compounds in cancer chemotherapy. Boston: Martinus Nijhoff, 1988:178–196.

58. Reed E, Ormond P, Bohr VA, Budd J, Bostick-Bruton F. Expression of the human DNA repair gene ERCC-1 relates to cisplatin drug resistance in human ovarian cancer cells. Proc Am Assoc Cancer Res 1989;30:488.

59. Popoff SC, Beck DJ, Rupp WD. Repair of plasmid DNA damaged in vitro with cis- or trans-diamminedichloroplatinum (II) in Escherichia coli. Mutat Res 1987;183:129–137.

60. van Duin M, de Wit J, Odijk H, et al. Molecular characterization of the human excision repair gene ERCC1: cDNA cloning and amino acid homology with the yeast DNA repair gene RAD10. Cell 1986;44:913–923.

61. Eastman A, Schulte N. Enhanced DNA repair as a mechanism of resistance to cis-diamminedichloroplatinum (II). Biochemistry 1988;27:4730–4734.

62. Shebani N, Jennerwein MM, Eastman A. DNA repair in cells sensitive and resistant to cis-diamminedichloroplatinum (II): Host cell reactivation of damaged plasmid DNA. Biochemistry 1989;28:3120–3124.

63. Chen G, Pan Q. Potentiation of the antitumor activity of cisplatin in mice by 3-aminobenzamide and nicotinamide. Cancer Chemother Pharmacol 1988;22:303–307.

64. Pera MF, Friedlos F, Mills J, Roberts JJ. Inherent sensitivity of cultured human em-

bryonal carcinoma cells to adducts of *cis*-diamminedichloroplatinum (II). Cancer Res 1987;47:6810–6813.

65. Bedford P, Fichtinger-Schepman AMJ, Shellard SA,. Differential repair of platinum-DNA adducts in human bladder and testicular tumor continuous cell lines. Cancer Res 1988;48:3019–3024.

66. Swinnen LJ, Barnes DM, Fisher SG, et al. 1b-D-Arabinofuranosylcytosine and hydroxyurea production of cytotoxic synergy with *cis*-diamminedichloroplatinum (II) and modification of platinum-induced DNA interstrand cross-linking. Cancer Res 1989;49:1383–1389.

67. Masuda H, Tanaka T, Matsuda H, Kusaba I. Increased removal of DNA-bound platinum in a human ovarian cancer cell line resistant to *cis*-diamminedichloroplatinum (II). Cancer Res 1990;50:1863–1866.

68. Zhen W, Link CJ, O'Connor PM, Bohr VA. Formation and repair of cisplatin lesions in specific genes in cisplatin sensitive and resistant human ovarian cancer cell lines. Proc Am Assoc Cancer Res [Abstract] 1991;32:7.

69. Tomita K, Tsuchiya H. Enhancement of cytocidal and antitumor effect of cisplatin by caffeine in human osteosarcoma. Clin Ther 1989;11:43–52.

70. Cantwell BMJ, Veale D, Rivett C, Ghani S, Harris AL. Cisplatin with high-dose infusions of hydroxyurea to inhibit DNA repair. Cancer Chemother Pharmacol 1989;23:252–254.

71. Cheung Y, Cradock JC, Vishnuvajjala BR, Flora K. Stability of cisplatin, iproplatin, carboplatin, and tetraplatin in commonly used intravenous solutions. Am J Hosp Pharm 1987;44:124–130.

72. Gormley PE, Bull JM, LeRoy AF, Cysyk R. Kinetics of *cis*-dichloro-diammineplatinum. Clin Pharmacol Ther 1979;25:351–357.

73. Himmelstein KJ, Patton TF, Belt RJ, et al. Clinical kinetics of intact cisplatin and some related species. Clin Pharmacol Ther 1981;29:658–664.

74. Corden BJ, Fine RL, Ozols RF, Collins JM. Clinical pharmacology of high-dose cisplatin. Cancer Chemother Pharmacol 1985;14:38–41.

75. Weiner MW, Jacobs C. Mechanism of cisplatin nephrotoxicity. Fed Proc 1983;42:2974–2978.

76. Casper ES, Kelson DP, Alcock NW, Young CW. Platinum concentrations in bile and plasma following rapid and 6-hour infusions of *cis*-dichloro-diammineplatinum (II). Cancer Treat Rep 1979;63:2023–2035.

77. Bajorin DF, Bosl GH, Alcock NW, et al. Pharmacokinetics of *cis*-diamminedichloroplatinum (II) after administration in hypertonic saline. Cancer Res 1986;46:5969–5972.

78. Myers CE. The use of intraperitoneal chemotherapy in the treatment of ovarian cancer. Semin Oncol 1984;11:275–284.

79. Ozols RF. Intraperitoneal chemotherapy in the management of ovarian cancer. Semin Oncol 1985;12:75–80.

80. Howell SB, Pfeifle CE, Wung W, et al. Intraperitoneal cisplatin with systemic thiosulfate protection. Ann Intern Med 1982;97:845–851.

81. Curt GA, Grygiel JJ, Corden BJ, et al. A phase I and pharmacokinetic study of diamminecyclobutane-dicarboxylatoplatinum (NSC 241240). Cancer Res 1983;43:4470–4473.

82. Reece PA, Bishop JF, Olver IN, et al. Pharmacokinetics of unchanged carboplatin (CBDCA) in patients with small cell lung carcinoma. Cancer Chemother Pharmacol 1987;19:326–330.

83. Oguri S, Sakakibara T, Mase H, et al. Clinical pharmacokinetics of carboplatin. J Clin Pharmacol 1988;28:208–215.

84. Van Echo DA, Egorin MJ, Aisner J. The pharmacology of carboplatin. Semin Oncol 1989;16(suppl 5):1–6.

85. Ozols RF. Intraperitoneal therapy in ovarian cancer: Time's up. J Clin Oncol 1991;9:197–199.

86. DeGregorio MW, Gandara DR, Holleran WM. High-dose cisplatin with diethyldithiocarbamate (DDTC) rescue therapy: Preliminary pharmacologic observations. Cancer Chemother Pharmacol 1989;23:276–278.

87. Qazi R, Chang AYC, Borch RF, et al. Phase I clinical and pharmacokinetic study of diethyldithiocarbamate as a chemoprotector from toxic effects of cisplatin. JNCI 1988;80:1486–1488.

88. Rothenberg ML, Ostchega Y, Steinberg SM, et al. High-dose carboplatin with diethyldithiocarbamate chemoprotection in treatment of women with relapsed ovarian cancer. JNCI 1988;80:1488–1492.

89. Glover D, Grabelsky S, Fox K, et al. Clinical trials of WE-2721 and *cis*-platinum. Int J Radiat Oncol Biol Phys 1989;16:1201–1204.

90. van der Hoop RG, Vecht CJ, van der Burg MEL, et al. Prevention of cisplatin neurotoxicity with an ACTH(4–9) analogue in patients with ovarian cancer. N Engl J Med 1990;322:89–94.

91. Terheggen PMAB, van der Hoop RG, Floot BGJ, Gispen WH. Cellular distribution of *cis*-diamminedichloroplatinum (II)-DNA binding in rat dorsal root spinal ganglia: Effect of the neuroprotecting peptide ORG.2766. Toxicol Appl Pharmacol 1989;99:334–343.

92. Parker RJ, Gill I, Tarone R, et al. Platinum-DNA damage in leukocyte DNA of patients receiving carboplatin and cisplatin chemotherapy, measured by atomic absorption spectrometry. Carcinogenesis 1991;12:1253–1258.

93. Reed E, Ozols RF, Tarone R, Yuspa SH, Poirier MC. Platinum-DNA adducts in leukocyte DNA correlate with disease response in ovarian cancer patients receiving platinum-based chemotherapy. Proc Natl Acad Sci USA 1987;84:5024–5028.

94. Reed E, Ozols RF, Tarone R, Yuspa SH, Poirier MC. The measurement of cisplatin-DNA adduct levels in testicular cancer patients. Carcinogenesis 1988;9:1909–1911.

95. Reed E, Ostchega Y, Steinberg SM, et al. Evaluation of platinum-DNA adduct levels relative to known prognostic variables in a cohort of ovarian cancer patients. Cancer Res 1990;50:2256–2260.

96. Reed E, Gupta-Burt S, Katz D, Poirier MC. Platinum-DNA adduct measured at autopsy in multiple human tissues. Proc Proc Am Assoc Cancer Res [Abstract] 1989;30:276.

97. Fichtinger-Schepman AMJ, van der Velde-Visser SD, van Dijk-Knijnenburg HCM, van Oosterom AT, Baan RA, Berends F. Kinetics of the formation and removal of cisplatin-DNA adducts in blood cells and tumor tissue of cancer patients receiving chemotherapy: Comparison with *in vitro* adduct formation. Cancer Res 1990;50:7887–7894.

98. Safirstein R, Winston J, Goldstein M, Moel D, Dikman S, Guttenplan J. Cisplatin nephrotoxicity. Am J Kidney Dis 1986;8:356–367.

99. Fjeldborg P, Sorensen J, Helkjaer PE. The long-term effect of cisplatin on renal function. Cancer 1986;58:2214–2217.

100. Tanaka H, Ishikawa E, Teshima S, Shimizu E. Histopathological study of human cisplatin nephropathy. Toxicol Pathol 1986;14:247–257.

101. Finley RS, Fortner CL, Grove WR. Cisplatin nephrotoxicity: A summary of preventative interventions. Drug Intell Clin Pharm 1985;19:362–367.

102. Coons HL, Leventhal H, Nerenz DR, Love RR, Larson S. Anticipatory nausea and emotional distress in patients receiving cisplatin-based chemotherapy. Oncol Nurs Forum 1987;14:31–35.

103. Aasebo U, Slordal L, Prytz PS, Aarbakke J. High-dose metoclopramide and chlorpromazine in the treatment of cisplatin-induced emesis. Pharmacol Toxicol 1987;60:337–339.

104. Legha SS, Dimery IW. High-dose cisplatin administration without hypertonic saline: Observation of disabling neurotoxicity. J Clin Oncol 1985;3:1373–1378.

105. Kobayashi H, Ohashi N, Watanabe Y, Mizukoshi K. Clinical features of cisplatin vestibulotoxicity and hearing loss. ORL J Otorhinolaryngol Relat Spec 1987;49:67–72.

106. Rothmann SA, Paul P, Weick JK, McIntyre WR, Fantelli F. Effect of *cis*-diamminedichloroplatinum on erythropoietin production and hematopoietic progenitor cells. Int J Cell Cloning 1985;3:415–423.

107. Kumar L, Dua H. Cisplatin induced anaemia. NZ Med J [letter] 1987;100(817):81.

108. Wilding G, Caruso R, Lawrence TS, et al. Retinal toxicity after high-dose cisplatin therapy. J Clin Oncol 1985;3:1683–1689.

109. Miller DF, Bay JW, Lederman RJ, Purvis JD, Rogers LR, Tomsak RL. Ocular and orbital toxicity following intracarotid injection of BCNU (carmustine) and cisplatinum for malignant gliomas. Ophthalmology 1985;92:402–406.

109a. Osanto S, Bukman A, Hoek F, Sterk PJ, DeLaat JAPM, Hermans J. Long-term effects of chemotherapy in patients with testicular cancer. J Clin Oncol 1992;10:574–579.

110. Pogliani EM, Pioltelli P, Rossini F, Lanzi E, Corneo G. Acute leukaemia following cisplatin for ovarian cancer. Haematologica (Pavia) [Letter] 1987;72:184–185.

111. Bassett WB, Weill RB. Acute leukemia following cisplatin for bladder cancer. J Clin Oncol [Letter] 1986;4:614.

112. Doll DC, List AF, Greco FA, et al. Acute vascular ischemic events after cisplatin-based combination chemotherapy for germ-cell tumors of the testis. Ann Intern Med 1986;105:48–51.

113. Talcott JA, Herman TS. Acute ischemic vascular events and cisplatin. Ann Intern Med [Letter] 1987;107:121–122.

114. Lederman GS, Garnick MB. Pulmonary emboli as a complication of germ cell cancer treatment. J Urol 1987;137:1236–1237.

115. Canobbio L, Fassio T, Gasparini G, et al. Cardiac arrythmia: Possible complication from treatment with cisplatin. Tumori 1986;72:201–204.

116. Frustaci S, Barzan L, Comoretto R, Tumolo S, Lo Re G, Mondardini S. Local neurotoxicity after intra-arterial cisplatin in head and neck cancer. Cancer Treat Rep 1987;71:257–259.

117. Scherini E, Biggiogera M, Bernocchi G, Mares V. Damage and repair of the immature rat cerebellum after *cis*-dichlorodiammineplatinum II (*cis*-DDP) treatment: An ultrastructural study. Acta Neuropathol (Berl) 1987;72:218–228.

118. Goldstein RS, Mayor GH, Rosenbaum RW, Hook JB, Santiago JV, Bond JT. Glucose intolerance following *cis*-platinum treatment in rats. Toxicology 1982;24:273–280.

119. Bunin N, Meyer WH, Christensen M, Pratt CB. Pancreatitis following cisplatin: A case report. Cancer Treat Rep [Letter] 1985;69:236–237.

120. Kelsen DP, Alcock N, Young CW. Cisplatin nephrotoxicity: Correlation with plasma platinum concentrations. Am J Clin Oncol 1985;8:77–80.

121. Nanji AA, Stewart DJ, Mikhael NZ. Hyperurioemia and hypoalbuminemia predispose to cisplatin-induced nephrotoxicity. Cancer Chemother Pharmacol 1986;17:274–276.

122. De Santo NG, Capasso G, Capodicassa G, Tancredi F, Nuzzi F, Giordano C. Acute renal failure due to cisplatin. Int J Pediatr Nephrol 1986;7:145–150.

123. Bodenner DL, Dedon PC, Keng PC, Borch RF. Effect of diethyldithiocarbamate on *cis*-diamminedichloroplatinum(II)-induced cytotoxicity, DNA cross-linking, and gamma-glutamyl transpeptidase inhibition. Cancer Res 1986;46:2745–2750.

124. Reed E, Gupta-Burt S, Yuspa SH, et al. Platinum-DNA adduct levels in malignant and nonmalignant tissues of cancer patients correlate with disease response. Clin Res 1988;36:499A.

125. Reed E, Poirier MC, Young RC, Ozols RF. High-dose cisplatin in hypertonic saline: Toxicity versus therapeutic benefit. In: Hacker MP, Lazo JS, Tritton TR, eds. Organ-directed toxicities of anti-cancer drugs. Boston: Martinus Nijhoff, 1988:203–213.

126. Ozols RF, Corden BF, Jacob J, et al. High-dose cisplatin in hypertonic saline. Ann Intern Med 1984;100:19.

127. Zwelling L, Kohn KW: Platinum complexes. In: Chabner BA, ed. Pharmacologic principles of cancer treatment. Philadelphia: WB Saunders, 1982:309–339.

127a. Trugman J, Hogenkamp HP, Roelofs R, Hrushesky WJ. Cisplatin neurotoxicity: Failure to demonstrate vitamin B_{12} inactivation. Cancer Treat Rep 1985;69:453–455.

128. Schweitzer VG, Dolan DF, Abrams GE, Davidson T, Snyder R. Amelioration of cisplatin-induced ototoxicity by fosfomycin. Laryngoscope 1986;96:948–958.

129. Boheim K, Bichler E. Cisplatin-induced ototoxicity: Audiometric findings and experimental chochlear pathology. Arch Otorhinolaryngol 1985;242:1–6.

130. Becouarn Y, Nguyen BB, David M, Lakdja F, Brunet R, Chauvergne J. Improved control of cisplatin-induced emesis with a combination of high doses of methylprednisolone and metoclopramide: A single-blind randomized trial. Eur J Cancer Clin Oncol 1986;22:1421–1424.

SECTION **8**

NATHAN A. BERGER

Alkylating Agents

Alkylating agents were among the first compounds identified to be useful in cancer chemotherapy and, because of their variety and relative tumoricidal selectivity, they remain important components of many modern chemotherapeutic regimens. They are useful as single agents. They serve as important components in combination chemotherapy regimens in which they are employed with other agents with different toxicities or mechanisms of actions, or both. The alkylating agents have also served as the basis for dose escalation studies in which their use has been extended from conventional to high-dose regimens with bone marrow transplant. In the latter approach, alkylating agents also have been employed therapeutically in ex vivo processes to purge tumor cells from bone marrow before it is reinfused into an autologous donor.

Although the alkylating agents are a diverse series of chemical compounds, they all have the common property of dissociating a positively charged, electrophillic, alkyl group capable of attacking negatively charged, electron-rich, nucleophilic sites on most biologic molecules, thereby adding alkyl groups at oxygen, nitrogen, phosphorous, or sulfur atoms. Their chemotherapeutic usefulness derives from their ability to form a variety of DNA adducts that sufficiently alter DNA structure or function, or both, so as to have a cytotoxic effect.[1] Figure 18–27 shows the activation of a simple alkylating agent

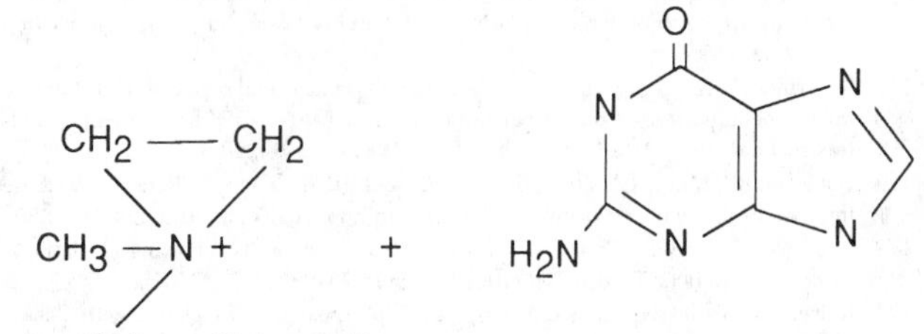

FIGURE 18–27. Spontaneous activation of nitrogen mustard to an imonium ion that forms a covalent bond with nucleophilic sites, such as the N7 position of guanine. The remaining free chloroethyl arm of nitrogen mustard can repeat the same sequence of reactions to form DNA crosslinks.

by formation, in aqueous solution, of a positively charged carbonium ion, which subsequently forms an adduct at a nucleophilic site on a guanine base. Many of the pharmacologically useful agents undergo a more complex activation process. For example, cyclophosphamide must undergo several steps of metabolic processing before it can generate a reactive intermediate. Agents containing chloroethyl alkylating groups must undergo a preliminary cyclization to form an unstable imonium ion with subsequent opening of the three-member ring to form the alkylating intermediate. Once generated, the positively charged alkylating intermediate attacks the different nucleophilic nitrogen, oxygen, or phosphorous groups in DNA with somewhat different specificity, depending on the chemistry of the agent. Different consequences ensue pending the sites and frequency of attack. In addition, because the reaction of alkylating agents with proteins or low-molecular-weight compounds, such as glutathione, serve to consume or inactivate the alkylating agents, this occurrence may contribute to drug resistance.

The most common site of DNA alkylation is the N-7 position of guanine, with fewer adducts occurring at the N-1 and O-6 positions of guanine, the N-1, N-3, and N-7 positions of adenine, the N-3 position of cytosine, and the O-4 position of thymidine.[1] Alterations at the N-7 of guanine are relatively silent in their effect on DNA function, because these adducts do not interfere with the base-pairing scheme. In contrast, adducts at the N-3 position of cytosine, the O-6 position of guanine, and the O-4 position of thymine interfere with the Watson-Crick base-pairing scheme and therefore are likely to interfere with fidelity of replication and transcription leading to mutagenicity and cytotoxicity. In addition to direct interference with replication and transcription, the formation of DNA adducts leads to a variety of structural lesions, including ring openings, base deletions, and strand scissions.[2,3] Many of the DNA adducts and lesions are further acted on by repair enzymes that can restore the integrity of the DNA, or if the repair process is only partially completed, it can cause additional DNA damage, such as the creation of apurinic sites or DNA strand breaks. If DNA adducts occur at the N-3 position of adenine or the N-7 position of guanine, the altered purine can be removed by a glycosylase that cleaves the bond between the altered base and the deoxyribose moiety resulting in a depurinated or apurinic site (AP) on the DNA.[4] The absence of a purine or pyrimidine base is detected by an AP or apyrimidinic endonuclease that excises the AP site along with several nucleotides on either side of the lesion.[2,3,5] The gap in one strand of the DNA is repaired by the sequential action of a DNA polymerase to fill in the defect using the opposite DNA strand as a template. This repair synthesis is followed by action of a DNA ligase to join the newly synthesized patch to the original DNA.[6] Topoisomerases are also involved in this process to make the damaged DNA available to repair enzymes.

In the absence of a faithful repair process, the persistence of an AP site may lead to mutations due to altered template specificity of the damaged strand and insertion of the wrong base on the opposite strand of newly synthesized DNA. If the nucleotide excision process is not completed by resynthesis and ligation, the persistent strand break can lead to chromosomal rearrangement or breakage. DNA strand breaks also lead to activation of the chromosomal enzyme poly(ADP-ribose) polymerase, which cleaves nicotinamide adenine dinucleotide (NAD+) and uses the adenosine diphosphoribose moiety to form poly(ADP-ribose), which serves to facilitate the DNA repair process.[7] In the presence of high levels of unrepaired DNA strand breaks, activation of this enzyme can consume NAD+, interfere with ATP generation, and cause cell death because of failure of energy-dependent processes.[8]

Bifunctional alkylating agents, such as melphalan and chlorambucil, with the capacity to generate two electrophilic groups and form two adducts with DNA, are capable of forming DNA-interstrand crosslinks that interfere directly with DNA replication, repair, and transcription.[9] In addition, the adducts can undergo many of the repair reactions outlined earlier that can result in restoration of integrity or further damage and cytotoxicity if not repaired with complete fidelity.

The enzymes involved in the DNA repair process provide rational targets for modulators to enhance the cytotoxic effects of alkylating agents. For example, the use of novobiocin to inhibit topoisomerase II potentiates the cytotoxic effects of several alkylating agents.[10] Furthermore, because DNA repair processes can be saturated, it seems likely that increasing doses of alkylating agents may exceed the capacity of cellular repair processes and contribute to the increased effectiveness of high-dose therapy.[11]

Formation and repair of O^6-alkylguanine adducts have recently received considerable attention. Although adducts at this position are relatively infrequent, they are highly cytotoxic and mutagenic because of their interference with the base-pairing scheme, resulting in the substitution of A-T base pairs in place of G-C.[12] Adducts at the O-6 guanine position are readily repaired by a protein, O^6-alkylguanine-DNA alkyltransferase, which transfers these adducts from the O-6 position on the base to an irreversible, covalent complex with a sulfhydryl group in the protein, restoring the normal guanine structure to DNA and causing inactivation of the protein.[12] This reaction is important for repairing O^6-guanine adducts before they can exert their mutagenic potential. The O-6 position of guanine also serves as the initial site for BCNU attachment before it forms a DNA crosslink.[12] Removal of these O-6 adducts can prevent formation of nitrosourea-induced crosslinks and cytotoxicity.[13] Alterations in the cellular susceptibility to nitrosoureas is affected directly by cellular levels of O^6-alkylguanine-DNA alkyltransferase, with higher levels of the protein leading to increased drug resistance, whereas inactivation of the protein leads to increased susceptibility to nitrosoureas.[14]

Cellular thiols, including glutathione, provide nucleophilic targets for covalent adduct formation by alkylating agents. Because these compounds serve to consume and inactivate the alkylating agents, alterations in their concentration and localization modify alkylating agent efficacy.[15] Overexpression of the sulfhydryl-rich protein, metallothionein, in transfected cells has been shown to confer resistance to several alkylating agents.[16] Alterations in glutathione transferase may also affect activity of alkylating agents. Buthionine sulfoxamine (BSO), which inhibits γ-glutamyl cysteine synthetase, the first enzyme in the glutathione synthesis pathway, drastically reduces cellular levels of glutathione and significantly increases susceptibility to alkylating agent cytotoxicity.[17] On the other hand, the radioprotective agent WR2721 has demonstrated a capacity to preserve thiol pools in normal tissue and is currently being tested for its protective effects against alkylating agent cytotoxicity.[18]

The alkylating agents show a common mechanism of action and are all potentially cytotoxic, mutagenic, and carcinogenic. However, variations in their structures are associated with differences in their pharmacokinetic features, lipid solubility, chemical reactivity, requirement for metabolic activation, alkylation sites on DNA, and membrane transport properties. Because of these differences, alkylating agents do not necessarily exhibit cross-resistance in clinical situations.[19] Tumors resistant to cyclophosphamide or phenylalanine mustard are not necessarily resistant to nitrosoureas. Multidrug resistance, which encompasses doxorubicin, etoposide, and vincristine, usually has no effect on alkylating agent sensitivity. In experimental systems, acquired alkylating agent resistance may be lost over a period during which there is no exposure to the alkylating agent. Although this effect has not been exploited in the clinical situation, the potential for reusing an alkylating agent should be considered when long periods exist between acquisition of resistance and rechallenge.

Alkylating agents are cell cycle dependent but not cell cycle specific. They exert their cytotoxic effects on cells throughout the cell cycle but have quantitatively greater activity against rapidly proliferating cells, possibly because the cells have less time to repair damage before entering the vulnerable phase of the cell cycle.[20] Cells in which DNA crosslinks occur accumulate and die in the G_2 phase of the cell cycle. Persistent DNA strand breaks may result in lethal chromosomal damage in the mitotic phase of the cell cycle.

Figure 18–28 shows the structure of the commonly used alkylating agents. Unique aspects of their clinical pharmacology and optimal clinical use are described in the following sections.

NITROGEN MUSTARD

Nitrogen mustard (see Fig. 18–28), originally studied for its potential as a vesicant in chemical warfare, is a highly reactive analog of sulfur mustard and was the first alkylating agent introduced into clinical therapy.[21] Its biologic activity resides in the presence of two chloroethyl groups attached to a common nitrogen. The compound is highly reactive in aqueous solution in which it undergoes spontaneous intramolecular rearrangement to form a quarternary ammonium compound with generation of two reactive chloroethyl groups.

Nitrogen mustard is usually administered by the intravenous route where, because of its high reactivity, it disappears from the circulation within minutes. It is sometimes applied topically for treatment of cutaneous malignancies or by intracavitary injection for treatment of malignant effusions associated with the presence of metastatic tumor deposits. Intracavitary administration is usually preceded by drainage of most of the effusion, so that the alkylating agent can be dispersed in the remaining fluid to gain access to tumor deposits implanted throughout the cavity.

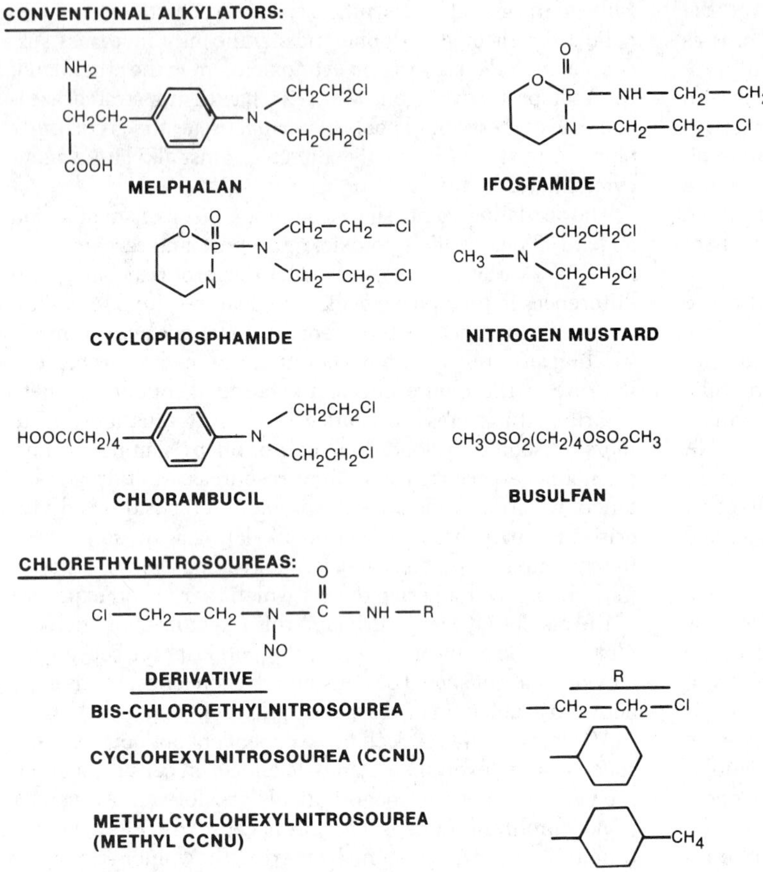

CONVENTIONAL ALKYLATORS:

MELPHALAN

IFOSFAMIDE

CYCLOPHOSPHAMIDE

NITROGEN MUSTARD

CHLORAMBUCIL

BUSULFAN

CHLORETHYLNITROSOUREAS:

DERIVATIVE
BIS-CHLOROETHYLNITROSOUREA

CYCLOHEXYLNITROSOUREA (CCNU)

METHYLCYCLOHEXYLNITROSOUREA
(METHYL CCNU)

FIGURE 18–28. Structures of commonly used alkylating agents and chloroethylnitrosoureas.

Nitrogen mustard is actively transported into cells by the choline transport system.[22] Exposure to this alkylating agent results in formation of simple DNA adducts, DNA-interstrand crosslinks, and DNA-protein crosslinks.[1,23] Resistance to nitrogen mustard at the cellular level is associated with alterations in kinetics of DNA crosslink formation and repair. This alteration may occur as a result of decreased drug uptake, increased drug conjugation with intracellular sulfhydryl groups, and increased DNA repair activity.[23–29] Nitrogen mustard causes nausea and vomiting after administration. It may cause thrombophlebitis and sclerosis of the veins through which it is administered, and it causes severe inflammation and tissue necrosis if extravasation occurs during administration. Under these conditions, prompt management measures need be instituted to prevent severe, permanent tissue damage.[26] Myelosuppression usually occurs after nitrogen mustard administration, with anemia and granulocytopenia predominating and variable degrees of thrombocytopenia occurring. Immunosuppression also may occur because of the lympholytic effect of nitrogen mustard.

The major use for nitrogen mustard currently is in the treatment of lymphomas, especially as part of the nitrogen mustard, vincristine, procarbazine, prednisone (MOPP) combination chemotherapy regimen for Hodgkin's disease. It is also used by topical application for treatment of cutaneous lymphomas, such as mycoses fungoides. It is sometimes administered by direct intracavitary injection for control of malignant pleural or peritoneal effusions.

MELPHALAN

Melphalan (see Fig. 18–28), a phenylalanine derivative of nitrogen mustard, was synthesized with the notion that it would be selectively concentrated in tumors, such as melanin-producing malignancies, that actively use phenylalanine or tyrosine.[27] The drug is relatively stable in media containing high concentrations of chloride ion and at acid pH. Melphalan is actively transported into cells by a high-affinity carrier, the L amino acid transport system, which also transports the amino acids leucine and glutamine.[28] In some tumor cells, a second transport system (which also carries alanine, serine, and cysteine) contributes to melphalan uptake but is less effective than the L system at high drug concentrations. High concentrations of leucine and glutamine can reduce melphalan toxicity in bone marrow colony-forming units in vitro and in tumor cells.[29] The ability of amino acids to protect against melphalan cytotoxicity appears related to their effects on the leucine carrier. Amino acid concentrations in plasma or ascitic fluid may influence the uptake and cytotoxicity of melphalan. The antiestrogen tamoxifen inhibits melphalan uptake by breast cancer cells.[30] Melphalan accumulation can also be impaired by doxorubicin, aminophylline, chlorpromazine. and indomethacin. Nicotinamide potentiates the cytotoxic effects of melphalan.[31] This reaction may result from nicotinamide inhibition of poly(ADP-ribose) polymerase or prolongation of plasma half-life.[31] Increasing tissue oxygenation potentiates the cytotoxic effects of melphalan, and in model systems its antitumor effects are enhanced by administration of oxygen-transporting perfluorocarbons and breathing of high oxygen concentration.[32]

Melphalan is administered orally, intravenously, or intraperitoneally. Absorption from the gastrointestinal tract is variable, and doses by this route must be adjusted according to bone marrow tolerance.[33] Food slows its absorption. Systemic availability is increased when the drug is administered in the fasting state, whereas a large meal may enhance melphalan degradation at alkaline pH in the proximal small intestine. After oral administration, between 20% and 50% of the drug is excreted in the stool. Despite the variation in bioavailability, the ease of oral administration makes this one of the most common routes for using melphalan in the chronic treatment of multiple myeloma.

After intravenous administration, the parent compound disappears from plasma with a half-life of approximately 1 to 2 hours, a rate consistent with the rate of hydrolysis of the chloride groups in plasma. Monohydroxy and dihydroxy metabolites and alkylated proteins are found in plasma soon after intravenous drug administration. About 15% of the drug is excreted intact in the urine.[33,34] The drug should be used cautiously in patients with severe renal failure, and doses should be reduced initially in patients with greater than 50% reduction in creatinine clearance.

In conventional doses, melphalan has a broad spectrum of activity, including antitumor effects against lymphomas, breast and ovarian cancer, and multiple myeloma. It has been used successfully in the adjuvant setting for breast cancer. Melphalan is used in high-dose regimens, with or without bone marrow transplant, in the treatment of acute myeloid leukemia, multiple myeloma, breast and colon cancer, Ewing's sarcoma, melanoma, and neuroblastoma.[35] After high-dose therapy, cerebrospinal fluid concentrations may reach 10% of the corresponding melphalan plasma levels.[35]

Because the parent compound does not irritate peritoneal surfaces, and it does not require hepatic activation, melphalan has been employed for treatment of intraperitoneal malignancies by direct intraperitoneal instillation.[36] A 100 to 1 gradient in drug concentration between peritoneal fluid and plasma is achieved by this route with little systemic toxicity. Although this schedule produces antitumor responses, its usefulness in ovarian cancer and other intraperitoneal tumors has not been established.

Melphalan routinely causes myelosuppression, with equal suppression of granulocyte and platelet production. Nadir counts usually occur at 28 to 35 days. Production of moderate leukopenia is an important target in gauging adequacy of melphalan dosage and systemic availability. Nausea and vomiting are infrequent with this agent. Alopecia is common during extended courses of treatment. Melphalan appears to be more carcinogenic than cyclophosphamide. An analysis of acute leukemia in women with ovarian cancer revealed a 93-fold increase in incidence compared with the general age-matched population and a two- to threefold increase relative to patients treated with cyclophosphamide.[37]

CHLORAMBUCIL

Chlorambucil (see Fig. 18–28) is a benzene butanoic acid derivative of nitrogen mustard and is a close structural congener of melphalan. It is stable in aqueous solution, is completely absorbed from the gastrointestinal tract, and reaches peak plasma levels within 1 hour of an oral dose, but has a delayed onset of action. Because of its convenience, ease of administration, and predictable myelotoxicity, it is the alkylating agent of choice for treatment of chronic lymphocytic leukemia.[38] It is usually administered on a daily basis for prolonged periods, with dose adjustments to avoid severely suppressing normal blood elements. It has few other side effects, but like other alkylating agents, chronic chlorambucil use has been implicated in production of pulmonary fibrosis and with the development of acute myeloid leukemia.[39,40]

BUSULFAN

Busulfan (see Fig. 18–28) is a bifunctional alkylating agent whose activity is mediated by two labile methane-sulfonate groups attached at opposite ends of a four-carbon alkyl chain. Hydrolysis of the methane sulfonates leads to the formation of carbonium ions that bind to nucleophilic sites on DNA and may result in DNA crosslinks.[1] The drug also binds extensively to sulfhydryl groups and proteins; however, the DNA adducts formed by busulfan account for its major antitumor effect. The drug is well absorbed from the gastrointestinal tract, and it is commonly used by daily oral administration for the treatment of chronic myelogenous leukemia, where its strong myelosuppressive action provides a smooth, long-term regulation of the leukocyte count. However, myelosuppression produced by busulfan is not quickly reversible and may last indefinitely if excessive doses are used. Busulfan is also an important component of high-dose preparative chemotherapy regimens preceding allogeneic and autologous bone marrow transplants, especially in the busulfan, cyclophosphamide regimen.[41] Chronic busulfan administration can result in increased pigmentation, especially over bony prominences in an Addisonian distribution but without abnormalities of adrenal function.[42] Busulfan also can cause pulmonary fibrosis resembling that seen after pulmonary irradiation, and it may also cause testicular atrophy and hepatocellular dysfunction. In high-dose transplantation regimens, busulfan can cause hepatic veno-occlusive disease, mucositis, hemorrhagic cystitis, seizures, rash, pneumonitis, and diarrhea.[43,44]

CYCLOPHOSPHAMIDE

Cyclophosphamide (see Fig. 18–28) differs from the previously noted alkylating agents in that it requires a multistep activation process before it can function as an antitumor alkylating agent.[45] In liver cells, the microsomal oxidase system converts the original compound to 4-hydroxycyclophosphamide, which reenters the circulation and is subsequently taken up into peripheral tissues and tumor, where it undergoes tautomerization to aldophosphamide (Fig. 18–29). The latter intermediate undergoes spontaneous decomposition to acrolein and phosphoramide mustard, both of which are available to react with nucleophilic groups. Aldophosphamide also can be inactivated by aldehyde dehydrogenase, and elevated levels of this enzyme have been associated with resistance to cyclophosphamide.[46] Phosphoramide mustard is considered to be the major cytotoxic derivative of cyclophosphamide. Acrolein also is a reactive agent capable of depleting cellular glutathione and causing DNA alkylation.[47]

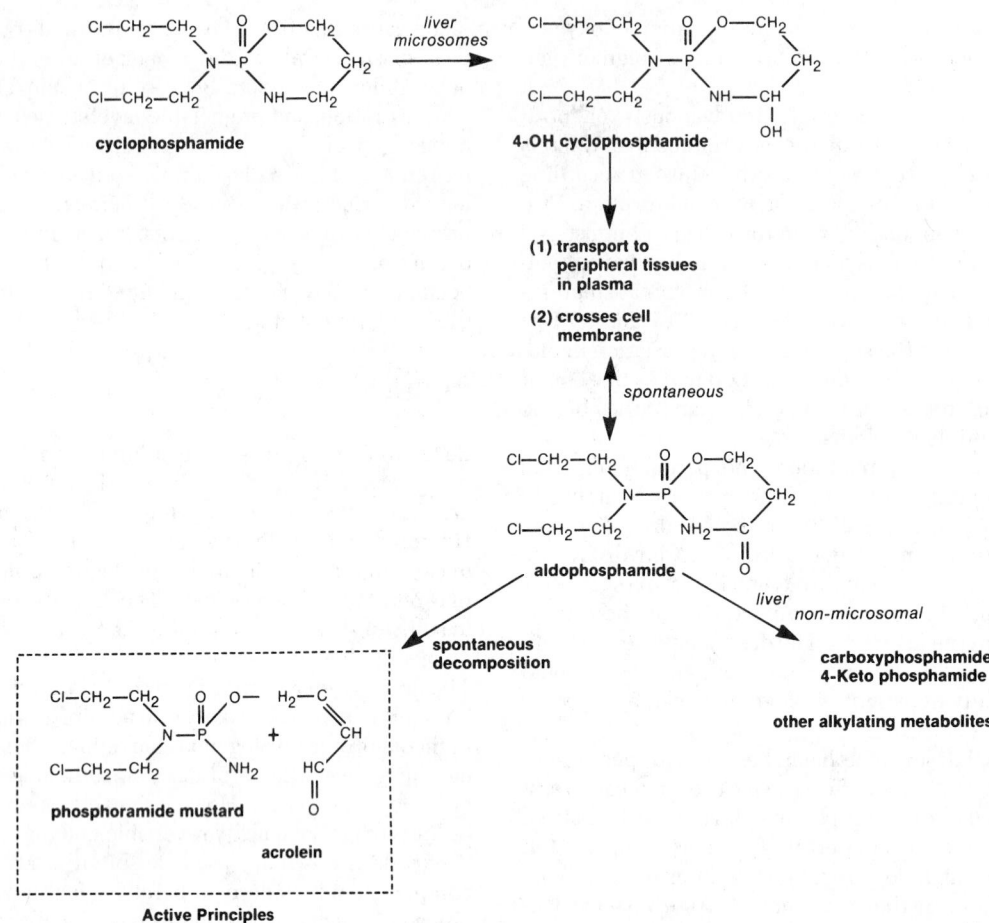

FIGURE 18–29. Metabolism of cyclophosphamide by hepatic mixed-function oxidase, and transformation into active intermediates.

Cyclophosphamide plays a major role in therapy of breast cancer for metastatic disease and in the adjuvant setting. It is used in various combinations for the treatment of lymphoid and myeloid malignancies and for therapy of nonneoplastic conditions, such as necrotizing systemic vasculitis and Wegener's granulomatosis. It also has an important use in bone marrow transplant regimens in which its immunosuppressive effects may help prevent graft rejection.[48]

Cyclophosphamide commonly is used orally and intravenously. It is stable as the parent compound, is well absorbed orally (90% bioavailability), and does not cause local irritation if infiltrated during attempted intravenous infusion. Cyclophosphamide produces significant leukopenia and immunosuppression but only mild thrombocytopenia. Nausea, vomiting, and alopecia are common side effects and are more common with high-dose intravenous therapy.[45] Immunosuppression may be associated with the development of *Pneumocystis carinii* pneumonia. Excretion of active metabolites, especially acrolein, in the urine can lead to hemorrhagic cystitis in as high as 10% of patients.[49] Recurrent episodes of cyclophosphamide-induced cystitis may lead to fibrosis and malignant transitional cell tumors.[50] Drug-induced hemorrhagic cystitis may be avoided by encouraging adequate hydration with 3 to 4 L of fluid per day and encouraging frequent urination for 24 hours after administration of cyclophosphamide. Other approaches to prevent this problem attempt to inactivate urine metabolites by providing elevated levels of

thiols in the urine. This includes the use of *N*-acetylcysteine, sodium-2-mercaptoethane sulfonate (MESNA).[51] A syndrome of inappropriate secretion of antidiuretic hormone and direct effects on the renal tubule can occur with cyclophosphamide and cause severe hyponatremia, seizures, and death. This possibility necessitates close monitoring of serum and urine electrolytes and patient intake and output. This toxicity can be prevented with furosemide.[52] As with most of the other alkylating agents, cyclophosphamide causes sterility in men and women and frequently induces amenorrhea accompanied by menopausal symptoms in premenopausal women. Cyclophosphamide is carcinogenic in animals and leukemogenic in humans.

High-dose cyclophosphamide (>100 mg/kg) is capable of producing all the toxicities noted earlier. In addition, cardiotoxicity, including acute cardiac necrosis, is a unique toxicity of cyclophosphamide seen primarily in patients receiving high-dose cyclophosphamide (>1.55 g/m²).[53] Myocardial toxicity appears to be associated with increased pharmacokinetic clearance of cyclophosphamide from the circulation, suggesting that patients with greater uptake and metabolism of this drug are at higher risk for toxicity.[54] The pharmacokinetics of cyclophosphamide and its metabolites have been studied to a limited extent; because the active metabolites are generated intracellularly from 4-hydroxycyclophosphamide, it is difficult to relate these studies to clinical toxicity. However, it has been suggested that monitoring plasma levels of the parent drug may be useful in titrating the antitumor dose and preventing toxicity in high-dose regimens.[54] Cyclophosphamide and its 4-hydroxymetabolite can be assayed in plasma by gas chromatography with nitrogen phosphorous detection.[55] The half-life of the parent compound is 5.3 hours in adults, with somewhat more rapid clearance in children. The half-life of 4-hydroxycyclophosphamide is 1.5 to 6 hours and is primarily a function of its rate of formation in liver.[56] Of possible relevance to the selective action of cyclophosphamide is the longer half-life repair of phosphoramide mustard adducts of DNA (8.5 hours) compared with 1.6 hours for nitrogen mustard adducts. In patients with renal or hepatic failure, the serum half-life of cyclophosphamide is prolonged and correlates with increased myelosuppression.[57]

IFOSFAMIDE

Ifosfamide (see Fig. 18–28), a drug closely related to cyclophosphamide by virtue of its oxazaphosphorine ring structure, differs from cyclophosphamide in that the 2-chloroethyl group is shifted from the exocyclic mustard-nitrogen to the nitrogen atom of the oxazaphosphorine ring. Like cyclophosphamide, it is activated by hepatic P-450 mixed function oxidase.[58] The change in structure alters the process and the pharmacokinetics such that hepatic drug activation is significantly slower, more inactive metabolites are produced, and approximately four times more drug is required to produce equal antitumor or toxic effects.[59] More chloroacetaldehyde is produced from ifosfamide than from cyclophosphamide, which may contribute to its greater level of urologic and neurologic toxicity.[60]

Ifosfamide is well absorbed orally (100% bioavailability) and has a plasma half-life of 5 to 6 hours after oral or intravenous administration.[61] It is usually administered as a continuous 5-day infusion of doses as high as 2400 mg/m^2/day with equivalent milligram doses of MESNA or in doses as high as 3 g/m^2 daily for two doses every 14 to 28 days, with 600 mg/m^2 MESNA every 4 hours for 48 hours. Patients should be hydrated so that the urine specific gravity is lower than 1.010 before drug administration.

Ifosfamide and cyclophosphamide have a similar spectrum of antitumor activity. Ifosfamide has not been proven to be clinically superior to cyclophosphamide in randomized trials at equitoxic doses. Nonetheless, it has been incorporated into combination chemotherapy regimens that are curative for testicular cancer, and it is effectively used in the treatment of soft tissue sarcomas and lung and ovarian cancer.[62–65] Ifosfamide is currently being evaluated in high-dose chemotherapy regimens given in association with bone marrow transplantation.

Ifosfamide differs somewhat from cyclophosphamide in its pattern of toxicity, causing less myelosuppression but dose-limiting cystitis. Alkylating metabolites are excreted in the urine, and MESNA effectively prevents cystitis even in patients with a history of cyclophosphamide- or ifosfamide-related cystitis.[66] Other significant toxicities include cerebellar dysfunction, seizures, and altered mental status in as many as 30% of patients treated with high doses of ifosfamide (1.6 g/m^2/d for 5 days or >5 g/day as a single dose). Ifosfamide given in a polypharmacy setting has also been associated with extrapyramidal neurotoxicity, including myoclonus and muscular spasticity.[67] The risk of neurotoxicity appears related to

hepatic dysfunction. High levels of a potentially neurotoxic metabolite, such as chloroacetaldehyde, have been detected in patients by gas chromatography.

4-HYDROPEROXYCYCLOPHOSPHAMIDE

A cyclophosphamide derivative, 4-hydroperoxycyclophosphamide, which can be directly activated by tumor cells, is used in bone marrow purging procedures in association with high-dose chemotherapy programs and autologous bone marrow rescue.[68] In these programs, the patients are treated systemically with high-dose chemotherapy to eliminate leukemic cells. Portions of bone marrow are removed before the high-dose therapy and treated ex vivo with 4-hydroperoxycyclophosphamide selectively to remove leukemic cells.[68] The purged autologous marrow, presumably free of occult leukemic cells, is reinfused to rescue the host from the side effects of severe chemotherapy-induced marrow aplasia.

NITROSOUREAS

The chloroethylnitrosoureas (see Fig. 18–28), including BCNU (1,3-bis(2-chloroethyl)-1-nitrosourea) and CCNU (1-(2-chloroethyl)-3-cyclohexyl-1-nitrosourea) are highly lipid soluble and chemically reactive compounds that are clinically active against a variety of tumors. Many derivatives that incorporate this basic nitrosourea structure but differ in their lipid solubility, side-group substitution, and aqueous stability have been synthesized in an effort to improve their therapeutic index.[69] Chlorozotocin, streptozotocin, and other glycosylated nitrosoureas have less bone marrow toxicity.

Chemical decomposition of these agents in aqueous solution (Fig. 18–30) yields two reactive intermediates, a chloroethyldiazohydroxide (II) and an isocyanate group (III).[70] The latter react with amine groups in a carbamoylation reaction. The isocyanates are believed to deplete glutathione, inhibit DNA repair, and alter maturation of RNA. Although carbamoylation may contribute to the overall effects of the nitrosoureas, compounds such as chlorozotocin that lack significant carbamoylating activity still preserve antitumor activity. The chloroethyldiazohydroxide undergoes further decomposition to yield reactive chloroethyl carbonium ions (IV) that form a variety of adducts with all four bases and the phosphate groups in DNA. Of major importance in the antitumor effects of nitrosoureas is the formation of DNA interstrand crosslinks as demonstrated by the close correlation between crosslink formation and cytotoxicity.[71] Alkylation seems to be the more important feature of nitrosourea action.

The mechanism of crosslink formation involves formation of a chloroethyl adduct at the position of guanine that subsequently undergoes an intramolecular rearrangement to produce unstable intermediate that reacts with cytosine in the opposite DNA strand. An N-1-guanine, N-3-cytosine-ethanol crosslink results. Development of the interstrand crosslink can be prevented by the repair protein, O-6-alkylguanine-DNA-alkyltransferase, which can remove the initial O-6-chloroethyl adduct or bind to the O-6 portion of the ethano-guanine adduct.[72,73] The first reaction removes the alkyl group leaving intact DNA, whereas the second reaction results in the formation of a protein-DNA crosslink.[72,73] Susceptibility

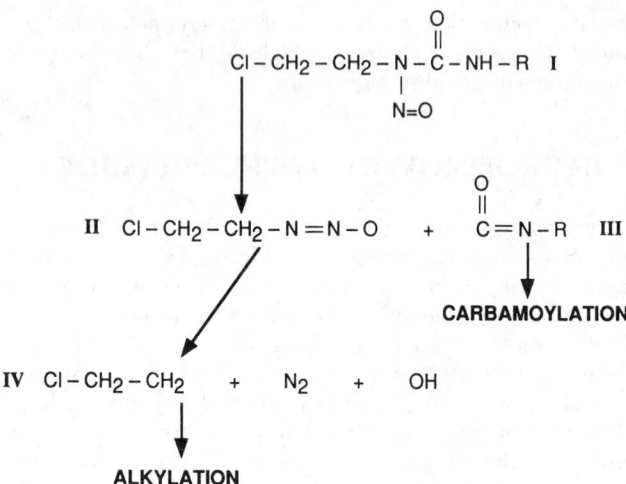

FIGURE 18–30. Decomposition of chloroethylnitrosoureas to form chloroethyl carbonium ion and a carbamoylating isocyanate group.

to the cytotoxic and mutagenic effects of nitrosoureas is modulated by cellular levels of the alkyltransferase protein.[74,75]

The nitrosoureas have many of the same features as classic alkylating agents. Their activity is enhanced by nitroimidazoles, hyperthermia, theophylline, and glutathione depletion.[76,77] However, in many experimental systems they do not share cross-resistance with classic alkylators. Nitrosourea resistance is associated with increased levels of glutathione-S-transferase and O-6-alkylguanine-DNA alkyltransferase.[74,75,78]

As a result of the extreme clinical reactivity of these compounds in aqueous solution, they disappear rapidly from the blood after absorption from the gastrointestinal tract or intravenous infusion. CCNU can be given in a single oral dose, whereas BCNU must be given intravenously. BCNU has a half-life of 22 minutes, whereas the orally administered CCNU is not detectable as parent drug in plasma because of complete conversion to monohydroxylated derivatives during its first pass through the liver.[79–81] CCNU metabolites reach peak plasma concentrations between 3 and 4 hours after administration and have plasma half-lives of 1.3 to 2.9 hours.[81] The high lipid solubility of the nitrosoureas may account for their activity against experimental and clinical intracranial tumors; the chloroethyl portion of CCNU crosses readily into the central nervous system (CNS), reaching concentrations that are 30% of those of the combined parent drug and metabolites in the plasma, and BCNU appears in the cerebrospinal fluid almost immediately after intravenous administration.[82]

The nitrosoureas are clinically active against Hodgkin's and non-Hodgkin's lymphoma, malignant melanoma, brain neoplasms, multiple myeloma, and gastrointestinal carcinomas. In high-dose regimens, given in association with bone marrow transplant, nitrosoureas have shown activity against melanoma, lung cancer, glioblastoma multiforme, and colon cancer.[83]

The most notable and consistent toxicity associated with nitrosoureas is delayed myelosuppression, which reaches a nadir 4 to 6 weeks after treatment and prevents the repetition of cyclic therapy at intervals shorter than 6 to 8 weeks. Severe and protracted leukopenia and thrombocytopenia may occur in patients receiving conventional doses of BCNU, CCNU, or methyl-CCNU, particularly in those who have received extensive prior chemotherapy. Prolonged use of these drugs

leads to cumulative bone marrow toxicity and, in some patients, to an aplastic bone marrow. Acute myeloid leukemia has been reported after therapy with nitrosoureas.[84] This is probably related to formation of the highly mutagenic O-6-alkylguanine adducts and their failure to be repaired due to low levels of O-6-alkylguanine-DNA alkyltransferase in myeloid precursors.[85]

Prolonged courses of treatment with BCNU and methyl-CCNU have been associated with pulmonary fibrosis, and this may occur at delayed intervals after therapy.[86] The total dose of BCNU was 1000 mg/m² or greater in all cases reported and was 2733 mg/m² for one reported case of pulmonary fibrosis induced by methyl-CCNU.[87] Chronic renal failure has been reported in children receiving methyl-CCNU for the treatment of brain tumors.[88] Azotemia or elevated serum creatinine levels developed after treatment was stopped in 5 of 6 patients who received more than 1500 mg/m² methyl-CCNU, and a decrease in kidney size was observed in all 6 patients. Total doses greater than 1200 mg/m² of BCNU or methyl-CCNU are associated with an increased risk of renal failure. High-dose BCNU is associated with cardiovascular toxicity, including hypotension, tachycardia, and flushing,[79] and with other fatal toxicities, including interstitial pneumonitis, encephalomyelopathy, hepatic necrosis, and cardiac necrosis.[83]

THIOTEPA

Thiotepa, N,N',N''-triethylenethiophosphoramide, is an example of the aziridine group of drugs (Fig. 18–31). It is relatively stable at physiologic and alkaline pH but is unstable in acid medium. Thiotepa is a complex, polyfunctional alkylating agent capable of producing a variety of DNA lesions. Incubation of thiotepa with L1210 cells produces a dose-dependent increase in DNA interstrand crosslinks, whereas inclusion of hepatic microsomes in the incubation system results in the formation of alkali label sites in the DNA.[89] Under these conditions, thiotepa undergoes oxidative desulfuration and is converted to its major in vivo metabolite triethylenephosphoramide (TEPA) (see Fig. 18–31).[90]

Cellular accumulation of thiotepa is biphasic, characterized by an initial, rapid phase of simple diffusion followed by a second, slower uptake phase requiring metabolic activity.[91] The initial, rapid diffusion phase results in wide tissue distribution.[91] After systemic administration of thiotepa, the parent drug and its derivative TEPA rapidly appear in the circulation.[90,92] This metabolic conversion most likely occurs in the liver, because it can be reproduced in vitro with hepatic cytochrome P-450 and NADPH.[89,93] After intravenous bolus injection of thiotepa, the peak serum concentration of TEPA reaches approximately 20% of that of the parent drug. TEPA remains in the circulation longer than the parent drug and the mean area under the curve for TEPA exceeds that of the parent drug.[92] The terminal half-life of thiotepa ranges from 1.2 to 2 hours and for TEPA ranges from 4.3 to 5.6 hours.[92] Agents such as clofibrate and phenobarbital, which induce hepatic cytochrome P-450 metabolism, accelerate thiotepa clearance by increasing metabolism to TEPA.[93] Although TEPA is the major in vivo circulating metabolite of thiotepa, variations in its pharmacokinetics do not correlate with toxicity. This suggests that TEPA may not be a pharmacologically

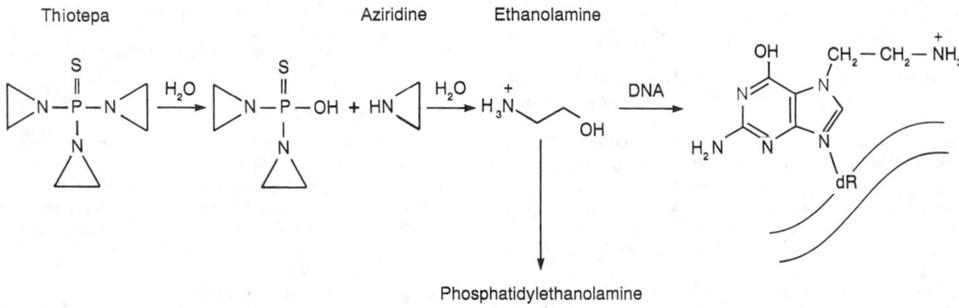

FIGURE 18–31. Schematic illustration showing metabolism of thiotepa to generate aziridine, which is hydrolyzed to ethanolamine, which is then incorporated into phosphatidyl ethanolamine or can react with DNA to produce base adducts, such as 7-alkylguanine, as shown in the schema. (Modified from Egorin MJ, Snyder SW. Characterization of nonexchangable radioactivity in L1210 cells incubated with [^{14}C]thiotepa: Labeling of phosphatidylethanolamine. Cancer Res 1990;50:4044–4049)

important component of the activity of thiotepa.[90] Additional support for this concept is the observation that thiotepa is capable of causing DNA damage and cytotoxicity in cells that cannot convert the parent drug to TEPA.[89]

Figure 18–31 presents a more recently defined pathway to explain the activity of thiotepa.[94] According to this scheme, thiotepa serves as a prodrug to enter cells rapidly by simple diffusion. An aziridine moiety is liberated from the prodrug by a spontaneous or enzymatic process, followed rapidly by loss of the remaining aziridine moieties. The highly reactive aziridines generate ethyleneimines that serve as monofunctional alkylating agents. These lead to the formation of DNA adducts, which are further metabolized to produce DNA strand breaks. Support for this pathway as the mechanism of thiotepa action derives from the demonstration that incubation of DNA with ethyleneimine or thiotepa generates the identical DNA adducts.[95] Further support for this pathway is provided by the observation that derivatives of radioactive thiotepa are incorporated into phosphotidylethanolamine. This is explained by hydrolysis of some of the aziridine molecules to ethanolamine, which are subsequently incorporated into phosphatidylethanolamine, accounting for the slow metabolic component of thiotepas cellular accumulation.[94] The ability of thiotepa to act as a monofunctional-DNA alkylating agent producing DNA adducts and strand breaks may be useful in situations in which cells have become resistant to DNA crosslinking agents.

Thiotepa is administered by the intravenous or intracavitary route; in the latter, it is has been used by intrapleural, intraperitoneal, or intravesical instillation.[96,97] It is not a vesicant and does not produce inflammation on intravenous infiltration. Both thiotepa and TEPA show excellent penetration into the cerebrospinal fluid, producing CSF concentrations almost identical to simultaneous plasma concentrations.[92]

In conventional doses, thiotepa is used for refractory ovarian cancer, especially by the intraperitoneal route.[97] It is used systemically for refractory breast cancer and by intravesical administration for superficial bladder cancer. More recently, thiotepa has been used extensively, alone and in combination, as part of high-dose therapy regimens in association with autologous bone marrow transplants.[98] In the high-dose setting, thiotepa has shown activity against melanoma, carcinoma of the breast, ovary and colon, soft tissue sarcomas, glioblastoma, non-small cell lung cancer, and neuroblastomas.

After conventional dose administration, the major toxic effect of thiotepa is myelosuppression, with nadir granulocytopenia and thrombocytopenia usually occurring at approximately 2 to 3 weeks.[91] In the conventional dose range, thiotepa is associated with mild nausea, vomiting, and headache. Alopecia is rare. Additional toxicities that occur with high-dose regimens include mucositis, cutaneous changes, and a dose-limiting CNS toxicity similar to an organic brain syndrome. The mucositis associated with high-dose thiotepa has components of severe esophagitis and enteritis. The cutaneous toxicities include an acute erythroderma followed by dry desquamation of the palms and soles. High-dose thiotepa has also been associated with a more chronic darkening or bronzing of the skin. The CNS toxicity associated with high-dose thiotepa has been characterized by inappropriate behavior, confusion, forgetfulness, and somnolence.[98] The latter toxicity is apparently related to the high lipid solubility and excellent CNS penetration of thiotepa.

REFERENCES

1. Ludlum DB. Alkylating agents and the nitrosoureas. In: Becker FF, ed. Cancer: A comprehensive treatise. vol 5. New York: Plenum Press, 1977:285–307.
2. Hanawalt PC, Cooper PK, Ganesan AK, Smith CA. DNA repair in bacteria and mammalian cells. Annu Rev Biochem 1979;48:783–836.
3. Bohr VA, Phillips DH, Hanawalt PC. Heterogeneous DNA damage and repair in the mammalian genome. Cancer Res 1987;47:6426–6436.
4. Cathcart R, Goldthwait DA. Enzymatic excision of 3-methyladenine and 7-methylguanine by a rat liver nuclear fraction. 1981;20:273–280.
5. Bose K, Karran P, Strauss B. Repair of depurinated DNA in vitro by enzymes purified from human lymphoblasts. Proc Natl Acad Sci USA 1978;75:794–798.
6. Söderhäll S, Lindahl T. DNA ligases of eukaryotes. FEBS Lett 1976;67:1–8.
7. Berger NA, Sikorski GW, Petzold SH, Kurohara KK. Association of poly(adenosine diphosphoribose) synthesis with DNA damage and repair in normal human lymphocytes. J Clin Invest 1979;63:1164–1171.
8. Berger, NA, Berger, SJ, Gerson SL. DNA repair, ADP-ribosylation and pyridine nucleotide metabolism as targets for cancer chemotherapy. Anticancer Drug Res 1987;2:203–210.
9. Lawley PD, Brookes P. Molecular mechanism of the cytotoxic action of difunctional alkylating agents and of resistance to this action. Nature 1965;206:480–483.
10. Eder JP, Teicher BA, Holden SA, Cathcart NS, Schnipper LE. Novobiocin enhances alkylating agent cytotoxicity and DNA interstrand crosslinks in a murine model. J Clin Invest 1987;79:1524–1528.
11. Ahmed FE, Stelow RB. Saturation of DNA repair in mammalian cells. Photochem Photobiol 1979;29:983–989.
12. Pegg AE. Mammalian O⁶alkylguanine-DNA alkyltransferase: Regulation and importance of response to alkylating carcinogenesis and therapeutic agents. Cancer Res 1990;50:6119–6129.
13. Brent TP, Remack JS. Formation of covalent complexes between human O⁶alkylguanine-DNA alkyltransferase and BCNU-treated defined length synthetic oligodeoxynucleotides. Nucleic Acids Res 1988;16:6779–6788.
14. Gerson SL, Berger NA, Arce C, Petzold SJ, Willson JKV. Modulation of nitrosourea resistance in human colon cancer by O⁶methylguanine. Biochem Pharmacol 1992;43:1101–1107.

15. Crook TR, Souhami RL, Whyman GD, McLean AEM. Glutathione depletion as a determinant of sensitivity of human leukemia cells to cyclophosphamide. Cancer Res 1986;46:5035–5038.

16. Lohrer H, Robson T. Overexpression of metallothionein in CHO cells and its effect on cell killing by ionizing radiation and alkylating agents. Carcinogenesis 1989;10:2279–2284.

17. Somfai-Relle S, Suzukake K, Vistica BP, Vistica DT. Reduction in cellular glutathione by buthionine sulfoximine and sensitization of murine tumor cells resistant to L-phenylalanine mustard. Biochem Pharmacol 1984;33:485–490.

18. Glick JH, Glover DJ, Weiler C, et al. Phase I clinical trials of WR-2721 with alkylating agent chemotherapy. Int J Radiat Oncol Biol Phys 1980;8:575–580.

19. Bergasagel DE. Treatment of plasma cell myeloma with cytotoxic agents. Arch Intern Med 1975;135:172–176.

20. Tannock IF. Cell kinetics and chemotherapy: A critical review. Cancer Treat Rep 1978;62:1117–1133.

21. Goodman LS, Wintrobe MM, Dameshek W, et al. Nitrogen mustard therapy: Use of methylbis(B-chorethyl)-aminohydrochloride for Hodgkin's disase, lymphosarcoma, leukemia and certain allied and miscellaneous disorders. JAMA 1946;132:126–132.

22. Lyons RM, Goldenberg GJ. Active transport of nitrogen mustard and chloine by normal and leukemic human lymphoid cells. Cancer Res 1972;32:1679–1685.

23. Ewig RAG, Kohn KW. DNA damage and repair in mouse leukemia L1210 cells treated with nitrogen mustard, 1,3-bis(2-chloroethyl)-1-nitrosourea, and other nitrosoureas. Cancer Res 1977;37:2114–2122.

24. Klatt O, Stehlin JS Jr, McBride C, Griffin AC. The effect of nitrogen mustard treatment on the deoxyribonucleic acid of sensitive and resistant Ehrlich tumor cells. Cancer Res 1969;29:286–290.

25. Hansson J, Lewensohn R, Ringborg U, et al. Formation and removal of DNA crosslinks induced by melphalan and nitrogen mustard in relation to drug-induced cytotoxicity in human melanoma cells. Cancer Res 1987;47:2631–2637.

26. Schneider SM, Distelhorst CW. Chemotherapy-induced emergencies. Semin Oncol 1989;16:572–578.

27. Bergel F, Stock JA. Cytotoxic alpha amino acids and endopeptides. Br Emp Cancer Camp Annu Rep 1953;31:6.

28. Vistica DT. Cytotoxicity as an indicator for transport mechanism: Evidence that melphalan is transported by two leucine-preferring carrier systems in the L1210 murine leukemia cell. Biochem Biophys Acta 1979;550:309–317.

29. Vistica DT, Toal NJ, Rabinovitz M. Amino-acid conferred protection against melphalan: Interference with leucine protection of melphalan cytotoxicity by the basic amino acids in cultured murine L1210 leukemic cells. Mol Pharmacol 1978;14:1136–1142.

30. Goldenberg GJ, Froese EK. Antagonism of the cytocidal activity and uptake of melphalan by tamoxifen in human breast cancer cells in vitro. Biochem Pharmacol 1985;34:763–770.

31. Brown DM, Horsman MR, Hirst DG, Brown JM. Enhancement of melphalan cytotoxicity in vivo and in vitro by inhibitors of poly(ADP-ribose) polymerase. Int J Radiat Oncol Biol Phys 1984;10:1665–1668.

32. Teicher BA, Crawford JM, Holden SA, Cathcart KNS. Effects of various oxygenation conditions on the enhancement by fluosol-DA of melphalan antitumor activity. Cancer Res 1987;47:5036–5041.

33. Tattersall MN, Jarman M, Newlands ES, et al. Pharmacokinetics of melphalan following oral or intravenous administration in patients with malignant disease. Eur J Cancer 1978;14:507–514.

34. Alberts DS, Change SY, Chen HSG, et al. Kinetics of intravenous melphalan. Clin Pharmacol Ther 1979;26:73–80.

35. Lazarus HM, Herzig RH, Graham-Pole J, et al. Intensive melphalan chemotherapy and cryopreserved autologous bone marrow transplantation for the treatment of refractory cancer. J Clin Oncol 1983;1:359–367.

36. Howell SB, Pfeifle CE, Olshen RA. Intraperitoneal chemotherapy with melphalan. Ann Intern Med 1984;101:14–20.

37. Greene MH, Harris EL, Gershenson DM, et al. Melphalan may be a more potent leukemogen than cyclophosphamide. Ann Intern Med 1986;105:360–367.

38. Alberts DS, Chang SY, Chen HS, et al. Pharmacokinetics and metabolism of chlorambucil in man: A preliminary report. Cancer Treat Rep 1979;6:9.

39. Cole SR, Myers TJ, Klatsky AU. Pulmonary disease with chlorambucil therapy. Cancer 1978;41:455.

40. Berk PD, Goldberg JD, Silverstein MN, et al. Increased incidence of acute leukemia in polycythemia vera associated with chlorambucil therapy. N Engl J Med 1981;304:441.

41. Santos GW, Tutschka PJ, Brookmeyer R, et al. Marrow transplantation for acute nonlymphocytic leukemia after treatment with busulfan and cyclophosphamide. N Engl J Med 1983;309:1347.

42. Kyle RA, Schwartz RS, Oliner HL, Dameshek W. A syndrome resembling adrenal cortical insufficiency associated with long-term busulfan (Myleran) therapy. Blood 1961;18:497.

43. Jones RJ, Lee KSK, Beschorner WE, et al. Venoocclusive disease of the liver following bone marrow transplantation. Transplantation 1987;44:778.

44. Peters WP, Henner WD, Grochow LB, et al. Clinical and pharmacologic effects of high dose single agent busulfan with autologous bone marrow support in the treatment of solid tumors. Cancer Res 1987;47:6402.

45. Colvin M. A review of the pharmacology and clinical use of cyclophosphamide. In: Pinedo HM, ed. Clinical pharmacology of antineoplastic drugs. Amsterdam: Elsevier-North Holland, 1978:245–261.

46. Hilton J. Role of aldehyde dehydrogenase in cyclophosphamide-resistant L1210 leukemia. Cancer Res 1984;44:5156–5160.

47. McDiarmid MA, Iype PT, Kolodner K, Jacobson-Karm D, Strickland PT. Evidence for acrolein-modified DNA in peripheral blood leukocytes of cancer patients treated with cyclophosphamide. Mutat Res 1991;248:93–99.

48. Santos GW, Sensenbrenner LL, Burke PJ, et al. The use of cyclophosphamide for clinical marrow transplantation. Transpl Proc 1972;4:559.

49. Droller MJ, Saral R, Santos G. Prevention of cyclophosphamide-induced hemorrhagic cystitis. Urology 1982;20:256.

50. Manohoran A. Carcinoma of the urinary bladder in patients receiving cyclophosphamide. Aust NZ J Med 1984;14:507–512.

51. Brock N, Phol J. Prevention of urotoxic side effects by regional detoxification with increased selectivity of oxazaphosphorine cytostatistics. IARC Sci Publ 1986;78:269.

52. Green TP, Mirken BL. Prevention of cyclophosphamide-induced antidiuresis by furosemide infusion. Clin Pharmacol Ther 1981;29:634.

53. Braverman AC, Antin JH, Plappert MT, Cook EF, Lee RT. Cyclophosphamide cardiotoxicity in bone marrow transplantation: A prospective evaluation of new dosing regimens. J Clin Oncol 1991;9:1215–1223.

54. Ayash LJ, Wright JE, Tretyakov O, et al. Cyclophosphamide pharmacokinetics: Correlation with cardiac toxicity and tumor response. J Clin Oncol 1992;10:995–1000.

55. El-Yazigi A, Martin CR. Improved analysis of cyclophosphamide by capillary gas chromatography with thermionic (nitrogen-phosphorus)-specific detection and silica sample purification. J Chromatogr Biomed Appl 1986;374:177–182.

56. Sladek NE, Powers JF, Grage GM. Half-life of exazaphosphorines in biological fluids. Drug Metab Dispos 1984;12:553–559.

57. Juma FD. Effect of liver failure on the pharmacokinetics of cyclophosphamide. Eur J Clin Pharmacol 1984;26:591–593.

58. Brock N, Hilgard P, Peukert M, et al. Basis and new developments in the field of oxazaphosphorines. Cancer Invest 1988;6:513–532.

59. Colvin M. The comparative pharmacology of cyclophosphamide and ifosfamide. Semin Oncol 1982;9(suppl 1):2–7.

60. Goren MP, Wright RK, Pratt CB, et al. Dechloroethylation of ifosfamide and neurotoxocity. Lancet 1986;2:1219–1220.

61. Carny T, Margison JM, Thatcher N, et al. Bioavialability of ifosfamide in patients with bronchial carcinoma. Cancer Chemother Pharmacol 1986;18:261–264.

62. Buckner CD, Clift RA, Fefer A, et al. High-dose cyclophosphamide (NSC-26271) for the treatment of metastatic testicular neoplasms. Cancer Chemother Rep 1974;58:709–714.

63. Elias A, Ryan L, Sulkes A, et al. Response to mesna, doxorubicin, ifosfamide, and dacarbazine in 108 patients with metastatic or unresectable sarcoma and no prior chemotherapy. J Clin Oncol 1989;7:1208–1216.

64. Ettinger DS. Ifosfamide in the treatment of non-small cell lung cancer. Semin Oncol 1989;16(suppl 3):31–38.

65. Sutton GP, Blessing JA, Homesley HD, et al. Phase II trial of ifosfamide and mesna in advanced ovarian carcinoma: A gynecologic oncology group study. J Clin Oncol 1989;7:1672–1676.

66. Andriole GL, Sandlund JT, Miser JS, et al. The efficacy of MESNA (2-mercaptoethane sodium sulfonate) as a uroprotectant in patients with hemorrhagic cystitis receiving further oxazaphosphorine chemotherapy. J Clin Oncol 1987;5:799–803.

67. Anderson NR, Tandon DS. Ifosfamide extrapyramidal neurotoxicity. Cancer 1991;58:72–75.

68. Yeager AM, Kaizer H, Santos GW, et al. Autologous bone marrow transplantation in patients with acute nonlymphocytic leukemia using ex vivo marrow treatment with 4-hydroperoxycyclophosphamide. N Engl J Med 1986;315:141–147.

69. Heal JM, Franza BR, Schein PS. Pharmacology of nitrosourea antitumor agents. In: Pinedo HM, ed. Clinical pharmacology of antineoplastic drugs. Amsterdam: Elsevier-North Holland, 1978:263–275.

70. Montgomery JA. Chemistry and structure-activity studies of the nitrosoureas. Cancer Treat Rep 1976;60:651–664.

71. Ewig RAG, Kohn DW. DNA-protein cross-linking and DNA interstrand crosslinking by haloethylnitrosoureas in L1210 cells. Cancer Res 1978;38:3197–3203.

72. Brent TP, Remack RS, Smith DG. Characterization of a novel reaction by human O⁶alkylguanine-DNA alkyltransferase with 1,3-bis(2-chloroethyl)-1-nitrosourea-treated DNA. Cancer Res 1987;47:6185–6188.

73. Ludlum DB. DNA alkylation by the haloethylnitrosoureas: Nature of modifications produced and their enzymatic repair of removal. Mutat Res 1990;233:117–126.

74. Gerson SL, Trey JE, Miller K. Potentiation of nitrosourea cytotoxicity in human leukemic cells by inactivation of O⁶alkylguanine-DNA alkyltransferase. Cancer Res 1988;48:1521–1527.

75. Futscher BW, Micetich KC, Barnes DM, Fisher RI, Erickson LC. Inhibition of a specific DNA repair system and nitrosourea cytotoxicity in resistant human cancer cells. Cancer Commun 1989;1:65–73.

76. Siemann DW. Modification of chemotherapy by nitroimidazoles. Int J Radiat Oncol Biol Phys 1984;19:1585–1594.

77. DeWys WD, Bathina SH. Synergistic antileukemic effect of theophylline and 1,3-bis(2-chloroethyl)-1-nitrosourea. Cancer Res 1980;40:2202–2208.

78. Waxman DJ. Glutathione S-transferases: Role in alkylating agent resistance and possible target for modulation chemotherapy—a review. Cancer Res 1990;50:6449–6454.

79. Henner WD, Peters WP, Eder JP, et al. Pharmacokinetics and immediate effects of high-dose carmustine in man. Cancer Treat Rep 1986;70:877–880.

80. Levin VA, Hoffman W, Weinkam RJ. Pharmacokinetics of BCNU in man: A preliminary study of 20 patients. Cancer Treat Rep 1978;62:1305–1312.

81. Lee FYF, Workman P, Roberts JT, Bleehen MN. Clinical pharamacokinetics of oral CCNU (lomustine). Cancer Chemother Pharmacol 1985;14:125–131.

82. DeVita VT, Denham C, Davidson JD. The physiological disposition of the carcinostatic 1,3-bis(2-chloroethyl)-1-nitrosourea (BCNU) in man and animals. Clin Pharmacol Ther 1967;8:566.

83. Phillips GL, Fay JW, Herzig GP, et al. Intensive 1,3-bis(2-chloroethyl)-1-nitrosourea (BCNU), NSC #4366650 and cyropreserved autologous marrow transplantation for refractory cancer: A phase I-II study. Cancer 1983;52:1792–1802.

84. Greene MH, Biole JD, Strike TA. Carmustine as a cause of acute nonlymphocytic leukemia. N Engl J Med 1985;313:579.

85. Gerson SL, Mller K, Berger NA. O[6]alkylguanine-DNA alkyltransferase activity in human myeloid cells. J Clin Invest 1985;76:2106–2114.

86. O'Driscol BR, Hasleton PS, Taylor PM, et al. Active lung fibrosis up to 17 years after chemotherapy with carmustine (BCNU) in childhood. N Engl J Med 1990;232:378–382.

87. Hundley R, Lukens JN. Nitrosourea-associated pulmonary fibrosis. Cancer Treat Rep 1979;63:2128–2130.

88. Harmon WE, Cohen JH, Schneeberger EE, et al. Chronic renal failure in children treated with methyl CCNU. N Engl J Med 1979;300:1200–1203.

89. Cohen NA, Egorin MJ, Snyder SW, et al. Interaction of N,N',N''-triethylethiophosphoramide and N,N',N''-triethylenephosphoramide with cellular DNA. Cancer Res 1991;51:4360–4366.

90. Hagen J. Pharmacokinetics of thio-TEPA and TEPA in the conventional dose-range and its correlation to myelosuppressive effects. Cancer Chemother Pharmacol 1991;27:373–378.

91. Egorin MJ, Synder SW, Pan S-S, Daly C. Cellular transport and accumulation of thiotepa in murine, human, and avian cells. Cancer Res 1989;49:5611–5617.

92. Heideman RL, Cole DE, Balis F, et al. Phase I and pharmacokinetic evaluation of thiotepa in the cerebrospinal fluid and plasma of pediatric patients: Evidence for dose-dependent plasma clearance of thiotepa. Cancer Res 1989;49:736–741.

93. Ng S-F, Waxman DJ. N,N',N''-triethylenethiophosphoramide (thio-TEPA) oxygenation by constitutive hepatic P450 enzymes and modulation of drug metabolism and clearance in vivo by P450-inducing agents. Cancer Res 1991;51:2340–2345.

94. Egorin MJ, Snyder SW. Characterization of nonexchangeable radioactivity in L1210 cells incubated with [14C]thiotepa: Labeling of phosphatidylethanolamine. Cancer Res 1990;50:4044–4049.

95. Musser SM, Pan S-S, Callery PS. Liquid chromatography-thermospray mass spectrometry of DNA adducts formed with mitomycin C, porfiromycin and thiotepa. J Chromatogr 1989;474:197–207.

96. Lokich JJ, Egorin MJ, Cohen BE, et al. A phase I study of thiotepa administered by short-term and protracted continuous intravenous infusion. Cancer 1989;63:46–50.

97. Kirmani S, McVey L, Loo D, Howell SB. A phase I clinical trial of intraperitoneal thiotepa for refractory ovarian cancer. Gynecol Oncol 1990;36:331–334.

98. Wolff SN, Herzig RH, Fay JW, et al. High-dose N,N',N''-triethylenethiophosphoramide (thiotepa) with autologous bone marrow transplantation: Phase I studies. Semin Oncol 1990;17:2–6.

SECTION 9

ROSS C. DONEHOWER
ERIC K. ROWINSKY

Anticancer Drugs Derived From Plants

Many of the currently used antineoplastic agents are natural products initially isolated from plants. Although the search for new anticancer agents includes programs for the rational synthesis of compounds aimed at particular chemotherapeutic targets, it seems likely that many important chemotherapeutic leads will continue to be identified by systematic screening of the natural products of plants, fungi, and marine animals. In this section of the chapter, the pharmacology of the vinca alkaloids, epipodophyllotoxins, and taxanes is reviewed.

VINCA ALKALOIDS

The vincas are natural alkaloids present in minute quantities in the common periwinkle plant (*Catharanthus roseus*). Although a number of these compounds have been investigated clinically, only vincristine and vinblastine have been approved currently for clinical use in the United States. The vincas are dimeric alkaloids formed from two different multiringed units (Fig. 18–32), an indole nucleus (catharanthine portion) and a dihydroindole nucleus (vindoline portion). Vincristine and vinblastine are structurally identical, with the exception of a single substitution on the vindoline nucleus, where vincristine possesses a formyl group and vinblastine a methyl group. Despite this small difference, these two agents differ dramatically in their antitumor spectrum and clinical toxicities. Desacetyl vinblastine (vindesine), initially identified as a metabolite of vinblastine, was introduced into clinical trials in the 1970s (see Fig. 18–32). Its developmental status remains uncertain, despite demonstrated antitumor activity in several malignancies, including non-small cell lung cancer. Two other semisynthetic derivatives of vinblastine have also entered clinical trial: vinzolidine and navelbine. These compounds are available in oral and intravenous formulations in contrast with the other vincas, which can only be administered intravenously. There is investigative interest in navelbine (Fig. 18–33) because of the encouraging activity observed in early clinical trials. The developmental status of vinzolidine remains uncertain.

The vinca alkaloids have an unusually broad spectrum of antitumor activity. Vincristine is an essential part of combination chemotherapy regimens for pediatric and adult acute lymphocytic leukemia.[1] Vincristine has also played an important role in the combination chemotherapy of Hodgkin's and non-Hodgkin's lymphoma.[2] Vincristine is commonly used in combination with other agents in the treatment of Wilms' tumor, Ewing's sarcoma, neuroblastoma, and rhabdomyosarcoma in children and multiple myeloma, breast cancer, and small cell lung cancer in adults.[3]

Vinblastine has been an integral component of curative chemotherapy regimens for germ cell cancers of the testis and advanced Hodgkin's disease and is commonly used for several other diseases.[3]

Vindesine has been most thoroughly evaluated in non-small

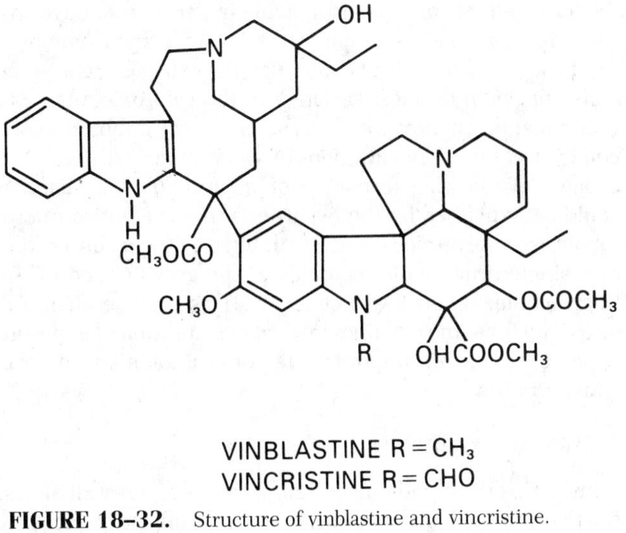

VINBLASTINE R = CH₃
VINCRISTINE R = CHO

FIGURE 18–32. Structure of vinblastine and vincristine.

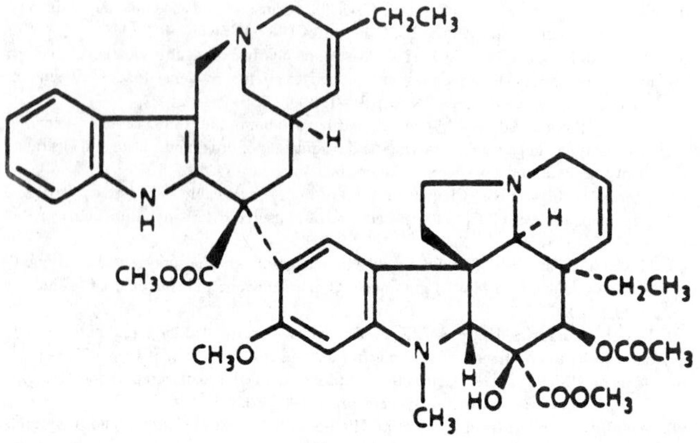

FIGURE 18–33. Structure of navelbine.

cell lung cancer in which the cumulative response rates from all studies approach those reported for the other vincas.[3]

Navelbine is currently undergoing extensive clinical testing in the United States in the hope that the encouraging results observed in early clinical trials in breast cancer and lung cancer in Europe will be sustained.[4]

MECHANISM OF ACTION

Microtubules are ubiquitous in eukaryotic cells and are vital to the performance of many critical cellular functions, such as the maintenance of cell shape and intracellular transport, in addition to mitosis. Many of the unique functional aspects of microtubules are the result of their existence in a dynamic equilibrium with tubulin dimers and their ability to polymerize and depolymerize in response to critical physiologic messages in the cell, including those related to cell cycle traverse. Vinca alkaloids exert their cytotoxic effects by binding to a specific site on tubulin and preventing polymerization of tubulin dimers, disrupting the formation of microtubules. This binding occurs at sites that are distinct from the binding sides of other antimicrotubule agents, such as colchicine, podophyllotoxin, and taxol.[5] The binding of vincas to tubulin prevents the polymerization of the tubulin subunits into microtubules; microtubule structures eventually disappear with continued drug exposure. Although the primary cytotoxic effect of vinca alkaloids is putatively by mitotic arrest, there is evidence that the lethal effects may be attributable in part to other actions. They appear to induce major cytolytic effects in vivo on non-proliferating cells in the G1 phase of the cell cycle, and some cells appear to be most sensitive to the cytotoxic effects of these agents when exposed in the G1 or the S phase of the cell cycle.[6] Low concentrations of vincristine (0.1 μmol) are capable of blocking formation of microtubules, a fact that could be explained by the hypothesis that the entire microtubule assembly process can be inhibited by the incorporation of a single drug-tubulin complex at the growing end of the microtubule.[6] Even lower concentrations may result in cytotoxicity for some cell lines in vitro, but duration of exposure appears to be an important factor, in addition to drug concentration.[7]

PHARMACOKINETICS

Considering the broad range of clinical uses of vinca alkaloids, relatively limited pharmacologic data are available, principally because of a lack of a suitably sensitive assay to quantitate the extremely low concentrations of drug that possess pharmacologic activity. Early studies were generally performed with radiolabeled compounds, with subsequent chromatographic separation of parent drug and metabolites. However, recently developed radioimmunoassays (RIAs) and enzyme-linked immunosorbent assays (ELISAs) with sensitivities in the picomolar range have the requisite sensitivity, perhaps at the expense of specificity.

After conventional doses of vincristine (1.4 mg/m²) given as a brief infusion or bolus, peak plasma concentrations approach 0.4 μmol.[8] The drug is extensively bound by serum proteins (48%) and the formed elements of blood, particularly platelets. After an intravenous bolus, the plasma disposition of vincristine is triphasic. Initial half-lives ($t_{1/2}$-α) in adults are less than 5 minutes because of extensive tissue uptake and binding.[9,10] β-Phase half-lives range from 50 to 155 minutes, and the terminal γ half-lives vary widely from 23 to 85 hours. Similar pharmacokinetic parameters are noted in children.[11] When pharmacokinetics have been studied using [³H]-vincristine with purification by high-performance liquid chromatography, the mean terminal half-life has been 64 minutes; α and β half-lives have been 0.85 and 7.4 minutes, respectively.[8] A direct linear relation between the maximum clinically tolerated dose of the vinca alkaloids, vincristine, vinblastine, and vindesine and their serum clearance has also been noted.[9,10] Vincristine has been demonstrated to enter the central nervous system of subhuman primates rapidly after intravenous injection, and concentrations above 1 nmol have been maintained in cerebrospinal fluid for longer than 72 hours after an intravenous bolus.[12] However, other studies with rats, dogs, monkeys, and humans have indicated that vincristine penetrates the human blood–brain barrier poorly.[13] Spinal fluid concentrations have been 20- to 30-fold lower than concurrent plasma levels and never exceeded 1.1 nmol in humans.[13]

Vincristine is metabolized primarily by the liver and excreted in the stool and, to a lesser extent, in urine. Seventy-two hours after the administration of radiolabeled vincristine, 12% of the radiolabel is excreted in urine (50% of which consists of metabolites) and approximately 70% is excreted in feces (40% of which consists of metabolites).[9] Vincristine concentrates rapidly in the bile with an initial bile to plasma vincristine concentration ratio of 100 to 1 that declines to 20 to 1 at 72 hours after a bolus dose.[14] In addition, metabolic products appear rapidly in the bile with only 46.5% present as the parent unmetabolized drug at 2 hours after infusion. Although not carefully studied, modifications in the doses of vincristine should be considered for patients with hepatic dysfunction, especially patients with obstructive liver disease.

The clinical pharmacology of vinblastine is similar to that of vincristine with extensive binding to serum proteins and the formed elements of blood.[15] After intravenous bolus injections of vinblastine, peak plasma concentrations reach 0.5 μmol.[9,10,16] As with vincristine, the plasma disposition of vinblastine is triphasic. The initial distribution phase is rapid with a $t_{1/2}$-α of less than 5 minutes, presumably secondary to extensive binding to tissues and the formed elements of blood. Vinblastine appears to be more avidly sequestered in tissues than vincristine, with 73% of labeled drug retained in the body 3 days after drug administration. Values reported for β and γ half-lives have ranged from 53 to 99 minutes and 20 to 24 hours, respectively.[9,10,16] Excretion of vinblastine is principally through the biliary tract, which again suggests that toxicity may be exaggerated in patients with hepatic insufficiency. Less than 15% of an administered dose is excreted in the urine, and fecal excretion of the parent compound is also low, suggesting extensive metabolism. The metabolic fate of vinblastine has not been fully characterized, but one metabolite, vindesine, appears to be as active as the parent compound. When vinblastine is administered by continuous intravenous infusion for 5 days at dosages from 1 to 2 mg/m²/day, steady-state drug concentrations of 1.1 to 6.6 nmol have been observed.[17]

Peak plasma vindesine concentrations of 0.1 to 1.0 μmol are reached after bolus intravenous injections of this agent, and levels typically decrease to less than 0.1 μmol by 1 to 2 hours. As with the other vincas, the plasma disappearance of vindesine is characterized by triexponential pharmacokinetics. Vindesine is rapidly distributed to body tissues, and its $t_{1/2}$-α is typically less than 5 minutes. β and γ half-lives range from 55 to 100 minutes and 20 to 24 hours, respectively. This prolonged elimination suggests that drug accumulation may occur with repeated doses at short intervals.[9,10,18] Vindesine has a large volume of distribution (600 L for the terminal phase) and negligible renal clearance, with 1% to 12% of the parent compound measured in the urine of patients on bolus or infusion schedules.[19] The liver is the principal organ responsible for the disposition of vindesine as determined in animal studies and in humans.[19,20] In a patient with a biliary T-tube, the measured renal clearance of vindesine was low (12 ml/min), but the biliary clearance was 29 ml/min, and biliary concentrations were significantly higher than simultaneously measured plasma levels.

The pharmacokinetic behavior of navelbine is similar to that of other vinca alkaloids, with drug disposition exhibiting biexponential or triexponential behavior. After intravenous administration, there is an initial rapid distribution phase (5–9 minutes) and a long elimination half-life of 20 to 49 hours.[21,22] Like the other vincas, the principal route of excretion is through the biliary tract (70–80%), and there is limited urinary excretion of the drug. Principal metabolites appear to be deacetylated forms, although other unidentified metabolites are also present in urine. Human studies of oral navelbine administered in a powder-filled capsule have shown the bioavailability of the parent compound to be approximately 40%, with peak plasma levels achieved 1 to 2 hours after an oral dose.[23] Similar studies of a liquid-filled gelatin capsule demonstrated 23% to 30% bioavailability.[24]

DRUG INTERACTIONS

Methotrexate accumulation in tumor cells is enhanced in vitro in the presence of vincristine or vinblastine,[25] an effect mediated by a vinca-induced blockade of drug efflux from cells. The minimal concentrations of vincristine required to achieve this effect occur only transiently in vivo, and experimental chemotherapy studies in mice have not demonstrated superiority of this sequence of administration. Pharmacokinetic interactions of vinca alkaloids and other drugs have not been studied in detail.

TOXICITY

Despite similarities in structure, the vinca alkaloids differ significantly in their clinical toxicity profiles. Peripheral neurotoxicity is the most frequent and dose-limiting toxic effect of vincristine.[26] It frequently occurs in patients who are older than 40 years and is related to cumulative dose. Initially, only symmetric sensory impairment and paresthesias may be encountered. However, neuritic pain and motor dysfunction may then develop, and loss of deep tendon reflexes, foot drop, wrist drop, ataxia, and paralysis can occur with continued administration. Patients may also complain of bone, back, and limb pain. Vincristine-induced peripheral neuropathic effects are usually first noted in adults who have received a total dose of 5 to 20 mg. Children tolerate this toxicity better than adults, and the elderly are particularly prone. Patients with lymphomas appear to be more highly predisposed to developing neurotoxicity when compared with patients with other malignancies, and particular care is warranted in treating patients with antecedent neurologic disorders, such as Charcot-Marie Tooth disease, or a history of poliomyelitis. The principal pathologic finding is primary axonal degeneration. Peripheral nerve conduction velocities are usually normal, although diminished amplitude of sensory and motor nerve action potentials and prolonged distal motor latencies are observed.[27] Motor, sensory, cranial, and autonomic nerves may all be affected by vincristine, resulting in hoarseness, diplopia, jaw pain, facial palsies, paralytic ileus, urinary retention, and postural hypotension. Fortunately, these complications are uncommon. Convulsions and altered mental status have also been reported.[3] Currently, the only known treatment for vincristine neurotoxicity is discontinuation of the drug or reduction of the dose or frequency of administration. A number of antidotes have been proposed, including thiamine, vitamin B_{12}, folinic acid, and pyridoxine, but none has been shown to be effective. However, coadministration of glutamic acid to patients receiving vincristine appears to decrease neurotoxicity in a randomized, prospective, double-blind trial.[28] The mechanism by which glutamic acid exerts this protective effect and whether this effect will be confirmed in subsequent trials are not known. Although neurotoxicity also occurs during therapy with vindesine, it is dose limiting in less than 10% of patients. Significant neurotoxicity occurs infrequently at the usual clinical doses of vinblastine. Mild paresthesias have been reported in as many as 30% of patients in phase II trials of navelbine.

Myelosuppression, in particular neutropenia, is the principal dose-limiting toxicity of vinblastine, vindesine, and navelbine. Thrombocytopenia and anemia are typically less common and less severe. The timing of the onset of neutropenia is usually 7 to 11 days after an intravenous bolus of one of these agents with recovery by day 14 to 21. Hematologic toxicity has not been cumulative. Gastrointestinal side effects have been noted with all the vinca alkaloids. Mucositis, pharyngitis, and stomatitis are commoner with vinblastine than with vincristine, but may occur with any of these agents. Other gastrointestinal effects (which are probably the result of autonomic neuropathy), such as constipation, ileus, bloating, and abdominal pain, are seen most commonly with vincristine or high doses of vinblastine or vindesine. Nausea, vomiting, and diarrhea may also occur. All the vinca alkaloids are potent vesicants and may cause significant tissue damage if extravasation occurs. Phlebitis may occur along the course of an injected vein with resultant sclerosis. Mild and reversible alopecia is a common finding, seen in as many as 20% of patients treated with vincristine. A variety of other side effects have been reported, including the syndrome of inappropriate antidiuretic hormone secretion, acute cardiac ischemia, fever without an obvious source, acute pulmonary edema, Raynaud's phenomenon, and liver damage.[3]

RESISTANCE

Resistance to the vinca alkaloids develops rapidly in vitro and has been ascribed to two mechanisms. The first involves mutations of the α or β subunits of the tubulin heterodimer leading to decreased vinca alkaloid binding.[29] The second, more well-characterized mechanism involves the multidrug resistance phenotype that confers broad resistance to many unrelated classes of bulky natural-product antineoplastic agents. There has been considerable interest in using pharmacologic agents in vivo to reverse multidrug resistance. Responses have been seen in multiple myeloma and lymphoma using verapamil in combination with a vinca alkaloid-containing regimen after the identical regimen was found to be inactive without verapamil.[29a]

EPIPODOPHYLLOTOXINS

Extracts of the mandrake plant (*Podophyllum peltatum*) have been used for medicinal purposes for centuries as cathartics or as treatment for parasites or venereal warts. Podophyllotoxin, an antimitotic agent that binds to a site on tubulin distinct from that occupied by the vinca alkaloids, was identified as the main constituent possessing cytostatic activity as early as the 1940s. These early podophyllotoxin derivatives possessed a prohibitive degree of clinical toxicity. However, two glycosidic derivatives of podophyllotoxin, etoposide (VP-16) and teniposide (VM-26), have demonstrated highly significant clinical activity against a wide variety of neoplasms, including non-Hodgkin's lymphomas, germ cell malignancies, leukemias, and small cell lung carcinoma.[30] These compounds have a complex structure consisting of a multiringed moiety, known as an *epipodophyllotoxin,* linked to a sugar, glucopyranoside, by an ether linkage. The structures of etoposide and teniposide differ only by the substitution of a methyl group (etoposide) for the thenylidine (teniposide) on the glucopyranoside sugar (Fig. 18–34). These agents possess a number of basic similarities in their pharmacologic characteristics, toxicities, and spectrum of antineoplastic action.

Teniposide is not approved for general use in the United States, although it is widely available in other countries. Extensive clinical trials have been performed with this drug, and it is clear that teniposide is an active antitumor agent, particularly in childhood monocytic leukemia. A major problem has been an assessment of what degree of activity teniposide possesses relative to etoposide.

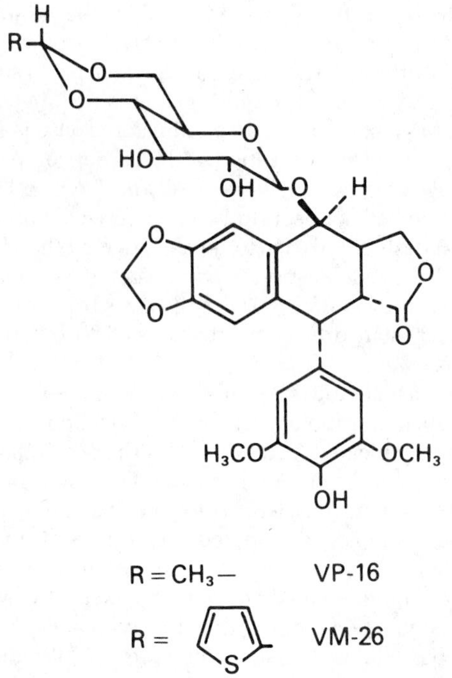

FIGURE 18–34. Structure of VP-16 and VM-26.

MECHANISM OF ACTION

The epipodophyllotoxins were initially thought to exert their cytotoxic effects by binding to tubulin and inhibiting microtubule assembly in a manner similar to the parent compound, podophyllotoxin. However, it was noted that these agents had no effect on microtubule assembly at concentrations that were highly cytotoxic.[31] By cell cycle analysis, the epidophyllotoxins were found to arrest cells in late-S or early-G2 phase of the cell cycle, rather than the G2/M border that would have been expected of an antimicrotubule agent.[32] It was subsequently found that these drugs produced DNA strand breaks in intact cells but that these effects were not seen when the epipodophyllotoxins were incubated in vitro with purified DNA, suggesting that direct chemical cleavage in DNA was not occurring.[33] The epipodophyllotoxins most likely exert their cytotoxic effects by interfering with the scission-reunion reaction of the enzyme topoisomerase II by stabilizing the putative cleavable enzyme-DNA complex in a cleavable state[34] (see Fig. 18–18). The enzyme then covalently binds to DNA, forming single-strand, protein-associated breaks. On a molar basis, teniposide is approximately tenfold more effective than etoposide at inducing RNA strand breaks.[35] Besides forming a cleavable complex, the epipodophyllotoxins inhibit the catalytic or "strand-passing" activity of topoisomerase II that permits the enzyme to catenate DNA circles and disentangle topologically constrained DNA.

Etoposide is also able to inhibit transport of nucleosides across the plasma membrane in a manner similar to podophyllotoxin, an action that may influence the efficacy of combinations of etoposide with antimetabolites.[31]

PHARMACOKINETICS

In adults with normal hepatic and renal function, the disposition of etoposide in plasma is best described as a biphasic process with an initial half-life of approximately 1.5 hours and a terminal half-life that ranges from 3 to 11 hours.[36] Peak plasma levels and areas under the plasma concentration versus time curve (AUC) increase linearly with doses over a 100 to 600 mg/m^2 dose range.[37] Mean peak plasma concentrations after a single intravenous dose of 290 mg/m^2 are approximately 30 μg/ml.[37,38] Etoposide does not accumulate in plasma after daily administration of 100 mg/m^2 for 5 consecutive days. In addition, plasma and renal clearances are independent of dose. Estimates of plasma clearance range from 16 ± 7 to 28 ± 9.7 ml/min/m^2, whereas the urinary clearance of etoposide ranges from 7.4 to 13.6 ml/min/m^2 and accounts for approximately 25% to 48% of total disposition. Using a two-compartment open model, the volume of distribution for etoposide at steady state ranges from 7 to 29 L/m^2.[36] After administration of radiolabeled etoposide to humans, 41.9% to 87.5% of the total radioactivity is recovered in the urine within 48 hours, with 66.8% in the form of unmetabolized drug. After an 80 mg/m^2 intravenous bolus, the mean urinary excretion over 48 hours is 39.8%, and fecal recovery ranges from 0% to 16% of administered radioactivity.[39] Only 6% or less of an intravenous dose is recovered in the bile as the parent compound. Therefore, biliary excretion appears to be a minor route of drug elimination, and metabolism probably accounts for most of the nonrenal clearance of etoposide in humans.

In children, approximately 55% of a dose of etoposide is excreted in the urine over 24 hours, and renal clearance accounts for approximately 35% of total body clearance over a dose range of 80 to 600 mg/m^2.[40] In one study of patients with hepatic and renal dysfunction, stepwise multiple linear regression analysis of patient-specific variables identified creatinine clearance and serum albumin as the best predictors of systemic clearance of etoposide, whereas hepatic function appeared to be an insignificant factor.[41] The excess risk of hematologic toxicity in patients with abnormal renal function can be managed by dose modification based on serum creatinine[42] or by adaptive control dosing based on measured plasma concentrations.[43] For patients with hepatic dysfunction, clearance rate, volume of distribution, and half-lives of etoposide are not significantly prolonged in patients with obstructive jaundice when compared with patients with normal hepatic function. Such patients appear to have a compensatory increase in renal excretion, and dose modification may therefore not be necessary.[44] However, total plasma etoposide concentrations may not accurately reflect the magnitude of systemic exposure to active drug because of the increased fraction of unbound drug in patients with liver dysfunction due to displacement by bilirubin. Caution is therefore justified in dosing such patients. A mathematical model to estimate the fraction of unbound etoposide has been developed that will require prospective pharmacodynamic validation but may prove useful in this situation.[45] Etoposide is metabolized by opening of its lactone ring, yielding its principal urinary metabolite, the hydroxy acid.[41] A *cis*-lactone is also identifiable in plasma and urine.[41] In addition, glucuronide or sulfate conjugates, or both, are excreted in urine in several species and represent 5% to 22% of the total dose in humans.[46] These metabolites do not have significant antineoplastic activity. After intravenous or oral administration, peak plasma etoposide concentrations and AUC values exhibit marked intrapatient and interpatient variability that confounds reliable estimates of absolute oral

bioavailability.[36,47] Bioavailability appears to be approximately 50% using the currently available formulation, although the range of value noted in individual patients varies widely (25–75%).

Preclinical and several well-conducted clinical trials have shown that the cytotoxic effects of etoposide are highly schedule dependent. In a study that examined the pharmacokinetic basis for this observation, a dramatic difference in response rates (10% versus 89%) was observed in untreated patients with extensive small cell lung cancer randomized to receive the same etoposide dose as a 24-hour infusion or as five consecutive daily 2-hour infusions. Pharmacokinetic analysis of the study arms revealed that levels of 1 μg/ml were maintained for twice as long a period in the 5-day arm.[48]

Instantaneous peak plasma concentrations of teniposide at a dose of 67 mg/m^2 range from approximately 20 to 30 μg/ml.[36,39] The plasma disposition of teniposide has been characterized as a biphasic process in some studies and as a triphasic process in others.[36,49] Values reported for the elimination half-life of teniposide vary according to the pharmacokinetic model used to fit the data: 6 to 10 hours in studies demonstrating biexponential decal and between 20 and 48 hours in those demonstrating triphasic characteristics. The pharmacokinetic behavior of teniposide does not differ significantly between children and adults.[36,46,50] Volume of distribution at steady state ranges from 8 to 30 L/m^2 in adults and 3 to 10 L/m^2 in children.[36] The volume of distribution at steady state has been calculated to be approximately 28.5% of body weight with a mean central compartment of 3.5 L.[50] Total plasma clearance has been 7 to 17 ml/min/m^2, and the renal clearance of the drug has been reported to be less than that of etoposide, 1 to 3 ml/min/m^2. Urinary excretion of the parent compound comprises 4% to 14% of the administered dose.[49]

Teniposide is more extensively metabolized than etoposide. Only 5% to 20% of the administered dose of teniposide is excreted as unchanged drug. Information pertaining to the metabolism of teniposide is scant, and only the hydroxy acid formed by opening of the lactone ring, the picro-lactone isomer, and the aglycone glucuronide metabolites have been identified in plasma and urine.[36,46,49] Only the aglycone has been demonstrated to possess anti-DNA activity. Etoposide has a threefold increased plasma clearance and sixfold increased renal clearance over teniposide in humans. Teniposide has a more complete metabolism and a lower renal clearance than etoposide, which account for its slower elimination. In addition, another factor that influences the slower elimination rate of teniposide may be its higher degree of protein binding (>99% for teniposide versus 94% for etoposide).

DRUG INTERACTIONS

Agents with diverse mechanisms of action, such as cyclophosphamide, carmustine, cisplatin, vincristine, cytosine arabinoside, 5-fluorouracil, and hydroxyurea, have demonstrated synergistic interaction with epipodophyllotoxins.[51] The epipodophyllotoxins also appear to be synergistic with methotrexate and enhance net cellular accumulation of methotrexate and methotrexate polyglutamates in vitro at clinically relevant concentrations.[52]

TOXICITY

The principal dose-limiting toxicity of the epipodophyllotoxins has been a dose-related myelosuppression. Granulocytopenia predominates, with nadir counts occurring 7 to 14 days after initiation of a course of therapy. Nadir granulocyte counts on the daily oral schedule of etoposide occur somewhat later, days 17 to 21. Thrombocytopenia occurs less frequently, and nadir counts are observed 9 to 16 days after etoposide. Hematologic recovery is usually complete by day 20 after standard doses, and cumulative toxicity is not usually observed. Patients who have received extensive prior myelosuppressive therapy by chemotherapy or irradiation to marrow-bearing areas of the skeleton are at increased risk for developing severe myelosuppression and should receive reduced doses. Nausea and vomiting occur in approximately 30% to 40% of patients and are more frequent with oral than intravenous administration. Discontinuation of treatment because of adverse gastrointestinal effects is rarely required. Constipation, diarrhea, dysphagia, aftertaste, abdominal pain, stomatitis, and anorexia have been reported, but are infrequent at conventional doses. Mucositis is a prominent toxicity at high doses and appears to be the dose-limiting nonhematologic toxicity of etoposide; severe hepatotoxicity also has been associated with high-dose etoposide.[53,54]

Etoposide induces transient hypotension after rapid intravenous administration that usually responds to slowing or cessation of the infusion and administration of fluids or other appropriate supportive therapies. Anaphylactic-like symptoms, characterized by chills, fever, tachycardia, bronchospasm, and dyspnea, may be associated with hypotension and occur in approximately 0.7% to 2% of patients. These reactions are usually observed during or immediately after administration of etoposide and often respond promptly to the cessation of the infusion and administration of pressor agents, corticosteroids, antihistamines, and volume expanders. Similar acute hypersensitivity reactions (*e.g.,* hypotension, flushing, bronchospasm) may develop if teniposide is infused rapidly. Teniposide is formulated in the same cremophor vehicle as taxol, and these reactions are believed to result from to the effects of the excipient.[55] Reversible alopecia, sometimes progressing to total baldness, occurs in at least 8% to 20% of patients. Increased pigmentation, pruritis, and, rarely, radiation recall dermatitis have been observed.[56] Therapy with epipodophyllotoxin has also been associated with subsequent development of acute nonlymphocytic leukemias.[57] Minor toxicities have included chemical phlebitis and local irritation with extravasation.

RESISTANCE

Malignant cells develop resistance to epipodophyllotoxins through several mechanisms, and in most instances this resistance generally includes etoposide and teniposide, regardless of which agent has been used for selection. In some cells, resistance is associated with decreased intracellular concentrations of etoposide and teniposide because of amplification of the *MDR* gene and increased cellular levels of the P-170 glycoprotein, the multidrug resistance efflux pump.[58,58a] A second mechanism of resistance is an enhanced ability to repair DNA strand breaks. Resistance to etoposide can be in-

duced by prior treatment with radiation, and inhibition of DNA repair can block the development of etoposide resistance.[59,60] Altered topoisomerase activity because of low cellular enzyme concentrations or structural alterations in the protein that may affect binding has also been identified as a cause of resistance in cells that demonstrate cross-resistance to other topoisomerase-II inhibitors, such as amsacrine and doxorubicin.[60a,60b] The predominant clinical mechanism of etoposide resistance has not been established.

TAXOL

The clinical development of taxol began in 1983 and for the first few years proceeded slowly. However, the unique chemical structure of this agent and its unique mechanism of action coupled with the significant antitumor activity observed in early clinical trials has made taxol perhaps one of the most important new agents to emerge in cancer therapy in the last decade. Interest in taxol began in the 1960s when a crude extract of bark from the Pacific yew, *Taxus brevifolia,* was shown to have broad antitumor activity in preclinical experimental tumor models in screening performed by the National Cancer Institute. In 1971, Wall and coworkers identified taxol as the active constituent of the bark extract.[60c] Taxol is composed of a complex 15-membered taxane ring system and an ester side chain attached at the C-13 position of the ring, which is essential for antitumor activity (see Fig. 18–3). The development of taxol was initially hampered by the difficulties inherent in large-scale isolation, extraction, and preparation of bulk compound for a natural product and the poor aqueous solubility of taxol. Interest in the drug was maintained during this time by the elucidation of the novel mechanism of action by which taxol exerts its cytotoxic effect and the ultimate availability of adequate drug supply for the necessary preclinical testing.[61,62] Should the clinical development of taxol continue to be successful, the issue of drug supply will become increasingly important. The current method of obtaining taxol depends on a process of extraction from tree bark. Because the tree is found principally in ancient forests of the Pacific northwest, this is an environmentally important issue. A renewable source of drug supply will be needed for the drug to be available for broad clinical use, and a number of options are under active exploration, including total synthesis or semisynthesis from a precursor. A taxol precursor, 10-deacetyl-baccatin III, has been isolated from the needles of other yew species, and this compound can be converted by semisynthesis to taxol or analogs by addition of the appropriate side chains. One of these analogs, taxotere, has also been selected for clinical development on the basis of its antitumor activity and improved solubility.[63]

The most impressive clinical antitumor activity of taxol has been observed in advanced ovarian cancer and metastatic breast cancer. The initial activity reported in refractory ovarian cancer[64] has been confirmed in three subsequent studies, with response rates ranging from 21% to 40%.[65–67] A phase III trial in the Gynecologic Oncology Group should help clarify the role of taxol in advanced ovarian cancer. Significant activity (56–62%) has also been observed in metastatic breast cancer patients.[68] Preliminary results from phase I studies of taxotere suggest that this agent also has activity in cancers of the ovary and breast.[69]

MECHANISM OF ACTION

The laboratory of Horwitz and coworkers initially demonstrated that taxol promotes microtubule assembly in vitro and that taxol stabilizes microtubules in mouse fibroblast cells exposed to the drug.[61,62] Taxol binds preferentially to microtubules rather than to tubulin dimers, with a binding constant of approximately 1 μmol.[70] Although the binding site for taxol on microtubules is distinct from the binding sites for exchangeable guanosine triphosphate (GTP) and for colchicine, podophyllotoxin, and vinblastine, the specific binding site for taxol on microtubules has not been identified. Unlike other antimicrotubule agents, such as colchicine and the vinca alkaloids, which induce microtubule disassembly, taxol shifts the equilibrium toward microtubule assembly and stabilizes microtubules at concentrations as low as 0.05 μmol/L, which can be easily achieved in patients. Overall, taxol decreases the critical concentration of tubulin required for microtubule assembly in the presence or absence of factors that are usually essential for assembly, such as exogenous GTP or microtubule-associated proteins.[71] Taxol-treated microtubules are stable even after treatment with calcium or low temperatures, conditions that usually promote disassembly.[72] This unusual stability inhibits the normal dynamic reorganization of the microtubule network. Concentrations of taxol (0.1–10 μmol) produce two distinct morphologic effects on cellular microtubules. During all phases of the cell cycle, cells form abundant arrays of disorganized microtubules aligned in parallel bundles.[62,73–75] Additionally, although taxol-treated cells show evidence of entry into mitosis as manifested by chromosomal condensation and breakdown of the nuclear membrane, they lack normal mitotic spindle apparatus. Instead of forming two mitotic spindle asters enucleated by bipolar centrioles, large numbers of abnormal asters that do not require centrioles for enucleation are formed.[73–75] These distinct morphologic effects suggest that taxol may adversely affect critical microtubule functions during interphase and mitosis, but the precise reasons for cell death are unclear.

PHARMACOKINETICS

The pharmacology of taxol has been studied in a number of phase I trials, and the results reported have been consistent.[76] Peak plasma concentrations achieved with brief infusions (6 hours) range from 1.3 to 13.0 μmol at the recommended dose of 175 to 250 mg/m^2.[77,78] On the more conventional 24-hour infusion schedule, steady-state plasma concentrations of 0.6 to 3.5 μmol have been maintained.[79] The disposition of taxol in plasma has been best characterized by a biexponential model. α and β half-lives have ranged from 0.27 to 0.31 hours (mean 0.29) and 1.3 to 8.6 hours (mean 5.0), respectively. Mean values for steady-state volumes of distribution have been large (55–183 L/m^2; mean, 110 L/m^2). Systemic clearances have ranged from 100 to 993 ml/min/m^2, but the principal mechanisms of systemic clearances have not been fully elucidated. When cisplatin administration precedes taxol in combination chemotherapy, taxol clearance has been demonstrated to decrease by approximately 30% and plasma concentrations to increase accordingly.[80] Total urinary excretion has been insignificant (range, 1.4–6.6%; mean, 4.8%). The importance of hepatic metabolism and biliary excretion in taxol disposition has been emphasized by a recent study in rats demonstrating that 12% and 29% of an injected dose are recovered in bile as unchanged taxol and metabolites, respectively.[81] The principal metabolites are derivatives hydroxylated at the *m* position of the benzoate at C-2 or the phenyl group at C-3' of the ester side chain, both of which have significantly diminished cytotoxic activity. Preliminary data suggest that human metabolism is qualitatively similar.[82]

DRUG INTERACTIONS

Interactions of other drugs with taxol have not yet been studied in detail at the level of plasma pharmacokinetics or cellular effects. Administration of cisplatin before a taxol infusion decreases the plasma clearance of taxol, significantly increasing systemic exposure. The resultant myelosuppression has been shown to be greater than for the reverse sequence. In vitro cytotoxicity of the combination of these two agents appears to be greater for the sequence of taxol followed by cisplatin rather than the reverse sequence or simultaneous exposure.[83]

TOXICITY

The principal dose-limiting toxicity of taxol is neutropenia.[76] The neutropenia is dose dependent and is not influenced by the schedule of administration, nor is it cumulative. Onset of neutropenia has usually occurred by day 8 after treatment, nadir neutrophil counts are observed by day 8 to 11, and recovery occurs by day 15 to 18. Episodes of fever during neutropenia have not been frequent, perhaps because of the short duration of taxol-induced myelosuppression. The major risk factor for neutropenia appears to be the extent of prior myelotoxic chemotherapy or irradiation. Anemia and thrombocytopenia have been uncommon.

A major concern during early clinical studies of taxol was the frequent occurrence of hypersensitivity reactions[84] consisting of hypotension, bronchospasm, dyspnea, urticaria, abdominal and extremity pain, and diaphoresis. It has been assumed that these reactions represent a nonimmunologically mediated release of histamine and other vasoactive substances induced by the drug or, more likely, its cremophor vehicle. With prolonged infusions (24 hours) and premedication with corticosteroid, diphenhydramine, and H_2 antagonists, the incidence has decreased to less than 10% of infusions. An important study ongoing in Canada and Europe will address the question of whether the cumbersome 24-hour infusion is necessary to prevent this toxicity when premedication is given.

Clinically significant neurologic toxicity has been uncommon when taxol is given as a single agent at doses less than 170 mg/ml, although mild neurosensory changes have been frequent with numbness and paresthesias occurring in the characteristic "glove and stocking" distribution. Neurologic examinations reveal distal sensory loss and loss of deep tendon reflexes. Electrophysiologic studies support axonal degeneration and demyelination as mechanisms for taxol neurotoxicity.[76,80,85] Transient myalgias and arthralgias, which are occasionally painful, have been observed in patients treated at higher doses. When taxol and cisplatin are given in combination chemotherapy, neurotoxicity becomes more prominent and is dose limiting when G-CSF is used to limit the neutropenia.[80,86]

Other toxicities that have been observed with taxol include nausea and vomiting, mucositis, total body alopecia, and rare local venous toxicity. Cardiac effects include bradycardia and rare instances of atrioventricular block, ventricular tachycardia, and myocardial infarction.[87]

RESISTANCE

Investigations with cell lines made resistant to taxol have characterized two potential mechanisms of acquired drug resistance. Some resistant cells have mutations in tubulin, resulting in impaired microtubule assembly. Continuous exposure to taxol is required for polymerization to proceed normally, thereby promoting the formation of functional microtubules.

A second well-documented mechanism of acquired taxol resistance involves the MDR phenotype that confers cross-resistance to vincristine, doxorubicin, and etoposide.[88] The multidrug resistance is more fully discussed in the section on drug resistance in this chapter.

REFERENCES

1. Aur RJA, Simone JV, Verzosa MS, et al. Childhood acute lymphocytic leukemia: Study VIII. Cancer 1978;42:2123–2134.
2. DeVita VT, Serpick AA, Carbone PP. Combination chemotherapy in the treatment of advanced Hodgkin's disease. Ann Intern Med 1970;73:891–895.
3. Rowinsky EK, Donehower RC. The clinical pharmacology and use of antimicrotubule agents in cancer chemotherapeutics. Pharmacol Ther 1991;52:35–84.
4. Depierre A, Lemarie E, Dabouis G, et al. A phase II study of navelbine in the treatment of non-small cell lung cancer. Am J Clin Oncol 1991;14:115–119.
5. Bryan J. Definition of three classes of binding sites in isolated microtubule crystals. Biochemistry 1972;11:2611–2616.
6. Madoc-Jones H, Mauro F. Interphase action of vinblastine and vincristine: Differences in their lethal action through the mitotic cycle of cultured mamalian cells. J Cell Physiol 1968;72:185–196.
7. Jackson DV, Bender RA. Cytotoxic thresholds of vincristine in a murine and human leukemia cell line in vitro. Cancer Res 1979;39:4346–4349.
8. Bender RA, Castle MC, Margileth DA, et al. The pharmacokinetics of [³H]-vincristine in man. Clin Pharmacol Ther 1977;22:430–438.
9. Nelson RL. The comparative clinical pharmacology and pharmacokinetics of vindesine, vincristine, and vinblastine in human patients with cancer. Med Pediatr Oncol 1982;10:115–127.
10. Nelson RL, Dyke RW, Root MA. Comparative pharmacokinetics of vindesine, vincristine, and vinblastine in patients with cancer. Cancer Treat Rev 1980;7(Suppl):17–24.
11. Sethi VS, Kimball JC. Pharmacokinetics of vincristine sulfate in children. Cancer Chemother Pharmacol 1981;6:111–115.
12. El Dareer SM, White VM, Chen FP, et al. Distribution and metabolism of vincristine in mice, rats, dogs and monkeys. Cancer Treat Rep 1977;61:1269–1277.
13. Jackson DV, Sethi VS, Spurr CL, et al. Pharmacokinetics of vincristine in the cerebrospinal fluid of humans. Cancer Res 1981;41:1466–1468.
14. Jackson DV, Castle MC, Bender RA. Biliary excretion of vincristine. Clin Pharmacol Ther 1978;24:101–107.
15. Owellen RJ, Hartke CA, Hains FO. Pharmacokinetics and metabolism of vinblastine in humans. Cancer Res 1977;37:2597–2602.
16. Creasey WA, Scott AI, Wei CC, et al. Pharmacological studies with vinblastine in the dog. Cancer Res 1975;35:1116–1120.
17. Lu K, Yap HY, Wetts S, et al. Comparative clinical pharmacology of vinblastine in patients with advanced breast cancer. Proc Am Soc Clin Oncol 1979;20:371.
18. Hande K, Gay J, Gover J, et al. Toxicity and pharmacology of bolus vindesine injection and prolonged vindesine infusion. Cancer Treat Rev 1980;7:25–30.
19. Jackson DV, Sethi VS, Long TR, et al. Pharmacokinetics of vindesine by bolus and infusion. Cancer Chemother Pharmacol 1984;13:114–119.
20. Rahmani R, Zhou XJ, Placidi M, et al. In vivo and in vitro pharmacokinetics and metabolism of vinca alkaloids in rat: I. Vindesine. Eur J Drug Metab Pharmacokinet 1990;15:49–55.
21. Jehl F, Quoix EM, Leveque D, et al. Pharmacokinetic and preliminary metabolic fate of navelbine in humans as determined by high performance liquid chromatography. Cancer Res 1991;51:2073–2076.
22. Rahmani R, Bruno R, Iliadis A, et al. Clinical pharmacokinetics of the antitumor drug, navelbine. Cancer Res 1987;47:5796–5799.
23. Armand JP, Marty M. Navelbine: A new step in cancer therapy. Semin Oncol 1989;16(Suppl.4):41–45.
24. Lucas VS, Donehower RC, Rowinsky EK, et al. Clinical results of the absolute bio-

availability and pharmacokinetics of weekly navelbine liquid-filled soft gelatin capsules at full therapeutic doses in patients with solid tumors. Proc Am Soc Clin Oncol 1992;11:111.
25. Bender RA, Bleyer WA, Frisby SA, et al. Alteration of methotrexate uptake in human leukemia cells by other agents. Cancer Res 1975;35:1305–1308.
26. Legha SS. Vincristine neurotoxicity: Pathophysiology and management. Med Toxicol 1986;1:421–427.
27. Bradley WG, Lassman LP, Pearce GW, et al. The neuropathy of vincristine in man: Clinical, electrophysiological and pathological studies. J Neurol Sci 1970;10:107–131.
28. Jackson DV, Wells HB, Atkins JN, et al. Amelioration of vincristine neurotoxicity by glutamic acid. Am J Med 1988;84:1016–1022.
29. Cabral FR, Brady RC, Schiber MJ. A mechanism of cellular resistance to drugs that interfere with microtubule assembly. Ann NY Acad Sci 1986;46:748–756.
29a. Meltzer PS, Dalton WS, Grogan TM, et al. Drug-resistance in multiple myeloma and non-Hodgkin's lymphoma: Detection of P-glycoprotein and potential circumvention by addition of verapamil to chemotherapy. J Clin Oncol 1989;7:415–424.
30. O'Dwyer PJ, Leyland-Jones B, Alonso MT, et al. Etoposide (VP-16-213): Current status of an active anticancer drug. N Engl J Med 1985;312:692–700.
31. Loike D, Horwitz SB. Effects of podophyllotoxin and VP-16 on microtubule assembly in vitro and nucleoside transport in HeLa cells. Biochemistry 1976;15:5435–5442.
32. Krishan A. Paika K, Frei E. Cytofluorometric studies on the action of podophyllotoxins and epipodophyllotoxins (VM-26, VP-16-213) on the cell cycle traverse of hyman lymphoblasts. J Cell Biol 1975;66:521–530.
33. Wozniak AJ, Ross WE. DNA damage as a basis for 4'demethylepipodophyll 9-(4, 6-0-ethylidine-β-D-glucopyranoside) (etoposide) cytotoxicity. Cancer Res 1983;43:120–124.
34. Yang L, Rowe TC, Liu LF. Identification of DNA topoisomerase II as an intracellular target of antitumor epipodophyllotoxins in Simian virus 40-infected monkey cells. Cancer Res 1985;45:5872–5876.
35. Long BH, Brattain MG. The activity of etoposide (VP16-213) and teniposide (VM-26) against human lung tumor cells in vitro: Cytotoxicity and DNA breakage. In: Issell BF, Muggia FM, Carter SK, eds. Etoposide (VP16): Current status and new developments. Academic Press, 1984:63–86.
36. Clarke PI, Slevin ML. The clinical pharmacology of etoposide and teniposide. Clin Pharm 1987;12:223–252.
37. Hande KR, Wedlund PJ, Noone RM, et al. Pharmacokinetics of high-dose etoposide (VP-16-213) administered to cancer patients. Cancer Res 1984;44:379–382.
38. D'Incalci M, Farina P, Sessa C, et al. Pharmacokinetics of VP-16-213 given by different administration schedules. Cancer Chemother Pharmacol 1982;7:141–145.
39. Creaven PJ. The clinical pharmacology of VM-26 and VP-16-213: A brief overview. Cancer Chemother Pharmacol 1982;7:133–140.
40. Sinkule JA, Hutson P, Hayes FA, et al. Pharmacokinetics of etoposide in children and adolescents with refractory solid tumors. Cancer Res 1984;44:3109–3113.
41. Arbuck SG, Douglas HO, Crom WR, et al. Etoposide pharmacokinetics in patients with normal and abnormal organ functions. J Clin Oncol 1986;4:1690–1695.
42. Simon J, Clark D, Slevin M. Renal function and etoposide pharmacokinetics: Is dose modification necessary? Proc Am Soc Clin Oncol 1991;10:281.
43. Mick R, Ratain M. Modeling interpatient pharmacodynamic variability of etoposide. Proc Am Soc Clin Oncol 1991;10:274.
44. Hande KR, Wolff SN, Greco FA, et al. Etoposide kinetics in patients with obstructive jaundice. J Clin Oncol 1990;8:1101–1107.
45. Stewart CF, Arbuck SG, Fleming RA, et al. Changes in the clearance of total and unbound etoposide in patients with liver dysfunction. J Clin Oncol 1990;8:1874–1879.
46. Evans WE, Sinkule JA, Crom WR, et al. Pharmacokinetics of teniposide (VM-26) and etoposide (VP-16-213) in children with cancer. Cancer Chemother Pharmacol 1982;7:147–152.
47. Harvey VJ, Stein ML, Smithe, MM, et al. Variable bioavailability following repeated oral doses of etoposide. Eur J Cancer Clin Oncol 1985;21:1315–1319.
48. Slevin ML, Clark PL, Joel SP, et al. A randomized trial to evaluate the effects of schedule on the activity of etoposide in small-cell lung cancer. J Clin Oncol 1989;7:1333–1340.
49. O'Dwyer PJ, Alonso MT, Leyland-Jones B, et al. Teniposide: A review of 12 years' experience. Cancer Treat Rep 1984;68:1455–1464.
50. Crom WR, Glynn-Barnhart AM, Rodman JH, et al. Pharmacokinetics of anticancer drugs in children. Clin Pharm 1987;12:168–213.
51. Ratain MJ, Schilsky RL, Wojack BR, et al. Hydroxyurea and etoposide: In vitro synergy and phase I clinical trial. JNCI 1988;6:1412–1416.
52. Yalowich JC, Fry DW, Goldman ID. Teniposide (VM-26) and etoposide (VP-16-213)-induced augmentation of methotrexate transport and polyglutamation in Ehrlich ascites tumor cells in vitro. Cancer Res 1982;42:3648–3653.
53. Wolfe SN, Fer M, McKay CM. High-dose VP-16-213 and autologous bone marrow transplantation for refractory malignancies: A phase I study. J Clin Oncol 1983;1:701–705.
54. Johnson DH, Greco FA, Wolfe SN. Etoposide-induced hepatic injury: A potential complication of high-dose therapy. Cancer Treat Rep 1983;67:1023–1024.
55. O'Dwyer PJ, King SA, Fortner CL, Leyland-Jones B. Hypersensitivity reactions to teniposide (VM-26): An analysis. J Clin Oncol 1986;4:1262–1269.
56. Fontana JA. Radiation recall associated with VP-16-213 therapy. Cancer Treat Rep 1979;63:224–225.
57. Winick N, McKenna R, Bowman WP, et al. Secondary acute myeloid leukemia in children with B-lineage acute lymphoblastic leukemia treated with an epipodophyllotoxin. Proc Am Soc Clin Oncol 1992;11:279.
58. Lee T, Roberts D. Flux of teniposide (VM-26) across the plasma membrane of teniposide resistant sublines of L1210 cells. Cancer Res 1984;44:2986–2990.

58a. Gupta RS. Genetic, biochemical and cross-resistance studies with mutants of Chinese hamster ovary cells resistant to the anticancer drugs VM-26 and VP-16-213. Cancer Res 1983;43:1568–1574.

59. Hill BT, Bellamy AS. Establishment of an etoposide-resistant human epithelial tumor cell line in vitro: Characterization of patterns of cross-resistance and drug sensitivities. Int J Cancer 1984;33:599–608.

60. Arnold A, Whitehouse J. Interaction of VP-16-213 with the DNA repair antagonist chloroquine. Cancer Chemother Pharmacol 1984;7:123–126.

60a. Glisson B. Characterization of acquired epipodophyllotoxin-resistant Chinese hamster ovary cell line: Loss of drug-stimulated DNA cleavage activity. Cancer Res 1986;46:1934–1938.

60b. Pommier Y, Kerrigan D, Schwartz RE, et al. Altered DNA topoisomerase II activity in Chinese hamster cells resistant to topoisomerase II inhibitors. Cancer Res 1986;46:3075–3081.

60c. Wani MC, Taylor HL, Wall ME, Coggon P, McPhail AT. Plant antitumor agents: VI. The isolation and structure of taxol, a novel antileukemic and antitumor agent from *Taxus brevifolia*. J Am Chem Soc 1971;93:2325–2327.

61. Schiff PB, Fant J, Horwitz SB. Promotion of microtubule assembly in vitro by taxol. Nature 1979;22:665–667.

62. Schiff PH, Horwitz SB. Taxol stabilizes microtubules in mouse fibroblast cells. Proc Natl Acad Sci USA 1980;77:1561–1563.

63. Bissery MC, Guenard D, Gueritte-Voegelein F, et al. Experimental antitumor activity of taxotere (RP 56976, NSC 628503), a taxol analogue. Cancer Res 1991;51:4845–4852.

64. McGuire WP, Rowinsky EK, Rosenshein NB, et al. Taxol: A unique antineoplastic agent with significant activity in advanced ovarian epithelial neoplasma. Ann Intern Med 1989;111:273–279.

65. Thigpen T, Blessing J, Ball H, et al. Phase II trial of taxol as a second-line therapy for ovarian carcinoma: A gynecologic oncology group study. Proc Am Soc Clin Oncol 1990;9:604.

66. Einzig AI, Wiernik P, Sasloff J, et al. Phase II study of taxol in patients with advanced ovarian cancer. Proc Am Assoc Cancer Res 1990;31:1114.

67. Sarosy G, Kohn E, Link C, et al. Taxol dose intensification in patients with recurrent ovarian cancer. Proc Am Soc Oncol 1992;11:226.

68. Holmes FA, Walters RS, Thieriault RL, et al. Phase II trial of taxol: An active drug in metastatic breast cancer. JNCI 1991;83:1797–1805.

69. Pazdur R, Newman RA, Newman BM, et al. Phase I trial of taxotere (RP56976) Proc Am Soc Clin Oncol 1992;11:111.

70. Parness J, Horwitz SB. Taxol binds to polymerized microtubules in vitro. J Cell Biol 1981;91:479–487.

71. Hamel E, del Campo AA, Lowe MC, et al. Interactions of taxol, microtubule-associated proteins and guanine nucleotides in tubulin polymerization. J Biol Chem 1981;256:11187–11894.

72. Thompson WC, Wilson L, Purich DL. Taxol induces microtubule assembly at low temperature. Cell Motil 1981;1:445–454.

73. Rowinsky EK, Donehower RC, Jones RJ, et al. Microtubule changes and cytotoxicity in leukemic cell lines treated with taxol. Cancer Res 1988;48:4093–4100.

74. Roberts JR, Rowinsky EK, Donehower RC, et al. Demonstration of the cell cycle positions for taxol-induced "asters" and "bundles" by measurement of flourescence, Feulgen-DNA content, and autoradiographic labeling of the same cells. J Histochem Cytochem 1989;37:1659–1665.

75. Roberts JR, Allison DC, Dooley WC, et al. Effects of taxol on cell cycle traverse: Taxol-induced polyploidization as a marker for drug resistance. Cancer Res 1990;50:710–716.

76. Rowinsky EK, Cazenave LA, Donehower RC. Taxol: A novel investigational antimicrotubule agent. JNCI 1990;82:1247–1259.

77. Longnecker SM, Donehower RC, Cates AE, et al. High-performance liquid chromatographic assay for taxol in human plasma and in the pharmacokinetics in a phase I trial. Cancer Treat Rep 1986;71:53–59.

78. Wiernik PH, Schwartz EL, Strauman JJ, et al. Phase I clinical and pharmacokinetic study of taxol. Cancer Res 1987;47:2486–2493.

79. Rowinsky EK, Burke PJ, Karp JE, et al. Phase I and pharmacodynamic study of taxol in refractory acute leukemias. Cancer Res 1989;49:4640–4647.

80. Rowinsky EK, Gilbert M, McGuire WP, et al. Sequences of taxol and cisplatin: A phase I and pharmacologic study. J Clin Oncol 1991;9:1692–1703.

81. Monsarrat B, Mariel E, Cros S, et al. Taxol metabolism, isolation and identification of three major metabolites of taxol in rat bile. Drug Metab Disp 1990;18:895–901.

82. Monsarrat B, Alvinerie P, Gares M, et al. Hepatic metabolism and bilary excretion of taxol. J Cell Pharmacol 1992 (in press).

83. Citardi M, Rowinsky EK, Schaefer KL, et al. Sequence-dependent cytotoxicity between cisplatin and the antimicrotubule agents taxol and vincristine. Proc Am Assoc Cancer Res 1990;31:2431.

84. Weiss R, Donehower RC, Wiernik PH, et al. Hypersensitivity reactions from taxol. J Clin Oncol 1990;8:1263–1268.

85. Lipton RB, Apfel SC, Dutcher JP, et al. Taxol produces a predominantly sensory neuropathy. Neurology 1989;39:368–373.

86. Forastiere AA, Rowinsky EK, Chaudry V, et al. Phase I trial of taxol and cisplatin plus G-CSF in solid tumors. Proc Am Soc Clin Oncol 1992;11:117.

87. Rowinsky EK, McGuire WP, Guarnieri T, et al. Cardiac disturbances during the administration of taxol. J Clin Oncol 1991;9:1704–1712.

88. Greenberger LM, Williams SS, Horwitz SB. Biosynthesis of heterogeneous forms of multidrug resistance-associated glycoproteins. J Biol Chem 1987;262:1–5.

Cancer: Principles & Practice of Oncology, Fourth Edition,
edited by Vincent T. DeVita, Jr., Samuel Hellman, Steven A. Rosenberg.
J.B. Lippincott Co., Philadelphia © 1993.

Richard Simon

CHAPTER **19**

Design and Conduct of Clinical Trials

This chapter highlights principles for the design and conduct of valuable therapeutic clinical trials in oncology. Many of these studies are one of the following types:

1. *Phase I studies.* Determine the relation between toxicity and dose-schedule of treatment.
2. *Phase II studies.* Identify tumor types for which the treatment appears promising.
3. *Phase III studies.*
   a. Determine the effects of a treatment relative to the natural history of the disease.
   b. Determine whether a new treatment is more effective than a standard therapy.
   c. Determine whether a new treatment is as effective as a standard therapy but is associated with less morbidity.

These classes of studies include evaluation of surgical procedures, radiotherapeutic treatments, chemotherapeutic drugs, immunostimulants, biologic response modifiers, antibiotics, antiemetics, and pain control agents. Each of the objectives stated previously is meaningful, however, only within the context of a defined patient population.

The experimental approach plays an important role in clinical oncology currently. In the experimental approach, there are roughly two components: clinical results rather than deductive reasoning are required for the evaluation of a treatment,[1] and the experimental approach requires that preplanned therapeutic interventions be administered to specified types of patients under conditions that are controlled to enable well-defined medical questions to be answered directly. Comparing the survival rates of breast cancer patients treated with mastectomy to those of patients receiving mastectomy plus

postoperative radiotherapy based on regional tumor registry data is an example of a nonexperimental survey. In such surveys, the investigators are passive observers, and they abstract the records they hope will provide information about the phenomena they want to study. Treatment assignments, diagnostic tests, and follow-up procedures are determined by the patients and physicians independently of the investigator. The statistical associations resulting from such studies are in themselves a weak basis for causal inferences about the relation between treatments administered and results observed. Treatments usually are selected based on subjective assessment of prognosis for the patient, capabilities of the physician, and variable diagnostic evaluations. It is generally impossible to identify and eliminate all the biases inherent in survey data.[2,3]

Surveys are sometimes called "observational studies," although this is inaccurate because all knowledge is based on observations. Surveys generally are the only feasible mechanisms for epidemiologic assessment of disease etiology, and when performed by highly trained and critical investigators, they can contribute greatly to public welfare.[4] Acute observations in poorly structured therapeutic settings can also lead to immensely valuable ideas to be pursued and tested in the laboratory and clinical trials. Surveys are, however, sometimes proposed as easy alternatives to planned clinical trials for the evaluation of treatments. For this purpose, the survey is distinctly inferior with regard to inherent reliability of conclusions concerning therapeutic effects. MacMahon and Pugh[4] point out the following:

Only a minority of statistical associations are causal. . . . Once a statistical association has been demonstrated, how can it be determined whether or not it is causal. . . . The most satisfactory procedure is a direct experiment. . . . The evaluation of the causal nature of a relationship, in the absence of direct experiment, is neither easy nor objective. . . . The field of cancer therapy is replete with examples of new modalities that were taken up with enthusiasm and proved worthless only after they had resulted in many years of futile cost and suffering.[4]

The difficult problems in analysis of survey data are discussed elsewhere. Improvements in computer technology have increased the ease of conducting medical surveys but have not had a major role in solving the basic weaknesses of this approach.

This chapter addresses principles for the design and conduct of therapeutic clinical trials in oncology. Such studies can be direct and easily interpretable mechanisms for answering important medical questions. To achieve this objective, however, certain principles must be followed in planning the study. The following sections address certain key aspects of this planning process.

The first result of the planning process is a written protocol. Typical subject headings for the protocol are shown in Table 19–1. This document should be self-contained, consistent, and carefully prepared. It should define uniform treatment and evaluation policies for a well-defined set of patients and should not leave important decisions to the discretion of the physician or the study chairperson. The protocol should define the questions to be answered by the study and should directly justify that the number of patients and nature of controls are adequate to answer these questions definitively. It is easy to embark on a futile or trivial study and to write the protocol merely as a guideline for clinical management supplemented by lofty objectives of no scientific meaning. Rushing the protocol development process and not being sufficiently critical of what is written or omitted contribute to this tendency. From the presentation of scientific background through the definition of data forms, the protocol should show clear, precise, and practical thinking.

STUDY OBJECTIVES

It is important to describe the study objectives specifically in the protocol. This description helps orient the protocol to represent a clearly thought-out research plan rather than merely a guide for clinical management. Clearly stated objectives are

TABLE 19–1. Subject Headings for a Protocol

1. Introduction and scientific background
2. Objectives
3. Selection of patients
4. Design of study (including schematic diagram)
5. Treatment plan
6. Drug information
7. Toxicities to be monitored and dosage modifications
8. Required clinical and laboratory data and study calendar
9. Criteria for evaluating the effect of treatment and endpoint definition
10. Statistical considerations
11. Informed consent and regulatory considerations
12. Data forms
13. References
14. Study chairperson, collaborating participants, addresses, and telephone numbers

necessary to ensure that the size of the study, the nature of the controls, and the plans for patient management are adequate and unbiased with regard to the questions posed.

Many studies in the social sciences are fishing expeditions that include numerous batteries of tests and result in exhaustive analyses. Such unstructured investigations are likely to result in some erroneous conclusions because of the multiplicity of the questions addressed.[5] Therapeutic studies in oncology generally have a more specific natural focus. Nevertheless, it is useful to describe the objectives in terms of specific questions to be answered by the study. Some protocols state that the objective is to "improve treatment," and some list numerous objectives that are not feasible within the size of study planned or for which there are inadequate controls. These characteristics often are an indication that insufficient critical thinking has been done in the planning stage to permit clear interpretation of the results that will be obtained.

The realities of numbers of patients required dictate that most studies should be restricted to one major question. It is best when positive or negative results are informative for patient management and for developing better treatments. Two examples of such studies are comparison of mastectomy to tumor resection for patients with stage I breast cancer and comparison of high-dose versus conventional-dose therapy with an effective drug. Many current studies provide no leads to build on when the results are negative.

Many current studies also fail to address the most important medical questions. The most important studies are often the most difficult to initiate. They may involve withholding a treatment established by tradition, potentially transferring patient management responsibility across specialties, standardizing procedures among people who believe their way is best, and sharing recognition with a large group of collaborators.

PATIENT ELIGIBILITY

Phase I studies generally are conducted with previously treated patients. However, the organ systems that are the expected targets of toxicity should be competent in patients selected for the study. Otherwise, the relations between dose-schedule and toxicity found in the study will not be relevant to the treatment of less debilitated patients.

Whereas phase I studies need not be performed separately by histologic tumor type, this is not the case for phase II studies. In phase II studies, the biologic response of major interest is that of the tumor itself. Because chemosensitivities vary among histologic types, it is important to study enough patients so that the evaluation of tumor response can be made separately by type.

When a drug enters phase II trials, it should be tested in the patient group that is most likely to show a favorable effect, provided that it is ethically permissible to do so. Otherwise, the chances of missing the activity of the drug are increased. This criterion is best fulfilled by patients with maximum performance status and the minimum extent of disease and prior chemotherapy. Although drugs active against tumors resistant to current agents are needed, testing in these patients should not be the primary basis for evaluating drug activity. Full-dose chemotherapy is often impossible in these patients, and lack of activity in previously treated patients is often not a predictor of lack of clinical usefulness in earlier disease. The deleterious effect of prior therapy on the probability of response was illustrated by etoposide in small cell carcinoma of the lung and has been documented more generally by Wittes and colleagues.[6,7] For the less sensitive cancers, chemotherapy offers little or no palliative benefit, and initial phase II trials should be limited to patients with no prior chemotherapy. In more sensitive tumors, such as breast, small cell lung, ovarian cancer or non-Hodgkin's lymphoma, it is desirable to evaluate new drugs on patients with no more than one previous treatment. Phase II evaluation is not appropriate in instances when treatment with curative potential is available. The "window of opportunity" design is being increasingly used in which nonpreviously treated patients with sensitive tumor types are given one or two courses of a phase II drug and then switched to a standard combination.[6] This approach does not mean that heavily pretreated patients should be denied the potential benefits of new active agents. The agents should be shown to be active in a favorable population of patients, however, before they are given to a less favorable group. It will save patients with advanced disease from exposure to inactive agents for which the likelihood of toxicity is much greater than the chance of benefit.

Eligibility criteria for phase III trials must accommodate two important considerations. First, all eligible patients should be expected to tolerate all of the treatments being compared. If one treatment is intensive, then debilitated patients who are not expected to tolerate full doses should not be included. The second consideration, however, is that the results of the trial may be applied on a national or international scale to select treatments. The fact that clinical trials performed on a small minority of selected patients determine treatment decisions for broad populations is a serious problem. The proportion of adults with cancer who participate in clinical trials is much less than 10%. Some studies have indicated that only a small minority of such patients would be eligible for clinical trials, even if they or their physicians wanted to participate.[8,9] It seems important, therefore, that efforts be made to place more emphasis on broadening eligibility criteria for confirmatory studies of national importance to better ensure that results that are meaningful for the general population of patients are obtained.

ENDPOINT

The term *endpoint* refers to the criterion by which patient benefit is measured. A meaningful and reliable endpoint is essential for a worthwhile study. In some of the social sciences, lack of an adequate endpoint is a major impediment to progress. For clinical oncology, there is often controversy about what endpoints reflect meaningful patient benefit. Explicit definition of the endpoint(s) is important for determining the size and duration of the trial and for ensuring that the proper measurements are taken and follow-up evaluations are performed without bias.

The major endpoints for evaluating the effectiveness of a treatment should be measures of patient welfare. Duration of survival and quality of life are two such endpoints. Quality of life has been used infrequently, because sufficiently simple and reproducible measures of important aspects of quality of life were not available. The development of such measures

that can be used broadly by clinicians in the conduct of therapeutic evaluations is an important area that is receiving increasing attention.

Survival generally is the most meaningful measure of benefit for phase III studies. The endpoints commonly used as alternatives to survival are degree of tumor shrinkage and duration for which the tumor is below the level of clinical detection. These endpoints are basically subjective measures. Whether a patient has a partial response depends on who is doing the measuring and what the response criteria are.[10–13] The more closely one looks, the fewer complete remissions are obtained, and the more rapidly recurrent disease is detected. Consequently, it is important that follow-up procedures be standardized in the protocol to ensure that the study is not jeopardized by biased evaluation of response. Subjectivity and missing data in defining "date of recurrence" is a major problem for the acceptance of disease-free survival as an unbiased endpoint in adjuvant clinical trials.

It cannot be assumed that response rates, duration of response, or disease-free intervals are proper endpoints for drawing conclusions about therapeutic efficacy, because they are not direct measures of patient welfare. There are examples, however, in which improvements in cure rates have followed major improvements in complete response rates and durations. The situation is more mixed with regard to partial responses. A treatment that causes partial responses is not necessarily beneficial to the patient. Even if it is demonstrated that partial responders live longer than nonresponders, it cannot be concluded that the treatment is beneficial.[14–16] Comparisons of survivals between responders and nonresponders are biased in several ways. First, responders, by definition, have lived long enough to achieve that status. Second, responders may have more favorable prognostic factors that would result in their living longer than would nonresponders, even in the absence of any treatment. Finally, it cannot be assumed that the difference in survival does not result from the shortening survival of the treatment for the nonresponders. To demonstrate that the treatment extends survival, the comparison of survival between responders and nonresponders is not relevant. It must be demonstrated that the treated group as a whole lives longer than an appropriate control group of similar prognosis.

For some kinds of cancer, partial responses are of substantial duration, are associated with improved palliation, and have been demonstrated to represent the effect of treatment on prolonging life by comparison to an appropriate control group. For other kinds of cancer, however, partial responses are of minimal duration and have not been demonstrated to represent a beneficial therapeutic effect for the patient. Increases in partial response rates without corresponding improvements in survival or palliation for the treated group should not be viewed as therapeutic improvements. However, partial responses are useful indicators of biologic activity for phase II studies, even in diseases where direct patient benefit cannot be demonstrated.

TREATMENT ALLOCATION

PHASE I STUDIES

Phase I trials involve estimation of the relation between dose and toxicity for a specified schedule and mode of administration. Such studies usually are performed by starting with a low dose not expected to produce serious toxicity in any patients. A starting dose of one tenth the LD_{10} expressed as milligrams per square meter of body surface area in the most sensitive species is usually used.[17] The dose is increased for subsequent patients according to a series of preplanned steps. Dose escalation for subsequent patients occurs only after sufficient time has passed to observe acute toxic effects for patient treated at lower doses. Cohorts of 3 to 6 patients are treated at each dose level. Often, if no dose-limiting toxicity (DLT) is encountered at a dose level, the dose is escalated for the next cohort. If the incidence of DLT is one third, then 3 more patients are treated at the same level. If no further cases of DLT are seen in the additional 3 patients, then the dose level is escalated for the next cohort. Otherwise, dose escalation stops. If the incidence of DLT is greater than one third in the initial 3 patients treated at a level, then dose escalation stops. The phase II recommended dose is often taken as the highest dose for which the incidence of DLT is less than 33%. Usually 6 or more patients are treated at the recommended dose.

The dose levels themselves are commonly based on a modified Fibonacci series.[18] The second level is twice the starting dose; the third level is 67% greater than the second; the fourth level is 50% greater than the third; the fifth level is 40% greater than the fourth; and each subsequent step is 33% greater than that preceding it. Escalating doses for subsequent courses in the same patient is generally not performed, except at low doses because of concern about cumulative toxicity. Many phase I studies that escalate doses within patients are not analyzed in a way that distinguishes patients from courses of therapy.

There is no compelling scientific basis for the approach described previously, except that experience has shown it to be safe and reasonably effective. In some instances, it results in having to explore many dose levels before the maximum tolerated dose (MTD) is reached. It also may provide an imprecise estimate of the MTD.[19] More precise estimates, however, may require much larger sample sizes in the dose range at which toxicity occurs. This approach also provides little information about how the MTD varies among patients. Other approaches have been proposed for specifying the dose levels, the number of patients treated per dose level, the dose escalation or deescalation criteria, and the method of estimating the MTD or recommended phase II dose.[19-21]

There also has been substantial interest in using serum concentrations of drugs to improve the conduct of phase I trials. Collins and associates[22] proposed basing dose escalation on the hypothesis that the area under the serum concentration versus time curve (AUC) at the human MTD equals the AUC at the LD_{10} for other species. One method of escalation proposed involved doubling the dose for cohorts of new patients until the AUC value equals 40% of the target AUC. Subsequently, modified Fibonacci escalation would be used. This approach is being explored for new drugs. In some instances, however, it cannot be used because important active metabolites are unknown, an adequate assay is unavailable, or the AUC hypothesis is of questionable validity based on interspecies animal toxicology data. There remains a strong motivation to improve the methodology of phase I trials conducted without serum concentration targets.

Some phase I trials evaluate more than one schedule, mode of administration, or approach to hematopoietic support.

There is often a comparative intent, although no formal statistical comparisons are planned. It is not generally recognized that the small sample sizes of 3 to 6 patients per dose level used in phase I trials usually results in an imprecise estimate of the MTD. Also, the comparison of two MTDs determined in this way is not reliable unless the differences are large. An additional problem is the fact that phase I trials generally have broad eligibility requirements and that the patients entered late in the trial may be different in ability to tolerate chemotherapy than those entered early. Like other studies with comparative intent, randomization is an important mechanism for ensuring comparability of patients. Phase I trials with comparative intent are not really phase I trials. The comparative objectives require careful consideration and detailed planning if they are to be taken seriously. This also applies to phase I trials of hematopoietic growth factors used in conjunction with a fixed chemotherapy regimen. In addition to determination of the MTD of the growth factor, there is sometimes interest in determining the "optimum biologic dose." Such studies are best designed as randomized phase III trials of two or more dose levels of the growth factor conducted after the MTD is determined.

For any phase I trial, the definition of DLT and the criteria for dose escalation and deescalation should be specified in the protocol. Active monitoring of results by the study chair is essential for a safe trial.

PHASE II STUDIES

The results of phase II studies can be misleading in two ways.[7] First, little antitumor effect may be seen, but the patients may be so debilitated or extensively pretreated that the results do not reflect true potential usefulness of the agent. Second, because of patient selection or inadequately rigorous response criteria, more favorable results are obtained than will be substantiated by further trials. To deal with these potential problems, it has been suggested that phase II studies involve a randomization between the experimental agent and a treatment known to have antitumor value.[23-26] The purpose of randomization would not be for determining which treatment was better, but for having a baseline response rate of similar patients treated with a known therapy. Peto[23] has suggested that two thirds of the patients should be randomized to the new treatment. When it is possible, this design can deal effectively with the false-positivity problem. Adequate standardization of response criteria or recognition of the limitation of partial response for reflecting patient benefit usually would be just as effective, however. The randomized design deals with the false-negativity problem by alerting us that the patient population is not responsive even to a regimen considered active for the disease. A better safeguard against false-negative results, however, is to use previously untreated patients in phase II studies when it is ethically possible.

For cooperative groups with sufficient patients simultaneously to conduct several phase II studies in a disease, randomization among the new agents is desirable.[27] There is no question that patient selection can influence results.[28] Such selection can lead to bias in the ranking of new agents. Differences among institutions in evaluation of response can make the problem even severer. The conduct of one master phase II study with randomized treatment assignment helps alleviate these problems.

Phase II trials may be designed with crossover to a specified treatment (another experimental agent or an established drug) when the patient fails the initial therapy. This aspect of the design usually supplies little information because so few patients make it through the secondary treatment, because there are so few responses, and because the condition of the patient has changed.

PHASE III STUDIES

Controls

The interpretation of most phase III studies involves some type of comparison of results. In some instances, the basis of comparison will be the natural history of the disease, and in others it will be another treatment. The term *control* will be used to represent the basis against which treatment is to be evaluated. Rarely, if ever, do researchers want to know only whether a treatment is better or worse than the control— they want to estimate the degree of difference. All measurement, ultimately, is comparative, and the categorization of a treatment as "good" or "bad" involves an implicit comparison.

To determine whether a new treatment cures any patients with a disease that is uniformly and rapidly fatal, history is a satisfactory control. In this situation, the patient population is completely homogenous with regard to cure in the absence of the new therapy. If 20% of patients are cured by conventional therapy and researchers can identify them by patient and tumor characteristics measured at diagnosis, they can restrict a study to the remaining 80% and have complete homogeneity. After they leave the setting of complete homogeneity with regard to the chosen endpoint, the definition of an adequate nonrandomized control becomes problematic.

In many studies the controls are numbers determined from publications or patients treated in nonexperimental settings in which the information is abstracted from tumor registries, data banks, or medical records. The meaningfulness of such controls is questionable. Often diagnostic and staging procedures, supportive care, secondary treatments, and methods of evaluation and follow-up are different for the controls and the current treatment group. There generally is differential bias in the selection of patients to be treated resulting from judgements by the physicians, self-selection by the patients, and differences in referral patterns. There may be bias in treatment ineligibility rates. Current patients are sometimes excluded from analysis for not meeting eligibility criteria, not receiving "adequate" treatment, refusing treatment, or a major protocol violation. The controls, on the other hand, generally contain all the patients. There may be differences in the distribution of known and unknown prognostic factors between the controls and the current treatment group. Often there is inadequate information to determine whether such differences are present, and current known prognostic factors may not have been measured or recorded for the controls. It generally is difficult to tell whether the controls would have been eligible for the current study and in what way they represent a selection of all eligible patients.

In the best circumstances, historical controls will be patients treated within the previous few years at the same institution or institutions performing the new study. The controls would be treated on a protocol having exactly the same eligibility requirements, workup, follow-up, and response evaluation procedures as the current study, referral patterns and accrual rate would be static, no patients in either group would be excluded from analysis because of ineligibility or nonevaluability, and an exhaustive demonstration of similarity in distribution of all suspected prognostic factors would be presented. These circumstances rarely are encountered in practice. Pocock[29] has reported 19 unselected instances under circumstances approaching these where a cooperative group carried one treatment over two successive studies. Even here, for 4 of 19 pairs of trials, the differences in outcome were statistically significant at the $p < 0.02$ level.

Formation of the control group by random assignment of treatment as an integral part of the planned study can avoid most of the systematic biases mentioned previously.[30-35] The random assignment should not be performed until the patient is found eligible, and then a truly random or nondecipherable mechanism should be used. Alternation, day of the week, or other predictable procedures are not adequate, because they allow bias in the decision of whether to enter a patient into a study based on knowledge beforehand of what treatment the patient will receive. Randomization does not ensure that the study will include a representative sample of all patients with the disease, but it does help ensure an unbiased evaluation of the relative merits of the two treatments for the types of patients entered.

Some of the advantages of randomization are subtle and not widely understood. For example, it is sometimes said that randomization is unnecessary, because matched historical or concurrent controls can be selected. But matches can be done only with regard to known prognostic factors, and these generally explain only a minor portion of the variability in prognosis among patients.[36] Matching with regard to known factors gives no assurance that the distributions of unknown factors are similar between the treatment groups. It also is sometimes said that randomization is not effective in ensuring that the treatment groups are similar with regard to unknown prognostic factors, unless the number of patients is large. This is true but reflects a misunderstanding of randomization. Randomization does not ensure that the groups are medically equivalent, but it distributes the unknown biasing factors according to a known random distribution so that their effects can be rigorously allowed for in significance tests and confidence intervals. This is true regardless of the study size. A significance level represents the probability that differences in outcome can be the result of random fluctuations. Without randomized treatment allocation, a "statistically significant difference" may be the result of a nonrandom difference in the distribution of unknown prognostic factors.

Randomization (or stratified randomization, to be discussed later) is inherently the method of treatment assignment that results in the most reliable basis for inference. This is not to say that all randomized studies are good or that all nonrandomized are bad, but that, everything else being equal, randomization adds considerably to the ease of interpretability of the study, because one need not worry about conscious or inadvertent systematic biases in patient selection or treatment assignment. Gehan and Freireich[37] and Pocock[38] have listed conditions under which nonrandomized studies may be considered reliable. Most nonrandomized studies do not meet these conditions. The oncology literature is filled with reports of nonrandomized studies in which scant attention is paid to comparability with regard to known prognostic factors. At this point, the major advantages of randomization are not the subtle aspects mentioned but avoidance of the major biases of most of poorly done, nonrandomized studies. If nonrandomized studies were scrupulously conducted and critically reported under the conditions described earlier for consecutive trials, the subtle advantages that randomization will always have might be less decisive. Modern alternative approaches based on nonexperimental data bases and tumor registries having concurrent nonrandomized controls are a poor alternative to either method.

Are randomized trials necessary for identifying major advances in treatment? No. There are many examples of therapeutic breakthroughs that were recognized without randomized trials. For the most part, however, these occurred in diseases in which the prognosis was 100% predictable before the advent of the new therapy, and there was no possibility of bias with regard to patient selection. False innovations are much more numerous than real breakthroughs, and it is difficult to distinguish one from the other.[39] There certainly is a role, however, for innovative, nonrandomized studies in diseases with uniformly bleak prognoses.

Some physicians are uncomfortable with the notion of randomization, believing that they have an obligation to develop an opinion about the relative merits of alternative possible treatments and to recommend a therapy to their patients accordingly.[40] This position is understandable, but it must be tempered by the following considerations. Different competent physicians often hold widely divergent opinions about the relative merits of alternative treatments for the same patient.[41,42] The little research done indicates that experienced, well-educated adults are likely to overrate the correctness of their opinions and hunches.[43] The experimental treatment generally is neither much better nor much worse than the control, and researchers have little real basis for selecting between the treatments before the trial. Gilbert and colleagues[43] point out the following:

> Much of current popular discussion of ethical issues takes the position that physicians should use their best judgement in prescribing for a patient. To what extent the physician is responsible for the quality of the judgement is not much discussed, except to say that he must keep abreast of the times. Some physicians will feel an obligation to find out that goes beyond the mere holding of an opinion. Such physicians will feel a responsibility to contribute to the research. In similar fashion, some current patients may feel a responsibility to contribute to the better care of future patients. The current model of the passive patient and the active outgoing physician is not the most effective one for a society that not only wants cures rather than sympathy, but insists on them—a society that has been willing to pay in patient cooperation and material resources for the necessary research.[43]

Korn and Baumrind described a hybrid approach to randomized clinical trials.[44] They propose that patients be randomly allocated a treatment only when there is clinical disagreement about the treatment of choice for that patient and, in those instances, the patient be assigned to a clinician who had thought that the regimen allocated is the one most appropriate for that patient.

If randomization is used, it generally should take place as late as possible before effecting treatment of the patient.[45,45a,46] For example, in evaluating a chemotherapeutic regimen as a postsurgical adjuvant treatment, randomization should take place after the surgery has been completed and the patient

has recovered sufficiently to begin receiving chemotherapy. This approach serves to reduce bias in the surgery administered and possible bias in disqualifications of randomized patients because of surgical findings, morbidity, or mortality.

Protocols for nonrandomized phase III studies should describe the control group used. The control group should consist of patients for whom records are available for detailed evaluation of comparability.

Stratified Randomization

When important prognostic factors are known for patients in a randomized study, it is often advisable to stratify the randomization to ensure equal distribution of these factors. This usually is accomplished by preparing a separate randomization list (or set of cards in sealed envelopes) for each distinct subset of patients (stratum). Each list must be balanced so that after each block of 4 to 10 patients within the stratum the treatment groups contain equal numbers of patients. Within the blocks, the sequence of treatment assignments is random. The stratification factors must be known for each patient at the time of randomization.

It generally is best to limit stratification to those factors definitely known to have important independent effects on response. If two factors are closely correlated, one, at most, should be included in the stratification. Peto and coworkers[45,45a] believe that stratification is an unnecessary complication, because adjustment for imbalances of known factors can be made in the analysis. For small studies, however, such adjustments should not be relied on. Stratification may obviate the chance of gross imbalances that cannot be adjusted for and ensures that the treatment comparisons are not totally dependent on statistical adjustment methods.[47,48] Also, stratified randomization serves to specify the important prognostic factors that may play a role in the analysis of the results. This can be used to limit the amount of post hoc "data dredging" that might be attempted, that is, subset analysis and covariate adjustments should be limited to prespecified stratification variables. Simon[49] and Kalish and Begg[50] have reviewed the various stratification methods available. Kalish and Begg[51] studied analytic aspects of adaptive stratification methods.

Crossover Designs

Crossover designs are often used in settings such as the comparative evaluation of antiemetics and antipain treatments. For example, patients might be randomized to receive an antiemetic during the first course of chemotherapy and a placebo during the second, or the alternate sequence. This design is motivated by the desire to increase the sensitivity of a study by using each patient as his or her own control and thereby to reduce the number of patients required. The usefulness of this approach is limited, because the condition of the patient changes with time, patients go off study before completing both periods, doses are reduced in the second period based on first period results, and the effect of a treatment may be influenced by previous treatments or conditioned by previous responses.

Crossover designs in which there are more than two treatment periods per patient are almost always difficult or impossible to interpret clearly. Such studies are often analyzed and reported in a manner that fails to distinguish distinct patients from multiple treatment episodes of the same patient. Useful methods for analyzing a two-period crossover design are described by Hills and Armitage[52] and by Koch.[53] Use of the crossover design is controversial and has been discouraged by the Food and Drug Administration (FDA).[54] If the relative efficacy of the treatments in the second period differs from that in the first period or is conditioned by first period response, it is not possible to use each patient as his or her own control. To determine whether such an interaction exists requires as many patients as a noncrossover design, and researchers should seriously weigh these considerations before adopting the crossover design.[55–57] The design should be mainly restricted to situations in which conditions of the treatment remain fixed and few patients will fail to complete both periods.

It is always best to administer a treatment in a clinical trial the way that it would be recommended for administration in the general medical practice. The crossover design is artificial in this regard. Less structured designs that repeatedly rerandomize the same patients are subject to this criticism and suffer from the introduction of additional correlations that generally are impossible to account for properly in the analysis.

Common Control Designs

In randomized multiinstitution studies, it is sometimes difficult to obtain agreement among all participants concerning the treatments to be used. A compromise design sometimes suggested is to allow each institution to select between doing a randomized study of treatments A and B or doing a randomized study of B and C. These two studies are conducted simultaneously, but at different institutions. It usually is recognized that this design is inferior to a simple randomization among all treatments A, B, and C within each institution, but it is hoped that it is better than a totally nonrandomized design. Schoenfeld and Gelber[58] have shown that unless one can assume that there are no differences among institutions in response to treatment, this design is inefficient. With three treatments (one being the common control), this design requires twice as many patients as a straightforward three-way, randomized design. Consequently, the common control design is not a good alternative.

Factorial Designs

In a 2×2 factorial design there are actually four treatments under study. The first factor represents two alternative treatment interventions, such as amputation and resection. The second factor represents two other alternative interventions superimposed on the first factor, such as adjuvant chemotherapy and no further treatment. Although there are actually four treatment groups (amputation alone, resection alone, amputation plus chemotherapy, resection plus chemotherapy), in some instances, the effect of each treatment factor can be evaluated using all of the patients and pooling with regard to the other factor (or with the influence of the other factor accounted for in the analysis, but not separate analysis for each level of the other factor).[23,59] The validity of such an analysis depends on the following types of assumptions: if adjuvant chemotherapy is beneficial for amputees, it is also

beneficial for resected patients. Similarly, the relative efficacy of the two surgical procedures does not depend on whether the patient receives adjuvant chemotherapy. If these assumptions are not satisfied, the study must be analyzed by the simultaneous comparison of all four treatment groups. If the sample size is computed assuming that these assumptions are true, however, then the study will not include enough patients to test adequately the assumptions or to be analyzed as a four-arm study. The factorial design offers the possibility of answering two questions for the price of one, but there is a risk of difficulty in interpretation.[60–62] For situations in which interactions are unlikely or in which both factors are unlikely to have a significant effect, the factorial design can provide a substantial improvement in the efficiency of clinical trials.

Combining Randomized and Historical Controls

Randomized studies are sometimes conducted weighted 2 to 1 in favor of new treatment, with the intent of incorporating historical controls in the analysis if their outcomes are similar to those of the randomized controls. This design rarely provides enough randomized controls for an adequate comparison with results for the historical control group. Pocock[38] has investigated other methods of combining controls from two successive studies, but he assumes that the expected difference between outcomes from the control groups is zero. A 2 to 1 randomization sometimes is reasonable, but not for the purpose of including historical controls.

SIZE AND DURATION OF THE STUDY

PHASES I AND II TRIALS

The size of phase I studies cannot be completely determined in advance. Guidelines that exist for planning size of such studies have been presented in a previous section.

Simon[63] has recently reviewed the statistical designs that have been developed for phase II trials. With any of the proposed designs, the accrual plan and decision rules are applied separately to each subset of patients for whom inferences are to be made (*e.g.*, previously untreated advanced colon cancer patients). The oldest approach is Gehan's two-stage design.[64] If the target activity level of interest is 20%, then 14 patients are accrued in the first stage. If no responses are obtained, the trial is terminated for such patients, and the drug is considered inactive for that subset. The basis for this conclusion is that if the true response rate is at least 20%, then the probability of obtaining 0 responses in 14 patients is less than 0.05. If researchers reject the drug for this subset when no responses are seen in the first 14 patients, the rejection error is 5%, for a true activity of 20%.

A second stage of the trial is essential to better estimate the response rate of the drug. The number of patients required for the second stage depends strongly on the precision desired for the estimated response rate. For a standard error of 10%, about 25 total patients are required (*e.g.*, 14 in the first stage, 11 in the second). For a standard error of 5%, the required total number of patients is generally in the range of 50 to 90. Gehan's design is often applied with 14 patients in the first stage and 25 total if any responses are obtained. A sample of 25 patients, however, generally provides a poor estimate of the true response probability, and a study of 35 to 40 patients is often preferable.

Gehan's plan frequently is misapplied by having too heterogenous a set of patients in the first stage. If no responses are observed among 14 patients of diverse tumor types or previous treatment experiences, no conclusion can be reached for any single well-defined class of patients. Researchers usually should strive for separate evaluation of results by whether the patient has received chemotherapy previously. If previously untreated patients are to be included, to minimize the number of patients exposed to an ineffective drug, it is advisable to delay entry of previously treated patients until the drug has demonstrated activity.

Gehan's plan also is frequently misapplied by failure to conduct the second stage for strata that exhibit at least one response in the first 14 patients. The second stage usually is essential, because even a drug with a 5% response rate has a 51% chance of producing at least one response in 14 patients.

Simon[65] has developed an optimized modification of Gehan's design. It is a two-stage design with n_1 patients in the first stage and n patients total. If the observed response rate

at the end of the first stage is $\leq r_1/n_1$, then the trial terminates and the drug is rejected as being of little interest. Otherwise, accrual continues to a total of n patients. At the end of the second stage, the drug is rejected if the observed response rate is $\leq r/n$.

Tables 19–2 and 19–3 show some of these optimized designs. To select a design, researchers must specify a target activity level p_1 of interest and also a lower activity level p_0. The first row of each triplet of optimal designs in Tables 19–2 and 19–3 provide probability ≤ 0.10 of accepting drugs worse than p_0 and probability ≤ 0.10 of rejecting drugs better than p_1. Subject to these two constraints, the optimal designs minimize the average sample size as functions of n_1, r_1, n, and r. The average sample size is calculated at the activity level p_0. Hence, the optimal designs are optimized for screening out poor drugs. Tables 19–2 and 19–3 show for each design the decision criteria, the average sample size, and the probability of stopping after the first stage for a drug with activity level p_0.

Tables 19–2 and 19–3 also show the "minimax" design for each situation. The minimax design is that design with the

TABLE 19–2. Simon Two-Stage Phase II Designs for $p_1 - p_0 = 0.20$*

		Optimal Design					Minimax Design			
		Reject Drug if Response Rate					Reject Drug if Response Rate			
p_0	p_1	$\leq r_1/n_1$	$\leq r/n$	EN (p_0)	PET (p_0)		$\leq r_1/n_1$	$\leq r/n$	EN (p_0)	PET (p_0)
0.05	0.25	0/9	2/24	14.5	0.63		0/13	2/20	16.4	0.51
		0/9	2/17	12.0	0.63		0/12	2/16	13.8	0.54
		0/9	3/30	16.8	0.63		0/15	3/25	20.4	0.46
0.10	0.30	1/12	5/35	19.8	0.65		1/16	4/25	20.4	0.51
		1/10	5/29	15.0	0.74		1/15	5/25	19.5	0.55
		2/18	6/36	22.5	0.71		2/22	6/33	26.2	0.62
0.20	0.40	3/17	10/37	26.0	0.55		3/19	10/36	28.2	0.46
		3/13	12/43	20.6	0.75		4/18	10/33	22.3	0.50
		4/19	15/54	30.4	0.67		5/24	13/45	31.2	0.66
0.30	0.50	7/22	17/46	29.9	0.67		7/28	15/39	35.0	0.36
		5/15	18/46	23.6	0.72		6/19	16/39	25.7	0.48
		8/24	24/63	34.7	0.73		7/24	21/53	36.6	0.56
0.40	0.60	7/18	22/46	30.2	0.56		11/28	20/41	33.8	0.55
		7/16	23/46	24.5	0.72		17/34	20/39	34.4	0.91
		11/25	32/66	36.0	0.73		12/29	27/54	38.1	0.64
0.50	0.70	11/21	26/45	29.0	0.67		11/23	23/39	31.0	0.50
		8/15	26/43	23.5	0.70		12/23	23/37	27.7	0.66
		13/24	36/61	34.0	0.73		14/27	32/53	36.1	0.65
0.60	0.80	6/11	26/38	25.4	0.47		18/27	24/35	28.5	0.82
		7/11	30/43	20.5	0.70		8/13	25/35	20.8	0.65
		12/19	37/53	29.5	0.69		15/26	32/45	35.9	0.48
0.70	0.90	6/9	22/28	17.8	0.54		11/16	20/25	20.1	0.55
		4/6	22/27	14.8	0.58		19/23	21/26	23.2	0.95
		11/15	29/36	21.2	0.70		13/18	26/32	22.7	0.67

* For each value of (p_0, p_1), designs are given for three sets of error probabilities (α, β). The first, second, and third rows correspond to error probability limits (0.10, 0.10), (0.05, 0.20), and (0.05, 0.10), respectively. α is the probability of accepting a drug with response probability p_0. β is the probability of rejecting a drug with response probability p_1. For each design, EN (p_0) and PET (p_0) denote the expected sample size and the probability of early termination when the true response probability is p_0.

TABLE 19-3. Simon's Two-Stage Phase II Designs for $p_1 - p_0 = 0.15$*

		Optimal Design					Minimax Design			
		Reject Drug if Response Rate					Reject Drug if Response Rate			
p_0	p_1	$\leq r_1/n_1$	$\leq r/n$	EN (p_0)	PET (p_0)		$\leq r_1/n_1$	$\leq r/n$	EN (p_0)	PET (p_0)
0.05	0.20	0/12	3/37	23.5	0.54		0/18	3/32	26.4	0.40
		0/10	3/29	17.6	0.60		0/13	3/27	19.8	0.51
		1/21	4/41	26.7	0.72		1/29	4/38	32.9	0.57
0.10	0.25	2/21	7/50	31.2	0.65		2/27	6/40	33.7	0.48
		2/18	7/43	24.7	0.73		2/22	7/40	28.8	0.62
		2/21	10/66	36.8	0.65		3/31	9/55	40.0	0.62
0.20	0.35	5/27	16/63	43.6	0.54		6/33	15/58	45.5	0.50
		5/22	19/72	35.4	0.73		6/31	15/53	40.4	0.57
		8/37	22/83	51.4	0.69		8/42	21/77	58.4	0.53
0.30	0.45	9/30	29/82	51.4	0.59		16/50	25/69	56.0	0.68
		9/27	30/81	41.7	0.73		16/46	25/65	49.6	0.81
		13/40	40/110	60.8	0.70		27/77	33/88	78.5	0.86
0.40	0.55	16/38	40/88	54.5	0.67		18/45	34/73	57.2	0.56
		11/26	40/84	44.9	0.67		28/59	34/70	60.1	0.90
		19/45	49/104	64.0	0.68		24/62	45/94	78.9	0.47
0.50	0.65	18/35	47/84	53.0	0.63		19/40	41/72	58.0	0.44
		15/28	48/83	43.7	0.71		39/66	40/68	66.1	0.95
		22/42	60/105	62.3	0.68		28/57	54/93	75.0	0.50
0.60	0.75	21/34	47/71	47.1	0.65		25/43	43/64	54.4	0.46
		17/27	46/67	39.4	0.69		18/30	43/62	43.8	0.57
		21/34	64/95	55.6	0.65		48/72	57/84	73.2	0.90
0.70	0.85	14/20	45/59	36.2	0.58		15/22	40/52	36.8	0.51
		14/19	46/59	30.3	0.72		16/23	39/49	34.4	0.56
		18/25	61/79	43.4	0.66		33/44	53/68	48.5	0.81
0.80	0.95	5/7	27/31	20.8	0.42		5/7	27/31	20.8	0.42
		7/9	26/29	17.7	0.56		7/9	26/29	17.7	0.56
		16/19	37/42	24.4	0.76		31/35	35/40	35.3	0.94

* For each value of (p_0, p_1), designs are given for three sets of error probabilities (α, β). The first, second, and third rows correspond to error probability limits (0.10, 0.10), (0.05, 0.20), and (0.05, 0.10), respectively. α is the probability of accepting a drug with response probability p_0. β is the probability of rejecting a drug with response probability p_1. For each design, EN (p_0) and PET (p_0) denote the expected sample size and the probability of early termination when the true response probability is p_0.

smallest maximum sample size n that satisfies the two constraints described previously. If there are several such designs, the one with the minimum average sample size (calculated at activity level p_0) is shown. Although minimax designs have somewhat larger average sample sizes than do optimal designs, in some instances, they are preferable, because the small increase in average sample size is more than compensated for by a large reduction in maximum sample size.

When there are sufficient numbers of patients available and several treatments to test, there are advantages to randomized phase II trials.[27] Although phase II trials are not comparative, in selecting the most promising treatment to pursue in phase III trials it is advantageous to evaluate the candidates on comparable patients. Table 19–4 from Simon and associates shows the number of patients required per treatment to ensure that the best treatment will have the highest observed response rate.[27] This calculation assumes that the true response probability for the best treatment is 15 percentage points better than for the others. This selection approach is not an alter-

TABLE 19-4. Number of Patients per Treatment for Randomized Phase II Selection Designs*

Smallest Response Probability	Number of Treatments		
	2	3	4
0.10	21	31	37
0.20	29	44	52
0.30	35	52	62
0.40	37	55	67
0.50	36	54	65
0.60	32	49	59
0.70	26	39	47
0.80	16	24	29

* Probability that the best treatment will have the largest observed response rate is 0.90 when the true response probability for the best treatment is 15 percentage points larger than that for the second best treatment.

native to phase III trial testing of a null hypothesis, but it is sometimes useful when one treatment will be carried forward, and the treatments are similar with regard to cost and toxicity.

PHASE III TRIALS

The protocol for a phase III study should specify the number of patients and duration of follow-up planned. These plans should be based on the specific study objectives and endpoints used. If the same protocol includes plans for treating distinct subsets of patients, it is desirable to accrue sufficient numbers of patients of each type for separate analyses, because the relative merits of the treatments may vary substantially. Because of unforeseen complications or larger than expected treatment differences, patient accrual may have to be terminated prematurely. Nevertheless, target sample sizes are essential to ensure that the study is feasible and to know when to stop in the absence of premature termination. If too few patients are studied, the results may be ambiguous or erroneous, which often happens.[66-69] The protocol should document that the target sample size can be accrued within a reasonable period of time (usually 3–4 years).

The usual statistical methods of sample size determination in comparative trials are oversimplified as rigid models of the complete analysis, but are useful for planning purposes. These methods are based on the assumption that, at the conclusion of the trial, a statistical significance test will be performed comparing the treatment groups with regard to a primary endpoint. A statistical significance level of 0.05 resulting from a treatment comparison has the following meaning: If there is no true difference in treatment efficacy, the probability of obtaining a difference in outcomes as extreme as that observed in the data is 0.05. The significance level does not represent the probability that the null hypothesis is true; it represents a probability of an observed difference, assuming that the null hypothesis is true. Conventional statistical theory ascribes no probabilities to hypotheses, only to data. With few patients in each of the treatment groups being compared, the difference in observed outcomes must be very extreme for the significance level to be as small as 0.05. As sample size increases, smaller differences in outcome will be statistically significant at the 0.05 level. In comparing proportions, 10 of 10 compared with 7 of 10 (a difference of 30%) is not statistically significant at the 0.05 level, whereas 40 of 40 compared with 35 of 40 (a difference of 12%) is.

For comparing two proportions, the usual method of sample size determination is as follows. It is assumed that after n patients have been observed on treatment A and n patients have been observed on treatment B, a statistical significance test will be performed. We want to determine n to be just large enough so that if the true response rate for A is p_A (*i.e.*, the response rate that would be observed in an infinite number of patients receiving A) and the true response rate for B is p_B, 80% of the time the significance level will be no greater

TABLE 19–5. Number of Patients in Each of Two Treatment Groups (One-Sided Test)

Smaller Success Rate	Larger Minus Smaller Success Rate									
	0.05	0.10	0.15	0.20	0.25	0.30	0.35	0.40	0.45	0.50
0.05	512*	172	94	62	45	35	28	23	19	16
	381†	129	72	48	35	27	22	18	15	13
0.10	786	236	121	76	54	40	31	25	21	17
	579	176	91	58	41	31	24	20	16	14
0.15	1026	292	144	88	60	44	34	27	22	18
	752	216	108	66	46	34	26	21	17	14
0.20	1231	339	163	98	66	48	36	29	23	19
	900	250	121	73	50	37	28	22	18	15
0.25	1402	377	178	105	70	50	38	29	23	19
	1024	278	132	79	53	38	29	23	18	15
0.30	1539	407	189	111	73	52	38	30	23	19
	1122	300	141	83	55	39	30	23	18	15
0.35	1642	429	197	114	74	52	38	29	23	18
	1196	315	146	85	56	40	30	23	18	14
0.40	1711	441	201	115	74	52	38	29	22	17
	1246	324	149	86	56	39	29	22	17	14
0.45	1745	446	201	114	73	50	36	27	21	16
	1271	327	149	85	55	38	28	21	16	13
0.50	1745	441	197	111	70	48	34	25	19	15
	1271	324	146	83	53	37	26	20	15	12

* Upper figure: Significance level 0.05, power 0.90.
† Lower figure: Significance level 0.05, power 0.80.

than 0.05. The 80% figure is called *the power of the test for detecting the difference,* $p_B - p_A$.

If we think of a study resulting in a significance level of less than 0.05 for the major comparison as a positive study, the power represents the probability of getting a true positive result when the actual response rates are p_A and p_B. If treatment A is a standard treatment, p_A is estimated from past data. The absolute magnitude $|p_B - p_A|$ is viewed as a difference that researchers want to have a power of 80% (for example) for detecting. For comparing two proportions, Tables 19–5 and 19–6 can be used to determine the number of patients to be assigned each of two treatments to achieve a specified power as a function of the true response rates. Table 19–5 is for obtaining one-sided significance levels less than 0.05, and Table 19–6 is for two-sided significance levels of less than 0.05. A one-sided significance level represents the probability by chance alone of obtaining a difference as large as and in the same direction as that actually observed. A two-sided significance level represents the probability by chance alone of obtaining a difference in either direction as large in absolute magnitude as that actually observed. Controversy exists over the appropriateness of one-sided or two-sided significance levels. This is discussed later in the chapter. A two-sided significance level of 0.05, however, has become widely accepted as a standard level of evidence. Suppose that based on past data, researchers estimate the success rate for treatment A to be 30% and that they want to have 80% power for

detecting a true success rate of treatment B of 55%. For a two-sided statistical significance test, Table 19–6 shows that 68 patients for each of the two treatments are needed (136 patients total). If a power of 80% is desired for detecting a true success rate of treatment B of 50%, 103 patients per treatment are needed. The required number of patients increases rapidly as the size of the difference to be detected decreases. Almost all phase III studies should be at least large enough to detect reliably a difference of 20% in success rate. Usually, a difference of 10% to 15 % is more realistic to expect and will still be clinically important if the success rate in question is a cure rate or long-term survival rate. The "not statistically different" results of smaller comparative studies often are mistakenly interpreted as saying something about the treatments, whereas they may be just a consequence of the inadequate numbers of patients.[66-69]

Tables 19–5 and 19–6 were constructed according to the methods of Casagrande and coworkers and are considered more accurate than tables previously published based on other approximations.[70] When the smaller success rate is thought to exceed 50%, the Tables given in this chapter should be used to compare failure rates (100% minus response rate).

When an unbalanced K/1 randomization is contemplated for comparing two treatments, the total sample size obtained from Tables 19–5 and 19–6 should be multiplied by $(K + 1)^2/4K$. For example, a 2 to 1 randomization requires 12.5% more total patients than an equally weighted design of the same

TABLE 19–6. Number of Patients in Each of Two Treatment Groups (Two-Sided Test)

Smaller Success Rate	Larger Minus Smaller Success Rate									
	0.05	0.10	0.15	0.20	0.25	0.30	0.35	0.40	0.45	0.50
0.05	620*	206	113	74	54	42	33	27	23	19
	473†	159	88	58	43	33	27	22	18	16
0.10	956	285	146	92	64	48	38	30	25	21
	724	218	112	71	50	38	30	24	20	17
0.15	1250	354	174	106	73	53	41	33	26	22
	944	269	133	82	57	42	32	26	21	18
0.20	1502	411	197	118	79	57	44	34	27	22
	1132	313	151	91	62	45	34	27	22	18
0.25	1712	459	216	127	84	60	45	35	28	23
	1289	348	165	98	65	47	36	28	22	18
0.30	1880	495	230	134	88	62	46	36	28	22
	1414	375	175	103	68	48	36	28	22	18
0.35	2006	522	239	138	89	63	46	35	27	22
	1509	395	182	106	69	49	36	28	22	18
0.40	2090	537	244	139	89	62	45	34	26	21
	1571	407	186	107	69	48	36	27	21	17
0.45	2132	543	244	138	88	60	44	33	25	19
	1603	411	186	106	68	47	34	26	20	16
0.50	2132	537	239	134	84	57	41	30	23	17
	1603	407	182	103	65	45	32	24	18	14

* Upper figure: Significance level 0.05, power 0.90.
† Lower figure: Significance level 0.05, power 0.80.

power. Weightings more extreme than 2 to 1 are rarely desirable.

For comparative trials of proportions using historical controls, appropriate tables are given by Makuch and Simon and are summarized in Table 19–7.[71] This table is for achieving 80% power with a one-sided significance level of 0.05. If the historical control group of 50 patients showed a success rate of 30% and 80% power is wanted for detecting a true success rate of 50% for the new treatment, Table 19–7 indicates that 69 new patients should be treated with the new experimental therapy. If there were 100 appropriate historical controls, Table 19–7 indicates that 48 new patients should be treated with the experimental therapy. It is assumed that all new patients will be given the experimental therapy. Tannock and Warr[72] have pointed out that "phase II" trials of combinations of drugs already known to be active are best viewed as historically

controlled phase III trials and that the endpoint should reflect true patient benefit. For this reason and for reasons of study efficiency, it is often advisable to use complete response or survival as the endpoint. Thall and Simon[73] have extended the results of Table 19–7 in two ways. First, they take into account the degree of consistency obtained in multiple studies with the control treatment. Second, they determine the optimum proportion of new patients that should be assigned to the control group. This model assumes, however, that the historical controls are "comparable."

Tables for comparing proportions are useful when the endpoint can be dichotomized as success or failure, which can be done for the complete response rate. The tables also can be used when survival and continuous disease-free survival are compared. In such instances, the table is used with regard to the proportion of patients who survive (or remain without evidence of disease) for some meaningful period (*e.g.*, 5 years). The number of patients required must then be observed for this period. The final analysis of such studies, however, generally consists of a comparison of the entire survival curves rather than just the proportions surviving 5 years. It is not possible to produce general tables of required number of patients for comparing survival curves, because the results depend on the form of the survival distributions, accrual rates, and the follow-up period.

George and Desu[74] and Rubinstein and associates[75] have developed useful methods for determining the required number of patients and the duration of follow-up when the survival distributions have an exponential form. Exponential survival corresponds to a constant force of mortality, that is, a constant percentage of the remaining patients die each month. For exponential survivals, the number of deaths required to achieve a specified power depends only on the ratio of median survivals to be detected and not on the actual median values. For example, Table 19–8 shows the number of total deaths required to have 90% statistical power for detecting a specified ratio of median survivals. It must be remembered, however, that for a disease in which the probability of dying by the final analysis is 50%, the number of patients required is twice the tabulated value. Table 19–8 is actually valid whenever the "hazard ratio," the ratio of forces of mortality for the two treatment groups, is constant over time. The translation of number of deaths, or "events," required to number of patients

TABLE 19–7. Number of Patients Needed in an Experimental Group for 80% Power to Detect (One-Sided $\alpha = 0.05$) a Specified Difference in Success Rates

Proportion of Success for Historical Controls	Number of Historical Controls						
	20	30	40	50	75	100	200
0.10	*	223†	108	80	58	50	42
	116	53‡	40	35	29	27	24
	39	27§	23	21	18	18	16
	22	17‖	15	14	13	13	12
0.20	*	*	285	167	101	83	65
	385	98	67	55	44	40	35
	67	40	33	30	26	24	22
	31	23	21	19	18	17	16
0.30	*	*	554	259	137	108	80
	882	137	87	69	54	48	42
	86	49	39	35	30	29	26
	31	27	24	22	20	19	18
0.40	*	*	699	303	153	120	88
	913	147	92	74	58	52	44
	85	50	41	36	32	30	27
	36	27	24	22	21	20	19
0.50	*	*	538	267	145	115	86
	455	122	83	68	55	50	43
	67	44	37	34	30	28	26
	30	24	22	20	18	18	17
0.60	*	*	295	185	117	97	76
	179	83	63	55	46	42	38
	45	33	29	27	25	24	22
	22	19	17	17	15	15	15

* Required sample size >1000.
† Number of patients needed for the new treatment to detect a difference in success rate of 15 percentage points.
‡ Number of patients needed to detect a difference in success rate of 20 percentage points.
§ Number of patients needed to detect a difference in success rate of 25 percentage points.
‖ Number of patients needed to detect a difference in success rate of 30 percentage points.

TABLE 19–8. Number of Events Needed for Comparing Survival Curves

Percentage Reduction in Hazard of Death	Ratio of Median Survival for Exponential Distributions	Number of Total Deaths to Observe*
20	1.25	846
30	1.43	330
33	1.50	257
40	1.67	162
50	2.0	88

* Total number of deaths in both groups to have power 0.90 for detecting ratio of median survival. Type I error $\alpha = 0.05$ (two sided).

required depends on the actual survival distributions, the rate of accrual, and the duration of follow-up after accrual. Sample size planning for historically controlled studies with a survival or disease-free survival endpoint is discussed by Dixon and Simon.[76]

The kinds of methods described are useful for ensuring that sufficient numbers of patients are treated so that an improvement in response is not missed because of the random fluctuations of small numbers. Numerous published "negative" results are actually uninterpretable for this reason.[66] For studies comparing a standard treatment to a more conservative or less invasive therapy, it is particularly important that the sample size be large, because otherwise clinically significant reductions in effectiveness will not be statistically significant. In the usual statistical formulation, the null hypothesis specifies that the two treatments are equivalent. Acceptance of the null hypothesis may result in erroneous adoption of a new, more conservative therapy. The burden of proof for studies of this type should be on showing that results are similar, not on demonstrating that they are dissimilar. Consequently, accepting the null hypothesis based on a significance test of low power is inappropriate. Large numbers of patients are required to ensure that important differences can be ruled out in the analysis, which should consist of calculating confidence intervals for the true difference in efficacy. The confidence interval provides a much clearer picture of what differences in efficacy are consistent with the data than a significance test. Makuch and Simon[77] and Durrleman and Simon[78] discuss this approach for planning the size and duration of therapeutic equivalence trials.

INTERIM ANALYSES OF PHASE III TRIALS

The methods described previously for determining the required number of patients assume that statistical analysis will be performed only at the conclusion of the trial. If statistical significance tests are performed repeatedly throughout the trial, the probability that the difference in outcomes will be statistically significant at the 0.05 level at some point by chance alone is greater than 5%.[79] This probability is called the *type I error* of the design. For example, in a study that reports a significance level of less than 0.05 for the major comparison as a positive study, the type I error represents the probability of getting a false-positive result. Fleming and associates have shown that the type I error can be as great as 26% or more if a significance test is performed every 3 months of a 3-year trial comparing two identical treatments.[80]

Interim analyses can be misleading, because they may be dominated by differences in treatment efficacy for minor subsets of patients of poorer prognosis and by transient differences in the distribution of prognostic factors.[68] Interim analyses also may influence the types and numbers of patients subsequently entered and even cause undesirable changes in patient management and evaluation of response. For these reasons, it has become increasingly common in multicenter clinical trials to have interim results reviewed only by a data monitoring committee rather than by the participating physicians. This approach helps protect the patients by having interim results carefully evaluated by a multidisciplinary committee and helps protect the study from damage resulting from misinterpretation of interim results. It also permits phy-

sicians to deal honestly with their patients about participation in the clinical trial without being concerned about the frequently occurring transient trends or lack of trends in the interim data. For these same reasons, it generally is inappropriate to present interim results at national meetings or in journals.[81]

A number of useful statistical designs have been developed for monitoring and interpreting interim results. Perhaps the simplest are those of Haybittle[82] and Peto.[23] They suggest that interim differences be discounted unless the difference is statistically significant at the two-sided $p < 0.0025$ level. If the interim differences are not significant at this level, the trial continues until its originally intended size. The final analysis is performed without regard to the interim analyses, and the type I error is almost unaffected by the monitoring.

Pocock,[83] O'Brien and Fleming,[84] Fleming and colleagues,[85] and others have developed group-sequential methods for interim monitoring based on a prespecified number of planned analyses. The critical p value for determining whether an interim difference should be judged statistically significant depends on the number of analyses that will be performed during the study. For a five-stage trial—four interim analyses and one final analysis—the critical p values are shown in Table 19–9. These designs are further discussed by Geller,[86] Fleming and Watelet,[87] Emerson and Fleming,[88] and DeMets and Gail.[89]

Extreme treatment differences at an interim analysis are unusual in cancer clinical trials. It is commoner to find that interim results do not support the hypothesis that the experimental treatment is substantially better than the control. The method of stochastic curtailment[90] was developed for evaluating such a circumstance. At any interim analysis, the probability of rejecting the null hypothesis at the end of the trial is calculated. This probability is calculated conditional on the data already obtained and on the assumption that the alternative hypothesis of superiority of the experimental treatment, used in designing the trial, is true. If this "conditional power" is less than about 0.20, then the trial may be terminated with acceptance of the null hypothesis. Stochastic curtailment can also be used as a basis for early rejection of the null hypothesis, if the probability of rejecting the null hypothesis at the end, conditional on current data and calculated under the null hypothesis, exceeds 0.80. With stochastic curtailment, interim analyses need not be equally spaced and the number of interim analyses need not be specified in advance; in fact, monitoring may be continuous. Stochastic curtailment is also useful for

TABLE 19–9. Nominal Two-Sided Significance Levels for Interim Monitoring Methods That Maintain an Overall Type I Error Level of 0.05

Analysis Number	Pocock[83]	Peto et al[83] and Haybittle[82]	O'Brien and Fleming[84]	Fleming, et al[85]
1	0.016	0.0027	0.00001	0.0051
2	0.016	0.0027	0.0013	0.0061
3	0.016	0.0027	0.008	0.0073
4	0.016	0.0027	0.023	0.0089
Final	0.016	0.049	0.041	0.0402

indicating when the actual failure rate in the control group is so much less than the planned failure rate that the clinical trial is no longer feasible. Halperin and colleagues,[91] Anderson,[92] and Cantor[93] have shown how to compute the conditional power needed to employ stochastic curtailment.

Several investigators have developed other designs for early termination of the clinical trial, if results are not promising for the experimental treatment.[94–98] For example, Table 19–10 shows some of the two-stage designs developed by Thall and coworkers for clinical trials with a dichotomous endpoint.[95] The first two columns show the hypothesized success rates for the control and experimental treatments. The remaining columns show the first-stage sample size per treatment and the maximum sample size per treatment. In all instances, the clinical trial is terminated after the first stage, and the experimental treatment is rejected as superior if the one-sided significance level for comparing success rates is not less than approximately 0.38. If the one-sided significance level is less than 0.38, then a second stage of patient accrual is completed to give the maximum sample size per group shown. When the treatments are equivalent, the probability of early termination is generally 60% to 65% with this design.

Schaid and associates developed designs for early termination when results are not promising in survival studies.[97] It provides for multiple experimental treatment arms, as do the designs of Thall and colleagues.[99,100] Such designs have been reviewed by Simon.[61] Jennison and Turnbull have presented methods for calculating confidence intervals for treatment differences at interim analyses.[101] Such confidence intervals can be useful in deciding when to terminate the trial.

The sequential designs that have been developed are useful tools for the difficult decisions sometimes presented by interim monitoring. Important clinical trials can be easily ruined by poorly based decisions to terminate early. Such errors are sometimes the result of inadequate recognition of the variability of sequentially accumulating data and sometimes of incomplete or poor quality data. Resulting publications foist unreliable conclusions on the medical community. The protocol should generally specify the target number of patients to be accrued, the duration of follow-up, and an interim monitoring plan that is soundly based statistically. It is usually inappropriate to present interim results at professional meetings or to publish results before accrual is complete and sufficient patient follow-up has occurred to ensure stability of conclusions.

EPIDEMIOLOGY OF CLINICAL TRIALS

Staquet and coworkers[102] and Zelen[103] have pointed out that many of the positive results reported from small trials can be expected to be false positives. In 100 trials, suppose there are 10 in which the experimental treatment is enough better than the control to have an 80% chance of detecting the difference in a small- or moderate-sized clinical trial. Of these 10 trials, obtaining a statistically significant difference in 8 cases (0.80 × 10) is expected. Of the remaining 90 trials, it is assumed that the treatments are approximately equivalent. Researchers expect to obtain a statistically significant difference in 5% (4.5) of these cases. Hence, of the 12.5 (8 + 4.5) trials that yield statistically significant results, the finding is a false-positive result in 4.5 of 12.5, or 36%, of the time. The 36% false-positive result is striking. It does depend on the assumption that only 10% of the trials actually represent important advances, but this assumption does not seem overly conservative. An additional factor to consider is that of publication bias.[104] This denotes the preference of journals to publish positive rather than negative results. A negative result from a small trial may not be published at all, and if it is, it is likely to be published in a less widely read journal than if the result were positive. Hence, even if the results of false positives are contradicted by the results of true negative trials comparing the same treatments, the existence of the latter may not be known.

These results should not be interpreted as contradicting the value of innovative single-institution clinical trials. Eliminating such trials would eliminate much of the possibility of real advances and the false-positive claims. It is important to re-

TABLE 19–10. Two-Stage Early Termination Designs

Success Rate Control	Success Rate Experimental Treatment	Power 0.80		Power 0.90	
		Stage 1 Sample Size per Treatment	Maximum Sample Size per Treatment	Stage 1 Sample Size per Treatment	Maximum Sample Size per Treatment
0.2	0.35	48	116	73	157
0.2	0.40	28	68	43	92
0.3	0.45	56	137	85	185
0.3	0.50	33	78	48	106
0.4	0.55	61	146	92	197
0.4	0.60	33	82	51	110
0.5	0.65	59	143	89	193
0.5	0.70	33	78	49	106
0.6	0.75	53	128	81	173
0.6	0.80	28	68	42	72

member, however, that results in the medical literature cannot generally be accepted at face value, and it is essential to recognize that "positive" results need confirmation in multicenter randomized clinical trials before they can be believed and applied to the general population.[105]

DATA MANAGEMENT

Data management is an important part of the conduct of a clinical trial. Obtaining reliable data requires the same planning and professional expertise as do the other aspects of the study. Some general guidelines for data management follow, although these are not applicable to all situations:

1. Data forms should be as simple and unambiguous as possible.
2. Relatively extensive initial information about patients should be collected, but the follow-up information should generally be limited to the major endpoints and serious complications.
3. Details of treatment administration should be reviewed continuously so that errors and misinterpretations can be corrected for future patients quickly.
4. Forms should be completed only by fully qualified persons. Uniformity of subjective evaluations should be ensured.
5. Whenever possible, an existing computerized data management system should be used rather than hiring programmers to start from scratch.
6. Data management should be treated seriously, and problems quickly resolved.

Physicians often design more extensive data forms than are actually needed, which results in unnecessary complexity in the conduct of the study, increased expense, and reduced reliability of the most important data elements. When expense is not an issue, it is difficult to argue against the potential value of data. But expense is generally an important issue, and collecting extensive data reliably is expensive. The development of good forms and procedures should occupy a prominent role in the planning process. If it is not treated with due respect by the trial organizers or supported adequately, the consequences are severe. The European Organization for Research on Treatment of Cancer Study Group on Data Management have compiled a book that describes the many important substantive, logistic, and administrative aspects of data management.[106]

ETHICS

INFORMED CONSENT

The basic principle of a clinical trial is to give patients the best known treatment in a preplanned manner that allows reliable conclusions to be drawn that can benefit future patients. The United States has adopted regulations for the protection of human subjects in research.[107] One of the regulations of the U.S. Department of Health and Human Services is that the investigator obtain informed consent of the patient or the patient's legally authorized representative. The three

major elements of informed consent are information, comprehension, and voluntariness. The regulation specifies that the consent must be sought under conditions that provide the patient an opportunity to consider whether to participate and that minimize the possibility of coercion. The information must be presented in language the patient can understand. Informed consent must be documented by use of a form signed by the patient. The basic required elements of informed consent are as follows:

1. A statement that the study involves research, an explanation of the purposes and procedures of the research, and identification of experimental procedures to be used.
2. A description of reasonably foreseeable risks to the patient.
3. A description of any benefits to the patient or others that may result from the research.
4. A disclosure of appropriate alternative procedures or treatments.
5. A statement concerning confidentiality of records and the possibility that the FDA may inspect the records.
6. An explanation of whether compensation or treatment is available if injury occurs.
7. An explanation of whom to contact concerning further information on the research or patients' rights and whom to contact in the event of a research-related injury.
8. A statement that participation is voluntary and that refusal will involve no loss of benefits to which the patient is otherwise entitled.

Informed consent is required in the United States for clinical trials. Some physicians believe that the process may be detrimental to the mental health of patients who do not want to know all of the potential, although perhaps unlikely, complications of therapy. For randomized studies, informed consent should be sought before the randomization is performed. Consequently, the patient must agree to accept any of the treatments being compared. This condition makes clear to the patient that the physician does not reliably know which treatment is best. This may be embarrassing to the physician and unsettling to the patient.

Many people have pointed out that informed consent is often not really informed, because most patients have neither the educational background nor the psychologic composure to be truly informed. Some people believe that the process of informed consent is "a legalistic trick to devolve what should properly be the doctor's responsibility onto the patient."[23] Informed consent is important. However, it is likely that most abuses of information occur outside clinical trials.

PRERANDOMIZATION

Zelen[108] proposed a design in which patients are randomized *after* being found eligible for the protocol but before consent to participate is sought. With one version of his proposal, consent is sought only for patients randomized to an experimental therapy. This version was controversial with regard to ethical considerations. The other version of Zelen's proposal involves seeking consent for both randomized groups of patients. Because the treatment assignment is known and can be presented at the time consent is sought, it was thought that physicians would approach more patients for participation in the trial, and patients would be more likely to participate. To avoid the possibility of bias in analysis of results, patients must be compared "as randomized" rather than "as treated." That is, a patient randomized to treatment A who refused and then received treatment B must be considered in the group A for analysis. Otherwise, the treatment comparison can be biased by a possible relation among prognosis, treatment, and refusal rate. Because the analysis must be performed as randomized, refusals dilute the differences in outcome that can be observed. To counteract this effect, the number of patients must be increased compared with a conventional trial in which most refusals occur before randomization and can be excluded from the analysis. The relation between refusal rate and increased sample size required for a prerandomization design is dramatic and is shown in Table 19–11. For a 15% refusal rate, the number of patients required is twice that of a conventional randomized trial. Even though the informed consent process may be more comfortable for the physician, it seems unlikely that prerandomization would often result in a doubling of accrual.

Two other concerns have been expressed about prerandomization.[109] First is the ethical issue of whether patients are really fully informed about possible alternative treatments when randomization has already occurred. The second issue is that there will be demand to analyze results as randomized and as treated. The results may differ, ruining credibility of the trial. Prerandomization is attractive to some physicians, although there is a lack of awareness of the earlier-mentioned problems. The limited experience to date with this design has given mixed results. Refusal rates have ranged from 10% to 30%. Accrual generally has increased, but not always by an amount sufficient to compensate for the inefficiency of the design.[109]

ACCUMULATING INFORMATION

Many researchers have struggled with the following question: Although it may be ethical to initiate a randomized clinical trial, does not the accumulation of interim results favoring one treatment make it unethical for a physician to continue entering patients? If the rate of patient entry is rapid compared with the time required to observe the major endpoints (*e.g.,* survival or duration of remission), this problem does not arise. A strong impetus for the development of sequential analysis methods has been to enable a reliable conclusion to be reached as early as possible for trials with slower accrual. Statistical methods of sequential analysis, however, are not, in themselves, substitutes for the human monitoring of interim results. Chalmers and others have suggested that the decision of when a trial should stop should be in the hands of a small monitoring committee that contains people who are not themselves entering patients into the study.[31,81] The physicians entering patients do not see interim results; hence, in a multiinstitution study, their opinions about the relative value of the treatments would remain essentially unchanged. With this approach, clinical trials are less likely to be terminated prematurely based on concern about transient trends or decreased accrual due to failure to see trends. This approach is used widely in fields other than oncology. Many cancer cooperative groups have now established study-specific data monitoring committees for all of their phase III trials, and they keep interim results blinded from other physicians. Because of the number of trials involved, completely independent committees have not been feasible.

The focus on ethical problems of accumulating information in randomized clinical trials derives to some extent from an oversimplified view of such studies. Most major trials are complex, requiring large sample sizes and long-term follow-up for evaluation of survival and complications. It is often difficult to evaluate the treatments thoroughly, even when accrual is completed, and to interpret the results in the context of other studies. This type of reliable evaluation usually is impossible during accrual with limited follow-up on limited numbers of patients and incomplete data, even for those already entered. In addition, few randomized studies result in treatments that differ so greatly in efficacy and with such slow accrual as to require early termination.

ANALYSIS

This section addresses several general aspects of analysis that are important for interpreting the researcher's own results and those of others.

SIGNIFICANCE LEVELS AND HYPOTHESIS TESTS

Medical decision making is complicated, and clinicians frequently misinterpret statistical significance tests in search of clear-cut answers from ambiguous data. A statistical significance level for comparing outcomes represents the probability of obtaining a difference as large as that actually obtained if the treatments were actually of equal efficacy and differences occur merely by chance. If differences in either direction as large in absolute value as the one actually obtained are included, the significance level is called *two sided*. If the probability is calculated only for differences in the same direction as that actually obtained, the significance level is called *one sided*. Generally, the two-sided significance level is twice the one-sided level.

TABLE 19–11. Prerandomization Sample Size Inflation Factor According to Overall Refusal Rate[96]

Refusal Rate	Inflation Factor
0.02	1.09
0.05	1.23
0.10	1.56
0.15	2.04
0.20	2.78
0.25	4.00
0.30	6.25
0.35	11.11
0.40	25
0.45	100
0.50	*

* If half the patients on each arm refuse to receive the other treatment, determination of differences in treatment effect is impossible, regardless of the sample size.

After significance tests had been used for many years, Neyman and Pearson[110] formalized a mathematic theory of "hypothesis testing." In this theory, before it is implemented, the study specifies a null hypothesis, an alternative hypothesis, and a decision rule for accepting one hypothesis and rejecting the other, based on the data obtained. The fraction of the time that the null hypothesis will be rejected in hypothetical repetitions of the experiment when it is in fact true is called the *type I error*. Similarly, the *type II error* is the fraction of the time that the alternative hypothesis would be rejected when it is true. The theory appeals to clinicians, because it simplifies complex medical decision making by providing "yes" or "no" answers: either the difference is "statistically significant" or it is not—period. The distinction between one- and two-sided decision rules becomes crucial because a one-sided $p = 0.05$ is simply "nonsignificant" if a type I error of 0.05 based on a two-sided decision rule is prespecified. Consideration of hypotheses suggested by the data is strictly forbidden in this framework.

The concept of prespecification of hypotheses is important for medical experimentation. But the accept-reject nomenclature of the Neyman-Pearson theory provides an oversimplified and sometimes misleading interpretation of the data. Significance levels can serve as useful aids to interpretation of results, but quibbling about whether a one-sided $p = 0.04$ is significant makes little sense. Significance levels are influenced by sample sizes, and failure to reject the null hypothesis does not mean that the outcomes are not different. There is no simple index of truth for interpreting results. Many physicians attempt to use the notion of statistical significance in this way, but the attempt has an unsound basis. Thorough presentation, skeptical evaluation, and cautious interpretation of results are always required.

Confidence intervals are generally much more informative than significance levels or the declaration of statistical significance. A confidence interval for the size of the treatment difference provides a range of effects consistent with the data. The significance level tells little about the size of the treatment effect, because it depends critically on the sample size. However, it is the size of the treatment effects, as communicated by confidence intervals, that should be used in weighting the costs and benefits of clinical decision making. Many "negative" results are actually "noninformative," and confidence intervals help determine when this is the case. Simon[69] has presented a nontechnical discussion of how to calculate confidence intervals for treatment differences with different types of endpoints.

EXCLUSIONS

Excluding patients from analysis because of treatment deviations, early death, or patient withdrawal can severely distort the results.[23,45,45a,111,112] Often, excluded patients have poorer outcomes than those not excluded. Researchers can rationalize that patients not receiving treatment as specified in the protocol did worse because of that fact, but this is just a rationalization, which may be erroneous. The poor prognosis of these patients may have led directly or indirectly to their exclusion. For example, in the Coronary Drug Project,[113] the 5-year mortality for poor adherers to placebo was 28.3%, significantly greater than the 15.1% for good adherers to placebo

($p = 4.7 \times 10^{-16}$). In randomized trials, there may be more potential exclusions in one treatment group, or the reasons for potential exclusion may differ among treatments. Excluding patients (or "analyzing them separately," which is equivalent to excluding them) for reasons other than that they did not satisfy the eligibility criteria of the study is a major problem in interpreting many studies. In randomized trials, the "intention-to-treat" analysis with all eligible randomized patients included should be the primary analysis. It is the result that is meaningful for broad-scale applicability of the results. If the conclusions of a study depend on exclusions, then these conclusions are suspect. Eligibility criteria for patients and collaborators should be established in such a way that there will be few protocol deviations. Generally, the treatment plan should be viewed as a policy to be evaluated. The treatment intended to be administered cannot be delivered uniformly well for all patients, but all eligible patients should generally be evaluable in phase III studies.

PROGNOSTIC FACTORS AND MULTIPLE ANALYSES

If major prognostic factors are known beforehand, it is often desirable to incorporate these factors into the analysis to correct for imbalances or to improve the precision of the estimates of treatment differences. It is common in clinical trial results for investigators to document that there are no statistically significant differences between the treatment groups with regard to prognostic factors. Although the documentation of comparability is important, the lack of statistical significance of any differences is irrelevant.[114] Nonstatistically significant imbalances for important prognostic factors can have a large effect on the comparisons of treatments with regard to outcome. It is generally desirable to incorporate major prognostic factors as stratification variables in the randomization. This method avoids the subjectivity that results from determining post hoc which variables to adjust for.[115]

Multiple subset analyses are often carried too far, however.[116,117] Table 19–12 shows the probability of obtaining at least one statistically significant ($p < 0.05$) difference by chance alone as a function of the number of independent comparisons of two equivalent treatments. With only five comparisons, the chance of at least one false-positive conclusion is 22.6%. When the number of endpoints, interim anal-

TABLE 19–12. Probability of Obtaining at Least One Statistically Significant ($p < 0.05$) Difference by Chance Alone in Multiple Comparisons of Two Equivalent Treatments

Number of Comparisons	Probability of at Least One "Significant" Difference (%)
1	5
2	9.7
3	14.3
4	18.5
5	22.6
10	40
20	64.1

yses, and subsets are considered in the analysis of clinical trials, these results should be disturbing. The comparisons performed in clinical trials are not entirely independent, but this does not have a major effect on ameliorating the problem. Fleming and Watelet[87] performed a computer simulation to determine the chance of obtaining a statistically significant treatment difference when two equivalent treatments in six subsets determined by three dichotomous variables are compared. The chance of a statistically significant difference between treatments in at least one subset was 20% at the final analysis and 39% in the final or one of the three interim analyses. Subset analysis, comparison of treatments with regard to multiple endpoints, and multiple interim analyses are common sources of erroneous conclusions. The primary endpoint should be defined in the protocol. Subset analyses and analyses with regard to other endpoints should be specified in advance as defined secondary analyses, and statistical significance should be declared only for significance levels much more extreme than the conventional 0.05. The simplest approach to multiple comparisons is to declare statistical significance only if the *p* value is less than 0.05/n, where n denotes the number of comparisons to be made. For example if n = 5, then 0.01 should be used; if n = 10, then 0.005 should apply. *Interaction tests* are statistical procedures that test for lack of homogeneity of treatment effect across subsets of patients. A statistically significant interaction should be documented before claiming that treatment effects vary among subsets. Such tests are described by Simon[117,118] and Gail and Simon.[119]

Generally, it is not valid to subset or to adjust the analysis by characteristics measured after the start of treatment (*e.g.,* treatment compliance, dose delivered, or toxicity). Analyses not restricted to the widely recognized endpoints and the few major subset hypotheses specified at the outset should be interpreted generally as hypothesis generation to be tested in a subsequent study.

ESTIMATION OF SURVIVAL FUNCTIONS

Representation of the distribution of survivals for a group of patients is a commonly encountered problem. The problem of representing the distribution of remission duration or time until disease progression is mathematically identical, although survivals are referred to in this discussion. The usual elementary methods of plotting histograms or calculating means and medians generally are not applicable, because some patients will not have died at the time of analysis. The data contain censored observations in the sense that survivals are known only to be at least as great as the observed values for the living patients.

The most satisfactory way of representing such data is to estimate the survival function S(t). This function represents the probability of surviving more than t time units. Time t is measured from diagnosis, start of treatment, or some other meaningful time-point. For randomized studies, it is best to measure time from the date of randomization. There are basically two satisfactory methods for estimating S(t). The first is the life table or actuarial method. It frequently is attributed to Berkson and Gage[120] or Cutler and Ederer[121] and is appropriate when the number of patients is large. The other method is the product limit method of Kaplan and Meier.[122] This method is appropriate for any number of patients, but it involves more effort than the life table method when the number of patients is large.

The first step in the application of either method is the calculation of survival time for all patients. Survival is the duration from the chosen baseline (*e.g.,* date of randomization) until death or date last known to be alive for patients who are not known to have died. To use the life table method, intervals for the grouping of survival times are determined. The life table, shown in Table 19–13, is then filled out. This sample life table is prepared with yearly intervals in the first column. The number of patients alive at the beginning of the interval is entered in column 2. The number who died in the interval is entered in column 4. Patients dying exactly at a time that represents a boundary between two intervals (*e.g.,* 365 days) are considered to have died in the preceding interval (*e.g.,* 0–1 year). Column 3 contains the number of patients who are lost to follow-up during the interval or are alive with maximum follow-up duration included in the interval. These latter patients are referred to as *withdrawn alive* in the conventional life table terminology. The life table method assumes that patients lost to follow-up or withdrawn alive during the interval are at risk of death for half of the interval. Hence column 5, the number alive at the start of the interval minus half the

TABLE 19–13. Life Table Method for Estimating a Survival Distribution

Years After Randomization $x - 1$ to x	No. Alive at Beginning of Interval 1_x	No. Lost to Follow-up or Withdrawn Alive During Interval w_x	No. Died During Interval d_x	Effective No. Exposed to Risk of Dying During Interval (Col 2 – ½ Col 3)	Proportion Dying (Col 4/Col 5) q_x	Proportion Surviving (Col 1 – Col 6) p_x	Cumulative Proportion Surviving From Randomization Through End of Interval $(p_1 \times p_2 \times \cdots \times p_x)$ S_x
0–1	252	38	94	233	0.40	0.60	0.60
1–2	120	34	10	103	0.10	0.90	0.54
2–3	76	30	4	61	0.07	0.93	0.50
3–4	42	18	4	33	0.12	0.88	0.44
4–5	20	12	0	14	0.00	1.00	0.44
5–6	8	8	0	4	0.00	1.00	0.44

Col, column.

number lost or withdrawn during the interval, represents an approximate number of patients at risk of death during the interval. Column 6 gives the ratio of the number of patients who died during the interval to the number at risk during the interval. Column 7 gives the estimated probability of surviving the interval for patients alive at the start of the interval. Column 8 should be studied carefully, because it provides the life table estimate of the survival distribution and indicates the logic behind the method. The probability of surviving more than 3 years after randomization, for example, equals the entry in the third row of column 8 (0.50). The logic is as follows: To survive 3 full years, the patients must survive through the first year, and given that the patients have survived the first year, they must survive the second year; and given that they have survived the second year, they must survive the third year. Consequently, the probability of surviving for at least 3 years is estimated by the product $p_1 \times p_2 \times p_3$ of factors in column 7. By using this product, the life table method takes maximal advantage of the mortality experience of patients with limited follow-up. The entry S_x in column 8, row x, represents the life table estimate of the probability of surviving more than x years from randomization. Computational shortcuts to observe are that for column 8, S_x equals p_x times S_{x-1}, and for column 2, $1_{x+1} = 1_x - w_x - d_x$.

The product limit method of Kaplan and Meier is similar in concept to the life table method. With the Kaplan-Meier approach, however, the intervals are defined by the actual survival times of patients who have died. Suppose, for example, that the survivals are 3, 3, 3+, 5, 6, 8+, 8+, 10, 10, and 12+ months, where a plus follows survivals for patients still alive. Then the intervals are 0 to 3, 3 to 5, 5 to 6, and 6 to 10 months, as shown in Table 19–14. With the Kaplan-Meier method, deaths occur only at the end of intervals. The entry 1_x in column 5 equals $1_x - w_x$ rather than $1_x - \frac{1}{2}w_x$ for the life table method. This is because deaths occur only at the ends of intervals here, and the number of patients at risk of death just before the interval end is $1_x - w_x$. In the entry w_x in column 3 for the Kaplan-Meier method, patients who are lost to follow-up or withdrawn alive at the end of an interval are considered not lost or withdrawn until the following interval. These differences between the Kaplan-Meier and life tables methods render the former more appropriate for studies with smaller numbers of patients.

After the values S_x have been calculated for the Kaplan-

Meier method, they may be graphed with time on the horizontal axis. The graph is a step function that starts at time zero and ordinate 1.0. It drops to value S_x at time x, where x is the time at the right end of an interval. The survival curve corresponding to Table 19–14 is shown in Figure 19–1. The tic marks are placed on the curve at 3, 8, and 12 months to represent the follow-up times of living patients. The step function is extended horizontally out to 12 months to represent follow-up of the last patient. The estimator S_x is approximately normally distributed in large samples. If m patients remain alive at time x, the standard error of S_x can be conservatively estimated as[45,45a]

$$S_x \sqrt{(1 - S_x)/m}$$

More extensive, but fairly nontechnical, discussions of statistical methods for the analysis of clinical trial data are given by Anderson and colleagues[123] and Harrington and Anderson.[124]

REPORTING RESULTS OF CLINICAL TRIALS

Effective reporting of results is an integral part of good research. Unfortunately, numerous reviews have indicated that the quality of reporting of clinical trial results is poor.[111,112,125–129] Pocock and associates concluded that "overall, the reporting of clinical trials appears to be biased toward an exaggeration of treatment differences."[127] Barr and Tannock have given a clear illustration of how this is easily done.[111] Simon and Wittes developed a set of methodologic guidelines for reports of clinical trials, and these guidelines have been adopted by major cancer journals worldwide.[130] The nine guidelines are listed as follows, with brief comments:

1. Authors should discuss briefly the quality control methods used to ensure that the data are complete and accurate. A reliable procedure should be cited for ensuring that all patients entered on study are actually reported on. If such procedures are not in place, their absence should be noted. Any procedures employed to ensure that assessment of major endpoints is reliable (*e.g.*, second-party review of responses) should be mentioned or their absence noted.

TABLE 19–14. Kaplan-Meier Method for Estimating a Survival Distribution

Months After Random- ization	No. Alive at Beginning of Interval 1_x	No. Lost to Follow-up or Withdrawn Alive During Interval w_x	No. Died During Interval d_x	Effective No. Exposed to Risk of Dying Just Before End of Interval (Col 2 – Col 3)	Proportion Dying (Col 4/Col 5) q_x	Proportion Surviving (1 – Col 6) p_x	Cumulative Proportion Surviving From Randomization Through End of Interval $(p_1 \times p_2 \times \cdots \times p_x)$ S_x
0–3	10	0	2	10	0.2	0.8	0.8
3–5	8	1	1	7	0.14	0.86	0.68
5–6	6	0	1	6	0.17	0.83	0.57
6–10	5	2	2	3	0.67	0.33	0.19

Col, column.

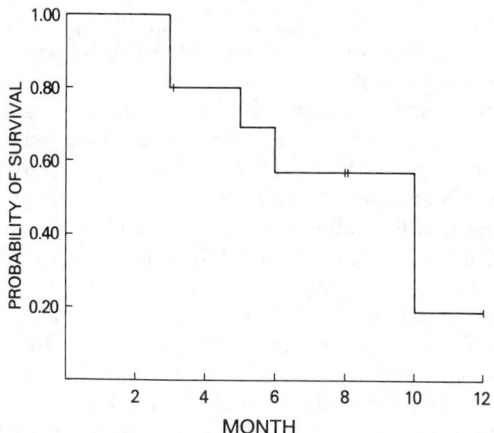

FIGURE 19–1.   Example of estimated survival distribution.

Comment. The intent is that a report make clear the extent to which the major data of the study rest on a firm and verifiable foundation. To ensure that all patients entered on a study are in fact included in the final report, there should be a formal registration mechanism for study entry. Quality control of response assessment requires much greater attention than it usually receives. Currently, numerous response criteria are employed, and the interobserver reliability of these is almost totally unknown. In any instance in which such procedures are in place, they should be explicitly cited in the methods section of the manuscript.

2. All patients registered on study should be accounted for. The report should specify for each treatment the number of patients who were not eligible, died, or withdrew before treatment began. The distribution of follow-up times should be described for each treatment, and the number of patients lost to follow-up should be given.

   Comment. Differences in policies for excluding patients from analysis are a source of variation in results among similar studies. Regardless of how response rates are calculated, all patients must be accounted for. This inclusion permits readers to recalculate rates as they want.

3. The study should not have an inevaluability rate for major endpoints of greater than 15%. Not more than 15% of eligible patients should be lost to follow-up or considered inevaluable for response due to early death, protocol violation, missing information, or other reasons.

   Comment. The 15% figure is somewhat arbitrary, but inevaluability rates of ≥20% usually reflect inappropriate patient selection. For phase III studies, disqualifications are a source of potential bias; when the disqualification rate approaches the magnitude of the difference in outcomes being tested, the results are not sufficiently reliable.

4. In randomized studies, the report should include a comparison of survival and other major endpoints for all eligible patients as randomized, that is, with no exclusions other than those not meeting eligibility criteria.

   Comment. Comparisons of outcomes in randomized studies that exclude eligible randomized patients are subject to potential bias. Patients who refuse further treatment, for example, may be prognostically fa-

vorable or unfavorable. This observation has been demonstrated for placebo patients in major cardiovascular trials. Consequently, the analysis of randomized trials should contain comparisons of all eligible randomized patients. The report may also contain other comparisons.

5. The sample size should be sufficient to establish or conclusively rule out the existence of effects of clinically meaningful magnitude. For "negative" results in therapeutic comparisons, the adequacy of sample size should be demonstrated by presenting confidence limits for true treatment differences or calculating statistical power for detecting differences.

   Comment. This point is basic but often not recognized. Small studies that find no statistically significant differences between treatments are generally indeterminate, not negative. Unfortunately, such studies are usually erroneously interpreted as negative. The problem is that the statistical power of small studies (*i.e.*, the probability of obtaining a statistically significant difference if the two treatments are truly different) is low. Reporting confidence limits in addition to or instead of significance levels clarifies the distinction between indeterminate and negative results.[69] For example, suppose the response rate for treatment A is 10 of 20 (50%) and for treatment B is 8 of 20 (40%). This difference is not significant ($p = 0.75$). But approximate 95% confidence limits for the true differences in response rates are −20.7% to +40.7%, so the data are consistent with a moderate difference favoring treatment B and a tremendous difference favoring treatment A. The trial is not negative but indeterminate; the *p* value is misleading, and the number of patients is inadequate.

   A sample size that is insufficient to answer the question originally posed by the trial is a serious problem. Oncologists and cancer patients are not well served by the publication of results that are inconclusive because of avoidable flaws in trial execution. The trial that does not accrue an adequate number of patients is a failed experiment; unless the reason for the poor accrual is itself illuminating, the field is no wiser after the trial than before.

6. Authors should state whether there was an initial target sample size and if so, what it was. They should specify how frequently interim analyses were performed and how the decisions to stop accrual and report results were arrived at.

   Comment. This refers to the sequential analysis of data as they are accumulating. It is not appropriate to interpret significance levels and confidence intervals at face value if accumulating data are repeatedly analyzed. That is, stopping accrual and publishing results as soon as a *p* value falls below 0.05 is a procedure with a high probability of producing erroneous conclusions. Generally, it is necessary to perform interim evaluation of results, but premature termination and reporting of the study should be based on *p* values much smaller than 0.05, if unreliable results are to be avoided.

7. Controls are generally not required for single-agent phase II trials, because no claims of therapeutic efficacy are (or should be) made. Such trials attempt to evaluate

only antitumor activity. Phase III trials, however, require controls. Nonrandomized studies should be performed as well as possible using explicit controls for which comparability can be thoroughly evaluated on a patient-by-patient basis. Comparison of survival between responders and nonresponders is not a valid way of establishing therapeutic efficacy.[14-16] This comparison can be biased in several ways. First, patients who die quickly are, by definition, nonresponders. Hence, there is a time bias. Second, responders may have more favorable prognoses, regardless of treatment. They may have less disease, less prior treatment, and better performance status. They may also be more favorable with regard to unknown prognostic factors. To evaluate the impact of a treatment on survival or disease-free survival, outcomes for all of the treated patients should be compared with those for an appropriate control group.

8. The patients studied should be adequately described. Applicability of conclusions to other patients should be carefully dealt with. Claims of subset-specific treatment differences must be carefully documented statistically as more than the random results of multiple-subset analyses.

    Comment. Care should be employed in extrapolating results to the general population of patients. Only a small fraction of patients enter clinical trials, and they are not a random sample. Proper statistical methodology is necessary to distinguish true subset-specific treatment differences from the random results of multiple-subset analyses. It is not generally recognized that, by chance alone, there is a 40% probability of finding at least one statistically significant false-positive treatment difference in the evaluation of ten disjoint subsets.

9. The methods of statistical analysis should be described in detail sufficient that a knowledgeable reader could reproduce the analysis if the data were available.

META-ANALYSIS

A meta-analysis is a quantitative summary of research in a particular area. It is distinguished from the traditional literature review by its emphasis on quantifying results on individual studies and on combining results across studies. Traditional reviews are often selective and subjective. Meta-analysis originated in the social sciences. It has become extremely popular in the fields of psychology and education, but the value of the approach remains controversial.[131] A major point of concern is the tendency to combine dissimilar studies and to overemphasize average results.

Research reviews in medical therapeutics are often limited by unavailability of actual study data to compare, reanalyze, and perhaps combine. During the past few years, a new type of review method has appeared in the medical literature.[132] Key components of this method are to include only randomized clinical trials; include all relevant randomized trials that have been initiated anywhere in the world, whether completed, published, or not; exclude no randomized patients from analysis; and assess therapeutic effectiveness based on the average results pooled across trials.

With this approach, attention is restricted to randomized trials, because potential bias from nonrandomized comparisons may swamp out small to moderate therapeutic effects. Including all relevant randomized trials that have been initiated anywhere in the world represents an attempt to avoid publication bias and ensures that all relevant evidence is available. Physicians tend to focus on "positive" results and discount "negative" results of related but nonidentical clinical trials. Publication bias[104] results from the tendency of journals to accept positive rather than negative studies. Avoiding exclusion of any randomized patient for reasons such as protocol compliance is also to avoid bias, because patients excluded from one treatment may be prognostically different than those excluded from another. Assessing therapeutic effectiveness based on average pooled results is an attempt to make recommendations based on the totality of evidence rather than on extreme but irreproducible isolated reports. In calculating average results, a measure of difference in outcome between treatments is calculated separately for each study. A weighted average of these study-specific differences is then computed.

A major issue of concern is the reasonableness of the calculation of average effect.[132] When the studies being pooled are similar with regard to the therapy delivered, patient population, and data quality, then averaging the results makes sense. In this situation, pooling could be valuable for detecting moderate treatment effects and may be essential for examining patient subsets. Often, however, the studies will not be similar. These studies will differ with regard to the therapeutic interventions compared. Generally, even if two studies plan to employ the same interventions, the doses actually delivered may differ grossly. Such differences may be accentuated by including all worldwide studies. Studies may also differ with regard to the kinds of patients included, and these differences can influence results. For example, older patients may tolerate intensive chemotherapy less well and have higher rates of death from other causes. Studies may also differ greatly with regard to degree of protocol compliance, adequacy of follow-up, and reliability of data.

When the studies differ substantially, it must be recognized that the average results may not be representative of the components making up the average. For example, substantial effectiveness of one treatment or one class of patients may be masked by pooling with ineffective treatments or unresponsive types of patients. Peto[133] argued that, although the degree of effectiveness may vary, unanticipated reversals of outcome differences ("qualitative interactions") are unlikely, That is, if one subset of patients benefits from the experimental treatment, then the other subsets may benefit more or less, but will not be harmed by the treatment. When dealing with toxic or expensive treatments, however, differences of degree, even without reversals, may severely limit the extent to which the results are useful for patient care purposes.

Unfortunately, the database available in a meta-analysis is often insufficient to answer the question of whether different classes of treatments have different levels of effects relative to a control or whether effects differ substantially among subsets of patients. This should not necessarily be viewed as a license to pool results across classes of treatment or patients on grounds of practicality. Although the average result can be of interest in itself, the overview should identify when the data are inadequate as a basis for reaching strong conclusions. If results are inconclusive because of lack of data or substantial interstudy variability, then that should be a primary conclusion.

In reporting a meta-analysis, it is important to display the results of individual trials in a manner that permits assessment of whether they are consistent with one another or whether there are outliers that dominate the averages. Although formal interaction tests may not be sufficiently powerful to test homogeneity of results, graphic display is important. The apparent outliers may provide leads to follow-up. The meta-analysis should attempt to understand major interstudy differences in results, not just average the outcomes. This process requires substantial knowledge of the disease and therapeutic modalities involved.

Meta-analysis can be useful in certain circumstances. It may permit researchers to have sufficiently large samples from randomized trials to identify small to moderate treatment effects and to examine relative treatment efficacy for subsets of patients. Some investigators dismiss this approach as important only for identifying trivial differences. However, a 10% difference in long-term survival rate for common solid tumors is clinically important, yet requires larger sample sizes than are used for many multiinstitution phase III clinical trials. For diseases such as primary breast cancer in which there are several subsets that warrant separate analysis, the sample size problem is even severer. Meta-analysis is not a substitute for properly designed and sized clinical trials, but if several similar major trials have been performed, meta-analysis can complement the individual trials.[134]

REFERENCES

1. Bull JP. The historical development of clinical therapeutic trials. J Chronic Dis 1959;10: 218–248.
2. Byar DP. Why data bases should not replace randomized clinical trials. Biometrics 1980;36:337–342.
3. Dambrosia JM, Ellenberg JH. Statistical considerations for a medical data base. Biometrics 1980;26:323–332.
4. MacMahon B, Pugh TF. Epidemiology: Principles and methods. Boston: Little, Brown, 1970.
5. Tukey JW. Some thoughts on clinical trials, especially problems of multiplicity. Science 1977;198:679–684.
6. Ettinger DS. Evaluation of new drugs in untreated patients with small-cell lung cancer: Its time has come. J Clin Oncol 1990;8:374–377.
7. Wittes, RE, Marsoni S, Simon R, et. al. The phase II trial. Cancer Treat Rep 1985;69: 1235–1239.
8. Antman K, Amato D, Wood W, et al. Selection bias in clinical trials. J Clin Oncol 1987;3:1142–1147.
9. Begg CA, Engstrom PF. Eligibility and extrapolation in cancer clinical trials. J Clin Oncol 1987;5:962–968.
10. Schneiderman MA. The clinical excursion into 5-fluorouracil. Cancer Chemother Rep 1962;16:107–118.
11. Moertel CG, Hanley JA. The effect of measuring error on the results of therapeutic trials in advanced cancer. Cancer 1976;38:388–394.
12. Gurland J, Johnson RO. How reliable are tumor measurements? JAMA 1965;29:973–978.
13. Warr D, McKinney S, Tannock I. Influence of measurement error on response rates. Cancer Treat Rep 1985;69:1127–1130.
14. Weiss GB, Bunce H, Hokanson JA. Comparing survival of responders and non-responders after treatment: A potential source of confusion in interpreting cancer clinical trials. Controlled Clin Trials 1983;4:43–52.
15. Anderson JR, Cain KC, Gelber RD. Analysis of survival by tumor response. J Clin Oncol 1983;1:710–719.
16. Simon R, Makuch RW. A nonparametric graphical representation of the relationship between survival and the occurrence of an event: Application to responder versus non-responder bias. Stat Med 1984;3:1–9.
17. Leventhal BG, Wittes RE. Research methods in clinical oncology. New York: Raven Press, 1988.
18. Schneiderman MA. Mouse to man: Statistical problems in bringing a drug to clinical trial. In: Proceedings of the Fifth Berkeley Symposium on Mathematical Statistical Probability, University of California. 1967;4:855–866.
19. Storer BE. Design and analysis of phase I clinical trials. Biometrics 1989;45:925–937.
20. O'Quigley J, Pepe M, Fisher L. Continual reassessment method: A practical design for phase I clinical trials in cancer. Biometrics 1990;46:33–48.
21. Edler L. Statistical requirements of phase I studies. Onkologie 1990;13:90–95.
22. Collins JM, Zaharko DS, Dedrick RL, Chabner BA. Potential roles for preclinical pharmacology in phase I clinical trials. Cancer Treat Rep 1986;70:73–80.
23. Peto R. Clinical trial methodology. Biomedicine 1978;28:24–36.
24. Herson J, Carter SK. Calibrated phase II clinical trials in oncology. 1986;Stat Med 5:441–447.
25. Chalmers TC. Randomization of the first patient. Med Clin North Am 1975;59:1035–1038.
26. Lee YJ, Wesley RA. Statistical considerations to phase II clinical trials in cancer: Interpretation, analysis and design. Semin Oncol 1981;8:403–416.
27. Simon R, Wittes RE, Ellenberg SS. Randomized phase II clinical trials. Cancer Treat Rep 1985;69:1375–1381.
28. Moertel CG, Schutt AJ, Hahan RG, et al. Effects of patient selection on results of phase II chemotherapy trials in gastrointestinal cancer. Cancer Chemother Rep 1974;59: 257.
29. Pocock SJ. Randomized clinical trials. Br Med J [Letter] 1977;1:1161.
30. Lasagna L. The controlled clinical trial: Theory and practice. J Chron Dis 1955;1: 353–367.
31. Chalmers TC, Block JB, Lee S. Controlled studies in clinical cancer research. N Engl J Med 1972;287:75–78.
32. Byar DP, Simon RM, Friedewald WT, et al. Randomized clinical trials: Perspectives on some recent ideas. N Engl J Med 1976;295:74–80.
33. Pocock SJ. Allocation of patients to treatment in clinical trials. Biometrics 1979;35: 183–197.
34. Hill AB. The clinical trial. Br Med Bull 1951;7:278–282.
35. Saks H, Chalmers TC, Smith H. Randomized versus historical controls for clinical trials. Am J Med 1982;72:233–240.
36. Simon R. The importance of prognostic factors in cancer clinical trials. Cancer Treat Rep 1984;68:185–192.
37. Gehan EA, Freireich EJ. Non-randomized controls in cancer clinical trials. N Engl J Med 1974;290:198–203.
38. Pocock SJ. The combination of randomized and historical controls in clinical trials. J Chronic Dis 1976;29:175–188.
39. Silverman WA. The lesson of retrolental fibroplasia. Sci Am 1977;236(6):100–107.
40. Hellman S, Hellman DS. Of mice but not men—problems of the randomized clinical trial. N Engl J Med 1991;324:1585–1589.
41. Shapiro AR. The evaluation of clinical predictions. N Engl J Med 1977;296:1509–1514.
42. Moore MJ, O'Sullivan, Tannock IF. How expert physicians would wish to be treated if they had genitourinary cancer. J Clin Oncol 1988;6:1736–1745.
43. Gilbert JP, McPeek B, Mosteller F. Statistics and ethics in surgery and anesthesia. Science 1977;198:684–689.
44. Korn EL, Baumrind S. Randomised clinical trials with physician-preferred treatment. Lancet 1991;337:149–152.
45. Peto R, Pike MC, Armitage P, et al. Design and analysis of randomized clinical trials requiring prolonged observation of each patient: I. Introduction and design. Br J Cancer 1976;34:585–612.
45a. Peto R, Pike MC, Armitage P, et al. Design and analysis of randomized clinical trials requiring prolonged observation of each patient: II. Analysis and examples. Br J Cancer 1977;35:1–39.
46. Durrleman S, Simon R. When to randomize. J Clin Oncol 1991;9:116–122.
47. Pocock SJ, Simon R. Sequential treatment assignment with balancing for prognostic factors in the controlled clinical trial. Biometrics 1975;31:103–115.
48. Brown BW Jr. Statistical controversies in the design of clinical trials. Controlled Clin Trials 1980;1:13–27.
49. Simon R. Restricted randomization designs in clinical trials. Biometrics 1979;35:503–512.
50. Kalish LA, Begg CB. Treatment allocation methods in clinical trials: A review. Stat Med 1985;4:129–144.
51. Kalish LA, Begg CB. The impact of treatment allocation procedures on nomial significance levels and bias. Controlled Clin Trials 1987;8:121–135.
52. Hills M, Armitage P. The two period cross-over clinical trial. Br J Clin Pharmacol 1979;8:7–20.
53. Koch GG. The use of non-parametric methods in the statistical analysis of the two-period change-over design. Biometrics 1972;28:577–584.
54. Brown BW Jr. The crossover experiment for clinical trials. Biometrics 1980;36:69–79.
55. Willan AR, Pater JL. Carryover and the two-period crossover clinical trial. Biometrics 1986;42:593–599.
56. Olver IN, Simon RM, Aisner J. Antiemetic studies: A methodological discussion. Cancer Treat Rep 1986;70:555–564.
57. Koch GG, Gitomer SL, Skalland l, et al. Some nonparametric and categorical data analyses for a change-over design study and discussion of apparent carry-over effects. Stat Med 1983;2:397–412.
58. Schoenfeld DA, Gelber RD. Designing and analyzing clinical trials which allow institutions to randomize patients to a subset of the treatments under study. Biometrics 1979;35:825–830.
59. Byar DP, Piantadosi S. Factorial designs for randomized clinical trials. Cancer Treat Rep 1985;69:1055–1064.
60. Simon R. A critical assessment of approaches to improving the efficacy of cancer clinical trials. In: Baum M, Kay R, Scheurlen H, eds. Recent results in cancer research. Vol III. Heidelberg: Springer-Verlag, 1988:18–26.
61. Simon R. Designs for efficient clinical trials. Oncology 1989;3:34–49.
62. Brittain E, Wittes J. Factorial designs in clinical trials: The effects of non-compliance and subadditivity. Stat Med 1989;8:161–171.

63. Simon R. How large should a phase II trial of a new drug be? Cancer Treat Rep 1987;71:1079–1085.

64. Gehan EA. The determination of the number of patients required in a preliminary and follow-up trial of a new chemotherapeutic agent. J Chronic Dis 1961;13:346–353.

65. Simon R. Optimal two-stage designs for phase II clinical trials. Controlled Clin Trials 1989;10:1–10.

66. Freiman JA, Chalmers TC, Smith H Jr, et al. The importance of beta, the type II error and sample size in the design and interpretation of the randomized control trial: Survey of 71 "negative" trials. N Engl J Med 1978;299:690–694.

67. Simon R. The size of phase III cancer Clinical Trials. Cancer Treat Rep 1985;69:1087–1092.

68. Pocock SJ. Size of cancer clinical trials and stopping rules. Br J Cancer 1978;38:757–766.

69. Simon R. Confidence intervals for reporting results from clinical trials. Ann Intern Med 1986;105:429–435.

70. Casagrande JT, Pike MC, Smith PG. An improved formula for calculating sample sizes for comparing two binomial distributions. Biometrics 1978;34:483–486.

71. Makuch RW, Simon R. Sample size considerations for nonrandomized comparative studies. J Chronic Dis 1980;33:171–175.

72. Tannock I, Warr D. Nonrandomized clinical trials of cancer chemotherapy: Phase II or III? JNCI 1988;80:800–801.

73. Thall PF, Simon R. Incorporating historical control data in planning phase II clinical trials. Stat Med 1990;9:215–228.

74. George SL, Desu MM. Planning the size and duration of a clinical trial studying the time to some critical event. J Chron Dis 1974;27:15–24.

75. Rubinstein LV, Gail MH, Santner TJ. Planning the duration of a comparative clinical trial with loss to follow-up and a period of continued observation. J Chronic Dis 1981;34:469–479.

76. Dixon DO, Simon R. Sample size considerations for studies comparing survival curves using historical controls. J Clin Epidemiol 1988;41:1209–1213.

77. Makuch R, Simon R. Sample size requirements for evaluating a conservative therapy. Cancer Treat Rep 1978;62:1037–1040.

78. Durrleman S, Simon R. Planning and monitoring of equivalence studies. Biometrics 1990;46:329–336.

79. McPherson K. Statistics: The problem of examining accumulating data more than once. N Engl J Med 1974;290:501–502.

80. Fleming TR, Green SJ, Harrington DP. Considerations of monitoring and evaluating treatment effects in clinical trials. Controlled Clin Trials 1984;5:55–66.

81. Green SJ, Fleming TR, O'Fallon JR. Policies for study monitoring and interim reporting of results. J Clin Oncol 1987;5:1477–1484.

82. Haybittle JL. Repeated assessment of results in clinical trials of cancer treatment. J Radiol 1971;44:793–797.

83. Pocock SJ. Interim analyses for randomized clinical trials. Biometrics 1982;38:153–162.

84. O'Brien PC, Fleming TR. A multiple testing procedure for clinical trials. Biometrics 1979;35:549–556.

85. Fleming TR, Harrington DP, O'Brien PC. Designs for group sequential Tests. Controlled Clin Trials 1984;5:348–361.

86. Geller N. Planned interim analysis and its role in cancer clinical trials. J Clin Oncol 1987;5:1485–1490.

87. Fleming TR, Watelet L. Approaches to monitoring clinical trials. JNCI 1989;81:188–193.

88. Emerson SS, Fleming TR. Interim analyses in clinical trials (with discussion by Simon R). Oncology 1990;4:126–136.

89. DeMets DL, Gail MH. Use of logrank tests and group sequential methods at fixed calendar times. Biometrics 1985;41:1039–1044.

90. Lan KKG, Simon R, Halperin M. Stochastically curtailed tests in long-term clinical trials. Commun Stat Sequent Anal 1982;1:207–219.

91. Halperin M, Lan KKG, Ware JH, Johnson MJ, DeMets DL. An aid to data monitoring in long-term clinical trials. Controlled Clin Trials 1982;3:311–323.

92. Anderson PK. Conditional power calculations as an aid in the decision whether to continue a clinical trial. Controlled Clinical Trials 1987;8:67–74.

93. Cantor AB. Power estimation for rank tests using censored data: Conditional and unconditional. Controlled Clin Trials 1991;12:464–473.

94. Ellenberg SS, Eisenberger MA. An efficient design for phase III studies of combination chemotherapies. Cancer Treat Rep 1985;10:1147–1152.

95. Thall PF, Simon R, Ellenberg SS, Shrager R. Optimal two-stage designs for clinical trials with binary response. Stat Med 1988;7:571–579.

96. Storer BE. A sequential phase II/III trial for binary outcomes. Stat Med 1990;9:229–235.

97. Schaid DJ, Wieand S, Therneau TM. Optimal two-stage screening designs for survival comparisons. Biometrika 1990;77:507–513.

98. Wieand S, Therneau T. A two-stage design for randomized trials with binary outcomes. Controlled Clin Trials 1987;8:20–28.

99. Thall PF, Simon R, Ellenberg SS. Two-stage selection and testing designs for comparative clinical trials. Biometrika 1988;75:303–310.

100. Thall PF, Simon, Ellenberg. A two-stage design for choosing among several experimental treatments and a control in clinical trials. Biometrics 1989;45:537–548.

101. Jennison C, Turnbull BW. Repeated confidence intervals for group sequential clinical trials. Controlled Clin Trials 1984;5:33–45.

102. Staquet MJ, Rosencweig M, Von Hoff DD, et al. The delta and epsilon errors in the assessment of cancer clinical trials. Cancer Treat Rep 1984;63:1917–1921.

103. Zelen M. Strategy and alternate randomized designs in cancer clinical trials. Cancer Treat Rep 1982;66:1095–110.

104. Begg CB, Berlin JA. Publication vias and dissemination of clinical research. JNCI 1989;81:107–115.

105. Simon R. Randomized clinical trials and research strategy. Cancer Treat Rep 1982;66:1083–1087.

106. Rotmensz N, ed. Data management and clinical trials: EORTC study group on data management. New York: Elsevier, 1989.

107. Fed Register, Vol 46, No 17: 8951. January 27, 1981.

108. Zelen M. A new design for randomized clinical trials. N Engl J Med 1979;300:1242–1245.

109. Ellenberg SS. Randomization designs in comparative clinical trials. N Engl J Med 1984;310:1404.

110. Neyman J, Pearson ES. On the use and interpretation of certain test criteria. Biometrika 1928;201:175–240.

111. Barr J, Tannock I. Analyzing the same data two ways: A demonstration model to illustrate the reporting and misreporting of clinical trials. J Clin Oncol 1989;7:969–978.

112. Tannock I, Murphy K. Reflections on medical oncology: An appeal for better clinical trials and improved reporting time of their results. J Clin Oncol 1983;1:66–70.

113. Coronary drug project research group. Influence of adherence to treatment and response of cholesterol on mortality in the coronary drug project. N Engl J Med 1981;303:1038–1041.

114. Senn SJ. Covariate imbalance and random allocation in clinical trials. Stat Med 1989;8:467–475.

115. Canner PL. Covariate adjustment of treatment effects in clinical trials. Controlled Clin Trials 1991;12:359–366.

116. Pocock SJ. Current issues in the design and interpretation of clinical trials. Br Med J 1985;290:39–42.

117. Simon R. Patient subsets and variation in therapeutic efficacy. Br J Clin Pharmacol 1982;14:473–482.

118. Simon R. Statistical tools for subset analysis in clinical trials. In: Baum M, Kay R, Scheurlen H, eds. Recent results in cancer research. Vol III. Heidelberg, Springer-Verlag, 1988:55–66.

119. Gail M, Simon R. Testing for qualitative interactions between treatment effects and patient subsets. Biometrics 1985;41:361–372.

120. Berkson J, Gage RP. Calculations of survival rates for cancer. Proc Mayo Clin 1950;25:270–286.

121. Cutler SJ, Ederer F. Maximum utilization of the life table method in analyzing survival. J Chronic Dis 1958;8:6990712.

122. Kaplan EL, Meier P. Nonparametric estimation from incomplete observations. J Am Stat Assoc 1958;53:457–481.

123. Anderson JR, Crowley JJ, Propert KJ. Interpretation of survival data in clinical Trials. (With discussion by Simon R). Oncology 1991;5:104–114.

124. Harrington DP, Anderson JW. Common methods of analyzing response data in clinical trials (with discussion by Simon R). Oncology 1990;4:95–113.

125. Begg CB, Pocock SJ, Freedman L, Zelen M. State of the art in comparative cancer clinical trials. Cancer 1987;60:2811–2815.

126. Begg CB. Quality of clinical trials. Ann Oncol 1990;1:319–320.

127. Pocock SJ, Hughes MD, Lee RJ. Statistical problems in the reporting of clinical trials. A survey of three medical journals. N Engl J Med 1987;317:426–432.

128. Oye RK, Shapiro MF. Reporting results from chemotherapy trials: Does response make a difference in patient survival? JAMA 1984;252:2722–2725.

129. Zelen M. Guidelines for publishing papers on cancer clinical trials: Responsibilities of editors and authors. J Clin Oncol 1983;1:164–169.

130. Simon R, Wittes RE. Methodologic guidelines for reports of clinical trials. Cancer Treat Rep 1985;69:1–3.

131. Slavin R. Meta-analysis in education: How has it been used? Educ Res 1984;6–15.

132. Yusuf S, Simon R, Ellenberg S. Proceedings of the workshop on the methodologic issues in overviews of randomized clinical trials. Stat Med 1987;6:217–409.

133. Peto R. Statistical aspects of cancer trials. In: Halnan KE, ed. Treatment of cancer. London: Chapman and Hall, 1982:867–871.

134. Simon R. Meta-analysis and cancer clinical trials. Princ Pract Oncol Update 1991;6:1–10.

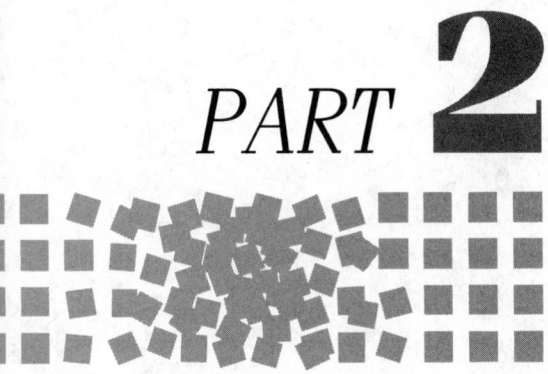

PART **2**

PRACTICE OF ONCOLOGY

Cancer: Principles & Practice of Oncology, Fourth Edition,
edited by Vincent T. DeVita, Jr., Samuel Hellman, Steven A. Rosenberg.
J.B. Lippincott Co., Philadelphia © 1993.

CHAPTER **20**

Cancer Prevention

SECTION **1**

PETER GREENWALD
CAROLYN CLIFFORD

Dietary Fat and Cancer

Recommending a major change in diet, particularly from the currently typical high-fat diet of Americans to diets substantially lower in fat, has required a substantial program of research on the possible effects of diets on disease incidence and mortality. Although there are some inconsistencies in the data relating dietary fat to cancer incidence, animal studies support a cancer-promoting role for fat and international epidemiologic studies strongly suggest that increased total dietary fat intake may be associated with increased incidence and mortality of cancers of the breast, the colon, the rectum, and the prostate. Cancers of the ovaries, the endometrium, and the pancreas also have been related to total fat intake, but the evidence is not conclusive.[1-3] Debate continues as to whether the observed associations between dietary fat and risk for certain cancers are due to dietary fat, to a few specific types of fat, or to excessive calories.

Cancers of the breast, the prostate, the colon, and the rectum, those most strongly associated with dietary fat intake, have considerable public health significance in the United States as evidenced by current incidence and mortality data.[4] For example, the breast cancer rate has been increasing since 1980; in 1992, more than 180,000 breast cancers will be diagnosed and approximately 46,000 women will die from the disease.[4] Cancer of the prostate, primarily a disease of the elderly, continues to be the commonest cancer among men;

it is estimated that 132,000 men will be diagnosed with prostate cancer in 1992. Almost 14% of all cancer diagnoses in 1992 will be cancer of the colon or rectum and these cancers will claim approximately 58,300 lives.[4] Incidence and mortality rates for breast, colon, and prostate cancers vary widely among countries worldwide. Rates are highest in North America and Western Europe and lowest in Asia with dramatic differences observed between countries with highest and lowest rates.[2,5,6] Diet, including fat intake, has been implicated as a contributing factor to these variations. Figure 20–1 illustrates the great differences in breast cancer mortality among countries and the direct correlation of breast cancer mortality with dietary fat intake.[7]

There is strong evidence that breast cancer risk decreases with increased parity and increases with age at first pregnancy, with history of benign breast disease, and in women who have female relatives with breast cancer. However, these factors are not readily modified. Currently, our practical knowledge related to reducing breast cancer risk rests largely in the area of dietary change; factors to be considered are presented in Table 20–1. Scientific evidence supports the view that dietary intervention may be an effective approach to prevent breast cancer and, possibly, to inhibit breast cancer recurrence. Dietary approaches to breast cancer prevention may be considered at different levels, including dietary recommendations for the general population, dietary intervention in the management of women at high risk for breast cancer, and dietary therapy as a component of regimens to reduce risk of recurrence after primary treatment of breast cancer.[8] This section discusses the epidemiologic and experimental evidence linking dietary fat to cancer risk; relevant clinical-metabolic studies; and past, current, and future clinical intervention studies for reducing cancer risk.

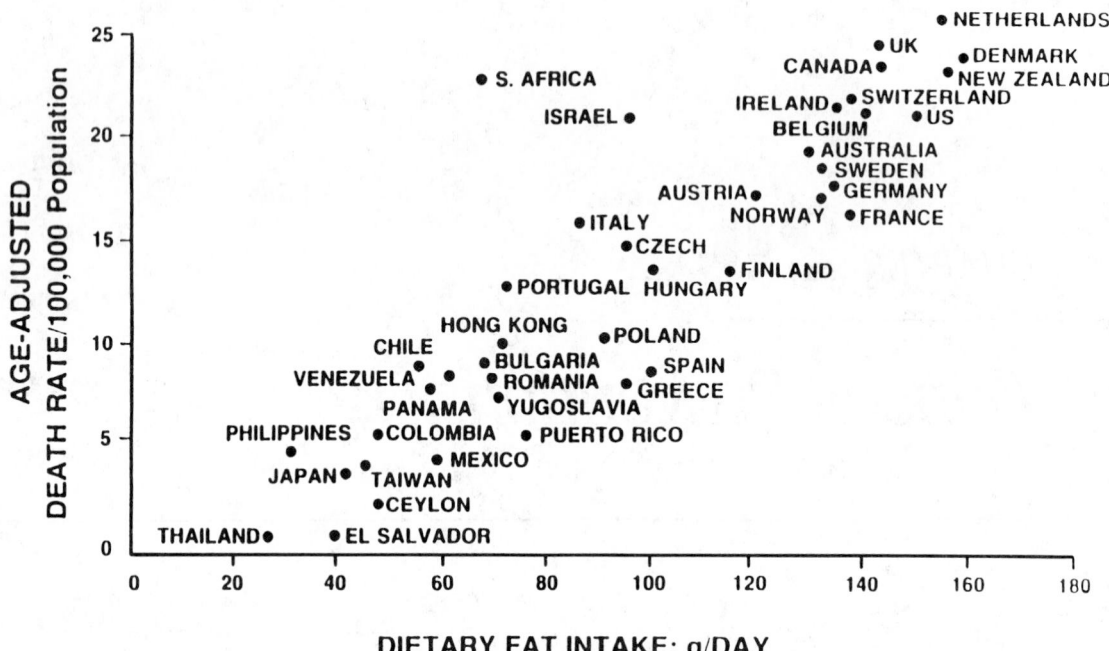

FIGURE 20–1.   International breast cancer age-adjusted mortality rates correlated with dietary fat intake.

EPIDEMIOLOGIC EVIDENCE

Epidemiologic evidence suggests an association between total dietary fat or type of fat consumed and increased cancer risk at several sites, including breast, colon, rectum, and prostate. However, a causal relation between dietary fat intake and cancer incidence still is debated.[3,9–15]

INTERNATIONAL, MIGRANT, AND TIME-TREND STUDIES

Despite certain limitations, international, migrant, and time-trend studies are an important approach to dietary fat epidemiologic studies.[9,11,14,15] These studies provide the strongest support for a high-fat diet as a risk factor for certain cancers, in particular breast and colon cancer.[10–12,15] Weaker international evidence also suggests a relation between dietary fat intake and cancers of the rectum and the prostate.[12,16]

Several international studies have demonstrated strong positive associations between total fat intake and breast, colon, and prostate cancers, even after adjustment for total caloric intake.[2,3,16–18] Strong direct associations were found between

TABLE 20–1.   Dietary Fat and Breast Cancer: Related Factors

Percentage of calories from fat
Grams of fat
Type of fat
Calories and energy expenditure
Obesity/overweight
Weight gain
Body size
Age, duration, level of exposure

---

saturated fat intake and the incidence of breast, colon, and prostate cancers and between consumption of total polyunsaturated fats and incidence of breast and prostate cancers.[3] High-fiber intake reduced the magnitude of the fat intake relation and cancer incidence, particularly for colon cancer.[3] Countries in which olive oil consumption was high had a lower risk for breast cancer than other countries.[2] Prentice and associates reported a strong positive correlation between the incidence of breast cancer and consumption of fat in 21 countries.[11] Data showed a 5.5-fold difference in breast cancer incidence between countries with the lowest (15%) and highest (45%) fat intakes and indicated that consumption of fat accounted for approximately 58% of the variation in incidence rate compared with a 14% contribution from total calories.[11]

In addition to the amount of fat, the type of fat consumed may be an important risk factor in cancer development. Consumption of the longer chain, highly polyunsaturated σ-3 fatty acids found in certain fish may offer protection against cancer. This finding has been indicated by studies of populations such as Greenland Eskimos who consume large amounts of fat derived from fish, but who are at low risk for cancer, including breast cancer.[19,20] In a study of 32 countries, a strong inverse association was found between breast cancer incidence and mortality and percentage of calories from saltwater fish after adjustment for fat intake.[21] Overall, the results of international studies indicate that total fat and different types of fatty acids may have various site-specific tumor-promoting or tumor-inhibiting properties.

The association between dietary fat and cancer incidence and mortality rates has been evaluated in diet-related studies of migrant populations that move from low- to high-cancer incidence areas. These studies show that, with time, migrant populations exhibit the higher cancer incidence rates of their adopted country for several cancers, including breast and colon.[15,22–27] Significant changes in dietary habits often occur soon after migration, providing a means of studying relative risk for disease development as a function of age and time at dietary changes.[28] Examination of individual diet surveys indicated that as Italian immigrants to Australia adopted the regional high-fat diet, their age-adjusted breast cancer mortality rates doubled over a 17-year period compared with Australian rates.[11,29] Major shifts in breast, prostate, and endometrial cancer incidence rates among four migrant groups to Hawaii—Japanese, Chinese, Filipinos, and whites—were found to be significantly associated with total fat, animal fat, and saturated and unsaturated fat intakes.[30,31] Unfortunately, most migrant studies fail to examine dietary habits before and after migration, limiting their usefulness in evaluating the causal link between diet and cancer risk.[15]

Time-trend studies support an association between consumption of fat and cancer mortality, particularly for breast cancer. Within-country time-trend studies generally control for several factors that confound international studies, such as the lack of standardized dietary assessment methods; however, because time-trend analyses usually report cancer deaths rather than incidence, they may significantly underestimate relative risk.[13] A time-trend study that followed Japanese dietary habits and cancer deaths found that the mean per capita fat intake, which increased from 23 g/day in 1957 through 1959 to 52 g/day in 1973, was accompanied by a doubling of the total number of annual breast cancer deaths between 1957 and 1973.[32] Time-trend analyses performed by Kurihara and colleagues[6] examined age-adjusted breast cancer mortality rates for 24 countries between 1950 and 1979. The overall trend for most countries was an increase in breast cancer deaths. A relation between per capita fat intake and time-related changes in breast cancer deaths was supported after regression analysis of mortality rates and food disappearance data from 14 countries, although this analysis indicated that about one half of the associations between breast cancer and dietary fat observed in international studies were due to confounding factors.[11,28] Prentice and coworkers[11] concluded that time-trend analyses suggest a relative risk estimate of approximately 0.3 to 0.4 (after adjusting for weight and age at menarche) for a reduction in dietary fat to 20% of caloric intake; these data were used to guide the feasibility phase of the Women's Health Trial, discussed later in this chapter.

CASE-CONTROL AND COHORT STUDIES

In contrast to international, migrant, and time-trend studies, most case-control (retrospective) and cohort (prospective) studies, which examine the association between diet and cancer at the level of the individual, have found only a small or no relation between cancer risk and total fat intake or consumption of fat-containing foods.[9,12–14] Rogers and Longnecker[12] reviewed 16 case-control and follow-up studies in which total fat intake was examined as a risk factor for breast cancer. Six of these studies showed a strong relation between a high-fat diet and breast cancer risk; eight others exhibited a weaker but still positive association. The relation between fat intake and breast cancer risk in the two studies with the largest direct association may be confounded by factors other than fat, such as reproductive determinants and some westernization of diet[32] or inconsistencies in assessment instruments.[33] The data from these 16 studies indicated that breast cancer risk was not related to menopausal status or to the type of fat consumed.

A meta-analysis of 12 of 14 case-control studies of diet and breast cancer showed a strong positive association between breast cancer risk and total fat and saturated fat intake in postmenopausal but not premenopausal women[10]; however, a reexamination of these studies by other authors questioned this analysis.[34] Goodwin and Boyd[35] and Graham and colleagues[34] concluded in their reviews of 14 and 13 case-control studies, respectively, that the relation between fat intake and risk for breast cancer is equivocal. Results of the largest cohort study of breast cancer risk to date, the Nurses Health Study, which included nearly 90,000 women, found no association between intake of total fat, saturated fat, linoleic acid, or cholesterol and breast cancer incidence or mortality.[36] Some investigators have concluded, based on the current epidemiologic case-control evidence obtained from western populations, that a moderate reduction in fat intake by adult women will have no detectable influence on risk for breast cancer.[12,36]

Results of case-control studies that examine fat intake as a risk factor for colorectal cancer suggest a small direct association.[37] Several studies indicate a much stronger direct relation between fat intake and rectal cancer than colon cancer; increased risk for large bowel cancers appears to be related to consumption of saturated fat rather than polyunsaturated or monounsaturated fat intake in most but not all studies.[38–44] Several other studies suggest that subjects who consume large amounts of meat, particularly beef, are at greatest risk for developing colorectal cancer[12,45]; data from the Nurses Health Study by Willett and associates support this suggestion and indicate that colon cancer incidence and animal fat intake are strongly correlated, even after adjustment for total calorie intake.[46] Women who consumed red meat daily, compared with once a month, had a 2.5 times greater risk for colon cancer, whereas frequent consumption of fish and skinless chicken was associated with decreased colon cancer risk. Several other studies found either no association or an inverse relation between fat intake and risk for large bowel cancer.[47–50] A protective effect of monounsaturated fat and linoleic acid has been indicated in some cases.[47,48] It has been suggested that the negative and inverse associations found in some case-control and cohort studies of fat intake and colorectal cancer risk may have resulted in part from methodologic problems.[37]

Several dietary studies of prostate cancer risk indicated a small to moderate positive relation between risk and consumption of fat or high-fat foods; however, these studies are not considered definitive.[12,37,51,52] Similarly, a small number of case-control studies of ovarian, pancreatic, and lung cancer risk demonstrated a small to moderate direct association between fat or high-fat food intake and risk, but these associations were weakened because of confounding factors such as the use of surrogate foods for fat intake; adjustment for caloric intake; or, in the case of lung cancer, adjustment for smoking.[12]

INTERPRETATION OF DATA FROM EPIDEMIOLOGIC STUDIES

The various designs associated with different types of epidemiologic studies influence the type of potential bias introduced into the study and the interpretation of the data being analyzed may contribute to the inconsistencies found in examining the role of diet in cancer incidence and mortality.[9,11–14,28,53,54] For example, international correlation, time-trend, and migrant studies of disease and eating habits generally are limited by the quality of available dietary data, the ability to control for confounding factors, and the observation that well-established disease risk factors may not be associated with variations in disease rates across countries or for certain periods within a country. As a result, international and geographic epidemiologic studies are useful for generating and adding indirect support for hypotheses but not for formal testing of prevention hypotheses. In the study of diet and disease, case-control and cohort studies may be relatively insensitive to a true dietary effect because often they are done in homogenous populations, for example, groups that have a narrow range of fat intake. In addition, the reliability of the major dietary assessment tools used in case-control and cohort studies is often considered a major source of bias, even in well-designed studies. Prentice and Sheppard concluded that no reliable epidemiologic methods currently exist for studying the role of diet in the development of cancers that are most critical to public health. They acknowledge, however, the important role of consistently positive or negative data from epidemiologic studies of diet and cancer and the potential of carefully selected and conducted large-scale randomized intervention trials.[28]

EXPERIMENTAL EVIDENCE

Most experimental studies suggest that dietary fat acts as a tumor promoter or enhancer, but some evidence indicates that fat may have a role in cancer initiation.[55–59] Early studies using mouse mammary tumors showed that the amount of dietary fat consumed after, but not before, exposure to a chemical carcinogen led to enhanced tumorigenesis and to the suggestion that fat affected the promotion process of carcinogenesis rather than the initiation.[55,60] The role of fat in tumor initiation is suggested by more recent experimental data.[57,61–63] Additional studies of mammary tumors suggest that fat may exert its tumor-enhancing effects either (1) directly, by influencing a variety of membrane characteristics, such as fluidity, transport, permeability, membrane-bound enzyme activities, and the status of hormone receptors or by affecting prostaglandin metabolism; or (2) indirectly, through mechanisms that involve neuroendocrine systems.[56,63–65] With respect to colon cancer, it has been postulated that total dietary fat influences the metabolic activity of fecal microflora and the concentration of sterol substrates in the large intestine. As a consequence, tumor-promoting substances (secondary bile acids) may be produced from bile acids within the lumen of the colon.[2] A mechanism linking dietary fat to prostate cancer has not been hypothesized; however, the endocrine system has been implicated as a mediator of dietary influences including fat.[66] As suggested by some epidemiologic data, experimental studies indicate that degree of saturation and chain length of dietary fats can influence tumorigenesis.[56,58,67–70] In animals, diets high in σ-6 or n-6 polyunsaturated fatty acids (linoleic acid) appear to be more potent enhancers of mammary, pancreatic, and probably colon tumors than diets con-

taining similar amounts of saturated fats derived from animal fats and tropical oils.[7,57,58,69–71] In contrast, fish oils containing eicosopentaneoic acid, an σ-3 polyunsaturated fatty acid, and olive oil, which contains large amounts of the monounsaturated fatty acid oleic acid, tend to have an inhibitory effect on tumor development in animals.[57,58,69,70] The tumor-promoting effects of fat are directly related to length of time that animals are fed high-fat diets[60,69,72–74] and appear to be reversible.[72,74] In addition, as demonstrated in several studies and discussed in more detail in other sections of this chapter, the promoting effect of dietary fat can be modified by other dietary components, most notably fiber.[3,12,69,75]

TOTAL CALORIC INTAKE AND CANCER RISK

Although a decrease in total caloric intake reduces tumor incidence in laboratory animals,[59,76–78] epidemiologic studies have not confirmed that reduction below optimum weight is beneficial against cancer in humans.[12,67,78] Several international correlation studies failed to find a significant relation between calories consumed and cancer risk,[2,3] and the results of case-control and cohort studies are mixed.[12,79] Rogers and Longnecker discuss the need for investigators to consider not only total caloric intake but also determinants of caloric intake, such as physical activity, body size, caloric balance, and metabolic efficiency, to assess adequately the relation between calories and cancer risk.[12]

In general, experimental studies show that animals fed high-fat diets develop mammary, pancreatic, colon, and other intestinal tract tumors more readily than animals consuming a low-fat diet ad libitum.[64,65,80–82] Animal studies also demonstrate that caloric restriction without essential nutrient deficiency slows biologic aging and the development of chemically induced tumors in laboratory animals.[59,63,67,77,83,84] An analysis of more than 100 animal experiments involving nearly 8000 mice and rats found that high-fat intake and high-caloric intake independently increased the incidence of mammary tumors.[85] A dose-related increase in tumor incidence is seen in animal experiments as total dietary fat intake increases from approximately 10% to 40% of calories.[60,63,67,80,86] Similarly, Albanes found dose-related decreases in site- and fat-adjusted tumor incidence when calories were reduced as much as 58%; even moderate restrictions in total caloric intake, that is, 7% to 20%, were associated with a significant decrease in tumor incidence compared with incidence rates for noncalorie-restricted animals.[76]

CLINICAL METABOLIC STUDIES

The role of dietary fat in cancer prevention is being evaluated in clinical metabolic studies that reflect specific human dietary changes. These studies may be used to assess nutrient levels proposed as compliance markers in intervention studies, to evaluate potential mechanisms of action for specific nutrients, or to monitor markers of biologic activity before and after controlled dietary manipulations.[87] No single parameter or battery of measurements has been identified at this time to monitor total fat intake; however, these studies are expected to contribute to the clinical monitoring of dietary modification and adherence. To determine the effect of fat and other dietary factors on human metabolism, cooperative research efforts between the U.S. Department of Agriculture's Beltsville Human Nutrition Research Center and the National Cancer Institute (NCI) have been developed.

Studies examining the metabolic effects of changes in dietary fat have been conducted separately in premenopausal women, postmenopausal women, and men. The effect of eating a controlled diet containing 40% or 20% fat calories at two different ratios of polyunsaturated to saturated (P:S) fats was investigated in premenopausal women. Results analyzed to date indicate that the low-fat diet was associated with a significant increase in serum triglycerides, decreased serum estradiol levels, a lengthening of the menstrual cycle, lower plasma levels of cortisol and higher levels of plasma insulin, changes in bile acid levels specific to the P:S ratio, cycle phase- and fat level-dependent changes in lipoproteins and red blood cell fluidity, and a reduction in percentage of body fat. A second study compared a variety of metabolic parameters in healthy men on a controlled high-fat, low-fiber reference diet with the same group of subjects consuming a controlled low-fat, high-fiber experimental diet. Results of lipid determinations indicate that total cholesterol, low-density lipoprotein (LDL) cholesterol, and high-density lipoprotein (HDL) cholesterol were 17% to 20% lower in men on the experimental diet compared with the reference diet, regardless of initial cholesterol level. Results also supported the hypothesis that changes in dietary lipids can substantially alter the in vivo production of E-series prostaglandins. A third study of low-fat diets with differing P:S ratios compared serum lipids and hormones in free-living postmenopausal women on an uncontrolled diet with those on a controlled 20% of calories from fat diet. Total analysis of lipid values indicated that the low-fat diets resulted in an average total cholesterol decrease of 7% (P:S = 1.0) to 10% (P:S = 0.57), whereas the HDL cholesterol and LDL cholesterol fraction decreased an average of 11% to 17%. Blood hormone responses were not significantly different between low- and high-fat diets.

The effect of a fat-modified diet on sex hormones during adolescence is being investigated by the NCI for early life-cycle hormone responses to fat intake. This is an ancillary study to the Diet Intervention Study in Children, which is being sponsored by the National Heart, Lung, and Blood Institute. The NCI study will characterize factors of adolescents that influence sex hormone levels and bioavailability, such as age, Tanner stage, anthropometric measures, physical activity, and diet, and will evaluate the effect of dietary intervention on sex hormone levels in parents of the participants.

CLINICAL INTERVENTION STUDIES

CHANGING TO A LOW-FAT DIET AS A MIDDLE-AGED ADULT

Although strong evidence for an effect of diet on cancer has been shown through epidemiologic, clinical, and laboratory studies, these studies do not offer the type of conclusive evidence that can be drawn only from a prospective trial; nor do these types of studies quantify the potential benefits of midlife dietary modification. Findings from animal studies cannot be extrapolated to humans directly; even indirect extrapolations

have enormous uncertainties because of critical differences in metabolism, physiology, duration of exposure (lifespan), and other potential confounders. Because of the large number and poorly characterized effects of confounding factors, clinical and epidemiologic, particularly case-control, studies are difficult to interpret. Although controlled metabolic studies, such as those conducted in a closed hospital metabolic unit or other supervised environment, may provide important information, for practical reasons they are short-term with small numbers of subjects who are not broadly representative of the population.

Cancer often has an insidious onset and lead times of many years. Optimally, reliable, direct evidence of the effect of diet on human health requires a field trial in which dietary changes can be instituted and maintained in a well-characterized set of subjects who are followed prospectively for a long enough time to determine changes in the frequency of disease incidence or death from suspect causes. This requires large numbers of subjects (several tens of thousands); a matched control group; and a close, frequent monitoring of current diet and health status. What influence or effect on disease endpoints can be expected from a midlife dietary modification is a critical question in need of a scientifically based rational response.

VANGUARD FEASIBILITY TRIAL

To examine the feasibility of a nationwide, randomized, multicenter intervention trial, the Women's Health Trial Vanguard Study was conducted to test the hypothesis that a low-fat diet followed for 10 years will reduce the risk for breast cancer. Three clinical sites were used to conduct the feasibility study, with a focus on addressing two primary questions. First, is it possible to recruit women aged 45 to 69 years into a clinical trial with a low-fat dietary intervention? Second, can or will these women adhere to such a long-term dietary intervention?

The overall conclusion from the Vanguard Study is that women recruited to this study can succeed in lowering mean dietary fat intake to below 25% of energy and can maintain this diet for 2 years. The reasonable nature of the dietary changes reported by the women and the agreement between expected and observed plasma total cholesterol levels at 12 and 24 months provide compelling evidence that the women's dietary records reflect their actual dietary intake. These data are among the first demonstrations that substantial dietary changes can be fostered and maintained in free-living people, thereby providing support that a randomized trial with a low-fat dietary intervention is a reasonable and feasible undertaking.[88]

WOMEN'S INTERVENTION NUTRITION STUDY

The Women's Intervention Nutrition Study (WINS) is a multiinstitutional clinical trial to test the effects of a low-fat diet in stage II breast cancer patients. The study will examine adherence to a dietary modification program for 300 postmenopausal stage II breast cancer patients in conjunction with chemotherapy or hormonal therapy. The primary objective of this study is to determine the degree to which patients will adhere to the dietary modification. The secondary objectives include identifying a set of behavioral and psychosocial variables that can be used as predictors of dietary change. This study is believed to be a critical intermediate step in the effort to determine whether a full-scale outcome study evaluating dietary modification as an adjunct to standard breast cancer therapy is justified.

WOMEN'S HEALTH INITIATIVE

On the strength of multiple studies from epidemiology and carcinogenesis research, the National Institutes of Health (NIH) is planning a major women's health initiative to address the prevention of health problems of women. This study will take a comprehensive approach to three major sources of morbidity and mortality—cancer, cardiovascular disease, and osteoporosis—in women of all races and all socioeconomic strata. Although distinctly different problems, these diseases are now linked through potential preventive regimens. The NIH proposes to address these issues by a study of the effects on disease risk of changes in diet, the use of hormones, and calcium supplementation. Components of this study include a large intervention trial with an associated cohort epidemiologic study and a community study. Coordinated by the NIH Office of Research on Women's Health and conducted by the NIH Associate Director for Prevention, the NCI, the National Heart, Lung, and Blood Institute, the National Institute on Aging, the National Institute of Arthritis and Musculoskeletal and Skin Diseases, and the National Institute of Child Health and Human Development, the Women's Health Initiative (WHI) will be the largest community-based clinical prevention and intervention trial ever conducted in the United States.

Insufficient knowledge about the feasibility of such a comprehensive trial for underserved populations has led the NCI to request proposals for a low-fat dietary intervention study mostly in underserved minority populations. The results of this minority study should help refine the WHI and be useful in other efforts aimed at dietary modification in minority groups. The overall objective of the study is to determine whether a low-fat diet (less than 20% of calories from fat) with increased intake of vegetables, fruits, and grain products reduces the incidence of breast and colon cancer and the mortality from cardiovascular disease in this study population.

ALCOHOL AND CANCER

Associations between alcohol consumption and cancer vary by site and type of alcoholic beverage. Alcohol intake is reported to be directly associated with cancers of the oral cavity, pharynx, esophagus, and larynx where alcohol interacts synergistically with smoking to increase risk. Primary liver, rectal, pancreatic, and breast cancer also have been linked with alcohol intake. The relative risks reported for these associations are reported as weak to modest.[37]

A review of the epidemiologic studies published between 1977 and 1989 examining breast cancer risk and alcohol intake reported that results from 10 of 16 case-control studies and 5 of 6 cohort studies support a weak positive association.[89] Recently, a meta-analysis of six dietary case-control studies (one each in Argentina, Australia, Canada, and Greece and two in Italy) investigating the association between alcohol and breast cancer risk found a statistically significant modest re-

lation between women who consumed 40 or more grams of alcohol per day and increased breast cancer risk. No association was seen between consumption of less than 40 grams of alcohol per day and breast cancer risk.[90] This finding differs slightly from that of another meta-analysis that consists of 12 case-control and 4 cohort studies[91] that include the Nurses' Health Study, a large prospective study of nearly 90,000 U.S. nurses.[92] This meta-analysis demonstrated a dose-response relation, or a continuous increase in risk with increasing alcohol intake.[91] However, several studies, such as a recent Canadian study of breast cancer risk and alcoholic beverage consumption, have concluded that there is no association.[93] The NCI Dietary Guidelines recommend that if alcoholic beverages are consumed at all, it should be done in moderation.

CONCLUSION

A recent analysis of 1985 to 1987 mortality data from 34 countries published by the World Health Organization showed significant correlations between the per person supply of fat from dairy products and lard and cancers of the breast, prostate, rectum, colon, and lung. The level of saturated fat intake was the most plausible link for the relation between the cancers considered and for ischemic heart disease mortality.[94] Although the data from this analysis and multiple animal experiments and human correlation studies strongly support the dietary fat-breast cancer hypothesis,[15] negative findings have been reported from several other investigations.[95] Much time and effort has been expended to determine the strength of this body of evidence as a basis for conducting a large-scale low-fat dietary intervention trial. When the NCI set dietary objectives several years ago based on information then available, recommendations to reduce the intake of calories from fat by about one third were prudent and they remain prudent as the research continues.[96] However, the research to assess the quantitative benefits of such changes has not been performed and the public response to changes in dietary practice remain far short of these recommendations. What kinds and how much dietary change will reduce the risk for diet-related cancers?

Reliable, direct evidence of the effect of diet on human health requires a field trial in which subjects can be monitored for individual consumption and educated to make and maintain dietary changes for 10 or more years to determine changes in the frequency of disease incidence or mortality from suspected risk factors. The extensive effort made for the Women's Health Trial Vanguard Study demonstrated that the intervention group made substantial dietary changes to reduce the intake of calories from fat from 40% to 20%—about half of the national norm.[88] Establishing the feasibility of a randomized low-fat dietary trial was an important milestone for the follow-through being planned as a nationwide multicenter study by the NIH WHI. Whether subjects will comply with a low-fat dietary modification for a prolonged period has been demonstrated for a subset of subjects through the assessment of dietary records, chemical analysis of dietary intake, and serum cholesterol measurements.[97,98] These methods for monitoring compliance, although subject to questions of precision, may be refined as the WHI trial proceeds. The large sample size and the associated costs have been major concerns for policymakers; however, the potential for reducing cancer risk, heart disease, and osteoporosis may provide significant public health benefits.

REFERENCES

1. Public Health Service, Office of the Surgeon General. The Surgeon General's report on nutrition and health. PHS Publication 88-50210, Washington, DC: US Government Printing Office, 1988.
2. Rose DP, Boyar AP, Wynder EL. International comparisons of mortality rates for cancer of the breast, ovary, prostate, and colon and per capita food consumption. Cancer 1986;58: 2363–2371.
3. Hursting SD, Thornquist M, Henderson MM. Types of dietary fat and the incidence of cancer at five sites. Prev Med 1990;19:242–253.
4. Miller BA, Ries LAG, Hankey BF, Kosary CL, Edwards BK, eds. Cancer Statistics Review: 1973–1989. Bethesda, MD: National Cancer Institute; NIH Pub. No. 92-2789, 1992.
5. Muir CS, Waterhouse J, Mack TM, Powell J, Whelan S. Cancer incidence in five continents. Vol V. Lyon, France: WHO International Agency for Research in Cancer, 1987.
6. Kurihara M, Aoki K, Tominaga S. Cancer mortality statistics in the world, Nagoya, Japan: University of Nagoya Press, 1984.
7. Carroll KK, Khor HT. Dietary fat in relation to tumorigenesis. Prog Biochem Pharmacol 1975;10:308–353.
8. Rose DP, Connolly JM. Dietary prevention of breast cancer. Med Oncol Tumor Pharmacother 1990;7:121–130.
9. Hebert JR, Miller DR. Methodologic considerations for investigating the diet-cancer link. Am J Clin Nutr 1988;47:1068–1077.
10. Howe GR, Hirohata T, Hislop TG, et al. Dietary factors and risk of breast cancer: Combined analysis of 12 case-control studies. JNCI 1990;82:561–569.
11. Prentice RL, Kakar F, Hursting SD, Sheppard L, Klein R, Kushi LH. Aspects of the rationale for the Womens' Health Trial. JNCI 1988;80:802–814.
12. Rogers AE, Longnecker MP. Biology of disease: Dietary and nutritional influences on cancer—a review of epidemiologic and experimental data. Lab Invest 1988;59:729–752.
13. Prentice RL, Pepe M, Self SG. Dietary fat and breast cancer: A quantitative assessment of the epidemiological literature and a discussion of methodological issues. Cancer Res 1989;49:3147–3156.
14. Willett WC. Epidemiologic studies of diet and cancer. Med Oncol Tumor Pharmacother 1990;7:93–97.
15. Schatzkin A, Greenwald P, Byar DP, Clifford CK. The dietary fat-breast cancer hypothesis is alive. JAMA 1989;261:3284–3287.
16. Armstrong B, Doll R. Environmental factors and cancer incidence and mortality in different countries, with special reference to dietary practices. Int J Cancer 1975;15:617–631.
17. Zaridze DG. Environmental etiology of large bowel cancer. JNCI 1983;70:389–400.
18. McKeown-Eyssen GE, Bright-See E. Dietary factors in colon cancer: International relationships. Nutr Cancer 1984;6:160–170.
19. Bang HO, Dyerberg J, Hjorne N. The composition of food consumed by Greenland Eskimos. Acta Med Scand 1976;200:69–73.
20. Kromann N, Green A. Epidemiological studies in the Upernavik District, Greenland: Incidence of some chronic diseases, 1950–1974. Acta Med Scand 1980;208:401–406.
21. Kaizer N, Boyd NF, Tritchler D. Fish consumption and breast cancer risk: An ecological study. Nutr Cancer 1989;12:61–68.
22. Smith RL. Recorded and expected mortality among Japanese of the United States and Hawaii with special reference to cancer. JNCI 1956;17:459–473.
23. Haenszel W. Cancer mortality among foreign-born in the United States. JNCI 1961;26:37–132.
24. Staszewski J, Haenszel W. Cancer mortality among Polish born in the United States. JNCI 1965;35:292–297.
25. Haenszel W, Kurihari M. Studies of Japanese migrants: I. Mortality from cancer and other diseases among Japanese in the United States. JNCI 1968;40:43–68.
26. Staszewski J, McCall MG, Stenhouse NS. Cancer mortality in 1962–1966 among Polish migrants to Australia. Br J Cancer 1971;25:599–610.
27. McMichael AJ, McCall MG, Hartshorne JM, et al. Patterns of gastro-intestinal cancer in European migrants to Australia: The role of dietary change. Int J Cancer 1980;25:431–437.
28. Prentice RL, Sheppard L. Validity of international, time trend, and migrant studies of dietary factors and disease risk. Prev Med 1989;18:167–179.
29. Armstrong BK. Nutrient intakes in Italian migrants and Australians in Perth. Food Nutr 1981;38:7–10.
30. Kolonel LN, Hankin JH, Lee JS, et al. Nutrient intakes in relation to cancer incidence in Hawaii. Br J Cancer 1981;44:332–339.
31. Kolonel LN, Nomura AMY, Ward-Hinds M, Hirohata T, Hankin JH, Lee JS. Role of diet in cancer incidence in Hawaii. Cancer Res 1983;43:2397S–2402S.
32. Hirayama T. Epidemiology of breast cancer with special reference to the role of diet. Prev Med 1978;7:173–195.
33. Lubin F, Wax Y, Modan B. Role of fat, animal protein, and dietary fiber in breast cancer etiology: A case-control study. JNCI 1986;77:605–612.
34. Graham S, Hellman R, Marshall J, et al. Nutritional epidemiology of postmenopausal breast cancer in Western New York. Am J Epidemiol 1991;134:552–556.
35. Goodwin PJ, Boyd NF. Critical appraisal of the evidence that dietary fat intake is related to breast cancer risk in humans. JNCI 1985;79:473–485.
36. Willett WC, Stampfer MJ, Colditz GA, Rasner BA, Hennekens CH, Speizer FE. Dietary fat and the risk of breast cancer. N Engl J Med 1987;316:22–28.
37. National Academy of Sciences, National Research Council, Commission on Life Sciences, Food and Nutrition Board. Diet and health: Implications for reducing chronic disease risk. Washington, DC: National Academy Press, 1989.
38. Whittemore AS, Wu-Williams AH, Lee M, et al. Diet, physical activity, and colorectal cancer among Chinese in North America and China. JNCI 1990;82:915–926.
39. Dales LC, Friedman GD, Ury HK, Grossman S, Williams SR. A case-control study of relationships of diet and other traits to colorectal cancer in American blacks. Am J Epidemiol 1979;109:132–144.
40. Miller AB, Howe GR, Jain M, Craib KJP, Harrison LW. Food items and food groups as risk factors in a case-control study of diet and colorectal cancer. Int J Cancer 1983;32:155–161.
41. Kune S, GA, Watson LF. Case-control study of dietary etiological factors: The Melbourne Colorectal Cancer Study. Nutr Cancer 1987;9:21–42.
42. Potter JD, McMichael AJ. Diet and cancer of the colon and rectum: A case-control study. JNCI 1986;76.557–569.
43. Jain M, Cook GM, Davis FG, Grace MG, Howe GR, Miller AB. A case control study of diet and colorectal cancer. Int J Cancer 1980;26:757–768.
44. West DW, Slattery ML, Robinson LM, et al. Dietary intake and colon cancer: Sex- and anatomic site-specific associations. Am J Epidemiol 1989;130:883–894.
45. Manousos O, Day NE, Trichopoulos D, Gerovalis F, Tzonou A, Polychronopoulou A. Diet and colorectal cancer: A case-control study in Greece. Int J Cancer 1983;32:1–5.
46. Willett WC, Stampfer MJ, Colditz GA, Rosner BA, Speizer FE. Relation of meat, fat, and their fiber intake to the risk of colon cancer in a prospective study among women. N Engl J Med 1990;323:1664–1672.
47. Macquart-Moulin G, Riboli E, Cornee J, Charnay B, Berthezene P, Day NE. Case-control study on colorectal cancer and diet in Marseilles. Int J Cancer 1986;38:183–191.
48. Tuyns AJ, Haelterman M, Kaaks R. Colorectal cancer and the intake of nutrients: Oligosaccharides are a risk factor, fats are not—A case-control study in Belgium. Nutr Cancer 1987;10:181–196.
49. Haenszel W, Locke FB, Segi M. A case-control study of large bowel cancer in Japan. JNCI 1980;64:17–22.
50. Stemmerman GN, Nomura AM, Heilbrun LK. Dietary fat and the risk of colorectal cancer. Cancer Res 1984;44:4633–4637.
51. Heshmat MY, Kaul L, Kovi J, et al. Nutrition and prostate cancer: A case-control study. Prostate 1985;6:7–17.
52. Kolonel LN, Yoshizawa CN, Hankin JH. Diet and prostatic cancer: A case-control study in Hawaii. Am J Epidemiol 1988;127:999–1012.
53. Gray-Donald K, Kramer MS. Causality inference in observational versus experimental studies: An empirical comparison. Am J Epidemiol 1988;127:885–892.
54. Vogel VG, McPherson RS. Dietary epidemiology of colon cancer. Hematol Oncol Clin North Am 1989;3:35–63.
55. Ip C. Ability of dietary animal fat to overcome the resistance of mature female rats to 7,12-dimethylbenz(a)anthracene-induced mammary tumorigenesis. Cancer Res 1980;40:2785.
56. Cohen LA. Dietary fat and mammary cancer. In: Reddy BS, Cohen LA, eds. Diet, nutrition, and cancer: A critical evaluation. Volume 1. Boca Raton, FL: CRC Press, 1986:77–100.
57. Cohen LA, Thompson DO, Maeura Y, Choi K, Blank ME, Rose DP. Dietary fat and mammary cancer: I. Promoting effects of different dietary fats on N-nitrosomethylurea-induced rat mammary tumorigenesis. JNCI 1986;77:33–42.
58. Cannizzo F Jr, Broitman SA. Postpromotional effects of dietary marine of safflower oils or large bowel or pulmonary implants of CT-26 in mice. Cancer Res 1989;49:4289–4294.
59. Birt DF, Pelling JC, White LT, Dimitroff K, Barnett T. Influence of diet and calorie restriction on the initiation and promotion of skin carcinogenesis in the Sencar mouse model. Cancer Res 1991;51:1851–1854.
60. Carroll KK, Khor TT. Effects of level and type of dietary fat on incidence of mammary tumors induced in female SpragueDawley rats by 7, 12-dimethylbenz(a)anthracene. Lipids 1971;6:415–520.
61. Welsch CW, DeHoog JV. Influence of caffeine consumption on 7,12-dimethyl-benz(a)anthracene-induced mammary gland tumorigenesis in female rats fed a chemically defined diet containing standard and high levels of unsaturated fat. Cancer Res 1988;48:2074–2077.
62. Reddy BS, Burill C, Rigotty J. Effects of diets high in omega-3 and omega-6 fatty acids on initiation and postinitiation stages of colon carcinogenesis. Cancer Res 1991;51:487–491.
63. Clinton SK, Visek WJ. The macronutrients in experimental carcinogenesis of the breast, colon, and pancreas. In: Ip C, Birt DF, Rogers AE, Mettlin C, eds. Dietary fat and cancer. New York: Alan R Liss, 1986:377–401.
64. Reddy BS, Cohen LA, McCoy D, Hill P, Weisburger JH, Wynder EL. Nutrition and its relationship to cancer. Adv Can Res 1980;32:237–345.
65. Hopkins GJ, Carroll KK. Role of diet in cancer prevention. J Environ Pathol Toxicol Oncol 1985;5:279–298.
66. Bosland MC. The etiopathogenesis of prostatic cancer with special reference to environmental factors. Adv Can Res 1988;51:1–106.
67. Palmer S. Diet, nutrition and cancer. Prog Food Nutr Sci 1985;9:283–341.
68. Carroll KK, Braden LM. Dietary fat and mammary carcinogenesis. Nutr Cancer 1985;6:254–259.
69. Carroll KK. Summation: Which fat/how much fat-animals. Prev Med 1987;16:510–515.

70. Carroll KK, Hopkins GJ. Dietary polyunsaturated fat versus saturated fat in relation to mammary carcinogenesis. Lipids 1979;14:155–158.

71. Chan PC, Ferguson KA, Dao TL. Effects of different dietary fats on mammary carcinogenesis. Cancer Res 1983;43:1079–1083.

72. Aylsworth CF, Jone C, Trosko JE, Meites J, Welsch CW. Promotion of 7,12-dimethylbenz(a)anthracene-induced tumorigenesis by high dietary fat: Possible role of intercellular communication. JNCI 1984;72:637–645.

73. Dao TL, Chan PC. Effects of duration of high-fat intake on enhancement of mammary carcinogenesis in rats. JNCI 1983;71:201–205.

74. Ip C, Ip MM. Inhibition of mammary tumorigenesis by a reduction of fat intake after a carcinogen treatment in young versus adult rats. Cancer Lett 1980;11:35–42.

75. Cohen LA, Kendall ME, Zang E, et al. Modulation of N-nitrosomethylurea-induced mammary tumor promotion by dietary fiber and fat. JNCI 1991;83:496–500.

76. Albanes D. Total calories, body weight, and tumor incidence in mice. Cancer Res 1987;47:1987–1992.

77. Tannenbaum A. The initiation and growth of tumors: Introduction: I. Effects of underfeeding. Am J Can 1940;38:335–350.

78. Albanes D. Caloric intake, body weight, and cancer: A review. Nutr Cancer 1987;9:199–217.

79. Knekt P, Albanes D, Seppanen R, et al. Dietary fat and risk of breast cancer. Am J Clin Nutr 1990;52:903–908.

80. Tannenbaum A. The genesis and growth of tumors: III. Effects of a high fat diet. Cancer Res 1942;2:468–475.

81. Welsch CW, House JL, Herr BL, Eliasberg SJ, Welsch MA. Enhancement of mammary carcinogenesis by high levels of dietary fat: A phenomenon dependent on ad libitum feeding. JNCI 1990;82:1615–1620.

82. Cohen LA, Choi K, Wang CX. Influence of dietary fat, caloric restriction, and voluntary exercise on N-nitrosomethylurea-induced mammary tumorigenesis in rats. Cancer Res 1988;48:4276–4283.

83. Weindruch R, Albanes D, Kritchevsky D. The role of calories and caloric restriction in carcinogenesis. Hematol Oncol Clin North Am 1991;5:79–89.

84. Ruggeri BA, Klurfeld DM, Kritchevsky D, Furlanetto RW. Caloric restriction and 7,12-dimethylbenz(a)anthracene-induced mammary tumor growth in rats: Alterations in circulating insulin, insulin-like growth factors I and II, and epidermal growth factor. Cancer Res 1989;49:4130–4134.

85. Freedman LS, Clifford CK, Messina M. Analysis of dietary fat, calories, body weight, and the development of mammary tumors in rats and mice: A review. Cancer Res 1990;50:5710–5719.

86. Silverstone H, Tannenbaum A. The effect of proportion of dietary fat on the rate of formation of mammary carcinoma in mice. Cancer Res 1950;10:448–453.

87. Taylor PR, Schatzkin A, Patterson BH, Schiffman MH, Albanes D. Clinical metabolic studies in cancer research. Prev Med 1989;18:194–202.

88. Henderson MM, Kushi LH, Thompson DJ, Gorbach SL, Clifford CK, Insull W Jr. Feasibility of a randomized trial of a low-fat diet for the prevention of breast cancer: Dietary compliance in the Women's Health Trial Vanguard Study. Prev Med 1990;19:115–133.

89. Hiatt RA. Alcohol consumption and breast cancer. Med Oncol Tumor Pharmacother 1990;7:143–151.

90. Howe G, Rohan T, Decarli A, et al. The association between alcohol and breast cancer risk: Evidence from the combined analysis of six dietary case-control studies. Int J Cancer 1991;47:707–710.

91. Longnecker MP, Berlin JA, Orza MJ, Chalmers TC. A meta-analysis of alcohol consumption in relation to risk of breast cancer. JAMA 1988;260:652–656.

92. Willett WC, Stampfer MJ, Colditz GA, Rosner BA, Hennekens CH, Speizer FE. Moderate alcohol consumption and the risk of breast cancer. N Engl J Med 1987;316:1174–1180.

93. Rosenberg L, Palmer JR, Miller DR, Clarke EA, Shapiro S. A case-control study of alcoholic beverage consumption and breast cancer. Am J Epidemiol 1990;131:6–14.

94. Kesteloot H, Lesaffre E, Joossens JV. Dairy fat, saturated animal fat, and cancer risk. Prev Med 1991;20:226–236.

95. Sun M. Debate rages over breast cancer study. Science 1988;239:17–18.

96. Greenwald P, Sondik E. Cancer control objectives for the nation: 1985–2000. NCI Monogr 1986;2:ix-74.

97. Boyd NF, Cousins M, Beaton M, Kriukiv V, Lockwood G, Tritchler D. Quantitative changes in dietary fat intake and serum cholesterol in women: Results from a randomized, controlled trial. Am J Clin Nutr 1990;52:470–476.

98. Boyd NF, Cousins M, Lockwood G, Tritchler D. The feasibility of testing experimentally the dietary fat-breast cancer hypothesis. Br J Cancer 1990;62:878–881.

SECTION **2**

PETER GREENWALD

Dietary Fiber and Cancer

The interest in defining the relation between dietary fiber and cancer can be traced to the early 1970s, when Burkitt cited international epidemiologic data indicating that fiber-rich diets played a protective role in cancer of the large bowel.[1] This study and others found that the lowest rates of colon cancer are in African and Asian countries, where high-fiber diets are consumed, and that the highest colon cancer rates are in western societies, where refined carbohydrates have commonly replaced naturally occurring fiber-rich foods and where intake of fiber is consequently low. For example, the Chinese diet contains three times more fiber than the typical American diet, and the colon cancer incidence rate in China is approximately two thirds lower than that of the United States.[2] The Chinese also consume about 33% less protein, 50% as much fat, and 30% more calories based on reference body weights than do Americans, indicating that these factors may influence colon cancer risk. The protective role of dietary fiber in colon cancer can be seen when comparing populations that consume relatively comparable high levels of fat (more than 30% of total calories), but whose diets differ with regard to fiber intake. Studies comparing rural Finland and New York[3] and Finland and Denmark[4] found that Finnish populations, with an average intake of approximately 31 g of fiber per day,[5] had a lower risk for developing colon cancer than the other two populations, which consumed no more than 17 g of fiber per day,[5] despite a similar high intake of fat (34–37% of total calories). Within-country regional differences have been observed, for example in Seventh-Day Adventists who are lacto-ovo-vegetarians and have significantly lower rates of colon cancer than are found in the overall U.S. population.[6]

The epidemiologic, experimental, and clinical studies conducted since Burkitt's observations suggest that the risk for colon cancer and possibly other cancers may be lowered by increasing the intake of dietary fiber and other dietary components associated with high intakes of grains, vegetables, and fruits.[7] With an estimated worldwide annual incidence rate of more than 1 million new cases of colorectal and breast cancer and an estimated 337,000 new cases in the United States anticipated in 1992, the public health implications for risk reductions are enormous.[8,9]

WHAT IS FIBER?

All dietary fiber is of plant origin and may be considered as a heterogenous mixture of components, including cellulose, hemicellulose, pectin, gums, and lignins. These fiber components can be divided into soluble fibers, which include gums, mucilages, pectins, and certain hemicelluloses, and insoluble fibers, which consist of cellulose, lignin, and some hemicelluloses. A general definition of fiber is the endogenous dietary components of plants that are resistant to digestion by human enzymes.[10] A more precise chemical definition includes the nonstarch polysaccharides in foods and the phenylpropane polymer lignin.[11] Fiber fractions also may be classified as to physiologic function, which is based on solubility. Insoluble fiber components appear to increase fecal bulk and decrease intestinal transit time. The soluble fraction primarily delays gastric emptying, slows glucose absorption, and lowers serum cholesterol; it has a lesser effect on bulk and transit time.

ESTIMATING FIBER CONTENT

Estimating the total fiber content of foods is difficult, primarily because the analytic methods available do not satisfactorily quantify all fiber components. As a result of this limitation, many of the older food tables give fiber values for crude fiber, which is an approximate measure of cellulose plus lignin, and no national food tables exist that provide data for individual food fractions.[11,12] A study of the relation between crude fiber and dietary fiber in diets of American college students indicated that crude fiber represents approximately one fourth to one third of total dietary fiber.[13]

FOOD SOURCES, FIBER TYPE, AND CANCER

Foods such as whole-grain breads and cereals, fruits, vegetables, legumes, and nuts contain large amounts of fiber. However, these foods differ markedly in the quantitative and qualitative nature of the fiber they provide. For example, the insoluble fiber fractions cellulose and hemicellulose are found chiefly in cereals and grains[14]; high levels of cellulose are present in roots, leafy vegetables, legumes, and certain fruits. Lignin is found primarily in fruits, especially berries, and pectin content is highest in citrus fruits and apples. The bran layer of cereal grains, fruit skins, seeds, and berries contain high levels of insoluble fiber components.[14] A summary of the major benefits and sources of the various soluble and insoluble fiber components is presented in Table 20–2.

Several studies attempt to compare the protective effect from grain and cereal fiber with that observed from vegetable and fruit fiber. McKeown-Eyssen and Bright-See[15] concluded that only cereal fiber had an inverse correlation with colon cancer mortality, whereas Rosen and associates[16] and Jensen[17] found that high intakes of total fiber and cereals appeared to provide protection against colon cancer.[12] In contrast, Slattery and colleagues[18] noted that high intakes of vegetables and fruits—but not grains—decreased the risk for colon cancer in men and women. A few studies have reported an apparent increased relative risk for cancer in the distal colon and rectum with high intakes of cereal fiber.[19,20]

DIETARY FIBER AND COLORECTAL CANCER

EPIDEMIOLOGIC STUDIES

Evidence that environmental and dietary factors may play an important role in colon cancer risk is derived in part from early cross-cultural studies, which show marked variability in colon cancer incidence among different nations and migrant groups. Persons from countries with low risk for colon cancer who immigrate to countries with high risk have a tendency to adopt the colon cancer risk of their new geographic location.[10,21] Studies of migrant populations indicate that the colon cancer incidence rates for Hawaiians and Filipinos are low compared with whites, but when these groups migrated to San Francisco, the differences in rates became less noticeable. Colon cancer mortality rates increased to U.S. levels for Japanese, Polish, and Norwegian populations who migrated to this country.[22-25] Conversely, populations that moved from an area of relatively higher risk for colon cancer, Scotland, to an area with lower risk, Australia, experienced a lower incidence rate after migration.[25] Although these studies did not necessarily evaluate dietary components, they suggested the possibility that diet may be associated with increased colon cancer risk after migration, and an assessment of diet and cancer in international, national, and regional populations ensued.

A review by Greenwald and coworkers of data from 40 epidemiologic studies published between 1970 and 1986 found that 32 studies (80%) demonstrated an inverse association between the incidence of colon cancer and the amount of fiber consumed; in 20 (63%) of these 32 studies, the inverse association was statistically significant.[21] No relation was seen in 6 of 40 studies, and the remaining 2 studies showed a direct association between fiber intake and risk for colon cancer.[21] In a recent assessment of 32 epidemiologic studies conducted since 1980 (16 of which were reviewed by Greenwald and colleagues), 24 studies (75%) demonstrated an inverse relation between the incidence of colon cancer and dietary fiber.[12] Four of these studies showed no association; three suggested a direct relation between fiber consumption and colon cancer risk; and one was not evaluated as to risk associated with fiber intake, but indicated an increased risk with high intakes of fat, meat, or energy. An important aspect of this review was an examination of a subset of eight case-control studies that used a quantitative food frequency questionnaire to quantitate the amount of food consumed and a quantitative measure of fiber intake; of these eight studies, six showed a strong protective effect of fiber and two indicated no relation.[12] This quantitative approach to estimating fiber consumption is found more frequently in recent studies and provides a more reliable estimate of fiber intake than the methods used in most earlier studies using food groups or derived-fiber food indices.

A rigorous assessment of 37 observational epidemiology studies published between 1970 and 1988 found that most of the studies (21 [57%]) showed a strong to moderate protective effect for high-fiber intake with regard to colon cancer risk.[7] Of these 21 studies, 16 showed a protective effect for at least one of the following: total dietary fiber; high fiber or high-fiber foods or breads; crude fiber; cereals; fiber from vegetables; cellulose, uronic acid, or other fiber subtypes; rice and wheat; and whole-grain bread and pasta. In many of these studies, high intakes of vegetables were inversely related to colon cancer risk. In the remaining five studies, a protective dietary effect was associated with vegetables only. These latter associations could occur, because some study populations get most of their fiber from vegetables and have a homogenous low cereal fiber intake.

Additional epidemiologic studies or repeated analyses of such studies are not likely to enhance the understanding of the relation between fiber and colon cancer unless coupled with better measurement of fiber intake or clinical-metabolic measures. Intervention trials that test specific fiber fractions, for example, wheat bran fiber, may be more helpful in resolving etiologic questions and evaluating the efficacy of such substances.[26]

In a case-control study of persons in New York State, food sources of fiber were examined in relation to risk for colon

TABLE 20–2.   Benefits and Examples of Good Sources of Soluble and Insoluble Fiber

	Soluble Fiber	*Insoluble Fiber*
Natural Fiber Components	Gums, mucilages, pectins, some hemicelluloses	Cellulose, lignins, some hemicelluloses
Benefits	May help in reducing blood cholesterol and controlling blood glucose levels	May help prevent colon cancer; helps prevent constipation
Good Sources	Oat bran, beans (navy, kidney, pinto, or lima), barley, vegetables, and fruits	Whole-wheat bread, beans (navy, kidney, pinto, or lima), cereals, and the skins of vegetables and fruits

and rectal cancer.[27] In persons with primary cancer of the colon confirmed histopathologically, cancer risk decreased with grain fiber intake for women and men and vegetable and fruit fiber intake for men only; insoluble grain fiber was more strongly associated with decreased risk than was soluble grain fiber. For rectal cancer cases, total fiber intake and consumption of fiber derived from vegetables and fruits was associated with decreased risk; however, consumption of grain fiber had no effect on risk. Rectal cancer risk was significantly reduced when intakes of soluble and insoluble fiber components from vegetables and fruits were high. A Utah population-based, case-control study indicated that crude fiber, but neither total dietary fiber nor neutral detergent fiber, was consistently associated with a decreased risk for colon cancer in men and women.[18] The protective fiber fractions in this study, particularly with regard to cancer in the ascending colon, were mannose and galactose in men and galactose and uronic acid in women. Bingham and colleagues[28] found that although total fiber intake did not correlate with colon cancer rates in England and Wales, cancer mortality was inversely associated with cellulose and uronic acid (pectins), which are derived primarily from vegetables and fruits.[7,21] Based on data from the Nurses Health Study, Willett and associates reported that a low intake of fruit fiber appeared to contribute to increased colon cancer risk; this association, however, was not statistically independent of red meat intake.[29]

ANIMAL CARCINOGENESIS STUDIES

The results of a number of animal studies support the protective role of fiber on tumor induction in colon cancer.[30,31] Pilch reviewed 44 experiments that examined the effects of dietary fiber on chemically induced colon cancer in animals and found that 22 of these studies demonstrated a protective effect of fiber.[10] The remaining studies indicated no effect or an enhancing effect on colon tumors. Differences between studies in part reflect variable susceptibility of animals to the different carcinogens used to induce benign adenomas and malignant carcinomas of the colon, for example, 1,2-dimethylhydrazine (DMH), azoxymethane (AOM), 3,2-dimethyl-4-aminobiphenyl, and methylnitrosourea (MNU)[32]; to the amounts, type, and route of administration of the carcinogen; and to variation in the amount and type of fiber consumed over time.[10] Other findings indicate that the possible protective effects of fiber in colon carcinogenesis are overridden by the promoting effect of high-fat diets.[10,31]

A study by Watanabe and colleagues[33] assessed two carcinogens (MNU and AOM) and various combinations and amounts of pectin, wheat bran, and fat. Diets were administered to rats during the initiation and promotion stages of carcinogenesis. AOM-induced colon tumors were greatly inhibited by pectin and wheat bran in diets. However, pectin did not protect against MNU-induced tumors. MNU is a direct-acting carcinogen, whereas AOM must be activated by liver and colon enzymes. In a study by Freeman and coworkers,[34] cellulose inhibited the development of DMH-induced tumors in rats but pectin did not. Wynder and Reddy[35] noted that rats fed diets high in wheat bran, citrus fiber, citrus pectin, cellulose, or lignin developed fewer chemically induced colon tumors than rats fed low- or no-fiber diets. When other studies using corn bran, rice bran, soybean bran, or oat bran were evaluated, no protective effect was evident.[10,35] In reviewing these and other animal studies, Pilch concluded that the type of fiber is an important protective or enhancing factor on outcome; the chemical and physical properties of the fiber component are of importance for the effects of various fibers; and wheat bran, when compared with other fiber sources, appears most consistently to inhibit tumor development in animals.[10]

MECHANISTIC STUDIES

Several mechanisms by which dietary fiber is believed to protect against colon cancer have been suggested: (1) by increasing fecal bulk, which, in turn, dilutes the concentrations of carcinogens in the feces; (2) by changing bacterial composition in the colon, which leads to deactivation of carcinogenic metabolites by binding to carcinogens, cocarcinogens, or both, or promoters in the bowel; (3) by inducing structural and functional chemical changes in the gut mucosa, including altering rates of cell proliferation; (4) by inhibiting the production of butyric acid, a differentiating agent that also serves as an energy source for cell proliferation; (5) by altering bile acid metabolism; (6) by reducing fecal pH; and (7) by accelerating the transit time of fecal material through the intestinal tract so that carcinogens from food or other sources have less contact with colon mucosa.[30,31,36–38]

Clinical metabolic investigations have studied fecal mutagenic activity and concentrations of secondary bile acids in various populations for a range of fiber intakes and found lower mutagen levels and reduced bile acids (deoxycholic acid and lithocholic acid) associated with high-fiber intake.[21,39] As a result of these investigations, fecal bile acids and fecal mutagenic activity are being studied as possible bioindicators of colon cancer incidence. In a study with healthy subjects, Reddy and colleagues examined the effects of types of dietary fiber on fecal mutagens and bile acids.[39] Subjects given 10 g dietary wheat bran or cellulose per day exhibited significantly decreased levels of fecal secondary bile acids and fecal mutagenic activity. Oat fiber supplementation had no effect on these fecal entities. A potentially protective effect by wheat fiber also was observed by Reddy and colleagues, who found that 21 of 72 subjects on a high-fat, moderately low-fiber diet excreted high levels of fecal mutagens thought to be important in the induction of malignant polyps.[40] When subjects with elevated fecal mutagen levels were fed diets supplemented with 10 g of wheat bran or cellulose per day, fecal mutagenic activity and secondary bile acids were significantly reduced; in contrast, the addition of 10 g of oat bran per day to the diet did not reduce either parameter.

Fecal bile acids also are being studied in a double-blind, placebo-controlled trial with wheat bran fiber in patients with adenomatous polyps.[40a] After 9 months of fiber treatment, patients receiving 13.5 g of wheat bran per day had a significant decrease in total fecal bile acid concentration and a concomitant increase in dry fecal weight. This clinical study has the strength of a double-blind, placebo-controlled design in high-risk patients and demonstrates a physiologic effect of fiber on fecal bile acid concentrations.

The rate at which tritium-labeled thymidine is incorporated into the DNA of epithelial cells of the rectal mucosa is much higher in patients with a history of resected colon or rectal cancer than in healthy persons.[41] Increases in the rate or pattern, or both, of colonic epithelial cell proliferation, which can be measured using [3H] thymidine labeling, may suggest a predisposition for gastrointestinal cancer.[42] As a result of these findings, an altered rate or pattern of [3H] thymidine labeling of cells is being studied as a potential biomarker to monitor proliferation. A recent study has investigated the effects of dietary wheat bran fiber on rectal epithelial cell proliferation in patients with resection for colorectal cancer.[41] In this study, 6 of 8 patients with initially elevated [3H] thymidine cell labeling demonstrated a significant decrease in labeling after treatment with 13.5 g of wheat bran fiber per day for 8 weeks; the mean reduction in labeling for all 16 patients in the study was 22%. Dietary supplementation with the wheat bran was well tolerated by the subjects, who were between 54 and 70 years of age.

Genetic factors also appear to influence the development of colon cancer. The contribution of inherited and somatic genetic mutations to colon cancer is unknown, but estimates provided by Kinzler and associates indicate that nearly 1 in 10,000 Americans, Britons, and Japanese are affected by familial adenomatous polyposis (FAP).[43] In their review of the role of heredity and cancer, Levine and colleagues report that even when families with a history of FAP are excluded, close relatives of patients with colon cancer are at a two to three times greater risk for developing cancer of the large bowel than are the general population.[44] A study of 389 patients with colorectal cancer indicated that approximately 15% to 20% of those patients had at least one first-degree relative who was affected by malignancies of the large bowel; the trend was strongest for siblings, but an excess of malignancies was found in parents.[45] These data suggest a strong genetic component in colorectal cancer.

Recent reports suggest that at least one gene on chromosome 5 is important in inherited (FAP and Gardner syndrome) and noninherited forms of colorectal cancer.[43,46,47] The two genes on chromosome 5 that are linked currently with colorectal cancers include the adenomatous polyposis coli and "mutated in colon cancer" (MCC) genes. MCC mutants have been found in approximately 15% of tumor tissue in nonhereditary colon cancers.[46] Other studies in animals and humans suggest that alterations in epithelial cell proliferation are indicative of a predisposition for colorectal cancer. Genetic markers that may serve as indicators for these proliferative disorders include chromosome 17 deletions, p53 gene mutations, and high levels of RAS oncogene expression in colon cancer cells.[42] The role of fiber in reducing colonic epithelial cell proliferation and polyp formation and decreasing mutagenic activity may be particularly important to patients with a genetic predisposition to colon cancer.

CLINICAL TRIALS

The protective effect of dietary fiber on colon cancer risk in humans is under study in a number of National Cancer Institute (NCI)-sponsored intervention trials. Evidence of inhibition of benign polyps in patients with FAP, a heritable disease that progresses to cancer in nearly all cases if left untreated, has been reported.[48] In a 4-year, randomized, double-blind, placebo-controlled study, the effect on rectal polyps of 4 g of ascorbic acid (vitamin C) plus 400 mg α-tocopherol (vitamin E), alone or with a supplement that provided approximately 11 g of grain fiber per day (total fiber from diet and supplement, 22.5 g/day), was studied in 58 patients with FAP; 20 patients were included in the high fiber-supplemented group. The number and size of the polyps decreased in patients consuming 22.5 g of wheat bran fiber per day (i.e., their normal diet plus the 11 g/day fiber supplement). No protective effect was observed for the vitamin supplements. A colon cancer prevention trial based on the protective evidence for fiber and calcium currently is in progress and is evaluating the effects of 2, 5, or 13.5 g of wheat bran fiber per day plus 1.25 or 0.1 g of calcium carbonate per day in patients at high risk for colon cancer.

As a result of the consistently strong evidence suggesting the role of diet in large bowel cancer, the NCI is implementing the Polyp Prevention Trial, a multiinstitutional randomized control study designed to determine whether a low-fat, high-fiber, and vegetable- and fruit-enriched eating plan prevents the recurrence of large bowel adenomatous polyps in otherwise healthy women and men who have had polypectomy. This clinical trial is based on the fact that large bowel adenomas are highly prevalent, occurring in 30% of middle-aged and older adults; the polyp recurrence rate is high in those people who have undergone surgical polyp removal; and there is a strong association between colon polyps and the development of colon cancer. This dietary intervention trial will enroll a total of 2000 male and female patients older than the age of 35 at ten clinical centers across the United States. Half of the subjects will be randomized to a control group with no intervention. The other half will be randomized to the diet intervention group, which will be given a diet including

20% of calories from fat, 18 g fiber/1000 cal, and five to eight servings of fruits and vegetables per day. The subjects in the Polyp Prevention Trial will be followed for 4 years, and the recurrence of polyps will be assessed in both groups at years 1 and 4 to determine the effect of this dietary intervention on the polyp recurrence rate.

DIETARY FIBER AND BREAST CANCER

A number of studies have investigated the role of fiber-rich foods in protecting against breast cancer. Case-control studies generally support a protective role of fiber in the development of breast cancer. Of seven case-control studies reviewed by Shankar and Lanza, six demonstrated an inverse association between risk of breast cancer and consumption of fiber and fiber-rich foods; three of these studies indicated that diets high in fiber or cereals, or both, reduced the risk of breast cancer; and an additional study suggested a weak protective effect of the fiber constituents of vegetables.[12] In five of these seven studies, the relation between fiber or vegetable consumption, or both, and breast cancer was stronger than the association with dietary fat intake. One study of 818 breast cancer patients demonstrated that dietary intakes high in animal protein and animal fat and low in fiber were associated with elevated risk for breast cancer; this association was strongest for women younger than 50 years of age but was weakened when nondietary factors were considered.[49]

Some international studies suggest that high intakes of cereals may be inversely related to breast cancer incidence. In a study of 37 countries, a high correlation was observed between the incidence rates of colon and breast cancer[50]; in countries with high incidence rates of these types of cancer, a weak inverse correlation between cereal consumption and cancer incidence and a direct relation between high intakes of fat and animal protein were found.[10,51,52] However, there was no association between total fiber intake and cancer.[10,52] In a comparison of 133 breast cancer patients and 218 healthy subjects, it was found that women with breast cancer had a lower energy-adjusted intake of dietary fiber than women in the control group.[53] More specifically, women in the lowest quartile for consumption of cereal products, but not total fiber, beta-carotene, fruits, vegetables, or all vegetable products combined, were at greatest risk for developing breast cancer. Another study indicated that consumption of fiber from grains appeared to decrease breast cancer risk in premenopausal and postmenopausal women; however, results of this study also suggested that for postmenopausal women, high intakes of vegetables and fruits were associated with an increased risk for breast cancer.[54] Other studies suggest that diets rich in high-fiber vegetables and fruits reduce the risk for breast cancer[55,56]; however, they failed to define an association between fiber and cancer incidence, making it difficult to distinguish between the effects of fiber and the many other constituents in these foods.

Few animal studies describing the relation between dietary fiber and breast cancer have been conducted. An early study by Carroll and Khor demonstrated that animals given cereal-based diets after exposure to 7,12-dimethylbenz[a]anthracene developed fewer mammary tumors than did rats consuming a casein-based semipurified diet.[57] Two additional reports

suggest that a high-fiber diet reduces the incidence of mammary tumors in rats[58,59]; one indicated that a high-fiber diet may aid in preventing breast cancer when a high-fat diet is consumed.[58] In contrast, the addition of fiber to a low-fat diet had essentially no effect on tumor incidence when compared with a fiber-unsupplemented, low-fat diet.

It is postulated that fiber may assist in preventing breast cancer by lowering circulating levels of estrogen. A review of several studies examining the connection between diet and systemic sex hormone patterns in women indicated that high intake of total fiber and high intakes of vegetable fiber, grain fiber, and fiber from fruits and berries were associated with low levels of testosterone, estrone, and androstenedione, with low levels of plasma free estradiol and free testosterone, and with elevated levels of sex hormone-binding globulin (SHBG), the protein to which estradiol is bound.[60] The overall reduction in the bioavailability of these hormones suggests that a fiber-enriched diet theoretically could reduce the risk of hormone-dependent cancer.

The primary mechanism by which dietary fiber influences estrogen levels involves enterohepatic circulation: The intestinal reabsorption of estrogen conjugates secreted in the bile requires deconjugation by the bacterial enzymes β-glucuronidase and sulfatase. These enzymes are induced by intraluminal fat, but their activity is reduced in the presence of high fiber.[61] Other studies have demonstrated that unconjugated estrogens bind to various natural fibers, particularly insoluble fiber constituents and fibers in vegetarian diets, interfering with enterohepatic cycling.[62,63] Additional evidence is provided by several small clinical studies that have investigated the relation between fiber intake and circulating androgens in healthy women and women with breast cancer. Adlercreutz and colleagues studied three groups of postmenopausal women: healthy omnivores, healthy vegetarians, and breast cancer patients.[64] The women with breast cancer consumed significantly less total fiber, nongrain fiber, and grain calories than did women in the two other groups; also, the breast cancer patients consumed about half as much grain fiber as vegetarians. Women in the cancer group had markedly higher plasma levels of androstenedione, testosterone, and free testosterone and lower plasma concentrations of SHBG than vegetarians. A positive association between plasma estrogens and fat consumption and an inverse relation between hormone levels and fiber consumption were found in a comparative study of premenopausal and postmenopausal white American women and Asian women who had migrated to Hawaii[65]; the Asian women, who had a markedly lower risk for breast cancer than did their American counterparts, consumed 20% less fat and significantly more fiber than the white women in the study. Another study in which the fat content of all diets was between 32% and 36% demonstrated a significant reduction in serum estrone and estradiol levels in premenopausal women whose diets were supplemented with approximately 15 g of wheat bran per day (total fiber 29 g/day) for 2 months.[66] Levels of fecal bacterial β-glucuronidase were reduced in these women. However, serum progesterone levels remained unaffected. The addition of corn bran or oat bran to the diet had no effect on circulating hormone levels or fecal bacterial enzymes.

Another mechanism by which fiber may interfere with the development of breast tumorigenesis is through the formation of mammalian lignans, estrogen-like compounds that result from the structural modification of plant lignans such as matairesinol and secoisolariciresinol by intestinal microflora.[60] Urinary excretion of the lignans enterolactone and enterodiol has been found to be positively associated with fiber intake and is reduced significantly in breast cancer patients.[67] Additional studies have demonstrated a positive correlation between urinary lignan excretion and plasma levels of SHBG and an inverse relation between urinary enterolactone concentrations and plasma levels of free testosterone.[68] It has been suggested that lignans stimulate the synthesis of SHBG in the liver, thereby indirectly reducing the amount of freely circulating unbound estrogen.[60] Although low levels of SHBG have been associated with increased breast cancer risk,[61] plasma levels of SHBG were unaffected in healthy premenopausal women given diets high in wheat, corn, or oat bran,[66] and no changes in circulating 17-β-estradiol were observed in rats given a high-fiber diet after exposure to the mammary tumor-inducing carcinogen NMU.[58] These latter data suggest that the apparent protective effect of fiber against breast cancer may not be mediated by SHBG or reductions in serum estradiol. Review of the limited number of studies investigating the relation between dietary fiber and breast cancer indicates that the degree of protection afforded by fiber is unclear and that the exact mechanism by which fiber may act is not known.

DIETARY FIBER AND OTHER CANCERS

Of the few studies of fiber intake and cancers of the esophagus, the mouth, the pharynx, the stomach, the endometrium, and the ovary, most indicate a protective effect from high fiber.[10-12] However, it is difficult currently to assess if this protective effect has its origin in fiber components or other dietary components, such as low fat or the microcomponents found in these complex mixtures.

ACHIEVING THE GUIDELINES FOR DIETARY FIBER

The role of dietary fiber as a significant factor that may decrease the incidence and mortality of colorectal cancer and possibly several other cancers is important to clinicians and their patients. Over the past 15 years, numerous scientific organizations in the United States have issued dietary recommendations to the public with an aim of reducing cancer risk, including the recommendation to increase fiber consumption.[52] The NCI suggests that healthy adults consume 20 to 30 g of dietary fiber per day, using a variety of food sources. This represents an increase over the 11 to 13 g/day that the average American now consumes.[69] The NCI also recommends a reduction in total fat intake from its present level of about 38% of calories to 30% or less. These guidelines are consistent with recommendations from other organizations, including the American Cancer Society and the American Heart Association.

The fiber contents of some foods in the major fiber-containing food groups—grains, vegetables, and fruits—are provided in Table 20–3; the foods are listed in descending order by fiber content per typical serving size. The source of

these data is the Nutrition Coding Center in Minneapolis, Minnesota. As an illustration of how to incorporate these foods to meet the guidelines, a sample 1-day menu was constructed (Fig. 20–2). Note that the guidelines can be easily met with a variety of commonly available foods. Although it is possible to meet the guidelines by relying on large portions of one or two fiber-dense foods (*e.g.*, high-fiber cereals or beans), this is not recommended because a limited diet may not provide

TABLE 20–3. Fiber Content of Selected Foods

Food Item (Amount)	Fiber (g)
Grain Products	
Cereals	
All bran (½ c)	13.1
40% Bran Flakes (1 c)	5.1
Raisin Bran (1 c)	5.0
Oatmeal, cooked (1 c)	3.6
Shredded Wheat (1 biscuit)	2.2
Cheerios (1 c)	1.9
Cornflakes (1 c)	0.5
Rice Krispies (1 c)	0.5
Breads	
Whole wheat bread (1 slice)	2.1
Rye bread (1 slice)	1.9
Bagel, plain (1 medium)	1.2
Italian bread (1 slice)	0.8
White bread (1 slice)	0.5
Pasta and Rice	
Brown rice, cooked (1 c)	3.3
Macaroni/spaghetti, cooked (1 c)	2.2
White rice, cooked (1 c)	1.0
Vegetables (Including Legumes)	
Baked beans (½ c)	7.0
Refried beans (½ c)	6.3
Lima beans (½ c)	4.2
Potato, baked, with skin (1 medium)	3.9
Peas, green, cooked (½ c)	3.3
Corn, cooked (½ c)	3.0
Broccoli, cooked (½ c)	2.6
Carrots, cooked (½ c)	2.4
Spinach, cooked (½ c)	2.1
Green beans, cooked (½ c)	2.0
Tomato juice (1 c)	1.9
Zucchini, cooked (½ c)	1.2
Fruits and Juices	
Strawberries, fresh (1 c)	3.9
Applesauce (1 c)	3.9
Orange, fresh (1 medium)	3.1
Apple, raw with skin (1 medium)	2.8
Banana (1 medium)	2.2
Cantaloupe (¼ medium)	1.9
Grapefruit, fresh (½ medium)	1.8
Orange juice (1 c)	0.8
Apple juice (1 c)	0.3

(The Nutrition Coding Center, Minneapolis, MN, 1990)

MEAL	FOOD (AMOUNT)	FIBER (g)
Breakfast	40% Bran Flakes (1 c)	5.1
	Skim milk (1 c)	
	Whole wheat toast (1 slice)	2.1
	Margarine (1 pat)	
	Orange, fresh (1 medium)	3.1
Lunch	Bean soup (1 c)	3.9
	Sandwich:	
	Turkey (3 oz)	
	Lettuce (1 leaf)	0.2
	Tomato (2 slices)	0.4
	Mayonnaise (2 tsp)	
	Whole wheat bread (2 slices)	4.2
	Apple, fresh, with skin (1 medium)	2.8
Dinner	Chicken breast (3 oz)	
	Baked potato, with skin (1 medium)	3.9
	Margarine (2 tsp)	
	Broccoli, cooked (½ c)	2.6
	Tossed salad (1 c)	0.2
	French dressing (1 tsp)	
Snack	Milk (1 c)	
	Graham crackers (4 squares)	0.8
	Total	**29.3**

FIGURE 20–2. A sample menu for 1 day (approximately 1800 calories) that meets the dietary recommendations for fiber.

adequate amounts of essential nutrients and other chemopreventive substances.

REFERENCES

1. Burkitt DP. Epidemiology of cancer of the colon and rectum. Cancer 1971;28:3–13.
2. Chen JC, Campbell JC, Li J-Y, Peto R. Diet, life-style, and mortality in China: A study of the characteristics of 65 Chinese counties (in English and Chinese). Ithaca, NY: Cornell University Press, 1990.
3. Reddy BS, Hedges AR, Laakso K, Wynder EL. Metabolic epidemiology of large bowel cancer: Fecal bulk and constituents in high-risk North American and low-risk Finnish populations. Cancer 1978;42:2832–2838.
4. Jensen OM, MacLennan R, Wahrendorf J. Diet, bowel function, fecal characteristics, and large bowel cancer in Denmark and Finland. Nutr Cancer 1982;4:5–19.
5. IARC, International Agency for Research on Cancer. Dietary fibre, transit-time, faecal bacteria, steroids, and colon cancer in two candinavian populations. Lancet 1977;2:207–211.
6. Phillips RL, Kuzma JW, Lotz TM. Cancer mortality among comparable members versus nonmembers of the Seventh-Day Adventist church. In: Cairns J, Lyons JL, Skolnick M, eds. Banbury report 4: Cancer incidence in defined populations. Cold Spring Harbor, NY: Cold Spring Harbor Laboratory, 1980:93–108.
7. Trock B, Lanza E, Greenwald P. Dietary fiber, vegetables, and colon cancer: Critical review and meta-analyses of the epidemiologic evidence. JNCI 1990;82:650–661.
8. Miller BA, Ries LAG, Hankey BF, Kosary CL, Edwards BK, eds. Cancer Statistics Review: 1973–1989. Bethesda, MD: National Cancer Institute, NIH Pub. No. 92-2789, 1992.
9. Parkin DM, Laara E, Muir CS. Estimates of the world-wide frequency of twelve common cancers in 1980. Int J Cancer 1988;36:184–197.
10. Pilch S. Physiological effects and health consequences of dietary fiber. Bethesda, MD: Federation of American Societies for Experimental Biology, Life Sciences Research, 1987.
11. Lanza E, Greenwald P. The role of dietary fiber in cancer prevention. PPO Updates, Sept. 1989;1–9.
12. Shankar S, Lanza E. Dietary fiber and cancer prevention. Hematol Oncol Clin North Am 1991;5:25–41.
13. Marlett JA, Bokram RL. Relationship between calculated dietary and crude fiber intakes of 200 college students. Am J Clin Nutr 1981;34:335–342.
14. Lanza E, Butrum RR. A critical review of food fiber analysis and data. J Am Diet Assoc 1986;86:732–743.
15. McKeown-Eyssen GE, Bright-See E. Dietary factors in colon cancer: International relationships. Nutr Cancer 1984;6:160–170.
16. Rosen M, Nystrom L, Wall S. Diet and cancer mortality in the countries of Sweden. Am J Epidemiol 1988;127:42–49.
17. Jensen OM. Cancer risk among Danish male Seventh-Day Adventists and other temperance society members. JNCI 1983;70:1011–1014.
18. Slattery ML, Sorenson AW, Mahoney AW, et al. Diet and colon cancer: Assessment of risk of fiber type and food source. JNCI 1988;80:1474–1480.
19. Martinez I, Torres R, Friaz Z, et al. Factors associated with adenocarcinomas of the large bowel in Puerto Rico. Rev Latinam Oncol Clin 1981;13:45.
20. Potter JD, McMichael AJ. Diet and cancer of the colon and rectum: A case-control study. JNCI 1986;76:557–569.
21. Greenwald P, Lanza E, Eddy GA. Dietary fiber in the reduction of colon cancer risk. J Am Diet Assoc 1987;87:1178–1188.
22. Haenszel W. Cancer mortality among foreign-born in the United States. JNCI 1961;26:37–132.
23. Haenszel W, Kurihari M. Studies of Japanese migrants: I. Mortality from cancer and other diseases among Japanese in the United States. JNCI 1968;40:43–68.
24. Smith RL. Recorded and expected mortality among Japanese of the United States and Hawaii with special reference to cancer. JNCI 1956;17:459–473.
25. McMichael AJ, McCall MG, Hartshorne JM, et al. Patterns of gastro-intestinal cancer in European migrants to Australia: The role of dietary change. Int J Cancer 1980;25:431–437.
26. MacLennan R. Rationale for intervention trials of dietary fiber and adenomatous polyps. In: Kritchevsky D, Bonfield C, Anderson JW, eds. Dietary fiber: Chemistry, physiology, and health effects. New York: Plenum Press, 1990:481–488.
27. Freudenheim JL, Graham S, Horvath PJ, et al. Risks associated with source of fiber and fiber components in cancer of the colon and rectum. Cancer Res 1990;50:3295–3300.
28. Bingham SA, Williams DRR, Cummings JH. Dietary fiber consumption in Britain: New estimates and their relation to large bowel cancer mortality. Br J Cancer 1985;52:399.
29. Willett WC, Stampfer MJ, Colditz GA, Rosner BA, Speizer FE. Relation of meat, fat, and their fiber intake to the risk of colon cancer in prospective study among women. N Engl J Med 1990;323:1664–1672.
30. Reddy BS. Diet and colon cancer: Evidence from human and animal model studies. In: Reddy BS, Cohen LA, eds. Diet, nutrition and cancer: A critical evaluation. Vol 1. Boca Raton, FL: CRC Press, 1986:47–65.
31. Reddy BS. Dietary fiber and colon cancer: Animal model studies. Prev Med 1987;16:559–565.
32. Shamsuddin AKM. Carcinoma in the large intestine: Animal models and human disease. Hum Pathol 1986;17:451–453.
33. Watanabe K, Reddy BS, Weisburger JH, et al. Effects of dietary alfalfa, pectin, and wheat bran on azoxymethane- or methylnitrosourea-induced colon carcinogenesis in F344 rats. JNCI 1979;63:141–145.
34. Freeman HJ, Spiller GA, Kim YS. A double-blind study on the effects of differing purified cellulose and pectin fiber diets on 1, 2-dimethyhydrazine-induced rat colonic neoplasia. Cancer Res 1980;40:2661–2665.

35. Wynder EL, Reddy BS. Dietary fat and fiber and colon cancer. Semin Oncol 1983;10: 264–272.

36. Cummings JH, Bingham SA. Dietary fibre, fermentation and large bowel cancer. Cancer Surv 1987;6:601–621.

37. Doll R, Peto R. The causes of cancer: Quantitative estimates of avoidable risks of cancer in the United States today. JNCI 1981;66:1192–1308.

38. Reddy BS. Dietary fat and its relationship to large bowel cancer. Cancer Res 1981;41: 3700–3705.

39. Reddy BS, Sharma C, Simi B, et al. Metabolic epidemiology of colon cancer: Effect of dietary fiber on fecal mutagens and bile acids in healthy subjects. Cancer Res 1987;47: 644–648.

40. Reddy BS, Engle A, Katsifis S, et al. Biochemical epidemiology of colon cancer: Effects of types of dietary fiber on fecal mutagens, acid, and neutral sterols in healthy subjects. Cancer Res 1989;49:4629–4635.

40a. Alberts, personal communication, 1991.

41. Alberts DS, Einspahr J, Rees-McGee S, et al. Effects of dietary wheat bran fiber on rectal epithelial cell proliferation in patients with resection for colorectal cancer. JNCI 1990;82:1280–1285.

42. Lipkin M. Biomarkers of increased susceptibility to gastrointestinal cancer: New application to studies of cancer prevention in human studies. Cancer Res 1988;48:235–245.

43. Kinzler KW, Nilbert MC, Su LK, et al. Identification of FAP locus genes from chromosome 5q21. Science 1991;253:661–665.

44. Levine EG, King RA, Bloomfield CD. The role of heredity in cancer. J Clin Oncol 1989;7:527–540.

45. Ponz de Leon M, Sassatelli R, Sacchetti C, et al. Familial aggregation of tumors in the three-year experience of a population-based colorectal cancer registry. Cancer Res 1989;49:4344–4348.

46. Marx J. Zeroing in on individual cancer risk: News and comment. Science 1991;253: 612–616.

47. Nishisho I, Nakamura Y, Miyoshi Y, et al. Mutations of chromosome 5q21 in FAP and colorectal cancer patients. Science 1991;253:665–669.

48. Decosse JJ, Miller HH, Lesser ML. Effect of wheat fiber and vitamins C and E on rectal polyps in patients with familial adenomatous polyposis. JNCI 1989;81:1290–1297.

49. Lubin F, Wax Y, Modan B. Role of fat, animal protein, and dietary fiber in breast cancer etiology: A case-control study. JNCI 1986;77:605–612.

50. Drasar B, Irving D. Environmental factors and cancer of the colon and breast. Br J Cancer 1973;27:167–172.

51. Irving D, Drasar B. Fibre and cancer of the colon. Br J Cancer 1973;28:462–463.

52. Havas S. Macronutrients and cancer. Clin Nutr 1990;9:49–55.

53. Van't-Veer P, Kilb CM, Verhoef P, et al. Dietary fiber, beta-carotene and breast cancer: Results from a case-control study. Int J Cancer 1990;45:825–828.

54. Pryor M, Slattery ML, Robison LM, et al. Adolescent diet and breast cancer in Utah. Cancer Res 1989;49:2161–2167.

55. LaVecchia CL, Decarli A, Franceschi S, et al. Dietary factors and the risk of breast cancer. Nutr Cancer 1987;10:205–214.

56. Katsouyanni K, Willett W, Trichopoulos D, et al. Risk of breast cancer among Greek women in relation to nutrient intake. Cancer 1988;61:181–185.

57. Carroll KK, Khor TT. Effects of level and type of dietary fat on incidence of mammary tumors induced in female Sprague-Dawley rats by 7,12-dimethylbenz(a)anthracene. Lipids 1971;6:415–520.

58. Cohen LA, Kendall ME, Zang E, et al. Modulation of N-nitrosomethylurea-induced mammary tumor promotion by dietary fiber and fat. JNCI 1991;83:496–500.

59. Magrane D, van Sant J, Butler B. Effect of high fat, fiber and caloric restriction on mammary tumorigenesis. Fed Proc [Abstract] 1986;45:5426.

60. Adlercreutz H. Western diet and Western diseases: Some hormonal and biochemical mechanisms and associations. Scand J Clin Lab Invest 1990;50:3–23.

61. Rose DP, Connolly JM. Dietary prevention of breast cancer. Med Oncol Tumor Pharmacother 1990;7:121–130.

62. Shultz TD, Howie BJ. In vitro binding of steroid hormones by natural and purified fibers. Nutr Cancer 1986;8:141–147.

63. Whitten CG, Shultz TD. Binding of steroid hormones in vitro by water-insoluble dietary fiber. Nutr Res 1988;8:1223–1235.

64. Adlercreutz H, Hamalainen E, Gorbach SL, Goldin BR, Woods MN, Dwyer JT. Diet and plasma androgens in postmenopausal vegetarian and omnivorous women and postmenopausal women with breast cancer. Am J Clin Nutr 1989;49:433–442.

65. Goldin BR, Adlercreutz H, Gorbach SL, et al. The relationship between estrogen levels and diets of Caucasian American and Oriental immigrant women. Am J Clin Nutr 1986;44:945–953.

66. Rose DP, Goldman M, Connolly JM, et al. High-fiber diet reduces serum estrogen concentrations in premenopausal women. Am J Clin Nutr 1991;54:520–525.

67. Adlercreutz H, Fostis T, Heikkinen R, et al. Excretion of the lignans enterolactone and enterodiol and of equol in omnivorous and vegetarian postmenopausal women and in women with breast cancer. Lancet 1982;2:1295–1299.

68. Adlercreutz H, Fostis T, Bannwort C, et al. Determination of urinary lignans and phytoestrogen metabolites, potential antiestrogens and anticarcinogens in urine of women on various habitual diets. J Steroid Biochem 1986;25:791–797.

69. Lanza E, Jones DY, Block G, et al. Dietary fiber intake in the US population. Am J Clin Nutr 1987;46:790–797.

SECTION **3**

PETER GREENWALD

Micronutrients and Chemoprevention

The sum of evidence gathered from population and experimental studies indicates that the factors that determine most cancer incidence are largely lifestyle and environmental. Therefore, if it were possible to identify all these factors, many types of cancer could be prevented.[1–3] Limiting human exposure to environmental carcinogens and the early detection of precancerous lesions dominated the field of cancer prevention research of the 1950s and 1960s and was followed by a substantial investment in the 1970s and 1980s by the National Cancer Institute (NCI) in the search for environmental influences of cancer. Because cancer is expected to become the leading cause of death in the United States by the year 2000 unless present trends can be reversed, there is a public health responsibility to accelerate the progress in the prevention and control of this disease.[4,5]

There is a strong possibility that preventive approaches may greatly impact cancer incidence. The study of micronutrients and chemoprevention is one approach that seeks to develop chemical agents that have the potential to slow or prevent the initiation of or progression to cancer in humans. Various naturally occurring micronutrients and synthetic compounds are observed to have anticarcinogenic properties.[1,6–8] These compounds appear to prevent the initiation, promotion, and progression of neoplastic development before or during the preneoplastic period. The more recent advances in molecular and cellular biology that underlie understanding multistage carcinogenesis are providing further support for new research strategies to prevent and treat cancer.[9,10]

EPIDEMIOLOGIC EVIDENCE

Epidemiology has been the major population research discipline used to evaluate causal hypotheses in human cancer, despite certain limitations of interpretation that can be made from these studies.[3] Findings from case-control, cohort, international, and migrant studies have provided an extensive body of data as the initial research leads for suggesting chemopreventive agents for human interventions.[11] The 1982 National Research Council Report on Diet and Cancer commissioned by the NCI concluded that sufficient epidemiologic evidence existed to suggest associations between incidence rates for certain cancers and specific dietary constituents, such as the macronutrients fat and fiber, and plant foods, such as vegetables, fruits, legumes, and whole grain products.[12] Since 1982, other studies have supported these conclusions and generated additional research leads for testing the chemopreventive potential of candidate agents.[13–15] Hundreds of diverse anticarcinogenic compounds currently are being tracked from experimental studies; most need further preclinical testing for possible development in clinical interventions.

Epidemiologic studies generally show an inverse relation between cancer incidence and intake of foods high in several specific antioxidant nutrients, such as beta-carotene, selenium, and vitamins C and E.[16-19] Other population studies have focused on the consumption of vegetables and fruits and their association with cancer risk. Ziegler[20,21] and Menkes and associates[22] observed in analyzing prospective and retrospective studies that low intakes of vegetables and fruits containing vitamin A, carotenoids, and other cancer-inhibiting micronutrients are consistently associated with increased risk for lung cancer. The evidence from a population-based case-control study in Hawaii showed stronger inverse associations for lung cancer risk with low intakes of vegetables (in particular, dark green and cruciferous) than for beta-carotene alone. This study suggests that other micronutrients in vegetables may be protective against lung cancer in humans and need to be characterized.[23] A few prospective and retrospective studies suggest that vegetable and fruit intake may reduce the risk of cancers of the mouth, the pharynx, the larynx, the esophagus, the stomach, the colon, the rectum, the bladder, and the cervix.[21] Other data suggest that selenium may reduce cancer risk but the results are not conclusive.[8,24] Although the epidemiologic data on the associations between soybeans and cancer risk are limited, rates of breast and colon cancer are considerably lower in Japan and China, where the consumption of products derived from soybeans is high. Soybeans contain several classes of important anticarcinogens, such as protease inhibitors, phytosterols, and isoflavones.[25-28]

Other human studies support the role of dietary calcium in decreasing excess proliferation and differentiation of colonic epithelial cells. Several case-control, cohort, and international correlation studies suggest that high intakes of dietary calcium reduce the risk for colon or colorectal cancer.[29-32] However, other epidemiologic studies indicate a weak or no relation, or a relation confounded by other dietary factors such as fat and fiber.[13,33] The strongest evidence for a protective role of calcium is found in experimental studies[34,35] and small clinical trials with persons at high risk for colorectal cancer, which generally show that calcium supplementation significantly reduces colonic cell proliferation.[34,36,37]

The specific agents and mechanisms for most of these factors may not be known, partly because the biologic activity of these dietary complexes is difficult to determine from population studies alone.[13] Further, multiple micronutrient deficiencies may be involved, which is consistent with the geographic pattern of esophageal cancer endemic in regions with nutrient-deficient diets. However, the contributions of well-designed classic epidemiologic studies that examine the strength of the evidence for protective or anticarcinogenic agents have proved crucial for the initial leads for designing intervention trials that can support or refute these hypotheses.

MECHANISMS OF CARCINOGENESIS AND CHEMOPREVENTION RESEARCH

Despite an incomplete definition of the biologic concepts involved, new studies are yielding approaches for mediating the events that contribute to malignant transformation. The key mechanisms involved in the delay or the prevention of carcinogenesis are more clearly understood today as a result of research developments on the multistages of carcinogenesis. These mechanistic studies have the potential to target specific events that increase the possibility for the treatment and control of biologic carcinogenesis.[38]

Promising chemopreventive agents under evaluation include several antioxidants; antiinflammatory agents; inhibitors of cellular proliferation; and agents that counteract prostaglandin, ornithine decarboxylase, and other tumor promoting activity.[8,38] Modulation of the key cellular regulatory pathways is a common strategy for chemoprevention.[11] Ornithine decarboxylase (ODC), for example, is greatly elevated in colorectal neoplasia and is a rate-limiting enzyme in the polyamine biosynthetic pathway known to be essential for the maintenance of cell growth and function.[38,39] Inhibition of polyamine biosynthesis has been shown to be chemopreventive in experimental models, possibly by blocking the induction of ODC.[39] Compounds such as difluoromethylornithine, certain retinoids, and the pharmaceutical piroxicam all block the promotion or progression, or both, of ODC activity.[38,40] Experimental studies and a limited amount of epidemiologic evidence suggest that aspirin and other nonsteroidal antiinflammatory drugs (NSAIDs) may offer protection against colon cancer.[41] Three epidemiologic studies indicate that the risk for colorectal cancer is reduced with regular aspirin use.[42-44] The largest report to date, a prospective study of 662,424 adults conducted by the American Cancer Society, found that mortality from colon cancer was reduced by approximately 40% in men and women who used aspirin more than 15 times a month for a minimum of 1 year compared with nonusers.[44] The mechanism for the proposed cancer-preventive action of aspirin and other NSAIDs is not known, but may be related to the ability of these compounds to inhibit the synthesis of prostaglandins that affect immune function and neoplastic and nonneoplastic cellular proliferation.[38] Many other promising chemopreventive agents act mechanistically by enhancing enzyme activity that can catalyze electrophilic detoxification and modify the oxidative metabolism of carcinogens.[6,8,45]

Other classes of compounds are being sought that may act by modifying or inactivating the expression of oncogenes or their protein products; tumor-suppressive compounds that can control the expression of oncogenes and receptors of certain peptide growth factors are also of interest to chemoprevention. These and similar research efforts are under investigation with the hope of directing chemoprevention at the molecular foundation of cancer prevention.[46,47] Transforming growth factor-β (TGFβ) is an example of a potent cellular antiproliferative agent with multiple actions and potential clinical applications. Several pharmacologic agents enhance TGFβ activity that normally acts to suppress the proliferation of epithelial cells.[48] Based on the work on multistage carcinogenesis, it is currently possible to design specific compounds for testing some aspect of tumor inhibition. Experimental evidence suggests that additive or synergistic effects of multiple inhibitors may provide greater anticarcinogenic activity than a single inhibitor.[49-51] Selecting effective combinations is mostly dependent on what is known about the agent's mechanism(s) of action for purposes of targeting different stages of carcinogenesis.[51]

BIOLOGIC MARKERS

The modulation of key biochemical or biologic indicators, the intermediate endpoints of the carcinogenic process, is being assessed as an early indicator of the reversal or prevention of malignancy. Currently, there are several intermediate biomarker endpoints that are of interest to clinicians as possible indicators of cancer risk, including premalignant lesions, histologic markers, and cytopathologic markers.[52] Their reliability for use in chemoprevention trials to reveal detectable changes as a result of a unique intervention remains unknown. If clinicians are to rely on the sensitivity of an intermediate endpoint as a valid cancer surrogate, a major effort is needed to validate biologic marker reliability. Identifying and assessing intermediate or surrogate marker endpoints is a program emphasis at the NCI, because fewer trial subjects would be required to achieve statistical power, and a greater number of agents could be evaluated over a shorter period with the use of a surrogate rather than a cancer endpoint. The ultimate use of a marker endpoint is dependent on the prospective analysis of clinical data from multiple studies. Markers of interest to chemopreventive studies include reversal of abnormal cytology, prevention or reversal of nuclear aberrations, modulation of enzyme activity such as ODC or prostaglandin synthetase inhibition, and DNA ploidy alterations. The products of genetic changes reported by Vogelstein and other investigators are of great experimental interest.[37,53–55]

THE CHEMOPREVENTION PROGRAM AT THE NCI

Chemoprevention research was first established at the NCI in the Laboratory of Chemoprevention in the 1970s. The early investigations conducted in this laboratory on the specificity of the retinoids in the control of cell differentiation and growth have directly influenced the planning and development of this research area. In 1982, the work on chemoprevention research was extended under the multidisciplinary NCI Chemoprevention Program (1) to identify and characterize new agents with efficacy observed in epidemiologic and animal studies and with a high probability of preventing cancer in humans, (2) to conduct preclinical efficacy and toxicity testing of candidate agents, and (3) to conduct clinical prevention trials with the least toxic and most efficacious agents for the suppression of tumorigenesis in humans.[56,57] To accomplish this agenda, the NCI developed a staged strategic system for preclinical drug development and phases I, II, and III human interventions. In many ways, this program parallels chemotherapeutic interventions in the use of pharmacokinetic and toxicity studies for drug development. Defined criteria and decision points for the continued evaluation of promising candidates are based on agent efficacy, toxicity, tolerance, and safety and provide the framework for preclinical and clinical evaluations, as shown in Figure 20–3.

PRECLINICAL CHEMOPREVENTIVE DRUG DEVELOPMENT

Agents considered for preclinical evaluation strongly suggesting efficacy and low toxicity are rapidly screened in various in vitro transformation systems. Systems selected are relevant to the human cancer problem, for example, cells of epithelial origin for evaluating the agent's activity specific to human cell substrates, available organ cultures in a particular differentiated organ, and systems that allow differentiation of the carcinogenesis stages of initiation and promotion. Table 20–4 indicates the battery of chemoprevention in vitro screens currently used in the NCI program to increase the predictive value of this stage of drug development.

Agents for human testing are further assessed in animals. Dose-response relations and the initial evidence of agent acceptability, toxicity, and tolerance are established.[56,58] The histopathology of lesions induced in the experimental model should be similar to the disease observed in humans. A battery of in vivo screens shown in Table 20–5 has been selected and represents target organs of primary relevance to the human cancer problem, including lung, breast, colon, bladder, skin, and connective tissue. Results from the in vivo assays are used to prioritize promising compounds for extended efficacy, preclinical toxicity, and clinical testing. The use of multiple models allows for observations of the tissue specificity difference characteristic of many chemopreventive agents. Toxicity studies conducted for select compounds parallel the preclinical chemotherapeutic toxicology and safety evaluations required by the U.S. Food and Drug Administration to ensure that an investigational agent is safe for chronic human trials. The toxicity studies, conducted in animals under the chemoprevention program, include acute oral toxicity; subchronic 30-day oral toxicity; chronic 1- and 2-year carcinogenic evaluations; reproductive toxicity studies; multigenerational developmental evaluations; neurobehavioral evaluations; and pharmacokinetic studies, including drug absorption and metabolism studies. Compounds found to have high efficacy and low toxicity after this phase of assessment are prioritized for clinical evaluation.

CLINICAL CHEMOPREVENTION RESEARCH

The first chemoprevention clinical trials at the NCI were begun in 1981 with a few well-characterized agents believed potentially efficacious and nontoxic for evaluation in humans. One measure of the opportunities being generated by chemoprevention research is that approximately 40 clinical chemoprevention trials are being sponsored by the NCI currently, including 13 phase I and 26 phases II and III trials. Selected chemoprevention clinical studies are shown in Table 20–6. The phase I intervention trial is undertaken in subjects studied at several levels of intake of the intervention to determine the feasibility of the clinical study. Endpoints for the phase I study are pharmacokinetic determinations of biologic activity, dose range, absorption, and metabolism. In brief, a phase I study is primarily a safety study in a small group of humans for determining a safe dose. Phase II trials are concerned with determining whether the agent demonstrates biologic activity that modulates a specified endpoint. Phase II studies accrue subjects at high risk for specific cancers and evaluate agent efficacy using some surrogate or intermediate endpoint of disease rather than the onset of malignancy. These limited trials also characterize dose, safety, and toxicity in the selected sub-

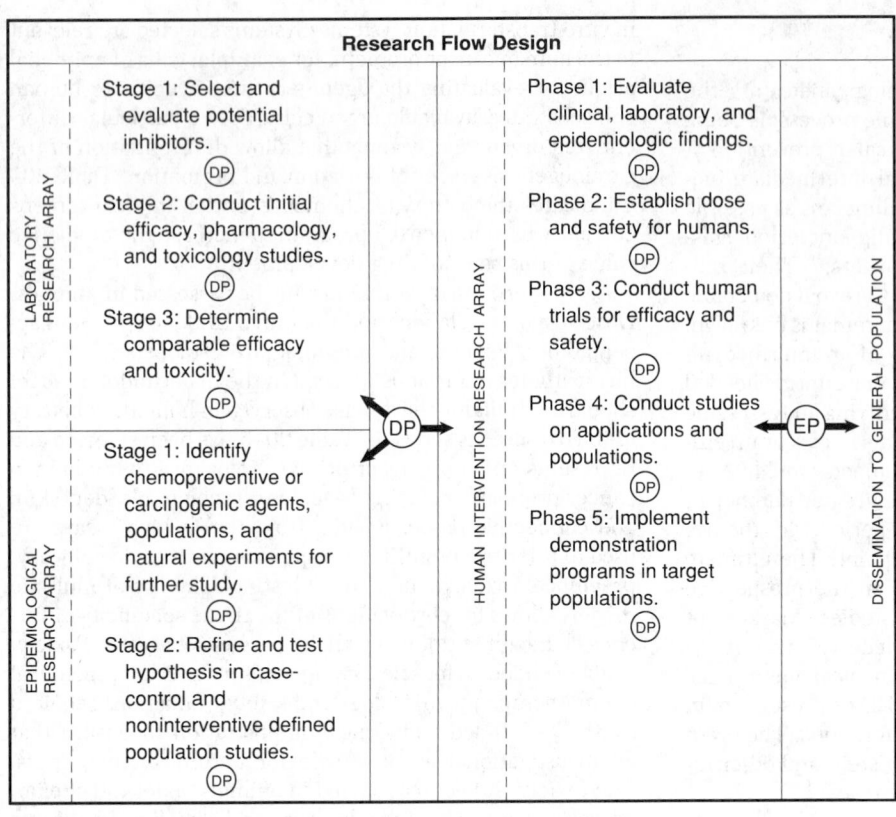

Research Flow Design

LABORATORY RESEARCH ARRAY

Stage 1: Select and evaluate potential inhibitors.
(DP)

Stage 2: Conduct initial efficacy, pharmacology, and toxicology studies.
(DP)

Stage 3: Determine comparable efficacy and toxicity.
(DP)

EPIDEMIOLOGICAL RESEARCH ARRAY

Stage 1: Identify chemopreventive or carcinogenic agents, populations, and natural experiments for further study.
(DP)

Stage 2: Refine and test hypothesis in case-control and noninterventive defined population studies.
(DP)

HUMAN INTERVENTION RESEARCH ARRAY

(DP)

Phase 1: Evaluate clinical, laboratory, and epidemiologic findings.
(DP)

Phase 2: Establish dose and safety for humans.
(DP)

Phase 3: Conduct human trials for efficacy and safety.
(DP)

Phase 4: Conduct studies on applications and populations.
(DP)

Phase 5: Implement demonstration programs in target populations.
(DP)

(EP)

DISSEMINATION TO GENERAL POPULATION

DP Decision Point
EP Evaluation Point

FIGURE 20–3. Research flow design of NCI Chemoprevention Program. DP = decision point; EP = evaluation point.

population. The degree of toxicity should be minimal. Once a candidate is found to have high efficacy and low toxicity in the phase II clinical study, prospective trials are planned as controlled phase III studies in a larger number of well-defined subjects over an extended period. Endpoints in these studies are the incidence of specific cancers, neoplastic changes, and changes in cellular or biochemical parameters associated with tumor progression but considered as surrogate or intermediate indicators of disease. For example, several controlled clinical trials sponsored by the NCI shown in Table 20–6 currently are in progress to evaluate the effects of calcium, calcium carbonate, or calcium plus fiber in persons with previous colon polyps at high risk for the recurrence of colorectal adenomas or subsequent colorectal carcinomas.

Randomized placebo-controlled clinical studies are in progress evaluating the effects of chemopreventive agents on

TABLE 20–4. In Vitro Chemoprevention Screening Systems

Cell System	Initiator	Promoter	Endpoint Inhibition of
Mouse epidermal cells (JB-6)	None	TPA	Growth of colonies in soft agar
Human primary epidermal cells (HFT)	Propane sultone	None	Calcium tolerance
Tracheal cell culture (RTE)	B (a) P	None	Colonies of morphologically transformed cells that are tumorigenic
Mammary organ culture (MMOC)	DMBA	TPA	Colonies of morphologically transformed cells that are tumorigenic
Human tumor cells (A427)	None	None	Growth of colonies in soft agar

B (a) P, Benzo(a)pyrene; DMBA, 7,12-Dimethylbenz(a)anthracene; TPA, 12-0-Tetracecanoylphorbol-13-acetate.
(National Cancer Institute, Division of Cancer Prevention and Control, Chemoprevention Branch, Bethesda, MD)

TABLE 20–5. In Vivo Chemoprevention Screening Systems (Animals)

Species	Carcinogen	Target Organ	Endpoint Inhibition of
Mouse	DMBA/TPA	Skin	Papillomas and carcinomas
Hamster	MNU or DEN	Lung and trachea	Squamous cell carcinomas
			Adenocarcinomas
Mouse	OH-BBN	Bladder	Transitional cell carcinomas
Rat	MNU or DMBA	Mammary gland	Adenocarcinomas
Rat	AOM	Colon	Adenocarcinomas

DMBA, 12-dimethylbenz(a)anthracene; TPA, 12-0-tetradecanoyl-phorbol-13-acetate; MNU, n-methyl-n-nitrosourea; DEN, n-nitroso-diethylamine; OH-BNN, n-butyl-n-(4-hydroxybutyl)nitrosamine; and AOM, azoxymethane.
(National Cancer Insitute, Division of Cancer Prevention and Control, Chemoprevention Branch, Bethesda, MD)

cancer endpoints or intermediate endpoints such as bronchial metaplasia and dysplasia, dysplasia of the cervix, regression of colon polyps, hyperproliferation of the colonic epithelial mucosa, and levels of ODC and prostaglandin synthetase activity. Published results of several chemoprevention trials include a study in smokers treated with folate and vitamin B_{12} that showed significant improvement of bronchial squamous metaplasia[59] and a study of the rate of polyp recurrence associated with vitamin C and E supplementation that showed a small effect and requires a larger study to ensure this was not a chance finding.[60]

Subsequently, protocols for these studies have improved, as have the underlying interpretations of positive and negative results. For example, prolonged use of beta-carotene has been found in some studies to cause declines in plasma levels of alpha-tocopherol.[60a] If targeted sites cannot receive effective levels of the test compound, negative results may not indicate lack of efficacy but lack of tissue maintenance or other clinical metabolic effects that could cloud the research findings. Measurements of blood and tissue levels, drug interactions, drug resistance, and patient sensitivity are data analysis issues of great interest for future trial designs. Several long-term studies discussed consider some of these parameters as the trials proceed.

LUNG CANCER PREVENTION TRIAL

The Alpha-Tocopherol, Beta-Carotene Lung Cancer Prevention Study is being conducted by the NCI in collaboration with the National Public Health Institute of Finland.[10] Although the primary endpoint of the trial is lung cancer incidence, other cancer and noncancer endpoints will be examined in relation to the intervention. This alliance offers a unique opportunity for prevention research among a high-risk Finnish population, which has marginal per capita intakes of several micronutrients and one of the highest incidence rates of lung cancer in the world. Oral administration of beta-carotene and alpha-tocopherol is being tested in a population of 29,000 men, ages 50 to 69, who are heavy smokers. This randomized, placebo-controlled, double-blind study has four treatment groups being evaluated using a 2×2 factorial design. Incident cancers will be identified through chest radiograph during intervals of the intervention and at the conclusion of the 6-year clinical follow-up procedures. A reduction in cancer incidence as demonstrated in the trial will be compared with national trends by monitoring Finland's Government-operated cancer registry.

NUTRITION INTERVENTION STUDIES OF ESOPHAGEAL CANCER IN LINXIAN, CHINA

Two intervention trials, expected to conclude active intervention in 1991, use large doses of vitamin-mineral supplements to evaluate the relation between the supplements and esophageal cancer mortality in a high-risk population.[61] The current trials are being conducted in the rural county of Linxian, China, selected because it has the highest rate of esophageal cancer in the world and because there is suspicion that the population's chronic deficiencies of multiple nutrients may be involved etiologically. The General Population Trial randomized 30,252 subjects beginning in 1986, and the Dysplasia Trial randomized 3393 subjects with cytologic evidence of esophageal dysplasia in a simple multivitamin versus placebo two-arm design. The General Population Trial uses a more complicated fractional factorial design to allow evaluation of four separate factors, including vitamin A plus zinc, riboflavin plus niacin, vitamin C plus molybdenum, and vitamin E plus selenium plus beta-carotene. Analyses of samples collected during these examinations include assessment of esophageal cytology, histology, cell proliferation, and DNA contents and measures of immune function and other studies. Pretrial sera and dietary assessments collected offer the opportunity to examine micronutrient and other variables prospectively in the trial cohorts.

COMMUNITY CLINICAL ONCOLOGY PROGRAM OF THE NCI

The speed and efficiency with which resulting scientific knowledge can be translated into health practices for the community has become increasingly important for the prevention and treatment of cancer. The NCI's Community Clinical Oncology Program (CCOP), a network of more than 1000 community physicians participating with their patients in NCI-approved research, is an example of a network designed to increase accrual of patients to trials and to increase adoption of state-of-the-art cancer therapies. Chemoprevention research in the medical setting is a high priority of the CCOP. Clinical studies being conducted within the CCOP include a double-blind trial to test the effects of a low dose of 13-*cis*-retinoic acid on the prevention of second primary tumors in stages I and II head and neck cancer, a pilot trial with alpha-tocopherol assessing oral leukoplakia remission, and the tamoxifen chemoprevention trial implemented in 1992 to evaluate the effectiveness of this antiestrogen to prevent the development of breast cancer in women at increased risk. Aspects of tamoxifen pharmacology, laboratory research, and clinical experience have been reviewed recently, and it has

TABLE 20–6. Selected Current Chemoprevention Intervention Trials

Target Site	Study Population	Study Agent(s)
All	Physicians	Beta-carotene 50 mg qod
Breast	High risk	4-HPR (fenretinide) 200 mg/d
Breast	High risk	Tamoxifen 20 mg/d
Cervix	Women, mild and moderate dysplasia	β-trans-Retinoic acid 0.372%
Cervix	Women, cervical dysplasia	Folic acid 5 mg/d
Cervix	Women, cervical dysplasia	Beta-carotene 30 mg/d
Colon	Previous colon adenoma	Beta-carotene 30 mg/d
		Ascorbic acid 1 g/d
		Alpha-tocopherol 400 mg/d
Colon	Previous colon adenoma	Calcium carbonate 3 g/d
Colon	Previous colon adenoma	Wheat bran 13, 5, or 2 g/d
		Calcium carbonate 1.25 or 0.1 g/d
Colon	Previous colon adenoma	Piroxicam 20, 10, 7.5, or 5 mg/d
Colon	High risk	Difluoromethylornithine (DFMO)
Colon	High risk	Calcium carbonate 3 or 5 g/d
Colon	Familial adenomatous polyposis	Sulindac 150 mg bid
Colon	Previous colon cancer	Beta-carotene 30 mg/d
Colon	Previous colon polyp	Calcium 1200 mg
Lung	Men, exposed to asbestos	Retinol 25,000 IU qod
		Beta-carotene 50 mg/d
Lung	High-risk women	Beta-carotene 50 mg qod
		Retinol 25,000 IU/d
Lung	Chronic smokers	13-cis-Retinoic acid 1 mg/kg/d
Lung	Cigarette smokers	Beta-carotene 30 mg/d
		Retinol 25,000 IU/d
Lung	High-risk women	Beta-carotene 50 mg qod
		Vitamin E 600 mg qod
Oral cavity	Oral leukoplakia	13-cis-Retinoic acid 1.5 mg/kg for 3 mo, then 0.5 mg/kg/d for 9 mo
		Beta-carotene 30 mg/d for 9 mo
Oral cavity	Oral leukoplakia	Bowman Birk inhibitor
Skin	Albinos in Tanzania	Beta-carotene 100 mg/d
Skin	Previous BCC of skin	Beta-carotene 50 mg/d
Skin	Previous BCC of skin	Retinol 25,000 IU/d
		13-cis-Retinoic acid 0.15 mg/kg
Skin	Actinic keratosis patients	Retinol 25,000 IU/d

BCC, basal cell carcinoma.
(National Cancer Institute, Division of Cancer Prevention and Control, Bethesda, MD)

been concluded that tamoxifen may be an especially attractive prevention option to women at increased risk for breast cancer.[62–64] Approximately 16,000 women will be randomized to receive 20 mg/day of tamoxifen or placebo for 5 years. The trial including follow-up is expected to last 10 years.

FUTURE DIRECTIONS

For the past 10 years the evidence has been accumulating for the role of micronutrients in modulating cancer risk. Quantified guidance is anticipated from the clinical study of micronutrients, although in many instances the evidence is not clear and in most cases it is not possible to implicate any specific factor to give public guidance regarding the avoidance or increased intake of a specific factor. Evaluation of the preventive effects of agents to a level of confidence for prescribing

their use in selected high-risk subgroups and, when appropriate, broad populations appears possible by the year 2000. A continuing scientific challenge is to resolve issues of individual variations in agent efficacy, toxicity, and bioavailability.

It may be feasible, in a relatively short time, for the molecular epidemiologist to develop a profile of individual risk that provides a strong rationale for defining specific interventions to modulate that risk in otherwise asymptomatic persons.[65] As a result of the work of molecular geneticists, individual risk tendencies for certain heritable cancers such as retinoblastoma, Wilms' tumor, and familial polyposis, currently can be predicted by genetic probes.[66,67] The ultimate test for predictability is how consistently a genetic abnormality can be demonstrated in the clinical evolution of malignant transformation.[68] The next step is to modify the transformation by applying these insights to new clinical approaches that benefit prevention and treatment. With the advent of the capability to predict individual risk, prevention strategies with chemopreventive agents can make a vital contribution to the reduction of cancer morbidity and mortality for those who can benefit most.[69]

REFERENCES

1. Bertram JS, Kolonel LN, Meyskens FL. Rationale and strategies for chemoprevention of cancer in humans. Cancer Res 1987;47:3012–3031.
2. Doll FRS, Peto R. The causes of cancer. New York: Oxford University Press, 1981.
3. Higginson J. Changing concepts in cancer prevention: Limitations and implications for future research in environmental carcinogenesis. Cancer Res 1988;48:1381–1389.
4. Meyskens FL. Coming of age: The chemoprevention of cancer. N Engl J Med 1990;323:825–826.
5. Weinstein IB. Cancer prevention: Recent progress and future opportunities. Cancer Res 1991;51:5080s.
6. Wattenberg LW. Inhibitors of chemical carcinogenesis. JNCI 1978;6:11–18.
7. Wattenberg LW. Chemoprevention of cancer. Cancer Res 1985;5:1–8.
8. Boone CW, Kelloff GJ, Malone WF. Identification of candidate cancer chemopreventive agents and their evaluation in animal models and human clinical trials: A review. Cancer Res 1990;50:2–9.
9. Weinstein IB. The origins of human cancer: Molecular mechanisms of carcinogenesis and their implications on cancer prevention and treatment: Twenty-seventh GHA Clowes Memorial Award Lecture. Cancer Res 1988;48:4135–4143.
10. Albanes D, Virtamo J, Rauta-Iahti M, et al. Pilot study: The U.S.-Finland lung cancer prevention trial. J Nutr Growth Can 1986;3:207–214.
11. Meyskens FL. Thinking about cancer causality and chemoprevention. JNCI 1988;80:1278–1281.
12. National Academy of Sciences, National Research Council, Committee on Diet Nutrition and Cancer. Diet, nutrition and cancer. Washington, DC: National Academy Press, 1982.
13. National Academy of Sciences, National Research Council, Commission on Life Sciences, Food and Nutrition Board. Diet and health: Implications for reducing chronic disease risk. Washington, DC: National Academy Press, 1989.
14. Rogers AE, Longnecker MP. Biology of disease: Dietary and nutritional influences on cancer: A review of epidemiologic and experimental data. Lab Invest 1988;59:729–752.
15. Palmer S. Diet, nutrition and cancer. Prog Food Nutr Sci 1985;9:283–341.
16. Hirayama T. Diet and cancer. Nutr Cancer 1979;1:67–81.
17. Kromhout D. Essential micronutrients in relation to carcinogenesis. Am J Clin Nutr 1987;45:1361–1367.
18. Block G. Vitamin C and cancer prevention: The epidemiologic evidence. Am J Clin Nutr 1991;53:270s–282s.
19. Knekt P, Aromaa A, Maatela J, Aaran RK, et al. Vitamin E and cancer prevention. Am J Clin Nutr 1991;53:283s–286s.
20. Ziegler RG. A review of epidemiologic evidence that carotenoids reduce the risk of cancer. J Nutr 1989;119:116–122.
21. Ziegler RG. Vegetables, fruits, and carotenoids, and the risk of cancer. Am J Clin Nutr 1991;53:251s–259s.
22. Menkes MS, Comstock GW, Vuilleumier JP, Helsing KJ, Rider AA, Brookmeyer R. Serum beta-carotene, vitamins A and E, selenium, and the risk of lung cancer. N Engl J Med 1986;315:1250–1254.
23. LeMarchand L, Yoshizawa CN, Kolonel LN, Hankin JH, Goodman MT. Vegetable consumption and lung cancer risk: A population-based case-control study in Hawaii. JNCI 1989;81:1158–1164.
24. Shamberger RJ, Tylko SA, Willis CE. Antioxidants and cancer: VI. Selenium and age-adjusted human cancer mortality. Arch Environ Health 1976;31:231–235.
25. Troll W, Kennedy AR. Workshop report from the Division of Cancer Etiology, National Cancer Institute, National Institutes of Health: Protease inhibitors as cancer chemopreventive agents. Cancer Res 1989;49:494–502.
26. St Clair WH, Billings PC, Carew JA, Keller-McGandy C, Newberne PM, Kennedy AR. Suppression of dimethylhydrazine-induced carcinogenesis in mice by dietary addition of the Bowman-Birk protease inhibitor. Cancer Res 1990;50:580–586.
27. Billings PC, Newberne PM, Kennedy AR. Protease inhibitor suppression of colon and anal gland carcinogenesis induced by dimethylhydrazine. Carcinogenesis 1990;11:1083–1086.
28. Messina M, Barnes S. The role of soy products in reducing risk of cancer. JNCI 1991;83:541–546.
29. Stemmermann GN, Nomura A, Chyou PH. The influence of dairy and nondairy calcium on subsite large-bowel cancer risk. Dis Colon Rectum 1990;33:190–194.
30. Slattery ML, Sorenson AW, Ford MH. Dietary calcium intake as a mitigating factor in colon cancer. Am J Epidemiol 1988;128:504–514.
31. Garland C, Shekelle RB, Barrett-Connor E, Criqui MH, Rossof AM, Paul O. Dietary vitamin D and calcium and risk of colorectal cancer: A 19-year prospective study in men. Lancet 1985;1:307–309.
32. Sorenson AW, Slattery ML, Ford MH. Calcium and colon cancer: A review. Nutr Cancer 1988;11:135–145.
33. Negri E, LaVecchia CL, D'Avanzo B, Franceschi S. Calcium, dairy products, and colorectal cancer. Nutr Cancer 1990;13:255–262.
34. Wargovich MJ, Lynch PM, Levin B. Modulating effects of calcium in animal models of colon carcinogenesis and short-term studies in subjects at increased risk for colon cancer. Am J Clin Nutr 1991;54:202S–205S.
35. Newmark HL, Lipkin M, Maheshwari N. Colonic hyperproliferation induced in rats and mice by nutritional-stress diets containing four components of a human Western-style diet (series 2). Am J Clin Nutr 1991;54:209S–214S.
36. Lipkin M, Newmark HL. Effect of added dietary calcium on colonic epithelial-cell proliferation in subjects at high risk for familial colon cancer. N Engl J Med 1985;313:1381–1384.
37. Lipkin M, Friedman E, Winawer SJ, Newmark HL. Colonic epithelial cell proliferation in responders and nonresponders to supplemental dietary calcium. Cancer Res 1989;49:248–254.
38. Kelloff GJ, Malone WF, Boone CW, Sigman CC, Fay JR. Progress in applied chemoprevention research. Semin Oncol 1990;17:438–455.
39. Luk GD, Moshier JA, Ehrinpreis MN. Ornithine decarboxylase as a marker for colorectal polyps and cancer. In: Steele G, Burt RW, Winawer SJ, Karr JP, eds. Basic and clinical perspectives of colorectal polyps and cancer. New York: Alan R. Liss, 1988:227–239.
40. Tempero MA, Nishoka K, Knott K, Zetterman RK. Chemoprevention of mouse colon tumors with difluoromethylornithine during and after carcinogen treatment. Cancer Res 1989;49:5793–5797.
41. Baron JA, Greenberg ER. Could aspirin really prevent colon cancer? N Engl J Med 1991;325:1644–1646.
42. Kune GA, Kune S, Watson LF. Colorectal cancer risk, chronic illnesses, operations, and medications: Case control results from the Melbourne colorectal cancer study. Cancer Res 1988;48:4399–4404.
43. Rosenberg L, Palmer JR, Zauber AG, Warshauer ME, Stolley PD, Shapiro S. A hypothesis: Nonsteroidal anti-inflammatory drugs reduce the incidence of large-bowel cancer. JNCI 1991;83:355–358.
44. Thun MJ, Namboodiri MM, Heath CW Jr. Aspirin use and reduced risk of fatal colon cancer. N Engl J Med 1991;325:1593–1596.
45. Sparnins VL, Wattenberg LW. Enhancement of glutathione S-transferase activity of the mouse forestomach by inhibitors of benzo(a)pyrene-induced neoplasia of the forestomach. JNCI 1981;66:796–771.
46. Friend SH, Dryja TP, Weinberg RA. Oncogenes and tumor-suppressing genes. N Engl J Med 1988;318:618–622.
47. Taylor JA. Oncogenes and their applications in epidemiologic studies. Am J Epidemiol 1989;130:6–13.
48. Sporn MB, Roberts AB. Transforming growth factor-β multiple actions and potential clinical applications. JAMA 1989;262:938–941.
49. Reddy BS, Nayini J, Tokumo K, Rigotty J, Zang E, Kelloff GJ. Chemoprevention of colon carcinogenesis by concurrent administration of piroxicam, a nonsteroidal antiinflammatory drug with D,L-α-difluoromethylornithine, an ornithine decarboxylase inhibitor in diet. Cancer Res 1990;50:2562–2568.
50. Ip C, Thompson HJ. New approaches to cancer chemoprevention with DFMO and selenite. JNCI 1989;81:839–843.
51. Ip C, Ganther HE. Combination of blocking agents and suppressing agents in cancer prevention. Carcinogenesis 1991;12:365–367.
52. Lippman SM, Lee JS, Lotan R, Hittelman W, Wargovich MJ, Hong WK. Biomarkers as intermediate endpoints in chemoprevention trials. JNCI 1990;82:555–560.
53. Stich HF, Stich W, Rosin MP, et al. Use of the micronucleus test to monitor the effect of vitamin A, beta-carotene and canthaxanthin on the buccal mucosa of betel nut/ tobacco chewers. Int J Cancer 1984;34:745–750.
54. Vogelstein B, Fearon ER, Hamilton SR, et al. Genetic alterations during colorectal-tumor development. N Engl J Med 1988;319:525–532.
55. Lippman SM, Peters EJ, Margovich MJ, et al. Bronchial micronuclei as a marker of an early stage of carcinogenesis in the human tracheobronchial epithelium. Int J Cancer 1990;45:811–815.
56. Greenwald P, Sondik E, Lynch B. Diet and chemoprevention in NCI's research strategy to achieve national cancer control objectives. Am Rev Public Health 1986;7:267–291.
57. Greenwald P, Nixon DW, Malone WF, Kelloff GJ, Stern HR, Witkin KM. Concepts in cancer chemoprevention research. Cancer 1990;65:1483–1489.
58. Malone WF, Kelloff GJ, Boone CW, Nixon DW. Chemoprevention and modern cancer prevention. Prev Med 1989;18:553–556.
59. Heimburger DC, Alexander DB, Birch R, et al. Improvement in bronchial squamous metaplasia in smokers treated with folate and B$_{12}$. JAMA 1988;259:1525–1530.
60. McKeown-Eyssen GE, Holloway C, Jazmaji V, Bright-See E, Dion P, Bruce WR. A randomized trial of vitamins C and E in the prevention of recurrence of colorectal polyps. Cancer Res 1988;48:4701–4705.
60a. Alberts, personal communication, 1991.
61. Li JY, Taylor PR, Li GY, et al. Intervention studies in Linxian, China: An update. J Nutr Growth Can 1986;3:199–206.
62. Love RR. Antiestrogens as chemopreventive agents in breast cancer: Promise and issues in evaluation. Prev Med 1989;18:661–671.
63. Love RR. Prospects for antiestrogen chemoprevention of breast cancer. JNCI 1990;82:18–21.
64. Prentice RL. Tamoxifen as a potential preventive agent in healthy postmenopausal women. JNCI 1990;82:1310–1311.
65. Shields PG, Harris CC. Molecular epidemiology and the genetics of environmental cancer. JAMA 1991;266:631–687.
66. Marx J. Many gene changes found in cancer. Science 1989;146:1386–1388.
67. Marx J. Zeroing in on individual cancer risk: News and comment. Science 1991;253:612–616.
68. Nowell PC. Molecular events in tumor development. N Engl J Med 1988;319:575–577.
69. Harris CC. Chemical and physical carcinogenesis: Advances and perspectives for the 1990s. Cancer Res 1991;51:5023s–5044s.

JULIE E. BURING
CHARLES H. HENNEKENS

SECTION **4**

Retinoids and Carotenoids

One promising area of current research in nutrition and cancer is the possibility that micronutrients, in particular retinoids or carotenoids, may decrease the incidence of epithelial cell cancers, which account for more than 90% of all cancer deaths, and in particular lung cancer, which causes 25% of all cancer deaths in the United States.[1-3] If retinoids or carotenoids yield even small to moderate reductions in cancer risk, about 20% to 30%, which is the magnitude of the most plausible benefits, the numbers of cancer deaths prevented each year and the public health impact would be substantial.

VITAMIN A ANALOGS AND PRECURSORS

Among micronutrients postulated as late-stage inhibitors of human cancer, vitamin A analogs and precursors have been studied extensively in basic research and in a numerous epidemiologic studies of cancer in humans. The term *vitamin A* can refer to retinol (preformed vitamin A) and its synthetic analogs, which include all-*trans*-retinoic acid and 13-*cis*-retinoic acid, or to the carotenoids (provitamin A), chief among which is beta-carotene, which are converted to retinol in the body as needed. From a nutritional viewpoint, it seems to make little difference whether intake consists of retinol, which is found in liver, egg yolks, and other animal products, fortified cereals, and vitamin pills, or of carotenoids, which are found in deep green and orange vegetables and fruits. Because retinoids and carotenoids behave differently in the body, if they have anticancer effects each may act by different mechanisms. It is important to distinguish among the various forms of vitamin A in assessing their possibilities for cancer chemoprevention.

RETINOIDS

FUNCTION AND MECHANISM AND LABORATORY AND ANIMAL STUDIES

Retinol and the other retinoids have potent hormone-like effects on cell growth and differentiation of epithelial tissues.[4,5] Most types of epithelial tissues depend on retinoids to control normal cell growth and differentiation. Data from numerous in vitro studies have indicated that retinoids inhibit the process of malignant transformation induced in cultured cells by various agents, including radiation,[6] sarcoma growth factor,[7] testosterone,[8] phorbol esters,[9-11] and other chemical carcinogens.[12-14] Retinoids can also reverse keratinization and other premalignant changes.[12,13,15-20] Although vitamin A deficiency has been shown to lead to premalignant changes in epithelia,[21-24] retinoid administration has been shown to cause regression of tumors induced by chemicals[4,25-27] or viruses[28] and delay the appearance of transplanted tumors.[29,30]

HUMAN STUDIES

Evidence on the relation of retinoids with human cancer is derived primarily from observational epidemiologic research, including case-control and cohort studies and blood-based investigations of serum retinol levels. Although some of these studies have suggested a benefit of retinol, others have not found an effect nor suggested a possible adverse effect. The totality of available epidemiologic evidence does not support any clear protective effect of retinol on cancer risk.

With respect to the observational epidemiologic studies, one[31] reported that intake of liver was significantly inversely related to risk for prostate cancer, whereas another[32] found protective effects from higher intakes of dietary retinol. However, four other studies reported no clear overall reduction in prostate cancer risk with increased retinol intake.[33-36] Three of these[33,35,36] found positive relations in age-specific subgroups but differed as to whether increased risks were in younger[33] or older[35,36] men. Among studies of lung cancer, two found protective effects in men but not women.[37,38] Two other investigations reported nonsignificant protective effects of higher retinol intake[39] and total vitamin A consumption,[40] whereas six studies found no effect of retinol on lung cancer risk.[41-46] Studies of breast cancer have been inconsistent, reporting protective,[47] adverse,[48] and null[49-53] effects of retinol intake. Studies of colorectal[54-61] and gastric[62-67] cancers show similarly inconsistent results. Of the investigations of female reproductive cancers, none that studied cervical neoplasia[68-72] or ovarian cancer[73-76] reported a significant association between retinol intake and cancer risk. Regarding cancer at other sites, two studies of pancreatic cancer[77,78] have reported statistically significant increased risks associated with high retinol intake, and a third[79] found no effect. Four studies of esophageal cancer[80-83] have reported statistically significant increased risks from high retinol intake, and investigations of mesothelioma,[84] melanoma,[85] and cancer of the larynx[86] showed no association. One study of bladder cancer[38] reported slightly lower total vitamin A intake among cases, and another found no effect.[87] For cancer of the pharynx, one investigation reported significant positive associations among white men[88] and black men,[89] and a second found no relation with retinol intake.[90] Finally, a study of all cancers in an elderly cohort[91] found no overall association with dietary vitamin A intake or supplement use, but did report a significant trend toward increased risk for prostate cancer with greater use of vitamin A supplements.

Many case-control studies that collected and analyzed blood specimens after the cancer was diagnosed have found lower retinol levels among cases than among controls.[92-98] However, these data have been difficult to interpret because of possible metabolic consequences of the disease itself or effects of the illness on the patient's appetite. Thus, the observed lowered levels of serum retinol in cases may be a consequence rather than a cause of disease. One methodologic approach that has the potential to address this limitation is to conduct prospective cohort studies in which blood specimens are drawn before the diagnosis of cancer. Using a nested case-control approach, baseline specimens are analyzed from all subsequent cases and a matched sample of control subjects. In these studies possible effects of preclinical disease on serum levels must be considered.

Studies of prediagnostic serum retinol levels and subsequent cancer are summarized in Table 20–7. Three such studies initially suggested protective effects of high serum retinol on overall cancer risk.[99–101] However, when cases from the first 2 years of follow-up were excluded[99] or additional cases from continued follow-up included,[102,103] the effects were markedly attenuated, suggesting that, as with blood-based case-control studies, low serum retinol levels may be a consequence rather than a cause of the cancer. Two studies[104,105] found decreased prostate cancer risks with increasing levels of serum retinol, although in one,[105] overall median values in cases and controls were similar. Three studies that found no overall association reported protective effects of high serum retinol levels on gastrointestinal cancer,[106,107] stomach malignancies,[108]

TABLE 20–7. Prediagnostic Serum Retinol Levels and Subsequent Cancer

Investigations	Site	Population	Mean Retinol		Units	p Value
Knekt[99]	All	766 Cases	Men	64.5	µg/dl	<0.01
			Women	58.7		
		1419 Controls	Men	66.7		0.08
			Women	60.4	IU/dl	
Wald[100]	All	86 Cases	214			<0.025
		172 Controls	229			
	Lung	14 Cases	187			<0.005
		172 Controls	229			
Kark[101]	All	85 Cases	41.3		µg/dl	0.003
		162 Controls	46.9			
Wald[102]	All	227 Cases	67.0		µg/dl	>0.05
		454 Controls	68.8			
Peleg[103]	All	61 Cases	51.3		µg/dl	>0.05
		111 Controls	51.7			
Reichman[104]	Prostate	84 Cases	59.4		µg/dl	<0.01
		2356 Controls	65.1			
Hsing[105]	Prostate	103 Cases	61*		µg/dl	>0.05
		103 Controls	64*			
Willett[106,107]	All	111 Cases	67.3		µg/dl	>0.05
		210 Controls	68.7			
Stahelin[108]	All	204 Cases	2.81		µmol/L	>0.05
		2421 Controls	2.81			
Salonen[109]	All	51 Cases	48.3		µg/dl	0.084
		51 Controls	52.4			
Nomura[110]	All	284 Cases	61.3*		µg/dl	>0.05
		304 Controls	59.6*			
Coates[111]	All	134 Cases	57		µg/dl	>0.05
		245 Controls	59			
Friedman[112]	All	151 Cases	82.2		µg/dl	>0.05
		302 Controls	82.4			
Russell[113]	Breast	30 Cases	54.9		µg/dl	>0.05
		288 Controls	55.3			
Connett[114]	All	156 Cases	69.8		µg/dl	>0.05
		311 Controls	70.8			
Criqui[115]	All	136 Cases	65.3		µg/dl	>0.05
		238 Controls	67.0			
Helzlsouer[116]	Bladder	35 Cases	55.2		µg/dl	>0.05
		70 Controls	56.4			
Schober[117]	Colon	72 Cases	59.1		µg/dl	>0.05
		143 Controls	51.8			
Menkes[118]	Lung	99 Cases	60.6		µg/dl	>0.05
		196 Controls	61.3			
Burney[119]	Pancreas	22 Cases	2.22		µmol/L	>0.05
		44 Controls	2.14			
Kok[120]	All	69 Cases	60.2		µg/dl	>0.05
		138 Controls	59.8			

* Median values.

TABLE 20–8.   Questionnaire Studies of Beta-Carotene Intake and Lung Cancer

Investigations	Cases	RR*	p Value
Hawaii[38]	364	0.45 Males	<0.05
		1.67 Females	>0.05
Italy[39]	47	0.34	>0.05
Texas[40]	308	0.85 (vs decedent controls)	>0.05
		0.45 (vs living controls)	<0.05
New York[41]	296 Males	0.55	<0.05
	154 Females	0.77	>0.05
Toronto[42]	839	0.89	>0.05
Hawaii[43]	230 Males	0.53	<0.05
	102 Females	0.37	<0.05
United Kingdom[44]	96	0.45	0.048 (trend)
New Jersey[45]	763	0.77	<0.05
Australia[46]	71	1.18	>0.05
Norway[138]	36	0.38	<0.05
Norway[139]	153	0.62	<0.05
Buffalo[140]	292	0.59	<0.05
Singapore[141]	233	0.45	<0.05
Japan[142]	611 Males	0.77	<0.05
	196 Females	0.72	<0.05
Chicago[143]	33	0.14	<0.05
Hawaii[144]	364	0.45	<0.05
New Mexico[145]	342	0.67	<0.05
Italy[146]	417	0.50	<0.05
Louisiana[147]	1253	0.88	0.29

* Relative risk in highest intake category of beta-carotene or carotene-rich foods compared with lowest category.

and lung cancer.[109] Numerous studies have reported no effect.[110–120] Results of prospective blood-based investigations, like those of case-control studies using questionnaires or blood specimens, have not supported a clear protective effect of serum retinol on subsequent cancer risk.

POTENTIAL OF RETINOIDS FOR CANCER CHEMOPREVENTION

Even if they were documented to reduce cancer risks, the transport and storage of retinoids in the body present a major drawback to their possible use as prophylactic agents by the general population. Within well-nourished populations, in whom deficiency is rare, blood levels of retinol appear to be largely unrelated to intake of vitamin A.[121–123] Moreover, excess unbound retinol is stored in the liver, so that long-term high intake can lead to hepatotoxicity or other symptoms of hypervitaminosis A. Although synthetic retinoids seem to be able to raise serum levels while bypassing the homeostatic mechanism, their side effects are substantial so their use may be limited to high-risk patients.

CAROTENOIDS

FUNCTION AND MECHANISM AND LABORATORY AND ANIMAL STUDIES

Some dietary beta-carotene is converted to retinol in the body so that ingestion of large amounts of beta-carotene could reduce cancer risk indirectly by preventing retinoid defi-

ciency.[124] However, most dietary carotenoids are absorbed directly from the intestine without undergoing transformation to retinol. Two intriguing properties of beta-carotene with respect to its potential for chemoprevention are its ability to trap certain organic free radicals[125,126] and to deactivate excited molecules, particularly excited or singlet oxygen[127–129] which is generated as a by-product of many normal metabolic processes. It is possible that carotene could have a direct protective effect against carcinogenesis, independent of its conversion to retinol, by deactivating these types of molecules[130] or by otherwise preventing damage caused by oxidation.[130–133] There have been few experiments performed to

TABLE 20–9.   Questionnaire Studies of Beta-Carotene Intake and Esophageal Cancer

Investigations	Cases	RR*	p Value
France[80]	743	0.53	>0.05
Buffalo[81]	178	0.66	>0.05
South Carolina[82]	207	0.80	>0.05
Italy[83]	105	0.23	<0.05
Iran[148]	344	0.59	<0.05
Buffalo[149]	122	0.68	<0.05
California[150]	275	0.44	<0.05
Uruguay[151]	261	0.56	0.05
Japan[152]	343	0.18	<0.05

* Relative risk in highest intake category of beta-carotene or carotene-rich foods compared with lowest category.

test the anticancer properties of beta-carotene in laboratory animals. Among mice[134-136] and rats,[137] however, highly significant protective effects of diets containing large amounts of beta-carotene (*e.g.*, 90 mg/kg) have been reported.

HUMAN STUDIES

Overall, the epidemiologic studies of beta-carotene are remarkably consistent in suggesting a protective effect on cancer risk. To date, more than 85 questionnaire studies of intake of fruits and vegetables rich in beta-carotene in relation to risks for cancer have been published, including more than 15,000 cases of cancer at 16 different sites, conducted in more than a dozen locations within the United States and in 20 other countries.

The strongest and most consistent evidence of a protective effect of high intake of carotene-rich foods comes from studies of lung cancer, most of which have suggested beneficial effects (Table 20–8).[38-45,138-147] Only one study reported an overall increased risk, but this was small and not statistically significant.[46]

Studies of beta-carotene and cancer at other sites have been less consistent. Most still suggest a protective effect, although individually many did not achieve statistical significance. Studies of cancer of the esophagus (Table 20–9)[80-83,148-152] and gastrointestinal tract (Table 20–10),[153,154] and most[62-67,155-157] but not all[158] studies of stomach cancer

TABLE 20–10. Questionnaire Studies in Beta-Carotene Intake and Gastric and Gastrointestinal Tract Cancer

Investigations	Cases	RR*	p *Value*
Gastric Cancer			
Pennsylvania[62]	111	0.58 (total vitamin A)	<0.05
New York[63]	293	0.43	<0.05
Italy[64]	206	0.39	<0.001 (trend)
China[65]	564	0.5	<0.05
Louisiana[66]	71 Whites	0.68	>0.05
	101 Blacks	1.08	>0.05
Canada[67]	246	0.33	<0.05
Norway[155]	228	0.59	<0.05
Minnesota[155]	83	0.67	<0.05
Japan[155]	1823	0.91	>0.05
Poland[156]	110	0.24	<0.05
Greece[157]	110	0.11	<0.001 (trend)
Japan[158]	139	1.3	>0.05
Gastrointestinal Tract			
Israel[153]	406	0.77	>0.05
United Kingdom[154]	514	0.59	<0.05

* Relative risk in highest intake category of beta-carotene or carotene-rich foods compared with lowest category.

TABLE 20–11. Questionnaire Studies of Beta-Carotene Intake and Colorectal Cancer

Investigations	Cases	RR*	p *Value*
Australia[55]	715	0.50	<0.01 (trend)
Belgium[56]	453 Colon	0.98	>0.05 (trend)
	365 Rectum	0.82	>0.05 (trend)
New York State[57]	227 males	0.59	<0.05
	145 Females	0.70	>0.05
Singapore[58]	203	0.85	>0.05
Australia[59]	Colon: 121 males	0.8	>0.05
	99 females	2.2	0.05
	Rectum: 124 males	0.9	>0.05
	75 females	0.5	>0.05
Hawaii[60]	102 colon	0.72	>0.05
	61 Rectum	0.83	>0.05
France[61]	399	0.58	0.004 (trend)
Norway[155]	278	0.71	<0.05
Minnesota[155]	373	0.71	<0.05
Buffalo[159]	193 Colon	0.57	<0.05
	260 Rectum	0.62	
Seventh-Day Adventists[160]	41	0.50	<0.05
China[161]	111	0.11	<0.05
Utah[162]	112 Males	0.6 †	>0.05
	119 Females	0.3†	<0.05
Utah[163]	112 Males	0.4	<0.05
	119 Females	0.5	0.05
Wisconsin[164]	353	0.81	>0.05
California[165]	147	0.85	>0.05

* Relative risk in highest intake category of β-carotene or carotene-rich foods compared with lowest category.
† Assessed overall vegetable intake.

(Table 20–10) have found inverse relations between dietary carotene or carotene-rich vegetable intake and cancer risk. Studies of colorectal cancer have been largely supportive of a protective effect of beta-carotene intake (Table 20–11),[55–61,155,159–165] as is the case with studies of prostate cancer (Table 20–12).[31,32,34–36,166–170] Studies of cancers in women have been less consistent (Tables 20–13 and 20–14). Many report findings in the direction of a protective effect of beta-carotene against cancers of the breast,[47–53,171–174] cervix,[68–72,175,176] and ovary,[73–76] but most do not achieve statistical significance. Studies of beta-carotene and cancers of other sites are summarized in Table 20–15.[77,78,84–90,177–185]

In prospective cohort studies assessing overall cancer risk, findings differed in two studies in the elderly in the United States, with one[91] showing no association with beta-carotene intake and another[186] reporting a statistically significant reduction in risk associated with high intake of carotene-rich vegetables. A large cohort study in Japan found a protective effect against total cancer from greater intake of carotene-containing vegetables.[187]

Further support for the carotene-cancer hypothesis is derived from blood-based studies. Studies relating blood levels of carotene drawn after the diagnosis of cancer consistently have found lower levels among cases than among controls.[92,94–97] Several prospective blood-based studies have indicated a protective effect of high serum carotene levels at baseline and subsequent total cancer risk (Table 20–16).[99,108,188] Four studies indicated a protective effect on lung cancer.[110,114,118,188] A study of rectal cancer suggested a possible adverse effect of high serum carotene,[189] whereas several others found no effect on all cancer or cancers of a variety of other sites.[105–107,116,117,119,189] In one of these studies,[189] in which median values were identical in melanoma cases and matched controls, the control distribution was strongly skewed toward higher values. In another of the investigations that reported no effect,[106,107] total carotenoids were measured rather than beta-carotene specifically.

TABLE 20–12. Questionnaire Studies of Beta-Carotene Intake and Prostate Cancer

Investigations	Cases	RR*	p Value
Minnesota[31]	182	0.45	<0.05
Japan[32]	100	0.47	<0.05
California[34]	142 Whites	1.0	>0.05
	142 Blacks	0.6	>0.05
Hawaii[35,168]	452	1.5 ≥70 years old	>0.09
		1.0 <70 years old	>0.55
United States[36]	149	0.9	>0.05
Japan[155]	63	0.50	<0.05
Buffalo[166]	371	0.6	<0.05
United States[167]	180	0.68 (green salad)	>0.05
		0.57 (tomatoes)	<0.05
Japan[169]	100	0.5	>0.05
Italy[170]	166	1.20	>0.05

* Relative risk in highest intake category of beta-carotene or carotene-rich foods compared with lowest category.

TABLE 20–13. Questionnaire Studies of Beta-Carotene Intake and Breast Cancer

Investigations	Cases	RR*	p Value
Greece[47]	120	0.56	>0.05
France[48]	924	1.0	>0.05
New York[49]	83	0.73	>0.05
Australia[50]	451	0.76	>0.05
Italy[51]	214	1.2	>0.05
Italy[52]	1108	0.83	>0.05
Italy[53]	250	1.0	>0.05
Buffalo[171]	2024	0.75	<0.05
Singapore[172]	200	0.33 (premenopausal women)	<0.05
Argentina[173]	150	0.92	>0.05
Holland[174]	133	0.91	>0.05

* Relative risk in highest intake category of beta-carotene or carotene-rich foods compared with lowest category.

POTENTIAL OF BETA-CAROTENE FOR CANCER CHEMOPREVENTION

If beta-carotene reduces risk for cancer, one main advantage as a potential chemopreventive agent among large populations is its metabolic properties. In contrast with retinol, dietary intake of beta-carotene appears to be directly related to blood levels.[122] Further, excess carotene is stored in adipose tissues rather than in the liver, so that consumption of even high doses for long periods does not seem to cause toxic symptoms.[190]

TABLE 20–14. Questionnaire Studies of Beta-Carotene Intake and Cervical and Ovarian Cancer

Investigations	Cases	RR*	p Value
Cervical Cancer			
Buffalo[68]	513	0.50	<0.05
Australia[69]	117	1.0	>0.05
Italy[70]	392 Invasive	0.18	<0.05
	247 Intraepithelial	1.09	>0.05
Washington State[71]	189	0.6	>0.05
United States[72]	271	0.98	>0.05
Chicago[175]	102	0.50	>0.05
Utah[176]	266	0.99	>0.05
Ovarian Cancer			
Utah[73]	85	0.5	0.05
Italy[74]	455	0.94	>0.05
Buffalo[75]	274	0.77	>0.05
China[76]	172	1.1	>0.05

* Relative risk in highest intake category of beta-carotene or carotene-rich foods compared with lowest category.

TABLE 20–15. Questionnaire Studies of Beta-Carotene Intake and Cancer at Various Sites

Investigations	Cases	RR*	p Value
Pancreatic Cancer			
Australia[77]	104	0.45	<0.05
Louisiana[78]	203 Males	0.82	>0.05
	160 Females	1.65	>0.05
Sweden[177]	99	0.3	<0.05
California[178]	490	0.7	<0.05
California[179]	40	>1	>0.05
Baltimore[180]	201	0.58	<0.05
Laryngeal Cancer			
Texas[86]	151	0.48	<0.05
Buffalo[181]	374	0.48	<0.05
Bladder Cancer			
Canada[87]	826	0.95	>0.05
Buffalo[182]	569	0.31	<0.05
Germany[183]	340 Males	0.59	<0.05
	91 Females	0.90	>0.05
Oral Cancer			
Brazil[184]	232	0.4	0.05
Mesothelioma			
Louisiana[84]	37	0.28	>0.05
Melanoma			
Boston[85]	204	0.7	>0.05
Pharyngeal Cancer			
United States[88]	871	0.8 Males	>0.05
		0.8 Females	>0.05
United States[89]	42 Males	0.2	<0.05
	48 Females	1.5	>0.05
Washington State[90]	166	1.0	>0.05
North Carolina[185]	227	0.7	>0.05

* Relative risk in highest intake category of beta-carotene or carotene-rich foods compared with lowest category.

THE NEED FOR RANDOMIZED TRIALS

Despite many laboratory-based and observational epidemiologic studies that have been conducted in an effort to elucidate the relations of both retinoids and carotenoids with the risk for developing cancer, the evidence remains inconclusive. Although current evidence does support a protective effect of carotene intake, it is not clear whether the observed reductions in risk associated with the highest intake levels are due to the carotene content of the vegetables. For example, although most studies did control for cigarette smoking, other dietary or nondietary factors associated with consuming a diet rich in beta-carotene could account for any apparent protective effect. Several studies[42,45,64,74] found stronger protective associations with intake of specific vegetables and fruits than with a computed carotene index, suggesting that carotene may be a marker for some other preventive factor or that other components of fruits and vegetables may, in addition to carotene, have chemopreventive properties. The best, if not the only, way to assess directly whether any vitamin A analog has the ability to reduce cancer risk in humans is through large-scale, randomized trials of sufficient duration of treatment and follow-up. If the trial is well designed and achieves an adequate sample size, the random allocation of treatments will, on average, distribute both known and unknown confounding factors equally between the groups, thereby increasing the likelihood that any differences that emerge are due to the treatment itself.[191]

Current trial data on beta-carotene and retinol administration are limited. Early clinical studies showed topical retinoids to be effective in reversing skin keratosis,[191] carcinoma of the skin,[192,193] and melanoma metastases[194] and oral administration of retinoids to confer a beneficial effect on oral leukoplakia,[195] bronchial metaplasia,[196] and many other cancerous and precancerous conditions.[197–199] A randomized trial of supplements containing both retinol and beta-carotene[200] showed a threefold decrease in chromosome breakage in oral mucosal cells of Filipino betel nut and tobacco chewers. Benefits on various premalignant markers of cancer have been reported in some[201–203] but not all[204] randomized trials testing carotene, retinol, and synthetic retinoids, either alone or in combination. A small randomized trial of lung cancer patients after tumor resection found lower recurrence rates among those receiving beta-carotene than those receiving placebo,[205] whereas a large multicenter trial found no effect of beta-carotene on recurrence of skin cancer after 5 years of treatment and follow-up.[206]

ONGOING TRIALS

Many randomized trials funded by the National Cancer Institute (NCI) are currently being conducted to evaluate the potential for secondary and primary prevention of cancer by beta-carotene and various retinoids (Table 20–17). Secondary prevention trials include studies of persons with previous diagnoses of skin, head and neck, and colon cancer. Many trials are being conducted among populations at high risk due to the presence of precancerous conditions, such as dysplasia, or risk factors, such as cigarette smoking and occupational asbestos exposure. One of the largest ongoing trials in high-risk groups is a collaborative investigation being conducted by the NCI and the Cancer Institute of the Chinese Academy of Medical Sciences. This trial is testing combinations of beta-carotene, retinol, and many other micronutrients to prevent esophageal cancer in persons with esophageal dysplasia in poorly nourished villages in Linxian, China, an area with unusually high incidence rates. A primary prevention trial in persons without dysplasia is also being conducted in this region using the same agents.

Two primary prevention trials are being conducted in healthy, well-nourished populations. The Physicians' Health Study (PHS), is a nationwide, randomized trial of beta-carotene in the prevention of cancer and of aspirin in the reduction of cardiovascular disease among 22,071 U.S. male physicians with no history of cancer or cardiovascular disease.[207,208] To address the need for long duration of treatment for an effect to emerge, the average duration of treatment

TABLE 20–16. Predignostic Serum Beta-Carotene Levels and Subsequent Cancer

Investigations	Site	Population	Mean BC	Units	p Value
Knekt[99]	All	766 Cases	72.3 Males	µg/L	<0.05 Males
			119.5 Females		
		1419 Controls	84.1 Males		>0.05 Females
			126.5 Females		
Hsing[105]	Prostate	103 Cases	24*	µg/dl	>0.05
		103 Controls	24*		
Willett[106,107]	All	111 Cases	114.5	µg/dl	>0.05
		210 Controls	111.6 (total carotenoids)		
Stahelin[108]	All	204 Cases	0.342	µmol/L	<0.05
		2421 Controls	0.428		
Nomura[110]	All	284 Cases	23.4*	µg/dl	>0.05
		304 Controls	29.0*		
	Lung	74 Cases	20.0*		<0.05
		304 Controls	29.0*		
Connett[114]	All	156 Cases	9.8	µg/dl	>0.05
		311 Controls	10.4		
	Lung	66 Cases	9.0		0.07
		131 Controls	11.6		
Helzlsouer[116]	Bladder	35 Cases	36.2	µg/dl	>0.05
		70 Controls	32.7		
Schober[117]	Colon	72 Cases	32.9	µg/dl	>0.05
		143 Controls	34.4		
Menkes[118]	Lung	99 Cases	25.1	µgdl	<0.05
		196 Controls	29.1		
Burney[119]	Pancreas	22 Cases	0.73	µmol/L	>0.05
		44 Controls	0.70		
Comstock[189]	Melanoma	20 Cases	0.33*	µmol/L	>0.05
		40 Controls	0.33*		
	Rectum	34 Cases	0.44*		>0.05
		68 Cases	0.38*		
	Basal cell skin	21 Cases	0.30*		>0.05
		42 Controls	0.32*		
	Breast	30 Cases	0.37*		>0.05
		59 Controls	0.41*		
Wald[188]	All	271 Cases	19.8	µg/dl	<0.05
		533 Controls	22.1		
	Lung	50 Cases	15.8		<0.05
		99 Controls	20.3		

* Median values.
BC, beta-carotene level.

and follow-up in this trial will be longer than 10 years. A further strategy for increasing the power of the PHS to detect a protective effect of beta-carotene was the collection of pre-randomization blood samples from 15,000 of the participants. Samples of those participants who develop cancer during the trial and a matched comparison group of controls who remained disease-free will be analyzed for baseline levels of carotene, retinol, and retinol-binding protein. The availability of this blood-based epidemiologic study within the randomized trial will improve the chances of detecting whether any protective effect of beta-carotene is limited to participants with lower levels at baseline. Among women, a nationwide, multifactorial trial of beta-carotene, vitamin E, and aspirin in ap-

parently healthy nurses began in 1992. This trial plans to enroll more than 40,000 women with no history of cancer or cardiovascular disease to test beta-carotene and vitamin E, alone and in combination, in reducing risks for cancer and cardiovascular disease.[209,210]

CONCLUSION

The availability during the next several years of data from these and other carefully designed and conducted randomized trials should provide definitive answers to the questions of whether supplementation with any natural or synthetic reti-

TABLE 20–17. Current NCI-Supported Clinical Trials of Beta-Carotene and Vitamin A

Investigations	Site	Population	Protocol
Secondary Prevention			
Chemoprevention of skin and oral cancer	Skin	Patients with previous basal cell skin cancer	Retinol 25,000 IU/d 13-*cis*-Retinoic acid 0.15 mg/kg
Chemoprevention of aerodigestive epithelial cancers	Head and neck	Patients with previous head and neck cancer, leukoplakia	13-*cis*-Retinoic acid Beta-carotene
Effects of beta-carotene on colonic cell proliferation	Colon	Patients with previous colon cancer	Beta-carotene 30 mg/d
High-Risk Groups			
Chemoprevention of lung cancer with retinoids and beta-carotene	Lung	Cigarette smokers	Beta-carotene 30 mg/d Retinol 25,000 IU/d
Beta-carotene clinical trial monitoring cervical dysplasia	Cervical		Beta-carotene 30 mg/d
Chemoprevention of esophageal cancer in China	Esophagus	Persons with esophageal dysplasia	Beta-carotene, Retinol, and other micronutrients
Cancer prevention with retinol and beta-carotene in persons with asbestosis	Lung	Men with asbestosis	Beta-carotene 30 mg/d Retinol 25,000 IU/d
Chemoprevention efficacy trial of beta-carotene and retinol	Lung	Heavy smokers	Beta-carotene 30 mg/d Retinol 25,000 IU/d
Chemoprevention of skin cancer in albinos	Skin	Albinos in Tanzania	Beta-carotene 100 mg/d
Chemoprevention of skin cancer by vitamin A	Skin	Actinic keratosis patients	Retinol 25,000 IU/d
Nutritional prevention of polyps in the large bowel	Colon	Previous colon adenoma	Beta-carotene 30 mg/d Ascorbic acid 1 g/d Alpha-tocopherol 400 mg/d
Primary Prevention			
Chemoprevention of esophageal cancer in China	Esophagus	Residents of area with high incidence	Beta-carotene, Retinol, and other micronutrients
A randomized trial of aspirin and beta-carotene in U.S. physicians	All sites	22,071 U.S. male physicians	Beta-carotene, 50 mg qod
Women's Health Study	All sites	40,000 U.S. female nurses (anticipated enrollment)	Beta-carotene 50 mg qod Vitamin E 600 IU qod

(Courtesy of Dr. Winfred Malone, National Cancer Institute, Chemoprevention Branch, Bethesda, MD)

noids or with beta-carotene will reduce the risk for cancer in humans. Despite the many published studies reviewed earlier, preventing cancer with beta-carotene or retinoids currently remains a promising hypothesis that requires rigorous testing in large-scale randomized trials of sufficient duration of treatment and strong follow-up measures.

REFERENCES

1. Cairns J. Cancer: Science and society. San Francisco: WH Freeman, 1978:173.
2. Doll R, Peto R. The causes of cancer: Quantitative estimates of avoidable risks of cancer in the United States today. JNCI 1981;66:1192–1308.
3. Hennekens CH. Vitamin A analogues in cancer chemoprevention. In: DeVita VT, Hellman S, Rosenberg SA, eds. Important advances in oncology. Philadelphia: JB Lippincott, 1986:23–25.
4. Wolback SB, Howe PR. Tissue changes following deprivation of fat soluble A vitamin. J Exp Med 1925;42f:753–777.
5. Moore T. Effects of vitamin A deficiency in animals: Pharmacology and toxicology of vitamin A. In: Sebrell WH, Harris RS, eds. The vitamins. Vol 1. New York: Academic Press, 1967:280–294.
6. Harisiadis L, Miller RC, Hall FJ, Borek C. A vitamin A analogue inhibits radiation-induced oncogenic transformation. Nature 1977;269:511–512.
7. Todaro GJ, DeLarco JE, Sporn MB. Retinoids block phenotypic cell transformation produced by sarcoma growth factor. Nature 1978;276:272–274.
8. Chopra DP, Wilkoff LJ. Effect of retinoids and estrogens on testosterone-induced hyperplasia of mouse prostate explants in organ culture. Proc Soc Exp Biol Med 1979;162:229–234.
9. Lichti U, Patterson E, Yuspa SH. Retinoic acid differentially inhibits the induction of ornithine decarboxylase by 12-0-tetradecanoylphorbol-13-acetate and by germicidal ultraviolet light. Proc Am Assoc Cancer Res 1979;20:105.
10. Kensler TW, Mueller GC. Retinoic acid inhibition of the comitogenic action of mezerein and phorbol esters in bovine lymphocytes. Cancer Res 1979;38:771–775.
11. Kensler TW, Verma AK, Boutwell RK, Mueller GC. Effects of retinoic acid and juvenile hormone on the induction of ornithine decarboxylase activity by 12-0-tetradecanoyl-phorbol-13-acetate. Cancer Res 1978;38:2986–2989.
12. Lasnitski I. Growth pattern of the mouse prostate gland in organ culture and its response to sex hormones, vitamin A and 3-methylcholanthrene. NCI Monogr 1963;12:381–403.
13. Sporn MB, Dunlop NM, Newton DL, Henderson NR. Relationships between structure and activity of retinoids. Nature 1976;263:110–113.
14. Merriman RL, Bertram JS. Reversible inhibitor by retinoids of 3-methyl-cholanthrene-induced neoplastic transformation in C3H/10T1/2 clone 8 cells. Cancer Res 1979;39:1661–1666.
15. Lasnitski I. Hypovitaminosis A in the mouse prostate gland cultured in chemically defined medium. Exp Cell Res 1962;28:40–51.
16. Chopra DP, Wilkoff LJ. Reversal by vitamin A analogues (retinoids) of hyperplasia induced by N-methyl-N'-nitro-N-nitrosoguanidine in mouse prostate organ cultures. JNCI 1977;58:923–930.

17. Lasnitski I. Reversal of methylcholanthrene-induced changes in mouse prostates in vitro by retinoic acid and its analogues. Br J Cancer 1976;23:239–248.

18. Sporn MB, Clamon GH, Dunlop NM, Newton DL, Smith JM, Saffiotti U. Activity of vitamin A analogs in cell cultures of mouse epidermis and organ cultures of hamster trachea. Nature 1975;253:47–50.

19. Clamon GH, Sporn MB, Smith JM, Saffiotti U. Alpha- and beta-retinyl acetate reverse metaplasias of vitamin A deficiency in hamster trachea in organ culture. Nature 1974;250:64–66.

20. Dickens MS, Sorof S. Prevention of transformation of mammary gland by retinoid in whole organ culture. Proc Am Assoc Cancer Res 1979;20:71.

21. Hennekens CH, Stampfer MJ, Willett WC. Micronutrients and cancer prevention. Cancer Prev Detect 1984;7:147–158.

22. Fujimaki Y. Formation of gastric carcinoma in albino rats fed on deficient diets. J Cancer Res 1925;10:469–477.

23. Mori S. The changes in the para-ocular glands which follow the administration of diets low in fat-soluble A: With notes on the effect of the same diets on the salivary glands and mucosa of the larynx and trachea. Bull Johns Hopkins Hosp 1922;33:357–359.

24. Wolbach SB, Howe PR. Vitamin A deficiency in the guinea-pig. Arch Pathol 1928;5:239–253.

25. Bollag W. Therapeutic effects of an aromatic retinoic acid analog on chemically induced skin papillomas and carcinomas of mice. Eur J Cancer 1974;10:731–737.

26. Verma AK, Shapas BG, Rice HM, Boutwell RK. Correlation of the inhibition by retinoids of tumor promoter-induced mouse epidermal ornithine decarboxylase activity and of skin tumor promotion. Cancer Res 1979;39:419–425.

27. Mayer H, Bollag W, Hanni R, Ruegg R. Retinoids, a new class of compounds with prophylactic and therapeutic activities in oncology and dermatology. Experientia 1978;34:1105–1119.

28. Frankel JW, Horton EJ, Winters AL, Samis HV, Ito Y. Inhibition of viral tumorigenesis by a retinoic acid analog: XI. Int Conf Chemother (Boston) [Abstract] 1979:850.

29. Trown PW, Buck MJ, Hansen R. Inhibition of growth and regression of a transplantable rat chondrosarcoma by three retinoids. Cancer Treat Rep 1976;60:1647–1653.

30. Kistler GS, Peter HJ. Wirkung von zwei reinoiden auf menschliche bronchuskarzinome in vivo (nu/nu-maus) und in vitro. Schweiz Med Wochenschr 1979;109:847–850.

31. Schuman LM, Mandell JS, Radke A, Seal U, Halberg F. Some selected features of the epidemiology of prostatic cancer: Minneapolis-St. Paul, Minnesota, case-control study, 1976–1979. In: Magnus K, ed. Trends in cancer incidence: Causes and practical implications. Washington, DC: Hemisphere 1982:345–354.

32. Oishi K, Okada K, Yoshida O, et al. A case-control study of prostatic cancer with reference to dietary habits. Prostate 1988;12:179–190.

33. Heshmat MY, Kaul L, Kovi J, et al. Nutrition and prostate cancer: A case-control study. Prostate 1985;6:7–17.

34. Ross RK, Shimizu H, Paganini-Hill A, Honda G, Henderson BE. Case-control studies of prostate cancer in blacks and whites in Southern California. JNCI 1987;78:869–874.

35. Kolonel LN, Hankin JH, Yoshizawa CN. Vitamin A and prostate cancer in elderly men: Enhancement of risk. Cancer Res 1987;47:2982–2985.

36. Hsing AW, McLaughlin JK, Schuman LM, et al. Diet, tobacco use, and fatal prostate cancer: Results from the Lutheran Brotherhood Cohort Study. Cancer Res 1990;50:6836–6840.

37. Gregor A, Lee PN, Roe FJC, Wilson MJ, Melton A. Comparison of dietary histories in lung cancer cases and controls with special reference to vitamin A. Nutr Cancer 1980;2:93–97.

38. Kolonel LN, Hinds MW, Nomura AMY, Hankin JH, Lee JS. Relationship of dietary vitamin A and ascorbic acid intake to the risk for cancers of the lung, bladder, and prostate in Hawaii. NCI Monogr 1985;69:137–142.

39. Pastorino U, Pisani P, Berrino F, et al. Vitamin A and female lung cancer: A case-control study on plasma and diet. Nutr Cancer 1987;10:171–179.

40. Bond GG, Thompson FE, Cook RR. Dietary vitamin A and lung cancer: Results of a case-control study of chemical workers. Nutr Cancer 1987;9:109–121.

41. Byers TE, Graham S, Haughey BP, Marshall JR, Swanson MK. Diet and lung cancer risk: Findings from the Western New York Diet Study. Am J Epidemiol 1987;125:351–363.

42. Jain M, Burch JD, Howe GR, Risch HA, Miller AB. Dietary factors and risk of lung cancer: Results from a case-control study, Toronto, 1981–1985. Int J Cancer 1990;45:287–293.

43. LeMarchand L, Yoshizawa CN, Kolonel LN, Hankin JH, Goodman MT. Vegetable consumption and lung cancer risk: A population-based case-control study in Hawaii. JNCI 1989;81:1158–1164.

44. Harris RWC, Key TJA, Silcocks PB, Bull D, Wald NJ. A case-control study of dietary carotene in men with lung cancer and in men with other epithelial cancers. Nutr Cancer 1991;15:63–68.

45. Ziegler RG, Mason TJ, Stemhagen A, et al. Dietary carotene and vitamin A and risk of lung cancer among white men in New Jersey. JNCI 1984;73:1429–1435.

46. Pierce RJ, Kune GA, Kune S, et al. Dietary and alcohol intake, smoking pattern, occupational risk, and family history in lung cancer patients. Results of a case-control study in males. Nutr Cancer 1989;12:237–248.

47. Katsouyanni K, Willett W, Trichopoulos D, et al. Risk of breast cancer among Greek women in relation to nutrient intake. Cancer 1988;61:181–185.

48. Richardson S, Gerber M, Cenee S. The role of fat, animal protein and some vitamin consumption in breast cancer: A case control study in Southern France. Int J Cancer 1991;48:1–9.

49. Potischman N, McCulloch CE, Byers TE, et al. Breast cancer and dietary and plasma concentrations of carotenoids and vitamin A. Am J Clin Nutr 1990;52:909–915.

50. Rohan TE, McMichael AJ, Baghurst PA. A population-based case-control study of diet and breast cancer in Australia. Am J Epidemiol 1988;128:478–489.

51. Marubini E, Decarli A, Costa A, et al. The relationship of dietary intake and serum levels of retinol and beta-carotene with breast cancer. Cancer 1988;61:173–180.

52. LaVecchia CL, Decarli A, Franceschi S, et al. Dietary factors and the risk of breast cancer. Nutr Cancer 1987;10:205–214.

53. Toniolo P, Riboli E, Protta F, Charrel M, Cappa APM. Calorie-providing nutrients and risk of breast cancer. JNCI 1989;81:278–286.

54. Tomkin GH, Scott L, Ogbuah C, O'Shaughnessy M. Carcinoma of the colon: Association with low dietary vitamin A in females— preliminary communication. J Roy Soc Med 1986;79:462–464.

55. Kune S, Kune GA, Watson LF. Case-control study of dietary etiological factors: The Melbourne Colorectal Cancer Study. Nutr Cancer 1987;9:21–42.

56. Tuyns AJ, Haelterman M, Kaaks R. Colorectal cancer and the intake of nutrients: Oligosaccharides are a risk factor, fats are not—a case-control study in Belgium. Nutr Cancer 1987;10:181–196.

57. Freudenheim JL, Graham S, Marshall JR, Haughey BP, Wilkinson G. A case-control study of diet and rectal cancer in Western New York. Am J Epidemiol 1990;131:612–624.

58. Lee HP, Gourley L, Duffy SW, Esteve J, Lee JS, Day NE. Colorectal cancer and diet in an Asian population—a case-control study among Singapore Chinese. Int J Cancer 1989;43:1007–1016.

59. Potter JD, McMichael AJ. Diet and cancer of the colon and rectum: A case-control study. JNCI 1986;76:557–569.

60. Heilbrun LK, Nomura AMY, Hankin JH, Stemmermann GN. Diet and colorectal cancer with special reference to fiber intake. Int J Cancer 1989;44:1–6.

61. Macquart-Moulin G, Riboli E, Cornee J, Charnay B, Berthezene P, Day NE. Case-control study on colorectal cancer and diet in Marseilles. Int J Cancer 1986;38:183–191.

62. Stehr PA, Gloninger MF, Kuller LH, Marsh GM, Radford EP, Weinberg GB. Dietary vitamin A deficiencies and stomach cancer. Am J Epidemiol 1985;121:65–70.

63. Graham S, Haughey BP, Marshall JR, et al. Diet in the epidemiology of gastric cancer. Nutr Cancer 1990;13:19–34.

64. LaVecchia CL, Negri E, Decarli A, D'Avanzo B, Franceschi S. A case-control study of diet and gastric cancer in Northern Italy. Int J Cancer 1987;40:484–489.

65. You WC, Blot WJ, Chang YS, et al. Diet and high risk of stomach cancer in Shandong, China. Cancer Res 1988;48:3518–3523.

66. Correa P, Fontham ETH, Pickle LW, Chen V, Lin Y, Haenszel W. Dietary determinants of gastric cancer in South Louisiana inhabitants. JNCI 1985;75:645–654.

67. Risch HA, Jain M, Choi NW, et al. Dietary factors and the incidence of cancer of the stomach. Am J Epidemiol 1985;122:947–959.

68. Marshall JR, Graham S, Byers TE, Swanson M, Grasure J. Diet and smoking in the epidemiology of cancer of the cervix. JNCI 1983;70:847–851.

69. Brock KE, Berry G, Mock PA, MacLennan R, Truswell AS, Brinton LA. Nutrients in diet and plasma and risk of in situ cervical cancer. JNCI 1988;80:580–585.

70. LaVecchia CL, Decarli A, Fasoli M, et al. Dietary vitamin A and the risk of intraepithelial and invasive cervical neoplasia. Gynecol Oncol 1988;30:187–195.

71. Verreault R, Chu J, Mandelson M, Shy K. A case-control study of diet and invasive cervical cancer. Int J Cancer 1989;43:1050–1054.

72. Ziegler RG, Brinton LA, Hamman RF, et al. Diet and the risk of invasive cervical cancer among white women in the United States. Am J Epidemiol 1990;132:432–445.

73. Slattery ML, Schuman KL, West DW, French TK, Robison LM. Nutrient intake and ovarian cancer. Am J Epidemiol 1989;130:497–502.

74. LaVecchia CL, Decarli A, Negri E, et al. Dietary factors and the risk of epithelial ovarian cancer. JNCI 1987;79:663–669.

75. Byers TE, Marshall JR, Graham S, Mettlin C, Swanson M. A case-control study of dietary and nondietary factors in ovarian cancer. JNCI 1983;71:681–686.

76. Shu XO, Gao YT, Yuan JM, Ziegler RG, Brinton LA. Dietary factors and epithelial ovarian cancer. Br J Cancer 1989;59:92–96.

77. Baghurst PA, McMichael AJ, Slavotinek AH, Baghurst KI, Boyle P, Walker AM. A case-control study of diet and cancer of the pancreas. Am J Epidemiol 1991;134:167–179.

78. Falk RT, Pickle LW, Fontham ETH, Correa P, Fraumeni JF. Life-style risk factors for pancreatic cancer in Louisiana: A case-control study. Am J Epidemiol 1988;128:324–336.

79. Farrow DC, Davis S. Diet and the risk of pancreatic cancer in men. Am J Epidemiol 1990;132:423–431.

80. Tuyns AJ, Riboli E, Doornbos G, Pequignot G. Diet and esophageal cancer in Calvados (France). Nutr Cancer 1987;9:81–92.

81. Graham S, Marshall JR, Haughey BP, et al. Nutritional epidemiology of cancer of the esophagus. Am J Epidemiol 1990;131:454–467.

82. Brown LM, Blot WJ, Schuman SH, et al. Environmental factors and high risk of esophageal cancer among men in coastal South Carolina. JNCI 1988;80:1620–1625.

83. Decarli A, Liati P, Negri E, Franceschi S, LaVecchia CL. Vitamin A and other dietary factors in the etiology of esophageal cancer. Nutr Cancer 1987;10:29–37.

84. Schiffman MH, Pickle LW, Fontham ETH, et al. Case-control study of diet and mesothelioma in Louisiana. Cancer Res 1988;48:2911–2915.

85. Stryker SW, Stampfer MJ, Stein EA, et al. Diet, plasma levels of beta-carotene and alpha-tocopheral, and risk of malignant melanoma. Am J Epidemiol 1990;131:597–611.

86. MacKerras D, Buffler PA, Randall DE, Nichaman MZ, Pickle LW, Mason TJ. Carotene intake and the risk of laryngeal cancer in coastal Texas. Am J Epidemiol 1988;128:980–988.

87. Risch HA, Burch JD, Miller AB, Hill GB, Steele R, Howe GR. Dietary factors and the incidence of cancer of the urinary bladder. Am J Epidemiol 1988;127:1179–1191.

88. McLaughlin JK, Gridley G, Block G, et al. Dietary factors in oral and pharyngeal cancer. JNCI 1988;80:1237–1243.

89. Gridley G, McLaughlin JK, Block G, et al. Diet and oral and pharyngeal cancer among blacks. Nutr Cancer 1990;14:219–225.

90. Rossing MA, Vaughan TL, McKnight B. Diet and pharyngeal cancer. Int J Cancer 1989;44:593–597.

91. Paganini-Hill A, Chao A, Ross RK, Henderson BE. Vitamin A, beta-carotene, and the risk of cancer: A prospective study. JNCI 1987;79:443–448.

92. Atukorala S, Basu TK, Dickerson JWT, Donaldson D, Sakula A. Vitamin A, zinc, and lung cancer. Br J Cancer 1979;40:927–931.

93. Basu TK, Donaldson D, Jenner M, Williams DC, Sakula A. Plasma vitamin A in patients with bronchial carcinoma. Br J Cancer 1976;33:119–121.

94. Abels JC, Gorham AT, Pack GT, Rhoades CP. Metabolic studies in patients with cancer of the gastrointestinal tract: I. Plasma vitamin A levels in patients with malignant neoplastic disease, particularly of the gastrointestinal tract. J Clin Invest 1941;20:749–764.

95. Wahi PN, Bodkhe RR, Arora S, Srivastava MC. Serum vitamin A studies in leukoplakia and carcinoma of the oral cavity. Indian J Pathol Bacteriol 1962;5:10–16.

96. Ibrahim J, Jafarey NA, Zuberi SJ. Plasma vitamin A and carotene levels in squamous cell carcinoma of the oral cavity and oropharynx. Clin Oncol 1977;3:58–63.

97. Basu TK, Raven RW, Dickerson JWT, Williams DC. Vitamin A nutrition and its relationship with plasma cholesterol level in the patient with cancer. Int J Vitam Nutr Res 1974;44:14–18.

98. Capel ID, Williams DC. The relationship between zinc and vitamin A in cancer patients. IRCS J Med Sci 1979;7:361.

99. Knekt P, Aromaa A, Maatela J, et al. Serum vitamin A and subsequent risk of cancer: Cancer incidence follow-up of the Finnish Mobile Clinic Health Examination Survey. Am J Epidemiol 1990;132:857–870.

100. Wald NJ, Idle M, Boreham J, Bailey A. Low serum-vitamin A and subsequent risk of cancer: Preliminary results of a prospective study. Lancet 1980;2:813–815.

101. Kark JD, Smith AH, Switzer BR, Hames CG. Serum vitamin A (retinol) and cancer incidence in Evans County, Georgia. JNCI 1981;66:7.

102. Wald NJ, Boreham J, Bailey A. Serum retinol and subsequent risk of cancer. Br J Cancer 1986;54:957–961.

103. Peleg I, Heyden S, Knowles M, Hames CG. Serum retinol and risk of subsequent cancer: Extension of the Evans County, Georgia, study. JNCI 1984;73:1455–1458.

104. Reichman ME, Hayes RB, Ziegler RG, et al. Serum vitamin A and subsequent development of prostate cancer in the first National Health and Nutrition Examination Survey Epidemiologic Follow-up Study. Cancer Res 1990;50:2311–2315.

105. Hsing AW, Comstock GW, Abbey H, Polk BF. Serologic precursors of cancer: Retinol, carotenoids, and tocopherol and risk of prostate cancer. JNCI 1990;82:941–946.

106. Willett WC, Polk BF, Underwood BA, et al. Relation of serum vitamins A and E and carotenoids to the risk of cancer. N Engl J Med 1984;310:430–434.

107. Willett WC, Polk BF, Underwood BA, Hames CG. Hypertension detection and follow-up program study of serum retinol, retinol-binding protein, total carotenoids, and cancer risk: A summary. JNCI 1984;73:1459–1462.

108. Stahelin HB, Gey KF, Eichholzer M, et al. Plasma antioxidant vitamins and subsequent cancer mortality in the 12-year follow-up of the Prospective Basel Study. Am J Epidemiol 1991;133:766–775.

109. Salonen JT, Salonen R, Lappetelainen R, Haenpaa PH, Alfthan G, Puska P. Risk of cancer in relation to serum concentrations of selenium and vitamins A and E: Matched case-control analysis of prospective data. Br Med J 1985;290:417–420.

110. Nomura AMY, Stemmermann GN, Heilbrun LK, Salkeld RM, Vuilleumier JP. Serum vitamin levels and the risk of cancer of specific sites in men of Japanese ancestry in Hawaii. Cancer Res 1985;45:2369–2372.

111. Coates RJ, Weiss NS, Daling JR, Morris JS, Labbe RF. Serum levels of selenium and retinol and the subsequent risk of cancer. Am J Epidemiol 1988;128:515–523.

112. Friedman GD, Blander WS, Goodman DS, et al. Serum retinol and retinol-binding protein levels do not predict subsequent lung cancer. Am J Epidemiol 1986;123:781–789.

113. Russell MJ, Thomas BS, Bulbrook RD. A prospective study of the relationship between serum vitamins A and E and risk of breast cancer. Br J Cancer 1988;57:213–215.

114. Connett JE, Kuller LH, Kjelsberg MO, et al. Relationship between carotenoids and cancer: The Multiple Risk Factor Intervention Trial (MRFIT) Study. Cancer 1989;64:126–134.

115. Criqui MH, Bangdiwala S, Goodman DS, et al. Selenium, retinol, retinol-binding protein, and uric acid: Associations with cancer mortality in a population-based prospective case-control study. Ann Epidemiol 1991;1:385–393.

116. Helzlsouer KJ, Comstock GW, Morris SJ. Selenium, lycopene, alpha-tocopherol, beta-carotene, retinol, and subsequent bladder cancer. Cancer Res 1989;49:6144–6148.

117. Schober SE, Comstock GW, Helsing KJ, et al. Serologic precursors of cancer: I. Prediagnostic serum nutrients and colon cancer risk. Am J Epidemiol 1987;126:1033–1041.

118. Menkes MS, Comstock GW, Vuilleumier JP, Helsing KJ, Rider AA, Brookmeyer R. Serum beta-carotene, vitamins A and E, selenium, and the risk of lung cancer. N Engl J Med 1986;315:1250–1254.

119. Burney PGJ, Comstock GW, Morris JS. Serologic precursors of cancer: Serum micronutrients and the subsequent risk of pancreatic cancer. Am J Clin Nutr 1989;49:895–900.

120. Kok FJ, van Duijn CM, Hofman A, et al. Micronutrients and the risk of lung cancer. N Engl J Med [Letter] 1987;316:1416.

121. Vahlquist A, Michaelsson G, Tuhlin L. Acne treatment with oral zinc and vitamin A: Effects on the serum levels of zinc and retinol binding protein (RBP). Acta Derm Venereol (Stockholm) 1978;58:437.

122. Willett WC, Stampfer MJ, Underwood BA, Taylor JO, Hennekens CH. Vitamins A, E and carotene: Effects of supplementation on their plasma levels. Am J Clin Nutr 1983;38:559–566.

123. Willett WC, Stampfer MJ, Underwood BA, et al. Vitamin A supplementation and plasma retinol levels: A randomized trial among women. JNCI 1984;73:1145.

124. Peto R, Doll R, Buckley JD, et al. Can dietary beta-carotene materially reduce human cancer rates? Nature 1981;290:201–208.

125. Krinsky NI, Deneke SM. Interaction of oxygen and oxy-radicals with carotenoids. JNCI 1982;69:205–210.

126. Packer JE, Mahood JS, Mora-Arellano VO, Slater TF, Willson RL, Wolfenden BS. Free radicals and singlet oxygen scavengers: Reaction of a peroxy-radical with beta-carotene, diphenyl furan and 1,4-diazobicyclo(2,2,2)-octane. Biochem Biophys Res Commun 1981;98:901–906.

127. Foote CS. Photosensitized oxidation and singlet oxygen: Consequences in biological systems. In: Pryor WA, ed. Free radicals in biology. Vol 2. New York: Academic Press, 1976:85–133.

128. Krinsky NI. Carotenoid protection against oxidation. Pure Appl Chem 1979;51:649–660.

129. Foote CS, Chang YC, Denny RW. Chemistry of singlet oxygen: X. Carotenoid quenching parallels biological protection. J Am Chem Soc 1970;92:5216–5219.

130. Oberley LW, Buettner GR. Role of superoxide dismutase in cancer: A review. Cancer Res 1979;39:1141–1149.

131. Demopoulos HB, Pietronigro DD, Flamm ES, Seligon ML. The possible role of free radical reactions in carcinogenesis. J Environ Pathol Toxicol 1980;3:273–303.

132. Reddy JK, Azarnoff DL, Hignite CE. Hypolipidaemic hepatic peroxisome proliferators form a novel class of chemical carcinogens. Nature 1980;283:397–399.

133. Shamberger RJ. Increase of peroxidation in carcinogenesis. JNCI 1972;48:1491–1497.

134. Epstein JH. Effects of beta carotene on UV-induced cancer formation in the hairless mouse skin. Photochem Photobiol 1977;25:211–213.

135. Matthews-Roth MM. Anti-tumor activity of beta-carotene, canthaxanthin, and phytoene. Oncology 1982;39:33–37.

136. Rettura G, Stratford P, Levenson SM, Seifter E. Prophylactic and therapeutic actions of supplemental beta-carotene in mice innoculated with C3HBA adenocarcinoma cells. JNCI 1982;69:73–77.

137. Rettura G, Duttagupta C, Listowsky P, Levenson SM, Seifter E. Dimethylbenz(a) anthracene (DMBA) induced tumors: Prevention by supplemental beta-carotene. Fed Proc 1983;42:786.

138. Bjelke E. Dietary vitamin A and human lung cancer. Int J Cancer 1975;15:561–565.

139. Kvale GX, Bjelke E, Gart JJ. Dietary habits and lung cancer risk. Int J Cancer 1983;51:397–405.

140. Mettlin C, Graham S, Swanson M. Vitamin A and lung cancer. JNCI 1979;62:1435–1438.

141. MacLennan R, DeCosta J. Risk factors for lung cancer in Singapore Chinese, a population with high female incidence rates. Int J Cancer 1977;20:854–860.

142. Hirayama T. Diet and cancer. Nutr Cancer 1979;1:67–81.

143. Shekelle RB, Liu S, Raynor WJ, et al. Dietary vitamin A and risk of cancer in the Western Electric Study. Lancet 1981;2:1185–1190.

144. Hinds MW, Kolonel LN, Hankin JH, Lee JS. Dietary vitamin A, carotene, vitamin C and risk of lung cancer in Hawaii. Am J Epidemiol 1984;119:227–237.

145. Samet JM, Skipper BJ, Humble CG, Pathak DR. Lung cancer risk and vitamin A consumption in New Mexico. Am Rev Respir Dis 1985;141:198–202.

146. Pisani P, Berrino F, Macaluso M, Pastorino U, Crosignani P, Baldasseroni A. Carrots, green vegetables and lung cancer: A case-control study. Int J Epidemiol 1986;15:463–468.

147. Fontham ETH, Pickle LW, Haenszel W, Correa P, Lin Y, Falk RT. Dietary vitamins A and C and lung cancer risk in Louisiana. Cancer 1988;62:2267–2273.

148. Cook-Mozaffari P, Azordegan F, Day NE, Ressicaud A, Sabai C, Aramesh B. Oesophageal cancer studies in the Caspian littoral of Iran: Results of a case-control study. Br J Cancer 1979;39:293–309.

149. Mettlin C, Graham S, Priore R, Marshall JR, Swanson M. Diet and cancer of the esophagus. Nutr Cancer 1981;2:143–147.

150. Yu MC, Garabrant DH, Peters JM, et al. Tobacco, alcohol, diet occupation, and carcinoma of the esophagus. Cancer Res 1988;48:3843–3848.

151. DeStefani E, Munoz N, Esteve J, et al. Mate drinking, alcohol, tobacco, diet, and esophageal cancer in Uruguay. Cancer Res 1990;50:426–431.

152. Nakachi K, Imai K, Hoshiyama Y, et al. The joint effects of two factors in the aetiology of oesophageal cancer in Japan. J Epidemiol Comm Health 1988;42:355–364.

153. Modan B, Cudde H, Lubin F. A note on the role of dietary retinol and carotene in human gastrointestinal cancer. Int J Cancer 1981;28:421–424.

154. Stocks P. Cancer incidence in North Wales and Liverpool region in relation to habits and environment. In: British Empire Cancer Campaign 35th Annual Report, Part II (Supplement). 1958:111–113.

155. Bjelke E. Dietary factors and the epidemiology of cancer of the stomach and large bowel. In: Aktuelle probleme der klinischen diatetik, Suppl ZU Aktuelle Ernahrungsmedizin. Stuttgart, Germany: George Theime Verlag, 1978:10–17.

156. Jedrychowski W, Wahrendorf J, Popiela T, Rachtan J. A case-control study of dietary factors and stomach cancer risk in Poland. Int J Cancer 1986;37:837–842.

157. Trichopoulos D, Ouranos G, Day NE, et al. Diet and cancer of the stomach: A case-control study in Greece. Int J Cancer 1985;36:291–297.

158. Kono S, Ikeda M, Tokudome S, Kuratsune M. A case-control study of gastric cancer and diet in Northern Kyushu, Japan. Jpn J Cancer Res 1988;79:1067–1074.

159. Graham S, Dayal H, Swanson M, Mittelman A, Wilkinson G. Diet in the epidemiology of cancer of the colon and rectum. JNCI 1978;61:709–714.

160. Phillips RL. Role of life-style and dietary habits in risk of cancer among Seventh-Day Adventists. Cancer Res 1975;35:3513–3522.

161. Hu J, Liu Y, Yu Y, Zhao T, Liu S, Wang Q. Diet and cancer of the colon and rectum: A case-control study in China. Int J Epidemiol 1991;20:362–367.

162. Slattery ML, Sorenson AW, Mahoney AW, et al. Diet and colon cancer: Assessment of risk of fiber type and food source. JNCI 1988;80:1474–1480.

163. West DW, Slattery ML, Robison LM, et al. Dietary intake and colon cancer: Sex- and anatomic site-specific associations. Am J Epidemiol 1989;130:883–894.

164. Young TB, Wolf DA. Case-control study of proximal and distal colon cancer and diet in Wisconsin. Int J Cancer 1988;42:167–175.

165. Peters RK, Garabrant DH, Yu MC, Mack TM. A case-control study of occupational and dietary factors in colorectal cancer in young men by subsite. Cancer Res 1989;49:5459–5468.

166. Mettlin C, Selenskas S, Natarajan N, Huben R. Beta-carotene and animal fats and their relationship to prostate cancer risk: A case-control study. Cancer 1989;64:605–612.

167. Mills PK, Beeson WL, Phillips RL, Fraser GE. Cohort study of diet, lifestyle, and prostate cancer in Adventist men. Cancer 1989;64:598–604.

168. LeMarchand L, Hankin JH, Kolonel LN, Wilkens LR. Vegetable and fruit consumption in relation to prostate cancer risk in Hawaii: A reevaluation of the effect of dietary beta-carotene. Am J Epidemiol 1991;133:215–219.

169. Mishina T, Watanabe H, Araki H, Nakao M. Epidemiological study of prostatic cancer by matched-pair analysis. Prostate 1985;6:423–436.

170. Talamini R, LaVecchia CL, Decarli A, Negri E, Franceschi S. Nutrition, social factors and prostatic cancer in a Northern Italian population. Br J Cancer 1986;53:817–821.

171. Graham S, Marshall JR, Mettlin C, Rzepka T, Nemoto T, Byers TE. Diet in the epidemiology of breast cancer. Am J Epidemiol 1982;116:68–75.

172. Lee HP, Gourley L, Duffy SW, Esteve J, Lee JS, Day NE. Dietary effects on breast-cancer risk in Singapore. Lancet 1991;337:1197–1200.

173. Iscovich JM, Iscovich RB, Howe GR, Shiboski S, Kaldor JM. A case-control study of diet and breast cancer in Argentina. Int J Cancer 1989;44:770–776.

174. Van't-Veer P, van Leer EM, Rietdijk A, et al. Combination of dietary factors in relation to breast-cancer occurrence. Int J Cancer 1991;47:649–653.

175. van Eenwyk J, Davis FG, Bowen PE. Dietary and serum carotenoids and cervical intraepithelial neoplasia. Int J Cancer 1991;48:34–38.

176. Slattery ML, Abbott TM, Overall JC, et al. Dietary vitamins A, C and E and selenium as risk factors for cervical cancer. Epidemiology 1990;1:8–15.

177. Norell SE, Ahlbom A, Erwald R, et al. Diet and pancreatic cancer: A case-control study. Am J Epidemiol 1986;124:894–902.

178. Mack TM, Yu MC, Hanisch R, Henderson BE. Pancreas cancer and smoking, beverage consumption, and past medical history. JNCI 1986;76:49–60.

179. Mills PK, Beeson WL, Abbey DE, Fraser GE, Phillips RL. Dietary habits and past medical history as related to fatal pancreas cancer among Adventists. Cancer 1988;61:2578–2585.

180. Gold EB, Gordis L, Diener MD, et al. Diet and other risk factors for cancer of the pancreas. Cancer 1985;55:460–467.

181. Graham S, Mettlin C, Marshall JR, Priore R, Rzepka T, Shedd D. Dietary factors in the epidemiology of cancer of the larynx. Am J Epidemiol 1981;113:675–680.

182. Graham S, Mettlin C. Dietary risk factors in human bladder cancer. Am J Epidemiol 1979;110:255–263.

183. Claude J, Kunze E, Frentzel-Beyme R, Paczkowski K, Schneider J, Schubert H. Life-style and occupational risk factors in cancer of the lower urinary tract. Am J Epidemiol 1986;124:578–589.

184. Franco EL, Kowalski LP, Oliveira BV, et al. Risk factors for oral cancer in Brazil: A case-control study. Int J Cancer 1989;43:992–1000.

185. Winn DM, Ziegler RG, Pickle LW, Gridley G, Blot WJ, Hoover RN. Diet in the etiology of oral and pharyngeal cancer among women from the Southern United States. Cancer Res 1984;44:1216–1222.

186. Colditz GA, Branch LG, Lipnick RJ, et al. Increased green and yellow vegetable intake and lowered cancer deaths in an elderly population. Am J Clin Nutr 1985;41:32–36.

187. Hirayama T. A large scale cohort study on cancer risk by diet, with special reference to the risk reducing effects of green-yellow vegetable consumption. In: Hayashi Y, Nagao M, Sugimura T, et al, eds. Diet, nutrition, and cancer. Tokyo, Japan: Japan Scientific Societies Press, 1986:41–53.

188. Wald NJ, Thompson SG, Densem JW, Boreham J, Bailey A. Serum beta-carotene and subsequent risk of cancer: Results from the BUPA Study. Br J Cancer 1988;57:428–433.

189. Comstock GW, Helzlsouer KJ, Bush TL. Prediagnostic serum levels of carotenoids and vitamin E as related to subsequent cancer in Washington County, Maryland. Am J Clin Nutr 1991;53:260s–264s.

190. Neiman C, Obbink HJR. The biochemistry and pathology of hypervitaminosis A. Vitam Horm 1954;12:69–99.

191. Hennekens CH, Buring JE. Epidemiology in medicine. Boston: Little, Brown, 1987.

192. Bollag W, Ott F. Therapy of actinic keratoses and basal cell carcinomas with local application of vitamin A acid. Cancer Chemother Rep 1971;55:59–60.

193. Ott F. Retinoic acid in the treatment of precancerous disorders and carcinoma of the skin. Ther Umsch 1972;20:607–609.

194. Levine N, Meyskens FL. Topical vitamin-A-acid therapy for cutaneous metastatic melanoma. Lancet 1980;2:224–225.

195. Koch HF. Biochemical treatment of precancerous oral lesions: The effectiveness of various analogues of retinoic acid. J Maxillofac Surg 1978;6:59–63.

196. Gouveia J, Hercend T, Lemaigre G, et al. Degree of bronchial metaplasia in heavy smokers and its regression after treatment with a retinoid. Lancet 1982;2:710–712.

197. Ryssel HJ, Brunner KW, Bollag W. Die perorale anwedung von vitamin-A-saure bei leukoplakien, hyperkeratosen und plattenepithelkarzinomen. Ergebnisse und vertraglichkeit. Schweiz Med Wochenschr 1971;101:1027–1030.

198. Evard JP, Bollag W. Konservative behandlung der rezidivierenden hardblasenpapillomatose mit vitmain-A-saure. Schweiz Med Wochenschr 1972;102:1880–1883.

199. Peck GL, Olsen TG, Butkus D, et al. Treatment of basal cell carcinomas with 13-cis-retinoic acid. Proc Am Assoc Cancer Res 1979;20:56.

200. Stich HF, Rosin MP, Vallejera MO. Reduction with vitamin A and beta-carotene administration of the proportion of micrinucleated buccal mucosal cells in Asian betel nut and tobacco chewers. Lancet 1984;2:1204–1206.

201. Stich HF, Rosin MP, Hornby AP, Mathew B, Sankaranarayanan R, Krishnan-Nair M. Remission of oral leukoplakias and micronuclei in tobacco/betel seed chewers treated with beta-carotene and with beta-carotene plus vitamin A. Int J Cancer 1988;42:195–199.

202. Stich HF, Hornby P, Dunn BP. A pilot beta-carotene intervention trial with Inuits using smokeless tobacco. Int J Cancer 1985;36:321–327.

203. Hong WK, Endicott J, Itri LM, et al. 13-cis-retinoic acid in the treatment of oral leukoplakia. N Engl J Med 1986;315:1501–1505.

204. Munoz N, Wahrendorf J, Bang LJ, et al. No effect of riboflavine, retinol, and zinc on prevalence of precancerous lesions of oesophagus. Lancet 1985;2:111–114.

205. Pastorino U, Soresi E, Clerici M, et al. Lung cancer chemoprevention with retinol palmitate. Acta Oncol 1988;27:773–782.

206. Greenberg ER, Baron JA, Stukel TA, et al. A clinical trial of beta carotene to prevent basal-cell and squamous cell cancers of the skin. N Engl J Med 1990;323:789–795.

207. Hennekens CH, Eberlein KA. A randomized trial of aspirin and beta-carotene among U.S. physicians. Prev Med 1985;14:165–168.

208. Steering Committee of the Physicians' Health Study Research Group. Final report on the aspirin component of the ongoing Physicians' Health Study. N Engl J Med 1989;321:129–135.

209. Women's Health Study Research Group. The Women's Health Study: Summary of the study design. J Myocardial Ischemia 1992;4:27–29.

210. Women's Health Study Research Group. The Women's Health Study: Background and rationale. J Myocardial Ischemia 1992;4:30–40.

BRIAN E. HENDERSON
LESLIE BERNSTEIN
RONALD ROSS

SECTION 5

Hormones

A substantial body of experimental, clinical, and epidemiologic evidence indicates that hormones play a major role in the cause of several human cancers.[1] This concept has been refined to epidemiologic hypotheses that relate specific hormones to cancers of the breast, the endometrium, and the prostate and the process of ovulation induced by gonadotropin release to cancer of the ovary. A key element of these hypotheses is that excessive hormonal stimulation of the particular target organ increases the number of cell divisions; random genetic errors accumulate during the process of repeated cell divisions and can lead to neoplastic phenotypes.[2,3]

Cancers of hormone-responsive tissues currently account for more than 20% of all newly diagnosed male and more than 40% of all newly diagnosed female cancers in the United States. Because of the evidence that endogenous hormones directly affect the risk for these cancers, chemoprevention through administration of "antihormones" has become an important focus of cancer prevention research. A summary of chemopreventive agents for hormone-induced cancers is shown in Table 20–18. The acceptability of any such agent

TABLE 20–18. Hormone Chemopreventive Agents Currently in Clinical Use

Chemopreventive Agent	Cancer Site	Mechanism of Action
Oral contraceptives	Endometrium	Antiestrogen
	Ovary	Cease ovulation
Progestogens (HRT)	Endometrium	Antiestrogen
LHRH agonist	Breast	Eliminate ovarian steroid hormone production
	Endometrium	
	Ovary	Cease ovulation
Tamoxifen	Breast	Antiestrogen

HRT, hormone replacement therapy; LHRH, luteinizing-hormone-releasing-hormone.

for widespread use in the prevention of cancer relies on the balance of the health benefits versus the health risks of such usage.

The prototype antihormone is progesterone, which has a natural antiestrogenic effect on endometrial cell proliferation. During the follicular phase of the ovulatory menstrual cycle, endometrial cells divide in response to estrogen stimulation that is unopposed by progesterone. During the luteal phase, further estrogen-induced endometrial cell proliferation ceases in the presence of progesterone. Epidemiologic evidence shows that events or circumstances that increase estrogen stimulation in the absence of progesterone increase endometrial cancer risk, whereas those that decrease unopposed estrogen exposure decrease risk.[4] The application of these principles to chemoprevention of endometrial cancer has been amply demonstrated through the use of oral contraceptives and through the addition of progestogens to estrogen replacement therapy.

ORAL CONTRACEPTIVES

ENDOMETRIAL CANCER

During the time when the association of prolonged use of estrogen replacement therapy and endometrial cancer was being established, case series reports suggested a similar as-

sociation between sequential oral contraceptives and endometrial cancer.[5] It is not surprising that sequential formulations had this effect on the endometrium, because they induced a menstrual cycle that began with a 14- to 16-day proliferation phase (administration of unopposed estrogen), followed by a short 7-day secretory phase (administration of estrogen-progestogen combination), and ending with a 5- to 7-day period without treatment. Three case-control studies that accumulated sufficient data on the use of sequential oral contraceptives showed a twofold increased risk for endometrial cancer among women who had used these preparations.[6-8] This association with endometrial cancer was partly responsible for the removal of sequential oral contraceptives from the sales market in the United States in 1976.[9]

In contrast to the adverse effects on the endometrium of sequential oral contraceptives, use of combination oral contraceptives has been reported consistently in case-control studies to decrease the risk of endometrial cancer by approximately 50% (Table 20–19).[7,8,10-14] Prospective cohort studies have demonstrated similar decreases in risk.[15,16] A protective effect of combination oral contraceptives is biologically plausible, because the presence of a progestogen, in combination with estrogen, for 21 days of the cycle followed by 7 days with no treatment minimizes endometrial mitotic activity.

In the large Cancer and Steroid Hormone (CASH) study sponsored by the Centers for Disease Control and the National Institute of Child Health and Human Development, the protective effect of combination oral contraceptives on endometrial cancer risk was the same for both short-term users (fewer than 5 years) and longer-term users (5 years or more),[6] although very short-term users (less than 1 year) were not protected.[13] In contrast, Henderson and colleagues observed a clear decrease in risk with increasing duration of use.[7] Among women with 6 or more years of use, the risk of endometrial cancer was less than one sixth that of women who had never used oral contraceptives. Whether the protective effect of combination oral contraceptives is long-lasting is an important question and study results have been mixed. In the CASH study, the protective effect of pill use persisted for women who discontinued using oral contraceptives 15 years before participation in the study.[6]

Results are mixed with regard to the ideal estrogen and progestogen potencies of these preparations for optimal pro-

TABLE 20–19. Case-Control Studies of Combination Oral Contraceptives and Endometrial Cancer

Investigations	Age Range	Relative Risk	No. of Patients Using Oral Contraceptives
Kaufman, 1980[10]	≤59	0.5	16
Weiss, 1980[8]	34–54	0.5	17
Hulka, 1982[11]	≤59	0.4	5
Kelsey, 1982[12]	45–74	0.6	6
Centers for Disease Control (CASH), 1983[6,13]	20–54	0.6	70
Henderson, 1983[7]	≤45	0.5	43
WHO Collaborative Study, 1988[14]	25–59	0.6	12

CASH, Cancer and Steroid Hormone Study; WHO, World Health Organization.

tection against endometrial cancer. No consistent, differential effects on endometrial cancer risk were demonstrated by specific formulations of oral contraceptives in the CASH study[13] or by examining the risk associated with relative potencies of estrogen and progestogen in the study by Henderson and colleagues.[7] Hulka and associates ranked products by their progestogen content and found the greatest reduction in risk for women using products with the highest progestogen dose.[11]

OVARIAN CANCER

In addition to their chemopreventive action on endometrial cancer risk, combination oral contraceptives suppress gonadotropins and ovulation and thereby reduce a woman's risk for epithelial ovarian cancer. The results of 13 case-control studies that have examined this issue are summarized in Table 20–20.[17–29] Except for a small series of women in Utah reported by Risch and associates, all studies have shown a decreased risk among oral contraceptive users that averages approximately 40%.[26] Reports from cohort studies of oral contraceptive use are consistent with these results.[15,16,30]

Because epithelial ovarian tumors are more common in less fertile women, this factor must be considered when interpreting results of studies, because it could lead to a spurious protective effect of pill use. Recent studies indicate that this explanation is unlikely to account for the lower risk among oral contraceptive users. The risk for ovarian cancer decreases with increasing duration of oral contraceptive use[18,25,28] and this dose-response effect appears to be independent of parity.[31] Protection appears to be long-lasting.[24,25,28] In the CASH study, women who first used oral contraceptives 10 years or longer before participating in the study had approximately one half the ovarian cancer risk of nonusers.[25]

BREAST CANCER

Unlike the antiestrogenic effects of progesterone on the endometrium, evidence is accumulating that progesterone increases the rate of cell division in the breast beyond that induced by estrogen.[32] As a result, the simultaneous presence of estrogen and progesterone in combination oral contraceptives is not protective against breast cancer as is the case for cancers of the endometrium and ovary.[33] Use of oral contraceptives during the postmenarchal and perimenopausal periods, when the naturally produced levels of estrogen and progesterone may decrease below the levels supplied by oral contraceptive formulations, may be associated with an increased risk for breast cancer.[33] Using a similar line of reasoning (*i.e.*, measuring the effect of oral contraceptive use relative to the woman's "normal" hormonal state), the more recently introduced low-dose oral contraceptives could hypothetically protect against breast cancer in regularly ovulating women by replacing natural levels of ovarian steroids with smaller amounts of the same hormones.

HORMONE REPLACEMENT THERAPY

ENDOMETRIAL CANCER

Case reports of endometrial cancer occurring in women after the use of estrogens have appeared in the medical literature for more than 30 years, but only since 1975 have there been

TABLE 20–20. Case-Control Studies of Oral Contraceptives and Epithelial Carcinoma of the Ovary

Investigations	Age Range	Relative Risk	No. of Patients Using Oral Contraceptives
Newhouse, 1977[17]	All ages	0.6	19
Casagrande, 1979[18]	25–49	0.8	41
McGowan, 1979[19]	Mean, 52	0.7	NP
Hildreth, 1981[20]	45–74	0.5	3
Willett, 1981[21]	30–55	0.8	13
Cramer, 1982[22]	≤59	0.4	34
Franceschi, 1982[23]	≤69	0.7	17
Rosenberg, 1982[24]	≤59	0.6	29
Centers for Disease Control (CASH), 1983[25]	20–54	0.6	90
Risch, 1983[26]			
Washington	34–74	0.4*	NP†
Utah	20–74	1.1*	NP†
LaVecchia, 1984[27]	≤59	0.6	18
Wu, 1988[28]	18–85	0.7	111
Booth, 1989[29]	≤64	0.5	35

* Estimated.
† Study provides percentage of patients exposed to oral contraceptives adjusted to age distribution of controls: 10.6% of 216 Washington patients and 10.9% of 68 Utah patients were exposed to oral contraceptives.
NP, not provided; CASH, Cancer and Steroid Hormone Study.

serious, controlled efforts to study this relation. Within 5 years of the initial studies, more than 20 studies appeared in the literature that examined this association. Nearly all studies demonstrated a strong association between estrogen use and disease risk that was related to dose and duration of use.[34-36]

The benefit of adding a progestogen to estrogen replacement therapy to reduce endometrial mitotic activity has been established.[37,38] Therefore, in response to the "epidemic" of endometrial cancer that followed the introduction of estrogen use, progestogens were added to estrogen in various doses using a wide spectrum of monthly regimens. Such combination therapy has been shown to reduce the estrogen-enhanced risk for endometrial cancer,[39] although there are serious concerns about the potential of the added progestogen to increase further the small risk of breast cancer in estrogen users[33,40] and to reduce the associated arteriosclerotic vascular benefit.[41]

LUTEINIZING-HORMONE-RELEASING-HORMONE AGONISTS

Among premenopausal women, a proposed strategy for retaining the benefit of oral contraceptives on the risk for endometrial and ovarian cancer while possibly preventing breast cancer is to eliminate ovarian estrogen and progesterone production by using luteinizing-hormone-releasing-hormone (LHRH) agonists. Experimentally, these drugs cause regression of estrogen-dependent dimethylbenzanthracene-induced rat mammary tumors[42]; clinically, they suppress ovulation and cause regression of metastatic breast cancer in premenopausal women.[43-45]

As a primary means for preventing breast cancer, the use of LHRH agonists is designed to exploit the preventive aspect of early menopause on breast cancer risk.[46] By totally eliminating ovarian steroid hormone production, LHRH agonists induce a reversible "bilateral oophorectomy."[47,48] It is predicted that such a regimen taken for 5 years during the premenopausal years would lead to a reduction in breast cancer risk of 38%, and such a regimen taken for 15 years could reduce risk by as much as 80%.[46] By preventing ovulation, as in the case with combination oral contraceptives, such a regimen markedly reduces endometrial and ovarian cancer risk.

The beneficial effect of eliminating ovarian steroid hormone production is associated with adverse side effects.[47,48] These adverse consequences are primarily those related to a hypoestrogenic state, both acutely and in the long term. Particular examples are hot flashes, bone loss, and probably a significantly increased risk for cardiovascular disease resulting at least in part from an increase in low-density lipoprotein cholesterol.[41] Extensive experience suggests that these harmful side effects can be eliminated by the addition of low-dose estrogen replacement therapy to the regimen. Such a regimen (LHRH agonist plus low-dose estrogen replacement therapy) does not affect the protective effect of LHRH agonists alone on ovarian cancer risk; Pike and colleagues have argued that the estrogen replacement therapy dose required to eliminate these side effects is sufficiently low to retain the major part of the benefit on breast cancer risk.[46] Intermittent regular addition of a progestogen to the regimen could avoid any increased risk for endometrial hyperplasia (or carcinoma) associated with low-dose estrogen replacement therapy. Med-

roxyprogesterone acetate given every 3 to 4 months for 13 days of one monthly cycle at a dose of 5 to 10 mg/day is one possible regimen.

This proposed regimen is a highly effective hormonal contraceptive method. In addition to the advantages related to breast cancer risk, such a regimen may provide other notable advantages over low-dose oral contraceptives in terms of long-term health effects. Although data are sparse, the addition of a low-dose estrogen replacement therapy to the LHRH regimen would appear to create a favorable lipid profile, particularly with regard to high-density lipoprotein cholesterol levels, and would be expected to have a favorable influence on cardiovascular disease risk.[46]

TAMOXIFEN

The first proposal for the hormonal chemoprevention of breast cancer was introduced by Cuzick and colleagues in 1986.[49] The goal was to treat healthy postmenopausal women at high risk for breast cancer using the antiestrogenic drug, tamoxifen. The rationale for this proposal was based partly on the extensive evidence that the amount of estrogen available to breast tissue is a critical factor in the cause of human breast cancer. Two years later, a summary analysis of 28 ongoing U.S., Canadian, and European randomized clinical trials showed a significant reduction in the mortality from breast cancer of women older than 50 years of age treated with tamoxifen.[50] This beneficial effect appears to extend to women who are lymph node positive or lymph node negative at diagnosis and to women regardless of the initial estrogen receptor status of their tumors.

The most compelling argument to extend the use of tamoxifen to healthy women at high risk for breast cancer is the lower risk for contralateral primary breast cancer observed among women receiving adjuvant tamoxifen therapy for breast cancer. Nayfield and colleagues[51] have summarized these data in tamoxifen patients compared with control patients from eight randomized trials (Table 20–21),[52-59] which show a 35% reduction in risk for contralateral breast cancer.

An ongoing concern that has guarded the optimism about the probable efficacy of such a regimen in primary breast cancer prevention is the possible adverse antiestrogenic effect of tamoxifen on other organ systems.[60] Tamoxifen shows highly selective antiestrogenic properties and appears to be an estrogen agonist in most other tissues. Of particular concern has been the possible antiestrogenic effect of tamoxifen on lipid and bone metabolism. There is strong evidence that menopause is associated with a substantial increase in heart disease risk and that this effect is most likely due to the loss of ovarian estrogen production.[61] Low-dose orally administered estrogen replacement therapy is associated with a substantial reduction in heart disease risk[62,63] and possibly stroke mortality.[64] These effects are likely mediated in part by the favorable effect of estrogen replacement therapy on lipid profiles; estrogen replacement therapy substantially increases high-density lipoprotein cholesterol levels and substantially reduces low-density lipoprotein cholesterol levels.

Tamoxifen appears to create a somewhat favorable lipid profile. The most authoritative article on this topic was published by Love and colleagues.[65] As part of a 2-year randomized, double-blind, placebo-controlled toxicity trial of tamoxifen in 140 postmenopausal women with a history of node-negative breast cancer (70 of whom were treated with tamoxifen), these investigators found that low-density lipoprotein cholesterol levels declined approximately 18% and that this decline persisted for at least 1 year of treatment. High-density lipoprotein cholesterol levels remained unchanged for the first 6 months of therapy but, compared with baseline values, were reduced significantly by 7% at 1 year. Total cholesterol was reduced significantly in the tamoxifen-treated group. Overall, because of the large declines in low-density lipoprotein cholesterol, the relative amount of high-density lipoprotein cholesterol (*i.e.*, high-density lipoprotein/total cholesterol ratio) increased among women treated with tamoxifen.

Nonetheless, the effect of long-term tamoxifen use with regard to heart disease risk remains uncertain; because the pattern of lipid changes with tamoxifen is different from that induced by estrogen replacement therapy, mechanisms other than lipid changes may be involved in the cardioprotective effect of estrogen replacement therapy, and there are few data in women regarding the potential benefits of reducing low-density lipoprotein cholesterol with regard to cardiovascular disease risk. The Scottish Adjuvant Tamoxifen Trial provides some preliminary evidence that tamoxifen may have a beneficial effect on coronary heart disease risk.[66] In this randomized trial, a group of women received 20 mg tamoxifen daily for at least 5 years and follow-up ranged from 5 to 11 years. Among postmenopausal women, those treated with tamoxifen had a statistically significant reduction in mortality due to acute myocardial infarction compared with control patients.

Available evidence on the effects of tamoxifen on bone mineral density is encouraging. Two studies evaluating this issue have reported slight increases in the density of the lumbar spine during tamoxifen treatment for postmenopausal breast cancer.[67,68] Although osteoporotic fracture rates have not been studied after tamoxifen use, these data suggest that, as with estrogen replacement therapy, fracture risk may be reduced.

Other lingering issues suggest caution in the initiation of a full-scale tamoxifen chemoprevention trial. There are reports that tamoxifen is associated with a substantially elevated risk for endometrial cancer of a magnitude comparable with that related to estrogen replacement therapy.[51] Although not every tamoxifen trial has reported such an effect, experimental evidence and the biochemical activity of tamoxifen support a causal relation.

Another concern is that tamoxifen may have estrogen-like effects on the liver. In rats, estrogens act as promoters of liver carcinogenesis.[69] Jordan reports that in large doses or with extended exposure, tamoxifen has produced rat liver tumors.[60] No increase in liver tumor incidence has been reported among tamoxifen-treated patients in any clinical trial, although Fornander and colleagues observed two cases of hepatocellular carcinoma among their patients receiving tamoxifen.[70]

A possible increased risk of thromboembolic disease has been suggested,[71,72] but has not been well documented. Among postmenopausal women receiving long-term adjuvant tamoxifen therapy, small decreases in the levels of antithrombin III have been reported,[73] although these values are generally within the normal range. As a result, a history of clotting disorders may be a contraindication to tamoxifen treatment.

Although tamoxifen probably reduces certain acute menopausal effects, such as vaginal dryness, the drug has no beneficial effect on hot flashes (there are data to suggest the opposite may be true) and the relation between tamoxifen and other acute menopausal symptoms is largely unstudied.

TABLE 20–21. Tamoxifen Effects on the Risk of Primary Contralateral Breast Cancer in Women With Stage I or II Breast Cancer*

Clinical Trial	Median Follow-Up (mo)	Tamoxifen-Treated Patients: No. Cancers/ No. Patients (%)	Controls: No. Cancers/ No. Patients (%)
NATO[52]	66	15/564 (2.7)	17/567 (3.0)
Scottish[53]	47	9/661 (1.4)	12/651 (1.8)
Stockholm[54]	84	29/931 (3.1)	47/915 (5.1)
Copenhagen[55]	78	3/164 (1.8)	4/153 (2.6)
Toronto/Edmonton[56]	70	3/198 (1.5)	3/202 (1.5)
ECOG 1178[57]	55	1/91 (1.1)	3/90 (3.3)
NSABP B-14[58]	59	23/1419 (1.6)	32/1428 (2.2)
CRC[59]	40	7/947 (0.7)	18/965 (1.9)
Total		90/4975 (1.8)	136/4971 (2.7)

* Biopsy-proved second primary breast cancers in contralateral breast; results from eight randomized controlled clinical trials.
NATO, Novaldex and Adjuvant Trial Organization; ECOG, Eastern Cooperative Oncology Group; NSABP, National Surgical Adjuvant Breast and Bowel Project; CRC, Cancer Research Campaign.
(Adapted from Nayfield SG, Karp JE, Ford LG, Dorr A, Kramer BS. Potential role of tamoxifen in prevention of breast cancer. JNCI 199;83:1450–1459—[with exception of the Stockholm trial, based on data presented by the ICI Pharmaceuticals Group at the Food and Drug Administration Oncology Drugs Advisory Committee Meeting, Bethesda, MD, June 29, 1990])

In summary, existing evidence regarding bone and lipid effects of tamoxifen is reassuring. Endometrial cancer, thromboembolic disease, and hot flashes continue to be legitimate concerns. However, tamoxifen has few other acute side effects, enhancing the feasibility of long-term compliance in large-scale trials. A chemoprevention trial of tamoxifen in American women at increased risk for breast cancer is currently being planned with accrual to begin in early 1992.

CHEMOPREVENTION OF PROSTATE CANCER

Testosterone is essential for the maintenance of prostatic tissue, but there are no studies in men relating variation in circulating testosterone levels to the rate of cell proliferation in the prostate. Epidemiologic support for an association of increased testosterone levels and increased prostatic cancer risk is inconsistent.[74] Prostatic adenocarcinomas can be produced by testosterone administration in rats and such treatment increases proliferation of the glandular cells in the prostate, which give rise to prostatic cancer.[75] Testosterone may increase the mitotic activity of prostatic cells in men and such an increase in mitotic activity would increase the risk of prostatic cancer.

Diethylstilbestrol and LHRH agonists are effective therapeutically in metastatic prostate cancer, presumably because of their indirect effect on testosterone production, by decreasing luteinizing hormone secretion. These drugs in their usual therapeutic doses produce impotence and other side effects that are unacceptable when considered as chemopreventive agents.

Despite the dependence of the prostate on testosterone for normal growth and maintenance, testosterone has no direct effects on prostatic epithelium requiring metabolic activation to dihydrotestosterone for these functions. Conversion of testosterone to dihydrotestosterone in the prostate requires activity of the enzyme 5-α-reductase.

Japanese and Chinese men have among the lowest prostate cancer rates in the world. Recent data strongly suggest that both of these populations have much reduced 5-α-reductase activity relative to U.S. blacks and whites.[76,77] These findings may provide a hormonal basis for the low levels of prostate cancer in these Asian populations and emphasize the need to clarify further the role of 5-α-reductase activity in prostatic carcinogenesis. If such enzymatic activity proves crucial, then chemoprevention of prostate cancer using the still experimental 5-α-reductase inhibitor category of drugs may be feasible. These drugs, which selectively block production of dihydrotestosterone from testosterone in the prostate, reduce prostatic size without affecting testosterone-dependent processes such as fertility, muscle strength, and libido.

REFERENCES

1. Henderson BE, Ross RK, Pike MC, Casagrande JT. Endogenous hormones as a major factor in human cancer. Cancer Res 1982;43:3232–3239.
2. Henderson BE, Ross RK, Bernstein L. Estrogens as a cause of human cancer: The Richard and Hinda Rosenthal Foundation Award Lecture. Cancer Res 1988;48:246–253.
3. Preston-Martin S, Pike MC, Ross RK, Jones PA, Henderson BE. Increased cell division as a cause of human cancer. Cancer Res 1990;50:7415–7421.
4. Key TJA, Pike MC. The role of estrogens and progestagens in the epidemiology and prevention of breast cancer. Eur J Cancer Clin Oncol 1988;24:29–43.
5. Silverberg SG, Makowski EL. Endometrial carcinoma in young women taking oral contraceptive agents. Obstet Gynecol 1975;46:503–506.
6. Centers for Disease Control. Oral contraceptive use and the risk of endometrial cancer. JAMA 1983;249:1600–1604.
7. Henderson BE, Casagrande JT, Pike MC, et al. The epidemiology of endometrial cancer in young women. Br J Cancer 1983;47:749–756.
8. Weiss NS, Sayvetz TA. Incidence of endometrial cancer in relation to the use of oral contraceptives. N Engl J Med 1980;302:551–554.
9. Piper JM, Kennedy DL. Oral contraceptives in the United States: Trends in content and potency. Int J Epidemiol 1987;16:215–221.
10. Kaufman DW, Shapiro S, Slone D, et al. Decreased risk of endometrial cancer among oral contraceptive users. N Engl J Med 1980;303:1045–1047.
11. Hulka BS, Chambless LE, Kaufman DG, et al. Protection against endometrial carcinoma by combination-product oral contraceptives. JAMA 1982;247:475–477.
12. Kelsey JL, LiVolsi VA, Holford TR, et al. A case-control study of cancer of the endometrium. Am J Epidemiol 1982;116:333–342.
13. Centers for Disease Control. Combination oral contraceptive use and the risk of endometrial cancer. JAMA 1987;249:796–800.
14. World Health Organization (WHO). WHO collaborative study of neoplasia and steroid contraceptives: Endometrial cancer and combined oral contraceptives. Int J Epidemiol 1988;17:263–269.
15. Ramcharan S, Pellegrin FA, Ray R, Hsu JP. A prospective study of the side effects of oral contraceptive use. Washington, DC: U.S. Government Printing Office, 1981.
16. Beral V, Hannaford P, Kay C. Oral contraceptive use and malignancies of the genital tract. Lancet 1988;2:1331–1335.
17. Newhouse ML, Pearson RM, Fullerton JM, et al. A case control study of carcinoma of the ovary. Br J Prev Soc Med 1977;31:148–153.
18. Casagrande JT, Louie EW, Pike MC, et al. Incessant ovulation and ovarian cancer. Lancet 1979;2:170–173.
19. McGowan L, Parent L, Lednar W, Norris HJ. The woman at risk for developing ovarian cancer. Gynecol Oncol 1979;7:325–344.
20. Hildreth NG, Kelsey JL, LiVolsi VA, et al. An epidemiological study of epithelial carcinoma of the ovary. Am J Epidemiol 1981;114:398–405.
21. Willett WC, Bain C, Hennekens CH, et al. Oral contraceptives and risk of ovarian cancer. Cancer 1981;48:1684–1687.
22. Cramer DW, Hutchinson GB, Welch WR, et al. Factors affecting the association of oral contraceptives and ovarian cancer. N Engl J Med 1982;307:1047–1051.
23. Franceschi S, LaVecchia CL, Helmrich SP, et al. Risk factors for epithelial ovarian cancer in Italy. Am J Epidemiol 1982;115:714–719.
24. Rosenberg L, Shapiro S, Slone D, et al. Epithelial ovarian cancer and combination oral contraceptives. JAMA 1982;247:3210–3212.
25. Centers for Disease Control. Oral contraceptive use and the risk of ovarian cancer. JAMA 1983;249:1596–1599.
26. Risch HA, Weiss NS, Lyon JL, et al. Events of reproductive life and the incidence of epithelial ovarian cancer. Am J Epidemiol 1983;177:128–139.
27. LaVecchia CL, Franceschi S, Decarli A. Oral contraceptive use and the risk of epithelial ovarian cancer. Br J Cancer 1984;50:31–34.
28. Wu ML, Whittemore AS, Paffenbarger RS, et al. Personal and environmental characteristics related to epithelial ovarian cancer: I. Reproductive and menstrual events and oral contraceptive use. Am J Epidemiol 1988;128:1216–1227.
29. Booth M, Beral V, Smith P. Risk factors for ovarian cancer: A case-control study. Br J Cancer 1989;60:592–598.
30. Harlow BL, Weiss NS, Roth GL, et al. Case-control study of borderline ovarian tumors: Reproductive history and exposure to exogenous female hormones. Cancer Res 1988;48:5849–5852.
31. Centers for Disease Control. The reduction in risk of ovarian cancer associated with oral-contraceptive use. N Engl J Med 1987;316:650–655.
32. Key TJA, Pike MC. The dose-effect relationship between "unopposed" oestrogens and endometrial mitotic rate: Its central role in explaining and predicting endometrial cancer risk. Br J Cancer 1988;57:205–212.
33. Bernstein L, Henderson BE. Hormone intake: Relationship to cancer risk. In: DeVita VT, Hellman S, Rosenberg SA, eds. Cancer prevention. Philadelphia: JB Lippincott, 1990:1–17.
34. Smith DC, Prentice R, Thompson DJ, Herrmann W. Association of exogenous estrogen and endometrial cancer. N Engl J Med 1975;293:1164–1167.
35. Ziel HK, Finkle WD. Increased risk of endometrial carcinoma among users of conjugated estrogens. N Engl J Med 1975;293:1167–1170.
36. Mack TM, Pike MC, Henderson BE, et al. Estrogens and endometrial cancer in a retirement community. N Engl J Med 1976;294:1262–1267.
37. Gal D, Edman CD, Vellios F, Forney JP. Long-term effect of megestrol acetate in the treatment of endometrial hyperplasia. Am J Obstet Gynecol 1983;146:316–321.
38. Gambrell RD. Clinical use of progestins in the menopausal patient: Dosage and duration. J Reprod Med 1982;27:531–538.
39. Voigt LF, Weiss NS, Chu J, et al. Progestogen supplementation of exogenous oestrogens and risk of endometrial cancer. Lancet 1991;338:274–277.
40. Hoover R, Gray LA, Cole P, MacMahon B. Menopausal estrogens and breast cancer. N Engl J Med 1976;295:401–405.
41. Henderson BE, Ross RK, Lobo RA, et al. Re-evaluating the role of progestogen therapy after the menopause. Fertil Steril 1988;49(suppl):9s–15s.
42. Nicholson RI, Walker KJ, Maynard PV. Anti-tumor potential of a new potent luteinizing hormone releasing hormone analogue, ICI 118630. Eur J Cancer 1980;1(suppl):295–299.
43. Harvey HA, Lipton A, Max DT, et al. Medical castration produced by the GnRH analogue leuprolide to treat metastatic breast cancer. J Clin Oncol 1985;3:1068–1072.

44. Williams MR, Walker KJ, Turkes A, et al. The use of an Lh-Rh agonist (ICI118360, Zoladex) in advanced premenopausal breast cancer. Br J Cancer 1986;53:629–636.

45. Dixon AR, Robertson JFR, Jackson L, et al. Goserelin (Zoladex) in premenopausal advanced breast cancer: Duration of response and survival. Br J Cancer 1990;62:868–870.

46. Pike MC, Ross RK, Lobo RA, et al. LHRH agonists and the prevention of breast and ovarian cancer. Br J Cancer 1989;60:142–148.

47. Gudmundsson JA, Nillius SJ, Bergquist C. Intranasal peptide contraception by inhibition of ovulation with the gonadotrophin-releasing hormone superagonist nafarelin: Six months clinical results. Fertil Steril 1986;45:617–623.

48. McLachlan RI, Healy DL, Burger HG. Clinical aspects of LHRH analogues in gynaecology: A review. Br J Obstet Gynaecol 1986;45:617–623.

49. Cuzick J, Wang DY, Bulbrook RD. The prevention of breast cancer. Lancet 1986;1:83–86.

50. Early Breast Cancer Trialists' Collaborative Group. Effects of adjuvant tamoxifen and of cytotoxic therapy on mortality in early breast cancer. N Engl J Med 1988;319:1681–1692.

51. Nayfield SG, Karp JE, Ford LG, Dorr A, Kramer BS. Potential role of tamoxifen in prevention of breast cancer. JNCI 1991;83:1450–1459.

52. Nolvadex and Adjuvant Trial Organization (NATO). Controlled trial of tamoxifen as a single adjuvant agent in the management of early breast cancer. Br J Cancer 1988;57:608–611.

53. Breast Cancer Trials Committee, Scottish Cancer Trials Office MRC. Adjuvant tamoxifen in the management of operable breast cancer: The Scottish trial. Lancet 1987;2:171–175.

54. Rutqvist LE, Cedermark B, Glas U, et al. Contralateral primary tumors in breast cancer patients in a randomized trial of adjuvant tamoxifen therapy. JNCI 1991;83:1299–1306.

55. Palshof T, Mourisden HT, Daehnfeldt JL, et al. Adjuvant endocrine therapy in pre- and postmenopausal women with operable breast cancer. Rev Endocr Rel Cancer 1985;17(suppl):43–50.

56. Pritchard KI, Meakin JW, Boyd NF, et al. Adjuvant tamoxifen in postmenopausal women with axillary node positive breast cancer: An update. In: Salmon SE, ed. Adjuvant therapy of cancer. Vol V. New York: Grune and Stratton, 1987:391–400.

57. Cummings FJ, Gray R, Davis TE, et al. Tamoxifen versus placebo: Double-blind adjuvant trial in elderly women with stage II breast cancer. In: Proceedings of the NIH Consensus development conference on adjuvant chemotherapy and endocrine therapy for breast cancer. Bethesda, MD: National Institutes of Health, 1986:119–123.

58. Fisher B, Constantino J, Redmond C, et al. A randomized clincial trial evaluating tamoxifen in the treatment of patients with node-negative breast cancer who have estrogen-receptor-positive tumors. N Engl J Med 1989;320:479–484.

59. CRC Adjuvant Breast Trial Working Party. Cyclophosphamide and tamoxifen as adjuvant therapies in the management of breast cancer. Br J Cancer 1988;57:604–607.

60. Jordan VC. Tamoxifen for the prevention of breast cancer. In: DeVita VT, Hellman S, Rosenberg SA, eds. Cancer prevention. Philadelphia: JB Lippincott, 1990:1–16.

61. Kannel WB, Hjortland MC, McNamara PM, et al. Menopause and risk of cardiovascular disease. Ann Intern Med 1976;85:447–452.

62. Ross RK, Pike MC, Mack TM, Henderson BE. Oestrogen replacement therapy and cardiovascular disease. In: Drife JO, Studd JWW, eds. HRT and osteoporosis. London: Springer-Verlag, 1990:209–222.

63. Barrett-Connor E, Bush TJ. Estrogen and coronary heart disease in women. JAMA 1991;265:1861–1867.

64. Paganini-Hill A, Ross RK, Henderson BE. Postmenopausal oestrogen treatment and stroke: A prospective study. Br Med J 1988;297:519–522.

65. Love RR, Newcomb PA, Wiebe DA, et al. Effects of tamoxifen therapy on lipid and lipoprotein levels in postmenopausal patients with node-negative breast cancer. JNCI 1990;82:1327–1332.

66. McDonald CG, Stewart HJ. Fatal myocardial infarction in the Scottish adjuvant tamoxifen trial. Br Med J 1991;303:435–437.

67. Love RR, Mazess RB, Torney DC, et al. Bone mineral density in women with breast cancer treated with adjuvant tamoxifen for at least two years. Breast Cancer Res Treat 1988;12:297–301.

68. Turken S, Siris E, Seldin D, et al. Effects of tamoxifen on spinal bone density in women with breast cancer. JNCI 1989;8:1086–1088.

69. Yager JD, Yager R. Oral contraceptive steroids as promoters of hepatocarcinogenesis in female Sprague-Dawley rats. Cancer Res 1980;40:3680–3685.

70. Fornander T, Rutqvist LE, Cedermark B, et al. Adjuvant tamoxifen in early breast cancer: Occurrence of new primary cancers. Lancet 1989;1:117–120.

71. Lipton A, Harvey HA, Hamilton RW. Venous thrombosis as a side effect of tamoxifen treatment. Cancer Treat Rep 1984;68:887–889.

72. Falkson HC, Gray R, Wolbert WH, et al. Adjuvant trial of 12 cycles of CMFPT followed by observation or continuous tamoxifen versus four cycles of CMFPT in postmenopausal women with breast cancer: An ECOG Phase III study. J Clin Oncol 1990;8:599–607.

73. Jordan VC, Fritz NF, Tormey DC. Long-term adjuvant therapy with tamoxifen effects on sex hormone binding globulin and antithrombin III. Cancer Res 1987;47:4517–4519.

74. Ross RK. Prostate cancer. In: Schottenfeld D, Fraumeni J, eds. Cancer epidemiology and prevention. 2nd ed. Cambridge, England: Oxford University Press, 1992 (in press).

75. Noble RL. The development of prostatic adenocarcinoma in Nb rats following prolonged sex hormone administration. Cancer Res 1977;37:1929–1933.

76. Ross RK, Bernstein L, Lobo RA, et al. Evidence for reduced 5-alpha-reductase activity in Japanese compared to U.S. white and black males: Implications for prostate cancer risk. Lancet 1992;339:887–889.

77. Lookingbill DP, Demers LM, Wang C, et al. Clinical and biological parameters of androgen action in normal healthy Caucasian versus Chinese subjects. J Clin Endocrinol Metab 1991;72:1242–1248.

SECTION **6**

Curtailing the Tobacco Pandemic

ALAN BLUM

By all rights, lung cancer should have been included along with smallpox as one of the diseases that was eradicated in the 20th century. Instead, to the undying shame of the health professions—and due to the untiring energy of the transnational tobacco conglomerates—the production, distribution, marketing, and use of tobacco continue to grow in every corner of the world. Deaths from lung cancer are expected to exceed 3 million a year by the turn of the century.[1]

Since U.S. Surgeon General Leroy E. Burney issued a policy statement in 1957 that accepted the cause-effect relation between cigarette smoking and lung cancer,[1a] each succeeding Surgeon General has been committed to curbing the use of tobacco. In 1964 the Report of the Advisory Committee to the Surgeon General on Smoking and Health reviewed and summarized the devastating scientific case against smoking.[2] This document and an analysis produced in the United Kingdom in 1962 by the Royal College of Physicians galvanized the medical community and the public alike. The Surgeon

General's report was written by ten eminent biomedical scientists who had been selected by Surgeon General Luther Terry from a list of 150 people (none of whom had taken a public position on the subject of smoking and health) approved by major health organizations and the tobacco industry.

Concerns about smoking had long been raised in the scientific community. In 1928 Lombard and Doering[3] reported a higher incidence of smoking among patients with cancer than among controls. Ten years later Pearl[4] reported that persons who smoked heavily had a shorter life expectancy than those who did not smoke. In 1939 Ochsner and DeBakey began reporting their observations on the relation between smoking and lung cancer.[5] They and other outspoken opponents of smoking, such as Dwight Harkin and William Overholt, were met with derision by the medical profession, more than two thirds of whom smoked.

Not until the epidemiologic work in the 1950s of Doll and Hill[4a] in the United Kingdom and Hammond and Horn[6] in the United States did the medical profession begin to take the problem seriously. Cigarette advertisements continued to appear in the *Journal of the American Medical Association* and other medical journals until the mid-1950s. A Viceroy cigarette advertisement published in medical journals in 1954 thanked the 64,985 doctors who visited Viceroy exhibits at medical conventions that year. Such scientific displays existed at various state medical society meetings until the 1980s. In

1978 the American Medical Association (AMA) issued a report, "Tobacco and Health," which summarized research projects that confirm the findings of the 1964 Surgeon General's report and cemented the association between smoking and heart disease.[6a] This report was entirely underwritten by the tobacco industry, which in effect had succeeded in muting any official action-oriented stance on the part of the AMA for 14 years.

Nonetheless, since 1985 when it first called for a ban on tobacco advertising, the AMA and its publications have become increasingly outspoken in the effort to curtail the use and promotion of tobacco. The AMA has funded two national conferences on tobacco and has made the subject of smoking and health one of its four top priorities. Pressure by the AMA led the Joint Commission on Accreditation of Healthcare Organizations to institute a policy mandating that accredited health facilities be smoke-free environments as of 1992.

Considering its $350 million annual income, the American Cancer Society (ACS) has been cautious and conservative in challenging the tobacco industry. Not until 1983 did the organization begin to address the subject of cigarette advertising. On the other hand, the ACS *has* made several major contributions, including the adoption of the annual stop-smoking day known as the Great American Smokeout, the sponsorship of world conferences on smoking and health (which currently draw 1000 people and are held every 3 years), and the creation of Globalink (a worldwide electronic communication network to aid the sharing of antitobacco strategies). The American Academy of Family Physicians has led medical specialty organizations in confronting tobacco problems by means of training for physicians in smoking cessation and financial support for antitobacco advocacy groups such as Doctors Ought to Care (DOC). Various chapters of the American Lung Association have done substantive lobbying and taken aggressive public stances in accelerating the passage of local clean indoor air legislation.

Governmental agencies, public health organizations, and academic institutions have not exerted much leadership on this issue. A remarkable grassroots antismoking movement that arose in the 1970s with the goal to create smoke-free public places impelled more traditional organizations to action. These groups—Action on Smoking and Health, Group Against Smoking Pollution, and Americans for Nonsmokers' Rights—paved the way for measures such as the federal ban on smoking in aircrafts and local laws that restrict smoking, remove cigarette vending machines, and ban the distribution of free tobacco samples.

Although numerous prospective studies conducted over the past 40 years have documented multifarious disease risks associated with smoking,[7] cancer has been linked to tobacco use for more than two centuries. In 1761, John Hill,[8] a London physician, reported an association between the use of snuff and cancer of the nose. The first U.S. Surgeon General's Report on Smoking and Health in 1964 concluded that cigarette smoking was the major cause of lung cancer in men and was causally related to laryngeal cancer and oral cancer in men.[2] More than 57,000 subsequent studies and 20 additional reports of the Surgeon General have documented the impact of tobacco use on morbidity and mortality in the United States and abroad. It is now understood that approximately 40% of all cancer deaths are attributable to cigarette smoking; smoking is thus responsible for more than 434,000 deaths per year in the United States, or 18% of all deaths.[9]

Smoking is the major cause of cancers of the lung, larynx, oral cavity, and esophagus and is a contributory factor in cancers of the pancreas, bladder, kidney, stomach, and uterine cervix (Table 20–22). Overall, cigarette smoking has been identified as the chief preventable cause of deaths due to cancer in the United States.[7]

LUNG CANCER

The most prominent conclusion of the 1964 Surgeon General's Report was the determination that cigarette smoking is the major cause of lung cancer in men.[2,10,11] There is a clear dose-response relation between lung cancer risk and daily cigarette consumption, and those people who smoke more than a pack of cigarettes a day have a risk that is at least 20 times that of nonsmokers.[7] The four major histologic forms of lung cancer—squamous cell, adenocarcinoma, small cell, and large cell—are all associated with smoking. Squamous cell cancer is the commonest form among men; in women, adenocarcinoma predominates.[12]

The identification of cigarette smoking as the major causative factor in the development of lung cancer led the tobacco industry to respond to such reports with the promotion of "less hazardous" cigarettes, including filtered, low-tar, and low-nicotine cigarettes, creating the illusion that the risk had been eliminated or diminished.[13–15,16] This recalled the multimillion dollar advertising campaigns developed in the 1940s to allay the public's concerns about cigarette smoking, including R. J. Reynolds' slogan, "More doctors smoke Camels than any other cigarette," American Tobacco Company's boast, "Lucky Strike is less irritating to sensitive or tender throats," and Philip Morris' claim, published in countless magazines, newspapers, and medical journals, "Every case of irritation of the nose and throat due to smoking cleared completely or definitely improved."[17] Lorillard's Kent cigarettes, one of the most widely promoted "health-oriented" brands of the 1950s, contained a filter that was made of asbestos.[17]

Over the years, such purported innovations in the design of the product have been met with overwhelming consumer acceptance. For example, between 1976 and 1982 sales of low-tar cigarettes, which offer few if any safety advantages, increased from 17% to 59% of total cigarette sales.[14] Currently, the tobacco industry continues to suggest health benefits to consumers through the use of words such as "light," "ultra-light," "mild," "medium," "slims," and "superslims." Because lung cancer risk is related to years of smoking and to the frequency and depth of inhalation,[18,19] those people who switch to buying allegedly less hazardous cigarette brands often smoke more and inhale more deeply to attain the satisfied level of nicotine.

Tragically, while smoking rates have declined by an average of 0.5% per year over the past 10 years, and while the incidence of lung cancer among black and white men has leveled off, the incidence of lung cancer continues to rise at a rate of 5% per year among women. Moreover, early detection hardly improves survival; the 5-year survival rate has remained at less than 10% since the 1960s.[9] Although there is a gradual

TABLE 20-22. Summary of Smoking and Cancer Mortality

Type of Cancer	Gender	Relative Risk Among Smokers		Mortality Attributable to Smoking	
		Current*	Former*	Percentage*	Number†
Lung	Male	22.4	9.4	90	82,800
	Female	11.9	4.7	79	40,300
Larynx	Male	10.5	5.2	81	2400
	Female	17.8	11.9	87	700
Oral cavity	Male	27.5	8.8	92	4900
	Female	5.6	2.9	61	1800
Esophagus	Male	7.6	5.8	78	5700
	Female	10.3	3.2	75	1900
Pancreas	Male	2.1	1.1	29	3500
	Female	2.3	1.8	34	4500
Bladder	Male	2.9	1.9	47	3000
	Female	2.6	1.9	37	1200
Kidney	Male	3.0	2.0	48	3000
	Female	1.4	1.2	12	500
Stomach	Male	1.5	?	17‡	1400
	Female	1.5	?	25	1300
Leukemia	Male	2.0§	?	20§	2000
	Female	2.0	?	20	1600
Cervix		2.1	1.9	31‡	1400
Endometrium		0.7	1.0	—	—

* Except as noted, data from The Health Consequences of Smoking; A Report of the Surgeon General, 1982,[7] 1989,[11] 1990.[20]
† Data based on Boring et al, 1991.[43]
‡ Data from Centers for Disease Control, MMWR, 1991.[79]
§ Data from Mills et al, 1990,[94] and Severson, 1987.[50]

decrease in risk for death from lung cancer after cessation of cigarette smoking, this message is perceived by many of those who smoke to mean that the risk for developing lung cancer will diminish immediately on quitting. This misunderstanding may lead to postponement of cessation in the belief that it does not matter when one stops. Although a diminished risk for lung cancer is experienced among former smokers after 5 years of cessation, the risk among former smokers remains higher than that of nonsmokers for as long as 25 years.[20] Any early reduction of health risk after cessation applies only to heart disease,[20] whereby a decline in risk for heart problems appears to occur within 1 year of cessation; even then, the remaining decline in excess risk for heart disease is more gradual, approaching those of persons who have never smoked only after many years of smoking abstinence.[16]

When people who smoke are exposed to other carcinogens at the workplace (*e.g.*, pipefitters and asbestos and uranium miners and radon), their risk for lung cancer is dramatically higher than those who do not smoke; moreover, the combined effects of smoking and occupational exposure to carcinogens is greater than the risk for either alone.[20a,20b,31]

LARYNGEAL CANCER

Cigarette smoking is the major cause of cancer of the larynx.[7,21] The 3650 deaths from laryngeal cancer in 1991 in the United States constituted 1% of all deaths from cancer.

Approximately 82% of the 12,500 new cases of laryngeal cancer diagnosed in 1991 were directly attributable to cigarette smoking. In three of the six major prospective studies that have investigated the relation between smoking and cancer of the larynx,[7,21-26] mortality ratios could not be calculated because all of the deaths from laryngeal cancer occurred in people who had smoked cigarettes.[21] Overall, deaths from cancer of the larynx were found to have occurred at a rate 6 to 13 times greater among persons who smoked cigarettes compared with nonsmokers. A similar risk for cancer of the larynx has been found among those people who smoke cigars or pipes;[27] because 80% of new cases of laryngeal cancer occur in men, it is essential to explode the myth that switching to a pipe or cigar conveys a reduced risk for cancer.

Williams and Horn[28] reported a strong dose-response relation between the number of cigarettes smoked per day and the risk for developing cancer of the larynx; other reports have confirmed that people who smoke more than 25 cigarettes a day have cancer mortality ratios 20 to 30 times greater than those who do not smoke.[7,21] There appears to be a synergistic effect between smoking and drinking, possibly as the result of alcohol acting as a solvent of carcinogens in tobacco smoke or as the result of an alteration in liver metabolism.[29] The risk for developing cancer of the larynx is as much as 75% higher in people who use tobacco and alcohol compared with people with exposure to either substance alone.[21,29] One study describes a typical patient with cancer of the larynx as a 50- to 60-year-old man who smoked cigarettes and was a moderate-to-heavy alcohol drinker.[30]

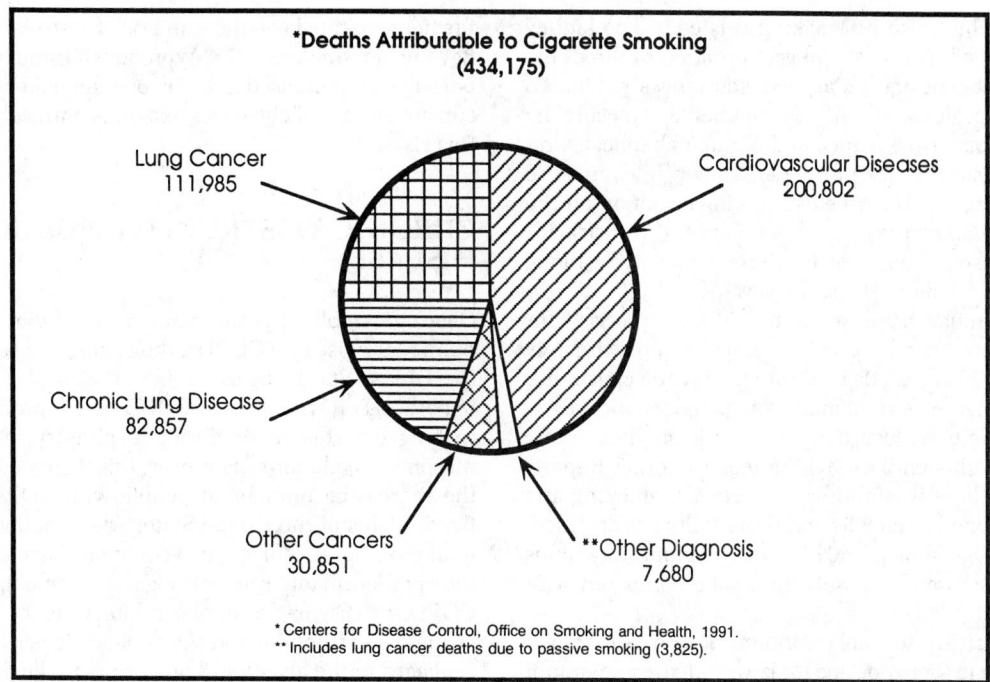

*Deaths Attributable to Cigarette Smoking
(434,175)

Lung Cancer
111,985

Cardiovascular Diseases
200,802

Chronic Lung Disease
82,857

Other Cancers
30,851

**Other Diagnosis
7,680

* Centers for Disease Control, Office on Smoking and Health, 1991.
** Includes lung cancer deaths due to passive smoking (3,825).

ORAL CANCER

There is a dose-response relation between the number of cigarettes smoked per day and cancers of the lip, tongue, salivary gland, floor of the mouth, mesopharynx, and hypopharynx.[7] The use of pipes, cigars, and spitting tobacco in its various forms (plug tobacco, loose leaf tobacco, twist tobacco, and moist snuff) is also associated with the development of cancers of the oral cavity; the risk of using these forms is of the same magnitude as that of using cigarettes.[7,21,32] Tobacco use is responsible for more than 90% of tumors of the oral cavity among men and 60% among women.[11]

There is a 27-fold increase in the rate of oral cancer among men who smoke cigarettes, pipes, or cigars and a sixfold increase among women who smoke.[11] Spitting tobacco is a significant cause of leukoplakia,[32–35] an abnormal thickening and keratinization of the oral mucosa that is recognized as a precursor of malignancy. The combination of alcohol and tobacco use produces an increase in risk for cancer of the oral cavity on a dose-related basis.[36]

ESOPHAGEAL CANCER

Prospective and retrospective epidemiologic studies have demonstrated that cigarette smoking is the major cause of cancer of the esophagus in men and women.[7,21] More than 15,000 Americans die each year from carcinoma of the esophagus (including a disproportionate number of blacks), 80% of which are attributable to smoking.[11] Death rates for esophageal cancer are as much as ten times greater among persons who smoke cigarettes, cigars, or pipes compared with those who do not.[27] As with laryngeal and oral cancer, alcohol consumption acts synergistically with smoking to increase by 25% to 50% the risk for developing esophageal cancer.[28,37,38]

In explaining a mechanism for tobacco-induced esophageal

cancer, Newcomb and Carbone note that carcinogens from tobacco smoke have extensive contact with the esophagus because they are swallowed after condensing on the mucous membranes of the mouth and pharynx and as mucus is cleared from the lungs.[39]

CANCER OF THE UTERINE CERVIX AND OVARY

Recent evidence has strengthened the association between cigarette smoking and cancer of the uterine cervix.[7,40–42] As many as one third of the 12,000 new cases of cervical cancer in the United States each year are attributable to cigarette smoking.[43] Women who smoke cigarettes have four times the risk of nonsmokers for developing cervical cancer.[42] The finding of nicotine and cotinine in the cervical secretions of cigarette smokers and of the mutagenic activity of these constituents of tobacco smoke in the cervical mucus further supports the epidemiologic findings.[44,45] It is hypothesized that these carcinogenic metabolites may interact with human papilloma viruses.[46]

OTHER CANCERS

A relation between smoking and bladder cancer was noted in the 1964 Surgeon General's Report.[2] The 1982 Surgeon General's Report concluded that cigarette smoking is a contributing factor for bladder and kidney cancer. In 1992, researchers at the National Cancer Institute (NCI) reported the results of a large population-based case-control study of cancer of the renal pelvis and ureter that confirms that cigarette smoking is the major cause of these tumors.[47] Forty percent of bladder cancers (or more than 4000 new cases in the United States each year) and kidney cancers (more than 3600 cases) currently are believed to be smoking related.[11] The kidney and bladder are subject to the longest duration of direct exposure to carcinogens and radioactive substances in tobacco smoke of any organ system.[48] Occupational exposure by smokers to various dyes, paints, and organic chemicals dramatically increases the risk of bladder cancer. In contrast to the beneficial effects over time of smoking cessation on the incidence of all other tobacco-related cancers, the risk for genitourinary cancer appears to remain elevated among former smokers for more than 15 years.[48,49]

People who smoke have two to three times the risk for pancreatic cancer that nonsmokers have[11]; approximately 30% of the 25,000 annual deaths from pancreatic cancer are attributable to cigarette smoking.[7] This pathogenetic mechanism may relate to exposure to tobacco metabolites in bile acids or blood. Although the 1964 Surgeon General's Report[2] concluded that there was no relation between smoking and stomach cancer, and although overall mortality has declined, recent evidence has shown a 50% increase in mortality ratios from this disease among those who smoke compared with those who do not.[7]

The fact that cigarette smoke contains at least two known causes of leukemia (benzene and ionizing radiation polonium 210) may explain the epidemiologic association between smoking and lymphoid and myeloid leukemia.[7] Currently, 20% to 30% of cases of leukemia are attributable to smoking.[50,50a]

Although there appears to be no relation between smoking and cancers of the colon and rectum, cancers of the liver, anus, penis, and vulva are commoner in persons who smoke than in those who do not.[39] An antiestrogenic effect of tobacco smoke is believed to explain the 30% less frequent occurrence of cancer of the uterine endometrium among postmenopausal women who smoke compared with those who do not;[51] in contrast, a 75% increased risk for breast cancer has been found among women who smoke heavily and who began smoking at a young age.[40]

CORONARY HEART DISEASE

Cigarette smoking is a primary risk factor for coronary heart disease (CHD). Overall, persons who smoke have a 70% greater CHD death rate, a twofold to fourfold greater incidence of CHD, and a twofold to fourfold greater risk for sudden death than nonsmokers.[52] Although women experience lower CHD rates than men, cigarette smoking is a major determinant of CHD in women.[53] Cigarette smoking is associated with coronary artery disease and aortic atherosclerosis.[52] In addition to such chronic conditions, cigarette smoking exerts acute effects, including coronary artery spasm, increased platelet aggregation, and a decreased ventricular fibrillation threshold.[52,54,55] The risk for myocardial infarction is proportional to the number of cigarettes smoked.[52]

CEREBROVASCULAR DISEASE

Stroke is the third leading cause of death in the United States.[11] The risk for stroke increases with the number of cigarettes smoked and declines after cessation of smoking; in 5 years former smokers have the same risk for stroke as persons who have never smoked.[20,52,56] Women who smoke cigarettes experience an increased risk for subarachnoid hemorrhage; the concurrent use of cigarettes and oral contraceptives magnifies this risk.[52]

CHRONIC OBSTRUCTIVE PULMONARY DISEASE

Cigarette smoking is the main cause of chronic obstructive pulmonary disease (COPD), the leading cause of disability in the United States. In the 1960s, the most widely advanced hypothesis on the cause of COPD linked progressive decline in lung function to recurrent respiratory infection and atmospheric pollution.[57] However, this theory could not explain the increasing number of people with COPD living in the Great Plains of the United States where pollution was a minimal risk. Epidemiologic investigations have since confirmed the predominant role of cigarette smoking in causing COPD.[11,58] Cigarette smoke inhibits ciliary activity of the bronchial epithelium and the phagocytic activity of the macrophages in the alveoli.[57] This results in the decreased clearance of foreign material and bacteria from the lung, which leads to increased infection, tissue destruction, and decreased lung function.

WOMEN AND SMOKING

In 1964, at the time of the first Surgeon General's Report discussing the smoking epidemic, lung cancer was the leading cause of death due to cancer in men and the fifth leading cause of cancer mortality among women.[2] This difference in lung cancer mortality rates can be explained by the fact that until the 1920s, it was socially unacceptable—and in some states illegal—for women to smoke.[58a] Men had taken up cigarette smoking in large numbers toward the end of the 19th century—in part because antispitting ordinances to curtail the spread of tuberculosis had led the tobacco companies to switch from the promotion of chewing tobacco and cigars to the inhalation of tobacco smoke by means of the cigarette. Smoking did not take hold among women until the 1920s when the American Tobacco Company began a mass media advertising campaign with the slogan, "To keep a slender figure, reach for a Lucky Strike instead of a sweet." At that time women did not smoke as many cigarettes or take as many puffs per cigarette as men.[58b] The appearance by motion picture heroines, athletes, and socialites in cigarette advertisements in the 1930s led to an increase in smoking among women so that by World War II a third of American women were smoking.

In 1968 cigarette maker Philip Morris began to associate smoking with the women's liberation movement by launching its Virginia Slims brand on a massive scale in the broadcast and print media with the slogan, "You've come a long way, baby." The brand name also underscored the constant pressure on women to be thin. When overt cigarette advertising was no longer permitted on television in 1971, the company created the Virginia Slims Tennis Circuit, telecasts of which circumvent the tobacco advertising ban by featuring players as young as 14 amid dozens of courtside billboards for Virginia Slims.

In 1981, in an article in an advertising journal headlined, "Women top cigarette target," the chief executive officer of R. J. Reynolds described the women's market as "probably the largest opportunity" for the tobacco company.[59] Currently, women continue to be a primary target for cigarette advertisers.

Smoking rates among less educated young women are increasing, as is the amount they smoke.[11] In 1990, the marketing plan for a new brand of R. J. Reynolds cigarettes, Dakota, identified a specific target: "virile females" ages 18 to 20 who have no education beyond high school and who aspire "to have fun with [their] boyfriends and partying."[60] Other "female" brands include Eve (Liggett), Style (Loews), Satin (Loews), Capri (BAT), More (R. J. Reynolds), and Misty (American Tobacco). The manufacturers sponsor a host of activities, including fashion shows, art exhibitions, and family reunions and offer T-shirts, diaries, and fashion accessories free of charge or in exchange for proof of purchase.

Such promotional efforts have undermined all efforts to educate young women about the adverse effects of cigarette smoking. The emphasis of public health campaigns on the dangers of smoking has failed to address the ubiquitous, sophisticated, and carefree appeal of tobacco advertising. Currently, lung cancer has surpassed breast cancer as the leading cause of cancer deaths among women,[11] a fact that is virtually unreported in women's magazines, of which only a handful do not accept tobacco advertising. The issue receives scant coverage on television, probably due to the advertising clout of the subsidiaries of tobacco conglomerates.

Cigarette smoking results in other problems for women, especially during pregnancy. There is a confirmed association between maternal smoking and low-birth-weight infants, and there is an increased incidence of premature birth, spontaneous abortion, stillbirth, and neonatal death.[61]

Although there has been a dramatic decline in smoking among physicians, medical students, and most other health professionals during the past several decades, smoking among nurses has not declined. Jacobson attributes this to anger by nurses at their subordination within a health service dependent on women but controlled by men.[62]

ETHNIC MINORITIES

Black and Hispanic Americans have the highest rates of lung cancer and cardiovascular disease in the United States.[63] The disproportionately high rates of smoking-related diseases among ethnic minorities can be attributed to the successful marketing of tobacco products to minority communities.[64] Billboards advertising cigarettes appear four to five times more often in inner city neighborhoods than in middle class suburbs.[65] Tobacco and alcohol constitute as much as 80% to 90% of the products advertised on billboards in inner city areas. Cigarette advertising in black and Hispanic magazines and newspapers represents a major source of revenue for these publications.[64,66,67] In more than 40 years of publication, the leading black-oriented magazine, *Ebony*, has carried few articles on smoking; not surprisingly, cigarette companies are a leading source of revenue. Major black and Hispanic civic

organizations, such as the National Association for the Advancement of Colored People, the Urban League, the United Negro College Fund, and La Raza, receive funding from tobacco companies; an exception is the National Coalition of Hispanic Health and Human Services Organizations.

The result of such successful marketing targeted to ethnic minorities is a higher rate of smoking among blacks[68] and an increase in smoking among Hispanic women.[69,70] Recent data from the 1987 National Health Interview Survey reveals that 32.9% of blacks smoke compared with 25% among the white middle class population.[69] Little if any change can be expected in smoking-related mortality among blacks and Hispanics, given the paucity of mass media efforts to counter tobacco use and promotion.

"LESS HAZARDOUS" CIGARETTES

In the 1950s, confronted with declining cigarette sales after the publication of studies linking smoking to lung cancer, tobacco companies began producing filter-tipped brands that were claimed to remove certain components of smoke, which manufacturers have never acknowledged to be harmful.[15] Brown & Williamson purchased advertising space in the Medicine section of *Time* to claim that Viceroy cigarettes offered "double-barrel health protection" and advertisements for Liggett & Myers' filter L & Ms claimed they were "Just what the doctor ordered." Until the 1960s tobacco companies promoted cigarettes at meetings of the AMA and other health organizations by means of scientific exhibits that sought to demonstrate the alleged benefits of one brand over another. Consumer demand soared. Currently, 97% of those who smoke buy filtered brands.

In the 1960s, to allay public anxiety about cancer after the publication of the first Surgeon General's Report on Smoking and Health, tobacco companies began marketing brands with purportedly lower levels of "tar" and nicotine. Throughout the 1970s the ACS, the NCI, and most major health organizations promoted the concept of a safer cigarette in the belief that most people who smoke cannot stop.[15] Persons who switch to allegedly low-tar cigarettes have been found to employ compensatory smoking, whereby they inhale more frequently

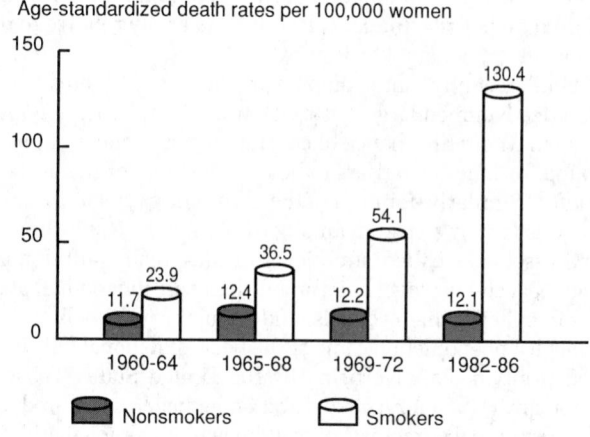

Age-standardized death rates per 100,000 women

Source: Cancer Prevention Studies I and II, American Cancer Society

and more deeply to maintain a satisfied level of nicotine.[14,15,71,72] More simply, "low tar" can be translated as "low poison."[73] Tar is a composite of more than 4000 separate solid poisons, including at least 43 known carcinogens.[11,71] Cigarettes with reduced yields of tar, nicotine, and carbon monoxide are not safer. A recommendation to switch to such brands is misguided.

Not until 1980 did the NCI drop its research effort to develop a less hazardous cigarette, choosing instead to concentrate on efforts to educate heavy smokers to stop.[74]

SPITTING TOBACCO

Snuff-dipping, the practice of placing a pinch of powdered flavored tobacco in the cavity between gum and cheek and sucking on the "quid," has increased dramatically among adolescents in the past 20 years. The consumption of chewing tobacco, the use of which involves a "chaw" that is held in the inner cheek area, has also increased.[75] Both forms of tobacco require continual expectoration, hence the term *spitting tobacco*. The manufacturers of these products prefer the term *smokeless tobacco*, implying that it is a safe alternative to smoking. After the publication in 1964 of the Surgeon General's Report on Smoking and Health, sales of spitting tobacco began to increase.[2] Between 1960 and 1970 sales of snuff and chewing tobacco increased 25% and between 1970 and 1980 sales doubled again. Connolly estimates that there are 16 million users of these products in the United States alone, of whom 3 million are younger than the age of 16.[76]

Snuff can appreciably accelerate a litany of destructive changes, including gingival recession, tooth abrasion, and periodontal bone destruction. Leukoplakia (also called *snuff-dipper's keratosis*), a nonspecific white patch involving the epithelium of the oral mucosa, is most often attributed to the use of tobacco and is found in 18% to 64% of users.[76] About 1 in 20 cases of leukoplakia will undergo malignant transformation into an epidermoid carcinoma. *N*-nitrosonornicotine, one of four tobacco-specific nitrosamines that have been isolated from snuff, has been shown to be tumorigenic in experimental animals.[75] Snuff has been found to contain other potent carcinogens, including polycyclic aromatic hydrocarbons and radiation-emitting polonium.

In India, where there is widespread chewing of betel nut and tobacco in combination, Jayant and colleagues found a sixfold higher risk for cancer of the oral cavity relative to the nonchewer, nonsmoker.[77]

Until recently, snuff dipping in the United States was a practice confined largely to black women in the rural Southeast, in whom the chance of contracting oral cancer has been found for long-term users to be 50 times that of nonusers of snuff.[78] Similarly, for most of the 20th century, tobacco chewing was largely a custom among rural men. In 1980 Christen and associates called attention to widespread snuff-dipping and tobacco-chewing habits among baseball and football players in colleges, high schools, and elementary schools.[79]

Such a phenomenon came at the heels of national television and print media advertising by the United States Tobacco Company (UST) for its Skoal and Copenhagen snuff products that featured testimonials of well-known professional athletes and country music performers. A pioneer in the practice of offering free samples of snuff by mail and at concerts and sporting events, UST boasted in a tobacco trade journal in 1984 that its advertisements in such publications as *The National Enquirer, Playboy, Sports Illustrated,* and *The New York Times Magazine* generated 400,000 written requests for samples in just 3 months.[80] Although television advertising for spitting-tobacco products was prohibited by the Comprehensive Smokeless Tobacco and Education Act of 1986, the promotion of these products on television has continued virtually unabated in the form of sponsored sporting events. In 1991, the Federal Trade Commission acted to limit the violations of the law by the Pinkerton Tobacco Company, sponsors of the televised "Red Man Chew Tractor Pulling Series," but it remains to be seen if other companies' brand names, such as UST's Skoal, equally visible in televised auto racing and rodeo, will disappear from the airwaves. (The Justice Department, which is entrusted with enforcement of the law that since 1971 has prohibited cigarette advertising on television, has never challenged the ubiquitous presence of tobacco promotion in sports on television; in contrast, the Federal government in Australia, following the lead of the states of Victoria and New South Wales, banned tobacco sponsorship of sports in 1992.)

Efforts of Connolly[76] and others have led to a ban on spitting tobacco in New Zealand (1987), Ireland (1988), Hong Kong (1988), and Australia (1990). In 1991, the European Bureau for Action on Smoking Prevention successfully campaigned for a ban on these products in the European Economic Community.

INVOLUNTARY (PASSIVE) SMOKING

Two thirds of the smoke from a burning cigarette never reaches the smoker's lungs, but instead goes directly into the air.[81] The 1986 Report of the Surgeon General, dedicated to a discussion of involuntary or passive smoking, defined environmental tobacco smoke (ETS)—also called *secondhand smoke*—as the combination of sidestream smoke that is emitted into the air from a burning cigarette between puffs and the fraction of mainstream smoke that is exhaled by one who smokes.[81]

An increasing number of studies has explored the health risks of the nonsmoker who is exposed to ETS.[11,81,82] The toxic and carcinogenic effects of ETS are similar to those of tobacco smoke inhaled by active smokers. The National Research Council has estimated that ETS is responsible for as many as 6000 lung cancer deaths among nonsmokers per year.[82]

At least 14 studies have demonstrated a risk of lung cancer in nonsmoking wives exposed to the secondhand smoke of their husbands.[9] Passive smoking has been found to increase the risk of leukemia, lymphoma, and cancer of the breast and uterine cervix.[8,42]

The risks of passive smoking extend beyond cancer. It is estimated that tobacco smoke in the home and workplace could be responsible for the deaths of 46,000 nonsmokers annually in the United States.[31,82a,82b] Most of these (32,000) are due to heart disease, making passive smoking the third leading preventable cause of death after smoking and the consumption of alcohol. Additionally, children of parents who smoke have an increased incidence of cough, bronchitis, otitis media, and pneumonia.[11] Children exposed to their parents' cigarette smoke have six times the average number of respiratory infections.[9]

EFFORTS TO CURTAIL TOBACCO USE

Although there is hardly a child or adult who has not heard that smoking is dangerous to health, the prevalence of smoking has declined by only 0.5% per year in the United States during the past 10 years.[11] By repeatedly citing seemingly improving prevalence figures and mentioning the 40 million Americans who have stopped smoking since 1964, health agencies underemphasize the fact that the number of current smokers has remained virtually constant at more than 55 million. Women, blue-collar workers, and minority groups in general are not appreciably reducing their cigarette consumption, and smoking rates among adolescents appear to be approaching the rates found in adolescents in the mid-1970s.[83] Although physicians and other health professionals should be working to end the tobacco pandemic, comparatively few are taking concerted action.[9,16,84,85] One obstacle is complacency stemming from the belief by some health professionals and some of the public that the war on smoking has been won.

The remaining discussion in this chapter concerns the challenge to health care professionals to reexamine their approaches, their attitudes, and their vocabulary and to begin looking at the tobacco problem as much in terms of promoting a consumerist message of not *buying* cigarettes as in terms of promulgating a health behavior of not smoking. Such a view may lead to a better understanding of why tobacco advertising has been more successful than health education and why the tobacco companies could be considered among the leading health educators.

INITIAL EFFORTS: PUBLIC INFORMATION AND SMOKING CESSATION

In the late 19th century and early 20th century, the crusading efforts of people such as Lucy Page Gaston led to the enactment of numerous laws prohibiting smoking in public places. Much of this success was undone by efforts on college campuses to portray smoking as a symbol of women's emancipation and by medical societies that raised money to send cartons of cigarettes to the soldiers during World War I. Although the impact of publicity that surrounded the release of the Surgeon General's Report in 1964 was demonstrated by an increased awareness of smoking-related health risks, this short-term dissemination of information did little to solve the problem.[16] Although programs emerged to help adults in their efforts to stop smoking, comparatively few resources have been devoted to primary prevention. The longstanding focus of tobacco control activities on cessation assumes that the major determinants of smoking behavior are within the individual person; the propaganda that promotes the initiation of tobacco use and helps perpetuate it has been ignored largely by government health agencies and researchers.

Approximately 300 cessation methods have been reported in the literature.[86] Popular techniques in the 1960s and 1970s included 5-day plans, group therapy, hypnosis, conditioning-

based approaches such as rapid smoking and satiation, self-help manuals, special filters, and over-the-counter pharmaceutical products containing either nicotine analogs or aversive chemicals. Approaches that were popularized in the 1980s included acupuncture, nicotine chewing gum, and physician counseling. In 1992, the introduction of transdermal nicotine patches through extensive promotional efforts aimed at pharmacists, physicians, and the lay public has created intense interest in smoking cessation. As with previous pharmacologic aids, the great expectations for the patch are unlikely to be fulfilled.

"Quit clinics" have been developed in the past 10 years by the ACS (FreshStart Program) and the American Lung Association (Freedom From Smoking) designed to be implemented in small-group sessions to help participants understand why people smoke, to handle withdrawal symptoms, and to manage stress. Such methods focus on cognitive and behavioral approaches, mostly neglecting attitudinal objectives.

In 1982, the NCI initiated its Smoking, Tobacco, and Cancer Program (STCP) as part of a restructuring of its cancer control activities. Out of the STCP, the NCI developed the Community Intervention Trial for Smoking Cessation (COMMIT), the largest smoking intervention trial in the world. The project, which includes 11 pairs of matched communities (one community in each pair serves as the intervention site and one as the control site), focuses on interventions primarily among heavy smokers. Changes in community smoking prevalence rates are being monitored throughout the trial.

More recently, the NCI (with logistic support from the ACS) has embarked on a major tobacco control project called the *American Stop Smoking Intervention Study for Cancer Prevention* (ASSIST). The project, which provides funds to the health departments in 17 states, began in 1991 and concludes in 1998. Each of the 17 funded states has assembled a coalition to disseminate materials through specific channels of intervention, including health care agencies, worksites, schools, media, and community networks. The ambitious goal of this $120 million project is to assist the NCI in achieving its goal of reducing cancer mortality rates by 50% by the end of the century. Because the tobacco industry will spend more than $28 billion on advertising and promotion during the years of ASSIST, critics decry this goal as overly optimistic.

Although 1.5 million Americans stop smoking each year, a similar number of adolescents begin smoking. At the same time, tobacco companies have maintained and increased efforts to promote smoking. Their appeals to freedom, wealth, glamour, manliness, athletic prowess, and sexual attractiveness undermine public health efforts.

Smoking cessation programs for the individual person cannot truly succeed in the absence of both workplace smoking bans and multimedia counter-advertising strategies that weaken the influence of the tobacco industry and reinforce the physician's office-based efforts.

Although cigarette smoking becomes an addiction, it is first a learned behavior. The "peer pressure" cited by tobacco companies as the reason for adolescent smoking is as much a manufactured product as the cigarette. The purpose of advertising is to sell cigarettes, to promote and reinforce the social acceptability of smoking, and to encourage complacency toward the enormous social and health toll taken by smoking-caused diseases. Cigarette manufacturers spend more money annually to promote smoking than is spent to advertise any other consumer product, including automobiles and food. More money is spent in 1 day in the United States to advertise cigarettes—$10 million—than the entire annual budget of the Office on Smoking and Health.

A CONSUMERIST APPROACH TO SMOKING CESSATION

Ideally, the validity of the success rate of a smoking cessation method should rest on the results of a controlled, double-blind study for which there is a follow-up of at least 6 months' duration of all participating subjects.[86,87] Few published outcome evaluations meet such criteria. Despite insufficient evidence to back up advertised claims, expensive commercial aids and clinics for smoking cessation proliferate. Many methods are costly, but having to pay a high fee for an alleged smoking cure may be the most motivating aspect of the method's success.

The physician's active involvement in smoking cessation, akin to his or her role in the prevention of smoking among adolescents and children, can be extremely crucial. More than 10 years ago, at a time when efforts to discourage smoking were much less widespread and accepted, Russell and colleagues found that 1 or 2 minutes of simple but unequivocal advice to stop smoking on the part of the physician resulted in a cessation rate of more than 5% measured at 1 year compared with 0.3% in the control group.[88]

Although many people say they have stopped on their own, such persons may not consciously attribute their success to the increasing social pressures that reinforced their decision. Not only has organized medicine become united in the past few years on the need for more assertive office-based and community-wide strategies to end smoking, but other forces in society, including large corporations and governmental agencies, have implemented smoke-free policies.

OFFICE-BASED STRATEGIES

Many factors may inhibit physician involvement in smoking cessation, such as time constraints, the lack of reimbursement by third-party payers for such counseling, and the absence of peer group reinforcement in a technologically oriented, tertiary care-centered health care system.

There is much the physician can do to become a better teacher about smoking in lieu of relegating this role to ancillary personnel, a smoking cessation clinic, or a pamphlet. The physician can develop an innovative strategy beginning outside the office or building. A bus bench, billboard, or sign in the parking lot with a straightforward or humorous health promotion message helps establish a thought-provoking and favorable image.

Magazines with cigarette advertisements should not appear in the physician's office in the absence of prominent stickers or rubber-stamped messages calling patients' attention to the deceptive, often absurd nature of such ads. Although responsibility for the office-based smoking cessation strategy should rest with the physician, it is invaluable to include all office staff as positive reinforcers for patients. Labeling each chart with a small no-smoking sticker to indicate the need for such

reinforcement may be helpful, although care must be taken to avoid stigmatizing the patient as a "smoker."

The key to successful smoking cessation efforts is a positive approach. A discussion about the diseases caused by smoking and the harmful constituents of tobacco smoke is essential—the physician would do well to impart, through graphic posters, pamphlets, slides, and other audiovisual aids, the gruesome consequences of smoking—but the benefits of not smoking must be emphasized as strongly. Educating patients about the facts of smoking in a single office visit is unlikely to result in behavioral change.

Through the use of creative analogies related to the patient's occupation, hobbies, or romantic interest, the physician can succeed in changing the patient's attitude toward smoking. For example, naming a partial list of the poisons and irritants in tobacco smoke, such as hydrocyanic acid (cyanide), ammonia, formaldehyde, and carbon monoxide, may mean little at first. By noting that cyanide is the substance used in the gas chamber in executions, that formaldehyde is used to preserve cadavers, and that ammonia is the predominant smell in urine, the physician is likely to make the patient think differently about cigarettes.

METAPHORS THAT MOTIVATE

A change in vocabulary on the part of the physician is essential for making progress in office-based smoking cessation. Instead of *pack-year history,* a more relevant term is the *inhalation count.* A pack-a-day smoking patient will breathe as many as 1 million doses of cyanide, ammonia, carcinogens, and carbon monoxide in less than 15 years, not including the inhalation of other peoples' smoke. Another way to emphasize the enormous amount smoked is to state the amount smoked in financial terms: a pack-a-day cigarette buyer will spend in excess of $800 a year (calculated at $2.25 a pack)—or in excess of $10,000 in 10 years if that money were put into a savings account or bond.

Although patient education and smoking cessation rest on the knowledge of the deleterious aspects of adverse health behavior, the cognitive component alone is insufficient. Both the physician and the patient must be motivated to succeed. Three keys to office-based smoking cessation are to *personalize, individualize,* and *demythologize.*

The physician can learn to personalize approaches to smoking cessation by carefully screening existing pamphlets and other audiovisual aids or by producing one's own handout. It is essential to scrutinize all such material, as one would with a new drug or medical device. Personally handing a brochure to the patient while pointing out and underlining certain passages or illustrations provides an important reinforcing message. The pamphlets, posters, and signs should be changed or otherwise updated every few weeks or months.

Individualizing the message to the patient is the cornerstone of success in patient education. The same cigarette counseling method cannot be used for a high school student, a construction worker, and an executive already showing signs or symptoms of heart disease. In the case of a high-school student, the physician should focus not only on such topics as emphysema and lung cancer, but also should emphasize the cosmetic unattractiveness of yellow teeth, bad breath, the loss of athletic ability, and the financial drain that results from buying cigarettes. To the construction worker, the physician might suggest the likelihood of fewer lost paydays, greater physical strength, and a greater ability to work if he or she should stop smoking.

In talking with the concerned executive, one should de-mythologize certain beliefs about smoking, such as that the ultra-low-tar cigarettes being smoked are safe. To the contrary, use of so-called low-tar brands may result in compensatory deeper inhalation of greater concentrations of chemical additives and noxious gases that increase the risk for heart attack.

DEBUNKING COMMON MYTHS

An important myth surrounding smoking is that it relieves stress. This idea can be debunked by pointing out that the stress that is relieved is that which resulted from being dependent on nicotine—this is the essence of addiction. At the same time, deep breathing has a relaxing effect. The physician can suggest that the patient try to postpone for 5 minutes every time he or she intends to light up, then inhale deeply for 5 minutes, then reconsider whether the cigarette is important.

Another myth reinforced in advertisements for Virginia Slims and other cigarettes aimed at women and girls is that smoking keeps weight off. One need not gain weight on stopping smoking if one will relearn to enjoy walking and running as much as one relearns the taste of food. By no means will all persons who stop smoking gain weight. Even among those who do, the average weight gain is less than 5 lb.[89]

Perhaps the biggest myth that has been encouraged in the medical literature is that the patient must be "ready to quit." Although common sense dictates that those who express a greater interest in smoking cessation will have a greater success rate, those patients who do not express an interest in smoking cessation symbolize the overall challenge to be faced in curing the pandemic. One of the reasons for the lack of motivation of patients may be their sense of inevitability of failure. It is conceivable that by not educating the nonmotivated smoking patient, the physician is reinforcing the notion that it may be too difficult to stop smoking.

Setting a quit date, the essential element of the smoking cessation literature, may rationalize the continuation of an adverse health practice and may strengthen denial. It is helpful to remind patients that they can stop now. If they do not stop, this does not mean the physician will not treat them the next time, but it is important to give encouragement and not reinforce excuses. It is helpful to give patients a few written reminders such as lists of the advantages and disadvantages of smoking, a set of rewards for not smoking and penalties for lighting up, the situations and environmental influences that encourage one to smoke, and the myths of smoking and smoking cessation. A prescription with a no-smoking symbol signed by the physician and included with the other prescriptions is a thoughtful gesture. The physician should not advise "cutting down," switching to a low-tar cigarette, or changing to a pipe or cigar.

CONSUMER ADVOCACY ROLE

Traditional office-based approaches begin by asking, "Do you smoke?" "How much do you smoke?" and "When did you start smoking?" Although this may provide the physician with relevant data for charting purposes, this approach is too often a signal for the patient to become defensive and resistant to further discussion, especially if the patient had no intention to stop smoking. There are alternative ways of obtaining information and at the same time piquing the patient's interest in the subject. By using and identifying with the vocabulary used by the consumer of cigarettes, the physician can adopt (and be perceived in) the role of consumer advocate as opposed to medical finger-wagger. The most important and nonthreatening questions to ask are, "What brand do you buy?" and "How much do you spend on cigarettes?" The patient is likely to be surprised and intrigued by these questions, which can be asked at any time in the course of the interview, because they appear to be nonjudgmental. They serve to suggest that the physician is not a know-it-all and a polemist. A question about the cost of cigarettes shows concern for the patient's financial well-being.

Promotions for various pharmacologic agents, mail order gadgets, and clinics in smoking cessation reinforce the notion that cigarette smoking is primarily a medical problem with a simple, easy to prescribe for, nonindividualized solution. When a patient requests a "drug that will help me stop smoking," the physician must confront the dilemma of not wanting to dash the patient's expectation while emphasizing that a drug or device is, at best, an adjunct and not a means of smoking cessation.

It is an unfortunate fact that many patients will not stop smoking until they have gone to a smoking cessation clinic.

APPROACH TO ADOLESCENTS

Children and adolescents who smoke cigarettes pose a special challenge, because they represent the market most carefully nurtured by tobacco advertisers. It is essential to avoid emphasizing the adult and dangerous nature of smoking. Smoking should be referred to as the self-decepting and short-sighted practice that it is. The single most important statement the physician can make to an adolescent is, "Come on, you're too old to smoke. That's for 11- and 12-year-old children who are trying to look grown up." Another strategy is for the physician to ask the adolescent who smokes to help think of ideas for talking to junior high school and primary school students who are just taking up smoking.

As a general rule in approaching the subject of smoking cessation with a patient, time and commitment on the part of the physician will result in greater success. The biggest obstacle to smoking cessation is complacency on the part of the physician.

ENDING THE TOBACCO PANDEMIC

In 1977, a physician-based organization, DOC,* was founded to educate the public, especially young people, about the major preventable causes of poor health and high medical costs. Its primary goal is to tap the highest possible level of commitment from every physician, resident, and medical student in ending the tobacco pandemic.

For more information about DOC and its programs, write to DOC, c/o Department of Family Medicine, Baylor College of Medicine, 5510 Greenbriar, Houston, TX 77005.

TABLE 20–23. Thirteen Steps to End the Cigarette Pandemic

1. Paid mass media counteradvertising
2. Dedicated excise tax to purchase counteradvertising
3. Clean indoor air legislation
4. Removal of tax exemptions from tobacco advertisers
5. Advertising and promotion bans
6. School-based campaigns to engender ridicule toward tobacco companies and cigarette advertising
7. Lawsuits against tobacco advertisers by relatives of dead and dying smokers
8. Enforcement of existing financial penalties for violating 1969 Public Health Smoking Act ban on TV cigarette advertising: $10,000 per violation; enforcement of criminal conspiracy laws
9. Divestment of tobacco stocks by universities, hospitals, health groups, insurance companies, and teacher pension funds
10. Legislation to reduce adolescent access to tobacco through bans on vending machines, free samples
11. Worldwide coordination of efforts to curtail U.S. and U.K. cigarette exports and promotion
12. Agricultural changes to end tobacco subsidies and World Bank support of tobacco growing
13. Smoking cessation programs

DOC's unique, multilayered approach involves the creation of strategies for the clinic, the classroom, and the community (Table 20–23). Although there have been significant strides made by the NCI and the AMA during the 1980s to encourage greater involvement of physicians with tobacco control, most programs have underused physicians, physicians-in-training, and other health professionals.

To begin to realize a smoke-free society, physicians and other health care professionals must expand their vision beyond the stream of individual patients passing through their examining rooms to a concern for proactively and systematically dealing with the health needs of the larger community.

REFERENCES

1. Peto R. Report on smoking-attributable mortality. World Conference on Smoking or Health, Buenos Aires, Argentina, April 1992.
1a. Burney LE. Policy over politics: The first statement on smoking and health by the Surgeon General of the United States Public Health Service. NY State J Med 1983;83:1252–1253.
2. US Department of Health, Education, and Welfare. Smoking and health: Report of the Advisory Committee to the Surgeon General. Atlanta, GA: Centers for Disease Control (PHS) 1103, 1964.
3. Lombard HL, Doering CR. Cancer studies in Massachusetts: Habits, characteristics, and environment of individuals with and without cancer. N Engl J Med 1928;198:481–487.
4. Pearl R. Tobacco smoking and longevity. Science 1938;87:216–217.
4a. Doll R, Hill AB. Lung cancer and other causes of death in relation to smoking: Second report on mortality of British doctors. Br Med J 1956;2:1071–1081.
5. Ochsner A, DeBakey ME. Primary pulmonary malignancy: Treatment by total pneumonectomy: Analysis of 79 collected cases and presentation of 7 personal cases. Surg Gynecol Obstet 1939;68:435.
6. Hammond EL, Horn D. Smoking and death rates—Report on forty-four months of follow-up of 187,783 men. JAMA 1958;166:1294–1308.
6a. American Medical Association Committee for Research on Tobacco and Health. Tobacco and health. Chicago: American Medical Association Education and Research Foundation (AMA-REF), 1978.
7. US Department of Health and Human Services. The Health Consequences of Smoking: Cancer: A Report of the Surgeon General. Washington, DC: US Department of Health and Human Services, Public Health Service, Office on Smoking and Health. DHHS (PHS) 82-50179, 1982.
8. Redmond DE. Tobacco and cancer: The first clinical report, 1761. N Engl J Med 1970;282:18–23.
9. Rakel RE, Blum A. Nicotine addiction. In: Rakel RE, ed. Textbook of family practice. 4th ed. Philadelphia: WB Saunders, 1990:1612–1623.
10. Royal College of Physicians. Smoking and Health: Summary and Report of the Royal College of Physicians of London on smoking in relation to cancer of the lung and other diseases. New York: Pitman, 1962.
11. US Department of Health and Human Services. Reducing the health consequences of smoking—25 Years of Progress: A report of the Surgeon General. Washington, DC: US Department of Health and Human Services, Public Health Service, Centers for Disease Control, Office on Smoking and Health. DHHS (CDC) 89-8411, 1989.
12. Damber LA, Larsson LG. Smoking and lung cancer with special regard to type of smoking and type of cancer. Br J Cancer 1986;53:673.
13. Kaufman DW. Constituents of cigarette smoke and cardiovascular disease. NY State J Med 1983;83:1267–1268.
14. Rickert WS. "Less hazardous" cigarettes: Fact or fiction? NY State J Med 1983;83:1269–1272.
15. Miller GH. The "less hazardous" cigarette: A deadly delusion. NY State J Med 1985;85:313–317.
16. US Department of Health and Human Services. Strategies to control tobacco use in the United States: A blueprint for public health action in the 1990s. Washington, DC: US Department of Health and Human Services, National Cancer Institute. DHHS (NIH) 92-3316, 1991.
17. Blum A. When "more doctors smoked Camels": Cigarette advertising in the journal. NY State J Med 1983;83:1347–1352.
18. Lubin JH, Blot WJ, Berrino F, et al. Modifying risk of developing lung cancer by changing habits of cigarette smoking. Br Med J 1984;288:1953–1956.
19. Lubin JH, Blot WJ, Berrino F, et al. Patterns of lung cancer risk according to type of cigarette smoked. Int J Cancer 1984;3:569–576.
20. US Department of Health and Human Services. The health benefits of smoking cessation: A report of the Surgeon General. Washington, DC: US Department of Health and Human Services, Public Health Service, Centers for Disease Control, Office on Smoking and Health. DHHS (CDC) 90-8416, 1990.
20a. Berry G, Newhouse ML, Antonis P. Combined effect of asbestos and smoking on mortality from lung cancer and mesothelioma in factory workers. Br J Med 1985;42:12–18.
20b. Selikoff IJ, Seidman H, Hammond EC. Mortality effects of cigarette smoking among amosite asbestos factory workers. JNCI 1980;65:507–513.
21. US Department of Health, Education, and Welfare. Smoking and health: A report of the Surgeon General. Washington, DC: Public Health Service, Office of the Assistant Secretary for Health, Office on Smoking and Health. DHEW (PHS) 79-50066, 1979.
22. Doll R, Peto R. Mortality in relation to smoking: 20 years observation on male British doctors. Br Med J 1976;2:1525–1536.
23. Kahn HA. The Dorn study of smoking and mortality among U.S. veterans: Report on eight and one-half years of observation. In: Haenszel W, ed. Epidemiological approaches to the study of cancer and other chronic diseases. Washington, DC: National Cancer Institute Monograph No. 19, US Department of Health, Education, and Welfare, Public Health Service, National Cancer Institute, 1966:1–125.
24. Hammond EC. Smoking in relation to the death rates of one million men and women. In: Haenszel W, ed. Epidemiological approaches to the study of cancer and other chronic diseases. Washington, DC: National Cancer Institute Monograph No. 19, US Department of Health, Education, and Welfare, Public Health Service, National Cancer Institute, 1966:127–204.
25. Weir JM, Dunn JE. Smoking and mortality: A prospective study. Cancer 1970;25:105–112.
26. Hirayama T. Smoking in relation to the death rates of 265,118 men and women in Japan: A report on five years of follow-up. Clearwater Beach, FL, American Cancer Society's Fourteenth Science Writers' Seminar, March 24–29, 1972:1–4.
27. Cullen JW. Principles of cancer prevention: Tobacco. In: DeVita VT, Hellman S, Rosenberg S, ed. Cancer: Principles and practice of oncology. 3rd ed. Philadelphia: JB Lippincott 1989:181–195.
28. Williams RR, Horn JW. Association of cancer sites with tobacco and alcohol consumption and socioeconomic status of patients: Interview study from the Third National Cancer Survey. JNCI 1977;58:525–547.
29. Flanders WD, Rochman KJ. Interaction of alcohol and tobacco in laryngeal cancer. Am J Epidemiol 1982;115:371–379.
30. Marks RD, Putney FJ, Scruggs HJ, et al. Management of cancer of the larynx. J SC Med Assoc 1975;71:333–336.
31. US Department of Health and Human Services. The health consequences of smoking: Cancer and chronic lung disease in the workplace: A report of the Surgeon General. Washington, DC: US Department of Health and Human Services, Public Health Service, Centers for Disease Control, Office on Smoking and Health. DHHS (PHS) 85-50207, 1985.
32. US Department of Health and Human Services. The health consequences of using smokeless tobacco: A report of the Advisory Committee to the Surgeon General. Washington, DC: US Department of Health and Human Services, Public Health Service. NIH Publication No. 86-2874, 1986.
33. Banoczy J, Sugar L. Progressive and regressive changes in Hungarian oral leukoplakias in the course of longitudinal studies. Commun Dentist Oral Epidemiol 1975;3:194–197.
34. Roed-Petersen B, Banoczy J, Pindborg JJ. Smoking habits and histological characteristics of oral leukoplakias in Denmark and Hungary. Br J Cancer 1973;28:575–579.
35. Sugar L, Banoczy J. Follow-up studies in oral leukoplakia. Bull WHO 1969;41:289–293.

36. Blot WJ, McLaughlin JK, Winn DM, et al. Smoking and drinking in relation to oral pharyngeal cancer. Cancer Res 1988;48:3282–3287.

37. Schottenfeld D, Gantt RC, Wynde EL. The role of alcohol and tobacco in multiple primary cancers of the upper digestive system, larynx, and lung: A prospective study. Prev Med 1974;3:277–293.

38. Schottenfeld D. Epidemiology of cancer of the esophagus. Semin Oncol 1984;11:92–100.

39. Newcomb PA, Carbone PP. The health consequences of smoking. Med Clin North Am 1992;76:305–331.

40. Baron JA, Byers T, Greenberg, ER, et al. Cigarette smoking in women with cancers of the breast and reproductive organs. JNCI 1986;77:677–680.

41. Brinton LA, Schainer C, Haenszel W, et al. Cigarette smoking and invasive cervical cancer. JAMA 1986;255:3265–3269.

42. Slattery ML, Robison LM, Schuman K, et al. Cigarette smoking and exposure to passive smoke are risk factors for cervical cancer. JAMA 1989;261:1593–1598.

43. Boring CC, Squires TS, Tong T. Cancer statistics 1991. CA 1991;41:19.

44. Sasson IM, Haley M, Hoffman D, et al. Cigarette smoking and neoplasia of the uterine cervix: Smoke constituents in cervical mucus. N Engl J Med 1985;312:315–316.

45. Holly EA, Petrakis NL, Friend NF, et al. Mutagenic mucus in the cervix of smokers. JNCI 1986;76:983–986.

46. Koutsky LA, Galloway D, Holmes KK. The epidemiology of genital papilloma virus infection. Epidemiol Rev 1988;10:120.

47. McLaughlin, Silverman DT, Hsing AW, Ross RK. Cigarette smoking and cancers of the renal pelvis and ureter. Cancer Res 1992;52:254–257.

48. Hartge P, Silverman D, Hoover R, et al. Changing cigarette habits and bladder cancer risk: A case-control study. JNCI 1987;78:1119.

49. Burch JD, Rohan TE, Howe GR, et al. Risk of bladder cancer by source and type of tobacco exposure: A case-control study. Int J Cancer 1989;141:622.

50. Severson RK. Cigarette smoking and leukemia. Cancer 1987;60:141.

50a. Mills PK, Newell GR, Beeson WL, et al. History of cigarette smoking and risk of leukemia and myeloma: Results from the Adventist health study. JNCI 1990;82:1832–1836.

51. Baron JA. Smoking and estrogen related disease. Am J Epidemiol 1984;119:9.

52. US Department of Health and Human Services. The Health consequences of smoking: Cardiovascular disease: A report of the Surgeon General. Washington, DC: US Department of Health and Human Services, Public Health Service, Office on Smoking and Health. DHHS (PHS) 84-50204, 1983.

53. Willett WC, Green A, Stampfer MJ, et al. Relative and absolute risks of coronary heart disease among women who smoke cigarettes. N Engl J Med 1987;317:1303–1309.

54. Martin JL, Wilson JR, Ferraro N, et al. Acute coronary vasoconstrictiveness effects of cigarette smoking in coronary heart disease. Am J Cardiol 1984;54:56–60.

55. Fitzgerald GA, Oates, JA, Nowak J. Cigarette smoking and hemostatic function. Am Heart Jl 1988;115:267–271.

56. Wolf PA, D'Agostino RB, Kasnel WB, et al. Cigarette smoking as a risk factor for stroke: The Framingham study. JAMA 1988;259:1025–1029.

57. Stuart-Harris CH. The epidemiology and evolution of chronic bronchitis. Br J Tuberculosis Dis Chest 1954;48:169–178.

58. Stuart-Harris CH. Chronic bronchitis: I. Abstr World Med 1968;42:649–669.

58a. Sobel R. They satisfy: The cigarette in American Life. New York: Anchor Press/Doubleday, 1978.

58b. Einster V. Mixed messages for women: A social history of cigarette smoking and advertising. NY State J Med 1985;85:335–340.

59. O'Conner JJ. Women top cigaret target. Advertising Age 1981;52:9, 93.

60. Trone Advertising Inc. V. F. Year: I. Promotion recommendations. North Carolina: Trone Advertising, 1989.

61. US Public Health Service. The Health Consequences of Smoking: 1969 Supplement to the 1967 Public Health Service Review. Washington, DC: US Department of Health, Education and Welfare, Public Health Service. PHS Publication No. 1696-2 (Supplement), 1969.

62. Jacobson B. The lady killers. London: Pluto Press 1981:53.

63. US Department of Health and Human Services. Report of the task force on black and minority health. Washington DC: US Department of Health and Human Services, 1985.

64. Blum A. The targeting of minority groups by the tobacco industry. In: Jones LA, ed. Minorities and cancer. New York: Springer-Verlag, 1989:153–162.

65. Citizens action handbook on tobacco and alcohol billboard advertising. Washington, DC, Scenic America, 1990.

66. Cooper R, Simmons B. Cigarette smoking and ill health among black Americans. NY State J Med 1985;85:344–347.

67. Ramirez A. A cigarette campaign under fire. The New York Times, January 12, 1990: D1, D4.

68. Romano PS, Bloom J, Syme SL. Smoking, social support, and hassles in an urban African-American community. Am J Public Health 1991;81:1415–1422.

69. US Department of Health and Human Services. Smoking tobacco, and cancer programs: 1985–1989 status report. Washington, DC: Public Health Service, National Institutes of Health, National Cancer Institute. NIH Publication No. 90-3107, 1990.

70. McGraw S, Smith K, Schensal J, Carrillo E. Sociocultural factors associated with smoking behavior by Puerto Rican adolescents in Boston. Soc Science Med 1991;33:1355–1364.

71. US Department of Health and Human Services. The health consequences of smoking: The changing cigarette: A report of the Surgeon General. Washington, DC: US Department of Health and Human Services, Public Health Service, Office on Smoking and Health, DHHS (PHS) 81-50156, 1981.

72. Benowitz NL, Hall SM, Herning RI, et al. Smokers of low-yield cigarettes do not consume less nicotine. N Engl J Med 1983;309:139–142.

73. Blum A. Cigarettes are so Kool—teenagers and the smoking epidemic. In: Encyclopaedia Britannica, Medical Annual, 1982.

74. Blum A. "Safe" cigarettes and other cons. Phys Assist Health Pract 1980;4:48.

75. Blum A. Smokeless tobacco. JAMA 1980;244:192.

76. Connolly G. personal communication, 1992.

77. Jayant K, Balakrishnan V, Sanghvi LD, et al. Quantification of the role of smoking and chewing tobacco in oral, pharyngeal, and esophageal cancer. Br J Cancer 1977;35:232–235.

78. Blum A. Using athletes to push tobacco to children: Snuff-dippin' cancer-lipped men. NY State J Med 1983;83:1365–1367.

79. Christen AG, McDaniel RK, Doran JE. Snuff dipping and tobacco chewing in a group of Texas college athletes. TX Dent J 1979;97:6–10.

80. Abrams R. Attorney General Abrams speaks out against smokeless tobacco. NY State J Med 1985;85:471.

81. US Department of Health and Human Services. The health consequences of involuntary smoking: A report of the Surgeon General. Washington, DC: Public Health Service, Centers for Disease Control, Office on Smoking and Health, Department of Health and Human Services, (CDC) 87-8398, 1986.

82. National Research Council, National Academy of Sciences. Environmental tobacco smoke: Measuring exposures and assessing health effects. Washington, DC: National Academy Press, 1986.

82a. Steenland K. Passive smoking and the risk of heart disease. JAMA 1992;267:94–99.

82b. Repace JL, Lowrey AH. Risk assessment methodologies for passive smoking-induced lung cancer. Risk Anal 1990;10:27–37.

83. Centers for Disease Control. Tobacco use among high school students—United States, 1990. MMWR 1991;40:617–619.

84. Every physician as a (potential) prevention specialist. In: The health care system and drug abuse prevention. Washington, DC: US Department of Health and Human Services, National Institute on Drug Abuse, 1981.

85. Blum A. Medicine vs. Madison Avenue: Fighting smoke with fire. JAMA 1980;243:739–740.

86. Schwartz JL. Review and evaluation of smoking cessation methods: The United States and Canada, 1978–1985. Washington, DC: US Department of Health and Human Services, Public Health Service, National Institutes of Health, NCI. NIH Publication No. 87-2940, 1987.

87. Schwartz JL. A critical review and evaluation of smoking control methods. Public Health Rep 1969;84:483–506.

88. Russell MA, Wilson C, Taylor C. The effects of general practitioners' advice against smoking. Br Med J 1979;2:231–235.

89. US Department of Health, Education, and Welfare. The health consequences of smoking: 1977–1978. Washington, DC: Office of the Assistant Secretary for Health, Office on Smoking and Health. DHEW Publication No. (PHS) 79-50065, 1979.

Cancer: Principles & Practice of Oncology, Fourth Edition,
edited by Vincent T. DeVita, Jr., Samuel Hellman, Steven A. Rosenberg.
J.B. Lippincott Co., Philadelphia © 1993.

CHAPTER **21**

Specialized Techniques of Cancer Management and Diagnosis

ROBERT C. KURTZ
CHARLES J. LIGHTDALE
ROBERT J. GINSBERG

SECTION **1**

Endoscopy

Endoscopy is one of the most rapidly advancing fields in medicine. Video or electronic instruments use microchip technology to capture endoscopic images that are clear and detailed, enabling more accurate diagnoses and greater ease in documentation with photographs and video tape. Many internal organs can be examined by endoscopy with video documentation, biopsy, cytology, and sonographic evaluation to determine diagnosis, operability, and staging.

Although diagnostic endoscopic procedures remain the major component of any endoscopy unit, therapeutic endoscopy is rapidly catching up. Endoscopic removal of polyps, tumor ablation with laser therapy, control of hemorrhage, relief of obstructive jaundice, and enteral nutritional support through endoscopically placed gastrostomy tubes are a few of the therapeutic endoscopic procedures available at most large medical centers.

UPPER GASTROINTESTINAL ENDOSCOPY

Upper gastrointestinal endoscopy is the procedure of choice for the diagnosis of esophagogastric neoplasia. Benign conditions that mimic or complicate cancer are also accurately diagnosed. Performance of biopsy or brush cytology during endoscopy provides a tissue diagnosis to complement observation and photography. Upper gastrointestinal endoscopy is increasingly used as the initial diagnostic test rather than as a follow-up to x-ray examination.[1]

Several developments have contributed using endoscopy for the diagnosis of esophagogastric tumors. Endoscopes have become so thin and maneuverable that there are no longer any blind areas to endoscopic evaluation. Until about a decade ago, the gastric fundus and cardia were difficult to see in their entirety, as was the lesser curvature of the antrum behind the angularis.[2] These areas are now routinely examined with retroflexion techniques. The patients usually require only mild sedation. The thin, forward-viewing endoscopes are passed under direct vision through the upper esophageal sphincter, making this a safer and more comfortable step than in the past. A barium roentgenographic "road map" is rarely necessary.

Upper gastrointestinal endoscopy is perhaps more invasive than a barium series, but it is more accurate. Endoscopy is more expensive, but it avoids test duplication and exposure to radiation, an issue of increasing concern. Complications of diagnostic upper gastrointestinal endoscopy are rare, and modern video endoscopic systems have solved the problem of high-quality images for documentation, analysis, and permanent record.[3]

DIAGNOSTIC
UPPER GASTROINTESTINAL ENDOSCOPY

The diagnostic accuracy of upper gastrointestinal endoscopy and biopsy for primary and metastatic upper gastrointestinal cancer is in the range of 95%.[1] Infiltrating cancer, as seen in some gastric adenocarcinomas and lymphomas, is less successfully biopsied, although a tissue diagnosis is still achieved in most cases with large biopsy forceps and needle aspiration cytology.[4]

Endoscopy is recommended for most patients with gastric ulcers found on upper gastrointestinal series before medical management, because a small percentage of benign-appearing ulcers are malignant.[1] If suspicion remains, repeat endoscopy is indicated in 6 to 8 weeks. This is not the case in duodenal ulcer disease, which is only rarely due to cancer. However, in patients with malignancies known to metastasize to the gastrointestinal tract, endoscopic evaluation of the duodenum may be warranted. Patients at high risk for upper gastrointestinal cancer, such as those with proven Barrett's esophagus or prior gastric adenomas, may be considered for periodic screening endoscopy, although the benefits of such screening remain controversial.[5]

There are areas of the world, most notably in northern China, where chronic esophagitis and epidermoid carcinoma of the esophagus are endemic.[6] Population screening programs for esophageal cancer have been carried out on a large scale in these areas with promising results. Screening has been based on esophageal cytologic specimens obtained by having patients swallow a thin tube with a brush or abrasive balloon on the tip, which is then pulled up the esophagus. If dysplastic or malignant cells are obtained, endoscopy with biopsy is performed.[7] Using these methods, early-stage esophageal cancers have been detected in asymptomatic persons with good probability for surgical cure. Similar screening programs carried out among heavy smokers and drinkers in the United States have not proven effective.[8] Another group at risk are patients with cancers of the head and neck, which are also related to use of tobacco and alcohol.[9] Early esophageal cancer has been found in as many as 5% of these patients who have no dysphagia. Endoscopic staining of the esophagus with Lugol's iodine solution may help in detecting small areas of malignancy.[9]

In Japan, where gastric cancer is a leading cause of death, mass population screening with radiographs and endoscopy has greatly improved the detection of early disease and subsequent survival.[10] In America and Europe, the overall incidence of gastric cancer is decreasing, but the percentage of cancers affecting the proximal stomach is increasing, as is the incidence of early gastric cancer detection.[11,12] Mass screening is not practical in relatively low-incidence Western countries. The increased frequency of detection of early gastric cancer has been attributed to greater a sensitivity to suggestive symptoms and a more aggressive application of improved radiologic and endoscopic methods.[13]

Whether patients with partial gastrectomy for benign disease are at long-term risk for gastric cancer and merit endoscopic screening is an open question, but in patients who have dysplasia detected by gastric biopsy, endoscopic surveillance seems indicated.[14]

Benign and malignant tumors are much less common in the small intestine than the stomach. The duodenum is the most frequent small intestine location for the development of adenomas and adenocarcinomas. Adenomas of the duodenum are particularly common in patients with familial adenomatous polyposis (FAP). In such cases, the adenomas tend to be flat and numerous.[15] Carcinoma of the duodenum, most often periampullary, is a major cause of death in patients with FAP who have had colectomies. The proximal duodenum is routinely examined during upper gastrointestinal endoscopy, and abnormalities are biopsied. Periodic endoscopic surveillance of the stomach and duodenum in patients with FAP is recommended, including the use of a side-viewing duodenoscope for better visualization of the ampulla of Vater.

Although endoscopy is most effective in evaluating intraluminal disease, it is less effective in assessing motility, extrinsic compression by contiguous structures, and the degree of luminal obstruction. Barium x-ray films and computed tomography (CT) scans provide better evaluation of extrinsic lesions causing compression and contour defects in the gastrointestinal tract and can better assess the degree of obstruction.

In managing patients with cancer, upper gastrointestinal endoscopy is the procedure of choice for diagnosing the source of gastrointestinal bleeding.[19] Barium x-ray studies are not effective for this purpose. Angiography is useful only in cases of massive bleeding. When the gastrointestinal bleeding source is uncertain, nuclear medicine scans may help. Upper gastrointestinal endoscopy should be done first and performed with ease and accuracy. Lesions identified can be treated at once with the endoscope.[18] In immunosuppressed patients with cancer and dysphagia, occult monilial or herpetic esophagitis is best diagnosed by upper gastrointestinal endoscopy, and the results can be confirmed by biopsy and cytologic examinations.[20,21]

THERAPEUTIC
UPPER GASTROINTESTINAL ENDOSCOPY

Therapeutic applications of upper gastrointestinal endoscopy include the placement of guide wires, stents, and balloons for dilation of benign and malignant strictures, removal of foreign bodies, removal of polyps by electrocautery, vaporization and coagulation of cancerous tissues with neodymium:yttrium-aluminum-garnet (Nd:YAG) laser, control of bleeding with electrocautery, heat, or laser probes, and the injection of epinephrine or sclerosing solutions by needle-tipped catheters for tumor necrosis or treatment of bleeding.[16–18]

In patients with advanced, unresectable cancer of the esophagus or gastric cardia that is unresponsive to primary treatment, endoscopic therapy has assumed a major role in the palliation of dysphagia. The mainstays of endoscopic palliation have been the plastic endoprosthesis and the Nd:YAG laser.[16] There are advantages and disadvantages to both methods. In about 70% of patients, laser therapy is much more likely to allow a normal diet, but it must be repeated at monthly intervals to avoid recurrent dysphagia. Although outpatient treatment is possible, laser sessions become increasingly time consuming and uncomfortable for the patient as the cancer progresses.[17] Esophageal stents ideally provide a longer lasting palliation, and they are the treatment of choice for tumors that are primarily infiltrating, submucosal, or extrinsic. Endoluminal stents are also useful for sealing fistulas into the tracheobronchial tree.[16] In most centers where an Nd:YAG laser is available, laser therapy is performed first, particularly if there is bulky intraluminal tumor.[17] However, some groups preferentially palliate esophageal and esophagogastric malignant stenoses with stents. The best results have been achieved with stents handmade from polyvinyl tubing, specifically tailored for the individual patient. These stents have a larger bore than the 10 to 11 mm usually provided by commercial stents, allowing a more normal diet.

Complications, mostly perforations, occur in about 5% of those treated with laser and 5% to 18% of those treated with stents.[16,17] The lowest complication rates are from the most experienced centers. For tight stenoses, gradual dilation over several sessions has been recommended to avoid perforation associated with rapid dilation to the diameter required for stent insertion. Self-expanding, membrane-sealed metal stents, potentially easier to insert, are in development. Photodynamic therapy using photochemical sensitizers and low-power laser light activation for more selective and safer laser therapy is being studied.[16]

COMPLICATIONS
OF UPPER GASTROINTESTINAL ENDOSCOPY

Upper gastrointestinal endoscopy in experienced hands is atraumatic and a safe procedure with few contraindications and only rare complications. The procedure can be performed safely even in patients on anticoagulants or with nadir blood counts, although therapeutic options in these patients are limited. In weakened or comatose patients, there is an increased risk of aspiration pneumonia. With modern endoscopes passed under direct vision, the probability of perforation is less than 0.1%.[3]

ENDOSCOPIC ULTRASONOGRAPHY

PRINCIPLES

Endoscopic ultrasonography is an important new extension of diagnostic gastrointestinal endoscopy. Using this modality, it is possible for the endoscopist to assess visible mucosal lesions, intramural disease processes deep to the mucosa, and extrinsic abnormalities in proximity to the wall of the gastrointestinal tract.[22-24]

Endoscopic ultrasonography uses high frequency ultrasound (>7 MHz) for high resolution, producing uniquely detailed views of the gut wall and surrounding structures that are unmatched by other imaging methods. The higher the frequency, the shorter is the penetration depth of ultrasound and the more limited is the field of view. However, a limited field is acceptable with endoscopic ultrasonography, because the transducer can be placed immediately adjacent to the area of interest.

Using endoscopic ultrasonography, the wall of the gastrointestinal tract can be imaged as a five-layer structure of alternating bright (*i.e.,* hyperechoic, echogenic) and dark (*i.e.,* hypoechoic) bands (Fig. 21–1). The histologic correlates of the five layers were the object of intense in vitro and in vivo studies.[25] It is now recognized that the echogenic layers consist in part of interface echoes produced as the sound waves travel between tissues of different density. For clinical purposes, the first two layers correspond to the superficial and deep mucosa, the third layer to the submucosa, the fourth to the muscularis propria, and the fifth to the serosa or adventitia.

Most clinical studies have been carried out using mechanical

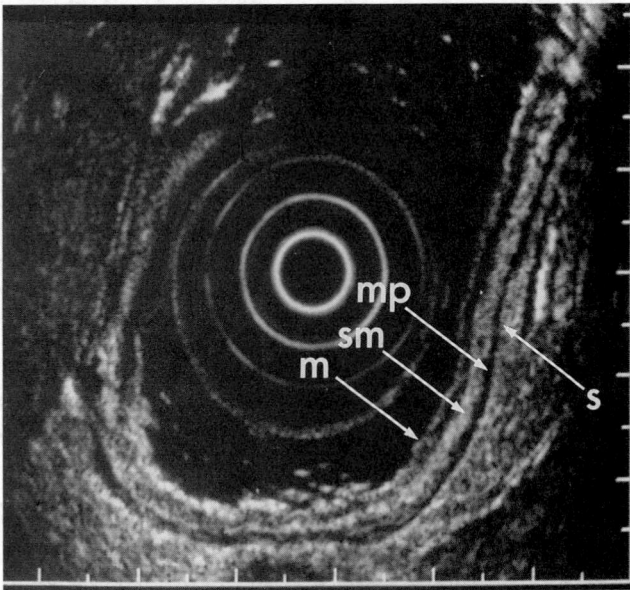

FIGURE 21–1. Endosonographic image of the normal gastric wall. The concentric circles in the center represent the transducer and water-filled balloon in the lumen of the stomach. From the lumen, the first two wall layers correlate with the superficial and deep mucosa (m), the third wall layer represents the submucosa (sm), the fourth layer is the muscularis propria (mp), and the fifth layer is the serosa (s).

sector scan instruments manufactured by the Olympus Corporation, principally the instrument designated GF-UM3. These instruments are combination endoscopes and ultrasound probes, which use an acoustic mirror rotating around a transducer with switchable 7.5- and 12-MHz frequencies.[22-24] An important advantage of this type of instrument is the 360° image produced. In the tubular gastrointestinal tract, this greatly facilitates orientation of the image. Optics are forward oblique, useful in locating lesions in the stomach and in guiding the instrument through the pylorus. The 4-cm rigid tip and the 13-mm diameter make the instrument somewhat difficult to use and limit passage through stenotic areas. A forward-viewing colonoscope with standard biopsy channel has recently been made, but the 15-mm tip diameter limits its use to the distal large bowel. A new duodenoscope has side-viewing optics and a tip diameter of 10.4 mm, but it is limited to one frequency of 7.5 or 12 MHz. A prototype EUS-20 system features a digital receiver, providing more sophisticated image management.

Instruments using linear or phased-array technology have the advantages of forward-viewing optics and no moving parts, but they provide a slice-like image, which makes orientation more difficult. The addition of Doppler ultrasound technology to evaluate vascularity and blood flow is easily obtained on all electronic instruments. Blind endosonography probes, rigid or flexible and mechanical or electronic, have been used mainly in the rectum. There is recent interest in ultrathin miniprobes that can pass through an endoscope biopsy channel. Initial testing of these probes indicates that they have a restricted field of view and often produce less than satisfactory images. They have been used to image focal lesions under direct vision and to image the bile ducts.[24]

INDICATIONS AND RESULTS

Endoscopic ultrasonography has been applied to a variety of clinical problems. It is most extensively used in the staging of esophageal, gastric, and rectal cancer. The accumulating data suggest that endoscopic ultrasonography is the most accurate imaging modality for staging depth of tumor invasion (T), with preoperative accuracy in the 80% to 90% range when compared with surgical pathology.[26-30]

Esophageal and gastric T1 cancers invade the mucosa or submucosa (Fig. 21–2) and are imaged as a disruption of the first three endosonographic wall layers. T2 cancers invade the muscularis propria to the subserosa and show a hypoechoic invasion of the fourth layer. T3 cancers invade through the serosa and penetrate the fifth layer. T4 cancers directly invade adjacent organs or structures.

At Memorial Sloan-Kettering Cancer Center, we prospectively used endoscopic ultrasonography in 50 patients for preoperative staging of esophageal cancer (Fig. 21–3) and in 50 patients for preoperative staging of gastric cancer (Fig. 21–4).[27,28] Results were compared for accuracy with surgical pathology and with computed tomography using rapid scanners, oral contrast, and dynamic technique. CT was performed after endoscopic ultrasonography and reviewed independently to avoid bias. Endoscopic ultrasonography was significantly more accurate than state-of-the-art dynamic CT in T staging of esophageal and gastric cancer. Most studies comparing endoscopic ultrasonography with CT for staging esophageal, gastric, and rectal cancer have found endoscopic ultrasonography superior for evaluating tumor extent.[26-30]

The greatest strength of endoscopic ultrasonography is in locating tissues. Histologic analysis is still required for the diagnosis of any abnormality. Endoscopic ultrasonography cannot reliably differentiate an inflammatory from a neoplastic process. For example, the method is not useful in de-

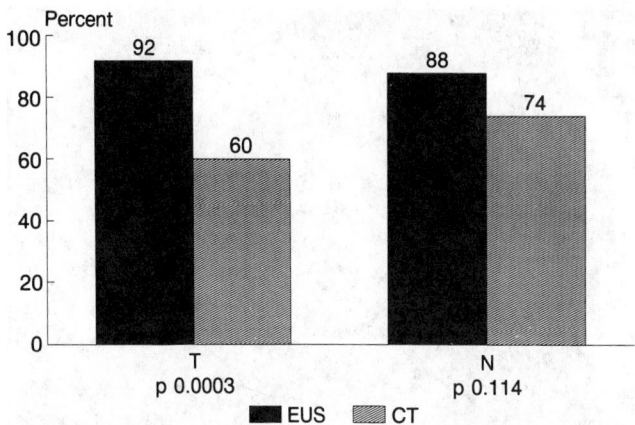

FIGURE 21–3.   Esophageal cancer staging concordance with surgical pathology. Results of preoperative staging in 50 consecutive patients who had surgery for esophageal cancer at Memorial Sloan-Kettering Cancer Center.

termining if a gastric ulcer is benign or malignant. In staging lymph nodes (N), endosonography has proven less accurate than in staging depth of tumor invasion, because the node must be located and characterized as benign or malignant. Lymph nodes 2 to 3 mm in diameter can be detected with endoscopic ultrasonography. Some investigators use the echo character of nodes for staging.[26-27] Nodes that are rounded, sharply defined, and hypoechoic are more likely to be malignant (Fig. 21–5). Using these criteria, staging regional lymph node metastases has been more accurate than other imaging modalities (*e.g.*, CT scan) and is accurate in the range of 70% to 80%.[26-30] Endoscopic ultrasonography also appears to be a sensitive method of detecting recurrent upper gastrointestinal cancer in an area of surgical anastomosis.[31] There have been false positives due to inflammation, and specificity needs to be improved. Endoscopic ultrasonography-directed needle biopsy and computer analysis for tissue characterization are areas of active research.

Endoscopic ultrasonography can easily differentiate extrinsic from intramural structures. There are characteristic images for cysts, leiomyomas, and lipomas, but it is not always

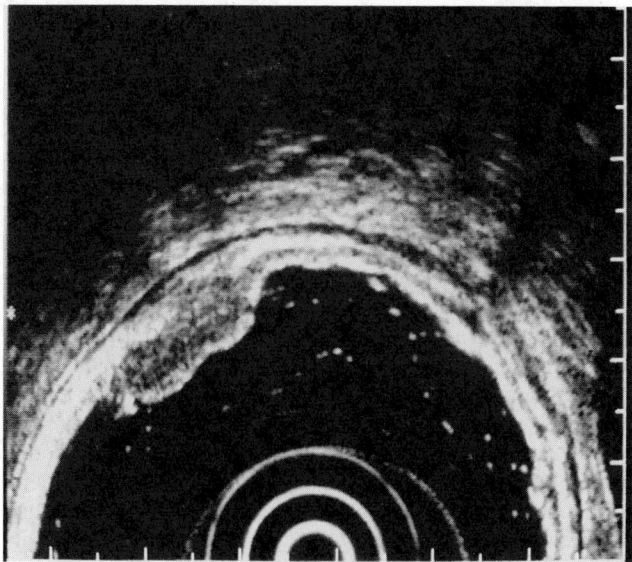

FIGURE 21–2.   Endosonographic image shows a polypoid hypoechoic disruption involving only the first three wall layers of the stomach at the angularis. A T1 cancer invading to the submucosa, but not involving the muscularis propria, was confirmed by surgical pathologic examination.

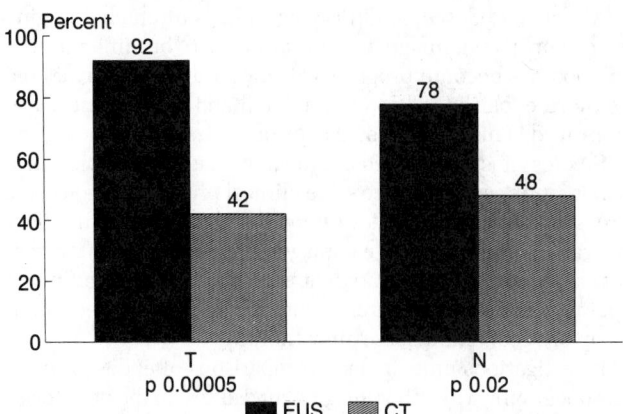

FIGURE 21–4.   Gastric cancer staging concordance with surgical pathology. Results of preoperative staging in 50 consecutive patients who had surgery for gastric cancer at Memorial Sloan-Kettering Cancer Center.

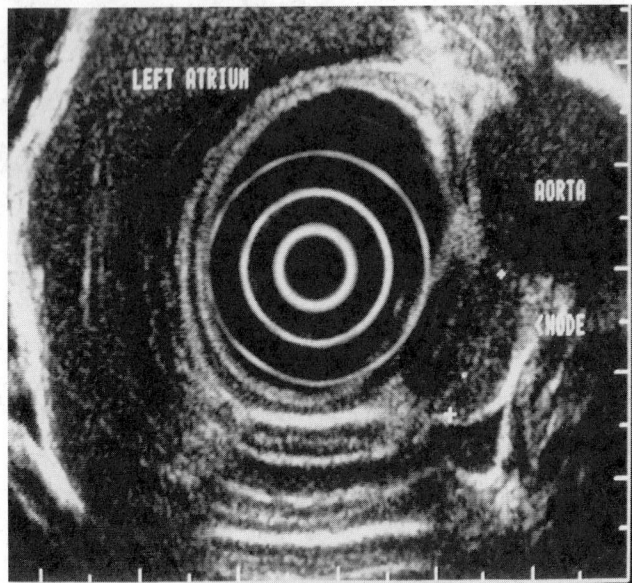

FIGURE 21-5. A round, hypoechoic sharply defined lymph node measuring 1.4 cm is imaged through the distal esophagus. The posterior node lies between the aorta and azygos vein. The relation of the esophagus to the left atrium is evident posteriorly. The node in a patient with cancer of the esophagogastric junction was malignant at the time of surgical resection.

possible to differentiate benign from malignant lesions.[32] Large gastric folds due to benign gastropathy can usually be differentiated from malignant infiltration by carcinoma or lymphoma, which tend to destroy normal tissue architecture.[33] Varices may be readily identified and assessed.[24] The method appears to offer a new approach to defining colon fistulas and abscesses in Crohn's disease.

Imaging the pancreas through the wall of the stomach and duodenum provides a highly detailed image, allowing detection of tumors even smaller than 1 cm.[34] Changes due to pancreatitis can be identified, but it is not possible to reliably differentiate neoplastic from inflammatory pancreatic masses.[35,36] Staging pancreatic, biliary, and ampullary cancer preoperatively and localizing neuroendocrine tumors have been carried out successfully with endoscopic ultrasonography.[36–38]

Although endoscopic ultrasonography is often challenging to perform and image interpretation can be difficult, the method has become progressively easier and more available as more experience has accumulated and instruments have improved. This trend should continue.

Studies must be carried out to show that endoscopic ultrasonography can be used to solve clinical problems. Promising areas of application include tumor staging for decisions about operative or nonoperative management or about local or radical resection, administration of preoperative or neoadjuvant therapy, assessment of treatment response, and detection of early or recurrent disease after therapy.

Investigations must include comparisons of endoscopic ultrasonography with other imaging modalities. In the near term, endoscopic ultrasonography will probably facilitate patient management if accurate tumor staging is important, if submucosal, intramural, and extrinsic processes require definition, and if detailed evaluation of the pancreas is needed.

The pace of various technologic advances cannot be predicted with certainty. However, despite its complexity and expense, endoscopic ultrasonography provides information so unique that its clinical role in the foreseeable future seems assured, particularly in applications involving the staging and management of gastrointestinal neoplasia.

SIGMOIDOSCOPY

PRINCIPLES

Rigid and flexible sigmoidoscopies are important endoscopic techniques for evaluating the distal colon and rectum. Rigid sigmoidoscopes are usually 25 cm long, and flexible instruments are 35 cm or 60 cm long. Although rigid sigmoidoscopes are less expensive to purchase and maintain and somewhat easier to use than their flexible counterparts, the flexible instruments offer greater depth of insertion, patient comfort, and acceptance.

INDICATIONS AND RESULTS

Colorectal cancer screening represents one of the most common indications for sigmoidoscopy, because the procedure is highly sensitive and specific. Because of its length, sigmoidoscopy misses proximal colon cancers and polyps. Sigmoidoscopic screening of large population groups remains controversial because most clinical trials have been uncontrolled and because the proposed goal of mortality reduction has not been met. In a case-control trial of rigid sigmoidoscopy, the investigators used data from 261 patients who died of distal colon and rectal cancer. Only 8.8% of these patients had had sigmoidoscopies, compared with 24.2% in a control population without cancer. The control patients who had sigmoidoscopies within the preceding 10 years had a 60% to 70% reduction in colorectal cancer mortality.[39] The use of sigmoidoscopy as part of a periodic comprehensive health evaluation to prevent the lethal complications of advanced cancer is case finding and should not be confused with population screening.[40] Case finding is based on physician assessment of a patient's risk factors and the use of clinical judgment in ordering appropriate diagnostic tests. The American Cancer Society recommends the use of sigmoidoscopic evaluation for average-risk, asymptomatic patients every 3 to 5 years, beginning at 50 years of age.[41]

Another indication for sigmoidoscopy is to complement air-contrast barium enema studies performed to evaluate colonic symptoms such as rectal bleeding. In a comparative study of flexible sigmoidoscopy with other diagnostic techniques, the combination of sigmoidoscopy and barium enema was almost as effective in identifying colon cancer as colonoscopy. The identification of small and medium-sized polyps was better with colonoscopy.[42] Sigmoidoscopy is also useful in following inflammatory bowel disease patients to assess therapy. It may be therapeutic for sigmoid volvulus, and it is used to follow patients with FAP after colectomy and ileorectal reconstruction and to evaluate family members for phenotypic expression of FAP.

Sigmoidoscopy is a safe procedure. Flexible sigmoidoscopy can be easily taught to primary care physicians.[43] Complications such as perforation of the colon during rigid or flexible sigmoidoscopy are possible but extremely rare. In a series of 5000 flexible sigmoidoscopies, no perforations occurred.[44]

COLONOSCOPY

DIAGNOSTIC COLONOSCOPY

During the past 20 years, colonoscopic examination of the large bowel has become the established method of evaluating and treating diseases of the large intestine. Modern colonoscopes are easier and safer to use, and complete evaluation by direct observation of the rectum and colon to the cecum is the rule. Abnormalities seen may be photographed, biopsied, and in the case of polypoid lesions, often entirely removed. Using lavage preparations for bowel cleansing, patients can often be prepared for colonoscopy within 24 hours.

Evaluation of abnormal findings after barium enema continues to be an important indication for colonoscopy. The type of barium enema examination performed influences the detection of neoplastic lesions. If a single-column barium enema study is performed, most adenomatous polyps and about half of the cancers are missed, as determined by subsequent colonoscopy. Double or air-contrast barium enema examinations identify most lesions larger than 2 cm in diameter, but smaller lesions are often missed. When a possible neoplastic lesion is identified on barium enema examination, colonoscopy is needed to determine the precise nature of the lesion, to remove it if it proves to be a benign-appearing polyp, for biopsy it if it can not be removed, and to confirm there are no synchronous lesions elsewhere in the colon. Synchronous adenomas occur in approximately 50% of patients with colon cancer, and separate synchronous colon cancers occur in 1.5% to 5% of patients.[45]

One of the most difficult areas in barium enema interpretation is differentiation of diverticular disease from colon cancer. Barium enema may underestimate the degree and intensity of diverticular inflammation. Colonoscopy, with associated biopsy and cytology, is the most important tool to use in making this distinction.[46] In 44 patients with diverticular disease, Hunt found 6 (13%) with unexpected cancer, and he was unable to adequately examine the colon in a similar number of patients.[47]

Hematochezia and melena thought not to be from an upper gastrointestinal source should be evaluated by colonoscopy. Cancer of the large bowel, particularly in the rectum and left colon, often cause rectal bleeding. Cancers involving the right colon are more likely to produce melanotic stools or occult bleeding with the gradual onset on iron deficiency anemia. Brand and colleagues studied more than 300 patients with recent rectal bleeding by colonoscopy.[48] They found that the bleeding was due to cancer in approximately 8% of their patients, but in more than 20%, it was due to benign colon polyps. Angiodysplasia was also an important cause of large bowel hemorrhage in their patient population. Tedesco and colleagues performed colonoscopy in 258 patients with rectal bleeding and negative proctosigmoidoscopy and barium enemas that were negative or showed only diverticula.[49] In 29 (11.2%) patients, cancer was found by the colonoscopic examination.

Asymptomatic patients with positive fecal occult blood tests should undergo colonoscopy. Data from the New York occult blood screening trial show that approximately 50% of patients tested for occult blood for the first time have a colonic neoplastic lesion.[50] About 12% of these lesions are cancers, and the rest are adenomatous polyps. These rates increase as the age of the study population increases.

Patients who have had a colon cancer or adenomatous polyp resected are at high risk for additional or metachronous lesions. Various estimates have placed the risk for metachronous cancer between 5% and 10%, but the risk of developing a metachronous adenoma can be as high a 60%, as defined in a study of 383 patients by Fowler and Hedberg.[51] The National Polyp Study, a multicenter randomized trial, demonstrated a polyp recurrence rate of 29% to 35%, depending on the number of endoscopic procedures performed and the time from the last procedure. These patients should be under colonoscopic surveillance.[52] Although precise follow-up intervals have not been established, after assuring a "clean" colon, repeat examinations at 3-year intervals seems prudent.

If there is a surgical anastomosis after colon cancer resection, attention to this area during colonoscopy is important for the early detection of a treatable anastomotic recurrence. Biopsy or brush cytology of the anastomosis should be part of each surveillance colonoscopy.

Surveillance for colon cancer in patients with longstanding chronic ulcerative colitis represents a special problem. Although there is disagreement about the magnitude of the cancer risk in ulcerative colitis, most investigators agree that it is unusual for cancer to develop within the first 8 to 10 years of the disease and that the estimated cumulative incidence thereafter is about 5% at 20 years and 12% at 25 years.[53] Annual surveillance colonoscopy should begin after 10 years. The aim of colonoscopy is to identify patients who are especially likely to develop colon cancer by finding dysplastic changes in the colonic mucosa on endoscopic biopsy. Multiple biopsies are obtained throughout the colon at approximately 10-cm intervals. The areas usually sampled are the cecum, ascending colon, hepatic flexure, transverse colon, splenic flexure, descending colon, sigmoid colon and rectum. Dysplasia is clear-cut neoplastic change in the colonic mucosa, and high-grade dysplasia triggers intervention. Several studies of colonoscopic surveillance were summarized by Waye.[54] Fifteen percent of patients studied were found to have dysplasia, and 20% of these were found to have colon cancer. Unfortunately, 10% of colitis patients with cancer had no evidence of dysplasia.

Recent studies have confirmed that colorectal cancer occurs in first-degree relatives (*i.e.*, parents, children, siblings) of patients with colorectal cancer about with three to four times the frequency expected by chance. There is also an increased risk for adenomatous polyps in first-degree relatives of patients with bowel cancer and an increased risk for colorectal cancer in first-degree relatives with adenomatous polyps.[55,56] Many physicians are now recommending colonoscopy in conjunction with fecal occult blood testing as the primary diagnostic tool for first-degree relatives in colon cancer families.

Screening colonoscopy has been studied in average-risk, asymptomatic patients with negative fecal occult blood studies. In one study, adenomatous polyps were detected at a rate that was twice that expected from flexible sigmoidoscopy alone.[57]

Fifty-three (25%) of 210 patients had adenomas, and 2 had cancers. The larger adenomas and both cancers were found in patients older than 60 years of age. Although routine screening colonoscopy cannot yet be recommended in average-risk, asymptomatic patients, the results of this study are intriguing.

THERAPEUTIC COLONOSCOPY: POLYPECTOMY

After a polyp is identified, colonoscopic polypectomy is performed. If possible, the polyp is totally removed and submitted for pathologic assessment. Complete colonoscopy should be performed at the time of polypectomy to identify and remove any synchronous polyps. Biopsy of polyps is not recommended, because the results may be misleading. Small polyps (≤7 mm in diameter) are often removed by "hot-biopsy" technique. Electric current is passed through a special biopsy forceps to cauterize the base of the polyp. The tissue in the forceps is sent to pathology. Larger polyps are removed by snare-cautery technique. A wire-loop is passed around the polyp base, and an electric current transects and cauterizes the polyp base. The entire polyp is retrieved and submitted to pathology for analysis. Most colonic polyps can be managed in this fashion. Large sessile polyps may need to be removed in a piecemeal approach. A small number of large sessile polyps (>2 cm in diameter) may not be removable safely during colonoscopy, and surgical resection is necessary. Marking the polypectomy site with an injection of a dilute solution of sterile India ink has been recommended as an accurate and permanent way for future endoscopic or surgical identification.[58]

COMPLICATIONS OF COLONOSCOPY

The major complications of colonoscopy are bowel perforation and hemorrhage. The rates of occurrence are different for diagnostic and therapeutic colonoscopy. In 4713 diagnostic colonoscopies reported on by the American Society for Gastrointestinal Endoscopy (ASGE), perforation occurred in 0.17%.[59] These perforations are usually the result of the mechanical force of the colonoscope shaft on the sigmoid colon, especially a sigmoid colon affected by diverticular disease or adhesions. In 1901 polypectomy patients reported by the ASGE, the perforation rate was 0.11%. In this group, perforation almost always occurred at the polypectomy site, usually related to the removal of a sessile polyp. Hemorrhage occurred more commonly after polypectomy than diagnostic colonoscopy (2.16% versus 0.01%). The syndrome of pain, leukocytosis, and fever after polypectomy does not always represent bowel perforation and may be due to a colonic transmural electrocautery burn. Conservative management in this setting is appropriate.[60]

LAPAROSCOPY

PRINCIPLES

Laparoscopy or peritoneoscopy involves the creation of a pneumoperitoneum and the insertion of a thin telescope through a puncture in the anterior abdominal wall. Additional punctures are commonly used for insertion of probes, biopsy needles, and other instruments. For diagnosis and for guided biopsy, laparoscopy can be performed using local anesthesia

and monitored sedation, similar to other endoscopic procedures. This type of laparoscopy should be differentiated from the operative manipulations involved in laparoscopic cholecystectomy or in gynecologic practice, which require general anesthesia.[61]

During laparoscopy, the anterior peritoneal space is visualized, with a view of the parietal peritoneum on the anterior abdominal wall and the diaphragm.[62] More than two thirds of the liver surface can be examined with the gallbladder, much of the greater omentum, and serosal surfaces of the stomach, small bowel, and colon. The internal pelvic organs can also be visualized. Less completely seen are posterior structures, such as the porta hepatis, pancreas, and spleen. The retroperitoneal lymph nodes and renal system are not evaluable.

INDICATIONS AND RESULTS

The ability to see large areas of parietal and visceral peritoneum and to evaluate the cause of ascites have been major indications for laparoscopy. CT scans have a low yield in imaging small peritoneal metastases. Paracentesis and blind peritoneal biopsy are frequently nondiagnostic. Deposits of even a few millimeters on the peritoneum are readily identified and biopsied at laparoscopy to differentiate between metastatic cancer, mesothelioma, or infections such as tuberculosis.[63]

Because so much of the liver surface can be examined in fine detail, laparoscopy has been used for diagnosis of liver disease and for precision biopsy. Primary and metastatic liver cancer is diagnosed with an accuracy in the range of 90%.[64,65] The ability to see and biopsy small lesions on the liver and peritoneum makes laparoscopy particularly useful in staging the extent of malignant disease. Benign focal conditions, such as fibrosis, cirrhosis, and hemangiomas, can be differentiated from malignant disease with high accuracy. Larger biopsy specimens are obtained at laparoscopy than by scan-guided aspiration biopsy. Enough material can be obtained to permit special histopathologic studies. Direct vision biopsy allows avoidance of vascular areas, and bleeding after biopsy can usually be controlled.[66]

Laparoscopy has been used for preoperative cancer staging, even if CT scans are negative. Experience with laparoscopic staging has been reported in patients with cancer of the pancreas, esophagus, stomach, gallbladder, and rectum.[67-70] Laparoscopy can increase the diagnostic yield of liver biopsy in Hodgkin disease and non-Hodgkin lymphoma.[71-73] Negative CT, ultrasound, or magnetic resonance imaging scans do not exclude the possibility that laparoscopy may detect liver or peritoneal malignancy.[74]

Laparoscopy has been diagnostic in fever of unknown origin, for chronic abdominal pain, after abdominal trauma, and in appendicitis. Examination of the female pelvic organs is a major indication for laparoscopy. Therapeutic and operative maneuver, such as lysis of adhesions, foreign-body removal, and abscess drainage, can be performed.

COMPLICATIONS OF LAPAROSCOPY

Laparoscopy is contraindicated in acute or unstable cardiopulmonary states, although there is a continuum of relative risk in chronic situations. Coagulation disorders that cannot be corrected are contraindications, but mild abnormalities may be acceptable. A history of generalized peritonitis is an absolute contraindication because of multiple dense adhesions, increasing the risk and decreasing the effectiveness of the procedure. Prior abdominal surgery, also associated with adhesions, represents a relative contraindication.[63]

An uncooperative patient should not have laparoscopy under local anesthesia, nor should patients have the procedure performed if skin infections interfere with sterile insertion of the laparoscope or if there are intestinal obstructions and dilated bowel loops. A small amount of ascites does not present a problem, but tense ascites must first be decreased by diuresis or paracentesis.[75]

The overall complication rate from laparoscopy is in the range of 1%, with serious complications delaying discharge or requiring surgery occurring in about 0.2% and with a mortality rate of 0.05%.[63] Subcutaneous emphysema and pneumoomentum are not serious and require no treatment. Mediastinal emphysema, pneumothorax, and air embolism are rare. Abdominal wall bleeding and laceration of blood vessels, organs, or bowel occur uncommonly, but they may require surgical management. Biopsy, especially of the liver, accounts for the most complications. Infection is rare, as is tumor implantation at the insertion site in malignant ascites.[63]

ENDOSCOPIC RETROGRADE CHOLANGIOPANCREATOGRAPHY

DIAGNOSTIC ENDOSCOPIC RETROGRADE CHOLANGIOPANCREATOGRAPHY

The technique of endoscopic retrograde cholangiopancreatography (ERCP) was first reported in 1968 and has been an important diagnostic tool for more than 20 years.[76] The skilled endoscopist working with a cooperative patient can often perform a diagnostic ERCP in less than 20 minutes. Success rates for cannulating the common bile duct and pancreatic duct are greater than 90%.

A side-viewing duodenoscope is used to afford excellent visualization of the ampulla. Cannulization of the ducts is then performed, and a contrast agent such as Renograffin-60 is injected into the desired duct under fluoroscopic control for subsequent x-ray films of the duct anatomy. Material for cytologic evaluation can be obtained from the biliary or pancreatic duct system, and biopsy of the ampulla, duodenum, and stomach can also be performed.

Evaluation of the jaundiced patient is one of the more important indications for ERCP. Noninvasive imaging procedures such as sonography and CT scans should be obtained first in the diagnostic workup. If obstruction of the biliary system is demonstrated, ERCP is then performed to identify the level of the obstruction and the probable cause. ERCP frequently leads directly to a therapeutic procedure: endoscopic sphincterotomy, removing bile duct gallstones, or placement of a biliary stent into the obstructed duct.

ERCP is a sensitive and specific diagnostic test for pancreatic cancer. At Memorial Sloan-Kettering Cancer Center, ERCP had a sensitivity of 92% and a specificity of 97% in the evaluation of 116 patients. For 530 patients with pancreatic cancer, normal pancreatograms were seen in only 15 (2.5%).[77] Typical findings include complete occlusion or stenosis of the main pancreatic duct, narrowing or obstruction of the intrapancreatic portion of the common bile duct, and the "double-duct" sign of stenosis or obstruction of the main

pancreatic duct and the common bile duct. There may also be endoscopic abnormalities, such as a duodenal mass or ulcer, for which biopsies document pancreatic cancer.

ERCP is useful if the patient's symptoms suggest pancreatic cancer but the sonogram or CT scan are equivocal. Frick and colleagues, using ERCP to evaluate 26 patients with indeterminant CT scans, found that ERCP aided the preoperative diagnosis in 25.[78] One pancreatic cancer was missed by ERCP. In an English study of 140 patients with undiagnosed severe chronic abdominal pain, the pancreatogram was abnormal in 25 (18%). For approximately one quarter of the patients, diagnoses were made.[79] These diagnoses included gallstones, peptic ulcer disease, pancreatic cancer, and chronic pancreatitis. ERCP may be difficult to interpret in the setting of chronic pancreatitis, and cancers can be missed.

Although recent studies suggest that ERCP can help in determining tumor size and the prognosis in carcinomas of the head of the pancreas, most clinicians do not use this technique in this way.

THERAPEUTIC ENDOSCOPIC RETROGRADE CHOLANGIOPANCREATOGRAPHY

The therapeutic use of ERCP is rapidly expanding. At Memorial Sloan-Kettering Cancer Center, the number of therapeutic ERCPs doubled during the last 5 years, and they now constitute almost 50% of all ERCPs performed. The major therapeutic procedures performed are endoscopic sphincterotomy and placement of endobiliary stents for the nonsurgical treatment of biliary obstruction.

Endoscopic sphincterotomy is performed by inserting a specialized cannula containing an electrosurgical cutting wire into the distal common bile duct. When an electrical current is passed through the exposed monopolar wire, a controlled incision is made in the sphincter, opening the distal bile duct and allowing the endoscopic removal of bile duct stones or the placement of endobiliary stents. Biopsy of ampullary tumors is facilitated by endoscopic sphincterotomy, and the associated obstructive jaundice may be temporarily relieved by this procedure. Bourgeois and colleagues obtained the correct histologic diagnosis in all 55 patients with periampullary cancer after endoscopic sphincterotomy but in only half before sphincterotomy.[80]

Nonsurgical biliary drainage has become an important tool in the palliative management of patients with malignant biliary obstruction. Endoscopic biliary drainage (EBD) is supplanting percutaneous biliary drainage (PTD) as the initial procedure of choice. A combined approach or rendezvous method has been used in patients for whom EBD has not been successful.[81]

In a prospective, randomized study comparing EBD with PTD in high-risk patients with malignant biliary obstruction, EBD was more successful in relieving jaundice (81% versus 61%) and had a significantly lower 30-day mortality rate (15% versus 33%). The morbidity of EBD was 19% and that with PTD was 67%.[82]

The location or level of the malignant biliary stricture is important in determining success and complication rates with EBD. Seventy patients with malignant hilar strictures were stratified by Deviere and associates into three groups. Twenty patients had common hepatic duct lesions (type I), and 50 patients had bifurcation or intrahepatic strictures (types II and III). Type I patients required only one stent, and their ducts were likely to be completely drained. Approximately 50% of the type II and III patients could have only one stent placed. These patients had a higher 30-day mortality, a higher rate of early cholangitis, a higher death rate from sepsis, and a shorter postprocedure survival than patients in whom adequate drainage was established. Success in adequately draining common bile duct and common hepatic duct strictures should be about 90% with large-bore endoprostheses. The success rate for establishing drainage in bifurcation or intrahepatic strictures in much lower. Using an aggressive approach, with multiple attempts and a combination of percutaneous and endoscopic techniques, the success rate of insertion of two or more stents is about 50% in patients with hilar strictures.[83]

EBD has been prospectively compared with surgical biliary bypass. Fifty-two patients with distal common bile duct obstruction were randomized to EBD or surgical biliary bypass.[84] Survival data for both groups was similar, as was the 90% success rate in relieving jaundice. Patients treated with EBD had a significantly shorter initial hospital (5 versus 13 days; $p < 0.002$). Readmissions to the hospital were more frequent in the EBD group, but the total hospital stay in days per patient until death was less in the EBD group (8 versus 13 days; $p < 0.01$). In patients with pancreatic cancer and jaundice, who are not candidates for surgical resection because of advanced disease or other medical problems, EBD should be the biliary drainage procedure of choice (Figs. 21–6 and 21–7).

COMPLICATIONS OF ENDOSCOPIC RETROGRADE CHOLANGIOPANCREATOGRAPHY

The most common complication of ERCP is cholangitis and sepsis. The rate of cholangitis and sepsis depends on the reason for the ERCP and the underlying pathology. For example,

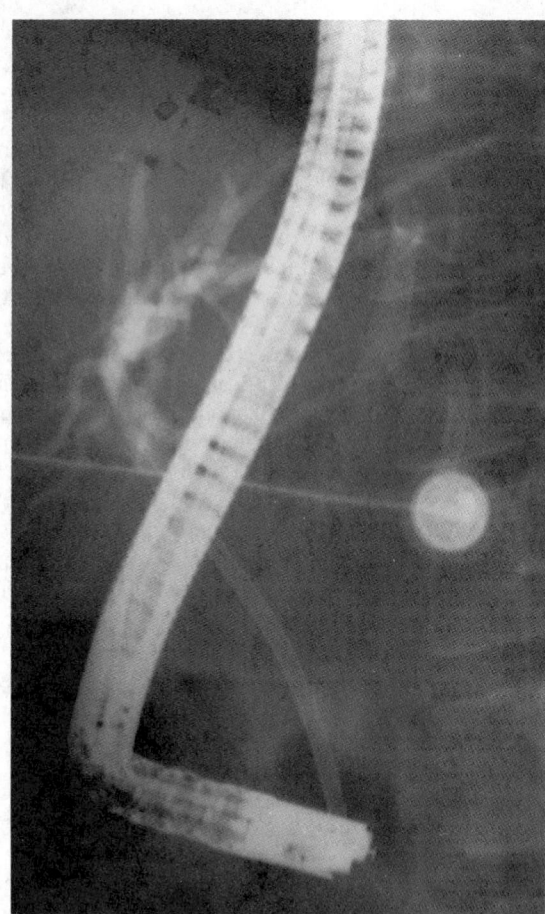

FIGURE 21–7. An endoscopically placed biliary stent is seen in the common bile duct across the malignant stricture shown in Figure 21–6.

therapeutic ERCP done for biliary obstruction may have a sepsis rate as high as 14%.[85]

The level of the biliary obstruction affects the rate of sepsis. In a Memorial Sloan-Kettering Cancer Center series looking at PTD after failed EBD, the rate of sepsis for patients with intrahepatic and bifurcation strictures was significantly greater than for those with common hepatic or common bile duct strictures (75% versus 17%; $p = 0.04$).[86] Another Memorial Sloan-Kettering Cancer Center study reviewed the microbiologic data for septic episodes after EBD and compared them with septic episodes after PTD.[87] Although enteric gram-negative organisms predominated in both groups, there were significantly more gram-positive organisms noted in the PTD group ($p < 0.0005$). Analysis of the antibiotic sensitivities revealed that the combination of ticarcillin clavulanate and gentamicin covered 91% of the EBD organisms.

Acute pancreatitis is another common complication of ERCP, and it is related to the injection of contrast material into the pancreatic duct. It usually occurs in fewer than 7% of patients. It is usually self-limited and rarely presents as a serious clinical problem.

SMALL INTESTINAL ENDOSCOPY: ENTEROSCOPY

Evaluation of the small intestine distal to the third portion of the duodenum was previously done by barium studies and an-

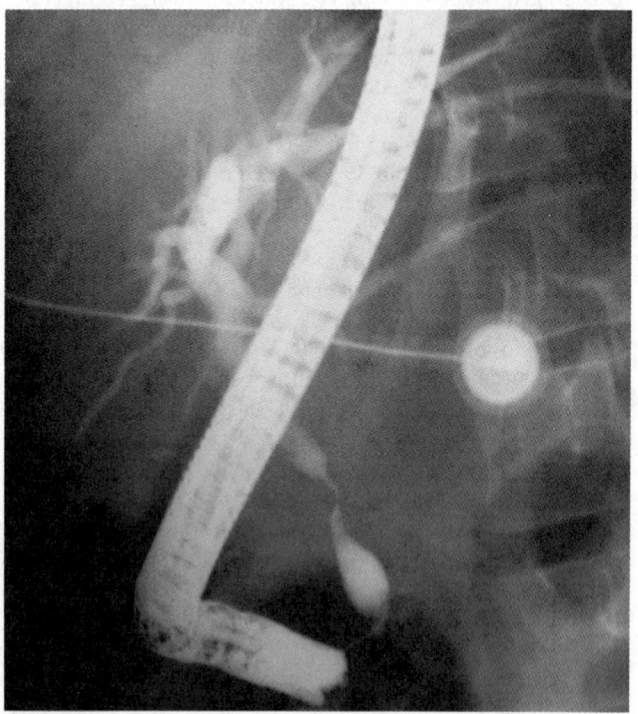

FIGURE 21–6. An endoscopic, retrograde cholangiogram demonstrating a short distal common bile duct stricture caused by a primary bile duct cancer.

giography. Two new endoscopic techniques for studying the small bowel have been developed.

PUSH ENTEROSCOPY

Peroral insertion of a standard disinfected or sterilized colonoscope has been used for endoscopy of the proximal 50 to 60 cm of small bowel. As with colonoscopy, biopsies may be performed for suspect areas. A new dedicated push enteroscope often can be passed rapidly to about 100 cm distal to the ligament of Treitz. Biopsy can be performed through this instrument, but fluoroscopy is often needed to assist its passage.

SONDE-TYPE ENTEROSCOPY

The sonde-type enteroscope is a slender endoscope approximately 2.7 m long. It has an inflatable balloon at its tip that helps in passage through the small intestine. There are several disadvantages to this instrument: no biopsy channel, the need for fluoroscopy, and the 8 hours needed for its use.

The major use for enteroscopy is evaluation of obscure causes of gastrointestinal bleeding. One study of push enteroscopy identified the source of bleeding in 15 (38%) of 39 patients.[88] The most common cause found was an arteriovenous malformation. The diagnostic yield in a study of 35 patients with obscure gastrointestinal bleeding using a sonde enteroscope was 26%.[89] A study of 258 patients identified nine malignant and four benign tumors to be the cause of the obscure bleeding in 13 (5%) patients.[90] In all of these studies, routine x-ray, endoscopic, and radionuclide techniques were negative. As the number of clinical centers offering enteroscopy increases, a more defined role for it can be established.

PERCUTANEOUS ENDOSCOPIC GASTROSTOMY

Since its original description by Ponsky and Gauderer in 1981, percutaneous endoscopic gastrostomy (PEG) has become a routine procedure done in an outpatient setting without general anesthesia in patients unable to take oral feedings or in whom parenteral nutritional support is not feasible.[91] PEG and percutaneous endoscopic jejunostomy (PEJ) placement

are rapid and safe and can eliminate the need for long-term nasal feeding tubes. Although the original use of PEGs was in neurologically impaired adults and children, the potential of this procedure in cancer patients was quickly realized. In one study of 42 patients with dysphagia and cancers of the head and neck, successful placement of PEGs and PEJs were achieved in 39.[92] No immediate complications occurred. After a mean follow-up period of 4.5 months, only 1 patient developed pneumonia, presumed to be caused by aspiration. Complication rates for surgical gastrostomies are reported to be as high as 75%.[93]

In patients who have had previous total or subtotal gastric resections, PEJs may be used. Shike and colleagues demonstrated an 83% success rate with PEJs.[94] The PEJs allowed infusions of significant amounts of fluids and between 900 and 2400 calories per day.

BRONCHOSCOPY

Bronchoscopy (Table 21–1) is the single most useful modality for accurately diagnosing lung cancer. With the advent of fiberoptic equipment introduced more than 20 years ago, this procedure has been used for diagnosis with increasing frequency.[95,96]

INDICATIONS AND RESULTS

The commonest oncologic indication for bronchoscopy is to diagnose and assist in staging lung cancer by direct observation and obtaining cytologic and histologic material for laboratory examination.[97] In investigating other upper aerodigestive tumors, bronchoscopy can rule out extension of laryngeal and esophageal carcinomas to the upper airway. Fiberoptic bronchoscopy has been especially important in identifying occult sites of malignancy if sputum cytology indicates malignant cells.

Therapeutically, bronchoscopy has been extensively used to remove retained secretions in the postoperative period, relieve obstructed airways due to malignancy (in conjunction with laser destruction), and to arrest bleeding. This technique is employed to deliver therapy (*i.e.,* photocoagulation, brachytherapy) in the definitive or palliative treatment of endobronchial malignancies.[98,99]

TABLE 21–1. Comparison of Rigid and Flexible Fiberoptic Bronchoscopy Techniques

Characteristics	*Rigid Bronchoscopy*	*Flexible Fiberoptic Bronchoscopy*
Biopsy	Generous specimen	Minute specimen
Visualization of bronchi	Excellent	Excellent
Visualization of segmental bronchi	With angled lenses only	Excellent
Biopsy of peripheral lesions	No	Yes
Anesthesia required	General	Local
Suctioning of secretions	Excellent	Good
Complications	Perforation and bleeding reported	Rare
Durability of instrument	Durable	Delicate
Training to perform examination	Extensive	Minimal
Management of airway obstruction	Yes	No

The rigid bronchoscope is also used to insert intraluminal stents required to maintain airway patency.

TECHNIQUE
Rigid Bronchoscopy

The open-tube rigid bronchoscope, although used less frequently for diagnosis in recent years, remains a valuable therapeutic tool. It is especially important in controlling airway hemorrhage and is favored by most endoscopists for laser coagulation.

The rigid bronchoscope can be introduced under local anesthesia, but the preferred approach is general anesthesia. Ventilation is maintained by intermittent insufflation through the bronchoscope or by continuous cyclical ventilation through a side port.

The rigid bronchoscope has the advantages of a large lumen, allowing suctioning of blood or fumes developing during laser coagulation and acquisition of larger biopsies (Fig. 21–8).

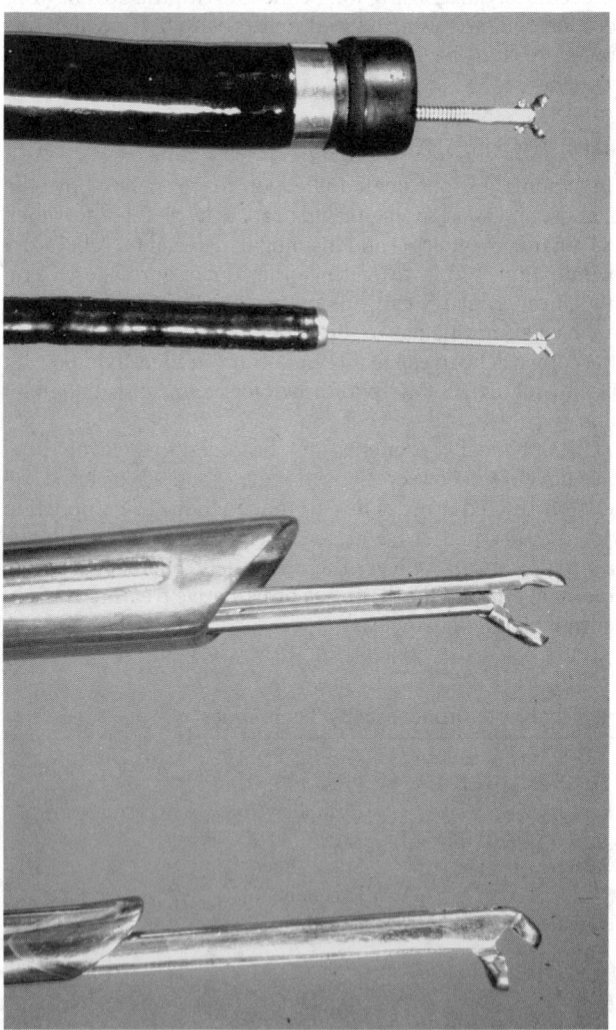

FIGURE 21–8. Comparison of flexible and rigid equipment and of biopsy potential. This photograph illustrates a flexible esophagoscope (*top*), flexible bronchoscope, rigid esophagoscope, and rigid bronchoscope (*bottom*) and the biopsy forceps that can be used with each endoscope.

Flexible Bronchoscopy

With the development of flexible fiberoptic bundles, flexible bronchoscopy has rapidly become the mainstay of endoscopic airway examination. The flexible equipment is small enough to be introduced transnasally or transorally under local anesthesia with or without sedation. Because of its small diameter (≤0.6 cm), the average fiberoptic bronchoscope can enter all segmental orifices of the tracheobronchial tree (Fig. 21–9). Newer instruments with external diameters as small as 2.0 mm can extend the visible range to the periphery of the lung and are being investigated for diagnosing peripheral nodules.[100] Miniaturization of video equipment has allowed endoscopy to improve the resolution and diagnostic abilities.

Most instruments have a suctioning port that is also used to pass brushes and biopsy forceps to obtain pathologic material for examination. The common specimens obtained include regional washings, brushings of observable lesions for exfoliative cytology, and direct biopsies of suspicious mucosal abnormalities.

Wang popularized the technique of transbronchial needle aspiration for diagnosis of malignancy in mediastinal lymph nodes and submucosal lesions inaccessible to direct biopsy or brushing.[101]

Although used less frequently than rigid bronchoscopy for laser coagulation therapy, flexible fibers can be passed through the operating channel for Nd:YAG laser treatment and argon-

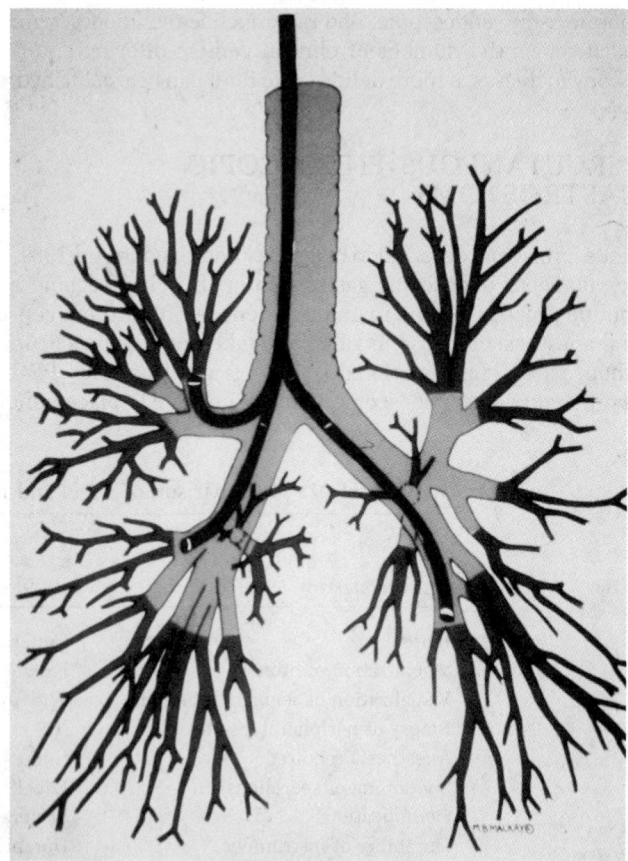

FIGURE 21–9. The range of the flexible bronchoscope within the tracheobronchial tree. The second order of branchings of the tracheobronchial tree can be inspected and biopsied.

beam excitation of hematoporphyrins to induce photocoagulation of malignant tissue.

The versatility and ease of use of the flexible bronchoscope has allowed this procedure to be performed in an out-patient setting with minimal inconvenience to the patient. It is used with increased frequency to aid the diagnosis of suspected lung cancer or other aerodigestive tumors.

THERAPEUTIC BRONCHOSCOPY

Bronchoscopy has been used with success in relieving endobronchial obstruction in dealing with significant airway hemorrhage. Most frequently, rigid bronchoscopy is the technique of choice.

Endobronchial tumors can be mechanically debrided using the tip of the rigid bronchoscope or large biopsy forceps.[109] Newer techniques of tumor coagulation and destruction avoid unnecessary or excessive bleeding. These techniques include cryosurgery, eletrocautery, and carbon dioxide, Nd:YAG, or argon destruction.[110] The lasers require significant training. These techniques are best applied to endobronchial tumors. Extrinsic compression caused by enlarged mediastinal lymph nodes does not respond to this type of treatment.

If extrinsic compression is a major problem, endobronchial stents can be inserted; they are similar to those employed for obstructing esophageal lesions. A variety of Silastic and expanding metallic stents have been devised for this treatment (Fig. 21–10).

Whether endobronchial tumor destruction or stents are used to maintain the airway, longer periods of palliation will be achieved if radiotherapy can be added after these procedures with external-beam radiation or internal brachytherapy.[99] With these newer techniques, approximately 80% of patients can be relieved of their obstructing symptoms for a median of 3 months.

Photodynamic therapy (*i.e.,* photoactivation of malignant cells using hematoporphyrin derivatives) has been employed to destroy endobronchial tumors. This technique is most applicable to in situ carcinoma and is effective in totally destroying tumors in approximately 50% of patients.[98] It can also be employed to destroy inoperable tumors obstructing the airway.[111] Most tumors respond to this therapy to some degree, and as many as 90% of patients achieve some palliation.

COMPLICATIONS OF BRONCHOSCOPY

The complications of rigid and flexible bronchoscopy are minimal, with fewer than 1.0% of patients experiencing any significant problems. Rigid bronchoscopy has the disadvantage of trauma to the teeth, lips, mouth, and larynx, which is usually avoided by using flexible fiberoptic bronchoscopy. Biopsy of lesions can lead to hemorrhage, although rarely excessive.[106] As with any other surgical procedure, care must be taken to select patients and avoid unnecessary hemorrhage. Transbronchial biopsy can lead to pneumothorax, albeit rarely, if routine precautions are taken to avoid a biopsy of the extreme

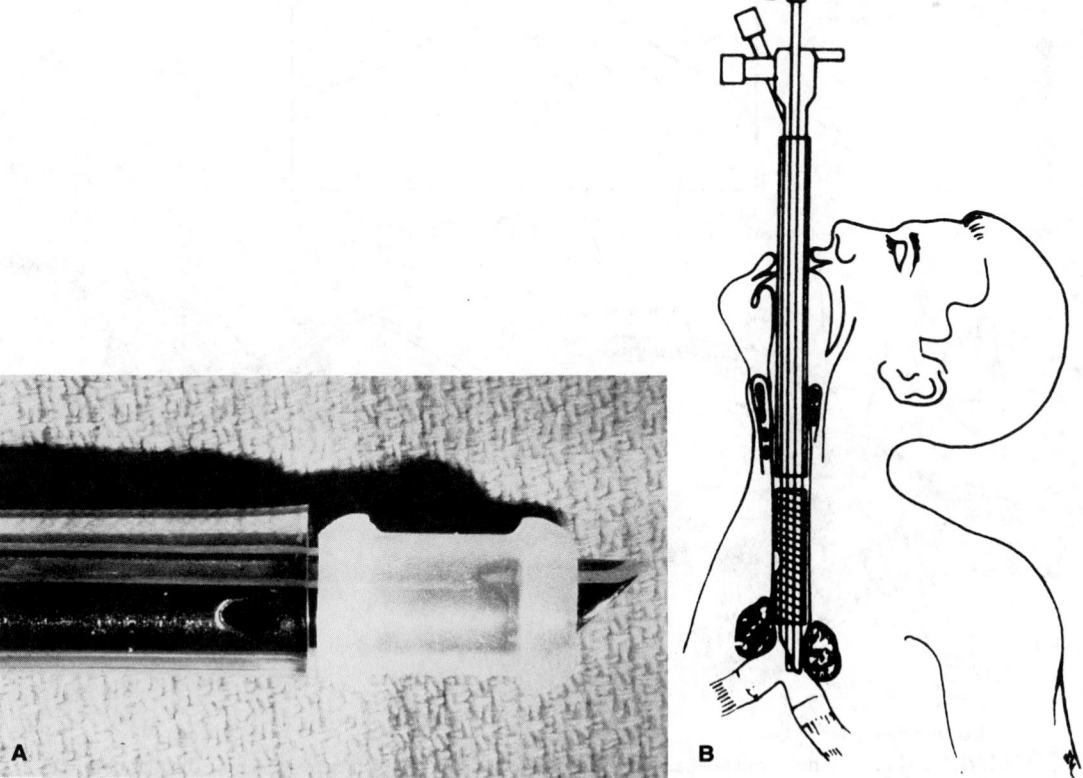

FIGURE 21–10. **(A)** An endobronchial stent "loaded" on the end of a rigid bronchoscope uses a chest tube as an inserter. **(B)** Illustration of the usefulness of an endobronchial stent in extrinsic compression.

periphery of the lung. Complications related to monitored sedation or general anesthesia can occur when these are used.

At the Cleveland Clinic, only 58 episodes of bleeding occurred in almost 7000 flexible bronchoscopies. Transbronchial biopsy showed a higher incidence of bleeding. No deaths ensued.[106] In two large series of bronchoscopies, the death rate was 0.1 and 0.3%.[107,108]

MEDIASTINOSCOPY

INDICATIONS

Mediastinoscopy is used most frequently to obtain lymph nodes from the superior mediastinum to assist in clinical staging. It is extremely valuable in identifying metastatic malignancy in these lymph nodes, providing histologic evidence of N2 and N3 (stage IIIA and IIIB) disease during the investigation of patients with lung cancer.[102] Less frequently, this technique is used to diagnose malignancies of the superior mediastinum presenting with mediastinal adenopathy. Lymphoma, primary lung cancers with mediastinal involvement, and a host of benign lesions can be diagnosed by this technique.

The procedure can also be used to identify mediastinal invasion by primary tumor and, by extending the mediastinal dissection, can biopsy lesions in the anterior mediastinum. Either pleural space can be entered through the mediastinum to detect abnormalities, especially in the paramediastinal regions.

TECHNIQUE

The technique of mediastinoscopy (Fig. 21–11) is simple and safe in the hands of well-qualified thoracic surgeons. A short suprasternal transverse incision is made, dissecting down to the pretracheal fascia, which is opened. Finger dissection in the paratracheal plane precedes the insertion of the mediastinoscope. Direct visualization of all areas of the superior mediastinum enables biopsies of the various mediastinal nodal stations.

Mediastinoscopy is performed under general anesthesia but can be performed on an out-patient basis. Frequently, it is employed just before thoracotomy for final clinical staging in patients suspected of harboring inoperable disease because of mediastinal spread.

RESULTS

Because of the ability to directly biopsy mediastinal lymph nodes, the accuracy of mediastinoscopy approaches 90% in staging the mediastinal involvement of lymph nodes in lung cancer.[103] Virtually no false-positive examinations occur. Because of the inaccessibility of certain areas of the medias-

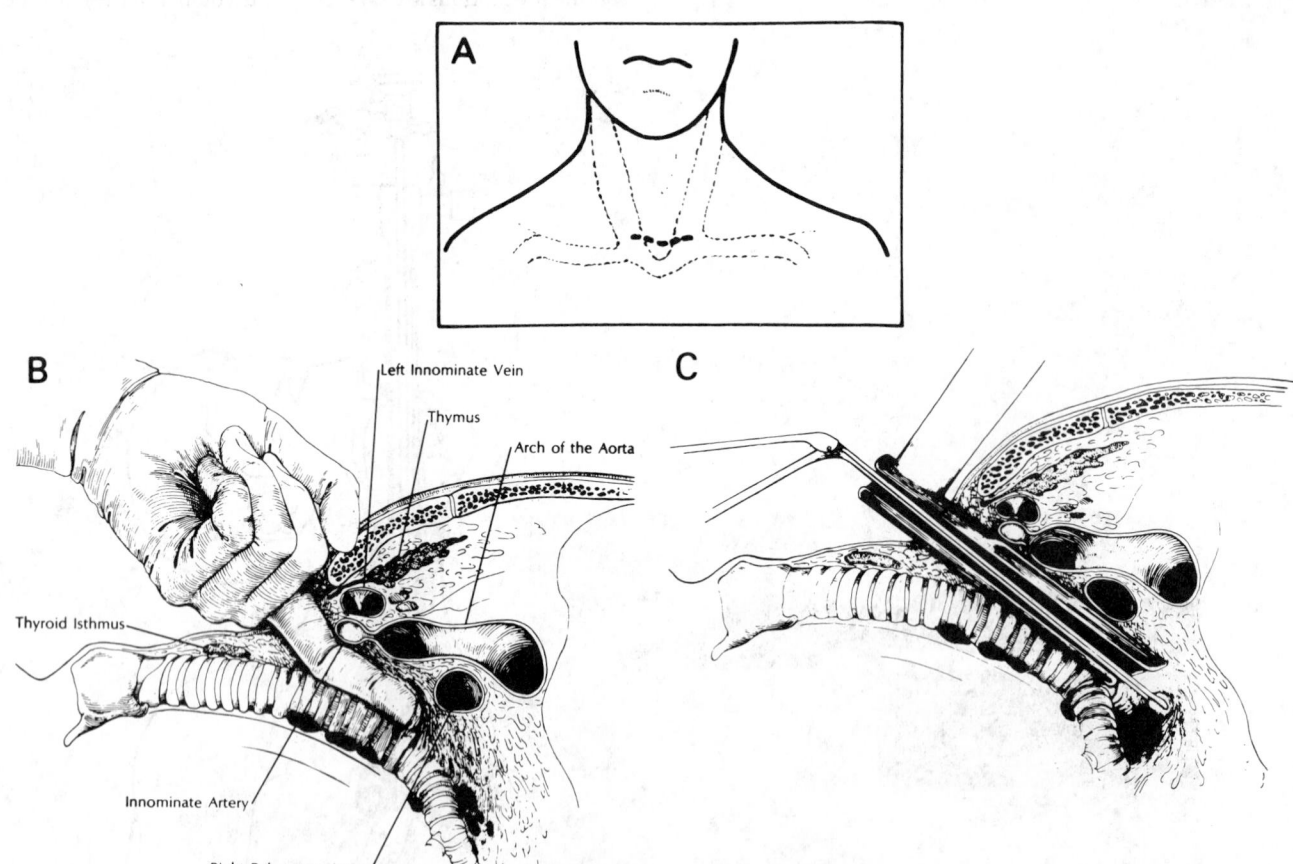

FIGURE 21–11. Technique of mediastinoscopy. **(A)** Make a 3- to 4-cm incision just above the manubrium. **(B)** Use the finger to dissect bluntly the loose fibrofatty tissue in front of the trachea down to the level of the pulmonary artery. **(C)** Introduce the endoscope, and take biopsies of suspicious tissues. Needle aspiration of structures before biopsy help to reduce hemorrhagic complications. (Modified from Kerschner PA. Transcervical approach to the superior mediastinum. Hosp Pract 1970;5:61–70)

tinum, a 10% false-negative rate can be expected. However, the inaccessible mediastinal lymph nodes are usually resectable at the time of surgery. If mediastinoscopy fails to reveal metastatic disease in patients with otherwise operable lung cancer, the resectability rate approaches 95%. Mediastinoscopy remains the most accurate method of assessing mediastinal involvement by lung cancer and remains a valuable tool in diagnosing other superior mediastinal lesions.

THORACOSCOPY

Until recently, thoracoscopy (pleuroscopy) was used to investigate and treat pleural effusions after simple thoracentesis failed. In most instances, open-tube instruments (*e.g.*, mediastinoscope) were used for inspection and biopsy. The use of thoracoscopy has been extended significantly with the introduction of miniaturized video equipment and improved instruments. Learning from the experience developed with laparoscopic surgery, thoracoscopic surgery has become a burgeoning enterprise.[104,105] As surgeons further explore the latitude of this procedure, thoracoscopy will be employed for diagnosis of pleural disease, assessing mediastinal spread of lung cancer, diagnosing lung disease and peripheral nodules, and excision of peripheral nodules. The newly developed thoracoscopic techniques can allow partial and total lung resection and dissection of mediastinal structures (*e.g.*, esophagus, thymus gland, mediastinal lymph nodes). The ultimate indications for video-assisted thoracoscopy await further investigation.

TECHNIQUE

Simple thoracoscopy can be performed using a small incision and inserting an open-tube scope (*e.g.*, mediastinoscope) for removal of fluid and simple biopsy of abnormal lesions on the pleural surface. Video-assisted thoracoscopy requires three to four small intercostal incisions and the development of a pneumothorax using one-lung anesthesia and inserting multiple trocars to allow the introduction of a videoscope plus a variety of instruments for surgical dissection. With this technique, the total visceral and parietal pleural surfaces can be examined and biopsied; the mediastinum can be entered, dissected, and biopsied; and portions of the lung can be removed, taking advantage of mechanical stapling devices.

INDICATIONS AND RESULTS

Thoracoscopy is an excellent tool for diagnosing pleural disease. Pleural lesions of the lung can be resected for diagnosis, avoiding a major thoracotomy and its attendant morbidity. Hospital stays are shortened, diminishing the use of expensive medical resources. The results of thoracoscopic resection for oncologic disease have yet to be determined. In employing this technique for cancer treatment, surgeons must be wary of inadequate resections.

REFERENCES

1. Takasu S. Recent advances in endoscopic diagnosis of esophagogastric cancer. In: Oguro Y, Takagi K, eds. Endoscopic approaches to cancer diagnosis and treatment. London: Taylor & Francis, 1990:19–27.

2. Winawer SJ, Posner G, Lightdale CJ, Fortner JG, Sherlock P, Melamed M. Endoscopic diagnosis of advanced gastric cancer. Factors influencing yield. Gastroenterology 1975;69:1183–1187.
3. Silvis SE, Nebel O, Rogers G, Sugawa C, Mandelstam P. Endoscopic complications. Results of the 1974 ASGE survey. JAMA 1976;235:928–930.
4. Iishi H, Yamamoto R, Tatsuta M, Okuda S. Evaluation of fine needle aspiration biopsy under direct vision gastrofiberscopy in diagnosis of diffusely infiltrative carcinoma of the stomach. Cancer 1986;57:1365–1369.
5. Lightdale CJ, Winawer SJ. Screening diagnosis and staging of esophageal cancer. Semin Oncol 1984;11:101–112.
6. Li FP, Shiang EL. Screening for esophageal cancer in 62,000 Chinese. Lancet 1979;2:804.
7. Yang CS. Research on esophageal cancer in China: A review. Cancer Res 1980;40:2633–2644.
8. Jacob P, Kahrilas PJ, Desai T, et al. Natural history and significance of esophageal squamous cell dysplasia. Cancer 1990;65:2731–2739.
9. Shiozaki H, Tahara H, Kobayashi K, et al. Endoscopic screening of early esophageal cancer with the Lugol dye method in patients with head and neck cancers. Cancer 1990;66:2068–2071.
10. Kaibara N, Kawaguchi H, Nishidoi H, et al. Significance of mass survey for gastric cancer from the standpoint of surgery. Am J Surg 1981;142:543–545.
11. Blot WJ, Devesa SS, Kneller RW, Fraumeni JF Jr. Rising incidence of adenocarcinoma of the esophagus and gastric cardia. JAMA 1991;265:1287–1289.
12. Green PHR, O'Toole KM, Slonim D, Wang T. Increasing incidence and excellent survival of patients with early gastric cancer: Experience in a United States medical center. Am J Med 1988;85:658–661.
13. Hallissey MT, Allum WH, Jewkes AJ, Ellis DJ, Fielding JW. Early detection of gastric cancer. Br Med J 1990;301:513–515.
14. Craanen ME, Dekker W, Ferwerda J, Blok P, Tytgat GNJ. Early gastric cancer: A clinicopathologic study. J Clin Gastroenterol 1991;13:274–283.
15. Kurtz RC, Sternberg SS, Miller H, DeCosse JJ. Upper gastrointestinal neoplasia in familial polyposis. Dig Dis Sci 1987;32:459–465.
16. Bown SG. Palliation of malignant dysphagia: Surgery, radiotherapy, laser, intubation alone or in combination. Gut 1991;32:841–844.
17. Lightdale CJ, Zimbalist E, Winawer SJ. Outpatient management of esophageal cancer with endoscopic Nd:YAG Laser. Am J Gastroenterol 1987;82:46–50.
18. Hamilton FA, Benjamin SB, Castell DO. Proceedings of the Consensus Conference in Therapeutic Endoscopy in Bleeding Ulcers. Gastrointest Endosc 1990;36:S1–S69.
19. Lightdale CJ, Kurtz RC, Boyle CC, Sherlock P, Winawer SJ. Cancer and upper gastrointestinal tract hemorrhage. Benign causes of bleeding demonstrated by endoscopy. JAMA 1973;226:139–141.
20. Eras P, Goldstein MJ, Sherlock P. *Candida* infection of the gastrointestinal tract. Medicine (Baltimore) 1972;51:367–379.
21. Lightdale CJ, Wolf DJ, Marcucci RA, Aalyer WR. Herpetic esophagitis in patients with cancer: Ante mortem diagnosis by brush cytology. Cancer 1977;39:223–226.
22. Tio TL, Tytgat GNJ. Atlas of transintestinal ultrasonography. Aalsmeer, The Netherlands: Drukkenj Mur Kostverloren BV, 1986.
23. Kawai K, ed. Endoscopic ultrasonography in gastroenterology. Tokyo: Igaku-Shoin, 1988.
24. Sivak MV Jr, Boyce GA, eds. Endoscopic ultrasonography. Gastrointest Endosc 1990;36: S1–S46.
25. Kimmey MB, Martin RW, Haggitt RC, Wang KY, Franklin DW, Silverstein FE. Histologic correlates of gastrointestinal ultrasound images. Gastroenterology 1989;96:433–441.
26. Tio TL, Coene PPLO, Schouwink MH, Tytgat GNJ. Esophagogastric carcinoma: Preoperative TNM classification with endosonography. Radiology 1989;173:411–417.
27. Botet JF, Lightdale CJ, Zauber AG, Gerdes H, Urmacher C, Brennan MF. Preoperative staging of esophageal cancer: Comparison of endoscopic US and dynamic CT. Radiology 1991;181:419–425.
28. Botet JF, Lightdale CJ, Zauber AG, et al. Preoperative staging of gastric cancer: Comparison of endoscopic US and dynamic CT. Radiology 1991;181:426–432.
29. Rosch T, Lorenz R, Suchy R, Dancygier H, Classen M. Colonic endoscopic ultrasonography: First results of a new technique. Gastrointest Endosc 1990;36:382–386.
30. Tio TL, Tytgat GNJ. Comparison of blind transrectal ultrasonography with endoscopic transrectal ultrasonography in assessing rectal and perirectal disease. Scand J Gastroenterol 1986;21(suppl 123):104–111.
31. Lightdale CJ, Botet JF, Kelsen DP, Turnbull AD, Brennan MF. Diagnosis of recurrent upper gastrointestinal cancer at the surgical anastomosis by endoscopic ultrasound. Gastrointest Endosc 1989;35:407–412.
32. Yasuda K, Nakajima M, Yoshida S, Kiyota K, Kawai K. The diagnosis of submucosal tumors of the stomach by endoscopic ultrasonography. Gastrointest Endosc 1989;35:10–15.
33. Tio TL, den Hartog Jager FCA, Tytgat GNJ. Endoscopic ultrasonography of non-Hodgkin lymphoma of the stomach. Gastroenterology 1986;91:401–408.
34. Yasuda K, Mukai H, Fujimoto S, Nakajima M, Kawai K. The diagnosis of pancreatic cancer by endoscopic ultrasonography. Gastrointest Endosc 1988;34:1–8.
35. Lees WR. Endoscopic ultrasonography of chronic pancreatitis and pancreatic pseudocysts. Scand J Gastroenterol 1986;21(suppl 123):123–29.
36. Rosch T, Lorenz R, Braig C, et al. Endoscopic ultrasound in pancreatic tumor diagnosis. Gastrointest Endosc 1991;37:347–352.
37. Tio TL, Cheng J, Wijers OB, Sars PRA, Tytgat GNJ. Endosonographic TNM staging of extrahepatic bile duct cancer: Comparison with pathological staging. Gastroenterology 1991;100:1351–1361.
38. Lightdale CJ, Botet JF, Woodruff JM, Brennan MF. Localization of endocrine tumors of the pancreas with endoscopic ultrasonography. Cancer 1991;68:1815–1820.

39. Schottenfeld D, Winawer SJ. Large intestine. In: Schottenfeld D, Fraumeni JF, eds. Cancer epidemiology and prevention. Philadelphia: WB Saunders, 1982.

40. Selby JV, Friedman GD, Quesenberry CP, Weiss NS. A case-control study of screening sigmoidoscopy and mortality from colorectal cancer. N Engl J Med 1992;326:653–657.

41. Winawer SJ, Kerner JF. Sigmoidoscopy: Case finding versus screening. Gastroenterology 1988;95:527–530.

42. American Cancer Society. Guidelines for the cancer-related checkup: Recommendations and rationale. CA 1980;34:130–176.

43. Winawer SJ, Leidner SD, Kurtz RC. Comparison of flexible sigmoidoscopy with other diagnostic techniques in the diagnosis of colorectal neoplasia. Dig Dis Sci 1979;24:277–281.

44. Baskin WN, Greenlaw RL, Fraker JT, et al. Flexible sigmoidoscopy training for primary care physicians. Gastrointest Endosc 1984;30:141–146.

45. Traul DG, Davis CB, Pollock JC, et al. Flexible fiberoptic sigmoidoscopy—the Monroe Clinic experience. A prospective study of 5000 examinations. Dis Colon Rectum 1983;26:161–166.

46. Marks G, Moses ML. The clinical application of flexible fiberoptic colonoscopy. Surg Clin North Am 1973;53:735–756.

47. Hunt RH. The role of colonoscopy in complicated diverticular disease. Acta Chir Belg 1979;78:349–353.

48. Brand EJ, Sullivan BH Jr, Sivak MV Jr, et al. Colonoscopy in the diagnosis of unexplained rectal bleeding. Ann Surg 1980;192:111–113.

49. Tedesco FJ, Waye JD, Raskin JB, et al. Colonoscopic evaluation of rectal bleeding. Ann Intern Med 1978;89:907–1002.

50. Winawer SJ, Schottenfeld D, Flehinger BJ. Colorectal cancer screening. JNCI 1991;83:243–253.

51. Fowler DL, Hedberg SE. Follow-up colonoscopy after polypectomy. Gastrointest Endosc [Abstract] 1980;26:67.

52. Winawer SJ, Zauber A, Diaz B, et al. The National Polyp Study: Overview of program and preliminary report of patient and polyp characteristics. In: Steele G, Burt R, Winawer SJ, Karr J, eds. Basic and clinical perspectives of colorectal polyps and cancer. New York: Alan R. Liss, 1988.

53. Butt J, Lennard-Jones JE, Ritchie J. A practical approach to the cancer risk in inflammatory bowel disease. Med Clin North Am 1980;64:1203–1220.

54. Waye JD. Screening for cancer in ulcerative colitis. Front Gastrointest Res 1986;10:243–256.

55. Burt RW, Bishop DT, Cannon LA, et al. Dominant inheritance of adenomatous colonic polyps and colorectal cancer. N Engl J Med 1985;312:1540–1544.

56. Cannon-Albright LA, Skolnick MH, Bishop T, et al. Common inheritance of susceptibility to colonic adenomatous polyps and associated colorectal cancers. N Engl J Med 1988;319:533–537.

57. Rex DK, Lehman GA, Hawes RH, et al. Screening colonoscopy in asymptomatic average-risk persons with negative fecal occult blood test. Gastroenterology 1991;100:64–67.

58. Lightdale CJ. India ink colonic tattoo: Blots on the record. Gastrointest Endosc 1991;37:99–100.

59. Gilbert GA, Hallstrom AP, Shaneyfelt SL, et al. The national ASGE colonoscopy survey: Complications of colonoscopy. Gastrointest Endosc [Abstract] 1984;30:156.

60. Waye JD. The post-polypectomy coagulation syndrome. Gastrointest Endosc 1981;27:184.

61. Lightdale CJ: Laparoscopy in gastroenterologic practice. In: Sherlock P, Jerzy-Glass G, eds. Progress in gastroenterology. New York: Grune & Stratton, 1983;461–475.

62. Beck K: Color atlas of laparoscopy. Philadelphia: WB Saunders, 1984.

63. Lightdale CJ. Indications, contraindications and complications of laparoscopy. In: Sivak M, ed. Gastroenterological endoscopy. Philadelphia: WB Saunders, 1987:1030.

64. Lightdale CJ, Winawer SJ, Kurtz RC, Knapper WH. Laparoscopic diagnosis of suspected liver neoplasms. Value of prior liver scans. Dig Dis Sci 1979;24:588–593, 1979.

65. Riemann JF. Peritoneoscopy in the diagnosis of liver metastases. In: Weiss L, Gilbert H, eds. Liver metastasis. Boston: Hall Medical Publishers, 1982;244–254.

66. Boyce HW Jr. Laparoscopy. In: Schiff L, Schiff ER, eds. Diseases of the liver. 6th ed. Philadelphia: JB Lippincott, 1987;443–456.

67. Warshaw AL, Tepper JE, et al. Laparoscopy in staging and planning of therapy for pancreatic cancer. Am J Surg 1986;151:76.

68. Dagnini G, Martin G, et al. Laparoscopy in the diagnosis of primary carcinoma of the gall bladder. Gastrointest Endosc 1984;30:289.

69. Dagini G, Caldironi MW, et al. Laparoscopy in abdominal staging of esophageal carcinoma. Gastrointest Endosc 1986;32:400.

70. Kriplani AK, Kapur ML. Laparoscopy for preoperative staging and assessment of operability in gastric carcinoma. Gastrointest Endosc 1991;37:441–443.

71. Devita VT, Bagley CM, Goodell B, et al. Peritoneoscopy in the staging of Hodgkin's disease. Cancer Res 31:1746–1750, 1971.

72. Coleman M, Lightdale, CJ, Vinciguerra VP, et al. Peritoneoscopy in Hodgkin's disease. Confirmation of results by laparotomy. JAMA 1976;236:2634–2636.

73. Chabner BA, Johnson RE, Young RC, et al. Sequential nonsurgical and surgical staging of non-Hodgkin's lymphoma. Ann Intern Med 85:149–154.

74. Brady PG, Pebbles M, Goldschmid S. Role of laparoscopy in the evaluation of patients with suspected hepatic or peritoneal malignancy. Gastrointest Endosc 1991;37:27–30.

75. Vilardell F, Seres I, Marti-Vicente A: Complications of peritoneoscopy: A survey of 1455 examinations. Gastrointest Endosc 1968;14:178–180, 1968.

76. McCune WS, Short PE, Moscovitz H. Endoscopic cannulation of the ampulla of Vater. Ann Surg 1968;167:752–756.

77. Freeney PC. Radiology of the pancreas: Two decades of progress in imaging and intervention. AJR 1988;150:975–981.

78. Frick MP, Feinberg SB, Goodale RL. The value of endoscopic retrograde cholangiopancreatography in patients with suspected carcinoma of the pancreas and indeterminant computed tomographic results. Surg Gynecol Obstet 1982;155:177–182.

79. Ruddell WSJ, Linott DJ, Axon ATR. The diagnostic yield of ERCP in the investigation of unexplained abdominal pain. Br J Surg 1983:70:74–75.

80. Bourgeois N, Dunham F, Verhest A, et al. Endoscopic biopsies of the ampulla of Vater at the time of endoscopic sphincterotomy: Difficulties in interpretation. Gastrointest Endosc 1984;30:163–166.

81. Dowsett JF, Vaira D, Hatfield ARW, et al. Endoscopic biliary therapy using the combined percutaneous and endoscopic technique. Gastroenterology 1989;96:1180–1186.

82. Speer A, Russell RCG, Hatfield A, et al. Randomized trial of endoscopic vs percutaneous stent insertion for malignant obstructive jaundice. Lancet 1987;2:57–61.

83. Deviere J, Baize M, de Toeuf J, et al. Long-term follow-up of patients with hilar malignant strictures treated by endoscopic biliary drainage. Gastrointest Endosc 1988;34:95–101.

84. Sheperd HA, Royle G, Ross APR, et al. Endoscopic biliary endoprosthesis in the palliation of malignant obstruction of the distal common bile duct: A randomized trial. Br J Surg 1988;75:1166–1168.

85. Kurtz, RC. Preoperative biliary decompression. In: Jacobson IM, ed. ERCP: Diagnostic and therapeutic applications. New York: Elsevier, 1989.

86. Kurtz RC, Botet JB, Gerdes H, et al: Percutaneous biliary drainage following failed endoscopic drainage in malignant biliary obstruction. Gastroenterology [Abstract] 1988;34:A189.

87. Levine JG, Kurtz RC, Botet J. Microbiological analysis of sepsis complicating nonsurgical biliary drainage in malignant obstruction. Gastrointest Endosc 1990;36:364–368.

88. Foutch PG, Sawyer R, Sanowski RA. Push enteroscopy for diagnosis of patients with gastrointestinal bleeding of obscure origin. Gastrointest Endosc 1990;36:337–340.

89. Gostout CJ, Schroeder KW, Burton DD. Small bowel enteroscopy: An early experience in gastrointestinal bleeding of unknown origin. Gastrointest Endosc 1991;37:5–8.

90. Lewis BS, Kornbluth A, Waye JD. Small bowel tumors: Yield of enteroscopy. Gut 1991;32:763–765.

91. Ponsky JL, Gauderer MWL. Percutaneous endoscopic gastrostomy: A non-operative technique for feeding gastrostomy. Gastrointest Endosc 1981;27:9–11.

92. Shike M, Berner YN, Gerdes H, et al. Percutaneous endoscopic gastrostomy and jejunostomy for long-term feeding in patients with cancer of the head and neck. Otolaryngol Head Neck Surg 1989;101:549–554.

93. Wasiljew BK, Ujiki GT, Beal JM. Feeding gastrostomy: Complications and mortality. Am J Surg 1982;143:194–195.

94. Shike M, Schroy P, Ritchie MA, et al. Percutaneous endoscopic jejunostomy in cancer patients with previous gastric resection. Gastrointest Endosc 1987;33:372–374.

95. Ikeda S, Eni Yanai T, Ishikawa S. Flexible bronchofiberscope. Keio J Med 1968;17:1–118.

96. Zavala DC, Richardson RH, Mukerjee PK, et al. Use of the bronchofiberscope for bronchial brush biopsy: Diagnostic results and comparisons with other brushing techniques. Chest 1973;63:889–892.

97. Shure D. Fiberoptic bronchoscopy: Diagnostic application. Clin Chest Med 1987;8:1–13.

98. Cortese DA. Bronchoscopic photodynamic therapy of early lung cancer. Chest 1986;90:629–631.

99. Seagren SL, Harrell JH, Horn RA. High-dose-rate intraluminal irradiation in recurrent endobronchial carcinoma. Chest 1985;88:810–814.

100. Tanaka M, Kawanami O, Satoh M. Endoscopic observation of peripheral airway lesions. Chest 1988;93:228–233.

101. Wang KP, Marsh BR, Summer WR, et al. Transbronchial needle aspiration for diagnosis of lung cancer. Chest 1980;80:48–50.

102. Ginsberg RJ. Evaluation of the mediastinum by invasive techniques. Surg Clin North Am 1987;67:1025–1035.

103. Luke WP, Pearson FG, Todd TRJ, et al. Prospective evaluation of mediastinoscopy for assessment of carcinoma of the lung. J Thorac Cardiovasc Surg 1986;91:553–556.

104. Nathanson LK. Basic instrumentation and operative technique for laparoscopic surgery. In: Cuschieri A, ed. Laparoscopic biliary surgery. London: Blackwell Scientific, 1990: 33.

105. Nathanson LK, Shimi SM, Wood RAB, Cuschieri A. Video thoracoscopic ligation of bulla and pleurectomy for spontaneous pneumothorax. Ann Thorac Surg 1991;52:316–319.

106. Cordasco EM, Mehta AC, Ahmad M. Bronchoscopically induced bleeding—a summary of 9 years' Cleveland clinical experience and review of a literature. Chest 1991;100:1141–1147.

107. Credle WF, Smiddy JF, Elliot RC. Complications of fiberoptic bronchoscopy. Ann Rev Respir Dis 1974;109:67–72.

108. Surratt DM, Smiddy JF, Bruber B. Deaths and complications associated with fiberoptic bronchoscopy. Chest 1976;69:747–751.

109. Mathisen DJ, Grillo HC. Endoscopic relief of malignant airway obstruction. Ann Thorac Surg 1989;48:469–473.

110. Goldberg M. Endoscopic laser for bronchogenic carcinomas. Surg Clin North Am 1988;68:635–644.

111. McCaughan JS, Williams TE Jr, Bethel BH. Photodynamic therapy of endobronchial tumors. Lasers Surg Med 1986;6:336–345.

RONALD A. CASTELLINO
ROBERT L. DELAPAZ
STEVEN M. LARSON

SECTION **2**

Imaging Techniques in Cancer

This chapter provides an overview of the currently available imaging modalities, highlights their advantages and disadvantages, and discusses their use in the management of cancer patients. The recommendations for using diagnostic imaging studies for specific tumors are addressed in other chapters.

Medical imaging is less than 100 years old. It has undergone major technologic enhancements during the past 25 years, resulting in markedly improved anatomic and physiologic information about sites previously inaccessible to the diagnostic imaging process. Therefore, although chest radiographs allow evaluation of the contours between the mediastinum and the aerated lung, computed tomography (CT) and magnetic resonance (MR) scans depict the structures that lie within this envelope, such as cardiac chambers, great vessels, lymph nodes, and the thymus. Likewise, although an upper gastrointestinal study provides indirect evidence about the size of the pancreas and subselective arteriography provides a more detailed assessment of pancreatic vascular anatomy, cross-sectional imaging techniques depict with great success the contour and internal texture of this elusive retroperitoneal organ.

There are frequently several diagnostic imaging tests that can be used to evaluate an organ or anatomic region, but at times, there is no agreement about which test is superior in its diagnostic accuracy and in which sequence the various tests should be used. Patients commonly undergo duplicate studies because of this uncertainty. Because significant improvements in these emerging technologies occur with surprising frequency, comparative clinical studies evaluating the accuracy of these technologies are quickly outdated.

Technologic innovations in diagnostic imaging studies have been remarkable and have been accompanied by enormous gains in the more precise evaluation of specific organs and anatomic regions. However, one must understand the limitations and advantages of these techniques for the best use of this information for patient management.

Close interaction between the diagnostic radiologist and the attending physician should provide the optimal environment for the judicious use of diagnostic radiology and nuclear medicine testing. A general understanding of the physical principles related to how images are generated by the various technologies is important to understand what inherent information (besides anatomy) such images may contain. The oncologist ordering an imaging study should define specific questions that need to be answered, in order to more appropriately choose and sequence the various imaging tests available. An understanding of the descriptive terms defining "accuracy" in diagnostic imaging is necessary to apply the information to patient management. These issues and other broad aspects of the diagnostic imaging process are presented in this chapter.

EXPECTATION VERSUS REALITY

The physical examination was once the only method for evaluating the physical status of a patient. Diagnostic imaging tests have greatly extended this assessment by displaying the structure and function of sites not evaluable by palpation, percussion, or auscultation. The increasing use of other types of diagnostic studies like endoscopy further extends the physical examination by employing sophisticated instrumentation. With endoscopy, the anatomy is directly "imaged" with visible light and recorded by the eye. Diagnostic radiotherapy and nuclear medicine studies use other radiant energy, such as x-rays, γ rays, ultrasound waves, and radiofrequency signals, which are recorded with film, scintillation counters, ultrasound transducers, or radiofrequency coils (Fig. 21–12).

With continued improvement of spatial resolution generated by current imaging technologies, there appear to be increased expectations by attending physicians of perfection of the imaging examination. Unfortunately, however, this is often not necessarily the case. It is understandable that expectations are raised based on the clarity of the generated images, and, to some extent, this has been contributed to by high levels of enthusiasm from groups who are positioned, by their access to emerging imaging technologies, to initially evaluate these techniques in a clinical setting. Furthermore, highly precise demonstration of lesions that frequently cannot be detected even at open surgical procedures by external palpation of the organ, tends to generate unrealistic levels of confidence that such information always provides meaningful information for managing the patient.

This understandable enthusiasm must be tempered, however, by constantly remembering that although a lesion may be depicted with a high degree of accuracy regarding size and location, the etiology of the lesion is frequently impossible to predict with the confidence levels sufficient to influence patient care (Fig. 21–13). Increasingly, the diagnostic radiology community is attempting to characterize lesions encountered on imaging studies in order to provide a higher level of confidence regarding the precise etiology of such lesions.

Observations made on imaging studies can be used to evaluate patients in much the same way that findings from the history and physical examination of the patient and laboratory data are assessed by the clinician to arrive at a diagnosis and develop a therapeutic plan. Similar criteria are used to determine that lymph nodes are pathologic by physical examination (*e.g.*, nodal enlargement, textural changes, fixation to adjacent tissues) and by imaging studies (*e.g.*, nodal enlargement based on "textural" changes determined by areas of nonhomogeneity on CT and ultrasound, or signal changes on magnetic resonance imaging [MRI] pulse sequences). Within the context of the known presentation and progression of the disease, this information is accepted as useful for patient management decisions. Only after these sites are subjected to biopsy and microscopic examination is it possible to determine the accuracy of the examination. Imaging studies are increasingly subjected to histopathologic confirmation to determine accuracy.

Pushing evaluation techniques to detect earlier stages of disease increases the number of false-positive results. However, adjusting the criteria to reduce the false-positive rate

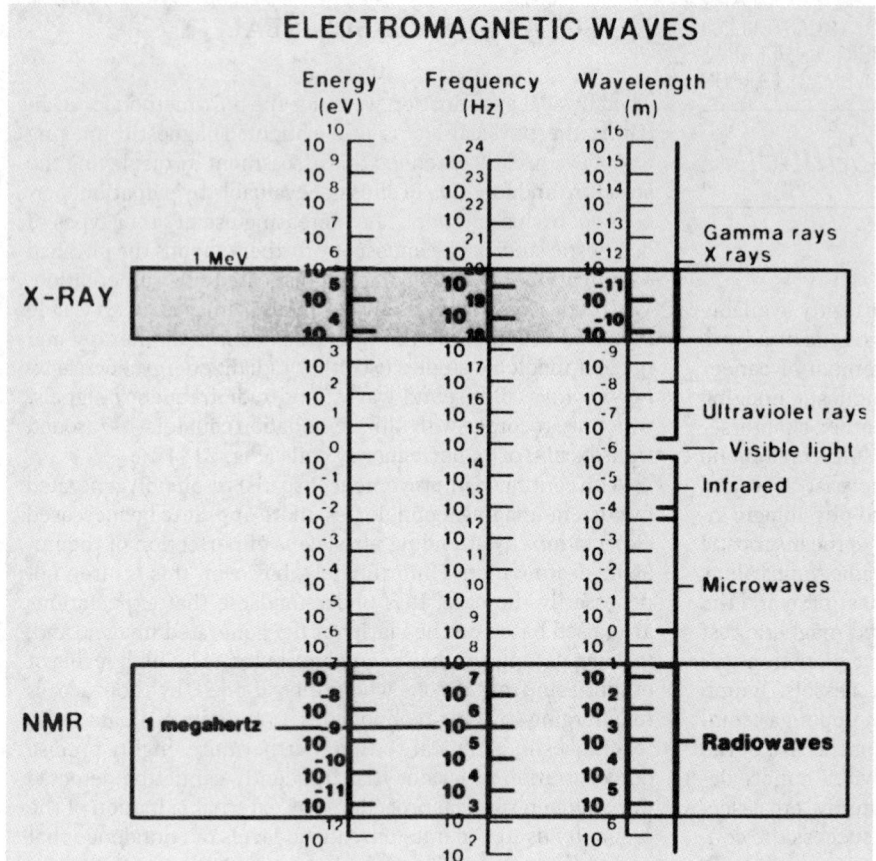

FIGURE 21–12. The electromagnetic spectrum is a continuum of electromagnetic waves. X-rays and γ rays, visible light, and radio waves are useful in medical diagnosis. (Young SW. Magnetic resonance imaging. Basic principles. 2nd ed. New York: Raven Press, 1988)

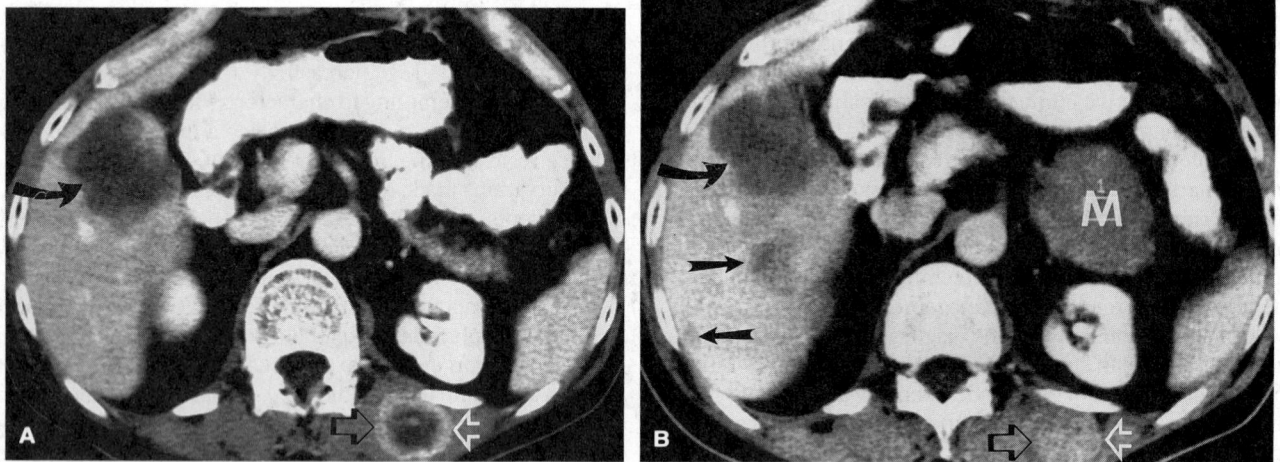

FIGURE 21–13. Contrast-enhanced CT scan of the upper abdomen of a 53-year-old man. **(A)** Staging study demonstrated a 5-cm, low-attenuation mass in the liver (*curved arrow*) and a 3-cm, low-attenuation mass with an "enhancing rim" (*open arrow*) in the left psoas muscle. Subsequent evaluation by dynamic CT scanning and percutaneous needle biopsies demonstrated that the liver mass was a cavernous hemangioma and the psoas mass was an unrelated neurofibroma, rather than suspected metastasis. **(B)** Ten months later, because of vague abdominal discomfort, a repeat CT study demonstrated the stable cavernous hemangioma (*curved arrow*) and left psoas neurofibroma (*open arrows*). However, new intrahepatic low-attenuation masses (*straight arrows*) and a mass (M) in the pancreatic tail had appeared. Percutaneous needle aspirations confirmed suspected disease relapse.

inevitably increases the number of false-negative studies, losing precious opportunities for early intervention. The ideal diagnostic criteria should allow the highest level of sensitivity (*i.e.*, ability to detect disease) and specificity (*i.e.*, ability to predict the absence of disease) attainable within the limitations of that technique. This level can be evaluated by developing a receiver operating characteristic (ROC) curve, which displays the changing ratios of sensitivity and specificity as the criteria change. This is a valuable technique for comparing the performance of different imaging modalities for the same clinical assessment.

Depiction of a lesion does not necessarily provide its etiology. Some diagnostic imaging criteria provide high levels of confidence for interpreting certain types of masses, such as those that contain water (*e.g.*, renal and hepatic cysts), fat (*e.g.*, renal angiomyolipomas, benign lipomas), calcifications suggesting benignity (*e.g.*, uterine leiomyomas, granulomas involving lung, liver, and spleen), and functional attributes (*e.g.*, vascularity in hepatic hemangiomas). It should not be surprising, however, that many masses cannot be further characterized on imaging studies when recognizing that the pathologist, with specimen in hand, although frequently able to suggest the etiology of a mass, will nonetheless need to confirm this impression by microscopic examination of the lesion. This level of evaluation is clearly far beyond the current capabilities of diagnostic imaging studies. Notice, however, that more precise information could be derived from some imaging studies, such as with the use of monoclonal labeled antibodies to identify with high selectivity tissues sharing common antigens, or the use of MRI with spectroscopy to characterize metabolism/function, and thereby provide a more precise understanding of etiology.

A "negative" examination does not exclude the presence of disease. As long as an estimation of size or volume remains the mainstay of diagnosis, false-negative studies will continue to hamper evaluation of the cancer patient. Even after correctly identifying a "radiologic" micrometastasis (*e.g.*, metastatic deposit of 5 mm in a lymph node opacified at lymphography or a punctate pulmonary metastasis seen on chest CT scans), this "micrometastasis" still represents an already large colony of viable cancer cells.

USES OF DIAGNOSTIC IMAGING

The choice of which imaging modality to use depends on at least three factors.

First, what information is being sought? Is the examination being used for screening, for initial staging of the patient, or to assess response to treatment and freedom from relapse? Is the intent of the study to detect whether there may be disease at a specific site or to delineate precisely the anatomic extent of involvement?

Second, what is the availability and quality of the imaging technology employed for the study? Is MRI or single photon emission computed tomography (SPECT) available? If so, can the study be readily scheduled, or are there long delays due to overcommitments? Are the available imaging units able to provide high quality, diagnostic studies?

Third, what is the level of familiarity and expertise with this technology by the diagnostic radiologist and nuclear medicine consultants? Are they equally adept in the supervision and interpretation of the technology compared with another?

SCREENING

Mammography is the only diagnostic imaging modality currently used in the United States to detect cancers in an asymptomatic population. This has occurred because of substantial advances in technology over the past decade that resulted in improved diagnostic images with lower radiation doses and because mammography has been supported by increasing expertise in interpreting the resultant images. Chest radiographs to screen for lung carcinoma or barium studies to screen for stomach and colon carcinomas are not employed in the general population, although there is sporadic use in groups at high risk for these diseases.

The ideal imaging test for screening large populations should possess a high level of sensitivity and an acceptable rate of specificity, employ technology that is widely available and relatively inexpensive, be noninvasive or minimally invasive (including an acceptable radiation burden), and be supported by competent technical and professional staff to obtain optimal images for subsequent interpretation.

STAGING STUDIES

After a histologic diagnosis of cancer is established, and depending on the tumor histology and other preexistent information about the extent of disease, several imaging studies can be employed to determine the stage of disease and guide patient management. During this initial evaluation, decisions about which tests to use for staging should be based on the information needed, the impact of the information on patient management, the need for baseline studies, the accuracy of the imaging studies, and the expertise of local consultants.

Detecting or Delineating Disease

Imaging studies should be employed if they possess a reasonable likelihood of providing sufficiently accurate information to predict the presence or absence of disease at a specific site. Oncologists are aware of the natural history of various primary cancers to order tests to evaluate specific anatomic sites at risk for involvement.

There are important distinctions between *detection of disease* at a specific site and *delineating the anatomic extent of disease* at the same site. For example, the choice of tests for detecting liver involvement is considerably different from the choice if it is important to know the number and locations of metastatic deposits (*e.g.*, for resection). For detection of hepatic metastasis, carefully performed CT or MRI studies, with careful attention to methods of intravenous contrast administration in the former and pulse sequence selection in the latter, appear to be relatively equivalent, with perhaps a slight advantage (statistically insignificant) for MRI.[1] However, if delineation of the extent of disease is required, the more complex performance of CT arterial portography, which requires catheter cannulation of the mesenteric vessels for infusion of iodinated contrast media, is significantly superior to other studies.[2]

Impact on Patient Management

Although imaging studies may accurately detect or delineate disease, it is important to balance this information with how useful it will be in the initial or subsequent management of the patient. Increasingly, studies evaluating diagnostic imaging tests try to assess their impact on patient management. These studies are more difficult to perform and require close cooperation with the attending physician groups. Even when such information is available, it is at times unclear as to how the results are to be used in a patient population. For example, a study of the impact of routinely performed chest CT scans of patients with newly diagnosed Hodgkin's disease indicated that the incremental information from such scans altered patient management for approximately 10% of patients.[3] Some researchers argue that a test impacting only 1 in 10 patients might not be worth the effort or expense, whereas others argue that a change in management for 1 of every 10 patients is well worth performing. If there is general agreement that a 10% yield is worthwhile, at what percentage level (*e.g.*, 5% or 2%) would a routinely performed study not be appropriate to perform, and how does the researcher determine the level below which such tests are not efficacious?

Baseline Imaging Studies

Although it may appear redundant to obtain studies that identify disease but do not influence management, baseline information can help to monitor the effects of treatment more efficiently. Imaging studies obtained before initiation of treatment serve as important monitors of response to treatment or detection of relapse. A baseline study is essential because subtle variations reflecting clinically significant changes can frequently only be assessed by careful comparison of sequential studies. Which imaging test is ordered for baseline purposes is influenced by cost, patient convenience, availability, degree of invasiveness, and inherent accuracy.

Diagnostic Accuracy of Imaging Studies

A large body of literature addresses sensitivity, specificity, and predictive values of various imaging modalities used for assessment of a specific organ or anatomic site. Studies of diagnostic accuracy of various imaging modalities are extremely difficult to perform, are frequently associated with the expected biases encountered in clinical investigation, and depend on the status of technology employed and expertise of the diagnostic radiologist or nuclear medicine group. This issue is addressed more fully later.

Local Expertise

The oncologist must develop an understanding of the skills available to his patients from the diagnostic radiology and nuclear medicine consultants. Certain imaging modalities have undergone (and continue to undergo) major enhancements in image production, and there may be extraordinary differences between the quality of the generated image and its subsequent interpretation compared with the same modality using less developed technology, or with other imaging modalities that are more "mature" (*i.e.*, technologically static).

For example, most radiology groups produce good-quality radiographs of the chest and extremities because optimal equipment and technical expertise are widely available. However, CT, MRI, ultrasound, or nuclear medicine studies often show extreme variations in quality, based in part on the level of technology available, the level of technical skills (from both the technologist and radiologist), and the level of expertise in interpreting the images. This is not surprising, because the oncologist also deals with disparate levels of expertise when relying on consultations from the surgical pathologist, the accuracy of clinical laboratory tests, and consultations from other subspecialties of the clinical oncology group (radiotherapy, medical/pediatric oncology, or surgical oncology), or other nononcologic medical consultants who are used to providing a comprehensive evaluation of the patient.

Although state-of-the-art equipment can provide superior images, careful tailoring of the study for the specific patient is necessary to enhance the resultant information. This is perhaps most obvious in diagnostic ultrasound, for which the skill of the technologist or physician scanning the patient is pivotal to a successful examination. Also critical is the appropriate use of technical parameters, such as the timing and method of injecting intravenous contrast material and the choice of slice thickness when performing CT and MRI examinations. Comparison of imaging studies from two different facilities using identical equipment often demonstrates substantial differences in image quality.

Equally important to the technical quality of the study are the skills of the diagnostic radiologist and nuclear medicine physician in interpreting the images and formulating an impression meaningful to the clinical problem at hand. Frequent consultation between the oncologist and the radiologist helps to tailor the examination to the clinical problem and to formulate a diagnostic consultative report.

Serendipitously Discovered Masses

As advances in technology have yielded images of greater spatial and contrast resolution, there has been a corresponding increase in cases in which abnormalities are detected (most typically masses, but also areas of abnormal uptake on radionuclide studies) as a part of staging and surveillance studies (Figs. 21–13 and 21–14). If the abnormalities occur at sites compatible with the known natural behavior of the tumor being evaluated, the information is usually accepted as important in managing the patient. However, if this information might initiate a significant change in patient management (*e.g.*, if a lesion compatible with a metastasis is found, so that the patient would be excluded from "curative" approaches, or be managed in a significantly different way, such as with systemic rather than local therapy) or if it is discordant with the expected patterns of disease for a particular tumor, then efforts to determine the etiology of such a finding are often pursued.

The first step in evaluating an abnormality discovered on an imaging study is to obtain prior imaging studies, if available. Therefore, findings on a chest radiograph of one or several pulmonary nodules, or a worrisome prominence of a mediastinal contour, can be disregarded if a chest radiograph from several years earlier also demonstrated these findings without

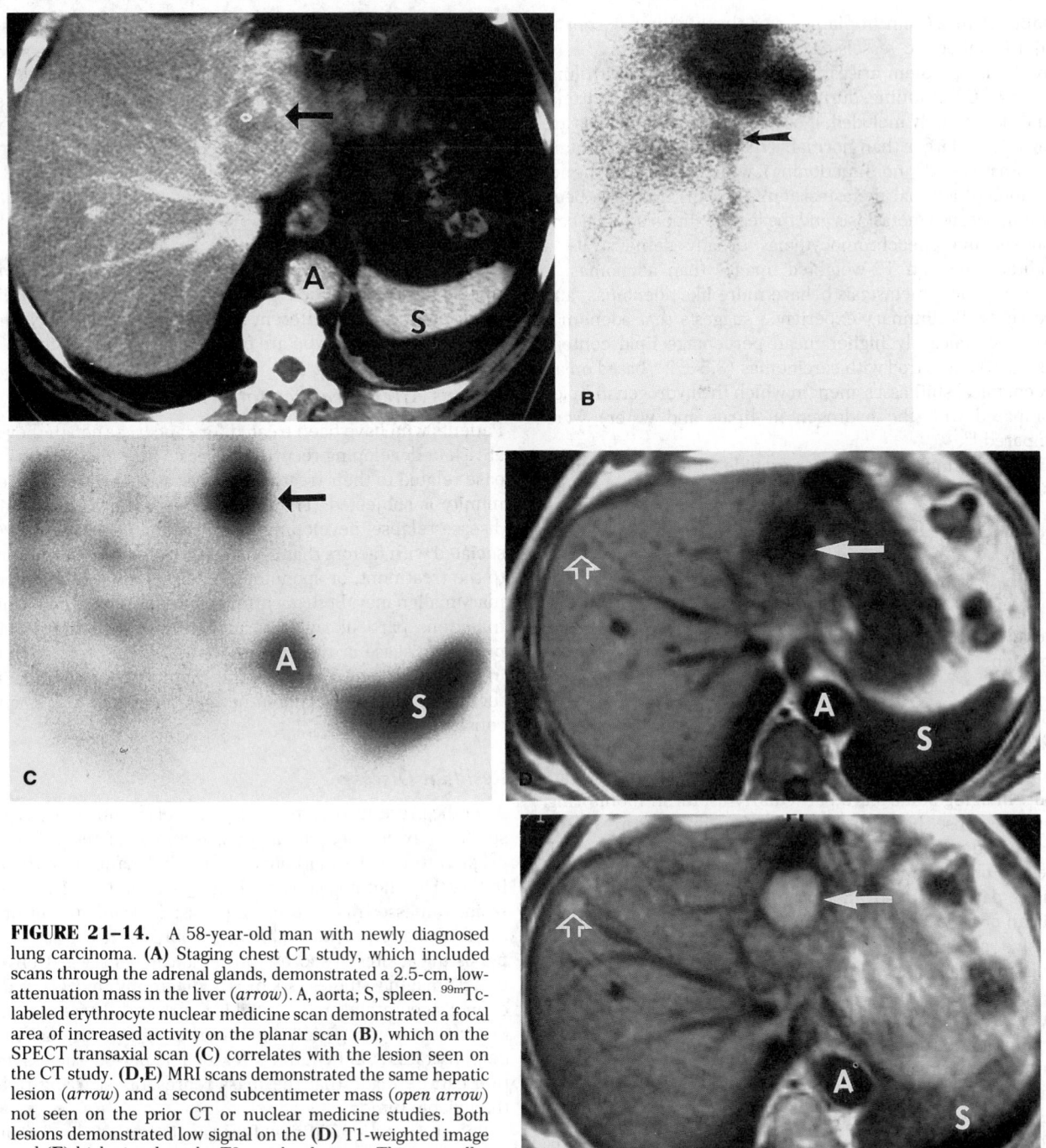

FIGURE 21–14. A 58-year-old man with newly diagnosed lung carcinoma. **(A)** Staging chest CT study, which included scans through the adrenal glands, demonstrated a 2.5-cm, low-attenuation mass in the liver (*arrow*). A, aorta; S, spleen. ^{99m}Tc-labeled erythrocyte nuclear medicine scan demonstrated a focal area of increased activity on the planar scan **(B)**, which on the SPECT transaxial scan **(C)** correlates with the lesion seen on the CT study. **(D,E)** MRI scans demonstrated the same hepatic lesion (*arrow*) and a second subcentimeter mass (*open arrow*) not seen on the prior CT or nuclear medicine studies. Both lesions demonstrated low signal on the **(D)** T1-weighted image and **(E)** high signal on the T2-weighted image. This constellation of findings is characteristic of a carcinous hemangioma.

interval change. However, most patients have not had a prior CT, ultrasound, or MRI study that can be used to evaluate an abnormality encountered on a similar study. When this occurs, other imaging modalities are often used as "problem solvers."

For example, detection of a low-density lesion within the liver by CT scanning occurs in 17% of patients, and many of these lesions are due to clinically inconsequential hepatic cysts or cavernous hemangiomas.[4] On nonenhanced and conventionally enhanced CT studies, cavernous hemangiomas can mimic metastasis. The classic changes observed on serial CT scans performed during bolus administration of intravenous contrast media (*e.g.*, contrast filling from the periphery to the center), although characteristic of hemangiomas, may also be seen with malignant liver masses. The characteristic ultrasound features of cavernous hemangiomas (*e.g.*, lesions with relatively high echogenicity) can also be seen with metastasis. It appears that hepatic cavernous hemangiomas are best identified with radionuclide scans of ^{99m}Tc-labeled erythrocytes and MRI scans of the liver (Fig. 21–14B to E).[5,6] Because the radionuclide study is more readily available and less costly than MRI studies, indeterminant lesions should first be studied with this technique. Important exceptions are lesions smaller than 2.0 cm in diameter or those lying adjacent to major intrahepatic vessels or cardiac chambers.

A similar problem arises in evaluating patients with lung cancer by CT scanning, during which a survey of the adrenal glands is routinely included, if one or both adrenal glands are shown to be larger than normal. The adrenals often contain adenomas (usually nonfunctioning), which can mimic the appearance of adrenal metastasis on CT scans. MRI has been helpful, because metastasis and the less common adrenal carcinomas and pheochromocytomas usually demonstrate a brighter signal on T2-weighted images than adenomas.[7-9] However, some metastasis behave more like adenomas, and vice versa. Preliminary experience suggests that adenomas have a significantly higher mean percentage lipid content (13.4 ± 8) compared with carcinomas (3.5 ± 2), based on an MR chemical shift assessment in which the hydrogen in lipids (compared with the hydrogen in lipids and water) were compared.[10]

If imaging modalities cannot provide sufficient assurance of the etiology of serendipitously discovered masses, the lesions can be further evaluated with image-guided percutaneous needle aspiration or biopsy. These procedures are widely available and require close cooperation between diagnostic radiologists skilled with these techniques and cytopathologists with expertise in preparing and evaluating the often small amounts of tissue provided with this relatively noninvasive approach.

SURVEILLANCE IMAGING STUDIES

After the patient is staged and treatment initiated, imaging studies are frequently employed to assess response to treatment. Imaging studies are particularly useful in monitoring tumor response, because the imaging techniques are reproducible and comparing baseline and subsequent studies provides an objective assessment of change in tumor volume. This is particularly advantageous if a noninvasive imaging test can provide information similar to that provided by more invasive assessments (*e.g.,* serial bone marrow aspirates). Imaging studies avoid the more subjective physical examination, which relies on periodic written summaries of the findings.

After treatment is completed, imaging studies are also used to monitor for relapse. There are few studies investigating appropriate intervals for evaluating the patient during or after treatment, the results of which could affect patient management. However, methodology does exist for determining the optimal timing and frequency in monitoring for relapse with tests for patients with specific tumors.[11] The follow-up imaging studies usually coincide with the follow-up visits to the oncologist's office, for which there is also little rationale for timing such patient visits. Instead, much of this appears to have evolved empirically, based on the oncologist's concerns about closely monitoring the patient or the patient's expectation of continued surveillance by his physician. If the patient develops signs or symptoms suspicious for relapse, or develops definite evidence of relapse, imaging studies are again used to evaluate the possibility of relapse or to restage the patient.

Baseline Studies

Comparison with serial prior studies (and not just with the most recent prior examination) is crucial in identifying early evidence of disease. It is important that these surveillance studies are performed with a similar technique, because the various imaging modalities and the tailoring of these studies can present information that is not readily comparable. For example, intraorgan masses may appear to have changed size based on the imaging technology used or how the study was conducted (*e.g.,* with or without contrast agents).

Routine Surveillance and Studies Prompted by Signs or Symptoms

If a patient develops a worrisome sign or symptom, appropriate imaging tests should be requested to help formulate a clinical assessment. This is different from using routinely performed studies for patients who are otherwise asymptomatic.

Lesions After Treatment of Primary Cancers

Patients who have been treated for cancer, although they are at risk of developing recurrent disease, may also develop disease related to their treatment or diseases to which the community is subjected. The emergence of a mass may reflect disease relapse, development of a second primary tumor associated with factors that initiated the initial tumor or related to the treatment, or spontaneous development of a new primary malignancy. Both opportunistic and community-acquired infections, particularly the former, are seen in patients whose primary disease or therapy has caused a compromise in the immune system. Acute or chronic manifestations of radiation therapy and various chemotherapeutic agents also require consideration.

Residual Disease

After the prescribed course of treatment is completed, imaging studies may demonstrate a persistent mass at the site of the original tumor that, although definitely smaller than before initiation of therapy, persists (Figs. 21–15 and 21–16). These residual masses may represent persistent viable tumor or be a manifestation of nonviable (*e.g.,* fibrosis, necrosis) tissue persisting at sites of successfully eradicated disease. Conventional imaging studies, such as radiography and CT scans, cannot accurately predict which is present. If treatment is discontinued and periodic monitoring of the residual mass demonstrates stability after a reasonable period, the assumption can be made that the mass represents scarring rather than viable tumor.

Because at times additional therapy is available to continue treating patients with partial responses, a precise determination of the cause of the residual mass is important to patient care. Imaging studies have addressed this issue with limited success. Initial expectations that patterns of enhanced CT scanning after intravenous bolus injections of iodinated contrast material could predict the etiology of residual lesions have been disappointing. Radionuclide studies using tracers, such as gallium citrate, that are concentrated by actively metabolizing cells are helpful if the tumor demonstrated uptake before treatment. After treatment, persistent radioisotope accumulation in the residual mass is consistent with persistent viable tumor, an assessment more accurately made with SPECT scanning. This approach is validated in Hodgkin disease but still needs to be evaluated for most other tumor types. Thallium is useful for detecting persistent low-grade lymphomas.

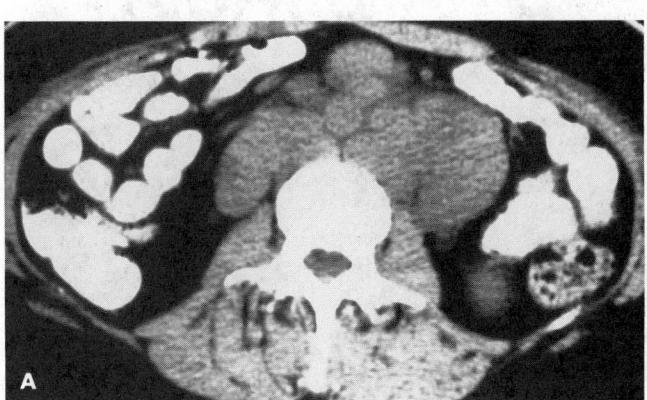 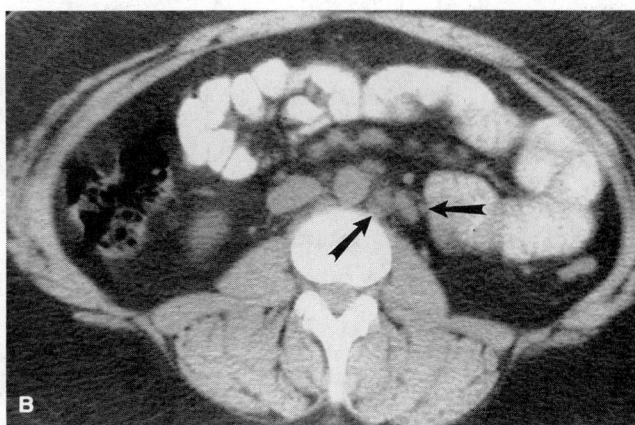

FIGURE 21–15. Patient with follicular non-Hodgkin's lymphoma. **(A)** Staging CT scan demonstrates bulky retroperitoneal and mesenteric lymphadenopathy. **(B)** After treatment, there is a marked decrease in size of the lymphadenopathy. However, residual soft-tissue "masses" persist in the left paraaortic region (*arrows*), which may represent persistent tumor or the residua of successfully treated disease.

Preliminary experience with MRI in evaluating the post-treatment residual mass is encouraging, based on an analysis of the signal characteristic of the mass with various pulse sequences.[12] Mature fibrosis is acellular or extremely hypocellular, and it contains little water compared with viable tumor cells. T2-weighted images of persistent tumor have high (*i.e.*, bright) signal compared with the low (*i.e.*, dark) signal of mature fibrosis. However, immature fibrosis, which is often present after recently completed radiotherapy or surgery, contains numerous cells and frequently edema, which produces a bright signal on T2-weighted images. It appears that differentiation based on T2-weighted images is useful only 6 to 9 months after cessation of treatment.

The use of ultrasound to "characterize" the composition of masses, compared with simply displaying their presence, can be useful in some settings. Evaluation of residual mediastinal masses in patients with lymphoma by transthoracic ultrasound suggests that an analysis of the "echo texture" within the mass can often predict whether there is viable tumor or fibrosis.[13]

ACCURACY

Assessment of accuracy for diagnostic imaging studies is increasingly expressed in terms of sensitivity, specificity, and positive and negative predictive values.[14–17] These parameters are also useful in studying other diagnostic tests, such as laboratory values, electrocardiographic interpretation, or assessment of the patient by physical examination. The use of "overall accuracy," which represents a percentage of correct positive and negative diagnoses of the total group of diagnosis, can provide misleading information, because it does not take into account the incidence or prevalence of the disease occurring in that population or the site being studied.

The accuracy of a diagnostic imaging test must be considered in the context in which the test is being performed. An important distinction that must be made is whether the test is being performed in a *screening* (*i.e.*, asymptomatic population) context or in a *diagnostic* (*i.e.*, symptomatic population) context. The accuracy of the test may be quite different in

these two circumstances. In most cases, the size of the lesion differs significantly and is likely to be much smaller in the asymptomatic patient being screened for disease than in the symptomatic patient. The prior probability of disease (*i.e.*, disease prevalence) is also different in these two patient groups; it is smaller in the general population being screened for disease. Unfortunately, in many studies of diagnostic images used for both purposes, such as mammography, a mixture of diagnostic and screening cases are included, clouding the statistical analysis of test accuracy.

Accuracy can be defined for a diagnostic imaging test with some precision, assuming a valid reference standard is available.[17] The relevant data from a study can be presented in a 2×2 grid (Fig. 21–17), in which true positive (TP), false positive (FP), false negative (FN), and true negative (TN) represent the frequencies of occurrence of the cross-tabulations of the test results (R+ or R−) and the definitive reference ("gold standard") diagnosis (D+ or D−).

The *sensitivity* is the proportion of diseased patients (or anatomic sites) that are correctly classified as being diseased [TP/(TP + FN)]. The *specificity* is the proportion of normal or nondiseased patients who are correctly classified as normal [TN/(FP + TN)]. It is desirable that both of these values be as large as possible. Two related measures are also useful in evaluating imaging tests: the *positive predictive value* [TP/(TP + FP)] and the *negative predictive value* [TN/(FN + TN)], which are the probabilities of correctly predicting true disease status based on the test result. A test is accurate to the extent that it leads to a correct classification, namely, TP or TN. The term *accuracy* is used to define the proportion of correct classifications [(TP + TN)/(TP + FP + FN + TN)]. However, this measure has been criticized on statistical grounds for being heavily dependent on the composition of the sample (*i.e.*, relative frequencies of D+ and D− patients), which emphasizes the importance of considering the context and prior probability of disease when the "overall accuracy" of an imaging test is assessed.

A cautionary note should be added here, concerning the use of this Bayesian terminology for diagnostic imaging studies. These precise definitions apply to tests that are binary—positive or negative. However, for most clinical imaging studies,

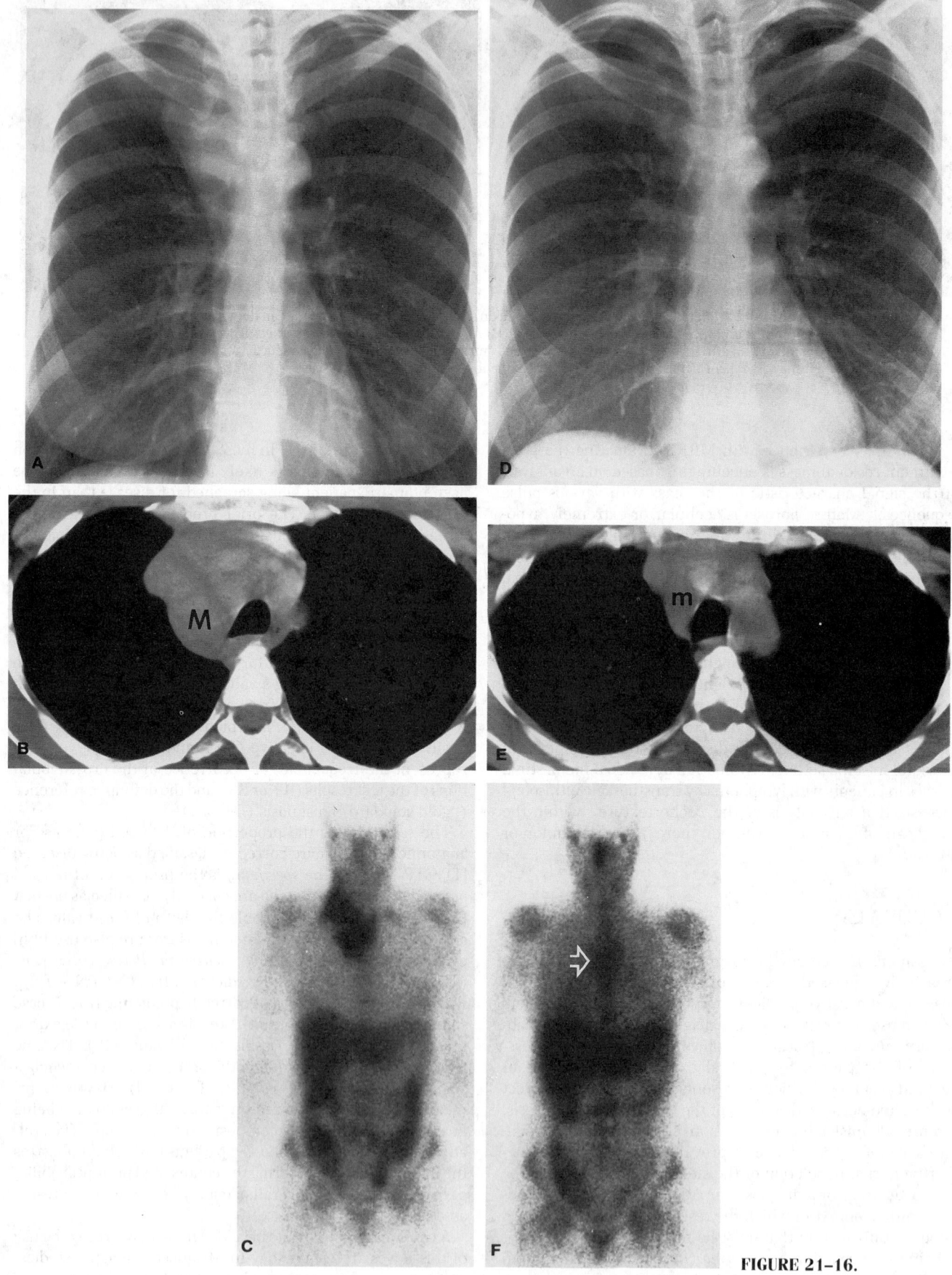

FIGURE 21–16.

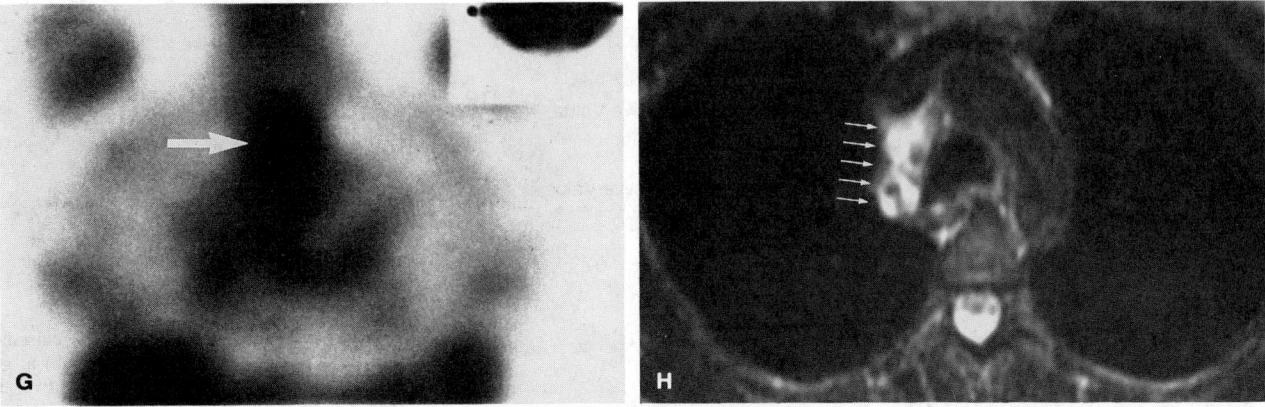

FIGURE 21–16. *(Continued)*

this is not the case. In practice, the calculation of sensitivity and specificity involves the arbitrary selection of positive criteria or a "cut-off" value. There are also differences between tests that are subjectively interpreted, which includes most diagnostic imaging studies, and those that are objectively or quantitatively interpreted, as is the case for laboratory assays and some nuclear medicine studies. The results of tests that are subjectively interpreted may be organized in a series of ordinal judgments, such as positive, probably positive, equivocal, probably negative, or negative, providing a semiquantitative approximation of the objective results of a truly quantitative measure. In either case, possible test results range from most positive to most negative, depending on the cut-off criterion selected. These outcomes reflect a range of disease likelihood ratios from most to least probable. In this context, individual estimates of sensitivity and specificity are of limited usefulness, because of the arbitrariness of the choice of the cut-off value. For example, if the sensitivity is higher for one test and the specificity is higher for another, which test is the better test?

To answer these kinds of questions, *receiver operator characteristic* (ROC) analysis is often used for comparing imaging tests. ROC analysis allows comparison between imaging tests when their cut-off values are not quantitative (*i.e.*, classification of studies based on subjective judgments about the findings). The ROC curve itself is a plot of sensitivity and specificity pairs (Fig. 21–18). By convention, the horizontal axis is the false-positive ratio (1 − the specificity), rather than the specificity itself. An accurate test is one for which the sensitivity is high and false-positive ratio is low, so that the ROC curve lies close to the left vertical and upper horizontal axes. Conversely, an ROC curve that lies close to the

45° line is no better than random and represents a study with no diagnostic value.

To determine sensitivity, specificity, and predictive values, a reference standard must be available by which to judge the test in question. Ideally, it should be a microscopic examination of the organ being studied. In the clinical setting, this is frequently not available, so that alternate gold standards might be used, such as comparison with other imaging studies with known sensitivities and specificities, correlation with "clinical assessment" such as the surgeon's observations during exploratory surgery, or correlation with clinical outcome. Clearly, these latter gold standards possess serious inherent flaws.

Even if tissue is available, various methodologic problems might be present that can seriously damage the results. Was the tissue removed from the same site as that identified as abnormal on the imaging study? How does one analyze cases in which inappropriate or no tissue was obtained or cases in which the imaging diagnosis was "equivocal," rather than positive or negative? Did the investigators include all cases or exclude those in which the study could not be performed (*e.g.*, medical contraindications, patient unwillingness to cooperate) or were technically suboptimal examinations? Were the patients in a consecutive, nonselected group, and was the clinical stage of their disease eventually identified; or were the patients selected and perhaps biased toward patients with more advanced disease, in which case an imaging study would be more likely to "succeed" because the patients often have more readily demonstrable sites of primary and secondary involvement? Were the interpreters of these studies "blinded" to other information, such as results of other imaging studies or the eventual pathologic findings, that would bias their re-

◄ **FIGURE 21–16.** A 37-year-old woman with Hodgkin's disease. **(A)** Staging chest radiographs and **(B)** chest CT demonstrated a right superior mediastinal mass (M). **(C)** The staging gallium scan demonstrated right superclavicular lymphadenopathy in addition to the right superior mediastinal mass. Approximately 6 months later, **(D)** a repeat chest radiograph demonstrated complete resolution of the mass after therapy. **(E)** However, chest CT at that time demonstrated a markedly smaller, but persistent, soft-tissue mass (m) in the right superior mediastinum. Gallium study with **(F)** planar and **(G)** SPECT coronal imaging showed persistent, although decreased, activity in the right superior mediastinum. **(H)** MR scan, performed with a pulse-sequence designed to suppress signal from fat and increase the conspicuity of tissues containing water, demonstrated a bright signal in the right superior mediastinum (*arrows*). Although highly suspicious for persistent viable tumor, such findings can be seen on MR scans 6 to 9 months after cessation of treatment.

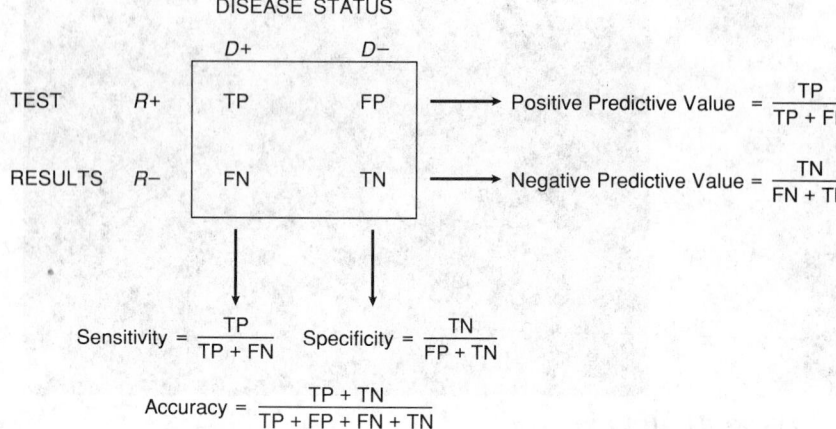

FIGURE 21–17. Bayesian 2 × 2 classification table of test results compared with a "gold standard" of diagnosis. TP, true positive; FP, false positive; FN, false negative; TN, true negative; D, disease status; and R, test result.

sults? In comparing two or more imaging modalities, was the level of sophistication of equipment and expertise of the radiology group equivalent, or was one of the evaluated modalities performed with less expertise and perhaps suboptimal equipment so that the other would perform better in a comparative study? These are some of the concerns in assessing the reported results of diagnostic imaging studies, and they apply to the performance of clinical research in all medical specialties.

Data on accuracy are essential for planning patient management. Even more important is whether the resultant changes in patient management favorably affect patient outcome, which can be viewed as affecting the quantity (*i.e.,* survival) or quality of life.[18] This important information is usually difficult and sometimes impossible to derive. To do so, an investigator would have to construct a clinical trial in which the results of a specific imaging test that might affect patient management would be randomized for use or nonuse and then observe the outcomes. This probably would not be accepted by patients, their physicians, and institutional review boards; during the period of the trial, technologic improvements could outdate the study before the analysis was complete.

Even if specific tests are identified as being sufficiently accurate to impact patient management and improve outcome, issues about cost and availability remain. Studies of cost effectiveness and assigning resources have been suggested to provide a rational basis for allocating increasingly limited health care resources.

The formation of the Radiology Diagnostic Oncology Group (RDOG) studies, sponsored by the National Institutes of Health and the National Cancer Institute, has been an important step toward development of carefully designed, prospective, multiinstitutional clinical research protocols for evaluating the accuracy of various imaging studies in oncology.[19] These protocols receive strong statistical support and careful attention to study designed to maximize information. Completed studies have evaluated CT and MRI in staging bronchogenic carcinoma and MRI and ultrasonography in staging prostate cancer.[20,21] Studies evaluating CT and MRI for staging patients with pancreatic carcinoma and colorectal tumors are nearing completion.[22,23] Recently initiated studies include evaluation of head and neck tumors and soft tissue and osseous sarcomas. Not surprisingly, the studies will need to be repeated to assess technologic enhancements. An ongoing study is reevaluating imaging of prostate cancer with

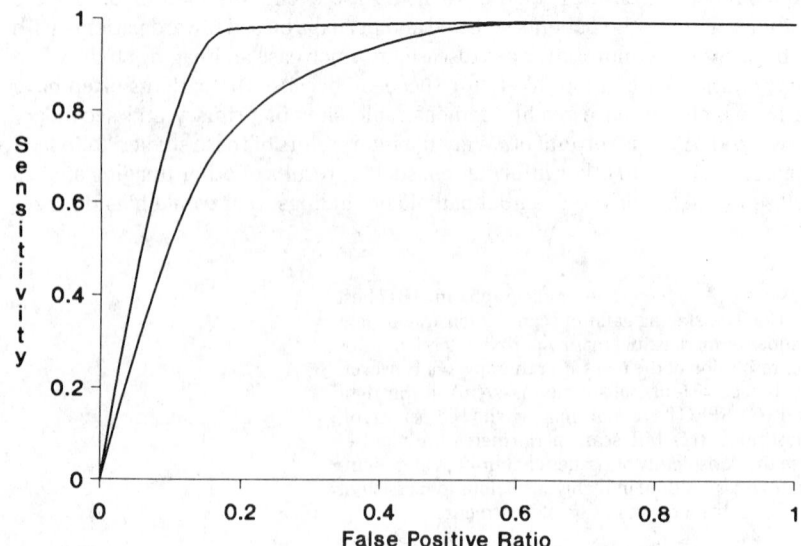

FIGURE 21–18. Receiver operator characteristic (ROC) curves for comparing two imaging tests. The more accurate test is shown by the curve with the higher sensitivity and lower false-positive ratio (*i.e.,* the curve closest to the left vertical and upper horizontal axes). (Rummeny EJ, Wernecke K, Saini S, et al. Comparison between high field strength MR imaging and CT for screening of hepatic metastases: a receiver operating characteristic analysis. Radiology 182:879–886, 1992)

endorectal ultrasound (compared with conventional pelvic ultrasound) and specialized endorectal radiofrequency coils for MR studies (compared with conventional body coils). The accuracy data for evolving imaging technologies must be continually refined until the technology reaches some plateau of maturity.

IMAGING MODALITIES

X-RAY TECHNOLOGIES

When electrons interact with matter, the ionizing electromagnetic radiations (*i.e.*, photons) emitted are called x-rays. (Photons which are emitted during the spontaneous natural decay of unstable elements are called α, β, or γ rays.) These generated photons interact with matter in a highly predictable fashion, because they are attenuated by absorption or scattering proportional to the atomic number (*i.e.*, electron density) of the materials being irradiated. These interactions occur with atoms, electrons, and nuclei, depending on the energy of the x-ray beam.

X-rays are the radiation energy used to produce most medical images, including plain film radiography, fluoroscopy, and x-ray CT. In x-ray imaging, the photons *transmitted* through a patient are recorded by some type of detector (*e.g.*, x-ray film, fluoroscopic screen, detectors in image intensifiers and CT gantries). Other imaging modalities record radiant energy *emitted* from within the patient by detecting the reflected sound waves in ultrasound, the radiofrequency waves in MRI, and γ rays (photons) in nuclear medicine.

X-ray images are based on the atomic numbers of the various atoms that compose the structures that lie within the anatomy being imaged. Structures of high attenuation coefficient (*e.g.*, bone, metallic-containing contrast media) absorb more photons than "water density" tissues (*e.g.*, organs, blood), which absorb more than fat-containing and finally air-containing structures. The exiting photons, which are "captured" on film or screen recorders or x-ray detectors, represent the summation of the atomic composition of the objects in the path of the photon. A projection image (*e.g.*, chest radiograph) superimposes all of the traversed three-dimensional anatomy on the two-dimensional image plane of the x-ray film. Tomographic techniques provide three-dimensional images, as in x-ray CT scanning.

Radiographic technique (*i.e.*, kilovoltage, milliamperage, and time), positioning, collimation of the x-ray beam in plain radiography or slice thickness in CT, and radiographic film and film processing have profound influences on the resultant image. Close attention to these and other factors is critical for optimizing the resultant image and minimizing radiation exposure to the patient. Periodic technologic refinements that improve contrast or spatial resolution lead to enhanced lesion detection (Fig. 21–19).

Frontal and lateral chest radiographs still account for almost half of all medical images. Characteristics of a well-exposed chest radiograph include proper positioning of the patient and coning to expose only the necessary areas within the thorax; using relatively high kilovoltage to maximize penetration through the mediastinum and diaphragmatic domes to increase detectability of pulmonary lesions that would be obscured with lower energies; performance in as deep an inspiratory effort as possible; and sharp detail, as evidenced by

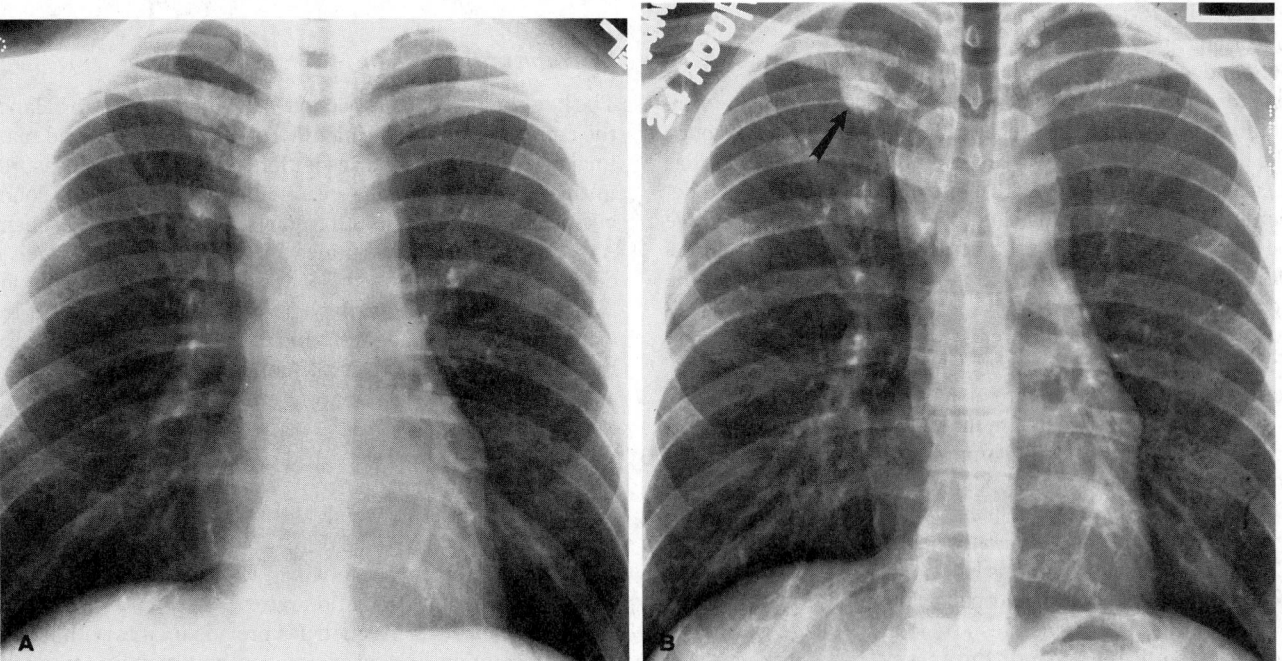

FIGURE 21–19. These two frontal chest radiographs were performed on the same patient within 24 hours of each other. **(A)** The conventional chest radiograph, performed with high-kV technique, demonstrated a superior mediastinal mass. **(B)** The chest radiograph performed with a technique that optimizes the amount of photons necessary to penetrate tissues of various thicknesses (notice the improved visualization of lung behind the heart and diaphragms) shows in addition a right apical pulmonary mass (*arrow*), which is suggested only on retrospective review of the conventional chest radiograph.

crisply delineated margins between pulmonary vessels and aerated lung.

X-ray CT studies are frequently employed for cancer patients. As with chest radiography, there are a variety of technical factors that greatly affect the quality of the resultant CT image. These include the choice of radiographic factors; patient positioning within the gantry; choice of an appropriate body norm and slice thickness, which may vary in the same examination from 10 mm to 5 mm or even 1.5 mm, depending on the area that is being evaluated; the judicious use of intravenous iodinated contrast material and the method of its administration, which increasingly is a bolus injection technique, because the drip infusion technique can obscure lesions; photography of the same scans at various window and level settings to provide soft-tissue, lung, liver, or bone windows; and choice of specific reconstruction algorithms to provide enhanced detail, such as prospective high-resolution scanning of bones and lungs.

Because x-ray CT images are obtained from a series of projections, this data can be manipulated to create image reconstructions in various planes, which can improve understanding of the anatomic relations within the patient. In dealing with computer-generated images, the possible introduction of misleading artifacts should be recognized.

ULTRASOUND

Unlike other imaging techniques, ultrasound uses sound waves rather than electromagnetic energy for image formation. Sound waves are categorized by the number of wave cycles passing a point in one second (*i.e.,* frequency measured in Hertz or cycles per second). Audible sound is in the range of 20 Hz to 20 kHz, and ultrasound includes frequencies above 20 kHz. Typical frequencies for most clinical ultrasound applications are 2.5, 3.5, 5.0, and 7.5 MHz.

Sound waves are mechanical phenomena that generate oscillatory vibrations in tissue, and tissue elasticity and deformability are required for propagation of sound waves through the body. As the sound waves pass through tissue, they act as a series of pressure waves that alternately compress and decompress the tissue, causing it to oscillate around its average position. In water and soft tissues, the predominant direction of sound waves is longitudinal, away from the source of the sound waves, with oscillatory motion of the tissue in the direction of the sound wave propagation. In solids such as bone, transverse or "shear" waves may be generated perpendicular to the longitudinal wave direction.

Ultrasound transducers are made of anisotropic piezoelectric crystals that expand or compress when voltage is applied to them, depending on the polarity of the electric current. Oscillation of the current polarity and application of the transducer to the body generates sound waves in the tissue. Conversely, when the transducer crystal is mechanically compressed or expanded, as occurs with sound waves reflected back from tissue, it generates an electric voltage that is recorded and processed to form the image. The same transducer element is used to generate and receive ultrasound waves. There are an assortment of transducers tailored to address specific imaging problems by offering a range of frequency characteristics, beam shaping, focal lengths, and other characteristics.

The energy of sound waves interacts with tissue through transmission, reflection, refraction, diffraction, scattering, and absorption. The precise nature of these interactions is determined by the characteristics of the tissue, the frequency of the ultrasound, the wavelength of the ultrasound relative to the object size, the orientation of the ultrasound beam to acoustic interfaces, and the acoustic impedance of the tissue. The acoustic impedances (Z), which depend on the density and elasticity of tissue, are greater in solids than in liquids, which are greater than in gasses. For example, the Z values for solid materials vary widely (*e.g.,* steel = 40.00, bone = 7.80, plastic = 3.20), those for tissue vary over a narrow range (mean soft tissue = 1.63, liver = 1.65, kidney = 1.62, water = 1.48, fat = 1.38), and those for gases are much lower (air = 0.0004).[24]

The junction between materials of different acoustic impedances forms an acoustic interface, which generates reflections of the sound beam. It is these returning reflections, or echoes, received by the transducer that are the data from which ultrasound images are generated. The spatial location of the acoustic interface is determined by the length of time required for the echo to be received; the longer the time, the farther it is from the transducer head. In general, the greater the acoustic impedance difference between materials, the greater is the fraction of the sound beam reflected and the smaller is the fraction transmitted through the interface. For example, at the water-fat interface, 3.5% of the sound is reflected and 96.5% is transmitted; at water-bone, 68% is reflected and 32% is transmitted; and at tissue-air, virtually 100% is reflected. Visualization of tissue beyond a tissue-bone interface is severely limited, and tissue-air interfaces are opaque, explaining the masking of structures in abdominal scanning created by bowel gas.

Instrumentation

The key challenge to ultrasound instrumentation is to balance the competing needs of maximal spatial resolution and maximal tissue penetration. Resolution in ultrasound is measured in the axial or depth dimension along the axis of the sound beam and lateral or azimuth resolution across the sound beam. Axial resolution is determined by the wavelength, which is determined by the transducer frequency. Lateral resolution is determined by the beam width, which is a function of the transducer size, focal length, and frequency. Sensitivity to the returning, reflected echoes also influences resolution. Typical axial resolutions in tissue are 2 mm at 2.5 MHz, 1 mm at 5 MHz, and 0.6 mm at 7.5 MHz. Lateral resolution is best at the focal distance of the transducer, where the beam width is the least. With many current applications, sector scanning is commonly used in which the transducer, or an array of transducers (*e.g.,* sequenced linear and phased arrays), generate a triangular image in which lateral resolution depends on lateral sweep or oscillation rate.

Higher transducer frequencies provide images with higher spatial resolution. However, the depth of penetration of the ultrasound beam is decreased at higher transducer frequencies. To obtain images of higher spatial resolution, the transducer needs to be of high frequency and close to the organ being studied. This is possible with superficial organs, such as ultrasound examinations of the thyroid and testes. Innovations in instrumentation have allowed placement of small, high-frequency transducers within the body for transvaginal and transrectal pelvic sonography, endoluminal ultrasonography after endoscopy of the upper gastrointestinal tract, transesophageal cardiac sonography, and intravascular applications.[25] These techniques provide remarkably detailed images of adjacent tissues, but only to a depth of several centimeters.

Doppler shift, which occurs when reflected sound waves return from moving objects, like erythrocytes in flowing blood, allows quantitation of flow phenomena in the body. Objects moving toward the transducer produce an upward frequency shift, and those moving away produce a shift to a lower frequency than those emitted by the transducer. The degree of these shifts can be quantitated and blood flow velocity measured. The angle of incidence of the ultrasound beam to the moving blood also influences these measurements, making them operate in a dependent and variable manner. Despite this variability, Doppler ultrasound examinations of major arteries and veins are common and valuable clinical applications.

Practical Imaging Considerations

The generation of an ultrasound image is highly operator dependent. Similar to barium gastrointestinal fluoroscopy and angiography, the skill of the person performing the study directly affects image quality and the degree of diagnostic information. Ultrasound examinations are frequently "tailored" to a specific problem or set of problems, which is a major advantage with this technology. Because ultrasound imaging represents real-time information, it is extremely useful in guiding biopsy and other interventional procedures.

The appearance of structures on ultrasound images depends on acoustic interfaces. Internal echogenicity is useful for determining tissue types and characteristics, especially with recently developed image analysis techniques. In general, echogenic tissues have complex structure and multiple acoustic interfaces, such as masses with areas of necrosis, edema, septations, or different tissue constituents. Echolucent zones are homogenous tissues with few or no acoustic interfaces. Therefore, free fluid in the bladder, in cystic structures, and in pleural and peritoneal spaces is echolucent and consequently does not attenuate the sound beam by reflection or scatter. In cysts, this results in the characteristic enhanced reflection off the far wall of the cyst, with enhanced through

transmission and prominent echoes beyond the far wall of the cyst. This definitive appearance of cysts is one of the most clinically useful signs in ultrasound gray-scale imaging. Conversely, the marked reflections that occur at the near interface of calcified objects create an absence of echoes beyond the object, known as an acoustic shadow. This pattern of high focal echogenicity and distal acoustic shadowing is characteristic of gallstones and renal calculi.

MAGNETIC RESONANCE IMAGING

Principles

MRI is a cross-sectional and three-dimensional imaging technique employing the principles of nuclear magnetic resonance (NMR). NMR is based on the behavior of certain atomic nuclei that are formed by an odd number of protons and neutrons (*i.e.*, odd atomic mass number), which behave like microscopic bar magnets with north and south poles. When these nuclei are placed in an externally applied magnetic field, their rotation around their internal axis, a property called *spin*, causes them to wobble around the axis of the external magnetic field, much like a spinning top, a behavior called *precession*. The frequency of precession or Larmor frequency is specific for each species of nuclear spin (*e.g.*, hydrogen, ^{1}H) and increases as the applied magnetic field increases. The advantage of higher magnetic fields is the recruitment of more nuclei that can be used to generate signal for imaging and the consequent improved signal-to-noise ratio. The relation between the frequency of precession (in MHz) and the applied magnetic field strength (in Tesla, T) is given by the *gyromagnetic ratio*. The specificity of the gyromagnetic ratio for the nuclear species and its variation with magnetic field strength are the key properties that allow magnetic resonance images to be formed.

Hydrogen is the nucleus used in most clinical MRI because it has the greatest sensitivity (*i.e.*, highest gyromagnetic ratio) compared with other biologically relevant nuclei such as phosphorus (^{31}P), sodium (^{23}Na), or carbon (^{13}C). Fortunately, it is also the most abundant atom with nuclear spin in tissues, making it an excellent choice for clinical imaging (Table 21–2).[26]

Magnetic resonance images are formed by placing the patient in an external magnetic field and observing the behavior of the sensitive nuclear spins as the properties of the magnetic field are manipulated (Fig. 21–20). This is done by transmitting a radiofrequency (RF) wave at precisely the Larmor

TABLE 21–2. Magnetic Species in Biologic Systems

NMR Species	Relative Abundance (%)	Gyromagnetic Ratio (MHz/10 kg)	Relative Sensitivity*	Applications
^{1}H, ^{13}C	100, 1	42.6, 10.7	1, 0.25	All
^{31}P	100	17.2	0.41	Nucleotides, phospholipids, phosphorylated metabolites
^{14}N, ^{15}N, ^{33}S	99.6, 0.4, 0.7	3.1, 4.3, 3.3	0.2, 0.1, 0.384	Amino acids, peptides, proteins
^{19}F, ^{2}H	100, 0.2	40.1, 6.5	0.94, 0.41	Isotopic label substituting for ^{1}H

* At constant frequency.

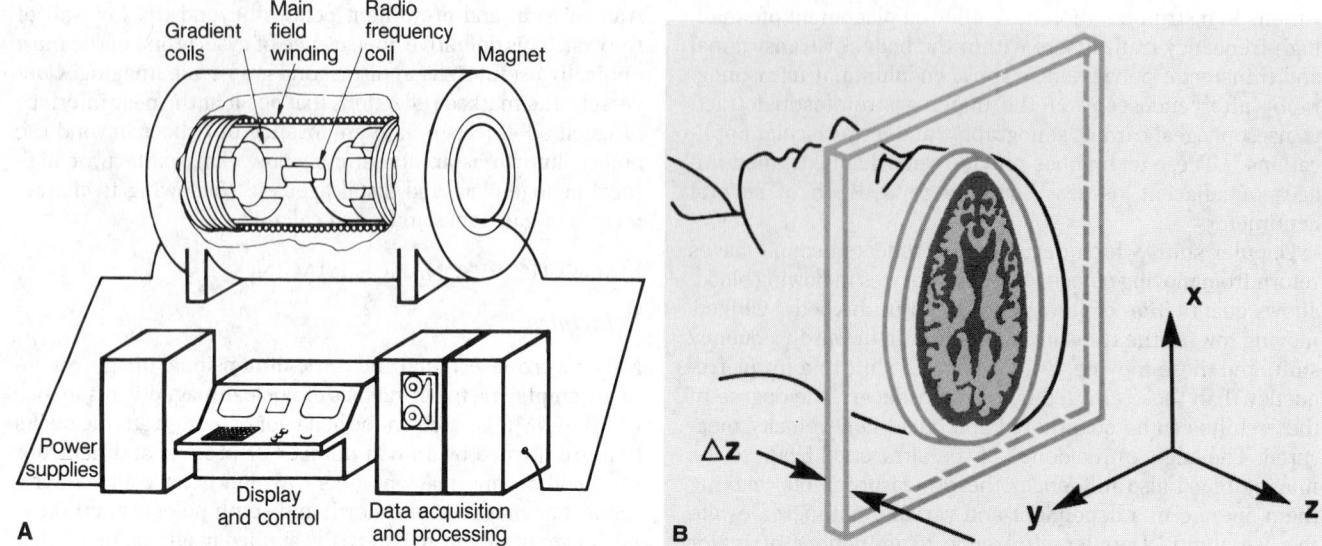

FIGURE 21–20. **(A)** The basic components of the MRI system. The patient is positioned at the center of the magnetic field within the magnet housing and various coils. (Bradley WG, Newton TH, Crooks LE. Physical Principles of Nuclear Magnetic Resonance. In: Newton TH, Potts GD. *Modern Neuroradiology Volume Two. Advanced Imaging Techniques.* Clavadel Press, San Anselmo, 1983) **(B)** MR images are formed by applying magnetic field gradients in x, y, and z axes of the imaging system (z is along the bore of the magnet, with x and y transverse to it). These allow spatial localization by selecting a frequency range along the gradients using radiofrequency pulses. In this case, the frequency range Δ_z (slice selection) determines the axial slice thickness and spatial localization in x and y form the image. Other slice orientations can be obtained without moving the patient by electronically switching slice-selection and image-formation planes (*e.g.,* slice-selection in x produces coronal images, and in y, produces sagittal images). (NMR: A perspective on imaging. General Electric Company, 1982)

frequency of the targeted nuclei (usually hydrogen). Because the RF matches the Larmor frequency, it is in resonance with it, and the transmitted energy is absorbed by the precessing nucleus. This RF pulse selectively tilts the angle of precession away from the axis of the external magnetic field. When the RF pulse is turned off, the precessing nuclei emit the energy absorbed as a signal of precisely the same frequency as they relax back to equilibrium, and the signal is received by the RF coils and used for image formation (Fig. 21–21). The time it takes to return (*i.e.,* relax) toward the axis of the external magnetic field can be measured and is profoundly affected by the immediate chemical milieu of the nucleus. The relaxation characteristics are different for the hydrogen nucleus (proton) associated with water (HOH) or with fat (-CH$_2$-), and these differences can be enhanced by manipulation of the RF pulse sequences.

Determining the position of each nucleus within the patient (*i.e.,* spatial encoding) to create an image is accomplished by applying a magnetic field gradient across the object being imaged and observing the change in gyromagnetic ratio along that gradient. Gradients applied along the major axis of the magnetic field (Z axis) are usually used to define image slice location and thickness for forming axial images. Gradients applied perpendicular to the Z axis define the in-plane X and Y axes coordinates of the image itself. Because slice location and orientation in MRI are controlled electronically by varying these gradients, orthogonal image slices can be obtained in axial, coronal, and sagittal planes without a change in patient position (see Fig. 21–20).

MR images reflect the intrinsic behavior of nuclear spins within tissues and the extrinsic variables that are manipulated during the acquisition of MR images. The intrinsic properties include nuclear spin density (*i.e.,* proton density for most clinical imaging), longitudinal relaxation (T1), and transverse relaxation (T2).

The *spin density* is the density of nuclei available for imaging within the tissue. For most clinical MRI, this is equivalent to the density of ^{1}H spins in water molecules and, to a lesser extent, ^{1}H spins in lipid molecules.

Longitudinal or T1 relaxation refers to the tendency of precessing nuclei to return to their prior orientation parallel to the Z axis of the magnetic field after being manipulated by a RF pulse (Figs. 21–21 and 21–22). The T1 relaxation time is used to quantitate this exponential increase in signal along the Z axis. T1 is the time for the signal to rise to 63% of the maximal equilibrium value and is approximately 200 to 800 msec for most tissues.

Transverse or T2 relaxation refers to the time required for loss of signal in the XY plane due to a loss of synchronous precession (*i.e.,* loss of phase coherence) between the protons generating signal for imaging (see Fig. 21–21). The T2 relaxation time is used to quantitate the exponential decline in signal that occurs with the loss of phase coherence. T2 is the time for the signal to decline to 63% of the original, coherent signal and is approximately 50 to 100 msec in most tissues.

The extrinsic variables manipulated in the acquisition of MR images include the parameters of the RF pulse sequence, such as the repetition time (TR), echo time (TE), and flip angle, and the image format parameters, such as the acquisition matrix (typically 256 × 256, 192, or 128 pixels), field of view (FOV, typically 16–24 cm), and slice thickness (typically 3, 5, or 10 mm). The RF pulse sequence is the active

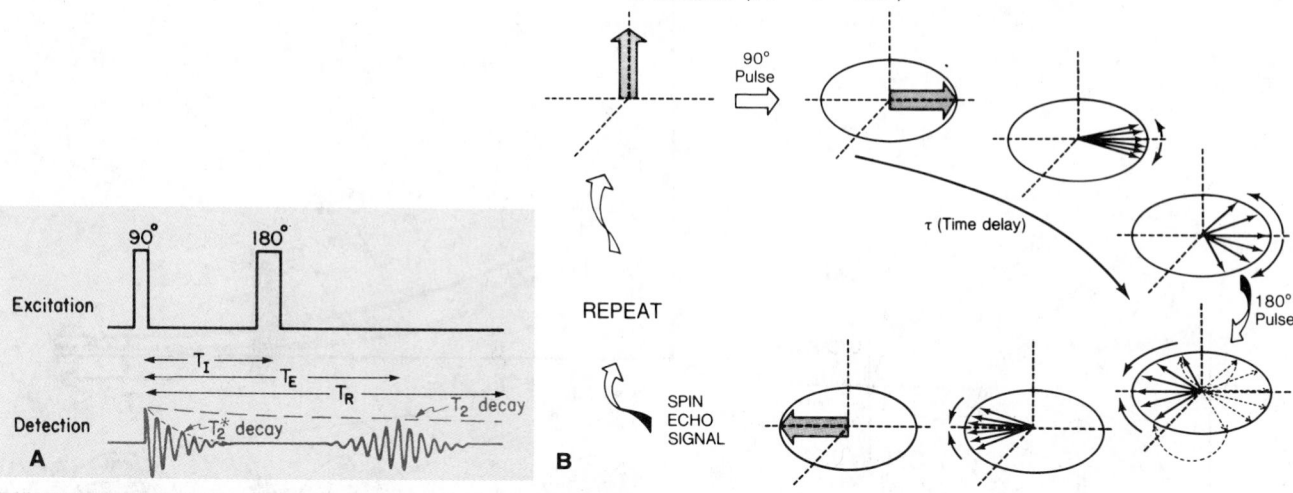

FIGURE 21–21. **(A)** Spin echo pulse sequence and pulse-timing diagram. The 180° pulse, applied TI milliseconds after the initial 90° pulse, generates a spin echo at time t = 2TI = TE. The amplitude of the echo is a function of the echo delay and the transverse (spin-spin) relaxation time T2. By contrast, the free induction signal decays with a time constant T2*, the effective transverse relaxation time. Notice that T2* ≤ T2. The repetition time (TR) of the pulse sequence is the interval between successive 90° radiofrequency (RF) pulses. (Wehrlic FW, MacFall JR, Newton TH. Parameters Determining the Appearance of NMR Images. In: Newton TH, Potts GD. *Modern Neuroradiology Volume Two. Advanced Imaging Techniques.* Clavadel Press, San Anselmo, 1983) **(B)** In the spin echo sequence, a 90° pulse rotates the net magnetization into the xy plane. The nuclear magnets, which are initially phase coherent, begin to spin out of phase. After a time period, τ, a 180° pulse is applied. After the second pulse, the magnetization partially refocuses to form an echo signal after a time, τ. **(C)** A 90° RF pulse produces a net magnetization in the xy plane. The loss of this magnetization occurs by two distinct relaxation processes, longitudinal (spin-lattice) and transverse (spin-spin) relaxation. Longitudinal relaxation is the return of magnetization to equilibrium with the applied magnetic field (z direction). The time for this decay is characterized by the time constant T1. Transverse relaxation is the loss of nuclear spin phase coherence. With a loss of phase coherence, the net magnetization in the xy plane decays to zero. The time for this process to occur is characterized by the time constant T2. (Harmes, et al. Principles of NMR. RadioGraphics 1984;4:34–39)

process by which image signals are generated in temporal coordination with the gradient applications used for spatial localization (see Fig. 21–21).

The RF pulses are delivered as oscillating currents that are synchronized with the Larmor frequency of precession of the nuclei under investigation (*e.g.,* ¹H). This produces resonance with the precessing nuclei, which results in a transfer of energy to them and widening of the precessing angle, moving the magnetic vector away from the Z axis and into the XY plane (a 90° pulse) or using a longer or higher amplitude pulse into the opposite orientation along the Z axis (a 180° pulse). The change in precession angle produced by the RF pulse is referred to as the *flip angle,* and in some image acquisition techniques, partial flip angles of less than 90° may be used.

A typical spin echo pulse sequence is shown in Figure 21–21. The RF sequence begins with a 90° pulse, flipping the nuclear magnetic vector into the XY plane, which is followed after a short interval by the 180° pulse, flipping the magnetic vector into the opposite orientation in the XY plane and rephasing the component microscopic vectors. This rephasing

corrects any dephasing that has occurred after the 90° pulse and produces a coherent signal called a spin echo. The *spin echo* is the signal returning from the resonating nuclei that is used for image formation. The time from the 90° pulse to the spin echo is the *echo time* (TE), typically 20 to 80 msec, but it can be as short as 5 msec or as long as 120 msec in some specialized pulse sequences. The complete image must be produced by multiple repetitions of the pulse sequence in conventional spin echo imaging (*i.e.,* 128, 192, or 256 times). The time between each set of RF pulses (*e.g.,* time from one 90° pulse to the next in spin echo imaging) is the *repetition time* (TR).

A slightly different type of pulse sequence, a *gradient echo* (GRE) technique, is used for some fast imaging studies that use partial flip angle RF pulses and gradient shifts instead of the 180° pulse to produce the signal echo. Faster techniques are currently under development that allow image acquisition in less than a minute to a few hundred milliseconds. These techniques use various approaches, including GRE with short TR (*e.g.,* 25 msec) and sequences in which larger segments of the image are obtained with each pulse cycle, such as fast

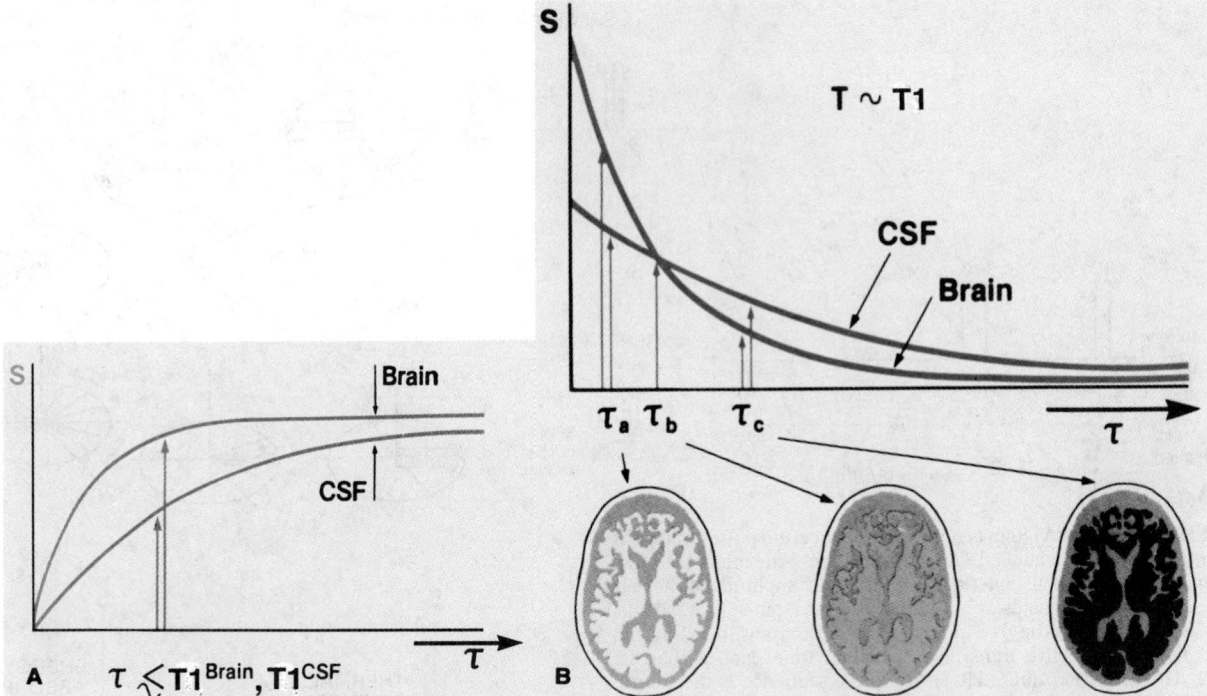

FIGURE 21–22. **(A)** T1 relaxation is illustrated here as the exponential rise in signal (S in y axis) over time (τ) for brain and CSF. The steep rise in the brain signal indicates a shorter T1 (faster relaxation) than the slow rise in the CSF signal. The maximum difference between these curves is at a time point marked by the up arrows. Using this short time interval for the TR of an SE pulse sequence produces a T1-weighted image with high signal intensity in brain and low signal intensity in CSF. **(B)** T2 relaxation is illustrated as the exponential decline in signal over time for brain and CSF. The time delays (τ_a, τ_b, τ_c) represent successively longer TE intervals in an SE pulse sequence. At τ_a, the brain has a higher signal than CSF, similar to a T1-weighted image. At τ_b, the brain and CSF are isointense, producing "balanced" image contrast. At τ_c, the brain has a lower signal than CSF, producing a T2-weighted image (see Fig. 21–11B). This complex relation between signal decay and TE is the result of "partial saturation" of the nuclear spins (producing different starting points for T2 curves along the y axis) when the TR time (T) is similar to T1, which is common in clinical MRI. (NMR: A perspective on imaging. General Electric Company, 1982)

spin echo, or in which the complete image is obtained in a single pulse cycle, as in echo-planar imaging. A detailed discussion of these techniques is available in sources listed in the references.[27–29]

Image Contrast

The final appearance of the MR image, the signal contrast between the different structures in the image plane, is largely determined by the choice of the RF pulse sequence (*i.e.*, TR and TE) for spin echo images and by the RF sequence and the flip angle for GRE images. Although the effect of these variables may be complex, there are guidelines for analyzing four types of images (Fig. 21–23).

First, images in which the signal difference between tissues (*i.e.*, image contrast) primarily depends on T1 relaxation are referred to as T1-weighted images (Figs. 21–22 and 21–24). These are acquired using short TR and TE times with spin echo images (*e.g.*, TR = 500 msec, TE = 20 msec) and large flip angles with GRE techniques (*e.g.*, 70°–90°). T1 differences between tissues are in the range between the long T1 of free water such as CSF (low signal) and the short T1 of

fat (high signal). In general, T1-weighted images primarily provide anatomic information and are used for images enhanced with gadolinium, which produces marked T1 shortening (high signal).

Second, there are images for which the signals between tissues depend primarily on T2 relaxation time differences, which are called T2-weighted images (see Figs. 21–22 and 21–24). These are acquired using long TR and TE times with spin echo images (*e.g.*, TR = 2000 msec, TE = 80 msec) and lower flip angles with GRE images (*e.g.*, 5°–30°). T2 differences reflect tissue water content and are in the range between the long T2 of free water such as CSF (high signal) and the short T2 of fat (low signal). T2-weighted images are more sensitive than T1-weighted images to early pathologic changes in most tissues.

Third, images acquired with intermediate TR and TE times (*e.g.*, TR = 2000 msec, TE = 20 msec) and intermediate flip angles tend to have balanced, or mixed, contrast that depends on T1 and T2 relaxation times. Although these images are commonly called proton density images because of the relatively flat appearance of the image contrast, this is a misleading term because the image contrast depends on a complex

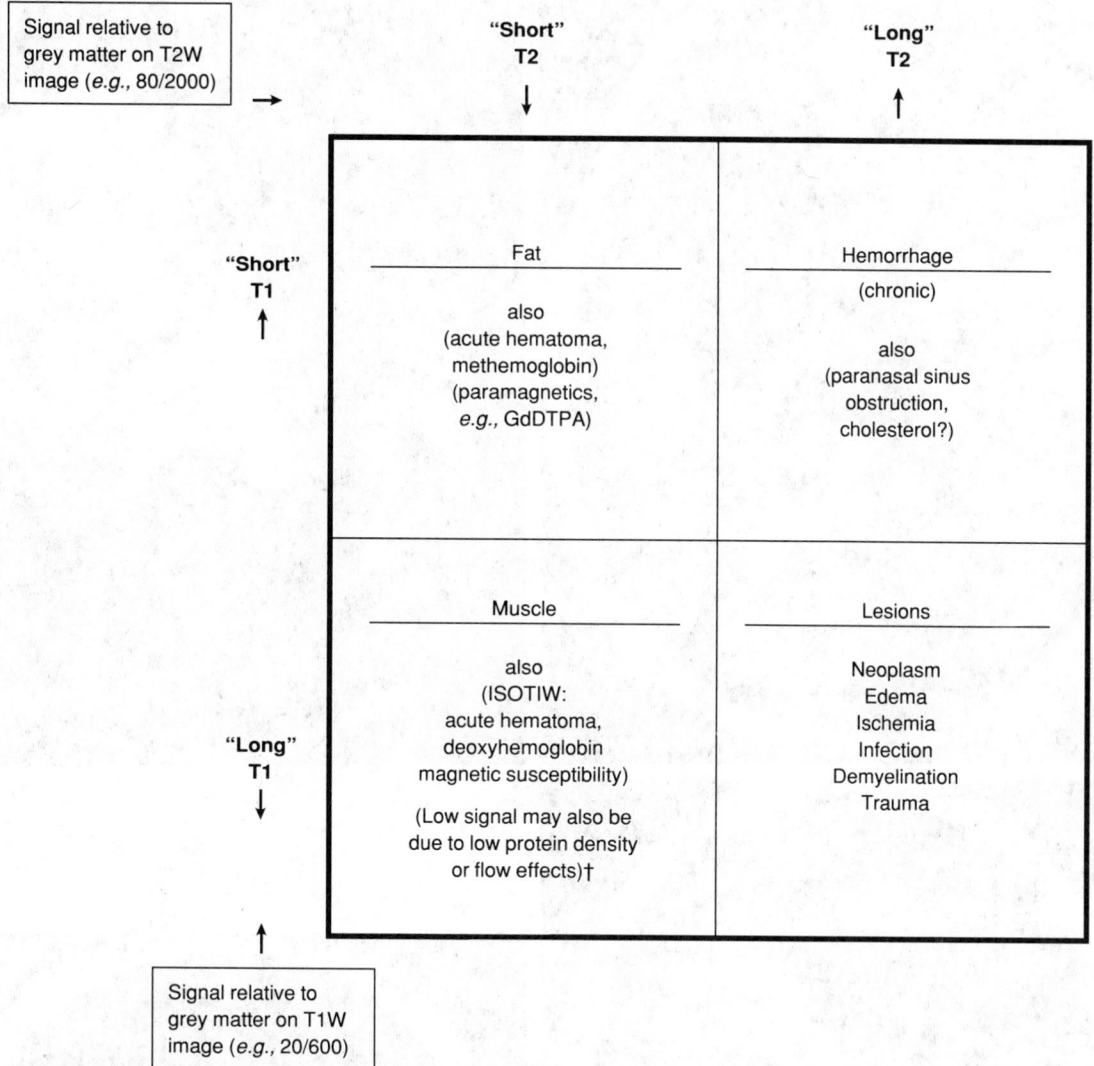

Signal relative to grey matter on T2W image (*e.g.*, 80/2000) →

"Short" T2 ↓

"Long" T2 ↑

"Short" T1 ↑

Fat

also
(acute hematoma, methemoglobin)
(paramagnetics, *e.g.*, GdDTPA)

Hemorrhage

(chronic)

also
(paranasal sinus obstruction, cholesterol?)

"Long" T1 ↓

Muscle

also
(ISOTIW:
acute hematoma, deoxyhemoglobin magnetic susceptibility)

(Low signal may also be due to low protein density or flow effects)†

Lesions

Neoplasm
Edema
Ischemia
Infection
Demyelination
Trauma

↑

Signal relative to grey matter on T1W image (*e.g.*, 20/600)

FIGURE 21–23. This 2 × 2 figure is a nonexhaustive guide to tissue classification using typical spin echo MR images 1.5T. This type of cross-comparison of tissue signal between T1-weighted and T2-weighted images to "sort out" classes of tissue is a common initial step for MRI interpretation. ↑, high signal; ↓, low signal; T1W, "T1-weighted" SE TE/TR; T2W, "T2-weighted" SE TE/TR.
* ISOTIW, isointense with normal brain or TIW image, hypointense on T2W image.
† Small or diffuse calcification is usually isointense with brain.
Dense calcification: low signal from low proton density and susceptibility gradients.
Relaxation times are approximate and are compared with grey matter.
Range of values: "Short" T1, 250–300 ms; "Short" T2, 40–50 ms; "Long" T1, 1000–1100 ms; "Long" T2, 120–130 ms.

interaction of proton density and relaxation times. This sequence may be clinically useful by providing tissue contrast not seen on T1-weighted or T2-weighted images.

Fourth, other properties of tissue contribute to image contrast, such as *fluid motion* (*e.g.*, blood, cerebrospinal fluid) and *magnetic susceptibility*. The effects of fluid motion tend to produce spin dephasing and signal loss on standard clinical pulse sequences. Techniques called MR angiography (MRA) that use vascular flow effects allow the formation of images of intravascular flow. Two general phenomena are used to generate MRA studies: inflow or time-of-flight effects and the phase shift effect caused by moving spins producing phase-contrast images. Time-of-flight effects occur if protons move

into an image during the time between the 90° RF flip and the signal echo. Because these protons have not experienced previous RF flips, they produce maximal signal from the echo, higher than the surrounding static tissue that has received multiple RF flips. A group of sequentially offset images can be used to trace the time-of-flight effect along the length of a vessel and produce an MR angiogram with a bright vessel lumen and dark surrounding tissue. The use of phase-shift effects for MRA is analogous to radiographic subtraction. Two images are obtained at slightly different times, and the shift in phase produced by moving blood is used to differentiate it from the static tissue that has not shifted between the images. Mathematic "subtraction" of the two images removes the

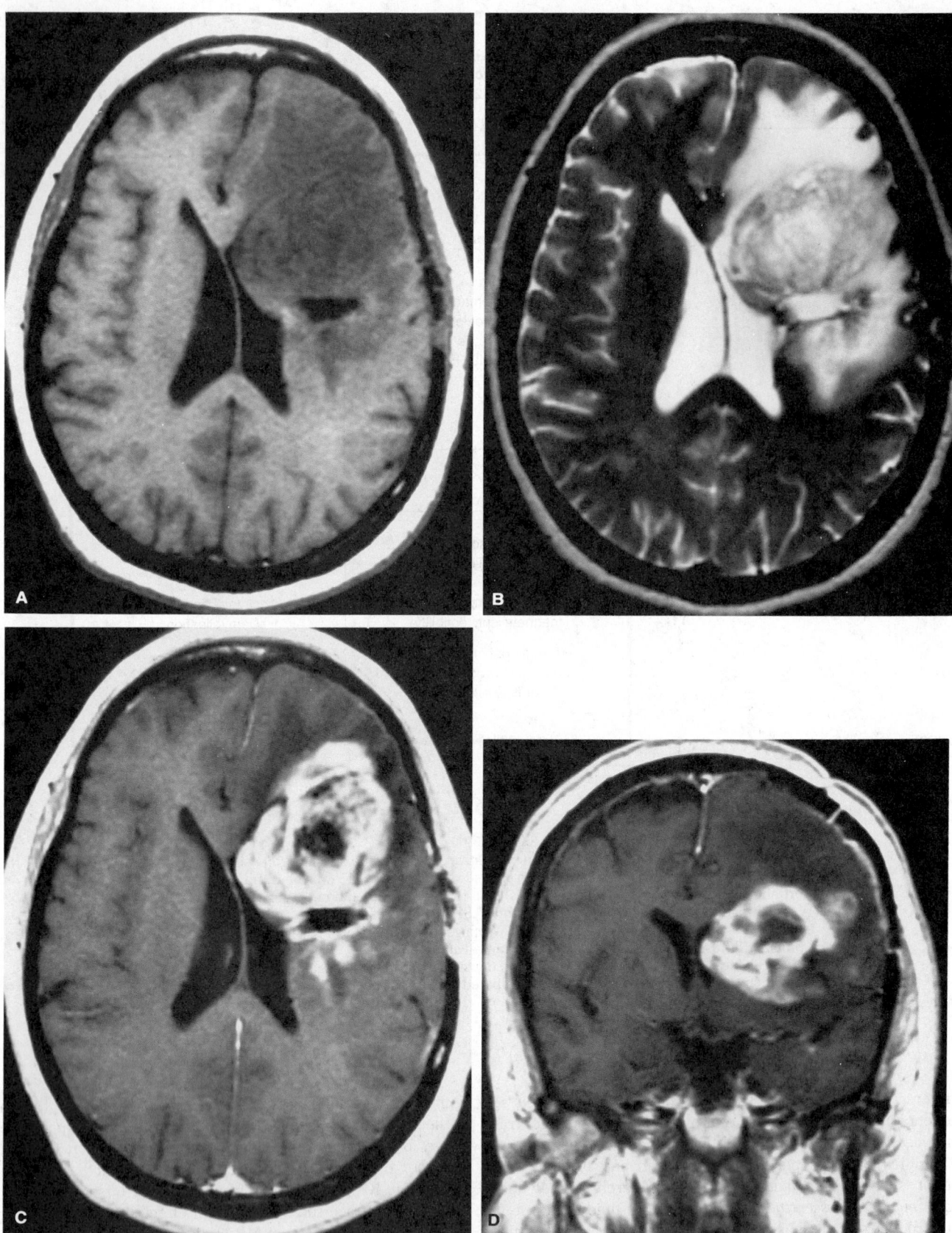

FIGURE 21–24. **(A)** T1-weighted noncontrast axial image of a primary brain tumor (glioblastoma multiforme) producing reduced signal (from prolonged T1) and mass effect in the left frontal lobe. CSF in the lateral ventricles is dark (very long T1). **(B)** T2-weighted axial image at the same level as **(A)** shows a complex, increased signal (prolonged T2) in the central tumor area and higher signal in the surrounding white matter edema; CSF is bright (very long T2). **(C)** T1-weighted axial image after intravenous GdDTPA infusion shows high signal intensity (short T1) in areas of blood-brain barrier breakdown in the central tumor. **(D)** T1-weighted coronal image also shows the enhancing lesion. The combination of axial, coronal, and sagittal views of a lesion is often helpful for precise localization and surgical or radiation therapy planning.

static tissue and produces an image of the vessel lumen, a phase-contrast MR angiogram (Fig. 21–25). In practice, time-of-flight MRA tends to be used in larger vessels with stenoses and zones of turbulent flow, such as the carotid artery bifurcation. Phase-contrast MRA tends to be used for smaller vessels, such as in the intracranial circulation, and if precise velocity quantitation and flow direction information are needed.

Magnetic susceptibility is the inherent ability of a substance to become magnetized. In tissue, magnetic susceptibility varies at the microscopic level; it is homogenous in fluids and inhomogenous in complex tissues. At interfaces between cellular structures or tissues with different magnetic susceptibilities, small magnetic field gradients are produced. These subtle, microscopic magnetic gradients cause a loss of phase coherence within image voxels and as water protons diffuse across them during image acquisition. The protons in different magnetic environments within the voxel precess at different rates, resulting in rapid phase dispersion and loss of signal from the voxel. The longer the interval between signal acquisitions (*i.e.*, echoes) in a pulse sequence, the more time is allowed for loss of phase coherence and consequent loss of signal. The time constant for this loss of phase coherence is T2*, which is a measure of transverse magnetization and is a function of magnetic field inhomogeneities and the T2 of tissue. T2* effects differ from T2 relaxation in that they strongly depend on field strength. Images sensitive to T2* are often used clinically to identify small areas of hemorrhage (*e.g.*, occult cerebral arteriovenous malformations). A potential application is measurement of tissue perfusion, based on the magnetic susceptibility gradients across capillary walls produced by the passage of a bolus of intravascular paramagnetic contrast material.[28]

The importance of magnetic field strength to MRI is primarily improved signal-to-noise ratio at higher fields. There is a fairly consistent appearance of MR images across the range of magnetic field strengths currently in use (0.15–1.5 T), with greater signal-to-noise ratio at high field strength and specific technical differences between imaging systems. However, subtle field-dependent effects on relaxation times (*e.g.*, T1 prolongation), inherent magnetic properties of the tissue (*e.g.*, magnetic susceptibility), and proton-electron interactions (*i.e.*, paramagnetic effects) may be more apparent on MR images obtained at higher magnetic fields.

Contrast Agents

As in CT scanning, intravascular contrast agents are used with MRI, especially for identifying blood-brain barrier breakdown and evaluating perfusion (enhancement) of neoplastic, inflammatory, and fibrotic tissues throughout the body. Intraluminal bowel contrast agents are also used to improve abdominal MRI.

All current MRI contrast agents produce marked T1 relaxation time shortening in the tissues where they localize in sufficient concentrations. This produces high signal on T1-weighted images. As of 1992, the only FDA-approved clinical intravascular contrast agent is the chelate gadolinium-DTPA (gadopentetate). Gadolinium is used because it has an especially strong paramagnetic effect on adjacent water protons, which causes marked T1 relaxation acceleration (*i.e.*, relaxation time shortening). In the central nervous system, this produces highly conspicuous enhancement in areas of blood-brain barrier breakdown, meningeal inflammation, and primary or metastatic tumor (see Fig. 21–24).

Nuclear Magnetic Resonance Spectroscopy

The techniques of experimental NMR can be applied to patients in vivo to generate clinical MR spectroscopy (MRS) studies.[30-32] The major difference between clinical MRS and experimental NMR spectroscopy is the lower magnetic field strength at which MRS is performed (*i.e.*, maximum of 1.5 T) compared with experimental NMR field strengths five to eight times higher. The value of the higher field strength used in NMR is improved signal-to-noise ratio and consequently better spectral discrimination between signals from specific chemical species.

With clinical MRS, this information is obtained in the intact patient, instead of from samples of tissue or fluid, and it is spatially localized within the image plane being studied, rather than being the sum of all components of the sample in the NMR spectrometer. Clinical MRS has provided useful biochemical information, initially with ^{31}P spectral data about

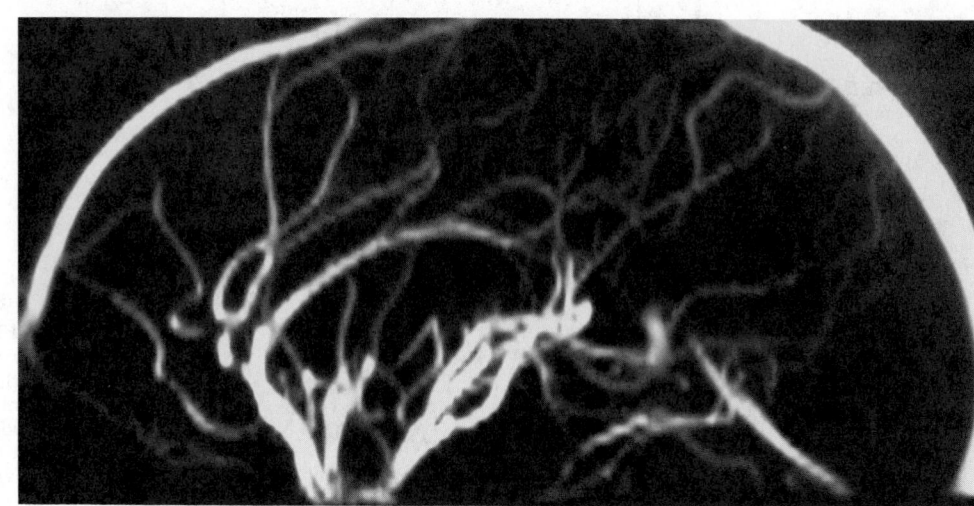

FIGURE 21–25. A phase contrast MR angiogram of the cerebral circulation is displayed as a lateral projection image (anterior is to the left of the image). Flow in the major branches of the anterior cerebral and middle cerebral arteries is apparent. Flow in the major venous structures is also seen, including the sagittal sinus and straight sinus.

cellular energy metabolism and more recently with ¹H spectra of proton-containing metabolites. Phosphorus MRS has been used to monitor energy metabolites such as ATP terminal phosphates, phosphocreatine, phosphomonoesters and phosphodiesters, and free phosphates (Fig. 21–26). Cellular pH can also be measured with ³¹P spectra. Characteristic changes in phosphorus spectra in muscle have been used to diagnosis enzymatic disorders such as McArdle's disease. Hydrogen MRS is currently being used to study proton moieties in cellular metabolites, especially in brain and brain tumors, such as lactate, N-acetyl-aspartate, choline, and creatine.

Current acquisition techniques used for clinical MRS require volume elements (voxels) approximately 64 cm³ (*i.e.,* a cube 4 cm on each side) for phosphorus and 8 cm³ (*i.e.,* a cube 2 cm on each side) for hydrogen, within the practical time limitation of under 30 minutes acquisition time. This is analogous to images with 2- to 4-cm resolution compared with the 1-mm resolution of current proton images. The major challenges to researchers attempting to expand the clinical application of MRS are improving the signal-to-noise ratio and localization techniques. Improved signal-to-noise ratio will allow more reliable discrimination between chemical species and acquisition from smaller voxels, improving the spatial resolution and therefore anatomic specificity of spectral data. Localization techniques are progressing away from the single voxel acquisition toward multivoxel techniques and presentation of spectral data in an image format with a separate image for each major metabolite.

NUCLEAR MEDICINE

Nuclear medicine uses radioisotopes as tracers to assess normal and abnormal physiology of living tissues. The results are usually displayed as an image that represents a regional body function rather than simple anatomy. "Hot spots" are detected when the process concentrates the radioactivity, as with tumors concentrating gallium 67, thallium 201, or radiolabeled monoclonal antibodies. "Cold spots" occur when tumors displace normal structures and tissues, such as space-occupying liver lesions on ⁹⁹ᵐTc-sulfur colloid scans.

Conventional nuclear medicine methods depend on the use of specific radiotracers and radiation detectors to create functional images of physiologic and pathophysiologic processes occurring in vivo in human patients. Most nuclear medicine methods in common use in oncology are qualitative in nature, rather than absolute rates of a physiologic process. Although availability is still limited, positron emission tomography images in a quantitative manner, greatly extending the power of these techniques for research and diagnosis in oncology.

Therapy using radioisotopic sources is of growing importance in oncology. Common radioisotopes used for imaging and therapy are listed in Table 21–3. PET isotopes are listed in Table 21–4.

Instrumentation

Most procedures are performed using an Anger type *gamma camera* system. This instrument detects the γ rays coming from the radiotracer within the patient. Over time, a two-dimensional projection image of the three-dimensional distribution of radioactivity in the patient is built up in a computer matrix, and it is usually recorded for display and interpretation on a CRT screen or x-ray film. These planar gamma camera images have the same disadvantage as planar x-ray images (*e.g.,* chest radiographs), because radioactivity is overlapping, often obscuring significant information. A three-dimensional representation of radioactivity distribution is often preferable.

Single photon emission computed tomography (SPECT)

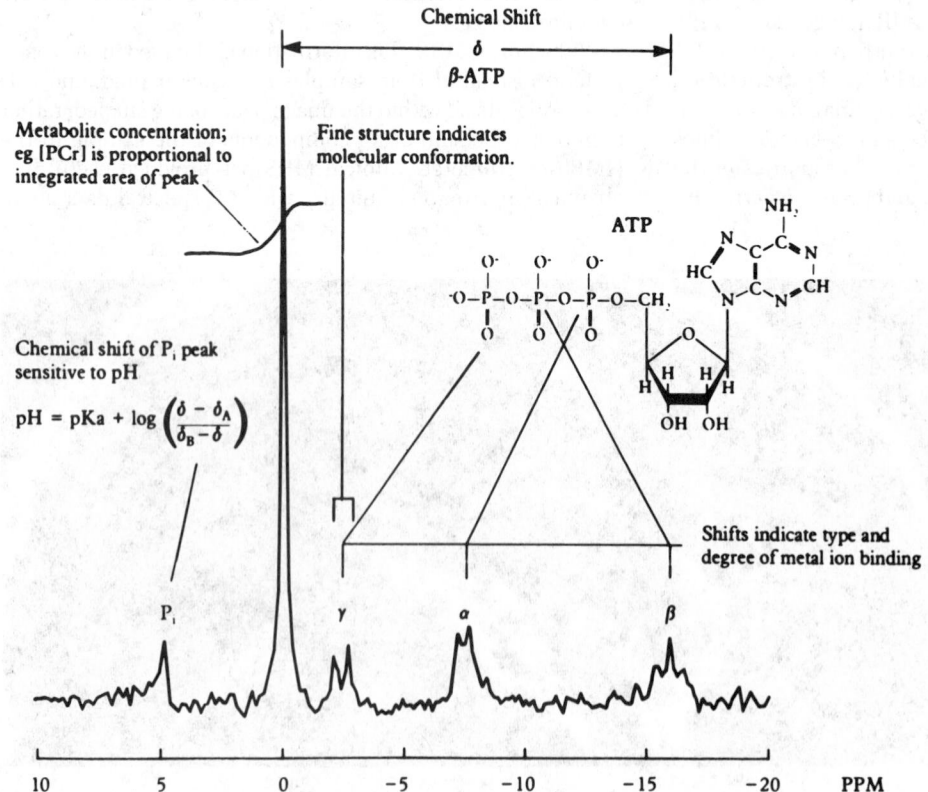

FIGURE 21–26. This ³¹P phosphorus spectrum illustrates the relation of the spectral frequency (in ppm) and molecular structure. (Shaw D. In vivo topical magnetic resonance. In: Partain CL, James A, Rollo FD and Price RR. *Nuclear Magnetic Resonance (NMR) Imaging.* W.B. Saunders Company, 1983)

TABLE 21-3. Common Radionuclides Used in Diagnosis and Therapy

Radionuclide	Half-Life	Decay Type, Energy
Iodine 131	8.0 d	Beta minus, 0.693 MeV Gamma rays, 360 keV
Iodine 123	13 h	Gamma rays, 159 keV
Iodine 125	60.2 d	Electron capture x-rays, 35 keV
Technitium 99m	6.0 h	Isomeric transition gamma rays, 140 keV
Indium 111	67.3 h	Electron capture gamma rays, 173, 247 keV
Rhenium 186	91. h	Beta minus (95%), 1.07 MeV electron capture (5%) gamma rays, 137 keV
Gallium 67	78.3 h	Electron capture gamma rays, 93, 185, 296 keV
Krypton 81m	13 sec	Isomeric transition gamma rays, 190 keV
Xenon 133	5.25 d	Beta minus, 0.346 MeV
Thallium 201	73 h	Electron capture x-rays, 80 keV
Phosphorus 32	14.3 d	Beta minus, 1.71 MeV
Yttrium 90	64 h	Beta minus, 2.7 MeV

TABLE 21-4. Common Positron Emitters Used in Nuclear Medicine

Emitter	Half-Life	Decay Type, Energy
Oxygen 15	123 sec	Beta plus, 1.74 MeV
Carbon 11	20 min	Beta plus, 0.97 MeV
Nitrogen 13	10 min	Beta plus, 1.20 MeV
Fluorine 18	110 min	Beta plus, 0.635 MeV
Iodine 124	4.15 d	Beta plus (26%), 2.4 MeV electron capture gamma rays, 605 keV

cameras create tomographic or cross-sectional images of conventional radiopharmaceutical activity distributions in vivo.[33] A specially designed gamma camera rotates about the patient, collecting a series of projection images that are mathematically processed, using computer techniques similar to x-ray CT or MRI, into a three-dimensional display. In the past decade, SPECT has become a routine clinical diagnostic procedure. Continuing advances in basic electronics, computing speed, and collimation design have led to higher resolution and easier use.[34]

Positron emission tomography (PET) provides quantitative tomographic images from a three-dimensional distribution of concentrations of radioactivity within the body. PET images are generated in a similar way to other tomographic methods, but the signal used to create the three-dimensional image comes from the radioactive decay of a positron-emitting radionuclide and the resultant γ rays which are released in the process. The physics of positron decay permits an "electronic collimation" as a basis for mapping the site of the radiotracer, which is superior to that used for planar or SPECT imaging.[35]

PET greatly enhances the study of radiotracer distributions. It can measure and map the nanomolar concentrations of biomolecules that participate in biochemical reactions in vivo. In some ways, PET is the biochemical analysis analog of a powerful microscope. Biologic studies of tumors, which before PET could only be done in the artificial environment of the test tube, can now be done at the tumor site within the body of the patient.[36]

A major disadvantage of PET is the requirement of positron-emitting radionuclides produced in a cyclotron, which must be close to the PET camera site because many radionuclides (*e.g.*, ^{11}C, ^{15}O, ^{18}F, ^{13}N) have short half-lives (see Table 21-2). However, PET extends the tracer principle for noninvasive use in diagnosis and research of cancer, based on two essential features of the method: the ability to detect absolute concentrations of radioactivity in vivo with high resolution and the use of tracer elements that are isotopes of the most important elements in biology.

Applications in Oncology

Most routine scanning in oncology is performed with the Anger camera in conventional (planar) mode, because this is the most efficient method of imaging large regions of the body. For more detailed knowledge about the three-dimensional distribution of the radiotracer, SPECT imaging may be performed. The greater contrast, anatomic clarity, and improved differentiation of normal from abnormal structures with SPECT scanning often leads to better diagnoses, but PET is of growing importance.

Bone scanning, a highly sensitive technique for detecting metastasis to bone, is usually performed with planar gamma camera imaging, using ^{99m}Tc-phosphanate compounds (Fig. 21-27). The physiologic principle is that a bone metastasis provokes an osteoblastic reaction, resulting in new bone formation, and the ^{99m}Tc-phosphanate compound is laid down in the hydroxyapatite crystal near the metastasis. If there is pain, and the planar bone scan is normal or equivocal, SPECT scanning should be performed, because SPECT may detect an early metastasis although the planar imaging is negative.[37]

^{67}Ga-citrate, a ferric ion analog, is bound to transferrin and transported into the cells of rapidly proliferating tissues after binding by transferrin receptors present on the cell surface. Two thirds of the administered ^{67}Ga is normally retained in the body in liver, spleen, and bone marrow for several days, and the remaining one third is excreted by the kidney and bowel. ^{67}Ga imaging is useful for monitoring the response of the gallium-avid malignant lymphomas to therapy (see Fig. 21-16). A ^{67}Ga-negative mass supports a positive therapeutic response and the absence of viable tumor.[38] SPECT scanning is particularly important for these tumors.[39] However, false-negative scans may be obtained if ^{67}Ga scanning is performed too soon after therapy. The optimal time for follow-up gallium scanning in treated patients remains to be determined. Persistent ^{67}Ga uptake 6 to 8 weeks after the cessation of therapy is a reliable indicator for active disease, and it is especially useful for patients with residual masses whose disease is thought to be inactive and no longer requiring therapy. Lung cancer, melanoma, osteosarcoma, and hepatocellular carcinoma have demonstrated ^{67}Ga uptake, but its use in these tumors is limited.

Thallium 201 scanning, using thallous ions injected intravenously, is a test of tumor viability (Fig. 21-28).[40] The ^{201}Tl

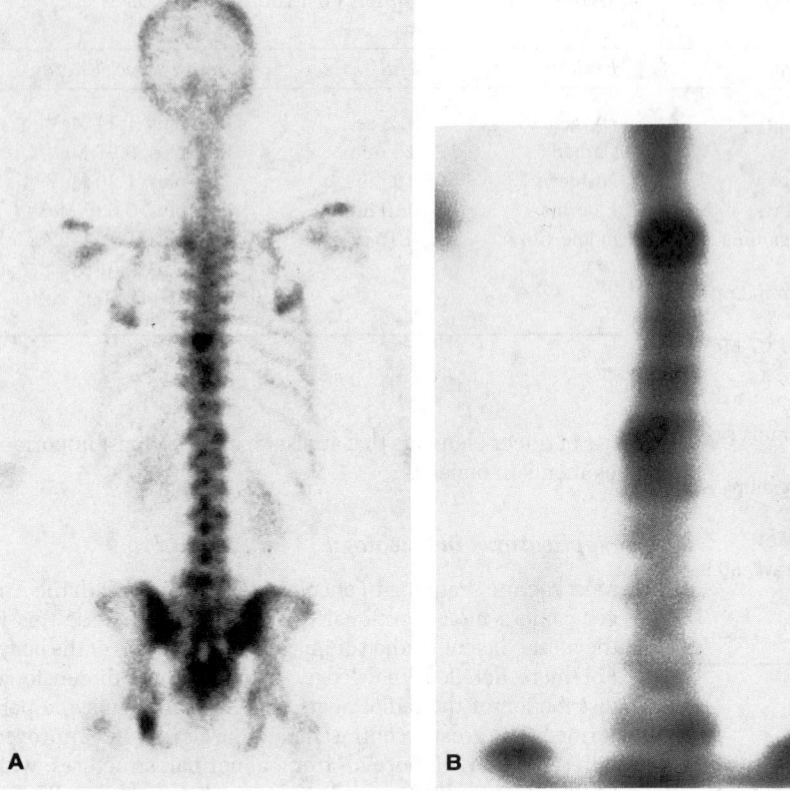

FIGURE 21–27. A premenopausal woman developed pain in her lower back 5 years after a modified radical mastectomy for breast cancer. **(A)** A technetium 99m methylene diphosphanate bone scan with planar imaging showed multiple sites of increased uptake in the sternum, left third rib, midthoracic spine, left ischium, and femoral necks bilaterally. **(B)** Coronal SPECT scan showed multiple additional sites of increased uptake in the lower thoracic spine and L5 vertebra, which were not evident on the planar bone scan.

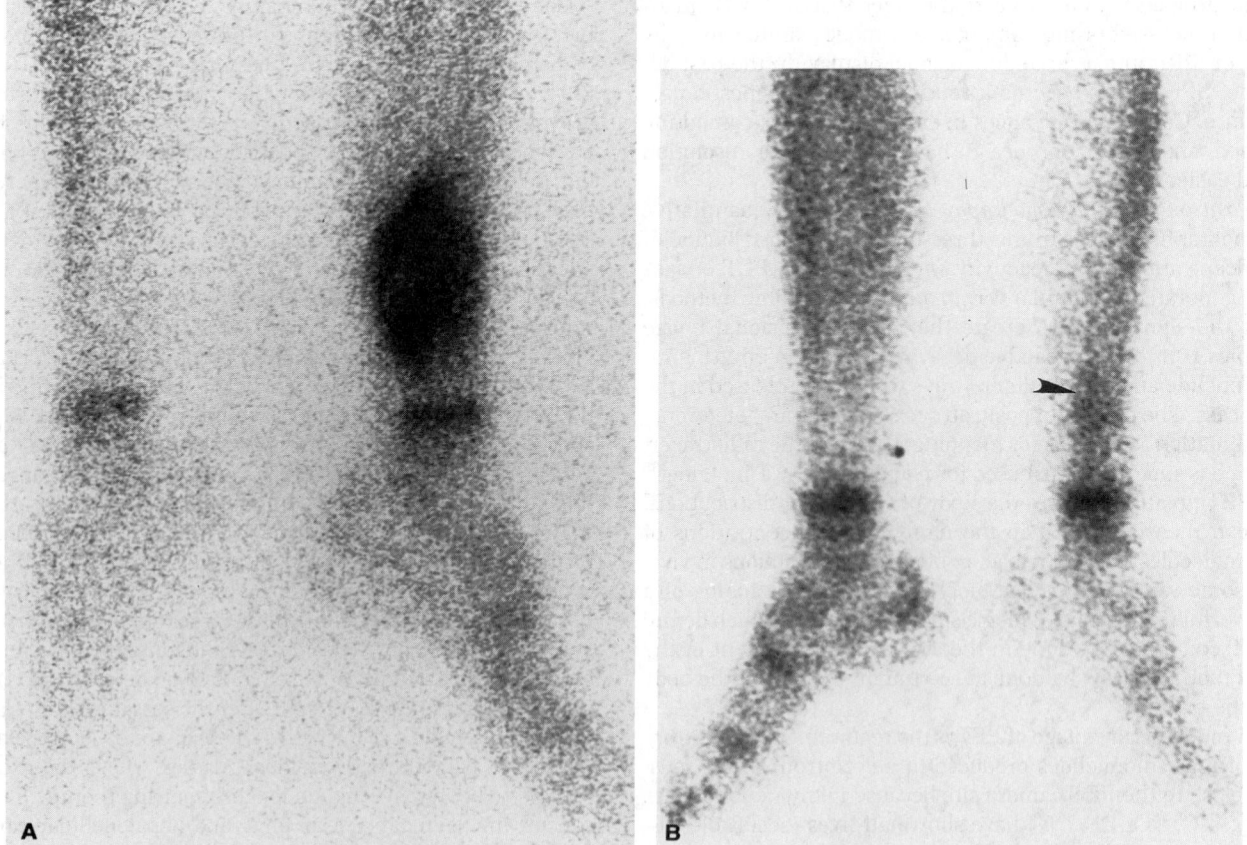

FIGURE 21–28. An adolescent with Ewing's sarcoma of the left lower leg. **(A)** In the staging thallium 201 scan, there is intense activity. **(B)** After therapy, the uptake has disappeared, and only a tiny residual soft-tissue blush is seen (*arrow*). After treatment, the biopsy showed that all visible cells were necrotic.

is concentrated by the sodium-postassium pump by tumors, has been successfully used to image lung cancer, thyroid cancer, breast cancer, and brain tumors, and appears to be useful in differentiating tumors from benign masses. There is usually substantial ^{201}Tl uptake in primary and metastatic cerebral tumors, with little uptake in normal brain tissue. Thallium uptake does not rely on breakdown of the blood-brain barrier, and the intensity of ^{201}Tl uptake correlates with the grade of tumor; the more malignant the tumor, the more avid it takes up [201]Tl.

Hepatic Scanning

Planar imaging of the liver for metastases has been largely supplanted by CT, ultrasound, and MRI. SPECT, by increasing image contrast in a three-dimensional, functional display that eliminates influences of overlapping radioactivity, can provide a practical alternative. However, SPECT imaging of the liver is a second-line test in further characterizing space-occupying hepatic lesions discovered on other imaging tests. If a mass seen on CT, MRI, or ultrasound cannot be differentiated as a tumor or hemangioma, radioisotope liver scanning using SPECT has an important role.[5] For lesions greater than 2.5 cm in diameter, SPECT ^{99m}Tc-labeled erythrocyte scintigraphy is sensitive and specific for hemangiomas (see Fig. 21–14). Delayed images reveal accumulation of the tracer within a dilated capillary network, which fills in centrally, unlike the adjacent liver. Caution should be exercised in interpretation of lesions that lie near large vessels and of smaller lesions.

Liver scanning can assess the adequacy of perfusion by intrahepatic arterial catheters for localized chemotherapy, such as in isolated colorectal metastases to the liver.[41] ^{99m}Tc-labeled microaggregated albumin (30–80-μm particles) is injected through the infusion pump into the hepatic artery. Extrahepatic perfusion may occur if the catheter tip position changes, perfusing the stomach, pancreas, or spleen and producing toxic effects. The resultant images map the areas of perfusion (Fig. 21–29).

2-Fluoro-2-deoxy-D-glucose PET Scanning

Early studies in animal tumors suggested a characteristic metabolism of malignancy, which resulted in sufficiently active retention of biochemical radiotracers in tumors to serve as a basis for PET imaging of tracers for glycolysis and RNA or DNA synthesis. The positron-labeled tracer 2-fluoro-2-deoxy-D-glucose (FDG) seemed promising for tumor detection. Initial observations in patients with primary brain tumors suggested that glucose metabolism increased with histologic grade, that radiation necrosis could be differentiated from tumors based on glucose metabolism, that an association existed between increasing metabolic rate and reduced prognosis, that visual symptoms correlated with alteration in glucose metabolism along optic pathways, that meningiomas could be categorized according to aggressiveness, that a profound metabolic change in low-grade gliomas accompanies malignant degeneration to higher grade tumors, and that brain tumors are less affected than normal cerebral cortex, which has a markedly reduced glucose metabolism in barbiturate coma. Other tumor types have not been as well studied as brain tumors, but it appears that the same general increase in metabolism of glucose affects non-CNS malignancies.

FDG has been used for imaging primary and metastatic breast cancers (Fig. 21–30),[42] and FDG PET imaging has been employed for differential diagnosis of colorectal recurrences from scar formation observed on CT.[43] PET images

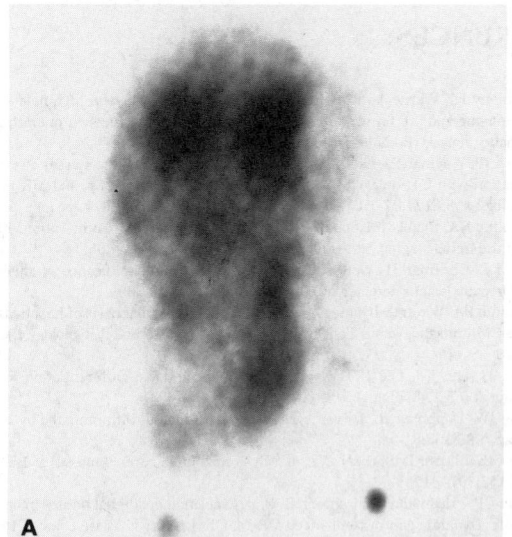
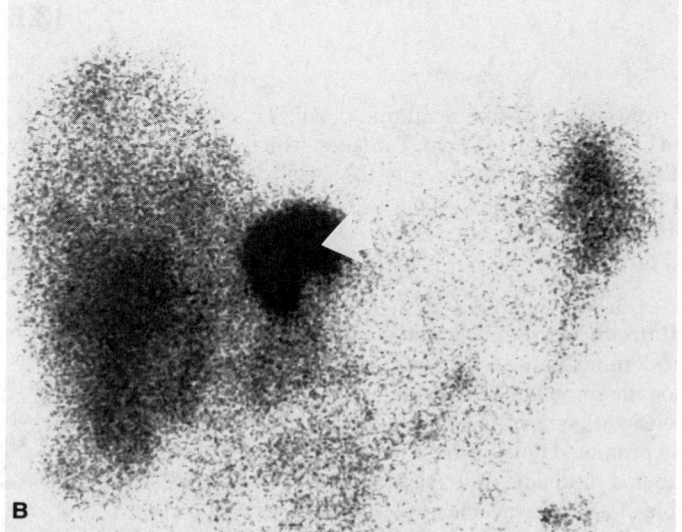

FIGURE 21–29. A 56-year-old man with metastatic colorectal carcinoma to liver was treated by chemotherapy infusion through an indwelling right hepatic artery catheter. **(A)** After injection of ^{99m}Tc microaggregated albumin (MAA) into the sideport of an infused pump, it is distributed throughout the right lobe of liver, indicating desired, selective perfusion. Areas of more intense uptake surround the metastatic lesions. **(B)** Five months later, a repeat ^{99m}Tc MAA study through the same port shows intense uptake at a site in the midline, near the terminus of the hepatic artery catheter (*arrow*), the diffuse activity throughout the entire liver and spleen, indicating movement of the catheter tip into the celiac artery.

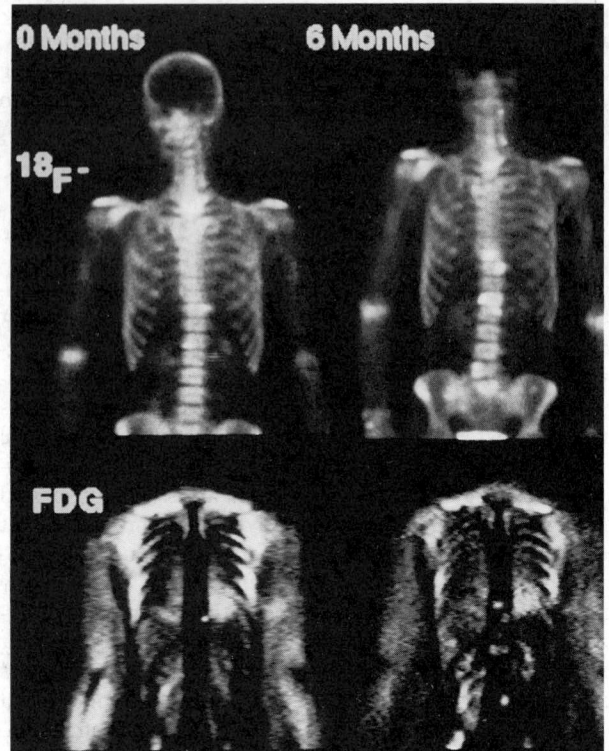

FIGURE 21-30. A breast cancer patient with progressive metastatic disease. In the upper row of images, the patient received ^{18}F fluoride, a bone seeking element, and high resolution planar bone scans were performed as a series of projection images at 0 and 6 months of follow-up. The bone scan shows progressive disease with increasing uptake in the cervical, lower thoracic, and upper and lower lumbar spine. PET scans after injection of FDG, a tracer of glucose metabolism, showed metabolic glucose images of the same region at 0 and 6 months after therapy (lower row). Sites of bony reaction demonstrated by the ^{18}F scan and glucose metabolism for the multiple metastatic lesions are readily seen. (Courtesy of Dr. Randall A. Hawkins, MD, PhD, Radiological Sciences, UCLA, Los Angeles, California)

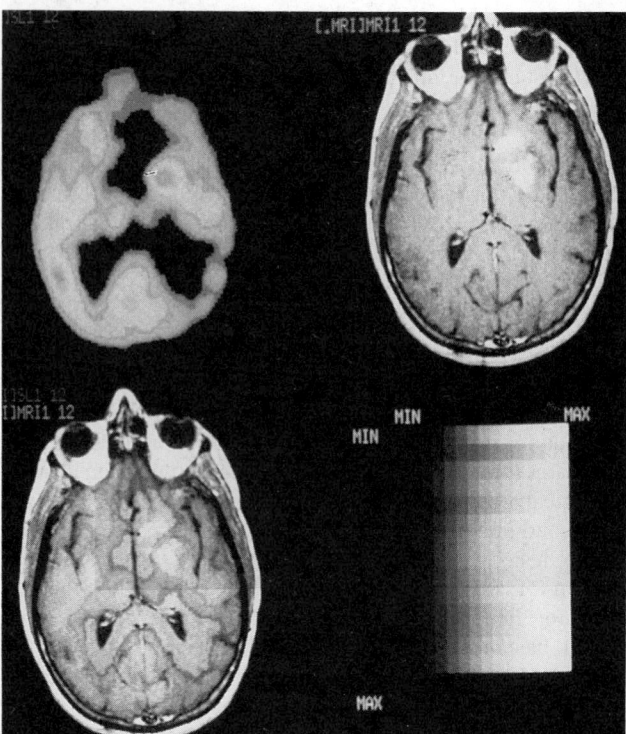

FIGURE 21-31. Combination image created from an MRI and an FDG PET scan. Areas of contrast enhancement on the MR image correspond to high and low metabolic activity on the PET image. These "fusion images" provide improved information about the spatial location of lesions and their metabolic state.

suffer from a lack of fine anatomic detail. This can be addressed by "fusion" of MRI or CT images, which possess high spatial and contrast resolution, with the metabolic information from PET images. These fusion images provide improved information about the location of lesions and their metabolic state (Fig. 21-31).

Radioimmunodiagnosis and Radioimmunotherapy

The identification of tumor-associated antigens, such as carcinoembryonic antigen, which can provide targets for radiolabeled antibodies, and the development of the hybridoma method promoted development of the clinical application of radiolabeled antibodies for diagnosis and therapy.[44,45] The principle of immunospecific targeting has been reaffirmed in multiple clinical trials using radiolabeled antibodies against many human tumors. The methods used are essentially nontoxic. Occult tumor has been identified in clinical studies of colorectal and ovarian cancers, melanoma, lymphoma, and neuroblastoma. Some tumors, particularly lymphoma, have had significant responses to radioantibody treatment alone. Additional development and evaluation are needed before the

role of radioimmunodiagnosis and therapy in oncology is defined, but the prospects for long-term success are excellent.

REFERENCES

1. Rummeny EJ, Wernecke K, Saini S, et al. Comparison between high-field strength MR imaging and CT for screening of hepatic metastasis: A receiver operating characteristic analysis. Radiology 1992;182:879–886.
2. Heiken JP, Weyman PJ, Lee JKT, et al. Detection of focal hepatic masses: Prospective evaluation with CT, delayed CT, CT during arterial photography, and MR imaging. Radiology 1989;171:47–51.
3. Castellino RA, Blank N, Hoppe RT, et al. Hodgkin's disease: Contributions of chest CT in the initial staging evaluation. Radiology 1986;106:603–605.
4. Jones EC, Chezmar JL, Nelson RC. The frequency and significance of small (≤15 mm) hepatic lesions detected by CT. AJR 1992;158:535–539.
5. Birnbaum BA, Weinreb JC, Megibow AJ, et al. Definitive diagnosis of hepatic hemangiomas: MR imaging versus Tc-99m-labeled red blood cell SPECT. Radiology 1990;176:95–101.
6. Brown JJ, Lee JM, Lee JKT, et al. Focal hepatic lesions: Differentiation with MR imaging at 0.5 T. Radiology 1991;179:675–679.
7. Reinig JW, Doppman JL, Dwyer AJ, et al. Adrenal masses differentiated by MR. Radiology 1986;158:81–84.
8. Baker ME, Blinder R, Spritzer C, et al. MR evaluation of adrenal masses at 1.5 T. AJR 1989;153:307–312.
9. Krestin GP, Friedmann G, Fischbach R, et al. Evaluation of adrenal masses in oncologic patients. Dynamic contrast-enhanced MR vs. CT. J Comput Assist Tomogr 1991;15:104–110.
10. Lenay-Willig A, Bittoun J, Luton JP, et al. In vivo MR spectroscopic imaging of the adrenal glands: Distinction between adenomas and carcinomas larger than 15 mm based on lipid content. AJR 1989;153:771–773.
11. Chang PJ, Parker BR, Donaldson SS, et al. Dynamic probabilistic model for determination of optimal timing of surveillance chest radiography in pediatric Hodgkin disease. Radiology 1989;173:71–75.
12. Lee JKT, Glazer HS. Controversy in the MR imaging appearance of fibrosis. Radiology 1990;177:21–22.
13. Wernecke K, Vassallo P, Hoffmann G, et al. Value of sonography in monitoring the

therapeutic response of mediastinal lymphoma: Comparison with chest radiography and CT. AJR 1991;156:265–272.

14. Begg CB, McNeil BJ. Assessment of radiologic tests: Control of bias and other design considerations. Radiology 1988;167:565–569.

15. Chang PJ. Bayesian analysis revisited: A radiologist's survival guide. AJR 1989;152:721–727.

16. Phillips WC, Scott JA. Medical decision making: Practical points for practicing radiologists. AJR 1990;154:1149–1155.

17. Begg C. Statistical issues in diagnostic medicine. Course syllabus (lecture 7). New York: Memorial Sloan-Kettering Cancer Center, 1990.

18. Hillman BJ. The value of imaging technology to patients' health. AJR 1988;150:1191–1192.

19. Gatsonis C, McNeil BJ. Collaborative evaluations of diagnostic tests: Experience of the Radiology Diagnostic Oncology Group. Radiology 1990;175:571–575.

20. Webb WR, Gatsonis C, Zerhouni EA, et al. CT and MR imaging in staging non-small cell bronchogenic carcinoma: Report of the Radiologic Diagnostic Oncology Group. Radiology 1991;178:705–713.

21. Rifkin MD, Zerhouni EA, Gatsonis C, et al. Comparison of magnetic resonance imaging and ultrasonography in staging early prostate cancer: Results of a multiinstitutional cooperative trial. New Engl J Med 1990;323:621–626.

22. Megibow AJ, Walsh SJ, Francis IF, et al. Comparison of CT and MR imaging in evaluation of patients with pancreatic adenocarcinoma: Report of the Radiologic Diagnostic Oncology Group. Presented at the Radiological Society of North America, Chicago, IL, December 1991.

23. Zerhouni EA, et al. CT and MR imaging in the staging of colorectal carcinoma: Report of the Radiologic Diagnostic Oncology Group 2 trial. Presented at the Radiological Society of North America, Chicago, IL, December 1991.

24. Sarti DA. Diagnostic ultrasound: Text and cases. 2nd ed. Chicago: Year Book Medical Publishers, 1987.

25. Botet JF, Lightdale C. Endoscopic sonography of the upper gastrointestinal tract. AJR 1991;156:63–68.

26. Young SW. Magnetic resonance imaging: Basic principles. 2nd ed. New York: Raven Press, 1988.

27. Cohen MS, Weisskoff RM. Ultra-fast imaging. Magn Reson Imaging 1991;9:1–37.

28. Rosen BR, Belliveau JW, Vevea JM, Brady TJ. Perfusion imaging with NMR contrast agents. Magn Reson Imaging 1990;14:249–265.

29. Wehrli FW. Fast-scan magnetic resonance: Principles and applications. New York: Raven Press, 1991.

30. Bottomley PA. Human in vivo NMR spectroscopy in diagnostic medicine: Clinical tool or research probe? Radiology 1989;170:1–15.

31. Semmler W, Gademann G, Bachert-Baumann P, Zabel HJ, Lorenz WJ, van Kaick G. Monitoring human tumor response to therapy by means of P-31 MR spectroscopy. Radiology 1988;166:533–539.

32. Glickson JD. Clinical NMR spectroscopy of tumors. Invest Radiol 1989;24:1011–1014.

33. Holman BL, Tumeh SS. Single photon emission computed tomography (SPECT). JAMA 1990;263:561–564.

34. Buddinger TF. Single photon emission computed tomography. In: Gottschalk A, Hoffer PB, Potchen EJ, eds. Diagnostic nuclear medicine. 2nd ed. Baltimore: Williams & Wilkins, 1988:108–127.

35. Mandelkern MA, Phelps ME. Methods and instrumentation for positron emission tomography. In: Gottschalk A, Hoffer PB, Potchen EJ, eds. Diagnositic nuclear medicine. 2nd ed. Baltimore: Williams & Wilkins, 1988:128–149.

36. Larson SM. Positron emission tomography in oncology and allied diseases. In: DeVita VT, et al, eds. Principles and Practice of Oncology Updates 1989;3:1–12.

37. Collier BD, Hellman RS, Krasnow AZ. Bone SPECT. Semin Nucl Med 1987;17:247–266.

38. Kaplan WD. Residual mass and negative gallium scintigraphy in treated lymphoma: When is the gallium really negative? J Nucl Med [Editorial] 1990;31:369–371.

39. Tumeh SS, Rosenthal DS, Kaplan WD, English RJ, Holman BL. Lymphoma: Evaluation with Ga-67 SPECT. Radiology 1987;164:111–114.

40. Kim KT, Black KL, Marciano D, et al. Thallium 201 SPECT imaging of brain tumors: Methods and results. J Nucl Med 1990;31:965–969.

41. Kemeny N. Is hepatic infusion of chemotherapy effective treatment for liver metastases? Yes. In: DeVita VT, Hellman S, Rosenberg SA, eds. Important advances in oncology. Philadelphia: JB Lippincott, 1991:207–227.

42. Wahl RL, Cody RL, Hutchins GD, Mudgett EE. Primary and metastatic breast carcinoma: Initial clinical evaluation with PET with radiolabeled glucose analogue 2-[F-18]-fluoro-2-deoxy-d-glucose. Radiology 1991;179:765–770.

43. Strauss LG, Conti PS. The applications of PET in clinical oncology. J Nucl Med 1991;32:623–648.

44. Kramer EL, Larson SM. Tumor Targeting with radiolabeled antibody for diagnosis and therapy. In: Oettgen HF, ed. Human cancer immunology, II. 11th ed. Philadelphia: WB Saunders, 1991:301–339.

45. Kohler G, Milstein C. Continuous cultures of fused cells secreting antibody of predefined specificity. Nature 1975;256:495–497.

SECTION 3

MORTON K. SCHWARTZ

Cancer Markers

As understanding of the pathophysiology of cancer increases, the role of tumor markers becomes more important in the management of cancer patients. Biochemical measurements of substances in blood and other body fluids have been used for these purposes for more than a century. In 1847, Sir Henry Bence Jones described in the urine of a patient what is referred to as the Bence Jones protein. It is a useful marker in patients with myeloma. This protein is now known to be identical with the light chain IgG, and most patients with myeloma excrete it in their urine whether or not the traditional "heat-cool" test is positive.[1] In 1867, Sir Michael Foster reported the presence of amylase in human blood, and urinary amylase was proposed even earlier as a marker for pancreatic cancer.[2]

In the 1930s, acid phosphatase was used in evaluating men with cancer of the prostate, and serum alkaline phosphatase gained wide acceptance in diagnosis of osteogenic sarcoma and other bone cancers.[2] Urinary chorionic gonadotropin became a standard test in evaluating and monitoring choriocarcinoma; vanillylmandelic acid and catecholamines became essential markers in neuroblastoma and pheochromocytoma; and 5-hydroxy indole acetic acid was used in carcinoid and a variety of hormones in neuroendocrine tumors.[3] In the 1950s, glycolytic and other enzymes were adopted as indicators of liver metastases.[2] However, it was only after the availability of immunoassays that cancer-related or cancer-specific tests were proposed, and the tumor marker era began. The introduction of carcinoembryonic antigen in 1965 and the report of its high sensitivity and specificity in colon cancer led to an ever-increasing number of tumor-associated antigens that were proposed by their developers as useful in cancer diagnosis and therapy.[4,5]

Tumor markers are substances that can be measured quantitatively by biochemical or immunochemical means in tissue or body fluids to detect a cancer and possibly the organ where it resides, to establish the extent of tumor burden before treatment, and to monitor the response to therapy. This definition excludes qualitative procedures such as fecal occult blood, the Papanicolaou smear, or immunocytostaining of cells in tissue sections or by continuous flow cytometry. With this definition, many substances can be identified as tumor markers. These include tumor-associated antigens, enzymes, specific proteins, metabolites, and oncogenes and oncogene products.

Measurement of tumor markers may be useful in screening total populations and high-risk groups, in diagnosis as aides in staging or confirmation of histopathology, and in therapy by predicting drug response, predicting prognosis, and monitoring for relapse. In the research laboratory, tumor markers yield a great deal of information about the natural history of the cancer.[2]

Some terms are essential to an understanding of the clinical use of tumor markers. Analytically, *sensitivity* is the lowest amount of analyte that can be detected, and epidemiologically, it is a measure of the ability to detect the cancer. Analytically, *specificity* means the degree of interference in the assay by extraneous substances that may be present in the sample, and epidemiologically, it is the ability of the test to identify the population without cancer. In any evaluation of tumor markers, the prevalence of the cancer in a given population and the analytic precision of the assay must be known.

The calculated predictive value can give information concerning clinical utility and cost effectiveness. The positive predictive value of a test is the number of true positive values divided by the sum of the true positives and false positives. The negative predictive value is the number of false negatives divided by the sum of the false negatives and true negatives. For a population of 100,000 in whom the prevalence of the cancer is 10% (*i.e.,* 10,000 expected cases) and for whom the test has a sensitivity of 75% and a specificity of 95%, the positive predictive value (*i.e.,* probability) of the marker is 7500 true positives/(7500 true positives + 4500 false positives) = 62.5%. The negative predictive value is 2500 false negatives/(2500 false negatives + 85,500 true negatives) = 2.8%.[6]

SERUM MARKERS

Table 21–5 lists the common serum tumor markers and their recommended use.

ALPHA-FETOPROTEIN

Alpha-fetoprotein (AFP) is synthesized by the fetal yolk sac, liver, and intestine and serves in the fetus as as a carrier protein and preserves oncotic pressure. Serum levels peak during the weeks 12 to 14 of gestation, and after week 16 week, the levels begin to fall and are essentially nondetectable during the first year of life and thereafter in healthy persons.

AFP is a glycoprotein with a single asparagine linked sugar chain. The 70-kd molecule has a half-life in serum of 4.5 days.[7,8] AFP of yolk sac origin binds concanavalin A, but there is no binding of concanavalin A by AFP of liver origin.[9] AFP is a serum marker in hepatocellular carcinoma (HCC) and in cancers involving yolk sac elements, and it has been successfully used in screening for HCC.[10,11] Although serum AFP

TABLE 21–5. Circulating Serum Tumor Markers

Cancer	Tumor Markers	Recommended Use†
Breast	CEA,* CA 15-3, CA 549, CA M26, M 29, CA 27.29, MCA	4
Gastrointestinal (colorectal, pancreas, stomach)	CEA*	3, 4
	CA 19-9, CA 195, CA 72-4, CA 50	4
Prostate	PSA,*	1(?), 3, 4
	PAP*	3, 4
Hepatocellular	AFP,*	1–4
	CEA*	4
Ovary	CA 125,*	3, 4
	Galactosyl transferase	4
Testicular (germ cell tumors)	AFP,*	2–4
	β-hCG,	2–4
	LDH,* placental-like AP* (seminoma)	3, 4
Trophoblastic	β-hCG	2–4
Lung (small cell)	NSE, CK-BB	4
Neuroblastoma	VMA,* Catecholamines,*	1–4
	NSE	4
Thyroid	Thyroglobulin,*	1, 4
	Calcitonin* (medullary)	2, 4
Head and neck	SCC	3, 4
Myeloma	Immunoglobulins* (Bence Jones protein)	2, 3
Carcinoid	5-HIAA	2
Neuroendocrine	Variety of hormones	2
Bone	Alkaline phosphatase	2–4
Nonspecific markers	Lipid-bound sialic acid, tissue polypeptide antigen, ferritin, sialyltransferase	3, 4
Liver metastases	Glycolytic enzymes, alkaline phosphatase, 5′-nucleotidase	3, 4

* FDA approved.
† 1, screening; 2, diagnosis; 3, prognosis; 4, monitoring course of disease or response to therapy.

is modestly abnormal in hepatitis and other benign liver diseases, elevated values are highly diagnostic for HCC. In Southeast Asia and Southern Africa, where hepatitis B is epidemic, AFP screening programs have been useful in detecting and confirming cases. AFP is essential for monitoring treatment. In high-risk patients, AFP values between 100 ng/ml and 350 ng/ml suggest a diagnosis of HCC, and levels over 350 ng/ml usually indicate the disease.[12]

If AFP is used for screening, the analytic sensitivity of the procedure must be considered. A more sensitive analytic technique may compromise the ability of the test to differentiate HCC from other forms of liver disease in which modest elevations of AFP are found. Radioimmunoassay for AFP is about 40,000 times more sensitive than the original immunodiffusion procedure. Differences in method sensitivity affect the reported clinical usefulness of the assay. In a comparison of AFP specificity between an agar diffusion assay and a more sensitive immunoradioautography method, specificity increased from the detection of 84 (71%) of 118 patients with HCC to 90 (78.3%) of 118. In the control group, the number of false positives increased from 10 (2.7%) of 366 patients to 80 (22.6%) of 354 cases. The increase in positive values in the cancer population was more than offset by the increase in the number of false positives in the control population. The less sensitive test was more appropriate for screening the population, but the more sensitive test would be necessary in day-to-day monitoring of a patient. In a collaborative screening study in which all laboratories used an agarose double diffusion technique, positive values were reported in 105 (70.9%) of 148 patients with HCC and in 12 (2.1%) of 555 of control patients, but in whites in the United States and Europe, elevations were observed to a much lesser extent: 178 (53.7%) of 331 of those with HCC.[13]

In an early summary of the Chinese experience, 143 positive persons were found among 394,000 tested.[14] After clinical and surgical review, 53 cases of HCC were documented. Of these, 33 (62%) would not have been found without the AFP assay. In a subsequent review of AFP screening of more than 5,000,000 Chinese, 1000 cases of HCC were detected.[15] The use of AFP in early detection of HCC is warranted because surgical removal of the tumor can improve 1-year survival rates from 14.8% to 79.1% and 3-year survival rates from 5.5% to 61.6%.[15] High levels of serum AFP indicate a poor prognosis. Sequential serum levels can be used to monitor the effects of therapy.

CHORIONIC GONADOTROPIN

Human chorionic gonadotropin (hCG) has been used for decades in diagnosis and more recently in monitoring the progress of gestational trophoblastic diseases (*i.e.*, hydatidiform mole, invasive mole, choriocarcinoma).[16] It exists in the serum of all patients with these diseases, and changes in serum or urine levels accurately reflect the course of the tumor. Urinary hCG can be a prognostic factor; markedly elevated concentrations indicate a poor prognosis. If the marker is used during chemotherapy, transient elevations may be observed after therapy is initiated, presumably due to tumor tissue breakdown and release of the hormone into the circulation.[17]

Human chorionic gonadotropin is a 45-kd glycoprotein

consisting of two subunits. The alpha subunit is indistinguishable from the alpha subunit of other pituitary hormones. The unique subunit of hCG is the 24- to 34-kd beta subunit. The half-life in serum is between 16 and 24 hours. The clearance pattern from the serum is bimodal, with a rapid component ($T_{\frac{1}{2}} = 5.97 \pm 0.63$ hours) and a slow component ($T_{\frac{1}{2}} = 35.6 \pm 8.0$ hours).[18] The fall off of hCG during therapy at a half-life rate indicates good success of therapy and excellent prognosis.

BETA SUBUNIT OF CHORIONIC GONADOTROPIN WITH ALPHA-FETOPROTEIN

In germ cell tumors, β-hCG and AFP are essential markers in clinical management.[19] These markers are found in serum of patients with embryonal malignant teratoblastomas of the testes and ovary, but they are not usually in the serum of patients with other embryonal tumors (*i.e.*, seminomas, chorioepitheliomas, neuroblastoma, Wilms tumor). In nonseminomatous testicular cancers, AFP and β-hCG permit effective assessment of the rate of tumor growth, help predict prognosis, and enable staging by the pathologist and clinician. Sequential assays are essential in the management of the patient. Both AFP and β-hCG must be measured, because either or both may be elevated.[20] During therapy, the tumor-cell population may change and express a different β-hCG and AFP pattern from that initially observed.

Elevations of AFP, β-hCG, or both occur in approximately 90% of patients with nonseminomatous testicular cancers. In fewer than 20% of patients with seminomas, β-hCG is elevated due to the presence of syncytiotrophoblast cells that are responsible for its biosynthesis. Positive marker values are presumptive evidence of a cancer, but a negative value should not be used to rule out disease. After the tumor is successfully removed, blood levels should fall, with a half-life of 16 to 24 hours for β-hCG and about 4.5 days for AFP. Successful therapy may be defined as a return of both markers to normal levels. Different methods may yield different normal reference ranges, and it is essential for each laboratory to establish its own normal range.

At Memorial Sloan-Kettering Cancer Center, clinical, laboratory, and histopathologic factors were subjected to multivariate analysis in an effort to predict the probability of response to therapy of patients with testicular cancer.[21] In the multivariate analysis, lactic dehydrogenase (LDH) and β-hCG were the most significant biochemical parameters. Carcinoembryonic antigen and AFP did not add to the ability to differentiate responders from nonresponders. The only other factor of statistical value was the total number of metastatic sites (TOTMET). When these factors were used, the probability (p) for complete response is $p = e^h/1 + e^h$. A value greater than 0.5 indicates response, and h is calculated as follows:

$$h = 8.514 - 1.973 \log (LDH + 1)$$
$$- 0.530 \log (hCG + 1) - 1.111 \text{ TOTMET.}$$

In 171 patients, the equation predicted that 121 patients would respond to therapy. Of these 121 patients, 114 (94%) actually responded. It also predicted that 50 patients would not respond, but of these, only 28 (56%) did not respond. The overall prediction rate was 142 (83%) of 171 patients. With an independent set of data collected at another institution, the model correctly predicted responses in 36 (86%) of 42 patients and in 5 of 7 patients who did not respond, giving an overall prediction rate of 41 (84%) of 49.

The usefulness of the model in a highly curable disease is the identification of patients who are unlikely to do well and who should be considered for alternate or additional therapy. If the probability equation is used, a less toxic chemotherapeutic regimen may be chosen for patients predicted to experience a response.[22] Response to therapy has been correlated with β-hCG and AFP levels in patients with advanced germ cell tumors (*i.e.*, stage III and bulky unresectable stage II nonseminomatous germ cell tumors). In 100 patients, 12 (92%) of 13 who had normal marker levels had a complete remission compared with 15 (54%) of 28 patients who had only β-hCG elevations, 10 (42%) of 23 who had only AFP elevations, and 25 (69%) of 36 who had both markers elevated.

For patients with values of AFP or β-hCG greater than 1000 ng/ml, prognosis was poor.[23] Survival was related to the size of the tumor and to the serum AFP and β-hCG concentrations.[24] Low levels of markers were defined as AFP levels less than 500 ng/ml and hCG values less than 1000 IU/ml. In patients with small tumors (<2 cm) and low marker levels, the 3-year survival rate was 91%, compared with 69% for those with elevated marker levels. For patients with large tumors (2–5 cm), the survival rates were 80% for patients with low marker levels and 70% for those with high marker levels. For patients with very large tumors (>5 cm), the 3-year survival rates were 69% for those with low concentrations of markers and 47% for those with high marker concentrations. Survival after therapy has been related to the rate of disappearance of the markers.[25] A satisfactory $T_{1/2}$ for AFP was defined as 7 days or less, and for β-hCG, it was 3 days or less. Of 156 patients with satisfactory half-lives, 129 (83%) survived at least 10 years, but only 12 of 42 patients with prolonged half-life levels survived this long. Only 6 were alive more than 24 months from the start of therapy ($p = 0.001$). Complete remission was observed in 139 (89%) of 156 of the patients with satisfactory half-lives.

PLACENTAL ALKALINE PHOSPHATASE

Placental alkaline phosphatase (PLAP) is a heat-stable form of alkaline phosphatase of placental origin. It has been proposed that PLAP can be used to confirm the diagnosis of seminoma and to monitor the disease.[26] In early studies of PLAP (*i.e.*, Regan isoenzyme), elevations of the enzyme occurred in 20% to 30% of patients with cancer of the breast or ovary, particularly serous cystadenocarcinoma of the ovary.[27] In ovarian cancer, PLAP may be a useful adjunct to the use of CA 125.[28] In seminoma, PLAP was elevated in 9 (43%) of 21 men at primary diagnosis and 9 (75%) of 12 men with metastatic disease.[26] A survey of the literature indicated that elevations were observed in 183 (40%) of 457 patients with stage I seminoma. In a comparison of PLAP, LDH, β-hCG, and AFP, PLAP and LDH were elevated in 10 (50%) of 20 of stage I seminoma patients and 6 (100%) of 6 men with stage II or III seminoma, and β-hCG was elevated in 67% of the stage I

patients and 67% of patients with more advanced disease. AFP was not elevated in any of the patients. Although PLAP is occasionally elevated in stage I nonseminomatous disease, an elevation of PLAP with a normal level of AFP suggests seminoma.[29]

URINARY GONADOTROPIN PEPTIDE

A peptide fragment of chorionic gonadotropin is found in urine.[29-31] This fragment has been called beta-core fragment, urinary gonadotropin fragment, or urinary gonadotropin peptide and has been proposed as a marker in ovarian cancer useful as an adjunct to CA 125. In one study, urinary gonadotropin fragment was elevated in the urine of 50% of women with stage I disease, 62% with stage II, 75% with stage III, and 86% with stage IV ovarian cancer.[29] Elevations were observed in only 4 (1.2%) of 323 of healthy women or those with benign gynecologic diseases. Sensitivity was 66% for all nontrophoblastic gynecologic cancers and 82% for ovarian cancer.[30] When urinary gonadotropin peptide and CA 125 were used to differentiate malignant from benign pelvic masses, the incidence of false positives was 1.2% among 169 patients with disease and 1% among 385 controls.[31]

CA 125

Serum CA 125 assays are useful in the management of patients with ovarian cancer. CA 125 is a 200-kd glycoprotein found as a surface protein on ovarian cancer cells. The monoclonal antibody used in the assay was raised against the antigen OVCA 433, prepared from a cell line of a papillary serous cystadenocarcinoma of the ovary.[32,33] The FDA approval of CA 125 is limited to use in monitoring second-look surgery in patients treated for ovarian cancer. It is indicated for use as an aid in the detection of residual ovarian carcinoma in patients who have undergone first-line therapy and would be considered for diagnostic second-look procedures. A level of 35 U/ml is predictive of residual disease, provided that alternative causes of an elevated CA 125 value can be excluded.[32,37] CA 125 elevations above 35 U/ml were observed in 1% of 888 normal women, 6% of 42 women with benign disease, in 86 (82%) of 105 of women with ovarian cancer, 21% of patients with colorectal cancer, 12% of women with breast cancer, 32% of those with lung cancer, and in 59% of patients with pancreatic cancer. Most of these patients had advanced disease. It is not clear in the report how early in the course of the ovarian cancer the CA 125 was elevated.[33]

There is a question about using CA 125 in screening or in diagnosis. This could not be done if a cutoff between normal and abnormal of 35 U/ml is used. If an attempt is made to eliminate interference by other cancers or benign disease by raising the normal-abnormal cutoff, other effects are observed. If the cutoff level is raised to 65 U/ml, or 7.6 standard deviations above the normal mean, elevations are observed in only 0.2% of normals and 2% of patients with benign disease. The detection of ovarian cancer is reduced from 82% to 73%, and significant numbers of positive values are still observed for other cancers. At 200 U/ml, there are no abnormal values found for normal persons or those with benign disease, but the detection of cancer of the ovary for those who have elevated values is reduced to 62%.[33]

If the patient with confirmed cancer is being monitored, a lower cutoff level is preferable, and comparison with the patient's own baseline value is recommended. If CA 125 is used to monitor patients, rising and falling levels correlate well with progression or regression of disease. In one report, progression was indicated by a rising CA 125 in 28 of 31 patients. Regression of disease was accompanied by a fall in CA 125, except in 2 women in whom there was clinical regression but CA 125 remained unchanged.[34] Data was compiled for 293 women who had second-look surgery. There were 120 women with elevated CA 125 values. Of these, 119 (99.1%) had residual tumor. The one woman with a positive CA 125 and no residual tumor at the time of surgery experienced a recurrence between the time the report was submitted and published.[35] In 173 women with CA 125 values within normal limits, 82 (48%) were found at laparotomy to have residual tumor. A most important caveat in the use of tumor markers is exemplified by these findings. A positive CA 125 value indicates the presence of the residual cancer, but a normal value should not give a false sense of security that all tumor has been removed.

The size of the tumor influences CA 125 elevation. Abnormal values were seen in 60% of women with tumors smaller than 2 cm but in 90% of women with tumors larger than 2 cm.[36] A study compared the use of various procedures in 20 patients to detect residual tumor after debulking surgery in patients receiving chemotherapy.[37] CA 125 alone indicated the presence of tumor in 17 (85%) of 20 of the patients. Clinical information did not increase the positive findings. When computed tomography (CT) findings were added to CA 125, residual tumor was detected in 1 additional patient. Clinical evaluation alone detected 8 (40%) of 20, and CT alone detected 12 (60%) of 20 of the patients. When CT scans and clinical evaluations were combined, only 13 (65%) of 20 of patients were identified. CA 125 was the most important individual marker of tumor. CT scan in combination with CA 125 minimally increased the ability to detect residual tumor before debulking surgery.

Other tumor markers have been evaluated in ovarian cancer, including carcinoembryonic antigen, other ovarian antigens, PLAP, lipid-associated sialic acid, galactosyltransferase, tissue polypeptide antigen, and ferritin.[38] None has the sensitivity or specificity of CA 125. Except PLAP, they do not appear to be useful as adjuncts to CA 125. CA 125 elevations can occur during pregnancy, in pelvic inflammatory disease, and in endometriosis. It has been recommended that CA 125 assays be obtained for all women who present with pelvic tumors. Limited data is available on the role of CA 125 in the management of women with endometrial cancer. Elevated values decreased in each of 10 women who experienced complete responses to therapy and in 10 patients with partial responses or stable disease. Rising titers were observed in each of 9 patients who had relapses. In one patient with progressive disease, there was no concomitant rise in CA 125.[39]

CARCINOEMBRYONIC ANTIGEN

In 1965, carcinoembryonic antigen (CEA) was identified in fetal intestine, liver, and pancreas during the first 6 months of pregnancy and in cancerous liver, colon, or pancreas but not in normal or benign adult tissue.[4] CEA is a cell-surface 200-kd glycoprotein, and much is known about its structure. In 1969, it was reported that plasma CEA was elevated in 35 of 36 patients with adenocarcinoma of the colon and that CEA titers decreased after successful surgery. Normal levels were observed in all patients with other forms of cancer or benign diseases.[5] Subsequent studies have not confirmed these initial findings, and it is now appreciated that CEA elevations are found in many cancers. Elevations are observed in more than 30% of patients with cancer of the lung, liver, pancreas, breast, colon, head or neck, bladder, cervix, and prostate.[3] The antigen can be found in normal tissues, and elevated plasma levels are related to the stage and extent of the disease, the degree of differentiation of the tumor, and the site of metastasis.[3]

The most complete study of CEA is a compilation of collaborative studies in which CEA values in 35,000 samples from more than 10,000 patients and controls were analyzed. Of 1425 normal persons who did not smoke, 98.7% had values less than 5.0 ng/ml. In 857 healthy persons with a smoking history, elevations were observed in 33%. There were 576 persons without clinical evidence of disease who underwent barium enema examination; 23 were found to have colon cancer and of these, CEA values of greater than 2.5 ng/ml were detected in 18. CEA elevations were related to the stage of disease. Elevations (>5 ng/ml) were observed in approximately 4% of patients with Dukes' stage A disease, 25% of those with stage B, 45% with stage C, and 65% with metastatic colon cancer, particularly disease metastatic to liver, lung, or bone.[40] CEA is not specific enough to be used in screening or diagnosis.

Patients who have levels of CEA greater than 10 ng/ml before treatment have much poorer prognosis than patients with values less than this.[41,42] In 358 patients with Dukes' stage B colon cancers, the mean time to recurrence was 19 months for those with CEA values between 10 and 70 ng/ml and 10 months for those with values greater than this. For patients with normal CEA values, the mean time to recurrence was 30 months. Declining concentrations of CEA are monitors of effective therapy, and rising levels indicate recurrence or lack of response to therapy. A National Cancer Institute (NCI) consensus panel concluded that "CEA is the best presently available noninvasive technique for postoperative surveillance of patients to detect disseminated recurrence of colorectal cancer. Declining concentrations of CEA are indicative of effective therapy, and rising levels indicate disease activity, though the increased CEA may precede clinical symptoms of recurrence by months."[43] A similar statement could be made for patients with lung or breast cancer.

Elevations of CEA do not occur in all patients who experience recurrences. Two patients with equally fulminating liver metastases may present completely different patterns. One may have a crescendo-like rise in CEA, and the other may exhibit no rise at all.[41] A positive and rising value is significant, but a normal value does not necessarily indicate the recurrence of tumor.

A summary of reports in the literature indicated that CEA elevations are observed in 60% to 94% patients with metastatic and recurrent colorectal cancer.[44] Normal values were reported for 53 of 225 patients, a false-negative rate of 24%. Immunostaining has indicated that CEA is not produced by poorly differentiated tumors, and this may account for the lack of elevation of serum CEA in some patients. Two groups of patients with gastric cancer who developed progressive, recurrent disease were sequentially followed over a 12-month period. In the one group of 47 patients with undifferentiated cancer, the CEA values were not elevated during the entire course of their disease. The mean preoperative value was 0.8 times the upper limit of normal (ULN), and the mean value at the end of 12 months was 0.4 times the ULN. In the patients with differentiated tumors, the preoperative value was 2.1 times the ULN and rose at a rapid rate thereafter. At 6 months, it was 4.7 times the ULN; at 9 months, it was 7 times the ULN; and at 12 months, the mean of the CEA values was 22.4 times the ULN.[45]

In patients with elevations, the rising CEA is the earliest sign of recurrence in approximately 50%. Several investigators have proposed that second-look surgery for colon cancer should be considered if there is a rising CEA titer and no other clinical or laboratory indications of recurrence. A group at Ohio State University has had the most experience with CEA-related second-look surgery in colorectal cancer.[46–48] In a retrospective study, 19 of 22 patients or 86% of those undergoing surgery were found to have recurrences, but only 6 (27%) had resectable tumors.[46] The results were much better in a prospective study; 17 (94%) of 18 patients had recurrent cancer, and 13 (72%) of these had a resectable tumor.[47] In most CEA-directed second-look studies, recurrent tumor is found on laparotomy (78–100% of patients), but the number of resectable cases is small (7–43%). In a review of the literature that included 363 patients, tumor was found in 272 (90%), but only 140 (46%) were suitable for second curative resections. Although CEA-directed surgery can identify patients with recurrent tumor, there are few studies on the effects of second-look surgery on overall survival. In one such study, 130 of 400 patients had recurrences identified by elevations in CEA or clinical findings, and 75 of these underwent second-look surgeries. In 43 patients, surgery was CEA directed, and in 32, it was based on clinical judgment. In the CEA group, 15 (37%) were alive and free of disease, 7 (16%) were alive with cancer, and 20 (46%) died. In the clinically directed group, 11 (34%) were alive and free of disease, 7 (22%) were alive with cancer, and 12 (38%) were dead. There was a significant difference in survival ($p = 0.03$) between those who elected second-look surgery and those who did not, but there was no difference between the CEA-directed and clinically directed groups. Survival was significantly longer ($p = 0.03$) for patients with preoperative CEA values less than 11 ng/ml.[48]

The role of CEA in monitoring response to chemotherapy is not clear. Conflicting reports may be due to the time sequence in collecting specimens. In a study in which the baseline for comparison was the average of several multiple assays over the first 3 months of therapy, there was a significant difference in survival ($p = 0.0001$) between patients with sequential values below the mean of the baseline and those with values above the baseline measurement.[49]

CEA is an important marker in breast cancer and is elevated in about 60% of women with metastatic disease.[3] In women who have marker elevations, values correlate with the course of the disease. As in colon cancer, CEA elevations in breast cancer are related to the extent of disease and the site of metastasis. A review of data from four studies indicated ab-

normal values in 9% of 194 patients with stage I breast cancer (range, 0–15%); 23% of 237 patients with stage II disease (range, 0–43%); 45% of 102 patients with stage III cancer (range, 31–64%), and 58% of 2171 patients with stage IV cancer (range in 22 studies, 29–100%).[50] The differences in the numbers of positive patients in these studies may be due to the selection of patients, the cutoff values when different CEA methods are used, or differences in collecting clinical information and in staging the patients.

A summary of CEA in evaluating recurrence included 13 studies of 1626 breast cancer patients. Of these women, 312 (19%) experienced recurrences. The site of recurrence or whether the recurrence was local or disseminated was not stated. Of these 312 patients, 107 (47%) exhibited an elevated CEA level 1 to 31 months before the recurrence. In 120 (53%) other patients, there was neither elevated or rising CEA values before documentation of the recurrence. These patients were declared to be "false negatives."[50]

The problems in using CEA in monitoring breast cancer during chemotherapy may be related to the kinetics of the changes in serum CEA levels, and this may explain discrepancies between reports about use of CEA in monitoring patients. In a study of 30 patients receiving chemotherapy, increases or decreases in CEA of more than 25% were considered significant. Clinical response to therapy was defined as at least a 50% reduction in tumor size; lack of response was at least a 25% increase in initial tumor size. There were four patterns in the sequential CEA values. Two of the four were expected: a steady increase in CEA concentrations during tumor progression or a steady decrease in the value in those who responded ($T_{\frac{1}{2}} = 22.8 \pm 4.1$ days; range, 12–23 days). The other two patterns were more difficult to understand. In 6 patients who had favorable clinical responses, there was an initial upward surge within 8 days of therapy, and the doubling time accelerated from 84.0 ± 13.1 days before therapy to 21.7 ± 6.1 days. There was then a sharp decline at a rate equal to a $T_{\frac{1}{2}}$ of 33.5 ± 6.2 days. In another group of 7 patients who did not have clinical responses, there was an immediate and rapid decline in CEA levels ($T_{\frac{1}{2}} = 6.8 \pm 1.2$ days) for 6 to 7 days. After this, the CEA level rapidly increased.[51]

It has been suggested that during chemotherapy decreases in marker level may reflect reduced tumor volume, reduced CEA synthesis, reduced release of CEA into the circulation, or increased CEA catabolism. Immediate and rapid decreases in CEA levels in breast cancer patients may not reflect successful response to therapy nor rapid increases indicate a lack of response. For 167 patients with metastatic breast cancer who received chemotherapy, pretreatment CEA values were significant in predicting response rate or remission.[52] Eighty-three of the 167 women had normal CEA values before treatment, and 73 (87%) of these responded to therapy. Of the 73 who responded, 35 relapsed, but increases in plasma CEA occurred in only 5 (15%). In 84 women with elevated pretreatment CEA levels, there were clinical responses in 70 (85%), reflected in 66 by decreased CEA levels. CEA levels returned to normal in 17 of 21 patients who responded completely and in 31 of 50 women with partial responses. Remission was significantly longer for patients whose CEA levels became normal. In 27 (82%) of 37 of patients whose disease progressed, CEA levels became elevated. In 24 of these, elevated CEA levels were observed 1 to 13 months before there was clinically documented evidence of recurrence. A paradoxical rise in serum CEA during the first 4 to 8 weeks of treatment was seen in many of the responding patients. In breast cancer, CEA monitoring is useful for patients who have pretreatment elevations, but CEA values obtained during the first 8 weeks of therapy may be related to factors other than clinical response and should probably be ignored.[51]

GASTROINTESTINAL CANCER MARKERS

Several antigens have been suggested as serum markers in gastrointestinal cancer. Attempts have been made to use them alone or as adjuncts to CEA. These mucin-type glycoproteins include CA 19-9, CA 195, TAG 72, and CA 50. CA 19-9 has received the most attention.

Although CA 19-9 is derived from a colon cancer cell line, it is not elevated in the sera of many patients with colorectal cancer.[53] CEA was elevated in 125 (72%) of 174 of patients, but CA 19-9 was elevated in 74 (42%) of these. CA 19-9 was elevated in 13 (87%) of 15 patients with pancreatic cancer, and CEA was elevated in only 10 (67%) of these. In a larger study of patients with pancreatic cancer, CA 19-9 was elevated in 32 (87%) of 37 patients, and CEA was elevated in only 15 (48%) of 31.[54] A combination of the CEA and CA 19-9 was not useful. Many patients with benign disease exhibited elevations. Elevations were observed in 3 (6%) of 48 persons with benign pancreatic disease and in 11 (19%) of 58 patients with liver disease. CA 19-9 is a better indicator of pancreatic or gastric disease than CEA. Extremely high levels are seen in pancreatic cancer, and CA 19-9 may be the best available marker for confirmation of disease and monitoring these patients.

CA 195 is a marker similar to CA 19-9. We have observed that CEA was elevated in 55 (76%) of 72 of patients with metastatic colon cancer, but CA 195 was elevated in only 42 (58%) of these patients. The combined markers detected 60 (83%) of the 72 patients. In pancreatic cancer, CA 195 was elevated in 16 (70%) of 23 patients and CEA in 8 (36%). The combination of CA 195 and CEA increased the yield by only 1 patient.[55] In another study, CEA was abnormal in 82 (57%) of 144 patients with active colon cancer, compared with 50 (61%) of 82 who had elevations of CA 19-9 and 63 (72%) of 88 with elevations of CA 195.[56] In patients with cancer of the upper gastrointestinal tract, elevations of CA 19-9 were seen in 54 (61%) of 88 of the patients, compared with 63 (72%) of 88 who had elevations of CA 195. There were elevations of CA 19-9 in 23% of persons with benign diseases and elevations of CA 195 in 10%.

TAG 72 is a high-molecular-weight glycoprotein that reacts with the monoclonal antibody B72.3. As a serum marker, it was elevated in 42% of 199 patients with gastric cancer and 38% of 104 patients with colon cancer. Elevations were also reported for patients with ovarian, breast, and prostate cancer. It was elevated in 55% of 77 patients with advanced gastric cancer and in 54% of 41 patients with advanced colon cancer.[57] TAG 72 was elevated in 15 (22%) of 68 of patients with pancreatic cancer and 16 (59%) of 27 of those with gastric cancer. The addition of CA 19-9 increased the positive ratio to 19 (70%) of 27 for gastric cancer patients and to 19 (28%) of 68 of those with pancreatic cancer.[58]

A fourth antigen of this group that has received little atten-

tion in the United States is CA 50. Clinical results are similar to those observed with CA 19-9.[59]

BREAST CANCER ANTIGENS

Although CEA has been used to monitor and manage patients with breast cancer, there is a need for markers with greater sensitivity and specificity. Many breast cancer antigens have been studied, including CA 15-3, CA 549, CAM 26, CAM 29, CA 26.27, and MCA. They are all high-molecular-weight glycoproteins (*i.e.*, mucins).

The marker that has caused the most interest and for which there is the most information is CA 15-3, a 300- to 450-kd glycoprotein. The antigen is identified by two antibodies (*i.e.*, DF3 and 115DB), one from human milk fat globules and the other from membranes of a human metastatic breast carcinoma cell line. CA 15-3 is elevated in only about 20% of women with primary breast cancer, but elevations between 61% and 84% have been recorded for women with metastatic breast cancer, particularly those with bone metastases.[60,61] In 158 patients with metastatic breast cancer, elevations of CA 15-3 were seen in 63% of the patients, compared with elevations of CEA in 41% of these women.[60] Elevations of 79% for CA 15-3 and 75% for CEA were seen in 24 patients with liver metastases, and CA 15-3 was elevated in 71% of 34 patients with bone metastases, compared with CEA elevations in 44% of the women.

Elevations of CA 15-3 were observed in approximately 8% of women with benign breast cancer and in 30% of patients with hepatitis. When the standard cutoff (<25 U/L) was used, the sensitivity in 134 patients was 31% and the specificity in 1208 patients was 86%. The diagnostic accuracy was 81%. CA 15-3 is also elevated in a significant number of patients with other cancers. It cannot be used for screening or for initial diagnosis, but it is an exceptionally good marker to monitor patients with recurrent disease. It falls during successful therapy, and elevations occur before clinical evidence of recurrence. Levels increased in 19 (91%) of 21 of women with progressive disease, decreased in 7 (78%) of 9 with regressive diseases, and did not change in 16 (59%) of 27 of patients with stable disease. If the definition of regression or progression was a change in CA 15-3 of 50% or more in either direction, progression would have been predicted in 14 (67%) of 21 patients and regression in 6 (67%) of 9 of the patients.

In women with advanced breast cancer, CA 15-3 was elevated in 130 of 173, and CEA was elevated in 97 of 103. CA 15-3 was significantly related to extent of metastases, the number of metastatic sites, and survival. CEA only correlated with the extent of disease.[61] When these two markers were evaluated for detecting progression of disease and a 25% change was considered significant, CA 15-3 was predictive for 26 of 54 patients and CEA for 19 of 26.[62]

Longitudinal studies of CEA and CA 15-3 have been conducted using 39 patients followed for 1 to 6 years.[63] Recurrent disease was documented by objective criteria in 33 (85%) of these women. At the time of recurrence, 23 (70%) exhibited abnormal CA 15-3 levels, and 19 (59%) had elevated CEA levels. During the studies, CA 15-3 progressively increased in 21 of 22 patients, and CEA levels rose in 14 of 22. In a study of 205 women who had recurrences 8 to 289 months after initial treatment, neither marker was elevated in 46

(22%), CA 15-3 in 57 (28%), CEA in 10 (5%), and both markers in 92 (45%). At a cutoff value of 25 U/L, the sensitivity (n = 134) was 31%, the specificity (n = 1208) was 86%, and the total accuracy was 81%[64]

In addition to CA 15-3, there are many other milk fat globule breast cancer membrane antigens under evaluation as serum markers, including CA 549, CA M26, CA M29, CA 27.29, and MCA. In comparing CA 15-3, CA 549, CEA, CA M26, and CA M29, it was found that they all exhibited negative predictive values of 50% to 52% and positive predictive values between 88% and 100%.[65,66] The use of two or more resulted in a better combined sensitivity at the expense of specificity. The best sensitivity for any two markers was 88% for CA 15-3 and CEA, compared with 79% for CA 15-3 alone and 68% for CEA alone. There may be an advantage in using panels in the follow-up of breast cancer patients at high risk for recurrence or during therapy, but it is difficult to assess the cost effectiveness because the optimal tumor marker panel may differ among patients.

PROSTATE-SPECIFIC ANTIGEN AND ACID PHOSPHATASE

Since 1939, acid phosphatase has been used in evaluating prostate cancer. Acid phosphatase is elevated in only 20% of men with early prostate cancer and in 80% of men with metastatic cancer.[2] It is not particularly useful in monitoring the course of the cancer. Similar observations have been reported whether immunochemical methods or older, catalytic enzyme assays that use specific substrates are employed.

Prostate-specific antigen (PSA) is a single-chain, 33-kd glycoprotein consisting of 240 amino acids. It is a kallikrein serine protease that may be identical to the p30 protein found in semen.[67-69] A 1987 NCI consensus meeting concluded that, in the management of prostate cancer, "biochemical evaluation is critical to the initial staging assessment. Serum alkaline phosphatase and acid phosphatase are helpful in identifying patients with metastatic disease. Serum prostate-specific antigen (PSA) is elevated more frequently in men with prostate cancer than is the acid phosphatase. PSA can be used to monitor response to local and systemic therapies. PSA is specific for prostate tissue but not for prostate cancer, precluding its use in screening."[70]

When a normal reference level of more or less than 4 ng/ml was used, PSA was elevated in 14 (35%) of 40 of men with stage A prostate cancer, 57 (60%) of 95 men with stage B, 44 (86%) of 51 of those with stage C disease, and 54 (77%) of 70 of those with stage D prostate cancer.[3] Elevations were also seen in 53 (28%) of 192 of men who attended a cancer detection clinic and had clinically diagnosed benign prostatic hypertrophy (BPH).[3] When acid phosphatase was determined in these patients by immunochemical or catalytic methods, the elevations in stage A cancer were, respectively, 13% and 20%, 25% and 20% in stage B, 45% in stage C by either method, and 57% and 63% in stage D. The two acid phosphatase methods gave statistically identical data, but the number of patients with elevations were fewer than observed with PSA.[3] In the men with BPH, elevations in acid phosphatase were seen in only 6% (immunochemical assay) and 3% (catalytic assay) of the patients.

The question is whether changing the normal-abnormal cutoff for PSA can separate men with cancer from those with BPH. If 10 ng/ml is used as the cutoff, only 15 (8%) of the 192 of the BPH patients had elevations. With a 10 ng/ml cutoff, the detection of patients with cancer would be 10 (25%) of 40 patients with stage A disease, 35 (37%) of 95 with stage B, 32 (52%) of 61 with stage C, and 45 (64%) of 70 with stage D. In a more extensive study, 122 (20%) of 597 men with BPH had abnormal values between 4 and 10 ng/ml, and 19 (3%) had values greater than this. In the cancer population, 119 (37%) of 319 had levels between 4 and 10 ng/ml, and 64 (20%) of 319 had values above 10 ng/ml. At a level greater than 4 ng/ml, the sensitivity was 23% and the specificity was 96%.[71]

The question has been raised about using PSA in screening.[72,73] In a large study, 1653 men without clinical symptoms of prostate disease were recruited through newspaper advertisements.[74] PSA tests were performed for all the men (*i.e.,* two assays, 6 months apart). Those with values less than 4.0 ng/ml (1516 men or 92%) were not subjected to further follow-up. In 107 (6%) men, the PSA level was between 4.1 and 10 ng/ml. Rectal examinations and ultrasonography were offered to these men. If either or both were abnormal or suspicious, a needle biopsy under ultrasound guidance was performed. There were 85 biopsies, and 19 (22%) of these were positive for prostate cancer. In 30 (2%) men whose PSA was greater than 10 ng/ml, a rectal examination, ultrasonography, and biopsy were offered. Of 27 biopsies performed, 18 (67%) were positive for prostate cancer.

The control group for this study was 235 men with urinary symptoms who presented at a urology clinic. Each of these patients had a digital rectal examination, ultrasonography, PSA determination, and a biopsy. Thirteen (11%) of 116 men who had PSA values less than 4 ng/ml were biopsy-proven positive, as were 19 (26%) of 74 who had PSA values between 4.1 and 9.9 ng/ml and 29 (64%) of 45 men with PSA values greater than 10 ng/ml.

The percentage of biopsy-positive men in the study group and the control group were identical. It may be concluded from these studies that screening with PSA detected prostate cancer in 37 (2.2%) of 1653 men, but 78% of the men with PSA values between 4.1 and 10 ng/ml and 33% of men with values greater than 10 ng/ml had negative biopsies. This means that 75 (67%) men with abnormal PSA values would undergo the additional studies without a confirmation of cancer and would be considered false positives. Based on the experience in the control group, 11% (13 of 116) of those with biopsy-proven prostate cancer would not be detected. If only the men with PSA values greater than 10 ng/ml were evaluated, a value that eliminates interference from BPH, 30 (2%) of 1653 would have elevations, and of these, 18 (67%) of 27 would be biopsy positive. During Prostate Cancer Awareness Week in 1990, 565 men presented themselves at screening clinics in Madison County, New York. Of these men, 447 had negative PSA and rectal examinations. Among 24 with elevated PSA and positive rectal examinations, 11 of 16 who had biopsies were positive. Of 35 with positive PSA and normal rectal examinations, 4 of 17 who had biopsies were positive, and in 59 with normal PSA but abnormal rectal examinations 5 of 21 who had biopsies were positive.[75] There is little doubt that PSA can detect a proportion of men with disease and is very useful adjunct in screening high-risk groups. In 287 patients who had bladder overflow obstruction, there were 19 biopsy-proven prostate cancers. Of these, 17 (89%) had PSA values greater than 10 ng/ml.[76]

PSA is widely used as a monitoring tool, and serum levels reflect response to therapy. Elevations may predict recurrence many months before clinical confirmation.[77-79] After surgery, a fall to "female" levels has been used to confirm removal of the cancer, and increases after surgery may indicate recurrence. A close correlation has been observed between tumor volume and PSA values, and there is an association between androgen concentrations and PSA.[80,81] PSA has not been a reliable marker in evaluating men with hormone-refractory prostate cancer.[82] In using PSA, it is important to consider a number of factors.[71,83,84] The $T_{1/2}$ of PSA is 2 to 3 days (3.15 $\pm$ 0.09 days), and after removal of all tumor, it may take 2 to 3 weeks for serum values to return to normal or baseline.[83] Elevations may occur after prostate manipulation, ultrasound, or biopsy. There is no circadian variation, but there may be 6% to 7% variation between values in several specimens collected from the same patient during the day; ambulatory values are higher than sedentary values, and values may fall as much as 50% (mean, 18%) within 24 hours of hospitalization. Different assays may yield different numbers, some of which may be 1.4 to 1.8 times higher than the others.

Is acid phosphatase testing needed if PSA is used? We reviewed 1445 patients at Memorial Sloan-Kettering Cancer Center in whom both assays were ordered. In 916 (63%) patients, there were elevations of PSA and acid phosphatase, and in 319 (29%), only PSA was elevated. However, there were 116 (8%) men who demonstrated elevations of acid phosphatase although the PSA was within normal levels (<4.0 ng/ml). In some of these patients, the acid phosphatase was markedly elevated or remained elevated during therapy although PSA was normal or fell to normal levels.

NEURON-SPECIFIC ENOLASE

Neuron-specific enolase (NSE) is one of the three dimeric isoenzymes of enolase, the glycolytic enzyme that catalyzes the conversion of 2-phosphoglycerate to phosphoenol pyruvate. This enzyme in serum is a specific marker of neuroendocrine tumors, including neuroblastoma, medullary carcinoma of the thyroid, and small cell carcinoma of the lung (SCCL). In initial studies, elevations were observed in 90% of patients with neuroblastoma and in 70% of patients with SCCL.[85] Elevations are primarily seen in patients with extensive disease. In SCCL, abnormal values were observed in 90% of patients with extensive disease, compared with 40% to 60% of persons with limited disease.[86]

NSE is useful in monitoring patients. Falls reflect response to successful therapy, and subsequent elevations reflect exacerbations. Longitudinal studies using 57 patients receiving chemotherapy indicated an excellent correlation between disease state and enzyme concentration.[87] In 40 of 50 patients who responded to therapy, there was a fall toward normal, but in 5 of 7 who had progressive disease, there was a rising level of NSE.

OTHER ENZYME MARKERS

Numerous enzymes have been proposed as markers. Creatine kinase BB (CK-BB), the brain isoenzyme, has been proposed

as a marker for SCCL, breast carcinoma, and prostate cancer. In SCCL, 27 (26%) of 105 of patients had elevations of CK-BB.[88] Its low sensitivity and specificity preclude its general use.

LDH and its isoenzyme (LDH_5) have been successfully used as prognostic markers for melanoma, various types of leukemia, testicular cancer, and some solid tumors. It has been used to stratify patients for treatment protocols.[89]

Galactosyltransferase has been used in monitoring ovarian cancer, and sialyltransferase has been proposed as a general marker. An isoenzyme of galactosyltransferase (galactosyltransferase II) has been used as a general marker.[90] The difficulty in assaying the glycotransferases has discouraged any clinical use of these markers.

Terminal deoxynucleotidyl transferase (TdT) is a DNA polymerase that does not require a template. Blast cells of patients with acute lymphocytic leukemia contain large amounts of TdT, but lymphocytes from persons without leukemia or with nonlymphoid leukemia have low or no detectable activities of this enzyme. Its presence in lymphocytes has been useful for differentiating acute lymphoid from acute myeloid leukemia, and it may be useful in classifying non-Hodgkin lymphoma. There are conflicting reports about whether TdT is useful in monitoring recurrence or remission.[91]

MULTIPLE MARKER PANELS

There have been many attempts to use multivariate and discriminant analyses to improve the sensitivity and specificity of tumor markers. One or two markers usually give results that are at least as good as those for a larger group of markers. In a multicenter study, a variety of markers, each of which had been reported to be elevated in patients with cancer of the lung, were combined to see if multivariate analysis would yield information not available by the use of one marker alone.[92] Of the analytes studied, none alone was of value, except CEA, which was elevated in 54% of the patients. Ferritin was elevated in 29%, lipid-bound sialic acid in 22%, total sialic acid in 25%, β_2-microglobulin in 4%, lipotropin in 27%, β-hCG in 18%, α-hCG in 5%, parathyroid hormone in 6%, and calcitonin in 17%.

Linear discrimination was used to see if a group of these markers would be effective in differentiating patients with lung cancer from healthy persons or those with benign lung disease. In the first part of the experiment, patients with advanced lung cancer were studied. Statistical analysis indicated that CEA and total sialic acid allowed the best separation of these groups. Lipid-bound sialic acid was almost as useful as total sialic acid. With this combination of markers, there was clear distinction between normal persons and those with advanced lung cancer. Similar separation was observed when the discriminant equation was used to compare the patients with lung cancer and those with benign lung disease. The next part of the study applied the statistical equations to patients with early lung cancer. The best combination of markers was ferritin plus CEA, but there was no significant separation of the lung cancer patients from normal persons. The conclusion from these studies was that more than two markers in combination do not add to the ability to identify cancer patients and that the currently available markers for lung cancer cannot be used successfully to identify patients with early cancer.

BODY FLUIDS OTHER THAN BLOOD

Attempts have been made to use assays of markers in ascitic fluid, gallbladder bile, breast cyst fluid, saliva, and cerebrospinal fluid. Opinions vary on the validity of CEA measured in ascitic fluid for helping to differentiate malignant and benign ascites. CEA levels in gallbladder bile are proposed as useful for establishing the presence of liver metastases in colorectal cancer. CA 125 measured in saliva may have greater specificity in detecting ovarian cancer than the assay of CA 125 in serum. The measurement of markers in breast cyst fluid has been proposed as a method to identify high-risk breast cancer patients.

In cerebrospinal fluid, a variety of markers have been useful in differentiating central nervous system tumors from other forms of central nervous system (CNS) disease.[93] The most useful battery has been CEA, LDH isoenzymes, and the enzyme β-glucuronidase. These are elevated in cerebrospinal fluid in leptomeningeal metastases but not in intraparenchymal brain metastases or epidural spinal metastases. They may also assist in differentiation of neoplastic meningitis from subacute or chronic infectious meningitis and may be useful in monitoring the effectiveness of therapy in meningeal metastases. They are more effective as markers in meningeal metastases related to solid tumors than to lymphoma or leukemia. The assay of β-hCG and AFP in cerebrospinal fluid may allow confirmation of CNS metastases in cases of uterine choriocarcinoma and testicular germ cell carcinomas and help to identify the histopathologic type in surgically inaccessible cancers.

NUCLEAR MAGNETIC RESONANCE

In 1986, Foessel and his associates reported that water-suppressed proton nuclear magnetic resonance (NMR) spectra of plasma correlated with the presence or absence of cancer.[94] The spectra were presumably dominated by the resonance of plasma lipoprotein lipids. The basis of the assay was the measurement of the line width of the relevant spectrum peak at half of the peak height. In 81 patients with biopsy-proven cancer, there was a significant difference ($p < 0.0001$) between their plasma and plasma from normal persons, those with benign disease except benign prostatic hypertrophy ($p < 0.001$), and those with diseases other than cancer ($p < 0.0001$). Numerous workers have attempted to substantiate this finding. Wilding and colleagues were unable to differentiate normal persons from patients with cancer.[95] However, they demonstrated a significant correlation of the NMR line width and triglyceride concentration. There was an inverse relationship between fasting triglyceride levels and the NMR spectral line widths. Several other investigators attributed the findings of Foessel and his associates to triglyceride concentration and concluded that analysis of line widths cannot be used as a cancer-detection test.[96–99] Engnn and coworkers evaluated the procedure in 104 patients with untreated cancer

and 164 healthy controls.[100] Although there was a significant difference between the mean values of the line widths in the two groups ($p < 0.001$), there was considerable overlap, and the researchers concluded that NMR is not generally reliable as a cancer test.

Foessel commented that deviance from his original report may be due to methodology differences, such as the use of optimal field strength, careful control of sample temperature, methods for magnet shimming, and collection of the sample.[101] Chumurny and his associates in a multicenter study evaluated many of the possible variables in the performance of the NMR test and concluded that, if all the variables are carefully controlled, the test is reproducible but does not have predictive values high enough to be used as a general screening test for cancer.[102] Pregnant women had patterns similar to patients with cancer. The mean line width was 39.5 ± 1.6 Hz in 44 normal controls, 29.5 ± 2.5 Hz in the 81 patients with cancer, and 36.1 ± 2.6 Hz in patients with nonmalignant disease. In the cancer patient, the HDL cholesterol was lower than in the other two groups.

In an attempt to sharpen the use of NMR spectra as a cancer test, Sletlen and his associates used multivariate analysis for several peaks.[103] In their evaluation, 71 and 76 data points of the methyl and methylene lipoprotein spectra, respectively, were used rather than the conventional approach of measuring the line width of a single peak at half-height. They claim to have successfully identified 27 of 29 specimens from patients with cancer and 54 of 55 from noncancer controls.

In an attempt to circumvent triglyceride interference in water-suppressed proton NMR, Foessel and colleagues used ^{13}C NMR.[104] This procedure, although time consuming, is not sensitive to triglyceride interference. In 480 blood bank donors and 208 women who were to have breast biopsies, the sensitivity of the ^{13}C NMR was 94%, and the specificity was 99%. The positive predictive value was 96%, and the negative predictive value was 98%. Because the ^{13}C NMR technique is time consuming, Foessel has recommended that the proton method be used first and positive or borderline results confirmed with the ^{13}C NMR procedure.

COST AND ACCEPTANCE OF USING TUMOR MARKERS

Although tumor markers can provide information on regression or progression of disease. There are still questions about whether the cost of the assays and the cost of other diagnostic procedures initiated by positive marker results are justifiable in the treatment of ultimately incurable disease and about what level of intervention is acceptable among false positives.[105] In a study of the use of CEA in monitoring of patients with colorectal cancer, it was conservatively estimated that the additional testing after a positive assay would be almost $600 and positive test-related surgery would cost about $6000 per patient. The monthly testing itself would cost about $500 annually.

Acceptance or rejection of these costs is related to individual definitions of cost effectiveness. Is cost effectiveness the expenditure of whatever is necessary to achieve the best possible result for the patient, or is it taking the most economic course consistent with good medical practice? The acceptance of a procedure as cost effective may also be culture related. HCC screening is accepted in China. In Japan, newborns are screened for neuroblastoma despite the fact that there are only 220 cases of neuroblastoma annually and that the cost per positive result is about $10,000. The cost of a biochemical or immunochemical test is usually less than other diagnostic procedures. The nihilist may say that marker assays are not useful or necessary until absolute therapy is available. I contend that markers provide clinically useful information, and whenever there is even the remotest possibility of altering the clinical course in a positive way, they should be included in the treatment plan.

REFERENCES

1. Kahn SN. Dear Dr. Bence Jones. Clin Chem 1991;37:1557–1558.
2. Schwartz MK. Enzymes in cancer. Clin Chem 1973;19:10–22.
3. Schwartz MK. Tumor markers in diagnosis and screening. In: Ting SW, Chen JS, Schwartz MK, eds. Human tumor markers. Amsterdam: Elsevier Science, 1987:3–16.
4. Gold P, Freedman SO. Demonstration of tumor specific antigen in human colonic carcinomata by immunologic tolerance and absorption techniques. J Exp Med 1965;127: 439–462.
5. Thompson DPM, Krupey J, Freedman SO, et al. The radioimmunoassay of circulating carcinoembryonic antigen of the human digestive system. Proc Natl Acad Sci USA 1969;64:161–167.
6. Sox HC. Probability theory in the use of diagnostic tests. Ann Intern Med 1986;104: 60–66.
7. Abelev GI. Alpha-fetoprotein as a marker of embryo-specific differentiation in normal and human tissues. Transplant Rev 1974;20:3–37.
8. Hirai H. Alpha fetoprotein. In: Chu TM, ed. Biochemical markers for cancer. New York: Marcel Dekker, 1982:23–59.
9. Chan DW, Miao YC. Affinity chromatographic separation of alpha-fetoprotein variants: Development of a mini-column procedure and application to cancer patients. Clin Chem 1986;32:2143–2146.
10. Sell S. Cancer markers of the 1990s. Clin Lab Med 1990;10:1–37.
11. Tatarinov YS. Detection of embryonic-specific globulin in the blood serum of patients with primary liver tumor. Vopr Med Khim 1964;10:90–91.
12. Okuda K. Early recognition of hepatocellular carcinoma. Hepatology 1986;6:729–738.
13. Bates SE. Clinical applications of serum tumor markers. Ann Intern Med 1991;115: 623–638.
14. Hirai H, Nishi S, Watabe H et al. Some chemical, experimental and clinical investigations on α-fetoprotein. In: Hirai H, Miyaji T, eds. Alpha-fetoprotein and hepatoma. Gann Monogr 1973;14:19–34.
15. Tang Z. Screening and early treatment of primary liver cancer with special reference to the east part of China. Ann Med Singapore 1989;9:203–205.
16. Bagshawe KD. Clinical application of hCG. Adv Exp Med Biol 1965;76:313–324.
17. Ross GT, Goldsein DP, Hertz R, et al. Sequential use of methotrexate and actinocycin D in the treatment of metastatic choriocarcinoma and related trophoblastic diseases in women. Am J Obstet Gynecol 1965;93:223–229.
18. Wehmann RE, Nisula BC. Metabolic and renal clearance rates of purified human chorionic gonadotropin. J Clin Invest 1981;68:184–194.
19. Schwartz MK. Biochemical and immunological diagnosis of cancer. Germ cell tumors. Tumor Biol 1987;8:106–108.
20. Nisselbaum JS, Bosl GJ, Golbey D, et al. Changes in serum alpha-fetoprotein and chorionic gonadotropin in response to cancer therapy. Ann Clin Lab Sci 1984;14:178–188.
21. Bosl GJ, Geller NL, Cirrincione C, et al. Multivariate analysis of prognostic variables in patients with metastatic testicular cancer. Cancer Res 1983;43:3403–3407.
22. Bajorin DF, Geller NL, Weisen SF, et al. Two-drug therapy in patients with metastatic germ cell tumors. Cancer 1991;67:28–32.
23. Vugrin D, Whitmore WF Jr, Nisselbaum J, et al. Correlation of serum tumor markers and lymphangiography with degrees of nodal involvement in surgical stage II testis cancer. J Urol 1982;2:683–684.
24. Report from the Medical Research Council Working Party: Prognostic factors in advanced non-seminomatous germ cell testicular tumors: Results of two multicenter studies. Lancet 1985;1:8–11.
25. Toner GC, Geller NC, Tan C, et al. Serum tumor marker half-life during chemotherapy allows early prediction of complete response and survival in nonseminomatous germ cell tumors. Cancer Res 1990;50:5904–5910.
26. Jeppson A, Wahren B, Stigbrand T, et al. A clinical evaluation of serum placental alkaline phosphatase in seminoma patients. Br J Urol 1983;55:73–78.
27. Nathanson L, Fishman WH. New observations on the Regan isoenzyme of alkaline phosphatase in cancer patients. Cancer 1971;27:1388–97.
28. Nouwen EJ, Pollet DE, Schelstraete JB, et al. Human placental alkaline phosphatase in benign and malignant ovarian neoplasia. Cancer Res 1985;45:892–302.
29. O'Connor J, Schlatterer JP, Briken S, et al. Development of highly sensitive immunoassays to measure human chorionic gonadotropin, its β-subunit and β-core fragment in the urine: Application of malignancies. Cancer Res 1988;48:1361–1366.
30. Cole LA, Wang Y, Elliot M, et al. Urinary human chorionic gonadotropin free beta-subunit and beta-core fragment: A new marker for gynecological cancers. Cancer Res 1988;48:1356–1360.
31. Cole LA, Nam JH, Chambers JT, et al. Urinary gonadotropin fragment, a new tumor marker II. For differentiating a benign from a malignant pelvic mass. Gynecol Oncol 1990;36:391–392.
32. Davis HW, Zurawski VR, Bast RC, et al. Characterization of the CA 125 antigen associated with epithelial ovarian carcinomas. Cancer Res 1986;46:6143.
33. Bast RC Jr, Klug TL, St. John E, et al. A radioimmunoassay using a monoclonal antibody to monitor the course of epithelial ovarian cancer. N Engl J Med 1983;309:883–887.
34. Klug TL, Bast RC Jr, Niloff JM, et al. Monoclonal antibody immunoradiometric assay for an antigenic determinant (CA 125) associated with human epithelial ovarian carcinomas. Cancer Res 1984;44:1048–1053.
35. Rubin SC, Hoskins WJ, Hakes TB, et al. CA 125 levels and surgical findings in patients undergoing secondary operations for epithelial ovarian cancer. Am J Obstet Gynecol 1989;160:667–671.
36. Canney PA, Moore M, Wilkinson PM, et al. Ovarian cancer antigen CA 125: A prospective clinical assessment of its role as a tumor marker. Br J Cancer 1984;50:765–769.
37. Ngan HYS, Wong LC, Chan SGW et al. Role of CA 125 and abdominal pelvic computerized axial tomogram in the monitoring of chemotherapy treatment of ovarian cancer. Cancer Invest 1990;8:465–470.
38. Jacobs I, Bast RC Jr. Immunodiagnosis of ovarian tumors. In: Herberman RB, Mercer DW, eds. Immunodiagnosis of cancer. 2nd ed. New York: Marcel Dekker, 1990:323–333.
39. Fanning J, Piver MS. Serial CA 125 levels during chemotherapy for metastatic recurrent endometrial cancer. Obstet Gynecol 1991;77:278–280.
40. Hansen HJ, Snyder JJ, Miller E, et al. Carcinoembryonic antigen (CEA) assay: A laboratory adjunct in the diagnosis and management of cancer. Hum Pathol 1974;5: 139–147.
41. Ladenson JH, McDonald JM, Schwartz MK. Colorectal cancer and carcinoembryonic antigen (CEA). Clin Chem 1980;26:1213–1220.
42. Wanebo HJ, Rao B, Pinsky CM, et al. Preoperative carcinoembryonic antigen level as a prognostic indicator in colorectal cancer. N Engl J Med 1978;229:448–451.
43. Goldenberg DM, Neville A, Carter A, et al. CEA (carcinoembryonic antigen): Its role as a marker in the management of cancer. J Cancer Res Clin Oncol 1981;101:239–242.
44. Sandler RS, Freund DA, Herbst CA Jr, et al. Cost effectiveness of postoperative carcinoembryonic antigen monitoring in colorectal cancer. Cancer 1984;53:193–198.
45. Maehara Y, Surgimachi K, Akagi M, et al. Serum carcinoembryonic antigen level increases correlate with tumor progression in patients with differentiated gastric carcinoma following noncurative resection. Cancer Res 1990;50:3952–3955.
46. Martin EW Jr, James KK, Hurtutise PE, et al. The use of CEA as an early indicator for gastrointestinal tumor recurrence and second-look procedures. Cancer 1977;39: 440–446.
47. Minton JP, James KK, Hurtubise PE, et al. The use of serial carcinoembryonic antigen determinations to predict recurrence of carcinoma of the colon and the time for a second-look operation. Surg Gynecol Obstet 1978;147:208–210.
48. Minton JP, Hoehn JL, Gerber DM, et al. Results of a 400 patient carcinoembryonic antigen second-look colorectal cancer study. Cancer 1985;55:1284–1290.
49. Quentmeier A, Schlag P, Holenberger P, et al. Assessment of serial carcinoembryonic antigen: Determinations to monitor the therapeutic progress and prognosis of metastatic liver disease treated by regional chemotherapy. J Surg Oncol 1989;40:112–118.
50. Beard DB, Haskell CM. Carcinoembryonic antigen in breast cancer. Clin Rev Am J Med 1986;80:241–245.
51. Kiang DT, Greenberg LJ, Kennedy BJ. Tumor marker kinetics in the monitoring of breast cancer. Cancer 1990;65:193–199.
52. Mughal AW, Hoctobagyi GN, Fritsche HA, et al. Serial plasma carcinoembryonic antigen measurements during treatment of metatastic breast cancer. JAMA 1983;249:1881–1886.
53. Koprowski H, Herlyn M, Steplewize Z, et al. Specific antigen in serum of patients with colon cancer. Science 1981;212:53–55.
54. Steinberg W, Gelfand R, Anderson K, et al. Comparison of the sensitivity and specificity of the CA 19-9 and CEA assays in detecting cancer of the pancreas. Gastroenterology 1986;90:343–349.
55. Schwartz MK, Schwartz D, Smith C, et al. Comparison of CEA and CA 195. Proc Am Assoc Cancer Res 1988;24:176.
56. Bhargava AK, Petrelli NJ, Kavna A, et al. Circulating CA 195 in colorectal cancer. J Tumor Marker Oncol 1987;2:319–327.
57. Gero EJ, Colcher D, Ferroni P, et al. CA 72-4 radioimmunoassay for the detection of the TAG 72 carcinoma-associated antigen in serum of patients. J Clin Lab Ann 1989;3: 360–369.
58. Heptner G, Domschke A, Domschke B. Comparison of CA 72-4 with CA 19-9 and carcinoembryonic antigen in the serodiagnosis of gastrointestinal malignancies. Scand J Gastroenterol 1989;24:745–750.
59. Holmgren J, Lindholm L, Pusson B, et al. Detection by monoclonal antibody of carbohydrate antigen CA 50 in serum of patients with carcinoma. Br Med J 288:1479–1482.
60. Hayes DF, Zurawski VR Jr, Kufe DW. Comparison of circulating CA 15-3 and carcinoembryonic antigen levels in patients with breast cancer. J Clin Oncol 1986;4:1542–1550.
61. Colomer R, Ruibal A, Salvador L. Circulating tumor marker levels in advanced breast

carcinoma correlate with the extent of metastatic disease. Cancer 1989;64:1674–1681.

62. Tondini C, Hayes DF, Gellman R, et al. Comparison of CA 15-3 and carcinoembryonic antigen in monitoring the clinical course of patients with metastatic breast cancer 1988;48:4107–4112.

63. Dnistrian AM, Schwartz MK, Greenberg EJ, et al. CA 15-3 and carcinoembryonic antigen in the clinical evaluation of breast cancer. Clin Chim Acta 1991;200:81–94.

64. Safi F, Kohler I, Rottinger E, et al. The value of the tumor marker CA 15-3 in diagnosing and monitoring breast cancer. Cancer 1991;68:574–582.

65. Dnistrian AM, Schwartz MK, Greenberg EJ, et al. Evaluation of CA M26, CA M29, CA 15-3 and CEA as circulating tumor markers in breast cancer patients. Tumour Biol 1991;12:82–90.

66. Dnistrian AM, Schwartz MK, Greenberg EJ, et al. CA 549 as a marker in breast cancer. Int J Biol Markers 1991;6:139–143.

67. Watt KWK, Lee PJ, McTimkula T, et al. Human prostate-specific antigen: Structural and functional similarity with serine protease. Proc Natl Acad Sci USA 1986;83:3166–3170.

68. Lilja H. A kallikrein-like serine protease in prostatic fluid cleaves the predominant seminal vesicle protein. J Clin Invest 1985;76:1899–1903.

69. Graves HC, Kamarei M, Stamey TA. Identification of prostate-specific antigen and serum protein P30 purified by a rapid chromatography technique. J Urol 1990;144:1510–1515.

70. Livingston RB, Bartolocci A, Becker JA, et al. Consensus conference: The management of clinically localized prostate cancer. JAMA 1988;258:2727–2730.

71. Oesterling JE. Prostate-specific antigen: A valuable clinical tool. Oncology 1991;5:4,107–126.

72. Schwartz MK. Can prostate-specific antigen be used in screening? In: Lange PH, ed. Tumor markers in prostate cancer. Princeton: Excerpta Medica, 1986:47–51.

73. Schwartz MK. The role of the laboratory in the prevention and detection of chronic disease. Clin Chem 1992;38:1539–1546.

74. Catalona WJ, Smith DS, Ratliff TL, et al. Measurement of prostate-specific antigen in serum as a screening test for prostate cancer. N Engl J Med 1991;324:1156–1161.

75. Muschenheim F, Omarbasha B, Kardjian PM, et al. Screening for carcinoma of the prostate with prostate-specific antigen. Ann Clin Lab Sci 1991;21:371–380.

76. Powell CS, Fielding AM, Rosser K, et al. Prostate-specific antigen—a screening test for prostatic cancer? Br J Urol 1986;64:504–506.

77. Osterling JE, Chan DW, Epstein JI, et al. Prostate-specific antigen in the preoperative and postoperative evaluation of localized prostatic cancer treated with radical prostatectomy. J Urol 1988;139:766–772.

78. Stamey TA, Yang N, Hay AR, et al. Prostate-specific antigen as a serum marker for adenocarcinoma of the prostate. N Engl J Med 1987;317:909–916.

79. Lange PH, Ercole CJ, Lightner DJ, et al. The value of serum prostate-specific antigen determinations before and after radical prostatectomy. J Urol 1989;141:873–879.

80. Stamey TA, Kabalin JW, McNeal JE, et al. Prostate-specific antigen in the diagnosis and treatment of adenocarcinoma of the prostate II radical prostatectomy treated patients. J. Urol 1989;141:1076–1083..

81. Arai Y, Yoshiki T, Yoshida O. Prognostic significance of prostate-specific antigen in endocrine treatment for prostatic cancer. J Urol 1990;144:1415–1419.

82. Scher HI, Curley T, Geller N, et al. Trimetrexate in prostatic cancer: Preliminary observations on the use of prostate-specific antigen and acid phosphatase as a marker in measurable hormone refractory disease. J Clin Oncol 1990;8:1830–1838.

83. Deijter SW Jr, Martin JS, McPherson RA, et al. Daily variability in human serum prostate-specific antigen and prostatic acid phosphatase: A comparable evaluation. Urology 1988;32:288–292.

84. Mannini D, Maver P, Aiello E, et al. Spontaneous circadian fluctuations of prostate-

specific antigen and prostatic acid phosphatase serum activities in patients with prostatic cancer. Urol Res 1988;16:9–12.

85. Notami T, Morikaw J, Kata K, et al. Radioimmunoassay development for human neuron-specific enolase: With some clinical results in lung cancers and neuroblastoma. Tumour Biol 1985;6:57–66.

86. Carney DN, Mararyos PH, Idhe DC, et al. Serum neuron-specific enolase: A marker for disease extent and response to therapy of small cell lung cancer. Lancet 1982;1:583–585.

87. Johnson DH, Marangos PJ, Forbes JT, et al. Potential utility of serum neuron-specific enolase levels in small cell carcinoma of the lung. Cancer Res 1984;44:5409–5414.

88. Carney DH, Zweig MH, Ihke DC, et al. Elevated serum creatine kinase BB levels in patients with small cell lung cancer. Cancer Res 1984;44:5399–5403.

89. Schwartz MK. Lactic dehydrogenase: An old enzyme reborn as a cancer marker? Am J Clin Pathol 1991;96:441–443.

90. Podolsky DK, Weiser MM, Isselbacher KJ, et al. A cancer-associated galactosyltransferase isoenzyme. N Engl J Med 1978;229:703–710.

91. Fleisher M, Stankievic R, Schwartz D, et al. Solid phase enzyme immunoassay of terminal deoxynucleotidyl transferase evaluated. Clin Chem 1987;33:293–296.

92. Gail MH, Nuenz L, McIntire KR, et al. Multiple markers for lung cancer diagnosis: Validation of models for localized lung cancer. JNCI 1988;80:97–101.

93. Wasserstrom WR, Schwartz MK, Fleisher M, et al. Cerebrospinal fluid biochemical markers in central nervous system tumors: A review. Ann Clin Lab Sci 1981;11:239–251.

94. Foessel ET, Carr JM, McDonagh J, et al. Detection of malignant tumors. Water suppressed proton nuclear magnetic resonance spectroscopy of plasma. N Engl J Med 1986;315:1369–1377.

95. Wilding P, Senior MB, Inubushi T, et al. Assessment of proton nuclear magnetic resonance spectroscopy for detection of malignancy. Clin Chem 1988;34:505–511.

96. Mims MP, Morrisett JD, Mattioli CA, et al. Effect of triglyceride levels on methyl and methylene envelope line widths in proton nuclear magnetic resonance spectroscopy of human plasma. N Engl J Med 1989;320:1452–1457.

97. Berger S, Pfluger KH, Etzel WA, et al. Detection of tumors with nuclear magnetic resonance spectroscopy of plasma. Eur J Cancer Clin Oncol 1989;25:535–543.

98. Okunieff P, Zietman A, Kahn J, et al. Lack of efficiency of water suppressed nuclear magnetic resonance spectroscopy of plasma for the detection of malignant tumors. N Engl J Med 1990;322:953–958.

99. Otvos JD, Jeyarajah EJ, Hayes LW, et al. Relationship between the proton nuclear magnetic resonance properties of plasma lipoproteins and cancer. Clin Chem 1991;37:369–376.

100. Engnn T, Krane J, Klepp O, et al. Proton nuclear magnetic resonance spectroscopy of plasma from healthy subjects and patients with cancer. N Engl J Med 1990;322:949–953.

101. Foessel ET. Commentary on "Detection of tumors with nuclear magnetic resonance spectroscopy of plasma" by Berger, KH Pfluger, WA Etzel and J Fischer. Eur J Clin Oncol 1989;25:925–927.

102. Chumurny GN, Hilton BD, Halverson D, et al. An NMR blood test for cancer: A critical assessment. NMR Biomed 1988;1:136–150.

103. Slelten E, Kvalheim OM, Kruse S, et al. Detection of malignant tumors by multivariate analysis of proton magnetic resonance spectra of serum. Eur J Cancer 1990;25:615–618.

104. Foessel ET, Hall FM, McDonagh J. C-13 NMR spectroscopy of plasma reduces interference of hypertriglyceridemia in the H-1 NMR detection of malignancy. Applications in patient with breast lesions. Breast Cancer Res Treat 1991;18:99–110.

105. Schwartz MK. Tumor markers: What is their role? Cancer Invest 1990;8:439–440.

SECTION **4**

DONALD L. MILLER
JOHN L. DOPPMAN

Interventional Radiology in Oncology

Interventional radiology procedures employ radiologic guidance to direct needles or catheters for invasive diagnosis or treatment of various disorders. Many of these procedures represent alternatives to surgery. The surgeon uses direct vision as a guide, while the radiologist relies on indirect vision with a variety of imaging methods.

The techniques of the interventional radiologist can be divided into five categories: diagnostic procedures to obtain material for histologic, cytologic, or other laboratory analysis and four broad categories of therapeutic intervention—drainage procedures for abscesses and occlusions of the biliary and urinary tracts, vascular and nonvascular balloon dilation, chemotherapy administration, and embolotherapy.[1] All the paraphernalia and procedures used in modern interventional radiology can be considered adaptations or applications of these basic concepts.

A simpler classification is appropriate for oncologic interventional radiology. This chapter reviews procedures used for cancer diagnosis, for cancer therapy, and as adjuncts in the management of cancer patients. This classification excludes several types of procedures, such as stone extraction and transluminal angioplasty, that have no direct application in oncologic practice.

PERCUTANEOUS BIOPSY FOR CANCER DIAGNOSIS

Percutaneous needle biopsy is an important technique in the diagnosis and staging of cancer.[2-4] Its increased use in the past decade is a consequence of the availability of safer needles, newer imaging techniques, and advances in cytology. The procedure is used to diagnose and stage malignancies, confirm metastases, and diagnose certain benign lesions.

TECHNIQUE

Radiologically guided percutaneous needle biopsy is usually performed with thin ("skinny") needles of 20 to 23 gauge, which are designed to yield aspirates of cells for cytologic examination. Some of these needles are also designed to yield small cores of tissue.[5,6] Regardless of which needle is used, the technique is usually referred to as fine-needle aspiration biopsy (FNAB).[4] Larger needles can be used to obtain larger cores of tissue and are most commonly used in the evaluation of bone tumors, hepatic lesions, and lymphomas, for which the larger needles produce more tissue, may yield higher accuracy rates, and do not appear to have a higher complication rate.[2,5,7-12] Some radiologists prefer a spring-loaded biopsy "gun" with an 18-gauge needle for almost all percutaneous needle biopsies.[13,14] Needle choice depends on the size, type, and location of the lesion and the preferences of the radiologist and cytopathologist.[7,15] Pathologists with less experience in cytology may require larger tissue samples for a confident diagnosis.

The role of the pathologist is critical, because skill and experience in cytology are the most important factors in reaching an accurate diagnosis. Pathologists vary in their preferences for different methods of tissue sampling, tissue fixation, and sample handling.[7,16] It is wise to follow the pathologist's preferences in this regard. It is often possible to arrange for a cytologist or cytotechnologist to be present during the biopsy, and this is helpful because specimens can be prepared on the spot and the radiologist can be given virtually instant information about their adequacy.[2,17] Additional needle passes can be made if the specimen is inadequate, and unnecessary additional passes can be avoided if the initial specimen is satisfactory. Johnsrude and colleagues[18] found that immediate cytologic review reduced the incidence of pneumothorax by 50% in patients undergoing percutaneous biopsy of intrathoracic lesions, but Miller and coworkers[19] found no increase in accuracy or decrease in the complication rate. Nevertheless, most radiologists and pathologists believe that this sort of close cooperation produces clear benefits.

A variety of imaging techniques can be used for needle guidance during biopsy.[3,4] Fluoroscopy is useful for lesions that are visible on plain films, such as pulmonary nodules, some bone lesions, and lymph nodes opacified by lymphangiography. Ultrasound and computed tomography (CT) have extended our ability to visualize lesions in the mediastinum, abdomen, pelvis, and head and neck, and they are commonly used to guide biopsies of these areas (Fig. 21–32). Magnetic resonance imaging (MRI) can also be used for guidance if the biopsy needle is fabricated from a stainless steel alloy that does not produce artifacts on MR images and does not move in a magnetic field. Mueller and colleagues performed MR-guided liver biopsies, and Duckwiler and associates biopsied lesions in the head and neck with MR guidance.[20,21] The choice of imaging modality is based on lesion size, position, and visibility; equipment availability; and the skills and preference of the radiologist. The radiologist who performs the biopsy must be the final arbiter.

CLINICAL ADVANTAGES

Much of the appeal of percutaneous biopsy is based on the use of this technique as a substitute for surgical biopsy, with attendant decrease in patient morbidity and costs.[22-26] In a review of 82 percutaneous biopsies performed in patients with

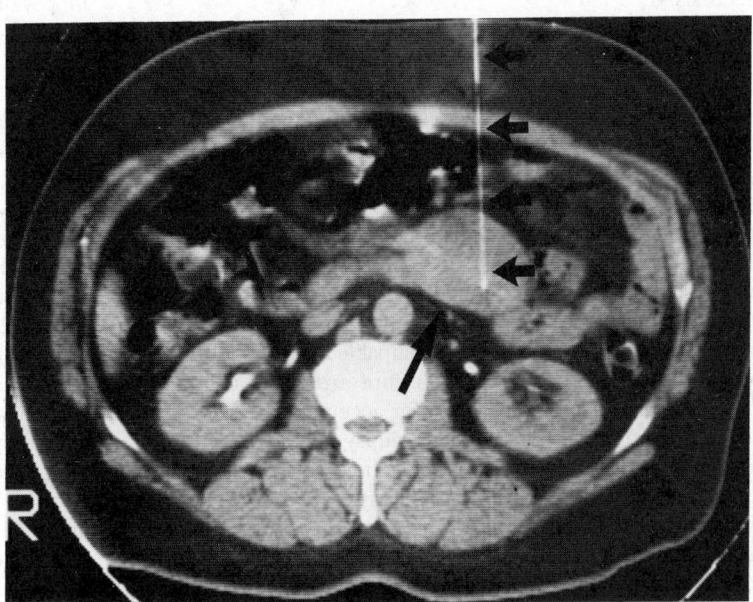

FIGURE 21–32. CT-guided biopsy of an abdominal mass. The needle is visible as a thin white line (*short black arrows*) terminating in the mass (*long black arrow*). The needle passes through gas-containing bowel. With thin needles, this is safe. The patient had no complications from the biopsy.

gynecologic malignancies and extrapelvic lesions, biopsy was highly cost effective, and it permitted surgery to be avoided in many patients.[23] In 72 patients undergoing percutaneous biopsy of thoracic lesions, biopsy shortened the time from admission to diagnosis, reduced the total number of thoracotomies, shortened the length of hospital stay, and resulted in a significantly reduced average and total hospitalization charge.[24] In a series of 422 patients with 400 proven pulmonary lesions, Westcott found that percutaneous biopsy established the diagnosis in 191 patients and made mediastinoscopy or thoracotomy unnecessary.[25] In a series of 53 patients with a clinical diagnosis of carcinoma of the pancreas, 30 laparotomies were avoided in 37 patients with positive biopsies.[26]

Most biopsies in adults can be performed as outpatient procedures under local anesthesia. In a series of 1000 consecutive CT-guided biopsies, the average procedure lasted only 22 minutes.[27] Percutaneous biopsy procedures are also appropriate for pediatric patients. Sedation or regional anesthesia may be necessary, but general anesthesia is usually not required.[28] In one series of 69 percutaneous diagnostic procedures in children 2 days to 17 years of age, general anesthesia was never necessary.[29] In another series, core biopsies were obtained with 14-gauge needles in 39 patients from 20 months to 18 years of age. Some of these patients were sedated, but none required general anesthesia.[30]

ACCURACY

The accuracy of percutaneous biopsy depends on the skill of the radiologist and the cytopathologist. Accuracy varies depending on the tumor type and the biopsy site. Seventy-five percent of initial needle passes into malignant lesions yield specimens containing malignant cells.[31] Additional needle passes can increase sensitivity, but more than four passes are rarely necessary, and each additional pass increases the risk of the procedure to some degree. Large masses should be biopsied near their periphery to avoid possible areas of necrosis.

A negative biopsy report does not necessarily mean that malignancy has been excluded. The wrong site may have been sampled, or the sample may be inadequate. Only positive biopsies documenting cancer or a specific benign lesion should influence therapeutic decisions.

FNAB of the breast occasionally produces small, transient hematomas, but these do not interfere with interpretation of subsequent mammograms. It has a sensitivity of approximately 90% and a false-negative rate of 3% to 10% for palpable breast cancers.[32] Hypercellular benign lesions and radiation-induced changes can mimic carcinoma, but most recent series report a specificity of 100% for FNAB of palpable masses.[33,34] Results of FNAB of nonpalpable breast lesions are not as good, and rigid criteria must be adhered to for acceptable results.[32]

The sensitivity of percutaneous biopsy for the detection of malignancy in lung nodules is as high as 90% to 98%, with accuracies of 80% to 98%.[2,4,17,35] Biopsy of the hilum and mediastinum is equally sensitive, although lymphoma can be difficult to diagnose with FNAB.[2,16,17,36]

Welch and colleagues prospectively studied 1000 consecutive CT-guided FNAB procedures, 266 of which were liver biopsies. Accuracy in the liver was 98.5%.[27] In other series, FNAB has an accuracy of about 95% for the diagnosis of liver metastases.[4,8,10,37] Sbolli and coworkers reported a sensitivity of 95% and a specificity of 100% for 138 patients with cirrhosis and hepatocellular carcinoma who underwent FNAB of the liver.[38] FNAB is also highly accurate for evaluating retroperitoneal lymph nodes in patients with locally recurrent or metastatic abdominal malignancies.[37]

Pancreatic biopsy is somewhat less useful, with an average reported sensitivity of 80% to 85% and accuracy of 85% to 90%.[27,39] It may be more appropriate to biopsy associated liver metastases or abdominal masses in patients with pancreatic lesions than to biopsy the pancreas directly. However, Del Maschio and colleagues studied 81 consecutive patients with chronic pancreatitis or pancreatic cancer and determined that FNAB of the pancreas had positive and negative predictive values of 100% in this setting.[40]

An adrenal mass in a patient with cancer may be biopsied to differentiate an adrenal metastasis from a nonfunctioning adrenal adenoma ("incidentaloma"). These are seen as serendipitous findings on approximately 1% of abdominal CT scans.[41,42] Adrenal FNAB is successful in 80% to 95% of enlarged glands.[27,43]

The diagnostic accuracy of retroperitoneal and pelvic lymph node biopsies varies from 65% to 90%, depending on the tumor type.[11,27,37,44,45] In most series, accuracy is higher in patients with nodal metastases from carcinoma than in patients with lymphoma, because the diagnosis of lymphoma may require a much larger tissue sample for accurate evaluation of cell patterns. However, diagnosis and subclassification can be accomplished by FNAB in many patients with non-Hodgkin lymphoma because the cytologic material obtained is suitable for DNA flow cytometry, cytogenetic and molecular studies, and immunocytochemical analysis.[11,16]

Percutaneous bone biopsy has an overall accuracy of about 80% in the diagnosis of primary bone tumors and 95% in the diagnosis of osseous metastases.[9,12,46] Large needles are usually required for the diagnosis of primary bone tumors and for biopsy of blastic lesions.[12] The blood from a bone biopsy specimen should also be sent for cytologic analysis, especially in patients with osseous metastases.[47]

CONTRAINDICATIONS AND COMPLICATIONS

The only absolute contraindication to FNAB is an intractable bleeding diathesis. Thrombocytopenia and coagulation disorders should be corrected before biopsy. FNAB maybe technically impossible in a patient who is unable or unwilling to remain still and suspend respiration, and the risk is also increased in these patients.

Overall, FNAB is a remarkably safe technique. The potential complications of the procedure are summarized in Table 21–6. The most common cause of death is hemorrhage from the liver, but this probably reflects the frequency of liver biopsies.[27,48,53] There is an increased risk of hemorrhage with biopsy of subcapsular lesions, unlike those deep in the hepatic parenchyma.[48] Fatalities may also occur from hemorrhagic pancreatitis after FNAB of the pancreas, asphyxiation due to

TABLE 21–6. Complications of Fine-Needle Aspiration Biopsy

Complication	Frequency (%)
Death[48,49,53] *	<0.05
Hemorrhage[27,48,49,53]	<1
Infection[48]	Rare
Tumor seeding[48]	<0.01
Syncope (biopsy of the breast)[50]	1
Pancreatitis (biopsy of the pancreas)[4,27,39]	<3
Pneumothorax (biopsy of lung or mediastinum)[2,4,17,35]	10–35
Pneumothorax requiring treatment (biopsy of lung or mediastinum)[2,4,17,35]	5–15

* Markedly increased risk for biopsy of pheochromocytoma.[51,52]

hemoptysis, or rarely, air embolism after lung biopsy.[2,48] Rarely, deaths have resulted from massive hormone release after biopsy of functioning endocrine tumors, such as carcinoids or pheochromocytomas.[48,54] Sepsis after biopsy is uncommon and is rarely fatal.[48]

Despite the theoretical risk of seeding tumor cells along the needle track, reports of needle-track tumor implants are uncommon, with fewer than 0.01% in a series of 16,381 biopsies,[48] and animal studies have shown the phenomenon to be highly unlikely.[55] Almost half of all reported episodes of tumor seeding occurred after biopsy of the pancreas, with fewer episodes occurring after kidney and liver biopsies.[48]

The most common complication of FNAB is pneumothorax, which is associated with biopsies that transgress the pleural space. Pneumothorax occurs in 10% to 35% of these patients, with chest tube drainage required in 5% to 15% of patients undergoing biopsy.[2,4,17,35] Preexisting lung disease (especially chronic obstructive pulmonary disease), greater number of needle passes, greater distance of lesion from the skin, and increased patient age increase the risk of pneumothorax.[2] In one series of 673 transthoracic needle biopsies, 98% of all pneumothoraces, including all those that required treatment, were detected on chest radiographs obtained at 1 hour after biopsy, and all were apparent on chest radiographs obtained at 4 hours after biopsy.[56] With 4 hours of observation after biopsy, the procedure can be safely performed on an outpatient basis.[2,17,35,56] Many pneumothoraces can also be managed on an outpatient basis, with a 7- or 9-French chest tube placed percutaneously by the radiologist.[2,17,35,56]

The risk of pancreatitis after pancreatic FNAB appears to be increased if the biopsied lesion is smaller than 3 cm in diameter or the biopsy is from a normal pancreas.[39,48,57,58] This may be due to leakage of pancreatic enzymes from normal pancreas; pancreatic adenocarcinomas generally do not produce enzymes.[39]

Biopsy of most adrenal masses is probably no more dangerous than biopsies of other parts of the body.[27,43,48,57] However, unintentional FNAB of a pheochromocytoma is potentially lethal. Several cases of severe hypertension, hypotension, and massive hemorrhage have been reported.[51,52]

CANCER TREATMENT

The application of intravascular catheter techniques to the therapy of tumors can be divided into two major modalities, regional chemotherapy delivered through selectively positioned catheters, and infarction of tumor by embolization. Both modalities have benefited by the development of highly selective catheter techniques and suitable embolizing agents. The most recent development is chemoembolization, a combination of both methodologies in which the blood supply to the tumor is occluded with a mixture of embolic material and a chemotherapeutic agent, providing ischemic and cytotoxic components to the therapy.

INTRAARTERIAL CHEMOTHERAPY

Selective intraarterial infusion of chemotherapeutic agents is based on the principle that tumor response increases with drug exposure. The narrow therapeutic index of many anticancer drugs limits the systemic dose of chemotherapeutic agent and provides a rationale for selective intraarterial chemotherapy.[59–61] Infusion of chemotherapeutic agents directly into the arterial supply of a neoplasm can produce higher drug concentrations in the tumor-bearing region without corresponding increases in systemic concentration.[62] The most common target has been metastatic disease in the liver, but primary bone sarcomas, pelvic tumors, and head and neck tumors have been treated in this way.[63–67]

Broad experience, meticulous technique, and persistent efforts are required of the angiographer to complete many of these treatment courses. Before treatment of hepatic tumors, angiographic occlusion of accessory hepatic arteries or the gastroduodenal artery may be required (Fig. 21–33).[68] Occlusion of the hepatic artery frequently complicates prolonged or repeated infusions, and collateral vessels may have to be used for later cycles.[69] Narrowing of the extrahepatic and intrahepatic bile ducts due to cholangitis induced by the chemotherapeutic agent occurs with distressing frequency.[70] In the brain, severe unilateral retinal toxicity complicates internal carotid artery infusions proximal to the opthalmic artery.

Because infusion rates for chemotherapeutic agents are invariably slow, uniform perfusion may not occur because of the tendency for streaming when slow infusions are performed into a rapidly moving blood stream.[70–72] Techniques for determining perfusion patterns have been developed, and various pumps have been developed to improve the uniformity of distribution of the chemotherapeutic agent.[72,73]

EMBOLIZATION

Transcatheter embolization seeks to induce necrosis of tumor by obstructing its arterial supply. This usually entails deliberate sacrifice of the organ harboring the tumor, as in embolization of renal cell cancers. In the liver, with its dual blood supply, a tumor can be embolized through the hepatic artery while the normal hepatic parenchyma is sustained by portal venous inflow.[74]

Embolizing agents can be categorized on the basis of the duration of vascular occlusion (*e.g.*, temporary versus long-acting) and site of occlusion (peripheral versus proximal).

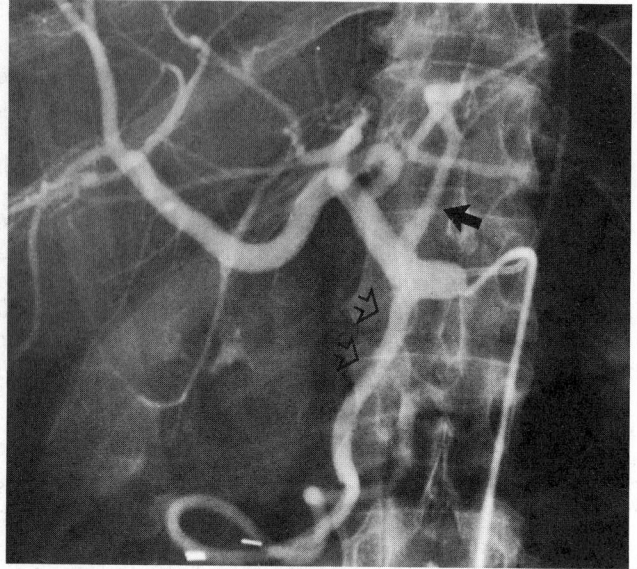

A

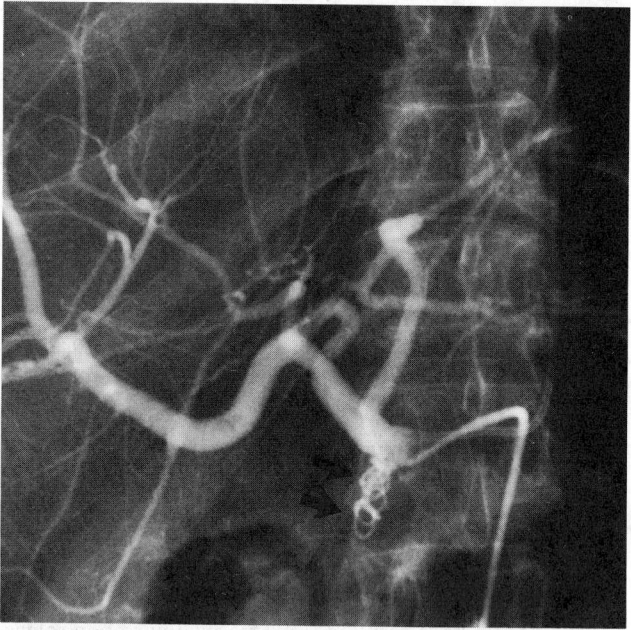

B

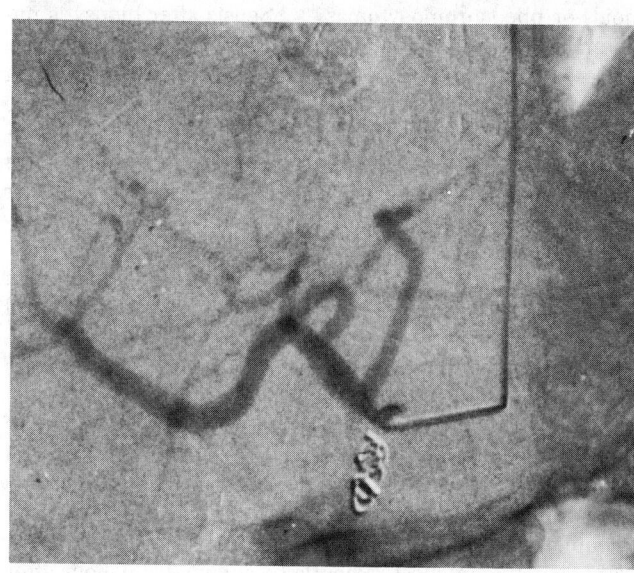

C

FIGURE 21–33. Hepatic artery infusion chemotherapy may require the use of interventional radiologic techniques. **(A)** A common hepatic artery angiogram before infusion reveals that the gastroduodenal artery (*open arrows*) arises almost opposite the left hepatic artery (*solid arrow*). The origin of the gastroduodenal artery must be blocked or drug will enter its vascular territory and cause gastric, duodenal, and pancreatic toxicity. **(B)** The gastroduodenal artery was occluded at its origin with Gianturco-Wallace-Anderson coils (*arrows*) delivered through the angiographic catheter. Retrograde filling of the gastroduodenal artery from the superior mesenteric artery by means of the pancreatic arcades maintains blood supply to the duodenum and pancreas. **(C)** Contrast material administered through the infusion catheter fills the right and left hepatic arteries but not the gastroduodenal artery. The effect is equivalent to surgical ligation of the gastroduodenal artery.

Temporary agents, such as absorbable gelatin sponge (Gelfoam dental packs) (Fig. 21–34), microfibrillar collagen hemostat (Avitene), and autologous clot are resorbed over a period of days to weeks. Permanent agents, such as polyvinyl alcohol foam (Ivalon) and Gianturco-Wallace-Anderson coils (see Fig. 21–32) are not metabolized, although the embolic effects may not be permanent in all cases.[75]

Even more important than the choice between temporary and permanent agents is the choice between peripheral and proximal occluding agents. Alcohol (dehydrated alcohol injection, USP) that acts as far peripherally as the capillary level and absorbable gelatin powder (Gelfoam sterile powder) that lodges in arterioles (see Fig. 21–32) cause vascular occlusion at a level distal to any possible collateral anastomoses and cause necrosis of the embolized territory. Gelfoam pledg-

ets, which are cut into small pieces before use and fragment further as they pass through the angiographic catheter, and Ivalon cause occlusion proximal to the most distal level of vascular anastomoses. They produce a peripheral embolic effect without infarction. At the most proximal level, coils occlude vessels 1 to 8 mm in diameter. In action and effect, they are identical to surgical ligation.

Temporary agents are rarely used as the sole agent for tumor embolization. Proximal occlusion of major feeding arteries is generally ineffective in tumor embolization because of the rapidity with which collateral channels develop. Peripheral embolizing agents occlude the arterial bed of a tumor and delay the development of collateral flow. Most angiographers seek to achieve peripheral occlusion of the vascular bed of the tumor with a permanent agent and, if indicated, follow

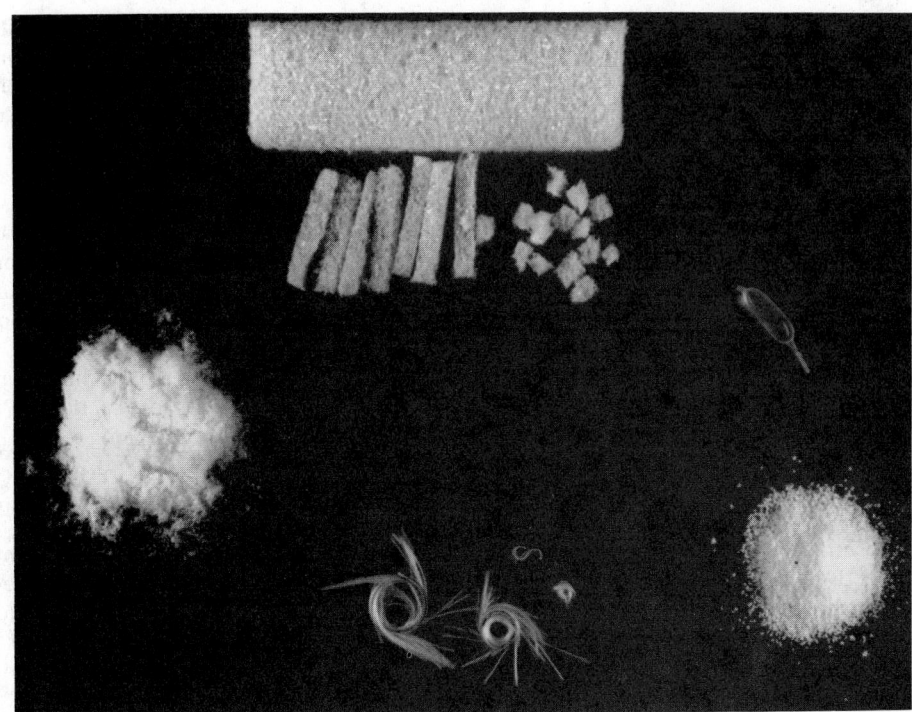

FIGURE 21-34. A variety of devices and materials are available as embolic agents. Shown here are (clockwise from top) a Gelfoam (Upjohn, Kalamazoo, MI) pledget, cut into segments and cubes, a detachable balloon, Ivalon (polyvinyl alcohol foam; Pacific Medical Industries, San Diego, CA) particles, stainless steel coils with strands of synthetic fiber attached to the coil, and Gelfoam powder. Gelfoam cubes are loaded into a syringe with saline and contrast material and injected into the artery for peripheral embolization. They are guided by blood flow in the vessel (flow-guided embolization). Detachable balloons are most commonly used in the central nervous system. Ivalon particles are a relatively permanent occluding agent compared with Gelfoam cubes. Coils come in many sizes and configurations. The largest (shown here) is 8 mm in diameter. The attached fibers help promote thrombus formation. Gelfoam powder contains very small particles and produces necrosis by occlusion of arterioles. Other particulate and liquid agents are also available.

with proximal large vessel occlusion to prolong the efficacy of the peripheral occlusion.

Applications

In many respects, tumors of the liver are ideal targets for embolic therapy. The liver has a dual blood supply from the hepatic artery (30%) and the portal vein (70%). Because primary and secondary hepatic neoplasms receive their blood supply exclusively from the hepatic artery with minimal peripheral contributions from the portal vein and because the liver can survive on its portal venous inflow alone, the hepatic artery can be embolized with a great margin of safety.[76] Carrasco and associates listed relative contraindications to hepatic artery embolization.[77] However, the major contraindication is the presence of main portal vein occlusion due to tumor or thrombus.[78] When first-order or second-order branches of the portal vein are occluded, hepatic artery embolization increases the risk of segmental hepatic infarction, but there is less risk of hepatic failure. Nakao and colleagues attempted to produce complete tumor ischemia by deliberately embolizing the segmental hepatic arterial and portal venous branches leading to a tumor, deliberately infarcting the hepatic segment in an attempt to achieve more complete tumor necrosis.[79]

Embolization of renal cell cancers is performed preoperatively to facilitate surgical resection and decrease intraoperative blood loss. It may also be used to control massive hematuria or to reduce the bulk of inoperable tumors and control pain. No convincing evidence exists that embolization of renal tumor stimulates an immune response. Infarction with absolute alcohol has replaced particulate embolization in many institutions.[80,81] Reflux of ethanol into the adrenal artery or

the aorta may lead to complications.[82,83] Infusion through an occluding balloon catheter in the renal artery is essential.

Control of pain from bony metastases may be achieved with some success with selective embolization.[84,85] Hepatic embolization is helpful for palliation of endocrine syndromes due to liver metastases from hormonally active tumors, such as islet cell tumors and carcinoids.[86,87] Transcatheter embolization has also been recommended to control massive hemorrhage from radiation cystitis or pelvic neoplasms and to reduce the vascularity of hypervascular bone metastases before stabilization operations and in bony tumors of the spine and pelvis, particularly unresectable giant cell tumors or aneurysmal bone cysts.[85,88,89,90–92]

Complications

All embolization procedures involve the risk of inadvertently embolizing nontargeted, critical organs. Cutaneous and mucosal injury during embolization of external carotid or internal iliac arteries has occurred, as has nerve damage, particularly with peripheral occluders such as cyanoacrylate or neurotoxic agents like alcohol. The use of intraarterial digital subtraction arteriography to monitor the embolic process has reduced the incidence of renal failure associated with high doses of contrast material.

Approximately 50% of patients experience a postembolization syndrome consisting of pain, fever, and sometimes nausea and vomiting.[93] Narcotics can control the pain, and the syndrome is self-limited (24–48 hours). Delayed complications, such as abscess formation in the infarcted tumor or organ, are surprisingly rare, but they usually require percutaneous or surgical drainage. Gas within the infarcted tumor or organ, usually demonstrated by CT, occurs routinely due to tumor necrosis or to air introduced at the time of embolization. In the absence of clinical signs of sepsis, the demonstration of gas does not indicate infection, and antibiotic therapy is not required.[94]

CHEMOEMBOLIZATION

Chemoembolization combines the benefits of intraarterial high-dose chemotherapy with obstruction of the tumor vascular bed. The goal is to prolong exposure time of the tumor to the chemotherapeutic agent and to add an ischemic component to enhance tumor necrosis.[63] One method uses particulate carriers, with chemotherapeutic agents bound to microspheres or contained within microcapsules (*e.g.*, liposomes).[95] The Japanese have used a different approach to treat hepatocellular carcinoma, taking advantage of the prolonged sequestration of intraarterially injected iodized oil within primary and secondary hepatic tumors. The iodinated ethyl ester of poppy seed oil (Lipiodol, Ethiodol) is sequestered in primary and secondary hepatic tumors after being injected selectively into the hepatic artery.[96,97] This technique was originally developed to increase the visibility and detectability of small hepatomas and liver metastases on CT. The mechanism of prolonged retention of these iodized oils within tumors has not been fully explained. In hepatic tumor models in rabbits, iodized oil accumulates within the tumor vasculature and the abnormal hepatic sinusoids surrounding the tumor.[98]

In a series of 99 patients with hepatocellular carcinoma studied by Takayasu and coworkers, the results suggest that iodized oil by itself is an ineffective embolizing agent despite its prolonged persistence in these tumors. Efficacy is improved by combining iodized oil with a chemotherapeutic agent, but the best results are obtained with a combination of iodized oil, chemotherapeutic agent, and peripheral embolization with Gelfoam.[99] This increases the contact time between tumor and chemotherapeutic agent. Yamashita and colleagues, in a prospective study of 275 patients with hepatocellular carcinoma, also found that the use of Gelfoam increased the initial response rate to chemoembolization with iodized oil and a chemotherapeutic agent.[100] However, the choice of treatment method was much less important in determining survival at 1 and 2 years.[100] Although this therapy is promising, not all hepatocellular carcinomas retain iodized oil. Van Beers and associates found that the likelihood of survival is related to the amount of iodized oil retained in the tumor.[101]

The effectiveness of hepatic chemoembolization with iodized oil also depends to a great degree on whether the tumor has a well-defined capsule. Small hepatocellular carcinomas are less susceptible to this form of therapy than larger, well-encapsulated lesions.[102] Small hepatocellular carcinomas, both primary and daughter lesions, do not have capsules, nor do hepatic metastases.[103] Encapsulated tumors are supplied exclusively by arterial feeders, but unencapsulated tumors receive significant blood supply from portal vein branches.[103] This difference in blood supply accounts for the difference in response to arterial chemoembolization.

There is still little experience with chemoembolization for the treatment of liver metastases. Metastases do retain iodized oil in some instances.[96] Although a poor response rate would be predicted due to the absence of a capsule around liver me-

tastases, Taniguchi and colleagues reported some responses to chemoembolization with a multidrug regimen.[104]

Chemoembolization should be used with caution in patients who are candidates for surgical resection. Nagasue and coworkers operated on 31 patients with hepatocellular carcinoma who had undergone preoperative chemoembolization.[105] Fifteen patients had severe adhesions, infarction of the liver or gallbladder, or intrahepatic abscess identified at surgery. Intraoperative ultrasonography was unable to visualize the tumor in 5 patients. Among 107 patients with hepatocellular carcinoma who had not undergone preoperative embolization, none had adhesions, infarctions, or abscesses identified at surgery, and intraoperative ultrasonography visualized the lesions in all patients. Preoperative chemoembolization did not improve long-term survival rates.

DIRECT PERCUTANEOUS TUMOR ABLATION

Several groups have investigated direct intratumoral injections of alcohol.[106–109] The most common tumor treated in this fashion is hepatocellular carcinoma.[106,108,109] The optimal tumor size is 3 cm or smaller. Absolute ethanol is injected through a fine needle directly into the tumor, usually under ultrasound guidance. Ethanol destroys tissue because of its dehydrating and protein degenerative effects and to a lesser extent because of its thromboembolic effects.[106] The end result is tumor necrosis, which often leaves no viable tumor.[109] The procedure is appropriate for patients who have small tumors but are poor candidates for surgery.[108] Patients with unresectable large tumors or multiple lesions should also undergo chemoembolization because ethanol cannot perfuse larger lesions uniformly and because some lesions may not be detected by ultrasound.[106]

Percutaneous ethanol injection has been used in a limited number of patients with small hepatic metastases.[107] As with treatment of hepatocellular carcinoma, more than one injection is usually required for each lesion, and these injections are given at separate sessions, once or twice each week. Livraghi and colleagues reported complete response in 11 of 21 lesions treated, but because of the natural history of metastatic disease, this treatment is appropriate only for patients with single, metachronous, inoperable lesions.[107] The procedure is contraindicated for patients with ascites, clotting abnormalities, or extrahepatic metastases.[106] Injection of ethanol into subcapsular hepatic lesions may result in alcohol leakage into the peritoneal cavity. Major complications are uncommon.

ADJUNCTS IN THE MANAGEMENT OF CANCER PATIENTS

BILIARY INTERVENTIONS

Although interventional radiology has a prominent role in the management of biliary stones and strictures, the major indication for biliary intervention in cancer patients is obstruction of the biliary tree. The obstructing lesion may be proximal in the biliary tree, as is seen with Klatskin tumors, metastases to the porta hepatis, and carcinoma of the gallbladder, or it may be distal, as in carcinoma of the pancreas and carcinoma of the ampulla. The intent is always to relieve the obstruction and either divert the flow of bile externally or bypass the obstruction with a catheter internally.

Indications

Palliation

Biliary drainage is performed for palliation or as a prelude to surgery. Palliative biliary drainage procedures are as effective as palliative surgical bypass procedures for the relief of jaundice, and the choice of therapy (surgery versus interventional drainage) does not appear to affect survival. In two large retrospective studies[110,111] and one prospective study,[112] there was no difference in the mortality rates at 30 days or in median survival. The choice between surgery and biliary drainage is probably best based on predicted survival and the patient's overall physical status.[113,114]

Biliary drainage performed as a palliative procedure should be reserved for patients with symptoms related to jaundice (*e.g.*, pruritus, anorexia, nausea) and for patients with biliary sepsis, in whom it is a relatively low-risk procedure and potentially lifesaving.[115,116] The procedure is associated with discomfort, and an external catheter, if one is left in place, is a visible reminder to the patient of the underlying malignancy. Some patients find an external catheter psychologically unbearable. For the patient with minimal symptoms due to biliary obstruction, it is wise to remember that it is difficult to make an asymptomatic patient feel better.

Preoperative Drainage

Guidelines for the use of biliary drainage as a prelude to surgical bypass, rather than as the sole palliative procedure, are somewhat ambiguous. Two retrospective studies[117,118] reported a reduction in surgical mortality and morbidity when preoperative biliary decompression was used, but four prospective studies[116,119–121] concluded that preoperative decompression conferred no advantage. Most surgeons base their approach on the results of the prospective studies, and preoperative biliary decompression is now reserved for selected patients.[122]

Choice of Technique

Access to the biliary tree may be obtained percutaneously with percutaneous transhepatic biliary drainage (PTBD) or endoscopically with endoscopic retrograde biliary drainage (ERBD). (It is also possible, although rarely necessary, to enter the biliary tree by a radiologically guided percutaneous transjejunal approach in patients who have Roux-en-Y jejunobiliary anastomoses.[123,124])

The choice of ERBD or PTBD is based on several factors, not the least of which is the skill and experience of the local radiologist and endoscopist. ERBD requires specialized equipment and is not universally available. In patients with unfavorable anatomy due to previous gastric or duodenal surgery, the endoscopist may be unable to pass the endoscope to the level of the papilla of Vater. Very distal common bile duct obstruction may sometimes prevent cannulation of the biliary tree, and firm proximal lesions in the common hepatic duct may not permit passage of an endoprosthesis.[125,126] In experienced hands, ERBD is successful in approximately 85% to 90% of patients.[125,127,128]

PTBD has an initial success rate close to 100%, and the anatomic problems that make ERBD difficult or impossible in some patients are not a factor with PTBD.[110,128–130] However, ERBD is associated with fewer bleeding complications than PTBD and better patient acceptance.[128] Ascites, coagulopathies, and intrahepatic metastases are relative contraindications to PTBD, but not to ERBD.

Another consideration is the use of an endoprosthesis (*i.e.*, entirely internal biliary stent) or a catheter that extends outside the patient. Biliary drainage devices eventually occlude due to tumor ingrowth or to accumulation of biliary sludge, which is composed in large part of a bacterial biofilm.[131] Patency rates are related to the diameter of the stent and to its position.[132,133] The major advantage of catheters for biliary drainage is that they can be irrigated daily to help maintain patency, and changing them is a relatively simple matter because access to the biliary tree is maintained. Catheters, which can be used for internal and external drainage, must be placed percutaneously.

There are two types of endoprostheses. The original type is a plastic tube that is placed across the obstruction. Bile flows through the lumen of the endoprosthesis. There are several devices of this type designed for placement by PTBD or ERBD.[134–137] These plastic stents typically have outer diameters of 12 to 14 Fr and inner diameters of 3 to 4 mm.[133] A newer type of endoprosthesis is the expandable metallic stent (Fig. 21–35). Several types are approved for use in the United States.[138–143] None of these metallic stents require an introducer larger than a 14-Fr outer diameter (one can be placed through a 7-Fr introducer), but they expand to an inner diameter of 10 mm or more in the biliary tree. The large lumen is their major advantage, but it may be offset by their higher cost, the frequent need for placement of multiple stents, the risk of occlusion due to tumor ingrowth, and the inability to demonstrate significantly improved patency rates in early series.[133] Some researchers think that metallic stents are well suited for the treatment of patients with malignant biliary obstruction.[143,144]

Plastic endoprostheses can be placed by PTBD and ERBD, and occasionally, both techniques are used simultaneously.[145,146] Most metallic stents must be placed by PTBD, but the Wallstent may be placed endoscopically.[147] Both types of endoprostheses have the major advantage of providing relief of obstruction without a protruding external catheter, which may be uncomfortable and psychologically unsettling.[134] However, because access to the biliary tree is lost after the endoprosthesis is placed, ERBD or PTBD must be repeated if the endoprosthesis becomes occluded. Plastic endoprostheses may be removed and replaced, but metallic stents are permanent.[148] Occluded metallic stents can be redilated, or a catheter or plastic stent can be placed through them.

Patients with malignant disease and a life expectancy of less than 4 months may be best served by placement of an endoprosthesis with ERBD, if possible.[126,132,134,137,149–151] A randomized prospective trial of endoprosthesis placement by ERBD or PTBD in 75 patients with malignant obstructive jaundice demonstrated a statistically significant higher success rate for relief of jaundice and a significantly lower 30-day

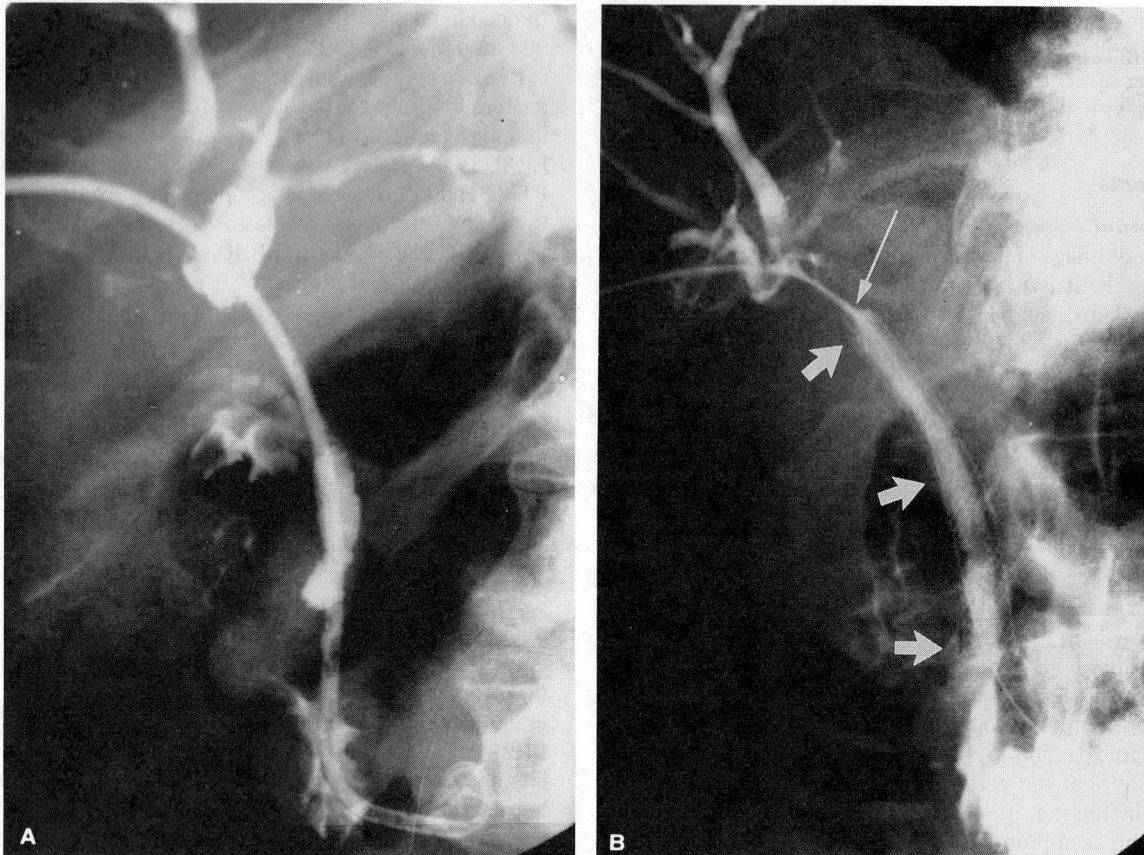

FIGURE 21–35. Placement of a metallic biliary stent in a man with pancreatic cancer. (Courtesy of Arina van Breda, MD, Alexandria Hospital, Alexandria, VA) **(A)** Cholangiogram after percutaneous transhepatic biliary drainage demonstrates marked narrowing of the common bile duct. **(B)** After placement of a self-expanding Wallstent (*short arrows*), contrast material injection through a transhepatic catheter demonstrates a much larger lumen in the stented area. The long arrow indicates the tip of the transhepatic catheter.

mortality for ERBD.[150] In other patients, the choice between endoprosthesis and catheter drainage depends mostly on the patient's preference and the technical feasibility and availability of ERBD.

Regardless of the method used to enter the biliary tree and relieve the obstruction, bile samples should be obtained for culture and cytology. In the setting of biliary obstruction, Suzuki and associates demonstrated infected bile in 89% of patients with fever and 39% of afebrile patients.[152] *Escherichia coli* and *Klebsiella* were the most frequent aerobic species. Anaerobes were much less frequent. Muro and colleagues obtained 10-ml samples of bile during the course of PTBD.[153] Bile cytology was positive in 34 of 100 patients with malignant obstruction of the biliary tree. If desired, brush, screw, and core biopsies of the obstructing lesion can also be obtained through the biliary tree.[154]

Efficacy

Biliary drainage procedures are unquestionably effective for the relief of obstruction and cholestasis. Internal biliary drainage reduces pressures in the biliary tree to normal and permits removal of bile pigments from liver tissue.[155] In one series, mean serum bilirubin decreased from 15.7 mg/dl be-

fore drainage to 4.9 mg/dl 10 days after drainage.[149] In another study, decrease in bilirubin showed a negative exponential correlation with the duration of drainage.[110] In a third study, the rate of decrease in bilirubin ranged from 0.23 to 4.9 mg/dl/day (mean, 1.4 mg/dl/day) and had no relation to the initial bilirubin value.[156] In patients with proximal obstruction of the biliary tree, at or above the level of the bifurcation of the common hepatic duct, relief of jaundice still occurs, even if only a portion of the biliary tree is drained. However, cholangitis may develop in the undrained segment, and placement of a second catheter may be required. Obstructive jaundice causes depression of immune system function, and one animal study demonstrated that relief of biliary obstruction by internal drainage was followed by recovery of hepatocellular function, cell-mediated immunity, and mononuclear phagocyte function in less than 7 days.[157] However, other studies indicate that liver function abnormalities persist for at least 10 days after relief of the obstruction.[158]

Complications

PTBD and ERBD are associated with different types of complications that occur with different frequencies.[128] PTBD results in death in fewer than 2% of patients.[129,130,159] Major complications, including septic shock, pleural effusions, bile peritonitis, hepatic abscess, pancreatitis, and major hemorrhage, occur in an additional 10% to 15%.[129,130,159,160] Cholangitis is the most common complication, occurring acutely in approximately 20% of patients. In debilitated cancer patients, cholangitis may occur early or late in as many as 47% of those undergoing PTBD.[161] Tumor spread as a result of PTBD has been reported.[162]

ERBD is considerably safer, because it is unnecessary to transgress the liver capsule or push catheters through the hepatic parenchyma. Hemorrhage and bile leakage from the liver is avoided.[150,151] Mortality is 1%.[125] Major acute complications are seen in 2% to 10% of patients, and the overall complication rate is 10% to 18%.[125,126,128,135] The primary risk is that associated with endoscopic sphincterotomy, which is often required to ease insertion of the endoprosthesis into the common bile duct.[126,127,135] Sphincterotomy has a mortality rate of 1% to 2% and a major complication rate of 7%, although occult bleeding may occur in as many as 36% of patients.[127,163]

Intervention in the Gallbladder

Among some critically ill, high-risk patients, standard surgical therapy for cholecystitis, gallbladder abscess, and malignant obstruction of the gallbladder may carry high morbidity and mortality rates. Other patients may present with jaundice, common bile duct obstruction, normal-sized intrahepatic bile ducts, and a distended gallbladder.[164] These patients are candidates for percutaneous cholecystostomy.[164–168] The gallbladder can be punctured percutaneously with a fine needle and bile obtained for culture.[166,168] The gallbladder can be opacified with contrast material to diagnose obstruction, and drainage can be instituted for empyema, acute calculous or acalculous cholecystitis, or common bile duct obstruction.[164,165,167] The procedure can be guided by ultrasound or CT. If a portable real-time ultrasound unit is used, the entire intervention can be performed as a bedside procedure. The complication rate is low, with no major complications in three series totalling 80 patients.[164,165,167] Serious vagal reactions have been reported in some patients, especially those with acutely inflamed gallbladders.[169] Although this procedure does not provide access to the entire biliary tree, it is a useful and minimally invasive adjunct in critically ill patients with gallbladder disease.

URINARY TRACT INTERVENTIONS

Since the first report of percutaneous nephrostomy (PCN) in 1955, the number of conditions treated in this fashion has greatly expanded as a result of the development of interventional radiology and endourology.[170–175] Nonetheless, the primary indication for PCN in oncology patients continues to be urinary diversion, and it has replaced operative nephrostomy tube placement for this purpose.

Guidance for PCN can be provided by fluoroscopy, ultrasound, CT, or a combination of these methods.[171] The skin entry site is usually along the posterior axillary line, below the twelfth rib, and the needle is directed toward the posterolateral cortex of the kidney.[174,175] More cephalad entry sites risk pneumothorax and injury to the spleen or liver. Ad-

justments in technique are required for splenomegaly, scoliosis, and anomalous rotations and positions of the kidney.

Types of Urologic Prostheses

There are three basic types of prostheses for urinary drainage: nephrostomy catheters, internal stents, and external stent catheters. Nephrostomy catheters are short catheters placed in the renal pelvis or upper collecting system to divert urine externally. They do not stent the ureter and cannot be used for internal drainage. They are the simplest devices to place and to change.

Double-J or double-pigtail stents have largely replaced other designs for entirely internal ureteral stents.[176,177] The end in the renal pelvis and the end in the bladder have J or pigtail shapes to reduce mucosal irritation and prevent migration (Fig. 21–36). These catheters can be placed using an antegrade (percutaneous) approach or a retrograde (cystoscopic) approach.[176,177]

The third type of urologic prosthesis is the ureteral stent with external drainage or access port (*e.g.*, nephroureterostomy).[178] In some ways, this is the most versatile of the urologic prostheses. The external port may be used for external drainage or can be capped off for internal drainage, and it provides easy accessibility when the catheter needs to be changed.

Each type of urologic prosthesis has advantages and disadvantages. Simple nephrostomy diversion uses a urine collection appliance that requires daily maintenance, and it is unsuitable for patients who are poorly motivated or who have altered mental status. Some patients find it socially unacceptable. Internal stents obviate many of these inconveniences, but require cystoscopy for removal or replacement of the stent. Because there is no outward indicator of stent function, stent failure can be insidious, and permanent renal damage may occur before it is recognized (see Fig. 21–34). Nephrostomy tube failure is readily identified by decreased urine volume, leakage around the catheter, fever, or flank pain that leads the patient to seek prompt attention. All urologic prostheses should be changed prophylactically on a regular basis.[179–181]

Complications

The mortality associated with PCN is less than 0.2%, and significant complications occur at the rate of only 4% to 5%.[171,182] Mortality for surgical urinary diversion in the oncology patient is about 3% to 8%, and the complication rate is 25% to 45%.[183,184]

Serious complications associated with PCN are primarily related to septicemia and hemorrhage. Bacteriuria is virtually universal in patients with external catheters, but it causes no clinical symptoms.[185] Septicemia, including septic shock, occurs in 1% to 2% of patients, most often those with preexisting infection.[186] Minor bleeding is common, but it clears within a few days. Clinically significant hemorrhage occurs at a rate of 1% to 2%.[171,187] Bleeding may be into the collecting system, the renal parenchyma and subcapsular tissue, or the perinephric space and retroperitoneum.[188,189] Hemorrhage may be delayed rather than immediate, because the nephrostomy tube may initially tamponade the injured vessel.[190]

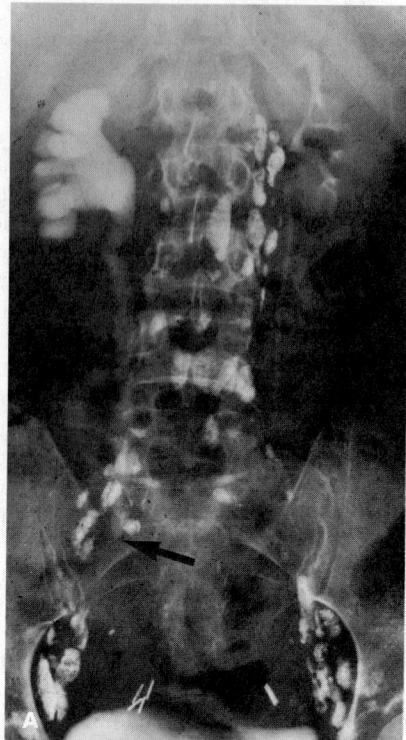 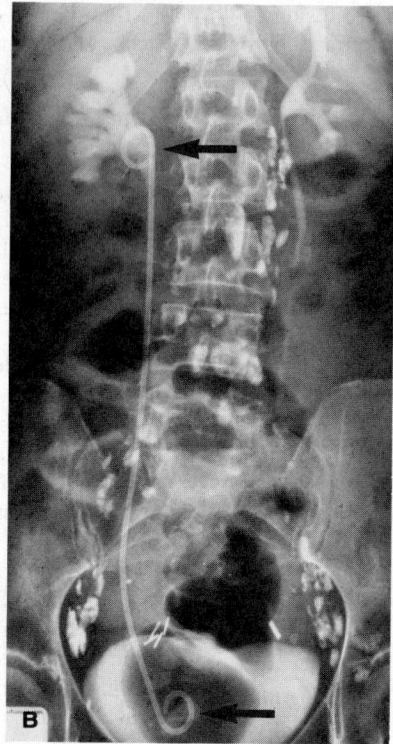 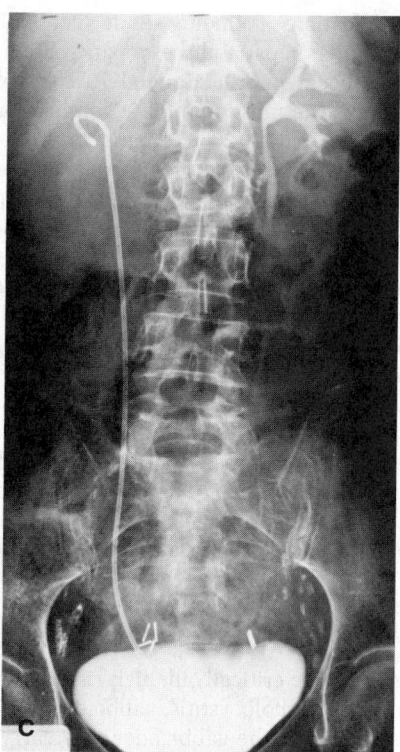

FIGURE 21–36.   Complete obstruction of the right ureter in a woman with ovarian carcinoma. **(A)** The initial intravenous urogram demonstrates hydronephrosis of the right kidney and complete obstruction of the right ureter (*arrow*). **(B)** The patient refused any drainage device that was not completely internal. A double pigtail internal ureteral stent was placed percutaneously. One pigtail is in the renal pelvis, and the other is in the bladder (*arrows*). **(C)** The patient returned for a routine follow-up intravenous urogram 2 months later. She was asymptomatic, but the urogram revealed complete obstruction of the right kidney. The internal stent was removed cystoscopically and a new one placed. The lumen of the original stent was completely blocked by encrustations.

Permanent injury to the kidney from PCN is rare. In a study of 36 patients 3 years or more after PCN, only 1 patient had a focal cortical scar that appeared to be related to PCN.[191]

PERCUTANEOUS PLACEMENT OF INFERIOR VENA CAVA FILTERS

Cancer is a frequent cause of hypercoagulable states and a common indication for placement of inferior vena cava filters.[192,193] Several filters designed for percutaneous placement have become available in the United States, including the bird's nest filter, the Vena-tech filter, the Simon nitinol filter, and a new version of the Greenfield filter, constructed of titanium.[194] All of these filters are permanent. Removable inferior vena cava filters have been under development for several years, but their design is difficult because modifications that make the filter easier to remove also make it more likely that the filter will migrate in the venous system.

The original Greenfield filter could be inserted surgically or percutaneously through the femoral vein or the jugular vein, using a carrier system. However, percutaneous insertion required use of a sheath with an outer diameter of 29.5 Fr and was associated with a 2% to 10% incidence of femoral vein thrombosis.[195–197] Newer filters use sheaths with a maximum outer diameter of only 7 Fr (*i.e.,* Simon nitinol filter) to 14 Fr (*i.e.,* Greenfield titanium filter) and cause fewer in-

sertion-site problems.[198] Although metastatic cancer may be a relative contraindication to surgical placement of an inferior vena cava filter, this is not true for percutaneously placed filters.[192,193] An experienced angiographer can insert a Greenfield filter percutaneously in 10 to 20 minutes with little discomfort to the patient.[199]

PLACEMENT AND REPOSITIONING OF VENOUS ACCESS DEVICES

Maintaining venous access can be very difficult in oncology patients, and placement of implantable central venous access devices is frequently required. This is most often done in the operating room, but it can also be done by an interventional radiologist in the radiology department.[200–202] Placement by the radiologist has several advantages. The fluoroscopy equipment in the interventional suite is far superior to that in the operating room, and ultrasound equipment is also readily available to guide the venous puncture.[201] Radiologic placement takes less time and costs less than surgical placement of these devices.[200] Catheter placement by unusual routes and into unusual sites, such as the translumbar approach to the inferior vena cava, is also possible using routine techniques of interventional radiology.[203,204] After all standard venous access sites have been exhausted, these uncommon sites and approaches may be the only alternative.

A central venous catheter may be placed with the tip malpositioned. Temporary central venous catheters can be removed and replaced if this occurs, but this is a more serious undertaking with an implanted central venous access device. An interventional radiologist can reposition the tips of temporary central venous catheters and implanted venous access devices without disturbing the remainder of the catheter or device. This is done with fluoroscopic guidance, using a guidewire inserted through the lumen of the venous access device or a second catheter, usually inserted through a femoral vein.[205,206] In either case, the malpositioned tip is redirected into the correct position, but the remainder of the access device is not affected.

MISCELLANEOUS PROCEDURES

The patient with cancer often has other medical problems, and radiologic interventions of many types may be useful. New forms of radiologic intervention and new methods for better accomplishing existing interventions are always being developed. Abscess drainage, management of gastrointestinal bleeding, transluminal angioplasty, intraarterial and intravenous thrombolysis, treatment of biliary and urinary stones and strictures, and removal of intravascular foreign bodies can all be accomplished by a well-trained interventional radiologist. Radiologic intervention will continue to have a major impact on the practice of oncology.

REFERENCES

1. White RI Jr. Interventional radiology: Reflections and expectations. The 1985 Eugene P. Pendergrass New Horizons Lecture. Radiology 1987;162:593–600.
2. Westcott JL. Percutaneous transthoracic needle biopsy. Radiology 1988;169:593–601.
3. Welch TJ, Reading CC. Imaging-guided biopsy. Mayo Clin Proc 1989;64:1295–1301.
4. Mueller PR, van Sonnenberg E. Interventional radiology in the chest and abdomen. N Engl J Med 1990;322:1364–1374.
5. Haaga JR, LiPuma JP, Bryan PJ, Balsara VJ, Cohen AM. Clinical comparison of small- and large-caliber cutting needles for biopsy. Radiology 1983;146:665–667.
6. Gazelle GS, Haaga JR. Biopsy needle characteristics. Cardiovasc Intervent Radiol 1991;14:13–16.
7. Böcking A. Cytological vs histological evaluation of percutaneous biopsies. Cardiovasc Intervent Radiol 1991;14:5–12.
8. Pagani JJ. Biopsy of focal hepatic lesions: Comparison of 18- and 22-gauge needles. Radiology 1983;147:673–675.
9. Mink J. Percutaneous bone biopsy in the patient with known or suspected osseous metastases. Radiology 1986;161:191–194.
10. Lüning M, Schröder K, Wolff H, Kranz D, Hoppe E. Percutaneous biopsy of the liver. Cardiovasc Intervent Radiol 1991;14:40–42.
11. Lawrence DD, Carrasco CH, Fornage B, Sniege N, Wallace S. Percutaneous lymph node biopsy. Cardiovasc Intervent Radiol 1991;14:55–62.
12. Carrasco CH, Wallace S, Richli WR. Percutaneous skeletal biopsy. Cardiovasc Intervent Radiol 1991;14:69–72.
13. Parker SH, Hopper KD, Yakes WF, Gibson MD, Ownbey JL, Carter TE. Image-directed percutaneous biopsies with a biopsy Gun. Radiology 1989;171:663–669.
14. Jennings PE, Donald JJ, Coral A, Rode J, Lees WR. Ultrasound-guided core biopsy. Lancet 1989;1:1369–1371.
15. Hall-Craggs MA, Lees WR. Fine Needle biopsy: Cytology, histology, or both? Gut 1987;28:233–236.
16. Suhrland MJ, Wieczorek R. Fine needle aspiration biopsy in the diagnosis of lymphoma. Cancer Invest 1991;9:61–68.
17. Perlmutt LM, Johnston WW, Dunnick NR. Percutaneous transthoracic needle aspiration: A review. AJR 1989;152:451–455.
18. Johnsrude IS, Silverman JF, Weaver MD, McConnell MD. Rapid cytology to decrease pneumothorax incidence after percutaneous biopsy. AJR 1985;144:793–794.
19. Miller DA, Carrasco CH, Katz RL, Cramer FM, Wallace SF, Charnsangavej C. Fine needle aspiration biopsy: The role of immediate cytologic assessment. AJR 1986;147:155–158.
20. Mueller PR, Stark DD, Simeone JF, et al. MR-guided aspiration biopsy: Needle design and clinical trials. Radiology 1986;161:605–609.
21. Duckwiler G, Lufkin RB, Teresi L, et al. Head and neck lesions: MR-guided aspiration biopsy. Radiology 1989;170:519–522.
22. Bret PM, Fond A, Casola G, et al. Abdominal lesions: A prospective study of clinical efficacy of percutaneous fine-needle biopsy. Radiology 1986;159:345–346.
23. Fortier KF, Clarke-Pearson DL, Creasman WT, Johnston WW. Fine-needle aspiration in gynecology: Evaluation of extrapelvic lesions in patients with gynecologic malignancy. Obstet Gynecol 1985;65:67–73.
24. Gobien RP, Bouchard EA, Gobien BS, Valicenti JR, Vujic I. Thin-needle aspiration biopsy of thoracic lesions: Impact on hospital charges and patterns of patient care. Radiology 1983;148:65–67.
25. Westcott JL. Direct percutaneous needle aspiration of localized pulmonary lesions: Results in 422 patients. Radiology 1980;137:31–35.
26. Mitty HA, Efremidis SC, Yeh H-C. Impact of fine-needle biopsy on management of patients with carcinoma of the pancreas. AJR 1981;137:1119–1121.
27. Welch TJ, Sheedy PF II, Johnson CD, Johnson CM, Stephens DH. CT-guided biopsy: Prospective analysis of 1,000 procedures. Radiology 1989;171:493–496.
28. Diament MJ, Boechat MI, Kangarloo H. Interventional radiology in infants and children: Clinical and technical aspects. Radiology 1985;154:359–361.
29. van Sonnenberg E, Wittich GR, Edwards DK, et al. Percutaneous diagnostic and interventional radiologic procedures in children: Experience in 100 patients. Radiology 1987;162:601–605.
30. Klose K-C, Mertens R, Alzen G, Löer F, Böcking A. CT-guided percutaneous large-bore biopsies in benign and malignant pediatric lesions. Cardiovasc Intervent Radiol 1991;14:78–83.
31. Ferrucci JT Jr, Wittenberg J, Mueller PR, et al. Diagnosis of abdominal malignancy by radiologic fine-needle aspiration biopsy. AJR 1980;134:323–330.
32. Fornage BD. Percutaneous biopsies of the breast: State of the art. Cardiovasc Intervent Radiol 1991;14:29–39.
33. Saunders G, Lakra Y, Libcke J. Comparison of needle aspiration cytologic diagnosis with excisional biopsy tissue diagnosis of palpable tumors of the breast in a community hospital. Surg Gynecol Obstet 1991;172:437–440.
34. Nicastri GR, Reed WP, Dziura BR. The accuracy of malignant diagnoses established by fine needle aspiration cytologic procedures of mammary masses. Surg Gynecol Obstet 1991;172:457–460.
35. Gardner D, van Sonnenberg E, D'Agostino HB, Casola G, Taggart S, May S. CT-guided transthoracic needle biopsy. Cardiovasc Intervent Radiol 1991;14:17–23.
36. Herman SJ, Holub RV, Weisbrod GL, Chamberlain DW. Anterior mediastinal masses: Utility of transthoracic needle biopsy. Radiology 1991;180:167–170.
37. Butler JA, Smith C. Fine-needle aspiration biopsy in the diagnosis of recurrent and metastatic intraabdominal malignancies. Am J Surg 1989;158:589–592.
38. Sbolli G, Fornari F, Civardi G, et al. Role of ultrasound guide fine needle aspiration biopsy in the diagnosis of hepatocellular carcinoma. Gut 1990;31:1303–1305.
39. Neuerburg J, Günther RW. Percutaneous biopsy of pancreatic lesions. Cardiovasc Intervent Radiol 1991;14:43–49.
40. Del Maschio A, Vanzulli A, Sironi S, et al. Pancreatic cancer versus chronic pancreatitis: Diagnosis with CA 19-9 assessment, US, CT, and CT-guided fine-needle biopsy. Radiology 1991;178:95–99.
41. Mitnick JS, Bosniak MA, Megibow AJ, Naidich DP. Non-functioning adrenal adenomas discovered incidentally on computed tomography. Radiology 1983;148:495–499.
42. Belldegrun A, Hussain S, Seltzer SE, Loughlin KR, Gittes RF, Richie JP. Incidentally discovered mass of the adrenal gland. Surg Gynecol Obstet 1986;163:203–208.
43. Vassiliades VG, Bernardino ME. Percutaneous renal and adrenal biopsies. Cardiovasc Intervent Radiol 1991;14:50–54.
44. Tikkakoski T, Siniluoto T, Ollikainen A, Päivänsalo M, Lohela P, Apaja-Sarkkinen M. Ultrasound-guided aspiration cytology of enlarged lymph nodes. Acta Radiol 1991;32:53–56.
45. Chagnon S, Cochand-Priollet B, Gzaeil M, et al. Pelvic cancers: Staging of 139 cases with lymphography and fine-needle aspiration biopsy. Radiology 1989;173:103–106.
46. Ayala AG, Zornosa J. Primary bone tumors: Percutaneous needle biopsy. Radiologic-pathologic study of 222 biopsies. Radiology 1983;149:675–679.
47. Hewes RC, Vigorita VJ, Freiberger RH. Percutaneous bone biopsy: The importance of aspirated osseous blood. Radiology 1983;148:69–72.
48. Smith EH. Complications of percutaneous abdominal fine-needle biopsy: A review. Radiology 1991;178:253–258.
49. Nolsøe C, Nielsen L, Torp-Pedersen S, Holm HH. Major complications and deaths due to interventional ultrasonography: A review of 8000 cases. J Clin Ultrasound 1990;18:179–184.
50. Helvie MA, Ikeda DM, Adler DD. Localization and needle aspiration of breast lesions: Complications in 370 cases. AJR 1991;157:711–714.
51. McCorkell SJ, Niles NL. Fine-needle aspiration of catecholamine-producing adrenal masses: A possibly fatal mistake. AJR 1985;145:113–114.
52. Casola G, Nicolet V, van Sonnenberg E, et al. Unsuspected pheochromocytoma: Risk of blood-pressure alterations during percutaneous adrenal biopsy. Radiology 1986;159:733–735.
53. Fornari F, Civardi G, Cavanna L, et al. Complications of ultrasonically guided fine-needle abdominal biopsy. Scand J Gastroenterol 1989;24:949–955.
54. Bissonnette RT, Gibney RG, Berry BR, Buckley AR. Fatal carcinoid crisis after percutaneous fine-needle biopsy of hepatic metastasis: Case report and literature review. Radiology 1990;174:751–752.
55. Eriksson O, Hagmar B, Ryo W. Effects of fine-needle aspiration and other biopsy procedures on tumor dissemination in mice. Cancer 1984;54:73–78.
56. Perlmutt LM, Braun SD, Newman GE, Oke EJ, Dunnick NR. Timing of chest film follow-up after transthoracic needle aspiration. AJR 1986;146:1049–1050.
57. Gazelle GS, Haaga JR. Guided percutaneous biopsy of intraabdominal lesions. AJR 1989;153:929–935.
58. Mueller PR, Miketic LM, Simeone JF, et al. Severe acute pancreatitis after percutaneous biopsy of the pancreas. AJR 1988;151:493–494.

59. Eckman WW, Patlak CS, Fenstermacher JD. Critical evaluation of principles governing the advantages of intra-arterial infusion. J Pharmacokinet Biopharm 1974;102:221–229.

60. Chen HG, Gross JK. Intra-arterial infusion of anticancer drugs; theoretical aspects of drug delivery and review of response. Cancer Treat Rep 1980;64:31–40.

61. Dedrick RL. Arterial drug infusion: Pharmacokinetic problems and pitfalls. JNCI 1988;80:84–89.

62. Goldberg JA, Kerr DJ, Watson DG, et al. The pharmacokinetics of 5-fluorouracil administered by arterial infusion in advanced colorectal hepatic metastases. Br J Cancer 1990;61:913–915.

63. Wallace S, Carrasco CH, Charnsangavej C, Richli WR, Wright K, Gianturco C. Hepatic artery infusion and chemoembolization in the management of liver metastases. Cardiovasc Intervent Radiol 1990;13:153–160.

64. Hohn DC, Stagg RJ, Friedman MA, et al. A randomized trial of continuous intravenous versus hepatic intraarterial floxuridine in patients with colorectal cancer metastatic to the liver: The Northern California Oncology Group trial. J Clin Oncol 1989;7:1646–1654.

65. Kashdan BJ, Sullivan KL, Lackman RD, et al. Extremity osteosarcomas: Intraarterial chemotherapy and limb-sparing resection with 2-year follow-up. Radiology 1990;177:95–99.

66. Jacobs SC, Menashe DS, Mewissen MW, Lipchik EO. Intraarterial cisplatin infusion in the management of transitional cell carcinoma of the bladder. Cancer 1989;64:388–391.

67. LaPolla JP, Roberts WS, Greenberg H, et al. Treatment of advanced gynecologic malignancies with intraarterial chemotherapy and accelerated fractionation radiation therapy: A preliminary report. Gynecol Oncol 1990;37:55–59.

68. Cho KJ, Andrews JC, Williams DM, Doenz F, Guy GE. Hepatic arterial chemotherapy: Role of angiography. Radiology 1989;173:783–791.

69. Charnsangavej C, Chuang VP, Wallace S et al. Angiographic classification of hepatic arterial collaterals. Radiology 1982;144:485–494.

70. Lutz RJ, Miller DL. Mixing studies during hepatic artery infusion in an in vitro model. Cancer 1988;62:1066–1073.

71. Blacklock JB, Wright DC, Dedrick R, et al. Drug streaming during intra-arterial chemotherapy. J Neurosurg 1986;64:284–291.

72. Saris SC, Blasberg RG, Carson RE, et al. Intravascular streaming during carotid artery infusions: Demonstration in humans and reduction using diastole-phased pulsatile administration. J Neurosurg 1991;74:763–772.

73. Wright KC, Wallace S, Kim EE, et al. Pulsed arterial infusions: Chemotherapeutic considerations. Cancer 1986;57:1952–1956.

74. Allison DJ, Booth A. Arterial embolization in the management of liver metastases. Cardiovasc Intervent Radiol 1990;13:161–168.

75. Miller DL. Failure of Ivalon to provide permanent hepatic arterial occlusion. Cardiovasc Intervent Radiol 1987;10:111–113.

76. Lin G, Hägerstrand I, Lunderquist A. Portal blood supply of liver metastasis. AJR 1984;143:53–55.

77. Carrasco CH, Charnsangavej C, Ajani J, Samaan NA, Richli W, Wallace S. The carcinoid syndrome. Palliation by hepatic artery embolization. AJR 1986;147:149–154.

78. Yamada R, Sato M, Kawabata M, et al. Hepatic artery embolization in 120 patients with unresectable hepatoma. Radiology 1983;148:397–401.

79. Nakao N, Miura K, Takahashi H, et al. Hepatocellular carcinoma: Combined hepatic arterial and portal venous embolization. Radiology 1986;161:303.

80. Ekelund L, Ek A, Forsberg L, et al. Occlusion of renal arterial tumor supply with Absolute Ethanol. Experience with 20 cases. Acta Radiol 1984;25:195–201.

81. Klinberg I, Hunter P, Hawkins IF, et al. Preoperative angioinfarction of localized renal cell carcinoma using absolute ethanol. J Urol 1985;133:21–23.

82. Fink IJ, Girton M, Doppman JL. Absolute ethanol injection of the adrenal artery: Hypertensive reaction. Radiology 1985;154:357–358.

83. Siniluoto TMJ, Hellström PA, Päivänsalo MJ, Leinonen ASS. Testicular infarction following ethanol embolization of a renal neoplasm. Cardiovasc Intervent Radiol 1988;11:162–164.

84. Chuang VP, Wallace S, Swanson D, et al. Arterial occlusion in the management of pain from metastatic renal carcinoma. Radiology 1979;133:611–614.

85. Bowers TA, Murray JA, Charnsangavej C, et al. Bone metastasis from renal carcinoma. J Bone Joint Surg 1982;64:749–754.

86. Ajani J, Carrasco CH, Charnsangavej C, et al. Islet cell tumors metastatic to the liver: Effective palliation by sequential hepatic artery embolization. Ann Intern Med 1988;108:340–344.

87. Marlink RG, Lokich JJ, Robins JR, Clouse ME. Hepatic arterial embolization for metastatic hormone-secreting tumors. Technique, effectiveness, and complications. Cancer 1990;65:2227–2232.

88. Kobayashi I, Kusano S, Matsubayashi T, et al. Selective embolization of the vesical artery in the management of massive bladder hemorrhage. Radiology 1980;136:345–348.

89. Pisco JM, Martins JM, Correia MG. Internal Iliac artery: Embolization to control hemorrhage from pelvic neoplasms. Radiology 1989;172:337–339.

90. Sundaresan N, Choi IS, Hughes JEO, Sachdev VD, Berenstein A. Treatment of spinal metastases from kidney cancer by presurgical embolization and resection. J Neurosurg 1990;73:548–554.

91. Wallace S, Granmayeh M, de Santos LA, et al: Arterial occlusion of pelvic bone tumors. Cancer 1979;43:322–328.

92. Suby-Long T, Bos GD, Rösch J. Biopsy-proven eradication of an aneurysmal bone cyst treated by superselective embolization: A case report. Cardiovasc Intervent Radiol 1988;11:292–295.

93. Hemingway AP, Allison DJ. Complications of embolization: Analysis of 410 procedures. Radiology 1988;166:669–672.

94. Carroll BA, Walter JF. Gas in embolized tumors. An alternate hypothesis for its origin. Radiology 1983;147:441–444.

95. Willmott N. Chemoembolisation in regional cancer chemotherapy: A rationale. Cancer Treat Rev 1987;14:143–156.

96. Nakakuma K, Tashiro S, Hiraoka T, et al. Hepatocellular carcinoma and metastatic cancer detected by iodized oil. Radiology 1985;154:15–17.

97. Yumoto Y, Jino K, Tokuyama K, et al. Hepatocellular carcinoma detected by iodized oil. Radiology 1985;154:19–24.

98. Miller DL, O'Leary TJ, Girton M. Distribution of iodized oil within the liver after hepatic arterial injection. Radiology 1987;162:849–852.

99. Takayasu K, Shima Y, Muramatsu Y, et al. Hepatocellular carcinoma: Treatment with intra-arterial iodized oil with and without chemotherapeutic agents. Radiology 1987;162:345–351.

100. Yamashita Y, Takahashi M, Koga Y, et al. Prognostic factors in the treatment of hepatocellular carcinoma with transcatheter arterial embolization and arterial infusion. Cancer 1991;67:385–391.

101. Van Beers B, Roche A, Cauquil P, et al. Transcatheter arterial chemotherapy using doxorubicin, iodized oil and gelfoam embolization in hepatocellular carcinoma. Acta Radiol 1989;30:415–418.

102. Kuroda C, Sakurai M, Monden M, et al. Limitation of transcatheter arterial chemoembolization using iodized oil for small hepatocellular carcinoma: A study of resected cases. Cancer 1991;67:81–86.

103. Wakasa K, Sakurai M, Kuroda C, et al. Effect of transcatheter arterial embolization on the boundary architecture of hepatocellular carcinoma. Cancer 1990;65:913–919.

104. Taniguchi H, Takahashi T, Yamaguchi T, Sawai K. Intraarterial infusion chemotherapy for metastatic liver tumors using multiple anti-cancer agents suspended in a lipid contrast medium. Cancer 1989;64:2001–2006.

105. Nagasue N, Galizia G, Kohno H, et al. Adverse effects of preoperative hepatic artery chemoembolization for resectable hepatocellular carcinoma: A retrospective comparison of 138 liver resections. Surgery 1989;106:81–86.

106. Shiina S, Tagawa K, Unuma T, Terano A. Percutaneous ethanol injection therapy for the treatment of hepatocellular carcinoma. AJR 1990;154:947–951.

107. Livraghi T, Vettori C, Lazzaroni S. Liver metastases: Results of percutaneous ethanol injection in 14 patients. Radiology 1991;179:709–712.

108. Livraghi T, Salmi A, Bolondi L, et al. Small hepatocellular carcinoma: Percutaneous alcohol injection—results in 23 patients. Radiology 1988;168:313–317.

109. Shiina S, Yasuda H, Muto H, et al. Percutaneous ethanol injection in the treatment of liver neoplasms. AJR 1987;149:949–952.

110. Passariello R, Pavone P, Rossi P, et al. Percutaneous biliary drainage in Neoplastic jaundice: Statistical data from a computerized multicenter investigation. Acta Radiol 1985;26:681–688.

111. Bonnell D, Ferrucci JT Jr, Mueller PR, Lacaine F, Peterson HF. Surgical and radiological Decompression in malignant biliary obstruction: A retrospective study using multivariate risk factor analysis. Radiology 1984;152:347–351.

112. Bornman PC, Harries-Jones EP, Tobias R, Van Stiegmann G, Terblanche J. Prospective controlled trial of transhepatic biliary endoprosthesis versus bypass surgery for incurable carcinoma of the head of the pancreas. Lancet 1986;1:69–71.

113. Hatfield ARW. Palliation of malignant obstructive jaundice—surgery or stent? Gut 1990;31:1339–1340.

114. Bear HD, Turner MA, Parker GA, et al. Treatment of biliary obstruction Caused by metastatic cancer. Am J Surg 1989;157:381–385.

115. Pessa ME, Hawkins IF, Vogel SB. The treatment of acute cholangitis: Percutaneous transhepatic biliary drainage before definitive therapy. Ann Surg 1987;205:389–392.

116. Thomas JH, Connor CS, Pierce GE, MacArthur RI, Iliopoulos JI, Hermreck AS. Effect of biliary decompression on morbidity and mortality of pancreaticoduodenectomy. Am J Surg 1984;148:727–731.

117. Gobien RP, Stanley JH, Soucek CD, Anderson MC, Vujic I, Gobien BS. Routine preoperative biliary drainage: Effect on management of obstructive jaundice. Radiology 1984;152:353–356.

118. Gundry SR, Strodel WE, Knol JA, Eckhauser FE, Thompson NW. Efficacy of preoperative biliary tract decompression in patients with obstructive jaundice. Arch Surg 1984;119:703–708.

119. Pitt HA, Gomes AS, Lots JF, Mann LL, Deutsch LS, Longmire WP Jr. Does preoperative percutaneous biliary drainage reduce operative risk or increase hospital cost? Ann Surg 1985;201:545–553.

120. McPherson GAD, Benjamin IS, Hodgson HJF, Bowley NB, Allison DJ, Blumgart LH. Preoperative percutaneous transhepatic biliary drainage: The results of a controlled trial. Br J Surg 1984;71:371–375.

121. Hatfield ARW, Tobias R, Terblanche J, et al. Preoperative biliary drainage in obstructive jaundice: A prospective controlled clinical trial. Lancet 1982;2:896–899.

122. Hamlin JA, Friedman ML. Interventional radiology in malignant biliary obstruction. Semin Oncol 1991;18:123–130.

123. Maroney TP, Ring EJ. Percutaneous transjejunal catheterization of Roux-en-Y biliary-jejunal anastomoses. Radiology 1987;164:151–153.

124. Martin EC, Laffey KJ, Bixon R. Percutaneous transjejunal approaches to the biliary system. Radiology 1989;172:1031–1034.

125. Soehendra N, Grimm H, Berger B, Nam VC. Malignant jaundice: Results of diagnostic and therapeutic endoscopy. World J Surg 1989;13:171–177.

126. Marks WM, Freeny PC, Ball TJ, Gannan RM. Endoscopic retrograde biliary drainage. Radiology 1984;152:357–360.

127. McLean GK, Burke DR. Nonoperative therapy of biliary obstruction. In: DeVita VT Jr, Hellman S, Rosenberg SA, eds. Important advances in oncology, 1987. Philadelphia: JB Lippincott, 1987:279–292.

128. Stanley J, Gobien RP, Cunningham J, Andriole J. Biliary decompression: An institutional comparison of percutaneous and endoscopic methods. Radiology 1986;158:195–197.

129. Günther RW, Schild H, Thelen M. Percutaneous transhepatic biliary drainage: Experience with 311 procedures. Cardiovasc Intervent Radiol 1988;11:65–71.
130. Akiyama H, Okazaki T, Takashima I, et al. Percutaneous treatments for biliary diseases. Radiology 1990;176:25–30.
131. Speer AG, Cotton PB, Rode J, et al. Biliary stent blockage with bacterial biofilm: A light and electron microscopy study. Ann Intern Med 1988;108:546–553.
132. McLean GK, Burke DR. Role of endoprostheses in the management of malignant biliary obstruction. Radiology 1989;170:961–967.
133. Mueller PR. Metallic endoprostheses: Boon or bust? Radiology 1991;179:603–605.
134. Dick R, Platts A, Gilford J, Reddy K, Irving JD. The Carey-Coons percutaneous biliary endoprosthesis: A three-centre experience in 87 patients. Clin Radiol 1987;38:175–178.
135. Walta DC, Fausel CS, Brant B. Endoscopic biliary stents and obstructive jaundice. Am J Surg 1987;153:444–447.
136. Kiil J, Kruse A, Rokkjaer M. Endoscopic biliary drainage. Br J Surg 1987;74:1087–1090.
137. Dick BW, Gordon RL, LaBerge JM, Doherty MM, Ring EJ. Percutaneous transhepatic placement of biliary endoprostheses: Results in 100 consecutive patients. J Vasc Intervent Radiol 1990;1:97–100.
138. Lammer J, Flueckiger F, Hausegger KA, Klein GE, Aschauer M. biliary expandable metal stents. Semin Intervent Radiol 1991;8:233–241.
139. Coons HG. Self-expanding stainless steel biliary stents. Radiology 1989;170:979–983.
140. Yoshioka T, Sakaguchi H, Yoshimura H, et al. Expandable metallic biliary endoprosthese: Preliminary clinical evaluation. Radiology 1990;177:253–257.
141. Lammer J, Klein GE, Kleinert R, Hausegger K, Einspieler R. obstructive jaundice: Use of expandable metal endoprosthesis for biliary drainage. Radiology 1990;177:789–792.
142. Adam A, Chetty N, Roddie M, Yeung E, Benjamin IS. Self-expandable stainless steel endoprostheses for treatment of malignant bile duct obstruction. AJR 1991;156:321–325.
143. Laméris JS, Stoker J, Nijs HGT, et al. Malignant biliary obstruction: Percutaneous use of self-expandable stents. Radiology 1991;179:703–707.
144. Dawson SL, Lee MJ, Mueller PR. Metal endoprostheses in malignant biliary obstruction. Semin Intervent Radiol 1991;8:242–251.
145. Tsang T-K, Crampton AR, Bernstein JR, Ramos SR, Wieland JM. Percutaneous-endoscopic biliary stent placement: A preliminary report. Ann Intern Med 1987;106:389–392.
146. Chespak LW, Ring EJ, Shapiro HA, Gordon RL, Ostroff JW. Multidisciplinary approach to complex endoscopic biliary intervention. Radiology 1989;170:995–997.
147. Neuhaus H, Hagenmüller F, Griebel M, Rotter M, Classen M. Endoskopische und perkutane Implantation selbstexpandierender Endoprosthesen bei biliären Stenosen. Dtsch Med Wochenschr 1990;115:1299–1306.
148. Lee MJ, Mueller PR, Saini S, Morrison MC, Brink JA, Hahn PF. Occlusion of biliary endoprostheses: Presentation and management. Radiology 1990;176:531–534.
149. Lammer J, Neumayer K. Biliary drainage endoprostheses: Experience with 201 placements. Radiology 1986;159:625–629.
150. Speer AG, Cotton PB, Russell RCG, et al. Randomised trial of endoscopic versus percutaneous stent insertion in malignant obstructive jaundice. Lancet 1987;2:57–62.
151. Summerfield JA. Biliary obstruction is best managed by endoscopists. Gut 1988;29:741–745.
152. Suzuki Y, Kobayashi A, Ohto M, et al. Bacteriological study of transhepatically aspirated bile: Relation to cholangiographic findings in 295 patients. Dig Dis Sci 1984;29:109–115.
153. Muro A, Mueller PR, Ferrucci JT Jr, Taft PD. Bile cytology: A routine addition to percutaneous biliary drainage. Radiology 1983;149:846–847.
154. Cope C, Marinelli DL, Weinstein JK. Transcatheter biopsy of lesions obstructing the bile ducts. Radiology 1988;169:555–556.
155. Frederiks WM, Schellens JPM, Marx F, Vreeling-Sindelárová H, Lygidakis NJ. The effect of internal biliary drainage on bile pigment accumulation and acid phosphatase activity in human liver during obstructive jaundice. Hepatogastroenterology 1991;38:39–44.
156. Clark RA, Mitchell SE, Colley DP, Alexander E. Percutaneous catheter biliary decompression. AJR 1981;137:503–509.
157. Megison SM, Dunn CW, Horton JW, Chao H. Effects of relief of biliary obstruction on mononuclear phagocyte system function and cell mediated immunity. Br J Surg 1991;78:568–571.
158. Fraser IA, Shaffer P, Tuttle SV, Lessler MA, Ellison EC, Carey LC. Hepatic recovery after biliary decompression of experimental obstructive jaundice. Am J Surg 1991;158:423–427.
159. Gazzaniga GM, Faggioni A, Bondanza G, Bagarolo C, Filauro M. Percutaneous transhepatic biliary drainage—twelve years' experience. Hepatogastroenterology 1991;38:154–160.
160. Savader SJ, Venbrux AC, Robbins KV, Gittelsohn AM, Osterman FA. Pancreatic response to percutaneous biliary drainage: A prospective study. Radiology 1991;178:343–346.
161. Carrasco C, Zornoza J, Bechtel WJ. Malignant biliary obstruction: Complications of percutaneous biliary drainage. Radiology 1984;152:343–346.
162. Chapman WC, Sharp KW, Weaver F, Sawyers JL. Tumor seeding from percutaneous biliary catheters. Ann Surg 1989;209:708–713.
163. Mellinger JD, Ponsky JL. Bleeding after endoscopic sphincterotomy as an underestimated entity. Surg Gynecol Obstet 1991;172:465–469.
164. van Sonnenberg E, D'Agostino HB, Casola G, Varney RR, Taggart SC, May SR. The benefits of percutaneous cholecystostomy for decompression of selected cases of obstructive jaundice. Radiology 1990;176:15–18.
165. McGahan JP, Lindfors KK. Percutaneous cholecystostomy: An alternative to surgical cholecystostomy for acute cholecystitis? Radiology 1989;173:481–485.
166. van Sonnenberg E, D'Agostino HB, Casola G, Varney RR, Ainge GD. Interventional radiology in the gallbladder: Diagnosis, drainage, dissolution, and the management of stones. Radiology 1990;174:1–6.
167. Vogelzang RL, Nemcek AA Jr. Percutaneous cholecystostomy: Diagnostic and therapeutic efficacy. Radiology 1988;168:29–34.
168. Teplick SK. Diagnostic and therapeutic interventional gallbladder procedures. AJR 1989;152:913–916.
169. van Sonnenberg E, Wing VW, Pollard W, Casola G. Life-threatening vagal reactions associated with percutaneous cholecystostomy. Radiology 1984;151:377–380.
170. Goodwin WE, Casey WC, Woolf W. Percutaneous trocar (needle) nephrostomy in hydronephrosis. JAMA 1955;157:891–894.
171. Reznek RH, Talner LB. Percutaneous nephrostomy. Radiol Clin North Am 1984;22:393–406.
172. Coleman CC, Kimura Y, Lange P, et al. Percutaneous nephrostomy: Indications, contraindications, preparation, and complications. Semin Intervent Radiol 1984;1:38–41.
173. Lee WJ, Smith AD, Cubelli V, Vernace FM. Percutaneous nephrolithotomy: Analysis of 500 consecutive cases. Urol Radiol 1986;8:61–66.
174. Rickards D, Jones SN. Percutaneous interventional uroradiology. Br J Radiol 1989;62:573–581.
175. Dunnick NR, Illescas FF, Mitchell S, Cohan RH, Saeed M. Interventional uroradiology. Invest Radiol 1989;24:831–841.
176. Mazer MJ, LeVeen RF, Call JB. Permanent percutaneous antegrade ureteral stent placement without transurethral assistance. Urology 1979;14:413–419.
177. Rozenblit G, Tarasov E, Srur MF, Neithamer CD Jr, Sumers EH, Sos TA. Druy ureteral stent set: Clinical experience in 25 patients. Radiology 1986;160:737–740.
178. Brazzini A, Castaneda-Zuniga WR, Coleman CC, et al. Urostent designs. Semin Intervent Radiol 1987;4:26–35.
179. Finney RP. Double-J and diversion stents. Urologic Clin North Am 1982;9:89–94.
180. Mardis HK. Evaluation of polymeric materials for endourologic devices. Emerging importance of hydrogels. Semin Intervent Radiol 1987;4:36–45.
181. LeRoy AJ, Williams J Jr, Segura JW, Patterson DE, Benson RC Jr. Indwelling ureteral stents: Percutaneous management of complications. Radiology 1986;158:219–222.
182. Stables DP, Ginsberg NJ, Johnson ML. Percutaneous nephrostomy: A series and review of the literature. AJR 1978;130:75–82.
183. Holden S, McPhee M, Grabstald H. The rationale of urinary diversion in cancer patients. J Urol 1979;121:19–21.
184. Sharer W, Grayhack JT, Graham J. Palliative urinary diversion for malignant ureteral obstruction. J Urol 1978;120:162–164.
185. Cronan JJ, Marcello A, Horn DL, Robinson A, Dorfman GS, Opal S. Antibiotics and nephrostomy tube care: Preliminary observations. Part I. Bacteriuria. Radiology 1989;172:1041–1042.
186. Barbaric ZL. Percutaneous nephrostomy for urinary tract obstruction. AJR 1984;143:803–809.
187. Cope C, Zeit RM. Pseudoaneurysms after nephrostomy. AJR 1982;139:255–261.
188. Cronan JJ, Dorfman GS, Amis ES, Denny DF Jr. Retroperitoneal hemorrhage after percutaneous nephrostomy. AJR 1985;144:801–803.
189. Harris RD, Walther PC. Renal arterial injury associated with percutaneous nephrostomy. Urology 1984;23:215–217.
190. Gavant ML, Gold RE, Church JC. Delayed rupture of renal pseudoaneurysm: Complication of percutaneous nephrostomy. AJR 1982;138:948–949.
191. Hruby W, Marberger M. Late sequelae of percutaneous nephrostomy. Work in progress. Radiology 1984;152:383–385.
192. Walsh DB, Downing S, Nauta R, Gomes MN. Metastatic cancer: A relative contraindication of vena cava filter placement. Cancer 1987;59:161–163.
193. Cohen JR, Tenenbaum N, Citron M. Greenfield filter as primary therapy for deep venous thrombosis and/or pulmonary embolism in patients with cancer. Surgery 1991;109:12–15.
194. Dorfman GS. Percutaneous inferior vena cava filters. Radiology 1990;174:987–992.
195. Pais SO, Mirvis SE, De Orchis DF. Percutaneous insertion of the Kimray-Greenfield filter: Technical considerations and problems. Radiology 1987;165:377–381.
196. Rose S, Simon DC, Hess ML, Van Aman ME. Percutaneous transfemoral placement of the Kimray-Greenfield vena cava filter. Radiology 1987;165:373–376.
197. Denny DF Jr, Dorfman GS, Cronan JJ, Greenwood LH, Morse SS, Yoselevitz M. Greenfield filter: Percutaneous placement in 50 patients. AJR 1988;50:427–429.
198. Hicks ME, Middleton WD, Picus D, Darcy MD, Kleinhoffer MA. Prevalence of local venous thrombosis after transfemoral placement of a bird's nest vena caval filter. J Vasc Intervent Radiol 1990;1:63–68.
199. Tadavarthy SM, Castaneda-Zuniga W, Salomonowitz E, et al. Kimray-Greenfield vena cava filter: Percutaneous introduction. Radiology 1984;151:525–526.
200. Robertson LJ, Mauro MA, Jaques PF. Radiologic placement of Hickman catheters. Radiology 1989;170:1007–1009.
201. Laméris JS, Post PJM, Zonderland HM, et al. Percutaneous placement of Hickman catheters: Comparison of sonographically guided and blind techniques. AJR 1990;155:1097–1099.
202. Andrews JC, Walker-Andrews SC, Ensminger WD. Long-term central venous access with a peripherally placed subcutaneous infusion port: Initial results. Radiology 1990;176:45–47.
203. Denny DF Jr, Greenwood LH, Morse SS, et al. Inferior vena cava: Translumbar catheterization for central venous access. Radiology 1989;170:1013–1014.
204. Lund GB, Lieberman RP, Haire WD, et al. Translumbar inferior vena cava catheters for long-term venous access. Radiology 1990;174:31–35.
205. Recht MP, Burke DR, Meranze SG, et al. Simple technique for redirecting malpositioned central venous catheters. AJR 1990;154:183–184.
206. Lois JF, Gomes AS, Pusey E. Nonsurgical repositioning of central venous catheters. Radiology 1987;165:329–333.

SECTION **5**   H. RICHARD ALEXANDER

Vascular Access and Other Specialized Techniques of Drug Delivery

The use of chronic indwelling venous access catheters has translated into improved safety and quality of life for cancer patients undergoing prolonged intravenous therapy. For physicians, the availability of continuous, reliable intravenous catheterization has provided an opportunity to design and deliver more complex and potentially more effective multidrug regimens. Because of the increasing use of chronic indwelling venous access catheters since their introduction into clinical practice almost 20 years ago, it is essential for all health care personnel involved with their use to have an understanding of appropriate catheter selection, routine maintenance procedures, and treatment options for catheter-related complications.[1,2] Long-term venous catheters are available as external devices, such as Hickman, Broviac, or Groshong catheters, or implanted ports, such as Port-A-Cath and Infusaport. Both types are available with single or double lumens; external catheters are also available as triple-lumen devices.

PATIENT SELECTION AND PREOPERATIVE PREPARATION

There are no established criteria for deciding which patients would benefit most from chronic indwelling venous catheters. The decision to place a catheter depends on the nature and duration of intravenous therapy, the anticipated need for repeated blood sample analyses, and patient preference. Typical candidates for chronic venous catheters include patients undergoing intensive therapy, such as autologous bone marrow transplant or aggressive combination chemotherapy, and patients needing protracted intravenous therapy. It has been estimated that more than 500,000 chronic indwelling venous catheters are inserted annually in the United States.[3] This represents an enormous expenditure of hospital resources for the device, insertion, and routine maintenance. The placement and presence of a chronic indwelling vascular access device in a patient is not free of risk, and the decision to place a catheter for any patient should be carefully considered.

Patients who are suitable candidates for placement of a long-term catheter are frequently already receiving potentially toxic intravenous therapy. Therefore, the optimal timing of catheter insertion should be planned for the interval in which the patient has recovered from treatment-related blood dyscrasias or other adverse treatment-related effects. The general condition of the patient should be carefully assessed to maximize the safety of the procedure. A prior history of thoracic procedures, active mediastinal disease such as Hodgkin's disease, previous irradiation to the chest, or multiple previous bilateral central lines should alert the physician to the possibility that the venous anatomy of the chest may be abnormal. In these situations, preoperative evaluation of venous patency may be

useful for selecting an appropriate insertion site. Successful imaging of thoracic venous anatomy can be performed with digital subtraction angiography, duplex Doppler ultrasound, computed tomography (CT), or magnetic resonance imaging.[4–6]

A knowledge of the patient's pulmonary reserve, particularly with respect to the presence of malignant pleural effusions, prior pulmonary resection, or extent of metastatic disease to the lung, may help in directing on which side a long-term venous catheter may be most safely inserted. The insertion of a catheter into an area of prior surgery with extensive skin-flap dissection, such as mastectomy or through irradiated skin, should be avoided, because it may predispose the patient to infectious complications.

The past administration of chemotherapeutic agents may have produced subclinical organ impairment, which should be appreciated before catheter placement. A clinical situation that occurs more frequently is significant neutropenia or thrombocytopenia secondary to recently administered chemotherapeutic agents. The insertion of long-term venous access catheters should be considered an elective procedure and performed when conditions are optimal for the patient. Recovery of absolute neutrophil counts greater than 1500/mm³ typically indicates the return of host immunocompetence and represents a time when catheter insertion can be performed without concerns that the development of febrile neutropenia or severe line sepsis may necessitate early catheter removal.[7] Patients whose catheters are inserted during periods of neutropenia have a higher incidence of septic episodes than in those without neutropenia.[8] Patients with infection should not undergo catheter placement until appropriate antibiotic treatment has been initiated and clinical evidence of infection has resolved.

Thrombocytopenia is frequently encountered in cancer patients and secondary functional platelet disorders may exacerbate a relatively mild low platelet count. Long-term venous access catheters can be safely inserted despite thrombocytopenia, and platelet transfusion perioperatively to 50,000/ml usually minimizes the incidence of postoperative hemorrhagic complications.[9] Some patients with refractory thrombocytopenia who do not respond well to platelet transfusion need long-term venous catheters. Venous cutdown on the external jugular, cephalic, or internal jugular vein may be the safest approach for them.

Malnutrition, other medications, or concurrent illnesses such as human immunodeficiency virus infection can prolong prothrombin or partial thromboplastin time. Although mild abnormalities of one parameter (*e.g.*, 1–2 seconds) does not necessarily require correction, preoperative administration of fresh frozen plasma or vitamin K may be necessary for more severe abnormalities.

CATHETER SELECTION

The selection of an external catheter or subcutaneous port and the decision to use a single- or dual-lumen catheter depends on the intensity of treatment, need for close monitoring of blood samples, and patient preference (Table 21–7).

For patients receiving intermittent bolus injections of chemotherapy as an outpatient, the subcutaneous port may be

TABLE 21–7. Features of Hickman and Broviac and Totally Implantable Venous Access Catheters

Hickman and Broviac Catheters	*Implantable Ports*
Double-lumen catheter easily inserted	Double lumen available but port is large
Regular maintenance requirements	Minimal maintenance
Wound care	No dressings
Heparin flushing	Monthly heparin flush
Restricts some activities like swimming	Cosmetically superior, minimal interference with life style
Maximal reliability for safe continuous intravenous therapy and blood sampling	Best suited for intermittent or maintenance chemotherapy; requires access with needle
Higher maintenance costs	Higher initial costs
Easy to remove	Requires second procedure to remove device

most suitable. Although most implanted ports are single lumen, a double-lumen port is available. The advantages of a subcutaneously implanted port are the ease of maintenance and cosmetic appearance (Fig. 21–37). Implantable ports are routinely flushed with dilute heparin solution biweekly or monthly and, when not in use, are completely contained under the skin, do not require a bandage, and minimally interfere with lifestyle. The port is anchored to underlying fascia in a subcutaneous pocket and accessed with a noncoring Huber needle that minimizes the potential for cracking the port diaphragm. Although the subcutaneous ports may be used for continuous infusion therapy, the potential for the access needle to dislodge and deliver chemotherapy to the subcutaneous space is not inconsequential. If a patient is receiving contin-

uous infusion therapy through an implanted port, the Huber access needle should be adequately secured and assessed at frequent intervals to ensure that it has not become dislodged.

Patients best suited for the Hickman and Broviac catheters include those receiving potentially toxic regimens given as prolonged continuous infusions, frequent supplemental intravenous fluids or blood products, medications for control of therapy-induced nausea and vomiting, frequent monitoring of blood counts, or total parenteral nutrition (Fig. 21–37). There are routine maintenance requirements for external catheters, including regular flushing with dilute heparin solutions, exit site care, and dressing changes.

Several studies have compared subcutaneous ports and external devices with respect to functional stability, infectious complications, and cost effectiveness.[10–15] May and Davis pooled data from available published reports, reviewing experience in adults and children with ports and catheters.[10] Although the pooled studies varied considerably with respect to patient characteristics, catheter maintenance schedules, and criteria for diagnosis of infection, the overall mean infection rate per 100 catheter days was 0.21 for catheters and 0.04 for ports. Wurzel reported a nonrandomized prospective comparison of overall infectious complications in 62 pediatric oncology patients with Hickman or Broviac catheters or implantable venous devices.[11] Although the relative risk of developing an infectious complication with external catheters was 1.5 compared with ports, this was not a statistically significant difference. In other reports of pediatric oncology patients, a significantly longer infection-free and overall failure-free interval was observed with implantable ports than with Hickman or Broviac catheters.[12,14,15] A prospective study of 43 patients randomly assigned to receive Hickman or Portacath catheters did not detect any significant differences in overall rates of infection between the groups.[16] There has not been any consistent data to indicate that the rate of catheter obstruction is different between ports and external catheters.[3,15] The initial cost of insertion is less for catheters than ports, but the cost of routine maintenance is higher, and the

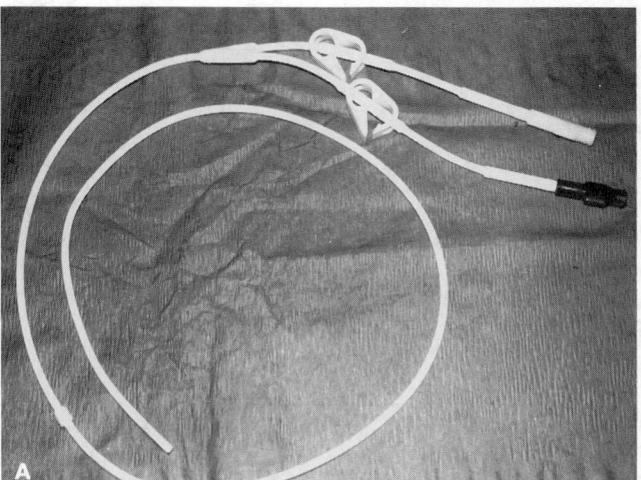
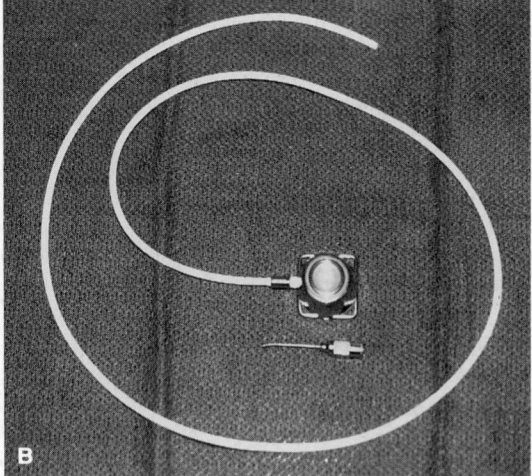

FIGURE 21–37. **(A)** A dual lumen 10 Fr Hickman catheter showing the Dacron cuff that facilitates fibrosis and secures the catheter in place. Hubs are color coded. **(B)** An implantable venous access device. The port is anchored to underlying fascia in a subcutaneous pocket and is accessed with a noncoring Huber needle to prevent damage to the diaphragm.

overall expense for the two types of devices is roughly comparable after 6 months of use.[12]

The data appear to indicate that in children and adults the overall complication rate from ports appears to be lower than for external catheters.[10,13,17] Some of these differences may represent bias in catheter selection based on diagnosis and intensity of treatment. With careful routine care, external devices are safe and provide reliable access to the venous system.

A comprehensive program of patient education, catheter maintenance, and surveillance is essential to provide the longest benefit from chronic venous access catheters.[3] At the National Cancer Institute, all patients receive instruction preoperatively about all aspects of catheter function, care, and maintenance. Some hours after the procedure and before discharge from the day hospital, the patient, a relative, or a responsible friend must demonstrate proficiency in catheter care techniques.

TECHNIQUE OF INSERTION

Most procedures can be performed safely on an outpatient basis, typically in an operating room suite to maximize sterile conditions. Fluoroscopy is used to confirm appropriate catheter placement. Catheters can be inserted using a local anesthetic with monitored anesthesia sedation. The preferred technique and most accessible site of insertion is the percutaneous method of Seldinger, using the subclavian vein. Percutaneous placement can be performed more quickly than and with comparable safety to an open venous cutdown.[15,18]

The patient is placed supine with a rolled towel between the scapulae to extend the shoulders. The precordium is prepared sterilely, and a local anesthetic is infiltrated infraclavicularly. With the patient in the Trendelenburg's position, a needle is advanced into the subclavian vein with the bevel up while gently aspirating on the attached 6-ml syringe (Fig. 21–38). Entry into the vein is confirmed by flow of venous blood into the syringe, at which time the needle is rotated 90°, the syringe is disconnected taking care not to allow air to be entrained into the vein through the needle, and a flexible guide wire is advanced through the needle. If pulsatile backflow of blood is observed through the needle, the subclavian artery has been cannulated, and after removal of the needle, direct pressure for several minutes should produce adequate hemostasis. If resistance is encountered after the flexible wire has been advanced 2 to 3 cm, the needle is probably not in the vein. This is illustrated occasionally by observing the wire coiled in the subcutaneous tissue on fluoroscopy during attempted advancement. In this situation, the needle should be withdrawn with the wire to avoid the possibility of shearing the wire. After successfully advancing the wire, its appropriate position can be confirmed with fluoroscopy.

A site on the precordium is selected for the exit site, infiltrated with anesthetic, and the catheter is tunneled through the subcutaneous tissue to the insertion site so that the Dacron cuff is situated subcutaneously just above the insertion site. The skin adjacent to the wire insertion site is then incised slightly, and the peel away sheath and vessel dilator is gently advanced over the wire. It is important to ensure that the sheath and dilator are threading over the wire by intermittently advancing and withdrawing the wire slightly and checking for

resistance (Fig. 21–38 inset). It is possible for the dilator to bend the wire and for the surgeon to advance the dilator through the mediastinal vascular structures. This could injure the mediastinal vascular structures and can result in fatality.[19] Ideally, the catheter tip should lie at the superior vena cava and right atrial junction or just inside the right atrium. A higher rate of catheter failure because of occlusive or thrombotic complications has been documented when the catheter tip was high in the superior vena cava or subclavian vein compared with catheter tips located in the right atrium.[17,20] The catheter is cut to its estimated desired length, determined from external bony landmarks. Typically, the right superior vena cava and right atrial junction lies approximately 4 to 6 cm inferior to the angle of Louis (Fig. 21–39). By approximating the course of the catheter through the vein on the patient's chest, the correct length can be determined.

If the subclavian vein is not suitable for catheter insertion, the external jugular or internal jugular vein may be used

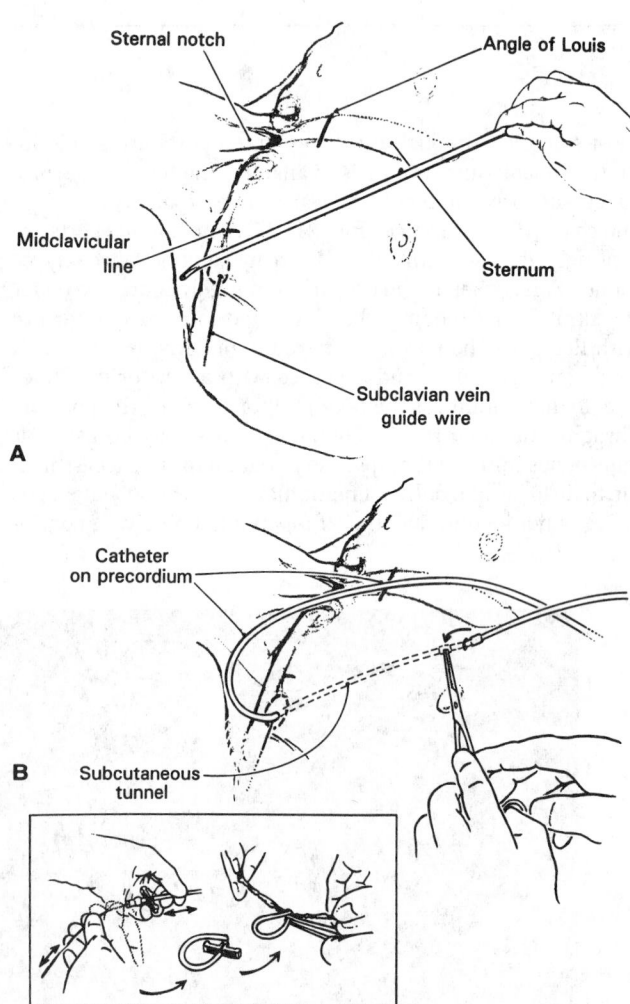

FIGURE 21–38. Insertion of a chronic venous catheter into the subclavian vein using the percutaneous technique. **(A)** After insertion of the guidewire, the catheter is tunneled from the chosen exit site to the venous cannulation site. **(B)** The Dacron cuff is placed subcutaneously just above the exit site. Inset illustrates that as the sheath and dilator are advanced over the guidewire, care is taken to ensure that the sheath and dilator are advancing along the course of the wire by intermittently moving wire back and forth. After trimming the catheter to a proper length, it is advanced through the peel-away sheath.

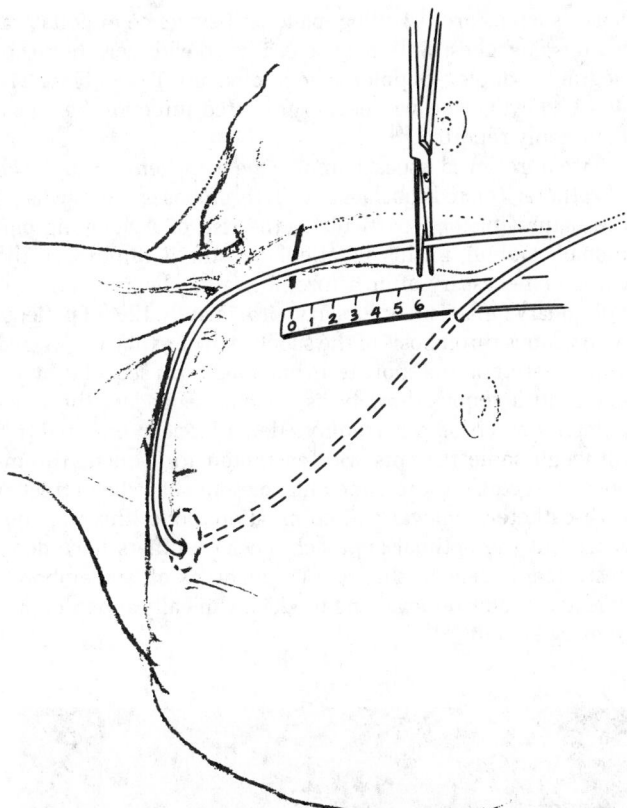

FIGURE 21–39. The length of the catheter can be estimated by simulating its course through the subclavian vein and superior vena cava along the clavicle and right border of the sternum. If the catheter is cut 6 cm inferior to the angle of Louis, it approximates a final position at the superior vena caval and right atrial junction.

through a short transverse cervical incision. Occasionally, patients with a protracted history of multiple venous access lines, extensive mediastinal tumor involvement, or previous radiation therapy or chest surgery may not have any access options in the previously described sites. In patients with occlusive superior central vein thrombosis, a technique involving a combined angiographic and operative approach has been described in which a guidewire or Dormia basket is inserted into the femoral vein and advanced retrograde through the occluded superior vena cava to a peripheral vein in the neck or arm. A cutdown is made over the wire or Dormia basket, and a Hickman or Broviac catheter is guided through the occlusion to the right atrium.[21]

The reported complication rate with catheters positioned in the inferior vena cava appears acceptably low, and chronic venous access with catheters in this position may represent the next most suitable site if others are not available.[22] Alternate insertion sites for chronic venous catheters include the saphenous vein, gonadal vein, intercostal vein, azygous vein, or direct placement into the inferior vena cava.[21–25]

ROUTINE POSTOPERATIVE MAINTENANCE

Careful attention to maintenance of line patency and care of the insertion site prolong the useful life of the catheter. There is considerable variability in the concentration of heparin and the frequency of flushing used in different institutions.[26] Typically, if external catheters are not being used, they are flushed daily or every other day with a dilute heparin solution, and implanted ports do not appear to require routine flushing.[27–29] One study reported that only 15% of Hickman catheters became occluded without any routine heparin flush.[30] Of seven occluded catheters, six were restored to patency with a short infusion of urokinase. Others reported that luminal clots can be detected in 15% to 30% of chronic indwelling venous catheters despite daily heparin flushing or the administration of low-dose Coumadin.[31,32] There is the potential danger of contamination with regular heparin flushes over time. The optimal schedule of catheter flushing and the need for heparin in the flush solution remain to be defined.

COMPLICATIONS

CATHETER OCCLUSION AND PERSISTENT WITHDRAWAL OCCLUSION

The inability to infuse fluids or withdraw blood from longterm indwelling venous access catheters can be a result of catheter-tip malposition, catheter kinking, fibrin sheath around the catheter, luminal occlusion due to blood clot or precipitation of drugs solutions, or catheter tip abutment against the venous wall.[4,33]

Luminal occlusion can be quickly recognized by the inability to infuse or withdraw fluids, and it occurs in as many as 20% to 30% of catheters.[4,31] If there is an inability to infuse through the catheter, a chest x-ray film should be obtained to rule out catheter malposition or kinking. If there is no catheter migration, the cause is probably catheter lumen occlusion. The ability to infuse but not aspirate from the catheter is called withdrawal occlusion, and it has been attributed to the development of a fibrin sheath around the tip of the catheter acting as a flap valve that does not interfere with infusion but does prevent aspiration.[34] The incidence of fibrin sheath in subclavian venous catheters has been reported to occur in up to 80% of patients.[35]

After confirming the appropriate location of the catheter on chest x-ray films, attempts to restore patency of occluded catheters or manage persistent withdrawal occlusion can be tried with a variety of thrombolytic agents that have been successful. Administration of urokinase (250,000 U in 150 ml D_5W), infused over 90 minutes, can resolve withdrawal occlusion in more than 90% of the catheters.[34] For catheter lumen occlusion, 2 ml of urokinase (2500–5000 U/ml), infused and left in the catheter for 30 minutes to 2 hours, is effective.[30] Alternately, a commercially available combination of streptokinase and streptodornase can be administered in a volume equal to the estimated internal volume of the catheter.[36] Tissue plasminogen activator has been used successfully in the treatment of occluded central venous catheters.[37] Although there is some possibility of embolizing a small luminal clot into the lungs, the clinical consequences are unknown but do not appear significant.[38]

CATHETER-RELATED VENOUS THROMBOSIS

A chronic indwelling catheter in the subclavian vein and the associated intimal injury at the insertion site predispose patients to the development of subclavian vein thrombosis. Thrombosis has occurred in as many as 40% of patients by clinical assessment or autopsy.[39–41] More than 60% of critically ill patients with indwelling internal jugular hemodynamic monitoring devices developed asymptomatic venous thromboses in one prospective study, indicating that the actual incidence in patients with long-term indwelling subclavian vein catheters may be higher than reported, because many thromboses may be clinically inapparent.[5] Central venous catheters may account for almost half of all deep venous thromboses of the upper extremity.[42]

The time course of catheter-related thrombosis can be 2 weeks to 2 years after catheter insertion, and the incidence of thromboses appears to increase with the duration of catheterization.[43,44] However, the development of catheter-related venous thrombosis does not appear related to age, sex, or coagulation status.[43] A higher incidence of catheter-related venous thromboses have been reported in patients with a blood hemoglobin greater than 127 g/L and patients with adenocarcinoma of the lung, versus patients with squamous tumors of the lung, head and neck, or esophagus.[41,45] Patients who develop symptoms compatible with subclavian vein thrombosis, such as arm swelling, pain, and evidence of collateral venous flow chest wall, may be evaluated with peripheral venography, duplex Doppler sonography, or CT scan (Fig. 21–40).[4–6] Fever even without documented infection has been commonly reported.[46]

Two unresloved issues dominate the management approach of catheter-related subclavian vein thromboses. First, what is the natural history, particularly the risk of developing pulmonary emboli, in this situation? Second, is removal of the catheter necessary after a thrombosis has been diagnosed? Pulmonary embolism occurs in approximately 12% of patients with venous thrombosis of the subclavian or axillary vein, and after treatment, the short-term and long-term sequelae of upper central venous thrombosis, such as secondary thrombophlebitis or chronic extremity edema, appear minimal.[42,46] Although some patients with asymptomatic venous thromboses detected on screening phlebography have been treated with catheter removal and observation alone, this may not represent the optimal approach, because others have demonstrated that sleeve thromboses can break off and embolize during catheter removal and produce clinically apparent pulmonary emboli.[40,44]

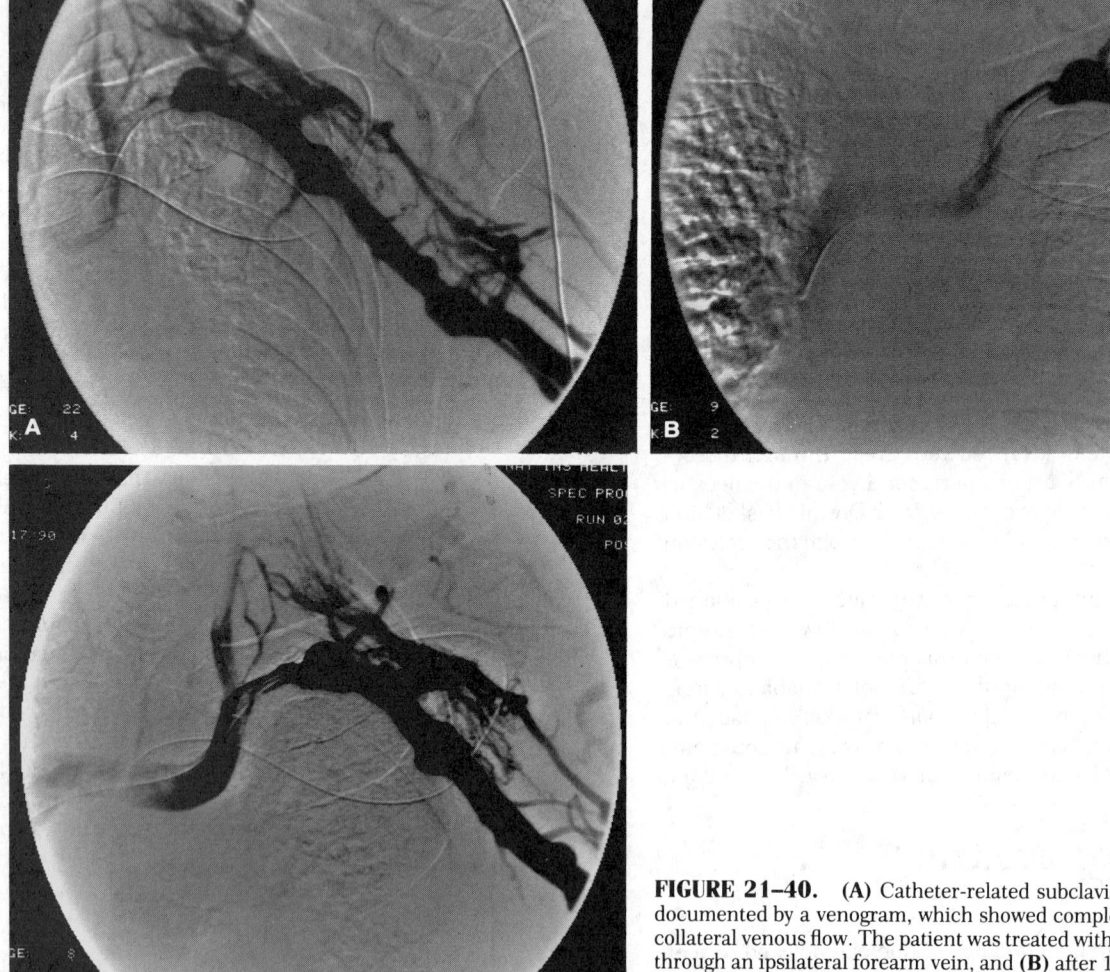

FIGURE 21–40.   **(A)** Catheter-related subclavian vein thrombosis documented by a venogram, which showed complete obstruction and collateral venous flow. The patient was treated with urokinase infusion through an ipsilateral forearm vein, and **(B)** after 16 hours and **(C)** 39 hours of urokinase infusion, he showed progressive resolution of thrombosis.

The ability to successfully treat a subclavian vein thrombosis with thrombolytic therapy is related to the duration of symptoms. Dissolution of thrombi can be achieved in more than 90% of patients who have a short interval of symptoms but in only 56% of patients with symptoms of longer than 1 week.[47]

After a diagnosis of subclavian vein thrombosis is made, particularly if it is symptomatic, prompt treatment is indicated. Initial supportive measures include arm elevation and analgesia for pain. In the past, systemic anticoagulation with heparin, catheter removal, and subsequent Coumadin was a standard approach for catheter-related thrombosis.[40,46] Although removal of the offending catheter is intuitive, recent reports have demonstrated highly successful treatment with anticoagulation or thrombolytic agents while the catheter remains in situ.[43,47–50] For adults, an intravenous bolus of streptokinase (250,000 U), followed by a 24- to 72-hour infusion at 100,000 U/hour, has been highly effective in completely resolving subclavian vein thrombosis despite failed heparin therapy.[51] Close patient monitoring for hemorrhagic complications is essential. Another approach is to infuse a thrombolytic agent directly into the site of subclavian vein thrombosis through an ipsilateral vein. Local infusion of urokinase has resulted in dissolution in 25 of 30 thrombi within 4 days with minimal morbidity (see Fig. 21–40).[47]

Several studies reported attempts to prophylactically treat patients with indwelling venous or pulmonary artery catheters to reduce the incidence of thrombus formation. In patients receiving total parenteral nutrition (TPN) through polyvinyl chloride central venous catheters, the addition of low-dose heparin to the TPN solution reduced the incidence of asymptomatic catheter-related thrombosis to one third of the rate observed in patients without heparin.[52] Heparin administration in patients with long-term venous access may also be indicated because the incidence of fibrin sheath formation is higher.[53] In patients with indwelling pulmonary artery catheters for hemodynamic monitoring during cardiopulmonary bypass, the use of heparin-bonded catheters significantly reduced the incidence of thrombus formation on the catheter.[54] A prospective, randomized trial evaluated the use of low-dose warfarin in cancer patients with long-term indwelling venous catheters.[55] The incidence of venous thrombosis, most of which were symptomatic in this study, was significantly reduced from 38% in untreated controls to 9.5% in patients receiving warfarin. Virtually all thromboses in both groups were symptomatic, and the addition of warfarin had no effect on coagulation parameters and was well tolerated. These results indicate that the incidence of catheter-related thromboses can be substantially reduced in patients at risk for thromboses. Methods to more accurately predict which patients will benefit from prophylactic treatment may allow more judicious use of this approach.

CATHETER-RELATED INFECTIONS

Because most patients with cancer who have long-term indwelling venous catheters experience periods of immunocompromise secondary to their disease or its treatment, infectious complications represent the most serious and potentially life-threatening effects of these devices. Reported overall infection rates are 3% to 60%.[8,13,27] The risk of developing septic complications is higher in patients with prolonged neutropenia, in patients younger than 2 years, and with external catheters than ports.[11,13,27]

Catheter-related infections can be divided into three types. *Exit site infections* are localized at the point where an external device exits the skin and are manifested by localized erythema and induration without systemic signs of infection. Most exit site infections are secondary to *Staphylococcus epidermidis*.[56–59] Initial management with local wound care and appropriate oral antibiotics without removing the catheter is indicated and frequently successful.[58,60,61] However, if there is evidence of developing bacteremia associated with an exit site infection, particularly if the isolated pathogen is *Staphylococcus aureus,* catheter removal may be necessary in as many as 90% of the patients.[62] Deciding exactly when a catheter should be removed is difficult, and many reports on this topic do not have standardized criteria for catheter removal.

The second type of infectious complication occurring with external catheters or implanted ports is called *tunnel or pocket infection.* It represents a suppurative and indurated process through the subcutaneous portion of a catheter or around the implanted port housing. These infections are frequently associated with varying degrees of surrounding cellulitis and systemic signs of infection may be present. The diagnosis is based on erythema, induration, and tenderness along the subcutaneous tunnel tract or around the subcutaneous port pocket. Frequently, purulent fluid can be expressed from the subcutaneous tunnel or aspirated from the port pocket. Because these infections are suppurative, occur in the presence of a foreign body, and are accompanied by local cellulitis, it is necessary to remove the catheter or implanted port and use appropriate antibiotics. Adequate drainage of any abscesses is necessary. If Gram stain of purulent fluid does not reveal bacteria, acid-fast staining should be done. Rapidly growing atypical mycobacterial infection of the tunnel or exit site is a rare but virulent type of infection. In these instances, catheter removal, excision of infected tissue, and antibiotic therapy appear important in resolving infection.[63]

Line sepsis or catheter-related bacteremia is the most serious and potentially life-threatening infectious complication of chronic indwelling venous catheters. It is manifested by clinical signs and symptoms of bacteremia, with no other source of infection identified by clinical and laboratory tests. The cause of line sepsis is unknown but may be secondary to the chronic colonization of the intravascular portion of the catheter from external sites on the catheter or the exit site.[64–66] With electron microscopy, bacterial colonization has been observed in an adherent glycocalyx biofilm on 13 (87%) of 15 chronic venous catheter lumens in cancer patients with a history of septicemia.[64] These findings indicate that adherent microorganisms may provide a source of recurring infection. In 41 patients in whom catheters were removed for catheter-associated bacteremia documented by subsequent catheter tip cultures (≥15 colonies per blood agar plate), direct Gram staining of the catheter tip revealed adherent microorganisms in all instances.[65] Because of the sensitivity and specificity of the Gram stain technique, it has been proposed as a rapid diagnostic method for catheter-associated infection.

For many patients the in situ diagnosis of catheter-associated infection is desirable to avoid premature or unnecessary line removal. Other sources of infection should be excluded based on clinical and laboratory findings. If positive blood cultures collected through the catheter show a fivefold to tenfold increase in colony count compared with peripheral quantitative blood cultures or, if peripheral cultures are not collected, a count of 100 colony-forming units per 1 ml or more from the indwelling venous catheter are identified, there is line sepsis.[61,67] Others have shown that semiquantitative cultures of blood drawn through the catheter hub have a 100% positive predictive value for catheter-tip colonization when more than 1000 colony-forming units per 1 ml are obtained.[68] Cercenado studied the value of exit site and hub cultures in diagnosing catheter-associated infection.[69] Of 53 infected catheters (≥15 colony-forming units per plate), 50 had positive cultures of identical microorganisms isolated from superficial sites (*e.g.*, exit site, catheter hub). When negative superficial cultures were obtained, the diagnosis of catheter-associated infection appeared unlikely because no tip culture was positive.

The major question in the treatment of catheter-related bacteremia is under what conditions should the infected catheter be removed? A number of studies have reported successful treatment of line sepsis while the catheter remains in situ.[7,8,16,61,67,70] Hartman reported the successful treatment of line-related septicemia in 25 (89%) of 28 children, including gram-negative, gram-positive, multiple-organism septicemia, and *Candida* fungemia.[8] Catheter-related bacteremia was defined as a positive blood culture obtained from the central venous catheter in a patient with fever and no localizing signs. Only 30% of patients had additional peripheral blood cultures, indicating that some of these septic episodes were not actually caused by line sepsis. Two studies of children with venous catheters used comparative semiquantitative blood cultures taken from the catheter and a peripheral site to diagnose catheter-related bacteremia.[67,70] The criteria for a diagnosis of catheter-related bacteremia in these studies were positive blood cultures taken through the catheter with sterile peripheral cultures or a greater than fivefold concentration of bacteria in catheter blood compared with peripheral blood. Antibiotic therapy with catheters in situ was successful in 12 (57%) of 21 patients and 11 (65%) of 17 patients. In another series of adults with chronic indwelling venous catheters and documented catheter-related sepsis, treatment was successful in 33 (61%) of 54 patients with antibiotics alone.[61]

The in situ treatment of catheter-related candidemia appears contraindicated because the rates of treatment failure, secondary complications, and mortality are higher than in children whose catheters are removed.[71,72] *Staphylococcus aureus* bacteremia in adults with Hickman catheters is not successfully treated without catheter removal.[62] Therefore, catheter-related infection secondary to *Candida* or *S. aureus* should be treated with early catheter removal and appropriate antibiotics. In other patients with catheter-related infection, the decision to remove the catheter should be based on the clinical assessment of the patient and response to initial antibiotic therapy. If there is persistent evidence of infection or any deterioration in the condition of the patient, the catheter should be removed.

DRUG DELIVERY SYSTEMS

Infusion devices used in conjunction with chronic indwelling catheters enable systemic or site-directed infusional therapy with antineoplastics, analgesics, or antibiotics in an ambulatory outpatient setting. Costs are reduced, and quality of life is improved because hospitalization is avoided.

Because implantable ports are used to access various intracorporeal sites, do not assume that any subcutaneously positioned port is a venous access device. Infusion devices are available in two basic types: a completely implantable subcutaneous version or an externally worn ambulatory device.[73] The first implantable pump in clinical use was the Infusaid, which weighs slightly less than 200 g empty and is contained in a subcutaneous pocket, usually on the upper abdominal wall. It has been most widely used to deliver continuous hepatic intraarterial therapy. The pump delivers a constant rate determined by internal flow resistors and is powered by the pressure generated from the expansion of a liquid fluorocarbon to the gaseous phase at body temperature. As the drug reservoir is filled percutaneously through a septum, the surrounding fluorocarbon chamber is recharged because gas is compressed and condensed into a liquid. Newer versions have a side-access septum that bypasses the infusion system and allows direct delivery of medications. Programmable, battery-powered implantable pumps use a peristaltic or solenoid pump mechanism. A telemetry system transmits or receives signals from the totally implanted device, which can turn the pump on or off, adjust delivery rate, and determine battery voltage.[74] The advantages of the subcutaneously implanted systems are cosmetic appearance, low risk of infection, and ease of maintenance. However, each unit is designed for single-patient use, and the cost can be substantial.

External infusion devices can connect to indwelling catheters and provide continuous infusion or intermittent bolus therapy.[75] The pumps are usually small and lightweight, and they can be comfortably worn without encumbering an ambulatory outpatient. Some models can be programmed to deliver a range of volumes for continuous infusion or intermittent bolus therapy. Ambulatory pumps are reusable because drug is contained in a syringe, bag, or cassette. The drug must be stable in solution for the calculated duration of infusion. The ambulatory infusion devices also provide an element of complexity to drug administration. There are a variety of features available on ambulatory infusion devices, such as audible or visual alarms or automatic shutoff in the event of a malfunction or completion of drug delivery. The programming contains lock levels that are tamper-resistant so that the patient does not inadvertently change the infusion rate. The patient or a family member should be intimately familiar with the pump and able to recognize and potentially address several problems, such as a kinked catheter, low battery, or completed infusion. Many patients are taught to check the residual volume display to ensure that it is decreasing at the anticipated rate. Some devices combine continuous infusion with patient-initiated intermittent bolus injections, which are delivered within preset time and dose limitations. This has been particularly useful for patients on continuous narcotic analgesic therapy.

CONCLUSIONS

The use of chronic indwelling venous access catheters, implantable ports, and ambulatory infusion devices have provided a dimension of independent living for many patients while they receive lifesaving therapy as outpatients. For the physician, these devices have provided an opportunity to develop a new level of sophistication in planning effective therapy for a variety of neoplastic conditions. Although significant problems can occur, careful patient monitoring, education, and prompt intervention by health care personnel can frequently resolve these complications and ensure the continued safe use of the devices.

REFERENCES

1. Broviac JW, Cole JJ, Schribner BH. A silicone rubber atrial catheter for prolonged parenteral alimentation. Surg Gynecol Obstet 1973;136:602–606.
2. Hickman RO, Buckner CD, Clife RA, Sanders JE, Stewart P, Thomas ED. A modified right atrial catheter for access to the venous system in marrow transplant recipients. Surg Gynecol Obstet 1979;148:871–875.
3. Groeger JS, Lucas AB, Coit D. Venous access in the cancer patient. PPO Updates 1991;5: 1–14.
4. Cassidy FP Jr, Zajko AB, Bron KM, Reilly JJ Jr, Peitzman AB, Steed DL. Noninfectious complications of long-term central venous catheters: Radiologic evaluation and management. AJR 1987;149:671–675.
5. Chastre J, Cornud F, Bouchama A, Biau F, Benacerraf R, Gibert C. Thrombosis as a complication of pulmonary-artery catheterization via the internal jugular vein. N Engl J Med 1982;3066:278–281.
6. Falk RL, Smith DF. Thrombosis of upper extremity thoracic inlet veins: Diagnosis with duplex Doppler sonography. AJR 1987;149:677–682.
7. Brar KA, Murray DL, Leader I. Central venous catheter infections in pediatric patients in a community hospital. Infection 1988;16:86–90.
8. Hartman GE, Shochat SJ. Management of septic complications associated with Silastic catheters in childhood malignancy. Pediatr Infect Dis J 1987;6:1042–1047.
9. Thompson WR, Alexander HR, Martin AJ, Fletcher JR, Ghosh BC. Percutaneous subclavian catheterization for prolonged systemic chemotherapy. J Surg Oncol 1985;29: 184–186.
10. May GS, Davis C. Percutaneous catheters and totally implantable access systems. Journal of Intravenous Nursing 1988;11:97–103.
11. Wurzel CL Halom K, Feldman JG, Rubin LG. Infection rates of Broviac-Hickman catheters and implantable venous devices. Am J Dis Child 1991;142:536–540.
12. Ross MN, Haase GM, Poole MA, Burrington JD, Odom LF. Comparison of totally implanted reservoirs with external catheters as venous access devices in pediatric oncologic patients. Surg Gynecol Obstet 1988;167:141–144.
13. Shaw JHF, Douglas R, Wilson T. Clinical performance of Hickman and Portacath atrial catheters. Aust N Z J Surg 1988;58:657–659.
14. Mirro J Jr, Rao BN, Stokes DC, et al. A prospective study of Hickman/Broviac catheters and implantable ports in pediatric oncology patients. J Clin Oncol 1989;7:214–222.
15. Mirro Jr, Rao BN, Kumar M, et al. A comparison of placement techniques and complications of externalized catheters and implantable port use in children with cancer. J Pediatr Surg 1990;25:120–124.
16. Kappers-Klunne MC, Degener JE, Stijnen T, Abels J. Complications from long-term indwelling central venous catheters in hematologic patients with special reference to infection. Cancer 1989;64:1747–1752.
17. Stanislav GV, Fitzgibbons RJ Jr, Bailey RT Jr, Mailliard JA, Johnson S, Feole JB. Reliability of implantable central venous access devices in patients with cancer. Arch Surg 1991;122: 1280–1283.
18. Jansen RFM, Wiggers T, van Geel BN, van Putten WLJ. Assessment of insertion techniques and complication rates of dual-lumen central venous catheters in patients with hematological malignancies. World J Surg 1990;14:101–106.
19. Pessa ME, Howard RJ. Complications of Hickman-Broviac catheters. Surg Gynecol Obstet 1985;161:257–260.
20. Stanislav GV, Fitzgibbons RJ Jr, Bailey RT, Mailliard JA, Johnson S, Feole JB. Reliability of implantable central venous access devices in patients with cancer. Arch Surg 1987;122: 1280–1283.
21. Torosian MH, Meranze S, Mullen JL, McLean G. Central venous access with occlusive superior central venous thrombosis. Ann Surg 1986;203:30–33.
22. Williard W, Coit D, Lucas A, Groeger JS. Long-term vascular access via the inferior vena cava. J Surg Oncol 1991;46:162–166.
23. Lammermeier D, Steiger E, Cosgrove D, Zelch M. Use of an intercostal vein for central venous access in home parenteral nutrition: A case report. JPEN 1986;10:659–124.
24. Pokorny WJ, McGill CW, Harberg FJ. Use of azygous vein for central catheter insertion. Surgery 1984;97:362.
25. Knox MF, Holton JC, Morris WD, Flippin TA. Translumbar inferior vena cava Groshong catheter placement in a patient with superior vena cava occlusion. J Arkansas Med Soc 1989;85:325–326.
26. Goldberg N, Koontz DP. Hickman-type catheters: A retrospective study of nursing care and flush procedures. Oncol Nurs Forum [Abstract] 1991;345(suppl A):215.
27. Greene FL, Moore W, Strickland G, McFarland J. Comparison of a totally implantable access device for chemotherapy (Port-A-Cath) and long-term percutaneous catheterization (Broviac). South Med J 1988;81:580–603.
28. Strum S, McDermed J, Korn A, Joseph C. Improved methods for venous access: The Port-A-Cath, a totally implanted catheter system. J Clin Oncol 1986;4:596–603.
29. Niederhuber JE, Ensminger W, Gyves JW, Lipeman M, Doan K, Cozzi E. Totally im-

30. planted venous and arterial access system to replace external catheters in cancer treatment. Surgery 1982;92:706–712.
30. Gillies H, Rogers HJ, Johnston J, Harper PG, Rudge CJ. Is repeated flushing of Hickman catheters necessary? Br Med J 1985;290:1708.
31. Anderson AJ, Krawnow SH, Boyer MW, et al. Hickman catheter clots: A common occurrence despite daily heparin flushing. Cancer Treat Rep 1987;71:651–653.
32. Anderson AJ, Krasnow SH, Boyer MW, Wadleigh RG, Cohen MH. Clots can frequently be aspirated from Groshong catheters. Am Assoc Cancer Res [Abstract] 1988;29:A907: 228.
33. Lazarus HM, Lowder JN, Herzig RH. Occlusion and infection in Broviac catheters during intensive cancer therapy. Cancer 1983;52:2342–2348.
34. Tschirhart JM, Rao MK. Mechanism and management of persistent withdrawal occlusion. Am Surg 1988;54:326–328.
35. Peters WR, Bush WH Jr. The development of fibrin sheath on indwelling venous catheters. Surg Gynecol Obstet 1973;137:43–47.
36. Hurtubise MR, Bottino JC, Lawson M, McCredie KB. Restoring patency of occluded central venous catheters. Arch Surg 1980;115:212–213.
37. Atkinson JB, Bagnall HA, Gomperts E. Investigational use of tissue plasminogen activator (t-PA) for occluded central venous catheters. JPEN 1990;14:310–311.
38. Anderson AJ, Krasnow SH, Boyer MW, et al. Hickman catheter clots: A common occurrence despite daily heparin flushing. Cancer Treat Rep 1987;71:6651–6653.
39. McDonough JJ, Altemeier WA. Subclavian venous thrombosis secondary to indwelling catheters. Surg Gynecol Obstet 1971;133:397–400.
40. Lokich JJ, Becker B. Subclavian vein thrombosis in patients treated with infusion chemotherapy for advanced malignancy. Cancer 1983;52:1586–1589.
41. Anderson AJ, Krasnow SH, Boyer MW, et al. Thrombosis: The major Hickman catheter complication in patients with solid tumor. Chest 1989;95:71–75.
42. Horattas MC, Wright DJ, Fenton AH, et al. Changing concepts of deep venous thrombosis of the upper extremity: Report of a series and review of the literature. Surgery 1988;104: 561–567.
43. Moss JF, Wagman LD, Riihimaki DU, Terz JJ. Central venous thrombosis related to the Silastic Hickman-Broviac catheters in an oncologic population. JPEN 1989;13:397–400.
44. Brismar B, Hardstedt C, Jacobson S. Diagnosis of thrombosis by catheter phlebography after prolonged central venous catheterization. Ann Surg 1981;194:779–783.
45. Jacobsen S, Brisman B. Blood hemoglobin: A possible predictor of central venous catheter-related thrombosis in parenteral nutrition. JPEN 1985;9:471–473.
46. Smith VC, Hallett JW Jr. Subclavian vein thrombosis during prolonged catheterization for parenteral nutrition: Early management and long-term follow-up. Thromb Parenter Nutr 1983;76:603–606.
47. Fraschini G, Jadeja J, Lawson M, Holmes FA, Carrasco HC, Wallace S. Local infusion of urokinase for the lysis of thrombosis associated with permanent central venous catheters in cancer patients. J Clin Oncol 1987;5:672–678.
48. Kramer FL, Goodman J, Allen S. Thrombolytic therapy in catheter-related subclavian venous thrombosis. J Can Assoc Radiol 1987;38:106–108.
49. Lacey SR, Zartisky AL, Azizkhan RG. Successful treatment of *Candida*-infected caval thrombosis in critically ill infants by low-dose streptokinase infusion. J Pediatr Surg 1988;23:1204–1209.
50. Lewis JA, LaFrance R, Bower RH. Treatment of an infected silicone right atrial catheter with combined fibrinolytic and antibiotic therapy: Case report and review of the literature. JPEN 1989;13:92–98.
51. Rubenstein M, Creger WP. Successful streptokinase therapy for catheter-induced subclavian vein thrombosis. Arch Intern Med 1980;140:1370–1371.
52. Fabri PJ, Mirtallo JM, Ruberg RL, et al. Incidence and prevention of thrombosis of the subclavian vein during total parenteral nutrition. Surg Gynecol Obstet 1982;155:238–240.
53. Wagman LD, Kirkemo A, Johnston MR. Venous access: A prospective randomized study of the Hickman catheter. Surgery 1984;95:303–308.
54. Hoar PF, Wilson RM, Mangano DT, Avery GJ, Szarnicki RJ, Hill JD. Heparin bonding reduces thrombogenicity of pulmonary-artery catheters. N Engl J Med 1981;305:993–995.
55. Bern MM, Lokich JJ, Wallach SR, et al. Very low doses of warfarin can prevent thrombosis in central venous catheters. Ann Intern Med 1990;112:423–428.
56. Press OW, Ramsey PG, Larson EB, Fefer A, Hickman RO. Hickman catheter infections in patients with malignancies. Medicine (Baltimore) 1984;63:189–200.
57. Krog MPM, Ekborn A, Nystrom-Rosander C, Rudberg CR, Simonsson NOB. Central venous catheters in acute blood malignancies. Cancer 1987;59:1358–1361.
58. Harvey MP, Trent RJ, Joshua DE, Ramsey-Stewart G, Storey DW, Kronenberg H. Complications associated with indwelling venous Hickman catheters in patients with hematological disorders. Aust N Z J Med 1986;16:211–215.
59. Schuman ES, Winters V, Gross GF, Hayes JF. Management of Hickman catheter sepsis. Am J Surg 1985;149:627–628.
60. Raaf JH. Results from use of 826 vascular access devices in cancer patients. Cancer 1985;55:1312–1321.
61. Benezra D, Kiehn TE, Gold JWM, Brown AE, Turnbull ADM, Armstrong D. Prospective study of infections in indwelling central venous catheters using quantitative blood cultures. Am J Med 1988;85:495–498.
62. Dugdale DC, Ramsey PG. *Staphylococcus aureus* bacteremia in patients with Hickman catheters. Am J Med 1990;89:137–141.
63. Flynn PM, van Hooser B, Gigliotti F. Atypical mycobacterial infections of Hickman catheter exit sites. Pediatr Infect Dis J 1991;1988:510–513.
64. Tenney JH, Moody MR, Newman KA, et al. Adherent microorganisms on luminal surfaces of long-term intravenous catheters. Arch Intern Med 1986;146:1949–1954.
65. Cooper GL, Hopkins CC. Rapid diagnosis of intravascular catheter-associated infection by direct Gram staining of catheter segments. N Engl J Med 1985;312:1142–1147.

66. Stillman RM, Soliman F, Garcia L, Sawyer PN. Etiology of catheter-associated sepsis. Arch Surg 1977;112:1497–1499.
67. Flynn PM, Shenep JL, Stokes DC, Barrett FF. In situ management of confirmed central venous catheter-related bacteremia. Pediatr Infect Dis J 1987;6:729–734.
68. Andremont A, Paulet R, Nitenberg G, Hill C. Value of semiquantitative cultures of blood drawn through catheter hubs for estimating the risk of catheter tip colonization in cancer patients. J Clin Microbiol 1988;26:2297–2299.
69. Cercenado E, Ena J, Rodriguez-Creixems M, Romero I, Bouza E. A conservative procedure for the diagnosis of catheter-related infections. Arch Intern Med 1990;150:1417–1420.
70. Viscoli C, Garaventa A, Boni L, et al. Role of Broviac catheters in infections in children with cancer. Pediatr Infect Dis J 1988;7:556–560.
71. Eppes SC, Troutman JL, Gutman LT. Outcome of treatment of candidemia in children whose central catheters were removed or retained. Pediatr Infect Dis J 1989;8:99–104.
72. Dato VM, Dajani AS. Candidemia in children with central venous catheters: Role of catheter removal and amphotericin B therapy. Pediatr Infect Dis J 1990;9:309–314.
73. Rohde TD, Buchwald H, Blackshear PJ. Implantable infusion pumps. In: Tyle P, ed. Drug delivery devices. New York: Marcel Dekker, 1988:235–260.
74. Fischell RE. A programmable implantable medication system (PIMS) as a means for intracorporeal drug delivery. In: Tyle P, ed. Drug delivery devices New York: Marcel Dekker, 1988:261–284.
75. Lukacsko P, May GS. Ambulatory infusion devices. In: Tyle P, ed. Drug delivery devices. New York: Marcel Dekker, 1988:178–211.

SECTION 6

ANTHONY B. MILLER

Cancer Screening

Of the approaches to cancer control that can reduce mortality—prevention, treatment, and screening—screening holds the greatest promise for a rapid and major impact, but because of practical and organizational difficulties, its potential may not be achieved. There are several scientific reasons why the early detection of cancer does not automatically guarantee reduced cancer mortality.[1] This chapter reviews the scientific basis for screening and considers the evidence on screening for several major cancers.

GENERAL PRINCIPLES OF SCREENING

There are benefits and disadvantages in screening for cancer.[2] The benefits include improved prognoses for some patients whose disease is detected by screening, but not for all. Those who benefit are primarily those who would have died from their disease without screening. This is the major benefit sought in screening programs. A second benefit of screening is that less radical treatment may be needed to cure some patients of their disease because it is detected at an early stage. A third benefit is reassurance for those with negative test results. Many people participate in screening programs for reassurance. A fourth benefit is resource savings, especially lower treatment cost if less radical treatment is instituted, and lower costs for treating patients who otherwise would have died from their disease, because these costs can be substantial.

The list of disadvantages is somewhat longer. The first is a longer period of morbidity because of earlier detection for patients whose prognosis is unaltered. A second disadvantage is overtreatment of borderline abnormalities. Many abnormalities discovered by screening might never have been recognized without a positive screening test. A third disadvantage is false reassurance for those with false-negative screening tests. In such cases, the subsequent development of symptoms may be ignored, with postponement of the diagnosis and a poorer prognosis than if the symptoms had led to prompt diagnosis. A fourth disadvantage is unnecessary morbidity for those with false-positive screening tests, which may initiate a complex series of diagnostic tests. A fifth disadvantage is the potential hazard of the test itself. There are also resource costs from administering the screening test, from the diag-

nostic tests induced by false positives, and from the overtreatment of borderline abnormalities.

Because of these disadvantages, it is important to insist on appropriate evaluation of the effectiveness of screening. This process begins with evaluation of the test itself, which should have adequate sensitivity (*i.e.*, proportion of those with the disease who test positive) and specificity (*i.e.*, proportion of those free of the disease who test negative) and be acceptable to those who are invited to be screened. The process continues with evaluation of the screening program. The ideal approach is the randomized controlled trial, in which participants are randomized to be screened and their outcome in terms of mortality from the cancer is compared with the randomized control group.[2] Although expensive, these trials are the only way to avoid the biases that accompany other methods to evaluate the effectiveness of screening, especially those that attempt to use numbers of cases detected, stage distribution, or survival as the principal endpoints. The biases are lead time, the time by which diagnosis is advanced by screening; length bias, the tendency of screening to detect cases of disease with a more prolonged natural history and a better prognosis than normal; selection bias, reflecting the recruitment of volunteers to screening who tend to have different risks of disease or death from disease than the general population; and overdiagnosis bias, the tendency of screening to bring to light and label as disease lesions that might never have been diagnosed in the patient's lifetime.[1]

If a precursor of cancer is identified by the screening test, treatment of this lesion may interrupt the natural history of the cancer and reduce the reported incidence of disease in the screened population. However, if the cancer is detected through screening, the incidence of the disease is increased (because of lead time and possibly overdiagnosis), and mortality from the disease in the population screened is the only valid outcome measure. Designs other than the randomized trial that use mortality in the population screened as the endpoint can avoid lead time, length bias, and overdiagnosis bias, but they cannot avoid selection bias, and they may overestimate or underestimate the effectiveness of screening. This especially affects the case-control approach, in which the screening history of cases (*i.e.*, deaths or patients with advanced disease) are compared with those of controls drawn from the same population.[3]

Even though screening has been judged to be effective, the programs introduced should be monitored to ensure that they achieve the expected benefits and that changes are not required in their organization. Reasons for failure include poor sensitivity of the test in routine practice or failure to screen those in the population at greatest risk for the disease. There may be a failure of the process of diagnosis or treatment that should follow a positive test. Screening should not be introduced unless there are adequate facilities for diagnosis and treatment of the detected abnormalities and effective treatment for detected disease. Even if these exist, failure of the referral process for diagnosis or treatment can result in failure of screening.

SCREENING FOR CERVICAL CANCER

Because screening for cervical cancer was introduced before there was recognition of the need to evaluate programs by randomized trials, other mechanisms have been used to evaluate the effectiveness of screening for this disease. They include geographic comparisons of screened and unscreened populations combined with studies of the trends of incidence and mortality that followed introduction of screening,[4] studies that correlated the intensity of screening with reduction in mortality from the disease,[5] and case-control studies.[6] Because a precursor is detected by screening (*e.g.*, carcinoma in situ, severe dysplasia), reduction in the incidence of the disease and reduction in mortality are valid endpoints.

Few countries have observed a dramatic reduction of the incidence or mortality from the disease that could be directly related to the introduction of screening. The exceptions to this are largely the Nordic countries, where organized programs were introduced and an impressive reduction in incidence and mortality followed within 6 to 10 years.[5] In North America and much of Europe, where organized screening was not introduced and screening was largely opportunistic (*i.e.*, using approaches that depend on the physician or the woman herself), reductions have not been dramatic, and it has often been difficult to determine the extent to which screening has been responsible. There is increasing interest in introducing organized programs in these countries, as indicated by a workshop report in Canada.[7]

The essential features of organized programs have been described[6]:

The women in the target population are identifiable.

Measures are available to guarantee high coverage and attendance, such as a personal letter of invitation.

There are adequate field facilities for taking the smears and adequate laboratory facilities to examine them.

An organized quality control program on taking of the smears and on interpreting them;

Adequate facilities exist for diagnosis and for appropriate treatment of confirmed neoplastic lesions.

There is a carefully designed and agreed referral system for management of any abnormalities found and for providing information about normal screening tests.

Evaluation and monitoring of the total program is organized.

One of the most controversial issues in cervical cancer screening is the frequency of rescreening. The American Cancer Society (ACS),[8] largely echoing an earlier report by a Canadian Task Force,[9] recommended screening every 3 years. This proved intensely controversial, especially to several clinical interests, and the recommendation was later changed back to one that could be interpreted as approving annual smears, although the physician has the discretion to perform tests less frequently.[10,11] This change was reflected in the Early Detection Working Guidelines of the National Cancer Institute (NCI) (Table 21–8).[12]

The changed guidelines failed to reflect the natural history of the disease. Several studies, including one from British Columbia, showed that the progression to invasive cancer from preclinical disease could take several years or decades.[13] The British Columbia and other data had been used in a mathematical model, the findings of which largely underlay the earlier ACS recommendations.[14] These data, together with data from other studies largely from Europe, were combined by a working group of the International Agency for Research on Cancer.[15] The analysis documented the expected degree of benefit from a negative screening test. Protection was maximal in the first 3 years after a negative test and persisted to some degree for at least 5 years. On the basis of this analysis, it was possible to compute the expected degree of benefit from different schedules of rescreening (Table 21–9). Almost as much benefit is obtained from tests conducted at 3-year

TABLE 21–8. Screening Recommendations for Major Cancer Sites

Site	UICC[3]	ACS[11]	NCI[49]	NCI[12]
Cervix	Smear ever 3 y from age 25–64	Annual smear from age 18; after 3 negative smears, less frequently at discretion of physician	Smear every 3 y from age 20–70	Annual smear from age 18; after 3 negative smears, less frequently at discretion of physician
Breast	MX +/− Px every 2 y age 50–69	Px every y from age 40; Mx every 1–2 y from age 40, every y from age 50; BSE every mo from age 20–40	Mx + Px every y from age 50	Px with each periodic exam; Mx every 1–2 y from age 40, every y from age 50; BSE every mo
Colon, rectum	NR	FOBT every y; sigmoidoscopy every 3–5 y from age 50; annual rectal from age 40	NR	FOBT every y; sigmoidoscopy every 3–5 y from age 50; annual rectal from age 40
Lung	NR	NR	NR	NC
Stomach	NR (except Japan)	NR	NR	NR
Prostate	NR	NC	NR	Annual rectal from age 40

Mx, mammography; Px, physical examination; NR, no recommendation; FOBT, fecal occult blood test; NC, not considered; BSE, breast self-examination.

TABLE 21–9. Effect of Different Screening Policies for Cervical Cancer

Screening Schedule	Cumulative Incidence of Cervical Cancer per 100,000 Women, 20–64 y	Percent Reduction in Cancer Incidence	No. of Tests
1. No screening	1575		
2. Screening every 5 y, ages 20–64	257.6	83.6	9
2a. Screening every 5 y, ages 25–64	286.7	81.8	8
2b. Screening every 5 y, ages 35–64	478.8	69.6	6
2c. Screening every year, ages 20– 34 then every 5 y, ages 35–64	232.3	85.5	21
2d. Screening at age 25, 26, 30, then every 5 y	274.5	82.6	9
3. Screening every 3 y, ages 20–64	137.8	91.2	15
3a. Screening every 3 y, ages 26–64	161.0	89.8	13
3b. Screening every 3 y, ages 35–64	352.8	77.6	10
3c. Screening every year, ages 20– 34, then every 3 y, ages 35–64	131.2	91.7	25
3d. Screening at age 25, 26, 29, then every 3 y	156.6	90.1	14
4. Screening every year, ages 20–64	105.0	93.3	45

(From IARC Working Group on Cervical Cancer Screening. Summary chapter. In: Hakama M, Miller AB, Day NE, eds. Screening for cancer of the uterine cervix. IARC Scientific Publications, No. 76. Lyon: International Agency for Research on Cancer, 1986:133–142)

intervals as from annual screening, at a considerable saving of resources.

The analysis assumes that the test is of high sensitivity and that a high proportion of at risk women attend for screening. Adequate sensitivity of the test can only be achieved by high-quality laboratory services and good compliance with an organized program; both are prerequisites for effective screening programs.[7] However, defects in either of these parameters can not be overcome by increasing the frequency of rescreening. Instead, actions must ensure an effective and cost-effective program.[6] The difficulty with annual screening, even in a wealthy country, is that it places emphasis on rescreening of women already in programs, but the emphasis needs to shift to bring women who are poorly screened or not screened at all into programs if failures of screening policies are to be avoided.[9,16]

Two other features of cervical cancer screening have proven controversial: the age range over which screening should be performed and the management of the preclinical lesions found as a result of screening. Table 21–9 indicates that initiating screening for patients 25 years of age is almost as effective as initiating screening at 20 years, but that postponing initiation of screening until age 35 is less effective, although not markedly so. Most jurisdictions in North America recommend initiation of screening of sexually active women between the ages of 18 to 20, because of a high frequency of preclinical lesions in young women.[7] One advantage of such a policy is that it can capitalize on the attendance of young women for contraceptive advice or antenatal care. However, many successful screening programs in Europe do not initiate screening until age 25.[3,6] Concentrating all screening on special health services for young women is not wise, because in most countries, those most at risk for the disease are women in their fifties and sixties who have not been screened or who

have lapsed from screening. It is one of the main purposes of organized programs of screening to ensure that these women are screened.

Screening is stopped for women who are 70 years old in Canada,[7] and screening every 3 years has been determined to be cost-effective for women older than 65 in the United States.[17] The International Union Against Cancer (UICC) Project on Evaluation of Screening for Cancer pointed out that "the protective effect at ages older than 65 is largely unknown in women who have been previously screened. Because of problems in taking smears, attendance for screening and possibly a lesser protection at older ages . . . it may be appropriate not to extend screening beyond the age of 65 for women who have had several negative smears in the previous 10 years and no positive smears."[3] A possibly more acceptable compromise for these women was adopted in Canada by extending the upper age to 69, although this was a research program issue.[7] However, there is little disagreement with the rest of the UICC recommendation for older women: "Women older than 65 who have not had several negative smears should continue to be screened until they have achieved such a record (at least two negative smears)."[3]

There has been concern expressed about substantial observer disagreement in classifying less severe forms of dysplasia and its importance in indicating increased risk of invasive cancer. The role of human papillomavirus-associated lesions in management is also controversial. Attempts to reduce the confusion about classification by setting up a two-stage system (*i.e.,* the Bethesda system[18]) was not judged in Canada to be helpful.[7] Reinforced by data confirming a low probability of progression for mild dysplasia, the Canadian group recommended cytologic surveillance for women with these lesions every 6 months for as long as 2 years unless there was cytologic evidence of progression. For cytologic abnormalities compatible with moderate or severe dysplasia, immediate referral for colposcopy for diagnosis was recommended.[7]

"Screening for cancer of the cervix is effective in reducing the incidence and mortality from the disease and is applicable as public health policy."[3] Maximal effectiveness is achieved by an organized program with broad coverage that initiates screening of women at the age of 25 and continues with screening every 3 or 5 years until the age of 60. Variations from this approach should only be considered if maximal coverage has been obtained, the resources are available, and the marginal cost effectiveness of the change has been evaluated.

SCREENING FOR BREAST CANCER

Much is known about screening for breast cancer, largely because this is a site for which several controlled trials and other studies have been completed or are in progress. The initial studies were in the United States, and subsequently, much of the activity has been in Europe.

UNITED STATES

The first trial of screening was that of the Health Insurance Plan (HIP) of greater New York. Approximately 62,000 women between the ages of 40 and 64 were randomized in the early 1960s to screening by annual mammography and physical examination of the breasts to a total of four screens or to a control group. Of those invited to be screened, 65% were screened at least once. The early (5-year) mortality results indicated a significant reduction in breast cancer mortality but was restricted to those between the ages of 50 and 64.[19] Subsequent follow-up (eventually completed at 18 years) suggested a benefit in younger women, commencing much later than that in older women, but the accrual numbers for the different age groups were small, and there is controversy about whether a real benefit was observed in the younger women.[20,21] The HIP study was conducted in the early years of mammography, and only 33% of breast cancer cases were detected by mammography alone with only 25% in women between the ages of 40 and 49. Physical examination conducted by carefully trained surgeons made a substantial contribution to case detection, and some have estimated that as much as 70% of the benefit from the screen may have been derived from the physical examinations.[21]

The HIP study was followed by the Breast Cancer Detection Demonstration Project (BCDDP). In the project, the combination of annual mammography, thermography, and physical examination of the breasts was used for 280,000 women 35 years of age and older. Because there was no control group, it was difficult to evaluate its effectiveness.[22] It was clear that thermography was not sensitive nor specific enough to be a viable screening test. Mammography had higher sensitivity than in the HIP study, especially for women younger than 50. Extensive data on case detection and survival have been published for this study that cannot be used to infer effectiveness of the screen because of the biases reviewed earlier in this chapter.[23,24] The breast cancer mortality rates for as long as 9 years in the study population have been compared with those expected in the general population.[25] Results indicate little

benefit for younger women, but in those 50 years of age or older who were recorded in the study files as asymptomatic on entry, a 40% reduction of breast cancer mortality below expectation was computed.

Two case-control studies evaluating the possible role of breast self-examination (BSE) in reducing advanced breast cancer have been reported.[26,27] Both were negative, although in one, there appeared to be some benefit for those who performed BSE.[26]

EUROPEAN STUDIES

Three population breast screening programs, two in the Netherlands and one in Italy, were evaluated with the case-control approach.[28–30] All three showed an effect of screening in reducing deaths in women older than 50 but no effect for younger women.[29,30] Two projects used mammography alone,[29,30] and the other used mammography plus physical examination.[28]

Four randomized trials are ongoing in Sweden. The largest, the two-county trial, used single mediolateral oblique view mammography every 21 months for women 40 to 49 years old and every 33 months for women 50 to 74. A significant reduction in breast cancer mortality in women 50 to 69 years of age was seen, starting at about 4 years after the initiation of screening and persisting through 10 years, but there was no effect for women 40 to 49 years old.[31,32] The other long-running trial (10 years) was in Malmö and used double-view mammography for women 45 to 69.[33] The effect was small and restricted to women older than 55. In younger women, there was a nonsignificant excess breast cancer mortality in the mammography group in the first 5 years after initiation of screening.

The third Swedish trial in Stockholm shows at 7 years an apparent effect for older women but not for those between 40 and 49 years of age.[34] The results of these trials are summarized in Table 21-10 and compared with the 10-year results of the HIP trial. Mortality results have not yet been reported from the fourth Swedish trial. An overview analysis of the four Swedish trials is in progress. This is expected to be completed in 1992. It may resolve the controversy that arose over the apparent differences in the findings in the two-county and Malmö trials.

In the United Kingdom, an ongoing study is comparing women 45 to 64 years of age who are screened by biennial mammography and annual physical examinations with a randomized component in one center (Edinburgh). Initial mortality results have been reported from the main study, and breast cancer mortality was reduced at years 6 and 7 in the two screening centers compared with the four control areas, but not in the two areas where only BSE teaching was offered, although an independent evaluation of BSE in one of these centers suggested some benefit.[35,36] In the Edinburgh randomized trial, no benefit was seen (Table 21–10).[37]

ONGOING STUDIES

A screening test for which there is little evidence of effectiveness is BSE. Several ongoing studies may eventually provide the evidence needed.[38] Only BSE has the potential to improve the outlook for interval cancers. The World Health

TABLE 21–10. Reduction of Breast Cancer Mortality by Age in the Randomized Screening Trials

Investigations	Patient Age at Entry	Study Group (Popn./Deaths)		Control Group (Popn./Deaths)		Percent Reduction in Study Group* (95% CI)
HIP	40–49	13682	39	13804	51	24 (−16; 50)
	50–59	12756	42	12967	61	31 (−2; 54)
	60–64	3698	14	3797	21	33 (6; 53)
Two-county	40–49	19844	28	15604	24	8 (−60; 48)
	50–59	23485	45	16805	54	40 (10; 60)
	60–69	23412	52	16269	58	35 (5; 36)
	70–74	10339	35	7307	31	23 (−24; 49)
Malmö	45–54	7981	28	8082	22	−29 (−125; 26)
	55–69	13107	35	13113	44	21 (−24; 49)
Stockholm	40–49	14375	16	7142	8	−7 (−116; 47)
	50–64	24789	23	12840	22	36 (−8; 62)
Edinburgh	45–54	11914	31	11148	31	7 (−28; 42)
	55–64	11312	37	10756	45	14 (−6; 52)

* A negative value indicates an increase in breast cancer mortality in the study group.
(Rutqvist LE, Miller AB, Andersson I, et al. Reduced breast cancer mortality with mammography screening—an assessment of currently available data. Int J Cancer Suppl 1990;5:76–84)

Organization concluded that only BSE can provide early diagnosis of breast cancer in many parts of the world.[39] Three studies are evaluating the effect of BSE. One is a cohort study of the Mama BSE program introduced by Gastrin in Finland in 1973.[40] The records of almost 30,000 women who enrolled in the program from 1973 to 1975 and who returned BSE calendars to Dr. Gastrin have been identified, and passive follow-up was conducted by record linkage to the Finnish Cancer Registry. The analysis shows elevated breast cancer incidence but reduced breast cancer mortality compared with that expected from the Finnish population.[41] The other two studies are randomized trials. The first, being conducted with group randomization by factory in Moscow and polyclinic in St. Petersburg has enrolled almost 200,000 women, half of whom have been instructed in BSE. Follow-up is expected to last at least through 1998.[42] The other trial, planned to enroll about 300,000, is underway in Shanghai.

There are two ongoing trials designed to evaluate the effect of screening for women between the ages of 40 and 49. The first, the National Breast Screening Study (NBSS) in Canada, has for women between the ages of 40 and 49 at entry the objective of determining the benefit of the combination of annual mammography, physical examination, and BSE instruction.[43] For women between the ages of 50 and 59 on entry, the trial is evaluating the incremental effect of mammography over and above physical examination and BSE instruction. Preliminary data on advanced breast cancers suggest no early mortality reduction in women between the ages of 40 and 49 and no difference for women 50 to 59 years old.[44] The other trial designed to evaluate the role of mammography screening in younger women is in its pilot phase in the United Kingdom. Women between the ages of 40 and 41 will be enrolled, randomized to annual mammography screening or no screening, and maintained on these allocations until they

reach the age of 50, when they will enter the U.K. National Screening Program. This will be a very large trial, and it may be many years before results are available.

An additional ongoing trial in the United Kingdom is designed to compare mammography screening every 1 or 3 years.

POLICY IMPLICATIONS

The UICC project on screening for cancer recently updated its conclusions on breast cancer screening.[3] The main conclusion was that screening by mammography every 1 to 3 years can reduce breast cancer mortality substantially in women between the ages of 50 and 70. In women younger than 50, there is little evidence of a benefit, at least in the first 10 years after initiation of screening.

The reason for the difference in the effects of screening younger and older women is not clear. Three reasons have been considered: reduced sensitivity of the screening tests in younger women, biologic difference in breast cancer premenopausally and postmenopausally, and the relative failure of therapy in younger women. The first two explanations achieved partial support from the Swedish two-county study,[45] and the latter was supported by the preliminary results of the Canadian NBSS.[44] Whatever the reason, breast cancer screening in younger women is less cost effective than in older women. This conclusion, first raised as a result of mathematical modeling of results available until about 1987, is confirmed by the failure of the more recently published studies to show a benefit in younger women.[46] Even if a benefit is eventually seen after follow-up of women in existing trials beyond 10 years from entry, the lack of benefit in the early years combined with the lower breast cancer mortality for women in their forties means that screening younger women is far less cost effective than screening older women. Although the Canadian NBSS was planned in the late 1970s with adequate power to detect a 40% reduction in breast cancer mortality in women between the ages of 40 and 49 at entry, the U.K. trial using women between the ages of 40 and 41 was planned in the late 1980s with power to detect a 20% reduction in breast cancer mortality, a figure believed to be more realistic in view of the evidence that had accumulated in the 1980s.

These considerations dispute the appropriateness of the updated recommendations of the ACS,[11] those of the American College of Radiology,[47] and the NCI Working Guidelines[12] that mammography be offered every 1 to 2 years for women age 40 to 49. The Canadian working group made no recommendation for screening this age group. In Table 21–8, the UICC recommendations for screening are compared with those of the ACS and the two sets of recommendations from the NCI.[8,11,12,49]

The radiation dosage required for mammography has fallen substantially from the 8-cGy surface dose used in the HIP study to 3 to 1 cGy used in the BCDDP, to 0.6 to 0.2 cGy used in the NBSS. Several analyses have confirmed that the benefit to be derived from low-dose modern mammography substantially exceeds any possible hazard, especially for women older than 40.[50–52]

Many groups have emphasized the importance of high-quality mammography and skillful interpretation of mammograms to localize and diagnose impalpable lesions.[3,40,53,54] The UICC project considers that screening every 2 years of women older than 50 is satisfactory, but screening of younger women many require shorter intervals.[3,40] These conclusions are reflected in the Swedish and Canadian programs,[48,55] although in the United Kingdom the program is restricted to women 50 to 69 years of age and given as single-view mammography every 3 years.[56] These approaches are different from those advocated by the ACS and the NCI (see Table 21–8), although not from the recommendations of the U.S. Preventive Services Task Force, which does not recommend mammography screening before the age of 50.[57] The Task Force also accepts mammography screening over the age of 50 every 1 or 2 years. This is supported by a Dutch analysis, which suggests that annual screening for women older than 50 may not be cost effective.[58]

SCREENING FOR COLORECTAL CANCER

Colorectal cancer is an important cause of morbidity and mortality in both sexes, and its natural history may make it amenable to control by screening.[59] There are two screening tests available: sigmoidoscopy and tests for occult blood in the feces. The initial evaluation of screening was by uncontrolled studies, such as that of Gilbertsen, who thought he had demonstrated a reduction in incidence and mortality from colorectal cancer after performing annual proctosigmoidoscopy on 21,150 men and women and following them for 5 years.[60,61] However, he failed to include the prevalent cases detected in his calculation of incidence, and considering the selective nature of the population screened, the improved survival demonstrated may simply have reflected screening biases.[62]

Several controlled trials of colorectal cancer screening have been conducted or are in progress. The earliest evaluated dig-

ital rectal examination and rigid sigmoidoscopy as part of multiphasic health screen offered annually. The control group was offered "usual care" and could request screening. Although a reduction in mortality from colorectal cancer was seen in the study group at 11 years, evaluation of the 16-year results suggested this was probably due to chance and not due to the effect of sigmoidoscopy.[63,64]

The other trials are evaluating the effect of the fecal occult blood test (FOBT). Two trials in the United States have been running long enough for results on mortality to be expected, but incomplete results have been presented for one, and no results have been published for the other. The trial in New York is evaluating the effect of the addition of the FOBT to routine sigmoidoscopic screening.[65] It was not randomized, and the results are difficult to interpret.[66] The trial in Minnesota used the FOBT alone, annually in one group and biennially in another. Because a decision was made to resume screening in that trial (stopped by design a few years ago), mortality results can not be expected for several years.[67]

A major difficulty with screening using the FOBT is a lack of specificity, especially if the test sample is rehydrated.[68] There seems to be a lack in sensitivity for detection of adenomas. The evidence for this is somewhat indirect but relates to the postulated adenoma-cancer sequence. If an appreciable proportion of cancers arise from adenomas and if the FOBT is capable of detecting adenomas, a reduction in incidence of colorectal cancer should be seen after FOBT screening, but this has so far not been observed in the trials.[3,68]

There has been a tendency to make recommendations on screening for colorectal cancer largely on the basis of the results from mathematical models.[8] The UICC project reviewed the mathematical models and carefully considered the assumptions that underlay them.[68] We concluded that the models should not be used as a basis for policy decisions unless and until their assumptions about benefit are based on actual data from controlled trials.

Without evidence that screening for colorectal cancer can reduce mortality, screening for colorectal cancer or its precursors is not recommended by the UICC project as public health policy.[3,68] The same conclusion was reached by the NCI Year 2000 Screening Committee.[49] The current trials should provide answers to some of the uncertainties, but results cannot be expected for 4 to 5 years. In the meantime, the ACS recommends that screening should start at age 50, with FOBT annually and sigmoidoscopy every 5 years.[11] The NCI Working Guidelines call for annual FOBT and sigmoidoscopy every 3 to 5 years after the age of 50 (see Table 21–8).[12] However, because compliance with these procedures is low, there may have to be major public and professional educational programs to accept the programs. Flexible sigmoidoscopy may have a role, if compliance can be demonstrated to be satisfactory, and there are plans to evaluate it as part of a major multicenter trial.[69]

OTHER SCREENING PROGRAMS

LUNG CANCER

Several early studies suggested that screening for lung cancer by means of semiannual chest radiographs with or without sputum cytology did not improve the prognosis of lung cancer in the populations studied.[2] In the 1970s, three randomized trials of lung cancer screening were initiated in the United States. Although chest radiographs and sputum cytologic analyses are capable of detecting cases in high-risk male heavy smokers, sputum cytology at 4-month intervals adds a small proportion of cases to those discovered by annul chest radiographs and does not demonstrably reduce lung cancer mortality. Chest radiographs at 4-month intervals confer no mortality advantage over routine care that includes annual chest radiographs.

The UICC group recommended assessing the value of the annual chest radiograph and suggested that case-control studies might have promise in this regard.[2] A study performed in the German Democratic Republic evaluated the role of mass miniature radiographs obtained at 2-year intervals and found no evidence that radiologic screening reduced the mortality from lung cancer.[70]

The UICC project[2] and the ACS[8] concluded that screening with sputum cytology and or chest radiographs could not be recommended. The negative conclusions from the three American controlled trials were such that the NCI Working Guidelines do not discuss screening for this site (see Table 21–8).[12] All organizations agree that the emphasis for control of lung cancer must be on prevention.

However, there are still concerns that the annual chest radiograph may have some value, because only one of the U.S. trials randomized 4-monthly chest radiographs, and a small reduction in lung cancer mortality could have been missed. The proposed multicenter trial will evaluate annual chest radiographs with a large enough population to ensure adequate power.[69]

BLADDER CANCER

Urinary cytology is capable of detecting urinary bladder cancers in persons in high-risk occupations and those living in areas where urinary schistosomiasis is endemic.[2] Improved survival of patients with screening-detected bladder cancer has been demonstrated, but it is unknown if a reduction in mortality will follow. Screening-detected cases in areas where urinary schistosomiasis is endemic are discovered at an earlier stage and require less extensive therapy than those diagnosed by routine measures. However, if bladder cancer screening is to play a role in cancer control, further research is needed. The role of urinary cytology in reducing mortality from bladder cancer in high-risk occupational groups and in areas of urinary schistosomiasis must be evaluated, preferably by means of controlled trials. An important prerequisite is to undertake treatment trials of early lesions found by screening.[71]

Until the results of controlled trials prove otherwise, screening for bladder cancer is not recommended as public health policy.[2]

ORAL CANCER

Visual examination is capable of identifying presymptomatic oral cancers. Exfoliative cytology is less sensitive than visual examination.[2] Neither test has been shown to reduce mortality from oral cancer. In technically advanced countries, it is difficult to evaluate the role of routine dental examinations, because they tend to be undertaken on people at low risk; high-

risk persons often avoid dental care. In developing countries where the disease incidence is high, programs have been proposed based on inspection for oral epithelial dysplasia by allied health professionals.[72] These have not been fully evaluated. Primary prevention could be combined with an oral cancer screening program. Oral examination as part of the periodic health examination is recommended by the NCI, especially for those at high risk due to tobacco and alcohol addiction, although no guidance is offered for ensuring that those most at risk for the disease can be persuaded to accept the examinations.[12]

OVARIAN CANCER

Ovarian cancer is common in Western countries and has a relatively high mortality rate, now in excess of cervical cancer because of the inaccessibility of the ovaries and the late stage of diagnosis of many ovarian cancers. Several screening tests are being developed, and tests for CA 125 and vaginal ultrasound are being evaluated.[3,6] One of the difficulties is the low specificity of the tests in premenopausal women. High specificity of the tests is essential, because diagnostic confirmation is invasive. In premenopausal women, the incidence of ovarian cancer is also low. This has led to the restriction of studies to postmenopausal women, in whom the disease incidence and the specificity of the tests are higher. It is still unknown whether the tests are sufficiently sensitive to produce a major benefit. Although using two or more tests can increase sensitivity if a positive result in either is acted on, this leads to a loss of specificity and increases costs and morbidity. Several issues must be addressed before ovarian cancer screening can be considered as public health policy. The proposed multicenter trial of other cancer sites has been expanded to include screening for ovarian cancer as a major component.[69]

ENDOMETRIAL CANCER

Although endometrial cancer is relatively common in Western countries, the person-years saved by screening may be limited, because it is largely a disease of elderly women. Available screening tests are based on endometrial samples subjected to cytologic analysis. These are not simple tests, and they require considerable care in their application.[6] Much more research into the effectiveness of endometrial cancer screening is required before it can be determined whether screening is likely to play a role in controlling the disease.

STOMACH CANCER

Screening programs for stomach cancer were introduced in Japan more than 20 years ago.[68] The screening test used has gradually been standardized and now comprises a photofluorographic barium meal technique with six standard views. In one area of Finland, screening using an immunologic test on gastric juice has been conducted.[73]

The UICC project concluded that considerable observational evidence had accumulated, including time trend and correlational analyses and one case-control study, and that the widespread application of screening in Japan had contributed to decreased mortality, although its contribution is probably smaller than that from declining incidence.[3,68,74,75] Because of uncertainty about its effectiveness, screening for gastric cancer in countries other than Japan cannot be recommended as public health policy. In the United States, no organization advocates screening for gastric cancer.

LIVER CANCER

Screening by means of serum α-fetoprotein levels is being evaluated in some parts of China where the risk of liver cancer is very high.[68] There is some evidence that small liver cancers can be successfully treated, but pending further research, screening for liver cancer cannot be recommended as public health policy.[68]

ESOPHAGUS

A similar conclusion was reached by the UICC group on esophageal cancer screening.[68] Although a test is available that involves cytologic examination of cells from possible precancerous lesions obtained with the aid of a balloon, there are difficulties associated with the cytologic diagnosis of esophageal dysplasia. Another concern is the unavailability of suitable treatment for any abnormalities found. Research into chemoprevention may provide a solution.

PROSTATE CANCER

Prostate cancer is the most frequently diagnosed cancer in men in the United States and second (after lung) in Canada, and in these countries, it is second only to lung cancer as a cause of mortality.[76,77] The incidence of prostate cancer rises steeply with increasing age relatively late in life, and it therefore has less importance as a cause of potential years of life lost; in Canada, it is number three after lung and colorectal cancer.[77] Nevertheless, it can be an important cause of morbidity, and there is increasing interest in the possibility of screening for prostate cancer using the digital rectal examination (DRE) or the prostate-specific antigen (PSA) and possibly transrectal ultrasound, although the latter may be of more value as a diagnostic test.[78] Screening for prostate cancer using the DRE is recommended by the ACS and in the early-detection guidelines of the NCI (see Table 21–8), but this may not be a valid screening test, because its sensitivity for early prostate cancer appears to be low.

There are many obstacles in the way of an effective screening program for prostate cancer. An acceptable and valid screening test must be available, and it must be matched by an acceptable and effective treatment for the preclinical lesions found.[3] This problem is particularly acute for prostate cancer because of the increasing frequency of latent prostatic carcinoma with increasing age and the morbidity and mortality of the radical procedures commonly used to treat prostate cancer.

Few data are available on the sensitivity and specificity of the screening tests that have been proposed.[69] Part of the difficulty is that studies have generally not been performed in screening circumstances, and the inferences drawn from clinical series may not be replicated in a screening program. A Toronto study suggested that ultrasound alone had the lowest sensitivity and positive predictive value.[78] DRE and PSA used alone had equivalent sensitivity, but PSA had better positive predictive value than DRE. The addition of PSA to DRE with ultrasound used to decide on a biopsy if either was negative marginally increased sensitivity but at a cost of a reduced positive predictive value. In this series, the PSA was the best screening test, and ultrasound was the worst.

Thompson and Fair reviewed the results of their own studies and those of others.[79] Although serum tumor markers (*e.g.*, PSA) have great appeal for mass screening, statistical analysis suggests that most patients with localized prostate carcinoma remain undetected, most detected cancers have progressed beyond local disease, and most patients with positive tests are subjected unnecessarily to expensive and potentially morbid diagnostic procedures. Currently, serum tumor markers cannot be advocated for mass screening for carcinoma of the prostate.[79]

In a Swedish study of DRE, there were 13 confirmations among 45 men suspected of having cancer of the prostate.[80] This worked out as a prevalence of 11.2 cancer cases per 1000 screened, with a positive predictive value of the test of 29% and a specificity of the order of 97.2%. This detection rate is about nine times the expected annual incidence, which is a much larger excess than expected for other sites, suggesting that symptomatic men preferentially volunteered or that a large number of latent cancers were detected.[78] Cancer of the prostate is frequently found at autopsy, especially in elderly men. Although it is not certain that the DRE or the PSA will be particularly sensitive to these lesions, a substantial proportion of the cancers found, especially at the upper end of the age range likely to be included in screening, may have such lesions. The cost of the treatment in terms of postoperative mortality could easily overwhelm any possible benefit of screening in delaying mortality for a few.[81]

The crucial distinction between screening and normal medical diagnosis and care is that the encounter is not originated by the individual who is the subject of screening; the provider of screening initiates the process.[82] The screener believes that the health of the community will be better as a result of screening. It is not possible to be certain that the health of everyone offered screening will be better, but the screener at least has an obligation to minimize the possibility of harm. These conditions cannot yet be met for screening for prostate cancer, and therefore screening for this condition should only be offered in the context of a properly designed randomized trial with validly constituted informed consent forms. Trials must be completed before a recommendation for including screening in a program of cancer control could be developed.[3] We are probably at least a decade away from such a recommendation. Prostate cancer screening is an important component of the multicenter trial under consideration.[69]

OTHER CANCERS

The UICC project has considered screening for melanoma, neuroblastoma, and nasopharyngeal carcinoma.[3] For none of these conditions is screening recommended as public health policy. For melanoma, the issue is the lack of documented effectiveness of screening, although self-examination and referral to skin clinics as part of public education campaigns have been advocated and are being assessed in some areas.[3] Some have advocated screening for those with the dysplasia nevus syndrome.[83]

The NCI Working Guidelines recommend testicular self-examination and routine palpation of the testicles as part of the periodic health examination.[12] However, no data uncontaminated by screening biases are offered in support of this recommendation.

FUTURE PERSPECTIVES

There are several obstacles to a major contribution from screening to cancer control.[84] These include an unfavorable natural history of many cancers, particularly lung cancer; poor organization of screening programs; and poor compliance of those at risk, especially for cancer of the cervix. Poor compliance may be exacerbated by economic barriers, and economic factors may be one of the reasons that only 37% of physicians followed the ACS guidelines on mammography screening for breast cancer in 1989.[85] For several cancers, a valid and effective screening test is not available. One class of screening test under development is based on monoclonal antibody technology, and such tests are already being considered for ovarian cancer.[3,6] There must be sensitive diagnostic tests to localize the small cancers detected by screening, unless the screening test can serve both functions, as with the use of radiolabeled antibodies. Continued research is also needed to reduce the cost and morbidity of treatment after false-positive tests (*e.g.*, screening for colorectal cancer).

In considering the potential contribution of screening to reduced cancer mortality by the year 2000, only screening breast and cervical cancers is judged likely to make an impact, and even the relatively small impact envisaged (*i.e.*, 3% reduction in overall cancer mortality) would require substantial increases in the proportion of women being screened.[49] For the other sites, it seems unlikely that any major impact will be achieved before the year 2000 (Table 21–11). I have lowered my estimate of a possible effect for screening colorectal cancer from that previously reported because of a lack of evidence of effectiveness accruing in the last 5 years.[84] However, even the impact envisaged must be regarded as temporary palliation, because continued effect demands continued

TABLE 21–11. Potential for Reduction in Mortality From Cancer With Screening by the Year 2000

Cancer Site	Percent Reduction in Mortality
Cervix	60
Breast	25
Lung	0
Colon/rectum	10
Bladder	5
Oral	5
Stomach (Japan)	30
Ovary	0
Endometrium	0
Other	5*

* A possible efffect of melanoma early-detection programs.

screening programs. Screening is a less productive approach to the control of cancer than prevention. Nevertheless, prevention may require many decades to achieve its full potential, and screening, which offers a fairly rapid return from appropriate investment, should remain part of our armamentarium for cancer control.

Several principles govern the introduction of screening programs:

The disease should be an important health problem.

The disease should have a detectable preclinical phase.

The natural history of the lesions identified by screening should be known.

There should be an effective treatment for the lesions.

The screening test should be acceptable and safe.

Ethics and economics also affect the possibility of cancer control by screening. Critical issues include the population to be included in screening programs and whether or not it is possible to introduce an organized screening program. It should not be assumed that a screening program for cancer will benefit the population to which it is applied. Ethics demand that only programs with proven effectiveness be widely disseminated, and it is also necessary to ensure that the program is continually monitored to ensure effectiveness. The benefits derived from the program must not exceed the financial resources nor the costs morbidity induced by the test and accompanying procedures.

Despite of these caveats, screening carries the potential for a fairly rapid and important impact on cancer mortality, often exceeding what can currently be anticipated from other approaches to cancer control.

REFERENCES

1. Miller AB. General principles of evaluation of screening. In: Miller AB, ed. Screening for cancer. Orlando, FL: Academic Press, 1985:3–24.
2. Prorok PC, Chamberlain J, Day NE, et al. UICC workshop on the evaluation of screening programmes for cancer. Int J Cancer 1984;34:1–4.
3. Miller AB, Chamberlain J, Day NE, Hakama M, Prorok PC. Report on a workshop of the UICC project on evaluation of screening for cancer. Int J Cancer 1990;46:761–769.
4. Hakama M. Trends in the incidence of cervical cancer in the Nordic countries. In: Magnus K (ed), Trends in cancer incidence. Washington, DC: Hemisphere, 1982:279–292.
5. Miller AB, Lindsay J, Hill GB. Mortality from cancer of the uterus in Canada and its relationship to screening for cancer of the cervix. Int J Cancer 1976;17:602–612.
6. Hakama M, Chamberlain J, Day NE, et al. Evaluation of screening programmes for gynaecological cancer. Br J Cancer 1985;52:669–673.
7. Miller AB, Anderson G, Brisson J, et al. Report of a National Workshop on screening for cancer of the cervix. Can Med Assoc J 1991;145:1301–1325.
8. American Cancer Society. Guidelines for the cancer-related check-up. Recommendations and rationale. CA 1980;30:193–240.
9. Task Force. Cervical cancer screening programs. The Walton Report. Can Med Assoc J 1976;114:1003–1033.
10. Fink DJ. Change in American Cancer Society checkup guidelines for early detection of cervical cancer. CA 1988;38:127–128.
11. Mettlin C, Dodd GD. The American Cancer Society guidelines for the cancer-related checkup: An update. CA 1991;41:279–282.
12. Early Detection Branch. Working guidelines for early cancer detection. Bethesda: Division of Cancer Prevention and Control, National Cancer Institute, 1987.
13. Boyes DA, Morrison B, Knox EG, et al. A cohort study of cervical cancer in British Columbia. Clin Invest Med 1982;5:1–29.
14. Eddy D. Screening for cancer: Theory, analysis, and design. Englewood Cliffs, NJ: Prentice Hall, 1980.
15. IARC Working Group on Cervical Cancer Screening. Summary chapter. In: Hakama M, Miller AB, Day NE, eds. Screening for cancer of the uterine cervix. IARC Scientific Publications, No. 76. Lyon: International Agency for Research on Cancer, 1986:133–142.
16. Chamberlain J. Reasons that some screening programmes fail to control cervical cancer. In: Hakama M, Miller AB, Day NE, eds. Screening for cancer of the uterine cervix.

IARC Scientific Publications no 76. Lyon: International Agency for Research on Cancer, 1986:161–168.

17. Muller C, Mandelblatt J, Schechter CB, et al. Costs and effectiveness of cervical cancer screening in elderly women—background paper. US Congress, Office of Technology Assessment, OTA-BP-H-65. Washington, DC: US Government Printing Office, 1990.

18. National Cancer Institute Workshop. The 1988 Bethesda system for reporting cervical/vaginal cytological diagnoses. JAMA 1989;262:931–934.

19. Shapiro S, Strax P, Venet L. Periodic breast cancer screening in reducing mortality from breast cancer. JAMA 1971;215:1777–1785.

20. Shapiro S, Venet W, Strax P, Venet L. Periodic screening for breast cancer. The Health Insurance Plan Project and its sequelae, 1963–1986. Baltimore: Johns Hopkins University Press, 1988.

21. Miller AB. Breast cancer screening. Who should be included? J Gen Intern Med 1990;5: S19–S22.

22. Beahrs OH, Shapiro S, Smart C, et al. Report of the working group to review the National Cancer Institute, American Cancer Society Breast Cancer Detection Demonstration Projects. JNCI 1979;62:640–709.

23. Baker LH. Breast cancer detection demonstration project: Five-year summary report. CA 1982;32:194–225.

24. Seidman H, Gelb SK, Silverberg E, et al. Survival experience in the Breast Cancer Detection Demonstration Project. CA 1987;37:258–290.

25. Morrison AS, Brisson J, Khalid N. Breast cancer incidence and mortality in the breast cancer detection demonstration project. JNCI 1988;80:1540–1547.

26. Newcomb PA, Weiss NS, Storer BE, et al. Breast self-examination in relation to occurrence of advanced breast cancer. JNCI 1991;83:260–265.

27. Muscat JE, Huncharek MS. Breast self-examination and extent of disease: A population-based study. Cancer Detect Prevent 1991;15:155–159.

28. Collette HJA, Day NE, Rombach JJ, et al. Evaluation of screening for breast cancer in a non-randomized study (the DOM project) by means of a case-control study. Lancet 1984;1:1224.

29. Verbeek ALM, Hendriks JHCL, Holland R, et al. Mammographic screening and breast cancer mortality age specific effects in the Nijmegen project, 1975–1982. Lancet [Letter] 1985;1:865.

30. Palli D, del Turco MR, Buiatti E, et al. A case-control study of the efficacy of a non-randomised breast cancer screening program in Florence (Italy). Int J Cancer 1986;38: 501–504.

31. Tabar L, Fagerberg CJG, Gad A, et al. Reduction in mortality from breast cancer after mass screening with mammography: Randomized trial from the breast cancer screening working group of the Swedish National Board of Health and Welfare. Lancet 1985;1: 829–832.

32. Tabar, L, Fagerberg G, Duffy SW, Day NE. The Swedish two county trial of mammographic screening for breast cancer: Recent results and calculation of benefit. J Epidemiol Community Health 1989;43:107–114.

33. Andersson I, Aspergren K, Janzon L, et al. Mammographic screening and mortality from breast cancer: The Malmö mammographic screening trial. Br Med J 1988;297: 943–948.

34. Rutqvist LE, Miller AB, Andersson I, et al. Reduced breast cancer mortality with mammography screening—an assessment of currently available data. Int J Cancer Suppl 1990;5:76–84.

35. United Kingdom Trial of Early Detection of Breast Cancer Group. First results on mortality reduction in the UK Trial of Early Detection of Breast Cancer. Lancet 1988;2:411–416.

36. Locker AP, Caseldine J, Mitchell AK, et al. Results from a seven-year programme of breast self-examination in 89,010 women. Br J Cancer 1988;60:401–405.

37. Roberts MM, Alexander FE, Anderson TJ, et al. Edinburgh trial of screening for breast cancer: Mortality at seven years. Lancet 1990;335:241–246.

38. Day NE, Baines CJ, Chamberlain J, et al. UICC project on screening for cancer: Report of the workshop on screening for breast cancer. Int J Cancer 1986;38:303–308.

39. Miller AB, Chamberlain J, Tsechkovski M. Self-examination in the early detection of breast cancer. A review of the evidence, with recommendations for further research. J Chron Dis 1985;38:527–540.

40. Gastrin G. Breast cancer control. Stockholm: Almqvist & Wiksell, 1981.

41. Gastrin G, Miller AB, To T, et al. Mortality from breast cancer in the Mama program for breast screening in Finland, 1973 to 1986. (in preparation).

42. Koroltchouk V, Stanley K, Stjernswärd J. The control of breast cancer. A World Health Organization perspective. Cancer 1990;65:2803–2810.

43. Miller AB, Howe GR, Wall C. The national study of breast cancer screening. Clin Invest Med 1981;4:227–258.

44. Miller AB, Baines CJ, To T, Wall C. The Canadian National Breast Screening Study. In: Miller AB, Chamberlain J, Day NE, et al, eds. Cancer screening. Cambridge: Cambridge University Press, 1991:45–55.

45. Day NE, Walter SD, Tabar L, et al. The sensitivity and lead time of breast cancer screening. A comparison of the results of different studies. In: Day NE, Miller AB, eds. Screening for breast cancer. Toronto: Hans Huber, 1988:105–109.

46. Eddy DM, Hasselblad V, McGivney W, et al. The value of mammography screening in women under age 50 years. JAMA 1988;259:1512–1519.

47. American College of Radiology. New ACR guidelines on mammography. Am Coll Radiol Bull 1982;38:6–7.

48. The Workshop Group. Reducing deaths from breast cancer in Canada. Can Med Assoc J 1989;141:199–201.

49. Greenwald P, Sondik EJ, eds. Cancer control objectives for the nation: 1985–2000. NCI Monogr 1986;2:27–32.

50. Howe GR, Sherman GJ, Semincew RM, Miller AB. Estimated benefits and risks of screening for breast cancer. Can Med Assoc J 1981;124:399–403.

51. Gohagen JK, Darby WP, Spitznagel EL, et al. Radiogenic breast cancer effects of mammographic screening. JNCI 1986;77:71–76.

52. Miller AB, Howe GR, Sherman GJ, et al. Mortality from breast cancer after irradiation during fluoroscopic examinations in patients being treated for tuberculosis. N Engl J Med 1989;321:1285–1289.

53. Miller AB, Bulbrook RD. Screening, detection and diagnosis of breast cancer. Lancet 1982;1:1109–1111.

54. Miller AB, Tschkovski M. Imaging technologies in breast cancer control: Summary report of a world health organization meeting. AJR 1987;148:1093–1094.

55. National Board of Health and Welfare. Mammographic screening for early detection of breast cancer. Guidelines from the National Board of Health and Welfare of Sweden, Stockholm: National Board of Health and Welfare, 1986:3.

56. Working Group. Breast cancer screening: Report to the Health Ministers of England, Wales, Scotland and Northern Ireland. London: H.M. Stationery Office, 1987.

57. U.S. Preventive Services Task Force. Guide to clinical preventive services. Washington, DC: Department of Health and Human Services, 1989:26.

58. Department of Public Health and Social Medicine. The costs and effects of screening for breast cancer. Final report. Rotterdam: Erasmus University, April 1990.

59. Winawer SJ, Fath RB, Scottenfeld D, et al. Screening for colorectal cancer. In: Miller AB, ed. Screening for cancer. Orlando, FL: Academic Press, 1985:347–366.

60. Gilbertsen VA. Proctosigmoidoscopy and polypectomy in reducing the incidence of rectal cancer. Cancer 1974;34:936–939.

61. Gilbertsen VA, Nelms JM. The prevention of invasive cancer of the rectum. Cancer 1978;41:1137–1139.

62. Miller AB. Review of sigmoidoscopic screening for colorectal cancer. In: Chamberlain J, Miller AB, eds. Screening for gastrointestinal cancer. Toronto: Hans Huber, 1988:3–7.

63. Dales LG, Freidman GD, Collen MF. Evaluating periodic multiphasic health check-ups: A controlled trial. J Chron Dis 1979;32:385.

64. Selby JV, Friedman GD, Collen MF. Sigmiodoscopy and mortality from colorectal cancer: The Kaiser Permanente multiphasic evaluation study. J Clin Epidemiol 1988;41:427–434.

65. Flehinger BJ, Herbert E, Winawer SJ, et al. Screening for colorectal cancer with fecal occult blood test and sigmoidoscopy: Preliminary report of the colon project of Memorial Sloan-Kettering cancer center and PMI-Strang clinic. In: Chamberlain J, Miller AB, eds. Screening for gastrointestinal cancer. Toronto: Hans Huber, 1988:9–16.

66. Miller AB. Colorectal cancer screening. JNCI [Letter] 1991;83:1111–1112.

67. Mandel JS, Bond J, Snover D, et al. The University of Minnesota's colon cancer control study: Design and progress to date. In: Chamberlain J, Miller AB, eds. Screening for gastrointestinal cancer. Toronto: Hans Huber, 1988:17–24.

68. Chamberlain J, Day NE, Hakama M, et al. UICC workshop of the project on evaluation of screening programmes for gastrointestinal cancer. Int J Cancer 1986;37:329–334.

69. Prorok PC, Byar DP, Smart CR, et al. Evaluation of screening for prostate, lung and colorectal cancers: The PLC trial. In: Miller AB, Chamberlain J, Day NE et al, eds. Cancer screening. Cambridge: Cambridge University Press, 1991.

70. Ebeling K, Nischan P. Screening for lung cancer: Results from a case-control study. Int J Cancer 1987;40:141–144.

71. Cartwright RA. Screening for bladder cancer with particular reference to individual groups. In: Prorok PC, Miller AB, eds. Screening for cancer: 1. General principles on evaluation of screening for cancer and screening for lung, bladder and oral cancer. Geneva: International Union Against Cancer, 1984:144–160.

72. Warnakulasuriya KAAS, Ekanayake ANI, Sivayoham S, et al. Utilization of primary health care workers for early detection of oral cancer and precancer cases in Sri Lanka. Bull World Health Organ 1984;62:243–250.

73. Hakama M, Pukkala E. Evaluation of an immunological screening for stomach cancer. In: Chamberlain J, Miller AB, eds. Screening for gastrointestinal cancer. Toronto: Hans Huber, 1988:71–75.

74. Hirayama T. Screening for gastric cancer. In: Miller AB, ed. Screening for cancer. Orlando, FL: Academic Press, 1985:367–376.

75. Oshima A, Hirata N, Ubukata T, et al. Evaluation of a mass screening program for stomach cancer with a case-control study design. Int J Cancer 1986;38:829–833.

76. National Cancer Institute of Canada. Canadian cancer statistics, 1991. Toronto: , 1991.

77. Boring CC, Squires TS, Tong T. Cancer statistics, 1992. CA 1992;42:19–38.

78. Miller AB. Issues in screening for prostate cancer. In: Miller AB, Chamberlain J, Day NE, et al. Cancer screening. Cambridge: Cambridge University Press, 1991:289–293.

79. Thompson IM, Fair WR. Screening for carcinoma of the prostate: Efficacy of available screening tests. World J Surg 1989;13:65–70.

80. Pedersen KV, Carlsson P, Varenhorst E, et al. Screening for carcinoma of the prostate by digital rectal examination in a randomly selected population. Br Med J 1990;300: 1041–1044.

81. Chodak GW, Schoenberg HW. Progress and problems in screening for carcinoma of the prostate. World J Surg 1989;13:60–64.

82. Miller AB. The ethics, the risks and the benefits of screening. Biomed Pharmacother 1988;42:439–442.

83. National Institutes of Health. Consensus Conference. Precursors to malignant melanoma. JAMA 1984;251:1864–1866.

84. Miller AB. Screening for cancer: Issues and future directions. J Chron Dis 1986;39: 1067–1077.

85. American Cancer Society. 1989 Survey of physicians' attitudes and practices in early cancer detection. CA 1990;40:77–101.

Cancer: Principles & Practice of Oncology, Fourth Edition,
edited by Vincent T. DeVita, Jr., Samuel Hellman, Steven A. Rosenberg.
J.B. Lippincott Co., Philadelphia © 1993.

CHAPTER **22**

Cancer of the Head and Neck

STIMSON P. SCHANTZ
LOUIS B. HARRISON
WAUN KI HONG

SECTION **1**

Tumors of the Nasal Cavity and Paranasal Sinuses, Nasopharynx, Oral Cavity, and Oropharynx

Cancers of the upper aerodigestive tract represent a diverse number of diseases. Each bears its own unique set of epidemiologic, anatomic, pathologic, and treatment considerations. This section reviews such considerations based on four anatomically defined regions: the nasal cavity and paranasal sinuses, the nasopharynx, the oral cavity, and the oropharynx.

There are general principles regarding these cancers that may be considered. Such principles involve anatomy (*i.e.,* anatomy primarily of the regional lymph nodes within the head and neck), pathology, staging and screening, and general principles of treatment involving single-modality or multimodality therapy, which are relevant to all sites.

ANATOMY

An understanding of the regional lymph node anatomy is critical to the care of head and neck cancer patients. There are several major lymphatic chains in the neck containing nearly 200 lymph nodes that run parallel to the jugular veins, spinal accessory nerve, and facial artery and into the submandibular

triangle (Fig. 22–1). To facilitate communication regarding cervical lymph node anatomy, the regions of the neck have been characterized by levels (Fig. 22–2).[1,2]

Level I includes nodes within the submental triangle and the submandibular triangle. The submental triangle extends from the midline anteriorly to the anterior belly of the digastric muscle posteriorly. Its third border is formed by the hyoid bone inferiorly. The submandibular triangle is bounded by the mandible superiorly. The anterior and the posterior belly of the digastric muscle complete the triangle.

Level II includes the jugular nodes extending from the subdigastric area down to the carotid bifurcation and the nodes surrounding the spinal accessory nerve from the jugular foramen to the posterior border of the sternocleidomastoid muscle. It includes the lymph nodes in the upper posterior cervical triangle above the entrance of the spinal accessory nerve into this triangle.

Level III represents the nodal area principally along the jugular vein between the carotid and its bifurcation, the posterior border of the sternocleidomastoid muscle, and the omohyoid muscle.

Level IV constitutes nodal areas below the omohyoid muscle above the level of the clavicle and between the carotid vessels anteriorly and the omohyoid muscle posteriorly.

Level V represents nodes in the posterior cervical triangle. Its borders are formed by the posterior edge of the sternocleidomastoid muscle, the level of the entrance of the spinal accessory nerve, the trapezius muscle, and the posterior belly of the omohyoid muscle.

Specific sites within the aerodigestive tract have a predetermined drainage pattern. A knowledge of this pattern aids in diagnosis and impacts on therapy. Drainage patterns are addressed in each of the anatomic subsites detailed in this chapter.

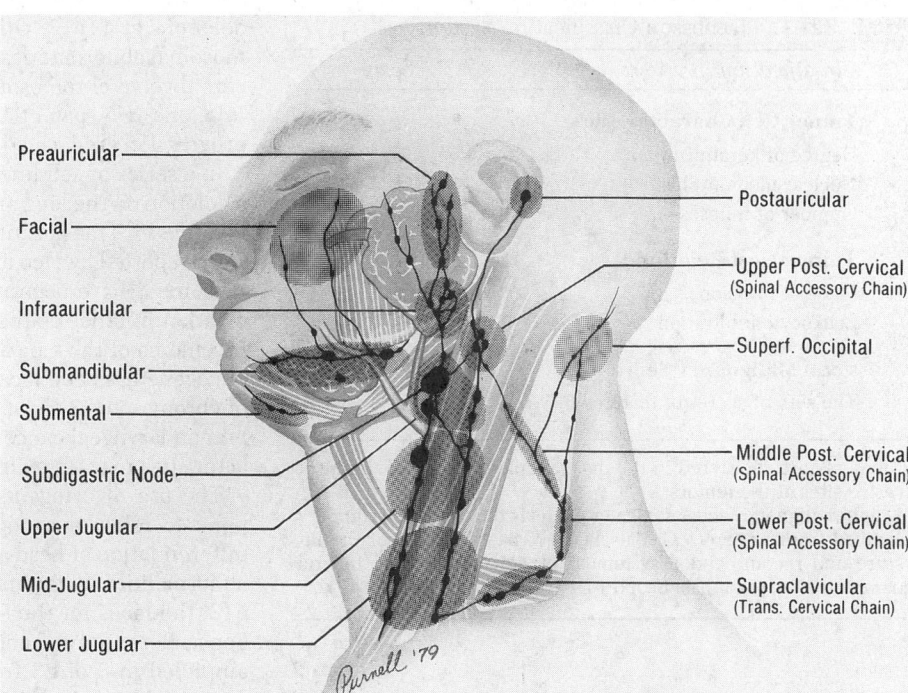

FIGURE 22–1. Superficial and deep cervical lymph nodes of the head and neck. (Shah JP. A color atlas of head and neck surgery. Orlando: Grune and Stratton, 1987)

PATHOLOGY

The predominant lesion within these anatomically defined regions is squamous cell carcinoma. Squamous cell carcinoma can be categorized into three classic differentiations: well-differentiated disease shows greater than 75% keratinization; moderately differentiated disease contributes to the bulk of squamous cell carcinoma and is characterized by 25% to 75% keratinization; and poorly differentiated disease demonstrates less than 25% keratinization. Other variants of squamous cell carcinoma include verrucous carcinoma, sarcomatoid squamous cell carcinoma, and lymphoepithelioma. Additional pathologic criteria of squamous cell carcinoma that is believed to be clinically relevant were developed by Jacobsson and others.[3–6] This includes the number of mitoses, presence of vascular invasion, size of nuclei, degree of inflammatory infiltrate, and pushing or infiltrating borders (Table 22–1).

PREMALIGNANCY

A series of pathologic changes from premalignant disease to frank malignancy can occur in the upper aerodigestive tract. Among the premalignant diseases are leukoplakia, erythoplakia, hyperplasia, and dysplasia. Each of these types has a propensity for malignant transformation.[7] Histopathologic assessment of leukoplakia reveals hyperparakeratosis that is variably associated with an underlying epithelial hyperplasia. Leukoplakia without underlying dysplastic changes is rarely associated with progression to malignancy, that is, less than 5% probability of malignant changes.[8,9] Erythroplakia is a condition within the oral cavity and pharynx characterized by red superficial patches adjacent to normal mucosa. Distinct from leukoplakic lesions as identified previously, erythroplakia is commonly associated with underlying epithelial dysplasia. It can be associated with carcinoma in situ to frank malignancy in nearly 40% of lesions.[8,10]

Dysplasia compared with the previous two clinical descriptives is a true histopathologic term that is characterized by several morphologic changes, including the presence of mitoses, pleomorphism, and prominent nucleoli. When dysplasia involves the entire thickness of the mucosa, it is commonly referred to as *carcinoma in situ*. Dysplasia has been associated

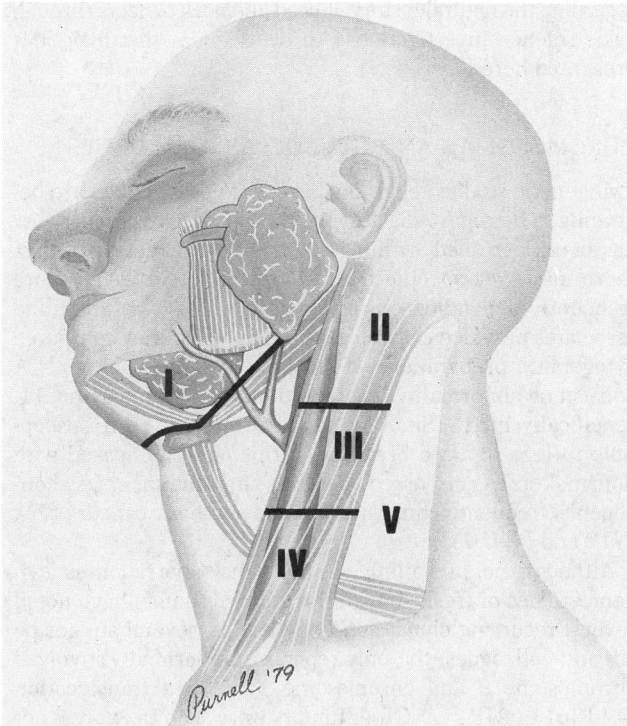

FIGURE 22–2. Level classification of regional cervical lymph nodes (see text for description). (Shah JP. A color atlas of head and neck surgery. Orlando: Grune and Stratton, 1987)

TABLE 22–1. Jacobsson Classification System

Classification	Score
Tumor Cell Characteristics	
Degree of keratinization	1–4
Nuclear pleomorphism	1–4
Number of mitoses	1–4
Tumor-Host Relations	
Mode of invasion	1–4
Leukocyte infiltration	1–4
Total Malignancy Score*	
The sum of scores of features 1–5	

All features are registered in the most anaplastic areas of the most invasive sites of the tumors.
* A high malignancy score indicates a poorly differentiated tumor.
(Modified from Anneroth G, Batsakis J, Kyba N. Review of the literature and recommended system of malignancy grading in oral squamous cell carcinomas. Scand J Dent Res 1987;95:229–249)

with a subsequent risk of progression to frank malignancy ranging from 15% to 30% of cases.[11,12]

NATURAL HISTORY

The clinically defined natural history of these cancers is considered in the respective subsites identified in this chapter. However, in the coming years, we will witness newer insight regarding the natural history of head and neck cancers through basic science investigations. An overview of that insight is presented here.

CHROMOSOMAL AND GENETIC ABNORMALITIES

Cytogenetic studies regarding head and neck cancers are beginning to be reported. Although no constitutive abnormality has been identified within head and neck cancer patients, there may exist specific fragile sites that are affected more frequently depending on tobacco exposures. Kao-Shan and associates provided critical information when they compared cytogenetic preparations of smokers and nonsmokers.[13] A consistent abnormality was identified on chromosome 11, specifically 11q13. Smokers were shown to be more susceptible to lung-induced breakage at this point compared with nonsmokers. As discussed later, this site contains several oncogenes frequently amplified in head and neck cancers (*i.e.,* INT2 and PRAD1).

Although no prevailing chromosomal aberration is evident, studies of fresh short-term-cultured tumors have noted several recurring clonal abnormalities. In several studies by Jin and colleagues, the only repeating abnormality involved chromosome 9 and chromosome 11 (*i.e.,* a translocation [9;11][p13;q21]).[14–16] Other tumors were seen to express abnormalities at 11q13. Additionally, Carey and colleagues[17] and Sacks and associates[18] identified deletions on chromosome 11 on long-term cell lines. Specifically, both investigators noted

deletions at 11p13. Other more commonly occurring chromosomal abnormalities identified within head and neck cancers involve chromosome 1.[19] Three oncogenes, L-*MYC*, N-*RAS,* and *JUN,* potentially relevant to head and neck cancer progression are located within that area (Fig. 22–3).

In a series of cell lines investigated by Heo and coworkers, a deletion on the long arm of chromosome 3 was consistently identified.[20] Translocations involving chromosome 11 (11q14) were reported by Heo and coworkers.[20] Aberrations on chromosome 3 have been noted as a primary chromosomal aberration in other epithelial cancers, for example, small cell carcinoma of the lung and renal cell carcinoma. The c-*RAF1* oncogene has been localized to the same short-arm segment of chromosome 3 and it is associated with a radiation-resistant human laryngeal cancer.[21] Specific genetically defined characteristics may ultimately govern the choice of therapies.

The use of cytogenetic analyses in many circumstances point to relevant oncogenes that modulate the growth and differentiation of head and neck cancer. As noted previously, abnormalities in chromosome 11 are identified frequently at q13, the locus for the *INT2, HST1, BCL1,* and *PRAD1* oncogenes. Berenson and colleagues noted that the *BCL1* gene was amplified in 8 of 23 fresh head and neck cancers.[22] These same authors noted that some of the tumors showed amplification of the c-*MYC* or H-*RAS* genes. Zhou and associates noted amplification in the *INT2* and *HST1* gene in head and neck cancers.[23]

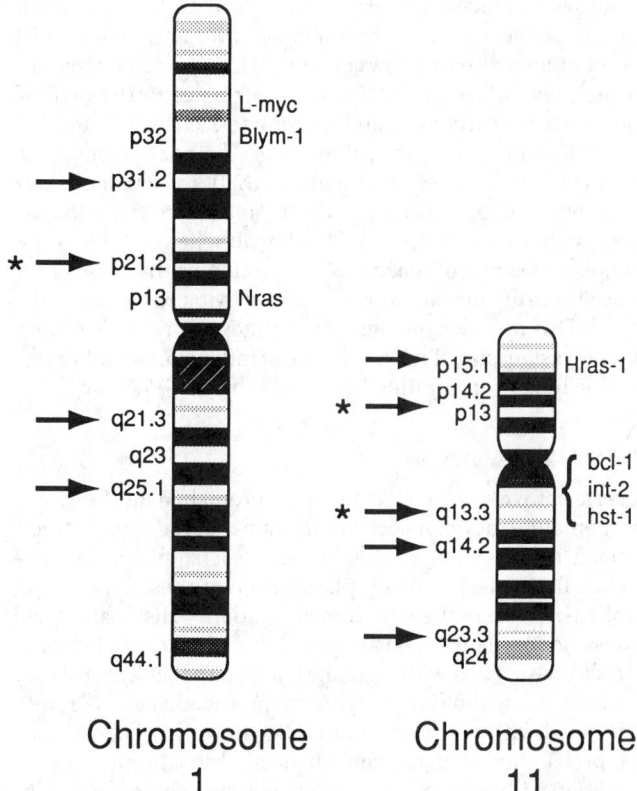

FIGURE 22–3. Frequently observed cytogenetic abnormalities in squamous cell cancers of the head and neck. The *arrow* in left column represents constitutive fragile sites in human chromosome analyses. The *asterisk* represents the site of frequently observed chromosomal anomalies in head and neck cancers. The right column lists oncogenes that are located near these breakpoints.

Studies of oncogene expression have otherwise failed to identify any consistent genetic alteration. The reason for discrepancies in oncogene expression may, in part, reflect the causal factor responsible for disease development and the afflicted population. Saraneth and coworkers examined oral cavity cancers occurring in the Indian population.[24] They determined the prevalence of amplification of c-*MYC*, N-*MYC*, L-*MYC*, H-*RAS*, Ki-*RAS*, and N-*RAS* in 23 cases.[24] Five- to tenfold amplification of c-*MYC*, N-*MYC*, Ki-*RAS* and N-*RAS* were identified in 56% of tumors. Most tumors that showed gene abnormalities had multiple genes amplified. Tumors from populations in Japan and the United States have failed to identify *RAS* gene abnormalities.[25,26] The underlying habit of betel nut chewing in the Indian population may account for the difference in these results. Inherited genetic predisposition may also be relevant. In regard to genetic predisposition, Saraneth and associates studied the L-*MYC* oncogene loci for genetic polymorphisms in cancer patients and control subjects.[27] The authors identified three common genotypes of the L-*MYC* gene that they termed *L-L*, *L-S*, and *S-S*. The relative ratio of these genotypes did not vary between cancer patients or controls. However, people with the S-S genotype had poorly differentiated tumors and those with the L-L genotype were associated with well-differentiated disease. The authors provided evidence that characteristics of head and neck cancer can be governed by the constitutive genetic make-up of the host.

The differences in oncogene abnormalities may reflect extent of disease and responsiveness to specific therapeutic modalities.[28–33] The most illustrative example is c-*MYC* abnormalities. Many authors have reported c-*MYC* expression in advanced stage disease.[24,31] *RAS* oncogene expression has been identified in more advanced disease. Field and colleagues identified a worse prognosis in patients whose tumors contained high levels of the c-*MYC* oncoprotein.[31] *RAS* gene expression may also relate to tumor therapeutic responsiveness. Clugston and associates noted no *RAS* mutations in 22 primary squamous cell carcinomas of the upper aerodigestive tract.[33] However, three of six recurrent cancer patients who had received radiation therapy contained a *RAS* mutation. *RAS* mutations may have conveyed radiation resistance. *RAF* gene abnormalities have already been associated with lack of response to radiation.[21] The study of oncogenes in head and neck cancer patients may provide insight to determinants of growth and progression of disease and to determinants of response to therapy.

GROWTH FACTORS
AND TUMOR SECRETORY PRODUCTS

The natural history of head and neck cancer is reflected in its growth patterns. Most head and neck oncologists recognize the implications of tumors that grow in an exophytic or an ulcerative-infiltrative pattern. The latter method of tumor growth is considered to be associated with a worse clinical outcome. As mentioned earlier, the concept of pushing versus infiltrative tumor borders has been identified as a histopathologic variable that governs prognosis. Research efforts have focused on factors that may account for this more aggressive growth tendency. Undoubtedly, no single mechanism exists. Recently, Meghji and coworkers have identified a 16,000 molecular weight substance secreted by head and neck cancers

that induces bone resorption and may facilitate tumor expansion.[34] These authors called this factor *osteoclastic bone resorption factor* and showed that it identified with interleukin-1 (IL-1). Huang and associates had shown previously that head and neck cancers were capable of secreting protein degradation products, such as protease, necessary for tumor invasion.[35] This substance was more apparent in well-differentiated disease. This corresponds to studies by Bauer and colleagues that showed that well-differentiated laryngeal tumors had an infiltrating tumor pattern and poorly differentiated tumors tended to have pushing borders.[36] Further characterization of collagenase associated with head and neck cancers have been performed.[37] Prostaglandin E_2 production, known to be a characteristic of head and neck cancer, may promote secretion of protein degradation products contained only within a tumor mass.[38]

Other characteristics associated with a more advanced rate of malignancy relate to the capacity for autocrine growth. Autocrine growth implies that the necessary growth factor receptors and growth factor products are contained only within a tumor mass. Autocrine growth may explain why researchers have observed that head and neck cancers with increased clonagenic potential in vitro and an increased capacity to proliferate in nude mice are generally associated with a worse prognosis. Numerous reports have demonstrated the increased expression of epidermal growth factor receptors (EGF-R) on head and neck cancers, in some instances reaching levels higher than the 1431 cell line standard.[26,39–43] The EGF-R expressed on head and neck cancers binds with great affinity to transforming growth factor-α (TGF-α). The latter is a strong mitogenic factor capable of inducing epithelial proliferation.[44] Studies by Partridge and associates have shown that oral cancer cells express high levels of TGF-α.[45] The autocrine axis of head and neck cancer can be related to the production of TGF-α and the expression of EGF-R.

Novel strategies designed to interfere with this process will arise. Yoneda and coworkers have shown the potential impact of using monoclonal antibodies, such as antibody 108, to the EGF-R.[46] Human tumors shown to induce the paraneoplastic syndrome were transplanted into nude mice by Yoneda and coworkers. Hypercalcemia and cachexia resulted within the animal. Reversal of hypercalcemia and inhibition of tumor growth was demonstrated by infusing the animal with the 108 antibody. Currently, human studies are planned.

HOST RESPONSE

The association between deficient immune response and the growth and development of head and neck cancer has been well documented.[47–52] Several features reinforce this notion compared with other processes.[47,48] First, deficiency in immune response occurs in patients independent of tumor stage. Second, deficiencies persist after disease treatment, suggesting that abnormal host response is more a determinant than a result of cancer progression. Many reviews on the subject have been published previously.[49–52] The defect in these patients has been related to humoral and cellular immune response.

Defects in cellular immunity were first reported in the early 1970s. At that time, absence of skin test reactivity to recall antigens was observed in some but not all patients.[53] Although not universally confirmed, such impaired skin test response was associated with a greater probability of disease progression. Further studies have characterized impaired response in vitro by means of many assays, including blastogenesis response to mutagens, phenotypic and quantitative subset analysis of lymphocyte populations, and immune functional assays.[54–58] More recent studies have focused on various immune effector mechanisms such as cytotoxic lymphocytes (major histocompatibility complex [MHC]-restricted effector mechanisms) and natural killer cell cytotoxicity.[58,59] The latter effector mechanism represents a more primitive immune defense mechanism and is characterized by its capacity to lyse tumor cells without regard to MHC restriction. Which effector mechanism is involved in head and neck cancer basis depends on phenotypic characteristics of the tumor in question. Head and neck cancers are noted to express multiple antigenic determinant. Esteban and associates reported that 30% of tumors lack MHC class I antigens.[60] Such MHC-lacking tumors have been reported as having a greater tendency to metastatic spread and to crossing anatomic barriers.[61]

The significance of immune response in head and neck cancer is becoming reinforced by recent clinical trials using biologic response modifiers. Ishikawa and colleagues have focused on adoptive transfer of lymphokine-activated killer cells.[59] Lymphocytes from these patients are cultured in the presence of IL-2 and autologous tumor. After expansion and activation, selective arterial catherization and perfusion with autologous lymphocytes are performed. Ishikawa and colleagues have reported that several patients treated in such fashion demonstrated antitumor response.[59]

The role of recombinant IL-2 given systemically to enhance natural immune function has been reported. Studies are preliminary and are handicapped by the associated toxicity of high-dose IL-2 infusions. Schantz and associates were able to document antitumor response in selected patients, although none had complete response (CR) (Fig. 22–4).[183] The role of biologic response modifiers as an adjuvant to standard therapy to prevent disease recurrence needs further attention.

Parameters of humoral immunity within head and neck cancer patients have also undergone extensive analysis.[61,62]

STAGING AND SCREENING

STAGING

The staging of head and neck cancer represents a standardized approach by which clinicians and researchers communicate the extent of disease within the individual patient. It is based on the TNM classification. *T stage* represents the extent of primary disease, *N* represents the extent of regional lymph node metastasis, and *M* is a measure of distant metastasis. The American Joint Committee on Cancer (AJCC) staging system, used for classifying TNM status, is revised periodically.[63]

The most recent clinical staging system, although based principally on physical examination, has incorporated specific radiographic observations of disease status. Invasion *through* cortical bone by an oral cavity tumor will upstage a T2 or T3 lesion to T4, that is, from stage II or III to stage IV.

Radiographic assessment of cervical lymph node metastases has not been integrated into clinical staging. The benefits of

these diagnostic techniques beyond that provided by standard physical examination is under investigation.[64–66]

The criteria for T staging within the upper aerodigestive tract differs depending on the primary site. N staging and M staging, however, are uniform and are considered.

REGIONAL LYMPH NODES

NX	Regional lymph nodes cannot be assessed.
N0	No regional lymph node metastasis.
N1	Metastasis in a single ipsilateral lymph node 3 cm or less in greatest dimension.
N2	Metastasis in a single ipsilateral lymph node more than 3 cm but not more than 6 cm in greatest dimension, in mulitple ipsilateral lymph nodes, or in bilateral or contralateral lymph nodes not more than 6 cm in greatest dimension.
N2A	Metastasis in a single ipsilateral lymph node more than 3 cm but not more than 6 cm in greatest dimension.
N2B	Metastasis in multiple ipsilateral lymph nodes not more than 6 cm in greatest dimension.
N2C	Metastasis in bilateral or contralateral lymph nodes not more than 6 cm in greatest dimension.
N3	Metastasis in a lymph node more than 6 cm in greatest dimension.

DISTANT METASTASIS

MX	Presence of distant metastasis cannot be assessed.
M0	No distant metastasis.
M1	Distant metastasis.

Table 22–2 represents the most recent stage classification defined by the AJCC.[63]

SCREENING

The significance of screening is emphasized by reports that most oral cancer lesions could have been detected several months earlier by appropriate dental examination.[67,68] The most extensively studied screening procedure has been oral exfoliative cytology, which has been recommended by the American Dental Association.[69] A high proportion of false-negative examinations have been reported with this procedure.[70,71] Those people who are most at risk, such as people with high tobacco and alcohol consumption patterns, are least likely to participate voluntarily in such efforts. This fact has been emphasized by a recent report by the Metropolitan Detroit Oral Cancer Screening Control Program in which 5679 people were evaluated in a 27-month period and 18 cancers were identified.[72] High-risk populations were believed not to benefit from screening.

Another screening method used frequently has been toluidine blue staining of aerodigestive mucosa.[73,74] Toluidine blue is a metachromatic nuclear stain that is taken up by dysplastic and cancerous epithelium. Mashberg has detailed extensively the appropriate use of toluidine blue and has reported false-positive results to approximate 9% and false-negative results approaching 5%.[74] Its value is that it is quick, inexpensive, and noninvasive.

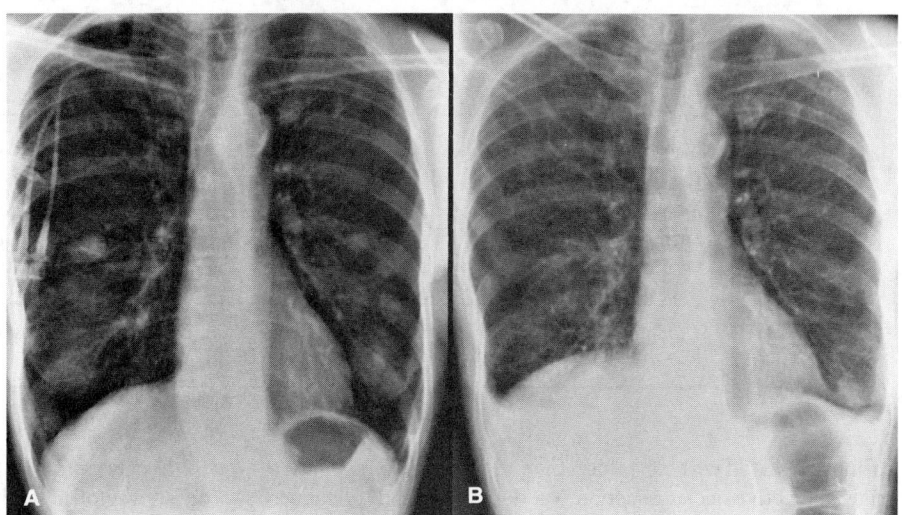

FIGURE 22–4. Interleukin-2- and interferon-α-induced regression of pulmonary metastases of poorly differentiated squamous cell carcinoma of the tongue. **(A)** Pretreatment. **(B)** Posttreatment after one course of therapy. Patient performance status precluded further therapy, and disease was noted to progress within 1 month of treatment cessation. (Schantz SP, Clayman GL, Dimery I, Morice D. Combination interleukin-2 and interferon-α in head and neck cancer. Cancer Bull 1991;43:133–138)

Standardized physical examination is the best means of detecting lesions of the upper aerodigestive tract. The care and thoroughness of the examiner is paramount.[75,76] The need for careful assessment was emphasized by Jesse and associates in their report on patients who present with regional metastatic disease from a presumed unknown primary.[75] Many patients examined carefully were found subsequently to have a primary cancer.

TREATMENT

GENERAL PRINCIPLES OF SURGERY

In the execution of effective surgical management, the single most significant principle is the adequate preoperative assessment of disease extent. Precise and methodic physical examination of the patient is extremely important. Such examination allows for the assessment of adequate extent of surgical excision, which remains for most cancers the fundamental tenet for achieving cure.

An extension of adequate preoperative assessment is optimal intraoperative exposure of disease. The surgeon should consider appropriate means to achieve operative exposure. The choice of incision and the ability to mobilize surrounding anatomic structures to achieve exposure are considered later

in the section for each anatomic subsite. Exposure is facilitated by careful hemostasis. In addition to allowing for better operative exposure, minimizing blood loss prevents potential sequela associated with blood transfusion. Weber and associates have reported expected blood loss for various surgical procedures involving cancers of the upper aerodigestive tract (Table 22–3).[77] Electrocautery dissection had been used by Weber and associates, which may explain the relatively infrequent need for blood transfusion. Electrocautery dissection has been adopted by many experienced surgeons as the preferred extirpative technique.

Additional methods of surgical excision have included the use of the Mohs technique and laser ablation.[81–83] However, these techniques cannot be considered standard surgical procedure currently.

General principles of surgery exist involving regional lymph node disease. The radical neck dissection is the standard in the surgical control of cervical metastases by which various procedures are judged. The radical neck dissection involves complete removal of the lymphatic pathways within the neck. To ensure complete extirpation, anatomic structures, including the sternocleidomastoid muscle, spinal accessory nerve, and jugular vein, are routinely sacrificed.

Recent developments in the management of cervical lymph node disease involve more conservative surgical procedures.[2,84–86] These procedures differ from the classic radical neck dissection primarily in sparing specific anatomic structures, such as the spinal accessory nerve and the sternocleidomastoid muscle. Table 22–4 provides a classification of selective neck dissections used currently and it details removed lymph node regions. Figures 22–5 through 22–7 depict surgical incision, resected lymph nodes, and preserved regional anatomy of one selective neck dissection (*i.e.*, a supraomohyoid neck dissection).

Controversy exists about the value of elective neck dissection in the face of clinically not defined (N0) disease. Arguments in favor of such procedures are based on the finding that more than 20% of clinically negative necks harbor histopathologic evidence of metastases.[87–89] Whether resection of this disease improves survival beyond that afforded by delayed neck dissection when disease becomes clinically evident

TABLE 22–2. Stage Grouping Based on AJCC Criteria[63]

Stage	Classification		
	T	*N*	*M*
0	Tis	N0	M0
I	T1	N0	M0
II	T2	N0	M0
III	T3	N0	M0
	T1	N1	M0
	T2	N1	M0
	T3	N0	M0
IV	T4	N0	M0

TABLE 22–3. Mean Blood Loss and Transfusion Requirements

Procedure	No. of Patients	No. With Neck Dissections	Estimate Blood Loss (ml) Mean ± 1 SD
Neck dissection	47	47	103 ± 152
Larynx/pharynx	57	29	236 ± 194
Maxillectomy	21	3	506 ± 386
Parotid/thyroid	54	28	126 ± 111
Oral cavity/oropharynx	68	50	203 ± 214

(Adapted from Weber RS, Lichtiger B, Byers RM, et al. Electrosurgical dissection for reducing blood loss in head and neck surgery. Head Neck Surg 1989;11;318–324)

cannot be stated with certainty. In one of the few prospective trials of elective neck dissection, Vandenbrouck and colleagues failed to find survival benefit in oral cavity cancer patients randomized to receive elective dissection.[90] The study is limited by the small number of subjects entered and more conclusive studies are necessary. In those patients who are not likely to receive careful postoperative assessment, it is recommended that elective neck dissection be performed.

GENERAL PRINCIPLES OF RADIATION THERAPY

For early-stage disease, both radiation and surgery are frequently curative and can produce similar rates of cure. Selection of treatment must be individualized to each patient and issues such as cosmetic and functional outcome, speed with which treatment can be completed, sequelae of each modality, patient reliability, risk for subsequent cancers, and capacity of salvage therapy must be considered should there be a recurrence.

For advanced head and neck cancer, surgery and radiation are combined frequently. There are proponents of preoperative radiation and postoperative radiation. Tupchong and associates reported the Radiation Therapy Oncology Group (RTOG) experience comparing preoperative radiation therapy

(5000 cGy) with postoperative radiation therapy (6000 cGy) for supraglottic and hypopharynx cancers.[91] Locoregional control was significantly better for the postoperative radiation group. The results were most significant for the supraglottic cancers. Marcial and coworkers analyzed the surgical complications in patients who received 5000 cGy preoperative radiation therapy for advanced but resectable head and neck cancer.[92] This group was compared with another group of patients who had surgery without preoperative radiation. There was no significant difference between the two groups in terms of the overall complication rate.

When making decisions about postoperative radiation, it is important to consider the local site and the regional volume. In terms of the local site, reasons to add postoperative radiation include inadequate margins, significant local invasion, and a large tumor in the T3 or T4 category. Studies have demonstrated that adequate doses of well-delivered postoperative radiation therapy can sterilize cancer-positive surgical margins.[93,94]

Regional issues that determine the need for postoperative radiation therapy include the presence of involved lymph

TABLE 22–4. Classification of Neck Dissections

Classification	Level of Lymph Nodes Removed
I. Standard radical dissection	I, II, III, IV, V
II. Modified radical neck dissection	I, II, III, IV, V
III. Modified neck dissection	
A. Functional neck dissection	II, III, IV, V (+I)
B. Selective neck dissection	
1. Submandibular triangle dissection	IB
2. Suprahyoid neck dissection	IA, IB
3. Anterior neck dissection	IIA, III, IVA
4. Posterior neck dissection	IIB, V
5. Supramohyoid neck dissection	IIA, IIB, III, V (+IB)
IV. Extended neck dissection	

(Adapted from Robbins KT, Medina JE, Wolfe GT, et al. Standardizing neck dissection terminology: Official report of the Academy's Committee for Head and Neck Surgery and Oncology. Arch Otolaryngol Head Neck Surg 1991;117:601–605)

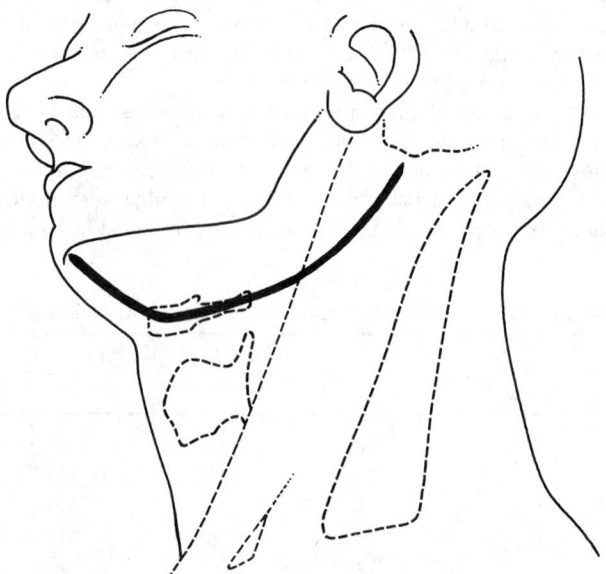

FIGURE 22–5. A standard apron incision used for a supraomohyoid neck dissection. This neck dissection is commonly used in patients with cancers of the oral cavity who are clinically N0. (Shah JP. A color atlas of head and neck surgery. Orlando: Grune and Stratton, 1987)

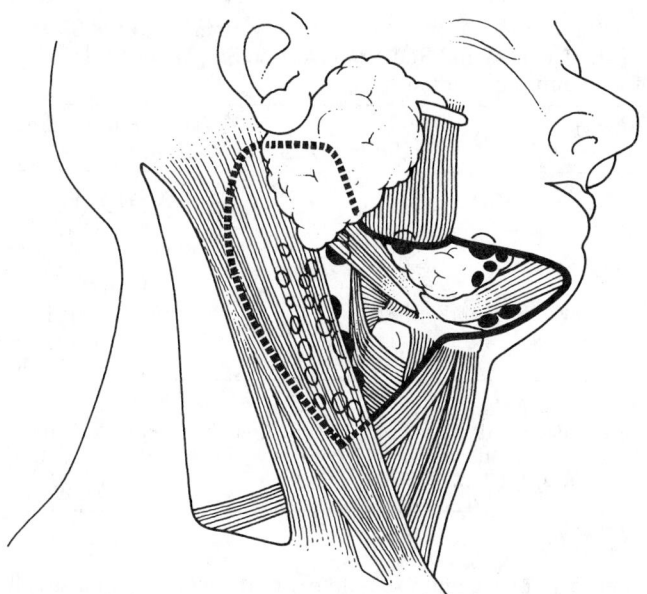

FIGURE 22–6. Cervical lymph nodes removed in a supraomohyoid neck dissection.

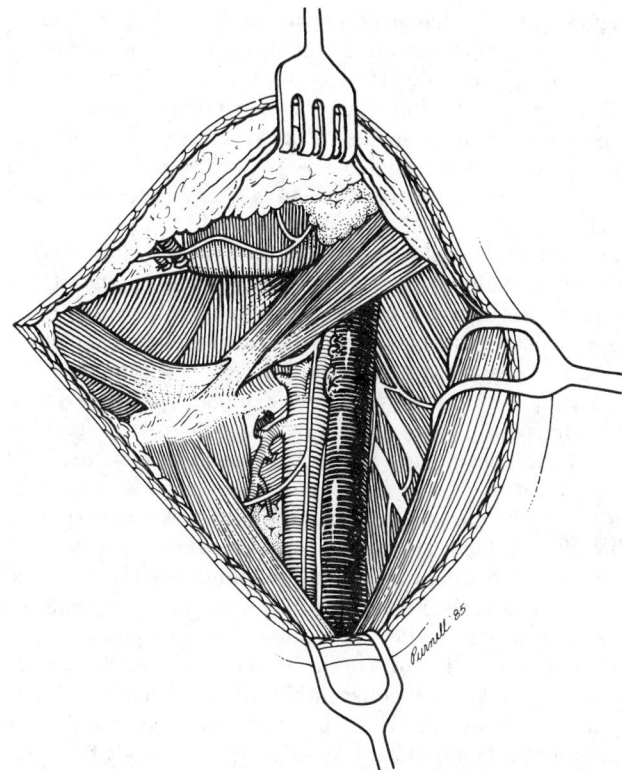

FIGURE 22–7. Regional anatomy after a supraomohyoid neck dissection. Major structures of the neck are preserved, including jugular vein and spinal accessory nerve. (Shah JP, Shemen LJ, Strong EW. Surgical therapy of oral cavity tumors. In: Thawley SE, Panje WR, eds. Comprehensive management of head and neck tumors. Philadelphia: WB Saunders, 1987:556)

nodes at one or more levels, extracapsular extension, the risk for contralateral nodal metastases requiring elective irradiation to the contralateral neck, risk for disease in undissected nodal areas such as the retropharyngeal region, and risk for disease in the lower neck.

Side effects of radiation therapy usually are separated into acute and late effects. Acute effects generally are related to inflammatory reactions in the tissues, epidermitis and mucositis, within the radiation field. Such effects include the following: loss or diminution of taste caused by irradiation of tissue including the taste buds; xerostomia caused by irradiation of the salivary glands; dryness in the eye caused by irradiation of the lacrimal glands; and epilation caused by irradiation of hair-bearing skin. Whether these effects are temporary or permanent is usually dose related and site related. Because radiation therapy to the salivary glands and oral cavity can have significant impact on dentition, all patients receiving this treatment should be seen by a dentist before radiation therapy. Any required dental work should be done before the initiation of radiation and patients should be placed on dental prophylaxis with fluoride applications. It has been shown that fluoride application significantly reduces dental sequelae after radiation therapy.[95] It has also been shown that dental extractions in an irradiated mandible can lead to osteonecrosis.[96]

New radiation therapy techniques have been significant in the treatment of head and neck cancer patients. For external-beam treatments, three-dimensional (3D) conformal radiation therapy is a particularly exciting new area because it allows the physician to plan radiation therapy based on 3D reconstruction of the target area and makes 3D planning of the radiation beams possible. As a result, it is frequently possible to lower the dose to surrounding normal tissue while potentially escalating the dose to the tumor.[97] Efforts to use this technique in nasopharyngeal cancer have been particularly interesting and are discussed in the section on nasopharyngeal cancer. The development of multileaf collimators and on-line

portal imaging techniques should make the delivery of 3D radiation therapy more efficient. There has been considerable interest in using twice-a-day (bid) radiation programs.[98–100] Whether these fractionation programs produce better tumor control than conventional radiation remains unproved. However, considerable retrospective data suggest a benefit that may be significant in patients with more advanced disease.[98,100] A prospective randomized trial by the RTOG failed to show a benefit to the bid program but was faulted by the fact that the total dose in the bid group was too low and significantly below the dose level in the conventional group. There are also new developments in the area of brachytherapy. The use of new isotopes, such as palladium 103, newly developed temporary implant techniques with iridium 192 and iodine 125, and emerging capabilities for intraoperative radiation therapy offer potential advances and therapeutic opportunities.

External-beam irradiation is usually delivered once a day, 5 days per week, continuous course until the desired dose is achieved. For postoperative radiation, the optimal dose has not yet been defined. In general, doses in the 6000- to 6500-cGy range in 6 to 7 weeks are delivered to the primary site and involved regions of the neck. Doses of 5000- to 5400-cGy in 5 to 6 weeks are given to areas at risk for microscopic disease that have not been operated on. Fletcher has shown that doses of 5000 cGy in 5 weeks are effective in sterilizing microscopic disease in areas at risk that have not had surgery.[101] Because the anatomic separation in the head and neck region is thinner than in other parts of the body, a low-energy linear accelerator is preferred. This means that cobalt 60, 4 mV or 6 mV photons will usually be preferred. Electron beams will also be used for the posterior neck or other regions where it is preferable to treat superficial structures and avoid irradiating deeper ones. Higher-energy linear accelerators have too much skin sparing to be useful in treating most head and neck cancers.

Patients with involved nodal metastases are usually managed by a combination of surgery and radiation. Although the N1 neck can frequently be managed by surgery or radiation (Table 22–5), those patients with more advanced disease are better served by combined treatment. Table 22–5 summarizes the regional control rates with radiation alone or combined with neck dissection. Table 22–6 shows neck control as a function of radiation dose. Hirabayashi and associates have reported that 31% of the N1 patients in their series had evidence of extracapsular spread.[102] Snyderman and coworkers reported that 38% of their N1 patients had extracapsular spread.[103] A similar cohort will be found to have multiple positive nodes. Therefore, it is clear that a significant percentage of patients who have neck dissection for N1 disease require postoperative radiation anyway because of the presence of these prognostic features. Vikram and colleagues have compared the results of surgery alone with those of combined surgery and postoperative radiation therapy in a retrospective study from the case material at the Memorial Sloan-Kettering Cancer Center.[104] Neck recurrence was analyzed as a function of the number of involved levels of nodes. When surgery was the only treatment to the neck, 37% of patients with one nodal level involved and 71% of patients with multiple levels involved developed neck failure. When postoperative radiation is added, neck failure is reduced to 16% in patients with one level and 13% in those with multiple levels. Radiation should be delivered beginning 4 to 6 weeks after surgery. The impact of delay beyond 6 weeks on tumor control is unclear, but probably not significant.[104–107]

PRINCIPLES OF CHEMOTHERAPY (RECURRENT DISEASE)

The survival for patients with local or disseminated recurrent squamous cell carcinoma of the head and neck is usually 6 to 10 months and has not been affected by the use of chemo-

TABLE 22–5. Control of Regional Lymph Node Metastases as a Function of Treatments*

Treatment	Classification			
	N0	N1	N2	N3
Radiation	10/57	2/26	10/34	15/36
Surgery	1/6	1/7	0/5	0/4
Combined	—	0/4	0/23	2/10

* Patients with squamous cell cancer of the tonsillar fossa and base of tongue, 1948 to 1967.
(Adapted from Barkley HT, Fletcher GH, Jesse RH, et al. Management of cervical lymph node metastases in squamous cell carcinoma of the tonsillar fossa, base of tongue, supraglottic larynx, and hypopharynx. Am J Surg 1972;124:462–467)

TABLE 22–6. Control Rates* As a Function of the Size of the Node(s) and Radiation Dose in Squamous Cell Carcinomas of the Laryngopharynx

Size of Node (cm)	Radiation Dose		Control Rate No./ Total No. (%)
<3	≤65 Gy >65 Gy	>0.001	15/26 (58) 86/95 (91)
3–5	≤70 Gy >70 Gy	<0.005	3/9 (33) 11/13 (85)
>5	≤70 Gy >70 Gy	<0.002	1/9 (11) 11/15 (73)

* Determinate group.
(From Bataini JP, Bernier J, Brugère J, et al. In: Pinel J, Leroux-Robert J, eds. Adenopathies Cervicales les Malignes. Paris: Masson Publishers, 1982:129–135)

therapy. Consequently, patients with recurrent squamous cell carcinoma of the head and neck are candidates for phase I and II trials of new drugs and new combinations of agents.

Single-Agent Chemotherapy Trials

The most active agents and their response rates are listed in Table 22–7[108–120] and include methotrexate, bleomycin, cisplatin, 5-fluorouracil (5-FU), and carboplatin.

METHOTREXATE. Methotrexate is the standard palliative therapy for recurrent metastatic squamous cell carcinoma of the head and neck. The standard dose for initiation is 40 mg/m^2/week to be escalated to 60 mg/m^2/week until dose-limiting toxicity or an objective response is reached. Therapy with this drug is relatively nontoxic, inexpensive, and convenient. Higher doses of methotrexate in single-arm studies were shown to produce higher response rates.[108–111] Five randomized trials have shown no significant difference in survival rates between higher doses of methotrexate with leucovorin (as much as 5000 mg) and standard-dose methotrexate (Table 22–8).[110–114]

BLEOMYCIN. Bleomycin has been studied extensively as a single agent and in combination in recurrent-metastatic squamous cell carcinoma of the head and neck. Response rates as a single agent vary from 6% to 45%, with a pooled average of 21%.[115] Because of its distinct toxicity (skin, mucous membranes, and lung tissue toxicity without any significant myelosuppression), it has an advantage in combination chemo-

TABLE 22–7. Single Agent in Recurrent and Metastatic Head and Neck Squamous Cell Carcinoma

Chemotherapeutic Agent	No. of Patients	Response Rate (%)
Methotrexate[115]	988	31
Bleomycin[115]	347	21
Cisplatin[115]	288	28
Carboplatin[119]	169	22
5-FU[115]	118	15

TABLE 22–8. Randomized Trials of Standard-Dose Versus High-Dose Methotrexate With Leucovorin in Recurrent and Metastatic Head and Neck Squamous Cell Carcinoma

Investigations	Dose of Methotrexate mg/m^2/wk*	Repsonse Rate (%)	Median Survival
Levitt, 1973[110]	(a) 40–115	44	Not reported
	(b) 120–540	60	
Vogl, 1979[111]	(a) 60 I.V.	34	
	(b) 60 po	27	
	(c) 500 po	27	
Woods, 1981[112]	(a) 50	31	≈42 wk
	(b) 500	21	≈21 wk
	(c) 5000	50	≈28 wk
Deconti, 1981[113]	(a) 40–60	26	≈22 wk
	(b) 120	24	≈19 wk
Taylor, 1984[114]	(a) 40 IM	22	4.2 mo
	(b) 1500 I.V.	32	4.2 mo

* (a), (b), (c) represent patient arm of randomized trial receiving indicated therapy.

therapy. It can be given in full dosage in combination with other agents with a different spectrum of toxicity. Continuous infusion of bleomycin produces less pulmonary toxicity than do bolus injections.

CISPLATIN. Cisplatin is perhaps the most important chemotherapeutic agent in squamous cell carcinoma of the head and neck. Most of the studies have used a dose of 80 to 100 mg/m^2 every 3 to 4 weeks as a standard dose. Response rates have ranged from 14% to 41%, with a pooled average of 28%.[115] Whether there is a dose-response relation is not yet proved. Single-agent, high-dose cisplatin in single-arm studies produced higher response rates,[116,117] but a randomized trial comparing 60 mg/m^2 doses with 120 mg/m^2 doses found no difference in response or survival.[118]

5-FLUOROURACIL. 5-FU was studied initially in recurrent squamous cell carcinoma of the head and neck as second- or

third-line chemotherapy to be used after other drugs failed. Response rates reported ranged from 0% to 33%, with an average of only 15%.[115] In these studies, 5-FU was usually given as an intravenous bolus daily for 5 days or weekly. The dose-limiting toxicity of this method of administration was myelosuppression. In the 1970s, 5-FU was studied as a prolonged infusion for 90 to 120 hours. The dose-limiting toxicity was found to be mucositis; myelosuppression was significantly lower. When 5-FU was used as an infusion instead of a bolus administration, it was found to have increased activity in squamous cell carcinoma of the head and neck and to have a synergistic interaction with cisplatin and enhanced cytotoxicity with modulators such as leucovorin. 5-FU remains under intense study in squamous cell carcinoma of the head and neck.

Other Single Agents

CISPLATIN ANALOGS. Carboplatin has been tested actively against recurrent squamous cell carcinoma of the head and neck. It has significantly less renal, otologic, neurologic, and gastrointestinal toxicity than does cisplatin. Response rates obtained have been in the range of 14% to 30%, with an average of 26%. Iproplatin trials have yielded much lower response rates and major toxicity in early phase II trials.[119,120]

Miscellaneous Drugs

METHOTREXATE ANALOGS. The methotrexate analogs trimetrexate, piritrexim, and edatrexate have all been tested and seem to be active.[121–124] Ifosfamide is another agent that deserves mention. In a recent study, ifosfamide was found to have a single-agent response rate of 17% in heavily pretreated patients,[125] enough to warrant further study. Etoposide has yielded poor response rates in early phase II trials.[126,128]

Combination Chemotherapy Trials

Different combination chemotherapy regimens have been tried in recurrent squamous cell carcinoma of the head and neck. Non-cisplatin-containing regimens have been reported to have response rates from 11% to 100% (Table 22–9).[128–139] In the 1970s and 1980s, studies focused on cisplatin combinations (Table 22–10).[140–169] It seems, based on single-arm trials, that cisplatin-based regimens lead to higher response rates, especially higher CR rates. In the early 1980s,

TABLE 22–9. Non-Cisplatin Regimens in Recurrent and Metastatic Head and Neck Squamous Cell Carcinoma[128,130–139]

Regimen	Response Range (%)	Average Response Rate (%)
BCMF	11–69	45
VBM	25–54	36.6
Price-Hill regimen*	13–41	35.5
MTX + 5-FU	16–100	49

C, cyclophosphamide; M, MTX, methotrexate; F, 5-FU, 5-fluorouracil; V, vincristine; B, bleomycin.
* Price–Hill regimen: combination of vincristine, methotrexate, bleomycin, 5-fluorouracil, hydrocortisone, and folinic acid.

TABLE 22–10. Cisplatin-Containing Regimens in Recurrent and Metastatic Head and Neck Squamous Cell Carcinoma[140–169]

Chemotherapy Combinations	Response Rate (%)	Average Response Rate (%)
PB	13–55	25.7
PAC	7–64	43.5
PVB	30–50	38.1
PBM	27–100	58.8
PBVe	45–63	50
PF	11–75	45

P, cisplatin; B, bleomycin; A, doxorubicin; C, cyclophosphamide; V, vincristine; M, methotrexate; Ve, velban; F, 5-fluorouracil.

TABLE 22–11. Cisplatin and 5-FU Combinations in Recurrent and Metastatic Head and Neck Squamous Cell Carcinoma

Chemotherapy Combinations	Response Rate (CR + PR)
PFL[170]	56 (6 + 30)
PBF[171]	50 (5 + 45)
PFBM[168,172]	63 (7 + 54), 87 (26 ± 67)
PFIL-2[173]	35 (5 + 30)
PFIFN[174]	30 (4 + 26)

P, cisplatin; F, 5-fluorouracil; L, leucovorin; B, bleomycin; M, methotrexate; IL-2, interleukin-2; IFN, interferon.

researchers at Wayne State reported a response rate of 70% and a CR rate of 27% using a cisplatin and 5-FU (PF) regimen. Other centers have since reported lower response rates. Newer combinations in which another active agent was added to the PF regimen have been attempted (Table 22–11).[170–175] No significant improvement in response rates or survival has been achieved to date.

Randomized Trials of Single and Multiagent Regimens

Eight randomized trials have been reported comparing methotrexate with other chemotherapeutic agents.[130,176–181] All ex-

TABLE 22–12. Randomized Trials of Methotrexate Against Other Chemotherapeutic Agents in Recurrent and Metastatic Head and Neck Squamous Cell Carcinoma

Investigations	Chemotherapy Regimens	Response Rate (%)	Median Survival (mo)
Hong, 1983[175]	M	24	6.1
	P	29	6.3
Drelichman, 1983[176]	M	33	5.6
	POB	41	4
Grose, 1985[177]	M	6	5
	P	8	4.5
Vogl, 1985[178]	MTX	35	5.6
	MBP	48	5.6
Williams, 1986[179]	M	16	7.3
	PVB	24	6.8
Campbell, 1987[180]	M	19	2.7
	P	40	8.7
	PM	31	5.3
	PF	33	6.7
Eisenberger, 1989[181]	M	25	6
	CpM	25	6
Forastiere, 1989[129]	M	11	5.6
	CpF	8	5.2
	PF	30	6.6

M, MTX, methotrexate; P, cisplatin; O, oncovin; B, bleomycin; V, vincristine; F, 5-fluorouracil; Cp, carboplatin.

cept one have failed to show any significant survival benefit (Table 22–12).

Six randomized trials have compared PF regimens with other chemotherapeutic agents (Table 22–13). The first of these compared PF infusion to PF bolus. The response rates were significantly higher in the infusion group. Patients on the infusion arm had a median survival of 27 weeks compared with 20 weeks for those on the bolus arm. In the other five trials, PF has been compared with other chemotherapeutic agents. In their latest analysis, Jacobs and colleagues compared PF in combination with cisplatin and 5-FU as single agents.[169] The response rate was the highest in the PF group; however, the median survival was not significantly different in the three arms.

Biologic Therapy for Recurrent Squamous Cell Head and Neck Cancer

Patients with head and neck cancer characteristically have moderate to severe depression of cellular and hormonal immunity, which may be reduced even further by surgery or radiation therapy. Early clinical trials adding nonspecific immunoadjuvant therapy (BCG or levamisole) were negative. An evaluation of thymosine as adjuvant therapy is still in progress. Cytokines (interferon-α, [IFN-α], interleukin-2 [IL-2], and combination IL-2 and IFN-α) have been used in squamous cell head and neck cancer. Results of the trial of IFN-γ against nasopharyngeal carcinoma were disappointing.[182]

Several human squamous cell head and neck cancer cell lines express high-affinity IL-2 receptors and are growth inhibited by IL-2 in vivo and in vitro. It has been shown in squamous cell head and neck cancer that tumor-infiltrating lymphocytes can be increased 30,000-fold by IL-2. Systemic

TABLE 22–13. Randomized Trials of Cisplatin and 5-FU Versus Other Agents in Recurrent and Metastatic Head and Neck Squamous Cell Carcinoma

Investigations	Agents	Response Rate (CR + PR) (%)	Median Survival (mo)
Kish, 1985[156]	PF (CI)	72 (22 + 50)	6.3
	PF (bolus)	20 (10 + 10)	4.6
Forastiere, 1989[129]	PF		6.6
	CpF		5.2
	M		5.6
Amrein, 1990[168]	Pf	46 (0 + 46)*	6
	PFBM	63 (7 + 56)*	6
Liverpool Study, 1990[162]	PF	24*	
	P	28*	
	M	12*	
	PM	22*	
Jacobs, 1991[169]	PF	40	5.5
	P	18	5
	F	15	6.1

* Not significant.

P, cisplatin; F, 5-fluorouracil; Cp, carboplatin; M, methotrexate; B, bleomycin; O, oncovin; CI, continuous infusion.

IF-2 and IFN-α have produced antitumor activity but with substantial toxicity.[183]

Retinoids have been studied in recurrent squamous cell head and neck cancer in two trials for a total of more than 30 heavily treated patients; in one, 13-*cis*-retinoic acid (13-cRA) produced a 15% response rate.[184] Research currently focuses on the best way to combine cytokines, retinoids, cytotoxic agents, and radiation therapy. A small series using combinations of the biologic agents IFN-α and IL-2 and another using IFN-α and retinoids have reported objective responses in advanced squamous cell head and neck cancer.[183–185]

Plasmapheresis followed by cytotoxic or biologic therapy is an interesting and provocative strategy that is currently under clinical investigation. The integration of biologic agents into cytotoxic regimens (IL-2 plus PF, IFN-α plus PF) have been studied. So far, it is not clear that the therapeutic indices of the IFN-α or IL-2 plus PF are greater than chemotherapy alone. A new area of highly specific therapy using antiepidermal growth factor monoclonal antibodies is under study in early clinical trials.

PRINCIPLES OF CHEMOTHERAPY (PREVIOUSLY UNTREATED DISEASE)

Neoadjuvant Chemotherapy

Chemotherapy may be given before or after ablative surgery or radiation therapy. The main advantages of induction chemotherapy (*i.e.*, chemotherapy before surgery or radiation therapy) are better tumor control and preservation of organ function. Induction chemotherapy eliminates the pharmacologic sanctuary problems (*i.e.*, poor vascularity leading to poor concentration of chemotherapy) after surgery or radiation therapy. Initial chemotherapy results in delivery of chemotherapy to the best possible host, resulting in increased compliance, responsiveness, and tolerance of higher doses. It results in better locoregional control and eliminates distant micrometastases (see Chap. 22, section 2 for a discussion on laryngeal cancer).

Nonrandomized Trials of Neoadjuvant Chemotherapy

Many induction trials have been reported in which the single agents methotrexate, bleomycin, or cisplatin were used.[186–194] The CR rate with single agents was low (< 5%). In the late 1970s, a combination of cisplatin and bleomycin used by Randolph and associates obtained a 71% response rate with a 19% CR rate.[195] Many other investigators since then have used the regimen and have confirmed the high overall response rate, but reported lower CR rates.[196–200] To achieve higher response rates, investigators added methotrexate[201–208] or vinca alkaloids[209–215] to the cisplatin and bleomycin regimen. The CR rate improved from 7% with cisplatin and bleomycin to 16% with cisplatin, bleomycin, and methotrexate and to 20% with cisplatin and bleomycin and a vinca alkaloid.

The next major advance occurred in the early 1980s when Wayne State investigators reported induction trials with a PF regimen.[216] They achieved a response rate of 88% (CR = 19%)[216] with two courses and 93% (CR = 54%) with three courses of the same regimen. Since then, many other investigators have used this regimen and reported partial response

(PR) rates of 63% to 98% and CR rates of 0% to 54% (Table 22–14).[216–234] This remains the most active regimen in previously untreated patients.

Trials with a modification of this regimen have been conducted or are in progress in an effort to increase CR rates (Table 22–15).[235–243] One of the newer regimens is cisplatin, 5-FU, and leucovorin (PFL). Vokes and coworkers treated 29 patients with oral leucovorin plus intravenous PF, and obtained a CR in 9 and PR in 17 patients after two cycles.[235] Dreyfuss and associates reported a 66% CR and 14% PR rate with the three cycles of the PFL regimen with leucovorin administered intravenously as a continuous infusion.[240]

A few non–cisplatin-containing chemotherapy combinations have been tried as induction therapy, but CR rates with these remain low. Hill and coworkers used a combination of vincristine, bleomycin, methotrexate (VBM), 5-FU, and hydrocortisone in 200 untreated patients with advanced disease.[244] They described a 66% response rate after two cycles (CR not mentioned). The CR rate after local therapy was significantly greater in chemotherapy responders (78%) than in chemotherapy nonresponders (49%). Overall survival duration was 32 months for all patients, 37 months for chemotherapy responders, and 69 months for all patients achieving CR after all therapy. Hill and coworkers also reported that oral cavity and nasopharyngeal cancer responded better to initial chemotherapy. Survival was longer in patients with nasopharyngeal and laryngeal tumors. Toxicity was minimal with this regimen.

Randomized Trials

Many randomized trials have been conducted to determine if the addition of chemotherapy improves survival. Thirteen randomized trials (Table 22–16) compared chemotherapy and surgery with or without radiation therapy with surgery only with or without radiation therapy only, and 12 randomized

TABLE 22–14. Cisplatin Plus 5-FU Induction Chemotherapy

Investigations	No. of Patients	RR (CR + PR) (%)
Kish[216]	26	88 (19 + 69)
Kish[217]	85	93 (54 + 39)
Kies[219]	60	87 (37 + 50)
Amrein[220]	31	84 (23 + 61)
Clark[221]	53	73 (30 + 43)
Khojasteh[222]	8	63 (0 + 63)
Loeffler[223]	27	96 (44 + 52)
Toohill[224]	27	86 (19 + 67)
Johnson[225]	21	76 (14 + 62)
Jacobs[226]	30	83 (43 + 40)
VA Larynx[227]	117	98 (49 + 49)
Thyss[228]	103	87 (35 + 52)
Paccagnella[229]	110	70 (29 + 41)
Martin[230]	37	68 (46 + 22)
Joveniaux[231]	40	38 (13 + 25)
Scherpe[232]	30	57 (20 + 37)
Dasmahapatra[233]	19	84 (26 + 58)
Verweij[234]	76	66 (17 + 49)

TABLE 22–15. 5-FU Plus Cisplatin Combinations as Neoadjuvant Chemotherapy

Investigations	Regimens	No. of Patients	RR (CR + PR) (%)
Vokes, 1990[235]	PFL (po)	29	90 (31 + 59)
Greenberg, 1987[236]	PF allopurinol	33	100 (45 + 55)
Ensley, 1988[237]	PF alt MLF	39	95 (51 + 44)
Kramer, 1988[238]	PBF		
Vokes, 1989[239]	PFM	34	88 (26 ± 62)
Dreyfuss, 1990[240]	PFL (I.V.)	35	80 (66 ± 14)
Kish, 1988[241]	High-dose PF	11	90 (45 + 45)
Vokes, 1991[242]	PFL po + IFN	20	100 (70 + 30)
Urba, 1990[243]	High-dose PF + MGBG	34	82 (44 + 38)

P, cisplatin; F, 5-fluorouracil; L, leucovorin; M, methotrexate; B, bleomycin; MGBG, mitoguazone; IFN, interferon; alt, alternating with.

trials (Table 22–17) compared chemotherapy and radiation therapy with radiation therapy alone.[245–263] The first group of trials were in operable patients who were randomized to receive the standard therapy of surgery with or without radiation therapy or induction chemotherapy followed by surgery with or without radiation therapy (see Table 22–16). None of the trials reported any survival benefit. The following criticisms undermine the validity of these trials: (1) there were too few patients in many of the trials; (2) relatively inactive regimens were used in most of the trials; (3) the trials used a heterogenous study population with mixed primary sites; (4) there was too improper stratification based on TN stage to have similar patient groups in both arms; (5) too few courses of chemotherapy were used before surgery in many trials; (6) there were extremely low CR rates; and (7) there were possible compromises of surgery and radiation therapy combinined in the experimental arm. Four of the trials used the most active regimen PF. For two of these trials, final results are not yet available.

In the second group of trials, patients were randomized between sequential chemotherapy and radiation therapy or radiation therapy alone (see Table 22–17). Many of these trials were conducted with patients with unresectable tumors. Only two of the trials reported a significant survival benefit. Arcangeli and colleagues reported a benefit with intraarterial methotrexate mainly in oral cavity tumors.[257] Merlano and coworkers recently reported on alternating chemotherapy of cisplatin and 5-FU with radiation therapy and found a significant survival benefit in the chemotherapy and radiation therapy group.[262] The remaining trials did not report any survival benefit.

Nevertheless, several important issues were resolved from these induction trials, including the following:

1. Induction chemotherapy can result in significant tumor regression in 60% to 90% and complete regression in 20% to 50% of patients with locally advanced head and neck squamous cell carcinoma.

TABLE 22–16. Randomized Trials of Neoadjuvant Chemotherapy

Investigations	Regimens	No. of Patients	CR + PR (%)	Survival Benefit
Stolwijk, 1985[245]	VBMCF	58	NR	None
Taylor, 1985[189]	ML	82	6 + 34	None
Rentschler, 1987[246]	M	55	NR	None
HN Contracts, 1987[200]	PB	443	3 + 34	None
Kun, 1986[247]	BCMF	83	5 + 63	None
Toohill, 1987[224]	PF	60	19 + 66	None
Richard, 1984[248]	VB	225	NR	None
Martin, 1988[249]	PFBM	107	6 + 43	None
Schuller, 1988[250]	PBMV	158	19 + 51	None
Martin, 1989[249]	PF	75	46 + 22	None
Paccagnella, 1990[229]	PF	221	29 + 41	NR
VA Study, 1991[227]	PF	332	49 + 49	None

P, cisplatin; M, methotrexate; V, vincristine; C, cyclophosphamide; F, 5-fluorouracil; L, leucovorin; B, bleomycin.

TABLE 22–17.　Randomized Trials of Sequential Chemotherapy Plus Radiation Therapy Versus Radiation Therapy

Investigations	Regimens	No. of Patients	Survival Benefit
Von Essen, 1968[251]	(a) MTX	87	None
	(b) 5-FU		
	(c) IUDR		
Richard, 1974[252]	MTX (IA)	39	None
Knowlton, 1975[253]	MTX	96	None
Lustig, 1976[255]	MTX	75	None
Fazekas, 1980[255]	MTX	638	None
Petrovich, 1981[256]	VM	23	None
Arcangeli, 1983[257]	MTX (IA)	142	Yes (oral cavity tumors)
Stell, 1990[258]	Price-Hill regimen*	80	None
Shetty, 1985[260]	VBMFUC	42	? None
Szpirglas, 1987[261]	DOBP	114	? None
Jaulerry, 1989[262]	PBVM	100	None
Merlano, 1991[263]	DDP + 5-FU alt with XRT	150	Yes

M, MTX, methotrexate; F, 5-FU, 5-fluorouracil; IUDR, iododeoxyuridine; V, vincristine; B, bleomycin; C, cyclophaosphamide; D, doxorubicin; O, oncovin; P, cisplatin; IA, intraarterial; alt; alternating; XRT, radiation therapy.
* Price–Hill regimen: combination of vincristine, methotrexate, bleomycin, 5-fluorouracil, hydrocortisone, and folinic acid.

2. Patients who achieve CR with chemotherapy have much better survival than do partial and nonresponders.
3. Chemotherapy response continues to increase through at least three courses of treatment.
4. Pathologic CR has been documented by biopsy or surgery in 30% to 70% of clinical complete responders.
5. Chemotherapy responders respond further to radiation therapy and chemotherapy nonresponders do not.
6. Radiation therapy alone may be enough for locoregional control in patients who achieve CR to chemotherapy.
7. Induction chemotherapy does not significantly increase surgical or radiation therapy complications.
8. TN stage and type of chemotherapy regimen are important prognostic factors for response to chemotherapy, whereas performance status, tumor site, TN stage, and response to chemotherapy are predictors for survival.
9. Although all sites of head and neck are lumped together in almost all the studies, there is growing evidence that different sites show different biologic behavior.
10. There is strong evidence for a definite decrease in distant metastases when chemotherapy is part of combined modality treatment of head and neck cancer.
11. Survival and quality of life (*i.e.*, organ preservation) should both be considered the endpoints rather than survival alone.

Concurrent Chemoradiotherapy

The purpose of simultaneous chemoradiotherapy is to increase locoregional control and prevent distant metastases. The possible synergistic effect has been explained by supposing that the drugs (*e.g.*, bleomycin, cisplatin, and others) interfere with cell repair after sublethal or potentially lethal damage or with tumor cell synchronization. Many clinical trials testing simultaneous chemoradiotherapy have been conducted since the 1960s (Table 22–18). All the agents active in head and neck cancer have been combined with radiation therapy to enhance its effect and possibly prevent distant metastases.

METHOTREXATE. Methotrexate has been used with concomitant radiation therapy based on its high single-agent activity in head and neck cancer. Two randomized trials have been published with opposing results. Condit[263] reported no improvement in the combined chemotherapy and radiation therapy group, whereas Gupta and colleagues[264] reported a significantly better primary control and survival, especially in oropharyngeal cancers. In the study by Gupta and colleagues, there was more cutaneous and mucosal toxicity in the chemotherapy and radiation therapy group, but no patients had their treatment interrupted or required nasogastric tube or intravenous feedings.[264] There was no increase in late toxicity.

BLEOMYCIN. Bleomycin has been combined with radiation therapy frequently in head and neck cancer. Many studies of bleomycin and radiation therapy report CR rates in the range of 38% to 79%.[265] There are at least eight randomized trials[266–275] comparing bleomycin and radiation therapy with radiation therapy alone. Three of the trials showed a benefit in response rate or survival or both.[266,267,274] However, the other five trials, including the large European Organization for Research on Treatment of Cancer (EORTC) randomized trial, did not reveal any significant benefit in the bleomycin and radiation therapy arm. Most of the studies did report increased acute toxicity, especially mucositis and skin reaction.

TABLE 22–18. Randomized Trials of Simultaneous Chemotherapy Plus
Radiation Therapy Versus Radiation Therapy

Investigations	Chemotherapy	No. of Patients	Response Benefit	Survival Benefit
Richards, 1969[239]	HU	40	Yes	NR
Stefani, 1980[278]	HU	150	No	No
Condit, 1968[263]	MTX	40	No	NR
Gupta, 1987[264]	MTX	313	Yes	Yes
Kapstad, 1978[266]	Bleomycin	29	Yes	NR
Shanta, 1980[267]	Bleomycin	157	Yes	Yes
Morita, 1980[268]	Bleomycin	45 (tongue)	No	No
Scandolaro, 1982[269]	Bleomycin	30	No	No
Pauinen, 1985[270]	Bleomycin	46	No	No
Shetty, 1985[271]	Bleomycin	38	NR	No
Vermund, 1985[272]	Bleomycin	222	No	No
Fu, 1987[274]	Bleomycin	104	Yes	Yes – DFS
Eschwege, 1988[275]	Bleomycin	199	No	No
Shigematsu, 1971[276]	5-FU	63	NR	Yes – DFS
Lo, 1976[277]	5-FU	163	Yes	Yes
Weissberg, 1989[279]	Mitomycin-C	117	Yes	Yes
Haselow, 1990[283]	CDDP	319	Yes	NR
Keegan, 1988[286]	CDDP + 5-FU	25	NR	Not yet

HU, hydroxyurea; M, MTX, methotrexate; F, 5-FU, 5-fluorouracil; CDDP, cisplatin; DFS, disease-free survival.

5-FLUOROURACIL. Many studies have used 5-FU with concurrent radiation therapy. Two randomized trials have been reported. In the study from Japan, intraarterial 5-FU was used with radiation therapy in maxillary sinus carcinoma.[276] Disease-free survival was better, but overall survival was similar in both groups. In the study by Lo and associates, 5-year survival was significantly better only in the oral cavity group.[277] 5-FU did increase the acute and late tissue toxicity of radiation therapy.

OTHER AGENTS. Hydroxyurea has been used concurrently as a radiosensitizer in some trials.[278] One randomized trial from Yale used mitomycin-C with radiation therapy and showed disease-free survival benefit.[279] Overall survival was better, but statistical significance was not reached. A high incidence of pulmonary complications was reported in the experimental arm.

CISPLATIN AND ITS COMBINATIONS. Recently, cisplatin has been used with increasing frequency concurrently with radiation therapy. CR rates ranging from 52% to 94% have been reported. Preliminary results of a randomized trial comparing cisplatin (20 mg/m^2 weekly) during radiation with conventional radiation were reported.[283] The CR rate in the concomitant arm was only 34%, which is in marked contrast to CR rates reported in other pilot studies.

Cisplatin in a dosage of 100 mg/m^2 every 3 weeks concomitant with radiation therapy has been evaluated in a phase II trial and seems to be promising.[284] In 124 patients treated with this schedule, the CR rate was 71% and the 3-year survival was 43%. Acute and chronic toxicity were acceptable. This result is supported by other pilot trials reported.[279-282]

Recently, some trials have been reported using combination chemotherapy concurrent with radiation therapy. The major advantage of this, in addition to controlling locoregional dis-

ease, would be to reduce distant metastases. Taylor and coworkers administered a regimen of concomitant cisplatin and 5-FU with conventional radiation every other week for seven cycles.[285] Results from 53 unresectable patients indicate a high clinical CR rate of 55% and PR rate of 43%. Overall, median survival was 37 months. Harrison and colleagues reported 24 patients treated with concomitant cisplatin and radiation therapy using combined conventional and hyperfractionated radiation therapy for unresectable disease.[373] CR was 64%, and PR was 32%. Keegan and coworkers reported on a randomized trial of cisplatin 100 mg/m^2 on day 1 and 5-FU 1000 mg/m^2/24 hours on days 1 to 4 during radiation every 28 days for two cycles versus radiation alone.[286] Toxicity was greater in the chemotherapy-radiation therapy group. Follow-up and patient numbers were too small to detect any significant difference in survival in the preliminary report, but the final report may show a difference. The concomitant PF combinations with radiation therapy in pilot trials have produced excellent CR rates.[287-290] However, normal tissue toxicity was markedly increased. These innovative concomitant approaches await confirmation of efficacy in randomized trials. Preliminary data indicate that carboplatin with radiation therapy leads to high CR rates (50–70%).[291-293] Further studies are needed to confirm the data and to establish the optimal dose and schedule of carboplatin.

Comparison of Different Strategies of Combining Chemotherapy and Radiation Therapy

Three different modes of combining chemotherapy and radiation therapy have been studied: sequential (*i.e.*, chemotherapy followed by radiation therapy); simultaneous (chemotherapy and radiation therapy concurrently); and alternating (*i.e.*, chemotherapy and radiation therapy given one after the other).

The mode of combining the two therapies is an important issue. The response rate may be better with concurrent chemotherapy and radiation therapy, but toxicity is definitely enhanced. To minimize normal tissue toxicity, it may be necessary to administer chemotherapy and radiation therapy in a sequential manner; however, this strategy can be detrimental to the control of some cancers. In head and neck cancer, the radiation dose needed for tumor control was more when the treatment duration was longer than 4 weeks.[294] This was thought to be due to accelerated repopulation of tumor cells surviving the initial treatment. The failure of induction chemotherapy to show any survival benefit in randomized trails may have a similar cause. If researchers considered radiation therapy a non-cross-resistant tumor killing agent and alternated it with chemotherapy, they might circumvent the problem of heterogenous tumor cell population and primary drug resistance. This hybrid of chemotherapy alternating with radiation therapy would reduce normal tissue toxicity compared with the simultaneous approach.

At least four randomized trials compare sequential chemotherapy and radiation therapy with simultaneous chemotherapy and radiation therapy.[226,295-298] Southeastern Cooperative Oncology Group (SECOG) randomized 262 patients to receive synchronous or sequential chemotherapy of VBM with or without 5-FU and radiation therapy.[295] They found disease-free survival to be better ($p = 0.07$) for the synchronous group, especially for laryngeal cancer patients. Treatment did not present serious problems of toxicity. Shetty and associates randomized 61 patients with base of tongue cancers to radiation therapy alone; to radiation therapy and bleomycin concurrently; and to VBM and mitomycin-C and 5-FU followed by radiation therapy.[260] There was no significant difference in disease-free survival in the three groups. Cognetti and colleagues randomized 60 patients with locally advanced squamous cell carcinoma of the head and neck to sequential PF and radiation therapy and simultaneous cisplatin and radiation therapy.[296] The 2-year overall survival was 38% for sequential and 46% for simultaneous chemotherapy and radiation therapy ($p = 0.56$). Toxicity was acceptable for both, indicating the feasibility of both approaches. Vannetzel and colleagues compared sequential PF and radiation therapy with concomitant cisplatin and 5-FU and radiation therapy every other week. Median time to failure was 9.8 months for the sequential group compared with more than 16 months for the concomitant group ($p < 0.07$). However, there was no overall survival difference in their last report.[298] Adelstein and coworkers randomized 48 patients to sequential PF and radiation therapy and simultaneous PF and radiation therapy.[297] The toxicities of the simultaneous and sequential arms were equivalent, except for mucositis, and resultant weight loss was more severe in the simultaneous arm. Relapse-free survival was significantly better in the simultaneous arm, although an overall survival advantage has not yet been demonstrated. The last three trials used the most active regimen of PF in the studies. Longer follow-up is needed before any conclusions are made.

Two interesting trials were reported recently by Merlano et al.[262,299] In the first trial, 116 patients were randomized to receive induction VBM chemotherapy followed by radiation therapy compared with alternating VBM chemotherapy and radiation therapy. The 4-year survival was 10% in the sequential arm compared with 12% in the concomitant arm. Mucosal tolerance was worse in the alternating group. In the

other trial reported, patients were randomized between alternating PF and radiation therapy and radiation therapy alone.[262a] There was a 46% CR rate in the chemotherapy arm compared with 28% in the radiation arm. There was a statistically significant ($p < 0.05$) difference in survival in favor of the chemotherapy arm. This mode of combination definitely needs more study.

Neoadjuvant and Adjuvant Chemotherapy

Several studies have used induction and postoperative adjuvant chemotherapy. However, there are several trials where patients were randomized to see if adjuvant therapy would benefit patients who had induction chemotherapy.

The Head and Neck Contracts Program had three arms in their randomized trial: induction chemotherapy followed by standard therapy, induction chemotherapy followed by standard therapy followed by adjuvant chemotherapy, and standard therapy alone.[300] There was no significant difference in overall and disease-free survival among the three arms. However, there was a decrease in distant metastases in the group that received maintenance adjuvant chemotherapy. Subset analysis reveals better disease-free or overall survival, or both, in three subgroups: oral cavity, T1–2 primary lesions, and N1–2 regional disease adenopathy group with adjuvant chemotherapy.

Ervin and associates randomized 46 patients who had induction chemotherapy and standard treatment to receive adjuvant chemotherapy rather than no chemotherapy.[207] The adjuvant arm showed significantly improved failure-free survival. Updated results revealed an improved 2-year disease-free survival (76% versus 41%; $p = 0.06$) for patients who had PR to induction chemotherapy. It did not benefit those patients who had CR to induction therapy.

Adjuvant Chemotherapy

A few nonrandomized trials evaluating postoperative adjuvant chemotherapy have been conducted. Two of these trials used PF.[300-302] All suggest benefit for high-risk patients receiving postoperative chemotherapy. There have been four randomized trials of adjuvant chemotherapy (Table 22–19).[304-307]

There is some evidence that adjuvant chemotherapy after surgery and radiation may benefit selected subgroups of patients (*e.g.*, those with oral cavity tumors, especially small bulk disease, and those who achieve PR to induction chemotherapy). The final results of the intergroup study were recently reported. The intergroup study's randomized trial had two arms: surgery and radiation therapy versus chemotherapy using cisplatin and 5-FU, three cycles between surgery and radiation therapy. A total of 442 patients were treated, and the median follow-up period was 45.7 months. There was no significant difference in overall and disease-free survival.[307] The two most important findings from the intergroup trial were reduction of distant metastases and improved survival rates in a high-risk group that received chemotherapy.

PRINCIPLES OF CHEMOPREVENTION OF UPPER AERODIGESTIVE TRACT CANCERS

Patients at increased risk for developing upper aerodigestive tract cancer may be identified by a history of previous head and neck cancer or exposure to risk factors such as alcohol

TABLE 22–19. Randomized Trials of Adjuvant Chemotherapy

Investigations	No. of Patients	Sites	Regimens	Comment
Bitter, 1981[304]	33	Oral cavity	XRT	3 yr, 29%
			MBV	3 yr, 65%
Huang, 1987[305]	126	Any head and neck	No treatment	58% NED
			MBVl	72% NED
Domenge, 1988[306]	144	Any with extracapsular	No treatment	Chemotherapy arm
	143	spread	PBM + MB	worse
Laramore, 1989[307]	442	Any head and neck	No treatment	Overall survival at 4 years was identical reduction of distant metastases in chemotherapy group

XRT, radiation therapy; M, methotrexate; B, bleomycin; V, vincristine; Vl, velhan; P, cisplatin.

and tobacco. Because alcohol and tobacco are avoidable risks, there has been considerable interest in developing effective prevention strategies for these patients. Because the progression to malignancy of these cancers is typically gradual, prevention therapy at early stages has also received considerable attention. One approach currently being tested is chemoprevention, which is the administration of drugs before the development of an invasive cancer to block the carcinogenic process. Chemoprevention trials in the upper aerodigestive tract, guided by epidemiologic studies, have often evaluated dietary constituents, such as beta-carotene and retinol. The retinoids, natural and synthetic analogs of vitamin A, have been studied extensively as chemopreventive agents.[308-311] Data from epidemiologic, in vitro, and animal studies strongly support the role of retinoid in suppressing epithelial carcinogenesis.[311-314] Retinoids can modulate the growth and differentiation of normal, premalignant, and malignant epithelial cells in culture and can suppress carcinogenesis in vivo in various human epithelial tissues.[311-318]

FIELD CARCINOGENESIS

Slaughter and colleagues reported the presence of histologic abnormalities and multiple tumor foci within surgical specimens after resection of squamous cell head and neck cancers.[319] Of the 783 oral cancer specimens they examined, all had epithelial hyperplasia and keratinization at the tumor margins and 11.2% contained multiple tumors. The authors hypothesized that carcinogen exposure placed the entire epithelial lining of the upper aerodigestive tract at increased risk for cancer, resulting in a "condemned mucosa," by a process they called *field cancerization*. The field cancerization hypothesis is supported by the occurrence of biochemical and cytologic changes throughout the upper aerodigestive tract in persons with carcinogen exposure. The occurrence of premalignant changes within the epithelium and the risk for multiple primary tumors support the field cancerization hypothesis.

Aerodigestive tract epithelial carcinogenesis is an extremely complex, multistep process. The process begins with genetic alterations and proceeds to altered expressions of regulatory gene products and dysregulated tissue growth, or proliferation, and dysregulated differentiation.[310] Gross histologic and clinical markers of this process are observable but not until late in the process. Researchers are incapable of detecting the subtle cellular, molecular, and biochemical changes that occur in the earliest, preneoplastic phases.[320] Nevertheless, advances in the biology of carcinogenesis are leading to the development of new markers of subtle intermediate stages, or endpoints, of the multistep process called *intermediate endpoint biomarkers*. These markers may provide far earlier and more specific indicators of cancer risk and drug efficacy in prevention trials than are currently possible with standard clinical and histologic evaluations.

CHEMOPREVENTION OF ORAL PREMALIGNANCY

Carotenoid Trials

The first chemointervention studies in oral premalignancy began in the mid-1950s and used high doses of topical and systemic vitamin A (Table 22–20). These early studies reported clinical and histologic activity and response, relapse, and toxicity patterns that are still relevant currently. One dramatic trial produced a response rate of 90% with systemic vitamin A.[321] Despite early promising results and insights, however, further study in this area was suspended for more than two decades. In 1988, Stich and coworkers conducted a small, randomized trial of single-agent systemic retinol and reported a remarkable 57% clinical complete remission rate with histologic documentation, confirming results of the earlier trial.[325]

Single-agent beta-carotene has been evaluated in four nonrandomized trials that included a total of almost 100 subjects. The clinical response rates varied widely, from 0 to 71%. In the mid-1980s, Stich and coworkers reported the first beta-carotene trials in Asian betel nut chewers with oral premalignant lesions.[323] No clinical activity was detected in the initial trial of a 10-week course of beta-carotene. This study was expanded to include canthaxanthine, a synthetic carotenoid not converted to retinol in vivo, and no clinical response was

TABLE 22–20. Natural-Agent Chemoprevention Trials in Oral Premalignancy

Investigations	Agents	No. of Patients	Clinical Response (%)
Wulf, 1957[321]	Vitamin A	20	90
Silverman, 1965[322]	Vitamin A*	503†	57
Stich, 1985[323]	Beta-carotene	23	0
Stich, 1988[324]	Beta-carotene	27	15‡·§
	Beta-carotene plus vitamin A	51	18‡·§
Stich, 1988[325]	Vitamin A	21	57‡
Toma, 1990[327]	Beta-carotene	24	27
Garewal, 1990[326]	Beta-carotene	24	71
Toma, 1990[327]	Selenium	25	33

* Topical only.
† Total from this report and literature review.
‡ Only complete resolution reported.
§ The rates of lesion resolution and *new* lesion development during therapy were identical (15% in the beta-carotene arm (vs placebo, *p* = 0.16); the respective rates in the beta-carotene plus vitamin A arm were 28% (resolution) and 8% (new lesion) (vs placebo, *p* = 0.004).

produced. The next pair of trials compared a 6-month intervention of beta-carotene with beta-carotene plus retinol. In the single-agent beta-carotene group, lesion response (15%) was countered equally by new lesion development (15%). The retinol and beta-carotene combination produced a CR rate of 18%, two times greater than that of beta-carotene alone and nine times greater than placebo.[324] Recent data from this group suggest that low-dose retinol (and, to a lesser degree, beta-carotene) can partially maintain a decrease in number of biomarkers of genetic damage, induced initially by combined retinol and beta-carotene. Stich's and coworkers' high-risk trial subjects were unique by virtue of intense localized carcinogen exposure and uniform lifestyle and diet (often deficient in vitamin A and carotenoids). Because they come from undeveloped countries, the applicability of the results to populations at risk in more industrialized nations is not clear. For example, micronuclei frequencies were higher in the groups in the study by Stich and coworkers than those indicated by the data from all other aerodigestive tract (lung, esophagus, head and neck) studies.

In a pilot trial, Garewal and colleagues reported a remarkable response rate of 71% in 24 patients with oral leukoplakia treated with beta-carotene at 30 mg/day for 3 months.[326] Fewer than half of these subjects developed dysplastic lesions, none of which were severe. In contrast, Toma and associates recently reported a response rate of 8% at 3 months (27% at 6 months) in 15 patients with oral leukoplakia who were treated with a higher dose of beta-carotene (90 mg/day).[327] Although these trials hold much promise, none were randomized and none of the beta-carotene studies included systematic histologic assessments. Therefore, beta-carotene's clinical value remains unproved.

The only other natural agent with published clinical results in oral premalignancy is selenium (an agent with proved activity in the lingual model), which has a 33% response rate

at 3 months in 25 subjects.[327] No toxicity has been reported in this or any of the natural-agent trials.

Retinoid Trials

Eight synthetic-agent trials limited to retinoids at daily doses of 1 mg/kg/day or greater consistently produced objective response rates in leukoplakia of 60% to 90%, with a median response rate of more than 75% (Table 22–21).[329-333] Compared with the limited and recent data with nontoxic natural agents, synthetic retinoid trials began more than two decades ago and include more than 200 treated patients. In the first of his two comparative trials, Koch treated 75 patients for 2 months with 70 mg/kg/day of 13-cRA, all-*trans*-retinoic acid, or etretinate.[328] Response rates were 87%, 59%, and 91%, respectively. On the basis of these results (etretinate was the most active and the least toxic), Koch designed a second study to compare oral etretinate alone with oral etretinate plus topical etretinate paste.[329] Response rates were high and roughly equivalent in the two study arms.

The variable natural history of oral premalignancy and lack of histologic confirmation of retinoid results led to the most recently reported final data from a randomized, placebo-controlled trial of 13-*cis*-retinoic acid (1–2 mg/kg/day for 3 months) conducted by Hong and coworkers.[332] The clinical objective response rate was 67% in the treated group compared with only 10% in the placebo group (*p* = 0.0002). This was the first study to assess histologically all patients before and after therapy. Pretreatment biopsies of 63% of the retinoid-treated group and 40% of the placebo group showed various degrees of dysplasia. Reversal of dysplasia occurred in 54% of the retinoid-treated group, including three severely dysplastic lesions, and only a 10% spontaneous reversal occurred in the placebo group (*p* = 0.01).

Toxicity was significant in those patients receiving 2 mg/kg. Cheilitis, facial erythema, and skin dryness and peeling occurred in 88% and conjunctivitis in 76% of patients. Forty-

TABLE 22–21. Synthetic Retinoid Chemoprevention Trials in Oral Premalignancy

Investigations	Agents	No. of Patients	Clinical Response (%)
Koch, 1978[328]	β-all *trans*-Retinoic acid	27	59
	13-*cis*-Retinoic acid	24	87
	Etretinate	24	92
Koch, 1981[329]	Etretinate*	4	83
	Etretinate	21	71
Cordero, 1981[330]	Etretinate	3	100
Shah, 1983[331]	13-*cis*-Retinoic acid†	11	100
Hong, 1985[332]	13-*cis*-Retinoic acid	24	67
Lippman, 1990[333]	13-*cis*-Retinoic acid	70	55
Total		214	75‡

* Oral and topical.
† Topical.
‡ Median complete response rate is 15%.

seven percent in this group required dose reduction to 1 mg/kg/day. With 1 mg/kg/day, 57% experienced mild skin toxicity and 29% had conjunctivitis. All subjects at this lower dose completed the 3-month therapy.

Response rates were not significantly different between patients receiving the lower (1 mg/kg/day) and the highest (2 mg/kg/day) doses. The study was terminated prematurely, after only 44 patients, because of highly significant response differences between treated and placebo subjects.

Although this randomized trial established the efficacy of 13-cRA in premalignant oral lesions, the following two serious problems were encountered: significant toxicity with high-dose 13-cRA and a relapse rate of higher than 50% within 3 months after stopping the drug. This relapse rate is a consistent finding in all oral premalignancy trials reported to date. Hong and coworkers designed a second study to prolong remission with less toxic maintenance therapy. After 3 months' induction with high-dose 13-cRA (1.5 mg/kg/day), responding (or stable) patients were randomized to a 9-month maintenance program with low-dose 13-cRA (0.5 mg/kg/day) or beta-carotene (30 mg/day).[334] Clinical, histologic, and biomarker endpoints were analyzed before therapy and after the induction and maintenance phases. Two thirds of subjects had dysplastic lesions, which were severe in more than 20%. This trial's high-dose induction phase produced a response rate consistent with the overall response rate of higher than 60% established in the earlier definitive trial. Data from the randomized maintenance phase indicate that low-dose 13-cRA is significantly more effective than beta-carotene in maintaining clinicopathologic remission and low micronuclei counts. Relapse rates after the 9-month maintenance phase were 10% in the 13-cRA group and 54% in the beta-carotene group (2-sided $p < 0.01$). This trial included laboratory analyses of the genomic biomarker micronuclei. Micronuclei results correlated generally with the clinical data—that is, lowered counts present in the clinically active retinoid arm and increased counts present in the clinically less active beta-carotene arm. The data, however, did not establish a significant one-to-one correlation between micronuclei changes and clinical results. Nevertheless, low-dose 13-cRA maintained remission effectively and further improved lesion and micronuclei response.

In addition to skin yellowing, no toxic effects occurred in the beta-carotene study. Low-dose 13-cRA also was well tolerated, although grade 2 or greater skin or lip dryness appeared in both groups. Low-dose 13-cRA was associated with mild and reversible toxicities. These data indicate that low-dose 13-cRA is an effective and well-tolerated maintenance therapy for oral premalignancy.

CHEMOPREVENTION OF SECOND PRIMARY TUMORS

Regardless of their initial treatment, head and neck cancer patients remain at significantly increased risk for second primary tumor (SPT) development. SPTs occur after treatment for all stages of head and neck cancers, but their impact is most striking in patients treated for early disease.[334]

The Connecticut Tumor Registry, multicenter oncology groups, and cancer centers indicate that SPTs, either synchronous or metachronous, develop conservatively at a constant yearly rate of 2% to 5% in previously treated patients

and contribute to a 6% to 8% excess annual mortality rate for them. These rates are higher in prospective studies.[334–336]

Multistep field carcinogenesis of multiple independent sites within the aerodigestive tract, significant activity of 13-cRA in reversing oral premalignancy, modest activity in advanced disease, and the constant high rate of SPTs in squamous cell carcinoma of the head and neck led to the design of an adjuvant trial in 13-cRA in squamous cell carcinoma of the head and neck.[338]

Patients were stratified by site (oral cavity, oropharynx, hypopharynx, or larynx) and treatment (surgery, radiation, or both) and were randomized in a double-blind fashion to receive 13-cRA (50–100 mg/m² of body weight/day) or placebo for 12 months.

The primary endpoint of this adjuvant study was the emergence of new disease and its development into either of two major pattern types: (1) progression (local recurrence and regional or distant metastasis) and (2) SPTs. The definition of SPTs was based on a modification of that given by Warren and Gates (Table 22–22).[339] Table 22–23 shows the pattern of treatment failures within the retinoid and placebo groups at a median follow-up of 42 months. The difference between the percentage of patients developing SPTs in the two patient groups was highly significant: 6% (3/49) in the 13-cRA group compared with 28% (14/51) in the placebo group ($p < 0.005$). Figure 22–8 shows the time-adjusted SPT rates in the two study groups.

No patient developed an SPT while on retinoid intervention. The SPT rate in the placebo arm of this prospective study (10% per year) was higher than the 3% to 6% per year reported from retrospective studies and tumor registries. Toxicity, however, from high-dose 13-cRA contributed to a high dropout rate in the treatment arm and represents a significant factor in future trial designs.

NASAL CAVITY AND PARANASAL SINUSES

EPIDEMIOLOGY

Cancers of the nasal cavity and paranasal sinuses are relatively infrequent cancers, with an incidence of 0.75 per 100,000 persons in the United States.[342] Lesions of the maxillary antrum are twice as frequent as those of the nasal cavity. Cancers of the ethmoid and sphenoid sinuses are the least frequently observed. Disease occurs more frequently in men than women (2:1 ratio) and primarily involves people in the sixth decade of life. Cancer of the paranasal sinuses are more frequently

TABLE 22–22. Criteria for Second Primary Tumor

A new cancer with different histology
Any cancer, regardless of site, occurring after 3 or more years
In the head and neck, a distinct lesion separated from the primary site by more than 2 cm of normal epithelium
In the lung, if histology is squamous cell cancer (within 3 years)
Lesion must present as a solitary mass
Must be free of locoregional recurrence of original tumor
Histologic findings of dysplasia or carcinoma in situ in bronchial epithelium

TABLE 22–23. Primary Treatment Failures by Study Group*

Type of Failure	13-cis-Retinoic Acid Group (N = 49) (%)	Placebo Group (N = 51) (%)	P Value†
No. of Relapse	15 (31)‡	17 (33)‡	NS
Local	4 (8)	7 (14)	NS
Regional	8 (16)	7 (14)	NS
Distant	8 (16)	5 (10)	NS
No. of Second Primary Tumors	3 (6)	14 (28)§	<0.005
Total	18 (37)	31 (61)	<0.05

* Median follow-up 42 months.
† By chi square test without Yates correction.
‡ Some patients had disease relapse in more than one site category.
§ Four patients developed more than one second primary tumor.
NS, not significant.

observed in other regions of the world, including Japan and South Africa.[343]

Etiologic factors involved in disease development are multifold. Exposure to nickel has been attributed to cancer development in the nasal cavity.[343,344] Occupations associated with a high incidence of nasal cavity cancers include those within the furniture, textile, and boot and shoe industries.[345–347] Other workers considered at risk include those involved with production of chromium, mustard gas, isopropyl alcohol, and radium.[342] When considering cancers of the paranasal sinuses, the most frequently cited agent has been Thoratrast.[348] Some authors have attributed maxillary sinus carcinoma to chronic sinusitis.

ANATOMY

The nasal cavity comprises the nasal vestibule, nasal antrum, and turbinates. The paired nasal cavities are separated by septal cartilage. The nasal vestibule is the triangular region of the nasal cavity bounded by the palatine processes of the maxilla inferiorly, the nasal septum medially, and the fibrofatty tissue called the *nasal ala* laterally. The nasal vestibule represents that portion of the nasal cavity composed of skin, that is, tissue that bears hair follicles and sweat glands. Its posterior border is demarcated by transition from skin to mucosa.

The nasal antrum represents the remaining portion of the nasal cavity and contains the inferior, middle, and superior turbinates. The superior and middle turbinates are composed of highly vascular tissue overlying fragile bony projections that inset onto the ethmoid air cell bony framework. The inferior turbinate is composed of a separate bone.

The paranasal sinuses include the maxillary, ethmoid, sphenoid, and frontal sinuses. More detailed anatomy of this region is provided in other references.[349]

Primary lymphatic drainage of the maxillary sinuses is into the submandibular nodal basin. The ethmoid sinuses drain into the submandibular and the retropharyngeal nodes. The

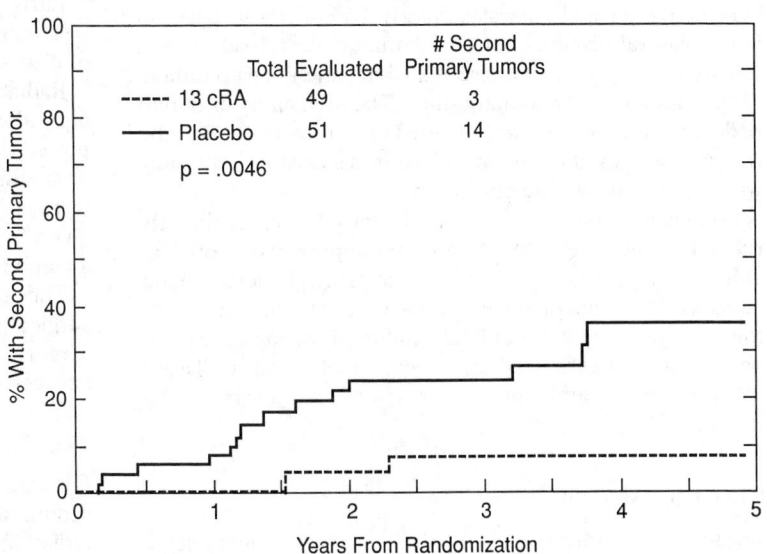

FIGURE 22–8. Adjuvant high dose 13-cRA trial, March 18, 1991. Time-adjusted second primary tumor rate in patients with squamous cell carcinoma of the upper aerodigestive tract. Patients were randomized to receive 13-*cis*-retinoic acid (cRA) or placebo after treatment of their index cancer (see text). Patients treated with cRA had significantly fewer second primary tumors.

nasal cavity drains into the above regions and along the course of the facial blood vessels into the submandibular triangle and to periparotid nodes.

PATHOLOGY

Most tumors of the nasal cavity and paranasal sinus are squamous cell carcinomas. Squamous cell carcinoma, distinct from other sites within the upper aerodigestive tract, is less predominant. A great variety of histopathologically distinct cancers occur in this region. Tumors found in the superior portion of the nasal cavity include adenocarcinoma and esthesioneuroblastoma. In the paranasal sinuses, additional neoplasms are tumors of minor salivary gland origin, including adenocarcinoma, adenoid cystic carcinoma, and mucoepidermoid carcinoma. Rare tumors of this region are lymphoma, mucosal melanoma, teratocarcinomas, angiosarcomas, and various odontogenic and bone tumors.

NATURAL HISTORY

The commonest cancers, that is, squamous cell carcinomas, are usually well differentiated and slow growing, and the tendency to metastasize is infrequent. Common presenting symptoms include a nonhealing ulcer, occasional bleeding, and unilateral nasal obstruction.

Given the anatomic limitations in making early diagnosis, disease is usually far advanced at the time of initial presentation. Other symptoms may reflect growth into the oral cavity causing dental pain, loose teeth, or ill-fitting dentures, or into the orbit leading to ocular symptoms such as diplopia, proptosis, and epiphora. Severe pain and trismus may occur with extension into the pterygoid fossa. Tumors in the superior nasal antrum and paranasal sinuses may invade the cribriform plate and extend into the anterior cranial fossa, causing anosmia or headache.

The regional lymph nodes most frequently involved with metastatic disease are nodes within the periparotid region or within the submandibular triangle. The propensity for spread to regional lymph nodes is dependent on the subsite in which primary disease may occur.[350–352] Approximately 20% of patients with cancers of the nasal vestibule develop clinically evident lymph node disease. Nearly 15% of these patients have bilateral disease. Regional lymph node spread is seen less frequently (approaching 10–15% of patients) with tumors of the ethmoid and maxillary sinus. The probability of lymph node spread increases with extension of tumors outside the normal confines of the nasal and paranasal cavities, especially with extension into the oral cavity.

Prognosis of patients with nasal cavity lesions is directly related to the size of the lesion and approximates 60% of afflicted patients at 5 years.[352,353] The principle determinant of survival is the presence of local recurrence, which is the most frequent site of disease failure. Prognosis for paranasal sinus cancers depends on extent of primary disease at presentation and approximates 30% for advanced T4 lesions.[350,354,355]

STAGING AND SCREENING

Because of the infrequency in which primary cancers occur in the nasal cavity region, AJCC classification has been adopted only within the maxillary sinus. *The definition of the TNM system for the maxillary sinus is as follows:*

PRIMARY TUMOR

TX	Primary tumor cannot be assessed.
T0	No existence of primary tumor.
Tis	Carcinoma in situ.
T1	Tumor limited to antral mucosa with no erosion or destruction of bone.
T2	Tumor with erosion of the infrastructure including the hard palate or middle nasal meatus.
T3	Tumor invades any of the following: skin of cheek, posterior wall of maxillary sinus, floor or medial wall of orbit, or anterior ethmoid sinus.
T4	Tumor invades contents of or any of the following: cribriform plate, posterior ethmoid or sphenoid sinuses, nasopharynx, soft palate, pterygomaxillary or temporal fossae, or base of skull.

The regional lymph node (N) and distant metastases (M) staging are identical to other sites within the upper aerodigestive tract and are as stated in the beginning of the chapter.

Careful examination of patients presenting with symptoms referable to the midface may minimize delay in diagnosis of these cancers. The advent of computed tomography (CT) has facilitated pretreatment evaluation of these tumors. Before the use of radioisotopic evaluation, extent of disease was underestimated frequently, becoming apparent only at the time of surgery.

TREATMENT

Treatment of Tumors of the Nasal Cavity

For tumors of the nasal cavity, the appropriate surgical procedure depends on the location of the primary disease. Tumors of the nasal septum can be approached through a lateral rhinotomy or by a midface degloving technique.[356] Cancers of the superior or lateral nasal cavity can be resected by a medial maxillectomy and an en bloc ethmoidectomy.[357]

Early tumors of the nasal cavity do not require elective treatment of regional lymph nodes because regional spread of disease is relatively infrequent.

Radiation therapy and surgical resection yield roughly equivalent results for early lesions. Wong and Cummings reported that most patients present with lesions that are 5 cm or smaller, and less than 10% present with lymph node metastases.[358] When radiation therapy is used, treatment can be given by external-beam techniques, interstitial implants, or a combination of both.

The difficulty with advanced tumors is in obtaining adequate surgical margins. Combined modality therapy consisting of surgery and radiation should be used in most circumstances because of the high propensity for local recurrence.

TREATMENT OF PARANASAL SINUS CANCERS

For cancers of the maxillary sinus, maxillectomy is the procedure of choice and usually is combined with postoperative radiation. For most lesions, maxillectomy entails a standard Weber-Ferguson incision through skin of the anterior face.

Which bone cuts are used depends on the decision whether to preserve or to resect the orbital floor and orbital contents.

Debate in the management of paranasal sinus cancers centers on extent of surgical resection and what constitutes resectability. Further, the management of the eye in patients with paranasal sinus cancer remains controversial. For T1 or T2 lesions of the maxilla, the eye can be preserved. Surgeons advocate resection of orbital contents in patients whose tumors transgress the orbital floor and infiltrate orbital contents. In certain circumstances, however, invasion of the orbital floor by maxillary sinus cancers cannot be determined preoperatively.

Should disease involve orbital floor but not extend into the orbit, resection of the bony floor may be entertained with preservation of the globe. However, ocular motion may be impaired, and diploplia can result from such a procedure secondary to loss of structural support of orbital contents. This complication has led to numerous procedures for reconstructing the resected orbital floor, including median galeal-pericranial flaps.[359] The value of one surgical approach compared with another is limited by the relative infrequency of these tumors. If periosteum of the floor is preserved, reconstruction is not usually indicated.

Factors that classically preclude surgical excision include cancer extending to the base of skull, nasopharynx, or sphenoid sinus.[360] Extensive involvement of the infratemporal fossa from tumors of the maxillary sinus has not been considered amenable to surgical resection for cure. Each of the decisions regarding resectability should be tempered by the skill of the primary surgeon and the availability of neurosurgical and reconstructive expertise.

A major decision in the treatment of paranasal sinus involves reconstruction of the surgical defects. The methods of reconstruction that have been advocated include temporal muscle slings, skin grafts, and composite flaps containing bone.

In general, elective treatment of regional lymph nodes in patients without clinical evidence of lymph node metastases is not indicated.

TREATMENT RESULTS

NASAL CAVITY

Spiro and associates have reviewed the results of therapy for 27 patients with squamous cell carcinoma of the nasal cavity.[361] Surgery alone was the treatment in 21 instances. Five-year determinate cure for nasal cavity lesions were 43%. Failure occurs most frequently at the local site in the surgery group. This failure occurs at rates ranging from 10% to more than 40%, emphasizing the need for effective multimodality therapy.[352,353,361,362]

Levendag and Pomp reported a series of 63 consecutive patients with squamous cell carcinoma of the nasal vestibule who were managed with radiation therapy, principally with interstitial implantation.[363] A mean dose of 62 Gy for T1 and 64 Gy for T2 lesions was used. Patients with nasal cavity lesions were grouped according to the classification system proposed by Wang.[364] Local control was obtained in 97% of T1N0 patients, and 79% of T2N0 patients. Similar results have been observed by other researchers.[358,365] Factors associated with an adverse outcome to primary radiation therapy include the presence of nodal metastases and local tumor extension into surrounding anatomic structures such as skin, lip, cartilage, and bone.

PARANASAL SINUS

Results of surgical resection of paranasal sinus cancer have demonstrated local control rates ranging from 10% to 90%, depending on disease stage.[360,361] Surgical series demonstrated that limits of surgical resection could be extended into the anterior and the middle cranial fossa, with 5-year survival rates approaching 50%.[366,367]

Parsons and colleagues reported on the success of radiation therapy against malignant tumors of the nasal cavity, ethmoid sinus, or sphenoid sinus.[368] The 10- and 15-year actuarial local control for all patients except the adenoid cystic histologies was 52% and 42%, respectively. A 10-year actuarial local control rate for stage I (7 patients) was 100%. The 10-year actuarial local control rate for stage II was 53% and for stage III it was 30%. Results were dependent on histology, with only a 17% local control in patients with adenoid cystic carcinoma. Although these data support the use of radiation alone for the occasional stage I patient, the results with more advanced stages is suboptimal. Treatment with surgery and postoperative radiation is preferred.[368–370]

Other adverse prognostic factors may relate to site of disease within the paranasal sinuses. Suprastructure lesions in the maxillary antrum, for instance, appear more readily controlled with radiation therapy than do infrastructure lesions.[369]

Yu-Hua and coworkers compared preoperative and postoperative radiation therapy in a cohort of patients with maxillary sinus carcinoma.[371] They reported 64% 5-year survival in the preoperative group compared with 26% in the postoperative group. The complication rate was higher (29% versus 14%) in the preoperative compared with the postoperative groups, but the authors concluded that preoperative radiation was better. However, preoperative radiation therapy is seldom used in resectable lesions. Zaharia and associates reported 149 patients treated with surgery and postoperative radiation therapy for cancer of the maxillary sinus.[372] Patients were treated at 180 to 200 cGy per day, 5 days per week, to a total dose in the 5500- to 6000-cGy range. Megavoltage equipment was used. Two patients had T1 lesions, 12 had T2 lesions, 117 had T3 lesions, and 198 had T4 lesions. The 5-year actuarial survival, corrected for death not due to cancer, was 42%. Clinical stage was an important prognostic feature, with survival being 75%, 36%, and 11% for stages II, III, and IV, respectively.

The reported local control rates for paranasal sinus tumors are suboptimal. Future results may be improved through the use of CT-based treatment planning. Figure 22–9 demonstrates a typical radiation technique for paranasal sinus tumors.

Chemotherapy of Cancer of the Paranasal Sinuses

Information on the role of chemotherapy in treating paranasal sinus cancers is limited, because it is usually reported as a subset of a larger study on head and neck cancer.

One form of chemotherapy that has been used for more than 20 years against head and neck cancers is intraarterial chemotherapy. The concentration of chemotherapy attainable

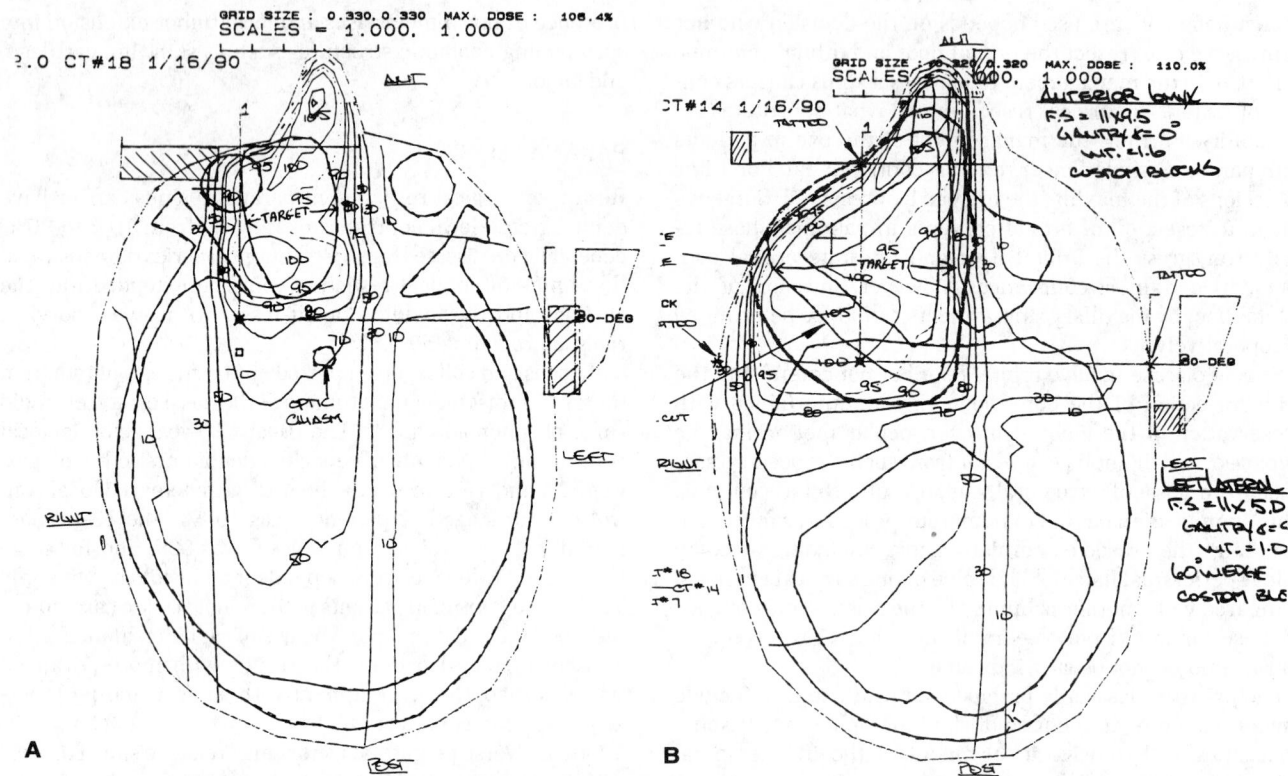

FIGURE 22–9. A patient with squamous cell carcinoma of the right maxillary antrum, with disease extension toward the medial portion of the right eye. He underwent a complete resection with close margin near the globe. He was treated with postoperative radiation therapy. The plan is shown here. **(A)** A representative cut through the level of the orbit. The plan calls for an AP field and a left lateral field. The anterior field is weighted over the lateral field 1.6 to 1. The target volume is seen, and the isodose curves show that the 90% isodose line covers the target volume well. The anterior field has a block for the lateral aspect of the orbit, thereby protecting the lacrimal gland. The medial aspect of the eye is in the target volume. The left lateral field has blocking for the spinal cord, the optic chiasm, and the left eye. The dose to the left orbit is less than 10%. A total of 6300 cGy was given, prescribed to the 90% line. This keeps the dose to the optic chiasm well within tolerance. **(B)** The same patient, with a cut through a level below the orbits but through the maxillary antrum. The target volume and isodose curves are seen.

at the site of the tumor is considerably more when delivered intraarterially, with less systemic toxicity. A number of trials of intraarterial chemotherapy in these tumors have been reported to improve the local control rate and prolong disease-free survival in previously untreated patients and to palliate patients with recurrent disease (Table 22–24). Sato and colleagues treated 68 patients who had paranasal sinus cancers with intraarterial 5-FU and radiation therapy.[374] In 57 patients, 38 showed disappearance of tumor, and among these, 22 required no further treatment. In 19 cases of residual tumor after therapy, partial resection of the maxilla and intracavitary irradiation were effective in eradicating the tumor. The 2-year survival was 57% compared with 41% in the historic controls treated with surgery and postoperative radiation therapy. Similar results were reported by Goepfert and coworkers with intraarterial 5-FU or methotrexate and radiation therapy.[375] Many patients avoided radical surgery, which resulted in better cosmesis.

Moseley and associates reported 10 patients treated with intraarterial bleomycin and methotrexate followed by radiation therapy and surgery.[376] Four patients had no residual disease, 1 had a single microscopic focus, and 2 had extensive necrosis in their resected specimens. Six of the 9 resected patients were alive and free of disease at 17 to 51 months.

Shibuya and colleagues reported that multimodality therapy with intraarterial 5-FU plus radiation therapy did not improve local control or survival.[377] In a randomized trial by Nervi and coworkers, 12 patients with maxillary sinus cancer were treated with intraarterial methotrexate followed by radiation therapy and 13 patients were treated by radiation alone.[378] No statistically significant difference in survival was found. However, many of the patients in both groups had T2 lesions.

In a recent study at the M.D. Anderson Cancer Center, intraarterial cisplatin and bleomycin, and intravenous 5-FU infusion were used as an induction regimen in 30 patients with advanced paranasal sinus cancers.[379] Of 28 evaluable patients, 6 had CR and 13 had PR. After chemotherapy, 13 patients had radiation therapy alone and 11 had surgery followed by radiation therapy. Overall, 21 patients were rendered free of disease. Of 18 patients who were initially judged to need orbital exenteration, only 7 required it. The median disease-free survival was 42 months.

Even though these pilot trials reported good results, there is no definite evidence that intraarterial chemotherapy is better than intravenous therapy. Wayne State reported its 10-year experience with intravenous cisplatin-based chemotherapy in 24 patients.[380] The response rate was 82% (CR, 44%; PR, 38%) for previously untreated patients and 88% (CR,

TABLE 22–24. Chemotherapy of Paranasal Sinuses

Investigations	Regimens	No. of Patients	Survival
Sato, 1970[374]	IA 5-FU + XRT ± surgery	57	2 y = 57%
	XRT + surgery	37	2 y = 47%
	Surgery + XRT	60	2 y = 41%
Goepfert, 1973[375]	IA 5-FU/MTX and XRT	23	2 y = 48%
			5 y = 26%
Nervi, 1978[378]	IA MTX + XRT	12	4 y = 30%
	XRT	13	4 y = 30%
Knegt, 1985[381]	XRT + surgery + XRT + topical 5-FU	60	2 y = 76%
			5 y = 65%
LoRusso, 1988[380]	I.V. chemotherapy (POB, PF, PFM)		MS CR 21 + mo (untreated) PR 13.5 mo
			MS CR 16 mo (treated) PR 13.5 mo
Dimery, 1988[379]	IA PB + I.V. 5-FU + XRT ± Surgery	30	Median DFS = 42 mo

F, 5-FU, 5-fluorouracil; M, MTX, methotrexate; C, cyclophosphamide; O, oncovin; I.V., intravenous; B, bleomycin; P, cisplatin; IA, intraarterial; XRT, radiation therapy; MS, median survival; DFS, disease-free survival.

38%; PR, 50%) for patients with recurrent disease. The median survival of untreated patients who achieved CR was 21 months; for those achieving PR it was 13 months, and for those achieving no response (NR) it was 3 months. For patients treated for recurrent disease who achieved a CR, the median survival was 16 months; for those who achieved a PR it was 13.5 months, and for those who achieved NR it was 5 months.

Based on the information published to date, it seems that intraarterial chemotherapy with radiation therapy in locally advanced maxillary sinus tumors can achieve results similar to surgery and radiation therapy without the effects of major surgery. For patients with paranasal sinus cancer who need orbital exenteration or major craniofacial resection, the option of intraarterial chemotherapy as induction therapy to preserve the eye can be considered as an alternative treatment.

Harrison and associates reported the results of a prospective study evaluating concomitant chemotherapy with radiation therapy for advanced unresectable head and neck cancer.[373] Eight of the 10 patients with unresectable paranasal sinus tumors had a CR to the combined chemotherapy and radiation therapy treatment program. None of the complete responders have had a local recurrence, although median follow-up is only 1 year. These encouraging results for unresectable paranasal sinus cancer raise the issue as to whether this combined modality approach could be successful in earlier-stage disease. Larger numbers of patients and longer follow-up are needed before this could be considered an alternative to standard treatment with surgery and radiation therapy.

NASOPHARYNX

EPIDEMIOLOGY

The epidemiology of nasopharyngeal carcinoma suggests multiple determinants, including diet, viral agents, and genetic susceptibility.[381,382] Endemic areas include Southern China, North Africa, and regions within the far northern hemisphere. The diet of the populations in these regions is what contributes a link to disease development.[383] Populations in endemic areas are characterized by intake of salt-cured fish and meat. The cooking of such food releases volatile nitrosamines that distribute over the nasopharyngeal mucosa when carried by steam.

In addition to diet, considerable epidemiologic evidence incriminates Epstein-Barr virus (EBV) in nasopharyngeal carcinoma development. Old and colleagues first demonstrated the presence of anti-EBV antibodies within the sera of nasopharyngeal carcinoma patients.[384] Knowledge about EBV serology has progressed rapidly, reinforcing the potential causal relation. More recent advances in molecular biology have provided more direct evidence of the carcinogenic properties of this herpesvirus, including the identification of EBV-related peptides capable of inducing malignant transformation of lymphoblastoid cell lines in vitro.[385,386]

Potential genetic determinants of nasopharyngeal carcinoma have been suggested by the increased incidence of disease in persons with specific major histocompatibility complex (MHC) profiles.[387] Loci associated with increased relative risk include the H2 locus antigen. Simons and colleagues reported that the so-called Singapore antigen, BW46, was associated with a high risk for nasopharyngeal carcinoma.[388] The risk for disease increases significantly in people with the H2 and Bw46 antigens. An increased odds ratio of disease was demonstrated in people who carry the B17 antigen.[387] In the latter instance, the disease is associated with an earlier age of onset.

The peak incidence of disease occurs in the fourth and fifth decades. The male to female ratio is 2.2:1.

ANATOMY

The nasopharynx is a cuboidal structure covered by stratified mucociliary columnar epithelium. Anteriorly, it is in continuity to the nasal cavity by way of the posterior choanae. The roof is formed by the basisphenoid, the basiocciput, and the anterior arch of the atlas. The roof gradually slopes inferiorly to become the posterior wall. The latter is formed by the first two cervical vertebrae. The lateral walls of the nasopharynx contain the eustachian tube openings that lie within the elevations of the torus tubarii, that is, the cartilaginous portions of the internal auditory canal. Behind the torus is the lateral pharyngeal recess or fossa of Rosenmuller, which is the commonest site of nasopharyngeal carcinoma development. The floor of the nasopharynx is the upper surface of the soft palate.

Lymphatic drainage from the nasopharynx encompasses all levels within the neck as it proceeds along the jugular vein and spinal accessory nerve. Extensive lymphatics within the nasopharynx drain into the retropharyngeal nodes medial to the carotid artery. Involvement of these nodes rarely can be detected clinically. Radiologic assessment, either CT or magnetic resonance imaging (MRI), is the most sensitive diagnostic technique for detecting retropharyngeal node enlargement.

PATHOLOGY

The World Health Organization (WHO) has divided nasopharyngeal carcinoma into three types: type 1, keratinizing squamous cell carcinoma; type 2, nonkeratinizing carcinoma; and type 3, the undifferentiated carcinoma.[389] The last is the most frequently identified neoplasm. It characteristically is associated with a lymphoid infiltrate, which accounts for its more familiar description, lymphoepithelioma. The proportion of type 1 nasopharyngeal carcinoma among the North American population is higher than that found in other locales.

Additional cancer types noted include lymphoma, juvenile angiofibroma, plasmacytoma, and adenocarcinomas. The last is of minor salivary gland origin.

NATURAL HISTORY

Nasopharyngeal cancer grows by infiltration or by expansion, with the former growth pattern predominating. Mucosal abnormalities frequently may reflect only a small portion of tumor extent. Occasionaly, no abnormalities of the mucosa are identifiable. In such instances, tumors may exist submucosally and extend into sites outside the confines of the nasopharynx proper.

The commonest presenting complaint of nasopharyngeal carcinoma is a mass in the neck, occurring in nearly 90% of patients. Additional frequently encountered symptoms include alterations in hearing associated with serous otitis media, tinnitus, nasal obstruction, and pain. Patients may present with symptoms that reflect growth of the disease into the many significant surrounding anatomic structures. Tumors can access the parapharyngeal space through the sinus of Morgagni, an opening in the lateral nasopharyngeal wall through which the eustachian tube courses. Infiltration laterally into paranasopharyngeal space may lead to pterygoid muscle involvement and trismus. Cranial nerve involvement often manifests with more extensive growth into the skull base. Growth into the cavernous sinus under such circumstances can lead to impairment of cranial nerves II to VI. Additionally, cancer may break through the pharyngeobasilar fascia and spread along vascular sheaths, that is, fascial planes surrounding the

jugular vein and carotid artery. Disease extending along these planes may also extend within the skull base and lead to cranial nerve involvement.

Any description of the natural history of nasopharyngeal carcinoma must take into account its metastatic potential. The metastatic potential of these tumors is governed by the WHO histopathologic classification. WHO type I has a greater propensity for uncontrolled local tumor growth and a lower potential for metastatic spread than the WHO type II and III cancers. Clinically advanced nodal metastases from WHO type I approximates 60%.[390-392] For WHO types II and III disease, clinical evidence of metastatic disease ranges from 80% to 90%. Distinct from cancers of the oral cavity and oropharynx, metastatic disease frequently presents itself in the posterior triangle. Metastasis of bilateral neck nodes are present in 53% of patients.[393] Another common location for metastatic disease is in the lymph nodes in the retropharyngeal space, the so-called nodes of Rouviere. Multiple nodal chains can be involved with disease, including chains along the special accessory nerve, the jugular vein, and the retropharyngeal pathway.

Prognosis for the various WHO classifications of nasopharyngeal carcinoma vary from approximately 15% 5-year survival for type I lesions to 60% for type III lesions depending on disease stage.[393,394] The 5-year survival for stage I approximates 67% and decreases to 15% for stage IV.

STAGING

PRIMARY TUMOR

TX   Primary tumor cannot be assessed.

T0   No evidence of primary tumor.

TIS: CARCINOMA IN SITU

T1   Tumor limited to one subsite of the nasopharynx.

T2   Tumor invades more than one subsite of the nasopharynx.

T3   Tumor invades nasal cavity or oropharynx or both.

T4   Tumor invades skull of cranial nerves or both.

The regional lymph node (N) and distant metastases (M) staging are identical to other sites within the upper aerodigestive tract and are as stated in the beginning of this chapter.

TREATMENT

Radiation therapy is the standard treatment of almost all nasopharyngeal carcinomas. Surgery is usually not feasible and cannot provide adequate margins of resection. There is considerable morbidity to nasopharyngeal surgery, even in the most carefully selected patients.

Modern imaging techniques, including CT and MRI, have changed radiation therapy for this disease dramatically. Yu and associates and other researchers have shown that CT scans upstage more than 50% of T2 and T3 patients.[395,396] These investigators found that CT identified parapharyngeal extension in more than 60% to 80% of patients. Celai and coworkers attempted to study the effect that CT staging and treatment planning had on therapeutic results.[397] They found that patients who were treated with CT treatment plans had improved local control and 5-year survival. This result will not surprise most radiation oncologists. Because CT and MRI scanning have identified disease extensions that were not known previously, the radiation therapy plans currently can be modified accordingly. An example is shown in Figure 22–10. The patient in the figure has parapharyngeal extension. A standard, bilateral opposed field arrangement for the nasopharynx and upper neck would significantly compromise the treatment to the parapharyngeal space. In particular, when the spinal cord block was added, the parapharyngeal extension was under the block and thereby underdosed. It is not surprising that this leads to treatment failure.

In addition to the benefits of target volume delineation that these new imaging techniques have provided, the advent of 3D radiation therapy treatment planning has been vital. Kutcher and colleagues and the experience at Memorial Sloan-Kettering Cancer Center revealed that multifield conformal plans were able to achieve excellent coverage of tumors while reducing the normal tissue doses compared with standard treatment techniques.[398] An example of a treatment plan is shown in Figure 22–11; this approach becomes complicated radiation therapy. Seven to ten fields might be necessary to provide the best dose distribution to the primary site. These need to be matched to upper neck fields, which then need to be matched to lower neck fields. The spinal cord must be protected at each junction. Electron beams are required for the posterior neck, and these are matched to the photon fields. The result is that as many as 15 fields might be required in a single patient.

Radiation therapy can control neck disease without the need for neck dissection. Neck control is high, even in patients with bulky cervical lymphadenopathy. All patients with nasopharyngeal disease require radiation treatment to regional cervical lymph nodes. Patients with N0 necks are usually treated with up to 5000 cGy to the entire neck in 180- to 200-cGy daily fractions. Patients with involved necks received at least 6000 cGy to the region of the involved neck, with a boost to higher doses to the gross disease itself. For N1 disease, an additional 500 to 1000 cGy is given. For bulkier necks, doses in the 1000- to 1500-cGy range are added. These additional boost dosages usually are done with electron beams.

Treatment of Recurrent Disease

For patients with local recurrence, a second course of radiation therapy can usually be delivered to the nasopharynx. This can be rewarding in selected patients. Wang has shown the importance of high-dose reirradiation in obtaining good results.[400] Five-year survival was 45% in patients who received 6000 cGy or more compared with 0% 5-year survivors in those who received less than or equal to 5000 cGy. The interval of time between the original treatment and the recurrence was of prognostic significance. For patients who recurred more than 2 years after their original treatment, 5-year survival could be obtained in 66%. Only 13% of patients who failed within 2 years of the original treatment were 5-year survivors. Wang emphasizes the importance of combining external-beam irradiation and brachytherapy in the management of recurrent disease.[400]

Brachytherapy alone has been used for selected patients with local recurrence. Harrison and others have reported the use of permanent ^{125}I implants for discrete local recurrences in the nasopharynx.[401,402] Either the transoral or the transpalatal approach can be used. Figure 22–12 shows a transpalatal approach; the transnasal approach can also be used.[403] If patients are selected with localized, discrete lesions that are limited to the mucosa, permanent implants can be successful. Permanent implants also have the advantage of limiting the normal tissue that is reirradiated.

In most situations, because the recurrent lesion is not discrete and localized, a combination of external-beam and intracavitary irradiation is important. The field size should be kept as small as possible, preferably smaller than 8 cm in maximum diameter.[404] A dose of 4500 to 5000 cGy is typically delivered with external-beam, followed by a boost to the nasopharynx with an intracavitary implant of an additional 1000 to 1500 cGy. The techniques for these different brachytherapy approaches have been reviewed by Harrison and coworkers.[405] It is important to tailor the implant to the specific location within the nasopharynx that must be irradiated. This can help maximize the dose to the target area and minimize the dose to the surrounding normal tissue. Stereotactic radiosurgery and combined chemotherapy and radiation therapy have been reported.[406] The relative roles of these techniques for patients with recurrent nasopharyngeal carcinoma remain to be determined.

The role for surgery in nasopharyngeal carcinoma is limited principally to treatment of residual or recurrent disease. Small, locally recurrent disease within the nasopharynx has been shown to be amenable to surgical resection with 5-year survival rates of 50% in small patient series.[406] Several approaches have been described, including the lateral infratemporal approach and the intraoral transpalatal approach.[406,407] Complications of such surgery include injury to cranial nerves, cerebral spinal fluid leaks, and hemorrhage secondary to vessel injury.

Management of regional recurrence entails the same considerations as regional recurrence from squamous cell carcinomas elsewhere within the upper aerodigestive tract. If the disease is resectable, an attempt at surgical ablation is indicated. In most instances, this requires a radical neck dissection. Brachytherapy can supplement the neck surgery if there is concern about residual disease.

Chemotherapy of Nasopharyngeal Carcinoma

For recurrences of nasopharyngeal carcinoma at the primary site or in the neck and distant metastases, systemic chemotherapy is usually indicated. Most reports on chemotherapy in head and neck cancer include only a small number of patients with nasopharyngeal cancer and, therefore, information is limited (Table 22–25). Nevertheless, several chemotherapeutic agents, especially those used primarily in combination treatment, have been tested. Among those agents tested are methotrexate, cyclophosphamide, nitrosourea, cisplatin, bleomycin, and doxorubicin.

Generally, combination chemotherapy has yielded better overall response rates and more CRs. A few trials in small numbers of patients have been reported in which combinations of bleomycin, cytoxan, methotrexate, and 5-FU (BCMF) produced 50% to 83% response rates.[408–410] Huang and colleagues reported 8 patients treated with bleomycin, methotrexate,

(text continues on page 602)

A
B

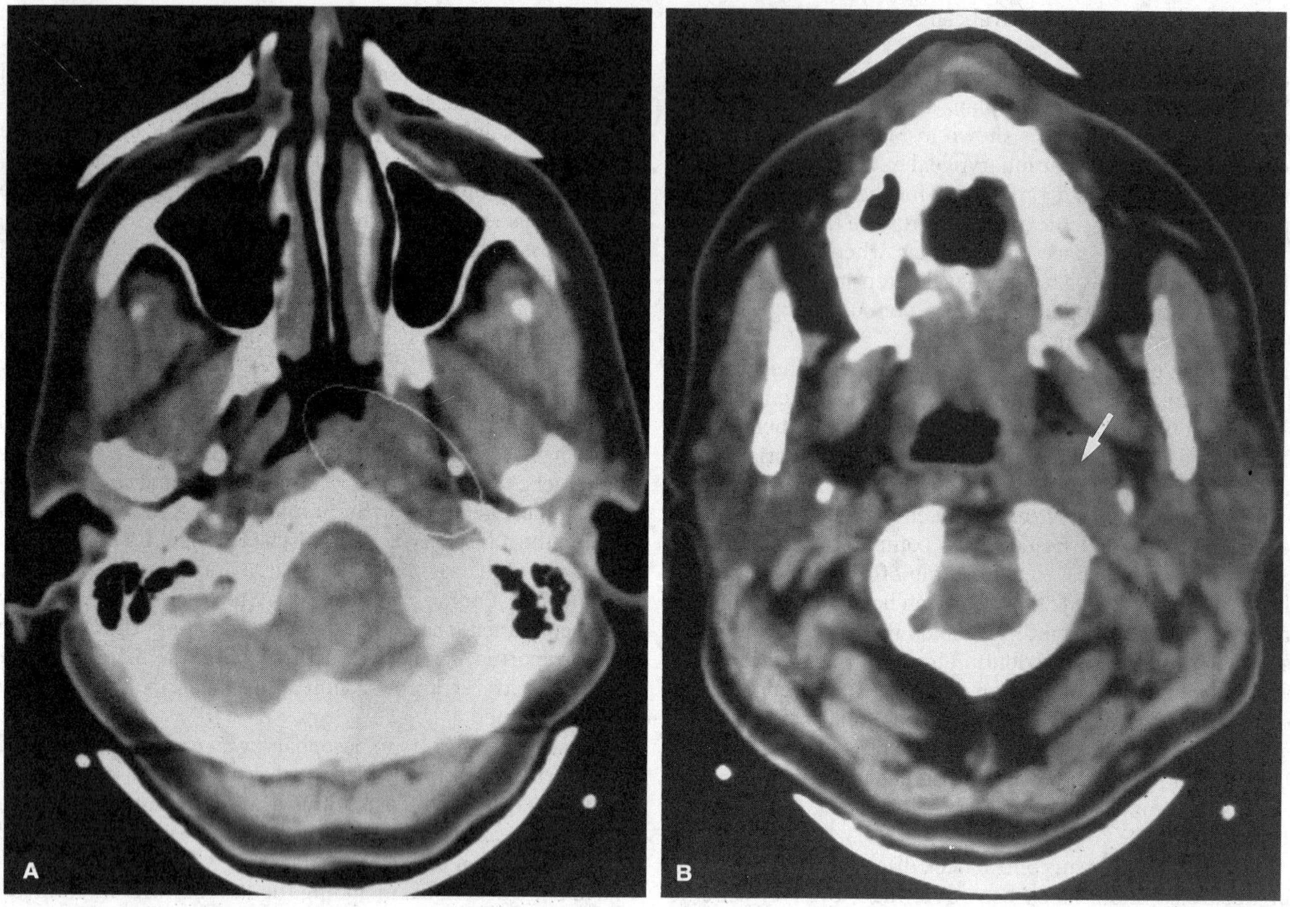

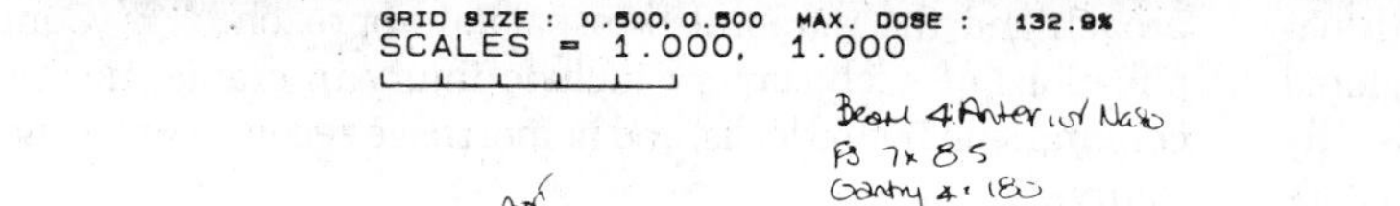

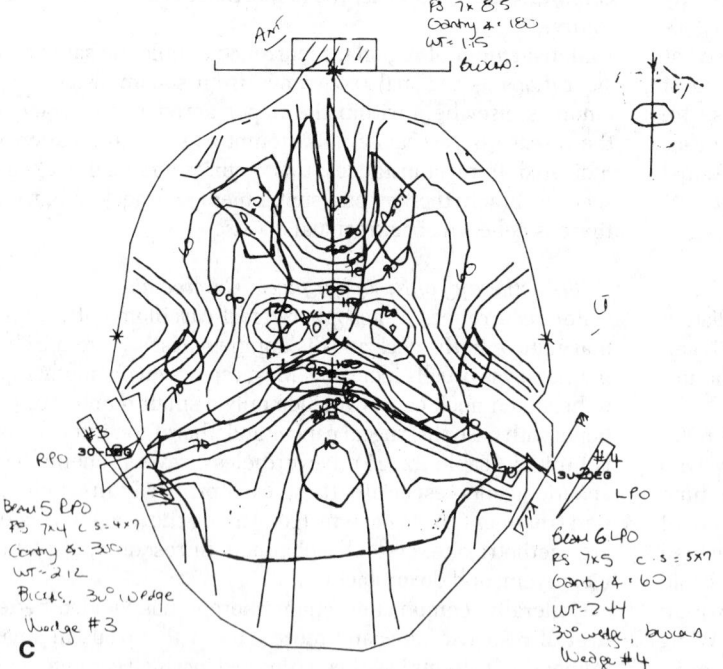

GRID SIZE : 0.500, 0.500 MAX. DOSE : 132.9%
SCALES = 1.000, 1.000
RPO
LPO
Wedge #3
Wedge #4
C

FIGURE 22–10. A patient with a squamous cancer of the nasopharynx that was staged as T2N0. **(A)** CT scan shows disease extension posteriorly in the parapharyngeal space. If bilateral opposed portals were used for the nasopharynx, the posterior extent of disease would be undertreated when the spinal cord block is placed. This demonstrates the need for CT scan in all nasopharynx patients. **(B)** Another CT scan shows retropharyngeal adenopathy. Again, this disease would be undertreated significantly by conventional, opposed lateral portals with a spinal cord block. **(C)** This patient was treated before there was 3D treatment planning. A three-field arrangement was used, which included two posterior oblique portals that protected the spinal cord, but treated the posterior extent of disease. A small portion of the posterior aspect of the disease is underdosed by 20%, even with this plant. This area was boosted with an I-125 implant. The patient remains NED at 3 years.

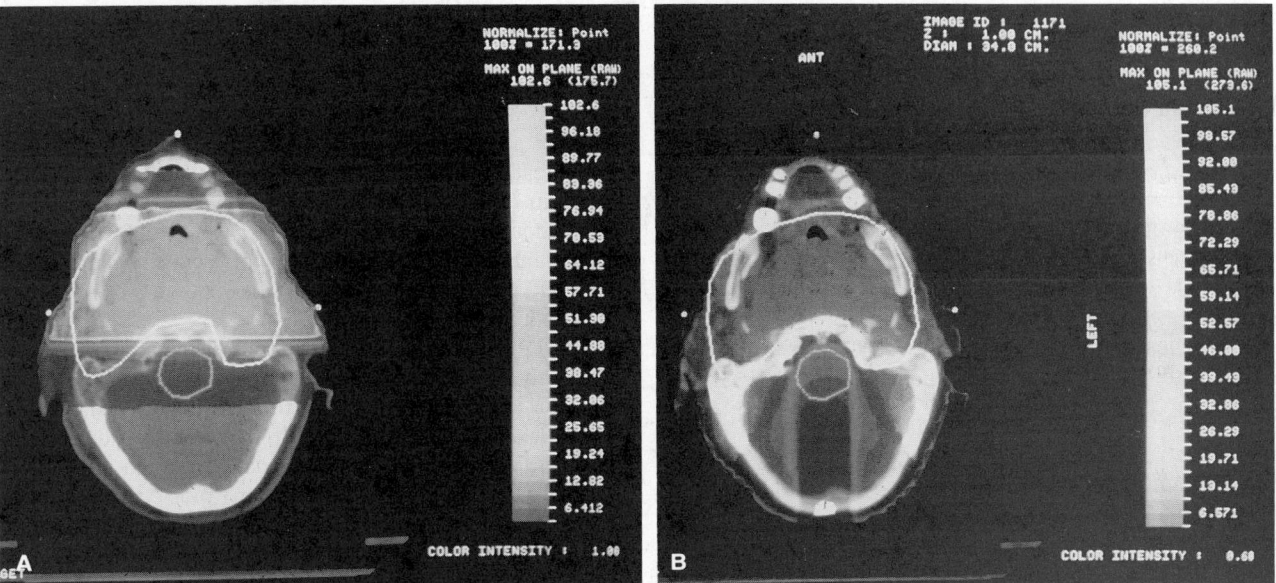

FIGURE 22-11. A patient with a T4N0 squamous carcinoma of the nasopharynx. The patient had bulky disease, extending into both retropharyngeal areas. **(A)** CT scan shows that target volume outlined. If bilateral opposed lateral portals were used to treat the nasopharynx, and a spinal cord block was placed at 4500 cGy, the posterior aspect of the target volume is underdosed. The retropharyngeal disease cannot be treated with this technique. **(B)** Using a 3D treatment plan, it is possible to encompass the entire retropharyngeal area adequately and still protect the brain stem and the spinal cord. This patient has a complete response to radiation therapy and is doing well 10 months after the completion of treatment.

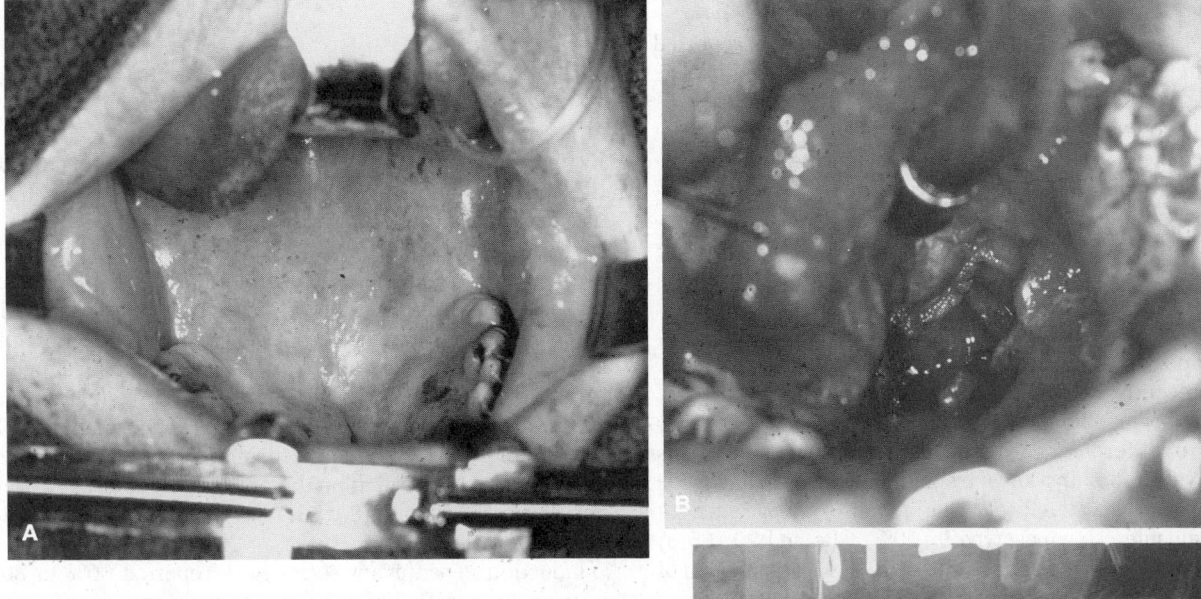

FIGURE 22-12. A patient with a discrete mucosal recurrence of a nasopharynx cancer. The recurrence was superficial and at the roof of the nasopharynx. It was not accessible through the opened mouth or through the nose. He was treated with an I-125 implant via the transpalatal approach. **(A)** This view looks into the mouth from above the patient's head, under general endotracheal anesthesia. A mouth retractor holds the mouth open. The tongue is at the top of the figure retracted by the tongue blade. The soft palate is exposed for the incision. **(B)** The soft palate has been incised and reflected to expose the interior of the nasopharynx. The torus tubarius is seen, and the glistening mucosa of the nasopharynx is directly visualized. Using this access, I-125 seeds are directly implanted into the roof of the nasopharynx. **(C)** Localization films of the implant show the position of the seeds in the roof of the nasopharynx.

TABLE 22–25. Chemotherapy and Biologic Therapy of Recurrent Nasopharyngeal Carcinoma

Investigations	No. of Patients	Chemotherapy Regimens	RR (CR) (%)
Geopfert, 1981[409]	18	BCMF or CAB	61
Huang, 1981[411]	8	BMVC	50
Decker, 1983[412]	17	P-based regimens	53 (18)
Lai, 1986[414]	10	PF	83 (14)
Cvitkovic, 1988[415]	17	BEP	88 (41)
Airoldi, 1989[413]	32	Different chemotherapy regimens	53 (16)
Leung, 1991[416]	22	CpF	55 (45)
Marchini, 1991[417]	26	PF	69 (27)
Cvitkovic, 1991[418]	21	PFMiE	76 (5)
Boussen, 1991[420]	44	PBF	86 (20)
Dimery, 1989[419]	14	IFN-γ	—*

* 4 minor response.
B, bleomycin; C, cyclophosphamide; E, epirubicin; Mi, mitomycin; M, methotrexate; F, 5-fluorouracil; V, vincristine; P, cisplatin; Cp, carboplatin; A, doxorubicin; IFN-γ, interferon-gamma.

vinblastine, and lomustine.[411] Dramatic tumor regression was seen in 4 patients. In 1983, Decker and coworkers reported a 10 year experience during which different chemotherapy regimens were used.[412] They reported 18% CR and 35% PR rates, for an overall response rate of 53%. In 1989, Airoldi and associates reviewed their experience using various chemotherapy regimens for recurrent and metastatic nasopharyngeal carcinoma.[413] The overall response rate for all combinations was 53.2%. However, PF was the most effective regimen, achieving 33.3% CR and 50% PR rates, for an overall response of 83.3%. The median duration of response was 7.2 months. Two other trials with PF have reported response rates of 73% and 83% and CR rates of 14% and 23%, respectively.

More recently, Boussen and colleagues from Gustave Roussy reported the first homogenous series of metastatic and recurrent undifferentiated nasopharyngeal cancer patients treated with a combination of cisplatin, bleomycin, and 5-FU (PBF) on a prospective trial.[420] Of a total of 49 patients, 44 were evaluable. They observed 9 (19%) CRs and 29 (60%) PRs, for an objective response rate of 79%. Mean duration of survival for complete responders was 25 months. Four patients were alive without evidence of disease more than 52 months. IFNs have antiviral activity against EBV and are immunomodulators. Clinical results with IFN-γ have been uniformly disappointing. IFN as a single agent appears to be inactive in head and neck squamous cell carcinoma and nasopharyngeal carcinoma.[419]

Based on these reports, it can be concluded that the highest response rates occur with platinum-containing combinations. Therefore, for palliation in patients who present with recurrent tumors, it is reasonable to give platinum-based regimens or to encourage participation in a clinical trial.

RESULTS OF TREATMENT

External-beam irradiation therapy alone has been shown to provide excellent local control for T1 and T2 lesions of the nasopharynx.[421–424] Wang reported better results when intracavitary radiation therapy is added to external-beam treatment alone.[421] However, results with external-beam plus intracavitary treatment are equivalent to the results of external-beam alone in other large centers. Well-delivered external-beam irradiation therapy should provide local control in at least 90% of patients with T1 lesions and between 85% and 90% of patients with T2 lesions. Doses in the 6500- to 7000-cGy range are used.

For T3 and T4 disease, local control rates have been significantly lower than the earlier stages, ranging from 62% to 73% for T3 lesions and 44% to 71% for T4 lesions.[422–424] There is a suggestion of a dose-response curve for radiation therapy. Vikram and coworkers have reported a 90% local control rate for T4 patients receiving more than 6700 cGy, although few patients have been followed more than 4 years.[426] With the use of 3D treatment planning and delivery, dose escalation to 7500 cGy and higher may be feasible. This may improve the local control and outcome for the T3 and T4 patients.

Results from M.D. Anderson Cancer Center show control of neck disease in all of 35 N0 patients, 27 of 30 (90%) N1 patients, 24 of 26 (92%) N2A patients, and 28 of 33 (85%) N2B patients.[399] However, patients with N3A metastases in the neck did worse, with only 10 of 16 (63%) achieving control.

Adjuvant Chemotherapy in Advanced Nasopharyngeal Carcinoma

Even though high survival rates can be achieved with radiation therapy alone for early stage lesions, the control of advanced nasopharyngeal carcinoma is poor, with most studies reporting a 5-year survival of 10% to 40%.[427] Advanced disease at the primary site presents problems in local control, and the risk for distant metastases is known to be particularly high with extensive nodal disease. With recent trials in induction chemotherapy for cancers of other head and neck sites, neoadjuvant or adjuvant chemotherapy has been investigated in an attempt to improve results obtained by local treatment. To date, numerous nonrandomized pilot studies of sequential chemotherapy and radiation therapy (cisplatin based, 7 trials; non-cisplatin regimen, 8 trials) have been reported (Tables 22–26 and 22–27).

Induction neoadjuvant series have reported 60% to 80% response rates (10–40% CR) with cisplatin and non-cisplatin-based regimens. After radiation therapy, the CR rate increased to more than 80%. Survival data from pilot trials are heterogenous and conflicting because of comparisons of their survival with histologic control. No firm conclusion about survival benefit can be drawn. There has not yet been a randomized trial report comparing induction chemotherapy followed by radiation therapy versus radiation therapy in locally advanced nasopharyngeal carcinoma. A randomized trial is underway at the Institut Gustave Roussy, and an International Cooperative study has been initiated.

Two trials addressed issues of concomitant chemotherapy and radiation therapy for advanced nasopharyngeal carcinoma.[437,441] In the U.S. Intergroup (RTOG and Southwest Oncology Group [SWOG]) randomized trial, disease-free survival and overall survival in patients treated with concomitant cisplatin and radiation therapy were encouraging compared with

TABLE 22–26. Adjuvant Chemotherapy in Locally Advanced Nasopharyngeal Carcinoma

Investigations	No. of Patients	Methods	Comments
Galligioni, 1982[428]	6	ABVD + XRT	CR 100% MS = 28 + mo
Rahuma, 1986[429]	66	XRT alone	S (3 y) = 61%
	16	XRT + CMF XRT + CMB	S (3 y) = 83%
Hill, 1987[430]	20	Price Hill regimen* + XRT	CR = 85% MS = 46
Khoury, 1987[431]	52	XRT alone	S (3 y) = 35%
	14	PB or PF + XRT	S (3 y) = 86%
Clark, 1987[432]	22	P-based chemotherapy + XRT	CR = 77% S (2 y) = 71% FFS (2 y) = 57%
Dimery, 1987[433]	69	XRT alone	CR = 91% MS = 67 mo
	21	Chemotherapy + XRT	CR = 81% ⎫ MS = >111 mo
	13	XRT ± chemotherapy	CR = 85% ⎭
Tannock, 1987[434]	140	XRT alone	Actuarial S (3 y) = 48%
	51	MBC + XRT	Actuarial S (3 y) = 48%
Zidan, 1987[435]	15	BMP + XRT	CR = 87% S (2.5 y) = 80%
Rossi, 1988[436]	116	XRT alone	RFS (4 y) = 56% S (4 y) = 67%
	113	XRT + OCA	RFS (4 y) = 58% S (4 y) = 58%

S, survival; O, vincristine; C, cyclophosphamide; A, doxorubicin; B, bleomycin; F, 5-fluorouracil; CR, complete response; MS, median survival; RFS, relapse-free survival; FFS, failure-free survival; M, methotrexate; V, vinblastine; P, cisplatin; D, DTIC; XRT, radiation therapy.
* Price–Hill regimen: combination of vincristine, methotrexate, bleomycin, 5-fluorouracil, hydrocortisone, and folinic acid.

TABLE 22–27. Adjuvant Chemotherapy in Locally Advanced Nasopharyngeal Carcinoma

Investigations	No. of Patients	Methods	Comments
Souhami, 1988[437]	30	MiFM + XRT concomitant	CR = 75% S (4 y) = 49% DFS (4 y) = 35%
En-Pee, 1989[438]	696	CVF + XRT	S (10 y) = 33%
	604		S (10 y) = 33%
Atichartakarn, 1988[439]	28	PF + XRT	CR = 82%
Tsujii, 1989[440]	22	XRT + CMU	RFS (5 y) = 50%
	26	XRT alone	RFS (5 y) = 31%
	29	XRT alone (higher dosage)	RFS (5 y) = 35%
Al Sarraf, 1990[441]	78	XRT alone	CR = 81%
	26	P + XRT	CR = 88%
Dimery, 1991[442]	43	PF + XRT	CR = 86% MS = 31 + m
Leung, 1991[416]	13	CpF + XRT	CR = 94%
Boussen, 1991[443]	30	ABP + XRT	CR = 64%
	30	AP + XRT	CR = 57%
Bachouchi, 1991[444]	61	BEP + XRT	CR = 98% DFS (2 y) = ?

S, survival; U, UFT (5-FU analogue); P, cisplatin; F, 5-fluorouracil; M, methotrexate; C, cyclophosphamide; V, vincristine; B, bleomycin; E, epirubicin; Mi, mitomycin-C; Cp, carboplatin; A, doxorubicin; DFS, disease-free survival; RFS, relapse-free survival; XRT, radiation therapy.

historical control groups.[441] Two trials of radiation therapy followed by chemotherapy have produced conflicting results.

Because most studies were relatively small and uncontrolled, no definite conclusions can be drawn about disease-free and overall survival rates. Therefore, initial or simultaneous chemotherapy and radiation therapy should not be used routinely in the management of nasopharyngeal cancer unless they are part of a clinical trial.

ORAL CAVITY

EPIDEMIOLOGY

Oral cavity cancer represents many diseases. Epidemiology as it relates to each of these disease processes differs. Because squamous cell carcinoma represents the preponderance of cancers that occur in this region, greater attention will be focused on its etiologic determinants than on etiologic determinants of cancers of other histology.

It is estimated that 30,000 new cases of oral cavity cancer occurred in 1991.[446,447] The relation between tobacco exposure and disease development has been demonstrated.[448,449] A clear dose–response relation has been identified, with a greater risk being directly proportional to intensity and duration of exposure. Alcohol has been identified as a coagent, most probably through a topical effect.[450] The mucosal areas that are exposed to prolonged contact with alcohol are at greatest risk for cancer development. Readers are referred to reviews on mechanisms of tobacco-induced carcinogenesis for an in-depth understanding.[451] Likewise, reviews regarding the role of alcohol in cancer development are available.[450,452]

Cigarette smoking cannot be considered the sole etiologic agent for oral cavity cancer. This fact is made evident by the observation that more than 50 million people in the United States consume cigarettes. The percentage of the total population using tobacco in its various forms is even greater. As mentioned, however, only 30,000 people develop oral cavity cancer annually. Therefore, other factors must be considered. Arguably, it is genetic susceptibility that may be the most significant variable. Genetic factors associated with increased risk include mutagen sensitivity, which is potentially reflective of an underlying DNA repair deficiency.[453] Syndromes that are characterized by mutagen sensitivity, including xeroderma pigmentosum, Fanconi anemia, and ataxia telangiectasia, have all been associated with oral cavity cancers.[454] Other relevant genetic markers may include inducibility of the cytochrome P-450 enzyme system.[455]

Additional risk factors for oral cavity cancer include diet.[456,457] Patients with vitamin A deficiency have been considered at high risk for malignant transformation of oral mucosa. High dietary consumption of fruits and vegetables have been found to provide a protective effect. Chronic irritants have been considered an etiologic factor, including mouthwash, poor dental hygiene, and syphilis.[458,459] Recent reports have incriminated marijuana smoking as a contributing factor to oral cavity cancer.[460]

Recent studies have focused on the viral etiology of cancers within the upper aerodigestive tract. Herpes simplex virus-type 1 (HSV-1) has long been considered an etiologic agent. The inability to identify HSV-1-related proteins within oral cavity cancers, however, has raised questions about the sig-

nificance of this virus.[461] Recent investigations have identified human papilloma virus within head and neck cancers, specifically types 2, 11, and 16.[462–465] Papilloma transcriptional factors, when inserted within human DNA, can alter normal gene replicative control mechanisms.

ANATOMY

The anatomy of the oral cavity is discussed in relation to each specific site.

STAGING

T staging for oral cavity cancer applies to all subsites within the oral cavity unless otherwise stated.

For the oral cavity, the definition of T staging is as follows:

	PRIMARY TUMOR
TX	Primary tumor cannot be assessed.
T0	No existence of primary tumor.
	TIS: CARCINOMA IN SITU
T1	Tumor 2 cm or less in greatest dimension.
T2	Tumor more than 2 cm but not more than 4 cm in greatest dimension.
T3	Tumor more than 4 cm in greatest dimension.
T4 (lip)	Tumor invades adjacent structures (*e.g.,* through cortical bone, tongue, skin of neck).
T4 (oral cavity)	Tumor invades adjacent structures (*e.g.,* through cortical bone, into deep [extrinsicl] muscle of tongue, maxillary sinus, and skin).

The regional lymph node (N) and distant metastases (M) staging are identical to other sites within the upper aerodigestive tract and are as stated in the beginning of this chapter.

PATHOLOGY

The commonest cancer within the oral cavity is squamous cell carcinoma. Additionally, cancers can arise from minor salivary glands; these latter cancers include adenoid cystic carcinoma, mucoepidermoid carcinoma, and adenocarcinoma. Rare soft tissue neoplasms include mucosal melanoma, plasmacytoma, and soft tissue sarcomas. Also found within the oral cavity are cancers arising from bone, including osteosarcomas.

There also exist neoplastic lesions that are not truly malignant disorders of bone growth, such as ameloblastoma. However, these lesions have a propensity for local expansion and destruction. The principles of sound oncologic surgery and radiation apply to these latter processes.[483]

NATURAL HISTORY

Earliest changes associated with squamous cell carcinoma are associated with erythema and slight mucosal surface irregularities. A punctate lesion often is identified. As disease progresses, several growth patterns emerge that can be characterized typically as exophytic or infiltrative. The latter is more characteristically associated with destruction of surrounding anatomic structures. The exophytic lesions have a less aggressive growth pattern. Both patterns are capable of producing metastasis and disease progression, and therapy should be planned accordingly.

Characteristics of the disease are reflected in certain histopathologic criteria. When tumor differentiation has been considered, it has been reported that poorly differentiated disease has a greater propensity for metastasis than does well-differentiated disease. This conclusion, however, has not been accepted universally. Jacobsson's criteria as outlined in Table 22–2 reflects the natural history of the disease. More specific information regarding natural history is discussed in relation to each anatomic subsite.

LIP

Epidemiology

Carcinoma of the lip is second only to skin cancer as a site of neoplasia within the head and neck region. It is reported to occur in approximately 3600 cases per year, or 1.8 persons per 100,000 population annually.[446] Most of these lesions occur on the lower lip and 95% occur in men. A principal etiologic factor, similar to other upper aerodigestive cancer, has been the use of tobacco, including pipes and cigars.[466] Sun exposure has been incriminated and may represent the most significant factor. The latter fact is of potential relevance, because of the increased incidence of other skin cancers and lip cancer. Patients who are genetically susceptible to skin cancers after sun exposure, that is, patients with xeroderma pigmentosum, are susceptible to lip cancer.[454] Such an observation emphasizes ultraviolet radiation as an etiologic agent. Disease has also been noted in renal and homograft recipients, implicating immunosuppression as a determinant.[467]

Anatomy

The lip is composed of the orbicularis oris muscle and is delineated by the junction of the vermillion border with the skin. Blood supply and sensory nerve supply are by means of the labial artery (a branch of the facial artery) and by cranial nerve V, respectively. The primary lymph node drainage is to levels I and II.

Pathology

The principal cancer involving the lip is squamous cell carcinoma. Other lesions include basal cell carcinoma. Rarely, minor salivary gland cancers can occur.

Natural History

Patients most frequently present with an exophytic or ulcerative lesion of the lower lip. Occasionally, these lesions are associated with bleeding and pain. The latter symptom, however, is a late feature of the disease. These lesions are typically slow growing. With progression, there may be associated numbness of the skin of the chin secondary to involvement of the mental nerve, a branch of the third division of cranial nerve V. Progression of disease along the mental nerve may extend into the mental foramen of the mandible. Such involvement leads to enlargement of the foramen with bone destruction and widening of the inferior alveolar canal. A Panorex examination of the mandible is recommended as part of each diagnostic evaluation.

Lymphatic spread occurs relatively infrequently in lip cancer; approximately 5% to 10% of patients develop evidence of nodal involvement.[468–470] Lymph node spread is typically to submandibular nodes or submental nodes. Lesions in the midline may spread bilaterally. The incidence of metastases have been related to histologic grading, with high-grade lesions being at greatest risk. The upper lip tends to metastasize earlier than the lower lip. Upper lesions will metastasize to periparotid nodes (*i.e.,* preauricular nodes) in addition to submandibular nodes.

The prognosis from lip cancer principally depends on the size of the primary tumor.[471–473] T1 lip cancers have a 5-year survival of 90%. T2 survival is 84%. With evidence of lymph node metastases, survival decreases to 50%. Perineural invasion represents a poor prognostic sign.[474] Prognosis appears worse in younger adults.[475] Tumors have a greater tendency to metastatic spread in these latter patients.

Treatment

Early Disease

Surgery or radiation therapy is the mainstay of therapy. Dysplasias and carcinoma in situ can be handled by lip shave, which is vermilionectomy with advancement of a mucosal flap. Those lesions that involve less than 30% of the lip can be resected with a V excision and primary closure of resulting defects. For larger lesions, transposition flaps are required for reconstruction.

Undoubtedly, the challenge in the surgical management of lip cancer resides in the best means of reconstruction. Oral competence remains the primary goal. Those lesions that require resection of 30% to 50% of the lip can be handled best with a transposition flap drawn from the uninvolved opposing lip. This reconstruction technique is termed *Abbe-Estlander*.[476–478] A detailed description of the Abbe-Estlander flap has been provided.[482] When the near total lip (50–75%) is involved, the Karapandzic advancement flap can be used.[479] This procedure has the benefit of providing a competent oral sphincter with an associated neurovascular integrity.

The problem with the Karapandzic reconstruction is that the reconstructed lip is tight and significantly foreshortened. Other methods have been devised, varying from simple nasolabial flaps based inferiorly or superiorly to more formal fan-type flaps, such as the Gillies flap and Webster cheek advancement flap.[480–482]

Most T1 to T3 squamous cell carcinomas of the lip can be managed by radiation therapy or surgery. The choice of radiation or surgery may depend on the size and location of disease. If the lesion is small and can be excised easily without functional sequelae, surgery would be the chosen treatment. Lesions involving commissures can be irradiated without the functional sequelae of surgery. However, involvement of the commissure under such circumstances is rare. Brachytherapy alone can be used for early T1 and small T2 lesions. Temporary implantation with ^{192}Ir is the treatment of choice. Doses in the 6000-cGy range are usually adequate, with the dose rate being in the 40- to 60-cGy/hour range. Figure 22–13 shows a clinical example of the brachytherapy procedure. Similarly, external-beam can be used alone or with an implant for T3 lesions.

Because of the infrequency in which early cancers spread to regional lymph nodes, elective treatment of the neck is not necessarily required.

Advanced Disease

Stages III and IV lip disease are managed optimally with combined surgery and postoperative radiation therapy. Reconstructive options are as described earlier. Doses in the 6000- to 6300-cGy range, delivered at 180 to 200 cGy per fractions for 6 to 7 weeks, is preferred. If the patient has

lymph node metastases in the neck, a neck dissection is performed along with the resection of the primary site. The postoperative radiation therapy is then delivered to the neck and the primary site. Even if the patient were N0, elective radiation therapy or elective node dissection should still be used as part of the management because of the increased risk for microscopic lymph node metastases in these patients.

For patients with T1 to T3 disease who have had an operation, sometimes the radiation oncologist is faced with a positive margin of resection. This situation can be managed with brachytherapy alone or localized superficial external-beam irradiation, with similar doses and techniques as when radiation therapy alone is used.

Results of Treatment

The radiation therapy results are similar to the reported results of surgical management.[483] Heller and Shah reported approximately 90% local control for T1, T2, and T3 lesions

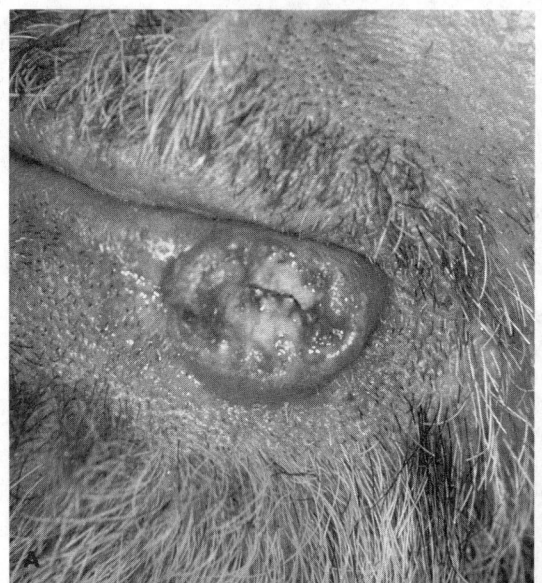

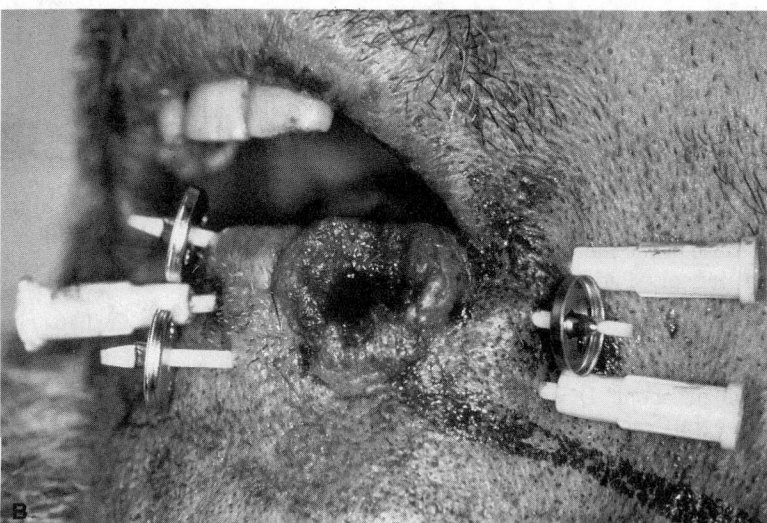

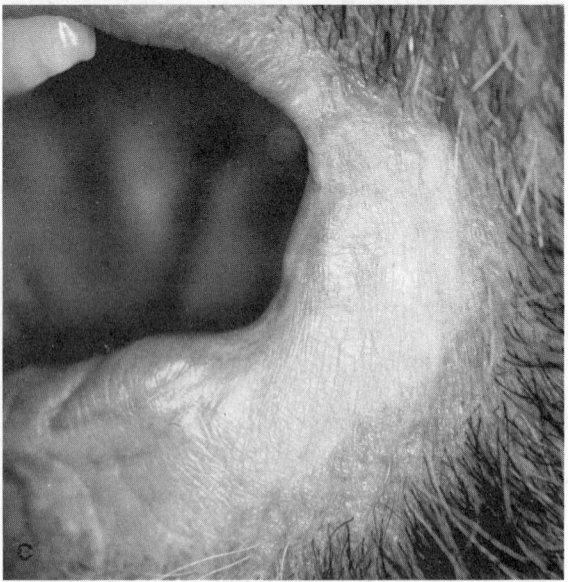

FIGURE 22–13. **(A)** A patient with a T1N0 squamous cancer of the lower lip. The lesion measured 2 cm in greatest diameter and involved the commissure. **(B)** An implant was used as treatment. Under local anesthesia with 2% lidocaine, 14-gauge angiocatheters were placed through the lesion. After localization and planning films were done, Ir-192 was loaded into these catheters. A total of 6000 cGy in 6 days was delivered. **(C)** The patient remains NED at 3 years. (Harrison L, Fass D. Radiation therapy for oral cavity cancer. Dental Clin North Am 1990;34:205–222)

treated with surgery alone.[471] A significant problem in surgical management is local recurrence, which may approach 40% for T3 and T4 lesions.[469] Fitzpatrick reported that the results of radiation therapy and surgery are basically equivalent.[484]

Jorgensen and associates reported a series of 869 lip cancers.[485] In 766 patients, treatment was performed entirely with brachytherapy. The remaining cases had external-beam irradiation, mainly with orthovoltage beams. Most patients had T1 or T2 lesions, with only 75 having T3 lesions. Local control was in the 90% range.

External-beam irradiation can also be used. Petrovich and coworkers reported on 250 patients, most receiving 5100 cGy in 3 weeks with daily fractions of 300 cGy.[486] There were 896 patients in the study, most of whom were treated with orthovoltage beams. Local control was obtained in 94% of T1 and T2 lesions and in 90% of T3. For T4 disease, 47% of the patients obtained local control with radiation alone, indicating the need for combined modality treatment for this subset.

ALVEOLAR RIDGE AND RETROMOLAR TRIGONE

Epidemiology

Cancers of the alveolar ridge and retromolar trigone constitute approximately 10% of all oral cancers.[487] Men are more frequently affected than women at a ratio of 4:1. An increased frequency in rural women of the Southeastern United States has been reported.

Anatomy

The alveolar ridge consists of an upper and a lower portion. The lower alveolar ridge has as its structural basis the alveolar process of the mandible extending from ascending ramus to ascending ramus, not inclusive of the retromolar trigone. Its borders extend from the gingival-labial sulcus to the free mucosa of the floor of the mouth. The alveolar process of the maxillary bone constitutes the upper alveolar ridge. The retromolar trigone is a triangular area that is composed principally of mucosa overlying the ascending ramus of the mandible. It is bounded superiorly by the hard palate, inferiorly by the alveolar ridge, medially by the anterior tonsillar pillar, and laterally by the gingival buccal sulcus.

Lymphatic drainage of the alveolar ridge and retromolar trigone is principally to levels I and II.

Pathology

Squamous cell carcinoma represents almost all the lesions in this area. Minor salivary gland lesions (*i.e.,* mucoepidermoid carcinomas and adenoid cystic carcinomas) can occur.

Natural History

Squamous cell carcinoma of the alveolar ridge grows in patterns similar to other squamous cell carcinomas of the oral cavity, which are as exophytic lesions or as infiltrative disease. The latter is commonly associated with bone destruction, which occurs in as many as 58% of cases. The presenting symptom primarily is pain that is exacerbated by chewing. Other symptoms include intermittent bleeding and loose teeth. In those patients who are edentulous, the principal complaint relates to ill-fitting dentures. The lower alveolus is affected most often in the molar and premolar region. Delay in diagnosis is characteristic because of confusion with inflammatory conditions, such as gingivitis or periodontitis.

These lesions have a higher probability of regional lymph node metastases than do other cancers within the oral cavity, with the exception of tongue cancer. Overall, the probability of lymph node metastases increases directly with the size of the primary tumor and averages 30%.[488-492] It may increase as much as 70% for T4 cancers. However, lymph node metastases tend to occur more frequently from mandibular alveolar ridge cancers than from maxillary alveolar ridge disease. Metastatic disease is primarily to lymph nodes in levels I and II. Byers and colleagues noted that less than 5% of patients develop disease in the posterior cervical triangle.[492]

The prognosis from alveolar ridge carcinoma is reflected by the extent of primary and regional lymph node metastatic disease.[489-492] T1 cancer of the alveolar ridge can be expected to have an 85% survival. T2 lesions and T3 lesions are associated with 80% and 60% survival, respectively. Prognosis with T4 lesions is poor, approximating 20%.

Treatment

Early Disease

Surgical management of carcinomas of the alveolar ridge reflects the management principles of cancers of other sites within the oral cavity. The fundamental feature remains the achievement of tumor-free surgical margins with the preservation of critical anatomic structures.

Early T1 or T2 lesions of the alveolar ridge can be managed successfully by surgery alone. With minimal cortical involvement or with involvement by cancer confined to the mucoperiosteum, resection may include a marginal (coronal) mandibulectomy that preserves the structural integrity of the mandible. The ability to preserve segments of the mandible is, in part, dependent on dental status. Not infrequently, edentulous patients present with thin "pipestem" mandibles that preclude all but a segmental resection.

The tendency for bone invasion by alveolar ridge carcinomas through thin mucoperiosteum or through tooth sockets makes primary radiation less feasible. In general, lesions of the gingiva are best managed by surgery.

A secondary benefit of neck dissection for alveolar ridge carcinomas results from the tendency of regional nodal spread. The considerations for elective neck dissection and the type of neck dissection have been discussed previously in this section. The infrequency of tumor spread of levels IV and V has led to acceptance of selective neck dissection of levels I to III in instances of a clinically N0 neck.

Advanced Disease

Advanced-stage tumors generally require multimodality therapy, including surgery and radiation. Segmental mandibulectomy is required. Advances in the management of such disease have related to improved reconstructive techniques, principally the use of osteomyocutaneous free-tissue transfer.[493]

Treatment Results

In those studies that report primary surgery results, the actuarial survival for stages I and II was 77% at 5 years compared with approximately 60% for stage III and 24% for stage IV.[492,494]

There are relatively few patients reported in the literature with gingival carcinoma that have been managed with primary radiation therapy.[494,495] Early retromolar trigone tumors can be treated successfully by primary radiation, especially when they are superficial. Figure 22–14 shows a clinical example.

FLOOR OF THE MOUTH

Epidemiology

The annual incidence of cancers of the floor of mouth is 0.6 cases per 100,000 in the United States.[446] It occurs in men approximately three times as frequently as it does in women.

Recent reports, however, have shown an increasing incidence of the disease among women.[495a] The median age of people developing squamous cell carcinoma is approximately 60 years.

Anatomy

The floor of the mouth is delineated by the free margin of the mucosa as it extends from the junction of the mobile tongue to the alveolar process. This margin extends from one anterior tonsillar pillar to the other. Within the floor of the mouth anteriorly are the openings of bilaterally located submandibular salivary glands known as *Wharton ducts*. These ductal openings are significant because anterior lesions of the floor

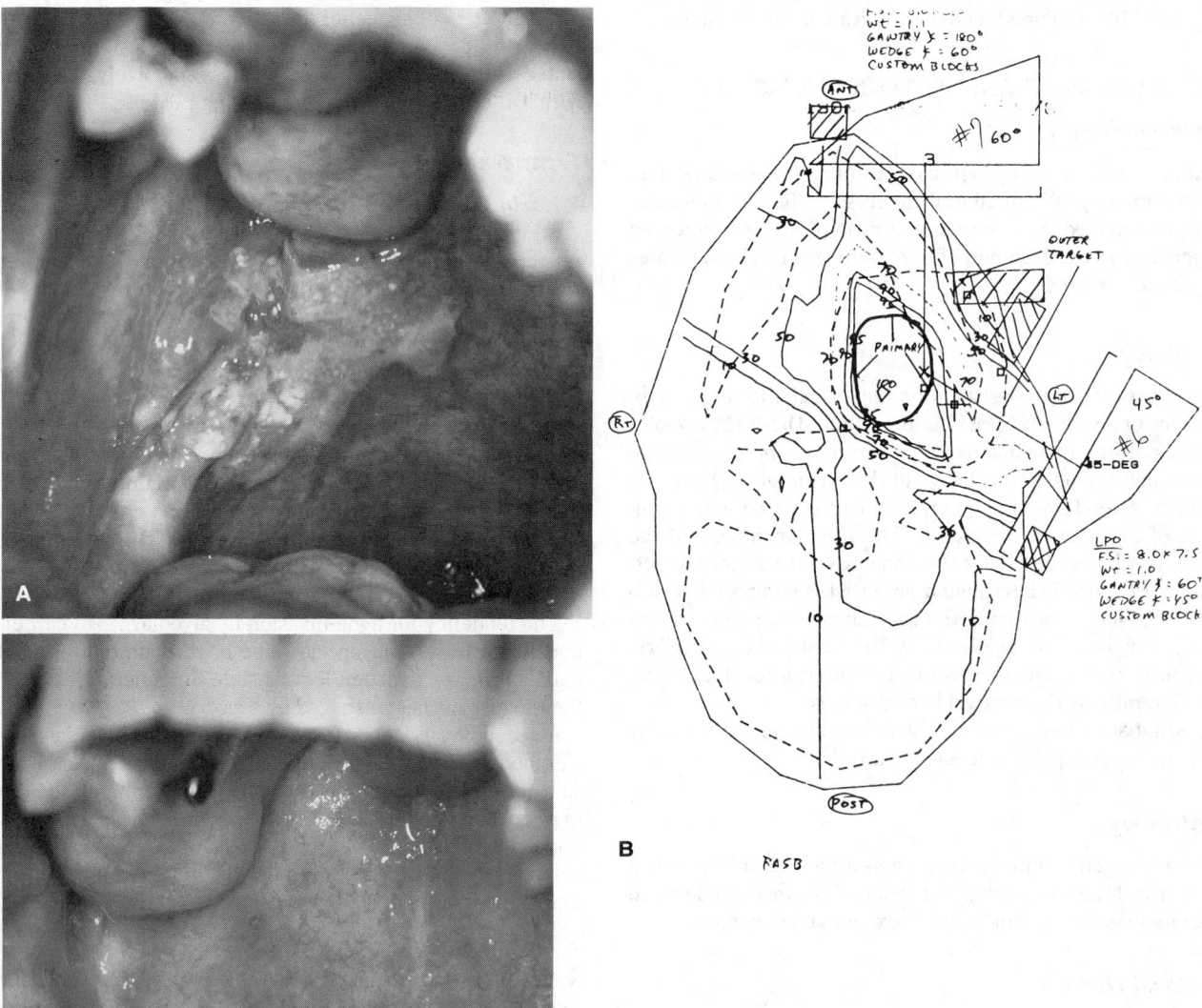

FIGURE 22–14. **(A)** A patient with a T2N0 squamous cancer of the right retromolar trigone. The patient was treated with definitive external beam radiation therapy to the primary and ipsilateral neck. **(B)** The treatment plan involved a wedged photon pair. The boost field is shown. The contralateral parotid area receives less than 10% of the dose, thereby avoiding xerostomia. The primary site received 7020 cGy, at 180 cGy per fraction. The right low neck received 5000 cGy/5 weeks with an ipsilateral low neck field (not shown). **(C)** The patient remains NED at 4.5 years.

of the mouth can frequently obstruct associated salivary flow leading to tenderness and enlargement of the respective submandibular gland. Also within the floor of the mouth are minor salivary glands and the sublingual glands. Distinct from mucosa of the tongue, mucosa of the floor of the mouth is nonkeratinizing stratified squamous epithelium under nonpathologic situations. Musculature constituting the floor of the mouth include the genioglossus, geniohyoid, and mylohyoid muscles. Blood and nerve supplies are principally from the paired lingual arteries and lingual nerves, respectively.

Pathology

Cancers of the floor of the mouth account for approximately 10% to 15% of all oral cavity cancers. Squamous cell carcinoma constitutes the commonest type of lesions within the floor of the mouth, with most of these lesions being moderate to well differentiated. There are several variants of squamous cell carcinoma of the floor of the mouth, including verrucous and sarcomatoid squamous cell carcinomas. Cancers derived from salivary gland tissue are encountered, including mucoepidermoid carcinomas, adenocarcinomas, and adenoid cystic carcinomas.

Natural History

Squamous cell carcinomas of the floor of the mouth typically present as infiltrative lesions that are characteristically painful. These lesions may extend anteriorly to invade bone, deeply to infiltrate muscles of the floor of the mouth, or posteriorly to invade the tongue. Occasionally, an enlarged lymph node in the neck is the presenting symptom.

Floor of the mouth cancers can grow to massive size without metastasizing to cervical lymph nodes. Approximately 12% of T1 lesions are associated with occult metastatic disease, depending on the thickness of the lesion.[171,176] Metastatic rates to cervical lymph nodes occur in 30%, 47%, and 53% of T2, T3, and T4 cancer, respectively.[172] Lymph nodes in the submandibular and submental triangles represent the first echelon of metastatic sites. Distant metastases are observed infrequently in patients who present with previously untreated disease.

Prognosis is influenced principally by disease stage and presence or absence of histopathologically confirmed regional lymph node metastases. The overall 5-year survival for stage I disease approximates 85% to 90%.[496,497] For stages II, III, and IV disease, 80%, 66%, and 32% of patients, respectively, are alive at 5 years. Other factors considered to reflect a worse prognosis include evidence of perineural invasion, depth of primary tumor invasion, and poor tumor differentiation.[498-500] The latter factor, however, has not been universally accepted as having prognostic significance.

Treatment

Early Disease

Treatment of floor of mouth cancers has been principally surgical resection but may be surgery or radiation alone. As is true for cancers of the alveolar ridge, superficial involvement of the mandible can be handled by marginal mandibulectomy (Fig. 22-15).

When radiation is used for early disease, results are improved when at least a portion of the treatment is delivered by an interstitial implant.[501,502] Interstitial implant alone also can be used.[503] Lesions that abut or are tethered to the periosteum of the mandible are not good candidates for primary radiation therapy. Implants against the mandible can lead to osteonecrosis.

The treatment of the neck for early cancer of the floor of mouth is controversial. Most authors would advocate elective neck treatment for clinically N0 disease. The value of this approach compared with the outcome with neck dissection and radiation therapy being performed for clinically developing disease remains unproved. Some authors have advocated performing neck dissection depending on the thickness of the primary lesion, that is, if the lesion is more than 4 mm thick.

Advanced Disease

For advanced lesions, combined therapy of surgery and radiation is the treatment of choice. Surgical resection generally entails partial glossectomy and segmental mandibulectomy. Identification of the inferior alveolar nerve and frozen-section histopathologic assessment should be performed during the operation to ensure that disease has not extended beyond surgical margins by perineural spread. Resection for most ad-

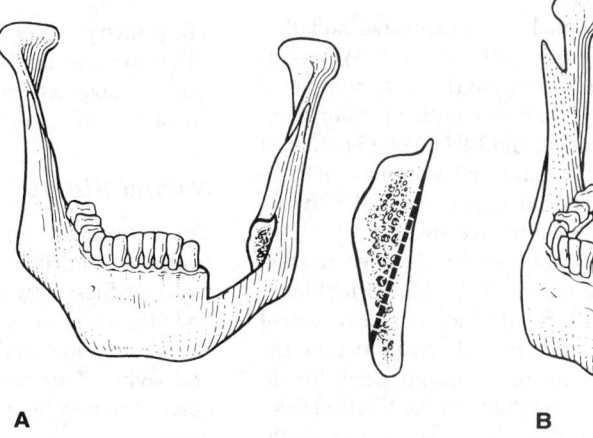
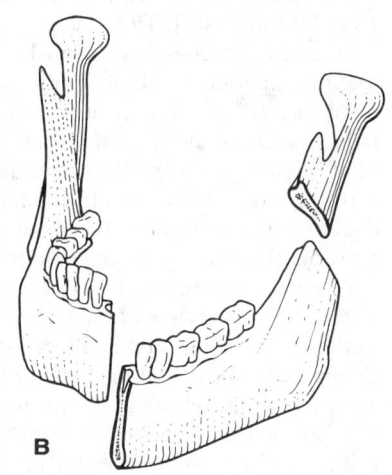

FIGURE 22–15. Types of mandibular resection for squamous cell carcinomas of the floor of mouth. **(A)** marginal resection that preserves mandibular continuity. **(B)** segmental mandibulectomy in which the entire segment of mandible is removed and mandibular continuity is lost. (Shah JP, Shemen LJ, Strong EW. Surgical therapy of oral cavity tumors. In: Thawley SE, Panje WR, eds. Comprehensive management of head and neck tumors. Philadelphia: WB Saunders, 1987:558)

A   **B**

vanced lesions requires removal of the entire thickness of the floor of the mouth.

New reconstructive techniques have greatly facilitated rehabilitation after surgical excision of advanced tumors. Techniques include myocutaneous flaps and osteomyocutaneous free flaps with microvessel anastomoses.[504]

Elective or therapeutic neck dissections, or both, are considered necessary in each case. Bilateral neck dissections are indicated for those lesions that approach or cross the midline.

Postoperative radiation entails doses of 6000 to 6300 cGy at the primary site. In instances of positive surgical margins, the author's policy is to treat the area of positive margins to 6300 cGy. Patients are treated with opposed lateral fields for the primary site and upper neck, which junctions to a low neck field at approximately the thyroid notch. A midline block is used for the low neck field to protect the larynx and the spinal cord. The dose to the low neck is usually 5000 cGy given in 5 weeks. The upper neck and primary site are generally treated with up to 4500 cGy in 5 weeks, after which a spinal cord block is placed. The primary site and upper neck are generally treated with 5400 cGy, after which a boost to the primary site and the involved region of the neck is increased to approximately 6300 cGy. Electron fields are used posterior to the spinal cord block, as needed, to bring the posterior neck to the appropriate dose.

Results of Treatment

Local recurrences after surgical resection of T1 and T2 floor of mouth cancers are noted in about 10% of the patient population.[496,497,505] As tumors increase in size, the pattern for failure becomes predominantly a regional problem. Nearly 40% of failures are solely within regional cervical lymph nodes.[496]

Mazeron and coworkers have reported a large recent radiation therapy series.[503] Most patients were treated with up to 6500 cGy with ^{192}Ir brachytherapy alone. Local control was 94% for T1N0 and 74% for T2N0 lesions and it was dependent on the size of the lesion and the presence or absence of gingival extension.

Wang and associates have reported excellent results with the use of intraoral cone electron boost and no brachytherapy.[506] The daily dose of radiation with the cone is frequently greater than the conventional 180- to 200-cGy range. Local control was obtained in all 13 patients with T1 lesions and in 19 of 20 (95%) with T2 lesions.

Fu and colleagues have published an extensive radiation therapy experience with floor of mouth cancer.[507] When implant was the only treatment or a part of the treatment, local failure occurred in 2% (1 of 39 patients) with T1 lesions, 7% (4 of 54 patients) with T2 lesions, and 14% (5 of 35 patients) with T3 lesions. The use of primary radiation may be associated with improved functional outcome compared with surgery, but this relation requires more investigation.[508]

When examining results of treatment for advanced disease, a retrospective review of the results at the Memorial Sloan-Kettering Cancer Center highlights the fact that local control is improved with combined surgery and radiation therapy, compared with surgery alone, for patients with stages III and IV head and neck lesions.[94] In a prospective randomized trial, Kramer and associates compared preoperative radiation (5000 cGy) plus surgery, surgery plus postoperative radiation (6000 cGy), and radiation therapy alone (6500–7000 cGy) with surgical salvage for patients with certain stage II and all stage III and IV squamous cancers of the oral cavity and the oropharynx.[509] There was no difference in the 4-year actuarial survival, or locoregional control, regardless of treatment type. However, this study did not stratify the results by anatomic subsite within the oral cavity and the oropharynx.

A recent report from Memorial Sloan-Kettering Cancer Center[94] highlights the importance of analyzing treatment results by anatomic subsite in patients with advanced disease. With a median follow-up of 6 years, the 5-year actuarial local control was 74%. However, the local failure rate was 38% for oral tongue (29 patients) compared with 11% for floor of mouth (22 patients); the difference was statistically significant.

TONGUE

Epidemiology

Tongue cancer is estimated to occur in 6200 persons each year in the United States.[446] Excluding the lip, the tongue exceeds all other sites in the oral cavity. The median age for persons with tongue cancer is approximately 60 years. The ratio of men to women is similar to other disease sites, approximately 3:1. An increase in tongue cancer has been reported among young adult men.[510,511] Some authors have suggested marijuana use as a contributing factor in this latter population.[460]

Anatomy

The oral tongue represents the mobile portion of the tongue musculature that extends from the line demarcated by the circumvallate papilla posteriorly to the junction of the floor of mouth anteriorly. It comprises the genioglossus, hyoglossus, styloglossus, and palatoglossus muscles. All the muscles are innervated by the hypoglossal nerves. Taste and sensation within the tongue are provided by the lingual nerve, a branch of the third division of cranial nerve V. Blood is supplied principally from the external carotid artery through the paired lingual arteries. Lymphatic drainage is principally to levels II, III, and I in decreasing order.

Pathology

The primary cancer of the tongue is squamous cell carcinoma. Other cancers are frequent and include minor salivary gland cancers, such as adenoid cystic carcinoma and adenocarcinoma. Myeloblastoma represents a rare tumor of the tongue.

Natural History

Tongue cancers can grow in an exophytic and an infiltrative fashion. The primary presenting symptom is pain, although many of these lesions can be painless. Difficulty in speech and deglutition occasionally is elicited. Tongue cancers tend to be more rapid in their onset than other cancers within the oral cavity. There may be a history of longstanding leukoplakia before the development of symptoms, especially in younger women.

Compared with other cancers within the oral cavity, tongue cancers have a greater propensity for lymph node metastases. This occurrence ranges from 15% to 75%, depending on the extent of primary disease.[472,512,513] Lymph nodes most frequently involved lie within level II, the jugulodigastric nodes. Nodes within levels I, III, and IV are involved in decreasing order; however, all nodes can be involved. The incidence of bilateral nodal metastases is as high as 25% of cases. Contralateral nodal metastases are present in 3% of cancers.

Prognosis is principally reflected in the extent of nodal metastases, ranging from 75% in early-stage node negative disease to 30% in those patients with advanced lesions. Other factors portending more aggressive disease include perineural and vascular invasion and infiltrative versus pushing borders.[514,515] Depth of invasion also has been considered significant. Whether tongue cancer in young adults represents a worse disease has not been demonstrated.[516]

Treatment

Early Disease

Disease control rates for early disease when using surgery or radiation therapy are equivalent, depending on treatment bias. Early-stage I and II lesions usually can be removed intraorally. Excision usually entails a hemiglossectomy. Special attention to surgical margins should be exercised, because disease may spread along muscle bundles beyond that expected by clinical assessment.

Most T1 lesions can be managed with brachytherapy alone. This generally consists of an ^{192}Ir implant. Although radium needles are still used by some groups, this is really an outdated technique that should be avoided. It introduces unnecessary exposure to the physicians, nurses, and other staff members and it does not allow the physician to optimize the dose distribution of the brachytherapy procedure.

Iridium 192 is inserted through afterloading catheters. The catheters are placed in the operating room with the patient under general anesthesia. The ^{192}Ir is loaded 1 or 2 days postoperatively. Localization films are taken, and computerized dosimetry is performed. The usual dose rate is in the 40- to 60-cGy/hour range, and the usual total dose is 6000 to 7000 cGy. The patient wears a tongue prosthesis during the dwell time of the implant to protect the hard and soft palate as much as possible.

Because the lesion increases in size when radiation is used as the primary therapy, combining external-beam irradiation with implant is preferred. First, the external-beam can be used as elective neck irradiation simultaneously with irradiation to the tongue. The implant then serves as the boost to the tongue. Second, the external-beam allows a wider margin of tongue to be treated than does the implant. In these situations, it is typical to treat the primary site and the neck to doses in the 5000-cGy range, followed by a 2000- to 3000-cGy implant boost to the tongue.

For N0 patients, this treatment program manages the primary site and the neck. For those patients with palpable neck nodes, a neck dissection can be performed at the same anesthesia as the implant, thereby completing the treatment to the primary site and the neck. This procedure can usually be done about 3 weeks after the completion of the external-beam irradiation.

Radiation therapy is suitable for most T1 lesions. For T2 and T3 lesions, it is most suitable for those tumors that are exophytic or have minimal infiltration. Tumors that are deeply infiltrative are preferably managed with a primary surgical approach, usually with postoperative radiation therapy.

Advanced Disease

The surgical management of more extensive lesions requires a mandibulotomy or a lingual-releasing procedure to gain access to disease. The latter procedure entails the removal of neck contents before primary cancer resection. The tongue is delivered into the neck by releasing musculature attachments posteriorly and mucosal attachments within the oral cavity. Large lesions with mandibular involvement require composite resection. The term *composite resection* refers to the removal of tissue involving multiple anatomically defined structures, one of which includes the mandible (Fig. 22–16). Typically, it refers to resection of a portion of the tongue, the floor of the mouth, and a segment of the mandible.

For patients who require postoperative radiation therapy to the primary site alone, brachytherapy often is appropriate. This is especially true for smaller lesions. The decision of how to deliver this irradiation is integrated with the management of the neck. The author prefers to use neck dissection as part of the management of all deeply infiltrative or advanced tongue lesions. For the N0 patients, this generally means a staging procedure or a functional neck dissection. For patients who have involved lymph nodes, this means a radical neck dissection or one of its modifications.

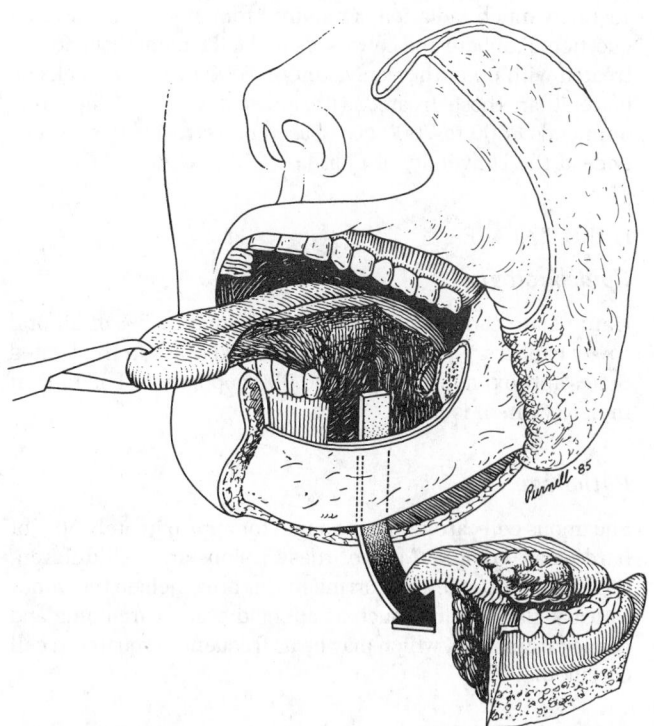

FIGURE 22–16. Composite resection of tongue, floor of mouth, and margin of mandible. (Shah JP, Shemen LJ, Strong EW. Surgical therapy of oral cavity tumors. In: Thawley SE, Panje WR, eds. Comprehensive management of head and neck tumors. Philadelphia: WB Saunders, 1987:558)

Results of Therapy

Decroix and Ghossein from the Curie Institute in Paris have reported on more than 600 patients treated with primary radiation therapy for T1, T2, or T3 squamous cell carcinoma of the oral tongue.[517] Although most of the patients had implants alone, a large cohort had combined external-beam irradiation plus implant. Almost all patients at this center received radiation therapy as their primary treatment. Primary control was obtained at 86% for T1, 80% for T2, and 68% for T3. These data compare favorably with the results obtained with partial glossectomy.

Spiro and Strong[518] and others have reviewed the Memorial Sloan-Kettering Cancer Center experience using partial glossectomy as primary management.[519,520] As was true for the Curie Institute series, the Memorial Hospital series is relatively unselected, with primary surgery being offered to most of the patients at that institution. Local control was obtained in 85% for T1, 77% for T2, and 50% for T3. These data serve to highlight the similarity in local control rates for surgery or irradiation for most early tongue lesions.

Relatively few recent studies report the results of therapy for surgery alone for advanced disease.[518,520,521] Radiation therapy is usually used in the postoperative setting. Failure is most often within regional lymph nodes and leads to a 5-year determinate survival of 35% for stages III and IV disease.[519,522]

Ange and associates have reviewed their experience using implants after excisional biopsy for patients with positive or close margins.[523] Local control was obtained in nearly 100% of the cases. Similar results have been reported by others. When the primary site and the neck require postoperative radiation therapy, external-beam techniques must be used. Just how much radiation is required remains an unanswered question. Bamberg and coworkers make the point that patients treated with up to the equivalent of 7000 cGy in 7 weeks do better than those treated with lower doses.[524] Million recommends 6500 to 7000 cGy, based on retrospective experience at the University of Florida.[525]

HARD PALATE

Epidemiology

Hard palate cancers constitute approximately 5% of all oral cavity cancers.[526] The incidence of the disease in the United States approximates 0.4 per 100,000 population. The ratio of men to women is 8:1.

Pathology

Squamous cell carcinoma accounts for approximately 50% of hard palate tumors. Most of these lesions are well differentiated. Other cancers occurring in this area include the minor salivary gland lesions such as adenoid cystic carcinoma and adenocarcinomas, which may be as frequent as squamous cell carcinoma.

Natural History

Cancers of the hard palate grow in a multiplicity of patterns, including deeply infiltrating, destructive lesions compared with diffuse, superficial lesions associated with microscopic invasion.

When considering metastatic squamous cell carcinoma of the hard palate, lymph node metastases is encountered less frequently from cancers of other sites within the oral cavity, ranging clinically from 6% to 29%.[87] Likewise, distant metastasis is infrequent. Prognosis in patients with squamous cell carcinoma is 75%, 46%, 36%, and 11% for stages I to IV disease, respectively.[527]

Treatment

Early Disease

Surgical management of early disease involves infrastructure maxillectomy, which is resection of the palatine process of the maxillary bone. Exposure for such resections is generally obtained through a Weber-Fergusson-type incision.

As stated earlier, carcinoma in situ and microinvasive disease can involve a significant portion of the hard palate with extension of disease onto the soft palate and retromolar trigone. Under such circumstances, primary radiation may be used.

Elective treatment of the neck is not generally required unless disease extends beyond the anatomic confines of the hard palate. Selective neck dissection under such circumstances is adequate. Such dissection includes removal of lymph nodes in levels I, II, and III.

Advanced Disease

Surgical resection of advanced disease may involve a near-total palatectomy. Generally, however, lesser operations are required. Advances in the surgical therapy of hard palate cancers involve the immediate use of prosthetic obturators that allow for early restoration of adequate speech and swallowing. The need for postoperative radiation is based on the closeness or involvement of tumor margins by tumor, perineural involvement, and presence of regional lymph node metastases.

Results of Treatment

Generally incorporating the treatment philosophy described earlier, Evans and Shah report an overall survival of 75% for stage I, 46% for stage II, 36% for stage III, and 11% for stage IV, respectively.[527] Most patients who die with disease do so as a result of advanced local recurrence.[527–529]

BUCCAL MUCOSA

Epidemiology

Cancer of the buccal mucosa accounts for approximately 8% of oral cavity cancers in the United States.[526] The disease may be seen much more frequently in other parts of the world, such as India, depending on tobacco consumption patterns. In the southeastern United States, the incidence of buccal mucosal cancer is much higher in women than in men, an observation attributed to the common use of snuff. The median age of persons with buccal mucosal cancer may be slightly higher than reported in patients with cancers of other sites within the oral cavity.

Anatomy

The buccal mucosa is composed of a mucous membrane that extends from the lips anteriorly to the retromolar trigone posteriorly. Inferiorly, it extends from the lateral alveolar sulcus of the mandible to the lateral sulcus of the maxillary alveolar ridge. Its blood and nerve supplies are from the facial artery and the third division of cranial nerve V. Lymphatics from the buccal mucosa drain primarily into level II and level I in decreasing order.

Pathology

As in other sites within the oral cavity, squamous cell carcinoma is the predominant neoplasm. The verrucous variant of squamous cell carcinoma is observed frequently. Only rarely are other cancers such as minor salivary gland tumors observed.

Natural History

Cancers of the buccal mucosa are more frequently exophytic than other cancers within the oral cavity. They are also relatively silent in their presentation and rarely present as a T1 lesion. Pain is the initial presenting complaint and subsequently is followed by bleeding and difficulty chewing. With extension of the disease outside the confines of the buccal mucosa into the pterygoid musculature, patients may present with trismus. Disease frequently invades the mandible or maxillary alveolar ridge, or both.

Lymph node metastases are observed most frequently within levels I and II and are observed clinically in 10% of presenting patients.[530]

Five-year survival ranges from 77% to 18%, depending on stage of disease.[531] Urist and colleagues have shown that tumor thickness is a significant prognostic factor.[530] Patients with tumors less than 6 mm in thickness have significantly better survival rates in their series than those with tumors more than 6 mm in thickness, regardless of tumor stage.

Treatment

Early Disease

Small lesions (T1 and early T2) can be managed with equal effectiveness by surgery or radiation therapy. If the tumor can be excised easily through the open mouth with minimal functional sequelae, then small lesions are probably best managed in that fashion. Larger T1 lesions and lesions that approach the commissure are best managed with radiation therapy. T2 lesions can be managed with radiation therapy if they are exophytic or relatively superficial. Deeper lesions are probably best managed by surgery.

In patients with small lesions and a clinically negative neck, the neck can be observed. Neck failure occurs in fewer than 10% of patients. However, for more advanced lesions, the neck is treated electively with the same therapeutic modality that is used for the primary lesion.

Radiation therapy can be used with various techniques. Interstitial brachytherapy, ipsilateral electrons, intraoral cone, or external-beam photon irradiation can all be employed. The exact technique selected depends on the clinical situation and the expertise of the radiation oncologist.

Advanced Disease

More advanced disease requires surgery as the principal therapeutic modality, usually with postoperative radiation. The initial factor in such treatment relates to adequate operative exposure. This is usually facilitated by dividing the lip in the midline and resecting the check posterolaterally to gain optimal exposure.

Care must be taken in assessing the need for resection of surrounding anatomic structures, such as the skin of the face, the upper alveolar ridge, and the mandible. Invasion of tumor into the buccal fat pad and into the dermis of cheek skin occurs frequently. Such invasion generally requires full-thickness resections, including oral mucosa and cheek skin. Such defects can be repaired with myocutaneous flaps. Free tissue transfer represents recently developed options for reconstruction.

Ipsilateral neck dissection is advocated in all instances of T3 or T4 primary disease, regardless of the nodal status.

Results of Treatment

Nair and colleagues have reported on 234 patients with buccal mucosa cancer treated with radiation therapy.[532] Disease-free survival at 3 years was 85% for stage I, 63% for stage II, 41% for stage III, and 15% for stage IV. All 13 patients with T1N0 disease were controlled with radiation therapy. Fifty percent of patients with T4 disease failed locally. The presence of nodal metastases clearly influenced the locoregional failure rate.

Bloom and Spiro reported the results for 90 patients with buccal mucosa cancer treated by surgery.[531] The 5-year survival rate by stage was 77%, 65%, 27%, and 18% more for stages I, II, III, and IV, respectively. Local failure was noted in 47% of patients, and regional failure was observed in 37%. These data are similar to the radiation therapy results[532] and to other primarily surgical series.[533]

OROPHARYNX

EPIDEMIOLOGY

The pharynx is divided into three regions: the nasopharynx, the oropharynx, and the hypopharynx. The discussion in this section is limited to the oropharynx and its encompassing sites, which are the base of the tongue, the tonsil and tonsillar fossa, the soft palate, and the posterior pharyngeal wall. Cancer of the oropharynx is expected to occur in approximately 4000 patients annually in the United States.[447] Most commonly, the disease involves patients in the fifth through seventh decades of life. Men are afflicted three to five times as frequently as women. The etiology of the disease, to the greatest extent, cannot be distinguished from cancers of the oral cavity. Tobacco and alcohol abuse constitute the most significant risk factors.

STAGING

As was true for staging of oral cavity cancers, staging of tumors of the oropharynx relies on physical examination and various imaging procedures, including CT scan.

Staging of the primary tumor is as follows:

T1	Tumor 2 cm or less in greatest dimension.
T2	Tumor more than 2 cm but not more than 4 cm in greatest dimension.

T3   Tumor more than 4 cm in greatest dimension.

T4   Tumor invades adjacent structures (*e.g.*, through cortical bone, soft tissues of neck, and deep [extrinsic] muscle of the tongue.

The regional lymph nodes (N) and distant metastases (M) staging are identical to other sites within the upper aerodigestive tract and are as stated earlier in this chapter.

BASE OF THE TONGUE

Anatomy

The base of the tongue is bounded anteriorly by a line demarcated by the circumvallate papillae. Posteriorly, it ends with the epiglottis. Laterally, it extends to the glossopalatini sulcus and includes the pharyngoepiglottic and glossoepiglottic folds. Tongue musculature comprises the genioglossus, styloglossus, palatoglossus, and hyoglossus muscles. The blood and nerve supplies are identical to that of the oral tongue and consist of the lingual artery and the hypoglossal nerve, respectively.

Lymphatics are extensive within the base of tongue. Drainage is into numerous node levels, including levels II, III, IV, and V in decreasing order. Disease may involve retropharyngeal lymph nodes in certain instances, such as with progression to the lateral pharyngeal wall.

Pathology

Base of tongue cancers occur less frequently than do cancers of other anatomically defined areas of the tongue. Squamous cell carcinoma represents nearly 95% of those cancers that occur in this subsite. Other cancers in this area include those of minor salivary gland origin, which are adenoid cystic and mucoepidermoid carcinomas and lymphomas.

Natural History

Cancers of the base of tongue are advanced frequently at the time of presentation. This observation is partly a reflection of the relatively silent location of such disease and its aggressive tendencies. Patients usually present with symptoms of pain and dysphagia. As in nasopharyngeal carcinomas, patients often present with a mass in the neck. A history of weight loss is common. Likewise, referred otalgia secondary to cranial nerve involvement is common. With progressive laryngeal involvement, a "muffled" quality of the voice may become apparent.

As in other squamous cell carcinomas of the head and neck, cancers of the base of the tongue can grow in an infiltrative or an exophytic pattern. Careful physical examination delineates such growth. An important component of that evaluation should include digital and bimanual palpation, which delineates the extent of base of tongue involvement and determines whether disease has infiltrated into the preepiglottic space. Figure 22–17 shows the routes of spread for squamous cell cancers for the base of the tongue.

Base of tongue tumors have a high propensity for metastatic spread to lymph nodes. Nearly 70% of patients with T1 lesions have clinically palpable disease in the neck. The risk for nodal

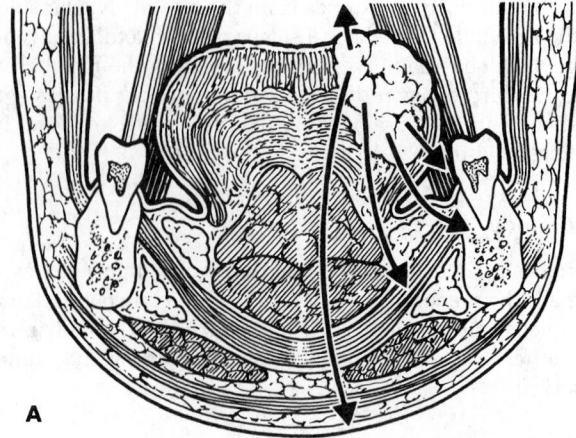

A

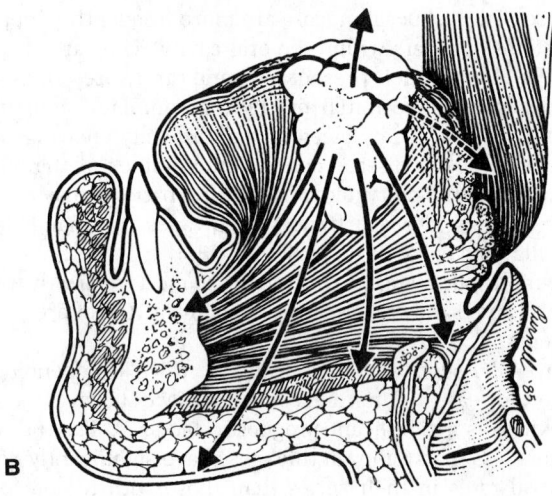

B

FIGURE 22–17.   Routes of spread of squamous cell carcinoma of the base of tongue. **(A)** Coronal view. **(B)** Lateral view. (Shah JP, Shemem LJ, Strong EW. Surgical therapy of oral cavity tumors. In: Thawley SE, Panje WR, eds. Comprehensive management of head and neck tumors. Philadelphia: WB Saunders, 1987:553)

metastases increases with T stage, approaching 85% for T4 cancers.[87] Likewise, tumors of the base of tongue have a high propensity for bilateral cervical lymph node spread, occurring in approximately 30% of patients.[87,534] Therapy should account for this propensity even in circumstances of early primary disease. Lymph nodes commonly involved include levels II and III. Levels IV, V, and VI, however, are more frequently involved than many other cancers of the head and neck, such as oral cavity lesions.

Prognosis for tongue base tumors is generally poor secondary to their advanced stage at presentation.[534–546] Stages I and II 5-year survival approximates 60% and 40%, respectively. Five-year survival for patients with stage III disease approximates 30%. For stage IV disease, survival diminished to 15% at 5 years.

Treatment

Early Disease

Early-stage cancer of the base of the tongue is treated readily by surgery or radiation therapy. Results are equivalent. Surgery for early unilateral lesions entails a hemiglossectomy. Surgical approaches can be transoral or by lateral pharyngotomy. The former approach entails a midline labiolingual split.

Radiation therapy has a high prospect of cure without the functional deficit that occurs with surgery. In general, treatment consists of 5000 to 5400 cGy with external-beam irradiation and 2000 to 3000 cGy boost to the base of the tongue by an ^{192}Ir implant. There is debate in the radiation oncology literature about whether to use an interstitial implant as the boost treatment.

Regional lymphadenectomy is recommended regardless of the primary size because of the high propensity of metastatic spread. Bilateral neck dissection is recommended for those lesions approaching midline structures.

Advanced Disease

For larger lesions involving the tongue base, primarily T4 lesions, total resection of tongue base and total laryngectomy may be required. The addition of total laryngectomy may be dictated for several reasons. Tumor may infiltrate through the relatively thin hyoepiglottic ligament and extend well into the preepiglottic space. Laryngectomy is required as part of an en bloc procedure necessary to ensure complete extirpation of disease. The removal of tongue and soft tissues of the neck (the preepiglottic space) impairs normal deglutition. With such surgery, chronic aspiration represents a major long-term complication. Total laryngectomy may represent the only means to isolate critical air-exchange passages from oral secretions. The need for laryngectomy is increased in patients with diminished cardiopulmonary reserve. Restoring bulk of the base of the tongue with myocutaneous flaps or free-tissue transfer may minimize aspiration problems.[537]

Extended supraglottic laryngectomy may be performed for smaller lesions involving the vallecula (disease in such circumstances should not extend along the pharyngoepiglottic fold to involve the lateral pharyngeal wall). In all the circumstances in which such a procedure is performed, pretreatment assessment must confirm adequate cardiopulmonary reserve.

The need for mandibulectomy as part of the surgical procedure for tongue base tumors is controversial. The traditional surgical management involves the composite (jaw, tongue, neck) resection. Such an en bloc procedure ensures more adequate tumor removal, including tumor within surrounding lymphatics. Further, closure of surgical defect is facilitated by such resection, that is, soft tissues are able to collapse with the removal of the mandible.

Recent advances in surgical technique and in the understanding of patterns of tumor spread militate against the need for mandibulectomy. Soft tissue defects can be repaired with free-tissue transfer, thereby facilitating wound closure. Studies of lymphatic spread of oropharyngeal tumors have shown that cancer not approximating periosteum rarely infiltrates the mandible.[538] Therefore, resection of bone is not required for oncologic reasons.

Results of Treatment

Surgical results of early base of tongue cancers have been encouraging, with local control rates approximating 85%.[534,539] The major determinant of the control rate is the tumor growth patterns. Exophytic tumors are controlled in 84% of instances compared with 58% with ulcerative and infiltrative disease.[540] With advanced disease, initial surgery is associated with a high probability of positive margins (25%), emphasizing the need for combined modality therapy.[535]

Data from Harrison and colleagues,[541,542] Goffinet and colleagues,[543] and Puthawala and colleagues[544] show that the local control rate for T1 and T2 base of tongue tumors is in the 90% range when treated with external-beam plus implant. Harrison and coworkers reported 36 previously untreated patients with squamous cancer of the base of the tongue treated at Memorial Sloan-Kettering Cancer Center between January 1981 and June 1990.[542] In general, treatment consisted of 5000 to 5400 cGy with external-beam irradiation and 2000 to 3000 cGy boost to the base of the tongue with an ^{192}Ir implant. Figure 22–18 shows a clinical example. Necks were generally managed with elective radiation alone in the N0 group (5 patients) or with radiation plus neck dissection in those patients with palpable lymph node metastases (31 patients). The median follow-up was 22 months. Crude local control was as shown in Table 22–28. Actuarial local control is 87.5%. Of the four local failures, two have been salvaged by surgery, yielding an overall local control, including salvage, of 94%. In addition, there has been only 1 patient who has failed in the neck, and this patient was regionally salvaged with neck dissection. This outcome yields an overall regional control rate of 100%. Goffinet and associates have reported similar results using nearly identical techniques.[543]

External-beam irradiation therapy alone has its advocates.[540,545] However, the only study that sought to compare external-beam alone, external-beam plus implant, and surgery plus postoperative radiation was done by Housset and colleagues.[546] They found that the local control rate for external-beam plus implant or surgery plus postoperative radiation was in the 80% range for T1 and T2 lesions compared with 50% for external-beam alone. Survival for external-beam alone was 17% compared with more than 50% for the other two approaches.

Well-delivered, high-dose external-beam irradiation therapy can be highly curative without brachytherapy. However, in the author's experience, high-dose hyperfractionated irradiation, as currently performed in some institutions, has greater acute morbidity than the lower dose external-beam plus implant.[547] In addition, the functional outcome of brachytherapy is excellent. Harrison and associates performed a function analysis in an effort to determine the quality of life for patients treated with external-beam plus brachytherapy.[542] The performance status scale reported by List and colleagues was used.[548] Patients analyzed their eating in public, speech articulation, and normalcy of diet. The mean scores were 83%, 93%, and 75%, respectively. The speech articulation scores are particularly encouraging.

Implants have been used for patients who have received prior radiation therapy to the oropharynx, who developed recurrent base of tongue cancers or an SPT in the base of tongue. Housset and coworkers reported on 55 patients who had received prior irradiation and in whom they performed ^{192}Ir implants.[549] One group of patients received a single implant delivering 6000 cGy, and a separate group received two split-course implants, receiving 3500 and 3000 cGy, respectively. The purpose of the split-course treatment was an attempt to minimize complications. There was no difference in the local

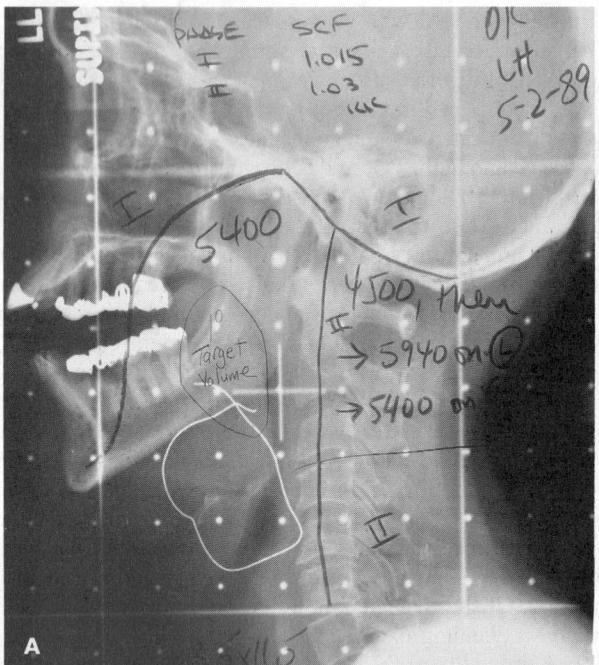

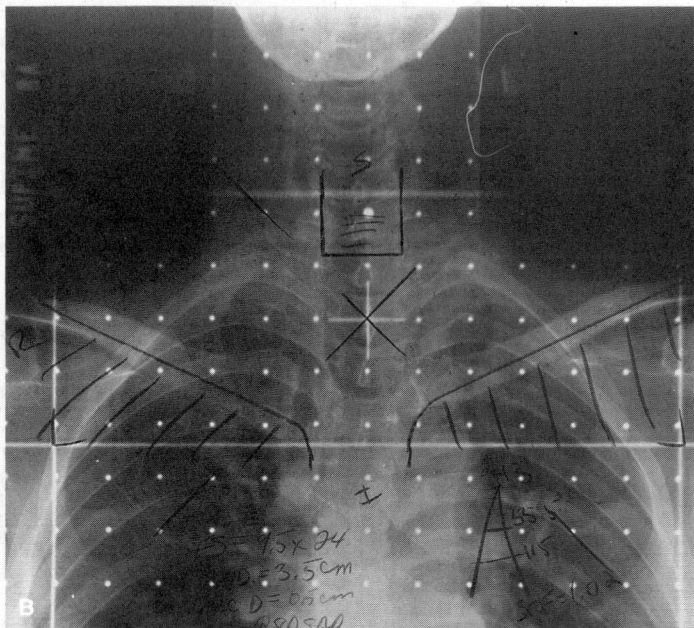

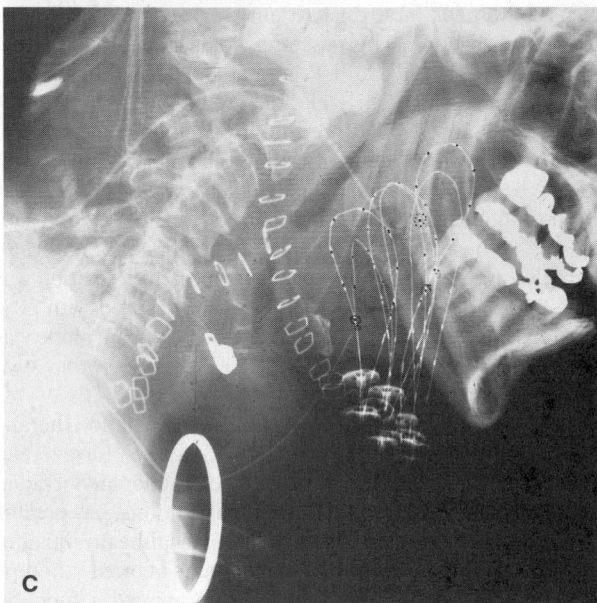

FIGURE 22–18. A patient with a T2N2 squamous cancer of the left side of the base of the tongue. The treatment plan consisted of initial external beam radiation therapy to the primary site and the entire neck bilaterally. This was followed by a left radical neck dissection and an implant, both done with the same anesthesia. **(A)** The simulation film shows the primary site outlined and the neck node with wire around it. A bite block is in place. A total of 4500 cGy was given to the primary site and both upper necks, after which a spinal cord block was placed. The primary and upper neck was then treated with 5400 cGy. Fraction size was 180 cGy/day. After that, the bed of the lymph node in the left neck was boosted with electrons to 6000 cGy. The posterior neck was boosted to 5400 cGy on the right and to 5940 cGy on the left. **(B)** The low neck was treated with a single anterior field to 5000 cGy/5 weeks. A midline block protects the spinal cord at the field junction. **(C)** Approximately 3 weeks after the external radiation was completed, the patient was taken to the operating room and a left radical neck dissection and an Ir-192 implant were done. The figure shows the catheters looped through the base of tongue by the submental approach. Also visible are the skin staples from the neck surgery. The implant delivered an additional 2800 cGy. The neck specimen was histologically negative. The patient remains NED at 2 years. He had a soft tissue ulcer in the tongue that healed with conservative management.

TABLE 22–28. Treatment of Carcinoma of the Base of the Tongue With External-Beam Irradiation Plus Brachytherapy*

T Stage	Crude Local Control†	Surgical Salvage†	Overall Crude Control†
T1	10/11	1/1	11/11
T2	13/14	1/1	14/14
T3	8/10	—	8/10
T4	1/1	—	1/1

* Crude local control, including salvage, by T stage.
† No. of patients controlled/Total no. of patients.

failure rate in either group, which ranged from 40% to 50%. However, there was a significant decrease in the incidence of muscosal necrosis in the split-course group compared with the single-course group, being 43% and 16%, respectively. Also, the researchers found that local failure in the split-course group corresponded to the degree of response after the first implant. Those patients who had a greater than 75% reduction after the first implant had an ultimate local failure rate of 14%. This finding is compared with a 70% local failure rate in patients who had less than 75% regression after the first implant. The use of the split-course technique made it possible to select patients who might have a better result, and it significantly decreased the rate of complication. Vikram and associates reported 10 patients who had been treated previously for base of tongue lesions.[547] All 10 received implants in an attempted salvage maneuver. Local control was obtained in 60% of the patients, with size being the most important prognostic feature. No local failures occurred in patients who had lesions 4 cm or smaller, whereas most of the patients with lesions larger than 4 cm were not salvaged. Overall survival in the entire group was poor, mainly because of uncontrolled recurrent neck disease.

TONSIL, TONSILLAR PILLAR, AND SOFT PALATE

Anatomy

The tonsillar pillars anteriorly (the palatoglossal muscle) and posteriorly (the palatopharyngeal muscle) and the glossopalatini sulcus inferiorly constitute a triangular region that houses the lymphoid tonsillar tissue. Extending from the tonsillar pillars is the soft palate. The latter demarcates the oral cavity from the oropharynx and the oropharynx from the nasopharynx. It is composed of the following muscles: palatoglossus, palatopharyngeus, levator veli palatine, tensor veli palatine, and the musculus uvulae.

Nerve supply to this region is by the trigeminal nerve. Lymphatics from the tonsillar region drain into the jugulodigastric basin and the submandibular triangle. Lympatics from the soft palate drain into the upper jugulodigastric lymph nodes and the retropharyngeal lymph nodes.

Pathology

As in other sites within the upper aerodigestive tract, the near-total lesions involving this region are squamous cell carcinoma. Occasionally lymphoepitheliomas have been identified within the tonsillar fossa. Other cancers include lymphomas and those derived from minor salivary glands.

Natural History

Cancers of the tonsil, tonsillar pillar, and soft palate may present and spread in various ways. Cancers of the tonsillar pillar tend to be more superficial than those of the tonsillar fossa. Tonsillar pillar cancers progress over a broad region, including the lateral soft palate, the retromolar trigone and buccal mucosa, the tonsillar fossa, and the glossopalatini sulcus.

Tonsillar fossa cancers present more often in advanced-stage disease than do cancers of the tonsillar pillar or the soft palate. Approximately 75% of patients present as stage III or stage IV disease. Disease in this area tends to be bulky and can progress to involve the base of the tongue and the lateral pharyngeal wall. Symptoms include pain, dysphagia, weight loss, and a mass in the neck. Should disease extend posteriorly and involve the pterygoid muscles, trismus may be a presenting sign.

Primary disease of the soft palate may behave in a more indolent manner. Tumors in this region may remain in the early stages, and disease may remain superficial, presenting as diffuse erythroplakia extending into the hard palate or inferiorly along the tonsillar pillar.

Tonsillar pillar cancers metastasize less frequently to regional lymph nodes than do cancers of the tonsillar fossa. Patients present with clinical evidence of nodal metastases

in 38% of T2 tonsillar pillar cancers, whereas 68% of T2 tonsillar fossa lesions are associated with clinically evident lymph node disease at presentation. Contralateral metastases are common for tonsillar fossa cancers. Nodal disease in tonsillar fossa cancer most often presents in an advanced stage, with nearly 55% of patients presenting with N2 or N3 disease.[87] Soft palate tumors are more commonly associated with bilateral lymph node metastases. Approximately 20% of patients present with bilateral disease.[87]

Prognosis for tonsillar fossa cancers range from 93% for stage I disease to 17% for stage IV disease.[550–553] For soft palate lesions, 5-year survival rates range from 21% to 85%, depending on disease stage.[554–556]

Treatment

Early Disease

Except in circumstances of early disease, the distinction between cancers arising in the tonsillar fossa and those arising in the tonsillar pillar cannot be made. Early cancers of this region can be treated by single-modality therapy of surgery or radiation therapy.

Surgical resection of early disease can occasionally be done transorally. Such an approach should be performed only in circumstances in which free surgical margins can be ensured. Better exposure to early cancers of this region may be obtained through a combined lipsplitting incision coupled with an anterior midline or lateral mandibulotomy. Careful dissection proceeds first by identifying anterior lateral margins. If tumors extend to the periosteum of the mandible but remain superficial, partial mandibulectomy may be performed. Partial mandibulectomy includes a coronal resection that leaves the body and the ascending ramus of the mandible in continuity.

Early squamous cell carcinomas of the tonsillar region can be treated with radiation therapy. Radiation can be delivered with external-beam, interstitial implant, or a combination of both.

Because of the high propensity for even early cancers of this region to metastasize to cervical lymph nodes, cervical lymphadenectomy should be included as part of the surgical resection. The various types of neck dissections that can be used have been discussed.

The author's choice for early lesions in which cervical lymph nodes are not clinically involved with disease would include a modified supraomohyoid neck dissection. Debate exists as to whether such dissection should be performed in continuity with extirpation of the primary disease. When possible, in-continuity dissection should be advocated.

When applying radiation therapy as the primary treatment modality, it is usually possible to treat the ipsilateral neck alone and to avoid contralateral neck irradiation. With such treatment, radiation dosage to the contralateral salivary gland is minimized, thereby reducing the incidence of xerostomia. It is standard practice to radiate the neck in all patients because of the rich lymphatic network in the orophayngeal region.

Early-stage soft palate tumors are treated readily with radiation therapy. Treatment can be delivered with external-beam, brachytherapy, or a combination of both. Figure 22–19 shows the external-beam technique in a typical patient. Most patients will not have palpable cervical lymph node metastases on presentation. It is unclear whether all patients

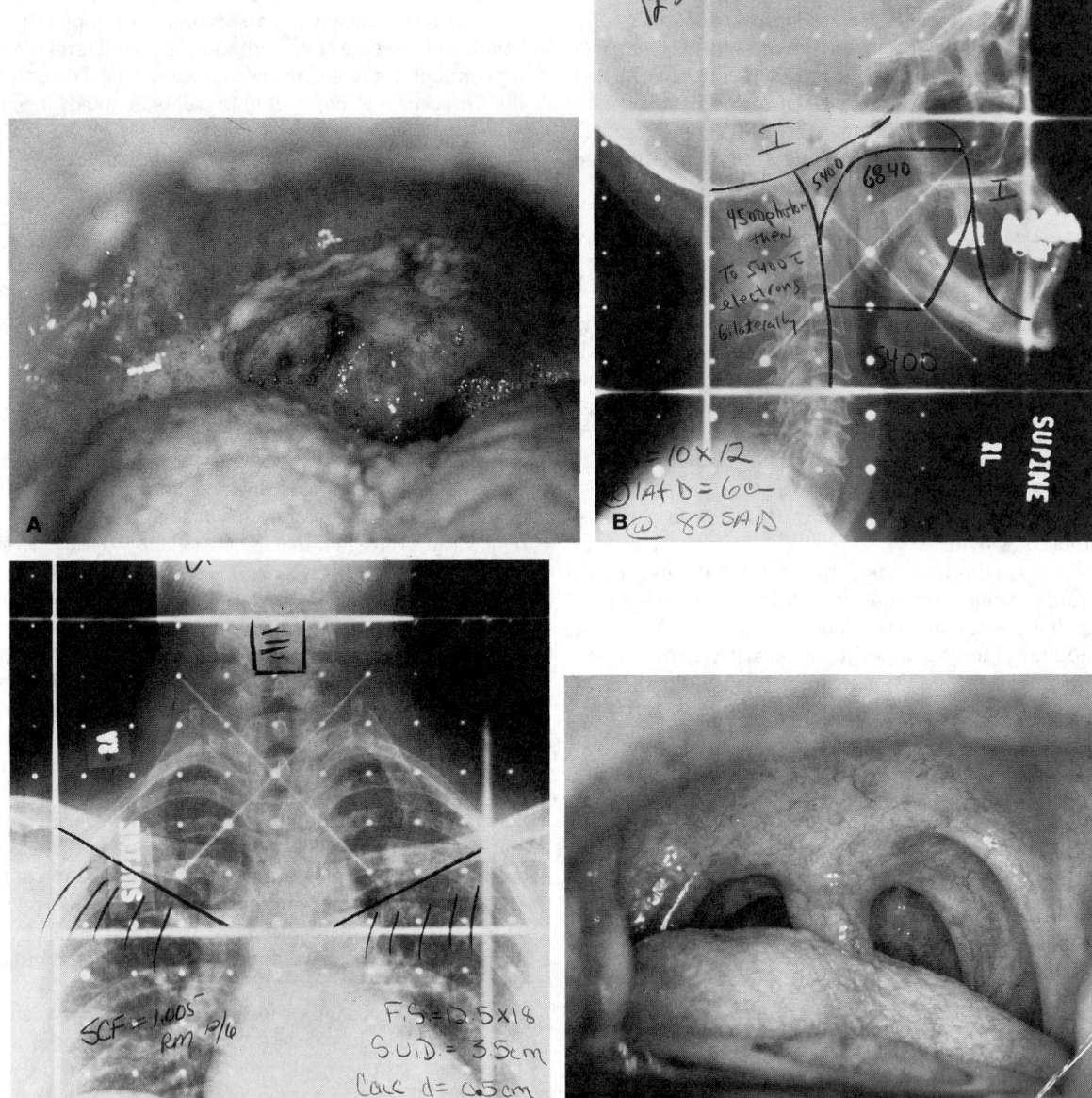

FIGURE 22–19. **(A)** A patient with a T2N0 squamous cancer soft palate. He was treated with external beam radiation therapy to the primary site and to both necks. Opposed lateral portals were used with a low anterior necks field. **(B** and **C)** The simulated fields are shown. The primary site and both upper necks received 4500 cGy, after which a spinal cord block was placed. The primary site and upper necks were then treated to 5400 cGy, including the retropharyngeal nodes up to the skull base. This completed the elective neck irradiation to the upper neck and retropharyngeal nodes. The primary site was treated to a total of 6840 cGy. The patient is asked not to swallow during treatment, so his palate remains in position. Adequate margin is placed around the palate in its plane of motion to avoid geographic miss. Fraction size is 180 cGy/day. The lower neck is treated with an anterior portal to 5000 cGy/5 weeks, thereby delivering elective nodal irradiation to that site. The posterior necks are boosted with electrons to 5400 cGy to protect the spinal cord. The spinal cord is protected at the junction of the lateral fields with the low anterior neck field by a midline block in the low neck field. This block also protects the larynx. For this purpose, the field is purposely junctioned above the thyroid notch but below the hyoid bone. **(D)** The patient remains NED at 2.5 years.

require prophylactic neck treatment. Prophylactic neck irradiation and observation alone have been used by various authors with a successful outcome.[557,558] Of course, this is retrospective and subject to the selection factors inherent in retrospective reviews. Small, superficial lesions can probably be treated locally, with observation of the neck. Larger T1 and most T2 lesions should receive elective neck treatment.

Advanced Disease

Advanced cancers (*i.e.*, stages III and IV disease) usually require combined modality therapy, including surgery and postoperative radiation therapy. This is especially true for tumors that are infiltrative rather than exophytic in nature. The extent of surgical resection should be governed by the size of the primary disease and its pattern of spread. Tumor-free surgical margins usually entail a segmental mandibulectomy in most circumstances of advanced disease in the tonsillar region.

Results of Treatment

Tonsillar Pillars and Fossa

Surgical resection as the sole modality of therapy for early disease is not often used in most series. However, studies have demonstrated that when resection is used, local control rates are excellent.[559] Even for advanced tumors in highly selected instances, effective local control can approach 80%.[559] The degree to which local control can be obtained depends on disease extension outside the tonsillar fossa. When disease extends to the lateral pharyngeal wall or the base of the tongue, local recurrence approaches 33% and 47%, respectively.[559-561]

Wong and colleagues have reported the results of definitive external-beam irradiation for 150 patients with previously untreated squamous cell carcinoma of the tonsillar fossa.[562] Most patients were treated with conventional fractionation, with total doses in the 6400- to 7200-cGy range. Local control was obtained in 15 of 16 patients (94%) with T1 lesions and in 51 of 52 patients (79%) with T2 lesions. Other series have reported local control rates for T2 lesions approximating 60%.[563,565-567] When surgical salvage is added, local control was 100% for T1 and 85% for T2. Wang has used an accelerated hyperfractionation program for oropharyngeal tumors.[564] During an earlier period, patients received 1.6 cGy per fraction, 2 fractions per day, to a total of 38.4 cGy. Because of acute toxicity, a 2-week break was then given. Treatment was then resumed at 1.8 cGy per fraction, 1 fraction per day, to a total of 65 cGy. This was called the *bid-qd program*. Recently, the treatment regimen was changed. The initial treatment remained the same, as did the 2-week break. However, when the patients returned for the second part of the treatment, they were resumed at 1.6 cGy per fraction, 2 fractions per day, to a total of 64 cGy. This was called the *bid-bid program*. For tonsil lesions (T1-4), the 36-month actuarial local control after irradiation therapy was 93% compared with 64% for the bid-qd program.

There has been increasing interest in brachytherapy for selected tonsillar lesions.[568,569] Puthawala and coworkers reported the results of 80 patients with previous untreated squamous cell carcinoma of the tonsillar region who received 4500 to 5000 cGy with external-beam irradiation, followed by an interstitial ^{192}Ir implant.[568] Patients with T1 or T2 disease received an implant boost of 2000 to 2500 cGy, and those with T3 to T4 lesions received a boost of 3000 to 4000 cGy. Overall, local control was 84%, and absolute 3-year disease-free survival was 72%. When looked at by stage, all 3 T1 patients obtained local control. For T2, T3, and T4 patients, local control was obtained in 14 of 15 (93%), 32 of 43 (74%), and 11 of 19 (58%), respectively.

For T3 lesions, the rate of local control with external-beam irradiation decreases considerably. However, it would appear that the subset of T3 tumors with tongue involvement have the highest local failure rate. Tong and coworkers reported that 18 of 39 (46%) of T3 patients ultimately developed failure in the primary site after external-beam irradiation.[560] Interestingly, all 18 patients who failed had lesions that extended into the base of tongue. Million reported that the addition of interstitial implant to the base of tongue, after external-beam irradiation, can improve the local control.[525] In the T3 patients

with base of tongue extension, 5 of 9 patients were controlled with external-beam alone compared with 13 of 17 who had full-dose external-beam plus a localized base of tongue implant. Puthawala and associates reported local control in 16 of 19 patients with T3N0 lesions and 5 of 6 patients with T3N1 lesions, all treated with external-beam and implant.[568] Wong and associates reported local control in 58% of patients with T3 treated with external-beam alone.[562] It would therefore appear that the results of external-beam irradiation alone for T3 tonsillar cancer are suboptimal. The addition of an interstitial implant may improve the results in selected patients. There may also be a role for a combination of surgery and radiation.

For T1-T2N0-N1 patients, it is usually possible to treat the ipsilateral neck alone and avoid contralateral neck irradiation. By doing this, the radiation dosage to the contralateral salivary gland tissue is minimized and the incidence of xerostomia is significantly reduced. Murthy and Hendrickson[571] reported that none of their 20 patients with N0 or N1 disease failed in the untreated contralateral neck when the primary and ipsilateral neck were controlled. Tong and coworkers reported that none of their patients with T1N0 or T2N0 lesions failed in either neck, despite the fact that approximately 40% of the cases had ipsilateral treatment only.[560] It is considered safe to omit contralateral neck treatment in most of these early lesions, as long as there is no extension into the base of the tongue or significant extension onto the soft palate.

The management of patients with more advanced lesions is somewhat controversial.[570-574] There are advocates of radiation therapy alone,[570] reserving surgery for salvage only. Other authors advocate an approach involving surgery and postoperative radiation.[572,573] Perez and colleagues analyzed 296 patients with epidermoid carcinoma of the tonsillar fossa.[565] In this group, 127 received radiation alone, 133 were planned to have preoperative radiation therapy plus surgery, and 36 received surgery plus postoperative radiation. There was no statistically significant difference in 3-year disease-free survival for T1-T2N0-N2 patients with radiation alone compared with radiation combined with surgery. In patients with T4 or N3 disease, there was an advantage to combined treatment over radiation alone, suggesting a benefit for those patients who had surgery. The authors concluded that radiation alone was the treatment of choice for early-stage lesions, but there might be an advantage in selected advanced-stage patients for a combination of surgery and postoperative irradiation. Dasmahapatra and associates reported that the 5-year survival for patients who had combined radiation and surgery was better than those who had radiation alone in the stages III and IV categories.[572] Spiro and Spiro could not demonstrate a benefit in survival when patients with stages III and IV disease were treated with radiation therapy alone, surgery alone, or combined surgery and irradiation.[574] This may be a reflection of selection bias, with more advanced and less favorable patients being treated with surgery and radiation combined. The RTOG has performed a prospective, randomized trial and analyzed various combinations of radiation and surgery for patients with advanced squamous cell cancer of the oropharynx.[509] Patients with oropharynx tumors were randomized to receive preoperative radiation therapy (5000 cGy) plus surgery, surgery plus postoperative radiation therapy (6000 cGy), or radiation therapy alone (6500 to 7000 cGy) with surgery reserved for salvage. This study revealed that the overall survival and the estimated 4-year locoregional control rate were not statistically different in any of the arms. One of the weaknesses of this study is that it did not stratify the results by subsite within the oropharynx. Therefore, it is impossible to determine what the specific results would be for tonsil patients.

Soft Palate

Recently, data has emerged that indicates support for the use of brachytherapy for small soft palate lesions.[557,576,577] Mazeron and colleagues reported 59 patients with T1 and T2 squamous cancer of the soft palate and uvula treated with definitive irradiation.[557] Sixteen patients had external-beam irradiation alone, 14 had ^{192}Ir implantation alone, and 29 had a combination of external-beam irradiation plus brachytherapy. Local failure occurred in 4 of 16 patients (25%) after external-beam irradiation alone, in 5 of 19 (18%) after combined external-beam irradiation and implant, but in 0 of 14 (0%) in the group selected for ^{192}Ir implant alone. These authors preferred the plastic tube technique over the guide gutter technique for implantation. It is unclear exactly how the patients were selected for each of the treatment strategies. The authors believed that severe dry mouth was less frequent in those patients who received all or part of the treatment by implantation compared with those who had external-beam irradiation alone. Similarly, Sealy and associates reported excellent control rates in patients with early squamous cell cancer of the soft palate and uvula treated with ^{192}Ir implants.[576]

Pernot and colleagues recently reported 277 patients treated with carcinoma of the oropharynx by exclusive radiation therapy.[558] The group (212 patients) of soft palate tonsil and posterior pillar lesions were lumped together in the reporting of results. Nine percent of these patients had soft palate lesions. In this group, 8 of 121 patients (7%) with T1 and T2 lesions exhibited recurrence. In the T3 category, 23 of 85 (27%) recurred. The overall local control at 5 years was 83%.

Amdur and coworkers reported an analysis of 75 patients with squamous cell carcinoma of the soft palate or uvula treated with radiation therapy alone or in combination with neck dissection.[578] Most patients received 6000 to 7500 cGy. Local control was obtained in all 8 patients with T1 disease and 14 of 19 patients with T2 disease. Including surgical salvage, 16 of 19 T2 patients obtained ultimate local control (84%). The results were far worse for T3 and T4 disease, with local control being 45% and 25%, respectively, for continuous-course external-beam irradiation. This series highlights the poor results achieved with radiation therapy for advanced disease, with good results for early-stage disease with external-beam alone. There is no definitive proof that brachytherapy is required for early-stage soft palate tumors. However, there may be a rationale for using implant as all or part of the treatment in an effort to improve the functional outcome with regard to salivary gland function. Brachytherapy spares the major salivary glands from receiving significant doses of radiation and decreases the risk for xerostomia. Proper patient selection is required, and the radiation oncologist must have expertise in performing a palatal implant.

Although the local control is excellent for early-stage disease, the overall survival may not necessarily reflect the high local control rate. Intercurrent illness and the problem of

SPTs represent a significant cause of mortality in this population.[557,577]

Complications from radiation therapy occur at a rate of about 10%, with severe complications, principally osteonecrosis of the mandible requiring surgical resection, occurring in 5% or less.[557,577,578]

Whether elective neck treatment is required has not been determined. The probability of neck recurrence in patients with early disease is low regardless of whether the neck is treated prophylactically.[557]

Most advanced soft palate tumors should be treated with combined surgery and postoperative radiation. Amdur and coworkers reported that the results of external-beam irradiation therapy alone for T3 and T4 disease were suboptimal.[578]

PHARYNGEAL WALL

Epidemiology

Epidemiologic considerations are as discussed for oropharyngeal cancers.

Anatomy

The pharyngeal wall within the oropharynx extends from the nasopharynx at a line demarcated by the soft palate to the level of the vallecular. It constitutes the posterolateral surfaces of the oropharynx. The pharyngeal constrictor muscles constitute the structural framework of the pharyngeal wall. Newer supply is from the pharyngeal branches of the ninth and tenth cranial nerves. Blood supply is largely from the ascending pharyngeal and superior thyroid arteries, emanating from the external carotid artery.

The pharyngeal wall is rich in lymphatics. Primary drainage is to retropharyngeal lymph nodes and nodes in levels II and III.

Pathology

Almost all lesions on the pharyngeal wall are squamous cell carcinomas. Occasional minor salivary gland lesions have been identified.

Natural History

Tumors of the posterior pharyngeal wall are usually identified in the late stages because of the silent location in which they develop. Symptoms at presentation include pain and bleeding. Weight loss is common. Patients may present with a mass in the neck as their initial symptom. Disease spread can be superiorly to involve the nasopharynx. Posteriorly, disease may infiltrate the prevertebral fascia. Inferiorly, disease spreads to involve the pyriform sinuses and hypopharyngeal walls.

Pharyngeal wall tumors have a propensity for cervical lymph node metastases. Clinically, palpable disease is identified in 25% of patients with T1 lesions, 30% of patients with T2 lesions, 66% of patients with T3 lesions, and more than 75% of patients with T4 disease. Given that most pharyngeal wall tumors extend past the midline, bilateral cervical metastases are common. Prognosis for pharyngeal wall cancers ranges from 75% for stage I disease, 70% for stage II, and 42% for stage III to 27% for stage IV disease.[579–581]

Treatment

Early Disease

Early-stage disease of the pharyngeal wall can be treated by surgery or radiation. Radiation therapy is preferred because of the functional impairment that may result from surgical resection. Surgical resection usually entails a transhyoid approach to gain access to the lesion.[580] Wide excision lesions include underlying prevertebral fascia. Split-thickness skin graft coverage is required. A significant morbidity after surgical resection is imparied swallowing secondary to resection of pharyngeal wall musculature.

Bilateral modified neck dissections are indicated in patients with early pharyngeal wall cancers.

An important issue in planning the radiation therapy for posterior pharyngeal wall tumors is the proximity of the spinal cord to the primary tumor volume. When opposed lateral fields are used and the spinal cord block is placed, the posterior edge of the field is dangerously close to the posterior aspect of the tumor. A sharp beam edge must be used to avoid underdosing the posterior aspect of the tumor, which can fall in the penumbra of the beam. This is best accomplished by avoiding cobalt 60 and using a 4 mV or 6 mV photon beam. Cerrobend blocks are used to define the posterior border. This border must be made as posterior as possible. It has been the practice of these authors to place this border at the anterior most aspect of the spinal cord. This is much closer to the spinal cord than in most other head and neck situations. Frequent portal films must be taken to ensure the accuracy of this field and to guarantee maximal spinal cord protection. This situation represents a difficult challenge to the radiation oncologist. One of the potential advantages to brachytherapy is the delivery of high doses to the tumor with relative sparing of the spinal cord. For this technique to be useful, tumors have to be relatively small and discrete, which is not often the situation.

Advanced Disease

Advanced disease of the posterior pharyngeal wall is best handled by multimodality therapy. Surgery involves a total laryngopharyngectomy reconstruction that, under such circumstances, includes a pectoralis major myocutaneous flap, a gastric pull-up, or a free-flap transposition with microvascular anastomoses. The last procedure, which entails a jejunal interposition, is becoming the procedure of choice. Rehabilitation and swallowing with the last procedure are hastened. This allows for more expeditious use of postoperative radiation therapy.

The use of radiation therapy postoperatively is recommended. The high incidence of retropharyngeal lymph node metastases and the associated increased locoregional failure rate mandates aggressive multimodality treatment.

Results of Treatment

Guillamondegui and associates reported on the surgical management of pharyngeal wall carcinomas.[579] Twenty-eight percent of the entire patient population developed locoregional recurrence. Local recurrence predominated. Salvage therapy in that series consisting of surgery or radiation was successful in 9 of 22 patients. The success of therapy was governed by the presence of retropharyngeal nodes with only 25% of such patients disease free at 2 years.

Meoz-Mendes and colleagues reported 164 patients with squamous cell carcinoma of the pharyngeal walls who were treated with definitive radiation at the M.D. Anderson Cancer Center.[582] The report included patients with oropharynx and hypopharynx lesions. The primary sites were irradiated to a dose of 7000 to 7500 cGy in 7 to 7.5 weeks. Local control was 71% for T1, 73% for T2, 61% for T3, and 37% for T4 lesions. The authors recommended radiation therapy alone for T1 and T2 lesions. They concluded that resectable T3 and T4 lesions should be treated with combined surgery and radiation.

Marks and coworkers reported from Washington University on 51 patients with pharyngeal wall cancer treated between 1964 and 1974.[583] Survival was no different for patients treated with low-dose preoperative radiation plus surgery compared with those treated with high-dose radiation alone. However, this was not randomized, and the surgical techniques were not standardized. Survival was poor with an actuarial 3-year survival rate of 17%. There was a greater complication rate in the patients receiving surgery, with 31% having pharyngocutaneous fistula and 14% carotid rupture; operative mortality was 14%. Marks and coworkers updated this series with a total of 89 patients treated between 1964 and 1981.[584] The update led to the suggestion that combined surgery and radiation might yield better results than high-dose radiation alone. Definitive conclusions are difficult to make.

Spiro and associates reported a 12-year study from the Memorial Sloan-Kettering Cancer Center.[585] Various operations were used during this time. There was no standardized treatment and at least eight different treatment approaches were used during the study period, representing various combinations of surgery, radiation therapy, and chemotherapy. This heterogeneity of treatment approaches highlights the uncertainty of the optimal management of this disease. Five-year survival was 32%, and the overall complication rate was 50%. A small group of patients was treated with ^{125}I implant to the primary site, followed by external-beam irradiation therapy. The implants were done using surgery for access. Local control in this small group of patients was excellent. Son and Kacinski reported 14 patients treated with a combination of implant and external-beam irradiation.[586] Twelve patients had locoregional control, and 2 patients developed reversible soft tissue and mucosal injury as a result of the radiation therapy. It would appear that this technique deserves further investigation. It represents a mechanism for delivering definitive radiation therapy with high doses to the tumor. However, it is clear that optimal therapy for tumors in this site have yet to be defined.

REFERENCES

1. Shah JP, Strong E, Spiro RH, Vikram B. Neck dissections: Current status and future possibilities. Clin Bull 1981;11:25–31.
2. Suen JY, Goepfert H. Editorial standardization of neck dissection nomenclature. Head Neck Surg 1987;10:75.
3. Jacobsson PA, Eneroth CM, Killander D, Moberger G, Martensson B. Histologic classification and grading of malignancy in carcinoma of the larynx. Acta Radiol Ther Phys Biol 1973;12:1–8.
4. Eneroth CM, Moberger G. Histological malignancy grading of squamous cell carcinoma of the palate. Acta Otolaryngol 1973;75:293–295.
5. Anneroth G, Batsakis J, Kyba N. Review of the literature and recommended system

of malignancy grading in oral squamous cell carcinomas. Scand J Dent Res 1987;95: 229–249.

6. Byrne M, Koppang HS, Lilling R, et al. New malignancy grading is a better prognostic indicator than Broder's grading in oral squamous cell carcinomas. J Oral Pathol Oral Med 1989;18:432–437.

7. Pindborg JJ. Oral precancer. In: Barnes L, ed. Surgical pathology of the head and neck. Vol 1. New York: Marcel Dekker, 1985:279–331.

8. Pindborg JJ. Oral cancer and precancer. Bristol: John Wright and Sons, 1980.

9. Cawson RA. Premalignant lesions in the mouth. Br Med Bull 1975;31:164–171.

10. Shafer WG, Waldron CA. Erythroplakia of the oral cavity. Cancer 1975;36:1021–1028.

11. Mincer HH, Coleman SA, Hopkins KP. Observations on the clinical characteristics of oral lesions showing histologic epithelial dysplasia. Oral Surg 1972;33:389–399.

12. Silverman S, Gorsky M, Lozada F. Oral leukoplakia and malignant transformation: A follow-up study of 257 patients. Cancer 1984;53:563–568.

13. Kao-Shan CS, Fine RL, Whang-Peng J, Lee EC, Chabner BA. Increased fragile sites and sister chromatid exchanges in bone marrow and peripheral blood of young cigarette smokers. Cancer Res 1987;47:6278–6282.

14. Jin Y, Heim S, Mandahl N, Biorklund A, Wannerberg J, Mitelman F. Multiple clonal chromosome aberrations in squamous cell carcinomas of the larynx. Cancer Genet Cytogenet 1990;44:209–216.

15. Jin YS, Mandahl N, Heim S, et al. t(6,7) (q23; p 22) as the sole chromosomal anomaly in a vocal cord carcinoma. Cancer Genet Cytogenet 1988;32:305–307.

16. Jin Y, Heim S, Mandahl N, et al. Multiple apparently unrelated clonal chromosomal abnormalities in a squamous cell carcinoma of the tongue. Cancer Genet Cytogenet 1988;32:93–101.

17. Carey TE, Van Dyke DL, Worsham MJ, et al. Characterization of human laryngeal primary and metastic squamous cell carcinoma cell lines UM-SCC-17A and UM-SCC-17B. Cancer Res 1989;49:6098–6107.

18. Sacks PG, Parnes SM, Gallick GE, et al. Establishment and characterization of two new squamous cell carcinoma cell lines derived from tumors of the head and neck. Cancer Res 1988;48:2858–2866.

19. Jin T, Higashi K, Mandahl N, et al. Frequent rearrangement of chromosomal bonds 1p 22 11q 13 in squamous cell carcinoma of the head and neck. Genes Chrom Cancer 1990;2:198–204.

20. Heo DS, Snyderman C, Gollin SM, et al. Biology, cytogenetics and sensitivity to immunological effector cells of new head and neck squamous cell carcinoma lines. Cancer Res 1989;49:5167–5175.

21. Kasid U, Pfeifer A, Weichselbaum R, et al. The *raf* oncogene is associated with a radiation resistant-human laryngeal cancer. Science 1987;237:1039–1041.

22. Berenson JR, Yang J, Mickel RA. Frequent amplification of the *bcl*-1 locus in head and neck squamous cell carcinomas. Oncogene 1989;4:1111–1116.

23. Zhou DJ, Casey G, Cline MJ, et al. Amplification of human int-2 in breast cancers and squamous cell carcinomas. Oncogene 1988;2:279–282.

24. Saraneth D, Panchal RG, Nair R, et al. Oncogene amplification of squamous cell carcinoma of the oral cavity. Jpn J Cancer Res 1989;80:430–437.

25. Hirano T, Steele PE, Gluckman JC. Low incidence of point mutation at codon 12 of K-*ras* proto-oncogene in squamous cell carcinoma of the upper aerodigestive tract. Ann Otol Rhinol Laryngol 1991;100:597–599.

26. Yamamoto T, Kamata N, Kawano H, et al. High incidence of amplification of the epidermal growth factor receptor gene on human squamous carcinoma cell lines. Cancer Res 1988;46:414–416.

27. Saranath D, Panchal RG, Nair R, et al. Restriction fragment length polymorphism of the L-*myc* gene in cancer patients. Br J Cancer 1990;61:530–533.

28. Field JK, Lamothe H, Spandidos DA. Clinical relevance of oncogene expression in head and neck tumors. Anticancer Res 1986;6:596–600.

29. Friedman WH, Rosenblum BN, Thornton H, et al. Oncogenes: Their presence and significance in squamous cell cancer of the head and neck. Laryngoscope 1985;95:313–316.

30. Pillai R, Reddiar KS, Balaram P. Oncogene expression and oral cancer. J Surg Oncol 1991;47:102–108.

31. Field JK, Spandidos DA, Stell PM, et al. Elevated expression of the c-*myc* oncoprotein correlates with poor prognosis in head and neck squamous cell carcinoma. Oncogene 1989;4:1463–1468.

32. Yokata J, Tsunetsugu-Yokota Y, Baltitora H. et al. Alterations of myc, myb, and ras-Ha proto-oncogene in cancers are frequent and show clinical correlation. Science 1986;231:261–265.

33. Clugston C, Keith N, Brown R. Does carcinogen exposure affect resistance of induced tumors to therapy? Proc Am Assoc Cancer Res 1991;32:A604.

34. Meghji S, Sandy JR, Scult AM, et al. Macromolecular osteolytic factor synthesized by squamous carcinoma cell lines from the head and neck in-vitro vs interleukin I. Br J Cancer 1988;58:17–21.

35. Huang CC, Blitzer A, Abramson M, Wu C. Collagenase and protease activities in head and neck tumors. Otolaryngol Head Neck Surg 1988;88:749–752.

36. Bauer WC. Concomitant carcinoma in situ and invasive carcinoma of the larynx. Can J Otolaryngol 1974;3:533–542.

37. Antonelli AR, Nicolai P, Capiello J, et al. Basement membrane components in normal, dysplastic neoplastic laryngeal tissue and metastatic lymph nodes. Acta Otolaryngol 1991;111:437–443.

38. Blitzer A, Huang CC. The effect of indomethacin on the growth of epidermoid carcinoma of the palate in rats. Arch Otolaryngol 1983;109:719–723.

39. Santini J, Formento JL, Francoual M, et al. Characterization, quantification, and potential clinical value of epidermal growth factor receptor in head and neck squamous cell carcinomas. Head Neck 1991;13:132–139.

40. Ishitoya J, Toriyanna M, Oguchi N, et al. Gene amplification and overexpression of EGF receptor in squamous cell carcinomas of the head and neck. Br J Cancer 1989;59:559–562.

41. Kamata N, Clida K, Rikimaru K, et al. Growth-inhibitory effects of epidermal growth factor and overexpression of its receptors on human squamous cell carcinomas in culture. Cancer Res 1986;46:1648–1653.

42. Eisbuch A, Blick M, Lee JS, Gutterman J. Analysis of the epidermal growth factor receptor gene in fresh human head and neck tumors. Cancer Res 1987;47:3603–3605.

43. Shirasuma K, Hayashido Y, Sugiyarma M, et al. Immunohistochemical localization of epidermal growth factor (EGF) and EGF receptor in human oral mucosa and its malignancy. Virchows Arch 1991;418:349–353.

44. Todd R, Chon MY, Matossian K, et al. Cellular sources of transforming growth factor-alpha in human oral cancer. J Dental Res 1991;70:917–923.

45. Partridge M, Green MR, Langdon JD, Feldman M. Production of TGF-x and TGF-B by cultured herakirocytes, skin and oral squamous cell carcinomas—potential autocrine regulation of normal and malignant epithelial cell proliferation. Br J Cancer 1989;60:542–548.

46. Yoneda T, Alsina MM, Watatani K, et al. Dependence of a human squamous carcinoma and associated paraneoplastic syndromes in the epidermal growth receptor pathway in nude mice. Cancer Res 1991;51:2438–2443.

47. Catalona WJ, Sample WF, Chretien PB. Lymphocyte reactivity in cancer patients: Correlation with tumor histology and clinical stage. Cancer 1973;31:65–71.

48. Lichtenstein A, Zighelborium J, Dorey F, Brossman S, Fahey JL. Comparison of immune derangements in patients with different malignancies. Cancer 1980;45:2090–2095.

49. Parkinson DR, Schantz SP. The immunobiological therapy of head and neck cancer. In: Clark J, ed: Head and neck oncology. Georg Thieme Verlog 1992:147–159.

50. Schantz SP, Guillamondegui OM. Developing perspectives in head and neck tumor immunology. Prob Gen Surg 1988;5:99–113.

51. Scully C. The immunology of cancer of the head and neck with particular reference to oral cancer. Oral Surg Oral Med Oral Pathol 1982;53:157–169.

52. Wolf GT. Tumor immunology, immune surveillance and immunotherapy of head and neck squamous carcinoma. In: Wolf GT, ed: Head and neck oncology. Boston: Martinus Nijhoff, 1984:430–441.

53. Eilber FR, Morton DL, Ketcham AS. Immunologic abnormalities in head and neck cancer. Am J Surg 1974;128:534–538.

54. Wanebo HJ, Jun MY, Strong EW, Oettgen H. T-cell deficiency in patients with squamous cell cancer of the head and neck. Am J Surg 1975;130:445–451.

55. Olkowski LL, Wilkins SA. T-lymphocyte levels in the peripheral blood of patients with cancer of the head and neck. Am J Surg 1975;130:440–444.

56. Wolf GT, Schamatz S, Hudson J, et al. Alterations in T-lymphocyte subpopulations in patients with head and neck squamous carcinoma: Correlations with prognosis. Arch Otolaryngol 1987;113:1200–1206.

57. Huang HT, Mold NG, Fisher SR, et al. A prospective study of squamous head and neck carcinoma: Immunologic aberrations in patients who develop recurrent disease. Cancer 1987;59:1721–1726.

58. Schantz SP, Brown BW, Lira E, Taylor DL, Beddingfield N. Evidence for the role of natural immunity in the control of metastatic spread of head and neck cancer. Cancer Immunol Immunother 1987;25:141–145.

59. Ishikawa T. Immunotherapy for head and neck cancer with killer cells induced by stimulation with autologous or allogeneic tumor cells and recombinant interleukin-2. Acta Otolaryngol 1989;107:346–351.

60. Esteban F, Concha A, Delgado M, et al. Lack of MHC class I antigens and tumor aggressiveness of the squamous cell carcinoma of the larynx. Br J Cancer 1990;62:1047–1051.

61. Katz AE. Immunolobiologic staging of patients with carcinoma of the head and neck. Laryngoscope 1983;93:445–463.

62. Schantz SP, Savage HE, Lee NK. Head and neck tumor immunology: II. Humoral immunity. In: Jacobs C, ed: Head and neck oncology. 3rd ed. Norvall, MA: Kluwer, 1990:243–264.

63. American Joint Committee on Cancer. Manual for staging of cancer. 3rd ed. Philadelphia: JB Lippincott, 1988:27.

64. Close LG, Merkel M, Vuittch MF, Reisch J, Schaefer SD. Computed tomographic evaluation of regional lymph node involvement in cancer of the oral cavity and oropharynx. Head Neck 1989;11:309–317.

65. Brekel van den MWM, Castelijns JA, Croll GA, et al. Magnetic resonance versus palpation of cervical lymph node metastasis. Arch Otolaryngol Head Neck Surg 1991;117:666–673.

66. Brekel van den MWM, Stel HV, Castelijns JA, Croll GJ, Snow GB. Lymph node staging in patients with clinically negative neck examinations by ultrasound and ultrasound-guided aspiration cytology. Am J Surg 1991;162:362–366.

67. Selbach GJ, von Hamm E. Clinical value of oral cytology. Acta Cytol 1963;7:337–341.

68. Baden E. Prevention of cancer of the oral cavity and pharynx. CA 1987;37:49–62.

69. Oral Cytology. J Am Dent Assoc [Editorial] 1967;74:899.

70. Mashberg A, Sanirt AM. Early detection, diagnosis, and management of oral and oropharyngeal cancer. CA 1989;39:67–89.

71. Folsam TC, White CP, Bromer L, Canby HF, Garrington GE. Oral exfoliative study: Reviews of the literature and report of a three-year study. J Oral Surg 1972;33:61.

72. Eckert M, Bloom HJ, Ross CS. A review of oral cancer screening and detection in the Metropolitan Detroit cancer control program. Prog Clin Biol Res 1982;83:195–206.

73. Strong MS, Vanghan CW, Incze IS. Toluidine blue in the management of carcinoma of the oral cavity. Arch Otolaryngol 1968;87:101–105.

74. Mashberg A. Re-evaluation of toluidine blue application as a diagnostic adjunct in the detection of asymptomatic oral squamous cell carcinoma: A continuing prospective study of oral cancer. Cancer 1980;46:758–763.

75. Jesse RH, Perez CA, Fletcher GH. Cervical lymph node metastasis: Unknown primary cancer. Cancer 1973;31:854–859.

76. Galtry RR, Ayer WA. Head, neck, and oral abnormalities in dentists participating in the health assessment program. J Am Dent Assoc 1986;112:338–341.

77. Weber RS, Lichtiger B, Byers RM, et al. Electro-surgical dissection for reducing blood loss in head and neck surgery. Head Neck Surg 1989;11:318–324.

78. Looser KG, Shah JP, Strong EW. The significance of "positive" margins in surgically resected epidermoid carcinomas. Head Neck Surg 1978;1:107–111.

79. Scholl P, Byers RM, Batsakis JG, et al. Microscopic cut-through of cancer in the surgical treatment of squamous carcinoma of the tongue: Prognostic and therapeutic implications. Am J Surg 1986;152:354–360.

80. Loree TR, Strong EW. Significance of positive margins in oral cavity squamous carcinoma. Am J Surg 1990;160:410–414.

81. Panje WR, Sher N, Karnell M. Transoral carbon dioxide laser ablation of cancers, tumors and other disease. Arch Otolarngol Head Neck Cancer Surg 1981;115:681–688.

82. Gluckman JL, Waners M, Shumrick K, et al. Photodynamic therapy: A viable alternative to conventional therapy for early lesions of the upper aerodigestive tract. Arch Otolaryngol Head Neck Surg 1986;112:949–956.

83. Mohs FE, Snow SN. Microscopically controlled surgical treatment of squamous cell carcinoma of the lower lip. Surg Gynecol Obstet 1985;160:37–41

84. Bocca E, Pignataro O. A conservation technique in radical neck dissection. Ann Otol Rhinol Laryngol 1967;76:975–985.

85. Medina JE. A rational classification of neck dissections. Otolaryngol Head Neck Surg 1989;100:169.

86. Robbins KT, Medina JE, Wolfe GT, et al. Standardizing neck dissection terminology: Official report of the Academy's Committee for Head and Neck Surgery and Oncology. Arch Otolaryngol Head Neck Surg 1991;117:601–605.

87. Lindberg RD. Distribution of cervical lymph node metastasis form squamous cell carcinoma of the upper respiratory and digestive tracts. Cancer 1972;29:1446–1450.

88. Byers RM, Wolf PF, Ballantyne AJ. Rationale for elective modified neck dissection. Head Neck Surg 1988;10:160–167.

89. Ali S, Tiwari RM, Snow GB. False positive and false negative neck nodes. Head Neck Surg 1985;8:78–82.

90. Vandenbrouck C, Sancho-Garnier H, Chassange D, et al. Elective versus therapeutic radical neck dissection in epidermoid carcinoma of the oral cavity: Results of a randomized clinical trial. Cancer 1980;46:386–390.

91. Tupchong L, Scott C, Blitzer P, et al. Randomized study of pre-operative vs post-operative radiation therapy in advanced head and neck carcinoma: Long-term follow-up of RTOG study 73-03. Int J Radiat Oncol Biol Phys 1991;20:21–28.

92. Marcial V, Delber R, Kramer S, Snow J, Davis L, Vallecillo L. Does pre-operative irradiation decrease the rate of surgical complications in carcinoma of the head and neck? Cancer 1982;49:1297–1301.

93. Vikram B, Strong E, Shah J, Spiro R. Failure at the primary site following multi-modality treatment in advanced head and neck cancer. Head Neck Surg 1984;6:720–723.

94. Zelefsky M, Harrison L, Fass D, et al. Post-operative radiotherapy for oral cavity cancers: Impact of anatomic subsite on treatment outcome. Head Neck 1990;12:470–475.

95. Regezi JA, Courtney RM, Kerr DA. Dental management of patients radiated for oral cancer. Cancer 1976;38:994–1000.

96. Moorish RB, Chan E, Silverman S, et al. Osteonecrosis in patients irradiated for head and neck carcinoma. Cancer 1981;47:1980–1983.

97. Leibel SA, Kutcher TJ, Harrison LB, et al. Improved dose distributions for 3-D conformal boost treatment in carcinoma of the nasopharynx. Int J Radiat Oncol Biol Phys 1991;20:823–833.

98. Wang CC, Blitzer TH, Suit HD. Twice-a-day radiation therapy for cancer of the head and neck. Cancer 1985;55:2100–2104.

99. Parsons JT, Mendenhall WM, Cassisi NJ, et al. Hyperfractionation for head and neck cancer. Int J Radiat Oncol Biol Phys 1988;14:649–658.

100. Cox JD, Pajak PF, Marcial VA, et al. Dose-response for local control with hyperfractinated radiation therapy in advanced carcinomas of the upper aerodigestive tracts: Preliminary report of Radiation Therapy Oncolgoy Group Protocol 83-13. Int J Radiat Oncol Biol Phys 1990;18:515–521.

101. Fletcher GH. Elective irradiaiton of subclinical disease in cancers of the head and neck. Cancer 1972;29:1450–1454.

102. Hirabayashi H, Koshii K, Uno K, et al. Extracapsular spread of squamous cell carcinoma in neck lymph nodes: Prognostic factor of laryngeal cancer. Laryngoscope 1991;101:502–506.

103. Synderman N, Johnson J, Schramm V, Myers E, Bedetti C, Thearle T. Extracapsular spread of carcinoma in cervical lymph nodes—Impact upon survival in patients with carcinoma of the supraglottic larynx. Cancer 1985;56:1597–1599.

104. Vikram B, Shah J, Spiro R. Failure in the neck following multi-modality treatment for advanced head and neck cancer. Head Neck Surg 1984;6:724–729.

105. Schiff P, Harrison L, Strong E, et al. Impact of the time interval between surgery and post-operative radiation therapy on locoregional control in advanced head and neck cancer. J Surg Oncol 1990;43:203–208.

106. Zelefsky MJ, Harrison LB, Fass DE, et al. Postoperative radiation therapy for advance oropharyngeal carcinoma: Long-term treatment results. Cancer (in press).

107. Amdur R, Parsons J, Mendenhall W, Million R, Tessess N. Post-operative irradiation for squamous cell carcinoma of the head and neck: An analysis of treatment results and complications. Int J Radiat Oncol Biol Phys 1989;16:25–36.

108. Mitchell MS, Wawro NW, DeConti RC, et al. Effectiveness of high-dose infusion of methotrexate followed by leucovorin in carcinomas of the head and neck. Cancer Res 1968;28:108–109.

109. Kirkwood JM, Miller D, Pitman S, et al. Initial high dose methotrexate-leucovorin in advanced squamous carcinoma of the head and neck. Proc Am Assoc Cancer Res 1978;19:398.

110. Levitt M, Mosher MB, DeConti RC, et al. Improved therapeutic index of methotrexate with "leucovorin rescue." Cancer Res 1973;33:1729–1734.

111. Vogle WR, Jacobs J, Moffitt S, et al. Methotrexate therapy with or without citrovorum factor in carcinoma of the head and neck, breast and colon. Cancer Clin Trials 1979;2:227–236.

112. Woods RL, Fox RM, Tattersall MHN. Methotrexate treatment of advanced head and neck cancers: A dose-response evaluation. Cancer Treat Rep 1981;65:155–159.

113. DeConti RC, Schoenfeld D. A randomized prospective comparison of intermittent methotrexate, methotrexate with leucovorin, and a methotrexate combination in head and neck cancer. Cancer 1981;48:1061–1072.

114. Taylor SG IV, McGuire WP, Hauck WW, et al. A randomized comparison of high-dose infusion methotrexate versus standard-dose weekly therapy in head and neck squamous cancer. J Clin Oncol 1984;2:1006–1011.

115. Al-Sarraf M. Chemotherapeutic management of head and neck cancer. Cancer Metast Rev 1987;6:191–198.

116. Havlin KA, Kuhn JG, Myers JW, et al. High-dose cisplatin for locally advanced or metastatic head and neck cancer: A phase II pilot study. Cancer 1989;63:423–427.

117. Forastiere AA, Takasugi BJ, Baker SR, Wolf GT, Kudla-Hatch V. High-dose cisplatin in advanced head and neck cancer. Cancer Chemother Pharmacol 1987;19:155–158.

118. Veronesi A, Zagonel V, Rirelli U, et al. High-dose versus low-dose cisplatin in advanced head and neck squamous carcinoma: A randomized study. J Clin Oncol 1985;3:1105–1108.

119. Al-Sarraf M. Management strategies in head and neck cancer: The role of carboplatin. In: Bunns PA Jr, Canetta R, Ozols RF, Rozencqeig M, eds. Carboplatin (JM-8): Current perspectives and future directions. Philadelphia: WB Saunders, 1990.

120. Abele R, Clavel M, Rossi A, et al. Iproplatin (CHIP, JM-9) in advanced squamous cell carcinoma of the head and neck: A phase II study of the EORTC early clinical trials group. Proc Am Soc Clin Oncol [Abstract #575] 1986;5:147.

121. Chabner BA, Collins JM. Cancer chemotherapy: Principles and practice. Philadelphia: JB Lippincott, 1990.

122. Al-Sarraf M, Metch B, Kish J, et al. Platinum analogs in recurrent and advanced head and neck cancer: A Southwest Oncology Group and Wayne State University Study. Cancer Treat Rep 1987;71:723–726.

123. Robert F. Trimetrexate as a single agent in patients with advanced head and neck cancer. Semin Oncol 1988;15:22–26.

124. Schornagel J, Cappelaere P, Verwey J, et al. A randomized phase II study of 10-ethyl-10-deaza-aminopterin (10-EdAM) and methotrexate (MTX) in advanced head and neck squamous cell cancer (AHNC), an EORTC study. Proc Am Soc Clin Oncol [Abstract #679] 1989;8:174.

125. Kish JA, Tapazoglou E, Ensley J, et al. Activity of ifosfamide (NSC-109724) in recurrent head and neck cancer patients. Proc Am Assoc Cancer Res [Abstract] 1990;31:190.

126. Cobleigh MA, Hill JH, Lad TE, et al. Phase II study of etoposide in previously untreated squamous cell carcinoma of the head and neck. Cancer Treat Rep 1987;71:321–322.

127. Shiu WC, Tsao SY. Etoposide (VP16-213) in the treatment of advanced nasopharyngeal carcinoma. Eur J Cancer Clin Oncol 1988;24:797–798.

128. Holoye PY, Byers RM, Gard DA, et al. Combination chemotherapy of head and neck cancer. Cancer 1978;42:1661–1669.

129. Forastiere A, Metch B, Schuller D, et al. Randomized comparison of cisplatin and 5-fluorouracil versus carboplatin +5-Fu versus methotrexate in advanced squamous cell carcinoma of the head and neck. J Clin Oncol 1992;10:1245–1251.

130. Cortes EP, Kalra J, James R, et al. Chemotherapy for head and neck cancer in relapse after prior radiotherapy and evaluation of method of bleomycin (Bleo) administration of anti-tumor effect. Proc Am Soc Clin Oncol 1980;21:364.

131. Amer MH, Al-Sarraf M, Vaitkevicius VK. Factors that affect response to chemotherapy and survival of patients with advanced head and neck cancer. Cancer 1979;43:2202–2206.

132. Wheeler RH, Liepman MK, Baker SR, et al. Cancer Treat Rep 1980;64:943–949.

133. Raafat J, Oster MW. Combination chemotherapy for advanced squamous cell carcinoma of the head and neck. Cancer Treat Rep 1980;64:187–189.

134. Hill BT, Shaw HJ, Dalley VM, et al. 24-hour combination chemotherapy without cisplatin in patients with recurrent or metastatic head and neck cancer. Am J Clin Oncol 1984;7:335–340.

135. Ringborg U, Ewert G, Kinnman J, et al. Sequential methotrexate and 5-fluorouracil treatment of squamous cell cracinoma to the head and neck. Cancer 1983;52:971–973.

136. Pitman SW, Kowal CD, Papac RJ, et al. Sequential methotrexate-5-fluorouracil in sequence in squamous head and neck cancer. Semin Oncol 1983;10(suppl 2):15–19.

137. Jacobs C. Use of methotrexate and 5-FU for recurrent head and neck cancer. Cancer Treat Rep. 1982;66:1925–1928.

138. Browman GP, Archibald SD, Young JEM, et al. Prospective randomized trial of one-hour sequential versus simultaneous methotrexate plus 5-Fluorouracil in advanced and recurrent squamous cell head and neck cancer. J Clin Oncol 1983;1:787–792.

139. Coates AS, Tatersall MHN, Swanson C, et al. Combination therapy with methotrexate and 5-Fluorouracil: A prospective randomized clinical trail of order of administration. J Clin Oncol 1984;2:756–761.

140. Elias EG, Chretien PB, Monnard E, et al. Chemotherapy prior to local therapy in advanced squamous cell carcinoma of the head and neck. Cancer 1979;43:1025–1031.

141. Wittes RE, Brescia F, Young CW, et al. Combination chemotherapy with *cis*-diamminedichloroplatinum (II) and bleomycin in tumors of the head and neck. Oncology 1975;32:202–207.

142. Creagan ET, Fleming TR, Edmonson JH, et al. Cyclophosphamide, adriamycin, and *cis*-diamminedichloroplatinum (II) in the treatment of patients with advanced head and neck cancer. Cancer 1981;47:240–244.

143. Creagan ET, Fleming TR, Edmonson JH, et al. Chemotherapy for advanced head and neck cancer with the combination adriamycin, cyclophosphamide, and *cis*-diamminedichloroplatinum (II): Preliminary assessment of a one-day vs. three-day drug regimen. Cancer 1981;47:2549–2551.

144. Amer MH, Izbicki RM, Vaitkevicius VK, et al. Combination chemotherapy with *cis*-diamminedichloroplatinum, oncovin, and bleomycin (COB) in advanced head and neck cancer: Phase II. Cancer 1980;45:217–223.

145. Amrein PC, Fingert H, Weitzman SA. Cisplatin-vincristine-bleomycin therapy in squamous cell carcinoma of the head and neck. J Clin Oncol 1983;1:421–427.

146. Caradonna R, Paladine W, Ruchdeschel JC, et al. Methotrexate, bleomycin, and high-dose *cis*-dichlorodiammineplatinum (II) in the treatment of advanced epidermoid carcinoma of the head and neck. Cancer Treat Rep 1979;63:489–491.

147. Ervin TJ, Weichselbaum R, Miller D, et al. Treatment of advanced squamous cell carcinoma of the head and neck with cisplatin, bleomycin, and methotrexate (PBM). Cancer Treat Rep 1981;65:787–791.

148. Kaplan BH, Vogl SE, Chiuten D, et al. Chemotherapy of advanced cancer of the head and neck (HNCa) with methotrexate (M), bleomycin (B) and *cis*-diamminedichloroplatinum (D) in combination—"MBD." Proc Am Soc Clin Oncol 1979;20:384.

149. Murphy WK, Valdivieso M, Bodey GP, et al. *Cis*-diamminedichloroplatinum-II (DDP), methotrexate (MTX) and bleomycin (BLM) chemotherapy for patients with advanced squamous cell carcinoma (SCC) of the head and neck (H&N). Proc Am Assoc Cancer Res [Abstract] 1980;21:166.

150. Vogl SE, Kaplan BH. Chemotherapy of advanced head and neck cancer with methotrexate, bleomycin, and *cis*-diamminedichloroplatinum II in an effective outpatient schedule. Cancer 1979;44:26–31.

151. Van Hoff DD, Alberts DS, Mattox DE, et al. Combination chemotherapy with cisplatin, bleomycin, and methotrexate in patients with advanced head and neck cancer. Cancer Clin Trials 1981;4:215–218.

152. Brown AW Jr, Blom J, Butler WM, et al. Combination chemotherapy with vinblastine, bleomycin, and *cis*-diamminedichloroplatinum (II) in squamous cell carcinoma of the head and neck. Cancer 1980;45:2830–2835.

153. Williams SD, Velez-Garcia E, Essessee I, et al. Chemotherapy for head and neck cancer: Comparison of cisplatin + vinblastine + bleomycin versus methotrexate. Cancer 1986;57:18–23.

154. Kish JA, Weaver A, Jacobs J, et al. Cisplatin and 5-fluorouracil infusion in patients with recurrent and disseminated epidermoid cancer of the head and neck.

155. Paredes J, Hong WK, Felder TB, et al. Prospective randomized trial of high-dose cisplatin and fluorouracil infusion with or without sodium diethyldithiocarbamate in recurrent and/or metastatic squamous cell carcinoma of the head and neck. J Clin Oncol 1988;6:955–962.

156. Kish JA, Ensley JF, Jacobs J, et al. A randomized trial of cisplatin (CACP) + 5-fluorouracil (5-FU) infusion and CACP + 5-FU bolus for recurrent and advanced squamous cell carcinoma of the head and neck. Cancer 1985;56:2740–2744.

157. Amrein PC, Weitzman SA. Treatment of squamous-cell carcinoma of the head and neck with cisplatin and 5-Fluorouracil. J Clin Oncol 1985;3:1632–1639.

158. Choksi AJ, Hong WK, Dimery IW, et al. Continuous cisplatin (24-hour) and 5-fluorouracil (120-hour) infusion in recurrent head and neck squamous cell carcinoma. Cancer 1988;61:909–912.

159. Creagan ET, Ingle JN, Schutt AJ, et al. A phase II study of *cis*-diamminedichloroplatinum and 5-fluorouracil in advanced upper aerodigestive neoplasms. Head Neck Surg 1984;6:1020–1023.

160. Merlano M, Tatarek R, Grimaldi A, et al. Phase I-II trial with cisplatin and 5-FU in recurrent head and neck cancer: An effective outpatient schedule. Cancer Treat Rep 1985;69:961–964.

161. Rowland Jr KM, Taylor SG IV, Spiers ASD, et al. Cisplatin and 5-FU infusion chemotherapy in advanced, recurrent cancer of the head and neck: An Eastern Cooperative Oncology Group pilot study. Cancer Treat Rep 1986;70:461–464.

162. Liverpool Head and Neck Oncology Group: A phase III randomized trial of cisplatinum, methotrexate, cisplatinum + methotrexate and cisplatinum + 5-FU in end stage squamous carcinoma of the head and neck. Br J Cancer 1990;61:311–315.

163. Dasmahapatra KS, Citrin P, Hill GJ, et al. A prospective evaluation of 5-fluorouracil plus cisplatin in advanced squamous-cell cancer of the head and neck. J Clin Oncol 1985;3:1486–1489.

164. Sridhar KS, Hirsch R, Fountzilas G, et al. Sequential cisplatin and 5-fluorouracil in advanced squamous cell head and neck cancer. Proc Am Soc Clin Oncol [Abstract] 1985;4:150.

165. Raymond MG, Lyman GH. Treatment of unresectable/recurrent epidermoid carcinoma of head and neck with cisplatin plus 5-fluorouracil infusion. Proc Am Soc Clin Oncol [Abstract] 1985;4:133.

166. Fosser VP, Paccagnella A, Venturelli E, et al. Cisplatin plus 5-fluorouracil 120 hour infusion in patients with recurrent and disseminated head and neck cancer. Proc Am Soc Clin Oncol [Abstract] 1985;4:150.

167. Khojasteh A, Reynolds RD, Ruble K. The comparison of regimen-dependent schedules of 5-fluorouracil and cisplatin in head and neck cancer. Proc Am Soc Clin Oncol [Abstract] 1986;6:126.

168. Amrein PC. Cisplatin and 5-fluorouracil vs. the same plus bleomycin and methotrexate in recurrent squamous cell carcinoma of the head and neck (SCC H&N). Proc Am Soc Clin Oncol [Abstract] 1990;9:175.

169. Jacobs C, Lyman G, Velez-Garcia E, et al. A phase III study comparing cisplatin (CP) and fluorouracil (5FU) as single agents and in combination for advanced squamous cell carcinoma (SCCA) of the head and neck—A final report. Proc Am Soc Clin Oncol [Abstract] 1991;10:197.

170. Vokes EE, Choi KE, Schilsky RL, et al. Cisplatin, fluorouracil, and high-dose leucovorin for recurrent for metastatic head and neck cancer. J Clin Oncol 198;6:618–626.

171. Guthrie TH, Brubaker LH, Porubsky ES, et al. Circadian cisplatin (C), bleomycin (B) and 5-fluorouracil (F) in advanced squamous cell carcinoma of the head and neck (SCCH). Proc Am Soc Clin Oncol [Abstract] 1990;9:178.

172. Hamm JT, Joseph G, Blumenreich MS, et al. Phase II trial of high-dose cisplatinum (CDDP), 5-fluorouracil (5FU), bleomycin, and methotrexate in advanced/recurrent head and neck cancer. Proc Am Soc Clin Oncol [Abstract] 1990;9:175.

173. Dimery I, Martin T, Bradley E, et al. Phase I trial of interleukin-2 (rIL-2) plus cisplatin (CDDP) and 5-fluorouracil (5-FU) in recurrent or advanced squamous cell carcinoma of the head and neck. Proc Am Soc Clin Oncol [Abstract] 1989;8:170.

174. Shirinian M, Choksi AJ, Dimery I, et al. Phase I/II study of cisplatin (P) + 5-fluorouracil (F) + α-interferon (IFN) for recurrent squamous cell carcinoma of the head and neck (SCCHN). ASCO [Abstract] 1992;

175. Hong WK, Schaefer S, Issell B, et al. A prospective randomized trial of methotrexate versus cisplatin in the treatment of recurrent squamous cell carcinoma of the head and neck. Cancer 1983;52:206–210.

176. Drelichman A, Cummings G, Al-Sarraf N, et al. A randomized trial of the combination of *cis*-platinum, oncovin and bleomycin (COB) versus methotrexate in patients with advanced squamous cell carcinoma of the head and neck. Cancer 1983;52:399–403.

177. Grose WE, Lehane DE, Dixon DO, et al. Comparison of methotrexate and cisplatin for patients with advanced squamous cell carcinoma of the head and neck region: A Southwest Oncology Group study. Cancer Treat Rep 1985;69:577–581.

178. Vogl SE, Schoenfeld DA, Kaplan BH, et al. A randomized prospective comparison of methotrexate with a combination of methotrexate, bleomycin, and cisplatin in head and neck cancer. Cancer 1985;56:432–442.

179. Williams SD, Velez-Garcia E, Essessee I, et al. Chemotherapy for head and neck cancer: Comparison of cisplatin plus vinblastine plus bleomycin versus methotrexate. Cancer 1986;57:18–23.

180. Campbell JB, Dorman EB, McCormick M, et al. A randomized phase III trial of cis-platinum, methotrexate, cisplatinum + methotrexate, and cisplatinum + 5-Flourouracil in end-stage head and neck cancer. Acta Otolaryngol (Stockh) 1987;103:519–528.

181. Eisenberger M, Krasnow S, Ellenberg S, et al. A comparison of carboplatin plus methotrexate versus methotrexate alone in patients with recurrent and metastatic head and neck cancer. J Clin Oncol 1989;7:1341–1345.

182. Dimery IW, Jacobs C, Tseng A, et al. Recombinant interferon-gamma in the treatment of recurrent nasopharyngeal carcinoma. J Biol Resp Modif 1989;8:221–226.

183. Schantz SP, Clayman GL, Dimery I, Morice R. Combination interleukin-2 and interferon-alpha in head and neck cancer patients. Cancer Bull 1991;43:133–145.

184. Lippman SM, Kessler JM, Al-Sarraf M, et al. Treatment of advanced squamous cell carcinoma of the head and neck with isotretinoin. Invest New Drugs 1988;6:51–56.

185. Hong WK, Bromer R. Chemotherapy in head and neck cancer. N Engl J Med 1983;308:75–79.

186. Tarpley JL, Chretien PB, Alexander JC Jr, et al. High-dose methotrexate as a preoperative adjuvant in the treatment of epidermoid carcinoma of the head and neck: A feasibility study and clinical trial. Am J Surg 1975;130:481–486.

187. Taylor SG IV, Bytell DE, DeWys WD, et al. Adjuvant methotrexate and leucovorin in head and neck squamous cancer: Two-year follow-up of a pilot project. Arch Otolaryngol 1978;104:647–651.

188. Ervin TJ, Kirkwood J, Weichselbaum RR, et al. Improved survival for patients with advanced carcinoma of the head and neck treated with methotrexate-leucovorin prior to definitive radiotherapy or surgery. Laryngoscope 1981;91:1181–1190.

189. Taylor SG IV, Applebaum E, Showel JL, et al. A randomized trial of adjuvant chemotherapy in head and neck cancer. J Clin Oncol 1985;3:672–679.

190. Popkin JD, Hong WK, Bromer RH, et al. Induction bleomycin infusion in head and neck cancer. Am J Clin Oncol 1984;7:199–204.

191. Jacobs C, Bertino JR, Goffinet DR, et al. 24-hour infusion of *cis*-platinum in head and neck cancers. Cancer 1978;42:2135–2140.

192. Wittes R, Heller K, Randolph V, et al. *cis*-Dichlorodiammineplatinum (II)-based chemotherapy as initial treatment of advanced head and neck cancer. Cancer Treat Rep 1979;63:1533–1538.

193. Schaefer SD, Middleton R, Reisch J, et al. Cisplatinum induction chemotherapy in the multi-modality initial treatment of advanced stage IV carcinoma of the head and neck. Cancer 1983;51:2168–2174.

194. Gad-El-Mawla N, Abul-Ela M, Mansour MA, et al. Preoperative adjuvant chemotherapy in relatively advanced head and neck cancer. Am J Clin Oncol 1984;7:195–198.

195. Randolph VL, Vallejo AM, Spiro RH, et al. Combination therapy of advanced head and neck cancer: Induction of remissions with diamminedichloroplatinum (II), bleomycin and radiation therapy. Cancer 1978;41:460–467.

196. Hong WK, Bhutani R, Shapshay SM, et al. Induction chemotherapy of advanced previously untreated squamous cell head and neck cancer with cisplatin and bleomycin. In: Preytayko A, Crooke S, Carter S, eds. Cisplatin: Current status and new developments. San Diego: Academic, 1980:431–444.

197. Glick JH, Marcial V, Richter M, et al. The adjuvant treatment of inoperable stage III and IV epidermoid carcinoma of the head and neck with platinum and bleomycin infusion prior to definitive radiotherapy: An RTOG pilot study. Cancer 1980;46:1919–1924.

198. Israel L, Aguilera J, Soudant J, et al. Bleomycin and cisplatinum with or without mitomycin-C in 110 previously untreated patients with head and neck cancer. Am J Clin Oncol 1983;5:305–311.

199. Coughlin CT, Grace M, O'Donnell JF, et al. Combined modality approach in the management of locally advanced head and neck cancer. Cancer Treat Rep 1984;68: 591–597.

200. Head and Neck Contracts Program. Adjuvant chemotherapy for advanced head and neck squamous carcinoma: Final report of the Head and Neck Contracts Program. Cancer 1987;60:301–311.

201. Elias EG, Chretien PB, Monnard E, et al. Chemotherapy prior to local therapy in advanced squamous cell carcinoma of the head and neck: Preliminary assessment of an intensive drug regimen. Cancer 1979;43:1025–1031.

202. Tannock I, Cummings B, Sorrenti V, et al. Combination chemotherapy used prior to radiation therapy for locally advanced squamous cell carcinoma of the head and neck. Cancer Treat Rep 1982;66:1421–1424.

203. Vogl SE, Lerner H, Kaplan BH, et al. Failure of effective initial chemotherapy to modify the course of stage IV (MO) squamous cancer of the head and neck. Cancer 1982;50:840–844.

204. Kies MS, Pecaro BC, Gordon LI, et al. Preoperative combination chemotherapy for advanced stage head and neck cancer: Promising early results. Am J Surg 1984;148: 521–524.

205. Mohit-Tabatabai MA, Rush BF Jr, Hill GJ, et al. Multimodality preoperative treatment for advanced cancer of the head and neck. Am J Surg 1984;148:521–524.

206. Adelstein DJ, Hines JD, Sharan VM, et al. Combination chemotherapy prior to definitive local therapy in squamous cell carcinoma of the head and neck. Oncology 1985;42: 80–85.

207. Ervin TJ, Clark JR, Weichselbaum RR, et al. An analysis of induction and adjuvant chemotherapy in the multidisciplinary treatment of squamous-cell carcinoma of the head and neck. J Clin Oncol 1987;5:10–20.

208. Zidan J, Kuten A, Cohen Y, et al. Multidrug chemotherapy using bleomycin, methotrexate, and cisplatin combined with radical radiotherapy in advanced head and neck cancer. Cancer 1987;59:24–26.

209. Al-Sarraf M, Drelichman A, Jacobs J, et al. Adjuvant chemotherapy with *cis*-platinum, oncovin, and bleomycin followed by surgery and/or radiotherapy in patients with advanced previously untreated head and neck cancer: Final report. In: Jones SE, Salmon SE, eds. Adjuvant therapy of cancer. 3rd ed. Philadelphia: Grune & Stratton, 1981:145–152.

210. Amrein PC, Fingert H, Weitzman SA. Cisplatin-vincristine-bleomycin therapy in squamous cell carcinoma of the head and neck. J Clin Oncol 1983;1:421–427.

211. Kukla LJ, Mantravade RVP, Applebaum EL, et al. Preirradiation chemotherapy for advanced head and neck carcinomas. Arch Otolaryngol 1984;110:78–81.

212. Schuller DE, Wilson H, Hodgson S, et al. Preoperative reductive chemotherapy for stage III or IV operable epidermoid carcinoma of the oral cavity, oropharynx, hypopharynx, or larynx, phase III: A Southwest Oncology Group Study [Abstract]. In: Proceedings of International Conference on Head and Neck Cancer, Chemotherapy II, Baltimore, July 22–27, 1984.

213. Perry DJ, Davis RK, Zajtchuk JR, et al. Vinblastine, bleomycin, and cisplatin in the treatment of squamous carcinoma of the head and neck. In: Jones SE, Salmon SE, eds. Adjuvant therapy of cancer. 4th ed. Philadelphia: Grune & Stratton, 1984:135–143.

214. Spaulding M, Ziegler P, Sunquist N, et al. Induction therapy in head and neck cancer. Cancer 1986;57:1110–1114.

215. Spaulding MB, Lore J, Klotch D, et al. Long-term follow-up of induction chemotherapy in advanced resectable head and neck cancer [Abstract]. In: Proceedings of the 2nd International Head and Neck Oncology Research Conference, Arlington, VA, September 10–12, 1987.

216. Kish J, Drelichman A, Jacobs, et al. Clinical trial of cisplatin and 5-FU infusion as initial treatment for advanced squamous cell carcinoma of the head and neck. Cancer Treat Rep 1982;66:471–474.

217. Kish JA, Ensley JF, Weaver A, et al. Improvement of complete response rate to induction adjuvant chemotherapy for advanced squamous cell carcinoma of the head and neck. Cancer Treat Rep 1982;66:471–474.

218. Shirinian M, Weber R, Dimery I, et al. Laryngeal preservation using induction chemotherapy followed by definitive XRT for patients with advanced stage head and neck squamous cell carcinoma requiring total laryngectomy. Proc Am Soc Clin Oncol [Abstract] 1992;

219. Kies MS, Lester EP, Gordon LI, et al. Cisplatin and infusion 5-fluorouracil (5-FU) in stage III and IV squamous cancer of the head and neck. Proc Am Soc Clin Oncol [Abstract] 1985;4:139.

220. Amrein PC, Witzman SA. Treatment of squamous-cell carcinoma of the head and neck with cisplatin and 5-fluorouracil. J Clin Oncol 1985;3:1632–1639.

221. Clark J, Fallon B, Norris C, et al. A randomized trial of two induction regimens for advanced squamous cell carcinoma of the head and neck (SCCHN)—Preliminary results. Proc Am Soc Clin Oncol [Abstract] 1986;5:132.

222. Khojasteh A, Reynolds RD, Ruble K. The comparison of sequence-dependent schedules of 5-fluorouracil (5FU) and cisplatin (CDDP) in head and neck cancer (H&N Ca). Proc Am Soc Clin Oncol [Abstract] 1987;6:126.

223. Loeffler TM, Lindemann J, Luckhaupt, et al. Split-dose cisplatin (DDP), folinic acid (FA) and 5-FU (FU) in advanced squamous cell cancer of the head and neck (SCCHN): An outpatient phase-II trial. Proc Am Soc Clin Oncol [Abstract] 1987;6:137.

224. Toohill RJ, Anderson T, Byhardt RW, et al. Cisplatin and fluorouracil as neoadjuvant therapy in head and neck cancer. Arch Otolaryngol Head Neck Surg 1987;113:758–761.

225. Johnson JT, Mayernik DG, Nyers EN, et al. Cisplatin-5-fluorouracil chemotherapy for advanced inoperable squamous carcinoma of the head and neck. Head Neck Surg 1987;9:336–340.

226. Jacobs C, Goffinet DR, Goffinet L, et al. Chemotherapy as a substitute for surgery in the treatment of advanced resectable head and neck cancer. Cancer 1987;60:1178–1183.

227. Department of Veterans Affairs Laryngeal Cancer Study Group. Induction chemotherapy plus radiation compared with surgery plus radiation in patients with advanced laryngeal cancer. N Engl J Med 1991;324:1685–1690.

228. Thyss A, Schneider M, Santini J, et al. Induction chemotherapy with *cis*-platinum and 5-fluorouracil for squamous cell carcinoma of the head and neck. Br J Cancer 1986;54:755–760.

229. Paccagnella A, Cavaniglia G, Zorat PL, et al. Chemotherapy (CT) before loco-regional treatment (LRT) in stage III + IV head and neck cancer: Intermediate results of an ongoing randomized phase III trial—A GSTIC study. Proc Am Soc Clin Oncol [Abstract] 1990;9:173.

230. Martin M, Hazan A, Vergnes L, et al. Randomized study of 5-fluorouracil (5-FU) and *cis*-platinum (DDP) as neoadjuvant therapy in head and neck cancer: A preliminary report. Proc Am Soc Clin Oncol [Abstract] 1989;8:175.

231. Joveniaux A, Caty A, Adenis L. L'association de cislatine et de 5 fluro-uracil dans le traitement primaire des carcinomes evolues des voies aerodigestive superieures. Bull Cancer 1984;71:390.

232. Scherpe A, Schroder M, von Heyden HW, Nagel GA. Chemotherapieergebnisse mit cisplatin and 5-fluorouracil bei plattenepithelkarzinomen des kopf-hals-bereiches. Onkologie 1984;7:302.

233. Dasmahapatra KS, Citrin P, Hill G, et al. A prospective evaluation of 5-fluorouracil plus cisplatin in advanced squamous-cell cancer of the head and neck. J Clin Oncol 1985;3:1486–1489.

234. Verweij J, de Jong PC, de Mulder PHM, et al. Induction chemotherapy with cisplatin and continuous infusion 5-fluorouracil in locally far-advanced head and neck cancer. Am J Clin Oncol 1989;12:420–424.

235. Vokes EE, Schilsky RL, Weichselbaum RR, et al. Induction chemotherapy with cisplatin, fluorouracil, and high-dose leucovorin for locally advanced head and neck cancer: A clinical and pharmacologic analysis. J Clin Oncol 1990;8:241–247.

236. Greenberg B, Ahmann F, Garewal H, et al. Neoadjuvant therapy for advanced head and neck cancer with allopurinol-modulated high dose 5-fluorouracil and cisplatin: A phase I–II study. Cancer 1987;59:1860–1865.

237. Ensley J, Kish J, Tapazoglou E, et al. An intensive, five-course, alternating combination chemotherapy induction regimen used in patients with advanced, unresectable head and neck cancer. J Clin Oncol 1988;6:1147–1153.

238. Kramer A, Choksi A, Dimery I. Induction chemotherapy using cisplatin, bleomycin and 5-fluorouracil (PBF) in advanced squamous cell carcinoma of the head and neck (SCCHN). Proc Am Soc Clin Oncol [Abstract] 1988;7:157.

239. Richards GL Jr, Chambers RG. Hydroxyurea: A radiosensitizer in the treatment of neoplasms of the head and neck. Am J Roentgen Rad Ther Nucl Med 1969;105:555.

240. Dreyfuss AI, Clark JR, Wright JE, et al. Continuous-infusion high-dose leucovorin with 5-fluorouracil and cisplatin for untreated stage IV carcinoma of the head and neck. Ann Intern Med 1990;112:167–172.

241. Kish JA, Ensley JF, Jacobs JR, et al. Evaluation of high-dose cisplatin and 5-Fu infusion as initial therapy in advanced head and neck cancer. Am J Clin Oncol 1988;11:553–557.

242. Vokes EE, Weichselbaum RR, Ratain MJ, et al. PFL with escalating doses of interferon-alpha-2B (IFN) as neoadjuvant chemotherapy for sage IV head and neck cancer (HNC): A clinical and pharmacokinetic analysis. Proc Am Soc Clin Oncol [Abstract] 1991;10: 20.

243. Urba S, Forastiere AA, Wolf GT. Induction chemotherapy (CT) with intensive continuous infusion high dose cisplatin (CDDP), 5-fluorouracil (5FU) and mitoguazone (MGBC) for advanced head and neck cancer (H&N CA). Proc Am Soc Clin Oncol [Abstract] 1990;9:171.

244. Hill BT, Price LA, MacRae K. Importance of primary site in assessing chemotherapy response and 7-year survival data in advanced squamous-cell carcinomas of the head and neck treated with initial combination chemotherapy without cisplatin. J Clin Oncol 1986;4:1340–1347.

245. Stolwijk C, Wagener DJ, van den Broek Levendaj PC, et al. Randomized adjuvant chemotherapy trial for advanced head and neck cancer. Neo-Neth J Med 1985;28: 347–351.

246. Rentschler RE, Wilbur DW, Petti GH, et al. Adjuvant methotrexate escalated to toxicity for resectable stage III and IV squamous head and neck carcinomas—A prospective, randomized trial. J Clin Oncol 1987;5:278–285.

247. Kun KE, Toohill RJ, Holoye PY, et al. A randomized study of chemotherapy for cancer of the upper aerodigestive tract. Int J Radiat Oncol Biol Phys 1986;12:173–178.

248. Richard J, Molinari R, Sancho-Garnier H, et al. A randomized trial comparing surgery preceded or not by intra-arterial chemotherapy in squamous cell carcinomas of the head and neck [Abstract]. In: Proceedings of the International Conference on Head and Neck Cancer, Baltimore, MD, 1984:113.

249. Martin M, Mazeron JJ, Brun B, et al. Neo-adjuvant polychemotherapy of head and neck cancer: Results of a randomized study. Proc Am Soc Clin Oncol [Abstract] 1988; 152:7.

250. Schuller DE, Metch B, Stein DW, et al. Preoperative chemotherapy in advanced resectable head and neck cancer: Final report of the Southwest Oncology Group. Laryngoscope 1988;98:1205–1211.

251. von Essen CF, Joseph LB, Simon GT, et al. Sequential chemotherapy and radiation therapy of buccal mucosa carcinoma in South India: Methods and preliminary results. Am J Roentgenol Rad Ther Nucl Med 1968;102:530–540.

252. Richard JM, Sancho H, Lepintre Y, et al. Intra-arterial methotrexate chemotherapy and telecobalt therapy in cancer of the oral cavity and oropharynx. Cancer 1974;34: 491–496.

253. Knowlton AH, Percarpio B, Bobrow S, et al. Methotrexate and radiation therapy in the treatment of advanced head and neck tumors. Radiology 1975;116:709–712.

254. Lustig RA, DeMare PA, Kramer S. Adjuvant methotrexate in the radiotherapeutic management of advanced tumors of the head and neck. Cancer 1976;37:2703–2708.

255. Fazekas JT, Sommer C, Kramer S. Adjuvant intravenous methotrexate or definitive radiotherapy alone for advanced squamous cancers of the oral cavity, oropharynx, supraglottic larynx or hypopharynx. Int J Radiat Oncol Biol Phys 1980;6:533–541.

256. Petrovich Z, Block J, Kuishk H, et al. A randomized comparison of radiotherapy with a radiotherapy-chemotherapy combination in stage IV carcinoma of the head and neck. Cancer 1981;47:2259–2264.

257. Arcangeli G, Nervi C, Righini R, et al. Combined radiation and drugs: The effect of intra-arterial chemotherapy followed by radiotherapy in head and neck cancer. Radiother Oncol 1983;1:101–107.

258. Stell PM, Dalby JE, Strickland P, et al. Sequential chemotherapy and radiotherapy in advanced head and neck cancer. Clin Radiol 1990;34:463–467.

259. Vokes EE, Moran WJ, Mick R, et al. Neoadjuvant and adjuvant methotrexate, cisplatin, and fluorouracil in multimodal therapy of head and neck cancer. J Clin Oncol 1989;7:838–845.

260. Shetty P, Mehta A, Shinde S, et al. Controlled study in squamous cell carcinoma of base of tongue using conventional radiation, radiation with single drug and radiation with multiple drug chemotherapy. Proc Am Soc Clin Oncol [Abstract] 1985;4:152.

261. Szpirglas H, Nizri D, Marneur M, et al. Neo-adjuvant chemotherapy: A randomized trial before radiotherapy in oral and oro-pharyngeal carcinomas: End results. In: Proceedings of the 2nd International Head and Neck Oncology Research Conference. Arlington VA, September 10–12, 1987:261–264.

262. Merlano M, Rosso R, Benasso M, et al. Alternating chemotherapy (CT) and radiotherapy (RT) vs RT in advanced inoperable SCC-HN: A cooperative randomized trial. Proc Am Soc Clin Oncol 1991;10:198.

262a. Jaulerry C, Mosseri V, Brunin F, et al. Induction chemotherapy in advanced head and neck cancer: Final results of a randomized trial. Int J Radiat Oncol Biol Phys 1989;15(suppl 1):137.

263. Condit PT. Treatment of carcinoma with radiation therapy and methotrexate. MO Med 1968;65:832–835.

264. Gupta NK, Pointon RCS, Wilkinson PM. A randomized clinical trial to contract radiotherapy with radiotherapy and methotrexate given synchronously in head and neck cancer. Clin Radiol 1987;38:575–581.

265. Fu KK. Clinical results of simultaneous chemotherapy and radiotherapy in head and neck cancer. In: Jacobs JR, Crissman JD, Valeriote FA, et al, eds. Head and neck cancer: Scientific perspectives in management and strategies for cure. New York: Elsevier, 1987:321–333.

266. Kapstad B, Bang G, Rennaes S, et al. Combined preoperative treatment with cobalt and bleomycin in patients with head and neck carcinoma—a controlled clinical study. Int J Radiat Oncol Biol Phys 1978;4:85–89.

267. Shanta Y, Krishnamurthi S. Combined bleomycin and radiotherapy in oral cancer. Clin Radiol 1980;31:617–620.

268. Morita K. Clinical significance of radiation therapy combined with chemotherapy. Strahlentherapie 1980;156:228–233.

269. Scandolaro L, Bertoni F. Tolleranza cutanea e mucosa e risposte cliniche a breve termine nella associazione tra radioterapia e bleomycina per tumori del distretto cervico-cefalico. Acta Otorhinol Ital 1982;2:213–220.

270. Pauinen LM, Parvinem M, Nordman E, et al. Combined bleomycin treatment and radiation therapy in squamous cell carcinoma of the head and neck region. Acta Radiol Oncol 1985;24:487–489.

271. Shetty P, Mehta A, Shinde S, et al. Controlled study in squamous cell carcinoma of base of tongue using conventional radiation, radiation with single drug and radiation with multiple drug chemotherapy. Proc Am Soc Clin Oncol [Abstract] 1985;4:152.

272. Vermund H, Kaalhus O, Winther F, et al. Bleomycin and radiation therapy in squamous cell carcinoma of the upper aerodigestive tract: A phase III clinical trial. Int J Radiat Oncol Biol Phys 1985;11:1877–1886.

273. Vermund H, Kaalhus O, Winther F, et al. Bleomycin and radiation therapy in squamous cell carcinoma of the upper aerodigestive tract: A phase III clinical trial. Int J Radiat Oncol Biol Phys 1985;11:1877–1886.

274. Fu KK, Phillips TL, Silverberg IJ. Combined radiotherapy and chemotherapy with bleomycin and methotrexate for advanced inoperable head and neck cancer: Update of a Northern California Oncology Group randomized trial. J Clin Oncol 1987;5:1410–1418.

275. Eschwege F, Sancho-Garnier H, Gerard JP, et al. Ten-year results of randomized trial comparing radiotherapy and concomitant bleomycin to radiotherapy alone in epidermoid carcinomas of the oropharynx: Experience of the European Organization for Research and Treatment of Cancer. NCI Monogr 1988;6:275–278.

276. Shigematsu Y, Sakai S, Fuchihata H. Recent trials in the treatment of maxillary sinus carcinoma with special reference to the chemical potentiation of radiation therapy. Acta Otolaryngol 1971;71:63–70.

277. Lo TCM, Wiley AL Jr, Ainfield FJ, et al. Combined radiation therapy and 5-fluorouracil for advanced squamous cell carcinoma of the oral cavity and oropharynx: A randomized study. AJR 1976;126:229–235.

278. Stefani S, Chung TS. Hydroxyurea and radiotherapy in head and neck cancer—long term results of a double-blind randomized prospective study. Radiat Oncol Biol Phys 1980;6:1398.

279. Weissberg JB, Son YH, Papac RJ, et al. Randomized clinical trial of mitomycin C as an adjunct to radiotherapy in head and neck cancer. Int J Radiat Oncol Biol Phys 1989;17:3–9.

280. Al-Sarraf M, Pajak TF, Marcial VA, et al. Concurrent radiotherapy and chemotherapy with cisplatin in inoperable squamous cell carcinoma of the head and neck: An RTOG study. Cancer 1986;59:259–265.

281. Crispino S, Tancini G, Barni S, et al. Simultaneous cisplatinum (CDDP) and radiotherapy in patients with locally advanced head and neck cancer. Proc Am Soc Clin Oncol [Abstract] 1987;6:123.

282. Wheeler R, Salter M, Stephens S, et al. Simultaneous high-dose cisplatin (HDCP) and radiation therapy (RT) for unresectable squamous cancer of the head and neck (SCH&N): A phase I/II study [Abstract]. In: Proceedings of the 2nd International Head and Neck Research Conference, Arlington, VA, September 10–12, 1987.

283. Haselow RE, Warshaw MG, Oken MM. Radiation alone versus radiation with weekly low dose cisplatinum in unresectable cancer of the head and neck. In: Fee WE Jr, Goepfert H, Johns ME, et al, eds. Head and Neck Cancer. Vol 2. Philadelphia: BC Decker 1990:279–281.

284. Al-Sarraf M, Pajak TF, Marcial VA, et al. Concurrent radiotherapy and chemotherapy with cisplatin in inoperable squamous cell carcinoma of the head and neck: An RTOG study. Cancer 1987;59:259–265.

285. Taylor SG IV, Murthy AK, Caldarelli DD, et al. Combined simultaneous cisplatin/fluorouracil chemotherapy and split course radiation in head and neck. J Clin Oncol 1989;7:846–856.

286. Keegan P, Pillsbury HR, Weissler M, et al. Simultaneous cisplatinum-5FU and radiotherapy alone in advanced squamous cell carcinoma of the head and neck. Proc Am Soc Clin Oncol [Abstract] 1988;7:157.

287. Wendt TG, Hartenstein RC, Wustrow TPU, et al; Improved two years survival and local control rate in locally advanced squamous cell carcinoma (SCC) of the head and neck by simultaneous chemo (CT)-radiotherapy (RT): Progress report. Proc Am Soc Clin Oncol [Abstract] 1987;6;126.

288. Murphy AK, Showel J, Taylor SG, et al. Treatment of advanced head and neck cancer with concomitant radiation and chemotherapy [Abstract]. In: Proceedings of the 2nd International Head and Neck Research Conference, Arlington, VA, September 10–12, 1987.

289. Gandia D, Wibault P, Recondo G, et al. High-volume advanced head and neck squamous cell cancer (HVA H+N SCC) treated with full dose simultaneous 7 weeks (wks) chemoradiotherapy (CH-RT). Proc Am Soc Clin Oncol [Abstract] 1991;10:201.

290. Schmotzer JA, Massouh M, Adelstein D, et al. Simultaneous (STM) chemoradiotherapy (CRT) with continuous infusion (CI) cisplatin (DDP) and 5-fluorouracil (5FU) for locally advanced squamous cell carcinoma of the head and neck (SCCHN). Proc Am Soc Clin Oncol [Abstract] 1991;10:202.

290. Parvinen LM, Parvinen M, Nordman E, et al. Combined bleomycin treatment and radiation therapy in squamous cell carcinoma of the head and neck region. Acta Radiol Oncol 1985;24:487–489.

291. Osoba D, Flores AD, Jay JH, et al. Phase I study of concurrent carboplatin and radiotherapy in previously untreated patients with stage III and IV head and neck cancer. Head Neck 1991;31:217–223.

292. Schnabel T, Zamboglou N, Pape H, et al. Phase II trial with carboplatin and simultaneous radiation in previously untreated advanced squamous cell carcinoma of the head and neck (SCCHN). Proc Am Soc Clin Oncol [Abstract] 1990;9:176.

293. Volling P, Mueller RP, Staar S, et al. Pilot study with carboplatin (CBDCA) and simultaneous accelerated radiation (RT) in advanced squamous cell carcinoma of the head and neck (SCCHN). Proc Am Soc Clin Oncol [Abstract] 1990;9:176.

294. Wallner JE, Li GC. Effect of cisplatin resistance on cellular radiation response. Int J Radiat Oncol Biol Phys 1987;13:587–591.

295. Interim report from the SECOG participants: A randomized trial of combined multidrug chemotherapy and radiotherapy in advanced squamous cell carcinoma of the head and neck. Eur J Surg Oncol 1986;12:289–295.

296. Cognetti F, Carlini P, Pinnaro P. Prospective randomized trial of neoadjuvant cisplatin and 5-FU followed by radiotherapy versus concurrent cisplatin and radiotherapy in locally advanced head and neck squamous cell cancer: Preliminary results [Abstract]. In: Proceedings of the 2nd International Conference on Head and Neck Cancer, Boston, MA, July 31–August 5, 1988.

297. Adelstein DJ, Sharan VM, Earle S, et al. Simultaneous versus sequential combined technique therapy for squamous cell head and neck cancer. Cancer 1990;65:1685–1691.

298. Vannetzel JM, Dray M, Murtley AK, et al. T and N patterns of failure with cisplatin 15-FU infusion chemotherapy and radiation in unresectable head and neck cancer. Proc Am Soc Clin Onc [Abstract] 1990;9:173.

299. Merlano M, Bargarino G, Benasso M, et al. Combined chemotherapy and radiation therapy in advanced inoperable squamous cell carcinoma of the head and neck. Cancer 1991;67:915–921.

300. Jacobs C, Makuch R. Efficacy of adjuvant chemotherapy for patients with resectable head and neck cancer: A subset analysis of the head and neck contracts program. J Clin Oncol 1990;8:838–847.

301. Johnson JT, Myers EN, Schramm VL, et al. Adjuvant chemotherapy for high-risk squamous-cell carcinoma of the head and neck. J Clin Oncol 1987;5:456–458.

302. Axelrod RS, Mohr R, Abayomi O, et al. CDDP, 5FU, RT in advanced head and neck cancer. Proc Am Soc Clin Oncol [Abstract] 1987;6:133.

303. Weaver A, Jacobs J, Al-Sarraf M, et al. Postoperative chemotherapy followed by radiotherapy in patients with advanced and resectable head and neck cancer [Abstract]. In: Proceedings of the International Conference on Head and Neck Cancer: Chemotherapy II, Baltimore, July 22–27, 1984.

304. Bitter K. Postoperative chemotherapy versus postoperative cobalt 60 radiation in patients with advanced oral carcinoma—report on a randomized study. Head Neck Surg 1981;264.

305. Huang AT, Fisher SR, Cole TB, et al. A study of postoperative and/or postradiation adjuvant chemotherapy [Abstract]. In: Proceedings of the 2nd International Head and Neck Oncology Research Conference, Arlington, VA, September 10–12, 1987.

306. Domenge C, Marandas P, Vignoud J, et al. Post-surgical adjuvant chemotherapy in extracapsular spread invaded lymph node (N+ R+) of epidermoid carcinoma of the head and neck: A randomized multicentric trial [Abstract #108]. In: Proceeding of the 2nd International Conference on Head and Neck Cancer: Combined Therapy, Boston, 1988.

307. Laramore G, Scott CB, Al-Sarraf M, et al. Adjuvant chemotherapy for resectable head and neck cancer: Report on intergroup study 0034. Int J Rad Oncol Biol Phys 1992;23: 705–713.

308. Lippman SM, Hong WK. Retinoid chemoprevention of upper aerodigestive carcinogenesis.

309. Lippman SM, Hong WK. Second malignant tumors in head and neck squamous cell carcinoma: The overshadowing threat for patients with early-stage disease. Int J Radiat Oncol Biol Phys 1989;17:691–694.

310. Sporn B. Approaches to prevention of epithelial cancer during the preneoplastic period. Cancer Res 1976;36:2699–2702.

311. Sporn B, Dunlop N, Newton D, et al. Prevention of chemical carcinogenesis by vitamin A and its synthetic analogs (retinoids). Fed Proc 1976;35:1332–1338.

312. Lotan R. Effects of vitamin A and its analogs (retinoids) on normal and neoplastic cells. Biochim Biophys Acta 1980;605:33–91.

313. Bollag W. Vitamin A and retinoids: From nutrition to pharmacotherapy in dermatology and oncology. Lancet 1983;1:860–863.

314. Lippman SM, Kessler JF, Meyskens FL Jr. Retinoids as preventive and therapeutic anticancer agents. Cancer Treat Rep 1987;71:391–405, 493–515.

315. Evans RM. The steroid and thyroid hormone receptor superfamily. Science 1988;240: 889–895.

316. Warrell RP Jr, Frankel S, Scheinberg DA, et al. All *trans* retinoic acid in acute promyelocytic leukemia: Preliminary U.S. clinical experience. Blood 1990;76(10, Suppl 1):1327.

317. Kraemer KH, DiGiovana JJ, Moshell AN, et al. Prevention of skin cancer in xeroderma pigmentosum with the use of oral isotretinoin. N Engl J Med 1988;318:1633–1637.

318. Wolbach SB, Howe PR. Tissue changes following deprivation of fat soluble A vitamin. J Exp Med 1925;42:753–777.

319. Slaughter DP, Southwick HW, Smejkal W. "Field cancerization" in oral stratification squamous epithelium: Clinical implications of multicentric origin. 1953;Cancer 6: 963–968.

320. Lippman SM, Lee JS, Lotan R, et al. Biomarkers as intermediate endpoints in chemoprevention trials. JNCI 1990;82:555–560.

321. Wulf K. Zur vitamin A behandlung der leukoplakien. Arch Klin Exp Derm 1957;206–495.

322. Silverman S, Eisenberg E, Renstrup G. A study of the effects of high doses of vitamin A on oral leukoplakia (hyperkeratosis), including toxicity, liver function and skeletal metabolism. J Oral Ther Pharm 1965;2:9–23.

323. Stich HF, Hornby AP, Dunn BP. A pilot beta-carotene intervention trial with inunits using smokeless tobacco. Int J Cancer 1985;36:321–327.

324. Stich HF, Rosin MP, Hornby AP, et al. Remission of oral leukoplakias and micronuclei in tobacco/betal quid chewers treated with beta-carotene and with beta-carotene plus vitamin A. Int J Cancer 1988;42:195–199.

325. Stich HF, Hornby AP, Mathew B, et al. Response of oral leukoplakias to the administration of vitamin A. Cancer Lett 1988;40:93–101.

326. Garewal HS, Meyskens FL, Killen D, et al. Response of oral leukoplakia to beta-carotene. J Clin Oncol 1990;8:1715–1720.

327. Toma S, Albanese E, De Lorenz M, et al. Aspetti biologici e prospettive applicative della chemioprevenzione nel cancro delle vie aerodigestive superiori. Acta Otorhinol Ital 1990;10:41–54.

328. Koch HF. Biochemical treatment of precancerous oral lesions: The effectiveness of various analogues of retinoic acid. J Maxillofac Surg 1978;6:59–63.

329. Koch HF. Effect of retinoids on precancerous lesions of oral mucosa. In: Orfanos CE, et al, eds. Retinoids: Advances in basic research and therapy. Berlin: Springer-Verlag, 1981:307–312.

330. Cordero AA, Allevato MAJ, Barclay CA, et al. Treatment of lichen planus and leukoplakia with the oral retinoid RO 10–9359. In: Orfanos CE, et al, eds. Retinoids: Advances in basic research and therapy. Berlin, Springer-Verlag, 1981:273–278.

331. Shah JP, Strong EW, DeCosse JJ, et al. Effect of retinoids on oral leukoplakia. Am J Surg 1983;146:466–470.

332. Hong WK, Endicott J, Itri LM, et al. 13-*cis*-Retinoic acid in the treatment of oral leukoplakia. N Engl J Med 1986;315:1501–1505.

333. Lippman SM, Toth BB, Batsakis JG, et al. Phase III trial to retain remission in oral premalignancy: Low-dose 13-cRA versus beta carotene. Proc Am Soc Clin Oncol [Abstract] 1992;11:781.

334. Cooper JS, Pajak TF, Rubin P, et al. Second malignancies in patients who have head and neck cancers: Incidence, effect on survival and implications for chemoprevention based on the RTOG experience. Int J Radiat Oncol Biol Phys 1989;17:449–456.

335. Tepperman BS, Fitzpatrick PJ. Second respiratory and upper aerodigestive tract cancers after oral cancer. Lancet 1981;2:547–549.

336. Vikram B. Changing patterns of failure in advanced head and neck cancer. Arch Otolaryngol 1984;110:564–565.

337. Lippman SM, Kessler JF, Al-Sarraf M, et al. Treatment of advanced squamous cell carcinoma of the head and neck with isotretinoin: A phase II randomized trial. Invest New Drugs 1988;6:51–56.

338. Hong WK, Lippman SM, Itri LM, et al. Prevention of second primary tumors with isotretinoin in squamous cell carcinoma of the head and neck. N Engl J Med 1990;323: 795–801.

339. Warren S, Gates O. Multiple primary malignant tumors: A survey of the literature and statistical study. Am J Cancer 1932;51:1358–1403.

Nasal Cavity and Paranasal Sinuses

342. Rousch GC. Epidemiology of cancer of the nose and paranasal sinuses: Current concepts. Head Neck Surg 1979;2:3–11.

343. Torjussen W, Haug FMS, Olsen A, Andersen I. Concentration and distribution of heavy metals in nasal mucosa of nickel-exposed workers. Acta Otolaryngol 1977;86: 449–463.

344. Pedersen EA, Hogetveit AC, Andersen A. Cancer of the respiratory organs among workers at a nickel refinery in Norway. Int J Cancer 1973;12:32–41.

345. Ironside P, Matthews J. Adenocarcinoma of the nose and paranasal sinuses in woodworkers in the state of Victoria, Australia. Cancer 1975;36:1115–1121.

346. Acheson ED, Hadfield EH, Macbeth RG. Carcinoma of the nasal cavity and accessory sinuses in woodworkers. Lancet 1967;1:311–312.

347. Acheson ED, Cowdell RH, Jolles B. Nasal cancer in the Northamptonshire boot and shoe industry. Br Med J [Clin Res] 1970;1:385–393.

348. Buda JA, Conley JJ, Rankow R. Carcinoma of the maxillary sinus following thoratrast instillation. Am J Surg 1963;106:868–873.

349. Moss-Salentijn L. Anatomy and embryology. In: Blitzer A, Lawson W, Friedman WH, eds. Surgery of the paranasal sinuses. Philadelphia: WB Saunders, 1985:1–23.

350. Sisson GA, Bytell DE, Becker SP, Ruge D. Carcinoma of the paranasal sinuses and cranial-facial resection. J Larynogol Otol 1976;90:59–70.

351. Robin PE, Powell DJ. Regional node involvement and distant metastasis in carcinoma of the nasal cavity and paranasal sinuses. J Laryngol Otol 1980;94:301–309.

352. Jackson RT, Fitz-Hugh GS, Constable WC. Malignant neoplasms of the nasal cavities and paranasal sinuses: A retrospective study. Laryngoscope 1977;87:726–736.

353. Bosch A, Vallecillo L, Frias Z. Cancer of the nasal cavity. Cancer 1976;37:1458–1463.

354. Sisson GA, Johnson NE, Amiri CS. Cancer of the maxillary sinus: Clinical classification and management. Ann Otol Rhinol Laryngol 1963;72:1050–1059.

355. Birt BD, Braint TDR. The management of malignant tumors of the maxillary sinus. Otolaryngol Clin North Am 1976;9:249–262.

356. Price JC, Holliday MJ, Johns ME, et al. The versatile midface degloving approach. Laryngoscope 1988;98:291–299.

357. Sessions RB, Humphrey DH. Technical modifications of the medial maxillectomy. Arch Otolaryngol 1983;109:575.

358. Wong GY, Cummings B. The place of radiation therapy in the treatment of squamous cell carcinoma of the nasal vestibule. Acta Oncol 1988;27:203–207.

359. Kirchner JC, Sasaki CT. Reconstructive surgery of the sinuses. In: Thawley SE, Panje WR, Batsakis JG, Lindberg RD, eds. Comprehensive management of head and neck tumors. Philadelphia: WB Saunders, 1987:433–444.

360. Jesse RH, Butler JJ, Healey JE, et al. Paranasal sinuses and nasal cavity. In: MacComb WS, Fletcher GH, eds. Cancer of the head and neck. Baltimore, Williams & Wilkins, 1967:329–356.

361. Spiro JD, Soo KC, Spiro RA. Squamous carcinoma of the nasal cavity and paranasal sinuses. Am J Surg 1991;158:328–332.

362. Lewis JS, Castro EB. Cancer of the nasal cavity and paranasal sinuses. J Laryngol Otol 1972;86:255–262.

363. Levendag P, Pomp J. Radiation therapy of squamous cell carcinoma of the nasal vestibule. Int J Radiat Oncol Biol Phys 1990;19:1363–1367.

364. Wang CC. Treatment of carcinoma of the nasal vestibule by irradiation. Cancer 1976;38:100–106.

365. Wang C, Cummings B, Elhakim T, et al. External irradiation for squamous cell carcinoma of the nasal vestibule. Int J Radiat Oncol Bio Phys 1986;12:1943–1946.

366. Ketcham AS, Chretien PB, Van Buren JM, et al. The ethmoid sinuses: A re-evaluation of surgical resection. Am J Surg 1973;126:469–476.

367. Terz JJ, Young HF, Lawrence W. Combined craniofacial resection for locally advanced carcinoma of the head and neck. Am J Surg 1980;140:618–622.

368. Parsons J, Mendenhall W, Mancuso A, et al. Malignant tumors of nasal cavity and ethmoid and sphenoid sinuses. Int J Radiat Oncol Biol Phys 1988;14:11–22.

369. Frich J. Treatment of advanced squamous carcinoma of the maxillary sinus by irradiation. Int J Radiat Oncol Biol Phys 1982;8:1453–1459.

370. Amendola B, Eisert D, Hazra T, et al. Carcinoma of the maxillary antrum: Surgery or radiation therapy? Int J Radiat Oncol Biol Phys 1981;7:743–746.

371. Yu-Hua H, Gui-Yi T, Yu-Quin Q, et al. Comparison of pre-and post-operative radiation in the combined treatment of carcinoma of the maxillary sinus. Int J Radiat Oncol Biol Phys 1982;8:1045–1049.

372. Zaharia M, Salem L, Travezan R, et al. Post-operative radiation therapy in the management of cancer of the maxillary sinus. Int J Radiat Oncol Biol Phys 1989;17:967–971.

373. Harrison L, Pfister D, Fass D, et al. Concomitant chemotherapy-radiation therapy followed by hyperfractionated radiation therapy for advanced unresectable head and neck cancer. Int J Radiat Oncol Biol Phys 1991;21:703–708.

374. Sato Y, Morita M, Takahashi H, et al. Combined surgery, radiotherapy, and regional chemotherapy in carcinoma of the paranasal sinuses. Cancer 1970;25:571–579.

375. Goepfert H, Jesse RH, Lindberg RD. Arterial infusion and radiation therapy in the treatment of advanced cancer of the nasal cavity and paranasal sinuses. Am J Surg 1973;126:464–468.

376. Moseley HS, Thomas LR, Everts EC, et al. Advanced squamous cell carcinoma of the maxillary sinus: Results of combined regional infusion chemotherapy, radiation therapy and surgery. Am J Surg 1981;141:522–525.

377. Shibuya H, Suzuki S, Horiuchi JI, et al. Reappraisal of trimodal combination therapy for maxillary sinus carcinoma. Cancer 1982;50:2790–2794.

378. Nervi C, Arcangeli G, Badaracco G, et al. The relevance of tumor size and cell kinetics as predictors of radiation response in head and neck cancer: A randomized study on

the effect of intraarterial chemotherapy followed by radiotherapy. Cancer 1978;41: 900–906.

379. Dimery IW, Lee YY, VanTassel P, et al. Combined intra-arterial (I.A.) and systemic chemotherapy (CT) for paranasal sinus carcinoma (PNSC). Proc Am Soc Clin Oncol [Abstract] 1988;7:150.

380. LoRusso P, Tapazoglou E, Kish JA, et al. Chemotherapy for paranasal sinus carcinoma: A 10-year experience at Wayne State University. Cancer 1988;62:1–5.

381. Knegt PP, Jong PC, van Angel JG, et al. Carcinoma of the paranasal sinuses: Results of a prospective pilot study. Cancer 1985;56:57–62.

Nasopharynx

381. Miller D. The etiology of nasopharyngeal cancer and its management. Otolaryngol Clin North Am 1980;13:167–175.

382. Henderson BE, Louie E, Jing JSH, Buell P, Gardner M. Risk factors associated with nasopharyngeal carcinoma. N Engl J Med 1976;295:1101–1106.

383. Yu MC, Ho JHC, Lai SH, Henderson BE. Cantonese-style salted fish as a cause of nasopharyngeal carcinoma: Report of a case-control study in Hong Kong. Cancer Res 1986;46:956–961.

384. Old LJ, Boyse EA, Oettgen HF, et al. Precipitating antibody in human serum to an antigen present in cultured Burkitt's lymphoma cells. Proc Natl Acad Sci USA 1966;56: 1699–1704.

385. Zur Hausen H, Schulte-Holthausen H, Klein G, et al. Epstein-Barr virus DNA in biopsies of Burkitt tumors and anaplastic carcinoma of the nasopharynx. Nature 1970;228:1056–1059.

386. Fahraeus R, Fu HL, Ernberg I, et al. Expression of Epstein-Barr virus-encoded proteins in nasopharyngeal carcinoma. Int J Cancer 1988;42:329–338.

387. Chan SH, Day HE, Kunaratnam N, Chia KB, Simons MJ. HLA and nasopharyngeal carcinoma in Chinese—a further study. Int J Cancer 1983;32:171–176.

388. Simons MJ, Wee GB, Goh EH, et al. Immunogenetic aspects of nasopharyngeal carcinoma: IV. Increased risk in Chinese of nasopharyngeal carcinoma associated with a Chinese related HCA profile (A2, Singapore 2). JNCI 1976;57:977–980.

389. International Histological Classification of Tumors, No. 19. Histological Typing of Upper Respiratory Tract Tumors. Geneva: World Health Organization, 1978:32–33.

390. Baker SR. Nasopharyngeal carcinoma: Clinical course and results of therapy. Head Neck Surg 1980;3:8–14.

391. Mesic JB, Fletcher GH, Goepfert H. Megavoltage irradiation of epithelial tumors of the nasopharynx. Int J Radiat Oncol Bio Phys 1981;7:447–453.

392. Neel HB III. Nasopharyngeal carcinoma: Clinical presentation, diagnosis, treatment, and prognosis. Otolaryngol Clin North Am 1985;18:479–493.

393. Chen KY, Fletcher GH. Malignant tumors of the nasopharynx. Radiology 1971;99: 165–171.

394. Hoppe RT, Williams J, Warnke R, et al. Carcinoma of the nasopharynx: Significance of histology. Int J Radiat Oncol Biol Phys 1978;4:199–205.

395. Yu Z, Xu G, Huang Y, et al. Value of computed tomography in staging the primary lesion (T-staging) of nasopharyngeal carcinoma (NPC): An analysis of 54 patients with special reference to the parapharyngeal space. Int J Radiat Oncol Biol Phys 1985;11:2143–2147.

396. Sham JST, Choy D. Prognostic value of paranasopharyngeal extension of nasopharyngeal carcinoma on local control and short term survival. Head Neck 1991;13: 298–310.

397. Celai E, Olmi T, Chiavacci A, et al. Computed tomography in nasopharyngeal carcinoma: II. Impact on survival. Int J Radiat Oncol Biol Phys 1990;19:1177–1182.

398. Kutcher GJ, Kuks Z, Brenner H, et al. Three-dimensional photon treatment planning for carcinoma of the nasopharynx. Int J Radiat Oncol Biol Phys 1991;21:169–182.

399. Mesic JB, Fletcher GH, Goepfert H. Megavoltage irradiation of endothelial of the nasopharynx. Int J Radiat Oncol Biol Phys 1981;7:447–453.

400. Wang CC. Re-irradiation of recurrent nasopharyngeal carcinoma: Treatment techniques and results. Int J Radiat Oncol Biol Phys 1987;13:953–956.

401. Harrison LB, Weissberg JB. A technique for interstitial nasopharyngeal brachytherapy. Int J Radiat Oncol Biol Phys 1987;13:451–453.

402. Harrison LB, Sessions RB, Fass DE, et al. Nasopharyngeal brachytherapy using access via a transpalatal flap. Am J Surg (in press).

403. Vikram B, Hilaris B. Transnasal permanent interstitial implantation of carcinoma of the nasopharynx. Int J Radiat Oncol Biol Phys 1984;10:153–155.

404. McNeese MB, Fletcher GH. Re-treatment of recurrent nasopharyngeal carcinoma. Radiology 1981;138:191–193.

405. Harrison LB, Nori B, Hilaris B, et al. Nasopharynx. In: The Interstitial Collaborative Working Group, ed. Interstitial brachytherapy. New York, Raven Press, 1990;95–109.

406. Fee WE, Gilmer PA, Goffinet DR. Surgical management of recurrent nasopharyngeal carcinoma after radiation failure at the primary site. Laryngoscope 1988;98:1220–1226.

407. Fisch U. The infratemporal fossa approach for nasopharyngeal tumors. Laryngoscope 1983;93:36–44.

408. Holoye PY, Byers RM, Gard DA, et al. Combination chemotherapy of head and neck. Cancer 1978;42:1661.

409. Goepfert H, Moran MG, Lindberg R, et al. Chemotherapy of advanced nasopharyngeal carcinoma [Abstract]. Proc Am Soc Clin Oncol 1981;22:427.

410. Cortes EP, Kalra J, Amin VC, et al. Chemotherapy for head and neck cancer relapsing after radiotherapy. Cancer 1981;47:1966–1970.

411. Huang AT, Cole TB, Fishburns R, et al. Chemotherapy for nasopharyngeal carcinoma. In: Grundman E, Krueger GRF, Ablashi DV, eds. Nasopharyngeal carcinomas, Cancer campaign. Vol 5. Stuttgart: Gustav Fischer Verlag, 1981.

412. Decker DA, Drelichman A, Al-Sarraf M. Chemotherapy for nasopharyngeal carcinoma: A ten-year experience. Cancer 1983;52:602–605.

413. Airoldi M, Pedani F, Gabriele P, et al. Combined chemotherapy for recurrent and metastatic nasopharyngeal carcinoma. J Chemother 1989;1:272–276.

414. Lai GM, Ng KT. High-dose 5-fluorouracil plus cis-platinum in treatment of advanced nasopharyngeal carcinoma (NPC). Proc Am Soc Clin Oncol [Abstract] 1986;5:143.

415. Cvitkovic E, Boussen H, Azli N. Increased complete response percentage with BEC (bleomycin -bleo-, epirubicin -epi-, cisplatinum -cddp-) in metastatic/advanced (ms/adv) undifferentiated carcinoma nasopharyngeal type (ucnt). Proc Am Soc Clin Oncol [Abstract] 1988;7:155.

416. Leung WT, Shiu W, Tao M, et al. Phase II study of carboplatin and 5-FU combination chemotherapy in treatment of advanced NPC (nasopharyngeal carcinoma). Proc Am Soc Clin Oncol [Abstract] 1991;10:199.

417. Marchini S, Licitra L, Grandi C, et al. Cisplatin and fluorouracil in recurrent and/or disseminated nasopharyngeal carcinoma (NPC). Proc Am Soc Clin Oncol [Abstract] 1991;10:202.

418. Cvitkovic E, Mahjoubi R, Lianes P, et al. 5-Fluorouracil (FU), mitomycin (M), epirubicin (E) cisplatin (P), in recurrent and/or metastatic (REC/MTS) undifferentiated nasopharyngeal carcinoma (UCNT): Preliminary activity/toxicity report. Proc Am Soc Clin Oncol [Abstract] 1991;10:200.

419. Dimery IW, Jacobs C, Tseng A, et al. Recombinant interferon-gamma in the treatment of recurrent NPC. J Biol Resp Modif 1989;8:221–226.

420. Boussen H, Cvitkovic E, Wendling JL, et al. Chemotherapy of metastatic and/or recurrent undifferentiated nasopharyngeal carcinoma with cisplatin, bleomycin, and fluorouracil. J Clin Oncol 1991;9:1675–1681.

421. Wang CC. Improved local control of nasopharyngeal carcinoma after intracavitary brachytherapy boost. Am J Clin Oncol 1991;14:5–8.

422. Hoppe R, Goffinet B, Bagshaw M. Carcinoma of the nasopharynx—eighteen years experience with megavoltage radiation therapy. Cancer 1976;37:2605–2617.

423. Bedwinek JM, Perez CA, Keys DJ. Analysis of failure after definitive irradiation for epidermoid carcinoma of the nasopharynx. Cancer 1980;45:2725–2729.

424. Mesic JB, Fletcher GH, Goepfert H. Megavoltage Irradiation of epithelial tumors of the nasopharynx. Int J Radiat Oncol Biol Phys 1981;7:447–453.

425. Million RR, Cassisi NJ. Nasopharynx. In: Million RR, Cassisi NJ, eds. Management of head and neck cancer—a multidisciplinary approach. Philadelphia: JB Lippincott, 1984:445–465.

426. Vikram B, Strong E, Manolatos S, et al. Improved cervical and carcinoma of the nasopharynx. Head Neck Surg 1984;7:123–128.

427. Peters LJ, Batsakis JG, Goepfert H, et al. The diagnosis and management of nasopharyngeal carcinoma in caucasians. In: Williams CJ, Krikorian JG, Green MR, et al, eds. Textbook of uncommon cancer. New York: John Wiley & Sons, 1988:975–1006.

428. Galligioni E, Carbone A, Tirelli U, et al. Combined chemotherapy with doxorubicin, bleomycin, vinblastine, dacarbazine and radiotherapy for advanced lymphoepithelioma. Cancer Treat Rep 1982;66:1207–1210.

429. Rahuma M, Rakowsky E, Barzilay J, et al. Carcinoma of the nasopharynx: An analysis of 91 cases and a comparison of differing treatment approaches. Cancer 1986;58: 843–849.

430. Hill BT, Price LA, MacRae KD. The promising role of safe initial non-cisplatin-containing combination chemotherapy in nasopharyngeal tumors. Cancer Invest 1987;5: 517–522.

431. Khoury GG, Paterson ICM. Nasopharyngeal carcinoma: A review of cases treated by radiotherapy and chemotherapy. Clin Radiol 1987;38:17–20.

432. Clark JR, Norris CM Jr, Dreyfuss AI. Nasopharyngeal carcinoma: The Dana-Farber Cancer Institute experience with 24 patients treated with induction chemotherapy and radiotherapy. Ann Otol Rhinol Laryngol 1987;96:608–614.

433. Dimery IW, Legha SS, Peters LJ, et al. Adjuvant chemotherapy for advanced nasopharyngeal carcinoma. Cancer 1987;60:943–949.

434. Tannock I, Payne D, Cummings B, et al. Sequential chemotherapy and radiation for nasopharyngeal cancer: Absence of long-term benefit despite a high rate of tumor response to chemotherapy. J Clin Oncol 1987;5:629–634.

435. Zidan J, Kuten A, Cohen Y, et al. Multidrug chemotherapy using bleomycin, methotrexate, and cisplatin combined with radical radiotherapy in advanced head and neck cancer. Cancer 1987;59:24–26.

436. Rossi A, Molinari R, Boracchi P, et al. Adjuvant chemotherapy with vincristine, cyclophosphamide, and doxorubicin after radiotherapy in local-regional nasopharyngeal cancer: Results of a 4-year multicenter randomized study. J Clin Oncol 1988;6:1401–1410.

437. Souhami L, Rabinowits M. Combined treatment in carcinoma of the nasopharynx. Laryngoscope 1988;98:881–883.

438. En-Pee Z, Pei-Gun L, Kuang-Long C, et al. Radiation therapy of nasopharyngeal carcinoma: Prognostic factors based on a 10-year follow-up of 1302 patients. Int J Radiat Oncol Biol Phys 1989;16:301–305.

439. Atichartakarn V, Kraiphibul P, Clongsusuek P, et al. Nasopharyngeal carcinoma: Result of treatment with cis-diamminedichloroplatinum II, 5-fluorouracil, and radiation therapy. Int J Radiat Oncol Biol Phys 1988;14:461–469.

440. Tsujii H, Kamada T, Tsuji H, et al. Improved results in the treatment of nasopharyngeal carcinoma using combined radiotherapy and chemotherapy. Cancer 1989;63:1668–1672.

441. Al-Sarraf M, Pajak TF, Cooper JS, et al. Chemo-radiotherapy in patients with locally advanced nasopharyngeal carcinoma: A Radiation Therapy Oncology Group study. J Clin Oncol 1990;8:1342–1351.

442. Dimery IW, Goepfert H, Peters LJ, et al. Survival update of advanced nasopharyngeal

carcinoma (NPC) treated with neoadjuvant chemotherapy (CT). Proc Am Soc Clin Oncol [Abstract] 1991;10:197.

443. Boussen H, Benna F, Jallouli M, et al. Primary chemotherapy (CT) with ADR-BLE-CDDP (PROT 1) versus ADR-PLAT (PROT II) before radiotherapy (RT) in undifferentiated nasopharyngeal carcinoma (UNPC): Two years analysis and natural history after CT. Proc of Am Soc Clin Oncol [Abstract] 1991;10:203.

444. Bachouchi M, Lianes P, Armand JP, et al. Two years follow up on bleomycin (B), epirubicin (E), cisplatin (P) in locally advanced undifferentiated carcinoma nasopharyngeal type (UCNT). Proc Am Soc Clin Oncol [Abstract] 1991;10:201.

Oral Cavity

446. Menck HR, Garfinkel L, Dodd GD. Preliminary report of the National Cancer Data Base. CA 1991;41:7–39.

447. Cancers of the oral cavity and pharynx: A statistics review. Monograph 1973–1987. Bethesda, MD: U.S. Department of Health and Human Services, 1991.

448. Wynder EL, Stellman SD. Impact of long-term filter cigarette usage on lung and larynx cancer risk: A case-control study. JNCI 1979;62:471–477.

449. Spitz MR, Fueger JJ, Goepfert H, Hong WK, Newell GR. Squamous cell carcinoma of the upper aerodigestive tract: A case comparison analysis. Cancer 1988;61:203–208.

450. Mashberg A, Garfinkel L, Harris S. Alcohol as a primary risk factor in oral squamous carcinoma. CA 1981;31:146–155.

451. Hoffmann D, Hecht SS. Nicotine-derived N-nitrosamines and tobacco-related cancer—current status and future directions. Cancer Res 1985;45:935–944.

452. Schottenfeld D. Alcohol as a co-factor in the etiology of cancer. Cancer 1979;43:1962–1966.

453. Schantz SP, Hsu TC. Head and neck cancer patients express increased clastogen-induced chromosome fragility. Head Neck 1989;11:337–343.

454. German J, ed. Chromosome mutation and neoplasia. New York: Alan R. Liss, 1983.

455. Guengerich FP. Roles of cytochrome p-450 enzymes in chemical carcinogenesis and cancer chemotherapy. Cancer Res 1988;48:2946–2954.

456. McLaughlin JK, Gridley G, Block G, et al. Dietary factors in oral and pharyngeal cancer. JNCI 1988;80:1237–1243.

457. Winn DM, Ziegler RG, Pickle LW, Gridley G, Blot WJ, Hoover RN. Diet in the etiology of oral and pharyngeal cancer among women from the Southern United States. Cancer Res 1984;44:1216–1222.

458. Wynder EL, Hultberg S, Jacobsson F, et al. Oral cancer and mouthwash. JNCI 1983;70:255–260.

459. Spitz MR, Newell GR. Descriptive epidemiology of squamous cell carcinoma of the upper aerodigestive tract. Cancer Bull 1987;39:79–81.

460. Donald PJ. Marijuana smoking—possible cause of head and neck carcinoma in young patients. Otolaryngol Head Neck Surg 1986;94:517–521.

461. Shillitoe EJ, Greenspan D, Greenspan JS, et al. Immunoglobulin class of antibody to herpes simplex virus in patients with oral cancer. Cancer 1983;51:65–71.

462. DeVilliers EM, Weidauer H, Otta H, et al. Papillomavirus DNA in human tongue carcinomas. Int J Cancer 1985;36:575–579.

463. Dekmezian RH, Batsakis JG, Goepfert H. In situ hybridization of papillomavirus DNA in head and neck squamous cell carcinomas. Arch Otolaryngol Head Neck Surg 1987;113:819.

464. Watts SL, Brewer EE, Fry TL. Human papillomavirus DNA types in squamous cell carcinomas of the head and neck. Oral Surg Oral Med Oral Pathol 1991;7:701–707.

465. Bradford CR, Zacks SE, Androphy EJ, et al. Human papillomavirus DNA sequences in cell lines derived from head and neck squamous cell carcinomas. Otolaryngol Head Neck Surg 1990;104:303–310.

466. Baker SR. Risk factors in multiple carcinoma of the lip. Otolaryngol Head Neck Surg 1980;88:248–258.

467. Berger HM, Goldman R, Gonick HC, Waisman J. Epidermoid carcinoma of the lip after renal transplantation: Report of two cases. Arch Intern Med 1971;128:609–612.

468. Sack JG, Ford CN. Metastatic squamous cell carcinoma of the lip. Arch Otolaryngol 1978;104:282–286.

469. Baker SR, Krause CJ. Carcinoma of the lip. Laryngoscope 1980;90:19–27.

470. Nuutinen J, Karja J. Local and distant metastases in patients with surgically treated squamous cell carcinoma of the lip. Clin Otolaryngol 1980;6:415–421.

471. Heller KS, Shah JP. Carcinoma of the lip. Am J Surg 1979;138:600–603.

472. Mendenhall WM, Million RR, Bova EJ. Analysis of time-dose factors in clinically positive neck nodes treated with irradiation alone in squamous cell carcinoma of the head and neck. J Radiat Oncol Biol Phys 1984;10:639–650.

473. Frierson HF Jr, Cooper PH. Prognostic factors in squamous cell carcinoma of the lower lip. Hum Pathol 1986;17:346–351.

474. Byers RM, O'Brien J, Waxler J. The therapeutic and prognostic implications of nerve invasion in cancer of the lower lip. Int J Radiat Oncol Biol Phys 1978;4:215–217.

475. Boddie HW, Fisher EP, Byers RM. Squamous carcinoma of the lower lip in patients under 40 years of age. South Med J 1977;70:711–712.

476. Baker SR, Krause CJ. Carcinoma of the lip. Laryngoscope 1980;90:19–27.

477. Abbé R. A new plastic operation for the relief of deformity due to double hairlip. Med Rec 1898;53:477.

478. Estlander JA. Eine Methods aus der einen Lippe Sulstanzverluste der Anderen zu Ersetzen. Arch Klin Chir 1872;14:622–628.

479. Karapandzic M. Reconstruction of lip defects by local arterial flaps. Br J Plast Surg 1974;27:93–99.

480. Baker SR, Krause CJ. Pedicle flaps in reconstruction of the lip. Facial Plast Surg 1983;1:61–69.

481. Webster JP. Crescenteric peri-alar cheek excision for upper flap advancement with a short history of upper lip repair. Plast Reconstr Surg 1935;27:434–444.

482. Jackson IT, ed. Local flaps in head and neck reconstruction. St. Louis: CV Mosby, 1985:327–412.

483. Harrison L, Fass D. Radiation therapy for oral cavity cancer. Dent Clin North Am 1990;34:205–222.

484. Fitzpatrick P. Cancer of the lip. J Otolaryngol 1984;13:32–36.

485. Jorgensen K, Elbrond O, Anderson A. Carcinoma of the lip—A series of 869 cases. Octaradiol Ther Phys Biol 1973;12:177–190.

486. Petrovich Z, Parker R, Luxten G, Kuisk H, Jepson J. Carcinoma of the lip in selective sites of head and neck skin: A clinical study of 896 patients. Radiol Ther Oncol 1987;8:11–17.

487. Cady B, Catlin D. Epidermoid carcinoma of the gum: A 20-year survey. Cancer 1969;23:551–569.

488. Euch JB, Kragh LV. Results of treatment of squamous cell carcinoma arising in mandibular gingiva. Arch Surg 1979;79:100–105.

489. Willen R, Nathanson A. Squamous cell carcinoma of the gingiva. Acta Otolaryngol 1973;75:299–300.

490. Torabinejad M, Rick GM. Squamous cell carcinoma of the gingiva. J Am Dent Assoc 1980;100:870–872.

491. Nathanson A, Jakobson A, Wersall J. Prognosis of squamous cell carcinoma of the gums. Acta Otolaryngol 1973;75:301–303.

492. Byers RM, Newman R, Russell N, et al. Results of treatment for squamous carcinoma of the lower gum. Cancer 1981;47:2236–2238.

493. Hidalgo, DA. Aesthetic improvements in free-flap mandible reconstruction. Am Soc Plast Reconstr Surg 1991;88:574–585.

494. Soo KC, Spiro RH, King W, et al. Squamous carcinoma of the gingiva: An update. Am J Surg 1988;156:281.

495. Million R, Cassisi N. Oral cavity. In: Million RR, Cassissi NJ, eds. Management of head and neck cancer—a multi-disciplinary approach. Philadelphia: JB Lippincott, 1984:295.

495a. Chen J, Katz RV, Krutchkoff DJ. Intraoral squamous cell carcinoma: Epidemiologic patterns in Connecticut from 1935 to 1985. Cancer 1990;66:1288–1296.

496. Shaha JP, Spiro RH, Shah JP, Strong EW. Squamous carcinoma of the floor of the mouth. Am J Surg 1984;148:455–461.

497. Guillamondegui OM, Oliver B, Hayden R. Cancer of the anterior floor of mouth: Selective choice of treatment and analysis of failures. Am J Surg 1980;140:56.

498. Soo K, Carter RC, O'Brien CJ, et al. Prognostic implications of perineural spread in squamous carcinoma of the head and neck. Laryngoscope 1986;96:1145.

499. Spiro RH, Huvos AG, Wong GY, et al. Predictive value of tumor thickness in squamous carcinoma confined to the tongue and floor of the mouth. Am J Surg 1986;152:351.

500. Arthur K, Farr HW. Prognostic significance of histologic grade in epidermoid carcinoma of the mouth and pharynx. Am J Surg 1972;124:489.

501. Gilbert E, Goffinet D, Bradshaw M. Carcinoma of the oral tongue and floor of mouth: Fifteen years' experience with linear excellarator therapy. Cancer 1975;35:1517–1524.

502. Mendenhall W, Van Ase W, Bover F, Million R. Analysis of time-dose factors in squamous cell carcinoma of the oral tongue and floor of mouth treated with radiation therapy alone. Int J Radiat Oncol Biol Phys 1981;7:1005–1011.

503. Mazeron J, Grimard L, Raynal M, et al. Iridium—192 curietherapy for T_1 and T_2 epidermoid carcinomas of the floor of mouth. Int J Radiat Oncol Biol Phys 1990;18:1299–1306.

504. Salibian AH, Rappaport I, Furnas DW, Auchauer BM. Microvascular reconstruction of the mandible. Am J Surg 1980;140:499–502.

505. Guillamondegui OM, Jesse RH. Surgical treatment of advanced carcinoma of the floor of the mouth. AJR 1976;126:1256–1259.

506. Wang CC, Doppke K, Biggs P. Intra-oral cone radiation therapy for selected carcinomas of the oral cavity. Int J Radiat Oncol Biol Phys 1983;9:1185–1189.

507. Fu K, Lichter A, Galante M. Carcinoma of the floor of mouth: An analysis of treatment results and the sites and causes of failure. Int J Radiat Oncol Biol Phys 1976;1:829–837.

508. Teichgraber J, Bowman J, Goepfert H. New test series for the functional evaluation of oral cavity cancer. Head Neck Surg 1985;8:9–20.

509. Kramer S, Gelber R, Snow J, et al. Combined radiation therapy and surgery in the management of advanced head and neck cancer: The final report of study 73-03 of the radiation therapy oncology group. Head Neck Surg 1987;10:19–30.

510. Shemen LJ, Klotz J, Shottenfeld D, Strong EW. Increase of tongue cancer in young men. JAMA 1984;252:1857.

511. Schantz SP, Byers RM, Goepfert H. Tobacco and cancer of the tongue in young adults. JAMA 1988;259:1943.

512. Lindberg R. Distribution of cervical lymph node metastases from squamous cell carcinoma of the upper respiratory and digestive tracts. Cancer 1972;29:1446–1449.

513. Strong EW. Carcinoma of the tongue. Otolaryngol Clin North Am 1979;12:107–113.

514. Yamamoto E, Mijakawa, Kohama G. Mode of invasion and lymph node metastasis in squamous cell carcinoma of the oral cavity. Head Neck Surg 1984;6:938.

515. Poleksic S, Kalwaic HJ. Prognostic value of vascular invasion in squamous cell carcinoma of the head and neck. Plast Reconstr Surg 1978;61:234.

516. Schantz SP, Byers RM, Goepfert H, Shallenberger RS, Beddingfield N. The implication of tobacco use in the young adult with head and neck cancer. Cancer 1988;62:1374–1380.

517. Decroix Y, Ghossein N. Experience of the Curie Institute in treatment of cancer of the mobile tongue: I. Treatment policy and results. Cancer 1981;47:496–502.

518. Spiro RH, Strong EW. Surgical treatment of carcinoma of the tongue. Surg Clin North Am 1974;54:233–239.

519. Callery CD, Spiro RH, Strong EW. Changing trends in the management of squamous carcinoma of the tongue. Am J Surg 1984;148:449.

520. Martin ME, Munster M, Sugarbaker ED. Cancer of the tongue. Arch Surg 1940;41:888-936.

520. Spiro R, Strong E. Epidermoid carcinoma of the mobile tongue—treatment by partial glossectomy alone. Am J Surg 1971;122:707-710.

521. Frazell EL, Lucas JC. Cancer of the tongue: Report of the management of 1554 patients. Cancer 1962;15:218-232.

522. Vikram B, Strong EW, Shah JP, Spiro R. Failure at the primary site following multimodality treatment in advanced head and neck cancer. Head Neck Surg 1984;1:720-723.

523. Ange D, Lindberg R, Guillamondegui O. Management of squamous cell carcinoma of the oral tongue and floor of mouth after excisional biopsy. Radiology 1975;116:143-146.

524. Bamberg M, Schulz U, Scherer E. Post-operative split course radiotherapy of squamous cell carcinoma of the oral tongue. Int J Radiat Oncol Biol Phys 1979;5:515-519.

525. Million R. Squamous cell carcinoma of the head and neck: Combined therapy: Surgery and post-operative radiation. Int J Radiat Oncol Biol Phys 1979;5:2161-2162.

526. Kroll SO, Hoffman S. Squamous cell carcinoma of the oral soft tissues—a statistical analysis of 14,253 cases by age, sex, and race of patients. J Am Dent Assoc 1976;92:571-574.

527. Evans JF, Shah JP. Epidermoid carcinoma of the palate. Am J Surg 1981;142:451.

528. Eneroth CM, Hjertman L, Moberger G. Squamous cell carcinoma of the palate. Acta Otolaryngol 1972;7:418-427.

529. Chung CK, Rahman SM, Lim ML, et al. Squamous cell carcinoma of the hard palate. Int J Radiat Oncol Biol Phys 1979;5:191-196.

530. Urist MM, O'Brien CJ, Soong SJ, et al. Squamous carcinoma of the buccal mucosa: Analysis of prognostic factors. Am J Surg 1987;154:411.

531. Bloom NO, Spiro RH. Carcinoma of the cheek mucosa: A retrospective analysis. Am J Surg 1980;140:556-559.

532. Nair M, Sankaranarayanan R, Padmanavhan T. Evaluation of the role of radiation therapy in the management of carcinoma of the buccal mucosa Cancer 1988;61:1326-1331.

533. Vegers J, Snow G, Van Der Wall I. Squamous cell carcinoma of the buccal mucosa—a review of 85 cases Archives of Otol. 1979;105:192-195.

Oropharynx

534. Whicker JH, DeSanto LW, Devine UD. Surgical treatment of squamous cell carcinoma of the base of the tongue. Laryngoscope 1972;82:1853-1861.

535. Harrold CC. Surgical treatment of cancer of the base of tongue. Am J Surg 1971;122:487-491.

536. Riley RW, Fee WE, Goffinet D, Cox R, Goode RI. Squamous cell carcinoma of the base of the tongue. Otolaryngol Head Neck Surg 1983;91:143-146.

537. Sessions DG. Surgical resection and reconstruction for cancer of the base of tongue. Otolaryngol Clin North Am 1983;16:309-322.

538. Marchetta FC, Sako K, Murphy JB. The periosteum of the mandible: An intraoral carcinoma. Am J Surg 1991;122:711-718.

539. Dupont J, Guillamondegui O, Jesse R. Surgical treatment of advanced carcinoma of the base of tongue. Am J Surg 1978;136:501-503.

540. Weber R, Gidley P, Morrison W, et al. Treatment selection for carcinoma of the base of tongue. Am J Surg 1990;160:415-419.

541. Harrison L, Sessions R, Strong E, et al. Brachytherapy as part of the definitive management of squamous cancer of the base of tongue. Int J Radiat Oncol Biol Phys 1989;17:1309-1312.

542. Harrison L, Zelefsky M, Sessions R, et al. The oncologic and functional outcome of base of tongue cancer treated with external beam radiation plus iridium-192 implant. Radiology 1992;184:267-270.

543. Goffinet D, Fee W, Wells J, et al. Iridium-192 pharyngoepiglottic fold implant—the key to successful treatment of base tongue carcinoma by radiation therapy. Cancer 1985;55:941-948.

544. Puthawala A, Syed A, Eads D, et al. Limited external beam and interstitial iridium-192 irradiation in the treatment of carcinoma of the base of tongue: A ten-year experience. Int J Radiat Oncol Biol Phys 1988;14:839-848.

545. Foote R, Parsons, J, Mendenhall W, et al. Interstitial implantation essential for successful radiotherapeutic treatment of base of tongue carcinoma? Int J Radiat Oncol Biol Phys 1990;18:1293-1298.

546. Housset M, Baillet F, Dessard-Diana B, et al. A retrospective study of three treatment techniques for T1/T2 base of tongue lesions: Surgery plus post-operative radiation, external radiation plus interstitial implantation, and external radiation alone. Int J Radiat Oncol Biol Phys 1987;13:511-516.

547. Vikram B, Strong E, Shah J, et al. An non-looping afterloading technique for base of tongue implant. results of the first 20 patients. Int J Radiat Oncol Biol Phys 1985;11:1853-1855.

548. List M, Ritter-Sterr C, Lansky S. A performance status scale for head and neck cancer patients. Cancer 1990;66:564-569.

549. Housset M, Baillet F, Delanian S, et al. Split-course interstitial brachytherapy with a source shift: The results of a new iridium implant technique vs single course implant for salvage irradiation of base of tongue cancers in 55 patients. Int J Radiat Oncol Biol Phys 1991;20:965-971.

550. Givens CD, Johns ME, Cantrell RW. Carcinoma of the tonsil. Arch Otol 1981;107:730.

551. Whicker JH, DeSanto LW, Devine UD. Surgical treatment of squamous cell carcinoma of the tonsil. Laryngoscope 1974;84:90-97.

552. Healy GB, Strong MS, Uchmakli A, et al. Carcinoma of the palatine arch: The rationale of treatment selection. Am J Surg 1976;132:498-502.

553. Barrs DM, DeSanto LW, O'Fallon WM. Squamous cell carcinoma of the tonsil and tongue—base region. Arch Otolaryngol 1979;105:479-485.

554. Eneroth CM, Hjertman L, Moberger G. Squamous cell carcinoma of the palate. Acta Otolaryngol 1972;73:418.

555. Fee WE, Schoeppel SL, Rubenstein R, et al. Squamous cell carcinoma of the soft palate. Arch Otolaryngol 1979;105:710-720.

556. Russ JE, Applebaum EL, Sisson GA. Squamous cell carcinoma of the soft palate. Laryngoscope 1977;87:1151-1156.

557. Mazeron J, Marinello G, Crook J, et al. Definitive radiation treatment for early stage carcinomas of the soft palate and uvula: The indications for iridium-192 implantation. Int J Radiat Oncol Biol Phys 1987;13:1829-1837.

558. Pernot M, Malissard L, Hoffstetter S, et al. Velotonsillar squamous cell carcinoma—277 cases treated by combined external irradiation and brachytherapy: Results according to localization, extension and dose rate. Int J Radiat Oncol Biol Phys 1991;1:142.

559. Remmler D, Medina JE, Byers RM, Meoz R, Pfalzgraf K. Treatment of choice for squamous cell carcinoma of the tonsillar fossa. Head Neck Surg 1985;7:206.

560. Tong D, Laramore G, Griffen T, et al. Carcinoma of the tonsil region. Cancer 1982;49:2007-2014.

561. Maltz R, Shumrick D, et al. Carcinoma of the tonsil: Results of combined therapy. Laryngoscope 1974;84:2172-2180.

562. Wong C, Ang K, Fletcher G, et al. Definitive radiotherapy for squamous cell carcinoma of the tonsillar fossa. Int J Radiat Oncol Biol Phys 1989;16:657-662.

563. Tong D, Laramore G, Griffin T, et al. Carcinoma of the tonsillar region-results of external irradiation. Cancer 1982;49:2009-2014.

564. Wang CC. Local control of oropharyngeal carcinoma after two accelerated hyperfractionation radiation therapy schemes. Int J Radiat Oncol Biol Phys 1988;14:1143-1146.

565. Perez C, Carmichael T, Devinenni V, et al. Carcinoma of the tonsilla fossa—a nonrandomized comparison of irradiation alone or combined with surgery: Long-term results. Head Neck 1991;13:282-290.

566. Perez, C, Purdy J, Breaux S, et al. Carcinoma of the tonsillar fossa—a non-randomized comparison of preoperative radiation and surgery or irradiation alone: Long-term results. Cancer 1982;50:2314-2322.

567. Perez C, Lee F, Ackerman L, et al. Carcinoma of the tonsillar fossa: Significance of dose irradiation and volume treated in the control of the primary tumor and metastatic nodes. Int J Radiat Oncol Biol Phys 1976;1:817-827.

568. Puthawala A, Syed A, Eads D, et al. Limited external irradiation and interstitial iridium-192 implant in the treatment of squamous cell carcinoma of the tonsillar fossa. Int J Radiat Oncol Biol Phys 1985;11:1595-1602.

569. Mazeron J, Lusinchi A, Marinello G, et al. Interstitial radiation therapy for squamous cell carcinoma of the tonsillar region: The Creteil experience. Int J Radiat Oncol Biol Phys 1986;12:895-900.

570. Mendenhall W, Parsons J, Cassisi N, et al. Squamous cell carcinoma of the tonsillar area treated with radical irradiation. Radiother Oncol 1987;10:23-30.

571. Murthy A, Hendrickson F. Contralateral neck treated necessary in early carcinoma of the tonsil? Int J Radiat Oncol Biol Phys 1980;6:91-94.

572. Dasmahapatra K, Mohit-Tabatabai M, Rush B, et al. Cancer of the tonsil—improved survival with combination therapy. Cancer 1986;57:451-455.

573. Zelefsky M, Harrison L, Armstrong J, Fass D. Post-operative radiation therapy for advanced oropharyngeal carcinoma: Long-term results. Cancer (in press).

574. Spiro J, Spiro R. Carcinoma of the tonsillar fossa—an update. Arch Otol Head Neck Surg 1989;115:1186-1189.

575. Gluckman J, Zitsch R. Current management of carcinoma of the oropharynx. Oncology 1990;4:23-30.

576. Sealy R, LeRoux T, Hering E, et al. The treatment of cancer of the uvula and soft palate and interstitial radioactive wire implants. Int J Radiat Oncol Biol Phys 1984;10:1951-1955.

577. Esche B, Haie C, Gerbaulet A, et al. Interstitial and external radiotherapy in carcinoma of the soft palate and uvula. Int J Radiat Oncol Biol Phys 1988;15:619-625.

578. Amdur R, Mendenhall W, Parsons J, et al. Carcinoma of the soft palate treated with irradiation: Analysis of results and complications. Radiother Oncol 1987;9:185-194.

579. Guillamondegui OM, Meoz R, Jesse RH. Surgical treatment of squamous cell carcinoma of the pharyngeal walls. Am J Surg 1978;136:474.

580. Ballantyne AJ. Principles of surgical management of cancer of the pharyngeal walls. Cancer 1967;20:663-669.

581. Cunningham MP, Catlin D. Cancer of the pharyngeal wall. Cancer 1967;20:1859.

582. Meoz-Mendez R, Fletcher G, Guillamondegui O, et al. Analysis of the results of irradiation in the treatment of squamous cell carcinomas of the pharyngeal walls. Int J Radiat Oncol Biol Phys 1978;4:579-585.

583. Marks J, Freeman R, Lee F, et al. Pharyngeal wall cancer: An analysis of treatment results, complications, and patterns of failure. Int J Radiat Oncol Biol Phys 1978;4:587-593.

584. Marks J, Smith P, Sessions D. Pharyngeal wall cancer—reappraisal after comparison of treatment methods. Arch Otol 1985;111:79-85.

585. Spiro R, Kelly J, Vega A, et al. Squamous carcinoma of the posterior pharyngeal wall. Am J Surg 1990;160:420-423.

586. Son Y, Kacinski B. Therapeutic concepts of brachytherapy/megavoltage in sequence for pharyngeal wall cancers: Results of integrated dose therapy. Cancer 1987;59:1268-1273.

ROY B. SESSIONS
LOUIS B. HARRISON
WAUN KI HONG

SECTION 2

Tumors of the Larynx and Hypopharynx

LARYNX

Considering that cancer occurs in the larynx 13 times less frequently than in the lung, 10 times less frequently than in the breast, and 9 times less frequently than in the prostate gland, the number of publications that have appeared in the North American literature on laryngeal cancer during the previous 5 years seems excessive. This considerable body of writing probably reflects the perceived importance of this disease relative to its potential impact on people's communicative and functional skills in society. A new attitude seems to exist among oncologists that is characterized by a keener concern for quality of life and death, and this applies especially to laryngeal cancer, for which any threat to a patient's "voice box" is associated with profound psychological overtones. Curing the cancer at any cost is no longer accepted casually, and now more than ever before, a premium is placed on return to a productive and useful lifestyle after cancer treatment. Nowhere in the oncology community is this change more vividly demonstrated than in the treatment of larynx cancer. Therefore, investigations continue into the methods of conservation laryngeal surgery, different radiation therapy strategies, and recently, combined chemotherapy and radiation therapy protocols designed for larynx preservation.[1-3] Although the cure rates of the various laryngeal malignancies have not changed dramatically during recent years,[4] the treatment options and the sequencing of those options have, and a higher percentage of laryngeal cancer patients are retaining their larynx in the process.

EPIDEMIOLOGY AND ETIOLOGY

Even though considerable differences between countries exist in the incidence of larynx cancer, its distribution within each country is consistent. For example, the disease most commonly affects middle-aged or older men who have smoked tobacco[5,6] and have drunk alcohol.[7,8] Laryngeal cancer rarely occurs in people who have done neither. In the United States during 1990, more than 12,000 new larynx cancers were diagnosed, and about 10,000 of those were in men. Even though this disease has always been more common in men, the current 4.5:1 ratio of men to women seems to be changing as the smoking habits of the sexes change—in 1956, this ratio was 15:1.[7] The peak incidence of larynx cancer is in the sixth decade. The disease occurs in young people only rarely.[8]

The following etiologic factors have been implicated in laryngeal cancer: voice abuse and chronic laryngitis[9,10]; certain dietary factors[11-13]; chronic gastric reflux[14]; and exposure to wood dust,[15] nitrogen mustard, asbestos, and ionizing radiation.[15-18] Most consistently seen, however, is the association between larynx cancer and smoking, whether by pipe, ciga-

rette, or cigar.[15] There seems to be an association with heavy alcohol intake and larynx cancer, and an enhancement of the already present risk factors associated with smoking.[19] On the other hand, some studies have failed to demonstrate an interdependent causal effect for alcohol intake and larynx cancer.[20] The issue of alcohol, smoke, and carcinogenesis is complicated by the nutritional deficiencies that usually occur in alcoholics.[13] In the larynx, this complex issue is more specifically defined by the fact that whatever the role of alcohol, it is apparently more significant in supraglottic than in glottic cancers.[21-24] As the current generation of those youngsters using smokeless tobacco matures, there may be some alteration of the relative incidence of supraglottic and glottic cancers. Those worldwide data that show large variations of laryngeal cancer statistics consistently reflect the smoking and drinking habits of the individual countries.[25] Also, the sites within the larynx affected by cancers vary considerably between countries. This distribution is shown in Table 22–29,[9,24,26-28] which represents a compendium of worldwide data that addresses the relative distributions of cancer within the larynx.

SURGICAL AND DEVELOPMENTAL ANATOMY

The larynx is a uniquely complicated organ that is strategically located so that significant alteration of its anatomy by either surgery or cancer can have a noticeable impact on digestive and respiratory physiology. The organ consists of three subsites, which are the glottis (paired true vocal cords), the supraglottis, and the subglottis. Because of different embryologic development and different lymphatic patterns that are subsite specific, discussing larynx cancers without specific reference to the exact location(s) within that structure invites inaccuracies in staging and miscalculations in treatment planning.

The larynx consists of five cartilages: the cricoid, the epiglottis, the paired arytenoids, and the shield-like thyroid cartilage. Suspended within the endolarynx are the mobile true vocal cords, which are collectively known as the *glottis*. That portion above the glottis, the supraglottis, consists of the false vocal cords, the epiglottis, and the aryepiglottic folds. These folds form the junction with the hypopharynx. The medial wall of the aryepiglottic fold is within the endolarynx, and its

TABLE 22–29. Geographic Variations in Larynx Cancer Sites*

Country	No. of Patients n	Site		
		Supraglottic (%)	Glottic (%)	Subglottic (%)
Japan[9]	6360	49	50	0.9
Finland[24]	638	67	32	1
Yugoslavia[26]	722	62	35	3.5
USA[27]	1645	34	65	1
Sweden[28]	578	11	87	2

* Relative incidence of larynx cancer by anatomic site and country. Notice variation between supraglottic and glottic incidence relative to different countries, but the relative consistency of subglottic occurrence.

lateral wall makes up the medial wall of the adjacent pyriform sinus (Fig. 22–20). Those lesions that arise on the rim of the aryepiglottic folds, therefore, have been appropriately referred to as *marginal cancers,* because they bridge the junction between the larynx and the hypopharynx. Those marginal lesions that extend predominantly into the endolarynx behave more like supraglottic cancers, whereas those lesions that spill into the pyriform sinus tend to follow the natural history of the hypopharynx. The subglottis is that portion of the larynx between the underedge of the true vocal cords and the cephalic border of the cricoid cartilage.[29]

The true vocal cords are a marvel of engineering and are attached anteriorly to the inner lamina of the thyroid cartilage and posteriorly to the arytenoids. The muscles of the vocal cords are complex in their activity and the relation between them and the overlying mucosa is critical to voice production. Any loss of mucosal mobility relative to the underlying muscle, such as that produced by surgery or, to a lesser extent, by radiation therapy, alters the voice. An appreciation of this fundamental fact is an important component in the selection of treatment of vocal cord cancer.

The lining of the endolarynx consists of respiratory epithelium except on the vibratory edges of the true vocal cords, which typically are lined with pseudostratified squamous epithelium.

The paired arytenoid cartilages each sit on the cephalic rim of the cricoid cartilage and rotate horizontally around a central pivot point. Each arytenoid is attached anteriorly to a true vocal cord, and the clockwise and counter-clockwise rotation of these cartilages drags the respective vocal cord attachment with it, causing abduction and adduction of those structures. Any or all of the muscles that are responsible for arytenoid rotation and also the branches of the recurrent laryngeal nerve fibers that innervate them can be damaged by invading cancer. The posterolateral aspect of the larynx is particularly vulnerable to the invasion of cancer because of the adjacency of the medial wall of the pyriform sinus. When cancers of this part

of the hypopharynx extend through the mucosa, they gain direct access to the important laryngeal compartment known as the *paraglottic space,* which leads to all parts of the endolarynx, including the vocal muscles and the preepiglottic space (Fig. 22–21). Treatment options for such a tumor are altered significantly because of the paraglottic space involvement. Tumors that invade the endolaryngeal muscles or the nerve fibers that innervate them usually create a noticeable effect on vocal cord motion. Of all the findings on laryngeal examination during cancer evaluation, the state of endolaryngeal mobility is probably one of the most important, a fact that has been substantiated by the separate designation that the American Joint Committee on Cancer (AJCC) has ascribed to the immobile vocal cord in this disease.[30]

Another type of motion alteration pertains to the anatomic relation between the vocal cord musculature and the overlying mucosa. This knowledge has only recently become available and has enhanced our understanding of early glottic cancer.[31] The vibratory mechanism that produces the voice comes partly from the mobility of the mucous membrane overlying the musculature of the vocal cord. The free edge of the true vocal cord consists of a pseudostratified squamous epithelium, under which is a lamina propria of fibroelastic and gelatinous consistency. This arrangement allows a sliding motion of the mucous membrane that creates a mucosal wave, the fluidity of which is a direct reflection of mucosal freedom from the underlying muscle. Any surface cancer that invades through the basement membrane, such as any depth deeper than carcinoma in situ, affects the mucosal wave by creating a tethering effect. These subtle differences are hardly appreciated by routine laryngeal examination but are obvious with laryngostroboscopic evaluation. An appreciation of these subtleties translates into the practical matter of determining whether to radiate or microscopically excise certain minimal vocal cord cancers.

Because of the different embryologic origins of the supraglottic from the glottic and subglottic larynx, and also because

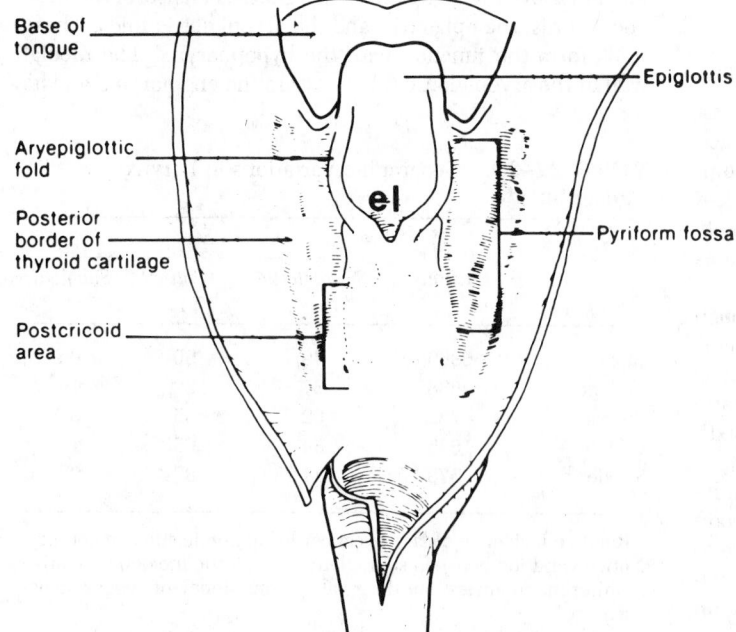

FIGURE 22–20.   Diagram of internal laryngeal and pharyngeal anatomy as viewed posteriorly. Note the entrance into the endolarynx (*el*).

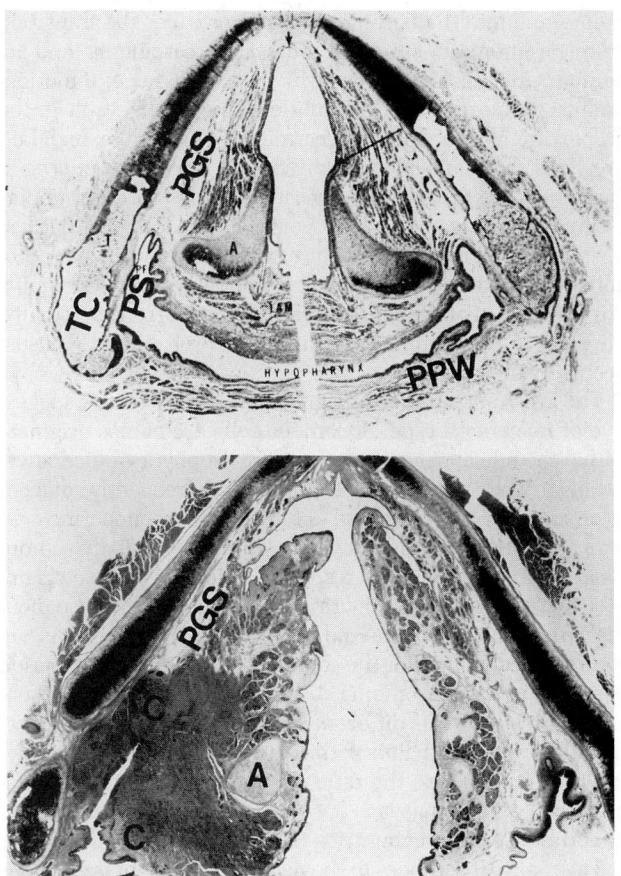

FIGURE 22–21. Axial sections of the human laryngopharynx at the level of the glottis. (*Upper*) Notice the relation of the pyriform sinus (PS) to the paraglottic space (PGS) of the endolarynx; the proximity of the lateral wall of the pyriform sinus to the thyroid cartilage (TC); and the relation of the pyriform sinus to the arytenoid (A). Ossification of the area of the thyroid cartilage shown in the axial section renders it vulnerable to skeletal invasion of cancer in this area. The posterior pharyngeal wall (PPW) acts as an extension of the lateral pharyngeal wall and the pyriform sinuses. (*Lower*) Cancer (C) of the pyriform sinus invades the endolarynx (PGS). (Courtesy of John Kirchner, MD)

of the independent lymphatic drainage patterns from each of these subsites, the larynx can be thought of as a compartmentalized structure. These features are important influences in determining the spread of various cancers within that organ.[32]

The lymphatics of the supraglottic larynx are profuse, and the frequency of metastasis associated with cancers of this subsite reflects that fact.[33] Lymphatic spread from the epiglottis is to the false cords, and these channels are directed bilaterally. The drainage from the false cords and the remainder of the supraglottic larynx is lateral and superior, and these channels exit the larynx bilaterally through the thyrohyoid membrane. They then proceed to the adjacent deep cervical nodes. The lymphatics of the infraglottic larynx drain laterally and inferiorly, out the cricothyroid membrane into the lower deep cervical lymph nodes. The true vocal cords, on the other hand, are unique in that they possess little or no lymphatic drainage.[32] From a lymphatic drainage standpoint, the left half of the larynx is essentially independent from the right and the supraglottic larynx is independent from the structures below. These facts are clinically demonstrated; in

their early stages, supraglottic cancers have little affinity for extension into the lower structures, and those beginning below do not tend to extend cephalad.[34,35] Knowledge of this unique pathogenesis has substantial impact on our ability to predict metastasis into various parts of the neck and on our planning of the various partial laryngectomies, that is, those conservation operations that allow removal of laryngeal parts while preserving vocal and swallowing functions. Additionally, radiation therapy planning, especially for occult cervical metastasis, is predicated on a thorough knowledge of these and other drainage tendencies of laryngeal cancers.

PATHOLOGY, PATHOGENESIS, AND NATURAL HISTORY

General Considerations

A variety of malignancies, most of which are primary to the larynx and others that are metastatic from distant sites, have been reported to occur in the larynx; a comprehensive classification is shown in Table 22–30.

More than 95% of all primary laryngeal malignancies are squamous cell carcinomas, with the remainder being sarcomas, adenocarcinomas, neuroendocrine tumors, and other types.[36]

It should be noted that knowledge and recognition of the neuroendocrine family of malignancies has changed considerably during recent years, and the exact percentage of these within the overall population of larynx cancers is unknown. In the past, certain tumors were vaguely classified as poorly differentiated malignancies, when they actually were neuroendocrine in origin. Modern techniques of immunohistochemical and morphologic analysis will almost certainly lead to the recognition and accrual of more of these tumors in the future.[37,38]

Seperate consideration must be given to the spectrum of premalignant squamous lesions, carcinoma in situ, and su-

TABLE 22–30. Classification of Laryngeal Malignancies by Histologic Type

Primary Malignancies	Melanoma
Epithelial Cancers	Nonepithelial Cancers
Squamous cell carcinoma	Sarcomas
Carcinoma in situ	Fibrosarcoma
Superficially invasive	Chondrosarcoma
Verrucous carcinoma	Rhabdomyosarcoma
Pseudosarcoma	Leiomyosarcoma
Anaplastic	Hemangiosarcoma
Transitional cell	Giant cell sarcoma
Lymphoepithelial	Lymphosarcoma
Adenocarcinoma	
Mucoepidermoid carcinoma	**Metastatic Malignancies**
Adenocarcinoma	Renal cell carcinoma
Adenoid cystic carcinoma	Thyroid carcinoma
Neuroendocrine tumors	Breast
Small cell carcinoma (oat cell)	Lung
Paraganglioma	Prostate
Carcinoid	Gastrointestinal tract
Oncocytic carcinoma	

perficial invasive carcinomas. To discuss the epithelial changes that precede and probably lead to carcinoma of the larynx is of considerable importance, because it is with this group of lesions that cancer prevention and conservative management are most effective. As our knowledge of this subject has increased, so too has our sophistication in applying the minimal techniques necessary to achieve excellent cure rates in these disorders.

Investigators have studied the occurrence of aberrant squamous epithelium in various areas of the larynx, and there seems to be a correlation between that metaplasia and the predilection for carcinogenesis in those respective sites;[39] however, because only lesions that began on the true vocal cords produce early symptoms and signs, the opportunity to treat early disease is largely limited to that structure, a fact that leads to spectacular cure rates for lesions of that site. The mucosal changes that lead to cancer take years to develop, and that evolution probably follows a consistent pattern. Most laryngeal squamous cell carcinomas result from prolonged exposure to recognized carcinogens that stimulate mucosal hyperplasia and metaplasia. Some of these changes are associated with keratosis and others are not. In some situations, epithelial atypia or dysplasia may exist, the degree of which probably determines whether a lesion is destined to become malignant.[40-42] In one large study by Slamniker, 3% of those patients who demonstrated vocal cord keratosis without atypia and 7% with mild atypia developed invasive carcinoma;[43] however, in those patients with moderate and severe atypia, 18% and 24%, respectively, developed carcinoma. Another study by Hjslet and colleagues showed a similar probability of cancer evolution in the group with less dysplasia and a strikingly higher probability in those patients with severe atypia.[44]

In addition to the morphologic appearance of mucosal alteration, DNA changes seem to show a correlation between cancer potential and cellular aneuploidy. In a study by Munck-Wirland and coworkers, for instance, all of those patients with dysplastic laryngeal lesions that later went on to become carcinoma demonstrated an aneuploid DNA pattern.[45]

These surface lesions, whether premalignant or not, have an inconsistent gross appearance. Some of these lesions are white and others are hyperemic. Many investigators believe the risk for cancer development is substantially higher in lesions that are soft and red in appearance.[42] Without histologic study, even the most experienced diagnostician cannot consistently predict the presence of cancer or the likelihood of its evolution in any of these surface lesions. Any given spot within a lesion does not necessarily represent the balance of that lesion. The facts that carcinoma in situ is often surrounded by dysplastic epithelium and that many areas of invasive carcinoma are surrounded by zones of carcinoma in situ and dysplastic epithelium[46] lend credence to the concept that each of these morphologic categories of epithelial disturbance is but part of a dynamic spectrum of disorders, each probably related and representing different stages of the same process. This means that dysplasia leads to carcinoma in situ, which leads to invasive carcinoma.

It is unknown whether those lesions that have achieved the status of carcinoma continue to grow at the same rate as they did during their premalignant state or whether their growth is accelerated. The growth of a cancer through the basement membrane into the lamina propria constitutes the transition from carcinoma in situ to microinvasive carcinoma, and accompanying this is a tethering of vocal cord mucosal motion. Failure to appreciate these subtle changes can result in the employment of suboptimal treatment. For example, high failure rates that have been reported with mucosal *stripping* in carcinoma in situ patients almost certainly represent underestimation of these lesions.[47] Some of those lesions that had been classified in the prestrobe era as carcinoma in situ probably contained areas of invasive carcinoma, and the stripping left behind foci of cancer that resulted in recurrence. Actually, pure vocal cord carcinoma in situ is probably an unusual occurrence.

The gross appearance of a given laryngeal lesion is suggestive of its general type. Squamous cell carcinomas originate within the mucous membrane and are exophytic or ulcerative, are of surface origin (Fig. 22–22), and are frequently adjacent to or surrounded by mucosal keratoses. Neuroendocrine cancers and tumors metastatic to the larynx are usually submucosal and, as such, do not resemble lesions of surface origin. Metastatic and neuroendocrine tumors are seen throughout the various subsites within the larynx, although the latter group shows a predilection for the supraglottic area. The distribution of squamous cell carcinoma within the various laryngeal subsites varies between different countries, a fact that reflects the different social habits within those cultures. For example, in the United States, the ratio of supraglottic to glottic squamous cell carcinomas is 2/3:1/3, whereas the reverse is true in certain European countries (see Table 22–29).

The major differences in the natural histories of the various squamous cell carcinomas of the larynx are related largely to the area anatomy and to the lymphatic drainage patterns of the respective subsite(s).

Cellular characteristics vary by site; in the supraglottis, lesions are more likely to be nonkeratinizing and poorly differentiated and, in general, they have more aggressive local behavior. Those lesions of the true vocal cords, on the other

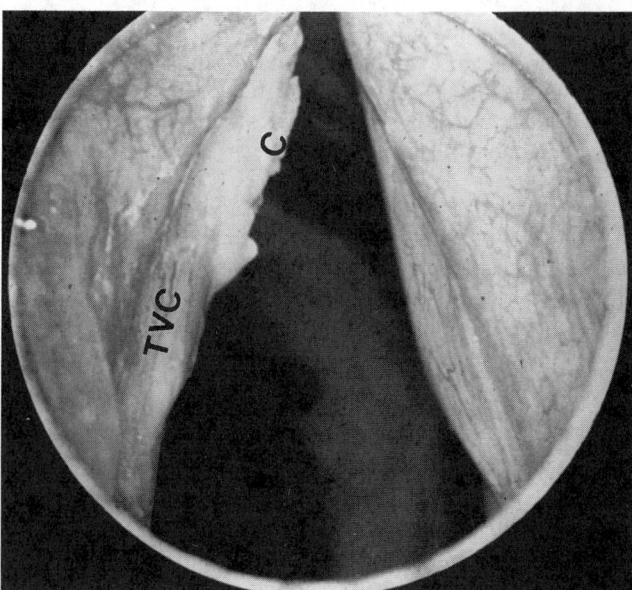

FIGURE 22–22. Squamous cell carcinoma (C) of the true vocal cord (TVC). Notice the "surface" appearance of the lesion.

hand, are more often well differentiated and tend to be less aggressive locally. Overall, although the degree of cellular differentiation is not thought to be the most significant fact in tumor grading, it does seem to correlate with the probability of cervical metastasis,[24,35,51,52] which in turn strongly impacts on survival.[53-55] Other local characteristics, such as tumor-host interface,[35,51,56] peritumor inflammatory response,[57] and vascular and perineural invasion[56] also seem important in determining performance. Finally, the actual tumor thickness and depth of invasion almost certainly have an influence on metastasis and, ultimately, on survival.

As in other sites in the aerodigestive tract, a multifactorial analysis of a variety of parameters, as well as patient performance status, may produce a more predictable prognostic indicator than the standard TNM staging outlined by the AJCC.[58]

Specific Subsites

Supraglottis

Lesions of the supraglottic larynx tend to spread locally. If they begin on the epiglottis, they can extend onto the false vocal cords and into the ventricle where inferior extension is initially thwarted. Often, however, these cancers penetrate into the paraglottic space from which they gain full access to the length of the endolarynx. These cancers often exit the paraglottic space cephalad and caudad to enter directly into the neck.

Most supraglottic lesions arise on the epiglottis, with fewer being seen on the false vocal cords and aryepiglottic folds. Those lesions that occur on the suprahyoid or upper part of the epiglottis are more often exophytic, whereas those that occur on the lower portion of that structure are likely to be endophytic or ulcerative.[48,49] The characteristic of endophytic growth is especially significant in this particular area of the epiglottis, because there are foramina here that lead directly through the cartilage into the preepiglottic space, which is a compartment that leads to the base of the tongue. What would appear to be a localized tumor in the endolarynx, therefore, can actually involve considerable unrecognized extralaryngeal extension.[50] Tumors are confined initially to the preepiglottic space by the ligamentous boundaries of that compartment, but once those barriers are overcome, the loosely arranged skeletal muscle fibers of the tongue provide no restriction to further tumor extension.[59] Modern imaging has greatly improved the ability to recognize tumor extension into the preepiglottic space and base of tongue.

Those lesions that occur on the laryngeal surface of the epiglottis are capable of invading and destroying that structure. The thyroid cartilage, on the other hand, is almost never destroyed by supraglottic cancers.[60,61] This feature has an influence on the design of treatment plans; for example, an ossified and invaded thyroid cartilage poses a substantial problem for surgeons attempting to perform partial laryngectomy and also for radiation oncologists attempting to deliver curative therapy.

Aryepiglottic fold cancers are somewhat different in their behavior, following more the tendencies of the pyriform sinus lesions, that is, spreading in a more diffuse fashion and metastasizing more frequently than their endolaryngeal counterparts. The more ominous natural history of these lesions relates to the more abundant and multidirectional lymphatic drainage of the area rather than to individual cellular peculiarities.[50]

Because of the profuse lymphatic network of the area, supraglottic carcinomas metastasize frequently to the cervical lymph nodes, and failure of treatment is usually a result of metastasis rather than local disease.[33,62-64] The incidence of patients with clinically positive lymph nodes at the time of diagnosis is 23% to 50% for all supraglottic sites and stages combined.[49,65,66-69] A substantial number of those patients with clinically negative necks turn out to have histologic disease if a neck dissection is done, or if left untreated, convert to clinically positive necks.[62,63] In supraglottic cancers, the probability of cervical metastasis and the probability of delayed contralateral metastasis increase in direct proportion to the size of the primary (*i.e.*, the T stage).[48,70,71] Lindberg reported impressive overall metastatic rates with various supraglottic carcinomas: T1 had 63%; T2 had 70%; T3 had 79%; and T4 had 73%.[33]

In that group of patients with supraglottic lesions that present with a clinically positive cervical node 2 cm in diameter or more, the possibility for contralateral neck metastasis is 40% or higher.[72] The epiglottis is particularly prone to bilateral metastasis, and even in smaller lesions of that site, the incidence of contralateral metastasis is more than 20%.[70] Much of the data on clinically positive necks and on occult metastasis were compiled before the routine employment of computed tomography (CT) and magnetic resonance imaging (MRI) of the neck. With the employment of these more sophisticated staging methods added to the already 75% to 85% accuracy of physical examination,[73-76] the overall incidence of metastasis noted at the time of diagnosis will probably be higher than that reported previously.

Glottis

Glottic or true vocal cord carcinoma is the commonest of all laryngeal cancers encountered in the United States. Although these lesions are usually well differentiated, they often demonstrate an infiltrative growth pattern, even when they appear exophytic and well organized. Most true vocal cord cancers occur on the anterior two thirds of that structure, a small percentage of them develop on the anterior commissure, and they rarely occur on the posterior commissure.[77]

To a large extent, growth characteristics and the natural history of glottic carcinomas are determined by the unique anatomy of the true vocal cords. First, the sparcity of the lymphatic drainage of the true vocal cords in all areas other than the posterior commissure makes metastasis of early lesions extremely unlikely. Second, the elastic layers (conus elasticus) within the larynx often divert cancers that begin on the free edge of the vocal cord and continue into the underlying vocalis muscle and paraglottic space, which is an inferolateral pathway that leads out of the larynx through the cricothyroid space. With penetration into the underlying tissues, all degrees of motion impairment, from subtle mucous membrane stiffness to frank fixation of the vocal cord, can follow. That increasing impairment of motion has a telling effect on local control and survival data, a fact that is reflected in AJCC staging designations. Much discussion continues about mobility change and its therapeutic implications, and it is in the group of glottic cancers that demonstrate this in which the clinical judgment of the physician is tested most.

The final anatomic factor unique to the glottis that influences the growth pattern of certain cancers is the anterior commissure ligament that forms the bridge between the anterior ends of the true vocal cords. This structure lies immediately against the inner lamina of the thyroid cartilage, and its presence initially retards penetration of cancers of that area, often causing their diversion upward onto the epiglottis or downward onto the cricothyroid membrane. From there, these lesions can escape the larynx into the anterior neck. If the cancer overcomes the ligamentous barrier at the anterior commissure, the cartilage is penetrated.[60,78] This event is particularly likely in thyroid cartilages that are ossified, and when this does occur, there are substantial therapeutic implications that compromise the radiotherapist and dictate certain surgical approaches.[79,80]

Subglottis

Carcinomas of the subglottic larynx are unusual, making up only about 1% to 8% of all laryngeal cancers.[81] These lesions tend to be poorly differentiated and often demonstrate an infiltrative growth pattern unrestricted by tissue barriers. These tumors are, therefore, frequently circumferential and can extend down the trachea. The incidence of cervical metastasis in this group of cancers is reported to be 20% to 30%, but that figure is somewhat obscured by the fact that the primary drainage pattern of these lesions is to the less detectable pretracheal and paratracheal nodes. The actual incidence of metastasis may, therefore, be significantly higher.[82,83]

Unusual and Rare Neoplasms

The pathology and pathogenesis of verrucous carcinoma is unique and deserves special consideration. This unusual tumor is poorly understood, and its origin, classification, and response to treatment are controversial.[84,85] Verrucous carcinoma is described as a distinct neoplastic entity of squamous origin that occurs in the oral cavity, larynx, esophagus, nose, and on the genitalia.[86-88] Some authorities have suggested the human papilloma virus as its cause.[90] Even though there are views to the contrary, most investigators consider verrucous carcinoma to be an entity unto itself.[89] Just because some tumors originally thought to be verrucous carcinoma are discovered to have features of squamous cell carcinoma and can become metastatic does not, in their opinion, justify combining the two diagnoses; actually, they think that such tumors were low-grade squamous cell carcinomas rather than verrucous carcinoma.[88] Other investigators, although conceding verrucous carcinoma to be unique, believe it to be only a variant of well-differentiated squamous cell carcinoma. Different authors believe that because verrucous carcinomas neither fulfill the histologic and cytologic criteria of malignancy nor possess the capability to metastasize, they should be renamed *verrucous acanthoma* rather than carcinoma.[91] When this lesion does occur in the larynx, it usually is on the true vocal cord, where it grows slowly and can cause significant local destruction by expanding gradually. Even though these lesions often destroy cartilage, they do not tend to metastasize; aggressiveness is directed locally.

Verrucous carcinoma is consistently difficult to diagnose, even when the clinical index of suspicion is high. This observation relates to the fact that these tumors microscopically demonstrate an exuberant and keratinizing hyperplasia that is benign by pure histologic and cytologic criteria.[92] The diagnosis is largely a clinical one and is most effectively achieved by concert between pathologist and surgeon, but usually only after multiple biopsies have been taken.

This tumor is typically a slow growing but relentless mass, exophytic and warty in appearance, and broad based at its interface with the mucosa (Fig. 22–23). Its surface is often necrotic and infected, and the associated inflammation of adjacent tissues can be remarkable. This tendency to cause inflammation can erroneously influence treatment planning. For example, the patient with verrucous carcinoma can demonstrate enlarged adjacent cervical lymph nodes that are worrisome, when in fact the adenopathy is only secondary to the inflammatory process. Even though this finding has been described in other aerodigestive tumors,[93] the mere presence of lymphadenopathy in the primary drainage area of an impressive primary tumor is worrisome, no matter how benign looking its histology. In such a circumstance, clinical judgment is enhanced greatly by modern imaging and cytopathologic techniques.

This discussion of the nature of verrucous carcinoma has substantial therapeutic implications, especially when the lesion occurs in the larynx. Essentially, squamous cell carcinoma is a radiosensitive cancer, a fact that provides treatment options to the physician. On the other hand, verrucous carcinoma seems to be somewhat radioresistant, whether found in the mouth or the larynx.[84] Additionally, there is anecdotal information suggesting radiation induced dedifferentiation into anaplastic cancer in these lesions. This transformation seems to occur in fewer than 10% of verrucous carcinoma[65,94-97] and may involve alteration of the DNA that facilitates the integration of the human papilloma virus into host cells.[90] Both the concept of radiation resistance and the transformation into anaplastic cancers are vigorously disputed.[88,98-100]

The neuroendocrine family of tumors represents an evolving data base. This is true largely because recent diagnostic

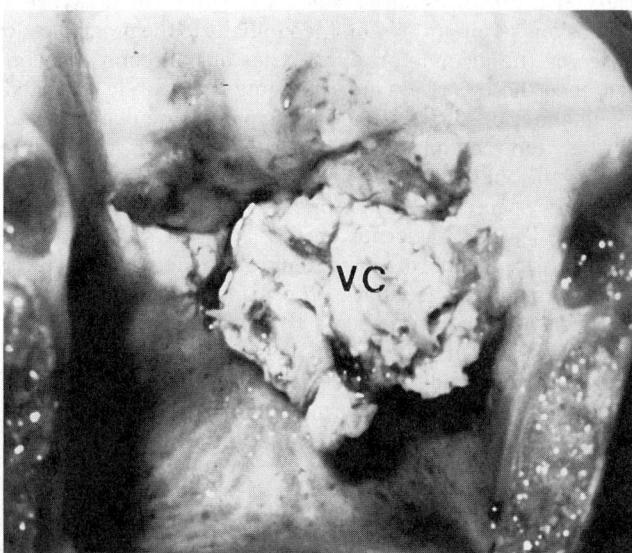

FIGURE 22–23. Total laryngectomy specimens demonstrate verrucous carcinoma (*VC*) of the true vocal cord as viewed posteriorly. Note exophytic, warty appearance of lesion and its sessile base on the cord.

techniques have allowed pathologists specifically to label as neuroendocrine in origin a variety of previously undefined cancers. Almost certainly, an immunohistochemical reexamination of laryngeal cancers previously diagnosed as atypical or undifferentiated malignancies would result in the reclassification of many as neuroendocrine tumors. The small cell tumors look and act much like their counterpart oat cell lung lesions, and as such, generally are managed by chemotherapy and radiation therapy.[37] Surgical procedures do not seem to enhance the likelihood of survival in patients with these tumors.[101-103] The other neuroendocrine tumors that occur in the larynx and that are rare are carcinoids and paragangliomas, which are best managed surgically.[104,105]

Cartilaginous malignancies,[106] malignant fibrous histiocytomas,[107] plasmacytomas,[108] granular cell tumors,[109] and primary lymphomas[110] have all been reported but are rare. Primary melanomas of the larynx are equally rare; of all of the larynx cancers reported from Memorial Sloan-Kettering Cancer Center between 1949 and 1983, only three were melanomas.[111]

DIAGNOSIS AND EVALUATION

Cancers of the supraglottic larynx usually do not produce early symptoms or signs, and it is common for the first hint of such a cancer to be cervical adenopathy. When symptoms do occur, they are often subtle; pain perceived in the primary site or in the ear (otalgia), a scratchy sensation when swallowing, or merely an alteration of one's tolerance for hot or cold foods may be all that is noticeable. Airway alteration, hoarseness, or a tendency to aspirate liquids are all produced by more advanced lesions.

Cancers of the glottis, on the other hand, are often detected early in the course of the disease because even a slight alteration of the vibratory surface of the true vocal cord(s) produces voice change. Heavy smokers are often hoarse, however, and

such alteration of the voice may not alarm them. Anyone with a voice change that does not resolve within several weeks ought to have a laryngeal examination. It is unusual for glottic cancer patients to seek medical attention because of cervical adenopathy. In such lesions, metastasis generally occurs late in the course of the disease, long after the early warning signals.

Fortunately, subglottic cancers are uncommon, but when they occur, they fail to produce early symptoms; therefore, the disease is often advanced by the time of diagnosis.

Most larynx cancers are squamous carcinomas, and as such, are surface lesions. Most are visible with routine laryngeal inspection, but a small percentage are obscure. The modern generation of flexible endoscopes (Fig. 22–24) has provided for a broad range of physicians the capability to examine the larynx; and although the optical resolution of these instruments is not as good as that achieved by traditional methods of mirror examination, the overall process of screening and follow-up after treatment has been enhanced by this technology. Importantly, these methods allow the occasional laryngeal examiner to see areas that previously have been visually inaccessible.

It is fundamental that the larynx be examined in the awake patient who is sitting upright. Direct laryngoscopy should be reserved for biopsy and a more detailed tumor mapping (Fig. 22–25). Even when done under local anesthesia, the introduction of a direct laryngoscope distorts the natural position and the relaxed motion of the larynx, and by doing so, tends to disguise subtle motion changes that are important in staging of these tumors. Certain subtleties of contour, such as bulging and tethering, are visually not appreciable during direct laryngoscopy.

The earliest stage of invasive glottic carcinoma through mucosa into the underlying lamina propria is visible as a tethering of the mucous membrane sliding over the underlying structures, meaning there is a loss of the membrane wave.[31]

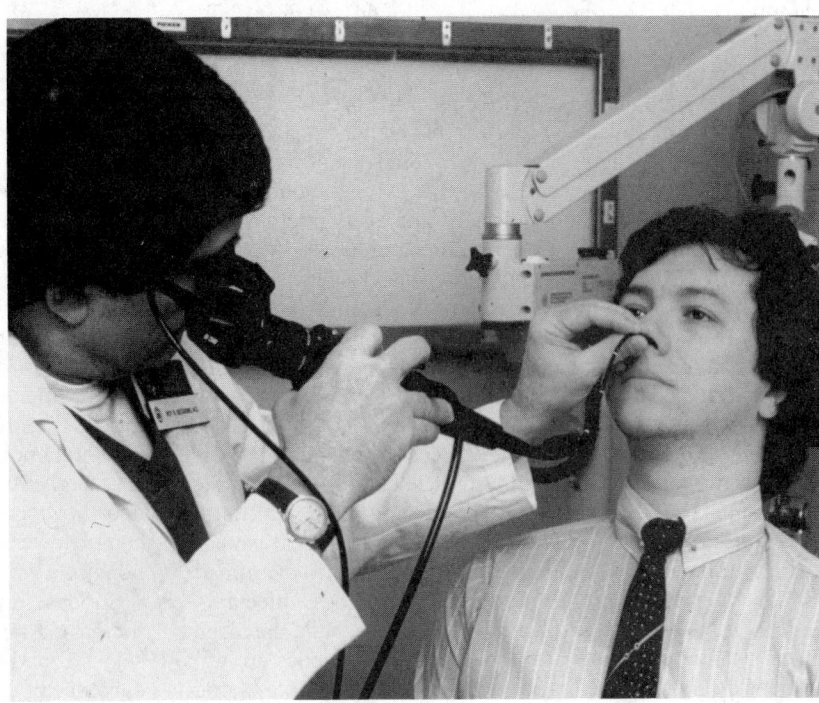

FIGURE 22–24. Flexible laryngeal endoscope in use.

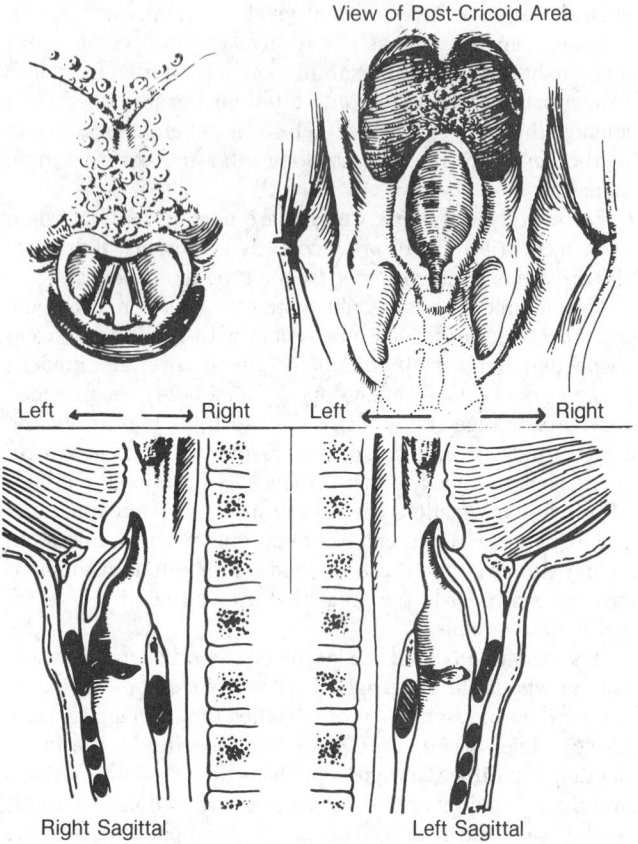

View of Post-Cricoid Area

Left ← → Right   Left ← → Right

Right Sagittal   Left Sagittal

FIGURE 22–25. Diagrams of laryngopharynx used for mapping and recording tumors.

The gross abductive capabilities of the vocal cord may be intact, but the early invasive character of a lesion can be appreciated only when the stroboscope is employed. As the process of invasion continues into the vocalis muscle, the actual lateral excursion of the vocal cord is limited and eventually lost. The ability of the clinician to view and interpret this scenario is critical to the sophisticated management of larynx cancer in general and vocal cord cancer in particular. Essentially, lesions of the true vocal cord that do not transgress the basement membrane, (*i.e.*, surface lesions) do not cause tethering of the membrane, and those that enter the underlying lamina propria do.[112] Benign lesions and even carcinoma in situ, therefore, may look extensive topographically, but their lack of depth is revealed by appropriate diagnostic technology. Even though contemporary methods of staging tend to emphasize the bulk and topographic size of tumors rather than depth, recent thinking has begun to focus more on this third dimension. As data are accumulated, more emphasis will be placed on this important matter.

Imaging should not be used to detect early larynx cancer, because the routine methods of physical examination are far more suitable. The primary care physician should not, therefore, initially resort to CT or MRI when a laryngeal cancer symptom persists. Instead, that patient should be examined by someone skilled in the appropriate techniques. Once a lesion is discovered, the evaluation of its depth, bulk, cartilage invasion, and the status of the regional lymph nodes are enhanced by CT or MRI. It is not clear which of the two imaging methods is better for larynx cancer evaluation. Both methods have certain advantages over the other, and both are of limited usefulness in evaluating the radiated larynx.[106] CT of the larynx is most effectively achieved in the axial plane, and because of this, the images show well the lateral tumor extension and the relation of that extension to cervical nodal disease. The axial projection is effective in demonstrating the important paraglottic space. CT effectively demonstrates the vertical extension of tumor, especially in the subglottic and anterior commissure areas. MRI offers the advantages of multiplane visualization of the larynx and, therefore, is especially valuable in evaluating the preepiglottic space and the adjacent base of tongue.

Invasion of laryngeal cartilage is important in most treatment planning. Determining whether this has occurred has always been difficult because of the inconsistency of the ossification that occurs in the laryngeal framework. Generally, cartilage is vulnerable to tumor invasion in those areas where it is ossified and somewhat resistant where it is not. Recent writings by Castelijns and associates[113,114] and by Towler and Young[115] have suggested that MRI is the method of choice for delineating this important finding. Other investigators would dispute this. One recent study has correlated MRI findings of cartilage invasion with the effectiveness of radiation treatment, and in so doing, the authors found a surprising number of the small glottic lesions with foci of cartilage invasion.[116] Significantly, it was from this group that most of the radiation failures of the series occurred. Other imaging methods such as tomography and laryngography have been surpassed by more elaborate technology and are mainly of historic interest.

STAGING

The AJCC last updated larynx staging in 1983, and that version is presented in Table 22–31.[30] Staging provides a commonality of language that is essential for effective outcome analysis. The larynx is a complex structure, because it involves many anatomic and physiologic factors that impact on performance and, therefore, on staging. Although it is essential that pathologic findings are always compared with preoperative analysis, it should be remembered that the staging referred to and that the AJCC has reported is a clinical one that is based on performance. The accuracy of clinical staging is periodically updated on the basis of better recognition of performance. For example, Pillsbury and Kirchner studied this question by comparing whole organ sections of nonradiated larynges and compared the actual pathologic findings with the preoperative staging.[117] They found that 40% had been categorized incorrectly, most inaccuracies being attributable to understaging. Most commonly, the depth of invasion had been underestimated, and the frequency of cartilage invasion was much higher than had been realized previously. Certainly, as imaging technology improves, so will the ability to stage more accurately. As clinicians employ treatment protocols that use neoadjuvant chemotherapy and in which the assessment of complete versus partial response is required, modern imaging hopefully will enhance the accuracy of that assessment.

Survival in larynx cancer decreases in a linear fashion with increasing stage. The most remarkable change is between stages II and III, the zone that generally represents the occurrence of cervical metastasis.

TABLE 22–31. American Joint Committee on Cancer Staging for Laryngeal Cancer (1988)

Tumor Size (T)

Supraglottis

Tis	Carcinoma in situ
T1	Tumor confined to site of origin with normal mobility
T2	Tyumor involves adjacent supraglottic site(s) or glottis without fixation
T3	Tumor limited to larynx with fixation or extension to involve postcricoid area, medial wall of pyriform sinus, or preepiglottic space
T4	Massive tumor extending beyond larynx to involve oropharynx, soft tissues of neck, or destruction of thyroid cartilage

Glottis

Tis	Carcinoma in situ
T1	Tumor confined to vocal cord(s) with normal mobility (includes involvement of anterior or posterior commissures)
T2	Supraglottic or subglottic extension of tumor with normal or impaired cord mobility
T3	Tumor confined to the larynx with cord fixation
T4	Massive tumor with thyroid cartilage destruction or extension beyond the confines of the larynx

Subglottis

Tis	Carcinoma in situ
T1	Tumor confined to the subglottic region
T2	Tumor extension to vocal cords with normal or impaired cord mobility
T3	Tumor confined to larynx with cord fixation
T4	Massive tumor with cartilage destruction or extension beyond confines of larynx, or both

Stage Grouping

Stage I	T1, N0, M0
Stage II	T2, N0, M0
Stage III	T3, N0, M0
	T1, T2, T3; N1, M0
Stage IV	T4, N0, N1; M0
	Any T, N2, N3; M0
	Any T, any N, M

TREATMENT AND SURVIVAL

Supraglottis

Because the supraglottic larynx is composed of multiple sites, speaking of it when discussing treatment results is not always accurate. Because each of the subsites are intimately related, and because the supraglottis is continuous with its neighboring hypopharynx, glottic larynx, and oropharynx, it can be difficult to determine the exact site of origin for many larger cancers. For example, when one encounters a lesion that involves the pharyngoepiglottic fold, aryepiglottic fold, and pyriform sinus, it can be difficult to know whether this is a primary hypopharynx cancer extending superiorly or a primary supraglottic cancer extending inferiorly.

Unlike glottic cancer in which cervical metastasis is relatively uncommon for early-stage disease, the probability of nodal spread in all supraglottic lesions is substantial.[33,48] There is a significant probability of contralateral metastasis in these lesions and that increases with increasing primary size.[70] This is especially true for epiglottic lesions, which make up most of the supraglottic carcinomas. It is essential to recognize that the site of treatment failure in supraglottic cancer is usually the neck; therefore, treatment strategies require neck management for virtually all lesions. For the N0 neck, this implies selective neck dissection or elective radiation, and for patients with clinically positive neck(s), this implies neck dissection(s) or therapeutic radiation, or a combination of both.

Early-stage primary disease is highly curable by partial laryngeal surgery or by radiation therapy. More advanced lesions, on the other hand, usually are treated with combined modalities and often require total laryngectomy. Wang and associates have reported an extensive experience with radiating early lesions dating back to 1973.[118] They have reported 5-year actuarial disease-free survival of 73% and 50% for T1 and T2 lesions, respectively. When surgical salvage was added, this survival increased to 80% and 58%, respectively. A total of 92% of T1 patients and 86% of T2 patients survived with their larynx. Mendenhall and colleagues reported local control of 100% of T1 and 81% of T2 lesions.[119] When surgical salvage was added, local control for T2 cancers increased to 88%. Importantly, the study by Mendenhall and colleagues revealed no significant differences in local control by anatomic subsite. Olofsson and coworkers reported a 47% 3-year survival for T1–2 lesions.[120] Lederman reported a 53% control rate for T1 and 64% for T2 tumors at 5 years.[121] Fletcher and associates reported local control in 94% of T1 and 89% of T2 lesions, with no difference noted by anatomic subsite within the supraglottis.[122] Vermund compared the 5-year survival for primary surgery with primary radiation for T1–4N0 supraglottic carcinoma.[123] The results for T1–3N0 disease were identical for both groups, but there was an advantage (56% versus 14%) for T4N0 treated by primary surgery.

Those smaller lesions of the supraglottis (*i.e.*, T1–2) are equally well treated with surgical procedures that remove only the upper portion of the larynx. The so-called supraglottic laryngectomy is physiologic and allows retention of vocal and swallowing functions. Because of the unique lymphatic drainage patterns of the organ and the presence of certain natural anatomic barriers to tumor spread, this operation is oncologically sound, yielding the same local control rates as achieved by total laryngectomy in comparable lesions.[26,49,124] Some authors described a 68% 5-year control rate with supraglottic laryngectomy[72]; Ogura and Biller reported an 85% 3-year control for epiglottis cancers treated with supraglottic laryngectomy, but this decreased to 71% with extension onto the false cords.[124]

Because of the complications associated with persistent swelling, swallowing difficulty, and wound healing, supraglottic laryngectomy usually is not recommended in patients who have had full-course radiation therapy. The decision to irradiate primarily a supraglottic laryngeal lesion should be made with the realization that the backup operation for failure of therapy is almost always a total laryngectomy.

Management of the neck is critical to successful therapy

of supraglottic cancer. Lavendag and Vikram studied elective surgical management of the neck in a group of patients with stages I and II supraglottic carcinomas treated with surgery alone at the Memorial Sloan-Kettering Cancer Center.[125] In those patients who underwent elective neck dissection, that is, the group with clinically negative necks, 32% were found to have histologically positive cervical lymph nodes. Half the patients with involved nodes eventually failed in the dissected neck. Additionally, 19% of patients with negative elective neck dissections failed in the contralateral neck. Finally, in a group of 48 patients who did not have elective neck dissection, 29% failed in the neck. Therefore, a total of 35% of the T1–2N0 patients ultimately developed cervical lymph node metastases. Importantly, nearly two thirds of those who relapsed in the neck eventually died from their cancer. On the other hand, none of the patients without neck relapse died from supraglottic cancer. Levendag and Vikram compared this experience with a similar patient group from the Rotterdam Radiotherapy Group and showed a similar 30% to 40% neck failure with surgery alone and a 19% failure when radiation therapy was administered to the necks.[125] Harwood and coworkers reported a 3% failure rate in the electively radiated neck.[126] These reports indicate that even the smallest supraglottic tumors require elective neck management.

A relative advantage of radiation therapy in the treatment of early-stage disease is that bilateral elective neck treatment can be done with minimal morbidity. If an adequate dose of elective neck radiation is given, neck relapse should be less than 5%. If surgery is chosen as the treatment for a T1 or T2 supraglottic lesion, the supraglottic laryngectomy should be combined with bilateral selective neck dissections. Radiation therapy is required in addition to surgery in the one third or so of these patients who are expected to have histologic disease in the neck(s). The obvious disadvantage to this approach is that it becomes necessary to employ two different treatment modalities compared with the strategy in which radiation therapy is employed primarily to primary and necks. The disadvantage of the latter plan is that when failure occurs, total laryngectomy is needed.

Although surgery and radiation appear to yield comparable results for small supraglottic lesions with negative necks, the effectiveness of radiation diminishes markedly in controlling advanced lesions.[65] Various studies of this group reported dismal survival statistics with radiation therapy management alone; Siirala and Paavolainen reported a 20% 5-year survival[127]; Vermund reported a 32% 5-year survival[123]; and Wang and colleagues reported a 5-year actuarial survival of 37% for T3 and 23% for T4 lesions.[128] Mendenhall and colleagues reported local control in 61% and 33% of radiated T3 and T4 lesions, respectively.[119] These numbers increase to 83% and 66% with surgical salvage.

Although selected T3 patients with small tumor volume can be radiated successfully, most patients with advanced disease require total laryngectomy. Postoperative radiation is employed routinely in those patients with bulky primary disease, histologically involved lymph nodes, and concerns about resection margins. The tracheal stoma is at risk for recurrence in patients who have subglottic extension and those with nodal metastases that involve the lower neck.

Hyperfractionated radiation has been used by some groups in an effort to improve results. For early-stage disease, there is no definitive evidence that hyperfractionation improves local control. However, Wang and coworkers report local control of 66% for T3–4 patients treated with twice per day therapy compared with 33% for those treated once per day.[118] This difference was statistically significant but was not generated in a randomized trial. The potential benefit to hyperfractionation was particularly noticable in patients with nodal metastases. Patients with nodal metastases who were treated with twice per day techniques had an actuarial local control of 76%, and this was a significantly better control rate than the 28% achieved with a once-a-day program. Prospective trials are needed to determine the relative benefit of hyperfractionation.

When surgery is combined with radiation, the issue arises as to whether preoperative or postoperative radiation is preferable. Tupchong and associates reported the results of a Radiation Therapy Oncology Group (RTOG) randomized trial that concluded that postoperative radiation is preferable to preoperative treatment for advanced supraglottic cancer.[129]

It is not the mission of this text to describe elaborately the various surgical techniques that are used to manage supraglottic laryngeal cancer; however, the student of this disease and its management should have at least a summary knowledge of the precise methods known collectively as *conservation* (not conservative) *laryngeal surgery*.

The compartmentalization of the larynx and the directional drainage patterns of the lymph channels within it provide the surgeon with a unique setting for removing that portion of the larynx above the true vocal cords, and with proper reconstruction, to allow retention of the swallowing and vocal functions of the patient. Because of the consistent drainage patterns of the area cancers, the so-called supraglottic laryngectomy is associated with the same cure rates as would be associated with a total laryngectomy in the same lesion. Essentially, this procedure is a horizontially directed hemilaryngectomy in which the surgeon removes the upper half of the thyroid cartilage and the contents within it, namely the false vocal cords, the epiglottis, and the aryepiglottic folds. The edge of the thyroid cartilage is brought up to and approximated to the transected base of the tongue. Because the motor nerve supply of the vocal cords comes from below (recurrent laryngeal nerves), the important glottic function of abduction and adduction are retained; because of this, voice and the important function of glottic closure that is critical to preventing aspiration are retained.

This operation is physiologically challenging, and patients with chronic pulmonary disease do not tolerate the aspiration that follows. Although this technique is oncologically sound in appropriate tumors, certain patients are not good candidates for its implementation. The correct use of the supraglottic laryngectomy is accomplished only by surgeons properly trained in this complex methodology and who have the experience to apply the right methods in the right situation. A succinct discussion of the method of selection for conservation procedures and which patients are suitable for them was developed by Sessions and Parish.[130] Although there have been certain chemoradiotherapy options popularized since that discussion was published, the fundamental principles are the same and can be applied to the philosophy of 1992.

There are a variety of conservation surgery procedures that are applied to variations of laryngeal cancer, but a description of each is beyond the scope of this text. A classification of these operations should be helpful to the reader in placing this important surgical methodology into the proper perspective. Such a classification is the following:

CLASSIFICATION OF CONSERVATION LARYNGEAL PROCEDURES

  I. Hemilaryngectomy
    a. Horizontal hemilaryngectomy (supraglottic)
    b. Vertical hemilaryngectomy
      1. Lateral hemilaryngectomy
      2. Frontal hemilaryngectomy
  II. Cordectomy
  III. Partial laryngopharyngectomy

Regarding specific techniques of definitive radiation for supraglottic carcinoma, all patients require a larynx contour. A larynx compensator may be required for maximum dose homogeneity. For T1–2 lesions, a total dose of 6500 to 6800 cGy is used at 180 cGy/fraction. For more advanced lesions, doses in the range of 7000 cGy are used. The severe complication rate for definitive irradiation is between 2% and 6%. The commonest complication is laryngeal edema requiring prolonged or permanent tracheostomy.

Hyperfractionated radiation has been used by some clinicians, but for early-stage supraglottic cancer there is no definitive evidence that hyperfractionation improves local control. Prospective trials are needed to determine the relative benefit of hyperfractionation.

Glottis

Early Lesions

Carcinoma in situ of the true vocal cord is highly curable. It can be cured with equal efficiency by microexcision, laser vaporization,[131,132] or radiation therapy.[133,134] Although pure carcinoma in situ lesions are unusual, there is a frequent association between carcinoma in situ and invasive carcinoma. Those series that have been reported in which there were numerous recurrences after stripping of vocal cord carcinoma in situ lesions almost certainly consisted of a heterogenous group that included lesions containing areas of invasive cancer. True carcinoma in situ, by definition, remains superficial to the basement membrane, and if mucosal excision techniques are confined to that group of patients, the cure rate should be the same as the best that can be achieved by radiation therapy. The advantages of radiation therapy are that the voice probably is better than with surgery, it is a more definitive treatment for invasive cancer that may exist within the lesion, there is no requirement for general anesthesia, and when treatment fails, a conservation surgical procedure can salvage most patients. The advantage of surgery, whether it be microexcision or laser vaporization, is that it is simpler, and radiation therapy is held in reserve for future use. As long as the integrity of the submucosa is not violated, the voice results with microexcision or laser vaporization are probably comparable with that achieved with radiation. All things considered, if the diagnosis of pure carcinoma in situ of the vocal cord(s) is fairly certain, microexcision or laser vaporization is probably the treatment of choice. The consistent problem is that many of these so-called carcinoma in situ lesions have been understaged and are riddled with areas of superficial invasive carcinoma. Also, certain carcinoma in situ lesions,

such as those on the anterior commissure, in the subglottis, or some that extend into the laryngeal ventricle, do not lend themselves to these surgical methods; in these, radiation is probably a better means of treatment.

For early glottic cancer (T1–2), excellent local control is achieved by radiation or partial laryngectomy. The relative advantage of radiation over surgery relates to function. With radiation, the voice is unquestionably better. After this treatment, the voice is normal or near normal most of the time. Harrison and coworkers have analyzed the impact on vocal quality by radiation therapy for T1 and T2 glottic lesions and their conclusion corroborated this tenet.[135] In contrast, all patients are hoarse to a varying degree after hemilaryngectomy or cordectomy. Hemilaryngectomy can be used successfully for salvage in many patients who fail radiation therapy.[136–138] In a carefully selected subset of those patients in whom the initial treatment is radiation therapy, there is a second line of defense against glottic cancer that does not involve sacrifice of the larynx.

The actual survival results for primary surgery for T1 glottic cancer are 84% to 98% with laryngofissure and cordectomy.[138–141] Various series have reported similar results with hemilaryngectomy, which is considered to be a better operation, oncologically and functionally, than a cordectomy. Essentially, the 5-year survival rates for primary surgery and primary radiation for T1 lesions are comparable.[142–146] Local control obtained in this same stage glottic group using conservation surgical procedures is reported to be 78% by Kirchner and Owen[65] and 87% by Ogura and associates.[147] Results obtained for comparable (T1) lesions treated by radiation therapy show local control of 91% by Harwood[133] and 93% by Pellitteri and colleagues.[146]

As is true with any treatment, the local control rate decreases with increasing tumor bulk. This finding is especially true for radiation therapy of early glottic cancer. Dickens and coworkers have reported the results for early glottic tumors of various sizes and extent.[148] The lesions were categorized by the type of surgical procedure that would have been necessary had surgery been used. This type of analysis provides an excellent basis for comparing the results of surgery and radiation. The local control with radiation alone in patients suitable for cordectomy was 97% and in patients who needed hemilaryngectomy it was 94%. In both categories, local control increased to 100% when surgical salvage was added. On the contrary, for patients managed by radiation therapy who would have required total laryngectomy, local control was only 65%, but increased to 91% when surgical salvage was added. Extension of these glottic carcinomas onto the anterior and posterior aspects of the larynx lessens the local control rates achieved with radiation therapy.[149] The surgical procedure required for salvage usually was a total laryngectomy rather than a hemilaryngectomy.

Specifically, with anterior commissure involvement, Sessions and associates reported a 5-year survival of 74% for T1 and T2 lesions,[150] and usually found that survival and recurrence rates of anterior commissure lesions correlate with the size and stage of the tumor.[151] Results with radiation therapy for early-stage glottic carcinomas that involve the anterior commissure are reported by Olofsson and colleagues[152] to be 80% survival at 5 years (including those recurrences salvaged by surgery) and Kirchner and Fischer,[78] who reported a local control rate of 85%. Those anterior commissure lesions that are thin and of low volume and that do not have substantial subglottic extension probably are treated with equal efficiency by partial laryngectomy or radiation therapy. As lesions become more advanced, the natural barrier of the anterior commissure ligament is overcome and the thyroid cartilage is invaded;[153] therefore, radiation therapy becomes less appealing than surgery as the front-line treatment. Most tumors involving the anterior commissure occur as a result of spread from the true vocal cord. Lesions actually arising in the anterior commissure are unusual, making up 1% to 2% of glottic cancers.[151,153]

In most centers, most T1 glottic cancers are treated with radiation therapy, and partial or total laryngectomy is used as a salvage operation in those patients who fail irradiation.

The management of T2 lesions is more complicated, because this is a somewhat heterogenous group. Surgical management usually consists of vertical hemilaryngectomy and is associated with 3-year survival rates of 83%[150] and 82%[147] in two major series. Primary radiation therapy with surgical salvage yields a net 5-year survival rate of 92% in Pellitteri's and associate's series,[146] 72% in Wang's series,[143] 90% in Fletcher's and colleague's series,[145] and 72% in Jorgensen's series.[144] Because of the heterogeneity of the T2 group, Wang has suggested subdividing these lesions into those with normal mobility (T2A) and those with impaired mobility (T2B).[143] He showed that local control was obtained in 86% of the former and 63% of the latter when primary radiation was used. Similar observations were made by Harwood,[133] whose series yielded 77% and 51% local control rates for T2A and T2B lesions, respectively. Essentially, T2B lesions seem to behave more like T3 than T2 lesions.

Radiation therapy usually is recommended as the primary treatment modality for T2 lesions with no vocal cord mobility impairment (T2A); however, in those lesions that demonstrate impairment of motion (T2B), hemilaryngectomy usually is preferred. The overall 5-year survival for T1 glottic carcinomas is 82% to 96%, and for T2 lesions it is 51% to 85%.[138,154–156]

Those conservation surgery procedures that can be applied to the management of glottic cancer are time honored and

tested, and when used in the properly selected case of laryngeal cancer, they consistently yield excellent results functionally and oncologically. The most commonly employed of these procedures is the vertical hemilaryngectomy (see the Classification of Conservation Laryngeal Procedures outlined earlier) in which the surgeon bisects the larynx and, to a varying degree, removes a portion or all of the true and false vocal cord along with the respective half of the thyroid cartilage. Because most of the lesions for which this operation is employed are located on the anterior two thirds of the vocal cord, the posterior-most resection line usually is in front of the arytenoid cartilage. In those circumstances in which the cancer extends onto the posterior larynx, this cartilage can be resected (Fig. 22–26). By using the perichondrium from the external surface of the half of the thyroid cartilage that has been removed, the operated side of the larynx heals in the midline, forming a firm buttress (pseudocord) against which the opposite and normal true vocal cord vibrates.

Although a variety of radiation therapy techniques for early-stage lesions have been reported, the most commonly used technique is opposed lateral fields. The patient is simulated in the supine position with maximal head extension. A head cast is made to ensure immobilization, and small portals are designed that treat the larynx alone. Field size is an important prognostic factor. The local recurrence rate is substantially higher for those patients whose field size is 25 cm² or larger. Actually, it would seem that field size is best at 5.5 × 5.5 cm to 6 × 6 cm.

Another important factor is the daily fractionation schedule. Fraction sizes of 200 cGy or greater should be used. Fraction sizes less than 200 cGy per day should be avoided, because the local recurrence rate is higher when this is done. Although there are variations of this theme, such as increasing each fraction dose and thereby achieving the ultimate goal sooner, the general goal of 200 cGy/day is to achieve a total of 6600 cGy in 33 fractions over 6.5 weeks. The authors recommend obtaining a larynx contour during each simulation and evaluating the dose distribution. A wedge is added to keep the inhomogeneity of dose within 10% of the prescription.

Treatment is delivered with cobalt 60 or 4 MeV linear accelerator. Because the neck can be relatively thin at the level

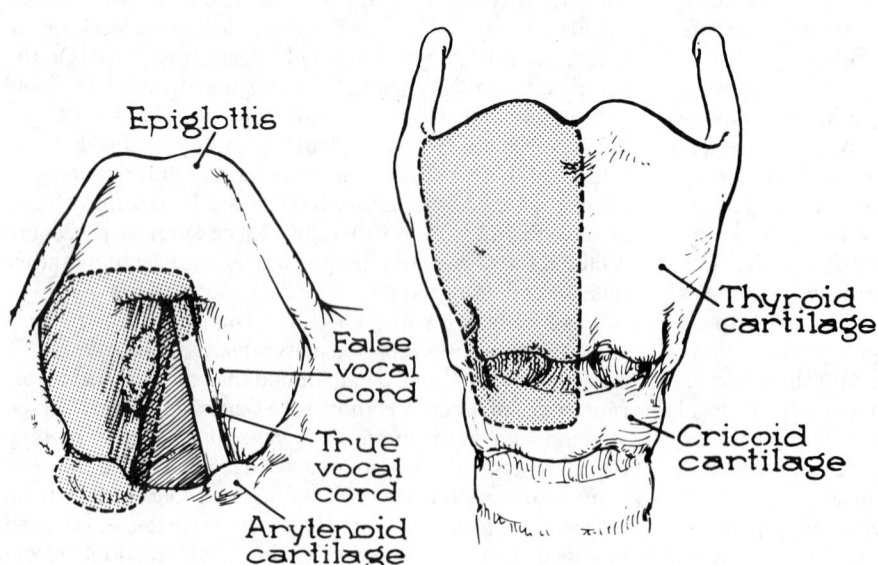

FIGURE 22–26. Axial and frontal views of larynx shows that portion of the organ removed by a horizontal hemilaryngectomy (*shaded*).

of the larynx and anterior neck, higher-energy linear accelerators may provide an inadequate dose distribution. A contour must be taken and proper dosimetry performed before using a higher energy beam.

Advanced Lesions

Glottic cancers that cause vocal cord or hemilaryngeal immobilization or fixation, or both (*i.e.*, T3), are substantially more ominous than are lesions that do not. At a minimum, such motion impairment reflects vocalis muscle invasion; however, there is often further tumor extension into the paraglottic space, opening the entire larynx and adjacent exit areas to cancer spread. Many of these lesions are associated with thyroid or cricoid cartilage destruction, and there is a tendency to underestimate glottic lesions with vocal cord fixation.[60] In Olofsson's and colleagues' study,[60] a significant number of tumors originally had been understaged as T3 cancers, but were actually T4 lesions with extralaryngeal extension. With the unpredictable extent of the disease and the overall high probability of cartilage destruction in mind, surgery traditionally has been favored over radiation therapy for the primary management of T3 lesions. Because of these same features, total laryngectomy is usually advised. The overall 5-year survival for T3 glottic cancers treated with total laryngectomy is reported to be 55% to 72% in four major series.[65,123] However, it has been shown by Kirchner and Som[157-159] that in carefully selected vocal cord lesions that are clearly limited to the vocalis muscle, and in which there is no associated cartilage destruction, hemilaryngectomy can be performed with oncologic safety. In their series of 22 patients, they demonstrated a 60% cure rate. In another similar study, Som reported a 58% curability in 26 patients with selected T3 glottic tumors treated by partial laryngectomy.[160] It should be noted that both of these significant studies were done before the use of CT or MRI. Such technology would have made the evaluation of these lesions and the delineation of their dimensions easier and more accurate. Even with this limitation lessened by contemporary technology, the reader should not be led to underestimate the difficulty of judging correctly the small subset of T3 lesions that is suitable for hemilaryngectomy. This is a judgment appropriately left only to those surgeons with considerable experience in partial laryngeal surgery.

Although there seems to be a deserved preference for primary surgery in the management of T3 glottic cancers, there also appears to be a subset of patients who can be cured without operation. Van den Bogaert[161] reported a local control rate of 53% in a group of patients with operable T3 lesions who had refused surgery. Harwood and colleagues reported a 45% 5-year local control for T3 glottic patients,[162] and Wang reported a 36% 5-year actuarial local control, which increased to 57% when surgical salvage was added.[163]

There is a suggestion of improvement of these results with hyperfractionated radiation therapy. In his group of 53 T3 glottic cancer patients, Mendenhall and coworkers reported a trend toward improved local control in patients treated with twice-daily radiation.[164] In this group, local control was obtained in 71% compared with 53% with once-daily treatment. Terhaard and associates[165] noticed the same trend as Mendenhall and coworkers, reporting an actuarial 3-year local control of 53% overall, but 67% in the subset of patients who were treated with twice-daily radiation therapy. These particular studies suggest that twice-daily radiation may control between 60% and 70% of patients with T3 glottic cancer. These data need further maturation and investigation.

There has been some interest in using radiation therapy to select those patients who might have radioresponsive tumors. In this strategy, radiation therapy is delivered up to a total dose of 4000 to 5000 cGy. At that point, the patient is critically reassessed. If there has been significant regression of disease with return of vocal cord mobility, then definitive radiation is continued. However, if the tumor has not responded satisfactorily, radiation is aborted, and a laryngectomy is performed. Terhaard and associates reported success using this method.[165] Mendenhall and coworkers,[164] however, found no correlation between the return of vocal cord mobility and eventual local control.

T4 tumor designation denotes cartilage destruction or extension of the tumor outside of the confines of the larynx. This grouping together of all T4 lesions is misleading, however, because it fails to account for the more favorable tumor of lesser thickness and volume that has achieved a T4 status only because it originated on a marginal zone and extended to an adjacent area, such as pyriform sinus or base of the tongue. There are favorable and unfavorable T4 lesions, and that determination is made appropriately on the basis of tumor volume, depth, and thickness. With this exception in mind, the performance of the group of T4 glottic lesions is expectedly poorer than that of lesser stages. Traditionally, most of these lesions are treated with total laryngectomy and some sort of a neck dissection and, depending on the status of the neck nodes, they may or may not receive postoperative radiation. The concept of organ preservation by induction chemotherapy identifying those lesions likely to respond to radiation therapy is a recent addition to the treatment armementarium. Those encouraging results of the nonrandomized trials and the results of the Veterans Administration Cooperative Study Group[1-3,166,167] include as part of the studies a number of patients with T4 lesions. Induction chemotherapy integrated larynx preservation protocols are still investigational and experimental, and although the initial results are encouraging, dogma about replacing standard therapy stratagies must be monitored sternly.

Those advanced lesions that have destroyed cartilage, an unfavorable subgroup, have been analyzed by Jesse,[168] who demonstrated an ominous pattern; of the 48 patients, 6% had distant metastasis at presentation, 39% had cervical metastasis, and 30% required an emergency tracheostomy at the time of diagnosis. With total laryngectomy and radiation in some patients, the 4-year cure rate was 54%; however, in that subset of patients who required tracheostomy or who had pharyngeal wall extension, the survival decreased to 38%. Other studies have demonstrated 5-year survival rates of 25% to 30%.[155,156]

Harwood and colleagues[162] reported local control in 56% of T4N0 glottic lesions treated with radical radiation therapy. Five-year survival for radiation with surgical salvage was 49%. Within this group, the local control for patients classified as T4 from cartilage invasion was 67% at 5 years. This was significantly better than those T4 patients who had pyriform sinus involvement. In this latter group, actuarial local control was only 19%. It does not seem that the T4 patients with hypopharyngeal involvement are good candidates for radical

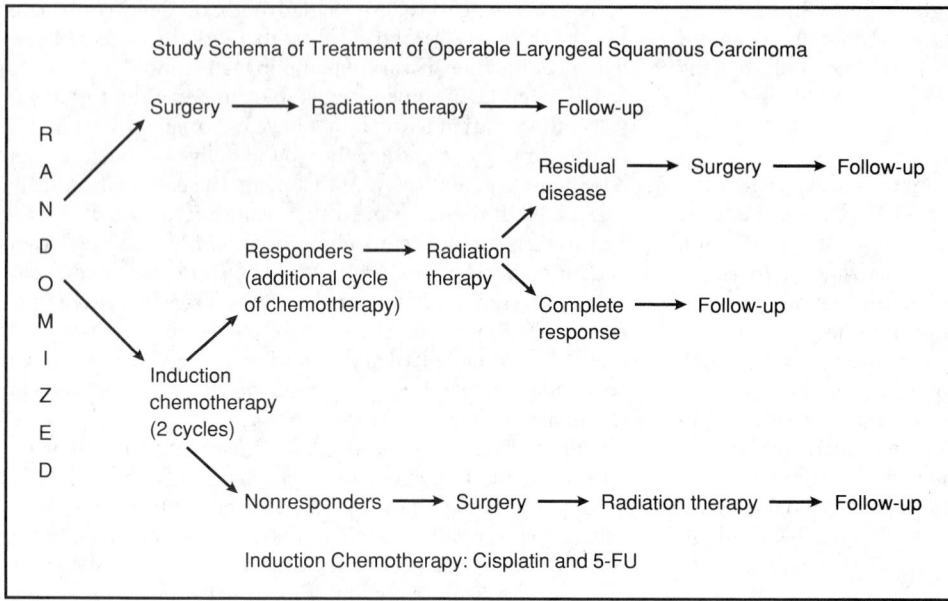

FIGURE 22–27. General treatment schema for organ preservation protocols as conceptualized by Hong and colleagues.[1]

radiation therapy. This circumstance parallels the dismal performance of a similar group treated surgically and reported by Jesse.[168] It also is similar to a comparably poor performance for those larynx cancer patients with hypopharyngeal extension noted by Pfister and colleagues[2] in their larynx preservation (induction chemotherapy) study. The same trend of poor performance for those larynx cancer patients with hypopharyngeal extension was noted by Karp and coworkers.[3] Whatever the treatment variation, this subset of patients consistently seems to do poorly.

In those T3 and T4 glottic cancer patients who are destined for laryngectomy, induction chemotherapy has been used recently in what is collectively referred to as the *larynx preservation protocols*. Hong and coworkers[1] conceptualized that significant tumor regression to induction chemotherapy seems to predict a favorable response to subsequent radiation therapy. The general schema for the various studies that have tested the concept of organ preservation for larynx cancer is shown in Figure 22–27. Various nonrandomized pilot trials and the Veterans Administration Laryngeal Study Group[167] have shown that the larynx can be preserved successfully in most patients with this induction chemotherapy and radiation therapy plan (Table 22–32). Laryngectomy is reserved for those patients who do not respond adequately or who have recurrence of disease. In these studies, laryngeal preservation was achieved without compromising the overall survival rate that would be expected with laryngectomy and postoperative radiation therapy. The results of the various Non-Randomized Organ Preservation Trials that followed this general plan are listed in Table 22–31.[1–3,166,169–174] The student of laryngeal cancer is cautioned to accept these early data for what they are: the encouraging results of investigational and experimental treatment strategies.

Several studies of organ preservation induction strategies should be discussed. Karp and colleagues[3] recently have reported a study that consisted of 35 previously untreated patients with advanced stage III and IV squamous cell carcinomas of the larynx and hypopharynx who received cisplatin-based induction chemotherapy with definitive radiation therapy for cure. All patients ordinarily would otherwise have been treated with total laryngectomy. After radiation therapy, complete response was achieved in 20 of 35 patients. Fifty percent of patients have survived 2 years and longer. Generally, patients with hypopharyngeal primaries had a lower rate of long-term survival and local control.

Another provocative strategy for organ preservation was investigated by Jacobs and coworkers[166] who reported on 35 head and neck squamous cell carcinoma patients who were treated with a cisplatinum and 5-fluorouracil protocol. This

TABLE 22–32. Various Nonrandomized Organ Preservation Trials for Laryngeal Cancer

Investigations	No. of Patients	Site	Organ Preservation (%)
Hong, 1985[1]	35	Larynx	57
Karp, 1991[3]		Hypopharynx	
Jacobs, 1987[166]	30	Any head and neck	40
Pinto, 1991[169]			
Hill, 1986[170]	73	Larynx	70
Urba, 1989[171]	38	Any head and neck	42
Demard, 1990[172]	45	Larynx	40
	26	Hypopharynx	46
Pfister, 1991[2]	40	Larynx Hypopharynx Oropharynx	85
Leyvrax, 1991[173]	58	Any head and neck	62
Shirinian, 1992[174]	64	Larynx Hypopharynx Oropharynx	64

study demonstrated for the first time that in patients who achieve a pathologic complete response to induction chemotherapy, eliminating surgery and substituting primary radiation therapy is feasible and does not compromise survival.

Pfister and associates[2] reported on Memorial Sloan-Kettering's experience with organ preservation strategies. Forty patients with resectable squamous cell carcinoma of the head and neck who would have required a total laryngectomy by standard regimens were treated with platinum-based induction chemotherapy. After completion of chemotherapy, patients with less than a major response were referred for surgery. All patients who had a major response to chemotherapy at the primary site were referred for radiation therapy. Those patients who had residual neck nodes underwent neck dissection also. Of the 40 patients, 26 who achieved a major response to chemotherapy and 8 who refused surgery were treated with radiation only. The 2-year overall actuarial survival was 58%. Pfister and colleagues concluded that larynx preservation with chemotherapy and radiation therapy is feasible in advanced resectable head and neck cancer without an adverse effect on survival.

In 1985, the Cooperative Studies Program of the Department of Veterans Affairs began a multiinstitutional, randomized clinical trial to determine whether induction chemotherapy and definitive radiation, with laryngectomy reserved for salvage, represented a better initial treatment approach for patients with stage III or IV laryngeal cancer than did total laryngectomy and postoperative radiation therapy. The results from the large Veterans Administration Cooperative Studies Program trial indicate that sequential induction chemotherapy and definitive radiation therapy can be an effective strategy for achieving laryngeal preservation in a high percentage of patients without compromising overall survival.[167] The Veterans Administration trial demonstrated no differences in survival between glottic and supraglottic patients. There was no reduction in survival of patients who did not have a substantial response to induction chemotherapy, as has been reported in head and neck cancers arising from other sites.

Because the results of radiation therapy alone have not been compared with induction chemotherapy plus radiation therapy in similarly staged patients, the precise contribution of chemotherapy in these schema remains uncertain, particularly in patients with more limited laryngeal cancer. Although there have been several pilot studies that have shown some enhancement of survival after induction chemotherapy and subsequent definitive radiation therapy,[175-177] this has not been significantly demonstrated in randomized trials.

The selection of a treatment strategy for T4 glottic cancers is dependent on a variety of factors, including the following:

1. If there is bulky neck disease, convention dictates laryngectomy, neck dissection, and postoperative radiation therapy, with both necks being included in the treatment plan.
2. If there is bulky neck disease and if the primary tumor does not have extensive hypopharyngeal extension, induction chemotherapy followed by radiation therapy to primary and neck can be employed in chemosensitive tumors. This would be followed by a neck dissection. In such lesions that are not chemoresponsive, laryngectomy

and neck dissection plus postoperative radiation therapy would be done.
3. If there is substantial hypopharyngeal extension, a conventional approach with laryngectomy or laryngopharyngectomy plus neck dissection and postoperative radiation therapy is recommended.
4. If there is no clinical neck disease present (*i.e.*, T4N0), induction chemotherapy followed by radiation therapy to primary and necks in chemoresponsive tumors should be considered. If such a lesion fails to respond adequately to induction chemotherapy, indicating the probability of relative radioresistance, then the logical course should be a laryngectomy. The laryngectomy probably should be accompanied by appropriate staging selective neck dissection(s)[178] and, depending on the result of the histologic analysis of the neck nodes harvested, postoperative radiation therapy.
5. In these large lesions, especially lesions that demonstrate subglottic extension, radiation must be directed to the tracheal stoma, because recurrence here can be seen in a substantial percentage of these patients. Other indications for postoperative radiation are cartilage and extensive soft tissue invasion.

Subglottis

Even though the preponderance of subglottic tumors are squamous cell carcinomas, adenocarcinomas and adenoid cystic carcinomas are seen occasionally.[82] The cure rate for these tumors is poor, despite combination therapy. Total laryngectomy and appropriate neck surgery, including thyroidectomy, is probably the surgical treatment most recommended and should be followed by radiation therapy.[179,180] Mediastinal dissection of the paratracheal nodal groups does not seem to add substantially to survival rates.[82]

Considerations for Neck Surgery

There are a variety of neck operations currently used in the various treatment plans for laryngeal cancer: the classic radical neck dissection, the modified radical neck dissection, and a group of regional dissections collectively known as *selective neck dissections*. This group of operations recently has been standardized and endorsed by the American Academy of Otolaryngology—Head and Neck Surgery, the Society for Head and Neck Surgeons, and the American Society for Head and Neck Surgery. The monograph outlining the recommended terminology should be studied and used to facilitate interinstitutional data recording and comparison.[178]

There is considerable diversity in the surgical community as to which of these operations should be applied to which situation. Exact guidelines are not consistently substantiated by the data available. Generalizations are applicable, however. The radical neck dissection is almost never used in the clinically negative neck, even though the probability for metastasis is extraordinary. This procedure is usually reserved for necks in which there is gross metastasis. The selective neck dissections often are applied when there is gross disease, but more often they are used as staging procedures in which the goal of the procedure is to harvest and sample the nodal groups at highest risk for metastasis. This philosophy has evolved as a result of our increasing reliance on radiation therapy as the second half of neck treatment whenever disease is discovered in the neck.

The choice of the appropriate selective neck dissection in larynx cancer is based on a knowledge of the consistent pattern of metastasis that is exhibited by the various subsites within the larynx; for example, lesions of the supraglottis are prone to metastasis bilaterally and to levels II and III. However, they rarely spread to level I of the neck.[33] Based on this knowledge, the logical staging operation for a supraglottic laryngeal cancer with a clinically negative neck would be tailored specifically to clean out those various compartments.

ALARYNGEAL REHABILITATION

The philosophy that emphasizes a maximal rehabilitative effort to return the patient to a functional role in society is exemplified vividly in the efforts currently being expended on vocal restoration after total laryngectomy. When laryngectomy is done, the normal method of vocal communication is lost. Since the first total laryngectomy by Bilroth,[181] an ideal method of artificially providing voice has been sought.[182–191] Until recently, most laryngectomy patients have had to rely on mechanical vibratory devices, esophageal speech, or written communication.

Only about 20% to 40% of patients master esophageal speech.[192] It is those postlaryngectomy patients with ineffec-

tive or no esophageal speech who are least likely to reenter their social and family environments as full participants. Even laryngectomy patients who have mastered esophageal speech are hampered by certain mechanical problems and stigmas that create difficulty with their ability to communicate well. Even when mastered, esophageal speech produces only short sentences or monotonal words of limited volume, and its production requires swallowing techniques that are often accompanied by facial grimacing, distortions, and embarrassment. The electrovibratory devices are helpful for intermittent use during the immediate postoperative period and as a back-up system, but are of limited value because one hand is occupied during their use (Fig. 22–28). With these instruments, the voice is mechanical and often distracting, and it is difficult for the user to be heard in a noisy environment.

The state of the art of vocal rehabilitation involves the employment of air shunting from the trachea to the neogullet, thereby setting up a vibratory column that produces noise that comes out of the mouth where it is articulated as speech. This is accomplished by a tracheoesophageal puncture (TEP) and placement of a silicone valve-like device that is structured to allow air into the neogullet, but not allow food or liquids out (Fig. 22–29). What is produced is a form of esophageal speech and voice, but one that is vastly superior to the traditional method of swallowing and burping. The tones produced are less monotonal, the volume of air is limited only by the inspiratory lung volume capacity (just as normal speech is) rather than by how much air is swallowed and burped, and the product has a more fundamental resemblance to normal voice than other methods. After the establishment of an ap-

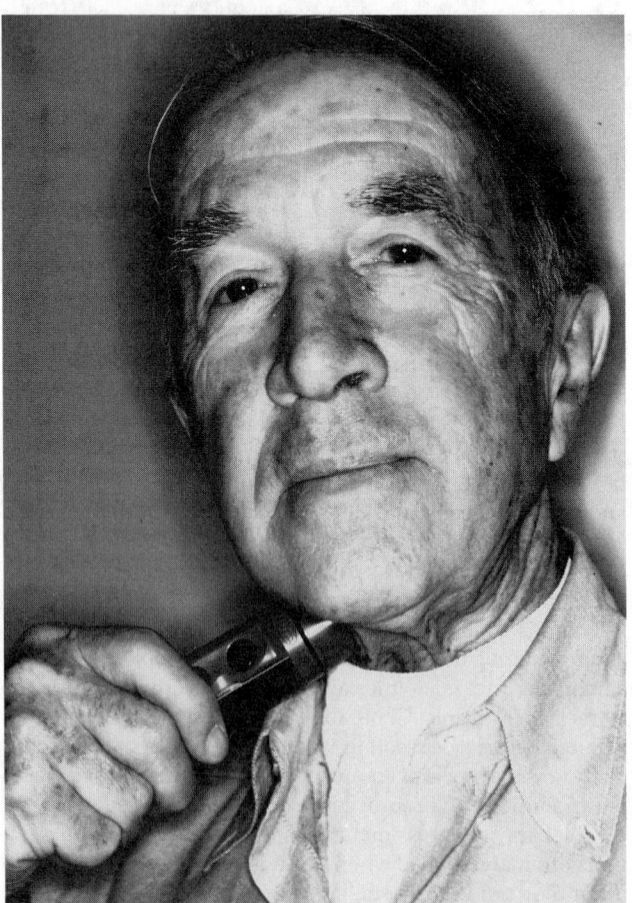

FIGURE 22–28.   Electrovibratory device for alaryngeal speech production in use.

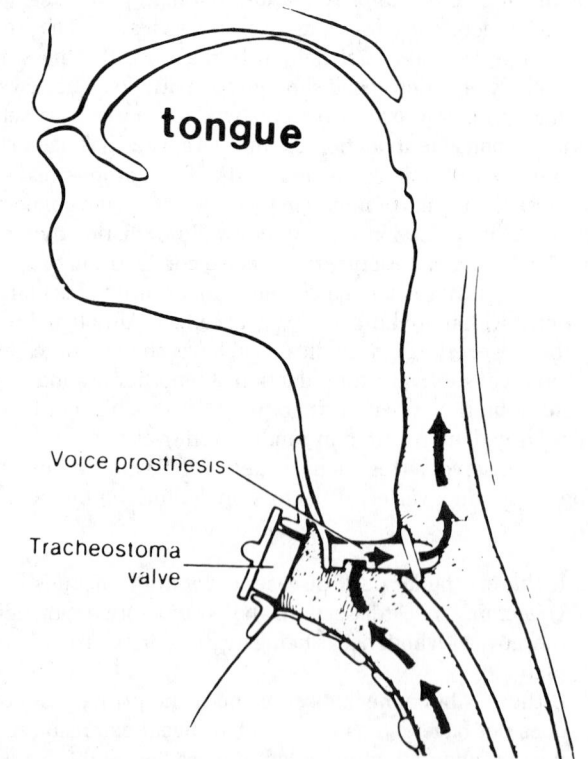

FIGURE 22–29.   Saggital diagram of head and neck depicts tracheoesophageal prosthesis in place in the posterior aspect of the tracheal stoma. Notice the external tracheostoma valve for use with prosthesis.

propriate fistula and the placement of the TEP prosthesis, a tracheostoma valve and external housing device is used (Fig. 22–29). This device allows normal breathing, but shunts the air into the underlying TEP prosthesis. With the increased airflow of voice production, air is routed into the esophagus and up the neogullet that vibrates and causes sound that comes out of the mouth as articulated speech. When an external valve is placed over the stoma with the TEP in place, the final product is a laryngectomized person who usually has exceptional speech with normal articulation and who can dress with clothing that allows complete coverage of the device.[193]

Patients can be returned to work and a relatively normal social life with a functional method of communication. This method effectively achieves voice in about 80% to 90% of patients.[194] There are other surgical methods of vocal rehabilitation,[195,196] but none with the extensive record of clinical application and success as that achieved by the tracheoesophageal phonation as developed and popularized by Singer and Blom[194] and others.[197]

The TEP procedure can be done with equal results at the time of laryngectomy (primary TEP) or as a secondary procedure after radiation. The matter of alaryngeal rehabilitation should be undertaken in concert between the head and neck surgeon and the speech pathologist. The patient who has been rushed to laryngectomy without adequate preoperative preparation (*i.e.*, education, counseling) is usually more difficult to rehabilitate. On the other hand, the patient who is well prepared usually achieves successful speech rehabilitation. It is our approach to take the patient methodically through a series of experiences after the determination is made that a laryngectomy is necessary. The laryngectomy patient should have multiple communication options; therefore, the authors endeavor to teach them how to use the electrovibratory device (see Fig. 22–28), esophageal speech, and TEP phonation (in a selected subset). The speech pathologist is involved at the outset, giving an in-depth description of the anatomy, the operation, and the proposed plan for rehabilitation. The team relies heavily on video demonstrations of the whole subject and patient volunteers who have had similar procedures. At this point, an attempt is made to incorporate family members in the instructional sessions, because a constructive support system contributes to a successful outcome. Additionally, the patient is taught how to use the eletrovibrating device before surgery so that he or she will be able to communicate during convalescence in the hospital. Contacts are also made with the American Cancer Society and various laryngectomy clubs. During this preoperative educational period, the initial training for esophageal speech is begun. After laryngectomy, the speech pathologist visits the patient in the hospital and encourages the use of the mechanical vibrating devices. The patient's perception of a continuum of rehabilitative effort is well served by this comprehensive approach in which the various members of the team communicate and function toward preestablished goals.

There is an ongoing controversy regarding primary versus secondary TEP. The authors favor the latter; however, others believe the procedure ought be done at the time of the laryngectomy. The primary approach shortens the time of rehabilitation, lessens overall expense and, according to the advocates of this approach, the patients have more immediate positive reinforcement in the critical perioperative period.

On the other hand, the advocates of the secondary placement of the TEP argue that by delaying the procedure, more time is allowed for the patient to adapt to and learn to care for the new laryngectomy stoma, the wound is allowed to mature, postoperative radiation therapy is completed, and the patient is allowed to begin learning skills of esophageal speech. The authors believe that the motivation to learn esophageal speech is lessened when a TEP is in place. If the patient is properly prepared psychologically and educationally, this orderly step-by-step approach to rehabilitation is more efficient. Finally, healing is a dynamic phenomenon, and the precise placement and angle of the prosthesis is better ensured by a secondary or delayed placement.

There are circumstances that make patient selection critical to the success of rehabilitation with TEP. To function at a practical level of phonation, the patient must have the cognitive skills and the dexterity necessary to care for the stoma and the TEP site. Patients who have had laryngopharyngectomies with reconstruction of the gullet have a somewhat unpredictable tracheoesophageal voice rehabilitation. Those patients who undergo free jejunal interposition procedures have a somewhat better and more predictable voice than those who have had a gastric transposition for reconstruction. The experience in voice rehabilitation in both of these groups is limited, and the vocal results achieved to date must be viewed as preliminary. Whether employed primarily or secondarily, the enormous contribution made to the laryngectomy patient by the current methods of TEP phonation cannot be underrated. There is a considerable experience currently with this method, and as the plastics technology continues to improve, the process of this type of vocal rehabilitation should be enhanced. It is hoped that the reader appreciates that the current concern among oncologists for quality of life is reflected by the considerable effort being devoted to saving the larynx with conservation operations, innovative radiation strategies, larynx-sparing chemoradiotherapy protocols, and, when these methods fail and laryngectomy is required, a vigorous and thoughtful effort to communications rehabilitation.

HYPOPHARYNX

DEFINITIONS

The hypopharynx is that area of the pharynx that lies behind and below the oropharynx, just out of the view provided by tongue blade and flashlight; as such, it is visually inaccessible by routine office examination. Cancers in the hypopharynx are usually aggressive in their behavior, grow in an area of abundant lymphatic drainage, fail to produce early symptoms or signs of disease, and usually occur in people who are depleted nutritionally and are immunologically compromised. It is not surprising then, that the survival rates for these cancers are poor, and at best, the treatment of them is difficult.

The hypopharynx extends from the oropharynx above to the esophageal inlet below, is cone shaped, and consists of three regions or subsites: the paired pyriform sinuses; the posterior pharyngeal wall; and the postcricoid area. The larynx is located at the anterior aspect of the hypopharynx, indenting it to create the two lateral sulci that are the pyriform sinuses. Even though these sulci lie partially within the framework of the thyroid cartilage, they are actually part of the hypopharynx, and cancers that develop within them behave differently than do those of the larynx. The lateral wall of the pyriform sinuses is continuous with the posterior pharyngeal wall, which extends around to be continuous with the lateral wall of the opposite pyriform sinuses. The apex of the sinus extends down to a level just inferior to those endolaryngeal muscles that make up the adjacent true vocal cord. Above, the medial wall of the pyriform sinuses forms the pharyngeal side of the aryepiglottic fold, which is the partition between hypopharynx and endolarynx. Laterally, the pyriform sinus extends superiorly to the glossoepiglotic fold. The posterior aspect of the pyriform sinus is open and connects with the hypopharyngeal cavity; each pyriform sinus is a three-walled space that opens into the general cavity (Figs. 22–20 and 22–21).

The funnel-shaped postcricoid area begins just below the arytenoids and extends to the level of the cricopharyngeus muscle below. It is lined with the mucosa that overlies the posterior lamina of the cricoid cartilage and that continues into the cervical esophagus. Laterally, the postcricoid mucosa blends with that of the pyriform sinuses and, because of this, these two areas are often affected by the same cancers.

Approximately 70% of hypopharyngeal lesions occur in the pyriform sinuses and the remaining 20% to 30% occur on the posterior pharyngeal and in the postcricoid area.[198] Postcricoid cancers make up a small percentage of the latter group. There are approximately 2500 new hypopharyngeal cancers diagnosed in the United States each year. Overall, these lesions occur more often in men by a significant ratio, but there does seem to be a higher incidence of lower hypopharyngeal, or postcricoid, cancers in women. The upper hypopharyngeal lesions are more common in men.[199] Those lower lesions are more often associated with nutritional abnormalities, whereas the lesions in the remainder of the hypopharynx seem to be associated with heavy smoking and drinking.[200] Those ratios vary somewhat internationally and change in accordance with the incidence of vitamin deficiencies.[201] For example, there is a higher incidence of carcinoma of the postcricoid area in patients with Plummer-Vinson syndrome, a condition in which there is an iron-deficiency anemia. This condition is especially prevalent in northern Europe and is seen in nonsmoking women. Also, other metabolic deficiencies, such as vitamin B_{12} malabsorption, may play a role in the development of these lesions.[202]

PATHOLOGY, PATHOGENESIS, AND NATURAL HISTORY

Almost all hypopharynx malignancies are squamous cell carcinomas that have developed in an environment of deranged mucosa. The generalized effects of the carcinogens encountered over a lifetime can lead to the occurrence of multiple mucosal sites of epithelial disturbances that range from dyskeratosis to frank cancer. The concept of *field cancerization* is in part responsible for the multiple, synchronous primary malignant lesions that occur in approximately 12% to 20% of hypopharyngeal cancers.[198,203–205]

Cancers of the hypopharynx are generally aggressive in their behavior and demonstrate a natural history that is characterized by diffuse local spread, early metastasis, and a relatively high rate of distant spread. The anatomy of the area is such that once a cancer has penetrated the mucosa, there are few barriers to diffuse tumor extension in the submucosal plane. Because of this and also because of the abundant lymphatic network of the region, a localized hypopharyngeal tumor is the exception rather than the rule. An important study by Harrison[205] demonstrated pathologically that in 40% of hypopharynx lesions, the true extent of the cancer had been underestimated initially. Tumors of the pharyngeal walls are more often ulcerative than exophytic and are particularly prone to an insidious and deceptive growth pattern that is characterized by skip metastasis and ill-defined margins; once submucosal, these lesions can resurface at various locations remote from the primary site. They can extend upward in this fashion and can travel all the way to the base of the skull. Cancers of the postcricoid area tend to spread laterally also and can cause vocal cord paralysis by invading fibers of the recurrent laryngeal nerve just as those fibers enter the larynx. Postcricoid lesions can extend downward creating *skip metastases* in the cervical esophagus. Gross involvement of the esophagus with postcricoid cancer is uncommon. These lesions usually do not produce early symptoms and, when discovered, they often have caused cricoid cartilage destruction.

It is significant that the lateral wall of the pyriform sinuses lies against that area of the thyroid cartilage that is often ossified, a state that renders it vulnerable to tumor invasion[61,206] (see Fig. 22–21). In Kirchner's and Owen's series of 500 whole-organ larynx sections, more than 50% of the pyriform sinus cancers demonstrated cartilage invasion.[65] This fact is relevant to the planning of radiation oncologists and surgeons, because cancer involvement in the cartilage lessens radiocurability and substantially compromises safe conservation or partial laryngeal surgery. Depending on the degree of ossification present, tumor that has invaded the thyroid or cricoid cartilage in one area can permeate the entire framework, even extending to the opposite lamina of that structure.

Overall, the distribution of metastatic hypopharynx cancer is to all levels of the neck, with the level II (*jugulodiagastric*) nodes being the commonest site, level III the next commonest site, and levels I, IV, and V the least likely sites.[33] Overall, the risk for cervical metastasis from pyriform sinus cancer is 75%, from posterior pharyngeal wall 60%, and from postcricoid 40%. Only 10% of pyriform sinus lesions present with bilateral metastasis. It occurs more commonly in postcricoid cancers and it is the norm in posterior pharyngeal lesions.[207] Approximately 60% of posterior pharyngeal wall lesions demonstrate bilateral cervical nodes at the initial examination.[208] Metastasis occurs early in the course of hypopharynx cancers. Approximately 60% of pyriform sinus lesions have clinically positive necks at the time of diagnosis, and many of those that have clinically negative necks turn out to have occult metastasis in the thyroid gland or in the paratracheal node chain.[70,209]

Because a significant number of postcricoid and pyriform sinus apical lesions metastasize to the less obvious paratracheal and thyroid gland lymphatics, the incidence of unobvious metastasis from those sites is somewhat greater than in the higher pyriform sinus and posterior pharyngeal wall lesions that typically metastasize to the deep jugular nodes.[210,211] Because of this, calculating occult metastatic rate is a problem in hypopharyngeal cancers.

Because the retropharyngeal lymph nodes that are located high in the neck are primary drainage sites for hypopharyngeal cancers and are involved in more than 40% of patients with posterior pharyngeal wall and pyriform sinus lesions,[212] it is especially important in the staging and treatment of this particular group of tumors to include these nodes in the field of dissection or radiation, or both. These lymphatics are part of the deep jugular chain, are outside of the constrictor muscles, and are readily visible by imaging (Fig. 22–30). Involvement of the retropharyngeal nodes may produce a symptom complex characterized by pain and stiffness in the neck, with pain radiating to the ipsilateral eye and forehead.

The incidence of distant metastasis from hypopharyngeal cancer is substantial, occurring in 24% of all sites and in all stages. This incidence is initially lower, rising in those subpopulations who live longest.[213,214]

DIAGNOSIS, EVALUATION, AND STAGING

Early diagnosis is not often achieved in hypopharyngeal cancer and most treatment series include few T1 lesions. In part, relatively late diagnosis can be blamed on the fact that many patients with these cancers have abused their health by smoking and drinking heavily, and because of that, they have a high tolerance for throat symptoms; however, it is also true that these lesions are often indolent and produce few symptoms until they are substantial in size. This is especially true for posterior pharyngeal wall cancers. More than 50% of patients with hypopharyngeal cancer have clinically obvious cervical metastasis at the time they are first encountered, and in half of these, the neck mass is actually the presenting symptom.[215-218] Pyriform sinus and posterior pharyngeal wall lesions can cause a sensation of irritation and mucus retention that is felt only with swallowing. Otalgia is characteristic of

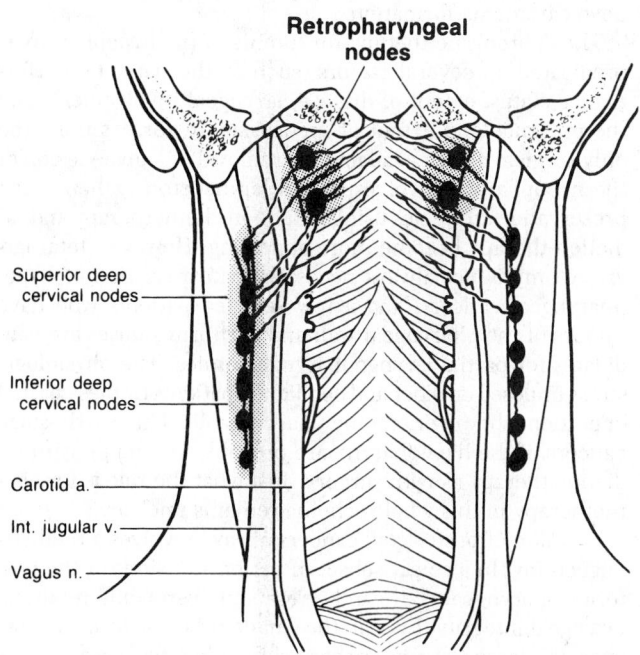

Retropharyngeal Lymph Nodes

FIGURE 22–30. Posterior view of pharynx and great vessels shows retropharyngeal nodes commonly involved in hypopharyngeal cancer.

pyriform sinus lesions and is a manifestation of cancer compromising the sensory fibers of the superior laryngeal nerve, the axons of which synapse with sensory nerves of the external auditory canal. The pain generated is typically dull and is perceived by the patient in the posterior and inferior aspects of the canal and on the posterior aspect of the auricle. In the absence of ear findings, persistent pain in these areas must be viewed with suspicion and a careful examination of the upper aerodigestive tract done by someone skilled in the appropriate methods. Voice change associated with pyriform sinus or postcricoid lesions is a late symptom and usually represents impairment of vocal cord function by invasion into the endolarynx or of a recurrent laryngeal nerve. Patients have often lost their ability to swallow comfortably or have a lack of willingness to swallow because of fear of aspiration. Because of this, they often become debilitated during the course of this disease.

Many patients with hypopharyngeal cancer are chronically ill before the development of their lesion, having the pulmonary and hepatic diseases that accompany a lifetime of tobacco and alcohol excesses. A recognition of the compounding nature of this association with hypopharyngeal cancer is essential in the formulation of an appropriate treatment plan.

Physical examination of the hypopharynx has become much less problematic since the development of the flexible, fiberoptically lighted endoscopes that are easily included in the basic outpatient facilities (see Fig. 22–24). The crevices and partially hidden areas of the laryngopharynx are well visualized using these instruments; however, the conventional handheld mirror examination is still the state of the art when used by the experienced head and neck diagnostician. For the infrequent examiner, however, the benefits of the flexible endoscope are significant. What is most essential is that the primary care physician not be reassured falsely by a normal routine tongue blade and light examination of the mouth and oropharynx. In those patients with persistent symptoms of swallowing alteration or discomfort, otalgia, or voice change, such an examination is totally inadequate, because only a small part of the hypopharynx and none of the larynx is visualized.

Examination of the hypopharynx can demonstrate pooling of secretions in all lesions of the area, but this finding is especially impressive in postcricoid and pyriform sinus cancers because of impairment of the passage of food and secretions into the esophagus. Often, such pooling is the only sign of a small lesion. In larger tumors, the abundance of secretions sometimes obscures the actual presence of the lesion. Occasionally, small and less obvious lesions of the medial wall and apex of the pyriform sinuses cause subglottic edema in the adjacent larynx. Postcricoid carcinomas generally produce esophageal obstructive symptoms sooner than tumors in other areas of the hypopharynx.

In deeply invasive postcricoid or posterior pharyngeal wall cancers, fixation of the larynx and the pharyngeal wall to the prevertebral fascia is often associated with a loss of normal laryngeal crepitation when the thyroid cartilage is manipulated from side to side. As with other sites in the head and neck, the importance of lesion thickness and depth is becoming more and more obvious, especially as the search continues for nonsurgical means of treating these cancers. The thickness or third dimension of hypopharyngeal tumors, their lateral extension into the neck, and, finally, the status of the adjacent lateral cervical and retropharyngeal nodes are visualized well by CT or MRI.[219,220]

Barium esophagogram is an effective tool for detecting second primary cancers in the esophagus and also in evaluating postcricoid lesions[221]; however, this study is of limited value because it visualizes only the surface of the area and does not demonstrate well the total tumor volume. Because of tissue edema and the resulting image distortion that can be caused by instrumentation, these studies should be obtained before endoscopy and biopsy whenever possible.

Each hypopharyngeal cancer should be examined, staged, and carefully mapped on a permanent record (see Fig. 22–25); importantly, this should be accomplished on the awake and upright patient. Direct endoscopy and biopsy should then be done on all patients under general anesthesia where adequate tissue can be sampled and the third-dimensional "feel" for the tumor is better appreciated. Finally, considering the significant incidence of multiple synchronous primary tumors that occur with hypopharyngeal cancer, esophagoscopy and bronchoscopy should be done at this time.

Staging System

As with most cancers, a workable staging system is critical to the evaluation of treatment methods and for the comparison of data between institutions. This is especially true now that the employment of sophisticated imaging allows a relative quantification of tumor volume and extension. Although staging based on physical examination alone is fairly accurate, imaging is especially important in those lesions that are treated by nonsurgical means, because pathologic positivity or negativity of the neck is never proved unless there is a recurrence. Although considerable effort has been expended to develop workable and descriptive terminology, there continue to be limitations to current staging for hypopharyngeal cancers. For example, the system is satisfactory for disease of the pyriform sinuses, but it cannot be applied completely to lesions of the posterior pharyngeal wall, because they usually do not invade the larynx, and fixation is not part of the natural history. Rather, posterior pharyngeal wall tumors would be more appropriately staged by tumor diameter, as is the case with oropharyngeal lesions. According to the current system, a 5×4 cm posterior pharyngeal lesion without laryngeal fixation would still be classified as a T1 lesion, but in fact, it would have a prognosis similar to that for a T3 lesion.[222] The most recent AJCC staging for hypopharyngeal cancer is as follows:[30]

Tis	Carcinoma in situ.
T1	Tumor confined to one subsite (*i.e.,* pyriform fossa or posterior pharyngeal wall).
T2	Extension of tumor to adjacent region or site, N0 hemilarynx fixation.
T3	Extension of tumor to adjacent region or site, with hemilarynx fixation.
T4	Massive tumor invading cartilage, bone, or soft tissue of the neck.

The nodal staging and the stage grouping for the hypopharynx are the same as with other head and neck sites.

TREATMENT AND SURVIVAL

A variety of prognostic factors have been identified for squamous carcinomas of the hypopharynx. Women and patients younger than 50 years of age seem to have a more favorable outcome.[223] Because these tumors can affect swallowing, significant weight loss can occur, and extreme nutritional deficiency and debilitation may even prevent the delivery of curative therapy. Because many of the symptoms of this disease result from an advanced state, most patients will be stage III or IV when diagnosed and, therefore, most are candidates for combined modality treatment. This involves surgery and radiation therapy and, more recently, investigational chemotherapy programs. There must be close collaboration between surgeon, radiation oncologist, and medical oncologist in the multidisciplinary evaluation and treatment of patients with hypopharyngeal cancer.

The fact that most patients with hypopharyngeal cancers currently are managed with combined treatment modalities probably should not suggest an inherent biologic difference between these tumors and other squamous cell carcinomas in the upper aerodigestive tract; rather, it is testimony to the fact that only a small number of these patients present with T1 or T2 disease. There are higher percentages of poorly differentiated carcinomas seen in the hypopharynx, but cell for cell, it is not clear that these cancers are any different than other poorly differentiated squamous cell carcinomas found in other sites. What makes hypopharyngeal cancers uniquely ominous is related instead to the anatomy of the area that allows extensive spreading of these tumors. Additionally, poor performance relates to debilitated patients, the extensive lymphatic drainage of the area, and to the fact that the diffuse carcinogenic effects that led to the initial problem also create an environment of condemned mucosa, multifocality, and de novo carcinoma formation.

The appropriate therapy for tumors of the hypopharynx is predicated on several factors, such as the patient's performance status, extent of disease, laryngeal involvement, and the presence and extent of metastasis. If, for example, the only surgical option available for removal of a given lesion of the hypopharynx involves a total laryngectomy, then organ preservation strategies using induction chemotherapy and radiation therapy become more appealing. However, total laryngectomy is not always necessary with resection of hypopharyngeal cancers, and a few selected patients who have tumors of the pharyngeal wall and pyriform sinuses are candidates for partial laryngopharyngectomies. The physiologic stress imposed on older and debilitated patients by these partial operations, however, can be unacceptable. Thin, early-stage cancers of the hypopharynx are probably as curable with radiation therapy as with surgery. Just what the role is for chemotherapy in this whole schema remains unclear.

Excision of postcricoid cancers always involves a total laryngectomy. In a select subset of patients, lesions of the posterior pharyngeal wall can be resected even while retaining laryngeal integrity. Even in the smaller of these lesions, however, the larynx can be preserved in only a few cases.[207] Because of the tendency of pharyngeal wall lesions to have ill-defined margins, generous resections are necessary; with such liberal tissue removal, much of the sensory innervation normally employed in the act of swallowing is violated. With large T3 and with T4 tumors, laryngectomy is mandatory to achieve adequate surgical margins and to avoid the significant chronic aspiration that usually follows pharyngectomy in these cases, and which is often incompatible with life. With the contemporary techniques of reconstruction in head and neck surgery being as sophisticated as they are, the limitations to this form of surgery do not relate to anatomic realignment; rather, they are physiologic, and an ill-conceived larynx preservation procedure may cure the cancer but condemn the patient to an unacceptable lifestyle. There are newer techniques of hypopharyngeal reconstruction being developed that employ reinnervated free flaps. This reconstitution of the sensory apparatus so important to deglutition may counteract, to some extent, the problems currently limiting the ability to resect this area radically.[224]

Limited T1 and T2 lesions on the medial wall of the pyriform sinus may be removed by partial laryngectomy, but either extension to the apex of the sinus or involvement of the adjacent postcricoid area dictates total laryngectomy. These medial wall lesions are particularly prone to penetrate the paraglottic space of the larynx (see Fig. 22–21), and when this occur, partial laryngectomy becomes oncologically unsafe. In a pyriform sinus lesion, any motion change noticed in the vocal cord suggests invasion into the larynx. There are notable surgeons who are skeptical of any indication for the employment of partial laryngectomy for cancers of the pyriform sinuses. However, whatever the indications, the point is that it is fundamental that any attempt to remove a pyriform sinus cancer with less than a total laryngectomy should be done only by those surgeons with considerable experience in making the subtle judgments so often involved in this type of laryngeal surgery. With the alternatives to surgery that are now available to treat these tumors, and considering our consistent ability to restore voice function after laryngectomy, any oncologic gamble associated with inadvisably trying to save the larynx is unacceptable. Overall, partial laryngopharyngectomy with preservation of voice and swallowing can be justifiably employed in fewer than 5% of all hypopharyngeal cancers.[225]

Radiation therapy is effective for early lesions of the hypopharynx, especially when they are exophytic.[226,227] Hypopharyngeal cancers are not always homogenous, however, and although part of the lesion may fit this description, there may exist an ulcerative component that is associated with an impressive depth and with skip metastasis. Modern imaging has helped in the pretreatment evaluation of these tumors, and a reasonable appraisal of thickness and overall tumor volume is often achieved by MRI. Mendenhall and associates report local control in 79% of T1 and 71% of T2 lesions treated with radiation; however, the 5-year survival in this group was only 60%.[227] Vandenbrouck and coworkers reported 5-year survival of only 40% in an extensive series of smaller lesions treated with radiation therapy.[226] These data are similar to those achieved surgically for early disease. For instance, Shah and colleagues reported 5-year survival of 43% and 38%, respectively, for surgically managed T1 and T2–3 (N0) hypopharyngeal disease.[228]

Disease control drops significantly for more advanced lesions. In both the series by Mendenhall and Bataini and their colleagues, T3 lesions treated with primary radiation therapy had approximately a 40% local control rate, but a dismal 5

year-survival of less than 20%.[227,229] Unfortunately, results of surgery for advanced disease are not any better. Shah and coworkers reported a 16% 5-year survival for patients with T3 disease.[228] When comparing single-modality therapy of hypopharyngeal cancers, results of surgery and radiation therapy are roughly equivalent, with both yielding suboptimal outcomes.

Because of the consistently poor survival data associated with the single-modality methods of treating more advanced hypopharyngeal cancer, combined therapy consisting of radiation administered after pharyngectomy or laryngopharyngectomy is the method currently being practiced in most centers.[227,230,231] The sequencing of the modalities is fairly standard, with the radiation generally employed postoperatively in all but selected circumstances. Essentially, this sequence allows the safe delivery of radiation doses in the 6000- to 7000-cGy range. Data from the M.D. Anderson Cancer Center revealed that postoperative radiation therapy in hypopharyngeal cancer had reduced their failure rate above the clavicle to 11% compared with 39% with surgery alone. Various trials from RTOG and others have compared preoperative with postoperative therapy, and that data suggest better locoregional control and a trend toward better survival in the group treated with postoperative therapy.[232,233] Select circumstances exist, however, in which radiation therapy is recommended before surgery. For example, in those circumstances in which the primary tumor is small and exophytic, and is therefore suitable for definitive radiation therapy, but in which a degree of neck disease precludes management with radiation alone, curative therapy to both the primary and neck followed by neck dissection is an acceptable treatment plan. Mendenhall and associates have reported an 80% 2-year control rate for disease above the clavicle in patients with advanced neck disease and early primary tumors that have been treated in this fashion.[227] Just as with other head and neck sites, the clonal progeny in cervical metastasis is often more prominent than in the primary tumor.

Several groups have reported results of a treatment strategy that consisted of primary radiation with surgery being used only for salvage. Kean and associates[234] reported 41% disease control using this approach. Most patients (75%) in this series had been staged as T3 and T4; approximately two thirds had palpable nodal metastases; and the 5-year survival was only 15%.

Traditional treatment programs of surgery and radiation therapy for hypopharyngeal carcinomas have been augmented by organ preservation induction-chemotherapy strategies. Although the hypopharynx has not been singled out for study, the results in three separate clinical trials have been extracted from a heterogenous group of tumors.[2,3,166] Within these trials, patients with tumors originating in the hypopharynx demonstrated a lower rate of long-term survival and local control than did patients in whom primary tumors arose at other sites of the upper aerodigestive tract. The value of induction chemotherapy in the treatment of squamous cell carcinoma of the hypopharynx has not been tested adequately, and its exact role is uncertain.

Survival data vary considerably between sites within the hypopharynx. Few postcricoid cancers are treated by radiation, but anecdotal experience suggests that a small subset of patients with smaller thin lesions are treatable with curative therapy. In almost all postcricoid lesions, extensive surgery consisting of laryngopharyngectomy or laryngopharyngo-esophagectomy with reconstruction is followed by postoperative radiation and yields a 20% to 25% 5-year survival.[235,236] Posterior pharyngeal wall lesions of earlier stages can be treated with equal effectiveness by radiation or by surgery. More advanced lesions are best treated by combined surgery followed by postoperative radiation.[237] Meoz-Mendes and colleagues reported that 91% of T1 and 73% of T2 lesions of the pharyngeal wall can be controlled with primary radiation.[237] This required a dosage greater than 6500 cGy. For T3–4 disease, similar doses controlled 61% and 37%, respectively. Pyriform sinus lesions of early stage are curable by radiation, whereas the much more common advanced lesions are best treated by combined therapy. Data recently accumulated by Vandenbrouck and coworkers[232] showed a 3-year survival rate of 48%, which dropped to 33% at 5 years for lesions treated with total and partial laryngectomy plus postoperative radiation therapy. In that same series, the 3-year survival rate was 67% in the group treated by partial laryngectomy plus postoperative radiation therapy. This latter statistic probably reflects the increased survival expected in lesser staged disease.

All treatment plans for hypopharynx cancer must consider certain facts: the overwhelming majority of these lesions metastasize to cervical lymph nodes, and in the case of the posterior pharyngeal wall, bilateral metastasis is the rule rather than the exception; 40% of posterior pharyngeal wall lesions and probably an equal number of upper pyriform sinus lesions metastasize to the retropharyngeal nodes; in those patients with clinically negative necks, the incidence of occult metastasis is substantial; and between 20% to 30% of pyriform sinus, and probably an equal number of posterior pharyngeal wall, lesions are associated with distant metastasis. Even in the lesser-stage hypopharyngeal lesions, the high rate of regional metastases requires inclusion of the neck(s) in all management plans.

Specific Treatment Methods

Patients treated with primary radiation therapy require treatment to the primary site and both necks. The primary site and upper neck fields are treated with bilateral opposed portals, and the low neck fields are treated with anterior portals. If lymph nodes are involved, a neck dissection usually is added. If no neck dissection is planned, the node-bearing regions must be treated to higher doses.

When patients who have had a total laryngectomy are receiving postoperative radiation, it is important to irradiate the tracheal stoma. For postoperative radiation, the total doses recommended to the primary site and involved areas of the neck are between 6000 and 6500 cGy in 6.5 to 7.5 weeks. The tracheal stoma is treated to a total dose of 5000 to 5500 cGy.

Lesions of the hypopharynx often require laryngopharyngectomy, or laryngopharyngoesophagectomy, after which the means of reconstruction consist of either free jejunal graft with microvascular anastomosis,[238] various myocutaneous flaps, or in the cases that include esophagectomy, gastric transposition.[239] Reconstruction of the hypopharynx has been enhanced greatly by the interposition free jejunal graft, which is less morbid than gastric transposition and is associated with a high rate of success.

Surgical management of the neck is similar to other sites in the upper aerodigestive tract. In those patients with substantial and multilevel disease, radical neck dissection usually is employed in continuity with the primary resection, unless the primary tumor has been treated with curative radiation. In those patients with minimal neck disease or with clinically negative necks, radiation alone can suffice or any of a variety of selected neck dissections can be employed as a means of removing gross disease from the neck in preparation for radiation.[178]

REFERENCES

1. Hong W, O'Donoghue G, Sheetz S. Sequential response patterns to chemotherapy and radiotherapy in head and neck cancer. In: Wagener D, Bligham G, Sweets V, Wils J, eds. Primary chemotherapy in cancer medicine. Vol 201. New York: Alan Liss, 1985: 191–197.
2. Pfister D, Strong E, Harrison L. Larynx preservation with combined chemo and radiotherapy in advanced head and neck cancer. J Clin Oncol 1991;9:830–859.
3. Karp D, Vaughan C, Carter R, et al. Larynx preservation with induction chemotherapy plus radiation as alternative to laryngectomy. Am J Clin Oncol 1991;14:273–279.
4. Barclay T, Rao N. The incidence and mortality rates for laryngeal cancer from total cancer registries. Laryngoscope 1975;83:254.
5. Krajina Z, Kucar Z, Zonic-Carnelutti V. Epidemiology of laryngeal cancer. Laryngoscope 1975;85:11–33.
6. Iwai H, Koike Y. Primary laryngoplasty. Laryngoscope 1975;85:929.
7. Lowry W. Alcoholism in cancer of the head and neck. Laryngoscope 1975;85:1275.
8. Austen D. Larynx. In: Schottenfeld P, FR Aumeni J, eds. Cancer epidemiology and prevention, Philadelphia: WB Saunders, 1982:554.
9. Iwamoto H. An epidemiological study of laryngeal cancer in Japan (1960–1969). Laryngoscope 1975;85:1162.
10. Krajina Z, Kucar Z, Konic-Carnelatti V. Epidemiology of laryngeal cancer. Laryngoscope 1975;85:1155.
11. Hiranandani L. Panel on epidemiology and etiology of laryngeal carcinoma. Laryngoscope 1975;85:1197.
12. DeStefani E, Correa P, Oreggia F. Risk factors for laryngeal cancer. Cancer 1987;60: 3087.
13. Graham S, Mettlin C, Marshall J. Dietary factors in the epidemiology of cancer of the larynx. Am J Epidemiol 1981;113:675.
14. Morrison M. Is chronic gastroesophageal reflux a causative factor in glottic carcinoma? Otolaryngol Head Neck Surg 1988;99:370–373.
15. Wynder E, Bross I, Day E. Epidemiological approach to the etiology of cancer of the larynx. JAMA 1956;160:1384.
16. Kurozumi S, Harada Y, Sugimoto Y, Saaski H. Airway malignancy in poisonous gas workers. Laryngol Otol 1977;91:217.
17. Morgan R, Shettigara P. Occupational asbestos exposure, smoking, and laryngeal carcinoma. Ann NY Acad Sci 1976;271:308.
18. Goolden A. Radiation cancer of the pharynx. Br Med J 1951;2:1110.
19. Lowry W. Alcoholism in cancer of the head and neck. Laryngoscope 1975;85:1275.
20. Spitz M, Fvegers J, Goepfert H, Hong W, Newell G. Squamous cell carcinoma of the upper aerodigestive tract. Cancer 1988;61:203–208.
21. Segi M. Age-adjusted death rates for cancer for selected sites in 46 countries in 1977, p. 13. Tokyo, Japan: Segi Institute for Cancer Epidemiology, 1982:13.
22. Ramadan M, Morton R, Stell P, Phawah P. Epidemiology of laryngeal cancer. Clin Otolaryngol 1982;7:417.
23. Pietramtoni L, Fior R. Clinical and surgical problems of cancer of the larynx and hypopharynx. Acta Otolaryngol 1958;142:1.
24. Lauerma S. Treatment of laryngeal cancer: A study of 638 cases. Acta Otolaryngol 1967;225:140.
25. Wynder E. Toward the prevention of laryngeal cancer. Laryngoscope 1975;85:1190.
26. Jankovic I, Merkas Z. Radiotherapy as the primary approach in the treatment of laryngeal cancer. In: Alberti P, Bryce D, eds. Workshops from the Centennial Conference on laryngeal cancer. East Norwalk, CT: Appleton-Century-Crofts, 1976:881.
27. Smith R, Caulk R, Frazell E. Revision of the clinical staging system for cancer of the larynx. Cancer 1973;31:72.
28. Martensson B. Indications for transconiscopy. In: Alberti P, Bryce D, eds. Workshops from the Centennial Conference on laryngeal cancer. East Norwalk, CT: Appleton-Century-Crofts, 1976:668.
29. Kirchner J. Growth and spread of laryngeal cancer—as related to partial laryngectomy. In: Alberti P, Bryce D, eds. Workshops from the Centennial Conference on laryngeal cancer. East Norwalk, CT: Appleton-Century-Crofts, 1976:54.
30. American Joint Committee on Cancer. Manual for staging of cancer. 3rd ed. Philadelphia: JB Lippincott, 1988.
31. Hirano M. Structure of the vocal fold in normal and disease states. In: Ludlow C, O'Connell H, eds. Proceedings of the Conference on the assessment of vocal pathology. Report No. 11. Rockville, MD: American Speech and Hearing Association 1981;11: 11–27.
32. Pressman J, Simon M, Moncel C. Anatomical studies related to the dissemination of cancer of the larynx. Trans Am Acad Ophthalmol Otolaryngol 1970;64:628.

33. Lindberg R. Distribution of cervical lymph nodes from squamous cell carcinoma of upper respiratory and digestive tracts. Cancer 1972;29:1446–1449.

34. Sekula J, Horzela T. Studies on the cervical lymph nodes utilizing iodinated I13, serum albumin in patients with carcinoma of the larynx. Arch Otolaryngol 1971;94:118.

35. Kashima H. The characteristics of laryngeal cancer correlating with cervical lymph node metastasis. In: Alberti P, Bryce D, eds. Workshops from the Centennial Conference on laryngeal cancer. East Norwalk, CT: Appleton-Century-Crofts, 1976:855.

36. Clinical evaluation of the larynx. In: Thawley S, Panje W, Batsakis J, Lindberg R, eds. Comprehensive management of head and neck tumors. Vol 1. Philadelphia: WB Saunders, 1987:874.

37. Milroy C, Rode J, Moss E. Laryngeal paragangliomas and neuroendocrine carcinomas. Histopathology 1991;18:201–209.

38. Laccourreye O, Chabardes E, Weinstein G, Carnot F, Brasnu R, Laccourreye H. Synchronous arytenoid and pancreative neuroendocrine carcinomas. Laryngol Otol 1991;105:573–575.

39. Arold-Schneider M, Schall H. Occurrence of non-metaplastic squamous epithelium within the larynx and its relation to the development of cancer. Laryngol Rhinol Otol 1990;69:91–97.

40. Crissman J. Laryngeal keratosis preceding laryngeal carcinoma. Arch Otolaryngol 1982;108:445.

41. Crissman J. Laryngeal keratosis and subsequent carcinoma. Head Neck Surg 1979;1:386.

42. Hellquist H, Lundgren J, Olofsson J. Hyperplasia, keratosis, dysplasia and carcinoma-in-situ of the vocal cords. Clin Otolaryngol 1982;7:11.

43. Sllamniku B, Bauer W, Painter C, Sessions D. The transformation of laryngeal keratosis into invasive carcinoma. Am J Otolaryngol 1989;10:42–54.

44. Hjslet P, Nielsen P, Palvio P. Premalignant lesions of the larynx. Acta Otolaryngol 1989;107:130–135.

45. Munck-Wirland E, Krylenstierna R, Lindholm J, Amer G. Image cytometry DNA analysis of dysplastic squamous epithelial lesions of the larynx. Anticancer Res 1991;11:597–600.

46. Bauer W. Concomitant carcinoma in situ and invasive carcinoma of the larynx. In: Alberti P, Bryce D, eds. Workshops from the Centennial Conference on laryngeal cancer. East Norwalk, CT: Appleton-Century-Crofts, 1976:127–136.

47. Miller A, Fisher H. Clues to the life history of carcinoma in situ of the larynx. Laryngoscope 1971;81:1475.

48. McGavran M, Bauer W, Ogura J. The incidence of cervical lymph node metastases from epidermoid carcinoma of the larynx and their relationship to certain characteristics of the primary tumor. Cancer 1961;14:55.

49. Kirchner J, Cornog J, Holmes R. Transglottic cancer: Its growth and spread within the larynx. Arch Otolaryngol 1974;99:247.

50. Spiro R, Alfonso A, Farr H, Strong E. Cervical node metastases for epidermoid carcinoma: A critical assessment of current staging. Am J Surg 1974;128:566.

51. Reid A, Robin P, Powell J, McConkey C, Rockley J. Staging carcinoma: Its value. J Laryngol Otol 1991;105:456–458.

52. Hirabayshi H, Koshi K, Uno K. Extracapsular spread of squamous carcinoma in neck nodes: Prognostic factors in laryngeal cancer. Laryngoscope 1991;101:502–506.

53. Staley C, Herzon F. Elective neck dissection in carcinoma of the larynx. Otolaryngol Clin North Am 1970;3:543.

54. Mohit-Tabatabai M, Sobel H, Rush B, Mashberg R. Relationship of thickness of floor of mouth stage I and II cancers to regional metastasis. Am J Surg 1986;152:351.

55. Molinari R. Clinical classification of laryngeal carcinoma critique of existing classifications and proposals of a new working classification. Acta Otorhinolaryng 1991;10:579–591.

56. Cachin Y. Supraglottic carcinomas: The early cases. Laryngoscope 1975;83:1617.

57. Coates H, DeSanto L, Devine K, Elveback L. Carcinoma of the supraglottic larynx: A review of 221 cases. Arch Otolaryngol 1976;102:686.

58. Gregor K. The preepiglottic space revisited—is it significant? Am J Otolaryngol 1990;11:161–165.

59. Micheau C, Luboinski B, Sancho H, Cachin Y. Modes of invasion of cancer of the larynx: A statistical, histological, and radioclinical analysis of 120 cases. Cancer 1976;38:346.

60. Olofsson J, Lord I, VanNostrand A. Vocal cord fixation in laryngeal carcinoma. Acta Otolaryngol 1973;75:486.

61. Kirchner J. One hundred laryngeal cancer studies by serial section. Ann Otol Rhinol Laryngol 1969;78:689.

62. Ogura J, Biller H, Wette R. Elective neck dissection for pharyngeal and laryngeal cancers. Ann Otol Rhinol Laryngol 1971;80:646–651.

63. Putney F. Elective versus delayed neck dissection in cancer of the larynx. Surg Gynecol Obstet 1961;112:736–742.

64. Fletcher G. Elective irradiation of subclinical disease in cancers of the head and neck. Cancer 1972;29:1450–1454.

65. Kirchner J, Owen J. Five hundred cancers of the larynx and pyriform sinus. Laryngoscope 1977;87:1288.

66. Ogura J, Sessions D, Spector G. Conservation surgery for epidermoid carcinoma of the supraglottic larynx. Laryngoscope 1975;85:1808.

67. Fayov J. Carcinoma of the endolarynx: Results of irradiation. Cancer 1975;35:1525.

68. Hansen H. Supraglottic carcinoma of the aryepiglottis fold. Laryngoscope 1975;85:1667.

69. Shah J, Tollefsen H. Epidermoid carcinoma of the supraglottic larynx. Am J Surg 1974;128:494.

70. Biller H, Davis W, Ogura J. Delayed contralateral cervical metastasis with laryngeal and laryngopharyngeal cancers. Laryngoscope 1971;81:1499.

71. Ogura J, Spector G, Sessions D. Conservation surgery for carcinoma of the marginal area. Laryngoscope 1975;85:1801.

72. Som M. Conservation surgery for carcinoma of the supraglottis. J Laryngol Otol 1970;84:655.

73. Colombo A, Bimbi G, Gelosa G, Brusamolino R. Cervical metastasis of N0 laryngeal cancer. Acta Otorhinolaryng 1990;10:121–127.

74. Sako K. Fallibility of palpation in diagnosis of metastasis to nodes. Surg Gynecol Obstet 1964;118:989.

75. Spiro R. Cervical node metastasis from epidermoid carcinoma of the oral cavity and oropharynx. Am J Surg 1974;128:562.

76. DeSanto L. Neck dissection: Is it worthwhile? Laryngoscope 1982;92:502.

77. Lawson W, Biller H, Suen J. Cancer of the larynx. In: Myers G, Suen J, eds. Cancer of the head and neck. 2nd ed. New York: Churchill Livingstone 1989:533–592.

78. Kirchner J, Fischer J. Anterior commissure cancer. In: Alberti P, Bryce D, eds. Workshops from the Centennial Conference on laryngeal cancer. East Norwalk, CT: Appleton-Century-Crofts, 1976:679–681.

79. Jesse R, Lindberg R, Horiot J. Vocal cord cancer with anterior commissure extension: Choice of treatment. Am J Surg 1971;122:437.

80. Sessions D, Ogura J, Fried M. Laryngeal carcinoma involving anterior commissure and subglottis. In: Alberti P, Bryce D, eds. Workshops from the Centennial Conference on laryngeal cancer. East Norwalk, CT: Appleton-Century-Crofts, 1976:674–678.

81. Lawson W, Biller H, Suen J. Cancer of the larynx. In: Myers G, Suen J, eds. Cancer of the head and neck. 2nd ed. New York: Churchill Livingstone 1989:558.

82. Stell P. The subglottic space. In: Alberti P, Bryce D, eds. Workshops from the Centennial Conference on laryngeal cancer. East Norwalk, CT: Appleton-Century-Crofts, 1976:682.

83. Harrison D. The pathology and management of subglottic cancer. Ann Otol Rhinol Laryngol 1971;80:6.

84. Kraus F, Perez-Mesa C. Verrucous carcinoma: Clinical and pathological study of 105 cases involving oral cavity, larynx, and genitalia. Cancer 1966;19:26.

85. Van Nostrand A, Olofsson J. Verrucous carcinoma of the larynx. Cancer 1972;30:691.

86. Biller H, Ogura J, Bauer W. Verrucous cancer of the larynx. Laryngoscope 1971;81:1323.

87. Ackerman L. Verrucous carcinoma of the oral cavity. Surgery 1948;23:670.

88. Batsakis J, Hybels R, Crissman J, Rice D. The pathology of head and neck tumors: Verrucous carcinoma: XV. Head Neck Surg 1982;5:29.

89. Abramson A, Brandsma J, Steinberg B, Winkler B. Verrucous carcinoma of the larynx. Arch Otolaryngol 1985;111:709–715.

90. Vesely J, Sibl O, Kudrmann J, Kremar M. Verrucous carcinoma of the larynx. Otolaryngology 1989;38:284–288.

91. Glanz H, Kleinasser O. Verrucous carcinoma of the larynx—a misnomer. Arch Otorhinolaryng 1987;244:108.

92. Myers E, Sobol S, Ogura H. Hemilaryngectomy for verrucous carcinoma of the glottis. Laryngoscope 1980;90:693.

93. Sessions R, Hudkins C. Malignant cervical adenopathy. In: Cummings C, ed. Otolaryngology: Head and neck surgery. 2nd ed. St. Louis: CV Mosby, 1992:1605–1625.

94. Biller H, Ogura J, Bauer W. Verrucous cancer of the larynx. Laryngoscope 1971;81:1323.

95. Fonts E, Greenlaw R, Rush B, Rovin S. Verrucous squamous cell carcinoma of the oral cavity. Cancer 1969;23:152.

96. Perez C, Kraus F, Evans J. Anaplastic transformation in verrucous carcinoma of the oral cavity after radiation therapy. Radiology 1966;86:108.

97. Elliott G, MacDougall J, Elliott J. Problems of verrucous squamous carcinoma. Ann Surg 1973;177:21.

98. Rider W. Toronto experience of verrucous carcinoma of the larynx. In: Alberti P, Bryce D, eds. Workshops from the Centennial Conference on laryngeal cancer. East Norwalk, CT: Appleton-Century-Crofts, 1976:460–461.

99. Medina J, Dichtel W, Luna M. Verrucous-squamous carcinomas of the oral cavity. Arch Otolaryngol 1984;110:437.

100. Burns H, Van Nostrand A, Bryce D. Verrucous carcinoma of the larynx: Management by radiotherapy and surgery. Ann Otol Rhinol Laryngol 1976;85:538–543.

101. Myerowitz R, Barnes E, Myers E. Small cell anaplastic (oat cell) carcinoma of the larynx. Laryngoscope 1978;88:1697.

102. Gould V, Linnoila R, Memoli V, Warren W. Neuroendocrine components of the bronchopulmonary tract. Lab Invest 1983;49:519.

103. Jakobsson P. Histologic grading of malignancy and prognosis in glottic carcinoma of the larynx. Can J Otolaryngol 1975;4:885.

104. Mullins J, Newman R, Coltman C. Primary oat cell carcinoma of the larynx. Cancer 1979;43:711.

105. Goldman N, Hood C, Singleton G. Carcinoid of the larynx. Arch Otolaryngol 1969;90:90.

106. Huizenga C, Balogh K. Cartilaginous tumors of the larynx. Cancer 1970;26:201.

107. Blitzer A, Lawson W, Biller H. Malignant fibrous histiocytoma of the head and neck. Laryngoscope 1977;87:1479.

108. Maniglia A, Xue J. Plasmacytoma of the larynx. Laryngoscope 1983;93:741.

109. Booth J, Osborn D. Granular cell myoblastoma of the larynx. Acta Otolaryngol 1970;70:279.

110. Anderson H, Maisel R, Cantrell R. Isolated laryngeal lymphoma. Laryngoscope 1976;86:1251.

111. Reuter V, Woodruff J. Melanoma of larynx. Laryngoscope 1986;96:389–393.

112. Sessions R, Miller S, Martin G, Solomon B, Harrison L, Stackpole S. Videostroboscopy in assessment of early glottic carcinomas. Trans Am Laryngol Assoc 1989;100:56–59.

113. Castelijns J, Gerristen G, Kaiser M, et al. Invasion of laryngeal cartilage by cancer: Comparison of CT to MR. Radiology 1989;167:199–206.

114. Castelijns J, Kaiser M, Valk J. MR imaging of laryngeal cancer. J Comput Asst Tomogr 1987;11:134.

115. Towler C, Young S. MRI of the larynx. Magn Reson 1989;5:228–241.

116. Castelijns J, Golding R, Van-Schaik C, Valk J, Snow G. MR findings of cartilage invasion by laryngeal cancer: Value of predicting outcome of radiation therapy. Radiology 1990;174:669–673.

117. Pillsbury H, Kirchner J. Clinical vs. histologic staging in laryngeal cancer. Arch Otolaryngol 1979;105:157.

118. Wang CC, Suit H, Bhitzer P. Twice/day radiation for supraglottic carcinoma. Int J Radiat Oncol Biol Phys 1986;12:3–7.

119. Mendenhall W, Parsons J, Stringer S. Carcinoma of the supraglottic larynx: A basis for comparing the results of radiotherapy and surgery. Head Neck 1990;12:204–209.

120. Olofsson J, Williams G, Bryce D, Rider W. Radiotherapy vs. conservation surgery in the treatment of selected supraglottic carcinomas. Arch Otolaryngol 1972;95:240.

121. Lederman M. Radiotherapy of cancer of the larynx. J Laryngol Otol 1970;84:867.

122. Fletcher G, Lindberg R, Hamberger H, et al. Reasons for irradiation failure in squamous cell carcinoma of the larynx. Laryngoscope 1975;85:987.

123. Vermund H. Role of radiotherapy in cancer of the larynx as related to the TNM system of staging. A review. Cancer 1970;5:485.

124. Ogura J, Biller H. Conservative surgery in cancer of the head and neck. Otolaryngol Clin North Am 1969;2:641.

125. Levendag P, Vikram B. The problem of neck relapse in early stage supraglottic cancer—results of different treatment modalities for the clinically negative neck. Int J Radiat Oncol Biol Phys 1987;13:1621–1624.

126. Harwood A, Beale F, Cummings B. Supraglottic laryngeal carcinoma: An analysis of dose-time-volume factors in 410 patients. Int J Radiat Oncol Biol Phys 1983;9:311–319.

127. Siirala V, Paavolaine M. The problem of advanced supraglottic carcinoma. Laryngoscope 1975;85:1633.

128. Wang CC, Schulz M, Miller D. Combined radiotherapy and surgery for carcinoma of the supraglottis and pyriform sinus. Am J Surg 1972;124:551.

129. Tupchong L, Scott C, Blitzer P. Randomized study of pre-operative vs. post-operative radiotherapy in advanced head and neck carcinoma: Long-term follow up of RTOG study 73-03. Int J Radiat Oncol Biol Phys 1991;20:21–28.

130. Sessions R, Parish R. How are patients chosen for conservation surgery of the larynx? In: Harrison DFN, ed. Dilemmas in otorhinolaryngology. London: Churchill Livingstone, 1988:283–301.

131. Strong M. Laser management of premalignant lesions of the larynx. In: Alberti P, Bryce D, eds. Workshops from the Centennial Conference on laryngeal cancer. East Norwalk, CT: Appleton-Century-Crofts, 1976:154–157.

132. McGuirt WF, Kaufman JA. Endoscopic laser surgery: An alternative in laryngeal cancer treatment. Arch Otolaryngol Head Neck Surg 1987;113:501.

133. Harwood A. Cancer of the larynx—the Toronto experience. J Otolaryngol 1982;11:1–21.

134. Ellman A, Goodman M, Wang C, Pilch B, Busse J. In situ carcinoma of the vocal cords. Cancer 1979;43:2422–2428.

135. Harrison L, Solomon B, Miller S, Fass D, Armstrong J, Sessions R. Prospective computer assisted voice analysis for patients with early stage glottic cancer; A preliminary report of the functional result of laryngeal irradiation. Int J Radiat Oncol Biol Phys 1990;19:123–127.

136. Biller H, Barnhill F, Ogura J, Perez C. Hemilaryngectomy following radiation failure for carcinoma of the vocal cords. Laryngoscope 1970;80:249.

137. Sorenson H, Hansen H, Thomsen K. Partial laryngectomy following irradiation. Laryngoscope 1980;90:1344.

138. Daly C, Strong E. Carcinoma of the glottic larynx. Am J Surg 1975;130:489.

139. Leroux-Robert J. A statistical study of 620 laryngeal carcinomas of the glottic region personally operated upon more than five years ago. Laryngoscope 1975;85:1440.

140. Sessions D, Maness G, McSwain B. Laryngofissure in the treatment of carcinoma of the vocal cord. Laryngoscope 1964;75:490.

141. Southwick H. Cancer of the larynx: Surgical management. In: Seventh National Cancer Conference proceedings. Philadelphia: JB Lippincott, 1973.

142. Constable W, White R, ElMakdi A, Fitz-Hugh G. Radiotherapeutic management of cancer of the glottis, University of Virginia, 1956–1971. Laryngoscope 1975;85:1494.

143. Wang CC. Treatment of glottic carcinoma by megavoltage radiation therapy and results. Am J Roentgenol Rad Ther Med 1974;120:157.

144. Jorgensen K. Carcinoma of the larynx: III. Therapeutic results. Acta Radiol 1974;13:446.

145. Fletcher G, Lindbert R, Hamberger A, Horiot J. Reasons for irradiation failure in squamous cell carcinoma of the larynx. Laryngoscope 1975;85:987.

146. Pellititteri P, Kennedy T, Vrabec D, Beiler D, Hellstrom M. Radiotherapy, the mainstay in the treatment of early glottic carcinoma. Arch Otolaryngol Head Neck Surg 1991;117;297–301.

147. Ogura J, Sessions D, Spector G. Analysis of surgical therapy for epidermoid carcinoma of the laryngeal glottis. Laryngoscope 1975;85:1522.

148. Dickens W, Cassisi N, Million R, Bova F. Treatment of early vocal cord carcinoma: A comparison of apples and apples. Laryngoscope 1983;93;216–219.

149. Wang CC. Treatment of squamous cell carcinoma of the larynx by radiation. Radiol Clin North Am 1978;16:209.

150. Sessions D, Ogura J, Fried M. The anterior commissure in glottic carcinoma. Laryngoscope 1974;85:1624.

151. Sessions D, Ogura J, Fried M. Laryngeal carcinoma involving the anterior commissure and subglottis. In: Alberti P, Bryce D, eds. Workshops from the Centennial Conference on laryngeal cancer. East Norwalk, CT: Appleton-Century-Crofts, 1976:674–678.

152. Olofsson J, Williams G, Rider W, Bryce D. Anterior commissure carcinoma: Primary treatment with radiotherapy in 57 patients. Arch Otolaryngol 1972;95:230.

153. Olofsson J. Specific features of laryngeal carcinoma involving the anterior commissure and subglottic region. In: Alberti P, Bryce D, eds. Workshops from the Centennial

Conference on laryngeal cancer. East Norwalk, CT: Appleton-Century-Crofts, 1976:626.

154. Ennuyer H, Bataini P. Laryngeal carcinomas: VI. Laryngoscope 1975;85:1467.

155. Hawkins N. The treatment of glottic carcinoma: An analysis of 800 cases: VIII. Laryngoscope 1975;85:1485.

156. Stewart J, Brown J, Palmer M, Cooper A. The management of glottic carcinoma by primary irradiation with surgery in reserve: VII. Laryngoscope 1975;85:1477.

157. Kirchner J, Som M. Clinical significance of fixed vocal cord. Laryngoscope 1971;81:1029.

158. Marchetta F, Sako K, Mattick W. Squamous cell carcinoma of the larynx. Am J Surg 1968;116:491.

159. Martensson B, Jacobsson F. Aspects on treatment of cancer of the larynx. Ann Otol Rhinol Laryngol 1967;156:313.

160. Som M. Cordal cancer with extension to vocal process. Laryngoscope 1975;85:1298.

161. Van den Bogart W, Ostyn F, Vander Schuerren E. The primary treatment of advanced vocal cord cancer: Laryngectomy or radiotherapy? Int J Radiat Oncol Biol Phys 1983;9:329–334.

162. Harwood A, Hawkins V, Beale F. Management of advanced glottic cancer: A 10-year review of the Toronto experience. Int J Radiat Oncol Biol Phys 1979;5:899–904.

163. Wang C. Radiation therapy of laryngeal tumors. In: Thawley S, Panje W, Batsakis J, Lindberg R, eds. Comprehensive management of head and neck tumors. Philadelphia: WB Saunders, 1987:906–919.

164. Mendenhall W, Parsons J, Stringer S. Stage T3 squamous cell carcinoma of the glottic larynx: Irradiation compared to laryngectomy. Int J Radiat Oncol Biol Phys 1991;21 (Suppl 1):142.

165. Terhaard C, Karim A, Hoogenraad S. Local control in T3 laryngeal cancer treated with radical radiotherapy: Time-dose relationship—the concept of nominal standard dose and linear quadratic model. Int J Radiat Oncol Biol Phys 1991;20:1207–1214.

166. Jacobs C, Goffinet D, Goffinet L. Chemotherapy as a substitute for surgery in the treatment of advanced resectable head/neck cancer. Cancer 1987;60:1178–1183.

167. Department of Veterans Affairs Laryngeal Cancer Study Group. Induction chemotherapy plus radiation compared with surgery plus radiation in patients with advanced laryngeal cancer. N Engl J Med 1991;324:1685–1690.

168. Jesse R. The evaluation of treatment of patients with extensive squamous cancer of the vocal cords. Laryngoscope 1975;85:1424.

169. Pinto H, Jacobs C, Goffinet D. Long-term follow-up or organ preservation in advanced head and neck cancer. Proc Am Soc Clin Oncol 1991;10:690.

170. Hill B, Price L, MacRae K; Importance of primary site in accessing chemotherapy response. J Clin Oncol 1986;4:1340–1347.

171. Urba S, Forastiere H, Wolf G. Intensive continuous infusion high dose cisplatin, 5—flurouracil, and mitognazone induction chemotherapy for advanced head and neck cancer. Proc Am Soc Clin Oncol [Abstract] 1989;8:172.

172. Denard F, Chauvel P, Santini J. Response to chemotherapy as justification for modification of the therapeutic strategy for pharyngolaryngeal carcinoma. Head Neck 1990;12:225–231.

173. Leyvrax S. Radio-chemotherapy combination to avoid major surgery and preserve organ function in advanced HNSCC. Proc Am Soc Clin Oncol [Abstract] 1991;10:677.

174. Shirinian M, Weber R, Dimery I. Laryngeal preservation using induction chemotherapy followed by definitive XRT for patients with advanced stage head and neck squamous cell carcinoma requiring total laryngectomy. Proc Am Soc Clin Oncol [Abstract] 1992;11:242.

175. Kies M, Gordon L, Hank W. Pre-operative chemotherapy in advanced resectable head and neck cancer: Final report of the Southwest Oncology Group. Laryngoscope 1988;98:1205–1211.

176. Ensley J, Jacobs J, Weaber A. Correlation between response to cisplatinum-combination chemotherapy and subsequent radiotherapy in previously untreated patients with advanced squamous cell cancers of the head and neck. Cancer 1984;54:811–814.

177. Price L, MacRae I, Hill B. Integration of safe initial combination chemotherapy for stage III and IV epidermoid carcinoma of the head and neck: 5-year survival data. Cancer Treat Rep 1983;67:535–539.

178. Robbins T, Medina J, Wolfe G, Levine P, Sessions R, Pruet C. Standardizing neck dissection terminology. Arch Otol Head Neck Surg 1991;117:601–605.

179. Harrison D. Laryngectomy for subglottic lesions. Laryngoscope 1975;85:1208.

180. Harrison D. Pathology and management of subglottic cancer. Ann Otol Rhinol Laryngol 1971;80:6.

181. Gussenbauer C. Veber die erste durch Th. Billroth Am Men schen ausgefuhrte Kehlkopf-Exstirpation und die anwendung eines Kunstlichen Kokopfes. Arch Klin Chir 1874;17:343.

182. Goode R. The development of an improved artificial larynx. Trans Am Acad Ophthalmol Otolaryngol 1969;73:279.

183. Fredrickson J, Charles D, Bryce D. An implantable electromagnetic sound source. In: Shedd D, ed. Surgical and prosthetic approaches to speech rehabilitation. Boston: GK Hall, 1980:247–257.

184. Briana A. Riabilitazione fonetica di laringectomizati a mezzo della corrente aerea expiratoria polmonare. Arch Ital Otol Rhinol Laryngol 1952;63:469.

185. Conley J, DeAmesti F, Pierce M. A new surgical technique for vocal rehabilitation of the laryngectomized patient. Am Otol Rhinol Laryngol 1958;67:655.

186. Asai R. Asai's new voice production method. Eighth International Congress of otorhinolaryngology. Tokyo, 1965.

187. Montgomery W, Toohill R. Voice rehabilitation after laryngectomy. Arch Otolaryngol 1968;88:499.

188. Calcaterra T, Jafek B. Tracheo-esophageal shunt for speech rehabilitation after total laryngectomy. Arch Otolaryngol 1971;94:124.

189. Taub S, Spiro R. Vocal rehabilitation of laryngectomy patients. Am J Surg 1972;124: 87.

190. Sisson G, McConnell F, Logeman J, Yeh S. Vocal rehabilitation after laryngectomy. Arch Otolaryngol 1975;101:178.

191. Arslau M, Serafini I. Restoration of laryngeal functions after total laryngectomy. Laryngoscope 1972;82:1349.

192. Gates G, Ryan W, Cooper J. Current status of laryngectomy rehabilitation: Results of therapy. Am J Otolaryngol 1982;3:1.

193. Blom E, Singer M, Hamaker R. Tracheostoma valve for post laryngectomy voice rehabilitation. Ann Otol Rhinol Laryngol 1982;91:576.

194. Singer M, Blom E, Hannaker R. Further experience with voice restoration after total laryngectomy. Ann Otol Rhinol Laryngol 1981;90:498.

195. Mozolewski E, Zietek E, Wysocui R. Arytenoid vocal shunt in laryngectomized patients. Laryngoscope 1975;85:853.

196. Iwai H, Koike Y. Primary laryngoplasty. Laryngoscope 1975;85:929.

197. Johns M, Cantrell R. Voice restoration of the total laryngectomy patient: The singer blom technique. Otolaryngol Head Neck Surg 1981;89:82.

198. Carpenter R III, DeSanto L. Cancer of the hypopharynx. Surg Clin North Am 1977;57: 7–23.

199. Ahlbom H. The results of radiotherapy of hypopharyngeal cancer at the radium hemmer, Stockholm, 1930–1939. Acta Radiol 1941;22:155.

200. Wynder E, Hultberg S, Jacobsson F, Bross I. Environmental factors in cancer of the upper alimentary tract. Cancer 1957;10:470.

201. Higginson J, Terracini B, Agthe C. Nutrition and cancer: Ingestion of foodborne carcinogens. In: Schottenfeld D, ed. Cancer epidemiology and prevention. Springfield, IL: Charles C. Thomas, 1975:177.

202. Larsson L, Sandstrom A, Westling P. Relationship of phenomenon—Vinson disease to cancer of the upper alimentary tract in Sweden. Cancer Res 1975;3:3308.

203. Cunningham M, Catlin D. Cancer of the pharyngeal wall. Cancer 1967;20:1859.

204. DeJong P. Intubation and tumor implantation in laryngeal carcinoma. Pract Otolaryngol 1969;31:119.

205. Harrison D. Pathology of hypopharyngeal cancer in relation to surgical management. J Laryngol Otol 1970;84:349.

206. Harrison D. Significance and means by which laryngeal cancer invades thyroid cartilage. Ann Otol Rhinol Laryngol 1984;93:392.

207. Guillamondegui O, Meoz-Mendez R, Jesse R. Surgical treatment of squamous cell carcinoma of the pharyngeal walls. Am J Surg 1978;136:474.

208. McGavarvan M, Bauer W, Spjut H. Carcinoma of the pyriform sinus. Arch Otolaryngol 1963;78:826.

209. Ogura J, Biller H, Wetti R. Elective neck dissection for pharyngeal and laryngeal cancers. Ann Otol Rhinol Laryngol 1971;80:646.

210. Ogura J, Jurema H, Watson R. Partial laryngopharyngectomy and neck dissection for pyriform sinus cancer. Laryngoscope 1960;70:1399.

211. Byers R, Wolf P, Ballantyne A. Rationale for elective modified neck dissection. Head Neck Surg 1988;10:160.

212. Ballantyne A. Methods of repair after surgery for cancer of the pharyngeal wall, post cricoid area, and cervical esophagus. Am J Surg 1971;122:482.

213. Marks J, Freeman R, Lee F, Ogura J. Pharyngeal wall cancer: An analysis of treatment results, complications, and patterns of failure. Int J Radiat Oncol Biol Phys 1978;4: 587.

214. Merino O, Landberg R, Fletcher C. An analysis of distant metastases from squamous cell carcinoma of the upper respiratory and digestive tracts. Cancer 1977;40:1415.

215. Keane T. Carcinoma of the hypopharynx. J Otolaryngol 1982;11:227.

216. Horwitz S, Caldarelli D, Hendrickson F. Treatment of carcinoma of the hypopharynx. Head Neck Surg 1979;2:107.

217. Lee D, Harris A, Gillette A. Carcinoma of the cervical esophagus. South Med J 1984;77: 1365.

218. Willatt D, Jackson S, McCormick M. Vocal cord paralysis and tumor length in staging post cricoid cancer. Eur J Surg Oncol 1987;13:131.

219. Friedman M, Shelton V, McFee M. Metastatic neck disease: Evaluation by computed tomography. Arch Otolaryngol 1984;110:443.

220. Mancuso A, Harnsberger H, Muraki A, Stevens M. Computed tomography of cervical and retropharyngeal lymph nodes: II. Pathology. Radiology 1983;148:709.

221. Grossman T, Kita M, Toohill R. The diagnostic accuracy of pharyngoesophagram compared to esophagoscopy of patients with head and neck cancer. Laryngoscope 1987;97: 1030.

222. Million R, Cassissi N. Management of head and neck cancer: A multidisciplinary approach. Philadelphia: JB Lippincott, 1984.

223. DeSanto L, Lillie J, Devine K. Surgical salvage after radiation for larynx cancer. Laryngoscope 1976;86:649–653.

224. Urken ML, Weinberg H, Vickery C, et al. The combined sensate radical forearm and iliac crest free flaps for reconstruction of significant glossectomy–mandibulectomy defects. Laryngoscope 1992;102:543–558.

225. Million R, Cassissi N. Radical irradiation for carcinoma of the pyriform sinus. Laryngoscope 1981;91:439.

226. Vandenbrouck C, Eschwege F, DeLaRochfordiere A. Squamous cell carcinoma of the pyriform sinus: Retrospective study of 351 cases treated at the Institut Roussy. Head Neck Surg 1987;10:4.

227. Mendenhall W, Parsons J, Devine J. Squamous cell carcinoma of the pyriform sinus treated with surgery and/or radiotherapy. Head Neck Surg 1987;10:88.

228. Shah J, Shaha A, Spiro R, Strong E. Carcinoma of the hypopharynx. Am J Surg 1976;132: 439.

229. Bataini P, Brugere J, Vernier J. Results of radical radiotherapy treatment of carcinoma of the pyriform sinus: Experience of the Institute Curie. Int J Radiat Oncol Biol Phys 1982;8:1276–1277.

230. Donald P, Hayes H, Dhalival R. Combined treatment for pyriform sinus cancer using postoperative irradiation. Otolaryngol Head Neck Surg 1980;88:738.

231. Hong W, Dimery I, Kramer A. The role of induction chemotherapy in the treatment of advanced head and neck cancer. In: Salmon S, ed. Adjuvant therapy of cancer. 5th ed. Orlando: Grune & Stratton, 1987:79.

232. Vandenrouck C, Sancho A, LeFur R. Results of a randomized clinical trial of preoperative irradiation versus post operative in treatment of tumors of the hypopharynx. Cancer 1977;39:1445–1449.

233. Kramer S, Gelber R, Snow J. Combined radiation therapy in the management of advanced head and neck cancer: Final report of study 73-03 of the radiation therapy oncology group. Head Neck Surg 1987;10:19–30.

234. Keane T, Hawkins N, Beal F. Carcinoma of the hypopharynx: Results of primary radical radiation therapy. Int J Radiat Oncol Biol Phys 1983;9:659–664.

235. Harrison D, Thompson A. Pharyngolaryngoesophagectomy with pharyngogastric anastomosis for cancer of the hypopharynx. Head Neck Surg 1986;8:418.

236. Griffiths J, Shaus H. Cancer of the laryngopharynx and cervical esophagus: Radical resection with repair of colon transplant. Arch Otolaryngol Head Neck Surg 1973;97: 340.

237. Meoz-Mendez R, Fletcher G, Guillamondegui O, Peters L. Analysis of the results of irradiation in the treatment of squamous cell carcinoma of the pharyngeal walls. Int J Radiat Oncol Biol Phys 1978;4:579.

238. Kato H, Iizuka T, Watanabe H. Reconstruction of the esophagus by microvascular surgery. Jpn J Clin Oncol 1984;14:379.

239. Theile D, Robinson D, McCafferty G. Pharyngolaryngectomy reconstruction by revascularized free jejunal graft. Aust NZ J Surg 1986;56:849.

ROY B. SESSIONS
LOUIS B. HARRISON
WAUN KI HONG

SECTION 3

Tumors of the Salivary Glands and Paragangliomas

The same group of neoplasms affect all salivary gland tissue, but with a predictable difference in type for the different anatomic sites. The major salivary glands consist of paired parotids in the preauricular area, paired submandibulars under the mandible, and paired sublinguals in the floor of the mouth. The minor salivary glands, on the other hand, are ubiquitous in the upper aerodigestive tract, occurring especially throughout the oral and nasal cavities and the paranasal sinuses. The likelihood of a neoplasm being malignant is highest in the sublingual and minor salivary glands, least in the parotids, and intermediate in the submandibular glands. Overall, salivary gland cancers make up about 3% of all head and neck malignancies diagnosed in North America each year, most of which are in the parotid gland. Overall, sublingual and minor salivary gland cancers are unusual.[1]

ANATOMY

The parotid gland is tightly compacted in the area immediately anterior and inferior to the external ear. It is best thought of in a three-dimensional sense, with the deep portion extending medially around the posterior rim of the ascending ramus of the mandible into the parapharyngeal space. The superficial part of the gland lies on the masseter muscle and extends inferiorly to overlie the sternocleidomastoid and diagastric muscles (Fig. 22–31). The fascia that engulfs both of these muscles forms a substantial glandular capsule around the parotid and submandibular glands that helps confine tumors to their site of origin. The most inferior extent of the parotid gland extends a variable distance, and, in those necks in which this extension is exaggerated, the glandular tail overlies the transverse process of C2 and the deep jugular lymph nodes at the level of C2. Not infrequently, a prominent transverse process or an enlarged lymph node in this area is misinterpreted as a parotid tail mass. To a great extent, modern imaging has helped avoid this misdiagnosis.

The facial nerve leaves the stylomastoid foramen at the base of the skull and almost immediately penetrates the parotid capsule posteriorly. Once within the gland, the nerve divides into five main branches, temporal, zygomatic, buccal, mandibular, and cervical, all extending in a consistent direction and depth and all gradually becoming more superficial as they extend anteriorly. Although there are no actual lobes defined by fascial planes, that part of the parotid gland superficial to the facial nerve is arbitrarily referred to as the *superficial lobe.* The gland that lies deep to the nerve is called the *deep lobe.* This fact has considerable bearing on the surgical anatomy and any dissection done within the parotid gland (see Fig. 22–31).

The deep lobe of the parotid gland extends into the parapharyngeal space, and as such, tumors of that portion of the gland can come into contact with the carotid artery, which forms the posterior boundary of that space. These tumors can press against the constrictor muscles of the pharynx that normally form the medial wall of that compartment (Fig. 22–32). Larger deep lobe parotid tumors can, therefore, present as a bulging tonsil pillar, a finding that is easily misinterpreted as an oropharyngeal neoplasm by the inexperienced diagnostician (Fig. 22–33). The distinction between a deep lobe parotid tumor and an oral lesion becomes clear on either magnetic resonance imaging (MRI) or computed tomography (CT) scans. There is some difficulty, however, in distinguishing deep lobe neoplasms from tumors that have their origin in the parapharyngeal space. This diagnosis depends on the presence or absence of a fat plane between the deep lobe and the tumor. The distinction between the two is important, because the differential diagnosis of tumors that originate in the parapharyngeal space must include lymphomas, neurogenic tumors, and paragangliomas,[2-4] none of which are likely to occur in the parotid gland. Most parotid tumors originate in the superficial lobe, probably because that portion of the gland is considerably larger than the deep lobe. Because there are no identifiable histologic differences between deep and superficial lobes, there is no reasonable explanation for this distribution of tumors other than the amount of salivary gland tissue available for tumor development. The distribution of different types of tumors is probably the same in the various parts of the gland.

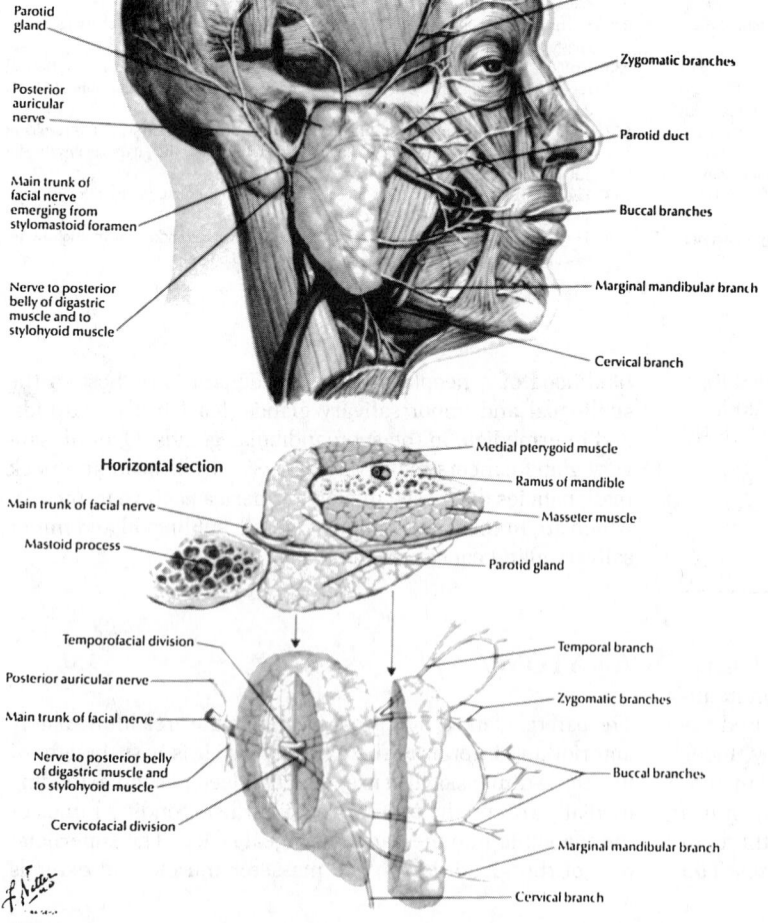

FIGURE 22–31. Representation of parotid gland and facial nerve anatomy. The lower part of diagram shows the details of the relation of the nerve to the surrounding gland. Various branches of the nerve are directed to various parts of the facial musculature. (CIBA Collection, Frank Netter, Artist)

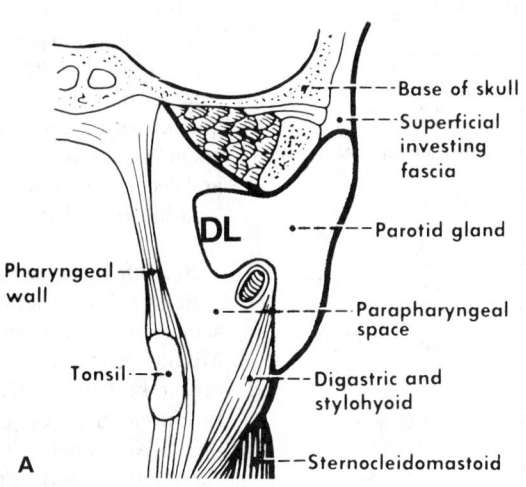

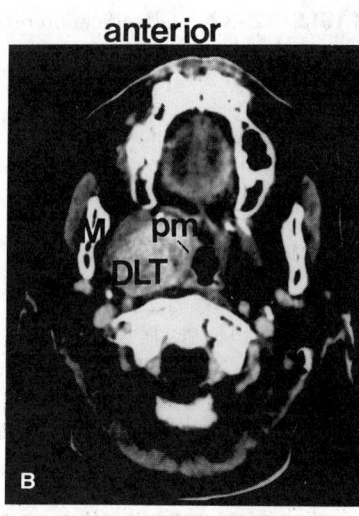

FIGURE 22–32. Presentation of deep lobe parotid gland tumors. **(A)** Schematic diagram shows frontal view just posterior to mandible where the deep lobe (*DL*) enters paraphryngeal space. Notice the proximity of the deep lobe to the pharyngeal muscles and the palate. **(B)** An axial CT scan of the skull shows the deep lobe tumor (*DLT*) occupying parapharyngeal space and pressing against pharyngeal constrictor muscles (*pm*). The retromandibular tunnel extends the deep lobe behind the mandible (*M*).

The lymphatics in and around the parotid gland consist of two groups. A knowledge of that nodal distribution is essential to an understanding of the natural history of tumors of the area. The preauricular (*periparotid*) nodes lie superficial to the gland capsule and serve to drain the external auditory canal, the facial and auricular skin, and the temple scalp. They are especially important drainage sites for squamous carcinomas and melanomas of adjacent skin. Parotid gland cancers usually do not drain into these nodes. The second group consist of five to seven *intraparotid* nodes that do play a role in the pathogenesis of parotid cancer. The efferents of the superficial nodes drain into the superficial jugular chain, and the intraglandular nodes drain into the upper and middle deep jugular lymph nodes.[1,5,6] The extraparotid (periparotid) nodes are readily palpable and are distinguished easily from primary parotid tumors. However, those nodes within the substance of the gland are not easily palpated, and only when they are enlarged do they become noticeable. Distinguishing them from primary parotid gland tumors can be difficult.

The submandibular gland lies in the submandibular triangle of the neck with its posterior extent adjacent to, but not continuous with, the parotid gland. Its deep surface lies against the muscular diaphragm of the floor of the mouth and is best examined bimanually, with one finger in the mouth and the external hand on the surface of the gland. Lymph nodes do not exist within the submandibular gland, but they lie around its surface. A mass outside the submandibular gland may represent a metastatic node from some other site, for example, the lateral tongue or the floor of the mouth. Drainage from the submandibular gland is into the adjacent nodes and upper deep jugular chain.[1]

The sublingual glands are located submucosally in the floor of the mouth, just superficial to the muscular diaphragm. They are oval in shape and lie along the inner table of the mandible. Lymphatic drainage from the sublingual glands is into submandibular lymphatics and then into the deep jugular nodes.

ETIOLOGY, PATHOLOGY, AND CLASSIFICATION

The causes of salivary gland cancer have not been determined. The following associated factors have been noted: low-level ionizing radiation with all salivary cancers[7–10]; a familial predisposition in parotid cancer[11]; and an association between wood dust inhalation and the development of adenocarcinoma of the minor salivary glands in the nose and paranasal sinuses.[12,13] Although these various associations have been described consistently, proof of cause and effect does not exist, and most salivary gland cancers remain unassociated with obvious etiologic factors.

There are different classifications of salivary gland neoplasms, but the one that seems to be the most consistently workable is shown in Table 22–33.

BENIGN TUMORS

Benign Mixed Tumor

Overall, most salivary gland neoplasms are benign, a fact that reflects an overwhelming predominance of parotid tumors, three fourths of which are nonmalignant. The benign mixed tumor is the commonest of the neoplasms that originate in

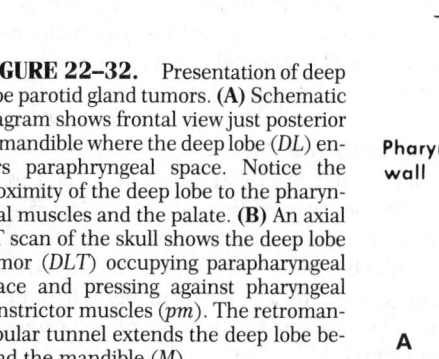

FIGURE 22–33. Intraoral photograph of soft palate mucosal bulge caused by parotid gland deep lobe tumor (*DLT*) as depicted in Figure 22–21. (Courtesy of Ronald Spiro, MD)

TABLE 22–33. Classification of Salivary Gland Neoplasms

Benign
Benign mixed tumor (pleomorphic adenoma)
Warthin's tumor (papillar cystadenoma lymphomatosum)
Benign lymphoepithelial lesion
Oncocytoma
Monomorphic adenoma

Malignant
Mucoepidermoid carcinoma
Adenoid cystic carcinoma
Adenocarcinoma
Malignant mixed tumor
Acinic cell carcinoma
Epidermoid carcinoma

the major salivary glands.[14,15] This tumor frequently is called a *pleomorphic adenoma*, a term that describes its multiple histologic components, including myxoid, mucoid, chondroid, and other elements. Although these lesions can occur in all salivary gland tissues, they are most commonly seen in the parotid gland.

The distinction between benign and malignant mixed tumors is often difficult, but those histologic features that most reliably separate the two include a tendency for perivascular and perineural invasion and significant cellular atypia and mitosis. Malignant lesions can be underinterpreted and their true nature not appreciated until metastasis occurs; even then, the metastatic site(s) may appear histologically benign.[16–18] At the opposite extreme, a benign but extremely cellular pleomorphic adenoma can be "overinterpreted" as a malignant mixed tumor. These factors must be critically considered when doing retrospective interinstitutional outcomes research.

The natural history of benign mixed tumor is one of slow growth and few symptoms. Despite assuming large proportions, those lesions that remain benign rarely affect facial nerve function clinically. In such tumors, however, the nerve is often chronically stretched around the mass and seems to become more fragile; tumor removal may be more readily associated with postoperative nerve weakness.

There is controversy regarding the evolution of a benign mixed tumor into its malignant counterpart. Many authors believe that the latter originates in a preexisting benign setting, which is the reason for the term *carcinoma expleomorphic adenoma*. Other researchers, however, believe that malignant mixed tumor arises de novo.[16–19]

Warthin's Tumor
(Papillary Cystadenoma Lymphomatosum)

This slow-growing, often cystic, and usually innocuous tumor almost always occurs in older men, seems to favor the tail of the parotid gland, and is noted to occur bilaterally in 10% of the cases. Because of the benign nature of this tumor, and because it can be easily diagnosed cytologically, surgical removal is not always necessary, especially in older or unhealthy patients.

Monomorphic Adenoma

The monomorphic adenomas are a group of benign lesions that can have a variety of growth patterns, including trabecular, cystic, and canilicular types. The commonest monomorphic adenomas are the basal cell and the oxphyllic adenomas (oncocytoma). Other lesions include sebaceous lymphadenomas and sebaceous adenomas. The parotid gland is the commonest location for the occurrence of these lesions.

Benign Lymphoepithelial Lesion

Benign lymphoepithelial lesion was first described in association with inflammatory conditions such as Sjögren's and Mikulicz's syndromes.[20] Recently, however, an apparent increase in its incidence has been seen in patients with human immunodeficiency virus (HIV). The term benign lymphoepithelial lesion now encompasses a spectrum of cystic changes seen in the parotid glands of HIV-infected persons, with atypical lymphoid hyperplasia being the common denominator. It is thought that these changes occur directly as a result of HIV infection of intraparotid lymph nodes.[21,22]

There are several reports of HIV-associated malignancies of the parotid, including non-Hodgkin's lymphoma,[23,24] Kaposi's sarcoma,[25,26] and adenoid cystic carcinoma.[27] Some of these have arisen in a background of a benign lymphoepithelial lesion. Malignancy after benign lymphoepithelial lesion, however, was described before the acquired immunodeficiency syndrome (AIDS) epidemic,[28] and it remains unclear whether HIV infection predisposes benign lymphoepithelial lesion to malignancy.

Treatment of benign lymphoepithelial lesion in HIV-infected patients is controversial. Some clinicians cite the association of malignancy as justification for parotidectomy.[29] Others have touted observation with intermittent fine-needle aspirations for decompression of cysts[30] or low-dose radiation therapy.[31] Optimal therapy should be individualized, depending on the clinical and diagnostic suspicion of malignancy, the status of the patient's HIV infection (asymptomatic versus AIDS-related complex versus AIDS), and risk-benefit analysis for patient and surgeon.

MALIGNANT TUMORS

Spiro and Spiro[1] have developed a compendium of the most extensive series of salivary gland cancer reported, and in their survey they have outlined the relative occurrence rates of the various cancers in both the parotid and submandibular glands. The various reports from nine studies total 1778 parotid gland tumors, the distribution of which is abbreviated and summarized in Table 22–34.[32–40] Summarized in Table 22–35 are comparable data for the submandibular gland that are taken from eight studies and that, when combined, reflect the relative distribution of 383 submandibular gland cancers by type.[33,41–47]

Acinic Cell Carcinoma

Acinic cell carcinoma is an uncommon tumor, in most series accounting for fewer than 10% of all salivary gland cancers.[48] Although acinic cell lesions usually are seen in the parotid gland, they occasionally are encountered in the submandibular gland.[49] These are low-grade malignancies that infrequently

TABLE 22–34. Relative Incidence* of Histologic Types of Parotid Gland Cancer

Histologic Type	Percentage
Mucoepi	32
Adeno	16
MMT	14
Adenoid C	11
Acinic C	11
Undiff + sq cell	16

* Total of 1778 cases from Memorial Sloan-Kettering Cancer Center. Mucoepi, mucoepidermoid; Adeno, adenocarcinoma; MMT, malignant mixed tumor; C, carcinoma; Undiff + sq cell, undifferentiated plus squamous cell.
(Adapted from Spiro R, Spiro J. Cancer of the salivary glands. In: Meyers E, Sven J, eds. Cacner of the head and neck. 2nd ed. London: Churchill Livingstone, 1984:645)

TABLE 22–35. Relative Incidence* of Histologic Types of Submandibular Gland Cancer

Histologic Type	Percentage
Adenoid cystic	41
Acinic cell	17
Mucoepi	12
MMT	10
Sq Cell	9
Undiff	9
Adeno	2

* Total of 383 cases from Memorial Sloan-Kettering Cancer Center. Mucoepi, mucoepidermoid; MMT, malignant mixed tumor; Sq cell, squamous cell; Undiff, undifferentiated; Adeno, adenocarcinoma.
(Adapted from Spiro R, Spiro J. Cancer of the salivary glands. In: Meyers E, Sven J, eds. Cancer of the head and neck. 2nd ed. London: Churchill Livingstone, 1984:645)

invade the facial nerve and are late to metastasize. When they do metastasize, however, it is usually to the lungs. Because of their slow growth, survival data are good when generous surgical excision is performed.[50,51]

Mucoepidermoid Carcinoma

Mucoepidermoid carcinoma occurs more frequently than any other in the major salivary glands. It is relatively more common in the parotid than in the submandibular gland, where it is third in occurrence after adenoid cystic carcinoma and adenocarcinoma (see Tables 22–34 and 22–35). Mucoepidermoid carcinoma is unique in that it demonstrates a broad spectrum of aggressiveness from the low-grade version that rarely kills to the high-grade lesion that frequently does kill. Low-grade mucoepidermoid carcinomas tend to create mostly local problems and can have a long natural history. A locally aggressive surgical approach is usually rewarded with cure. Although metastasis can occur from these lesions, it is the exception rather than the rule. There is such a performance gradient between low- and high-grade mucoepidermoid tumors that some investigators believe that the low-grade version should be referred to as *mucoepidermoid tumor* rather than carcinoma. When low-grade mucoepidermoid cancer metastasizes, however, it can be lethal.[52–54] The high-grade, and to a great extent the intermediate-grade mucoepidermoids, are often troublesome, because they are locally aggressive and are prone to invasion of nerves and vessels and to early metastasis. Spiro and others have reported that 44% of the previously untreated patients with intermediate- or high-grade mucoepidermoid parotid tumors develop nodal involvement at some stage. Analysis of high-grade mucoepidermoids alone reveals an incidence of nodal metastasis from all salivary gland sites that seems to be even higher.[52,55–57] Because of the propensity for regional nodal metastasis in high-grade mucoepidermoid carcinomas, a regional nodal dissection combined with a generous local or primary resection plus postoperative radiation therapy are important in the treatment of these lesions.

Grading of mucoepidermoid lesions relates in part to the ratio between epidermoid and glandular elements, with the high-

grade tumors having a higher proportion of the former.[56,57] It is common for those higher grade tumors that demonstrate little glandular component on routine hematoxylin and eosin stains to be misinterpreted as epidermoid or squamous cell carcinomas.

Adenocarcinoma

Adenocarcinomas make up about 16% of the parotid gland and 9% of the submandibular gland cancers (see Tables 22–34 and 22–35). These lesions are encountered with relatively greater frequency in the minor salivary glands of the nose and paranasal sinuses. A difference in survival seems to correlate with grade; high-grade tumors having a poor prognosis and the low-grade ones performing much more favorably.[16,48,58] In the higher grade tumors, the treatment failures result predominantly from distant spread. Along with the overall poor performance, this fact is important in helping to judge the degree of radicality with which locoregional disease should be treated.

Squamous Cell Carcinoma

Squamous cell carcinomas are uncommon in salivary tissue, making up about 7% of parotid gland and 10% of submandibular gland cancers.[48] The high-grade tumors do poorly and usually present with an advanced stage of cancer.[59,60] Squamous cell carcinomas of the parotid gland frequently are not primary to that gland but instead represent metastasis into parotid nodes from adjacent sites, such as temple, auricular, and facial skin. Skin lesions that come from virtually any site on the face tend to metastasize to the superficial lymph nodes that lie external to the parotid capsule.[61,62]

Malignant Mixed Tumor

Malignant mixed tumors make up about 14% of parotid gland and 12% of submandibular gland cancers (see Tables 22–34 and 22–35). The diagnosis is often difficult because of the similarities with malignant mixed tumors' benign counterpart. Many of the malignant mixed tumors seem to originate in previous pleomorphic adenomas, but just how often they occur de novo is unknown. This controversy has continued for some time. These authors believe that the evolution of a malignant mixed tumor in the existing site of a pleomorphic adenoma (*i.e.*, benign mixed tumor) is a reasonable explanation for the occurrence that is periodically seen in which a longstanding and stable tumor begins to grow significantly. In this circumstance, the assumption of malignant development should be made and management tailored accordingly. The exact probability of any given benign mixed tumor becoming a malignant mixed tumor is unknown. Survival from malignant mixed tumor must be measured over a lengthy period, because the natural history of this lesion can be characterized by long-term but inexorable growth. Metastasis to regional lymph nodes occurs in more than one fourth of the cases.[35,37,48,58,63]

Adenoid Cystic Carcinoma

Adenoid cystic carcinoma makes up almost one fourth of the malignant salivary gland tumors treated in most series and constitutes about 10% to 15% of all parotid gland malignancies (see Table 22–34). This cancer is relatively more common in minor than in major salivary gland tissue. It is unique because of a prolonged natural history, even when there has been local recurrence or distant metastasis. For instance, patients are known to live for 10 to 15 years despite pulmonary metastasis, which is the most frequent site of distant spread. When visceral or bone metastasis occurs, however, death usually follows quickly.[1] The actual cure rate of adenoid cystic carcinoma is poorly defined, because long-term follow-up is often not included in data analyses. Also clouding the issue of cure is the fact that some 10- to 20-year studies have shown disease-related deaths that continue to occur for as long as follow-up was done.[57,64] Some investigators believe that most adenoid cystic carcinomas will recur if followed long enough. Overall, the rate of pulmonary metastasis from these cancers is about 40%.

Adenoid cystic carcinoma has an exceptional capability to invade nerve tissue, and when this does occur, local control and survival are compromised. Such a morphologic finding is the rule rather than the exception in adenoid cystic carcinoma, and a recognition of this consistent tendency is essential in planning treatment, which usually consists of wide surgical excision and radiation therapy. Treatment failure most often occurs in the primary tumor site. Some authors have drawn a correlation between histologic patterns of adenoid cystic carcinoma and clinical behavior.[65,66] Others, although conceding certain behavior pattern differences in the different histologic variants of adenoid cystic carcinoma, do not believe any such correlation exists between these features and long-term outcome.[64]

NATURAL HISTORY, BEHAVIOR, AND TREATMENT

Malignant tumors of major salivary gland origin are a heterogenous group of diseases; there are three primary sites and at least eight different histologies of a relatively uncommon group of cancers. For this reason, studies reporting treatment results have often grouped primary sites and histologic types.

This is a flawed methodology, however, and when the problem is compounded by analyzing short-term results in diseases that often have a long natural history, many questions remain unanswered.

Most patients with benign tumors present with an asymptomatic swelling of the lip or the parotid, the submandibular, or the sublingual glands. Neurologic signs such as mucosal or tongue numbness associated with a floor of mouth mass usually indicate a malignancy. In the presence of a lip mass, a numb lower lip can result from tumor involvement of the submental nerve. Facial nerve weakness that is associated with a parotid or submandibular tumor is an ominous finding. Even in huge tumors of the parotid gland that are benign, the facial nerve usually is unaffected. Essentially, any compromise in nerve function greatly heightens concern for malignancy. The most significant symptom that suggests malignancy in a salivary gland tumor is persistent pain.

The commonest benign tumor, benign mixed tumor, can be troublesome. There is usually a pseudocapsule around this lesion and, importantly, finger-like projections of tumor penetrate into the surrounding glandular parenchyma, whether it is parotid or submandibular. Enuculeation of these lesions tends to leave behind foci of tumor that result in local recurrence in a substantial percentage of patients. Invariably, the overall patient management is complicated by recurrence, because having to deal with recurrent tumor adjacent to facial nerve always places that structure in considerable jeopardy.

A special problem exists with tumors of the parotid deep lobe, because frequently they are not surrounded by much glandular parenchyma, and even the best of operations consist largely of their enucleation. In both of these circumstances in which the probability for leaving behind histologic disease is high, the employment of postoperative radiation therapy must be considered. It should be remembered that benign mixed tumor, although not classified as malignant, can ultimately cause great hardship for a patient. Multiple recurrences, skull base involvement, facial nerve paralysis, malignant transformation, and, ultimately, incurable disease can all result from a casual early approach to this neoplasm. This tumor should be thought of as locally malignant, and any operation done should allow for a wide berth of normal tissue.

Malignant tumors of the parotid can be locally aggressive, demonstrating invasiveness that leads to involvement of the facial nerve, skin, bone, and surrounding soft tissue. Prognosis is related to tumor size and is affected by histologic grade. In general, however, decreasing survival occurs for many years, especially in patients with adenoid cystic carcinoma and malignant mixed tumor. Distant metastasis may not always represent a terminal event, and treatment of primary disease is not necessarily precluded by lung metastasis, especially in adenoid cystic carcinoma.

Another general principal of management that applies particularly to higher grade adenocarcinomas, malignant mixed tumor, and adenoid cystic carcinoma is that their failure is frequently at a distant site, and by combining postoperative radiation therapy with "moderate locoregional" surgery, marked mutilation and physiologic comprimise are often avoided. The liberal resection of facial nerve, mandible, and other important structures solely because they are in the field is no longer the predominant surgical philosophy; surgical minimalism applies in which such structures are rarely sacrificed unless obviously invaded by tumor. The surgeon's reliance on postoperative radiation therapy to manage histologic disease has dramatically altered the surgical feats required to deal with these malignant salivary gland tumors.

Overall, the prognosis for parotid cancer is better than submandibular gland cancer; 50% to 81% 5-year survival in the former and 30% to 50% for the latter are reported.[34,37,41,42,44-47,55,67] The 10-year survival rate declines in both sites. The lessened survival rate in the submandibular gland group probably relates to the larger proportion of adenoid cystic carcinoma in that group.

Differences in histology impact on natural history, with the prognosis for acinic cell carcinoma being the most favorable of the major salivary cancers; more than 75% 5-year and more than 65% 10-year survivals are reported in various series.[36,37,52,63] Low-grade mucoepidermoid carcinomas show 76% to 95% 5-year survival rates, whereas only 30% to 50% of those with high-grade tumors are alive at 5 years.[35,36,52,59] The survival data for intermediate grade mucoepidermoids are in between the low and high grades. Adenoid cystic carcinoma, on the other hand, must be analyzed with the realization that 5-year survival rates are always better than they are at 10 years, which are better than 15 years, and so on. Most series show 50% to 90% 5-year survival rates, 30% to 67% 10-year survival rates, and 25% 15-year survival rates for treated adenoid cystic carcinoma.[35-37,64-67] Patients with adenocarcinomas of major salivary glands show gradual deterioration of survival statistics with the passage of time: 76% to 85% survival at 5 years and 34% to 71% at 10 years.[35,36,58,65] Patients with malignant mixed tumors do not do well, with only 31% to 65% surviving at 5 years and 23% to 30% surviving at 10 years.[11,35-37,65,67]

Distant metastasis is a significant concern in most higher grade salivary gland malignancies, with at least 40% of the patients with adenoid cystic carcinoma demonstrating this feature,[64] and 26% to 32% with malignant mixed tumor demonstrating it. Even in lower grade tumors such as acinic cell carcinoma, there is a measurable incidence of distant metastasis.[16,52] In all of these lesions, the site of distant metastasis is most commonly the lungs. Overall, the likelihood of this occurrence is almost double in the submandibular gland over the parotid gland.[48]

Regional lymphatic metastasis is a subject of considerable importance in malignant salivary gland tumors. In the extensive series reported from Memorial Sloan-Kettering Cancer Center, 14% of these patients presented with palpable nodal metastases. Thirty-four percent of the patients with high-grade as opposed to only 2% with low-grade tumors demonstrated this finding. Additionally, in the group of patients that had clinically negative necks but who had elective neck dissections, 49% of the high-grade and 7% of the low-grade tumors turned out to have histologically positive necks.[70] These statistically significant figures suggest that the incidence of occult and clinically positive nodal disease are increased in high-grade malignant salivary gland tumors.

Spiro and associates believed that the most important prognosticator for survival is tumor stage. Accordingly, in 1975, they proposed a staging system that was later incorporated into the current American Joint Committee on Cancer (AJCC) staging system.[55,71] This system addresses primary size and the presence or absence of fixation or facial nerve dysfunction.

It was first applied only to parotid sites, but seems to serve all salivary sites. Figure 22–34 describes the AJCC staging system. According to Spiro, the cumulative survival exceeds 90% at 10 years in patients with stage I and II disease, whereas only 22% of stages III and IV patients are alive at 10 years.[48]

CLINICAL EVALUATION AND WORKUP

Short of surgical exploration, physical examination remains the most important tool in diagnosis. A hard mass with fixation or nerve palsy is a suspicious finding and, importantly, the diagnostician's general sense is predictive for malignancy. However, any malignancy can masquerade in a more benign appearance and presentation. Cytologic analysis achieved through fine-needle aspiration is helpful in certain selected circumstances, especially when the index of suspicion for malignancy is high or when the patient is not a good candidate for surgery. In the latter circumstance, the patient is somewhat reassured by benign cytology and more secure with a non-surgical approach. In a patient with disseminated cancer and a salivary gland mass, being able to easily make a diagnosis with a fine-needle aspiration can be of considerable value to the patient. The heterogeneity of salivary gland tissue is such, however, that a negative fine-needle aspiration does not substantially alter the treatment plan in most circumstances. Finally, if an older male patient with bilateral tumors has a fine-needle aspiration suggestive of Warthin's tumor, surgery can be avoided.

CT scan and MRI are helpful in analyzing the important third dimension of larger tumors, especially those that involve the deep lobe of the parotid gland. These imaging technologies are important in studying malignant tumors. However, these expensive methods are not necessary for evaluation of all parotid or submandibular gland tumors. One other imaging technology, sialography, is of historic interest only as it pertains to tumors.

TREATMENT OF MAJOR SALIVARY GLAND TUMORS

Surgery of parotid, submandibular, and sublingual gland tumors should be excisional rather than incisional whenever possible. The diagnosis of parotid tumors usually is established by removal of that part of the gland in which the tumor exists. In the case of a lesion of the parotid superficial lobe, for instance, the least extensive or most conservative operation should be a superficial parotidectomy, which also serves as a diagnostic procedure. Before surgery, the surgeon must have a sense of whether the tumor is benign or malignant. This is achieved by physical examination, history, and technologic aids such as fine-needle aspiration and imaging. Sacrifice of the facial nerve or any of its branches usually is reserved for direct involvement by malignant tumor. Occasionally, the nerve or one of its branches is encased within but not invaded by a benign tumor, and a tedious removal of the neoplasm, while sparing the nerve branch, is necessary. Radiation therapy usually is not used as part of the primary management with benign lesions; however, for a lesion that encases the nerve, for recurrent lesions, and in the circumstance in which

Primary Tumor

TO   No evidence of primary tumor.

T1   Tumor 2 cm or less in greatest dimension.

T2   Tumor more than 2 cm but not more than 4 cm in greatest dimension.

T3   Tumor more than 4 cm but not more than 6 cm in greatest dimension.

T4   Tumors more than 6 cm in greatest dimension.

Note: All categories are subdivided: (A) no local extension, (B) local extension, defined as clinical evidence of skin, soft tissue, bone, or nerve invasion.

Lymph Nodes

N0   No regional lymph node metastasis.

N1   Metastasis in a single ipsilateral lymph node, 3 cm or less in greatest dimension.

N2A   Metastasis in a single ipsilateral lymph node more than 3 cm but not more than 6 cm in greatest dimension.

N2B   Metastasis in multiple ipsilateral lymph nodes, none more than 6 cm in greatest dimension.

N2C   Metastasis in bilateral or contralateral lymph nodes, none more than 6 cm in greatest dimension.

N3   Metastasis in a lymph node more than 6 cm in greatest dimension.

Distant Metastasis

M0   No distant metastasis.

M1   Distant metastasis.

Stage Grouping

Stage I	T1A	N0	M0
	T2A	N0	M0
Stage II	T1B	N0	M0
	T2B	N0	M0
	T3A	N0	M0
Stage III	T3B	N0	M0
	T4A	N0	M0
	Any T (except T4B)	N1	M0
Stage IV	T4B	Any N	M0
	Any T	N2, N3	M0
	Any T	Any N	M1

FIGURE 22–34. 1988 revision of AJCC staging for salivary gland cancer.

there is incomplete gross tumor removal, it is often recommended.[72] Postoperative radiation therapy is probably important in recurrent deep lobe parotid tumors, whether benign or malignant, even though all gross tumor has been removed. To add radiation after the routine and uncomplicated removal of a benign tumor of the superficial lobe of the parotid or from the submandibular gland seems unwarranted.

A *lumpectomy and radiation* initial approach to benign disease does not seem advisable in light of our consistent ability to remove these tumors successfully and safely. Dawson and Orr[72] reported 311 patients managed with local excision plus radiation therapy. The local recurrence rate at 10 years was 1.5%, and the cumulative risk for recurrence was 8% at 20 years. Most of these late recurrences were malignant. One of 4 patients developed malignant recurrence at 15 years and 3 at 18 years, raising the possibility of radiation-induced tumors rather than malignant dedifferentiation as part of the natural history of the disease.

The indications for adding radiation to surgery in the management of malignant tumors include positive margins, advanced primary tumor stage, including facial nerve involvement, positive neck nodes, high-grade histology, deep lobe involvement, and tumor spillage during the operation.

Data that show the benefits of adding radiation therapy are abundant. Armstrong and coworkers[73] recently compiled stastics from a retrospective matched-pair analysis that use historical controls from Memorial Sloan-Kettering Cancer Center, and their data strongly suggested a statistically significant locoregional control and survival enhancement with the addition of postoperative radiation therapy for all patients with positive nodes and all patients with stage III or IV disease. The 5-year determinant survival for patients with high-grade histology was better in the surgery plus radiation patients (57% versus 28%), as was the 5-year local control rate (63% versus 44%). There were no benefits achieved for lower-grade or lower-staged tumors.

Other series consistently have shown an improvement in locoregional control in patients with major salivary gland cancers who received postoperative radiation therapy.[63,68,74–78] These consistent data are a marked improvement over the substantial local failure of 39% for parotid gland and 60% for submandibular gland that have been reported in patients treated by surgery alone.[48]

Other recent data suggest that in those lesions that are locally advanced at the time of initial treatment, and in those patients with involved margins, intraoperative brachytherapy in addition to surgery and postoperative external-beam irradiation therapy might be useful in improving local control.[75] Fu and associates showed that patients with positive resection margins had improved local control with the addition of radiation.[79] Overall, only 14% of those with microscopic disease at or close to the surgical margin experienced local failure when postoperative radiation therapy was given compared with 54% who failed locally in the surgery-only group. Most patients in this series received total doses between 5000 and 7500 cGy.

Although a detailed technical description of parotid surgery is inappropriate to this text, several points should be made about this meticulous but safe surgical technique. Were it not for the presence of the facial nerve within the actual substance of the parotid gland, the procedure would be far less worrisome. However, this important motor nerve, along with all of its branches, transects the parotid parynchyma in such a manner that almost all parotid tumor operations involve nerve identification, isolation, and dissection. The approaches to these vary somewhat, but consistent to all is the fundamental surgical tenant of a generous and well-planned incision, flap elevation, and wide exposure. When well designed, the parotidectomy incision, even though long, leaves little obvious scar. The incision usually is begun anterior to the auricle, above the tragus of that structure, extends behind the edge of the external ear canal to minimize its exposure, then swings along the lower edge of the ear lobe, down to the first horizontal crease of the cervical skin, and then anteriorly for a variable distance. A skin flap is then lifted anteriorly to an extent that exposes the entire external surface of the parotid gland (Fig. 22–35). The gland is separated from the anterior border of the sternocleidomastoid muscle, and the posterior belly of the diagastric muscle is identified lying deep to the sternocleidomastoid muscle. Using the diagastric muscle and the cartilaginous ear canal as landmarks, the main trunk of the facial nerve is identified as it exits the stylomastoid foramen and extends anteriorly. The various branches of the nerve are dissected out and, in the case of the tumors within the superficial lobe of the parotid gland, that lobe and the tumor contained within are removed, with keen attention being paid to not violating the capsule of the neoplasm. To remove tumors that are within the deep lobe, various manipulations of the nerve are often necessary after the superficial lobe has been removed. Often, the oncologic principles of wide excision with ample surrounding normal parynchyma are not achievable in deep lobe tumors, and the adequacy of the surgery must be judged with stern reservations; a liberal consideration is given to the employment of postoperative radiation therapy. In situations of a large deep lobe neoplasm, other techniques of deep lobe exposure, such as submandibular gland excision and mandibulotomy, may be necessary to accomplish safely and effectively the important goal of en bloc tumor removal. Modern imaging provides the means with which the surgeon can be forewarned about deep lobe involvement size and the probability of needing extended methods to extricate the tumor from the parapharyngeal space. Whether a partial or a total parotidectomy is done, the defect incurred usually is reasonable. With proper attention to detail, the dissection of the facial nerve and the removal of most tumors can be accomplished with minimal risk for facial weakness postoperatively. The closure of the skin incision usually is followed by a good esthetic result.

Radiation therapy techniques should include treatment planning simulation and CT scan in all patients with major salivary gland tumors. A variety of treatment plans are possible. The most commonly employed technique involves a wedged photon pair or a mixed plan combining ipsilateral photon and electron beams. When the primary site and the neck are treated, the upper neck usually is irradiated along with the primary site. The low neck is treated with a separate field that is generally junctioned at approximately the level of the thyroid notch.

The exact dose required for postoperative radiation therapy has not been determined. Harrison and colleagues analyzed

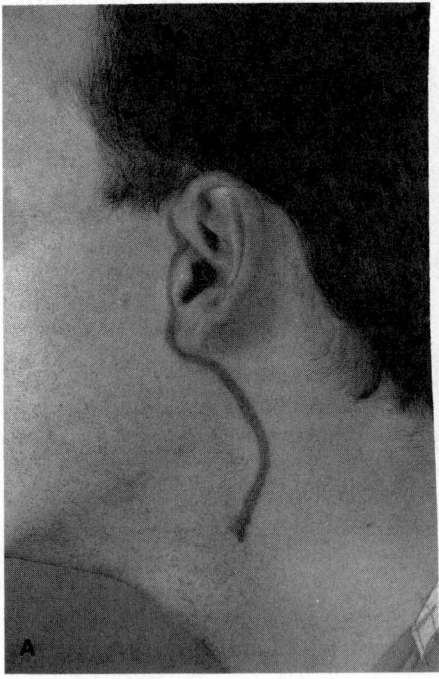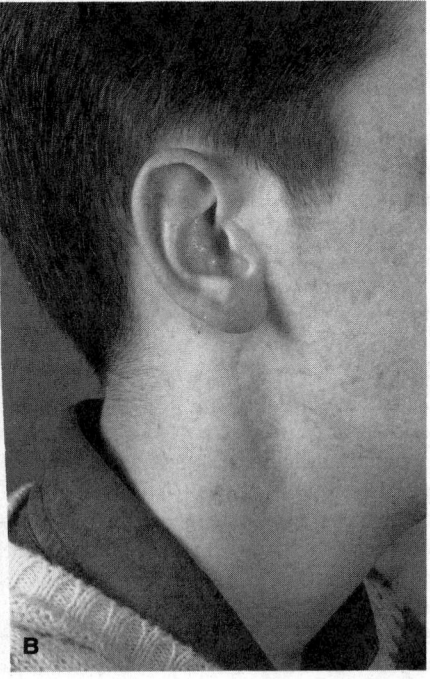

FIGURE 22–35. Typical parotidectomy incision. **(A)** The drawing of the incision is designed to blend into natural skin folds and minimize visibility. **(B)** One-year postoperative result of an actual parotidectomy incision done using the same incision design as depicted in A.

the radiation dose compared with the outcome.[75] Patients who received doses of at least 5750 cGy were compared with patients receiving lower doses. The 10-year local control rate for the higher dose group was 72% compared with 53% for those in the lower-dose group. Although a trend in favor of high doses was suggested, the difference was not statistically significant. McNaney and coworkers reviewed treatment failure and the total dose for patients receiving less than 6000 cGy or greater.[77] The doses that were associated with treatment failure did not lend themselves to a specific dose-response relation. In general, doses in the 6000- to 6500-cGy range in 6 to 7 weeks are used for postoperative radiation therapy, except in patients with involved margins or T4 disease who may require even higher doses. The high local failure rate experienced previously at the Memorial Sloan-Kettering Cancer Center with T4 patients has led to an intensification of local treatment in that institution. Such patients are treated with surgery, intraoperative brachytherapy, plus postoperative external-beam irradiation.

Because of the unique natural history of adenoid cystic carcinoma and because of its affinity for neural involvement, this tumor bears special and separate consideration. Data from three studies consistently show that postoperative radiation therapy should be added for almost all adenoid cystic carcinomas.[75,80,81] If there had been involved neck nodes, then the neck should be included as well. Elective neck irradiation is generally not recommended.

Regarding the general management of the neck, the influence of T stage and grade are important. In a study by Armstrong and associates, 474 patients with major salivary gland cancers were reviewed.[73] High-grade tumors had a 49% risk for occult metastases compared with only 7% for intermediate- or low-grade tumors. Epidermoid cancers had a risk of 41% compared with only 10% for all other histologies combined. Submandibular tumors had a higher risk for occult metastases (21%) compared with parotid tumors (9%). Occult disease was found in 7% of T1 and T2 tumors, 16% of T3, and 24% of T4 tumors. Essentially, in those patients with clinically positive nodes, postoperative radiation therapy is needed. The question of how to manage the clinically negative neck best is aided by the data of Armstrong and associates cited earlier. In patients who would otherwise need postoperative radiation therapy due to concerns about the primary site, elective neck treatment with radiation can be used. It is appropriate to dissect electively the necks of high-risk patients as a means of staging the nodes. If there is histologic disease present, postoperative radiation therapy to the neck should be added. In this study, the periparotid nodes were the ones most commonly involved. However, if node dissection was limited to the periparotid and level II nodes, 25% of the node-positive patients would have had nodes missed at levels III and IV. This was because of skip metastases to levels III and IV without level II metastases. This point emphasizes the need for treatment of the entire neck in patients found to have positive nodes.

In patients with a clinically positive neck, surgery and postoperative radiation therapy are indicated. Unlike squamous cell carcinoma of the head and neck, where nodal disease in one neck frequently places the contralateral neck at risk, this does not appear to be the case with major salivary gland cancers. King and Fletcher[82] and Harrison and associates[75] have shown in two separate studies that elective contralateral neck radiation is not necessary in this circumstance.

Chemotherapy trials have been limited by the heterogeneity and rarity of the disease. Nevertheless, several single-agent trials have been conducted. Promising results have been achieved with doxorubicin, 5-fluorouracil (5-FU), methotrexate, cyclophosphamide, and cisplatin. Combinations of chemotherapy also have been studied in a number of trials.[83–96] Cyclophosphamide plus doxorubicin plus cisplatin (CAP), the most studied regimen, has produced responses from 22% to 100% and complete response rates of 0% to 40%.[89,92,96] Response durations, however, have been short, lasting from 5 to 9 months. The addition of 5-FU to CAP (FACP) in a recent study did not increase the response rate.[95] Low patient numbers and heterogenous histologies in these studies make it difficult to objectively compare the results of single-agent with combination trials. It seems that patients with adenocarcinoma, adenoid cystic carcinoma, acinic cell carcinoma, and malignant mixed tumor have similar chemosensitivity to doxorubicin and cyclophosphamide combinations. Patients with mucoepidermoid and undifferentiated tumors respond better to drugs active against squamous cell carcinoma (*e.g.*, cisplatin, 5-FU, and methotrexate).[88] The current standard chemotherapy options for recurrent or metastatic salivary gland tumors are all palliative. The activity of combinations, especially CAP regimens, in patients with metastatic disease provides a rationale for using the same regimen in neoadjuvant or postoperative adjuvant settings in patients with high-grade tumors. To date, reports on this regimen have appeared only sporadically.

There continues to be a need for trials of newer agents for these cancers. Future phase II and phase III studies should be developed as cooperative multiinstitutional mechanisms to achieve answers within a reasonable period. Hormonal or biologic therapies have not been studied adequately either.

MINOR SALIVARY GLAND TUMORS

Minor salivary gland tumors can occur in any age group and they have no particular sex predilection. Minor salivary glands are ubiquitous in the upper aerodigestive tract, so tumors of these glands can occur anywhere in the head and neck; however, the palate is the commonest site for benign and malignant growths. Ectopic salivary gland tissue can lead to tumors in such diverse locations as the middle ear or the thyroid area. Table 22–36 shows the distribution by the sites of origin in the Memorial Sloan-Kettering Cancer Center's experience with these tumors.[1] These lesions occur in the nasal cavities and paranasal sinuses, nasopharynx, larynx, lip, floor of mouth, and other sites in the head and neck, but overall, they are most frequently seen in the oral cavity. It is often impossible to differentiate between a primary sublingual tumor and a minor salivary gland tumor in the anterior floor of the mouth.

Between 65% and 88% of all of these tumors are malignant.[97] Adenoid cystic carcinoma is the commonest histology, occurring in as many as 55% of patients with minor salivary gland tumors.[98] Otherwise, the representing histologies are the same as for major salivary gland tumors, including mucoepidermoid cancer, adenocarcinoma, malignant mixed tumor, and anaplastic carcinoma. Small cell (oat cell) carcinoma of minor salivary gland origin has also been reported.[99] These tumors tend to present as painless submucosal masses and can be present for many years without change. Malignant

TABLE 22–36. Incidence of Various Sites of Origin of Minor Salivary Gland Tumors*

Site	Benign	Malignant	Total
Palate	58	114	172
Tongue	2	62	64
Cheek	9	38	47
Maxillary sinus	1	43	44
Nasal cavity	3	20	23
Gingiva	0	22	22
Floor of mouth	0	21	21
Lip	5	11	16
Larynx	0	15	15
Tonsil	1	9	10
Retromolar trigone	0	9	9
Nasopharynx	0	6	6
Ethmoid sinus	0	5	5
Pharynx	2	3	5
Total	81	378	459

* Total of 459 cases from the Memorial Sloan-Kettering Cancer Center.
(Adapted from Spiro R, Spiro J. Cancer of the salivary glands. In: Meyers E, Sven J, eds. Cancer of the head and neck. 2nd ed. London: Churchill Livingstone, 1984:645)

tumors can persist without change, but more commonly increase in size over time.

Any submucosal mass should be considered a minor salivary gland tumor until proved otherwise. The malignancies can spread to invade local tissue, including bone and nerve. Tumors of the floor of the mouth or the tongue can extend into the neck and into the mandible. Adenoid cystic cancer has a particular predilection to grow along the perineural sheaths and extend to great distances from the primary tumor along nerve pathways. It is important for the surgeon to realize that skip areas of tumor involvement can occur along the nerve trunks. For instance, when this lesion occurs in the lateral aspect of the soft palate, it can infiltrate the branches of the greater palatine nerve, extend centrally, and can ultimately occupy the gasserian ganglion in the middle cranial fossa. This potential occurrence should be included in any treatment planning to include that ganglion. The presence of a negative frozen section taken from the nerve trunk proximal to the originally discovered peripheral nerve involvement does not rule out the possibility that the nerve is involved with tumor more centrally. This leads to the need to include the ganglion in treatment planning. Adenoid cystic carcinomas can spread along the haversian canals of bone. Therefore, when there is questionable involvement of mandible with floor of mouth lesions, the surgeon must be prepared to deal with further extension than is obvious.

Fewer than 20% of patients with minor salivary gland malignancies present with lymph node metastases, and approximately 10% who demonstrate clinically negative necks have the subsequent appearance of nodal metastases. As is true with the major salivary gland tumors, the incidence of nodal metastases is related to grade and tumor size (*i.e.*, stage).

There is no uniform staging system for minor salivary gland

tumors. It is most useful to use the system for the anatomic site in which the tumor arises. Survival seems to correlate with clinical stage. Olsen and coworkers showed that tumor size was significant for mucoepidermoid carcinoma of the oral cavity.[100] In their study, patients with lesions larger than 2 cm did much worse than those with lesions smaller than 2 cm. In the latter group, there were no deaths from mucoepidermoid cancer.

TREATMENT OF MINOR SALIVARY GLANDS TUMORS

Surgery is usually the treatment of choice for minor salivary gland tumors. Enucleation is considered inadequate therapy and is associated with a recurrence rate as high as 93%[100]; therefore, wide excision or regional excision must be performed when possible. Few data exist on primary radiation treatment. Ellis and colleagues have reported their results for minor salivary gland tumors.[101] A total of 20 patients with minor salivary gland malignancies received only radiation therapy for their disease; 7 had early and 13 had advanced stage tumors. Local control was obtained in 6 of 7 (86%) of early-stage lesions, a result that is comparable with surgical management. For the more advanced lesions, however, radiation alone controlled only 2 of 13 (15%), which is a result considerably inferior to a combined surgery and irradiation strategy. Although this and other limited studies suggest that radiation can be effective for small tumors, surgery usually is considered the treatment of choice whenever possible. In certain early lesions in which the operation would induce significant cosmetic or functional sequelae, a radiation alternative is reasonable. Advanced lesions should always be treated initially with surgery, usually followed by postoperative radiation therapy. Exactly which patients should receive postoperative radiation therapy remains unclear. These authors tend to recommend the guidelines that have been established for major salivary gland tumors; patients with advanced stage disease, lymph node metastases, high-grade tumors, or inadequate surgical margins are treated with postoperative irradiation. Many patients will have a combination of these factors.

Eapen and colleagues reported 70 patients with salivary gland carcinomas.[102] Approximately one third had minor salivary gland tumors, and the indications for postoperative radiation therapy were inconsistent; however, there was a significant decrease in locoregional failure in patients who were given postoperative radiation therapy. The actuarial risk of locoregional failure in the nonradiated patients was 62% compared with 20% in the radiated group. Ninety percent of the patients received between 5500 and 6590 cGy in 5 to 6.5 weeks. In 95% of irradiated patients, the regional lymph nodes were treated along with the primary site.

Tran and coworkers reviewed the University of California at Los Angeles experience with salivary gland tumors of the oral cavity.[98] A total of 62 patients with previously untreated lesions were analyzed, all of whom were treated with primary surgical resection. Twenty-four patients received postoperative radiation therapy due to advanced local disease or involved margins of resection, or both. Most of the patients in this series had adenoid cystic histology, and the palate was the commonest primary site. Local tumor control in patients with positive margins was 50% for surgery alone compared with 71% with combined surgery and postoperative radiation therapy. There was a trend toward lower disease control and survival for patients with adenoid cystic carcinoma compared with the other histologies.

The experience with minor salivary gland tumors of the nasal cavity and paranasal sinuses has also been reported by Tran and coworkers.[98] Thirty-five patients seen and treated between 1962 and 1985 were included, most of whom (68%) had adenoid cystic carcinoma. Adenocarcinoma was seen in about half the ethmoid and nasal cavity lesions. Local control for the combined surgery and irradiation group was 62% compared with 18% for surgery alone and 9% for radiation alone. This benefit of radiation was present despite the fact that the irradiated group had higher stage disease and more patients with inadequate surgical margins. For those with positive margins, local failure was seen in 67% with surgery alone and 30% with postoperative radiation therapy.

Just as in the major salivary gland, the data on the treatment of adenoid cystic cancer of minor salivary gland origin clearly demonstrate a local control advantage for patients receiving combined surgery and postoperative radiation therapy compared with surgery alone. These authors recommend this strategy for almost all adenoid cystic carcinomas of minor salivary gland origin. A young patient with a small lesion that is resected completely may be an exception to this rule. All treatment decisions must be individualized.

Koss and associates reported 14 patients with small cell carcinoma of the minor salivary gland origin.[99] Although there are no conclusive data from this or other series, these lesions may be managed optimally with resection, chemotherapy, and local radiation therapy.

The technique of radiation therapy for minor salivary gland tumors is similar to the technique for squamous cancer at the corresponding primary site. For postoperative irradiation, doses in the 6000- to 6500-cGy range in 6 to 7 weeks are used. Wide portals are required, especially for adenoid cystic cancer. The nerve pathways up to and including the base of skull should be included in the treated portals. When radiation therapy alone is used for early-stage disease, doses of at least 7000 cGy in 7 to 7.5 weeks should be used. Brachytherapy can be used for a portion of the treatment, especially in oral cavity lesions. Elective nodal irradiation usually is not indicated except in selected circumstances, such as the occasional patient with minor salivary gland tumors of the nasopharynx. Whether elective nodal irradiation is required here is unclear, but it can certainly be justified on the basis of the rich lymphatic drainage of the nasopharynx.

SPECIFIC TREATMENT AND SPECIAL SITUATIONS

Deep lobe parotid tumors, whether benign or malignant, are often inaccessible by standard parotidectomy. In such a circumstance, a variety of mandibulotomy techniques are available to surgeons that provide excellent exposure to the whole parapharyngeal space, the parotid tumor, and the carotid sheath.[103] Because deep lobe tumors are often not surrounded by parotid gland parenchyma, removing the lesion without fragmentation often is made possible by this method of exposure.

In cancers that involve the facial nerve or branches of it, the involved segment is best resected and grafted with an interposition of nerve harvested from another site. Often,

however, nerve can be dissected off a tumor surface and, with the employment of postoperative radiation therapy, control results similar to a more radical approach are achievable. Fortunately, the need to sacrifice the facial nerve is encountered infrequently, but when it does become necessary, the consequence of the surgery and the gravity of the prognosis takes on an added dimension.

The functional and esthetic results of correctly done nerve grafting, although not perfect, are good in a substantial percentage of cases. Essentially, clinicians are working in an era of surgical minimalism in which the tendency is to sacrifice the facial nerve only in extreme circumstances. The increasing body of knowledge showing the value of postoperative radiation therapy has in large part been responsible for this more conservative philosophy in dealing with the facial nerve in parotid gland surgery. There have been no studies done that document the effectiveness of this approach, which has evolved from considerable anecdotal information.

Not infrequently, a particular situation arises in which a patient with a submandibular mass was explored, and for various reasons, only a gland resection was done at the initial operation. The glandular pathology later revealed the existence of a malignancy. The literature is not clear in its recommendations, but the value of reoperation usually lies in the removal of gross disease, such as that left behind at the primary site or metastatic nodes. To reoperate and radically remove regional nerves such as cranial nerve XII or to remove mandible in the absence of such gross disease does not seem warranted. A neck dissection of some sort usually is recommended, and postoperative irradiation to the primary bed and neck should be conducted. Considering the potential for locoregional control with this plan, and considering that more radical measures at the locoregional site do nothing to prevent distant metastasis, this moderate approach seems appropriate.[104]

Regarding radiation therapy, neutrons have been suggested as preferable to photons, especially for advanced salivary gland malignancies. Griffin and colleagues reported a prospective randomized trial that demonstrated improved complete response, improved locoregional control, and a potential survival advantage for neutron- versus photon-treated patients.[105] The lack of availability of neutrons, however, precludes most patients from receiving this therapy.

PARAGANGLIOMAS

The paragangliomas have been known historically by a variety of names including, *glomus tumors, chemodectomas, non-chromaffin paragangliomas, glomerocytomas, carotid body* and *tympanic body tumors,* and *receptomas.* These names and others make up a heterogenous and confusing list that addresses certain individual characteristics of various tumors, but which fails to achieve a necessary consistency of classification.[106–108] Essentially, these tumors make up a family of neoplasms that develop from the paraganglia tissues, which are themselves chemoreceptor organs that are distributed throughout the body. These organs are of neural crest origin and have similar functions and similar histologic appearances.[109] Their cells of origin are part of the *diffuse neuroendocrine system* (DNES), a name that has replaced the term *amine precursor uptake and decarboxylase system.* The new terminology acknowledges that the primary products of these cells, neuropeptides and catecholamines, may serve as neurotransmitters, neurohormones, hormones, and parahormones.[110]

The chief cell is probably the principal component involved and seems to be the actual chemoreceptor of the paraganglia, containing acetylcholine, catecholamines, and serotonin. This cell is of neural crest origin, and therefore neuroendocrine in nature. It renders the paraganglia receptive to hypoxia and pH changes and to fluctuations in the blood carbon dioxide concentration.[111]

These chief cells migrate with autonomic ganglion cells; they are in close association with sympathetic ganglia and the aorta and its main branches.[112] Many head and neck paraganglia, and their respective neoplasms, are distributed in relation to the vessels and cranial nerves of the primitive branchial arches. Because of this, they are called *branchiomeric paraganglia*.[106,113,114] For example, the jugulotympanic paragangliomas are related to the third gill arch, but the intravagal paragangliomas are not associated with the gill arches or their arterial derivatives.[106] Although paragangliomas can be seen in a variety of head and neck locations such as the orbit, the maxilla, the larynx, and the trachea, most are found on the carotid body, the vagus nerve, or in the jugulotympanic area. Throughout the body, the paraganglia are consistent in their locations and can be classified as follows[116]:

I. Branchiomeric paraganglia
   a. Temporal bone (tympanicum, jugulare)
   b. Carotid body
   c. Other head and neck (orbit, laryngeal, nasal)
   d. Subclavian, aortic, pulmonary
II. Intravagal (upper mediastinal) paraganglia
III. Aorticosympathetic (retroperitoneal) paraganglia
IV. Visceral (pelvic, vagal, mesenteric) paraganglia

The term *glomus* was applied to paragangliomas because it was believed that the chief cells within the paraganglia were derived from specialized pericytes or from blood vessel walls, as is seen in true arteriovenous glomus complexes.[106] Depending on whether they began in the ear or on the jugular bulb, those tumors that develop in the jugulotympanic paraganglia usually are referred to as *glomus tympanicum* or *glomus jugulare tumors*.[116] The paraganglia from which this group of neoplasms arises are associated with the tympanic branch of the glossopharyngeal nerve and the auricular branch of the vagus nerve, respectively.[116] The paragangliomas of the intravagal area often are referred to as *glomus intravagal*,[117] or *vagal body tumors*.[118] The term *glomus*, while enjoying considerable name recognition, is deceiving, because it suggests a pathologic uniqueness. Such is not the case, however, because all the head and neck paragangliomas have similar histologic, ultrastructural, and cytochemical features.[106,109,114] The first description of a temporal bone glomus tumor by Lubbers referred to a *carotid body-like tumor* that was thought to be metastatic from a contralateral carotid body tumor.[119] What separates these tumors from each other is the location in which they develop and their functional capabilities.

PATHOGENESIS

The word *functional* is used as a prefix to describe those paragangliomas that secrete catecholamines (epinephrine and norepinephrine) and serotonin. Even though the capacity for catecholamine synthesis and secretion has been documented for both jugulotympanic and intravagal paragangliomas, this particular group of tumors actually has the lowest catecholamine content of all paragangliomas.[106,117,118,120,121] Other functional capabilities have been documented in these tumors, but the significance of any secretory activity should be evaluated by its clinical impact. The incidence of clinically functional paragangliomas is only 1% to 3%[122]; however, because of the potentially serious consequences of a catecholamine crisis during manipulations of a functional tumor, the evaluation of patients with paragangliomas should include screening for symptoms and signs of catecholamine secretion and the measurement of the appropriate blood and urine products.[123]

Overall, paragangliomas are uncommon neoplasms. They occur as nonfamilial and familial tumors, with the former developing more frequently in women and the latter in men. The mode of inheritance is thought to be autosomal dominant.[114,124-127]

Multiple paragangliomas occur synchronously in 25% to 50% of the familial and in as many as 10% of nonfamilial tumors.[125,127-130] Individual tumors vary in this regard; for example, carotid body tumors are reported to occur in 50% of nonfamilial and 30% of familial cases. Any combination of two, three, or more locations of synchronous tumors can occur, but the most frequent combination involves concurrent carotid body and jugulotympanic tumors.[126] Synchronous occurrence is seen between paragangliomas and other DNES lesions such as pheochromocytomas.[125,129] Even though this occurrence is unusual, the serious consequences of not being warned before surgery mandates a compulsive screening for this tumor in all paragangliomas. Specifically, in those patients with certain catecholamine profiles, the existence of a pheochromocytoma must be ruled out before any surgery is undertaken. Parathyroid adenomas, thyroid carcinomas, and certain other neural crest tumors are seen concurrently with jugulotympanic, intravagal, and carotid body paragangliomas.[114,131,132] Essentially, this group of neoplasms must always be thought of as a potentially systemic affliction, especially in those patients with a family history of such tumors.

CLINICAL BEHAVIOR AND NATURAL HISTORY

The clinical behavior of paragangliomas is largely determined by cellular characteristics and tumor location. Regarding the former, malignancy occurs rarely and is typically defined by the existence of metastasis rather than by cellular characteristics. Metastasis is usually to lungs, lymph nodes, liver, bone, and spleen[132-134]; because paraganglia tissue is not usually found in any of these organ systems, its presence within them constitutes metastasis. Metastasis apparently occurs more frequently in intravagal and jugulotympanic paragangliomas than it does in carotid body tumors.[135] This is probably the case because of the relation of these tumors to the jugular vein.[136,137] Other authors have, anecdotally, used local invasion characteristics alone as criteria to classify paragangliomas as malignant.[138-140] There is a suggestion that the status of DNA ploidy might be useful in determining malignancy. In the final analysis, however, there are no consistent criteria other than metastasis that can be used to gauge aggressiveness.[141] Much like the primary paragangliomas, which are late to metastasize, metastatic sites are characterized by a restrained natural history; some patients with known lung and bone metastases can live as many as 25 years after discovery.[140] In addition, spontaneous remission of metastatic paraganglioma has been reported.[142]

The natural history of primary paragangliomas usually is characterized by slow and inexorable growth, and the alterations of those structures into which or around which they grow determines the symptoms and signs that occur. The jugulotympanic tumors extend into the skull, the eustachian tubes, and the normal cracks and furrows of the ear space. If they begin in the hypotympanicum, or if they start in the jugular bulb, they often can be seen through the tympanic membrane, but only by appropriate imaging can the true extent of the tumor be determined. A bluish-red mass behind the tympanic membrane or a polyp in the external ear canal can be but the tip of an extensive paraganglioma, and a casual biopsy or a myringotomy can lead to troublesome bleeding. These tumors initially create a sense of fullness in the ear, along with a conductive hearing loss and pulsatile tinnitus. Destruction of the temporal bone can lead to facial nerve weakness, vertigo, deafness, and intracranial complications, such as cerebrospinal fluid leak and meningitis. When a tumor occurs in the jugular area, its otologic manifestations can precede or be preceded by vagal nerve signs. Paragangliomas of the vagus nerve, on the other hand, almost always create vocal cord paralysis before otologic symptoms and signs.[143] Overall, only about 3% of paragangliomas are associated with the vagus nerve.[144] These slowly growing tumors occur most often at the base of the skull and in the parapharyngeal space, but may arise anywhere along the course of the vagus nerve and its branches. When they are located high in the neck, vagal paragangliomas tend to displace the internal carotid artery anteriorly. Cervically located paragangliomas most commonly present as asymptomatic masses,[145] and in the absence of unusually aggressive local behavior, neurogenic signs such as those caused by involvement of the sympathetic trunk and cranial nerves X, XI, and XII usually occur only after extensive growth.

Carotid body paragangliomas actually can grow to impressive dimensions without creating neurologic or vascular findings. These facts are important in determining treatment philosophy, especially in older, asymptomatic patients. These tumors begin in the adventitia of the artery, usually at or around the bifurcation of the internal and external carotid arteries. Because they generally develop from the medial aspect of the arterial system, they tend to displace the arteries laterally, causing a typical appearance of splayed and lateralized vessels (Fig. 22–36). This finding is important in diagnosis, because it is unique. As these neoplasms become larger, they can occupy the parapharyngeal space, actually presenting as a bulge in the tonsil area. Encroachment into this area can produce dysphagia. Also, large tumors can occasionally produce compressive carotid artery symptoms.

EVALUATION

The diagnostic workup of paragangliomas should consist of CT or MRI and, in selected situations, angiography. Imaging should delineate bone destruction and complete tumor extension intracranially and extracranially. CT is traditionally thought to be more effective in imaging bone, but MRI has added a superior capability in accessing intracranial extension and the relation of tumor to bone. With proper enhancement

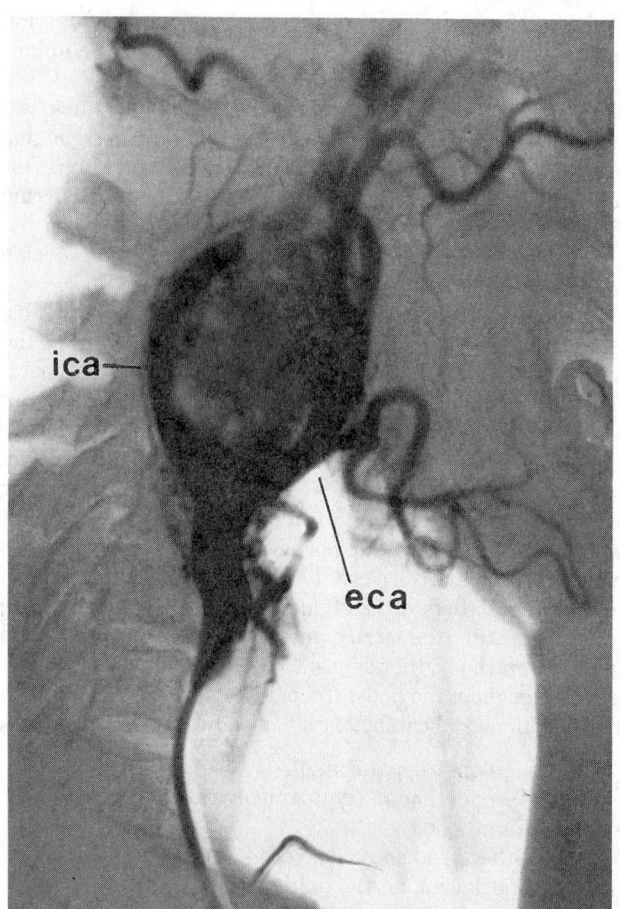

FIGURE 22–36. Arteriogram shows carotid body paraganglioma in a 44-year-old woman. Notice the splaying of internal (*ica*) and external carotid (*eca*) arteries and the extreme vascularity of the tumor.

techniques, one or both of these images plus clinical evaluation can provide sufficient information to plan treatment in most paragangliomas. This is a point relevant to overall management strategy; if radiation therapy is the planned treatment, the radiation oncologist must be comfortable enough with the diagnosis to proceed without a biopsy. Fine-needle aspiration and cytologic analysis can be helpful, but because of the location medial to the carotid artery, and because of the dense vascularity of most of these lesions, this may not always be practical. Open biopsy becomes necessary when the diagnosis is not achieved by these other means.

The main value of invasive arteriography is in preoperative preparation, such as tumor embolization done just before surgery or for studying contralateral crossover blood supply. Because of the potential for excessive bleeding, biopsy should be avoided whenever possible.

Paragangliomas are usually rich in their blood supply. When surgery is planned, intraluminal embolization of the main arterial supply and the tumor bed is helpful in safe and less morbid removal of large tumors. In 1992, the growing concern for the purity of the blood supply is such that surgeons should avoid transfusion whenever possible. Preoperative embolization can be extremely helpful in pursuing this goal. This technique has its most impressive impact in the removal of larger carotid body and jugular bulb tumors and is probably unnecessary in most small tumors. There are researchers who specifically recommend that embolization not be employed in carotid body tumor surgery, because it can cause an inflammatory response that may make the dissection more difficult.[144] These authors do not share this view, however, and believe that embolization greatly aids in this operation. The techniques of embolization are beyond the scope of this chapter, and the reader is referred to the literature on that subject; however, it must be emphasized that the employment of this technology is accompanied by some risks and should be undertaken only by an experienced interventional radiology team. Additionally, embolization of paragangliomas is only an adjunct to surgery and should not be considered as the primary treatment of these highly vascular tumors, no matter how successful the devascularization results are with embolization. If embolization is not promptly followed by tumor removal, undesirable collateral circulation and vascular shunting occurs, ultimately complicating an already tedious surgical process. Actually, the sooner the surgery follows the embolization, the more effective the hemostasis during surgery. If surgery is not to be the treatment of choice, then embolization should not be done.

TREATMENT AND RESULTS

Paragangliomas usually are considered benign, and although metastasis and aggressive local behavior can occur, they are the exception rather than the rule. Traditionally, the mainstay of treatment has been surgical removal,[146,147] but repeated series of cases treated by radiation therapy have demonstrated its effectiveness in achieving local control of these tumors.[148–150,152] Other investigators have reviewed the literature and have compared surgical results with radiation therapy results. Based on these studies, there is no difference in local control achieved by either modality. Accordingly, the decision of whether to operate should be based on a formula that considers tumor size, patient age and general health, symptoms and signs present before treatment, treatment related morbidity, and the expertise of those involved in the planned treatment.

The reluctance to use radiation therapy probably results from a historic bias against treating benign tumors with this modality. The definition of local control is somewhat different between radiation therapists and surgeons. In traditional cancer thinking, sustained complete response after radiation is the criterion by which local control usually is judged. Proponents of treating these tumors with radiation therapy argue that this is not the case with paragangliomas, because these lesions are predominantly vascular, with only a proportion of cells having the ability to proliferate. Even if the proliferative element is sterilized by radiation therapy, they point out, the nonproliferative vascular mass often remains, left to be misinterpreted as persistent disease. They emphasize that the resolution of the clinical symptoms, or in the case of the originally asymptomatic patient, the lack of rapid progression of symptoms are what constitute local control; as long as the tumor does not grow and cause increasing local morbidity, the goals of treatment have been satisfied. Those series that compare the two treatment modalities may be somewhat biased against radiation therapy, because many tumors radiated were not favorable lesions by virtue of their size and recurrent state. Ideally, an accurate comparison of treatment methods should analyze comparable tumors.

Cummings and coworkers have reported 45 patients radiated for glomus tumors.[148] Only 3 patients (6.6%) have had symptomatic recurrences. In 2 of these patients, it was believed that recurrence was due to a "geographic miss." The radiation therapy was effective in relieving the presenting symptoms of most patients. For example, 27 of 35 (77%) patients who received 3500 cGy in 3 weeks had complete relief of their tinnitus. The remaining 23% had partial relief or stabilization of symptoms. All patients with pain, vertigo, discharge, bleeding, and abnormalities of the fifth cranial nerve had complete relief of their symptoms with radiation therapy. All patients with cranial nerve IX through XII abnormalities had partial relief or stabilization of their cranial nerve abnormalities. The authors noted that symptomatic improvement often did not occur until many months after radiation therapy. This highlighted the need to follow these patients closely over a long period. As long as there was no clinical progression, the authors believed there would be no need to intervene in the postradiation setting.

Kim and associates have analyzed the dose-response relation for irradiation of paragangliomas.[149] The literature was reviewed, and the rate of failure was correlated with dose. Overall, recurrence was 25% when the radiation dose was less than 4000 cGy. With doses greater than 4000 cGy, local recurrence was rare. Overall, only 2 of 142 patients (1.4%) who received more than 4000 cGy had local recurrence. The authors recommended doses in the 4000- to 4500-cGy range, delivered in 4 to 4.5 weeks. In the study by Cummings and coworkers, only 3500 cGy was used, but was given over 3 weeks.[148] This is a hypofractionation technique that delivers a greater dose per fraction than conventional radiation therapy. The biologic effects of this dose would be greater than 4000 cGy with conventional fractionation.

On the other hand, surgeons are skeptical of the persistence of chief cells years after radiation therapy and the viability of this tissue and its capacity to proliferate 20 to 30 years after dormancy.[153] Further, malignant transformation of tissue secondary to radiation has been reported in these tumors,[140] and although unusual, this occurrence is of concern.

There are complications associated with both methods of treatment, with most series showing the rate to be higher in those patients managed by surgery.[154] It should be pointed out, however, that most series have studied cases accumulated over many years, and in many of the earlier surgical cases, modern temporal bone and carotid artery bypass techniques had not yet been developed. The contemporary methods of reducing intraoperative bleeding by preoperative embolization usually are not included in these series. The intraoperative precision achieved by using these contemporary methods surely makes the previous complication data invalid. The complications associated with radiation therapy are dose related. Bone and brain necrosis and abscess are the most serious of those reported. Each of these has occurred in approximately 1% of treated patients. All these complications should not occur as long as doses in the 4000- to 4500-cGy range are used. Fuller and colleagues reported one fibrosarcoma in their series that was considered a radiation-induced malignancy.[155] There are no other radiation-induced malignancies reported to date.

The decision to operate or radiate should be based on a formula that considers tumor size and location, patient age and health, symptoms or signs present before treatment, potential morbidity, and the expertise and availability of those involved in treatment. The decision should be made in concert between the head and neck surgeon and the radiation oncologist, and with an appreciation for the fact that this group of tumors is one of the most complex and dangerous to treat in the head and neck. To do nothing is an acceptable option in some patients, because these lesions are often tolerated well for long periods.

A reasonable plan in patients with head and neck paragangliomas is to operate and remove those lesions, whether jugulotympanic, intravagal, or carotid body, that are smaller and less likely to be associated with significant operative morbidity. For large tumors that demonstrate extensive bone destruction or intracranial involvement, or both, or in which considerable operative morbidity is expected, radiation therapy is probably the method of choice for achieving local control. In young patients, radiation therapy tends to be avoided if a reasonable surgical option is available. On the other hand, the risk for radiation-induced cancer is small, and these authors do not hesitate to recommend it to young patients if the surgical procedure required is likely to be associated with unreasonable morbidity. Older patients are especially suited for radiation therapy, because local control usually is sustained throughout the balance of their lifetime.

The surgery of carotid body tumors is fraught with hazards, and only those head and neck surgeons trained in vascular techniques should attempt to remove these lesions, especially in the circumstance of recurrence. Carotid artery bypass or shunt, or even artery resection and reconstruction, are sometimes necessary to achieve complete tumor removal. Any clinician attacking one of these lesions should be prepared to use these techniques. Likewise, removal of jugulotympanic lesions should only be attempted by surgeons trained in otologic and skull base techniques. Those intravagal paragangliomas that are located high in the neck are often the most challenging to be dealt with surgically, being too high to approach by a conventional cervical exposure and too low to be handled from an intracranial approach. These are true skull base lesions, often having an epicenter within the jugular foramen. This mostly inaccessible location is best approached by complex but precise and well-described skull base techniques.[147]

Overall, the most accepted treatment for paragangliomas is surgical extirpation; however, radiation therapy is an effective alternative to surgery for achieving local control in certain patients. The definition of cure in paragangliomas is illusive and, in this regard, the patient's age is important in the decision process. The existence of an asymptomatic paraganglioma in an elderly patient or a patient in ill health is of questionable concern and, therefore, consideration for observation only should be given.

REFERENCES

1. Spiro R, Spiro J. Cancer of the salivary glands. In: Meyers E, Suen J, eds. Cancer of the head and neck. 2nd ed. London: Churchill Livingstone, 1984:645.
2. Som P, Biller H, Lawson W. Tumors of the parapharyngeal space. Ann Otol Rhinol Laryngol 1981;90(Suppl 80):3–15.
3. Som P, Braun I, Shapiro M. Tumors of the parapharyngeal space: MR imaging. Radiology 1987;164:823.
4. Work W, Gates G. Tumors of the parotid gland and parapharyngeal space. Otol Clin North Am 1969;2:497.
5. Cassissi N, Dickerson D, Million R. Squamous cell cancer of the skin metastatic to parotid nodes. Arch Otol 1978;104:336–339.
6. Conley T. Salivary glands and the facial nerve. New York: Grune & Stratton, 1975.
7. Takeichi N, Hirose F, Yamamoto H. Salivary gland tumors in atomic bomb survivors, Hiroshima, Japan: Epidemiologic observation. Cancer 1976;38:2462.
8. Maxon H, Saenger E, Buncher C. Radiation-associated carcinoma of the salivary glands. Ann Otol Rhinol Laryngol 1981;90:107.
9. Katz A, Preston-Martin S. Salivary gland tumors and previous radiation therapy to the head and neck. Am J Surg 1984;147:345.
10. Schneider A, Favus M, Stachura M. Salivary gland neoplasms as a late consequence of head and neck radiation. Ann Intern Med 1977;87:160.
11. Hollander L, Cunningham M. Management of cancer of the parotid gland. Surg Clin North Am 1973;53:113.
12. Klintenber C, Olofsson J, Hellquist H, Sokjer H. Adenocarcinoma of the ethmoid sinuses: A review of 28 cases with special reference to dust exposure. Cancer 1984;54:482.
13. Hadfield E, Macbeth R. Adenocarcinoma of the ethmoids in furniture workers. Ann Otol Rhinol Laryngol 1971;80:699.
14. Evans R, Cruckshank A; Epithelial tumors of the salivary glands. Philadelphia: WB Saunders, 1970.
15. Foote FM, Frazell E. Tumors of the major salivary glands. Cancer 1953;6:1965.
16. Batsakis J, Regezi T, Bloch D. The pathology of head and neck tumors: III. Head Neck Surg 1979;1:260.
17. Livolsi V, Perzin K. Malignant mixed tumors arising in salivary glands: Carcinomas arising in benign mixed tumors. Cancer 1971;39:2209.
18. Gerughty R, Scofield H, Brown F, Hennigar C. Malignant mixed tumors of salivary origin. Cancer 1969;24:471.
19. Spiro R, Huvos A, Strong E. Malignant mixed tumor of salivary gland origin. Cancer 1978;41:924.
20. Godwin J. Benign lymphoepithelial lesion of the parotid gland. Cancer 1952;5:1089–1103.
21. Smith F, Rajdeo H, Danesar N, Bhuta K, Stahl R. Benign lymphoepithelial lesion of the parotid gland in intravenous drug users. Arch Pathol Lab Med 1988;112:742–745.
22. Bruner J, Cleary K, Smith F, Batsakis J. Immunocytochemical identification of HIV antigen in parotid lymphoid lesions. J Laryngol Otol 1989;103:1063–1066.
23. Colebunder R, Frances H, Marmon J, Bila K, Kandi K. Parotid swelling during human immunodeficiency virus infection. Arch Otolaryngol Head Neck Surg 1988;114:330–332.
24. Ioachim H, Ryan J, Blangrund S. Salivary gland lymph nodes: The site of lymphadenopathies and lymphomas associated with human immunodeficiency virus infection. Arch Pathol Lab Med 1988;112:1224–1228.
25. Yeh C, Fox P, Fox C, Travis W, Lane H, Baum B. Kaposi's sarcoma of the parotid gland in acquired immunodeficiency syndrome. Oral Surg Oral Path Oral Med 1989;67:308–312.
26. Reath D, Noone R, Columbus M, Murphy J. Primary Kaposi's sarcoma of the intraparotid lymph nodes with AIDS. Plast Reconstr Surg 1987;80:615–618.
27. McShane D, Vellend H, Dayal V. AIDS, otolaryngology and a case of adenoid cystic carcinoma of the parotid arising in a patient with AIDS-related complex. J Otolaryngol 1987;16:10–15.
28. Gravanis M, Giansanti J. Malignant histopathologic counterpart of the benign lymphoepithelial lesion. Cancer 1970;26:1332–1342.
29. Finfer M, Schinella R, Rothstein S, Persky M. Cystic parotid lesions in patients at risk for the acquired immunodeficiency syndrome. Arch Otolaryngol Head Neck Surg 1988;114:1290–1294.
30. Sperling N, Lin P. Parotid disease associated with HIV infection. Ear Nose Throat J 1990;69:475–477.
31. Terry J, Lorec T, Thomas M, Marti J. Major salivary gland lymphoepithelial lesions and the acquired immunodeficiency syndrome. Am J Surg 1991;162:324–329.
32. Spiro R. Tumors of the parotid gland. In: Chretien P, Johns M, Sheod D, eds. Head and neck cancer. Philadelphia: Marcel Dekker, 1985:223.
33. Eneroth C. Salivary gland tumors in the parotid gland, submandibular gland, and the palatal region. Cancer 1971;27:1415.
34. Hodgkinson D. The influence of facial nerve sacrifice in surgery of malignant parotid tumors. J Surg Oncol 1976;8:425.
35. Friedman M, Levin B, Grybanskas V. Malignant tumors of the major salivary glands. Otolaryngol Clin North Am 1986;19:625.
36. Guillamondegni O, Byers R, Luna M. Aggressive surgery in treatment for parotid cancer: The role of adjunctive postoperative radiotherapy. Am J Roentgenol Rad Ther Med 1975;123:49.
37. Tu G, Hu Y, Jiang P, Qin D. The superiority of combined therapy in parotid cancer. Arch Otolaryngol 1982;108:710.
38. Rajla S. Malignant parotid tumors. Cancer 1977;40:136.
39. Hollander L, Cunningham M. Management of cancer of the parotid gland. Surg Clin North Am 1973;53:113.
40. Hugo N, McKinney P, Griffith B. Management of tumors of the parotid glands. Surg Clin North Am 1973;53:105.
41. Spiro R, Hajdu S, Strong E. Tumors of the submaxillary gland. Am J Surg 1976;132:463.
42. Conley J, Myers E, Cole R. Analysis of 115 patients with tumors of the submandibular gland. Ann Otol Rhinol Laryngol 1972;81:323.
43. Simons J, Beahrs O, Woolner L. Tumors of the submaxillary gland. Am J Surg 1964;108:485.
44. Byers R, Jesse R, Guillamondegni O, Luna M. Malignant tumors of the submaxillary gland. Am J Surg 1973;126:458.
45. Lowe J, Farmer J. Submaxillary gland tumors. Laryngoscope 1974;84:542.

46. Trail M, Lubritz J. Tumors of the submandibular gland. Laryngoscope 1974;84:1225.

47. Rajla S. Submaxillary gland tumors. Cancer 1970;26:821.

48. Spiro R. Salivary neoplasms: Overview of 25 years' experience with 2,807 patients. Head Neck Surg 1986;8:177.

49. Perzin K, Livoisi V. Acinic cell carcinoma arising in ectopic salivary gland tissue. Cancer 1980;45:967.

50. Spiro R, Huvos A, Strong E. Acinic cell carcinoma of salivary origin. Cancer 1978;41: 924.

51. Chong GC, Beahrs O, Woolner L. Surgical management of acinic cell carcinoma of the parotid gland. Surg Gynecol Obstet 1974;136:65.

52. Spiro R, Huvos A, Berk R, Strong E. Mucoepidermoid carcinoma of salivary gland origin. Am J Surg 1978;136:461.

53. Eneroth C, Hertman L, Moberger G, Soderberg G. Mucoepidermoid carcinoma of the salivary glands with special reference to the possible existence of a benign variety. Acta Otolaryngol 1972;73:68.

54. Thoryaldsson S, Beahrs O, Woolner L, Simons J. Mucoepidermoid tumors of major salivary glands. Am J Surg 1970;120:432.

55. Spiro R, Huvos A, Strong E. Cancer of the parotid gland. Am J Surg 1975;130:452.

56. Healey W, Perzin K, Smith L. Mucoepidermoid carcinoma of salivary gland origin. Cancer 1970;26:368.

57. Nasomento A, Amarol A, Prado L. Mucoepidermoid carcinoma of salivary glands. Head Neck Surg 1986;8:409.

58. Spiro R, Huvos A, Strong E. Adenocarcinoma of salivary gland origin. Am J Surg 1982;144:423.

59. Eneroth C. Facial nerve paralysis: A sign of malignancy in parotid tumors. Arch Otolaryngol 1972;95:300.

60. Conley T, Hamaker R. Prognosis of malignant tumors of the parotid gland with facial paralysis. Arch Otolaryngol 1975;101:39.

61. Conley J, Arena S. Parotid gland as a focus of metastasis. Arch Surg 1963;87:757.

62. Nicholas R, Pinnock L, Szymanowski R. Metastases to parotid nodes. Laryngoscope 1980;90:1324.

63. Borthune A, Kjellevold K, Kaalhus O, Vermurad H. Salivary gland malignant neoplasms: Treatment and prognosis. Int J Rad Oncol Biol Phys 1986;12:747.

64. Spiro R, Huvos H, Strong E. Adenoid cystic carcinoma of salivary gland origin. Am J Surg 1974;128:512.

65. Eneroth C, Hamberger C. Principles of treatment of different types of parotid tumors. Laryngoscope 1974;84:1732.

66. Matsuba H, Simpson J, Mauney M, Thawley S. Adenoid cystic salivary gland carcinoma: A clinicopathologic correlation. Head Neck Surg 1986;8:200.

67. Cohen J, Guillamondegui O, Batsabis J, Medina J. Cancer of the minor salivary glands of the larynx. Am J Surg 1985;150:513.

68. Johns M, Coulthard S. Survival and follow-up in malignant tumors of the salivary glands. Otolaryngol Clin North Am 1977;10:455.

69. Spiro R, Huvos A, Strong E. Malignant mixed tumor of salivary origin. Cancer 1977;39: 388.

70. Armstrong J, Harrison L, Thaler H, et al. The indications for elective treatment of the neck in cancer of the major salivary glands. Cancer 1992;69:615–619.

71. American Joint Committee for Cancer Staging and End Results. Manual for staging of cancer. Chicago: American Joint Committee for Cancer, 1978.

72. Dawson A, Orr J. Long-term results of local excision and radiotherapy in pleomorphic adenoma of the parotid. Int J Rad Oncol Biol Phys 1985;11:451–455.

73. Armstrong J, Harrison L, Sprio R, Strong E, Fass D, Fuks Z. The role of postoperative radiation therapy in malignant salivary gland tumors: A matched pain analysis using historic controls. Int J Rad Oncol Biol Phys 1988;15:176.

74. Fitzpatrick P, Theriault C. Malignant salivary gland tumors. Int J Rad Onc Biol Phys 1986;12:1743–1747.

75. Harrison L, Armstrong J, Spiro R, Fass D, Strong E. Post-operative radiation therapy for major salivary gland malignancies. J Surg Oncol 1990;45:52–55.

76. North C, Lee D, Piantadosi S, Zahurak M, Johns M. Carcinoma of the major salivary glands treated by surgery or surgery plus post-operative radiotherapy. Int J Rad Oncol Biol Phys 1990;18:1319–1326.

77. McNaney D, McNeese M, Guillamondegui O. Postoperative irradiation in malignant epithelial tumors of the parotid. Int J Rad Oncol Biol Phys 1983;9:1289.

78. Elkon D, Coleman M, Hendrickson F. Radiation therapy in the treatment of malignant salivary gland tumors. Cancer 1978;41:502.

79. Fu K, Leibel S, Levine M. Cancer of the major and minor salivary glands. Cancer 1977;40:2882.

80. Simpson J, Matsuba H, Thawley S. Improved treatment of salivary gland adenocarcinoma planned confirmation surgery and irradiation. Laryngoscope 1986;96:904–907.

81. Vikram B, Strong E, Shah J, Spiro R. Radiation therapy in adenoid cystic carcinoma. Int J Rad Oncol Biol Phys 1984;10:221–223.

82. King J, Fletcher G. Malignant tumors of the major salivary glands. Radiology 1971;100: 381–384.

83. Alberts D, Manning M, Coulthard S. Adriamycin/cisplatinum/cyclophosphamide combination chemotherapy for advanced carcinoma of the parotid gland. Cancer 1981;47:645–648.

84. Dreyfuss A, Clark J, Fallon B. Cyclophosphamide, doxorubicin, and cisplatin combination chemotherapy for advanced carcinomas of salivary gland origin. Cancer 1987;60:2869–2872.

85. Belani C, Eisenberger M, Gray W. Preliminary experience with chemotherapy in advanced salivary gland neoplasms. Med Pediatr Oncol 1988;16:197–202.

86. Licitra L, Bonfante V, Spinazze S. Cyclophosphamide, doxorubicin, and cisplatin (CAP) for advanced salivary gland carcinoma. Proc Am Soc Clin Oncol [Abstract] 1991;10: 204.

87. Tannock I, Sutherland D. Chemotherapy for adenocystic carcinoma. Cancer 1980;46: 452–454.

88. Schramm V Jr, Srodes C, Myers E. Cisplatin therapy for adenoid cystic carcinoma. Arch Otolaryngol 1981;107:739–741.

89. Creagan E, Woods J, Rubin J. Cisplatin-based chemotherapy for neoplasms arising from salivary glands and contiguous structures in the head and neck. Cancer 1988;62: 2313–2319.

90. Venook A, Tseng A Jr, Meyers F. Cisplatin, doxorubicin, and 5-fluorouracil chemotherapy for salivary gland malignancies: A pilot study of the Northern California Oncology Group. J Clin Oncol 1987;5:951–955.

91. Sessions R, Lehane D, Smith R. Intra-arterial cisplatin treatment of adenoid cystic carcinoma. Arch Otolaryngol 1982;108:221–224.

92. Kaplan M, Johns M, Cantrell R. Chemotherapy for salivary gland cancer. Otolaryngol Head Neck Surg 1986;95:165–170.

93. Dimery I, Legha S, Shirinian M. Fluorouracil, doxorubicin, cyclophosphamide, and cisplatin combination chemotherapy in advanced or recurrent salivary gland carcinoma. J Clin Oncol 1990;8:1056–1062.

94. Triozzi P, Brantley A, Fisher S. 5-Fluorouracil, cyclophosphamide, and vincristine for adenoid cystic carcinoma of the head and neck. Cancer 1987;59:887–890.

95. Posner M, Ervin T, Weichselbaum R. Chemotherapy of advanced salivary gland neoplasms. Cancer 1982;50:2261–2264.

96. Suen J, Johns M. Chemotherapy for salivary gland cancer. Laryngoscope 1982;92: 235–239.

97. McKenna R. Tumors of the major and minor salivary glands. CA 1984;34:24–39.

98. Tran L, Sidrys J, Sadeghi A, Ellerbroek N, Hanson D, Parker R. Salivary gland tumors of the oral cavity. Int J Rad Oncol Biol Phys 1990;18:413–417.

99. Koss L, Spiro R, Hajdu S. Small cell (oat cell) carcinoma of minor salivary gland origin. Cancer 1972;30:737–741.

100. Olsen K, Devine D, Weiland L. Mucoepidermoid carcinoma of the oral cavity. Otol Head Neck Surg 1981;89:783–791.

101. Ellis E, Million R, Mendenhall W, Parsons J, Cassisi N. The use of radiation therapy in the management of minor salivary gland tumors. Int J Rad Oncol Biol Phys 1988;15: 613–617.

102. Eapen L, Gerig L, Catton G, Danjoux C, Girard A. Impact of local radiation in the management of salivary gland carcinomas. Head Neck Surg 1988;10:239–245.

103. Biller H, Shugar J, Krespi Y. A new technique for wide-field exposure of the base of the skull. Arch Otolaryngol 1981;107:698.

104. Sessions R, Ward P, Johns M, Goeffinet D. Carcinoma of the submaxillary gland, radiation and or surgery? Head Neck Surg 1987;10:129–132.

105. Griffin T, Pajak T, Laramore G, et al. Neutron vs. photon irradiation of inoperable salivary gland tumors: Results of an RTOG-MRC cooperative randomized study. Int J Rad Oncol Biol Phys 1988;15:1085–1090.

106. Glenner G, Grimley P. Tumors of the extra-adrenal paraganglion system (including chemoreceptors). In: Atlas of tumor pathology. 2nd series, Part 9. Washington, DC: Armed Forces Institute of Pathology, 1974:1–90.

107. Mulligan R. Chemodectoma in the dog. Am J Pathol [Abstract] 1950;28:680–681.

108. Rosenwasser H. Glomus jugulare tumors. Arch Otolaryngol 1968;88:29–66.

109. Zak F. An expanded concept of glomus tissue. NY State J Med 1954;54:1153.

110. Pearse A. The diffuse neuroendocrine system: Historical review. Front Horm Res 1984;12:1–7.

111. Bleau H, Rougues L, Gerard P. L'angiome du rocher et son aspect radiographique. Presse Med 1950;58:1141.

112. Case 14-1975. Case records of the Massachusetts General Hospital. N Engl J Med 1975;292:741–745.

113. Kohn A. Uber den Bau und die entwickling der sogenannten caotisdruse. Arch Mikr Anat Mika Anat 1903;62:263.

114. Batsakis J. Paragangliomas of the head and neck. In: Tumors of the head and neck: Clinical and pathological considerations. 2nd ed. Baltimore: Williams & Wilkins, 1979: 369–380.

115. Smith P, Schwaber, M, Goebel, J. Clinical evaluation of glomus tumors of the ear and the base of the skull. In: Thawley S, Panje W, Batsakis J, Lindberg R, eds. Comprehensive management of head and neck tumors. Philadelphia: WB Saunders, 1987:207.

116. Guild S. The glomus jugulare, a nonchromaffin paraganglion, in man. Ann Otol Rhinol Laryngol 1953;62:1045–1071.

117. Conley J, Clairmont A. Glomus intravagale. Laryngoscope 1977;87:2096–2100.

118. Kahn L. Vagal body tumor (nonchromaffin paraganglioma, chemodectoma, and carotid body-like tumor) with cervical node metastases and familial association. Cancer 1976;38: 2367–2377.

119. Lubbers J. Fezwel van her os petrum met gecombineerede hersenzenuw verlanning. Ned Tijdschr Gencesk 1937;81:2566.

120. Cantrell R, Kaplan M, Winn H, Atuk N, Jahrsdoerfer R. Catelcholamine-secreting inframtemporal fossa paraganglioma. Ann Otol Rhinol Laryngol 1984;93:583–588.

121. Brown J. Glomus jugulare tumors revisited: A ten-year statistical follow-up of 231 cases. Laryngoscope 1985;95:284–288.

122. Schwaber M, Glasscock M, Jackson C, Nissen A, Smith P. Diagnosis and management of catecholamine secreting glomus tumors. Laryngoscope 1984;94:1008–1015.

123. Million R, Cassisi, N, Wittes R. Cancer of the head and neck. In: DeVita V, Hellman S, Rosenberg S, eds. Cancer: Principles and practice of oncology. 2nd ed. Philadelphia: JB Lippincott, 1985:407.

124. Brown J. Glomus jugulare tumors: Methods and difficulties of diagnosis and surgical treatment. Laryngoscope 1967;77:26–67.

125. Parkin J. Familial multiple glomus tumors and pheochromocytomas. Ann Otol Rhinol Laryngol 1981;90:60–63.

126. Van Baars F, Van den Broek P, Cremers C, Veldman J. Familial non-chromaffinic paragangliomas (glomus tumors): Clinical aspects. Laryngoscope 1981;91:988–996.

127. Van Baars F, Cremers C, Van den Broek P, Veldman J. Familiar non-chromaffinic paragangliomas (glomus tumors): Clinical and genetic aspects (abridged). Acta Otolaryngol 1981;91:589–593.

128. Spector G, Ciralski R, Maisel R, Ogura J IV. Multiple glomus tumors in the head and neck. Laryngoscope 1975;85:1066–1075.

129. Irons G, Weiland L, Brown W. Paragangliomas of the neck. Clinical and pathologic analysis of 116 cases. Surg Clin North Am 1977;57:575–583.

130. Bickerstaff E, Howell J. The neurological importance of tumors of the glomus jugulare. Brain 1953;76:576–593.

131. Revak C, Morris S, Alexander G. Pheochromocytoma and recurrent chemodectomas over a 25-year period. Radiology 1971;100:53–54.

132. El Fiky F, Paparella M. A metastatic glomus jugulare tumor: A temporal bone report. Am J Otol 1984;5:197–200.

133. Borsanyi S. Glomus jugulare tumors. Laryngoscope 1962;72:1336–1385.

134. Taylor M, Alford B, Greenberg S. Metastasis of glomus jugulare tumors. Arch Otolaryngol 1965;82:5–13.

135. Crouzet G, Vasdev A, Lambrinidis M, et al. Spinal metastasis of carotid paragangliomas. J Neuroradiol 1989;16:172–178.

136. Spector G, Sobol S, Thawley S, Maisel R, Ogura J. Panel discussion: Glomus jugulare tumors of the temporal bone. Laryngoscope 1979;89:1628–1639.

137. Druck N, Spector G, Ciralsky R, Ogura J. Malignant glomus vagale. Arch Otolaryngol 1976;102:634–36.

138. Pantanowitz D, Sareli P. Multiple malignant paragangliomas. S Afr Med J 1989;76:441–443.

139. Odze R, Begin L. Malignant paragangliomas of the posterior mediastinum. Cancer 1990;65:564–569.

140. Johnstone P, Ross R, Desiletz D. Malignant jugulotympanic paragangliomas. Arch Pathol Lab Med 1990;114:976–979.

141. Granger J, Houn H. Head and neck paragangliomas: A clinicopathologic study with DNA flow cyometry. South Med J 1990;83:1407–1412.

142. Nixon D, York R, McConnel F. Spontaneous remission of metastatic paraganglioma. Am J Med 1987;83:805–806.

143. Leonetti N, Brackman D. Glomus vagale tumor: The significance of early vocal cord paralysis. Otolaryngol Head Neck Surg 1989;100:533–537.

144. Hirsch B, Johnson J, Black F, Meyers E. Paraganglioma of vagal origin. Otolaryngol Head Neck Surg 1982;90:708.

145. Nunez D, Lang N, Pollack J. Associated carotid body tumor and pharyngeal pouch. J Laryngol Otol 1989;103:531–532.

146. Mischkle R, Balkany T. Skull base approach to glomus jugulare tumors. Laryngoscope 1987;90:89–94.

147. Glasscock M, Harris P, Newsome G. Glomus tumors: Diagnosis and treatment. Laryngoscope 1974;84:2006–2032.

148. Cummings B, Beale F, Garrell P. The treatment of glomus tumors in the temporal bone by megavoltage radiation. Cancer 1984;53:2635–2640.

149. Kim J, Elkon D, Lim M. Optimum dose of radiotherapy for chemodectomas of the middle ear. Int J Rad Oncol Biol Phys 1980;6:815–819.

150. Boyle J, Shimm D, Coulthard S. Radiation therapy for paragangliomas of the temporal bone. Laryngoscope 1900;8:896–901.

151. Valdagni P, Amichett M. Radiation therapy of carotid body tumors. Am J Clin Oncol 1990;13:45–48.

152. Peyzant P, Chow J, Easley J. 25 years experience with radiation therapy for temporal bone chemodectomas. Int J Rad Oncol Biol Phys 1989;17:1303–1307.

153. Schwaber M, Gussack G, Kirkpatrick W. The role of radiation therapy in the management of catacholamine secreting glomus tumors. Otolaryngol Head Neck Surg 1988;98:150–154.

154. Wang M, Hussey D, Doornbos J, Vigliotti A, Wen B. Chemodectomas of the temporal bone: A comparison of surgery and radiotherapeutic results. Int J Rad Oncol Biol Phys 1988;14:643–648.

155. Fuller A, Brown H, Harrison E. Chemodectomas of the glomus jugulare tumors. Laryngoscope 1967;77:218.

Cancer: Principles & Practice of Oncology, Fourth Edition,
edited by Vincent T. DeVita, Jr., Samuel Hellman, Steven A. Rosenberg.
J.B. Lippincott Co., Philadelphia © 1993.

CHAPTER **23**

Cancer of the Lung

ROBERT J. GINSBERG
MARK G. KRIS
JOHN G. ARMSTRONG

SECTION **1**

Non-Small Cell Lung Cancer

EPIDEMIOLOGY

INCIDENCE AND MORTALITY

In the United States, lung cancer is the leading cause of cancer death in men and has surpassed breast cancer as the leading cause of cancer death in women in the latter part of the 1980s.[1] The incidence of lung cancer currently exceeds 70 per 100,000 men. In 1992, there will be 161,000 new cases and 146,000 deaths from this disease. Only 13% of persons with lung cancer will survive 5 years (Fig. 23–1).

SMOKING AND LUNG CANCER

The Evidence for a Causal Association

The epidemiologic data on smoking and lung cancer fulfill the criteria for causal association, including consistency of results across studies, the strength of the relation, its specificity, the correct temporal sequence between exposure and disease, and the coherence of the association as evidenced by a dose-response relation.[2–4]

It has been estimated that the lung cancer mortality attributable to smoking is 80% among men (about 65,000 deaths per year) and 75% among women (about 27,000 deaths per year).[5] Mattson and colleagues calculated that a 35-year-old man who smokes 25 cigarettes or more per day has a 13% risk of dying from lung cancer before the age of 75, a 10%

chance of dying from coronary heart disease, and a 28% chance of dying from smoking-related disease.

There is evidence for a dose-response relation for smoking and lung cancer. The risk for lung cancer increases with the number of cigarettes smoked, the duration of smoking, earlier age at onset of smoking, degree of inhalation, the tar and nicotine content, and the use of unfiltered cigarettes.[4] It decreases in proportion to the number of years after smoking cessation.[7–13] Passive smoking increases the lung cancer risk.[14–17] Recent investigations suggest that cigarette smoke constituents are carcinogenic (Table 23–1).[6,18–22]

OCCUPATION AND LUNG CANCER

Increases in lung cancer risk accompany exposure to carcinogens such as asbestos, radon, bis(chloromethyl)ether, polycyclic aromatic hydrocarbons, chromium, nickel, and inorganic arsenic compounds.[23,24] The association with occupational exposure to these agents appears to be independent of cigarette smoking.

Several other occupations are associated with increased risk for lung cancer. This association appears to depend in part on high rates of smoking and their interaction with known and suspected carcinogens in the workplace. Occupations with a high smoking prevalence have increased cancer risk. Women who work as waitresses, cashiers, nurses' aides, and orderlies have smoking prevalence in excess of 40%, as do men who work as drivers, construction workers, painters, mechanics, and watchmen.[25]

Asbestos

The component fibers of asbestos, particularly crocidolite, are known carcinogens with a proved ability to cause lung cancer as observed in shipyard workers, insulation workers, cement

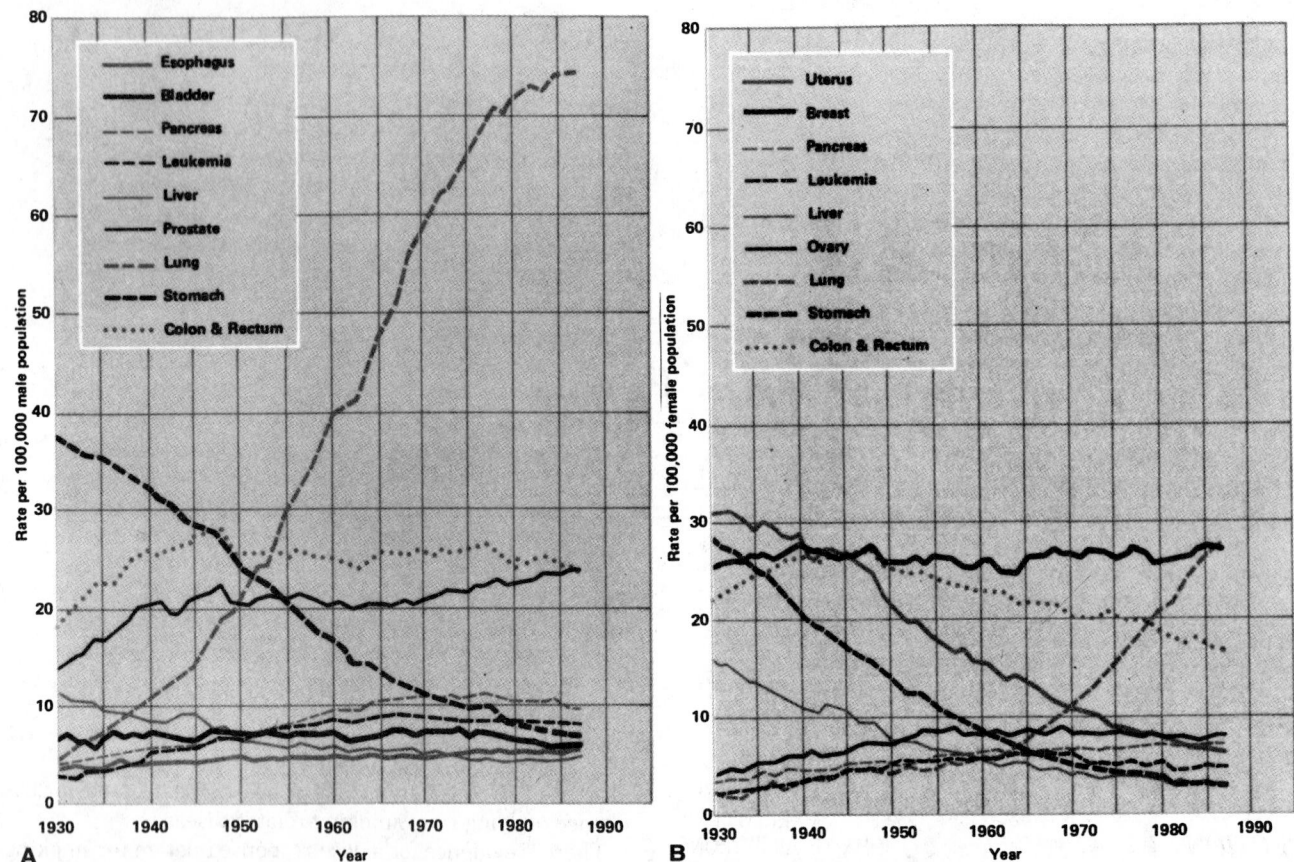

FIGURE 23–1.   The age adjusted cancer death rates for selected sites in **(A)** males and **(B)** females in the United States from 1930 to 1987. It appears that lung cancer deaths from smoking is leveling off in males but is continuing to rise in females. Data adjusted to the age distribution of the 1970 US Census Population. (US National Center for Health Statistics and US Bureau of the Census)

workers, boiler workers, and probably in people with non-occupational exposures. There is a dose-response effect of asbestos exposure[26] and a synergism between asbestos and smoking is evident.[27,28] If asbestos exposure is analyzed with controls for smoking, the relative risk for lung cancer ranges from 1.5 to 13.1.[26,29–34] Unlike other causal agents, short-lived exposure to asbestos can be a risk factor if the intensity of exposure is high.[34] It is estimated that between 4000 to 6000 cases of lung cancer (approximately 3–4% of all cases) are caused by asbestos.[35] If no asbestos exposure occurred, even greater reductions in lung cancer incidence might result because of the synergism between the two agents.[36]

Radon

Radon is a naturally occurring chemically inert gas and is a decay product of uranium-238. Radon undergoes radioactive decay to short-lived daughter products, two of which emit heavily ionizing α-particles. Inhaled α-particles can deliver intense radiation to a depth of 41 to 71 μm in the epithelial lining of the airway. The carcinogenic effect results from nonlethal events in the nuclei. Radon has been recognized as a potentially important carcinogen because it is present in soil and rocks and seeps into homes and office buildings. If ventilation is restricted, it can accumulate in the atmosphere. Although miners who are exposed to higher radon concen-

trations than those prevailing in U.S. homes have an increased risk for lung cancer, the degree of risk associated with indoor radon exposure is unknown.[37–43]

DIET AND LUNG CANCER

The role of dietary antioxidant micronutrient deficiency in the etiology of lung cancer is reviewed in Chapter 20. The presumed method of prevention of carcinogenesis by these nutrients is that antioxidant micronutrients including carotenoids, vitamins C and E, and selenium have an important role in scavenging free radicals produced endogenously and exogenously by tobacco smoke, solvents, and pollutants. Carotenoids and vitamins C and E trap free radicals and reactive oxygen molecules, whereas selenium is a component of antioxidant enzymes.[44–50]

Analysis of the role of nutrients in the cause of lung cancer is confounded by methodologic problems and the conflicting results of studies.[45]

THE EVIDENCE FOR A GENETIC PREDISPOSITION

There is increasing evidence that genetic factors can contribute to lung cancer risk, because the metabolites of carcinogens cause the malignancy and the pathways to create these metabolites are genetically determined.[55] Several approaches

TABLE 23–1. Major Mutagens, Carcinogens, and Related Substances in Tobacco Smoke

Substance	Effect	Model
Particulate Phase		
A. Neutral Fraction	C	Rodents
Benzo[*a*]pyrene	C	
Dibenz[*a*]anthracene	C	
B. Basic Fraction	C	
Nicotine		
Tobacco-specific nitrosamines	C	Rodents
C. Acidic Fraction	CC + TP	
Cathecol		
Unidentified	TP	
D. Residue	C	
Nickel	C	
Cadmium	C	
^{210}Po	C	
Gaseous Phase	C + M	
Hydrazine	C	Mice
Vinyl chloride	M	Ames

C, carcinogen; CC, cocarcinogen; TP, tumor promoter; M, mutagen. (Modified from Loeb LA, Ernster VL, Warner KE, Abbotts J, Lazlo J. Smoking and lung cancer: An overview. Cancer Res 1984;44:5940–5958; and from United States Public Health Service. The health consequences of smoking—Cancer: A report of the Surgeon General. Rockville, MD: US Dept. of Health and Human Services, Office on Smoking and Health, 1982)

have been adopted to detect a genetic association, including studies of familial clustering, of naturally occurring antigens, and of drug metabolism. Studies of familial clustering are inconclusive and have been interpreted as showing a substantial effect and no effect.[55] Heighway observed that the allele a4 Aa-*RAS* occurred in 29% of patients with non-small cell lung cancer (NSCLC) compared with 15% of control patients (*p* = 0.03).[56] Numerous other chromosomal abnormalities (rearrangements and deletions) are present in lung cancer, particularly small cell lung cancer (SCLC).[57] It is unclear whether these abnormalities cause the lung cancer or result from the genetic instability observed in malignant transformation. The metabolism of the antihypertensive drug debrisoquin is determined by a single gene. The metabolisms of more than 20 drugs and chemicals correlate with that of debrisoquin.[55] This correlation may also apply to carcinogenic components of cigarette smoke, although this is not proved for any one substance.[55,58–61]

The molecular and genetic events underlying the pathogeneses of lung cancer are an active area of investigation, but there is no conclusive genetic abnormality defining the risk for lung cancer.

BIOLOGY OF LUNG CANCER

The tracheobronchial tree develops from a pharyngeal bud. By the 10th week of embryogenesis, a branched structure has formed. This structure is lined by a single layer of cells that

eventually gives rise to the entire respiratory mucosa. All lung tumors appear to be derived from cells developing from this primitive endodermal structure, with the various histologic subtypes displaying different morphologic and functional characteristics.[62,63] For example, epithelial carcinoma is characterized by stratification of cells with extracellular keratinization. If cells originally derived from this mucosa later undergo malignant transformation, NSCLC develops, possibly due to DNA damage.[65,66]

CARCINOGEN METABOLISM AND DNA DAMAGE

Hereditary variation in the manner in which carcinogens are activated or inactivated appears to be a factor in defining the risk for developing lung cancer.[67–71]

Debrisoquine Metabolic Phenotype

Cytochrome P-450 (CYP2D6) hydroxylates compounds such as debrisoquine and a tobacco-specific *N*-nitrosamine.[67] The activity of P-450 is polymorphic, inherited in a recessive manner, and linked to lung cancer risk.[58] It has been proposed that P-450 activates a chemical carcinogen in tobacco smoke. The rate of 4-hydroxylation of debrisoquine varies several hundredfold. A strong association has been noted between the high metabolic phenotype for 4-debrisoquin hydroxylase and the development of lung cancer, with lung cancer patients more likely to have the extensive metabolizer phenotype compared with normal controls.[58,72,73] This phenotype increases the risk for developing lung cancer eightfold. This increased risk is primarily for histologic types other than adenocarcinoma.[74] Rapid metabolizers of debrisoquine who are occupationally exposed to high levels of asbestos or polycyclic aromatic hydrocarbons have an 18- or 35-fold risk for developing lung cancer.[59]

Glutathione-S Transferase Isozyme Activity

Wide genetic variations in the detoxification of enzymes may define the risk for developing lung cancer. Glutathione-S transferases (GSTs) are multifunctional proteins that catalyze the conjugation of glutathione to electrophiles[75] detoxifying carcinogenic polycyclic aromatic hydrocarbons.[76] The isozymes differ in their activity and have low *GST-8,25* activity, which is inherited as an autosomal dominant trait and may increase the risk for developing lung cancer caused by smoking.[77,78]

DNA Repair Rates

Once chromosomal damage has occurred, inherited variations in the ability to repair DNA damage may be important in the progression to frank malignancy. The activity of O^6-methylguanine-DNA methyl transferase was measured in fibroblast cultures taken from a group of lung cancer patients who presented at a young age or who had a family history of the disease. The activity of this enzyme was shown to be significantly reduced or absent compared with normal controls.[79] O^6-methylguanine-DNA methyl transferase is required for the repair of DNA, and an impaired ability to remove DNA adducts produced by carcinogens may result in the development of stable mutations, permitting the progressive accumulation of genetic damage. This may explain the increased incidence of lung cancer in this group of patients.[80]

CHROMOSOMAL DELETIONS, ONCOGENES, AND TUMOR SUPPRESSOR GENES

Loss of chromosomal material has been observed in many lung cancer cells.[81] Prominent among these losses is the deletion of material from chromosome region 3p21. These deletions have been seen in all types of lung cancer, suggesting that the deletion may represent an early stage in the pathogenesis or a prerequisite for its development.[83] The specific deleted genes involved in lung cancer have not been identified.[84]

The p53 gene, which has been studied extensively in SCLC, is mutated in all types of lung cancer.[85,86] Different point mutations are observed in NSCLC and SCLC. Different mutations of p53 have been observed for different primary sites of cancer.[87] Specific base-pair transversions (G:C to T:A) occur with increased frequency among p53 mutations in NSCLC and invariably occur on the nontranscribed strand.[87] Transversions are more frequent than substitutions among the p53 mutations in esophageal cancer, another tobacco-related malignancy. These observations may reflect specific events initiating neoplastic transformation of lung or esophageal tissues brought on by exposure to tobacco smoke. Altered expression of the retinoblastoma gene has been identified in SCLC and NSCLC.[84]

Tumorigenesis may arise from point mutations or changes in the level of expression of protooncogenes. Many activated protooncogenes have been associated with human lung cancer, including *RAS, RAF, FUR, NEU, JUN, MYC, SIS, FES, FMS, FPS, FOS* and c-*ERBB2*.[64,88,89] Some patterns have been identified. For example, the highest level of p21^ras has been seen in squamous cell carcinomas,[90] whereas mutations in the K-*RAS* gene appear specific for adenocarcinoma.[1,92] Certain protooncogenes (*e.g.,* c-*ERBB2*, c-*SIS*, and c-*FES*) are expressed more frequently on NSCLC than on SCLC.[88] Although N-*MYC* appears restricted in its expression to SCLC, c-*MYC* and L-*MYC* can be expressed in both SCLC and NSCLC.[66] The metastatic behavior of several histologic subtypes of lung cancer has been related to certain L-*MYC* types.[93] Some of these protooncogenes are more widely expressed. Constitutive expression of c-*RAF1* has been identified in all histologic types of lung cancer[94] and the nuclear oncogene product c-*JUN* has been shown to be expressed at high levels in NSCLC, SCLC, and normal lung tissue.[95]

GROWTH FACTORS

The uncontrolled production of multiple growth factors has been identified in human lung cancer cell lines. These peptides can promote and inhibit the proliferation by paracrine and autocrine loops by way of specific receptors. The cells of most tissues affected by the action of peptide growth factors contain specific protein receptors that, when activated, demonstrate tyrosine kinase activity.[96] An example is the product of the protooncogene c-*ERBB2*, which is a sequence homologous to the intracellular portion of the epidermal growth

factor receptor[88,92] and is expressed at high levels in epidermoid carcinoma.[97]

Epidermal growth factor receptors are expressed by normal bronchial epithelial cells as well.[98] Blocking epidermal growth factor receptors by using monoclonal antibodies can inhibit the growth of these cells. Insulin-like growth factor-1 stimulates the growth of NSCLC cell lines in vitro.[99]

The importance of these events in carcinogenesis has been demonstrated in experimental systems. For example, transfecting a mutated *RAS* gene into small cell cancer cell lines changes the phenotype to that suggestive of NSCLC.[100] If Ha-*RAS*, Ki-*RAS*, or the combination of c-*MYC* and c-*RAF* are transferred into SV40-10 immortalized human bronchial epithelial cells (BEAS-2B), these cells have a reduced response to growth inhibition by transforming growth factor-β or serum and have gained a selective clonal advantage.[64]

APPLICATIONS OF ADVANCES IN LUNG CANCER BIOLOGY TO CLINICAL PRACTICE

Advances in our understanding of the biology of lung cancer have the potential to impact on all areas of lung cancer management. The identification of specific mutations related to tobacco exposure has elucidated the possible molecular foundation for the association of cigarette smoking and lung cancer and may allow better identification of at-risk persons for chemoprevention programs. The presence of autocrine growth factor receptors, specific mutations, or chromosomal deletions may provide additional or more accurate means for diagnosis, staging, choosing therapies, and establishing prognosis for persons with lung cancer. The presence of K-*RAS* point mutations has been associated with a shortened survival in patients with completely resected NSCLC.[101] Clinical trials targeting adjuvant therapies for resected NSCLC patients with K-*RAS* point mutations have been designed.

These developments have already led to new therapeutic approaches. Monoclonal antibodies blocking the action of epidermal growth factor are in clinical trial.[102] The activation of cellular receptors for virtually all autocrine growth factors involves the activation of a protein kinase.[96] This observation has provided a new therapeutic target and the search for agents specifically inhibiting this enzyme is underway. The mutated sequences of p53 provide a unique, tumor-specific antigen at which to direct immunologic attacks.

PATHOLOGY OF LUNG CANCER

The World Health Organization (WHO) classification of lung cancer is accepted worldwide (Table 23–2). NSCLC includes the major headings of carcinoma, adenocarcinoma, and large cell (undifferentiated) carcinoma.

HISTOGENESIS

There is increasing evidence that lung cancer is derived from a pluripotent stem cell that is capable of expressing various phenotypes. This epithelial stem cell, in normal histogenesis, differentiates to those cells found in the tracheobronchial tree, including pseudostratified reserved cells, ciliated goblet columnar cells, neuroendocrine cells, and type I and type II

TABLE 23–2. World Health Organization Histologic Classification of Epithelial Bronchogenic Carcinoma

  I. Benign
 II. Dysplasia and carcinoma in situ
III. Malignant
    A. Squamous cell carcinoma (epidermoid) and spindle (squamous) carcinoma
    B. Small cell carcinoma
       1. Oat cell
       2. Intermediate cell
       3. Combined oat cell
    C. Adenocarcinoma
       1. Acinar
       2. Papillary
       3. Bronchoalveolar
       4. Mucus-secreting
    D. Large cell carcinoma
       1. Giant cell
       2. Clear cell

pneumocytes that line the alveoli. Those cells that are capable of division can express hyperplastic, metaplastic, or neoplastic change.[103]

Frequently, lung cancer exhibits two or more histologic patterns. The frequency of this occurrence depends on the assiduousness of the pathologist and the number of sections examined. In one study, in which at least 10 blocks from each tumor were examined, 45 of the 100 cases demonstrated heterogeneity and 10% of cases showed elements of squamous cell carcinoma and adenocarcinoma.[104]

SQUAMOUS CELL CARCINOMA

Squamous cell carcinoma, once the most frequent (*i.e.,* in North America) of all lung cancers, has not seen the marked increase that has been observed with adenocarcinoma. The latter tumor accounts for most of the recent increased incidence of lung cancer and accounts for approximately 30% of all lung cancer. Squamous cell carcinoma arises most frequently in proximal bronchi. It is associated with squamous metaplasia and, in its earliest form, carcinoma in situ, in which stratified squamous epithelium is replaced by malignant squamous cells without invasion through the basement membrane. Because of the ability of these cells to exfoliate, this tumor can be detected by cytologic examination at its earliest stage. With further growth, the tumor invades the basement membrane and extends into the bronchial lumen producing obstruction with resultant atelectasis or pneumonia.

Histologically, the squamous cell tumor is composed of sheets of epithelial cells that may be well or poorly differentiated. Most well-differentiated tumors demonstrate keratin pearl. The more poorly differentiated tumors, if determined to be squamous cell carcinoma, have positive keratin staining (Fig. 23–2).

These tumors tend to be slow growing and it is estimated that up to 3 or 4 years are required from the development of in situ carcinoma to a clinically apparent tumor.

ADENOCARCINOMA

Adenocarcinoma is the most frequently occurring tumor in North America and accounts for 40% of all lung cancer. Some

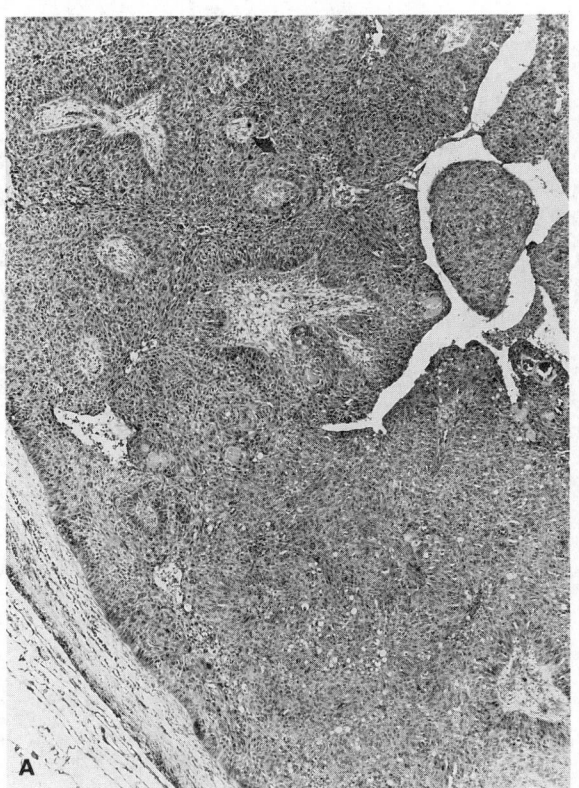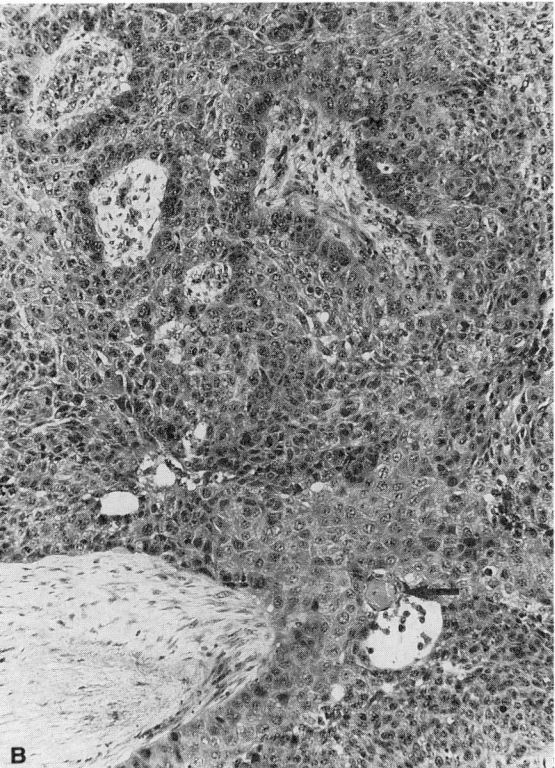

FIGURE 23–2. Moderately differentiated squamous cell carcinoma. Sheets of tumor cells with variable amounts of cytoplasm and moderate nuclear atypia are present. Focal keratinization is evident (*arrow*). **(A)** Low power magnification. **(B)** High power magnification.

of the increase in occurrence of adenocarcinoma is due to better identification and fewer tumors being classified as undifferentiated large cell tumors. Worldwide, a similar increase in adenocarcinoma is being seen.[105] Most of these tumors are peripheral in origin and arise from surface epithelium or bronchial mucosal glands and as peripheral scar tumors (Fig. 23–3).

Histologically, these tumors form glands and produce mucin. Although they can be subdivided by light microscopy into the four types defined by the WHO Histologic Classification, it appears that bronchoalveolar carcinoma is a distinct clinicopathologic entity (Fig. 23–4).[106] This latter tumor appears to arise from type II pneumocytes, grows along alveolar septa by lapidic growth, and shows little if any desmoplastic or glandular change. These tumors are interesting in that they may present as a solitary peripheral nodule, a multifocal disease, or a rapidly progressive pneumonic form that appears to spread from lobe to lobe, ultimately encompassing both lungs. Other than T1N0 tumors, adenocarcinoma has a worse prognosis stage for stage than squamous cell carcinoma.

With increasing frequency, immunohistochemistry and electron microscopy have been used by pathologists to identify adenocarcinoma more accurately.[107] Using these techniques, adenocarcinoma cells stain positive for carcinoembryonic antigen and keratin. Recently, specific monoclonal antibodies that recognize adenocarcinoma have been identified.[108]

LARGE CELL CARCINOMA

Large cell carcinoma is the least common of all NSCLC, accounting for approximately 15% of all lung cancers. Using histochemical staining, electron microscopy, and monoclonal antibodies, many tumors that were diagnosed previously as undifferentiated large cell carcinoma can currently be classified more appropriately as poorly differentiated adenocarcinoma or squamous cell carcinoma. For this reason, the incidence of this type of tumor continues to decrease (Fig. 23–5).

Although the WHO Classification divides this group into giant cell and clear cell varieties, these classifications have little clinical relevance. Few true giant cell tumors have been identified, although they do represent a poorly differentiated subtype with what appears to be a poorer prognosis. The prognosis of large cell undifferentiated carcinoma appears to be similar to that of adenocarcinoma, and these two histologic types are grouped together in most clinical trials.

METHODS OF SPREAD

After a period of time as a primary tumor growing within lung parenchyma or within the bronchial wall, the tumor invades the vascular and lymphatic channels and results in spread to regional draining lymph nodes and distant metastatic sites. Occasionally, airway-borne metastases can be seen in lung parenchyma near the primary tumor.

In most instances, lymphatic spread occurs earlier than spread to metastatic sites elsewhere. The regional lymphatic drainage of the lung is outlined in Figure 23–6. In the lung tissue, lymphatic drainage follows the bronchoarterial branching pattern with lymph nodes situated at the origin of these branchings. Ultimately, these lymphatic channels coalesce, draining into lymph nodes situated around segmental

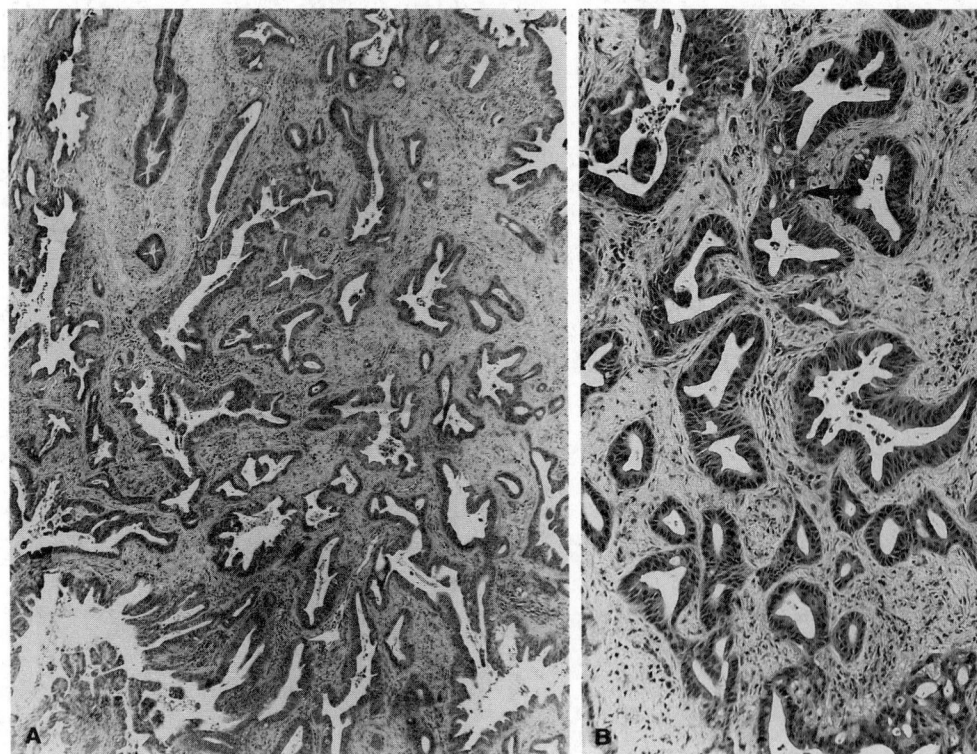

FIGURE 23–3. Well-differentiated adenocarcinoma. Well-formed glands with a focal cribriform arrangement (*arrows*) are surrounded by a cellular stroma. **(A)** Low power magnification. **(B)** High power magnification.

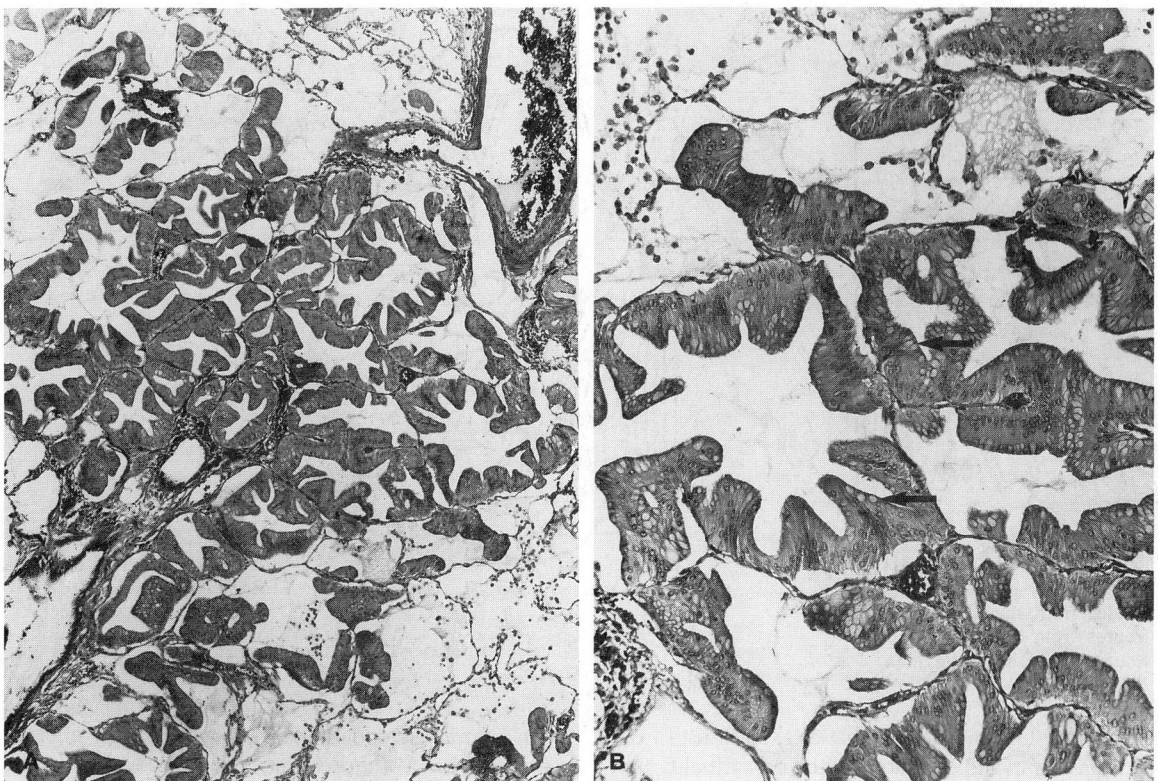

FIGURE 23–4.   Bronchoalveolar carcinoma. Columnar cells with minimal nuclear atypia are arranged along intact alveolar septae. The lepidic growth pattern is associated with no stromal reaction. Mucin vacuoles are present in the apical cytoplasm (*arrows*). (**A**) Low power magnification. (**B**) High power magnification.

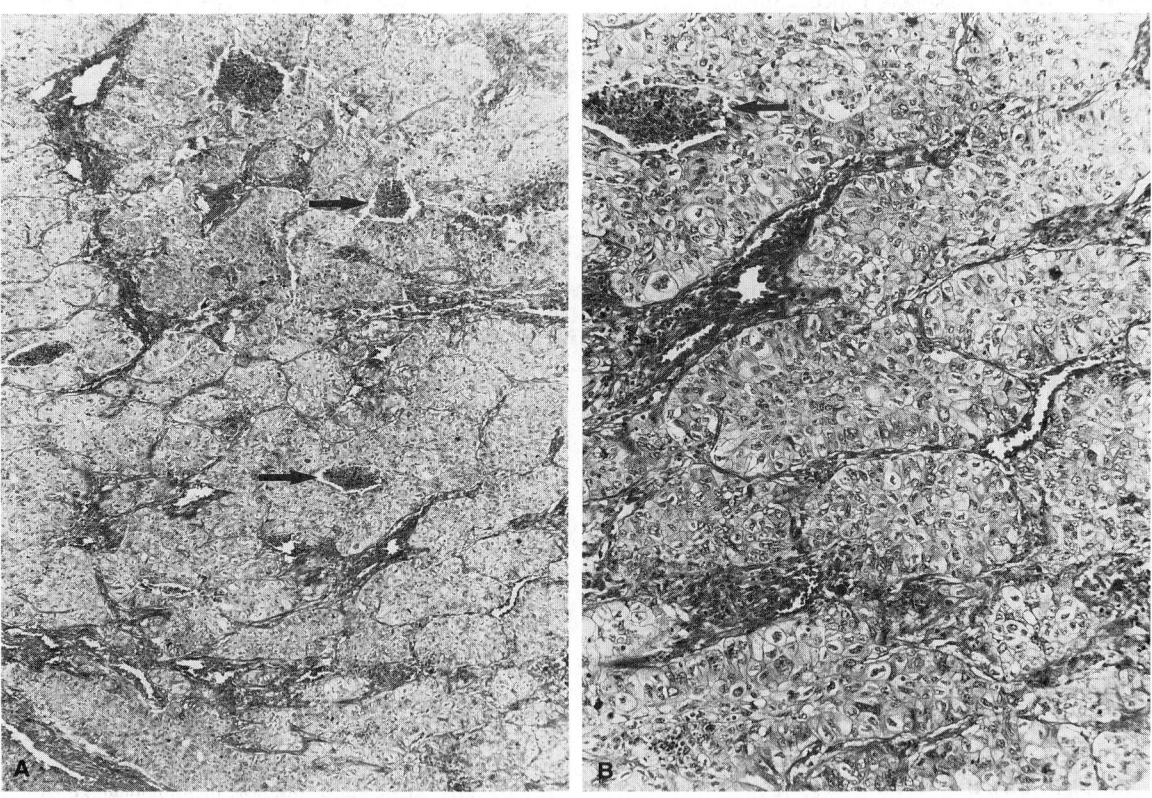

FIGURE 23–5.   Large-cell undifferentiated carcinoma. Sheets of highly atypical cells with focal necrosis (*arrows*) are present. There is no evidence of keratinization of gland formation. (**A**) Low power magnification. (**B**) High power magnification.

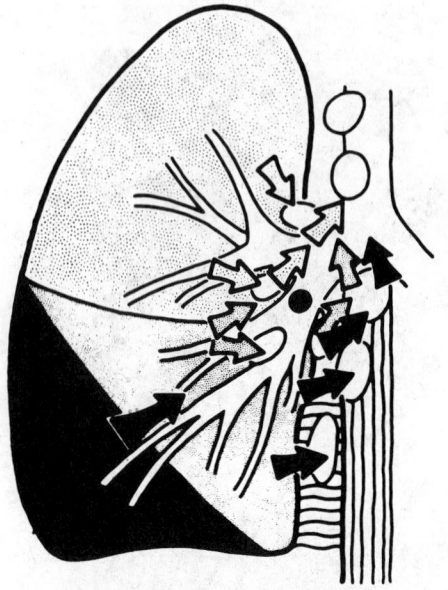

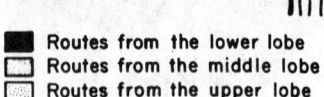

■ Routes from the lower lobe
□ Routes from the middle lobe
▨ Routes from the upper lobe

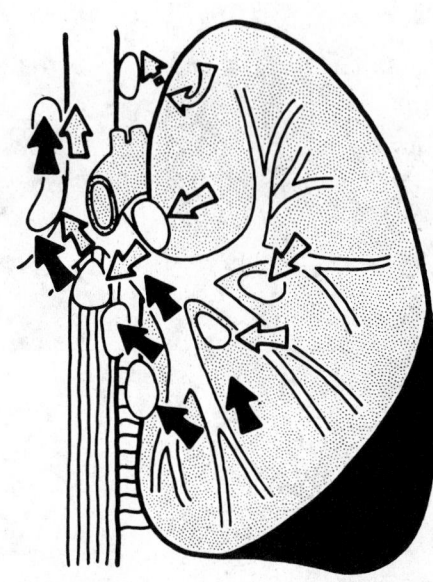

FIGURE 23–6. The regional lymphatic drainage of the lung as described by Noel. Most of the lymphatic drainage ultimately reaches the right superior mediastinum and right supraclavicular regions.

and lobar bronchi. Lower lobe lymphatics then drain to the posterior mediastinum and ultimately to the subcarinal lymph nodes. In the right upper lobe, lymphatics drain toward the superior mediastinum. In the left upper lobe, lymphatic channels run along the great vessels (aorta and subclavian artery) in the anterior mediastinum and in one third of cases along the main bronchus into the superior mediastinum.

Ultimately, all these lymphatic channels drain to the right lymphatic and left thoracic ducts. Metastatic lymphatic spread of lung cancer follows these lymphatic channels with tumor involving bronchopulmonary (N1), mediastinal (N2, N3), and supraclavicular (N3) lymph nodes.

Retrograde lymphatic spread to the pleural surface can occur, especially in peripheral tumors. The primary tumor can spread locally to contiguous structures, including mediastinal pleura or organs and the chest wall or diaphragm. Once vascular invasion occurs, metastatic spread to distant sites is common. The organs involved most frequently are the bone, liver, adrenals, and brain. As demonstrated in autopsy studies, lung cancer metastases can be found in every organ system.[109]

CLINICAL FEATURES

The signs and symptoms manifested by patients who have lung cancer depend on the location of the tumor, its locoregional spread, and the effects of metastatic growth. Lung cancer is associated with paraneoplastic syndromes more frequently than any other tumor (Table 23–3). Many patients present with an asymptomatic lesion discovered incidentally on a chest x-ray film.

LOCOREGIONAL MANIFESTATIONS

Tumors arising in the larger airways produce symptoms related to the growth of the tumor. Frequently, patients present with a persistent cough. In larger airways, with encroachment of the lumen, a wheeze or stridor may develop. As the tumor grows, areas of necrosis may develop resulting in bleeding. Massive hemoptysis is rare with most patients experiencing blood-streaked sputum.

With continued growth, distal airways become obstructed

TABLE 23–3. Common Signs and Symptoms of Lung Cancer

Symptoms secondary to central or endobronchial growth
  of the primary tumor
    Cough
    Hemoptysis
    Wheeze and stridor
    Dyspnea from obstruction
    Pneumonitis from obstruction (fever, productive cough)
Symptoms secondary to peripheral growth of the primary tumor
    Pain from pleural or chest wall involvement
    Cough
    Dyspnea on a restrictive basis
    Lung abscess syndrome from tumor cavitation
Symptoms related to regional spread of the tumor in the thorax
  by contiguity or by metastasis to regional lymph nodes
    Tracheal obstruction
    Esophageal compression with dysphagia
    Recurrent laryngeal nerve paralysis with hoarseness
    Phrenic nerve paralysis with hemidiaphragm elevation
      and dyspnea
    Sympathetic nerve paralysis with Horner syndrome
    Eighth cervical and first thoracic nerves with ulnar pain
      and Pancoast syndrome
    Superior vena cava syndrome from vascular obstruction
    Pericardial and cardiac extension with resultant tamponade,
      arrhythmia, or cardiac failure
    Lymphatic obstruction with pleural effusion
    Lymphangitic spread through lungs with hypoxemia and dyspnea

(Cohen MH. Signs and symptoms of bronchogenic carcinoma. In: Straus MJ, ed. Lung cancer: Clinical diagnosis and treatment. (New York; Grune & Stratton, 1977:85–94)

resulting in atelectasis, pneumonia, and occasionally abscess formation. These obstructive complications often result in fevers and the signs and symptoms of pulmonary infection. If pleural surfaces are involved in the infection, pleuritic pain may develop with or without a detectable pleural effusion. Increasing shortness of breath can ensue when endobronchial obstruction and the failure of ventilation of segments, lobes, or an entire lung occurs.

Depending on the location of the primary tumor, adjacent structures such as the chest wall or mediastinum may ultimately become involved by direct spread and then radicular chest wall pain develops. With apical tumors, the classic Pancoast's syndrome (lower brachial plexopathy, Horner's syndrome, and shoulder pain) may become manifest due to local invasion of the lower brachial plexus (T1 and C8 nerve roots), chest wall, and stellate ganglion. Similarly, tumors located near the mediastinum may invade local structures and interfere with the phrenic nerve, vagus nerve, or recurrent nerve and result in malfunction of the specific end organs (*e.g.,* vocal cord, diaphragm). It is not uncommon for patients to present initially with symptoms of a recurrent nerve palsy including hoarseness and cricopharyngeal dysphagia. Superior vena caval syndrome usually results from mediastinal lymphadenopathy encroaching on this structure rather than primary invasion. Direct invasion of the pericardium can occur and lead to a malignant pericardial effusion with signs and symptoms of pericardial tamponade. Pleural invasion ultimately results in a pleural effusion. Pleuritic pain or increasing shortness of breath due to a massive pleural effusion can ensue. Nodal involvement in the posterior mediastinum, usually from lower lobe tumors, can produce partial or complete obstruction of the esophagus resulting in dysphagia and, occasionally, symptoms of a tracheoesophageal fistula. Involvement of the superior mediastinum often causes a nonproductive cough. Nonspecific and vague chest pains, generally referred to the ipsilateral hemithorax, are frequent occurrences in patients with lung cancer. These pains are visceral and unrelated to invasion of local structures. Other nonspecific symptoms including weight loss and a general unwell feeling are common.

METASTATIC MANIFESTATIONS

Nearly all persons with advanced inoperable NSCLC demonstrate symptoms referable to their disease at the time of initial presentation.[110,111] Most patients have more than one symptom at the onset of their illness.[111] The frequency of lung cancer symptoms in persons with advanced (stages III and IV) NSCLC are presented in Table 23–4.[112] Fatigue and decreased activity were reported by more than 80% and most patients also experienced cough, dyspnea, decreased appetite, and weight loss. The high incidence of lung cancer symptoms, the occurrence of multiple symptoms in most patients, and the severity of these complaints demand prompt treatment of the lung cancer and careful attention to the management of each symptom while definitive therapy is in progress.

Although lung cancer can metastasize to virtually any organ, the most common sites of spread that are clinically apparent include pleura, lung, bone, brain, adrenal, pericardium, and liver.[109] The presenting complaints of a person with metastatic spread are largely determined by the specific metastatic organ

TABLE 23–4. Frequency of Lung Cancer Symptoms in a Group of 69 Patients With Inoperable Non-Small Cell Lung Cancer

Symptom	Percentage
Fatigue	84
Decreased activity	81
Cough	71
Dyspnea	59
Decreased appetite	57
Weight loss	54
Pain	48
Hemoptysis	25

(Hollen PJ, Gralla RJ, Kris MG, et al. Quality of life assessment in individuals with lung cancer: Lung cancer symptom scale. Eur J Cancer 1992 [in press])

site involved. For example, lung metastases can cause cough, dyspnea, sputum production, pain, or hemoptysis. Bone metastases present with pain and limitation of use of the affected bone. The management of specific metastatic complications is discussed in Chapter 61.

We cannot explain the high prevalence of adrenal metastases in NSCLC detected in 41% of patients at autopsy.[109] Most adrenal metastases are asymptomatic and discovered incidentally during a staging evaluation or at autopsy. If symptomatic, adrenal metastases present with unilateral pain in the flank, abdomen, or costovertebral angle. The computed tomographic (CT) scan is the most reliable method of diagnosis. Fine-needle aspiration of the adrenal provides a safe method to confirm the presence of metastatic disease in the adrenal if pathologic documentation is necessary. Adrenal hormone insufficiency due to adrenal metastases from lung cancer can occur.[113]

Pericardial complications due to direct invasion, metastatic spread, or cancer-associated but nonmalignant pericardial effusion[114] are a frequent and underdiagnosed complication of lung cancer. The presenting complaints of dyspnea, cough, and chest discomfort are identical to those of pulmonary tumors or pleural metastases. Signs of pericardial tamponade often are absent. Electrocardiograms generally show only sinus tachycardia. Changes in voltage are often subtle and recognizable only on careful scrutiny of multiple previous tracings. Similarly, enlargement of the cardiac silhouette on chest x-ray film is often subtle and apparent only on review of multiple previous studies. The frequent association of a pleural effusion in patients with pericardial involvement further impedes the prompt diagnosis of this condition.[115] The echocardiogram provides a safe and rapid diagnostic test for this condition and also provides information on the presence and severity of associated cardiac compromise. Pericardial involvement should be considered in any lung cancer patient with dyspnea, cough, or chest discomfort.

NONMETASTATIC FEATURES

A variety of systemic complications of epithelial lung cancer not caused by metastases have been identified. Many of these conditions are not specific to lung cancer but appear to occur frequently in lung cancer patients because of the large number of persons with this disease. The anorexia-cachexia syndrome and generalized weakness and fatigue are the most common and most poorly understood nonmetastatic complications of lung cancer. The management of metabolic emergencies is discussed in Chapter 60.

Hypertrophic pulmonary osteoarthropathy most frequently is seen in lung cancer patients. Symptoms of bone and joint pain herald the onset of this condition and can be the presenting signs of lung cancer. Clubbing of the digits is observed. The alkaline phosphatase level is commonly elevated and serum hepatic enzyme levels are normal. Plain x-ray films of affected bones demonstrate periosteal inflammation and elevation and radionuclide bone scans reveal an intense and symmetric generalized increased uptake of the radiolabel, particularly in the long bones. Symptoms respond dramatically to aspirin and nonsteroidal antiinflammatory agents and disappear after effective definitive treatment of the primary lesion. Clubbing of the digits may persist.

STAGING OF LUNG CANCER

In 1985, the American Joint Committee on Cancer (AJCC), the Union Internationale Contra Cancer (UICC), and the Japanese Cancer Committee (JCC) agreed to a worldwide TNM staging system.[116] This has been accepted rapidly and is used extensively in the management of lung cancer.

The primary tumor is subdivided into four T categories depending on size, site, and local involvement (T1–4). Lymph node spread has been subdivided into bronchopulmonary (N1), ipsilateral mediastinal (N2) and contralateral or supraclavicular disease (N3), and metastatic spread is absent or present (M0 or M1; Table 23–5).

Four stages of lung cancer have been identified with significant differences found in 5-year survival depending on the stage of disease at diagnosis (Fig. 23–7). The accuracy of these stages in predicting survival have been confirmed by many authors (Fig. 23–8).

Although the new staging system lacks accuracy in defining certain subsets of locally advanced disease (T4 and N3),[117] it is a functional system that should be used for all patients. Although the system is accurate even in SCLC, most practitioners grossly divide SCLC into limited (stages I, II, and III) and extensive (stage IV) disease only. The TNM staging includes clinical, surgical, and pathologic assessment. Using pretreatment minimal invasive techniques only, a significant percentage of patients are clinically understaged compared with the ultimate stage identified by surgical and pathologic staging. Despite these inadequacies, it is clinically relevant to stage all lung cancer patients before treatment (clinical) and after therapy (surgical and pathologic).[118,119]

DIAGNOSTIC AND STAGING PROCEDURES

In a patient suspected of harboring lung cancer, an accurate diagnosis with confirmatory cytology or histology and an estimate of the stage of the disease are extremely important

TABLE 23–5. TNM Staging System for Lung Cancer

Stage	Descriptors	5-Year Survival (%)
I	T1–2N0M0	60–80
II	T1–2N1M0	25–50
IIIA	T3N0–1M0	25–40
	T1–3N2M0	10–30
IIIB	Any T4 or any N3M0	<5
IV	Any M1	<5

T Descriptor	Definition
TX	Positive malignant cell; no lesion seen
T1	<3 cm diameter
T2	>3 cm diameter
	Distal atelectasis
T3	Extension to pleura, chest wall diaphragm, or pericardium
	<2 cm from carina or total atelectasis
T4	Invasion of mediastinal organs
	Malignant pleural effusion

N Descriptor	Node Involvement
N0	No involvement
N1	Ipsilateral bronchopulmonary or hilar
N2	Ipsilateral or subcarinal mediastinal
	Ipsilateral supraclavicular nodes
N3	Contralateral mediastinal hilum or supraclavicular

M Descriptor	Metastatic Involvement
M0	None
M1	Metastases present

(Figs. 23–9 and 23–10). The modalities used for diagnosis and clinical staging are discussed together.

HISTORY AND PHYSICAL EXAMINATION

A detailed history and accurate physical examination remain the most important steps in assessing a patient with lung cancer. Smoking history, past exposure to environmental carcinogens, and family history may suggest a higher probability of lung cancer. New symptomatology such as a change in cough, hemoptysis, or history of recurrent respiratory infection are suggestive. Symptoms suggesting locoregional spread include chest pain, symptoms of recurrent nerve palsy, or superior vena caval obstruction. Those symptoms suggestive of metastatic disease frequently include symptoms of cerebral metastases, bone pain, or weight loss. Occasionally, patients suffering from NSCLC present with symptoms and signs of a paraneoplastic syndrome, but not as frequently as with small cell tumors.

Physical examination should be directed toward the chest in search of signs of partial or complete obstruction of airways, atelectasis or pneumonia, and pleural effusions. Examination of the head and neck that includes draining regional lymph node areas may demonstrate lymphadenopathy indicating regional lymphatic (N3) spread.

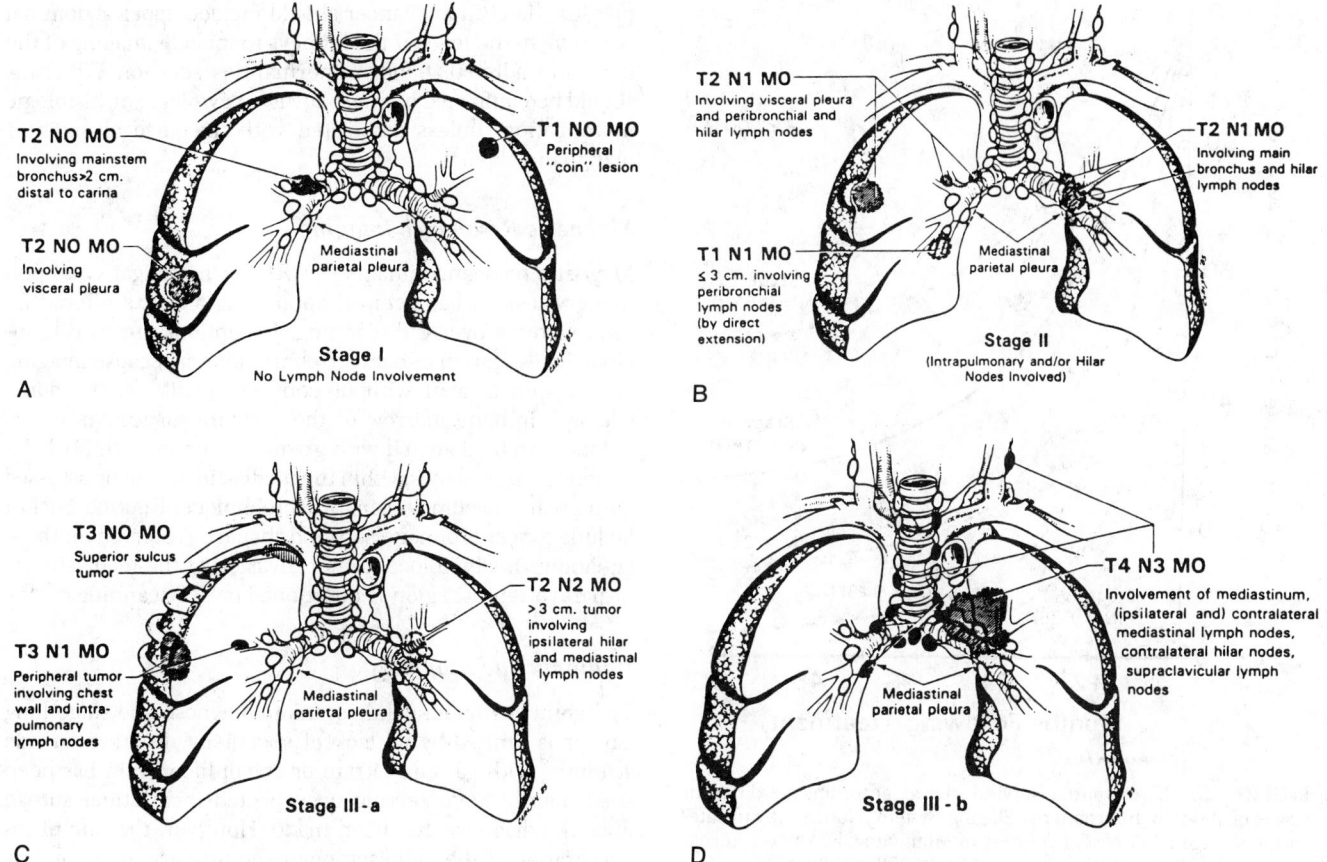

FIGURE 23–7.   New International Staging System (ISS) **(A)** Categories of stage I disease; **(B)** Categories of stage II disease; **(C)** Categories of stage IIIA disease; **(D)** Categories of stage IIIB disease. (Courtesy of Mountain CF. A new international staging system for lung cancer. Chest 1986;89:225S)

SPUTUM CYTOLOGY

Once the disease is suspected, a simple and effective method for obtaining a positive diagnosis of lung cancer is sputum cytology. The yield from sputum cytology depends on many factors, including the ability of the patient to produce sufficient sputum, the size of the tumor, the proximity of the tumor to major airways, and to a lesser extent the histologic type of the tumor.

With three sputum samples, up to 80% of central tumors can be diagnosed. The yield is much smaller for peripheral tumors, dropping to less than 20% for peripheral tumors less than 3.0 cm in diameter. A 3-day collection of early morning sputa preserved in Saccamano solution appears to be the optimal method of assessment. Squamous cell tumors are diagnosed more frequently by cytology than adenocarcinoma or large cell tumors. Another factor affecting the ability of sputum cytology to diagnose malignancy is the experience and training of the cytopathologist. Viral infections can produce cellular changes difficult to distinguish from malignancy, especially adenocarcinoma. Frequently, severe dysplasia is misinterpreted as a malignancy and vice versa. Tockman and colleagues recently have described a monoclonal antibody staining technique that may diagnose more accurately the presence or absence of malignancy in severely dysplastic cells.[120]

IMAGING STUDIES

Chest X-Ray Film

The chest x-ray film is probably the most valuable tool in the diagnosis of lung cancer. A perfectly normal chest x-ray film rules out this diagnosis in most instances, except for the rare occult tumor.[121] Plain chest radiography can reveal peripheral nodules or hilar and mediastinal changes suggestive of lymphadenopathy or pleural effusions, which are all suggestive of possible malignancy (Fig. 23–11). Areas of subsegmental, segmental, lobar, or lung collapse suggest an endobronchial obstruction. Recent advances in plain radiography (*e.g.*, AMBER x-ray films) may improve the diagnostic yield of this modality.[122,123]

Computed Tomography

With the introduction of computed tomography (CT) in the late 1970s, a giant step was taken in the ability to diagnose and stage lung cancer using noninvasive imaging techniques. CT imaging can confirm abnormalities seen on plain chest x-ray film and can often detect lesions that cannot be resolved on chest x-ray film. CT scans play an important role in staging of lung cancer, especially spread to areas of the mediastinum undetected on plain films. Normal mediastinal lymph nodes

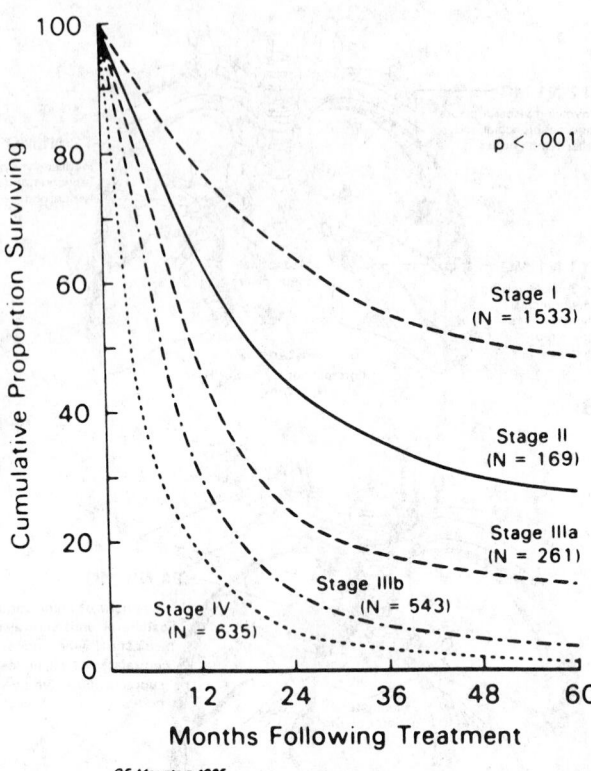

FIGURE 23–8. Actuarial survival curves according to different stages of the new International Staging System. Notice the subcategories of stage III disease. (Courtesy of Mountain CF. A new international staging system for lung cancer. Chest 1986;89:225S)

are less than 1.0 cm in transverse diameter. Any larger lymph node suggests lymphadenopathy and should be investigated further by more invasive techniques.[124,125] CT scanning suggests possible areas of local invasion of the primary tumor to chest wall or vertebral or mediastinal structures. Small pleural effusions or pleural nodules, often undetected on plain films, may be evident on CT scans. An advantage of CT scanning is the ability to detect abnormalities below the diaphragm, especially metastases to liver and adrenal. CT scanning for the

investigation of lung cancer should include upper abdominal scanning to the level of the kidneys to include imaging of the liver and adrenal gland. Abnormalities seen on CT scans should be confirmed by more invasive cytologic or histologic investigation, unless associated with unequivocal signs of malignancy.[126]

Magnetic Resonance Imaging

Magnetic resonance imaging (MRI) for investigation of pulmonary lesions has been disappointing and has offered no improvement over CT scanning. Exceptions to this rule include investigation of paravertebral tumors, because imaging of the spinal canal without contrast media can be done. Changes in bone marrow of the vertebra suggestive of carcinoma can be detected with greater accuracy with MRI. Invasion of tissue planes within the mediastinum can be assessed with greater accuracy using MRI technique. Routine MRI of all lung cancer is unnecessary and should be reserved for those situations in which local tumor invasion of the mediastinum or paravertebral region is questioned on CT scanning.[127–129]

Radionuclide Scanning

The ability of radionuclide scans to diagnose and stage lung cancer is limited by its lack of specificity. Routine nuclide scanning with gallium citrate or cobalt-bleomycin has been used mainly for detecting unsuspected mediastinal spread once the diagnosis has been made. However, the rate of incorporation of the radioisotope by the primary tumor and its metastatic foci is variable and has limited its clinical use in diagnosis and staging.[130,131] Recently, isotope-labeled monoclonal antibodies have been investigated as a technique for staging and hopefully diagnosing this disease. Specific monoclonal antibodies directed to lung cancer cells may prove valuable as diagnostic and staging modalities in the future. Routine radionuclide bone scanning to rule out asymptomatic unsuspecting bone metastases in early-stage disease has never been shown to be cost effective but is still advocated by many practitioners. Bone scans are more valuable in clinical stage III disease if considering curative therapy .[132]

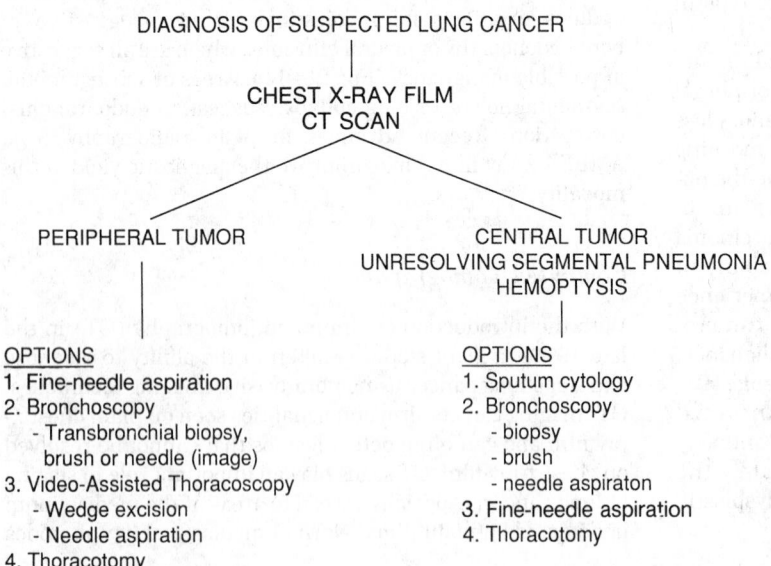

FIGURE 23–9. A schema to indicate the diagnostic procedures depending on the presenting lesion.

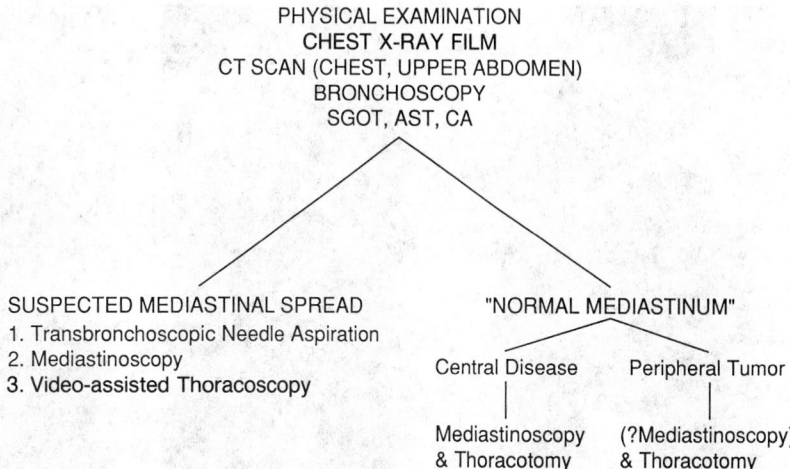

FIGURE 23–10.   Clinical staging of lung cancer: a schema to indicate extent of disease evaluation.

Percutaneous Fine-Needle Aspiration

Fine-needle aspiration biopsy of pulmonary nodules is an excellent method of obtaining cytologic or histologic material for positive identification of malignancy. This is performed using fluoroscopic or CT-guided techniques. The positive yield in experienced hands can be as high as 95%. However, an indeterminate biopsy cannot be accepted as negative. False-negative examinations are frequent and must be considered indeterminate unless a positive benign diagnosis (*e.g.*, hamartoma, tuberculosis) can be made.[133] Abnormalities of bone, liver, or adrenal glands suggesting metastatic disease frequently can be confirmed by fine-needle aspiration biopsy using ultrasonography or CT-guided biopsies.

Bronchoscopy

Although rigid bronchoscopy was used for many years to confirm the diagnosis of lung cancer, the introduction of flexible fiberoptic bronchoscopy more than 20 years ago has revolutionized this approach. Although invasive, the procedure can be performed under local anesthesia with or without sedation with minimal morbidity and exceptional safety. Using flexible fiberoptic instruments, the proximal tracheobronchial tree can be examined up to the second or third subsegmental division and cytology or histologic specimens can be obtained from abnormal lesions identified. Diagnostic yield of fiberoptic bronchoscopy with cytologic brushing and biopsy for histology when a visible lesion is identified is more than 90%. Even with no visible lesion, the area of suspicion can be irrigated and lavaged obtaining cytologic material. Using fiberoptic bronchoscopy and image intensification, peripheral lesions can be reached by cytology brushes, needles, or biopsy forceps and specimens can be obtained. This is especially effective in lesions of more than 2.0 cm in diameter. After a bronchoscopic procedure, the yield of sputum cytology appears to increase, making this technique of value as an added diagnostic tool.

The bronchoscope is a valuable tool for staging. The site of the primary tumor in a major airway may affect its stage (T3 versus T2 versus T1). Transbronchoscopic needle aspiration through the airway wall, as popularized by Wang,[134,135] can confirm the presence of a malignancy in mediastinal lymph nodes (N3 versus N2 versus N1). Care must be taken with this latter technique, because false-positive examinations have been reported and differentiation between resectable N2 versus unresectable N2 or N3 disease cannot be determined by needle aspiration alone. A more invasive approach (*e.g.*, mediastinoscopy, thoracoscopy) may be required.[136]

Mediastinoscopy and Mediastinotomy

Mediastinoscopy was developed by Carlens 30 years ago to facilitate staging of superior mediastinal lymph nodes (N2 or N3) before consideration of therapy in patients with lung cancer. It remains the most accurate lymph node staging technique to assess superior mediastinal lymph nodes, which are involved frequently in this disease. The procedure is simple, safe, and effective in experienced hands. In two recent large series, the mortality rate was 0 and the major morbidity rate less than 1.0%.[137,138] In patients suspected of having inoperable disease by virtue of mediastinal involvement as detected by CT scanning, confirmation by mediastinoscopy is indicated. Depending on the philosophy of management of patients with minimal mediastinal involvement, mediastinoscopy can be used to a greater or lesser extent by individual practitioners. If induction (neoadjuvant, primary) chemotherapy is to be used in the management of patients, then mediastinoscopy is extremely valuable for accurate staging of the disease before such induction treatment. Involvement of anterior mediastinal lymph nodes, which occurs frequently in left upper lobe tumors, can be assessed by the extended mediastinoscopy technique[139] or an anterior mediastinotomy as advocated by Chamberlain.[140] Because these are the first level of mediastinal lymph nodes to be involved in disease, many practitioners defer this examination if cervical mediastinoscopy fails to reveal metastatic disease in the superior mediastinum. Patients without superior mediastinal involvement have a good prognosis after resection even with involvement of anterior mediastinal (first level) nodes.[141]

Thoracoscopy

More recently, video-assisted thoracoscopy has been used in the diagnosis and staging of lung cancer. Peripheral nodules can be identified and biopsied or excised using video-assisted minimally invasive techniques and mediastinal lymph nodes

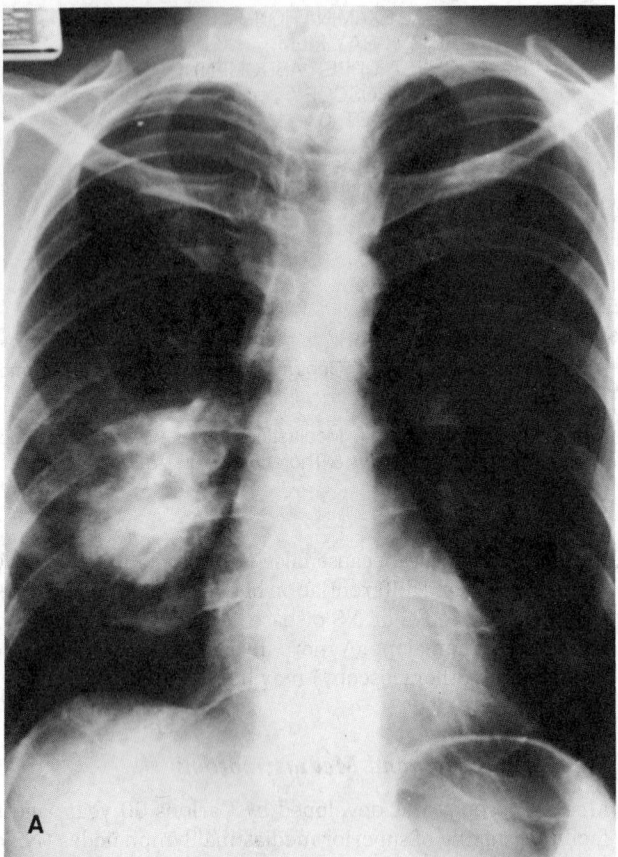 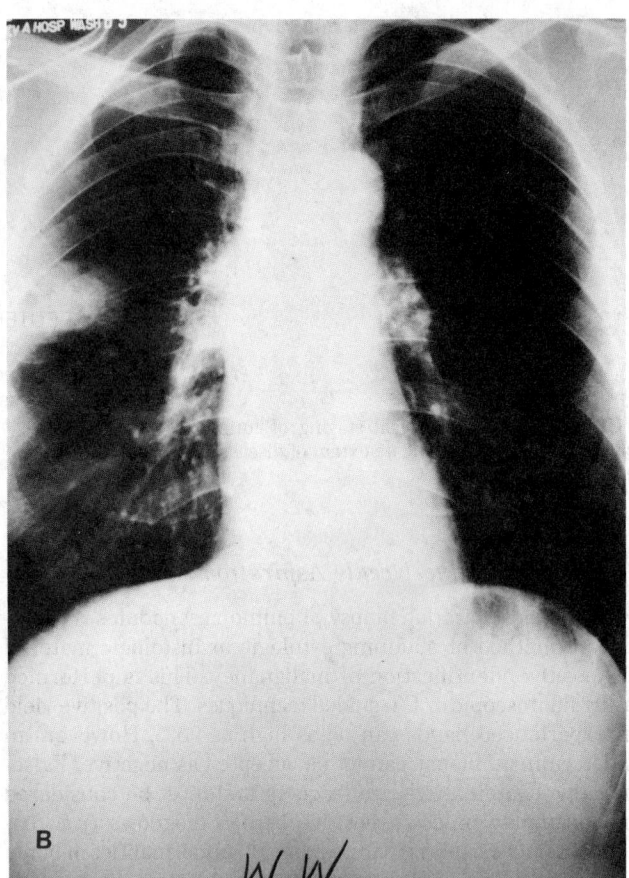

FIGURE 23–11. Chest radiographs of patients with different presentations of lung cancer. **(A)** A centrally located tumor on cavitation suggestive of squamous cell carcinoma. **(B)** A peripherally located nodule with possible pleural involvement. **(C)** A large hilar mass in mediastinal adenopathy suggesting stage IIIB disease. **(D)** Multiple bilateral pulmonary nodules of bronchoalveolar carcinoma. **(E)** Patient with small cell lung cancer involving a large, bulky central mass with hilar and mediastinal adenopathy and obstruction of the right upper lobe.

can be sampled for histologic examination. This technique identifies suspected pleural disease and has the ability to accurately assess the status of pleural effusions. The exact indications and use of this minimally invasive technique awaits prospective studies. Video-assisted thoracoscopy remains an investigative tool.[142–144]

Thoracotomy

Diagnostic thoracotomies continue to be used in the diagnosis and staging of lung cancer. With less invasive procedures, more than 95% of tumors can be accurately diagnosed and staged without thoracotomy. There remain a few patients in whom there is a high suspicion of cancer without a diagnosis before thoracotomy. At the time of thoracotomy, a diagnosis can be made by fine-needle aspiration biopsy, incisional or preferably excisional biopsy, and frozen-section analysis. All of these techniques can provide tissue that can be rapidly assessed by pathologists. At the time of thoracotomy, further staging is mandatory by the surgeon by mediastinal lymph node sampling or complete lymph node dissection. Not infrequently, unsuspected involvement of adjacent structures is recognized only at the time of surgery, identifying a T3 or T4 tumor.

EXTENT OF DISEASE EVALUATION

Once the diagnosis of lung cancer has been made, and before consideration of definitive therapy, a clinical extent of disease evaluation is required. Frequently, history and physical examination suggest lymphatic or distant metastatic spread. These symptoms or signs should be confirmed by appropriate radiologic studies directed at the organs suspected to be involved. In those patients suspected to have disease localized to the hemithorax, there has been significant debate about the minimum required investigations to prove or disprove metastatic spread. After an accurate history and physical examination, routine studies should include chest x-ray films, routine hematologic survey, and specific biochemical markers including serum calcium, alkaline phosphatase, and aspartate amino-transferase (AST). Elevated levels of these biochemical markers indicate the need for investigation for bony or liver metastases.

In the United States, virtually all patients considered for curative treatment of lung cancer undergo routine CT scanning of the chest and upper abdomen to detect mediastinal lymph node enlargement, unsuspected pulmonary metastases, and unsuspected liver and adrenal metastases. Whether the use of CT scans is cost effective in detecting these unsuspected

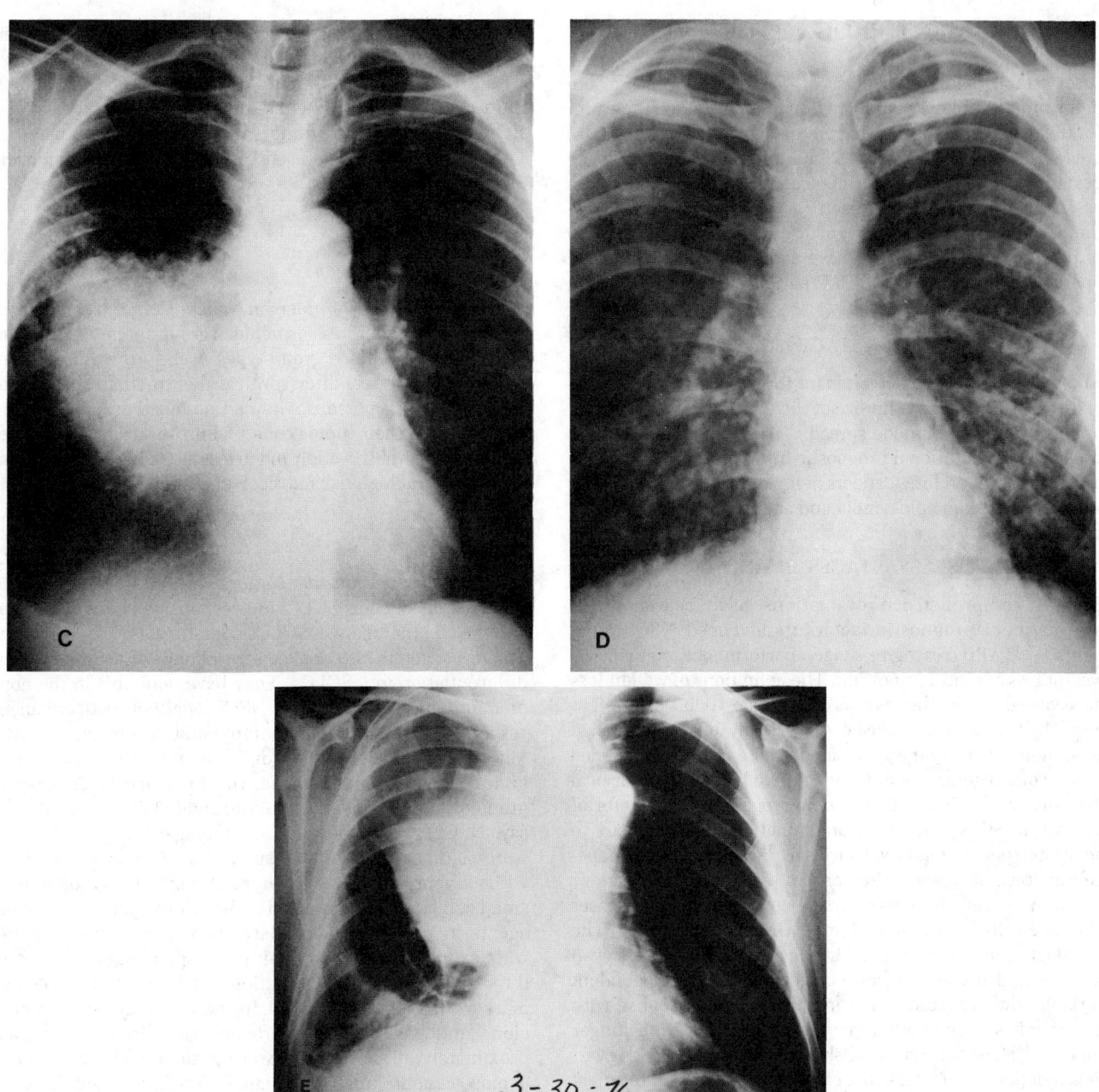

FIGURE 23–11. *(Continued)*

metastases is a moot point. Frequently, abnormalities found with this examination lead to further invasive testing ultimately revealing a false-positive investigation. Similarly, the routine use of bone scans despite the absence of clinical or biochemical abnormalities can be questioned.

The routine use of mediastinoscopy before surgical intervention for the treatment of lung cancer is hotly debated. With mediastinoscopy, inoperable superior mediastinal disease can be identified, thereby avoiding some unnecessary thoracotomies. About 5% of patients harbor inoperable unsuspected mediastinal disease if mediastinoscopy is not used as a routine staging operation, despite the use of CT scans.

For peripheral nodules less than 3 cm in diameter with no other abnormalities detected on chest x-ray film, physical examination, or biochemical screening, it is probably not cost effective to pursue all of these investigations in clinical practice. In those patients with more locally advanced disease (clinical stages II and III) or patients with suggestive adverse prognostic signs (*e.g.*, weight loss) a more complete metastatic survey should be performed.

The routine use of CT or MRI scanning of the brain to detect asymptomatic cerebral metastasis has not been settled, but is probably not cost effective in early stages (I and II) of disease.

PRETREATMENT PROGNOSTIC FACTORS

After establishing the diagnosis of NSCLC, it is necessary to determine the likely course and outcome. This is important for the patient and the treating physician because this estimate guides the choice of therapy. Such information is vital for the design and interpretation of clinical trials in which it is necessary to discriminate between the effectiveness of a new therapy and the natural history of disease for a particular group of patients.[145] Several trials have addressed these issues for operable and inoperable NSCLC patients.

EARLY-STAGE DISEASE: STAGES I AND II

The major prognostic determinant for this group is the stage of disease, particularly the size of the tumor and the presence or absence of lymph node spread.[116] Histologic subtype may provide some additional prognostic information with the outcome in large cell lung cancers being different from that observed in resected epidermoid and adenocarcinomas.[146]

ADVANCED DISEASE: STAGES III AND IV

Several comprehensive evaluations have searched for pretreatment prognostic factors in advanced NSCLC patients.[147–152] Pretreatment stage, performance status, and weight loss are most important. The definitions of weight loss have varied among the reviews (more than 10 lb,[149] % weight loss,[148–152] presence or absence).[147] Many of the trials had small numbers of women evaluated. Those trials that included more women generally found women to have longer survival than men.[150,151] Serum lactate dehydrogenase, a predictor of survival in SCLC and many other malignancies, appears to be an independent survival variable.[151,152] Whether any specific metastatic disease site confers a survival advantage or disadvantage remains controversial. Bone and liver metastases have been cited most often as predicting shorter survival. The histologic subtype of NSCLC has little influence on survival in advanced disease. When considered as an independent variable, the occurrence of a major objective response with cisplatin-based chemotherapy was associated with a longer survival.[151] There is no established model combining the various independent factors that can be recommended to select appropriate therapy or to predict outcome for individual patients.

NEW APPROACHES TO DETERMINE PROGNOSIS

Ploidy

Several trials evaluating tumor ploidy have shown that patients with diploid tumors have had a longer survival than those with aneuploid tumors.[153,154] A recent trial found aneuploidy a significant negative prognostic factor for squamous cell carcinoma only.[155] Further study is necessary to define the significance of ploidy in NSCLC.

Epidermal Growth Factor Receptors

After the identification of the presence and often increased numbers of epidermal growth factor receptors (EGFR) on lung cancer cells, trials have assessed the impact of EGFR expression on survival. In one trial, operable patients with EGFR-positive tumors survived significantly longer than those with EGFR-negative tumors (median survival 71 and 28 months, respectively).[156] In a second trial, overexpression of EGFR in primary lung tumors was associated with poor survival.[157] Currently, the presence of EGFR on lung cancer cells is a common finding but its prognostic significance remains uncertain.

Blood Group Antigen

Investigators at M. D. Anderson Cancer Center have reported recently that the expression of blood group antigen A in tumors of patients with blood group types A and AB was associated with longer survival after surgical therapy than those blood group A and AB persons who had no blood group antigen A expressed on their tumor cells.[158] Further trials are planned to confirm this observation and to test its usefulness in defining a population at high risk for recurrence and shortened survival.

Neuroendocrine Markers

After the observation that tumors with neuroendocrine differentiation, such as SCLC, are responsive to chemotherapy and the fact that many NSCLCs contain SCLC elements, several investigators have looked for evidence of neuroendocrine differentiation in NSCLCs. They have done this in the hope of identifying a population of NSCLC patients with enhanced responsiveness to chemotherapy and improved survival. Markers of neuroendocrine differentiation include chromogranin, L-dopa decarboxylase, the presence of dense core granules, neuron-specific enolase, and Leu-7. Using a dye assay, NSCLC cells lines with neuroendocrine differentiation were significantly more sensitive than non-small cell lines without neuroendocrine differentiation.[159] In a group of non-small cell lung cancer treated with various chemotherapeutic agents, neuron-specific enolase, Leu-7, and chromogranin were expressed more commonly in responding patients.[160] In the same study, responding patients with two or more positive markers had superior survival. In another study using a monoclonal antibody to define neuroendocrine differentiation, approximately 30% of tumors were positive and the presence of biopsies containing more than 50% positively staining cells was associated with shortened survival in a multivariable analysis.[161] Neuron-specific enolase positivity has been noted in approximately 20% of patients with inoperable adenocarcinoma of the lung; this has been associated with improved response, but has had no effect on survival.[162] Although they remain an area of investigation, neuroendocrine markers cannot be used as a determinant of response or survival in NSCLC.

Genetic Markers

The intensive study of the role of oncogenes in the pathogenesis of human malignancy has led to an investigation of oncogene activation in lung cancer. K-*RAS* point mutations occur in almost one third of human lung adenocarcinomas,[91] and the presence of K-*RAS* point mutations define a subgroup of operable NSCLC patients at high risk for relapse and shortened survival.[101] Another genetic abnormality with potential prognostic implication is chromosomal deletion. After observations of the loss of DNA sequences on the short arm of chromosome 3 in all SCLC specimens studied, investigators at the National Cancer Institute (NCI) studied 15 persons with NSCLC. Loss of 3p alleles was documented in 4 patients.[163] The prognostic significance of this observation has not been tested.

OCCULT LUNG CANCER

An occult lung cancer is defined as a tumor in an asymptomatic patient without radiographic findings. In most instances, this cancer is detected by finding abnormal cells on sputum cytologic examination. On occasion, an occult lung cancer may be identified serendipitously at bronchoscopy performed for other reasons (*e.g.*, screening persons with other aerodigestive tract abnormalities). These occult tumors are usually found at an early stage, either as in situ disease or early T1N0 tumors. A truly occult lung cancer, undetected by radiography and asymptomatic, is almost always at this early stage of disease. An extremely high proportion (>90%) of such tumors can be totally cured by surgical removal.

LUNG CANCER SCREENING

In the hope that the screening of high-risk population groups by sputum cytology and chest x-ray films would improve the identification of early-stage lung cancer, the NCI Cooperative Early Lung Cancer Group was formed more than 20 years ago and developed protocols for screening high-risk persons (male cigarette smokers of more than 45 years of age). More than 30,000 male volunteers at three centers were recruited and followed, half underwent intensive screening with four monthly sputum examinations and an annual chest x-ray film and the other half was a control group. Each center had different methods of following the control group, but initial chest x-ray films were performed by all study groups. The results of this trial demonstrated that lung cancers identified by screening methods were more frequently early-stage tumors (40% versus 15%) and patients developing lung cancer during the screening period had an overall 5-year survival of 35% versus 13% in the general population. Despite these findings, there was no impact in overall survival of the two groups when all deaths were considered.[164,165] It was found that sputum cytology can identify squamous cell carcinomas, and yearly chest x-ray films can identify with modest accuracy squamous cell carcinomas and adenocarcinomas. Small cell carcinoma is rarely detected at an early stage no matter what the screening technique. Screening trials performed in Europe have failed to alter the total death rate in screened versus control groups. All trials demonstrated an improved ability to diagnose lung cancer early. Because these screening interventions fail to alter mortality rates, mass screening for lung cancer cannot be recommended. Despite the failure of mass screening, most investigators involved in these studies continue to believe that a person with a high risk for developing lung cancer would be prudent to have an annual chest x-ray film. Sputum cytology may be worthwhile as an initial screen, limiting further follow-up to those patients demonstrating dysplasia. Tockman and

colleagues have developed a monoclonal antibody which, in early trials, has had the ability to identify sputum abnormalities in those persons who develop lung cancer at a very early stage. This approach is the subject of an ongoing trial to further evaluate the role of monoclonal antibody screening.

EARLY DETECTION

Early detection of lung cancer depends on imaging and sputum cytology techniques.

Chest X-Ray Film

Although there are no specific recommendations from cancer agencies, plain posteroanterior and lateral chest x-ray films have been used on a yearly basis in high-risk persons in an attempt to provide an earlier diagnosis of lung cancer. Important in this approach is the ability to compare previous x-ray films with recent films to detect subtle changes. Routine CT scans of high-risk persons have not been performed as a screening technique and the impact of digitized AMBER chest radiography has not been assessed.

Sputum Cytology

The routine use of annual sputum examination for cytologic assessment has not been demonstrated to be effective in the detection of early lung cancer. Dysplastic changes identified at sputum cytology should be followed. Severe dysplasia indicates a significant chance of ultimately developing into lung cancer.[166] Persons with severe dysplasia should be followed extremely closely.[167] The monoclonal antibody developed by Tockman and colleagues may improve the yearly detection rate of lung cancer by using specific monoclonal antibodies.[120]

Bronchoscopy

Bronchoscopy can identify early mucosal changes suggestive of lung cancer. In situ and T1N0 proximal tumors can be identified with relative ease. The improved acuity of video equipment used with bronchoscopy will probably increase this yield.[168] Hematoporphyrins are preferentially taken up by rapidly dividing cells, and using hematoporphyrin excitation by specific wave lengths (630 nm or 410 nm) of light. A characteristic fluorescence occurs in tissue containing the hematoporphyrin sensitizer. Bronchoscopy can be used to detect occult neoplasms but has the disadvantage of false-positive results due to fluorescence of cellular atypia or metaplasia and to a lack of easy availability of this technique. Only two or three centers are pursuing the diagnostic technique.[169,170] A new approach, without using drugs, exploits spectral differences of autofluorescence (LIFE = lung imaging fluorescent endoscopy) and is being investigated in the detection and localization of early lung cancer.[171]

MANAGEMENT OF OCCULT CANCER

The management of occult lung cancer depends on the stage of disease at diagnosis. Because most of these tumors are early T1N0 carcinomas, many are treated by surgical excision. If surgery is contraindicated in such patients, curative radiotherapy is indicated. With proximal early-stage tumors, the role of brachytherapy to augment the total dose is unknown but curative treatment can be applied in this fashion.

In those patients identified as having in situ carcinomas, hematoporphyrin destruction of such lesions can be attempted. Hayata[172] found that early lesions should be less than 1 cm square in total surface area. Only a complete endobronchial response to such therapy is acceptable in such patients. After such a response, local recurrences are rare. Recommendations for primary treatment with photodynamic therapy in minimal occult tumor awaits further definition.[172,173] Only those patients who have had complete responses should be maintained on this type of treatment protocol. If possible, surgical treatment is indicated for this early-stage disease and for all in situ lesions persisting after nonsurgical treatment (*e.g.*, phototherapy, radiotherapy).

SURGERY FOR NON-SMALL CELL LUNG CANCER

In stages I and II NSCLC, if the tumor has not extended beyond the bronchopulmonary lymph nodes, a complete excision is almost always possible and surgery provides the best chance for cure (Fig. 23–12). Controversy arises in the management of stage IIIA disease. In the international classification, T3 disease indicates a primary tumor with local invasion of surrounding structures but that is still excisable and curable. Ipsilateral (N2) mediastinal lymph node involvement, despite being potentially resectable, remains a contentious issue when indications for surgery are discussed. Again, if a complete excision occurs, the patient is afforded a chance of cure. In clinical staging, the surgeon must assess the possibility of completely removing the tumor and its involved nodes at operation. N2 disease identified preoperatively (clinical staging) by imaging studies or mediastinoscopy affords a much poorer prognosis.

Except for a few unusual circumstances, stage IIIB disease by virtue of unresectable lymph node spread (N3) or primary tumor invasion of vital structures denotes inoperability with a small likelihood of success after surgical excision. Similarly, lung cancer that has metastasized to distant organs is beyond the realm of surgical excision. However, there has been a renewed interest in removing the primary tumor and a solitary metastatic focus. In selected persons, this affords long term disease-free control.

PATIENT SELECTION

The preoperative assessment of patients considered for surgical treatment of lung cancer includes clinical staging of the disease to assess its resectability, assessment of the cardiopulmonary reserve of the patient to determine whether the intended pulmonary resection is possible, and assessment of the patient with regard to the perioperative risk of the procedure. Traditionally, patients are suitable candidates for pneumonectomy if the ultimate forced expiratory volume in 1 second (FEV_1) is greater than 1.2 L, the patient does not suffer from hypercarbia, and cor pulmonale is not present.[174-176] Pulmonary function studies best suited to assess these parameters include spirometry, arterial blood gases, diffusion/ capacity, and, if indicated, ventilation-perfusion scans to estimate the proportions of functioning pulmonary tissue to be excised. Patients requiring lobectomy or lesser resections require similar postoperative pulmonary function parameters.[177,178] Recent prospective analyses have failed to show differences in pulmonary volumes and FEV_1 after lobectomy or lesser resections.[179,180] The amount of functioning pulmonary tissue removed by lobectomy or lesser resection rarely interferes with ultimate recovery.

More important in the preoperative assessment of patients is the ability of the patient to tolerate a general anesthetic and the rigors of the early postoperative period. To prevent postoperative cardiopulmonary complications and decrease

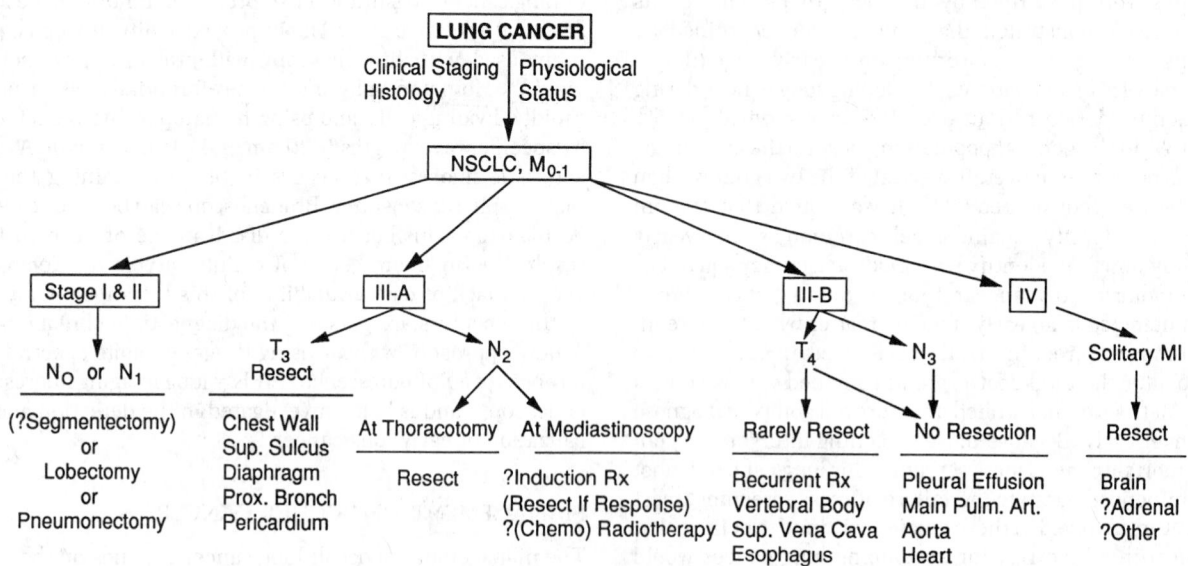

SCHEMA FOR ROLE OF CURATIVE SURGERY IN LUNG CANCER

FIGURE 23–12. A schema for operability at the various stages of non-small cell lung cancer.

the chance of other major postoperative problems, care must be taken to determine accurately the patient's cardiopulmonary status preoperatively. Cardiopulmonary exercise studies, gaited cardiac radionuclide studies, and echocardiography have been introduced with the hope of improving the estimation of these risks. The ability of patients to perform the necessary pulmonary toilet (*e.g.*, coughing, deep breathing) after such procedures requires intensive preoperative instruction and a period of rehabilitation if necessary. Pulmonary complications increase remarkably if the ratio of FEV_1 to forced vital capacity (FVC) is below 75% of that predicted, indicating significant airway obstruction. FEV_1/FVC ratios that are less than 50% of those predicted lead to unacceptable postoperative morbidity and mortality.

POSTOPERATIVE CARE

A major insult in cardiopulmonary reserve reflected by pulmonary resection demands that patients undergoing such procedures require intensive care and monitoring in the postoperative period. This is best served by a 24- to 48-hour period in a monitored setting. With newer forms of pain control (*e.g.*, epidural narcotic analgesia, patient controlled analgesia, intrathoracic analgesia) it is hoped that less morbidity will occur after pulmonary resection.

SURGICAL PROCEDURES

Until 40 years ago, pneumonectomy was considered the surgical excision of choice in managing lung cancer.[181] If complete excision can be obtained by lobectomy, it has been the preferred resection with what appears to be equal opportunity for long-term success.[182] In the past 20 years, there has been a resurgence of interest in lesser resections and lung-conserving operations. Jensik has been the major proponent of segmentectomy for Tl/2N0 peripheral tumors.[183] Survival after such a limited resection and the morbidity and mortality of the operation appear at least equivalent to lobectomy in retrospective analyses.[184] Except in a few isolated centers, resections other than segmentectomy (*e.g.*, wedge excision, precision cautery dissection) have been reserved for situations in which it is believed that the patient cannot tolerate a lobectomy because of poor cardiopulmonary condition. In proximally situated tumors, in which a pneumonectomy may be required for total excision, lung-conserving operations using bronchoplastic procedures to preserve uninvolved lobes (*e.g.*, sleeve lobectomy) have results equivalent to the more extensive pneumonectomy.

Morbidity and Mortality of Surgical Procedures

With improved surgical and anesthetic techniques and perioperative care, the postoperative mortality for surgical resections has decreased remarkably over the past 50 years. The mortality rate for pneumonectomy is less than 6%, for lobectomy less than 3%, and for lesser resections 1% or less. These mortality figures are affected significantly by the age of the patient, the stage of the disease, and the extent of resection.[185] The commonest complications after resectional surgery are not technical failures of the operation but cardiopulmonary problems. Improved preoperative assessment and postoper-

ative care to identify high-risk patients and decrease these complications ultimately lead to lessened operative risks for the patient (Table 23–6).[186]

LOCALIZED NON-SMALL CELL LUNG CANCER: STAGES I AND II

Stages I and II lung cancer denotes disease limited to the hemithorax with tumor extension no further than the visceral pleura peripherally (T2) or hilar nodes proximally (N1). In such cases, surgical excision is the treatment of choice. In most instances, lobectomy is the resectional procedure required. If the primary tumor or lymph nodes involve the proximal bronchus, proximal pulmonary artery, or cross the major fissure such that a complete resection is only possible by pneumonectomy, this more extensive procedure should be performed.

The role of mediastinal lymphadenectomy as part of the surgical procedure remains hotly debated. The proponents of complete mediastinal lymphadenectomy argue that complete removal of mediastinal lymph nodes improves survival. This dissection provides the best possible surgical staging by removing all lymph nodes, which can then be analyzed pathologically for metastatic involvement. At minimum, for accurate final surgical-pathologic staging, lymph node sampling of all draining areas should be performed at the time of surgical resection.[187,188] A recently completed randomized trial comparing mediastinal lymphadenectomy with mediastinoscopy combined with intraoperative lymph node sampling shows no difference in survival, locoregional recurrence, or accuracy of the two staging procedures as applied to stage I or II lung

TABLE 23–6. Postoperative Mortality for Surgical Resections

	Mortality (%)	Complications (%)
Type of Resection		
Segment or wedge	1.3	10.4
Lobectomy	2.9	15
Pneumonectomy	6.2	15
Age		
<50	1.3	3
50–59	1.3	10.7
60–69	4.1	13.0
70–79	7.0	24.5
>80	8.1	20
Pulmonary Function		
FEV_1 < 1.2	NS	22
FEV_1 1.2–2.0	NS	14
FEV_1 > 2	NS	14
Disease Stage		
I	NS	10.6
II	NS	11.2
III	NS	18.6

NS, not stated.

cancer. In peripheral T1N0 tumors, the role of lesser resection (segmentectomy, wedge excision, or precision cautery dissection) has yet to be defined completely. A recent randomized trial conducted by the Lung Cancer Study Group[180] shows that after short-term follow-up, the locoregional recurrence rate with limited resection is twofold to threefold greater than with lobectomy (15% versus 5%). Mortality, morbidity, and pulmonary function were equal in both arms of the study. For this reason, limited resection should be reserved for compromise situations in which the surgeon believes that lobectomy is contraindicated and a complete excision can be performed by a lesser resection (Table 23-7). If a complete surgical excision can be obtained with lung-conserving bronchoplastic procedures, it should be performed. In retrospective analyses, the cure rate after sleeve resection of proximal bronchi or pulmonary arteries, thereby preserving uninvolved lung tissue, is no different than that after pneumonectomy for similar early (N0) stage patients. The quality of life allowed by such lung-preserving operations makes this the preferable approach (Fig. 23-13).

After surgical resection for stages I and II lung cancer, the 5-year survival without recurrence exceeds 50% in stage I and 35% in stage II disease. In completely resected T1N0 tumors, 5-year survival exceeds 70%. Approximately 25% of patients who do not survive are tumor-free at death, suggesting that surgical resection in early-stage lung cancer renders 80% of patients tumor-free.

LOCALLY ADVANCED LUNG CANCER: STAGE IIIA DISEASE

Stage IIIA disease includes T3 tumor or N2 nodal spread or both. Surgical resection of locally advanced primary tumors (T3) yields a higher survival rate than that seen if mediastinal lymph nodes (N2) are involved. There is a significant difference in prognosis between patients with T3N0 disease and patients with N2 disease. In either instance, the goal of surgery is to perform a complete resection. Preclinical staging and an extensive extent of disease work-up is required before offering surgery to ensure that a complete resection is anticipated and no metastatic disease is present.

T3 Tumors

Those tumors invading the chest wall, the diaphragm, and the mediastinal pleura or pericardium and those tumors sit-

uated within 2 cm of the carina constitute the designation of T3. Naruke at the Japan National Cancer Center reported an overall 5-year survival of 26% in 327 patients treated with this stage of disease.[188] At Memorial Sloan-Kettering Cancer Center, 77 patients with completely resected tumors had a 42% 5-year survival, but of 48 patients with incomplete resections, none survived beyond 2½ years.[189] It appears that up to 50% of patients with T3N0 lesions resected completely survive 5 years. Once lymph nodes are involved, the prognosis is much worse. Even with the tumor resected completely, only 20% of 32 patients with lymphatic metastases in T3 lesions survived 5 years and few if any did not survive when mediastinal nodes were involved.

CHEST WALL INVASION. Involvement of parietal pleura, chest wall muscle, or rib constitutes a T3 tumor. The deeper the invasion, the worse the prognosis. In all instances, the tumor should be resected en bloc with the involved chest wall and a minimum of 2 cm of normal chest wall removed in all directions beyond the tumor. Prognosis is related to the completeness of resection, with no patients surviving 5 years after an incomplete resection (Table 23-8).

The role of preoperative or adjuvant therapy after resection of chest wall tumors has not been delineated clearly. There are no prospective trials and only gathered reports of retrospective trials with varying results.[190-192]

SUPERIOR SULCUS TUMORS. Henry Pancoast described a tumor in the apex of the lung invading the first rib with associated involvement of the brachial plexus and stellate ganglion, creating Pancoast's syndrome (rib erosion, shoulder pain radiating down the arm, and Horner's syndrome). Shaw and Paulson were the first to report a curative resection in this disease. Since that initial report, most surgeons treat a documented superior sulcus tumor with preoperative radiotherapy of 3000 to 4500 cGy followed by en bloc resection of the involved lung, chest wall, and frequently the T1 nerve root. Residual disease at the time of resection is treated with postoperative radiotherapy or intraoperative brachytherapy.[193] The overall survival for patients with resected tumors has been reported in the range of 40% (Table 23-9). Adverse prognostic factors include involved mediastinal lymph nodes, bony erosion, and adenocarcinoma on histology. Contraindications to surgery for superior sulcus tumors include a T4 tumor (vertebral body invasion, subclavian artery or vein invasion) or unresectable N2 disease. Occasionally, palliative resection of such lesions may be required for pain relief.

TABLE 23-7. Results of Limited Pulmonary Resection Performed as an Intentional Procedure, Mainly for T1N0 Tumors

Investigations	No. of Patients	Estimated 5-year Survival (%)	Operative Mortality (%)	Local Recurrence (%)
Jensik[442]	296	52	1	12
Read[443]	113	70	4.4	4.4
Wain[444]	164	<50	5	5
Lung Cancer Study Group[445]	123	70	1	17.5

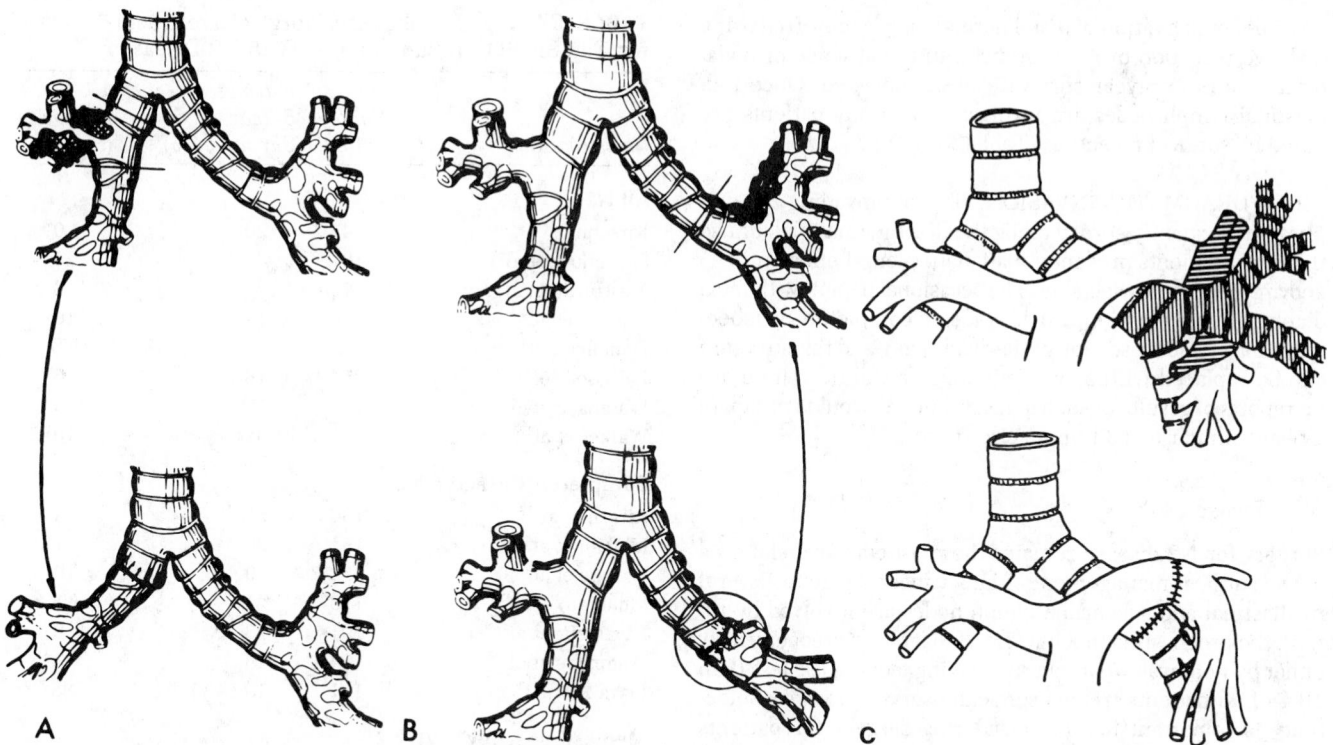

FIGURE 23–13. Bronchoplastic and bronchovascular sleeve resections to preserve pulmonary function. **(A)** Right upper lobe sleeve resection. **(B)** Left upper lobe sleeve resection. **(C)** Left upper lobe bronchovascular sleeve resection.

MEDIASTINAL INVASION. Invasion of the mediastinal pleura, pericardium, or mediastinal fat constitutes T3 disease. In many instances, en bloc resection of the involved mediastinal tissue can be accomplished yielding a complete resection. The results of such mediastinal invasion are not well known. At Memorial Sloan-Kettering Cancer Center only approximately 10% of such patients, completely resected, survived 5 years.[194] This review of 225 patients with mediastinal invasion indicates that once mediastinal invasion occurs, major structures frequently are involved (T4) or concomitant mediastinal lymph node disease is present (N2 or N3). In such patients, technical resectability should be determined preoperatively if possible.

MRI scanning to detect mediastinal invasion is of no more value than CT scanning to detect mediastinal invasion and mediastinoscopy is indicated before resection of any of these tumors. Of 225 patients analyzed in the Memorial series, only 22% could be completely resected, 44% were totally unresectable, and 34% were incompletely resected. In this report of the results of mediastinal invasion, brachytherapy was used in incomplete resections with a surprising 22% survival rate in this small subset of patients.

PROXIMAL AIRWAY INVOLVEMENT. Tumors within 2 cm of the carina can be resected by pneumonectomy, but, if

TABLE 23–8. Results After Surgical Treatment for Non-Small Cell Lung Cancer With Chest Wall Invasion (T3)

Investigations	No. of Patients (Total CR)	Estimated 5-Year Survival (%) (Total)	Mortality (%)
Paone et al[446]	32 (28)	35	3
Patterson et al[447]	35 (30)	38	9
Piehler et al[448]	93 (66)	33*	15
McCaughan et al[449]	125 (77)	40*	4
Van de Wal et al[450]	16 (NS)	12	6
Allen et al[451]	52 (NS)	26	4

* Survival of patients with completely resected tumors.
CR, complete resection; NS, not stated.

TABLE 23–9. Results After Surgical Treatment for Non-Small-Cell Lung Cancer With a Superior Sulcus Lesion (T3)

Investigations	No. of Patients	Estimated 5-Year Survival (%)	Mortality (%)
Paulson[452]	79	31	3
Anderson et al[453]	28	34	7
Devine et al[454]	40	10	8
Rice et al[455]	36	28	0
Miller[456]	36	31	NS
McKneally[457]	25	51	NS
Ricci et al[458]	41	34	5
Carrel et al[459]	37	29	NS
Dartevelle et al[460]	24	32 (2-y)	4
Komaki et al[461]	25	40	NS

NS, not stated.

possible, preservation of distal normal lung is preferred using a sleeve resection of main bronchi. In the absence of nodal disease, a 50% 5-year survival can be expected. Once mediastinal lymph nodes are involved, few if any patients are cured by surgical resection (Table 23–10).[195]

DIAPHRAGMATIC INVASION. Tumors invading the diaphragm frequently spread along the diaphragmatic pleura so that most patients present a malignant pleural effusion (T4) and are usually unresectable. The occasional patient with focal diaphragmatic invasion can be resected completely by lobectomy and en bloc resection of the diaphragm, and this structure can be replaced with a synthetic mesh or fabric. There are no reports of results of such surgery, but one would anticipate a result similar to T3 tumors elsewhere.

N2 Disease

Surgery for N2 disease remains the most controversial area in the surgical management of lung cancer. Once ipsilateral mediastinal and subcarinal lymph nodes are involved by tumor, the prognosis is much worse. If diagnosed preoperatively either by noninvasive or invasive staging techniques, less than 10% of all patients treated surgically survive 5 years. Selectivity is important before considering surgery for patients preoperatively identified with N2 disease. Adverse prognostic factors include multiple levels of N2 disease, multiple lymph nodes at one level involved with tumor, adenocarcinoma, and extranodal spread of disease. More than 75% of patients with N2 disease are discovered with disease extending beyond one lymph node station.

MINIMAL N2 DISEASE. Single-station lymph node involvement with microscopic foci of disease not clinically apparent on noninvasive staging constitutes this subset. Patients with this very early stage usually are discovered at the time of thoracotomy or at pretreatment mediastinoscopy. Five-year survival rates after surgical resection are reported in the range of 10% to 20% and are somewhat higher if a complete resection is performed (Table 23–11). Incomplete resection results in a noncurative treatment with few if any survivors beyond 3 years. The criteria for resection of minimal N2 disease includes a normal CT scan with regard to mediastinal involvement or mediastinoscopy identifying one station of lymph nodes involved with only microscopic disease. For this stage of disease, a complete mediastinal lymph node dissection is warranted. Proponents of mediastinal lymph node dissection, versus lymph node sampling, in all patients treated by surgical resection for lung cancer believe that this extended dissection identifies patients with N2 disease who would have benefited by the complete nodal dissection. One retrospective study suggests a doubling of 5-year survival (15.9% versus 6.7%) when lymph node dissection is carried out in patients with this stage of disease.[196]

ADVANCED N2 DISEASE. Those tumors with mediastinal involvement beyond that described in minimal N2 disease constitute this large segment of patients presenting with stage IIIA disease. This more advanced "bulky" N2 disease, which is usually discovered preoperatively and is termed *clinical N2*, is considered by most surgeons to be inoperable and there are few 5-year survivals identified after surgical resection.[197–199] It is this group of patients in whom induction therapies using chemotherapy or chemoradiotherapy has been tested (see discussion later in this chapter). Standard therapy for this stage of disease must still be considered primary chemoradiotherapy.

TABLE 23–11. Results After Surgical Treatment for Non-Small Cell Lung Cancer With N2 Disease

Investigations	No. of Patients	Estimated 5-Year Survival (%)	Mortality (%)
All N2			
Kirschner[469]	45	20	0
Sawamura et al[470]	107	?	25
Mastrorilli et al[471]	108	?	2
Naruke et al[472]	426	14	10
Deneffe et al[473]	42	9	NS
Lavasseur et al[474]	254	18	6
Watanabe et al[475]	153	17	3
Walker et al[476]	70	32*	10
Completely Resected N2			
Kirsch et al[477]	136	21	4
Martini et al[478]	151	30*	1
Naruke et al[472]	252	19	10
Mountain et al[479]	118	21†	NS
Lavasseur et al[474]	191	23	6
Watanabe et al[475]	84	24	3
Frytak et al[480]	101	19 (4-y)	NS
Mediastonoscopy + VE N2			
Pearson et al[481]	79	9	NS
Coughlin et al[482]	28	18	NS

* Adjusted for noncancer deaths.
† Excluding operative deaths.
NS, not stated.

TABLE 23–10. Results After Surgical Treatment for Non-Small Cell Lung Cancer With Proximal Airway Involvement (T3)

Investigations	No. of Patients	Estimated 5-Year Survival (%)	Mortality (%)
Van Den Bosch et al[462]	50	41	8
Ungar et al[463]	99	54*	7
Eschapasse[464]	31	42	7
Keszler[465]	76	22*	6
Maeda et al[466]	23	13*	5
Vogt-Moykopf et al[467]	97	12	15
Naruke[468]	62	39	1

* Crude survival.

LOCALLY ADVANCED LUNG CANCER: STAGE IIIB DISEASE

T4 Lesions

Stage IIIB includes patients with a T4 or N3 lesion, both of which usually are considered unresectable disease. Radiation therapy or chemotherapy or a combination of both remains the standard treatment for these patients. In general, they are not referred for surgical treatment. In a large retrospective study, resected stage IIIB patients had an overall 5-year survival of 6%.[200] Occasionally, such patients can be totally cured of their disease.

T4 Tumors

T4 tumors are the invading mediastinal structures (the carina and trachea, the heart and great vessels, the esophagus or vertebral body) and the presence of a malignant pleural effusion. Naruke and colleagues reported a 5-year survival in 8% of 104 selected patients after resection of such a T4 lesion.[200]

CARINAL INVASION. Primary lung cancer invading the carina is generally considered unresectable. Pneumonectomy with tracheal sleeve resection and direct reanastomosis of the trachea to the contralateral mainstem bronchus can be accomplished with reported 5-year survivals approaching 20% (Table 23–12).

Anastomotic dehiscence with bronchial fistula formation and postoperative pulmonary insufficiency are major postoperative problems and are the main causes of the high operative mortality, which varies from 11% to 27%. Only selected persons without N2 disease should be offered such a resection.

INVASION OF SUPERIOR VENA CAVA. Involvement of the superior vena cava (SVC) has been treated occasionally by resection and graft replacement. Long-term survivors are limited to case reports.[201,202] In our retrospective analysis, there were no 5-year survivors after resection in 18 patients with SVC invasion.[194] Preoperative distinction of SVC invasion by the tumor itself (T4) or its involved mediastinal lymph nodes (N2) can be difficult. Reported series include few cases, so that the significance of this finding cannot be assessed; however, it appears likely that only T4 and not N2 lesions can be cured with resection.

INVASION OF MYOCARDIUM, AORTA, ESOPHAGUS, AND VERTEBRAL BODY. Surgical resection resulting in complete excision of a primary tumor with mediastinal organ invasion is usually not possible. Palliative incomplete resections have not demonstrated survival or palliation benefit. In a series from Memorial Sloan-Kettering Cancer Center, there were no 5-year survivors in 19 patients with involvement of aorta or in 3 patients with invasion of the atrium, although not all patients underwent resection of the primary tumor or part of the invaded organ. One patient out of 7 (14%) with invasion of the esophagus lived beyond 5 years.[194] Despite these results, limited invasion of the atrial wall can occasionally be resected completely with the hope of an occasional cure. En bloc resection of the lung with part of the involved aorta, esophagus, or vertebral body, not uncommon in treatment of superior sulcus tumors, may result in long-term survival for selected patients. Postoperative radiotherapy to augment local control may be of benefit in these situations.

PLEURAL EFFUSION. Approximately 5% to 10% of the patients with lung cancer present with a nonmalignant pleural effusion, a result of atelectasis, obstructive pneumonitis, lymphatic or venous obstruction, or a pulmonary embolus. Although nonmalignant, this type of effusion defines a poor prognosis. The Mayo Clinic demonstrated that even cytologically negative pleural effusions were predictive of surgical unresectability in 95% of these patients. They concluded that, in patients with cytologically negative pleural effusions, unresectability must be documented surgically.[500] Naruke reported a 40% 5-year survival of 112 patients with a nonmalignant effusion, identical to the 5-year survival in 1298 patients without effusion. Even with malignant pleural effusions, occasional 5-year survivals have been documented when all disease has been eradicated.[200,203] In general, malignant pleural effusions indicate incurable disease by a surgical approach.

STAGE IV DISEASE: SURGERY FOR SOLITARY METASTASES

M1 Lung

To differentiate between a second primary lung cancer and a metastasis in synchronous lung lesions, or among a local recurrence, a new primary lung cancer, and a pulmonary metastasis from a previous resected lung cancer in metachronous lung lesions can be difficult. A second or recurrent lung lesion is considered a metastasis if the histology is identical to the primary tumor and occurs in the opposite lung or in a noncontiguous area of the ipsilateral lung. Deslauriers and colleagues found that the presence of satellite nodules discovered at surgery, clearly separated from the primary tumor but with identical histologic characteristics, is a poor prognostic fac-

TABLE 23–12. Results After Surgical Treatment for Non-Small Cell Lung Cancer With Carinal Invasion (T4)

Investigations	No. of Patients	Estimated 5-Year Survival (%)	Mortality (%)
Deslauriers[483]	26	23*	27
Fujimura et al[484]	15	0	NS
Faber[485]	33	15*	24
Dartevelle et al[486]	55	23	11
Mastrorilli et al[487]	11	20	0
Tsuchiya et al[488]	20	59 (2-y)	15
Vogt-Moykopf et al[489]	59	30 (2-y)	14
Mathisen et al[490]	37	19	19

* Crude survival.
NS, not stated.

tor.[204] In patients with satellite nodules from all stages of lung cancer, 5-year survival was 21.6% compared with 44% if no nodules were present. The mechanism of tumor spread in the lung is not well known, but may develop as a result of a blood-borne or airway-borne metastasis from a primary bronchogenic carcinoma. The new TNM staging system fails to classify specifically these synchronous lung lesions. The same criteria in selecting patients for surgical resection of a pulmonary metastasis from a primary lung cancer should be maintained in patients with metastatic carcinoma to the lung from other primaries.[205] If a solitary synchronous lesion is discovered in a different lobe from the primary tumor, resection of both lesions is the treatment of choice.

M1 Brain

Brain metastases constitute more than 25% of all observed recurrence in patients with resected NSCLC and are seen with greater frequency at autopsy.[206] In a review by the Lung Cancer Study Group, the brain was the only site of first recurrence in 6.4% of patients with completely resected NSCLC and accounted for approximately 20% of all recurrences.[207] Nearly half of the patients seen with brain metastases have solitary lesions on CT scan. When symptomatic, the median survival without therapy is limited to 1 month. Corticosteroids and whole-brain irradiation can offer effective palliation of symptoms but only modestly increase survival up to 6 months.[208] A solitary brain metastasis is best treated by surgical resection, if possible, with 5-year survival in the range of 10% to 20% (Table 23–13). Surgical excision of a brain metastasis, no matter the primary site (approximately 75% from NSCLC), followed by radiation has been shown to be superior to radiotherapy alone in prolonging median survival (9.2 versus 3.4 months), in preventing local recurrence, and in providing a better quality of life.[209]

M1 Adrenal

Adrenal metastases from bronchogenic carcinoma are found in approximately one third of the patients at autopsy. Routine preoperative upper abdominal CT scanning may reveal an adrenal mass in approximately 10% of patients.[210]

There have been a few case reports of adrenalectomy for solitary adrenal metastasis and there has been long-term sur-

vival after combined excision of the primary lung tumor and its metastatic lesion.[211-213] The ultimate role of such an approach has yet to be defined.

M1 Liver, Bone, Skin

There have been no reports of long-term survival after combined surgical excision of a primary lung cancer with a solitary liver, bone, or skin mestastasis. It is rare that these lesions are truly solitary metastatic foci.

PATTERNS OF FAILURE AFTER POTENTIALLY CURATIVE RESECTION OF LUNG CANCER

Recognition of prognostic and surgical factors that predict for specific anatomic failure patterns can allow selection of patients for local, systemic, or combined therapy. The survival and anatomic patterns of failure after surgical therapy of early-stage NSCLC are presented in Table 23–14. After surgical resection, patients with pathologic stage T1–2N0 tumors who have negative resection margins have survival rates in excess of 40% to 50%. For such patients, isolated mediastinal or primary site recurrences are unusual and there is no rationale for the routine use of postoperative radiation therapy. Patients with T1N1 tumors have an isolated local failure rate of 12% (8/67). The rate of isolated distant failure for patients with T1N1 tumors is 33% (22/67) and points to the need for developing effective prophylactic therapy for systemic and central nervous system spread. For patients with T2N1 tumors, the isolated local failure rate is 14% (8/58) and the distant failure rate is 36% (21/58), again demonstrating the need for effective adjuvant systemic therapy.[214] Because isolated N1 metastases are rare in these large surgical series, adjuvant local therapy should be considered in patients with documented N1 disease if the mediastinal nodes were neither sampled nor dissected, because occult N2 disease may be present.

Survival rates decrease for those with T3 or N2 tumors discovered intraoperatively. When no adjuvant therapy is used for these more advanced patients, there is thoracic recurrence in approximately 20% of patients even if the resection margins are negative and distant metastases become even more common, suggesting that both failure patterns need to be addressed if survival is to be improved.[215] Increasingly, conservative re-

TABLE 23–13. Results After Combined Resection for Primary Non-Small Cell Lung Cancer With a Single Brain Metastasis (M1)

Investigations	Year	No. of Patients	Estimated 5-Year Survival (%)	Mortality (%)
Salerno et al[491]	1979	23	13	22
Winston et al[492]	1980	22	9 (2-y)	10
White et al[493]	1981	38	15 (2-y)	6
Mussi et al[494]	1985	20	34	0
Ehrenhaft[495]	1986	40	12	2
Magilligan et al[496]	1986	41	21	2
Read et al[497]	1989	27	21	0
Macchiarini et al[498]	1991	37	30	0
Burt et al[499]	1991	185	13	3

TABLE 23–14. Survival and Anatomic Failure Patterns After Surgery Alone for Early Stage Non-Small Cell Lung Cancer

Investigations	Stage	No. of Patients	Survival (y)	Patterns of Failure Thorax Only	Thorax + DM	DM Only
Pairolero	T1N0	170	71% (5)	6% (10/170)	?	15% (25/170)
Pairolero	T2N0	158	59% (5)	6% (9/158)	?	23% (37/158)
Pairolero	T1N1	18	33% (5)	28% (5/8)	?	39% (7/18)
Mountain	T3N0/1	69	36% (5)	12% (8/69)	4% (3/69)	25% (14/69)
Mountain	T1/3N2	92	26% (5)	1% (1/92)	5% (5/92)	32% (29/92)
Martini	T1N1	17	56% (5)	0%	?	47% (8/17)
Martini*	T2N1	58	48% (5)	14% (8/58)	?	36% (21/58)
Iascone*	T1N0	16	NS	19% (3/16)	?	6% (1/16)
Iascone*	T2N0	20	NS	25% (5/20)	?	5% (1/20)
Iascone*	T3N0	11	NS	36% (4/11)	?	18% (2/11)
Feldt†	T1N0	162	NS	9% (15/162)	?	17% (28/162)
Feldt†	T2N0	196	NS	11% (22/196)	?	30% (59/196)
Feldt†	T1N1	32	NS	9% (3/32)	?	22% (7/32)

* Few patients received adjuvant radiation therapy and/or chemotherapy.
† Failure patterns are for first relapse only.
DM, distant metastases; NS, not stated.

sections are being performed for early-stage lung cancers, although they have not been proved equally effective. For sleeve lobectomies, isolated local failures are more common than distant failures (ranging from 30–52%) and are particularly high if the procedure is performed to conserve parenchyma in patients with compromised pulmonary function.[501–503] This high incidence of isolated local failure provides a basis for the selective use of postoperative radiation therapy after sleeve lobectomy. Second primary lung cancers occur frequently in all surviving patients at a rate of approximately 1% per year.[216,217]

ADJUVANT THERAPIES AFTER SURGICAL RESECTION

POSTOPERATIVE RADIATION THERAPY

Considerable controversy surrounds the use of postoperative radiation therapy for NSCLC. Although postoperative radiotherapy reduces local recurrences in selected patients after complete resection, it does not impact on survival because distant metastases are common regardless of the control of intrathoracic disease.[215] Many issues need to be confronted when considering the appropriateness of postoperative radiation therapy, including the influence of histology, the benefit of preventing thoracic recurrence compared with the treatment of symptomatic recurrence, the toxicity of radiation, and the possibility that patients with mediastinal spread may derive a survival advantage.

The analysis of failure patterns suggests that routine postoperative radiation therapy is unlikely to benefit patients with completely resected T1–2N0 disease. The randomized trial of Van Houtte demonstrated that isolated local failure for T1–2N0 patients was low regardless of the use of 6000 cGy of radiation and no survival advantage resulted.[218] Bangma ran-domized 73 patients to receive postoperative radiation (4300–4600 cGy) or no further therapy. Approximately 75% of the patients in both arms of the study had T1–2N0 tumors and no survival advantage was present.[219] Both of these studies suggest that postoperative radiation therapy may be detrimental. It is possible that the delivery of a major proportion of the radiation dose through oblique fields causes pneumonitis, which contributes to overall mortality.

The prospective trial of the Lung Cancer Study Group compared the outcome of 108 patients with completely resected squamous cancer who received surgery and postoperative radiation (5000 cGy) with that of 102 patients treated with definitive surgery alone. Approximately 62% of the combined surgery and radiation group and 65% of the surgery alone group had T2N1 (stage II) tumors. The addition of radiation did not result in an overall survival advantage. However, radiation significantly reduced local failure as the site of first failure for all patients (1% versus 21%).[215] The principal toxicity of postoperative radiation was esophagitis (24%) and was usually mild. Neurologic toxicity in the radiation group was surprisingly frequent, occurring in 10% of patients.

Chung compared 29 patients with T1–2 primary tumors and node-positive disease (79% N1, 21% N2) treated with surgery alone with 38 similarly staged patients (76% N1, 24% N2) who received an average of 4600 cGy postoperative radiation in addition to surgery. For the group with surgery alone, survival at 3 years was 10% compared with 40% with radiation and local control was 51% compared with 91% with radiation.[220] Ferguson reported a median survival of 13 months for 11 T1–2N1 patients treated with surgery alone, compared with 19 months for 7 patients who had surgery plus radiation and 46 months for 16 patients who received postoperative radiation and combination chemotherapy.[221] In contrast, Choi noted that for a group of T1–2N1 squamous carcinoma patients, 1-year disease-free survival was 8/21 for surgery alone compared with 12/22 when radiation was added ($p = 0.14$).[222]

In a retrospective analysis, Green demonstrated that only 3% (1/30) of resected patients with T1 or T2 primary lesions with resected positive hilar or mediastinal lymph nodes treated with surgery alone survived to 5 years compared with 35% (23/65) when radiation was added. One third of these node-positive patients had mediastinal disease. The survival rate of these patients and its dependence on radiation was not compared with that of the patients with only hilar involvement.[223] Overall, the retrospective data do not provide a clear picture of the impact of postoperative radiation on local control or survival of patients with stage II NSCLC.

Few data specifically address postoperative radiation therapy for T3 tumors. Piehler reported that postoperative radiation therapy did not improve survival (54% at 5 years) when used selectively for "some" of 31 patients with T3N0 tumors with chest wall invasion (not Pancoast tumors).[224] Trastek treated 73 patients with T3 (NX and N0/2) tumors involving the parietal pleura (not invading chest wall, not Pancoast tumors) and reported that postoperative radiation, which was used for 21% (15/73) of the patients, had no influence on survival.[225] In both these reports neither the selection factors for the use of radiation nor the therapeutic details were stated.

The prospective trial of the Lung Cancer Study Group included 22 patients with ipsilateral mediastinal lymph node involvement in each arm. In contrast to other groups, these patients with mediastinal spread receiving radiation had significantly fewer recurrences of any type (6/22) than those who did not receive radiation (13/22). Although radiotherapy appeared to prolong the disease-free interval for these patients, overall survival was not enhanced. These results are not conclusive but do raise the possibility that radiation may prolong the disease-free interval.[215] Israel randomized patients to receive 4500 to 5500 cGy mediastinal postoperative radiation rather than no radiation. Patients in both arms of the study were randomized to no additional treatments or to treatment with bacillus Calmette-Guérin (BCG), chemotherapy alone, or chemotherapy with BCG. The systemic therapy had no influence on outcome. The preliminary results showed that for node-positive patients disease-free survival was approximately 65% with radiation compared with approximately 40% without ($p = 0.26$).[226] This same trend was observed by Astudillo, who retrospectively compared the survival of 71 resected patients with mediastinal spread who received 4500 to 5000 cGy to the mediastinum and hila with that of 30 patients who did not. Although median survival was enhanced by 15 months compared with 6 months ($p = 0.07$), by 5 years the curves converged.[227] Several retrospective studies have addressed the role of postoperative radiation therapy but have not separated patients with mediastinal spread (stage IIIA) from those with hilar spread (stage II).[220,223] The retrospective analyses that have focused on patients with mediastinal lymph node involvement have suggested that postoperative radiation therapy may prolong survival.[228] Although retrospective reports raised the possibility that the survival of resected patients with mediastinal involvement at surgery could be enhanced by postoperative radiation, the prospective data do not support this.

After potentially curative resection of early-stage lung cancer, positive resection margins may occur at vascular margins, the chest wall, resected nodes, and most commonly the bronchial margin. Although the use of postoperative radiation therapy is the standard of care in this setting, it is not clear if it impacts on survival. Several factors may explain this; for example, most of these patients have positive nodes.[229] With or without adjuvant therapy, distant metastases are the predominant pattern of failure and as few as 33% of patients not receiving radiation may develop a clinically evident local recurrence.[230] Law reported that local failure occurred in 25% (3/12) of patients with positive margins who received between 4200 and 5000 cGy versus 29% (4/14) of those who did not.[230] This failure of radiotherapy to decrease the local recurrence rate may have been due to the low doses employed. Emami and colleagues reported a higher 4-year survival (28%) for 19 patients who received a higher dose of radiation including a cone down to the area of positive margin.[231]

Technique of Postoperative Radiation Therapy

Postoperative radiation for patients with microscopic residual disease or with resected hilar or mediastinal involvement needs to be planned carefully. The target volume is determined by correlating preoperative imaging studies, intraoperative findings, surgical clips, and the pathologic review of the resected specimen. The objective is to treat the ipsilateral hilum, the mediastinal nodes bilaterally, and the ipsilateral supraclavicular area. Peripheral primary tumors that do not abut the mediastinum or hilum and are not adjacent to the chest wall usually are removed with generous margins. After surgery, their preoperative location is occupied by relocated and uninvolved lung parenchyma, which does not need therapy. The commonest indications for irradiation of the primary tumor bed are central lesions or peripheral lesions abutting or involving pleura or chest wall. To determine the impact of surgical resection on the lung capacity, all patients should have repeat pulmonary function tests including flow rates, diffusing capacity, and arterial blood gases. This should be delayed until just before simulation to allow maximal recovery from postoperative pain, which can interfere with the patient's ability to perform these tests. The standard postoperative dose is 5040 cGy in 180-cGy fractions or 5000 cGy in 200-cGy fractions. Consequently, most of this dose can be given with energy greater than 6 MV using opposed anterior and lateral fields with appropriate attention to the spinal cord dose. Half-field wedges can be used to decrease the dose to the cord superiorly where the separation is less than at other levels. One approach is to deliver 4140 cGy to the target volume with these fields, which rarely deliver more than 4500 cGy to any portion of the cord, and to give the rest of the dose with fields that completely exclude the spinal cord (*i.e.,* opposed lateral fields for central or anterior tumors, and oblique fields for posterior or posterolateral tumors). It is important to deliver as much as possible of the total dose with anterior and posterior fields (while respecting cord tolerance), because all other field arrangements include more normal lung tissue. If the patient has a pneumonectomy, the dose to the remaining lung must be minimized. Oblique fields may be preferable. After penumonectomy it is important to take frequent beam films during therapy because the mediastinum shifts as the pneumonectomy cavity fills with fluid. More sophisticated planning using multiple fields from the start is advisable if it is necessary to treat a tumor bed that is adjacent to the vertebral column and spinal cord.

Adjuvant Chemotherapy After Complete Resection of NSCLC

Despite research over three decades, there is no proved role for any postoperative systemic therapy in stage I, II, or III NSCLC patients who have undergone complete surgical resections. No regimen has shown consistent improvements in either disease-free survival or overall survival in this setting. The use of adjuvant chemotherapy in patients with stage IIIA disease based on nodal spread remains unsettled. The accumulated experience in this area has laid the groundwork for future studies. This information, combined with the availability of more effective anticancer drugs, makes this a relevant area for study.

RATIONALE FOR ADJUVANT CHEMOTHERAPY. About one half of patients who develop NSCLC present with disease confined to the chest. Many of these patients can be technically resected; however, long-term survival rates are disappointing. Death in most resected patients is cancer-related and follows systemic recurrence. Because chemotherapy has been shown to induce objective regressions in NSCLC patients with metastatic disease, clinical trials have addressed the use of chemotherapy given postoperatively. It was theorized that the administration of chemotherapy after surgery could reduce treatment failures by eradicating circulating tumor cells and subclinical metastases not recognized at surgery. This approach has been successful in pediatric osteogenic sarcomas, Wilms' tumor, and breast cancer.

RESULTS OF COMPLETED ADJUVANT CHEMOTHERAPY TRIALS. Randomized prospective studies examining postoperative adjuvant chemotherapy in bronchogenic carcinoma were initiated in the 1960s. Initially, adjuvant single drug chemotherapy (nitrogen mustard and cyclophosphamide intrapleurally and intravenously) was used without any evidence of improved survival.[232,233] Two drug combinations were then tested (cyclophosphamide and methotrexate; lomustine and hydroxyurea), and again no significant difference in survival was observed when the treated group was compared with the untreated controls.[234] European studies confirmed the failure of single drug chemotherapy to influence survival after resection.[235,236]

In the 1980s, the Lung Cancer Study Group performed a series of randomized trials addressing the role of adjuvant therapy after surgery, testing intrapleural BCG, oral levamisole and intrapleural BCG, and cyclophosphamide, doxorubicin, and cisplatin (CAP) chemotherapy.[239,242,243]

Three recently completed trials have suggested some prolongation of disease-free survival rates with adjuvant treatment. When patients receive at least 50% of their planned chemotherapy dose, median survival seems to be prolonged.[241] The Lung Cancer Study Group demonstrated prolonged disease-free survival using CAP chemotherapy with radiotherapy in locally advanced incompletely resected disease.[242] However, the most recent Lung Cancer Study Group trial failed to demonstrate any advantage of CAP chemotherapy in early-stage disease.[243]

PREOPERATIVE (INDUCTION, PRIMARY, NEOADJUVANT) THERAPIES

Most stage III patients evaluated for resection other than T3 lesions have a disease extent that prohibits curative surgery or radiotherapy. Even if disease is confined to the chest at onset, most patients eventually develop metastases and die from systemic disease that largely cannot be addressed by surgery or radiotherapy alone or in combination. During the past decade, combination chemotherapy programs have been developed that produce reproducible rates of response in patients with stage IV NSCLC.[244] These same regimens have shown increased rates of response and better tolerability in patients with stage III disease in general and stage IIIA in particular.[244-246] The combination chemotherapy programs with the highest rates of response[244] and that have demonstrated modest but real improvements in survival[246,247] most often include cisplatin given at doses of 100 mg/m². In addition to causing regressions of intrathoracic tumors, combination chemotherapy has the potential to control systemic disease, the chief cause of mortality in this group. Regressions induced by chemotherapy can facilitate complete resections and theoretically can decrease the extent of radiotherapy fields required to provide lethal doses to the entire tumor volume. Chemotherapy given before surgery or radiation has the potential to allow the treatment of more advanced tumors and to facilitate the complete eradication of lesions. It may lessen treatment-related morbidity by decreasing the size of the "target" for the surgical or radiation oncologist.

Since the 1970s, investigators have tested the ability of combination chemotherapy before surgery to improve surgical and overall outcome. Three preoperative approaches employing primary chemotherapy have been tried—chemotherapy alone, chemotherapy with concomitant radiotherapy, and chemotherapy with sequential radiotherapy.

Preoperative radiation may improve resectability and destroy cancer cells beyond the margins of resection. The doses of radiation required preoperatively are generally lower than needed after surgery, when tissues become more hypoxic and therefore relatively radioresistant.

INDUCTION RADIATION THERAPY ALONE

The initial report of preoperative radiation for NSCLC was by Bromley and Szur in 1955.[248] From a large population of patients with early and intermediate stage disease, they selected 66 patients who responded to a median of 4700 cGy and performed resection and lymph node dissection. Complete tumor eradication in the primary tumor and nodes was detected in 47% (29/62) of evaluated patients. However, survival was poor, with approximately 17% alive at various follow-up times. This was accounted for in part by the 27% prevalence of bronchopleural fistula, all but one of which were fatal. Other groups have evaluated this approach and the results are summarized in Table 23–15. The accumulated data demonstrate no increase in resectability or survival with preoperative radiotherapy as the only induction treatment. Preoperative radiation is not recommended for stage I or II NSCLC patients who are appropriate candidates for complete surgical resection.

TABLE 23–15. Preoperative Radiation for Resectable Lung Cancer

Investigations	Dose (cGy)	No. of Patients	Resectable (%)	Tumor Eradication (%)	Fistula (%)	Survival (%) (y)
Bromley and Szur, 1955[248]	4700	66	100†	47	27	17 (?)
Bloedorn, 1964[504]	6000	83	55	35‡	25	16 (>1)
National Cancer Institute*	≥4000	290	61	?	9	14 (5)
Warram, 1975[505]	0	278	64	?	3	16 (5)
Veterans' Administration*	4000–5000	166	52	27	§	44 (1)
Shields, 1970[506]	0	165	55	0	§	69 (1)

* Randomized trial.
† Selected from a heterogenous population of 573 patients.
‡ Percentage applies to the resectable cases included in this table and the unresectable cases who received radiotherapy to render them resectable.
§ The incidence of fistula was comparable in both arms but was not enumerated.

INDUCTION CHEMOTHERAPY ALONE

Initial studies using various chemotherapy regimens suggested that preoperative chemotherapy could be administered and may be beneficial in this setting.[249,250] Martini demonstrated that otherwise resectable patients with ipsilateral mediastinal lymphadenopathy as their only site of distant spread could have 3-year survival of 43% and 5-year survival of 24% if both the primary tumor and ipsilateral mediastinal nodes were resected completely and followed by mediastinal irradiation.[251,252] In contrast, the same studies revealed that persons with ipsilateral mediastinal lymphadenopathy so large that it was clinically apparent on plain chest x-ray film had an 18% resectability rate and an 8% 3-year survival. Using combination chemotherapy with high-dose cisplatin (120 mg/m^2), vinca alkaloids, and mitomycin vinca alkaloid cisplatinum (MVP) preoperatively, a program was developed to use this regimen as primary chemotherapy in stage IIIA patients with clinically apparent ipsilateral mediastinal spread.[253] In a group of 73 patients, the objective major response rate to MVP chemotherapy was 77% with a 10% complete response rate. Overall, 60% of patients underwent complete resections and 12% had pathologic complete responses at surgery. The median survival was 19 months for all patients and 27 months for those with complete resections. The 3-year survival for the completely resected patients was 44%, a significant improvement over the previous surgery-only experience in which the 3-year survival was 8% ($p = 0.001$).[252] Two treatment-related deaths occurred. Using the MVP chemotherapy program before surgery, Burkes and colleagues reported a 69% chemotherapy response rate, a 49% complete resection rate, and a median survival of 19 months for all 35 patients studied.[254] Fossella recently has reported an ongoing randomized trial comparing surgery alone with the combined modality program of induction chemotherapy with etoposide, cyclophosphamide, and cisplatin before surgery.[255] He reports significant differences in 2-year survival and distant recurrence rate favoring the primary chemotherapy arm. A second randomized trial comparing surgery alone with cisplatin, mitomycin, and ifosfamide followed by surgery demonstrated a significant survival improvement among patients receiving induction chemotherapy.[255a]

INDUCTION CHEMOTHERAPY WITH CONCOMITANT RADIOTHERAPY

Cisplatin-based combination chemotherapy has been combined with concomitant radiotherapy in an effort to improve results. Faber and Bonomi have conducted two consecutive trials in clinical stage III NSCLC patients.[256] The first trial (FP) combined 5-fluorouracil (5-FU), cisplatin, and 4000 cGy of chest radiotherapy; the second (EFP) added etoposide to the regimen. The complete resection rate was 68% in the FC trial and 76% in the EFC program. Median survivals were 21 months and 34 months, respectively. The difference in survival was not significant. Four treatment-related deaths occurred in the two trials. The Lung Cancer Study Group combined 5-FU, cisplatin, and 3000 cGy of chest radiotherapy.[257] Overall, 42% of patients underwent a complete surgical resection, and a median survival of 11 months was observed overall. These results were similar to an earlier trial by the Lung Cancer Study Group employing CAP with 3000 cGy of chest irradiation in which a 33% resection rate and 11-month median survival were seen in stage III patients.[258] The Cancer and Leukemia Group B has tested the combination of 5-FU, vinblastine, cisplatin, and 3000 cGy in 32 stage IIIA patients.[259] The complete resection rate was 62% and three treatment-related deaths occurred. The Southwest Oncology Group (SWOG) has employed 4500 cGy with etoposide and cisplatin and has documented a 65% complete resection rate in a preliminary report.[260]

INDUCTION CHEMOTHERAPY WITH SEQUENTIAL RADIOTHERAPY

Skarin and colleagues have followed CAP chemotherapy with 3000 cGy of chest radiotherapy and surgical exploration in 41 patients with stage III NSCLC.[261] Complete resections were performed in 88% and the median survival for all patients was 32 months. Twenty-two of the 36 patients rendered disease-free have relapsed, 18 (66%) systemically. Sherman has reported the experience of the University of Massachusetts combining high-dose cisplatin and vindesine followed by 3000 cGy of radiotherapy.[262] The observed response rate with chemotherapy was 56%, the complete resection rate 62%, and the median survival was 27 months for the resected patients.

STATUS OF INDUCTION THERAPY PRECEDING SURGERY FOR STAGE III NON-SMALL CELL LUNG CANCER

As with all other therapies for patients with stages III and IV NSCLC, the optimal treatment of operable patients with stage IIIA NSCLC remains controversial. All patients should be encouraged to participate in prospective trials evaluating therapy for this stage of disease as their initial treatment program. The accumulated results of investigations in this area are extensive and can be used to define future research strategies and to guide the therapy of selected patients who cannot participate in prospective trials (Table 23–16).

Experience shows that this approach is feasible and that complication rates are not excessive when compared with rates of single-modality treatments for patients of similar stage. A variety of chemotherapy programs have been tried. A common thread is the drug cisplatin. The highest rates of response with chemotherapy alone employ cisplatin doses of 100 mg/m^2. Overall, response rates reported in all trials in stage IIIA patients generally exceed 50% and are higher than those seen for the same regimens in stage IV patients. The lowest response rates are seen with regimens containing cyclophosphamide, an agent with low single activity in this disease. Resection rates usually exceed 50% and median survivals range from 11 to 34 months, clustering around 20 months. The addition of radiation, concomitantly or sequentially, does not appear to substantially alter complete resection rates or

survival compared with chemotherapy alone in the trials reported. Outcomes in cooperative trials are inferior to those reported for the same programs initially tested in a single institution. Close cooperation among medical, radiation, and surgical oncologists is essential in the design and conduct of these combined modality trials. These studies demand the meticulous implementation of the optimal methods of supportive care (*i.e.*, prevention of cisplatin-induced nephrotoxicity and emesis, management of radiation-induced esophagitis and pneumonitis, and preoperative and postoperative pulmonary care), because most participants share the benefits and the adverse effects of each treatment modality employed.

What direction should future research in this area follow? One quarter or more of patients do not respond to induction chemotherapy regimens and most patients who do respond initially and undergo complete surgical resections relapse. Two thirds of the recurrences are systemic. This being the case, it appears unreasonable to look to further advances in surgery to improve survival. A review of the accumulated data suggests that adding radiotherapy to preoperative programs can add toxicity and does not appreciably improve resection rates or survival when compared with preoperative chemotherapy alone. The ability of a locoregional therapy modality like radiotherapy to control systemic relapse is inherently limited. Based on the accumulated results and relapse patterns, advancements in the chemotherapy regimens used in patients with clinical mediastinal lymphadenopathy are most likely to improve overall outcome.

Although response rates to chemotherapy are high in stage III patients, clinical and pathologic complete response rates generally are less than 20%. The overall experience with in-

TABLE 23–16. Induction Chemotherapy Programs Tested Preoperatively in Patients With Stage III Non-Small Cell Lung Cancer

	Investigations	No. of Patients	Chemotherapy	Response Rate (%)	Resection Rate (%)	Median Survival (Mo)
Induction Chemotherapy Only						
Memorial Hospital, NY	Pisters[253]	73	MVP	77	60	19
Toronto	Burkes[254]	39	MVP	64	46	19
M.D. Anderson Cancer Center	Fossella[255]	13	CEP	33	46	—
Barcelona	Rosell[255a]	22	MIP	63	77	18
Induction Chemotherapy With Concomitant Radiotherapy						
Rush-Presbyterian	Faber[256]	64	FP	56	68	20
Rush-Presbyterian	Faber[256]	29	EFP	—	76	34
Lung Cancer Study Group	Weiden and Piantados[257]	76	FP	51	42	11
Lung Cancer Study Group	Eagan[258]	42	CAP	51	33	11
Cancer and Leukemia Group B	Strauss[259]	41	FVP	51	59	16
Southwest Oncology Group	Albain[260]	65	EP	65	65	—
Induction Chemotherapy With Sequential Radiotherapy						
Dana-Farber	Skarin[261]	41	CAP	53	88	32
Worchester	Sherman[262]	21	VP	56	62	—

M, mitomycin; V, vinblastine or vindesine; P, cisplatin; C, cyclophosphamide; E, etoposide; F, 5-fluorouracil; A, doxorubicin (Adriamycin); I, ifosfamide.

duction chemotherapy has shown that persons with complete responses have the highest resection and survival rates. Complete response should be the initial major outcome evaluated in developing new induction programs. Regimens that do not increase the complete response rate are unlikely to affect long-term outcome and they should not be tested further. Another approach would be to develop strategies aimed at decreasing recurrence in patients rendered disease-free. Because 60% of recurrences occur in the first 2 years of treatment, therapies shown to improve this outcome could be identified in a short period.

PRIMARY RADIOTHERAPY FOR LUNG CANCER

STAGES I AND II NON-SMALL CELL LUNG CANCER

Some patients present with surgically resectable disease but have medical contraindications or refuse surgery. For such patients, primary radiation therapy offers an alternative and potentially curative approach.[263] The first published experience was from Hilton and Smart who gave 4000 to 5500 cGy using orthovoltage equipment to 38 patients. The crude survival was 17/38 (47%) at 2 years and 8/38 (17%) at 5 years.[264,265] Hong and colleagues treated 44 patients with 4000 cGy to the mediastinum and 5500 to 7000 cGy to the primary. The crude 5-year survival was 27% for the 22 patients receiving doses of less than 6100 cGy compared with 36% for the 22 patients receiving more than 6900 cGy, suggesting that high doses are superior.[266] Hafty and colleagues treated 43 patients, delivering a median of 5900 cGy in a continuous course to 11 patients and a median of 5400 cGy split course to 32 patients. Overall actuarial 5-year survival was 21%. Patients receiving continuous therapy had a lower thoracic failure rate and improved disease-free and overall actuarial survival rates compared with those receiving split-course radiation.[267] No other series with stages I and II NSCLC compare continuous and split-course treatment plans. Noordijk and colleagues used a 6000-cGy split course for 50 patients with surgically resectable well-staged T1–2N0M0 tumors. The fields were confined to the primary tumor. Permanent local control was achieved in 30% of patients (15/50) and the 5-year crude survival was 16%.[268] Both split and continuous courses are acceptable, with the split course being more practical and economical and the continuous course with smaller fractions being theoretically more sparing of late-responding normal tissues. For patients with poor pulmonary function, the potential benefit of elective nodal irradiation must be balanced against the possible damage induced by such therapy. Noordijk and colleagues, who treated patients without hilar adenopathy (T1–2N0), demonstrated that elective mediastinal irradiation may not be essential.[268] Therefore, radiation confined to the primary tumor alone appears to be acceptable for patients with N0 disease and pulmonary disease severe enough to preclude the safe use of elective mediastinal irradiation. There are no data addressing the omission of elective mediastinal irradiation for patients with N1 disease. In summary, primary external-beam irradiation therapy for early-stage NSCLC has acceptable morbidity, good local control, and good survival rates. Although the data are not conclusive, evidence supports the use of high doses to the primary tumor. The better results reported with surgery for early-stage disease may in part be due to the more favorable performance status of surgical patients and the fact that surgically treated patients are staged more rigorously and the results are reported by pathologic stage rather than clinical stage. Most patients who receive primary radiation therapy are not staged surgically and may have occult N2 (mediastinal) disease, and such patients may be excluded or reported separately in surgical series. An alternative approach, reported by Hilaris and colleagues, used brachytherapy with external radiotherapy in 55 patients with borderline pulmonary function.[269] Preoperatively, the patients had tumors considered resectable by lobectomy or a lesser procedure. At the time of surgery, however, a more radical procedure than the patient could tolerate was considered necessary. The gross tumor was implanted with intraoperative brachytherapy. After brachytherapy, 24 patients received a median dose of 4400-cGy external-beam irradiation therapy. The actuarial 5-year survival was 32%, suggesting that this approach was reasonable for patients who are found to be medically inoperable at the time of surgery.

STAGE IIIA (N2) NON-SMALL CELL LUNG CANCER

The conventional treatment of NSCLC with clinically evident ipsilateral mediastinal nodal metastases (N2 disease) has been radical radiation therapy. General considerations regarding the use of radical radiation therapy for locally advanced disease are addressed later in this chapter. Perez reported the outcome of patients with mediastinal disease treated on prospective Radiation Therapy Oncology Group (RTOG) protocols with doses of 4000 to 6000 cGy. The median survival was 12 months for T1N2 patients (n = 17), 10 months for T2N2 patients (n = 96), and 8 months for T3N2 patients. A subsequent RTOG study evaluated the effect of a range of doses of hyperfractionated radiation therapy (120 cGy given twice daily in a continuous course, 5 days per week). Survival at 1 year was 41% for T1–3N2 patients and 34% for T4N2 patients treated with 6960 cGy of hyperfractionated radiation. Patients with ipsilateral mediastinal lymph node involvement with a performance status of 80 or higher and weight loss of 5% or less (n = 50) who received 6960 cGy had a 1-year survival of 58% and 3-year survival of 20%, compared with 30% and 7% for similar patients (n = 59) treated with 6000 cGy on previous RTOG protocols. This promising preliminary experience suggests that this hyperfractionated approach may lead to long-term survival for selected patients. This program is being tested in an ongoing three-arm randomized trial comparing hyperfractionated radiotherapy (6960 cGy), standard fractionated (6000 cGy) radiotherapy, or standard radiotherapy preceded by cisplatin and vinblastine.

SELECTION OF PATIENTS

Generally accepted eligibility criteria for radical radiation therapy for lung cancer are based on extent and spread of tumor and on patient physiologic status. Distant metastases and pleural or pericardial effusions are contraindications. There are no strict tumor size criteria, but lesions (primary or nodal) in excess of 8 cm in diameter may not be suitable for treatment with radical intent.[271] A Karnofsky performance status of 60% or more is required, as is adequate pulmonary function. Bleehen and Cox have recommended that the vital capacity be 45% of predicted, the FEV$_1$ be 40% of predicted, the single breath diffusing capacity for carbon monoxide corrected for hemoglobin be 45% of predicted, the Pao$_2$ be greater than 60 mm Hg, and the Paco$_2$ be less than 49 mm Hg.[271] These figures should be used as guidelines rather than strict criteria, because radiation may improve performance status or relieve airway obstruction.

TECHNIQUE OF PRIMARY RADIATION THERAPY

The technical objectives of radical radiotherapy are to deliver a high dose (more than 6000 cGy) to gross disease, to give 5000 cGy to nodal drainage areas that are being treated electively, and to keep the dose to critical normal structures such as the spinal cord and lung parenchyma at or below safe levels. Pulmonary function tests are obtained before therapy. At initial simulation, patients are immobilized while supine in custom Alpha cradle molds (Smithers Medical Products, Akron, OH), which are used for all phases of planning and therapy. The arms are folded behind the head to allow the use of any oblique treatment angle. Anterior, posterior, lateral, and sometimes oblique films are taken. Next, CT scan slices are obtained at 1-cm intervals from the superior to the inferior extent of the simulated fields. On the hard copies of the CT scan (mediastinal and lung windows), the gross disease target volume is outlined by placing a 1-cm margin around radiographically visible primary tumor or nodal disease. Elective nodal target volumes are outlined using mediastinal windows by placing a 1-cm margin around the ipsilateral hilum and mediastinal drainage areas, the opposite mediastinum, the subcarinal region, and the ipsilateral supraclavicular area.

Computerized planning with lung density correction is used to select appropriate fields, wedges, compensators, beam weightings, and blocking to deliver the required doses to the target while keeping the spinal cord dose at approximately 4500 cGy and minimizing the dose to the lung (Fig. 23–14).

It is a mistake to deliver cord tolerance by anterior and posterior fields and then start the planning process. The latter approach may require posterior portions of the target volume to be excluded from further therapy (to avoid overdosing the cord) and consequently to be underdosed. This situation can be avoided by the use of appropriate oblique fields from the outset. Because the portion of treatment delivered off the spinal cord has to traverse normal lung, it is better to spread this dose over the entire course in lower doses per fraction. For radical cases, the total dose to gross disease should be more than 6000 cGy.

In deciding the total dose to gross disease, the patient's performance status, pulmonary function, and the proportion of dose delivered to lung tissue need to be taken into account. As discussed later in the chapter, there is a strong rationale for using doses as high as 7000 cGy, but this should not be done if the risk for pneumonitis is prohibitive. Unfortunately, there are no objective means of evaluating a plan to determine the actual risk for pneumonitis. Ongoing research correlating dose-volume histograms with quantitative changes in pulmonary function may provide a tool for this task.

THE IMPACT OF RADIATION ON THE NATURAL HISTORY OF LOCALLY ADVANCED NON-SMALL CELL LUNG CANCER

The principal question concerning radical radiation therapy for locally advanced lung cancer is whether it has sufficient impact on the natural history of the disease to justify its routine use as initial management.[272,273] The only prospective randomized trial that compared radiation therapy with no treatment was that performed by the Veterans Administration.[233] Between 4000 and 5000 cGy were delivered to 308 male patients with lung cancer with a variety of histologic subtypes (including SCLC), and 246 patients were treated with placebo. Although radiation had a significant influence on survival, the clinical impact was small with only 22% of radiation patients alive at 1 year compared with 16% of controls. Survival beyond

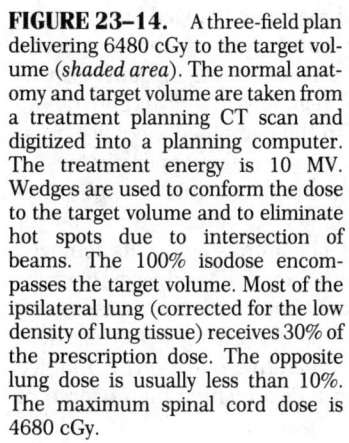

FIGURE 23–14. A three-field plan delivering 6480 cGy to the target volume (*shaded area*). The normal anatomy and target volume are taken from a treatment planning CT scan and digitized into a planning computer. The treatment energy is 10 MV. Wedges are used to conform the dose to the target volume and to eliminate hot spots due to intersection of beams. The 100% isodose encompasses the target volume. Most of the ipsilateral lung (corrected for the low density of lung tissue) receives 30% of the prescription dose. The opposite lung dose is usually less than 10%. The maximum spinal cord dose is 4680 cGy.

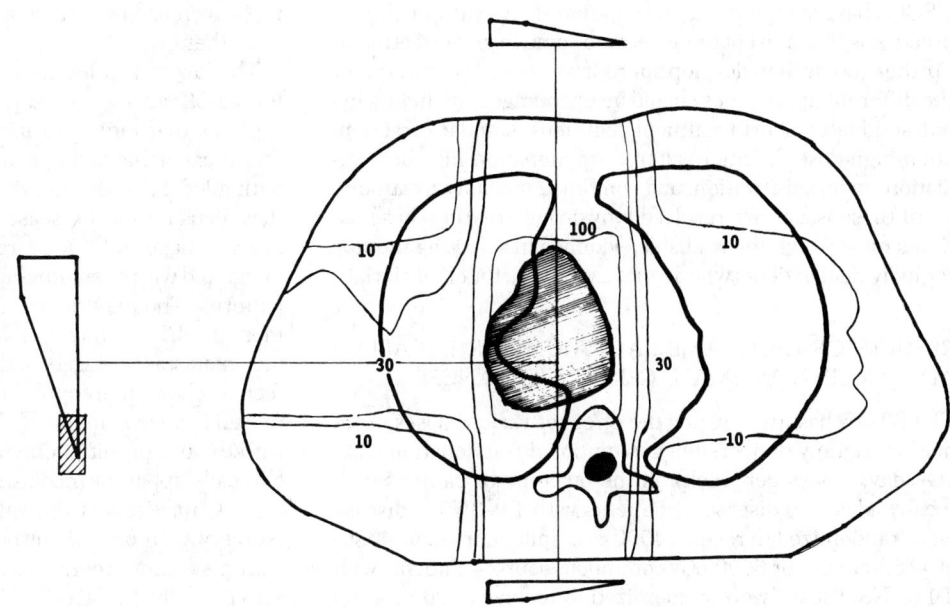

1 year was not reported. Unfortunately, this leaves many questions unanswered. The dose of radiation was small and was delivered with orthovoltage equipment. Most patients had a performance status of 70% or less. Such a low dose of radiation is unlikely to eradicate more than a small percentage of tumors, and significantly higher radiation doses and modern technique could impact on these results. Although these issues were first raised almost three decades ago, this basic question remains unanswered.

A subsequent trial begun in 1970 in the United Kingdom used similar doses of radiation for 48 patients.[273a] Survival was not increased compared with the control arms, which were treated with chemotherapy. Unfortunately, this trial had many of the same limitations as the Veterans Administration study. A recent multiinstitutional trial randomized over 300 patients to thoracic radiation, thoracic radiation with vindesine, or vindesine alone.[273b] Survival was comparable in all arms. In both radiotherapy-containing arms, however, 6000 cGy was delivered without the routine use of simulation, a standard procedure when administering radical radiation treatment. Even when simulation is used, and computer planning is applied, parts of the target volume can be underdosed significantly. By analyzing delivery of dose to target volumes on a three-dimensional (3D) system, Armstrong and colleagues demonstrated that underdosing of target volumes occurs in most patients treated with sophisticated conventional techniques.[274] This uncertainty about the actual tumor dose delivered, and the lack of a no-treatment control group, limits the strength of this study's conclusion. Using a different study design, Kubota and colleagues demonstrated improved survival in a group of patients receiving initial chemotherapy and then randomized to receive (n = 31) or not receive (n = 32) 5000 to 6000 cGy of thoracic radiation. Thoracic radiation significantly prolonged the time to progression and increased 2-year survival, which was 29% with radiation compared with 6% without radiation ($p < 0.05$).[275]

Although the impact of thoracic radiation on the natural history of locally advanced NSCLC remains unresolved, some practical considerations suggest that further efforts to address it are unlikely to be rewarding. Most patients with advanced NSCLC have symptoms at presentation. The reality of clinical practice is that most patients receive some form of treatment. Further research to develop appropriate selection criteria for the different approaches should be encouraged, including hypofractionated short-treatment regimens, standard fractionation high-dose radiation, altered fractionation high-dose radiation, radiosensitization, and combined modality treatment. Until these issues are resolved, physicians treating these patients must weigh the available evidence in selecting therapy for individual patients who are not candidates for clinical trials.

RESULTS OF HIGH-DOSE RADIATION FOR LOCALLY ADVANCED NON-SMALL CELL LUNG CANCER

The RTOG has investigated the effect of various doses of radiation therapy delivered in conventional fractionation (200 cGy/day, 5 days per week) on the outcome of patients with locally advanced disease.[276] Patients with T1–3N0–2 disease were randomized to receive 4000-cGy split courses, or 4000-cGy, 5000-cGy, or 6000-cGy continuous courses. Patients with T4 or N3 disease were randomized to receive 3000 or 4000

cGy continuous or split course. For patients with T1–3N0–2 disease (n = 379), overall median survival was approximately 9 months, and 5-year survival was 5%. Between 1 and 3 years the curves diverged showing a survival advantage for the use of 6000 cGy compared with lower doses. For stage T4 or N3 disease (n = 372), median survival was approximately 6 months and 3-year survival approximately 5%. There was no clear effect of dose on survival. For patients with T1–3N0–2 disease, complete response rates ranged from 9% with a 4000-cGy split course to 26% with a 6000-cGy continuous course. Similarly, major response rates (complete and partial) ranged from 47% with a 4000-cGy split course to 64% with a 6000-cGy continuous course. For patients with T4 or N3 disease, complete response rates occurred in approximately 15% for all doses and major response rates were approximately 45%.[276] The anatomic patterns of failure of 299 evaluable patients with T1–3N1–2 disease (78% of total) were reported by Perez. Patients treated with a 4000-cGy split course had a 53% failure rate within the irradiated lung. In 32% of the patients, infield failure was the only documented site of failure. Distant metastases occurred in 50% of the patients. Patients treated with 6000 cGy had a 35% failure rate within the irradiated lung. In 12% of patients, in-field failure was the only documented site of failure. Distant metastases occurred in 64% of patients.

The poor survival obtained with conventionally fractionated radiation therapy for locally advanced NSCLC cannot be attributed solely to the inability of a local treatment modality to control a disease with a marked propensity for distant spread. It may be due in part to the inadequacy of such therapy in achieving local control. A randomized trial that tested the value of chemotherapy added to 6500 cGy of external-beam irradiation demonstrates the failure of radiation to achieve local control.[277] By performing routine bronchoscopies during follow-up, Arriagada and colleagues showed that local control was less than 20% at 1 year in both arms. Possible reasons for the failure of radiation therapy to have a major impact on survival include the inadequate delivery of dose to target volumes, radioresistance, the deleterious effect of excessive toxicity on normal tissues, and the propensity for distant metastases overshadowing any beneficial effect of improvement in local therapy.

The low rate of local control does not detract from the potential of radiation therapy to improve outcome but rather suggests that efforts to increase its efficacy are justified so that it can achieve its primary objective of effectively eliminating local disease. Survival may be enhanced by strategies that focus on local disease control alone, as the experience of Cox suggests.[278] A more effective local modality can be integrated with chemotherapy regimens to address both failure patterns. The experience with the combined modality treatment of SCLC, which has an even greater propensity for distant metastases, suggests that the development of more effective chemotherapy is not likely to remove the need for radical local treatment.[279–281] The promising results achieved with the use of initial chemotherapy followed by surgery for clinically apparent mediastinal lymph node metastases from NSCLC may reflect the value of aggressive local treatment (surgery with or without postoperative radiation) combined with a systemic therapy with a documented high degree of activity against NSCLC.[282,283]

ALTERED FRACTION SCHEMES FOR NON-SMALL CELL LUNG CANCER: SPLIT-COURSE RADIATION THERAPY

There are several theoretical advantages to split-course radiation therapy. It is postulated that the interval between the courses (usually 2–4 weeks) allows for maximal recovery of acute toxicity. Normal cells may repopulate more quickly than cancer cells during the interval and reoxygenation and redistribution of cancer cells may occur, rendering them more radiosensitive during the second course. However, an accelerated repopulation of malignant cells may occur during this interval.[284] A significant number of patients develop metastases during this time, providing an opportunity to avoid unnecessary further local treatment. Several randomized trials have compared split-course with continuous radiation. Lee and colleagues treated patients with NSCLC that was considered unresectable and compared 5000 cGy given over 4 to 5 weeks (n = 86) to a split course of 5000 cGy given over 7 to 8 weeks (n = 102). They found no difference in response rates or survival.[285] Holsti randomized 158 patients to 5000 cGy in 5 weeks and 205 patients to a split course of 5500 cGy with a 2- to 3-week rest halfway through. Response rates, including minor responses, were increased slightly with split-course radiation (70% versus 56%), but survival was 40% at 1 year in both arms.[286] Both of these authors described less toxicity in the split-course arms. In a randomized trial of the RTOG, Simpson reported that a 4000-cGy continuous course gave response rates, palliation, and survival similar to the same dose delivered with larger fractions in a split course. Toxicity was similar in both arms with severe reactions occurring in 5% of the continuous-course patients and 8% of the split-course arm.[287] In a randomized trial that compared two split-course regimens, Guthrie reported that metastases occurred in 8% of patients during the interval.[288] These trials do not justify the routine use of split-course regimens. However, because the outcome is comparable with continuous courses, it is reasonable to use a split-course regimen with large fraction size to minimize the time and cost of treatment.

ACCELERATED RADIATION THERAPY FOR NON-SMALL CELL LUNG CANCER

Hyperfractionated radiation therapy is a method of intensifying radiation effect by delivering smaller dose fractions (*e.g.*, 120 cGy per fraction). This treatment often is given more than once per day, increasing the total daily dose to approximately 240 cGy or more. Consequently, if given in a continuous course 5 days per week, the treatment is described as *accelerated*. Theoretically, this approach has a greater effect against cancer cells and keeps chronic side effects at acceptable levels because of the low dose per fraction.

In a randomized phase I–II trial, Cox and colleagues used 6960 cGy of hyperfractionated radiation therapy for locally advanced NSCLC and reported a median survival of 13 months for patients with high performance status and minimal weight loss.[278] This improved survival over conventionally fractionated radiation therapy in standard doses provides the rationale for an ongoing randomized trial comparing standard fractionation treatment with or without chemotherapy. Saunders and colleagues from the United Kingdom have delivered 140 cGy

three times daily, 7 days per week, for a total dose of 5040 cGy over 12 days.[289] They reported complete responses in 46% (12/26) of evaluable patients with locally advanced disease. The major acute side effect was esophagitis, which necessitated a fluid diet but was usually minimal by 5 weeks after the start of therapy. The RTOG used an accelerated (not hyperfractionated) program and treated 56 patients with 180-cGy fractions to a volume containing gross disease and nodal areas and gave a simultaneous boost of 90 cGy to gross disease, thereby delivering 270 cGy per day to gross disease. The total dose to gross disease was 7500 cGy over 5.5 weeks. The overall response rate among the 44 patients who completed treatment was 73%, and acute toxicity was low. Only 20% of the 44 evaluable patients were alive between 1 and 3 years after therapy.[290] In conclusion, preliminary data suggest that accelerated fractionation may enhance local disease eradication and potentially impact on survival. There are no completed phase III trials addressing the value of this approach and it cannot be recommended for general use.

RADIOSENSITIZERS AND CONCOMITANT CHEMOTHERAPY AND RADIATION THERAPY

Radiosensitizers

Various agents have been used as radiosensitizers for locally advanced NSCLC with promising results in phase II trials. However, phase III randomized trials consistently have failed to demonstrate an increase in response rates or a survival advantage for several chemotherapy agents or for misonidazole. The role of cisplatin has been studied in three phase III randomized trials. The Hoosier Oncology Group failed to detect any advantage to cisplatin given at 3-week intervals during a course of 6000 cGy of radiation.[291] Minatel delivered 6 mg/m^2 of cisplatin daily with a modest dose of radiation (4500 cGy) and detected no advantage to the use of cisplatin.[292] In a three-arm randomized study involving 331 patients, the European Organization for Research for Treatment of Cancer compared no cisplatin, weekly low-dose (30 mg/m^2 weekly × 4) cisplatin, and daily low-dose (6 mg/m^2 daily × 20) cisplatin during 6600 cGy of radiation. The local control rates and survival were higher in the cisplatin arms and were highest in the daily cisplatin arm.[293] Lonidamine is a radiosensitizer and hyperthermia sensitizer that, in vitro, can inhibit the repair of potentially lethal damage induced in malignant cells by radiation.[294] In a phase II randomized trial, Privitera compared radiation (5500 cGy) with lonidamine or with placebo and found that response rates and survival were enhanced.[295] Because the number of patients was small, phase III trials are required to confirm these data. In summary, no conclusive data suggest that radiosensitizers have a favorable impact on the outcome of locally advanced NSCLC.

Combined Chemotherapy and Radiation Therapy

Because distant failure is common after radiation therapy for locally advanced NSCLC, attempts have been made to improve survival by adding chemotherapy to radiation therapy. Cyclophosphamide, 5-FU, nitrogen mustard, vinblastine, and vindesine have been used as single agents without improving survival.[296–305] Combination chemotherapy can produce higher response rates and potentially could be more efficacious in that setting.

The randomized trials comparing radiation with or without combination chemotherapy or other systemic treatment are detailed in Table 23–17. In a recent trial, the Cancer and Leukemia Group B randomized patients with locally advanced disease to receive 6000 cGy of thoracic radiation with (n = 78) or without (n = 77) induction chemotherapy with vinblastine (5 weekly courses of 5 mg/m²) and cisplatin (100 mg/m² twice). The patients were selected by having a performance status of greater than 80, weight loss of less than 5%, and a hematocrit of greater than 30%. Median survival was 14 months with chemotherapy compared with 10 months without chemotherapy (*p* = 0.006) and 3-year survival was 23% with chemotherapy compared with 11% without.[306] An ongoing intergroup study using similar selection criteria is attempting to confirm these data. A large randomized study from France tested the value of vindesine, cyclophosphamide, cisplatin, and lomustine added to 6500 cGy (split-course) of thoracic radiation. Survival was not increased by the addition of chemotherapy. Distant metastases were reduced significantly to 45% in the chemotherapy arm (n = 176) compared with 67% in the radiation alone arm (n = 177).[277] These data suggest a strong rationale for exploring the combined use of the most effective chemotherapy regimens with more effective thoracic radiation approaches. A combination of chemotherapy and radiotherapy was prospectively compared with the best supportive care in another randomized trial. The median

survival was 11 months for patients treated with 3 cycles of induction cisplatin (100 mg/m²) and etoposide (125 mg/m² intravenously day 1, 250 mg/m² orally days 2 and 3) followed by 4000 cGy of thoracic radiation (n = 53) compared with 7 months for best supportive care (n = 66; *p* = 0.05).[307] These findings suggest that combined therapy can alter the natural history of locally advanced NSCLC, although further studies are necessary.

TOXICITY OF RADIATION

Acute side effects begin during the second to third week of conventionally fractionated radiation. Dermatitis rarely is severe and can be minimized by avoiding trauma to and the use of cosmetics on treated skin. It is treated with aloe vera gel or perfume-free ointments containing petrolatum, mineral oil, mineral wax, and wool wax alcohol. Esophagitis usually presents as mild to moderate pain on swallowing, which may require a semisolid diet or analgesics (particularly in liquid form). Acute esophagitis generally does not progress to chronic esophagitis. Dry, nonproductive cough can be caused by a radiation effect in the trachea or bronchi and can persist for prolonged periods after radiation is completed.

Radiation pneumonitis is the commonest significant complication of radical radiation and can be fatal in a small percentage of patients. Its incidence is related to dose, fractionation, and volume of lung irradiated. Typically it manifests as fever, dyspnea, tachycardia, and hypoxia. The diffusing ca-

TABLE 23–17. Randomized Trials of Radiation Therapy With and Without Systemic Therapy for Locally Advanced Non-Small-Cell Lung Cancer

Investigations	Radiation Therapy (cGy) (No. of Patients)	Systemic Therapy (No. of Patients)	Median Survival (Mo)	
			Without Systemic Therapy	With Systemic Therapy
VALG Petrovich, 1977[507]	5000–6000 (171)	CCNU, hydroxyurea (174)	6	7
Southwest Oncology Group White, 1982[508]	6000 (49)	Adria, levamisole (33)	11	6
SECSG Krauss, 1984[509]	4000–6000 (118)	Levamisole (112)	11	10
Radiation Therapy Oncology Group Perez, 1988[510]	6000 (129)	Levamisole (131)	12	9
FSGLC Mattson, 1988[511]	5500 (119)	CAP (119)	10	11
North Central Cancer Treatment Group Morton, 1988[512]	6000 (53)	MACC (54)	9	10
Italy Trovo, 1990[513]	4500 (62)	CAMP (49)	11	10
Radiation Therapy Oncology Group Asbell, 1990[514]	6000 (81)	Thymosin (87)	ND	ND
Cancer and Leukemia Group B Dillman, 1990[246]	6000 (77)	Vbl, cis (78)	10	14
France Arriagada, 1991[277]	6500 (177)	Vnd, cyt, cis CCNU (176)	10	12

CCNU, lomustine; Adria, doxorubicin (Adriamycin); CAP, cyclophosphamide, doxorubicin, cisplatin; MACC, methotrexate, doxorubicin, cyclophosphamide, CCNU. CAMP, Cyclophosphamide, doxorubicin, methotrexate, procarbazine; Vnd, vindesine; Cyt, cyclophosphamide; Cis, cisplatin; Vbl, vinblastine, ND, no difference; VALG, Veterans' Administration Lung Group; FSGLC, Finnish Study Group for Lung Cancer; SECSG, Southeastern Cancer Study Group.

pacity may be decreased in the early phase and may be preceded by exercise-induced oxygen desaturation. Radiographs show diffuse, nonhomogenous opacification largely confined to the port. If it is symptomatic and if other processes have been excluded, it is treated with prednisone (1 mg/kg/day). Prophylaxis against *Pneumocystis carinii* pneumonia with trimethoprim sulfamethoxazole during prednisone therapy is recommended. Steroids should be tapered slowly to avoid exacerbations. Patients who have received thoracic radiation and have never exhibited any signs of pneumonitis and who are given high-dose steroids for other reasons can develop pneumonitis when the steroids are discontinued. Corticosteroids have little impact on radiation damage that has already progressed to fibrosis. There is no indication for the routine use of antibiotics or anticoagulants.

SUPERIOR SULCUS TUMORS

The management of superior sulcus tumors (Pancoast's tumors) is controversial. Radiation therapy is an essential component of treatment as sole therapy, preoperative therapy, postoperative therapy, or as intraoperative brachytherapy. The use of preoperative radiation therapy has been pioneered by Shaw and colleagues. Preoperative doses of 3000 to 3500 cGy were used to reduce the volume of tumor, thereby facilitating complete resection. Operations were performed 1 month after the completion of radiation to allow time for pain relief, improvement in performance status, and resolution of skin changes facilitating good wound healing and, in some patients, to exclude the emergence of distant metastases that would make radical local therapy inappropriate. In the initial report of this procedure, 5 of 9 patients followed for more than 1 year were disease-free.[308] Serious complications related to combined radiation and surgery include brachial plexus deficits, Horner's syndrome, postoperative respiratory problems, and myelitis.

A variety of preoperative doses of radiation have been used and survival figures range from 20% to 34% at 5 years. The usual technique is to use paired anterior and posterior fields. The dose received by the spinal cord must be calculated superiorly. If the dose exceeds 105% of the prescription dose, a half-field wedge is used as a cord dose-compensator. It is crucial to use CT scans or MRI scans or both to determine field borders. Because these tumors can extend superiorly in the paravertebral region, the upper border should be at the level of the thyroid notch and the larynx should not be blocked. The lateral border should cover the entire supraclavicular fossa

and be at least 3 cm lateral to gross disease. The medial border should be 2 cm beyond the contralateral border of the vertebrae. If mediastinoscopy is negative, the lower border should be just below the carina.

Radiation therapy has been used postoperatively for patients not receiving preoperative radiation and in those who have positive nodes or involved margins despite preoperative radiation. Hilaris used surgery with intraoperative brachytherapy for most of the 36 patients followed by postoperative radiation and reported 20% 5-year survival.[309]

Shahian treated 18 patients with 3000 to 4000 cGy preoperatively and gave 2000 to 3500 cGy postoperatively to 14 of these patients who had positive nodes or positive resection margins. The 5-year survival was 56%. The technique of postoperative radiation is similar to preoperative radiation until spinal cord tolerance is reached (approximately 4500–4600 cGy in 180-cGy fractions), at which point a block is added to exclude the spinal cord and opposite mediastinum with a total dose of approximately 5000 cGy.[310]

Generally accepted contraindications to surgery in patients with superior sulcus tumors include extensive involvement of the brachial plexus, involvement of the subclavian artery, vertebral bodies, esophagus, mediastinal node metastases, or distant metastases. Patients with unresectable T4 tumors or mediastinal nodal metastases can be treated with radical radiation. In general, fields are designed as described earlier in this chapter. After excluding the spinal cord at tolerance dose, the anterior and posterior fields are continued to more than 6000 cGy. Series of 20 patients or more receiving radical radiation alone are summarized in Table 23–18. It is difficult to compare these results with those of combined surgery and radiation because of the selection of patients with better performance status and less advanced disease for combined surgery and radiation. This has prompted many authors to question if combined therapy is better than radical radiation alone. Beyer reported 48% 5-year survival for 15 patients treated with radiation and surgery compared with 0% for 13 patients treated with radiation alone. However, the authors point out that there was a definite adverse selection bias for treatment with radiation alone.[311] Similarly, Komaki reported that survival at 2 years was 22% (13/60) without surgery compared with 52% (13/25) when surgery was a component of therapy. The survival advantage associated with the use of surgery was restricted to patients with weight loss of less than 5%.[312] Neal and colleagues reported that despite adverse selection for therapy with radical radiation alone there was no survival advantage with combined surgery and radiation but that severe

TABLE 23–18. Primary High-Dose Radiation Alone for Pancoast Tumors

Investigations	No. of Patients	Dose (cGy)	Severe Complications (%)	Survival (y)
Attar, 1979[515]	29	5500–6000	No data	7% (3)
Komaki, 1981[516]	36	4000–6400	0	23% (5)
Van Houtte, 1984[517]	31	2000–7000	0	18% (5)
Anderson[453]	27	4900 (mean)	No data	0% (5)
Komaki[312]	31	6000–6600	6	23% (5)
Neal[313]	32	5600–7500	3	13% (5)

complications were more frequent in the combined arm (21%, 6/29) compared with the radiation alone arm (3%, 1/32).[313] Because superior sulcus tumors are uncommon, it is unlikely that a randomized trial addressing this issue can be performed and it is not possible to determine the better approach. Surgery should be reserved for patients with clearly resectable disease, better performance status, and minimal weight loss. Radical radiation or investigational approaches may be considered for others.

INNOVATIVE RADIATION TECHNIQUES

Conformal Three-Dimensional Treatment Planning

Conformal three-dimensional (3D) treatment planning is a technique whereby precise anatomic data accumulated from high resolution CT scans are used to build a computerized 3D image of a patient's normal structures and the tumor. The optimal radiation beam parameters and orientation are selected by objectively comparing candidate plans using calculations and visual displays. This approach has the potential to maximize the delivery of the prescribed dose to target volumes while reducing the exposure of normal structures. Armstrong and colleagues compared the use of conventional and 3D planning for locally advanced lung cancer and demonstrated that the delivery of high-dose radiation to the target volume was significantly better with the 3D system. The 3D system reduced the dose to the lungs.[314] Future phase I–II trials will determine the clinical impact of this technologic advance.

Neutrons

Because neutrons deposit energy in a dense distribution, they can overwhelm the repair capacity of a cell and overcome the ability of a malignant cell to repair damage. Hypoxic tumors may be sensitive to neutron cell damage because such damage does not depend on the presence of molecular oxygen. Theoretically, neutron therapy should be useful for large lung tumors that contain resistant hypoxic components.

Schnabel randomized 48 patients to receive 1800 cGy (neutron) and compared the outcome with 67 controls receiving 5400 cGy (photon) and reported no advantage in local control or survival. With increased follow-up, patients treated with neutrons developed a higher incidence of pneumonitis.[315] The RTOG randomized patients to three arms: 6000 cGy of photons (n = 39), 1800–2000 cGy of neutrons (n = 29), or combined neutrons and photons (n = 34). Median survival was 8, 8, and 7 months, respectively. Severe toxicity rates (mostly pulmonary) were 5%, 31%, and 15%, respectively, confirming the increased risk of therapy with neutrons observed by Schnabel.[316] In an attempt to limit this late toxicity, Livingston and colleagues used smaller neutron fields that were limited to areas of residual disease after induction chemotherapy. The high rates of toxicity were avoided, but high rates of thoracic failure were noted, particularly outside the port.[317] The equipment used for these trials was not customized for patient treatment and had practical limitations that may have contributed significantly to overdosage and toxicity. An ongoing randomized trial of the RTOG uses modern neutron treatment facilities and is comparing the results with standard photon therapy.

Intraoperative Brachytherapy and Radiation

The implantation of radioactive isotopes has been investigated to allow the precise localization of dose in the tumor and to spare adjacent normal tissues because of the limited penetration of the low-energy emission. High total tumor dose in the range of 16,000 cGy is feasible because of the low dose rate (approximately 8 cGy/hour).[318] If there is gross residual disease greater than 1 cm in width, a volume implant is required using hollow needles and the Mick afterloader (Mick Industries, New York, NY). Plaques of residual disease or areas of possible microscopic disease are covered with a planar implant performed by direct suturing of iodine 125 seeds encapsulated in vicryl or by evenly spacing suture seeds in a premeasured polyglycolic acid mesh and suturing the mesh directly onto the area at risk.[319] The latter technique is well suited to areas such as the major vessels or paraspinal region.[314]

The results achieved with this approach for stages I and II medically inoperable tumors and Pancoast's tumors have previously been discussed. Hilaris reported on 101 patients with unresectable primary tumors invading major vessels, pericardium, or esophagus who were treated with biopsy only, brachytherapy, and external-beam irradiation. These patients had no evidence of mediastinal metastases at thoracotomy. Median survival was 11 months, and 2-year survival was 21%. Hilaris reported 100 patients with stage III disease. Iodine 125 implants were performed for unresected or incompletely resected primary tumors and iridium 192 implants were used for mediastinal disease. Local control was more than 70% at 5 years and survival was 22%.[320] Despite these results, intraoperative brachytherapy has not been adopted widely, because its superiority to external radiation alone has not been demonstrated clearly.

Intraoperative Radiation

Intraoperative radiation using linear accelerators with modified cones has been reported.[321] The cone is applied to the area at risk. Normal structures that are not involved by the cancer are retracted or covered with custom blocks. Electron energies are selected to cover the required depth appropriately. Doses in the range of 1000 to 2500 cGy are given in a single fraction in the operating room. The NCI reported that 2 of 4 patients died due to complications and the other 2 experienced life-threatening fistulae.[322] In Austria, 21 patients with negative nodes after mediastinal dissection received 1000 to 2000 cGy of intraoperative electron therapy to unresected primary tumors. This was supplemented postoperatively by 4500 to 4600 cGy external-beam irradiation. Responses were documented by CT scan as early as 4 weeks and improved with time, eventually leading to 33% complete response rate and a disease-free survival of 90% (19/21) at a median follow-up of 1 year. The good results in this group of patients may be due to the negative nodes and the fact that many of the tumors were resectable early-stage tumors in medically unfit patients. Only 1 patient died due to therapy.[323] Less favorable results were obtained in Spain, where 34 patients with unresected or incompletely resected primary or nodal tumors received an intraoperative dose of 1000 to 1500 cGy followed by 4600 to 5000 cGy external-beam irradiation postoperatively. Acute pneumonitis occurred in 35% (12/34), median survival was 12 months, and freedom from thoracic progression occurred in 30%.[324] The limited experience with intraoperative radiation for NSCLC fails to demonstrate that it is superior to radical external-beam irradiation therapy alone. In view of its frequent toxicity, use of intraoperative radiation remains experimental.

Prophylactic Cranial Irradiation for Locally Advanced Non-Small Cell Lung Cancer

The hypothesis that prophylactic cranial irradiation (PCI) can improve survival is based on the assumption that isolated brain failures occur commonly and lead to death and that these can be effectively prevented by tolerable doses of radiation. Isolated brain failures are not common and it is not possible to predict the patients at risk. Consequently, it is unlikely that survival would be improved significantly if effective prophylaxis were delivered to the entire population of resected patients. Of 1532 patients treated surgically on prospective trials of the Lung Cancer Study Group, only 6.8% (104/1532) had first recurrences in the brain. Seventy-one percent of the patients in this series had T1–2N0 tumors. Patients with locally advanced disease treated with thoracic radiation on the RTOG protocols had an initial brain failure rate of 7% for squamous histology, 19% for adenocarcinoma, and 13% for large cell carcinoma. Even for adenocarcinoma, the brain is a less common site of initial failure than bone (24%) and the opposite lung (21%).[325]

Four randomized trials of PCI added to chest radiation (with and without chemotherapy) have been reported for patients with locally advanced disease and have not demonstrated improved survival with PCI. Cox and colleagues reported that 2000 cGy of PCI reduced brain failures to 6% among 136 patients compared with 13% among 145 patients treated without PCI.[326] A randomized trial of PCI used 3000 cGy and reduced CNS metastases to 4% (of 46 patients) compared with 27% (of 51 patients) without PCI.[327] Similarly, a SWOG study of 254 patients showed that 3000 to 3750 cGy reduced brain failures from 11% without PCI to 0% with PCI.[338] The RTOG randomized patients with adenocarcinoma and large cell tumors and reported that PCI of 3000 cGy reduced brain failures to 9% (8/93) compared with 19% (18/94) without PCI ($p = 0.1$).[329] Because PCI reduces brain failure without affecting survival, the major issues are the optimal dose and fractionation schedule, whether initial PCI or delayed therapeutic cranial irradiation for selected patients improves ultimate neurologic status, and whether the advent of more effective thoracic and systemic therapy changes the anatomic pattern of failure and prompts a reappraisal of the role of PCI. Currently, PCI cannot be recommended for any stage of NSCLC and its use remains under investigation.

CHEMOTHERAPY FOR LUNG CANCER

CURRENT STATUS

Although chemotherapy programs induce predictable and reproducible responses in NSCLC patients and produce modest but real improvements in survival, no regimen is completely effective and none has led conclusively to cure. There is no standard chemotherapy program for this disease. All appropriate patients with inoperable NSCLC should be encouraged to participate in clinical trials as initial therapy. The improvements in response and survival achieved through investigations of chemotherapeutic agents over the past 15 years merit attention. Not only can this experience be used to guide the treatment of selected patients who cannot take part in clinical trials, but it has established study methodology and a foundation on which future treatment programs can be built.

WHO SHOULD RECEIVE CHEMOTHERAPY?

Performance status remains the single most important pretreatment factor that predicts response, response duration, and survival for NSCLC patients receiving chemotherapy.[331] Most trials have been conducted in persons with a Karnofsky performance status of 60% or greater, and there is no evidence of the usefulness of chemotherapy for persons with a performance status less than 50%. Response rates are lower for patients with a performance status of 60% to 70% compared with those with a status of 80% or greater.[331] When results in phase II trials are compared, persons who previously received chemotherapy demonstrate lower rates of response than patients without previous chemotherapy.[332] The toxicity of therapy can be appreciably greater in patients with lower performance status.[333] Available chemotherapy programs have been tested formally only in patients with normal cardiac, pulmonary, hematopoietic, hepatic, neurologic, and renal function and cannot be recommended for use in patients with significant dysfunction of any major organ system. The use of chemotherapy, particularly in these settings, remains under investigation.

DEVELOPMENT AND SELECTION OF CHEMOTHERAPY AGENTS

In 1949, Karnofsky and Burchenal defined endpoints in chemotherapy studies and established guidelines for the development of anticancer agents.[334] They stressed the evaluation of subjective and objective endpoints and cautioned against judging an agent's usefulness based on any single criterion. They established standards to guide agent development. First, they observed that only agents with demonstrated anticancer activity can possibly prolong survival or change the natural history of cancer in patients. Second, Karnofsky and Burchenal noted that even though most useful anticancer agents demonstrate a range of activity, overall response rates must be predictable and reproducible. Third, toxicity is an important concern and must be taken into account when considering any agent's usefulness. Fourth, because no single agent is likely to be curative in and of itself, drugs should be used in combination. A corollary of this last concept is that even from a drug's early development, its potential use in combination should be taken into account. If the degree of toxicity of a single agent precludes its use in combinations, it is unlikely to have a significant impact on any given cancer. The usefulness and validity of these concepts has been demonstrated in the development of every curative and uniformly effective chemotherapy program.

For NSCLC, a 15% or greater major objective response rate demonstrated in multiple single agent phase II trials is considered the threshold of clinical usefulness.[332] Agents with activity below this level are unlikely to have a significant impact on this disease. When designing combination regimens, each agent included should meet or exceed the 15% threshold of single-agent activity. When this approach is followed, each agent generally adds its activity to the regimen. For example, if cisplatin and vindesine, each of which has activity in the 15% to 20% range,[332] are combined, the two-drug combination yields a 43% major objective response rate.[335] If mitomycin is added, another drug with activity in the 20% range,[336] the observed response rate increases to 60%.[337] Conversely, when agents with activity less than 15%, such as cyclophosphamide, doxorubicin, and bleomycin, are added to the two-drug regimens, there is little or no improvement in response rates, and the toxicity of the regimen is heightened and often forces the attenuation of the active drugs in the regimen.[332,338]

When developing combination programs, component drugs should be selected to take advantage of their differing mechanisms of action and toxicities. Careful attention should be paid to the dose and schedule of the individual drugs because they should vary little from that used in the single agent-trials that proved the agent's effectiveness and safety in NSCLC patients. Dose attenuations should occur only in the face of toxicity that cannot be controlled by aggressive supportive care measures. Established supportive care measures, such as the use of combination antiemetics to control vomiting caused by cisplatin or the use of filgrastim (G-CSF) to lessen chemotherapy-induced neutropenia, are integral parts of chemotherapy regimens and should be standardized and built into chemotherapy programs as they are designed.

These guidelines are important considerations in selecting individual drugs for study and designing combination chemotherapy regimens. They also can assist the clinician who must choose a chemotherapy program for a patient from among the many regimens tested. The best results in advanced NSCLC patients are provided by regimens of individually active drugs with nonoverlapping toxicities that are given at dosages and schedules tested in phase II trials and according to proved methods of supportive care.

COMPLETED CHEMOTHERAPY TRIALS

Single Agents

More than 50 chemotherapeutic agents have been tested in NSCLC patients in the past two decades. Although the trials have varied and the true response rates for many agents in epithelial lung cancer cannot be determined conclusively, only five agents have response rates generally accepted to be 15% or greater after testing in at least 14 patients. These five agents are cisplatin, ifosfamide, mitomycin, vinblastine, and vindesine.[332] These same five agents also yielded the best results when used in combination chemotherapy trials in a meta-analysis of 100 reports involving more than 6000 NSCLC patients.[244]

Cisplatin has been crucial to the development of effective chemotherapy for advanced NSCLC. Only since its introduction have we been able to establish treatment programs that could reliably and reproducibly induce major objective regressions in this disease. Cisplatin is the foundation of virtually all the most effective combination chemotherapy programs

tested in advanced NSCLC patients. In ten single-agent trials of cisplatin in 497 patients, the overall major objective response rate was 21%.[339–348] These same single-agent trials suggest a dose-response relation for cisplatin in this disease with objective response rates of 15% or less at doses of 30 mg/m²/week,[339–345] 25% with cisplatin doses of 40 mg/m²/week,[346] and 38% with planned doses of 50 mg/m²/week.[347,348] In the meta-analysis of 100 completed combination chemotherapy studies, trials using cisplatin given at doses of 100 mg/m² in combination with other agents had higher response rates than trials employing cisplatin at doses of 70 mg/m².[244]

Although intravenous etoposide, carboplatin, 5-FU, doxorubicin, and cyclophosphamide commonly are used alone and in combination regimens in the treatment of NSCLC, each has an overall response rate of less than 15% when tested in single-agent phase II trials.[332] Intravenous etoposide alone has a pooled response rate of 8% in five trials evaluating 262 patients.[349,350] In a recent multicenter randomized trial comparing intravenous etoposide along with intravenous etoposide and cisplatin, the 7% observed major response rate with etoposide was inferior to the 26% response rate of the two-drug regimen ($p > 0.005$).[350] Activity may be improved by giving prolonged courses of oral etoposide.[351] Carboplatin has produced a 12% response rate in five trials studying 295 patients.[352–356] All trials reported leukopenia, thrombocytopenia, and vomiting. A multicenter randomized trial compared carboplatin with cisplatin when each was used in combination with etoposide. The major objective response rate was 16% with carboplatin and etoposide and 27% with cisplatin and etoposide.[357]

Combination Chemotherapy Regimens

General Considerations

During the past two decades, hundreds of articles have reported the testing of combination chemotherapy programs in patients with advanced NSCLC. A recent review by Donnadieu and colleagues analyzes the varying results.[244] They noted higher response rates in the following three cases: (1) combinations tested in stage III compared with stage IV patients; (2) combinations of cisplatin, vindesine, vinblastine, mitomycin, and ifosfamide; and (3) cisplatin used at doses of 100 mg/m². The more common chemotherapy regimens are presented in Table 23–19. For all regimens, response and survival information obtained in confirmatory studies shows a range of results that in general are lower than those presented in the original report. Cooperative groups usually report lower rates of response and shorter survival than rates seen in single institutions. Despite these differences, the most useful regimens show the highest and most consistent rates of response and survival. Results reported later in this chapter reflect testing of these regimens as the initial chemotherapy given to each patient.

CISPLATIN AND VINDESINE. Gralla and colleagues reported a 40% major objective response rate in 40 advanced NSCLC patients treated with vindesine and cisplatin (120 mg/m²).[355] The overall survival was 10 months. The group of patients treated with cisplatin at 120 mg/m² had significantly longer response durations and responding patients had longer survivals than those randomized to receive cisplatin at

TABLE 23–19. Combination Chemotherapy Programs for Advanced Non-Small Cell Lung Cancer Patients

Chemotherapy Program	Response Rates in Initial Report (%)	Range (%)
Cisplatin plus vindesine[335]	40	16–40
Cisplatin 120 mg/m² day 1, 29 then q 6 wk		
Vindesine 3 mg/m² day 1, 8, 15, 22, 29 then q 2 wk		
Cisplatin plus vinblastine[364]	41	13–52
Cisplatin 120 mg/m² day 1, 29 then q 6 wk		
Vinblastine 5 mg/m² day 1, 8, 15, 22, 29 then q 2 wk		
Cisplatin plus etoposide[370]	38	20–38
Cisplatin 60 mg/m² day 1 then q 3–4 wk		
Etoposide 120 mg/m² day 4, 6, 8 then q 3–4 wk		
Mitomycin plus vindesine[518]	36	10–36
Mitomycin 10 mg/m² day 1, 22 then q 6 wk		
Vindesine 3 mg/m² day 1, 8, 15, 22, 29 then q 2 wk		
Cisplatin plus vindesine plus mitomycin[374]	60	—
Cisplatin 120 mg/m² day 1, 29 then q 6 wk		
Vindesine 3 mg/m² day 1, 8, 15, 22, 29 then q 2 wk		
Mitomycin 8 mg/m² day 1, 29, and 71 only		
Cisplatin plus vinblastine plus mitomycin[376]	67	13–73
Cisplatin 120 mg/m² day 1, 29 then q 6 wk		
Vinblastine 4 mg/m² day 1		
2 mg/m² day 8		
4.5 mg/m² day 15, 22, 29 then q 2 wk		
Mitomycin 8 mg/m² day 1, 29, and 71 only		

doses of 60 mg/m². Since that report, at least seven trials have tested similar regimens employing vindesine and cisplatin at doses of 100 mg/m².[333,347,358–362] Major objective response rates have varied from 25% to 35% and median survivals from 6.5 to 11.0 months. Overall, a 26% rate of response (95% confidence interval 25% to 33%) has been observed among 691 patients enrolled in eight trials. Reported toxicities include myelosuppression, peripheral neuropathy, ototoxicity, vomiting, and alopecia.

VINBLASTINE AND CISPLATIN. The two-drug regimen combining cisplatin (120 mg/m²) with vinblastine was tested initially by two groups who reported response rates of 52% and 41%, and median survival of 5.5 and 12.3 months.[363,364] Four additional trials using vinblastine and cisplatin (100 mg/m²) report response rates ranging from 15% to 36% and median survivals ranging from 5.3 to 7.5 months.[246,365–367] The overall rate of response reported for these six trials is 26% (99/375) and the resulting 95% confidence interval is 22% to 31%. Toxicities are qualitatively similar to those of the vindesine-cisplatin regimen. Two trials tested cisplatin given at 60 mg/m² with vinblastine yielding an overall response rate of 16% and median survivals of 6.3 and 7.0 months.[368,355]

CISPLATIN AND ETOPOSIDE. The significant activity of this regimen was demonstrated by Sierocki and Wittes in SCLC.[369] Longeval and Klastersky tested this combination using cisplatin (60 mg/m²) in 94 patients with advanced NSCLC. They observed a 38% major objective response rate and a median survival of 7.5 months.[370] Since then, the program has been studied in at least seven trials with response rates ranging from 12% to 38% and median survivals ranging from 5.3 to 8.3 months.[333,350,357,361,371–373] The overall rate of re-

sponse for this regimen tested in 647 patients is 28% and the 95% confidence interval is 25% to 32%. Common adverse effects include leukopenia, thrombocytopenia, alopecia, vomiting, peripheral neuropathy, and ototoxicity.

Three trials tested etoposide with cisplatin given at a dose of 100 mg/m².[366,372,345] The pooled response rate was 21% and the median survival ranged from 5.3 to 7.0 months. One of these trials randomly assigned patients given the same dose of etoposide to receive cisplatin at 60 mg/m² or cisplatin at 120 mg/m². No significant differences in outcome were reported.

MITOMYCIN AND VINDESINE AND CISPLATIN. Kris and colleagues reported a 60% major objective response rate and 11-month median survival among 90 patients given cisplatin at 120 mg/m² with vindesine and mitomycin.[374] Two trials have tested regimens employing cisplatin 60 mg/m² with vindesine and mitomycin. Joss noted a 41% response rate and an 8-month median survival.[375] Einhorn reported a 20% major objective response rate and 4.3-month median survival.[360] Myelosuppression was more common and more severe than that seen in the two-drug vindesine and cisplatin trials. Mitomycin-induced pulmonary effects were seen in 2% of patients.[374]

MITOMYCIN AND VINBLASTINE AND CISPLATIN (MVP). Gralla and colleagues conducted a prospective trial to define a suitable dose of vinblastine when used in combination with mitomycin and cisplatin (120 mg/m²) given at doses and schedules tested in the previous trials with vindesine.[376] The best schedule tested reduced hospitalization for neutropenia and fever from 26% to 0% and the median leukocyte nadir from 1800/mm³ to 3300/mm³, while producing an overall response rate of 67% and median survival of 16 months. Five other trials have documented the effectiveness of this regimen with response rates ranging from 13% to 73%.[366,377-380] The overall response rate for this 3-drug regimen among 451 patients in six trials is 43% and the 95% confidence interval is 38% to 48%.

Other trials have tested three-drug chemotherapy programs combining mitomycin, vinblastine, and cisplatin at doses from 40 to 75 mg/m². Response rates have ranged from 20% to 46% with median survivals from 5.5 to 6.0 months.[355,381] The overall response rate for studies testing lower doses of cisplatin is 26% (112/427), less than the pooled rates for MVP programs using cisplatin at doses 100 mg/m² ($p > 0.0001$).

VINDESINE AND MITOMYCIN. In a group of 55 untreated patients with advanced NSCLC, the two-drug combination of vindesine and mitomycin produced a 36% major objective response rate and a median survival of 6.1 months.[381a] This outpatient regimen was well tolerated; significant myelosuppression and other serious toxicities were noted in less than 10% of patients. This regimen was tested in four other trials with response rates ranging from 10% to 36%.[362,382-384] Median survivals range from 5.5 to 10.2 months. Overall, this two-drug regimen has produced a 27% major objective response rate (95% confidence intervals of 22–32%) in 316 patients.

IFOSFAMIDE-CONTAINING COMBINATIONS. Less data have accumulated from trials testing ifosfamide in combination with other agents in advanced NSCLC patients. If used in combination with mitomycin and either 100 mg/m² of cisplatin[385] or 50 mg/m² of cisplatin,[386] response rates were 69% and 56% and median survivals 9.5 and 9.2 months, respectively. A randomized study comparing the three-drug combination of ifosfamide, etoposide, and cisplatin with the two-drug combination of etoposide and cisplatin revealed no differences in response rate or survival.[371]

DOES CHEMOTHERAPY IMPROVE SURVIVAL IN ADVANCED NON-SMALL CELL LUNG CANCER?

The results of combination chemotherapy trials described earlier show a median survival of treated patients ranging from 5 to 12 months. Although major objective response rates range from 13% to 73%, rates in most trials are less than 50%. Therefore, the likely magnitude of overall survival improvement using combination chemotherapy programs should be modest and measured in months. The four randomized trials comparing combination chemotherapy regimens with the best supportive care in patients with stages III and IV NSCLC confirm this expectation.[247,358,387,388]

The median survival in the arms using only best supportive care ranged from 2.3 to 5.3 months from start of study and the median survival among patients given chemotherapy ranged from 6.8 to 8.6 months. In each trial, patients receiving combination chemotherapy lived longer. The difference between the two study arms ranged from 2.5 to 5.5 months. The observed median survivals were significantly different at the $p = 0.05$ level in two of the four trials.[470,387] A recent meta-analysis including these four trials published in manuscript form and three other incomplete[365] or preliminary reports[389,390] compared overall survival among patients given

best supportive care alone or with chemotherapy in more than 600 patients with advanced NSCLC.[391] This review demonstrated an increased probability of survival for those patients randomized to the chemotherapy arms at 3, 6, and 9 months after study entry.[391]

Dillman and colleagues reported a multicenter, randomized trial in which patients with stage III NSCLC receiving radiotherapy with curative intent were randomized to receive no additional therapy or 5 weeks of chemotherapy before irradiation.[246] Chemotherapy consisted of two doses of cisplatin (100 mg/m²) and five doses of vinblastine, all given over a 5-week period. The median survival of patients receiving chemotherapy and irradiation was 13.8 months compared with 9.7 months for persons receiving irradiation alone, a 4.1 month difference ($p = 0.0066$). Survival at 1, 2, and 3 years was improved for the group receiving chemotherapy, and failure-free survival was significantly better ($p = 0.04$). A trial testing concomitant cisplatin and chest radiotherapy revealed improved survival at 2 and 3 years for persons given concomitant cisplatin and irradiation compared with irradiation alone.[293]

The completed trials and the meta-analysis of all studies show a modest but definite improvement in survival for advanced NSCLC patients receiving combination chemotherapy. The clinical significance of this improvement remains open to debate.

BENEFITS OF CHEMOTHERAPY ON LUNG CANCER SYMPTOMS, HOSPITALIZATION, AND COST

In a companion analysis to the trial by Rapp and colleagues comparing best supportive care to combination chemotherapy,[247] Jaakkimainen studied the cost and hospitalization rates for the two study arms.[392] The use of chemotherapy was associated with a cost saving over best supportive care alone, and the overall costs for chemotherapy treatment were comparable with those incurred by patients with other serious illnesses, such as heart disease. The group receiving best supportive care spent the most time in the hospital at an average of 24 days or 20% of their projected median lifespan. In contrast, persons receiving vindesine and cisplatin spent an average of 22 days in the hospital. This amount of time, which includes hospitalizations to receive chemotherapy, translates into 10% of their median lifespan spent in the hospital.

More than 80% of patients with advanced NSCLC have significant pulmonary and extrapulmonary symptoms of their disease at presentation.[110,111] In a trial prospectively measuring cough, pain, dyspnea, and hemoptysis, all these symptoms improved during chemotherapy treatment.[111] Most of these patients had their Karnofsky performance status maintained or improved and gained weight while receiving chemotherapy. Although the careful measurement and analysis of study endpoints other than response and survival in advanced NSCLC is currently in its infancy, the data collected suggest that combination chemotherapy can control lung cancer symptoms and decrease hospitalization at a reasonable cost.

NEW CHEMOTHERAPEUTIC AGENTS AND APPROACHES

Several individual drugs in completed phase II clinical trials have shown activity in NSCLC. These include epirubicin and vinorelbine and a pyrimidine antimetabolite, gemcitabine.[393–406] Newer agents that demonstrate some activity include taxol and chloroquinoxaline sulfonamide.[407–409] A new class of anticancer drugs, the differentiating agents, are under active study. These include retinoic acid derivatives and hexamethylene bisacetamide (HMBA).[410–412]

IMMUNOTHERAPY OF NON-SMALL CELL LUNG CANCER

Despite extensive investigation, immunotherapy has not demonstrated any effect as adjuvant treatment in NSCLC. Several trials have used intradermal and intrapleural BCG and levamisole without success.[413–418] Interferons have been tested alone and in combination with other drugs, and despite preclinical data demonstrating additive or synergistic effects when interferon is combined with cytotoxic agents such as 5-FU or cisplatin, trials have shown no significant activity in clinical settings.[419–422] The cytokine interleukin-2 has undergone limited testing without evidence of success.[423] Similarly, monoclonal antibodies directed at antigens on the surface of lung cancer cells, although under study, have no established role in the management of these patients.[424,425]

PALLIATION OF LUNG CANCER

In view of the poor survival of patients with locally advanced NSCLC and patients with metastatic disease, effective palliation is an important objective. Carroll followed 134 inoperable patients and reported that 64% needed immediate local palliation and of those with no thoracic symptoms at presentation half required subsequent local treatment.[429] Therefore, a watch and wait policy is appropriate for only a minority of patients and it is crucial that they be followed carefully to prevent the development of serious local complications of the disease, which may be more difficult to palliate. It is important to intervene before SVC obstuction, obstructive pneumonia, or lobar collapse occurs. The latter two conditions produce a radiographic picture in which tumor and other processes are not easily distinguishable and large radiation fields may be necessary for effective control.

RADIOTHERAPY FOR INTRATHORACIC DISEASE

External-Beam Irradiation

There are numerous randomized trials in which the palliative benefit of radiation therapy is well documented.[429a,429b,429c] Various regimens produce a high rate of palliation that often is sustained for a significant proportion of a patient's survival. A significant number of patients suffer recurrence of symptoms. There are few data reporting the result of retreatment with radiation. Jackson retreated 22 patients recurring after radical radiation and delivered between 2000 to 3000 cGy in 200-cGy fractions. Symptomatic improvement occurred in 52% and median survival was 5.4 months.[430] The randomized trials suggest that certain symptoms such as hemoptysis or pain are more effectively palliated, whereas dyspnea and poor performance status appear to be more refractory. However, investigators in Italy used either 550 cGy or 880 cGy once per week for a total dose of 4400 cGy and reported that 80% of 45 patients experienced an average improvement of 20 points on the Karnofsky performance status scale.[431] There are no conclusive data proving the palliative superiority of a more protracted low dose per fraction schedule or a rapid course of large fraction size. Theoretically, the use of large fractions may predispose patients to suffer higher rates of chronic complications. The RTOG trial shows that even the regimen with larger fraction sizes had a low prevalence of severe complications (8%). However, few patients live a long time, and protracted treatment is more time consuming and involves more expense and disruption of the normal lifestyle.

Intraluminal Brachytherapy

Direct permanent implantation of ^{125}I seeds into endobronchial tumors was developed at Memorial Sloan-Kettering Cancer Center in the 1960s. Relief of symptoms was achieved in approximately 60% of cases, but there was significant morbidity due to perforation of the airway, hemorrhage, and ventilatory arrest.[432] Subsequent workers avoided direct implantation into tissues and used temporary intraluminal placement of cobalt 60 or ^{192}Ir to deliver one or more large fractions over a few days.[433,434] High-dose-rate fractionated intraluminal therapy was developed to avoid such prolonged treatment times, which were uncomfortable for the patient and required hospitalization with attendant expense and radiation risk to personnel. The use of high-dose-rate intraluminal brachytherapy was pioneered at Memorial Sloan-Kettering Cancer Center.[432] The procedure typically is performed on an outpatient basis. The treatment catheter is positioned under bronchoscopic guidance and then connected to the remote afterloading machine, which contains a ^{192}Ir source (10 Ci) that travels along the catheter and is programmed to remain at specific locations to deliver a precisely controlled dose over several minutes. In a population of patients who previously had received radiation, this endoluminal brachytherapy yielded symptomatic improvement in 75% of patients, and there were a few long-term survivors.[435] Similar data were reported by Macha and colleagues, who obtained a response in 79% (44/56) of patients receiving 750 cGy at 1 cm from the source in four treatments. Radiologic improvement occurred in 88% (22/25) of patients with collapse or atelectasis and improvements in FEV_1 and vital capacity were well documented.[436] Burt and colleagues gave 1500 to 2000 cGy at 1 cm in one fraction of HDR-ILBRT and reported relief of hemoptysis in 86% (24/28), dyspnea in 64% (21/33), and cough in 50% (9/18).[437] Unlike other series, they did not use laser therapy before radiation. Laser treatment provides immediate relief of symptoms, facilitates catheter placement beyond the obstruction, and may increase response rates and duration. Seagren and colleagues reported significantly improved response rates among a population of 36 patients who received laser treatment compared with 14 who did not.[438] Because of the heterogeneity of reports, future trials must select with accuracy those patients who might benefit from endobronchial therapy.

Distant Metastases

NSCLC metastasizes to many organs. For asymptomatic metastatic disease, remote from critical locations, the usual approach is expectant management or chemotherapy. Isolated symptomatic lesions, such as bone metastases and spinal cord compression (even if asymptomatic), are managed with palliative courses of radiation (*e.g.,* 3000 cGy in 10 fractions; see Chapter 60).

Brain metastases are particularly common and can be debilitating. The standard therapy for multiple brain metastases in NSCLC is whole-brain irradiation therapy. This is accompanied by 4 mg of dexamethasone four times daily before and during radiation, and by anticonvulsants only if seizures occur. The RTOG has studied various dose and fractionation schemes for 1994 patients with brain metastases arising from several primary sites including lung (approximately 50% of patients). The schedules used were 2000 cGy in 1 week, 3000 cGy in 2 weeks, 3000 cGy in 3 weeks, 4000 cGy in 3 weeks, and 4000 cGy in 4 weeks. The shorter schedules tended to give more rapid relief of neurologic symptoms, but otherwise the schedules had a comparable palliative effect (50% overall), duration of improvement (9–13 weeks), and median survival (15–18 weeks).[439]

Surgical resection combined with postoperative radiation has been advocated for single metastases. At Memorial Sloan-Kettering Cancer Center, 104 patients with NSCLC were treated with surgery and radiation (n = 35) or radiation alone (n = 69). Median survival was 18 months for the combined arm compared with 4 months without it. The patients on the combined therapy arm had fewer metastases to other organs and tended to have controlled primary tumors or more aggressively managed primaries.[440] Patchell randomized 45 patients with resectable single brain metastases (82% NSCLC primaries) to receive radiation alone or combined resection and radiation to the whole brain. Median survival (40 weeks versus 15 weeks) and duration of functional independence (38 weeks versus 8 weeks) were significantly higher in the combined surgery and radiation arm.[441] The magnitude of the difference in survival has prompted an increasing acceptance of resection and postoperative radiation for solitary brain metastases arising from NSCLC.

SURGICAL PALLIATION OF LUNG CANCER

Even when surgery cannot lead to cure, it may afford the best palliation of symptoms. Palliative surgical intervention may include bronchoscopic removal of tumor to relieve endobronchial obstruction or hemoptysis, pleurodesis to relieve symptomatic malignant pleural effusions, pericardial fenestration for malignant pericardial effusions, endobronchial or endoesophageal stents for relief of obstruction, and, occasionally, surgical resection of primary tumors and lung parenchyma for relief of septic complications or massive hemoptysis. Occasionally, en bloc resection, albeit incomplete, may be an excellent palliative for painful invasion of bony structures such as vertebra or ribs.

Relief of Endobronchial Obstruction

Bronchoscopic removal of endobronchial tumor is an efficient way of relieving endobronchial obstruction. Simple mechanical débridement using the bronchoscope is often sufficient. More recently, coagulative techniques such as CO_2, argon or Nd-YAG laser, electrocautery, and cryotherapy have been used

in conjunction with mechanical débridement. All of the techniques can be effective. Massive hemorrhage from the lesion is rare but can be avoided by the judicious use of coagulative techniques. In most instances, endobronchial débridement and coagulation is best carried out by rigid bronchoscopy.

Pleurodesis of Malignant Pleural Effusions

Malignant pleural effusions associated with lung cancer can be difficult to treat. In most cases, a portion of the ipsilateral lung is atelectatic making pleurodesis more refractory. Before pleurodesis, a chest tube should be inserted to completely drain the pleural effusion and ensure that the lung is expandable. Occasionally, endobronchial removal of the tumor may allow such expansion. After confirmation that the visceral and parietal pleural can be opposed, pleurodesis can be effected using interpleural tetracycline, bleomycin, or talc. The latter chemical appears to be most effective, especially because tetracycline, usually used for this purpose, is no longer available in the United States.

Pericardial Effusions

Symptomatic pericardial effusion secondary to metastatic disease from lung cancer can be treated by simple pericardial drainage, by drainage followed by sclerosis of the pericardium, or by the creation of a pericardial window using the subxiphoid laparotomy approach, the anterior thoracotomy approach, or, most recently, the video-assisted thoracoscopic approach. In all surgical approaches, a pericardial window is created and a chest tube is inserted to complete the drainage of the pericardium.

Bronchial and Esophageal Obstruction

Extrinsic compression of major airway or the esophagus sometimes complicates lung cancer that has involved mediastinal lymph nodes. In minimal endobronchial disease, bronchoscopy or esophagoscopy to relieve obstruction yields only temporary relief. In such instances, insertion of endobronchial or endoesophageal stents may relieve the problem. Because of the proximity of the major airways to the esophagus, these stents may cause compression of the other organ. This is especially true when endoesophageal stenting is used with resultant major airway compression. Such treatment frequently yields good temporary palliation of symptoms.

Palliative Resection

It is rare that palliative resection for uncontrolled symptoms is indicated. Endobronchial obstruction with distal uncontrolled pneumonia or lung abscess can be treated by endoscopic removal of tumor, or, in lung abscess, percutaneous or transbronchoscopic drainage of the abscess. It is rare that a palliative, incomplete surgical resection is required for patients presenting with these complications. In most instances, lesser procedures afford excellent palliation.

Invasion of tumors into vertebral bodies or the spinal canal may, on rare occasions, require surgical resection of the primary tumor and involved vertebral body to relieve uncontrollable pain or impending spinal cord damage. In most instances, such surgery provides only short-term palliation.

REFERENCES

1. Epidemiology Cancer Statistics 1991. CA 1991;41:19–36.
2. Parkin DM. Trends in lung cancer worldwide. Chest 1989;96(Suppl):5–8.
3. Cullen JW. The National Cancer Institute's smoking, tobacco and cancer program. Chest 1989;96(Suppl):9–13.
4. Loeb LA, Ernster VL, Warner KE, Abbotts J, Laszlo J. Smoking and lung cancer: An overview. Cancer Res 1984;44:5940–5958.
5. Minna JD, Higgins GA, Glatstein EJ. Cancer of the lung. In: DeVita VT, Hellman S, Rosenberg SA, eds. Cancer: Principles and practice of oncology. 3rd ed. Philadelphia: JB Lippincott, 1989:597.
6. Mattson ME, Pollack ES, Cullen JW. What are the odds that smoking will kill you? Am J Public Health 1987;77:425–431.
7. Garfinkel L, Stellman SD. Smoking and lung cancer in women: Findings in a prospective study. Cancer Res 1988;48:6951–6955.
8. Cullen JW, Mckenna JW, Massey MM. International control of smoking and the US experience. Chest 1986;89(Suppl 4):2206–2218.
9. US Department of Agriculture, Economic Research Service. Tobacco situation and outlook, publication TS-210. April 1990.
10. Garfinkel L, Silverberg E. Lung cancer and smoking trends in the United States over the past 25 years. CA 1991;41:137–145.
11. Stellman SD, Garfinkel L. Smoking habits and tar levels in a new American Cancer Society prospective study of 1.2 million men and women. JNCI 1986;76:1057–1063.
12. Pierce JP, Fiore MC, Novotny TE. Trends in cigarette smoking in the United states: Projections to the year 2000. JAMA 1989;261:265.
13. Masironi R, Rothwell K. Trends in and effects of smoking in the world. World Health Stat Q 1988;41(3–4):228–241.
14. Hoffman D, Haley NJ, Brunnemann KD, Adams JD, Wynder E. Cigarette sidestream smoke: Formation, analysis and model studies on the uptake by non-smokers. Presented at the US–Japan meeting on new etiology of lung cancer, Honolulu, HI, March 21–23, 1983.
15. Wald NJ, Nanchahal K, Thompson SG, Cuckle HS. Does breathing other people's smoke cause lung cancer? Br Med J 1986;293:1217–1222.
16. Greenberg RA, Haley NJ, Etzel RA, Loda FA. Measuring the exposure of infants to tobacco smoke: Nicotine and cotinine in urine and saliva. N Engl J Med 1984;310:1075–1078.
17. Janerich DT, Thompson WD, Varela LR, et al. Lung cancer and exposure to tobacco smoke in the household. N Engl J Med 1990;323:632–636.
18. Florin I, Rutberg L, Curvall M, Enzell CR. Screening of tobacco smoke constituents for mutagenecity using the Ames' test. Toxicology 1980;18:219–223.
19. Phillips DH, Hewer A, Martin CN, Garner RC, King MM. Correlation of DNA adduct levels in human lung with cigarette smoking. Nature 1988;336:790–792.
20. Slebos RJC, Dalesio O, Mooi WJ, Offerhaus GJ, Rodenhuis S. Mutational activation of the K-ras oncogene is associated with smoking in adenocarcinoma of the lung. Proc Am Soc Clin Oncol 1991;10:244.
21. Hecht SS, Hoffman D. Tobacco-specific nitrosamines, an important group of carcinogens in tobacco and tobacco smoke. Carcinogenesis 1988;9:875–884.
22. Castonguay A, Stoner GD, Schut HAJ, Hecht SS. Metabolism of tobacco-specific nitrosamines by cultured human tissues. Proc Natl Acad Sci USA 1983;80:6694–6697.
23. Fraumeni JF Jr. Carcinogenesis: An epidemiological appraisal. JNCI 1975;55:1039–1046.
24. Fraumeni JF Jr, Blott WJ. Lung and pleura. In: Schottenfeld D, Fraumeni JF Jr, eds. Cancer epidemiology and prevention. Philadelphia: WB Saunders, 1982:564–582.
25. National Academy of Sciences. Environmental tobacco smoke: Measuring exposures and assessing health effects. Appendix D. Washington, DC: National Academy Press, 1986.
26. Seidman H, Selikoff I, Gelb S. Mortality experience of amosite asbestos factory workers: Dose-response relationships 5–40 years after onset of short-term work exposure. Am J Ind Med 1986;10:479–514.
27. Kjuus H, Langard S, Skjaerven R. A case-referent study of lung cancer, occupational exposure and smoking II: Role of asbestos exposure. Scand J Work Environ Health 1986;12:203–209.
28. Kjuus H, Langard S, Skjaerven R. A case-referent study of lung cancer, occupational exposure and smoking I: Comparison of title-based and exposure-based occupational information. Scand J Work Environ Health 1986;12:193–202.
29. Selikoff IJ, Hammond EC, Seidman H. Mortality experience of insulation workers in the United States and Canada, 1943–76. Ann NY Acad Sci 1979;330:91–116.
30. Robinson C, Lemen R, Wagoner JK. Mortality patterns, 1940–1975 among workers employed in an asbestos textile friction and packing products manufacturing facility. In: Lemen R, Dement JM III, eds. Dusts and disease. Park Forest South: Pathatox Publishers, 1979:131–143.
31. Armstrong BK, de Klerk NH, Musk AW, Hobbs MS. Mortality in miners and millers of crocidolite in Western Australia. Br J Ind Med 1988;5:5–13.
32. McDonald AD, Fry JS, Woolley AJ, McDonald JC. Dust exposure and mortality in American chrysotile asbestos friction products plant. Br J Ind Med 1984;41:151–157.
33. Finkelstein MM. Mortality among employees of an Ontario asbestos-cement factory. Am Rev Respir Dis 1984;129:754–761.
34. Talcott JA, Thruber WA, Kantor AF, et al. Asbestos-associated diseases in a cohort of cigarette-filter workers. N Eng J Med 1989;321:1220–1223.
35. Omenn G, Merchant J, Boatmann E, et al. Contribution of environmental fibres to respiratory cancer. Environ Health Perspect 1986;70:51–56.
36. Kjuus H, Langard S, Skjaerven R. A case-referent study of lung cancer, occupational

exposure and smoking III. Etiologic fraction of occupational exposures. Scand J Work Environ Health 1986;12:210–215.
37. Fabrikant J. Radon and lung cancer the BEIR IV report. Health Physics 1990;59:89–97.
38. Roscoe R, Steenland K, Halperin W, Beaumont J, Waxweiler R. Lung cancer mortality among nonsmoking uranium miners exposed to radon daughters. JAMA 1989;262:629–633.
39. Schoenberg J, Klotz J, Wilcox H, et al. Case-control study of residential radon and lung cancer among New Jersey women. Cancer Res 1990;50:6520–6524.
40. Blot W, Zhao-Yi X, Boice J, et al. Indoor radon and lung cancer in China. JNCI 1990;82:1025–1030.
41. Lubin J, Boice J. Estimating Rn-induced lung cancer in the United States. Health Physics 1989;57:417–427.
42. Nero A, Schwehr M, Nazaroff W, Revzan K. Distribution of airborne radon-222 concentrations in US homes. Science 1986;234:992–997.
43. Environmental Protection Agency. A citizen's guide to radon: What it is and what to do about it, publication OPA-86-004. Washington, DC: Environmental Protection Agency, 1986.
44. Dorgan JF, Schatzkin A. Antioxidant micronutrients in cancer prevention. Hematol Oncol Clin North Am 1991;5:43–68.
45. Block G. Vitamin C and cancer prevention: The epidemiologic evidence. Am J Clin Nutr 1991;53(Suppl):270–282.
46. Stahelin HB, Gey KF, Eichholzer M, Ludin E. Beta-carotene and cancer prevention: The Basel Study. Am J Clin Nutr 1991;53(Suppl 1):265–269.
47. Menkes MS, Comstock GW, Vuilleumier JP, Helsing KJ, Rider AA, Brookmeyer R. Serum beta-carotene, vitamins A and E, selenium, and the risk of lung cancer. N Engl J Med 1986;315:1250–1254.
48. Kvale G, Bjelke E, Gart JJ. Dietary habits and lung cancer risks. Int J Cancer 1983;31:397–405.
49. Knekt P, Aromaa A, Maatela J et al. Serum selenium and subsequent risk of cancer among Finnish men and women. JNCI 1990;82:864–868.
50. Salonen JT, Alfthan G, Huttenen JK. Association between serum selenium and the risk of cancer. Am J Epidemiol 1984;120:342–349.
51. Shekelle R, Lepper M, Liu S. Dietary vitamin A and risk of cancer in the Western Electric Study. Lancet 1981;2:1185.
52. Willet WC, Polk BF, Underwood BA. Relation of serum vitamins A and E and carotenoids to the risk of cancer. N Engl J Med 1984;310:430–434.
53. Nomura AMY, Stammermann GN, Heilbrun. Serum vitamin levels and the risk of cancer of specific sites in men of Japanese ancestry in Hawaii. Cancer Res 1985;45:2369–2372.
54. Kok FJ, van-Duijn CM, Hofman A, Vermeeren R, de-Bruijn AM, Valkenburg HA. Micronutrients and the risk of lung cancer. N Engl J Med [Letter] 1987;316:1416.
55. Law MR, Hetzel Mr, Idel JR. Debrisoquine metabolism and genetic predisposition to lung cancer. Br J Cancer 1987;59:686–687.
56. Heighway J, Thatcher N, Cerny T, Hasleton PS. Genetic predisposition to human lung cancer. Br J Cancer 1986;53:453.
57. Birrer MJ, Minna JD. Molecular genetics of lung cancer. Semin Oncol 1988;15:226–235.
58. Ayesh R, Idle JR, Ritchie JC, Crothers M, Hetzel MR. Metabolic oxidation phenotypes as markers for susceptibility to lung cancer. Nature 1984;312:169–170.
59. Caporaso N, Hayes RB, Dosemeci M, Hoover R, Ayesh R, Hetzel M, Idle J. Lung cancer risk, occupational exposure, and the debrisoquine metabolic phenotype. Cancer Res 1989;49:3675–3679.
60. Speirs CJ, Murray S, Davies DS, Mabadeje AFB, Boobis AR. Debrisoquine oxidation phenotype and susceptibility to lung cancer. Br J Clin Pharmacol 1990;29:101–109.
61. Benitez J, Ladero JM, Jara C, et al. Polymorphic oxidation of debrisoquine in lung cancer patients. Eur J Cancer 1991;27:158–161.
62. Ruff M, Pert C. Small cell carcinoma of the lung: Macrophage-specific antigens suggest hemopoietic stem cell origin. Science 1984;225:1034–1036.
63. Gazdar A, Bunn P, Minna J. Origin of human small cell lung cancer. Science 1985;229:679–680.
64. Harris CC. Chemical and physical carcinogenesis: Advances and perspectives for the 1990s. Cancer Res 1991;51:5023s–5044s.
65. Minna J, Bettey J, Birrer M. Genetic changes involved in the pathogenesis of human lung cancer including oncogene activation, chromosomal deletions, and autocrine growth factor production. In: Fortner J, Rhoads J. In: Accomplishments in cancer research—1987 General Motors Cancer Research Foundation. Philadelphia: JB Lippincott, 1988:155–182.
66. Minna JD, Battey JF, Birrer M, et al. Chromosomal deletion, gene amplification, alternative processing, and autocrine growth factor production in the pathogenesis of human lung cancer. Int Symp Princess Takamatsu Cancer Res Fund 1986;17:109–122.
67. Gonzalez FJ, Crespi CL, Gelboin HV. DNA-expressed human cytochrome P450s: A new age of molecular toxicology and human risk assessment. Mutat Res 1991;247:113–127.
68. Huberman E, Sachs L. Metabolism of the carcinogenic hydrocarbon benzo(a)pyrene in human fibroblast and epithelial cells. Int J Cancer 1973;11:412–418.
69. Belinsky S, Doan M, White C, et al. Cell specific differences in O-methylguanine-DNA methyltransferase activity and removal of O-methylguanine in rat pulmonary cells. Carcinogenesis 1988;9:2053–2058.
70. Autrup H, Harris C. Metabolism of chemical carcinogens by human tissues. In: Autrup H, Harris CC. Human carcinogenesis. New York: Academic Press, 1983:169–194.
71. Harris C. Human tissues and cells in carcinogenesis research. Cancer Res 1987;47:1–10.

72. Idle J, Mahgoub A, Sloan T, et al. Some observations on the oxidation phenotype status of Nigerian patients presenting with cancer. Cancer Lett 1981;11:331–338.

73. Kaisary A, Smith P, Jaczq E, et al. Genetic predisposition to bladder cancer: Ability to hydroxylate debrisoquine and mephenytoin as risk factors. Cancer Res 1987;47: 5488–5493.

74. Sugimura H, Caporaso N, Modali R, et al. Association of rare alleles of the harvey ras protooncogene locus with lung cancer. Cancer Res 1990;50:1857–1862.

75. Robertson I, Guthenberg C, Mannervik B, et al. The glutathione conjugation of benzo(a)pyrene diol-epoxide by human glutathione transferases. In: Cooke M, Dennis A. Polynuclear aromatic hydrocarbons: A decade of progress. Columbus: Battelle Press, 1988:799–808.

76. Ketterer B. Protective role of glutathione and gluthathione transferases in mutagenesis and carcinogenesis. Mutat Res 1988;202:343–361.

77. Seidegard J, Pero RW. The hereditary transmission of high glutathione transferase activity towards trans-stilbene oxide in human mononuclear leukocytes. Human Genet 1985;69:66–68.

78. Seidegard J, Pero RW, Miller DG, et al. A gluthathione transferase in human leukocytes as a marker for the susceptibility to lung cancer. Carcinogenesis 1986;751–753.

79. Rudiger H, Schwartz U, Serrand E, et al. Reduced O6-methylguanine repair in fibroblast cultures from patients with lung cancer. Cancer Res 1989;49:5623–5626.

80. Lawley P. Some chemical aspects of dose response relationships in alleylation mutagenesis. Mut Res 1974;23:283–295.

81. Solomon E, Borrow J, Goddard AD. Chromosome aberrations and cancer. Science 1991;254:1153–1160.

82. Brauch H, Johnson B, Hovis J, et al. Molecular analysis of the short arm of chromosome 3 in small-cell and non-small-cell carcinoma of the lung. N Engl J Med 1987;317: 1109–1113.

83. Kik K, Osinga J, Carritt B. Deletion of a DNA sequence at the chromosomal region 3p21 in all major types of lung cancer. Nature 1987;330:578–581.

84. Weinberg RA. Tumor suppressor genes. Science 1991;254:1138–1146.

85. Takahashi T, Nau M, Chiba I, et al. P53: A frequent target for genetic abnormalities in lung cancer. Science 1989;246:491–494.

86. Levine A, Momand J, Finlay C: The p53 tumour suppressor gene. Nature 1991;351: 453–456.

87. Hollstein M, Sidransky D, Vogelstein B, et al. p53 mutations in human cancers. Science 1991;253:49–53.

88. Bergh J. Gene amplification in human lung cancer. The myc family genes and other proto-oncogenes and growth factor genes. Am Rev Respir Dis 1990;142:20–26.

89. Slamon D, deKerion J, Verma I. Expression of cellular oncogenes in human malignancies. Science 1984;224:256–262.

90. Kurzrock R, Gallick G, Gutterman J. Differential expression of p21 ras gene products among histological subtypes of fresh primary human lung tumors. Cancer Res 1986;46: 1530–1534.

91. Rodenhuis S, van de Wetering ML, Mooi WJ, et al. Mutational activation of the K-RAS oncogene: A possible pathogenetic factor in adenocarcinoma of the lung. N Engl J Med 1987;317:929–937.

92. Slebos R, Rodenhuis S. The molecular genetics of human lung cancer. Eur Respir J 1989;2:1022.

93. Kawashima K, Shikama H, Imoto K. Close correlation between restriction fragment length polymorphism of the L-myc gene and metastasis of human lung cancer to the lymph nodes and other organs. Proc Natl Acad Sci USA 1988;85:2353–2356.

94. Kiefer P, Wegmann B, Bacher M, et al. T1 Different pattern of expression of cellular oncogenes in human SO. J Cancer Res Clin Oncol 1990;116:29–37.

95. Schutte J, Nau M, Birrer M, et al. Constitutive expression of multiple mRNA forms of the c-jun oncogene in human lung cancer cell lines. Proc Am Assoc Cancer Res [Abstract] 1988:455.

96. Aaronson SA. Growth factors and cancer. Science 1991;254:1146–1153.

97. Cerny T, Barnes D, Hasleton P. Expression of epidermal growth factor receptor (ECF-R) in human lung tumors. Br J Cancer 1986;54:265–269.

98. Sherwin SA, Minna JD, Gazdar AF, et al. Expression of epidermal and nerve growth factor receptors and soft agar growth factor production by lung cancer cells. Cancer Res 1981;41:3538–3542.

99. Natale R, Cuttitta F, Nakanishi Y, et al. IGF-1 can stimulate proliferation of non-small cell lung cancer cell lines cell lines in vitro. Proc Am Soc Clin Oncol [Abstract] 1988;7:197.

100. Mabry M, Nakagawak T, Gesell M, et al. Introduction of harvey murine sarcoma virus (Ha-MSV) into human small cell lung cancer (SCLC) is associated with phenotypic changes. Proc Am Assoc Cancer Res [Abstract] 1987;28:39.

101. Slebos R, Kibbelaar R, Dalesio O. K-RAS oncogene activation as a prognostic marker in adenocarcinoma of the lung. N Engl J Med 1990;323:561–565.

102. Divgi CR, Kris M, Real FX, et al. Phase I and imaging trial of indium 111–labeled anti-epidermal growth factor receptor monoclonal antibody 225 in patients with squamous cell lung carcinoma. JNCI 1991;83:97–104.

103. Linnoila I. Pathology of non-small cell lung cancer: New diagnostic approaches. Hematol Oncol Clin North Am 1990:1027–1051.

104. Roggli VI, Volmer RB, Greenberg ST, et al. Lung cancer heterogeneity: A blinded and randomized study of 100 consecutive cases. Hum Pathol 1985;16:569.

105. Percy C, Horm JW, Goffman TE. Trends in histologic type of lung cancer, SEER Program, 1973–1981. In: Mizell M, Korrea P, eds. Lung cancer causes and prevention. Deerfield Beach, FL: Verlag, Chemie International, 1984:153.

106. Clayton F. The spectrum and significance of bronchoalveolar carcinomas. Pathol Annu 1988;23:361.

107. Hammer SP, Bolan JW, Bockus D, et al. Ultrastructural and immunohistochemical features of common lung tumors: An overview. Ultrastruct Pathol 1985;9:283.

108. Souhami RL, Beverly PC, Bobrow LG. Antigens of small-cell lung cancer: First International Workshop. Lancet 1987;2:325.

109. Matthews MJ. Problems in morphology and behavior of bronchopulmonary malignant disease. In: Israel I, Chahanian P, eds. Lung cancer: Natural history, prognosis and therapy. New York: Academic Press, 1976:23–62.

110. Sorenson J, Badsberg J, Olsen J. Prognostic factors in inoperable adenocarcinoma of the lung: A multivariate regression analysis of 259 patients. Cancer Res 1989;49: 5748–5754.

111. Kris M, Gralla R, Potanovich L, et al. Assessment of pretreatment symptoms and improvement after edam + mitomycin + vinblastine (EMV) in patients (PTS) with inoperable non-small cell lung cancer (NSCLC). Proc Am Soc Clin Oncol 1990;9: 229.

112. Hollen PJ, Gralla RJ, Kris MG, et al. Quality of life assessment in individuals with lung cancer: Lung cancer symptom scale. Eur J Cancer 1992 (in press).

113. Redman BG, Pazdur R, Zingas AP, et al. Prospective evaluation of adrenal insufficiency in patients with adrenal metastasis. Cancer 1987;60:103–107.

114. Wade JL, Little AG, Vogelzang NJ, et al. Idiopathic pericardial effusions in patients with malignancy. Proc Am Soc Clin Oncol 1984;3:15.

115. Posner MR, Cohen AT, Skarin AT. Pericardial disease in patients with cancer. Am J Med 1981;71:407–413.

116. Mountain CF. A new international staging system for lung cancer. Chest 1986;89(Suppl):225–323.

117. Watanabe Y, Shimizu J, Oda M, et al. Proposals regarding some deficiencies in the new international staging system for non-small cell lung cancer. Jpn J Clin Oncol 1991;21:160–168.

118. Naruke T, Goya T, Tsuchiya R, Suemasu K. Prognosis and survival in resected lung carcinoma based on the new international staging system. J Thorac Cardiovasc Surg 1988;96:440–457.

119. Mountain CF. Value of the new TNM staging system for lung cancer. Chest 1989;97: 935–947.

120. Tockman MS, Gupa PK, Myers JD, et al. Sensitive and specific monoclonal antibody recognition of human lung cancer antigen on preserved sputum cells. J Clin Oncol 1988;6:1685–1693.

121. Melamed MR, Flehinger B, Zaman MB, et al. Detection of true pathologic stage I lung cancer in a screening program and the effect on survival. Cancer 1981;47:1182–1187.

122. Vlasbloem H, Schultz Kool LJ. AMBER: A scanning multiple-beam equalization system for chest radiography. Radiology 1988;169:29–34.

123. Wandtke JC, Plewes DB, McFaul JA. Improved pulmonary nodule detection with scanning equalization radiography. Radiology 1988;169:23–27.

124. Jolly PC, Hutchinson CH, Detterbeck F, et al. Routine computed tomographic scans, selective mediastinoscopy and other factors in evaluation of lung cancer. J Thorac Cardiovasc Surg 1991;102:226–271.

125. Dales RE, Stark RM, Sankaranarayan AN. Computed tomography to stage lung cancer. Am Rev Respir Dis 1990;141:1096–1101.

126. Fontana RS. Meta-analysis of computed tomography for staging non-small cell lung cancer. Am Rev Resp Dis [Editorial] 1990;141:1093–1094.

127. Heelan R, Martini N, Westcot JW, et al. Carcinomas involving the hilum and mediastinum: Computed tomographic and magnetic resonance evaluation. Radiology 1985;156:111–115.

128. Payne PY, Bronskill MJ, Henkelman RM, et al. Mediastinal lymph node metastases from bronchogenic carcinoma: Detection with MR imaging and CT. Radiology 1987;162:651–656.

129. Batra P, Brown K, Collins JD, et al. Evaluation of intrathoracic extent of lung cancer by plain chest radiography, computed tomography and magnetic resonance imaging. Am Resp Dis 1988;137:1456–1462.

130. Kies MS, Baker AW, Kennedy PS. Radionuclide scans in staging of carcinoma of lung. Surg Gynecol Obstet 1978;147:175–176.

131. Little AG, DeMeester TR, Ryan JW. The use of radionuclide scans in lung cancer: Gallium-67 scanning for preoperative staging. In: Kittle CF, ed. Current controversies in thoracic surgery. Philadelphia: WB Saunders, 1986:122–128.

132. Michel F, Soler M, Imhof E, Perruchoud AP. Initial staging of non-small cell lung cancer: Value of routine radioisotope bone scanning. Thorax 1991;46:469–473.

133. Wescott JL. Direct percutaneous needle aspiration of localized pulmonary lesions: Results in 422 patients. Radiology 1980;137:31–35.

134. Wong JP, Terri TB. Transbronchial needle aspiration in the diagnosis and staging of bronchogenic carcinoma. Am Rev Resp Dis 1983;127:344–347.

135. Harrow EM, Oldenburg FA, Lindenfelter MS, Smith AM. Transbronchial needle aspiration in clinical practice: A five year experience. Chest 1989;96:1268–1272.

136. Cripp AJ, DiMarco AF, Lankerani M. False-positive transbronchial needle aspiration in bronchogenic carcinoma. Chest 1984;85:696–697.

137. Luke WP, Pearson FG, Todd TRJ, et al. Prospective evaluation of mediastinoscopy for assessment of carcinoma of the lung. J Thorac Cardiovasc Surg 1986;91:53–56.

138. McCaughan JS, William TE Jr, Bethel BH. Photodynamic therapy of endobronchial tumors. Lasers Surg Med 1986;6:336–345.

139. Ginsberg RJ, Rice TW, Goldberg M, et al. Extended cervical mediastinoscopy-a single staging procedure for bronchial carcinoma of the left upper lobe. J Thorac Cardiovasc Surg 1987;94:673–678.

140. McKneal TM, Chamberlain JM. Diagnostic anterior mediastinotomy. Ann Thorac Surg 1966;2:523.

141. Patterson GA, Piazza D, Pearson FG, et al. Significance of metastatic disease in subaortic lymph node. Ann Thorac Surg 1987;43:155–159.

142. Mack M, Aronoff R, Acuff T. Present role of thoracoscopy in the diagnosis and treatment of diseases of the chest. Ann Thorac Surg 1992;54:403–409.

143. Miller DL, Allen MS, Trastek VF, et al. Video thoracoscopic wedge resections of the lung. Ann Thorac Surg 1992 (in press).

144. Lewis R. One hundred consecutive patients undergoing video-assisted thoracic operations. Ann Thorac Surg 54:421–426.

145. Aisner J, Hansen HH. Commentary: Current status of chemotherapy for non-small cell lung cancer. Cancer Treat Rep 1981;65:979–986.

146. Kayser K, Bulzebruk H, Probst G, et al. Retrospective and prospective tumor staging evaluating prognostic factors in operated bronchus carcinoma patients. Cancer 1987;59:355–361.

147. Green N, Kurohara SS, George FW. Cancer of the lung. An in-depth analysis of prognostic factors. Cancer 1971;28:1229–1233.

148. Lanzotti VJ, Thomas DR, Boyle LE, et al. Survival with inoperable lung cancer: An integration of prognostic variables based on simple clinical criteria. Cancer 1977;39:303–313.

149. Stanley KE. Prognostic factors for survival in patients with inoperable lung cancer. JNCI 1980;65:25–32.

150. Finkelstein DM, Ettinger DS, Ruckdeschel JC. Long-term survivors in metastatic non-small cell lung cancer. An Eastern Cooperative Oncology Group. J Clin Oncol 1986;4:702–709.

151. O'Connell JP, Kris MG, Gralla RJ, et al. Frequency and prognostic importance of pretreatment clinical characteristics in patients with advanced non-small cell lung cancer treated with combination chemotherapy. J Clin Oncol 1986;4:1604–1614.

152. Sorensen, JB, Badsberg JH, Olsen J. Prognostic factors in inoperable adenocarcinoma of the lung: A multivariate regression analysis of 259 patients. Cancer Res 1989;49:5748–5754.

153. Zimmerman PV, Bint MH, Hawson GAT, et al. Ploidy as a prognostic determinant in surgically treated lung cancer. Lancet 1987;530–533.

154. Volm M, Hahn EW, Mattern J, et al. Five-year follow-up study of independent clinical and flow cytometric prognostic factors for the survival of patients with non-small cell lung carcinoma. Cancer Res 1988;48:2923–2928.

155. Sahin A, Lee JS, Ro JY, et al. DNA flow cytometric (FCM) analysis of non-small cell lung cancer (NSCLC). Proc Am Soc Clin Oncol 1989;8:226.

156. Lee JS, Ro JY, Sahin A, et al. Expression of epidermal growth factor receptor (EGFR): A favorable prognostic factor for surgically resected non-small cell lung cancer (NSCLC). Proc Am Soc Clin Oncol 1989;8:226.

157. Hendler F, Shum-Siu A, Nanu L, et al. Increased EGF receptors and the absence of an alveolar differentiation marker predict a poor survival in lung cancer. Proc Am Soc Clin Oncol 1989;8:223.

158. Lee JS, Ro JY, Sahin AA, et al. Expression of blood-group antigen A: A favorable prognostic factor in non-small-cell lung cancer. N Engl J Med 1991;324:1084–1090.

159. Gazdar AF, Tsai CM, Park JG, et al. Relative chemosensitivity of non-small cell lung cancers (NSCLC) expressing neuroendocrine (NE) cell properties. Proc Am Soc Clin Oncol 1988;7:200.

160. Graziano SL, Mazid R, Newman N, et al. The use of neuroendocrine immunoperoxidase markers to predict chemotherapy response in patients with non-small-cell lung cancer. J Clin Oncol 1989;7:1398–1406.

161. Berendsen HH, de Leij L, Poppema S, et al. Clinical characterization of non-small cell tumors showing neuroendocrine differentiation features. J Clin Oncol 1989;7:1614–1620.

162. Sorensen JB, Skov BG, Hirsch FR, et al. Prognostic impact of neuron specific enolase (NSE) and chromogranin in adenocarcinoma of the lung (ACL). Proc Am Soc Clin Oncol 1989;8:220.

163. Brauch H, Johnson B, Hovis J, et al. Molecular analysis of the short arm of chromosome 3 in small-cell and non-small-cell carcinoma of the lung. N Engl J Med 1987;317:1109–1113.

164. Berlin NI, Buncher CR, Fontana RS, et al. Early lung cancer detection: Summary and conclusions. Am Rev Resp Dis 1984;30:565–570.

165. Berlin NI, Buncher CR, Fontana RS, et al. National Cancer Institute Cooperative Lung Cancer Detection Program: Results of initial screen (prevalence) early lung cancer detection—Introduction Am Rev Resp Dis 1984;130:545–549.

166. Pilotti S, Ralk EF, Gribaudi D, et al. Sputum cytology for the diagnosis of carcinoma of the lung. Acta Cytol (Baltimore) 1982;26:649–654.

167. Risse EKJ, Vooigis GP, Van't Hof MA. Diagnostic significance of "severe dysphagia" since sputum cytology. Acta Cytol (Baltimore) 1988;32:629–634.

168. Shure D. Fiberoptic bronchoscopy: Diagnostic application. Clin Chest Med 1987;8:1–13.

169. Lam S, Palcic D, McLean D, et al. Detection of early lung cancer using low dose Photofrin II. Chest 1990;97:333–337.

170. Kinse JH, Cortese DA. Endoscopic system for simultaneous visual examination and electronic detection of fluorescence. Rev Sei Instrum 1987;51:1403–1406.

171. Palcic B, Lam S, Hung J, Macauley C. Detection and localization of early lung cancer by imaging techniques. Chest 1991;99:742–743.

172. Hayata Y, Kato H, Komaka C, et al. Photoradiation therapy with hematoporhyrin derivative in early and stage I lung cancer. Chest 1984;86:169–177.

173. Edell ES, Cortese DA. Bronchoscopic localization and treatment of occult lung cancer. Chest 1989;96:919–921.

174. Reichl J. Assessment of operative risk of pneumonectomy. Chest 1972;62:570–576.

175. Taube K, Koniezko N. Prediction of postoperative cardiopulmonary function of patients undergoing pneumonectomy. J Thorac Cardiovasc Surg 1980;28:348–351.

176. Putman JB, Lammermeier DE, Colon R, et al. Predicted pulmonary function in survival after pneumonectomy for primary lung cancer. An Thorac Surg 1990;49:909–915.

177. Gass GD, Olsen GN. Preoperative pulmonary function testing to predict postoperative morbidity and mortality. Chest 1986;89:127–135.

178. Olsen GN, Block AJ, Swanson EW, et al. Pulmonary function evaluation of a lung resection candidate:A prospective study. Am Rev Resp Dis 1975;111:379–387.

179. Murphy TP, Casey MT. Determination of operability in candidates who undergo lung resection for bronchogenic carcinoma. Can J Surg 1990;33:470–473.

180. Ginsberg RJ, Rubinstein L (for the Lung Cancer Study Group). A randomized comparative trial of lobectomy vs limited resection for patients with Tl N0 non-small cell lung cancer. Lung Cancer [Abstract] 1991;7(Suppl):83, 304.

181. Graham EA, Sedal JJ. Successful removal of the entire lung for carcinoma of the bronchus. JAMA 1933;101:1371–1374.

182. Churchill ED, Sweet RH, Sutter L, Scannell JD. The surgical management of carcinoma of the lung. The study of cases treated at the Massachusetts General Hospital from 1930–50. J Thorac Cardiovasc Surg 1950;20:349–365.

183. Jensik RJ, Faber LD, Milloy FJ, Monson BO. Segmental resection for lung cancer: A 15 year experience. J Thorac Cardiovasc Surg 1973;66:563–572.

184. Jensik RJ. The extent of resection for localized lung cancer: Segmental resection. In: Kittle CF, ed. Current controversies in thoracic surgery. Philadelphia: WB Saunders, 1986:175–182.

185. Ginsberg RJ, Hill LD, Eagan RT, et al. Modern day operative mortality for surgical resection in lung cancer. J Thorac Cardiovasc Surg 1983;86:654–658.

186. Deslauriers J, Ginsberg RJ, Dubois P, Beaulieu M, et al. Modern operative morbidity for elective surgical resection in lung carcinoma. CJS 1989;32:335–339.

187. Martini N, Flehinger BJ. The role of surgery in N2 lung cancer. Surg Clin North Am 1987;67:1037–1049.

188. Naruke T, Goya T, Tsuchiya R, et al. The importance of surgery to non-small cell carcinoma of the lung with mediastinal lymph node metastases. An Thorac Surg 1988;46:603–610.

189. Martini N. Surgical treatment of non-small cell lung cancer by stage. Semin Surg Oncol 1990;6:248–254.

190. Carrel T, Nachbur B, Bleher A. Is radiotherapy prior to surgical resection indicated for bronchogenic carcinoma with chest wall infiltration and for Pancoast tumors? Lung Cancer [Abstract] 1988;4:80.

191. Patterson GA, Ilves R, Ginsberg RJ, et al. The value of adjuvant radiotherapy in pulmonary and chest wall resection for bronchogenic carcinoma. Ann Thorac Surg 1982;34:692–697.

192. Piehler JM, Pairolero PC, Weiland LH, et al. Bronchogenic carcinoma with chest wall invasion: Factors affecting survival following en bloc resection. Ann Thorac Surg 1982;34:684–691.

193. Hilaris BS, Martini N, Wong GY, Nori D. Treatment of superior sulcus tumor (Pancoast tumor). Surg Clin N Am 1987;67:965–977.

194. Burt ME, Pomerantz AH, Bains MS. Results of surgical treatment of stage III lung cancer invading the mediastinum. Surg Clin N Am 1987;67:987–1000.

195. Deslauriers J, Gaulin P, Beaulieu M, et al. Long term clinical and functional results of sleeve lobectomy for primary lung cancer. J Thorac Cardiovasc Surg 1986;92:871–879.

196. Naruke T, Goya T, Tsuchiya R, Suemasu K. The importance of surgery to non-small cell carcinoma of the lung with mediastinal lymph node metastasis. Ann Thorac Surg 1988;46:603–610.

197. Martini N, Flehinger BJ, Zaman MB, Beattie JB. Results of resection in non-oat cell carcinoma of the lung with mediastinal lymph node metastasis. Ann Surg 1983;198:386–397.

198. Martini N, Flehinger BJ. The role of surgery in N2 lung cancer. Surg Clin N Am 1987;67:1037–1049.

199. Shields TW. The significance of ipsilateral mediastinal lymph node metastasis (N2 disease) in non-small cell carcinoma of the lung. J Thorac Cardiovasc Surg 1990;99:48–53.

200. Naruke T, Goya T, Tsuchiya R, Suemasu K. Prognosis and survival in resected lung carcinoma based on the new international staging system. J Thorac Cardiovasc Surg 1988;96:440–447.

201. Dartevelle P, Chapelier A, Navajas M, et al. Replacement of superior vena cava with polytetrafluorethylene grafts combined with resection of mediastinal-pulmonary malignant tumors. J Thorac Cardiovasc Surg 1987;94:361–366.

202. Nakahara K, Ohno K, Mastumura A, et al. Extended operation for lung cancer invading the aortic arch and superior vena cava. J Thorac Cardiovasc Surg 1989;97:428–433.

203. Reyes L, Parvez Z, Regal AM, Takita H. Neoadjuvant chemotherapy and operations in the treatment of lung cancer with pleural effusion. J Thorac Cardiovasc Surg [Letter] 1991;101:946–947.

204. Deslauriers J, Brisson J, Cartier R, et al. Carcinoma of the lung: Evaluation of satellite nodules as a factor influencing prognosis after resection. J Thorac Cardiovasc Surg 1989;97:504–512.

205. McCormack P. Surgical resection of pulmonary metastasis. Semin Surg Oncol 1990;6:297–302.

206. Magilligan DJ, Duvernoy C, Malik G, et al. Surgical approach to lung cancer with solitary cerebral metastasis: Twenty–five years' experience. Ann Thorac Surg 1986;42:360–364.

207. Figlin RA, Piantadosi S, Feld R (for the Lung Cancer Study Group). Intracranial recurrence of carcinoma after complete surgical resection of stage I, II and III non-small cell lung cancer. N Engl J Med 1988;318:1300–1305.

208. Martini N. Rationale for surgical treatment of brain metastasis in non-small cell lung cancer. Ann Thorac Surg 1986;42:357–358.

209. Patchell RA, Tibbs PA, Walsh JW, et al. A randomized trial of surgery in the treatment of single metastases to the brain. N Engl J Med 1990;322:494–500.

210. Allard P, Yankaskas BC, Fletcher RH, et al. Sensitivity and specificity of computed tomography for the detection of adrenal metastatic lesions among 91 autopsied lung cancer patients. Cancer 1990;66:457–462.

211. Twomey P, Montgomery C, Clark O. Successful treatment of adrenal metastasis from large-cell carcinoma of the lung. JAMA 1982;248:581–583.
212. Raviv G, Klein E, Yellin A, et al. Surgical treatment of solitary adrenal metastases from lung carcinoma. J Surg Oncol 1990;43:123–124.
213. Reyes L, Parvez Z, Nemoto T, et al. Adrenalectomy for adrenal metastasis from lung carcinoma. J Surg Oncol 1990;44:32–34.
214. Martini N, Flehinger BJ, Nagasaki F, Hart B. Prognostic significance of Nl disease in carcinoma of the lung. J Thorac Cardiovasc Surg 1983;86:646–653.
215. Weisenburger TH (for the Lung Cancer Study Group). Effects of postoperative mediastinal radiation on completely resected stage II and stage III epidermoid carcinoma of the lung. N Engl J Med 1986;315:1377–1381.
216. Feld R, Rubinstein L, Weisenberger TH (for the Lung Cancer Study Group). Sites of recurrence in resected stage I non-small cell lung cancer: A guide for future studies. J Clin Oncol 1985;2:1352–1358.
217. Pairolero PC, Williams DE, Bergstralh MS, et al. Post–surgical stage I bronchogenic carcinoma: Morbid implications of recurrent disease. Ann Thorac Surg 1984;38:331–338.
218. Van Houtte P, Rocmans P, Smets P, et al. Postoperative radiation therapy in lung cancer: A controlled trial after resection of curative design. Int J Radiat Oncol Biol Phys 1980;6:983–986.
219. Bangma PJ. Postoperative radiotherapy. In: Deeley TJ, ed. Carcinoma of the bronchus (modern radiotherapy). New York: Appleton-Century-Crofts, 1971:163–170.
220. Chung CK, Stryker JA, O'Neill M, DeMuth WE. Evaluation of adjuvant postoperative radiotherapy for lung cancer. Int J Radiat Oncol Biol Phys 1982;8:1877–1880.
221. Ferguson MK, Little AG, Golomb HM, et al. The role of adjuvant therapy after resection of T1 N1 M0 and T2 N1 M0 non-small cell lung cancer. J Thorac Cardiovasc Surg 1986;91:344–349.
222. Choi NC, Grillo HC, Gardiello M, Scannell JG, Wilkins EW. Basis for new strategies in postoperative radiotherapy of bronchogenic carcinoma. Int J Radiat Oncol Biol Phys 1980;6:31–35.
223. Green N, Kurohara SS, George FW, Crews QE. Postresection irradiation for primary lung cancer. Radiology 1975;116:405–407.
224. Piehler JM, Pairolero PC, Weiland LH, Offord KP, Payne WS, Bernatz PE. Bronchogenic carcinoma with chest wall invasion: Factors affecting survival following en bloc resection. Ann Thorac Surg 1982;34:684–691.
225. Trastek VF, Pairolero PC, Piehler JM, et al. En bloc (non-chest wall) resection for bronchogenic carcinoma with parietal fixation. Factors affecting survival. J Thorac Cardiovasc Surg 1984;87:352–358.
226. Israel L, Bonadonna G, Sylvester R (for the EORTC Lung Cancer Group). Controlled study with adjuvant radiotherapy, chemotherapy, immunotherapy, and chemoimmunotherapy in operable squamous carcinoma of the lung. In: Muggia F, Rozencweig, eds. Lung cancer: Progress in therapeutic research. New York: Raven Press, 1979.
227. Astudillo J, Contill C. Role of postoperative radiation therapy in stage IIIa non-small cell lung cancer. Ann Thorac Surg 1990;50:618–623.
228. Kirsch MM, Sloan H. Mediastinal metastases in bronchogenic carcinoma: Influence of postoperative irradiation, cell type, and location. Ann Thorac Surg 1982;33:459–463.
229. Kaiser LR, Fleshner P, Keller S, Martini N. Significance of extramucosal residual tumor at the bronchial resection margin. Ann Thorac Surg 1989;47:265–269.
230. Law MR, Henk JM, Lennox SC, Hodson ME. Value of radiotherapy for tumour on the bronchial stump after resection for bronchial carcinoma. Thorax 1982;37:496–499.
231. Emami B, Kim T, Roper C, Simpson JR, Pilepich MV, Hederman MA. Postoperative radiation therapy in the management of lung cancer. Radiology 1987;164:251–253.
232. Slack NH. Bronchogenic carcinoma: Nitrogen mustard as a surgical adjuvant and factors influencing survival. University surgical adjuvant lung project. Cancer 1970;25:987–1002.
233. Higgins GA, Shields TW. Experience of the Veterans Administration surgical adjuvant group. In: Muggia F, Rozencweig M, eds. Lung cancer: Progress in therapeutic research. New York: Raven Press, 1979.
234. Shields TW, Higgins Jr GA, Humphrey EW, et al. Prolonged intermittent adjuvant chemotherapy with CCNU and hydroxyurea after resection of carcinoma of the lung. Cancer 1982;50:1713–1721.
235. Brunner KW, Marthaler T, Muller W. Effects of long-term adjuvant chemotherapy with cyclophosphamide (NSC-2627.2) for radically resected bronchogenic carcinoma. Cancer Chemother Rep 1973;4:125–132.
236. Girling DJ, Stott H, Stephens RJ, Fox W. Fifteen-year followup of all patients in a study of post-operative chemotherapy for bronchial carcinoma. Br J Cancer 1985;52:867–873.
237. Stanley K (for The Ludwig Lung Cancer Study Group [LLCSG]). Immunostimulation with intrapleural BCG as adjuvant therapy in resected non-small cell lung cancer. Cancer 1986;58:2411–1416.
238. Millar JW, Roscoe P, Pearce SJ, et al. Five-year results of a controlled study of BCG immunotherapy after surgical resection in bronchogenic carcinoma. Thorax 1982;37:57–60.
239. Holmes EC, Gail M (for the Lung Cancer Study Group). Surgical adjuvant therapy for stage II and stage III adenocarcinoma and large–cell undifferentiated carcinoma. J Clin Oncol 1986;4:710–715.
240. Ferguson MK, Little AG, Golomb HM, et al. The role of adjuvant therapy after resection of T1 N1 M0 and T2 N1 M0 non-small cell lung cancer. J Thorac Cardiovasc Surg 1986;91:344–349.
241. Ayoub J, Vigneault E, Hanley J, et al. The Montreal multicenter trial in operable non-small cell lung cancer (NSCLC): A multivariate analysis of the predictors of relapse. Proc Am Soc Clin Oncol 1991;10:247.

242. Lad T, Rubinstein L, Sadeghi A. The benefit of adjuvant treatment for resected locally advanced non-small cell lung cancer. J Clin Oncol 1988;6:9–17.
243. Holmes EC. Adjuvant therapy of non-small cell lung cancer. In: Salmon SE, ed. Adjuvant therapy of cancer VI. Philadelphia: WB Saunders, 1990:119–124.
244. Donnadieu N, Paesmans M, Sculier J. Chemotherapy of non-small cell lung cancer according to disease extent: A meta-analysis of the literature. Lung Cancer 1991;7:243–252.
245. Green M, Stoopler M, Anderson J, et al. Vinblastine (V) and cisplatin (CDDP) chemotherapy in advanced non small cell lung cancer (NSCLC). Proc Am Soc Clin Oncol 1985;4:176.
246. Dillman R, Seagren S, Proprert K, et al. A randomized trial of induction chemotherapy plus high–dose radiation versus radiation alone in stage III non-small cell lung cancer. N Engl J Med 1990;940–945.
247. Rapp E, Pater J, Willan A, et al. Chemotherapy can prolong survival in patients with advanced non-small cell lung cancer: Report of a Canadian multicenter randomized trial. J Clin Oncol 1988;6:633–641.
248. Bromley LL, Szur L. Combined radiotherapy and resection for carcinoma of the bronchus. Lancet 1955;5:937–941.
249. Takita H, Regal A, Antkowiak J, et al. Chemotherapy followed by lung resection in inoperable non-small cell lung carcinomas due to locally far-advanced disease. Cancer 1986;57:630–635.
250. Raut Y, Huu N, Clavier J, et al. Surgery and chemotherapy: A new method of treatment for squamous cell bronchial carcinoma. J Thorac Cardiovasc Surg 1984;88:754–757.
251. Martini N, Flehinger B, Zaman M, et al. Prospective study of 445 lung carcinomas with mediastinal lymph node metastases. J Thorac Cardiovasc Surg 1980;80:390–397.
252. Martini N, Flehinger B, Zaman M, et al. Results of resection in non-oat cell carcinoma of the lung with mediastinal lymph node metastases. Ann Surg 1983;198:386–397.
253. Pisters K, Kris M, Gralla R, et al. Preoperative chemotherapy in stage IIIA non-small cell lung cancer: An analysis of a trial in patients with clinically apparent mediastinal node involvement. In: Salmon S. Adjuvant therapy of cancer VI. Philadelphia: WB Saunders, 1990:133–137.
254. Burkes R, Ginsberg R, Shepherd F, et al. Induction chemotherapy with mitomycin, vindesine, and cisplatin for stage III unresectable non-small cell lung cancer: Results of the Toronto phase II trial. J Clin Oncol 1992;10:580–586.
255. Fossella F, Ryan B, Dhingra H, et al. Interim report of a prospective randomized trial of neoadjuvant chemotherapy plus surgery vs surgery alone for IIIA non-small cell lung cancer (NSCLC). Proc Am Soc Clin Oncol 1991;10:240.
255a. Rosell R, Gomez-Codina J, Camps C, et al. Favourable outcome and aneuploidy reversion following neoadjvant chemotherapy (CT) in stage IIIA non-small cell lung cancer (NSCLC). Proc Am Soc Clin Oncol 1992;11:287.
256. Faber L, Kittle C, Warren W, et al. Preoperative chemotherapy and irradiation for stage III non-small cell lung cancer. Ann Thorac Surg 1989;47:669–677.
257. Weiden P, Piantadosi S. Preoperative chemoradiotherapy in stage III non-small cell lung cancer (NSCLC): A phase II study of the lung study group (LCSG). Proc Am Soc Clin Oncol 1988;7:197.
258. Eagan R, Ruud C, Lee R, et al. Pilot study of induction therapy with cyclophosphamide, doxorubicin, and cisplatin (CAP) and chest irradiation prior to thoracotomy in initially inoperable stage III M0 non-small cell lung cancer. Cancer Treat Rep 198771:895–900.
259. Strauss GM, Herndon JE, Sherman DD, et al. Neoadjuvant chemotherapy and radiotherapy followed by surgery in stage IIIA non-small cell carcinoma of the lung: Report of a cancer and leukemia group B phase II study. J Clin Oncol 1992;10:1237–1244.
260. Albain K, Rusch V, Crowley J, et al. Concurrent cisplatin (DDP), VP–16, and chest irradiation (RT) followed by surgery for stages IIIa and IIIb non-small cell lung cancer (NSCLC): A Southwest Oncology Group (SWOG) Study (#8805). Proc Am Soc Clin Oncol 1991;10:244.
261. Skarin A, Jochelson M, Sheldon T, et al. Neoadjuvant chemotherapy in marginally resectable stage III M0 non-small cell lung cancer: Long-term follow-up in 41 patients. J Surg Oncol 1989;40:266–274.
262. Sherman D, Strauss G, Schwartz J, et al. Combined modality therapy for regionally advanced stage III non-small cell carcinoma of the lung (NSCLC) employing neoadjuvant chemotherapy (CT), radiotherapy (RT), and surgery (S). Proc Am Soc Clin Oncol 1987;6:167.
263. Armstrong JG, Minsky BD. Primary radiation therapy for stage I and II medically inoperable non-small cell lung cancer. Cancer Treat Rev 1989;16:247–255.
264. Hilton G. Present position relating to cancer of the lung: Results with radiotherapy alone. Thorax 1960;15:17–18.
265. Smart J. Can lung cancer be cured by irradiation alone? JAMA 1966;195:158–159.
266. Hong XZ, Wei BY, Li JZ, et al. Curative radiotherapy of early operable non-small cell lung cancer. Radiother Oncol 1989;14:89–94.
267. Hafty BG, Goldberg NB, Gerstley J, Fischer DB, Peschel RE. Results of radical radiation therapy in clinical stage I, technically operable non-small cell lung cancer. Int J Radiat Oncol Biol Phys 1988;15:69–73.
268. Noordijk EM, Poest CE, Hermans J, Wever AMJ, Leer JWH. Radiotherapy as an alternative to surgery in elderly patients with resectable lung cancer. Radiother Oncol 1988;13:83–89.
269. Hilaris BS, Nori D, Martini N. Intraoperative radiotherapy in stage I and II lung cancer. Semin Surg Oncol 1987;3:22–32.
270. Armstrong J, Martini N, Kris M, Harrison L. Induction chemotherapy for non-small cell lung cancer with clinically evident mediastinal nodal metastases: The role of postoperative radiotherapy. Int J Radiat Oncol Biol Phys 1992;23:605–613.
271. Bleehen NM, Cox JD. Radiotherapy for lung cancer. Int J Radiat Oncol Biol Phys 1985;11:1001–1007.

272. Cox JD, Komaki R, Byhardt RW. Is immediate radiation therapy indicated for patients with unresectable non-small cell lung cancer? Yes. Cancer Treat Rep 1983; 67:327–331.

273. Payne DG. Non-small-cell lung cancer: Should unresectable stage III patients routinely receive high-dose radiation therapy? J Clin Oncol 1988;6:552–558.

273a. Berry RJ, Laing AH, Newman CR, Peto J. The role of radiotherapy in treatment of inoperable lung cancer. Int J Radiat Oncol Biol Phys 1977;2:433–439.

273b. Johnson DH, Einhorn LH, Bartolucci A, et al. Thoracic radiotherapy does not prolong survival in patients with locally advanced, unresectable, non-small cell lung cancer. Ann Int Med 1990;113:33–38.

274. Armstrong J, Burman C, Leibel S, Fontenla D, Kutcher G, Fuks Z. Conformal three dimensional treatment planning may improve the therapeutic ratio of high dose radiation therapy for lung cancer. Int J Radiat Oncol Biol Phys 1991;21(1):146.

275. Kubota K, Furuse K, Kawahara M, Fukuoka M, Negoro S. Randomized trial of chemotherapy with or without thoracic radiation therapy for treatment of locally advanced non-small cell lung cancer. Pro Am Soc Clin Oncol 1990;9:226.

276. Perez CA. non-small cell carcinoma of the lung: Dose-time parameters. Cancer Treat Symp 1985;2:131–142.

277. Arriagada R, Le Chevalier T, Quoix E, et al. Chemotherapy effect on locally advanced non-small cell lung carcinoma: A randomized study on 353 patients. Proceedings of the 32nd annual ASTRO meeting, 1990. Int J Radiat Oncol Biol Physics 1990;19(Suppl l):195.

278. Cox JD, Azarnia N, Byhardt RW, Shin KY, Emami B, Pajak TF. A randomized phase I/II trial of hyperfractionated radiation therapy with total doses of 60.0 Gy to 79.2 Gy: Possible survival benefit with >69.6 Gy in favorable patients with stage III radiation therapy oncology group non-small-cell lung carcinoma: Report of radiation therapy oncology group 83-11. J Clin Oncol 1990;8:1543–1555.

279. Armstrong JG, Shank B, Scher H, Gaynor J, Martini N, Kris M. Limited small cell lung cancer: Do favorable short-term results predict ultimate outcome? Am J Clin Oncol 1991;14:285–290.

280. Turrisi A, Glover DJ, Mason B. A preliminary report: Concurrent twice-daily radiotherapy plus platinum-etoposide chemotherapy for limited small cell lung cancer. Int J Radiat Oncol Biol Phys 1988;15:183–187.

281. Johnson BE, Grayson J, Woods E, et al. Limited stage small cell lung cancer treated with concurrent etoposide/cisplatin plus bid chest radiotherapy. Proc Am Soc Clin Oncol 1989;8:228.

282. Martini N, Kris MG, Gralla RJ, et al. The effects of preoperative chemotherapy on the resectability of non-small cell lung carcinoma with mediastinal lymph node metastases (N2M0). Ann Thorac Surg 1988;45:370–379.

283. Burkes R, Ginsberg R, Shepherd F, et al. Neo-adjuvant trial with MVP (mitomycin-c + vindesine + cisplatin) chemotherapy for stage III (T1-3, N2, M0) unresectable non-small cell lung cancer (NSCLC). Proc Am Soc Clin Oncol 1989;8:221.

284. Withers HR, Taylor J, Maciejewski B. The hazard of accelerated tumor clongen repopulation during radiotherapy. Acta Oncol 1988;27:131–146.

285. Lee R, Carr D, Childs D. Comparison of split-course radiation therapy and continuous radiation therapy for unresectable bronchogenic carcinoma: 5 year results. AJR 1976;126:116–122.

286. Holsti L, Mattson K. A randomized study of split–course radiotherapy of lung cancer: Long-term results. Int J Radiat Oncol Biol Phys 1980;6:977–981.

287. Simpson JR, Francis ME, Perez-Tamayo R, Marks RD, Rao DV. Palliative radiotherapy for inoperable carcinoma of the lung: Final report of a RTOG multi-institutional trial. Int J Radiat Oncol Biol Phys 1985;11:751–758.

288. Guthrie R, Ptacek J, Hass C. Comparative analysis of two regimens of split course radiation in carcinoma of the lung. AJR 1973;117:605–608.

289. Saunders M, Dische S, Fowler J, et al. Radiotherapy employing three fractions on each of twelve consecutive days. Acta Oncologica 1988;27:163–167.

290. Emami B, Perez CA, Herskovich A, Hederman MA. Phase I/II study of treatment of locally advanced (T3,T4) non-oat cell lung cancer with high dose radiotherapy (rapid fractionation): Radiation Therapy Oncology Group Study. Int J Radiat Oncol Biol Phys 1988;15:1021–1025.

291. Tokars R, Ansari R, Mantravadi R, et al. A phase III study of thoracic radiation with or without concurrent cisplatinum chemotherapy in locoregional unresectable non-small cell carcinoma of the lung: A Hoosier Oncology Group Protocol. Int J Radiat Oncol Biol Phys 1991;21(1):136.

292. Minatel E, Trovo M, Franchin G, et al. Radiotherapy versus RT enhanced by cisplatin in stage III non-small lung cancer: Randomized trial. Int J Radiat Oncol Biol Phys 1991;21(1):136.

293. Schaake-Koning C, Van den Bogaert W, Dalesio O, et al. Effects of concomitant cisplatin and radiotherapy on inoperable non-small cell lung cancer. N Engl J Med 1992;326:524–530.

294. Kim JH, Alfieri A, Kim SH, Young C, Silvestrini R. Radiosensitization of meth-A fibrosarcoma in mice by lonidamine. Oncology 1984;41(1):36–38.

295. Privitera G, Battista CG, Patane C, et al. Phase II double-blind randomized study of lonidamine and radiotherapy in epidermoid carcinoma of the lung. Radiother Oncol 1987;10:285–290.

296. Brouet D. Results of a trial using radiotherapy and chemotherapy in bronchial cancer. Eur J Cancer 1968;4:437–445.

297. Host H. Cyclophosphamide as an adjuvant to radiotherapy in the treatment of unresectable bronchogenic carcinoma. Cancer Chemother Rep 1973;4:161–164.

298. Kaung D, Wolf J, Hyde L, et al. Preliminary report of the treatment of nonresectable cancer of the lung. Cancer Chemother Rep 1974;58:359–364.

299. Holsti L. Alternative approaches to radiotherapy alone and radiotherapy as part of a combined therapeutic approach for lung cancer. Cancer Chemother Rep 1973;4:165–169.

300. Hall TC, Dederick M, Chalmers T, et al. A clinical and pharmacologic study of chemotherapy and X-ray therapy in lung cancer. Am J Med 1967;43:186–193.

301. Benninghoff D, Alexander L. Treatment of lung carcinoma: Radiation versus radiation combined with 5–fluorouracil. NY State J Med 1967;68(1):532–534.

302. Krant MJ, Chalmers T, Dederick M, et al. Comparative trial of chemotherapy and radiotherapy in patients with nonresectable cancer of the lung. Am J Med 1963;35:363–373.

303. Durrant KR, Ellis F, Black J, et al. Comparison of treatment policies in inoperable cancer of the lung. Lancet 1971;1:715–719.

304. Coy P. A randomized study of irradiation and vinblastine in lung cancer. Cancer 1970;26:803–809.

305. Johnson DH, Einhorn LH, Bartolucci A, et al. Thoracic radiotherapy does not prolong survival in patients with locally advanced, unresectable, non-small cell lung cancer. Ann Intern Med 1990;113:33–38.

306. Dillman RO, Seagren SL, Propert KJ, et al. A randomized trial of induction chemotherapy plus high-dose radiation versus radiation alone in stage III non-small cell lung cancer. N Engl J Med 1990;14:940–945.

307. Leung W, Shiu W, Tsao S, et al. Combined chemotherapy and radiotherapy versus best supportive care in treatment of inoperable limited stage non-small cell lung cancer. Proc Am Soc Clin Oncol 1990;9:939.

308. Shaw R, Paulson D, Kee J. Treatment of the superior sulcus tumor by irradiation followed by resection. Ann Surg 1961;154:29–40.

309. Hilaris B, Martini N, Wong G, Nori D. Treatment of superior sulcus tumor (Pancoast tumor). Surg Clin North Am 1987;67(5):965–977.

310. Shahian D, Neptune W, Ellis H. Pancoast tumors: Improved survival with preoperative and postoperative radiotherapy. Ann Thorac Surg 1987;43:32–38.

311. Beyer D, Weisenburger T. Superior sulcus tumors. Am J Clin Oncol 1986;9(2):156–161.

312. Komaki R, Mountain C, Holbert J, et al. Superior sulcus tumors: Treatment selection and results for 85 patients without metastases (M0) at presentation. Int J Radiat Oncol Biol Phys 1990;91:31–36.

313. Neal C, Amdur R, Mendenhall W, Knauf D, Block A, Million R. Pancoast tumor: Radiation therapy alone versus preoperative radiation plus surgery. Int J Radiat Oncol Biol Phys 1991;21:651–660.

314. Armstrong JG, Fass DE, Bains M, et al. Paraspinal tumors: Techniques and results of brachytherapy. Int J Radiat Oncol Biol Phys. 1991;20:787–790.

315. Schnabel K, Vogt-Moykopf I, Berberich W, Abel U. Vergleich einer neutronen-mit einer photonenbestrahlung des bronchialkarzinoma. Strahlentherapie 1983;159:458–464.

316. Austin-Seymour M, Griffin T, Laramore G, Maor M, Parker R. High-LET radiation therapy of non-small cell lung cancer. Chest 1989;96(Suppl):72–73.

317. Livingston R, Griffin B, Higano C, et al. Combined treatment with chemotherapy and neutron irradiation for limited non-small cell lung cancer: A Southwest Oncology Group Study. J Clin Oncol 1987;5:1716–1724.

318. Hilaris BS, Martini N. The current state of intraoperative interstitial brachytherapy in lung cancer. Int J Radiat Oncol Biol Phys 1988;15:1347–1354.

319. Hilaris BS, Nori D, Anderson LL. Atlas of brachytherapy. New York: Macmillan, 1988:46–69.

320. Hilaris B, Gomez J, Nori D, Anderson L, Martini N. Combined surgery, intraoperative brachytherapy, and postoperative external radiation in stage III non-small cell lung cancer. Cancer 1985;55:1226–1231.

321. Abe M, Takahishi M, Yabumoto E, Adachi H, Yoshii M, Mori K. Clinical experiences with intraoperative radiotherapy of locally advanced cancers. Cancer 1980;45:40–48.

322. Pass HI, Sindelar W, Kinsella T, et al. Delivery of intraoperative radiation therapy after pneumonectomy: Experimental observations and early clinical results. Ann Thorac Surg 1987;44:14–20.

323. Juettner FM, Arian-Schad K, Porsch G, et al. Intraoperative radiation therapy combined with external irradiation in nonresectable non-small-cell lung cancer: Preliminary report. Int J Radiat Oncol Biol Phys 1990;18:1143–1150.

324. Calvo F, Ortiz de Urbina D, Abuchaibe O, et al. Intraoperative radiotherapy during lung cancer surgery: Technical description and early clinical results. Int J Radiat Oncol Biol Phys 1990;19:103–109.

325. Perez CA, Pajak TF, Rubin P, et al. Long-term observations of the pattern of failure in patients with unresectable non-oat cell carcinoma of the lung treated with definitive radiotherapy. Cancer 1987;59:1874–1881.

326. Cox J, Stanley K, Petrovich Z, Paig C, Yesner R. Cranial irradiation in cancer of the lung of all cell types. JAMA 1981;245:469–472.

327. Umsawadi T, Valdivieso M, Chen T, et al. Role of elective brain irradiation during combined chemoradiotherapy for limited disease non-small cell lung cancer. J Neurooncol 1984;2:253–259.

328. Mira J, Miller T, Crowley J. Chest irradiation (RT) vs. chest RT + chemotherapy +/− prophylactic brain RT in localized non small cell lung cancer: A Southwest Oncology Group randomized study. Int J Radiat Oncol Biol Phys 1990;19(Suppl 1):145.

329. Russel A, Pajak T, Selim H, et al. Prophylactic cranial irradiation for lung cancer patients at high risk for development of cerebral metastases: Results of a prospective randomized trial conducted by the Radiation Therapy Oncology Group. Int J Radiat Oncol Biol Phys 1991;21:637–643.

330. Pisters K, Divgi C, Kris M, et al. Phase I and imaging trial of radiolabeled anti–EGF receptor monoclonal antibody RG 83852 in non-small cell lung cancer. Proc Am Soc Clin Oncol 1991;10:265.

331. O'Connell J, Kris M, Gralla R, et al. Frequency and prognostic importance of pre-

treatment clinical characteristics in patients with advanced non-small cell lung cancer treated with combination chemotherapy. J Clin Oncol 1986;4:1604–1614.

332. Kris M, Cohen E, Gralla R. An analysis of 134 phase II trials in non-small cell lung cancer IV. Toronto: World Conference on Lung Cancer, 1985:39.

333. Ruckdeschel J, Findelson D, Ettinger D, et al. A randomized trial of the four most active regimens for metastatic non-small cell lung cancer. J Clin Oncol 1986;4:14–22.

334. Karnofsky D, Burchenal J. The clinical evaluation of chemotherapeutic agents in cancer. In: MacLoed C. Evaluation of chemotherapeutic agents. New York: Columbia University Press, 1949:191–205.

335. Gralla R, Casper E, Kelsen D. Cisplatin plus vindesine combination chemotherapy for advanced carcinoma of the lung: A randomized trial investigating two dosage schedules. Ann Intern Med 1981;95:414–420.

336. Kris M. Mitomycin in combination chemotherapy regimens for patients with advanced non-small cell lung cancer. In: Gralla R, Einhorn L. Treatment and prevention of small cell lung cancer and non-small cell lung cancer. London: Royal Society of Medicine Services, 1989:101–108.

337. Kris M, Gralla R, Wertheim M, et al. Trial of the combination of mitomycin, vindesine, cisplatin in patients with advanced non-small cell lung cancer. Cancer Treat Rep 1986;70:1091.

338. Kelsen D, Gralla R, Stoopler M. Cisplatin, doxorubicin, cyclophosphamide, and vindesine combination chemotherapy for non-small cell lung cancer. Cancer Treat Rep 1982;66:247–251.

339. Britell J, Eagan R, Ingle J, et al. Cis–Dichlorodiammineplatinum (II) alone followed by Adriamycin plus cyclophosphamide at progression versus cis-Dichlorodiammineplatinum (II), Adriamycin, and cyclophosphamide in combination for adenocarcinoma of the lung. Cancer Treat Rep 1978;62:1207–1210.

340. Rossof A, Bearden J, Coltman CJ. Phase II evaluation of Cis–diamminedichloroplatinum. Cancer Treat Rep 1976;66:1679–1680.

341. Vogel S, Berenzweig M, Camacho F. Efficacy study of intensive cisplatin therapy in advanced non-small bronchogenic carcinoma. Cancer 1982;50:24–26.

342. Casper ES, Gralla RJ, Kelson DP, et al. Phase II trials with high dose cis–dichlorodiammineplatinum (II) in the treatment of non-small cell lung cancer. Cancer Treat Rep 1979;63:2107–2109.

343. Panettiere F, Vance R, Stuckey W, et al. Evaluation of single-agent cisplatin in the management of non-small cell carcinoma of the lung: A Southwest Oncology Group Study. Cancer Treat Rep 1983;67:399–400.

344. Bhuchar VK, Lanzotti VJ. High dose cisplatin for lung cancer. Cancer Treat Rep 1982;66:375–376.

345. Klastersky J, Sculier J, Bureau G, et al. Cisplatin versus cisplatin plus etoposide in the treatment of advanced non-small cell lung cancer. J Clin Oncol 1989;7:1087–1092.

346. DeJager R, Longeval E, Klastersky J. Phase II clinical trials with high dose cisplatin with fluid and mannitol induced diuresis in advanced lung cancer: A phase II clinical trial of the EORTC Lung Cancer Working Party (Belgium). Cancer Treat Rep 1980;63:1341–1346.

347. Gandara D, DeGregorio M, Wold H, et al. High-dose cisplatin in hypertonic saline: Reduced toxicity of a modified dose schedule and correlation with plasma pharmacokinetics. A Northern California Oncology Group pilot study in non-small cell lung cancer. J Clin Oncol 1986;4:1793–1793.

348. Gandara D, Wold H, Perez E, et al. Cisplatin dose intensity in non-small cell lung cancer: Phase II results of a day 1 and day 8 high–dose regimen. JNCI 1989;81:790–794.

349. Itri L, Gralla R. A review of etoposide in patients with non-small cell lung cancer (NSCLC). Cancer Treat Rev 1982;9:115–118.

350. Rosso R, Salvati F, Ardizzoni A, et al. Etoposide versus etoposide plus high-dose cisplatin in the management of advanced non-small cell lung cancer. Cancer 1990;66:130–134.

351. Saxman S, Logie K, Stephens D, et al. Phase II trial of daily oral etoposide in patients with surgically unresectable non-small cell lung cancer (NSCLC). Proc Am Soc Clin Oncol 1990;9:238.

352. Olver I, Donehower R, Van Echo D, et al. Phase II trial of carboplatin (CBDCA) in non-small cell lung cancer (NSCLC). Proc Am Soc Clin Oncol 1985;4:182.

353. Kreisman H, Ginsberg S, Propert K, et al. Carboplatin or iproplatin in advanced non-small cell lung cancer: A cancer and leukemia group B study. Cancer Treat Rep 1987;71:1049–1052.

354. Gatzemeier U, Hossfeld D, Neuhauss R, et al. Phase II trial with carboplatin in patients with advanced unresectable non-small cell lung cancer. Proc Am Soc Clin Oncol 1989;8:237.

355. Bonomi P, Finkelstein D, Ruckdeschel J, et al. Combination chemotherapy versus single agents followed by combination chemotherapy in stage IV non-small cell lung cancer: A study of the Eastern Cooperative Oncology Group. J Clin Oncol 1989;7:1602–1613.

356. Micetich K, Creekmore S, Fisher R. A phase II trial of a 24-hour infusion of carboplatin in patients with non-small cell lung cancer. In: Bunn PJ, Ceretta R, Ozols R. Carboplatin: Current perspective and future directions. Philadelphia: WB Saunders, 1990: 317–322.

357. Klastersky J, Lacroix H, Dabouis G, et al. A randomized study comparing cisplatin or carboplatin with etoposide in patients with advanced non-small cell lung cancer: European Organization for Research and Treatment of Cancer Protocol 07861. J Clin Oncol 1990;8:1556–1562.

358. Woods R, Williams C, Levi J, et al. A randomized trial of cisplatin and vindesine versus supportive care only in advanced non-small cell lung cancer. Br J Cancer 1990;61:608–611.

359. Elliot J, Ahmedzao S, Hole D. Vindesine and cisplatin combination chemotherapy compared with vindesine as a single agent in the management of non-small cell lung cancer: A randomized trial. Eur J Cancer Clin Oncol 1984;20:1025–1032.

360. Einhorn L, Loehrer J, Williams S, et al. Random prospective study of vindesine plus high-dose cisplatin versus vindesine plus cisplatin plus mitomycin C in advanced non-small cell lung cancer. J Clin Oncol 1986;4:1037–1043.

361. Dhingra H, Valdivieso M, Carr D, et al. Randomized trial of three combinations of cisplatin with vindesine and/or VP–16–213 in the treatment of advanced non-small cell lung cancer. J Clin Oncol 1985;3:176–184.

362. Luedke D, Einhorn L, Omura G, et al. Randomized comparison of two combination regimens versus minimal chemotherapy in non-small cell lung cancer: A Southeastern Cancer Study Group Trial. J Clin Oncol 1990;8:886–891.

363. Woodcock T, Blumenreich M, Richman S, et al. Combination chemotherapy with cis–diammindichloroplatinum and vinblastine in advanced non-small cell lung cancer. J Clin Oncol 1983;1:247–250.

364. Kris M, Gralla R, Kalman L, et al. Randomized trial comparing vindesine plus cisplatin with vinblastine plus cisplatin in patients with non-small cell lung cancer with an analysis of methods of response assessment. Cancer Treat Rep 1985;69:387–395.

365. Ganz P, Figlin R, Haskell C, et al. Supportive care versus supportive care and combination chemotherapy in metastatic non-small cell lung cancer: Does chemotherapy make a difference? Cancer 1989;63:1271–1278.

366. Weick J, Crowley J, Natale R, et al. A randomized trial of five cisplatin-containing treatments in patients with metastatic non-small cell lung cancer: A Southwest Oncology Group Study. J Clin Oncol 1991;9:1157–1162.

367. Green M, Stoopler M, Anderson J, et al. Vinblastine (V) and Cisplatin (CDDP) chemotherapy in advanced non small cell lung cancer (NSCLC). Proc Am Soc Clin Oncol 1985;4:176.

368. Huberman M, Lokich J, Greene R, et al. Vinblastine plus cisplatin in advanced non-small cell lung cancer: Lack of advantage for vinblastine infusion schedule. Cancer Treat Rep 1986;70:287–89,

369. Sierocki J, Hilaris P, Hopfan S, et al. Cis-dichlorodiammineplatinum (II) and VP 16-213: An active induction regimen for small cell carcinoma of the lung. Cancer Treat Rep 1979;63:1593–1597.

370. Longeval E, Klastersky J. Combination chemotherapy with cisplatin and etoposide in bronchogenic squamous cell carcinoma and adenocarcinoma. Cancer 1982;50: 2751–2756.

371. Paccagnella A, Favaretto A, Brandes A, et al. Cisplatin, etoposide, and ifosfamide in non-small cell lung carcinoma: A phase II randomized study with cisplatin and etoposide as the control arm. Cancer 1990;65:2631–2634.

372. Klastersky J, Sculier J, Ravez P, et al. A randomized study comparing a high and a standard dose of cisplatin in combination with etoposide in the treatment of advanced non-small cell lung carcinoma. J Clin Oncol 1986;4:1780–1786.

373. Mitrou P, Fischer M, Weissenfels I, et al. Treatment of inoperable non-small cell bronchogenic carcinoma with etoposide and cis-platinum. Cancer Treat Rev 1982;9: 139–142.

374. Kris M, Gralla R, Wertheim M. Trial of the combination of mitomycin, vindesine and cisplatin in patients with advanced non-small cell lung cancer. Cancer Treat Rep 1985;70:1091–1096.

375. Joss R, Burki K, Dalquen P, et al. Combination chemotherapy with mitomycin, vindesine, and cisplatin for non-small cell lung cancer. Cancer 1990;11:2426–2434.

376. Gralla R, Kris M, Potanovich L, et al. Enhancing the safety and efficacy of the MVP regimen (mitomycin + vinblastine + cisplatin) in 100 patients with inoperable non-small cell lung cancer (NSCLC). Proc Am Soc Clin Oncol 1989;8:227.

377. Spain R. Neoadjuvant mitomycin C, cisplatin, and infusion vinblastine in locally and regionally advanced non-small cell lung cancer: Problems and progress from the perspective of long-term follow–up. Semin Oncol 1988;15:6–15.

378. Folman R, Rosman M. The role of chemotherapy in non-small cell lung cancer: The community perspective. Semin Oncol 1988;15:16–21.

379. Haedicke K, Camp B, Farber L, et al. Treatment of advanced non-small cell lung cancer (NSCLC) with mitomycin, velban, cisplatin (MVP) at Yale. Proc Am Soc Clin Oncol 1986;5:183.

380. Livingston R, Griffin B, Higano C, et al. Combined treatment with chemotherapy and neutron irradiation for limited non-small cell lung cancer: A Southwest Oncology Group Study. J Clin Oncol 1987;5:1716–1724.

381. Ruckdeschel J, Finkelstein D, Mason B, et al. Chemotherapy for metastatic non-small cell bronchogenic carcinoma: EST 2575. Generation V–a randomized comparison of four cisplatin-containing regimens. J Clin Oncol 1985;3:72–80.

381a. Kris MG, Gralla RJ, Kelsen DP, et al. Trial of vindesine plus mitomycin in stage 3 non-small cell lung cancer. An active regimen for outpatient treatment. Chest 1985;87: 368–372.

382. Shinkai T, Saijo N, Tominaga K, et al. Comparison of vindesine plus cisplatin or vindesine plus mitomycin in the treatment of advanced non-small cell lung cancer. Cancer Treat Rep 1985;69:945–951.

383. Gatzemeier U, Heckmayr M, Hossfeld D, et al. Chemotherapy of advanced NSCLC: A prospective randomized trial comparing DDP/VP with Mito/IFO and Mito/VDS. Lung Cancer [Abstract] 1988;4:125.

384. Klastersky J, Sculier J, Vandermoten G. Combination chemotherapy with mitomycin C and vindesine in the treatment of non-small cell lung carcinoma (NSCLC). Toronto: Proceedings of the Fourth World Conference on Lung Cancer, 1985.

385. Giron C, Ordonez A, Jalon I, et al. Combination chemotherapy with ifosfamide, mitomycin, and cisplatin in advanced non-small cell lung cancer. Cancer Treat Rep 1987;71:851–853.

386. Cullen M, Joshi R, Chetiyawardana A, et al. Mitomycin, ifosfamide and cisplatin in

non-small cell lung cancer: Treatment good enough to compare. Br J Cancer 1988;58: 359–361.

387. Cormier Y, Bergeron D, La Forge J, et al. Benefits of polychemotherapy in advanced non-small cell bronchogenic carcinoma. Cancer 1982;50:845–849.

388. Cellerino R, Tummarello D, Guidi F, et al. A randomized trial of alternating chemotherapy versus best supportive care in advanced non-small cell lung cancer. J Clin Oncol 1991;9:1453–1461.

389. Quoix E, Dietemann A, Charconneau J, et al. Disseminated non-small cell lung cancer (NSCLC): A randomized trial of chemotherapy (CT) versus palliative care (PC). Lung Cancer 1988;4(Suppl):127.

390. Kaasa S, Lund E, Host H, et al. Combination chemotherapy versus symptomatic treatment in patients with non-small cell lung cancer, extensive disease 0–0007. London: Fifth European Conference on Clinical Oncology, 1989.

391. Souquet P, Boissel J, Bernard J. Utility of the chemotherapy in advanced non-small cell lung cancer: Results of a meta-analysis. Lung Cancer 1991;7(Suppl):101.

392. Jaakkimainen L, Goodwin J, Pater J, et al. Counting the costs of chemotherapy in a National Cancer Institute of Canada randomized trial in non-small cell lung cancer. J Clin Oncol 1990;8:1301–1309.

393. Casazza A, DiMarco A, Bertazzoli C. Antitumor activity, toxicity, and pharmacological properties of 4'-epiadriamycin. In: Siegenthaler W, Luthy R. Current chemotherapy. Washington, DC: American Society of Microbiology, 1978:1257–1260.

394. Kalman J, Kris M, Gralla R, et al. Phase II trial of 4'-epi-doxorubicin in patients with non-small cell lung cancer. Cancer Treat Rep 1983;67:591–592.

395. Feld R, Wierzbicki R, Walde D, et al. High dose epirubicin (E) given as a daily × 3 schedule in patients (pts) with untreated extensive non-small cell lung cancer (NSCLC): A phase I–II study. Proc Am Assoc Cancer Res 1988;29:208.

396. Martoni A, Melotti B, Guaraldi M, et al. Activity of high dose epirubicin (HD EPI) in non small cell lung cancer (NSCLC). Proc Am Soc Clin Oncol 1990;9:237.

397. Depierre A, Lemarie E, Dabouis G, et al. Phase II study of navelbine (NVB) in non-small cell lung cancer (NSCLC). Proc Am Soc Clin Oncol 1988;7:201.

398. Giaccone G, Donadio M, Ferrati P, et al. Teniposide in the treatment on non-small cell lung carcinoma. Cancer Treat Rep 1987;71:83–85.

399. Shum K, Kris M, Gralla R, et al. Phase II study of 10-ethyl-10-deaza-aminopterin in patients with stage III and IV non-small cell lung cancer. J Clin Oncol 1988;6:446–450.

400. Lee J, Libshitz H, Murphy W, et al. Phase II study of 10-ethyl-10-deaza-aminopterin (10-EdAM; CGP 30 694) for stage IIIB or IV non-small cell lung cancer. Invest New Drugs 1990;8:299–304.

401. Souhami R, Hartley J, Allen R, et al. Phase II study of 10-EdAM (10-ethyl-10-deazamiopterin) in untreated advanced non-small cell lung cancer (NSCLC). Proc Am Soc Clin Oncol 1991;10:252.

402. Negoro S, Masahiro F, Masuda N, et al. Phase I study of weekly intravenous infusions of CPT-11, a new derivative of camptothecin, in the treatment of advanced non-small cell lung cancer. JNCI 1991;83:1164–1168.

403. Fukuoka M, Negoro S, Niitani H, et al. A phase II study of new camptothecin derivative, CPT-11 in previously untreated non-small cell lung cancer (NSCLC). Proc Am Soc Clin Oncol 1990;9:226.

404. Abbruzzese J, Grunewald R, Weeks E, et al. A phase I clinical, plasma, and cellular pharmacology study of gemcitabine. J Clin Oncol 1991;90:491–498.

405. Hertel L, Boder G, Kroin J, et al. Evaluation of the antitumor activity of gemcitabine (2',2'-difluoro-2'-deoxycytidine). Cancer Res 1990;50:4417–4422.

406. Anderson H, Lund B, Hansen HH, et al. Phase II study of gemcitabine in non-small cell lung cancer (NSCLC). Proc Am Soc Clin Oncol 1991;10:247.

407. Brown T, Havlin G, Weiss G, et al. A phase I trial of taxol given by a 6-hour intravenous infusion. J Clin Oncol 1991;9:1261–1267.

408. Rigas J, Kris M, Tong W, et al. Phase I trial of chloroquinoxaline sulfonamide (CQS): A unique agent with activity in NSCLC selected for study based on activity in an in vitro stem cell assay. Lung Cancer 1991;7:108.

409. Shoemaker R. New approaches to antitumor drug screening: The human tumor colony forming assay. Cancer Treat Rep 1986;70:9–12.

410. Hong W, Lippman S, Itri L, et al. Prevention of second primary tumors with isotretinoin in squamous-cell carcinoma of the head and neck. N Engl J Med 1990;323:795–800.

411. Warrell R, Frankel S, Miller W, et al. Differentiation therapy of acute promyelocytic leukemia with tretinoin (all-trans retinoic acid). N Engl J Med 1991;324:1385–1394.

412. Young C, Fanucchi M, Walsh D, et al. Phase I trial and clinical pharmacological evaluation of hexamethylene bisacetamide administration by ten-day continuous intravenous infusion at twenty-eight-day intervals. Cancer Res 1988;48:7304–7309.

413. Ruckdeschel J, Codish S, Stranahan A, et al. Postoperative empyema improves survival in lung cancer: Documentation and analysis of a natural experiment. N Engl J Med 1972;287:1013–1017.

414. McNeally M, Maver C, Kausel H. Regional immunotherapy of lung cancer with intrapleural B.C.G. Lancet 1976;1:377–379.

415. Stanley K. Ludwig Lung Cancer Study Group (LLCSG). Immunostimulation with intrapleural BCG as adjuvant therapy in resected non-small cell lung cancer. Cancer 1986;58:2411–2416.

416. Anthony H. Yorkshire trial of adjuvant therapy with levamisole in surgically treated lung cancer. In: Terry W, Rosenberg S. Immunotherapy of human cancer. New York: Elsevier North Holland, 1982:135–145.

417. Amery W, Cosemans J, Gooszen H, et al. Four year results from double-blind study of adjuvant levamisole treatment in resectable lung cancer. In: Terry W, Rosenberg S. Immunotherapy of human cancer. New York: Elsevier North Holland, 1982:123–133.

418. Holmes E, Gail M. Surgical adjuvant therapy for stage II and stage III adenocarcinoma and large–cell undifferentiated carcinoma. J Clin Oncol 1986;4:710–715.

419. Krown S, Stoopler M, Gralla R, et al. Phase II trial of human leukocyte interferon in non-small cell lung cancer: Preliminary results. In: Terry W, Rosenberg S. Immunotherapy of human cancer. Amsterdam: Elsevier North Holland, 1982:397–405.

420. Grunberg S, Kempf R, Itri L. Phase II study of recombinant alpha interferon in the treatment of advanced non-small cell lung carcinoma. Cancer Treat Rep 1985;69: 1031–1032.

421. Schiller J, Storer B, Dreicer R, et al. Randomized phase II–III trial of combination beta and gamma interferons and etoposide and cisplatin in inoperable non-small cell cancer of the lung. JNCI 1989;81:1739–1743.

422. Wadler S, Schwartz E. Antineoplastic activity of the combination of interferon and cytotoxic agents against experimental and human malignancies: A review. Cancer Res 1990;50:3473–3486.

423. Rosenberg S, Lotze M, Mule J. New approaches to the immunotherapy of cancer using interleukin-2. Ann Intern Med 1988;108:853–864.

424. Dillman R. Monoclonal antibodies for treating cancer. Ann Intern Med 1989;111: 592–603.

425. Dienhart D, Schmelter R, Lear J, et al. Imaging of non-small cell lung cancers with a monoclonal antibody, KC-4G3, which recognizes a human milk fat globule antigen. Cancer Res 1990;50:7068–7076.

426. Veale D, Kerr N, Gibson J, et al. Characterization of epidermal growth factor receptor in primary human non-small cell lung cancer. Cancer Res 1989;49:1313–1317.

427. Lee J, Ro J, Sahin A, et al. Expression of epidermal growth factor receptor (EGFR): A favorable prognostic factor for surgically resected non-small cell lung cancer (NSCLC). Proc Am Soc Clin Oncol 1989;8:226.

428. Hendler F, Shum-Siu A, Nanu L, et al. Increased EGF receptors and the absence of an alveolar differentiation marker predict a poor survival in lung cancer. Proc Am Soc Clin Oncol 1989;8:223.

429. Carroll M, Morgan SA, Yarnold JR, et al. Prospective evaluation of a watch policy in patients with inoperable non-small cell lung cancer. Eur J Cancer Clin Oncol 1986;22: 1353–1356.

429a. Bleehen N. Inoperable non-small cell lung cancer (NSCLC): A Medical Research Council randomized trial of palliative radiotherapy with two fractions or ten fractions. Br J Cancer 1991;63:265–270.

429b. Teo P, Tai T, Choy D, Tsui K. A randomized study on palliative radiation therapy for inoperable non-small cell carcinoma of the lung. Int J Radiat Oncol Biol Phys 1988;14: 867–871.

429c. Simpson J, Francis M, Perez-Tamayo R, Marks R, Rao D. Palliative radiotherapy for inoperable carcinoma of the lung: Final report of the RTOG multi-institutional trial. Int J Radiat Oncol Biol Phys 1988;11:751–758.

430. Jackson M, and Ball D. Palliative retreatment of locally recurrent lung cancer after radical radiotherapy. Med J Aust 1987;147:391–394.

431. Bindi M, Tucci E, Pepi F, Belezza A, Pirtoli L. Changes in performance status in patients with pulmonary carcinoma treated with mono-fractionation radiotherapy once a week. Giornale Italiano Di Oncologia 1990;10:89–92.

432. Nori D, Hilaris B, Martini N. Intraluminal irradiation in bronchogenic carcinoma. Surg Clin North Am 1987;67:1093–1101.

433. Schray M, McDougall J, Martinez A, Edmundson G, Cortese D. Management of malignant airway obstruction: Clinical and dosimetric considerations using an iridium-192 afterloading technique in conjunction with the Neodymium-YAG laser. Int J Radiat Oncol Biol Phys 1985;11:403–409.

434. Mehta M, Shahabi S, Jarjour N, Kinsella T. Endobronchial irradiation for malignant airway obstruction. Int J Radiat Oncol Biol Phys 1989;17:847–851.

435. Fass DE, Armstrong JG, Harrison LB, Nori D. Fractionated high dose endobronchial treatment for recurrent lung cancer. Endocurietherapy/Hyperthermia Oncology 1990;6:211–215.

436. Macha H, Coch K, Stadler M, Scumacher W, Krumacher E. New technique for testing occlusive and stenosing tumors of the trachea and main bronchi: Endobronchial irradiation by high dose iridium-192 combined with laser utilization. Thorax 1987;42: 511–515.

437. Burt P, O'Driscoll R, Notley M, Barber P, Stout R. Intraluminal irradiation for the palliation of lung cancer with the high dose rate micro-Selectron. Thorax 1990;45: 765–768.

438. Seagren S, Harrell J. Prospective trial of palliative high dose rate endobronchial irradiation with or without laser for recurrent non-small cell lung cancer. Proc Am Soc Clin Oncol 1990;9:224.

439. Borgelt B, Gelber R, Larson M, Hendrickson F, Griffin T, Roth R. Ultra-rapid high-dose irradiation schedules for the palliation of brain metastases: Final results of the first two studies by the Radiation Therapy Oncology Group. Int J Radiat Oncol Biol Phys 1981;7:1633–1638.

440. Mandell L, Hilaris B, Sullivan M, et al. The treatment of single brain metastasis from non-oat cell lung carcinoma: Surgery and radiation versus radiation therapy alone. Cancer 1986;58:641–649.

441. Patchell R, Tibbs P, Walsh J, et al. A randomized trial of surgery in the treatment of single metastases to the brain. N Engl J Med 1990;322:494–500.

442. Jensik RJ. The extent of resection for localized lung cancer: Segmental resection. In: Kittle CF, ed. Current controversies in thoracic surgery. Philadelphia: WB Saunders, 1986:175–182.

443. Read RC, Boop WC, Schaeffer RC. Survival after conservative resection for T1 N0 M0 non-small cell lung cancer. Ann Thorac Surg 1990;49:391–400.

444. Wain JC, Mathisen DJ, Hilgenberg AD, et al. Wedge and segmental resection for primary lung carcinomas. Proc Am Assoc Thorac Surg [Abstract] 1991;25:86.

445. Ginsberg RJ, Rubinstein L (for the Lung Cancer Study Group). A Randomized comparative trial of lobectomy vs limited resection for patients with T1 N0 non-small cell lung cancer. Lung Cancer 1991;7(Suppl):83, 304.

446. Paone JF, Spees EK, Newton CG, et al. An appraisal of en bloc resection of peripheral bronchogenic carcinoma involving the thoracic wall. Chest 1982;81:203–207.

447. Patterson GA, Ilves R, Ginsberg RJ, et al. The value of adjuvant radiotherapy in pulmonary and chest wall resection for bronchogenic carcinoma. Ann Thorac Surg 1982;34:692–697.

448. Piehler JM, Pairolero PC, Weiland LH, et al. Bronchogenic carcinoma with chest wall invasion: Factors affecting survival following en bloc resection. Ann Thorac Surg 1982;34:684–691.

449. McCaughan BC, Martini N, Bains MS, McCormack PM. Chest wall invasion in carcinoma of the lung: Therapeutic and prognostic implications. J Thorac Cardiovasc Surg 1985;89:836–841.

450. Van de Wal HJ, Lacquet LK, Jongerius CM. Chirurgische behandeling van longtumoren met doorgroei in de thoraxwand. (Belg) Tijdschr voor Geneeskunde 1987;43:91–96.

451. Allen MS, Mathisen DJ, Grillo HC, et al. Bronchogenic carcinoma with chest wall invasion. Ann Thorac Surg 1991;51:948–951.

452. Paulson DL. The "superior sulcus" lesion. In: Delarue NC, Eschapasse H. International trends in general thoracic surgery, vol 1: Lung cancer. Philadelphia: WB Saunders, 1985:121–131.

453. Anderson TM, Moy PM, Homes EC. Factors affecting survival in superior sulcus tumors. J Clin Oncol 1986;4:1598–1603.

454. Devine JW, Mendenhall WM, Million RR, Carmichael MJ. Carcinoma of the superior sulcus treated with surgery and/or radiation therapy. Cancer 1986;57:941–943.

455. Rice TW, Pringle JF, Sinclair JE, et al. Superior sulcus tumors: Results of treatment. Lung Cancer [Abstract] 1986;2:156–157.

456. Miller JI. Discussion of: Shahian DM, Neptune WB, Ellis FH. Pancoast tumors: Improved survival with preoperative and postoperative radiotherapy. Ann Thorac Surg 1987;43:32–38.

457. McKneally M. Discussion of: Shahian DM, Neptune WB, Ellis FH. Pancoast tumors: Improved survival with preoperative and postoperative radiotherapy. Ann Thorac Surg 1987;43:32–38.

458. Ricci C, Rendina EA, Venuta F. Surgical treatment of superior sulcus tumors. Lung Cancer [Abstract] 1988;4(Suppl):95.

459. Carrel T, Nachbur B, Bleher A. Is radiotherapy prior to surgical resection indicated for bronchogenic carcinoma with chest wall infiltration and for pancoast tumors? Lung Cancer [Abstract] 1988;4:80.

460. Dartevelle P, Marzelle J, Chapelier A, Loc'h F. Extended operations for T3-T4 primary lung cancers: Indications and results. Chest 1989;96(Suppl):51–53.

461. Komaki R, Mountain CF, Holbert JM, et al. Superior sulcus tumors: Treatment selection and results for 85 patients without metastasis (M0) at presentation. Int J Radiat Oncol Biol Phys 1990;19:31–36.

462. Van Den Bosch JMM, Bergstein PGM, Laros CD, Gelissen HJ, Schaepkens van Riempst ALEMS, Wagenaar SjSc. Lobectomy with sleeve resection in the treatment of tumors of the bronchus. Chest 1991;80:154–157.

463. Ungar I, Gyeney I, Scherer E, Szarvas I. Sleeve lobectomy: An alternative to pneumonectomy in the treatment of bronchial carcinoma. Thorac Cardiovasc Surg 1981;29:41–46.

464. Eschapasse H. Proceedings of the minisymposia. Toronto: Fourth World Conference on lung cancer, 1985:52–53.

465. Keszler P. Sleeve resection and other bronchoplasties in the surgery of bronchogenic tumors. Int Surg 1986;71:229–232.

466. Maeda M, Nanjo S, Nakamura K, Nakamoto K. Tracheobronchoplasty for lung cancer. Int Surg 1986;71:221–228.

467. Vogt-Moykopf I, Fritz T, Meyer G, et al. Bronchoplastic and angioplastic operation in bronchial carcinoma: Long term results of a retrospective analysis from 1973–1983. Int Surg 1986;71:211–220.

468. Naruke T. Bronchoplastic and bronchovascular procedures of the tracheobronchial tree in the management of primary lung cancer. Chest 1989;96(Suppl):53–56.

469. Kirschner PA. Lung cancer: Preoperative radiation therapy and surgery. NY State J Med 1981;81:339–342.

470. Sawamura K, Mori T, Hashimoto S, et al. Results of surgical treatment for N2 disease. Lung Cancer [Abstract] 1986;2:96.

471. Mastrorilli M, Bragaglia RB, Cipolla G, et al. Surgical management of N2 lung cancer. Lung Cancer [Abstract] 1988;4(Suppl):97.

472. Naruke T, Goya T, Tsuchiya R, Suemasu K. The importance of surgery to non-small cell carcinoma of the lung with mediastinal lymph node metastasis. Ann Thorac Surg 1988;46:603–610.

473. Deneffe G, Stalpaert G. Five year survival in resected T3/N2 lung cancer. Acta Chir Belg 1989;89:159–160.

474. Levasseur PH, Regnard JF. Long term results after surgery for N2 non small cell lung cancer. Bruges, Belgium: Presented at the International Association for the Study of Lung Cancer (IASLC) Workshop, June 17–21, 1990.

475. Watanabe Y, Shimizu J, Oda M, et al. Aggressive surgical intervention in N2 non-small cell cancer of the lung. Ann Thorac Surg 1991;51:253–261.

476. Walker WS, Carey F, Cameron EWJ, Lamb D. Results of surgery for N2 status bronchial carcinoma. Bruges, Belgium: Presented at the International Association for the Study of Lung Cancer (IASLC) Workshop, June 17–21, 1990.

477. Kirsch MM, Sloan H. Mediastinal metastasis in bronchogenic carcinoma: Influence of postoperative irradiation, cell type and location. Ann Thorac Surg 1982;33:459–463.

478. Martini N, Flehinger BJ. The role of surgery in N2 lung cancer. Surg Clin North Am 1987;67:1037–1049.

479. Mountain CF. The biological operability of stage III non-small cell lung cancer. Ann Thorac Surg 1985;40:60–64.

480. Frytak S, Eagan RT, Sawamura K, et al. Treatment of "limited" stage III non-small cell carcinoma of the lung. Cancer Invest 1988;6:193–207.

481. Pearson FG, Delarue NC, Ilves R, et al. Significance of positive superior mediastinal nodes identified at mediastinoscopy in patients with resectable cancer of the lung. J Thorac Cardiovasc Surg 1982;83:1–11.

482. Coughlin M, Deslauriers J, Beaulieu M, et al. Role of mediastinoscopy in pretreatment staging of patients with primary lung cancer. Ann Thorac Surg 1985;40:556–560.

483. Deslauriers J. Discussion of: Jensik RJ, Faber LP, Kittle CF, Miley RW, Thatcher WC, El-Baz N. Survival in patients undergoing tracheal sleeve pneumonectomy for bronchogenic carcinoma. J Thorac Cardiovasc Surg 1982;84:489–496.

484. Fujimura S, Kondo T, Imai T, et al. Prognostic evaluation of tracheobronchial reconstruction for bronchogenic carcinoma. J Thorac Cardiovasc Surg 1985;90:161–166.

485. Faber LP. Results of surgical treatment of stage III lung carcinoma with carinal proximity: The role of sleeve lobectomy versus pneumonectomy and the role of sleeve pneumonectomy. Surg Clin North Am 1987;67:1001–1014.

486. Dartevelle PG, Khalife J, Chapelier A, et al. Tracheal sleeve pneumonectomy for bronchogenic carcinoma: Report of 55 cases. Ann Thorac Surg 1988;46:68–72.

487. Mastrorilli M, Bragaglia RB, Cippola D'Abruzzo G, et al. The tracheo-bronchoplastic procedures for lung cancer. Lung Cancer [Abstract] 1988;4(Suppl):87.

488. Tsuchiya R, Goya T, Naruke T, Suemasu K. Resection of tracheal carina for lung cancer. J Thorac Cardiovasc Surg 1991;99:779–787.

489. Vogt-Moykopf I, Meyer G, Naunheim K, et al. In: Baue AE, Geha AS, Hammond GL, Luks H, Naunheim KS. Glenn's thoracic and cardiovascular surgery. 5th ed. New York: Appleton & Lange, 1991:403–417.

490. Mathisen DJ, Grillo HC. Carinal resection for bronchogenic cancer. J Thorac Cardiovasc Surg 1991;102:16–23.

491. Salerno TA, Little JR, Munro DD. Bronchogenic carcinoma with a brain metastasis: A continuing challenge. Ann Thorac Surg 1979;27:235–237.

492. Winston KR, Walsh JW, Fischer EG. Results of operative treatment of intracranial metastatic tumors. Cancer 1980;45:2639–2645.

493. White KT, Fleming TR, Laws ER. Single metastasis to the brain: Surgical treatment in 122 consecutive patients. Mayo Clin Proc 1981;56:424–428.

494. Mussi A, Janni A, Pistolesi M, et al. Surgical treatment of primary lung cancer and solitary brain metastasis. Thorax 1985;40:191–193.

495. Ehrenhaft JL. Discussion of: Magilligan DJ, Duvernoy C, Malik G, et al. Surgical approach to lung cancer with solitary cerebral metastasis: Twenty–five years' experience. Ann Thorac Surg 1986;42:360–364.

496. Magilligan DJ, Duvernoy C, Malik G, et al. Surgical approach to lung cancer with solitary cerebral metastasis: Twenty–five years' experience. Ann Thorac Surg 1986;42:360–364.

497. Read RC, Boop WC, Yoder G, Schaefer R. Management of non small cell lung carcinoma with solitary brain metastasis. J Thorac Cardiovasc Surg 1989;98:884–891.

498. Macchiarini P, Bonaguidi R, Hardin M, Angeletti CA. Results and prognostic factors of surgery in the management of non-small cell lung cancer (NSCLC) with solitary brain metastasis (SBM). Proc Am Soc Clin Oncol [Abstract] 1991;10:253.

499. Burt M, Wronski M, Galicich J, Martini N, Ginsberg R (Members of the Memorial Sloan–Kettering Cancer Center Thoracic and Neurosurgical Services). Solitary brain metastasis from non-small cell lung cancer: Results of therapy. Presented at the 71st Annual Meeting of the American Association for Thoracic Surgery, Washington, DC, May 6–8, 1991.

500. Decker DA, Diner DE, Pague WS, et al. The significance of a cytologically negative pleural effusion in bronchogenic carcinoma. Chest 1978;6:640–642.

501. Jensik RJ. The role of segmental resection in lung cancer. Chest 1986;89(5):335.

502. Perelman MI. Lumpectomy for lung cancer. Chest 1986;89(S):336.

503. Bennett WF, Smith RA. A twenty-year analysis of the results of sleeve resection for primary bronchogenic carcinoma. J Thorac Cardiovasc Surg 1978;76:840–845.

504. Bloedorn FG, Cowley RA, Cuccia CA, Mercado R, Wizenberg MJ, Linberg EJ. Preoperative irradiation in bronchogenic carcinoma. Am J Roent Rad Ther Nucl Med 1964;92:77–87.

505. Warram J. Preoperative irradiation of cancer of the lung: Final report of a therapeutic trial. Cancer 1975;36:914–925.

506. Shields TW, Higgins GA, Lawton R, Heilbrunn A, Keehn RJ. Preoperative x-ray therapy as an adjuvant in the treatment of bronchogenic carcinoma. J Thor Cardiovasc Surg 1970;59:49–61.

507. Petrovich Z, Mietlowski W, Ohanian M, Cox J. Clinical report on the treatment of locally advanced lung cancer. Cancer 1977;40:72–77.

508. White JE, Chen T, Reed R, Mira J. Stuckey WJ, Weatherall T, O'Bryan R, Samson M, Seydel G. Limited squamous cell carcinoma of the lung: A Southwest Oncology Group randomized study of radiation with or without doxorubicin chemotherapy and with or without levamisole immunotherapy. Cancer Treat Rep 1982;66:1113–1120.

509. Krauss S, Comas F, Perez C, et al. Treatment of inoperable non small cell carcinoma of the lung with radiation therapy, with or without levamisole: A randomized trial of the Southeastern Cancer Study Group. Am J Clin Oncol 1984;7:405–412.

510. Perez Ca, Bauer M, Emamai B, et al. Thoracic irradiation with or without levamisole in unresectable non-small cell carcinoma of the lung: A phase III randomized trial of the RTOG. Int J Radiat Oncol Biol Phys 1988;15:1337–1346.

511. Mattson K, Holsti LR, Holsti P, et al. Inoperable non-small cell lung cancer: Radiation with or without chemotherapy. Eur J Clin Oncol 1988;24:477–482.

512. Morton R, Jett J, Maher L, Therneau T. Randomized trial of thoracic radiation therapy with or without chemotherapy for treatment of locally unresectable non-small cell lung cancer. Proc Am Soc Clin Oncol 1988;7:200.

513. Trovo M, Minatel E, Veronesi A, et al. Combined radiotherapy and chemotherapy

versus radiotherapy alone in locally advanced epidermoid bronchogenic carcinoma. Cancer 1990;65:400–404.

514. Asbell S, Pajak T, Seydel H, et al. Phase III RTOG double blind lung cancer trial of XRT and subsequent thymosin or placebo. Proceedings Am Soc Clin Oncol 1990;9: 242.

515. Attar S, Miller J, Satterfield J, et al. Pancoast's tumor: Irradiation or surgery? Ann Thor Surg 1979;28:578–586.

516. Komaki R, Roh J, Cox J, Lopes da Conceicao A. Superior sulcus tumors: Results of irradiation of 36 patients. Cancer 1981;48:1563–1568.

517. van Houtte P, MacLennan I, Poulter C, Rubin P. External radiation in the management of superior sulcus tumor. Cancer 1984;54:223–227.

518. Kris MG, Gralla RJ, Kelsen DP, et al. Trial of vindesine plus mitomycin in stage 3 non-small cell lung cancer: An active regimen for outpatient treatment. Chest 1985;87: 368–372.

DANIEL C. IHDE
HARVEY I. PASS
ELI J. GLATSTEIN

SECTION **2**

Small Cell Lung Cancer

The principles of clinical management of small cell lung cancer (SCLC) diverge greatly from therapeutic approaches in patients with the other three major cell types. This section reviews the ways in which SCLC is distinct from non-small cell lung cancers (NSCLC) and then discusses the treatment of SCLC. The epidemiology, etiology, pathology, clinical features, staging, and prognostic features of epithelial lung cancers are presented comprehensively in section 1 of this chapter.

EPIDEMIOLOGY AND ETIOLOGY

Because of the propensity of SCLC to develop early regional and distant metastases, the proportion of lung cancers diagnosed as small cell carcinoma varies with the setting in which the data are obtained. This proportion ranges from 25% in autopsy series to 17% to 29% in biopsy and cytology diagnostic specimens to only 3% to 12% in surgically resected neoplasms.[1] In the National Cancer Institute's (NCI) population-based Surveillance, Epidemiology, and End Results (SEER) program, SCLC consists of 18% of all primary lung cancers.[2] Both institutional and population-based data suggest that SCLC is the most rapidly increasing cell type of lung cancer, especially in women.[3-5]

The predominant risk factor for lung cancer is cigarette smoking, and this particularly holds true for small cell and squamous carcinomas.[6] We have treated approximately 500 SCLC patients and less than 2% of these patients denied a history of cigarette abuse. Small cell carcinoma was the commonest type of pulmonary cancer found in uranium miners,[7] although all histologic types of lung cancer were increased. Radioactive radon daughters are thought to be the cause of excess lung cancer noted in underground miners throughout the world.[8] The magnitude of the carcinogenic effect of residential radon exposure has proved more difficult to estimate.[9] Although no overall excess lung cancer risk could be documented in a study in China in which household radon levels were monitored for 1 year, the relative risk associated with increasing radon exposure was greatest for small cell carcinoma.[10]

PATHOLOGY OF SMALL CELL LUNG CANCER

The epithelial origin of small cell carcinoma was first recognized in 1926 by Barnard.[11] Before that time, it was termed *oat celled sarcoma* of the mediastinum. The intramucosal site of origin of this carcinoma is often difficult to identify, but the tumor is thought to arise from basal neuroendocrine or Kulchitsky cells. These peptide hormone-secreting cells are uncommon in the adult but abundant in the fetal lung.[12] Small cell cancers infiltrate the submucosa in the early stages of disease, whereas squamous metaplasia or dysplasia is seen in the overlying bronchial mucosa. Normal bronchial markings may be obliterated by this process. In advanced stages, bronchial lumina may be obstructed by extrinsic compression or endobronchial tumor.[13] Silver stains are focally positive in about half of the cases, and neurosecretory granules usually are found on electron microscopic studies.[1] However, electron microscopic findings, including absence of neurosecretory granules, do not identify patients with differing responses to therapy, as long as light microscopic criteria for the diagnosis of SCLC are fulfilled.[14]

The 1981 World Health Organization classification divides SCLC into three subtypes: the oat cell or lymphocyte-like, the intermediate, and the combined (small cell carcinoma with squamous carcinoma or adenocarcinoma).[15] The classic oat cell type is characterized by small round or oval cells with darkly staining nuclei, indistinct or absent nucleoli, and scanty cytoplasm. The intermediate type consists of larger cells with a lower nuclear to cytoplasmic ratio and polygonal or fusiform nuclei. All subtypes of small cell carcinoma consist of cells that are at least two to three times the size of a mature lymphocyte and exhibit the characteristic features of salt-and-pepper distribution of chromatin, nuclear molding, areas of cellular necrosis, and deposition of DNA-derived material on elastic fibrils.[1] Numerous atypical mitoses may be identified. Mixtures of oat cell and intermediate subtypes of small cell cancer are seen frequently in a single tumor. The histologic distinction between SCLC and non-small cell lung cancers is of great clinical importance. The intermediate subtype of small cell cancer may sometimes be confused with poorly differentiated squamous carcinoma, large cell cancer, or poorly differentiated adenocarcinoma, particularly in metastatic sites. Some tumors form distinct tubules and rosettes and can be confused with adenocarcinomas. In some small cell tumors, prominent clusters of anaplastic large cells may be seen; in others, nests of squamous cells may be found.

Despite their submucosal location, small cell carcinomas often have malignant cells exfoliated into sputa and cytologic washings. Bronchoscopy yields malignant cytology in more than 90% of clinically apparent disease.[13] In well-preserved material, cytologic diagnosis appears as accurate as tissue diagnosis.[16,17] Other clinicopathologic features include the presence of marked osteoblastic activity in a few patients with bony metastases, associated focal acute pancreatitis from peripancreatic nodal disease, and a significant number of metastases to endocrine organs (*i.e.,* thyroid in 8%, pituitary in 15%, testes in 7%, and parathyroid in 1%).[1] In most surgically resected specimens, small cell cancer involves lymph nodes. Small cell tumors cavitate infrequently. The first principle of treatment is to procure an accurate histologic diagnosis. Quality and quantity of the histologic samples are important. Common problems for the clinical pathologist are crushing artifact, poor fixation, overstaining, or inadequate amounts of materials. Crushing artifact in a needle aspiration must not be mistaken for small cell carcinoma. A histologic (tissue block) diagnosis is preferred when doubts exist. A major problem in the use of histologic criteria is the degree of interobserver and intraobserver variability in reading the same specimens. The distinction between small cell and non-small cell carcinomas is consistent in 90% of cases if adequate material is reviewed by well-trained observers experienced in lung cancer pathology.[18] Concurrence among pathologists in the diagnosis of subtypes of small cell cancer is much less frequent.[19] If expert pathologists agree that a definite small cell component exists in a mixed lung cancer, the patient probably should be considered to have small cell carcinoma and should be treated as such.

To determine the clinical relevance of prospective subtyping of small cell carcinoma, several series of patients underwent systematic evaluations to assess the extent of tumor dissemination before intensive combination chemotherapy. In most instances, no difference was seen between oat cell and intermediate subtypes with respect to stage of disease, sites of metastases, response to therapy, or survival.[20–22] When histologic subtypes in the initial biopsy were compared with the subtype of other pathologic specimens in the same patient, concordance of the subtypes was present in only 71%.[22] Because of the lack of clinical implications, the marginal reproducibility of the pathologic distinction between oat cell and intermediate types, the greater frequency of the oat cell subtype in crushed specimens, and the failure of any small cell tumor cell lines to possess morphologic characteristics of the oat cell subtype,[23] a new pathologic classification of SCLC has been proposed. Subtypes are (1) small cell carcinoma (formerly oat cell and intermediate), which comprises more than 90% of cases; (2) a new mixed small cell and large cell variant; and (3) combined (small cell carcinoma combined with squamous or adenocarcinoma).[24]

The two less common histologic subtypes may be associated with a different prognosis. The mixed small cell and large cell variant occurs in 4% or more of patients. Two earlier single-institution studies reported diminished response to combination chemotherapy in this variant and inferior survival compared with small cell carcinoma without a large cell component.[20,25] This observation was not confirmed in a recent cooperative group trial.[26] A substantial fraction of patients with the initial diagnosis of small cell carcinoma have partially or exclusively large cell cancer and occasionally other lung cancer cell types at autopsy.[27,28] At the Finsen Institute, the 13% of small cell carcinoma patients with non-small cell

components at autopsy had shortened survival compared with patients with pure SCLC.[29] In a report from Vanderbilt University, 2% of small cell carcinoma patients had the combined subtype, with either squamous or adenocarcinoma elements admixed with small cell components histologically.[30] These patients tended to have more localized and sometimes surgically respectable disease, with a more favorable prognosis. These autopsy and clinical data support the concept that different pathologic types of lung cancer originate from a common bronchial mucosal stem cell that can differentiate along several pathways.

New findings in cellular biology should allow pathologists eventually to distinguish SCLC from NSCLC by tests other than light microscopy. Small cell tumors express markers of neuroendocrine differentiation much more frequently than non-small cell pulmonary tumors. As biochemical and immunologic reagents become generally available and these markers are studied in prospective clinical trials, their use in diagnosis and patient management can be assessed and documented.

CELLULAR AND MOLECULAR BIOLOGY

The neuroendocrine nature of SCLC was suggested initially by its association with such paraneoplastic syndromes produced by peptide hormones as the ectopic secretion of adrenocorticotrophic hormone and arginine vasopressin (antidiuretic hormone). Studies of fresh and fixed pathologic materials have documented the presence of neurosecretory dense-core granules, the metabolic apparatus for synthesis of numerous biogenic amines (present in amine precursor uptake and decarboxylation or *APUD cells*) and for elaboration of various peptide hormones and growth factors.[31]

The establishment of numerous continuously proliferating tumor cell lines from patients with small cell carcinoma has permitted sophisticated studies of this cancer's cellular and molecular biology.[32] Compared with cell lines of other types of lung cancer, most small cell lines express elevated levels of the critical APUD enzyme L-dopa decarboxylase, gastrin-releasing peptide (GRP), and neuron-specific enolase, all markers of neuroendocrine differentiation. They grow as floating spheric aggregates in culture, have slow doubling times, and exhibit neurosecretory dense-core granules on electron microscopy.[33] A few small cell lines of the *variant type* are larger cells with lower nuclear to cytoplasmic ratios, more rapid doubling times, and loss of some neuroendocrine features.[34] They may be derived from the mixed small cell and large cell subtype in patients.

GRP acts as a growth factor for normal bronchial epithelium[35] and for small cell carcinoma in vitro and in vivo in nude mice.[36–38] Small cell carcinoma in vitro synthesizes and secretes GRP and possesses GRP receptors on its cell surface. It therefore may produce a factor that stimulates its own growth, a so-called *autocrine growth factor.*[38] Both synthetic peptides with anti-GRP activity[39] and the monoclonal antibody 2A11 raised against bombesin, the amphibian analog of GRP,[38] have inhibited small cell carcinoma growth in experimental systems. The antibody is undergoing clinical evaluation.[40] In addition to GRP, several neuropeptides may play growth-regulatory roles in small cell carcinoma[41] and there is evidence that insulin-like growth factor-I functions as an in vitro autocrine growth factor.[42]

Numerous somatic genetic abnormalities have been documented in SCLC. Cytogenetic studies reveal multiple chromosomal abnormalities, the most consistent being a deletion of a portion of the short arm of chromosome 3, which is almost universally present.[43] Analyses of karyotypic and restriction fragment length polymorphism (RFLP) data also reveal frequent loss of genetic material on chromosomes 13q and 17p.[44] Sites of chromosomal deletion often pinpoint the location of a tumor suppressor gene (or antioncogene), the loss of normal expression of which is associated with malignancy. In almost all SCLCs, abnormalities of the retinoblastoma (*RB*) tumor suppressor gene, which is located on 13q,[45] and the p53 tumor suppressor gene, which is located on 17p,[46] are present. Mechanisms such as deletions, lack of expression, and point mutations are responsible for the absence of the normal gene product. The putative tumor suppressor gene on chromosome 3p has not been identified conclusively. Interestingly, many small cell carcinomas arising in extrapulmonary sites do not have loss of genetic material in the same region of 3p.[47]

Dominant oncogenes stimulate tumor growth through amplification, increased expression, translocation, or mutation. The best documented oncogene abnormalities in SCLC are in the *MYC* family. Amplification occurs in 30% to 50% of cell lines and 11% to 24% of tumors,[48] and overexpression may be much more frequent.[49] In one study, gene amplification was present in specimens from 28% of previously treated patients but in only 8% of previously untreated patients,[50] suggesting that this genetic event develops late in the natural history of the cancer. Amplification of c-*MYC* may have clinical implications because the time from initial chemotherapy to clinical relapse was significantly shorter in patients whose cell lines established at relapse had c-*MYC* amplification than in patients whose cell lines did not.[51] Point mutations of the *RAS* oncogene family, which are observed in many solid tumors including NSCLC, appear to be infrequent in small cell carcinoma.[52]

IN VITRO DRUG AND RADIATION SENSITIVITY TESTING

The ability to grow lung cancer cells in vitro has greatly simplified assessment of the sensitivity of small cell carcinoma to chemotherapeutic agents and radiotherapy. As in lung cancer patients, small cell carcinoma cell lines are much more sensitive to a variety of chemotherapeutic agents in vitro than are NSCLC lines.[53] One could reasonably question whether the tumor specimens from which the cell lines are established are representative of small cell tumors in general. Data from more than 60 uniformly treated, prospectively studied, extensive-stage SCLC patients indicate that the prognosis of patients from whom tumor specimens are obtained is similar whether or not a cell line eventually develops,[54] although this may not be true in specimens taken from the primary tumor.[55] Cell lines provide reagents for biochemical analysis of the basis of drug resistance. Studies of methotrexate and doxorubicin resistance have shown how complex and multifactorial drug resistance can be. Reduced sensitivity to methotrexate in individual cell lines has been correlated with elevated levels of dihydrofolate reductase due to gene amplication, decreased

intracellular accumulation due to reduced polyglutamation of the drug, and decreased thymidylate synthase activity.[56,57] In doxorubicin-resistant cells,[58] decreased intracellular drug levels, increased DNA repair, and altered doxorubicin-topoisomerase interaction were all noted. These findings may explain why certain cancer cells were resistant to certain drugs, but they do not address the common clinical problem (seen especially in patients with progressive tumor despite chemotherapy) of resistance to multiple drugs to which the patient has never been exposed. This multidrug-resistant (MDR) phenotype often is attributed to expression of a drug efflux pump, the p170 glycoprotein encoded by the *MDR1* gene.[59] However, the first large study of a panel of small cell carcinoma cell lines and tumors revealed that the *MDR1* gene was expressed infrequently. Furthermore, there was no correlation between gene expression and previous exposure to chemotherapy, response to chemotherapy, or in vitro drug sensitivity.[60] Other mechanisms of multidrug resistance are presumably relevant in SCLC, but they have not been defined unequivocally.

Radiation sensitivity testing has revealed that most small cell tumor lines exhibit greater sensitivity than most non-small cell lines or than large cell variants of SCLC.[61,62] There are only minimal data addressing whether radiation response patterns for individual tumors in vitro correlate with the clinical response exhibited by tumors in patients.

In a prospective clinical trial at the NCI,[63] attempts were made to obtain tumor biopsies for cell culture and drug sensitivity testing from 80 consecutive patients with extensive-stage SCLC. All patients received etoposide and cisplatin (EP) as their initial drug regimen, but their second regimen was either a three-drug program based on in vitro drug testing of the patient's own cancer or, if such data were unavailable, the standard three-drug cyclophosphamide, doxorubicin, vincristine (CAV) program. Tumor specimens were harvested from 75% of patients, and drug testing data were obtained in 33%. Drug sensitivity of the cell lines was highly correlated with clinical response to EP. Possibly because cell lines tended to be generally sensitive or generally resistant to the seven standard drugs tested in vitro, there was no significant difference in response rates between the standard second drug regimen and the regimen based on drug-sensitivity testing of the patient's own tumor. This suggests that cell lines taken directly from patients may be more useful for screening of potential new chemotherapeutic agents than for drug selection in individual patients. The NCI currently uses human lung cancer cell lines in its initial drug screen.[64]

CLINICAL FEATURES

CLINICAL PRESENTATION

Signs and symptoms of SCLC depend on the size and location of the primary tumor and the presence or absence of regional or distant metastases. With the exception of certain paraneoplastic syndromes, which are uncommon, most clinical signs are not explicitly associated with SCLC compared with NSCLC.[65] Because the primary tumor most often arises in a central endobronchial location, patients typically present with cough, dyspnea, wheezing, hemoptysis, chest pain, or postobstructive pneumonitis. Plain chest radiographs in SCLC, compared with NSCLC, more often demonstrate hilar and mediastinal adenopathy, atelectasis, and pneumonitis, and less often exhibit a peripheral tumor location, pleural effusion, and chest wall involvement. Cavitation is unusual.[66-68]

The usual submucosal location of small cell carcinoma accounts for the lower frequency of hemoptysis compared with squamous cell cancer.[69] Tumor extension to the mediastinum occurs almost invariably, accounting for the frequent occurrence of regional metastatic symptoms such as superior vena cava syndrome, hoarseness from recurrent laryngeal nerve paralysis, and dysphagia. Almost 10% of patients have superior vena cava syndrome at diagnosis, and judicious invasive diagnostic procedures usually can be performed safely. Survival is similar to patients of the same stage without the syndrome.[70]

The interval from symptoms to diagnosis in small cell carcinoma is shorter than in other types of lung cancer,[65] as is the interval from diagnosis to death in untreated patients.[71] Despite these facts and the high rate of tumor cell proliferation as assessed by tritiated thymidine incorporation into tumor cells, mean doubling time on chest radiographs is 91 days, shorter than in adenocarcinoma of the lung but much longer than in aggressive lymphomas or testicular cancer.[72] This apparent contradiction probably is best explained by the high rates of cell division and cell death. The latter is well documented by frequent areas of necrosis on microscopic examination.

Unfortunately, by the time the diagnosis of SCLC is established, dissemination to distant organ systems has almost always occurred. This fact was first clearly elucidated by autopsy data in patients dying from non-cancer-related causes within 30 days after complete surgical resection of lung cancer (Table 23–20). Almost 70% of small cell patients had metastatic cancer (to distant sites in 63%), far more than in any other cell type.[73] Autopsies in patients dying of advanced lung cancer reveal cancer confined to the thorax in 4% of small cell cancer patients compared with approximately 15% in large cell cancer and adenocarcinoma and 45% in squamous cancer.[74]

Patients may or may not be symptomatic from distant metastatic deposits. Radiographically detectable central nervous system (CNS) metastases are symptomatic in more than 90% of patients. Bone metastases usually are not painful and pathologic fractures are rare. Liver metastases cause usually mild abnormalities of laboratory tests in 50% to 60% of pa-

tients, but liver function is impaired seriously in a few of these patients. In occasional patients, jaundice may be due to extrahepatic biliary obstruction from pancreatic or nodal metastases rather than to tumor replacement of the liver; prognosis is not as dire in the former group.[75] Leukopenia or thrombocytopenia in less than extensive bone marrow involvement is uncommon.[76] During induction chemotherapy, patients with positive bone marrow have more severe infections and require more red blood cell transfusions than do patients without tumor in the marrow,[77] but differences in severity of leukopenia and thrombocytopenia are not impressive.

Elevated plasma concentrations of immunologically detected polypeptide hormones occur much more frequently in SCLC than do symptoms from the corresponding paraneoplastic syndromes,[78-80] because immunoassays detect both inactive precursors and the actual hormone. The syndrome of inappropriate secretion of antidiuretic hormone (SIADH), ectopic Cushing's syndrome, and the Eaton-Lambert, or myasthenia-like, syndrome are specifically associated with small cell carcinoma. The frequency of SIADH at presentation varies according to definition of the syndrome but in one large series[81] was present in 11% of patients. Only 27% of patients fulfilling the diagnostic criteria for SIADH, however, were symptomatic from hyponatremia. Presence of SIADH was not correlated with stage of disease or prognosis. Hyponatremia in some patients may be due to secretion of atrial natriuretic factor.[82]

Ectopic Cushing's syndrome with clinically recognizable hypercortisolism was present at diagnosis in 2.4% of patients in a recent report,[83] and was associated with short survival and frequent complications from chemotherapy. The cause of the uncommon Eaton-Lambert syndrome is impaired release of acetylcholine from nerve terminals at the neuromuscular junction, probably mediated by autoantibodies that impair calcium influx.[84] Autoantibodies cross-reacting with SCLC cells in vitro have been documented in the even rarer neurologic syndromes of subacute sensory neuronopathy, cerebellar ataxia,[85] and retinal degeneration.[86] In general, endocrinologic paraneoplastic syndromes are ameliorated by response to chemotherapy, but often this is not the case with neurologic syndromes. Diaminopyridine may be helpful in Eaton-Lambert syndrome.[84]

TABLE 23–20. Incidence at Autopsy of Persistent Tumor After "Curative" Surgical Therapy for Lung Cancer in Patients Dying of Other Causes Within 30 Days Postoperatively

Cell Type	No. of Patients	Percentage With Persistent Tumor		
		Total	Local Disease Only	Distant Metastases
Epidermoid carcinoma	131	34	17	17
Adenocarcinoma	30	43	3	40
Large cell carcinoma	22	14	0	14
Small cell carcinoma	19	69	6	63

(Modified from Matthews MJ, Kanhouwa S, Pickner J, et al. Frequency of residual and metastatic tumors in patients undergoing curative surgical resection of lung cancer. Cancer Chemother Rep 1973;[part 3];4:63–67)

EXTRAPULMONARY SMALL CELL CARCINOMA

Approximately 4% of small cell carcinoma patients present without an obvious pulmonary or mediastinal lesion on chest radiograph and computed tomographic (CT) scan of the thorax and on bronchoscopy or sputum cytology.[87,88] These cases fall into two groups—those with an obvious primary extrapulmonary tumor arising in sites such as the larynx, esophagus, or uterine cervix, and a smaller fraction with lymph nodal or disseminated metastases without any detectable primary tumor.[87,89] These neoplasms resemble SCLC morphologically. Some contain neurosecretory granules on electron microscopy (although data are not available in many reports), and are occasionally associated with the same endocrine paraneoplastic syndromes as pulmonary small cell tumors. Although there is heterogeneity among different primary sites, their clinical behavior is often aggressive, with median survival of less than 1 year and a tendency to develop nodal and disseminated metastatic disease. These unusual cancers are grouped collectively on morphologic grounds, but they probably represent several different neoplasms with disparate tumor biology.

The commonest sites of origin of extrapulmonary small cell carcinoma are the uterine cervix (although many reports do not distinguish between neuroendocrine and squamous variants), esophagus, larynx and pharynx, colon and rectum, prostate, and paranasal sinuses.[89] Merkel's cell carcinoma of the skin, although not strictly a small cell carcinoma, is difficult to distinguish from small cell cancer morphologically, contains neurosecretory granules, and exhibits more aggressive clinical behavior than other skin carcinomas.[90] Among all carcinomas arising in various organs in which extrapulmonary small cell carcinoma has been observed, the frequency of small cell carcinoma is estimated at 3.5% in the minor salivary glands, 1% in the pancreas, 0.9% in the esophagus, 0.3% in the larynx and pharynx, 0.2% in the colon and rectum, and from 0.2% to 14% in the uterine cervix, probably because of differing diagnostic criteria with inconsistent inclusion of the squamous cell variant.[89]

STAGING EVALUATION AND PROGNOSTIC FACTORS

STAGING EVALUATION

In patients with small cell carcinoma, the staging system and staging procedures frequently are different from those used in NSCLC because the primary treatment modality always includes chemotherapy. Because a few small cell tumors can be surgically extirpated, detailed TNM staging has proved valuable in identifying candidates for an operative approach and in estimating prognosis in this setting.[91] Nearly all investigators studying the treatment of SCLC have adopted the simple two-stage system of the Veterans Administration Lung Group.

In this system, limited-stage disease is defined as tumor confined to one hemithorax and the regional lymph nodes, whereas extensive-stage disease is defined as disease beyond these bounds. The definition of limited stage is based on a judgment as to whether all detectable tumor can be encompassed within a tolerable radiotherapy port, and therefore is

a physiologic and an anatomic definition. Ipsilateral pleural effusion and varying degrees of supraclavicular node involvement have been considered consistent with limited or extensive stage by different authors.

In the individual cancer patient, staging procedures are of value in selecting patients who can benefit from therapy that is efficacious in only certain stages. Most commonly, staging is used to identify patients who can be managed solely with locoregional treatment, to assign prognosis, and to identify areas of tumor involvement that can be monitored to determine response. In groups of patients, the staging process documents patterns of failure to a given form of treatment, suggesting new therapeutic strategies, and permits uniform communication in reporting the results of clinical trials. Because all patients with SCLC receive chemotherapy, staging procedures do not identify patients who can be given locoregional treatment alone. The staging process divides patients into those with limited-stage and extensive-stage disease, which is of clear prognostic significance and in most cases leads to administration of chest irradiation in the former group. Documenting initially involved sites of tumor aids in later identification of tumor response and of tumor progression, because initial tumor deposits are the areas in which progression usually occurs with the exception of the CNS.

The extent of the initial staging evaluation depends on clinical circumstances (Table 23–21). Outside a clinical trial setting, when distant metastases are evident or treatment is not affected by stage, simple screening tests followed only by those studies that have an increased likelihood of being positive[92,93] are performed. In a prospective clinical trial or when stage-specific therapy is to be administered, additional studies are appropriate. If the purpose of staging is to exclude patients with extensive disease from receiving chest irradiation, then no procedures beyond those indicated by initial screening tests need to be done after an unequivocal site of distant metastases is documented. Because of the frequent involvement of mediastinal lymph nodes in SCLC and the poor prognosis of node-positive patients who undergo surgical resection,[94] staging tests to evaluate the mediastinum are recommended in patients in whom surgical removal of the primary tumor is being considered.

The timing of restaging to assess response and the tests to be performed depend on the cost and availability of specific procedures and the philosophy of the treating physician. Tumor sites that are initially involved should be reevaluated. Any set of staging recommendations is somewhat arbitrary, and individualization of the process in different clinical circumstances is often appropriate.

Treatment for SCLC is, in some respects, as demanding as thoracotomy and pulmonary resection. In addition to anatomic staging, assessment of the patient's ability to tolerate therapy is required. The combined use of intensive chemotherapy and aggressive radiotherapy can produce treatment-associated mortality rates of 5% or more. The most important risk factor for treatment-related mortality is performance status. Many physicians believe that only those patients who are ambulatory more than 50% of the time and who have adequate cardiopulmonary, renal, and hepatic function should undergo aggressive, highly toxic, therapy.

The primary tumor and regional nodal spread are evaluated by chest x-ray films. Fiberoptic bronchoscopy with bronchial

TABLE 23–21. Staging Procedures for Small Cell
Lung Cancer

Minimum Survey (Screening Tests)

Complete history and physical examination
Chest x-ray film (with CT to assist in portal design if other than
  palliative chest irradiation is to be given)
Liver function tests and physical examination of liver (with
  radionuclide or CT liver scan if results are abnormal)
Bone pain/alkaline phosphatase (with radionuclide bone scan if
  results are abnormal)
Neurologic history and examination (with CT scan of brain if
  results are abnormal)
Platelet count or leukoerythroblastic peripheral blood smear (with
  bone marrow aspiration/biopsy if results are abnormal; also
  recommended if no other unequivocal distant metastatic disease
  has been documented or if all initial sites of involvement are to be
  reassessed to determine response)

Procedures for Patients in Clinical Trials or Receiving Stage-Dependent Therapy*

Complete history and physical examination
Chest x-ray film plus CT scan of chest to assist in portal design if
  chest irradiation (other than palliative) is to be employed; plus
  fiberoptic bronchoscopy if no evaluable tumor is found on chest
  film
Liver function tests/radionuclide or CT liver scan
Liver biopsy (peritoneoscopy or ultrasound guided) if either liver
  function tests or scan are abnormal and best information
  concerning liver status is required to select therapy
Radionuclide bone scan
CT scan of brain in presence or absence of neurologic
  abnormalities if brain irradiation is to be given to asymptomatic
  patients
Bone marrow aspiration/biopsy (bilaterally if best information
  concerning marrow status is required)

Procedures Before Attempted Surgical Resection if Patient Is Known to Have Small Cell Cancer

All staging procedures listed for patients in clinical trials
Fiberoptic bronchoscopy
Evaluation of mediastinum
  CT scan of chest
  Mediastinoscopy†

---

* Evaluation can be stopped after documentation of extensive disease
if staging is being used only to identify candidates for stage-specific
therapy.
† Unless thought unnecessary by operating surgeon.
(Modified from Ihde DC. Staging evaluation and prognostic factors
in small cell lung cancer. In: Aisner J, ed. Lung cancer. New York:
Churchilll Livingstone, 1985;241–268)

---

washings and biopsy are essential to document the extent of
disease and may be used to determine the degree of tumor
response during follow-up. Before treatment, fiberoptic bronchoscopy reveals evidence of cancer in more than 90% of
patients, including approximately 8% to 10% in whom the
tumor is not evaluable on chest films. Patients with evidence
of tumor by bronchoscopy after initial therapy have a much
higher relapse rate in the chest within 6 months than do patients with normal bronchoscopy.[13,95]

CT scans of the thorax provide more precise definition of
parenchymal, mediastinal, and pleural disease.[96,97] They are
probably most useful in design of radiotherapy portals and in
assessing persistence or early relapse of chest tumor. In a few

patients, abnormalities that appear after chemotherapy on
CT scan but not on chest radiograph later prove to be sites of
tumor recurrence.[97,98] In our experience, all patients with intrathoracic tumor resolution by chest radiograph and persistent endobronchial disease on bronchoscopy are identified as
not being in complete remission by CT scans. There is little
evidence that magnetic resonance imaging (MRI) provides
information not present on CT scan in assessing intrathoracic
disease.

The common sites of extrathoracic metastatic disease detected during pretreatment staging are bone in 19% to 38%
of cases, liver in 17% to 34%, bone marrow in 17% to 23%,
and the CNS in 0% to 14% (Table 23–22).[76,92,93] Radionuclide
bone scans are more sensitive than skeletal x-ray films in
identifying osseous metastases; the latter should be used to
confirm potential metastatic sites detected on bone scan. The
greater the number of bone scan abnormalities, the more
likely it is that sites of extraosseous metastatic disease will
be found. The principal problem with bone scans in small
cell carcinoma is false-positive examination due to benign
bone and joint disease.[99] Therefore, bone scans should not
serve as the sole basis for making therapeutic decisions, but
should alert the clinician to the need for further evaluation.
After treatment, osteoblastic changes sometimes can be seen
on bone radiographs, probably representing regeneration of
bone, not new metastases.[76]

Bone marrow involvement is assessed with bone marrow
aspiration and biopsy. Often the two procedures are complementary. An additional 10% of patients (30% of all positive
marrows) have bone marrow involvement if bilateral biopsies
are done.[76] Less than 5% of patients have bone marrow involvement as the sole site of extensive-stage disease.[77,100] A
positive marrow examination yields pathologic proof that extensive disease is present, providing assurance of extrathoracic
mestatases that cannot be obtained with equivocal imaging
studies. The results of bone scans and marrow examinations
are significantly correlated, but they are complementary because each can be positive when the other is unrevealing.[99,101]

TABLE 23–22. Involvement of Extrathoracic Sites
at Diagnosis After Pretreatment Staging Studies
in Small Cell Lung Cancer

	Patients With Finding (%)
Final stage	
Limited-stage	30–40
Extensive-stage	60–70
Bone	19–38
Liver	17–34
Bone marrow	17–23
Brain	0–14
Lymph nodes	7–25
Soft tissue	3–11

(Modified from Abrams J, Doyle LA, Aisner J. Staging, prognostic
features, and special considerations in small cell lung cancer. Semin
Oncol 1988;15:261–277; and from Ihde DC. Staging evaluation and
prognostic factors in small cell lung cancer. In: Aisner J, ed. Lung
cancer. New York: Churchill Livingstone, 1985:241–268)

Interestingly, the requirement for transfusion of blood products or dosage reductions during chemotherapy does not predict that bone marrow metastases will be found at autopsy.[102]

Although liver function tests are abnormal in 93% of patients whose livers are histologically positive for tumor, they also are abnormal in 41% of patients with histologically negative livers.[76] Both false-positive and false-negative liver CT and radionuclide scans are observed. If patients have a filling defect on liver scan and abnormal liver function tests, histologic proof of liver involvement can be obtained in almost 90% of cases, whereas patients in whom both scan and function tests are negative have positive liver biopsies less than 10% of the time. If either the scan or biochemical tests but not both are abnormal, the probability of liver involvement at biopsy is approximately 20%.[103] To prove or disprove liver involvement, the best method is peritoneoscopy with multiple biopsies.[103,104] Ultrasound-guided fine-needle aspiration of the liver is about as sensitive as peritoneoscopy in yielding pathologic confirmation of liver involvement.[105]

CNS metastases are very common, occurring in approximately 30% of SCLC patients at diagnosis or during the subsequent course of disease.[106] CT scans of the brain are superior to radionuclide scans in documenting brain metastases in patients with neurologic symptoms or signs, but both are abnormal in most cases. As screening examinations in asymptomatic patients, the yields of both are low in the range of 5% to 10% for CT scan and less than 5% for radionuclide scan.[107-109] The CT scan is the examination of choice, with greater sensitivity and positive predictive accuracy than the radionuclide scan.[109] Problematic CT examinations should be resolved with MRI. Many clinicians advocate screening CT scans at diagnosis of SCLC in asymptomatic patients, because brain irradiation would be administered if the test were positive. However, there is no evidence that detection of brain metastases in asymptomatic patients is associated with superior survival compared with patients whose metastases are diagnosed because of neurologic symptoms or signs.[109,110] Patients with brain metastases as the only site of extensive-stage disease have a median survival not markedly different from patients with limited disease, although long-term survival is rare and relapse in the brain after irradiation is frequent.[109,111,112] In asymptomatic patients with a negative neurologic examination, the most clear-cut indication for head CT scan is before administration of prophylactic cranial irradiation. If asymptomatic lesions were discovered, a higher dose of radiotherapy would be delivered.[113] Periodic brain CT scans during follow-up of asymptomatic patients did not produce better control of brain metastases or survival in a randomized trial.[114]

Metastases to the CNS can involve the spinal epidural or leptomeningeal space. Once one site of CNS metastatic disease is discovered, the probability of finding metastases at other CNS sites increases greatly. Clinically apparent multiple sites are discovered in 20% of patients with CNS metastases and in 73% of such patients at autopsy.[115] Screening asymptomatic patients with cerebrospinal fluid (CSF) cytology is unrewarding.[116] Patients suspected of having spinal cord compression should undergo MRI or a myelogram promptly. Likewise, patients with signs or symptoms of leptomeningeal involvement should have CSF cytology obtained. Brain imaging studies also should be performed in both situations. Back

pain and bone destruction on radiographs are found in most patients whose cord compression is present at the diagnosis of SCLC, but less often in patients whose epidural lesion is documented during the subsequent course of disease.[117] Occasional patients with symptoms of spinal cord dysfunction, often manifested as Brown-Séquard syndrome, prove to have intramedullary rather than epidural tumor.[118]

Because of the high frequency of intraabdominal metastases found at autopsy in the adrenals, pancreas, kidneys, and lymph nodes, pretreatment staging of these areas could be considered. CT scans frequently are used instead of radionuclide scans to image the liver, but otherwise abdominal CT scanning is not recommended. Although upper abdominal CT scans performed prospectively reveal evidence of metastases in 36% of patients and can demonstrate metastatic dissemination that cannot be identified by other means, they uncommonly demonstrate metastases in patients with otherwise limited disease.[119,120] Furthermore, when patients with normal adrenal glands by CT scan underwent percutaneous thin needle biopsy, 17% of the glands adequately sampled revealed metastases.[121] Negative CT scans provide only modest assurance of lack of involvement.

MRI has been compared with bone marrow examination, radionuclide bone scan, and CT scans of the brain and abdomen in a prospective study.[122] All sites identified by conventional staging were confirmed by MRI. One fifth of patients were advanced from limited to extensive stage, principally because of detection of marrow involvement. The clinical and financial implications of these findings need further evaluation.

Although imaging studies provide considerable staging and follow-up data, they are expensive and time consuming. Tumor markers requiring only periodic blood tests would be highly desirable if comparable utility could be documented. Unfortunately, no such tests are available. Potential candidates include neuron-specific enolase (NSE), creatine kinase-BB (CK-BB), chromogranin A (CGA, the matrix protein of neurosecretory granules), and carcinoembryonic antigen (CEA). Small cell carcinoma produces high levels of NSE, CK-BB, CGA, and often CEA intracellularly, and with tumor cell breakdown, these products are released into the serum where they can be measured by radioimmunoassay.[123-126]

Serum levels of NSE[124,127] and CEA[125] measured in many patients correlate with bulk of tumor and response (or lack thereof) to chemotherapy. A small number of observations indicate the same findings hold for CK-BB and CGA.[123,126] There has been no prospective controlled demonstration that use of any of these markers, or combinations thereof,[128] can substitute for more conventional staging procedures or improve therapeutic results.

PROGNOSTIC FACTORS

Numerous prognostic factors have been identified in patients receiving chemotherapy for SCLC. Most of these factors are either attributes of the patient or of the tumor or laboratory values obtained from serum or blood specimens. A review of five multivariate statistical analyses published since 1989 of patient groups ranging in size from 411 to more than 2500 provides considerable information about which factors are of independent importance (Table 23-23).[129-133] Ambulatory

TABLE 23–23. Important Prognostic Factors
in Small Cell Lung Cancer

Host Factors
Performance status
Gender (female favorable)

Tumor Factors
Stage of disease (limited or extensive)
Limited disease: absence of mediastinal or supraclavicular nodes
  and pleural effusion
Extensive disease: number of organ systems with metastases,
  absence of liver or brain involvement

Serum and Blood Tests
Elevated levels of lactate dehydrogenase and alkaline phosphatase
  unfavorable
Low sodium unfavorable

(Modified from Albain et al,[129] Dearing et al,[130] Rawson et al,[131] Sagman et al,[132] and Spiegelman et al[133])

---

performance status and female gender were consistently favorable host factors. Limited-stage disease was by far the most
important favorable tumor factor, but metastases limited to
a single organ system or absence of liver or brain involvement
in extensive disease and absence of mediastinal or supraclavicular nodal spread or of pleural effusion in limited disease
were sometimes associated with better outcome. Numerous
abnormalities in blood or serum tests conveyed a poor prognosis with elevations in lactate dehydrogenase and alkaline
phosphatase and low serum sodium values being identified
most often.

It is difficult to determine which of these prognostic factors
are most important, because few groups of investigators perform exactly the same pretreatment evaluations in their patients. The sensitivity of the staging procedure performed can
affect whether involvement of a specific organ influences
prognosis. Less sensitive tests, such as radionuclide tests
compared with CT brain scans and imaging studies of the
liver compared with liver biopsies, are more likely to be associated with impaired prognosis if positive, presumably because greater tumor volume is necessary to produce a positive
test.[130] Performing a larger number of more sensitive staging
tests does not influence prognosis, but the survival of both
limited-stage and extensive-stage patients is improved because
patients with minimal extrathoracic metastases are moved
from limited to extensive stage—the so-called Will Rogers'
effect.[134] Staging patients only on the basis of symptoms and
clinical severity of disease can partially correct for this bias
when comparing patient outcome from different eras in which
different staging techniques were used.[135]

Many of the prognostic factors identified in Table 23–23
are correlated. Performance status and disease stage are
somewhat correlated, in that extensive-stage patients have
worse performance status, although each variable exerts independent effects.[136] Abnormalities in lactate dehydrogenase
and liver function tests are correlated with the number of
organ systems involved by metastases in extensive disease.[130]
The favorable prognosis of limited-disease patients whose tu-

mor has been completely surgically resected before initiation
of chemotherapy is well known.[137,138]

Other host-related factors, some of which correlate with
performance status and some of which do not, may affect
prognosis. In some studies, weight loss is an unfavorable
prognostic factor independent of stage and performance status
for untreated patients[71] and for those given chemotherapy,[139]
particularly for more ambulatory cases with a lower tumor
burden. Impaired immune status as assessed by delayed hypersensitivity skin testing correlates with shorter survival, especially in patients with an otherwise favorable prognosis.[140]
Some recent studies of many patients suggest that younger
patients have a better outcome when receiving chemotherapy,
possibly because of greater tolerance for side effects of treatment.[129,141] An early study suggested that patients who discontinue cigarette smoking, particularly those who quit more
than a year before diagnosis, have a better outcome.[142] Although this finding was not confirmed in a subsequent analysis,[143] all patients should be encouraged to stop smoking.
Finally, as in all other cancers, patients with SCLC who develop tumor progression during or after administration of
chemotherapy have a poor prognosis, with median survival
of 8 weeks in one large cooperative group study.[144]

Virtually all of the information on prognostic factors in
SCLC has been derived from patients entered on prospective
clinical trials. Although there is no reason to believe such
factors do not predict prognosis in patients who do not participate in these studies, survival differences may exist between patients who are and are not entered onto clinical trials.
In a recent study of 215 consecutive cases of small cell carcinoma, only 20% of patients were placed on available chemotherapy protocols.[145] Survival in extensive-stage patients
placed on study was superior to survival in patients who were
managed "off protocol." In limited-stage patients, no survival
differences were noted. These results are consistent with the
conventional wisdom that poor performance status patients
or those with severe nonneoplastic illnesses are less often
entered into clinical trials. Because most limited-stage patients
are diagnosed while still in good medical condition, their survival is much less affected by whether the patient is judged
suitable for protocol entry.

TREATMENT OF SMALL CELL
CARCINOMA OF THE LUNG

SCLC differs from other cell types of lung cancer in its more
aggressive clinical course in the absence of treatment and in
its superior responsiveness to chemotherapy and thoracic irradiation. Median survival in surgically unresectable patients
randomized to supportive care alone in a clinical trial conducted during the 1960s was 12 weeks for patients with limited
and 5 weeks for those with extensive-stage disease.[71] Its natural history is characterized by relentless tumor progression
and the early development of distant metastatic deposits.
When compared with other types of lung cancer with comparable extent of tumor dissemination, a shorter duration of
symptoms before diagnosis and reduced survival once a diagnosis is established are evident.[71,146] In a study of 19 patients
subjected to potentially curative surgical resection and who

died within 30 days of operation of non-cancer-related causes, 70% had distant metastases at postmortem examination.[73] More than 70% of cases have mediastinal lymph node involvement at diagnosis, which in itself usually precludes surgical resection.[147,148] Approximately two thirds of newly diagnosed patients have evidence of distant metastases when systematic staging procedures are applied.[148] At autopsy, only 4% of patients demonstrate tumor dissemination beyond the thorax.[74]

These findings of frequent tumor spread to regional lymph nodes and distant extrathoracic sites by the time of initial clinical presentation indicate that small cell carcinoma is a systemic disease process early after inception in almost all patients. Therefore, it is not surprising that reliance on locoregional forms of treatment alone fails in most patients. In an early British study performed in the 1960s, patients considered candidates for surgical resection by the standards of the time were randomized to thoracotomy with the intent of tumor removal or to definitive irradiation of the primary tumor and regional lymphatics.[149] Although radiotherapy was shown to be superior to attempted surgical removal in terms of survival (Table 23–24), less than 4% of these apparently operable patients were alive 5 years after randomization.

In the original publication describing the TNM staging system for lung cancer by the American Joint Committee on Cancer,[150] the outcome of SCLC patients treated during the 1960s at American university medical centers was reported. Five-year survival in 368 patients was less than 1%. This figure amply documents the almost completely ineffective management of this neoplasm before the use of systemic chemotherapy. Shortly thereafter, a review of the outcome of a large number of American SCLC patients who were thought to be surgically operable revealed absolutely no differences in survival whether or not a thoracotomy was performed.[151] Until the 1980s, these data led most thoracic surgeons to abandon surgical therapy in patients with an established diagnosis of small cell carcinoma.

Chest irradiation rarely was administered as the sole treatment for SCLC after 1970. Long-term survival with irradiation in the era of chemotherapy and improving radiotherapy techniques can be assessed only in studies of patients who received initial thoracic radiotherapy, with chemotherapy often being administered when progressive disease developed. In this setting, reported survival rates for patients given radiotherapy as sole initial treatment include 2% at 2 years,[152] 7% at 30 months,[153] 4% at 3 years,[154] and 3% at 5 years.[155] Given expected additional relapses up to the 5-year point and poorly defined patient selection factors, long-term survival results with a policy of chest irradiation alone at diagnosis for limited-stage patients are grossly inadequate.

In 1969, an important randomized trial by the Veterans Administration Lung Cancer Study Group documented that three courses of cyclophosphamide more than doubled median survival compared with supportive care alone in extensive-stage SCLC.[156] This finding sharply contrasted with the results of similar studies of single-agent chemotherapy in other cell types of lung cancer and led to the rapid investigation of the role of chemotherapy in patients with small cell carcinoma. Randomized studies, which use what would be considered suboptimal chemotherapy, demonstrated that in most instances adjuvant chemotherapy given after surgical resection prolonged survival compared with no further treatment. Because of the small numbers of patients with small cell carcinoma enrolled in most of these trials, this becomes more evident when the data are pooled (Table 23–25).[157–160] Similarly, in most randomized clinical trials, the addition of chemotherapy to chest irradiation in patients with limited-stage SCLC yielded improved median or longer-term survival compared with a policy of irradiation as sole initial treatment followed by chemotherapy at the time of tumor progression (Table 23–26).[152,153,161–163] Once again, the drug therapy used in these trials, whether single agent or combination, was not optimal. These early trials of chemotherapy used as an adjuvant to locoregional treatments and multiple other studies using chemotherapy as the sole form of therapy quickly established that small cell carcinoma was by far the most responsive type of lung cancer to drug treatment.

The results of chemotherapy administration in SCLC are similar to the optimal methods of drug treatment in several adult cancers that can be cured with chemotherapy alone. For example, in small cell carcinoma, testicular carcinoma, Hodgkin disease, and diffuse aggressive lymphomas, numerous single agents induce objective responses. Combination chemotherapy produces superior survival compared with single-agent treatment, and responses to chemotherapy occur quickly. Increased drug doses, up to a point, are associated with improving survival, and maintenance chemotherapy in responding patients is of little or no value. Over the past two decades, therapeutic research has been built on the assump-

TABLE 23–24. Survival in Patients With Operable Small Cell Lung Cancer Randomized to Surgery or Radiotherapy

Group	No. of Patients	Mean Survival (mo)	Survival Rate (%)		
			1-Year	2-Year	5-Year
Surgery	71	6.5	21	4	1†
Radiotherapy	73	10*	22	10	4

* Significant survival differene ($p = 0.04$) in favor of radiotherapy.
† One patient unable to receive surgery; given irradiation.
(Modified from Fox, W, Scadding JG. Medical Research Council comparative trial of surgery and radiotherapy for primary treatment of small-celled or oat-celled carcinoma of bronchus. Lancet 1973;2: 63–65)

TABLE 23–25. Pooled Results From Randomized Surgical Adjuvant Studies in Small Cell Lung Cancer

Adjuvant Therapy	No. of Patients	2-Year Survivors (%)
Chemotherapy	92	26
Placebo	61	8

(Modified from Higgins et al,[157] Shields et al,[159] Wingfield,[160] and Karrer et al[158])

TABLE 23–26. Selected Randomized Trials of Radiotherapy Alone Versus Chemotherapy Plus Radiation Therapy in Limited-Stage Disease

Investigations	Radiotherapy Dose (cGy)	Chemotherapy†	No. of Patients	Survival Median (mo)	Survival 1-Year (%)	Survival 2-Year (%)
Seydel et al[152]	4500	None	110	10	NR	2
		C + CCNU	107	11*	NR	8
Medical Research Council[162]	3000	None	121	6	18	NR
		C + MTX + CCNU	115	10†	34	NR
Bergsagel et al[161]	4000–5000	None	14	5	NR	NR
		C	27	10‡	NR	NR
Petrovich et al[153]	5000–6000	None	33	5	28	12
		CCNU + HU	35	9†	28	5
Perez et al[163]	4500	None	23	11	36	15
		C + A + DTIC	24	8*	38	22

NR, not reported; C, cyclophosphamide; CCNU, lomustine; MTX, methotrexate; HU, hydroxyurea; A, doxorubicin; DTIC, dacarbazine.
* Survival differences between groups not statistically significant.
† Significantly improved survival with chemotherapy.
‡ Survival differences not analyzed.
(Modified from Bunn PA, Ihde DC. Small cell bronchogenic carcinoma; A review of therapeutic results. In: Livingston RB, ed. Lung cancer 1. Amsterdam: Martinus Nijhoff, 1981:169–208)

tions that SCLC is fundamentally a systemic disorder responsive to chemotherapeutic agents and that combination chemotherapy is the mainstay of treatment. Several detailed reviews summarizing the therapy of this neoplasm and critically evaluating which approaches yield optimal results have been published over the past decade.[48,146,164–166]

SINGLE-AGENT CHEMOTHERAPY

During the 1970s, seven chemotherapeutic agents that yielded reproducible response rates of at least 30% when given to newly diagnosed patients with SCLC were identified. In the past decade, using the less stringent criterion of reproducible response rates of 20% or greater, because fewer previously untreated patients received single-agent treatment, activity of five additional drugs was documented. These drugs are listed in Table 23–27, along with other agents with less well-confirmed activity. Complete response rates to single-agent therapy are less than 5% and impact on survival is modest.[167,168] Furthermore, only vincristine and altretamine among active drugs available in the United States do not have myelosuppression as a major dose-limiting toxicity. It is difficult to construct combination programs in which the full single-agent dose of each compound is used.

Etoposide (VP-16), cyclophosphamide, doxorubicin, cisplatin, and vincristine are probably the most commonly used agents. Scheduling of etoposide and probably vincristine is important in optimizing their efficacy. In an older randomized study comparing three different schedules of etoposide as sole therapy, schedules with 3 or 5 doses per week produced higher response rates than a weekly schedule.[169] Recently, a randomized trial using etoposide as the sole initial treatment confirmed that the identical dose was much more effective when administered over 5 days rather than over 24 hours.[170]

If given with other active agents in combination regimens, the efficacy of divided dosage administration is more difficult to establish.[171] Etoposide is usually given in three to five divided doses in week 1 every 3 weeks. More protracted 2- or 3-week schedules of daily oral etoposide are active in previously treated[172] and newly diagnosed[173] patients, although it is not known whether this schedule is superior to the more

TABLE 23–27. Chemotherapeutic Agents With Documented Activity Against Small Cell Lung Cancer

Group 1 (Activity Known Before 1980)

Cyclophosphamide
Mechlorethamine (nitrogen mustard)
Doxorubicin (Adriamycin)
Methotrexate
Altretamine (hexamethylmelamine)
Etoposide (VP-16)
Vincristine

Group 2 (Activity Documented After 1980)

Carboplatin (CBDCA)
Teniposide (VM-26)
Ifosfamide
Vindesine*
Epirubicin*

Group 3 (Less Reproducible or Lower Activity)

Cisplatin
Lomustine (CCNU)
Fluorouracil
Nimustine (ACNU)*
Prednimustine*
Lonidamine*

* Not commercially available in the United States.

standard 3 to 5 doses per week. Vincristine is usually administered every 3 weeks because of neurotoxicity, even though the best evidence for its single-agent activity was obtained on a weekly schedule.[174]

Drugs that are highly active in newly diagnosed patients may exhibit only marginal activity in patients with relapsed SCLC. Etoposide has a response rate of 40% to 80% in previously untreated patients,[175,176] but when given to 116 patients relapsing after modern combination chemotherapy it produced only 9% responses.[177] A similar differential is observed with the etoposide analog teniposide (VM-26), which yields 90% responses in untreated patients but only 15% responses in previously treated patients.[178] In one of the few randomized studies designed to evaluate a dose-response relation for a single agent in SCLC,[179] too few responses to permit analysis were seen with etoposide at any of three dose levels up to 900 mg/m^2 in 77 previously treated patients.

Of the five drugs first demonstrated to possess clear activity in phase II trials in SCLC during the 1980s (see Table 23–27), all but carboplatin (CBDCA) are analogs of drugs previously known to be useful. It is possible that some active drugs were among the many agents deemed inactive during the same era in studies that were principally conducted in previously treated patients. The single-agent response rate of cisplatin, commonly used in combination regimens given for initial treatment, is less than 15%.[175] It was evaluated as a single agent almost exclusively in previously treated patients, and probably has activity comparable with its analog carboplatin, which exhibited 60% responses in 30 previously untreated patients.[180] These considerations suggest that phase II trials should be performed in fully ambulatory but previously untreated patients with a poor prognosis, that is, in patients with extensive disease. If the patient fails to respond after a short time, a standard combination chemotherapy regimen could be administered. Such a strategy is acceptable when the phase II agent is active.[178,180,181]

Some phase II studies in untreated extensive-stage patients, including one using a doxorubicin analog, yielded shorter than anticipated survival.[182,183] With careful patient selection, patient survival is not likely to be compromised by initial therapy with an inactive investigational agent, as suggested by a recent phase II study[184] and a randomized trial in which patients received an experimental drug that proved inactive or standard combination chemotherapy.[185] Whether this approach more effectively selects new active drugs for SCLC remains to be seen. A recent review indicates that all known active drugs would have been identified when given to previously treated patients if the criteria for declaring efficacy had been lowered to a 10% response rate.[175] The complex issue of patient eligibility criteria for phase II trials has been discussed in detail.[186]

COMBINATION CHEMOTHERAPY

Aggressive combination chemotherapy regimens yield the best response rates (Fig. 23–15) and the highest percentage of long-term survivors in SCLC.[146,164] In limited disease, optimal regimens should produce 85% to 95% overall response rates, 50% to 60% complete response rates, median survival of 12 to 16 months, and 2-year disease-free survival of 15% to 25%. Corresponding results in patients with extensive disease are

overall response rates of 75% to 85%, complete response rates of 15% to 25%, and median survival of 7 to 11 months. Two-year disease-free survival in extensive disease is rare.

Although these therapeutic outcomes leave substantial room for improvement, they represent a fourfold to fivefold increase in median survival compared with survival of untreated patients. These outcomes have been made possible only by the development of effective combination chemotherapy programs. The principles of administration of combination drug regimens for SCLC are discussed in detail in this section.

Superiority to Single Agents

Response rates routinely seen with combination chemotherapy appear greatly superior to rates observed with single agents in previously untreated patients.[187] However, only a few prospective randomized trials conducted during the 1970s, when combination chemotherapy for SCLC was initially developed, directly compared combination regimens with single-agent regimens in the absence of chest irradiation (Table 23–28). In two trials in which two- or three-drug cyclophosphamide-containing programs were compared with cyclophosphamide alone,[188,189] response rates and survival were better with the combination regimen. Another study investigated whether administering four drugs simultaneously or as sequential single agents was the more effective approach and found modestly improved response rates with the former strategy.[190] These trials used drug doses that induced only mild myelosuppression and incorporated drugs such as lomustine (CCNU), procarbazine, and dacarbazine that are less active or of unproved efficacy in the combination regimen. Some minimally myelosuppressive combination programs result in inferior response and survival compared with regimens of the same drugs given in doses producing moderately severe hematologic toxicity.[191] It is not surprising that the randomized studies of combination compared with single-agent chemotherapy sometimes demonstrated real but less than overwhelming advantages of combination programs. Nonetheless, the response rates attained with appropriately delivered combination programs using only drugs of known activity are superior to the early data with single agents given in conventional doses (Table 23–29).[167] The principle of the advantage of combination chemotherapy for SCLC is considered firmly established.

Recently, good response rates and survival have been noted in elderly European patients given single-agent etoposide or teniposide as sole treatment.[176,192] These findings have brought under scrutiny the dogma that combination chemotherapy is unequivocally superior in all small cell carcinoma patients. Single-agent treatment is an acceptable option in patients with poor performance status or with other medical factors that increase the risk of treatment-related toxicities. Until this issue is evaluated in controlled clinical trials, combination chemotherapy should be considered standard treatment for patients at less than excessive risk from chemotherapy.

Number and Types of Drugs in Combination Regimens

Two prospective randomized trials (see Table 23–28) demonstrated a survival advantage with the addition of a third drug to a two-drug program[147] and of a fourth agent to a three-

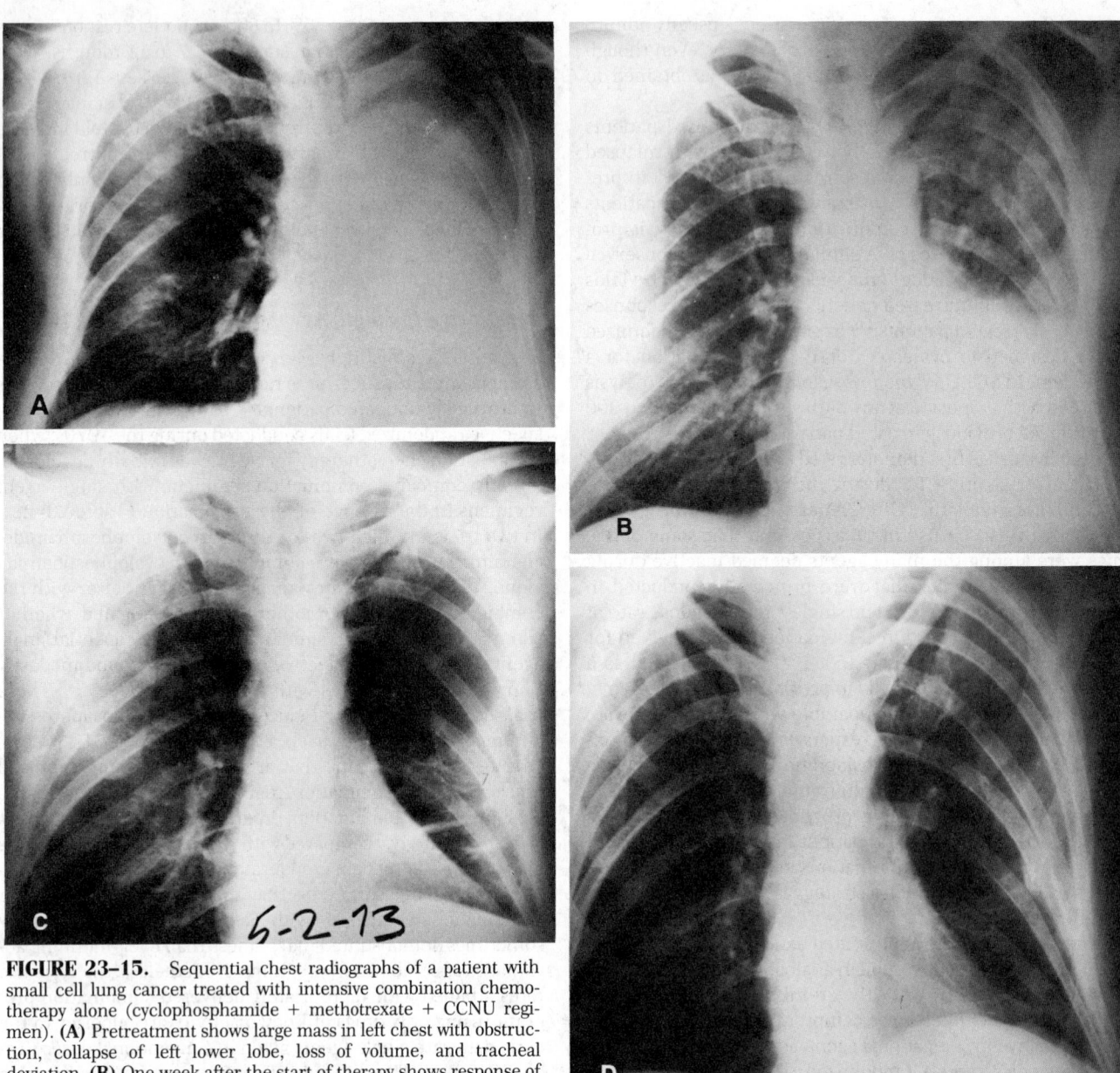

FIGURE 23–15. Sequential chest radiographs of a patient with small cell lung cancer treated with intensive combination chemotherapy alone (cyclophosphamide + methotrexate + CCNU regimen). **(A)** Pretreatment shows large mass in left chest with obstruction, collapse of left lower lobe, loss of volume, and tracheal deviation. **(B)** One week after the start of therapy shows response of tumor and remaining bulk of tumor in pulmonary parenchyma, hilar, and mediastinal nodes. **(C)** Three weeks after the start of therapy. Almost complete resolution of tumor; however, there is still some residual stranding and possible mediastinal adenopathy. **(D)** Five weeks after the start of treatment; no tumor visible by chest radiograph. Fiberoptic bronchoscopy with washings and biopsy at 6 weeks revealed no evidence of tumor.

drug program[21] in patients with extensive-stage disease given chemotherapy alone. Three-drug programs yielded better response rates than one- or two-drug programs in patients also given chest irradiation.[193] Regimens using greater numbers of agents simultaneously have been studied only infrequently, because the use of too many drugs concurrently necessitates compromises in dose that probably limit efficacy. There is little evidence to support giving more than three or four drugs simultaneously in the therapy of SCLC.[167]

The drug regimens given in randomized trials documenting the value of adding additional agents to a combination pro-

duced only modest degrees of myelosuppression. Increasing drug doses in the combination with the smaller number of drugs may be just as efficacious as increasing the number of drugs administered. Escalating the dose of even a single agent such as cyclophosphamide to levels that require hospitalization can yield complete response rates in limited-disease patients of 55%,[194] a rate as high or higher than that achieved with many combination programs. If different combination regimens are being compared, the specific agents being administered and the dose intensity with which they are delivered must be considered. For example, one

TABLE 23–28. Early Randomized Trials Evaluating the Optimal Number of Simultaneously Administered Chemotherapeutic Agents

Investigations	Drug and Dose (mg/m²)	No. of Patients	Complete and Partial Response Rate (%)	Median Survival	Comments
Combination Chemotherapy vs Single Agents					
Edmonson et al[189]	C 700 + CCNU 70	110	43	20 wk	Combination drugs better, $p < 0.01$ CR + PR, $p = 0.07$ survival
	C1000	118	22	17 wk	
Lowenbraun et al[188]	C 500 + A 50 + DTIC 250	207	57	31 wk	Combination drugs better, $p < 0.01$ CR + PR, $p = 0.01$ survival
	C 1100	34	12	18 wk	
Alberto et al[190]	MTX 40 + C420 + VCR 1.2 + PCZ 560*	59	65	NR	Simultaneous drugs better, $p = 0.1$ CR + PR; survival not different
	MTX → C → PCZ → VCR†	14	36	NR	
Three Drugs vs Two Drugs					
Hansen et al[147]	C 500 + MTX 20 + CCNU 50‡	33	56	33 wk	Three drugs better, CR + PR not different, $p = 0.17$ survival
	C 500 + MTX 20	29	38	23 wk	
Four Drugs vs Three Drugs					
Hansen et al.[21]	C 700 + MTX 20 + CCNU 70 + VCR 1.3§	52	78	7.7 mo	Four drugs better, CR + PR not different, $p < 0.01$ survival
	C 700 + MTX 20 + CCNU 70	53	75	6.0 mo	

CR, complete response; PR, partial response; VCR, vincristine; PCZ, procarbazine; A, doxorubicin; C, cyclophosphamide; CCNU, lomustine; MTX, methotrexate; DTIC, dacarbazine.
* Weekly doses given for 8 weeks.
† Sequential single agents each given for 2 weeks.
‡ C every 3 weeks, MTX twice weekly, CCNU every 6 weeks.
§ C and CCNU every 4 weeks, MTX × 2 in week 3, VCR weekly first cycle.
(Modified from Ihde DC, Bunn PA. Chemotherapy of small cell bronchogenic carcinoma. In: Williams CJ, Whitehouse JMA, eds. Recent advances in clinical oncology. Edinburgh: Churchill Livingstone, 1982;305–323)

randomized study found significantly improved response rates and survival in extensive-stage patients treated with cyclophosphamide, etoposide, and vincristine compared with cyclophosphamide and vincristine. These findings more convincingly demonstrated the contribution of etoposide to the three-drug program, because the cyclophosphamide dose

TABLE 23–29. Objective Tumor Responses to Single-Agent or Combination Chemotherapy in Previously Untreated Patients With Small Cell Lung Cancer (No Radiation Therapy)

Drug Treatment	No. of Patients	Response (%)	
		All Objective*	Complete
Single agent†	753	15–20	2.5
Combination	1236	70	31

* Objective tumor responses include partial and complete responses. Complete response rate data available for only 572 patients.
† Includes only data for cyclophosphamide, nitrogen mustard, doxorubicin, methotrexate, etoposide, hexamethylmelamine, and vincristine.
(Adapted from Bunn PA Jr, Ihde DC. Small cell bronchogenic carcinoma: A review of therapeutic results. In: Livingston RB, ed. Lung cancer: Advances in research and treatment. The Hague: Martinus Nijhoff, 1981:169–208)

was doubled in the two-drug combination so that the myelosuppression associated with each regimen was similar.[195]

Although many combination chemotherapy regimens for SCLC appear to possess similar efficacy, the CAV program (representative doses are cyclophosphamide 1000 mg/m², doxorubicin 45 mg/m², and vincristine 2 mg) was one of the most commonly used combinations during the 1980s and reproducibly yielded the optimal response rates, median survival, and long-term survival as outlined in limited-stage and extensive-stage disease. Until recently, it was considered the standard regimen against which to compare newer approaches. Etoposide was probably the most actively studied newer agent in the 1980s, and many randomized trials evaluated whether adding etoposide to or substituting it for one of the components of CAV is beneficial.

Three controlled trials keeping CAV doses identical compared CAV plus etoposide (CAVE) with CAV alone.[196-198] Two found significantly greater response rates with CAVE, but survival was not significantly improved. In an equitoxic comparison of standard dose CAV with etoposide versus higher dose CAV, there were no differences in response rates or survival.[199] Other randomized trials addressed the utility of substituting etoposide for one of the drugs in CAV. Median survival in extensive-stage patients was prolonged by 2 months when etoposide was substituted for doxorubicin[195] or vincristine,[200] although myelosuppression and perhaps drug dose intensity were greater with CAE in the latter trial. In neither study did the etoposide-containing program prove superior in limited-stage patients. In a large randomized study of 269 extensive-stage patients, etoposide was substituted for methotrexate at two different time points in a 4-week, four-drug regimen consisting of cyclophosphamide, methotrexate, lomustine, and vincristine.[201] Significantly improved survival was seen when etoposide was given earlier but not when given later in the chemotherapy cycle. Increased myelosuppression was observed only with early etoposide. These studies do not provide unequivocal evidence that etoposide-containing programs are superior to programs not containing this drug, although etoposide is among the most active agents in SCLC.

The combination EP exhibits therapeutic synergy in murine leukemia,[202] produces a fraction of long-term survivors in refractory testicular cancer,[203] and recently has been evaluated in many types of cancer. In previously treated SCLC, this two-drug program produced objective response rates of 50% or more in some recent studies,[204,205] in contrast to usual response rates of less than 10% for most other salvage regimens studied in the past decade. These encouraging results led to trials of EP as sole chemotherapeutic treatment[206,207] with acceptable therapeutic results in limited and extensive disease. Two groups of investigators[208,209] noted that after administration of two to four cycles of EP, further tumor regression was not observed with subsequent CAV.

Two recent studies randomized patients to CAV or EP as sole initial chemotherapy.[210,211] Patients given EP had marginally or significantly better response rates and similar survival compared with patients receiving CAV. Furthermore, EP given as salvage therapy to patients who failed to respond to CAV or developed tumor progression after CAV produced response rates twice as high as when CAV was given as salvage treatment after EP. Another trial randomized limited-stage patients to receive or not receive two cycles of EP after six cycles of CAV with or without chest irradiation. A 30-week improvement in median survival was demonstrated with the addition of EP,[212] implying that EP may be able to eradicate tumor cells resistant to CAV. EP has produced less neutropenia and infection than CAV in randomized trials.[210,211] In summary, EP is an effective combination that likely has the most favorable therapeutic index of current chemotherapy programs, thereby readily permitting the addition of a third myelosuppressive agent, should greater antitumor effects of the three-drug program be demonstrated. It is a commonly used regimen.

Substitution of carboplatin for cisplatin in the EP program has yielded an active combination with reduced gastrointestinal toxicity but greater myelosuppression.[213] In previously untreated patients, survival with EP was superior to results with etoposide combined with ifosfamide in a German study,[214] further supporting the value of the EP regimen. Doses and schedules of some effective, commonly used combination chemotherapy regimens for SCLC are provided in Table 23–30.[215]

Intensity of Initial Chemotherapy

Most drug programs for SCLC, with the probable exception of EP, are designed to produce moderately severe myelosuppression with leukopenia of 1000 to 2000 cells/μL in most patients. Such regimens do not require hospitalization but do

TABLE 23–30. Effective Commonly Used Combination Chemotherapy Programs for Small Cell Lung Cancer

Drug	Dose, Route, and Day(s) of Administration
CAV	
Cyclophosphamide	1000 mg/m² I.V. day 1
Doxorubicin	45 mg/m² I.V. day 1
Vincristine	2 mg I.V. day 1
Repeat cycle every 3 weeks	
CAE	
Cyclophosphamide	1000 mg/m² I.V. day 1
Doxorubicin	45 mg/m² I.V. day 1
Etoposide	50 mg/m² I.V. days 1–5
Repeat cycle every 3 weeks	
CAVE	
Cyclophosphamide	1000 mg/m² I.V. day 1
Doxorubicin	50 mg/m² I.V. day 1
Vincristine	1.5 mg/m² I.V. day 1
Etoposide	60 mg/m² I.V. days 1–5
Repeat cycle every 3 weeks	
EP	
Etoposide	100 mg/m² I.V. days 1–3
Cisplatin	25 mg/m² I.V. days 1–3
Repeat cycle every 3 weeks	
CMCcV	
Cyclophosphamide	700 mg/m² I.V. day 1
Methotrexate	20 mg/m² po days 18, 21
Lomustine	70 mg/m² po day 1
Vincristine	1.3 mg/m² I.V. days 1, 8, 15, 22
Repeat cycle every 4 weeks	first cycle and then day 1
CAV and EP	
Cycle of CAV as above alternating every 3 weeks with cycle of EP as above	

(Modified from Ihde DC. Chemotherapy in lung cancer. In: Brain MC, Carbone PP, eds. Current therapy in hematology–Oncology 3. Toronto: BC Decker, 1988:213–217)

mandate careful monitoring to avoid or ameliorate infectious or bleeding complications. One approach to overcoming drug resistance in this tumor has been to administer more intensive chemotherapeutic regimens, because the tenets of the dose-response relation in chemotherapy of cancer in animals and humans suggest that dose rate may be critical to tumor cell kill, particularly in more responsive neoplasms.[216] Although increases in drug doses may often increase tumor response rate and duration, this approach is limited by toxicity to normal host tissues.

Several randomized (Table 23–31) and nonrandomized trials have studied the concept of dose-response relations in SCLC. The first randomized trial addressing this question administered twofold higher doses of cyclophosphamide, methotrexate, and lomustine regimen (CMC) for the initial 6-week induction and demonstrated significantly improved response rates and survival with higher drug doses.[191] A much larger controlled trial using the CMC regimen studied the effects of a higher dose of only the cyclophosphamide component during the first 6 weeks of treatment and found modest but significant

TABLE 23–31. Completed Randomized Studies of Intensity of Initial Combination Chemotherapy in Small Cell Lung Cancer

Investigations	Drug and Dose (mg/m²)	No. of Patients	Complete and Partial Response Rate (%)	Median Survival (%)	Comments
Cohen et al[191]	C 1000 + MTX 15 + CCNU 100*	23	96	10.5	High doses better: $p < 0.05$
	C 500 + MTX 10 + CCNU 50	9	45	5.0	CR + PR, $p < 0.05$ survival
Mehta et al[217]	C 1500 + MTX 15 + CCNU 70*	175†	64	10.25	High dose better: $p = 0.04$
	700 + MTX 15 + CCNU 70	174	54	9	CR + PR, $p = 0.04$ survival
Johnson et al[219]	C 1200 + A 70 + VCR 1‡	101	63 (22 CR)	7	High dose better: $p = 0.04$
	C 1000 + A 40 + VCR 1	146	53 (12 CR)	8	CR; CR + PR and survival not different
Figueredo et al[220]	C 1560 + A 59 + VCR 0.9§	52	71 (21 CR LD, 8 ED)	14	No differences in CR,
	C 990 + A 50 + VCR 1.0	51	61 (22 CR LD, 8 ED)	12	response duration, or survival

CR, complete response; PR, partial rseponse; LD, limited disease; ED, extensive disease; C, cyclophosphamide; MTX, methotrexate; CCNU, lomustine; A, doxorubicin; VCR, vincristine.
* High-dose regimen for first 6 weeks.
† Approximate number.
‡ High-dose regimen for first 9 weeks.
§ Doses are actual doses given, not intended doses; high dose regimen for first 12 weeks.

increases in response rate and survival, particularly in patients with limited-stage disease.[217] Nonrandomized trials suggest that very high doses of cyclophosphamide (4.8 to 8.0 g/m²) given as a single agent produce a much higher than anticipated fraction of complete responses in limited[194] and extensive[218] disease.

Increasing doses of other standard chemotherapy programs or drugs in an outpatient setting has not yielded improved results. In two randomized studies of the CAV regimen, the doses of cyclophosphamide were increased 20% to 56% and the doses of doxorubicin were increased 18% to 75% during the first 9 to 12 weeks of chemotherapy.[219,220] Although the complete response rate was modestly improved in one trial, there was no effect on response duration or survival with higher doses of CAV in either study. Preliminary results of a smaller trial involving administration of 67% higher doses of EP for the first 6 weeks of therapy show no benefit for the high-dose program,[221] suggesting that in the outpatient setting, the maximal therapeutic effects of this combination may be attained at doses associated with a median leukocyte nadir of 2600 cells/μL. There appears to be no advantage of high-dose methotrexate with leucovorin rescue compared with standard-dose methotrexate when added to the CAV regimen.[222] It is probable that CMC is less effective at equitoxic doses than CAV or EP, explaining why benefits of higher than standard doses have been demonstrable in randomized trials only with the CMC program or its variants.

To obtain markedly increased tumor cell kill, multiple nonrandomized trials using even higher doses of cyclophosphamide, doxorubicin, etoposide, or cisplatin have been initiated. These studies, which require hospitalization of most or all patients and are occasionally given with autologous bone marrow transplant,[223] most often include patients with extensive-stage disease. Several early studies tested higher individual doses or more frequent administration of cyclophosphamide,

doxorubicin, and etoposide,[224–226] whereas more recent trials with similar philosophic intent used alternating drug combinations or regimens including high doses of etoposide and cisplatin.[227,228] Although high complete response rates sometimes have been observed, response duration and survival appear similar to results attained with many standard, less intensive programs. Intensive approaches requiring routine hospitalization of patients are appropriate only in the setting of a clinical trial.

A more recent strategy to increase the dose intensity of chemotherapy is to administer identical drug doses over a shorter time. Several groups have reported promising pilot studies of weekly chemotherapy, usually given on an outpatient basis, for 12 to 16 weeks.[229–231] This approach is being tested in randomized trials. A recent comprehensive meta-analysis used statistical techniques developed to assess the importance of dose-rate intensity, which accounts for dose and interval of chemotherapy administration. More dose-intense programs of CAV, CAVE, or EP could not be shown to be associated with consistently better therapeutic results.[232]

Late Intensification

Because most patients with SCLC ultimately relapse, several groups have proposed treating the smaller tumor burden in maximally responding patients with an intensive approach, rather than awaiting overt tumor progression. This strategy would administer intensive treatment only to responders, those most likely to derive benefit; allow therapy of a reduced tumor bulk, which would likely be less resistant to treatment than at time of relapse; and apply intensive therapy only to patients in the best possible medical condition. At least eight trials treating at least 5 patients with so-called *late intensification* have been published.[233–240] Most trials included patients with extensive-stage disease and did not restrict entry to patients in complete remission after standard therapy. The proportion of patients beginning standard therapy who actually received the planned late intensification ranged from 18% to 38%. The late intensification programs were diverse and included single-agent and combination chemotherapy with local-field or total-body irradiation in some cases. Autologous bone marrow infusions were given to some or all patients, although this was probably unnecessary except for those receiving total-body irradiation.

Treatment-associated deaths ranged from 15% to 30% in four of the trials. Although some patients not in complete response after standard therapy achieved complete response with late intensification, the duration of these responses was brief. The fraction of disease-free survivors has been small, and most of such patients are in complete remission before late intensive therapy. There has been no improvement in the outcome of all patients beginning standard chemotherapy with the intent of administering late intensification compared with patients given standard therapy without late intensification.[235,241] Late intensive therapies remain a suitable subject of clinical investigation, particularly in limited-stage patients who attain a complete response to standard therapy. Because markedly superior results cannot be expected with this approach using available drugs, randomized trials will probably be required to demonstrate efficacy convincingly.

Cyclic Alternating Combination Chemotherapy

As might be predicted from its rapid growth rate, in SCLC, responses to chemotherapy occur quickly. Symptomatic improvement is usual with the first cycle of treatment and it is uncommon for tumor masses to demonstrate further regression after 12 or sometimes even 6 weeks.[191,208,242,243] Early introduction of a new non-cross-resistant drug program before the development of tumor progression is conceptually attractive. Goldie and Coldman have provided a detailed mathematic model of the spontaneous origin of drug-resistant clones in malignant tumors at a mutation rate proportional to the number of actively dividing tumor cells.[244] This model predicts that as many active agents as possible should be given at full doses as quickly as possible to maximize the chance of eradication of the entire tumor cell population. Because myelosuppressive toxicity does not allow all possible drugs to be given simultaneously, another suitable strategy is to alternate the administration of two combination regimens that are equally effective and non-cross-resistant.[245] Alternating combinations are commonly used in the treatment of SCLC.

Although this point has not been demonstrated rigorously, most chemotherapy programs in small cell carcinoma appear to have about equal efficacy. If non-cross-resistance is defined as a second drug combination producing a substantial fraction of complete remissions if administered after tumor progression on a first drug combination, most if not all chemotherapy programs in SCLC are not non-cross-resistant. There has been, at best, minimal survival benefit from alternation of two or more combination regimens, although new complete responses sometimes occur with initiation of the second combination. The duration of initial remission has been prolonged by this strategy in some randomized trials.[246-248] Occasional randomized studies have shown improved survival with alternating combinations, but the magnitude of benefit has been modest, requiring randomization of more than 500 patients to be detectable[246] or using combinations that probably had unequal efficacy.[249]

Interest in the possible superiority of alternating chemotherapy regimens was reawakened when EP was shown to be an active salvage regimen in patients failing CAV treatment.[204,205] This raises the possibility that EP could be less cross-resistant with CAV than previously used combinations. A large study of 289 patients with extensive disease found an increased response rate, response duration, and survival with an alternating combination CAV and EP program compared with CAV alone, although the advantage in median survival was only 6 weeks.[250] This trial could not distinguish whether the superiority of the cyclic alternating treatment was due to the alternating strategy or to the fact that EP is superior to CAV. Two subsequent, similarly large trials from the United States and Japan have addressed this question.[210,211] The U.S. study was confined to extensive-stage patients. Response rates and response duration were significantly higher with the alternating combination CAV and EP program than with CAV alone in one study,[211] but there were no survival differences among extensive-stage patients in either. Among limited-stage patients in the Japanese study, the alternating regimen yielded better survival than EP or CAV given alone, although fewer than 150 patients of this stage were randomized. Taken together with the earlier randomized trial in limited-stage patients demonstrating better survival when EP was given after completing 6 cycles of CAV,[212] these results suggest that administration of more than one chemotherapy program might be more effective in patients with a lesser tumor burden.

Cyclic alternating administration of two active combination chemotherapy regimens is an acceptable but not mandatory treatment strategy in SCLC. At a minimum, this approach should reduce drug toxicities that depend on the total cumulative dose of a single agent, such as cardiac toxicity of doxorubicin and neurotoxicity of cisplatin and vincristine.

Duration of Chemotherapy Administration

In the 1970s, SCLC chemotherapy was based on treatment strategies for acute lymphoblastic leukemia, and chemotherapy in responding SCLC patients often continued for up to 2 years. Several early studies of CAV with chest irradiation for patients with limited-stage disease produced similar survival outcomes despite variations in the planned duration of chemotherapy from 3 or 4 months to 24 months (Table 23-32).[251-253] More recently, treatment programs based on CAV and chest irradiation intended to last for 61 and 18 weeks, respectively, had almost identical response rates and median and 2-year survival in consecutive large patient groups treated at a single institution.[254] These data suggest that a disproportionate fraction of the antitumor effects of chemotherapy occurs in the early cycles. This is consistent with the results of some randomized studies comparing higher and lower doses of the same drugs (see Table 23-31), in which higher doses given for only the first 6 to 9 weeks produce superior response rates or survival.

If most or all tumor regression from drug treatment occurs within the first few cycles of therapy, continuation of chemotherapy (or maintenance) would be of minimal benefit. Many chemotherapy programs used since the early 1980s are

TABLE 23–32. Early Studies of Combined-Modality Therapy (CAV + Chest RT) in Limited-Stage Disease With Various Durations of Maintenance Chemotherapy

Investigations	Duration of Therapy (mo)*	No. of Patients	Complete Response Rate (%)	Median Survival (mo)	2-Year Disease-Free Survival Rate (%)
Johnson et al[253]	3–4	36	75	18.5	28
Greco et al[252]	14	32	91	16	25
Einhorn et al[251]	25	19	89	17	26

CAV, cyclophosphamide + doxorubicin + vincristine; RT, radiation therapy.
* Total duration of chemotherapy planned in responding patients.
(Modified from Ihde DC, Bunn PA. Chemotherapy of small cell bronchogenic carcinoma. In Williams CJ, Whitehouse JMA, eds. Recent advances in clinical oncology. Edinburgh: Churchill Livingstone, 1982:305–323)

intended to be discontinued in responding patients after 4 to 6 months with therapeutic results similar to previously used 12- and 24-month regimens.

Only recently have randomized trials addressed the optimal duration of chemotherapy in SCLC. The results of most trials suggest that, as in most other cancers potentially curable with chemotherapy, there is little role for maintenance therapy (Table 23–33). A preliminary report of a large European trial demonstrated prolonged time to tumor progression in patients receiving 12 rather than 5 cycles of chemotherapy without survival differences,[255] as did two British studies of 6 versus 12 and 4 versus 8 cycles of treatment.[243,256] In one of these trials, patients were randomized to chemotherapy or supportive care alone after tumor progression. Survival was compromised with supportive care alone in patients who initially received only 4 chemotherapy cycles but not in those receiving 8, emphasizing that minimally treated patients in particular may benefit from further treatment at relapse. In another trial, in which only complete responders with extensive disease were randomized, those given maintenance chemotherapy had equivalent survival to patients in whom chemotherapy was discontinued.[246]

In summary, administering chemotherapy for only 4 to 6 months in stable responding patients is recommended, be-

cause this approach does not compromise survival and minimizes the toxicity and expense of chemotherapy.

Chemotherapy in Special Clinical Settings

SCLC is among the commonest underlying neoplasms in patients presenting with superior vena cava syndrome. Thoracic radiotherapy has been the traditional treatment for this problem. Chemotherapy was quickly recognized to be able to provide rapid palliation in small cell carcinoma[257] and in a randomized trial proved to be as effective as chemotherapy and chest irradiation in ameliorating the syndrome.[258] Chemotherapy alone is appropriate treatment for superior vena cava obstruction in patients in whom chest irradiation is not otherwise indicated. In our experience, combination chemotherapy alone leads to resolution of atelectasis and reduction in pleural effusions in 70% and 50% of extensive-stage patients, respectively.

Cranial irradiation is generally administered when brain metastases are diagnosed in SCLC patients. Recently, several investigators have observed regression of such metastases with chemotherapy alone.[259,260] There are insufficient data on duration of therapeutic effects to recommend this approach outside clinical trials, but patients with recurrent metastases after

TABLE 23–33. Recent Randomized Trials of Maintenance Chemothearpy in Small Cell Lung Cancer

Investigations	Response	Stage	Cycles of Chemotherapy*	No. of Patients	Significant Difference in	
					Time to Progressive Disease	Survival
Splinter[255]	CR/PR/NC	All	5/12	426	Yes	No
Ettinger et al[246]	CR	ED	NR*	73	Yes	No
Spiro et al[243]	CR/PR/NC	All	4/8	610	Yes	No†
Bleehan et al[256]	CR/PR	All	6/12	265	NR	No

* With or without maintenance.
† Provided chemotherapy given at relapse in patients randomized to no maintenance.
CR, complete response; PR, partial response; NC, no change; ED, extensive disease; NR, not reported.

previous brain irradiation can be candidates for a trial of chemotherapeutic management. Because the brain is a frequent site of subsequent relapse in patients responding to initial chemotherapy, drug treatment could be more effective for overt intracranial tumor because of disruption of the blood–brain barrier.

Toxicities of Combination Chemotherapy

The major acute toxicities produced by all combination chemotherapy programs used in SCLC are those related to myelosuppression, specifically neutropenia-associated fever and infection, and, to a lesser extent, thrombocytopenic bleeding. Patients with poor performance status or extensive-stage disease are at greater risk. Nausea, vomiting, and alopecia are associated with many drugs. Toxicities peculiar to specific agents, such as cardiomyopathy with doxorubicin, neurotoxicity with vincristine and cisplatin, and hemorrhagic cystitis with cyclophosphamide, are observed.

With most standard chemotherapy programs, the duration of neutropenia is short. Febrile episodes are reported in approximately 30% of patients, documented infections in approximately 5%, and infectious deaths in 2%.[261] Herpes zoster[262,263] and perirectal abscesses[264] occasionally develop during chemotherapy. Even more intensive chemotherapy programs can be delivered to selected patients in a hospital setting with a treatment-related death rate of approximately 5%, if there is strict adherence to meticulous supportive care.[265]

With more aggressive chemotherapy programs that induce febrile neutropenia in more than 75% of patients, administration of granulocyte colony-stimulating factor substantially ameliorates this complication, the frequency of documented infections, and the days of intravenous antibiotics and hospitalization.[266] Whether colony-stimulating factors become a common adjunct to the treatment of SCLC depends greatly on whether more toxic drug regimens can be shown to be superior. Their effectiveness should be compared with that of prophylactic oral antibiotics such as trimethoprim sulfamethoxazole, which in some randomized studies has significantly reduced the incidence of infection and time spent on antibiotics.[267]

If chemotherapy is combined with chest irradiation, and especially if the two modalities are given concurrently, the rate of infectious complications is increased due to significantly greater myelosuppression.[268,269] The addition of chest radiotherapy to chemotherapy significantly reduces the frequency of circulating granulocyte-monocyte precursor colony-forming units in the peripheral blood,[270] and even the small radiation portals used for brain metastases can increase the degree of myelosuppression from concurrent chemotherapy.[271]

Acute myeloblastic leukemia has been reported in a few long-term survivors who received chemotherapy for SCLC. The actuarial risk at 2 to 3 years is 2% to 4% in two large series,[272,273] and chromosomal deletions similar to those seen in treatment-associated leukemia after chemotherapy of Hodgkin disease have been reported.[273,274] Most affected patients received protracted chemotherapy including procarbazine or a nitrosourea or both; shorter durations of treatment and lesser use of nitrosoureas and procarbazine should further

reduce the frequency of this uncommon complication. Although several drugs administered to small cell carcinoma patients, including methotrexate, cyclophosphamide, and the nitrosoureas are associated with pulmonary toxicity, it occurs infrequently in patients not receiving chest irradiation. Serial pulmonary function studies in patients with tumor regression to chemotherapy alone generally show improvement.[275,276] Although acute tumor lysis syndrome with hyperkalemia, hyperphosphatemia, and hypocalcemia rarely has been reported,[277] routine administration of allopurinol and frequent monitoring of serum electrolyte levels is not necessary.

With standard chemotherapy regimens given with or without chest irradiation, anticipated treatment-associated death rates from all causes are 0% to 4% in limited-stage SCLC patients and 2% to 8% in extensive-stage SCLC patients. The potential for major morbidity and occasional mortality emphasizes that chemotherapy for this neoplasm should be administered only by physicians experienced in avoiding and managing drug-related toxicities. However, the survival benefits of therapy greatly exceed the decrements in lifespan produced by its side effects.

RADIOTHERAPY AND COMBINED-MODALITY THERAPY

Technical Aspects of Radiation Therapy

The most crucial problem in successfully irradiating the primary tumor complex in a patient with SCLC is the degree of pulmonary compromise already sustained as a consequence of heavy smoking. The patient is unlikely to have normal pulmonary function in either lung, and what the radiotherapist can accomplish is greatly determined by the patient's physical condition. Although no particular pulmonary function test is absolutely crucial, we prefer that the patient have an FEV_1 of greater than 1 L; a lesser value usually implies that definitive radiotherapy is contraindicated.

The key to this dilemma is the integration of the diagnostic evaluation of the extent of the neoplasm within the thorax with the simulation process, which defines the volume of irradiation. Simulation should occur before any treatment begins. The patient is placed supine on the simulator table and set up using an isocentric technique, encompassing all neoplasm with a margin of approximately 1.5 to 2 cm. If the neoplasm is in the upper portion of the thorax, we include the supraclavicular nodes bilaterally. If the upper mediastinum appears uninvolved, we usually omit supraclavicular nodes from the treatment volume. We use the isocentric rather than standard source-to-skin distance technique, because this facilitates the change to a posterior field angled obliquely off the spinal cord during the latter part of the treatment. A CT scan obtained on a flat surface in the treatment position is used to determine the target volume to be encompassed isocentrically.

The simulation process uses a diagnostic x-ray tube that duplicates the megavoltage treatment machine in terms of its geometric, mechanical, and optical properties. It allows visualization of internal structures on a diagnostic film and relates them to entrance fields on the patient's skin. A simulation film may be compared with a port verification film obtained on the treatment machine to ensure that desired structures are being encompassed accurately. Because megavoltage x-rays are absorbed similarly by soft tissue and bone, anatomic detail in the port verification film is poor and major structures are minimally delineated. However, the simulator film can still be compared reliably with the port film. We prefer to use gradicules to verify the center of the field and compare that with simulation films that identify the isocenter.

SCLC is so radioresponsive that we believe it is crucial to resimulate the patient once a week during treatment. If radiation treatment is begun on a Monday, which is typical, we resimulate the patient every Friday during treatment to shrink the field as quickly as possible. This process helps minimize radiation injury of uninvolved pulmonary tissue. Our scheme, using a concurrent combined-modality approach, dictates that the patient receive only 3 weeks of irradiation, so only two additional simulations are usually necessary.

If the brain is to be irradiated (prophylactically in complete responders or therapeutically in patients with detectable intracranial lesions), we generally treat the entire cranial vault and protect the ocular lenses and extend the field inferiorly to the second cervical vertebral level as the field cuts across the spinal cord. This method allows easy matching of fields should the patient subsequently require additional irradiation to the lower cervical spine or neck region.

The biologic effect of a given dose of irradiation varies markedly depending on how it is fractionated. Various formulas have been derived that attempt to relate the total dose, number of fractions, and days of exposure to some single numeric equivalent.[278–280] Fundamentally, they are based on estimates of normal tissue tolerance, of which the most important determinant is actually the volume of treatment, which most formulas neglect. Another important correlate to morbidity of normal tissue injury is the size of the individual fraction used. All other things being equal, the schedule that approaches tolerance and that uses larger individual fractions is more likely to give injury than one that uses smaller fractions.

If chemotherapy and irradiation are combined, as is virtually always the case in SCLC, some of the classic fractionation equations do not hold. A retrospective review of various fractionation schemes used at the NCI showed that more than 3 weeks of combined-modality treatment led to greater severity of morbidity and even mortality.[281] Our subsequent treatment programs of concurrent chemotherapy and radiation were limited to 3 weeks to attempt to optimize tumor control while limiting pulmonary toxicity.

Most normal tissues and cancers are characterized by radiation survival curves with demonstrable shoulders, implying a capacity to repair radiation damage.[282] In contrast, most small cell carcinomas, at least tumor cell lines studied in vitro, exhibit little or no shoulder.[62] This suggests that further fractionating the irradiation dose in SCLC patients might not impair antitumor effectiveness but would ameliorate pulmonary damage. In uncontrolled clinical trials, increasing the number of radiation fractions to twice daily appears to improve local tumor control while minimizing lung complications by decreasing individual fraction size.[283,284] This approach is under investigation.

We currently treat intrathoracic SCLC with 150 cGy twice a day to a total dose of 4500 cGy in 3 weeks. We allow at least 4 hours, and preferably 6, between treatments on each day.

Customized blocking limits the exposure to normal tissues as the treatment continues for 3 weeks. The initial portals are delivered anteroposteriorly and posteroanteriorly (AP/PA), switching to opposed oblique fields when necessary to limit the direct spinal cord dose to 4000 cGy. Occasionally, a patient's pulmonary function is so marginal that the decision is made to not shift to the oblique fields because of fear of expanding the total treatment volume, thereby risking radiation pneumonitis. In this setting, it becomes imperative that a spinal cord block be used, which is probably suboptimal from the standpoint of tumor control, because the block may also protect centrally located SCLC.

Some authors have advocated radiation doses of 5000 to 6000 cGy for SCLC.[285] We do not believe such doses are necessary in conjunction with combined-modality treatment, due to the impressive responsiveness of this neoplasm to chemotherapy and irradiation. For overt metastatic lesions in the central nervous system, we use 4500 cGy in 150-cGy fractions twice a day, because it is likely that the ability to sterilize intracranial metastases is considerably less than is the case with intrathoracic disease.[113] If there are only one or two clinically documented intracranial lesions, we may well boost them to doses beyond 5000 cGy in patients without other metastatic disease.

Chest Irradiation in Limited Disease

The systemic nature of SCLC even when it appears localized after careful staging precludes sole reliance on a locoregional form of therapy. Most patients with limited-stage disease given chest irradiation alone rapidly die of distant metastases, emphasizing the need for primary systemic treatment. After combination chemotherapy began to be used in the management of small cell carcinoma in the 1970s, the resulting high response rates and improved survival led to speculation that chest radiotherapy added toxicities while contributing little or no therapeutic advantage in chemotherapy-treated patients. However, this neoplasm is the most responsive of all cell types of lung cancer to thoracic radiotherapy with objective tumor regression occurring in 90% of patients.[286] The primary tumor complex is a site of tumor progression in up to 80% of relapsing limited-stage patients treated with chemotherapy alone.[165,242] Chest irradiation given in conjunction with chemotherapy might logically improve therapeutic results in patients with limited disease.

Retrospective reviews of nonrandomized trials using chemotherapy with or without chest irradiation for limited-stage disease suggested the following conclusions.[167,287] First, a lower rate of chest relapse is seen with combined-modality therapy, although the frequency still approaches 33%. Second, hematologic, pulmonary, and esophageal complications are increased with the use of both modalities. Third, whereas median survival appears similar, 2-year disease-free survival appears superior for combined-modality therapy than for chemotherapy alone. Retrospective data suffer from several deficiencies. Because chemotherapy alone is less toxic than combined-modality treatment, there may be a consistent bias against giving combined-modality therapy to poor-risk patients. If administration of radiotherapy is delayed for several chemotherapy cycles, patients with the worst prognosis who develop early failure are automatically excluded from combined-modality series. Analysis of local relapse rates can sometimes be misleading, because only an isolated chest recurrence in a completely responding patient might be expected to compromise survival and definitions of local relapse rates are heterogenous.[288] Variations in dose and schedule of irradiation and specific chemotherapy programs used further complicate comparison of chest relapse rates from different series. Less effective chemotherapy combined with effective irradiation reduces the frequency of first failures in the chest (because distant metastases will be more prone to develop), whereas more effective chemotherapy combined with less efficacious irradiation yields the opposite result. Using uncontrolled data, it is very difficult to determine the value of adding chest irradiation to combination chemotherapy.

In the past several years, this uncertainty has been clarified by the completion of several prospective randomized trials. Seven published mature trials in which at least 80 patients with limited disease were randomized to receive chemotherapy alone or the same chemotherapy with chest irradiation are summarized in Table 23–34. The temporal relations between chemotherapy and irradiation have been far from uniform in these studies. *Concurrent therapy* is defined as combined-modality therapy in which chemotherapy and radiotherapy are given simultaneously. In *alternating therapy*, radiotherapy is administered on days of the chemotherapy cycle in which no drugs are given without any delay in the subsequent chemotherapy cycle. *Sequential therapy* is defined as administration of chemotherapy and radiotherapy separately in time with delay in chemotherapy doses for delivery of irradiation or with one modality begun only after completion of the other. The trials also varied in the chemotherapy regimen used, the time at which chest radiotherapy was begun, the dose and schedule of irradiation, whether chemotherapy was given to all patients randomized to receive it or only to responders (or only to complete responders) to it, and whether prophylactic cranial irradiation was administered.

Four of the seven studies reported borderline or significantly improved survival with combined-modality treatment; two used concurrent radiotherapy,[269,289] one alternating radiotherapy[290] and one sequential irradiation during a chemotherapy hiatus.[291,292] The magnitude of the survival benefit was modest, ranging from 1 to 4 months improvement in median survival and increases in 2-year survival from 7% to 17%. The two studies with the longest follow-up demonstrate much less of an advantage beyond 5 years for patients given radiotherapy, at least partially because of intercurrent deaths and second lung cancers in the combined-modality arms.[269,292] Of the three studies not demonstrating improved survival with added chest irradiation, two[293,294] used sequential radiotherapy and one[295] a concurrent regimen in which only a single drug

TABLE 23–34. Randomized Prospective Trials of Combined-Modality Therapy Versus Chemotherapy Alone in Limited-Stage Small Cell Lung Cancer

Investigations	Drugs	Chest Radiation Therapy	No. of Patients	Median Survival CT	Median Survival CMT	Survival Differences	2-Year Disease-Free or Overall Survival (actual or projected) (%) CT	2-Year Disease-Free or Overall Survival (actual or projected) (%) CMT
Bunn et al[269]	CML/ VAP	40Gy/15Fx/wk 1/CONC/Cont	96	11.6	15.0	p = 0.035	12 6	28 (OS) 23 (DFS)
Perry et al[289]	CAEV	I: 50Gy/25Fx/wk 1/CONC/Cont	399	13.6	I: 13.1	p = 0.009	8	I: 15 (DFS)
		II: 50Gy/25Fx/wk 10/CONC/Cont			II: 14.6			II: 25
Perez et al[290]	CAV	40Gy/14Fx/wk 5, 8, 11/ALT/Split	291	11.2	14.0	p = 0.030	19	28 (OS)
Fox[291,292]	CAV	40Gy/20Fx/wk10/ SEQ/Cont	84	12.7	16.5	p = 0.003	2	15 (DFS)
Østerlind et al[295]	CMVL	40Gy/10Fx/wk 6, 10/CONC/Split	125	11.5	10.5	p = 0.240	8	5 (DFS)
Souhami et al[294]	AV/CM	40Gy/20Fx/wk 13/SEQ/Cont	130	R: 12.0 NR: 7.0	13.0 8.5	p > 0.05 p > 0.05	12 12	14 (OS) 4
Kies et al[293]	VMEAC	48Gy/22Fx/wk 13, 17/SEQ/ Split/CR only	93	16.0*	16.0*	p = 0.860	25*	35* (OS)

C, cyclophosphamide; M, methotrexate; L, lomustine, V, vincristine; A, doxorubicin; P, procarbazine; E, etoposide; P, cisplain
CT, chemotherapy alone; CMT, combined-modality therapy; R, responders; NR, nonresponders; CR, complete responders; CONC, concurrent with chemotherapy; SEQ, sequential administration of two modalities with delay of chemotherapy to administer radiation therapy; ALT, alternating chemotherapy and radiation therapy without delay of chemotherapy; Cont, continuous radiation therapy 5 fractions per week; Split, split-course radiation therapy; Fx, fractions; OS, overall survival; DFS, disease-free survival.
* Survival values for complete responders only.
(Modified from Seifter EJ, Ihde DC. Therapy of small cell lung cancer: A perspective on two decades of clinical research. Semin Oncol 1988;15:278–299)

was given simultaneously with irradiation. The negative sequential trial conducted exclusively in patients in complete remission from chemotherapy[293] was initiated because of earlier uncontrolled data suggesting marked improvement in disease-free survival when irradiation was given to complete responders at the completion of drug administration.[296] The lack of survival benefit from *consolidation treatment* with irradiation after chemotherapy is completed was confirmed recently in a small randomized trial.[297] Combined-modality treatment increased the complete response rate in three of the four trials for which this information was available and significantly reduced chest recurrence rates in five of seven trials.

A recent meta-analysis evaluated 13 randomized trials in which more than 2100 limited-stage SCLC patients were randomized to receive chemotherapy alone or with chest irradiation.[298] Patients given combined-modality therapy had a 14% reduction in death rate and a 5.4% improvement in 3-year survival compared with those receiving chemotherapy alone. Both differences were highly significant. This analysis reinforces the results of the larger individual studies (see Table 23–34), which demonstrated modest but statistically significant improvement in survival with combined-modality treatment.

Whether variations in the relation of the radiation and chemotherapy components of combined-modality therapy influence its antitumor effects is by no means resolved. Concurrent and alternating combined-modality programs that do not incorporate planned delays in chemotherapy for radiotherapy administration appear to possess superior efficacy. Among the randomized trials in Table 23–34, three of four concurrent or alternating programs yielded improved survival and one of three sequential programs produced a marginally significant improvement favoring irradiation. This apparent superiority of concurrent or alternating programs is consistent with the known dominance of distant metastases as the major determinant of survival in most patients and suggests these methods are preferable. No randomized comparisons of concurrent or alternating versus sequential strategies have been reported.

The dose of thoracic irradiation needed to control locoregional small cell carcinoma was initially thought to be reduced when chemotherapy was given with irradiation.[299] As improved drug treatment yielded better control of distant metastases, a high frequency of local failures with lower dose schedules such as 3000 cGy in 2 weeks became apparent.[300] Retrospective data in patients given combined-modality therapy suggested that doses above 5000 cGy were needed for optimal prevention of locoregional failure,[301] and one randomized trial demonstrated superior local tumor control with 3750 cGy compared with 2500 cGy.[302] Most authorities agree on the need for higher doses in the range of 4500 to 5000 cGy or more with conventional fractionation for optimal local control. Simply because a radiotherapy program reduces local recurrences does not mean it is optimal. Even more effective irradiation might be able to eradicate chest tumor completely in additional patients with intrathoracic neoplasm as their sole residual cancer, which would become evident only if survival is the endpoint analyzed.

Randomized trials have yielded conflicting results on whether concurrent irradiation is best given early or late in the chemotherapy program. A study by the Cancer and Leukemia Group B found better results with delayed irradiation, perhaps because a greater percentage of projected chemotherapy doses was actually administered,[289] whereas an NCI of Canada trial came to the opposite conclusion.[303]

Minimizing the toxicities of the combined-modality approach without compromising therapeutic efficacy is a pertinent objective needing further clinical research. The addition of chest irradiation has moderately to greatly increased myelosuppressive, pulmonary, and esophageal complications of treatment, particularly with concurrent regimens. In an NCI trial, 26% of combined-modality patients developed severe pulmonary toxicity requiring hospitalization a median of 2 months from beginning of treatment compared with 4% of patients given chemotherapy alone.[269,275] Five combined-modality patients in complete remission died from this complication. In completely responding patients, pulmonary function tests improved in patients given chemotherapy alone but did not improve in combined-modality cases.[275] The Finsen Institute (Denmark), which used concurrent chemotherapy and irradiation, reported 7% deaths from pulmonary and pericardial complications in complete responders.[295] This frequency of pulmonary complication in patients given combined-modality treatment is higher than that seen in patients given only chemotherapy and in patients receiving chest irradiation alone. Several trials report high rates of esophagitis, with occasional strictures, and weight loss in patients given combined-modality therapy.[269,295]

Not all concurrent combined-modality programs produce excessive pulmonary toxicity,[289] suggesting that the specific drugs combined with irradiation are influential in inducing this complication. EP may be an especially suitable regimen for concurrent chemoradiotherapy in SCLC. After two successive trials of sequential combined-modality treatment in limited-stage patients produced 4-year survival of approximately 10% in the Southwest Oncology Group (SWOG), a third trial in which EP was given concurrently with chest irradiation beginning on the first day of therapy resulted in 30% 4-year survival with severe pulmonary toxicity in only one patient.[304]

Although alternating regimens have been used less often, those interdigitating chemotherapy and irradiation appear to have reduced pulmonary toxicity while maintaining the therapeutic advantage of radiotherapy.[290,305] Studies of radiation toxicity in animals suggest that concurrent chemotherapy programs might be expected to be more toxic than alternating or sequential designs, and available clinical data are consistent with this hypothesis, particularly with regard to pulmonary injury. Unfortunately, the least toxic sequential approach has been shown only infrequently to possess a survival advantage in individual randomized trials.

Delivering chest irradiation in multiple daily fractions on experimental grounds might be expected to ameliorate pulmonary toxicity while retaining antitumor efficacy. Results from several pilot studies combining EP and twice-daily chest irradiation are promising with median survival of greater than 2 years in some trials and, in most cases, minimal treatment-associated pneumonitis.[284,306,307] Whether these excellent results are due to the concurrent use of EP and radiotherapy or to hyperfractionated irradiation is the subject of a large randomized trial.

In summary, some programs incorporating the addition of chest irradiation to chemotherapy in limited-stage SCLC improve survival, especially when radiotherapy is given in a concurrent or alternating fashion. Combined-modality therapy is a technically complex undertaking requiring close coordination between medical and radiation oncologists. Because not all combined-modality programs increase survival but essentially all increase toxicity, chest irradiation need not be considered mandatory in all patients, especially those with impaired pulmonary function or poor performance status. Investigational studies that do not include chest irradiation remain appropriate. Survival gains from the greater antitumor efficacy of combined-modality programs are partially compromised by the toxicities of treatment, the modification of which is under active investigation. If results of chemotherapy improve so that more patients have eradication of systemic but not of local tumor, chest radiotherapy could have survival impact in larger numbers of cases. However, distant metastases remain the predominant cause of failure, and most limited-stage patients who are irradiated still die from their small cell carcinoma. Better systemic treatment has much greater potential for producing survival gains than does increased efficacy of locoregional therapy.

Chest Irradiation in Extensive Disease

In retrospective reviews, the addition of chest irradiation to chemotherapy for patients with extensive-stage SCLC reduced the frequency of progressive disease in the thorax but did not alter overall response rates, median survival, or 2-year disease-free survival.[167,287] Because extensive-disease patients have complete response rates of only 15% to 30% with chemotherapy regimens and frequently relapse in distant metastatic sites, a localized form of treatment would be expected to have little survival impact. Successive large studies by the SWOG also confirm that although thoracic radiotherapy can substantially reduce the frequency of initial relapses at the primary tumor site, there is no apparent effect on survival.[308]

Three clinical trials have randomized patients with extensive disease to chemotherapy alone or chemotherapy with irradiation to the chest tumor and to some or all sites of overt distant metastases. In these studies, there were no worthwhile response or survival advantages with the addition of radiotherapy.[300,309,310] Except as part of a clinical trial, there is no role for chest irradiation in extensive-stage SCLC other than for symptomatic palliation.

Wide-Field Radiation Therapy

Pilot studies have examined the role of hemibody irradiation and total-body irradiation in this radioresponsive malignancy. Hemibody irradiation is an active agent in SCLC because it can induce complete responses in some patients who only partially respond after combination chemotherapy.[311] The initial treatment is usually given to the upper hemibody where the bulk of tumor is located. In some studies, treatment of the lower hemibody is administered after hematologic recovery from the upper hemibody dose. Recently, a controlled German trial confirmed that chemotherapy produced markedly better survival than hemibody irradiation in extensive-disease patients.[312] As an adjunct to combination chemotherapy in both limited and extensive disease, hemibody irradiation yielded substantial toxicity in several pilot studies without any benefit in tumor response or survival.[311,313] There is also no

evidence that low doses of total-body irradiation are of benefit as an adjuvant to chest irradiation or chemotherapy in limited-stage and extensive-stage patients.[314,315] In a large randomized trial in patients with limited disease given chemotherapy and chest irradiation, additional radiotherapy to upper abdominal potential sites of relapse produced no improvement in response duration or survival.[316] Wide-field irradiation has no role in the management of SCLC.

Prophylactic Cranial Irradiation

Brain metastases are detected in approximately 10% of SCLC patients at the time of presentation and are diagnosed later during life in another 20% to 25%.[115,317] The likelihood for development increases with lengthening survival. In the absence of therapy to the central nervous system (CNS), actuarial analysis reveals a probability of brain metastases of 50% to 80% in 2-year survivors.[317,318] At postmortem examination they are found in up to 65% of cases.[319] Because these metastases are sometimes the sole site of clinical relapse from complete remission and are frequently clinically disabling, prophylactic cranial irradiation (PCI) has been used for the past 10 to 15 years in an effort to curtail their development.

A review of 716 patients entered on nine prospective randomized trials assessed the benefit of PCI given at or within a few months of diagnosis in patients initially free of CNS involvement (Table 23–35).[193,316,320–326] When the results of these trials are considered together, doses of PCI ranging from 2000 to 4000 cGy reduced the frequency of clinically detected brain metastases from 22% to 6%.[327] In six of these trials, a significantly reduced risk for intracranial tumor spread was present. No significant impact of PCI on survival was observed in any of these studies. Retrospective analyses suggest that virtually all benefit in preventing intracranial metastases with PCI is confined to patients with a complete response to systemic therapy.[318,320] In actuarial analyses, partial or nonresponders had equivalent likelihood for recurrence in the brain whether or not PCI was administered.[318] This is not surprising, because residual systemic cancer could readily metastasize to the CNS after completion of PCI.

Only complete responders could potentially derive any survival benefit from PCI because in patients without complete response, systemic tumor is the predominant factor influencing survival. In both randomized and nonrandomized studies that addressed this question, there is no evidence that PCI influences survival in completely responding patients.[320,326] Some investigators have proposed dispensing with PCI in favor of therapeutic brain irradiation whenever indicated.[328] This policy assumes that in most instances cranial irradiation can effectively control symptoms from overt brain metastases for the duration of the patient's life. Because the duration of survival is short in most patients who develop brain metastases during the course of therapy, this assumption is not unreasonable. Other physicians have questioned the durability of palliation after therapeutic brain radiotherapy.[110,329]

Even if survival were not improved, there would be no reason other than expense and patient inconvenience not to offer PCI to completely responding patients if it were free of toxicity. With the advent of greater numbers of 5-year and longer survivors with SCLC, it has become evident that some patients have neurologic and intellectual impairment

TABLE 23–35. Randomized Trials of Prophylactic Cranial Irradiation (PCI)

Investigations	No. of Patients	Dose (cGy)	Initiation	Patients With Brain Relapse (%)		
				PCI	No PCI	p Value
Jackson[324]	29	3000	Day 1	0	27	<0.05
Maurer[193]	163	3000	Week 9	4	18	<0.01
Hansen[316]	109*	4000	Week 12	9	13	NS
Beiler[321]	54	2400	Week 3	0	16	<0.05
Cox[322]	45*	2000	Day 1	17	24	NS
Seydel[326]	219*	3000	Day 1	5	20	<0.005
Aroney[320]	32†	3000	At CR	0	27	NS
Eagan[323]	30*	3600	Week 20	13	73	<0.05
Katensis[325]	35	4000	Day 1	12	44	<0.05
Total	716			6	22	

NS, not significant; CR, complete response.
* Limited-stage patients only.
† Only complete responders randomized.
(Modified from Pedersen AG, Kristjansen PEG, Hansen HH. Prophylactic cranial irradiation and small cell lung cancer. Cancer Treat Rev 1988;15:85–103)

and abnormalities on brain CT scan that are potentially related to PCI.[330-333] In one study, both CT scan and CNS abnormalities were significantly more frequent in patients who had received PCI or therapeutic brain irradiation than in those who had not.[333] These findings are especially disturbing because complete responders, those most likely to benefit from PCI, live longer and are at greater risk for possible complications. Many deficits on neuropsychologic testing are unsuspected on casual examination, but a few patients have major impairments. CT scan abnormalities continue to worsen for several years after treatment is discontinued, although they may stabilize eventually.[334] Neurologic abnormalities were most prominent in one series in patients who were given PCI concurrently with high-dose chemotherapy or in individual radiation fractions of 400 cGy,[331] and some authorities suggest PCI should be administered only in standard fractions of 200 cGy after completion of chemotherapy.[335] These abnormalities may not be due solely to PCI. Chemotherapy, possible paraneoplastic syndromes, and effects of chronic cigarette abuse are several factors that might contribute to the abnormalities. Administration of methotrexate, procarbazine, and lomustine, agents less commonly used in therapy now than a decade ago, have been suggested to be incriminated.[333,336]

Opinions on whether PCI should be used in small cell carcinoma diverge widely, and no consensus is possible. Clinical trials randomizing completely responding patients to receive or not receive PCI should provide more conclusive documentation of toxicities and potential survival benefits of PCI. Until the results of such trials are available, we administer PCI under the following guidelines after a thorough discussion with the patient of potential risks and benefits.

1. Only complete responders are treated.
2. Radiotherapy fractions of 200 to 300 cGy are given over 2 to 3 weeks to a total dose of 2400 to 3000 cGy.
3. PCI should not be administered on days when chemo-

therapy is given, and the interval between drug and radiation treatments should be as long as possible.

Therapeutic Brain Irradiation

Brain metastases are a major source of morbidity in patients with SCLC.[106] Patients with brain metastases are at increased risk for spread to other areas of the central nervous system, especially epidural and meningeal tumor.[115] Because the prognosis of patients with brain metastases varies widely, the philosophy with which these metastases are approached depends on the clinical setting. In general, patients who are diagnosed at the time of presentation of small cell carcinoma have a better prognosis with little difference in median survival in some series between patients with limited disease and those with brain metastases as the sole site of extensive disease at diagnosis, although recurrence of brain metastases after irradiation is common and 2-year survival is poor.[109,111,112] Median survival is only 3 months if metastases develop during or after initial treatment. Prognosis is better if brain metastases are the only evidence of disease outside the thorax.[113] Two series report that neurologic symptoms at the time brain metastases are discovered have no impact on survival, probably because many patients have successful short-term palliation and widespread systemic cancer is present in most patients.[110,113]

Radiotherapy remains the treatment of choice for brain metastases in SCLC, although tumor regression can occur in previously untreated patients given chemotherapy alone.[259] Many radiation oncologists administer steroids (often dexamethasone 4 mg four times a day) with irradiation, especially if neurologic symptoms are present. After completion of irradiation, steroids are tapered to the lowest possible level that suppresses neurologic symptoms and often can be discontinued. Doses of cranial irradiation vary widely and are influenced by the patient's performance status, life expectancy, extent of tumor dissemination, and the likelihood of meaningful response of systemic tumor. A common palliative dose schedule is 3000 cGy in ten fractions over 2 weeks. Higher doses are administered in appropriate clinical settings and are associated with better results, although patient selection factors probably explain much of this association.

Immediate response to brain irradiation is usually reported in terms of relief of neurologic symptoms and varies from 60% to 85%.[110,113,328] In one series in which responses were confirmed by brain CT scans, complete and partial response rates were 32% and 31%, respectively.[113] Response duration is often short. Brain metastases were said to be symptomatic or a contributing cause of death after irradiation in 45% to 54% of patients in two studies.[110,329] In another report,[113] 24 of 37 responding patients had clinical evidence of progressive intracranial tumor before death. The actuarial median response duration was 10 months in complete responders and 5 months in partial responders, with patients who died without evidence of intracranial tumor progression being censored at the time of death. The actuarial likelihood of remaining in response at 12 months for all responding patients was 20%.

Despite these inadequacies in long-term control of brain metastases by irradiation, small cell carcinoma is a widely disseminated disease in most patients, and the effectiveness of treatment for brain metastases has little influence on survival in most patients. Therefore, short-term symptomatic control is an appropriate goal in most cases. It is those patients with prospects for more prolonged survival in whom the durability of therapeutic effects is relevant, including patients who are diagnosed with brain metastases as the only site of disseminated disease and those whose complete response to systemic therapy is terminated solely by brain metastases. Although there is no conclusive evidence of better efficacy, more aggressive radiation dose schedules, such as 4000 to 5000 cGy in 3 to 5 weeks given in one or two daily fractions, may be appropriate in these settings.

Treatment of Spinal Cord and Leptomeningeal Metastases

Patients with SCLC can experience cancer dissemination throughout the neuraxis, including the spinal cord and leptomeninges. At diagnosis, approximately 2% have spinal tumor and less than 0.5% have meningeal tumor, but a clinical diagnosis of spinal or meningeal cancer can be made at some time in the patient's course in an estimated 5% and 2.5% of cases, respectively.[106,115–117]

Early diagnosis is the key to successful therapy of spinal cord compression, because patients who are paraplegic by the time the diagnosis is established can only infrequently be restored to ambulatory status with any form of treatment. This is especially critical in small cell carcinoma, because a high proportion of patients with spinal cord metastases present at the time of initial diagnosis. If life expectancy is several months or longer when chemotherapy is given, preserving ambulation is critical.

Median survival from the clinical diagnosis of carcinomatous leptomeningitis in small cell carcinoma is less than 2 months. Almost 90% of patients have undergone chemotherapy and are afflicted with progressive or persistent systemic cancer at the time of diagnosis, so treatment has little influence on survival. The exceptions are those few cases with meningeal involvement at initial diagnosis or as the sole site of relapse from complete remission. Intrathecal methotrexate, often accompanied by irradiation to symptomatic areas of the neuraxis, is the most commonly used therapy. Patients receiving this combined treatment clear their cerebrospinal fluid of malignant cells about half the time but less often have complete resolution of neurologic symptoms and signs.[116] However, most poor-prognosis patients with rapidly advancing systemic tumor probably receive only palliative treatment. Because of the rarity of carcinomatous meningitis as the sole site of initial failure in completely responding patients, prophylactic therapy of the meningeal space with either intrathecal chemotherapy or irradiation is not indicated.

SURGICAL RESECTION OF SMALL CELL LUNG CANCER

Early efforts at surgical management of SCLC were characterized by incomplete staging before and during thoracotomy and by the absence of effective adjunctive chemotherapy. Nevertheless, some studies in the 1960s reported 5-year or longer survival in more than 10% of the patients.[337,338] These results were overshadowed by two studies in the 1970s that provided philosophic justification for not using a surgical approach in this disease. The British Medical Research Council published a trial of 144 patients that demonstrated the modest superiority of radiotherapy as primary treatment for SCLC considered operable (see Table 23–24).[149] Shortly thereafter, an American study compared the survival of 146 patients considered operable who were not resected with 41 resected patients and found no differences.[151]

The first hint that proper staging would lead to less bias in the interpretation of surgical results came from the subset of SCLC patients described by Higgins in his report of the management of the solitary pulmonary nodule.[339] In a 10-year follow-up of 15 small cell patients with solitary nodules (1% of total cases), 11 who would be classified as having stage I tumors[91] had a 5-year survival of 36%. Rejuvenation of interest in surgical resection for this cancer received its greatest support from the recognition that newly available chemotherapeutic agents could possibly provide effective adjunctive therapy. Meyer reported that of 10 pathologically staged stages I and II patients who were resected and given chemotherapy for at least 1 year, 80% remained well at 30 months.[94] Of greater significance were the carefully designed trials conducted by the Veterans Administration Surgical Oncology Group.[340] Of 148 small cell carcinoma patients entered on four trials, 132 who survived a potentially curative resection were randomized to receive preoperative adjuvant chemotherapy or surgery alone. A 23% overall 5-year survival was recorded with survival patterns that were more favorable in less advanced stages: T1–2N0, 28% to 60%; T1–2N1, 9% to 31%; and T3 or N2, 3.6%. Although survival was marginally better with the addition of postoperative chemotherapy, it was clear that the small group of patients with localized disease after sophisticated surgical staging techniques could enjoy much better survival with surgical resection alone than was appreciated previously.

Several factors have strengthened the rationale for incorporating surgical therapy into the total package of treatment for selected SCLC patients. Despite the high response rate to chemotherapy regimens, the rate of relapse in the thorax can approach 75% in the absence of properly administered radiotherapy. There has been a gradual shift toward identification of more localized potentially resectable subgroups of limited-disease patients with clinical staging. This has been encouraged by the use of invasive procedures, including Wang needle biopsy, mediastinotomy and mediastinoscopy, and by the recognition that the new international staging system for lung cancer can provide a common language for discussing these issues.[91]

The theoretical justifications for combining surgery with other therapies for SCLC as enumerated by Meyer are as follows[341]:

1. Because local relapse is a problem, surgical removal may offer a better chance for disease control.
2. Surgery used for local control, unlike radiotherapy, would not limit the intensity of chemotherapy that could be delivered.
3. By rendering the patient free of disease in the chest without affecting bone marrow reserves, surgery could possibly make the chemotherapy more effective.
4. Complete surgical staging could identify patients at higher risk of recurrence.

During the past few years, numerous uncontrolled reports have provided considerable insight into whether these theoretical considerations are valid.[341]

Only a modest quantity of data exist on how often surgical resection at the diagnosis of SCLC is possible. Prospective studies of the feasibility of initial thoracotomy by their nature cannot include cases discovered only at thoracotomy to have small cell carcinoma. As many as 16% of patients with SCLC have been said to be operative candidates,[342] but this is most likely an unrealistically high estimate because patients who have been evaluated by a thoracic surgeon constitute a highly selected group.

There does not seem to be a marked increase in mortality in patients who have operative removal of small cell carcinoma. In the few studies that describe operative risks after chemotherapy and radiotherapy, the mortality rate varies between 0% and 10%.[343–348] Many of these studies report no operative mortality or increased morbidity compared with expected outcomes in patients undergoing pulmonary resection for other indications. The extent of resection—pneumonectomy or lobectomy—generally has been dictated by the intraoperative findings rather than the original extent of the tumor in patients given preoperative chemotherapy.

Surgery Followed by Chemotherapy

The initial poor long-term survival rates with surgery of SCLC were obtained in patients with clinical stages I through III who for the most part underwent only minimal staging procedures by current standards. Only when results are categorized by tumor stages can the potential curative effects of surgery alone be demonstrated. One recent report, for example, documents 5-year survival of 35% in stage I and 23% in stage II patients.[346] The only randomized trials of surgery compared with surgery with postoperative chemotherapy were begun about 20 years ago and used inferior drug regimens. Nonetheless, taken together they did reveal a survival advantage from chemotherapy

(Table 23–6). In the 1990s, thoracic oncologists never recommend surgery as sole treatment for SCLC.[349]

Statements regarding the efficacy of combined-modality approaches for SCLC that include surgical resection can be evaluated only when stratified by the temporal relations among the different modalities. Table 23–36 presents representative results for programs of initial surgery followed by adjunctive chemotherapy after surgery; patients with multiple stages of tumor are included.[137,341,344,350–353] In general, modern combination chemotherapy programs, usually including cyclophosphamide, doxorubicin, vincristine, or etoposide, have been used. Survival experience is heterogenous ranging from 5-year survival of 9% in earlier studies to as high as 83% in more recent studies.

Nodal status and primary tumor (T) status have significant impact on the survival of patients with resected SCLC. These prognostic factors were addressed directly in a few studies. Angeletti[354] and Shepherd[353] reported increased survival of node negative compared with N1 and N2 patients after surgical resection and postoperative chemotherapy, whereas Macchiarini[351] found a decrease in 5-year survival with increasing T-category in surgically resected patients without nodal metastases. Five-year survival is rare in patients given postoperative chemotherapy after mediastinal node disease has been documented at initial surgical resection,[344,346] although this observation is not universal.[353] Nonetheless, most authorities believe any survival benefits of initial surgical resection are likely to be confined to patients with pathologic stages I and II, and conventional wisdom holds that surgical resection at diagnosis in patients with N2 disease is considered experimental.

All data on outcome of patients who receive surgery and modern postoperative chemotherapy are uncontrolled. One can only observe that the survival of such patients is better than the survival of patients with limited disease who receive chemotherapy alone and better than the reported outcome of all but a few series of patients, most of them recent, given chemotherapy and chest irradiation. An important point concerning initial surgical resection that remains unresolved is whether the superior outcome of more localized (*i.e.*, stages I and II) patients who undergo complete resection before initiation of chemotherapy is attributable to the resection itself

TABLE 23–36. Survival Data With Surgery Followed by Postoperative Chemotherapy in Small Cell Lung Cancer

Investigations	No. of Patients	Median Survival (mo)	Survival (y)
Østerlind[352]	52	NR	27% (2.5)
Meyer[341]	10	NR	83% (5)
Hayata[350]	106	NR	9% (5)
Shepherd[353]	63	19	31% (5)
Macchiarini[351]	42	33	36% (5)
Friess[137]	15	25	30% (4)
Hara[344]	19	NR	42% (5)

NR, not reported.

or to an inherently better prognosis in patients with a tumor burden small enough to permit resection.

Because a controlled trial to address this question cannot be done due to the impossibility of randomizing patients whose small cell carcinoma is diagnosed only at the time of thoracotomy to undergo or not undergo surgical extirpation of their cancers, institutional data on patients with similar tumor burden after clinical staging who do and do not proceed to thoracotomy may be relevant. In Denmark, survival of patients considered clinically operable is similar whether or not an operation with the intent of completing resecting the tumor is performed,[138] although both these groups live much longer than other limited-stage patients. At the University of Toronto, a similar analysis evaluating only patients without evidence of mediastinal metastases on chest radiograph or mediastinoscopy, produced similar conclusions.[355] Early-stage patients may benefit from surgical resection. If a resectable SCLC is documented for the first time at thoracotomy, we recommend that the surgeon proceed with the operation if mediastinal node metastases are absent. In patients with a proved pathologic diagnosis, thoracotomy for tumor resection in clinical stage I disease should be considered only after complete staging procedures, including mediastinoscopy or mediastinotomy, reveal no evidence of tumor spread.

The question of the SCLC presenting as a solitary pulmonary nodule is controversial. In a retrospective review of 408 small cell carcinoma patients, Quoix found that solitary pulmonary nodule cases have a median survival of 24 months.[356] The improved prognosis could be explained by many factors, not the least of which is simply early diagnosis, or lead time bias. Another possibility is that the solitary nodule may represent a fundamentally different category of SCLC or may not be small cell lung cancer at all. Warren reevaluated 50 cases of surgically resected SCLC.[357] Thirty-four were pathologically confirmed to be SCLC, and stage I cases had a surprisingly low 9% 2-year survival. Twelve cases were reclassified as well-differentiated neuroendocrine carcinoma, and 2-year survival

of these stage I patients was 75%. The significance of these findings is unclear.

Chemotherapy Followed by Surgery

Theoretically, surgical resection in SCLC might be more effective if performed after initial chemotherapy rather than at the time of diagnosis. Chemotherapy could be given in an immediate attempt to eradicate occult distant metastatic disease, the major cause of treatment failure. Only patients who respond to the chemotherapy, that is, those most likely to benefit, would undergo thoracotomy. Comprehensive initial preoperative staging procedures could be avoided, or at least be less rigorous, because chemotherapy would be the first treatment. After response to chemotherapy a larger fraction of patients might be surgical candidates.

There has been a steady increase since 1984 in the fraction of cases reported to be resectable after chemotherapy response. There is more uniformity in presurgical staging procedures, including mediastinoscopy, used to identify patients who might benefit from postchemotherapy surgery. As shown in Table 23–37, resection rates in some series can exceed 50% with estimated 5-year survivals in resected patients of 35% to 65%.[343,345,347,348,358,359] Factors that prevent thoracotomy include poor response to chemotherapy, poor pulmonary function or other medical problems, and patient refusal.[348] The selection criteria for potential surgical candidates often exclude those with such adverse prognostic factors as supraclavicular adenopathy, superior vena cava syndrome, bulky mediastinal involvement, and pleural effusions.

The use of chemotherapy followed by surgery has led to higher survival rates compared with chemotherapy (often with chest irradiation) in patients with stage I disease with median survival not yet reached in patients from Toronto.[347] Stages II and III patients had median survivals of 69 and 52 weeks, respectively, and significant differences in survival were noted in all resected patients compared with 19 eligible patients

TABLE 23–37. Survival Data With Chemotherapy Followed by Surgical Resection

Investigations	No. of Patients	Stage	Response Rate (%)	No. of Resected Patients	Median Survival (mo)	Survival (y)
Prager et al[359]	40	Limited	85	8 (20%)	NR	50% (1–2)
Holoye et al[358]	26*	Limited	100	17 (65%)	R: 61 U: 16	65% (5)
Baker et al[343]	37	Limited	73	20 (54%)	R: 26 U: 12	65% (2–3)
Johnson et al[345]	24*	Limited	100	17 (53%)	R: 20 U: 18	NR
Williams et al[348]	38	Limited	84	21 (55%)	R: 33 U: 10	48% (3–5)
Shepherd et al[347]	72	I, II, IIIA	80	33 (46%)	R: 21 U: 12	36% (5)

* Patients deemed surgical candidates only after response to chemotherapy.
NR, not reported; R, resected; U, unresectable.

who did not receive surgery after the chemotherapy. The median survival of stage II and III patients was no different than that of otherwise eligible patients not receiving thoracotomy (51 weeks). The best results, not surprisingly, are found in patients with no malignant cells in the surgical specimen.[348] Some authors report absence of long-term survival in patients with initial mediastinal node involvement who undergo post-chemotherapy resection.[360] Other studies do not confirm these findings.[347]

Survival of patients with surgery followed by chemotherapy and with chemotherapy followed by surgery was similar in Toronto.[361] The more fundamental question, whether post-chemotherapy surgery improves survival, cannot be regarded as settled, although in one institution survival was similar for limited-stage patients who were considered eligible or ineligible for eventual surgical resection should they respond to chemotherapy.[348] Preliminary results from the Lung Cancer Study Group trial in which 144 patients who responded to chemotherapy (42% of those beginning chemotherapy) were randomized to undergo or not undergo thoracotomy for attempted surgical resection did not reveal survival differences.[362] Mature results of this study should greatly influence future practice.

Local Recurrence Rates and Histologic Findings

One of the chief theoretical justifications for adding surgery to the treatment regimen for SCLC is the possibility of influencing relapse in the tumor bed or the mediastinum. Local recurrences are infrequent in patients who have had surgery at diagnosis, possibly because patients with stage I or II disease are overrepresented in this group.[353,354] Patients who have been pretreated with chemotherapy more often have clinical stage IIIA disease and their local relapse rate is higher, in the range of 18% to 28%.[347,348] These local relapse rates still appear considerably less than in patients given chemotherapy with or without radiation therapy with no surgical intervention. Patients given initial chemotherapy who have a negative biopsy of the primary tumor site at the time of surgery, and therefore do not have resection performed, have a high frequency of local recurrence.[345]

Histologically mixed disease is a not uncommon occurrence when SCLC is resected after chemotherapy. Non-small cell elements and mixed small cell and non-small cell elements occur in 5% to 35% of specimens.[343,348,358,361] Whether these pathologic findings may be attributable to selection by chemotherapy of non-small cell elements present in the original tumor, histologic changes induced by chemotherapy, the presence of a second lung cancer, or incorrect initial diagnosis is not resolved. Nevertheless, surgery may prove therapeutically efficacious if the only residual cancer is non-small cell in type. Because of this frequency of mixed histologies at the time of resection after chemotherapy, the Toronto group reported a retrospective analysis of salvage surgery in limited SCLC.[363] Twenty-eight selected patients underwent thoracotomy after lack of response to induction chemotherapy or relapse after initial response. A surprising resection rate of 82% was possible and 10 patients (36%) had mixed elements histologically. Projected 5-year survival is 23%. These findings must be verified in other patients who are prospectively iden-

tified by specific selection criteria before we can recommend such an approach.

TREATMENT OF RELAPSING OR PROGRESSIVE TUMOR

Although response rates to chemotherapy at diagnosis are high in SCLC, most patients eventually develop tumor recurrence. Results of salvage therapy for relapsing or progressing disease are poor with infrequent objective responses and a median survival from disease progression of only 2 to 3 months.[144] Long-term disease-free survival after relapse is virtually nonexistent. EP is the most commonly used salvage chemotherapy regimen in patients who have not previously received either of these agents. Although several studies have reported objective response rates of 50% or more with this treatment after failure of CAV chemotherapy, complete responses are uncommon and impact on survival is uncertain.[204,205] It is probable that the more recent practice of administering initial chemotherapy for only 4 to 6 months has allowed the activity of EP to be documented in the salvage setting, because patients receiving this program in two studies that reported high response rates had not received any chemotherapy for a median of 3 to 5 months before relapse.[204,205] In contrast, another trial of EP in patients who had received six previous drugs with a median time off chemotherapy of less than 1 month reported a 12% response rate.[364]

Patients whose tumors progress after a long period off chemotherapy demonstrate better response to salvage regimens than patients with little or no time off treatment.[172,365] Although the usual practice in small cell carcinoma patients with relapsing disease is to administer agents to which the patient's tumor has not been exposed previously, the same agents used for initial therapy can yield relatively durable response rates of more than 50% after a long complete remission in which maintenance chemotherapy was not given.[366] Similar results have been noted in the therapy of relapsing multiple myeloma and Hodgkin's disease.

Relapsed patients frequently undergo testing with investigational chemotherapeutic agents in phase I or phase II trials. The difficulties in identifying new active drugs in this setting were discussed earlier in the chapter. Restricting studies of investigational drugs to good performance status patients who have not received chemotherapy in the months preceding tumor progression may help alleviate this problem. Development of better second-line chemotherapy for small cell carcinoma is sorely needed.

Radiotherapy often is the most useful palliative agent in patients with progressive symptomatic small cell carcinoma. The objective response rates of 60% or more seen in patients receiving chest irradiation,[367] often with doses lower than those used for primary treatment, are consistently higher than can be obtained with chemotherapeutic agents in this setting. Thoracic radiotherapy should be considered strongly in patients with pulmonary symptoms or in those who relapse solely in the chest. In a small pilot study of highly selected patients with relapse confined to the thorax after administration of chemotherapy alone, twice-daily chest irradiation followed by a new chemotherapy regimen was associated with a 67% complete response rate and a median survival of 6 months.[368]

Radiotherapy is the treatment of choice for superior vena cava syndrome recurrent after chemotherapy, painful bone metastases, spinal cord compression, and brain metastases in patients without previous cranial irradiation. Radiotherapy often provides short-term symptomatic relief. Unfortunately, patients with brain metastases after PCI or previous therapeutic cranial irradiation have a poor prognosis and only occasionally derive palliative benefit.[113]

BIOLOGIC RESPONSE MODIFIERS AND OTHER TREATMENTS

Chemotherapy, radiotherapy, and, in selected cases, surgical resection are effective forms of therapy for SCLC. Other treatment modalities have been investigated but are not established. Impaired response to cutaneous delayed hypersensitivity testing has been associated with a poorer survival in some groups of patients with small cell carcinoma.[140] This and similar observations led to a series of trials of biologic response modifiers and other immunologic-based therapies as an adjunct to standard treatments.

Nonspecific immunostimulation with both bacillus Calmette-Guérin (BCG) vaccine and the methanol-extractable residue (MER) of BCG has been evaluated in several prospective randomized studies. In two large SWOG studies,[369,370] response rate, response duration, and overall survival were no different in patients receiving chemotherapy and chest irradiation randomized to receive or not receive BCG. At least three randomized trials failed to demonstrate benefit with the addition of MER to various standard treatments.[371–373]

Sixty-seven SCLC patients were randomized to receive or not to receive calf thymosin fraction V, a modulator of T-cell function capable of correcting some immunologic defects in inherited T-lymphocyte disorders. Doses of 60 mg/m^2, 20 mg/m^2, or no thymosin were administered twice weekly during the first 6 weeks of chemotherapy with or without chest irradiation.[374] Patients given thymosin 60 mg/m^2 had significantly improved survival, even after adjusting for other prognostic factors. A larger study conducted in 91 patients randomly given thymosin 60 mg/m^2 twice weekly for 16 weeks or no thymosin during initial combined-modality treatment could not confirm these findings.[375]

Reduced expression of major histocompatibility antigens on small cell carcinoma cells and increased expression in vitro in the presence of interferons[376] provide some rationale for clinical evaluation of these biologic response modifiers. In small phase II trials, α- and γ-interferons have not produced objective responses.[377,378] Preliminary results of a Finnish randomized trial suggest that interferon-α may prolong complete remission after completion of chemotherapy.[379] A confirmatory study is underway. There is insufficient evidence of direct antitumor efficacy of any biologic response modifier in SCLC for these agents to be used except in a research setting.

The nutritional status of small cell carcinoma patients is sometimes abnormal and weight loss is a negative prognostic factor in patients receiving chemotherapy.[139] Total parenteral nutrition given during chemotherapy can ameliorate weight loss, but weight gained with this maneuver is mostly fat or fluid and is not associated with total body nitrogen retention.[380] No improvements in response rate or survival with total par-

enteral nutrition were noted in a randomized study of 119 patients.[381]

Another adjunctive therapy evaluated because of antimetastatic effects in some animal tumor systems is systemic anticoagulation. A small randomized trial studied the addition of warfarin to combination chemotherapy and radiation therapy and demonstrated significantly longer survival.[382] A much larger controlled study could not confirm this observation, although response rates were improved.[383]

TREATMENT OF EXTRAPULMONARY SMALL CELL CARCINOMA

Because of their low incidence and origin in diverse anatomic sites, uniform recommendations for therapy of small cell carcinomas arising in extrapulmonary sites cannot be made. In patients with a documented primary site and regional lymph node metastases, prognosis is worse.[87] Partial and occasional complete responses to chemotherapy regimens used in SCLC are reported, although experience is insufficient to reliably estimate response rates.[87–89] Tumors arising in the esophagus, larynx and pharynx, and prostate have short median survival, and systemic chemotherapy as an adjunct to locoregional treatment can be considered. Complete responses to chemotherapy lasting up to 12 months have been reported anecdotally in esophageal tumors.[384,385] Because of frequent regional node metastases, radiation therapy is recommended for tumors of the uterine cervix. There are few data on the effects of chemotherapy in proved neuroendocrine small cell cervical carcinoma, but adjuvant chemotherapy in localized disease is sometimes suggested because of the common development of distant metastases.[89,386] Small cell carcinomas of the paranasal sinuses, minor salivary glands, colon, and rectum without nodal metastases have good prognoses with locoregional therapy, and chemotherapy has not been used.[89] In Merkel's cell tumors originating in the skin of the head and neck, elective and therapeutic node dissections have been recommended; durable responses to chemotherapy have been reported in a few cases of metastatic disease.[90,387] In patients who present with distant metastatic and perhaps with regionally recurrent extrapulmonary small cell carcinoma, with or without a known primary tumor site, combination chemotherapy used for SCLC should be considered.

SUMMARY OF THE PRINCIPLES OF PRIMARY THERAPY

The principles of initial treatment of the patient with SCLC and recommendations for their implementation are outlined in Table 23–38. As in any malignant neoplasm, correct pathologic diagnosis is imperative before therapy is initiated. Review of diagnostic material with an experienced pathologist is always appropriate, but especially so when the sole material available is from a fine-needle aspirate. The number of pretreatment staging procedures needed to determine the extent of tumor dissemination depends on the clinical situation. Procedures must be sufficient to identify tumor lesions and permit response assessment and to separate limited-stage from extensive-stage disease if chest radiotherapy is to be given to limited-stage patients. Determination of the patient's ability

TABLE 23–38. Principles of Initial Therapy
for Small Cell Lung Cancer

Correct histologic diagnosis on adequate pathologic material

Appropriate initial staging to determine extent of tumor
dissemination

Assessment of physiologic status and ability to tolerate therapy

Consideration of surgical resection in fully staged stage I patients

Moderately intensive combination chemotherapy with a published
regimen of proved efficacy consisting of two to four drugs

Capacity to provide good supportive care

Incorporation of chest irradiation into management of limited-stage
disease

Restaging to assess response

Discontinuation of chemotherapy in responding patients after 4 to
6 months

Use of cyclic alternating combination therapy acceptable but of
unproved survival benefit

Consideration of prophylactic cranial irradiation in complete
responders

to tolerate aggressive chemotherapy or combined-modality
treatment is important to avoid excessive morbidity and mortality in minimally ambulatory and other patients who derive
little benefit from more toxic therapy. In patients who have
stage I tumor after complete staging that includes pathologic
evaluation of the mediastinum, thoracotomy with attempted
surgical resection may be considered. Moderately intensive
combination chemotherapy with a published regimen of two
to four drugs documented to produce at least 10% to 15% 2-
year survival in limited-stage disease should be used. This
mandates the capacity to provide supportive care of myelosuppressive complications, particularly infection and bleeding.

In limited-stage patients, concurrent or alternating combined-modality programs of chemotherapy and chest irradiation are recommended, preferably a program shown to in-

crease survival in a prospective randomized trial. Reevaluation
of sites of initial disease to assess response should be performed after approximately 12 weeks. Chemotherapy probably should be discontinued in stable responding patients after
18 to 24 weeks. Known effective cyclic alternating combination chemotherapy regimens are appropriate treatment and
may well increase initial response duration, but their impact
on survival is not definite. Risk-benefit considerations for
prophylactic cranial irradiation are not defined. If PCI is to
be administered, we recommend that it be given only to complete responders, avoiding high doses per fraction of irradiation and of concurrent chemotherapy and irradiation.

There is no question that optimal treatments for SCLC have
made a major impact on survival (Table 23–39). Major gains
in median survival occurred with the introduction of chemotherapy into the management of this disease. This statistic
has improved fourfold to fivefold in both limited-stage and
extensive-stage disease, compared with results in patients receiving only supportive care. A fraction of patients with
limited-stage disease and rare patients with extensive-stage
disease attain 2- to 3-year disease-free survival. Nonetheless,
minimal improvement in therapeutic outcome has been documented since the early 1980s despite many modifications
and permutations of available drugs and other forms of treatment, and approximately 95% of patients with SCLC ultimately die of their affliction. Major advances in the understanding of the biology of this cancer have been forthcoming
at the same time that the pace of clinical advances has slowed.
These advances may lead to novel, more effective approaches
to prevention, diagnosis, and therapy.

LONG-TERM SURVIVAL AND CURE

Given the intensity and complexity of the staging and therapy
of SCLC, it is reasonable to ask if any patients can be cured
by applying the principles outlined in the preceding section.
In 1984, a compilation of nine reports describing 1343 SCLC

TABLE 23–39. Impact of Treatment on Survival in Small Cell Lung Cancer
According to Extent of Disease

| Therapy | Median Survival (mo) | | 2–3 Year Survival (%) | |
	Limited Disease*	Extensive Disease	Limited Disease	Extensive Disease
Supportive care	3	1.5	—	—
Surgery	5–6*	—	4–5*	—
	11†	—	30–35†	—
Thoracic radiotherapy	10*	—	10*	—
	3–9	—	2–7	—
Single-agent chemotherapy	6	4	—	—
Combination chemotherapy	10–14	7–11	5–15	1–3
Combination chemotherpy with chest irradiation	12–16	7–11	10–25	1–2

* Operable patients in prechemotherapy era.
† Selected, carefully evaluated, pathologically staged patients.
(Modified from Morstyn G, Ihde DC, Lichter AS, et al. Small cell lung cancer 1973–1983: Early
progress and recent obstacles. Int J Radiat Oncol Biol Phys 1984;10:515–539)

patients treated with combination chemotherapy with or without chest irradiation revealed that 90 patients (7%) were alive and disease-free 2 years or more from the start of therapy.[146] These 2-year disease-free survivors represented 13% of patients presenting with limited-stage disease but only 2% of those with extensive-stage disease. More than 80% of the 2-year survivors had received chest irradiation as part of their treatment, and almost all of the few extensive-stage patients had metastases confined to a single organ system. This duration of follow-up is not adequate to assess long-term survival, because relapses can still occur beyond this point.[273,388]

Sufficient time since the widespread use of chemotherapy for SCLC has elapsed to permit assessment of survival at 5 years and beyond. Most reported experience is summarized in Table 23–40.[273,388–393] Overall calculations reveal that 72 patients (4%) of 2006 cases beginning what would currently be regarded as standard treatment were alive 5 years later. One report excluded patients with stages I and II cancers, a prognostically more favorable group.[389] The actual 5-year survival for limited-stage patients is 7% and for extensive-stage patients it is 1%. These publications confirm that relapses of SCLC continue to occur between 2 and 5 years. About two thirds of patients who are disease-free after 2 years do not relapse, and the likelihood of relapse is 26% and 14%, respectively, in patients who are disease-free 30 months and 3 years from the beginning of treatment.[273,388] Only rare relapses occur 5 to 10 years after beginning initial therapy,[394] and small cell carcinoma is therefore similar to other types of lung cancer in that 5 years of follow-up is an appropriate time after which the curative potential of a treatment can be assessed.

TABLE 23–40. Studies Reporting Small Cell Lung Cancer Patients Living 5 Years or Longer

Investigations	Stage	5-Year Survivors (no./total) (%)	Survivors at 5-Years (%) (both stages)
Smith et al[392]	Limited	4/17 (24)	12
	Extensive	1/25 (4)	
Livingston et al[390]	Limited	11/103 (11)	5
	Extensive	6/270 (2)	
Vogelsang et al[393]	Limited	5/94 (5)	2
	Extensive	0/131	
Johnson et al[273]	Limited	17/103 (17)	8
	Extensive	4/149 (3)	
Jacobs et al* [389]	Limited	2/102 (2)	1
	Extensive	0/138	
Østerlind et al[388,391]	Limited	19/443 (4)	3
	Extensive	3/431 (1)	
Total	Limited	58/862 (7)	
	Extensive	14/1144 (1)	
Overall total		72/2006 (4)	

* Excluding patients with stage I or II carcinomas.
(Modified from Seifter EJ, Ihde DC. Therapy of small cell lung cancer: A perspective on two decades of clinical research. Semin Oncol 1988;15:278–299)

Even though the original SCLC can be eradicated in a small fraction of patients, the risk of death from other causes in long-term survivors is far higher than in the age-matched population. Development of second smoking-related malignancies, most notably NSCLC, represents a significant threat to these patients.[388,394] In the NCI series,[395] NSCLCs appeared in most instances to be second primary neoplasms by virtue of their occurrence in lobes of the lung that were not the site of the initial small cell cancer. After 3 years of disease-free survival, subsequent pulmonary cancers were more likely to be of a new non-small cell type than a recurrent small cell histology.[394] In long-term survivors who present with a pulmonary mass, confirmation of the pathologic diagnosis is required because an occasional patient has a surgically resectable non-small cell tumor. The risk for development of NSCLC beyond 2 years from the diagnosis of small cell carcinoma was 4.4% per person-year, about 10 times higher than the rate found in screening studies in smoking men over the age of 45.[395] Although a chemotherapy- or radiation-related contribution to this high risk cannot be excluded completely, patients with roentgenographically occult NSCLC managed only with surgical resection at the Mayo Clinic have a similar likelihood for developing a second lung cancer.[396] Whether these second lung cancers in long-term survivors can be prevented by retinoid therapy, as may be true in persons with initial squamous carcinomas arising in the head and neck region,[397] is a suitable subject for clinical investigation. Long-term survivors also have a sixfold increased risk of death from nonneoplastic causes, principally from cardiovascular and pulmonary diseases.[388]

Chronic pulmonary, esophageal, and neurologic complications of treatment can be present in long-term survivors of SCLC. Between 50% and 70% of these patients, however, are able to resume a lifestyle comparable to that which they led before the diagnosis of cancer.[388,394] Although the increased risks for second malignancies and late toxicities can be devastating in individual patients, they do not outweigh the therapeutic benefits of prolonged survival for most patients and the possibility of cure for a few patients.

REFERENCES

1. Matthews MJ, Gordon PR. Morphology of pulmonary and pleural malignancies. In: Straus MJ, ed. Lung cancer: Clinical diagnosis and treatment. New York: Grune & Stratton, 1977:49–69.
2. Ries LAG, Hankey BF, Miller BA, et al. Cancer statistics review, 1973–1988, NIH publication 91-2789. Bethesda, MD: National Cancer Institute, 1991.
3. El-Torky M, El-Zeky F, Hall JC. Significant changes in the distribution of histologic types of lung cancer. Cancer 1990;65:2361–2367.
4. Devesa SS, Shaw GL, Blot WJ. Changing patterns of lung cancer incidence by histological type. Cancer Epidemiol Biomark Prev 1991;1:29–34.
5. Wu AH, Henderson BE, Thomas DC, et al. Secular trends in histologic types of lung cancer. JNCI 1986;77:53–56.
6. Rosenow EC, Carr DT. Bronchogenic carcinoma. CA 1979;29:233–246.
7. Archer VE, Saccomanno G, Jones JH. Frequency of different histologic types of bronchogenic carcinoma as related to radiation exposure. Cancer 1974;34:2056–2060.
8. Radford EP, Renard KGSC. Lung cancer in Swedish iron miners exposed to low doses of radon daughters. N Engl J Med 1984;310:1485–1494.
9. Harley NH, Harley JH. Potential lung cancer risk from indoor radon exposure. CA 1990;40:265–275.
10. Blot WJ, Xu ZY, Boice JD, et al. Indoor radon and lung cancer in China. JNCI 1990;82:1025–1030.
11. Barnard WG. The nature of the "oat-celled sarcoma" of the mediastinum. J Pathol 1926;29:241–244.
12. Gazdar AF, Carney DN, Guccion JE, et al. Small cell carcinoma of the lung: Cellular origin and relationship to other tumors. In: Greco FA, Oldham RK, Bunn PA, eds. Small cell lung cancer. New York: Grune & Stratton, 1981:145–175.

13. Ihde DC, Cohen MH, Bernath AM, et al. Serial fiberoptic bronchoscopy during chemotherapy for small cell carcinoma of the lung: Early detection of patients at high risk of relapse. Chest 1978;74:531–536.

14. Copple B, Wright SE, Moatamed F. Electron microscopy in small cell lung carcinoma: Clinical correlation. J Clin Oncol 1984;2:910–916.

15. Organization World Health. The World Health Organization histological typing of lung tumours. 2nd ed. Am J Clin Pathol 1982;77:123–136.

16. Kanhouwa SB, Matthews MJ. Reliability of cytologic typing of lung cancer. Acta Cytol 1976;20:229–232.

17. Yesner R, Gerstl B, Auerbach O. Application of the World Health Organization classification of lung carcinoma to biopsy material. Ann Thorac Surg 1965;1:33–45.

18. Rilke F, Carbone A, Clemente C, et al. Surgical pathology of resectable lung cancer. In: Muggia FM, Rozencweig M, eds. Lung cancer: Progress in therapeutic research. New York: Raven Press, 1979:129–142.

19. Hirsch FR, Matthews MJ, Yesner R. Histopathologic classification of small cell carcinoma of the lung: Comments based on an interobserver examination. Cancer 1982;50:1360–1366.

20. Hirsch FR, Østerlind K, Hansen HH. The prognostic significance of histopathologic subtyping of small cell carcinoma of the lung according to the classification of the World Health Organization: A study of 375 consecutive patients. Cancer 1983;52:2144–2150.

21. Hansen HH, Dombernowsky P, Hansen M, et al. Chemotherapy of advanced small cell anaplastic carcinoma. Ann Intern Med 1978;89:177–181.

22. Carney DN, Matthews MJ, Ihde DC, et al. Influence of histologic subtype of small cell carcinoma of the lung on clinical presentation, response to therapy, and survival. JNCI 1980;65:1225–1230.

23. Gazdar AF, Linnoila RI. The pathology of lung cancer: Changing concepts and newer diagnostic techniques. Semin Oncol 1988;15:215–225.

24. Hirsch FR, Matthews MJ, Aisner S, et al. Histopathologic classification of small cell lung cancer: Changing concepts and terminology. Cancer 1988;62:973–977.

25. Radice PA, Matthews MJ, Ihde DC, et al. The clinical behavior of "mixed" small cell/large cell bronchogenic carcinoma compared to "pure" small cell subtypes. Cancer 1982;50:2894–2902.

26. Aisner SC, Finkelstein DM, Ettinger DS, et al. The clinical significance of variant-morphology small cell carcinoma of the lung. J Clin Oncol 1990;8:402–408.

27. Matthews MJ. Effects of therapy on the morphology and behavior of small cell carcinoma of the lung: A clinicopathologic study. In: Muggia FM, Rozencweig M, eds. Lung cancer: Progress in therapeutic research. New York: Raven Press, 1979:155–165.

28. Abeloff MD, Eggleston JC, Mendelsohn G, et al. Changes in morphologic and biochemical characteristics of small cell carcinoma of the lung: A clinicopathologic study. Am J Med 1979;66:757–764.

29. Sehested M, Hirsch FR, Østerlind K, et al. Morphologic variations of small cell lung cancer: A histopathologic study of pretreatment and posttreatment specimens in 104 patients. Cancer 1986;57:804–807.

30. Mangum MD, Greco FA, Hainsworth JD, et al. Combined small cell and non–small cell lung cancer. J Clin Oncol 1989;7:607–612.

31. Gazdar AF, Helman L, Israel MA, et al. Expression of neuroendocrine cell markers L-dopa decarboxylase, chromogranin A, and dense core granules in human tumors of endocrine and nonendocrine origin. Cancer Res 1989;48:4078–4082.

32. Gazdar AF, Carney DN, Russell EK, et al. Establishment of continuous, clonable cultures of small-cell carcinoma of the lung which have amine precursor uptake and decarboxylation cell properties. Cancer Res 1980;40:3502–3507.

33. Carney DN, Gazdar AF, Bepler G, et al. Establishment and identification of small cell lung cancer cell lines having classic and variant features. Cancer Res 1985;45:2913–2923.

34. Gazdar AF, Carney DN, Nau MM, et al. Characterization of variant subclasses of cell lines derived from small cell lung cancer having distinctive biochemical, morphological, and growth properties. Cancer Res 1985;45:2924–2930.

35. Willey JC, Lechner JF, Harris CC. Bombesin and the C-terminal tetradecapeptide of gastrin-releasing peptide are growth factors for normal human bronchial epithelial cells. Exp Cell Res 1984;153:245–248.

36. Alexander R, Upp J, Poston G, et al. Effects of bombesin on growth of human small cell lung carcinoma in vivo. Cancer Res 1988;48:1439–1441.

37. Carney DN, Cuttitta F, Moody TW, et al. Selective stimulation of small cell lung cancer clonal growth by bombesin and gastrin-releasing peptide. Cancer Res 1987;47:821–825.

38. Cuttitta F, Carney DN, Mulshine J, et al. Bombesin-like peptides can function as autocrine growth factors in human small-cell lung cancer. Nature 1985;316:823–826.

39. Woll PJ, Rozengurt E. [D-Arg[1],D-Phe[5],D-Tryp[7,9],Leu[11]] substance P, a potent bombesin antagonist in murine Swiss 3T3 cells, inhibits the growth of human small cell lung cancer cells in vitro. Proc Natl Acad Sci USA 1988;85:1859–1863.

40. Mulshine J, Avis I, Carrasquillo J, et al. Phase I study of anti-gastrin releasing peptide monoclonal antibody in patients with lung cancer. Proc Am Soc Clin Oncol [Abstract] 1990;9:230.

41. Sethi T, Rozengurt E. Multiple neuropeptides stimulate clonal growth of small cell lung cancer: Effects of bradykinin, vasopressin, cholecystokinin, galanin, and neurotensin. Cancer Res 1991;51:3621–3623.

42. Nakanishi Y, Mulshine JL, Kasprzyk PG, et al. Insulin-like growth factor-I can mediate autocrine proliferation of human small cell lung cancer cell lines in vitro. J Clin Invest 1988;82:354–359.

43. Whang-Peng J, Kao-Shan CS, Lee EC, et al. A specific chromosome defect associated with human small-cell lung cancer: Deletion 3p.[14-23] Science 1982;215:181–182.

44. Yokota AJ, Wad M, Shimosato Y, et al. Loss of heterozygosity on chromosomes 3, 13,

45. Harbour JW, Lai SL, Whang-Peng J, et al. Abnormalities in structure and expression of the human retinoblastoma gene in small cell lung cancer. Science 1988;241:353–357.

46. Takahashi T, Nau MM, Chiba I, et al. p53: A frequent target for genetic abnormalities in lung cancer. Science 1989;246:491–494.

47. Johnson BE, Whang-Peng J, Naylor SL, et al. Retention of chromosome 3 in extrapulmonary small cell cancer shown by molecular and cytogenetic studies. JNCI 1989;81:1223–1228.

48. Viallet J, Ihde DC. Small cell carcinoma of the lung: Clinical and biologic aspects. Crit Rev Oncol Hematol 1991;11:109–135.

49. Takahashi T, Obata Y, Sekido Y, et al. Expression and amplification of myc gene family in small cell lung cancer and its relation to biological characteristics. Cancer Res 1989;49:2683–2688.

50. Brennan J, O'Connor T, Makuch RW, et al. Myc family DNA amplification in 107 tumors and tumor cell lines from patients with small cell lung cancer treated with different combination chemotherapy regimens. Cancer Res 1991;51:1708–1712.

51. Johnson BE, Ihde DC, Makuch RW, et al. Myc family oncogene amplification in tumor cell lines established from small cell lung cancer patients and its relationship to clinical status and course. J Clin Invest 1987;79:1629–1634.

52. Mitsudomi T, Viallet J, Mulshine JL, et al. Mutations of ras genes distinguish a subset of non-small-cell lung cancer cell lines from small-cell lung cancer cell lines. Oncogene 1991;6:1353–1362.

53. Carmichael J, Mitchell JB, DeGraff WG, et al. Chemosensitivity testing of human lung cancer cell lines using the MTT assay. Br J Cancer 1988;57:540–547.

54. Stevenson HC, Gazdar AF, Linnoila RI, et al. Lack of relationship between in vitro tumor growth and prognosis in extensive-stage small-cell lung cancer. J Clin Oncol 1989;7:923–931.

55. Masuda N, Fukuoka M, Matsui K, et al. Establishment of tumor cell lines as an independent prognostic factor for survival time in patients with small-cell lung cancer. JNCI 1991;83:1743–1748.

56. Curt GA, Carney DN, Cowan KH, et al. Unstable methotrexate resistance in human small-cell carcinoma associated with double minute chromosomes. N Engl J Med 1983;308:199–202.

57. Curt GA, Jolivet J, Carney DN, et al. Determinants of the sensitivity of human small-cell lung cancer cell lines to methotrexate. J Clin Invest 1985;76:1323–1329.

58. Twentyman PR, Fox NE, Wright KA, et al. Derivation and preliminary characterization of Adriamycin-resistant lines of human lung cancer cells. Br J Cancer 1986;53:529–537.

59. Chen C, Chin JE, Ueda K, et al. Internal duplication and homology with bacterial transport proteins in the mdr1 (P-glycoprotein) gene from multidrug-resistant human cells. Cell 1986;47:381–389.

60. Lai SL, Goldstein LJ, Gottesman MM, et al. MDR1 gene expression in lung cancer. JNCI 1989;81:1144–1150.

61. Carmichael J, Degraff WG, Gamson J, et al. Radiation sensitivity of human lung cancer cell lines. Eur J Cancer Clin Oncol 1989;25:527–534.

62. Carney DN, Mitchell JB, Kinsella TJ. In vitro radiation and chemotherapy sensitivity of established cell lines of human small cell lung cancer and its large cell morphological variant. Cancer Res 1983;43:2806–2811.

63. Gazdar AF, Steinberg SM, Russell EK, et al. Correlation of in vitro drug-sensitivity testing results with response to chemotherapy and survival in extensive stage small cell lung cancer: A prospective clinical trial. JNCI 1990;82:117–124.

64. Boyd MR, Shoemaker RH, McLemore TL, et al. New drug development. In: Roth J, Ruckdeschel J, Weisenburger T, eds. Thoracic oncology. Philadelphia: WB Saunders, 1989:711–721.

65. Seifter EJ, Ihde DC. Small cell lung cancer: A distinct clinicopathologic entity. In: Bitran JD, Golomb HM, Little AG, Weichselbaum RR, eds. Lung cancer: A comprehensive treatise. Orlando: Grune & Stratton, 198:285–300.

66. Byrd RB, Carr DT, Miller WE, et al. Radiographic abnormalities in carcinoma of the lung as related to histologic cell type. Thorax 1969;24:573–575.

67. Cohen MH. Signs and symptoms and bronchogenic carcinoma. In: Straus MJ, ed. Lung cancer: Clinical diagnosis and treatment. New York: Grune & Stratton, 1977:85–94.

68. Green N, Kurohara SS, George FW, et al. The biologic behavior of lung cancer according to histologic type. Radiol Clin Biol 1972;41:160–170.

69. Cohen MH, Matthews MJ. Small cell bronchogenic carcinoma: A distinct clinicopathologic entity. Semin Oncol 1978;5:234–241.

70. Sculier JP, Evans WK, Feld R, et al. Superior vena cava syndrome in small cell lung cancer. Cancer 1986;57:847–851.

71. Zelen M. Keynote address on biostatistics and data retrieval. Cancer Chemother Rep [Part 3] 1973;4:31–42.

72. Brigham BA, Bunn PA, Minna JD, et al. Growth rates of small cell bronchogenic carcinoma. Cancer 1978;42:2880–2886.

73. Matthews MJ, Kanhouwa S, Pickren J, et al. Frequency of residual and metastatic tumor in patients undergoing curative surgical resection for lung cancer. Cancer Chemother Rep [Part 3] 1973;4:63–67.

74. Matthews MJ. Problems in morphology and behavior of bronchopulmonary malignant diseases. In: Israel L, Chahinian AP, eds. Lung cancer: Natural history, prognosis, and therapy. New York: Academic Press, 1976:23–62.

75. Johnson DH, Hainsworth JD, Greco FA. Extrahepatic biliary obstruction caused by small cell lung cancer. Ann Intern Med 1985;102:487–490.

76. Ihde DC, Hansen HH. Staging procedures and prognostic factors in small cell carcinoma of the lung. In: Greco FA, Oldham RK, Bunn PA, eds. Small cell lung cancer. New York: Grune & Stratton, 1981:261–283.

77. Ihde DC, Simms EB, Matthews MJ, et al. Bone marrow metastases in small cell carcinoma of the lung: Frequency, description, and influence on chemotherapeutic toxicity and prognosis. Blood 1979;53:677–686.
78. Hansen M, Hammer M, Hummer L. Diagnostic and therapeutic implications of ectopic hormone production in small cell carcinoma of the lung. Thorax 1980;35:101–106.
79. Hansen M, Hansen HH, Hirsch FR, et al. Hormonal polypeptides and amine metabolites in small cell carcinoma of the lung with special reference to stage and subtypes. Cancer 1980;45:1432–1437.
80. Gropp C, Havemann K, Scheuer A. Ectopic hormones in lung cancer patients at diagnosis and during therapy. Cancer 1980;46:347–354.
81. List AF, Hainsworth JD, Davis BW, et al. The syndrome of inappropriate secretion of anti-diuretic hormone in small cell lung cancer. J Clin Oncol 1986;4:1191–1198.
82. Bliss DP, Battey JF, Linnoila RI, et al. Expression of the atrial natriuretic factor gene in small cell lung cancer tumors and tumor cell lines. JNCI 1990;82:305–310.
83. Shepherd FA, Laskey J, Evans WK, et al. Cushing's syndrome associated with ectopic corticotropin production and small-cell lung cancer. J Clin Oncol 1992;10:21–27.
84. McEvoy KM, Winderbank AJ, Daube JR, et al. 3.4-Diaminopyridine in the treatment of Lambert-Eaton myasthenic syndrome. N Engl J Med 1989;321:1567–1571.
85. Anderson NE, Rosenblum MK, Graus F, et al. Autoantibodies in paraneoplastic syndromes associated with small-cell lung cancer. Neurology 1988;38:1391–1398.
86. Thirkill CE, FitzGerald P, Sergott RC, et al. Cancer-associated retinopathy (CAR syndrome) with antibodies reacting with retinal, optic-nerve, and cancer cells. N Engl J Med 1989;321:1589–1594.
87. Levenson RM, Ihde DC, Matthews MJ, et al. Small cell carcinoma presenting as an extrapulmonary neoplasm: Sites of origin and response to chemotherapy. JNCI 1981;67: 607–612.
88. Fer MF, Levenson RM, Cohen MH, et al. Extrapulmonary small cell carcinoma. In: Greco FA, Oldham RK and Bunn PA, eds. Small cell lung cancer. New York: Grune & Stratton, 1981:301–325.
89. Remick SC, Hafez GR, Carbone PP. Extrapulmonary small cell carcinoma: A review of the literature with emphasis on therapy and outcome. Medicine 1987;66:457–471.
90. Goepfert H, Remmler D, Silva E, et al. Merkel cell carcinoma (endocrine carcinoma of the skin) of the head and neck. Arch Otolaryngol 1984;110:707–712.
91. American Joint Committee on Cancer. Lung cancer. In: Beahrs O, Henson D, Hutter R, Myers M, eds. Manual for staging of cancer. 3rd ed. Philadelphia: JB Lippincott, 1988:115–121.
92. Abrams J, Doyle LA, Aisner J. Staging, prognostic features, and special considerations in small cell lung cancer. Semin Oncol 1988;15:261–277.
93. Ihde DC. Staging evaluation and prognostic factors in small cell lung cancer. In: Aisner J, ed. Lung cancer. New York: Churchill Livingstone, 1985:241–268.
94. Meyer JA. Effect of histologically verified TNM stage on disease control in treated small cell carcinoma of the lung. Cancer 1985;55:1747–1752.
95. Nakhosteen JA, Niederle N. Small cell lung cancer: Serial bronchofiberoscopy and photographic documentation: The bridge sign. Chest 1983;83:12–16.
96. Harper PG, Houang M, Spiro SG, et al. Computerized axial tomography in the pretreatment assessment of small-cell carcinoma of the bronchus. Cancer 1981;47:1775–1780.
97. Griffin CA, Lu C, Fishman EK, et al. The role of computed tomography of the chest in the management of small-cell lung cancer. J Clin Oncol 1984;2:1359–1365.
98. Whitley NO, Fuks JZ, McCrea ES, et al. Computed tomography of the chest in small cell lung cancer: Potential new prognostic signs. AJR 1984;141:885–892.
99. Levenson RM, Sauerbrunn BJL, Ihde DC, et al. Small cell lung cancer: Radionuclide bone scans for assessment of tumor extent and response. AJR 1981;137:31–35.
100. Campling B, Quirt I, DeBoer G, et al. Is bone marrow examination in small cell lung cancer really necessary? Ann Intern Med 1986;105:508–512.
101. Levitan N, Byrne RE, Bromer RH, et al. The value of bone scan and bone marrow biopsy in staging small cell lung cancer. Cancer 1985;56:652–654.
102. Kristjansen PEG, Osterlind K, Hansen M. Detection of bone marrow relapse in patients with small cell carcinoma of the lung. Cancer 1986;58:2538–2541.
103. Mulshine JL, Makuch RW, Johnston-Early A, et al. Diagnosis and significance of liver metastases in small cell carcinoma of the lung. J Clin Oncol 1984;2:733–741.
104. Dombernowsky P, Hirsch F, Hansen HH, et al. Peritoneoscopy in the staging of 190 patients with small-cell anaplastic carcinoma of the lung with special reference to subtyping. Cancer 1978;41:2008–2012.
105. Hansen SW, Jensen F, Pedersen NT, et al. Detection of liver metastases in small cell lung cancer: A comparison of peritoneoscopy with liver biopsy and ultrasonography with fine-needle aspiration. J Clin Oncol 1987;5:255–259.
106. Sculier JP, Feld R, Evans WK, et al. Neurologic disorders in patients with small cell lung cancer. Cancer 1987;60:2275–2283.
107. Wittes RE, Yeh SDJ. Indications for liver and brain scans: Screening tests for patients with oat cell carcinoma of the lung. JAMA 1977;238:506–507.
108. Johnson DH, Windham WW, Allen JH, et al. Limited value of CT brain scans in the staging of small cell cancer. AJR 1983;140:37–40.
109. Crane JM, Nelson MJ, Ihde DC, et al. A comparison of computed tomography and radionuclide scanning for detection of brain metastases in small cell lung cancer. J Clin Oncol 1984;2:1017–1024.
110. Cox JD, Komaki R, Byhardt RW, et al. Results of whole-brain irradiation for metastases from small cell carcinoma of the lung. Cancer Treat Rep 1980;64:957–961.
111. Giannone L, Johnson DH, Hande KR, et al. Favorable prognosis of brain metastases in small cell lung cancer. Ann Intern Med 1987;106:386–389.
112. Van Hazel G, Scott M, Eagan RT. The effect of CNS metastases on the survival of patients with small cell cancer of the lung. Cancer 1983;51:933–937.
113. Carmichael J, Crane JM, Bunn PA, et al. Results of therapeutic cranial irradiation in small cell lung cancer. Int J Radiat Oncol Biol Phys 1988;14:455–459.
114. Hardy J, Smith I, Cherryman G, et al. The value of computed tomographic (CT) scan surveillance in the detection and management of brain metastases in patients with small cell lung cancer. Br J Cancer 1990;62:684–686.
115. Nugent JL, Bunn PA, Matthews MJ, et al. CNS metastases in small cell bronchogenic carcinoma: Increasing frequency, description, and changing pattern with lengthening survival. Cancer 1979;44:1885–1893.
116. Rosen ST, Aisner J, Makuch RW, et al. Carcinomatous leptomeningitis in small cell lung cancer: A clinicopathologic review of the National Cancer Institute experience. Medicine 1982;61:45–53.
117. Pedersen AG, Bach F, Melgaard B. Frequency, diagnosis, and prognosis of spinal cord compression in small cell bronchogenic carcinoma: A review of 817 consecutive patients. Cancer 1985;55:1818–1822.
118. Murphy KC, Feld R, Evans WK, et al. Intramedullary spinal cord metastases from small cell carcinoma of the lung. J Clin Oncol 1983;1:99–106.
119. Ihde DC, Dunnick NR, Johnston-Early A, et al. Abdominal computed tomography in small cell lung cancer: Assessment of extent of disease and response to therapy. Cancer 1982;49:1485–1490.
120. Poon PY, Feld R, Evans WK, et al. Computed tomography of the brain, liver, and upper abdomen in the staging of small cell carcinoma of the lung. J Comput Assist Tomogr 1982;6:963–965.
121. Pagani JJ. Normal adrenal glands in small cell lung carcinoma: CT-guided biopsy. AJR 1983;140:949–951.
122. Jelinek JS, Redmond J, Perry JJ, et al. Small cell lung cancer: Staging with MR imaging. Radiology 1990;177:837–842.
123. Carney DN, Zweig MH, Ihde DC, et al. Elevated serum creatine kinase-BB levels in patients with small cell lung cancer. Cancer Res 1984;44:5399–5403.
124. Johnson DH, Marangos PJ, Forbes JT, et al. Potential utility of serum neuron-specific enolase in small cell carcinoma of the lung. Cancer Res 1984;44:5409–5414.
125. Sculier JP, Feld R, Evans WK, et al. Carcinoembryonic antigen: A useful prognostic marker in small cell lung cancer. J Clin Oncol 1985;3:1349–1354.
126. Sobol RE, O'Connor DT, Addison J, et al. Elevated serum chromogranin A concentrations in small cell lung carcinoma. Ann Intern Med 1986;105:698–700.
127. Carney DN, Marangos PJ, Ihde DC, et al. Serum neuron specific enolase: A marker for disease extent and response to therapy in patients with small cell lung cancer. Lancet 1982;1:583–585.
128. Aroney RS, Dermody WC, Aldenderfer P, et al. Multiple sequential biomarkers in monitoring patients with carcinoma of the lung. Cancer Treat Rep 1984;68:859–866.
129. Albain KS, Crowley JJ, LeBlanc M, et al. Determinants of improved outcome in small cell lung cancer: An analysis of the 2,580-patient Southwest Oncology Group data base. J Clin Oncol 1990;8:1563–1574.
130. Dearing MP, Steinberg SM, Phelps R, et al. Outcome of patients with small cell lung cancer: Effects of changes in staging procedures and imaging technology on prognostic factors over 14 years. J Clin Oncol 1990;8:1042–1049.
131. Rawson NSB, Peto J. An overview of prognostic factors in small cell lung cancer: A report from the Subcommittee for the Management of Lung Cancer of the United Kingdom Coordinating Committee on Cancer Research. Br J Cancer 1990;61:597–604.
132. Sagman U, Maki E, Evans WK, et al. Small-cell carcinoma of the lung: Derivation of a prognostic staging system. J Clin Oncol 1991;9:1639–1649.
133. Spiegelman D, Maurer LH, Ware JH, et al. Prognostic factors in small-cell carcinoma of the lung: An analysis of 1,521 patients. J Clin Oncol 1989;7:344–354.
134. Feinstein AR, Sosin DM, Wells CK. Stage migration and new diagnostic techniques as a source of misleading statistics for survival in cancer. N Engl J Med 1985;312: 1604–1608.
135. Pfister DG, Wells CK, Chang CK, et al. Classifying clinical severity to help solve problems of stage migration in nonconcurrent comparisons of lung cancer therapy. Cancer Res 1990;50:4664–4669.
136. Ihde DC, Makuch RW, Carney DN, et al. Prognostic implications of stage of disease and sites of metastases in patients with small cell carcinoma of the lung treated with intensive combination chemotherapy. Am Rev Respir Dis 1981;123:500–507.
137. Friess GG, McCracken JD, Troxell ML, et al. Effect of initial resection of small-cell carcinoma of the lung: A review of Southwest Oncology Group Study 7628. J Clin Oncol 1985;3:964–968.
138. Østerlind K, Hansen M, Hansen HH, et al. Treatment policy of surgery in small cell carcinoma of the lung: Retrospective analysis of a series of 874 consecutive patients. Thorax 1985;40:272–277.
139. DeWys WD, Begg C, Lavin PT, et al. Prognostic effect of weight loss prior to chemotherapy in cancer patients. Am J Med 1980;69:491–497.
140. Johnston-Early A, Cohen MH, Fossieck BE, et al. Delayed hypersensitivity skin testing as a prognostic indicator in patients with small cell lung cancer. Cancer 1983;52: 1395–1400.
141. Poplin E, Thompson B, Whitacre M, et al. Small cell carcinoma of the lung: Influence of age on treatment outcome. Cancer Treat Rep 1987;71:291–296.
142. Johnston-Early A, Cohen MH, Minna JD, et al. Smoking abstinence and small cell lung cancer survival: An association. JAMA 1980;244:2175–2179.
143. Bergman B, Sörenson S. Smoking and effect of chemotherapy in small cell lung cancer. Eur Respir J 1988;1:932–937.
144. Livingston RB, Trauth CJ, Greenstreet RL. Small cell carcinoma: Clinical manifestations and behavior with treatment. In: Greco FA, Oldham RK, Bunn PA, eds. Small cell lung cancer. Orlando: Grune & Stratton, 1981:285–300.
145. Quoix E, Finkelstein H, Wolkove N, et al. Treatment of small-cell lung cancer on protocol: Potential bias of results. J Clin Oncol 1986;4:1314–1320.
146. Morstyn G, Ihde DC, Lichter AS, et al. Small cell lung cancer 1973–1983: Early progress and recent obstacles. Int J Radiat Oncol Biol Phys 1984;10:515–539.

147. Hansen HH, Selawry OS, Simon R, et al. Combination chemotherapy of advanced lung cancer: A randomized trial. Cancer 1976;38:2201–2207.
148. Østerlind K, Ihde DC, Ettinger DS, et al. Staging and prognostic factors in small cell carcinoma of the lung. Cancer Treat Rep 1983;67:3–9.
149. Fox W, Scadding JG. Medical Research Council comparative trial of surgery and radiotherapy for primary treatment of small-celled or oat-celled carcinoma of the bronchus: Ten-year follow-up. Lancet 1973;2:63–65.
150. Mountain CF, Carr DT, Anderson WA. A system for the clinical staging of lung cancer. AJR 1974;120:130–138.
151. Mountain CF. Clinical biology of small cell carcinoma: Relationship to surgical therapy. Semin Oncol 1978;5:272–279.
152. Seydel HG, Creech R, Pagano M, et al. Small cell carcinoma: Combined modality treatment of regional small cell undifferentiated carcinoma of the lung. Int J Radiat Oncol Biol Phys 1983;9:1135–1141.
153. Petrovich Z, Ohanian M, Cox J. Clinical research on the treatment of locally advanced lung cancer: Final report of VALG protocol 13 limited. Cancer 1978;42:1129–1134.
154. Carr DT, Childs DS, Lee RE. Radiotherapy plus 5-FU compared to radiotherapy alone for inoperable and unresectable bronchogenic carcinoma. Cancer 1972;29:375–380.
155. Choi CH, Carey RW. Small cell anaplastic carcinoma of the lung: Reappraisal of current management. Cancer 1976;37:2651–2657.
156. Green RA, Humphrey E, Close H, et al. Alkylating agents in bronchogenic carcinoma. Am J Med 1969;46:516–525.
157. Higgins GA, Shields TW. Experience of the Veterans Administration Surgical Adjuvant Group. In: Muggia FM, Rozencweig M, eds. Lung cancer: Progress in therapeutic research. New York: Raven Press, 1979:433–442.
158. Karrer K, Pridun N, Denck H. Chemotherapy as an adjuvant to surgery in lung cancer. Cancer Chemother Pharmacol 1978;1:145–159.
159. Shields TW, Humphrey EW, Eastridge CE, et al. Adjuvant cancer chemotherapy after resection of carcinoma of the lung. Cancer 1977;40:2057–2062.
160. Wingfield HV. Combined surgery and chemotherapy for carcinoma of the bronchus. Lancet 1970;1:470–471.
161. Bergsagel DE, Jenkin RDT, Pringle JF, et al. Lung cancer: Clinical trial of radiotherapy alone vs. radiotherapy plus cyclophosphamide. Cancer 1972;30:621–627.
162. Medical Research Council Lung Cancer Working Party. Radiotherapy alone or with chemotherapy in the treatment of small-cell carcinoma of the lung. Br J Cancer 1979;40: 1–10.
163. Perez CA, Krauss S, Bartolucci A, et al. Thoracic and elective brain irradiation with concomitant or delayed multiagent chemotherapy in the treatment of localized small cell carcinoma of the lung. Cancer 1981;47:2407–2413.
164. Aisner J, Alberto P, Bitran J, et al. Role of chemotherapy in small cell lung cancer: A consensus report of the International Association for the Study of Lung Cancer workshop. Cancer Treat Rep 1983;67:37–43.
165. Johnson DH, Greco FA. Small cell carcinoma of the lung. CRC Crit Rev Oncol/Hematol 1986;4:303–336.
166. Seifter EJ, Ihde DC. Therapy of small cell lung cancer: A perspective on two decades of clinical research. Semin Oncol 1988;15:278–299.
167. Bunn PA, Ihde DC. Small cell bronchogenic carcinoma: A review of therapeutic results. In: Livingston RB, ed. Lung cancer 1. The Hague: Martinus Nijhoff, 1981:169–208.
168. Ihde DC, Bunn PA. Chemotherapy of small cell bronchogenic carcinoma. In: Whitehouse JMA, Williams CJ, eds. Recent advances in clinical oncology. Edinburgh: Churchill Livingstone, 1982:305–323.
169. Cavalli F, Sonntag R, Jungi F, et al. VP-16-213 monotherapy for remission induction of small cell lung cancer: A randomized trial using three dosage schedules. Cancer Treat Rep 1978;62:473–475.
170. Slevin ML, Clark PI, Joel SP, et al. A randomized trial to evaluate the effect of schedule on the activity of etoposide in small-cell lung cancer. J Clin Oncol 1989;7:1333–1340.
171. Mead GM, Thompson J, Sweetenham JW, et al. Extensive stage small cell carcinoma of the bronchus: A randomized study of etoposide given orally by one-day or five-day schedule together with intravenous adriamycin and cyclophosphamide. Cancer Chemother Pharmacol 1987;19:172–174.
172. Johnson DH, Greco FA, Strupp J, et al. Prolonged administration of oral etoposide in patients with relapsed or refractory small-cell lung cancer: A Phase II trial. J Clin Oncol 1990;8:1613–1617.
173. Clark PI, Cottier B, Joel SP, et al. Prolonged administration of single-agent oral etoposide in patients with untreated small cell lung cancer. Proc Am Soc Clin Oncol [Abstract] 1990;9:226.
174. Dombernowsky P, Hansen HH, Sorenson PG, et al. Vincristine in the treatment of small cell anaplastic carcinoma of the lung. Cancer Treat Rep 1976;60:239–242.
175. Grant SC, Gralla RJ, Kris MG, et al. Single agent chemotherapy trials in small-cell lung cancer, 1970–1990: The case for studies in previously treated patients. J Clin Oncol 1992;10:484–498.
176. Carney DN, Grogan L, Smit EF, et al. Single-agent oral etoposide for elderly small cell lung cancer patients. Semin Oncol 1990;17(Suppl 2):49–53.
177. Issell BF, Einhorn LH, Comis RL, et al. Multicenter Phase II trial of etoposide in previously treated small cell carcinoma of the lung. Cancer Treat Rep 1985;69:127–128.
178. Bork E, Hansen M, Dombernowsky P, et al. Teniposide (VM-26), an overlooked highly active agent in small-cell lung cancer: Results of a Phase II trial in untreated patients. J Clin Oncol 1986;4:524–527.
179. Wolff SN, Birch R, Sarma P, et al. Randomized dose-response evaluation of etoposide in small cell carcinoma of the lung: A Southeastern Cancer Study Group trial. Cancer Treat Rep 1986;70:583–587.
180. Smith IE, Harland SJ, Robinson BA, et al. Carboplatin: A very active new cisplatin analog in the treatment of small cell lung cancer. Cancer Treat Rep 1985;69:43–46.
181. Blackstein M, Eisenhauer EA, Wierzbicki R, et al. Epirubicin in extensive small-cell lung cancer: A phase II study in previously untreated patients: A National Cancer Institute of Canada Clinical Trials Group study. J Clin Oncol 1990;8:385–389.
182. Cullen MH, Smith SR, Benfield GFA, et al. Testing new drugs in untreated small cell lung cancer may prejudice the results of standard treatment: A phase II study of oral idarubicin in extensive disease. Cancer Treat Rep 1987;71:1227–1230.
183. Malik STA, Rayner H, Fletcher J, et al. Phase II trial of mitoxantrone as first-line chemotherapy for extensive small cell lung cancer. Cancer Treat Rep 1987;71:1291–1292.
184. Evans WK, Eisenhauer EA, Cormier Y, et al. Phase II study of amonafide: Results of treatment and lessons learned from the study of an investigational agent in previously untreated patients with extensive small-cell lung cancer. J Clin Oncol 1990;8:390–395.
185. Ettinger DS, Finkelstein DM, Abeloff MD, et al. Justification for evaluating new anticancer drugs in selected untreated patients with a chemotherapy-sensitive advanced cancer: An ECOG randomized study. Proc Am Soc Clin Oncol [Abstract] 1990;9:224.
186. Moore TD, Korn EL. Phase II trial design considerations for small-cell lung cancer. JNCI 1992;84:150–154.
187. Broder LE, Cohen MH, Selawry OS. Treatment of bronchogenic carcinoma II: Small cell cancer. Cancer Treat Rev 1977;4:219–260.
188. Lowenbraun S, Bartolucci A, Smalley RV, et al. The superiority of combination chemotherapy over single agent chemotherapy in small cell lung carcinoma. Cancer 1979;44:406–413.
189. Edmonson JH, Lagakos SW, Selawry OS, et al. Cyclophosphamide and CCNU in the treatment of inoperable small cell carcinoma and adenocarcinoma of the lung. Cancer Treat Rep 1976;60:925–932.
190. Alberto P, Brunner KW, Martz G, et al. Treatment of bronchogenic carcinoma with simultaneous or sequential combination chemotherapy, including methotrexate, cyclophosphamide, procarbazine and vincristine. Cancer 1976;38:2208–2216.
191. Cohen MH, Creaven PJ, Fossieck BE, et al. Intensive chemotherapy of small cell bronchogenic carcinoma. Cancer Treat Rep 1977;61:349–354.
192. Bork E, Ersbøll J, Dombernowsky P, et al. Teniposide and etoposide in previously untreated small-cell lung cancer: A randomized study. J Clin Oncol 1991;9:1627–1631.
193. Maurer LH, Tulloh M, Weiss RB, et al. A randomized combined modality trial in small cell carcinoma of the lung: Comparison of combination chemotherapy-radiation therapy versus cyclophosphamide-radiation therapy: Effects of maintenance chemotherapy and prophylactic whole brain irradiation. Cancer 1980;45:30–39.
194. Souhami RL, Finn G, Gregory WM, et al. High-dose cyclophosphamide in small cell carcinoma of the lung. J Clin Oncol 1985;3:958–963.
195. Hong WK, Nicaise C, Lawson R, et al. Etoposide combined with cyclophosphamide plus vincristine compared with doxorubicin plus cyclophosphamide plus vincristine and with high-dose cyclophosphamide plus vincristine in the treatment of small-cell carcinoma of the lung: A randomized trial of the Bristol Lung Cancer Study Group. J Clin Oncol 1989;7:450–456.
196. Jett JR, Everson L, Therneau TM, et al. Treatment of limited-stage small-cell lung cancer with cyclophosphamide, doxorubicin, and vincristine with or without etoposide: A randomized study of the North Central Cancer Treatment Group. J Clin Oncol 1990;8:33–39.
197. Jackson DV, Case LD, Zekan PJ, et al. Improvement of long-term survival in extensive small-cell lung cancer. J Clin Oncol 1988;6:1161–1169.
198. Messieh AA, Schweicker JM, Lipton A, et al. Addition of etoposide to cyclophosphamide, doxorubicin, and vincristine for remission induction and survival in patients with small cell lung cancer. Cancer Treat Rep 1987;71:61–66.
199. Lowenbraun S, Birch R, Buchanan R, et al. Combination chemotherapy in small cell lung carcinoma: A randomized study of two intensive regimens. Cancer 1984;54:2344–2350.
200. Einhorn L, Greco F, Wampler G, et al. Adriamycin, etoposide versus cytoxan, adriamycin, vincristine in the treatment of small cell lung cancer. Proc Am Soc Clin Oncol [Abstract] 1987;6:168.
201. Hirsch FR, Hansen HH, Hansen M, et al. The superiority of combination chemotherapy including etoposide based on in vivo cell cycle analysis in the treatment of extensive small cell lung cancer: A randomized trial of 288 consecutive patients. J Clin Oncol 1987;5:585–591.
202. Schabel FM, Trader MW, Laster WK, et al. Cisdichlorodiamineplatinum (II): Combination chemotherapy and cross-resistance studies with tumors of mice. Cancer Treat Rep 1979;63:1459–1473.
203. Hainsworth JD, Williams SD, Einhorn LH, et al. Successful treatment of resistant germinal neoplasms with VP-16 and cisplatin. J Clin Oncol 1985;3:666–671.
204. Evans WK, Osoba D, Feld R, et al. Etoposide (VP-16) and cisplatin: An effective treatment for relapse of small-cell lung cancer. J Clin Oncol 1985;3:65–71.
205. Porter LL, Johnson DH, Hainsworth JD, et al. Cisplatin and etoposide combination chemotherapy for refractory small cell carcinoma of the lung. Cancer Treat Rep 1985;69:479–481.
206. Boni C, Cocconi G, Bisagni G, et al. Cisplatin and etoposide (VP-16) as a single regimen for small cell lung cancer. Cancer 1989;63:638–642.
207. Evans WK, Shepherd FA, Feld R, et al. VP-16 and cisplatin as first-line therapy for small-cell lung cancer. J Clin Oncol 1985;3:1471–1477.
208. Sierocki JS, Hilaris BS, Hopfan S, et al. Cis-Dichlorodiamineplatinum (II) and VP-16-213: An active induction regimen for small cell carcinoma of the lung. Cancer Treat Rep 1979;63:1593–1597.
209. Woods RL, Levi JL. Chemotherapy for small cell lung cancer: A randomized study of maintenance chemotherapy with cyclophosphamide, adriamycin, and vincristine after

remission induction with cis-platinum, VP-16-213 and radiotherapy. Proc Am Soc Clin Oncol [Abstract] 1984;3:214.

210. Roth BJ, Johnson DH, Einhorn LH, et al. Randomized study of cyclophosphamide, doxorubicin, and vincristine versus etoposide and cisplatin versus alternation of these two regimens in extensive small-cell lung cancer: A Phase III trial of the Southeastern Cancer Study Group. J Clin Oncol 1992;10:282–291.

211. Fukuoka M, Furuse K, Saijo N, et al. Randomized trial of cyclophosphamide, doxorubicin, and vincristine versus cisplatin and etoposide versus alternation of these regimens in small-cell lung cancer. JNCI 1991;83:855–861.

212. Einhorn LH, Crawford J, Birch R, et al. Cisplatin plus etoposide consolidation following cyclophosphamide, doxorubicin, and vincristine in limited small-cell lung cancer. J Clin Oncol 1988;6:451–456.

213. Bishop JF, Raghavan D, Stuart-Harris R, et al. Carboplatin (CBDCA, JM-8) and VP-16-213 in previously untreated patients with small cell lung cancer. J Clin Oncol 1987;5:1574–1578.

214. Wolf M, Havemann K, Holle R, et al. Cisplatin/etoposide versus ifosfamide/etoposide combination chemotherapy in small-cell lung cancer: A multicenter German randomized trial. J Clin Oncol 1987;5:1880–1889.

215. Ihde DC. Chemotherapy in lung cancer. In: Brain MC, Carbone PP, eds. Current therapy in hematology–oncology 3. 3rd ed. Toronto: BC Dekker, 1988:213–217.

216. Frei E, Canellos GP. Dose: A critical factor in cancer chemotherapy. Am J Med 1980;69:585–591.

217. Mehta C, Vogl SE. High-dose cyclophosphamide in the induction therapy of small cell lung cancer: Minor improvements in rate of remission and survival. Proc Am Assoc Cancer Res [Abstract] 1982;23:155.

218. Ettinger DS, Karp JE, Abeloff MD, et al. Intermittent high-dose cyclophosphamide chemotherapy for small cell carcinoma of the lung. Cancer Treat Rep 1978;62:413–422.

219. Johnson DH, Einhorn LH, Birch R, et al. A randomized comparison of high-dose versus conventional-dose cyclophosphamide, doxorubicin, and vincristine for extensive-stage small-cell lung cancer: A Phase III trial of the Southeastern Cancer Study Group. J Clin Oncol 1987;5:1731–1738.

220. Figueredo AT, Hryniuk WM, Strautmanis I, et al. Co-trimoxazole prophylaxis during high-dose chemotherapy of small-cell lung cancer. J Clin Oncol 1985;3:54–64.

221. Ihde DC, Mulshine JL, Kramer BS, et al. Randomized trial of high vs. standard dose etoposide (VP16) and cisplatin in extensive stage small cell lung cancer. Proc Am Soc Clin Oncol [Abstract] 1991;10:240.

222. Hande KR, Oldham RK, Fer MF, et al. Randomized study of high-dose low-dose methotrexate in the treatment of extensive small cell lung cancer. Am J Med 1982;73:413–418.

223. Farha P, Spitzer G, Valdivieso M, et al. High-dose chemotherapy and autologous bone marrow transplantation for the treatment of small cell lung carcinoma. Cancer 1983;52:1351–1355.

224. Abeloff MD, Ettinger DS, Order SE, et al. Intensive induction chemotherapy in 54 patients with small cell carcinoma of the lung. Cancer Treat Rep 1981;65:639–646.

225. Brower M, Ihde DC, Johnston-Early A, et al. Treatment of extensive stage small cell bronchogenic carcinoma: Effects of variation in intensity of induction chemotherapy. Am J Med 1983;75:993–1000.

226. Valdivieso M, Cabanillas F, Keating M, et al. Effects of intensive induction chemotherapy for extensive-disease small cell bronchogenic carcinoma in protected environment-prophylactic antibiotic units. Am J Med 1984;76:405–412.

227. Markman M, Abeloff MD, Berkman AW, et al. Intensive alternating chemotherapy regimen in small cell carcinoma of the lung. Cancer Treat Rep 1985;69:161–166.

228. Johnson DH, DeLeo MJ, Hande KR, et al. High-dose induction chemotherapy with cyclophosphamide, etoposide, and cisplatin for extensive-stage small-cell lung cancer. J Clin Oncol 1987;5:703–709.

229. Miles DW, Earl HM, Souhami RL, et al. Intensive weekly chemotherapy for good-prognosis patients with small-cell lung cancer. J Clin Oncol 1991;9:280–285.

230. Murray N, Shah A, Osoba D, et al. Intensive weekly chemotherapy for the treatment of extensive-stage small cell lung cancer. J Clin Oncol 1991;9:1632–1638.

231. Taylor CW, Crowley J, Williamson SK, et al. Treatment of small-cell lung cancer with an alternating chemotherapy regimen given at weekly intervals: A Southwest Oncology Group pilot study. J Clin Oncol 1990;8:1811–1817.

232. Klasa RJ, Murray N, Coldman AJ. Dose-intensity meta-analysis of chemotherapy regimens in small-cell carcinoma of the lung. J Clin Oncol 1991;9:499–508.

233. Cunningham D, Banham SW, Hutcheon AH, et al. High-dose cyclophosphamide and VP-16 as late dosage intensification therapy for small cell carcinoma of the lung. Cancer Chemother Pharmacol 1985;15:303–306.

234. Humblet Y, Symann M, Bosly A, et al. Late intensification chemotherapy with autologous bone marrow transplantation in selected small-cell carcinoma of the lung: A randomized study. J Clin Oncol 1987;5:1864–1873.

235. Ihde DC, Deisseroth AB, Lichter AS, et al. Late intensive combined modality therapy followed by autologous bone marrow infusion in extensive stage small cell lung cancer. J Clin Oncol 1986;4:1443–1454.

236. Klastersky J, Nicaise C, Longeval E, et al. Cisplatin, adriamycin, and etoposide (CAV) for remission induction of small-cell bronchogenic carcinoma: Evaluation of efficacy and toxicity and pilot study of a "late intensification" with autologous bone-marrow rescue. Cancer 1982;50:652–658.

237. Sculier JP, Klastersky J, Strychmans P, et al. Late intensification in small cell lung cancer: A phase I study of high doses of cyclophosphamide and etoposide with autologous bone marrow transplantation. J Clin Oncol 1985;3:184–191.

238. Smith IE, Evans BD, Harland SJ, et al. High-dose cyclophosphamide with autologous bone marrow rescue after conventional chemotherapy in the treatment of small cell lung carcinoma. Cancer Chemother Pharmacol 1985;14:120–124.

239. Spitzer G, Farha P, Valdivieso M, et al. High-dose intensification therapy with autologous bone marrow support for limited small-cell bronchogenic carcinoma. J Clin Oncol 1986;4:4–13.

240. Stewart P, Buckner CD, Thomas ED, et al. Intensive chemoradiotherapy with autologous bone marrow transplantation in selected small cell carcinoma of the lung: A randomized study. Cancer Treat Rep 1983;67:1055–1059.

241. Harper PG, Souhami RL. Intensive chemotherapy with autologous bone marrow transplantation in small cell carcinoma of the lung. Recent Results Cancer Res 1985;97:146–156.

242. Cohen MH, Ihde DC, Bunn PA, et al. Cyclic alternating combination chemotherapy for small cell bronchogenic carcinoma. Cancer Treat Rep 1979;62:163–170.

243. Spiro SG, Souhami RL, Geddes DM, et al. Duration of chemotherapy in small cell lung cancer: A Cancer Research Campaign trial. Br J Cancer 1989;59:578–583.

244. Goldie JH, Coldman AJ. A mathematical model for relating sensitivity of tumours to their spontaneous mutation rate. Cancer Treat Rep 1979;63:1727–1735.

245. Goldie JH, Coldman AJ, Gudauskas GA. Rationale for the use of alternating non-cross resistant chemotherapy. Cancer Treat Rep 1982;66:439–449.

246. Ettinger DS, Finkelstein DM, Abeloff MD, et al. A randomized comparison of standard chemotherapy versus alternating chemotherapy and maintenance versus no maintenance therapy for extensive stage small-cell lung cancer: A Phase III study of the Eastern Cooperative Oncology Group. J Clin Oncol 1990;8:230–240.

247. Elliott J, Østerlind K, Hansen HH. Cyclic alternating non-cross-resistant chemotherapy in the management of small cell anaplastic carcinoma of the lung. Cancer Treat Rev 1984;11:103–113.

248. Østerlind K, Sörenson S, Hansen HH, et al. Continuous versus alternating combination chemotherapy for advanced small cell carcinoma of the lung. Cancer Res 1983;43:6085–6089.

249. Daniels JR, Chak LY, Sikic BL, et al. Chemotherapy of small cell carcinoma of the lung: A randomized comparison of alternating and sequential combination chemotherapy programs. J Clin Oncol 1984;2:1192–1199.

250. Evans WK, Feld R, Murray N, et al. Superiority of alternating non-cross-resistant chemotherapy in extensive small cell lung cancer. Ann Intern Med 1987;107:451–458.

251. Einhorn LH, Bond WH, Hornback W, et al. Long term results in combined modality treatment of small cell carcinoma of the lung. Semin Oncol 1978;5:309–313.

252. Greco FA, Richardson RL, Snell JD, et al. Small cell lung cancer: Complete remission and improved survival. Am J Med 1979;66:625–630.

253. Johnson RE, Brereton HD, Kent CH. "Total" therapy for small cell carcinoma of the lung. Ann Thorac Surg 1978;25:509–515.

254. Feld R, Evans WK, DeBoer G, et al. Combined modality induction therapy without maintenance chemotherapy for small cell carcinoma of the lung. J Clin Oncol 1984;2:294–304.

255. Splinter TAW, EORTC Lung Cancer Cooperative Group. Induction vs. induction plus maintenance chemotherapy in small cell lung cancer: Definitive evaluation. Proc Am Soc Clin Oncol [Abstract] 1988;7:202.

256. Bleehan NM, Fayers PM, Girling DJ, et al. Controlled trial of twelve versus six courses of chemotherapy in the treatment of small cell lung cancer. Br J Cancer 1989;59:584–590.

257. Dombernowsky P, Hansen HH. Combination chemotherapy in the management of superior vena cava obstruction in small-cell anaplastic carcinoma of the lung. Acta Med Scand 1978;204:513–516.

258. Spiro SG, Shah S, Harper PG, et al. Treatment of obstruction of the superior vena cava by combination chemotherapy with and without irradiation in small-cell carcinoma of the bronchus. Thorax 1983;38:501–505.

259. Lee JS, Murphy WK, Glisson BS, et al. Primary chemotherapy of brain metastases in small-cell lung cancer. J Clin Oncol 1989;7:916–922.

260. Twelves CJ, Souhami RL, Harper PG, et al. The response of cerebral metastases in small cell lung cancer to systemic chemotherapy. Br J Cancer 1990;61:147–150.

261. Feld R: Complications in the treatment of small cell carcinoma of the lung. Cancer Treat Rev 1981;8:5–25.

262. Feld R, Evans WK, DeBoer G. Herpes zoster in patients with carcinoma of the lung. Am J Med 1982;73:795–801.

263. Huberman MS, Fossieck BE, Bunn PA, et al. Herpes zoster and small cell bronchogenic carcinoma. Am J Med 1980;68:214–218.

264. Earle MF, Fossieck BE, Cohen MH, et al. Perirectal infections in patients with small cell lung cancer. JAMA 1981;246:2464–2466.

265. Markman M, Abeloff MD. Management of hematologic and infectious complications of intensive induction therapy for small cell carcinoma of the lung. Am J Med 1983;74:741–746.

266. Crawford J, Ozer H, Stoller R, et al. Reduction by granulocyte colony-stimulating factor of fever and neutropenia induced by chemotherapy in patients with small-cell lung cancer. N Engl J Med 1991;325:164–170.

267. De Jongh CA, Wade JC, Finley RS, et al. Trimethoprim/sulfamethoxazole versus placebo: A double-blind comparison of infection prophylaxis in patients with small cell carcinoma of the lung. J Clin Oncol 1983;1:302–307.

268. Abeloff MD, Klastersky J, Drings PD, et al. Complications of treatment of small cell carcinoma of the lung. Cancer Treat Rep 1983;67:21–26.

269. Bunn PA, Lichter AS, Makuch RW, et al. Chemotherapy alone or chemotherapy with chest radiation therapy in limited stage small cell lung cancer: A prospective randomized trial. Ann Intern Med 1987;106:655–662.

270. Abrams RA, Litcher AS, Bromer RH, et al. The hematopoietic toxicity of regional radiation therapy: Correlations for combined modality therapy with systemic chemotherapy. Cancer 1985;55:1429–1435.

271. Lee JS, Umsawasdi T, Dhingra HM, et al. Effects of brain irradiation and chemotherapy on myelosuppression in small cell lung cancer. J Clin Oncol 1986;4:1615–1619.

272. Johnson DH, Porter LL, List AF, et al. Acute nonlymphocytic leukemia after treatment of small cell lung cancer. Am J Med 1986;81:962–968.

273. Johnson BE, Ihde DC, Bunn PA, et al. Patients with small cell lung cancer treated with combination chemotherapy with or without irradiation: Data on potential cures, chronic toxicities, and late relapses after a five- to eleven-year follow-up. Ann Intern Med 1985;103:430–438.

274. Bradley EC, Schechter GP, Matthews MJ, et al. Erythroleukemia and other hematologic complications of intensive therapy in long-term survivors of small cell lung cancer. Cancer 1982;49:221–223.

275. Brooks BJ, Seifter EJ, Walsh TE, et al. Pulmonary toxicity with combined modality therapy for limited stage small cell lung cancer. J Clin Oncol 1986;4:200–209.

276. Sorensen PG, Østerlind K, Groth S, et al. Effects of intensive chemotherapy on respiratory function in patients with small cell carcinoma of the lung. Eur J Cancer Clin Oncol 1983;19:901–906.

277. Vogelzang NJ, Nelimark RA, Nath KA. Tumor lysis syndrome after induction chemotherapy of small cell bronchogenic carcinoma. JAMA 1983;249:513–514.

278. Ellis F. Dose, time and fractionation: A clinical hypothesis. Clin Radiol 1969;20:1–7.

279. Ellis F. Nominal standard dose and the ret. Br J Radiol 1971;44:101–108.

280. Fowler JF. What next in fractionated radiation therapy? Br J Cancer 1984;49(Suppl 6):285–300.

281. Catane R, Lichter AS, Lee YJ, et al. Small cell lung cancer: Analysis of treatment factors contributing to prolonged survival. Cancer 1981;48:1936–1943.

282. Hall EJ. Radiobiology for the radiologist. Philadelphia: JB Lippincott, 1988.

283. Turrisi AT, Glover DJ. Thoracic radiotherapy variables: Influence on local control in small cell lung cancer limited disease. Int J Radiat Oncol Biol Phys 1990;19:1473–1479.

284. Ihde DC, Grayson J, Woods E, et al. Twice daily chest irradiation an an adjuvant to etoposide/cisplatin therapy of limited stage small cell lung cancer. In: Salmon S, ed. Adjuvant therapy of cancer VI. Philadelphia: WB Saunders, 1990:162–165.

285. Ajaikumar BS, Barkley T. The role of radiation therapy in the treatment of small cell undifferentiated bronchogenic cancer. Int J Radiat Oncol Biol Phys 1979;5:977–982.

286. Salazar O, Rubin P, Brown J, et al. Predictors of radiation response in lung cancer: A clinico-pathobiological analysis. Cancer 1976;37:2636–2650.

287. Lichter AS, Bunn PA, Ihde DC, et al. The role of radiation therapy in the treatment of small cell lung cancer. Cancer 1985;55:2163–2175.

288. Ihde DC. How should we report results of clinical trials of combined chemotherapy and chest irradiation in limited stage small cell lung cancer? Antibiot Chemother 1988;41:65–69.

289. Perry MC, Eaton WL, Propert KJ, et al. Chemotherapy with or without radiation therapy in limited small-cell carcinoma of the lung. N Engl J Med 1987;316:912–918.

290. Perez CA, Einhorn L, Oldham RK, et al. Randomized trial of radiotherapy to the thorax in limited small-cell carcinoma of the lung treated with multiagent chemotherapy and elective brain irradiation: A preliminary report. J Clin Oncol 1984;2:1200–1208.

291. Fox RM, Woods RL, Brodie GN, et al. A randomized study: Small cell anaplastic lung cancer treated by combination chemotherapy and adjuvant radiotherapy. Int J Radiat Oncol Biol Phys 1980;6:1083–1085.

292. Rosenthal MA, Tattersall MHN, Fox RM, et al. Adjuvant thoracic radiotherapy in small cell lung cancer: Ten-year follow-up of a randomized study. Lung Cancer 1991;7:235–241.

293. Kies MS, Mira JG, Crowley JJ, et al. Multimodal therapy for limited small cell lung cancer: A randomized study of induction combination chemotherapy with or without thoracic radiation in complete responders; and with wide-field versus reduced-field radiation in partial responders: A Southwest Oncology Group study. J Clin Oncol 1987;5:592–600.

294. Souhami RL, Geddes DM, Spiro SG, et al. Radiotherapy in small cell cancer of the lung treated with combination chemotherapy: A controlled trial. Br Med J 1984;288:1643–1646.

295. Østerlind K, Hansen HH, Hansen HS, et al. Chemotherapy versus chemotherapy plus irradiation in limited small cell lung cancer: Results of a controlled trial with 5 years follow-up. Br J Cancer 1986;54:7–17.

296. Cox JD, Holoye PY, Libnoch JA. The role of consolidation irradiation in combined modality therapy of small cell carcinoma of the lung. Int J Radiat Oncol Biol Phys 1982;8:1271–1276.

297. Carlson RW, Sikic BI, Gandara DR, et al. Late consolidative radiation therapy in the treatment of limited-stage small cell lung cancer. Cancer 1991;68:948–958.

298. Johnson DH, Arriagada R, Ihde DC, et al. Meta-analysis of randomized trials evaluating the role of thoracic radiotherapy in limited-stage small cell lung cancer. Proc Am Soc Clin Oncol [Abstract] 1992;11:288.

299. Cox JD, Byhardt R, Komaki R, et al. Interaction of thoracic irradiation and chemotherapy on local control and survival in small cell carcinoma of the lung. Cancer Treat Rep 1979;63:1251–1255.

300. Williams C, Alexander M, Glatstein EJ, et al. The role of radiation therapy in combination with chemotherapy in extensive oat cell cancer of the lung: A randomized study. Cancer Treat Rep 1977;61:142–143.

301. Choi NC, Carey RW. Importance of radiation dose in achieving improved loco-regional tumor control in limited stage small-cell lung carcinoma: An update. Int J Radiat Oncol Biol Phys 1989;17:307–310.

302. Coy P, Hodson I, Payne DG, et al. The effect of dose of thoracic irradiation on recurrence in patients with limited stage small cell lung cancer: Initial results of a Canadian multicenter randomized trial. Int J Radiat Oncol Biol Phys 1988;14:219–226.

303. Murray N, Coy P, Pater J, et al. The importance of timing for thoracic irradiation in the combined modality treatment of limited stage small cell lung cancer. Proc Am Soc Clin Oncol [Abstract] 1991;10:243.

304. McCracken JD, Janaki LM, Crowley JJ, et al. Concurrent chemotherapy/radiotherapy for limited small cell lung carcinoma: A Southwest Oncology Group study. J Clin Oncol 1990;8:892–898.

305. Arriagada R, Le Chevalier T, Ruffie P, et al. Alternating radiotherapy and chemotherapy in 173 consecutive patients with limited small cell lung carcinoma. Int J Radiat Oncol Biol Phys 1990;19:1135–1138.

306. Turrisi AT, Glover DJ, Mason BA. A preliminary report: Concurrent twice-daily radiotherapy plus platinum-etoposide chemotherapy for limited small cell lung cancer. Int J Radiat Oncol Biol Phys 1988;15:183–187.

307. Turrisi A, Wagner H, Glover D, et al. Limited stage small cell lung cancer: Concurrent BID thoracic radiotherapy with platinum-etoposide: An ECOG study. Proc Am Soc Clin Oncol [Abstract] 1990;9:230.

308. Livingston RB, Mira JG, Chen TT, et al. Combined modality treatment of extensive small cell lung cancer: A Southwest Oncology Group study. J Clin Oncol 1984;2:585–590.

309. Livingston RB, Schulman S, Mira JG, et al. Combined alkylators and multiple-site irradiation for extensive small cell lung cancer: A Southwest Oncology Group study. Cancer Treat Rep 1986;70:1395–1401.

310. Wilson RB, Mira JG, Chen TT, et al. Comparison of chemotherapy alone versus chemotherapy and radiation therapy of extensive small cell carcinoma of the lung. J Surg Oncol 1983;23:181–184.

311. Urtasun RC, Belch A, Bodnar D, et al. Radiation as a non-cross-resistant systemic agent: Experience with hemibody and total body irradiation in patients with small cell lung cancer. Cancer Treat Symp 1985;2:41–47.

312. Hüttner J, Wiener N, Quadt C, et al. A randomized clinical trial comparing systemic radiotherapy versus chemotherapy versus local radiotherapy in small cell lung cancer. Eur J Cancer Clin Oncol 1990;25:933–937.

313. Powell BL, Jackson DV, Scarantino CW, et al. Sequential hemibody irradiation integrated into a chemotherapy-local radiotherapy program for limited disease in small cell lung cancer. Int J Radiat Oncol Biol Phys 1986;12:1951–1956.

314. Byhardt RW, Cox JD, Wilson JF, et al. Total body irradiation vs. chemotherapy as a systemic adjuvant for small cell carcinoma of the lung. Int J Radiat Oncol Biol Phys 1979;5:2043–2048.

315. Dillman RO, Seagren SL, Taetle R. Failure of low-dose, total-body irradiation to augment combination chemotherapy in extensive-stage small cell carcinoma of the lung. J Clin Oncol 1983;1:242–250.

316. Hansen HH, Dombernowsky P, Hirsch FR, et al. Prophylactic irradiation in bronchogenic small cell anaplastic carcinoma: A comparative trial of localized versus extensive radiotherapy including prophylactic brain irradiation in patients receiving combination chemotherapy. Cancer 1980;46:279–284.

317. Komaki R, Cox JD, Whitson W. Risk of brain metastases from small cell carcinoma of the lung related to length of survival and prophylactic irradiation. Cancer Treat Rep 1981;65:811–814.

318. Rosen ST, Makuch RW, Lichter AS, et al. Role of prophylactic cranial irradiation in preventing central nervous system metastases in small cell lung cancer: Potential benefit restricted to patients with complete response. Am J Med 1983;74:615–624.

319. Hirsch FR, Paulson OB, Hansen HH, et al. Intracranial metastases in small cell carcinoma of the lung: Correlation of clinical and autopsy findings. Cancer 1982;50:2433–2437.

320. Aroney RS, Aisner J, Wesley MN, et al. Value of prophylactic cranial irradiation given at complete remission in small cell lung carcinoma. Cancer Treat Rep 1983;67:675–682.

321. Beiler DD, Kane RC, Bernath AM, et al. Low dose elective brain irradiation in small cell carcinoma of the lung. Int J Radiat Oncol Biol Phys 1979;5:944–945.

322. Cox JD, Petrovich Z, Paig C, et al. Prophylactic cranial irradiation in patients with inoperable carcinoma of the lung. Cancer 1978;42:1135–1140.

323. Eagan RT, Frytak S, Lee RE, et al. A case for preplanned thoracic and prophylactic whole brain radiation therapy in limited small cell lung cancer. Cancer Clin Trials 1981;4:261–266.

324. Jackson DV, Richards F, Cooper MR, et al. Prophylactic cranial irradiation in small cell carcinoma of the lung. JAMA 1977;237:2730–2733.

325. Katsenis AT, Karpasitis N, Giannakakis D, et al. Elective brain irradiation in patients with small cell carcinoma of the lung. In: Lung cancer: International Congress Series 558. Amsterdam: Excerpta Medica, 1982:277–284.

326. Seydel HG, Creech R, Pagano M, et al. Prophylactic versus no brain irradiation in regional small cell lung carcinoma. Am J Clin Oncol 1985;8:218–223.

327. Pedersen AG, Kristjansen PEG, Hansen HH. Prophylactic cranial irradiation and small cell lung cancer. Cancer Treat Rev 1988;15:85–103.

328. Baglan RJ, Marks JE. Comparison of symptomatic and prophylactic irradiation of brain metastases from oat cell carcinoma of the lung. Cancer 1981;47:41–45.

329. Lucas CF, Robinson B, Hoskin PJ, et al. Morbidity of cranial relapse in small cell lung cancer and the impact of radiation therapy. Cancer Treat Rep 1986;70:565–570.

330. Fleck JF, Einhorn LH, Lauer RC, et al. Is prophylactic cranial irradiation indicated in small-cell lung cancer? J Clin Oncol 1990;8:209–214.

331. Johnson BE, Becker B, Goff WB, et al. Neurologic, neuropsychologic, and cranial computed tomography scan abnormalities in 2–10 year survivors of small cell lung cancer. J Clin Oncol 1985;3:1659–1667.

332. Laukkanen E, Klonoff H, Allan B, et al. The role of prophylactic brain irradiation in limited stage small cell lung cancer: Clinical, neuropsychologic, and CT sequelae. Int J Radiat Oncol Biol Phys 1988;14:1109–1117.

333. Lee JS, Umsawasdi T, Lee Y, et al. Neurotoxicity in long-term survivors of small cell lung cancer. Int J Radiat Oncol Biol Phys 1986;12:313–321.

334. Johnson BE, Patronas N, Hayes W, et al. Neurologic, computed cranial tomographic, and magnetic resonance imaging abnormalities in patients with small-cell lung cancer: Further follow-up of 6- to 13-year survivors. J Clin Oncol 1990;8:48–56.

335. Turrisi AT. Brain irradiation and systemic chemotherapy for small-cell lung cancer: Dangerous liaisons? J Clin Oncol [Editorial] 1990;8:196–199.

336. Frytak S, Shaw JN, O'Neill BP, et al. Leukoencephalopathy in small cell lung cancer patients receiving prophylactic cranial irradiation. Am J Clin Oncol (CCT) 1989;12: 27–33.

337. Lennox SC, Flavell G, Pollock DJ, et al. Results of resection for oat cell carcinoma of the lung. Lancet 1968;2:925–927.

338. Taylor AB, Shinton NK, Waterhouse JAH. Histology of bronchial carcinoma in relation to prognosis. Thorax 1963;18:178–181.

339. Higgins GA, Shields TW, Keehn RJ. The solitary pulmonary nodule: Ten-year follow-up of Veterans Administration-Armed Forces cooperative study. Arch Surg 1975;110: 570–575.

340. Shields TW, Higgins GA, Matthews MJ, et al. Surgical resection in the management of small cell carcinoma of the lung. J Thorac Cardiovasc Surg 1982;84:481–488.

341. Meyer JA. Indications for surgical treatment in small cell carcinoma of the lung. Surg Clin North Am 1987;67:1103–1115.

342. Sridhar KS, Hussein AM, Thurer RJ. Evolving role of surgical treatment in limited disease small cell lung carcinoma. J Surg Oncol 1989;40:155–161.

343. Baker RR, Ettinger DS, Ruckdeschel JC, et al. The role of surgery in the management of selected patients with small cell carcinoma of the lung. J Clin Oncol 1987;5:697–702.

344. Hara N, Ohta M, Ichinose Y, et al. Influence of surgical resection before and after chemotherapy on survival in small cell lung cancer. J Surg Oncol 1991;47:53–61.

345. Johnson DH, Einhorn LH, Mandelbaum I, et al. Postchemotherapy resection of residual tumor in limited stage small cell lung cancer. Chest 1987;92:241–246.

346. Prasad US, Naylor AR, Walker WS, et al. Long term survival after pulmonary resection for small cell carcinoma of the lung. Thorax 1989;44:784–787.

347. Shepherd FA, Ginsberg RJ, Patterson GA, et al. A prospective study of adjuvant surgical resection after chemotherapy for limited small cell lung cancer: A University of Toronto Lung Oncology Group Study. J Thorac Cardiovasc Surg 1989;97:177–186.

348. Williams CJ, McMillan I, Lea R, et al. Surgery after initial chemotherapy for localized small cell carcinoma of the lung. J Clin Oncol 1987;5:1579–1588.

349. Karrer K, Shields TW, Denck H, et al. The importance of surgical and multimodality treatment for small cell bronchial carcinoma. J Thorac Cardiovasc Surg 1989;97:168–176.

350. Hayata Y, Funatsu H, Suemasu K, et al. Surgical indications in small cell carcinoma of the lung. Jpn J Clin Oncol 1978;8:93–100.

351. Macchiarini P, Hardin M, Basolo F, et al. Surgery plus adjuvant chemotherapy for $T_{1-3}N_0M_0$ small cell lung cancer. Am J Clin Oncol (CCT) 1991;14:218–224.

352. Østerlind K, Hansen M, Hansen HH, et al. Influence of surgical resection prior to chemotherapy on the long-term results in small cell lung cancer: A study of 150 operable patients. Eur J Cancer Clin Oncol 1986;22:589–593.

353. Shepherd FA, Evans WK, Feld R, et al. Adjuvant chemotherapy following surgical resection for small cell carcinoma of the lung. J Clin Oncol 1988;6:832–838.

354. Angeletti CA, Macchiarini P, Mussi A, et al. Influence of T and N stages on long term survival in resectable small cell lung cancer. Eur J Surg Oncol 1989;15:337–340.

355. Shepherd FA, Ginsberg R, Evans WK, et al. "Very limited" small cell lung cancer: Results of non-surgical treatment. Proc Am Soc Clin Oncol [Abstract] 1984;3:223.

356. Quoix E, Fraser R, Wolkove N, et al. Small cell lung cancer presenting as a solitary pulmonary nodule. Cancer 1990;66:577–582.

357. Warren WH, Memoli VA, Jordan AG, et al. Reevaluation of pulmonary neoplasms resected as small cell carcinoma: Significance of distinguishing between well-differentiated and small cell neuroendocrine carcinomas. Cancer 1990;65:1003–1010.

358. Holoye PY, McMurtrey MJ, Mountain CF, et al. The role of adjuvant surgery in the combined modality therapy of small-cell bronchogenic carcinoma after a chemotherapy-induced partial remission. J Clin Oncol 1991;8:416–422.

359. Prager RL, Foster JM, Hainsworth JD, et al. The feasibility of adjuvant surgery in limited-stage small cell carcinoma: A prospective evaluation. Ann Thorac Surg 1984;38: 622–626.

360. Meyer JA, Gullo JJ, Ikins PM, et al. Adverse prognostic effect of N2 disease in treated small cell carcinoma of the lung. J Thorac Cardiovasc Surg 1984;88:495–501.

361. Shepherd FA, Ginsberg RJ, Feld R, et al. Surgical treatment for limited small-cell lung cancer: The University of Toronto Lung Oncology Group experience. J Thorac Cardiovasc Surg 1991;101:385–393.

362. Lad T, Thomas P, Piantadosi S. Surgical resection of small cell lung cancer: A prospective randomized evaluation. Proc Am Soc Clin Oncol [Abstract] 1991;10:244.

363. Shepherd FA, Ginsberg R, Patterson GA, et al. Is there ever a role for salvage operations in limited small cell lung cancer? J Thorac Cardiovasc Surg 1991;97:177–1989.

364. Batist G, Carney DN, Cowan KH, et al. Etoposide (VP-16) and cisplatin in previously treated small-cell lung cancer: Clinical trial and in vitro correlates. J Clin Oncol 1986;4: 982–986.

365. Giaccone G, Donadio M, Bonardi G, et al. Teniposide in the treatment of small-cell lung cancer: The influence of prior chemotherapy. J Clin Oncol 1988;6:1264–1270.

366. Batist G, Ihde DC, Zabell A, et al. Small-cell carcinoma of the lung: Reinduction therapy after late relapse. Ann Intern Med 1983;98:472–474.

367. Ochs JJ, Tester WJ, Cohen MH, et al. "Salvage" radiation therapy for intrathoracic small cell carcinoma of the lung progressing on combination chemotherapy. Cancer Treat Rep 1983;67:1123–1126.

368. Choi NC, Propert K, Carey R, et al. Accelerated radiotherapy followed by chemotherapy for locally recurrent small cell carcinoma of the lung. Int J Radiat Oncol Biol Phys 1987;13:263–266.

369. McCracken JD, Heilbrun L, White J, et al. Combination chemotherapy, radiotherapy, and BCG immunotherapy in extensive (metastatic) small cell carcinoma of the lung. Cancer 1980;46:2335–2340.

370. McCracken JD, Chen T, White J, et al. Combination chemotherapy, radiotherapy, and BCG immunotherapy in limited small-cell carcinoma of the lung: A Southwest Oncology Group study. Cancer 1982;49:2252–2258.

371. Aisner J, Wiernick PH. Chemotherapy versus chemoimmunotherapy for small-cell undifferentiated carcinoma of the lung. Cancer 1980;46:2543–2549.

372. Jackson DV, Paschal BR, Ferree C, et al. Combined chemotherapy-radiotherapy with and without the methanol-extraction residue of bacillus Calmette-Guérin (MER) in small cell carcinoma of the lung. Cancer 1982;50:48–52.

373. Maurer LH, Pajak T, Eaton W, et al. Combined modality therapy with radiotherapy, chemotherapy, and immunotherapy in limited small-cell carcinoma of the lung: A Phase III Cancer and Leukemia Group B study. J Clin Oncol 1985;3:969–976.

374. Cohen MH, Chretien PB, Ihde DC, et al. Thymosin fraction V prolongs the survival of small cell lung cancer patients treated with intensive combination chemotherapy. JAMA 1979;241:1813–1815.

375. Scher HI, Shank B, Chapman R, et al. Randomized trial of combined modality therapy with and without thymosin fraction V in the treatment of small cell lung cancer. Cancer Res 1988;48:1663–1670.

376. Doyle A, Martin WJ, Funa K, et al. Markedly decreased expression of class I histocompatibility antigens, protein, and mRNA in human small-cell lung cancer. J Exp Med 1985;161:1135–1151.

377. Olesen BK, Ernst P, Nissen MH, et al. Recombinant interferon A (IFN-rA) therapy of small cell and squamous cell carcinoma of the lung: A Phase II study. Eur J Cancer Clin Oncol 1987;23:987–989.

378. Newman HFV, Bleehan NM, Galazka A, et al. Small cell lung carcinoma: A Phase II evaluation of r-interferon-Γ. Cancer 1987;60:2938–2940.

379. Mattson K, Niiranen A, Holsti L, et al. Low-dose of natural α-interferon as maintenance therapy for small cell lung cancer: A Phase III study. Proc Am Soc Clin Oncol [Abstract] 1989;8:227.

380. Shike M, Russell DM, Detsky A. Changes in body composition in patients with small cell lung cancer: The effect of total parenteral nutrition as an adjunct to chemotherapy. Ann Intern Med 1984;101:303–309.

381. Clamon GH, Feld R, Evans WK, et al. Effect of adjuvant central IV hyperalimentation on the survival and response to treatment of patients with small cell lung cancer: A randomized trial. Cancer Treat Rep 1985;69:167–177.

382. Zacharski LR, Henderson WG, Rickles FR, et al. Effect of warfarin on survival in small cell carcinoma of the lung: Veterans Administration Study 75. JAMA 1981;245: 831–835.

383. Chahinian AP, Propert KJ, Ware JH, et al. A randomized trial of anticoagulation with warfarin and of alternating chemotherapy in extensive small-cell lung cancer by the Cancer and Leukemia Group B. J Clin Oncol 1989;7:993–1002.

384. Nichols GL, Kelsen DP. Small cell carcinoma of the esophagus: The Memorial Hospital experience from 1970 to 1987. Cancer 1989;64:1531–1533.

385. Van der Gaast A, Verwey J, Prins E, et al. Chemotherapy as treatment of choice in extrapulmonary undifferentiated small cell carcinomas. Cancer 1990;65:422–424.

386. van Nagell JR, Powell DE, Gallion HH, et al. Small cell carcinoma of the uterine cervix. Cancer 1988;62:1586–1593.

387. Feun LG, Savaraj N, Legha SS, et al. Chemotherapy for metastatic Merkel cell carcinoma. Cancer 1988;62:683–685.

388. Østerlind K, Hansen HH, Hansen M, et al. Mortality and morbidity in long-term surviving patients treated with chemotherapy with or without irradiation for small-cell lung cancer. J Clin Oncol 1986;4:1044–1052.

389. Jacobs RH, Greenberg A, Bitran JD, et al. A ten-year experience with combined modality therapy for stage III small cell lung carcinoma. Cancer 1986;58:2177–2184.

390. Livingston RB, Stephens RL, Bonnet JD, et al. Long-term survival and toxicity in small cell lung cancer. Am J Med 1984;77:415–417.

391. Østerlind K, Hansen HH, Hansen M, et al. Long-term disease-free survival in small-cell carcinoma of the lung: A study of clinical determinants. J Clin Oncol 1986;4:307–1313.

392. Smith IE, Sappino P, Bondy P, et al. Long-term survival five years or more after combination chemotherapy and radiotherapy for small cell lung carcinoma. Eur J Cancer Clin Oncol 1981;17:1249–1255.

393. Vogelsang GB, Abeloff MD, Ettinger DS, et al. Long-term survivors of small cell carcinoma of the lung. Am J Med 1985;79:49–56.

394. Johnson BE, Grayson J, Makuch RW, et al. Ten-year survival of patients with small cell lung cancer treated with combination chemotherapy with or without irradiation. J Clin Oncol 1990;8:396–401.

395. Johnson BE, Ihde DC, Matthews MJ, et al. Non-small cell lung cancer: Major cause of late mortality in small cell lung cancer patients. Am J Med 1986;80:1103–1110.

396. Cortese D, Pairolero PC, Bergstralh EJ, et al. Roentgenographically occult lung cancer: A ten-year experience. J Thorac Cardiovasc Surg 1983;86:373–380.

397. Hong WK, Lippman SM, Itri LM, et al. Prevention of second primary tumors with isotretinoin in squamous-cell carcinoma of the head and neck. N Engl J Med 1990;323: 795–801.

Cancer: Principles & Practice of Oncology, Fourth Edition,
edited by Vincent T. DeVita, Jr., Samuel Hellman, Steven A. Rosenberg.
J.B. Lippincott Co., Philadelphia © 1993.

J. C. Rosenberg

CHAPTER **24**

Neoplasms of the Mediastinum

Within the past decade, there have been technical advances in the fields of diagnostic imaging, pathology, and therapeutic oncology that have significantly altered the management of mediastinal malignancies and rendered some of the approaches recommended in the older literature obsolete. These developments are discussed in this chapter.

One thing that has not changed is the manner in which these lesions present to the clinician. Approximately half of all mediastinal masses are asymptomatic and are discovered only if a chest roentgenogram is obtained for a reason unrelated to the mediastinal abnormality (Fig. 24–1).[1] Asymptomatic mediastinal masses are usually benign, and those that are symptomatic manifest themselves in a wide variety of ways (Table 24–1).[1-5] This chapter concentrates on mediastinal masses that are of neoplastic origin. Approximately 30% of primary mediastinal masses are malignant, and all, except thymomas and thymic carcinomas, occur elsewhere in the body and are dealt with in greater detail in other chapters.

ANATOMIC CONSIDERATIONS

The boundaries of the mediastinum are the diaphragm inferiorly, the parietal pleura laterally, the sternum anteriorly, the vertebral column and adjacent ribs posteriorly, and the thoracic outlet superiorly. The thoracic outlet is at the level of the first thoracic vertebra and the first ribs. The volume of space encompassed by these boundaries is not large, but it has a dense concentration of many different kinds of anatomic structures that can give rise to many different kinds of mass lesions and neoplasms (Tables 24–2 to 24–4).

Despite the small volume, it is clinically relevant to divide the mediastinum into compartments because of the constancy with which anatomic structures are located within specific areas of the mediastinum and the relatively high frequency with which different lesions occur within certain mediastinal areas. Recommendations for dividing the mediastinum into compartments are summarized in Fig. 24–2. It is not reasonable to set precise limits on each of these divisions, because the anatomic limits of the confined area we are dealing with are difficult to differentiate clinically. Many tumors extend beyond the limits of a single compartment and overlap other parts of the mediastinum, making it difficult sometimes to determine the primary site of the tumor.

The most constant association between the location of a mediastinal tumor and a division of the mediastinum can be found in the anterosuperior mediastinum, where 90% of thyroid masses, thymomas, and germ cell neoplasms (*e.g.,* teratomas) are located. Eighty percent of neurogenic tumors are located in the posterior mediastinum, and 50% of mediastinal lymphomas occur in the middle mediastinum. There is some indication that there has been an increase in the overall number of malignant tumors of the mediastinum during the last 25 years, and differences in the frequency of various tumors have been reported.[1-7] Considerable improvement in the treatment of these malignancies has corresponded with increased survival during this time. Mediastinal tumors and cysts in the adult are distributed throughout the mediastinal compartments in the following manner: 55% in the anterosuperior compartment, 20% in the middle mediastinum, 25% in the posterior compartment, and 5% cannot be reasonably localized.[5] In children, the posterior mediastinum contains 63% of the lesions; 26% occur in the anterior mediastinum, and 11% occur in the middle compartment.[6]

The relative frequency of tumors and cysts in a large combined group of patients is shown in Table 24–5 and is similar to another large series of patients reviewed by Cohen and colleagues.[1,4] Data such as these can be distorted if the criteria used for including lymphomas in the tabulations are not strict.

759

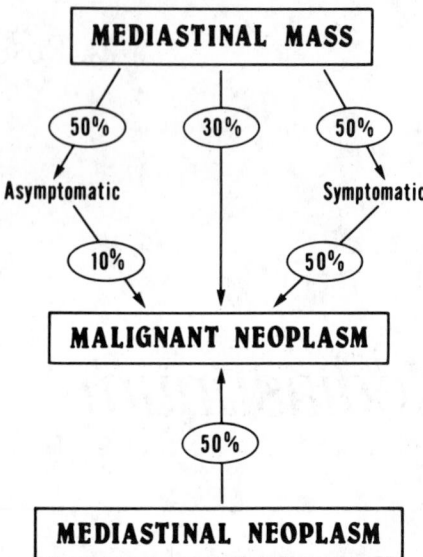

FIGURE 24–1. Symptomatic mediastinal masses are often malignant neoplasms. Half of all new growths of the mediastinum are malignant.

Only a lymphoma originating as a mediastinal mass should be considered a mediastinal tumor. Lymphomas with mediastinal involvement do not qualify as primary mediastinal neoplasms. Primary mediastinal lymphomas have some unique characteristics, but they are not sufficiently unique to merit separate consideration.[8,9] Table 24–6 lists the relative frequency of primary tumors in the anterior mediastinum in a combined series of 702 adults and 179 children.[7] The anterior mediastinum is the area with the highest number of mediastinal masses and the highest percentage of malignancies.

DIAGNOSIS

IMAGING TECHNIQUES

Roentgenographic examinations constitute the most important diagnostic studies that can be performed to define the location and extent of a mediastinal mass. Chest roentgenograms in posteroanterior and lateral projections can detect a mediastinal mass (Fig. 24–3). The value of comparing current films with previously obtained chest roentgenograms cannot be overemphasized. However, computed tomography (CT) using contrast enhancement is the best means of visualizing mediastinal tumors and is required for evaluating the abnormality seen on the chest roentgenogram.[10–17] Before the introduction of this valuable diagnostic tool in 1975, a long list of procedures were recommended and used to delineate a mediastinal mass.[10] They have all been replaced by CT of the mediastinum, which often can precisely identify the margins between the tumor and adjacent anatomic structures, defining the extent of involvement of the mediastinum by the tumor (Fig. 24–4).

Magnetic resonance imaging (MRI), unlike CT, can define vascular structures without the use of contrast material and

TABLE 24–1. Signs and Symptoms of Mediastinal Masses

Nonspecific
Chest discomfort—fullness, tightness, pain
Anorexia
Weight loss
Malaise

Secondary to Compression or Displacement of Adjacent Mediastinal Structures
Tracheobronchial compression—cough, wheezing, stridor, dyspnea, recurrent respiratory infections
Esophageal compression—dysphagia
Superior vena cava syndrome
Horner's syndrome
Vocal cord paralysis—dysphonia
Pulmonic stenosis—murmurs
Cardiac tamponade or arrhythmias

Secondary to Endocrine Function
Cushing's disease
Gynecomastia
Hypertension
Hypoglycemia

Systemic Syndromes
Thymoma*
  Myasthenia gravis
  Red cell aplasia
  Hypogammaglobulinemia
  Autoimmune diseases
Carcinoid of thymus
  Multiple endocrine abnormalities (type I)
  Cushing's syndrome
Neurofibroma
  Osteoarthritis
Lymphoma
  Alcohol-induced pain
  Fever
Teratoma
  Hypoglycemia—insulin-producing tumor

---

* See Table 24-7 for a complete list of systemic syndromes associated with thymomas.

---

can provide sagittal sections for further delineation of the anatomic associations of the tumor. It offers no other advantages and has the disadvantages of long scanning times, great expense, and limited availability.[14,15] However, the need to determine if the mediastinal mass in question is an aneurysm, hemangioma, or another form of vascular structure, such as a tortuous artery, cannot be overemphasized. MRI and arteriography assume greater importance in these situations.[15,16]

In the supraaortic, prevascular, pericardial, and paratracheal areas, sonography can be helpful in establishing the relation between the mass and the adjacent anatomy.[17]

If a thyroid scan is to be carried out to delineate a mass in the anterosuperior mediastinum, ^{131}I should be used rather

TABLE 24–2. Location of Anatomic Structures Within the Mediastinal Compartments

Superior Mediastinum

Transverse aorta and great vessels
Thymus gland

Anterior Mediastinum

Ascending aorta
Vena cava and azygos vein
Thymus gland
Lymph nodes
Fat and connective tissue

Posterior Mediastinum

Sympathetic chain
Vagus
Esophagus
Thoracic duct
Lymph nodes
Descending aorta

Middle Mediastinum

Heart and pericardium
Trachea and major bronchi
Pulmonary vessels
Lymph nodes
Fat and connective tissue

than technetium pertechnetate, which cannot identify mediastinal masses because of the high background of this nuclide in the vascular structures of the chest.[18] [131]I localizes in the thyroid in most patients with mediastinal thyroid tissue. As many as 10% of mediastinal masses may be goiters, 25% of which can be found in the posterior mediastinum.

ENDOSCOPY

Bronchoscopy and esophagoscopy should be performed if the radiographic abnormality could be caused by a lung or esophageal tumor or if symptoms suggest involvement of the aerodigestive tract in the mediastinum. The frequency of lung cancer requires that it be considered in patients with a mediastinal mass who have a history of smoking and who are 40 years of age or older. The role of mediastinoscopy in the evaluation of a mediastinal mass is discussed in the next section.

BIOPSY PROCEDURES

Palpable cervical or supraclavicular nodes should be biopsied. Mediastinoscopy and anterior mediastinotomy are worthwhile procedures if the mediastinal mass consists of enlarged lymph nodes that may be caused by lymphoma, metastatic cancer, or sarcoidosis. If lymph node biopsies are obtained, it is important that portions of the node be kept in sterile saline for culture and sensitivity studies for the determination of T-cell and B-cell subpopulations and for direct imprints. Biopsy of a mediastinal tumor by means of mediastinoscopy or anterior mediastinotomy is useful if resection of the mass is contraindicated because of its extent or the patient's general condition. However, mediastinal biopsies as isolated procedures may compromise an adequate resection if they are used routinely. This is especially true for thymomas. Germ cell tumors and lymphomas are not treated by excision as the primary therapy. Ferguson and colleagues emphasized the diminishing role of nonoperative therapy.[19] In their experience, 61% of anterior mediastinal masses did not require surgical therapy.

The dilemma of which lesions to biopsy and which to excise for diagnosis and therapy is being resolved by better localization techniques and interpretation of fine-needle aspiration cytologic preparations. Improved techniques and greater experience has rendered this procedure more accurate than it

TABLE 24–3. Mediastinal Masses and Their Distribution

Superior	*Anterior*	*Middle*	*Posterior*
Lymphomas	Lymphomas	Lymphomas	Neurogenic tumors
Thyroid masses	Teratomas	Bronchogenic cysts	Lymphomas
Thymic tumors or cysts	Thymic tumors or cysts	Pericardial cysts	Bronchogenic cysts
Thymoma	Thyroid masses	Sarcoidosis	Enteric cysts
Thymolipoma	Parathyroid tumors	Lipomas	Xanthogranulomas
Carcinoid	Germinal cell neoplasms	Lung cancers	Esophageal masses and diverticula
Lung cancers	Lung tumors	Plasma cell myeloma	Lung cancers
Parathyroid tumors	Lipomas	Vascular tumors	Thyroid masses
Aneurysm or ectasia of innominate or subclavian arteries	Lymphangiomas	Epicardial fat pads	Hiatal hernias
Myxomas	Fibromas	Hiatal hernias	Paravertebral abscesses
Cylindromas of trachea	Hemangiomas		Fibrosarcomas
Bronchogenic cysts	Chondromas		Meningoceles
Tumors arising in posterior mediastinum	Rhabdomyosarcomas		Myxomas
	Morgagni hernias		Chondromas
	Paragangliomas from carotid body		Pheochromocytomas
	Pericardial cysts		Aneurysms of descending aorta
	Lymph nodes		Enlargement of azygous and hemiazygous veins
			Thoracic duct cysts
			Tumors of spinal column

TABLE 24–4. Classification of Mediastinal Tumors

Neurogenic
Arising from peripheral nerves
   Neurofibroma
   Neurilemoma (Schwannoma)
   Neurosarcoma
Arising from sympathetic ganglia
   Ganglioneuroma
   Ganglioneuroblastoma
   Neuroblastoma
Arising from paraganglionic tissue
   Pheochromocytoma
   Chemodectoma (paraganglioma)

Thymic
Thymoma
Carcinoid
Thymolipoma

Lymphoma
Hodgkin's disease
Histiocytic lymphoma
Undifferentiated

Germ Cell Tumors
Seminoma
Nonseminomatous tumors
Pure embryonal cell
Mixed embryonal cell
   with seminomatous elements
   with trophoblastic elements
   with teratoid elements
   with entodermal sinus elements (yolk sac tumors)
Teratoma, benign

Aneurysms

Mesenchymal Tumors
Fibroma and fibrosarcoma
Lipoma and liposarcoma
Myxoma
Mesothelioma
Leiomyoma and leiomyosarcoma
Rhabdomyosarcoma
Xanthogranuloma
Mesenchymoma
Hemangioma
Hemangioendothelioma
Hemangiopericytoma
Lymphangioma
Lymphangiomyoma
Lymphangiopericytoma

Endocrine Tumors
Thyroid
Parathyroid

Cysts
Pericardial
Bronchogenic
Enteric
Thymic
Thoracic duct
Meningoceles

Hernias
Hiatal
Morgagni

Lymphadenopathy
Inflammatory
Granulomatous
Sarcoid

---

has been in the past. Fluoroscopic, CT, and ultrasonic guidance have been used to position the needle, which can be used to obtain tissue and cellular material.[20–22] These procedures interfere minimally with the ultimate resection of a malignancy and can be helpful in planning definitive surgical or nonsurgical therapy. Used in conjunction with electron microscopy and immunohistochemical studies, the sensitivity (*i.e.,* inversely related to the number of false negatives) can be in the range of 80%. Specificity (*i.e.,* inversely related to the number of false positives) is usually greater than 90%.

Ultimately, many mediastinal masses do require major surgery. Thoracotomy is required, using a median sternotomy or posterolateral incision. Large mediastinal masses that cause acute respiratory distress, especially in children, can present insurmountable problems during the induction of anesthesia and do not lend themselves to surgical therapy. These ad-

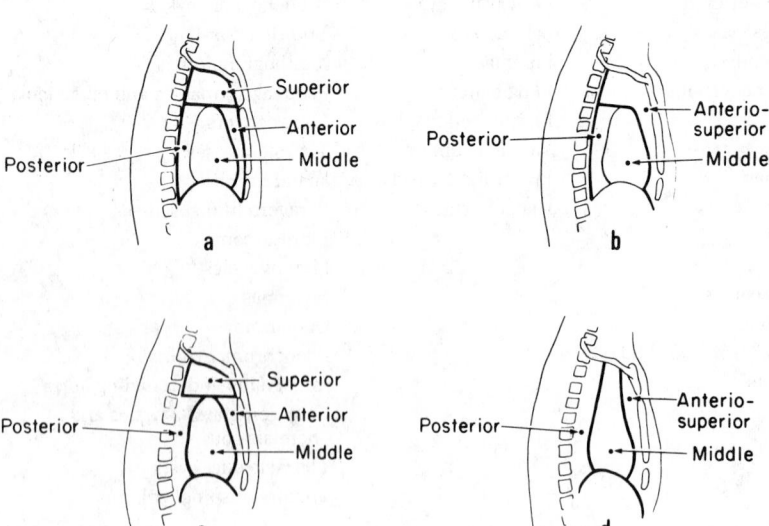

FIGURE 24–2. Recommendations for dividing the mediastinum into compartments.

TABLE 24–5. Relative Frequency (%) of Primary Mediastinal Tumors and Cysts

Tumor or Cyst	Adults (n = 1950)	Children (n = 437)
Neurogenic tumors	21	40
Thymomas	19	0
Lymphomas	13	18
Germ cell neoplasms	11	11
Mesenchymal tumors	7	9
Endocrine tumors (thyroid, parathyroid, and carcinoid)	6	0
Primary carcinomas	3	4
Cysts (pericardial, bronchogenic, enteric, and others)	20	18

(Silverman NA, Sabiston NC Jr. Mediastinal masses. Surg Clin North Am 1980;60:757)

TABLE 24–6. Relative Frequency (%) of Primary Anterior Mediastinal Tumors

Tumors	Adults (n = 702)	Children (n = 179)
Thymic lesions (cysts, hyperplasia, and thymoma)	47	17
Germ cell neoplasms	15	24
Lymphomas	23	45
Endocrine tumors (thyroid and parathyroid)	16	0
Mesenchymal tumors	0	15

(Mullen B, Richardson JD. Primary anterior mediastinal tumors in children and adults. Ann Thorac Surg 1986;42:338)

vanced lesions are best treated by chemoradiation, even in the absence of a tissue diagnosis. Even if tissue can be obtained, the biopsy specimen of a mass that cannot be completely removed occasionally leaves the pathologist confused if light microscopy alone is relied on. Electron microscopy and immunohistochemical studies are often required to define the true nature of the neoplasm. Accurate frozen-section diagnoses during the operation can be even more difficult to make and may mislead the surgeon to overtreat or undertreat the tumor.

HORMONAL ASSAYS AND TUMOR MARKERS

Hormonal assays and the determination of tumor markers are valuable in selected patients. Pheochromocytomas and some neurogenic tumors (*e.g.,* paragangliomas) are accompanied by elevated urinary catecholamine, homovanillic acid, or vanillylmandelic acid levels. Germ cell tumors, teratomas, and some carcinomas elaborate glycoproteins that act as oncofetal antigens (*e.g.,* carcinoembryonic antigen, α-fetoprotein). Chorionic gonadotropin levels may be elevated in some pa-

tients with germ cell tumors. These markers are most valuable in following patients after treatment and are less useful as diagnostic studies.

THYMIC NEOPLASMS

Several malignancies can arise from the tissue elements that make up the thymus, such as lymphomas, thymomas, germ cell tumors, carcinoids, and carcinomas. Benign neoplasms are also possible, although they occur less frequently than the cancers. The thymoma, thymic carcinoma, and thymolipoma are the only neoplasms found exclusively in the thymus.

THYMIC DEVELOPMENT AND FUNCTION

Although the fully developed thymus is considered a lymphatic organ, its embryologic origins are from the endoderm as epithelial outgrowths of the lower portion of the third pharyngeal pouches on each side. The upper parts of the third pharyngeal pouches give rise to the parathyroid glands that migrate into the neck. The right and left thyroid anlagen descend into the mediastinum to become a bilobed glandular structure that varies greatly in shape and size.[23,24]

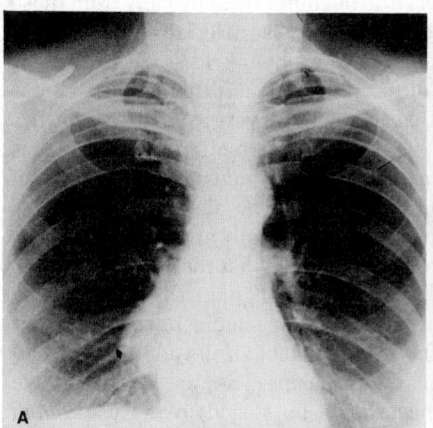 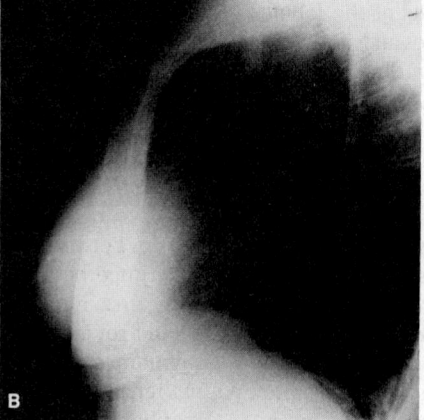 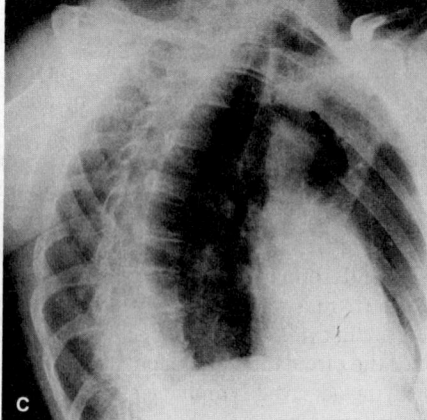

FIGURE 24–3. **(A)** Posteroanterior, **(B)** lateral, and **(C)** oblique views of an anterior mediastinal mass that was found to be an encapsulated thymoma on exploration of the mediastinum (see Fig. 24–4).

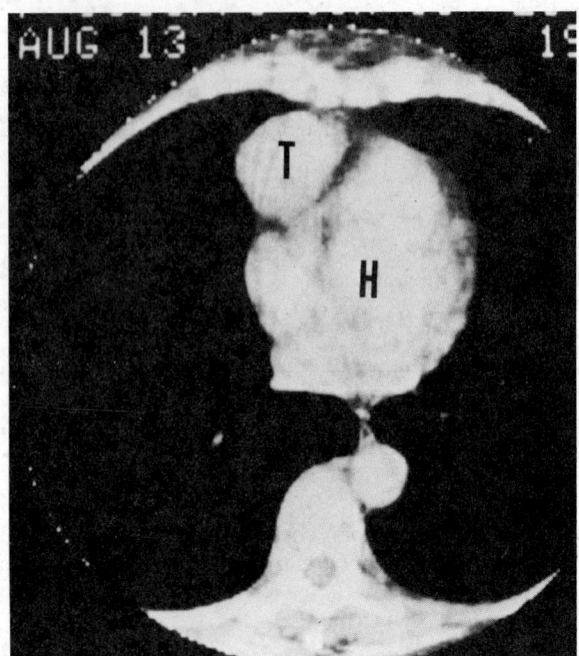

FIGURE 24–4. Computed tomography of the patient with the thymoma depicted in Figure 24–3. The thymoma (*T*) is located immediately anterior to the base of the heart (*H*).

The cords of epithelial cells that initially make up the thymus grow out into the surrounding mesenchyma. These cords subsequently constitute the medullary areas of the lobules of the thymus. The epithelial cells in the cords spread out to form a reticulum but never lose contact with each other. In some areas, the epithelial cells pile up and undergo keratinization and degeneration, forming distinctive structures known as the Hassall corpuscles. These structures are found in the medulla of the lobules.

As the epithelial cords proliferate and send out side branches into the mesenchyma, lymphocytes appear within the spaces between the epithelial cells of the cortex of the lobules. These lymphocytes are derived from hematopoietic stem cells that arise in the bone marrow and migrate to the thymus. The stem cells are concentrated in the periphery of the cortex of the thymic lobules. They give rise to the smaller lymphocytes located in the deeper cortex of the lobule and fill the spaces between the epithelial cells. Medullary areas of the lobules in the mature thymus contain few lymphocytes and are largely epithelial in character. Germinal centers and lymphoid follicles are normally lacking in the thymus.[25]

The process of lymphoblastic differentiation into mature lymphocytes requires humoral factors produced by the epithelial cells of the thymus. One preparation of the hormone (*i.e.*, thymosin) is a polypeptide that can support the development of precursor lymphocytes into thymocytes.

The differentiation of human lymphoblasts into thymocytes by the thymus takes place in fetal and early postnatal life. The thymocytes in the deeper cortex of the thymic lobules enter the circulation and populate all of the lymphatic tissue as thymus-derived lymphocytes (*i.e.*, T lymphocytes). They have characteristic surface markers and specialized immunologic functions but are morphologically similar to the other major subpopulations of lymphocytes.

Congenital absence of the thymus (DiGeorge's syndrome) or its removal early in life results in a deficiency of cellular immune function. Thymectomy in the adult decreases immunologic competence, but because the half-life of thymus-derived lymphocytes in humans is several years, the decrease in immunologic function due to the loss of T lymphocytes is gradual and less evident than when the thymus is removed at birth or shortly thereafter.

Although mature thymus glands vary greatly in size and shape, the size usually correlates well with the age of the patients. The thymus gland reaches a maximum size of 30 to 40 g in the adolescent, but its greatest size relative to the rest of the body is attained at approximately 4 years of age. After puberty, the thymus gradually involutes, and the lymphoid component disappears. The parenchyma is largely replaced by fat. The Hassall corpuscles remain to identify the gland, and the thymus never completely disappears.

In the adult, the thymus is usually beneath the upper part of the sternum. Its lower tip may end at any point between the first intercostal space and the costal cartilage of the seventh rib. In two thirds of the patients studied by Bell and colleagues, the caudal extent of the thymus was between the third and fourth ribs.[23] Almost all of the glands terminated above the xyphoid. The thoracic portion of the thymus is usually thickest where it rests on the pericardium. The cervical extent of the thymus is usually the least distinct of the gland's margins. The upper end of the thymus blends imperceptibly into the cervical fat and may extend up to the level of the sixth cervical vertebra. Thymic tissue can also be found in the anterior mediastinal and retrocarinal adipose tissue, which may explain the few ectopic thymomas and the failure of some patients with myasthenia gravis to respond to thymectomy.[26]

THYMOMA

The epithelium of the thymus is the site of origin of thymomas. Lymphocytic elements may be present and even dominate the histologic appearance of a thymoma, but it is always the epithelial elements that give rise to this tumor.[27] It is composed of bland cells that do not have the cytologic features of a malignancy.[25,28] However, some thymomas invade the surrounding tissues and metastasize to sites within the chest. Rarely do they spread to other organs. The tumors that are invasive and metastasize do not differ histologically from those that are encapsulated and noninvasive. Electron microscopic, immunohistochemical, and morphometric studies have not revealed consistent differences between thymomas that are invasive and those that are not. However, a distinction has been made between "benign" and "malignant" thymomas based on whether there is gross or microscopic evidence of invasion, although there is a consistent, albeit small, number of "benign" thymomas that recur locally and regionally (Fig. 24–5). Because there is no evidence that there is an intrinsic difference between benign and malignant thymomas other than invasiveness, this distinction should be discarded. It should replaced by the more clinically relevant view that all thymomas are malignant neoplasms. They are not aggressive malignancies, but they should be staged in the traditional manner of malignant tumors.

Staging should be based on the anatomic extent of involvement, as determined clinically and histopathologically. Local,

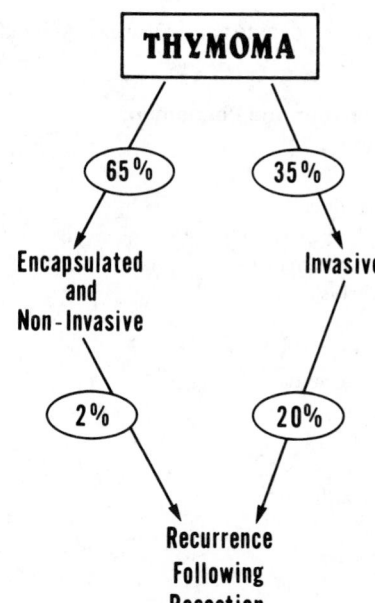

FIGURE 24–5. Although rates vary from series to series, approximately two thirds of thymomas are ``benign.'' The recurrence rate after removal of these tumors is low, unlike the higher recurrence rate after resection of invasive thymomas.

regional, and distant involvement should be specified rather than describing the tumors as as benign or malignant. Noninvasive and invasive thymomas are a reasonable way of describing thymomas, but the following staging system, modified by Masaoka and colleagues after one originally proposed by Bergh, is more precise and has gained wide acceptance since being introduced in 1981:[29,30]

Stage I	Intact capsule; no capsular invasion microscopically
Stage II	Macroscopic or microscopic invasion into or through the capsule into the surrounding fatty tissue or mediastinal pleura
Stage III	Invasive growth by direct extension into the pericardium, great vessels, or lungs
Stage IVA	Pleural or pericardial implants
Stage IVB	Lymphogenous or hematogenous metastasis

Pathology

The cut surface, traversed by fibrous septa, is usually fleshy and lobulated. Cystic areas are seen in 40% to 60% of specimens.[25,28]

Several classifications of thymomas have been devised based on the histopathology of these tumors. Rosai and Levine have reviewed this aspect of thymomas completely in their monograph, and the subject has been recently summarized by Walker et al.[25,28] The simplest classification designates three cell types, based on the predominant cell comprising the tumor. If 67% to 80% of the tumor consists of lymphocytes or epithelial cells, it is classified as lymphocytic or epithelial, respectively.[25,28] If these two cellular elements occur in equal numbers, the tumor is called mixed or lymphoepithelial. In

all instances of thymoma, the number of mitotic figures seen is low, regardless of the invasiveness of the tumor.[25,31–37]

The most common epithelial cell is a plump polygonal cell with a moderate amount of clear cytoplasm and a round nucleus. Some epithelial cells are spindle shaped with an elongated nucleus. If the spindle cell predominates, the thymoma is referred to as a spindle cell thymoma. Approximately one third of thymomas are lymphocytic. The other two thirds of thymomas are roughly equally distributed among the epithelial, lymphoepithelial, and spindle cell varieties. Some studies indicate that patients with epithelial and lymphoepithelial thymomas have lower survival rates than patients with lymphocytic or spindle cell varieties and are more likely to also have myasthenia gravis and other systemic syndromes.[34]

Another classification of thymomas is based on their postulated ontogeny. A cortical thymoma is one that is composed of the kind of polygonal cells that resemble those found in the cortex of the normal thymus. Spindle cells are thought to represent the neoplastic equivalents of normal thymic medullary cells, and if they predominate, the tumors are called medullary thymomas. Lesions containing both cell types are known as mixed corticomedullary thymomas. According to this classification, which places little emphasis on the lymphocytic component of the tumor, most thymomas are of the mixed type and, like the cortical thymomas, are associated with a poorer prognosis and a higher frequency of systemic syndromes.[38] There has been some enthusiasm about the prognostic value of this classification, especially if combined with the previously described staging system, which has not been universally shared because of the variability of histologic appearances in thymomas.[39,40]

Electron microscopic studies of the neoplastic cells reveal that they have the characteristic features of epithelial cells: prominent cytoplasmic processes, desmosomes, and cytoplasmic tonofilaments. Attention has recently focused on immunohistochemical studies of thymomas. Studies of lymphocytes have substantiated the nonneoplastic nature of these cellular elements.[27,41] The thymic epithelium expresses thymic hormones, HLA antigens, acetylcholine receptor epitopes, and cytokeratins. Recognition of the latter moieties in lymphocyte-predominant tumors can help to diagnose a thymoma. Flow cytometry and morphometry have provided insights into the biology of neoplastic thymic cells, but with inconclusive results. The tumor's invasiveness, confirmed histopathologically, remains the best indication of its malignant potential.

Thymomas are slow-growing tumors. Some have stayed the same size for as long as 15 years.[25] The most common form of metastatic involvement is the occurrence of pleural or pericardial implants. They are thought to result from the shedding of tumor cells from the primary thymoma. Metastases to regional nodes or distant organs is uncommon. Isolated reports of extrathoracic spread have mentioned the liver, bone, colon, kidney, brain, extrathoracic lymph nodes, and spleen.

Clinical Findings

Fortuitous discovery of a thymoma after a chest roentgenogram is obtained for reasons unrelated to the tumor occurs in 30% to 40% of patients with this neoplasm. Patients are usually between 40 and 60 years of age. Thymomas are more aggressive in children than in adults but rarely occur in the pediatric age group. There is little difference in the frequency with which men and women are affected, although some series report a slightly increased incidence among women.

Seventy-five percent of tumors develop in the anterior mediastinum, and they are the neoplasms most frequently found in this compartment. Approximately 15% occupy the anterior and superior mediastinum, and 6% are primarily in the superior mediastinum. No more than 5% to 10% of thymomas occur in other locations, such as the head and neck and middle and posterior mediastinum.

The lesion is characteristically located anterior to the junction of the ascending aorta with the heart. The great vessels may be displaced posteriorly by the tumor. More than 90% of the tumors can be seen on standard chest roentgenograms. Thymomas are round or oval with smooth or lobulated margins. The mass may protrude to one or both sides of the mediastinum, and calcifications may be seen in 20% of them.

CT is indispensable if a thymoma is suspected. It allows precise definition of the extent of involvement of the suspected thymoma (see Fig. 24–4). Cysts can be differentiated from solid tumors, and pleural and pericardial implants can be identified. MRI does not add significantly to the information gained by CT.[10]

Nonspecific symptoms characteristic of all mediastinal masses, such as cough, dyspnea, dysphagia, chest tightness, and chest pain, may occur. Chest pain may be a sign of an advanced malignant lesion. A superior vena cava syndrome may also result from an advanced lesion.

The most striking clinical manifestations of a thymoma are the systemic syndromes that can be anticipated in at least half of the patients with this neoplasm.

Thymoma-Associated Systemic Syndromes

The systemic syndromes that may be associated with a thymoma are listed in Table 24–7. Their occurrence often leads to the discovery of the tumor. Only the three most common are discussed here.

Because the parathyroid and thymus glands are derived from the third pharyngeal pouches, the group at the Mayo Clinic thought it would be reasonable to compare the incidence of diseases associated with thymomas and parathyroid adenomas, with the latter acting as a control group.[42] They reviewed the cases of 146 of their own patients with thymoma and 452 found in the literature with sufficient data to evaluate whether an associated disease occurred. The incidence of other diseases with thymoma was 71%, compared with a 12% incidence among 177 patients with parathyroid adenomas. The diseases associated with thymomas were categorized (see Table 24–7).

In some patients, more than one disease was associated with the thymoma, such as myasthenia gravis and thrombocytopenia. Almost 70% of the patients with a thymoma and other diseases had immunologic disorders. Approximately 10% had a malignancy and 5% had an endocrine disorder. The remaining 15% had severe infections or other seemingly unrelated conditions, such as megaesophagus. The most frequent association was between thymoma and myasthenia gravis. Thirty percent to 50% of patients with thymoma had myasthenia gravis. Some of the endocrine disorders, such as

TABLE 24–7. Syndromes and Diseases Associated With Thymomas

Autoimmune or Immune Phenomena

Myasthenia gravis
Cytopenias
Hypogammaglobulinemia
Polymyositis
Systemic lupus erythematosus
Rheumatoid arthritis
Thyroiditis
Sjögren's syndrome
Chronic ulcerative colitis
Pernicious anemia
Raynaud's disease
Regional enteritis
Rheumatic endocarditis
Sarcoid
Dermatomyositis
Scleroderma
Takayasu's syndrome

Endocrine Disorders

Hyperthyroidism
Addison's disease
Panhypopituitarism

Nonthymic Cancer

Severe Infections and Miscellaneous Diseases

Myocarditis
Megaesophagus
Chronic macrocutaneous candidiasis
Other

Cushing's syndrome, are concomitants of a carcinoid tumor of the thymus, which may be mistakenly diagnosed as a thymoma.

MYASTHENIA GRAVIS. The pathophysiologic characteristics of myasthenia gravis are the rapid exhaustion of voluntary muscular contractions and a slow return to a normal state. Repetitive stimulation of the motor nerve to a muscle in patients with myasthenia gravis results in progressive decrement of muscle action potentials. The major symptoms of patients with this disease are weakness and fatigue. Another characteristic is that these symptoms are relieved by drugs that inhibit acetylcholinesterase, an enzyme located within the synaptic junction (*i.e.*, end plate) between the motor neuron and striated muscle.

The disease is an abnormality of neuromuscular transmission caused by the autoimmune destruction of the acetylcholine receptors in the postsynaptic villi of voluntary muscle.[43,44] The immune response eliminates acetylcholine receptors and impairs postsynaptic structure and function. Patients with myasthenia gravis have 70% to 90% fewer acetylcholine receptors per neuromuscular junction than do normal people. Because there are fewer functioning acetylcholine receptors within the end plate of patients with myasthenia gravis, acetylcholine is less effective in transmitting the signal from nerve to muscle. The presence of antibodies to the receptors is diagnostic for myasthenia. Antistriated muscle antibodies are found in about a third of patients with myasthenia. They do not appear to be involved in the pathogenesis of the disease, but they are good markers for a possible thymoma.

An association between the thymus and myasthenia gravis was first suspected when pathologic changes were found in the thymus gland of 75% to 85% of patients with this neuromuscular disease (Fig. 24–6).[45] Germinal centers are not normally present in the thymus gland, but 70% of patients with myasthenia gravis and thymic abnormalities demonstrate this form of thymic lymphoid (follicular) hyperplasia. It is characterized by germinal center proliferation in the medullary and cortical areas of the thymus without necessarily increasing the gross appearance or weight of the thymus. Thymic hyperplasia may be difficult to detect by CT. It may require measuring the thickness of the thymic lobes to determine if they are within normal limits.

Approximately 15% of patients with myasthenia have gross or microscopic (occult) thymomas, depending on the frequency with which patients with myasthenia gravis have thymectomy or have an autopsy to search for the lesion. CT detects virtually all but the microscopic thymomas.

The association of the thymus, thymomas, and myasthenia gravis remains an enigma despite all that has been learned in the past decade. A virally induced "thymitis" could trigger the process in which antigenic components within the thymus are recognized by the T lymphocytes and the antigens cross-react with acetylcholine receptors.

Thymomas in patients with myasthenia gravis are usually smaller than those found in nonmyasthenic patients. This finding may be an artifact of serendipitous discovery when the thymus is removed. Invasive thymomas are in fewer myasthenic than nonmyasthenic patients.

There are no morphologic or immunohistochemical parameters of a thymoma that are specific for the concomitant or subsequent occurrence of myasthenia gravis, but some features are more frequently associated with myasthenia. Myasthenia gravis is more likely to accompany epithelial and lymphoepithelial lesions rather than spindle cell thymomas, but red cell aplasia is more likely to be associated with the spindle cell thymoma. Using the Marino Müller-Hermelink classification results in the finding that the cortical and mixed corticomedullary thymomas are more frequently associated with myasthenia than are the pure medullary thymomas.[38] Another pathologic feature of myasthenia gravis is the high frequency of lymphoid follicles with germinal centers in the thymic tissues surrounding the thymoma.

Myasthenia gravis is twice as common in young women (<40 years) than in men. In older patients, the distribution between the sexes favors the men. Patients with thymomas and the syndrome tend to be older (15–35 years) than myasthenic patients without thymoma. The response rate to thymectomy in the younger women with thymoma and myasthenia is better (60%) than in the older men (25%) with the same association of diseases.

A patient with a thymoma and myasthenia gravis has a poorer prognosis than a myasthenia patient without a thymoma, because improvement in muscle strength after thymectomy can be anticipated in only 25% of patients with myasthenia gravis and a thymoma, but a 40% to 60% response rate can be expected for myasthenia patients without thymomas. Approximately 20% of patients who respond have complete remissions. The remainder are improved. The salutary effect of thymectomy may be due to the removal of the source of antigenic stimulation to the production of antiacetylcholine receptors. Because significant improvement of myasthenic patients is seen after receiving immunosuppressive drugs, it is also possible that removal of the thymus benefits patients by virtue of an immunosuppressive effect.[46]

RED CELL APLASIA. Pure red cell aplasia is considered an autoimmune disorder and can be found in 5% of patients with thymomas. It is uncommon for myasthenia gravis and hypogammaglobulinemia to also exist in these patients, but such combinations have been reported. A third to half of the patients with red cell aplasia have thymomas.[47] This syndrome appears after the age of 40 in 96% of these patients. The diagnosis is based on examination of the bone marrow. Erythrocyte precursors are absent, but platelet and leukocyte elements are usually normal. An associated decrease in the number of platelets or leukocytes occurs in 30% of patients with red cell aplasia. Thymectomy has produced remissions of the disease in 38% of patients. The relation between thymoma and red cell aplasia is not understood.[48]

HYPOGAMMAGLOBULINEMIA. This abnormality occurs in 5% to 10% of patients with thymoma.[40] Patients with hypogammaglobulinemia have a 10% incidence of thymoma. More than a third of the patients also have red cell hypoplasia. Combined humoral and cellular immunodeficiencies exist, and thymectomy has not proved beneficial in this condition.

Treatment of Thymoma

SURGERY. Because of the propensity of thymomas to recur or develop local metastases after the integrity of the capsule is violated, incisional biopsies of these tumors should be

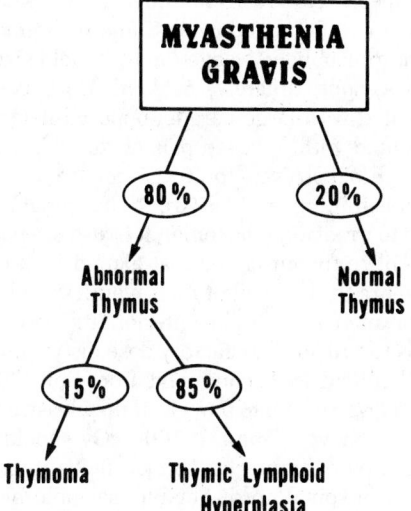

FIGURE 24–6. Thymic abnormalities are frequent in patients with myasthenia gravis. Thymic lymphoid hyperplasia and thymoma may exist in the same patient.

avoided. Incisional biopsy should be reserved for the patient who is unable to tolerate a resection or who has a tumor that cannot be removed because of its local extension into vital structures. Fine-needle aspiration cytology has not compromised curative resection and is an excellent alternative to incisional biopsy.

The most effective therapy of a thymoma is its complete removal. If a thymoma is encapsulated (stage I), it can easily be removed with the entire thymus without disturbing the integrity of the capsule. The thymus and surrounding tissue should be removed with every thymoma. Virtually all patients with stage I thymomas are cured of the tumor. No more than 2% develop recurrences, which usually take the form of pleural, pericardial, or diaphragmatic implants or of a localized mediastinal tumor.[36]

An aggressive surgical approach demands wide resection of invaded structures for stage II and III thymomas. Every effort should be made to preserve the phrenic nerves. Bilateral phrenic nerve interruption can be disastrous for a patient with myasthenia gravis. Pericardium, pleura, diaphragm, and lung should be resected if these structures are involved. Lobectomy or pneumonectomy may be required, depending on specific circumstances and extent of involvement. Resection of the innominate vein and portions or all of the superior vena cava has been performed because these vessels were invaded.[49] A patch of autogenous vein or prosthetic material or a vascular graft of Teflon or Dacron can bridge the resulting venous defect, with the expectation of a good functional result. If extensive involvement precludes complete resection (*e.g.*, invasion of the heart, great vessels, or trachea), as much tumor as can be safely resected should be removed to prevent cardiac tamponade or tracheal occlusion and asphyxiation.

Resection should also be undertaken for recurrences within the chest, and the same aggressive approach recommended for primary resections should be adopted.

A median sternotomy provides the best exposure of the anterior mediastinum for resecting the thymus and a thymoma unless the tumor is dominant in one of the thoracic cavities, for which standard right or left lateral thoracotomies are preferable. A bilateral submammary incision transecting the sternum may provide a more cosmetic result, but the exposure this incision provides is not optimal, and it may be more difficult to deal adequately with invasive lesions. The poor exposure provided by a cervical incision renders this approach unsatisfactory for the resection of a thymoma, although it has been used to perform a thymectomy if a thymoma is not thought to be a possibility.[50] The occurrence of myasthenia gravis after thymectomy for thymoma is related to recurrent disease or residual thymic tissue, emphasizing the importance of carrying out a thorough excision of this gland if a patient with myasthenia is to have a thymectomy. Monden and colleagues showed that the palliation and remission rates of myasthenia among patients with thymomas are significantly greater for extended thymectomy than for the more limited procedure.[51] Because radiation therapy for thymoma may be followed by clinical worsening of myasthenic symptoms, this adjuvant modality cannot be relied on to improve the results of thymectomy if the patient has myasthenia.[52]

The intricacies of managing the myasthenic patient's respiratory problems intraoperatively and postoperatively require an experienced, well-trained team of neurologists,

anesthesiologists, surgeons, and intensivists. Improved management of this phase of the procedure is responsible for reducing the mortality from a high of 27% to the current rate of less than 6%.[53]

RADIATION THERAPY. Thymomas are relatively radiosensitive. Postoperative radiation therapy constitutes excellent adjuvant therapy and is considered mandatory for all patients with invasive thymomas, with or without complete resection.[54–59] A review of the literature revealed that the recurrence rate was 28% for total resection of invasive thymomas not treated with postoperative radiotherapy. The recurrence rate was only 5% if postoperative irradiation was employed for a similar group of tumors.[54] Because these data are not from a prospective randomized study nor a meta-analysis, the low recurrence rate after irradiation could be influenced by the large number of patients with noninvasive thymomas. Nonetheless, there is general agreement that postoperative radiation therapy is beneficial, and the surgeon should therefore mark off the extent of the resected tumor and thymus with metallic radioopaque clips after performing a resection to facilitate treatment planning by the radiotherapist.

There is some disagreement concerning the role of adjuvant radiotherapy for patients with encapsulated noninvasive thymomas. Because the recurrence rate is approximately 2% and radiotherapy carries some morbidity, Rosai and Levine oppose the use of postoperative radiotherapy if these tumors are removed in toto.[25] At the other extreme is the view that no patient with thymoma can be considered to have been adequately treated unless he or she receives radiotherapy.[37] Preoperative radiation therapy was used by several groups with equivocal benefits. Efforts are underway to render unresectable thymomas resectable by using irradiation in combination with chemotherapy, with some encouraging results.

Radiotherapy as adjuvant therapy, as treatment of recurrences, or as treatment for unresectable primary thymomas usually consists of 3500 to 5000 cGy given over 3 to 6 weeks. Dosages in excess of 5000 cGy do not significantly increase response rates but do increase the risk of postirradiation complications if large fields are used. Doses greater than 4500 cGy require special care to avoid injury to the spinal cord. If the tumor is small, Penn and Hope-Stone recommend using two large anterior oblique wedge fields.[56] Field size in their experience was approximately 15×8 cm. More extensive lesions are treated with large parallel opposed fields that can be supplemented with a wedge pair or an additional direct anterior field. Field sizes up to 20×15 cm are used. The use of angled fields minimizes exposure to the spinal cord.[57]

In addition to irradiating the tumor, it is also often important to treat the entire thymus gland that extends from the sixth cervical vertebra to the level of the seventh costal cartilage. Skeggs recommends a single anterior and two posterior oblique fields to provide satisfactory dose distribution.[58]

Marks and colleagues recommend a dose of 4000 cGy to the tumor bed given over 4 to 5 weeks if the invasive thymoma is completely removed. The last 1000 cGy should be given by means of a pair of anterior oblique fields to reduce the total dose to the spinal cord. For unresectable or partially resected disease, a dose of 4500 cGy administered in 5 to 6 weeks is recommended. Shrinking fields should be used as the tumor responds. A split course of irradiation should be considered for large tumors to spare the spinal cord.[59] This approach has resulted in complete local tumor control in 9 patients when used in conjunction with resection.

Pneumonitis is a frequent (40%) side effect of radiotherapy after large fields are used.[56] To minimize radiation damage to the lungs in patients with pleural implants, Ariartnam and colleagues use a moving strip technique.[55] Mediastinitis, pericarditis, and myocarditis are additional but infrequent complications of thymic irradiation if unresectable or residual thymomas require large fields and high doses. If unresectable or residual tumors are carefully marked during resection, it should be possible to treat a small tumor volume to a high dose without undue complications.

CHEMOTHERAPY. Until recently, there was little experience with chemotherapy in the treatment of thymomas. Corticosteroids, alkylating agents, cisplatin, and doxorubicin have been used as single agents with modest results.[60]

Daugaard and colleagues reported complete responses that lasted a median of 37 months in 4 of 9 patients treated with vincristine, cyclophosphamide, lomustine, and prednisone. The overall response rate was 56%.[61] Partial remissions have been reported by others using combinations of cyclophosphamide and vincristine.[62] Chemotherapy combinations using doxorubicin and cisplatin yield higher response rates than other regimens. Response rates in the range of 70% can be expected, and half are complete responses.[63–68]

Thirty-two patients with stage III or IV invasive thymoma had a 91% overall clinical response rate and a 47% complete clinical remission rate using a 4-day course of cisplatin (50 mg/m^2) and doxorubicin (40 mg/m^2) on day 1, vincristine on day 3 (0.6 mg/m^2), and cyclophosphamide on day 4 (700 mg/m^2).[63] A median of five courses of therapy was administered. Complete responses were confirmed in 5 of 7 patients who underwent thoracotomy after the chemotherapy. The oncologists are now using this regimen preoperatively for all patients with thymomas.

Three cycles, 3 weeks apart, of cisplatin and epirubicin (75 and 100 mg/m^2, respectively) on day 1 and etoposide (120 mg/m^2) on days 1, 3, and 5 produced responses in all of the 7 patients with stage III thymomas who were treated. All subsequently underwent resection and postoperative radiation therapy.[69]

A neoadjuvant protocol for locally advanced unresectable or recurrent thymoma currently being tested in conjunction with radiotherapy and surgery by Komaki and colleagues with the Radiation Therapy Oncology Group uses three cycles of cyclophosphamide, doxorubicin, cisplatin, and prednisone (CAPPr regimen) at 3-week intervals. A dose of 500 mg of cyclophosphamide is given as an intravenous bolus on day 1. Doxorubicin (20 mg/m^2) and cisplatin (30 mg/m^2) are given intravenously on days 1 through 3. Prednisone (100 mg) is given orally on days 1 through 5.

RESULTS OF THERAPY. Masaoka and colleagues reported 5- and 10-year overall survival rates of 74% and 57%, respectively. Patients who underwent a total resection of the tumor had a 5-year survival rate of 89%. Five-year survival correlated with the stage of disease: stage I, 93%; stage II, 86%; stage III, 70%; stage IV, 50%.[29] An analysis of prognostic factors from the same institution 4 years later indicated that

an overall recurrence or persistence rate of 19% did not depend on age or sex but was lower in patients with myasthenia (11% versus 31%).[70] This association was generally true for tumors of the same stage. Recurrence rates increased as the stage of the disease increased.

Verley's report of the experience of a clinic in France revealed survival rates of 85% and 80% at 5 and 10 years, respectively.[37] Patients with invasive tumors had a survival rate of approximately 50% at 5 years and 35% at 10 years. Associated autoimmune diseases had no influence on survival. All patients were treated with irradiation postoperatively. Recurrences were found in 6% of patients with noninvasive tumors and in 36% of patients with invasive tumors.

In a series of 241 patients, 66% of whom had myasthenia gravis, the 5- and 10-year survival rates were 81% and 76%, respectively.[71] Survival was significantly higher ($p < 0.05$) for tumor patients with myasthenia (85% versus 78% at 5 years). This is a reversal of what was reported in the older literature, reflecting improvements in the care of patients with myasthenia gravis. Patients with other autoimmune manifestations had lower survival rates than the rest of the group.

The experiences at the Massachusetts General Hospital and Toronto General Hospital reflect the change in prognosis for patients with thymomas and myasthenia gravis. The overall 5- and 10-year survival rates for a group of 85 patients reported by Wilkins was 87% and 64%, respectively. The 10-year actuarial survival rate for thymoma patients with myasthenia gravis was 72%.[72] The overall 5-year survival rate at the Toronto General Hospital for patients without myasthenia was 71%. For patients with myasthenia, it was 92%.[73] The overall 5- and 10-year survival rates for the 283 patients reported from the Mayo Clinic was 67% and 53%, respectively.[74]

THYMIC CARCINOMA

Because thymic carcinomas most commonly occur in the anterosuperior compartment of the mediastinum, they were thought to arise from thymic epithelium or embryonic nests within the thymus. Several reviews of patients with this diagnosis support the view that these cancers arise from thymic epithelium but are far more malignant than thymomas that are also derived from thymic epithelium.[38,75] The cancers show frequent mitoses, nuclear atypia, polygonal cells, and spindle cells.

Thymic carcinomas are highly lethal and differ from thymomas morphologically and biologically. They should not be classified with the thymomas nor referred to as undifferentiated thymomas despite the fact that about half are highly undifferentiated. The others have adenocarcinomatous, sarcomatous (*i.e.*, spindle cell), or squamous cell appearances.

Lymphoepithelioma-like carcinomas similar to those seen in the nasopharynx have occurred in the thymus. The two neoplasms may have a common cause. Epstein-Barr viral (EBV) penetration and replication is thought to take place in the epithelial elements of the thymus and in the epithelial cells of the nasopharyngeal lymphoid tissue. A patient with a thymic carcinoma of the lymphoepithelioma type had the serologic profile of EBV, EBV-associated nuclear antigens in the carcinoma cells, and a high level of viral genomes of EBV detected in the DNA. All of this indicates that EBV is involved in the genesis of some thymic carcinomas and some undifferentiated nasopharyngeal carcinomas.[76] A link to EBV cannot be demonstrated in all lymphoepithelioma-like thymic carcinomas.[28,77] Unlike patients with the same tumor in the nasopharynx, patients with this cancer in the mediastinum fare poorly.

All of the variants of thymic carcinoma are highly lethal and should be approached aggressively by all modalities of therapy. A combination of cisplatin, vinblastine, and bleomycin has been effective in the treatment of thymic carcinomas.[78]

CARCINOID OF THE THYMUS

Until 1972, many carcinoid tumors of the thymus were not recognized as distinct lesions and were mistakenly labeled as variants of thymomas.[25,79–81] They have a similar morphology and similar malignant potential, and they respond to the same therapy, which probably accounts for the confusion between carcinoids and thymomas. However, significant morphologic and immunochemical differences exist between these two tumors, and they can now be readily differentiated.

Wick and Rosai consider this tumor to be derived from cells of the "diffuse neuroendocrine system" and classify the neoplasm with other mediastinal tumors such as intrathymic parathyroid tumors, oat cell carcinomas, and juxtavascular or paraspinal paragangliomas.[81,82] As of 1980, approximately 100 thymic carcinoids were reported.[80] Their gross appearance is similar to that of thymomas. The tumors are not usually encapsulated and may invade adjacent structures. Fibrous compartmentalization and cystic changes seen in thymomas do not occur in thymic carcinoids. The two tumors may have similar appearances by light microscopy, but electron microscopy and immunohistochemical studies can accurately differentiate carcinoid tumors from thymomas.

Carcinoid tumors are characterized by numerous cytoplasmic nonsecretory granules, as are other foregut carcinoids. Thymomas have desmosomes, tonofilaments, and elongated cytoplasmic processes not seen in carcinoids. Carcinoids contain argyrophil cells that can be detected by appropriate staining techniques. Invasiveness is seen in 50% of thymic carcinoids, compared with 35% of thymomas. Thymomas rarely have extrathoracic metastases, but thymic carcinoids metastasize to lymph nodes, bone, and other sites in as many as 70% of patients. The bone metastases are often osteoblastic. Metastases may appear as late as 8 years after initial diagnosis.[66]

Thymic carcinoids have been classified among the amine precursor uptake and decarboxylation tumors (*i.e.*, APUDomas), which are known to have the potential of elaborating peptide, amines, kinins, and prostaglandins.

The most frequent endocrine syndrome reported to be directly caused by thymic carcinoids is Cushing's syndrome. In these instances, the carcinoid produces elevated levels of ACTH that is not suppressible by exogenous dexamethasone and can therefore be confused with idiopathic adrenocortical hyperplasia or pituitary adenomas. Carcinoids of the thymus can produce calcitonin. Patients with the carcinoid syndrome caused by thymic carcinoids are extremely rare. Only 35% of carcinoid tumors of the thymus demonstrate endocrine activity or are part of a heredofamilial endocrine syndrome.[81] Patients with thymic carcinoids have been described with type I multiple endocrine neoplasias (MEN I; Werner's syndrome; pituitary, parathyroid, and pancreatic islet cell tumors). In two thirds of these patients the carcinoids showed a high degree of malignant potential. Carcinoid tumors of the thymus can coexist with medullary carcinomas of the thyroid (MEN II; Sipple's syndrome; medullary carcinoma of the thyroid; pheochromocytoma; and hyperparathyroidism).

Carcinoid tumors of the thymus are treated by wide excision of the thymus containing the tumor. The resection should include contiguous invaded structures that can be sacrificed or replaced. Postoperative radiation therapy is recommended for patients with persistent or recurrent tumor, but the therapeutic effects of irradiation and chemotherapy are uncertain.[81]

THYMOLIPOMA

Thymolipoma (*i.e.*, lipothymoma), a rare, benign neoplasm, is a curious mixture of fat and hyperplastic thymic tissue. Both components are present in increased amounts, resulting in an enlargement of the thymus gland so that its weight usually exceeds 500 g, 10 times the normal weight of the thymus.[25] Twenty-five percent of these tumors weigh more than 2000 g. The mass usually drapes itself around the heart, producing the radiographic appearance of cardiomegaly. This lesion is not merely a lipoma involving the thymus gland, because the normal thymic tissue is also hyperplastic and is interspersed with the fat. However, the thymus component has none of the characteristics of a thymoma, and thymolipomas have never been reported to recur after removal.

GERM CELL TUMORS

Extragonadal germ cell tumors are also covered in Chapter 37, which deals with testicular tumors. All types of germinal tumors found in the testes have been reported in the mediastinum. Approximately 10% of all mediastinal tumors are of germinal origin, and they are second only to thymomas in frequency. Only 1% of germ cell tumors are found in the mediastinum.

HISTOGENESIS

Extragonadal germ cell tumors usually develop along the body midline in the cranium, the mediastinum, and the retroperitoneal and presacral areas. The histogenesis of these tumors is uncertain. Those arising within the thymus presumably originate from germ cells that migrated into this gland during embryogenesis. Because the urogenital ridge extends from C6 to L4, its juxtaposition to the thymic anlage favors this possibility. However, the germ cells migrate posteriorly along the midline rather than anteriorly, and primordial germ cells in the absence of a germ cell neoplasm have not been found in the thymus.[83] Another possible origin of germ cell tumors is the maldevelopment of thymic anlage during embryogenesis or potentially biphasic germ cells left within the thymus or anterior mediastinum. These benign and malignant tumors of germ cell origin may have nothing to do with the thymus, but by convention, they have been classified with tumors of the thymus. Residual thymic tissue may be found surrounding benign teratomas, and malignant lesions usually obliterate all evidence of the thymus, making it difficult to ascertain the exact relation between these tumors and the thymus.[83]

There is always the possibility that a germ cell tumor of the mediastinum is not a primary lesion but represents a metastasis from a testicular or ovarian cancer. However, autopsies of patients with primary germ cell tumors of the mediastinum have enabled pathologists to examine multiple sections of the patients' gonads, and no evidence of testicular or ovarian involvement has been found in most patients with mediastinal germ cell tumors. Occasionally, there is evidence of an occult neoplastic lesion in the testes or scarring that could represent a primary germ cell tumor that had undergone spontaneous regression.[83,84] Other autopsies of patients with germ cell tumors of the testes have shown that metastases solely to the anterior mediastinum occur rarely. If anterior mediastinal metastases from a testicular tumor exist, middle and posterior mediastinal lymph nodes are also usually involved.[85]

There is an association between mediastinal germ cell neoplasms and Klinefelter's syndrome (*i.e.*, gynecomastia, testicular atrophy, increased levels of follicle-stimulating hormone). The karyotype characteristic of Klinefelter's syndrome, 47,XXY, was found in 4 of 22 patients with primary mediastinal germ cell tumors, although this karyotype is usually seen in only 1 of 600 newborn males.[86] Patients with Klinefelter's syndrome and germ cell tumors are generally diagnosed in the second rather than third decade of life.

Patients with mediastinal germ cell tumors, particularly nonseminomatous tumors containing yolk sac elements, have a higher incidence of hematologic neoplasms. These were originally thought to occur as a result of chemotherapy. The hematologic abnormalities appear to arise from the same malignant progenitor cell that gives rise to the germ cell tumor. Cytogenetic studies have revealed a high frequency of a single copy of isochrome 12p in these patients.[87]

INDICATIONS FOR TESTICULAR BIOPSY

In the past, it was recommended that the testes of all patients with mediastinal germ cell tumors be removed or biopsied to exclude the possibility of occult testicular primaries giving rise to mediastinal metastases. If a mass is palpated in the testes of a young male patient with an anterior mediastinal tumor, these procedures are indicated. A testicular biopsy is also indicated if CT demonstrates involvement of pelvic or retroperitoneal lymph nodes or if an isolated retroperitoneal germ cell tumor is discovered. However, testes that are normal on physical examination and on high-resolution ultrasonography need not be removed nor explored if a mediastinal germ cell tumor is found.[88]

CLASSIFICATION SYSTEMS

Several classifications of germ cell tumors have been devised, but none are satisfactory for the extragonadal varieties, because few mediastinal germ cell tumors are composed of a single type of cell. Most are mixtures of various kinds of germ cells. The seminomas are an exception. They can exist as a pure seminoma, but there are often seminomatous elements in embryonal carcinomas, teratocarcinomas, choriocarcinomas, and endodermal sinus tumors (*e.g.*, yolk sac tumors).

The most clinically relevant classification is one that divides germ cell tumors into pure primary seminomas or nonseminomatous tumors, recognizing that in the latter group seminomatous elements may exist with other cell types. Nonseminomatous tumors may also include germ cell neoplasms that are predominantly of one or another of the types of germ cell tumors listed previously. This classification system separates the tumors on the basis of their biologic behavior, response to therapy, and prognosis. Pure seminomas are less malignant, are far more radiosensitive, and have a better prognosis than mixed nonseminomatous tumors.

SEMINOMA

Primary pure seminomas (*e.g.*, dysgerminoma, germinoma) comprise half of all germ cell tumors of the mediastinum and occur principally in men 20 to 40 years of age. No more than 5% of these tumors occur in women.[89] The tumors usually cause symptoms by impinging on structures in the anterior mediastinum. Chest pain is the most common symptom, but cough, dyspnea, and superior vena cava obstruction can also occur. Approximately 20% of patients may be asymptomatic.[90] Chest roentgenograms usually reveal an anterior mediastinal mass with smooth, lobulated borders.

In a few patients, other germ cell elements occur in the malignancy in small amounts, resulting in mildly elevated levels of α-fetoprotein or β-chorionic gonadotrophin. If the levels are very high, the pathologic diagnosis of nonseminomatous tumor of the mixed type should be considered.

Most patients with mediastinal seminoma have extensive involvement of the great vessels when they are first seen. Only 20% of the tumors could be completely excised in the patients reported by the Memorial Hospital and the Mayo Clinic.[85,91] The role of preoperative cytoreductive surgery (*i.e.*, debulking) for mediastinal seminomas is questionable. If performed, it should be conservative and not add to the morbidity and mortality of the disease.

Because this tumor is extremely radiosensitive, local disease can usually be controlled with radiotherapy. The excellent response of seminomas to radiation therapy contrasts with the nonseminomatous germ cell tumors, which are relatively radioresistant. In a determination of the contribution of radiotherapy to outcome, 13 of 27 patients with pure seminomas had a 100% actuarial 5-year survival, but the survival of patients with other germ cell histologies was 8.8%.[92]

Radiation therapy should be administered by a shaped mediastinal field, using a midplane dose of up to 4500 cGy over 5 to 6 weeks.[93] This dose is larger than that recommended for gonadal seminomas, because it is the experience of some radiotherapists that lower doses may result in a higher frequency of local recurrences.[93] A split course of therapy with interruption after approximately 2000 to 3000 cGy is a possible alternative. A more conservative dose of approximately 3500 cGy has been recommended by others.[91,92]

Because the supraclavicular, infraclavicular, and low cervical lymph nodes can be easily included in the field of radiation, these areas should be treated as well. Prophylactic irradiation of the upper abdominal and paraaortic lymph nodes is recommended by some groups but deemed unnecessary by others.

Most patients with mediastinal seminomas present with bulky primary tumors and metastatic disease. Involvement of lymph nodes, bone, liver, spleen, tonsil, thyroid, skin, and the central nervous system has been reported. Patients with advanced disease should be treated with cisplatin-based combination chemotherapy in the same manner as patients with nonseminomatous germ cell tumors, and like the nonseminomatous cancers, excellent responses can be anticipated. Combination chemotherapy with vinblastine, bleomycin, and cisplatin (VBP regimen), with or without doxorubicin, can induce complete remissions (58%) and long-term disease-free survival.[94] It has been recommended that patients with extragonadal seminomas be treated initially with high-dose cisplatin-containing combination chemotherapy followed by surgical resection of any residual disease.[95] This approach has merit for treating locally advanced tumors.

Surgery plus irradiation produces 5-year survival rates of 58% to 82% for patients with limited disease.[93,94,96] Patients with advanced seminomas treated initially with chemotherapy and subsequently with surgery and chemotherapy also fare well, although long-term results are not available. Of 11 patients so treated, 10 had complete responses, 6 of which were confirmed postoperatively.[95]

NONSEMINOMATOUS PURE AND MIXED GERM CELL CARCINOMAS

Mixed nonseminomatous germ cell tumors can contain any combination of seminomatous, embryonal, endodermal sinus, teratomatous, or trophoblastic elements. The latter cell type has the appearance and functional characteristics of a choriocarcinoma. Alternatively, the nonseminomatous germ cell tumor can consist predominantly of one of these cell types. Teratocarcinomas can be cystic or solid and usually contain elements of embryonal cell carcinoma. Other malignant components, such as adenocarcinoma, squamous cell carcinoma, and sarcoma, may be present.[97]

Like seminomas of the mediastinum, this is a disease of young men. Pleuritic or substernal pain with dyspnea, cough, and hemoptysis are frequent presenting symptoms. Gynecomastia occurs in 33% to 50% of men with choriocarcinoma. Elevated levels of β-chorionic gonadotrophin may exist with choriocarcinoma and can be used to evaluate the efficacy of therapy and detect early recurrences and metastases. Elevated levels of β-chorionic gonadotrophin occur in 60% of patients with nonseminomatous germ cell tumors.

Serum levels of α-fetoprotein and carcinoembryonic antigen may be helpful in a similar fashion. If the tumors demonstrate a predominant pattern of endodermal sinus elements, serum α-fetoprotein levels are likely to be high. Approximately 70% of patients with nonseminomatous germ cell tumors have elevated levels of α-fetoprotein.

The mainstay of therapy for nonseminomatous germ cell tumors is intensive chemotherapy. VBP with or without doxorubicin resulted in complete remissions in approximately 65% of patients with nonseminomatous germ cell tumors. Patients with choriocarcinomas and pure endodermal sinus tumors had the poorest responses.[98] The most important prognostic indicator for mediastinal endodermal sinus tumors is whether they can be completely excised before or after chemotherapy.[99] Failure of tumor markers to return to normal after chemotherapy is another poor prognostic sign. A multimodality approach is currently recommended for mediastinal nonsem-

inomatous germ cell tumors. After intensive cisplatin-based chemotherapy with emphasis on normalizing serum tumor markers, aggressive resection of residual disease should be undertaken. This therapeutic regimen resulted in a 57% 5-year survival rate at Indiana University.[100]

BENIGN TERATOMAS IN ADULTS

Teratomas are true neoplasms that originate in pluripotent cells and are not to be considered malformations. They are composed of a wide diversity of tissues foreign to the organ or site in which they arise. Histologically, they are characterized by mature forms of one or more representative tissues from each of the embryonic germ layers of ectoderm, endoderm, and mesoderm.[25,83] Lesions that are cystic and contain hair and teeth have been called dermoid cysts. The tumors are most common in young adults, and unlike the malignant germ cell tumors, benign teratomas occur with equal frequency in both sexes.

After the gonads, the mediastinum is the second most frequent location of teratomas in adults. In children, the sacrococcygeal area is the most frequent site of teratomas, followed by the mediastinum. Mediastinal teratomas are most often found in the anterosuperior compartment, at the junction of the heart and the great vessels. Calcifications occur in 75% of the lesions. Occasionally, teratomas can be found in the pericardium or posterior mediastinum.

Most patients with teratomas are asymptomatic. Symptoms are usually caused by the large size of the tumor and compression of adjacent structures. Erosion into a bronchus is a uncommon complication, as is rupture into the pericardium. Insulin production by a teratoma may produce hypoglycemia.

Benign teratomas are easily excised after exposing them through a midline sternotomy or standard posterolateral thoracotomy.

NEUROGENIC TUMORS

Neurogenic tumors vie with thymomas as the most common neoplasm of the mediastinum in adults and are the most common neoplasms in children (see Table 24–5).[1,3,5,101]

HISTOGENESIS

Neural crest tissue gives rise to the nerve cells and the supporting sheath cells (*i.e.*, Schwann cells) that surround them. If Schwann cells undergo malignant transformation, they are called neurilemomas or schwannomas. Neurofibromas arise from Schwann cells, but contain neuronal elements as well.

Embryologists have been able to delineate several cell types as the neural crest cells progress into neurones (*i.e.*, ganglion cells). Sympathogonia are the first kinds of cells that can be recognized. Next in the progression are neuroblasts, the cells of origin of neuroblastomas. Neuroblasts can become a sympathicoblast or a pheochromocyte. The latter give rise to pheochromocytomas (*i.e.*, chromaffin positive) and paragangliomas or chemodectomas (*i.e.*, chromaffin negative). Sympathicoblasts give rise to ganglioneuroblastomas. Malignant neuroblastomas and ganglioneuroblastomas spontaneously revert to the benign, more differentiated ganglioneuroma in 25% of patients.

NEURILEMOMAS AND NEUROFIBROMAS

Neurilemomas (*i.e.*, schwannomas) and neurofibromas can arise from the intercostal nerves or the sympathetic ganglia in the posterior mediastinum. The vagus and phrenic nerves are rarely the sites of these neoplasms. Neurilemomas and neurofibromas make up at least 65% of all mediastinal neurogenic tumors, and approximately 65% to 75% are found in the upper half of the chest and on the right side.

The pathologist may have difficulty differentiating neurilemomas and neurofibromas. Occasionally, these tumors are mistaken for low-grade sarcomas. Electron microscopy and immunohistochemical staining reveal their neurogenic origin.[102] A type of neurilemoma characterized as a cellular neurilemoma may appear malignant but does not metastasize and only infrequently recurs.[103] In most series, neurilemomas predominate over neurofibromas and are considered the most frequently encountered neurogenic tumor.[104] Ganglioneuromas may have a histopathologic picture similar to nerve sheath tumors.

From 25% to 40% of patients with nerve sheath tumors have multiple neurofibromatosis (*i.e.*, von Recklinghausen's disease). If a patient with von Recklinghausen's disease presents with a posterior mediastinal mass, it is more likely to be a meningocele than a posterior mediastinal neurofibroma.

Neurilemomas and neurofibromas of the posterior mediastinum are readily removed surgically. In 10% of patients, they may extend through an intervertebral foramen and assume a dumbbell shape. Sixty-five percent of these patients have signs of spinal cord compression. Roentgenologic studies demonstrating erosion of vertebral pedicles or enlargement of the intervertebral foramina adjacent to a posterior mediastinal mass suggest the possibility of a dumbbell-shaped neurogenic tumor. A myelogram or MRI scan can establish whether there is an intraspinous component of the tumor.[105]

Neurofibrosarcomas and malignant neurilemomas constitute 10% to 20% of the tumors and are more frequently seen in patients with von Recklinghausen's disease. These lesions carry a poor prognosis. Recurrences may occur even if the lesion is originally thought to be benign. Patients operated on for neurogenic tumors should be followed closely for many years.[104] Resection of the tumor may be performed by two separate incisions, one for laminectomy and the other for thoracotomy, or by a combined approach. The spinal component should be dealt with first to minimize bleeding into the spinal canal. If this occurs with compression of the spinal cord, the patient can become paraplegic.

TUMORS OF NERVE CELLS

Neuroblastomas and ganglioneuroblastomas are poorly differentiated malignant tumors found predominantly in children (see Chapter 49). If occurring in the posterior mediastinum, their treatment is the same as for those encountered elsewhere in the body. These tumors are often unresectable.

The benign ganglioneuroma is easily excised at the time of thoracotomy.

Intrathoracic pheochromocytomas do not differ from those arising in the abdomen.

Paragangliomas of the mediastinum share many characteristics with neuroendocrine tumors like carcinoids. They can be classified into two types. Paravertebral paragangliomas are found in the posterior mediastinum and occur in patients at an average age of 29; 60% affect males.[83] Almost half of these tumors synthesize catecholamines. Aorticopulmonary paragangliomas are found in the anterior mediastinum in older patients (average age of 49) and demonstrate a slight predilection for women. Only 3% of these paragangliomas synthesize catecholamines. Aorticopulmonary paragangliomas are more invasive and have a poorer prognosis than those located in the posterior mediastinum. About half of patients with mediastinal paragangliomas die of the disease.[106] Paragangliomas that are more aggressive have the same pathologic picture as those that do not metastasize, and all paragangliomas should be considered malignant tumors that grow slowly and can recur or metastasize after many years. They should be removed as completely as possible. Recurrences may respond to radiation therapy.

SOFT TISSUE TUMORS

Most of the connective tissue tumors found in the soft tissues and discussed in Chapter 42 can also be found in the mediastinum.[1] They constitute 6% to 7% of mediastinal neoplasms. About half of these tumors are malignant. Benign tumors are permanently eradicated by surgical excision. Malignant mesenchymal tumors should be treated as other soft tissue sarcomas are, with combinations of excision, irradiation, and chemotherapy.

Seventy-five percent of mediastinal lipomas are located anteriorly and may present the same roentgenographic appearance as a pericardial cyst in the right cardiophrenic angle. Large lipomas can extend into adjacent mediastinal compartments in an unpredictable manner. Liposarcomas tend to occur in the posterior mediastinum, where they may be confused with neurogenic tumors and rare xanthogranulomas. Lipomatous tumors can be readily recognized by CT.

Mediastinal lymphangiomas can be difficult tumors to completely excise because they can become densely adherent to the great vessels and other mediastinal structures.[102] They are most often found in the anterior mediastinum.

Mesotheliomas may present as a mediastinal mass arising from the pleura or pericardium. If they are localized, resection is curative. Diffuse invasive lesions have a poor prognosis. Histologic criteria cannot predict the behavior of the tumor.

Mediastinal hemangiomas are rare lesions that have been reported in more than 100 patients.[107] They can be found in the anterosuperior or posterior mediastinum. CT and MRI reveal enhancing masses but are nondiagnostic for hemangiomas. Although successful subtotal resection of these tumors has been performed, the possibility of massive hemorrhage during the procedure should not be considered lightly. These tumors can invade contiguous structures, and total excision can be hazardous. Local recurrences are possible, but there has been no evidence of malignant degeneration of these slow-growing, benign tumors. Most of them remain stable without continued local invasion. Radical excision of these tumors is therefore not justifiable unless life-threatening hemorrhage has occurred.

REFERENCES

1. Silverman NA, Sabiston DC. Mediastinal masses. Surg Clin North Am 1980;60:757.
2. Adkins RB, Maples MD, Hainsworth JD. Primary malignant mediastinal tumors. Ann Thorac Surg 1984;38:648.
3. Wychulis AR, Payne WS, Clagett OT, et al. Surgical treatment of mediastinal tumors. J Thorac Cardiovasc Surg 1971;62:379.
4. Cohen AJ, Thompson L, Edwards FH, Bellamy RF. Primary cysts and tumors of the mediastinum. Ann Thorac Surg 1991;51:378.
5. Davis RD, Oldham HN, Sabiston DC. Primary cysts and neoplasms of the mediastinum: Recent changes in clinical presentation, methods of diagnosis, management and results. Ann Thorac Surg 1987;44:229.
6. Grosfeld JL, Weinberger M, Kilman JW, et al. Primary mediastinal neoplasms in infants and children. Ann Thorac Surg 1971;12:179.
7. Mullen B, Richardson JD. Primary anterior mediastinal tumors in children and adults. Ann Thorac Surg 1986;42:338.
8. Lichtenstein AK, Levin A, Taylor CR, et al. Primary mediastinal lymphomas in adults. Am J Med 1980;68:509.
9. Strickler JG, Kurtin PJ. Mediastinal lymphoma. Semin Diagn Pathol 1991;8:2.
10. Brown K, Aberle DR, Batra P, Steckel RJ. Current use of imaging in the evaluation of primary mediastinal masses. Chest 1990;98:467.
11. Pugatch RD, Foling LJ. Computed tomography of the thorax: A status report. Chest 1981;80:618.
12. Spizarny DL, Rebner M, Gross BH. CT evaluation of enhancing mediastinal masses. J Comput Assist Tomogr 1987;11:990.
13. Miller GA, Heaston DK, Moore AV, et al. CT differentiation of thoracic aneurysm from pulmonary masses adjacent to the mediastinum. J Comput Assist Tomogr 1984;8:437.
14. Webb WR, Gamou G, Stark DD, et al. Evaluation of magnetic resonance sequences in imaging mediastinal tumors. Am J Radiol 1984;143:525.
15. von Shulthess GK, McMurdo K, Tscholakoff D, et al. Mediastinal masses: MR imaging. Radiology 1986;158:289.
16. Schurawitzki H, Stiglbauer R, Klepetko W, Eckersberger F. CT and MRI in benign mediastinal hemangioma. Clin Radiol 1991;43:91.
17. Wernecke K, Vassallo P, Potter R, Luckner HG, Peters PE. Mediastinal tumors: Sensitivity of detection with sonography compared with CT and radiography. Radiology 1990;175:137.
18. Irwin RS, Braman SS, Arvanitidis AN, et al. Thyroid scanning in preoperative diagnosis of mediastinal goiter. Ann Intern Med 1978;89:73.
19. Ferguson MK, Lee K, Skinner DB, Little AG. Selective operative approach for diagnosis and treatment of anterior mediastinal masses. Ann Thorac Surg 1982;44:583.
20. Sawkney S, Jain R, Berry M. Tru-cut biopsy of mediastinal masses guided by real-time sonography. Clin Radiol 1991;44:16.
21. Herman SJ, Holub RV, Weisbrod GL, Chamberlain DW. Anterior mediastinal masses: Utility of transthoracic needle biopsy. Radiology 1991;180:167.
22. van Sonnenberg E, Lin AS, Deutsch AL, Mathey RF. Percutaneous biopsy of difficult mediastinal, hilar, and pulmonary lesions by computed tomographic guidance and a modified coaxial technique. Radiology 1983;148:300.
23. Bell RH, Knapp BI, Anson BJ, et al. Form, size, blood supply and relations of the adult thymus. Q Bull Northwest Univ Med School 1954;28:156.
24. Sloan HE Jr. The thymus in myasthenia gravis. Surgery 1943;13:154.
25. Rosai J, Levine GD. Tumors of the thymus. Atlas of tumor pathology, 2nd series, fascicle 13. Washington, DC: Armed Forces Institute of Pathology, 1976.
26. Fukai I, Funato Y, Mizuno T, Hashimoto T, Masaoka A. Distribution of thymic tissue in the mediastinal adipose tissue. J Thorac Cardiovasc Surg 1991;101:1099.
27. Lauriola L, Maggiano N, Marino M, Carbone A, Piantelli M, Musiani P. Human thymoma: Immunologic characteristics of the lymphocyte component. Cancer 1981;48:1992.
28. Walker AN, Mills SE, Fechner RE. Thymomas and thymic carcinomas. Semin Diagn Pathol 1990;7:250.
29. Masaoka A, Monden Y, Nakahara K, Tanioka T. Follow-up study of thymomas with special reference to their clinical stages. Cancer 1981;48:2485.
30. Bergh NP, Gatzinsky P, Larsson S, et al. Tumors of the thymus and thymic region: I. Clinicopathological studies of thymomas. Ann Thorac Surg 1978;25:91.
31. LeGolvan DP, Abell MR. Thymomas. Cancer 1977;39:2142.
32. Gray GF, Gutowski WT. Thymoma: A clinicopathologic study of 54 cases. Am J Surg Pathol 1979;3:235.
33. Gerein AN, Srivastava SP, Burgess J. Thymoma: A ten-year review. Am J Surg 1978;136:49.
34. Salyer WR, Eggleston JC. Thymoma: A clinical and pathological study of 65 cases. Cancer 1976;37:229.
35. Batata MA, Martini N, Huvos AG, et al. Thymomas: Clinicopathologic features, therapy and prognosis. Cancer 1974;34:398.
36. Fechner RE. Recurrence of noninvasive thymomas. Cancer 1969;23:1423.
37. Verley JM, Hollmann KH. Thymoma: A comparative study of clinical stages, histologic features and survival in 200 cases. Cancer 1985;55:1074.
38. Marino M, Müller-Hermelink HK. Thymoma and thymic carcinoma: Relation of thymoma epithelial cells to the cortical and medullary differentiation of thymoma. Virchows Arch [A] 1985;407:119.
39. Pescarmona E, Rendian EA, Venuta F, et al. Analysis of prognostic factors and clinicopathological staging of thymoma. Ann Thorac Surg 1990;50:534.
40. Kornstein MJ, Curran WJ, Turrisi AT, Brooks JJ. Cortical versus medullary thymomas: A useful morphological distinction? Hum Pathol 1988;19:1335.
41. Eimoto T, Techima K, Shirakusa T, et al. Heterogeneity of epithelial cells and reactive components in thymomas: An ultrastructural and immunohistochemical study. Ultrastruct Pathol 1986;10:157.
42. Souadjian JV, Enriquez P, Silverstein MN, et al. The spectrum of diseases associated with thymoma. Arch Intern Med 1974;134:374.
43. Seybold ME. Myasthenia gravis: A clinical and basic science review. JAMA 1983;250:2516.
44. Lindstron J. Autoimmune response to acetylcholine receptors in myasthenia gravis and its animal model. Adv Immunol 1979;27:1.
45. Alper LI, Papatestas A, Kark A, et al. Histologic reappraisal of thymus in myasthenia gravis. Arch Pathol 1971;91:55.
46. Shellito J, Khandekar JD, McKeever WP, et al. Invasive thymoma responsive to oral corticosteroids. Cancer Treat Rep 1978;62:1397.
47. Zeok JV, Todd EP, Dillon M, et al. The role of thymectomy in red cell aplasia. Ann Thorac Surg 1979;28:257.
48. Masaoka A, Hashimoto T, Shibata K, Yamakowa Y, Nakamae K. Thymomas associated with pure red cell aplasia: Histology and follow-up studies. Cancer 1989;64:1872.
49. Tanabe T, Kubo Y, Hashimoto M, et al. Patch angioplasty of the superior vena caval obstruction (case reports with long follow-up results). J Cardiovasc Surg 1979;20:519.
50. Papatestas AE, Pozner J, Genkins G, Kornfeld P, Matta R. Prognosis in occult thymomas in myasthenia gravis following transcervical thymectomy. Arch Surg 1987;122:1352.
51. Monden Y, Nakahara K, Kagotani K, Fuji Y, Masaoka A, Kawashima Y. Myasthenia gravis with thymoma: Analysis of and postoperative prognosis for 65 patients with thymomatous myasthenia gravis. Ann Thorac Surg 1984;38:46.
52. Moden Y, Nakahara K, Nanjo S, et al. Invasive thymoma with myasthenia gravis. Cancer 1984;54:2513.
53. Wilkins EW, Castleman B. Thymoma: A continuing survey at the Massachusetts General Hospital. Ann Thorac Surg 1979;28:252.
54. Curran WJ, Kornstein MJ, Brooks JJ, Turrisi AT. Invasive thymoma: The role of mediastinal irradiation following complete or incomplete surgical resection. J Clin Oncol 1988;6:1722.
55. Ariaratnam LS, Kalnicki S, Mincer F, et al. The management of malignant thymoma with radiation therapy. Int J Radiat Oncol Biol Phys 1979;5:77.
56. Penn CRH, Hope-Stone HF. The role of radiotherapy in the management of malignant thymoma. Br J Surg 1972;59:533.
57. Nakahara K, Ohno K, Hashimoto K, et al. Thymoma: Results with complete resection and adjuvant postoperative radiation in 141 consecutive patients. J Thorac Cardiovasc Surg 1988;95:1041.
58. Skeggs DBL. Complications associated with the radiotherapy of thymic tumors. Proc R Soc Med 1973;66:115.
59. Marks RD, Wallace KM, Petit HS. Radiation therapy control of 9 patients with malignant thymoma. Cancer 1978;41:117.
60. Boston B. Chemotherapy of invasive thymoma. Cancer 1976;38:49.
61. Daugaard G, Hansen HH, Rorth M. Combination chemotherapy for malignant thymoma. Ann Intern Med 1983;99:189.
62. Evans WK, Thompson DM, Simpson WJ, Feld F, Phillips MJ. Combination chemotherapy in invasive thymoma: Role of COPP. Cancer 1980;46:1523.
63. Chahinian AP, Bhardroj S, Meyer RJ, Jaffrey IS, Kirschner PA, Holland JF. Treatment of invasive or metastatic thymoma: Report of eleven cases. Cancer 1981;47:1752.
64. Goldel N, Boning L, Fredrick A, Holzel D, Hartenstein R. Chemotherapy of invasive thymoma: A retrospective study of 22 cases. Cancer 1989;63:1493.
65. Fornasiero A, Daniele O, Ghiotto C, et al. Chemotherapy of invasive thymoma. J Clin Oncol 1990;8:1419.
66. Fornasiero A, Danielo O, Ghiotto C, et al. Chemotherapy for invasive thymoma: A thirteen-year experience. Cancer 1991;68:30.
67. Loehrer PJ, Perez CA, Roth LM, Greco FA, Livingston RB, Einhorn LH. Chemotherapy for advanced thymoma: Preliminary results of an intergroup study. Ann Intern Med 1990;113:520.
68. Hy E, Levine J. Chemotherapy of malignant thymoma: Case report and review of the literature. Cancer 1986;57:1101.
69. Macchiarini P, Chella A, Ducci F, et al. Neoadjuvant chemotherapy, surgery and postoperative radiation therapy for invasive thymoma. Cancer 1991;68:706.
70. Monden Y, Nakahara K, Iioka S, et al. Recurrence of thymoma: Clinicopathological features, therapy and prognosis. Ann Thorac Surg 1985;39:165.
71. Maggi G, Casadio C, Cavallo A, Cianci R, Molinatti M, Ruffini E. Thymoma: Results of 241 operated cases. Ann Thorac Surg 1991;51:152.
72. Wilkins EW, Grillo HC, Scannell JG, Moncure AC, Mathisen J. Role of staging in prognosis and management of thymoma. Ann Thorac Surg 1991;51:888.
73. Shamji F, Pearson FG, Todd TR, Ginsberg RJ, Ilves R, Cooper JD. Results of surgical treatment for thymoma. J Thorac Cardiovasc Surg 1984;87:43.
74. Lewis JE, Wick MR, Scheithauer BW, Bernatz PE, Taylor WF. Thymoma: A clinicopathologic review. Cancer 1987;60:2727.
75. Wick MR, Weiland LH, Scheithauer BW, Bernatz PE. Primary thymic carcinomas. Am J Surg Pathol 1982;6:613.
76. Leysraz S, Henle W, Chahinian AP, et al. Association of Epstein-Barr virus with thymic carcinoma. New Engl J Med 1985;312:1296.
77. Hartmann A, Roth C, Minck C, Niedobitek G. Thymic carcinoma: Report of 5 cases and review of the literature. J Cancer Res Clin Oncol 1990:116:69.
78. Dy C, Calvo FA, Mindan JP, et al. Undifferentiated epithelial rich invasive malignant

thymoma: Complete response to cisplatin, vinblastine and bleomycin therapy. J Clin Oncol 1988;6:536.

79. Salyer WR, Salyer DC, Eggleston JC. Carcinoid tumors of the thymus. Cancer 1976;37:958.

80. Wick MR, Carney JA, Bernatz PE, Brown LR. Primary mediastinal carcinoid tumors. Am J Surg Pathol 1982;6:195.

81. Wick MR, Rosai J. Neuroendocrine neoplasms of the mediastinum. Semin Diagn Pathol 1991;8:35.

82. Wick MR, Scheithauer BW. Oat cell carcinoma of the thymus. Cancer 1982;49:1652.

83. Dehner LP. Germ cell tumors of the mediastinum. Semin Diagn Pathol 1990;7:266.

84. Luna MA, Valenzuela-Tamariz J. Germ-cell tumors of the mediastinum, postmortem findings. Am J Clin Pathol 1976;65:450.

85. Martini N, Golbey RB, Hajdu SJ, et al. Primary mediastinal germ cell tumors. Cancer 1974;33:763.

86. Nichols CR, Heerema NA, Palmer C, Loehrer PJ, Williams SD, Einhorn LH. Klinefelter's syndrome associated with mediastinal germ-cell neoplasms. J Clin Oncol 1987;5:1290.

87. Nichols CR, Roth BJ, Heerema N, Griep J, Tricot G. Hematologic neoplasia associated with primary mediastinal germ cell tumors. N Engl J Med 1990;322:1425.

88. Kirschling RJ, Krols LK, Charboneau JW, Grantham JG, Zinke H. High-resolution ultrasonographic and pathologic abnormalities of germ cell tumors in patients with clinically normal testes. Mayo Clin Proc 1983;58:648.

89. Polansky SM, Barwick KW, Ravin CE. Primary mediastinal seminoma. AJR 1979;132:17.

90. Aygun C, Slawson RG, Bajaj K, Salazar OM. Primary mediastinal seminoma. Urology 1984;23:109.

91. Hurt RD, Bruckman JE, Farrow GM, Bernatz PE, Hahn RG, Earle JD. Primary mediastinal seminoma. Cancer 1982;49:1658.

92. Kersh CR, Eisert DR, Constable WC, et al. Primary malignant mediastinal germ-cell tumors and the contribution of radiotherapy: A southeastern multi-institutional study. Am J Clin Oncol 1987;10:302.

93. Bush SE, Martinez A, Bagshaw MA. Primary mediastinal seminoma. Cancer 1981;48:1877.

94. Clamon GH. Management of primary mediastinal seminoma. Chest 1983;83:263.

95. Jain KK, Bosi GJ, Bains MS, Whitmore WF, Golbey RB. The treatment of extragonadal seminoma. J Clin Oncol 1984;2:820.

96. Economou JS, Trump PL, Holmes EC, Eggleston JE. Management of primary germ cell tumors of the mediastinum. J Thorac Cardiovasc Surg 1982;83:643.

97. Fox RM, Woods RL, Tattersall MH, et al. Undifferentiated carcinoma in young men. The atypical teratoma syndrome. Lancet 1979;1:1316.

98. Hainsworth JD, Einhorn LH, Williams SD, Stewart M, Greco FA. Advanced extragonadal germ cell tumors: Successful treatment with combination chemotherapy. Ann Intern Med 1982;97:7.

99. Truong LD, Harris L, Mattioli C, et al. Endodermal sinus tumor of the mediastinum. A report of seven cases and review of the literature. Cancer 1986;58:730.

100. Wright CD, Kesler KA, Nichols CR, et al. Primary mediastinal nonseminomatous germ cell tumors: Results of a multimodality approach. J Thorac Cardiovasc Surg 1990;99:210.

101. Gale AW, Jelihovsky T, Grant AF, et al. Neurogenic tumors of the mediastinum. Ann Thorac Surg 1974;17:434.

102. Swason P. Soft tissue neoplasm of the mediastinum. Semin Diagn Pathol 1991;8:14.

103. White W, Shiu MH, Rosenblum MK, Erlandson RA, Woodruff JM. Cellular schwannoma: A clinicopathologic study of 57 patients and 58 tumors. Cancer 1990;66:1266.

104. Hajula A, Mattila S, Luosto R, Kostianinen S, Mattila I. Mediastinal neurogenic tumors. Early and late results of surgical treatment. Scand J Thorac Cardiovasc Surg 1986;20:115.

105. Ricci C, Rendina EA, Venata F, Pescarmona EO, Gagliardi F. Diagnostic imaging and surgical treatment of dumbbell tumors of the mediastinum. Ann Thorac Surg 1990;50:586.

106. Olson JL, Salyer WR. Mediastinal paragangliomas (aortic body tumor): A report of 4 cases and a review of the literature. Cancer 1978;41:2405.

107. Cohen A, Sbaschnig RJ, Hochholzer L, Lough FC, Albus RA. Mediastinal hemangiomas. Ann Thorac Surg 1987;43:656.

Cancer: Principles & Practice of Oncology, Fourth Edition,
edited by Vincent T. DeVita, Jr., Samuel Hellman, Steven A. Rosenberg.
J.B. Lippincott Co., Philadelphia © 1993.

Jack A. Roth   Allen S. Lichter

Joe B. Putnam, Jr   Arlene A. Forastiere

CHAPTER **25**

Cancer of the Esophagus

INCIDENCE AND EPIDEMIOLOGY

Cancer of the esophagus has the greatest variation in geographic distribution of any malignancy. A 17-fold difference in age-adjusted mortality for males exists for countries with the highest and lowest incidence.[1] Data from the World Health Organization show that the mortality is highest in China, Puerto Rico, and Singapore. Geographic variation in incidence exists within countries. In China, the incidence in the county with the highest rate (Hebi) is 139.8 persons per 100,000 population, and in the county with the lowest rate (Hunyuan), the incidence is 1.43 persons per 100,000.[2]

Other areas have shown variation in the incidence over time. In the Transkei region of the Cape Province in South Africa, the incidence of esophageal cancer increased dramatically between 1940 and 1950. Before 1940, the incidence was low among black males 35 to 64 years of age, but by 1950 it had increased to 246 per 100,000. Other regions with high incidence include Iran, France, and Switzerland. The reason for these extreme geographic variations is not known, but environmental and nutritional factors are suspected.[2]

Esophageal cancer is uncommon in the United States. The overall age-adjusted incidence in 1987 was 3.9 persons per 100,000.[3] The age-adjusted overall mortality of 3.4 persons per 100,000 is similar to the incidence, indicating the high mortality rate for this cancer.

The incidence of esophageal cancer is much higher in blacks than in whites. The incidence for white males in 1987 was 5.5 per 100,000 and that for black males was 17.3 per 100,000. A similar trend was noted for black females (4.3/100,000) compared with white females (1.6/100,000). The age-adjusted mortality for blacks was correspondingly high (14.4/100,000 for males and 3.8/100,000 for females) compared with that for whites (5.0/100,000 for males and 1.2/100,000 for females).

The major histologic types of esophageal cancer are squamous (epidermoid) carcinoma and adenocarcinoma. Adeno-carcinoma of the esophagus frequently has been classified as a gastric carcinoma. However, esophageal adenocarcinomas arising in Barrett's epithelium are clearly esophageal in origin. Adenocarcinomas arising in the gastric cardia frequently metastasize to nodal groups in the drainage bed of the esophagus and spread submucosally along the esophagus. The treatment of these tumors is similar to that of squamous cancer, and their prognosis is similar.

The incidence of adenocarcinoma of the esophagus in whites is higher than in blacks.[4,5] Recently, an increase in the incidence of adenocarcinomas of the esophagus and gastric cardia was noted in white males. The increases among men from 1976 to 1987 ranged from 4% to 10% per year and exceeded those of other cancers during this period. This increase could not be explained by a change in the incidence of gastric cancer or squamous cancer. Excessive alcohol consumption and smoking increase the risk for developing esophageal cancer, and together they act synergistically. However, no specific risk factors have been implicated in the development of esophageal adenocarcinoma.

PREDISPOSING CONDITIONS

Tylosis

Tylosis is a disease characterized by hyperkeratosis of the skin of the palms and soles and papillomata of the esophagus. The syndrome is inherited in an autosomal dominant fashion. Squamous cell carcinomas of the esophagus develop with a high frequency in affected families.[6]

Achalasia

In patients with achalasia, the risk for developing esophageal carcinoma may be as high as 20%. Cancers can occur in the middle and lower third of the esophagus but are more common in the middle third. Cancers generally occur an average of 17 years after the diagnosis of achalasia.[7]

Barrett's Esophagus

Barrett's esophagus is a premalignant condition that may proceed to development of adenocarcinoma of the esophagus (see the section on adenocarcinoma).

Caustic Injury

Squamous carcinomas arising in lye strictures are responsible for 1% to 4% of esophageal carcinomas.[8,9] The carcinomas appear an average of 40 years after injury. The low incidence of carcinoma and the potentially high operative morbidity associated with resection of a chronically scarred esophagus argue against resection of these strictures. If repeated dilations fail, a bypass may relieve dysphagia in the absence of cancer.

Esophageal Diverticula

Infrequently, squamous cancers develop in esophageal diverticula. The incidence in 1249 patients was 0.4% in one series.[10] In this series, diverticulectomy alone was curative in the absence of full-thickness penetration, lymph node metastasis, or extension to the margin of resection.

Esophageal Webs

There are reports of cancer of the upper esophagus associated with upper esophageal webs.[11] The association of esophageal webs with iron deficiency anemia, glossitis, cheilosis, koilonychia, brittle fingernails, and splenomegaly is referred to as the Plummer-Vinson or Paterson-Kelly syndrome. This syndrome occurs more frequently in females than in males. Treatment of the webs consists of endoscopic rupture. Dilations may be necessary if endoscopic rupture is not successful. Iron replacement is indicated for the anemia.

SECOND PRIMARY TUMORS

Esophageal cancers may develop as second primary tumors in patients with other primary tumors of the upper aerodigestive tract. Patients with upper aerodigestive tract cancers develop second primary tumors at the rate of 4% of patients per year.[12,13] In patients with head and neck cancers, one third of the second primary tumors arise in the esophagus. Cancers of the tonsil and palate most frequently were associated with esophageal second primaries. The appearance of a second primary tumor adversely affects survival from the first cancer. Cancers developing in this region are associated with tobacco consumption. Most second primary tumors arise in upper aerodigestive epithelium that is exposed to a carcinogen such as cigarette smoke; this phenomenon is called field cancerization.

RARE CANCERS OF THE ESOPHAGUS

VARIANTS OF SQUAMOUS CELL CARCINOMA

Squamous Cell Carcinoma With Sarcomatoid Features

The variant of squamous cell carcinoma with sarcomatoid features has been called pseudosarcoma, carcinosarcoma, spindle cell carcinoma, carcinoma with spindle cell features,

and polypoid carcinoma. The tumor has an incidence between 0.5% and 15% and occurs primarily in men older than 60 years.[14,15] This tumor may have a more favorable prognosis than conventional esophageal cancer. Lymph node metastases are reported in 20% to 30% of cases.[16,17]

Adenoid Cystic Carcinoma

Adenoid cystic carcinoma is an uncommon tumor, with an incidence of 0.75% reported in a review of 792 primary esophageal malignancies.[18] Most of these tumors occur in men in the sixth decade of life. The symptomatology and aggressiveness of this cancer are similar to squamous carcinoma. The median duration of symptoms is 3 months before diagnosis. The median survival after diagnosis is 9 months.

Mucoepidermoid Carcinoma

Mucoepidermoid carcinoma, also called adenosquamous carcinoma, contains a mixture of squamoid, mucous, and intermediate cells. These tumors are aggressive and have survival rates similar to those of squamous carcinoma.[19] Although the histology is similar to its salivary gland counterpart, the esophageal tumor has a poor prognosis.

Small Cell Carcinoma

The prevalence of small cell carcinoma is 1.7% to 2.4%, and most patients are in their sixth to eighth decades of life.[20,21] The tumor occurs primarily in the middle and lower esophagus, and the symptoms are similar to those of squamous cell carcinoma. The cell of origin for small cell carcinoma is not definitively known. Most investigators believe the tumors originate from the argyrophilic cell located in the basal layer of the squamous epithelium.[22] Alternatively, these tumors may arise from a common stem cell.[21,23,24] The prognosis is poor for most patients. These tumors are responsive to chemotherapy, which is generally the recommended primary treatment.[25,26]

Sarcomas

Sarcomas of the esophagus are rare, with leiomyosarcoma the most common sarcoma. A variety of sarcomas have been described, including fibrosarcoma, osteosarcoma, synovial sarcoma, hemangiopericytoma, rhabdomyosarcoma, liposarcoma, and malignant mesenchymoma. Only one or two cases of each type of tumor have been reported. Gastrointestinal involvement with Kaposi's sarcoma occurs in 50% to 70% of patients with Kaposi's sarcoma and the acquired immunodeficiency syndrome (AIDS). On endoscopy, the lesions may appear as dark red mucosal maculas or submucosal violaceous nodules.[27] The disease generally is not symptomatic, although hemorrhage can occur.[28]

Malignant Lymphoma and Hodgkin's Disease

Esophageal involvement by lymphoma occurs in 1% to 8% of cases.[29,30] In most cases, esophageal involvement is secondary and caused by extension from other sites. Primary malignant lymphoma of the esophagus is rare. However, primary lymphomas associated with AIDS have been reported.[31-34]

Metastases

In most cases, involvement of the esophagus by another primary tumor is caused by direct extension of the primary tumor or its nodal metastases. Primary sites most often involved include stomach, lung, and thyroid. Patients with advanced breast cancer have a 9% prevalence of esophageal involvement, which may present as dysphagia.[16,17] Radiation therapy and chemotherapy may provide palliative relief of symptoms. Other cancers that have been reported to metastasize to the esophagus include cancers of the kidney, pancreas, cervix, and bladder, leukemia, and melanoma.

ANATOMY

The esophagus spans the interval between the hypopharynx and the stomach. Conventionally, the esophagus originates at the cricoid cartilage at the level of the cricopharyngeus muscle and topographically at the level of the sixth cervical vertebrae. The cervical esophagus is about 5 cm long, with the upper portion located behind the larynx. It lies just to the left of midline and extends to the thoracic inlet. The thoracic esophagus begins at the thoracic inlet and extends 20 to 25 cm to the gastroesophageal junction or to the esophageal hiatus of the diaphragm. Surprisingly, the intrathoracic component of the esophagus is short; however, its strategic location, nestled among all major thoracic structures, presents considerable technical challenge to the surgeon.

During endoscopy, lesions are localized in the esophagus by measuring the distance to the abnormality from the central incisors (Fig. 25–1). By this measure, the esophagus begins about 15 to 19 cm from the incisors at the cricopharyngeus muscle and terminates at the gastroesophageal junction, 38 to 40 cm distally. The thoracic inlet begins about 20 cm from the central incisors (at the level of T1). Esophageal tumors involving the larynx or the posterior membranous trachea require laryngectomy and esophageal resection.

The esophagus lies just to the left of midline behind the trachea and crosses the left main stem bronchus at its junction with the trachea. Tracheoesophageal fistulas generally occur at this point. Topographically, this occurs at the angle of Louis, anteriorly, or T4–5, posteriorly (about 23 to 25 cm from the incisors). The arch of the aorta passes in front of the esophagus at this level and may produce a shallow depression that pulsates during endoscopy. The esophagus, like other components of the gastrointestinal tract, distends, so that tumors may grow to considerable size and involve adjacent structures before discovery. Resection of the tumor when adjacent organs are involved may not be feasible.

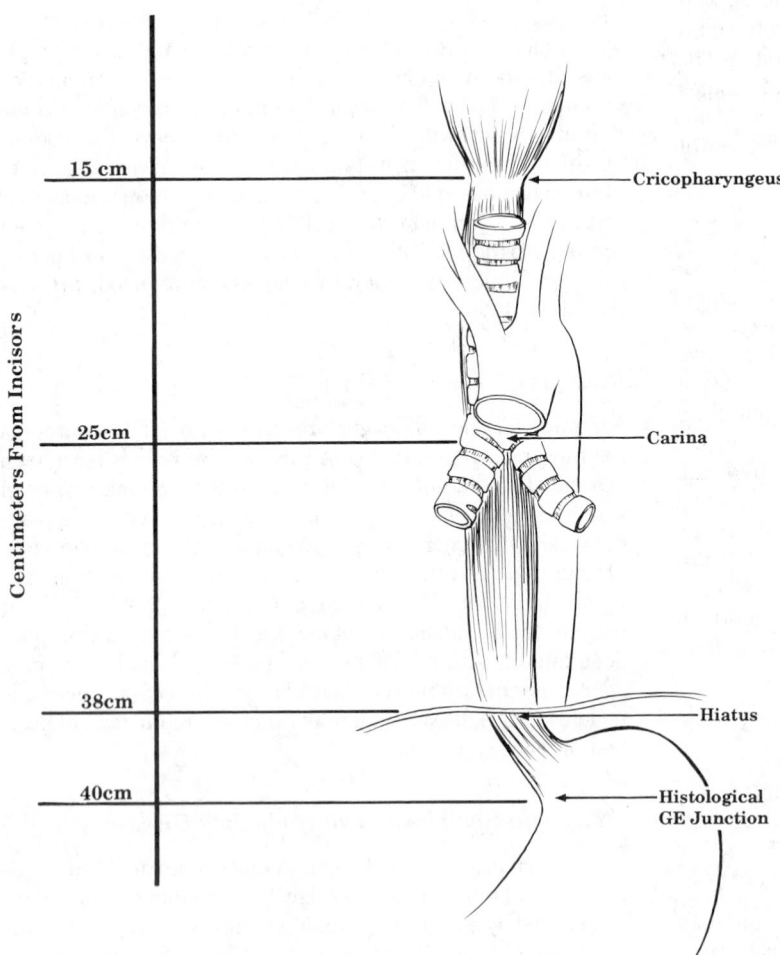

FIGURE 25–1. General anatomy of the esophagus with major landmarks identified.

The American Joint Committee for Cancer (AJCC) Staging and End Results Reporting divides the esophagus into three principal regions: the cervical esophagus, extending from the cricopharyngeus to the thoracic inlet; the upper and midthoracic esophagus, extending from the thoracic inlet (18 cm from the upper incisor teeth) to a point 10 cm above the esophagogastric junction, usually located at T8 (31 cm from the incisors); and the lower thoracic esophagus, which is the distal 10 cm of the esophagus.[35]

The AJCC standards are based on strict anatomic and length criteria. Most radiologists and surgeons divide the esophagus into "thirds" to correspond to the following: the upper third, from the superior portion of the aortic arch up; the middle third, from the inferior pulmonary vein up to the superior portion of the aortic arch; and the distal third, from the inferior pulmonary vein to the gastroesophageal junction. This is the simplest anatomic classification and the one most commonly used. About 15% of all esophageal cancers occur in the upper third of the esophagus, 50% in the middle, and 35% in the lower third. The numbers vary from series to series, and some report that the lower third lesions are the most common, as these are the tumors most amenable to therapy.

BLOOD SUPPLY

The blood supply to the esophagus is segmental, with three main arterial sources: inferior thyroid artery, the bronchial arteries at the level of the carina, and the left gastric and inferior phrenic artery (Fig. 25–2). Autopsy studies have revealed that all major vascular trees that supply the esophagus divide into minute branches some distance from the esophagus. This capillary network extends into the esophagus and supplies the submucosal area with the richest vascular supply. Because of this rich vascular plexus within the submucosa, the esophagus can be mobilized and remain viable. The transhiatal esophagectomy therefore can be performed without significant hemorrhage as long as the dissection is performed within this 1 cm capillary zone around the esophagus.[36] The blood supply of the cervical esophagus is the superior and inferior thyroid arteries. There may be small branches supplied from the subclavian artery. The thoracic esophagus is supplied by branches from the aorta to the esophagus just below the level of the carina. The lower esophagus and cardia are supplied by branches from the left gastric artery. The veins from the thoracic esophagus drain into the azygous and hemizygous system and the intercostal veins, which are tributaries of the azygous system (Fig. 25–3).

LYMPHATIC DRAINAGE

The lymphatic supply of the esophagus is extensive (Fig. 25–4). A dense network of lymphatic vessels within the mucosa and the submucosa communicate freely with lymphatic channels in the muscular layers of the esophagus and with those that extend through the esophagus into the thoracic nodes. Lymphatic fluids from any portion of the esophagus may travel to any other portion of the esophagus and may spread to any region of the thorax or draining nodal bed. Tumors and lymph from tumors from any portion of the esophagus may spread to any other portion of the esophagus because of the rich lymphatic supply and drainage system. Tumors of any portion of the esophagus may drain into the supraclavicular lymph

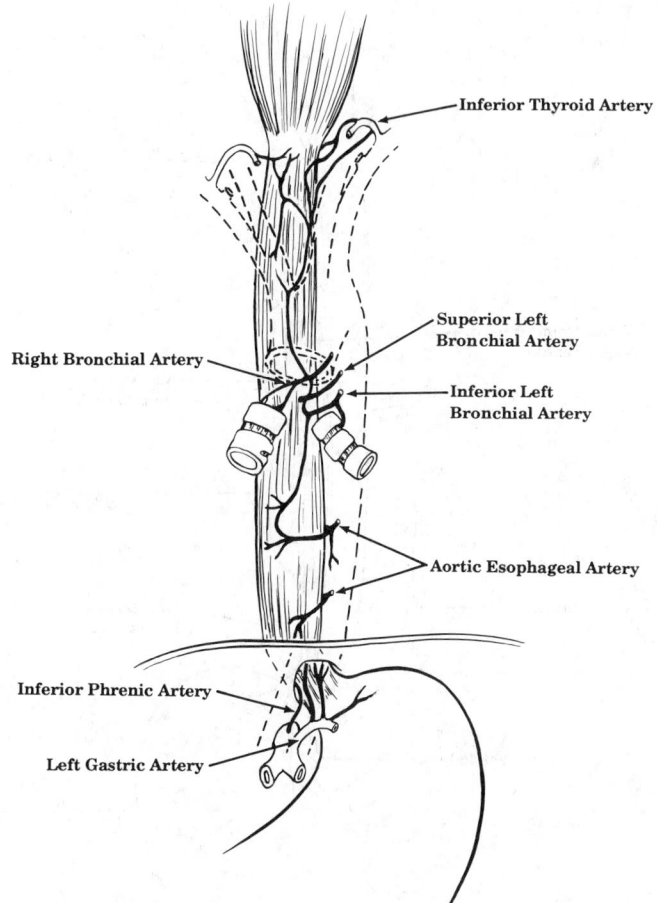

FIGURE 25–2. Blood supply of the esophagus.

nodes or into the cervical nodes. A careful physical examination must be performed to evaluate for the presence of metastatic disease to these nodes. A thorough palpation of both supraclavicular fossae, including the areas behind the sternocleidomastoid muscles and the clavicular heads, may yield positive results to the careful examiner. A histologic diagnosis may be obtained by node excision or by needle aspiration and cytologic examination.[37] A positive result demonstrates systemic spread of the disease and modifies subsequent treatment. Local control of esophageal cancers with surgery or radiation therapy must consider the potential for lymphatic involvement with tumor at the time of treatment. Although lymphatic flow is unpredictable, the pattern of the lymphatic drainage favors a longitudinal spread rather than a circumferential spread.

The lymph drains to several regional beds. For the upper third of the esophagus, the lymph drains to the internal jugular, cervical, and supraclavicular areas. For the upper and middle thirds, lymph drains to the paratracheal, hilar, subcarinal, and paraesophageal, periaortic, and pericardial regions. For the distal third, lymph drains to the lesser curvature, left gastric, and celiac axis.

Involvement of celiac nodes may occur in 10% of the esophageal cancers located in the cervical and upper thoracic esophagus. Up to 44% of patients with middle third esophageal tumors may have celiac nodal involvement.[38] Most commonly,

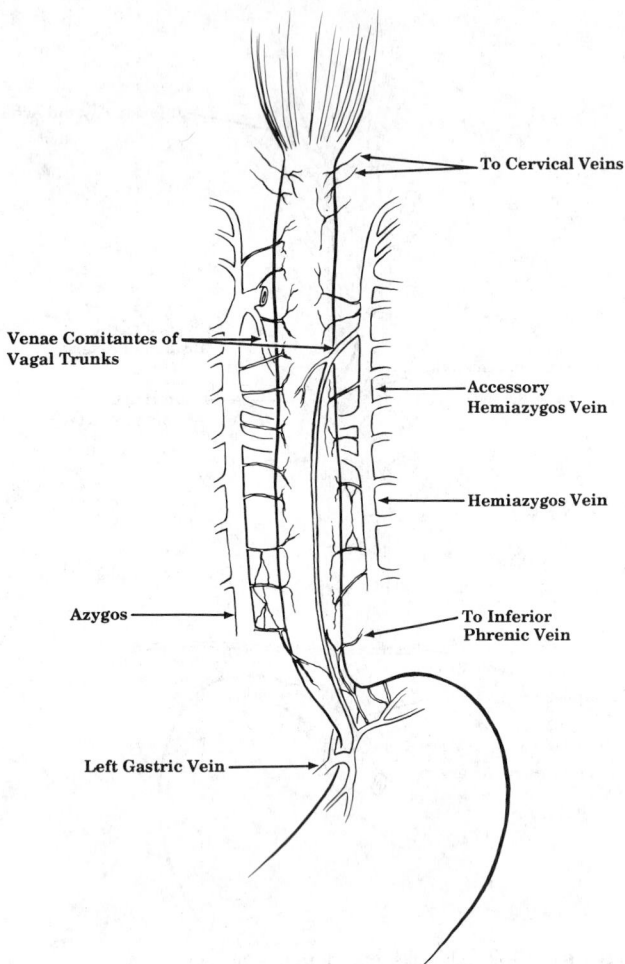

FIGURE 25–3.   Venous drainage of the esophagus.

the distal esophagus drains to these beds. The rich lymphatic drainage of the esophagus is responsible for spread throughout the entire esophagus, and this must be considered when resection is performed. Ten centimeters of esophagus beyond the tumor must be resected. Because the esophagus is short in the chest, a total esophagectomy usually is required for optimal surgical control. A lesser resection may be performed; however, so-called skip areas without total esophagectomy may increase the risk for local recurrence.[39,40]

CLINICAL PRESENTATION

The patient who presents with esophageal cancer usually is a man between 55 and 65 years of age with a long-standing history of cigarette abuse and heavy alcohol intake. Dysphagia and weight loss are the initial symptoms of carcinoma of the esophagus in 90% of patients. Difficulty in swallowing does not occur until the circumference of the esophagus is narrowed to less than 13 mm in diameter because the esophagus is distensible. Occasionally the onset of dysphagia is sudden, but most patients complain of a vague difficulty in swallowing for the preceding 3 to 6 months. Most patients complain of food sticking and point to their throat at the level of the sternal notch. This sticking of food may occur anywhere from the

midthoracic esophagus to the level of the cricopharyngeus and usually indicates a middle or upper third cancer. Patients who complain of food sticking in the epigastrium usually have cancers of the middle or lower third. Odynophagia (painful swallowing) is seen in about half of the patients with cancer of the esophagus. Bony metastases are identified when point tenderness is noted in the bones. Regurgitation of undigested food, retrosternal or epigastric pain, or aspiration pneumonia may be present. Advanced lesions may present with hematemesis, melena, cough from a tracheoesophageal fistula, hemoptysis, or problems related to nerve involvement, such as Horner's syndrome or paralysis of the recurrent laryngeal nerve (Table 25–1).[41–47] Tumors of the esophagus may present with superior vena cava syndrome, but this is rare in the absence of dysphagia. Erosion of the esophagus into the aorta may result in exsanguinating hemorrhage. Other signs of unresectable malignant disease may be found with malignant pleural effusion or malignant ascites. Palpable supraclavicular or cervical lymph nodes should be biopsied to exclude metastases.[37] Metastasis to the bones may produce a paraneoplastic syndrome from hypercalcemia.

Most patients who complain of dysphagia have a plain chest x-ray film (for evaluation of the thorax and mediastinum) and a barium swallow. The gross appearance of a carcinoma of

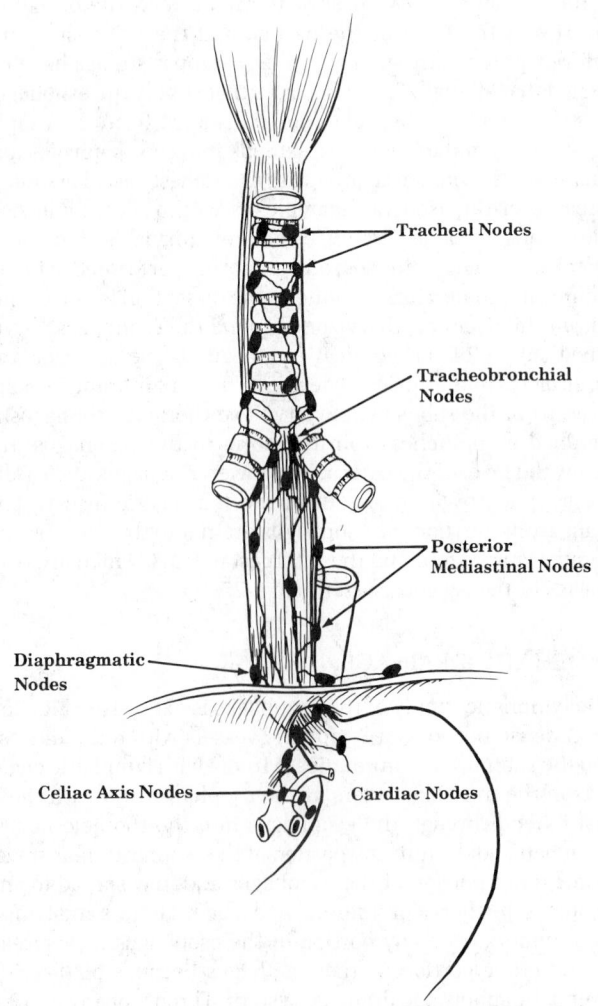

FIGURE 25–4.   Major lymphatic drainage areas of the esophagus.

TABLE 25–1. Symptoms of Advanced Carcinoma of the Esophagus

Investigations	Symptoms	Patients With Symptoms (%)
Akiyama, 1990[41] Ojala et al, 1982[42]	Dysphagia	80–96
Ojala et al, 1982[42] Pedersen et al, 1982[43]	Weight loss	42–46
Ojala et al, 1982[42] Stair and Brian, 1982[44] Sweet, 1948[45]	Pain	6–20
Ojala et al, 1982[42]	Cachexia	6
Ojala et al, 1982[42] Ojala et al, 1982[46]	Cough or hoarseness	3–4
Duranceau and Jamieson, 1984[47]	Tracheoesophageal fistula	1–13

the esophagus is best depicted by an esophagogram. Rarely do other lesions present with the characteristic appearance of cancer of the esophagus. Confirmation of the histologic type of tumor requires endoscopy with biopsy and brushings of the esophagus.

DIAGNOSIS

Any patient who complains of dysphagia and weight loss must be suspected of an esophageal carcinoma. A history and physical examination are performed and a chest x-ray film and barium swallow obtained. Particular attention should be paid to alcohol and tobacco abuse, weight loss, and other constitutional symptoms. Metastasis must be excluded initially by a physical examination and a chest x-ray film. A barium swallow provides the initial assessment of the extent of disease in the esophagus and may suggest the involvement of other thoracic structures.

Esophagoscopy is required for histologic examination of the primary tumor and to determine the presence of intramural metastasis. Flexible and rigid esophagoscopy are appropriate diagnostic modalities. Intramural metastasis (a negative prognostic factor for survival) may be identified in up to 11% of patients. Seventy percent of intramural metastases on the proximal side of the esophageal tumor may be detected during this examination.[40]

All lesions seen at the time of the esophagoscopy must be biopsied and brushed. The tumor, if it is located within the submucosa, may push normal mucosa in front of it, and biopsies of the bulge may reveal only normal mucosa. Brushings of the tumor are diagnostic in 90% of cases, whereas only 70% of biopsies are.[48,49] If both techniques are used and multiple biopsies are obtained, a diagnosis of malignancy is confirmed in more than 95% of patients.

Abrasive cytology may have diagnostic value. Clinicians at the Linxian County Hospital in the Hunan Province of China have developed a technique of abrasive cytology that uses a catheter and a balloon covered with cottonette to scrape loose esophageal mucosal cells. This cytologic examination has been 90% accurate in patients with early cancer of the esophagus.[50] In the United States, biopsies and brushings are used more often, whereas in Asia abrasive cytology is used more fre-

quently to detect the increasing incidence of esophageal carcinoma.

STAGING

Accurate clinical staging of esophageal carcinoma is difficult due to its location deep within the thorax. The main objectives of clinical staging of esophageal carcinoma are (1) to identify patients who may benefit from definitive treatment of their primary carcinoma; (2) to exclude patients with metastases from surgery, because their survival time is short (about 6 months)[44]; and (3) to assess responses to radiation therapy, chemotherapy, and surgical interventions. Because many esophageal cancers are being treated with preoperative radiation or chemotherapy, postsurgical evaluation may not accurately define the stage of the initial diagnosed cancer. The TNM staging system for the cervical and thoracic esophagus is outlined in Table 25–2. Stage grouping is given in Table 25–3.

Patients with metastases should not be subjected to surgical resection as their primary treatment modality. Patients with lymph node involvement have a shortened life expectancy because nodal metastases, even adjacent but separate nodal metastases, often represent systemic spread of tumor beyond the limits of the resection. Excellent palliation (but not cure) may be obtained with surgery in these patients, but improvement in survival rests with better adjuvant therapy. The recommendations for preoperative clinical staging are a chest x-ray film, a barium swallow, and computed tomographic (CT) scans of the chest and upper abdomen (to include the liver and adrenals). CT scans of the chest may identify accurately patients whose tumors involve the airways or aorta. CT is a poor way to detect abdominal lymph node metastases or small liver metastases.[52] A bone scan should be obtained in patients with complaints of bone pain, along with plain films of the abnormal areas. A bronchoscopy is mandatory for patients

TABLE 25–2. TNM Staging for Esophageal Cancer

Primary Tumor (T)

TX	Minimum requirements to assess the primary tumor cannot be seen
T0	No evidence of primary tumor
Tis	Preinvasive carcinoma (carcinoma in situ)
T1	Tumor invades into but not beyond the submucosa
T2	Tumor invades into but not beyond the muscularis propria
T3	Tumor invades into the adventitia
T4	Tumor invades contiguous structures

Regional Lymph Nodes (N)

Cervical Esophagus (Cervical and Supraclavicular Lymph Nodes)

NX	Lymph nodes cannot be assessed
N0	No demonstrable metastasis to regional lymph nodes
N1	Regional lymph nodes contain metastatic tumor

Thoracic Esophagus (Nodes in the Thorax, Not Those of the Cervical, Supraclavicular, or Abdominal Areas)

N0	No nodal involvement
N1	Nodal involvement

Distant Metastasis (M)

MX	Distant metastasis cannot be assessed
M0	No evidence of distant metastasis
M1	Distant metastasis present

TABLE 25–3. Stage Grouping for Esophageal Cancer

Stage I	Stage II	Stage III	Stage IV
T1N0M0	T2N0M0	T3N0M0	Any T, Any NM1
	T1N1M0	T3N1M0	
	T2N1M0	T4N1M0	

with a middle or upper third tumor. Bone scans and bronchoscopy may identify metastases not evident by CT scan.[53] Pulmonary function studies are helpful in assessing the patients physiologic reserves and ability to tolerate a thoracotomy.

NATURAL HISTORY AND PATTERNS OF SPREAD

Like other cancers within the gastrointestinal system, esophageal cancers are rarely found while small and more easily treated. More frequently, the patient presents late because the distensible esophagus compensates readily for partial obstruction of the lumen by a tumor. Patients with carcinoma of the esophagus commonly are not aware of their problem until the tumor is large and obstructive symptoms occur or it extends into adjacent structures.

Esophageal cancers are characterized by extensive local growth, lymph node metastases, and invasion of adjacent structures before becoming more widely disseminated. In patients with squamous cell carcinoma of the esophagus, early asymptomatic patients with in situ carcinoma have demonstrated that 3 to 4 years may pass before advanced cancer develops.[54] The unique lymphatic drainage of the esophagus and the long interval during which the tumor is asymptomatic account for the extensive involvement of lymph nodes and structures adjacent to the esophagus at the time of diagnosis. The poor prognosis of these patients is influenced by the proximity of the aorta and trachea and the absence of a serosal covering. In one series of 117 patients with esophagectomy and extensive lymph node dissection, mortality was less than 3%. Lymphatic metastases were identified in the neck of 32% of these patients, and in about half of the lymph nodes in the chest and abdomen.[55]

The length of the esophagus involved by the neoplasm correlated with the extent of involvement of adjacent structures and inversely related to curability. Tumors 5 cm long or less are more often localized (65% localized, 35% metastatic) than tumors greater then 5 cm in length (25% localized, 75% metastatic).[56]

Distant metastases are less often identified when patients present with dysphagia from carcinoma of the esophagus. Autopsies have shown that widespread distant metastases are almost always present at the time of death.[57] Esophageal carcinoma can spread to any viscera or site (liver, lung, pleura, stomach, peritoneum, kidney, adrenal gland, brain, and bone) and is most likely present as subclinical disease when the patient is first diagnosed.[58] Surgery for esophageal carcinoma should focus on palliation of the dysphagia and local control of the carcinoma. The risks of surgery (bleeding, infection, leak, death) are too high to perform esophagectomy for patients with unresectable disease or visceral metastases. Even

patients whose tumors were localized within the esophagus, 94% of patients in one study, have residual tumor at autopsy.[59]

ASSOCIATED MALIGNANCIES AT OTHER SITES

Synchronous or metachronous malignancies of the aerodigestive tract occur in 5% to 12% of patient with carcinoma of the esophagus. About half can be found in the head and neck areas. The oral cavity, pharynx, larynx, and lung are the most frequent sites. Oral and pharyngeal cancers are most often associated with cancer of the esophagus, and laryngeal cancers are most often associated with cancer of the lung. Direct laryngoscopy, bronchoscopy, and esophagoscopy in patients with head and neck cancer show that about 5% of patients have synchronous lung or esophageal cancer or both. Most of these patients (75%) are asymptomatic.[60,61]

THERAPY FOR CANCER OF THE ESOPHAGUS

The two primary treatments of clinically localized cancer of the esophagus are surgery and radiation therapy. Surgical resection is the treatment of choice for early lesions (stages I and II). For patients with more advanced localized cancers, neither treatment has been shown definitively to be superior. A comparison of the merits of these two primary treatment modalities is presented here. The low survival rates with single modality therapy have prompted numerous investigations into multimodality therapy, including preoperative radiation therapy, preoperative chemotherapy, and combined preoperative radiation therapy and chemotherapy. Cooperative group trials in progress will resolve some of these issues.

Palliation is the primary goal for patients with advanced local cancers or metastases. The primary goals of palliation are restoration of swallowing and relief of pain. Radiation therapy, chemotherapy, and endoscopic treatment all contribute to palliation and are discussed later in this chapter.

SURGICAL THERAPY FOR CARCINOMA OF THE ESOPHAGUS

With rare exceptions, carcinoma of the esophagus is, at diagnosis, a systemic disease.[62] It matters little which operation is done for the patient with carcinoma in situ or stage I esophageal cancer, because these patients have prolonged survival regardless of the magnitude of the operation performed. In most patients, surgery represents the best chance for cure and the best palliation for dysphagia and local control of their disease. Various methods of esophagectomy have been proposed, but it falls to the individual surgeon to evaluate the benefits of a particular approach in treating the patient with esophageal carcinoma.

Orringer has proposed four goals of esophagectomy[62]:

1. To relieve dysphagia
2. To achieve an operative mortality of less than 10%
3. To require hospitalization of 14 or fewer days
4. To minimize late complications and morbidity (*e.g.*, infection, stricture, reflux, and aspiration)

Patients with local or locoregional carcinoma of the esophagus usually are considered suitable candidates for resection of the esophagus and reestablishment of gastrointestinal continuity. Because of the surgery's extent, adequate cardiac and pulmonary reserves are needed. Patients for planned resection involving a right thoracotomy should have adequate pulmonary function and cessation of smoking for a *minimum* of 2 weeks before surgery. Advanced age alone is *not* a contraindication for resection.[63] Patients with alcoholic cirrhosis or portal hypertension may have abdominal venous varicosities that preclude any attempt at resection.

Surgery alone provides good palliation. It rarely results in cure, except in carcinomas in situ or in stage I carcinomas found serendipitously. Long-term survival is uncommon and has prompted numerous studies evaluating combined modality therapy in improving palliation and survival in patients with carcinoma of the esophagus.[64-67]

Katlic and others at the Massachusetts General Hospital examined the outcome of 701 patients with squamous cell carcinoma of the esophagus treated between 1950 and 1979. Tumor location was upper third in 25% of patients, middle third in 52%, and lower third in 23%. Resection was performed in 261 cases (37.2% overall). Postoperative mortality fell from 30% in the 1950s to 10% in the 1970s. Respiratory complications were the predominant cause of death. Five-year survival rates ranged from 7% to 20%.[68]

Preoperative Evaluation of the Patient With Esophageal Carcinoma

Any patient who presents with dysphagia and weight loss must be considered as having esophageal carcinoma until this diagnosis is excluded. A thorough history and examination can yield important clues to the extent of the tumor and potential for metastases. Symptoms produced by advanced esophageal cancers may indicate unresectable disease. Patients without evidence of extraregional spread of the disease may be excellent candidates for surgical resection or for various multimodality treatments for carcinoma of the esophagus.

The value of noninvasive studies rests in the evaluation of the patient for potential treatment options. Surgical resection and radiation therapy can provide good local control of the tumor. Radiation therapy causes a posttreatment stricture more often than surgery, particularly if the original tumor was long. In addition, the question of persistent tumor always exists. Metastases from the esophageal neoplasm require systemic chemotherapy or local palliation. In patients with locally resectable tumor and without metastatic disease, surgery provides excellent palliation.

A number of studies are required to evaluate the patient thoroughly for resectability, including a history and physical examination, barium swallow, and endoscopy for histologic diagnosis. Bronchoscopy is mandatory for patients with tumors involving the middle or upper third of the esophagus, because tumor invading the posterior membranous trachea or a tracheoesophageal fistula renders the patient surgically unresectable. The barium swallow and the esophagoscopy provide information about the length of the tumor, circumferential extent of the tumor, and character of the tumor (*e.g.*, whether it is bleeding, fungating, polypoid, and so forth). Patients with metastases from esophageal carcinoma have a shortened life expectancy, and surgical resection in these patients usually is not justifiable.[69] Patients should have a CT scan of the chest and upper abdomen and a bone scan, although skeletal surveys

in the absence of bony pain are not cost effective. Endoscopic ultrasonography of the esophagus has been used to assess the extent of the circumferential involvement of the esophageal carcinoma with the surrounding structures. This study is most valuable for tumors of the upper and middle third of the esophagus and may assist in clinical staging. The length of the esophagus involved by the cancer, infiltration of the cancer into adjacent organs, and involvement of lymph nodes may be assessed by this technique.[70-76]

The results of several studies involving CT in esophageal cancer have been reviewed recently.[53,70,77-79] Those using preoperative CT followed by surgical confirmation of stage have shown that CT is best at assessing local extensions of disease and at delineating liver or adrenal metastases. CT is less accurate in assessing the degree of periesophageal lymph node involvement or adjacent tissue invasion. CT underestimates the length of the esophageal lesion. CT scans are helpful in planning radiation therapy and may be useful in assessing the tumor response to radiation therapy and chemotherapy.

Lefor and colleagues examined 32 patients with CT scans of the chest to correlate preoperative staging with postoperative survival.[80] Lesion width of >3.0 cm and the presence of esophageal spread of tumor were the factors associated with poorer survival.

Nuclear magnetic resonance imaging (MRI) is used to determine precisely the extent of involvement of esophageal cancer. MRI has many of the same qualities as CT scans, but MRI scans may be better in assessing the relation of esophageal cancer to vascular structures such as the aorta or to the membranous trachea.

Endoscopy, using the rigid or flexible esophagoscope, is ideal for evaluating the mucosal extent of esophageal cancers. Flexible esophagoscopy is suitable for evaluating the entire esophagus and optimal for tumors of the distal esophagus. Flexible esophagoscopy may evaluate the stomach and duodenum for ulcer disease. Patients with tumors of the upper or middle third esophagus may benefit from rigid esophagoscopy and rigid bronchoscopy to better assess the extent of the tumor and the mobility of the esophagus and trachea, respectively.

Because of the high incidence of second malignancies within the aerodigestive tract, the mouth, pharynx, larynx, and tracheobronchial tree must be examined carefully (particularly in patients with upper and middle third lesions). Bronchoscopy is not often required in patients with a distal third tumor who have had a normal chest x-ray film and a normal CT scan of the chest. In patients with a middle third tumor, flexible bronchoscopy may screen for second primary tumors of the tracheobronchial tree. Patients with an upper third tumor must have bronchoscopy because of the intimate relation of the esophagus with the posterior membranous trachea. Rigid bronchoscopy is helpful to evaluate fixation of the posterior membranous trachea. Bulging of the posterior membranous trachea or the left mainstem bronchus or narrowing of the left mainstem bronchus imply abutting tumor. Biopsy and brushings of this area are mandatory.

Patients with clinically enlarged celiac nodes or apparently resectable histologically positive celiac nodes are suitable for surgery. Patients with histologic evidence of metastases usually do not benefit from surgery. Biopsy of the celiac and lesser curvature lymph nodes is valuable in planning therapy and providing prognostic data. These nodes are resected separately or en bloc with the primary tumor. Celiac node involvement occurs in 10% of patients with upper esophageal malignancies. With lower esophageal cancers, the incidence increases at least fivefold.[38]

If the patient has liver or bony metastases, or extensive and unresectable regional lymphadenopathy, then the patient may be better palliated by methods other than resection or bypass. The patient usually has less than 12 months to live and the advantages of an esophagectomy or bypass are rarely apparent.

Resectability

The presence of metastases (bone, liver, brain, or extensive and unresectable regional nodal metastases) precludes any attempt at resection for cure. Surgeons who attempt palliative esophageal resection or a bypass of the unresectable esophageal tumor should be experienced, and the risk of the procedure should be less than the anticipated 5-year survival rate (*e.g.*, if the 5-year survival rate is 10%, the mortality from the operation should be less than 10%).

In patients without obvious metastases, local control may be obtained with surgery. Patients with extensive middle third tumors may have a tumor adjacent or adherent to the prevertebral fascia, the posterior membranous trachea, or the aortic adventitia. Often preoperative studies suggest this involvement. A transthoracic approach by right thoracotomy may be performed first to assess resectability and to mobilize the esophagus. Should the mass be unresectable, the risk of the proposed esophagectomy is avoided; only the much lower risk of a thoracotomy is taken. Should the mass be resectable, the patient may gain an additional measure of safety from direct visualization afforded by thoracotomy. Thoracic nodal disease may be assessed and resected by thoracotomy.

In about 5% of patients undergoing a planned transhiatal esophagectomy, the tumor is fixed to an intrathoracic structure. In these patients, the tumor is assessed through a right thoracotomy after abdominal exploration and mobilization of the conduit.

Preparation of the Patient for Surgery

Proper evaluation and preparation of the patient and planning of the operation often makes the postoperative course of the esophagectomy patient stable and predictable.

Pulmonary Preparation

Patients are not permitted to smoke for a minimum of 2 weeks before surgery. Bronchorrhea from localized inflammation of the posterior membranous trachea after the esophageal resection, coupled with a right thoracotomy, can lead to prolonged intubation, increased secretions, atelectasis, poor pulmonary function, and pneumonia. Increased mucus production the first few days after cessation of cigarette smoking compounds the problem of adequate pulmonary hygiene with thick secretions. Reintubation may be required. Incentive spirometry is begun *before* surgery and continued throughout the postoperative course to minimize atelectasis.

Cardiac Preparation

Active patients with a normal electrocardiogram may not require further evaluation of cardiac function before surgery.

Patients older than 60 years, those with a history of heart disease or abnormal electrocardiograms, or those with atherosclerosis benefit from further evaluation before surgery. Preoperative loading with digoxin may be helpful in older patients to prevent rapid ventricular response in atrial fibrillation.

Nutrition Preparation

The patients nutritional status is optimized before surgery with enteral or intravenous alimentation. Patients who receive at least 5 days of preoperative nutritional support have fewer complications.[81] Fewer complications have been found in patients who receive preoperative total parenteral nutrition; however, the benefit was found only in those patients who were severely malnourished before surgery.[82]

Presurgical weight loss greater than 10% impacts negatively on subsequent survival. Roth and colleagues noted that patients with a weight loss of less than 10% responded better to chemotherapy and overall did better than patients with a weight loss greater than 10%, implying that those patients who lost less had less advanced disease.[64] Still, there is no evidence that correction of this weight loss before surgery improves prognosis.[64,83]

Enteral feedings are preferred. Soft silastic nasogastric feeding tubes may be placed blindly or under fluoroscopic guidance, even in patients with severe obstruction. Percutaneous gastrostomy may be required in these patients, particularly if several weeks of enteral nutrition are planned. Intravenous alimentation may be required in those patients in whom a feeding tube or gastrostomy cannot be placed.

All patients should be properly hydrated before surgery. Patients with esophageal cancer are prone to dehydration, even those with good oral fluid intake. All patients should be admitted to the hospital at least one night before surgery for hydration with IV fluids in preparation for the surgery the next day.

Dental Preparation

All patients should have a dental consult before surgery to evaluate periodontal health. Anaerobic bacteria within the mouth can cause fatal mediastinal infection; therefore, dental work or extraction should precede esophageal resection.

Antibiotic and Pulmonary Embolism Prophylaxis

Routine antibiotic coverage is usually a second generation cephalosporin, because most esophageal resections are clean-contaminated cases. Patients who have obstruction before surgery may require additional coverage for anaerobes.

All patients should have some type of prophylaxis from deep venous thrombosis or pulmonary embolism. Subcutaneous heparin (5000 U subcutaneously every 8 to 12 hours) is inexpensive and well tolerated. Other forms of prophylaxis, such as elastic stockings or intermittent compression stockings, may be effective.

Other Preparation

A preoperative mechanical catharsis and oral antibiotic may be valuable, particularly if the stomach is unsuitable for use as a conduit because of previous gastric surgery, extensive ulcer disease, or other conditions.

TABLE 25–4. Types of Resection

Ivor Lewis Esophagectomy[84]

Laparotomy and preparation of conduit (stomach preferred)
Right thoracotomy for esophageal mobilization and resection
Intrathoracic anastomosis

Radical En Bloc Esophagectomy

Laparotomy and preparation of conduit (colon)
Thoracoabdominal exploration with resection en bloc of
   thoracic esophagus
   mediastinal lymph nodes
   stomach
   spleen
   celiac and thoracic lymph nodes

Total Thoracic Esophagectomy[87]

Laparotomy and preparation of conduit (stomach preferred)
Neck exploration and mobilization of esophagus
Resection of head of left clavicle to widen thoracic inlet
Retrosternal placement of conduit
Cervical anastomosis
Right thoracotomy for esophageal mobilization and resection

Transhiatal Esophagectomy[88]

Laparotomy and preparation of conduit (stomach preferred)
Neck exploration and mobilization of esophagus
Transhiatal resection
Cervical anastomosis

Anesthesia

In the operating room, a radial artery catheter and at least two large-bore intravenous lines are placed to provide fluids and blood products. A central line may be placed in older patients or in those with underlying cardiac dysfunction. A Foley catheter is inserted. The patient is positioned and the operative field is prepared. An esophagoscopy is performed in the operating room by the surgeon before definitive resection. Flexible or rigid bronchoscopy is performed in the operating room by the surgeon in patients with esophageal carcinoma of the middle or upper third of the esophagus.

APPROACHES TO ESOPHAGEAL RESECTION

Esophagectomy for carcinoma of the esophagus poses considerable physiologic and technical challenges. Various techniques are used to resect the esophagus (Table 25–4).[84-88] The total thoracic esophagectomy and the Lewis procedure (also known as the Ivor Lewis procedure) require a thoracotomy and celiotomy. Transhiatal esophagectomy resects the entire esophagus through the esophageal hiatus and the thoracic inlet. A cervical anastomosis is used. A thoracotomy is avoided, and the stomach is placed into the esophageal bed. The Lewis procedure uses an abdominal exploration and intrathoracic anastomosis. A total thoracic esophagectomy also requires a thoracotomy. The stomach is mobilized and placed

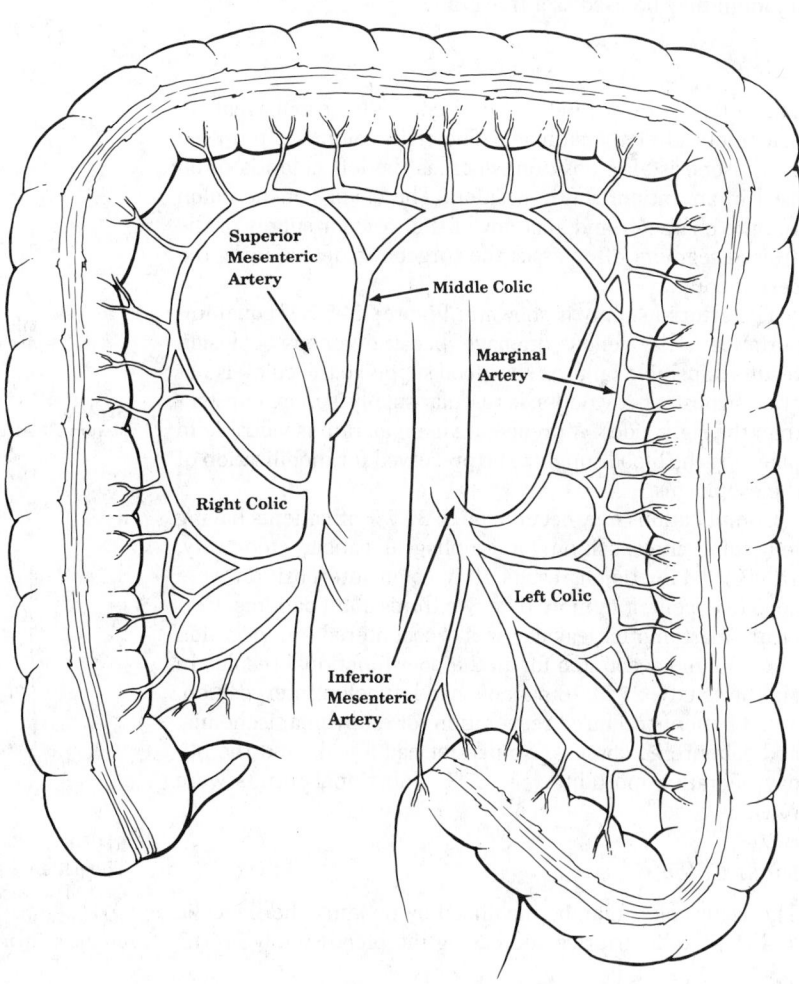

FIGURE 25–5. Arterial blood supply to the colon.

retrosternally. A cervical anastomosis is fashioned after removing the head of the left clavicle. A right thoracotomy is then performed to resect the total thoracic esophagus. The value of the more extensive operation (sometimes called an en bloc esophagectomy) in terms of morbidity and mortality[89] is no greater than that of the transhiatal esophagectomy, which is considered a more palliative procedure.[90] There are advantages and disadvantages to each procedure.

Patients with previous gastric resection often do not have sufficient stomach to serve as a conduit, but colon or jejunum may be used to reestablish gastrointestinal continuity. Blood supply to the colon is well documented and can be easily discerned on preoperative angiography or intraoperatively with finger palpation or Doppler probe. The use of colon for a conduit adds time and morbidity to the operation. Rarely used, but of historical interest, are external skin tubes or external appliances (tubes) that may be interposed for gastrointestinal continuity.

Jejunum

More recently, free jejunal graft interposition has been used successfully after resection for carcinoma of the upper cervical esophagus or hypopharynx that does not extend past the thoracic inlet. Once the esophagus is resected, the proximal and distal anastomoses are completed to stabilize the graft. Vascular access is usually obtained from the external carotid artery and the internal jugular vein. In this fashion, 15 to 20 cm of jejunum may be used as a free graft.

Colon

The colon is the second organ of choice for esophageal replacement after the stomach. The right colon is often used in an isoperistaltic position, whereas the left colon is often used in an antiperistaltic position. The quality of the colon and the character and anatomy of the vascular supply of the desired segment often assist the surgeon in determining the best conduit.

The arterial supply is shown in Figure 25–5. Of equal importance is the venous drainage, because venous occlusion results in pedicle failure. The blood supply to the colon is not always constant (the left-side vascular supply is more constant than the right side). A preoperative angiogram is valuable in planning the blood supply to be preserved for mobilization of the esophagus.

Complications may occur in up to 35.7% of patients having left colon interposition for esophageal cancer (mortality, 11.9%).[91] Functional results after colon interposition were good to excellent in more than two thirds of all patients. Cervical anastomotic leakage was encountered on occasion (13.5%) and accounted for all the poor functional results. In another study, 21 of 26 patients had left colon interposition, and 3 patients required reoperation for empyema, ischemia, and subphrenic abscess. No patient had a leak, and the 30-day operative mortality was 4.5%. Functional results were rated as good.[92]

Right Colon

The right colon may be mobilized by dividing the ileocolic and right colic arteries and basing the blood supply on the middle colic artery (Fig. 25–6). If the length is not sufficient because of a short ascending colon, the left colon may be preferable.

Transverse Colon

The transverse colon may be used in a peristaltic fashion. The right colic artery and the middle colic artery are divided and the colon pedicle is based on the left colic artery.

Left Colon

The left colon may have a more consistent blood supply than the right colon. The left colon and sigmoid may be mobilized and the left colic artery divided. Branches from the inferior mesenteric artery may be divided to mobilize the sigmoid colon further. At least 2 cm of mesentery is needed to protect the marginal artery. The left colon would be placed in an isoperistaltic position (Fig. 25–7).

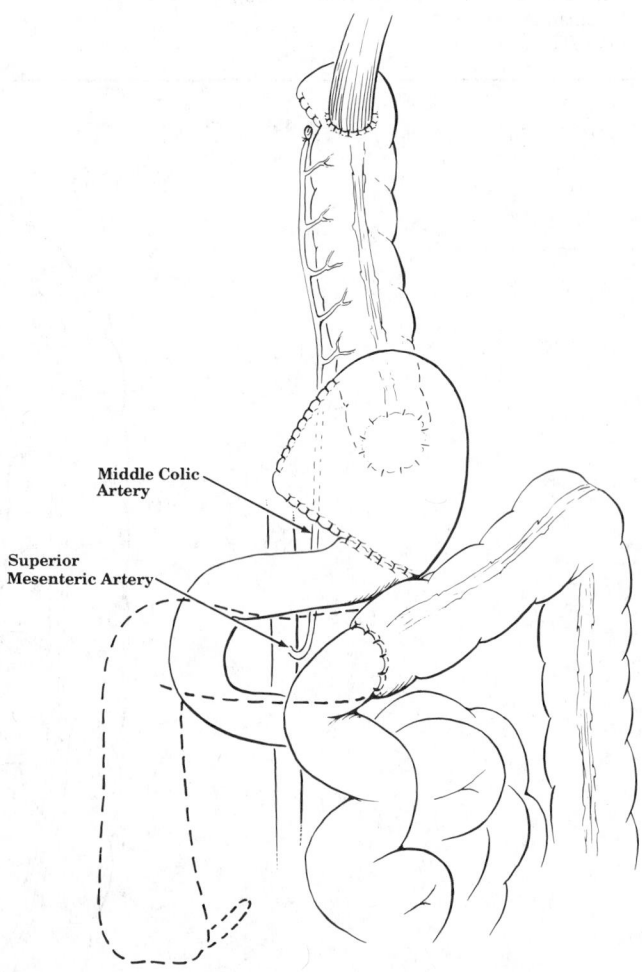

FIGURE 25–6. Use of the right colon in an isoperistaltic position. The patient had a prior vagotomy and antrectomy for peptic ulcer disease. The vascular supply to the colon is behind the transverse mesocolon and the stomach, and the cologastrostomy is placed posteriorly on the stomach.

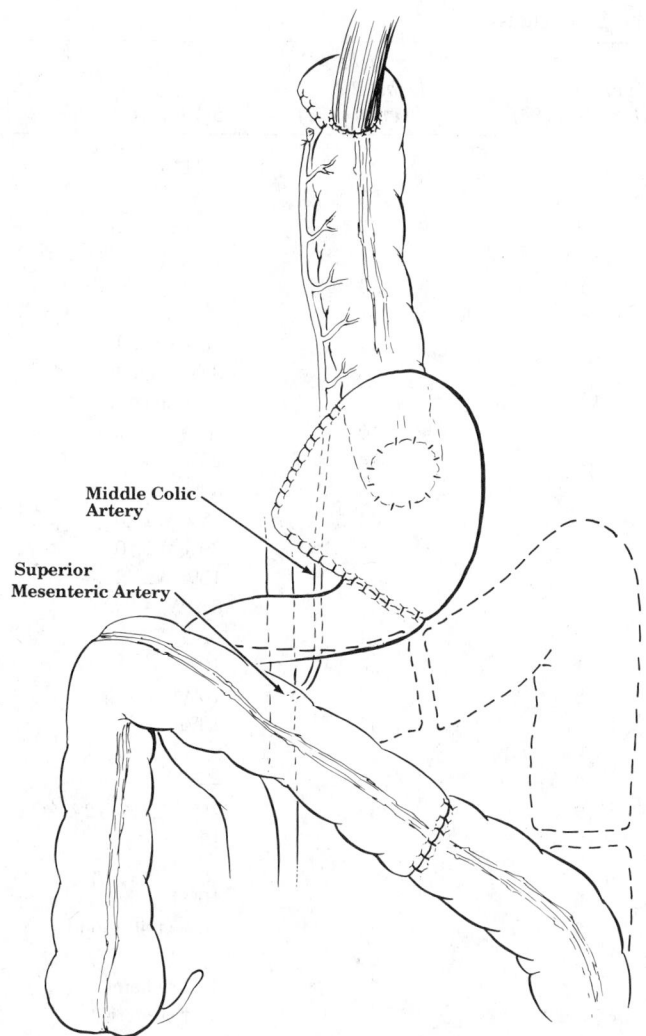

Middle Colic Artery

Superior Mesenteric Artery

FIGURE 25–7. Use of the left colon in an antiperistaltic position.

RESULTS OF SURGICAL RESECTION

Although overall survival after esophageal resection has remained fairly constant, operative mortality has slowly decreased over the past 30 years. The major problems of this operation are inadequate staging, intrathoracic extension of tumor, and reestablishment of alimentary tract continuity. Selection of conduit location and construction of the esophageal-conduit anastomosis, anastomotic leak, and postoperative respiratory compromise have been identified as problems in establishing alimentary tract continuity.[93] Various solutions have been proposed. In 1945, Sweet proposed a left thoracoabdominal approach for esophagectomy.[94] In 1946, Lewis proposed a combined laparotomy and right thoracotomy.[95] More recently, Orringer has revived the transhiatal or blunt esophagectomy, which avoids a thoracotomy and minimizes respiratory complications.[90,96] Each technique has particular advantages and disadvantages (Tables 25–4 and 25–5).[64,85,97–113]

Most surgeons develop expertise in and emphasize a single technique of esophagectomy. The decrease in operative mor-

tality reflects refinement in surgical technique due to increased experience in operative and perioperative care in the surgical treatment of carcinoma of the esophagus in various centers throughout the country.

Ellis described an 18-year experience with 275 patients who underwent resection with a 30-day mortality rate of only 2.2%. Intrathoracic esophagogastrostomy was performed in 196 patients, whereas cervical anastomosis was performed in 61 patients (53 of them had a transhiatal esophagectomy). Major complications (*e.g.,* prolonged hospital stay) occurred in 40 patients (14.5%). Tumor stage was the most important determinant of long-term survival. The actuarial 5-year survival rate was 20.8% for all patients and 23.3% for those patients in whom a curative resection was achieved.[98]

Mathisen and colleagues reported 104 patients with intrathoracic anastomoses after esophagectomy for carcinoma of the esophagus with nonanastomotic leaks. Sixty-four of the patients had a left thoracoabdominal incision, and 40 patients had a Lewis esophagectomy. All anastomoses were constructed by the two-layer inverting technique with interrupted silk sutures. Operative mortality was 2.9% (3 patients). Five percent (5 patients) required one to three dilations. Major complications included pneumonia (12 patients, 12%) and reexploration for bleeding (2 patients, 2%). Positive lymph node metastases were identified in 75% of patients. Anastomotic recurrence was documented in 6 patients (6%).[100]

Shao reported 6123 cases of carcinoma of the gastric cardia and esophagus for which the resectability rate was 89.9%. Overall mortality was 3%, and the complication rate was 10.3%. The 5-year survival rate was 36.8%, and 10-year survival rate was 17.2%.[114]

Age alone is not a contraindication to surgery. Patients older than 70 years have a postoperative mortality similar to that of other age groups (13%).[63]

Lewis Esophagectomy

In 1946, Lewis proposed a combined laparotomy (Fig. 25–8) and right thoracotomy (Fig. 25–9) approach that provided excellent exposure for preparation of the conduit and for resection of the esophagus and reanastomosis of the conduit in the chest.[95] In a recent series of 100 patients treated with a combined laparotomy and right thoracotomy, postoperative complications occurred in 27 patients (including pulmonary complications in 11 and anastomotic leak in 9). The 30-day operative mortality was 3%. The 5-year survival rate was 85% for patients with stage I tumors, 34% for patients with stage II tumors, and 15% for patients with stage III tumors. Thirty-one patients required postoperative dilations for some degree of dysphagia.[101] In another study of 100 patients undergoing Lewis esophagogastrectomy, 70 patients were cured and 30 were palliated. Operative mortality was 4% and morbidity 7% (due to anastomotic leakage). Fifteen patients had pulmonary complications. The 3-year survival rate was 25%; it was better in early stage disease (stage I or II, 68.4%) than in later stage disease (stage III, 23%).[87]

Mitchell had excellent results in a series of 40 esophagogastrectomies performed with laparotomy and right thoracotomy; there was no operative mortality, no anastomotic leak, and no major pulmonary complication.[102]

TABLE 25–5.   Results of Surgical Resection for Carcinoma of the Esophagus

Investigations	Resection Technique	No. of Patients	Operative Mortality (%)	Operative Morbidity (Overall) (%)	5-Year Survival
Lozac'h et al, 1991[97]	R Thor	100	4	22	25%*
Ellis, 1989[98]	R Thor	275	2.2	25	21%
Mansour and Downey, 1989[99]	R Thor	100	3	27	15% stage II
					10% stage III
Mathisen et al, 1988[100]	R Thor	40	2.9	13	33% SCCA; 8% ACA
	L Thor	64			
King et al, 1987[101]	R Thor	100	3	27	86% stage I
					34% stage II
					15% stage III
Mitchell, 1987[102]	R Thor	40	0	10	7%
Goldfaden et al, 1986[103]	R Thor	43	14	84	20%
DeMeester et al, 1988[104]	En bloc	14	7	—	53%
Altorki and Skinner, 1990[85]	En bloc	111	11	44	55% W1N0
					29% W1N0
					15% W2N2
					8% W1–2N2
Gupta, 1990[105]	THE	40	12	71†	—
Gotley et al, 1990[106]	THE	54	11	26	10%†
Hankins et al, 1989[107]	THE	26	8	85	10%†
Goldfaden et al, 1986[103]	THE	29	7	48	18%
Page et al, 1990[108]	L Thor	115	9	16	22%†
Pradhan et al, 1989[109]	L Thor	110	3	19	—
Matthews and Steel, 1987[110]	L Thor	75	12	33	28% SCCA; 12% ACA
Mannell and Becker, 1991[111]	Total	93	12	—	13%
	R Thor	34			
Hankins et al, 1989[107]	Total	52	6	75	10%†
Chasseray et al, 1989[12]	Total	43	9	51	30% at 40 months
	R Thor	49	14	39	
Roth et al, 1988[64]	Total	36	0	39	25%† chemo
					5%† surgery
Akiyama et al, 1976[113]	Total	130	1	5	—

SCCA, squamous cell carcinoma; ACA, adenocarcinoma; R Thor, right thoracotomy; L Thor, left thoracotomy; Total, total esophagectomy (retrosternal conduit with cervical anastamosis and thoracotomy for esophageal resection); En bloc, radical en bloc esophagectomy; Chemo, chemotherapy followed by surgery group; Surgery, surgery only group.
* Survival at 3 years.
† Includes pleural entry.

Radical En Bloc Esophagectomy

Radical resection for esophageal cancer can be compared with radical resection for breast cancer. The value of surgical resection lies in local control of the neoplasm. Although surgery may be considered curative for early stage disease in either instance, surgery cannot control the systemic spread or wide lymphatic spread in either disease. The survival rate after radical en bloc esophagectomy[89] is no greater than that after transhiatal esophagectomy.[96]

DeMeester and colleagues proposed an extended en bloc resection of carcinoma of the esophagus consisting of thoracic esophagectomy, mediastinal lymph node dissection, and gastrectomy with abdominal (celiac) lymph node dissection.[104] Alimentary tract continuity was reestablished using the left colon. Operative mortality was 7%, and actuarial survival rates were 53% at 5 years (stages I and II). In 111 patients treated with en bloc esophagectomy, operative mortality was 11% and complications occurred in 49 patients (44%). No recurrences were noted after 3 years. Survival was dependent on tumor stage.[115]

Total Thoracic Esophagectomy

A total thoracic esophagectomy (TTE), as described by Akiyama and colleagues,[113] consists of laparotomy for mobilization of the stomach (see Fig. 25–8) or colon with retrosternal placement of the conduit and cervical anastomosis (Figs. 25–10 and 25–11). The patient then has a right thoracotomy for esophageal resection.

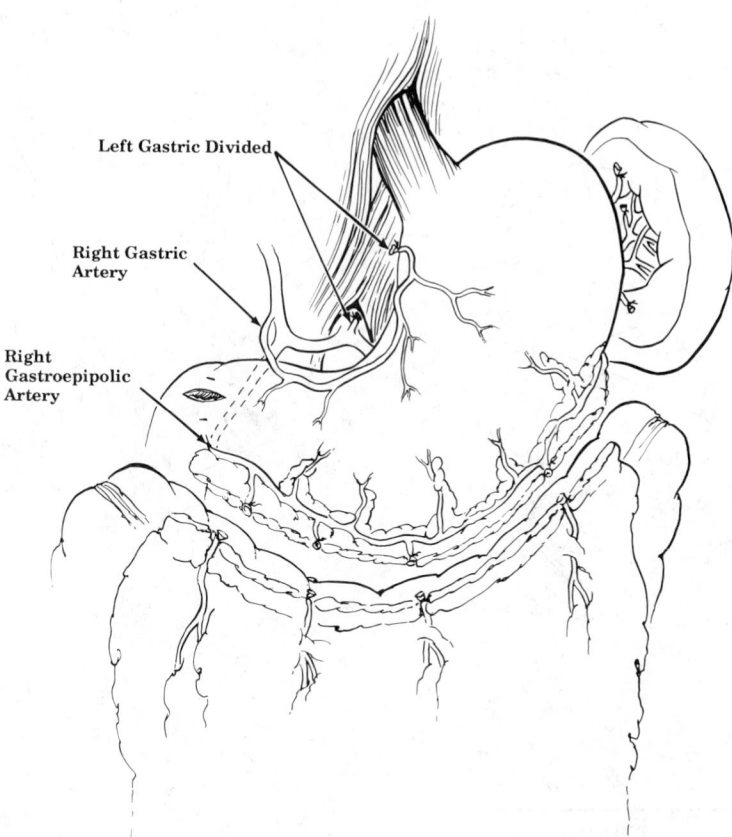

Left Gastric Divided

Right Gastric
Artery

Right
Gastroepipolic
Artery

FIGURE 25–8. Mobilization of the stomach. The stomach is used primarily as a conduit for esophageal replacement. The blood supply is based on the right gastric artery and gastroepiploic artery. The left gastric and the short gastric arteries are divided. Notice the pyloromyotomy.

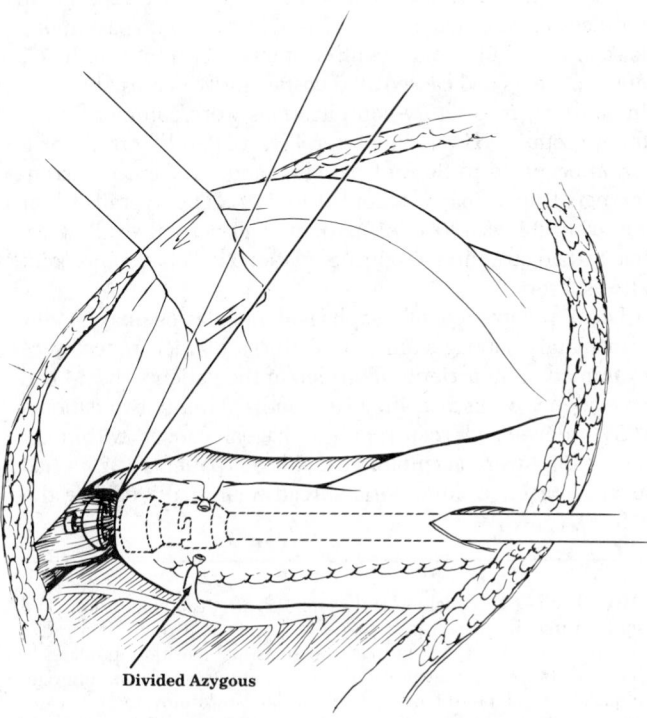

Divided Azygous

FIGURE 25–9. Right thoracotomy and intrathoracic anastomosis after the Lewis esophagectomy. A surgical stapling device is used to create an end-to-end anastomosis within the chest. The anastomosis is placed above the level of the azygous vein, and the suture line along the lesser curvature is oversewn.

A recent study compared TTE (21 patients) with the Lewis procedure (25 patients).[116] Overall mortality was 22% but decreased to 5% during the last 3 years. The 5-year survival rate was 20%. No differences in long-term survival were noted between the two groups, but there was better reflux control in patients undergoing TTE.

Transhiatal Esophagectomy

Transhiatal esophagectomy (THE) has been proposed as an alternative to transthoracic esophagectomy (Figs. 25–12 and 25–13). Critics of THE suggest that the operation is subjective, dangerous because it is done blind, and an inadequate cancer operation. Proponents suggest that THE minimizes physiologic trauma to the patient, pulmonary complications, operative time, and duration of hospitalization. This procedure provides good palliaton of dysphagia. Even with middle third tumors, operative mortality is similar to that of the transthoracic approach (9%).[117]

A learning curve for THE is apparent because surgeons with less experience have more complications that surgeons with more experience. The anatomy of structures important in performing THE has been described by Strano and Bremner.[118] Orringer reported 100 patients with mortality of 6% after THE and no mortality from anastomotic leaks.[90,96] Complications included pleural entry in two thirds of the patients, recurrent laryngeal nerve injury (transient) in 31 patients (4 patients required Teflon injection into the paralyzed cord),

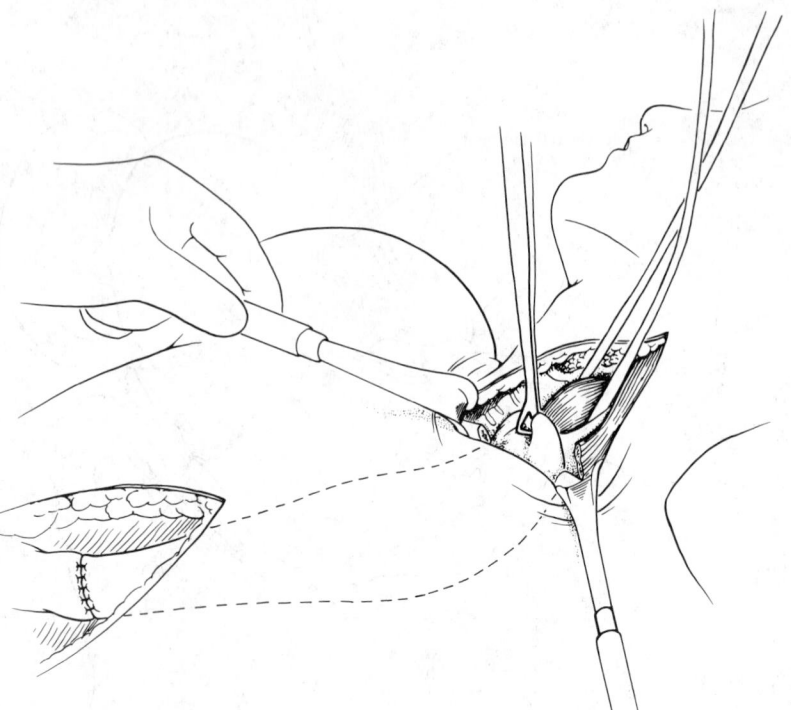

FIGURE 25–10. Reestablishment of alimentary continuity. The stomach is placed in a retrosternal position and a cervical anastomosis is fashioned. The proximal third of the clavicle and lateral portion of the manubrium is resected. A pyloroplasty has been created.

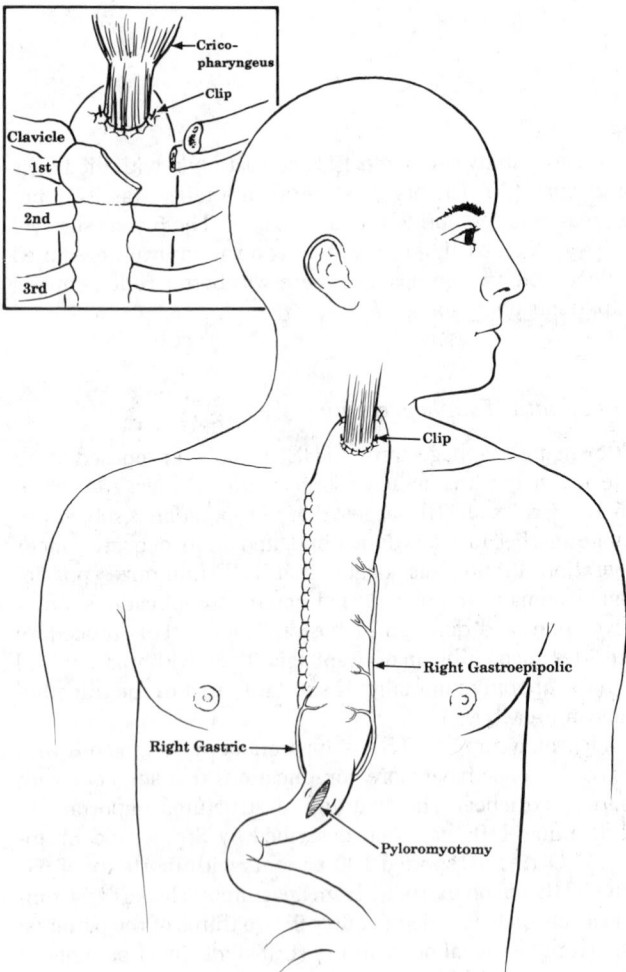

and, more rarely, tracheal laceration (2 patients), chylothorax (2 patients), or anastomotic leak (5 patients, 5%).

In contrast, other investigators describe THE performed in 40 patients with a 30-day mortality rate of 12%. Complications included intraoperative pneumothorax (71%) treated by tube thoracostomy, transient hoarseness (19%), and anastomotic leak (17%). Pulmonary complications occurred in only 7% of the patients and caused all 6 postoperative deaths (11%).[105] In contrast, respiratory complications were common in another group of 54 patients after THE (41%).[110] Atrial fibrillation occurred in 26% of patients, and transient recurrent laryngeal nerve palsy occurred in 11%. The overall 3-year survival rate was 10%. All patients had normal swallowing, but 11 had strictures requiring dilation (20%) at some point after surgery.[106]

Local recurrence of esophageal neoplasms may follow transhiatal esophagectomy.[119] Patterns of recurrence were examined in 35 patients. Thirteen of the patients (37%) had no evidence of disease after 18 months. Twenty-two patients (63%) developed recurrent esophageal cancer within 14 months; 13 were asymptomatic. Eleven patients (32%) had local recurrence. Metastatic spread was usually outside the

FIGURE 25–11. Position of the stomach after esophagectomy. The stomach may be placed in a posterior mediastinal route or a retrosternal route (*inset*). A posterior mediastinal position provides a shorter distance and may provide for better emptying after eating. The stomach is tacked to the prevertebral facia. A pyloromyotomy or pyloroplasty is created to prevent gastric stasis and enhance gastric emptying. The pyloromyotomy and the cervical anastomosis are marked with metal clips to enhance localization on postoperative radiographic studies. (*Inset*) The proximal third of the clavicle and the lateral portion of the manubrium and first rib may be resected to increase the diameter of the thoracic inlet for a retrosternal conduit.

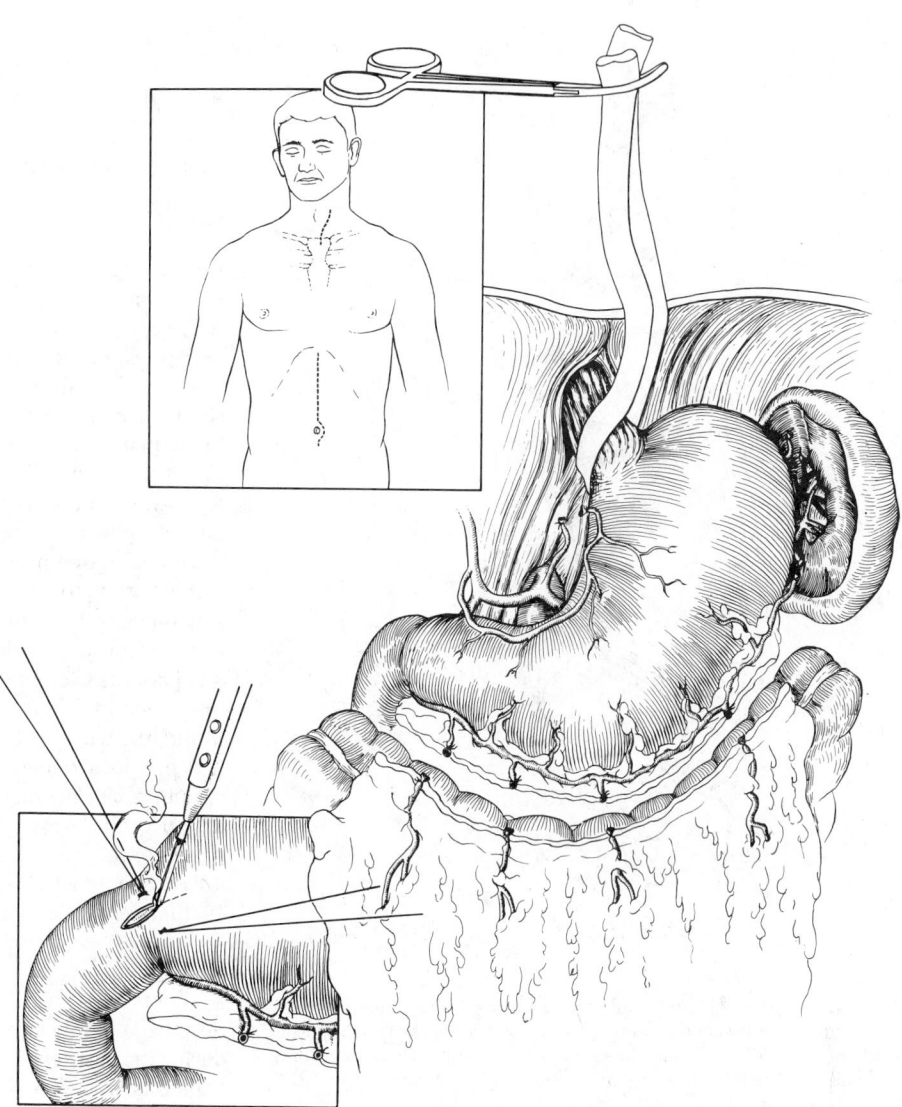

FIGURE 25–12. Mobilization of the stomach. The stomach is mobilized to preserve the gastroepiploic and the right gastric arteries. A pyloromyotomy or a pyloroplasty is fashioned. The spleen is not removed.

conduit, and CT scans were better than barium studies in detecting the recurrent tumor.[120]

Gastric emptying is impaired after THE. Fourteen patients were examined for rates of solid and liquid gastric emptying. Gastric emptying occurred best in upright patients and was dependent on an upright position for 1 to 2 hours after meals.[121]

Comparison of Transhiatal Esophagectomy and Transthoracic Esophagectomy

Transhiatal esophagectomy and transthoracic esophagectomy have been compared in several studies. In one study, 52 patients underwent TTE and 26 patients underwent THE. Five anastomotic leaks occurred in the THE group, and only one required hospitalization longer than 14 days. Three leaks occurred in patients in the TTE group, and the hospital stays of these 3 patients were extended by several weeks. Overall morbidity was high; it was 75% in the TTE group and 85% in the THE group (p = not significant). Overall mortality was

similar: 3 of the 52 TTE patients (6%) and 2 of the THE patients (8%) died. THE works as well as TTE without causing significant increases in hospitalization duration, mortality, or morbidity.[107] In another study, TTE was performed in 43 patients and THE in 29. The demographics of the two groups were similar. Fewer complications occurred in the THE group (48%) than in the TTE group (86%, $p < 0.05$). THE had a better mortality rate than TTE (7% versus 14%, $p < 0.05$), less intraoperative blood loss (1187 ml versus 2150 ml, $p < 0.05$), and shorter postoperative hospitalization (12.3 days versus 22.2 days, $p < 0.05$). There was no difference in survival rates.[103]

In a third review, 210 patients with middle or distal esophageal carcinoma underwent resection by THE (n = 38) or TTE (n = 172).[122] More complications occurred in the THE group, including excessive bleeding and perforation of the esophagus at the tumor in 7 patients (18%) and recurrent laryngeal nerve injury in 5 patients (13%). The survival was better in the TTE group. The fact that THE was performed infrequently may explain the higher rate of complications.

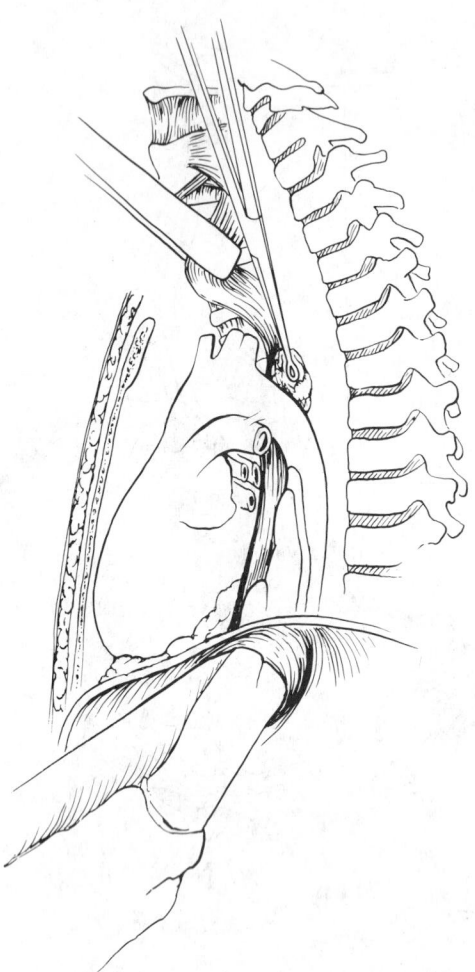

FIGURE 25–13.   Transhiatal esophagectomy. The surgeon's hand may be used to dissect the esophagus off the prevertebral facia posteriorly in the midline. When the esophagus is completely mobilized, it is divided in the neck with a surgical stapling device and removed. A cervical anastomosis is created.

Left Thoracotomy

The left thoracotomy approach has been used for carcinoma of the esophagus; resection is hampered, however, by the aortic arch. Pradhan and colleagues examined the left thoracotomy approach in 110 patients.[109] Postoperative mortality was 2.7% and morbidity was caused by respiratory complications, which occurred in 21 patients (19%). Page and colleagues noted the same results in 119 patients, with a perioperative mortality 8.7% (10 of 115 patients), a leakage rate of 1.7% (2 of 115), and benign stricture in 16 patients (14%).[108] The survival rate at 3 years was 22.1%.

Endothoracic Endoesophageal Resection

An endothoracic endoesophageal pull-through procedure cores out the mucosa of the esophagus with the tumor, theoretically eliminating bleeding, chylothorax, and membranous tracheal injury. In a study of 68 patients, this procedure resulted in no intraoperative deaths and an operative mortality rate of 13.2%

(9 patients). Overall leaks occurred in 13.3% of patients (8 of 68). The stomach was preferred for reconstruction, but the left colon was used if the stomach was not suitable.[123]

Laryngoesophagectomy

Esophageal neoplasms in the cervical esophagus may involve the posterior membranous trachea and the cricopharyngeus muscle. Tumors in the hypopharynx may extend to the cervical esophagus. In these patients, resection of the larynx and the esophagus is required. An anterior cervical tracheostomy with a *gastric interposition* is commonly performed. When the tumor involves more of the trachea, an anterior mediastinal tracheostomy may be constructed after removal of the breastplate. The esophagus is mobilized by means of a transhiatal approach.[124,125] Laryngoesophagectomy with gastric interposition offers the best chance for cure or palliation of advanced hypopharyngeal and laryngeal tumors. Patients who have undergone previous radiation therapy may be resected safely, although healing may be poor. Forty-one patients with squamous cell carcinoma of the esophagus were treated with laryngectomy, esophagectomy, and gastric pull-up. Twenty-one patients had undergone previous radiation therapy. Complications included one operative death (2.5%) and anastomotic leaks in 9 patients (22%). All 9 of these patients had had previous radiation therapy, and 3 required flap reconstruction. The average postoperative hospital stay was 31 days. The overall 2-year survival rate was 35%. In a study of 42 patients, mortality was 19% and the complication rate was 40%. The length of hospitalization ranged from 23 days (without complications) to 44 days (with complications).[126]

COMPLICATIONS OF SURGERY

Surgical complications of esophagectomy have decreased during the past several years. During the past decade, mortality from this procedure dropped from 31% to 8%. The cumulative 5-year survival rate remains unchanged at 21%. Extended resection held no survival advantage over conventional resection or transhiatal esophagectomy (THE) regarding long-term survival.[127] Of 202 patients undergoing esophageal resection, 21 patients died in the hospital (10.4%). Fourteen patients died of multisystem failure. Risk factors were postoperative respiratory failure ($p < 0.001$), emergency reoperation ($p < 0.001$), and leak ($p < 0.01$). Forty-two percent of survivors had complications. Gastric stasis occurred in 8%.[128]

An anastomotic leak in the chest is life threatening. Improvements in techniques for hand-sewn anastomoses and better mechanical stapling devices may eventually eliminate this complication. In one series, 14 of 242 patients who underwent intrathoracic anastomosis had leak, and 2 patients died. Hand-sewn anastomoses and single-layer anastomoses were more likely to leak than were mechanical or stapled anastomoses and double-layer suturing.[129]

Techniques, locations, and results for various anastomoses were evaluated in 221 patients (122 sutured and 99 stapled). Leaks occurred in 21 sutured anastomoses (17.2%) and 7 stapled anastomoses (7.1%) ($p < 0.05$). Strictures were more common in the stapled group (13 of 99, 13%) compared with the hand-sewn group (2 of 122, 1.6%).[130] The circular stapler was used in 85 patients, 19 of whom had the Lewis procedure and 66 of whom had a low left thoracotomy. The overall mortality rate was 20%. Mortality was related to leakage in 4.7% of the patients. Benign strictures were dilated in 22% of surgical patients.[131]

Chasseray and colleagues examined cervical or thoracic anastomosis from esophagectomy in a prospective trial.[112] Forty-nine patients underwent laparotomy and right thoracotomy with intrathoracic anastomosis (TA), and 43 patients underwent laparotomy, right thoracotomy, and cervical anastomosis (CA). Anastomotic leak was more frequent after CA (26%) than after TA (4%, $p < 0.002$). Respiratory complications were more frequent with TA than with CA (p = not significant). Thirty-day mortality rates were similar for the two groups (14.3% TA, and 9.3% CA). Strictures occurred in 14% of patients who had TA and in 23% of those who had CA. Duration of survival was related to extent of disease; the 2-year survival rate was 47%, and the 3.5-year survival rate was 30%.[112]

ADENOCARCINOMA OF THE ESOPHAGUS

Adenocarcinoma involving the stomach and esophagus may be described as a gastroesophageal junction tumor. Many of these tumors arise in Barrett's esophagus, a premalignant lesion.[132] Studies examining the treatment and survival of patients with these neoplasms of the distal esophagus or the gastric cardia (extending into the esophagus) often make no distinction between tumors arising primarily from the stomach extending into the esophagus and those arising primarily from the esophagus.

Primary adenocarcinoma of the esophagus is not as rare as was once thought. In a series of 163 patients with esophageal cancer seen between 1975 and 1982, 6.7% had a primary adenocarcinoma of the esophagus.[133] This figure is close to that reported from Denmark, in which 6.9% of the esophageal carcinomas were found to be adenocarcinoma.[134] Some studies have shown that esophageal adenocarcinomas accounted for 34% of all esophageal cancers and 60% of tumors confined to the lower third of the esophagus.[135]

More recently, rates of adenocarcinoma of the esophagus have increased 4% to 10% per year in contrast to declining rates of adenocarcinoma of the more distal portions of the stomach.[136–140] The Surveillance, Epidemiology, and End Results (SEER) program noted that the overall incidence of adenocarcinoma (0.4 persons per 100,000) increased more than 74% in white men between 1973 and 1982. Most of these tumors (79%) arise in the lower third of the esophagus.[138] This disease is one primarily affecting white males,[109,117,127,128,130] who have a greater frequency of hiatal hernia (40%) and smoking and alcohol use. *Helicobacter pylori* infections have been associated with an increased risk for gastric carcinoma, although the role of *Helicobacter pylori* as an etiologic agent in the pathogenesis of esophageal adenocarcinoma is not known.[140–143]

ORIGINS OF PRIMARY ADENOCARCINOMA

Adenocarcinoma of the esophagus may arise from three sources: superficial and deep glands of the esophagus, embryonic remnants of glandular epithelium in the esophagus, or metaplastic glandular epithelium. The superficial and deep glands of the esophagus are mucus-secreting cells indistinguishable in appearance from the cardiac glands of the stomach. Secretions from the superficial glands located within the mucosa enter the lumen of the esophagus through ducts lined by a single layer of mucus cells. The terminal portion of the ducts from these glands is lined with squamous cells. The deep esophageal glands are thought to give rise to the mucoepidermoid carcinomas occasionally found in the esophagus.[144]

Primary adenocarcinoma of the esophagus may arise from ectopic islands of columnar epithelium or submucosal glands. These glands may be congenital or may arise from Barrett's esophagus (columnar cell-lined epithelium). Aberrant gastric mucosa, particularly in the upper and middle third of the esophagus, may be Barrett's mucosa and give rise to primary adenocarcinoma.[145]

BARRETT'S ESOPHAGUS

Barrett's esophagus, or columnar cell-lined esophagus (CLE), may be found in up to 20% of patients undergoing esophagoscopy for esophagitis. The number of these patients who develop adenocarcinoma is unknown but may be as many as half of all patients.[146] The relation between Barrett's esophagus and adenocarcinoma is not completely clear, but 59% to 86% of all adenocarcinomas of the esophagus may arise in Barrett's mucosa. Therefore, Barrett's esophagus and adenocarcinoma may have a common etiology.[146–148]

Why Barrett's esophagus occurs is not clear. Repetitive chemical trauma from reflux may damage the squamous mucosa of the esophagus, which may be replaced by glandular epithelium growing up from the stomach. Submucosal esophageal glands from within the esophagus itself may proliferate and cover the injured esophageal surface.

The natural history of Barrett's esophagus has been studied at length.[149–152] Once Barrett's esophagus occurs, it is unlikely that it will resolve. Medical or surgical management have little influence on the subsequent development of malignancy. If esophagitis is found in a patient with Barrett's esophagus, it must be corrected and controlled. Routine annual or biannual screening should be performed for all patients with Barrett's esophagus, and any severe dysplasia should be resected.[153]

In a study of 241 patients with Barrett's esophagus, the prevalence of adenocarcinoma was 27% (65 patients).[72] Thirty percent of the patients were operated on for adenocarcinoma arising from Barrett's mucosa. In 8 patients, the carcinoma was discovered on routine endoscopy for a incidence of 3.3%, and in 4 other patients, disease progression from Barrett's esophagus to carcinoma was documented. The 65 patients with carcinoma underwent surgery; 61 (94%) had operable disease. The operative mortality rate was 3.3%, and the actuarial 5-year survival rate was 23.7%. Adenocarcinoma occurred in 6 patients who had previous antireflux surgery; this surgery did not consistently protect against the development of carcinoma in patients with a previous diagnosis of Barrett's esophagus. Surveillance must be continued for life.[150] In another study conducted over 10 years, 76 patients were identified as having Barrett's esophagus.[146] Fifty-six patients (74%) had complications relating to their reflux. Twenty-nine patients had carcinoma (38%). Antireflux surgery was performed in 35 patients. The resolution of Barrett's esophagus in the esophagus of these patients was not well documented.

Incidence of Adenocarcinoma in Barrett's Esophagus

Numerous investigators have examined the clinical and molecular changes that occur as Barrett's mucosa evolves from minimal or mild dysplasia to severe dysplasia or carcinoma in situ, and then to invasive malignancy. Barrett's esophagus frequently is identified at the periphery of the esophageal adenocarcinoma, suggesting that the tumor arises from Barrett's mucosa. However, Barrett's mucosa is not identified in all patients with esophageal adenocarcinoma. The apparent absence of Barrett's mucosa on histologic examination may be related to the overgrowth of adenocarcinoma in all areas previously occupied by the Barrett's mucosa; on the other hand, the neoplasm may arise in an area uninvolved by Barrett's mucosa.

In one study conducted over 6 years, 50 patients with Barrett's esophagus were identified.[154] Twelve patients had superficial adenocarcinoma arising in Barrett's esophagus, for a prevalence of 24%. High-grade dysplasia was identified in 6 of the 12 patients, but this diagnosis was later changed to adenocarcinoma.

Duhaylongsod and Wolfe examined 16 patients with adenocarcinoma arising in Barrett's esophagus, 34 patients with adenocarcinoma not related to Barrett's esophagus, and 30 patients with Barrett's esophagus without adenocarcinoma.[155] A marked male predominance was noted in malignant Barrett's esophagus. Most of the malignancies were located at the gastroesophageal junction. The 4-year survival rate in non-Barrett's adenocarcinoma was 35%, whereas that in Barrett's adenocarcinoma was 60%.[155]

Molecular Changes Associated With Barrett's Esophagus

As an identified premalignant lesion, Barrett's mucosa has been studied intensively for particular histologic and molecular changes that may predispose it to malignancy. Abnormalities have been demonstrated in Barrett's mucosa histologically and by flow cytometry.[156,157] Eighty-six specimens from 25 patients with Barrett's mucosa were so evaluated. Seventy-three had no dysplasia, and 13 had some dysplasia (7 low grade, 6 high grade). Eight patients without dysplasia were aneuploid, and 11 patients with dysplasia were aneuploid. Histologic dysplasia and aneuploidy did not occur together consistently and may reflect separate subgroups of patients at risk.[158] Electron microscopic examination of cytoplasmic organelles revealed an abnormal depletion of organelles required for mucus biosynthesis. These observations may be biologically significant in identifying a population at increased risk for developing adenocarcinoma of the esophagus.[159] Chromosomal abnormalities have been identified in patients with adenocarcinoma related to Barrett's mucosa.[160] Fifteen short-term cultures of Barrett's mucosa were grown in vitro, and 10 cases were evaluated. Nine of the 10 cultures had evidence of chromosome rearrangement, and the researchers demonstrated that Barrett's esophagus had clonal proliferation of karyotypically abnormal cells.

Ornithine decarboxylase (ODC) is the rate-limiting enzyme in polyamine biosynthesis and is usually induced during the G_1 phase of the cell cycle. An increase in cellular polyamine synthesis is a general characteristic of growing cells. ODC activity in Barrett's mucosa is elevated compared with that in the adjacent gastric or small intestinal epithelium, which suggests that the regulation of polyamine metabolism by this enzyme may be altered in this premalignant tissue.[161,162] In 15 patients with Barrett's mucosa, high-grade dysplasia had more ODC activity than low-grade dysplasia.[162] The retinoid 13-cis-retinoic acid produced no change in the extent of the lesion in 11 patients.[156,163]

Molecular techniques can probe for changes in the *RAS* oncogene or p53 tumor suppressor gene. In Barrett's esophagus, no expression of the c-Ha-*RAS* protooncogene, p53, or c-*MYC* was detected, and no amplification of c-Ha-*RAS* or of six other protooncogenes was detected.[164] Other researchers have confirmed that no *RAS* mutations or p53 mutations have been found in esophageal tumor samples.[165] However, p53 mutations were identified in 4 of 7 samples of Barrett's epithelium that had little or no dysplasia but were located adjacent to esophageal adenocarcinomas. This finding suggests that p53 mutations may be a marker for premalignant changes in Barrett's mucosa. Other molecular events are required for tumor development, because these p53 mutations are lost when adenocarcinoma develops.[165]

Management of Barrett's Esophagus

Medical Management

In one prospective randomized study, 67 patients with Barrett's esophagus were followed over 36 months. Medical management (predominantly H_2 blockers) did not result in consistent reduction in the extent of Barrett's epithelium over this period. Eighty-two percent of the patients had a change in length of the lesion at less than 1 cm per year.[166] Omeprazole (20 mg/day) reduced the percentage of time patients had an esophageal pH below 4 and reduced the number of reflux episodes longer than 5 minutes, but it had no effect on acid clearance. In patients with Barrett's esophagus, omeprazole lowered intragastric acidity.[135] Omeprazole may be more effective than H_2 blockers (*e.g.*, cimetidine, ranitidine) in causing regression of Barrett's esophagus.[167]

Surgical Management

Resection is the treatment of choice in patients with adenocarcinoma of the esophagus or gastroesophageal junction. Longitudinal spread of tumor along the rich lymphatic plexus is frequent and esophagectomy is required. Mahoney and Condon examined 37 patients with adenocarcinoma involving the distal esophagus.[168] Thirty-three patients had stage III or IV tumor at the time of operation. THE was performed in 27 patients. Three patients died, for a mortality of 8%, and anastomotic leak occurred in 9 patients. Dilations were performed on 11 patients one or more times. Mediastinal recurrence occurred in 3 patients (8%). Thirty-one percent of the patients were still alive after 2 years. Surgery is the treatment of choice in patients with Barrett's esophagus who have severe or high-grade dysplasia.[153,169-173] Some investigators have suggested that patients who are otherwise suitable candidates for esophagectomy but who have a single biopsy showing severe dysplasia should undergo resection.[173]

Surgical management of patients with high-grade dysplasia is identical to that for patients with carcinoma in situ. The management of high-grade (or severe) dysplasia was examined in 9 patients without evidence of carcinoma who had columnar lining of the esophagus extending orad from the cardia.[170] Eight patients underwent resection and colon interposition; the other patients had sleeve resection of the cervical esophagus. Multifocal carcinoma was found in 3 patients, and 1 patient had microinvasive carcinoma. No carcinoma was found in the remaining 4 patients. Esophagectomy is indicated in these patients, because 45% have esophageal carcinoma, and the potential for long-term survival is high. In another study in which 88 patients with Barrett's mucosa were identified, 19 underwent resection, including those with high-grade dysplasia (3 patients) or parietal cells in the esophagus (1 patient), those who did not undergo long-term surveillance (2 patients), and those for whom it was not possible to exclude adenocarcinoma preoperatively (2 patients). Five patients were resected for large penetrating ulcer, a complication of Barrett's esophagus.[170]

Antireflux Procedures for Treatment of Barrett's Mucosa

The role of gastroesophageal reflux in causing Barrett's esophagus is unknown, although the two are associated. The mechanisms of malignant degeneration of Barrett's esophagus to adenocarcinoma are unknown. Routine surveillance (esophagogastroscopy) in patients with Barrett's esophagus permits early detection of severe dysplasia or carcinoma in situ and, presumably, improves the selection of patients selection for esophagectomy and long-term survival. The recommendation is that patients with Barrett's esophagus should be examined at least once every 2 years by esophagoscopy with serial longitudinal biopsies and brushings.[151] Regression of Barrett's epithelium after antireflux surgery has been noted in some patients after antireflux surgery. Thirty-seven patients with Barrett's mucosa were identified from 241 patients who had an antireflux procedure. Four patients (11%) had partial regression of their reflux, but 3 of the 4 patients developed carcinoma (8.1%) over 16 years. Good reflux control was obtained in 92%. The authors suggest that antireflux procedures should be done for the usual reasons in patients with gastroesophageal reflux who have Barrett's esophagus (mild or moderate dysplasia), noting that some patients will have regression and some will develop carcinoma. They recommend yearly endoscopic and histologic surveillance for all patients.[174]

Surveillance for Patients With Barrett's Mucosa

Surveillance for Barrett's mucosa progressing to adenocarcinoma was conducted in 32 patients with Barrett's esophagus.[175] Adenocarcinoma developed in 3 patients during 166.1 patient years. Dysplasia was found in 2 of these patients 6 and 15 months before the diagnosis of adenocarcinoma. One patient had adenocarcinoma. Barrett's mucosa was unchanged in all but 3 patients despite operative or medical treatment over 3 to 12 years. Barrett's esophagus is a potential premalignant condition, and endoscopic surveillance is mandatory.

Sixty-two cases of Barrett's esophagus were identified among 707 patients with hiatal hernia (8.7%). Ten adenocarcinomas were associated with Barrett's changes, for a prevalence of 13.8%. Fifty-one patients had an antireflux procedure, whereas 11 underwent resection. Six patients had adenocarcinoma and 5 had severe dysphagia (an incidence of 1 new case per 274 patient-years [1.72%]).[176] It is not known whether correction of reflux by medical management or antireflux surgery influences progression to adenocarcinoma.

Some investigators suggest that annual screening for Barrett's is not effective. The incidence in one study was 1 new case in 170 patient-years, and the survival of patients with Barrett's esophagus was not different from an age- and sex-matched control population.[177] Others recommend endoscopic surveillance every 2 years as a better use of resources.[178]

RADIATION THERAPY IN THE TREATMENT OF ESOPHAGEAL CANCER

Radiation therapy continues to play an important role in the treatment of carcinoma of the esophagus. It is used in four different settings in the treatment of this disease: (1) as a single modality, curatively or palliatively; (2) combined with surgery, preoperatively or postoperatively; (3) combined with chemotherapy as definitive treatment; and (4) combined with chemotherapy and surgery. When used alone, radiation therapy frequently provides prompt relief of esophageal obstruction, often allowing patients to eat a normal or near-normal diet for the better part of their disease course. A major advantage of radiation therapy compared with surgery is that the treatment is rarely associated with acute mortality. Despite this apparent advantage over surgery, most surgical series report better long-term survival than do radiation therapy series. There are a number of problems with reports on esophageal cancer that must be kept in mind. Many surgical series report results not based on attempted surgical resections, but on *successful* surgical resections, eliminating those that were inoperable or those that were resected for palliative purposes only. This artificially inflates the surgical survival figures. Furthermore, surgical patients tend to be healthy enough to undergo the rigors of a radical operative procedure, and the surgeon is able to obtain complete and accurate clinical and pathologic staging data.

Radiation therapy series are, by definition, far different. They usually include patients who were treated for potentially curable disease *and* patients treated palliatively. The staging of radiated patients is never well defined, because it must be done with radiographic procedures in lieu of anatomic and pathologic data. Most radiation therapy series took place before CT scanning was in use to screen out patients with occult metastatic disease and to better plan the radiation therapy treatment volume itself. It is possible that in similar stage patients, the overall results of radiation therapy and surgery may be similar.[179] A prospective randomized clinical trial is necessary to resolve this issue. Newer treatment techniques combining radiation with chemotherapy, with or without the addition of surgery, are enhancing the effectiveness and importance of radiation therapy in esophageal carcinoma.

RADIATION THERAPY ALONE

Radiation therapy alone as a treatment for esophageal cancer is being used less frequently as programs combining radiation therapy with chemotherapy prove their worthiness (see the sections on combined modality therapy of carcinoma of the esophagus). Over time, it is likely that radiation therapy alone will be confined to elderly and infirm patients who are not candidates for aggressive combined modality therapy. In addition, radiation will continue to be used as a sole modality for the palliation of patients with known metastatic disease. Because significant numbers of patients present in a situation in which radical attempts at cure are inadvisable, radiation therapy as a sole treatment will always play a part in the management of this tumor.

Prognostic Factors and Patient Selection

A list of prognostic factors relevant to the radiotherapeutic management of esophageal cancer is presented in Table 25–6. Tumor size continues to be a powerful predictor of outcome in patients treated with radiation therapy alone.[180,181] When the tumor is 5 cm in length or smaller, especially if it is non-circumferential, the 5-year survival rate can reach 15% to 20%.[182,183] In combined modality programs, it can exceed 50%.[184] However, patients with tumors greater than 10 cm in length are rarely cured. Women invariably survive longer than do men, although women continue to make up a minority of the patient population with esophageal carcinoma.[182–185] Location of the tumor continues to be associated with outcome in some studies; tumors in the upper third of the esophagus have a slightly better outcome than tumors in the lower two-thirds.[183–185] An important predictor of radiation therapy outcome is pretreatment of swallowing function and weight loss. Patients who have high-grade obstruction and weight loss have a much worse outcome than do patients who do not have these pretreatment signs.[186,187] These factors are probably a surrogate for tumor size, because patients with smaller tumors are much less likely to have high-grade esophageal obstruction than are patients with large tumors. Finally, radiation dose appears to influence outcome: patients treated with higher radiation doses do better than patients treated with lower doses.[180,186,187] This factor may be a dependent variable because patients in the best clinical condition often receive the highest radiation doses, whereas more symptomatic patients receive lower doses and shorter courses of treatment.

Several factors remain relative contraindications to radiation therapy. Patients with a communication from the esophagus into the tracheobronchial tree have a very short survival and should be considered for palliation with a surgical bypass or an esophageal tube.[188] In some patients with tracheoesophageal fistulas, the fistulas close during a prolonged course of radiation. Survival time is still measured in months, however, and most of these months are taken up receiving the radiation itself.[189] Involvement of the trachea or bronchus by esophageal carcinoma without a detectable fistula often leads to fistula formation during radiation as the tumor shrinks.[190] These patients have a poor outcome with radiation and are best palliated with other measures. Established mediastinitis and hemorrhage from the tumor remain contraindications to radiation therapy.

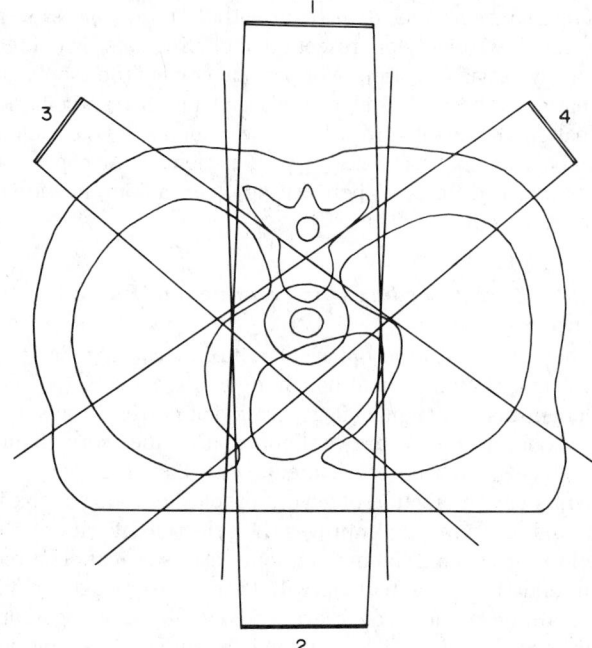

A

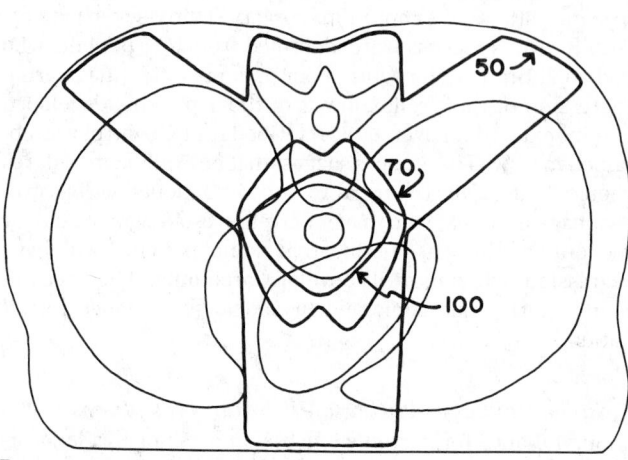

B

FIGURE 25–14. **(A)** The classic radiation field configuration for treatment of esophagus cancer. Two oblique fields are matched to an anterior field, with or without a posterior field. This three- or four-field plan produces a high-dose volume around the esophagus. The oblique fields spare the spinal cord so that dose to this structure can be kept below tolerance levels. **(B)** Isodose curves for this treatment technique. The 100% volume encompasses the tumor, whereas the spinal cord receives less than 70% of the dose.

TABLE 25–6. Prognostic Factors for Radiation Treatment of Esophageal Cancer

Better Prognosis	Worse Prognosis
Female	Male
< 5 cm length	> 10 cm length
Upper one-third	Lower one-third
Mild or no obstruction	High-grade obstruction and weight loss
High-dose radiation	Low-dose radiation

Technique of Radiation

External-Beam Irradiation

The intent of curative radiation therapy in any tumor site is to treat the primary tumor and its potential microscopic extension, along with the appropriate regional nodes with a cancerocidal dose while respecting the tolerance of adjacent normal tissue. The radiation oncologist must arrange the treatment fields and the patient's treatment position so that the set-up can be reproduced accurately each treatment day for 6 to 7 weeks. Reproducibility of daily set-up is greatly facilitated by immobilization on the treatment table with the aid of a custom-molded body cast or a foam cradle. Ideally, patients with carcinoma of the esophagus are treated in the prone position to maximize the separation between the esophagus and the spinal cord.[191-194] In many elderly patients, the prone position is too tiring and they are not able to old this position long enough to accomplish simulation and daily treatment. In that case, the supine position is used. In either treatment position, the arms are raised over the head to allow for easy access into the CT scanner so that scans can be obtained in the exact treatment position.

The normal structures must be taken into account during esophageal irradiation if complications are to be minimized.

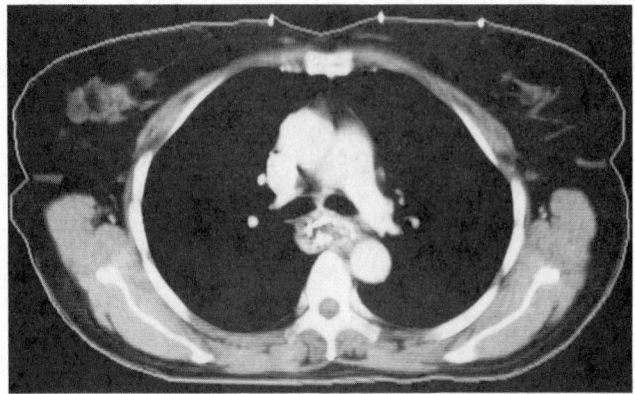

A

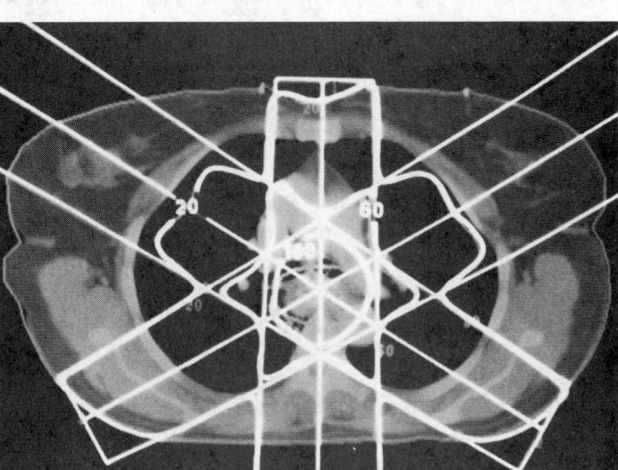

B

FIGURE 25-16.   (A) CT scan of a patient with esophageal cancer. The patient is in the supine position on a flat couch that duplicates the treatment couch. The esophageal tumor with thickening of the esophageal wall can be seen clearly. (B) Three-field plan (anterior and two posterior obliques) superimposed on the CT scan. The esophageal tumor is encompassed in the high-dose zone, and the spinal cord is partially spared radiation with the oblique portals.

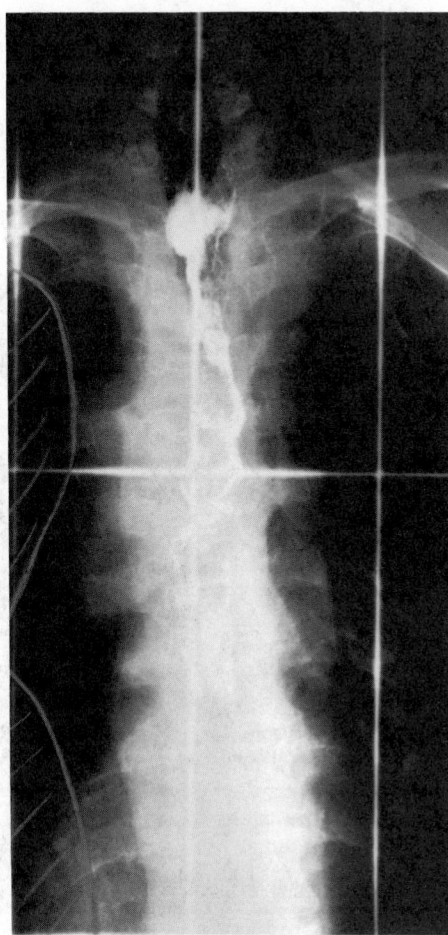

FIGURE 25-15.   A typical portal for the treatment of esophageal cancer. This field is 22 cm long and includes at least a 5-cm margin proximally and distally.

In esophageal carcinoma, there are two major dose-limiting structures. The first is the spinal cord, which lies in close proximity to the esophagus. The radiation tolerance of the spinal cord is in the range of 4500 to 5000 cGy, whereas esophageal carcinoma requires doses in excess of this for eradication. To spare the spinal cord, some of the radiation treatment must be administered through oblique fields that treat the esophagus while shielding the spinal cord. These oblique fields, coupled with anterior and posterior fields, make up the commonly used four-field esophageal treatment plan (Fig. 25-14).

The radiation field is designed to encompass the gross and microscopic extensions of tumor and regional lymph nodes. The radiographic extent of the tumor is covered with a 5- to 6-cm margin in the cephalad-caudad direction. Although esophageal cancer can spread more than 6 cm from the primary site in about 15% of cases,[195] such patients are rarely cured with radiation therapy alone. Because combined modality protocols using chemotherapy with or without surgery are frequently used, such microscopic distal extension is often effectively treated by the chemotherapy or the surgery. In addition, as the volume of the radiation field increases, complications of combined modality treatment can increase. There is a natural desire to try, if possible, to limit the size of the radiation portal to just what is necessary to treat. Pearson achieved the best results reported in the radiation literature by using a limited field size.[196] Even when a 5- to 6-cm margin is taken around the tumor, field sizes often are 15 to 20 cm or more in length, which is still a substantial volume (Fig. 25–15).

When treating the patient with radiation therapy alone, the field is usually 7 to 8 cm wide, enough to cover the esophagus and nearby structures such as the periesophageal lymph nodes. However, using CT scan information, there can be significant amounts of periesophageal soft-tissue extension that is difficult, if not impossible, to recognize on plain x-rays taken with barium contrast.[197] Furthermore, CT scans display the location, size, and density of pulmonary tissue. This allows for radiation treatment to be planned with a correction built in for the increased radiation transmission that occurs through low-density lung tissue.[198]

CT scanning can be used as a basis for radiation therapy treatment planning. The scan can be brought up on the treatment planning screen (Fig. 25–16A), and beams can be superimposed on this CT image. Dose calculations can be performed in the region of the esophagus, and periesophageal soft tissues can be encompassed within the high-dose volume (Fig. 25–16B). Furthermore, CT scans can be reformatted in the sagittal plane. This provides a view of the esophagus and spinal cord throughout the length of the treatment field. Such

displays are valuable in the treatment planning of esophageal cancer (Fig. 25–17).

The overall approach to radiation therapy for the patient with esophageal carcinoma involves several steps. First, the patient planned radiation fields for the simulated, and films of each treatment port are taken using barium contrast (see Fig. 25–15). The patient is then taken to the CT scanner, and CT slices throughout the esophageal bed are obtained while the patient lies in the previously fabricated immobilization cast. The CT scans are then viewed, and the target volume on each slice outlined. Using a graphics display tool called the *beam's-eye view*,[199] the CT target volumes can be superimposed onto the simulator films. One can then easily determine whether the target volumes included in the radiation field are adequate and whether the shielding blocks can be safely added to protect normal tissues (see Fig. 25–17). The ability to see tumor and normal tissue anatomy on CT scans and the increasing use of combined modality therapy has refocused attention onto regional lymph node treatment in the radiation therapy of esophageal cancer. Spread to regional nodes occurs in 40% to 60% of esophageal cancer patients,[200] and sterilization of this local lymph node spread is critical in the curative treatment of this disease. Several institutions routinely include supraclavicular nodes in their treatment of patients with upper esophageal lesions and celiac nodes in their threatment of patients with lower esophageal lesions.[201] The dose of radiation varies between institutions and depends on whether chemotherapy or surgery is used in the patient's treatment. Definitive dose schedules of radiation have ranged between 5000 cGy in 20 treatments over 4 weeks to 6600

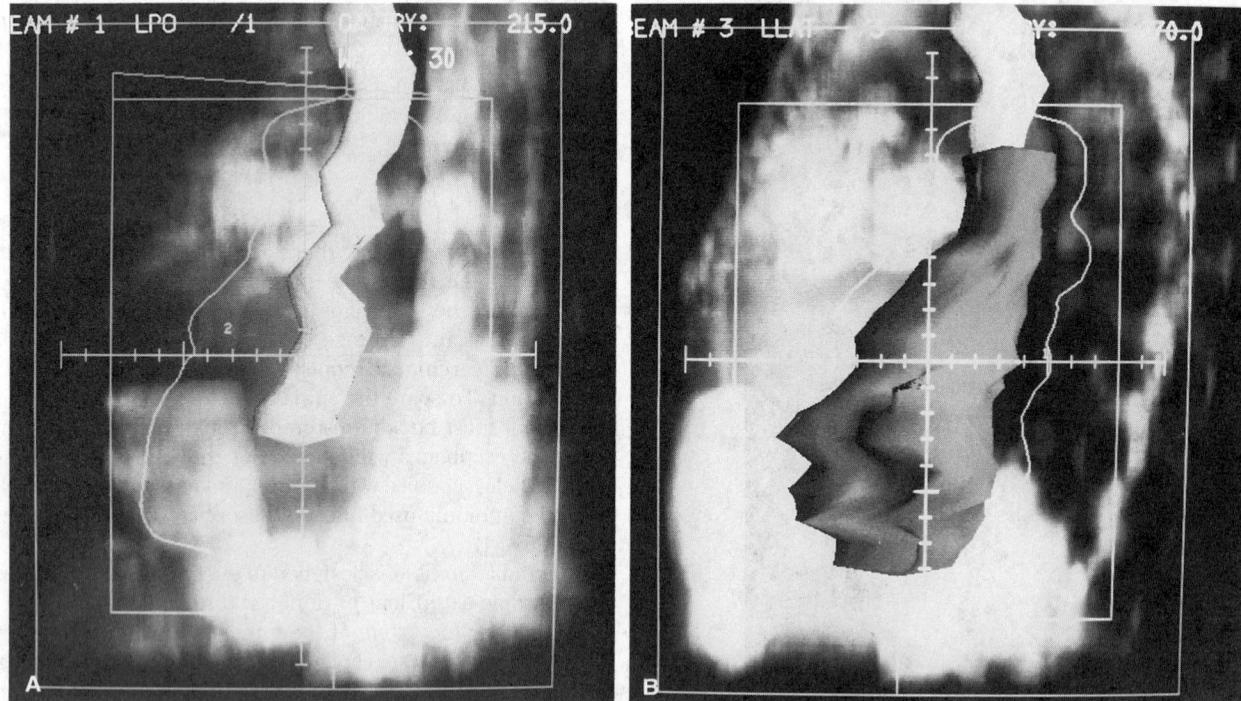

FIGURE 25–17. **(A)** A left posterior oblique view with the esophagus reconstructed from CT scan. The narrow barium-filled lumen can be seen. **(B)** The same esophagus shows the periesophageal extension of tumor. The tumor is much wider than the esophagus itself. The three-dimensional study visualizes tumors that otherwise might have been shielded from view.

cGy in 33 treatments over 7 weeks. Although no dose regimen has proved superior to any other, several studies have suggested that high-dose treatment is superior to low-dose treatment in the overall control of tumor and in the determination of ultimate survival.[180,186,187] The radiation oncologist should attempt to be as aggressive as possible with the radiation dose, remaining cognizant of the tolerance of normal tissues such as spinal cord and lung.

Intracavity Radiation

The implantation of radioactive sources within or around a tumor has a history in radiation oncology that is as old as the field itself. The first tumor to be treated in this fashion was probably carcinoma of the cervix, where the cervical canal represented a natural cavity for the radioactive source. Recognition that the lumen of the esophagus represented a natural opening for the introduction of radioactive material into the center of an esophageal cancer goes back decades, to the early part of this century.[202] Since that time, a number of intraluminal applicators have been tried. In 1969, Rider reported on a series of patients treated with external radiation followed by insertion of an intraluminal radium bougie.[203] These early results were encouraging, and the 3-year survival rate was 37%. Since that time, a number of reports have appeared concerning intraluminal radiation, the most recent of which used remote afterloading sources to eliminate exposure of hospital staff to radiation (Fig. 25–18).[204–206] The esophageal lesion suitable for such therapy must be relatively small, because the esophagus must be able to accept intubation, and the dose distribution from such therapy covers a small distance, about 1 to 1.5 cm in diameter. Nonetheless, reports of intraluminal therapy for rapid palliation of obstruction are encouraging, and this therapy is likely to find a place for the immediate relief of symptoms in the elderly[207] and debilitated patient.[208,209] Other reports are beginning to appear using intraluminal therapy as a boost before or after external-beam treatment.[204,205] The use of an intracavitary boost after external-beam therapy seems to be the most logical method. Once the external-beam therapy has an opportunity to shrink the tumor, residual macroscopic or microscopic disease can lie within or in close proximity to the esophageal wall. A high-dose boost can be applied to these sites without much additional radiation entering the spinal cord or lungs. In Hishikawa's series, local control was achieved in 65% of stage I or II patients and in 45% of stage III or IV patients.[205] Of the 148 patients treated, 42 (28%) had a posttreatment ulcer, 15 (10%) had stricture, and 6 (4%) had formed fistulas. The 2-year survival rate in the stage I or II cases was 43%, and the 5-year rate was 18%. There is a great deal of interest in intraluminal high-dose rate afterloading therapy in the radiation oncology community, and clinical research on this technique, especially as a boost dose in definitive radiation cases, is in progress.

Clinical Course After Irradiation of the Esophagus

The squamous epithelium of the esophagus has about the same radiosensitivity as that of the oral mucosa.[210] De-epithelialization leads to clinical symptoms of esophagitis that begin 1 to 2 weeks after the start of treatment and, in some patients, can be severe. Tumor response to radiation usually begins after 2 to 3 weeks. Improvement in swallowing and relief of tumor pain can help in making the discomfort of esophagitis more tolerable. Measures that can reduce the symptoms of esophagitis include systemic analgesics and viscous lidocaine. The possibility of *Candida* esophagitis should always be con-

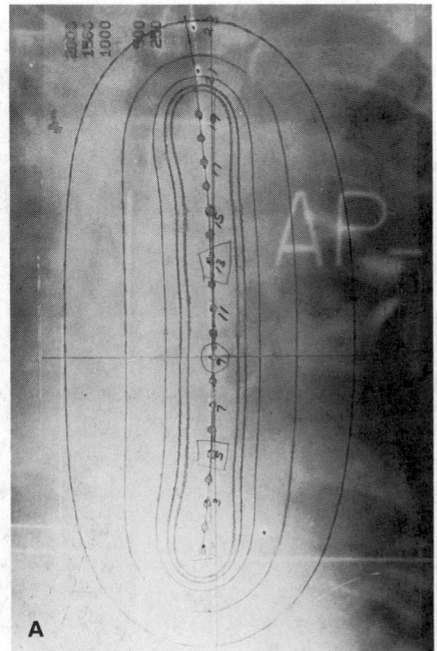
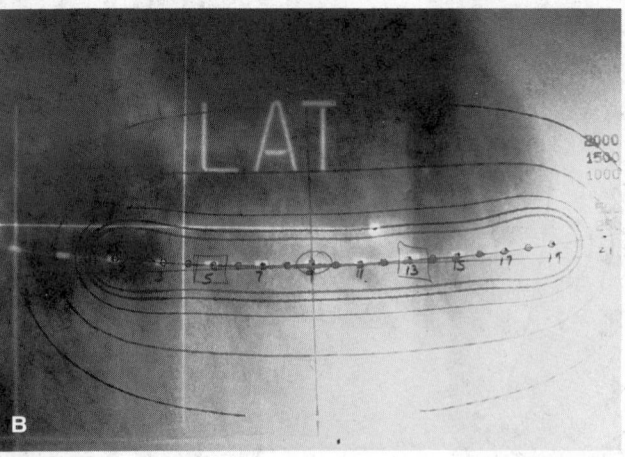

FIGURE 25–18. Radiation dose from an intracavitary esophageal treatment. **(A)** Anterior and **(B)** lateral views. Numbers indicate the total dose in cGy stemming from the application. The 1000-cGy dose falls 1 cm from 1 cm from the intraluminal source.

sidered, and a trial of antimonilial antibiotics can be of dramatic benefits in some patients. The radiation tolerance of the esophagus is generally regarded to be about 6500 cGy.[211] However, chemotherapeutic agents, especially doxorubicin, can dramatically increase the radiation sensitivity of the esophagus; care must be exercised in the concurrent administration of drugs with radiation. A fair amount of experience has been gained with the administration of 5000 cGy concurrent with cisplatin-based chemotherapy and 6000 cGy with 5-fluorouracil (5-FU) chemotherapy (see the sections on combined modality treatment). Clinical research is attempting to escalate the dose of external-beam irradiation to determine the maximum tolerated dose that can be given with chemotherapy.

Results of Radiation Therapy Alone

Relief of Symptoms and Tumor Response

Esophageal carcinoma is highly sensitive to the effects of radiation therapy. Fifty percent to 60% of patients respond radiographically, and 60% to 85% of patients achieve some palliative benefit with radiation, typically lasting a median of 5 to 10 months (Fig. 25–19).[212,213] A detailed study on the effect of radiation therapy on dysphagia was carried out by Caspers and colleagues.[186] Of 127 irradiated patients, 55% were completely obstructed or could swallow only liquids at the time of initiation of radiation therapy. Seventy-one percent of the patients who presented with significant dysphagia responded to radiation therapy; 76% of patients were able to eat at least semisolid food after treatment, whereas only 45% had been able to before treatment. The median dysphagia-free interval was 7.5 months, and 20% of patients were still dysphagia-free at 3 years. Of the 119 patients who sustained a tumor-related death, 63 (53%) died without any evidence of local progression. Forty-five of these 63 patients had a complete clearance of tumor on esophagogram and died without clinical evidence of local recurrence. Forty-five of the 119 patients (38%) died without clinical evidence of tumor. These results attest to the effectiveness of radiation therapy in providing relief of dysphagia, although only half the radiated population maintains swallowing function until the time of death.

Survival With Radiation Treatment Alone

In a number of series amounting to more than 450 patients with preoperative irradiation, local eradication of tumor (or the appearance of nonviable tumor) occurred in about 15% of patients whose tumors were resected after a course of radiation (Table 25–7).[213–215] The 15% figure might be an overestimation of the true tumor sterilization rate, because not all patients who were preoperatively irradiated were taken to surgery and not all who were taken were resectable. On the other hand, in some patients who had pathologically detectable tumor, the tumor cells were nonviable after radiation. The figure of 15% for known tumor eradication is probably not far from accurate. Because about 30% of esophageal carcinoma patients present with nonmetastatic disease, one might theorize that the cure rate of esophageal carcinoma treated with radiation therapy alone could be as high as 5%. This turns out to be the case in the many reported series including a large review of 8500 cases.[216] In several series of patients treated in the 1970s and 1980s, median survival was typically

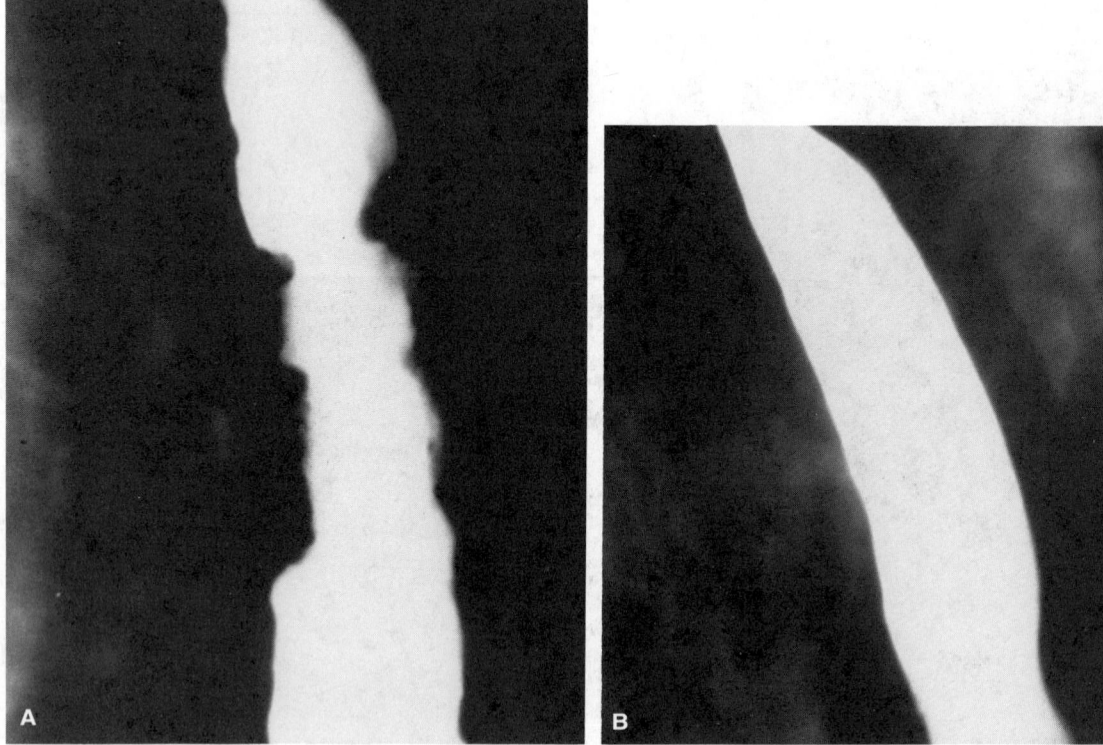

FIGURE 25–19. **(A)** A midesophageal lesion before treatment. **(B)** Esophagram after treatment. Swallowing was restored and the specimen was negative on pathologic examination.

TABLE 25–7. Effectiveness of Radiation Therapy in Sterilizing Esophageal Carcinoma

Investigations	No. of Patients Resected	No. of Tumor-Free Specimens
Kelsen et al, 1990[213]	31	1
Liu et al, 1986[214]	59	10
Marks et al, 1976[215]	101	12 (9 CIS)
Sugimachi et al, 1986[222]	104	15
Yadava et al, 1991[223]	68	8
Morita et al, 1985[212]	49	16
Hussey et al, 1980[190]	41	4
Doggett et al, 1970[224]	24	4
Total	478	70 (14.6%)

CIS, carcinoma in situ.

8 to 10 months, with a 1-year survival rate of about 35%, a 2-year survival rate of about 10% to 15%, and a 5-year survival rate of about 5%.[180,182,183,185,186]

Duration of survival after radiation is related to tumor stage. When tumors less than 5 cm are treated, long-term survival is increased. For example, Earlam and Johnson recently reported a series of 22 patients who were treated with radiation therapy for small, operable squamous cell carcinomas of the esophagus.[217] The 1-year survival rate was 46% and the 5-year survival rate was 14%, a result similar to many surgical series. With the enhanced effectiveness that chemotherapy adds to radiation (see the section on combined modality treatment), a nonsurgical approach remains a viable option in the curative treatment of carcinoma of the esophagus.

Complications of Radiation

Death or serious long-term morbidity due to esophageal irradiation is uncommon. Occasionally, patients have been reported with radiation pneumonitis, pericarditis, myocarditis, or spinal cord damage. The most frequent complication from esophageal irradiation is stricture. In a recent study by O'Rourke, 40% of patients developed a postradiation stricture, although combined modality therapy was used in more than half the patients.[218] The previous report from the Princess Margaret Hospital suggested that most postradiation strictures that did not quickly resolve with dilation were malignant.[219] In O'Rourke's experience, half the strictures were benign and the survival rate of patients with benign stricture actually exceeded that of patients who experienced no stricture.[218] Not all postradiation stricture heralds the development of recurrent disease; many of these patients can be managed successfully by conservative means.[220] Occasionally, patients present with nonmalignant ulceration in the esophagus,[221] and such events may increase in frequency as high-dose-rate intraluminal irradiation is used and more concurrent chemotherapy is undertaken. Occasionally, fistula formation, with or without hemorrhage, is seen; these complications usually result from rapid resolution of tumor that has invaded from the esophagus into neighboring trachea, bronchus, or aorta.

COMBINATIONS OF RADIATION AND SURGERY

Preoperative Radiation Therapy

Several groups of radiation oncologists and surgeons have tested the hypothesis that the results of treating esophageal carcinoma can be improved by delivering radiation therapy before a surgical resection.[212–215,222–230] Such efforts arose out of the hope that because radiation and surgery each have advantages and disadvantages that may be complementary, the two used together would be synergistic and reinforce their benefits. Radiation therapy carries a low morbidity and mortality and can, in high dosage, produce marked regression in tumor bulk, occasionally sterilize a primary tumor, and sterilize microscopic disease in areas that are not subjected to surgical resection. It is possible to treat a wider area surrounding the esophageal tumor by radiation therapy than can be reasonably accomplished by surgical means. In about 15% of cases, the tumor is sterilized by the preoperative radiation (see Table 25–7). On the other hand, esophagectomy can treat a great length of the esophagus contributing to local control of tumor while providing a better chance for long-term palliation, and possibly, for long-term cure. Reduction in tumor bulk from irradiation can increase resectability rates and decrease operative mortality by making the surgical procedure easier to perform. The final benefit of preoperative radiation is the prevention of metastasis and local recurrences that might stem from clonogenic tumor cells being liberated by the surgical manipulation.

In general, survival from preoperative radiation correlates with the extent of tumor destruction seen in the operative specimen. For example, Morita and colleagues found a 44% 2-year survival rate and a 28% 5-year survival rate when preoperative radiation showed extensive tumor destruction.[212] Survival rates were cut in half when this destructive effect was not seen. Sugimachi,[222] Hambraeus,[229] Yadava,[223] and Kelsen[213] report that responders to preoperative radiation survive longer than nonresponders.

The results of preoperative radiation are somewhat controversial. In some single institution reports, survival rates of 15% or more at 5 years are reported,[212,214,222,228] whereas the long-term survival rate in patients who received radiation therapy alone is about 2% to 5%. There are two points to make about this fact. First, these results may not be any better than might be achieved by treating the same population by surgery alone. In a well-conducted clinical trial of preoperative radiation therapy, with a crossover to chemotherapy after resection, Kelsen reported a median survival of 11 months and a 20% survival rate at the median follow-up of 34 months.[213] These results are not better than those seen with surgery alone. The second point is that many reports of preoperative radiation therapy do not specify whether survival rates are calculated based on the total number of patients evaluated, the total number of patients treated, the total number of patients taken to surgery, the total number of patient resected, or the total number of patients who survived the operation. By dropping out patients at each one of these branch points and reducing the denominator, long-term survival rates can be inflated artificially.

Two randomized trials of preoperative radiation versus surgery alone have been reported. The first study, by Launois and colleagues, studied 124 French patients treated from 1973 to 1976.[230] In this study, resection rates for the two treatment groups were similar, as was the operative mortality rate, which was more than 20%. The median and long-term survival rates were disappointing. Excluding patients who died during surgery, the average survival was only 4.5 months for those who received preoperative radiation and 8.2 months for those who had surgery alone. This difference was not statistically significant. The 5-year survival rates were similar (9.5% for the combined modality group and 11.5% for the patients treated with surgery alone). This study can be criticized, however. The radiation dose was not standard, and 4000 cGy was delivered over 8 to 12 days. This intense dose of radiation may account for the somewhat higher postoperative mortality rate seen in the irradiated patients. Resection was attempted only 8 days after completion of this high-dose radiation, when the inflammatory response secondary to therapy might still be present. The short interval between radiation and operation does not allow time for tumor shrinkage and may explain why the resectability rate was unaffected by radiation.

The second trial, performed by the European Organization for Research on the Treatment of Cancer (EORTC), compared preoperative radiation with chemotherapy.[226] This study treated patients from 1976 to 1982. Two hundred and one patients were treated; the radiation regimen was 3300 cGy, delivered in 10 fractions over 12 days. The resection rate was similar for the two groups, as was the operative mortality of about 19%. The overall survival rate was identical for both groups, as was the median survival of about 1 year. Local control was increased in the preoperative radiation group, 19 of whom had local recurrence with or without distant spread compared with 34 patients in the surgery alone group who had local recurrence. This study can be criticized because of the low dose of radiation and again because the surgery took place only 8 days after the radiation.

A more recent trial of preoperative irradiation has been reported from China by Huang and his colleagues [225] One hundred and sixty patients were treated with or without 4000 cGy before surgery; the 5-year survival rate was 45% for the preoperative radiation arm and 25% for the surgery alone arm. This study has not been reported fully in the peer-reviewed literature.

In summary, preoperative irradiation can shrink many tumors; 60% to 70% of patients have an objective response and about 15% of patients are rendered free of identifiable tumor at the time of surgery. It is unclear whether preoperative irradiation enhances survival over that obtained by surgery alone, and with the encouraging results coming from combined modality studies of chemotherapy in the treatment of esophageal carcinoma, preoperative radiation alone probably will not play an important role in the treatment of this disease in the future.

Postoperative Radiation Therapy

The rationale for radiation therapy after a curative resection of esophageal carcinoma is based on the hope that irradiation will eradicate residual microscopic or small amounts of macroscopic disease. Postoperative irradiation could, in theory, be effective in controlling implantation or seeding of the tumor, which may have occurred at the time of operation.

More effective radiation might be possible after surgery than before surgery. The surgeon can demarcate the extent of tumor with radiopaque clips at the time of operation, allowing the radiation oncologist to direct treatment accurately to the involved area. The tissue volumes to be treated with postoperative irradiation remain difficult to define. Once the esophagus and its lymphatics have been removed, it is almost impossible to define which lymph nodes and pathways of tumor spread should be addressed with irradiation. If the entire tumor bed from the upper esophagus down to the diaphragm needs to be addressed, the treatment can be extensive and debilitating. If the stomach has been brought up to replace the esophagus, the treatment dose must be limited to 4500 to 5000 cGy because of the stomach's sensitivity to radiation.

Nonetheless, occasional reports appear in the literature of patients who had positive tumor margins, received postoperative radiation, and turned out to be long-term survivors.[231-233] Overall, there is a paucity of data on the efficacy of postoperative radiation as an adjunct to surgery. Because of this, postoperative radiation therapy has never achieved a status as one of the standard treatments for this disease. Its use is probably best restricted to patients whose tumors have been resected with a positive tumor margin that can be clipped and treated with carefully designed radiation fields. It is unlikely that large-scale trials of postoperative radiation in esophageal carcinoma will be mounted.

COMBINATIONS OF RADIATION AND CHEMOTHERAPY

Treatment of carcinoma of the esophagus with combinations of radiation therapy and chemotherapy began about 15 to 20 years ago.[234-238] The rationale for this combined modality therapy is relatively straightforward. The problem with carcinoma of the esophagus is locoregional and systemic. A combination of a local modality such as radiation therapy and a systemic modality such as chemotherapy could address these problems simultaneously. By giving the drugs and radiation together, one immediately addresses both treatment problems from the outset of therapy. Finally, some chemotherapeutic agents such as 5-FU and cisplatin are known to enhance the effectiveness of radiation, and their administration might add to the local cell kill produced by radiation.

Some of the earliest experience with combined modality therapy in esophageal carcinoma came from Wayne State University, where treatment was based on the model of anal carcinoma, in which low doses of radiation (3000 cGy) and concurrent 5-FU plus mitomycin C produced startling results.[234] The results from the first esophageal study showed that complete responses could be obtained; the suggestion of a prolonged median survival of 18 months and a 2-year survival rate of 35% in those whose tumors were resected after chemotherapy was encouraging.[239] Over the next several years, a variety of studies were performed, either as single-institution experiences or as phase II pilot studies in cooperative groups.[240-250] The results from these studies are summarized in Table 25–8. In general, the median survival of 12 to 20 months and the 2-year survival rate of 35% to 40% seem encouraging. Patients with early disease, and patients who might be considered ideal surgical candidates, fared especially well.

TABLE 25–8. Results of Combined Chemotherapy and Radiation Therapy

Investigations	Drugs	Radiation Dose (cGy)	No. of Patients	Complete Response	Survival 1-Year	2-Year	Median
Nonrandomized Studies							
Chan et al, 1988[240]	5-FU/MMC/cisplatin	4000–5000	21	86%	64%	32%	13 mo
Coia et al, 1991[184]	5-FU/MMC	5000–6000	57	Stage I, II NS	74%	44%	18 mo
		5000–6000	33	Stage III, IV NS	NS	NS	8 mo
John et al, 1989[241]	5-FU/MMC/cisplatin/MTX	4000–5000	30	77%	53%	29%	11 mo
Keane et al, 1985[242]	5-FU/MMC	4500–5000	35	78%	47%	28%	NS
Leichman et al, 1987[243] Herskovic et al, 1988[244]	5-FU/cisplatin	5000	22	NS	77%	38%	22 mo
Richmond et al, 1987[245]	5-FU/cisplatin	5600–6000	27	NS	NS	39%	12 mo
Seitz et al, 1990[246]	5-FU-cisplatin	4000	35	71%	55%	45%	17 mo
Randomized Studies							
Araujo et al, 1991[247]	5-FU/MMC/cisplatin	5000	28	75%	64%	38%	NS
	Control	5000	31	58%	55%	22%	NS
Herskovic et al, 1991[248]	5-FU/cisplatin	5000	61	73%	50%	38%	12.5 mo
	Control	6400	59	60%	33%	10%	8.9 mo
Roussel et al, 1988[249]	MTX	5600	75	NS	31%	12%	9 mo
	Control	4500	69	NS	35%	6%	8 mo
Sischy et al, 1990[250]	5-FU/MMC	4000 + 2000	118	NS	NS	NS	Stage I, 22.3 mo
	Control	4000 + 2000	118	NS	NS	NS	Stage III, 11.6 mo

5-FU, 5-fluorouracil; MMC, mitomycin C; MTX, methotrexate; NS, not stated.
* Probable boost.

In Coia's series, patients with stage I nonobstructing, noncircumferential tumors (tumors less than 5 cm in length, without esophageal spread) had a 73% survival rate at 3 years with 100% local tumor control.[184] The 3-year survival rate in the patients with stages I and II tumors was 29%. Seitz and colleagues reported that 15 patients with stage I or II tumors had a median survival of 28 months.[246] When esophagectomy was added to combined modality therapy, 25% to 35% of patients showed a complete histologic clearance of tumor, a substantially higher rate than that seen when radiation therapy by itself was used preoperatively, as reported in Table 25–7.

Although results from small single institution and cooperative group studies are encouraging, data from randomized prospective trials are necessary to establish the superiority of radiation plus chemotherapy over radiation alone, if such a superiority exists. Three large randomized prospective trials have been completed recently comparing combined radiation therapy and chemotherapy with radiation alone, and two studies showed an advantage for the combined modality treatment (see Table 25–8).[247–249] The study by Roussel and colleagues used methotrexate as a single agent and saw no improvement over radiation alone.[249] The Eastern Cooperative Oncology Group (ECOG) randomized 130 patients to receive radiation therapy alone (4000 cGy) or the same dose of radiation with concurrent treatment with mitomycin C and 5-FU. The study, which was reported in abstract form in 1990,[235] showed a statistically significant improvement in outcome for patients treated with combined modality. The median survival improved from 9 months to 15 months with combined mo-

dality therapy, and the results were especially impressive in patients with stage I disease.

The other major study was performed by the Radiation Therapy Oncology Group (RTOG).[248] This trial began in January 1986 and randomized 129 patients to receive 5000 cGy with concurrent cisplatin/5-FU or 6400 cGy of radiation alone. A dose of 5-FU of 1000 mg/m^2/day was administered as a continuous intravenous infusion over the first 4 days of weeks 1, 5, 8, and 11. Cisplatin, at a dose of 75 mg/m^2/day, was given by rapid intravenous infusion on day 1 of each 5-FU course. Because the radiation took a full 5 weeks to deliver, concurrent chemotherapy was administered twice during the radiation therapy, and two additional courses were given after the conclusion of the radiation. Although the study was planned to include 150 patients, it was stopped after 129 patients were accrued, because the early stopping rule was satisfied and the survival rate of the patients who received combined modality was shown to be significantly superior. The median survival of 12.5 months in the combined modality group was higher significantly longer ($p = 0.009$) than the 8.9 months median survival in the radiation therapy alone arm. The differences in survival rates at 12 months (33% versus 50%) and 24 months (10% versus 38%) were statistically significant ($p = 0.0017$). The patterns of treatment failure also were significantly different in this study. In the radiation therapy alone group, 40% of patients had persistent disease at the end of the study, and an additional 24% of patients had a clinical local recurrence, for a total of 64% local failures. In contrast, the combined modality arm had a 27%

rate of persistent disease and a 16% subsequent local failure rate, for a total of 43% local failures. This difference was statistically significant ($p = 0.005$).

The RTOG trial shows that a combined chemoradiotherapy approach using cisplatin/5-FU is superior to radiation therapy alone in the treatment of nonmetastatic carcinoma of the esophagus. This result, and that of the ECOG trial, provide the first solid evidence that a combination of chemotherapy plus radiation therapy will emerge as the treatment of choice in patients who are being managed nonsurgically. Neither of these trials shows that combined chemotherapy and radiation therapy is superior to surgery alone as a single modality. Furthermore, with median survivals of 12 to 14 months and 2-year survival rates of about 35%, combined with a 40% local failure rate, both these studies leave considerable room for improvement. Studies of intensifying the therapy by increasing the dose of radiation, adding additional cycles of chemotherapy before radiation, or a combination of both, are under way. Another method of increasing the intensity of local therapy is to add a surgical esophagectomy to the combined radiation therapy and chemotherapy. This form of therapy is discussed below.

COMBINED CHEMOTHERAPY AND RADIATION THERAPY FOLLOWED BY SURGERY

Despite the encouraging results with combinations of chemotherapy plus radiation, and the knowledge that randomized trials are now showing that this combination is superior to radiation therapy alone in the curative treatment of esophageal carcinoma, local persistence and progression of disease still remain problems. In Coia's study, 14 of 29 failures (48%) were at least partly local.[184] In the combined modality arm of the randomized RTOG trial, 27% of patients never cleared their disease and an additional 16% progressed in the primary area after clearance of all recognizable tumor for a 43% local failure rate. Other studies report similar results despite improvements in combined modality therapy. It can be hypothesized that the addition of a surgical esophagectomy after maximal tumor clearance by chemotherapy plus radiation therapy could contribute to the local control of disease, improve the quality of life, and possibly improve survival. A

number of studies have been carried out to test this hypothesis, and they are summarized in Table 25–9.[119,239,243,245,251,252] The only randomized trial of this treatment strategy reported is by Anderson and colleagues.[251] Bleomycin as a single agent was chosen for the chemotherapy, and the dose of radiation administered to these patients was low. Results in both arms were equally poor. The largest study was reported by Poplin and colleagues for the Southwest Oncology Group (SWOG) and the RTOG.[252] Of 113 patients enrolled on the study, only 63% made it to the operating room and only 49% actually had tumor resections. The 1-year and 2-year survival rates and median survivals were not much different than those of effective surgical protocols or combination chemotherapy plus radiation therapy protocols without surgery.

At the University of Michigan, Forastiere and colleagues enrolled 43 patients on an intensive course of preoperative chemotherapy plus twice-daily radiation followed by a transhiatal esophagectomy.[119] One problem in previous experiences with combined preoperative chemotherapy and radiation therapy has been a high postoperative mortality rate. In the SWOG/RTOG study cited above, operative mortality was 11%,[252] and in the Leichman study, a full 30% of patients did not leave the hospital after their surgery.[253] In contrast, of the 41 patients in this series who had transhiatal (nonthoracotomy) esophagectomy, there was only one postoperative death (2.4%). In Forastiere's trial, surgery appeared safe and beneficial. In most other reported combined modality series using surgery, all the long-term survivors have been patients whose surgical specimens were pathologically disease free. In this trial, 26 of the 41 patients who had resections had positive specimens. The median survival for these patients was 26 months, and one third remained alive and disease free at 5 years. It appears that surgery can convert some patients' response from partial to complete. Of the 36 completely resected patients, only one has had a solitary local failure, and 4 others have had local failures concomitant with distant disease. Therefore, 75% of completely resected patients have remained free of local disease, a figure that appears better than that from combined modality studies from which surgery has been eliminated. This group of investigators initiated a randomized trial comparing their aggressive combined modality therapy with transhiatal esophagectomy alone.

Undoubtedly, additional research into preoperative chemotherapy and radiation therapy is warranted. As surgical

TABLE 25–9. Results of Chemoradiotherapy Followed by Surgery

Investigations	Drugs	Radiation Dose (cGy)	No. of Patients	No. of Operations	No. of Resections	Survival 1-Year	Survival 2-Year	Survival Median
Andersen et al, 1984[251]	Bleomycin	3000	65	38	35	NS	25%	6.5 mo
	Control	3500	59	36	28	NS	19%	6.5 mo
Forastieve et al, 1990[119]	5-FU + cisplatin + vinblastine	3750–4500	43	41	36	65%	55%	29 mo
Franklin et al, 1983[239]	5-FU + MMC	3000 + 2000	30	23	23	NS	NS	11 mo
Leichman et al, 1987[243]	5-FU + cisplatin	3000 + 2000	21	19	15	NS	NS	18 mo
Poplin et al, 1987[252]	5-FU + cisplatin	3000 + 2000	113	71	55	47%	28%	12 mo
Richmond et al, 1987[245]	5-FU + cisplatin	3000	15	15	15	NS	38%	13 mo

5-FU, 5-fluorouracil; MMC, mitomycin C; NS, not stated.

techniques improve, postoperative mortality will decrease, further enhancing the usefulness of the technique. As chemotherapeutic regimens become more successful, the importance of local disease control will increase. Combinations of radiation plus surgery may offer the best chance for local tumor sterilization, and this mode of therapy will continue to be pursued. Combinations of all three modalities—chemotherapy plus radiation plus surgery—must be considered investigational and are best pursued in the context of a clinical trial.

CHEMOTHERAPY

The poor survival of patients with clinically localized squamous cell or adenocarcinoma of the esophagus suggests that occult dissemination of disease is present in most patients at diagnosis. Studies of patterns of recurrence and data from autopsy series confirm the potential of these tumors to spread to all organs.[254-258] Five-year survival rates for patients who undergo total removal of all gross disease with negative margins of resection approach 20%.[259,260] When all operative candidates are considered, these figures fall to 5% to 10%. This provides a rationale for adding a systemic therapy to local treatments (surgery and radiation) or for systemic therapy as the primary treatment of patients with overt metastases at diagnosis. Chemotherapy has been used to palliate patients with recurrence or metastases; as an adjuvant to surgery, either preoperative or postoperative in potentially curable patients; and concomitantly with radiation therapy.

Clinical trials to determine the efficacy of a chemotherapy regimen use the standard response criterion of a 50% or greater decrease in tumor size. Measurement of such a decrease, however, requires a bidimensional lesion that can be examined serially. For the esophageal cancer patient with metastatic disease, this can be accomplished reliably using pulmonary nodules, soft tissue nodules, or liver nodules as indicators. If disease is limited to the primary tumor, CT scans of the chest and the barium esophagogram are of limited value in measuring change in tumor size and predicting histologic complete response.[261-263] Single agents have been tested in patients with recurrent or metastatic squamous cell carcinoma of the esophagus. These patients often have a high tumor burden and poor performance status. Although this makes them a difficult group to study with little prospect for prolonging survival, the results of clinical trials in this population have identified drugs with activity against these tumors.[264] Combination regimens tested in this patient group yielded higher response rates.[264] Duration of response to single-agent or combination chemotherapy is brief, lasting less than 3 months, and palliation of symptoms is minimal. A more promising approach is the use of chemotherapy in newly diagnosed patients before surgery or radiation, or concomitant with radiation therapy in which improvement in survival is the primary endpoint.

PREOPERATIVE CHEMOTHERAPY

The rationale for preoperative chemotherapy in the treatment of patients with esophageal cancer is based on the poor survival rates achieved with single modality therapy and the knowledge that systemic spread of disease occurs early.[255-258] Data from laboratory models suggest that chemotherapy given before surgery may be of greater benefit in eradicating micrometastatic disease and preventing the emergence of drug-resistant clones.[265-268] Theoretically, preoperative chemotherapy may facilitate resection and allow the treating physician to assess the effectiveness of the particular regimen in shrinking the tumor. In some trials, the decision of whether to administer postoperative adjuvant chemotherapy has been resolved by the response to preoperative chemotherapy.[269-273]

The objective assessment of response when disease is limited to the primary tumor mass with or without regional node enlargement requires special consideration. The barium esophagogram is the most frequently used examination to determine reduction in tumor size. Agha and colleagues showed that tumor measurements could be made with a degree of accuracy using the vertical length of tumor, depth, lumen size, and extent of ulceration as parameters for serial comparison when all examinations were performed and interpreted by the same radiologist.[262] In most hospital settings, radiographic studies provide the physician with an indication of change in tumor size, enabling one to classify tumor size change as a reduction to less than half the original size, reduction to more than half original size, no change, or increase in size. Because it is difficult to measure a response accurately with bidimensional measurements, many of the trials simply designate major response,[272-274] good response,[274] or clinical partial response[271,272] to represent substantial reduction of tumor (as detected by CT scan, barium esophagogram, or endoscopy) accompanied by improvement in symptoms of dysphagia. Kelsen, in a series of meticulously conducted trials evaluating preoperative chemotherapy, established the criteria that should be used to declare a response complete.[264] The patient should have no evidence of tumor by barium esophagogram, CT, or endoscopic evaluation. Brushings, washings, and biopsy specimens must be negative for tumor in patients who are not undergoing resection, and for operative candidates there should be no residual tumor in the resected esophageal specimen and nodal tissue.

The results of studies of preoperative chemotherapy in which most patients were surgical candidates are detailed in Table 25–10.[213,269-280] The first of a series of cisplatin-based trials was reported by Coonley and colleagues.[275] One course of cisplatin and infused bleomycin given preoperatively to 43 patients produced a 14% response rate with no histologically complete responses. Thirty-four patients were operative candidates, and of these, 53% had a potentially curative resection (all gross tumor removed and negative margins). The median survival of the 34 surgical patients was 10 months. In two subsequent trials, Kelsen tested two cycles of preoperative cisplatin, vindesine, and bleomycin.[213,276] In the earlier trial, a 63% response rate was observed, although there were no histologic complete responses.[276] Curative resections were performed in 47%, and the median survival for surgically treated patients was 16.2 months. Because of the high response rate and prolonged survival compared with historical controls, this regimen was pursued in a randomized comparison with preoperative radiation therapy.[213] Fifty-five percent of chemotherapy-treated patients responded; there were 3 patients with histologically complete responses. Although a crossover design resulted in most patients receiving all three

TABLE 25–10. Preoperative Chemotherapy Regimens

Investigations	Treatment Plan	Carcinoma Histology	No. of Patients	Response (Path CR)	Operative Candidates	Curative Resection Rate*	Median Survival† (mo)
Coonley et al, 1984[275]	Cisplatin/bleomycin cisplatin 3 mg/kg day 1 bleomycin 10 mg/m² day 3 + 10 mg/m² C.I.V.I. days 3–6 1 cycle preop, 1 cycle postop	Squamous	43	14%	34	53%	10 (34 patients analyzed)
Kelsen et al, 1983[276]	Cisplatin/vindesine/bleomycin cisplatin 3 mg/kg day 1 vindesine 3 mg/m² weekly bleomycin 10 mg/m² day 3 + 10 mg/m² C.I.V.I. day 3–6 2 cycles preop	Squamous	45	63%	34	47%	16.2 (34 patients analyzed)
Kelsen et al, 1990[213]	Cisplatin/vindesine/bleomycin (doses as above) versus preop radiation therapy	Squamous Squamous	38 48	55% (3) 64% (2)	36 37	NS NS	10.4 12.4
Schlag et al, 1988[274]	Cisplatin/vindesine/bleomycin (doses as above)	Squamous	42	45% (2)	40	55%	16
Roth et al, 1988[269]	Cisplatin/vindesine/bleomycin doses as above, 2 cycles preop, cisplatin/vindesine × 6 mo postop‡ versus surgery	Squamous Squamous	19 20	47% (1)	17 19	NS NS	8 9
Kelsen et al, 1986[277]	Cisplatin/vindesine/MGBG cisplatin 120 mg/m² day 1 vindesine 3 mg/m² weekly MGBG 500 mg/m² day 1 + 15 2 cycles preop	Squamous	20	42% (1)	13	NS	8.5
Forastiere et al, 1987[270]	Cisplatin/vinblastine/MGBG cisplatin 100 mg/m² day 1 vinblastine 1.6 mg/m² day 1–4 MGBG 500 mg/m² day 1 + 8 2 cycles preop, 3 cycles postop‡	Squamous Adeno	11 18	64% (1) 31%	25	80%	14
Carey et al, 1986[271] Hilgenberg et al, 1988[278] Carey et al, 1990[279]	Cisplatin/5-FU cisplatin 100 mg/m² day 4 5-FU 1000 mg/m² C.I.V.I. day 1–4 2 cycles preop, 4 cycles postop‡	Squamous	59	64% (1)	NS	NS	20
Kies et al, 1987[280]	Cisplatin/5-FU cisplatin 100 mg/m² day 1 5-FU 1000 mg/m² C.I.V.I. day 1–5 3 cycles	Squamous	26	42%	14	NS	17.8

(continued)

TABLE 25–10.   *(Continued)*

Investigations	Treatment Plan	Carcinoma Histology	No. of Patients	Response (Path CR)	Operative Candidates	Curative Resection Rate*	Median Survival† (mo)
Ajani et al, 1990[272]	Etoposide/5-FU/cisplatin etoposide 90 mg/m² day 1, 3, 5 5-FU 900 mg/m² C.I.V.I. day 1–5 cisplatin 20 mg/m² day 1–5 2 cycles preop, 3 to 4 cycles postop‡	Adeno	35	49% (1)	32	78%	23
Ajani et al, 1991[273]	Etoposide/doxorubicin/cisplatin etoposide 150 mg/m² day 1–3 doxorubicin 20 mg/m² day 1–3 cisplatin 35 mg/m² day 1–3 GM-CSF starting day 4 2 to 3 cycles preop, 2 to 3 cycles postop‡	Adeno	27	52%	25	80%	10

Adeno, adenocarcinoma; C.I.V.I., continuous intravenous infusion; 5-FU, 5-fluorouracil; GM-CSF, granulocyte-macrophage colony-stimulating factor; MGBG, methylglyoxal-bis-guanylhydrazone (methyl-GAG); NS, not stated; Path CR, pathologic complete response.
* All gross tumor removed and negative margins of resection.
† Represents survival of all study patients unless indicated otherwise.
‡ Postoperative chemotherapy given to preoperative responders only.

modalities, the median survival of those randomized to initial chemotherapy was only 10.4 months. Using the same preoperative cisplatin, vindesine, and bleomycin regimen, Schlag observed a 45% response rate after two cycles were administered to 42 patients.[274] Fifty-five percent had a potentially curative resection, and the median survival of all patients was 16 months.

Roth and colleagues conducted the only randomized trial of comparing preoperative chemotherapy and surgery.[269] Forty-seven percent of patients responded after two cycles of cisplatin, vindesine and bleomycin, including one histologically complete response. The actuarial survival curves for the two groups were not significantly different and the median survival for both groups was 9 months. However, patients who responded to preoperative chemotherapy had a significantly longer survival (median, greater than 20 months) then nonresponders (median, 6.2 months) and patients in the surgery alone treatment group. In a prognostic factor analysis, weight loss of less than 10% before randomization was the only factor predictive of longer survival. The response rates to the cisplatin, vindesine, and bleomycin combination in these four trials ranged from 45% to 63%; a total of 76 responses were observed in 141 patients (54%).[213,269,274,276] Dose-limiting toxic effects reported by all investigators were moderate myelosuppression and tolerable nausea and vomiting.

In a similar trial, Kelsen substituted the polyamine synthesis inhibitor mitoguazone (methyl-GAG or MGBG) for bleomycin.[277] Forty-two percent of 19 patients responded, including one who had a histologically complete response. The median survival duration of this small series was 8.5 months, which was not an improvement over previously tested combinations.[276]

Forastiere and colleagues tested the cisplatin, MGBG, and vinblastine regimen in 29 patients with adenocarcinomas of the esophagus and gastroesophageal junction and squamous cell carcinoma.[270] Responses were observed in 31% of the adenocarcinoma patients and 64% of the squamous cell cancers and included one histologically complete response. Curative resections were carried out in 80% of the responders, but the median survival time of all patients was only 14 months. Initial sites of recurrence correlated somewhat with histologic type: 66% of the recurrent squamous cell cancers were locoregional, and 78% of the recurrent adenocarcinomas were distant. Although postoperative chemotherapy was planned for the responders to preoperative treatment, it was not feasible in 50% of the candidates.

A preoperative regimen of cisplatin and infused 5-FU was evaluated by Carey and colleagues in 59 patients with squamous cell histology.[271,278,279] Thirty-eight patients (64%) had regression of tumor, including 23 in which no tumor was detected on barium esophagogram or endoscopy, but only one histologically complete response was documented. Forty-seven patients had resections; the median survival time of these patients was 23.7 months, and for all 59 patients it was

20 months. Thirty-one percent of the original 35 patients studied are alive at 5 years.[278,279] Kies and colleagues gave three cycles of cisplatin and 5-FU before surgery or radiation therapy to 26 patients with squamous cell cancer of the esophagus.[280] Eleven (42%) patients had reduction in tumor size by (CT, endoscopy, or barium esophagogram) and improvement in dysphagia. Three of these had no visible tumor and negative biopsies. Although only 14 patients had esophagectomy as their definitive treatment, the median survival time of all 26 patients was 17.8 months, suggesting possible benefit from a third cycle of chemotherapy.

Based on previously documented activity of methotrexate and cisplatin in squamous cell carcinoma of the head and neck, Advani and colleagues treated 44 patients with these two drugs and leucovorin before radiation therapy.[281] Response was categorized as good if serial esophagograms showed at least a 50% reduction in tumor length and a doubling or greater increase in lumen diameter. Responses were observed in 48% of the patients, suggesting that this regimen has short-term efficacy.

Two trials reported by Ajani focused entirely on adenocarcinoma of the esophagus and gastroesophageal junction.[272,273] Thirty-five potentially resectable patients received a regimen of etoposide, infused 5-FU, and cisplatin for two cycles before surgery and three or four after surgery if response occurred. Eleven patients had a marked reduction in tumor bulk, and 6 had no tumor evident by endoscopy and random mucosal biopsy. Only one patient proved to have a histologically complete response after resection. The median survival of all 35 patients was 23 months. The major toxic effect was moderate myelosuppression, which did not prevent 80% of the patients from receiving a total of five or six cycles of chemotherapy.

In a follow-up study, Ajani evaluated a regimen of high-dose etoposide, doxorubicin, and cisplatin with granulocyte-macrophage colony-stimulating factor (GM-CSF) in 29 adenocarcinoma patients.[273] Major responses were observed in 52% of the patients, but median survival was only 10 months. Severe myelosuppression was a frequent side effect, as were constitutional symptoms from the GM-CSF.

Because most preoperative chemotherapy trials accrued small numbers of patients to determine feasibility, there is little information on prognostic factors. In most studies, chemotherapy responders survived longer then nonresponders, and patients undergoing a curative resection lived longer than unresectable patients.[213,272,276,278-280] Two trials in which multivariate analyses were performed identified weight loss as the only predictive factor for survival.[269,272]

In summary, preoperative chemotherapy is tolerable and does not appear to increase surgical morbidity. Substantial reduction in tumor bulk occurs in 40% to 60% of patients, but histologically complete responses are infrequent. Because measurement of tumor response is difficult, survival and histologically complete response rates should be the parameters for comparison between studies, and improvement in these endpoints the ultimate goal. All but one trial limited preoperative chemotherapy to one or two cycles.[280] The impact of three or more cycles on survival has not been investigated. Only one small randomized trial with surgery as the control arm has been published.[269] Although this trial showed no advantage of surgery over chemotherapy, confirmation of these findings in large numbers of patients is needed. The optimal

treatment regimen and approach for adenocarcinoma is unknown. Because this histologic type is increasing in frequency, intergroup trials currently include this patient population. A multiinstitutional cooperative group trial is in progress that compares surgery alone with three preoperative cycles of cisplatin and 5-FU followed by surgery and two additional cycles of cisplatin and 5-FU. Until this intergroup trial is completed, multimodality treatment of esophageal cancer using preoperative chemotherapy must be considered investigational.

PALLIATION FOR CARCINOMA OF THE ESOPHAGUS

Patients with esophageal carcinoma may be surgically unresectable because of the extent of the tumor locally or metastases distally. These patients require relief from dysphagia and pain. Numerous modalities are available for palliation of symptoms of esophageal obstruction, including external-beam irradiation, intraluminal brachytherapy, intubation through the tumor with various prostheses, placement of stents, laser opening of the occluded esophagus, and simple dilation (Table 25–11).[69,282-293] The application of a given method of palliation depends to a great extent on the patient's physical condition and the expertise of the surgeon, oncologist, and radiation therapist.

RADIATION THERAPY

External-Beam Irradiation

The use of external-beam radiation therapy for local control of esophageal cancer is described earlier in this chapter.

Intraluminal Brachytherapy

Patients with symptomatic esophageal carcinoma not amenable to surgical resection and previously treated with external-beam irradiation may be candidates for intraluminal brachytherapy. In this procedure, a radioactive bead is placed through a catheter prepositioned through the area to be irradiated. This radiative source passes through the area in a given amount of time to provide a finite and controlled radiation dose to the local tissues. The depth of penetration of the radiation rarely exceeds 2 or 3 cm.

Sur and colleagues treated 9 patients with advanced squamous cell carcinoma of the middle third of the esophagus with intraluminal brachytherapy.[287] Even without previous external-beam irradiation, intraluminal brachytherapy may be effective. Fleischman and colleagues showed that 9 of 10 patients with advanced esophageal cancer treated with intraluminal brachytherapy achieved palliation equivalent to that of external-beam irradiation.[288] Most patients had already experienced failures of other palliative modalities. Holting and colleagues successfully used laser and intraluminal brachytherapy in 16 of 45 patients (previously treated with laser) to prolong palliation.[282]

SURGERY

All surgery for symptomatic carcinoma of the esophagus is palliative in the strictest sense, as tumors often have spread through the lymphatics. Because of the high attendant mor-

TABLE 25-11. Results of Procedures for Palliation of Obstructing Carcinoma of the Esophagus

Investigations	Techniques	No. of Patients	Mortality (%)	Morbidity (%)	Improvement or Relief of Dysphagia (%)	Median Survival
Holting et al, 1991[282]	Surgery	26	19	31	80	—
Hirai et al, 1989[283]	Surgery	93	36	33	60	6 mo
Segalin et al, 1989[284]	Surgery	49	20	46	71	6 mo
Mannell et al, 1988[285]	Surgery	124	11	50	82	5 mo
Orringer, 1984[69]	Surgery	37	24	59	25	6 mo
Lundell et al, 1989[286]	Dilation	41	0	5	100*	—
Sur et al, 1991[287]	Brachytherapy	9	0	0	100*	100% > 9 mo
Fleischman et al, 1990[288]	Brachytherapy	10	0	0	90	2 mo
Loizou et al, 1991[289]	Intubation	30	0	13	90	5 mo
Hahl et al, 1991[290]	Intubation	27	11	48	89	None at 1 y
Pattison et al, 1990[291]	Intubation	110	15	29	—	—
Segalin et al, 1989[284]	Intubation	254	10	17	0	4 mo
Buset et al, 1987[292]	Intubation	116	4	14	95	6 mo
Unruh et al, 1985[293]	Intubation	88	18	41	—	3–4 mo
Hahl et al, 1991[290]	Laser	69	0	9	55	12% at 1 y
Holting et al, 1991[282]	Laser	29	2	—	80	9 mo
	Laser + brachytherapy	16				
Loizou et al, 1991[289]	Laser	43	0	2	63	6 mo
Segalin et al, 1989[284]	Laser	50	0	0	83	4 mo
Buset et al, 1987[292]	Laser	28	0	4	100	7 mo

* Multiple procedures required.

tality and morbidity, resection or bypass of unresectable esophageal carcinoma should be carefully considered before being undertaken as a means of palliation.[285,294] Occasionally, patients undergo mobilization of the stomach or conduit and resection of the esophagus only to have remaining gross disease found. In these patients, surgery serves as excellent palliation, and this residual disease may be further controlled by radiation therapy or a combination of radiation therapy and chemotherapy. These patients have tumors that are considered resectable on preoperative studies.

The survival rate of patients with metastatic esophageal carcinoma is poor.[51] Such patients, already debilitated from malnutrition and tumor burden, poorly tolerate a lengthy operation and resection. Despite some advocates of this approach, most surgeons do not support bypass procedures for palliation of esophageal carcinoma because of the high attendant morbidity and mortality. Orringer examined the results in 37 patients who underwent gastric bypass for palliation of esophageal carcinoma.[69] Operative mortality was 24% (9 patients), and anastomotic leaks occurred in 19% (7 patients). Only 25% of patients (7 of 28) achieved good palliation. The average survival in patients who left the hospital alive was 5.9 months.

Other groups have examined the value of esophageal bypass alone and in comparison with other modes of palliation. Mannell examined 124 patients who underwent esophageal bypass for unresectable disease. Hospital mortality was 11% (11 patients). Median survival was 5 months and was improved by radiation therapy. Patients who survived the surgery (82%) had complete and lasting palliation of dysphagia.[285] Holting

and colleagues studied 71 patients who received surgical palliation (n = 26) or endoscopic laser palliation (n = 45).[282] Survival rates were the same in both groups. The stenosis-free interval was longer in the surgery group (24 weeks), and local reocclusion was more common the laser group. Hospital mortality was 19%, and complications occurred in 31%.

Segalin and colleagues examined patients treated with bypass, intubation, or laser. Overall mortality was 9.6%, and the 1-year survival rate was 29.1%. Excellent or good results were obtained in 78% of patients. In patients undergoing bypass (n = 49), the mortality rate was 20.4% and the median survival was 6.2 months. Intubation was performed in 254 patients; the 30-day mortality was 10.2% and the median survival 4.0 months. Laser therapy was performed in 50 patients with no operative mortality (median survival, 4.1 months).[284] Surgical treatment alone provides good results but with high operative morbidity and mortality. Better palliation may be obtained with intubation or laser.

Cervical esophagostomy (a "spit fistula") and gastrostomy do not palliate any patient with esophageal carcinoma. The stoma is difficult to manage, and the patients are social outcasts. Eating or drinking are possible, but oral alimentation is not possible.

DILATION

Simple dilation is less consistently effective in the treatment of esophageal carcinoma. The neoplasm continues to grow and narrow the lumen despite frequent dilations. Lundell examined the palliative effect of repeated endoscopic dilation in 41 patients. Dysphagia recurred in all patients, and most dilations had to be repeated at 4-week intervals. Most patients required three or fewer dilations during their remaining lifespan. The complication rate (perforation) was low (5%), and only a short hospital stay was required.[286]

ESOPHAGEAL INTUBATION

For many years, tubes of various sorts have been forced through the esophageal lumen partially obstructed with neoplasm in an attempt to relieve dysphagia. Complications from placement of tubes are high (≥10%), as is hospital mortality (≥10%). Pattison and colleagues examined 71 patients treated with pulsion intubation (11 patients, 15.5% mortality) and traction intubation (6 patients, 15.4% mortality).[291] Mortality is similar in other studies.[293] Esophageal intubation may be helpful in patients with tracheoesophageal fistula to prevent or limit soilage of the tracheobronchial tree.[295]

Kratz and colleagues compared three tubes: Celestin tubes, implanted by laparotomy and traction; Proctor-Livingston tubes, implanted by pulsion with laparotomy for staging; and Atkinson tubes, placed by pulsion.[296] Patients with the Atkinson tube had few complications and a low mortality rate (6% mortality) compared with the others (42% mortality). Patients undergoing laparotomy had an associated 41% hospital death rate.

Several studies have compared intubation with laser therapy for palliation. Most suggest that laser therapy is preferable because of its lower mortality and morbidity rates. Survival rates are equivalent.[297,298] Buset and colleagues treated 116 patients by intubation and 28 patients by laser. The morbidity rate for intubation was 13.8% and that for laser was 3.6%; the mortality rate was 4.3% for intubation and 0% for laser.[292] In a prospective and nonrandomized two-center trial, Loizou and colleagues treated 43 patients with laser and 30 patients with intraluminal intubation.[289] Relief of dysphagia (80%) and survival rates (5 to 6 months) were similar between the two groups. Laser-treated patients did better over the remainder of their lives but required more procedures.

Metallic expandable stents are being used with some success for the short-term palliative management of unresectable esophagogastric neoplasms.[299]

LASER

Laser ablation of obstructive lesions is effective in palliating more than 80% of patients with obstructing esophageal carcinoma in most series.[300–304] Laser therapy has been shown to have a lower mortality rate and fewer complications than tube insertion. Hahl and colleagues treated 69 patients with laser therapy and 27 patients with esophageal tube insertion.[290] Patients with laser treatment had no fatal complications, an overall complication risk of 8.7%, and a 1-year survival rate of 2%. Patients with tube insertion had a mortality rate of 11%, a complication rate of 48%, and no 1-year survivors. Laser therapy followed by intubation was not significantly better than laser therapy alone.[298]

Several factors may affect long-term outcome after laser therapy. Predictors of long-term survival include initial tumor length of less than 6 cm ($p < 0.01$),[297,305] improvement after the initial laser treatment ($p < 0.005$), and an adenocarcinoma histologic type ($p < 0.05$).[297]

Reed and colleagues conducted a prospective randomized trial examining esophageal intubation alone (n = 10), intubation plus radiation therapy (n = 8), and laser ablation plus intubation plus radiation therapy (n = 9). Eighty percent of patients who had a tube insertion had complications. Survival was not significantly different between groups.[306]

CHEMOTHERAPY

Single Agents

Several reviews[264,307,308] outline the results of single-agent studies, which are summarized in Table 25–12.[268,281,309–327] The cumulative response rate for any one drug is low, on the order of 15% to 20%, and there is no indication of survival benefit. Symptomatic improvement, if reported, is brief. Response data for many of the older, standard agents come from broad phase I–II trials with small numbers of esophageal cancer patients included. For bleomycin, one must rely on the cumulative results of multiple small trials to get an indication of the true response rate.

Bleomycin has been tested in 80 patients at doses in the range of 10 to 20 mg/m^2 daily or twice weekly, usually by the intravenous route.[309–315] Twelve responders were reported, for a 15% response rate. Continuous infusion bleomycin has not been studied. Bleomycin was the most widely used drug before the availability of cisplatin.

Lokich and colleagues administered 5-FU by continuous infusion for 6 weeks to 13 patients with newly diagnosed esophageal cancer.[317] Assessment with endoscopy and barium esophagogram demonstrated a complete response in one patient, partial responses in 10, and no response in two, for an 85% response rate. These results are in contrast to an ECOG trial, in which a 15% response rate was observed in previously treated patients given intermittent bolus 5-FU.[316] Similar results were reported for methotrexate: a 12% response rate in recurrent disease patients[316] and a 48% response rate in newly diagnosed patients.[281] Five studies of cisplatin have been reported.[268,318,321–323] Four used doses ranging from 50 to 120 mg/m^2 every 3 to 4 weeks; of the 86 patients treated, 20 responded, yielding a 23% complete and partial response rate.[318,321–323] A 73% response rate was reported by Miller and associates, who used a more dose-intense schedule of cisplatin, 120 mg/m^2 on days 1 and 15, in 15 patients before surgery.[268] Although no complete responses were observed, these data suggest that sensitivity to chemotherapy is greater in the newly diagnosed patient.

In contrast to the activity observed in phase II evaluations of cisplatin, carboplatin tested in a total of 59 patients with squamous cell cancer of the esophagus in three trials resulted in only a 5% cumulative response rate.[324–326] Steel and colleagues evaluated carboplatin in 14 patients with adenocarcinoma of the esophagus and observed no complete or partial responses.[328] Therefore, studies show little activity for this drug in squamous carcinoma or adenocarcinoma of the esophagus.

Etoposide, a drug with activity in a number of other solid tumors proved disappointing in phase I–II trials of squamous cell cancer of the esophagus. Coonley and associates saw no

TABLE 25–12. Single-Agent Chemotherapy Trials in Squamous Cell Carcinoma of the Esophagus

Investigation	Drug	Dose	Evaluable Patients	Complete and Partial Responses (%)	Response Duration
Clinical Screening Group, 1970[309]	Bleo	10–20 mg/m²/d I.V. or IM	5	1 (20)	NS
Bonnadonna et al, 1972[310]	Bleo	10–20 mg/m²/d or 15–30 mg/m² biw I.V.	10	2 (20)	NS
Yagoda et al, 1972[311]	Bleo	0.25 mg/kg/d I.V.	4	0	
Stephens, 1973[312]	Bleo	15 mg/d IM	3	1 (33)	NS
Ravry et al, 1973[313]	Bleo	20 mg/m²/d I.V.	14	0	
Tancini et al, 1974[314]	Bleo	10–20 mg/m²/d or 15–30 mg/m² biw I.V.	29	4 (14)	1–2 mo
Kolaric et al, 1976[315]	Bleo	15 mg/m² biw I.V.	15	4 (27)	1–4 mo
Ezdinli et al, 1980[316]	5-FU	500 mg/m² I.V. daily × 5 d	26	4 (15)	5–26 wk
Lokich et al, 1987[317]	5-FU	300 mg/m² continuous I.V. infusion × 6 wk	13*	11 (85)	NS
Engstrom et al, 1983[318]	MMC	20 mg/m² I.V. every 4–6 wk	24	10 (42)	12 wk
Whitington and Clos, 1970[319]	MMC	0.05 mg/kg I.V. daily × 10 d	7	1 (14)	NS
Kolaric et al, 1980[320]	DOX	40 mg/m² I.V. for 2 d	13	5 (38)	3.2 mo
Erdinli et al, 1980[316]	DOX	60 mg/m² I.V. q 3 wk	20	1 (5)	NS
Ezdinli et al, 1980[316]	MTX	40 mg/m² I.V. weekly	26	3 (12)	8–15 wk
Advani et al, 1985[281]	MTX	200 mg/m² I.V. q 10 d	44*	21 (48)	NS
Davis et al, 1980[321]	DDP	3 mg/kg I.V. q 4 wk	17	1 (6)	NS
Ravry and Moore, 1980[322]	DDP	90 mg/m² I.V. q 3 wk	10	4 (40)	2 mo
Panettiere et al, 1984[323]	DDP	50 mg/m² I.V. d 1 + 8 q 3 wk	35	9 (26)	3 mos
Engstrom et al, 1983[318]	DDP	50 mg/m² I.V. q 3 wk	24	6 (25)	11 wk
Miller et al, 1985[268]	DDP	120 mg/m² I.V. d 1 + 15	15*	11 (73)	NS
Sternberg et al, 1985[324]	CBP	400 mg/m² I.V. q 4 wk	30	2 (7)	11.5 mo
Mannell and Winters, 1989[325]	CBP	450 mg/m² I.V. q 4 wk	11	1 (14)	NS
Queisser et al, 1990[326]	CBP	130–160 mg/m² I.V. d 1, 3, 5 q 4 wk	18	0	
Coonley et al, 1983[327]	Etop	100–120 mg/m²/d I.V. d 1, 3, 5	20	0	

Bleo, bleomycin; CBP, carboplatin; DDP, cisplatin; DOX, doxorubicin; Etop, etoposide; 5-FU, 5-fluorouracil; MMC, mitomycin C; MTX, methotrexate; NS, not stated.
* Preoperative treatment.

responses in 20 patients,[327] and in two broad phase I trials, responses were observed in 2 of 4 patients.[329]

Two investigational agents have demonstrated moderate activity in squamous cell carcinoma of the esophagus. Kelsen tested the MGBG and vindesine and observed a 17% response rate to each drug.[330,331] Responders included patients previously treated with cisplatin-based combination chemotherapy. Both drugs were subsequently incorporated into combination regimens given preoperatively.

In summary, bleomycin, 5-FU, mitomycin, and cisplatin are commercially available agents with moderate activity in squamous cell carcinoma of the esophagus. There is no role for single agents for the palliation of advanced esophageal cancer because of the low order and brief duration of response. Higher response rates were achieved in several studies in which single-agent chemotherapy was administered to newly diagnosed patients before surgery or radiation therapy. This suggests that the evaluation of new drugs should be carried out in patients with minimal or no previous treatment.

Combination Chemotherapy

The results of single-agent studies led to the testing of combination regimens, primarily in patients with squamous cell carcinoma. Because this malignancy is uncommon, most studies included patients treated preoperatively and those with recurrent and metastatic disease. The results of platinum-based combination chemotherapy regimens are detailed in Table 25–13.[275–277,332–340] The evaluable patients listed in this data summary include only those who received palliative treatment for recurrent disease or incurable disease at diagnosis. Most series contain small numbers of patients, so that the 95% confidence intervals are large and overlapping. Nearly all responses are partial; there was only an occasional clinically complete response. Duration of response is variable but on average ranges from 3 to 6 months.

Kelsen and colleagues at Memorial Sloan-Kettering Cancer Center have the largest single-institution experience with platinum-based regimens.[276,277,330,340] Their first study evaluated cisplatin and infused bleomycin in 17 patients with recurrent or metastatic disease.[275] They observed a 17% response rate and a median survival time of 4 months. The addition of vindesine to the cisplatin and bleomycin combination produced brief responses in 33%.[276] Dinwoodie and colleagues evaluated this combination and reported a 29% response rate in 27 advanced esophageal cancer patients.[332] The combination of cisplatin, MGBG, and vindesine was tested by Kelsen in 20 patients and yielded partial responses in

TABLE 25–13.   Combination Chemotherapy for Advanced Inoperable and Metastatic Squamous Cell Carcinoma

Investigations	Chemotherapy	Evaluable Patients	Complete and Partial Response (%)	Medial Response Duration	Median Survival
Coonley et al, 1984[275]	Cisplatin + bleomycin	17	17	6 mo	4 mo
Kelsen et al, 1983[276]	Cisplatin + bleomycin + vindesine	24	33	7 mo	NS
Dinwoodie et al, 1986[332]	Cisplatin + bleomycin + vindesine	27	29	3 mo	NS
DeBasi et al, 1984[333]	Cisplatin + bleomycin + MTX	31	26	5 mo	5 mo
Vogl et al, 1981[334]	Cisplatin + bleomycin + MTX	9	44	6 mo	7.5 mo
Vogl et al, 1985[335]	Cisplatin + bleomycin + MTX + MGBG	9	55	5 mo	NS
Kelsen et al, 1986[277]	Cisplatin + MGBG + vindesine	20	40	3 mo	4 mo
Chapman et al, 1987[336]	Cisplatin + MGBG + vinblastine	36	11	13 wk	3.4 mo
Gisselbrecht et al, 1983[337]	Cisplatin + 5-FU + doxorubicin	21	33	NS	8 mo
DeBasi et al, 1986[338]	Cisplatin + 5-FU + allopurinol	37	35	9 mo	NS
Iizuka et al, 1991[339]	Cisplatin + 5-FU	35	34	NS	NS
Lovett et al, 1991[340]	Carboplatin + vinblastine	16	0		

5-FU, 5-fluorouracil; MGBG, mitoguazone (methyl-GAG); MTX, methotrexate; NS, not stated.

40%.[277] The three-drug combinations appeared to result in higher response rates, but median response durations, survival durations, and complete response rates were not improved. The primary toxic effect was myelosuppression that generally was well tolerated. The most recent report from the Memorial Sloan-Kettering group was a phase II trial of carboplatin and vinblastine.[340] No response was observed in 16 patients, even though 11 with advanced, inoperable cancer were previously untreated, and 15 patients had Karnofsky performance scores of 70% or better. The results of this trial and of phase II single-agent carboplatin trials[324–326] indicate that carboplatin and cisplatin do not have comparable activity in squamous cell carcinoma of the esophagus. The efficacy of carboplatin for the treatment of adenocarcinoma of the distal esophagus and gastroesophageal junction needs to be further evaluated.[326]

The combination of cisplatin, bleomycin, and methotrexate, with and without MGBG, was tested in phase II trials by Vogl and colleagues.[334,335] In each study, 9 patients with advanced inoperable or metastatic disease were evaluable. The group that received MGBG had a response role of 44%, and the group that did not receive MGBG had a rate of 55%; the durations of responses were similar. There was one death due to drug toxicity; it was presumed to be related to methotrexate, but no interstitial pneumonitis or azotemia was noted.

Gisselbrecht and colleagues treated 21 patients with the three-drug combination cisplatin, 5-FU, and doxorubicin.[337] Two complete responses and 7 partial responses were observed, for a response rate of 33%. Nausea and vomiting were the primary toxic effects.

The combination of cisplatin and infused 5-FU with allopurinol was evaluated by DeBasi and colleagues in 37 patients with advanced esophageal cancer.[338] Ten partial responses and 3 complete responses were observed, for a 35% overall response rate. About half of the patients had locally extensive unresectable disease; only one patient had received previous chemotherapy. The median survival time was 5 months. The results of two other trials using cisplatin and infused 5-FU in advanced squamous cell carcinoma of the esophagus have been reported as preliminary abstracts.[339,341] The EORTC conducted a randomized phase II trial evaluating single-agent cisplatin 100 mg/m^2 and the combination of cisplatin and 5-FU 1000 mg/m^2/day infused for 5 days.[341] The overall response rates for the 70 randomized patients were 11% for single-agent cisplatin and 38% for the combination. The characteristics of the patients were not fully described. Iizuka and colleagues reported a 34% objective response rate in 35 patients with advanced inoperable or recurrent squamous cell carcinoma.[339] The regimen consisted of cisplatin 70 mg/m^2 and 5-FU 700 mg/m^2/day as a 5-day infusion repeated every 3 weeks. These studies demonstrate that 25% to 35% of patients with recurrent or extensive inoperable squamous cell carcinoma of the esophagus respond to cisplatin-based combination chemotherapy. Response duration is brief, and most patients achieve only a partial response. Determining whether there is an advantage to combination chemotherapy over single-agent chemotherapy for this patient population requires a randomized trial. Only one preliminary report attempts to address this issue by a randomized phase II trial design.[341] Aggressive multiagent therapy should not be recommended for the patient with a poor performance status.

REFERENCES

1. Huang GJ, Wu YK. Carcinoma of the esophagus and gastric cardia. New York: Springer-Verlag, 1984.
2. Yang CS. Research on esophageal cancer in China: A review. Cancer Res 1980;40:2633–2644.
3. National Cancer Institutes. Cancer statistics review 1973–1987. Bethseda, MD: US Department of Health and Human Services, 1989.
4. Hesketh PJ, Clapp RW, Doos WG, Spechler SJ. The increasing frequency of adenocarcinoma of the esophagus. Cancer 1989;64:526–530.
5. Blot WJ, Devesa SS, Kneller RW, Fraumeni JF Jr. Rising incidence of adenocarcinoma of the esophagus and gastric cardia. JAMA 1991;265 (10):1287–1289.
6. Harper PS, Harper RMJ, Howel-Evans AW. Carcinoma of the oesophagus with tylosis. Quart J Med 1970;34:317.
7. MacFarlane SD. Carcinoma of the esophagus. In: Hill L, Kozarek R, McCallum R, Mercer CD, eds. The esophagus: Medical and surgical management. Philadelphia: WB Saunders, 1988:237–256.
8. Appelqvist P, Salmo M. Lye corrosion carcinoma of the esophagua: A review of 63 cases. Cancer 1980;45:2655–2658.

9. Hopkins JRA, Postlethwait RW. Caustic burns and carcinoma of the esophagus. Ann Surg 1992;194:146–148.
10. Huang B, Unni KK, Payne WS. Long-term survival following diverticulectomy for cancer in pharyngoesophageal (Zenker's) diverticulum. Ann Thorac Surg 1984;38:207–210.
11. Shamma MH, Benedict EB. Esophageal webs. N Engl J Med 1958;259:378–384.
12. Licciardello JTW, Spitz MR, Hong WK. Multiple primary cancer in patients with cancer of the head and neck: Second cancer of the head and neck, esophagus, and lung. Int J Radiat Oncol Biol Phys 1989;17:467–476.
13. Cooper JS, Pajak TF, Rubin P, et al. Second malignancies in patients who have head and neck cancer: Incidence, effect on survival and implications based on the RTOG experience. Int J Radiat Oncol Biol Phys 1989;17:449–456.
14. Xu L, Sun C, Wu LH. Clinical and pathological characteristics of carcinosarcoma of the esophagus: Report of four cases. Ann Thorac Surg 1984;37:197–203.
15. Turnball AD, Rosen P, Goodner JT. Primary malignant tumors of the esophagus other than typical epidermoid carcinoma. Ann Thorac Surg 1973;15:463–473.
16. Matsusaka T, Watanabe H, Enjoji M. Pseudosarcoma and carcinosarcoma of the esophagus. Cancer 1976;55:249–256.
17. Osamura RY, Shimamura K, Hata J. Polypoid carcinoma of the esophagus. A unifying term for "carcinosarcoma" and "pseudosarcoma." Am J Surg Pathol 1978;2:201–208.
18. Epstein JI, Sears DL, Tucker RS. Carcinoma of the esophagus with adenoid cystic differentiation. Cancer 1984;53:1131–1136.
19. Bell-Thomson J, Haggitt RC, Ellis Jr FH. Mucoepidermoid and adenoid cystic carcinoma of the esophagus. J Thorac Cardiovasc Surg 1980;79:438–446.
20. Reyes CV, Chejfec G, Jao W. Neuroendocrine carcinomas of the esophagus. Ultrastruct Pathol 1980;1:367–376.
21. Briggs JC, Ibrahim NBN. Oat cell carcinoma of the esophagus: A clinico-pathological study of 23 cases. Histopathology 1983;7:261–277.
22. Tateishi R, Taniguchi H, Wada A. Argyrophil cells and melanocytes in esophageal mucosa. Arch Pathol 1974;98:87–89.
23. Tanoue S, Shimoda T, Suzuki M. Anaplastic carcinoma of the esophagus. Acta Pathol Jpn 1983;33:831–841.
24. Ho KJ, Herrera GA, Jones JM. Small cell carcinoma of the esophagus: Evidence for a unified histogenesis. Hum Pathol 1984;15:460–468.
25. Kelsen DP, Weston E, Kurtz R. Small-cell carcinoma of the esophagus. Treatment by chemotherapy alone. Cancer 1980;45:1558–1561.
26. Rosenthal SN, Lemkin JA. Multiple small cell carcinoma of the esophagus. Cancer 1983;51:1944–1946.
27. Gelb A, Miller S. AIDS and gastroenterology. Am J Gastroenterol 1986;81:619–622.
28. Welch K, Fiunkbeiner W, Alpers CE. Autopsy findings in the acquired immune deficiency syndrome. JAMA 1984;252:1152–1159.
29. Druckrey H, Preussman R, Ivankovic SL. Organotropic carcinogenic effects of 65 various N-nitroso-compounds on BD rats. Z Krebsforsch 1967;69:103.
30. Li MH, Li P, Li PJ. Recent progress in research on esophageal cancer in China. Adv Cancer Res 1980;33:173–249.
31. Bernal A, del Junco GW. Endoscopic and pathologic features of esophageal lymphoma: A report of four cases in patients with acquired immune deficiency syndrome. Gastrointest Endosc 1986;32:96–99.
32. Worgan P, Baldock CR. Lymphosarcoma of the oesophagus. J Laryngol Otol 1976;90:207–210.
33. Berman MD, Falchuk KR, Trey C. Primary histiocytic lymphoma of the esophagus. Dig Dis Sci 1979;24:883–886.
34. Matsuura H, Saito R, Nakajima S. Non-Hodgkin's lymphoma of the esophagus. Am J Gastroenterol 1985;80:941–946.
35. American Joint Committee for Cancer Staging and End-Results Reporting. Manual for staging of cancer. Chicago: American Joint Committee for Cancer Staging and End-Results Reporting, 1978.
36. Liebermann-Meffert DMI, Luescher U, Neff U, Ruedi TP, Allgower M. Esophagectomy without thoracotomy: Is there a risk of intramediastinal bleeding? Ann Surg 1987;206:184–192.
37. Van Overhagen H, Lameris JS, Zonderland HM, Tilanus HW, van Pel R, Schutte HE. Ultrasound and ultrasound-guided fine needle aspiration biopsy of supraclavicular lymph nodes in patients with esophageal carcinoma. Cancer 1991;67:585–587.
38. Guernsey JM, Knudsen DF. Abdominal exploration in the evaluation of patients with carcinoma of the thoracic esophagus. J Thorac Cardiovasc Surg 1970;59:62.
39. Watson WL, Goodner JT, Miller TP, et al. Torek esophagectomy: The case against segmental resection for esophageal cancer. J Thorac Cardiovasc Surg 1956;32:347.
40. Takubo K, Sasajima K, Yamashita K, Tanaka Y, Fujita K. Prognostic significance of intramural metastasis in patients with esophageal carcinoma. Cancer 1990;65:1816–1819.
41. Akiyama H. Surgery for cancer of the esophagus. Baltimore: Williams & Wilkins, 1990.
42. Ojala K, Sorri M, Jokinin K, et al. Symptoms of carcinoma of the oesophagus. Med J Aust 1982;1:384–385.
43. Pedersen H, Hansen HS, Cederquist C, et al. The prognostic significance of weight loss and its integration in stage grouping of oesophageal cancer. Acta Chir Scand 1982;148:363–366.
44. Stair JM, Brian JE. The spectrum of esophageal carcinoma. J Ark Med Soc 1982;82:107–114.
45. Sweet RH. Carcinoma of the esophagus and stomach. JAMA 1948;137:1213–1215.
46. Ojala K, Sorri M, Jokinin K, et al. Symptoms and diagnostic delay in patients with carcinoma of oesophagus and gastric carcinoma: A retrospective study of 225 patients. Postgrad Med J 1982;58:264–267.
47. Duranceau A, Jamieson GG. Malignant tracheoesophageal fistula. Ann Thorac Surg 1984;37:346–354.
48. Kobayashi K, Kasugai T. Brushing cytology for the diagnosis of gastric cancer involving the cardia of the lower esophagus. Acta Cytol 1978;22:155.
49. Winaiwer SJ, Sherlock P, Belladonna JA, et al. Endoscopic brush cytology in esophageal cancer. JAMA 1975;232:1358.
50. Wu YK, Huang GJ, Shao LF, et al. Progress in the study and surgical treatment of cancer of the esophagus in China, 1940–1980. J Thorac Cardiovasc Surg 1982;84:325.
51. Skinner DB. Esophageal malignancies: Experience with 110 cases. Surg Clin North Am 1976;56:137–147.
52. Becker CD, Barbier P, Porcellini B. CT evaluation of patients undergoing transhiatal esophagectomy for cancer. J Comput Assist Tomogr 1986;10:607–611.
53. Inculet RI, Keller SM, Dwyer A, Roth JA. Evaluation of noninvasive tests for the preoperative staging of carcinoma of the esophagus: A prospective study. Ann Thorac Surg 1985;40:561–565.
54. Guanrei Y, He H, Sunghong Q, et al. Endoscopic diagnosis of 115 cases of early esophageal carcinoma. Endoscopy 1982;14:157.
55. Isono K, Ochiai T, Okuyama K, Onoda S. The treatment of lymph node metastasis from esophageal cancer by extensive lymphadenectomy. Jpn J Surg 1990;20:151–157.
56. Takagi I, Karasawa K. Growth of squamous cell esophageal carcinoma observed by serial esophagographies. J Surg Oncol 1982;21:57.
57. Mantravadi R, Ladd T, Briele H, et al. Carcinoma of the esophagus: Sites of failure. Int J Radiat Oncol Biol Phys 1982;8:1897.
58. Arbitol A, Straus M, Granklin G, et al. Infusional chemotherapy and cyclic chemotherapy for inoperable esophageal and gastric cardia carcinoma. Am J Clin Oncol 1983;6:195.
59. Anderson L, Ladd T. Autopsy findings in squamous cell carcinoma of the esophagus. Cancer 1982;50:1587.
60. Shibuya H, Tahogi M, Horiuchi J, et al. Carcinomas of the esophagus with synchronous or metachronous primary carcinoma in other organs. Acta Radiol Oncol 1982;21:39.
61. Shons AR, McQuarrie DG. Multiple primary epidermoid carcinomas of the upper aerodigestive tract. Arch Surg 1985;120:1007.
62. Orringer MB. Transthoracic versus transhiatal esophagectomy: What difference does it make? Ann Thorac Surg 1987;44:116–118.
63. Muehrcke DD, Kaplan DK, Donnelly RJ. Oesophagogastrectomy in patients over 70. Thorax 1989;44:141–145.
64. Roth JA, Pass HI, Flanagan MM, Graeber GM, Rosenberg JC, Steinberg S. Randomized clinical trial of preoperative and postoperative adjuvant chemotherapy with cisplatin, vindesine, and bleomycin for carcinoma of the oesophagus. J Thorac Cardiovasc Surg 1988;96:242–248.
65. Whittington R, Coia LR, Haller DG, Rubenstein JH, Rosato EF. Adenocarcinoma of the esophagus and esophago-gastric junction: The effects of single and combined modalities on the survival and patterns of failure following treatment. Int J Radiat Oncol Biol Phys 1990;19:593–603.
66. Orringer MB, Forastiere AA, Perez Tamayo C, Urba S, Takasugi BJ, Bromberg J. Chemotherapy and radiation therapy before transhiatal esophagectomy for esophageal carcinoma. Ann Thorac Surg 1990;49:348–354.
67. Roth JA, Ajani JA, Rich TA. Multidisciplinary therapy for esophageal cancer. Adv Surg 1990;23:239–260.
68. Katlic MR, Wilkins EW, Grillo HC. Three decades of treatment of esophageal squamous carcinoma at the Massachusetts General Hospital. J Thorac Cardiovasc Surg 1990;99:929–938.
69. Orringer MB. Substernal gastric bypass of the excluded esophagus: Results of an ill-advised operation. Surgery 1984;96:467–470.
70. Halvorsen RA, Thompson WM. Primary neoplasms of the hollow organs of the gastrointestinal tract: Staging and follow-up. Cancer 1989;63:1181–1188.
71. Rice TW, Boyce GA, Sivak MV. Esophageal ultrasound and the preoperative staging of carcinoma of the esophagus. J Thorac Cardiovasc Surg 1991;101:536–543.
72. Siewert JR, Holscher AH, Dittler HJ. Preoperative staging and risk analysis in esophageal carcinoma. Hepatogastroenterology 1990;37:382–387.
73. Tio TL, Coene PP, Luiken GJ, Tytgat GN. Endosonography in the clinical staging of esophagogastric carcinoma. Gastrointest Endosc 1990;36:S2–10.
74. Vilgrain V, Mompoint D, Palazzo L, et al. Staging of esophageal carcinoma: Comparison of results with endoscopic sonography and CT. AJR 1990;155:277–281.
75. Tio TL, Cohen P, Coene PP, Udding J, den Hartog Jager FC, Tytgat GN. Endosonography and computed tomography of esophageal carcinoma: Preoperative classification compared to the new (1987) TNM system. Gastroenterology 1989;96:1478–1486.
76. Tio TL, Coene PP, Schouwink MH, Tytgat GN. Esophagogastric carcinoma: Preoperative TNM classification with endosonography. Radiology 1989;173:411–417.
77. Sharma OP, Subnani S. Role of computerized tomography imaging in staging oesophageal carcinoma. Semin Surg Oncol 1989;5:355–358.
78. Duignan JP, McEntee GP, O'Connell DJ, Bouchier Hayes DJ, O'Malley E. The role of CT in the management of carcinoma of the oesophagus and cardia. Ann R Coll Surg Engl 1987;69:286–288.
79. Salonen O, Kivisaari L, Standertskjold Nordenstam CG, Somer K, Virkkunen P. Computed tomography in staging of oesophageal carcinoma. Scand J Gastroenterol 1987;22:65–68.
80. Lefor AT, Merino MM, Steinberg SM, et al. Computerized omographic prediction of extraluminal spread and prognostic implications of lesion width in esophageal carcinoma. Cancer 1988;62:1287–1292.
81. Daly JM, Massar E, Giacco G, et al. Parenteral nutrition in esophageal cancer patients. Ann Surg 1982;196:203.

82. The Veterans Affairs Total Parenteral Nutrition Cooperative Study Group. Perioperative total parenteral nutrition in surgical patients. N Engl J Med 1991;325:525–532.

83. Pedersen H, Hansen HS, Cederquist C, et al. The prognostic significance of weight loss and its integration in stage grouping of oesophageal cancer. Acta Chir Scand 1982;148:363.

84. Lewis I. The surgical treatment of carcinoma of the esophagus with special reference to a new operation for growth of the middle third. Br J Surg 1946;2:18–31.

85. Altorki NK, Skinner DB. En bloc esophagectomy: The first 100 patients. Hepatogastroenterology 1990;37:360–363.

86. Skinner DB. En bloc resection for neoplasms of the esophagus and cardia. J Thorac Cardiovasc Surg 1983;85:59–71.

87. Akiyama H, Hiyama M, Hashimoto C. Resection and reconstruction for carcinoma of the thoracic oesophagus. Br J Surg 1976;63:206–209.

88. Orringer MB. Transhiatal esophagectomy without thoracotomy for carcinoma of the esophagus. Adv Surg 1986;19:1–49.

89. Skinner DB. En bloc resection for neoplasms of the esophagus and cardia. J Thorac Cardiovasc Surg 1983;85:59–71.

90. Orringer MB. Transhiatal esophagectomy without thoracotomy for carcinoma of the thoracic esophagus. Ann Surg 1984;200:282–288.

91. Huang MH, Sung CY, Hsu HK, Huang BS, Hsu WH, Chien KY. Reconstruction of the esophagus with the left colon. Ann Thorac Surg 1989;48:660–664.

92. Lundell L, Olbe L. Colonic interposition for reconstruction after resection of cancer in the esophagus and gastroesophageal junction. Eur J Surg 1991;157:189–192.

93. Byth PL, Mullens AJ. Peri-operative care for oesophagectomy patients. Aust Clin Rev 1991;11:45–50.

94. Sweet RH. Surgical management of carcinoma of the midthoracic esophagus. N Engl J Med 1945;233:1–7.

95. Lewis I. The surgical treatment of carcinoma of the esophagus with special reference to a new operation for growth of the middle third. Br J Surg 1946;2:18–31.

96. Orringer MB. Transhiatal esophagectomy without thoracotomy for carcinoma of the esophagus. Adv Surg 1986;19:1–49.

97. Lozac'h P, Topart P, Etienne J, Charles JF. Ivor Lewis operation for epidermoid carcinoma of the esophagus. Ann Thorac Surg 1991;52:1154–1157.

98. Ellis FH Jr. Treatment of carcinoma of the esophagus or cardia. Mayo Clin Proc 1989;64:945–955.

99. Mansour KA, Downey RS. Esophageal carcinoma: Surgery without preoperative adjuvant chemotherapy. Ann Thorac Surg 1989;48:201–204.

100. Mathisen DJ, Grillo HC, Wilkins EW Jr, Moncure AC, Hilgenberg AD. Transthoracic esophagectomy: A safe approach to carcinoma of the esophagus. Ann Thorac Surg 1988;45:137–143.

101. King RM, Pairolero PC, Trastek VF, Payne WS, Bernatz PE. Ivor Lewis esophagogastrectomy for carcinoma of the esophagus: Early and late functional results. Ann Thorac Surg 1987;44:119–122.

102. Mitchell RL. Abdominal and right thoracotomy approach as standard procedure for esophagogastrectomy with low morbidity. J Thorac Cardiovasc Surg 1987;93:205–211.

103. Goldfaden D, Orringer MB, Appleman HD, Kalish R. Adenocarcinoma of the distal esophagus and gastric cardia: Comparison of results of transhiatal esophagectomy and thoracoabdominal esophagogastrectomy. J Thorac Cardiovasc Surg 1986;91:242–247.

104. DeMeester TR, Zaninotto G, Johansson KE. Selective therapeutic approach to cancer of the lower esophagus and cardia. J Thorac Cardiovasc Surg 1988;95:42–54.

105. Gupta NM. Transhiatal esophagectomy. Acta Chir Scand 1990;156:149–152.

106. Gotley DC, Beard J, Cooper MJ, Britton DC, Williamson RC. Abdominocervical (transhiatal) oesophagectomy in the management of oesophageal carcinoma. Br J Surg 1990;77:815–819.

107. Hankins JR, Attar S, Coughlin TR Jr, et al. Carcinoma of the esophagus: A comparison of the results of transhiatal versus transthoracic resection. Ann Thorac Surg 1989;47:700–705.

108. Page RD, Khalil JF, Whyte RI, Kaplan DK, Donnelly RJ. Esophagogastrectomy via left thoracophrenotomy. Ann Thorac Surg 1990;49:763–766.

109. Pradhan GN, Eng JB, Sabanathan S. Left thoracotomy approach for resection of carcinoma of the esophagus. Surg Gynecol Obstet 1989;168:49–53.

110. Matthews HR, Steel A. Left-sided subtotal oesophagectomy for carcinoma. Br J Surg 1987;74:1115–1117.

111. Mannell A, Becker PJ. Evaluation of the results of oesophagectomy for oesophageal cancer. Br J Surg 1991;78:36–40.

112. Chasseray VM, Kiroff GK, Buard JL, Launois B. Cervical or thoracic anastomosis for esophagectomy for carcinoma. Surg Gynecol Obstet 1989;169:55–62.

113. Akiyama H, Hiyama M, Hashimoto C. Resection and reconstruction for carcinoma of the thoracic oesophagus. Br J Surg 1976;63:206–209.

114. Shao LF, Gao ZG, Yang NP, Wei GQ, Wang YD, Cheng CP. Results of surgical treatment in 6,123 cases of carcinoma of the esophagus and gastric cardia. J Surg Oncol 1989;42:170–174.

115. Altorki NK, Skinner DB. En bloc esophagectomy: The first 100 patients. Hepatogastroenterology 1990;37:360–363.

116. Plukker JT, van Slooten EA, Joosten HJ. The Akiyama procedure in the surgical management of oesophageal cardiacarcinoma. Eur J Surg Oncol 1988;14:33–40.

117. Hurley JP, Keeling P. Transhiatal oesophagectomy: Its role for tumours of the middle third of the intrathoracic oesophagus. Ir Med J 1990;83:23–25.

118. Strano S, Bremner CG. Transhiatal blunt esophagectomy. Surg Gynecol Obstet 1988;166:541–544.

119. Forastiere AA, Orringer MB, Perez Tamayo C, et al. Concurrent chemotherapy and radiation therapy followed by transhiatal esophagectomy for local-regional cancer of the esophagus. J Clin Oncol 1990;8:119–127.

120. Becker CD, Barbier PA, Terrier F, Porcellini B. Patterns of recurrence of esophageal carcinoma after transhiatal esophagectomy and gastric interposition. AJR 1987;148:273–277.

121. Orringer MB, Stirling MC. Esophagectomy for esophageal disruption. Ann Thorac Surg 1990;49:35–42.

122. Fok M, Siu KF, Wong J. A comparison of transhiatal and transthoracic resection for carcinoma of the thoracic esophagus. Am J Surg 1989;158:414–419.

123. Saidi F, Abbassi A, Shadmehr MB, Khoshnevis Asl G. Endothoracic endoesophageal pull-through operation: A new approach to cancers of the esophagus and proximal stomach. J Thorac Cardiovasc Surg 1991;102:43–50.

124. Lam KH, Choi TK, Wei WI, Lau WF, Wong J. Present status of pharyngogastric anastomosis following pharyngolaryngo-oesophagectomy. Br J Surg 1987;74:122–125.

125. Baker JW, Schechter GL. Management of panesophageal cancer by blunt resection without thoracotomy and reconstruction with stomach. Ann Surg 1986;203:491–499.

126. Ujiki GT, Pearl GJ, Poticha S, Sisson GA, Shields TW. Mortality and morbidity of gastric 'pull-up' for replacement of the pharyngoesophagus. Arch Surg 1987;122:644–647.

127. Muller JM, Zieren U, Wolters U, Pichlmaier H. Results of esophagectomy and gastric bypass for cancer of the esophagus. Hepatogastroenterology 1989;36:522–528.

128. Griffin S, Desai J, Charlton M, Townsend E, Fountain SW. Factors influencing mortality and morbidity following oesophageal resection. Eur J Cardiothorac Surg 1989;3:419–423.

129. Peracchia A, Bardini R, Ruol A, Asolati M, Scibetta D. Esophagovisceral anastomotic leak: A prospective statistical study of predisposing factors. J Thorac Cardiovasc Surg 1988;95:685–691.

130. McManus KG, Ritchie AJ, McGuigan J, Stevenson HM, Gibbons JR. Sutures, staplers, leaks and strictures: A review of anastomoses in oesophageal resection at Royal Victoria Hospital, Belfast 1977–1986. Eur J Cardiothorac Surg 1990;4:97–100.

131. Smirniotis V, Morritt GG. EEA stapler in oesophagogastrectomies. Int Surg 1990;75:36–38.

132. Rogers EL, Goldkind SF, Iseri OA, et al. Adenocarcinoma of the lower esophagus: A disease primarily of white men with Barrett's esophagus. J Clin Gastroenterol 1986;8:613–618.

133. Steiger Z, Wilson RF, Leichman L, et al. Primary adenocarcinoma of the esophagus. J Surg Oncol 1987;36:68.

134. Cederquist C, Nielsen J, Berthelsen A, et al. Adenocarcinoma of the esophagus. Acta Chir Scand 1980;146:411.

135. Wang HH, Antonioli DA, Goldman H. Comparative features of esophageal and gastric adenocarcinomas: Recent changes in type and frequency. Hum Pathol 1986;17:482–487.

136. Powell J, McConkey CC. Increasing incidence of adenocarcinoma of the gastric cardia and adjacent sites. Br J Cancer 1990;62:440–443.

137. Lund O, Hasenkam JM, Aagaard MT, Kimose HH. Time-related changes in characteristics of prognostic significance in carcinomas of the oesophagus and cardia. Br J Surg 1989;76:1301–1307.

138. Yang PC, Davis S. Incidence of cancer of the esophagus in the US by histologic type. Cancer 1988;61:612–617.

139. Harvey JC, Kagan AR, Ahn C, Frankl H, Davidson W. Adenocarcinoma of the esophagus: A survival study. J Surg Oncol 1990;45:29–32.

140. Nomura A, Stemmermann GN, Chyou PH, Kato I, Perez Perez GI, Blaser MJ. *Helicobacter pylori* infection and gastric carcinoma among Japanese Americans in Hawaii. N Engl J Med 1991;325:1132–1136.

141. Parsonnet J, Friedman GD, Vandersteen DP, et al. *Helicobacter pylori* infection and the risk of gastric carcinoma. N Engl J Med 1991;325:1127–1131.

142. Loffeld RJ, Willems I, Flendrig JA, Arends JW. *Helicobacter pylori* and gastric carcinoma. Histopathology 1990;17:537–541.

143. Correa P, Fox J, Fontham E, et al. *Helicobacter pylori* and gastric carcinoma: Serum antibody prevalence in populations with contrasting cancer risks. Cancer 1990;66:2569–2574.

144. Ming, S.C. Tumors of the esophagus and stomach. In: Atlas of Tumor Pathology, 2nd series, fascicle 7. Washington, DC: Armed Forces Institute of Pathology.

145. Barrett N. The lower esophagus lined by columnar epithelium. Surgery 1957;41:881.

146. Rosenberg JC, Budev H, Edwards RC, et al. Analysis of adenocarcinoma in Barrett's esophagus utilizing a staging system. Cancer 1985;55:1353.

147. Molina JE, Lawton BR, Myers WO, et al. Esophagogastrectomy for adenocarcinoma of the cardia. Ann Surg 1982;195:146–151.

148. Kalish RJ, Clancy PE, Orringer MB, et al. Clinical, epidemiologic, and morphologic comparison between adenocarcinomas arising in Barrett's esophageal mucosa and in the gastric cardia. Gastroenterology 1984;86:461–467.

149. DeMeester TR, Barlow AP. Surgery and current management for cancer of the esophagus and cardia. Curr Probl Cancer 1988;12:243–328.

150. Streitz JM, Ellis FH, Gibb SP, Balogh K, Watkins E. Adenocarcinoma in Barrett's esophagus: A clinicopathologic study of 65 cases. Ann Surg 1991;213:122–125.

151. Altorki NK, Skinner DB. Adenocarcinoma in Barrett's esophagus. Semin Surg Oncol 1990;6:274–278.

152. Harvey JC, Kagan AR, Hause D, Sachs T, Frankl H. Adenocarcinoma arising in Barrett's esophagus. J Surg Oncol 1990;45:162–163.

153. Dent J. Approaches to oesophageal columnar metaplasia (Barrett's oesophagus). Scand J Gastroenterol Suppl 1989;168:60–66.

154. De Baecque C, Potet F, Molas G, Flejou JF, Barbier P, Martignon C. Superficial adenocarcinoma of the oesophagus arising in Barrett's mucosa with dysplasia: A clinicopathological study of 12 patients. Histopathology 1990;16:213–220.

155. Duhaylongsod FG, Wolfe WG. Barrett's esophagus and adenocarcinoma of the esophagus and gastroesophageal junction. J Thorac Cardiovasc Surg 1991;102:36–41.

156. Garewal HS, Sampliner RE, Fennerty MB. Flow cytometry in Barrett's esophagus: What have we learned so far. Dig Dis Sci [Editorial] 1991;36:548–551.

157. Haggitt RC, Reid BJ, Rabinovitch PS, Rubin CE. Barrett's esophagus: Correlation between mucin histochemistry, flow cytometry, and histologic diagnosis for predicting increased cancer risk. Am J Pathol 1988;131:53–61.

158. Fennerty MB, Sampliner RE, Way D, Riddell R, Steinbronn K, Garewal HS. Discordance between flow cytometric abnormalities and dysplasia in Barrett's esophagus [see comments]. Gastroenterology 1989;97:815–820.

159. Levine DS, Reid BJ, Haggitt RC, Rubin CE, Rabinovitch PS. Correlation of ultrastructural aberrations with dysplasia and flow cytometric abnormalities in Barrett's epithelium. Gastroenterology 1989;96:355–367.

160. Garewal HS, Sampliner R, Liu Y, Trent JM. Chromosomal rearrangements in Barrett's esophagus: A premalignant lesion of esophageal adenocarcinoma. Cancer Genet Cytogenet 1989;42:281–286.

161. Garewal HS, Gerner EW, Sampliner RE, Roe D. Ornithine decarboxylase and polyamine levels in columnar upper gastrointestinal mucosae in patients with Barrett's esophagus. Cancer Res 1988;48:3288–3291.

162. Garewal HS, Sampliner R, Gerner E, Steinbronn K, Alberts D, Kendall D. Ornithine decarboxylase activity in Barrett's esophagus: A potential marker for dysplasia. Gastroenterology 1988;94:819–821.

163. Garewal HS, Sampliner R. Barrett's esophagus: A model premalignant lesion for adenocarcinoma. Prev Med 1989;18:749–756.

164. Meltzer SJ, Zhou D, Weinstein WM. Tissue-specific expression of c-Ha-ras in premalignant gastrointestinal mucosae. Exp Mol Pathol 1989;51:264–274.

165. Bai SX. Primary esophageal adenocarcinoma: Report of 19 cases. Chung Hua Chung Liu Tsa Chih 1989;11:383–385.

166. Sampliner RE, Garewal HS, Fennerty MB, Aickin M. Lack of impact of therapy on extent of Barrett's esophagus in 67 patients. Dig Dis Sci 1990;35:93–96.

167. Fiorucci S, Santucci L, Farroni F, Pelli MA, Morelli A. Effect of omeprazole on gastroesophageal reflux in Barrett's esophagus. Am J Gastroenterol 1989;84:1263–1267.

168. Mahoney JL, Condon RE. Adenocarcinoma of the esophagus. Ann Surg 1987;205:557–562.

169. Altorki NK, Sunagawa M, Little AG, Skinner DB. High-grade dysplasia in the columnar-lined esophagus. Am J Surg 1991;161:97–99.

170. Altorki NK, Skinner DB, Segalin A, Stephens JK, Ferguson MK, Little AG. Indications for esophagectomy in nonmalignant Barrett's esophagus: A 10-year experience. Ann Thorac Surg 1990;49:724–7266.

171. Palley SL, Sampliner RE, Garewal HS. Management of high-grade dysplasia in Barrett's esophagus. J Clin Gastroenterol 1989;11:369–372.

172. Williamson WA, Ellis FH, Gibb SP, et al. Barrett's Esophagus. Prevalence and incidence of adenocarcinoma. Arch Intern Med 1991;151:2212–2216.

173. Starnes VA, Adkins RB, Ballinger JG, et al. Barrett's esophagus: A surgical entity. Arch Surg 1984;119:563–567.

174. Williamson WA, Ellis FH Jr, Gibb SP, Shahian DM, Aretz HT. Effect of antireflux operation on Barrett's mucosa. Ann Thorac Surg 1990;49:537–541.

175. Ovaska J, Miettinen M, Kivilaakso E. Adenocarcinoma arising in Barrett's esophagus. Dig Dis Sci 1989;34:1336–1339.

176. Ribet M, Mensier E, Pruvot FR. Barrett's esophagus and adenocarcinoma. Eur J Cardiothorac Surg 1987;1:29–32.

177. Van der Veen AH, Dees J, Blankensteijn JD, Van Blankenstein M. Adenocarcinoma in Barrett's oesophagus: An overrated risk. Gut 1989;30:14–18.

178. Achkar E, Carey W. The cost of surveillance for adenocarcinoma complicating Barrett's esophagus. Am J Gastroenterol 1988;83:291–294.

179. Earlam R. An MRC prospective randomized trial of radiotherapy versus surgery for operable squamous cell carcinoma of the esophagus. Ann R Coll Surg Engl 1991;73:8–12.

180. Petrovich Z, Langholz B, Formenti S, Luxton G, Astrahan M. Management of carcinoma of the esophagus: The role of radiotherapy. Am J Clin Oncol [CCT] 1991;14(1):80–86.

181. Yang Z, Gu X, Zhao S, et al. Long term survival of radiotherapy for esophageal cancer: Analysis of 1136 patients surviving more than 5 years. Int J Radiat Oncol Biol Phys 1983;9:1769–1773.

182. Langer M, Choi N, Orlow E, Hermes G, Wilkins E. Radiation therapy alone or in combination with surgery in the treatment of carcinoma of the esophagus. Cancer 1986;58:1208–1213.

183. Okawa T, Kita M, Tanka M, Ikeda M. Results of radiotherapy for inoperable locally advanced esophageal cancer. Int J Radiat Oncol Biol Phys 1989;17:49–54.

184. Coia L, Engstrom P, Paul A, Stafford P, Hanks G. Long-term results of infusional 5-FU, mitomycin-C, and radiation as primary management of esophageal carcinoma. Int J Radiat Oncol Biol Phys 1991;20:29–36.

185. Harrison L, Fogel T, Picone J, Fischer D, Weissberg J. Radiation therapy for squamous cell carcinoma of the esophagus. J Surg Oncol 1988;37:40–43.

186. Caspers R, Welvaart K, Verkes R, Hermans J, Leer J. The effect of radiotherapy on dysphagia and survival in patients with esophageal cancer. J Rad Ther Oncol 1988;12:15–23.

187. Welvaart K, Caspers R, Verkes R, Hermans J. The choice between surgical resection and radiation therapy for patients with cancer of the esophagus and cardia: A retrospective comparison between two treatments. J Surg Oncol 1991;47:225–229.

188. Little AG, Furguson MK, DeMeester TR, et al. Esophageal carcinoma with respiratory tract fistula. Cancer 1984;53:1322–1328.

189. Yamada S, Takai Y, Ogawa Y, Kakuto Y, Sakamoto K. Radiotherapy for malignant fistula to other tracts. Cancer 1989;64:1026–1028.

190. Hussey D, Barkley H Jr, Bloedorn F. Carcinoma of the esophagus. In: Fletcher GH, ed. Textbook of radiotherapy. Philadelphia: Lea & Febiger, 1980:688–703.

191. Corn B, Coia L, Chu J, Hwang C, Stafford P, Hanks G. Significance of prone positioning planning treatment for esophageal cancer. Int J Radiat Oncol Biol Phys 1991;31:1303–1309.

192. Lewinsky B, Annes G, Mann S, et al. Carcinoma of the esophagus: An analysis of results and treatment techniques. Radiol Clin N Am 1975;44:192–204.

193. Smoron G, O'Brien C, Sullivan C. Tumor localization and treatment technique for cancer of the esophagus. Radiology 1974;111:735–736.

194. Vijayakumar S, Muller-Runkel R. Irradiation of the thoracic esophagus: Prone versus supine treatment positions. Acta Radiol Oncol 1986;25:187–189.

195. Miller C. Carcinoma of the thoracic esophagus and cardia. Br J Surg 1962;49:597.

196. Pearson JG. The present status and future potential of radiotherapy in the management of esophageal cancer. Cancer 1977;39:882.

197. Lefor A, Merino M, Steinberg S, et al. Computerized tomographic prediction of extra-luminal spread and prognostic implications of lesion width in esophageal carcinoma. Cancer 1988;62:1287–1292.

198. McKenna G, Fraass BA, Van de Geijn Y, et al. Is correction for lung density in radiotherapy treatment planning necessary? Int J Radiat Oncol Phys Biol 1987;13:273–278.

199. McShan DL, Fraass BA, Lichter AS. Full integration of the beam's eye view concept into computerized treatment planning. Int J Radiat Oncol Biol Phys 1990;18:1485–1494.

200. Giuli R, Gignoux M. Treatment of carcinoma of the esophagus. Ann Surg 1980;192:44–52.

201. Fisher S, Brady L. Esophagus. In: Perez CA, Brady LW, eds. Principles and procedure of radiation oncology. Philadelphia: JB Lippincott, 1992:853–870.

202. Guisez J. Essais de traitement de quelques cas d'epithelioma de l'oesophage par les applications locales directes de radium. Le Bulletin Soc Med Hop (Paris) 1909;27:717–722.

203. Rider W, Mendoza R. Some opinions on the treatment of cancer of the oesophagus. Am J Radiol 1969;105:514.

204. Flores A, Nelems B, Evans K, Hay J, Stoller J, Jackson S. Impact of new radiotherapy modalities on the surgical management of cancer of the esophagus and cardia. Int J Radiat Oncol Biol Phys 1989;17:937–944.

205. Hishikawa Y, Kurisu K, Taniguchi M, Kamikonya N, Miura T. High-dose-rate intra-luminal brachytherapy for esophageal cancer: 10 years experience in Hyogo College of Medicine. Radiother Oncol 1991;23:107–114.

206. Burt P, Notley H, Stout R. A simple technique for intraluminal irradiation in oesophageal tumours using the high-dose-rate microelectron. Br J Radiol 1989;62:748–750.

207. Hishikawa Y, Kurisu K, Taniguchi M, Kamikonya N, Miura T. Radiotherapy for carcinoma of the esophagus in patients aged eighty or older. Int J Radiat Oncol Biol Phys 1991;20:685–688.

208. Fleischman E, Kagan R, Bellotti J, Streeter O, Harvey J. Effective palliation for inoperable esophageal cancer using intensive intracavitary radiation. J Surg Oncol 1990;44:234–237.

209. Rowland CG, Pagliero KM. Intracavitary irradiation in palliation of carcinoma of oesophagus and cardia. Lancet 1985;2:981–983.

210. Fajardo L. Pathology of radiation injury. New York: Masson, 1982:50–53.

211. Seaman W, Ackerman L. The effect of radiation on the esophagus. Radiology 1957;68:534.

212. Morita K, Takagi I, Watanabe M, Niwa K, Kanazawa H. Relationship between the radiologic features of esophageal cancer and the local control by radiation therapy. Cancer 1985;55:2668–2676.

213. Kelsen D, Minsky B, Smith M, Beitler J, Niedzwiecki D, et al. Preoperative therapy for esophageal cancer: A randomized comparison of chemotherapy versus radiation therapy. J Clin Oncol 1990;8(8):1352–1361.

214. Liu G, Huang Z, Rong T, Yang M, Chang E, Xiao Q. Measures for improving therapeutic results of esophageal carcinoma in stage III: Preoperative radiotherapy. J Clin Oncol 1986;32:248–255.

215. Marks R Jr, Scruggs H, Wallace K. Preoperative radiation therapy for carcinoma of the esophagus. Cancer 1976;38:84–89.

216. Earlam R, Cunha-Melo J. Oesophageal squamous cell carcinoma: II. A critical review of radiotherapy. Br J Surg 1980;67(7):457–461.

217. Earlam R, Johnson L. 101 Oesophageal cancers: A surgeon uses radiotherapy. Ann R Coll Surg Engl 1990;72:32–40.

218. O'Rourke I, Tiver K, Bull C, et al. Swallowing performance after radiation therapy for carcinoma of the esophagus. Cancer 1988;61:2022–2026.

219. Beatty J, Rider W. Carcinoma of the esophagus: Pretreatment assessment, correlation of radiation treatment parameters with survival and identification and management of radiation treatment failure. Cancer 1975;43:2254.

220. Levine M, Langer J, Laufer I, Kligerman M. Radiation therapy of esophageal carcinoma: Correlation of clinical and radiographic findings. Gastrointest Radiol 1987;12:99–105.

221. Yang Z, Hu Y, Gu X. Non-cancerous ulcer in the esophagus after radiotherapy for esophageal carcinoma—a report of 27 patients. Radiother Oncol 1990;19:121–129.

222. Sugimachi K, Matsufuji H, Kai H, et al. Preoperative irradiation for carcinoma of the esophagus. Surg Gynecol Obstet 1986;162(2):174–176.

223. Yadava O, Hodge A, Matz L, Donlon J. Esophageal malignancies: Is preoperative radiotherapy the way to go? Ann Thorac Surg 1991;51:189–193.

224. Doggett RLS, Guernsey J, Bagshaw M. Combined radiation and surgical treatment of carcinoma of the thoracic esophagus. Rad Ther Oncol 1970;5:147–154.

225. Huang G, Gu X, Want I, et al. Experience with combined preoperative irradiation and surgery for carcinoma of the esophagus. Gann Monogr Cancer Res 1986;31:159–164.

226. Gignoux M, Roussel A, Paillot B. The value of preoperative radiotherapy in esophageal cancer: Results of a study of the EORTC. World J Surg 1987;11:426–432.

227. Wilson S, Hiatt J, Stabile B, et al. Cancer of the distal esophagus and cardia: Preoperative irradiation prolongs survival. Am J Surg 1985;150:114–121.

228. Akakura I, Nakamura Y, Kakegawa T, et al. Surgery of carcinoma of the esophagus with preoperative radiation. Chest 1970;57:37–47.

229. Hambraeus G, Mercke C, Willen R, Ranstam J, et al. Prognostic factors influencing survival in combined radiotherapy and surgery of squamous cell carcinoma of the esophagus with special reference to a histopathologic grading system. Cancer 1988;62:895–904.

230. Launois B, DeLaRue D, Campion J, et al. Preoperative radiotherapy for carcinoma of the esophagus. Surg Gynecol Obstet 1981;153:690.

231. Fraser R, Wara W, Thomas A, et al. Combined treatment methods for carcinoma of the esophagus. Radiology 1978;128:461.

232. Goodner J. Surgical and radiation treatment of cancer of the thoracic esophagus. Am J Roentgenol Rad Ther Nucl Med 1969;105:523.

233. Gunnlaugson G, Wychulis A, Roland C, Ellis FH Jr. Analysis of the records of 1657 patients with carcinoma of the esophagus and cardia of the stomach. Surg Gynecol Obstet 1970;130:997.

234. Kolaric K, Maricic Z, Roth A, Dujmovic I. Combination of bleomycin and adriamycin with and without radiation in the treatment of inoperable esophageal cancer: A randomized study. Cancer 1980;45:2265–2273.

235. Byfield J, Barone R, Mendelsohn J, et al. Infusional 5-fluorouracil and x-ray therapy for non-resectable esophageal cancer. Cancer 1980;45:703–708.

236. Earle J, Gelber R, Moertel C, Hahn R. A controlled evaluation of combined radiation and bleomycin therapy for squamous cell carcinoma of the esophagus. Int J Radiat Oncol Biol Phys 1980;6:821–826.

237. Steiger Z, Franklin R, Wilson R, et al. Complete eradication of squamous cell carcinoma of the esophagus with combined chemotherapy and radiotherapy. Am Surg 1981;45:95–98.

238. Nigro ND, Vaitkevicius VK, Considene B Jr. Combined therapy for cancer of the anal canal: A preliminary report. Dis Colon Rectum 1974;17:354–356.

239. Franklin R, Steiger Z, Vaishampayan G, et al. Combined modality therapy for esophageal squamous cell carcinoma. Cancer 1983;51:1062–1071.

240. Chan A, Wong A, Arthur K. Concomitant 5-fluorouracil infusion, mitomycin C and radical therapy in esophageal squamous cell carcinoma. Int J Radiat Oncol Biol Phys 1988;16:59–65.

241. John M, Flam M, Mowry P, et al. Radiotherapy alone and chemoradiation for non-metastatic esophageal carcinoma: A critical review of chemoradiation. Cancer 1989;63:2397–2403.

242. Keane T, Harwood A, Elhakim T, et al. Radical radiation therapy with 5-fluorouracil infusion and mitomycin C for oesophageal squamous carcinoma. Radiother Oncol 1985;4:205–210.

243. Leichman L, Herskovic A, Leichman P, et al. Nonoperative therapy for squamous cell cancer of the esophagus. J Clin Oncol 1987;5(3):365–370.

244. Herskovic A, Leichman L, Lattin P, et al. Chemoradiation with and without surgery in the thoracic esophagus: The Wayne State experience. Int J Radiat Oncol Biol Phys 1988;15:655–662.

245. Richmond J, Seydel H, Bae Y, et al. Comparison of three treatment strategies for esophageal cancer within a single institution. Int J Radiat Oncol Biol Phys 1987;13:1617–1620.

246. Seitz J, Giovannini M, Padaut-Cesana J, et al. Inoperable nonmetastatic squamous cell carcinoma of the esophagus managed by concomitant chemotherapy (5-fluorouracil and cisplatin) and radiation therapy. Cancer 1990;66:214–219.

247. Araujo C, Souhami L, Gil R, et al. A randomized trial comparing radiation therapy versus concomitant radiation therapy and chemotherapy in carcinoma of the thoracic esophagus. Cancer 1991;67:2258–2261.

248. Herskovic A, Martz K, Al-Sarraf M, et al. Combined chemotherapy and radiotherapy compared with radiotherapy alone in patients with cancer of the esophagus. N Engl J Med 1992;326:1593–1598.

249. Roussel A, Bleiberg H, Dalesio O, et al. Palliative therapy of inoperable oesophageal carcinoma with radiotherapy and methotrexate: Final results of a controlled clinical trial. Int J Radiat Oncol Biol Phys 1988;16:67–72.

250. Sischy B, Ryan L, Haller D, et al. Interim report of EST 1282 phase III protocol for the evaluation of combined modalities in the treatment of patients with carcinoma of the esophagus, stage I and II [Abstract]. Proc Am Soc Clin Oncol 1990;9:105.

251. Andersen A, Berdal P, Edsmyr F, et al. Irradiation, chemotherapy and surgery in esophageal cancer: A randomized clinical study. Radiother Oncol 1984;2:179–188.

252. Poplin E, Fleming T, Leichman L, et al. Combined therapies for squamous cell carcinoma of the esophagus: A Southwest Oncology Group study (SWOG-8037). J Clin Oncol 1987;5(4):622–628.

253. Leichman L, Steiger Z, Seydel G, et al. Preoperative chemotherapy and radiation therapy for patients with cancer of the esophagus: A potentially curative approach. J Clin Oncol 1984;2(2):75–79.

254. Mantravadi R, Lad T, Briele H, et al. Carcinoma of the esophagus: Sites of failure. Int J Radiat Oncol Biol Phys 1982;8:1897.

255. Mandard AM, Chasle J, Marnay J, et al. Autopsy findings in 111 cases of esophageal cancer. Cancer 1981;48:329.

256. Attah E, Hadju S. Benign and malignant tumors of the esophagus at autopsy. J Thorac Cardiovasc Surg 1980;55:396.

257. Bosch A, Frias Z, Caldwell W, et al. Autopsy findings in carcinoma of the esophagus. Acta Radiol Oncol 1979;18:103.

258. Aisner JA, Forastiere A, Aroney R. Patterns of recurrence for cancer of the lung and esophagus. Cancer Treat Symposia 1983;2:87.

259. Skinner DB. Surgical treatment for esophageal carcinoma. Semin Oncol 1984;11:136.

260. Ellis FH Jr. Treatment of carcinoma of the esophagus or cardia. Mayo Clin Proc 1989;64:945.

261. Quint LE, Glazier GM, Orringer MB, et al. Esophageal carcinoma: CT findings. Radiology 1985;155:171.

262. Agha FP, Gennis MA, Orringer MB, et al. Evaluation of response to preoperative chemotherapy in esophageal and gastric cardia cancer using biphasic esophagrams and surgical-pathologic correlation. Am J Clin Oncol 1986;9:227.

263. Kelsen DP, Helan R, Coonley C, et al. Clinical and pathological evaluation of response to chemotherapy in patients with esophageal cancer. Am J Clin Oncol 1983;6:539.

264. Kelsen D. Chemotherapy of esophageal cancer. Semin Oncol 1984;11:159.

265. Pendergast WJ, Drake WP, Mardinary MR. A proper sequence for the treatment of B_{10} melanoma: Chemotherapy, surgery, and immunotherapy. JNCI 1976;57:539.

266. Fisher B, Gunduz N, Soffer EA. Influence of the interval between primary tumor removal and chemotherapy on kinetics and growth of metastases. Cancer Res 1983;43:1488–1492.

267. Goldie J, Coldam A. The genetic origin of drug resistance in neoplasms: Implications for systemic therapy. Cancer Res 1984;44:3643.

268. Miller JL, McIntyre MD, Hatcher CR. Combined treatment approach in surgical management of carcinoma of the esophagus: A preliminary report. Ann Thorac Surg 1985;40(3):289.

269. Roth JA, Pass HU, Flanagan MM, et al. Randomized clinical trials of preoperative and postoperative adjuvant chemotherapy with cisplatin, vindesine, and bleomycin for carcinoma of the esophagus. J Thorac Cardiovasc Surg 1988;96:242.

270. Forastiere A, Gennis MK, Orringer M et al. Cisplatin, vinblastine and mitoguazone chemotherapy for epidermoid and adenocarcinoma of the esophagus. J Clin Oncol 1987;15:1143.

271. Carey RW, Hilgenberg AD, Wilkins EW, et al. Preoperative chemotherapy followed by surgery with possible postoperative radiotherapy in squamous cell carcinoma of the esophagus; Evaluation of the chemotherapy component. J Clin Oncol 1986;4:697.

272. Ajani JA, Roth JA, Ryan B, et al. Evaluation of pre and postoperative chemotherapy for resectable adenocarcinoma of the esophagus or gastroesophageal junction. J Clin Oncol 1990;8:1231.

273. Ajani J, Roth J, Ryan B, et al. High-dose chemotherapy with GM-CSF for resectable adenocarcinoma of the esophagus. Proc Am Soc Clin Oncol [Abstract 472] 1991;10:151.

274. Schlag P, Herrmenn R, Raeth V, et al. Preoperative (neoadjuvant) chemotherapy in squamous cell cancer of the esophagus. Recent Results Cancer Res 1988;10:14.

275. Coonley DJ, Bains M, Hilaris B, et al. Cisplatin and bleomycin in the treatment of esophageal carcinoma: A final report. Cancer 1984;54:2341.

276. Kelsen DP, Hilaris B, Coonley C, et al. Cisplatin, vindesine and bleomycin combination chemotherapy of local-regional and advanced esophageal carcinoma. Am J Med 1983;75:645.

277. Kelsen DP, Fein R, Coonley C, et al. Cisplatin, vindesine and mitoguazone in the treatment of esophageal cancer. Cancer Treat Rep 1986;70:255.

278. Hilgenberg AD, Carey RW, Wilkins EW, et al. Preoperative chemotherapy, surgical resection and selective postoperative therapy for squamous cell carcinoma of the esophagus. Ann Thorac Surg 1988;45:357.

279. Carey RW, Hilgenberg AD, Grilow HC, et al. Esophageal carcinoma: Long-term followup of patients treated by neo-adjuvant chemotherapy, surgery and possible postoperative radiation and/or chemotherapy. Proc Am Soc Clin Oncol [Abstract 404] 1990;9:105.

280. Kies MS, Rosen ST, Tsang TK, et al. Cisplatin and 5-fluorouracil in the primary management of squamous esophageal cancer. Cancer 1987;60:2156–2160.

281. Advani SHI, Saikia TK, Swaroop S. Anterior chemotherapy in esophageal cancer. Cancer 1985;56:1502.

282. Holting T, Friedl P, Schraube N, Fritz P, Schlag P, Herfarth C. Palliation of esophageal cancer: Operative resection versus laser and afterloading therapy. Surg Endosc 1991;5:4–8.

283. Hirai T, Yamashita Y, Mukaida H, et al. Bypass operation for advanced esophageal cancer: An analysis of 93 cases. Jpn J Surg 1989;19:182–188.

284. Segalin A, Little AG, Ruol A, et al. Surgical and endoscopic palliation of esophageal carcinoma. Ann Thorac Surg 1989;48:267–271.

285. Mannell A, Becker PJ, Nissenbaum M. Bypass surgery for unresectable oesophageal cancer: Early and late results in 124 cases. Br J Surg 1988;75:283–286.

286. Lundell L, Leth R, Lind T, Lonroth H, Sjovall M, Olbe L. Palliative endoscopic dilatation in carcinoma of the esophagus and esophagogastric junction. Acta Chir Scand 1989;155:179–184.

287. Sur RK, Kochhar R, Singh DP, et al. High dose rate intracavitary therapy in advanced carcinoma esophagus [see comments]. Ind J Gastroenterol 1991;10:43–45.

288. Fleischman EH, Kagan AR, Belloti JE, Streeter OE Jr, Harvey JC. Effective palliation for inoperable esophageal cancer using intensive intracavitary radiation. J Surg Oncol 1990;44:234–237.

289. Loizou LA, Grigg D, Atkinson M, Robertson C, Bown SG. A prospective comparison of laser therapy and intubation in endoscopic palliation for malignant dysphagia. Gastroenterology 1991;100:1303–1310.

290. Hahl J, Salo J, Ovaska J, Haapiainen R, Kalima T, Schroder T. Comparison of endoscopic Nd:YAG laser therapy and oesophageal tube in palliation of oesophagogastric malignancy. Scand J Gastroenterol 1991;26:103–108.

291. Pattison CW, Griffin SC, Coker C, Townsend ER, Fountain SW. Palliative intubation of malignant oesophageal strictures. Scand J Thorac Cardiovasc Surg 1990;24:153–155.

292. Buset M, des Marez B, Baize M, et al. Palliative endoscopic management of obstructive esophagogastric cancer: Laser or prosthesis. Gastrointest Endosc 1987;33:357–361.

293. Unruh HW, Pagliero KM. Pulsion intubation versus traction intubation for obstructing carcinomas of the esophagus. Ann Thorac Surg 1985;40:337–342.

294. Hambraeus GM, Walther BS. Oesophagectomy without thoracotomy. Experiences from 30 cases. Scand J Thorac Cardiovasc Surg 1988;22:216–219.

295. Storms P, Pagliero KM. Self adjusting stent in the management of malignant tracheo-oesophageal fistula. Acta Chir Belg 1990;90:9–12.

296. Kratz JM, Reed CE, Crawford FA, Stroud MR, Parker EF. A comparison of endoesophageal tubes: Improved results with the Atkinson tube. J Thorac Cardiovasc Surg 1989;97:19–23.

297. Alderson D, Wright PD. Laser recanalization versus endoscopic intubation in the palliation of malignant dysphagia. Br J Surg 1990;77:1151–1153.

298. Barr H, Krasner N, Raouf A, Walker RJ. Prospective randomized trial of laser therapy only and laser therapy followed by endoscopic intubation for the palliation of malignant dysphagia. Gut 1990;31:252–258.

299. Song HY, Choi KC, Cho BH, Ahn D, SKim KS. Esophagogastric neoplasms: Palliation with a modified gianturco stent. Radiology 1991;180:349–354.

300. Isaac JR, Sim EK, Ngoi SS, Goh PM. Safe and rapid palliation of dysphagia for carcinoma of the esophagus. Am Surg 1991;57:245–249.

301. Siegel HI, Laskin KJ, Dabezies MA, Fisher RS, Krevsky B. The effect of endoscopic laser therapy on survival in patients with squamous-cell carcinoma of the esophagus: Further experience. J Clin Gastroenterol 1991;13:142–146.

302. Schulze S, Fischerman K. Palliation of oesophagogastric neoplasms with Nd:YAG laser treatment. Scand J Gastroenterol 1990;25:1024–1027.

303. Ahmed ME, Gustavsson S. Current palliative modalities for esophageal carcinoma: Clinical review. Acta Chir Scand 1990;156:95–98.

304. Brennan FN, McCarthy JH, Laurence BH. Endoscopic Nd-YAG laser therapy for palliation of upper gastrointestinal malignancy. Med J Aust 1990;153:27–31.

305. Naveau S, Chiesa A, Poynard T, Chaput JC. Endoscopic Nd-YAG laser therapy as palliative treatment for esophageal and cardial cancer: Parameters affecting long-term outcome. Dig Dis Sci 1990;35:294–301.

306. Reed CE, Marsh WH, Carlson LS, Seymore CH. Kratz JM. Prospective, randomized trial of palliative treatment for unresectable cancer of the esophagus. Ann Thorac Surg 1991;51:552–555.

307. Falkson G, Ckoetzer BJ, Jerblanch AP. Oesophageal cancer: Chemotherapy overview. S Afr Med J 1987;71:21.

308. Leichman L, Berry BT. Experience with cisplatin in treatment regimens for esophageal cancer. Semin Oncol 1991;18(Suppl 3):64.

309. Clinical Screening Group. Study of the clinical efficiency of bleomycin in human cancer. Br Med J 1970;2:643.

310. Bonadonna G, de Lena M, Monfardini S, et al. Clinical trial with bleomycin in lymphomas and solid tumors. Eur J Cancer Clin Oncol 1972;8:205–215.

311. Yagoda A, Mukherji B, Young C, et al. Bleomycin, an antitumor antibiotic: Clinical experience in 274 patients. Ann Intern Med 1972;77:861.

312. Stephens F. Bleomycin: A new approach in cancer chemotherapy. Med J Aust 1973;1:1277.

313. Ravry M, Moertel CG, Schutt AJ, et al. Treatment of advanced squamous cell carcinoma of the gastrointestinal tract with bleomycin (NSC 125066). Cancer Chemother Rep 1973;57:493.

314. Tancini G, Bajetta E, Bonadonna G. Therapy with bleomycin alone and in combination with methotrexate in epidermoid carcinoma of the esophagus. Tumori 1974;60:65–71.

315. Kolaric K, Moricic Z, Dujmovic I, et al. Therapy of advanced esophageal cancer with bleomycin, irradiation and combination bleomycin and irradiation. Tumori 1976;62:255.

316. Ezdinli E, Gelber R, Desai, et al. Chemotherapy of advanced esophageal carcinoma: Eastern Cooperative Oncology Group experience. Cancer 1980;46:2149.

317. Lokich J, Shea M, Chaffey, et al. Sequential infusional 5-fluorouracil followed by concomitant radiation for tumors of the esophagus and the gastroesophageal junction. Cancer 1987;60:275.

318. Engstrom P, Lavin P, Lassen D. Phase II evaluation of mitomycin and cisplatin in advanced esophageal carcinoma. Cancer Treat Rep 1983;67:713.

319. Whittington R, Clos H. Clinical experience with mitomycin C. Cancer Chemother Rep 1970;54:195.

320. Kolaric K, Maricic Z, Roth A, et al. Combination of bleomycin and adriamycin with and without radiation in the treatment of inoperable esophageal cancer. Cancer 1980;45:2265.

321. Davis S, Shanmugathasa M, Kessler W. Cis-dichlorodiammine platinum (I1) in the treatment of esophageal carcinoma. Cancer Treat Rep 1980;64:709.

322. Ravry M, Moore M. Phase II pilot study of cisplatinum (I1) in advanced squamous cell esophageal cancer. Proc Am Soc Clin Oncol 1980;21:353.

323. Panettiere F, Leichman L, Tilchen E, et al. Chemotherapy for advanced epidermoid carcinoma of the esophagus with single agent cisplatin: Final report on Southwest Oncology Group study. Cancer Treat Rep 1984;68:1023.

324. Sternberg C, Kelsen D, Dukeman M, et al. Carboplatin: A new platinum analog in the treatment of epidermoid carcinoma of the esophagus. Cancer Treat Rep 1985;69:1305.

325. Mannell A, Winters Z. Carboplatin in the treatment of oesophageal cancer. South Afr Med J 1989;76:213.

326. Queisser W, Preusser P, Mross KB, et al. Phase II evaluation of carboplatin in advanced esophageal carcinoma: A trial of the phase 1/II study group of the Association for Medical Oncology of the German Center Society. Onkologie 1990;13:190.

327. Coonley C, Bains M, Kelsen DP. VP-16-213 in the treatment of esophageal cancer: A phase II trial. Cancer Treat Rep 1983;67:397–398.

328. Steel A, Cullen MH, Robertson PW, et al. A phase II study of carboplatin in adenocarcinoma of the esophagus. Br J Cancer 1988;58:500.

329. Radice P, Bunn P, Ihde D. Therapeutic trials with VP-16 and VM-26. Cancer Treat Rep 1979;63:1231.

330. Kelsen DP, Chapman R, Bains M. Phase II study of methyl-GAG in the present treatment of esophageal carcinoma. Cancer Treat Rep 1982;66:1427–1429.

331. Kelsen DP, Bains MS, Cvitkovic E, et al. Vindesine in the treatment of esophageal carcinoma: A phase II study. Cancer Treat Rep 1979;63:2019–2021.

332. Dinwoodie WR, Bartolucci M, Lyman GH, et al. Phase II evaluation of cisplatin, bleomycin, and vindesine in advanced squamous cell carcinoma of the esophagus: A Southeastern Cancer Study Group trial. Cancer Treat Rep 1986;70:267.

333. DeBasi P, Salvagno L, Endrizi L, et al. Cisplatin, bleomycin and methotrexate in the treatment of advanced oesophageal cancer. Eur J Cancer Clin Oncol 1984;20:743.

334. Vogl SE, Greenwald E, Kaplan BH. Effective chemotherapy for esophageal cancer with methotrexate, bleomycin and cis-diamminedichloroplatinum 11. Cancer 1981;48:2555.

335. Vogl SE, Camacho F, Berenzweig M, et al. Chemotherapy for esophageal cancer with mitoguazone, methotrexate, bleomycin and cisplatin. Cancer Treat Rep 1985;69:21.

336. Chapman R, Fleming TR, Van Damme J, et al. Cisplatin, vinblastine, and mitoguazone in squamous cell carcinoma of the esophagus: A Southwest Oncology Group Study. Cancer Treat Rep 1991;71:1185.

337. Gisselbrecht C, Calvo F, Mignot L, et al. Fluorouracil, adriamycin and cisplatin combination chemotherapy of advanced esophageal carcinoma. Cancer 1983;52:974.

338. De Basi P, Sileni VC, Salvagno L, et al. Phase II study of cisplatin, 5-FU, and allopurinol in advanced esophageal cancer. Cancer Treat Rep 1986;70:909–910.

339. Iizuka T, Kakegawa T, Ide H, et al. Phase II study of CDDP + 5-FU for squamous esophageal carcinoma: JEOG Co-operative Study results. Proc Am Soc Clin Oncol [Abstract 496] 1991;10:157.

340. Lovett D, Kelsen D, Eisenbergsr M, et al. A phase II trial of carboplatin and vinblastine in the treatment of advanced squamous cell carcinoma of the esophagus. Cancer 1991;67:354.

341. Bleiberg H, Jacob JH, Bedenne L, et al. Randomized phase II trial of 5-fluorouracil (5FU) and cisplatin (DDP) versus DDP alone in advanced oesophageal cancer. Proc Am Soc Clin Oncol [Abstract 447] 1991;10:145.

Cancer: Principles & Practice of Oncology, Fourth Edition,
edited by Vincent T. DeVita, Jr., Samuel Hellman, Steven A. Rosenberg.
J.B. Lippincott Co., Philadelphia © 1993.

H. Richard Alexander
David P. Kelsen
Joel E. Tepper

CHAPTER **26**

Cancer of the Stomach

Until 1988, adenocarcinoma of the stomach was the leading cause of cancer death worldwide, and in the early 1980s, an estimated 670,000 new cases developed annually. At the beginning of this century, gastric cancer was the leading cause of cancer death in the United States, but the annual incidence of gastric cancer has decreased significantly from 33 of 100,000 persons in 1935 to 9 of 100,000 in the last decade. In 1991, 23,800 new cases were expected in the United States, with 13,400 patients dying from the disease.[1] Despite the overall decrease in gastric cancers, there is disturbing epidemiologic evidence that the number of patients with proximal gastric and gastroesophageal adenocarcinomas has markedly increased during the past 15 years.[2,3]

The decreased rate of gastric cancers in the United States has not been uniformly experienced in other countries. In Japan, Eastern Europe, and South America, especially in Chile and Costa Rica, gastric cancer is epidemic. In Japan, the incidence is highest (100:100,000), and stomach cancer represents the leading cause of death from all malignant diseases, the number one cause of death nationally.[4]

The prognosis for stomach cancer in the United States is extremely poor, with the 5-year survival rate ranging from 5% to 15%. Most cases are diagnosed at an advanced stage, and even after "curative" gastrectomy, locoregional and distant disease recurs in at least 80% of patients. This has motivated surgeons, medical oncologists, and radiation oncologists to explore innovative treatment approaches for gastric cancer to improve the outlook for patients afflicted with this disease.

EPIDEMIOLOGY

Stomach cancer occurs approximately twice as often in men than women, and the incidence is higher among U.S. black men than white men (1.5:1). Starting in the fourth decade, the incidence of stomach cancer increases with advancing age, reaching a peak incidence in the seventh decade in men and a slightly later peak incidence in women.[5,6]

The mortality rate for stomach cancer has decreased over the past 60 years from 31.5 of 100,000 white men in 1935 to 7.8 of 100,000 U.S. men of all races in 1983. However, this decline in mortality reflects the decreased incidence of the disease, because relative 5-year survival rates have not changed considerably over the past 30 years. Data from the National Cancer Institute (NCI) Surveillance, Epidemiology, and End Results (SEER) program indicate that there was a very slight but statistically significant improvement in 5-year relative survival among whites from 1979 to 1984 compared with the interval from 1974 to 1976 (16% versus 14%). From 1979 to 1984, blacks had a slight but statistically significantly better survival than whites (16.5% versus 15.7%). Practically speaking, these differences are negligible, and the data clearly show the extremely poor prognosis for patients diagnosed with gastric cancer.

In the past, the primary site for most gastric adenocarcinomas was in the distal stomach (*i.e.*, body or antrum), but during the last 10 to 15 years, proximal gastric cancers and distal esophageal adenocarcinomas have become significantly more common. The increase in the incidence of proximal tumors is particularly worrisome because of their poorer prognosis, stage for stage, compared with distal cancers.[7,8] In 1991, Blot and colleagues, reviewing the NCI SEER database for 1976 through 1987, reported that a shift to proximal gastric lesions occurred, with an annual increase in proximal gastric lesions of 4.3% for white men, 4.1% for white women, 3.6% for black men, and 5.6% for black women.[2] The incidence of adenocarcinoma elsewhere in the stomach was about the same or slightly lower. For 1984 through 1987, they reported that cancers of the cardia made up 47% of all gastric cancers in white men. The annual incidence of new proximal gastric and distal esophageal cancers on a percentage basis is increasing faster than the incidence of melanoma or lung cancer. Similar data have been reported by European investigators.[9] Paralleling the increased rate of adenocarcinomas of the distal esophagus is an apparent increase in Barrett's esophagus (*i.e.,* columnar cell-lined esophagus).

The incidence of stomach cancer is highest in Japan, South America, Eastern Europe, and portions of the Middle East. In most countries, the mortality approximates the incidence; in Chile and Costa Rica, the mortality rates for gastric cancer exceed 40 of 100,000 persons. In low-incidence areas, such as New Zealand and Australia, the mortality rate is less than 10 of 100,000 (Fig. 26–1).[6] In Japan, despite the epidemic incidence of gastric cancer, there has been a decline in mortality rates over the past 25 years as a result of mass screening.[10]

The study of migrant populations from areas of high to low risk have produced evidence of environmental influences on the development of gastric cancer.[11–16] Among Japanese migrating from the highest-risk prefectures in Japan to Hawaii, the risk for stomach cancer persisted, even after a Western diet was adopted. The high risk for stomach cancer was observed in second-generation offspring who continued to consume a Japanese diet but was low in those adopting a Western diet.[14] In Polish migrants living in the United States for 10 years, the incidence of gastric cancer decreased and became intermediate between the countries of origin and adoption.[13] These studies suggest that environmental exposure in early life is essential in determining risk but that other environ-

mental or cultural factors may continually influence the predisposition to cancer.

ETIOLOGY AND PATHOGENESIS

In 1965, Lauren described two distinct histologic types of stomach adenocarcinoma: intestinal and diffuse.[17] Classified in this way, the etiologic and epidemiologic factors of this disease become more understandable.[11]

The intestinal variant arises from precancerous areas such as gastric atrophy or intestinal metaplasia within the stomach, occurs more commonly in men than women, is more frequent in an older population, and represents the dominant histologic type in areas where stomach cancer is epidemic, suggesting a predominantly environmental cause. The diffuse form does not typically arise from recognizable precancerous lesions, represents the major histologic type in endemic areas, occurs slightly more frequently in women and in younger patients, and has a higher association with familial occurrence (blood type A), suggesting a genetic predisposition.[18] The most celebrated example of the genetic tendency for developing stomach cancer is illustrated in the Bonaparte family; Napoleon, his father, and grandfather all died from gastric carcinoma.[19] Changes in the incidence of gastric cancer within populations over time or between geographically distinct populations appear to reflect a difference or change in the incidence of the intestinal form.[12,20]

Most studies that have investigated the role of diet in the

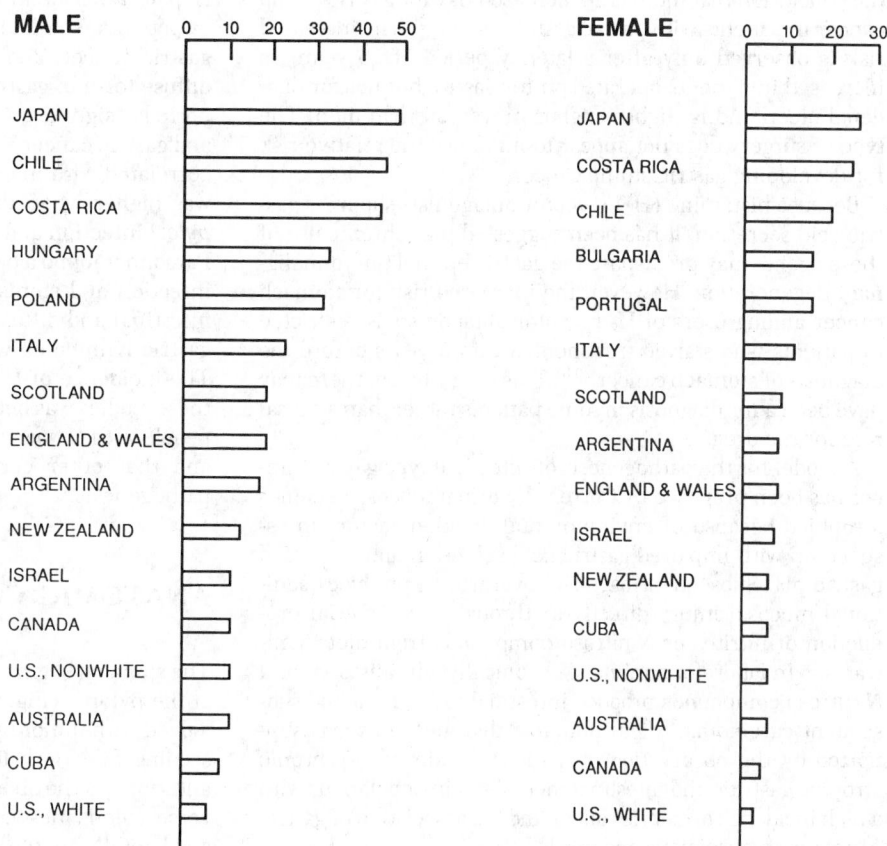

FIGURE 26–1. Age-adjusted stomach cancer mortality rates for selected countries, 1984. (Modified from Mettlin C. Epidemiologic studies in gastric adenocarcinoma. In: Douglass HO Jr, ed. Gastric cancer. New York: Churchill Livingstone, 1988:1–25)

development of stomach cancer agree that the consumption of raw (but not cooked) vegetables, fruit, citrus fruit, and high-fiber bread are inversely related to stomach cancer risk (Table 26–1).[11,16,21,22] Dietary habits that may be associated with an increased risk for stomach cancer include diets low in animal protein and fat, high in complex carbohydrates, high in salted meats or fish, and nitrates in drinking water. Diets rich in vitamin A and C are associated with a low risk for gastric cancer.[11]

The incidence of gastric cancer is inversely related to socioeconomic status, which probably reflects a number of social, occupational, or cultural factors associated with a high or low incidence of the disease.[16] A high incidence has been associated with the practice of smoking or salting meat and fish and a low incidence with the use of refrigeration and better food preparation. The use of well water that may contain high concentrations of nitrates or *Helicobacter pylori* is a risk factor for gastric cancer, but the risk associated with the use of a central water supply is lower.[23,24] Smoking tobacco increases the relative risk, but there is no consistent data to support that alcohol consumption affects the incidence of stomach cancer (see Table 26–1).[22]

In 1922, Balfour observed that there was an association between the development of gastric cancer and previous partial gastrectomy for benign disease.[25] A gastric stump cancer arises in the gastric remnant no less than 5 years after partial gastrectomy, differentiating a de novo gastric stump cancer from a locally recurrent tumor that was not recognized at the original operation.[26,27] There has been considerable controversy about whether previous gastric surgery should be considered a risk factor for gastric cancer. Two meta-analyses support the conclusion that there is an increased risk for gastric stump cancer in patients with partial gastrectomy.[28,29] The increased risk is observed only after a latency period of 15 years, is increased in patients operated on for gastric but not for duodenal ulcer, and is slightly higher in women than men. The type of surgery does not appear to influence the relative risk for developing gastric stump cancer.

Because histamine (H₂) receptor antagonists suppress gastric acid secretion, it has been suggested that chronic use of these agents may predispose the gastric epithelium to malignant degeneration. However, the increased risk for stomach cancer among users of H_2 receptor antagonists is restricted to patients who started treatment within 5 years before the diagnosis of stomach cancer.[30,31] This suggests that there may have been a misdiagnosis in some patients rather than a causal role for the drug.

A model for the pathogenesis of intestinal type gastric cancer has been proposed by Correa.[11] Normal mucosa becomes atrophied because of environmental or other factors in association with impaired gastric acid secretion and increased gastric pH. Subsequent bacterial overgrowth produces additional mucosal injury directly or through the bacterial production of nitrites or *N*-nitroso compounds from dietary nitrates.[23] In laboratory animals, chronically administered oral *N*-nitroso compounds produce intestinal metaplasia and subsequent carcinoma.[32,33] In humans, this mechanism is supported by the observation of a high prevalence of chronic atrophic gastritis and intestinal metaplasia in populations with a high incidence of gastric cancer and the association of gastric cancer with pernicious anemia.[20,34–36]

TABLE 26–1. Factors Associated With Increased Risk of Developing Stomach Cancer

Nutritional
Low fat and protein consumption
Salted meat or fish
High nitrate consumption
Low dietary vitamin A and C

Environmental
Poor food preparation (smoked foods)
Lack of refrigeration
Poor drinking water (well water)
Occupation (rubber, coal workers)
Smoking

Social
Low social class

Medical
Prior gastric surgery
Helicobacter pylori infection
Gastric atrophy and gastritis

The high incidence of *H. pylori* isolated in symptomatic and asymptomatic persons with gastritis indicates a possible contributory role for *H. pylori* in initiating mucosal injury and the subsequent development of chronic atrophic gastritis.[24,37] *H. pylori* was identified in noncancerous tissue in almost 90% of patients who had undergone resection for intestinal-type gastric cancer, and it was found in 32% of those with the diffuse form of gastric cancer.[38] Two case-control studies reported a significant association between *H. pylori* infection and gastric cancer.[39,40] The risk for developing gastric cancer correlated with increasing *H. pylori* IgG antibody levels and was higher when the interval between the diagnosis of *H. pylori* infection and gastric cancer was longer than 10 years. Parsonnet found a particularly strong association for *H. pylori* infection and stomach cancer in women and blacks.[39] The intestinal and diffuse types of stomach adenocarcinoma and gastric lymphoma were associated with *H. pylori* infection. The incidence of *H. pylori* infection in matched controls in these studies was between 61% and 76%, indicating that most people with *H. pylori* infection do not develop stomach cancer and that other contributing factors are important in its pathogenesis.

ANATOMIC CONSIDERATIONS

The stomach begins at the gastroesophageal junction and ends at the pylorus (Fig. 26–2). Adjacent organs may become involved with tumor by direct extension or localized peritoneal seeding. Superiorly lie the diaphragm and left lobe of the liver, anteriorly is the abdominal wall, and inferiorly are the transverse colon, mesocolon, and greater omentum. Posteriorly and laterally are the spleen, pancreas, left adrenal, left kidney, and splenic flexure of the colon. Extensive en bloc resection of adjacent organs directly involved by large primary tumors may be necessary to extirpate all disease. Cancers arising from the middle of the greater curvature may directly involve the splenic hilum and tail of the pancreas, and more distal tumors may invade the transverse colon. Proximal cancers may extend into the diaphragm or the left lateral segment of the liver.

The blood supply to the stomach is extensive and is based on vessels arising from the celiac axis (see Fig. 26–2). The right gastric artery, arising from the hepatic artery, and the left gastric artery, arising from the celiac axis directly, course along the lesser curvature. Along the greater curvature are the right gastroepiploic artery, which originates from the gastroduodenal artery at the inferior border of the proximal duodenum, and the left gastroepiploic artery branching from the splenic artery laterally. The short gastric arteries (*i.e.,* vasa brevia) arise directly from the splenic artery and make a relatively small contribution to the blood supply of the proximal portion of the stomach. The preservation of any of these vessels in the course of a subtotal gastrectomy for carcinoma is neither necessary nor possible if the operation is performed correctly, and the most proximal few centimeters of remaining stomach are well supplied by collateral flow from the lower segmental esophageal arcade. The rich submucosal blood supply of the stomach is an important factor in its ability to heal rapidly and produce a very low incidence of anastomotic disruption.

The venous supply of the stomach tends to parallel the arterial supply. Venous efflux is ultimately through the portal venous system, reflected in the fact that the liver is a primary site for metastatic spread.

The lymphatic drainage of the stomach is extensive, and distinct anatomic groups of perigastric lymph nodes have been defined according to their relation to the stomach and its blood supply (Fig. 26–3). There are six perigastric lymph node groups. Along the greater curvature are the subpyloric and gastroepiploic nodes, and along the lesser curvature are the suprapyloric and the lesser curvature lymph nodes. Proximally, there are the right and left pericardial nodes. The second-echelon (extraperigastric) nodes include the common hepatic, left gastric, splenic hilum, and splenic artery lymphatics, which drain into the celiac and periaortic lymphatics. Proximally there are lower esophageal lymph nodes; extensive spread of gastric cancer along the intrathoracic lymph channels may be manifested clinically by a metastatic lymph node in the left supraclavicular fossa (*i.e.,* Virchow's node) or left axilla (*i.e.,* Irish's node). As the submucosal lymphatic supply of the stomach becomes extensively involved with tumor, other routes of lymphatic drainage may be recruited. Tumor spread to the lymphatics in the hepatoduodenal ligament can extend along the falciform ligament and result in subcutaneous

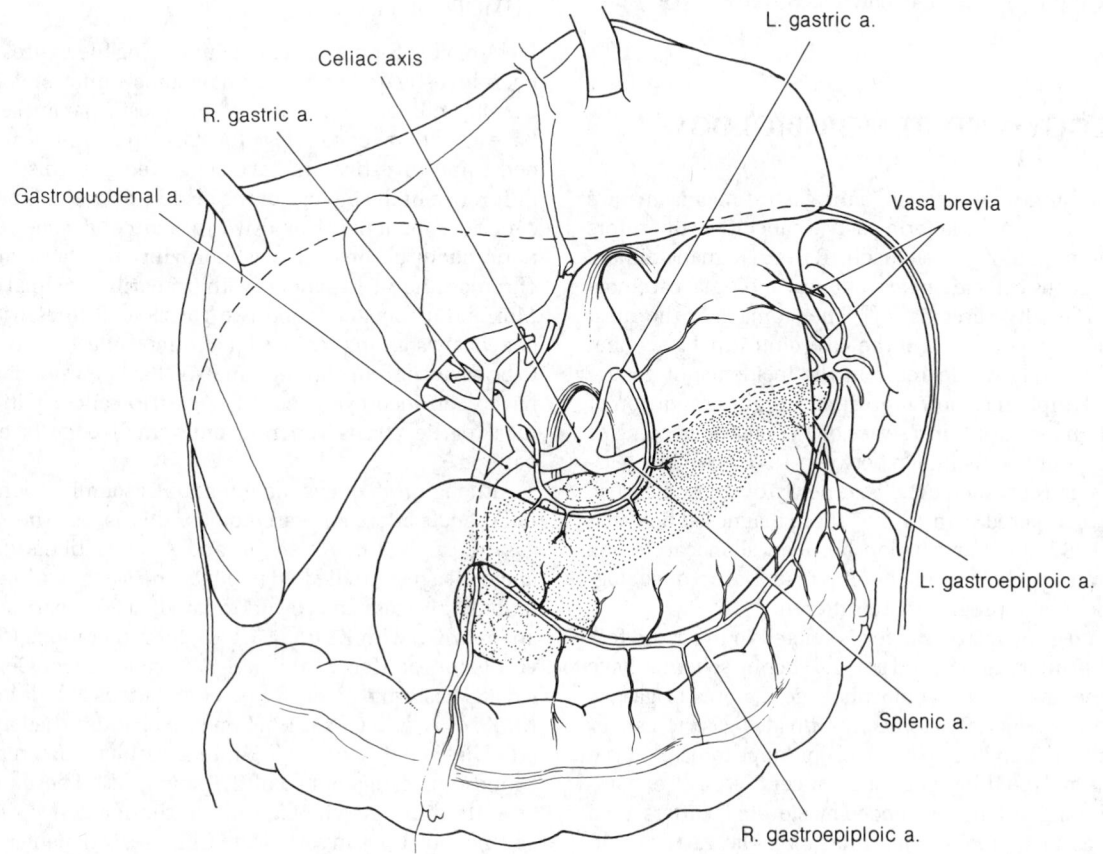

FIGURE 26–2.   Blood supply to the stomach and anatomic relations of the stomach with other adjacent organs likely to be involved by direct extension of a large gastric malignancy.

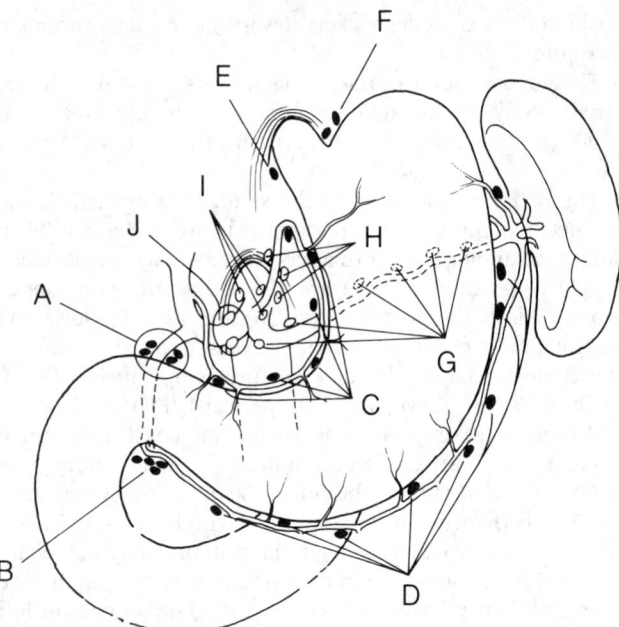

FIGURE 26–3.   Lymphatic drainage of the stomach. The six groups of perigastric lymph nodes: A, suprapyloric; B, infrapyloric; C, lesser curvature; D, greater curvature; E, right pericardial; F, left pericardial. Second-eschelon draining lymph nodes: G, splenic artery; H, proximal left gastric; I, celiac axis; J, hepatic artery.

periumbilical tumor deposits known as Sister Mary Joseph's nodes.

PATHOLOGY AND TUMOR BIOLOGY

Approximately 95% of all malignant gastric neoplasms are adenocarcinomas, and the term gastric cancer usually refers to adenocarcinoma of the stomach. Rare malignant tumors include squamous cell carcinoma, adenoacanthoma, carcinoid tumors, and leiomyosarcoma.[41-43] The stomach is the most common site for lymphoma of the gastrointestinal tract, and because of the relative decrease in the incidence of gastric carcinoma, lymphomas now represent a larger proportion of gastric malignancies.[41,44] In a series of 147 gastric neoplasms diagnosed at a single institution between 1978 and 1982, gastric lymphoma represented 2.8% of newly diagnosed gastric neoplasms, compared with 19% of those diagnosed between 1983 and 1987.[45] Differentiation between adenocarcinoma and lymphoma can be difficult, but it is essential because staging, treatment, and prognosis are different.[44,46]

The prognosis of gastric cancer is related to the gross features of the primary tumor, and several staging schemes have been proposed based on the morphologic features of gastric tumors. The Borrmann classification divides gastric cancer into five types, depending on macroscopic appearance.[47] Type I represents polypoid or fungating cancers, type II encompasses ulcerating lesions surrounded by elevated borders, type III represents ulcerated lesions infiltrating the gastric wall, type IV tumors are diffusely infiltrating tumors, and type V lesions are unclassifiable cancers. The gross morphologic ap-

pearance of gastric cancer and the degree of histologic differentiation are not independent prognostic variables.[4,5,48] Ming proposed a histomorphologic staging system that divides gastric cancer into a prognostically favorable expansive type or a poor-prognosis infiltrating type.[48] Based on an analysis of 171 gastric cancers, the expansive-type tumors were grossly uniformly polypoid or superficial, and the infiltrating tumors were usually diffuse. Grossly ulcerated lesions were equally divided between the expanding or infiltrating forms. Broders' classification of gastric cancer grades tumors histologically from 1 (well differentiated) to 4 (anaplastic). Bearzi and Ranaldi correlated the degree of histologic differentiation with the gross appearance of 41 primary gastric cancers seen on endoscopy.[49,50] Ninety percent of protruding or superficial cancers were well differentiated (grade 1), and almost half of all ulcerated tumors were poorly differentiated or diffusely infiltrating (grade 3 or 4).

The most widely used classification of gastric cancer was proposed in 1965 by Lauren and divides gastric cancer into intestinal or diffuse forms.[17] This classification scheme based on tumor histology effectively characterizes two varieties of gastric adenocarcinomas that manifest distinctively different pathologic, epidemiologic, etiologic, and prognostic factors. The intestinal variety represents a differentiated cancer with a tendency to form glands. This tumor typically arises in areas of preexisting intestinal metaplasia. The diffuse form exhibits little cell cohesion and has a predilection for extensive submucosal spread and early metastases.

TUMOR BIOLOGY

DNA ploidy, S-phase fraction, and oncogene expression have been investigated to better understand tumor biology and to develop clinical indicators of prognosis. Japanese patients have a better outcome, stage for stage, than American patients, and some investigators have suggested that this is due to a difference in the biology of the disease between Japanese and American patients. Houldsworth and colleagues reported a nonrandom chromosomal abnormality on the short arm of chromosome 11 in patients with primarily proximal tumors.[51] Mor and associates found two gastric cell lines with homogeneously staining regions on chromosome 11 that appeared to be derived from chromosome 10q26.[52] Few previous studies have examined cytogenetics in gastric cancer patients, and most earlier trials reported only small cohorts of 1 to 5 patients.

Although *RAS* oncogene mutation is seen frequently in colonic and pancreatic carcinomas, this is not the case with gastric cancers of American and Asian patients. Sakomoto and colleagues studied 26 patients and saw no *RAS* point mutations.[53] Nagata and coworkers studied 25 Japanese patients and found 2 with Ki-*RAS* (*KRAS*) point mutations (8%).[54] Investigators at Memorial Sloan-Kettering Cancer Center studied 28 Western patients for point mutations at H-*RAS* (*HRAS*), *KRAS*, or N-*RAS* (*NRAS*).[55] Two (7%) patients had mutations, one *NRAS* and one *KRAS*. Similar results were reported by Chinese investigators (0 of 27 patients).[56] There appears to be little difference biologically in the incidence of *RAS* oncogene mutations in American, Chinese, or Japanese patients. Although amplification is uncommon, protein overexpression has been reported in the absence of gene amplification.[57,58]

The p53 oncogene appears to be important in the development of many malignancies. Tamura and colleagues studied 24 gastric cancer patients, 9 of whom had p53 mutations between exons four and eight.[59] Flow cytometry was performed for these patients, and all those with mutations had aneuploid tumors. No mutations were seen in 10 patients with diploid cancers. Kim and colleagues studied 15 Japanese patients and saw a single mutation.[60]

Amplification or overexpression of *HER2/NEU* (*ERBB2*) has been reported to be of prognostic significance in several solid tumors, especially breast cancer. Many studies have determined its effect in gastric cancer (Table 26–2). In a total of 283 patient samples, 18 (7%) demonstrated gene amplification.[51,61–66] Although amplification is an uncommon event in gastric cancer, protein overexpression is seen substantially more frequently. Yonemura and colleagues reported that overexpression of *HER2/NEU* was seen in 31 of 260 (11.9%) Japanese patients and that this group had a poorer survival outcome.[67,68] Albino and colleagues found similar numbers of American patients have overexpression of this oncogene.[69] Kameda and colleagues studied 34 patients and found that 55% of them were immunohistochemically positive for the protein product.[70] However, Jain studied 93 patients and found only 11% had overexpression of *HER2/NEU*. These patients had a better outcomes than in most trials, showing that overexpression of *HER2/NEU* is a poor prognostic variable.[71]

Yasui and colleagues studied 122 patients with resected gastric cancer for overexpression of the EGF receptor protein and found that EGF receptor was more likely to be detected in advanced disease than in early gastric cancers.[72] Levels of EGF were significantly higher in tumor than in benign gastric tissue.

Other protooncogenes have also been studied including c-*MYC*, c-*RAF*, *RAF1*, c-*MOS*, c-*FOS*, c-*ERBB1* and c-*YES1*. Levels of oncogene amplification are similar to the low levels of amplification reported for *HER2/NEU* or have not been identified. Correlations with outcome for these other oncogenes have not yet been established.

Flow cytometry has been employed extensively for gastric cancer. Using this technique, potential biologic differences between proximal and distal gastric cancer was explored at Memorial Sloan-Kettering Cancer Center.[73] In 50 patients undergoing resection, 96% of the proximal tumors were aneuploid, and only half of distal tumors were aneuploid (*p* < 0.008). Aneuploidy was associated with a poorer disease-free survival rate in the group with distal tumors (Table 26–3). Because proximal tumors have a poorer clinical outcome, may have a different failure pattern, and may be biologically different from distal gastric cancers, the site of the primary tumor (*i.e.*, proximal or distal) should be a stratification variable in designing adjuvant gastric cancer trials.

None of the studies indicates that the biology of disease is different between Western and Japanese patients. The incidence of aneuploidy, the relative infrequency of *RAS* oncogene point mutation, and the frequency of *HER2/NEU* overexpression or amplification are similar in the two populations. Japanese investigators have not yet reported a cytogenetic analysis of chromosome 11, nor has a large enough series of American patients been studied to determine if observed similarities or differences in chromosomal abnormalities are real. Therapeutic advances in either country may therefore have equal applicability in the other.

PATTERNS OF SPREAD

Similar to the situation with most adenocarcinomas of the gastrointestinal tract, carcinomas of the stomach can spread by local extension to involve adjacent normal structures and can develop lymphatic, peritoneal, and distant metastases. These extensions occur by local invasion, lymphatic spread, or hematogenous dissemination. It is important to have an understanding of the patterns of spread, because a rational treatment approach should be based on the sites of tumor extension and newer approaches to therapy must address the failure patterns found after standard therapy. This is especially important in gastric cancer, for which the postsurgical failure pattern may direct additional local therapy (*e.g.*, radiation therapy) or a high incidence of intraabdominal disease may recommend the use of intraperitoneal therapy. A high incidence of systemic metastases favors the use of adjuvant chemotherapy.

Many of the studies that evaluated the patterns of tumor spread are from the older surgical literature. The tumor initially spreads by penetration into the gastric wall, extension through the wall, and involvement of an increasing percentage of the stomach. Therapeutic impact is greatest if the tumor has penetrated through the gastric serosa and there is a risk of tumor invasion of adjacent structures or if lymphatics are involved. Zinninger evaluated the spread in the gastric wall and found many variations.[74] Tumor often spreads through the intramural lymphatics in submucosal, intramuscular, or subserosal layers. The tumor can spread locally into the esophagus or the duodenum. Duodenal spread of the malignancy is principally through the muscular layer by direct infiltration and through the subserosal lymphatics, but it is not generally extensive. Spread into the esophagus can occur through any of the layers, but primarily through the submucosal lymphatics. Of 51 patients with prepyloric or antral primaries, 63% had duodenal extensions, and of 39 patients with primaries in the gastric fundus, 28% had esophageal extensions.[74]

TABLE 26–2. *HER2/NEU* (*ERB2*) Amplification or Overexpression in Primary Gastric Cancers

Investigations	No. of Patients	Amplification
Tsujino[61]	89	4/89 (4/19 advances)
Park[62]	51	4
Houldsworth[51]	28	3
Razani[63]	50	3
Kury[64]	3	0
Yokota[65]	43	5
Gutman[66]	19	1
Subtotal	283	18 (7%)
Kameda[70]	34	18 (55%)*
Jain[71]	93	11%*

* Overexpression.

TABLE 26–3. Flow Cytometry in Gastric Cancer

Investigations	Technique	No. of Patients	Aneuploid (%)	Correlation With Stage	Correlation With Survival
Yonemura[67]	Paraffin	422*	46	Positive†	Positive‡ (70% vs 40%)
Kimura[241]	Paraffin	127*	44	Positive	Positive‡ (77% vs 40%)
Baba[107]	Paraffin	93*	39.8	NS§	NS
deAretxabala[243]	Paraffin	58¶	67	NS	Positive‡ (57% vs 26%)
Korenaga[244]	Paraffin	254¶	40	Positive	Positive (91% vs 74%)
Ballantyne[245]	Paraffin	44*	64	NS	Negative‖
Nanus[73]	Fresh tissue	50¶	70	Positive	Positive†,#
Schneeberger[246]	Paraffin	92¶	65	NS	NS**

* All patients underwent potentially curative resections.
† Positive correlation with metastases to liver, peritoneum, lymph nodes. *P* values by metastatic site range from 0.01 to 0.05.
‡ Five-year survival.
§ NS, not stated.
‖ At 3 years of survival.
¶ Includes noncurative patients.
# Disease-free survival, 18 versus 5 months (median).
** At 18 months, 58% versus 31%.

Local extension occurs through the length of the stomach and by deep invasion through the wall to involve adjacent structures. Extension can occur through the gastric serosa to involve the omentum, spleen, kidney, liver, pancreas, or bowel. Serlin, reporting for the Veterans Administration Surgical Adjuvant Group, found that approximately 67% of their 903 patients had serosal penetration and approximately 62% of patients had lymphatic metastases.[75] Data for carcinomas of the body of the stomach from Memorial Sloan-Kettering demonstrated that in 49 (23%) of 213 patients the primary tumor had invaded adjacent organs, necessitating resection of those organs.[76] Papachristou, also from Memorial Sloan-Kettering, described resection of the transverse colon, liver, pancreas, kidney and adrenal, part of the diaphragm, and gallbladder in patients undergoing resection for gastric cancer.[77] Dupont reported on the extent of disease at presentation from 423 patients at Charity Hospital.[78] Only 11% of patients had disease grossly confined to the stomach, and 11% of patients had gastric primary and nodal disease. Extension to adjacent structures was demonstrated in 27% and distant visceral metastases in 31% of patients. The overall incidence of histologically positive nodes was 52%. Kennedy, in a review for the American Joint Commission on Cancer (AJCC) Staging, reported that 34% of patients had their primary tumor limited to the gastric wall, 59% had disease invading through the serosa with or without invasion of adjacent structures, and 7% had diffuse involvement of the entire stomach (linitis plastica).[79]

Lymphatic invasion occurs early, as evidenced by the fact that at least 50% of patients have evidence of lymphatic disease at the time of resection. In a review of 1241 patients, Kennedy reported a 76.5% incidence of nodal positivity.[79] However, the site of lymphatic metastasis varies widely, depending on the site of the primary tumor. The most common

analysis of lymphatic spread divides the stomach into proximal, middle, and distal gastric segments. Sunderland describes an 88% incidence of positive nodes, with the proximal lesions having the highest incidence of nodal involvement in the superior gastric region, but with a low (12%) incidence of nodal involvement in the subpyloric region.[80] The distal lesions have a low incidence of nodal involvement in the paracardial region (8.5%) and in the pancreaticolienal region (0%) near the hilum of the spleen.

Investigators from Japan evaluated the relation of nodal involvement and the site of the primary.[81] In a cohort of 1931 patients undergoing resection for gastric cancer, 71% had invasion into serosa or into neighboring organs, and 49% had nodal metastases. The nodal metastases were then analyzed by whether the primary originated in the proximal, middle, or distal third of the stomach and the location of the tumor in the lesser or greater curvature and anterior or posterior wall (Table 26–4). The incidence of metastases in a nodal group was highest if the tumor was located close to it, and the incidence of involvement of the immediately adjacent lymph nodes (N1 status) was substantially higher than that for more distant nodes (N2), although these more distant nodes were involved in a moderate percentage of patients. Peritoneal and distant metastases occur in a large percentage of patients. The results of several autopsy series are shown in Table 26–5.

The percentage of patients who are cured after surgical therapy is low, and disease recurs in multiple locoregional and systemic sites (Table 26–6). In two autopsy series, the rate of locoregional failure after potentially curative resection was 40% to 80%.[82,83] Locoregional relapse for gastric cancer is usually defined as tumor in perigastric tissues (*e.g.*, retroperitoneal "gastric bed," perigastric lymph nodes, gastric remnant). McNeer from Memorial Hospital found that 80.5%

TABLE 26–4. Pattern of Nodal Metastases From Gastric Cancer

| | Nodal Metastases (%) According to the Origin of the Primary | | |
Metastases	Upper Third of Stomach	Middle Third of Stomach	Lower Third of Stomach
Pericardia	22	9	4
Lesser or greater curvature	25	36	37
Right gastric artery suprapyloric	2	3	12
Infrapyloric	3	15	49
Left gastric artery	19	22	23
Common hepatic artery	7	11	25
Celiac axis	13	8	13
Splenic artery or hilum	11	3	2
Hepatoduodenal ligament	1	2	8
Others	0–5	0–5	0–5

(Maruyama K, Gunven P, Okabayashi K, Sasako M, Kinoshita T. Lymph node metastases of gastric cancer. Ann Surg 1989;210:596–602)

of patients had local failure after primary surgical therapy.[82] The local recurrences were primarily in the gastric remnant, the perigastric nodes, and gastric bed and duodenal stump. Many patients had multiple sites of local failure. Shiu found a 23% local recurrence rate for 169 patients treated for carcinoma of the body of the stomach.[76]

Although some of the larger multiinstitutional trials are harder to evaluate because patterns of failure are often not fully reported and because only the first site of failure is evaluated, the results of the Gastrointestinal Tumor Study Group (GTSG) are of interest.[84] In their adjuvant trial, approximately 10% of patients had local failures, 10% failed in the lung, 14% in the liver, 9% in the peritoneum, and 19% in other sites. Of the patients who entered the GTSG metastatic disease trials, 39% had peritoneal involvement, 44% had liver involvement, and 15% had both.

Gunderson reported a reanalysis of the reoperation series performed by Wangensteen at the University of Minnesota, in which patients had second-look laparotomies after resection of their primary tumors.[85] Of the patients with lymph node-positive disease at initial resection, 59 (87%) of 68 had a locoregional recurrence. Most local failures occurred in the gastric bed (78%), although some occurred in the anastomosis or stump (34%) or in the regional lymph nodes (68%). A recent trial from the British Stomach Cancer Group found an incidence of local failure in patients treated with surgery alone to be 37 (54%) of 69.[86] A series evaluating local failure patterns reported by Landry and associates from the Massachusetts General Hospital showed a total locoregional failure rate of 38%, with most of the recurrences in the gastric bed, the anastomosis, or the gastric stump (Table 26–7).[87] The incidence of local failure increased if the primary disease had extended through the gastric wall or lymph nodes were involved at the initial surgery. Liver metastases occurred in 30% of patients and peritoneal seeding in 23%. Extraabdominal failure was relatively rare and occurred in 13% of patients.

These data suggest that gastric cancer patients have disease recurrence because of inadequacy of surgical resection with resulting local failure and because of metastatic disease. However, the metastases have a high propensity to remain localized intraabdominally, and increased attention to methods of controlling this disease locally could result in improved long-term results.

CLINICAL PRESENTATION

SIGNS AND SYMPTOMS

Most patients with gastric cancer are diagnosed with advanced-stage disease, and this is reflected in the nonspecific symptoms that characterize the disease. Patients may have a combination of signs and symptoms such as weight loss, anorexia, fatigue, or epigastric discomfort, none of which unequivocally indicates gastric cancer. The clinical significance of weight loss in gastric cancer should not be underestimated. De Wys reported that more than 80% of 179 patients with advanced nonmeasurable gastric cancer had a greater than 10% decrease in body weight. Patients with weight loss had a significantly shorter survival than those without weight loss.[88]

In some patients, symptoms may suggest the presence of a

TABLE 26–5. Site of Metastases at Autopsy or Operation*

Site	Warwick[235] (n = 176)	DuPont[236] (n = 348)	Clarke[237] (n = 250)
Liver	38	54	40
Peritoneum	20	24	17
Omentum	13	21	
Lungs	12	22	19
Mesentery	9		
Pancreas	7	29	
Adrenals	5	15	12

* Other sites include bone and central nervous system.

TABLE 26–6. Patterns of Locoregional Failure in Clinical, Reoperative, and Autopsy Series

Site	MGH[87] (Clinical) (n = 130)*		University of Minnesota[85] (Reoperation) (n = 105)*		McNeer et al[82] (Autopsy) (n = 92)*	
	No.	%	No.	%	No.	%
Gastric bed	27	21	58	55	48	52
Anastomosis or stumps	33	25	28	27	55	60
Abdominal or stab wounds			5	5		
Lymph node(s)	11	8	45	43	48	52

Incidence—Any Component

* Number at risk.

lesion in specific locations. A history of dysphagia may indicate a tumor in the cardia with extension through the gastroesophageal junction. A complaint of early satiety is an infrequent symptom of gastric cancer but indicates a diffusely infiltrating tumor that has resulted in loss of distensibility of the gastric wall. Persistent vomiting is consistent with an antral carcinoma obstructing the pylorus. Significant gastrointestinal bleeding is uncommon with gastric cancer, but hematemesis does occur in about 10% to 15% of patients.[41] Unfortunately, many patients are diagnosed after the development of ascites, jaundice, or a palpable mass, indicating extensive and incurable disease.

Because the transverse colon is held close to the stomach by the gastrocolic ligament, it is a potential site of malignant fistula and large bowel obstruction from a gastric primary. Diffuse peritoneal spread of disease frequently produces other sites of intestinal obstruction. On pelvic or rectal examination, a large ovarian mass (Krukenberg's tumor) or a large peritoneal implant in the pelvis (Blumer's shelf), which can produce symptoms of rectal obstruction, may be felt.

A firm, smooth, enlarged liver or a distinct hepatic mass may indicate metastases. An epigastric mass may represent a large gastric cancer that has directly invaded or anteriorly displaced the left lateral segment of the liver.

Gastric cancer may metastasize to superficial lymph nodes, and a careful examination of the supraclavicular and axillary (particularly left) lymph nodes should be performed. Nodular metastases in the subcutaneous tissue around the umbilicus or in peripheral lymph nodes represent areas in which tissue diagnosis can be established with minimal morbidity.

EVALUATION

If gastric cancer is suspected, a barium study or flexible upper endoscopy with biopsy should be performed. Many physicians consider upper endoscopy the study of choice, because biopsy can be performed at the same setting. After the diagnosis is established, staging procedures involve careful physical examination, routine blood screening tests, and abdominal and chest computed tomography (CT) scanning. Barium contrast

TABLE 26–7. Failure Patterns After Resection for Gastric Cancer at Massachusetts General Hospital

Stage* Metastases	TNM Stage	No. of Patients	Locoregional Failure Alone (%)	Total Locoregional Failure (%)	Total Distant Failure (%)
A1	T1N0	4	0	0	0
B1	T1–2N0	16	1	19	31
B2	T3N0	12	1	50	50
B3	T4N0	5	0	40	60
C1	T1–2N4	17	12	24	29
C2	T3N4	44	23	36	55
C3	T4N4	32	22	56	67
Total		130	16	38	52

* Gunderson-Sosin modification of the Astler Coller system.
(Landry J, Tepper J, Wood W, Moulton E, Koerner F, Sullinger J. Patterns of failure following curative resection of gastric carcinoma. Int J Radiat Oncol Biol Phys 1990;19:1357–1362)

studies have limited accuracy for determining resectability, but using double-contrast techniques, a positive diagnosis of lesions between 5 and 10 mm can be made in 75% of patients.[89] Computed tomography of the chest, abdomen, and pelvis is useful for assessing the lateral extension of the tumor and systemic metastases (Fig. 26–4).[90-92] However, as many as 50% of patients have more extensive disease found at laparotomy than was predicted by preoperative CT.[93]

Since its introduction into clinical practice in the late 1960s, upper endoscopy has become routinely used for the initial diagnosis and staging of gastric adenocarcinoma and should be performed in any patient with localized disease for which surgical treatment is anticipated. Numerous reports have demonstrated that its accuracy for diagnosis is greater than 95%.[89,94-97] Visualization of the esophagus, stomach, and duodenum can provide direct and indirect information about the extent of disease. The size, location, and morphology of the tumor, including the proximal and distal extent of spread, and other mucosal abnormalities should be carefully evaluated. Decreased distensibility of the stomach, abnormal peristaltic activity, or abnormal pyloric function may indicate extensive submucosal infiltration or extramural extension of tumor into the vagi. The likelihood of a positive yield on biopsy is greater than 95% if six to ten tissue samples are obtained.[97-99]

A new staging technique involves endoscopic ultrasonography (EUS). EUS uses a high-frequency (7.5 or 12 MHz) transducer at the end of an endoscope. It allows highly accurate staging of the depth of invasion of the primary tumor (T stage) and is more accurate than CT scan for lymph node status, which are the key determinants in prognosis for patients with locoregional disease. Lightdale and colleagues performed a prospective evaluation of EUS in 50 patients with localized gastric cancer and found EUS superior to CT or magnetic resonance imaging (MRI) for assessing T and N stages.[100] Because EUS is capable of identifying small metastases in the left lobe of the liver or small amounts of ascites, it was superior to CT for M stage as well. Tio and coworkers demonstrated similar accuracy for determining T stage. EUS was less accurate for nodal status.[101] The major limitation of EUS is that the currently available instrument has a rather large (1.3 cm)

diameter; in 25% to 40% of patients, the endoscope cannot be passed through a tumor stricture of the proximal stomach or gastroesophageal junction. Because CT may identify metastases to distant sites (*e.g.*, liver, adrenal, ovaries), CT and EUS are complimentary tests.

SCREENING

Mass screening programs for gastric cancer have been most successful in high-risk areas, especially in Japan.[102] A variety of screening tests with a sensitivity and specificity of about 90% have been studied in Japanese patients, and screening frequently includes the use of double-contrast barium x-rays or upper endoscopy.[10] The yield in these screened populations has been substantial; in some Japanese studies, as many as 40% of newly diagnosed patients have early gastric cancer, and as many as 60% of patients are actively participating in routine mass screening programs (Fig. 26–5).[103] This is clinically important, because early gastric cancer has a very high cure rate if treated surgically. However, the fact that gastric cancer remains the number one cause of death in Japan may reflect the limitations of a mass screening program if the entire population at risk is not effectively screened.

STAGING AND PROGNOSIS

As with other neoplasms, the uniform and accurate staging of gastric cancer is essential to predict prognosis and assess response to treatment. The AJCC has recently revised the TNM classification for stomach cancer (Table 26–8). Modifications from the older staging system include a simplification of T stage (Fig. 26–6), and T4 now defines any tumor invading adjacent structures, and the N3 disease category has been eliminated. Under the current staging system, tumor involvement of the paraaortic, hepatoduodenal, retropancreatic, and

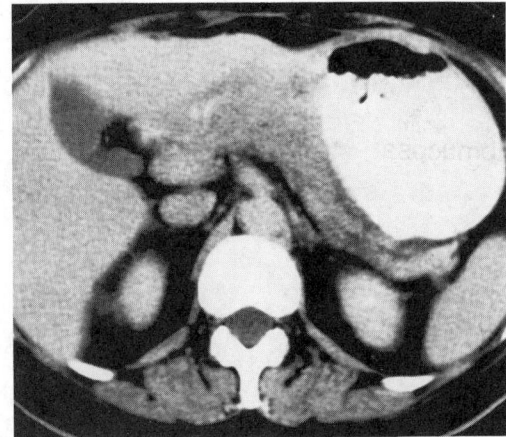

FIGURE 26–4. CT scan demonstrates a large antral adenocarcinoma, which is producing a partial gastric outlet obstruction and appears to be invading the pancreas and possibly the liver. At operation, the tumor was invading the body of the pancreas but not the liver.

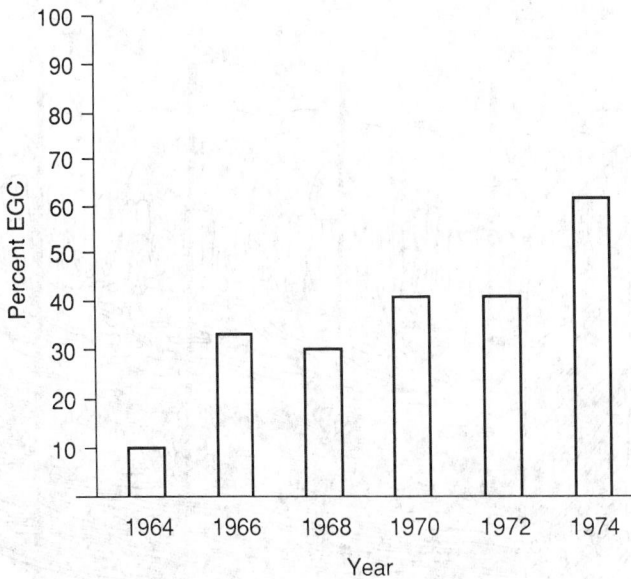

FIGURE 26–5. Increasing percentage of cancers diagnosed at an early stage (T1–2N0) in patients actively participating in a mass screening in Japan. (Modified from Kaneko E, Nakamura T, Umeda N, et al. Outcome of gastric carcinoma detected by gastric mass survey in Japan. Gut 1977;18:626–630)

TABLE 26–8. AJCC Staging of Gastric Cancer, 1988

Primary Tumor (T)

TX	Primary tumor cannot be assessed
T0	No evidence of primary tumor
Tis	Carcinoma in situ
T1	Tumor invades lamina propria or submucosa
T2	Tumor invades muscularis propria
T3	Tumor invades adventitia
T4	Tumor invades adjacent structures

Regional Lymph Nodes (N)

NX	Regional lymph node(s) cannot be assessed
N0	No regional lymph node metastasis
N1	Metastasis in perigastric lymph node(s) within 3 cm of edge of primary tumor
N2	Metastasis in perigastric lymph node(s) more than 3 cm from edge of primary tumor, or in lymph nodes along left gastric, common hepatic, splenic, or celiac arteries

Distant Metastasis (M)

MX	Presence of distant metastasis cannot be assessed
M0	No distant metastasis
M1	Distant metastasis

Stage Grouping

Stage 0	Tis	N0	M0
Stage IA	T1	N0	M0
Stage IB	T1	N1	M0
	T2	N0	M0
Stage II	T1	N2	M0
	T2	N1	M0
	T3	N0	M0
Stage IIIA	T2	N2	M0
	T3	N1	M0
	T4	N0	M0
Stage IIIB	T3	N2	M0
	T4	N1	M0
Stage IV	T4	N2	M0
	Any T	Any N	M1

mesenteric lymph nodes are now classified as metastatic disease. Although not a formal component of stage grouping, the histopathologic grade and type should be recorded.

There is considerable disparity between the survival of patients with stomach cancer in Japanese and Western series. Although early diagnosis, a higher incidence of intestinal-type tumors, and the use of radical surgery in Japan may explain some of the difference, a major contributing factor may be the extensive and meticulous surgical and pathologic staging of gastric cancer in Japan. Several reports from the United States, Japan, and Europe have demonstrated the significant prognostic impact of advancing T stage (Table 26–9).[104–110]

The General Rules for Gastric Cancer Study in Surgery and Pathology as published by the Japanese Research Society for Gastric Cancer (JRSGC) define the primary tumor stage based on the depth of invasion and the presence and extent of serosal (S) invasion (Table 26–10).[47,111] The S0 classification is further divided into m, (mucosa), sm (submucosa), and pm (muscularis propria) components. The ss (subserosa) and S1 tumors were reclassified to further stratify the degree and type of serosal invasion. Ssα is a subserosal tumor with expansive growth, ssβ is a subserosal tumor with intermediate growth, and ssγ is a subserosal tumor with infiltrating growth. S2 and S3 are now defined as se (cancer cells exposed to the peritoneal cavity), si (cancer cells infiltrating neighboring tissue), or sei (coexistence of se and si).[104,107]

The Japanese staging system extensively classifies 18 lymph node regions into four N categories depending on their relation to the primary tumor and anatomic location. The careful and complete prosection of the operative specimen may often be performed by the attending surgeon. Involvement with N1 and N2 lymph node groups represents regional disease, which is encompassed by en bloc resection of second-echelon lymph nodes, and N3 and N4 lymph nodes are considered distant metastases. The presence and extent of intraabdominal me-

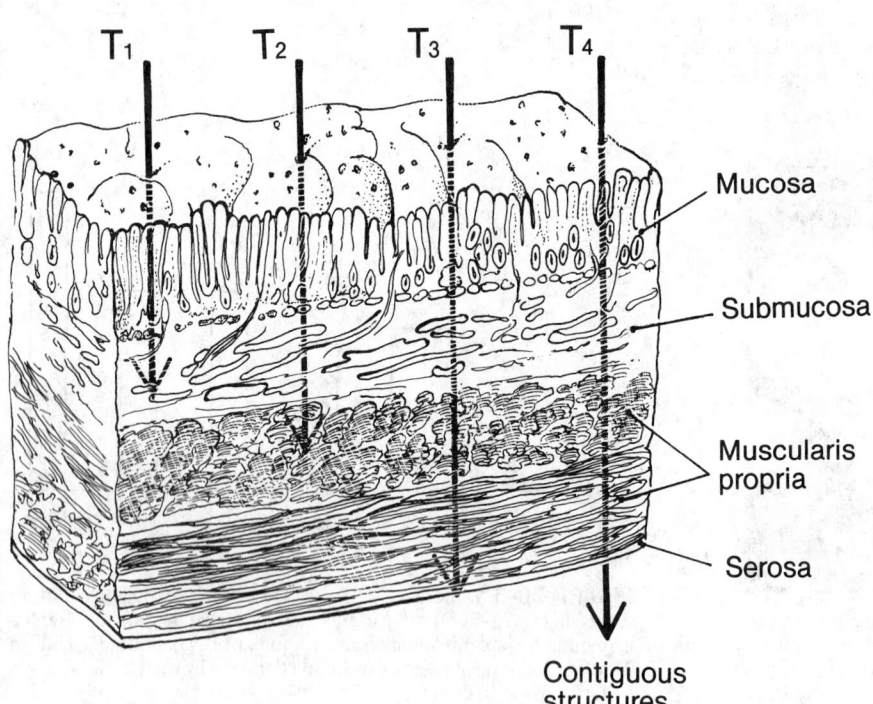

FIGURE 26–6. Definition of T stage based on depth of penetration of the gastric wall.

TABLE 26–9. Survival After Curative Resection for Gastric Cancer Analyzed by Depth of Invasion

		5-Year Survival (%)					
		T1		T2		T3	T4
Investigations	No. of Patients	m‡	sm	pm	ss	se	si/sei
Noguchi[104] (Japan)	3143	94	87	75	51	23 (S2)*	5
Maruyama[105] (Japan)	3176	95	87	82	65	34 (S2)	14
Boku[106] (Japan)	238	——————— 90 ———————				42 (S2)	29
Baba[107] (Japan)	142	——————— 55 ———————				34	32
Hermanck[108] (Germany)	977	84	75	73	40	24	25
Shiu[109] (USA)	246	——————— 56 ———————				32	
Bozetti[110] (Italy)	361	82		69		——— 38 ———	

* S2, serosal invasion.
† T stage of tumor.
‡ Depth of penetration; m, mucosa; sm, submucosa; pm, muscularis propria; ss, subserosa; se, cancer cells in peritoneal cavity; si, cancer cells infiltrating neighboring tissue; sei, coexistence of se and si.

TABLE 26–10. Japanese Surgical Staging System for Gastric Cancer

Staging System

S0	No serosal invasion
S1	Suspected serosal invasion
S2	Definite serosal invasion
S3	Adjacent organ involvement
N1	Perigastric lymph nodes
N2	Lymph nodes around the left gastric artery, common hepatic artery, splenic artery, and celiac axis
N3	Lymph nodes in the hepatoduodenal ligament, posterior aspect of pancreas, and root of mesentery
N4	Paraaortic and middle colic lymph nodes
P0	No peritoneal metastases
P1	Adjacent peritoneal involvement
P2	A few scattered metastases to distant peritoneum
P3	Many distant peritoneal metastases
H0	No liver metastases
H1	Metastases limited to one lobe
H2	A few bilateral metastases
H3	Numerous bilateral metastases

Stage Grouping

I	S0, N0, P0, H0
II	S1, N0–1, P0, H0
III	S2, N0–2, P0, H0
IV	S3, N3–4, P1–3, H1–3

(Nishi M, Nakajima T, Kajitani T. The Japanese research society for gastric cancer— the general rules for the gastric cancer study and an analysis of treatment results based on the rules. In: Preece PE, Cuschieri A, Wellwood JM, eds. Cancer of the stomach. New York: Grune & Stratton, 1986:107–121)

tastases to the peritoneum and liver are categorized (see Table 26–10). Lymph node metastases, including the N stage and number of positive lymph nodes, are strong predictors of outcome in gastric cancer (Table 26–11). Two studies assessed quantitative involvement of lymph nodes and survival after resection for gastric cancer and found that survival with as many as 3 to 4 metastatic lymph nodes is better than with more extensive lymph node involvement.[109,112] Japanese survival statistics are consistently better for patients with nodal metastases than for comparable American patients (see Table 26–11).

TREATMENT OF LOCALIZED DISEASE

SURGERY

Rationale

The only potentially curative modality for localized gastric cancer is surgery. However, there is disagreement among surgeons about the appropriate extent of resection, because improved outcome has not been conclusively linked with more radical surgery. Current areas of discussion include the potential therapeutic benefit from extended lymphadenectomy, the routine use of total versus subtotal gastrectomy for tumors of the body or antrum, and prophylactic splenectomy.

TABLE 26–11. Survival After Resection for Gastric Cancer Analyzed by Lymph Node Status

		5-Year Survival (%)				
Investigations	No. of Patients	N0	N1	N2	N3	N4
Noguchi[104] (Japan)	3145	80	53	26	10	3
Maruyama[105] (Japan)	3176	85	61	31	10	2
Bozetti[110] (Italy)	361	57	——— 43 ———			
Hermanek[108] (Germany)	977	74	36	20	10	
Shiu[109] (USA)	246	67	32	9		

There is considerable debate about whether the routine use of an extensive en bloc resection of second-echelon lymph nodes (R-2 resection) is superior to a more limited lymphadenectomy of the perigastric lymph nodes (R-1 resection). Approximately 30 years ago, the JRSGC proposed a standardized R-2 resection for patients undergoing curative gastrectomy.[113] As radical surgery for gastric cancer has become uniformly accepted in Japan, the operative mortality rate for R-2 resection has declined, and 5-year survival after curative resection has improved. Maruyama reported results from more than 20,000 cases from a nationwide registry for three periods, 1963 through 1966, 1969 through 1973, and 1971 through 1985.[105] The 30-day operative mortality declined from 3.8% in the first period to 1.0% in the latest. When patients are compared by stage, depth of tumor invasion, serosal invasion, and N1 or N2 nodal metastases, there was improved survival in the most recent period compared with the first (Table 26–12). However, radical R-2 resection did not improve survival for patients with extranodal disease, such as peritoneal metastases, distant lymph node metastases (N3 or N4), or diffusely infiltrating carcinomas (linitis plastica). In another retrospective review from Japan, Kodama compared survival among 254 patients undergoing simple resection or 454 patients undergoing extensive regional lymph node dissection for gastric carcinoma.[114] The therapeutic effect (*i.e.*, difference in 5-year survival) of extensive node dissection was limited to those patients with serosal invasion (T3) and those with positive lymph node metastases. The patients with T1,

T2, or T4 and N0 disease did not show a benefit from extensive node dissection. In both studies, groups that were operated on in different time periods were compared, and it is possible that other factors could be influencing the outcome of these patients.

Sowa, for a series of 486 patients who underwent curative (R-2) resection for gastric cancer, demonstrated that tumor size and depth of penetration were directly related to the incidence of lymph node metastases in gastric cancer and that the rate of skip metastases was less than 1%.[115] In this study and others, T1 or T2 lesions have metastases limited to perigastric lymph nodes in 15% to 40% of patients, suggesting that in selected cases of early gastric cancer, a limited lymphadenectomy may extirpate all nodal disease.[114,116] However, in a retrospective analysis of 210 patients who underwent R-1 or R-2 gastrectomies with curative intent, extensive lymphadenectomy that encompassed one echelon of pathologically uninvolved nodes in early gastric cancer (T1–3N0–1) was associated with better survival than those with a less extensive lymphadenectomy (60% versus 25%).[117] Irvin reported a similar 60% 5-year survival rate for 22 patients undergoing curative R-1 resection with pathologically negative nodes (T1–3N0).[118]

Because of the technical difficulty of an extended lymphadenectomy, some researchers addressed the possibility of employing selective lymph node dissection in gastric cancer with macroscopically suspicious nodes. However, Okamura reported that the mean size of metastatic lymph nodes in 370

TABLE 26–12. Changing Treatment Results After Resection for Gastric Cancer in Japan Over a 22-Year Interval

Standard for Comparison	5-Year Survival* (%)		
	1964–1966 (n = 6050)	1969–1973 (n = 12,535)	1971–1985 (n = 3176)
Depth of invasion			
Submucosa (T1)	90.3	95.5	87.4
Muscularis propria (T2)	70.2	80.1	82.2
Subserosa (T2)	49.8	57.1	64.5
Serosal invasion (T3)	22.1	30.0	34.1
Adjacent organ invasion (T4)	7.3	15.7	14.3
Lymph node metastases			
N0	79.5	87.4	85.4
N1	38.5	45.4	60.6
N2	22.8	26.9	30.9
Stage			
I	93.5	95.6	90.7
II	60.6	70.1	71.7
III	32.7	36.3	44.3
IV	5.8	10.5	9.0
Peritoneal metastases	9.1	10.0	5.1
Liver metastases	4.8	6.7	6.5
Curative resection	64.2	73.3	75.2
Palliative resection	10.4	11.6	9.3

* Five-year survival is relative (age-adjusted) for the periods 1963–1966 and 1969–1973 and cumulative for 1971–1985.
(Maruyama K, Okabayashi K, Kinoshita T. Progress in gastric cancer surgery in Japan and its limits of radicality. World J Surg 1987;11:418–425)

patients undergoing R-2 gastrectomy was 7 mm and that the ability to correctly diagnose metastatic involvement by intraoperative macroscopic examination was only 20%.[119] Although there is a direct correlation between lymph node size and the frequency of metastases, Noguchi found that 30% of all metastases to lymph nodes occur in nodes less than 3 mm.[104] Therefore, it is unlikely that selective lymphadenectomy based on gross appearance of lymph nodes is feasible or appropriate.

A single prospective randomized trial of R-1 versus R-2 gastrectomy was reported by Dent from Cape Town, South Africa (Table 26–13).[120] At surgery, only 43 of 403 patients were identified with potentially curable disease (T1–2N0–1) and randomized to receive R-2 or R-1 gastrectomy. There was no difference in survival with a median follow-up of 3 years. Patients undergoing R-2 resection had a significantly longer operating time, greater transfusion requirement, and longer hospital stay. However, in Japan where extended R-2 resection is performed routinely, operative mortality is minimal and does not appear related to the extent of lymphadenectomy.[121]

The retrospective reports from Japan indicate that the routine use of extended lymphadenectomy for potentially curable gastric cancer can be performed safely and can improve survival compared with the Western experience with more limited R-1 resection and to the period in Japan before the routine use of R-2 resection. In the United States and Europe, there is evidence from retrospective reports that the extended lymphadenectomy may improve the outcome in selected patients with limited disease (T1–3N0–1) but can result in substantial morbidity. A single prospective randomized trial with a limited number of patients did not support the routine use of extended R-2 gastrectomy. In the United States, the advanced stage of disease at surgery in most patients remains the key determinant of survival, and in Japan and the United States, peritoneal, hepatic, or unresectable nodal metastases portends a dismal prognosis despite R-2 resection. The routine application of lymphadenectomy is currently being evaluated in several random-assignment trials in Europe. Because it may have a therapeutic effect, the type of operation must also be taken into account in assessing the results of adjuvant trials, and such studies should prospectively address the issue of the surgical procedure to be performed.

Ideally, the extent of gastric resection should provide the optimal cancer procedure with the minimal morbidity. The

TABLE 26–13. Results of a Prospective Randomized Trial Comparing R-1 and R-2 Resection for Potentially Curable Gastric Carcinoma

Standards for Comparison	R-1	R-2	p Value
n	22	21	—
Operating time (h ± SEM)	1.7 ± 0.6	2.33 ± 0.7	<0.005
Transfusions (units/group)	4	25	<0.005
3-year survival (log rank test)	0.78	0.76	<0.77

(Dent DM, Madden MV, Price SK. Randomized comparison of R-1 and R-2 gastrectomy for gastric carcinoma. Br J Surg 1988;75:110–112)

rationale for the routine use of total gastrectomy is presumably based on the appreciation that extensive intramural extension of tumor may be present and that simultaneous multiple gastric cancers have been reported in almost 6% of patients.[122,123] Papachristou showed that patients with inadequate proximal margins of resection are predisposed to local recurrence.[124] The median margin of resection in patients who developed a stump recurrence after distal gastrectomy was 3.5 cm, compared with 6.5 cm for patients who did not develop stump recurrence ($p < 0.05$). Although older retrospective data suggest that survival is improved with total gastrectomy compared with subtotal gastrectomy, current evidence does not support this.[125,126]

A French cooperative prospectively randomized trial comparing total gastrectomy with subtotal gastrectomy has reported data on postoperative morbidity, mortality, and 5-year survival. Analysis was performed for 169 patients with adenocarcinoma of the antrum operated on with curative intent.[126] The groups were well matched for the usual prognostic variables. The overall complication rate and postoperative mortality was 32% and 1.3%, respectively, for total gastrectomy and 34% and 3.2%, respectively, for subtotal gastrectomy. There was no difference in cumulative 5-year survival rates between groups. Other series have reported an operative mortality after total gastrectomy ranging from 4% to 18%, and anastomotic leak is responsible for as many as 50% of these operative deaths.[127–130]

For patients with proximal lesions, total gastrectomy or proximal gastric resection are the two procedures necessary to extirpate disease. Carcinomas arising in the proximal one third of the stomach are frequently larger, ulcerated and diffuse, have a higher incidence of serosal penetration and lymph node metastases, and have a significantly worse prognosis than distal gastric lesions.[7,109] Although there is no evidence to indicate that proximal gastric resection or total gastrectomy is superior as a cancer operation for proximal gastric tumors, the functional sequelae and postoperative mortality of proximal gastric resection are worse than for total gastrectomy. In a series of 89 patients reported by Buhl who were treated with total gastrectomy, distal gastric resection, or proximal gastric resection, the latter group had a higher incidence of dumping, heartburn, and reduced appetite.[131] The quality of life and capacity to work were reduced in patients with proximal gastric resection.

The Norwegian Stomach Cancer Trial prospectively studied the incidence of postoperative complications and mortality in more than 1000 consecutive patients undergoing surgery for gastric cancer.[132] The postoperative mortality rate among more than 760 patients undergoing resection was 8.3% and was highest in patients undergoing proximal resection (16%) and lower in those with total gastrectomy (8%), subtotal gastrectomy (10%), or distal resection (7%). Factors significantly related to the incidence of postoperative complications included advancing age, male sex, no antibiotic prophylaxis, and splenectomy. Similar to the postoperative mortality, the complication rate was highest for proximal resections (52%), followed by total gastrectomy (38%), subtotal resection (28%), and distal resection (19%).

For proximal lesions, it appears that total gastrectomy using a variety of reconstructive options provides better functional results, fewer complications, and lower operative mortality than proximal gastric resection, and for more distal tumors, survival after subtotal gastrectomy is no worse than total gastrectomy and has less attendant morbidity.

The value of routine splenectomy during gastric resection for tumors not adjacent to or invading the spleen has been critically evaluated by several researchers.[104,132-134] Sugimachi reviewed more than 300 patients and found that 4-year survival was adversely affected by the use of "prophylactic" splenectomy (*i.e.,* tumors not adjacent to or infiltrating the spleen).[133] Noguchi, in an excellent review of surgery for gastric cancer in Japan, concluded that the evidence to support routine splenectomy with gastric resection in that country is conflicting and not well established.[104] The Norwegian Stomach Cancer Trial demonstrated a higher complication rate with the use of splenectomy in their prospective trial (42% versus 27%), and this has been supported by Brady in a retrospective analysis of more than 390 patients undergoing curative gastric resection at Memorial Sloan-Kettering Cancer Center.[132,134]

Operative Technique

A bilateral subcostal incision or a generous midline abdominal incision should be used to gain adequate exposure to the upper abdomen. Careful intraoperative staging of disease should be performed. At remote sites from the stomach, inspection for ascites, peritoneal seeding, disease in the pelvis such as drop metastasis, or ovarian involvement should be performed. In the upper abdomen, attention should be directed to the liver, greater omentum, root of the mesentery below the transverse colon, and the presence of paraaortic adenopathy. The stomach should be inspected to assess the location and extent of tumor. Careful palpation of large tumors may be necessary to determine whether there is direct invasion of adjacent structures like the pancreas. The extent of gastric resection is dictated by the size and location of the primary, and if the surgeon chooses, an R-2 lymphadenectomy can be performed for potentially curable tumors.

The R-2 radical subtotal gastrectomy commences with mobilization of the greater omentum from the transverse colon. It is usually easiest to continue to divide the gastrosplenic ligament as far laterally and superiorly as possible. The division of the vasa brevia can be done at any point during the procedure when it appears technically easiest. After the omentum is mobilized, the anterior peritoneal leaf of the transverse mesocolon is incised along the lower border of the colon to the head of the pancreas, and with a combination of blunt and sharp dissection, it is lifted off of the mesocolon and anterior surface of the pancreas to the level of the splenic artery. This can be a tedious maneuver, but theoretically, it provides additional protection against serosal spread of tumor to the local peritoneal surface.

The infrapyloric lymph nodes are dissected, and the origin of the right gastroepiploic artery and vein are ligated. The hepatic artery pulse is palpated in the hepatoduodenal ligament, and the overlying peritoneum is incised along the hepatic artery toward the celiac axis. The gastrohepatic ligament is divided close to the liver up to the gastroesophageal junction. The right gastric artery is identified and ligated. The lymph node-bearing tissue overlying the gastroduodenal artery and superior to the duodenum are mobilized. At this point, some surgeons prefer to divide the duodenum distal to the pylorus and reflect the stomach and omentum cephalad.

Starting near the splenic hilum and proceeding medially, the lymph nodes along the splenic artery are dissected; multiple small clips provide hemostasis. A similar dissection is performed along the hepatic artery, moving toward the celiac axis. Near the celiac axis, the lymph node-bearing tissue is dissected until the left gastric artery is visualized and can be divided at its origin. The proximal peritoneal attachments of the stomach and distal esophagus can then be incised, and the proximal extent of resection is chosen. After removal of the specimen, the extent of retroperitoneal dissection can be assessed (Fig. 26-7).

Despite the fact that the entire blood supply of the stomach has been interrupted, a cuff of proximal stomach will invariably show very good vascularization from the feeding distal esophageal arcade. Most surgeons prefer to anastomose jejunum to stomach versus esophagus because of the technical ease and excellent healing. Reconstruction using a variety of techniques has been described and is a matter of personal choice (Fig. 26-8).

ADJUVANT CHEMOTHERAPY

Rationale

Patients who are at high risk for recurrence after resection have stage T3 or T4, any N, and M0 tumors. Definitive staging currently is obtained postoperatively after pathologic evalu-

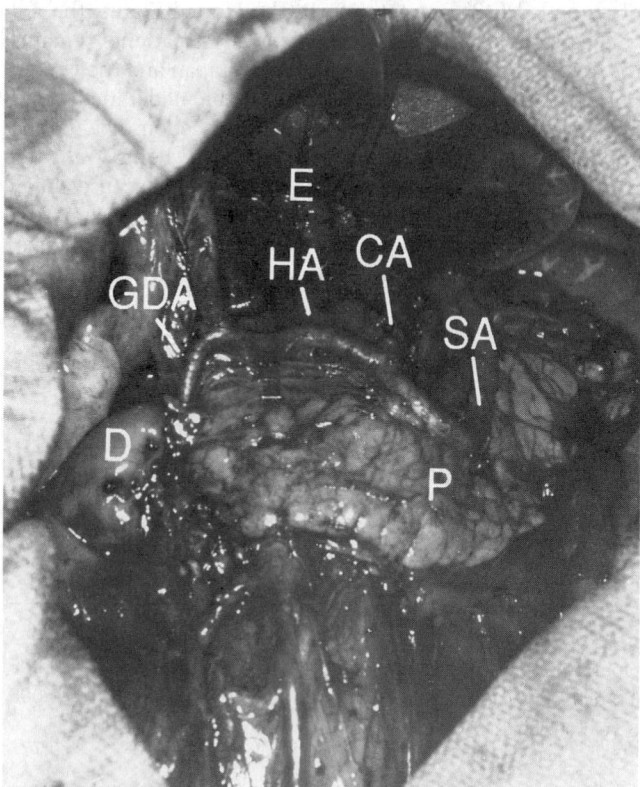

FIGURE 26-7.   Results of lymph node dissection after R-2 total gastrectomy. D, duodenum; P, pancreas; E, esophagus; SA, splenic artery; CA, celiac axis with ligated left gastric artery; HA, hepatic artery; GDA, gastroduodenal artery. (Courtesy of Daniel Coit, MD, New York, NY)

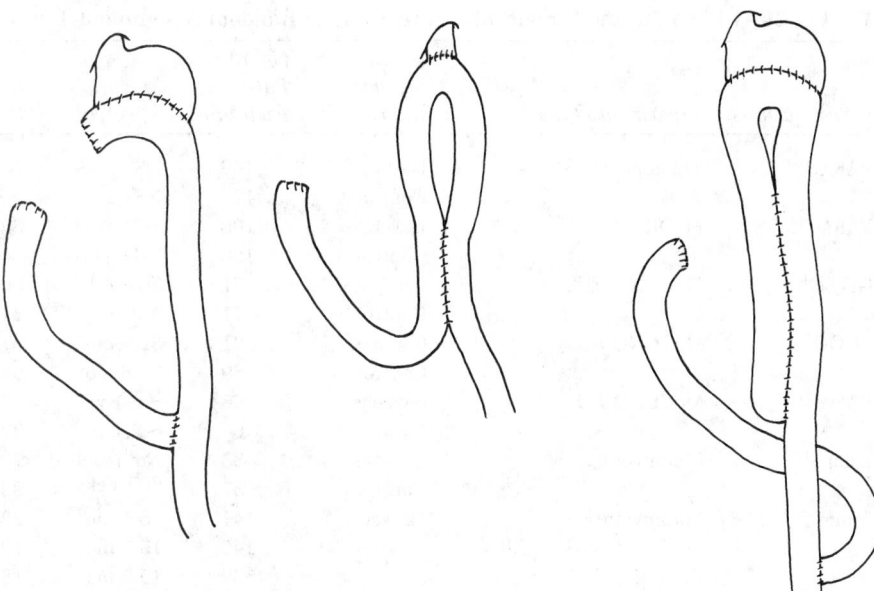

FIGURE 26–8. Variations in types of reconstruction after total or subtotal gastrectomy include (from left to right) the Roux-en-Y, Braun, and Lawrence techniques.

ation of the resected specimen. After curative surgery, even patients without nodal metastases (T3N0) have at least a 50% chance of dying within 5 years. Lymph node metastases have an even more ominous implication. Although 80% to 90% of American patients fall in the high-risk group, preoperative identification of patients at low risk for recurrence is difficult. In the United States, only 5% to 10% of newly diagnosed gastric cancer patients have early-stage disease. Nonetheless, until adjuvant programs of proven effectiveness are developed, sparing patients who have an excellent outcome with surgery alone from the potential toxicities of chemotherapy or chemotherapy plus irradiation is appropriate. Because routine preoperative tests currently used, including CT or MRI scans of the abdomen and chest, do not accurately stage the depth of tumor invasion (T stage) or identify regional nodal involvement (N stage), the low-risk patient is difficult to identify preoperatively.

The traditional approach to adjuvant therapy (especially for patients with gastric cancer) is the use of postoperative chemotherapy. Adjuvant therapy is usually considered to be additional treatment for patients who have already undergone potentially curative therapy; for gastric cancer, this is a surgical procedure in which all gross disease has been removed with no evidence of metastases. However, a recent large surgical series indicated that only 30% to 40% of patients with gastric cancer undergoing exploration had a potentially curative resection.[135] The remaining patients had unresectable disease or had a palliative resection with gross residual tumor or microscopically positive margins. In this situation, postoperative therapy should not be considered to be adjuvant.

The timing of postoperative therapy varies widely. In some centers, especially in Japan, postoperative therapy for gastric cancer patients begins immediately after surgery, but in the United States, treatment usually starts 4 to 6 weeks after resection. There are several reasons for starting adjuvant therapy soon after resection. Studies such as those by Fisher and colleagues showing an increased labeling index of metastasis after resection of the primary (suggesting a potential for in-

creased cell kill) have led some investigators to postulate that adjuvant treatment should begin immediately before or after resection.[136,137] Moreover, there is a high incidence of peritoneal failure for gastric cancer patients after resection, and data from several animal models indicate that the risks of peritoneal implantation and of intraabdominal tumor spread immediately after laparotomy are high.[138,139] Especially for intraperitoneal chemotherapy, a strong argument exists for immediate postoperative treatment. Delays of 4 to 8 weeks after surgery before beginning systemic therapy may allow metastatic disease to grow, making its eradication difficult or impossible. A number of investigational studies are now underway in gastrointestinal malignancies involving immediate postoperative adjuvant therapy, including the intraperitoneal route, to address the problem of peritoneal and hepatic metastases.

Adjuvant Protocols

Table 26–14 summarizes the results of several prospective random-assignment trials in gastric cancer, some of which began in the 1960s.

Two early trials from the Veterans Administration Surgical Adjuvant Study Group (VASAG) investigated the use of thiotepa or FUDR (floxuridine) after surgical resection.[140,141] The effectiveness of either agent in advanced disease patients has not been well explored. Neither demonstrated an improvement in survival, although survival details in the thiotepa study were not given. Toxicity in the thiotepa trial was substantial, requiring dose attenuation.

Three studies used a combination of 5-fluorouracil (5-FU) and the nitrosourea methyl-CCNU as adjuvant therapy after gastric resection. In advanced disease, 5-FU and methyl-CCNU had only modest effectiveness, and this combination was an inferior arm in a random-assignment trial using patients with advanced disease. The Gastrointestinal Tumor Study Group (GTSG) randomly assigned patients to no additional treatment or to 18 months (originally 2 years) of

TABLE 26–14. Adjuvant Therapy of Gastric Cancer: Random-Assignment Trials

Investigations	Treatment Groups	Surgery Interval*	No. of Patients Evaluable	Median Survival	5-Year Survival (%)	p Value	Treatment Mortality (%)
VASAG[140]	Thiotepa	Day 1	136	NS	NS	"No difference"	24¶
	Control		125	NS	NS		8¶
VASAG[141]	FUDR	Day 1	100	~18 mo†	32‡		13.6¶
	Control		129	~18 mo†	34‡	"Not significant"	12.4¶
GITSG[142]	MeCCNU-FU	6 weeks	71	56 mo	50	0.06	1.4
	Control		71	33 mo	31		
ECOG[143]	MeCCNU-FU	6 weeks	91	32.7 mo	57§	0.73	2.2
	Control		89	36.6 mo	57§		
VASAG[144]	MeCCNU-FU	6 weeks	66	~2.1 y	38.9‖	0.89	NS
	Control		68	~2.1 y	37.8‖		
Estape[145]	Mitomycin	4 weeks	33	Not reached	76*	0.001	0
	Control	60 weeks	37		30*		
Allum[146]	Mitomycin/FU	12 weeks	141	15.5 mo	28	0.98	
	Mitomycin/FU + CMFV		140	15.5 mo	10		8
	Control		130	15.5 mo	18		
Coombes[149]	FAM	6 weeks	133	>36 mo	45.7	0.17	2.2
	Control		148	>36 mo	35.4		
Nakajima[147]	Mitomycin-FU-Ara C	7–10 days	81	>5 y	68.4	0.09	0
	Mitomycin-Ftorafur-Ara C		83	>5 y	62.5		0
	Control		79	>5 y	51.4		
SWOG[150]	FAM	Not stated	39	25 mo	NS	0.5	0
	Control		36	25 mo	NS		
Krook[151]	FA	4–6 weeks	61	36	32	NS	3
	Control			64			
Estrada[152]	MeCCNU-FU-A	Not stated	31	NS	29	NS	3
	Control		35		37		

FU, fluorouracil; A, doxorubicin (Adriamycin); NS, not significant.
* Maximal interval between surgery and study entrance.
† Excludes operative mortality.
‡ Three-year survival.
§ Two-year survival.
‖ Survival of 3.5 years.
¶ Operative mortality.

methyl-CCNU and 5-FU.[142] A second cycle of 5-FU was given on days 36 through 40; cycles were repeated every 10 weeks. Patients were eligible to enter the study as late as 6 weeks after resection. At the time of the initial GTSG report, overall survival for the chemotherapy arm was superior to that of the control (p = 0.07). At a later analysis, the survival curves reached statistical significance, still in favor of the chemotherapy arm. However, an identical study using 5-FU and methyl-CCNU performed during the same period by the Eastern Cooperative Oncology Group (ECOG) using the same dose and schedule and including a total of 180 patients demonstrated no difference in disease-free or overall survival.[143] In a third study by VASAG, the same agents were used on a different schedule in patients after curative resection.[144] No difference in survival was seen. Because methyl-CCNU has a small but definite increased risk for inducing acute nonlymphocytic leukemia and there is a lack of confirmed adjuvant efficacy for the combination, use of 5-FU and methyl-CCNU as adjuvant treatment for gastric cancer is not appropriate.

One Western trial investigated the use of high-dose mitomycin C after surgical resection. Only 33 patients received chemotherapy; 37 patients were in a control group. A striking difference in survival was seen: 7 relapses in the treated arm and 23 in the control arm (p < 0.001). The chemotherapy dose schedule was mitomycin C (20 mg/m²) once every 6 weeks for four doses. Eighty percent of patients in the treated group remained free of disease after 5 years, and the median survival for the control group was approximately 60 weeks. A recent update continues to show a significant survival advantage after 10 years of follow-up for the mitomycin-treated group.[145] This study has not yet been repeated in larger numbers of patients.

Allum and associates reported the results of a three-arm random-assignment trial comparing postoperative 5-FU and mitomycin C with or without cyclophosphamide, 5-FU, vincristine, and methotrexate induction compared with surgery only.[146] The study allowed entrance up to 12 weeks after surgery. The surgery-only group received saline every 3 weeks;

140 patients received 5-FU and mitomycin C plus a 5-day induction course of cyclophosphamide, 5-FU, vincristine, and methotrexate; and 141 patients received 5-FU and mitomycin C alone. Therapy was continued for 2 years. With a median follow-up of 100 months, there was no significant survival difference between the treated or control groups. The median survival for patients receiving therapy was 43 days longer than that for those receiving no additional treatment.

Nakajima and colleagues treated a group of 243 patients with mitomycin C, 5-FU, and cytosine arabinoside, or with a similar regimen in which 5-FU was replaced by Ftorafur; the control patients had surgery only.[147] There were no statistical differences in survival at 5 years, although the 5-year survival rate for chemotherapy patients was somewhat better than for the control group ($p = 0.09$). Subgroup analyses indicated significant differences in survival for those with early-stage disease (stages I and II), but these were retrospective (unplanned). In a second study, Ochiai and colleagues compared chemotherapy with chemoimmunotherapy after resection.[148] The immunotherapy used was a *Nocardia* rubra cell wall skeleton extract. There was no surgery-only control; both groups received mitomycin, 5-FU, and cytosine arabinoside chemotherapy. Therapy was started perioperatively; patients received mitomycin during surgery and on day 1, and they then began weekly mitomycin, 5-FU, and cytosine arabinoside. There were 90 patients in the chemotherapy group and 97 in the chemoimmunotherapy group. No difference in survival for patients having curative resections was seen. A subgroup of 71 patients did not undergo a curative resection and were analyzed separately. A survival advantage for those receiving chemoimmunotherapy was seen.

The results of doxorubicin-containing combination chemotherapy regimens have been reported. Coombes and co-workers studied 315 patients with curatively resected gastric cancer who were randomized to receive 5-FU, doxorubicin, and mitomycin (FAM regimen) or no postoperative therapy.[149] Of the original group, 281 patients were evaluable for analysis. Chemotherapy could be started as late as 6 weeks from operation. Although 26% of patients in the control arm and 18% in the treated group had N2 disease, this difference was not statistically significant. With a median follow-up of 68 months, 56% of patients in the treated arm and 61% of those in the control arm had recurrence of disease. There was no statistically significant difference in disease-free survival nor in overall survival. A number of subgroup analyses were performed, the most positive of which was an effect for patients with T3 or T4 tumors who had positive lymph nodes ($p = 0.07$) in favor of the FAM group. This was an unplanned subgroup analysis. Three FAM patients died from suspected treatment-related complications. In a second FAM study, reported in abstract form, the Southwest Oncology Group failed to find an improvement in survival for the treated group.[150] Both groups of investigators have concluded that adjuvant chemotherapy using FAM should only be used in an investigational setting.

Krook and colleagues used a different doxorubicin-containing combination in the adjuvant setting.[151] After curative resection, 125 evaluable patients were randomized to observation alone or to three cycles of 5-FU (350 mg/m^2/day) for 5 days plus doxorubicin (40 mg/m^2) on day 1. Therapy was repeated on days 35 and 70. Treatment began between 4 and 6 weeks after resection. There were no differences in median survival between the two groups, and the 5-year survival rates were almost identical. Two deaths were caused by sepsis during treatment-related leukopenia.

Estrada and associates studied the use of methyl-CCNU, 5-FU, and doxorubicin in evaluable patients after resection.[152] Thirty-one patients received 12 to 18 months of adjuvant chemotherapy; 35 patients were observed. At 5 years, there was no difference in disease-free (29% treated versus 34% observed) or overall survival. There were two treatment-related deaths.

Because some gastric cancers are positive for estrogen receptor protein, Harrison and colleagues treated 100 patients in a random-assignment trial with tamoxifen as a single agent.[153] This study allowed entrance of patients who had residual gross disease and was therefore not truly adjuvant chemotherapy. In this group, 55.8% of tumors were estrogen receptor positive. There was no effect of tamoxifen on survival outcome; in fact, the control group did slightly better than the treated group.

Neoadjuvant Chemotherapy

Practical and theoretical considerations for the use of neoadjuvant (also called primary or preoperative) chemotherapy were reviewed by Muggia and Gill.[154] Primary chemotherapy can induce early tumor regression, potentially improve local control rates with subsequent surgery or irradiation, allows use of more conservative local measures, and may identify responding patients who could benefit from postoperative chemotherapy. However, early use of systemic treatment may allow emergence of a resistant clone of tumor cells, can delay effective local control, and can lead to uncertainty as to the extent of resection. Responding patients may refuse surgery or irradiation.

Neoadjuvant chemotherapy given for several cycles before definitive locoregional therapy allows a simultaneous assault on distant metastases and the primary tumor and is employed when the patient is best able to tolerate potential toxicities. Because current chemotherapy used in gastric cancer can have substantial toxic effects, preoperative identification of patients at high risk for recurrence with surgery alone would be valuable. Endoscopic ultrasonography is highly accurate in assessing T stage (*i.e.*, T1 versus T3), and may be very useful for identifying high risk patients best suited for neoadjuvant chemotherapy.

The use of systemic therapy early in the treatment plan is rational in a disease in which there is a high propensity for systemic failure with or without local recurrence. Neoadjuvant chemotherapy is an attractive concept in diseases such as gastric cancer for which complete resection of the primary tumor is difficult or impossible and systemic dissemination is common. The percentage of patients with proximal gastric cancers (*i.e.*, adenocarcinoma of the cardia or gastroesophageal junction) has increased, and proximal tumors result in a poorer survival than do distal (*i.e.*, body-antrum) lesions. The failure pattern for gastroesophageal junction and esophageal adenocarcinomas was studied in a group of 77 patients who had undergone potentially curative surgery, defined as removal of all gross disease, negative resection margins, and no evidence of distant visceral involvement (T1–3NanyM0).[155] Locoregional failure was uncommon, but distant metastases was seen in most patients. Sites of recurrence were determined clinically in most patients. The high rate of extraabdominal distant metastases was similar to that of epidermoid carcinoma of the esophagus and was greater than that usually reported for distal gastric cancers.

For gastric cancer, many patients cannot undergo potentially curative resections, systemic metastases are common, and the local failure rate despite resection ranges from 40% to 80%. These factors are the rationale for the use of neoadjuvant chemotherapy.

Intraperitoneal Chemotherapy

Because peritoneal and hepatic recurrences are common, the use of intraperitoneal postoperative chemotherapy is undergoing investigation at several centers. Japanese and some American investigators have long pointed out that such an approach is feasible, and the pharmacokinetic advantages to intraperitoneal chemotherapy have been described.[156] The theoretical advantages for using intraperitoneal treatment immediately after surgery have been reviewed by Sugarbaker and coworkers.[157] In preclinical studies, Archer and Grey, using rats, demonstrated that intraperitoneal chemotherapy is capable of treating peritoneal and liver micrometastasis.[158] In a second study, Murthy and colleagues demonstrated in mice that the frequency of tumor formation at sites of surgical trauma in the peritoneum ranged from 28% to 82%, depending on the type of incisions made in the peritoneal cavity, compared with a rate of 33% for formation of peritoneal tumors in nonoperated mice.[139] Eggermont and associates demonstrated that a laparotomy can enhance the rate of intraperitoneal tumor growth.[138] A random-assignment trial in colon cancer by Sugarbaker and colleagues demonstrated a change in the failure pattern, with a marked decrease in peritoneal metastasis with intraperitoneal chemotherapy compared with intravenous treatment, but with no change in survival.[158a]

These laboratory and small clinical trials of treating other gastrointestinal malignancies led to studies of gastric cancer. Western and Japanese investigators explored the role of intraperitoneal treatment with mitomycin, 5-FU or its analogs, or cisplatin in the postoperative period.

Schiessel and colleagues reported the results of a multicenter German study investigating the use of intraperitoneal chemotherapy.[159] This is not a truly adjuvant study, because some patients had only palliative resections that left gross residual tumor behind. Thirty-three patients received no additional therapy after surgery, and 31 patients received intraperitoneal cisplatin as a single agent. The cisplatin (90 mg/m²) was given with systemic thiosulfate. Therapy was begun within 4 weeks of therapy. Toxicity was acceptable, but there was no survival advantage for the intraperitoneal chemotherapy group.

Atiq and coworkers reported the preliminary results of a phase II trial using cisplatin and 5-FU intraperitoneally with simultaneous continuous intravenous infusion of 5-FU. All patients had undergone a curative gastric resection.[160] Treatment was started from 14 to 28 days after surgery. In a preliminary report of a group of 30 patients, toxicity was tolerable, primarily involving myelosuppression. Nonhematologic complications were mild. Only 7 of 28 patients at risk had

recurrent disease. The median follow-up time in this study was short.

Although many random-assignment trials have been performed with patients who have undergone potentially curative resection for gastric cancer, there are no confirmed Western trials in which systemic adjuvant therapy has been of proven benefit. Some Japanese trials reporting positive results have had serious methodologic flaws.[161] Although some Western trials have used therapy in the immediate postoperative period, most studies allow 6 to 8 weeks of delay before initiating systemic treatment. There are sound theoretical grounds for giving chemotherapy in the immediate postoperative period for patients with gastric cancer. Investigational trails involving the use of intraperitoneal chemotherapy are ongoing. Several recent studies indicate that with careful dose adjustment, toxicity of immediate postoperative chemotherapy is acceptable. For now, standard therapy in the United States remains observation only after surgical resection, but entrance of high-risk patients into carefully designed clinical trials is strongly recommended.

ADJUVANT RADIATION THERAPY

Rationale

The reason to consider adjuvant radiation therapy for the treatment of a malignancy is because the locoregional failure rate with conventional therapy is high enough that local failure can be a significant factor in preventing cure or that locoregional failures produce significant symptomatic problems for the patient. The data presented earlier in this chapter suggests that locoregional failure can occur in approximately 35% to 40% of some patient groups (although the range in reported series is very large). Despite the fact that some of these data have been available for many years, there is still only a small amount of data suggesting that radiation therapy has a major impact on the outcome of patients with gastric cancer.

Few studies have evaluated radiation therapy alone (with no concomitant chemotherapy) as an adjuvant to surgical resection of gastric cancer. The small amount of data available does not allow firm conclusions about the value of radiation therapy alone, although it does suggest much benefit. Most of the studies that have evaluated radiation therapy as an adjuvant have used concomitant 5-FU chemotherapy.

Some of the earliest data on radiation therapy of gastric cancer comes from the Mayo Clinic, where studies were performed in the 1960s on the use of radiation therapy and 5-FU for several gastrointestinal malignancies. Although these reports were based on patients with locally advanced tumors, they laid the groundwork for the subsequent adjuvant studies. Childs and colleagues reported a study of patients with advanced gastric cancer who were randomized to radiation therapy alone to a dose of approximately 4000 cGy or radiation therapy combined with 5-FU as a radiation sensitizer (bolus 5-FU for 3 days, 15 mg/kg/day).[162] There was a significant improvement in the survival with the combination of 5-FU and irradiation compared with irradiation alone. Because the dose of 5-FU was extremely low, most people have interpreted these data as showing an advantage for the use of 5-FU as a radiation sensitizer. This is consistent with the data that have been obtained in other gastrointestinal sites, such as rectal or pancreatic cancer, for which 5-FU has improved survival when combined with radiation therapy. It suggests that trials evaluating adjuvant radiation therapy alone would have much less likelihood of demonstrating a benefit than those that use combined modalities. Therefore, studies such as those from the British Stomach Cancer Group, which randomized patients to postoperative radiation therapy, to postoperative chemotherapy with 5-FU, doxorubicin, and mitomycin C, or to surgery alone, would be much less likely to show an advantage for radiation therapy. In fact, the British trial demonstrated no survival advantage from the use of adjuvant therapy, although the local recurrence rate was decreased by the use of radiation therapy: 54% with surgery alone and 32% with radiation therapy ($p < 0.01$).[86]

Two studies used chemotherapy plus concurrent irradiation. In one, noncuratively resected patients were included. Dent and colleagues treated 142 patients who were randomly assigned to no additional therapy or to 2000 cGy given in eight fractions over 10 days plus 5-FU (12.5 mg/kg) given daily for 4 days immediately before the beginning of irradiation.[163] A second cycle was given on day 28. Patients in "division one" had no residual gross disease but may have had incomplete resection. There were 31 patients in the control group and 35 in the chemotherapy and irradiation group. Even though this is not truly an adjuvant study, there was no difference in survival between the two groups. The control arm had a slight survival advantage. Moertel and associates from the Mayo Clinic reported the results of a randomized trial of radiation therapy (3750 cGy in 24 fractions) plus 5-FU (15 mg/kg/day × 3 days) versus surgery alone for poor-prognosis patients, including those with scirrhous carcinomas, metastases to regional lymph nodes, invasion of adjacent structures, or tumors originating in the cardia.[164] Eighty percent of patients had positive nodal disease, and approximately 25% had invasion of adjacent structures. The treated patients had a 5-year survival rate of 20%, and the surgery-only controls had a 4% 5-year survival rate. The issue is confused by the fact that there were 10 patients who were randomized to adjuvant treatment but who refused therapy. In this small cohort of patients, the 5-year survival rate was 30%. Locoregional recurrence was decreased from 54% in the surgery-alone arm to 39% in the combined-modality arm. The survival results in these studies are similar to those reported in nonrandomized series, such as that by Slot, in which 57 patients with poor prognostic factors received postoperative radiation therapy to a dose of 3000 to 5000 cGy combined with 5-FU.[165] The 5-year survival rate was 26%, with 16 patients having a locoregional recurrence as the first sign of relapse.

Although other studies have evaluated other combinations of chemotherapy with radiation therapy, there has not been any advantage shown for any drug regimen besides 5-FU chemotherapy.[166,167] The data do not allow a definite conclusion that radiation therapy is of value as adjuvant treatment for poor-risk gastric adenocarcinoma. It does suggest, however, that for patients with nodal positivity, serosal involvement, or close or positive surgical resection margins, that postoperative radiation therapy may be of value. This approach will be studied in a national intergroup trial evaluating two cycles of chemotherapy with 5-FU and leucovorin followed by radiation therapy to a dose of 4500 cGy with concurrent chemotherapy.

Newer approaches increasing the total radiation dose have been tried. An approach investigated at a few centers is the use of intraoperative electron-beam radiation therapy, which was pioneered by Abe.[168] With this technique, patients receive a single dose of high-energy electrons delivered to the tumor bed at the time of gastrectomy. Because most of the normal structures can be moved from the path of the radiation beam, the risk for producing significant bowel complications is much reduced. In a nonrandomized trial, Abe demonstrated an improved 5-year survival rate for patients with locally advanced disease (usually because of posterior infiltration) who were treated with intraoperative radiation therapy (Table 26–15). A small trial of a similar approach at the NCI did not demonstrate any significant survival advantage.[169] Whether the advantage demonstrated in the Japanese trial will hold up and whether the results could be obtained as well with external-beam irradiation is not defined. The exact role of this approach in the treatment of gastric cancer must still be determined.

Technique of Radiation Therapy

In delivering radiation therapy for gastric carcinoma, the radiation oncologist is significantly constrained by the normal tissues close to the tumor mass, which limit the radiation dose that can be delivered safely. The spinal cord, kidneys, small bowel, and liver are too close to be entirely avoided. The stomach itself is a radiation sensitive tissue, and a high dose (>5000 cGy) to a functional stomach tissue can produce ulceration and bleeding.

Irradiating the upper abdomen can produce several acute side effects, typically including nausea, weight loss, and fatigue. With properly planned radiation fields, the nausea is not generally severe, but given the prolonged course of radiation, if careful attention is not given to the patient's nutritional status, the therapy can produce more harm than good. A combination of antiemetics, multiple small feedings, and nutritional supplements is usually sufficient, but on occasion, feeding tubes are useful. If a patient cannot maintain his or her weight before the initiation of the radiation therapy, therapy will be difficult. The other acute side effects are relatively minor and easily managed. The possible late side effects that

TABLE 26–15. Surgery Alone Versus Surgery and Intraoperative Radiation Therapy in Japan

	5-Year Survival			
	Surgery		Surgery + IORT	
Stage	No.	%	No.	%
I	43	93	20	88.1
II	11	54.5	18	77.6
III	38	36.8	19	44.6
IV (no distant metastases)	18	0	27	19.5

(Abe M, Takashashi M. Intraoperative radiotherapy: The Japanese experience. Int J Radiat Oncol Biol Phys 1981;7:863–868)

must be considered include damage to spinal cord, liver, kidney, and stomach.

Late kidney and renal failure or radiation-induced spinal cord transection are possible complications from excess irradiation, but if proper attention is paid to these structures during treatment planning, they are rarely a problem. The tolerance dose of the stomach itself is approximately 5000 cGy, and doses above this level often produce gastric ulceration.

It is commonly the case that at least one kidney needs to be in the radiation field to a high dose (>3000 cGy), which usually causes significant renal injury. This is most commonly the left kidney, but the right kidney can also be at high risk. Studies have demonstrated that, for a patient with baseline renal function that is within the normal range, treating one kidney to high dose is unlikely to produce a renal injury that adversely affects the patient's quality of life.[170] The compensatory hypertrophy of the unirradiated kidney generates adequate renal function, and the risk for renovascular hypertension is low. If the equivalent of one kidney can be eliminated from the radiation field and the patient starts with a relatively normal creatinine clearance, the patient should tolerate the radiation course adequately. Standard radiation tolerance doses should be observed for the other normal tissues.

If radiation therapy is being used as an adjuvant or with curative intent, the patterns of spread of the tumor must be considered in planning the radiation field. In contrast to many other tumor sites, a standard radiation field is often inappropriate in treatment of this disease, because the spread patterns relate to the site of origin and the extension that is found on preoperative imaging studies and at surgery. The lymphatic pattern of spread was previously discussed, and it greatly influences the radiation fields that are appropriate. Although the oncologist usually wishes to encompass much of the stomach (or the gastric bed) for tumors that originated and remained limited to the gastric antrum, it is not necessary to irradiate the entire cardia of the stomach or to extend the radiation field to encompass the lower esophagus, but it is necessary to treat the periduodenal lymph nodes. For tumors originating in the cardia, it is essential that the field extend up into the esophagus and that there be full coverage of the bed of the gastric cardia and fundus, but it is possible to safely avoid irradiating the periduodenal nodes. Local failure from gastric cancer often occurs because of posterior extension of the primary tumor onto the pancreas and into other retroperitoneal tissues. Therefore, full coverage of these areas of posterior invasion is essential. An example of a typical radiation field is shown in Fig. 26–9. The radiation fields are primarily anteroposterior and posteroanterior fields, although lateral and oblique fields can be useful for the final boost. If lateral fields are used for a substantial portion of the large field treatment, care must be taken to avoid treating large segments of the liver to doses over 2000 to 2500 cGy.

The total radiation dose is determined primarily by the tolerance of the normal tissues. Generally, a dose of 4500 cGy given in 180-cGy fractions each day has a minimal chance of producing significant late complications. At doses over 5000 cGy, the risk of late complications increases, and doses greater than this should be limited to very small volumes. The data strongly suggest that the combination of 5-FU and irradiation

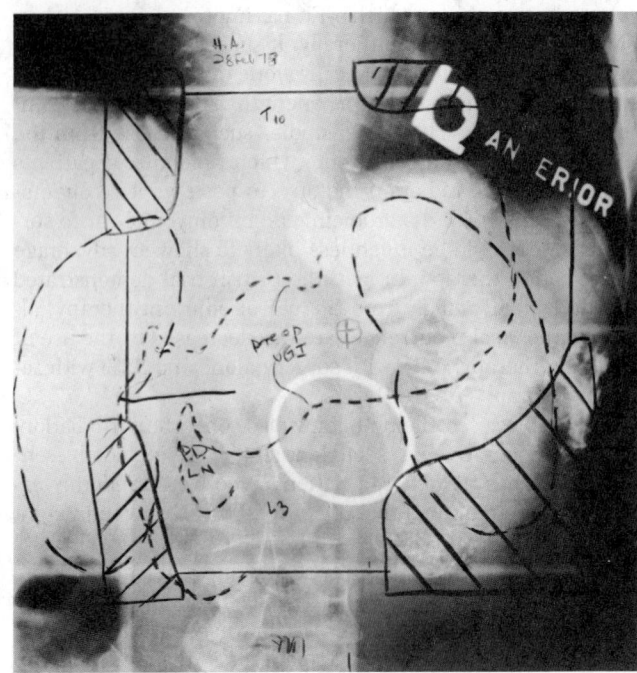

FIGURE 26–9. Typical treatment field for postoperative radiation therapy of a tumor in the body of the stomach. This field encompasses the entire tumor bed and virtually all regional lymphatic sites. For tumors that are located more proximally or distally in the stomach, the fields can be shaped to avoid regions at lower risk.

is more effective than radiation therapy alone. Although the optimal method of drug administration is unknown, it is appropriate to use, as a minimum, 3 days of bolus 5-FU during the first and last weeks of radiation therapy.

TREATMENT OF ADVANCED GASTRIC CANCER

During the last 20 years, many chemotherapeutic agents have been studied for treating gastric cancer. Although there have been recent reports of very high response rates with some of the newer combination chemotherapy regimens, the median survival of patients with advanced cancer continues to be dismal.

SINGLE-AGENT CHEMOTHERAPY

The objective response rates reported for single agents in patients with gastric cancer are shown in Table 26–16. 5-FU is the most extensively studied single agent in this disease; an overall objective response rate of 21% has been seen.[171,172] The two most commonly employed schedules for administering 5-FU as a single agent are daily intravenous injections for 5 consecutive days, repeated every 4 to 5 weeks, and weekly intravenous injections. Both schedules have similar response rates and have similar toxicity profiles. The major side effects of 5-FU are mucositis, diarrhea, myelosuppression, and (using a continuous infusion) the hand-foot syndrome. 5-FU has been a common element in most combination chemotherapy regimens for gastric cancer.

TABLE 26–16. Single-Agent Chemotherapy for Gastric Cancer

Drugs	Evaluable Patients	Response Rate (%)	95% Confidence Limits (%)
Antimetabolites			
5-Fluorouracil	416	21	17–25
Carmofur (oral)	31	19	5–33
Ftorafur (oral)	19	27	7–46
Methotrexate	28	11	0–22
Trimetrexate	26	19	4–34
Triazinate	26	15	2–29
Hydroxurea (oral)	31	19	5–33
Antibiotics			
Mitomycin C	211	30	24–36
Doxorubicin	141	17	11–23
Epirubicin	80	19	10–27
Heavy Metals			
Cisplatin	139	19	12–25
Carboplatin	41	5	0–12
Alkylating Agents			
BCNU	33	18	5–31
Methyl-CCNU	37	8	0–17
Chlorambucil	18	17	0–34
Miscellaneous			
Uracil (oral)	34	27	12–41
Etoposide	25	12	0–25
Amsacrine	125	0	0
Diaziquone	30	0	<14
Razoxane	19	0	<14
Bisantrene	26	4	0–11
Mitoguazone	31	3	0–9

Mitomycin C, an antitumor antibiotic, has been extensively used in the treatment of gastric cancer, especially in Japan. The overall objective response rate for mitomycin C has been approximately 30%.[173–175] Its major toxic effect is delayed and cumulative myelosuppression, and the drug is usually given on an intermittent basis every 4 to 8 weeks.

Doxorubicin (Adriamycin), an anthracycline antibiotic, is the next most studied single agent for gastric cancer. In 141 evaluable patients with advanced disease, it had an overall response rate of 17%.[173,174,176] Doxorubicin is a potent agent with significant but manageable early side effects. Its most critical toxicity is irreversible myocardial damage. Cisplatin has recently been studied by several groups. As a single agent, it has produced major responses in 19% of patients, including those previously treated.[177–184] Amsacrine caused no responses in gastric cancer patients.[185] Other chemotherapeutic agents that have been studied in advanced gastric cancer with modest or minimal activity are shown in Table 26–16.[186–200] Complete responses are extraordinarily uncommon with single agents, even with those having the highest reported activity. Responses are generally of brief duration and without a significant impact on survival.

COMBINATION CHEMOTHERAPY

Numerous attempts have been made to develop more effective multidrug regimens using known active drugs; some trials have included other agents that did not have substantiated activity. Phase II and prospective randomized phase III trials have been reported. In general, results from multicenter phase III trials have had lower response rates than single-institution phase II studies for the same drug regimens (Table 26–17).[201–211] Several combination chemotherapy regimens have shown response rates in the range of 3% to 50%, usually in phase II studies.

The combination of 5-FU, doxorubicin, and mitomycin C (FAM regimen) was introduced by Macdonald and colleagues in the late 1970s and was widely used in the 1980s.[212] In the initial report of this regimen, 26 (42%) of 62 patients achieved a partial response; there were no complete responses. The median duration of response was 9 months; the median survival for the whole group was 5.5 months, although the median survival for responding patients was 12.5 months. Results using FAM in various dose schedules were reported for more than 650 patients with a cumulative response rate of 30%; the complete remission rate was 2% (see Table 26–17).[175] The median remission duration was 5 to 10 months, with a median survival of 6 to 9 months for all patients treated. Variants of the FAM regimen (*e.g.*, increased doxorubicin dose) were given to 310 patients. The overall response rate of 28% for modified regimens is similar to the response rate reported for 346 patients treated with the original FAM combination. The median survival of patients treated on FAM variants was identical to the survival of those treated on the original FAM regimen.[175]

The GTSG performed two prospective randomized trials, including the FAM regimen in which patients with measurable and nonmeasurable disease were studied (Table 26–18). All patients were evaluable for survival outcome but not necessarily for objective response. The first study randomized patients to four treatment arms: 5-FU plus methyl-CCNU, 5-FU plus doxorubicin plus methyl-CCNU (FAMe), 5-FU plus doxorubicin plus mitomycin C (FAM), and 5-FU plus ICRF-159 plus methyl-CCNU.[202] In this study, FAM had a response rate of 25% with a median survival of 30 weeks, which was similar to the 30% response rate and 34-week median survival with FAMe. In the second GTSG study, patients were randomized to FAM, FAMe, and FA (5-FU plus doxorubicin).[205] The FA treatment arm was included to determine the relative contribution of mitomycin C and methyl-CCNU in treating this disease. The primary endpoint of this study was survival, with only 23% of all patients in this trial having measurable disease. Among the small number of patients evaluable for response, the FAMe regimen demonstrated a 25% response rate, and the FAM regimen had a 17% response; only 1 (5%) of the 19 patients in the FA arm obtained a partial remission. Although the median survival was longest with FAMe, there were no statistically significant differences between the three arms. However, the FAM regimen in this study was administered slightly differently from the original Georgetown program. The dosage schedules of selected chemotherapy regimens are shown in Table 26–19.

ECOG reported the results of a four-arm randomized, controlled trial in which the original FAM regimen was compared

TABLE 26–17. Combination Chemotherapy for Gastric Cancer

Drugs	Evaluable Patients	Response Rate (%)	95% Confidence Limits (%)	Median Survival (mo)
FU-Doxo-Mito (FAM)	656	30	27–33	6–9+
FAM (variants)	310	28	23–33	
FU-Doxo-Methyl-CCNU (FAMe)	141	25	18–32	5.5–8.5
FU-Doxo-BCNU (FAB)	194	41	34–48	6–8
FU-Doxo-CDDP (FAP)	234	34	28–40	6–13
FU-Epirub-Mito (FEM)	123	32	23–40	5–6
FU-Epirub-BCNU (FEB)	45	42	28–57	9
FU-Epirub-CDDP (FEP)	66	44	32–56	Not stated
FU-Methyl-CCNU	224	19	14–24	3.5–5.5
FAM-BCNU	41	22	9–35	6.0
FU-Mito-AraC	356	36	31–41	16–20 (mean)
Etop-CDDP	79	18	9–26	4.5
Etop-Doxo-CDDP (EAP)	173	53	46–61	6–9
FU-Etop-Leucovorin (ELF)	51	53	39–67	11.0
FU-Doxo-MTX (FAMTX)	364	41	36–46	3.5–10.5

FU, fluorouracil; Epirub, epirubicin; Doxo, doxorubicin; Ara-C, cytosine arabinoside; Mito, mitomycin; Etop, etoposide; CDDP, cisplatin; MTX, methotrexate.

directly with FAMe, with 5-FU plus methyl-CCNU, and with doxorubicin plus mitomycin C (see Table 26–18).[201] Using a proportional hazards model of survival, there was a significant improvement in median survival time with FAM compared with the other three regimens individually. The difference was greatest between FAM and 5-FU methyl-CCNU ($p < 0.0078$); the difference was borderline for FAM versus FAMe ($p < 0.0537$). ECOG concluded that the FAM regimen should be included in future studies based on its favorable response data and the toxicity profile. Of the patients entered on this trial, 17% were excluded from analysis for various reasons, and after 1 year, the survival advantage of FAM was lost.

The North Central Cancer Treatment Group compared single-agent 5-FU to 5-FU plus doxorubicin and to FAM.[213] The primary endpoint of this study was survival. Thirty-five of 151 patients in the study had measurable disease, making an assessment of true differences in response rate impossible. There was no difference in median survival among the three treatment arms. The investigators also failed to find any significant differences in the palliative effect among these three treatment regimens. Because of a lack of improvement in median survival and due to the expense and toxicity associated with FAM compared with single-agent 5-FU, the researchers recommended that 5-FU as a single agent be continued as the standard treatment of advanced gastric cancer to which all other new treatment regimens should be compared.

The in vitro synergy between cisplatin and 5-FU, the activity of cisplatin as a single agent in gastric cancer, and the bone marrow toxicity of mitomycin led several investigators to replace mitomycin in the FAM combination with cisplatin. The cumulative overall response rate for the FAP regimen was 34%, with 5% of the patients achieving complete remissions (see Table 26–17).[175,204,206] The median duration of survival was 6 to 13 months. Cisplatin and doxorubicin were given in

doses of 60 to 100 mg/m^2 and 30 to 60 mg/m^2 per cycle, respectively. The 5-FU dose and schedule varied in individual trials.

To assess the individual contribution of cisplatin, methyl-CCNU, and triazinate in combination with 5-FU and doxorubicin, the GTSG performed a prospective randomized trial comparing FAP, FAMe, and FAT (5-FU, doxorubicin, triazinate).[204] The primary endpoint was survival. Of 249 patients studied, 38% had measurable disease and were evaluable for response. The response rates for FAP, FAMe, and FAT were 19%, 15%, and 20%, respectively. Median survivals were 31 weeks (FAP), 24 weeks (FAMe), and 30 weeks (FAT). Severe toxicity was seen in 69% of patients treated with FAP, 62% of those on FAMe, and 42% of those on FAT.

Epirubicin, an analog of doxorubicin that in preclinical studies has less cardiac toxicity than, but equivalent, tumor activity to doxorubicin (see Table 26–16), was substituted for doxorubicin in a FAP-type regimen reported by Cunningham and coworkers.[214] Ten (71%) of 14 evaluable patients achieved an objective response. In a second trial involving 52 evaluable patients, the response rate was 37%, with a 17% complete remission rate.[215] Median durations of survival were not reported. These are preliminary results that must be confirmed in larger phase II and randomized phase III trials.

In a review of Japanese studies, Ogawa reported a cumulative response rate of 36% in 356 patients with a combination of 5-FU, mitomycin C, and cytarabine (see Table 26–17).[216] The mean survival was 16 to 20 months. However, in a randomized trial of 5-FU alone compared with 5-FU, mitomycin, and cytarabine, Cocconi and colleagues found no statistical difference between the response rate, duration of response, or median survival in the two arms.[172]

Because of evidence that etoposide and cisplatin may be synergistic and that the combination of the two may be helpful in overcoming multidrug resistance, the drugs have been

TABLE 26–18. Combination Chemotherapy: Prospective Randomized Trials in Advanced Gastric Cancer

Drugs	Evaluable Patients	Response Rate (%)	95% Confidence Limits (%)	Median Survival
FU	51	18	7–28	7.0 (NS)
vs				
FU-Doxo	49	27	14–39	7.0
vs				
FAM	51	38	24–51	7.0
FU-methyl-CCNU	44	14	3–24	3.4 ($p < 0.0078$)*
vs				
Doxo-Mito	46	29	15–41	5.0
vs				
FAM	46	39	25–53	7.4
vs				
FAMe	39	29	14–42	6.0
FU-Doxo	78	5	0–10	6.3 (NS)
vs				
FAM	78	17	8–25	6.4
vs				
FAMe	76	25	15–35	7.1
FU	41	15	4–25	7.0 (NS)
vs				
FAM-BCNU	41	22	9–35	6.0
Doxo	36	21	9–36	3.4 ($p = 0.04$)
vs				
FAMe	38	47	32–63	6.0
vs				
FU-Mito-AraC	36	14	3–25	3.2
Doxo	37	22	8–35	4.0 (NS)
vs				
FU-Mito	53	43	30–57	4.5
vs				
FU-methyl-CCNU	49	24	12–37	4.2
Doxo	93	13	6–20	5.0 (NS)
vs				
FAB	94	40	30–49	8.2
FU	95			9.0 (NS)
vs				
FU-methyl-CCNU	84			6.2
FAM	44	34	20–48	8.0 (NS)
vs				
CDDP-Doxo-Mito	43	23	11–36	7.0
FAMTX	30	33	16–50	7.0 (NS)
vs				
EAP	30	20	6–34	6.0
FAM	103	9	3–14	7.2 ($p = 0.004$)
vs				
FAMTX	105	41	32–50	10.5

FU, fluorouracil; Doxo, doxorubicin; Mito, mitomycin; Me, methyl-CCNU; Ara-C, cytosine arabinoside; NS, not significant; CDDP, cisplatin; FAMTX, fluorouracil, doxorubicin, and methotrexate.
* *p* value between FU-methyl CCNU versus FAM.

TABLE 26–19. Dosage Schedules of Selected Regimens for Gastric Cancer

Drugs	Dose/m^2 (mg)	Day
FAMTX		
Fluorouracil	1500	1
Methotrexate	1500	1
Doxorubicin	30	15
Repeat cycle on day 29		
EAP		
Etoposide	125	4, 5, 6
Doxorubicin	20	1, 7
Cisplatin	40	2, 8
Repeat cycle on day 29		
FAP		
Fluorouracil	300	1–5
Doxorubicin	40	1
Cisplatin	60	1
Repeat cycle every 5 weeks		
FAM		
Fluorouracil	600	1, 8, 29, 36
Doxorubicin	30	1, 29
Mitomycin	10	1
Repeat cycle every 8 weeks		
ELF		
Etoposide	120	1–3
Fluorouracil	500	1–3
Leucovorin	300	1–3
Repeat cycle every 3–4 weeks		

combined in the treatment of many tumors.[217,218] Two phase II trials of etoposide and cisplatin in advanced gastric cancer (including gastroesophageal junction adenocarcinoma) showed an 18% response rate in 79 evaluable patients (Table 26–20). Kelsen and associates reported only one major objective regression among 33 evaluable patients.[219] Cisplatin at a dose of 60 mg/m^2 was given on days 1 and 29 and every 6 weeks thereafter, with etoposide given at a dose of 100 mg/m^2 on days 3, 5, and 7 and on 31, 33, and 35. Toxicity was tolerable. In the second trial, Elliott and colleagues saw 13

responses in 46 evaluable patients.[220] Etoposide was given at a dose of 130 mg/m^2/day for 3 days plus cisplatin in a dose of 45 mg/m^2/day on days 2 and 3. Both drugs were given by continuous intravenous infusion, and the cycles were repeated every 4 weeks. Most patients experienced severe toxicity. The median duration of response was 4 months.

Preusser and coworkers used the combination of etoposide, doxorubicin, and cisplatin (EAP) and reported a 64% response rate among 67 patients, with a complete remission rate of 21%.[221] The median duration of survival for all patients was 9 months. Including patients with locoregional tumor treated in a separate trial, Preusser and colleagues treated 101 patients with EAP with a cumulative response rate of 57%.[222] Analyzing response as a function of extent of disease, patients with locoregional tumor had a response rate of 73%, with a 29% complete remission rate, and those with metastatic disease had a response rate of 49%, with a complete remission rate of 8%. The median survival time for patients with locally advanced disease was 17 months and 8.5 months for those with metastatic disease. In four subsequent phase II trials of EAP involving 173 evaluable patients, a cumulative response rate of 53% and a complete remission rate of 6% were seen (see Table 26–20).[223-225] However, in each of the subsequent trials after the initial study reported by Preusser, there was a treatment-related death rate of 10% to 14%.

In part because EAP had severe toxic effects in older patients, Wilke and colleagues devised a combination chemotherapy regimen of etoposide, leucovorin, and 5-FU (ELF) for patients older than 65 years of age with advanced gastric cancer (see Tables 26–17 and 26–19).[226] The rationale for this combination was that 5-FU and etoposide are active agents in gastric cancer that are well tolerated and have no cumulative organ toxicity, with the dose-limiting toxicity being overlapping myelosuppression; etoposide and 5-FU are synergistic and are not cross-resistant; and leucovorin enhances the cytotoxicity of 5-FU in other tumors. Fifty-one patients older than 65 years of age or with cardiac disease were treated. The overall response rate was 53%, including a complete remission rate of 12%. The response rate in patients with locally advanced disease was 70%, compared with 49% in patients with distant metastases. The median duration of response was 9.5 months. Twenty percent of patients experienced grade 3 or 4 myelosuppression. Nonhematologic toxicity was usually mild, with only 7 patients having grade 3 diarrhea. The researchers recommended ELF as a suitable regimen for high-

TABLE 26–20. EAP Regimen for Gastric Cancer

Investigations	No. of Patients	Response Rate (%)	95% Confidence Interval (%)	Median Survival (mo)	Toxic Death (%)
Preusser[221]	67	64	53–75	9	0
Katz[223]	25	72	56–75	6+	10
Taguchi[224]	29	44	24–64	8	10
Lerner[225]	22	43	25–61	Not stated	14
Kelsen[228]	30	20	6–34	6	13

(Kelsen D, Atiq O. Therapy of upper gastrointestinal tract cancers. In: Haskell CM, ed. Current problems in cancer. Chicago: Mosby Yearbook, 1991;15:239–294)

risk patients (*i.e.*, advanced age, cardiac risk factors). These early results must be confirmed in more patients in phase II and randomized phase III trials.

The concept of biochemical modulation of 5-FU involves the use of agents designed to increase the pool of phosphoribosyl pyrophosphate in tumor cells, resulting in increased 5-FU ribonucleotide metabolites and increasing the effectiveness of 5-FU-directed tumor cell death. Klein and associates studied sequential high-dose methotrexate followed by 5-FU, in combination with doxorubicin (FAMTX) in advanced gastric cancer (Table 26–21).[227] The interval between the administration of methotrexate and 5-FU is 1 hour in the original FAMTX regimen. Klein and colleagues reported a response rate of 59% for 100 evaluable patients, with a complete remission rate of 12%. In a review of his experience, Klein observed a 6% long-term (>5 years) survival rate for patients receiving FAMTX. In subsequent studies using FAMTX, 364 patients treated with this regimen had a cumulative response rate of 41%. In the follow-up studies, there were 4% treatment-related deaths, comparable to a 3% rate in the original Klein study.

Kelsen and coworkers reported the results of a random-assignment trial comparing EAP with FAMTX for advanced gastric cancer.[228] Sixty patients (30 in each arm) were entered into the study. The two arms were well balanced for the usual prognostic variables. The response rates were similar, with a 33% response rate for the FAMTX arm and a rate of 20% for EAP. Three (10%) patients had complete remission rates on the FAMTX arm; no complete responses were seen with EAP. Although there were no significant differences in the response rate, EAP was significantly more toxic than FAMTX for neutropenia, anemia, and thrombocytopenia. There were four (13%) treatment-related deaths on the EAP arm but none on the FAMTX arm (*p* = 0.04). An equal number of patients were admitted for toxic effects on both arms of the trial, but patients on EAP remained in the hospital for significantly longer periods than those on the FAMTX arm (median, 8 days versus 5 days). The study was initially designed for 65 patients per arm, but at an interim analysis performed at the 50% accrual point, it was determined that the EAP was highly unlikely to have more than 50% of the activity of FAMTX. Because of the significant toxic effects, the study was closed. The median durations of survival of all patients were similar: 7 months for FAMTX and 6 months for EAP 6. The research-

ers concluded that FAMTX was at least as active as EAP and was significantly less toxic.

The European Organization for Research on the Treatment of Cancer (EORTC) published the results of a multicenter prospective randomized trial comparing FAMTX with FAM (see Table 26–18).[229] For 208 evaluable patients, the response rate for FAMTX was significantly superior to FAM (*p* < 0.0001). There were 5 complete responders in the FAMTX arm, but none on the FAM regimen. Survival among FAMTX patients was also superior. The toxic death rate of the two combinations was similar: 4% for FAMTX and 3% for FAM. At 1 year, 41% of FAMTX and 22% of FAM patients were alive. There were no FAM-arm survivors at the 2-year, but 9% of the patients on the FAMTX arm survived. Severe hematologic toxicity was seen in more patients on FAM than on the FAMTX regimen. Although of great interest, a confirmatory trial has not yet been reported.

No combination chemotherapy has had decisively superior survival to 5-FU alone. The approaches of biochemical modulation of 5-FU, the identification of new active agents, and the subsequent development of effective combination therapy should be vigorously pursued. As is true for many other solid tumors, patients with advanced gastric cancer should be treated on well-designed trials that seek to address these issues.

SURGERY FOR PALLIATION

Based on preoperative assessment or intraoperative findings, an operation for gastric cancer may be performed with palliative intent. Because the survival for patients with advanced gastric cancer is so poor, any proposed operation should have a good chance of providing sustained symptomatic relief while minimizing the attendant morbidity and need for prolonged hospitalization. Ekbom reviewed the results of palliative resection compared with intestinal bypass (gastrojejunostomy) in 75 patients with advanced gastric cancer.[230] The most frequent symptoms for which patients underwent operation included pain, hemorrhage, nausea, dysphagia, or obstruction. Operative mortality was 25% for gastrojejunostomy, 20% for palliative partial or subtotal gastrectomy, and 27% for total or proximal palliative gastrectomy. The most common and often fatal complication was anastomotic leak. After gastrojejunostomy, 80% of patients had relief of symptoms for a mean of 5.9 months, compared with palliative resection,

TABLE 26–21. FAMTX Regimen for Gastric Cancer

Investigations	No. of Patients	Response Rate (%)	95% Confidence Interval (%)	Median Survival (mo)	Toxic Deaths (%)
Klein[227]	116	58	49–69	9	3
Weh[238]	50	34	21–47	7	0
Herrman[239]	20	0	0–17	3.5	10
Wils[240]	67	33	22–44	6	6
Wils[229]	81	41	30–52	10.5	4
Kelsen[228]	30	33	14–46	7	0

(Kelsen D, Atiq O. Therapy of upper gastrointestinal tract cancers. In: Haskell CM, ed. Chicago: Mosby Yearbook, 1991;15:239–294)

which provided palliation of symptoms in 88% of patients for a mean of 14.6 months. Although the duration of palliation was significantly longer after resection ($p < 0.01$), the selection criteria for resection or for bypass were not controlled, and some bias against performing a palliative resection in high-risk patients with more advanced disease may have existed.

Meijer reported a retrospective analysis of 51 patients undergoing palliative intestinal bypass or resection.[231] In 20 (77%) of 26 patients undergoing resection, palliation was considered moderate to good, with a mean survival of 9.5 months. After gastroenterostomy, there was some palliation in 8 (30%) of 25, and survival was 4.2 months. The results of total gastrectomy for palliation in 27 patients with advanced gastric cancer has been presented by Butler and colleagues.[127] Operative mortality was only 4%, but morbidity affected 48% of patients. Median survival was 15 months, with a survival rate of 38% at 2 years. This substantial survival at 2 years reflects the fact that, although all patients were symptomatic before surgery, only half had stage IV disease. Patients with linitis plastica present a serious therapeutic challenge. Resection may provide palliation of symptoms.[127] However, survival after total gastrectomy is exceedingly poor, ranging from 3 months to one year.[232]

Bozzetti reviewed the outcomes of 246 patients with advanced gastric cancer who underwent simple exploratory laparotomy alone, gastrointestinal bypass, or palliative resection at the National Cancer Institute of Milan.[233] When survival was compared for patients with similar type and extent of disease, there was a consistent trend for improved median survival with palliative resection in patients with local spread (4.4 versus 8 months) and distant spread of disease (3 versus 8 months). Boddie reported similar results for 45 patients undergoing palliative resection for advanced gastric cancer at the M.D. Anderson Hospital.[234] Operative mortality for resection was 22%. In 21 patients who had undergone a palliative bypass procedure, survival was significantly shorter than for those undergoing resection ($p < 0.01$).

In selected patients with symptomatic advanced gastric cancer, resection of the primary disease appears to provide symptomatic relief with acceptable morbidity and mortality, even if there is macroscopic residual disease. The criteria for deciding which patients may benefit from palliative surgery have not been established and the data available represent retrospective analyses of patients selected for operation. The choice of procedure in these studies may have been influenced by differences in opinion about the value of palliative surgery in patients with such a grave prognosis.

RADIATION THERAPY FOR PALLIATION

There have been no studies evaluating the use of radiation therapy in patients with locally recurrent or metastatic carcinoma of the stomach. Its use is likely to be limited to palliation of symptoms, such as bleeding or controlling pain secondary to local tumor infiltration. Although there are minimal data available, radiation therapy seems to be fairly effective (from anecdotal experience) in controlling bleeding, as is true in other sites. This can often be accomplished at relatively low radiation doses. Pain from local tumor invasion can be palliated, although the dose required is higher (4000 cGy).

Rarely, there may be a patient with a focal local recurrence without metastases that is amenable to relatively high-dose radiation therapy for prolonging survival or a patient in whom radiation therapy would be given as an adjuvant to surgical resection. However, there are no data to support this approach.

CONCLUSIONS

Despite the declining overall incidence of gastric cancer in the United States, there is an increase in the incidence of proximal gastric cancers, which are predominantly poorly differentiated. Worldwide, the incidence of gastric cancer varies, and it remains a significant cause of cancer death. Most patients with gastric cancer in the United States are found at the time of diagnosis to have advanced disease.

Gastric adenocarcinoma represents two distinct types of cancer with different pathogenesis, epidemiology, and prognosis. There is intense interest in the development of genetic data that can predict outcome. Studies involving cytogenetics, oncogene amplification, or overexpression are a high priority. Preliminary data for cytogenetic abnormalities in gastric cancer and gene overexpression are being amassed. Comparison of biologic data between Japanese and American patients can determine whether better outcome in Japanese patients is related to a different biology of the disease or to different therapeutic approaches. The use of endoscopic ultrasonography preoperatively may help identify patients at high risk for recurrence with surgery alone. Investigational trials involving neoadjuvant chemotherapy targeting this population may be feasible. Experimental evidence strongly supports the use of systemic therapy alone or regional plus systemic therapy in the immediate postoperative period. An intergroup trial addressing the value of adjuvant chemotherapy and concurrent radiation is in progress.

The role of radical surgery in the treatment of this disease has not been clearly defined. Retrospective data indicate that R-2 gastrectomy may benefit patients with limited disease, and prospective trials that may justify its routine use are currently underway. In patients who have undergone resection with curative intent, radiation therapy, external-beam or IORT, has been used to reduce the high incidence of local and regional failure. Intraperitoneal chemotherapy for gastric cancer is theoretically enticing in view of the failure pattern of the disease.

The development of regimens that are active in patients with advanced disease, particularly in their ability to induce complete remissions, are necessary to make progress in the adjuvant setting. Regimens involving biochemical modulation of 5-FU such as the FAMTX regimen are one major focus of investigation. The development of new active agents is equally important. No combination regimen has yet demonstrated its superiority over single-agent chemotherapy in confirmed trials, although the recent EORTC study comparing FAMTX to FAM is of considerable interest.

REFERENCES

1. Boring C, Squires T, Tong J. Cancer Statistics 1991. CA 1991;41:28–29.
2. Blot WJ, Devesa SS, Kneller RW, Fraumeni JF. Rising incidence of adenocarcinoma of the esophagus and gastric cardia. JAMA 1991;265:1287–1289.

3. Meyers WC, Damiano RJ, Postlethwait RW, Rotolo FS. Adenocarcinoma of the stomach. Ann Surg 1987;205:1–8.

4. Mishima Y, Hirayama R. The role of lymph node surgery in gastric cancer. World J Surg 1987;11:406–411.

5. Nagayo T. Background data to the study of advanced gastric cancer. In: Nagayo T, ed. Histogenesis and precursors of human gastric cancer. New York: Springer-Verlag, 1986:17–39.

6. Mettlin C. Epidemiologic studies in gastric adenocarcinoma. In: Douglass HO Jr, ed. Gastric cancer. New York: Churchill Livingstone, 1988:1–25.

7. Maehara Y, Miriguchi S, Kakeji Y, Orita H, Haraguchi M, Korenaga D, Sugimachi K. Prognostic factors in adenocarcinoma in the upper one-third of the stomach. Surg Gynecol Obstet 1991;173:223–226.

8. Hesketh P, Clapp R, Doos W, et al. The increasing frequency of adenocarcinoma of the esophagus. Cancer 1989;64:526–530.

9. Powell J, McConkey CC. Increasing incidence of adenocarcinoma of the gastric cardia and adjacent sites. Br J Cancer 1990;62:440–443.

10. Murakami R, Tsukuma H, Ubukata T, Nakanishi K, Fujimoto I, Kawashima T, Yamazaki H, Oshima A. Estimation of validity of mass screening program for gastric cancer in Osaka, Japan. Cancer 1990;65:1255–1260.

11. Hotz J, Goebell H. Epidemiology and pathogenesis of gastric carcinoma. In: Meyer HJ, Schmoll HJ, Hotz J, eds. Gastric carcinoma. New York: Springer-Verlag, 1989: 3–15.

12. Correa P, Cuello C, Duque E. Carcinoma and intestinal metaplasia in the stomach in Colombian migrants. JNCI 1970;44:297–306.

13. Staszewski J. Migrant studies in alimentary tract cancer. Recent Results Cancer Res 1972;39:85–97.

14. Haenszel W, Kurihara M, Segi M, Lee RKC. Stomach cancer among Japanese in Hawaii. JNCI 1972;49:969–988.

15. Correa P. Clinical implications of recent developments in gastric cancer pathology and epidemiology. Semin Oncol 1985;12:2–10.

16. Boeing H. Epidemiological research in stomach cancer: Progress over the last ten years. J Cancer Res Clin Oncol 1991;117:133–143.

17. Lauren P. The two histological main types of gastric carcinoma: Diffuse and so-called intestinal-type carcinoma. Acta Pathol 1965;64:31–49.

18. Aird I, Bentall HH. A relationship between cancer of stomach and the ABO glood groups. Br Med J 1953;1:799–801.

19. Sokoloff B. Predisposition to cancer in the Bonaparte family. Am J Surg 1938;40: 673.

20. Imai T, Kubo T, Watanabe H. Chronic gastritis in Japanese with reference to high incidence of gastric carcinoma. JNCI 1971;47:179–195.

21. Chyou P-H, Nomura AMYH, Hankin JH, Stemmerman GN. A case-cohort study of diet and stomach cancer. Cancer Res 1990;50:7501–7504.

22. Nomura A, Grove JS, Stemmermann GN, Severson RK. A prospective study of stomach cancer and its relation to diet, cigarettes, and alcohol consumption. Cancer Res 1990;50: 627–631.

23. Forman D. Are nitrates a significant risk factor in human cancer? Cancer Surg 1989;8: 443–458.

24. Burstein M, Monge E, León-Barúa R, Lozano R, Berendson R, Gilman RH, Legua H, Rodriguez C. Low peptic ulcer and high gastric cancer prevalence in a developing country with a high prevalence of infection by *Helicobacter pylori*. J Clin Gastroenterol 1991;13:154–156.

25. Balfour DC. Factors influencing the life expectancy of patients operated on for gastric surgery. Ann Surg 1922;76:405–408.

26. Lygidakis NJ. Gastric stump carcinoma after surgery for gastroduodenal ulcer. Ann R Coll Surg Engl 1981;63:203–205.

27. Giarelli L, Melato M, Stanta G, Bucconi S, Manconi R. Gastric resection: A cause of high frequency of gastric carcinoma. Cancer 1983;52:1113–1116.

28. Stalnikowicz R, Benbassat J. Risk of gastric cancer after gastric surgery for benign disorders. Arch Intern Med 1990;150:2022–2026.

29. Tersmette AC, Offerhaus, GJA, Tersmette KWF, Giardiello FM, Moore CW, Tytgat GNJ, Vandenbroucke, JP. Meta-analysis of the risk of gastric stump cancer: Detection of high risk patient subsets for stomach cancer after remote partial gastrectomy for benign conditions. Cancer Res 1990;50:6486–6489.

30. La Vecchia C, Negri E, D'Avanzo B, Franceschi S. Histamine-2-receptor antagonists and gastric cancer risk. Lancet 1990;336:355–357.

31. Schumacher MC, Jick SS, Jick H, Feld AD. Cimetidine use and gastric cancer. Epidemiology 1990;1:251–254.

32. Matsukura N, Kawachi T, Sasajima K, Sano T, Sugimura T, Hirota T. Induction of intestinal metaplasia in the stomachs of rats by N-methyl-N'-nitro-N-nitrosoguanidine. JNCI 1978;61:141–144.

33. Sasajima K, Kawachi T, Matsukura N, Sano T, Sugimura T. Intestinal metaplasia and adenocarcinoma induced in the stomach of rats by N-propyl-N'-nitro-N-nitrosoguanidine. J Cancer Res Clin Oncol 1979;94:201–206.

34. Morson BC. Carcinoma arising from areas of intestinal metaplasia in the gastric mucosa. Br J Cancer 1955;9:377–285.

35. Hoffman NR. The relationship between pernicious anemia and cancer of the stomach. Geriatrics 1970;25:90–95.

36. Correa P, Haenszel W, Cuello C, et al. Gastric precancerous process in a high-risk population: Cross-sectional studies. Cancer Res 1990;50:4731–4736.

37. Dooley CP, Cohen H, Fitzgibbons PL, Bauer M, Appleman MD, Perez-Perez GI, Blaser MJ. Prevalence of *Helicobacter pylori* infection and histologic gastritis in asymptomatic persons. N Engl J Med 1989;321:1562–1566.

38. Parsonnet J, Vandersteen J, Goates J, Sibley RK, Pritikin J, Chang Y. *Helicobacter*

pylori infection in intestinal- and diffuse- type gastric adenocarcinomas. JNCI 1991;83: 640–643.

39. Parsonnet J, Friedman GD, Vandersteen DP, Chang Y, Vogelman JH, Orentreich N, Sibley RK. *Helicobacter pylori* infection and the risk of gastric carcinoma. N Engl J Med 1991;325:1127–1131.

40. Nomura A, Stemmermann GN, Chyou P-H, Kato I, Perez-Perez GI, Blaser MJ. *Helicobacter pylori* infection and gastric carcinoma among Japanese Americans in Hawaii. N Engl J Med 1991;325:1132–1136.

41. Moertel CG. The stomach. In: Holland JF, Frei E III, eds. Cancer medicine. Philadelphia: Lea & Febiger, 1982:1760–1774.

42. Pack GT. Unusual tumors of the stomach. Ann NY Acad Sci 1964;114:985.

43. Phillips JC, Linsay JW, Kendall JA. Gastric leiomyosarcoma: Roentgenologic and clinical findings. Am J Dig Dis 1970;15:239.

44. Macon WL IV. Gastric lymphoma vs adenocarcinoma. Arch Surg 1979;114:305–306.

45. Hayes J, Dunn E. Has the incidence of primary gastric lymphoma increased? Cancer 1989;63:2073–2076.

46. Haber DA, Mayer RJ. Primary gastrointestinal lymphoma. Semin Oncol 1988;15: 154–169.

47. Nishi M, Nakajima T, Kajitani T. The Japanese research society for gastric cancer—the general rules for the gastric cancer study and an analysis of treatment results based on the rules. In: Preece PE, Cuschieri A, Wellwood JM, eds. Cancer of the stomach. New York: Grune & Stratton, 1986:107–121.

48. Ming S-C. Gastric carcinoma: A pathobiological classification. Cancer 1977;39:2475–2485.

49. Bearzi I, Ranaldi R. Early gastric cancer: A morphologic study of 41 cases. Tumori 1982;68:223–233.

50. Sakita T, Oguro Y, Takasu S, Lukutomi H, Mura T. The development of endoscopic diagnosis of early carcinoma of the stomach. Jpn J Clin Oncol 1971;1:113–128.

51. Houldsworth J, Cordon-Cardo C, Ladanyi M, Kelsen DP, Chaganti RSK. Gene amplification in gastric and esophageal adenocarcinomas. Cancer Res 1990;50:6417–6422.

52. Mor O, Messinger Y, Rotman G, et al. Novel DNA sequences at chromosome 10q26 are amplified in human gastric carcinoma cell lines: Molecular cloning by competitive DNA reassociation. Nucleic Acids Res 1991;19:117–123.

53. Sakamoto H, Mori M, Tara M, et al. Transforming gene from human stomach cancers and a noncancerous portion of human stomach mucosae. Proc Natl Acad Sci USA 1986;83:3997–4001.

54. Nagata Y, Abe M, Kobayashi K, et al. Glycine to asparatic acid mutations at codon 13 of the L-Ki-*ras* gene in human gastrointestinal cancers. Cancer Res 1990;50:480–482.

55. Nanus DM, Kelsen DP, Mentle IR, et al. Infrequent point mutations of *ras* oncogenes in gastric cancers. Gastroenterology 1990;98:955–960.

56. Jiang W, Kahn SM, Guillem JJ, et al. Rapid detection of *ras* oncogenes in human tumors: Applications to colon, esophageal and gastric cancers. Oncogene 1989;4: 923–928.

57. Okuchi N, Yao T, et al. Frequent overexpression, but not activation by point mutation of *ras* genes in primary human gastric cancers. Gastroenterology 1987;93:1339–1345.

58. Okuchi N, Hand P, Merlo G, et al. Enhanced expression of c-Ha-*ras* p21 in human stomach adenocarcinomas defined by immunoassays using monoclonal antibodies and in situ hybridization. Cancer Res 1987;47:1413–1420.

59. Tamura G, Kihana T, Nomura K, Terada M, et al. Detection of frequent p53 gene mutations in primary gastric cancer by cell sorting and polymerase chain reaction single-strand conformation polymorphism analysis. Cancer Res 1991;51:3056–3058.

60. Kim J, Takahashi T, Chiba I, et al. Occurence of small p53 gene abnormalities in gastric carcinoma tumors and cell lines. JNCI 1991;83:938–943.

61. Tsujino T, Yoshida K, Nakayama H, et al. Alterations of oncogenes in metastatic tumors of human gastric carcinomas. Br J Cancer 1990;62:226–230.

62. Park JB, Rhim JS, Park SC, et al. Amplification, overexpression and rearrangement of the *erb*B2 protooncogene in primary human stomach carcinomas. Cancer Res 1989;49:6605–6609.

63. Ranzani GN, Pellegata NS, Previderè C, et al. Heterogeneous protooncogene amplification correlates with tumor progression and presence of metastases in gastric cancer patients. Cancer Res 1990;50:7811–7814.

64. Kury FD, Schneeberger C, Sliutz G, et al. Determination of HER-2/*neu* amplification and expression in tumor tissue and cultured cells using a simple, phenol free method for nucleic acid isolation. Oncogene 1990;5:1403–1408.

65. Yokota J, Yamamoto T, Miyahima N, et al. Genetic alterations of the c-*erb*B-2 oncogene occur frequently in tubular adenocarcinoma of the stomach and are often accompanied by amplification of the v-*erb*A homologue. Oncogene 1988;2:283–287.

66. Gutman M, Asaf D, Skornick Y, et al. Sporadic amplification of c-*myc* and c-*erb*-B2 proto-oncogenes in solid tumors. Proc Am Assoc Cancer Res 1988;29:A1800.

67. Yonemura Y, Ninomiya I, Yamaguchi A, et al. Evaluation of immunoreactivity for *erb*-B2 protein as a marker of poor short-term prognosis in gastric cancer. Cancer Res 1991;51:1034–1038.

68. Yonemura Y, Ninomiya I, Ohoyama S, et al. Expression of c-*erb*B-2 oncoprotein in gastric carcinoma. Cancer 1991;67:2914–2918.

69. Albino A. Personal communication, 1991.

70. Kameda T, Yasui W, Yoshida K, et al. Expression of ERBB2 in human gastric carcinomas: Relationship between p185ERBB2 expression and the gene amplification. Cancer Res 1990;50:8002–8009.

71. Jain S, Filipe MI, Gullick WJ, et al. C-*erb*B-2 protooncogene expression and its relationship to survival in gastric carcinoma: An immunohistochemical study on archival material. Int J Cancer 1991;48:668–671.

72. Yasui W, Sumiyoshi H, Hata J, et al. Expression of epidermal growth factor receptor in human gastric and colonic carcinomas. Cancer Res 1988;48:137–141.

73. Nanus DM, Kelsen DP, Niedzwiecki D, Chapman D, Brennan M, Cheng E, Melamed M. Flow cytometry as a predictive indicator in patients with operable gastric cancer. J Clin Oncol 1989;7:1105–1112.

74. Zinninger M. Extension of gastric cancer in the intramural lymphatics and its relation to gastrectomy. Am Surg 1954;20:920–927.

75. Serlin O, Keehn R, Higgins G, Harrower H, Mendeloff G. Factors related to survival following resection for gastric carcinoma: Analysis of 903 cases. Cancer 1977;40:1318–1329.

76. Shiu M, Papachristou D, Kosloff C, Eliopoulos G. Selection of operative procedure for adenocarcinoma of the midstomach. Ann Surg 1980;192:730–737.

77. Papachristou D, Shiu M. Management by en bloc multiple organ resection of carcinoma of the stomach invading adjacent organs. Surg Gynecol Obstet 1981;152:483–487.

78. Dupont B, Cohn I Jr. Gastric adenocarcinoma. In: Hickey RC, ed. Current problems in cancer. Chicago: Year Book Medical Publishers, 1980;4:1–46.

79. Kennedy B. TNM classification for stomach cancer. Cancer 1970;26:971–983.

80. Sunderland D. The lymphatic spread of gastric cancer. In: McNeer G, Pack G, eds. Neoplasms of the stomach. Philadelphia: JB Lippincott, 1967:408–420.

81. Maruyama K, Gunven P, Okabayashi K, Sasako M, Kinoshita T. Lymph node metastases of gastric cancer. Ann Surg 1989;210:596–602.

82. McNeer G, Vandenberg H Jr, Donn F, Bowden L. A critical evaluation of subtotal gastrectomy for the cure of cancer of the stomach. Ann Surg 1951;134:2–7.

83. Wisbeck W, Becher E, Russel A. Adenocarcinoma of the stomach: Autopsy observations with therapeutic implications for the radiation oncologist. Radiother Oncol 1986;7:13–18.

84. Bruckner H, Stablein D. Sites of treatment failure: Gastrointestinal tumor study group analyses of gastric, pancreatic, and colorectal trials. Cancer Treat Symp 1983;2:199–210.

85. Gunderson L, Sosin H. Adenocarcinoma of the stomach: Areas of failure in a re-operative series (second or symptomatic look): Clinicopathologic correlation and implications for adjuvant therapy. Int J Radiat Oncol Biol Phys 1982;8:1–11.

86. Allum W, Hallissey M, Ward L, Hockey M. A controlled, prospective, randomized trial of adjuvant chemotherapy or radiotherapy in resectable gastric cancer: Interim report. Br J Cancer 1989;60:739–744.

87. Landry J, Tepper J, Wood W, Moulton E, Koerner F, Sullinger J. Patterns of failure following curative resection of gastric carcinoma. Int J Radiat Oncol Biol Phys 1990;19:1357–1362.

88. DeWys WD, Begg D, Lavin PT. Prognostic effect of weight loss prior to chemotherapy in cancer patients. Am J Med 1980;69:491–499.

89. Kurihara M, Shirakabe H, Yarita T, Izumi T, Miyasaka K, Maruyama T, Kobayasi S. Diagnosis of small early gastric cancer by x-ray, endoscopy, and biopsy. Cancer Detect Prev 1981;4:377–383.

90. Halvorson R, Thompson W. Primary neoplasms of the hollow organs of the gastrointestinal tract: Staging and follow-up. Cancer 1991;67:1181–1188.

91. Dehn TCB, Reznek RH, Nockler IB, White FE. The pre-operative assessment of advanced gastric cancer by computed tomography. Br J Surg 1984;71:413–417.

92. Moss AA, Schnyder P, Marks W, Margulis AR. Gastric adenocarcinoma: A comparison of the accuracy and economics of staging by computed tomography and surgery. Gastroenterology 1981;80:45–50.

93. Cook AO, Levine BA, Sirinek KR, Gaskil HV III. Evaluation of gastric adenocarcinoma. Arch Surg 1986;121:603–606.

94. Hatfield ARW, Slavin G, Segal AW, Levi AJ. Importance of the site of endoscopic gastric biopsy in ulcerating lesions of the stomach. Gut 1975;16:884–886.

95. Qizilbash AH, Castelli M, Kowalski MA, Churly A. Endoscopic brush cytology and biopsy in the diagnosis of cancer of the upper gastrointestinal tract. Acta Cytol 1980;24:313–318.

96. Kurtz RC, Sherlock P. The diagnosis of gastric cancer. Semin Oncol 1985;12:11–18.

97. Dekker W, Tytgat GN. Diagnostic accuracy of fiberendoscopy in the detection of upper intestinal malignancy. A follow-up analysis. Gastroenterology 1977;73:710–714.

98. Winawer SJ, Sherlock P, Hajdu SI. The role of upper gastrointestinal endoscopy in patients with cancer. Cancer 1976;37:440–448.

99. Graham DY, Schwartz JT, Cain GD, Gyorkey F. Prospective evaluation of biopsy number in the diagnosis of esophageal and gastric carcinoma. Gastroenterology 1982;82:228–231.

100. Lightdale C, Botet J, Brennan M, et al. Endoscopic ultrasonography compared to computerized tomography for preoperative staging of gastric cancer. Gastrointest Endosc 1989;67:1181–1188.

101. Tio T, Cohen P, Coene P, et al. Endosonography and computed tomography of esophageal carcinoma. Gastroenterology 1989;96:1478–1486.

102. Kaneko E, Nakamura T, Umeda N, et al. Outcome of gastric carcinoma detected by gastric mass survey in Japan. Gut 1977;18:626–630.

103. Kaneko E, Nakamura T, Umeda N, et al. A longer term follow-up study of patients with gastric cancer detected by mass screening. Cancer 1989;63:613–617.

104. Noguchi Y, Imada T, Matsumoto A, et al. Radical surgery for gastric cancer: A review of the Japanese experience. Cancer 1989;64:2053–2062.

105. Maruyama K, Okabayashi K, Kinoshita T. Progress in gastric cancer surgery in Japan and its limits of radicality. World J Surg 1987;11:418–425.

106. Boku T, Nakane Y, Minoura T, Takada H, Yamamura M, Hioki K, Yamamoto M. Prognostic significance of serosal invasion and free intraperitoneal cancer cells in gastric cancer. Br J Surg 1990;77:436–439.

107. Baba H, Korenaga D, Okamura T, Saito A, Sugimachi K. Prognostic factors in gastric cancer with serosal invasion. Arch Surg 1989;124:1061–1064.

108. Hermanek P. Prognostic factors in stomach cancer surgery. Eur J Surg Oncol 1986;12:241–246.

109. Shiu MH, Perrotti M, Brennan MF. Adenocarcinoma of the stomach: A multivariate analysis of clinical, pathologic and treatment factors. Hepatogastroenterology 1989;36:7–12.

110. Bozzetti F, Bonfanti G, Morabito A, et al. A multifactorial approach for the prognosis of patients with carcinoma of the stomach after curative resection. Surg Gynecol Obstet 1986;162:229–234.

111. Japanese Research Society for Gastric Cancer. General rules for gastric cancer study in surgery and pathology. Jpn J Surg 1981;11:127–139.

112. Okusa T, Nakane Y, Boku T, Takada H, Yamamura H, Hioki K, Yamamoto M. Quantitative analysis of nodal involvement with respect to survival rate after curative gastrectomy for carcinoma. Surg Gynecol Obstet 1990;170:488–494.

113. Japanese Research Society of Gastric Cancer. The general rules for the gastric cancer study in surgery and pathology. Jpn J Surg 1981;11:127–145.

114. Kodama Y, Sugimachi K, Soejima, K, Matsusaka, T, Inokuchi K. Evaluation of extensive lymph node dissection for carcinoma of the stomach. World J Surg 1981;5:241–248.

115. Sowa M, Kato Y, Nishimura M, Kubo T, Maekawa H, Umeyama K. Surgical approach to early gastric cancer with lymph node metastasis. World J Surg 1989;13:630–636.

116. Boku T, Nakane Y, Okusa T, Hirozane N, Imabayashi N, Hioki K, Yamamoto M. Strategy for lymphadenectomy of gastric cancer. Surgery 1989;105:585–592.

117. Shiu MH, Moore E, Sanders M, et al. Influence of the extent of resection on survival after curative treatment of gastric carcinoma. Arch Surg 1987;122:1347–1351.

118. Irvin TT, Bridger JE. Gastric cancer: An audit of 122 consecutive cases and the results of R1 gastrectomy. Br J Surg 1988;75:106–109.

119. Okamura T, Tsujitani S, Korenaga D, et al. Lymphadenectomy for cure in patients with early gastric cancer and lymph node metastasis. Am J Surg 1988;155:476–480.

120. Dent DM, Madden MV, Price SK. Randomized comparison of R1 and R2 gastrectomy for gastric carcinoma. Br J Surg 1988;75:110–112.

121. de Aretxabala X, Konishi K, Yonemura Y, et al. Node dissection in gastric cancer. Br J Surg 1987;74:770–773.

122. Collins WT, Gall EA. Gastric carcinoma: A multicentric lesion. Cancer 1952;5:62–72.

123. Kosaka T, Miwa K, Yonemura Y, et al. A clinicopathologic study on multiple gastric cancers with special reference to distal gastrectomy. Cancer 1990;65:2602–2605.

124. Papachristou DN, Fortner JG. Local recurrence of gastric adenocarcinomas after gastrectomy. J Surg Oncol 1981;18:47–53.

125. McNeer G, Bowden L, Booher RJ, McPeak CJ. Elective total gastrectomy for cancer of the stomach: End results. Ann Surg 1974;180:252–256.

126. Gouzi JL, Juguier M, Fagniez PL, et al. Total versus subtotal gastrectomy for adenocarcinoma of the gastric antrum. Ann Surg 1989;209:162–166.

127. Butler JA, Dubrow TJ, Trezona T, Klassen M, Nejdl RJ. Total gastrectomy in the treatment of advanced gastric cancer. Am J Surg 1989;158:602–605.

128. Kawaura Y, Mori Y, Nakajima H, Iwa T. Total gastrectomy with left oblique abdominothoracic approach for gastric cancer involving the esophagus. Arch Surg 1988;123:514–518.

129. Saario I, Salo J, Lempinen M, Kivilaakso E. Total and near-total gastrectomy for gastric cancer in patients over 70 years of age. Am J Surg 1987;154:269–270.

130. Paolini A, Tosato F, Cassese M, et al. Total gastrectomy in the treatment of adenocarcinoma of the cardia. Am J Surg 1986;151:238–243.

131. Buhl K, Schlag P, Herfarth C. Quality of life and functional results following different types of resection for gastric carcinoma. Eur J Surg Oncol 1990;16:404–409.

132. Viste A, Haugstvedt T, Eide GE, Soreide O. Postoperative complications and mortality after surgery for gastric cancer. Ann Surg 1981;207:7–13.

133. Sugimachi K, Kodama Y, Kumashiro R, Kanematsu T, Shoichi N, Inokuchi K. Critical evaluation of prophylactic splenectomy in total gastrectomy for the stomach cancer. Gann 1980;71:704–709.

134. Brady MS, Rogatko A, Dent LL, Shiu MH. Effect of splenectomy on morbidity and survival following curative gastrectomy for carcinoma. Arch Surg 1991;126:359–364.

135. Rohde H, Gebbensleben B, Bauer P. Has there been any improvement in the staging of gastric cancer? Findings from the German gastric cancer TNM study group. Cancer 1989;64:2465–2481.

136. Fisher V, Gunduz N, Saffer E. Influence of the interval between primary tumor removal and chemotherapy on kinetics and growth of metastasis. Cancer Res 1983;43:1488–1492.

137. Gunduz N, Fisher B, Saffer E. Effect of surgical removal on the growth and kinetics of residual tumor. Cancer Res 1979;39:1361–1365.

138. Eggermont A, Steller E, Sugarbaker P. Laparotomy enhances intraperitoneal growth and abrogates the anti-tumor effects of interleukin-II and lymphokine activated killer cells. Surgery 1987;102:71–77.

139. Murthy S, Goldschmidt R, Rao L, et al. The influence of surgical trauma on experimental metastasis. Cancer 1989;64:2035–2044.

140. VA Cooperative Surgical Adjuvant Study Group. Use of thiotepa as an adjuvant to the surgical management of carcinoma of the stomach. Cancer 1965;18:291–297.

141. Serlin O, Wolkoff J, Amadeo J, et al. Use of 5-fluorodeoxyuridine (FUDR) as an adjuvant to the surgical management of carcinoma of the stomach. Cancer 1969;25:223–228.

142. Gastrointestinal Tumor Study Group. Controlled trial of adjuvant chemotherapy following curative resection for gastric cancer. Cancer 1982;49:1116–1122.

143. Engstrom P, Labin P, Douglas H, et al. Postoperative adjuvant 5-fluorouracil plus methyl-CCNU therapy for gastric cancer patients. Cancer 1985;55:1868–1873.

144. Higgins G, Amadeo J, Smith D, et al. Efficacy of prolonged intermittent therapy with

combined 5-FU and methyl-CCNU following resection for gastric carcinoma. Cancer 1983;52:1105–1112.

145. Estape J, Grau J, Lcobendas F, et al. Mitomycin C as an adjuvant treatment to resected gastric cancer: A 10-year follow-up. Ann Surg 1991;213:219–221.

146. Allum W, Hallissey N, Kelly K. Adjuvant chemotherapy in operable gastric cancer: 5-year follow-up of first British Stomach Cancer Group trial. Lancet 1989;1:571–574.

147. Nakajima T, Takahashi T, Takagi K, et al. Comparison of 5-fluorouracil with Ftorafur in adjuvant chemotherapies with combined inductive and maintenance therapies for gastric cancer. J Clin Oncol 1984;2:1366–1371.

148. Ochiai T, Sato H, et al. A randomly controlled study of chemotherapy versus chemo immunotherapy in postoperative gastric cancer patients. Cancer Res 1983;43:3001–3007.

149. Coombes R, Schein P, Chilvers C, et al. A randomized trial comparing adjuvant fluorouracil, doxorubicin, and mitomycin with no treatment in operable gastric cancer. J Clin Oncol 1990;8:1362–1369.

150. Gagliano R, McCracken J, Chen T. Adjuvant chemotherapy with FAM in gastric cancer: A SWOG study. Proc Am Soc Clin Oncol 1983;2:114.

151. Krook J, O'Connell M, Wieand H, et al. A prospective randomized evaluation of intensive-course 5-fluorouracil plus doxorubicin as surgical adjuvant chemotherapy for resected gastric cancer. Cancer 1991;67:2454–2458.

152. Estrada E, Lacave L, Valle M, et al. Methyl-CCNU, 5-fluorouracil, and Adriamycin (MeFA) as adjuvant chemotherapy in gastric cancer. Proc Am Soc Clin Oncol 1988;7: 94.

153. Harrison J, Morris D, Ellis I, et al. The effect of tamoxifen and receptor status on survival in gastric carcinoma. Cancer 1989;64:1007–1010.

154. Muggia F, Gill I. Primary chemotherapy. PPO Updates 1990:2.

155. Fein R, Kelsen DP, Geller N, et al. Adenocarcinoma of the esophagus and gastroesophageal junction: Results of therapy and prognostic variables. Cancer 1985;56: 2512–2519.

156. Markman M. Intraperitoneal chemotherapy for malignant diseases of the gastrointestinal tract. Surg Gynecol Obstet 1987;164:89–93.

157. Sugarbaker P, Cunliffe W, Belliveau J, et al. Rationale for integrating early postoperative intraperitoneal chemotherapy into the surgical treatment of gastrointestinal cancer. Semin Oncol 1989;16:83–97.

158. Archer S, Grey B. Intraperitoneal 5-fluorouracil infusion for treatment of both peritoneal and liver micro-metastasis. Surgery 1990;108:502–507.

158a. Sugarbaker P, Gianola F, Speyer J, Wesley R, Barofsky I, Meyers C. Prospective randomized trial of intravenous versus intraperitoneal 5-fluorouracil in patients with primary colon or rectal cancer. Surgery 1985;98:414–421.

159. Schiessel R, Funovicks J, Schick B, et al. Adjuvant intraperitoneal cisplatin therapy in patients with operated gastric carcinoma: Results of a randomized trial. AMA 1989;16:68–69.

160. Atiq O, Kelsen D, Shiu M, et al. Postoperative adjuvant intraperitoneal and intravenous chemotherapy in poor-risk gastric cancer patients. Proc Am Soc Clin Oncol 1991;10: 137.

161. Nakajima T. Adjuvant chemotherapy for gastric cancer in Japan: Present status and suggestions for rational clinical trials. Jpn J Clin Oncol 1991;67:2588–2593.

162. Childs D, Moertel C, Holbrook M, Reitemeier R, Colby M. Treatment of unresectable adenocarcinomas of the stomach with a combination of 5-Fluorouracil and radiation. Am J Roentgenol Radium Ther Nucl Med 1968;102:541–544.

163. Dent D, Werner I, Novis B, et al. Prospective randomized trial of combined oncological therapy for gastric carcinoma. Cancer 1979;44:385–391.

164. Moertel C, Childs D, O'Fallon J, Holbrook M, Schutt A, Reitemeier R. Combined 5-fluorouracil and radiation therapy as a surgical adjuvant for poor prognosis gastric carcinoma. J Clin Oncol 1984;2:1249–1254.

165. Slot A, Meerwaldt J, van Putten W, Treurniet-Donker A. Adjuvant postoperative radiotherapy for gastric carcinoma with poor prognostic signs. Radiother Oncol 1989;16: 269–274.

166. Gunderson L, Sosin H. Combined modality treatment of gastric cancer. Int J Radiat Oncol Biol Phys 1983;9:965–975.

167. Caudry M, Escarmant P, Maire J, Demeaux H, Guichard F, Azaloux H. Radiotherapy of gastric cancer with a three field combination: Feasibility, tolerance, and survival. Int J Radiat Oncol Biol Phys 1987;13:1821–1827.

168. Abe M, Takashashi M. Intraoperative radiotherapy: The Japanese experience. Int J Radiat Oncol Biol Phys 1981;7:863–868.

169. Sindelar W, Kinsella T. Randomized trial of resection and intraoperative radiotherapy in locally advanced gastric cancer. Proc Am Soc Clin Oncol 1987;28:91.

170. Willett C, Tepper J, Orlow E, Shipley W. Renal complications secondary to radiation treatment of upper abdominal malignancies. Int J Radiat Oncol Biol Phys 1986;12: 1601–1604.

171. Comis S. Integration of chemotherapy into combined modality treatment of solid tumors. Cancer Treat Rep 1974;1:221–238.

172. Cocconi G, DeLisi V, Di Blasio B. Randomized comparison of 5-FU alone or combined with mitomycin and cytarabine (MFC) in the treatment of advanced gastric cancer. Cancer Treat Rep 1982;66:1263–1266.

173. Gastrointestinal Tumor Study Group. Phase II–III chemotherapy studies in advanced gastric cancer. Cancer Treat Rep 1979;63:1871.

174. Moertel CG, Lavin PT. Phase II–III chemotherapy studies in advanced gastric cancer. Cancer Treat Rep 1979;63:1863.

175. Preusser P, Achterrath W, Wilke H, et al. Chemotherapy of gastric cancer. Cancer Treat Rev 1988;15:257–277.

176. Levi JA, Fox RM, Tattersall MH. Analysis of a prospectively randomized comparison

177. Lacave AJ, Izarzugaza I, Aparicio IMAG, et al. Phase II clinical trial of *cis*-dichlorodiammineplatinum in gastric cancer. Am J Clin Oncol 1983;6:35–38.

178. Aabo K, Pedersen H, Rorth M. Cisplatin in the treatment of advanced gastric carcinoma: A phase II study. Cancer Treat Rep 1985;69:449–450.

179. Lacave AJ, Wils J, Diaz-Rubio E, et al. Cisplatinum as second-line chemotherapy in advanced gastric adenocarcinoma: A phase II study of the EORTC gastrointestinal tract cancer cooperative group. Eur J Cancer Clin Oncol 1985;21:1321–1329.

180. Perry MC, Green MR, Mick R, et al. Cisplatin in patients with gastric cancer: A cancer and leukemia group B phase II study. Cancer Treat Rep 1986;70:415–416.

181. Kantarjian H, Ajani JA, Karlin DA. *Cis*-diaminodichloroplatinum (II) chemotherapy for advanced adenocarcinoma of the upper gastrointestinal tract. Oncology 1985;42: 69–71.

182. Leichman L, McDonald B, Dindogru A, et al. Cisplatin: An active drug in the treatment of disseminated gastric cancer. Cancer 1984;53:18–22.

183. Vogl SE, Camacho FJ, Engstrom PF, Bennett JM. Phase II trial of cisplatin in advanced gastric cancer. Cancer Treat Rep 1984;68:1497–1498.

184. Beer M, Cocconi G, Ceci G, et al. A phase II study of cisplatin in advanced gastric cancer. Eur J Cancer Clin Oncol 1983;19:717–720.

185. The Southeastern Cancer Study Group. m-AMSA treatment of advanced colorectal, pancreatic, and gastric carcinoma. Proc Am Soc Clin Oncol 1981;22:454.

186. Grohn P, Heinonen E, Kumpulainen E, et al. Oral carmofur in advanced gastrointestinal cancer. Am J Clin Oncol 1990;13:477–479.

187. Bjerkeset T, Fjosne H. Comparison of oral Ftorafur and intravenous 5-fluorouracil in patients with advanced cancer of the stomach, colon, or rectum. Oncology 1986;43: 212–215.

188. Jin ML. Combined UFTM for 140 patients with advanced gastric cancer. Chung Hua Chung Liu Tsa Chih 1989;11:130–132.

189. Livingston RB, Carter SK. Single agents in cancer chemotherapy. New York: Plenum Press, 1970.

190. Wadler S, Green M, Muggia F. The role of anthracyclines in the treatment of gastric cancer. Cancer Treat Rev 1985;12:105–132.

191. Cazup E, Estevez R, Bruno M, et al. Phase II trial of 4'-epi-doxorubicin in locally advanced or metastatic gastric cancer. Cancer Treat Rev 1988;74:313–315.

192. Kelsen DP, Magill R, Cheng E, et al. Phase II trial of etoposide (VP-16) in the treatment of upper gastrointestinal tract malignancies. Cancer Treat Rep 1983;67:509–510.

193. Kovach JS, Moertel CG, Schutt AJ. A controlled study of combined 1,3-bis-2-chloroethyl-1-nitorsourea and 5-fluorouracil therapy for advanced gastric and pancreatic cancer. Cancer 1974;33:563.

194. Moertel CG, Mittelman JA, Bakermeier RF, et al. Sequential and combination chemotherapy of advanced gastric cancer. Cancer 1976;38:678.

195. Asbury RF, Cnaan A, Haller D. Eastern Cooperative Oncology Group (ECOG) phase II study of trimetrexate (TMTX) in metastatic gastric cancer. Proc Am Soc Clin Oncol 1990;9:126.

196. Bruckner HW, Lokich JJ, Stablein DM. Studies of Baker's antifol, methotrexate, and Razoxane in advanced gastric cancer: A gastrointestinal tumor study group report. Cancer Treat Rep 1982;66:1713–1717.

197. Kim DJ, Kim NK, Meng KH. Phase II trial of carboplatin (CBDCA) in patients with advanced adenocarcinoma of the stomach. Proc Am Soc Clin Oncol 1989;8:114.

198. De Simone P, Kramer B, Omura GA, Bartolucci AA. Phase II evaluation of diaziquone in gastric and pancreatic cancers. Am J Clin Oncol 1986;9:401–402.

199. Panettiere F, Jones S, Jischi N, et al. Bisantrene hydrochloride in gastric adenocarcinoma: A Southwest Oncology Group study. Med Pediatr Oncol 1986;14:78–80.

200. Moore G, Bross I, Ausman R, et al. Effects of chlorambucil (NSC 3088) in 374 patients with advanced cancer. Cancer Chemother Rep 1968;52:661.

201. Douglass H, Lavin P, Goudsmit A, et al. An Eastern Cooperative Oncology Group evaluation of combination of methyl-CCNU, mitomycin-C, Adriamycin, and 5-fluorouracil in advanced measurable gastric cancer (Est 2277). J Clin Oncol 1984;2: 1372–1381.

202. The Gastrointestinal Tumor Study Group. A comparative clinical assessment of combination chemotherapy in the management of advanced gastric carcinoma. Cancer 1982;1362:1366.

203. The Gastrointestinal Tumor Study Group. Randomized study of combination chemotherapy in unresectable gastric cancer. Cancer 1984;53:13–17.

204. Gastrointestinal Tumor Study Group. Triazinate and platinum efficacy in combination with 5-fluorouracil and doxorubicin: Results of a three-arm randomized trial in metastatic gastric cancer. JNCI 1988;80:1011–1015.

205. Lacave A, Wils J, Bleiberg H, et al. An EORTC gastrointestinal group phase III evaluation of combinations of methyl-CCNU, 5-fluorouracil, and Adriamycin in advanced gastric cancer. J Clin Oncol 1987;5:1387–1393.

206. Epelbaum R, Haim N, Stein M, et al. Treatment of advanced gastric cancer with DDP (cisplatin), Adriamycin, and 5-fluorouracil (DAF). Oncology 1987;44:201–206.

207. Schnitzler G, Queisser W, Heim ME, et al. Phase III study of 5-FU and carmdustine versus 5-FU, carmustine, and doxorubicin in advanced gastric cancer. Cancer Treat Rep 1986;70:477–479.

208. Lopez M, DiLauro L, Papaldo P, Conti EMS. Treatment of advanced measurable gastric carcinoma with 5-fluorouracil, Adriamycin, and BCNU. Oncology 1986;43: 288–291.

209. Janieson G, Gill P. A prospective trial of 5-FU and BCNU in the treatment of advanced gastric cancer. Aust N Z J Surg 1985;5:16–19.

210. Levi J, Dalley D, Aroney R. Improved combination chemotherapy in advanced gastric cancer. Br Med J 1979;2:1471–1473.

211. Levi J, Fox R, Tattersall M, et al. Analysis of a prospectively randomized comparison

of doxorubicin versus 5-fluorouracil, doxorubicin, and BCNYU in advanced gastric cancer: Implications for future studies. J Clin Oncol 1986;4:1348–1355.

212. Macdonald JS, Schein PS, Woolley PV, et al. 5-Fluorouracil, mitomycin-C, and Adriamycin (FAM): A new combination chemotherapy program for advanced gastric carcinoma. Ann Intern Med 1980;93:533.

213. Cullinan SA, Moertel CG, Fleming TR, et al. A comparison of three chemotherapeutic regimens in the treatment of advanced pancreatic and gastric carcinoma. JAMA 1985;253:2061–2067.

214. Cunningham D, Cahn A, Menzies-Gow N. Cisplatin, epirubicin, and 5-fluorouracil (CEF) has significant activity in advanced gastric cancer. Proc Am Soc Clin Oncol 1990;9:123.

215. Caccia G, Alasino C, Fein L. 5-Fluorouracil plus epirubicin in patients with advanced gastric cancer. Proc Am Soc Clin Oncol 1990;9:123.

216. Ogawa M. A recent overview of chemotherapy for advanced stomach cancer in Japan. Appl Cancer Chemother 1978;24:149–159.

217. Mabel JA, Little AD. Therapeutic synergism in murine tumors for combinations of *cis*-dichlorodiammine platinum with VP-16-213 or BCNU. Proc Am Assoc Cancer Res 1979;20:230.

218. Seeber S, Osieka R, Schmidt CG, et al. In vivo resistance towards anthracyclines, etoposide, and *cis*-diamminedichloroplatinum (II). Cancer Res 1982;67:4719–4725.

219. Kelsen DP, Buckner J, Einzig A, et al. Phase II trial of cisplatin and etoposide in adenocarcinomas of the upper gastrointestinal tract. Cancer Treat Rep 1987;71:329–330.

220. Elliot T, Moertel C, Wieand H, et al. A phase II study of the combination of etoposide and cisplatin in the therapy of advanced gastric cancer. Cancer 1990;65:1491–1494.

221. Preusser P, Wilke H, Achtermath W, et al. Phase II study with the combination etoposide, doxorubicin, and cisplatin in advanced measurable gastric cancer. J Clin Oncol 1989;7:1310–1317.

222. Wilke H, Preusser P, Fink U, et al. Preoperative chemotherapy in locally advanced and nonresectable gastric cancer: A phase II study with etoposide, doxorubicin and cisplatin. J Clin Oncol 1989;7:1318–1326.

223. Katz A, Gansl R, Simon S, et al. Phase II trial of VP-16, Adriamycin, and cisplatinum in patients with advanced gastric cancer. Proc Am Soc Clin Oncol 1989;8:98.

224. Taguchi T. Combination chemotherapy with etoposide, Adriamycin and cisplatin (EAP) for advanced gastric cancer. Proc Am Soc Clin Oncol 1989;8:108.

225. Lerner A, Steele GD, Mayer RJ. Etoposide, doxorubicin, and cisplatin for advanced gastric adenocarcinoma: Results of a phase II trial. Proc Am Soc Clin Oncol 1990;9:103.

226. Wilke H, Preusser P, Fink U, et al. New developments in the treatment of gastric carcinoma. Semin Oncol 1990;17:61–70.

227. Klein HO. Long-term results with FAMTX (5-fluorouracil, Adriamycin, methotrexate) in advanced gastric cancer. Cancer Res 1989;9:1025–1026.

228. Kelsen D, Atiq O, Saltz L, et al. FAMTX (fluorouracil, methotrexate, Adriamycin) is as effective and less toxic than EAP (etoposide, Adriamycin, cisplatin): A random assignment trial in gastric cancer. Proc Am Soc Clin Oncol 1991;10:137.

229. Wils JA, Klein HO, Wagener DJT, et al. Sequential high-dose methotrexate and fluorouracil combined with doxorubicin—a step ahead in the treatment of advanced gastric cancer: A trial of the European Organization for Research and Treatment of Cancer Gastrointestinal Tract Cooperative Group. J Clin Oncol 1991;9:827–831.

230. Ekbom GA, Gleysteen JJ. Gastric malignancy: Resection for palliation. Surgery 1980;88:476–481.

231. Meijer S, De Bakker OJGB, Hoitsma HFW. Palliative resection in gastric cancer. J Surg Oncol 1983;23:77–80.

232. Aranha GV, Georgen R. Gastric linitis plastica is not a surgical disease. Surgery 1989;106:758–763.

233. Bozzetti F, Bonfanti G, Audisio RA, et al. Prognosis of patients after palliative surgical procedures for carcinoma of the stomach. Surg Gynecol Obstet 1987;164:151–154.

234. Boddie AW Jr, McMurtrey MJ, Diacco GG, McBride CM. Palliative total gastrectomy and esophagogastrectomy. Cancer 1983;51:1195–1200.

235. Warwick M. Analysis of one hundred and seventy-six cases of carcinoma of the stomach submitted to autopsy. Ann Surg 1928;88:216.

236. Dupont JB Jr, Lee JR, Burton GR, Cohn I Jr. Adenocarcinoma of the stomach: Review of 1,497 cases. Cancer 1978;41:941–947.

237. Clarke JS, Cruze K, El Farra S, et al. The natural history and results of surgical therapy for carcinoma of the stomach: An analysis of 250 cases. Am J Surg 1961;102:143.

238. Weh H, Platz D, Garbrecth M, et al. Ergobnis eines modifzerten FAMeth chemotherapei protokolls beim metastasierten magenkarzinom. Dtsch Med Wochenschr 1989;114:1391–1396.

239. Hermann R, Fritz D, Queizer W, et al. Chemotherapei des magenkarzinom. Dtsch Med Wochenschr 1984;109:1463.

240. Wils J, Beliberg H, Blijham G, et al. An EORTC gastrointestinal evaluation of the combination of sequential methotrexate and 5-fluorouracil combined with Adriamycin in advanced measurable gastric cancer. J Clin Oncol 1986;4:1799–1803.

241. Kimura H, Yonemura Y. Flow cytometric analysis of nuclear DNA content in advanced gastric cancer and its relationship with prognosis. Cancer 1991;67:2588–2593.

242. Baba H, Korenaga D, Okamura T, et al. Prognostic significance of DNA content with special reference to age in gastric cancer. Cancer 1989;63:1768–1772.

243. de Aretxabala X, Yonemura Y, Sugiyama K, et al. DNA ploidy pattern and tumor spread in gastric cancer. Br J Surg 1988;75:770–773.

244. Korenaga D, Okamura T, Saito A, et al. DNA ploidy is closely linked to tumor invasion, lymph node metastasis and prognosis in clinical gastric cancer. Cancer 1988;62:309–313.

245. Ballantyne K, James P, Robins R, et al. Flow cytometric analysis of the DNA content of gastric cancer. Br J Cancer 1987;56:52–54.

246. Schneeberger A, Finley R, Trooster M, et al. The prognostic significance of tumor ploidy and pathology in adenocarcinoma of the esophagogastric junction. Cancer 1990;65:1206–1210.

Cancer: Principles & Practice of Oncology, Fourth Edition,
edited by Vincent T. DeVita, Jr., Samuel Hellman, Steven A. Rosenberg.
J.B. Lippincott Co., Philadelphia © 1993.

Murray F. Brennan

Timothy J. Kinsella

Ephraim S. Casper

CHAPTER **27**

Cancer of the Pancreas

Pancreatic cancer is the fourth largest cancer killer of adults in the United States. The incidence of new cases of the disease and the death rate each year remain close. In 1991, approximately 28,000 new cases were seen in the United States, and 25,200 deaths occurred. The incidence is exceeded only by lung, colorectal, skin, prostate, and breast cancers.[1]

EPIDEMIOLOGIC CONSIDERATIONS

Because most patients with pancreatic cancer die from the disease, mortality data are a good indicator of incidence, provided that diagnostic accuracy is high.[2] Diagnostic accuracy can be checked by comparing the number of cases histologically confirmed at operation, biopsy, or autopsy with the number of cases diagnosed. For cancer of the pancreas, this varies from 75% to 95%.[2]

The incidence of cancer of the pancreas is stable compared with other cancers, and age-specific death rates increase with age (Fig. 27–1).[2] Risk increases after age 30, with most cases occurring between 65 and 79.[3] The median age at presentation in national surveys from 1973 through 1977 is 69.2 years for men and 69.5 years for women.[4] Of 1179 patients suspected of having peripancreatic cancer presenting to Memorial Sloan-Kettering Cancer Center (MSKCC) from October 1983 to October 1990, the overall male to female ratio was 1.3:1.0. A male to female ratio of 1.7:1.0 for pancreatic cancer only was found in other series.[5] The male to female ratio differs according to age and has been reported for pancreatic cancer deaths, varying from 2:1 for patients younger than 40 years of age to 1:1 for patients older than 80 years. Current data suggest that the male to female ratios for age at presentation younger than 40 are 1.4:1, 1.5:1 for 41 to 50 years, 1.3:1 for 51 to 80 years; and 1.8:1 for patients older than 80.

The incidence of pancreatic cancer in several predomi-

nantly Spanish populations in the United States varies from 3.4 per 100,000 women in Puerto Rico to 9.3 per 100,000 Spanish men in New Mexico.[6] These racial differences are emphasized by the incidence in Korean men in Los Angeles (16.4 per 100,000), black men in Los Angeles (11.0 per 100,000), and Chinese men in the same city (3.7 per 100,000). Intermediate rates are seen for the United States white population, the Spanish population, and the Japanese population.

The incidence in countries of origin and in first-generation and second-generation immigrants has been examined. The rate in the first generation rapidly increases to the rate of U.S. whites. This is not solely due to smoking, although it may account for the effect in Japanese and Chinese populations.[7]

The influence of birthplace has been examined in Israel, and the incidence of carcinoma of the pancreas varies from 9.9 per 100,000 men born in Europe or America to 6.4 per 100,000 men born in Africa or Asia. In non-Jewish residents, the incidence is 3.1 per 100,000.

Similar wide variations can be demonstrated in male incidence at various sites within different countries. For example, incidences vary from 9.5 per 100,000 in Saskatchewan, Canada, to 2.2 in the Northwestern Territory of Canada. There has been a progressive international increase in the incidence of pancreatic cancer. In England and Wales from 1911 to 1971, the mortality from cancer of the pancreas in men and women increased at least fivefold.[8] The one exception is India, which shows the lowest incidence for men and women.[6] Rates in the United States appear stable.

ETIOLOGIC FACTORS

Several environmental factors have been associated with an increased risk of pancreatic carcinoma, although the exact

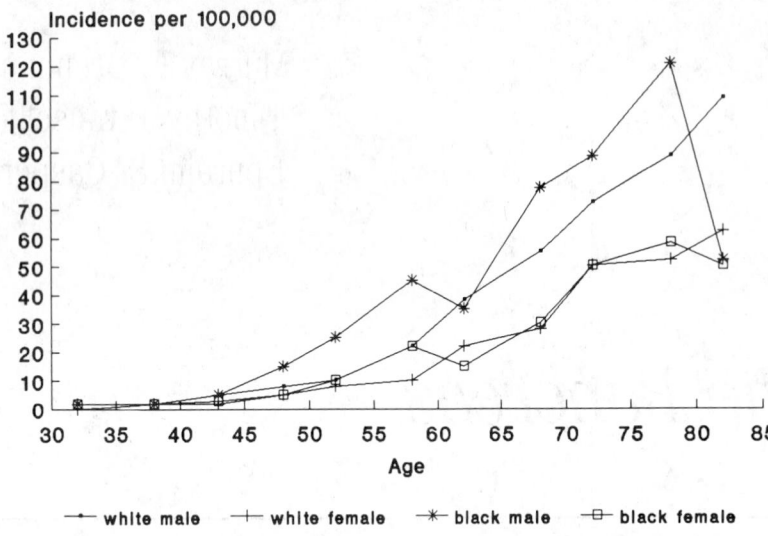

Incidence per 100,000

← white male   + white female   —*— black male   —□— black female

Levin DL. Cancer 31:1231, 1973

FIGURE 27–1. Epidemiology of pancreatic cancer from the Third National Cancer survey. Age-specific death rates increase with age. (Levin DL. Connelly RR. Cancer of the pancreas: Available epidemiologic information and its implications. Cancer 1973;31:1231)

cause remains unclear. Pancreatic carcinoma, like several other common malignancies, appears to be more prevalent among persons in lower socioeconomic groups.[9] Close scrutiny of the available epidemiologic studies shows that pancreatic carcinoma has less of a demographic association with social class than do other common malignancies, such as breast and lung carcinoma.[5,9] Several dietary factors have been implicated. At least one study showed a positive correlation between coffee consumption and pancreatic carcinoma.[10] In this case-control study, patients with carcinoma of the pancreas had a history of greater coffee consumption than the control group of patients with benign gastrointestinal disorders. Because the control group contained patients with peptic ulcer disease and had an overall average coffee intake below the level of consumption for the general population, it is difficult to confirm whether patients with cancer of the pancreas actually consumed more coffee than is considered average. There have been at least two other studies that have not confirmed the association of coffee intake and pancreatic carcinoma.[11,12]

One study suggested an association between alcohol consumption and an increased risk of carcinoma of the pancreas.[13] In Finnish men with a history of alcohol abuse, an excess of pancreatic carcinoma was found, compared with the overall Finnish population. At least three other studies have shown little or no correlation between alcohol consumption and pancreatic carcinoma.[14-16]

Cigarette smoking has been associated with an increased risk of pancreatic carcinoma.[2,17,18] A study from Veterans Administration hospitals showed almost twice the rate of pancreatic carcinoma for heavy cigarette smokers (*i.e.*, at least two packs daily) compared with nonsmokers.[19] Cigarette smoke contains carcinogens, including the nitrosamines that have induced pancreatic malignancies in laboratory animals.[20,21]

An increased incidence of pancreatic carcinoma occurs among patients with chronic pancreatitis.[22,23] Calcifications associated with chronic pancreatitis have been found in 3% of patients with documented pancreatic carcinoma.[24,25] However, there appears to be no association between biliary calcifications and carcinoma of the pancreas.[26] Epidemiologic

studies of patients have shown that almost 15% have a history of diabetes mellitus, which appears to be higher than expected.[27,28] In more than half of the patients with diabetes and pancreatic carcinoma, the onset of clinical diabetes preceded the diagnosis of pancreatic carcinoma by no longer than 3 months.[26,28] This suggests that the carcinoma may cause pancreatic endocrine insufficiency. Diabetes mellitus, presenting many months to years before the development of pancreatic carcinomas, would be better evidence for an etiologic correlation, but this type of temporal association is not commonly found.[27]

Long-term exposures to solvents and petroleum compounds appear to increase the risk of pancreatic carcinoma.[26] A prospective study of workers exposed to benzidine and β-naphthylamine showed a higher incidence.[29] The nitrosamines are recognized as potent pancreatic carcinogens in hamsters.[30] Azaserine has produced pancreatic tumors in rats.[31] Exposure for 10 years or longer to these industrial chemicals may increase the risk of pancreatic carcinoma by a factor of five.[26]

ANATOMIC CONSIDERATIONS

The pancreas lies transversely in the posterior peritoneum of the upper abdomen and weighs approximately 100 g. The superior part of the duodenum overlaps the pancreas and passes backward, upward, and to the right. The remaining parts are overlapped by the pancreas itself. The tail of the pancreas usually extends out to the splenic hilum, and it is approximately 15 cm long.

The surgically important lymphatic drainage is in intimate association with the surface and borders of the pancreas and indirectly with the celiac, preaortic, and superior mesenteric groups. Because of the diffuse, surrounding lymphatic drainage, it is thought that tumors in the pancreas can drain virtually to any of the surrounding node-bearing areas.

The diameter of the pancreatic duct varies. Within the head, it is 3 to 4.8 mm; within the body, 2 to 3.5 mm; and within the tail, 0.9 to 2.4 mm.[32] Two to 3 ml of contrast material can fill the main pancreatic duct, and 7 to 10 ml can fill the smaller ducts.[33]

The uncinate process can extend from just behind the vessels to the left of the superior mesenteric artery and is an important feature of transection during operation. Failure to remove this portion of the uncinate process completely in a pancreaticoduodenectomy can result in troublesome intraoperative and postoperative bleeding.

The most important anatomic abnormalities that influence pancreatic resection are those of vascular supply. There are usually variations in the hepatic artery; the most common abnormality is the right hepatic artery, arising from the superior mesenteric artery. The course is variable and usually proceeds behind the common duct and the portal vein. This can occur in as many as 25% of patients. The accessory left hepatic artery is rarely a problem, because it tends to rise from the common hepatic or left gastric artery and passes in the lesser omentum. Rarely, it may arise from the superior mesenteric or from the gastroduodenal artery. In 2% to 4% of patients, the common hepatic artery arises from the superior mesenteric and occasionally passes through the head of the pancreas, which can be a major problem during resection.[34]

The portal vein rarely lies anterior to the duodenum. Biliary tract abnormalities usually accompany this vascular abnor-mality. The portal vein may communicate with the superior vena cava, and rarely, a pulmonary vein joins the portal vein. Congenital strictures in the portal vein can occur, and the preduodenal portal vein is often associated with other abnormalities of the pancreas, including malrotation.

PATHOLOGIC CLASSIFICATION

Pancreatic cancers arise from the exocrine and endocrine parenchyma of the gland.[35,36] Approximately 95% occur within the exocrine portion of the pancreas and may arise from ductal epithelium, acinar cells, connective tissue, or lymphatic deposits. Only 2% of tumors of the exocrine pancreas are benign.[37]

The less common tumors of the endocrine pancreas arise from islet of Langerhans cells, and most are benign. An overview of the classification of benign and malignant tumors of the pancreas are presented in Table 27-1.

The most common pancreatic cancer is a ductal adenocarcinoma, which accounts for about 80% of all pancreatic cancers.[38] In a recent analysis of patients presenting to the MSKCC, 69% of 1192 admitted during 7 years with peripancreatic cancer had adenocarcinoma of the pancreas. Less

TABLE 27-1. Histogenic Classification of Pancreatic Neoplasms

Origin	Benign	Malignant
Duct Cell	Polyp	Duct cell carcinoma
	Papilloma	Giant cell carcinoma
	Adenoma	Adenosquamous carcinoma
	Cystadenoma	Microglandular adenocarcinoma
	Oncocytoma	Mucinous carcinoma
	Benign papillary cystic neoplasm	Cystadenocarcinoma
		Papillary cystic carcinoma
Acinar Cell	Acinar cell adenoma	Acinar cell carcinoma
	Acinar cell cystadenoma	Acinar cell cystadenocarcinoma
Connective Tissue	Lipoma	Malignant fibrous histiocytoma
	Leiomyoma	Fibrosarcoma
	Benign peripheral nerve tumor	Liposarcoma
	Hemangioma	Leiomyosarcoma
	Lymphangioma	Malignant peripheral nerve tumor
		Rhabdomyosarcoma
		Hemangiosarcoma
		Lymphangiosarcoma
		Hemangiopericytoma
		Malignant lymphoma
		Plasmacytoma
Islet Cell	Insulinoma	Malignant insulinoma
	Glucagonoma	Malingnant glucagonoma
	Gastrinoma	Malignant gastrinoma
	Adenoma, functionally inactive	Islet cell carcinoma, functionally inactive
		Islet cell carcinoma carcinoid type
Uncertain	Fibroadenoma	Pancreaticoblastoma

(Modified from Cubilla AL, Fitzgerald PJ. Tumors of the exocrine pancreas. Washington, DC: Armed Forces Institute of Pathology, 1984 and from Legg MA: Pathology of the pancreas. In: Brooks JR, ed. Surgery of the pancreas. Philadelphia; WB Saunders, 1983:41-77)

common ductal cancers include squamous cell carcinomas, giant cell carcinomas, and carcinosarcomas. Carcinomas of the pancreas usually arise in the proximal gland, which includes the head, neck, and uncinate process.[39] Carcinomas arise in the distal gland less commonly, with 20% of all carcinomas occurring in the body and 5% to 10% occurring in the tail. Grossly, carcinomas appear hard and gritty and are often whitish. Microscopic changes of acute and, more commonly, chronic pancreatitis often surround a pancreatic carcinoma and can make the diagnosis difficult, especially if small amounts of tissue are obtained with a percutaneous biopsy.

Because most pancreatic tumors are ductal in origin, pancreatic ductal obstruction is a common finding. Cancers in the pancreatic head often produce obstruction of the pancreatic and common bile ducts. Invasion of adjacent duodenum, with ulceration and partial or complete duodenal obstruction, occurs in as many as 25% of pancreatic head cancers.[39] Obstruction of the portal or superior mesenteric vein can result from local invasion of tumors of the proximal pancreas. Tumors of the distal gland are often larger at diagnosis (5–10 cm) than proximal gland tumors.[35,36] These distal tumors of the pancreatic body and tail can obstruct the splenic vein. A characteristic pathologic feature of pancreatic adenocarcinomas is the early development of subclinical metastases.[26,39] Fewer than 20% of patients have disease macroscopically confined to the pancreas at diagnosis; 40% of patients present with locally advanced disease, including involvement of regional lymph nodes and adjacent pancreatic tissue, and more than 40% have identifiable visceral metastases at presentation, usually involving the liver.[26] Peritoneal implants occur in 35% of patients at presentation. The natural history of pancreatic carcinomas is highlighted by widespread metastases to other abdominal viscera and extraabdominal spread to lung, bone, and brain.

Cystic neoplasms of the pancreas are rare tumors that have characteristic pathologic features.[35,36] These tumors are usually large, filled with mucinous secretions, and may be multilocular. Microscopically, the cysts are lined with columnar epithelium alone (*i.e.*, cystadenomas) or with a mixture of columnar epithelium and atypical malignant epithelial cells (*i.e.*, cystadenocarcinomas). These carcinomas are usually localized, and approximately 50% of patients can be cured with surgery alone. Papillary-cystic neoplasms are usually seen in young women and make up less than 0.5% of all peripancreatic cancers.[40] The tumors are usually large at the time of presentation, often with local invasion, but with a relatively indolent course. Other rare (<1%) tumors of the nonendocrine pancreas include acinar cell carcinomas, pancreatic sarcomas, and lymphomas.

CLINICAL FEATURES

STAGING

In 1981, the American Joint Committee for Cancer Staging and End Results Reporting published a staging system for pancreatic carcinoma based on the extent of the primary tumor, the status of regional lymph nodes, and the presence of metastatic disease.[41] This TNM staging system is presented in Table 27–2. The primary tumor status was defined by ex-

TABLE 27–2. Staging of Carcinoma of the Pancreas

TNM Classification

T1	No direct extension of the primary tumor beyond the pancreas
T2	Limited direct extension to duodenum, bile duct, or stomach
T3	Advanced direct extension, incompatible with surgical resection
TX	Direct extension not assessed
N0	Regional lymph nodes not involved
N1	Regional lymph nodes involved
NX	Regional lymph nodes not assessed
M0	No distant metastasis
M1	Distant metastasis present
MX	Distant metastasis not assessed

TNM Staging System

Stage I	T1–2, N0, M0
	No direct extension with no regional nodal involvement
Stage II	T3, N0, M0
	Direct extension into adjacent tissue with no lymph node involvement
Stage III	T1–3, N1, M0
	Regional lymph node involvement with or without direct tumor extension
Stage IV	T1–3, N0–1, M1
	Distant metastatic disease present

tension through the pancreatic capsule; nodal status was defined by the presence of regional pancreatic lymph node involvement; and metastatic disease status was defined by the presence of distal lymph node, peritoneal, or visceral metastatic disease. In the surgical staging system based on the TNM system, stage I disease is localized within the pancreatic capsule and amenable to surgical resection; stage II disease is locally advanced with invasion of the duodenum or peripancreatic soft tissue and not surgically resectable; stage III disease has regional lymph node involvement; and stage IV disease has distant metastases.

SIGNS AND SYMPTOMS

Cancer of the pancreas is a highly malignant disease. Most patients present with disease advanced beyond the scope of potentially curative treatment. The hallmarks of pancreatic carcinoma are pain and clinical wasting. Tumors in the head of the pancreas often cause biliary obstruction. Patients develop signs and symptoms of gastric outlet and duodenal obstruction because of local tumor invasion, with mechanical obstruction and motility problems, the cause of which is probably infiltration of the splanchnic nerves. Splanchnic nerve invasion produces severe pain, which is often difficult to eradicate by medication. Carcinoma of the body and tail rarely produces gastric obstruction because of local infiltration and is often asymptomatic until well advanced. Even without mechanical obstruction of the stomach and duodenum, marked loss of appetite is a common symptom. A typical patient with pancreatic carcinoma has lost more than 10% of his body weight at diagnosis, and wasting is progressive. Distant metastases, particularly to liver, occur early in the course of the disease.

The initial symptoms are nonspecific and insidious at onset. The typical patient reports a gradual onset of anorexia, nausea, upper to middle abdominal pain, and weight loss. Because of the nonspecific nature of these symptoms, early diagnosis of pancreatic cancer is difficult and requires a high index of suspicion on the part of the physician initially involved in the patient's care. A delay in diagnosis of several months from the initiation of symptoms is common. In a report from the Cancer of the Pancreas Task Force, fewer than 33% of patients experienced symptoms for 2 months or less before diagnosis.[41] Delays in diagnoses are reported in other large reviews.[39,42]

Pain is the most common symptom in patients with pancreatic cancer and is often the reason for seeking medical attention. Virtually all patients have pain at some point in the course of their disease. Typically, the pain is in the epigastrium or hypochondrium and is described as gnawing. Occasionally, pain may be relieved with meals, mimicking peptic ulcer disease. Radiation of pain to the low thoracic or upper lumbar back occurs in many patients, but back pain alone is an uncommon presentation of pancreatic carcinoma. Severe pain often indicates local tumor infiltration into the retroperitoneum and splanchnic nerve plexus and is often considered a sign of unresectability. Severe pain may be slightly more common with carcinomas of the pancreatic body and tail.[39]

Anorexia and weight loss are two other common symptoms. The cause of weight loss is unknown. A report of a small number of patients with pancreatic cancer and significant weight loss pointed to subclinical malabsorption, rather than inadequate caloric consumption, as the source of weight loss.[43] These patients responded to oral pancreatic enzyme supplements, but the theory of malabsorption requires additional study. The sudden onset of diabetes mellitus as a manifestation of pancreatic endocrine insufficiency is uncommon, but it is thought to be a sign of development of carcinoma of the pancreas.[44]

Obstructive jaundice is a common sign, particularly for lesions of the pancreatic head. Associated symptoms of dark urine and pale stools occur. Totally painless jaundice is not common in pancreatic carcinoma and occurs more often in ampullary carcinoma or a primary bile duct carcinoma.[45] Although the gallbladder is commonly distended at exploration, fewer than 33% of patients have a palpable gallbladder at presentation (Courvoisier's sign).[45] Splenomegaly, another uncommon physical finding, usually occurs with tumors of the distal gland involving splenic vein obstruction. Early spread of tumor to the liver and peritoneum occurs in 15% to 25% of patients and presents with the signs of a palpable liver or abdominal distension with ascites.[39]

Patients may have a higher risk for depression at diagnosis than patients with other abdominal tumors. One study reported depression in 67% of 46 patients with pancreatic carcinoma, compared with fewer than 10% of 64 patients with colon carcinoma.[46] Considering the delay in diagnosis of several months in most patients, a reactive depression may be expected. Patients with pancreatic carcinoma may have a higher frequency of venous thrombosis and migratory thrombophlebitis (Trousseau's sign).[47] Thrombophlebitis appears more commonly in patients with tumors of the distal pancreas, but there is no clear correlation between the development of thrombophlebitis with an underlying pancreatic carcinoma in an otherwise healthy patient.[45]

DIAGNOSIS

An algorithm for the diagnosis of adenocarcinoma of the pancreas is outlined in Figure 27–2. If pancreatic cancer is suspected because of nonspecific upper abdominal symptoms, weight loss, or jaundice, clinical confirmation is required. This is usually obtained by physical examination to confirm jaundice, ascites, palpable mass, or metastatic disease. Chemical

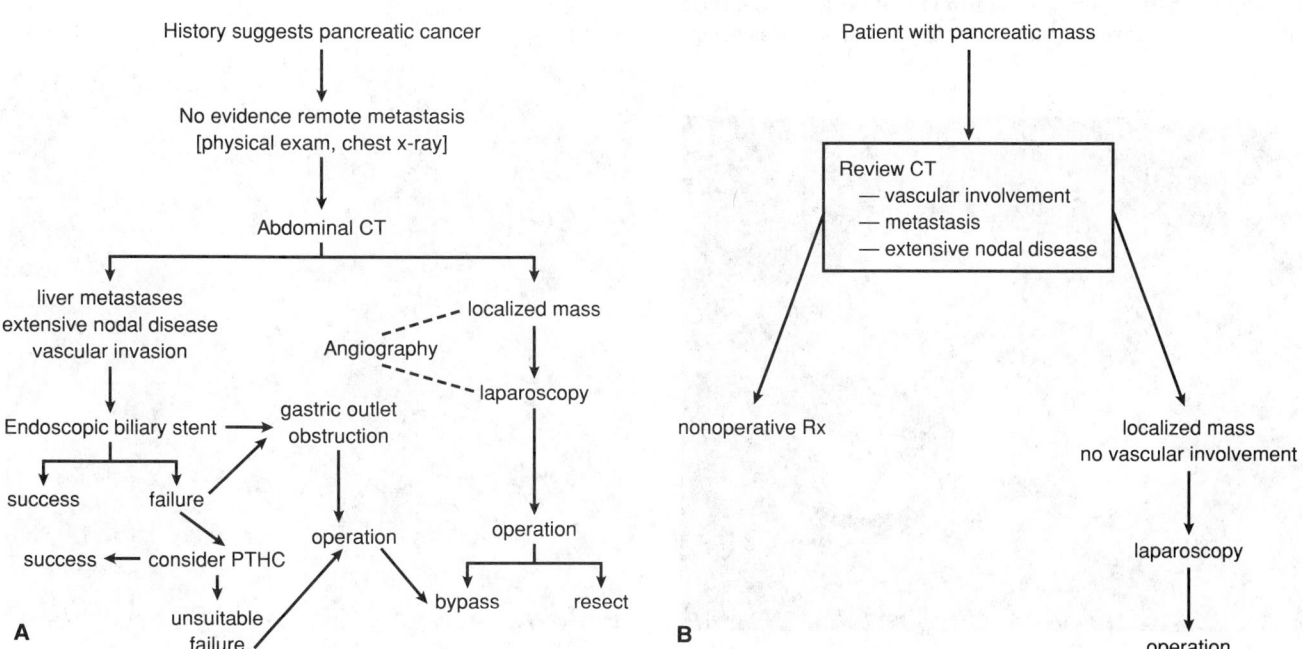

FIGURE 27–2. Algorithms for diagnosis of adenocarcinoma of the pancreas. **(A)** The jaundiced patient. **(B)** The nonjaundiced patient.

confirmation of the jaundice can be obtained by serum indices. Radiologic tests can evaluate the extent of the disease.

Computed tomography (CT) is the mainstay of diagnostic confirmation and evaluation of the extent of disease. CT can demonstrate the mass in the pancreas, metastatic disease in the liver and the periaortic and retropancreatic lymph nodes, and ascites. Enormous masses arising from the pancreas suggest lymphoma or sarcoma (Fig. 27–3). Clear identification of cystic changes, with or without calcification, suggests the possibility of cystadenoma or cystadenocarcinoma. Masses in young people suggest the possibility of pancreaticoblastoma.

Endosocopic retrograde cholangiopancreatography (ERCP) is a valuable tool in the diagnosis and in the localization of the tumor to the ampulla. The demonstration of obstructed, stenotic, or sclerosed ducts suggests adenocarcinoma (Fig. 27–4). A lesion seen on CT scan with a subsequently normal pancreatic duct may suggest an islet cell neoplasm and exclude pancreatic adenocarcinoma. Care must be taken not to misinterpret a normal duct as an islet cell tumor if the pancreatic lesion is an adenocarcinoma involving the uncinate process. CT results have positive identification rates from 63% to 100%, with an average of 65%. Ultrasound has a similar range, from 23% to 95%, and ERCP has a positive identification rate of 53% to 96%.[42]

If the tumor appears to be localized, the next step is to evaluate for resectability. CT plays a central role in determination of the involvement, particularly of superior mesenteric and celiac axis vessels.[42] If these vessels are not involved and a reasonable assessment can be made about obstruction of the portal vein on the basis of CT, resection can be considered. If the tumor is clearly unresectable or if metastatic disease is identified based on the CT scan, we proceed to pathologic confirmation. If there is concern about resectability and if there are compelling reasons not to explore the patient, we use angiography (Fig. 27–5).

Angiography is used to locate abnormal vasculature, such as a right hepatic artery arising from the superior mesenteric artery, and to determine unresectability based on encasement

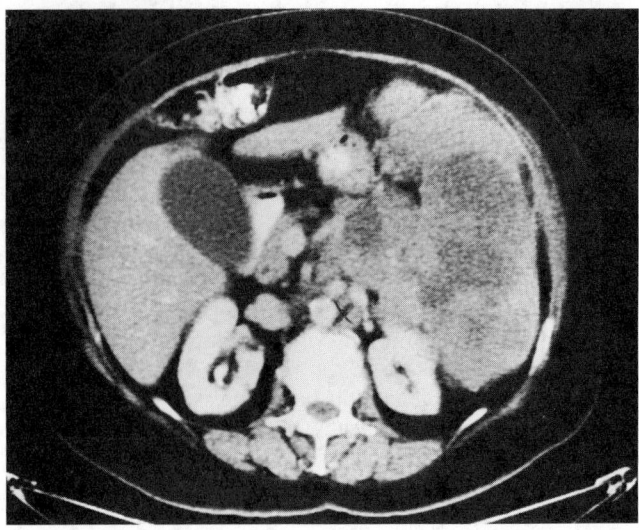

FIGURE 27–4. Large pancreatic mass shown subsequently to have a normal pancreatic duct by endoscopic retrograde cholangiopancreatography. The patient had a primary pancreatic lymphoma.

of the superior mesenteric or, rarely, hepatic or celiac axis arteries. The abnormal vasculature does not warrant the uniform use of angiography before surgery. The aberrant right hepatic artery can usually be detected in the porta hepatis at the time of resection and often runs behind the pancreas and porta hepatis, rather than directly through the pancreas. The complete encasement of the superior mesenteric or celiac arteries by adenocarcinoma is an absolute contraindication to resection.

If the tumor is deemed unresectable or metastatic disease is identified, histopathologic confirmation should be obtained by direct fine-needle biopsy of the pancreas or percutaneous biopsy of a liver metastasis.

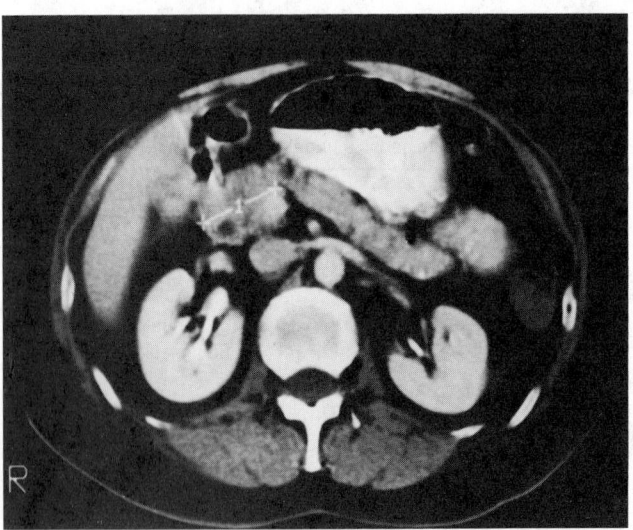

FIGURE 27–3. Obvious mass on CT scan, shown to have normal pancreatic duct and benign minimal enlargement by operation and long-term follow-up.

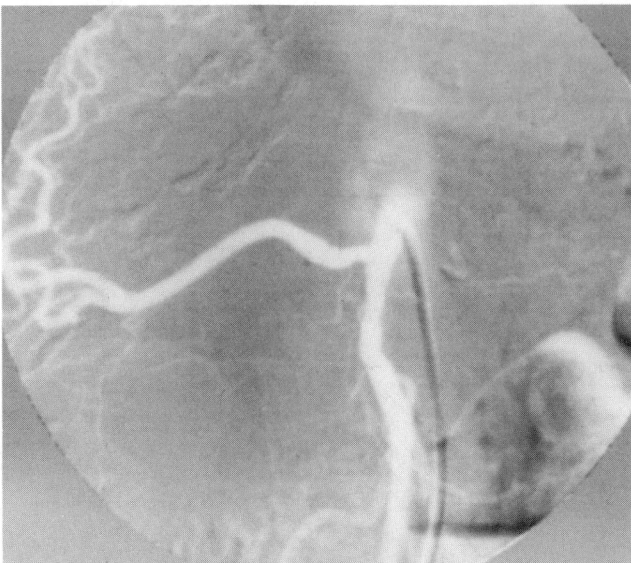

FIGURE 27–5. Angiography of pancreas shows encasement of an abnormal right hepatic artery arising from the superior mesenteric artery.

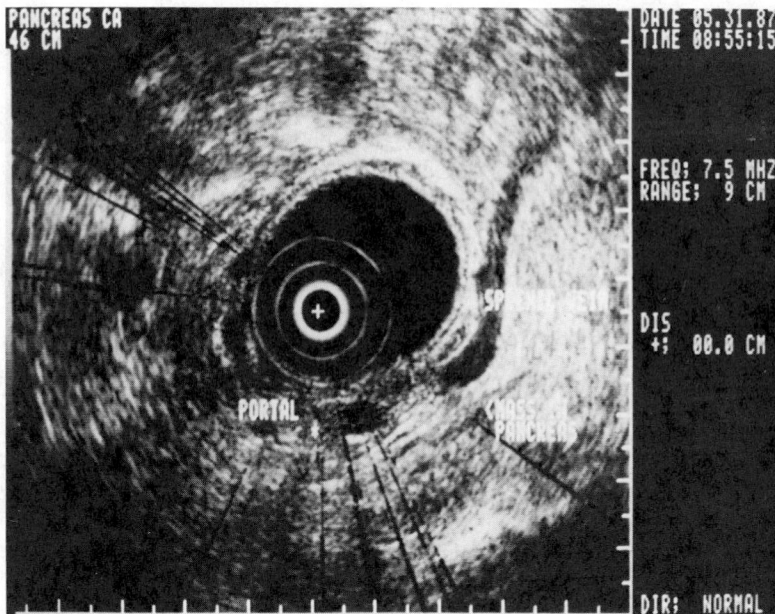

FIGURE 27–6.   Endoscopic ultrasound shows portal vein invasion by pancreatic cancer.

Upper gastrointestinal contrast studies are much less valuable than CT. The contrast study is redundant, because most patients have endoscopy as part of the ERCP. Magnetic resonance imaging (MRI) is only now undergoing serious evaluation for detecting pancreatic abnormalities. MRI may eventually displace CT, but CT is currently the procedure of choice.

A new modality is endoscopic ultrasound. It is used mainly for staging gastric and esophageal cancer but can demonstrate local invasion by pancreatic neoplasms into the portal vein (Fig. 27–6).

Percutaneous transhepatic cholangiograms are indicated on limited occasions. They are primarily used if there is concern about the proximal extent of any stenotic lesion of the common bile duct. It is appropriate at the time of ERCP, if the common bile duct can be entered, to place a stent or a nasobiliary catheter before considering further surgical intervention.

SEROLOGIC MARKERS

During the last several years, there has been increased clinical interest in defining a role for serologic markers in the diagnosis and management of patients with pancreatic carcinoma. The ideal serologic marker should have high specificity and sensitivity, should differentiate localized from metastatic disease at presentation, and should be a sensitive indicator of response to treatment or tumor recurrence. This ideal marker is not yet available for pancreatic carcinoma. A summary of the six available serologic markers for pancreatic carcinoma is given in Table 27–3.

Carcinoembryonic antigen (CEA), a high-molecular-weight glycoprotein found normally in fetal tissue, has been studied most extensively. It is elevated (>2.5 mg/ml) in only 40% to 50% of patients with pancreatic cancer. It may be used to differentiate pancreatic carcinoma from acute or chronic pancreatitis (≤10% of patients with elevated CEA), but CEA can be elevated significantly in many other benign upper intestinal disorders, including chronic hepatitis, cirrhosis, cho-

lelithiasis, and peptic ulcer disease. It can be elevated in biliary, gastric, hepatocellular, and colorectal carcinomas.[48,49]

Three other serologic markers for pancreatic carcinoma were developed as antibodies against tumor-associated antigens from human colorectal cancer cell lines: CA 19-9, CA 195, and a human epithelial ovarian cell line, CA 125.[50-54] These markers variably crossreact against pancreatic carcinoma (see Table 27–3). Similar to CEA, these markers may react with gastrointestinal and other cancers, such as CA 125 for ovarian and breast carcinomas. Based on available information, CA 19-9 and CA 195 have shown approximately twofold greater specificity for pancreatic carcinoma than CEA or CA 125.[55-61]

Two other antibodies, DU-PAN-2 and SPAN-1, have been screened in patients with pancreatic carcinoma. Both were raised against human pancreatic cancer cell lines. The specificity of these newer markers in patients with pancreatic cancer are comparable to CA 19-9.[62,63] However, they are reactive against several other types of cancer, principally gastrointestinal neoplasms, and many benign conditions previously listed for CEA.

TABLE 27–3.   Sensitivity and Specificity of Selected Serologic Markers in Pancreatic Carcinoma

		Elevated Levels (%)		
Marker	Normal Serum Level	Pancreatic Carcinoma	Other GI Cancers	Chronic Pancreatitis
CEA	≤2.5 mg/ml	40–45	10–50	10
CA 125	≤35 μ/ml	40–45	10–50	20
CA 19-9	≤37 μ/ml	75–80	20–70	20
CA 50	≤21 μ/ml	75–80	20–50	15
DUPAN-2	≤150 mg/ml	70–75	10–80	10
SPAN-1	≤30 μ/ml	75–80	20–60	15

There is no highly specific and highly sensitive serologic marker for screening and managing patients with pancreatic carcinoma. Some clinical series have demonstrated the value of using several markers to improve specificity.[57] One limitation to the applicability of these serologic markers in patients with pancreatic carcinoma is that any associated liver dysfunction (*e.g.,* extrahepatic cholestasis) can increase the markers. Intraoperative attempts to improve specificity by comparing portal and peripheral blood levels have not been worthwhile.[56]

PREOPERATIVE LAPAROSCOPY

With the increased use of peritoneal examination with the laparoscope, many patients with pancreatic cancer can be saved an unnecessary operation by preoperative evaluation. This is particularly true, because it is no longer necessary to operatively decompress the biliary tree for many patients. This can be done endoscopically or transhepatically; even in patients requiring gastric outlet obstruction relief, the obstruction is often incomplete and can be managed by dietary maneuvers. It is important to ensure that the patient does not undergo a significant operation if evidence of unresectability or metastasis is present. A report examining the use of peritoneoscopy in 352 patients with clinical suspicion of liver involvement with cancer, found that 90% of 112 patients could have a diagnostic liver biopsy.[64]

The application of this technique to the jaundiced patient has been examined by Irving.[65] This included hepatic puncture for cholangiography or contrast injection directly into the gallbladder, which would seem to be an inappropriate approach because of the ease with which radiologic investigation of the biliary tree can be performed.

A subsequent paper by the same group emphasized the diagnosis and staging of 23 patients with carcinoma of the pancreas or periampullary region who were examined laparoscopically.[66] Hepatic metastases were identified in 3 patients and metastatic deposits elsewhere in 2. In patients who had pancreatic adenocarcinoma involving the body and tail, the incidence of metastases was even higher (6 of 8 patients). A report of 73 patients with pancreatic adenocarcinoma undergoing laparoscopy suggested that 42 of 51 could be correctly staged as incurable or inoperable by laparoscopy.[67] Despite this, only 4 of 9 judged resectable by laparoscopy were found to be so on laparotomy. The diagnosis could be confirmed by laparoscopic fine-needle aspiration cytology in 92%. Laparoscopy was particularly valuable in finding unappreciated peritoneal implants. There is little doubt that the use of laparoscopy will expand and be of value in excluding patients from unnecessary laparotomy.

TREATMENT OF LOCALIZED DISEASE

Surgical resection remains the treatment of choice for pancreatic adenocarcinoma and is currently the only potentially curative therapy.

PREOPERATIVE BILIARY DECOMPRESSION
FOR OBSTRUCTIVE JAUNDICE

Preoperative biliary drainage before operation has been practiced for several years. Dr. Alan O. Whipple's early experience with a pancreaticoduodenectomy was preceded by relief of obstruction by bypass.[68] Retrospective studies suggested that preliminary decompression by cholecystectomy decreased operative mortality from 50% to 8%.[69]

Percutaneous transhepatic biliary drainage (PTBD) reduced operative mortality to 8.2%, compared with 28% in historical controls.[70] Several other retrospective studies using historical controls and other trials, including concurrent nonrandomized controls and no controls, suggested benefit.[71-74] The combined results of these studies suggested an operative mortality of 13.7% among patients undergoing preoperative PTBD, compared with 26% among patients undergoing surgery without it. Two of the five trials suggested a significant reduction in mortality and in morbidity. The apparent improvement associated with PTBD in these studies may be explained by other factors, such as the exclusion of high-risk patients from subsequent operations or the use of PTBD as the definitive form of palliation. In these studies, 98 (40%) of 246 patients undergoing PTBD did not proceed to subsequent laparotomy.

Prospective randomized trials challenged the value of PTBD. In 1982, the first prospective evaluation in a single-arm trial of 37 patients, 35 of whom had malignant obstruction, resulted in drainage-related morbidity of 54% and drainage-related mortality of 13.5%.[75] Postoperative mortality was 24%. In two well-controlled, randomized trials, 127 patients, 94% of whom had malignant disease, showed no benefit in morbidity or mortality, from PTBD.[76,77] Overall mortality was 14% with or without preliminary drainage. In-hospital mortality was 23% among patients drained and 16% among those not drained. In one of the trials, there was a 19% mortality among 31 patients not drained and 32% mortality among 34 patients drained, including five deaths before any operation and two additional deaths resulting from complications of drainage procedure. Five patients required early surgery for bile peritonitis.[77]

In all these trials, there were many complications related to PTBD. A prospective, controlled trial showed no benefit in operative mortality and a prolongation of hospital stay with the drainage procedure for patients with benign and malignant biliary obstruction.[78] No objective benefit other than decrease in bilirubin resulted from preoperative drainage. The high complication rate with the percutaneous procedure has obscured any potential benefit from the biliary decompression.

The alternative is endoscopically placed biliary drainage, which has theoretical appeal in providing similar drainage with less risk of complication. In a comprehensive series of 595 cases collected from six centers in Japan and Europe, a 97.5% success rate has been claimed.[79] This is far in excess of any success rate that most North American centers have been able to provide. Complication rates are small (4%). The principal complication is cholangitis. Mortality is less than 2%. Current trials examine benefits of preoperative nasobiliary drainage in alleviating the risks and complications of postoperative patients. In centers where the overall operative mortality is less than 5%, it is unlikely that any benefit in mortality can be shown by such studies without large numbers of patients. In a randomized trial comparing endoscopic and percutaneous stent insertion in 75 patients with malignant obstructive jaundice, the endoscopic route had a greater success rate in relieving jaundice and was associated with a significantly lower complication rate and 30-day mortality rate.[80]

Proponents of the percutaneous route have challenged this study because of a high percutaneous complication rate.[81]

RESECTION

Surgical resection remains the only possible chance for cure and allows confirmation of the histologic and site-specific subtypes. Candidates for resection can be carefully chosen by preoperative testing.

Incision and Evaluation

The bilateral subcostal incision with the extensive use of an upper-hand retractor to gain complete and adequate access to the upper abdomen is preferred. Rarely, an upper midline extension (Mercedes-Benz) is required.

Primary contraindications to resection are liver metastasis or extrapancreatic serosal implantation. It is important to examine the inferior surface of the mesocolon to be sure there is no tumor extending through it. For many patients, this is an indication of unresectability. In most patients, evidence of obvious nodal involvement with cancer in the portal area precludes subsequent resection.

After it is clear that the tumor, duodenum, and the head of the pancreas are mobile, the histopathologic diagnosis is obtained, if it has not been obtained preoperatively. This is done by a single pass of a transduodenal Tru-cut needle, holding the pancreas and tumor with the fingers and thumb of the left hand. Although difficulty may be encountered in obtaining a histologic diagnosis, most physicians have reported a low false-negative rate, and diagnoses were readily obtained.[39,82]

Rarely, a decision is made to proceed with a pancreatic resection although no histologic diagnosis of carcinoma can be obtained. Some surgeons advocate this approach, but if possible, a clear histologic diagnosis should be obtained. However, repetitive transduodenal or open biopsies should be discouraged. Greater difficulty is encountered with persistent attempts at aggressive biopsy with no subsequent progression to resection than if the surgeon proceeds with conventional resection because of the high likelihood that a pancreatic or periampullary carcinoma exists. If the issue of proceeding to resection without a definitive cancer diagnosis has been fully discussed with the patient preoperatively, operative resection can proceed based on the experienced surgeon's expectations.

If tumor invades or adheres to the celiac axis or origin of the common hepatic artery, it is a contraindication for resection. After the hepatic vessels are free, the suprapancreatic portal vein is dissected just medial to the curve of the hepatic artery. This can be easily identified between common duct and hepatic artery, and its freedom from any local tumor invasion should be established. This exposure is limited, and the vein is more easily demonstrated from the inferior approach.

The relation of the tumor to the portal vein is established inferiorly through the lesser sac. Gross and encompassing involvement and difficulty in obtaining dissection between vein and pancreas are limits to resection. Minimal adherence to the vein, however, does not prevent resection and can be dealt with by resection of the vein. The surgeon should assess whether the superior mesenteric artery is involved. It is rare that involvement of the origin of the superior mesenteric artery exists without encasement of the portal vein, often with obvious venous collaterals and varices.

Pancreaticoduodenectomy

The tissue to be resected includes the distal stomach, the gallbladder, the common bile duct, the head of the pancreas with the contained tumor, all four parts of the duodenum, and the first part of the small intestine. Procedures preserving the pylorus can, on rare occasions, be done for small lesions involving the ampulla. Cholecystectomy is performed, and if the duct enters low on the common duct, it can be done from fundus to duct, taking the gallbladder with the specimen.

Carefully remove the uncinate process. Many surgeons do not remove the uncinate process completely, but it is important to do so, because it can be a worrisome site of subsequent bleeding. In uncinate process tumors, unresectability may be encountered late in the procedure. If that is suspected by the early assessment, the uncinate process should be dissected before the small bowel is divided. If invasion of the portal vein is encountered, isolation above and below can be obtained and the vein transected if necessary. If the vein is resected, mobilization of the small intestine can easily make up several centimeters, allowing end-to-end approximation with vascular 4-0 sutures. This enables the specimen to be removed, and the tissue remaining is ready for reconstruction.

Reconstruction

Choledochojejunostomy is performed first, because it is the deepest anastomosis. A small longitudinal incision is made with cautery over the serosa of the small bowel, and the serosa is gently teased from the mucosa to allow a greater entry site for serosa. The mucosa protrudes, increasing the apparent size of the mucosal opening. The horizontal running everting mattress suture of 3-0 or 4-0 monofilament absorbable suture is used to the back wall, and a separate anterior line of running suture then placed (Fig. 27–7). By taking a larger bite on the

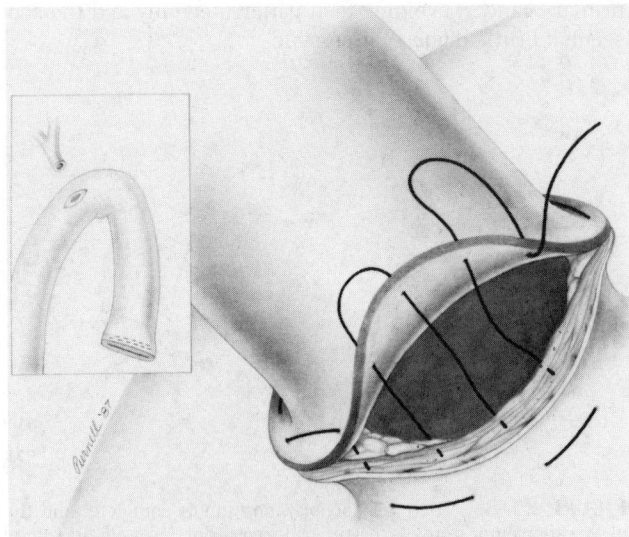

FIGURE 27–7. The choledochojejunostomy is performed by a running, everting, nonabsorbable, monofilament suture.

serosal side and a small bite on the mucosal side, a satisfactory mucosa-to-mucosa anastomosis can be obtained. If the duct is small, a series of interrupted sutures may be preferable.

The pancreaticojejunostomy is performed. A similar incision in the small intestine is made along the jejunal wall, and horizontal monofilament absorbable mattress sutures are placed to attach the pancreas to the small bowel. A direct duct-to-mucosa anastomosis is performed with three interrupted 5-0 monofilament sutures. A similar row of horizontal mattress sutures is placed anteriorly to approximate pancreas to the small intestine (Fig. 27–8). After this has been completed, the standard gastrojejunostomy is performed, usually with two continuous absorbable layers of sutures. The completed anastomoses appear as in Figure 27–9, although the gastrojejunostomy is sometimes retrocolic.

We prefer to use two low-pressure closed suction drains, one in the upper right quadrant and one from the left side of the pancreaticojejunostomy. The wound is closed in standard fashion with a running mass closure with absorbable No. 1 monofilament suture material.

Extended Resections

Extended pancreatic resections have been proposed to include resection of the portal vein, superior mesenteric artery, and celiac axis and an extended nodal dissection.[83] This "regional pancreatectomy" has undergone considerable evolution and refinement and now has an acceptable operative morbidity and mortality.

Current approaches to pancreatic resection for adenocarcinoma have evolved from major arterial resection, but they encompass more extensive nodal dissection and liberal use of portal vein resection, with primary reanastomosis if necessary.

The debate about total pancreatectomy as a preferred procedure over more limited resections is abating. Because the results in long-term survival do not clearly depend on the type of pancreatic resection, most experienced surgeons rely on the procedure that most easily and completely removes the primary cancer, avoiding total pancreatectomy and the subsequent brittle diabetes if possible.

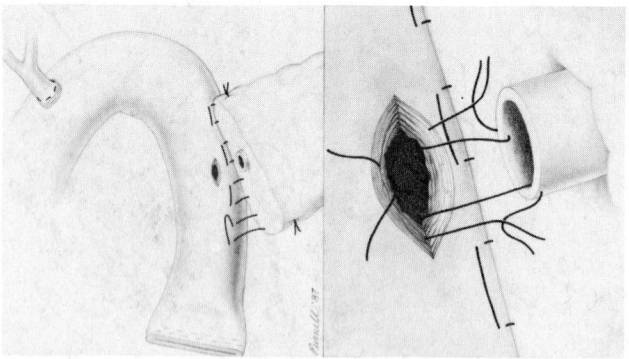

FIGURE 27–8.   The choledochojejunostomy is complete, and the pancreaticojejunostomy is begun. The posterior layer of horizontal mattress sutures fixes the pancreas to the jejunum and two or three interrupted 5-0 nonabsorbable prolene complete a mucosa-to-mucosa anastomosis of the pancreatic duct to the jejunum.

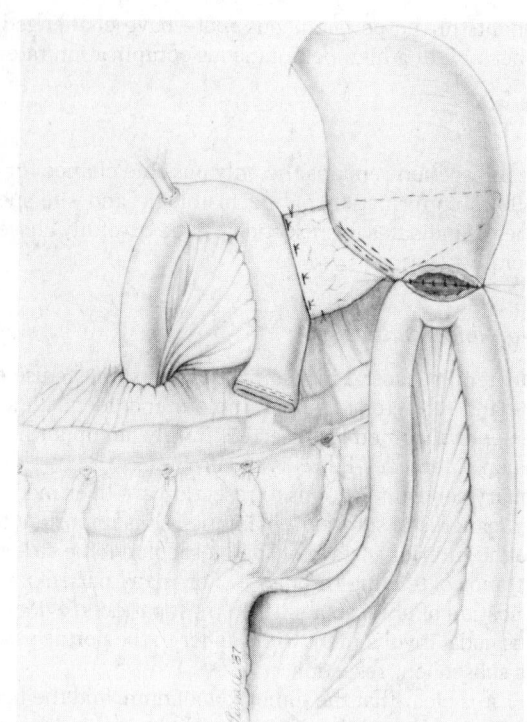

FIGURE 27–9.   The completed reconstruction, showing the pancreaticojejunostomy, the choledochojejunostomy, and gastrojejunostomy. The pancreatic and jejunal anastomosis is usually done retrocholic, and the gastrojejunostomy can be retrocholic, as shown here, or anticholic.

Results

Operative resection remains the only potentially curative approach, although the long-term survival results of surgical resection are still low. Adjuvant therapies have improved median survival only minimally, and palliative procedures provide limited benefit.

The number of patients who present with suspected adenocarcinoma of the pancreas is greater than the actual incidence. From 1983 to 1990, MSKCC admitted 1192 adult patients suspected of having peripancreatic carcinoma. Of these, 69% had adenocarcinoma of the pancreas. The remainder had bile duct cancer (12%), islet cell cancer (6%), or ampullary or duodenal cancer (8%). The age range for these patients was 27 to 90 years.

OPERABILITY.   Of 818 patients with adenocarcinoma of the pancreas, 602 (74%) underwent exploration and 151 (25%) were resected. Comparable figures for the resectability rate of other peripancreatic tumors are shown in Figure 27–10.

Most patients require a pancreaticoduodenectomy or total pancreatectomy. In 151 successive resections of patients with adenocarcinoma of the pancreas in 7 years, there were only 15 distal pancreatic resections, 10% of those resected. Operations lasted for an average of 7 hours (range, 1.5–14.5 hours), and the median intraoperative blood replacement was 750 ml (range, 0–6500 ml).

The results of resection, bypass, and pancreatic implantation have been previously reported from MSKCC.[84] Until

	n	Resected*	Explored	Resected†
Adenocarcinoma of the Pancreas	818	151 (18%)	602	151 (25%)
Bile Duct	144	27 (19%)	108	27 (25%)
Islet Cell	70	29 (41%)	54	29 (54%)
Ampulla	63	48 (76%)	57	48 (84%)
Duodenum	37	21 (57%)	33	21 (64%)
Other	60	25 (42%)	53	25 (47%)
Total	**1192**	**301 (25%)**	**907**	**301 (33%)**

MSKCC 1983–1990 * % of all patients † % of explored

FIGURE 27–10. Resectability rates for peripancreatic tumors at Memorial Sloan-Kettering Cancer Center.

1980, operative and in-hospital mortality was between 16% and 20% for resection, biopsy, or bypass (Tables 27–4 and 27–5).

This was similar to the operative mortalities of 15% to 25% reported before 1982. In a recent report of 50 cases of adenocarcinoma, patients operated on between 1969 and 1980 were compared with those operated on between 1981 and 1986.[108] The operative mortality rate fell from 24% in the first period to 2% in the second, remarkably similar to the operative mortality of 18% until 1980 at MSKCC and of 3% between 1983 and 1990, with similar numbers of patients (Fig. 27–11). Age has not been a barrier to resection. Patients who are older than 70 years of age have no greater operative mortality and similar survival rates compared with younger patients.

SURVIVAL. Operative morbidity and mortality have markedly decreased. Long-term survival, however, is little changed (see Tables 27–4 and 27–5). The MSKCC experience is shown in Figure 27–12. The apparent 20% 5-year survival should be interpreted with caution, because only a small number of patients are at risk beyond 5 years. For the 61 patients with adenocarcinoma of the pancreas resected more than 5 years ago, 10 (17%) are alive and 7 (12%) alive without disease. For the 23 patients with ampullary carcinoma, resected more than 5 years ago, 12 (52%) are alive; 10 (43%) without evidence of disease. The influence of brachytherapy on survival of unresected patients was shown to be a median of 8 months, with no in-hospital mortality. Current data show a significant improvement in those receiving brachytherapy (Fig. 27–13). Hospital stay was not affected by brachytherapy treatment.

TABLE 27–4. Results of Resection for Cure of Adenocarcinoma of the Pancreas

Investigations	Years of Treatment	No. of Patients	No. of Patients per Year	Operative Mortality (%)	Median Survival (mo)
Bowden[85]	26	51	2	31	9
Portland Surg. Coop[86]	10	27	2	22	22
Crile[87]	Selected	28		NS*	6
Feduska[88]	11	16	1	44	7
Wilson[89]	16	13	1	23	10
Brooks[90]	10	16	1	13	23
Shapiro[91]	Selected	24		8	11
Nakase[92]	25	430	17	22	12 (head)
				10 b + t,* 5 total	
Tepper[93]	10	31	3	16	11
Knight[94]	10	16	1	14	16
Moosa[95]	7	52	7	8	23
Longmire[96]	21	50	2	NS*	16
Edis[97]	25	162	6	16	10
Fortner[98]	9	36	4	15	NS*
Herter[99]	39	82	2	19	9
Morrow[84]	6	39	6	18	18
Trede[100]		59		1	5/59 5 y†
Gudjonsson[101]	37	2398			92/2398†
Michelassi[102]	41	79	2	20	
Trede[103]	4	53	13	0	
MSKCC‡	7	151	21	3	
Cameron[104]	21	89	5	9	11.9

* NS, not stated; b + t, body and tail of pancreas.
† Overall survival.
‡ Data not published.

TABLE 27–5. Bypass Procedures

Investigations	No. of Patients	Mortality (%)	Mean Survival (mo)
Bowden[85]	114	57	5
Portland Coop[86]	248	18	5.4
Crile[87]	28		8
Feduska[88]	60	33	6
Wilson[89]	80	14	6
Brooks[90]	35	15	5.8
Shapiro[91]	24	4	8
Nakase[92]	1791	21	5 head
			3 b + t*
			3 total
Knight[94]	155	22	7
Moosa[95]	31	6	6
Longmire[96]	103		6
Van Heerden[105]	151	6	6†
Brooks[106]	51	24	7
Herter[99]	152	17	6
DeRooij[107]	180	5	8

* b + t, body and tail of pancreas.
† This is a median figure.

ADJUVANT RADIATION THERAPY FOR RESECTABLE DISEASE

Radiation therapy in combination with surgical resection has been used to improve local disease control and survival. The pattern of failure after surgical resection by pancreaticoduodenectomy was analyzed for 31 patients from the Massachusetts General Hospital, in which survival (median, 10.5 months) and operative mortality (16%) were equivalent to other surgical series at that time (1963–1973).[93] Of 26 postoperative survivors, 22 patients died from recurrent or persistent pancreatic carcinoma, 13 cases of which were confirmed by reexploration for suspected recurrence or by autopsy. When the clinical and pathologic findings were combined, 13 (50%) patients were thought to have locoregional recurrence within the surgical bed. Only 4 (15%) of 26 patients demonstrated distant metastases without evidence of local failure.

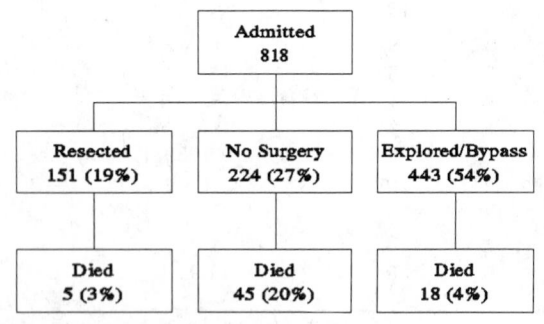

MSKCC 10/15/83 – 10/15/90

FIGURE 27–11. Thirty-day mortality rates for patients with adenocarcinoma of the pancreas. The mortality rate from resection is now less than 5%.

The problem of persistent locoregional disease after surgical resection of early clinical stage (stage I) disease was reflected in a recent autopsy series from Japan.[109] Of 8 patients with T1 or T2 tumors, 6 had microscopic metastases in grossly negative lymph nodes in the pancreatic bed, and 4 had microscopic involvement of regional paraaortic nodes. No distant metastases were found in this small series. Based on these two series and others, persistent local disease for early-stage pancreatic cancer is a problem that may be corrected with adjuvant radiation therapy.[93,109]

Preoperative radiation therapy for localized pancreatic carcinoma has been used in three small series. Pilepich and Miller used preoperative radiotherapy for 17 patients with localized, but unresectable, lesions.[110] Sixteen of the 17 patients had been explored and judged to be unresectable based on tumor extension through the pancreatic capsule (at least stage II disease). The primary tumor was less than 5 cm in 4 patients and 5 cm or larger in the remaining 13 patients. These patients received conventionally fractionated (200-cGy fractions) radiation therapy of 4000 to 5000 cGy in 4 to 5 weeks. Eleven of the 17 patients were reexplored, with 6 patients undergoing resection of tumors of the pancreatic head. Two patients remained disease free at 5 years. The second series involved 7 patients with tumor of the pancreatic head or periampullary area who received a pancreaticoduodenectomy procedure and 4500 cGy of radiation delivered preoperatively (5 patients) or postoperatively (2 patients).[111] Two patients survived for 5 years, and there were no clinically detected local recurrences. The third series involved a retrospective review of 18 patients with pancreatic head (12 patients) or periampullary tumors (6 patients) who received conventional fractionated irradiation to 5000 cGy approximately 1 month before exploration.[112] Although all tumors were judged to be resectable before irradiation, 16 patients (89%) underwent resection by a Whipple procedure (15 patients) or total pancreatectomy (1 patient). All 18 tumors responded to irradiation with an approximate 50% shrinkage (3.3 ± 0.8 cm before, to 2.0 ± 0.7 cm after) using CT and ultrasound. There was no difference in response between pancreatic head and periampullary cancers. Histopathologic examination of the 16 resected specimens showed "severely damaged" tumor cells (interpreted as nonviable) in more than one third of the resected specimens, particularly at the periphery. Only 2 patients developed postoperative complications (1 with anastomotic leak; 1 with gastrointestinal bleeding), and there were no postoperative deaths. With limited follow-up (2–39 months), only 1 patient died with liver metastases.

Although these limited data suggest that moderate dose preoperative radiation therapy may increase resectability and possibly survival with acceptable morbidity, the routine use of preoperative irradiation is not warranted. Weese and colleagues performed a small prospective study of neoadjuvant combined modality therapy consisting of 5000 cGy with concurrent continuous infusion 5-fluorouracil (5-FU) and mitomycin C.[113] Of 14 patients with locally advanced pancreas cancer, 9 patients were explored after clinical restaging within 3 weeks of this regimen, and 6 patients underwent curative resection. Five of the 6 patients with resected tumors remained free of recurrence for 4 to 40 months after diagnosis. Larger prospective trials are necessary to define a role for this neoadjuvant approach. Such a multiinstitutional approach

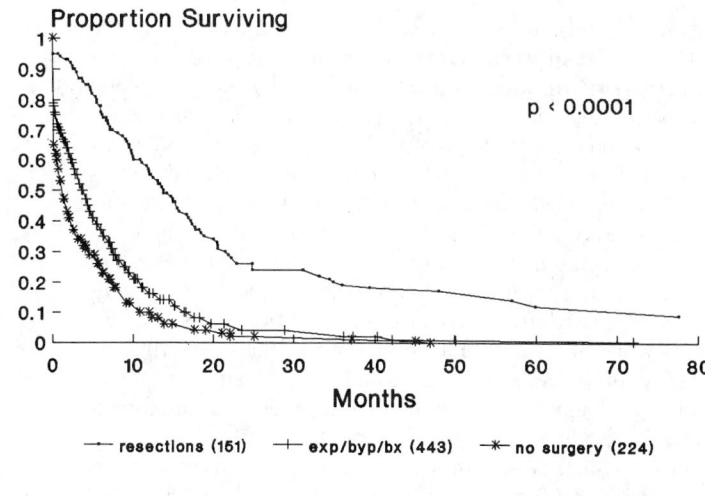

FIGURE 27–12. Survival of patients with adenocarcinoma of the pancreas having resection, bypass, or no surgery at Memorial Sloan-Kettering Cancer Center. Survival favors resection ($p < 0.0001$).

is being considered by the Eastern Cooperative Oncology Group.

Two groups performed randomized prospective trials of postoperative radiation therapy in patients with resected carcinoma of the pancreas. In a National Cancer Institute study, 32 patients with locally confined pancreatic carcinoma underwent total or regional pancreatectomy and were randomly allocated to receive intraoperative radiotherapy (IORT) as adjuvant treatment or conventional treatment.[114] The IORT group of 16 patients received 2000 cGy, using 9 to 12 MeV electrons to the tumor bed and regional nodal basins immediately after resection. The surgical and radiotherapeutic details of IORT are described elsewhere.[115,116] The control group of 16 patients received operation alone for stage I disease and external-beam radiation therapy (5000 cGy in 5–6 weeks) postoperatively for stage II and stage III disease. More than 90% of patients on both arms of this study had stage II or III disease.

Operative mortality was high (9 of 32 patients) but was similar in the IORT and control groups, as was the incidence of complications in the postoperative period. After operative deaths were excluded from analysis, the disease-free survival was increased in the IORT patients (20 months) compared with the control group (12 months, $p=0.1$), but overall survival was similar. Local disease control was significantly improved in the IORT group. Although the number of patients on this trial was modest, it appears that IORT can improve control of locally advanced disease after pancreatectomy but with significant morbidity.

The Gastrointestinal Tumor Study Group (GITSG) reported on a prospective randomized trial comparing surgery (usually pancreaticoduodenectomy) to operation plus postoperative adjuvant therapy with external-beam irradiation and 5-FU.[117] The radiation was given in two courses of 2000 cGy each, separated by 2 weeks for a total dose of 4000 cGy. At the beginning of each 2000-cGy course, 5-FU (500 mg/m²) was

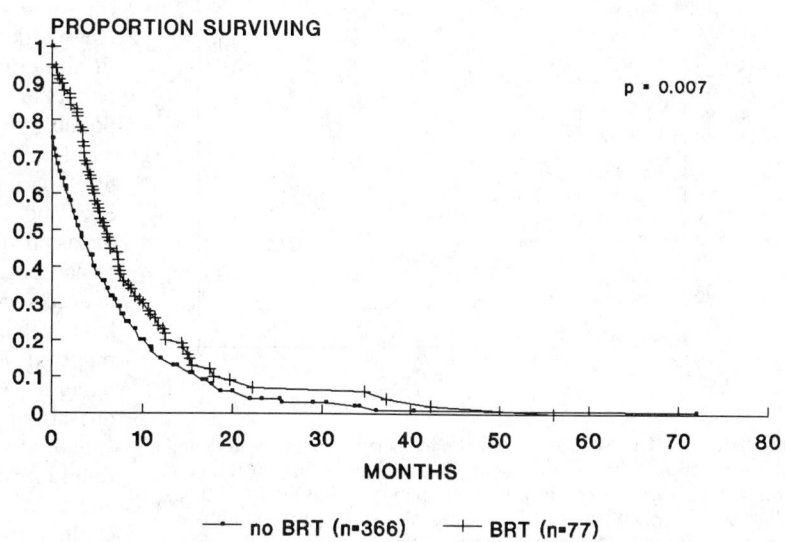

FIGURE 27–13. Survival favors patients receiving brachytherapy ($p = 0.007$) for adenocarcinoma of the pancreas.

given daily for 3 days. After completion of the radiation, the 5-FU was given weekly for 2 years or until progression of disease. Forty-three patients were randomized to surgery alone (22 patients) or postoperative adjuvant therapy (21 patients), with an equal distribution of patients with stage I, II, or III disease. There was a significant improvement in median survival (21 months versus 11 months, $p=0.05$) and 2-year survival (43% versus 18%, $p=0.05$) in patients receiving postoperative combined modality therapy (Fig. 27–14). Median disease-free survival was 9 months and 11 months in the control and treated groups, respectively, and the overall death rates were 86% and 71%, respectively. Subsequently, the GITSG entered an additional 30 patients with similar clinical and pathologic features into the postoperative combined-modality treatment arm.[118] In this study (Fig. 27–15), results similar to the treated arm were obtained. The survival curves are carried to 60 months in the earlier study (see Fig. 27–14), but in the latter study, results are only given for 24 months.

Although these reports from the National Cancer Institute and the GITSG support the use of postoperative adjuvant treatment, the routine use of external-beam irradiation with or without 5-FU cannot be routinely recommended.[119] Without studies of alternative therapies, postoperative radiation therapy with 5-FU appears to be the adjuvant therapy most likely to prolong survival, but the use of this therapy, because of the limited survival prolongation, requires individualization. A series of resected pancreatic carcinoma shows considerable variation in the median survival of 10 to 23 months, with the upper limit similar to the results of the adjuvant therapy trials.[84,95–97,99]

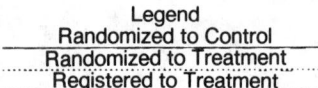

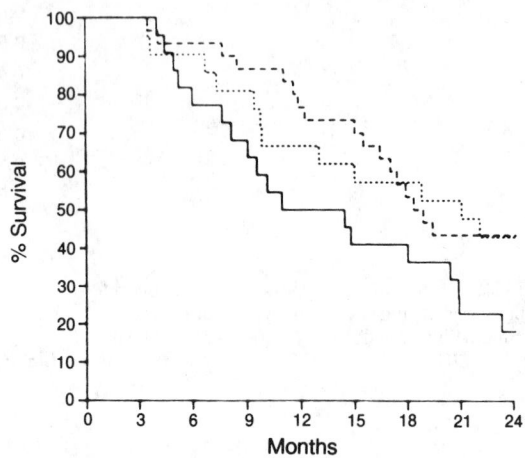

FIGURE 27–15. GITSG: probability of survival by treatment. (Gastrointestinal Tumor Study Group: Further evidence of effective adjuvant combined radiation and chemotherapy following curative resection of pancreatic cancer. Cancer 1987;59:2006–2010)

TREATMENT FOR LOCALIZED UNRESECTABLE AND METASTATIC DISEASE

BYPASS PROCEDURES

Between 1970 and 1979, 15,942 (34%) of 46,888 patients in England and Wales had operations for pancreatic cancer, and 95% of these were biliary bypasses for relief of jaundice. Only 5% of the 34% underwent resection; between 1970 and 1979, fewer than 800 pancreatic resections were performed in all of England and Wales, despite their very high incidence of pancreatic cancer.[7] The hospital mortality for pancreatic bypass was 20%, compared with 14% mortality for resection in the same series. From 1985 through 1990, 1458 patients in New York State had pancreatic resections for malignancies. Because more than 80% of the patients with carcinoma of the pancreas present with obstructive jaundice and resection is possible in only 25%, palliative bypass has received considerable attention.[105,106,108] In a collected series of more than 8000 patients with unresectable carcinoma of the pancreas, Sarr and Cameron showed that patients undergoing biliary bypass had a lower operative mortality rate (19%) than patients subjected to diagnostic laparotomy only (26%).[120] The overall survival was longer (5.4 months) for patients having bypass than for those subject to diagnostic laparotomy (3.5 months). For the 818 patients with adenocarcinoma of the pancreas admitted to MSKCC from 1983 through 1990, the operations performed are illustrated in Figure 27–16.

Palliative procedures involve diversion of the biliary tract, relief of gastric outflow obstruction, nutritional rehabilitation, and pain control. The choice of choledochojejunostomy or cholecystojejunostomy for bypass has long been debated. Cholecystojejunostomy is technically simpler and more ex-

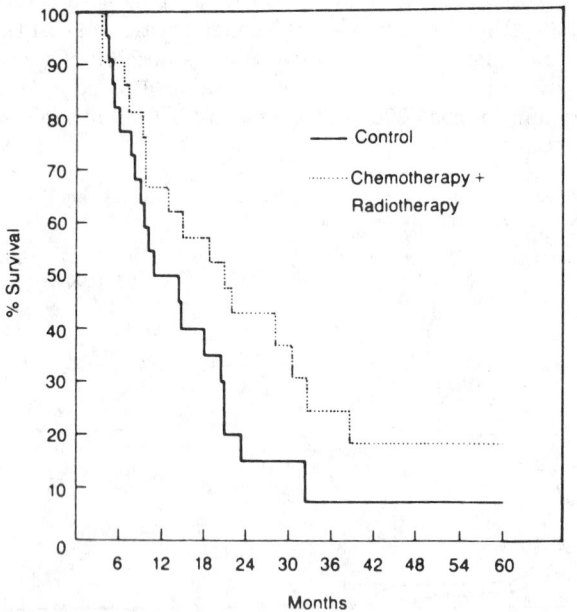

FIGURE 27–14. GITSG: comparison of survival in treated and control groups. Survival was greater in the treated than in the control groups throughout the follow-up period (adjusted $p = 0.03$) (Kalser MH, Ellenberg SS. Pancreatic cancer: Adjuvant combined radiation and chemotherapy following curative resection. Arch Surg 1985;120:901)

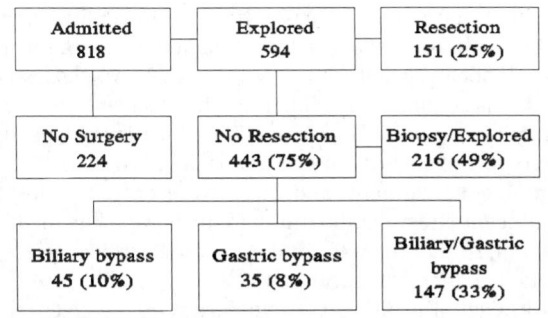

FIGURE 27–16. Types of operations performed for adenocarcinoma of the pancreas at Memorial Sloan-Kettering Cancer Center from 1983 to 1990.

peditious, and choledochojejunostomy is more difficult and, if a large tumor or extensive mesenteric infiltration exists, hazardous. The relative merits of adequacy of decompression of the biliary tree have been examined.[121–123] If cholecystojejunostomy is to be performed, the cystic duct must be patent and enter the common duct well above the site of malignant obstruction. A comparison of cholecystojejunostomy and choledochojejunostomy at MSKCC found no difference in time for the bilirubin to fall or overall mortality, and there was a minimal benefit in median survival for choledochojejunostomy (289 days versus 221 days) (Fig. 27–17).[107]

There have been questions about the merits in terms of survival.[120] In a collected series of over 900 patients, the operative mortality was identical among patients undergoing biliary drainage through the common duct (20%) to those undergoing cholecystojejunostomy (16%). Survival among

more than 1600 patients was similar after biliary decompression using either the common bile duct (6.5 months) or the gallbladder (5.3 months). These comparisons, although not addressing stage or extent of disease, suggest that the methods are equally acceptable.

The problem of recurrent jaundice is poorly addressed. At worst, fewer than 5% to 10% of patients with obstructive jaundice in which the cholecystojejunostomy was used as the decompression route have recurrent jaundice, which can be resolved with an endoscopic procedure. The particular methods of diversion include simple cholecystojejunostomy with a loop, Roux-en-Y cystojejunostomy, cholecystoduodenostomy, choledochoduodenostomy, and choledochojejunostomy by a loop or by the Roux-en-Y method. These have been compared for survival rates, and none seems to show a significant benefit. A review of 1114 patients showed all methods to give a range of survival between 4.8 and 7.8 months, with considerable overlap.[120]

Complete duodenal obstruction is an unusual presenting symptom of pancreatic cancer but is often a component of the disease. Many patients have some abnormality of the duodenal outlet detected by endoscopy or by upper gastrointestinal radiologic studies. Approximately 30% of patients present with nausea and vomiting, some of which is associated with duodenal obstruction.[39,124] There has been considerable debate about whether gastroenterostomy should be performed in all patients or only if there is apparently imminent obstruction. The objection to routine gastroenterostomy is based on the fact that most patients do not require it, that it increases morbidity due to increased operative time and additional anastomoses, and that some extrapolations suggested increased mortality. The possibility of subsequent stomal ulceration or

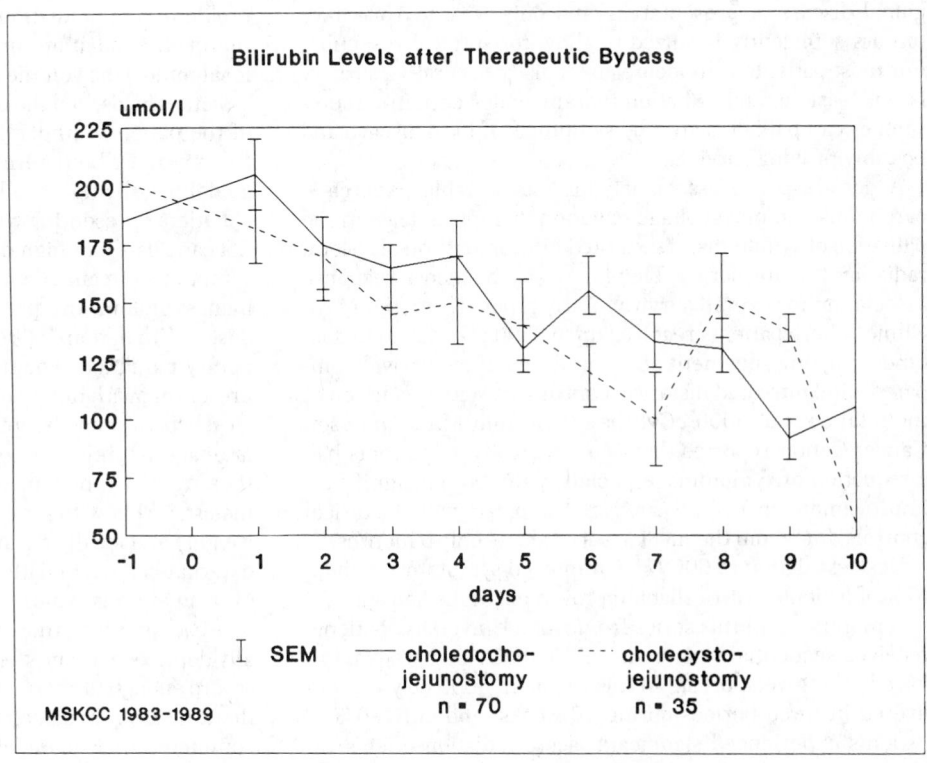

FIGURE 27–17. Comparison of cholecystojejunostomy and choledochojejunostomy, (DeRooij PD, Rogatko A, Brennan MF. Evaluation of palliative surgical procedures in unresectable pancreatic cancer. Br J Surg 1991; 78:1053–1058)

some contribution of the gastroenterostomy to functional gastric emptying delay has also been raised.

The rate of reoperations for subsequent duodenal obstruction in patients without previous gastroenterostomy appears to be quite high, ranging from 2% to 50%. Sarr and Cameron suggest that 13% of patients not undergoing gastroenterostomy at the time of initial operation subsequently required gastroenterostomy for development of duodenal obstruction.[120] One review reported that almost 50% of patients who did not have a gastric duodenal bypass initially and survived for 6 months or more were likely to develop duodenal obstruction and needed reoperation.[100] Others suggested a mortality of 10% to 20%.[125,126]

In a collected series of more than 500 patients, there was an average survival of 5.8 months for patients with gastroenterostomy and an average of 6.6 months for those not undergoing gastroenterostomy.[120] Similar figures for operative mortality are suggested in a review of 648 patients: 17% operative mortality with gastroenterostomy and 18% mortality without gastroenterostomy. The use of prophylactic gastric bypass at MSKCC was accompanied by increased morbidity, but it was associated with increased survival (medians, 249 versus 136 days).[107] This could be accounted for by extent of disease. The issue remains in doubt. If minimal gastric outlet obstruction exists and the disease is advanced, prophylactic gastric bypass appears not to be worth the increased morbidity.

RADIATION THERAPY FOR UNRESECTABLE LOCAL DISEASE

Radiation therapy continues to be a primary treatment for patients with locally advanced unresectable tumors. As many as 50% of patients with pancreatic carcinoma have locoregional disease at presentation, and only 10% to 15% have tumors sufficiently localized to allow for surgical resection. For most patients with locoregional disease, curative surgery is not feasible, and radiation therapy under certain circumstances can palliate signs and symptoms of local disease and possibly prolong survival.

A dose-response association for unresectable pancreatic carcinoma and megavoltage radiation therapy, at least in the palliation of symptoms, is suggested in a comparison of several radiation therapy series. There may also be a dose-response association for overall survival. Early reports from the Mayo Clinic, where patients received up to 3500 cGy, failed to document any improvement of symptom relief or survival compared with untreated historical controls.[127] With escalation of the total dose to 5000 cGy, the group from M.D. Anderson Cancer Center reported that as many as 33% of patients had a reduction of symptoms, especially pain, but no significant improvement in overall survival compared with historical controls, for whom the median survival was only 6 months.[128]

Dose escalation to 6000 cGy improved symptoms in about 67% of patients, with a slight improvement in median survival to 8 months.[129] In this series from Duke University, patients received sequential treatments of 2000 cGy in 2 weeks, followed by a 2-week break. In this regimen, 6000 cGy was delivered in three periods during 10 weeks, and only 10% of patients experienced significant, acute radiation effects requiring early cessation of treatment.

The group from Thomas Jefferson University treated patients with 7000 cGy over 9 weeks, using a combination of 45-mV photons and high-energy (15–40 MeV) electrons.[130,131] With this combination of photons and electrons, effective palliation was observed in 50% to 70% of patients, depending on the type and severity of symptoms. Thirty-six of 40 patients completed treatment, and there were only 2 patients with significant late radiation injury to the bowel. The median survival of 10 months was similar to some surgical series of resectable pancreatic carcinoma.[26,96]

Although it is difficult to compare retrospective treatment series because of dissimilar and often unknown patient selection factors, as the total dose of external-beam irradiation was increased from 3500 to 7000 cGy, a trend of an increased tumor response, as measured by palliation of signs and symptoms and by increased overall survival, was evident. However, even with doses as high as 7000 cGy, local tumor control was achieved clinically in only 50% of patients.[130,131] Many patients who initially respond favorably to the external-beam irradiation of unresectable pancreatic carcinoma later show evidence of tumor regrowth and the return of local signs and symptoms before death. Even with high-dose external-beam irradiation of 7000 cGy, patients rarely survive 5 years or more.[129,130] Because of these poor treatment results, experimental irradiation techniques have been used alone or in combination with conventional external-beam photon irradiation with or without chemotherapy in an attempt to improve local control and influence overall survival.

External-Beam Photon Irradiation

Selection of optimal treatment for a patient with a locally advanced unresectable pancreatic carcinoma poses a major problem to the radiation oncologist. Considerations in determining the radiation therapy technique include the extent of local tumor, the volume of normal tissues included within the radiation fields, and the baseline medical and nutritional status of the patient. Although the role of external-beam radiation therapy must be determined on an individual basis, certain guidelines should be followed.

Patients presenting with widespread metastatic disease are not candidates for high-dose external-beam irradiation. If local symptoms of pain and intestinal obstruction are the predominant symptoms in a patient presenting with metastasis, lower doses of radiation (5000 cGy) may be used to provide temporary palliation. For the patient with unresectable disease presenting with biliary obstruction and clinical jaundice, surgical bypass or endoscopic or percutaneous transhepatic biliary drainage is preferable to palliative external-beam radiation therapy. For a patient with no clinical evidence of visceral metastasis but with significant weight loss (>10–15% of body weight) and locally advanced unresectable disease, high-dose external-beam irradiation is not warranted, because this type of irradiation is typically complicated by acute symptoms of nausea, vomiting, anorexia, and diarrhea.[132] In the nutritionally depleted patient, the acute radiation symptoms are often severe enough to abort a planned course of high-dose radiation therapy. Even in selected patient series, at least 10% do not complete the planned course of high-dose radiation therapy.[129,130]

Patients with unresectable pancreatic carcinoma found suitable for aggressive external-beam radiation therapy should have locally advanced disease without evidence of dissemination and should demonstrate adequate nutritional status. In this patient group, the intent of external-beam irradiation is to deliver a dose of at least 6000 cGy to gross disease and 4500 to 5000 cGy to microscopic disease. A major concern in radiation treatment planning for this patient group is the amount of normal tissues included within the high-dose volume. Organs that limit upper abdominal irradiation include stomach, small bowel, large bowel, liver, kidney, and spinal cord. Although the tolerance of each of these organs is reasonably well defined, when using conventionally fractionated irradiation (180–200 cGy daily), factors such as previous surgical procedures or the use of concomitant chemotherapy may lower the threshold for acute and late radiation injury, particularly to the intestine.[132] Simple techniques at the time of treatment planning may significantly reduce the risk of radiation damage to dose-limiting tissues like the small bowel.[133] A typical external-beam radiation treatment plan for a patient with unresectable pancreatic carcinoma is illustrated in Figure 27–18.

Specialized Methods of Radiation Therapy

Because local control is achieved in fewer than 50% of patients, more specialized methods of radiation have been used, often in conjunction with external-beam therapy with or

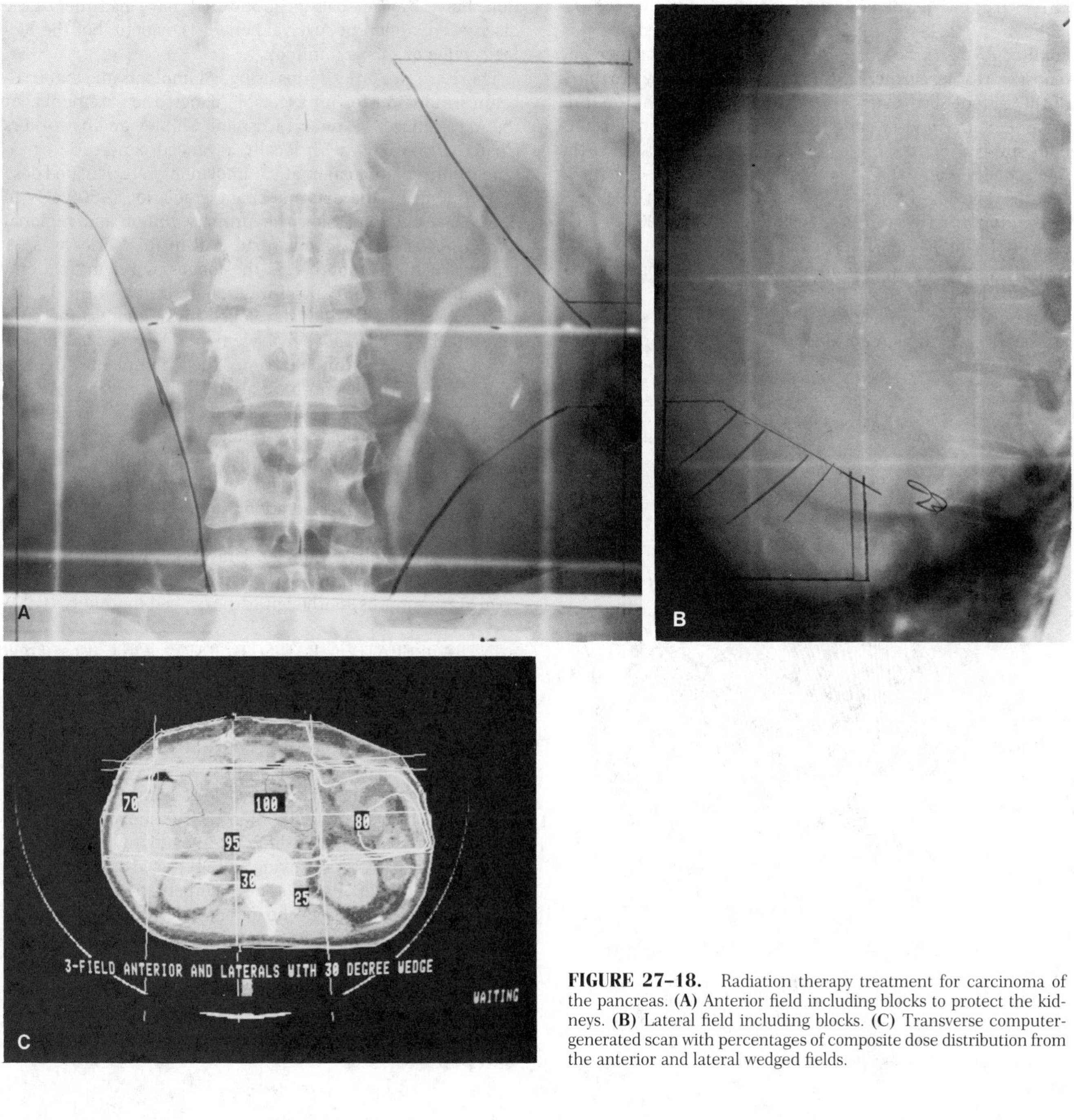

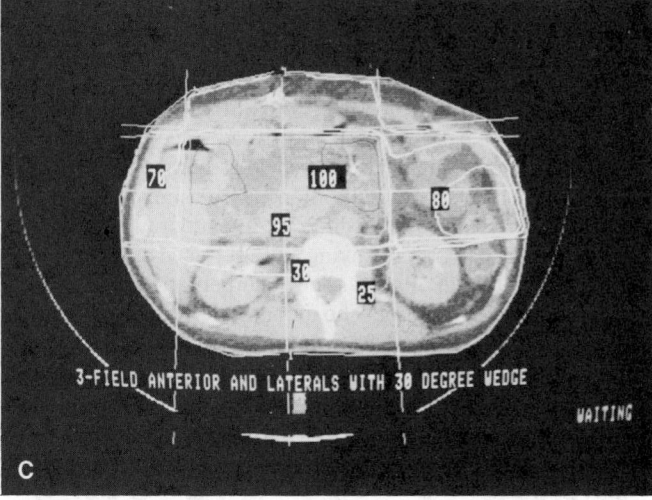

FIGURE 27–18. Radiation therapy treatment for carcinoma of the pancreas. **(A)** Anterior field including blocks to protect the kidneys. **(B)** Lateral field including blocks. **(C)** Transverse computer-generated scan with percentages of composite dose distribution from the anterior and lateral wedged fields.

without chemotherapy to deliver higher effective tumor doses. These specialized experimental techniques include the use of interstitial implants, IORT, high linear energy transfer (high LET) or fast-neutron therapy, and charged particle irradiation.

INTERSTITIAL THERAPY. Interstitial irradiation involves implantation of radioactive sources into the pancreatic parenchyma (Fig. 27–19).[134] The use of interstitial implants is attractive because of the rapid falloff in dose from a radioactive source and because of the low dose rate delivered (<100 cGy/hour), which can result in a greater biologic effectiveness.

The most commonly used isotope for pancreatic implants is iodine 125 (^{125}I). The largest published experience with ^{125}I implants in unresectable pancreatic carcinoma is from MSKCC between 1975 and 1980.[84,134] A total of 33 patients underwent interstitial implantation with ^{125}I seeds. Seven (21%) patients developed significant postoperative complications, although 4 of these may have been related to a concomitant bypass procedure or the result of multiple pancreatic biopsies creating a pancreatic fistula. Approximately two thirds of the patients had a surgical bypass, 11 patients at the time of implantation and 11 patients before implantation. The median survival for the entire group was 8 months, with the longest survivor alive and without evidence of disease at 33 months. The dose from the ^{125}I implant varied with the extent of the tumor but was in the range of 16,000 to 20,000 cGy delivered over 1 year. Twelve patients in this series also received external-beam photon irradiation using conventional fractionation to a dose of 3000 to 4000 cGy.

There was no significant difference in overall survival in the series of 33 implanted patients (median, 8 months) compared with a separate group of 39 patients (median, 18 months) who underwent resection at MSKCC during the same period.[84] In another study, 9 of 33 patients receiving ^{125}I implant had documented liver metastasis at the time of implantation, and the other 24 patients had locally advanced unresectable disease.[134] The 30-day mortality for this group was 0%, compared with 18% for the surgically resected patients. Theoretically, significant complications can result from this therapy, but in the MSKCC experience, hospital stay was not different for patients receiving or not receiving brachytherapy. Another series of ^{125}I pancreatic implants from MSKCC is illustrated in Figure 27–13. Between 1983 and 1990, a group of 77 patients underwent bypass surgery with ^{125}I implantation, and another 366 patients were explored without implantation. In this nonrandomized series, patients undergoing ^{125}I implantation had no evidence of metastatic disease at exploration, but the other patient group may have had metastatic disease. An apparent survival benefit is evident, but the biologic value of this is minimal.

There are two other series using ^{125}I implants and external-beam irradiation for unresectable pancreatic carcinoma. At the Massachusetts General Hospital, Shipley and coworkers treated 12 patients with locally advanced pancreatic carcinoma with a combination of ^{125}I implantation (calculated dose of 16,000 cGy) and external-beam irradiation (4500 cGy in 5 weeks), encompassing the primary tumor and regional lymph nodes.[135] The median survival in this series was 11 months, with 30 months for the longest surviving patient. Clinical local tumor control was achieved in 9 of the 12 patients. Pancreatic fistulas developed in 2 patients, and both responded to conservative management. The group at Thomas Jefferson University also combined the ^{125}I implant with postoperative external-beam irradiation.[131] In this series, 18 patients received a ^{125}I implant (12,000 cGy) and external-beam radiation therapy (6000 cGy); they had a median survival of 12 months, and only 1 patient was thought to have failed locally. Treatment complications included abscess formation in 3 patients, duodenal ulceration with perforation in 1 patient, and pancreatitis in 1 patient. A more recent analysis of this approach at Thomas Jefferson University, which integrated systemic chemotherapy, showed similar results (median survival, 12.5 months), although with reduced morbidity.[136]

INTRAOPERATIVE RADIOTHERAPY. IORT uses large, single doses of radiation delivered directly to an exposed tumor and potential areas of regional spread at the time of surgical exploration. High-energy electrons have been used most frequently in Japan and in the United States. IORT has been used alone in patients with locally advanced unresectable pancreatic carcinoma with little obvious therapeutic gain. The largest experience with IORT alone is from Japan, where 108 patients were treated at 14 different institutions.[137] There was pain relief in patients receiving an IORT dose of greater than 2000 cGy, although there was no documentation of the extent or duration of pain relief. The median survival was 6 months, and most patients died from progressive disease within 12 months. Ulceration and hemorrhage of the duodenum included within the IORT field occurred in 25% of the patients, but there were no treatment-related deaths. The investigators concluded that the IORT dose should be limited to less than 3000 cGy if a significant segment of duodenum must be in-

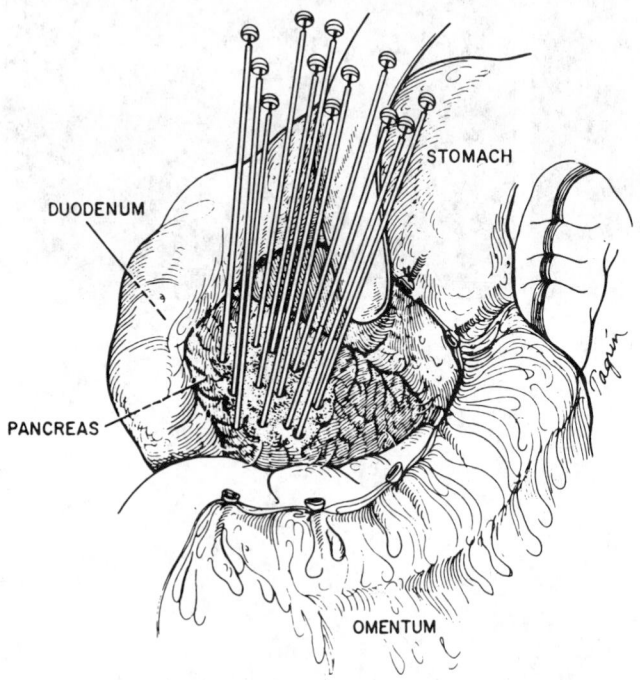

FIGURE 27–19. Interstitial implantation of the pancreas with radioactive sources for brachytherapy. (Shipley WU, Nardi GL, Cohen AM, et al. Iodine-125 implant and external beam irradiation in patients with localized pancreatic carcinoma. A comparative study to surgical resection. Cancer 1980;45:709–714)

cluded within the IORT field. In another study from two other Japanese centers, 33 patients received an IORT dose of 2000 to 4000 cGy, which gave prompt pain relief (within 1 week) for 50% of patients. There was a suggestion of an improved survival in IORT patients (median, 6 months) compared with patients treated with only surgical bypass (median, 2.5 months).[138]

A combination of intraoperative electron-beam irradiation and external-beam photon irradiation has been used in patients with unresectable pancreatic carcinoma at three major medical centers within the United States. A total of 63 patients with locally advanced disease were treated at the Massachusetts General Hospital between 1978 and 1985 on a single-arm pilot study.[139,140] All patients received preoperative external-beam irradiation of 1000 cGy delivered in five fractions during the week before exploration. At exploration, the patients received intraoperative electron-beam irradiation of 1500 to 2000 cGy, with most receiving 2000 cGy. Misonidazole, a hypoxic cell sensitizer, was given at a dose of 3.5 g/m² immediately before IORT in 41 of 63 patients. A surgical bypass of the bile duct or duodenum was performed as indicated. Postoperatively, the patients received an additional 3960 cGy of external-beam irradiation over 5 weeks. The median survival of the group was 14 months, with a 16.5-month median survival for patients receiving IORT without misonidazole and a 12-month median survival for patients receiving IORT with misonidazole. Approximately 60% of patients were alive at 1 year, and 25% were alive at 2 years. As determined clinically by follow-up CT scans, about 67% of patients had local control at 1 year, but only 40% continued to have local control at 2 years. The longest survival in the series was 52 months.

At the Mayo Clinic, a total of 52 patients with primary unresectable pancreatic carcinoma have been treated with a combination of IORT to 2000 cGy and external-beam radiation therapy of 4500 to 5000 cGy, using conventional fractionation.[141] Some patients also received 5-FU given intravenously for 3 consecutive days at 500 mg/m² during weeks 1 and 5 of the external-beam irradiation. These patients were compared with a group of 122 patients with locally advanced unresectable pancreatic cancer treated by external-beam irradiation alone (4000–6000 cGy), often with a similar 5-FU regimen during the same time period (1974–1985). Although there appeared to be a significant difference in clinical local control favoring external-beam irradiation and IORT rather than external-beam irradiation alone with 1 year (82% versus 48%) and 2 year follow-up (66% versus 20%), no differences in median (12–13 months) nor long-term survival were found.

In the National Cancer Institute study of IORT in patients with unresectable carcinoma of the pancreas, 32 patients with unresectable stage III disease or with limited stage IV disease (liver and peritoneal metastases detected at exploration) were entered into a prospectively randomized trial.[114] The patients in the treatment group received surgical biliary and gastric bypass followed by IORT to the primary tumor of 2500 cGy using 18- to 22-MeV electrons. These patients received postoperative external-beam radiation therapy of 5000 cGy over 6 to 7 weeks. The control group received the biliary and gastric bypass and postoperative external-beam irradiation of 6000 cGy delivered in split courses of 2000 cGy over 2 weeks, with cycles separated by a 2-week break. Both the experimental

and control groups received 5-FU, begun concomitantly with external-beam irradiation at 500 mg/m² for 3 days and repeated every 4 weeks for a year. In this study, in which most patients had stage IV disease, the median survival for the IORT and control patients was 8 months. All patients on the control arm died within 18 months, and patients on the IORT arm died within 24 months. Time to local disease progression was longer in the IORT arm, but more than 50% of patients failed locally. Four patients had complete autopsies. Radiation-related changes were seen, with widespread necrosis and little or no viable tumor identified in 2 patients.[142] Although the treatment-related complication rates were similar for the IORT and control groups, 3 patients receiving IORT developed severe, but not fatal, late duodenal hemorrhage. Exocrine pancreatic function appeared unaffected in the IORT and external-beam irradiation patients, although experimental canine data suggest that exocrine deficiency may be a late complication.[143]

Based on the published experience with IORT alone or with the combination of IORT and external-beam irradiation, there does not appear to be any major improvement in overall survival for patients with locally advanced unresectable pancreatic carcinoma. Although the initial experience of the contribution of misonidazole as a radiation sensitizer was positive, additional follow-up at Massachusetts General Hospital and the National Cancer Institute suggests that there is no benefit from the addition of the sensitizer to IORT.[114,139,140] Some of these series suggest a decrease in local failure, but the development of widespread metastatic disease during or shortly after treatment continues to be the major problem. Data from Japan using similar combinations of IORT and external-beam irradiation are no different from the results of United States institutions.[144]

HIGH LINEAR ENERGY TRANSFER RADIATION. The use of high LET radiation can theoretically improve tumor response because its ability to kill cells has little dependence on oxygen concentration. With photon irradiation, which is low LET radiation, cell kill can vary by a factor of 2.5 to 3.0, depending on the tissue concentration of oxygen. Fast-neutron irradiation is a type of high LET commonly used in the United States, although it is available only at a few centers.

Between 1980 and 1984, the Radiation Therapy Oncology Group (RTOG) conducted a small 3-arm randomized trial using patients with locally advanced pancreas carcinoma, comparing equivalent biologic doses of external-beam photon irradiation and neutron irradiation alone.[145] Only 49 patients were entered, with 23 patients receiving photons, 11 patients receiving mixed beam, and 15 patients receiving neutrons. No differences in local control nor survival (median, 6–8 months) were found, suggesting that neutrons alone or mixed with photon irradiation offer no benefit compared with the technically easier approach of photon irradiation.

CHARGED PARTICLE IRRADIATION. Helium ions and negative pi mesons have been used to treat locally advanced pancreatic carcinoma. Unlike photons or neutrons, for which the beam energy is attenuated continuously in tissue, the dose distribution of charged particles is characterized by a discrete stopping region called the Bragg peak, which depends on the initial beam energy. A relatively homogenous dose distribution can be obtained for a tumor volume using beam modulators. These charged particles are biologically more effective than photons, with factors of relative biologic effectiveness of 1.2 for helium ions and 1.5 for negative pi mesons, compared with 1.0 for photons.

The Northern California Oncology Group performed a randomized trial using patients with locally advanced pancreas cancer of helium ion radiation therapy to split-course photon irradiation (6000 cGy over 10 weeks).[146] All patients also received bolus infusions of 5-FU (500 mg/m²) on days 1 through 3 of helium ion irradiation and with each 2-week course of external-beam irradiation. The bolus 5-FU schedule was continued monthly for 2 years or until disease progression. Between 1978 and 1982, 49 patients were randomized. No significant differences in local control (10% versus 5%, favoring helium ion irradiation) nor median survival (7.8 months versus 6.5 months, favoring helium ion irradiation) were found. As with neutron irradiation, the use of charged particle irradiation is of no clinical benefit compared with conventional external-beam photon irradiation despite the biologic advantages.

COMPLICATIONS OF SURGICAL OR INTRAOPERATIVE IRRADIATION

Many physicians have argued against pancreatic resection for adenocarcinoma of the pancreas because of operative mortality in the range of 20% to 30%. The operative mortality in our hands is less than 5%, similar to other reported series. Estimated median operative blood loss in the 151 resections performed at MSKCC for adenocarcinoma of the pancreas from 1983 to 1990 was 2000 ml, with a median replacement of 750 ml (0–6500 ml). Mortality is usually associated with a leak of the pancreaticojejunal anastomosis, and the second most common complication is postoperative hemorrhage. The high frequency of leakage from pancreaticojejunostomy has been used as an argument in favor of performing total pancreatectomy. We think these complications are small and uncommon, and with operative mortality less than 5%, they should not be used as an argument against resection.

One early postsurgical complication is delayed gastric emptying, which is usually self-limiting and requires agents such as Reglan. If drainage is adequate, pancreaticojejunal leaks and biliary leaks can usually be treated conservatively. On rare occasions, reexploration for such anastomotic difficulties is justified. Later technical complications include stenosis at the choledochojejunal anastomosis. Stenoses are often associated with the development of cholangitis and with progressive deterioration in liver function. The symptoms are intermittent fever and chills, accompanied by mildly elevated liver function test findings. Diagnosis can be confirmed by ultrasound or CT scanning, which can demonstrate a dilated duct and intraductal stones. If sufficient doubt exists, transhepatic percutaneous cholangiography can clearly demonstrate the problem. This can be remedied by re-resection of the anastomosis, performed after all the biliary stones have been removed.

Metabolic complications include diabetes mellitus and pancreatic exocrine insufficiency. The development of insulin-dependent diabetes mellitus depends on the amount of normal pancreas left, and various tests of pancreatic reserve are being explored.[147,148] For most patients who do not have diabetes preoperatively and who require resection only of the head of the pancreas, no supplemental insulin is needed after the procedure.

Unless there was extensive antecedent pancreatitis or chronic obstruction and glandular obstruction, pancreatic insufficiency is usually mild. If there is significant diarrhea or fat malabsorption, add pancreatic enzyme supplementation before each meal. Other complications are usually indicators of recurrent disease. Most commonly, the recurrence of pain, jaundice from obstruction or intrahepatic metastases, and the development of ascites are harbingers of relatively imminent demise and require only symptomatic or palliative treatment.

Complications of intraoperative radiation therapy can be significant, with pancreatic leak, the development of pancreatic ascites, and occasionally, prolonged delays in return to normal gastrointestinal function. Despite this, we were not able to demonstrate prolonged hospital stays because of brachytherapy. In all of these situations, nutritional deficits are common, and perioperative use of nutritional support by the parenteral or enteral route is to be encouraged. An ongoing randomized trial of the benefit of postoperative total parenteral nutrition in these patients has not yet shown significance.[149]

SYSTEMIC THERAPY

Most patients with pancreatic cancer have obvious metastases or uncontrollable locally advanced disease at presentation or shortly thereafter. Although a few patients experience clinically meaningful responses to single agents or to combination chemotherapy, attempts to define a treatment that reproducibly induces response in even 20% of patients have been unsuccessful. Responses are partial and are usually 3 to 6 months long. In most phase II trials, the median survival of patients with metastatic pancreatic adenocarcinoma is in the range of 12 to 14 weeks, and even in the most optimistic of reports, overall survival results are dismal.

Patients with metastatic disease frequently present in a debilitated state. Because the median age of patients with pancreatic carcinoma is approximately 70 years, many have other complicating medical illnesses. Nausea, vomiting, cachexia, hepatic dysfunction, jaundice, ascites, intravascular volume depletion, and poorly controlled pain are common problems. Many patients postpone seeking medical attention while symptoms worsen insidiously, but many others do complain to their physicians for months before the necessary diagnostic studies are performed. A nihilistic approach on the part of primary care physicians, surgeons, and medical oncologists may contribute to the delay in diagnosis. The result is a self-fulfilling prophecy, because patients who present in a frail, medically unstable state at the end of a period of rapid clinical deterioration are unlikely to benefit from any available antineoplastic therapy.

The precarious physiologic condition of many patients with pancreatic carcinoma renders them poor candidates for clinical trials. When these patients are included in phase II studies, the likelihood of recognizing agents with real, if limited, activity is diminished. Moreover, toxicity is increased; it is often difficult to differentiate side effects of therapy from the natural progression of the disease. Inclusion of patients who are rapidly deteriorating in phase III studies almost certainly explains the invariable decline in response and survival compared with phase II findings. Improved diagnostic tools, combined with an awareness of potential therapeutic options, may lead to earlier diagnosis, when therapeutic intervention and participation in clinical trials is appropriate.

Evaluating response to therapy is often difficult in patients with pancreas cancer. Before the era of CT scanning, when most trials of the conventional chemotherapeutic agents were conducted, palpable abdominal masses were often used as indicator lesions. Lack of precision in measurements obtained by physical examination undoubtedly contributed to inaccurate estimates of therapeutic activity. Even with modern medical imaging techniques, the extent of disease is often underestimated, and assessment of response, as defined by classic criteria, is difficult. Primary pancreatic tumors often invade nearby structures and are associated with inflammation and fibrosis. Borders are usually indistinct, and true "bidimensionally measurable" primary disease is often an illusion. Changes can often be appreciated on CT scans, but measurement is subject to bias and interobserver variation. Patients may succumb to the metabolic effects of the cancer or to distant metastases without a substantial change in the size of the primary lesion. Liver metastases are often seen as discrete nodules on CT scan, but peritoneal disease is often clinically obvious, but difficult to measure. Changes in serum concentrations of tumor markers, such as CEA and CA 19-9, have not paralleled tumor burden precisely.

The assessment of tumor response is fundamental to phase II evaluations, but change in the size of a measurable mass is a surrogate endpoint. Improvement in the quality and quantity of life is the real objective of treatment, and recommendations for individual patients should be guided by the impact of therapy on these goals. Measurement of pain and "quality of life" is complex, and measurements are influenced by treatments directed at symptom control and specific antineoplastic therapy. The demonstration of modest improvements in these outcomes and in survival requires well-designed controlled clinical trials.

The obstacles encountered in evaluating antineoplastic regimens may be one reason for the lack of substantial progress in the therapy of pancreatic cancer. Relatively little is known about the biology of pancreas cancer. There are few laboratory models of this disease, and there is a lack of preclinical pharmacology that is specific to pancreas cancer and that might be used to guide clinical trials. Reasons for response or resistance to the agents that have been studied have not been elucidated. Recent insights regarding the pharmacology of available chemotherapeutic agents, the development of novel immunotherapeutic strategies, and new discoveries in the field of molecular biology hold potential for genuine advances in the therapy of this disease.

CHEMOTHERAPY

Activity of Individual Agents

Results of one-arm and randomized trials with single-agent chemotherapy using standard and experimental drugs in patients with adenocarcinoma of the pancreas are presented in Tables 27–6 and 27–7. 5-FU is the most studied and widely used agent. In 212 cases collected from the literature in 1975, a response of 28% was recorded.[150] In prospective randomized trials, fewer than 20% of patients have responded to 5-FU.[151,201,202] The optimal dose and schedule of 5-FU has not been defined. Continuous intravenous infusion of 1 g/m²/day for 5 days or intravenous injection of 400 to 500 mg/m² daily for 5 consecutive days every 4 to 5 weeks are popular schedules. Some physicians prefer once-weekly treatment with or without a 5-day loading dose. 5-FU is not absorbed reliably

TABLE 27–6. Activity of Individual Agents Used in the Treatment of Patients With Pancreatic Adenocarcinoma

Drug	Responders/Total No. of Patients	Percent Response (95% Confidence Interval)*	Investigations
5-Fluorouracil	60/212	28 (22–34)	Carter[150]
	5/31	16 (6–32)	Kovach[151]
	3/16	19 (1–43)	Hansen[152]
	0/14	0 (0–21)	Tajiri[153]
Mitomycin C	11/53	21 (10–32)	Crooke[154]
	6/18	33 (16–62)	Carter[155]
Streptozotocin	3/27	11 (3–27)	Carter[150]
Doxorubicin	2/25	8 (1–24)	Schein[156]
Nitrosoureas			
Semustine (methyl-CCNU)	1/68	6 (2–15)	Moertel[157]
Carmustine (BCNU)	0/37	0 (0–8)	Carter[150]
	0/21	0 (0–14)	Kovach[151]
Lomustine (CCNU)	3/19	16 (4–36)	Carter[150]
Chlorozotocin	3/57	5 (1–13)	GITSG[158]

* Estimated two-sided 95% confidence interval for responses.

TABLE 27–7.   Activity of Individual Agents Studied in Series of 10 or More Patients With Pancreatic Adenocarcinoma

Drugs	Responders/ Total No. of Patients	Percent Response (95% Confidence Interval)*	Investigations
Intercalators			
Amsacrine	0/54	0 (0–7)	Inamasu[159]
	0/27	0 (0–11)	Omura[160]
	0/27	0 (0–11)	Sternberg[161]
Idarubicin	2/32	6 (1–19)	Mittleman[162]
Epirubicin	3/16	19 (5–43)	Hochster[163]
	8/34	24 (11–41)	Wils[164]
	0/20	0 (0–14)	Loven[165]
	2/34	6 (1–18)	GITSG[166]
Esorubicin	0/16	0 (0–18)	Blayney[167]
	3/47	6 (2–17)	Vaughn[168]
Menogaril	2/38	5 (2–17)	Brown[169]
	0/15	0 (0–19)	Sternberg[170]
Mitoxantrone	0/14	0 (0–21)	Bedikian[171]
	0/30	0 (0–10)	DeSimone[172]
	2/24	8 (2–25)	Taylor[173]
Alkylators			
Melphalan	1/43	2 (1–7)	Horton[174]
	2/15	13 (2–37)	Smith[175]
Ifosfamide	6/10	60 (27–85)	Gad-El-Mawla[176]
	6/27	22 (10–41)	Loehrer[177]
	1/29	3 (0–17)	Bernard[178]
	3/30	10 (3–24)	GITSG[179]
	2/30	7 (1–21)	Ajani[180]
Diaziquone (AZQ)	0/17	0 (0–17)	DeSimone[181]
	0/21	0 (0–14)	Tilchen[182]
	0/21	0 (0–14)	GITSG[166]
Antimetabolites			
Methotrexate	1/25	4 (0–19)	Schein[156]
Metoprine	0/24	0 (0–12)	Sternberg[183]
Edatrexate	0/14	0 (0–20)	Casper[184]
Trimetrexate	0/14	0 (0–20)	Carlson[185]
Triazinate	0/31	0 (0–10)	GITSG[166]
Fludarabine	0/15	0 (0–19)	Kilton[186]
Fazarabine	0/14	0 (0–20)	Casper[184]
Gemcitabine	5/39	13 (3–23)	Casper[187]
Plant Alkyloids			
Etoposide	0/28	0 (0–11)	Horton[174]
	0/26	0 (0–11)	Sternberg[188]
Vinblastine	0/33	0 (0–8)	Guy[189]
Vindesine	1/15	6 (0–30)	Magill[190]
Miscellaneous			
Amonifide	0/14	0 (0–20)	Linke[191]
β-2'-deoxythioguanosine	2/32	6 (1–14)	GITSG[192]
Carmofur	0/38	0 (0–8)	Grohn[193]
Cisplatin	0/14	0 (0–20)	Kantarjian[194]
Iproplatin	3/30	10 (3–24)	Abbruzze[195]
Hexamethylmelamine	4/55	7 (1–18)	GITSG[192]
Dactinomycin	1/28	4 (1–17)	Schein[156]

(continued)

TABLE 27–7. *(Continued)*

Drugs	Responders/ Total No. of Patients	Percent Response (95% Confidence Interval)*	Investigations
Dianhydrogalactitol	1/40	2 (1–9)	GITSG[192]
L-Asparaginase	0/10	0 (0–27)	Lessner[196]
Maytansine	0/48	0 (0–5)	GITSG[158]
MGBG	2/33	6 (1–14)	Inamasu[197]
	2/36	6 (1–14)	Ravry[198]
Pibenzimol	0/26	0 (0–11)	Patel[199]
	0/23	0 (0–13)	Kraut[200]
Razoxane (ICRF159)	2/29	7 (1–21)	GITSG[192]

* Estimated two-sided 95% confidence interval for responses.

from the gut, and oral administration should not be used. In a random assignment trial, none of 14 patients who received 5-FU (15 mg/kg) orally had tumor regression (median survival, 53 days), whereas 3 of the 16 who received the same dose intravenously experienced partial responses (median survival, 110 days).[203] Prolonged continuous intravenous infusions of 5-FU in doses ranging from 170 to 300 mg/m^2/day have been advocated, but it is unclear that this method of administration is more efficacious or less toxic than older and less complicated schedules.[152,153] Different schedules of administration have not been extensively compared prospectively in patients with pancreas cancer, nor has a serious dose-intensity analysis been performed.

Other older agents that have been used in combination chemotherapy include mitomycin C, the nitrosoureas, doxorubicin (Adriamycin), and streptozotocin. Streptozotocin has been of special interest because of its toxic effects on normal pancreatic islet cells and ductal epithelium. The phase II data for these and other conventional agents are quite limited, and much of what is accepted regarding the antineoplastic activity of these agents has been extrapolated from combination chemotherapy trials. Doses of individual agents are often reduced in combinations because of overlapping toxicities, and few of the older agents have been studied at doses close to their maximally tolerated dose. Many of the trials were conducted exclusively or largely with previously treated patients. Given the difficulties encountered in assessing response to therapy, it can be stated that many agents with activity in other diseases have not been tested adequately in patients with pancreas cancer.

One exception is ifosfamide. An initial report in which 6 of 10 patients experienced major responses prompted a series of larger phase II trials.[176] Pooling all reported phase II studies, there have been 18 (14%) responders among 126 patients; excluding the unusually favorable results obtained in the initial report, the overall response in the literature is 10%. Although one group claimed a response of 22%, this observation was not been confirmed by others.[177–180] Furthermore, that same group saw a response of only 7% with the combination of ifosfamide plus FU, even though the dose of ifosfamide was similar in both studies.[204]

Several experimental agents were evaluated during the past 15 years. Many of these studies included poor-risk, previously treated patients. Few agents demonstrated sufficient activity in their initial evaluation to encourage further study. The results with the anthracyclines, however, are of interest. Preliminary data from MSKCC indicate that most pancreatic adenocarcinomas express the MDR1 (multidrug resistance) phenotype. Because a few patients do respond to anthracyclines, strategies to reverse multidrug resistance merit evaluation in patients with pancreas cancer. Gemcitabine (2′,2′-difluorodeoxycytidine) is the only recently evaluated agent that has demonstrated activity in this disease.[187] Objective responses associated with clinical improvement were seen with only minimal toxicity during the initial phase II evaluation, and additional study of this agent is underway.

Combination Chemotherapy

Initial combination chemotherapy trials in gastrointestinal cancer used combinations of 5-FU plus BCNU. Early encouraging reports of responses in limited numbers of patients with pancreas cancer led to larger trials using 5-FU plus nitrosourea combinations.[205] In a randomized trial comparing 5-FU alone, BCNU alone, and the combination of 5-FU plus BCNU in patients with pancreatic or gastric cancer, the response observed among the 82 patients with pancreas cancer to the combination (33%) was superior to that seen with 5-FU (16%) alone, but the difference was not statistically significant; there were no responses to single-agent BCNU.[151] Overall, there was no survival advantage for patients treated with combination chemotherapy over those treated with single agents. There were two randomized trials in which patients with pancreas cancer received 5-FU plus a nitrosourea or no specific anticancer therapy (Table 27–8). A small Danish study reported a median survival of 13 weeks for the group treated with 5-FU plus BCNU and 14 weeks for those who received no chemotherapy.[206] In a Veterans Administration study, 152 patients were randomized to 5-FU plus CCNU or to supportive care.[207] Toxicity was mild, but there was no evidence of benefit for the treated group. Median survival was 3.0 months in the treatment arm, and 3.9 months for those who received no chemotherapy.

Early reports of multidrug combinations suggested that higher response rates could be achieved with more than two drugs (Table 27–9). The combination of streptozotocin, mi-

TABLE 27–8. Randomized Trials of Chemotherapy Versus Supportive Care in Patients With Pancreatic Adenocarcinoma

Regimens	No. of Patients	Median Survival (mo)	Investigations
Fluorouracil + BCNU	20	3.0	Andersen[206]
Observation	20	3.3	
Fluorouracil + CCNU	65	3.0	Frey[207]
Observation	87	3.9	
Mallinson regimen	21	10.3	Mallinson[208]
Observation	19	2.1	

tomycin C, and 5-FU (SMF regimen) induced responses in 43% and 32% of patients in two independent trials using slightly different schedules.[209,210] Subsequently, the FAM regimen (5-FU, doxorubicin, and mitomycin C), which had demonstrated activity in gastric cancer, yielded responses in 10 (37%) of 27 of patients with pancreas cancer; 40% responded in a trial of a modified FAM program.[211,212] Similar results have been seen in other phase II trials of combination chemotherapy containing 5-FU and mitomycin C.[201,218–221] SMF given as described by Wiggans[209] and FAM (as described by Smith[211] were studied in two randomized trials. The Cancer and Leukemia Group B studied 184 patients; among the 133 patients with measurable disease, 14% of the patients treated

with FAM responded, compared with 4% of those treated with SMF. For all patients treated with FAM, the median survival was 6.1 months, and for SMF-treated patients, it was 4.2 months. None of these differences was statistically significant.[215]

As part of a larger randomized phase II program, the GITSG compared FAM with the original SMF (SMF I) and with a modified SMF schedule (SMF II). Eighty-four eligible patients were randomized to one of these three regimens as first therapy. The response to FAM was 14%, and to the two SMF regimens, it was 14% and 15%, respectively. The median survival for patients treated with FAM was 3 months, and for the original SMF regimen, 4.5 months.[216]

The North Central Cancer Treatment Group (NCCTG) conducted an important three-arm randomized trial comparing 5-FU alone, 5-FU plus doxorubicin (FA), and FAM in patients with advanced pancreatic or gastric cancer (see Table 27–9).[201] The primary endpoint of this trial was survival, and most patients did not have measurable disease. In the single-agent arm, 5-FU was given in a 5-day course at a dose of 500 mg/m^2/day every 4 weeks for two cycles and every 5 weeks thereafter. In the FA combination, 5-FU was administered in a 4-day course using a dose of 400 mg/m^2/day, with doxorubicin (40 mg/m^2) given on the first day of each cycle; chemotherapy was recycled every 4 weeks for two cycles and every 5 weeks thereafter. FAM was administered at the original doses and schedule. In the cohort of 144 patients with pancreas cancer, 33 had measurable disease; objective responses were documented in 3 of 10 patients treated with 5-

TABLE 27–9. SMF and FAM Regimens for Pancreas Cancer: Results of Single-Arm and Randomized Trials

Regimen*	No. of Patients	Responders/ Total Patients† (% Response)	Median Survival (mo)	Investigations
SMF	23	10/23 (43)	6.0	Wiggans[209]
SMF	22	7/22 (32)	6.0	Bukowski[210]
FAM	10	10/27 (37)	6.0	Smith[211]
FAM	15	6/15 (40)	3.7	Bitran[212]
FAM	72	10/45 (22)	4.4	Buroker[213]
FAMe	72	2/43 (5)	4.0	
MF	73	5/60 (8)	4.0	Bukowski[214]
SMF	72	19/56 (34)	4.2	
FAM	94	9/65 (14)	6.1	Oster[215]
SMF	94	3/68 (4)	4.2	
FAM	29	4/29 (14)	2.7	GITSG[216]
SMF I	28	4/28 (14)	4.0	
SMF II	27	4/27 (15)	3.1	
F	50	3/10 (30)	5.1	Cullinan[201]
FA	44	3/10 (30)	(no significant difference)	
FAM	50	1/13 (8)	(no significant difference)	
SMF	42	4/39 (10)	10.0	Kelsen[217]
CAC	40	2/36 (6)	5.0	

* F, fluorouracil; S, streptozotocin; A, doxorubicin (Adriamycin); M, mitomycin C; Me, methyl CCNU; CAC, cisplatin + ara-C + caffeine.
† Among patients with measurable disease.

FU, 3 of 10 treated with FA, and 1 of 13 treated with FAM. The Kaplan-Meier survival curves for all patients treated with each of the three regimens could be superimposed, with a median survival of 4.7 months. Predictors of improved survival included being female (*i.e.*, median survival of 29 weeks, compared with 14 weeks for men), having a better performance status, and having locoregional disease rather than distant metastases. In one small randomized trial, patients treated with a regimen consisting of 5-FU, cyclophosphamide, methotrexate, and vincristine followed by maintenance therapy with 5-FU plus mitomycin C, had a median survival of 10.3 months, compared with 2.1 months for patients who received no chemotherapy (see Table 27–8).[208] The NCCTG compared this regimen, the combination of 5-FU, doxorubicin and cisplatin (FAP),[222] and 5-FU alone in a recently reported phase II trial.[202] Median survival for the 5-drug regimen was 4.5 months compared with 3.5 months for 5-FU alone or FAP, and the survival curves were virtually identical.

The European Organization for Research on Treatment of Cancer has tried to build on observations made in recent phase II trials by studying the combinations of epirubicin plus 5-FU and epirubicin plus ifosfamide.[223,224] Neither regimen yielded results significantly different from their experience with epirubicin alone.[164]

The disappointing results with empirically selected phase II agents led the group at MSKCC to study a novel combination with activity against a human pancreatic cancer xenograft in the nude mouse.[225] The combination of cisplatin, ara-C, and caffeine (CAC regimen) was piloted in a disease-specific phase I study of the combination.[226] The doses achieved in the clinic were equivalent to the doses used in the mice, and 41% of

patients responded. In a randomized phase II trial, however, the response to CAC was 6%, with a median survival of 5 months, and the response to SMF was 10%, with a median survival of 10 months.[217]

The results of randomized trials in patients with pancreas cancer are summarized in Table 27–10. Several of the regimens studied are shown in Table 27–11.

Modulation of Fluorouracil

The occasional responses observed in patients with advanced disease treated with 5-FU-based chemotherapy and the results of combined 5-FU plus radiation therapy studies in patients with localized pancreatic carcinoma suggest that 5-FU can affect the natural history of pancreas cancer. Although the clinical benefit of such treatments appears to be limited, the fact that responses are seen at all suggests that there is an opportunity for improving therapy. The activity of 5-FU can be enhanced in experimental systems using drugs that alter the biochemical pathways involved in pyrimidine synthesis and degradation. Biochemical modulation appears to have been translated into clinical benefit in patients with colon cancer, and these results stimulated attempts to improve the efficacy of 5-FU in pancreas cancer.

The combination of 5-FU plus leucovorin was introduced to intensify the inhibition of thymidylate synthase by the 5-FU metabolite FdUMP. In 1985, the combination of 5-FU (30 mg/kg) plus leucovorin (100–200 mg) produced four durable responses among 8 patients with adenocarcinoma thought to be of pancreatic origin.[230] Unfortunately, the activity of this combination could not be confirmed in two subsequent phase

TABLE 27–10. Randomized Trials of Combination Chemotherapy in Patients With Pancreatic Adenocarcinoma

Regimen*	No. of Patients	Responders/ Total Patients† (% Response)	Median Survival (mo)	Investigations
FU	31	5/31 (16)	≈6.0	Kovach[151]
BCNU	21	0/21 (0)	(no significant	
FU + BCNU	30	10/30 (33)	difference)	
F	34	7/34 (21)	≈5.6	Awrich[227]
FS + tubercidin	39	3/39 (8)	≈4.4	
F	176		4.9	Moertel[228]
F + spironolactone	Total		3.5	
FS			4.2	
FS + spironolactone			3.7	
Melphalan	43	1/43 (2)	1.8	Horton[174]
FMe	41	4/41 (10)	3.3	
FMeS	43	3/43 (7)	2.8	
FS	42	5/42 (12)	3.0	Moertel[229]
CS	51	6/51 (12)	2.1	
F	64	1/14 (7)	3.5	Cullinan[202]
FAP	59	2/13 (15)	3.5	
CFMtxVM	61	3/14 (21)	4.5	

* F, fluorouracil; S, streptozotocin; A, doxorubicin (Adriamycin); Me, methyl CCNU; P, cisplatin; Mtx, methotrexate, V, vincristine; M, mitomycin C.
† Among patients with measurable disease.

TABLE 27–11. Combination Chemotherapy for Patients With Adenocarcinoma
of the Pancreas

Regimen and Protocol	Responders/ Total Patients	Percent Response (Two-Sided 95% Confidence Limits)	Median Survival (mo)	Investigations
SMF				
Streptozotocin 1 g/m² days 1, 8, 29, 36	10/23	43 (25–64)	6	Wiggans[209]
Mitomycin C 10 mg/m² day 1				
Fluorouracil 600 mg/m² days, 1, 8, 29, 36				
Recycle every 56 days				
SMF				
Streptozotocin 300 mg/m² daily, days 1–4, 29–33	7/22	32 (13–58)	6	Bukowski[210]
Mitomycin C 10 mg/m² day 1				
Fluorouracil 500 mg/m² daily, days 1–5, 29–33				
Recycle every 56 days				
FAM				
Fluorouracil 600 mg/m² days 1, 8, 29, 36	10/27	37 (20–57)	6.0	Smith[211]
Adriamycin 30 mg/m² days 1, 29				
Mitomycin C 10 mg/m² day 1				
Recycle every 56 days				
FAM				
Fluorouracil 500 mg/m² days 1, 8, 21, 28	6/15	40 (19–67)	3.7	Bitran[212]
Adriamycin 30 mg/m² days 1, 21				
Mitomycin C 10 mg/m² day 1				
Recycle every 42 days				
Mallinson Regimen				
Fluorouracil 500 mg days 1–5	—	—	10.3	Mallinson[208]
Cyclophosphamide 300 mg days 1, 5				
Vincristine 1 mg days 2, 5				
Methotrexate 20 mg days 1, 4 followed in 4 weeks by				
Fluorouracil 10 mg/kg days 1–5 every 6 weeks				
Mitomycin C 100 μg/kg days 1–5 every 6 weeks				
FAP				
Fluorouracil 300 mg/m² days 1–5	6/29	21 (9–37)	2.3	Moertel[222]
Adriamycin 40 mg/m² day 1				
Cisplatin 60 mg/m² day 1				
Recycle every 35 days				

II trials. Only two responses were seen among 27 patients treated on a weekly schedule using 5-FU (600 mg/m²) with leucovorin (500 mg/m²), and no responses were seen among 19 patients treated with a 6-day high-dose (500 mg/m²/day) leucovorin infusion with a daily bolus 5-FU (370 mg/m²) for 5 days.[231,232] Because the toxic effects of 5-FU plus leucovorin can be life-threatening, this combination should not be used outside the research setting. Other attempts at biochemical modulation have used PALA (phosphonacetyl-L-aspartate), an inhibitor of de novo pyrimidine biosynthesis, to increase the phosphorylation of 5-FU to FUMP, with the goal of increasing the incorporation of 5-FU into RNA. Two phase II trials demonstrated responses in 3 of 16 and 1 of 21 patients, respectively. In early results, the combination of PALA plus 5-FU plus leucovorin produced responses in 5 of 6 patients.[233–235]

Many of the regimens used in patients with pancreas cancer were selected for study after demonstrating activity in stomach cancer. In a randomized trial, the combination of 5-FU plus doxorubicin plus methotrexate (FAMTX regimen) showed superiority over FAM in patients with advanced gastric cancer.[236] This regimen employs the sequential administration of high-dose methotrexate plus 5-FU followed by leucovorin 24 hours later, a different biochemical strategy. Only modest activity was seen with this regimen in patients with pancreas cancer; among 25 evaluable patients, the response was 16%.[237] Investigators in the United States and in Europe are continuing to explore other combinations of 5-FU with leucovorin, PALA, and methotrexate.

No drug or combination chemotherapy program has demonstrated superiority over 5-FU alone in terms of palliation or prolonging survival, and 5-FU remains the "standard" in clinical practice, although few patients truly benefit from treatment. Combination chemotherapy is frequently more toxic than 5-FU, and its use outside of prospective clinical trials cannot be recommended.

Regional Chemotherapy

Pancreas cancer is often a problem confined to the region of the pancreas, the peritoneal cavity, or the liver. Although distant metastases are occasionally seen, they rarely are relevant to the clinical course of the patient. This led investigators to consider regional approaches to therapy. One is intraarterial therapy, by selective arterial infusion with or without radiotherapy or by the technique of isolation perfusion with extracorporeal chemofiltration.[238–240] In the latter technique, chemotherapy is administered through catheters placed in selected arteries or the abdominal aorta. During drug infusion, venous blood is circulated through a hemofiltration filter by means of a double-lumen filtration catheter placed in the inferior vena cava to remove drug before it enters the systemic circulation. Several small series that included patients with pancreas cancer claimed responses for strategies using 5-FU, mitomycin C, and cisplatin or using 5-FU and cisplatin. Although the techniques have been well documented, these approaches have not been studied systematically in terms of therapeutic efficacy.

At least 40% of patients with pancreas cancer have clinically relevant peritoneal metastases. One approach that has not been exploited in patients with pancreas cancer is intraperitoneal chemotherapy. The ideal setting for such treatment appears to be in the adjuvant setting in which the volume of any intraperitoneal disease is low. Most surgeons are reluctant to add intraperitoneal chemotherapy to patients who have undergone pancreatoduodenectomy because of the concern about disrupting biliary or pancreatic anastomoses. As operative care becomes less morbid, adjuvant intraperitoneal treatment may become more practical. Intraperitoneal therapy may find a role as an adjunct to irradiation, systemic chemotherapy, or intraarterial therapy.

COMBINED-MODALITY THERAPY FOR LOCALLY ADVANCED DISEASE

A role for 5-FU as a radiation sensitizer was proposed by Heidelberger in 1958.[241] This approach was evaluated at the Mayo Clinic, where preliminary results in patients with gastrointestinal cancer led to a small randomized trial in which patients with unresectable pancreas cancer were treated with radiation alone (3500–4000 rads) with a low dose of 5-FU (approximately 45 mg/kg) divided over the first 3 days of treatment or to the same dose of radiation with a saline placebo.[242,243] A statistically significant advantage in survival was observed in the patients who received 5-FU (Table 27–12).

In 1974, the GITSG initiated a series of prospective randomized trials using postoperative adjuvant therapy for patients with pancreas cancer. In the first study, treatment with high-dose radiation (6000 rads) alone was compared with treatment with the same dose of radiation with 5-FU and a lower dose of radiation (4000 rads) with 5-FU. Radiation was delivered in 2000-rad, 2-week courses, and in the 5-FU-containing arms, 5-FU was administered by rapid intravenous injection at a dose of 500 mg/m²/day on the first 3 days of each 2000-rad radiation course. Four weeks after completion

TABLE 27–12. Randomized Trials Using Patients With Locally Advanced Adenocarcinoma of the Pancreas

Investigations	Regimen*	No. of Patients	Median Survival (mo)	Estimated 1-Year Survival (%)
Moertel[243]	RT (3500–4000) with saline	32	5.5†	5
	RT (3500–4000) with FU 15 mg/kg daily × 3	32	10.4†	25
Moertel[244]	First cohort			
	RT (6000)	25	5.3	15
	RT (6000) with FU	30	9.4	40
	RT (4000) with FU	27	5.3	45
	Second cohort			
	RT (6000) with FU	86	11.5	50
	RT (4000) with FU	83	8.5	45
GITSG[245]	RT (6000) with FU + FU maintenance	73	8.6	35
	RT (4000) with doxorubicin + doxorubicin, FU maintenance	70	7.7	25
Klaasen[246]	RT (4000) with FU + FU maintenance	47	8.3	26
	FU	44	8.2	30
GITSG[247]	RT (4000) with FU + SMF maintenance	22	9.7	41
	SMF	21	7.4	19

* All radiation dosages are given in cGy. FU, fluorouracil; SMF, streptozotocin, mitomycin C, and fluorouracil.
† Mean survival.

of radiation, maintenance 5-FU was administered at a dose of 500 mg/m² weekly for 2 years or until progression of disease. In an analysis of the data early in the trial, the median survival in the no-chemotherapy arm (18 weeks) was considered sufficiently inferior to the median survival in the two 5-FU plus radiation therapy arms (35 weeks) that accrual to the radiation therapy only arm was terminated. Analysis of the data at the completion of the trial demonstrated no significant survival difference between the two remaining arms, although there was a nonsignificant advantage for the patients receiving the higher dose of radiation.[244]

In a subsequent GITSG trial, patients were randomized to receive radiation (6000 rads) with concurrent low-dose 5-FU, followed by maintenance weekly 5-FU, or to radiation (4000 rads) with concurrent weekly low-dose doxorubicin followed by maintenance doxorubicin until cardiotoxic doses were approached, followed by weekly 5-FU. Maintenance therapy was to be continued until the point of progressive disease. No significant difference in survival was seen.[245]

In an Eastern Cooperative Oncology Group (ECOG) trial, patients with locally advanced disease were randomized to treatment with irradiation (4000 rads) with 5-FU (600 mg/m²) given intravenously on the first 3 days of radiotherapy, followed by the same dose of 5-FU weekly, or to treatment with weekly 5-FU (600 mg/m²) alone. The median survival time was identical for patients treated in the two arms, and a similar proportion of patients were alive 1 year after starting therapy.[246] In contrast, a recent GITSG trial compared irradiation (5400 cGy in 180-cGy fractions) with concurrent low-dose 5-FU, followed by SMF chemotherapy (as given by Wiggans), to treatment with SMF alone. The survival with the combined modality therapy was superior to that same with chemotherapy alone. Interpretation of this trial is confounded by the small number of patients randomized from a large number of institutions and a high proportion of treatment violations. Local control of the pancreatic mass was not superior in the radiation therapy arm.[247] It is impossible to make a definitive statement about the relative roles of radiation and chemotherapy for locally advanced pancreas cancer at this time.

HORMONAL THERAPY

Rationale and Preclinical Data

There are several lines of evidence to suggest that pancreas cancer may be under the influence of sex hormones. The disease appears to be more prevalent in men than in women, especially those younger than 50. High concentrations of estrogen receptors and estrogen synthetic enzymes (*e.g.*, aromatase, 5-reductase) have been found in pancreatic adenocarcinomas. Serum testosterone concentrations are lower in men and women with pancreas cancer than in patients with other cancers or healthy persons.[248–250] Cyproterone acetate (*i.e.*, antiandrogen) inhibited the growth of human pancreatic adenocarcinoma xenografts in nude mice in one study, and a luteinizing hormone-releasing hormone (LHRH) analog, D-trp-6-LHRH, induced regression of nitrosamine-induced pancreatic cancers in hamsters.[251,252]

The possibility that other hormonal factors may affect the growth of pancreas cancer has also been explored. Cholecystokinin (CCK) and secretin stimulate the growth of the exo-

crine pancreas in animals. Although the role of these hormones in tumorigenesis is uncertain, CCK can stimulate the growth of a human pancreatic adenocarcinoma cell line.[253] Among the actions of somatostatin and its analogs is the inhibition of the secretion or action of gastrointestinal hormones, including CCK. In two human pancreatic adenocarcinoma cell lines, growth inhibition was seen with octreotide.[254] Experimental somatostatin analogs (*e.g.*, RC-160), but not octreotide, were shown to bind to normal human pancreas and pancreatic adenocarcinoma.[255] RC-160 and D-trp-6-LHRH, alone and in combination, inhibited the growth of the nitrosamine-induced hamster pancreas cancer.[256]

Clinical Trials

The response data for tamoxifen in patients with adenocarcinoma of the pancreas are limited (*i.e.*, no responses in a single trial involving 14 patients), but the effect of tamoxifen on survival was examined in several studies.[257] In three uncontrolled trials, survival appeared to be improved compared with historical controls.[258–260] In a prospective, randomized, double-blind trial, however, patients receiving tamoxifen had a median survival of 115 days, and the median survival in the placebo group was 122 days; the proportion of patients alive at 1 year was the same (8%) in both groups.[261] In a three-arm trial, similar outcomes were seen for groups of patients randomized to tamoxifen, cyproterone acetate, or no active therapy.[262]

Perhaps the first trial of hormonal therapy in gastrointestinal cancer was a combination chemotherapy and hormone therapy with 5-FU plus spironolactone or testololactone.[263] A dramatic improvement in survival of patients with pancreas cancer was reported. The lactones were selected for their possible inhibitory effects on purine synthesis, but testololactone is an inhibitor of aromatase and has demonstrated limited clinical activity in patients with breast cancer. Spironolactone was ultimately chosen for evaluation in patients with pancreas cancer in a prospective trial that demonstrated no advantage for the addition of this agent to 5-FU or to the combination of 5-FU plus streptozotocin.[228] In another randomized study, the addition of spironolactone to 5-FU plus BCNU also failed to show an advantage in response or survival.[264] The addition of aminoglutethimide to FAM chemotherapy did not appear to improve response or survival in a small randomized study.[265]

Among 14 patients with pancreas cancer treated with octreotide, there were no objective responses, but prolongation of survival over historical controls, and symptomatic benefit has been reported in patients treated with RC-160 or with D-trp-6-LHRH.[266–268] An objective response was reported in 1 of 17 patients treated with the latter agent. No responses were seen among 21 patients in a study of combination hormonal therapy with octreotide and leuprolide.[269] The possible impact of octreotide on survival is the subject of an ongoing NCCTG trial in which patients are randomized to receive this agent, 5-FU alone, or 5-FU plus leucovorin.

Progestational agents, such as megestrol acetate or medroxyprogesterone, have been used in patients with pancreas cancer, less for an anticipated antineoplastic effect than for their reported ability to relieve anorexia and improve patients' sense of well-being. Studies targeting patients with pancreas cancer have not been reported.

BIOLOGIC THERAPY

The interferons have not been studied extensively in patients with pancreas cancer. In a phase II trial of interferon-γ (INF-γ), no responses were seen among the 13 evaluable patients.[208] Although favorable results were reported initially in patients with colon cancer,[270] the combination of 5-FU with interferon yielded only 3 responses among 46 evaluable patients with pancreatic adenocarcinoma.[271] There has been considerable interest in the use of monoclonal antibodies for therapy in patients with pancreatic cancer. Monoclonal antibody (MoAb) 17-1A is a murine IgG2a that targets a 37-kd glycoprotein on the surface of many gastrointestinal adenocarcinomas.[272] Although MoAb 17-1A does not mediate complement-dependent lysis of tumor cells, it does participate in antibody-dependent cellular cytotoxicity (ADCC). In preliminary clinical studies of MoAb 17-1A, some responses were seen in patients with pancreatic carcinoma.[273,274] The demonstration of enhancement of ADCC by INF-γ led to a therapeutic trial of recombinant INF-γ (10^6 U/m^2) daily for 4 days with MoAb 17-1A (150 mg in autologous leukocytes) on days 2, 3, and 4 in patients with advanced pancreas cancer.[275] Immunologic studies documented enhanced ADCC and improved natural cytotoxicity in treated patients, but the only objective regression was a complete response of 4 months' duration among the 25 evaluable patients. Toxicity was tolerable, and fever and mild hepatic enzyme elevation were the most prominent toxic effects, although 1 patient with a history of congestive heart failure developed fulminant fatal heart failure with the first dose of interferon. A phase II trial of repetitive doses of MoAb 17-1A (500 mg) 3 times weekly for 8 weeks failed to show objective responses in any of 28 patients, including 16 who received the full 8-week course.[276]

Another monoclonal antibody, 494/32, has been studied clinically. This murine antibody is of the IgG1 isotype, binds strongly to human pancreatic cancer cells and mediates ADCC. A partial response was seen in a patient with pancreas cancer during the phase I–II evaluation of this antibody.[277] In a prospective randomized trial using patients who underwent pancreatic resection, median survival of the 29 patients who received postoperative 494/32 was 14.2 months, not statistically different from the 12.9-month median survival of the 32 control patients.[278]

Other antibodies of interest include B72.3 and CC49, directed at the TAG-72 tumor-associated antigen, a glycoprotein expressed by a variety of gastrointestinal cancers.[279] An antigen defined by B72.3 is expressed in human pancreas cancer, and ^{90}Y-labeled B72.3 localizes to human pancreatic cancer xenografts in nude mice.[280,281] CC49 is a second-generation, high-affinity antibody to the TAG-72 antigen, and it may possess superior properties as a carrier of therapeutic isotopes.[282] The intraperitoneal use of radiolabeled antibodies against the TAG-72 antigen is being explored clinically.

Pancreas cancer cells overexpress the epidermal growth factor (EGF) receptor.[283] This receptor is a transmembrane glycoprotein expressed by a variety of normal and malignant cells. Binding of EGF or transforming growth factor-α (TGF-α) to a site on the external surface of the plasma membrane activates the intracellular portion of the receptor, a tyrosine kinase, triggering growth regulatory mechanisms. In two human pancreatic adenocarcinoma cell lines, TGF-α stimulated growth, but the normal inhibitory effects of TGF-β were not seen.[284] An autocrine loop involving TGF-α and the EGF receptor in pancreas cancer has been proposed.[285,286] These observations suggest an opportunity for therapeutic intervention with antibodies against the EGF receptor.

A new biologic approach that merits intense study derives from the observation that more than 80% of pancreatic adenocarcinomas contain a mutated K-*RAS* gene.[287] It is likely that this oncogene plays an important role in the development or progression of pancreas cancer, and it is an obvious target for novel therapeutic strategies. The pathways important to the function of this growth regulatory gene are subject to pharmacologic intervention, and drugs directed at these functions are in preclinical development.

SUMMARY

The differences in survival seen among individual single-arm trials and within randomized trials are more likely a result of variation in pretreatment prognostic factors rather than a true difference in therapeutic efficacy. Inclusion of patients with locally advanced, nonmetastatic disease in some phase II trials may account for the frequent observation of "stable disease," and the relatively favorable survival results sometimes seen in preliminary studies but not confirmed in larger, randomized trials is probably a result of appropriately careful selection of metabolically stable patients for the phase II studies. The observed differences in outcome among the different regimens are insignificant, measured in weeks. Patients with advanced pancreas cancer who seek therapy should be offered the option of participation in trials of new drugs and strategies.

PAIN IN PATIENTS WITH PANCREAS CANCER

Abdominal pain is the most common symptom in patients with pancreatic carcinoma, and it is often what motivates the patient to seek medical attention. The natural history and mechanisms of pain in patients with pancreas cancer have not been studied extensively. In one report of pain prevalence among patients with lung, prostate, uterine, cervical, or pancreatic cancer, 60% of 25 patients with pancreatic cancer reported "moderate to bad" pain in the week before the history taking.[288] In a recent MSKCC study of patients awaiting exploratory laparotomy or chemotherapy for pancreas cancer, 45% had moderate or severe pain, but 38% had no pain. Among the patients who had pain, 90% complained of abdominal pain, but 48% reported pain in the chest, and 48% had lumbosacral pain.[289] Many patients with pancreas cancer experience other symptoms that are related to the disease or its treatment, including malaise, fatigue, and nausea. This constellation of symptoms, taken together with a patient's emotional reaction to the illness, result in "suffering" that goes beyond pain but that may intensify the perception of pain, making management more difficult.

There are several potential causes of pain in patients with pancreas cancer, and the symptoms experienced by individual patients are probably often related to multiple factors. The classic deep, severe pain is believed to result from tumor infiltration into the retroperitoneum and splanchnic nerve plexus.[290] Recent surgical operations, gastric or small bowel obstruction, bile duct dilatation, and peritoneal and hepatic metastases are recognized causes of local and referred pain. Many patients report crampy or poorly characterized diffuse abdominal pain associated with other gastrointestinal symptoms, such as eructation, constipation, and "gas." The relation of these symptoms to specific pathophysiologic mechanisms is not well understood.

In the many studies of external-beam radiation therapy in patients with pancreas cancer, only five series examined its impact on pain.[129,131,245,246,291] Symptom relief was reported in one third to three quarters of the patients, but the quality and duration of pain control was rarely stated. It is unknown if more innovative radiation techniques can produce more effective palliation. Reports regarding the effects of chemotherapy on pancreas cancer pain alone have been rare. Although recent NCCTG studies attempted to prospectively evaluate palliation in general, data on pain relief in patients receiving chemotherapy for advanced pancreatic carcinoma are limited.[201,202]

Pain management with oral or parenteral narcotic analgesics is adequate for many patients, although the side effects of these drugs may mimic or exacerbate the symptoms pancreas cancer, such as nausea and disturbances in bowel motility. The discomfort attributed to narcotic-induced obstipation can be so severe that patients discontinue the analgesic regimen. Many patients with pancreas cancer are elderly, and they may be more susceptible to oversedation and confusion.

If medical management is unsuccessful or associated with unacceptable side-effects, percutaneous chemical neurolysis can be useful.[292] The percutaneous injection of 50 ml of 50% alcohol after a diagnostic injection of Pontocaine was described in 1964.[293] Needle verification by radiographic techniques, particularly CT scanning, appears to reduce morbidity and improve efficiency.[294,295] The efficacy of celiac plexus block approaches 90%, but the quality and duration of analgesia has not been studied prospectively in a large group of patients with pancreas cancer.[296,297] Serious complications of a percutaneous nerve block are rare (<1%) and result from inadvertent injection into the peritoneal cavity, causing peritonitis, or into the subarachnoid space, causing paralysis. Transient hypotension as a result of splanchnic pooling after injection occurs more commonly and responds to supportive care. Intraoperative chemical neurolysis has been advocated by some investigators. At laparotomy, both sides of the celiac axis are directly injected with 50% alcohol or 6% phenol. No increased morbidity or mortality, compared with laparotomy and surgical bypass alone has been reported.[290]

There are no prospective studies comparing the effectiveness of radiation and nerve blocks in patients with pain refractory to medical management, nor is the optimal approach to treating the various types of pain experienced by patients well established. For this disease, in which the therapeutic options are limited, there is an opportunity and a serious need for careful study of symptom management.

REFERENCES

1. Boring CC, Squires TS, Tong T. Cancer statistics, 1991. CA 1991;41:19.
2. Levin DL, Connelly RR. Cancer of the pancreas: Available epidemiologic information and its implications. Cancer 1973;31:1231.
3. American Cancer Society. Cancer facts and figures—1990. Atlanta: American Cancer Society, 1990.
4. Pollack ES. The epidemiology of cancer and the delivery of medical care services. Public Health Rep 1984;99:476.
5. Buncher CR. Epidemiology of pancreatic cancer. In: Moosa AR, ed. Tumors of the pancreas. Baltimore: Williams & Wilkins, 1980:415.
6. World Health Organization. Cancer incidence in five continents, vol V. Lyon: IARC Science Publications, 1987.
7. Thomas DB, Karagas MR. Cancer in first and second generation Americans. Cancer Res 1987;47:5771.
8. Allen-Mersh TG, Earlam RJ. Pancreatic cancer in England and Wales: Surgeons look at epidemiology. Ann R Coll Surg Engl 1986;68:154.
9. Hoover R, Mason T, McKay F, et al. Geographic patterns of cancer mortality in the United States. In: Fraumeni JF, ed. Persons at high risk of cancer. An approach to cancer etiology and control. New York: Academic Press, 1975:343–360.
10. MacMahon B, Yen S, Trichopoulos D, et al. Coffee and carcinoma of the pancreas. N Engl J Med 1981;304:630.
11. Feinstein A, Horowitz R, Spitzer W, et al. Coffee and pancreatic cancer: The problems of etiologic science and epidemiologic case-control research. JAMA 1981;246:957.
12. Wynder E, Hall N, Polansky M. Epidemiology of coffee and pancreatic cancer. Cancer Res 1983;43:3900.
13. Hakulinen T, Lehtimaki L, Lehtonen M, et al. Cancer morbidity among two male cohorts with increased alcohol consumption in Finland. JNCI 1974;52:1711.
14. Wynder E, Mabuchi K, Maruchi N, et al. A case-control study of cancer of the pancreas. Cancer 1973;31:641.
15. Wynder E, Mabuchi K, Maruchi N, et al. Epidemiology of cancer of the pancreas. JNCI 1973;50:645.
16. Monson R, Lyon J. Proportional mortality among alcoholics. Cancer 1975;36:1077.
17. Wynder E. An epidemiologic evaluation of the causes of cancer of the pancreas. Cancer Res 1975;35:2228.
18. Krain L. The rising incidence of carcinoma of the pancreas. An epidemiologic appraisal. Am J Gastroenterol 1970;54:500.
19. Kahn H. The Dorn study of smoking and mortality among U.S. veterans: Report on eight and one-half years of observation. NCI Monogr 1966;19:1.
20. Pour P, Wilson R. Experimental tumors of the pancreas. In: Moosa A, ed. Tumors of the pancreas. Baltimore: Williams & Wilkins, 1980:37.
21. Sindelar W, Kurman C. Nitrosamine-induced pancreatic carcinogenesis in outbred and inbred Syrian hamsters. Carcinogenesis 1982;3:1021.
22. Bartholomew L, Gross J. Carcinoma of the pancreas associated with chronic relapsing pancreatitis. Gastroenterology 1958;35:473.
23. Lundh G, Nordenstam H. Pancreas calcification and pancreas cancer. A discussion of two cases. Acta Chir Scand 1970;136:493.
24. Robin A, Scott J, Rosenfeld D. The occurrence of carcinoma of the pancreas in chronic pancreatitis. Radiology 1970;94:289.
25. Mainz D, Webster P. Pancreatic carcinoma. A review of etiologic considerations. Am J Dig Dis 1974;19:459.
26. Brooks J. Cancer of the pancreas. In: Brooks JR, ed. Surgery of the pancreas. Philadelphia: WB Saunders, 1983:263.
27. Sasaki A, Kamado K, Horiuchi N. A changing pattern of causes of death in Japanese diabetics. Observations over fifteen years. J Chronic Dis 1978;312:433.
28. Karmody A, Kyle J. The association between carcinoma of the pancreas and diabetes mellitus. Br J Surg 1969;56:362.
29. Mancuso T, El-Attar A. Cohort study of workers exposed to beta-naphthylamine and benzidine. J Occup Med 1967;9:277.
30. Pour P, Althoff J, Kruger F, et al. The effect of N-nitrosobis-(2-oxopropyl)-almine after oral administration to hamsters. Cancer Lett 1977;2:323.
31. Longnecker D, Curphey T. Adenocarcinoma of the pancreas in azerine-treated rats. Cancer Res 1975;35:2249.
32. Skandalakis JE, Gray SW, Rower JS, et al. Anatomical complication of pancreatic surgery. Contemp Surg 1979;15:17.
33. Kasugai T, Kuno N, Kobayashi S. Endoscopic pancreatocholangiography. Gastroenterology 1972;63:217.
34. Michels NA. The hepatic, cystic and retroduodenal arteries and their relations in the biliary ducts. Ann Surg 1951;133:503.
35. Cubilla AL, Fitzgerald PJ. Surgical pathology of tumors of the exocrine pancreas. In: Moosa AR, ed. Tumors of the pancreas. Baltimore: Williams & Wilkins, 1980:159–193.
36. Cello JP. Carcinoma of the pancreas. In: Sleisenger MH, Fordtran JS, eds. Gastrointestinal disease: Pathophysiology, diagnosis, management, 3rd ed. Philadelphia: WB Saunders, 1983:1514–1527.
37. Cubilla AL, Fitzgerald PJ. Tumors of the exocrine pancreas. Washington, DC: Armed Forces Institute of Pathology, 1984.
38. Legg MA. Pathology of the pancreas. In: Brooks JR, ed. Surgery of the pancreas. Philadelphia: WB Saunders, 1983:41–77.
39. Howard JM, Jordan GL. Cancer of the pancreas. Curr Probl Cancer 1977;2:1.
40. Sclafani LM, Reuter VE, Coit DG, Brennan MF. The malignant nature of papillary and cystic neoplasms of the pancreas. Cancer 1991;68:153–158.
41. Cancer of the Pancreas Task Force: Staging of cancer of the pancreas. Cancer 1981;47:1631.
42. Gudjonsson B, Livestone EM, Spiro HM. Cancer of the pancreas. Diagnostic accuracy and survival statistics. Cancer 1978;42:2494.
43. Perez MM, Newcomer AD, Moertel CG, et al. Assessment of weight loss, food intake, fat metabolism, malabsorption, and treatment of pancreatic insufficiency in pancreatic cancer. Cancer 1983;52:346.

44. Go VLW, Taylor WF, DiMagno EP. Efforts at early diagnosis of pancreatic cancer: The Mayo Clinic experience. Cancer 1981;47:1698.

45. Moertel CG. Exocrine pancreas. In: Holland JF, Frei E, eds. Cancer medicine, 2nd ed. Philadelphia: Lea & Febiger, 1982:1792–1804.

46. Fras I, Litin EM, Pearson JS. Comparison of psychiatric symptoms in carcinoma of the pancreas with those in some other intra-abdominal neoplasms. Am J Psychiatry 1967;123:1553.

47. Sack GH, Levin J, Bell WR. Trousseau's syndrome and other manifestations of chronic disseminated coagulapathy in patients with neoplasms: Clinical, pathophysiologic, and therapeutic features. Medicine (Baltimore) 1977;56:1.

48. Moosa AR, Mackie CR, Gelder FB, et al. The value of tumor markers in the diagnosis and management of nonendocrine tumors of the pancreas. In: Moosa AR, ed. Tumors of the pancreas. Baltimore: Williams & Wilkins, 1980:355–380.

49. Cooper MJ, Mackie CR, Skinner DB, et al. A reappraisal of the value of carcinoembryonic antigen in the management of patients with various neoplasms. Br J Surg 1979;66:120.

50. Haglund C. Tumour marker antigen CA 12-5 in pancreatic cancer. A comparison with CA 19-9 and CEA. Br J Cancer 1986;54:897.

51. Bast RC, Klug TL, St John E, et al. A radioimmunoassay using a monoclonal antibody to monitor the course of epithelial ovarian cancer. N Engl J Med 1983;309:883.

52. Bast RC, Feeney M, Lazarus H, et al. Reactivity of a monoclonal antibody with human ovarian carcinoma. J Clin Invest 1981;68:1331.

53. Ritts RE, Del Villano BC, Go VLM, et al. Initial clinical evaluation of an immunoradiometric assay for CA 19-9 using the NCI serum bank. Int J Cancer 1984;33:339.

54. Habib NA, Herschman MJ, Haberland F, et al. The use of CA 50 radioimmunoassay in differentiating benign and malignant pancreatic disease. Br J Cancer 1986;53:697–699.

55. Basso D, Fabris C, DelFaver G, et al. Combined determination of serum CA19-9 and tissue polypeptide antigen: Why no improvement in pancreatic cancer diagnosis? Oncology 1988;45:24–29.

56. Talbot RW, Nagorney DM, Pemberton JH, et al. Comparison of portal and peripheral blood levels of carcinoembryonic antigen, CA 19-9 and CA 125 tumor-associated antigens in patients with colorectal and pancreatic cancer. Cancer Res 1989;49:542–543.

57. Lucarott ME, Habib NA, Kelly SB, et al. Clinical evaluation of combined use of CEA, CA 19-9, and CA 50 in the serum of patients with pancreatic carcinoma. Eur J Surg Oncol 1991;17:51–53.

58. Piantino P, Andriulli A, Gindro T, et al. CA 19-9 assay in differential diagnosis of pancreatic carcinoma from inflammatory pancreatic diseases. Am J Gastroenterol 1986;81:436.

59. Haglund C, Roberts PJ, Kuusela P, et al. Gastrointestinal cancer associated antigen CA 19-9 in histological specimens of pancreatic tumors and pancreatitis. Br J Cancer 1986;53:189.

60. Pasquali C, Sperti C, D'Andrea AA, et al. Evaluation of carbohydrate antigens 19-9 and 12-5 in patients with pancreatic cancer. Pancreas 1987;2:34.

61. Benini L, Cavallini G, Zordan D, et al. Prospective clinical evaluation of the diagnostic accuracy of monoclonal (CA 19-9, CA 50, CA 12-5) and polyclonal (CEA, TPA) antigens in respect to pancreatic cancer. Dig Dis Sci 1986;31:254.

62. Kiriyama S, Hayakawa T, Kondo T, et al. Usefulness of a new tumor marker, SPAN-1, for the diagnosis of pancreatic cancer. Cancer 1990;65:1557–1561.

63. Mahvi DM, Meyers WC, Bast RC, et al. Therapeutic efficacy as defined by a seriodiagnostic test utilizing a monoclonal antibody in carcinoma of the pancreas. Ann Surg 1985;202:440.

64. Bleiberg H, Rozencweig M, Mathieu M, Beyens M, Gompel C, Gerard A. The use of peritoneoscopy in the detection of liver metastases. Cancer 1978;41:863–867.

65. Irving AD, Cuschieri A. Laparoscopic assessment of jaundiced patients: Review of 53 patients. Br J Surg 1978;65:678–680.

66. Cuschieri A, Hall AW, Clark J. Value of laparoscopy in the diagnosis and management of pancreatic cancer. Gut 1978;19:672–677.

67. Cuschieri A. Laparoscopy for pancreatic cancer: Does it benefit the patient? Eur J Surg Oncol 1988;14:41–44.

68. Whipple AO, Parsons WB, Mullins CR. Treatment of carcinoma of the ampulla of Vater. Ann Surg 1935;102:763.

69. Maki T, Sato T, Kakizaki G. Pancreatoduodenectomy for periampullary carcinomas: Appraisal of a two-stage procedure. Arch Surg 1966;92:825.

70. Nakayama T, Ikeda A, Okuda K. Percutaneous transhepatic drainage of the biliary tract: Technique and results in 104 cases. Gastroenterology 1978;74:554.

71. Denning DA, Ellison EC, Carey LC. Preoperative percutaneous transhepatic biliary decompression lowers operative morbidity in patients with obstructive jaundice. Am J Surg 1981;141:61.

72. Norlander A, Kalin B, Sundblad R. Effect of percutaneous transhepatic drainage upon liver function and postoperative mortality. Surg Gynecol Obstet 1982;155:161.

73. Gundry SR, Strodel WE, Knol JA, et al. Efficacy of preoperative biliary tract decompression in patients with obstructive jaundice. Arch Surg 1984;119:703.

74. Dooley JS, Dick R, Olney J, et al. Non-surgical treatment of biliary obstruction. Lancet 1979;2:1043.

75. McPherson GAD, Benjamin IS, Habib NA, et al. Percutaneous transhepatic drainage in obstructive jaundice: Advantages and problems. Br J Surg 1982;62:261.

76. Hatfield ARW, Tobias R, Terblanche J, et al. Preoperative external biliary drainage in obstructive jaundice: A prospective controlled clinical trial. Lancet 1982;2:896.

77. McPherson GAD, Benjamin IS, Hodgson HJF, et al. Preoperative percutaneous biliary drainage: The best results of a controlled trial. Br J Surg 1984;71:371.

78. Pitt HA, Cameron JL, Postier RG, et al. Factors affecting mortality in biliary tract surgery. Am J Surg 1981;141:66.

79. Hagenmuller F, Classen M. Therapeutic endoscopic and percutaneous procedures for biliary disorders. Prog Liver Dis 1982;7:299.

80. Speer AG, Cotton PB, Russell RC, et al. Randomised trial of endoscopic versus percutaneous stent insertion in malignant obstructive jaundice. Lancet 1987;2:57.

81. Bornman PC, Terblanche J, Harries-Jones EP, et al. Endoscopic versus percutaneous stents for malignant jaundice. Lancet 1987;2:689.

82. Isaacson R, Weiland LH, McIlrath DC. Biopsy of the pancreas. Arch Surg 1974;109:227.

83. Fortner JG. Regional resection of the pancreas: A new surgical approach. Surgery 1973;73:307.

84. Morrow M, Hilaris B, Brennan MF. Comparison of conventional surgical resection, radioactive implantation, and bypass procedures for exocrine carcinoma of the pancreas 1975–1980. Ann Surg 1984;199:1.

85. Bowden L, McNeer G, Pack G. Carcinoma of the head of pancreas—Five-year survival in four patients. Am J Surg 1965;109:578.

86. Portland Surgical Society Cooperative Study: A ten-year experience with carcinoma of the pancreas. Arch Surg 1967;94:322.

87. Crile G. The advantages of bypass operations over radical pancreaticoduodenectomy in the treatment of pancreatic carcinoma. Surg Gynecol Obstet 1970;130:1049.

88. Feduska N, Dent T, Lindenauer S. Results of palliative operations for carcinoma of the pancreas. Arch Surg 1971;103:330.

89. Wilson S, Block G. Perimapullary carcinoma. Arch Surg 1974;108:539.

90. Brooks J, Culebras J. Cancer of the pancreas—palliative operation, Whipple procedure or total pancreatectomy? Am J Surg 1976;131:516.

91. Shapiro T. Adenocarcinoma of the pancreas: A statistical analysis of biliary bypass vs. Whipple resection in good-risk patients. Ann Surg 1975;182:715.

92. Nakase A, Matsumoto Y, Uchida K, et al. Surgical treatment of cancer of the pancreas and the periampullary region. Cumulative results in 57 institutions in Japan. Ann Surg 1977;185:52.

93. Tepper J, Nardi G, Suit H. Carcinoma of the pancreas: Review of MGH experience from 1963 to 1973. Cancer 1976;37:1519.

94. Knight R, Scarborough J, Goss J. Adenocarcinoma of the pancreas—A ten-year experience. Arch Surg 1978;113:1401.

95. Moosa A, Lewis M, Mackie C. Surgical treatment of pancreatic cancer. Mayo Clin Proc 1979;54:468.

96. Longmire W, Transero L. The Whipple procedure and other standard operative approaches to pancreatic cancer. Cancer 1981;47:1706.

97. Edis A, Kiernan P, Taylor W. Attempted curative resection of ductal carcinoma of the pancreas. Review of Mayo Clinic experience: 1951–1975. Mayo Clin Proc 1980;55:531.

98. Fortner J. Surgical principles for pancreatic cancer: Regional total and subtotal pancreatectomy. Cancer 1981;47:1712.

99. Herter F, Cooperman A, Ahlborn T, et al. Surgical experience with pancreatic and periampullary cancer. Ann Surg 1982;195:274.

100. Trede M. The surgical treatment of pancreatic carcinoma. Surgery 1985;97:28–35.

101. Gudjonsson B. Cancer of the pancreas: 50 years of surgery. Cancer 1987;60:2284.

102. Michelassi F, Erroiu F, Dawson PJ, et al. Experience with 647 consecutive tumors of the duodenum, ampulla, head of the pancreas, and distal common bile duct. Ann Surg 1989;210:544–556.

103. Trede M, Schwall G, Saeger HD. Survival after pancreatoduodenectomy: 118 consecutive resections without an operative mortality. Ann Surg 1990;211:447–458.

104. Cameron JL, Crist DW, Sitzmann JV, et al. Factors influencing survival after pancreaticoduodenectomy for pancreatic cancer. Am J Surg 1991;161:120–125.

105. Van Heerden J, Heath P, Alden C. Biliary bypass for ductal adenocarcinoma of the pancreas: Mayo Clinic experience, 1970–1975. Mayo Clin Proc 1980;55:537.

106. Brooks DC, Osteen R, Gray E, et al. Evaluation of palliative procedures of pancreatic cancer. Am J Surg 1981;141:430.

107. DeRooij PD, Rogatko A, Brennan MF. Evaluation of palliative surgical procedures in unresectable pancreatic cancer. Br J Surg 1991;78:1053–1058.

108. Crist DW, Sitzmann JV, Cameron JL. Improved hospital morbidity, mortality and survival after the Whipple procedure. Ann Surg 1987;206:358.

109. Nagai H, Kuroda A, Morioka Y. Lymphatic and local spread of T1 and T2 pancreatic cancer. Ann Surg 1986;204:65.

110. Pilepich MV, Miller HH. Pre-operative irradiation in carcinoma of the pancreas. Cancer 1980;46:1945.

111. Kopelson G. Curative surgery for adenocarcinoma of the pancreas/ampulla of Vater. The role of adjuvant pre- or post-operative radiation therapy. Int J Radiat Oncol Biol Phys 1983;9:911.

112. Ishikawa O, Ohhigashi H, Teshima T, et al. Clinical and histopathological appraisal of preoperative irradiation for adenocarcinoma of the pancreatoduodenal region. J Surg Oncol 1989;40:143–151.

113. Weese JL, Nussbaum ML, Paul AR, et al. Increased resectability of locally advanced pancreatic and periampullary carcinoma with neoadjuvant chemotherapy. Int J Pancreatol 1990;1:177–185.

114. Sindelar WF, Kinsella TJ. Randomized trial of intraoperative radiotherapy in resected carcinoma of the pancreas. Int J Radiat Oncol Biol Phys 1986;12(suppl 1):148.

115. Frass BA, Miller RW, Kinsella TJ, et al. Intraoperative radiation therapy at the National Cancer Institute: Technical innovations and dosimetry. Int J Radiat Oncol Biol Phys 1985;11:1299.

116. Sindelar WF, Hoekstra HJ, Kinsella TJ. Surgical approaches and techniques in intraoperative radiotherapy for intra-abdominal, retroperitoneal, and pelvic neoplasms. Surgery 1987;103:247–256.

117. Gastrointestinal Tumor Study Group. Pancreatic cancer: Adjuvant combined radiation and chemotherapy following curative resection. Arch Surg 1985;120:899.

118. Gastrointestinal Tumor Study Group. Further evidence of effective adjuvant combined radiation and chemotherapy following curative resection of pancreatic cancer. Cancer 1987;59:2006.

119. Kinsella TJ. Adjuvant radiotherapy in pancreatic carcinoma: A reappraisal. Cancer Invest 1988;6:745–746.

120. Sarr MG, Cameron JL. Surgical management of unresectable carcinoma of the pancreas. Surgery 1982;91:123.

121. Bufkin WJ, Smith PE, Krementz FT. Evaluation of palliative operations for carcinoma of the pancreas. Arch Surg 1967;94:240.

122. Blievernicht SW, Neifeld JP, Terz JJ, et al. The role of prophylactic gastrojejunostomy for unresectable periampullary carcinoma. Surg Gynecol Obstet 1980;151:794.

123. Elmslie RG, Slovatinek AH. Surgical objectives in unresected cancer of the head of the pancreas. Br J Surg 1972;59:500.

124. Hart PF, Gillett DJ. Non-functioning palliative gastroenterostomy. Aust N Z J Surg 1972;41:354.

125. Glantz G, Ozeran RS. Role of gastroenterostomy in management of pancreatic carcinoma. Am Surg 1966;32:670.

126. Collure DWD, Burns GP, Schenk WG JR. Clinical, pathological, and therapeutic aspects of carcinoma of the pancreas. Am J Surg 1974;128:683.

127. Billingsley JS, Bartholomew LG, Childs DS. A study of radiation therapy in carcinoma of the pancreas. Proc Staff Meet Mayo Clin 1958;33:426.

128. Miller TR, Fuller LM. Radiation therapy of carcinoma of the pancreas. Report on 91 cases. Am J Roentgenol Radium Ther Nucl Med 1958;80:787.

129. Haslam JB, Cavanaugh PJ, Stroup SL. Radiation threapy in the treatment of irresectable adenocarcinoma of the pancreas. Cancer 1973;32:1341.

130. Dobelbower RR, Borgelt BB, Strubler KA, et al. Precision radiotherapy for cancer of the pancreas: Technique and results. Int J Radiat Oncol Biol Phys 1980;6:1127.

131. Whittington R, Dobelbower RR, Mohiuddin M, et al. Radiotherapy of unresectable pancreatic carcinoma: A six-year experience with 104 patients. Int J Radiat Oncol Biol Phys 1981;7:1639.

132. Kinsella TJ, Sindelar WF, Bloomer WD. Radiation enteritis: Pathophysiology, clinical manifestations and management. In: Nyhus LM, Nelson RL, eds. Surgery of the small intestine. Norwalk, CT: Appleton-Century-Crofts, 1987:193–203.

133. Shanahan TG, Mehta MD, Kinsella TJ. Minimization of small bowel volume within treatment fields utilizing customized "belly boards." Int J Radiat Oncol Biol Phys 1990;19:469–476.

134. Hilaris B, Moorthy C, Kim J. Radiotherapeutic management of pancreatic cancer at Memorial Sloan-Kettering Cancer Center. In: Conn I, ed. Pancreatic cancer: New directions in therapeutic management. New York: Masson, 1980:251–262.

135. Shipley WU, Nardi GL, Cohen AM, et al. Iodine 125 implant and external beam irradiation in patients with localized pancreatic carcinoma. A comparative study of surgical resection. Cancer 1980;45:709.

136. Mohiuddin M, Cantor RJ, Biermann W, et al. Combined modality treatment of localized unresectable adenocarcinoma of the pancreas. Int J Radiat Oncol Biol Phys 1988;14:79–84.

137. Abe M, Takahashi M. Intraoperative radiotherapy: The Japanese experience. Int J Radiat Oncol Biol Phys 1981;7:863.

138. Nishamura A, Nakano M, Otsu H, et al. Intraoperative radiotherapy for advanced carcinoma of the pancreas. Cancer 1984;54:2375.

139. Shipley WU, Wood WC, Tepper JE, et al. Intraoperative electron beam irradiation for patients with unresectable pancreatic carcinoma. Ann Surg 1984;200:289.

140. Tepper JE, Shipley WU, Warshaw AL, et al. The role of Misonidazole combined with intraoperative radiation therapy in the treatment of pancreatic carcinoma. J Clin Oncol 1987;5:579.

141. Gunderson LL, Martin JK, Kvols LT, et al. Intraoperative and extenal beam irradiation ± 5-FU for locally advanced pancreatic cancer. Int J Radiat Oncol Biol Phys 1987;13:319.

142. Sindelar WF, Hoekstra H, Rstrepo C, et al. Pathological tissue changes following intraoperative radiotherapy. Am J Clin Oncol 1986;9:504.

143. Ahmadu-Sura F, Gillette EL, Withrow SJ, et al. Exocrine pancreatic function following intra-operative irradiation of the canine pancreas. Cancer 1988;6:1091–1095.

144. Shibamato Y, Manabe T, Baba M, et al. High dose external beam and intraoperative radiotherapy in the treatment of resectable and unresectable pancreatic cancer. Int J Radiat Oncol Biol Phys 1990;19:605–611.

145. Thomas FJ, Krall J, Hendrickson F, et al. Evaluation of neutron irradiation of pancreatic cancer: Results of a randomized Radiation Therapy Oncology Group clinical trial. Am J Clin Oncol 1989;12:283–289.

146. Lindstadt D, Quivey JM, Castro JR, et al. Comparison of helium-ion radiation therapy and split-course megavoltage irradiation from the unresectable adenocarcinoma of the pancreas. Radiology 1988;168:261,264.

147. Pisters PWT, Restifo NP, Cersosimo E, Brennan MF. The effects of euglycemic hyperinsulinemia and amino acid infusion on regional and whole body glucose disposal in man. Metabolism 1991;40:59–65.

148. Cersosimo E, Pisters PWT, Pesola G, et al. Insulin secretion and action in patients with pancreatic cancer. Cancer 1991;67:486–493.

149. Sclafani LM, Shike M, Queseda E, Posner M, Brennan MF. A randomized prospective trial of TPN following major pancreatic surgery. (submitted).

150. Carter SK. The integration of chemotherapy into a combined modality approach for cancer treatment: VI. Pancreatic adenocarcinoma. Cancer Treat Rev 1975;3:193.

151. Kovach JS, Moertel CG, Schutt AJ, et al. A controlled study of combined 1,3-bis-(2-chlorethyl)-1-nitrosorea and 5-fluorouracil therapy for advanced gastric and pancreatic cancer. Cancer 1974;33:563.

152. Hansen R, Quebbeman E, Ritch P, Chitambar C, Anderson T. Continuous 5-fluorouracil infusion in carcinoma of the pancreas: A phase II study. Am J Med Sci 1988;295:91–93.

153. Tajiri H, Yashimori M, Okazaki N, Miyaji M. Phase II study of continuous infusion of 5-fluorouracil in advanced pancreatic cancer. Oncology 1991;48:18–21.

154. Crooke ST, Bradner WT. Mitomycin C. A review. Cancer Treat Rev 1976;3:121.

155. Carter SK. Mitomycin C (NSC-26980) Clinical brochure. Cancer Chemother Rep 1968;1:99–114.

156. Schein PS, Lavin PT, Moertel CG, et al. Randomized phase II clinical trial of Adriamycin in advanced measurable pancreatic carcinoma: A Gastrointestinal Tumor Study Group report. Cancer 1978;42:19.

157. Moertel CG, Doublass HO, Hanlet J, et al. Phase II study of methyl-CCNU in the treatment of advanced pancreatic carcinoma. Cancer Treat Rep 1976;60:1659–1661.

158. Gastrointestinal Tumor Study Group. Phase II trials of maytansine, low-dose chlorozotocin, and high-dose chlorozotocin as single agents against advanced measurable adenocarcinoma of the pancreas. Cancer Treat Rep 1985;69:417.

159. Inamasu M, Oishi N, Chen T, et al. Phase II trial of amsacrine in pancreatic carcinoma: A Southwest Oncology Group study. Cancer Treat Rep 1984;68:1411.

160. Omura GA, Bartolucci AA, Lessner HE, et al. Phase II evaluation of amsacrine in colorectal, gastric, and pancreatic carcinomas: A Southeastern Cancer Study Group trial. Cancer Treat Rep 1984;68:929.

161. Sternberg CN, Magill GB, Sordillo PP, et al. Phase II evaluation of m-AMSA (4'-(9-acridinylamino)-methane-sulfon-m-anisidide) in patients with adenocarcinoma of the pancreas. Am J Clin Oncol 1983;6:459.

162. Mittelman A, Magill GB, Raymond V, et al. Phase II trial of Idarubicin in patients with pancreatic cancer. Cancer Treat Rep 1987;712:657.

163. Hochster H, Green MD, Speyer JL, et al. Activity of epirubicin in pancreatic cancer. Cancer Treat Rep 1986;70:299.

164. Wils J, Bleiberg H, Blijham G, et al. Phase II study of epirubicin in advanced adenocarcinoma of the pancreas. Eur J Cancer Clin Oncol 1985;21:191.

165. Loven D, Figer A, Vigler N, et al. Epirubicin in the treatment of advanced carcinoma of the pancreas. Proc Am Soc Clin Oncol [Abstract] 1989;9:113.

166. Gastrointestinal Tumor Study Group. Phase II trials of the single agents Baker's antifol, diaziquone, and epirubicin in advanced pancreas cancer Cancer Treat Rep 1987;71:865–867.

167. Blayney DW, Goldberg DA, Leong LA, et al. Phase II trial of esorubicin in advanced pancreatic carcinoma. Cancer Treat Rep 1986;70:683–684.

168. Vaughn CB, Salmon SE, Fleming TR. Phase II evaluation of esorubicin (4'deoxydoxorubicin) in pancreatic adenocarcinoma: A Southwest Oncology Group study. Invest New Drugs 1990;8:81–85.

169. Brown TD, Goodman PJ, Fleming TR, Baker LH, Macdonald J. Phase II trial of menogarol in adenocarcinoma of the pancreas: A Southwest Oncology Group study. Invest New Drugs 1991;9:77–78.

170. Sternberg CN, Magill GB, Cheng EW, Hollander P. Phase II trial of menogarol in the treatment of advanced adenocarcinoma of the pancreas. Am J Clin Oncol 1988;11:174–176.

171. Bedikian AY, Stroehlein J, Korinek J, et al. Phase II evaluation of dihydroxyanthracenedione (DHAD, NSC 301739) in patients with upper gastrointestinal tumors. A preliminary report. Am J Clin Oncol 1983;6:473.

172. DeSimone PA, Gams R, Bartolucci A. Weekly mitoxantrone in the treatment of advanced pancreatic carcinoma: A Southeastern Cancer Study Group trial. Cancer Treat Rep 1986;80:929.

173. Taylor SA, Fleming T, Von Hoff DD, et al. Phase II evaluation of mitoxantrone in advanced pancreatic carcinoma: A Southwest Oncology Group study. Invest New Drugs 1990;8:77–80.

174. Horton J, Gelber R, Engstrom P, et al. Trials of single agent and combination chemotherapy for advanced cancer of the pancreas. Cancer Treat Rep 1981;65:65.

175. Smith DB, Kenny JB, Scarffe JH, et al. Phase II evaluation of melphalan in adenocarcinoma of the pancreas. Cancer Treat Rep 1985;69:917.

176. Gad-el-Mawla N, Ziegler JL. Ifosfamide treatment of pancreatic cancer. Cancer Treat Rep 1981;65:357–358.

177. Loehrer PJ, Sr, Williams SD, Einhorn LH, Ansari R. Ifosfamide: An active drug in the treatment of adenocarcinoma of the pancreas. J Clin Oncol 1985;3:367–372.

178. Bernard S, Noble S, Wilcosky T, et al. A phase II study of ifosfamide (IFOS) plus N-acetyl cysteine (NAC) in metastatic pancreatic adenocarcinoma (pc). Proc Am Soc Clin Oncol [Abstract] 1986;5:328.

179. Gastrointestinal Tumor Study Group. Ifosfamide is an inactive substance in the treatment of pancreatic carcinoma. Cancer 1989;64:2010–2013.

180. Ajani JA, Abbruzzese JL, Goudeau P, et al. Ifosfamide and mesna: Marginally active in patients with advanced adenocarcinoma of the pancreas. J Clin Oncol 1988;6:1703–1707.

181. DeSimone P, Kramer B, Omura GA, et al. Phase II evaluation of diaziquone in gastric and pancreatic cancers: A Southeastern Cancer Study Group trial. Am J Clin Oncol 1986;9:401.

182. Tilchen EJ, Fleming T, Mills G, et al. Phase II evaluation of diaziquone in gastric and pancreatic cancers. A Southwest Oncology Group study. Cancer Treat Rep 1987;71:1309–1310.

183. Sternberg CN, Magill GB, Sordill0 PP, et al. Phase II evaluation of metoprine in advanced pancreatic adenocarcinoma. Cancer Treat Rep 1984;68:1053.

184. Casper ES, Schwartz GK, Johnson B, Kelsen DP. Phase II trials of fazarabine (arabinofuranosyl-5-azacytosine) and edatrexate in patients (pts) with pancreatic adenocarcinoma. Proc Am Soc Clin Oncol 1992;12:194.

185. Carlson RW, Doroshaw JH, Odujinrin OO, Flam MS, Malec M, Lamborn KR. Trimetrexate in locally advanced or metastatic adenocarcinoma of the pancreas: A phase

II study of the Northern California Oncology Group. Invest New Drugs 1990;8:387–389.

186. Kilton L, Benson A, Greenburg A, et al. Phase II trial of fludarabine phosphate (FAMP) in adenocarcinoma of the pancreas: An Illinois Cancer Council study. Proc Am Soc Clin Oncol [Abstract] 1988;7:1–3.

187. Casper ES, Green MR, Brown TD, et al. Phase II trial of gemcitabine (2'2'-difluoro-deoxycytidine) in patients with pancreatic cancer. Proc Am Soc Clin Oncol [Abstract] 1991;10:143.

188. Sternberg CN, Magill GB, Cheng EW, Applewhite A, Sordillo PP. Etoposide (VP-16) in the treatment of advanced adenocarcinoma of the pancreas. Am J Clin Oncol 1988;11:172–173.

189. Guy JT, Fleming T, Pollock TW, et al. 5-Day vinblastine infusion for pancreatic adenocarcinoma. A phase II Southwest Oncology Group study. Invest New Drugs 1990;8:205–206.

190. Magill GB, Cheng EW, Currie VE. Chemotherapy of pancreatic cancer with vindesine (DVA). Proceedings of the American Association for Cancer Research 1981;22:458.

191. Linke K, Pazdur R, Ajani A, et al. Phase II trial of amonifide in advanced pancreatic carcinoma. Proc Am Soc Clin Oncol [Abstract] 1991;10:146.

192. Gastrointestinal Tumor Study Group. Phase II trials of hexamethylmelamine, dianhydrogalactitol, razoxane, and beta-2'-deoxythioguanosine as single agents against advanced measurable tumors of the pancreas. Cancer Treat Rep 1985;69:713.

193. Grohn P, Heinonen E, Kumpulainen E, et al. Oral carmofur in advanced gastrointestinal cancer. Am J Clin Oncol 1990;13:477–479.

194. Kantarjian H, Ajani JA, Karlin DA. *Cis*-diaminochloroplatinum (II) chemotherapy for advanced adenocarcinoma of the upper gastrointestinal tract. Oncology 1985;42:69–71.

195. Abbruzzese J, Ajani JA, Faintuch J, et al. Phase II study of iproplatin (CHIP) in patients with advanced gastric and pancreatic carcinoma. Proc Am Soc Clin Oncol [Abstract] 1989;9:123.

196. Lessner HE, Valenstein S, Kaplan R, et al. Phase II study of L-asparaginase in the treatment of pancreatic carcinoma. Cancer Treat Rep 1980;64:1359.

197. Inamasu MS, Oishi N, Chen TT, et al. Phase II study of mitoguazone in pancreatic cancer: A Southwest Oncology Group study. Cancer Treat Rep 1986;70:531.

198. Ravry MJR, Omura GA, Hill GJ, et al. Phase II evaluation of mitoguazone in cancers of the esophagus, stomach, and pancreas: A Southeastern Cancer Study Group trial. Cancer Treat Rep 1986;70:533.

199. Patel SR, Kvols LK, Rubin J, et al. Phase I–II study of pibenzimol hydrochloride (NSC 322921) in advanced pancreatic carcinoma. Invest New Drugs 1991;9:53–57.

200. Kraut EH, Fleming T, Segal M, Neidhart JA, Behrens BC, Macdonald J. Phase II study of pibenzimol in pancreatic cancer: A Southwest Oncology Group study. Invest New Drugs 1991;9:95–96.

201. Cullinan SA, Moertel CG, Fleming TR, et al. A comparison of chemotherapeutic regimens in the treatment of advanced pancreatic and gastric carcinoma. JAMA 1985;253:2061.

202. Cullinan S, Moertel CG, Wieand HS, et al. A phase III trial on the therapy of advanced pancreatic carcinoma. Cancer 1990;65:2207–2212.

203. Stolinsky DC, Pugh RP, Bateman JR. 5-fluorouracil (NSC-19383) therapy for pancreatic carcinoma: Comparison of oral and intravenous routes. Cancer Chemother Rep 1975;59:1031.

204. Loehrer PJ, Sr, Williams SD, Nichols CR. Ifosfamide plus 5-fluorouracil for treatment of adenocarcinoma of the pancreas. Cancer Treat Rep 1987;71:1115–1116.

205. Lokich J, Chawla PL, Brooks J, et al. Chemotherapy in pancreatic carcinoma: 5-Fluorouracil (5-FU) and 1,3,bis-(2-chloroethyl)-1-nitrosourea (BCNU). Ann Surg 1974;179:450.

206. Andersen JR, Friis-Mollek A, Hancke S, et al. A controlled trial of combination chemotherapy with 5-FU and BCNU in pancreatic cancer. Scand J Gastroenterol 1981;16:973.

207. Frey C, Twomey P, Keehn R, et al. Randomized study of 5-FU and CCNU in pancreatic cancer. Cancer 1981;47:27.

208. Mallinson CN, Rake MO, Cocking JB, et al. Chemotherapy in pancreatic cancer: Results of a controlled, prospective, randomized, multicenter trial. Br Med J 1980;281:1589.

209. Wiggins RG, Wooley PV, MacDonald JS, et al. Phase II trial of streptozotocin, mitomycin C and 5-fluorouracil (SMF) in the treatment of advanced pancratic cancer. Cancer 1978;41:387.

210. Bukowski RM, Aberhalden RT, Hewlett JS, et al. Phase II trial of streptozotocin, mitomycin C, and 5-fluorouracil in adenocarcinoma of the pancreas. Cancer Clin Trials 1980;3:321.

211. Smith FP, Hoth DF, Levin B, et al. 5-Fluorouracil, Adriamycin and mitomycin C (FAM) chemotherapy for advanced adenocarcinoma of the pancreas. Cancer 1980;46:2014–2018.

212. Bitran JD, Desser RK, Kozloff MF, et al. Treatment of metastatic pancreatic and gastric adenocarcinoma with 5-fluourouracil, Adriamycin, and mitomycin C (FAM). Cancer Treat Rep 1979;63:2049.

213. Buroker T, Kim PN, Groppe C, et al. 5-FU infusion with mitomycin C vs. 5-FU infusion with methyl-CCNU in the treatment of advanced upper gastrointestinal cancer. A Southwest Oncology Group study. Cancer 1979;44:1215–1221.

214. Bukowski RM, Balcerzak SP, O'Bryan RM, Bonnet JD, Chen TT. Randomized trial of 5-fluorouracil and mitomycin C with or without streptozotocin for advanced pancreatic cancer. A Southwest Oncology Group Study. Cancer 1983;52:1577–1582.

215. Oster MW, Gray R, Panasci L, et al. Chemotherapy for advanced pancreatic cancer: A comparison of 5-fluorouracil, Adriamycin, and mitomycin-C (FAM) with 5-fluorouracil, streptozotocin and mitomycin-C (FSM). Cancer 1986;57:29.

216. Gastrointestinal Tumor Study Group. Phase II studies of drug combination in advanced pancreatic carcinoma: Fluorouracil plus doxorubicin plus mitomycin-C plus fluorouracil. J Clin Oncol 1986;4:1794.

217. Kelsen DP, Hudis C, Niedzwiecki D, et al. A phase II comparison trial of streptozotocin, mitomycin, and 5-fluorouracil with cisplatin, cytosine arabinoside, and caffeine in patients with advanced pancreatic carcinoma. Cancer 1991;68:965–969.

218. Bukowski RM, Schacter LP, Groppe CT, et al. Phase II trial of 5-fluuorouracil, Adriamycin, mitomycin-C and streptozotocin (FAM-S) in pancreatic cancer. Cancer 1982;50:197.

219. Smith FP, Rustgi VK, Schertz G, et al. Phase II study of 5-FU, doxorubicin, and mitomycin (FAM) and chlorozotocin in advanced measurable pancreatic cancer. Cancer Treat Rep 1982;66:2095.

220. Karlin DA, Stroehlein JR, Bennetts RW, et al. Phase I–II study of the combination of 5-FU, doxorubicin, mitomycin, and semustine (FAMMe) in the treatment of adenocarcinoma of the stomach, gastroesophageal junction, and pancreas. Cancer Treat Rep 1982;66:1613.

221. Sternberg C, Magill G, Sordillo P, et al. MiFA III (mitomycin, 5-fluorouracil, and Adriamycin) chemotherapy for advanced adenocarcinoma of the pancreas. Am J Clin Oncol 1984;7:529–533.

222. Moertel CG, Rubin J, O'Connell MJ, et al. A phase II trial of combined 5-fluourouracil, doxorubicin and cisplatin in the treatment of advanced upper gastrointestinal adenocarcinoma. J Clin Oncol 1986;4:1053.

223. Wils J, Bleiberg H, Dalesio O, et al. An EORTC Gastrointestinal Group phase II evaluation of epirubicin combined with 5-fluorouracil in advanced adenocarcinoma of the pancreas. Eur J Cancer Clin Oncol 1987;23:1017–1018.

224. Wils J, Bleiberg H, Buyse M, et al. An EORTC Gastrointestinal Group phase II evaluation of epirubicin combined with ifosfamide in advanced adenocarcinoma of the pancreas. Eur J Cancer Clin Oncol 1989;25:1119–1120.

225. Kyriazis AP, Kyriazis AA, Yagoda AA. Enhanced therapeutic effect of cis-diamminodichloroplatinum against nude mouse grown human pancreatic adenocarcinoma when combined with I-B-D-arabionfuranosylcytosine and caffeine. Cancer Res 1985;45:6083.

226. Dougherty JB, Kelsen D, Kemeny N, Magill G, Botet J, Niedzwiecki D. Advanced pancreatic cancer: A phase I–II trial of cisplatin, high dose cytarabine, and caffeine. JNCI 1989;81:1735–1738.

227. Awrich A, Fletcher WS, Klotz J, et al. 5-FU versus combination therapy with tubercidin, streptozotocin, and 5-FU in the treatment of pancreatic carcinomas: COG protocol 7230. J Surg Oncol 1979;12:267–273.

228. Moertel CG, Engstrom P, Lavin PT, et al. Chemotherapy of gastric and pancreatic carcinoma. A controlled evaluation of combinations of 5-fluorouracil with nitrosoureas and "lactones." Surgery 1979;85:509.

229. Moertel CG, Douglass HO Jr, Hanley J, et al. Treatment of advanced adenocarcinoma of the pancreas with combinations of streptozotocin plus 5-fluorouracil and streptozotocin plus cyclophosphamide. Cancer 1977;40:605, 1977

230. Bruckner HW, Crown J, McKenna A, Hart R. Leucovorin and 5-fluorouracil as a treatment for disseminated cancer of the pancreas and unknown primary tumors. Cancer Res 1988;48:5570.

231. DeCaprio JA, Arbuck SG, Mayer RJ. Phase II study of weekly 5-fluorouracil (5-FU) with folinic acid (FA) in previously untreated patients with unresectable measurable pancreatic adenocarcinoma. Proc Am Soc Clin Oncol [Abstract] 1989;8:388.

232. Crown J, Casper ES, Botet J, Murray P, Kelsen DP. Lack of efficacy of high-dose leucovorin and fluorouracil in patients with advanced pancreatic adenocarinoma. J Clin Oncol 1991;9:1682–1686.

233. Schilder RJ, Paul AR, Walczak J, DiFino SM, et al. Phase II trial of PALA/5-fluorouracil (5-FU) in pancreatic cancer. Proc Am Soc Clin Oncol 1990;9:422.

234. Morrell LM, Bach A, Richman SP, Goodman P, Fleming TR, MacDonald JS. A phase II multi-institutional trial of low-dose N-(phosphonacetyl)-L-aspartate and high dose 5-fluorouracil as a short term infusion in the treatment of adenocarcinoma of the pancreas. Cancer 1991;67:363–366.

235. Ardalan B, Sridhar K, Richman S, et al. Addition of high-dose leucovorin (LV) to high-dose infusion of 5-fluorouracil (5-FU) and low-dose PALA. Effective in pancreatic cancer therapy. Proc Am Soc Clin Oncol [Abstract] 1991;10:423.

236. Wils JA, Klein HO, Wagener DJT Bleiberg H, et al. Sequential high-dose methotrexate and fluorouracil combined with doxorubicin. A step ahead in the treatment of advanced gastric cancer. A trial of the EORTCG. J Clin Oncol 1991;9:827–831.

237. Scheitauer W, Funovics J, Mueller C, Ludwig H. Sequential high-dose methotrexate, 5-fluorouracil, and doxorubicin for treatment of advanced pancreatic cancer. J Cancer Res Clin Oncol 1990;116:132–133.

238. McCracken JD, Olson M, Cruz AB Jr, Leichman L, Oishi N. Radiation therapy combined with intra-arterial 5-FU chemotherapy for treatment of localized adenocarcinoma of the pancreas. A Southwest Oncology Group study. Cancer Treat Rep 1982;66:549–551.

239. Crist KA, Arredondo MA, Chaudhuri B, Thomford NR, Chaudhuri PK. Pharmacokinetic and toxicity of isolated perfusion of human pancreas-duodenum with mitomycin-C. Reg Cancer Treat 1991;3:305–307.

240. Aigner KR, Muller H, Bassermann R. Intra-arterial chemotherapy with MMC, CDDP, and 5-FU for nonresectable pancreatic cancer—a Phase II study. Reg Cancer Treat 1990;3:1–6.

241. Heidelberger C, Griesbach L, Montag BJ, et al. Studies on fluorinated pyrimidines: II. Effects on transplanted tumors. Cancer Res 1958;18:305–317.

242. Childs DS Jr, Moertel CG, Holbrook MA, Reitemeier RJ, Colby MY Jr. Treatment of malignant neoplasms of the gastrointestinal tract with a combination of 5-fluorouracil and radiation. Radiology 1965;84:843–847.

243. Moertel CG, Childs DS Jr, Reitermeier RJ, Colby MY Jr, Holbrook MA. Combined 5-

fluorouracil and supervoltage radiation therapy of locally unresectable gastrointestinal cancer. Lancet 1969;2:865–867.

244. Moertel CG, Frytak S, Hahn RG, et al. Therapy of locally unresectable pancreatic carcinoma: A randomized comparison of high dose (6000 rads) radiation alone, moderate dose radiation (4000 rads + 5-fluorouracil) and high dose radiation + 5-fluorouracil. Cancer 1981;48:1705–1710.

245. Gastrointestinal Tumor Study Group. Radiation therapy combined with Adriamycin or 5-fluorouracil for the treatment of locally unresectable pancreatic carcinoma. Cancer 1985;56:2563–2568.

246. Klaasen DJ, MacIntyre JM, Catton GE, Engstrom PF, Moertel CG. Treatment of locally unresectable cancer of the stomach and pancreas: A randomized comparison of 5-fluorouracil alone with radiation plus concurrent and maintenance 5-fluorouracil. An Eastern Cooperative Group study. J Clin Oncol 1985;3:373–378.

247. Gastrointestinal Tumor Study Group. Treatment of locally unresectable carcinoma of the pancreas: Comparison of combined modality therapy (chemotherapy plus radiotherapy) to chemotherapy alone. JNCI 1988;80:751–755.

248. Greenway B, Iqbal MJ, Johnson PJ, Williams R. Oestrogen receptor proteins in malignant and fetal pancreas. Br Med J 1981;283:751–753.

249. Iqbal MJ, Greenway BA, Wilkinson ML, Johnson PJ, Williams R. Sex-steroid enzymes, aromatase and 5-reductase in the pancreas: A comparison of normal adult, foetal, and malignant tissue. Clin Sci 1983;65:71–75.

250. Greenway B, Iqbal MJ, Johnson PJ, Williams R. Low serum testosterone concentrations in patients with carcinoma of the pancreas. Br Med J 1983;286:93–95.

251. Greenway B, Duke D, Pym B, et al. The control of human pancreatic adenocarcinoma xenografts in nude mice by hormone therapy. Br J Surg 1982;69:595.

252. Szende B, Srkalovic G, Schally AV, Lapis K, Groot K. Inhibitory effects of analogs of luteinizing hormone-releasing hormone and somatostatin on pancreatic cancer in hamsters. Cancer 1990;65:2279–2290.

253. Smith JP, Solomon TE, Bagheri S, Kramer S. Cholecystokinin stimulates growth of human pancreatic adenocarcinoma SW-1990. Dig Dis Sci 1990;35:1377–1384.

254. Upp JR Jr, Olson D, Poston GJ, et al. Inhibition of growth of two human pancreatic adenocarcinomas in vivo by somatostatin analog SMS 201-995. Ann Surg 1988;155:29.

255. Srkalovic G, Cai RZ, Schally AV. Evaluation of receptors for somatostatin in various tumors using different analogs. J Clin Endocrinol Metab 1990;70:661–669.

256. Zalatnai A, Schally AV. Treatment of N-nitorso-bis-(2-oxopropyl)-amine-induced pancreatic cancer in Syrian golden hamsters with D-Trp-6-LH-RH and somatostatin analog RC-160 microcapsules. Cancer Res 1989;49:1810–1815.

257. Crowson MC, Dorrell A, Rolfe EB, Fielding JWL. A phase II study to evaluate tamoxifen in pancreatic adenocarcinoma. Eur J Surg Oncol 1986;12:335–336.

258. Theve NO, Pousette A, Carlstrom K. Adenocarcinoma of the pancreas—a hormone sensitive tumor? A preliminary report on Nolvadex treatment. Clin Oncol 1983;9:193–197.

259. Tonnesen K, Kamp-Jensen M. Antiestrogen therapy in pancreatic carcinoma: A preliminary report. Eur J Surg Oncol 1986;12:69–70.

260. Wong A, Chan A, Arthur K. Tamoxifen therapy in unresectable adenocarcinoma of the pancreas. Cancer Treat Rep 1987;71:7.

261. Bakkevold KE, Petterson A, Arnesjo B, Espehaug B. Tamoxifen therapy in unresectable adenocarcinoma of the pancreas and the papilla of Vater. Br J Surg 1990;77:725–730.

262. Keating JJ, Johnson PJ, Cochrane AMG, et al. A prospective randomised controlled trial of tamoxifen and cyproteone acetate in pancreatic carcinoma. Br J Cancer 1989;60:789–792.

263. Waddell WR. Chemotherapy for carcinoma of the pancreas. Surgery 1973;74:420–429.

264. Stephens RL, Hoogstraten B, Haas C, et al. Pancreatic cancer treated with carmustine, fluorouracil and spironolactone. A randomized study. Arch Intern Med 1978;138:115.

265. Harvey H, Lipton A, Santen S, et al. Chemo-hormonal therapy of pancreatic carcinoma. Proc Am Soc Clin Oncol [Abstract] 1989;8:424.

266. Klijn JGM, Hoff AM, Plantig AST, et al. Treatment of patients with metastatic pancreatic and gastrointestinal tumours with the somatostatin analogue Sandostatin: A phase II study including endocrine effects. Br J Cancer 1990;62:627.

267. Poston GJ, Davies N, Schally AV, et al. Phase one B study of somatostatin analogue RC-160 in the treatment of patients with advanced exocrine pancreatic cancer. Digestion 1990;46:121.

268. Gonzalez-Barcena D, Ibarra-Olmas MA, Garcia-Carrasco F, Gutierrez-Samperio C, Comaru-Schally AM, Schally AV. Influence of D-Trp-6-LH-RH on the survival time in patients with advanced pancreatic cancer. Biomed Pharmacother 1989;43:313–317.

269. Suri P, Lipton A, Harvey HA, et al. Hormonal therapy of pancreatic carcinoma with GNRH and Somatostatin analogs. Proc Am Soc Clin Oncol 1991;10:1059.

270. Wadler S, Lembersky B, Atkins M, Kirkwood J, Petrelli N. Phase II trial of fluorouracil

271. Derderian P, Pazdur R, Ajani J, et al. Phase II study of 5-fluorouracil (5-FU) and recombinant alfa-2A interferon (rIFN) in the treatment of advanced pancreatic carcinoma. Proc Am Soc Clin Oncol [Abstract] 1991;10:453.

272. Gottlinger H, Funke I, Johnson JP, et al. The epithelial cell surface antigen 17-1A, a target for antibody mediated tumor therapy: Its biochemical nature, tissue distribution and recognition by different monoclonal antibodies. Int J Cancer 1986;38:47–53.

273. Herlyn DM, Steplewski Z, Herlyn MF, et al. Inhibition of growth of colorectal carcinoma in nude mice by monoclonal antibody. Cancer Res 1980;44:717.

274. Herlyn DM, Koprowski H. IgG2a monoclonal antibodies inhibit human tumor growth through interaction with effector cells. Proc Natl Acad Sci USA 1982;79:4761.

275. Tempero MA, Sivinski C, Steplewski Z, Harvey E, Klassen L, Kay HD. Phase II trial of interferon gamma and monoclonal antibody 17-1A in pancreatic cancer: Biologic and clinical effects. J Clin Oncol 1990;8:2019–2026.

276. Weiner LM, Halle DG, Kirkwood J, et al. Phase II trial of repetitive murine monoclonal antibody therapy in pancreatic carcinoma. An ECOG trial. Proc Am Soc Clin Oncol [Abstract] 1991;10:512.

277. Buchler M, Kubel R, Malfertheiner P, et al. Immuntherapie des fortgeschrittenen Pankreaskarzinoms mit dem monoklonalen Antikorper BW 494. Dtsch Med Wochenschr 1988;113:374–380.

278. Buchler M, Friess H, Schultheiss HK, Gebhardt C, et al. A randomized controlled trial of adjuvant immunotherapy (murine monoclonal antibody 494/32) in resectable pancreatic cancer. Cancer 1991;68:1507–1512.

279. Thor A, Ohuchi N, Szpak CA, Johnston WW, Schlom J. Distribution of oncofetal antigen tumor-associated glycoprotein-72 defined by monoclonal antibody. Cancer Res 1986;46:3118–3124.

280. Lyubsky S, Madariaga J, Lozowski M, et al. A tumor-associated antigen in carcinoma of the pancreas defined by monoclonal antibody b72. 3. Am J Clin Pathol 1988;89:160–167.

281. Mehta MP, Kubsad SS, Fowler JF, Verma AK, Hsieh JT, Kinsella TJ. ^{90}Y.B72.3 against pancreatic cancer: Dosimetric and biological analysis. Int J Radiat Oncol Biol Phys 1990;19:627–631.

282. Molinolo A, Simpson JF, Thor A, Schlom J. Enhanced tumor binding using immunohistochemical analyses by second generation anti-tumor-associated glycoprotein 72 monoclonal antibodies versus monoclonal antibody B72.3 in human tissue. Cancer Res 1990;50:1291–1298.

283. Korc M, Meltzer P, Trent J. Enhanced expression of epidermal growth factor receptor correlates with alterations of chromosome 7 in human pancreatic cancer. Proc Natl Acad Sci USA 1986;83:5141–5144.

284. Beauchamp RD, Lyons RM, Yang EY, Coffey RJ, Jr, Moses HL. Expression of and response to growth regulatory peptides by human pancreatic carcinoma cell lines. Pancreas 1990;5:369–380.

285. Smith JJ, Deryneck R, Korc M. Production of transforming growth factor alpha in human pancreatic cancer cells: Evidence for a superagonist autocrine cycle. Proc Natl Acad Sci USA 1987;84:7567.

286. Korc M. Autocrine regulation in human pancreatic cancer cells. Proc American Association for Cancer Research [Abstract] 1990;31:477.

287. Almoquera C, Shibata D, Forrester K, et al. Most human carcinomas of the exocrine pancreas contain mutant c-K-*ras* genes. Cell 1988;53:49.

288. Greenwald HP, Bonica JJ, Bergner M. The prevalence of pain in four cancers. Cancer 1987;60:2563.

289. Hudis C, Kelsen D, Niedzwiecki D, Banks W, Portenoy R, Foley K. Pain is not a prominent symptom (S) in most patients (PTS) with early pancreas cancer (PC). Proc Am Soc Clin Oncol 1991;10:326.

290. Flanigan D, Kraft R. Continuing experience with palliative chemical splanchniectomy. Arch Surg 1978;113:509.

291. Green N, Beron E, Melbye RW, et al. Carcinoma of pancreas—palliative radiotherapy. AJR 1973;117:620–622.

292. Saltzburg D, Foley K. Management of pain in pancreatic cancer. Surg Clin North Am 1989;69:629–649.

293. Bridenbaugh L, Moore D, Campbell D. Management of upper abdominal cancer pain: Treatment with celiac plexus block with alcohol. JAMA 1964;190:99.

294. Hanowell S, Kennedy S, MacNamara T, et al. Celiac plexus block. Diagnostic and therapeutic applications in abdominal pain. South Med J 1980;73:1330.

295. Buy JN, Moss A, Singler R. CT guided celiac plexus and splanchnic nerve neurolysis. J Comput Assist Tomogr 1982;6:315.

296. Jones J. Celiac plexus block with alcohol for relief of upper abdominal pain due to cancer. Ann R Coll Surg Engl 1977;59:46.

297. Thompson G, Moore D, Bridenbaugh L. Abdominal pain and alcohol celiac plexus nerve block. Anesth Analg 1977;56:1.

Cancer: Principles & Practice of Oncology, Fourth Edition,
edited by Vincent T. DeVita, Jr., Samuel Hellman, Steven A. Rosenberg.
J.B. Lippincott Co., Philadelphia © 1993.

Michael T. Lotze

John C. Flickinger

Brian I. Carr

CHAPTER **28**

Hepatobiliary Neoplasms

Tumors of the liver are among the most common malignancies in the world. The annual international incidence of the disease is about 1,000,000 cases, with a male to female ratio of about 4 to 1. In the United States, about 15,400 new tumors of the liver and biliary passages are diagnosed each year, with an estimated 12,300 deaths each year.[1] About half of these tumors are in the gallbladder, a third are in the intrahepatic and extrahepatic biliary ducts, and the remainder are primary hepatocellular carcinomas (HCCs), accounting for about 4000 to 6000 cases per year in the United States.[2–4] The death rates among males in low-incidence countries such as the United States are about 1.9 deaths per 100,000 per year. In intermediate areas such as Austria and South Africa, incidence rates range from 5.1 to 20.0 persons per 100,000 per year. In high-incidence areas such as China and Korea, rates are as high as 23.1 to 150 persons per 100,000 per year.[3] Little has changed in the last 5 years to alter these statistics, although better imaging studies have become available to define intrahepatic spread of hepatic malignancies, and transplantation increasingly has been applied and has a better defined role. The twin problems of major derangements in hepatic physiology associated with many neoplasms of the biliary tree and the high recurrence rate of most of these tumors will require new information about hepatobiliary biology and tumors to allow significant progress. Advances in the management of these malignancies probably will depend on immunization strategies for the hepatitis B and C viruses and on developing a means of decreasing cirrhosis of any origin.

LOBAR ANATOMY AND PHYSIOLOGY

Surgical approaches for the therapy of hepatobiliary neoplasms require an understanding of the complexities of the anatomy of the liver. The liver receives oxygenated blood from the portal vein, which arises from mesenteric veins draining the gut, the splenic vein, and the hepatic arterial inflow. Hepatic effluent includes blood exiting through three hepatic veins into the suprahepatic vena cava immediately below the right atrium and bile secreted into bile canaliculi by hepatocytes. Bile is passed into progressively larger ducts, finally exiting the liver in the proper hepatic duct. The common hepatic duct is formed after intersection of the cystic duct leading to and from the gallbladder. The common duct usually joins the pancreatic duct at the ampulla of Vater, where pancreatic and biliary secretions are excreted into the lumen of the duodenum. Variations of hepatic anatomy are particularly common. Although the liver appears to be morphologically divided by an umbilical fissure into a right and left lobe, the true division is based on hepatic arterial and portal inflow between these functional elements of the liver and occurs on a line roughly drawn between the superior vena cava and the gallbladder fossa. Further division of the liver into medial and lateral segments is demarcated by the falciform ligament on the left and into anterior and posterior segments on the right by the entrance of the portal structures. Division of the liver into a total of 8 segments by Couinaud reflects the underlying vascular complexity of the liver (Fig. 28–1). The numbering sequence starts with 1, the caudate or Spigelian lobe immediately to the left and posterior to the vena cava, and then circles to encompass segments 2 (superior) and 3 (inferior) within that portion of the liver to the left of the umbilical fissure, segment 4 (that portion of the left lobe immediately medial to the umbilical fissure), and segments 5 through 8, following in a clockwise fashion the medial, lateral-inferior, lateral, and medial superior segments, in that order. These considerations are crucial in performing a formal lobectomy (Fig. 28–2) or segmentectomy of the liver but are less important when considering nonanatomic resections.

883

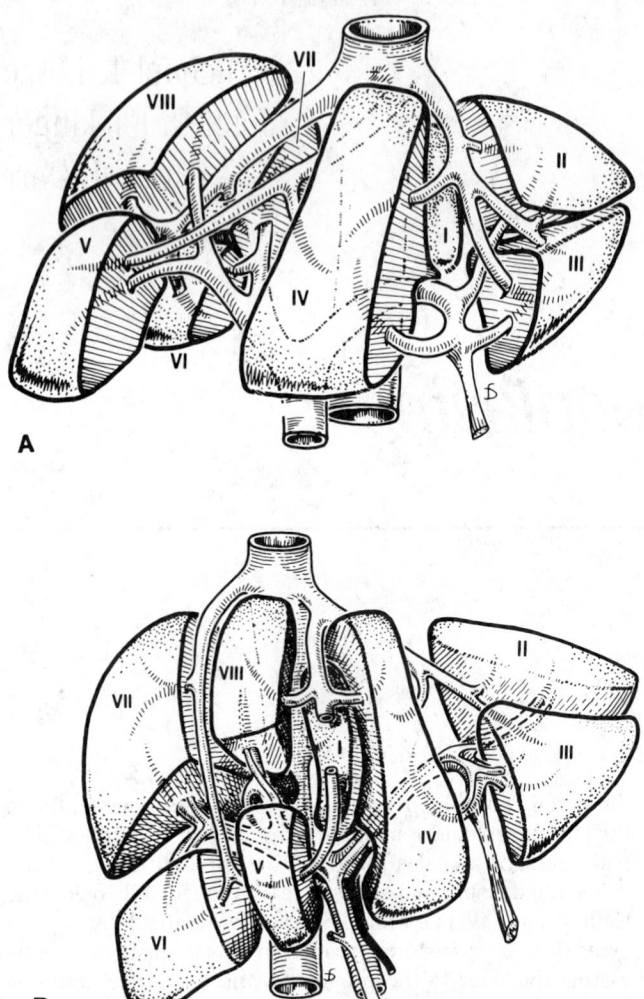

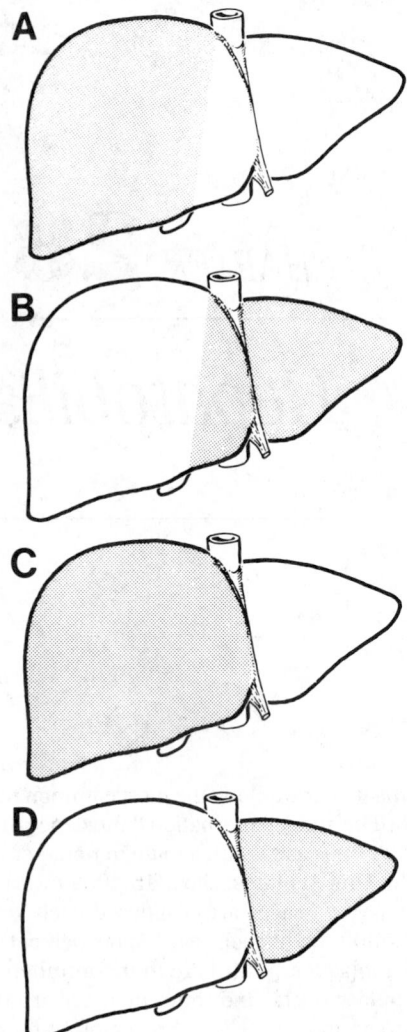

FIGURE 28–1.   The functional division of the liver and liver segment according to Couinaud's nomenclature, as seen (A) in the patient and (B) in ex vivo. (Blumgart LH. Surgery of the liver and biliary tract. Edinburgh: Churchill Livingstone, 1988)

FIGURE 28–2.   The four common hepatectomies. (A and B) Right and left hepatectomy as defined by the main portal scissura. (C and D) Right left lobectomy as defined by the umbilical fissure. (Blumgart LH. Surgery of the liver and biliary tract. Edinburgh: Churchill Livingstone, 1988)

LIVER REGENERATION

The liver is able to grow in size with increases in age. This is due in part to an increase from a single cell "liver plate" between endothelia to a double cell thickness after the age of 5 years.[5] The liver also is able to increase its number of cells after surgical removal of the liver or after damage by toxins or disease. There are several molecular signals that regulate liver growth.[6] Complete mitogens, which themselves cause hepatocyte proliferation, include EGF (epidermal growth factor), TGF-α (transforming growth factor-α), FGF (fibroblast growth factor), HGF (hepatocyte growth factor), and a small-molecular-weight lipid, hepatopoietin-B. EGF and TGF-α are products of platelets. FGF-α has been noted to increase in the serum of patients with HCC. HGF appears to be about 10 times more potent than EGF in causing hepatic mitogenesis and is one of a family of heparin-binding growth factors.[7–9] HGF is a member of a family of molecules that includes prothrombin and plasminogen and are defined as Kringle proteins because of the tertiary structure. Other hepatotropic sub-

stances include norepinephrine, another unidentified factor released into the serum after hepatectomy,[9] and factors produced by islets such as insulin and glucagon.[10] Vasopressin, angiotensin II, angiotensin III, and estrogens appear to have a role in hepatic regeneration. Retinoic acid receptor-α is markedly elevated in HCC. More differentiated cells are inhibited by the presence of retinoic acid, whereas less differentiated or fetal-appearing cell lines are stimulated by retinoic acid.[11] Retinoids inhibit the growth of transplanted rat hepatomas and induce maturation of fetal liver cells in culture. Recent studies demonstrate that mouse hepatocytes can migrate to the liver after intrasplenic injection, supporting their potential use as vehicles for gene therapy for metabolic and other disorders. Growth inhibitory substances include TGF-α, interleukin-1α (IL-1α), and an unidentified hepatocyte proliferation inhibitor. Liver regeneration may be stimulated by signals from outside the liver or from the liver cells themselves. The precise means by which liver regeneration stops (perhaps by a TGF-β-dependent mechanism) is unclear.

Various means have been used to demonstrate return of liver volume after hepatic resection in man. These include ultrasound and computed tomography (CT).[12-14] Most researchers agree that hepatic regeneration occurs within the first few weeks or months after resection, with essentially complete regeneration taking from 3 months to 1 year. Longer periods are observed primarily in patients with liver dysfunction and cirrhosis.

RETICULOENDOTHELIAL SYSTEM AND IMMUNE FUNCTION

Hepatic resident macrophages known as Kupffer's cells actively phagocytose and metabolize a variety of particles and macroaggregates. The liver responds rapidly to inflammation as a secondary response to circulating immunologic hormones and proinflammatory cytokines including IL-1, tumor necrosis factor (TNF-α), IL-6, and transforming growth factor-β (TGF-β).[15-19] Decreases in bile flow result in cholestasis and decreased production of albumin, and increased production of acute-phase reactants is observed after immune activation. The liver is a central target after systemic immune activation. Antichymotrypsin production by the liver is induced by IL-6, IL-1, TNF-α, and TGF-β. Some other factors are only induced by IL-6 and include fibrinogen, fibronectin, and haptoglobin. All four cytokines down-regulate α-fetoprotein (AFP) production. TNF infusion into patients with liver metastases has been associated with severe hypophosphatemia, presumably due to enhanced uptake, a finding also frequently observed after extensive hepatic resection.[17] Serum amyloid-A (SAA) increases up to 1000-fold during the acute-phase response and may be induced by IL-1 or IL-6. Enhanced transcription and translation of these acute-phase reactants is regulated by molecules binding to regulatory elements upstream of these individual genes. Regulation of hepatocyte protein production occurs through Kupffer's cells and hepatocyte production of nitric oxide.[20]

Immune recognition by T cells requires expression on targets of class I or class II major histocompatibility complex (MHC) antigens. Such antigens are poorly displayed on most normal hepatocytes[21] but are inducible by cytokines such as interferon-α or interferon-γ. HCCs appear to have increased expression of class I MHC antigens and variable expression of class II MHC markers.[21-23] No specific relations among individual HLA, B, C, or DR antigens and HCC have been noted in Chinese patients with HCC.[24] The immune response to hepatitis B, which appears to be mediated in large part by T cells,[24,25] is associated with expression of certain MHC types. The ability of the host immune response to react or not react (toleragenesis) may be related to induction of the carrier state associated with hepatitis B infection.[26] Some MHC alleles have been associated with genetic nonresponsiveness to the hepatitis B vaccine.[27] The ability of the liver to respond to infectious pathogens such as hepatitis and not to respond to other protein antigens undoubtedly requires fine regulation of the immune response. Both large granular lymphocytes and T cells can be demonstrated in the liver of experimental animals and are found to be increased after exogenous IL-2 administration.[28] Alloreactive lymphocytes responding to hepatic transplants[29] and lymphocytes infiltrating HCC[30] can be grown readily in combinations of cytokines including IL-2 and TNF. Such cells may have important antitumor effects, and their adoptive transfer represents a potential strategy for treatment of such tumors. Natural killer cell activity in the peripheral blood of patients with HCC appears to be reduced.[31-33]

HEPATOCELLULAR CARCINOMA

EPIDEMIOLOGY

Epidemiologic studies of HCC have been of two general types: those of country-based incidence rates (Table 28-1) and those of migrants (Table 28-2).[34,35] Table 28-1 shows a sampling of incidence rates of countries in South America, Asia, Africa and Europe. Hyperendemic hot spots occur in areas such as China and sub-Saharan Africa. In Asia and Africa, high incidence rates have been associated with high endemic hepatitis

TABLE 28-1. Age-Adjusted Incidence Rates for Hepatocellular Carcinoma

	No. of Persons per 100,000 per Year	
Country	Males	Females
Argentina	6.0	2.5
Peru	4.0	2.9
Brazil, Recife	9.2	8.3
Brazil, Sao Paulo	3.8	2.6
Colombia	2.8	1.4
Costa Rica	5.1	2.2
Mozambique	112.9	30.8
South Africa, Cape: Bantu	26.3	8.4
South Africa, Cape: White	1.2	0.6
Senegal	25.6	9.0
Nigeria	15.4	3.2
Swaziland	10.5	3.0
Algeria	1.6	1.4
Gambia	33.1	12.6
Burma	25.5	8.8
Phillipines	19.9	6.2
Japan	7.2	2.2
Korea	13.8	3.2
Thailand	6.8	2.3
China, Shanghai	34.4	11.6
India, Bombay	4.9	2.5
India, Madras	2.1	0.7
Israel, born in Europe	3.4	4.7
Israel, born in Africa	7.4	1.5
United Kingdom	1.6	0.8
France	6.9	1.2
Germany, Hamburg	4.5	1.7
Italy, Varese	7.1	2.7
Norway	1.8	1.1
Spain, Navarra	7.9	4.7

(Muir C, et al. Cancer incidence in five continents. IARC Scientific Publications. vol V. no. 88. Lyons, France: International Agency for Research in Cancer, 1989)

TABLE 28–2. Age-Adjusted Incidence Rates
for HCC Among Male Migrants

Population	No. of persons per 100,000 per year
Chinese	
People's Republic of China, Shanghai	31.7
Hong Kong	34.4
Singapore	32.2
United States	
San Francisco	18.1
Los Angeles	12.0
Hawaii	7.8
Jews	
Born in Israel	1.5
Born in Europe and USA	3.1
Born in Asia and Africa	3.6
Japanese	
Japan	
Osaka	5.5
Miyagi	2.5
United States	
Hawaii	5.7
San Francisco	3.0
Los Angeles	2.7

(Steinitz R. Cancer incidence: Jewish migrants to Israel 1961–1981. IARC Scientific Publication. no. 98. Lyon, France: International Agency for Research in Cancer, 1989)

B carrier rates and mycotoxin contamination of foodstuffs, stored grains, drinking water, and soil. Ethnic factors appear to be important, because incidence rates can vary in the same population according to ethnic origins. Examples of variations within a given population have been found in studies of this type in Los Angeles and Israel.[34–36]

ETIOLOGIC FACTORS

Causative agents for HCC have been studied along two general lines. First, there are those agents that have been found to be carcinogenic in experimental animals, particularly rodents, and which are thought to be present in the human environment (Table 28–3). Second, epidemiologic associations of hepatoma with various other human diseases have been identified (Table 28–4). Probably the best studied and most potent ubiquitous natural chemical carcinogen is aflatoxin B_1, a product of the *Aspergillus* fungus. *Aspergillus flavus* mold and aflatoxin product have been found in a variety of stored grains, particularly in hot humid parts of the world where grains such as rice stored in unrefrigerated conditions.[37] In the months after the monsoon in Southeast Asia, most village-based grains can be seen to be covered by a white layer. This layer contains high levels of aflatoxin and is consumed over the after months by most of the village. Data on aflatoxin contamination of food stuffs correlate well with incidence rates in Africa and to some extent in China. In hyperendemic areas of China, even farm animals such as ducks have HCC.

TABLE 28–3. Rodent Chemical Hepatocarcinogens Known to Exist in the Human Environment

Synthetic Materials and Medicines

Sex hormones (*e.g.*, androgens, estrogen)
Vinyl chloride
Aurothioglucose
Oxazepam
Phenobarbital
Thiouracil
Industrial dyes and colorants (*e.g.*, *p*-aminoazobenzene, *O*-aminotoluene)

General Environmental Pollutants

N-nitrosodimethylamine (*e.g.*, nitrite and nitrate-treated foods)
Polychlorinated biphenyls
Carbon tetrachloride
Chloroform
Vinyl chloride
DDT, aldrin, dieldrin, heptachlor (pesticides)
Bis-(2-choroethyl) ether (soil fumigant, insecticide)
Diallate (herbicide)
Dioxane (solvent)
Hydrazine (rocket fuel)
Trichoroethylene (dry cleaning solvent)

Natural Products

Aflatoxins
Sterigmatocystins (*Aspergillus versicolor*)
Luteoskyrin, cyclochlorotine (rice toxins)
Pyrrolizidine alkaloids (*Senecio* plants, bush tea)
Cycasin (cycad plants)
Safrole (sassafras oil)
Tannic acid, tannins
Griseofulvin

The most potent hepatocarcinogens appear to be natural products that occur in the environment and are synthesized by plants, fungi, and bacteria. In large areas of the world, rice toxins are eaten, as are the *Senecio* plants and bush teas containing pyrrollizidine alkaloid, tannic acid, safrole, and, in the Pacific, the cycad plants. Although hepatocarcinogens for rodents are used as medicinal compounds for humans (see Table 28–3), there is little evidence that any except the sex hormones have an important role in human hepatocarcinogenesis. A considerable literature exists on the hepatocarcinogenicity of anabolic steroids and the induction of benign hepatomas by estrogens.[38] Although estrogens are capable of causing HCC in rodents as promoting agents, an epidemiologic association in humans has never been shown. Complete carcinogens inducing HCC include aflatoxin B_1 and, for hepatic angiosarcoma, vinyl chloride, thorotrast, and possibly inorganic arsenic compounds. In an industrial society, a large number of environmental pollutants, particularly pesticides and insecticides, are known rodent carcinogens.[39]

Hepatitis and Hepatocellular Carcinoma

Case control studies and cohort studies have shown a strong association between chronic hepatitis B carriage rates and

TABLE 28–4. Conditions Associated
With Hepatocellular Carcinoma

Cirrhosis

Hepatitis B virus*
Alcohol*
Autoimmune chronic active hepatitis*
Cryptogenic cirrhosis†
Non-A, non-B†
Primary biliary cirrhosis‡‖

Metabolic Diseases

Genetic hemochromatosis*
Hereditary tyrosinemia*
Alpha$_1$-antitrypsin deficiency†
Ataxia telangiectasia†
Types 1 and 3 glycogen storage disease†
Galactosemia†
Citrullinemia†
Hereditary hemorrhagic telangiectasia†
Porphyria cutanea tarda†
Wilson's disease‡
Orotic aciduria†
Alagille's syndrome (congenital cholestatic syndrome)†

Environmental

Thorotrast†
Androgenic steroids†
Cigarette smokings§
Aflatoxin§
Pyrrolizidine alkaloids§
Cycasin§
N-nitrosylated compounds§

---

* High risk.
† Moderate risk.
‡ Low risk.
§ Risk not determined in humans.
‖ More typically associated with cholangiocarcinoma.

---

increased incidence of HCC (Table 28–5).[40,41] Although up to a 200-fold excess incidence of HCC was found in Taiwan,[42] the association of chronic HBV in different populations of Southeast Asia who have HCC is varied. An apparent increase with time of the incidence of HCC in Japan is associated with a stable incidence of chronic hepatitis B (Fig. 28–3).[43] This

increase in Japanese HCC incidence rates in the last three decades is thought to be due to previously undiagnosed hepatitis C (Table 28–6). The relative role of these two viruses is under examination. Several animal models are available for the study of hepatitis B virus such as the woodchuck, the Peking duck, or the ground squirrel, which are infected with hepatitis B-like viruses (hepadnaviruses) and which also develop HCC. A large scale intervention study sponsored by the World Health Organization is underway in Asia and involves hepatitis B virus vaccination of newborns. Ten percent to 15% of those populations have chronic hepatitis B, most of which is thought to be transmitted at birth through the vaginal canal. It will take another 40 years for evidence to indicate whether this intervention reduces the indigenous incidence rates of HCC.

Clinical Associations With Hepatocellular Carcinoma

The 60% to 80% association of HCC with underlying cirrhosis has been long recognized, most typically with macronodular cirrhosis in Southeast Asia, but also with micronodular cirrhosis in Southeast Asia, Europe, and the United States.[44,45] It is not clear whether cirrhosis itself is a predisposing factor to the development of subsequent HCC or whether the underlying causes of the cirrhosis are actually the carcinogenic factors. About 20% of North American patients with HCC do not have underlying cirrhosis, and probably not more than 70% have associated hepatitis B. Several underlying conditions are associated with an increased risk for the development of HCC (see Table 28–4).

TUMOR CLASSIFICATION

Tumors of the hepatobiliary system can be classified as benign or malignant (Table 28–7) and by the tissue of origin, whether the mesenchymal or the more common epithelial neoplasms.[5] Malignant epithelial neoplasms constitute 85% to 95% of all tumors of the liver. Six percent to 12% are benign, again largely of epithelial origin. Mixed HCC/cholangiocarcinoma can also be found, typically in 2% of our patient population

TABLE 28–5. Role of Hepatitis B in Case-Control of Hepatocellular Carcinoma

Study Population	No. of Patients		HBsAg-Positive		Relative Risk (95% CI)	Attributable Risk (%)
	HCC	Controls	HCC (%)	Controls (%)		
High-Risk Areas						
Senegal	165	328	61.2	11.3	12.4 (7.7–19.3)	56.3
South Africa	289	213	61.6	11.3	12.6 (7.7–20.1)	56.7
Hong Kong	107	107	82.0	22.0	21.3 (10.1–45.9)	78.5
People's Republic of China	50	50	86.0	22.0	17.0 (4.3–99.4)	77.9
Philippines	104	84	70.0	18.0	10.83 (5.3–20.9)	63.9
Intermediate-Risk Area						
Greece	194	451	45.9	7.3	10.7 (6.8–16.6)	41.6
Low-Risk Area						
United States	86	161	17.9	0.0	(10.0–100)	

(Data modified from Munoz N, Bosch X. Epidemiology of hepatocellular carcinoma. In: Okuda K, Ishak KA, eds. Neoplasms of the liver. New York: Springer-Verlag, 1987)

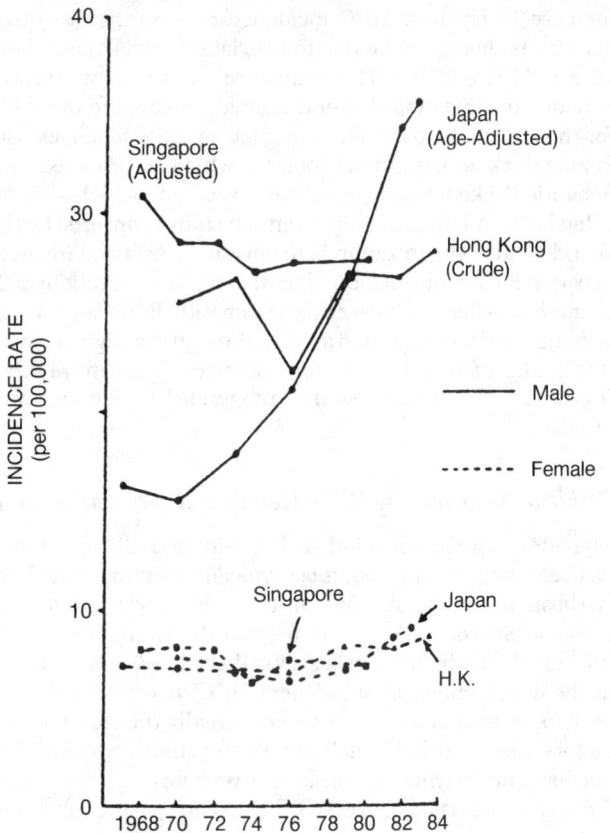

FIGURE 28–3. Trends in the incidence of primary liver cancer in Japan, Singapore, and Hong Kong. Although the age-adjusted or crude rate of primary liver cancer in males has been relatively constant during the past 15 years in Singapore and Hong Kong, it rose significantly in Japan. The incidence among females has been much lower in all of these countries. (Okuda K, Fujimoto I, Hannai A, Urano Y. Changing incidence of hepatocellular carcinoma in Japan. Cancer Res 1987;47:4967–4972)

in Pittsburgh. About 1% to 3% are malignant mesenchymal tumors.[5] About half of the hepatobiliary tumors in the United States arise in the gallbladder or in the extrahepatic biliary tree. Other distinctions made clinically and reflected in the staging system include the size of the tumor, with those smaller than 2 cm often representing tumor with the best

prognosis.[46] Those having a well-defined rim by CT scan or on subsequent pathologic examination have a better prognosis. Tumors arising in patients from the occident appear to be less aggressive than those in the orient. Rare inflammatory pseudomasses and pseudotumors associated with infarction or inflammation can be recognized and need to be differentiated from true tumors arising in the liver.[47,48]

Many other tumors have a propensity to metastasize to the liver or to the adjacent biliary tree. The tumors most frequently metastasizing to the liver during their natural course include melanoma (especially uveal melanoma with the clinical picture of one eye and an enlarged liver), and gallbladder, colon, pancreas, and breast carcinomas. By absolute number and in decreasing order of frequency, the most frequent tumors of nonhepatic origin in the liver include lung cancer, colon cancer, pancreatic cancer, breast cancer, and gastric carcinoma.[5] Metastases usually obtain access to the liver by hematogenous spread through the portal vein or the hepatic artery. In turn, metastases to the liver can travel from there to the regional lymph nodes. The lymphatics of the liver course between lobules and drain primarily through vessels surrounding the portal veins directly into the liver hilum and cisterna chyli. The remaining 20% is drained by vessels ascending along the vena cava.[49] Grossly, metastatic tumors are often peripheral, multiple, and cause umbilication of the surface of the liver, whereas primary tumors are more often central and solitary.

WORKUP OF HEPATIC TUMORS

In a patient presenting with a new abdominal mass or other indications of new hepatic decompensation, levels of carcinoembryonic antigen, B$_{12}$, AFP, or des-γ-carboxy prothrombin (or PIVKA-II, protein induced by vitamin K absence or alteration) should be measured. Prothrombin time (PT), partial thromboplastin time (PTT), and albumin levels reflect hepatic synthetic function and should be measured. Traditional liver function tests (*e.g.*, transaminases, lactic dehydrogenase, alkaline phosphatate) should be obtained (Table 28–8). Decreases in platelet and white blood cell counts may reflect portal hypertension and associated hypersplenism. Hepatitis A, B, C, and D serology should be evaluated. An ultrasound

TABLE 28–6. Global Epidemiology of Hepatocellular Carcinoma and Anti-Hepatitis C Virus (Anti-HCV)

Area, Country	Overall Anti-HCV Positivity Rate in HCC Patients (%)	Anti-HCV According to HBsAg Status		Anti-HCV in Controls Without HCC
		Positive (%)	Negative (%)	
Central Japan	73.5 (61/83)	35 (10/29)	94 (51/54)	0.9–1.2
North Italy	65 (86/132)	54 (22/41)	70 (64/91)	Not determined
Sicily, Italy	76 (152/200)	58 (18/31)	79 (134/169)	Not determined
Barcelona, Spain	75 (72/96)	55.5 (5/9)	77 (67/87)	7.3
Miami, USA	52.5 (31/59)	61.1 (11/18)	48.8 (20/41)	0.5
South Africa	28.9 (110/380)	25.5 (47/184)	32.1 (63/196)	0.7
Taiwan	33.3 (22/26)	16.7 (7/42)	62.5 (15/24)	0.95

(Data from Okuda K, Fujimoto I, Hannai A, Urano Y. Changing incidence of hepatocellular carcinoma in Japan. Cancer Res 1987;47:4967–4972)

TABLE 28–7. Hepatobiliary Neoplasms

Hepatic Tumors	**Extrahepatic Tumors**

Hepatic Tumors

Benign Epithelial Tumors and Tumor Bile Conditions

Hepatocellular hyperplasia: macroregenerative nodule, nodular hyperplasia, mixed hamartoma

Hepatocellular adenoma: typical; associated with anabolic steroids

Hepatic cysts: simple, polycystic

Bile duct adenoma

Benign mesenchymal tumors and tumor-like conditions: mesenchymal hamartoma, hemangioma, infantile hemangioendothelioma, lymphangiomatosis, lipoma, leiomyoma, fibroma, inflammatory pseudotumor, myxoma

Tumor of heterotopic tissue and uncertain origin: adrenal rest tumors, pheochromocytoma, pancreatic rests, carcinoid, neuroendocrine infantile sinusoidal tumor, teratoma, yolk sac tumor, malignant trophoblastic tumor, hepatic malignant mixed tumor

Primary Malignant Epithelial Tumors

Hepatocellular carcinoma

Hepatocellular carcinoma variants: childhood, fibrolamellar, combined, spindle cell, clear cell, giant cell, carcinosarcoma, sclerosing

Hepatoblastoma

Cholangiocarcinoma and Cholangiocellular Carcinoma

Hepatic cystadenocarcinoma, squamous cell carcinoma

Primary Malignant Mesenchymal Tumors

Angiosarcoma, hemangioendothelioma, leiomyosarcoma, malignant schwannoma, fibrosarcoma, malignant fibrous histiocytoma, lymphoma, osteosarcoma, rhabdomyosarcoma, mesenchymal sarcoma

Extrahepatic Tumors

Benign Tumors of the Gallbladder

Epithelial (adenoma, mixed tumor), mesenchymal (leiomyoma, hemangioma, lipoma), paraganglioma, neurofibroma, ganglioneurofibroma (in type 2B, multiple endocrine neoplasia syndrome)

Malignant Tumor of the Gallbladder

    Adenocarcinoma: well-differentiated, papillary, pleomorphic giant cell, intestinal type, small cell (poorly differentiated), signet-ring cell type, clear cell type with associated choriocarcinoma-like areas, colloid

    Squamous cell carcinoma and adenosquamous carcinoma

    Oat cell carcinoma (small cell)

    Carcinosarcoma

    Malignant lymphoma

    Malignant melanoma

    Malignant mesenchymal tumors: rhabdomyosarcoma, malignant fibrous histiocytoma, angiosarcoma, Kaposi's sarcoma (with AIDS), leiomyosarcoma.

Benign Tumors of the Extrahepatic Bile Ducts

Adenoma (papillary or tubular), cystadenoma (hamartoma), granular cell myoblastoma, paraganglioma; benign mesenchymal tumor (fibroma, lipoma, leiomyoma, neurilemoma), amputation neuroma, heterotopic rests.

Malignant Tumors of the Extrahepatic Bile Ducts

Adenocarcinoma: well-differentiated, pleomorphic giant cell, adenosquamous, oat cell, colloid

Malignant mesenchymal tumors: embryonal rhabdomyosarcoma, leiomyosarcoma, malignant fibrous histiocytoma

(Modified from Albores-Saavedra, J, Henson DE. Tumors of the gallbladder and extrahepatic bile ducts, 1986. In: Craig JP, Peters RL, Edwardson HA. Tumors of the liver and intrahepatic bile ducts. Washington, DC: Armed Forces Institute of Pathology, fascicles 22 and 26, 1989)

TABLE 28–8. Workup and Treatment of Suspected Hepatic Neoplasms

Screen	Alpha-fetoprotein, PIVKA-II (protein induced by vitamin K absence)
	Hepatitis B surface antigen and antibody
	Hepatitis C antibody
	LFTs, platelet, albumin, prothrombin time, partial thromboplastin time
Assess local extent	CT with angioportography or Lipiodol scan with CT or T1- and T2-weighted MRI
Make diagnosis	Needle biopsy or open biopsy (need corrected coagulation studies)
Assess metastatic sites	Head and chest CT scan
	Bone scan
	Evaluation of symptomatic sites on x-ray film
Treatment for resectable disease	Wedge or lobar resection (conventionally resectable) or Orthotopic liver transplant or Neoadjuvant chemotherapy IA or I.V. for 1–3 mo; then resect or consider transplantation

(IA, intraarterially; I.V., intravenously.

examination of the liver is an excellent screening tool to identify occult neoplasms.

Good quality CT scans with and without intravenous contrast or with coincident administration of contrast material delivered into the superior mesenteric artery (angioportography) should be performed to assess the local extent of tumor and to identify intrahepatic extension or metastases. Contrast administered through the superior mesenteric artery enters the portal circulation and, in the absence of severe portal hypertension, provides excellent contrast of normal tissue compared with intrahepatic tumors. Magnetic resonance imaging (MRI) also can provide this type of detailed information. An iodized oil emulsion (Lipiodol) can be delivered into the portal circulation (5–15 ml) and detected by late CT scan at 1 week, demonstrating retention in tumor. Celiac arteriography with selective lobar or superselective studies is occasionally useful to delineate the relation of the tumor to vessels and to differentiate it from the rare hypovascular pseudotumor (Fig. 28–4).[50] Hepatic tumors usually are hypervascular and show tortuosity of the vessels, vascular pooling, and hepatic staining. They often demonstrate rapid entry of contract into the associated hepatic veins. Arterial portal shunting in the presence of portal hypertension can be observed.

Ultrasonography in prospective studies has been shown to be more sensitive than repetitive AFP testing, especially for small tumors in high-risk patients.[51] Using transducers of 3.5 or 5.0 MHz, both diagnosis and biopsy of suspicious lesions

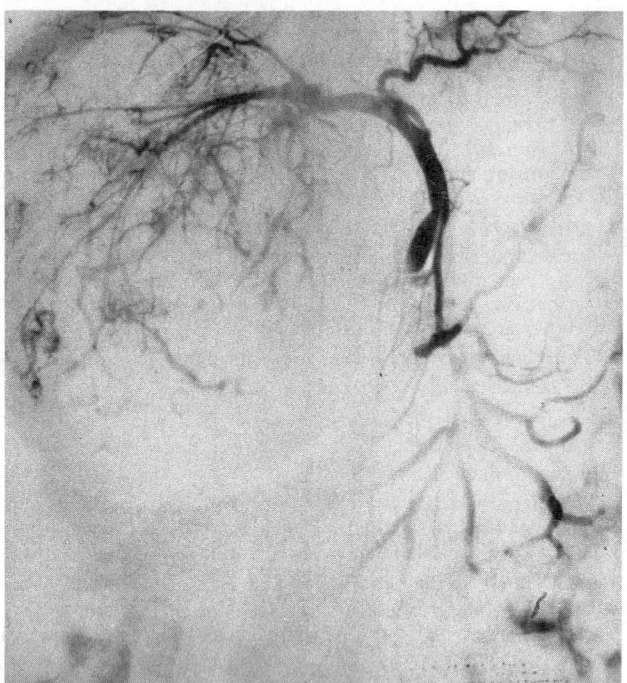

FIGURE 28–4.   Hypervascularity of a primary hepatocellular carcinoma as shown by arteriography. Notice the straightening of vessels within the tumor and early venous filling.

can be carried out. Ultrasound is widely used in the diagnosis of HCC, particularly in surveillance programs for patients with chronic liver disease who are at risk for the development of HCC. Ultrasonography is particularly useful for the diagnosis of portal venous thrombosis and is thought to be more sensitive in this respect than a CT scan or even an angiogram. Ultrasound helps differentiate HCC from metastatic tumors because HCC has a typical ring sign when smaller than 2 cm. If patients have only persistent elevation of liver enzymes, it is probably useful to obtain a blind-needle biopsy to establish the nature of the underlying disease.[52] Blind-needle biopsy is successful in establishing a diagnosis of HCC only in less than 40% of instances unless massive replacement of the liver is noted. For patients with suspected malignancy with a normal CT scan, laparoscopy may be helpful to direct biopsy.[53]

Questions that need to be addressed with imaging studies are the location and number of masses in the liver, whether there is evidence of extrahepatic tumor spread, and whether the vessels are patent or not. CT scan appears to display tumor extent better than sonography, but both imaging modalities often miss lesions smaller than 1 to 2 cm.[54] Angioportography, in which contrast material is directly infused into the mesenteric vessels, has been demonstrated to show small lesions and to be superior to conventional dynamic CT.[55–57] Direct comparisons of individual imaging modalities have been limited by the lack of a gold standard to define the number and size of lesions identified.[54,58,59] Studies done at the University of Pittsburgh using resected livers from individuals undergoing liver transplantation indicated that lesions were detectable by sonography in 81% of instances and by CT in 94%. Although vascular invasion was shown at pathology in 53% of instances, it was only detectable by CT in 31% and by sonography in

17%. It is particularly difficult in patients with underlying cirrhosis to make the fine distinctions regarding number of lesions and vascular invasion that are crucial in operative decision making. CT scanning can identify details regarding some tumors, such as the characteristic central scarring of fibrolamellar tumors.[60] The limitations of CT portography are its high sensitivity and the detection of small abnormalities such as flow voids or benign lesions. False-negative results have been identified,[61] especially in instances were there was fatty infiltration of the liver. MRI is particularly good at detecting intrahepatic lesions, especially in T2-weighted studies. Some difficulty in differentiating hemangiomas with a high T2 signal from HCC can be obviated because a less intense signal is observed with hepatomas.[61,62] One of the major problems with such techniques is the requirement for long data acquisition time and poor anatomic definition because of a low signal to noise ratio. The use of paramagnetic contrast agents such as gadolinium and the use of T1-weighted sequences appear to provide somewhat better contrast.[63] The T2-weighted spin echo sequences appear to be the most efficient to detect tumor. Studies at the National Cancer Institute comparing CT, ultrasound, and MRI indicated that the single best study was MRI.[63] In imaging 27 patients with known HCC, the short T1 inversion recovery (STIR sequence) appear to be the single best means to evaluate lesions, particularly in the porta hepatis.

Technetium 99m sulfur colloid is used for hepatic scintigraphy. This study is based on the uptake of the colloid by the hepatic reticulendothelial system. Scintigraphy results in photopenic areas in HCC images. A variation is SPECT (single-photon-emission CT), which uses a rotating gamma camera. This modality gives more precise spatial orientation and clearer images. Use of liver scintigraphy with ^{99m}Tc diisopropylimidodiacetic acid (IDA) showed tumor uptake in 75% of hepatoma lesions. The use of iodized oil as a contrast agent during angioportography allows early and delayed detection of tumor and potentially allows selective delivery of chemotherapeutic agents to such tumors.[64,65] Angiography often shows hypervascularity of the tumor in contrast to the appearance of metastases (see Fig. 28–4).

Obtaining a pathologic diagnosis can be treacherous in patients with HCC. Bleeding studies often are abnormal due to thrombocytopenia and decrease in liver-dependent clotting factors, and these tumors tend to be hypervascular. Spillage of tumor has been suggested as a problem after percutaneous biopsy. Percutaneous biopsy is usually recommended for patients undergoing neoadjuvant studies because it is critical to have an initial tissue diagnosis. Fine-needle aspirates often provide sufficient material for diagnosis.[65] In addition, laparoscopic approaches can be used.[53] Some surgeons elect to proceed with definitive resection if no contraindication exists, both for diagnosis and definitive therapy. Specialized immunohistochemical staining can differentiate primary tumors of the liver from metastatic deposits. The cellular origin of most cases can often be identified with fine-needle aspirates; 78% of HCCs are aneuploid and 22% are diploid. Elevated AFP levels are significantly associated with aneuploid tumors but appear to provide no information regarding survival.[67] In other gastrointestinal tumors, including gastric and esophageal cancers, clinical outcome is more clearly related to aneuploidy. The rapidity of proliferation of cells can be detected by in vitro incorporation of the thymidine analog 5-bromo-2'-deoxyuridine, which can provide prognostic information. Those individuals with low DNA synthetic capacity have a greater 2-year survival after surgery and a lesser incidence of intrahepatic metastases than do those with high DNA synthetic capacity.[68]

Positron emission tomography using nitrogen 13 ammonia as the positron donor is one of several techniques for imaging hepatomas that have been used at specialized centers.[69] The functional ability of liver tumors to perform at least some of the functions of normal liver is reflected in such studies and in studies using ^{99m}Tc-IDA derivatives.[70] These agents are normally taken up by hepatocytes and excreted into the bile canaliculi but can also be taken up by primary and metastatic hepatomas.[71,72] Computerized studies are available at most institutions and can demonstrate the rapidity of uptake and excretion from involved and noninvolved areas of the liver. The ability to use this as a functional test of the liver to assess which patients might most safely go through hepatic resection remains to be demonstrated.

More conventional studies include late indicators of hepatic dysfunction. Liver function tests include assays primarily of enzymes released by the liver such as aminotransferases and γ-glutamate transferase and tests of hepatic synthetic function. More sophisticated studies of liver function include the aminopyrine breath test, measures of serum bile acid concentrations, and indocyanine green clearance. Many of these studies reflect both hepatic blood flow and hepatocyte function.[73–75] Attempts to determine what the postoperative hepatic function will be after resection are particularly important in the cirrhotic patient population because most individuals with hepatoma have cirrhosis. In some centers, the presence of cirrhosis is considered a contraindication to resection, although many surgeons agree that limited resection is possible especially for portions of the liver composed of largely nonfunctioning tumor. The availability of liver transplantation in the event of hepatic insufficiency at an individual institution is particularly germane for surgeons willing to take on this difficult cadre of patients. Predictors of safe hepatic resection include indocyanine green (ICG) clearance.[76,77] Lesser procedures are better tolerated in patients with better overall ICG clearance.[78] Assessment of the amount of hepatic blood flow[79–81] or more precise evaluation of ICG clearance in the liver remnant remaining after resection are other methods.[82] With the greater availability of liver transplantation, patients with compromised liver function at our institution are considered for transplantation in most instances. Given the propensity for multicentricity and interhepatic spread, liver transplantation may be the most reasonable strategy for HCC.

SCREENING FOR HEPATOCELLULAR CARCINOMA

Many discrete patient populations are susceptible to hepatoma. Because of the availability of sensitive serum markers and the high prevalence of disease, it is possible that certain populations could be screened on a regular basis. In patient populations in which hepatitis B or C is prevalent, studies designed to determine whether early detection of the virus might help detect tumors would seem to be appropriate.[83–84] A recent workshop on screening for hepatocellular carcinoma was held at the National Cancer Institute to determine which patient populations might benefit.[85] Beasley and colleagues studied a group of Taiwanese male postal carriers who were positive for hepatitis B surface antigen (HBsAg) and found an annual incidence of HCC of 495 per 100,000.[86] This risk was 98 times that observed in individuals who were HBsAg-negative. The incidence of primary HCC in Alaskan natives also is markedly increased, again related to a high prevalence of hepatitis B virus infection.[87–89] By evaluating apparently asymptomatic HBsAg-positive blood donors at American Red Cross centers, a minimum relative risk of 12.7 was noted for liver cancer compared with HBsAg-negative individuals.[90] In HBsAg-positive men between the ages of 30 and 35, 3 deaths due to hepatoma were noted, which computes as a 248-fold greater risk compared with the general population. HBsAg-positive individuals at greatest risk are men, have a family history of the disease, are older than 45 years, or have cirrhosis.[85] Prospective studies in high-risk populations generally have concluded that ultrasound is more sensitive than elevations in AFP levels.[91–94] A study conducted in Italian patients with cirrhosis identified a yearly incidence of 3% but no appreciable increase in the rate of detection of potentially curable tumors.[93] Although high-risk patients continue to be screened as recommended by the recent workshop,[85] major changes in longevity with these disorders are more likely to result from prevention strategies, including universal vaccination against hepatitis B virus.[95]

SEROLOGIC ASSAYS FOR DETECTION OF HEPATOCELLULAR CARCINOMA

Serologic assays for detection and clinical follow-up of patients with HCC were developed after AFP was identified in the serum of animals bearing transplantable hepatomas[96] and later was detected in humans.[97] Improvements in the assay, including the development of radioimmunoassays for AFP,[98–102] allowed sequential studies in high-risk patients and patients being treated with surgical resection or chemotherapy (Fig. 28–5). Although AFP levels are elevated in about 80% to 90% of individuals from the Orient bearing hepatoma, it is only increased in about 60% to 70% of patients from the United States and Europe.[99] Although elevations in AFP levels can be detected early in the course of the disease, most clinical studies suggest that ultrasound is an even more sensitive modality. Still, increases in AFP levels are the gold standard against which other assays must be judged. The other most widely used assay is that for des-γ-carboxy prothrombin (PIVKA-II). Levels of this protein are increased in as many as 91% of patients with HCC but may be elevated in patients with vitamin K deficiency, chronic active hepatitis, or metastatic carcinoma.[103–106] The modest elevations in levels of AFP and PIVKA-II observed in chronic hepatitis and cirrhosis sometimes make it difficult to differentiate them from hepatoma. Although many other assays have been developed, these two have the greatest aggregate sensitivity and specificity.[107–120]

PRINCIPLES OF SURGICAL RESECTION AND TRANSPLANTATION

Although hepatic resection for tumors arising within the liver has been performed since 1886, hepatic resection has been

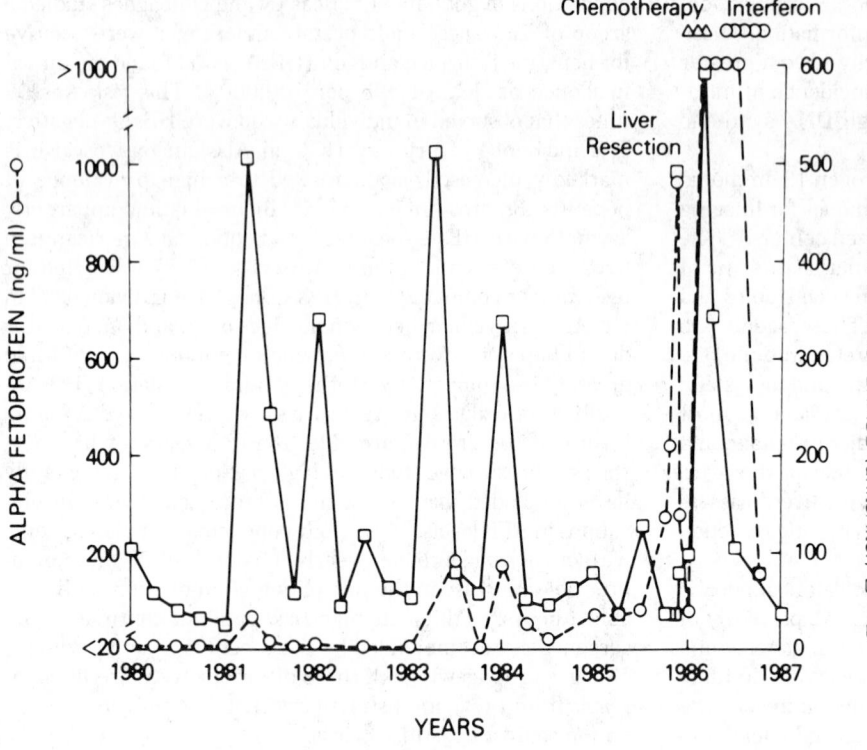

FIGURE 28–5. Sequential α-fetoprotein (AFP) and liver enzyme assays in a patient with chronic hepatitis B. Recurrent bouts of hepatitis associated with increases in aspartic amino transferase were occasionally associated with increases in AFP levels to approximately 200 ng/ml with prompt resolution when the hepatitis resolved. Increases in AFP levels of more than 200 ng/ml in the absence of significant hepatitis prompted ultrasonic examination and detection of a solitary hepatocellular carcinoma, which was resected. Chemotherapy-associated hepatitis was treated with interferon, which promptly decreased the transferase and AFP levels.

performed frequently and safely only in the last 30 years, with advances in the understanding of hepatic anatomy and physiology, surgical technique, anesthesia, and blood replacement.[121] As much as 80% to 90% of the liver can be removed during surgical resection with either a formal lobectomy or with segmentectomies wedge resection of individual lesions. The underlying function of the remaining liver and in particular the presence of cirrhosis dictates the ability of such lesions to be surgically excised.[122–124] Preoperative workup is designed to assess the local extent of the disease and to demonstrate no evidence of intrahepatic or extrahepatic metastatic disease. An arteriogram is obtained by many surgeons to demonstrate the highly variable hepatic arterial anatomy, although operative dissection is often sufficient for this purpose.

For a hepatectomy, the incision usually is made through a bilateral subcostal approach that can be extended into the right chest as necessary, especially for tumors invading the diaphragm or those that are extremely bulky. Early identification and ligation of structures within the porta hepatis coursing to the lobe to be resected is important. Alternatively, occlusion of hepatic portal and arterial inflow can be obtained by the so-called Pringle maneuver by encircling the structures of the porta hepatis with an umbilical tape or clamp. This maneuver can be performed safely for periods as long as 45 minutes to an hour during the course of hepatic resection and dramatically decreases blood loss. Controlled hypotension can decrease blood loss as well. More aggressive hepatic vascular exclusion is rarely performed except under circumstances of hepatic transplantation, in which bypass of the portal and inferior vena caval blood flow is frequently performed.[125] Division of the hepatic parenchyma is a time-consuming and tedious procedure requiring meticulous operative technique. A variety of means have been used, including so-called finger

fracture, electrocautery, an unsheathed suction catheter, sharp dissection, or the ultrasonic dissector.[126–128] The technique used depends on the experience of the individual surgeon. Several procedures have been developed for lobar resection and segmentectomy,[129,130] but the greatest mortality and difficulty are associated with extended hepatectomies or trisegmentectomies.[131–133] Hemorrhage is the main cause of death with technical misadventures related to protecting the left hepatic duct.[133] Problematic lesions are those presenting within the hilum of the liver, for which specialized techniques and anastomosis have been devised.[134–137] Anastomosis of divided hilar ducts to the bowel allows biliary drainage.[134] Combined portal vein and liver resection has been performed primarily for tumors arising in the gallbladder and biliary tract, with mortality rates reported at 8% to 17%.[137] For advanced carcinoma of the biliary tract, even more extensive procedures involving hepatopancreaticoduodenectomy (which combines the surgical equivalent of Whipple's procedure with partial or total hepatic resection) followed by liver transplantation have been performed, albeit with significant morbidity (92%) and mortality (13%).[138] These procedures perhaps are best used for patients with early slow-growing lesions extending along the biliary tract.

During formal hepatic lobar resection, the confluence of the hepatic veins at the suprahepatic vena cava needs to be examined. The middle and left hepatic veins are often fused. In addition to the right hepatic vein, direct drainage of the right lobe of the liver through posterior and inferior hepatic veins directly into the vena cava is noted.[139,140] Other major aids in performing hepatic surgery have been the development of rapid infusion systems to replace the blood loss that frequently occurs during major hepatic resections and transplantation procedures and the use of intraoperative ultrasonography.[141-148] The ability of the surgeon to palpate the liver and to apply a sterile ultrasonic probe directly to the liver surface allows detection of occult tumors (other intrahepatic lesions), tumor thrombi in the portal vein, and small lesions preoperatively identified but nonpalpable at the time of surgery. Manipulation of a cirrhotic macronodular liver and differentiation of regenerative nodules from intrahepatic lesions often is difficult.

The major complications after surgical resection are related to bleeding and massive blood infusion, to sepsis (reported to occur in as many as 10–15% of patients),[149] and to jaundice related to technical misadventures involving to the hepatic ducts or insufficient liver to sustain the individual.[150] The results of surgical resection are described below in sections on the individual tumors. Because of the high recurrence observed in many resected tumors of the liver, neoadjuvant or adjuvant therapies using chemotherapy or radiation therapy are being developed.[151,152] In some instances, previously unresectable tumors have been made operable with preoperative therapy, especially in children.[151] A recent report from Japan suggests that postoperative chemotherapy may prove beneficial.[152]

For patients whose tumors are deemed unresectable, management is primarily designed to provide portal venous decompression if necessary, to decompress the biliary tree, and to provide palliation by decreasing the size of the tumor, especially in patients with very large malignancies. Decompression of the biliary tree has been revolutionized by the development of percutaneous and endoscopic stent placement. Although it needs to be individualized in patients, a randomized trial demonstrated relative benefit for placement of endoscopic stents.[153] Such stents maintain biliary patency without the need for an external drainage catheter and the pain associated with a catheter traversing the abdomen or ribcage.[154-156] Exchange of the catheter is recommended at about 3- to 4-month intervals to prevent occlusion. Alternative approaches for such patients need to be considered. This includes placement of a subcutaneous portal or arterial reservoir to deliver chemotherapy[157] or alternatively using a completely implantable pump.[158] Cryosurgery of primary liver cancer has been associated with prolonged survival in some instances[159] and has been facilitated by the availability of the intraoperative ultrasound monitor.[160] The progression of liquid nitrogen freezing can be monitored using ultrasonic probes. Intraoperative radiation therapy (discussed later in this chapter), hyperthermia laser-mediated destruction, alcohol injection, and delivery of interstitial radiation therapy[161] have been suggested. Although local eradication of tumor can be demonstrated, the precise roles of these techniques in extending survival have not been demonstrated formally.

Recurrence after hepatic resection of a HCC at the previous resection margin or at a distant location within the liver suggests inadequate initial resection, metastatic spread, or a de novo malignancy. Some patients may benefit from repeat hepatic resection.[162-164] In a recent series from Japan in 62 patients subjected to resection, 41 were noted to have recurrences. Most of these recurrences (93%) were in the residual liver, with the remainder occurring in bone and lung. Among the patients who underwent local reexcision for their tumors, most recurrences (18 of 19) were found in the residual liver, often in the same segment or in the one adjacent to it. This suggests that larger initial hepatic resections should be per-

formed to prevent recurrence, a strategy that has been used by our group.

HEPATIC TRANSPLANTATION FOR PRIMARY TUMORS OF THE LIVER

Since the performance of the first human orthotopic liver transplant in 1963, extensive experience has been gained with this procedure, so that about 1600 to 2000 liver transplants are performed in the United States each year.[165,166] Most of the first patients to receive transplants had primary hepatic malignancy.[167,168] Some individuals with incidental malignancies were cured, and an occasional patient enjoyed prolonged disease-free survival. The National Institutes of Health Consensus Development Conference on liver transplantation in 1983 concluded that "primary hepatic malignancy confined to the liver but not amenable to resection may be an indication for transplantation. Results to date indicate a strong likelihood of recurrence of malignancy, nonetheless the procedure may achieve significant palliation."[169] This general conclusion persisted over the next decade with attempts to balance the dearth of organs available for transplantation and the palliative nature of hepatic transplantation for patients with hepatic malignancy.[170] Advances in transplantation include the use of extracorporal venovenous bypass techniques, development of duct-to-duct anastomosis to reconstruct the biliary tree, and means to use reduced liver segments, especially in small children.[165,166,171] The liver graft is only ABO typed for the recipient. Prevention of graft rejection has been revolutionized by the availability of the potent immunosuppressive agents cyclosporine and FK506.[166] Five-year survivals for nonmalignant disease after liver transplantation are routinely 80% to 90% at many centers. With the exception of neuroendocrine tumors, tumors metastatic to the liver are not treated with hepatic transplantation. Even with primary tumors of the liver, recurrence is the rule, occurring between 3 and 36 months after transplantation. More aggressive procedures such as combined upper abdominal exenteration and hepatic and visceral transplantation have been studied but are not widely used because of the nutritional problems observed in these patients.[172]

Many liver transplantations for HCC have been performed.[173-175] In a group of patients treated in Germany, 61 patients underwent transplantation as their primary operation and 6 after initial resection and recurrence.[174] At 2 years, 13 of 23 patients were alive at 1 year, half of them disease free. Although smaller numbers of patients were followed for longer periods, 3 individuals were noted to be alive at 5 years. The presence of tumor thrombosis in the portal vein and extrahepatic tumor adversely impacted on survival. Similarly, the size of the primary tumor, the presence of positive lymph nodes, evidence of distant metastases, advanced stage, and the presence of residual tumor all correlated with decreased survival in this patient population.

Some patients, such as those with fibrolamellar carcinoma, appear to have prolonged survival after transplantation. A recent report of the Transplant Tumor Registry suggests that the percentage of individuals with recurrence with fibrolamellar carcinoma (38%) is not dissimilar from the 40% recurrence rate (253 of 637) reported after transplantation for hepatoma and other primary and metastatic tumors of the liver.[175] Eighty-seven percent of the patients with recurrence had died at the time of that report. In addition to the problems associated with management of immunosuppression, immunosuppressive agents such as cyclosporine may have hepatotropic effects on the normal liver cells and potentially on the residual HCC.[176–178] Tumor doubling times may be shorter in patients with recurrent pulmonary metastatic disease who have undergone transplantation when compared with patients previously treated with conventional resection.[178]

RADIOBIOLOGY OF THE HEPATOBILIARY SYSTEM

Liver tolerance to ionizing radiation is critical factor to be considered if radiation therapy is used for tumors involving or adjacent to the liver or the biliary system. Radiation hepatitis has been reported with whole-liver irradiation doses above 2500 cGy, and the risk rises rapidly with doses above 3500 cGy if 200-cGy fractions are used.[179,180] Liver tolerance to radiation is highly dependent on the dose per fraction, with an estimated α to β ratio of 150 cGy.[181] If dose fractions of 250 or 300 cGy are used, whole-liver tolerance is limited to 2500 cGy in 10 fractions or 2100 cGy in 7 fractions. After reviewing dose-volume histograms in 11 patients receiving whole-liver irradiation and boost treatment to 5300 to 7000 cGy equivalent, Austin-Seymour and colleagues recommended that no more than 30% of the liver be irradiated to doses in excess of 3000 to 3500 cGy at 200-cGy fractions.[182]

In the acute phase of hepatic injury, congestion in the central veins and central lobular sinusoids is seen and followed by proliferation of epithelial cells in the central lobular zone and liver cell atrophy and degeneration.[179,183] Clinical laboratory tests of liver function affected by acute radiation hepatitis include elevated alkaline phosphatase, mildly elevated serum levels of glutamic-oxaloacetic transaminase (SGOT) and glutamic-pyruvic transaminase (SGPT), and decreased anionic dye (BSP or rose bengal) clearance.[179] Thrombocytopenia has been reported to accompany radiation hepatitis in children irradiated concurrently with dactinomycin administration.[184] Late changes in the liver are characterized by central lobular and periportal fibrosis with cirrhotic reconstruction of liver architecture.[84] Cell-to-cell interaction mediated through cytokines such as TGF-β1 may play an important role in radiation injury to the liver.[185]

The biliary ducts appear to have a greater tolerance to radiation than the liver parenchyma. In the treatment of cholangiocarcinoma, intracavitary brachytherapy boosts have been administered to doses as high as 10,600 cGy to a depth of 0.5 cm in combination with fractionated external-beam irradiation to 4000 to 5000 cGy.[186] No hepatic complications were observed, although duodenal ulcers did develop in some patients. In a study of 63 patients irradiated for primary biliary carcinomas, the actuarial risk of developing a symptomatic duodenal ulcer was 29% 2 years after radiation therapy.[187] This risk was not significantly related to external-beam irradiation dose or to intraluminal boost brachytherapy, and the contribution of external biliary drainage catheters was not determined. A study of intraoperative radiation to the liver hilum of rabbits found that doses of more than 3000 cGy were associated with the development of hepatic parenchymal atrophy and significant biliary fibrosis and necrosis.[188] Studies of intraoperative radiation of the extrahepatic bile duct in dogs identified fibrosis and stenosis occurring at doses of more than 2000 cGy.[189]

HEPATOCELLULAR CARCINOMA

CLINICAL FEATURES

Common symptoms in patients affected with HCC include the following: abdominal pain (91%), weight loss (35%), weakness (31%), fullness and anorexia (27%), abdominal swelling (43%), jaundice (7%), and vomiting (8%). Common physical signs are hepatomegaly (89%), hepatic bruit (28%), ascites (52%), splenomegaly (65%), jaundice (41%), wasting (15%), and fever (38%).[190,191] Abdominal swelling may occur as a consequence of ascites due to the underlying chronic liver disease or may be due to a rapidly expanding tumor. Occasionally, central necrosis or hemorrhage leads to massive peritoneal blood loss and death. It occurs in 10% to 20% of Asians and in about 6% of blacks and is rare among Europeans. Hemoperitoneum from bleeding HCC is a well-recognized complication of needle biopsy of vascular hepatomas. Unexplained weight loss in a known cirrhotic patient is a suspicious indicator of developing HCC. In countries such as Japan where there is an active surveillance program, HCC tends to be picked up at an earlier stage, when symptoms may be few or attributable only to the underlying disease. Jaundice is infrequent and usually due to the underlying liver disease. About 10% of patients have jaundice attributable to the HCC. This may be due to obstruction of the main intrahepatic ducts, to obstruction of the common hepatic duct at the porta hepatis, to infiltration into the biliary radicals or, extremely rarely, to blood in the biliary tree. Hematemesis typically occurs due to esophageal varices from the underlying portal hypertension and chronic liver disease. Bone pain may occur in 3% to 12% of patients, but necropsies show that about 20% of patients have pathologic bone metastases. Respiratory symptoms may occur on presentation but are rare. They are usually due to an elevated hemidiaphragm resulting from hepatomegaly or to pain from rib metastases. Pleural effusions may occur, but symptomatic lung metastases are rare.

EVALUATION OF THE HEPATOMA PATIENT

The history is important in evaluating putative predisposing factors including a past history of hepatitis or jaundice, blood transfusion, or use of intravenous drugs. A family history of HCC or hepatitis should be noted, and a detailed social history should include job descriptions to identify industrial exposure to possible carcinogenic drugs including sex hormones. Physical examination is important to evaluate underlying liver disease indicated by jaundice, ascites, peripheral edema, spider nevi, palmar erythema, and weight loss. Evaluation of the abdomen includes assessment of hepatic size, presence of masses, hepatic nodularity, and tenderness and presence of splenomegaly. Histologic proof of the presence of HCC is mandatory, and in our practice requires a core liver biopsy of the mass under ultrasound or CT guidance. Fine-needle aspiration is often insufficient to make the diagnosis, and core biopsies are obtained routinely.

It is important to ascertain the presence of ongoing alcohol consumption or acute active hepatitis B or hepatitis C viral infection. Ongoing alcohol consumption can make an impact on the toxicity of chemotherapy and the results of liver resection or transplantation. Ongoing active hepatitis in the posttransplant period is a major basis for chemotherapy toxicity.

The main objectives on workup are to ascertain whether there is extrahepatic disease or portal venous vascular invasion by tumor within the liver. Both are major adverse prognostic factors.[191a] Extrahepatic disease is diagnosed predominantly by chest CT scan and to a lesser extent with bone scan. Although cranial metastases are reported, they are rare. The focus of abdominal investigation is to detect spread of tumor within the liver and within the abdomen. The latter concerns peritoneal or lymph node spread. These are best ascertained with ultrasound, abdominal CT scan, and MRI. For reasons that are unclear, it is usually necessary to do all three because lesions can be picked up with one modality but not with another. The most sensitive tests are CT portography and lipiodol CT scanning. If resection is contemplated, these are considered mandatory in picking up small lesions in the apparently normal residual lobe and are reported to be capable of diagnosing 50% more lesions than with CT scan alone. In our practice, they are done at the same time. A mesenteric arteriogram is performed with a CT portogram and the catheter is then advanced into the hepatic artery, when 10 ml of lipiodol is injected. One week later, a repeat abdominal CT scan is obtained. The purpose of this delayed CT scan is that lipiodol is nonselectively taken up into the whole liver but nonspecific uptake is cleared over the ensuing 5 days. The CT scan performed 1 week later will normally detect lipiodol only in the hepatomas. This is also a very useful technique for assuring that a needle biopsy is obtained from correct lesions because the finding of lipiodol microscopically shows that the needle was actually in the visualized mass. The diagnosis of lymph node disease can be difficult in the region of the porta hepatis and cannot be made with any confidence or safety by nonsurgical techniques, even at laparoscopy. However, the combination of CT scan and MRI typically picks up most lymph nodes greater than 1 cm in diameter. Given the fact that hepatoma normally arises on the basis of cirrhosis with regenerative or hyperplastic nodules, biopsy-proof of the nature of the hepatoma is mandatory. Fine-needle aspirates are often insufficient for the diagnosis of hepatocellular carcinoma and core biopsy is normally accepted as necessary for the diagnosis. Staining with α-fetoprotein is helpful when positive, but 50% of our tumors are not positive. In situ hybridization for albumin mRNA in our hands is positive in greater than 90% of hepatomas, and accurately distinguishes hepatomas from tumors of nonhepatocyte origin. Our practice includes a biopsy of the nonhepatoma liver to ascertain the degree of severity of any underlying cirrhosis. This has practical implications in the consideration of the intensity of chemotherapy that may be tolerated as well as likelihood of this toleration of large resections. Again, in our experience, biochemical indices of liver reserve such as ICG clearance or caffeine antipyrene tolerance have not been helpful nor predictive of hepatic reserve. Tumor invasion of the portal vascular system can be inferred by obliteration of the right, left, or main branch portal veins on CT scan or on CT portography. In our hands, definitive presurgical evidence can be obtained by percutaneous biopsy of a thrombosed portal vein, because no bleeding is found in the presence of the thrombus. Although a theoretical possibility of tracking of tumor after needle biopsy has been considered, in our hands this is rare, and with the increased responses found with chemotherapy, we have seen no evidence in the last 300 biopsies of hepatocellular carcinoma. Any ascites needs to be examined for cytologic evidence of peritoneal tumor.

Physical Signs

Hepatomegaly is the most frequent physical sign and occurs in 50% to 90% of patients. The liver size may be massive, particularly in epidemic areas. Abdominal bruits arising from the HCC, presumably from the increased vascularity, vary in incidence from 6% to 25%. Ascites occurs in 30% to 60% of patients and is usually due to the underlying liver disease, although occasionally it may be caused by hemoperitoneum. It is important to tap the ascites of any HCC patient and send it for cytologic examination, because malignant ascites has a major adverse impact on prognosis. Splenomegaly occurs commonly, mainly due to the associated portal hypertension from the underlying liver disease. Acute splenomegaly may be due to portal vein occlusion by the tumor. Weight loss and muscle wasting are common, particularly with rapidly growing or large tumors. Fever is found in 10% to 50% of patients with HCC. The cause is not clear, although tumor necrosis has been invoked as an explanation. Signs of chronic liver disease often are present, including jaundice, dilated abdominal veins, palmar erythema, gynecomastia, testicular atrophy, and peripheral edema. The Budd-Chiari syndrome has been reported in several series due to HCC invasion of the portal veins and less frequently in the hepatic veins. This causes tense ascites and a large tender liver. Virchow-Trosier nodes occur in the supraclavicular region but are rare. Cutaneous metastasis has been reported as reddish blue nodules.

Paraneoplastic Syndromes

A variety of paraneoplastic syndromes have been described. Most of these are biochemical abnormalities without associated clinical consequences. The most important ones include hypoglycemia (also caused by end-stage liver failure), erythrocytosis, hypercalcemia, hypercholesterolemia, dysfibrinogenemia, carcinoid syndrome, increased thyroxine-binding globulin, sexual changes, and porphyria cutanea tarda. Hypoglycemia occurs in two settings. It appears as rapidly growing HCC among the Chinese, and as part of a terminal illness when it is mild. In the other setting, HCC is more slowly growing, but the hypoglycemia may be profound. Its pathogenesis is unclear. Erythrocytosis occurs in 3% to 12% of patients. Sexual changes are of three types: isosexual precocious puberty, gynecomastia, and feminization. The latter is thought to be due to the underlying liver disease. Hypercholesterolemia occurs in 10% to 40% of patients and is due to an absence of normal feedback control in hepatoma cells, the result of a deletion in β-hydroxy-methylglutaryl coenzyme A reductase.

Staging

A staging system for hepatic tumors has been developed by the Union Internationale Contra le Cancer (UICC) and is outlined in Table 28–9. The best prognosis is for stage I solitary

TABLE 28-9. TNM Staging System for Liver Tumors from the Union Internationale Contra le Cancer

Primary Tumor (T)

TX   Primary tumor cannot be assessed
T0   No evidence of primary tumor
T1   Solitary tumor 2 cm or less in greatest dimension without vascular invasion
T2   Solitary tumor 2 cm or less in greatest dimension with vascular invasion, or
     Multiple tumors limited to one lobe none more than 2 cm in greatest dimension without vascular invasion, or
     A solitary tumor more than 2 cm in greatest dimension without vascular invasion
T3   Solitary tumor more than 2 cm in greatest dimension with vascular invasion, or
     Multiple tumors limited to one lobe, none more than 2 cm in greatest dimension, with vascular invasion, or
     Multiple tumors limited to one lobe, any more than 2 cm in greatest dimension, with or without vascular invasion
T4   Multiple tumors in more than one lobe or tumor(s) involve(s) a major branch of portal or hepatic vein(s)

Lymph Node (N)

NX   Regional lymph nodes cannot be assessed
N0   No regional lymph node metastasis
N1   Regional lymph node metastasis

Distant Metastasis (M)

MX   Presence of distant metastasis cannot be assessed
M0   No distant metastasis
M1   Distant metastasis

Stage Grouping

I	T1	N0	M0
II	T2	N0	M0
III	T1	N1	M0
	T2	N1	M0
	T3	N0	M0
	T3	N0	M0
IVA	T4	Any N	M0
IVB	Any T	Any N	M1

tumors that are less than 2 cm in diameter and without vascular invasion. Adverse prognostic features include multiple tumors, vascular invasion, and lymph node spread. The latter is invariably associated with a dire prognosis and the incorporation of lymph node disease in stage III may need reclassification. Vascular invasion may be macroscopic or microscopic. In general, large tumors invariably have microscopic invasion that cannot be appreciated until after resection. As a consequence, full staging usually can be made only after surgical extirpation of the tumor. Stage II disease involves a solitary tumor 2 cm or smaller with vascular invasion, or multiple tumors limited to one liver lobe that are 2 cm or smaller without vascular invasion, or a solitary tumor larger than 2 cm and limited to one lobe without vascular invasion. Stage III disease contains a mixture of lymph node-positive and lymph node-negative tumors. That subset with lymph node-positive disease has a poor prognosis with few survivors at 1 year. This group includes solitary tumors larger than 2 cm with vascular invasion and multiple tumors limited to one lobe with or without vascular invasion and has a much poorer prognosis than stage II disease for all forms of resection or

transplantation (see discussion later in this chapter). Stage IVA disease includes multiple tumors in more than one liver lobe and tumors involving a major branch of the portal or hepatic vein, macroscopically or microscopically. The prognosis of such patients is poor after resection or transplantation, with few 1-year survivors. A working staging system based entirely on clinical grounds that incorporate the contribution of underlying liver disease has been developed by Okuda and colleagues.[190] Adverse prognostic signs include tumor size (>50% of liver), ascites (+), hypoalbuminemia (<3 g/dl) and hyperbilirubinemia (>3 mg/dl). A patient with Okuda stage III (advanced) tumors, namely with three or more positive features, has a dire prognosis because the liver usually cannot be resected curatively and typically does not tolerate chemotherapy.

SURGICAL MANAGEMENT OF HEPATOCELLULAR CARCINOMA

Small Hepatomas

With the increased and widespread use of surveillance programs in populations at risk, HCC increasingly is being diagnosed at a subclinical level before symptoms arise. Such lesions are typically smaller than 3 cm in diameter and are found because of the surveillance of serial AFP and ultrasound performed in patients with known chronic hepatitis or cirrhosis. An increasing literature from the Orient, particularly from Japan, has addressed the optimal management of these cases, and resection papers have indicated 5-year survival rates of 40% to 70%.[192] Increasingly, and particularly in Japan, ultrasound-guided ethanol injections and arterial or endoscopic embolization have become accepted means of treatment. As part of surveillance programs, more patients are being identified with asymptomatic HCCs smaller than 5 cm. The natural history of these tumors appears to be repeated recurrence after resection, with 5-year survival rates of about 50%.[193] Part of this poor survival is due to the underlying liver disease. Median survival for nontreated patients was 13 months compared with 29 months for resected patients in one study.[193]

Resection

Many studies have examined the immediate and long-term survival of various degrees of resection for HCC in cirrhotic and noncirrhotic patients.[194-196] Unfortunately, few studies have compared survival after resection by stage of disease. Studies that have attempted to analyze prognostic factors have reached a consensus on the important negative factors: lymph node involvement, vascular invasion, tumor thrombus, diffuse spreading type of HCC, absence of capsule, size larger than 5 cm, and multiple or bilobar tumors. These factors all appear to have adverse prognostic significance.[174] Two papers have analyzed a large number of resections by TNM rating system. In a study from the United States and Germany, 3-year survival was about 75% for TNM stage II disease, 50% for TNM stage III disease, and 10% to 20% for stage IVA (nonmetastatic) disease. Overall, stage for stage, survival appears better in the absence of cirrhosis than with cirrhosis. A multicenter analysis of surgical treatment by stage from Japan showed a 3-year survival of 50% for surgically resected stage I disease and 25% for stage II disease.[194] Similar results are reported from Europe and Japan.[194,198-200] Investigators have found high intrahepatic recurrence rates[201,202] that often are amenable to a secondary resection,[203] suggesting liver transplantation as a primary or secondary treatment modality. Reported results on neoadjuvant chemotherapy are limited and conflicting.[204,205]

Liver Transplantation

Liver transplantation has been used in the management of advanced bilobar HCC or in HCC in the presence of advanced cirrhosis. Until recently, survival rates after transplantation and resection for HCC stages III and IVA have been similar and poor, with about 20% survival after 2 years.[194,196] Two recent large series document the end results by stage of tumor, and average survival results are given in Table 28–10, which is a compilation of these two papers.[174,197] Other centers have had similar experience.[206-210] A combination of neoadjuvant and adjuvant chemotherapy may enhance survival in a number of patients.[211,212] The precise role of chemotherapy and liver transplantation should become clear in the next few years.

Optimal Treatment for Resectable Hepatocellular Carcinoma

The high recurrence rates after surgery for resectable stages I, II, and III HCC require a consideration of alternate approaches. One alternative is liver transplantation, considering the high survival rates for patients with stages I and II. Even though patients with these stages are technically resectable, transplantation may offer better long-term survival if organs are available and surgical risks are low. An alternate strategy may be the use of neoadjuvant or adjuvant chemotherapy coupled to resection. The only type of chemotherapy with a reproducible track record of responses is intraarterial. Therefore, preoperative cytoreduction or postresection chemotherapy by means of an implantable pump seem to be a logical choice for a controlled trial comparing chemotherapy and surgery with resection alone.

CHEMOTHERAPY OF HEPATOCELLULAR CARCINOMA

Systemic Chemotherapy

Several controlled and uncontrolled studies have been performed with most of the major classes of cancer chemother-

TABLE 28–10. Survival After Liver Transplantation for Hepatocellular Carcinoma

	1-Year	2-Year	3-Year	5-Year
Stage I	75	75	75	75
Stage II	80	70	60	60
Stage III	60	40	40	40
Stage IVA	50	30	15	10

(Data from Ringe B, Pichlmayr R, Wittekind C, Tusch G. Surgical treatment of hepatocellular carcinoma: Experience with liver resection and transplantation in 198 patients. World J Surg 1991;15:270–285; and from Iwatsuki S, Starzl TE, Sheahan DA, et al. Hepatic resection versus transplantation for hepatocellular carcinoma. Ann Surg 1991;214:221–229)

apy, given as single agents and in combination. Results of recent reviews[213,214] and some of the larger studies are outlined in Table 28–11. Despite initial encouraging reports of single-agent doxorubicin from Uganda, subsequent studies have failed to confirm initial enthusiastic reports of this or any other single agent. The consensus is that no single drug or combination of drugs given systemically leads to reproducible response rates of more than 25% or has any effect on survival. Drugs that appear to have no reproducible response when given systemically as single agents include 5-fluorouracil (5-FU), doxorubicin, cisplatin, VP-16, and neocarzinostatin. No combination of these drugs has been associated with survival beyond that of untreated controls. There appears to be little justification for treating patients with single or combination drugs in a systemic fashion outside cancer clinical trials, which probably will be phase II trials of new agents.

Regional Chemotherapy

In contrast to the dismal results of systemic chemotherapy for regional or metastatic HCC, many encouraging reports have appeared concerning regional chemotherapies for HCC confined to the liver (Table 28–12). Most experience, but not all,[212] comes from the Far East where, due to the numerous cases, systematic studies are able to be performed. Despite the increased hepatic extraction of chemotherapy demonstrated for a few drugs, drugs such as doxorubicin, cisplatin, mitomycin C, and possibly neocarzinostatin have produced substantial objective responses when administered regionally. In contrast to the Western experience of metastatic colon cancer to the liver, little data are available on continuous hepatic arterial infusion for HCC. Almost all studies have used bolus administration. Because few reports have stratified responses or survival based on TNM staging, it is difficult to know how long-term prognosis is related to tumor extent. Many studies on regional intrahepatic arterial chemotherapy use an embolizing agent such as iodized oil, gelatin sponges (Gelfoam), starch, microspheres, or even arterial ligation in addition to chemotherapy. Consistently higher objective response rates have been reported[225-242] compared with any form of systemic chemotherapy.[215-224] The widespread use of some form of embolization in addition to chemotherapy in the Orient has produced a significant literature on its toxicities. These include the almost universal presence of high fever (more than 95% of patients), abdominal pain (more than 60%) and anorexia (more than 60%). In addition, more than 20% of patients have increased ascites or transient elevation of transaminases. Cystic artery spasm and cholecystitis are not uncommon.

Current Procedure of Chemotherapy

Our current practice is to attempt cytoreduction of hepatocellular carcinoma within the liver before any plan for resection or transplantation. This is based on intrahepatic arterial chemotherapy with doxorubicin 40 mg/m² and cisplatinum 100 mg/m² given in 100 ml normal saline over 30 minutes every 4 weeks through the femoral artery.[213a,214a] The chemotherapy is usually given into either the right or the left lobe but not both at any one treatment session in order to minimize hepatic decompensation. For unilobular lesions, the

TABLE 28–11. Selected Recent Studies of Chemotherapy in Hepatocellular Carcinomas

Investigations	Drug	No. of Patients	Partial Responses (PR) (%)
Systemic Chemotherapy			
Sciarrino et al, 1985[215]	Doxorubicin	109	—
Chlebowski et al, 1984[216]	Doxorubicin	157	11
Ihde et al, 1977[217]	Doxorubicin	13	15
Falkson et al, 1984[218]	Doxorubicin + 5-fluorouracil + methyl-CCNU	192	19
Ravry et al, 1984[219]	Doxorubicin + bleomycin	60	16
Cavalli et al, 1981[220]	VP-16	26	13
Melia et al, 1983[221]	VP-16	22	18
Melia et al, 1981[222]	Cisplatin	13	1
Ravry et al, 1986[223]	Cisplatin	2	0
Falkson et al, 1987[224]	Cisplatin	35	17
Falkson et al, 1987[224]	Mitoxantrone	34	8
Intrahepatic Arterial Chemotherapy			
Onohara et al, 1988[225]	Cisplatin	33	55
Kajanti et al, 1986[226]	Cisplatin	10	40
Ando et al, 1987[227]	Epirubicin	54	15

PR, partial response.

TABLE 28–12. Intrahepatic Artery Combination Chemotherapy for Hepatocellular Carcinoma

Investigations	Agents	No. of Patients	Responses (%)
Sasaki et al, 1987[228]	Platinum + gelatin sponge	20	65
Kasugai et al, 1989[229]	Platinum + ethiodized oil	25	38
Ohnishi et al, 1984[230]	MMC + microcapsules	20	32
Lin et al, 1988[231]	5-FU + Ivalon	21	32
Fujimoto et al, 1985[232]	5-FU/MMC + starch	19	68
Audisio et al, 1990[233]	MMC + microcapsules	30	43
Kobayashi et al, 1986[234]	Doxorubicin + ethiodized oil	33	42
Kanematsu et al, 1989[235]	Doxorubicin + ethiodized oil	70	47
Shibata et al, 1989[236]	Platinum + ethiodized oil	71	47
Konno et al, 1983[237]	SMANCS + ethiodized oil	44	90
Pelletier et al, 1990[238]	Doxorubicin + gelatin sponge	42	17
Carr et al, 1991[239]	Doxorubicin/cisplatin	25	50
Venook et al, 1990[240]	Doxorubicin/cisplatin/MMC + gelatin sponge	50	24
Ohnishi et al, 1987[241]	MMC + microcapsules	32	28
Ohnishi et al, 1987[241]	MMC + gelatin sponge + microcapsules	34	57
Beppu et al, 1991[242]	Cisplatin + ethiodized oil + aclarubicin microspheres	62	50

5-FU, 5-fluorouracil; MMC, mitomycin C; SMANCS, styrene maleic acid conjugates of neocarzinostatin and mitomycin C.

treatment is repeated into that one lobe. For massive or bilobar lesions, often alternating treatment strategies will be considered or treatment into the artery feeding the main mass of the tumor initially or a nominal two or three cycles into each side. The treatment is well tolerated and patients can usually be discharged from the hospital 24 hours later. The artery for injection cannot always be inferred by CT scan, but must be ascertained directly by right and left hepatic arteriography. Addition of lipiodol to the chemotherapy has been shown by many groups, including ourselves, to influence response rates.[363,364] Although embolizing agents als increase responses, there is a significant risk of hepatocellular decompensation with their use in the presence of portal vein thrombus or bilirubin greater than 2.0 mg/dl. Cytotoxic chemotherapy is also hazardous with or without embolization in the presence of Child's C cirrhosis or a bilirubin greater than 2.5 mg/dl. We have found that use of low dose chemotherapy is not associated with responses. One practice approach is the use of escalating doses of chemotherapy, starting at 50% calculated of doses. This has proved useful in view of the unpredictable nature of hepatic decompensation.

Several newer embolizing agents currently are being evaluated which hold the promise for higher response rates, including Yttrium glass beads and degradable starch microspheres (Spherex). These studies are ongoing and results are preliminary to date.

MINUTE HCC

The results comparing local therapy with no therapy suggest a survival advantage to local therapy—ethanolization or local resection—in either noncirrhotic or cirrhotic liver. If necessary, repeated ethanol injections or re-resections may be appropriate and worthwhile.

HEPATOCELLULAR CARCINOMA, TNM STAGE I

Surgical resection for stage I HCC can be expected to give approximately 50% 3-year survivors, compared with less than 10% without treatment. Limited studies indicate a possible benefit of added regional chemotherapy. Whether neoadjuvant or adjuvant chemotherapy will be most useful in decreasing postresection recurrence, has yet to be determined. Either way, intraarterial chemothrapy is probably the only modality with a track record of effectiveness. For the patient with postresection recurrence, re-resection is feasible and is supported by several publications. However, because the HCC recurrence is often panhepatic, regional chemotherapy before any second resection, may be the better choice.

HEPATOCELLULAR CARCINOMA, TNM STAGE II

Tumors with vascular invasion or multiple unilobar tumors without vascular invasion have a typical postresection survival of 25% at 3 years. In this group of patients, the impact of preresection arterial chemotherapy (plus or minus embolization/lipiodolization) may be expected to have its greatest impact. Multiple tumors or vascular invasion can be expected to predict intrahepatic dissemination with postresection recurrence. A trial is needed comparing resection with resection

plus neoadjuvant intaarterial chemotherapy. In favor of preresection chemotherapy is the ability to evaluate an antitumor effect (CT scan, markers), and the risks of hepatic decompensation in the postresection period due to a small hepatic volume and reserve. Recent data on human liver regeneration postresection indicate that several months are necessary for substantial regeneration to occur. Adjuvant chemotherapy after regeneration may be too late, and if given early, may precipitate hepatic insufficiency.

HEPATOCELLULAR CARCINOMA, TNM STAGE III

Solarity or multiple tumors in one lobe of any size greater than 2 cm with vascular invasion have a poor postresection prognosis in all centers. Unfortunately, the TNM classification also includes node-positive patients in this group. The latter is a dire prognostic sign, and such patients should probably be reclassified in the future. Usually, the extended resection required in this group of patients needs experienced resectionists capable of doing trisegmentectomy. Recent perioperative mortality for this procedure has dropped below 10% among experienced groups. Reported survivorship in this group for node-negative disease can be as high as 50% at 3 years, but for patients with cirrhosis, less than 10% survival is reported. Therefore, the treatment choices in the cirrhotic patient would apper to be among intrarterial chemotherapy, resection and neoadjuvant artrial chemotherapy, or liver transplantation. Recent results with liver transplantation in this group are encouraging.

HEPATOCELLULAR CARCINOMA, TNM STAGE IVA

Patients with bilobar HCC or with a major portal or hepatic vein branch tumor thrombus are unresectable, and have had a poor prognosis with liver transplantation until recently. The addition of both neoadjuvant and adjuvant chemotherapy to liver transplantation has recently led to encouraging longer-term survival. Studies in several groups are onging. Curiously, aggressive intraarterial chemotherapy alone may also lead to long-term (1 year) survival in these unresectable patients, especially those with Child's A or B cirrhosis only, or without cirrhosis.

HEPATOCELLULAR CARCINOMA, TNM STAGE IVB

The management of patients with metastatic HCC or with localized by lymph-node positive disease resides entirely within the realm of phase II clinical trials, probably using novel agents. No data to date supports the use of currently available systemic chemotherapy in this patient group.

Future Directions in Chemotherapy

The presence of cell-surface receptors for various growth factors and hormones on hepatomas and hepatoma cell lines and the disparities in the gross male to female ratio of incidence suggest the possibility of hormonal manipulation.[243] Recent studies have shown no objective response to tamoxifen[244,245] or to the antiandrogen ketoconazole.[246] Results of an EORTC trial of an antiandrogen (Anandron) and a leutinizing hormone-releasing hormone agonist (Zoladex) are pending. However, interim analysis shows no survival advantage to Anandron treatment. A recent study suggests an effect of interferon.[247] Recent studies and studies in progress include phase I studies of antiangiogenic drugs, studies of degradable starch microspheres (Spherex) designed to reduce the toxicities of embolization, studies of LAK cells alone or in addition to chemotherapy, and the evaluation of immunosuppressive drugs such as rapamycin and its analogs, with growth inhibitory or antihepatotropic actions. The use of genetically engineered cells that overexpress lymphokines or growth inhibitory factors is under investigation.

FIBROLAMELLAR HEPATOCELLULAR CARCINOMA

Fibrolamellar HCC (FL-HCC) was originally described in 1956,[248] and the clinical implications of this more indolent form of HCC were determined later.[249,250] Unlike HCC, FL-HCC has a slight female preponderance and typically is not associated with fibrosis, hepatitis B or C, or elevated AFP levels. Des-γ-carboxy prothrombin typically is elevated and neurotensin levels often are elevated.[251] They show neuroendocrine differentiation and can stain for neuron-specific enolase, neurotensin, vasoactive intestinal peptide, and serotonin.[252] Longer survival rates have been reported in small series after resection and liver transplantation.[253] No series reports convincing data on chemotherapy-induced remissions. In our recent series of 12 patients, no responses were obtained with intraarterial chemoembolization with cisplatin or doxorubicin or with systemic 5-FU, folinic acid, and interferon-α.

HEPATOBLASTOMA

Hepatoblastoma affects about 1 child per 100,000 and is the most common primary malignant liver tumor in children, followed next by HCC.[254,255] It is usually diagnosed before the age of 3 years. Abdominal swelling is the most common presenting abnormality; there is a male predominance of almost 2 to 1.[255,256] Serum AFP is elevated in 75% to 96% of patients.[257] On CT scan, an enhancing tumor mass is identified that is solitary in 80% of cases with speckled calcifications present in more than 50% of cases.[257] Angiography is used for localization and assessment of resectability. On angiography, hepatoblastomas are usually hypervascular with irregular ill-defined tumor margins. Overall long-term survival ranges from 15% to 37%.[257–260] Poor prognosis is associated with aneuploidy and the anaplastic subtype of hepatoblastoma.[255,258,261] The Children's Cancer Study Group staging system is shown in Table 28–13.[262]

Complete resection is possible in 50% to 67% of children with hepatoblastoma and is associated with cure rates between 30% and 70%.[255-256] Preoperative chemotherapy has been used with some success in converting unresectable tumors to resectable lesions.[263,264] Adjuvant chemotherapy has been used after resection of hepatoblastoma.[175] Evans and colleagues reported that 20% of 24 hepatoblastomas were relapse free 8 to 42 months after surgical resection and adjuvant vincristine, doxorubicin, 5-FU, and cyclophosphamide.[262] Radiation therapy has been used to treat unresectable hepatoblastomas but its role is controversial.[255,265] Orthotopic liver transplan-

TABLE 28–13. Children's Cancer Study Group Staging for Hepatoblastoma

Group I	Complete resection of tumor by wedge, lobectomy, or extended lobectomy as initial treatment
Group IIA	Tumor rendered completely resectable by initial irradiation and chemotherapy
Group IIB	Residual tumor confined to one lobe
Group III	Tumor involving both lobes of the liver
Group IIIB	Regional lymph node involvement with tumor
Group IV	Distant metastases of tumor regardless of the extent of liver involvement

(Data from Evans AE, Land VJ, Newton WA, Randolph JG, Sather HN, Tefft M. Combination chemotherapy [vincristine, Adriamycin, cyclophosphamide, 5-fluorouracil] in the treatment of children with malignant hepatoma. Cancer 1982;50:821–826)

tation appears to have a role in children with unresectable hepatoblastoma if the tumor does not become resectable after preoperative chemotherapy. Penn reported on 18 patients undergoing liver transplantation for unresectable hepatoblastoma.[175] Tumors recurred in 6 patients and 5 survived disease free for more than 2 years with actuarial survival rates of about 50%.

CANCER OF THE BILIARY SYSTEM

EPIDEMIOLOGY

Biliary cancer is a relatively rare disease in the United States and Western hemisphere. More than 4000 deaths from biliary cancer occur in the United States each year.[266] The development of biliary cancer appears to be associated with inflammation of the biliary system. Worldwide, the greatest incidence of biliary cancer is associated with infestations of the liver flukes *Clonorchis sinensis*, *Opisthorchis viverrini*, and *Opisthorchis felineus*.[267] Less than 1% of patients with ulcerative colitis develop biliary tract cancer. Cholangiocarcinoma is associated with ulcerative colitis, Crohn's disease, biliary atresia, and congenital abnormalities of the intrahepatic bile ducts.[268] Cholangiocarcinoma occurs in 2% to 10% of patients with hepatolithiasis and in 8% of patients with Caroli's disease.[269,270] In patients with sclerosing cholangitis, cholangiocarcinoma is found in 9% of patients at the time of liver transplantation but in 33% to 42% at autopsy.[271,272] In patients with gallbladder carcinoma, the incidence of cholelithiasis varies from 70% to 90%. As many as 60% of patients with calcified or so-called porcelain gallbladders from chronic cholecystitis develop carcinomas of the gallbladder.[273,274]

CLASSIFICATION AND PATHOLOGY

Biliary cancers can occur anywhere in the hepatobiliary system and are classified according to location (Fig. 28–6). Peripheral or intrahepatic cholangiocarcinoma occurs in the parenchyma of the liver proximal to the bifurcation of the hepatic ducts and appears to arise from the proximal bile ducts, bile ductules, or intrahepatic peribiliary glands.[275] Although many authors use the term cholangiocarcinoma to refer to any primary cancer of the biliary system, others restrict its

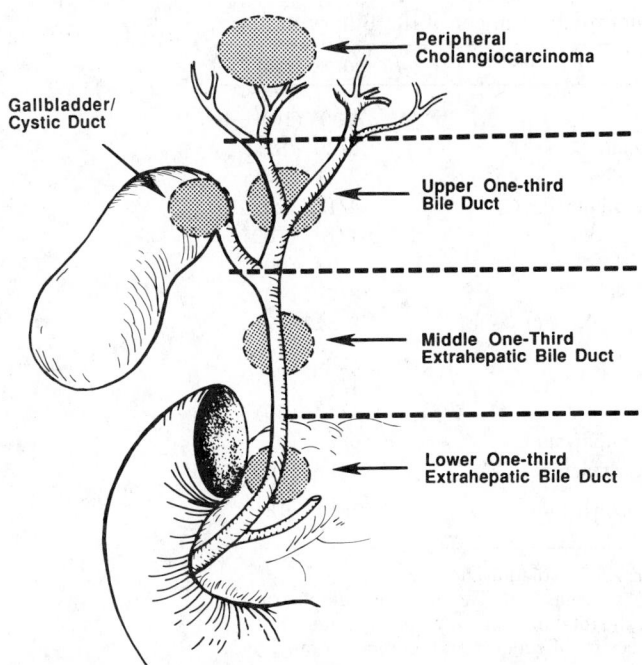

Gallbladder/
Cystic Duct

Peripheral
Cholangiocarcinoma

Upper One-third
Bile Duct

Middle One-Third
Extrahepatic Bile Duct

Lower One-third
Extrahepatic Bile Duct

FIGURE 28–6. Location of tumors involving the biliary system.

use to intrahepatic tumors and classify the remainder as biliary duct cancers or gallbladder cancers. The term extrahepatic biliary duct tumor excludes cancers of the ampulla of Vater, gallbladder tumors, and peripheral cholangiocarcinomas. Klatskin tumors are those tumors arising at the bifurcation of the right and left hepatic ducts.

More than 90% of primary biliary tumors are adenocarcinomas of varying degrees of differentiation.[276] Although primary biliary cancers can be further subclassified (see Table 28–7), most are ductal adenocarcinomas.[277] Mixed HCC/cholangiocarcinoma is not an uncommon intrahepatic tumor, and rare cases of pure HCC have been reported in the extrahepatic bile ducts.[278] Poorly differentiated small cell tumors

of the biliary system are rare aggressive tumors that sometimes respond to chemotherapy agents used in the treatment of small cell carcinoma of the lung.[279,280] Cholangiocarcinomas can be differentiated from HCCs by AFP staining, which is positive in 35% to 73% of hepatomas but never in cholangiocarcinomas, and by CA 19-9 or CA 50 staining, which is positive in 80% to 90% of cholangiocarcinomas but negative in hepatomas.[281] Expression of c-*MYC*, c-*RAS*, and c-*ERBB2* oncogenes may help differentiate cholangiocarcinomas from nonneoplastic lesions.[282] Hsu performed an immunohistochemical analysis of 15 gallbladder and 13 extrahepatic bile duct tumors and observed significantly poorer survival in patients with pure or predominant neuroendocrine differentiation.[279]

Several important pathologic factors must be taken into consideration in planning surgery or any other local therapy for these tumors. Cholangiocarcinomas are often accompanied by a zone of dysplastic tissue around the tumor and are multifocal in as many as 42% of patients.[283] Lymph node metastases occur in 30% to 50% of primary biliary cancers. Tumor seeding at surgery is possible with biliary tract cancers; prevention requires careful attention to surgical technique. Verbeek and colleagues reported a high incidence of tumor cells in cytologic examinations of bile fluid obtained during operation on intrahepatic duct tumors and described its possible consequence in 3 patients who developed implantation metastases.[284] Spread of cancer cells into connective tissue of the hepatoduodenal ligaments has been proposed as a mechanism for local recurrence of hilar cholangiocarcinoma in some patients after resection.[285]

CHEMOTHERAPY

Most reports of chemotherapy for cancers of the biliary system involve small numbers of patients. Response rates are similar for carcinomas of the gallbladder and bile duct and intrahepatic cholangiocarcinomas. As shown in Tables 28–14 and 28–15 the response rates for various systemic chemotherapy regimens vary widely among the small reported series, but the average response rates for single-agent and multiagent

TABLE 28–14. Single-Agent Systemic Chemotherapy for Cancer of the Biliary System

Investigations	Drug	Partial Response Rate (%)
Falkson et al, 1984[286]	5-Fluorouracil*	3/30 (10)
Davis et al, 1974[287]		3/23 (13)
Haskell, 1980[288]		4/17 (24)
Falkson et al, 1984[286]	Streptozocin*	0/14 (0)
Falkson et al, 1984[286]	Methyl-CCNU*	1/17 (6)
Crooke and Bradner, 1976[290]	Mitomycin C	7/15 (47)
Von Eyben et al, 1980[291]		0/10 (0)
Bukowski et al, 1983[292]	*m*-AMSA (amsacrine)	2/23 (9)
Haskell, 1980[288]	BCNU	2/2 (100)
Adolphson and Carpenter, 1982[293]	Doxorubicin	1/1 (100)
Bodey et al, 1981[294]	Neocarzinostatin	1/1 (100)
	Single-drug response rate	24/153 (16)

* Patients failing 5-fluorouracil were randomized between streptozocin and methyl-CCNU.

TABLE 28–15. Multiagent Systemic Chemotherapy for Cancer of the Biliary System

Investigations	Drug	Response Rate (%)
Falkson et al, 1984[286]	Oral 5-FU	3/30* (10)
Falkson et al, 1984[286]	Oral 5-FU + streptozocin	2/26 (8)
Falkson et al, 1984[286]	Oral 5-FU + methyl-CCNU	3/31 (10)
Harvey et al, 1984[295]	FAM (5-FU + DOX + mitomycin C)	4/14 (29)
Uchiyama et al, 1988[296]		1/1 (100)
Tavey and Hester, 1979[297]	DOX + bleomycin	1/5 (20)
Hall et al, 1974[298]	Ftotafur + DOX + BCNU	3/7 (43)
Stillwagon et al, 1991[299]	DOX + 5-FU + 2100 cGy XRT (1 cycle)	9/52† (17)
Shibata et al, 1990[300]	Etoposide + 5-FU	2/2 (100)
Koda et al, 1990[301]	UFT + DOX	1/4 (25)
Koda et al, 1990[301]	UFT + DOX + cisplatin	1/2 (50)
Novell et al, 1991[302]	Epirubicin + 5-FU + mitomycin C	0/1 (0)
Yamaguchi et al, 1991[303]	IL-2 + LAK + cyclophosphamide	1/1 (100)
	Overall multiagent response rate	17/94 (18)

DOX, doxorubicin; 5-FU, 5-fluorouracil; UFT, ftotafur; XRT, radiation therapy.
* Three-arm randomized Eastern Cooperative Oncology Group trial. The oral 5-FU alone arm was also reported in Table 28–14, but was not included in the total multiagent response rate.
† Not included in the total multiagent response rate because of concurrent radiation therapy.

regimens are 16% and 18%, respectively.[286–303] The response rates with hepatic artery infusion are generally higher and average 45% (Table 28–16).[302,304–310]

PERIPHERAL CHOLANGIOCARCINOMA

Peripheral or intrahepatic cholangiocarcinoma is rare in the United States and slightly more common in the Far East. It accounts for 10% to 20% of all primary liver tumors.[311] The clinical presentation of patients with peripheral cholangiocarcinomas is similar to that for HCC. Because the tumor is usually asymptomatic in early stages, most patients have advanced disease at presentation. The most common presenting complaints are dull, right upper quadrant pain, epigastric pain, and weight loss.[268,311] Jaundice occurs in only 24% of patients with peripheral cholangiocarcinoma compared with 71% of patients with hilar or Klatskin tumors.[311] The CT and MRI appearance of peripheral cholangiocarcinoma is similar to HCC. Intrahepatic ducts are more likely to be dilated and

angiography may show a characteristic picture of stretched, scanty, attenuated branches of the hepatic artery.[268]

Intrahepatic metastases and tumor growth along the biliary tract frequently occur. Lymph node involvement is more common with peripheral cholangiocarcinoma than in hilar bile duct tumors. In a series of 65 peripheral and 27 hilar cholangiocarcinomas (92 studied at autopsy), Nakajima and colleagues found lymph node involvement in 86% of peripheral compared with 33% of central tumors.[277] Intrahepatic and systemic metastases were found in 68% and 71%, respectively, of the autopsied patients with peripheral tumors. Cirrhosis is present in up to 15% of patients with cholangiocarcinoma, which is much less common than in patients with HCC.[268]

The TNM staging of intrahepatic or peripheral cholangiocarcinomas is the same as that for HCC (Table 28–17). Conventional surgical resection is possible in a few patients. Altaee and colleagues reported a series of 42 patients with peripheral cholangiocarcinoma seen at Kings College Hospital in London

TABLE 28–16. Hepatic Artery Infusion Chemotherapy for Cancer of the Biliary System Including Gallbladder Carcinoma

Investigations	Drug	Response Rate (%)
Massey et al, 1971[304]	5-Fluorouracil	1/3 (33)
Warren et al, 1972[305]	Floxuridine	9/15 (60)
Watkins et al, 1978[306]		5/11 (45)
Reed et al, 1981[307]		2/10 (20)
Seeger et al, 1989[308]		2/2 (100)
Garnick et al, 1979[309]	Doxorubicin	1/2 (50)
Wada et al, 1989[310]	Cisplatin + 5-fluorouracil + mitomycin C	1/1 (100)
Novell et al, 1991[302]	Epirubicin (Lipiodol suspension)	0/3 (0)
	Overall intraarterial response rate	21/47 (45)

TABLE 28–17. Extrahepatic Biliary Duct Cancers: TNM Clinical Classification From the UICC and AJCC

			Stage	*Grouping*
T: Primary Tumor				
TX	Primary tumor cannot be assessed		Stage 0	Tis N0M0
Tis	Carcinoma in situ		Stage I	T1N0M0
T1	Tumor invades mucosa or muscle layer		Stage II	T2N0M0
	T1A	Tumor invades mucosa		
	T1B	Tumor invades muscle layer		
T2	Tumor invades perimuscular connective tissue			
T3	Tumor invades adjacent structures: liver, pancreas, duodenum, gallbladder, colon, stomach		Stage III	T1N1M0
				T2N1M0
N: Regional Lymph Nodes				
NX	Regional lymph nodes cannot be assessed		Stage IVA	T3N0M0
				T3N1M0
N0	No regional lymph node metastasis			
N1	Regional lymph node metastasis		Stage IVB	T1–3N0–1M1
	N1A	Metastasis in cystic duct, pericholedochal, and/or hilar lymph nodes (*i.e.*, in the hepatoduodenal ligament)		
	N1B	Metastasis in peripancreatic (head only), periduodenal, periportal, celiac, and/or superior mesenteric lymph nodes		
M: Metastasis				
MX	Metastasis cannot be assessed			
M0	No metastasis			
M1	Metastasis present			

from 1969 to 1989.[312] Survival was indistinguishable from that of 70 patients with hilar cholangiocarcinomas, the median survival being 12 months in both groups. Although 13 of the 42 patients with peripheral cholangiocarcinoma underwent liver transplantation, no patient survived more than 42 months. Penn reported a 17% actuarial 5-year survival rate for a series of 109 intrahepatic and extrahepatic cholangiocarcinoma patients transplanted at various centers throughout the world; there is no significant difference between the recurrence rates of central and peripheral tumors.[175] Chen and colleagues reported on 20 patients with peripheral cholangiocarcinoma undergoing surgery in Taiwan from 1977 to 1987 who had a median survival of 20.5 months.[311] Four patients lived more than 3 years and 1 patient was alive 5 years after resection, intraluminal radiation therapy, and systemic chemotherapy. Because 16 of 20 tumors were diagnosed at the time of surgery for hepatolithiasis, early diagnosis may be responsible for the better survival in this series compared with others.

Stillwagon and colleagues reported a 5% complete response and 46% partial response (30% tumor reduction) for the treatment of peripheral cholangiocarcinoma with a regimen of initial whole-liver irradiation to 2100 cGy in 7 fractions, doxorubicin, cisplatin, and ^{131}I anti-CEA antibody.[299] Although the median survival was 14 months from diagnosis and 10 months from treatment, no patient survived more than 2 years from the start of treatment.

EXTRAHEPATIC BILIARY DUCT CANCER

Carcinoma of the extrahepatic biliary ducts occurs in less than 1% of patients in autopsy series and is encountered in 0.5%

to 1.4% of biliary tract operations.[313] The median survival for all patients with this disease averages 12 months.[187,314–317] Within the biliary duct, 57% of these tumors are located in the upper third, 15% in the middle third, and 18% in the lower third. Ten percent are diffuse.[314–316] The percentage of lymph node involvement from different surgical and autopsy series averages 41%.[318]

Although the diagnosis of extrahepatic biliary tract cancer can be suggested by its radiographic appearance, a tissue diagnosis should be established through brushings from endoscopic retrograde cholangiopancreatography (ERCP), percutaneous transhepatic cholangiography (PTC), CT-guided needle biopsy, open biopsy, or resection. Dalton-Clarke and colleagues reported a true-positive result on cytology with fine-needle aspiration biopsy in 88% of 17 patients with hilar cholangiocarcinoma, compared with a detection rate of 73% for brushings.[319] Rabinovitz and colleagues studied exfoliative cytology from biliary brushings of 37 patients with bile duct carcinomas and 28 patients with benign strictures and calculated the probability of detecting bile duct cancer after one, two, or three negative or suspicious brushings to be 43%, 32%, and 0% respectively.[320] Two of the 28 patients with benign strictures had one suspicious brushing sample. The differential diagnosis of an obstruction at the bifurcation of the hepatic ducts includes many possible causes.[321] Of a series of 98 patients with a preoperative radiographic diagnosis of Klatskin tumor, 68 cases were confirmed as sclerosing cholangiocarcinomas of the hepatic hilum, 5 were papillary bile duct carcinomas, 12 were gallbladder carcinomas invading the hilum, 5 were metastatic tumors to the bile duct, 2 were cases of Mirizzi's syndrome (a gallstone compressing the main hepatic duct), 3 were granulomas, and 3 had idiopathic focal stenosis.[318] The 8% incidence of benign biliary strictures in this series underscores the need for establishing a definitive diagnosis of malignancy in these patients before starting radiation therapy or chemotherapy.

NONOPERATIVE BILIARY DRAINAGE

The establishment of biliary drainage addresses the primary complaint of most patients with extrahepatic biliary tract tumors and is often the first step in treatment. Percutaneous transhepatic intubation can be performed at the time of transhepatic cholangiography. In addition to establishing biliary drainage, this provides easy access for biliary brushings to establish a tissue diagnosis. Cutaneous transhepatic biliary drainage tubes provide easy access for brachytherapy. Replacement of external biliary drainage catheters with internal stents is possible. In many cases, adequate biliary drainage can be established at the time of ERCP by placement of an internal stent without the necessity or discomfort of external biliary drainage catheters.

STAGING AND SURGICAL RESECTION

The TNM staging system for carcinomas of the extrahepatic bile duct is shown in Table 28–17. Median survival for surgically staged patients with extrahepatic biliary duct cancers in the French Surgical Association survey range from 64 months for T1 lesions to 6 months for patients with metastases.[314] Surgical resection is the treatment of choice for extrahepatic biliary duct tumors. The 5-year actuarial survivals after resection of upper, middle, and lower third lesions average 10%, 7%, and 39%, respectively, but vary among different institutions as do resection rates (Table 28–18). Median survival after resection of upper, middle, and lower third extrahepatic biliary cancers average 21, 12, and 46 months, respectively. Pancreaticoduodenectomy (Whipple's procedure) is normally required for successful resection of the lower third extrahepatic biliary tract tumors. Klatskin tumors involving only one hepatic duct can be resected by hepatic lobectomy on the involved side.

Vogt's review of 10 surgical series found resection rates varying from 10% to 61% (mean 35%), operative mortalities varying from 0 to 23% (mean 9%), and median survivals varying from 17 to 28 months (average 20 months).[324] Patients undergoing palliative rather than definitive resections in the same series experienced operative mortalities of 4% to 33% (mean 15%) and median survivals of 7.5 to 12 months (average 9 months). Reding and colleagues reviewed 552 carcinomas of the extrahepatic biliary ducts.[314] The overall median survival was 11 months. Patients undergoing surgical transtumoral intubation and those undergoing biliary and digestive anastomosis had similar mortality rates of 27% and similar median survivals of 9 months. Although this analysis was not stratified by tumor stage, operative mortality and long-term survival were similar regardless of whether hepatectomy was performed as part of the excision.

RADIATION THERAPY OF EXTRAHEPATIC BILIARY DUCT CANCER

Radiation therapy has been used both as the primary treatment of extrahepatic biliary cancers and an adjuvant therapy along with surgical resection. Many series indicate that radiation therapy improves the survival of patients with extrahepatic

TABLE 28–18. Survival After Surgical Resection of Extrahepatic Biliary Duct Tumors*

Location	Investigations	Years Treated	Resection Rate (%)	No. Resected	Median Survival* (mo)	5-Year Survival* (%)
Upper Third	Reding et al, 1991[314]	1955–1989	32	181	23	11†
	Chao and Greager, 1991[316]	1974–1987	14	14	18	0
	Cameron[322]	1973–1989	55	53	12	8
	Tompkins et al, 1990[315]	1954–1978	47	22	13	0
	Tompkins et al, 1990[315]	1978–1988	17	10	39	30
	Average value		46	320	20	10
Middle Third	Reding et al, 1991[314]	1955–1989	47	31	13	NR
	Chao and Greager, 1991[316]	1974–1987	67	15	13	0
	Pitt et al, 1987[323]	1954–1981	65	19	10	12
	Average value		57	65	12	7
Lower Third	Reding et al, 1991[314]	1955–1989	51	46	64	50†
	Chao and Greager, 1991[316]	1974–1987	57	7	16	0
	Pitt et al, 1987[323]	1954–1981	68	22	18	28
	Average value		57	75	46	39

NR, not reported.
* For patients undergoing surgical resection with or without postoperative radiation therapy.
† Figures estimated from published survival curves or other published data.

biliary duct cancers who have not undergone a complete re-section. Unfortunately, few patients live more than 5 years without surgical resection.[314,317,322–325] Grove and colleagues reported a median survival of 2.2 months in 9 patients with proximal bile duct cancer without metastatic disease who underwent operative stent placement without radiation therapy; the median survival was 12.2 months in 19 patients who received fractionated external-beam irradiation after operative stent placement ($p = 0.005$).[323] The role of postoperative radiation therapy after complete resection is controversial. Cameron and colleagues reviewed a series of 96 patients with proximal cholangiocarcinomas in whom the resection rate of 55% and postoperative radiation therapy was used in 66% of patients.[322] They found that radiation therapy significantly extended survival in patients undergoing palliative stenting, but not in those undergoing resection. The 5-year survival of resected patients was 8% compared with no 5-year survival in the stented group. In the French Surgical Association survey, there was no difference in survival between patients who underwent surgical resection with and without radiation therapy.[314] In patients undergoing palliative surgery, there was a trend for improved survival with radiation therapy (median survival of 13 versus 8 months; $0.05 < p < 0.10$), compared with those not receiving radiation therapy. In a multicenter study, Gonzales and colleagues compared 17 patients undergoing surgery alone with 38 patients undergoing surgery with postoperative radiation therapy and found median survivals of 8.25 and 19.0 months and 3-year survivals of 10% and 31%, respectively ($p = 0.0005$).[325] The median survival of 47 patients who underwent biliary drainage and radiation therapy was 12.3 months, and their 3-year survival was 12%. Because retrospective studies analyzing the effect of radiation therapy after complete surgical resection have not been stratified for factors such as tumor stage and the presence of microscopic or gross tumor at resection margins, it is difficult to make conclusions regarding the effect of radiation therapy because patients with poorer prognostic features could have been selected for radiation therapy.

Intraluminal brachytherapy techniques allow a high dose of radiation to be administered to a bile duct tumor with relative dose sparing of surrounding normal structures (Fig. 28–7). Although brachytherapy has been used alone, because of the short effective range of intraluminal radiation therapy (usually prescribed to a depth of 0.5 cm from the catheter), most radiation therapists favor using intraluminal brachytherapy as a boost after fractionated external-beam irradiation to fields encompassing the tumor and adjacent lymph nodes. Using intraluminal brachytherapy alone, Karani and colleagues reported a median survival of 17 months.[327] Many radiation therapists favor combining initial external-beam irradiation with intraluminal brachytherapy over either treatment modality alone. Johnson and colleagues reported a median survival of 9 months with intraluminal brachytherapy alone compared with 16 months with combination external-beam irradiation.[328] Meyers and Jones reported an average survival of 3.6 months for 5 patients who received intraluminal brachytherapy alone compared with 14.3 months in 22 patients who received external-beam irradiation plus brachytherapy.[329] Fields and Emami reported a median survival of 15 months in 8 patients receiving fractionated external-beam irradiation and brachytherapy compared with a median sur-

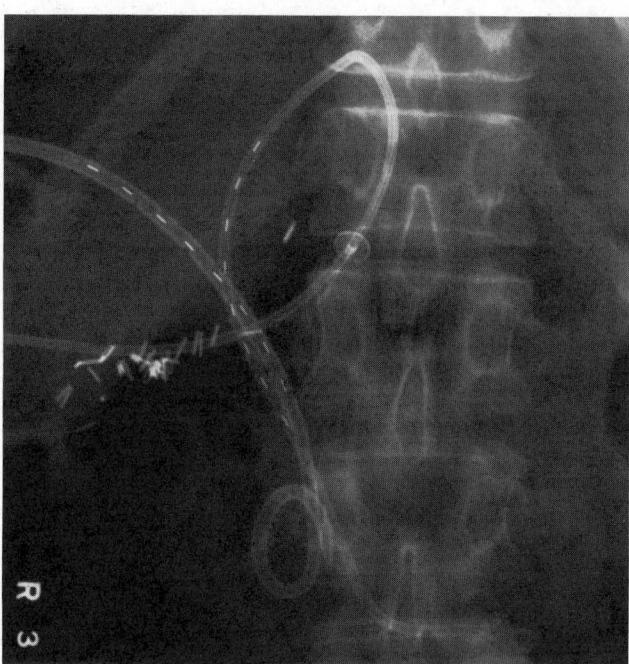

FIGURE 28–7. Radiograph of intraluminal brachytherapy sources (iridium 192) for treatment of a Klatskin tumor.

vival of 7 months in 9 patients receiving external-beam irradiation only ($p = 0.06$).[330] An analysis of the University of Pittsburgh experience in 63 biliary cancer patients suggested that the better survival observed with external-beam irradiation combined with intraluminal brachytherapy was due to patient selection.[187] Gonzales and colleagues were unable to verify any improvement in survival with the addition of brachytherapy to external-beam irradiation compared with external-beam irradiation alone for primary or postoperative treatment of Klatskin's tumors.[325] They did find improved survival (median 12.6 versus 6.6 months) with doses of more than 4000 cGy compared with lower doses ($p = 0.001$).

NEW TREATMENT APPROACHES

Intraoperative radiation therapy (IORT) is being evaluated for treatment of advanced bile duct carcinomas with microscopic or gross residual tumor after surgical resection. Because IORT is administered at the time of surgical exploration and resection, the radiation dose can be administered to the tumor bed, and normal tissue can be shielded or excluded from the radiation treatment field. Iwasaki and colleagues reported a series of 81 patients with bile duct tumors that included 13 patients who received a noncurative resection plus IORT, 6 patients who received IORT plus biliary drainage, and 21 patients who underwent biliary drainage alone.[331] Two-year survival rates of 17%, 20%, and 9%, respectively, were found, with only 1 patient living more than 3 years. Busse and colleagues reported on 12 patients who underwent IORT plus postoperative radiation therapy and on 15 patients with primary or recurrent carcinomas of the biliary tree.[332] Thirteen patients also received external-beam irradiation and 9 received chemotherapy. The median survival of the 12 patients with primary disease was 14 months with local control in the porta hepatis in 5 of 10 evaluable patients. Only 2 patients were alive at the time of the report. One patient was alive and free of disease 2 years after resection with IORT and external-beam irradiation for microscopic residual disease. A second patient whose tumor was not resected was alive and disease free 11 months after IORT and postoperative external-beam irradiation.

Minsky and colleagues reported encouraging preliminary results for combined 5-FU and mitomycin C chemotherapy with radiation therapy used to treat 8 patients with extrahepatic biliary duct tumors and 2 patients with gallbladder cancer.[333] External-beam irradiation was administered to 5000 cGy to the tumor bed and lymph nodes followed in 9 patients by 1500 cGy of external beam boost irradiation and by intraluminal brachytherapy in 6 patients. The 3-year actuarial survival was 50%, with 2 patients reported alive and free of disease at 48 and 52 months; unfortunately, these two long-term survivors had no tissue diagnosis.

Liver transplantation is an appealing new approach to the treatment of otherwise unresectable extrahepatic biliary duct tumors. Penn reported the results of liver transplantation for cholangiocarcinoma from the Cincinnati Transplant Tumor Registry, using data from liver transplantation centers throughout the world.[175] A total of 109 patients with peripheral or hilar cholangiocarcinoma were analyzed without separation of central and peripheral tumors. Eight patients had 5-FU or doxorubicin chemotherapy before or after transplantation and 6 had radiation therapy. Forty-eight of 109 tumors recurred; the 2- and 5-year actuarial survival rates were 30% and 17%, respectively, with 3 patients surviving more than 5 years. At the University of Pittsburgh, 53 patients with biopsy-proved cholangiocarcinoma involving the liver hilum were treated from 1981 to 1990. Figure 28–8 compares the survival rates of 26 patients who received fractionated radiation therapy to doses greater than 4500 cGy with 13 patients who underwent orthotopic liver transplantation and external-beam irradiation

alone and 9 patients who underwent orthotopic liver transplantation with neoadjuvant chemoradiotherapy (7 patients) or upper abdominal exenteration and cluster surgery or both (5 patients).[334] Neoadjuvant chemoradiotherapy consisted of radiation therapy to 5000 cGy administered twice daily in 150-cGy fractions with concurrent 5-FU, folinic acid, and interferon-α. Although these results are preliminary, the improved survival rate for the treatment group receiving neoadjuvant chemoradiotherapy warrants continued investigation.

CARCINOMA OF THE GALLBLADDER

Carcinoma of the gallbladder is an aggressive disease with overall survival rates of about 5% and median survivals of 6 months.[336–342] Because gallbladder tumors are usually asymptomatic until they reach advanced stages, most patients present with extensive disease. The most common presenting symptoms are abdominal pain (54%), jaundice (46%), weight loss (28%), anorexia (19%), and nausea and vomiting (19%).[338,339] As in cholecystitis, there is a female predominance with 61% to 75% female patients in most series. The median age at diagnosis in most series is about 70 years.[343,344]

PATHOLOGY AND STAGING

The predominant histology for cancer of the gallbladder is adenocarcinoma, which occurs in 85% of patients.[343,345] Guo and colleagues classified 21 of 284 cases of carcinoma of the gallbladder as undifferentiated and found that they were associated with a significantly shorter median survival (3 months versus 13 months) for adenocarcinomas.[344] Lymphadenopathy was found in about 40% of patients.[338,343,345,346] Liver invasion is reported in about 50% of patients in different surgical series.[338,345,346] Chao reported a 53% incidence of lymphade-

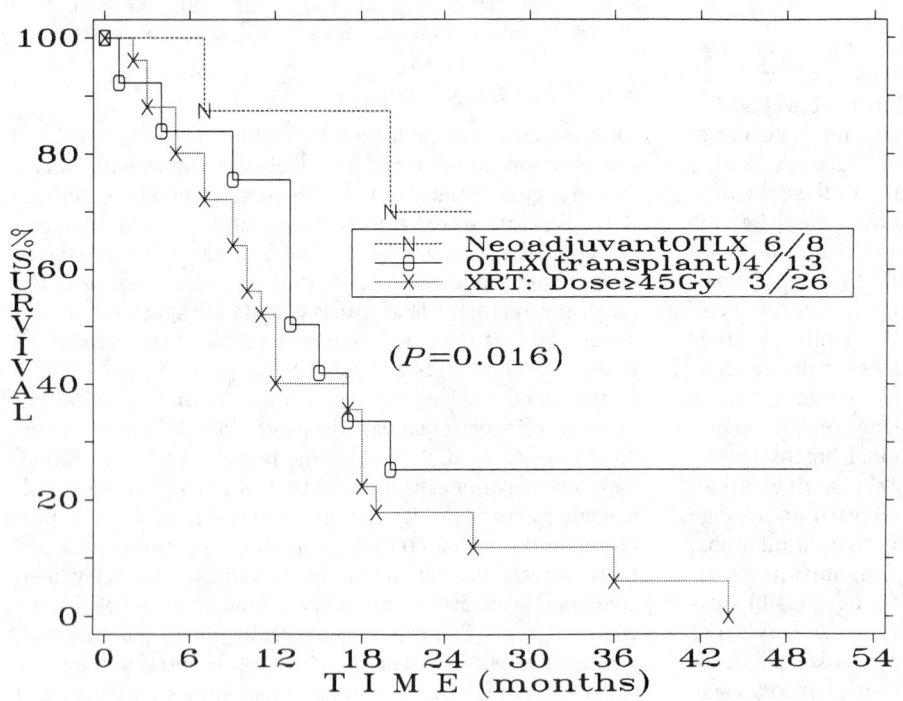

FIGURE 28–8.   Actuarial survival of patients with hilar cholangiocarcinoma treated by full-course radiation therapy of more than 4500 cGy, liver transplantation radiation therapy, or radical treatment with neoadjuvant chemoradiotherapy with liver or cluster transplantation.

nopathy in 74 cases, with the nodes involved being peripancreatic (22%), porta hepatis (18%), choledochal (8%), cystic (6%), periaortic (16%), and mesenteric (6%).[338] About 80% of gallbladder cancers are correctly diagnosed preoperatively by ultrasonography and 60% by CT.[347] Endoscopic ultrasonography can sometimes provide information on depth of tumor invasion, whereas direct cholangiography and angiography can be useful in evaluating tumor extent and resectability.[347]

The two commonly used staging systems are the TNM staging system of the UICC (Table 28–19) and the Nevin staging system. Ogura and colleagues analyzed a series of 1686 resected cases of gallbladder carcinoma from 172 hospitals in Japan with 5-year survivals of 83%, 73%, 37%, 15%, and 7% for T1A, T1B, T2, T3, and T4 tumors respectively.[348]

THERAPY

The primary treatment modality for carcinoma of the gallbladder is surgical resection. Tumors limited to the mucosa are usually incidental findings at the time of cholecystectomy for chronic cholecystitis. Cholecystectomy alone may be adequate in these patients.[348] Patients with gallbladder carcinomas invading beyond the mucosal layer may benefit from more radical procedures such as extended cholecystectomy with regional lymph node dissection and resection of the gallbladder bed, if appropriate. This is controversial, however, with many reports suggesting no improvement in survival with aggressive resection. Pancreaticoduodenectomy has been recommended by some investigators when lymphadenopathy posterior to the pancreas or duodenal invasion is present.[348]

The role of radiation therapy as primary or adjuvant postoperative treatment for carcinoma of the gallbladder is controversial. Because series are small, tumor response is difficult to assess, and patient selection factors vary in different series, it is difficult to evaluate the effect of radiation therapy in this disease. Pattern of failure studies show that local recurrence occurs in 86% of patients with gallbladder cancer after cholecystectomy, which suggests that local radiation therapy may

TABLE 28–19. TNM Staging for Carcinoma of the Gallbladder

Tis	Carcinoma in situ		
T1	Confined to mucosal or muscular layer		
	T1A Limited to mucosa		
	T1B Invades muscular layer		
T2	Invades perimuscular connective tissue		
T3	Invades serosa and/or one organ, liver less than 2 cm		
T4	Invades two or more organs, or liver more than 2 cm		
	N1A Hepatoduodenal ligament nodes: cystic duct, pericholedochal, or hilar		
	N1B Other regional nodes: peripancreatic (head only), periportal celiac, or superior mesenteric		
Stage 0	Tis	N0	M0
Stage I	T1	N0	M0
Stage II	T2	N0	M0
Stage III	T1	N1	M0
	T2	N1	M0
	T3	Any N	M0
Stage IV	T4	Any N	M0
	Any T	Any N	M1

be of use.[349] Vaittinen reported a median survival of 63 months for patients receiving postoperative radiation therapy compared with 29 months for patients undergoing surgery alone.[345] Bosset and colleagues reported 5 of 7 gallbladder cancer patients free of disease at 5, 9, 11, 31, and 58 months after complete resection and postoperative radiation therapy to 5400 cGy in 30 fractions.[350] Of 4 patients treated by Houry and colleagues with Nevin stage III or IV tumors that received 4500 to 5500 cGy radiation therapy after complete resection, one patient with stage III disease survived 84 months.[351] The median survival of the 16 other patients in their series who underwent radiation therapy with or without partial resection was 8 months, compared with median survivals of 1.5 to 2.0 months in historical control series without radiation therapy.[351]

Todoroki and colleagues reported on 17 patients with TNM stage IV gallbladder carcinomas who received 2000 to 3000 cGy of IORT (plus 3600 cGy of external-beam irradiation in 10 patients).[352] The 3-year survival was 10%, with the longest survivor free of disease at 3 years, which the authors compared with no 3-year survival among the 9 stage IV patients with resection alone at their institution.[352] Busse and colleagues treated 10 patients with IORT for gross residual gallbladder cancer and reported a median survival of 1 year with no long-term survivors.[353] The chemotherapy response rates for carcinoma of the gallbladder do not differ significantly from intrahepatic cholangiocarcinomas or extrahepatic bile duct cancers. The composite response rate for tumor confined to the mucosa is 59% but only 9% for those to the serosa, 7% for those with nodal disease, and 1% for liver metastases.[354]

OTHER TUMORS OF THE LIVER

BENIGN TUMORS

The various benign hepatobiliary neoplasms represent a minority of all tumors of the liver (see Table 28–7). For instance, only 0.5 to 1% of all cholecystectomies performed are associated with benign tubular or papillary adenomas.[5] Benign mesenchymal tumors are rarely seen. Adenomas of the extrahepatic bile ducts are rare and usually present with jaundice. Cystadenomas (or hamartoma) and granular cell tumors of the ducts have been described. The incidence of primary hepatic tumors in Los Angeles County revealed that about 12% of tumors presenting within the liver were benign, including focal nodular hyperplasia (7.8%), bile duct adenomas (3.0%), hepatocellular adenomas (0.9%), and inflammatory pseudotumor (0.2%).[5] Focal nodular hyperplasia is observed as a solitary mass often with a central fibrous scar and is the most common benign hepatic tumor. These are most frequently detected in women but generally are not associated with oral contraceptive use as are hepatocellular adenomas. Most patients are not advised to undergo treatment. Cessation of sex hormone therapy often is associated with regression. This tumor is only rarely believed to be associated with malignancy.

Hepatocellular adenomas may be single or multiple and often are associated with exogenous estrogen or androgen use. They are observed in tyrosinemia and glycogen storage disease. They may be associated with hemorrhage. Among women, the incidence increases from about 0.1 per 100,000 to 3.4 per 100,000 after beginning oral contraceptives. If a mass observed on an x-ray film regresses after stopping oral contraceptives, only observation is indicated.[122] Excision is usually advised for lesions that do not regress. In a recent series reported from Bismuth's group, 4 of 24 patients with liver cell adenomas seen between 1976 and 1989 had tumors associated with glycogen storage disease.[355] Eighty-three percent of their patients were women, of whom 87% had received oral contraceptives or other hormone therapy before diagnosis. Seventeen patients underwent surgical resection without operative mortality. Hemangiomas of the liver are usually small, may be multiple, and often present as cavernous variants that occasionally appear as masses. They have been observed more frequently with improvements in hepatic imagining modalities. Treatment is rarely needed except for patients with symptomatic enlargement.

EPITHELIOID HEMANGIOENDOTHELIOMA

Epithelioid hemangioendothelioma is a low-grade, malignant, soft tissue tumor of endothelial origin that follows a clinical course between a hemangioma and an angiosarcoma with metastases occurring in 28% of patients.[356-359] Factor VIII staining differentiates hemangiothelioma from other nonvascular tumors. It is unlikely to be confused with infantile hemangioendothelioma, which is benign, because of its different clinical presentation and pathologic features. This tumor may develop as a primary lung or soft tissue tumor. The patients range in age from 19 to 86 years with an average age of 50 years. The patient usually presents with nonspecific complaints and an abdominal mass, whereas only 12% of patients present with jaundice. In contrast to angiosarcoma, there is a female predominance (63% of patients).[357] Epithelioid hemangioendothelioma has been related to vinyl chloride exposure in some patients.[358]

Although some patients have survived as long as 28 years with no anticancer therapy, Weiss and Enzinger recommended radical surgery if possible.[359] Penn reported a series of 21 patients who underwent orthotopic liver transplantation for treatment of epithelioid hemangioendotheliomas; 7 of 21 patients recurred with tumor, with 4 dying from disease and 3 alive with disease.[175] The actuarial survival rate was 82% at 2 years and 43% at 5 years.

SARCOMAS OF THE LIVER

Angiosarcoma (also referred to as malignant hemangioendothelioma, hemangiosarcoma, or Kupffer's cell sarcoma), is a rare liver tumor that is the most common of the malignant mesenchymal tumors affecting the liver. About 25 cases occur in the United States each year.[356] Patients range in age from 24 to 93 years, with the peak in incidence in the sixth and seventh decades; 85% of patients are males.[266,360] The most common initial symptom is abdominal pain. Other common symptoms are abdominal swelling usually due to liver enlargement, liver failure, nausea, anorexia, occasional vomiting, and jaundice. Angiosarcoma has been associated with exposure to thorotrast, arsenic solutions, and vinyl chloride.

Angiosarcoma is an aggressive neoplasm, with most patients dying within 6 months of diagnosis. Distant metastases develop in 50% of patients. Surgical resection is usually unsuccessful because most patients present with advanced tumors. Some long-term survivors have been reported after a partial hepatectomy, but few patients survive more than 1 to 3 years after complete resection because of metastatic disease. Attempts to treat hepatic angiosarcomas with radiation therapy or chemotherapy have been disappointing.[360] The limited experience with orthotopic liver transplantation for treatment of angiosarcoma also has been disappointing. Penn reported development of tumor recurrences in 9 of 14 transplant patients with tumors classified as angiosarcomas or epithelioid hemangioendothelial sarcomas; the 2-year survival was 15% with no patient surviving more than 28 months after surgery.[175] Other soft tissue sarcomas involving the liver are extremely rare. Ishak and colleagues reported 2 cases and reviewed 14 cases of primary hepatic fibrosarcoma in adults and 6 cases of leiomyosarcoma involving the liver or ligamentum teres.[356] Hepatic metastases from a gastrointestinal or uterine primary need to be ruled out before the diagnosis of primary leiomyosarcoma of the liver can be made. Surgical resection is the treatment of choice for primary hepatic sarcomas.[356] The prognosis for unresectable tumors is poor. The liver can occasionally be the primary site for rhabdomyosarcoma, which is more common in children than adults. Treatment is similar to that for rhabdomyosarcoma in other locations—surgical excision, if possible, and chemotherapy. Undifferentiated sarcomas of the liver are rare and usually occur in children between the ages of the 6 and 15 years.[266,356,361,362] Most undifferentiated sarcomas of the liver are unresectable and poorly responsive to radiation therapy or chemotherapy.[266,361] In a report of 9 cases and a literature review by Leuschner and colleagues, the median survival was 12 months, and 37% of patients were disease free for an average of 37.5 months.[362] Other miscellaneous and rare malignant liver tumors include lymphoma of the liver, primary squamous cell carcinoma of the liver, which may arise from congenital hepatic cysts, carcinosarcoma, malignant mesenchymoma, and primary hepatic carcinoid.[266,356]

REFERENCES

1. Boring CC, Squires TS, Tong T. Cancer Statistics, 1992. CA 1992;42:19–38.
2. Tabor E, DiBiscegli AM, Purcell RH, eds. Etiology, pathology, and treatment of hepatocellular carcinoma in North America. Advances in applied biotechnology series, vol 13. Houston, TX: Gulf Publishing, 1991.
3. Simonetti RG, Camma C, Fiorella F, Politi F, D'Amico G, Pagliaro L. Hepatocellular carcinoma. Dig Dis Sc 1991;36:962–972.
4. DiBiscegli AM, Rustgi VK, Hoofnagle JH, Dusheiko GM, Lotze MT. Hepatocellular Carcinoma. Ann Intern Med 1988;108:390–401.
5. Albores-Saavedra J, Henson DE. Tumors of the gallbladder and extra-hepatic bile ducts, 1986. In: Craig JR, Peter Rl, Edwardson HA. Tumors of the liver and intrahepatic bile ducts. Washington, DC: Armed Forces Institute of Pathology, fascicles 22 and 26, 1989.
6. Michalopoulos GK. Liver regeneration: Molecular mechanisms of growth control. FASEB J 1990;4:176–193.
7. Matsuda H, Matsumoto M, Haraguchi S, Kanai K. Partial purification of a growth factor synthesized by a rat hepatoma cell line established in serum-free medium. Cancer Res 1989;49:2118–2122.
8. Zarnegar R, Michalopoulos G. Purification and biological characterization of human hepatopoietin A: A polypeptide growth factor for hepatocytes. Cancer Res 1989;49: 3314–3320.
9. Ove P, Francavilla A, Coetzee ML, Makowka L, Starzl TE. Response of cultured hepatocytes to a hepatomitogen after initiation by conditioned medium or other factors. Cancer Res 1989;49:98–103.
10. Ricordi C, Lacy PE, Callery MP, Pyong PW, Flye W. Trophic factors from pancreatic islets in combined hepatocyte-islet allografts enhance hepatocellular survival. Surgery 1988;105:218–219.
11. Sever CE, Locker J. Expression of retinoic acid α and β receptor genes in liver and hepatocellular carcinoma. Molecular Carcinogenesis 1991;4(2):138–144.

12. Zoli M, Marchesini G, Melli A, Viti G, Marra A, Marrano D, Pisi E. Evaluation of liver volume and liver function following hepatic resection in man. Liver 6:286–291.1986;

13. Nagasue N, Yukaya H, Ogawa Y, Kochno H, Nakamura T. Human liver regeneration after major hepatic resection. Ann Surg 206:30–39.1987;

14. Chen MF, Hwang TL, Hung CF. Human liver regeneration after major hepatectomy. Ann Surg 1991;213:227–229.

15. Lanser ME, Brown GE. Stimulation of rat hepatocyte fibronectin production by monocyte-conditioned medium is due to interleukin 6. J Exp Med 1989;170:1781–1786.

16. Mackiewica A, Speroff T, Ganapathi MK, Kushner I. Effects of cytokine combinations on acute phase protein production in two human hepatoma cell lines. J Immunol 1991;146:3032–3037.

17. Del Giglio A, Zukiwski AA, Ali MK, Mavligit GM. Severe, symptomatic, dose-limiting hypophosphatemia induced by hepatic arterial infusion of recombinant tumor necrosis factor in patients with liver metastases. Clin Exp Immunol 1991;83:488–491.

18. Raynes JG, Eagling S, McAdam PWJ. Acute-phase protein synthesis in human hepatoma cells: Differential regulation of serum amyloid A (SAA) and haptoglobin by interleukin 1 and interleukin 6. Clin Exp Immunol 1991 (83):448–491.

19. Won KI, Baumann H. NF-AB, a liver-specific and cytokine-inducible nuclear factor that interacts with the interleukin-1 response element of the rat α_1-acid glycoprotein gene. Mol Cell Biol 1991;11:3001–3008.

20. Curran RD, Billiar TR, Stuehr DJ, Hofmann K, Simmons R. Hepatocytes produce nitrogen oxides from L-arginie in response to inflammatory products of Kupffer cells. J Exp Med 1989;157:1769–1774.

21. Franco A, Barnaba V, Natali P, Balsano C, Musca A, Balsano F. Expression of class I and class II major histocompatibility complex antigens on human hepatocytes. Pathology 1988;3(3):449–454.

22. Sung CH, Hu CP, Hsu HC, et al. Expression of class I and class II major histocompatibility antigens on human hepatocellular carcinoma. J Clin Invest 1989;83:421–429.

23. Paterson AC, Sciot R, Kew MC, Callea F, Dusheiko Gm, Desmet VJ. HLA expression in human hepatocellular carcinoma. Br J Cancer 1988;57:369–373.

24. Lin DY, Liae F, Huang CC. The distribution of HLA-A, B, C, DR antigens in Chinese patients with hepatocellular carcinoma in Taiwan. Tumor Antigens 1987;29:110–114.

25. Barnaba V, Franco A, Alberti A, Benvenuto R, Balsano F. Selective killing of hepatitis B envelop antigen-specific B cells by class I-restricted, exogenous antigen-specific T Lymphocytes. Nature 1990;345:258–260.

26. Milich DR, Jones JE, McLaclan A, Houghten R, Thornton GB, Hughes JL. Distinction between immunogenicity and tolerogenicity among HBcAg T cell determinants. J Immunol 1989;143(10):3148–3156.

27. Alper CA, Kruskall MS, Marcus-Bagley D, et al. Genetic prediction of nonresponse to hepatitis B vaccine. N Engl J Med 1990;321(11):707–712.

28. Lafreniere R, Borkenhagen K, Bryant LD, Anton AR, Chung A, Poon MC. Analysis of liver lyphoid cell subsets pre- and post-*in vitro* administration of human recombinant interleukin 2 in a C57BL/6 murine system. Cancer Res 1990;40:1658–1666.

29. Saidman SL, Demetris AJ, Zeevi A, Duquesnoy RJ. Propagation of lymphocytes infiltrating human liver allografts. Transplantation 1990;49(1):107–111.

30. Shimizu Y, Iwatsuki S, Herberman R, Whiteside TL. Effects of cytokines on *in vitro* growth of tumor-infiltrating lymphocytes obtained from human primary and metastatic liver tumors. Cancer Immunol Immunother 1991;32:280–288.

31. Chuang WL, Liu HW, Chang WY. Natural killer cell activity in patients with hepatocellular carcinoma relative to early development and tumor invasion. Cancer 1990;65:926–930.

32. Nakajima T, Mizwsima N, Kanai K. Relationship between natural killer activity and development of hepatocellular carcinoma in patients with cirrhosis of the liver. Jpn J Clin Oncol 1987;17:327–332.

33. Brooks RH, Kew MC, Rabson AR. Depressed natural cytotoxicity but normal natural killer cytotoxic factor (NKCF) production by mononuclear cells derived from patients with hepatocellular carcinoma. Cancer Immunol Immunother 1987;25:149–152.

34. Muir C. Cancer incidence in five continents. IARC Scientific Publications. vol V. no. 88. Lyon, France: International Agency for Research in Cancer, 1987.

35. Steinitz R. Cancer incidence: Jewish migrants to Israel 1961–1981. IARC Scientific Publication. no. 98. Lyon, France: International Agency for Research in Cancer, 1989.

36. Di Bisceglie AM. Chronic viral hepatitis and hepatocellular carcinoma in the US. In: Tabor, E, Di Bisceglie AM, Purcell RH, eds. Etiology, pathology, and treatment of hepatocellular carcinoma in Northern America. Houston, TX: Gulf Publishing, 1991.

37. Linsell CA. Environmental chemical carcinogens and liver cancer. In: Lapis K, Johannesen JV, eds. Liver carcinogenesis. Hemisphere Publishing, 1979.

38. Henderson BE, Preston-Martin S, Edmondson HA. Hepatocellular carcinoma and oral contraceptives. Br J Cancer 1983;48:437.

39. U.S. Department of Health and Human Services. Sixth annual report on carcinogens. Washington, D.C.: U.S. Government Publication 92-12066. 1991.

40. Munoz N, Bosch X. Epidemiology of hepatocellular carcinoma. In: Okuda K, Ishak KA, eds. Neoplasms of the liver. New York: Springer-Verlag, 1987.

41. Lutwick LI. Relation between aflatoxins and hepatitis B virus and hepatocellular carcinoma. Lancet 1979;755.

42. Beasley RP, Hwang LY, Lin CC, et al. Hepatocellular carcinoma and hepatitis B virus: A prospective study of 22,707 men in Taiwan. Lancet 1981;2:1129.

43. Okuda K, Fujimoto I, Hannai A, Urano Y. Changing incidence of hepatocellular carcinoma in Japan. Cancer Res 1987;47:4967–4972.

44. Edmondson HA, Steiner PE. Primary carcinoma of the liver. Cancer 1954;7:462–503.

45. Tiribell C, Malato M, Croce LS, Giarelli L, Okuda K, Ohnishi K. Prevalence of hepatocellular carcinoma and relation to cirrhosis. Hepatology 1989;10:798–1002.

46. Beahrs OH, Henson DE, Hutter RV, Myers MH. Manual for staging of cancer. Philadelphia: JB Lippincott, 1988:87–103.

47. Haaga JR, Morrison SC, County J, Fanaroff AA, Shah M. Infarction of the left hepatic lobe in a neonate on serial CTs: Evolution of a pseudomass to atrophy. Pediatr Radiol 1991;21:150–151.

48. Schwartz RE, Lotze MT. Pseudo-pseudotumor of the liver. Submitted for publication, 1992.

49. Aspestrand F, Schrumpf E, Jacobsen M. Hanssen L, Endresen K. Increased lymphatic flow from the liver in different intra-and extrahepatic diseases demonstrated by CT. J Comput Assist Tomogr 1991;15:550–554.

50. Pokorny CS, Painter Dm, Waugh RC, McCaughan GW, Gallagher Nd, Tattersall MHN. Inflammatory pseudotumor of the liver causing biliary obstruction. J Clin Gastroenterol 1991;13(3):338–341.

51. Sheu JC, Sung JL, Chen DS, et al. Early detection of hepatocellular carcinoma by real-time ultrasonography. Cancer 1985;56:660–666.

52. Van Ness MM, Diehl AM. Is liver biopsy useful in the evaluation of patients with chronically elevated liver enzymes? Ann Intern Med 1989;111:473–478.

53. Brady PG, Peebles M, Goldschmid S. Role of laparoscopy in the evaluation of patients with suspected hepatic or peritoneal malignancy. Gastrointest Endosc 1991;37:27–30.

54. Miller WJ, Federle MP, Campbell WL. Diagnosis and staging of hepatocellular carcinoma. AJR 1991;157:303–306.

55. Merine D, Takayasu K, Wakao F. Detection of hepatocellular carcinoma: Comparison of CT during arterial portography with CT after intraarterial injection of iodized oil. Radiology 1990;175:707–710.

56. Matsui O, Kadoya M, Suzuki M, et al. Work in progress: Dynamic sequential computed tomography during arterial portography in the detection of hepatic neoplasm. Radiology 1983;146:721–727.

57. Hosoki T, Chatani M, Mori S. Dynamic computed tomography of hepatocellular carcinoma. AJR 1982;139:1099–1106.

58. Heiken JP, Weyman DJ, Lee JKT, et al. Detection of focal hepatic masses: Prospective evaluation with CT, delayed CT, CT during arterial portography, MR imaging. Radiology 1989;171:47–51.

59. Nelson RC, Chezmar JL, Sugarbaker PH, Bernardino ME. Hepatic tumors: Comparison of CT during arterial portography, delayed CT, MR imaging for preoperative evaluation. Radiology 1989;172:27–34.

60. Soyer P, Roche A, Levesque M, Legmann P. CT of fibrolamellar hepatocellular carcinoma. J Comput Assist Tomogr 1991;15(4):533–538.

61. Ohtomo K, Itai Y, Furui S, Yashiro N, Yoshikawa K, Iio M. Hepatic tumors: Differentiation by transverse relation time (T2) of magnetic resonance imaging. Radiology 1985;155:421–423.

62. Itai Y, Ohtomo K, Furui S, Minami M, Yoshikawa K, Yashiro N. MR imaging of hepatocellular carcinoma. J Comput Assist Tomogr 1986;10(6):963–968.

63. Feuerstein I, Miller DH, Dibesceglie, A et al. Radiologic findings in hepatocellular carcinoma. In: Tabor E, DiBisceglie AM, Purcell RH, eds. Etiology, pathology, and treatment of hepatocellular carcinoma in North America. Houston, TX: Gulf Publishing, 1991:255–272.

64. Anonymous. Lipiodol computed tomography for small hepatocellular carcinomas. Lancet 1991;337:333–334.

65. Novell R, Dusheiko G, Hilson A, Dick R, Begent R, Hobbs, K. Lipiodol computed tomography for small hepatocellular carcinomas. Lancet 1991;337(8743):729.

66. Houn HY, Sanders MM, Walker EM Jr, Pappas AA. Fine needle aspiration in the diagnosis of liver neoplasms: A review. Ann Clin Lab Sci 1991;21:2–11.

67. Chen MF, Hwang TL, Tsao KC, Sun CF, Chen TJ. Flow cytometric DNA analysis of hepatocellular carcinoma: Preliminary report. Surgery 1991;109:455–459.

68. Tarao K, Shimizu A, Harada M, et al. *In vitro* uptake of bromodeoxyuridine by human hepatocellular carcinoma and its relations to histopathologic findings and biologic behavior. Cancer 1991;68:1789–1798.

69. Hayashi N, Tamaki N, Yonekura Y, et al. Imaging of the hepatocellular carcinoma using dynamic positron emission tomography with nitrogen-13 ammonia. J Nucl Med 1985;26:254–257.

70. Gilbert SA, Brown PH, Krishnamurthy GT. Quantitative nuclear hepatology. J Nucl Med Tech 1987;15(1):38–43.

71. Drane WE, Krasicky GA, Johnson DA. Radionuclide imaging of primary tumors and tumor-like conditions of the liver. Clin Nucl Med 1987;12:569–582.

72. Pons F, Lomena F, Calvet X, et al. Uptake of technetium-99m DISIDA by bone metastasis from a hepatoma. Clin Nucl Med 1988;13:280–282.

73. McIntyre N. The limitations of conventional liver function tests. Sem Liver Dis 1983;3(4):265–274.

74. Gottlieb MC, Stratton HH, Newell JC, Shah DM. Indocyanine green: Its use as an early indicator of hepatic dysfunction following injury in man. Arch Surg 1984;119:264–268.

75. Monroe DS, Baker AL, Schneider JF, Krager PS, Klein PD, Schoeller D. The aminopyrine breath test and serum bile acids reflect histologic severity in chronic hepatitis. ABP Chron Hep 1982;2(3):317–322.

76. Takasaki T, Kobayashi S, Suzuki S, et al. Predetermining postoperative hepatic function for hepatectomies. Int Surg 1980;65(4):09–313.

77. Ikamoto E, Kyo A, Yamanaka N, Tanaka N, Kuwata K. Prediction of the safe limits of hepatectomy by combined volumetric and functional measurements in patients with impaired hepatic function. Surgery 1984;95(5):586–591.

78. Kanematsu T, Takenaka K, Matsumata T, Furuta T, Sugimachi K, Inokuchi K. Limited

hepatic resection effective for selected cirrhotic patients with primary liver cancer. Ann Surg 1984;199(1):51–56.

79. Yamanaka N, Okamoto E, Kuwata K, Tanaka N. A multiple regression equation for prediction of posthepatectomy liver failure. Ann Surg 1984;200(5):658–663.

80. Mimura H, Takakura N, Ohno Y, et al. Determination of the extent of feasible hepatic resection from hepatic blood flow. World J Surg 1986;10:302–310.

81. Stimpson RE, Pellegrini CA, Way LW. Factors affecting the morbidity of elective liver resection. Am J Surg 1987;153:189–195.

82. Matsumata T, Kanematsu T, Yoshida Y, Furuta T, Yanaga K, Sugimachi K. The indocyanine green test enables prediction of postoperative complications after hepatic resection. World J Surg 1987;2(5):678–681.

83. Laverero M, Tagger A, Balsano C, et al. Antibodies to hepatitis C virus in patients with hepatocellular carcinoma. J Hepatol 1991;12:60–63.

84. Di Bisceglie AM, Order SE, Klein JL, et al. The role of chronic viral hepatitis in hepatocellular carcinoma in the United States. Am J Gastroenterol 1991;86(3):335–338.

85. McMahon BJ, London T. National Cancer Institute workshop on screening for hepatocellular carcinoma. J Natl Cancer Inst 1991;83(13):916–919.

86. Beasley RP. Hepatitis B virus: The major etiology of hepatocellular carcinoma. Cancer 1988;61:1942–1954.

87. Heyward WL, Lanier AP, Bender TR, et al. Primary hepatocellular carcinoma in Alaskan natives. Int J Cancer 1981;28:47–50.

88. Heyward WL, Bender TR, Kilkenny S, et al. Early detection of primary hepatocellular carcinoma by screening for alpha-fetoprotein in high-risk families. Lancet 1983:1161–1162.

89. Popper H, Thung SN, McMahon BJ, Lanier AP, Hawkins I, Alberts SR. Evolution of hepatocellular carcinoma associated with chronic hepatitis B virus infection in Alaskan Eskimos. Arch Pathol Lab Med 1988;112:498–504.

90. Dodd RY, Nath N. Increased risk for lethal forms of liver disease among HBsAg-positive blood donors in the United States. J Virol Methods 1987;17:81–94.

91. Cattone M, Turri M, Caltagirone M, et al. Early detection of hepatocellular carcinoma associated with cirrhosis using ultrasound and alfa-fetoprotein: A prospective study. Hepatogastroenterology 1988;35:101–103.

92. Kanematsu T, Sonoda T, Takenada K, Matsumata T, Sugimachi K, Inokuchi K. The valve of ultrasound in the diagnosis and treatment of small hepatocellular carcinoma. Br J Surg 1985;72:23–25.

93. Colombo M, de Franchis R, Del Ninno E, et al. Hepatocellular carcinoma in Italian patients with cirrhosis. N Engl J Med 1991;325:675–680.

94. Colombo M, Mannucci PM, Brettler DB, et al. Hepatocellular carcinoma in hemophilia. Am J Hematol 1991;37:243–246.

95. Hoofnagle JH. Toward universal vaccination against hepatitis B virus. N Engl J Med 1989;9:1333–1334.

96. Abelev GI, Perova SD, Khramkova NI, Postnikova ZA, Irlin IS. Production of embryonal α-globulin by transplantable mouse hepatomas. Transplantation 1963;1:174–180.

97. Tatarinov, YS. Detection of embryospecific α-globulin in the blood sera of patients with primary liver tumor. Vopr Med Khim 1964;10:90–91.

98. Waldmann TA, McIntire KR. The use of a radioimmunoassay for alpha-fetoprotein in the diagnosis of malignancy. Cancer 1974;34:1510–1515.

99. Matsumoto Y, Suzuki T, Asada I, Ozawa K, Tobe T, Honjo I. Clinical classification of hepatoma in Japan according to serial changes in serum alpha-fetoprotein levels. Cancer 1982;49:354–360.

100. Bellet DH, Wands JR, Isselbacher KJ, Bohoun C. Serum α-fetoprotein levels in human disease: Perspective from a highly specific monoclonal radioimmunoassay. Proc Natl Acad Sci USA 1984;81:3869–3873.

101. McIntire KR, Vogel CL, Primack A, Waldmann TA, Kyalwazi SK. Effect of surgical and chemotherapeutic treatment on alpha-fetoprotein levels in patients with hepatocellular carcinoma. Cancer 1976;37:677–683.

102. Buamah PK, Cornell C, James OFW, Skillen AW, Harris AL. Serial serum AFP heterogeneity changes in patients with hepatocellular carcinoma during chemotherapy. Cancer Chemother Pharmacol 1986;17:182–184.

103. Liebman HA, Furie BC, Tong MJ, et al. DES-γ-carboxy (abnormal) prothrombin as a serum marker of primary hepatocellular carcinoma. N Engl J Med 1984;310(22):1427–1431.

104. Lefrere JJ, Gozin D, Soulier JP, et al. Specificity of increased des-gamma-carboxy prothrombin in hepatocellular carcinoma after vitamin K1 injection. J Hepatol 1987;5:27–29.

105. Fujiyama S, Morishita T, Hashiguchi O, Sato T. Plasma abnormal prothrombin (des-γ-carboxy prothrombin) as a marker of hepatocellular carcinoma. Cancer 1988;61:1621–1628.

106. Sakon M, Monden M, Gotoh M, et al. The effects of vitamin K on the generation of des-γ-Carboxy prothrombin (PIVKA-II) in patients with hepatocellular carcinoma. Am J Gastroenterol 1991;86(3):339–345.

107. Melia WM, Johnson PJ, Carter S, Munro-Neville A, Williams R. Plasma carcinoembryonic antigen in the diagnosis and management of patients with hepatocellular carcinoma. Cancer 1981;48:1004–1008.

108. Paradinas JF, Melia WM, Wilkinson ML, et al. High serum vitamin B12 binding capacity as a marker of the fibrolamellar variant of hepatocellular carcinoma. Br Med J 1982;285:840–842.

109. Collier NA, Bloom SR, Hodgson HJF, Weinbren K, Lee YC, Blumgart LH. Neurotensin secretion by fibrolamellar carcinoma of the liver. Lancet 1984;538–540.

110. Sawabu N, Nakagen M, Ozaki K, Wakabayashi T, Toya D, Hattori N, Ishii M. Clinical evaluation of specific γ-GTP isoenzyme in patients with hepatocellular carcinoma. Cancer 1983;51:327–331.

111. Melia WM, Bullock S, Johnson PJ, William R. Serum ferritin in hepatocellular carcinoma. Cancer 1983;51:2112–2115.

112. Kaneto A, Kubo Y, Nagasaki Y, et al. Clinical evaluation of serum ferritin in hepatocellular carcinoma and liver cirrhosis. Kanzo 1980;21(6):745–753.

113. Kew MC, Fisher JW. Serum erythropoietin concentrations in patients with hepatocellular carcinoma. Cancer 1986;58:2485–2488.

114. Yeh YC, Tsai JF, Chuang LY, et al. Elevation of transforming growth factor α and its relationship to the epidermal growth factor and α-fetoprotein levels in patients with hepatocellular carcinoma. Cancer Res 1987;47:896–901.

115. Derynck R, Goeddel DV, Ullrich A, et al. Synthesis of messenger RNAs for transforming growth factors α and β and the epidermal growth factor receptor by human tumors. Cancer Res 1987;47:707–712.

116. Ito N, Kawata S, Tamura S, et al. Elevated levels of transforming growth factor β messenger RNA and its polypeptide in human hepatocellular carcinoma. Cancer Res 1991;51:4080–4083.

117. Lee FY, Lee SK, Tsai YT, Wu JC, Lai KH, Lo KJ. Serum C-reactive protein as a serum marker for the diagnosis of hepatocellular carcinoma. Cancer 1989;63:1567–1571.

118. Grieco A, Stefano VD, Cassano A, et al. Hepatocellular carcinoma in cirrhosis: Is antithrombin III a neoplastic marker? Dig Dis Sci 1991;36(7):990–992.

119. Haglund C, Lindgren J, Roberts PJ, Nordling S. Difference in tissue expression of tumor markers CA 19-9 and CA 50 in hepatocellular carcinoma and cholangiocarcinoma. Br J Cancer 1991;63:386–389.

120. Fabris C, Basso DA, Leandro G, et al. Serum CA 19-9 and alpha-fetoprotein levels in primary hepatocellular carcinoma and liver cirrhosis. Cancer 1991;68:1795–1798.

121. Luis Gazz. Chir, 1896.

122. Malt R. Current concepts: Surgery for hepatic neoplasms. N Engl J Med 1985;313(25):1591–1596.

123. Guest J, Blumgart LH. Surgery of liver tumors. Clin Gastroenterol 1987;1(1):131–150.

124. Schwartz S. Hepatic resection. Ann Surg 1990;211(1):1–8.

125. Delva E, Barberousse JP, Nordlinger B, et al. Hemodynamic and biochemical monitoring during major liver resection with use of hepatic vascular exclusion. Surgery 1984;95(3):309–318.

126. Hodgson WJB, DelGuercio RM. Preliminary experience in liver surgery using the ultrasonic scalpel. Surgery 1984;95(2):230–234.

127. Ottow RY, Barbieri SA, Sugarbaker PH, Wesley RA. Liver transection: A controlled study of four different techniques in pigs. Surgery 1985;97(5):596–601.

128. Nagao R, Kawano N, Morioka Y. A new instrument for hepatic resection. Surg Gynecol Obstet 1988;166:269–271.

129. Couinaud CM. A simplified method for controlled left hepatectomy. Surgery 1985;97(3):358–361.

130. Franco D, Bonnet P, Smadja C, Grange D. Surgical resection of segment VIII (anterosuperior subsegment of the right lobe) in patients with liver cirrhosis and hepatocellular carcinoma. Surgery 1985;98(5):949–953.

131. Starzl TE, Koep LJ, Weil R III, Lilly JR, Putnam CW, Aldrete JA. Right trisegmentectomy for hepatic neoplasms. Surg Gynecol Obstet 1980;150:208–214.

132. Couinaud C. Exposure of the left hepatic duct through the hilum or in the umbilical of the liver: Anatomic limitations. Surgery 1989;105(1):21–27.

133. Carabasi RA III, Messerschmidt WH, Jarrell BE, Vernick JJ, Rosato FE. A method for protection of the left hepatic duct during right hepatic trisegmentectomy. Surg Gynecol Obstet 1986;162:190–198.

134. Bengmark S, Ekberg H, Evander A, Klofver-Stahl B, Tranberg KG. Major liver resection for hilar cholangiocarcinoma. Ann Surg 1988;207(2):120–125.

135. Hasegawa H, Makuuchi M, Yamazaki S, Gunven P. Central bisegmentectomy of the liver: Experience in 16 patients. World J Surg 1989;13:786–190.

136. Nimura Y, Hayadawa N, Kamiya J, et al. Combined portal vein and liver resection for carcinoma of the biliary tract. Br J Surg 1991;78:727–731.

137. Tashiro S, Uchino R, Hiraoka T, et al. Surgical indication and significance of portal vein resection in biliary and pancreatic cancer. Surgery 1991;109(4):481–487.

138. Nimura Y, Hayakawa H, Kamiya J, et al. Hepatopancreatoduodenectomy for advanced carcinoma of the biliary tract. Hepatogastroenterology 1991;38(2):170–175.

139. Qu QJ, Hermann RE. The role of hepatic veins in liver operations. Surgery 1984;95(4):381–391.

140. Makuuchi M, Hasegawa H, Yamazaki S, Takayasu K. Four new hepatectomy procedures for resection of the right hepatic vein and preservation of the inferior right hepatic vein. Surg Gynecol Obstet 1987;164:69–72.

141. Igawa S, Kinoshita H, Sakai K. Clinical significance of intraoperative sonography on hepatectomy in primary carcinoma of the liver. World J Surg 1984;8:772–777.

142. Sheu JC, Lee CS, Sung JL, Chen DS, Yang PM, Lin TY. Intraoperative hepatic ultrasonography: An indispensable procedure in resection of small hepatocellular carcinomas. Surgery 1985;97(1):97–103.

143. Castaing D, Emond J, Kunstlinger F, Bismuth H. Utility of operative ultrasound in the surgical management of liver tumors. Ann Surg 1986;204(5):600–605.

144. Machi J, Isomoto H, Yamashita Y, Kurohiji T, Shirouzu K, Kakegawa T. Intraoperative ultrasonography in screening for liver metastases from colorectal cancer: Comparative accuracy with traditional procedures. Surgery 1987;101(6):678–684.

145. Rifkin MD, Rosato FE, Branch HM, Foster J, Yang SL, Barbot DJ, Marks GJ. Intraoperative ultrasound for the liver: An important adjunctive tool for decision making in the operating room. Ann Surg 1987;205(5):466–472.

146. Makuuchi M, Hasegawa H, Yamazaki S, Takayasu K, Moriyama N. The use of operative ultrasound as an aid to liver resection in patients with hepatocellular carcinoma. World J Surg 1987;11:615–621.

147. Bismuth H, Castaing D, Garden J. The use of operative ultrasound in surgery of primary liver tumors. World J Surg 1987;11:610–614.
148. Takada T, Yasuda H, Uchiyama K, Hasegawa H, Shikata J. Contrast-enhanced intraoperative ultrasonography of small hepatocellular carcinomas. Surgery 1990;107: 528–532.
149. Yanaga K, Kanematsu T, Takenaka K, Sugimachi K. Intraperitoneal septic complications after hepatectomy. Ann Surg 1986;203(2):148–152.
150. Starzl TC, Putnam CW, Groth CG, Corman JL, Taubman J. Alopecia, ascites and incomplete regeneration after 85–90% liver resection. Am J Surg 1975;125:587–590.
151. Weinblatt ME, Siegel SE, Siegel MM, Stanley P, Weitzman JJ. Preoperative chemotherapy for unresectable primary hepatic malignancies in children. Cancer 1982;50: 1061–1064.
152. Nonami T, Isshiki K, Katoh H, et al. The potential role of postoperative hepatic artery chemotherapy in patients with high-risk hepatomas. Ann Surg 1991;213(3):222–226.
153. Spear AG, Cotton PB, Russell RCG. Randomized trial of endoscopic versus percutaneous stent insertion in malignant obstructive jaundice. Lancet 1987;1:57–62.
154. Matsuda Y, Shimakura K, Akamatsu T. Factors affecting the patency of stents in malignant biliary obstructive disease: Univariate and multivariate analysis. Am J Gastroenterol 1991;86(7):843–849.
155. Neuhaus H, Hagenmuller F, Griebel M, Classen M. Percutaneous cholangioscopic or transpapillary insertion of self-expanding biliary metal stents. Gastrointest Endosc 1991;37:31–37.
156. Jackson JE, Roddie ME, Chetty N, Benjamin IS, Adam A. The management of occluded metallic self-expandable biliary endoprosthesis. AJR 1991;157(2):291–292.
157. Akimaru K, Uchiyama K, Saito M, Ishimura Y, Kanauchi S, Shoji T. Subcutaneous portal reservoir for chemotherapy of metastatic carcinoma of the liver. Surg Gynecol Obstet 1984;158:93–94.
158. Schwarty SI, Jones LS, McCune CS. Assessment of treatment of intrahepatic malignancies using chemotherapy via an implantable pump. Ann Surg 1985;201(5):560–567.
159. Zhou XD, Tank ZY, Yu YQ, Ma ZC. Clinical evaluation of cryosurgery in the treatment of primary liver cancer. Cancer 1988;61:1889–1892.
160. Ravikumar TS, Kane R, Cady B, et al. Hepatic cryosurgery with intraoperative ultrasound monitoring for metastatic colon cancer. Arch Surg 1987;122:403–409.
161. Masters A, Steger AC, Bown SG. Role of interstitial therapy in the treatment of liver cancer. Br J Surg 1991;78:518–523.
162. Dagradi AD, Mangiante GL, Marchiori LAM, Nicoli NM. Repeated hepatic resection. Int Surg 1987;72:87–92.
163. Kanematsu T, Matsumata T, Takenada K, Yoshida Y, Higashi H, Sugimachi. Clinical management of recurrent hepatocellular carcinoma after primary resection. Br J Surg 1988;75:203–206.
164. Nagao T, Inoue S, Yoshimi F, et al. Postoperative recurrence of hepatocellular carcinoma. Ann Surg 1990;211(1):28–33.
165. Starzl TE, Demetris AJ, Van Thiel D. Liver transplantation, first of two parts. N Engl J Med 1989;321(15):1014–1022.
166. Starzl TE, Demetris AJ, Van Thiel D. Liver transplantation, second of two parts. N Engl J Med 1989;321(16):1092–1099.
167. Iwatsuki S, Klintmalm GBG, Starzl TE. Total hepatectomy and liver replacement (orthotopic liver transplantation) for primary hepatic malignancy. World J Surg 1982;6: 81–85.
168. Iwatsuki S, Gordon RD, Shaw BE Jr, Starzl TE. Role of liver transplantation in cancer therapy. Ann Surg 1985;202(4):401–407.
169. National Institutes of Health Consensus Development Conference Statement on Liver Transplantation, June 20–23, 1983. Hepatology 1984;4(1):107S–110S.
170. Diethelm AG. Ethical decisions in the history of organ transplantation. Ann Surg 1990;211(5):505–520.
171. Strong R, Ong TH, Pillay P, Wall D, Balderson G, Lynch S. A new method of segmental orthotopic liver transplantation in children. Surgery 1988;104(1):104–107.
172. Tzakis AG, Todo S, Madariaga J, Tzoracoeleftherakis E, Fung J, Starzl TE. Upper-abdominal exenteration in transplantation for extensive malignancies of the upper abdomen: An update. Transplantation 1991;51(3):727–728.
173. Busuttil RW, Goldstein LI, Danovitch GM, Ament ME, Memsic LDF. Liver transplantation today. Ann Intern Med 1986;104:377–389.
174. Ringe B, Pichlmayr R, Wittekind C, Tusch G. Surgical treatment of hepatocellular carcinoma: Experience with liver resection and transplantation in 198 patients. World J Surg 1991;15:270–285.
175. Penn I. Hepatic transplantation for primary and metastatic cancer of the liver. Surgery 1991;110(4):726–735.
176. Kim YI, Calne RY, Nagasue N. Cyclosporin A stimulates proliferation of the liver cells after partial hepatectomy in rats. Surg Gynecol Obstet 1988;166:317–322.
177. Mazzaferro V, Porter KA, Scotti-Foglieni CL, et al. The hepatotropic influence of cyclosporine. Surgery 1990;107:533–539.
178. Yokoyama I, Carr B, Saitsu H, Iwatsuki S, Starzl TE. Accelerated growth rates of recurrent hepatocellular carcinoma after liver transplantation. Cancer 1991;68:2095–2100.
179. Ingold JA, Reed GB, Kaplan HS, Bagshaw MA. Radiation hepatitis. AJR 1965;93:200–208.
180. Phillips R, et al. Roentgen therapy of hepatic metastases. Am J Roentgenol Radiat Ther Nucl Med 1954;71:826–834.
181. Hendry JH. Response of human organs to single (or fractionated equivalent) doses of irradiation. Int J Radiat Oncol Biol Phys 1989;(56)5:691–700.
182. Austin-Seymour MM, Chen GT, Castro JR, et al. Dose volume histogram analysis of liver radiation tolerance. Int J Radiat Oncol Biol Phys 1986;(12)1:31–5.
183. Lewin K, Millis RR. Human radiation hepatitis. A morphologic study with emphasis on the last changes. Arch Pathol 1973;96:21–26.
184. Tefft M, Mitus A, Jaffe N. Irradiation of the liver in children: Acute effects enhanced by concomitant chemotherapeutic administration. AJR 1971;111:165.
185. Anscher MS, Crocker IR, Jirtle RL. Transforming growth factor-beta-1 expression in irradiated liver. Radiat Res 1990;122(1):77–85.
186. Johnson DW, Safai C, Goffinet DR. Malignant obstructive jaundice: Treatment with external beam and intracavitary radiotherapy. Int J Radiat Oncol Biol Phys 1985;11: 411–416.
187. Flickinger JC, Epstein AH, Iwatsuki S, et al. Radiotherapy for primary carcinoma of the extrahepatic biliary system: An analysis of 63 cases. Cancer 1991;68:289–294.
188. Todoroki T. The late effects of single massive irradiation with electrons of the liver hilum of rabbits. Jpn J Gastroenterol Surg 1978;11:169.
189. Sindelar WF, Tepper J, Travis EL. Tolerance of bile duct to inoperative irradiation. Surgery 1982;92:533.
190. Okuda K, Obata H, Nakajima Y, Ohtsuki T, Okazaki N, Ohnishi K. Prognosis of primary hepatocellular carcinoma. Hepatology 1984;4:3S–6S.
191. Cheng EW-K, Lightdale CJ. Primary liver cancer: Diagnosis and laboratory findings. In: Wanebo HJ, ed. Hepatic and biliary cancer. New York: Marcel Dekker, 1987.
191a. Carr BI. J Surg Oncol 1993 (in press).
192. Ebara M, Ohto M, Shinegawa T, Sugiura N, Kimura K, et al. Natural history of minute hepatocellular carcinoma smaller than three centimeters complicating cirrhosis. Gastroenterology 1986;90:289–298.
193. Tang ZY. Subclinical hepatocellular carcinoma. Beijing: China Academic Publishing; Berlin: Springer-Verlag, 1985.
194. Okuda K, Ohtsuki T, Obata H, et al. Natural history of hepatocellular carcinoma and prognosis in relation to treatment: Study of 850 Patients. Cancer 1985;56:918–928.
195. Yamanaka N, Okamoto E, Foyosaka A, et al. Prognostic factors after hepatectomy for hepatocellular carcinoma. Cancer 1990;65:1104–1110.
196. Lee C-S, Sung J-L, Hwang L-Y, et al. Surgical management of 109 patients with symptomatic and asymptomatic hepatocellular carcinoma. Surgery 1986;99:481–490.
197. Iwatsuki S, Starzl TE, Sheahan DA, et al. Hepatic resection versus transplantation for hepatocellular carcinoma. Ann Surg 1991;214:221–229.
198. Franco D, Capussotti L, Smadja C, et al. Resection of hepatocellular carcinoma. Gastroenterology 1990;98:733–738.
199. Nagao T, Inoue S, Goto S, et al. Hepatic resection for hepatocellular carcinoma. Ann Surg 1987;205:33–40.
200. Nagorney DM, Van Heerden JA, Illstrup DM, Adson MA. Primary hepatic malignancy: Surgical management and determinants of survival. Surgery 1989;106:740–749.
201. Beghiti J, Panis Y, Farges, et al. Intrahepatic recurrence after resection of hepatocellular carcinoma complicating cirrhosis. Ann Surg 1991;241:114–117.
202. Nagao T, Inoue S, Yoshimi F, et al. Post-operative recurrence of hepatocellular carcinoma. Ann Surg 1990;211:28–33.
203. Nagasue N, Yukaya H, Chang Y-C, et al. Assessment of pattern and treatment of intrahepatic recurrence after resection of hepatocellular carcinoma. Surg Gynecol Obstet 1990;171:217–222.
204. Imaoka S, Sasaki Y, Shibata T, et al. A pre-operative chemoembolization therapy using lipiodol, cisplatin and gelatin sponge for hepatocellular carcinoma. Cancer Chemother Pharmacol 1989;23:S126–S128.
205. Nagasue N, Galizia A, Kohno H, et al. Adverse effects of preoperative hepatic artery chemoembolization for resectable hepatocellular carcinoma. Surgery 1989;106:81–86.
206. Ismail T, Angrisani L, Gunson BK, et al. Primary hepatic malignancy: The role of liver transplantation. Br J Surg 1990;77:983–986.
207. Bismuth H, Ericson BJ, Rolles K, et al. Hepatic transplantation in Europe. Lancet 1987;2:674–676.
208. Olthoff KM, Millis M, Rosove MH. Is liver transplantation justified for the treatment of hepatic malignancies? Arch Surg 1990;125:1261–1268.
209. O'Grady JG, Polson RJ, Rolles K, et al. Liver transplantation for malignant disease. Ann Surg 1987;207:373–379.
210. Yokoyama I, Todo S, Iwatsuki S, Starzl TE. Liver transplantation in the treatment of primary liver cancer. Hepatogastroenterology 1990;37:188–193.
211. Stone MJ, Klintmalm G, Polter D, et al. Neo-adjuvant chemotherapy and orthotopic liver transplantation for hepatocellular carcinoma. Transplantation 1989;48:344–347.
212. Carr BI, Starzl TE, Iwatsuki S, Van Thiel D. Aggressive treatment for advanced hepatocellular carcinoma: High response rates and prolonged survival. Hepatology 1991;14:243.
213. Lee Y-T N. Systemic and regional treatment of primary carcinoma of the liver. Cancer Treat Rev 1977;4:195–212.
213a. Carr BI. High objective response rates of advanced hepatocellular carcinoma to intra-arterial chemotherapy. Proc ASCO 1992;11:470.
214. Nerenstone SR, Ihde DC, Friedman MA. Clinical trials in primary hepatocellular carcinoma: Current status and future directions. Cancer Treat Rev 1988;15:1–31.
214a. Carr BI. A controlled prospective randomized trial comparing intra-arterial (I/A)cis-platinum, doxorubicin and S/Q interferon alpha, with or without lipiodol for hepatocellular carcinoma (HCC). Hepatology 1992;16:60.
215. Sciarrino E, Simonetti R, LeMoli S, et al. Adriamycin treatment for hepatocellular carcinoma: Experience with 109 patients. Cancer 1985;56:2751–2754.
216. Chlebowski RT, Brzechwa-Adjukiewica A, Cowden A, et al. Doxorubicin (75 mg/m²)

for hepatocellular carcinoma: Clinical and pharmacokinetic results. Cancer Treat Rep 1984;68:487–491.

217. Ihde DC, Kane RC, Cohen MH, et al. Adriamycin therapy in American patients with hepatocellular carcinoma. Cancer Treat Rep 1977;61:1385–1387.

218. Falkson G, MacIntyre JM, Moertel CG, et al. Primary liver cancer: An Eastern Cooperative Oncology Group trial. Cancer 1984;54:970–977.

219. Ravry JR, Omura GA, Bartolucci AA. Phase II evaluation of doxorubicin plus bleomycin in hepatocellular carcinoma: A Southeastern Cancer Study Group trial. Cancer Treat Rep 1984;68:1517–1518.

220. Cavalli F, Rozencweig M, Goldhirsch A, Hansen HH. Phase II study of oral VP-16–213 in hepatocellular carcinoma. Eur J Cancer Clin Oncol 1981;17:1079–1082.

221. Melia WM, Johnson PG, Williams R. Induction of remission in hepatocellular carcinoma. Cancer 1983;51:206–210.

222. Melia WM, Westaby D, Williams R. Diamminodichloride platinum (cisplatinum) in the treatment of hepatocellular carcinoma. Clin Oncol 1981;7:275–280.

223. Ravry JR, Onura GA, Bartolucci AA, et al. Phase II evaluation of cisplatinum in advanced hepatocellular carcinoma and cholangiocarcinoma: A Southeastern Cancer Study Group trial. Cancer Treat Rep 1986;70:311–312.

224. Falkson G, Ryan LM, Johnson LA, et al. A randomized phase II study of mitoxantrone and cisplatin in patients with hepatocellular carcinoma: An ECOG study. Cancer 1987;60:2141–2145.

225. Onohara S, Kobayashi H, Itoh Y, et al. Intra-arterial cis-platinum infusion with sodium thiosulfate protection and angiotensin II induced hypertension for treatment of hepatocellular carcinoma. Acta Radiologica 1988;29:197–202.

226. Kajanti M, Rissanen P, Virkkunen P, et al. Regional intra-arterial infusion of cisplatin in primary hepatocellular carcinoma. Cancer 1986;58:2386–2388.

227. Ando K, Hirai K, Kubo Y. Intra-arterial administration of epirubicin in the treatment of non-resectable hepatocellular carcinoma. Can Chemother Pharmacol 1987;19: 183–189.

228. Sasaki Y, Imacka S, Kasugai H, et al. A new approach to chemoembolization therapy for hepatoma using ethiodized oil, cisplatin, gelatin sponge. Cancer 1987;60:1194–1203.

229. Kasugai H, Kojima J, Tatsuta M, et al. Treatment of hepatocellular carcinoma by transcatheter arterial embolization combined with intraarterial infusion of a mixture of cisplatin and ethiodized oil. Gastroenterology 1989;97:965–971.

230. Ohnishi K, Tsuchiya S, Nakayama T, et al. Arterial chemoembolization of hepatocellular carcinoma with mitomycin C microcapsules. Radiology 1984;152:51–55.

231. Lin D. Liaw Y, Lee T, et al. Hepatic arterial embolization in patients with unresectable hepatocellular carcinoma: A randomized controlled trial. Gastroenterology 1988;94: 453–456.

232. Fujimoto S, Miyazaki M, Endoh F, et al. Biodegradable mitomycin C microspheres given intra-arterially for inoperable hepatic cancer. Cancer 1985;56:2404–2410.

233. Audisio RA, Doci R, Mazzaferro V, et al. Hepatic arterial embolization with microencapsulated mitomycin C for unresectable hepatocellular carcinoma occurring in cirrhosis. Cancer 1990;65:1211–1218.

234. Kobayashi H, Hidaka H, Kajiya Y, et al. Treatment of hepatocellular carcinoma by transarterial injection of anticancer agents in iodized oil suspension or of radioactive iodized oil solution. Acta Radiol Diagn 1986;27:139–147.

235. Kanematsu T, Furuta T, Takenaka K, et al. A 5-year experience of lipiodolization: Selective regional chemotherapy for 200 patients with hepatocellular carcinoma. Hepatology 1989;10:89–102.

236. Shibata J, Fujiyama S, Sata T, et al. Hepatic arterial injection chemotherapy with cisplatin suspended in an oily lymphographic agent for hepatocellular carcinoma. Cancer 1989;64:1586–1594.

237. Konno T, Maeda H, Iwai K, et al. Effect of arterial administration of high-molecular-weight anticancer agent SMANCS with lipid lymphographic agent on hepatoma: A preliminary report. Eur J Cancer Clin Oncol 1983;19:1053–1065.

238. Pelletier G, Roche A, Ink O. A randomized trial of hepatic arterial chemoembolization in patients with unresectable hepatocellular carcinoma. J Hepatology 1990;11:181–184.

239. Carr BI, Starzl TE, Iwatsuki S, et al. Aggressive treatment for advanced hepatocellular carcinoma (HCC): High response rates and prolonged survival. Hepatology 1991;14: 243.

240. Venook AP, Stagg RJ, Lewis BJ, et al. Chemoembolization for hepatocellular carcinoma. J Clin Oncol 1990;8:1108–1114.

241. Ohnishi K, Sugita S, Nomura F, et al. Arterial chemoembolization with mitomycin C microcapsules followed by transcatheter hepatic artery embolization for hepatocellular carcinoma. Am J Gastroenterol 1987;82:876–879.

242. Beppu T, Ohara C, Yamaguchi Y. A new approach to chemoembolization for unresectable hepatocellular carcinoma using aclarubicin microspheres in combination with cisplatin suspended in iodized oil. Cancer 1991;68:2555–2560.

243. Carr BI, Van Thiel DH. Hormonal manipulation of human hepatocellular carcinoma. J Hepatol 1990;11:287–289.

244. Farinati F, Salvagnini M, de Maria N, et al. Unresectable hepatocellular carcinoma: A prospective controlled trial with tamoxifen. J Hepatol 1990;11:297–301.

245. Engstrom PF, Levin B, Moertel CG, Schott A. A phase II trial of tamoxifen in hepatocellular carcinoma. Cancer 1990;65:2641–2643.

246. Gupta S, Korula J. Failure of ketoconazole as anti-androgen therapy in non-resectable primary hepatocellular carcinoma. J Clin Gastroenterol 1988;10:651–654.

247. Lai C-L, WU P-C, Lok A S-F, et al. Recombinant alpha-2 interferon is superior to doxorubicin for inoperable hepatocellular carcinoma: A prospective randomized trial. Br J Cancer 1989;60:928–933.

248. Edmonson, HB. Difficulty of diagnosis of tumors and tumor-like lesions of the liver in infancy and childhood. Am J Dis Child 1956;91:168–186.

249. Craig JP, Peters RL, Edmonson HB, Omaka M. Fibrolamellar carcinoma of the liver. Cancer 1980;46:312–319.

250. Berman, MM, Libbey NP, Faster JH. Hepatocellular carcinoma: Polygonal cell type with fibrous stroma—an atypical variant with favorable prognosis. Cancer 1980;46: 1448–1455.

251. Collier NA, Bloom SA, Hodgson HJF, Weinbren K, Lee TC, Blumgart LH. Neurotensin secretion by fibrolamellar carcinoma of the liver. Lancet 1986;1:538–569.

252. Wang J, Dhillon AP, Sanky EA, Wightman AK, Lewin JF, Scheuer PJ. Neuroendocrine differentiation in primary neoplasms of the liver. J Pathol 1991;163:61–67.

253. Starzl TE, Iwatsuki S, Shaw BW, et al. Treatment of fibrolamellar hepatoma with partial or total hepatectomy and transplantation of the liver. Surg Gynecol Obstet 1986;162:165–168.

254. Kingston JE, Herbert A, Draper GJ, Mann JR. Association between hepatoblastoma and polyposis coli. Arch Dis Child 1983;58:959–62.

255. Halpern E, Kun LE, Constine LS, et al. Pediatric radiation oncology. New York: Raven Press, 1989:280–288.

256. Stocker JT, Ishak KG. Hepatoblastoma. In: Okuda K, Ihak KG, eds. Neoplasms of the liver. New York: Springer-Verlag, 1987.

257. Lack EE, Neave C, Vawter GF. Hepatoblastoma: A clinical and pathologic study of 54 cases. Am J Surg Pathol 1982;6:693–705.

258. Mahour GH, Wogu GU, Siegel SE, Isaacs H. Improved survival in infants and children with primary malignant liver tumors. Am J Surg 1983;146:236–240.

259. Weinberg AG, Finegold MJ. Primary hepatic tumors of childhood. Human Pathol 1983;14:512–537.

260. Schmidt D, Harms D, Lang W. Primary malignant hepatic tumors in childhood. Virchows Arch A 1985;407:387–405.

261. Hata Y, Ishizu H, Ohmori K. Flow cytometric analysis of the nuclear DNA content of hepatoblastoma. Cancer 1991;68:2566–2570.

262. Evans AE, Land VJ, Newton WA, Randolph JG, Sather HN, Tefft M. Combination chemotherapy (vincristine, Adriamycin, cyclophosphamide, 5-fluorouracil) in the treatment of children with malignant hepatoma. Cancer 1982;50:821–826.

263. Filler RM, Ehrlich PF, Greenberg ML, Babyn PS. Preoperative chemotherapy in hepatoblastoma. Surgery 1991;110:591–597.

264. Habrand JL, Pritchard J. Role of radiotherapy in hepatoblastoma and hepatocellular carcinoma in children and adolescents: Results of a survey conducted by the SIOP Liver Tumour Study Group. J Med Pediatr Oncol 1991;19(3):208.

265. Ninane J, Perilongo G, Stalens JP, Guglielmi M, Otte JB, Mancini A. Effectiveness and toxicity of cisplatin and doxorubicin (PLADO) in childhood hepatoblastoma and hepatocellular carcinoma: A SIOP pilot study. J Med Pediatr Oncol 1991;19(3):199–203.

266. Ottow RT, August DA, Sugarbaker PH. Treatment of proximal biliary tract carcinoma: An overview of techniques and results. Surgery 1985;97:251–262.

267. Srivatanakul P, Parkin DM, Jiang Y, et al. The role of infection in *Opisthorchis viverrini*, hepatitis B virus, and aflatoxin exposure in the etiology of liver cancer in Thailand. Cancer 1991;68:2417.

268. Kew MC. Tumors of the liver. In: Rakim D, Boyer TD, ed. Hepatology: A textbook of liver disease. 2nd ed. Philadelphia: WB Saunders, 1990:1206–1240.

269. Chen MF, Jan YY, Wang CS, et al. Clinical experience in 20 hepatic resections for peripheral cholangiocarcinoma. Cancer 1989;64(11):2226–32.

270. Tsunoda T, Furui J, Yamada M, Eto T, et al. Caroli's disease associated with hepatolithiasis: A case report and review of the Japanese literature. Gastroenterol Jpn 1991;26(1)74–79.

271. Marsh JW, Iwatsuki S, Makowka L, et al. Orthotopic liver transplantation for primary sclerosing cholangitis. Ann Surg 1988;207:21–25.

272. Rosen CB, Nagorney DM, Wiesner RH, et al. Cholangiocarcinoma complicating primary sclerosing cholangitis. Ann Surg 1991;213:21–25.

273. Arnaud JP, Graf P, Granfort JL, et al. Primary carcinoma of the gallbladder: Review of 25 cases. Am J Surg 1979;138:403.

274. Polk HC. Carcinoma of the calcified gallbladder. Gastroenterology 1966;50:582.

275. Terada T, Nakanuma Y. Pathological observations of intrahepatic peribiliary glands in 1,000 consecutive autopsy livers. II. A possible source of cholangiocarcinoma. Hepatology 1990;12:92–97.

276. Goodnight JE. Bile duct carcinoma. Surg Clin North Am 1981;61:981–986.

277. Nakajima T, Konda Y, Miyazaki M, Okui K. A histopathologic study of 102 cases of intrahepatic cholangiocarcinoma: Histologic classification and modes of spreading. Hum Pathol 1988;19:1228–1234.

278. Park CM, Cha IH, Chung KB, et al. Hepatocellular carcinoma in extrahepatic bile ducts. Acta Radiologica 1991;32:34–36.

279. Hsu W, Deziel DJ, Gould VE. Neuroendocrine differentiation and prognosis of extrahepatic biliary tract carcinomas. Surgery 1991;110:065–611.

280. Guo K, Yamaguchi K, Enjoji M. Undifferentiated carcinoma of the gallbladder: A clinicopathologic immuno-histochemical study of 21 patients with a poor prognosis. Cancer 1988;61:1872–1879.

281. Haglund C, Lindgren J, Roberts PJ, Nordling S. Difference in tissue expression of tumor markers CA 19-9 and CA 50 in hepatocellular carcinoma and cholangiocarcinoma. Br J Cancer 1991;63(3):386–9.

282. Voravud N, Foster CS, Gilbertson JA, et al. Oncogene expression in cholangiocarcinoma and in normal hepatic development. Hum Pathol 1989;20:1163–1168.

283. Suzuki M, Takahashi T, Oouchi K, Matsuno S. The development and extension of hepatohilar bile duct carcinoma: A three dimensional tumor mapping in the intrahepatic

biliary tree visualized with the aid of a graphics computer system. Cancer 1989;64:658–666.

284. Verbeek PM, Van Der Heyde MN, Ramsoekh T, Bosma A. Clinical significance of implantation metastases after surgical treatment of cholangiocarcinoma. Semin Liver Dis 1990;2:142–140.

285. Tsuzuki T, Kuramochi S, Sugioka A, et al. Postresection autopsy findings in patients with cancer of the main hepatic duct junction. Cancer 1991;67:3010–3013.

286. Falkson G, MacIntyre JM, Moertel CG. Eastern Cooperative Oncology Group experience with chemotherapy for inoperable gallbladder and bile duct cancer. Cancer 1984;54:965–969.

287. Davis HL Jr, Ramirez G, Ansfield FJ. Adenocarcinoma of stomach, pancreas, liver, and biliary tracts: Survival of 328 patients treated with fluoropyrimidine therapy. Cancer 1974;33:193–197.

288. Haskell CM. Cancer of the liver. In: Haskell CM, ed. Cancer treatment. Philadelphia: WB Saunders, 1980:319–357.

289. Stillwagon GB, Order SE, Klein JL, et al. Multimodality treatment of nonresectable intrahepatic cholangiocarcinoma with ^{131}I anti-CEA—a Radiation Therapy Oncology Group study. Int J Radiat Oncol Biol Phys 1987;13:687–695.

290. Crooke ST, Bradner WT. Mitomycin-C: A review. Cancer Treat Rev 1976;3:121–139.

291. Von Eyben F, Hellekant C, Mattson M, Ljungquist V, Jonsson K. Mitomycin-C in advanced gallbladder carcinoma. Acta Radiol 1980;19:81–84.

292. Bukowski RM, Leichman LP, Rivkin SE. Phase II trial of m-ASMA in gallbladder and cholangiocarcinoma: A Southwest Oncology Group study. Eur J Cancer Clin Oncol 1983;6:721–723.

293. Adolphson CC, Carpenter JT Jr. Response to doxorubicin and mitomycin in cholangiocarcinoma: A case report. Cancer Treat Rep 1982;66:209–210.

294. Bodey GP, Bedikian AY, Valdivieso M, et al. Chemotherapeutic management of hepatobiliary and pancreatic cancer. In: Stroehlein JR, Romsdahl MM, eds. Gastrointestinal cancer. New York: Raven Press, 1981:279–292.

295. Harvey JH, Smith FP, Schein PS. 5-Fluorouracil, mitomycin, and doxorubicin (FAM) in carcinoma of the biliary tract. J Clin Oncol 1984;2(11):1245–1248.

296. Uchiyama K, Takada T, Yasuda H, et al. A case of intrahepatic bile duct cancer responding to 5-fluorouracil, Adriamycin, and mitomycin C chemotherapy. Gan To Kagaku Ryoho (English abstract) 1988;15:1987–1990.

297. Tavey M Jr, Hester M. Phase II study of Adriamycin plus bleomycin for the treatment of hepatocellular and biliary tract carcinoma. Proc Am Soc Clin Oncol 1979;20:415.

298. Hall SH, Benjamin RS, Murphy WK, et al. Adriamycin, BCNU, ftorafur chemotherapy of pancreatic and biliary tract cancer. Cancer 1974;44:2008–2013.

299. Stillwagon GB, Order SG, Haulk T, et al. Variable low dose rate irradiation (^{131}I-Anti-CEA) and integrated low dose chemotherapy in the treatment of nonresectable primary intrahepatic cholangiocarcinoma. Int J Radiat Oncol Biol Phys 1991;21:1601–1605.

300. Shibata T, Sato T, Konda H, Ootani I, et al. Two cases of obstructive jaundice due to extrahepatic carcinoma of the bile duct with marked response to daily oral administration of etoposide. Gan To Kagaku Ryoho 1990;17(12):2429–32.

301. Koda K, Nakazawa O, Morita K, Kure T, et al. Combination chemotherapy of UFT with Adriamycin (ADM) and cisplatin (CDDP) for advanced gastrointestinal cancer. Gan To Kagaku Ryoho 1990;17(9):1893–900.

302. Novell JR, Dusheiko G, Markham NI, Reddy K, et al. Selective regional chemotherapy of unresectable hepatic tumours using lipiodol. HPB Surg 1991;4(3):223–34.

303. Yamaguchi Y, Takayma T, Kawami H, Sato Y, et al. LAK cell adoptive immunotherapy and its problems. Nippon Geka Gakkai Zasshi 1991;92(9):1234–1236.

304. Massey WH, Fletcher WS, Judkins MP, Dennis DL. Hepatic artery infusion for metastatic malignancy using percutaneously placed catheters. Am J Surg 1971;121:160.

305. Warren KW, Mountain JC, Lloyd-Jones W. Malignant tumors of the bile-ducts. Br J Surg 1972;59:501.

306. Watkins E Jr, Oberfield RA, Cady B, Clouse ME. Arterial infusion chemotherapy of diffuse hepatic malignancies. Prog Clin Cancer 1978;7:235.

307. Reed ML, Vaitkevicius VK, Al-Sarraf M, Vaughn CB, et al. The practicality of chronic hepatic artery infusion therapy of primary and metastatic malignancies: Ten-year results of 124 patients in a prospective protocol. Cancer 1981;47:402.

308. Seeger J, Woodcock TM, Blumenreich MS, Richardson JD. Hepatic perfusion with FUdR utilizing an implantable system in patients with liver primary cancer or metastatic cancer confined to the liver. Cancer Invest 1989;7(1):1–6.

309. Garnick MB, Ensminger WD, Israel M. A clinical-pharmacological evaluation of hepatic arterial infusion of Adriamycin. Cancer Res 1979;39:4105.

310. Wada H, Sasaki Y, Imaoka S, Shibata T, et al. Intra-arterial and intraportal therapy combined with decollateralization in unresectable cholangiocellular carcinoma: A case report. Gan To Kagaku Ryoho 1989;16(8):2867–70.

311. Chen M, Jan Y, Wang C, et al. Clinical experience in 20 hepatic resections for peripheral cholangiocarcinoma. Cancer 1989;64:2226–2232.

312. Altaee MY, Johnson PJ, Farrant JM, Williams R. Etiologic and clinical characteristics of peripheral and hilar cholangiocarcinoma. Cancer 1991;68:2051–2055.

313. Mori W, Nagasato K. Cholangiocarcinoma and related lesions. In: Okuda K, Peters RL, eds. Hepatocellular carcinoma. New York: John Wiley & Sons, 1976:227–246.

314. Reding R, Buard JL, Lebeau G, Launois B. Surgical management of 552 carcinomas of the extrahepatic bile ducts (gallbladder and periampullary tumors excluded). Results of the French Surgical Association Survey. Ann Surg 1991;213(3):236–41.

315. Tompkins RK, Saunders KD, Roslyn JJ, Longmire WP. Changing patterns in diagnosing and management of bile duct cancer. Ann Surg 1990;211:614–621.

316. Chao TC, Greager JA. Carcinoma of the extrahepatic bile ducts. J Surg Oncol 1991;46(3):145–50.

317. Mahe M, Romestaing P, Talon B, et al. Radiation therapy in extrahepatic bile duct carcinoma. Radiother Oncol 1991;21:121–127.

318. Kopelson G, Harisiadis L, Tretter P. The role of radiation therapy in cancer of the extrahepatic biliary system: An analysis of thirteen patients and a review of the literature on the effectiveness of surgery chemotherapy and radiotherapy. Int J Radiat Oncol Biol Phys 1977;2:883–894.

319. Dalton-Clarke HJ, Pearse E, Krause T, et al. Fine needle aspiration cytology and exfoliative biliary cytology and exfoliative biliary cytology in the diagnosis of hilar cholangiocarcinoma. Eur J Surg Oncol 1986;12:143–145.

320. Rabinovitz M, Zajko AB, Hassanein T, et al. Diagnostic value of brush cytology in the diagnosis of bile duct carcinomas: A study in 65 patients with bile duct strictures. Hepatology 1990;12:747–752.

321. Wetter LA, Ring EJ, Pellegrini CA, Way LW. Differential diagnosis of sclerosing cholangiocarcinomas of the common hepatic duct (Klatskin tumors). Am J Surg 1991;161:57–63.

322. Cameron JL, Pitt HA, Zinner MJ, et al. Management of proximal cholangiocarcinomas by surgical resection and radiotherapy. Am J Surg 1991;159:91–97.

323. Pitt HA, Roslyn JJ, Tompkins RK. Surgical resection of bile duct cancer: The UCLA exprience. In: Wanebo HJ, ed. Hepatic and biliary cancer. New York: Marcel Dekker, 1987:339–355.

324. Vogt DP. Current management of cholangiocarcinoma. Oncology 1988;2:37–44.

325. Grove MK, Hermann RE, Vogt DP, Broughan TA. Role of radiation after operative palliation in cancer of the proximal bile ducts. Am J Surg 1991;161(4):454–458.

326. Gonzales DG, Gerard JP, Maners AW, et al. Results of radiation therapy in carcinoma of the proximal bile duct (Klatskin tumor). Semin Liver Dis 1990;10(2):131–141.

327. Karani J, Fletcher M, Brinkley D, Dawson JL, Williams R, Nunnerly H. Internal biliary drainage and local radiotherapy with iridium-192 wire in treatment of hilar cholangiocarcinoma. Clin Radiol 1985;36:603–606.

328. Johnson DW, Safai C, Goffinet DR. Malignant obstructive jaundice: Treatment with external beam and intracavitary radiotherapy. Int J Radiat Oncol Biol Phys 1985;11:411–416.

329. Meyers WC, Jones RS. Internal irradiation for bile duct cancer. World J Surg 1988;12:99–104.

330. Fields JN, Emami B. Carcinoma of the extrahepatic biliary system: Results of primary and adjuvant radiotherapy. Int J Radiat Oncol Biol Phys 1987;13:331–338.

331. Iwasaki Y, Todoroki T, Fukao K, et al. The role of intraoperative radiation therapy in the treatment of bile duct cancer. World J Surg 1988;12:91–98.

332. Busse PM, Stone MD, Sheldon TA, et al. Intraoperative radiation therapy for biliary tract carcinoma: Results of a 5-year experience. Surgery 1989;10:724–733.

333. Minsky BD, Wesson MF, Armstrong JC, et al. Combined modality therapy of extrahepatic biliary system. Int J Radiat Oncol Biol Phys 1990;18:1157–1163.

334. Flickinger JC, Carr BI. Radiotherapy alone compared to liver transplantation and neoadjuvant chemoradiotherapy for hilar cholangiocarcinoma. Proc Ann Meeting Amer Radium Soc, 1992 [abstract]: 4–5.

335. Starzl TE, Todo S, Tzakis A, et al. Abdominal organ cluster transplantation for the treatment of upper abdominal malignancies. Ann Surg 1990;210:374.

336. Burgess P, Murphy PD, Clague MB. Adenocarcinoma of the gallbladder: A 5-year review of outcome in Newcastle upon Tyne. J R Soc Med 1991;842:84–86.

337. Silk YN, Douglass HO, Nava HR, et al. Carcinoma of the gallbladder: The Roswell Park experience. Ann Surg 1989;210:751–757.

338. Chao TC, Greager JA. Primary carcinoma of the gallbladder. J Surg Oncol 1991;46(4):215–221.

339. Wanebo HJ, Castle WN, Fechner RE. Is carcinoma of the gallbladder a curable lesion? Ann Surg 1982;195:624–631.

340. Nevin JE, Moran TJ, Kay S et al. Carcinoma of the gallbladder. Cancer 1976;37:141–148.

341. Bergdahl L. Gallbladder carcinoma first diagnosed at microscopic examination of gallbladders removed for presumed benign disease. Ann Surg 1980;191:19–22.

342. Morrow CE, Sutherland DE, Florack G et al. Primary gallbladder carcinoma: Significance of subserosal lesions and results of aggressive surgical treatment and adjuvant chemotherapy. Surgery 1983;94:709–714.

342. Frierson HF, Fechner RE. Pathology of malignant neoplasms of the gallbladder and extrahepatic bile ducts. In: Wanebo HJ, ed. Hepatic and biliary cancer. New York: Marcel Dekker, 1987:281–297.

343. Sumiyoshi K, Nagai E, Chijiiwa K, Nakayama F. Pathology of carcinoma of the gallbladder. J Surg 1991;15(3):315–21.

344. Guo K, Yamaguchi K, Enjoji M. Undifferentiated carcinoma of the gallbladder: A clinicopathologic, histochemical, and immunohistochemical study of 21 patients with a poor prognosis. Cancer 1988;61:1872–1879.

345. Vaittinen E. Carcinoma of the gallbladder: A study of 390 cases diagnosed in Finland 1953–1967. Ann Chir Gynaecol Fenn 1970;59 (Suppl 168):7–31.

346. Fahim RB, McDonald JR, Richards JC, Ferris DO. Carcinoma of the gallbladder: A study of its modes of spread. Ann Surg 1962;156:114–124.

347. Chijiiwa K, Sumiyoshi K, Nakayama F. Impact of recent advances in hepatobiliary imaging techniques on the preoperative diagnosis of carcinoma of the gallbladder. J Surg 1991;15(3):322–7.

348. Ogura Y, Mizumoto R, Isaji S, Kusuda T et al. Radical operations for carcinoma of the gallbladder: Present status in Japan. World J Surg 1991;15(3):337–43.

349. Kopelson G, Harisiadis L, Tretter P, et al. The role of radiation therapy in cancer of the extra-hepatic biliary system: An analysis of thirteen patients and a review of the literature of the effectiveness of surgery, chemotherapy and radiotherapy. Int J Radiat Oncol Biol Phys 1977;2:883–894.

350. Bosset JF, Mantion G, Gillet M, et al. Primary carcinoma of the gallbladder: Adjuvant postoperative external irradiation. Cancer 1989;64:1843–1847.

351. Houry S, Schlienger M, Huguier M, Lacaine F, Penne F, Laugier A. Gallbladder carcinoma: Role of radiation therapy. Br J Surg 1989;76:448–450.

352. Todoroki T, Iwasaki Y, Orii K, Otsuka M et al. Resection combined with intraoperative radiation therapy (IORT) for stage IV (TNM) gallbladder carcinoma. World J Surg 1991;15(3):357–366.

353. Busse PM, Cady B, Bothe A Jr, Jenkins R et al. Intraoperative radiation therapy for carcinoma of the gallbladder. World J Surg 1991;15(3):352–356.

354. Falkson G, MacIntyre JM, Moertel CG. Eastern Cooperative Oncology Group experience with chemotherapy for inoperable gallbladder and bile duct cancer. Cancer 1984;54:965–969.

355. Leese T, Farges O, Bismuth H. Liver cell adenomas: A 12-Year surgical experience from a specialist hepato-biliary unit. Ann Surg 1988;208(5):558–564.

356. Ishak KG, Sesterhen IA, Goodman ZD, et al. Epithelioid hemangioendothelioma of the liver. Hum Pathol 1984;15:839.

357. Ishak KG, Sesterhen IA, Goodman ZD, et al. Epithelioid hemangioendothelioma of the liver. Hum Pathol 1984;15:839.

358. Shin MS, Carpenter JT Jr, Ho KJ. Epithelioid hemangioendothelioma: CT manifestations and possible linkage to vinyl chloride exposure. J Comp Assist Tomogr 1991;15(3):505–7.

359. Weiss SW, Enzinger FM. Epithelioid hemangioendothelioma: a vascular tumor often mistaken for a carcinoma. Cancer 1982;50:970–81.

360. Makk L, Delmore F, Creech JL et al. Clinical and morphological features of hepatic angiosarcoma in vinyl chloride workers. Cancer 1976;37:149.

361. Stocker JT, Ishak KG. Undifferentiated (embryonal) sarcoma of the liver. Ann Surg 1955;141:246.

362. Leuschner I, Schmidt D, Harms D. Undifferentiated sarcoma of the liver in childhood: Morphology, flow cytometry, and literature review. Hum Pathol 1990;21(1):68–76.

Cancer: Principles & Practice of Oncology, Fourth Edition,
edited by Vincent T. DeVita, Jr., Samuel Hellman, Steven A. Rosenberg.
J.B. Lippincott Co., Philadelphia © 1993.

Daniel G. Coit

CHAPTER **29**

Cancer of the Small Intestine

Malignant and benign small bowel tumors are unusual. It is estimated that small bowel tumors comprise fewer than 10% of all gastrointestinal tumors, although their incidence depends on whether autopsy data are included.[1] Approximately two thirds of all small bowel tumors are malignant.[2-16] These account for 0.1% to 0.3% of all malignancies.[17-19] There are 2100 to 2400 new cases of small bowel malignancies annually in the United States, which is 0.4 to 1.0 cases per 100,000 persons, with a slight male predominance.[9,20-24] There are fewer than 1000 deaths from primary malignant small bowel tumors annually in the United States, which is a rate of approximately 0.5 deaths per 100,000 persons.[25] Approximately one third of small bowel tumors are benign, and the tumors affect men and women roughly equally.

Patients presenting with small bowel tumors are usually in their seventh decade; patients with malignant tumors are slightly younger than those with benign tumors.[9] In a review of the Surveillance, Epidemiology, and End Results registries from 1973 to 1982, Weiss found the incidence of these tumors to be low among patients younger than 30, with a steady increase in incidence with increasing age for adenocarcinoma, carcinoid, and lymphoma. The incidence of sarcoma levels off after the seventh decade (Fig. 29-1).[24]

ETIOLOGY

CHARACTERISTICS OF THE SMALL BOWEL

The small bowel constitutes approximately 75% of the length of the gastrointestinal tract, and provides 90% of the absorptive surface. Despite this predominance in length and surface area, the small bowel appears quite resistant to developing malignancies. Small bowel malignancies account for only 1% to 3% of all gastrointestinal malignancies.[17,20-23,26,27] They oc-

cur 36 to 60 times less frequently than malignancies of the colon.[2,8,9,19,28] Several hypotheses have been formulated to explain this. There is relatively rapid transit through the small bowel compared with the colon, resulting in less exposure of the mucosa to potential carcinogens. Carcinogens are diluted by the large volume of enteric secretions. This liquid may be less mechanically irritating to the small bowel mucosa than solid stool is to the colonic mucosa. The small bowel contains a small, metabolically inactive bacterial population, which may not be capable of transforming potential procarcinogens to their active components.[19] The contribution of the alkaline pH to the resistance of small bowel neoplasms is unknown. The proximal small bowel contains several microsomal enzyme systems known to detoxify carcinogens, particularly benzopyrene hydroxylase.[29,30] There are increased numbers of T lymphocytes and B cells secreting IgA in the distal ileum. This may contribute to a local immunosurveillance system that prevents the development of malignancies. Evidence in support of this is derived from the immunocompromised patients—those with the acquired immunodeficiency syndrome or on chronic immunosuppression—who seem more prone to develop lymphoma and Kaposi's sarcoma in the distal small bowel.

The small intestine appears to be susceptible to carcinogens. Adenocarcinomas in the small intestine occur proximally, in a similar distribution as azoxymethane-induced adenocarcinoma in rats.[31] This distribution correlates with the length of contact of the small bowel mucosa with pancreaticobiliary secretions, implicating bile as a possible carcinogen.[32] Diversion of the bile in animals has been shown to decrease the incidence of experimentally induced small bowel malignancies.[33]

Lowenfels correlated dietary fat intake and the incidence of small bowel carcinoma for various countries around the

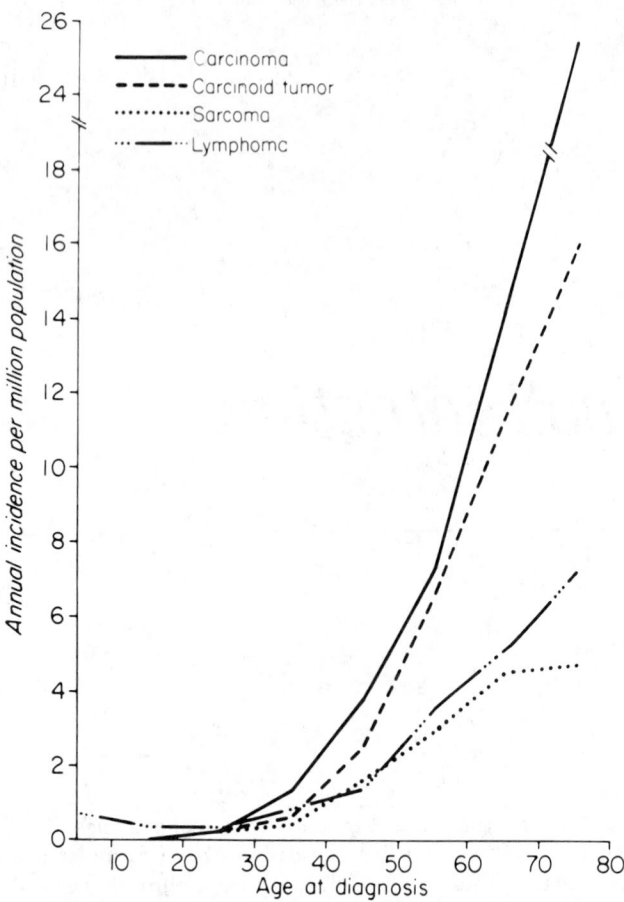

FIGURE 29–1. Incidence of small bowel malignancy by age at diagnosis for adenocarcinoma, carcinoid, lymphoma, or sarcoma. (Weiss NS, Yang C. Incidence of histologic types of cancer of the small intestine. JNCI 1987;78:653–656, with permission)

world (Fig. 29–2).[34] Pollard showed that the incidence of methylazoxymethanol acetate-induced intestinal carcinoma in rats could be markedly reduced by dietary restriction, further implicating oral intake as a possible promoter of intestinal malignancy.[35]

PREMALIGNANT LESIONS

There are several small bowel lesions that predispose to the development of small bowel malignancy. The adenoma-carcinoma sequence has been described.[36] Perzin and colleagues observed that 25% of primary small bowel carcinomas demonstrated adenomatous epithelium in the same lesion.[37] This finding has particular significance in patients with familial adenomatous polyps, for whom polyps of the upper gastrointestinal tract have been recognized with increasing frequency.[38–43]

Patients with chronic Crohn's disease are at increased risk for the development of small bowel carcinoma.[44–46] Malignancy in these patients is often preceded by dysplasia.[47,48] Differentiating clinically between distal small bowel malignancy and Crohn's disease without histologic confirmation can be exceedingly difficult.[49–52]

Patients with longstanding adult celiac disease (nontropical sprue), particularly patients unresponsive to dietary gluten withdrawal, are also at increased risk for harboring small bowel malignancy, particularly lymphoma, although adenocarcinomas also occur.[53–55]

Patients with Peutz-Jeghers syndrome develop primary carcinoma of the gastrointestinal tract.[56–59] The primary polyp of Peutz-Jeghers syndrome is a hamartoma, and the in situ transformation of a hamartomatous polyp to adenocarcinoma has not been clearly demonstrated. Because these patients often have an adenomatous component in their primarily hyperplastic and hamartomatous polyps, the development of malignancy more likely represents malignant evolution of the adenomatous component rather than transformation of the other hamartomatous elements.[58,59]

Patients with von Recklinghausen's neurofibromatosis have benign and malignant gastrointestinal involvement.[60–63] Although most of these small bowel tumors are benign neurofibromas and leiomyomas, malignant tumors of nerve tissue origin, adenocarcinomas, and carcinoid tumors have been reported.[64–66]

PATHOLOGY

More than 35 histologic variants of small bowel neoplasms have been described. These can be subdivided as benign and malignant and further classified according to their cell of origin (Table 29–1). Approximately two thirds of small bowel tumors are malignant, with their anatomic and histologic distribution shown in Table 29–2. The remaining one third are benign, with their anatomic and histologic distribution shown in Table 29–3.

Several researchers have commented on the inordinately high incidence of second primary malignant tumors in patients with primary small bowel malignancies, averaging 29% (range, 16–74%) in a collected series of 1016 patients.[3,4,21,23,25,26,67–73] The reason is unknown, although many have linked it to a defect in these patients' immune surveillance systems. The clinical implications of these observations are clear. Any patient who has had a primary small bowel malignancy should be watched closely for the development of a second malignant tumor.

PRESENTATION

There is no specific symptom complex that is diagnostic of benign or malignant small bowel tumors. The presentation depends on the location of the tumor and its growth pattern. Malignant lesions are more often symptomatic than benign lesions and for a shorter duration.[3,4,9–13,16] Although fewer than half of the patients with benign small bowel tumors develop symptoms, more than 90% of patients with malignant tumors of the small bowel are symptomatic before diagnosis.[2,9,21,69,75] There is often a significant delay between the onset of symptoms and the final diagnosis, which averages 6 to 8 months.[4–6,15] Maglinte, in a review of 77 patients with small bowel malignancy, found the average delay between onset of symptoms and presentation to the physician was 1 month,

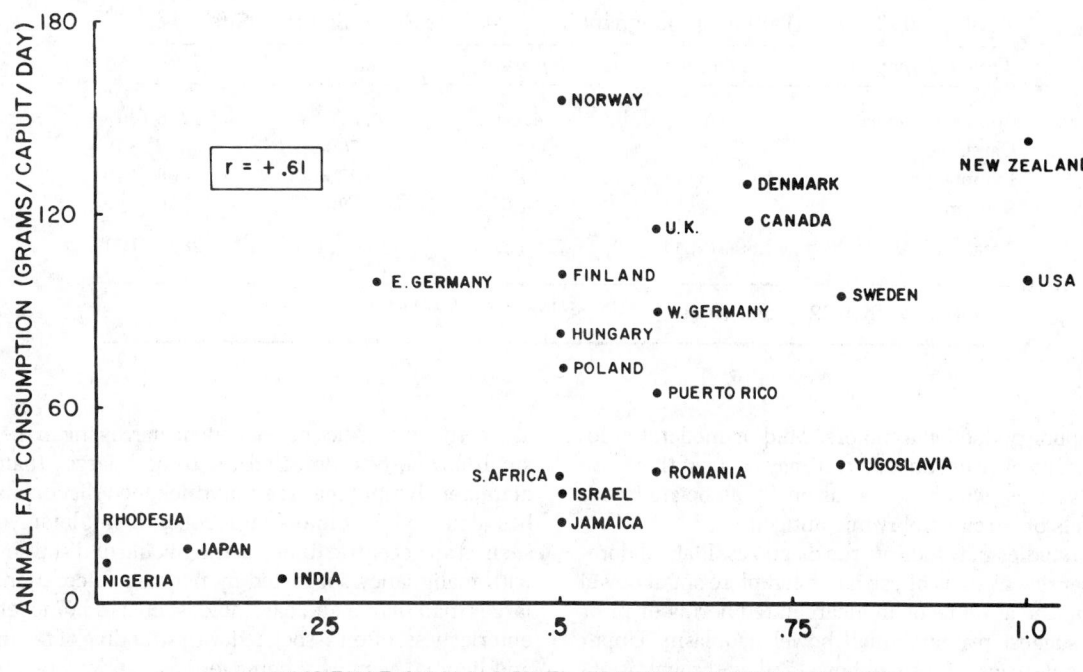

FIGURE 29–2. Incidence of carcinoma of the small bowel correlates with the average daily animal fat consumption. (Lowenfels AB, Sonni A. Distribution of small bowel tumors. Cancer Lett 1977;3:83–86, with permission)

but the average interval from seeing the physician to final diagnosis was 7.8 months.[74]

In patients with benign tumors, pain from obstruction is the most common symptom, occurring in 42% to 70%; bleeding, usually chronic, occurs in 20% to 53% of patients.[9,15,76] The most common cause of adult intussusception is a benign small bowel tumor. A palpable mass or perforation is rare.

In patients with malignant tumors, pain, not always associated with obstruction, occurs in 32% to 86% and weight loss in 32% to 67%.[3,9,15,76] Bleeding occurs somewhat less frequently than in patients with benign small bowel tumors.[7] Perforation, usually localized, occurs in approximately 10% of patients, usually those with lymphomas or sarcomas. A pal-

pable mass, which may represent dilated bowel proximal to an obstructing tumor, is appreciated in less than 25% of patients with malignant small bowel tumors.

DIAGNOSIS

The diagnosis of small bowel tumors is rarely made preoperatively. With the exception of an elevated 5-hydroxyindole-acetic acid (5-HIAA) in patients with carcinoid syndrome, the presenting signs and symptoms of small bowel tumors are nonspecific. Laboratory examination may reveal a mild anemia with chronic blood loss. Hyperbilirubinemia may occur

TABLE 29–1. Pathology of Primary Small Bowel Tumors by Cell of Origin

Cell of Origin	Benign Tumors	Malignant Tumors
Epithelium	Adenoma	Adenocarcinoma
Connective tissue	Fibroma	Fibrosarcoma
Smooth muscle	Leiomyoma	Leiomyosarcoma
Fat	Lipoma	Liposarcoma
Vascular endothelium	Hemangioma	Angiosarcoma
Lymphatics	Lymphangioma	Lymphangiosarcoma
Lymphoid tissue	Pseudolymphoma	Lymphoma
Nerve	Neurofibroma, ganglioneuroma	Neurofibrosarcoma, GAN tumor
Argentaffin cell		Carcinoid
Mixed	Hamartoma	

(Modified from Sindelar WF. Cancer of the small intestine. In: DeVita VT, Hellman S, Rosenberg SA, eds. Cancer: Principles and practice of oncology. Philadelphia: JB Lippincott, 1989:878)

TABLE 29–2.   Distribution of Malignant Tumors of the Small Bowel by Site

Tumor Type*	Duodenum	Jejunum	Ileum	Total (%)
Adenocarcinoma	559	413	276	1248 (45)
Carcinoid	55	73	709	837 (30)
Lymphoma	26	147	235	408 (14)
Sarcoma	54	143	129	326 (11)
Total (%)	694 (25)	776 (27)	1349 (48)	2819 (100)

* Information from 22 patient series.[2,3,5–10,13–16,18,19,23,24,27,32,68,69,75,131]

with periampullary duodenal tumors. Mild or moderate elevations of results of liver function test may occur if there are hepatic metastases, which are occasionally associated with elevated levels of carcinoembryonic antigen.

Radiologic studies may indicate the diagnosis. Plain abdominal films that reveal signs of partial or complete small bowel obstruction in the absence of an incarcerated hernia or prior laparotomy suggest primary small bowel neoplasm. Upper gastrointestinal series with small bowel follow through is abnormal in 53% to 83% of patients, delineating small bowel tumor in 30% to 44% of patients.[77,78] This diagnostic accuracy can be improved to greater than 90% using enteroclysis, with particular attention to the distensibility of the small bowel.[78–80] Barium enema can be useful in the diagnosis of small bowel disease, particularly lymphoma, where thickening of the distal ileum may be seen on refluxing contrast material into the distal small bowel. This finding is not specific and can be identical to the appearance of regional ileitis. Hyams suggested that a rectal biopsy revealing granulomatous disease can reliably differentiate inflammatory from neoplastic changes in the terminal ileum.[49]

Computerized tomography (CT) is more accurate in detecting small bowel tumors.[81–86] In a review of 35 patients with small bowel tumors, Laurent found CT scans to be abnormal for 97%, predicting tumor in 80%. The CT scan predicted tumor histology for 69% of patients and tumor stage for 61% of patients. CT scans predicted extramural invasion and liver metastases correctly for 75% of 18 patients with malignant tumors; CT scans were accurate in predicting regional lymph node status in only 25% of the patients. Laurent described characteristic CT findings for adenocarcinoma, seen as a partially obstructing concentric narrowing in the proximal small bowel, best detected for tumors larger than 3 cm in diameter; lymphoma, seen as thickened distal small bowel, best detected for tumors larger than 2 cm; leiomyosarcoma, seen as an eccentric tumor of the middle or distal small bowel, with malignancy suggested by necrosis, ulceration, and size larger than than 5 cm; carcinoid, seen as a homogenous mesenteric mass, often associated with stranding of the mesentery; and lipoma, seen as a homogenous, fat-density small bowel or mesenteric nodule.[82]

Other investigators have focused on small bowel thickness as measured by CT scan to predict enteric disease.[81,86] Although small bowel wall thickness indicates disease, it does not specify malignancy.

Angiography is rarely helpful in the diagnosis of small bowel tumors. Angiograms may be abnormal in vascular smooth muscle tumors of the small bowel and may help to define the source of occult but active upper gastrointestinal bleeding in patients with a small bowel hemangioma.[77] Alfidi found angiography helpful in diagnosing patients with small bowel arterial venous malformations, identifying lesions in 9 patients after negative laparotomy results.[87] Angiography may rarely demonstrate occlusion of the peripheral branches of the mesenteric circulation responsible for the syndrome of mesenteric ischemia seen occasionally in the carcinoid syndrome. Nuclear medicine scans using technetium-labeled erythrocytes may help define the source of occult chronic gastrointestinal blood loss after normal colonic and upper gastrointestinal endoscopy. Oliver suggested that the sensitivity of this test would be improved if more frequent images were obtained.[88]

With more sophisticated instrumentation, endoscopy is

TABLE 29–3.   Distribution of Benign Tumors of the Small Bowel by Site

Tumor Type*	Duodenum	Jejunum	Ileum	Total (%)
Leiomyoma	21	61	46	128 (35)
Polyp/Adenoma	31	17	17	65 (19)
Lipoma	10	13	27	50 (14)
Hemangioma	1	10	24	43 (12)
Fibroma	3	7	12	22 (6)
Other	27	8	13	48 (14)
Total (%)	93 (26)	124 (34)	139 (40)	356 (100)

* Data from 12 patient series.[2–7,9,10,13–16]

more frequently used in the investigation of small bowel disease. Upper gastrointestinal endoscopy with total duodenoscopy is the mainstay for detection, diagnosis, and occasionally, treatment of proximal neoplasms. There has been renewed interest in peroral enteroscopy.[89] With newer instrumentation, total small bowel enteroscopy can be achieved. Enteroscopy can help in diagnosing focal lesions and more diffuse lesions such as Mediterranean lymphoma.[90,91] It may be most useful in localizing the source of occult nongastric, noncolonic gastrointestinal bleeding.[92] Iida described the use of intraoperative enteroscopy to enhance the detection and removal of polyps in patients with familial adenomatous polyposis syndrome.[93] Intraoperative enteroscopy with transillumination of the bowel wall has been used in patients with identified arteriovenous malformations and gastrinomas that could not be otherwise localized at the time of operation.[89,94]

Colonoscopy with retrograde ileoscopy may be useful in the diagnosis of primary lymphoma of the ileum.[95] The small bowel in as many as 30% of patients can be visualized by retrograde ileoscopy in experienced hands.[95]

MANAGEMENT

BENIGN TUMORS OF THE SMALL BOWEL

The distribution of benign small bowel tumors by diagnosis and anatomic location is shown in Table 29–3. Most are leiomyomas, followed in frequency by adenomas, lipomas, vascular lesions, and fibrous lesions.

Leiomyomas

Leiomyomas of the small bowel account for 20% to 40% of all benign small bowel tumors and are the most common small bowel tumor according to a review by Wilson.[97] These tumors grow within or outside the bowel lumen, and the growth pattern determines the presenting symptoms. Perforation is unusual. It can be difficult to differentiate benign from malignant smooth muscle tumors of the gastrointestinal tract intraoperatively, even after histologic evaluation by frozen section. According to the comprehensive review by Skandalakis, malignancy in lesions smaller than 4.0 cm in diameter is unusual.[98] Histologic criteria of malignancy include necrosis, nuclear pleomorphism, and increased mitotic activity. Surgical management of small bowel leiomyomas includes segmental resection with grossly negative margins. Because lymph node metastases are unusual even for malignant leiomyosarcomas of the small bowel, extensive mesenteric lymphadenectomy is not required.

Villous Adenomas of the Duodenum

Small bowel polyps are categorized based on principles of management: villous adenomas of the duodenum, adenomas of the distal small bowel, and Peutz-Jeghers hamartomas.

Although villous adenomas of the duodenum are unusual, the duodenum is the most common location in the small bowel for these lesions. Their most common presenting sign is obstructive jaundice, and the diagnosis is made with upper gastrointestinal endoscopy. Most lesions are located in the second portion of the duodenum, usually on the medial wall, surrounding the ampulla of Vater. They are increasingly recognized as a component of the familial adenomatous polyposis syndrome.[38–43] Several reports of villous tumors of the duodenum have appeared in the last 10 years.[99–111] These tumors have a high propensity, averaging 45%, for malignant degeneration. Risk factors associated with malignancy include size greater than 5 cm, age over 50 years, and more distally situated polyps.[103,112] This propensity for malignant degeneration together with their location around the ampulla of Vater combine to make management decisions difficult. Although several physicians have advocated local excision for benign lesions, it is impossible to be certain of the benign nature of a tumor before complete histologic examination.[100,113] Local recurrence rates of 17% to 75% have been reported after local excision, occasionally with malignant degeneration of the recurrent tumors.[102,104,108,110,111] Ongoing endoscopic surveillance is mandatory after local excision of these lesions. Lesions in the third and fourth portion of the duodenum may be managed with wedge or sleeve resection. Lesions in the first or second portion of the duodenum should be managed with pancreaticoduodenectomy if there is any question about the diagnosis.

Survival after complete excision is excellent in patients with benign villous adenomas and carcinoma in situ. Patients with invasive carcinoma fare comparably to those with periampullary adenocarcinoma.

Small Bowel Adenomas

Adenomas in the remainder of the small intestine are rare. They are distributed more proximally, and case reports of malignant degeneration have appeared.[114] These tumors should be managed with segmental resection.

Peutz-Jeghers Hamartomas

Peutz-Jeghers hamartomas are always multifocal, occurring primarily in the small intestine.[115,116] Symptoms of chronic low-grade obstruction with recurrent intussusception usually become apparent in the second decade of life, and frequently warrant repeated surgical intervention.

Appropriate surgical management of these tumors includes enterotomy and polypectomy. If bowel resection is required, a minimal length of bowel should be sacrificed, because this disease is a chronic problem, and frequent reoperation can be anticipated. Gastrointestinal malignancy occurs in these patients with increased frequency, and it is important before laparotomy to verify the status of the stomach and colon, because intraoperative palpation of these structures can be unreliable.

Other Benign Lesions

Angiomas of the small bowel are rare and may be multifocal. They are usually discrete and well circumscribed, presenting most often as occult gastrointestinal bleeding. Management consists of segmental resection of the small bowel.[97,117,118]

Patients with small bowel lipomas usually present with symptoms of abdominal pain consistent with partial obstruction.[119] The difficulty in managing these lesions is that they may involve the small bowel diffusely.[120] Surgical management involves resection of the symptomatic segment of bowel.

Brunner's gland hamartomas are extremely rare, with fewer than 100 reports in the world literature. Symptoms at presentation depend on the size of the tumor and include a lack of symptoms, chronic upper gastrointestinal bleeding, and duodenal or biliary obstruction. Because these are submucosal tumors, preoperative diagnosis is rarely possible. Treatment involves endoscopic removal of pedunculated lesions or surgical resection of larger lesions.[121-123]

Upper digestive tract involvement by systemic neurofibromatosis (von Recklinghausen's syndrome) occurs in 2% to 25% of patients with this disease.[61] This may be an underestimate, because much of the involvement is asymptomatic and detected only on postmortem examination. Typically, involvement is characterized by submucosal neurofibromas. Duodenal paragangliomas have been associated with von Recklinghausen's disease.[62,63] Although these lesions are generally considered benign, Inai and colleagues reported a case of duodenal paraganglioma with regional lymph node metastases.[64]

Inflammatory polyps may occur at any point within the small bowel, from the duodenum through the ileum, and they are occasionally associated with preexisting Crohn's disease.[124-127] These are uniformly benign lesions arising from the submucosa, usually solitary, and presenting with symptoms of obstruction. Management consists of polypectomy or segmental small bowel resection.

MALIGNANT TUMORS OF THE SMALL BOWEL

The distribution of malignant small bowel tumors by diagnosis and anatomic location is shown in Table 29–2.

Adenocarcinoma

Adenocarcinomas comprise 25% of all small bowel tumors, and 45% of all malignant small bowel tumors. These tumors are distributed proximally in the small bowel, with almost 80% located in the duodenum or jejunum. For purposes of analyzing mode of presentation, diagnosis, management, and outcome, the tumors can be categorized as those of the duodenum and those of the jejunum and ileum.

DUODENUM. Approximately 45% of all adenocarcinomas of the small bowel arise within the duodenum. Approximately 15% of these are in the first portion of the duodenum, 40% in the second portion of the duodenum, and 45% in the distal duodenum, a distribution pattern that parallels the relative lengths of each portion.[72,132-136] The median age of these patients is 60 years. Symptoms are related to the size and site of the tumor. The most common symptom is upper abdominal pain related to partial duodenal obstruction.[132,135] Series that include periampullary tumors also report an incidence of biliary obstruction.[133] Anemia with guaiac-positive stools is frequent, although frank upper gastrointestinal hemorrhage is unusual.[135]

Diagnosis is usually suspected from the results of an upper gastrointestinal series (Fig. 29–3). Hypotonic duodenography may improve the accuracy of this test.[137] Histologic confirmation can be obtained preoperatively in most patients by upper gastrointestinal endoscopy with total duodenoscopy.

As outlined in Table 29–4, most patients who present with duodenal carcinoma are explored, and of those explored, most are resected. Patients with tumors of the first and second portions of the duodenum require pancreaticoduodenectomy; those with tumors of the third and fourth portions of the duodenum may be completely resected with segmental duodenectomy and primary anastomosis. Because 22% to 71% of patients with duodenal adenocarcinoma have positive nodes at presentation and there is a finite 5-year survival rate for regional nodal involvement, curative resection of duodenal carcinomas should always include a systemic regional lymphadenectomy, regardless of the primary tumor location.[132-136,150]

Outcome in these patients is determined by resectability, lymph node involvement, and histologic grade.[132-136] There is no clear evidence that pancreaticoduodenectomy results in superior survival to segmental resection if resection is technically feasible.[130,144]

The role of postoperative adjuvant therapy has not been clearly defined for this group of patients. In patients with advanced unresectable disease, palliative radiation therapy may help control chronic blood loss. Because these tumors behave more like gastric cancer than pancreatic cancer, participation in an investigational chemotherapy program incorporating 5-fluorouracil (5-FU) may be warranted.[150]

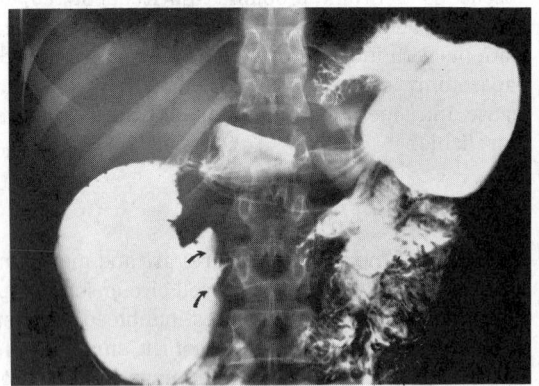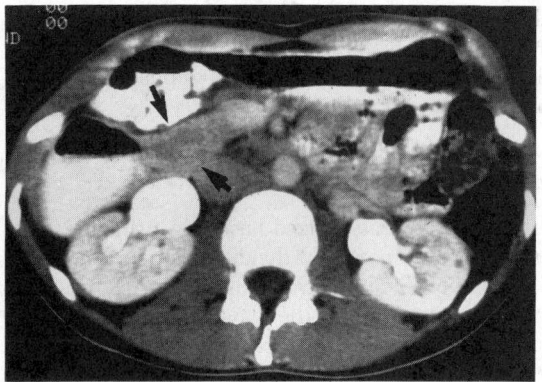

FIGURE 29–3.   Upper gastrointestinal series and CT scan of an obstructing adenocarcinoma of the third portion of the duodenum.

TABLE 29–4. Duodenal Adenocarcinoma

Investigations	No. of Patients	Explored n	Explored %	Operative* Mortality (%)	Resected† n	Resected† %	5-Year Survival (%)
Awlmark, 1980[136]	66	49	74	24	49	100	33
Lillemoe, 1980[138]	12	11	92	36	6	55	33
Joesting, 1981[135]	104	104	100	18	53	51	46
Cohen, 1982[139]	40						38
Herter, 1982[140]	38						27
Williamson, 1983[32]	26	26	100		18	69	17
Kellum, 1983[141]	3			0			33
Ouriel, 1984[72]	34	32	94		19	54	25
Gaddy, 1985[142]	5	5	100	0	2	40	0
Jones, 1985[143]	12	1	100	0	12	100	18
Grace, 1986[144]	5						60
Tarazi, 1986[145]	17						28
Gonzalez, 1987[146]	3	3	100	0	2	67	0
Sarma, 1987[147]	3	2	67	0	1	50	33
Crist, 1987[148]	9						33
Lai, 1988[132]	24	24	100	8	24	100	8
Michelassi, 1989[149]	16	10	63	10	10	100	10
Brennan, 1990[150]	32	29	91	0	18	62	60

* Mortality as a percent of those explored.
† Resected as a percent of those explored.

JEJUNUM AND ILEUM. The remainder of the small bowel, the jejunum and ileum, account for the remaining 55% of small bowel adenocarcinomas. As seen in Table 29–5, much of the information we have about these tumors is derived from small series collected over several years. The report by Adler is a collected series based on several large tumor registries.[129] Most reports are from institutions seeing fewer than 1 patient with small bowel adenocarcinoma annually.

Presenting signs or symptoms of obstruction occur in 50% to 74% of patients and of occult gastrointestinal bleeding in 33% to 64%.[32,68,129] Although the adenocarcinoma of the small bowel may be suspected based on a small bowel follow-through series or CT scan, neither examination is specific, and the diagnosis is frequently not made until laparotomy.[32]

At the time of operation, 77% to 100% of distal small bowel adenocarcinomas are resectable, although regional lymph node metastases are frequent.[32,68,72,73,151] The principles of surgical resection include attainment of negative surgical margins and wide resection of the corresponding mesentery of the involved segment of small bowel.

Survival of these patients is generally poor, with most series reporting only 20% to 30% of patients alive at 5 years (see Table 29–5). Prognostic factors include depth of tumor penetration and the presence of nodal or systemic metastases. Histologic grade of the tumor has been predictive of outcome.[72] After curative resection, survival rates of 45% to 70% have been reported for patients with negative nodes, falling to 12% to 14% for those with positive nodes.[72,129] Radiation therapy is difficult in these patients because of the mobile nature of the small bowel mesentery and the inability to localize the target field. The impact of chemotherapy in the management of these tumors is difficult to ascertain. Jigyasu reported one partial response among 14 patients treated with 5-FU-based combination chemotherapy, and those patients were accrued over 30 years.[153]

Carcinoid Tumors

Carcinoid tumors represent 30% of all small bowel malignancies (see Table 29–2) and 19% of all small bowel tumors, second only to adenocarcinoma in frequency. The small bowel

TABLE 29–5. Survival of Patients With Adenocarcinoma of the Small Intestine

Investigations	No. of Patients	Period (y)	5-Year Survival (%)
Awrich, 1980[69]	26	25	26
Mittal, 1980[8]	10	21	62
Norberg, 1981[10]	11	34	0
Waterhouse, 1981[12]	24	28	18
Adler, 1982[129]	338	43	17
Lanzafame, 1982[70]	29	40	35
Barclay, 1983[23]	74	30	22
Williamson, 1983[31]	68	64	14
Ouriel, 1984[72]	65	31	30
Cooper, 1985[152]	25	15	0
Johnson, 1985[22]	16	28	6
Zollinger, 1986[15]	18	20	17
Martin, 1986[27]	87	38	21
Cicarelli, 1987[20]	17	14	12
Brophy, 1989[75]	18	14	36
Lioe, 1990[73]	25	34	16
Desa, 1991[16]	7	15	20

is the second most common site of carcinoid tumors after the appendix. Ninety percent of all small bowel carcinoids arise in the ileum (see Table 29–2). These tumors are often silent, with many series including otherwise asymptomatic tumors discovered incidentally at laparotomy or autopsy. If present, the most common presenting symptom is vague, nonspecific abdominal pain.[71,154,155] This pain may be due to several causes. There is frequently an intense desmoplastic fibrous reaction around the primary tumor, with shortening of the small bowel mesentery, kinking of the bowel, and ileus or partial bowel obstruction, thought to be induced by the biochemical products of the tumor. Frequently, partial bowel obstruction may occur from the tumor itself. A syndrome of chronic mesenteric ischemia has been described in these patients, associated with a mesenteric angiopathy described as elastic vascular sclerosis.[156] On angiography, this is manifested by occlusion of the peripheral small vessels of the mesenteric arcade.

Although only 10% to 17% of patients with small bowel carcinoid present with carcinoid syndrome, as many as 67% develop features of the syndrome at some point during their course.[96,115,158,159] Symptoms include flushing of the head and neck and upper chest in 84% to 94% of patients, a watery secretory diarrhea in 70% to 86% of patients, with both symptoms occurring in 58% of patients. Right-sided valvular heart disease exists in 37% to 50% of patients, with bronchial asthma manifested in 17% to 23% of patients.[157,159-161] These symptoms are often prompted by emotion, alcohol intake, or the ingestion of tyramine-containing foods, such as blue cheese or chocolate.[160] Virtually all patients with evidence of carcinoid syndrome have bulky liver metastases and elevated urinary 5-HIAA levels.

Without the classic carcinoid syndrome, preoperative diagnosis of these tumors is unusual. Radiologic findings, even with small bowel follow-through studies, are inconclusive, revealing only an ileus-like or partial obstruction picture. CT scan may reveal a mass infiltrating the mesentery with or without liver metastases. Rarely, mesenteric angiography reveals occlusion of the peripheral mesenteric vessels.

At laparotomy these tumors appear as firm, tan, submucosal nodules, usually in the distal small bowel. Symptomatic tumors tend to be larger than those found incidentally or at autopsy.[154] The frequency of metastatic disease to regional lymph nodes and liver is related to the size of the tumor. Nodal metastases are unusual with tumors smaller than 1 cm in diameter but occur with 33% to 67% of tumors 1 to 3 cm and in 75% to 90% of tumors larger than 3 cm.[71,157,160,162-164] Most patients presenting with symptomatic small bowel carcinoids have metastatic disease at the time of operation.

Approximately 30% of small bowel carcinoids are multiple, mandating a careful search of the remainder of the small bowel before definitive surgical management.[71,154,155,158,161,162] Surgical management of the primary tumor includes wide resection of the primary tumor with complete resection of the supporting mesentery. Although the likelihood of regional lymph node metastases is known to increase with size, metastases have been reported in carcinoids smaller than 1 cm.[157,165]

Management of carcinoid tumors metastatic to liver is primarily directed toward controlling symptoms of the carcinoid syndrome. Prolonged remission of symptoms has been achieved after resection of bulky liver metastases, even if in-

complete.[96,157,163,166] For unresectable disease, short-term remission of symptoms has been observed with hepatic dearterialization.[157,166] Hepatic arterial infusion chemotherapy has been attempted without convincing reports of success.[159,163]

Medical management of the symptoms of carcinoid syndrome has employed a long list of drugs, all with limited success. The most effective drug in controlling these symptoms is the long-acting somatostatin analog SMS-201. Given as a subcutaneous injection, this drug controls the symptoms in most patients.[160]

Systemic chemotherapy has been disappointing. Active agents include 5-FU, streptozotocin, mitomycin C, cyclophosphamide, methotrexate, interferon-α, and doxorubicin (Adriamycin). The most active single agents are 5-FU and doxorubicin, and the most effective combination regimens reported are methotrexate with cyclophosphamide, 5-FU with streptozotocin, or streptozotocin with doxorubicin.[157] Although response rates of 30% to 55% are reported, none of these drugs, alone or in combination, has clearly demonstrated any impact on the generally indolent natural history of this disease.

The prognosis for patients with carcinoid tumors of the small intestine is better than for those with adenocarcinomas (Table 29–6), and depends on tumor size, depth of invasion, and lymph node or liver metastases.[71,154,155,157,167,169] Other factors that have been identified as prognostically significant by univariate analysis include female sex,[168] lack of symptoms, complete resectability,[71] and histologic growth pattern.[170] In advanced disease, two investigators looked at the association

TABLE 29–6. Survival of Patients With Carcinoid of the Small Intestine

Investigations	No. of Patients	Period (y)	5-Year Survival (%)
Awrich, 1980[69]	28	25	47
Mittal, 1980[8]	9	10	87
Norberg, 1981[10]	8	34	63
Waterhouse, 1981[12]	26	28	69
Lanzafame, 1982[70]	18	40	44
Collin, 1982[21]	16	15	33
Zeitels, 1982[167]	28	37	62
Barclay, 1983[23]	94	30	64
Peck, 1983[154]	30	10	31
Strodel, 1983[71]	82	20	59
Dawes, 1984[163]	32	18	80
Thompson, 1985[161]	66	10	62
Giuliani, 1985[14]	4	34	67
Olney, 1985[158]	75	44	33
Johnson, 1985[22]	22	28	50
Zollinger, 1986[15]	10	20	60
Martin, 1986[27]	89	38	51
O'Rourke, 1986[165]	43	10	52
Cicarelli, 1987[20]	20	14	35
Sjoblom, 1988[155]	48	19	77
Brophy, 1989[75]	8	14	83
Nwiloh, 1990[164]	11	22	44
McDermott, 1991[168]	42	18	66
Desa, 1991[16]	7	15	64

of DNA ploidy and prognosis, finding a trend toward better prognosis for patients with solely diploid tumors.[171,172] This tumor has a pattern of indolent growth. Without metastatic disease, complete resection of localized carcinoid tumors results in 75% to 94% 5-year survival rates.[160,168,169] With regional lymph node involvement, 5-year survival rates of 45% to 90% have been reported.[155,157,159,163,168,169] Five-year survival rates of 19% to 54% have been reported for patients with liver metastases.[155,157,159-161,168,169]

Lymphoma

Lymphoma may involve the gastrointestinal tract primarily or as a manifestation of disseminated systemic disease. Primary small bowel lymphoma comprises 1% to 4% of all gastrointestinal malignancies and 17% of all small bowel malignancies (see Table 29–2). The gastrointestinal tract is the most frequent site of extranodal lymphoma, the stomach being the most frequent site, followed by the small bowel and colon.[173] Within the small bowel, the incidence of lymphoma increases with progression distally, and the most frequent site is the ileum. This parallels the relative amount of lymphatic tissue in the wall of the small bowel at these locations.

The diagnosis of primary small bowel lymphoma must satisfy the criteria specified by Dawson.[174] There must be no peripheral or mediastinal lymphadenopathy. The peripheral blood smear must display a normal leukocyte absolute and differential count. Tumor involvement must be predominantly in the gastrointestinal tract. Most oncologists think that there should be no evidence of liver or spleen involvement.[152,175] Antecedent conditions associated with the development of primary small bowel lymphoma include nontropical sprue and Crohn's disease.[55,130,152]

Gastrointestinal lymphoma has been traditionally staged using a modification of the Ann Arbor staging system.[176] Because this was not a staging system originally designed for lymphomas of the gastrointestinal tract, Blackledge established a staging system incorporating the prognostic significance of perforation (Table 29–7).[177]

TABLE 29–7. Staging Systems for Small Bowel Lymphoma

Ann Arbor Staging System

I Involvement of a single nodal group or single nodal site (IE)
II Involvement of more than one nodal group on the same side of the diaphragm or involvement of a single extranodal site with one or more nodal groups on the same side of the diaphragm (IIE)
III Involvement of nodes on both sides of the diaphragm, with or without involvement of extranodal sites (IIIE), spleen (IIIS), or both (IIES)
IV Diffuse involvement of viscera or bone marrow

Blackledge Staging System

I Tumor confined to the gastrointestinal tract
II Tumor with local mesenteric nodal involvement
III Tumor with perforation
IV Tumor with distant (paraaortic and beyond) nodal involvement
V Tumor with visceral or bone marrow involvement

There are four major clinical presentations of primary small intestinal lymphoma: the Western type, the Mediterranean type, pediatric lymphoma, and Hodgkin's lymphoma.

The most common, the Western type, occurs primarily in adults at a median age of 54 to 61 years, and it has a distinct male predominance.[130,173-180] These lesions are usually focal and found in the distal small bowel. The most common presenting symptom is abdominal pain related to partial bowel obstruction. The most common physical finding is a mass. Anemia occurs in approximately 20% of these patients, and about 10% of patients with this type of lymphoma present with perforation.[130,178,180-182]

The diagnosis of Western-type lymphoma is often made only at laparotomy. Radiologic findings suggesting the diagnosis include a diffuse segment of thickened distal small bowel on small follow-through examination. This finding can often be better demonstrated by CT scan (Fig. 29–4). These radiologic findings may be easily confused with those of other segmental diseases of the distal small intestine, such as Crohn's disease.[183]

Several systems classify the pathology of small bowel lymphomas. Using the Rappaport system, approximately 60% of non-Hodgkin's lymphomas are diffuse histiocytic (40% diffuse large cell and 20% immunoblastic), 25% are lymphocytic, and the remainder are mixed types. The Kiel system uses morphology and cell-surface markers to classify lymphomas. Most small bowel lymphomas are intermediate or high grade.[152,179,184,185]

Management of these patients usually entails surgical exploration with resection of the affected segment of small bowel with its subjacent mesentery, and 50% to 78% of patients who present with lymphoma undergo complete surgical resection.[32,130,178,179] The role of adjuvant therapy for patients with completely resected disease is debated. Most physicians agree that any patient with evidence of incompletely resected disease or regional nodal metastases can benefit from adjuvant chemotherapy.[178] Some think that adjuvant chemotherapy is warranted after complete resection of all high-grade lymphomas, even if they are stage IE.[186,187] Auger reported 16 patients undergoing complete surgical resection. The median survival for those undergoing complete resection with chemotherapy was 34 months, compared with 14 months for patients undergoing complete surgical resection without adjuvant chemotherapy.[179] The results were not analyzed by the presence or absence of nodal metastases, and the issue of adjuvant chemotherapy remains unresolved in patients with lymphoma localized to the bowel.

Adjuvant radiation therapy had been advocated, although the long-term side effects of abdominal radiation therapy and the efficacy of contemporary combination chemotherapy make this option less attractive.[130,178,186]

Most recent series report 5-year survival rates in excess of 50% with aggressive multimodality therapy (Table 29–8). Prognostic factors include stage at presentation, complete response to therapy, complete resectability, histologic subtype, and the use of multimodality therapy.[152,173,178,179,183,185,187,192] Unlike the indolent course of carcinoid tumors, most deaths in patients with small bowel lymphoma occur within 2 years of diagnosis.[181,189]

Mediterranean lymphoma is the most common lymphoma encountered in Middle Eastern and African populations, oc-

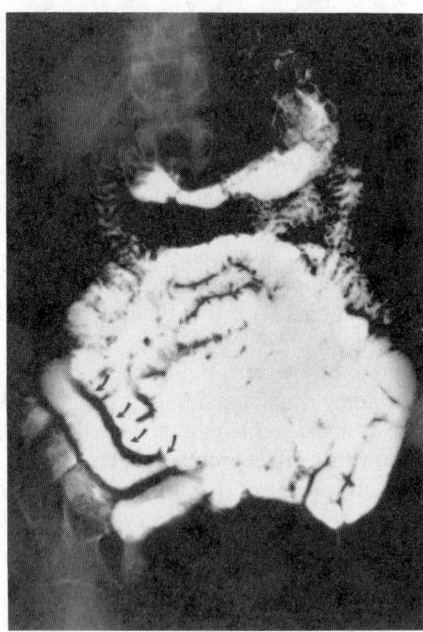 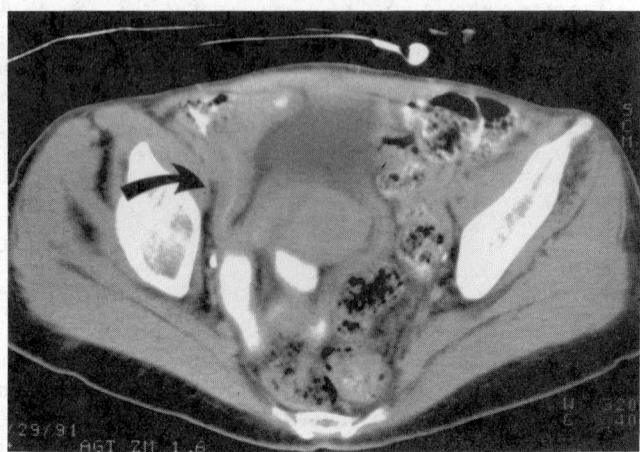

FIGURE 29–4. Small bowel follow-through series and CT scan of a primary small bowel lymphoma show a thickened terminal ileum.

curring with an equal sex distribution among young adults (median age, 30).[188,193] Typically, these patients present with the triad of pain, malabsorption (*i.e.*, weight loss and diarrhea), and clubbing of their nails.[188] Approximately 50% of these patients present with a mass. Although neither a specific nor diagnostic finding, approximately one third of patients with Mediterranean lymphoma have free alpha heavy chain protein in their serum and jejunal fluid. Mediterranean lymphoma generally involves the entire small bowel, manifested histologically by villous atrophy and an intense lymphoplasmacytoid infiltrate in the lamina propria of the small bowel. Diagnosis can often be made by peroral jejunal biopsy. Surgery is employed if the diagnosis is unclear or for complications such as obstruction or perforation. Grossly, the bowel appears to be involved by a diffuse thickening with some nodularity. Lymph nodes are involved in 85% of patients.

Management consists primarily of systemic chemotherapy, although reports of whole-abdominal radiation therapy have appeared.[186] Prognosis tends to be poor, with Al Bahrani reporting a 23% 5-year survival rate.[188]

Childhood lymphoma typically occurs in patients younger than 15 years of age, and the patient presents with symptoms of pain and physical findings of a mass in the right lower quadrant, often with associated intussusception. Histologically, almost half of these lymphomas resemble a Burkitt's lymphoma.[191] These patients often require resection before systemic therapy, because perforation during treatment is common. The prognosis is improving in the era of combined-modality therapy, with a survival of 76% reported by Fleming; all deaths in this series occurred within 10 months of diagnosis.[191] Outcome depends on stage at presentation and resectability.[152,188,193]

Primary Hodgkin's lymphoma of the small bowel accounts for fewer than 3% of all small bowel lymphomas.[152,184] In many reported cases, this diagnosis may represent impingement of mesenteric lymphadenopathy on the small bowel rather than primary visceral involvement.[194] Management consists of diagnostic and palliative surgery, followed by definitive systemic chemotherapy.

TABLE 29–8. Survival of Patients With Lymphoma of the Small Intestine

Investigations	No. of Patients	Period (yr)	5-Year Survival (%)
Awrich, 1980[69]	18	25	33
Mittal, 1980[8]	5	10	80
Contreary, 1980[178]	24	32	27
Rosenfelt, 1980[173]	12	9	40
Waterhouse, 1981[12]	8	28	12
Lanzafame, 1982[70]	4	40	50
Weingrad, 1982[185]	15	30	44
Collin, 1982[21]	3	15	33
Williamson, 1983[31]	41	64	15
Al-Bahrani, 1983[188]	132	14	23
Rao, 1984[181]	15	12	42
Skudder, 1985[189]	12	15	33
Giuliani, 1985[14]	14	34	40
Dragosics, 1985[190]	13	8	32
Martin, 1986[27]	8	38	62
O'Rourke, 1986[130]	36	10	56
Shepherd, 1988[186]	7	13	57
Sweetenhaus, 1989[175]	19	12	58
Brophy, 1989[75]	7	14	20
Fleming, 1990[191]	54	25	76
Auger, 1990[179]	22	8	50
Desa, 1991[16]	13	15	10

Sarcoma

Sarcomas of the small intestine are extremely unusual, comprising approximately 9% of all small bowel tumors and 11% of all small bowel malignancies (see Table 29–2). Most are of smooth muscle origin (*i.e.*, leiomyosarcomas and leiomyoblastomas), although case reports of other histologies have appeared. Recent reports grouped these tumors as gastrointestinal stromal tumors, from which another variant, the gastrointestinal autonomic nerve tumor, can be differentiated by immunohistochemistry and electron microscopy.[195,196] From a clinical and prognostic viewpoint, the tumors can be discussed together.

The tumors can present with several symptoms, depending on their growth pattern. Endoenteric lesions may present as bleeding or obstruction. An exoenteric lesion may present as an abdominal mass or perforation before any sense of obstruction is evident. Although the diagnosis may be suggested by upper gastrointestinal series with a small bowel follow-through study or enteroclysis, with or without abdominal CT scan, it is rarely made preoperatively. These tumors are vascular, with a plethora of tumor vessels visualized by arteriography. Intraoperatively, the tumors are usually appreciated as a firm, encapsulated mass arising from the bowel. It is difficult clinically and by frozen section examination to differentiate a small leiomyosarcoma from its benign counterpart, the leiomyoma.

The principles of surgical management include wide resection of the primary tumor, including any adjacent structures that may be invaded. Duodenal tumors involving the medial wall of the second portion of the duodenum require pancreaticoduodenectomy; smaller leiomyosarcomas of the duodenum may be treated with wedge or sleeve resection. For sarcomas of the jejunum and ileum, the involved segment of intestine is resected together with its supporting mesentery. Deliberate extended lymphadenectomy is unnecessary, because the tumors involve regional lymph nodes in fewer than 15% of patients.[197,198]

The prognosis depends on tumor size, histologic grade, local invasiveness, and resectability (Table 29–9).[197–201] Peritoneal and liver metastases are the most common causes of treatment failure, and there is no evidence that adjuvant chemotherapy or radiation therapy after complete resection diminishes this risk of subsequent relapse.[202] Standard treatment of symptomatic metastatic disease usually involves doxorubicin-based combination chemotherapy. Although response rates as high as 40% have been reported with these regimens, no convincing impact on the survival of patients with advanced metastatic gastrointestinal sarcoma has been demonstrated.

Metastatic Disease

The small bowel is frequently involved by metastatic disease. The most common tumor metastasizing to the gastrointestinal tract is melanoma, with 60% of the patients dying of melanoma found to have metastatic disease involving the gastrointestinal tract at autopsy.[203] Other extraabdominal tumors that are known to metastasize to the small intestine include lung, breast, cervix, and kidney.[204–211] Case reports of small bowel metastases from other tumors, including thyroid, Merkel cell carcinoma, and hepatoma, have appeared.[212–214] Intraabdominal tumors that may involve the small bowel by transperitoneal spread include colorectal carcinoma, ovarian carcinoma, gastric carcinoma, pancreatic carcinoma, and transitional cell carcinoma of the genitourinary system. The small bowel may also be involved by direct extension from any intraabdominal malignancy.

Symptoms of small bowel metastases include bleeding, obstruction, and perforation. Although surgery for local invasion of the small bowel can often be performed with curative intent, treatment is usually palliative for patients with hematogenous or transperitoneal metastases. Identification of obstructing metastatic lesions is usually possible, although these are rarely solitary. Identification of the bleeding metastasis among multiple small bowel lesions can be difficult.

The outcome in patients undergoing small bowel resection for metastatic melanoma has been summarized by several researchers. Median survivals of between 4.5 and 8.5 months are reported, with few long-term survivors.[203,215–218] Caputy identified small bowel involvement as an independent adverse prognostic indicator for patients with melanoma metastatic to the gastrointestinal tract.[216] Branum found a mean survival of 31 months for patients whose tumors were completely resectable, compared with 10 months for patients undergoing noncurative procedures. This was probably a reflection of the extent of tumor burden rather than the impact of therapy.[217]

TABLE 29–9. Survival of Patients With Sarcoma of the Small Intestine

Investigations	No. of Patients	Period (yr)	5-Year Survival (%)
Awrich, 1980[69]	10	25	38
Mittal, 1980[8]	3	10	33
Norberg, 1981[10]	9	34	11
Waterhouse, 1981[12]	12	28	50
Lanzafame, 1982[70]	15	40	33
Chiotasso, 1982[197]	28	30	42
Shiu, 1983[198]	18	25	32
Johnson, 1985[22]	12	28	25
Zollinger, 1986[15]	10	20	10
Martin, 1986[27]	33	38	18
Cicarelli, 1987[20]	8	14	12
McGrath, 1987[199]	14	34	40
Brophy, 1989[74]	11	14	40
Kimura, 1991[200]	16	24	50
Dougherty, 1991[201]	14	24	18

REFERENCES

1. Ellis H. Tumours of the small intestine. Semin Surg Oncol 1987;3:12–21.
2. Wilson JM, Melvin DB, et al. Primary malignancies of the small bowel: A report of 96 cases and review of the literature. Ann Surg 1974;180:175–179.
3. Silberman H, Crichlow RW, Caplan HS. Neoplasms of the small bowel. Am Surg 1974;180:157–161.
4. Treadwell TA, White R. Primary tumors of the small bowel. Am J Surg 1975;130:749–755.
5. Croom RD, Newsome JF. Tumors of the small intestine. Am Surg 1975;41:160–167.
6. Freund H, Lavi A, Pfeffermann R, Durst AL. Primary neoplasms of the small bowel. Am J Surg 1978;135:757–759.
7. Miles RM, Crawford D, Duras S. The small bowel tumor problem. Ann Surg 1979;189:732–740.
8. Mittal VK, Bodzin JH. Primary malignant tumors of the small bowel. Am J Surg 1980;140:396–399.
9. Herbsman H, Wetstern L, Rosen Y, et al. Tumors of the small intestine. Curr Probl Surg 1980;17:123–182.
10. Norberg K, Emas S. Primary tumors of the small intestine. Am J Surg 1981;142:569–573.
11. Ahlman H, Kjellstrom T. Clinically diagnosed small intestinal tumors in an urban Swedish area. Acta Chir Scand 1981;147:371–376.

12. Waterhouse G, Skudlarick J, Adkins RB. A clinical review of small bowel neoplasms. South Med J 1981;74:1202–1203.

13. Gupta S, Gupta S. Primary tumors of the small bowel: A clinicopathological study of 58 cases. J Surg Oncol 1982;20:161–167.

14. Giuliani A, Caporale A, Teneriello F, Alessi G, Serpieri P. Primary tumors of the small intestine. Int Surg 1985:331–334.

15. Zollinger RM, Sternfeld W, Schreiber H. Primary neoplasms of the small intestine. Am J Surg 1986;151:654–658.

16. Desa L, Bridger F, et al. Primary jejunoileal tumors: A review of 45 cases. World J Surg 1991;15:81–87.

17. Sager GF. Primary malignant tumors of the small intestine. Am J Surg 1978;135:601–602.

18. Coutsoftides T, Shibata HR. Primary malignant tumors of the small intestine. Dis Colon Rectum 1979;22:24–26.

19. Lowenfels AB. Why are small-bowel tumours so rare? Lancet 1973;1:24–26.

20. Cicarelli O, Welch JP, Kent G. Primary malignant tumors of the small bowel: The Hartford Hospital experience, 1969–1983. Am J Surg 1987;153:350–354.

21. Collin CF, Amerson JR, et al. Primary malignant small bowel tumors: Clinical imitators of benign disease. Surg Gastroenterol 1982;1:203–211.

22. Johnson AM, Harman PK, Hanks JB. Primary small bowel malignancies. Am Surg 1985;51:31–36.

23. Barclay THC, Schapira DV. Malignant tumors of the small intestine. Cancer 1983;51:878–881.

24. Weiss NS, Yang C. Incidence of histologic types of cancer of the small intestine. JNCI 1987;78:653–656.

25. Laws H, Han SY, Aldrete, J. Malignant tumors of the small bowel. South Med J 1984;77:1087–1090.

26. Goel JP, Didolkar MS, Elias EG. Primary malignant tumors of the small intestine. Surg Gynecol Obstet 1976;143:717–719.

27. Martin RG. Malignant tumors of the small intestine. Surg Clin North Am 1986;66:779–785.

28. Reyes EL, Talley RW. Primary malignant tumors of the small intestine. Am J Gastroenterol 1970;54:30–43.

29. Wattenberg LW. Carcinogen-detoxifying mechanisms in the gastrointestinal tract. Gastroenterology 1966;51:932–935.

30. Wattenberg LW. Studies of polycyclic hydrocarbon hydroxylases of the intestine possibly related to cancer effect of diet on benzpyrene hydroxylase activity. Cancer 1971;28:99–102.

31. Williamson RC, Welch CE, Malt RA. Adenocarcinoma and lymphoma of the small intestine. Ann Surg 1983;197:172–178.

32. Ross RK, Hartnett NM, Bernstein L, Henderson BE. Epidemiology of adenocarcinomas of the small intestine: Is bile a small bowel carcinogen? Br J Cancer 1991;63:143–145.

33. Scudamore CH, Freeman HJ. Effects of small bowel transection, resection, or bypass in 1,2-dimethylhydrazine-induced rat intestinal neoplasia. Gastroenterology 1983;84:725–731.

34. Lowenfels AB, Sonni A. Distribution of small bowel tumors. Cancer Lett 1977;3:83–86.

35. Pollard M, Luckert PH. Tumorigenic effect of direct and indirect acting chemical carcinogens in rats on a restricted diet. JNCI 1985;74:1347–1349.

36. Sellner F. Investigations on the significance of the adenoma-carcinoma sequence in the small bowel. Cancer 1990;66:702–715.

37. Perzin KH, Bridge MF. Adenomas of the small intestine: A clinicopathologic review of 51 cases and a study of their relationship to carcinoma. Cancer 1981;48:799–819.

38. Gahtan V, Nochomovitz LE, Robinson AM, Garcia VF, Smith LE. Gastroduodenal polyps in familial polyposis coli. Am Surg 1989;55:278–280.

39. Bulow S, Lauritsen KB, Johannsen A, Svendsen LB, Sondergaard JO. Gastroduodenal polyps in familial polyposis coli. Dis Colon Rectum 1985;28:90–93.

40. Jarvinen HJ, Sipponen P. Gastroduodenal polyps in familial adenomatous and juvenile polyposis. Endoscopy 1986;18:230–234.

41. Iida M, Yao T, Itoh H, Watanabe H, Matsui T, Iwashita A, Fujishima M. Natural history of duodenal lesions in Japanese patients with familial adenomatosis coli (Gardner's syndrome). Gastroenterology 1989;96:1301–1306.

42. Domizio P, Talbot IC, Spigelman AD, Williams CB, Phillips RKS. Upper gastrointestinal pathology in familial adenomatous polyposis: Results from a prospective study of 102 patients. J Clin Pathol 1990;43:738–743.

43. Kurtz RC, Sternberg SS, Miller HH, Decosse JJ. Upper gastrointestinal neoplasia in familial polyposis. Dig Dis Sci 1987;32:459–465.

44. Hawker PC, Gyde SN, Thompson H, Allan RN. Adenocarcinoma of the small intestine complicating Crohn's disease. Gut 1982;23:188–193.

45. Frank JD, Shorey BA. Adenocarcinoma of the small bowel as a complication of Crohn's disease. Gut 1973;14:120–124.

46. Morowitz DA, Block GE, Kirsner JB. Adenocarcinoma of the ileum complicating chronic regional enteritis. Gastroenterology 1968;55:397–402.

47. Petras RE, Mir-Madjlessi SH, Farmer RG. Crohn's disease and intestinal carcinoma. A report of 11 cases with emphasis on associated epithelial dysplasia. Gastroenterology 1987;93:1307–1314.

48. Simpson S, Traube J, Riddell RH. The histologic appearance of dysplasia (precarcinomatous change) in Crohn's disease of the small and large intestine. Gastroenterology 1981;81:492–501.

49. Hyams JS, Goldman H, Katz AJ. Differentiating small bowel Crohn's disease from lymphoma. Role of rectal biopsy. Gastroenterology 1980;79:340–343.

50. Ribeiro MB, Greenstein AJ, Heiman TM, Yamazaki Y, Aufses AH. Adenocarcinoma of the small intestine in Crohn's disease. Surg Gynecol Obstet 1991;173:343–349.

51. Bonacina E, Barbano PR, Barberis M, Rossi MV. Primary adenocarcinoma of terminal ileum with clinical and gross morphologic features simulating Crohn's disease. A case report. Tumori 1985;71:513–518.

52. Keller RJ, Hertz I, Zimmerman M, Geller S. Carcinoma of the ileum simulating Crohn's disease. AJR 1982;138:151–153.

53. Swinson CM, Coles EC, Slavin G, Booth CC. Coeliac disease and malignancy. Lancet 1983;1:111–115.

54. Holmes GKT, Dunn GI, Cockel R, Brookes VS. Adenocarcinoma of the upper small bowel complicating coeliac disease. Gut 1980;21:1010–1016.

55. Trier JS. Celiac sprue. N Engl J Med 1991;325:1709–1719.

56. Giardiello FM, Welsh SB, Hamilton SD, Offerhaus GJ, et al. Increased risk of cancer in the Peutz-Jeghers syndrome. N Engl J Med 1987;316:1511–1514.

57. Konishi F, Wyse NE, Muto T, Sawada T, et al. Peutz-Jeghers polyposis associated with carcinoma of the digestive organs. Dis Colon Rectum 1989;30:790–799.

58. Spigelman AD, Murday V, Phillips RKS. Cancer and the Peutz-Jeghers syndrome. Gut 1990;30:1588–1590.

59. Linos DA, Dozois RR, Dahlin DC, Bartholomew LG. Does Peutz-Jeghers syndrome predispose to gastrointestinal malignancy? Arch Surg 1981;116:1182–1184.

60. Hochberg FH, Dasilva AB, Galdabini J, Richardson EP. Gastrointestinal involvement in von Recklinghausen's neurofibromatosis. Neurology 1974;24:1144–1151.

61. Rutgeerts P, Hendrick H, Geboes K, Ponette E, Broeckaert L, Vantrappen G. Involvement of the upper digestive tract by systemic neurofibromatosis. Gastrointest Endosc 1981;27:22–24.

62. Williams SJ, Lucas RJ, McCaughey RS. Paraganglioma of the duodenum: A case report. Surgery 1980;87:454–458.

63. Kheir SM, Halpern NB. Paraganglioma of the duodenum in association with congenital neurofibromatosis. Cancer 1984;53:2491–2496.

64. Inai K, Kobuke T, Yonehara S, Tokuoka S. Duodenal gangliocytic paraganglioma with lymph node metastasis in a 17-year-old boy. Cancer 1989;63:2540–2545.

65. Kingston RD. Neurofibromatosis and small bowel adenocarcinoma—an unrecognized association. Gut 1988;29:134.

66. Wheeler MH, Curley IR, Williams ED. The association of neurofibromatosis pheochromocytoma, and somatostatin-rich duodenal carcinoid tumor. Surgery 1986;100:1163–1168.

67. Alexander JW, Altemeier WA. Association of primary neoplasms of the small intestine with other neoplastic growths. Ann Surg 1968;167:958–964.

68. Morgan DF, Busuttil RW. Primary adenocarcinoma of the small intestine. Am J Surg 1977;134:331–333.

69. Awrich AE, Irish CE, et al. A twenty-five-year experience with primary malignant tumors of the small intestine. Surg Gynecol Obstet 1980;151:9–13.

70. Lanzafame RJ, Long JE, Hinshaw JR. Primary cancer of the small bowel. NY State J Med 1982;8:1325–1329.

71. Strodel WE, Talpos G, Eckhauser F, Thompson N. Surgical therapy for small-bowel carcinoid tumors. Arch Surg 1983;118:391–397.

72. Ouriel K, Adams J. Adenocarcinoma of the small intestine. Am J Surg 1984;147:66–71.

73. Lioe TF, Biggart JD. Primary adenocarcinoma of the jejunum and ileum: Clinicopathological review of 25 cases. J Clin Pathol 1990;43:533–536.

74. Maglinte DDT, O'Connor K, Bessette J, Chernish SM, Kelvin FM. The role of the physician in the late diagnosis of primary malignant tumors of the small intestine. Am J Gastroenterol 1991;86:304–308.

75. Brophy C, Cahow CE. Primary small bowel malignant tumors. Am Surg 1989;55:408–412.

76. Ashley SW, Wells SA. Tumors of the small intestine. Semin Oncol 1988;15:116–128.

77. Ekberg O, Ekholm S. Radiography in primary tumors of the small bowel. Acta Radiol 1980;21:79–84.

78. Bessette JR, Maglinte DDT, Kelvin FM, Chernish SM. Primary malignant tumors in the small bowel: A comparison of the small-bowel enema and conventional follow-through examination. AJR 1989;153:741–744.

79. Maglinte DDT, Hall R, Miller RE, Chernish SM, Rosenak B, Elmore M, Burney BT. Detection of surgical lesions of the small bowel by enteroclysis. Am J Surg 1984;147:225–229.

80. Cohen ME, Barkin JS. Enteroscopy and enteroclysis: The combined procedure. Am J Gastroenterol 1989;84:1413–1415.

81. Schnyder PA, Candardjis G. CT detection of benign and malignant abnormalities of the small bowel. Eur J Radiol 1983;3:33–38.

82. Laurent F, Raynaud M, Biset JM, Boisserie-Lacroix M, Grelet P, Drouillard J. Diagnosis and categorization of small bowel neoplasms: Role of computed tomography. Gastrointest Radiol 1991;16:115–119.

83. James S, Balfe DM, Lee JKT, Picus D. Small bowel disease: Categorization by CT examination. AJR 1987;148:863–868.

84. Dudiak KM, Johnson CD, Stephens DH. Primary tumors of the small intestine: CT evaluation. AJR 1989;152:995–998.

85. Scatairge JC, Allen HA, Fishman EK. Computed tomography of the small bowel. Semin Ultrasound CT MR 1987;8:403–423.

86. Siegel MJ, Evans SJ, Balfe DM. Small bowel disease in children: Diagnosis with CT. Radiology 1988;169:127–130.

87. Alfidi RJ, Esselstyn CD, Tarar R, Klein HJ, Hermann RE, Weakley FL, Turnbull RB Jr. Recognition and angiosurgical detection of arteriovenous malformations of the bowel. Ann Surg 1971;174:573–582.

88. Oliver GC, Rubin RJ, Park YH, Ashton JK. Preoperative localization of intermittently bleeding small intestinal tumors using Tc-99m-labeled red blood cell scanning report of two cases. Dis Colon Rectum 1987;30:715–720.

89. Bowden TA. Endoscopy of the small intestine. Surg Clin North Am 1989;69:1237–1247.
90. Foutch PG, Sanowski RA, Kelly S. Enteroscopy: A method for detection of small bowel tumors. Am J Gastroenterol 1985;80:887–890.
91. Halphen M, Najjar T, Jaafoura H, Cammoun M, Tufrali G. Diagnostic value of upper intestinal fiber endoscopy in primary small intestinal lymphoma. Cancer 1986;58:2140–2145.
92. Gilbert DA, Buelow RG, Chung RSK, Cunningham JT, et al. Status evaluation: Enteroscopy. Gastrointest Endosc 1991;37:673–677.
93. Iida M, Yao T, Ohsato K, Itoh H, Watanabe H. Diagnostic value of intraoperative fiberscopy for small-intestinal polyps in familial adenomatosis coli. Endoscopy 1980;12:161–165.
94. Frucht J, Norton JA, London JF, Vinayek R, Doppman JL, Gardner JD, Jensen RT, Maton PN. Detection of duodenal gastrinomas by operative endoscopic transillumination. Gasteroenterology 1990;99:1622–1627.
95. Estrin HM, Farhi DC, Ament AA, Yang P. Ileoscopic diagnosis of malignant lymphoma of the small bowel in acquired immunodeficiency syndrome. Gastrointest Endosc 1987;33:390–391.
96. Moertel CG, Sauer WG, Dockerty MB, Baggenstoss AH. Life history of the carcinoid tumor of the small intestine. Cancer 1961;14:901–912.
97. Wilson JM, Melvin DB, Gray G, Thorbjornson B. Benign small bowel tumors. Ann Surg 1975;181:247–250.
98. Skandalakis JE, Gray SW. Smooth muscle tumors of the small intestine. In: Smooth muscle tumors of the alimentary tract: Leiomyomas and leiomyosarcomas, a review of 2525 cases. Springfield, IL: Charles C. Thomas, 1962:112–154.
99. Choctaw WT, Burbige EJ, McCandless CM. Duodenal villous adenoma. Am Surg 1980;640–643.
100. Everett GD, Shirazi SS, Mitros FA. Villous tumors of the duodenum. Am J Gastroenterol 1981;75:376–379.
101. Komorowski RA, Cohen EB. Villous tumors of the duodenum: A clinicopathological study. Cancer 1981;47:1377–1386.
102. Reddy RR, Schuman BM, Priest RJ. Duodenal polyps: Diagnosis and management. J Clin Gastroenterol 1981;3:139–145.
103. Delpy JC, Bruneton JN, Drouillard J, Leconte P. Non-vaterian duodenal adenomas: Report of 24 cases and review of the literature. Gastrointest Radiol 1983;8:135–141.
104. Haglund U, Fork FT, Genell S, Rehnberg O. Villous adenomas in the duodenum. Br J Surg 1985;72:26–27.
105. Ryan DF, Schapiro RH, Warshaw AL. Villous tumors of the duodenum. Ann Surg 1986;203:301–306.
106. Brian JE, Herring GF, Stair JM. Duodenal villous adenomas. J Surg Oncol 1986;33:203–206.
107. Celik C, Venditti JA, Satchidanand S, Freier DT. Villous tumors of the duodenum and ampulla of Vater. J Surg Oncol 1986;33:268–272.
108. Galandiuk S, Hermann RE, Jagelman DG, Fazio VW, Sivak MV. Villous tumors of the duodenum. Ann Surg 1988;207:234–239.
109. Krukowski ZH, Ewen SW, Davidson AI, Matheson NA. Operative management of tubulovillous neoplasms of the duodenum and ampulla. Br J Surg 1988;75:150–153.
110. Chappuis CW, Divincenti FC, Cohn I Jr. Villous tumors of the duodenum. Ann Surg 1989;209:593–599.
111. Bjork KJ, Davis CJ, Nagorney DM, Mucha P Jr. Duodenal villous tumors. Arch Surg 1990;125:961–965.
112. Kutin ND, Ranson JHC, Gouge TH, Localio SA. Villous tumors of the duodenum. Ann Surg 1975;181:164–168.
113. Schulten MF, Oyasu R, Beal JM. Villous adenoma of the duodenum—a case report and review of the literature. Am J Surg 1976;132:90–99.
114. Steinberg LS, Shieber W. Villous adenomas of the small intestine. Surgery 1972;71:423–428.
115. Dormandy TL. Gastrointestinal polyposis with mucocutaneous pigmentation (Peutz-Jeghers syndrome). N Engl J Med 1957;256:1186–1190.
116. Dormandy TL. Gastrointestinal polyposis with mucocutaneous pigmentation (Peutz-Jeghers syndrome). N Engl J Med 1957;256:1093–1103.
117. Bilton JL, Riahi M. Hemangioma of the small intestine. Am J Gastroenterol 1967;48:120–124.
118. Sivula A. Intestinal haemangioma. Acta Chir Scand 1966;131:485–491.
119. Brzezinski W, Bailey RJ, Besney M, Turner G. Small-bowel lipoma: An uncommon cause of obstruction. Can J Surg 1990;33:423–424.
120. Climie ARW, Wylin RF. Small-intestinal lipomatosis. Arch Pathol Lab Med 1981;105:40–42.
121. Silverman L, Waugh JM, Huizenga KA, Harrison EG. Large adenomatous polyp of Brunner's glands. Am J Clin Pathol 1961;36:438–443.
122. De Silva S, Chandrasoma P. Giant duodenal hematoma consisting mainly of Brunner's glands. Am J Surg 1977;133:240–243.
123. Maglinte DDT, Mayes SL, Ng AC, Pickett RD. Brunner's gland adenoma: Diagnostic considerations. J Clin Gastroenterol 1982;4:127–131.
124. Shimer GR, Helwig EB. Inflammatory fibroid polyps of the intestine. Am J Clin Pathol 1984;81:708–714.
125. Manning RJ, Lewis C. Inflammatory ileal polyps in Crohn's disease presenting as refractory iron deficiency anemia. Gastrointest Endosc 1986;32:122.
126. Ott DJ, Wu WC, Shiflett DW, Pennell TC. Inflammatory fibroid polyp of the duodenum. Am J Gastroenterol 1980;73:62–64.
127. Assarian GS, Sundareson A. Inflammatory fibroid polyp of the ileum. Hum Pathol 1985;16:311–312.
128. Nothinger F. Erfahrung mit 50 klinisch manifesten Dunndarmtumoren. Helv Chir Acta 1980;47:597–599.
129. Adler SN, Lyon DT, Sullivan PD. Adenocarcinoma of the small bowel clinical features, similarity to regional enteritis, and analysis of 338 documented cases. Am J Gasteroenterol 1982;77:326–330.
130. O'Rourke MGE, Lancashire RP, Vattoune JR. Lymphoma of the small intestine. Aust N Z J Surg 1986;56:351–355.
131. Taggart DP, Imrie CW. A new pattern of histologic predominance and distribution of malignant diseases of the small intestine. Surg Gynecol Obstet 1987;165:515–518.
132. Lai ECS, Doty JE, Irving C, Tompkins RK. Primary adenocarcinoma of the duodenum: Analysis of survival. World J Surg 1988;12:695–699.
133. Kerremans RP, Lerut J, Penninck FM. Primary malignant duodenal tumors. Ann Surg 1979;190:179–182.
134. Spira IA, Ghazi A, Wolff WI. Primary adenocarcinoma of the duodenum. Cancer 1977;39:1721–1726.
135. Joesting DR, Beart RW, vanHeerden JA, Weiland LH. Improving survival in adenocarcinoma of the duodenum. Am J Surg 1981;141:228–231.
136. Awlmark A, Andersson A, Lasson A. Primary carcinoma of the duodenum. Ann Surg 1980;191:13–18.
137. Chernish SM, Miller RE, Rosenak BD, Scholz NE. Hypotonic duodenography with the use of glucagon. Gastroenterology 1972;62:392–398.
138. Lillemoe K, Imbembo AL. Malignant neoplasms of the duodenum. Surg Gynecol Obstet 1980;150:822–826.
139. Cohen JR, Kuchta N, Geller N, Shires GT, Dineen P. Pancreaticoduodenectomy. Ann Surg 1982;195:608–617.
140. Herter FP, Cooperman AM, Ahlborn TN, Antinori C. Surgical experience with pancreatic and periampullary cancer. Ann Surg 1982;195:274–281.
141. Kellum JM, Clark J, Miller HH. Pancreatoduodenectomy for resectable malignant periampullary tumors. Surg Gynecol Obstet 1983;157:362–366.
142. Gaddy M, Max MH. Carcinoma of the duodenum. South Med J 1985;78:150–152.
143. Jones BA, Langer B, Taylor BR, Girotti M. Periampullary tumors: Which ones should be resected? Am J Surg 1985;149:46–52.
144. Grace PA, Pitt HA, Tompkins RK, DenBesten L, Longmire WP. Decreased morbidity and mortality after pancreatoduodenectomy. Am J Surg 1986;151:141–149.
145. Tarazi RY, Hermann RE, Vogt DP, Hoerr SO, Esselstyn DB, Cooperman AM, Steiger E, Grundfest S. Results of surgical treatment of periampullary tumors: A thirty-five year experience. Surgery 1986;100:716–722.
146. Gonzalez CD, Evans EC. Primary adenocarcinoma of the duodenum. Am Surg 1987;53:174–179.
147. Sarma DP, Weilbaecher TG. Adenocarcinoma of the duodenum. J Surg Oncol 1987;34:262–263.
148. Crist DW, Sitzmann JV, Cameron JL. Improved hospital morbidity, mortality, and survival after the Whipple procedure. Ann Surg 1987;206:358–365.
149. Michelassi F, Erroi F, Dawson PJ, Pietrabissa A, Noda S, Handcock M, Block GE. Experience with 647 consecutive tumors of the duodenum, ampulla, head of the pancreas, and distal common bile duct. Ann Surg 1989;210:544–556.
150. Brennan MF. Duodenal cancer. Asian J Surg 1990;13:204–209.
151. Koretz MJ, Graham R. Primary adenocarcinoma of the jejunum. Am Surg 1989;55:539–542.
152. Cooper BT, Read AE. Small intestinal lymphoma. World J Surg 1985;9:930–937.
153. Jigyasu D, Bedikian AY, Stroehlein JR. Chemotherapy for primary adenocarcinoma of the small bowel. Cancer 1984;53:23–25.
154. Peck JJ, Shields AB, Boyden AM, Dworkin LA, Nadal JW. Carcinoid tumors of the ileum. Am J Surg 1983;146:124–132.
155. Sjoblom SM. Clinical presentation and prognosis of gastrointestinal carcinoid tumors. Scand J Gasteroenterol 1988;23:779–787.
156. Makridis C, Oberg K, Juhlin C, Rastad J, Johansson H, Lorelius LE, Akerstrom G. Surgical treatment of mid-gut carcinoid tumors. World J Surg 1990;14:377–385.
157. Moertel CG. Treatment of the carcinoid tumor and the malignant carcinoid syndrome. J Clin Oncol 1983;1:727–740.
158. Olney JR, Urdaneta LF, Al-Jurf AS, Jochimsen PR, Shirazi SS. Carcinoid tumors of the gastrointestinal tract. Am Surg 1985;51:37–41.
159. Tilson MD. Carcinoid syndrome. Surg Clin North Am 1974;54:409–423.
160. Vinick AI, McLeod MK, Fig LM, Shapiro B, Lloyd RV, Cho K. Clinical features, diagnosis, and localization of carcinoid tumors and their management. Gastrointest Clin North Am 1989;18:865–896.
161. Thompson GB, vanHeerden JA, Martin JK Jr, Schutt AJ, Carney JA. Carcinoid tumors of the gastrointestinal tract: Presentation, management and prognosis. Surgery 1985;98:1054–1063.
162. Woods HF, Bax NDS, Smith JAR. Small bowel carcinoid tumors. World J Surg 1985;9:921–929.
163. Dawes L, Schulte WJ, Condon RE. Carcinoid Tumors. Arch Surg 1984;119:375–378.
164. Nwiloh JO, Pillarisetty S, Moscovic EA, Freeman HP. Carcinoid tumors. J Surg Oncol 1990;45:261–264.
165. O'Rourke MGE, Lancashire RP, Vattoune JR. Carcinoid of the small intestine. Aust N Z J Surg 1986;56:405–408.
166. Martin JK Jr, Moertel CG, Adson MA, Schutt AJ. Surgical treatment of functioning metastatic carcinoid tumors. Arch Surg 1983;118:537–542.
167. Zeitels J, Naunheim K, Kaplan EL, Straus F. Carcinoid tumors—a 37-year experience. Arch Surg 1982;117:732–737.
168. McDermott E, Guduric B, Brennan MF. Prognostic variables in gastrointestinal carcinoid tumors (submitted).
169. Godwin JD. Carcinoid tumors—an analysis of 2837 cases. Cancer 1975;36:560–569.
170. Johnson LA, Lavin P, Moertel CG, et al. Carcinoids: The association of histologic growth pattern and survival. Cancer 1983;51:882–889.

171. Nobin AP, Erhardt K, Auer G, Falkmer S, Martensson H. Nuclear DNA patterns and survival in metastasizing ileal carcinoids. World J Surg 1987;11:372–377.

172. Tsushima K, Nagorney DM, Weiland LH, Lieber MM. The relationship of flow cytometric DNA analysis and clinicopathology in small-intestinal carcinoids. Surgery 1989;105:366–373.

173. Rosenfelt F, Rosenberg SA. Diffuse histiocytic lymphoma presenting with gastrointestinal tract lesions—the Stanford experience. Cancer 1980;45:2188–2193.

174. Dawson IM, Cornes JS, Morson BC. Primary malignant lymphoid tumors of the intestinal tract: Report of 37 cases with a study of factors influencing prognosis. Br J Surg 1961;40:80–88.

175. Sweetenhaus JW, Mead GM, Wright DH, McKendrick JJ, Jones DH, Williams CJ, Whitehouse JMA. Involvement of the ileocaecal region by non-Hodgkin's lymphoma in adults: Clinical features and results of treatment. Br J Ca 1989;60:366–369.

176. Carbone PP, Kaplan HS, Mussoff K, Smithers DW, Tubiana M. Report of the committee on Hodgkin's disease staging classification. Cancer Res 1971;31:1860.

177. Blackledge G, Bush H, Dodge OG, Crowther D. A study of gastrointestinal lymphoma. Clin Oncol 1979;5:209–219.

178. Contreary K, Nance FC, Becker WF. Primary lymphoma of the gastrointestinal tract. Ann Surg 1980;191:593–598.

179. Auger MJ, Allan NC. Primary ileocecal lymphoma. Cancer 1990;65:358–361.

180. Gray GM, Rosenberg SA, Cooper AD, Gregory PB, Stein DT, Herzenberg H. Lymphomas involving the gastrointestinal tract. Gasteroenterology 1982;82:143–152.

181. Rao AR, Kagan AR, Potyk D, Nussbaum H, Chan P, Hintz BL, Wollin M, Ryoo MC. Management of gastrointestinal lymphoma. Am J Clin Oncol 1984;7:213–219.

182. ReMine SG, Braasch JW. Gastric and small bowel lymphoma. Surg Clin North Am 1986;66:713–722.

183. Sartoris DJ, Harell GS, Anderson MF, Zboralske FF. Small bowel lymphoma and regional enteritis: Radiographic similarities. Radiol 1984;152:291–296.

184. Morgan DR, Holgate CS, Dixon MF, Bird CC. Primary small intestinal lymphoma: A study of 39 cases. J Pathol 1985;147:211–221.

185. Weingrad DN, Decosse JJ, Sherlock P, Straus D, Lieberman PH, Filippa DA. Primary gastrointestinal lymphoma: A 30-year review. Cancer 1982;49:1258–1265.

186. Shepherd FA, Evans WK, Kutas G, Yau JC, et al. Chemotherapy following surgery for stages IE and IIE non-Hodgkin's lymphoma of the gastrointestinal tract. J Clin Oncol 1988;6:253–260.

187. Steward WP, Harris M, Wagstaff J, Scarfe JH, et al. A prospective study of the treatment of high grade histology non-Hodgkin's lymphoma involving the gastrointestinal tract. Eur J Cancer Clin Oncol 1985;21:1195–1200.

188. Al-Bahrani ZR, Al-Mondhiry H, Bakir F, Al-Saleem T. Clinical and pathologic subtypes of primary intestinal lymphoma. Cancer 1983;52:1666–1672.

189. Skudder PA Jr, Schwartz SI. Primary lymphoma of the gastrointestinal tract. Surg Gynecol Obstet 1985;160:5–8.

190. Dragosics B, Bauer P, Radaszkiewicz T. Primary gastrointestinal non-Hodgkin's lymphoma—a retrospective clinicopathologic study of 150 cases. Cancer 1985;55:1060–1073.

191. Fleming ID, Turk PS, Murphy SB, Crist WM, Santana VM, Rao BN. Surgical implications of primary gastrointestinal lymphoma of childhood. Arch Surg 1990;125:252–256.

192. Aozasa K, Ueda T, Kurata A, Kim CW, et al. Prognostic value of histologic and clinical factors in 56 patients with gastrointestinal lymphomas. Cancer 1988;61:309–315.

193. Haghighi P, Nasr K. Primary upper small intestinal lymphoma (so-called Mediterranean lymphoma). Pathol Ann 1973;8:231–255.

194. Monco A, Sartori C. Hodgkin's primary lymphoma of the small intestine. Haematologica 1984;69:568–571.

195. Antonioli DA. Gastrointestinal autonomic nerve tumors: Expanding the spectrum of gastrointestinal stromal tumors. Arch Pathol Lab Med 1989;113:831–833.

196. Herrera GA, Cerezo L, Jones JE, Sach J, et al. Gastrointestinal autonomic nerve tumors—plexosarcomas. Arch Pathol Lab Med 1989;113:846–853.

197. Chiotasso PJP, Fazio VW. Prognostic factors of 28 leiomyosarcomas of the small intestine. Surg Gynecol Obstet 1982;155:197–202.

198. Shiu MH, Farr GH, Egeli RA, Quan SHG, Hajdu SI. Myosarcomas of the small and large intestine: A clinicopathological study. J Surg Oncol 1983;24:67–72.

199. McGrath PC, Neifeld JP, Lawrence W, Kay S, Horsley JS III, Parker GA. Gastrointestinal sarcomas: Analysis of prognostic factors. Ann Surg 1987;206:706–710.

200. Kimura H, Yonemura Y, Kadoya N, Kosaka T, et al. Prognostic factors in primary gastrointestinal leiomyosarcoma: A retrospective study. World J Surg 1991;15:771–777.

201. Dougherty MJ, Compton C, Talbert M, Wood WJ. Sarcomas of the gastrointestinal tract: Separation into favorable and unfavorable prognostic groups by mitotic count. Ann Surg 1991;214:569–574.

202. Ng EH, Pollack RE, Romsdahl MM. Prognostic implications of patterns of failure for gastrointestinal leiomyosarcomas. Cancer 1992;69:1334–1341.

203. Ihde JK, Coit DG. Melanoma metastatic to the stomach, small bowel and colon. Am J Surg 1991;162:208–211.

204. McNeill PM, Wagman LD, Neifeld JP. Small bowel metastases from primary carcinoma of the lung. Cancer 1987;59:1486–1489.

205. Leidich RB, Rudolf LE. Small bowel perforation secondary to metastatic lung carcinoma. Ann Surg 1981;193:67–69.

206. Koos L, Field RE. Metastatic carcinoma of breast simulating Crohn's disease. Int Surg 1980;65:359–362.

207. Nyberg B, Sonnenfeld T. Metastatic breast carcinoma causing intestinal obstruction. Acta Chir Scand 1986;530:95–96.

208. Farmer RG, Hawk WA. Metastatic tumors of the small bowel. Gasteroenterology 1964;47:496–504.

209. Ngan H. Involvement of the duodenum by metastases from tumours of the genital tract. Br J Radiol 1970;43:701–705.

210. Haynes IG, Wolverson RL, O'Brien JM. Small bowel intussusception due to metastatic renal carcinoma. Br J Urol 1986;58:460.

211. Lawson LJ, Holt LP, Rooke HWP. Recurrent duodenal haemorrhage from renal carcinoma. Br J Urol 1966;38:133–137.

212. Phillips DL, Benner KG, Keefe EB, Traweek ST. Isolated metastasis to small bowel from anaplastic thyroid carcinoma. J Clin Gasteroenterol 1987;9:563–567.

213. Naunton Morgan TC, Henderson RG. Small bowel metastases from a Merkel cell tumor. Br J Radiol 1985;58:1212–1213.

214. Yang PM, Sheu JC, Yang TH, Chen DS, Yu JY, Lee CS, Hsu HC, Sung JL. Metastasis of hepatocellular carcinoma to the proximal jejunum manifested by occult gastrointestinal bleeding. Am J Gasteroenterol 1987;82:165–167.

215. Reintgen DS, Thompson W, Garbutt J, Seigler HF. Radiologic, endoscopic and surgical consideration of malignant melanoma metastatic to the small intestine. Curr Surg 1984;41:87–89.

216. Caputy G, Donohue JH, Goellner JH, Ilstrup DM. Metastatic melanoma of the gastrointestinal tract: The results of surgical management. Arch Surg 1991;126:1353–1358.

217. Branum GD, Seigler HF. Role of surgical intervention in the management of intestinal metastases from malignant melanoma. Am J Surg 1991;162:428–431.

218. Wilson BG, Anderson JR. Malignant melanoma involving the small bowel. Postgrad Med J 1986;62:355–357.

Cancer: Principles & Practice of Oncology, Fourth Edition,
edited by Vincent T. DeVita, Jr., Samuel Hellman, Steven A. Rosenberg.
J.B. Lippincott Co., Philadelphia © 1993.

Alfred M. Cohen
Bruce D. Minsky
Richard L. Schilsky

CHAPTER **30**

Colon Cancer

Adenocarcinoma of the large bowel affects about one person in 20 in the United States and in most Westernized countries. With more than 155,000 new cases diagnosed in the United States each year, representing 15% of all cancers, this disease constitutes a major public health problem. If diagnosed in its early stages, this common malignancy is highly curable by surgical treatment with minimal morbidity and mortality.

This chapter reviews recent advances in the biology and multidisciplinary treatment of primary colon cancer. Topics relevant to colon and rectal cancer are discussed. Treatment of patients with potentially curable cancers is discussed separately from treatment of patients with unresectable, recurrent, or metastatic disease. Management of patients with rectal cancer is covered in Chapter 31.

Figure 30–1 provides an overview of the end results of treatment of patients with colon and rectal adenocarcinoma. It demonstrates the need for improved earlier diagnosis and control of micrometastatic disease. Figure 30–2 suggests that efforts in these directions have reduced the overall death rate from this cancer. The 5-year relative survival rate from colon cancer increased from 41% in the 1950s to 54% in the 1980s; the rate for rectal cancer increased from 40% to 51.5% during the same period.[1]

ANATOMY

GROSS ANATOMY OF THE LARGE BOWEL

The large bowel is divided into the colon and rectum. For treatment purposes, the large bowel should be considered in terms of free intraperitoneal location versus extraperitoneal location. Locoregional treatment failure of intraperitoneal tumors is more likely to manifest as peritoneal seeding, whereas such failure of extraperitoneal tumors manifests as local recurrence. Extraperitoneal sites include the pelvis and the abdominal retroperitoneum.

The cecum, transverse colon, and sigmoid loop are mobile structures that lie free in the peritoneal cavity and are completely covered with serosa (visceral peritoneum). The dorsal or posterior aspect of the ascending and descending colon and both flexures are frequently without serosa. Tumor spread from these segments may involve the retroperitoneal soft tissues, kidney, ureter, and pancreas. Although the rectum frequently is considered to be extraperitoneal, the anterior surface of the upper third of the rectum is covered with serosa and is therefore intraperitoneal. Patterns of recurrence of high rectal cancer may depend on whether the location of the tumor is anterior or posterior.

ARTERIAL SUPPLY TO THE LARGE BOWEL

Although standard surgical treatment of large bowel cancer includes resection of the potentially involved node-bearing mesentery, the extent of mesenteric resection frequently depends on arterial supply (Fig. 30–3).

VENOUS DRAINAGE

The venous system of the colon and upper rectum drains into the portal circulation. The distal 5 to 7 cm of the rectum has a dual drainage. The superior hemorrhoidal vein drains into the portal circulation by way of the inferior mesenteric vein; the middle and inferior hemorrhoidal veins pass through pelvic veins directly into the inferior vena cava. Therefore, distal rectal cancers are more likely to produce isolated pulmonary metastases.

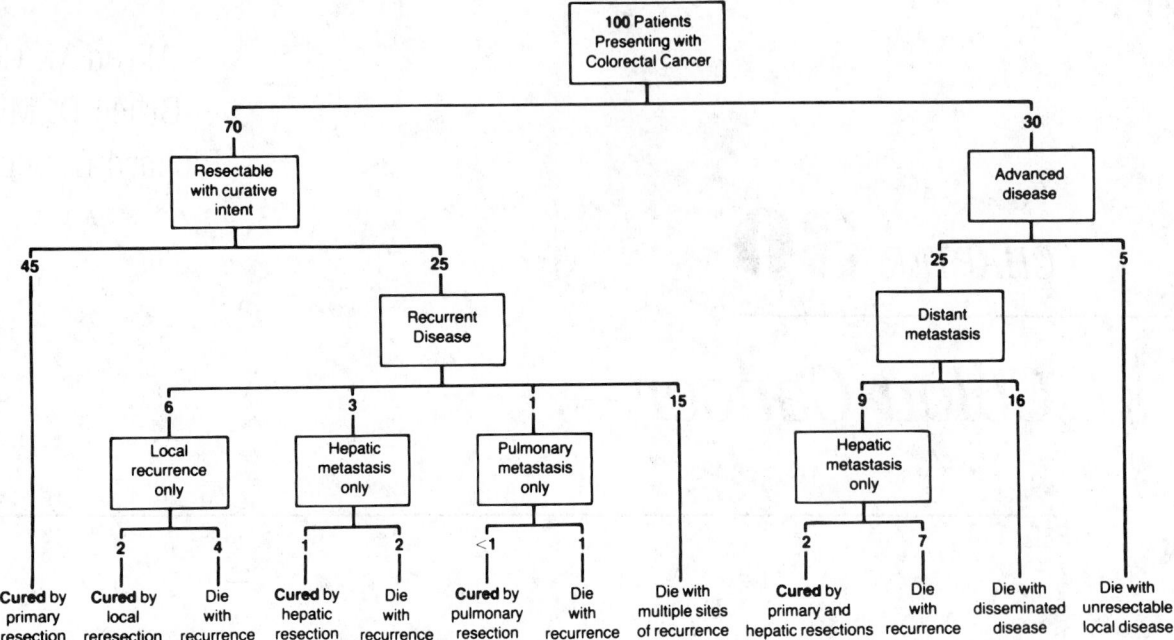

FIGURE 30–1. Patterns of failure in 100 patients presenting with large bowel cancer. (August DA, Ottow RT, Sugarbaker PH. Clinical perspectives on human colorectal cancer metastases. Cancer Metastasis Rev 1984;3:303–324)

LYMPHATIC DRAINAGE

Management of patients with colorectal cancer requires an understanding of the location of the lymphatics and the patterns of drainage to lymph nodes. Surgical resection of tumor-bearing lymph nodes may be curative. Surgical lymphadenectomy should be considered as a therapeutic and staging procedure.

The intramural lymphatics of the large bowel begin as a plexus beneath the lamina propria, superficial to the muscularis mucosa. This anatomic relation explains the absence of lymph node metastases associated with in situ tumors. The lymphatics pass into the submucosa, where they follow blood capillaries. Efferent lymphatic vessels proceed radially outward through the circular and longitudinal muscle layers to communicate with an intramuscular and subserosal lymphatic plexus. Some lymphatics drain into subserosal epicolic lymph nodes. Most extramural lymphatics enter the mesentery and

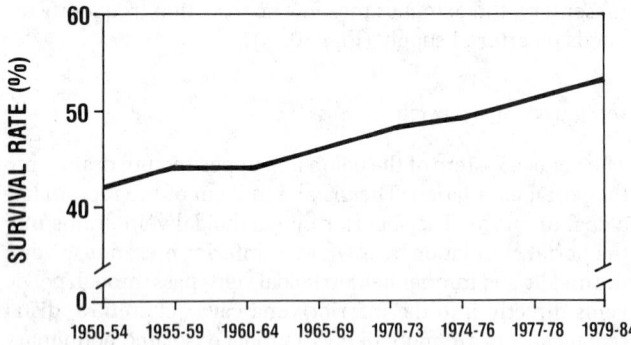

FIGURE 30–2. Improvement in 5-year relative survival rates from colorectal cancer (men and women).[2]

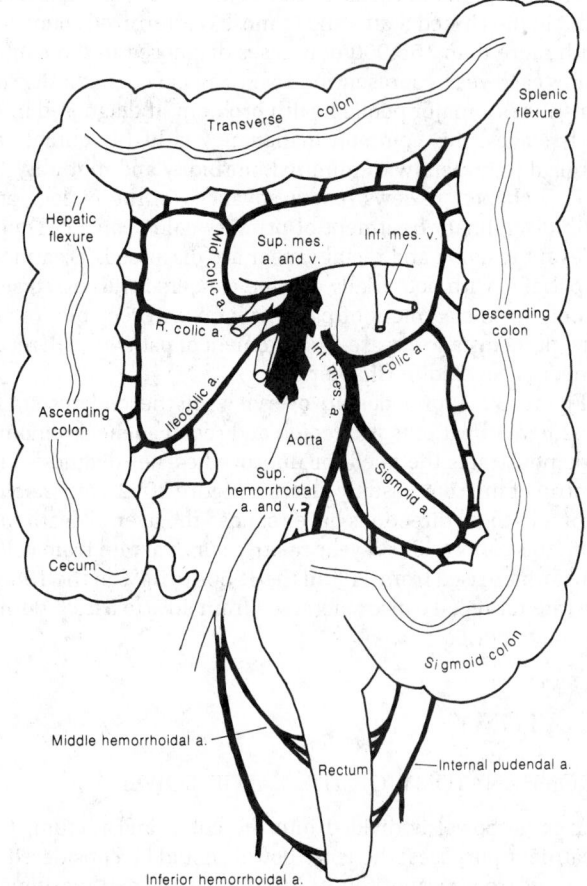

FIGURE 30–3. Anatomic segments and vascular supply to the colon and rectum. (Jones T, Shepard WC. A manual of surgical anatomy. Philadelphia: WB Saunders, 1945)

converge toward the major arterial trunks. The paracolic groups of lymph nodes along the marginal vascular arcades are the most numerous and are important sites of tumor metastases. The intermediate nodal groups are more proximal, involving the bifurcation of major arterial branches. Central or principal nodes are contiguous to the inferior mesenteric and superior mesenteric arteries and ultimately to the entire paraaortic chain.

EPIDEMIOLOGY

Worldwide, the incidence rates of colorectal cancer vary widely, from 3.4 cases per 100,000 population in Nigeria to 35.8 cases per 100,000 population in Connecticut.[2] In addition to North America, Australia, New Zealand, and portions of Northern and Western Europe have a high incidence of the disease.[3,4] In the United States, the Northeast has had a particularly high mortality from bowel cancer, with a marked clustering of cases in more densely populated areas. These trends are gradually becoming less apparent, but they still exist.[3] American immigrants originally from Germany, Ireland, Czechoslovakia, and Greece tend to have a higher incidence of disease than immigrants from other nations.[5,6]

The age-specific incidence of disease in the United States appears to rise steadily from the second to the ninth decade. Men have proportionately more rectal cancer than women, but both sexes are represented almost equally.[7]

In the United States, two religious groups have a diminished risk for large bowel cancer. Seventh-Day Adventists and Mormons have a standardized mortality ratio of 0.52 to 0.81 for bowel cancer at all sites, compared with geographic cohorts of other religions. Both groups refrain from using alcohol and tobacco and practice some form of dietary moderation.[8–11] The reasons for the 20% to 50% risk reduction are not clear; these populations continue to be the subjects of detailed studies.

Colorectal cancer is a dynamically changing disease entity.[3] There has been a progressive trend toward disease of the more proximal colon and away from disease of the rectosigmoid bowel.[2,12–14] Less than 60% of cases are endoscopically visible with rigid proctosigmoidoscopy.

ETIOLOGY

It has long been postulated that colorectal cancer is caused or promoted by environmental factors, especially by dietary factors that affect the enteric milieu.[15] It is suspected that carcinogens are present in feces.[16,17] Mutagens are present in the stools of many people who eat a Western diet.[18] The role of these mutagens as an etiologic factor in human colorectal cancer remains undefined. Although it is not possible to identify a specific cause of colon cancer, epidemiologic studies of nutritional habits and migration patterns are revealing. Studies with animal models of colon cancer strongly demonstrate that fat acts during the promotion stage of carcinogenesis and that both the type and quantity of fat are important determinants.[19] Both national and international studies reveal a clear association of human colorectal cancer with certain diets, such as those rich in animal fats and meat and poor in fiber, and with certain high-risk populations.[3,6,20,21]

Japanese in their native country have a low incidence of colorectal cancer, about 6 to 8 cases per 100,000 population.[2] However, first-generation Japanese emigrants to Hawaii have a 2.5-fold greater rate of large bowel cancer, similar to that of whites living in Hawaii.[22,23] Exposure to the typical American diet, which is rich in cholesterol and fat and low in fiber, appears to affect the risk even in first-generation immigrants.[24]

To identify the causative factors more precisely, at least six etiologic hypotheses are being tested preclinically, epidemiologically, or with clinical intervention, as described below.

FECAPENTAENES

Fecapentaenes are potent mutagenic compounds found in human feces and thought to be produced by gut microflora. They were active in the Ames *Salmonella* assay[25] and in mammalian cell systems.[26] There is a correlation between the level of stool fecapentaenes and tumor incidence in selected high-risk and low-risk populations in South Africa.[27] Bruce[28] and Correa and colleagues[29] have suggested a positive association between fecapentaene levels and the incidence of colon polyps. Intraluminal levels of fecapentaenes can be lowered by fiber, vitamin C, and vitamin E.[30,31]

3-KETOSTEROIDS

Presumed to be derived from metabolic products of cholesterol, 3-ketosteroids are potential tumor promoters or initiators. They induce genetic damage in cell cultures and rodent bowel.[32,33] At least two of these compounds have been identified in human feces and they may be present in higher concentrations in persons at higher risk for colon cancer.[34–36]

PYROLYSIS PRODUCTS

Compounds that result from the broiling or frying of meat at high temperatures, such as benzo[*a*]pyrene, have proved carcinogenic in rodents[37,38] and are suspected of contributing to gastric and esophageal cancers.[15]

NORMAL BILE ACIDS

Directly related to the intake of fat, bile acids such as deoxycholic and cholic acid are thought to induce gut lumen proliferation.[39,40] Populations that consume more fat have more bile acid secretion and an associated increased incidence of colon cancer. Removal of the gall bladder results in high levels of bile acids in the cecum, ascending colon, and stool[41,42] and may be associated with a greater frequency of right-sided colon cancer.[43] It is the free, not total, bile acid concentration that is most critical.[44,45]

INSUFFICIENT DIETARY CALCIUM

Calcium salts appear to modulate the damage described above by reducing the concentration of free bile acids through the formation of insoluble bile salt complexes.[44] At least one cohort study found that individuals with colon cancer tend to have a lower intake of calcium.[46]

FECAL pH

Alkaline environments support higher concentrations of free bile acids and other potential carcinogens.[47,48] In such an environment, bile acids are more soluble and carcinogens are more damaging in animal model systems.[48,49] Epidemiologic studies from South Africa and the United States reveal a higher incidence of colon cancer in subjects with a higher stool pH.[46,50,51]

PRIMARY PREVENTION

The prevention of colorectal cancer can be defined as primary or secondary.[52] Primary prevention is the identification and eradication of factors responsible for colorectal cancer. The focus of this approach involves dietary nutrients. Secondary prevention is the eradication of premalignant disease before its transformation into cancer.

Despite the inability to identify precisely the factor or factors responsible for colon cancer, a variety of dietary interventions have been considered and are being tested. Case control and population studies in Scandinavia, Israel, and the United States support the contention that increased dietary fiber is of value.[16,53-55] Of the many types of fiber, cellulose and bran fiber are more effective in reducing carcinogenesis than other fibers.[56-58] It remains unclear if the protective effect of bran fiber protects against rectal cancer.[59] Reddy and colleagues examined the effect of different types of dietary fiber and fiber fraction (wheat bran, oat fiber, and cellulose) on fecal mutagens and bile acids in a limited cohort of normal volunteers.[18] Compared with a control diet, there was a significant decrease in fecal mutagenic activity with cellulose and wheat bran. Changing the diet back to the control increased the fecal mutagenic activity significantly. Supplementation of the diet with cellulose or wheat bran decreased the concentration of fecal bile acids in the stool significantly. Oat bran had no major effect on these findings. Therefore, mutagen production and bile acid concentration may depend on the type of fiber consumed. The type of bran consumed also influences the type and activity of fecal bacterial enzymes.[60]

Limitation of total dietary fat and cholesterol has been proposed.[15] Studies of immigrant populations to Hawaii, populations in Nebraska,[6] and Seventh-Day Adventists[61] confirm that increased fat and cholesterol ingestion can be associated with increased risk for colorectal cancer. Persons with an increased intake of dietary vitamin D and calcium have a decreased risk for colon cancer.[62] In persons at increased risk for colon cancer, supplemental dietary calcium decreased the proliferation of epithelial cells in colon crypts.[63,64] However, the inhibitory effect of extracellular calcium appears to cease after a point in the progression of cancer.[65] The use of antioxidants is also being evaluated. Vitamin C, tocopherol, and selenium are micronutrients that have diverse biochemical effects but protect gut epithelium from fecapentaene and other carcinogenic (oxidative) damage.[66-68] Simple dietary supplementation with these agents has not proved to be of dramatic benefit.[69,70]

With the identification of many phenotypic "intermediate biomarkers" associated with colorectal cancer, such as colon-crypt-cell proliferation index, clinical prevention trials may generate useful insights without having to wait decades for the end results.[71]

SECONDARY PREVENTION

It is possible to identify some patients at high risk for developing colorectal cancer. Secondary prevention strategies in these patients may include removal of precancerous lesions (neoplastic polyps) or excising the entire end-organ at risk. Management of patients with precancerous diseases is discussed later in this chapter.

CLINICAL RISK FACTORS FOR COLORECTAL CANCER
(TABLE 30–1)

GENETIC

Familial Polyposis Syndromes

Several heritable syndromes are associated with adenomatous polyposis and a high risk for large bowel cancer.[72] The most important is the familial adenomatous polyposis (FAP) syndrome. Few colon cancer patients have this condition, because its incidence in the United States is between 1 person in 6850 and 1 person in 8300 population.[73] Without intervention, virtually all affected individuals develop colorectal cancer. The disease is inherited as an autosomal dominant trait, with greater than 90% penetrance. Affected persons develop pan-colon adenomatous polyposis. The polyps are not present at birth, but by late adolescence more than 1000 may be visualized. New mutations may arise in 20% to 30% of index cases of polyposis, and a careful evaluation of family members is necessary.[74-77] Gardner syndrome, inherited as an autosomal dominant trait, occurs with half the frequency of familial adenomatosis syndrome. The entire large and small bowel may be affected by adenoma.[72] Other mesenchymal abnormalities that may coexist include desmoid tumors of the mesentery

---

TABLE 30–1. Clinical Risk Factors for Colorectal Cancer

Genetic
    Familial adenomatous polyposis syndrome
    Gardner's, Oldfield's, or Turcot's syndrome
    Peutz-Jegher syndrome
Familial
    Familial colorectal cancer syndrome (Lynch I)
    Hereditary adenocarcinomatosis syndrome (Lynch II)
    Family history of colorectal cancer
Preexisting disease
    Inflammatory bowel disease
    Colorectal cancer
    Pelvic cancer after irradiation
    Neoplastic colorectal polyps
General
    All men and women over age 40

and abdominal wall,[78] lipomas, sebaceous cysts, osteomas, and fibromas. Because the full clinical spectrum may not be expressed in a given patient, an evaluation of family members is warranted.[79,80] Related to this clinical entity may be the Oldfield syndrome of multiple sebaceous cysts associated with polyposis and adenocarcinoma.[81] It is likely that all of these syndromes are variations of the same genetic defect and that FAP is the generic appellation for these groups. Less common is the Turcot syndrome, probably an autosomal recessive condition, which is associated with malignant central nervous system tumors in addition to bowel polyposis.[82]

Hereditable Syndromes Not Particularly Associated With Colon Cancer

Both the Peutz-Jeghers syndrome and generalized juvenile polyposis are characterized by hamartomatous polyps of the bowel. The patient with Peutz-Jeghers syndrome has multiple tumors, usually clustered more in the small bowel (duodenum) than in the large intestine, and mucocutaneous pigmented lesions.[83] There is only a small chance (2–3%) of malignant degeneration.[83] The juvenile polyposis syndrome also is characterized by multiple hamartomas of the entire bowel. The chance of malignancy is considered to be small.[83,84]

Familial Cancer Syndromes

Some families appear to have a high frequency of colon cancer without adenomatous polyposis of the bowel, termed *hereditary nonpolyposis colorectal cancer* (HNPCC). The clinical condition described by Lynch and Lynch, the Lynch I syndrome, is inherited as an autosomally dominant pattern with greater than 90% penetrance.[85] It has several unusual clinical features including the development of multiple colon cancers at an early age in several generations. Most of these cancers are located in the proximal colon. A more generalized condition, also inherited as an autosomal dominant trait, has been described by Lynch and colleagues[86,92] (Lynch II syndrome) and Law[87] for families with multiple colon and extracolon adenocarcinomas (familial adenocarcinomatosis). This syndrome is characterized by the early onset of adenocarcinomas of the colon, ovary, pancreas, breast, and bile duct and of the urologic (most commonly ureter and renal pelvis), endometrial, and gastric systems.[86]

In first-degree relatives of patients with Lynch type II hereditary nonpolyposis cancer syndrome, there is a sevenfold increase in colon cancer incidence.[93] Macklin has demonstrated that the relatives of persons with sporadic colon cancer have a twofold to threefold greater chance of developing large bowel cancer than the general population.[94] The clustering of colon and rectal cancer in those with a positive family history but without an excess number of polyps has not been characterized as a specific genetic disorder.[72] Rather, environmental and dietary factors may be of greater importance—or, more likely, the etiology lies in a subtle interplay of heredity and environmental factors.[95] Burt and colleagues analyzed a large family with multiple colon cancer cases but without a precisely definable pattern of inheritance and reported adenomatous polyps in 21% of 191 family members but in only 9% of 132 controls.[96] They proposed that this excess of polyps and colon cancer was the result of an unspecified autosomal dominant gene for susceptibility rather than chance occurrence. This group of patients is also the subject of investigation regarding genotypic changes.[97]

The hereditary flat adenoma syndrome (HFAS) has been described by Muto and colleagues[88] and by Lynch and colleagues.[89] Flat adenomas with diameters greater than 5 mm show aneuploidy in 80%.[90] The clinical features of these syndromes are compared in Table 30–2.[91]

Molecular Genetics of Colorectal Cancer

Only recently has the genetic basis of colorectal cancer and its precursors begun to be understood. The development of colorectal cancer is a multistep process that involves a successive loss of chromosomes. Rapid advances in molecular biology techniques have allowed characterization of the genetic changes thought to be responsible for this multistep process.

More definitive studies using genetic linkage were made possible when the locus for FAP was discovered. Using RFLP analysis and in situ hybridization of DNA from 13 families of patients with FAP, the location of the FAP gene was found to be close to a marker at 5q21-q22.[98] The gene for FAP has been cloned and sequenced independently by two groups.[99–101]

Colorectal cancer has provided a useful model for the understanding of the multistep process of carcinogenesis. The availability of numerous polymorphic DNA markers provides

TABLE 30–2. Clinical Features of Inherited Cancer Syndromes

Feature	FAP	HNPCC	FAS
Age of onset	Early	Early	Late
No. of adenomas	>100	<10	0–100
Adenoma distribution	Left of total	Mainly right side	Mainly right side
Cancer distribution	Random	Mainly right side	Mainly right side
Other cancers	Periampullary	Endometrial, other	Periampullary

FAP, familial adenomatosis polyposis; HNPCC, heriditary nonpolyposis colon cancer; FAS, flat adenoma syndrome.
(Modified from Lynch HT, Smyrk T, Watson P, et al. Hereditary colorectal cancer. Semin Oncol 1991;18:337–366)

a means for localization of other mutations associated with the somatic loss of heterozygosity in colon cancer and suggests that other tumor suppressor genes may be involved in colorectal oncogenesis more downstream from the formation of a polyp. Vogelstein and colleagues examined the genetic alterations in colorectal tumor specimens at various stages of neoplastic development and found that changes the 5q chromosome and the *RAS* oncogene tend to occur early in the pathway.[102] Frequent mutations have been found in K-*RAS* using RNAse protection assay[103] and DNA hybridization analysis.[104] Further downstream in the progression to malignancy is the deletion of a region of chromosome 18. This region was deleted frequently in carcinomas and advanced adenomas but only occasionally in early adenomas. This gene has been named *deleted in colon cancer* (DCC) and the primary structure of its protein product is homologous to the neural cell adhesion molecule (N-CAM). This suggests that it may play a role in cell–cell contact and that inactivation may be related to loss of contact inhibition and metastatic potential. Linkage of Lynch syndrome II to the Kidd blood group located near the region of the DCC gene suggests that mutations in DCC may be important in the pathogenesis of this syndrome.[105] Vogelstein and colleagues discovered a fourth tumor suppressor gene called *mutated in colon cancer* (MCC), also located at 5q21, that has loss of function mutations in sporadic colorectal cancer.[106]

INFLAMMATORY BOWEL DISEASE

There is a well-recognized increased risk (up to 30-fold) for colon cancer in patients with inflammatory bowel disease. For patients with ulcerative colitis, the incidence of malignancy increases with the extent of bowel involvement, age at onset, severity, and duration of the disease.[107–110] Among all patients diagnosed with colorectal cancer, only about 1% have an antecedent history of inflammatory bowel disease. Using an actuarial analysis, the cumulative incidence of cancer in patients with inflammatory bowel disease is 5% after 20 years and 12% after 25 years. Ekbom and colleagues found the incidence of colorectal cancer in patients with ulcerative colitis was 5.7 times that expected.[111] The relative risk for colorectal cancer was lowest for patients with proctitis (1.7) and left-sided colitis (2.8) and highest with pancolitis (18.8). Patients with pancolitis for 30 years have a more than 35% chance of developing bowel cancer.[112–115] At even greater risk are those persons in whom severe pancolitis began in childhood. Other atypical aspects of malignancy include multifocal disease (10–20% of cases) and proximal colon primary sites (40–50%).[109,116,117] The pathogenesis of cancer in ulcerative colitis is the same as in adenomatous polyps. The mucosa undergoes dysplasia, and as these changes progress the probability of cancer increases. Cell kinetic studies[118] and microspectrophometric measurement of DNA content[119] may help detect patients at high risk for developing colon cancer.

Granulomatous Colitis

Crohn's disease also carries an increased risk for large bowel and small bowel cancer.[120] Although granulomatous colitis is not associated with cancer as frequently as ulcerative colitis,

bowel adenocarcinomas with atypical presentations at younger ages are often reported.[117,121,122] Tumors usually arise in affected portions of the bowel, but also may be metachronous and may occur in sites of previous surgery.[123]

Previous Malignant Disease

Patients who have undergone treatment for a large bowel adenocarcinoma are at greater risk for developing a second colorectal tumor. The likelihood that a second primary bowel cancer will develop either coincident with the index lesion or at a later time is at least threefold.[124–126] The clear implication for the follow-up of patients after definitive resection is that regular reevaluation is required. Clustering of breast, ovarian, and colon cancer in the same patients has been demonstrated. The aggregation of multiple adenocarcinomas is similar to the pattern described for familial adenocarcinoma syndrome.[127]

Irradiation of the pelvis seems to enhance a person's risk for developing sigmoid cancer. Patients who have undergone radiation therapy for cervical, endometrial, or bladder cancer may be at enhanced risk for developing large bowel cancer, possibly irradiation-induced.[128,129]

Previous Noncancer Surgery

Patients who have undergone cholecystectomy or ureterosigmoidostomy have a higher incidence of large bowel cancer. A high concentration of inciting or promoting compounds in the secretions may account for the increased risk for neoplasia.[130–132]

Polyps

Neoplastic and inflammatory polyps occur in the large bowel. Adenomatous polyps may be tubular or villous. Tubular adenomas are four times more common than the villous adenomas and are usually smaller. In general, larger polyps are more likely to contain a malignant focus than the smaller ones; nearly half of polyps larger than 2 cm in diameter contain malignancy. About 25% of patients with one tubular polyp have others. Tubular adenomas are more evenly distributed throughout the large bowel, whereas villous tumors are more frequently found in the rectum.[133] Villous adenomas are reported to be 8 to 10 times more likely than tubular polyps to be cancerous.[133–136]

Predictably, the larger the number of these adenomas, the greater the chance that cancer will develop.[137] Although it is not necessary to have a polyp before or coincident with a cancer, this sequence occurs five times more frequently than cancer alone.[2]

GENERAL POPULATION

Men and women over the age of 40 constitute the largest population at risk for colorectal cancer. Although colorectal cancer sometimes is found in children, the incidence of disease increases steadily up to the eighth decade.[138,139]

DIAGNOSIS

Colorectal cancer may be diagnosed when a patient presents with symptoms or as the result of a screening program. Except for patients with obstructing or perforating cancers, the duration of symptoms does not correlate with prognosis.[137,140,141] Because early colorectal cancer produces no symptoms and because many of the symptoms of colorectal cancer are non-specific, aggressive efforts at detection through screening programs are essential.

We cannot adequately stress the vagueness of abdominal symptoms associated with colorectal cancer. Twelve percent of otherwise healthy patients without colorectal cancer complain of a change in bowel habits in the recent past and 11% report abdominal pain.[142] Even rectal bleeding has a low predictive value in the diagnosis of colorectal cancer.[143] Screening strategies are discussed later in the chapter.

EVALUATION OF THE SYMPTOMATIC PATIENT

Symptoms of colon cancer—intermittent abdominal pain, nausea, or vomiting—are secondary to bleeding, obstruction, or perforation. A palpable mass is common with right colon cancer. Bleeding may be acute and most commonly appears as red blood mixed with stool. Dark blood is most commonly secondary to diverticular bleeding. Occasionally, melena may be associated with a right colon cancer. Chronic occult blood loss with iron deficiency anemia occurs frequently. Such patients may present with weakness and high-output congestive heart failure. Lesser degrees of bleeding may be detected as part of a fecal occult blood test (discussed under screening). Rectal bleeding associated with anticoagulant use should be investigated to rule out colon cancer. Malignant obstruction of the large bowel is most commonly associated with cancer of the sigmoid. If the ileocecal valve is competent, such obstructions manifest as acute abdominal illness. If the ileocecal valve is incompetent, the illness is more insidious, with increasing constipation and abdominal distention noticed over many days. The major differential diagnosis in such cases includes cancer and diverticulitis. A limited barium enema examination may yield only suggestive data, and even fiberoptic endoscopy may not be diagnostic if associated edema precludes reaching the cancer with the endoscope. Cytology of a brush biopsy specimen obtained through the fiberoptic endoscope may be diagnostic.

Perforation of colon cancer may be acute or chronic. The clinical picture of acute perforation may be identical to that of appendicitis or diverticulitis, with pain, fever, and a palpable mass. In the presence of obstruction, there may be a perforation through the tumor or through proximal nontumorous colon (cecum). The distinction is important from a prognostic viewpoint. Chronic perforation with fistula formation into the bladder from sigmoid colon cancer is similar to diverticulitis. Gross pneumaturia may occur, or the patient may present with recurrent urinary tract infections only. The continued presence of cystitis with multiple enteric organisms on culture, despite repeated treatment, mandates diagnostic studies. Bladder cytologies, cystoscopy, brushings, and biopsies may not lead to the correct diagnosis. Fiberoptic endoscopy of the colon is the most valuable diagnostic procedure.

Metastatic Disease

Synchronous liver metastasis occurs in 5% to 10% of patients and occasionally is the presenting manifestation of colorectal cancer. The patient may complain of pain in the right upper quadrant, right hypochondrium, right posterior chest, or right shoulder. The pain may be a continuous ache, or it may be experienced as an acute episode related to hemorrhage or necrosis of a metastasis. Hepatomegaly may be detected on routine physical examination of an otherwise asymptomatic patient. It is important to evaluate the gastrointestinal tract in such patients, even if the fecal occult blood test is negative, before proceeding with a premature liver biopsy.

SCREENING

The early detection of colorectal cancer is potentially associated with a dramatic reduction in the disease-related mortality. The slow growth of most colorectal cancers and the high diagnostic sensitivity of colonoscopy and air-contrast barium enema justify aggressive screening strategies. In addition, some screening approaches may detect early cancers and benign neoplastic polyps. Endoscopic removal of such polyps may, to some extent, prevent subsequent colorectal cancer. Screening strategies must take into account the risk of the population being screened, the segments of the large bowel at greatest risk, cost-effectiveness of screening, patient compliance, and the availability of various technologies.[144-146]

HIGH-RISK GROUPS

Family History

In persons with a family history of colorectal cancer, screening should begin at age 35 to 40 years with yearly fecal occult blood and probably some type of endoscopic surveillance.[147] Flexible sigmoidoscopy (with the 60- to 65-cm instrument) every 3 to 5 years should be considered, with full colonoscopy if an adenomatous polyp is identified.[148,149] Autosomal dominant cancer families require frequent invasive screening with colonoscopy or sigmoidoscopy combined with air-contrast barium enema examination every 3 to 5 years beginning at age 40.[144]

Familial Adenomatous Polyposis

Once the diagnosis of FAP is made, many patients undergo a total colectomy with ileorectal anastomosis or a total proctocolectomy with ileostomy or ileal pouch-anal anastomosis. Those with retained rectum should undergo rigid proctoscopy with fulguration of polyps every 6 months for the rest of their lives.

Personal History of Cancer or Polyp

Endoscopic surveillance of the entire remaining bowel is appropriate every 1 to 3 years.[149,150] An air-contrast barium enema examination combined with limited endoscopy is also reasonable.[151] The National Polyp Study is prospectively gathering data on the frequency and type of follow-up appropriate for these patients.[152,153] Preliminary data indicate that patients with multiple polyps, particularly villous lesions, are at a greater risk for subsequent polyp formation.

Ulcerative Colitis

Patients who have a history of extensive ulcerative colitis (except patients with isolated ulcerative proctitis) for at least 10 years and who are not treated by proctocolectomy require colonoscopic surveillance every 1 to 2 years. Any worrisome area is biopsied, and multiple blind biopsies of seemingly normal mucosa are performed to detect dysplasia.[154–157]

SCREENING STRATEGIES FOR THE GENERAL POPULATION[145,146,158]

Digital Rectal Examination

The digital rectal examination is a traditional part of the annual physical examination. In addition to low rectal cancers, anal and prostatic cancers may be detected. A stool specimen is obtained for occult blood determination. The sensitivity of the digital rectal examination has decreased with the more proximal shift in the location of colorectal cancer. Although it is difficult to demonstrate a reduction in cancer mortality from periodic rectal digital examinations, the procedure should remain part of any regular physical examination.[159]

Rigid Sigmoidoscopy

Rigid sigmoidoscopy is comparatively inexpensive, but its usefulness is restricted by the length of bowel that can be examined and by patients' unwillingness to undergo the procedure. In a series of 26,000 patients over the age of 45 studied at the Strang Clinic, asymptomatic cancer was detected in 58.[160] The cure rate in these patients was 90%.

Flexible Sigmoidoscopy

Flexible proctosigmoidoscopes are available in 25 to 35 cm lengths and 60 to 65 cm lengths. The light source is provided by fiberoptic technology. Viewing may use fiberoptics or direct videoendoscopic technology. The shorter scopes are easy to learn to use, more comfortable for the patient, and more applicable for screening programs using nonphysician personnel.[161,162] The longer flexible sigmoidoscopes reach on the average 45 cm proximal to the anus, which is the junction of the descending colon and sigmoid, and they allow detection of about two thirds of colorectal cancers and polyps.[148,162–168] Any patient found to have a neoplastic polyp on screening endoscopy should be considered at high risk and should undergo complete examination of the remaining colon and more intense surveillance.

Fecal Occult Blood Testing

Guaiac-impregnated paper slide tests for fecal occult blood have been available for 20 years.[169–172] The relatively low cost and the potential for patient testing at home have generated considerable interest in this approach. All guaiac tests measure hemoglobin indirectly by the determination of its peroxidase activity. Two other approaches are being studied. The HemoQuant test (SmithKline Diagnostics, Sunnyvale, CA) is a quantitative assay for fecal hemoglobin based on the conversion of heme to fluorescent porphyrins.[173,174] The test is more costly and requires more complicated testing support. Data are not available comparing this test with existing guaiac-based systems in a large screening program. An immunochemical approach to the detection of human fecal hemoglobin is possible and would obviate false-positive tests associated with dietary hemoglobin and ingestion of peroxidase-containing foods.[175,176]

In considering the overall impact of fecal occult blood screening programs, a number of features must be stressed. False-positive tests are expensive and at best inconvenient for the patient. Patients with positive test results undergo extensive diagnostic testing, which may include sigmoidoscopy, barium enema, colonoscopy, and upper gastrointestinal endoscopy.[177] Patients with false-negative results may be inappropriately reassured and disregard subsequent symptoms.

All guaiac-based fecal occult blood tests are unreliable to some degree. Ahlquist and Beart reported positive Hemoccult test results with as little as 0.04 mg hemoglobin per gram of stool (normal, <2 mg/g) and negative results with as much as 42.5 mg/g.[178] Fecal occult blood testing as a screening technique assumes that colorectal cancers (many of which are ulcerated) are associated with detectable intraluminal blood loss. However, some colorectal cancers bleed intermittently, and others not at all. In several studies of patients with known colorectal cancer, 20% to 30% of patients had negative fecal occult blood tests.[179–181] Less than one third of patients with polyps have stools positive for occult blood.[181]

EVALUATION OF THE POSITIVE FECAL OCCULT BLOOD TEST. Because the predictive value of a positive test is less than 20%, the few dollars spent for the fecal occult blood test leads to a great expenditure of funds to identify patients with true-positive results.[177] Although a complete colonoscopy is probably the most direct way to exclude cancer and polyps, air-contrast barium enema examination may be the most cost-effective approach to the evaluation of the patient with a positive test result.[182] Rigid or flexible sigmoidoscopy must complement the barium study.

SCREENING PROGRAMS. Data from selected large series are presented in Table 30–3.[181,183–186] About 2.5% of tested patients are Hemoccult (or Hemoccult II) positive, with compliance rates ranging from 20% to 97%. Three large-scale prospective population-based programs are attempting to demonstrate a reduction in colorectal cancer mortality with fecal occult blood test screening and to define compliance and cost issues associated with this test. These studies are taking place at the University of Minnesota, at the Strang Clinic in New York, in Nottingham, England, and in Goteborg, Sweden.[172,181,185,187]

Screening Recommendations for the General Population

We recommend yearly fecal occult blood tests and sigmoidoscopy every 3 to 5 years beginning at age 40. We encourage the increased use of flexible sigmoidoscopy as part of a screening strategy.

TABLE 30–3. Screening Programs for Colorectal Cancer Using Fecal Occult Blood Tests

Investigations	No. of Patients	Compliance	Positive Tests (%)	Cancers Detected	Predictive Value (%)
Gilbertsen et al[183]	23,000	72	2.3	54	11.3
Winawer et al[184]	13,127	74	2.5	59	17.7
Winchester et al[185]	54,101	26	4.4	29	4.7
Sontag et al[186]	13,522	22	4.6	14	10.3
Cummings et al[683]	58,934	20	2.3	17	6.4
Hardcastle et al[181]	10,253	39	2.4	17	13.7

PATHOLOGY

GROSS APPEARANCE

Tumor configuration may be divided into fungating (exophytic), ulcerating, stenosing, and constricting (annular, circumferential). About two thirds of all tumors are ulcerating and one third are fungating.[188] Right-sided cancers are usually fungating in nature. They tend to grow more into the lumen and to extend along one wall, especially in the capacious cecum. Left-sided cancers tend to grow more into the bowel wall and circumferentially, having a typical "napkin-ring" configuration on barium enema examination. Growth along circumferential lymphatics may account for much of this behavior.

HISTOLOGIC TYPES

The major histologic type of large bowel cancer is adenocarcinoma, which accounts for 90% to 95% of all large bowel tumors.[189,190] It is the only histologic type further classified by grade, and a number of histologic types of large bowel cancer have been identified. The World Health Organization (WHO) has developed a classification of benign and malignant tumors.[191] The classification of malignant tumors is given in Table 30–4. Descriptions of most of these pathologic types

TABLE 30–4. World Health Organization Classification of Malignant Primary Tumors of the Large Intestine

Epithelial tumors
 Adenocarcinoma
 Mucinous adenocarcinoma
 Signet-ring cell adenocarcinoma
 Squamous cell carcinoma
 Adenosquamous carcinoma
 Undifferentiated carcinoma
 Unclassified carcinoma
Carcinoid tumors
 Argentaffin
 Nonargentaffin
 Composite
Nonepithelial tumors
 Leiomyosarcoma
 Others
Hematopoietic and lymphoid neoplasms
Unclassified

may be found in the Armed Forces Institute of Pathology Series;[192] illustrations of each may be found in that series and in the WHO series.[191]

Colloid or mucinous adenocarcinoma represents about 17% of large bowel tumors.[193] These adenocarcinomas are defined by large amounts of extracellular mucin retained within the tumor. A separate WHO classification is the rare signet-ring cell carcinoma (2–4% of mucinous carcinomas), which contains intracellular mucin pushing the nucleus to one side. Some signet-ring tumors appear to form a linitis plastica type tumor by spreading intramurally, usually not involving the mucosa.[194] Other rare variants of epithelial tumors include squamous cell carcinomas, of which about 40 cases have been reported,[195] and adenosquamous carcinomas, sometimes called adenoacanthomas.[190] Finally, there are the undifferentiated carcinomas, which contain no glandular structures or other features such as mucous secretions. Other designations for undifferentiated carcinoma include carcinoma simplex, medullary carcinoma, and trabecular carcinoma. Gibbs has emphasized that undifferentiated carcinomas are not necessarily anaplastic.[196] He describes undifferentiated carcinoma as a malignant epithelial neoplasm that does not differentiate into formed tubules but exhibits little nuclear pleomorphism and few bizarre mitoses.

From 4% to 17% of carcinoids may appear in the rectum, and 2% to 7% may appear in the colon.[197-199] These small, firm, polypoid nodules are covered by an intact mucosa and rarely produce the carcinoid syndrome. Sarcomas account for 0.1% to 0.3% of all malignancies of the colorectum.[200,201]

DEGREE OF DIFFERENTIATION

Broders was a pioneer in classifying the adenocarcinomas by their degree of differentiation.[202] He designated four grades, based on the percentage of differentiated tumor cells. In Broders' system, *well differentiated* meant well-formed glands resembling an adenoma. Broders included the mucinous carcinomas in his system, whereas Dukes considered mucinous carcinomas separately.[203] Because of the poor prognosis associated with mucinous carcinomas, others group them with the most undifferentiated tumors.

The Dukes grading system considered the arrangement of the cells rather than the percentage of differentiated cells. The initial Dukes approach has evolved into the three-grade system that is now the most widely used. Grade 1 is the most differentiated, with well-formed tubules and the least nuclear polymorphism and mitoses. Grade 3 is the least differentiated, with only occasional glandular structures, pleomorphic cells, and a high incidence of mitoses. Grade 2 is intermediate between Grades 1 and 3.[189,204]

Jass and colleagues use seven parameters in their grading criteria: histologic type, overall differentiation, nuclear polarity, tubule configuration, pattern of growth, lymphocytic infiltration, and amount of fibrosis.[205]

SPREAD OF COLORECTAL CANCER

Much of our knowledge about the local and distant spread of colorectal cancer is due to the meticulous and elegant studies of Cuthbert Dukes, a pathologist at St. Mark's Hospital in London, who did extensive studies on the local invasion of rectal cancer and on lymphatic involvement by this disease. In 1930, Dukes and his colleague Gordon-Watson described the spread of rectal cancer,[206] which Dukes expanded in later papers.[203,207,208] Much of this information applies to colon cancer as well.

LOCAL INVASION

After the initial mucosal growth, a tumor may progress in several directions, but usually it protrudes first into the lumen. Dukes found that subsequent lateral invasion was greater in the transverse rather than the longitudinal direction, leading to circumferential growth.[203,209] Black and Waugh found the same growth pattern in colon cancer.[196] Mural penetration may result in local failure or peritoneal seeding.

One way of examining histologic sections is with whole mounts of the cross-section of the bowel.[210,211] This histologic procedure defines the invasion profile of lateral transmural penetration. Although the procedure has not been used extensively, it may be of great use in future studies. An additional pattern of local spread is perineural invasion, or spread along the perineural spaces, which may reach as far as 10 cm from the primary tumor.[212]

LYMPHATIC EXTENSION

In 1930, Dukes concluded, incorrectly, that lymph node metastases occurred only after local tumor spread into the perirectal tissues.[206] The exceptions were generally with high-grade tumors. More recent studies have demonstrated a 10% to 20% incidence of nodal metastases from rectal cancer limited to the bowel wall.[213–225]

In 1935, Gabriel and colleagues described the orderly and predictable course of spread of lymphatic disease in rectal cancer.[226] First, disease metastasizes to the perirectal nodes at the level of the primary tumor or immediately above it. Then the chain accompanying the superior hemorrhoidal vessels is involved. Rarely are there discontinuous or skip metastases.[226–229] The pericolic lymph nodes along the mesenteric border of the pelvis usually are not involved by these rectal tumors unless there is extensive tumor with lymphatic blockage. Gabriel and colleagues pointed out that in late stages of the disease, when the hemorrhoidal lymphatics are blocked, there is lateral or downward spread.[226] Grinnell noted such retrograde flow in 34 (3.7%) of 913 cases of colon and rectum

tumors.[230] In colon carcinoma, the normal lymphatic flow is through the lymphatic channels along the major arteries, with three echelons of lymph nodes: pericolic, intermediate, and principal. If tumors lie between two major vascular pedicles, lymphatic flow may drain in either or both directions (Fig. 30–4). If the central lymph nodes are blocked by tumor, lymphatic flow can become retrograde along the marginal arcades proximally and distally.[231]

The risk for lymph node metastases increases with increasing tumor grade.[208] Dukes found that 30% of low-grade tumors were associated with positive lymph nodes compared with 81% of high-grade tumors. The number of lymph nodes involved also increased with grade: an average of 3.2 nodes were involved for low-grade tumors and 6.8 for high-grade tumors.

HEMATOGENOUS SPREAD

The liver is the primary site of hematogenous metastases, followed by the lung. In about 40% of autopsy studies, the liver is the only site involved.[232–234] Involvement of other sites in the absence of liver or lung involvement is rare.

The major venous drainage of the lower rectum occurs by a dual system: drainage from the superior hemorrhoidal veins

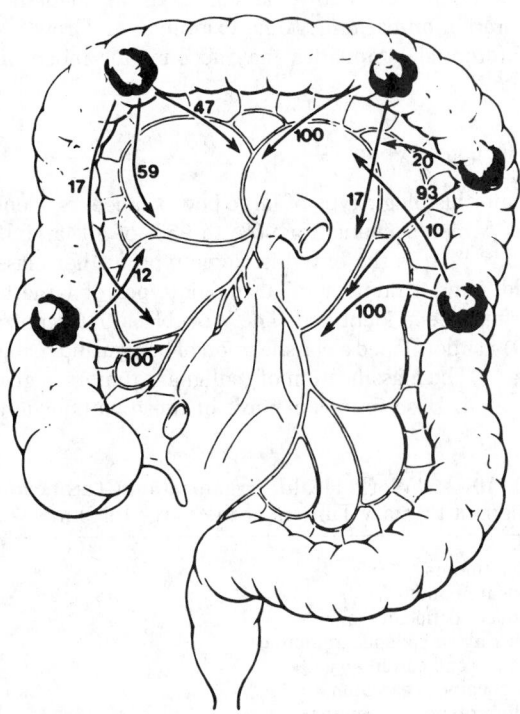

FIGURE 30–4.   For tumors that lie between two pedicles, lymphatic flow may drain in either or both directions. From a study of cleared specimens, it was possible to determine the preferential route by the location of lymphatic metastases. The numbers above signify the percentage of metastasizing carcinomas in the above locations that have demonstrated positive nodes along a given vascular route. For example, node-positive tumors lying between the ileocolic and right colic arcades metastasize along the ileocolic pedicle in 100% of cases and along the right colon in 12% of cases. (Hertzer FP, Slanetz CA. Patterns and significance of lymphatic spread from cancer of the colon and rectum. In: Weiss L, Gilbert HA, Ballon SC, eds. Lymphatic system metastasis. Boston: GK Hall, 1980:283)

enters the portal system to the liver, whereas drainage from the middle and inferior hemorrhoidal veins eventually reaches the vena cava to get to the lungs. Bone metastases in the sacrum and the vertebral bodies may occur through the vertebral venous plexus, as originally described by Batson.[235] In 1977, Vider and colleagues proposed that this system represented another mechanism of metastatic spread.[236] The portal mesenteric and caval systems offer low-pressure drainage to the liver and lungs, whereas the vertebral venous plexus is a high-pressure system that may open only during defecation, allowing metastases to go to the skeleton and central nervous system. Such a hypothesis accords with the early appearance of bone metastases in the sacrum, coccyx, pelvis, and lumbar vertebrae.

IMPLANTATION

Implantation refers to the release of tumor cells from the primary tumor and their deposition on another surface. Implantation has been reported with tumor cells shed intraluminally, from the serosal surface through the peritoneum, and by surgical manipulation and resultant deposition on wound surfaces.[237]

Intraluminal spread of tumor occurs by release of the tumor cells from the mucosal surface of the primary tumor and their deposition distally in the bowel, in fistulas, abscesses, or hemorrhoids. The mechanism of such implantation is considered to be the deposition of viable cells onto the surface of a fistula or an ulcerated or surgically treated hemorrhoid. There are many reports of tumor growth in hemorrhoids.[238–240] Peritoneal seeding is a frequent result of transmural penetration and tumor shedding.[241]

STAGING AND PROGNOSTIC FEATURES

The staging of colorectal carcinoma has been complicated by the fact that it has evolved over half a century. Various authors have developed systems that use the same descriptors to represent different stages. Even one common and simple staging system, the Dukes classification for cancer of the rectum, has been misinterpreted by various authors.[242] This is not surprising, because the definitions changed even in the series of publications by Dukes.[203,206] Because of these discrepancies in coding for the same stages, comparison of clinical studies is often impossible.

Most investigators agree that the most important independent pathologic factor for survival or recurrence after potentially curative surgery is the stage of cancer, which is determined by the depth of penetration through the bowel wall and the presence and number of positive lymph nodes.[224,225,243] Other independent factors for survival have included gross appearance,[244] lymphatic vessel invasion,[245] blood vessel invasion,[246] nucleolar organizer regions,[247] character of invasive margin and tumor type,[248] number of mast cells,[249] nuclear shape,[250] sedimentation rate and leukocytosis,[251] lymphocytic infiltration,[205] obstruction, perforation, and rectal bleeding,[252] character of invasive margin and peritumoral lymphocytic infiltration,[253] infiltrating border (lateral margins),[54] age, grade, venous invasion, gender, and obstruction,[246] ploidy,[255–259] and preoperative carcinoembryonic antigen.[260]

SURGICAL-PATHOLOGIC STAGING

Dukes' Classification and Its Modifications

The first practical staging system was the Dukes classification,[203] which classified rectal tumors from A to C, with stage A indicating penetration into but not through the bowel wall, stage B indicating penetration through the bowel wall, and stage C indicating involvement of lymph nodes, regardless of the extent of bowel wall penetration. This system, developed from an earlier clinical grouping by Lockhart-Mummery,[261] had the virtue of being simple and predictive of prognosis. It has been modified since then by many authors including Dukes[226] to reflect finer levels of penetration and nodal metastases, and has been extended to include the colon and the rectum. In 1935, Dukes' stage C was further subdivided into C1 (locally positive nodes) and C2 (positive nodes at the point of ligature).[226]

The most commonly used staging systems are shown in Figure 30–5. Kirklin and colleagues split the Dukes' stage A into a new stage A (mucosa only) and stage B1 (into but not through the muscularis propria) and changed Dukes' stage B to B2.[262] In the initial Dukes' staging classification, stage D was not formally designated.[203] In 1949, he reported a fourth stage characterized as disease beyond the limit of surgical resection.[263] This fourth stage was formally defined as *D* by Turnbull and colleagues in 1967.[264] The Astler-Coller staging system allowed separation of wall penetration and nodal status.[213] The Gunderson-Sosin modification of the Astler-Coller staging system subdivided T3 tumors into those with microscopic ($B2_m$ or $C2_m$) and gross ($B2_{m+g}$ or $C2_{m+g}$) penetration of tumor through the bowel wall.[214] The subscript designation $m + g$ indicates on gross inspection that the tumor is transmural and is confirmed on microscopic examination.

In a recent analysis of clinical trials in patients with colorectal cancer treated on their protocols, the National Surgical Adjuvant Breast and Bowel Project (NSABP) compared the prognostic abilities of modifications of the original Dukes' classification.[265] In Dukes' stage C, the level of positive node involvement was not predictive of ultimate survival. The depth of penetration and the number of positive nodes were significant predictors of survival, and the number of positive nodes was the strongest factor in this analysis. The number of positive nodes was independently prognostic in the multivariate analysis from the Large Bowel Cancer Project in London.[266] The number of positive nodes has been included in the Gastrointestinal Tumor Study Group (GITSG) classification[267] and the TNM systems of the American Joint Committee on Cancer (AJCC)[268] and the Union Internationale Contra le Cancer (UICC).[269] The data suggest that any future classification or staging system should consider the number of positive nodes as a predictive discriminant.

The TNM Classification

The AJCC[188] and the UICC[269] proposed staging systems using the TNM classification. There was not total agreement between the staging systems, and neither system specifically considered the number of positive nodes. In studies that examined the prognostic ability of pathologic TNM staging, survival was identical or even reversed for stages II and III.[270–272]

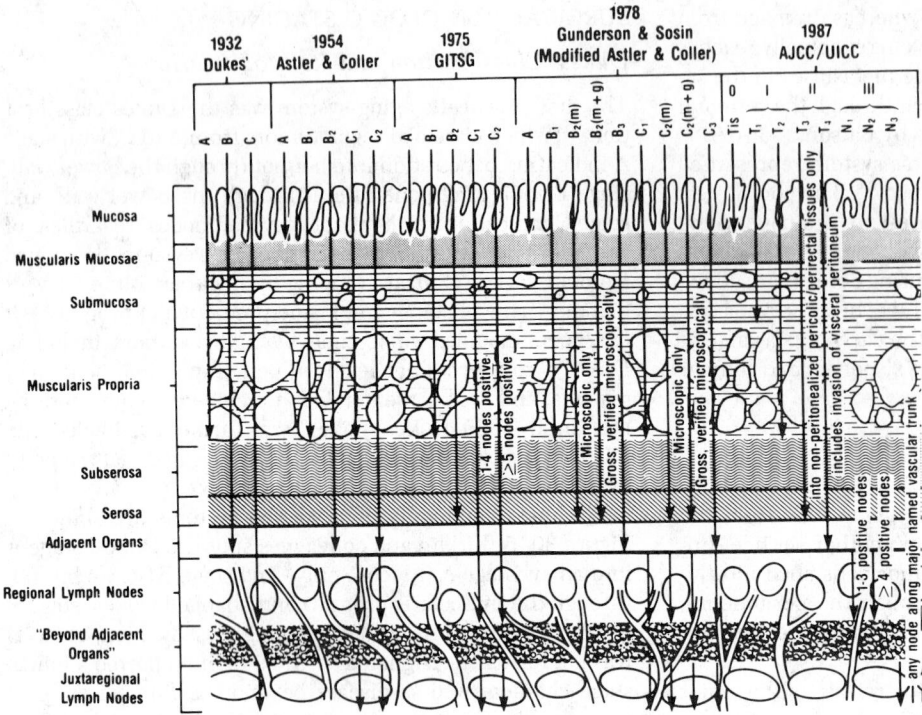

FIGURE 30–5. Comparison of various pathologic staging systems.

A revised, 1988 joint AJCC/UICC TNM staging system unified the two systems. The revised system is simpler and considers the important prognostic factor the number of positive nodes.[268,273,274] Free mesothelial penetration also is considered.[275] To determine the relative prognostic capability of the TNM, Astler-Coller, and Dukes' staging systems in patients with rectal cancer, the NSABP performed a separate analysis of the R-01 protocol.[276] Although neither the TNM or Astler-Coller staging systems improved the predictive capability of Dukes' A, the subdivision of Dukes' C into the Astler-Coller stages C1 and C2 increased the predictive capability.

Jass and colleagues have offered a new prognostic classification of rectal cancer.[253] Using a Cox regression analysis, they found that the number of positive nodes, whether the invasive border was pushing or infiltrative, the presence of a conspicuous lymphocytic infiltrate, and the absence or presence of transmural penetration were independent prognostic factors. The authors concluded that this prognostic classification was simple to use and superior to the Dukes system. The NSABP performed a comparison of the Dukes (and modified Dukes) and Jass staging systems using clinical information from the R-01 protocol.[277] The data further validated the Jass staging system. Due to the simple objectivity of the modified Dukes and TNM systems, the Jass staging system has not been formally incorporated by the NSABP or other major clinical groups.

The issue of which staging system to use remains unresolved. The 1987 UICC[278] and 1988 AJCC[279] TNM staging systems incorporate information regarding the number of positive nodes. In contrast to the GITSG[267] and Jass[253] staging systems, which stratify by 1 to 4 compared with 5 or more positive nodes, the UICC and AJCC staging systems stratify by 1 to 3 versus 4 or more positive nodes. This latter dichotomy is supported by data from Cohen and colleagues.[280]

Another important prognostic factor is the depth of serosal penetration by tumor. The Gunderson-Sosin modification of the Astler-Coller staging system subdivided T3 tumors into those with microscopic ($B2_m$ or $C2_m$) or gross ($B2_{m+g}$ or $C2_{m+g}$) penetration of tumor through the bowel wall.[214] In patients with rectal cancer, there was a nonsignificant improvement in survival in patients with microscopic compared with gross penetration of tumor through the bowel wall in stages B2 and C2.[221,224] In patients with colon cancer, this difference reached statistical significance[225] and has been confirmed by Newland and colleagues.[275]

Cawthorne and associates examined the extent of mesorectal spread in 167 patients with rectal cancer.[281] Slight mesorectal spread was defined as less than 4 mm and extensive mesorectal spread was defined as more than 4 mm. There was a significant decrease in 5-year survival in patients with extensive versus slight mesorectal spread (25% versus 55%, $p < 0.001$). By multivariate analysis, the extent of mesorectal spread was found to be an independent prognostic factor for survival.

In contrast to the modified Astler-Coller staging system, the UICC, AJCC, GTSG, and Jass staging systems do not incorporate information regarding the difference between microscopic and gross extension of tumor through the bowel wall. Despite this shortcoming, we strongly recommend the use of the AJCC/UICC TNM system for reporting results. Table 30–5 outlines the three most widely used systems: the Dukes, the modified Astler-Coller, and the TNM/UICC.

ADDITIONAL PROGNOSTIC VARIABLES

Clinical Features

AGE. Ever since Hoerner in 1958 reported the poor prognosis of colorectal cancer in the very young,[282] numerous ar-

TABLE 30–5. 1987 AJCC/UICC Staging Classification of Colorectal Cancer

Primary Tumor (T)

TX	Primary tumor cannot be assessed
T0	No evidence of tumor in resected specimen (prior polypectomy or fulguration)
Tis	Carcinoma in situ
T1	Invades submucosa
T2	Invade muscularis propria
T3–T4	Depends on whether serosa is present

Serosa present:

T3	Invades through muscularis propria into Subserosa
	Serosa (but not through)
	Pericolic fat within the leaves of the mesentery
T4	Invades through serosa into free peritoneal cavity or through serosa into a contiguous organ

No serosa (distal two thirds rectum, posterior left or right colon):

T3	Invades through muscularis propria
T4	Invades other organs (vagina, prostate, ureter, kidney)

Regional Lymph Nodes (N)

NX	Nodes cannot be assessed (*e.g.,* local excision only)
N0	No regional node metastases
N1	1–3 positive nodes
N2	4 or more positive nodes
N3	Central nodes positive

Distant Metastases (M)

MX	Presence of distant metastases cannot be assessed
M0	No distant metastases
M1	Distant metastases present

Dukes Staging System Correlated With TNM

Dukes' A = T1N0M0
T2N0M0
Dukes' B = T3N0M0
T4N0M0
Dukes' C = T(any)N1M0, T(any)N2M0
Dukes' C2 = T(any)N3M0
Dukes' D = T(any)N(any)M1

Modified Astler-Coller (MAC) System Correlated With TNM

MAC A = T1N0M0
MAC B1 = T2N0M0
MAC B2 = T3N0M0, T4N0M0
MAC B3 = T4N0M0
MAC C1 = T2N1M0, T2N2M0
MAC C2 = T3N1M0, T3N2M0
T4N1M0, T4N2M0
MAC C3 = T4N1M0, T4N2M0

Note: In all pathologic staging systems, particularly those applied to rectal cancer, the abbreviations (m) and (g) may be used: (m) denotes microscopic transmural penetration; (g) or (m + g) denotes transmural penetration visible on gross inspection and confirmed microscopically.
(Modified from American Joint Committee on Cancer. Manual for staging of cancer. 3rd ed. Philadelphia: JB Lippincott, 1988; and from Union Internationale Contre le Cancer. TNM Classification of Malignant Tumors. 4th ed. Geneva: UICC, 1987)

ticles have supported this conclusion in patients less than 40 years old. Various explanations have been offered, including delay in diagnosis of the disease and the large number of mucoid adenocarcinomas in this group. Dukes and Bussey suggested that the much higher rate of lymphatic metastases in patients under 40 years was due either to a delay in receiving treatment or to more rapid progression of the disease in young patients; they favored the latter explanation.[208] Their data indicated that the average age (62 years) of patients with low-grade malignancies was considerably higher than those with high-grade malignancies (55 years).[208] Recio and Bussey found that 53% of tumors in young patients were high grade, compared with only 20% of tumors in the older age groups in which colorectal carcinoma is more common.[283] They also noted an increased number of mucoid tumors in younger patients. Many authors have supported these findings.[283–285] Adolescent patients under 20 years have presented with high-stage, mucin-producing, and high-grade tumors and have had a poor survival as a result.[286] When stage-adjusted survival has been analyzed, in almost all reports there has been no difference in relative prognosis for the younger age group.[286–290]

GENDER. Women have a more favorable prognosis than men in terms of survival from colorectal cancer, just as they often survive better with other malignancies.[291,292] Four large analyses showed an improved survival for females.[246,293–295] Other studies have not shown a difference in prognosis by gender.[289,296–298] In women, risk for proximal colon cancer increases with null or low parity.[299]

SYMPTOMS. Beahrs and Sanfelippo reported that symptomatic colorectal cancer patients had a 5-year survival rate of 49%, compared with 71% for asymptomatic patients.[300] Patients in whom colorectal cancer is detected by a screening technique such as fecal occult blood testing or sigmoidoscopy may be treated at an earlier stage and therefore might have a greater chance for cure. Several reports note high survival rates in patients in whom colorectal cancer was detected by screening. In these studies, the number of patients with positive lymph nodes has been small and the survival rates high.

DURATION OF SYMPTOMS. In a study of 161 patients, Pescatori and colleagues found that patients with symptoms for more than 6 months had a significantly higher rate of radical operations, a lower postoperative mortality, and a higher 5-year survival rate—43% compared with only 32% for patients with symptoms of less than 6 months' duration.[301] They found no correlation between the duration of symptoms and pathologic stage.[301] This improved survival may reflect the slow growth rate of tumors in these patients. Copeland and colleagues analyzed 1084 patients and reported a slight improvement in the 5-year disease-free survival rate for patients with symptoms of 6 months' duration or less (31%) compared with 37% for patients who had symptoms for longer than 6 months.[302] By multivariate analysis, Chapuis and colleagues found that duration of symptoms had no effect on survival when stage was controlled.[246]

OBSTRUCTION AND PERFORATION. Obstruction and perforation appear to reduce survival.[223,246,252,303–311] In patients with colorectal cancer undergoing a potentially curative resection, the median 5-year survival (all stages combined) of those with obstruction is 40% compared with 30% for those with perforation.[312] Obstruction was the only symptom that had an independent effect in the multivariate analysis of 709 patients in Sydney.[246] A compilation of patients with colorectal cancer treated on NSABP clinical trials analyzed data from 1021 patients.[311] The presence of bowel obstruction strongly influenced the prognostic outcome. The GITSG used multivariate analysis to examine prognostic features in 572 patients with colon cancer.[252] Obstruction was an important indicator of prognosis, independent of Dukes' stage. Bowel perforation was important as a prognostic feature only for disease-free survival. In regard to perforating cancers, one should distinguish between perforation through the tumor and perforation proximal to an obstructing cancer.

HEMORRHAGE OR RECTAL BLEEDING. Hemorrhage or rectal bleeding has been associated with an improved prognosis. A possible explanation is that surface erosion manifests early and leads to early intervention, not that it is a symptom of tumor penetration.[313] In the GITSG colon cancer experience, the presence of melena or rectal bleeding marginally prolonged survival ($p = 0.08$) even after the effects of Dukes stage were considered.[252] In another study, symptomatic or asymptomatic anemia had no effect on prognosis.[302] In the analysis of the Sydney Hospital experience, patients with rectal bleeding had a significantly longer survival on univariate analysis; however, the significance of bleeding disappeared on multivariate analysis.[246]

LOCATION OF THE PRIMARY TUMOR. In general, the 5-year survival is lower for patients with cancer of the rectosigmoid and rectum than for patients with cancer elsewhere in the colon.[293,294,297,302,311,314] In regard to colon primaries, some authors suggest a worse prognosis for patients with lesions in the right colon.[293,311] Others find no difference;[289,295] still others report a worse prognosis for patients with disease in the left colon.[301] For rectal cancers, a decreased survival has been noted for patients with lesions below the peritoneal reflection, compared with patients with lesions above the perineal reflection.[315,316]

PRIMARY TUMOR SIZE. Colorectal cancer is unusual in that most studies find no significant adverse relation of tumor size to survival.[204,219,221,224,246,293,294,317,318] A few studies have shown improved survival with smaller tumors.[217]

PRIMARY TUMOR CONFIGURATION. As early as 1939, Grinnell reported that survival was higher in patients with tumors projecting into the lumen (83%) than in patients whose tumors were either intermediate (45% survival) or in-

filtrating (38%).[228] The reasons for such differences in survival include the lower frequency of penetration of the bowel wall by exophytic tumors compared with ulcerating tumors (24% versus 39%),[319] less frequent nodal metastases with exophytic tumors than with ulcerating lesions,[319–321] and fewer hematogenous metastases (23% versus 31%).[186] Overall, exophytic tumors are limited to the bowel wall (46%) more frequently than are ulcerating tumors (24%).[319] The recent GTSG colon adjuvant study looked at exophytic compared with nonexophytic tumors and found that the presence of an exophytic lesion had a significantly beneficial effect on survival.[252]

BLOOD TRANSFUSION. The association of perioperative blood transfusions with an increase in the recurrence rate of colorectal cancer is unclear, and conflicting data have been reported. Several authors have suggested that perioperative blood transfusions have a negative effect on disease-free interval in patients with colorectal or colon cancer.[322–324] Other prognostic variables were not considered in these studies. Other studies have shown no relation.[297,325–327]

Pathologic Features

ADJACENT ORGAN INVOLVEMENT. Adjacent organs or structures are involved in about 10% of colorectal cancer cases. Spratt and Spjut found that removal of a contiguous pathologically invaded organ did not alter 5- and 10-year survival rates.[293] Nathanson and colleagues, in a multivariate analysis of prognostic factors, indicated that the second most important factor was involvement of adjacent organs, which increased the relative risk of dying from colorectal cancer to 2.6.[328] Few series have examined the prognostic significance of pathologic confirmation of tumor invasion into an adjacent organ or structure, compared with adherence alone, in stages B3 and C3 colorectal cancer.[213,225,329,330] Eldar and colleagues found a significant decrease in survival in patients with stage B3 disease in whom tumor invasion was pathologically confirmed, but not in stage C3.[329] Minsky and colleagues analyzed patients with colon or rectal cancer according to whether they had stage B3 or C3 disease clinically or if the disease was verified microscopically.[224,225] Patients with stage B3 colon cancer verified pathologically had a 27% 5-year actuarial survival rate, significantly lower than the 88% survival in patients with B3 disease who were thought to have only clinical adjacent organ involvement.[225] This difference was not seen in patients with rectal cancer.[224]

LATERAL MARGINS. In general, when pathologists describe negative margins of resection, they are referring to the proximal and distal margins. Because the staging of rectal cancer depends on the penetration of tumor through the bowel wall, it would be logical to examine the lateral margin on resection. Quirke and colleagues examined the lateral margins in 52 patients with rectal cancer using whole mount sections and meticulous sectioning techniques.[254] For the total patient group, there was a significant increase in local failure in the 12 patients with positive lateral margins compared with those with negative lateral margins (85% versus 3%; $p < 0.001$).

DEGREE OF DIFFERENTIATION (GRADE). Dukes and others reported a correlation of grade with lymph node and distant metastases found at operation.[207,208,215] Grade also has been correlated with the likelihood of venous spread,[185,208] the risk for lymphatic penetration,[185] extent of local spread,[208] the number of lymph node metastases,[319,331] and increasing wall penetration.[319] In another study, grade was not associated with the extent of local invasion.[332]

Univariate analysis has shown a clear relation between survival and histologic grade in both colon and rectal cancer. In several recent multivariate analyses, grade was independently prognostic of survival.[246,252,266,295,315,333]

COLLOID (MUCINOUS) CANCER. In the broad sense, colloid carcinoma is an adenocarcinoma with an associated clear, gelatinous fluid, which may be either intracellular or extracellular. The intracellular variety, most commonly known as *signet cell* or *signet-ring cell carcinoma*, accounts for about 4% of colloid cancers and 1% to 2% of all colorectal cancers. Some signet-ring cell cancers form a linitis plastica appearance by spreading intramurally, usually not involving the mucosa.[208] In most series, the cancer has a poor prognosis.[334]

The most common variety of colloid is extracellular and is commonly referred to as *colloid* or *mucinous cancer*. Although there is a fairly uniform histologic definition of mucin, there is no consensus as to the location or percentage of the colloid pattern in adenocarcinoma that must be present to be defined as colloid carcinoma. Umpleby and colleagues defined moderate colloid adenocarcinoma as containing 60% to 80% of a colloid pattern, and high colloid as an adenocarcinoma containing more than 80% of a colloid pattern.[335] Symonds and Vickery defined colloid carcinoma as those tumors containing more than 60% colloid.[334] Minsky and colleagues defined colloid cancer as an adenocarcinoma of which more than two thirds was growing in a colloid pattern.[336] Many authors have reported a worse survival in patients with colloid cancers.[334,335,337] Some of the adverse prognosis is a function of the higher stage at presentation in most patients.[338,339]

VASCULAR INVASION. Since the initial report by Brown and Warren[232] in 1938 that demonstrated an increase in visceral metastasis in patients with rectal cancer with vascular invasion, investigators have examined the influence of vascular invasion by tumor in colon, rectal, and colorectal cancer. One would predict the presence of vascular invasion to be associated with an increased incidence of lymph node and distant metastasis and with a corresponding decrease in survival. This is not a consistent finding. Differences in the definition of vascular invasion, the methods of detection, and perhaps the metastatic potential of the cells once they have gained access to blood and lymphatic vessels may explain, in part, some of the variations observed.

Vascular invasion has two distinct components: blood vessel invasion (BVI) and lymphatic vessel invasion (LVI). In many series, *vascular invasion* is a general term used to define BVI or LVI or both. The use of elastic tissue stains are important to help identify BVI. If elastic tissue stains are not used, BVI will be correctly identified in only 16% of the cases.[340,341] In the series reported by Minsky and colleagues[340,341] and by Krasna and colleagues,[342] elastic tissue stains were used and BVI was identified clearly and scored separately from LVI. Unfortunately, most of the other series examining vascular

invasion did not use elastic tissue or other special stains, thereby introducing uncertainty both in the identification of BVI and in the differentiation of BVI from LVI.

BLOOD VESSEL INVASION. There are two types of BVI. Invasion of blood vessels within the bowel wall is defined as intramural BVI and invasion of blood vessels outside the bowel wall (pericolon fat or adventitia) is defined as extramural BVI. In general, BVI refers to vein invasion rather than arterial invasion. The overall incidence of arterial invasion is less than 1%.

Colon Cancer. The only series that specifically examines the influence of BVI in colon cancer is from Minsky and colleagues.[341] The overall incidence of BVI was 42% and the incidence of BVI increased with grade and stage. For the total group, patients whose tumors were BVI positive had a significant decrease in survival (BVI-positive tumors 74% versus BVI-negative tumors 85%; $p = 0.04$). When examined by the type of BVI, those patients whose tumors contained simultaneous extramural and intramural BVI had a significantly lower survival compared with patients with BVI-negative tumors (32% versus 85%). By proportional hazards analysis, BVI was not an independent prognostic factor for survival.

Rectal Cancer. In rectal cancer, the incidence of BVI varies from 17% to 61% and increases with stage and grade.[212,232,343–346] The first series to examine thoroughly both the intramural and extramural types of BVI was reported by Talbot and colleagues.[347] Of those tumors with BVI, 31% were intramural and 69% were extramural, compared with 61% and 23%, respectively, in the series from Minsky and colleagues.[341]

Minsky and colleagues found that the extramural component of BVI was responsible for the adverse impact on survival.[341] For the total patient group, actuarial 5-year survival was significantly decreased in patients who had tumors containing extramural BVI, (either as the only type of BVI [33%] or as a component of BVI [35%]) compared with patients who had tumors that were BVI negative (72%) or contained intramural BVI (either as the only type of BVI [72%] or as a component of BVI [77%]). By proportional hazards analysis, BVI was not an independent prognostic factor for survival.

Using a modification of Talbot's definition of BVI, Horn and colleagues found, by univariate analysis, a significant decrease in 5-year survival in patients with BVI (30% versus 69%; $p < 0.01$).[348] In an update of their results, BVI was found to be an independent prognostic factor for distant metastasis, although it was less significant than stage.[349]

Colorectal Cancer. In six series, tumors of the colon and rectum are not analyzed separately. The incidence of BVI varies from 25% to 81% and increases with stage and grade.[228,246,342,350–352] By multivariate analysis, Chapuis and colleagues found BVI to be an independent prognostic factor for survival.[246] This was not confirmed by Wiggers and colleagues.[350] The only series to use elastic tissue stains and score BVI separately from LVI was from Krasna and colleagues.[342] There was a significant decrease in 3-year survival in patients with BVI-positive compared with BVI-negative tumors (30% versus 62%; $p < 0.003$). The incidence of extranodal metastasis was also higher in patients with BVI-positive compared with BVI-negative tumors (60% versus 17%; $p < 0.0001$). The type of BVI did not influence the incidence of failure or survival.

LYMPHATIC VESSEL INVASION. The incidence of LVI varies from 8% to 73% and increases with stage and grade. All series report a lower survival for patients with LVI-positive tumors compared with LVI-negative tumors.

Michelassi and colleagues examined 110 patients with rectal cancer and found vascular or lymphatic microinvasion in 73%.[353] There was an increase in local failure in those patients with LVI-positive tumors (23% versus 0%). By multivariate analysis, LVI was an independent prognostic factor for survival.

In an analysis by Minsky and colleagues of 462 patients with colorectal cancer, a greater incidence of LVI was found in tumors of the colon compared with tumors of the rectosigmoid and rectum (15% versus 10%).[245] Tumors with intramural and extramural BVI had the highest incidence of LVI compared with BVI-negative tumors (52% versus 5%; $p = 0.05$). There was a significantly increased incidence and number of positive lymph nodes in LVI-positive tumors compared with LVI-negative tumors (59% versus 25%; $p = 0.0004$). The average number of positive nodes in patients with LVI-positive tumors was 4.8 compared with 2.2 in patients with LVI-negative tumors ($p = 0.0003$). There was a significant decrease in 5-year survival in patients with LVI-positive tumors compared with those with LVI-negative tumors in both the colon (57% versus 84%; $p = 0.0001$) and rectum (38% versus 71%; $p = 0.004$). By proportional hazards analysis, LVI was found to be an independent prognostic factor for survival. Therefore, both the Michelassi[353] and Minsky[245] series confirm that LVI is an independent prognostic factor for survival.

PERINEURAL INVASION. In general, the incidence of perineural invasion varies from 14% to 32%. The classic study of perineural invasion was reported by Seefeld and Bargen,[212] who noted that malignant spread by growth along perineural spaces occurred as far as 10 cm from the primary tumor. The incidence of perineural invasion was 30% in 100 cases, increasing with grade and Dukes' stage. Patients with perineural invasion had more local recurrences in the scar or anastomotic site than those free of perineural invasion (81% versus 30%). The 5-year survival rate was also lower in the former group (7% versus 35%). Spratt and Spjut confirmed this survival difference.[293] In a study of 77 patients with colorectal cancer, there was a significant decrease in survival in those patients whose tumors had neural invasion (30% versus 58%; $p < 0.003$).[354]

IMMUNE RESPONSE TO THE PRIMARY TUMOR. Considerable interest has been expressed in the prognostic value of local inflammatory reactions at the primary tumor site. Spratt and Spjut noted a decrease in survival with a lack of an inflammatory response around the tumor periphery.[293] Murray and colleagues reported an increased 5-year survival rate for patients with Dukes' B and C colon cancer when local inflammation was present (89% versus 46%).[355] Local inflammation has been found in about 50% to 75% of tumors.[204,355] Jass and colleagues demonstrated that lymphocytic infiltration was the most important factor in their grading

model (Cox regression analysis) and was also important in their "best" model with grade- and stage-related parameters.[205] Carlon and colleagues similarly noted that lymphocytic infiltrate around the primary and pattern of growth was the most significant prognostic feature.[356] Svennevig and associates reported a higher number of mononuclear cells in the peritumoral stroma and the tumor parenchyma in those patients cured by surgery.[357]

By univariate analysis, lymphatic stroma reaction was a prognostic factor for local failure in rectal cancer,[358] and lymphocytic infiltration was a prognostic factor for survival in colon cancer.[248] In an analysis of the NSABP R-01 rectal adjuvant protocol, survival was significantly decreased with increasing numbers of eosinophils and mast cells present at the tumor border.[359] By multivariate analysis, the number of mast cells was an independent prognostic factor for survival.

REACTIVE LYMPH NODES. Many investigators have shown that an apparent immunologic response in regional lymph nodes correlates with improved survival.[355,360–362] In sigmoid colon cancer, Patt and associates noted that sinus histiocytosis and paracortical immunoblastic activity individually correlated with an increased survival.[360] If both features were present, survival was even better. There was no benefit from increased germinal center activity in this study. Murray and colleagues also reported an increased survival with sinus histiocytosis of the draining lymph nodes, and an even greater increase in survival when this feature was present with a local inflammatory reaction to the primary.[355] Pihl and colleagues observed that paracortical lymph node hyperplasia occupying more than 15% of the lymph node section was favorably associated with survival.[362]

CARCINOEMBRYONIC ANTIGEN AND OTHER BIOMARKERS. The value of preoperative carcinoembryonic antigen (CEA) level as an independent prognostic indicator is unclear. The preoperative CEA levels reflect the tumor burden.[363–365] Many authors have reported that an increased level (5 ng/ml) indicates an increased risk for recurrence,[365–372] but others have not found it to be a good prognostic variable.[373–376] Steele and colleagues reported that an increased CEA level was prognostic for colon cancer but not for rectal cancer.[377] The Mayo Clinic reported that CEA level was strongly associated with survival but that within stages it was only independently prognostic for Dukes' C patients with four or more positive lymph nodes.

COLLAGEN. Interstitial collagen is a major component of the tumor matrix. In 54 patients with colorectal cancer, Wobbes and colleagues found no correlation between the amount of interstitial collagen and prognosis.[378] Offerhaus and colleagues found that by univariate analysis, expression of collagen type IV was associated with an improved prognosis in patients with colorectal cancer.[379] This was not confirmed with multivariate analysis. In node-positive colorectal cancer, patients with limited basement membrane deposition of type IV collagen had a lower survival compared with those with moderate to extensive deposition.[380]

NUCLEAR MORPHOLOGY. Several investigators have used morphometric measurements to determine if differences in nuclear size and shape correlate with survival in colorectal cancer. The results are conflicting. Mitmaker and colleagues found by multiple regression analysis that nuclear shape was the most highly significant predictor of survival in colorectal cancer.[250] In contrast, Heimann and colleagues reported that there was no correlation between nuclear morphometry and stage or survival.[381] A linear regression analysis showed a significant linear relation between the mean nuclear area and the number of positive nodes in colorectal cancer, although there was no correlation with survival.[382]

CELL CYCLE PARAMETERS AND PLOIDY. In colorectal cancer, there is an increasing loss of diploidy as cells progress from premalignant to malignant.[383] There is also a significant increase in tissue CEA levels in aneuploid compared with diploid tumors.[384]

As in other prognostic factors in colorectal cancer, the influence of DNA content on the patterns of failure and survival varies greatly. Most series report aneuploidy to be a poor prognostic factor for survival,[255,257,259,384-401] whereas others report little or no difference.[402-407] In those series in which aneuploidy is an independent prognostic factor, some find it less predictive than stage[259,385,393,401,408] and others find it more predictive than stage.[255,409]

In general, there is an increase in aneuploidy with increasing stage. Aneuploid tumors tend to have a less favorable and higher growth rate compared with diploid tumors. Often, aneuploid tumors are associated with other pathologic factors indicative of a poor prognosis.[390] By univariate and multivariate analyses, most series show that DNA content is an independent prognostic factor for survival. It still is not clear if the DNA index offers additional prognostic information beyond stage. Such data are being used as a determinant of high-risk node-negative patients.[409]

Additional Tumor Biologic Features

ONCOGENES. Most series report an increased expression of oncogenes in more aggressive colorectal cancers. For example, expression of c-*MYC* was increased in mucinous and high-grade tumors[410,411] and *RAS* in node-positive tumors.[412] By univariate analysis, Ha-*RAS* and Ki-*RAS* expression was independent of grade, stage, and ploidy status.[413] Mizoguchi and colleagues reported increased expression of *MDR1* with lower grade cancers.[414] Murnane and colleagues reported that cathepsin B gene expression is inversely related to stage.[415]

Allelic or genetic deletion of tumor suppressor genes may be pivotal in the development of metastases. Prognosis has been inversely correlated with loss of p53[416,417] and nm23-H1.[418]

GROWTH FACTORS. The level of transforming growth factor-α (TGF-α) in colon cancer is four times that seen in normal colon mucosa. The level does not appear to correlate with histology, stage, or grade.[419] Steele and colleagues found higher levels of epidermal growth factor receptor expression in node positive compared with node negative colorectal cancer.[420]

IMMUNOLOGY AND MARKERS. Many antigens have been associated with colorectal cancer cells. The CEA level was discussed earlier as a preoperative prognostic factor. In future years, monoclonal antibody technology will allow identification of multiple additional antigens. An overview of various antigens follows.

CARCINOEMBRYONIC ANTIGEN. CEA was referred to as an *oncofetal protein* after Gold and Freeman isolated it in 1965 from human adult colon cancer and fetal colon epithelium using adsorption and tolerance techniques.[421] It is a heavily glycosylated, single chain peptide of 200,000 daltons molecular weight. Electron microscopic immunochemical techniques demonstrate the protein in normal colon columnar and goblet cells.[422] Monoclonal antibody technology has indicated a large number of epitopes.[423,424] Studies with these epitopes are under way with the hope of improving the specificity of this antigen in the detection and treatment of colorectal cancer.

BLOOD GROUP ANTIGENS. Many investigators have confirmed the lack of expression of normal blood group ABH antigens in the distal colon and rectal mucosa and the presence of such antigens on cancers in these locations.[425-428] A recent report suggests that ABH antigens appear in neoplastic (adenomatous) polyps but not hyperplastic polyps.[429] Many of the tumor-associated antigens detected with monoclonal antibodies are modified blood-group glycolipids.[430] The modified Lewis antigens represent another group of oncofetal antigens associated with colorectal cancer.[431-433]

CA 19-9. Of the large number of antigens defined on colorectal cancers, albeit not exclusively, one of the most widely studied has been the carbohydrate cell surface antigen designated 19-9, which was identified by Koprowski and associates.[434] This antigen is a sialylated lacto-*N*-fucopentose that is related to the Lewis blood group substance.[435] CA 19-9 is released into the blood of cancer-bearing patients and is detected with the CA 19-9 assay system. The antigen recognized by this antibody appears to be a class 3 differentiation antigen.[436]

OTHER MONOCLONAL ANTIBODY-DEFINED ANTIGENS. Koprowski and colleagues identified another antigen with monoclonal antibody 17-1A.[437,438] This system has been of particular interest because immunologic inhibition of growth can result with infusion of this antibody. Johnson and associates defined a high molecular weight glycoprotein (TAG-72) using monoclonal antibody B72.3.[439] Although this antigen is present in 85% of colorectal cancers, there is considerable heterogeneity in its expression in the primary tumor, lymph nodes, and distant metastases.[440]

TREATMENT OF PRECANCEROUS COLORECTAL DISEASE

NEOPLASTIC POLYPS (ADENOMAS)

Histologically, neoplastic polyps are tubular, villous, or a combination of both. Villous tumors have a higher propensity to be associated with cancer in the polyp. In addition, patients with multiple villous polyps are more likely to develop additional polyps after removal of the initial lesions. Because the finding of a polypoid mass on endoscopy or barium enema examination does not connote benignity, such lesions should be removed except in the most infirm patients. Almost all pedunculated polyps can be removed by endoscopic snare polypectomy. Sessile lesions frequently can be removed piecemeal, but with an increased risk for perforation. Several sessions may be necessary. Large sessile villous lesions in the cecum and ascending colon may require colectomy for safe removal.

Data accruing from the National Polyp Study will define more precisely the appropriate follow-up strategies for patients with polyps. Data from several sources allow us to endorse the follow-up algorithms in Figures 30–6 and 30–7 as general guidelines.[441–444]

The large villous adenoma of the rectum can pose a difficult management problem. Transanal local excision at the level of the submucosa allows for complete histologic examination. About 75% of soft, nonulcerated tumors prove benign on subsequent examination, whereas 15% contain superficial cancer and only 10% contain invasive cancer.[445] Random biopsies of grossly benign-appearing lesions are unreliable and make subsequent surgical excision more difficult.[446] Electrocoagulation with cautery, piecemeal snare excision, and Nd:YAG laser ablation have been used but preclude complete histologic assessment. Very large tumors can be excised and mucosa closed by muscle plication and mucosal advancement.[447,448] Low anterior resection, coloanal procedures, and abdominoperineal resection play a role in the management of extensive benign rectal polyps.

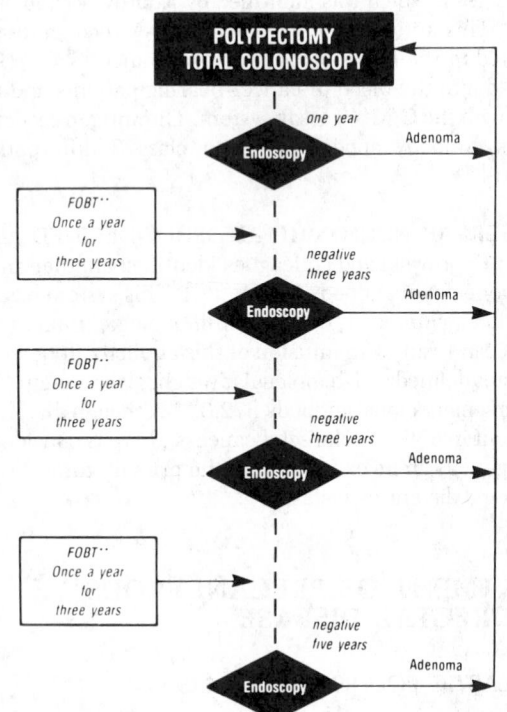

FIGURE 30–6.   Management of the minimal-risk patient with colorectal adenomas defined as the following: a solitary adenoma; ≤2 cm pedunculated; if sessile then having tubular histology with only mild or moderate dysplasia.[441]

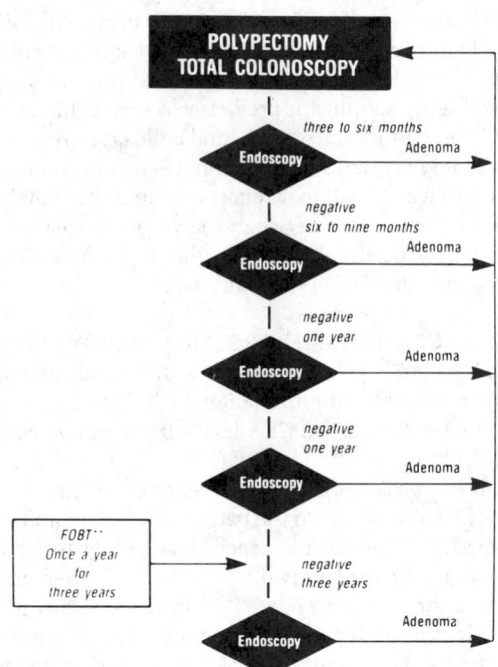

FIGURE 30–7.   Management of the high-risk patient with colorectal adenomas defined as the following: multiple adenomas; ≥2 cm; sessile; villous or tubulovillous; with severe dysplasia, carcinoma in situ, or invasive cancer.[441]

FAMILIAL ADENOMATOUS POLYPOSIS

There is continued controversy as to the appropriate surgical management of patients with FAP.[449,450] Because almost all untreated patients develop colorectal cancer by age 40, prophylactic surgery is warranted. Total abdominal colectomy with ileorectal anastomosis is usually the procedure of choice if the rectum is free of polyps. The rectal stump must be examined frequently (as often as every 6 months) for signs of cancer. Polyps must be regularly removed or fulgurated. Cancer has been reported to develop in the retained rectal stump in as few as 5% to over half of such patients. The results from the major centers are summarized in Table 30–6. Unquestionably, there is increased risk with increased duration of follow-up. The risk is considerably less if the rectum is not involved by the polyposis (20% of polyposis patients).[451] In patients not willing to risk developing cancer in the retained rectum, or in patients with a carpet of polyps in the rectum, total proctocolectomy is appropriate. In most younger patients, restorative proctocolectomy with a distal mucosal proctectomy and an ileal pouch-anal anastomosis enhances the quality of

TABLE 30–6.   Risk of Rectal Cancer After Abdominal Colectomy for Polyposis

Investigations	No. of Patients	Subsequent Rectal Cancer
St. Marks Hospital[684]	174	13% (at 25 years)
Mayo Clinic[685]	178	59% (at 23 years)
Memorial Sloan-Kettering[686]	27	10%
Cleveland Clinic[687]	133	7.5%

life.[452] Multiple aspects of the management of these patients are described in a recent monograph.[453]

ULCERATIVE COLITIS

As described in the section on screening, many patients with ulcerative colitis can be followed endoscopically, with selective surgery in those who develop high-grade dysplasia or cancer.[454–458] Restorative total proctocolectomy with distal submucosal proctectomy and ileal pouch-anal anastomosis should be considered in the younger patient undergoing elective surgery.[459,460]

TREATMENT OF POTENTIALLY CURABLE COLON CANCER

PRETREATMENT EVALUATION

The following are general guidelines for the pretreatment evaluation of patients with potentially curable colorectal cancer:

> *History:* In addition to the personal medical history, the family history of colorectal cancer, polyps, and other cancers should be obtained.
> *Physical Examination:* Check for hepatomegaly, ascites, lymphadenopathy. In women, rule out synchronous ovarian pathology and breast cancer.
> *Laboratory Data:* Blood count, CEA, liver chemistries.
> *Gastrointestinal:* Full colonoscopy or proctosigmoidoscopy and air-contrast barium enema (in the absence of obstruction or perforation).
> *Imaging:* A preoperative chest radiograph is appropriate. Colon cancer patients may benefit from a perioperative computed tomography (CT) scan or ultrasound study of their liver as a baseline. Only a small subset of patients have intrahepatic tumor not recognizable at laparotomy that will impact on the operative procedure. Although preferable, this study need not be performed preoperatively if liver chemistries are normal and hepatomegaly is not present.

GENERAL SURGICAL PRINCIPLES

The morbidity of elective colon surgery is directly related to the mechanical and oral antibiotic bowel preparation, the use of perioperative systemic antibiotics, and the skill of the surgical and anesthesia team.

Extent of Bowel Resection

Except for the occasional minimally invasive polypoid cancer, which frequently can be cured by endoscopic polypectomy, en bloc surgical resection is the primary treatment approach in patients with colon cancer. Fortunately, almost all of these cancers can be treated without a permanent or even temporary colostomy. This should be explained to the patient and family at an early point in the consultation, because concern about a colostomy frequently supersedes all other considerations of the patient. Surgical treatment of colon cancer requires excision of an adequate amount of normal colon proximal and distal to the tumor, of adequate lateral margins if the tumor is adherent to a contiguous structure, and of the regional lymph nodes. Pathologic studies indicate that tumor rarely spreads

more than 1.2 cm longitudinally beyond the area of gross involvement, and a 5-cm margin is more than adequate.[196] However, removal of intermediate and more central (principal) lymph nodes requires ligation and division of multiple main vascular trunks. Therefore, the extent of the colon resection for potentially curable colon cancer is determined by the biology of local tumor growth and by the associated lymphadenectomy.

Extent of Lymph Node Dissection

Patients with colon cancer metastatic to regional lymph nodes may still be cured with surgery. Hence, lymphadenectomy is not only necessary for staging but is also therapeutic. The paracolic and intermediate lymph nodes are resected routinely, but it is not clear to what extent removal of more central or principal lymph nodes is therapeutic. Enker and colleagues described excellent results in the treatment of colon cancer, which they believed were due in part to an extensive lymphadenectomy.[461] However, Grinnell reported that all 17 patients with carcinoma of the descending colon, sigmoid, or rectum with positive nodes around the origin of the inferior mesenteric artery died from cancer.[462]

Adequate regional lymph node dissection is part of effective therapy for colon cancer. Small segmental resections with removal of only the paracolic lymph nodes are suitable operations only in the presence of liver metastases or peritoneal seeding or in medically poor-risk patients. Relevant intermediate nodes should be removed routinely. The extent of resection of central nodes depends on the patient's age, body habitus, and overall medical condition, and on the operative findings.

No-Touch Technique

The discovery of numerous tumor cells within the portal vein associated with intraoperative manipulation of the tumor led to the suggestion that the lymphovascular pedicle be ligated before mobilization of the primary tumor.[264,463,464] Concepts of tumor biology suggest that in most patients with subsequent liver metastases, micrometastases are already established before the primary tumor is resected. Intraoperative vascular dissemination may play only a small role in the metastatic process. From a practical surgical viewpoint, it can be difficult and potentially dangerous to isolate vascular structures prematurely. A randomized prospective trial of the no-touch technique was performed in the Netherlands.[465] Results suggest a small benefit with preliminary vascular ligation only in the subset of patients with sigmoid colon cancer and histologic evidence of venous invasion.

Prevention of Intraluminal Spread

There appears to be little doubt that tumor cells are exfoliated into the intestinal lumen. It is likely that some of these cells are alive and capable of implanting on exposed cut surfaces of the bowel.[237,466] Isolated suture line recurrences are rare after right colectomy, occurring more often after left-sided colectomies and in rectal operations. The greater longitudinal bowel margins with right-sided colon cancers and the presence of active digestive enzymes and cytotoxic bile may explain some of this discrepancy. Stapled anastomoses do not seem to be any more susceptible to tumor implantation than those that are hand-sewn. Precautions to minimize the implantation of cancer cells have been suggested.[467-469] Those that have shown efficacy in animal studies include isolation of the tumor with proximal and distal ligatures, irrigation of the lumen, formaldehyde or electrocautery treatment of bowel edges, and use of iodized suture material. No randomized clinical trial has ever tested these hypotheses.

Prophylactic Oophorectomy

Because 2% to 8% of women with colorectal cancer have synchronous ovarian metastases[470-472] and 1% to 7% of those who undergo potentially curative resections develop subsequent ovarian metastases, prophylactic oophorectomy may be useful in the overall management of such patients. Such an approach would reduce the risk for primary ovarian cancer, which is about 1% for women over age 40 and is perhaps higher in colorectal cancer patients.[473] Extensive ovarian metastases are almost always part of widespread recurrent tumor. It remains unclear whether prophylactic removal of grossly normal ovaries containing micrometastatic colon cancer actually increases the cure rate. We recommend that women with colorectal cancer be asked preoperatively for permission to perform a bilateral oophorectomy. Certainly, if the ovaries are found to be grossly abnormal, they should be removed. A hysterectomy is not required in the treatment of ovarian metastases. If a premenopausal woman is considering childbirth, prophylactic oophorectomy is not warranted. However, in most perimenopausal and postmenopausal women with potentially curable colorectal cancer, consideration should be given to removal of grossly normal ovaries.

SITE-SPECIFIC SURGERY

General guidelines for appropriate operative resection for colon cancers involving the major locations are illustrated in Figures 30–8 and 30–9. The exact anastomotic techniques (*e.g.*, hand-sewn versus stapled anastomoses, use of different suture materials, one or two layers) are a function of the surgeon's preference.[474]

TREATMENT RESULTS

Many variables affect the curability of colorectal cancer. Multivariate analysis indicates the surgical-pathologic stage is the most important. This section examines expected end results after surgery for potentially curable colon cancer as a function of stage. The impact of the many other prognostic variables on outcome was discussed earlier in the chapter, and the management of patients with unresectable primary cancer or synchronous hematogenous metastases is discussed later.

The 5-year survival rates after surgical resection appear to have improved in recent years. Although the data may indicate the widespread application of appropriate surgical techniques in resecting these cancers, the use of perioperative CT scanning may have increased the ability to detect early liver metastases and, therefore, to define more accurately the patient population selected for potentially curative surgery. Whether one looks at a large experience of a single surgeon such as

that of E. S. R. Hughes in Australia[292] or the multicenter experience of the United Kingdom Large Bowel Cancer Project,[266] it appears that most patients with colon cancer resectable at the time of laparotomy are cured by surgical extirpation.

Cure Rates for Node-Negative Patients

The 5-year survival rate for patients with tumors involving the mucosa or submucosa is in excess of 90%. Muscle wall invasion decreases the 5-year survival rate slightly to 80%. Transmural penetration is still associated with cure in most patients, with survival in the 60% to 80% range. Data from selected series are listed in Table 30–7.

Cure Rates for Node-Positive Patients

The overall 5-year cure rate for patients with regional lymph node metastases is about one third. Patients with four or fewer involved lymph nodes have a good prognosis. The end results reported by the GITSG indicate a survival of 56% in patients with one to four positive nodes.[475] Results from NSABP[265] and the United Kingdom Large Bowel Cancer Project[266] support this distinction. Data from Memorial Sloan-Kettering Cancer Center suggest subgrouping into 1 to 3 nodes and 4 or greater nodes is more appropriate.[280] Data from selected series are summarized in Table 30–8.

Patterns of Recurrence

Recurrence occurs in local (direct extension), regional (lymphatic and nodal), and peritoneal seeding patterns. The major risk for recurrence in patients with colon cancer remains disseminated disease. The liver is involved in as many as two thirds of patients who die from colon cancer.[476] Ovarian metastases develop in up to 7% of women with colon cancer and are a symptomatic problem in about half of those patients.

The risk for locoregional failure varies with the pathologic stage of the primary tumor. In addition, posterior penetration in a portion of the colon devoid of serosa may increase local recurrence rate. In an autopsy series from the University of Florida, the local recurrence rate in patients who died from cancer was 27% in those with T3N0M0 disease, 21% in those with T2N1M0 disease, and 52% in those with T3N1M0 disease.[216] A similar analysis from the University of Washington identified a 27% recurrence rate in patients with transmural tumor with almost two thirds of these patients having retroperitoneal node recurrence.[477] The rate was 69% if the tumor adhered to or invaded adjacent structures. Only 19% of the 53 patients autopsied had isolated locoregional recurrences.

Recurrence patterns have been analyzed in a group of 533 patients with colon cancer treated at the Massachusetts General Hospital.[476,478] The overall locoregional failure rate was 19%, with only 6% isolated local failures. However, two thirds of the patients with disease recurrence at any site had some component of locoregional failure. The local recurrences correlated with gross transmural penetration of the primary tumor, and particularly with adherence to or invasion of surrounding organs. The local failure rate approached 50% in patients with five or more positive lymph nodes. These findings are supported by a report from the Peter Bent Brigham

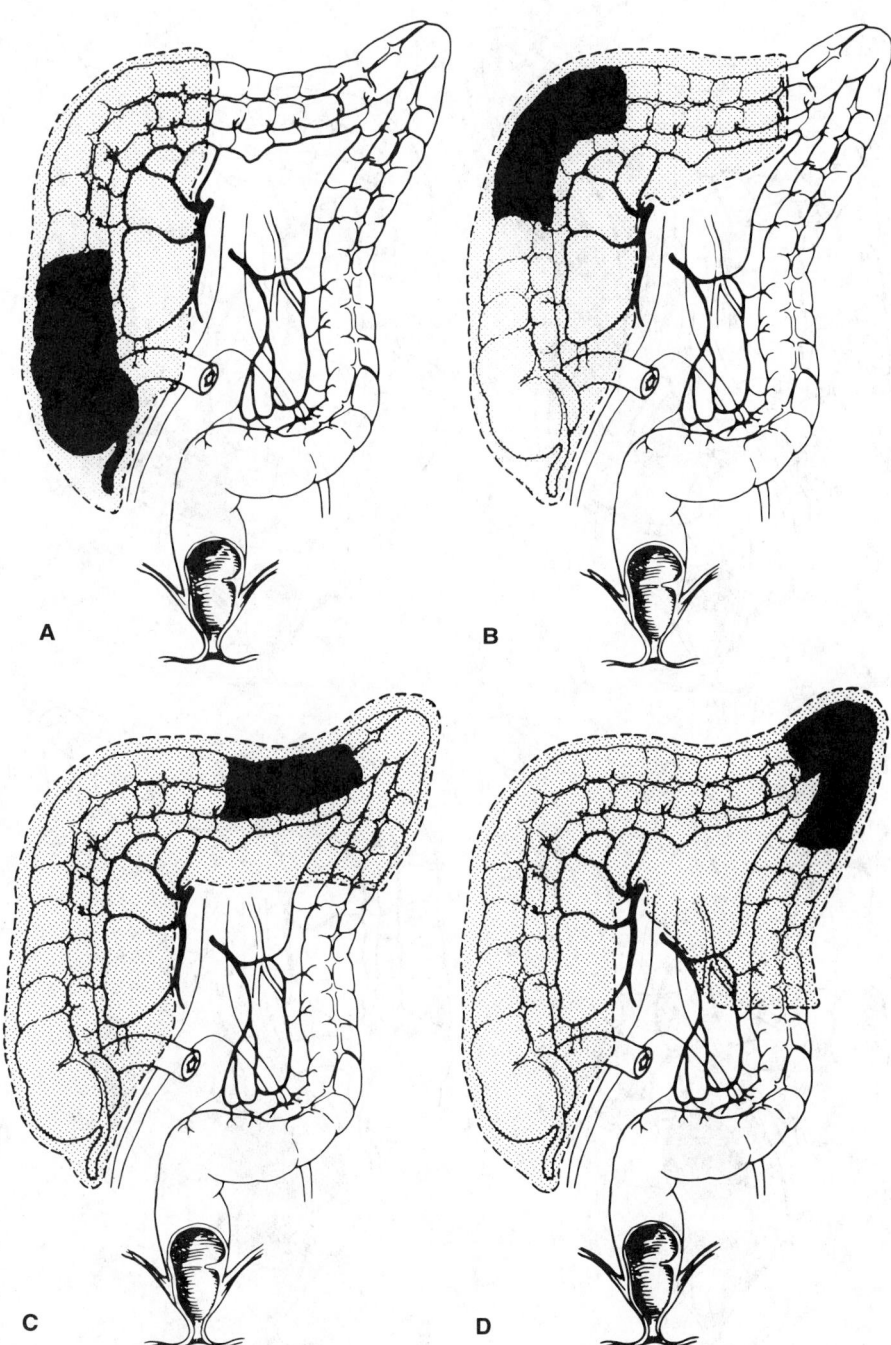

FIGURE 30–8. Surgical resection for ascending and transfer colon cancers. **(A)** Surgical resection for a cecal or ascending colon cancer. **(B)** Surgical resection for a cancer at the hepatic flexure. **(C)** Preferable surgical resection for cancer for the transverse colon. A segmental resection may be appropriate in poor-risk patients. **(D)** Preferred extensive resection for cancer at the splenic flexure. (Modified from Enker WE. Surgical treatment of large bowel cancer. In: Enker WE, ed. Cancer of the colon and rectum. Chicago: Yearbook, 1978:73–106)

Hospital, in which patients with sigmoid colon cancer had an overall regional recurrence rate of 18%.[217] This represented a two-thirds failure rate in patients with disease recurrence at any site. In half of these patients, failure was expressed as isolated regional recurrence.

The incidence of peritoneal seeding has not been well documented.[241] In the autopsy series reported from the University of Washington, treatment failure manifested as peritoneal seeding was identified in 36% of patients who died from colon cancer. Peritoneal seeding occurred in the absence of locoregional recurrence in 58% of those cases.[477] The Massachusetts General Hospital autopsy series has yielded a comparable 32% failure rate by peritoneal seeding.[479]

SPECIFIC MANAGEMENT PROBLEMS IN COLON CANCER

SYNCHRONOUS CANCERS

Synchronous colorectal cancers occur in 3% to 5% of patients.[480,481] In addition, about one third of cancer-bearing patients have associated benign neoplastic polyps. These data suggest that in the absence of obstruction, preoperative clearance of the remaining colon is recommended, either by air-contrast barium enema examination or, preferably, by colonoscopy.[482]

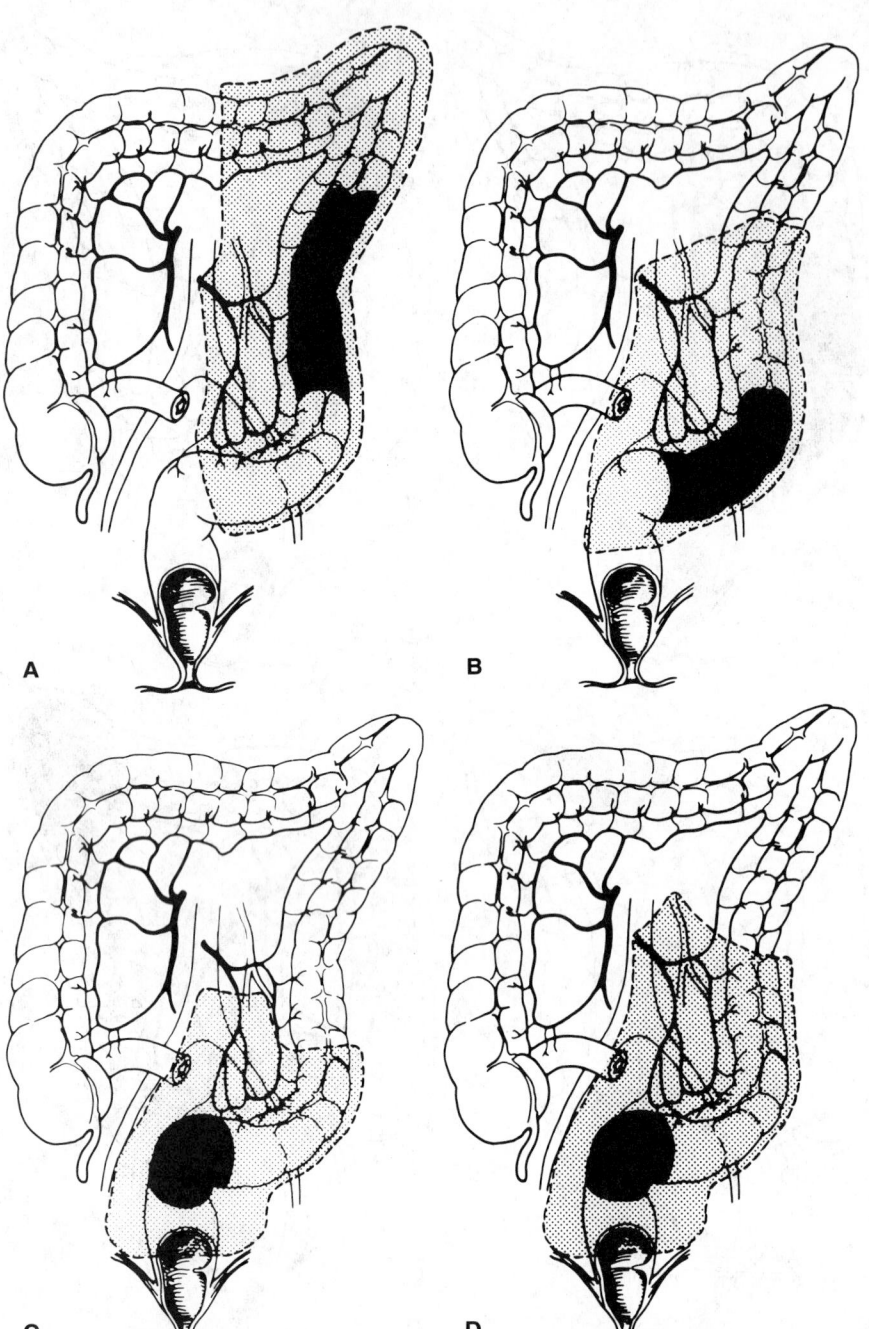

A

B

C

D

FIGURE 30–9. Surgical resection for distal colon cancer. **(A)** Surgical resection for a descending colon cancer. **(B)** Preferred surgical procedure for cancer of the middle and proximal sigmoid colon. In poor-risk patients the inferior mesenteric artery and the left colic artery may be preserved. **(C)** Surgical resection for cancer of the rectosigmoid. **(D)** A more radical surgical resection for cancer of the rectosigmoid. (Modified from Enker WE. Surgical treatment of large bowel cancer. In: Enker WE, ed. Cancer of the colon and rectum. Chicago: Yearbook, 1978:73–106)

OBSTRUCTING CANCERS

Left-sided colon obstruction traditionally was managed by a three-stage operative approach.[309] Initially, patients underwent a diverting transverse colostomy or occasionally a cecostomy. The second stage, undertaken 10 to 14 days later, involved tumor resection. As the final procedure, the colostomy was closed. However, unless the patient is very ill, a two-stage Hartmann procedure is more commonly used. The tumor is resected, with the proximal colon brought to the skin as an end-colostomy. The distal colon is sutured or stapled closed. The second operation reestablishes intestinal continuity. If a preliminary diverting colostomy is chosen, it is important at the time of initial surgery to examine the cecum

for perforation and the liver for metastases. Intraoperative whole-gut colon lavage may be used to mechanically clear the colon proximal to an obstruction. This may allow a one-stage resection.

The patient with an obstructing cancer of the ascending or transverse colon usually can be treated with a single-stage resection. An ileal-colon anastomosis is performed, which even in the absence of bowel preparation usually heals without complication.

PERFORATING CANCERS

Perforation of the colon can occur proximal to an obstructing cancer. Recognition of this catastrophe and the timely per-

TABLE 30–7. Five-Year Survival Rates in Node-Negative Colon Cancer

Investigations	Stage	Survival (%)
Willet et al[476]	T1N0M0	97
	T2N0M0	90
	T3N0M0	78
	T4N0M0	63
Eisenberg et al[296]	Dukes' A	82
	Dukes' B	73
GITSG[688,689]	T3N0M0	80

TABLE 30–8. Five-Year Survival Rates in Node-Positive Colon Cancer

Investigations	Stage	Survival (%)
Willet et al[476]	T2N1M0	74
	T3N1M0	48
	T4N1M0	38
Eisenberg et al[296]	Dukes' C	40
GITSG[688,689]	Dukes' C (1–4 nodes)	56
	Dukes' C (>4 nodes)	26
Cohen et al[280]	Dukes' C (1–3 nodes)	60
	Dukes' C (>3 nodes)	30

formance of radical surgical resection, peritoneal cavity irrigation, drainage, and antibiotic administration have lessened the morbidity and mortality. Chronic perforations into a contiguous organ with or without fistula formation are discussed later in the chapter. Acute free perforations into the peritoneal cavity leading to generalized peritonitis or localized abscess formation can be catastrophic. The differential diagnosis primarily includes appendicitis, diverticulitis, or perforated gastroduodenal ulcer.

CONTIGUOUS ORGAN INVOLVEMENT

Direct involvement of adjacent organs occurs in about 10% of patients. Extended surgery in such patients is associated with cure rates of 20% to 50%.[310,483,484] The tumor-bearing colon may be adherent due to inflammatory adhesions or it may be attached by direct penetration of tumor. Penetration into an adjacent hollow organ such as bladder or small bowel may lead to a fistula. Almost one half of clinically adherent or invaded viscera are attached by inflammatory adhesions only.[484] All such attachments should be presumed to be due to direct tumor penetration and should not be divided and biopsied. If such attachments are torn inadvertently, the survival, albeit retrospective analysis, is half that associated with direct multivisceral resection.[484,485]

CANCER IN POLYPS

Cancer is present in about 5% of adenomatous polyps.[486] Cancers invasive to the level of the muscularis mucosa do not have access to the lymphatic pathways and can be cured by endoscopic or surgical polypectomy. This section considers the treatment of cancer that is invasive at least through the muscularis mucosa in an otherwise benign adenomatous or villous polyp. The extent of invasion and whether the polyp is pedunculated or sessile must be considered. After endoscopic polypectomy of such lesions, one must address the risk for residual localized or nodal cancer compared with the risk for definitive colectomy.[487] Decision analysis theory can be applied for help with this troublesome problem.[488]

Figure 30–10 defines the various levels of invasion and helps in conceptualizing the problem.[491] In addition to the level of invasion, additional histopathologic data to be taken into account include the degree of differentiation (grade), the presence of lymphatic or blood vessel invasion, and adequacy of endoscopic resection (margin). Patients at high risk for

local residual or nodal metastatic cancer have polyps containing one or several of the following features: poorly differentiated cancer, lymphatic vessel invasion, tumor invasive to level 3 or 4, or a positive or close polypectomy margin.[489–492]

The major issue is the risk for lymph node metastases. Colacchio and colleagues have documented what they believe is an unacceptable risk associated with conservative (nonresective) management of most of these patients.[493] The overall risk for nodal metastases is reported by these authors to be 10%. Nivatvongs looked only at patients who subsequently underwent surgical resection and defined subsets based on polyp configuration and gross extent of invasion.[694] His data and review of the literature provide the most realistic appraisal of the risk for lymph node metastases (Table 30–9). Because about half of the patients with lymph node metastases die from cancer, the incremental survival benefit from surgery for cancer limited to the head of a polyp is only 1.5%.

In summary, polypectomy alone can cure almost all patients with a moderately or well-differentiated cancer limited to the head of a pedunculated adenomatous polyp, with clear margins on the stalk, and no histopathologic evidence of lymphatic vessel invasion.[487] The polypectomy site should be examined endoscopically in 4 to 6 months to confirm the absence of mucosal recurrence.

Not all polyps can be removed endoscopically. Large sessile lesions, particularly of the thin-walled ascending colon, pose a major therapeutic challenge. Large villous tumors have a high likelihood (up to 40%) of containing carcinoma in the polyp. Therefore, limited biopsies are subject to extensive sampling error false-negatives. If endoscopic removal is attempted, piecemeal removal with the snare cautery over several sessions is required. Such patients should be observed as inpatients for 1 to 2 days to rule out a perforation. Large benign sessile adenomas may require surgical resection as the least morbid approach to removal.

ADJUVANT THERAPIES

ADJUVANT RADIATION THERAPY FOR COLON CANCER

Rationale

The rationale of the use of adjuvant radiation therapy in colon cancer is based on the patterns of failure after potentially

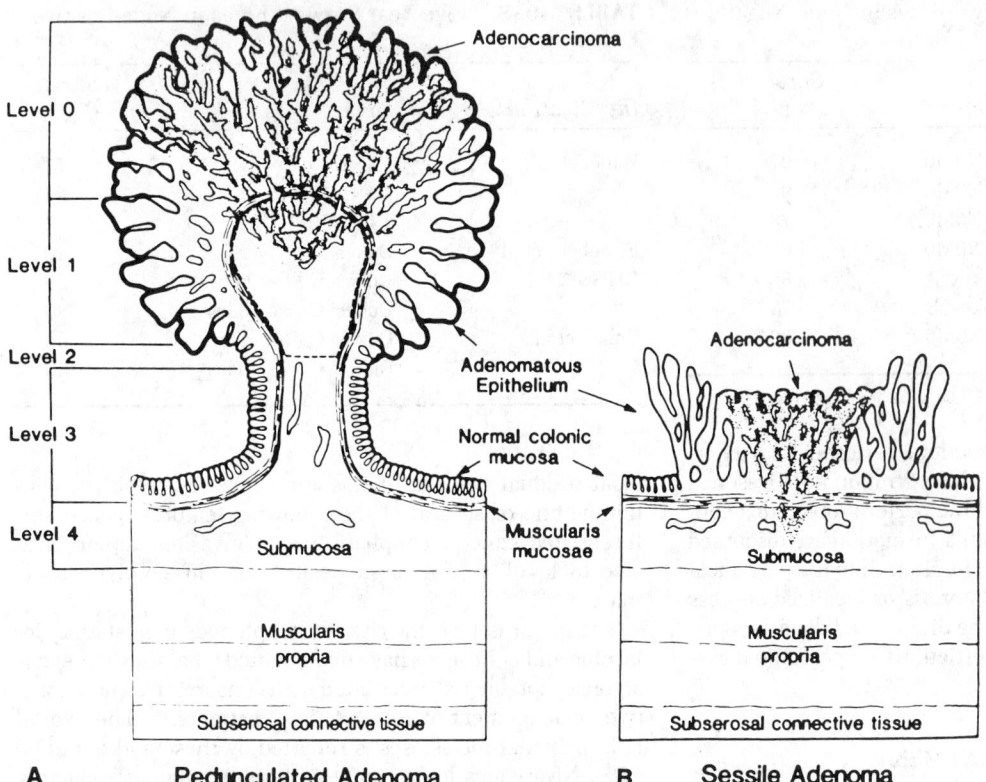

A   Pedunculated Adenoma

B   Sessile Adenoma

FIGURE 30–10. Levels of invasion in a pedunculated adenoma **(A)** and a sessile adenoma **(B)**. The stippled areas represent zones of carcinoma. Any invasion below the muscularis mucosae in a sessile lesion represents level 4 invasion (submucosa). In contrast, invasive carcinoma in a pedunculated adenoma must traverse a considerable distance before it reaches the submucosa of the underlying bowel wall. However, any cancer that penetrates the muscularis mucosae is at risk for dissemination. (Haggitt RC, Glotzbach RE, Soffer EE, et al. Prognostic factors in colorectal carcinomas arising in adenomas: Implications for lesions removed by endoscopic polypectomy. Gastroenterology 1985;89:328–336)

curative surgery. The primary determinant of failure patterns in colorectal cancer is the location of the tumor in reference to the peritoneal reflection. In contrast to tumors located at or below the peritoneal reflection (rectosigmoid and rectum), tumors located above the peritoneal reflection (cecum-sigmoid), have a higher incidence of failure within the abdominal cavity.[225,476,478,494]

Results of Whole Abdominal Radiation

Based on the high incidence of abdominal failure, phase II trials were designed to examine the efficacy of whole abdominal radiation therapy (Table 30–10).[495–498] This discussion is limited to the four trials in which patients were treated in the adjuvant setting. Excluded are the series by Patanaphan and colleagues,[499] which included patients with rectal cancer, and by Ghossein and associates,[497] which included patients with residual disease.

In general, patients received 2000 to 3000 cGy to the whole abdomen with or without a boost to the primary tumor bed. In three of the series, bolus 5-fluorouracil (5-FU) was delivered with a variety of doses and schedules. The combined preliminary results revealed an in-field (abdominal) failure rate of 14% to 50% and a 3-year survival of about 50%. Significant toxicity varied from 5% to 38%. Although the initial phase II results appeared promising, these preliminary data have not been updated and randomized trials are required to confirm any possible benefit.

The use of whole abdominal radiation therapy is limited by dose considerations. To treat the volume at risk with a potentially curative dose of radiation required for microscopic disease, the whole abdomen would need to receive 4500 cGy.

Although limited portions of the abdomen can tolerate this dose, the tolerance of the whole abdomen with conventional fractionation is 3000 cGy. Given the dose limitations of whole abdominal radiation and the randomized data, which reveal a significant impact of systemic chemotherapy on survival, the use of whole abdominal radiation therapy is of limited interest.

Rationale of Local Radiation Therapy

Although the overall incidence of local failure is low in colon cancer, data based on anatomic location and selected pathologic features suggest that there are subsets of patients who have a higher incidence of local failure. There is no agreement as to how to define these subsets. In the Gunderson report, the highest incidence of local failure occurred in the cecum (30%) and the transverse colon had one of the lowest rates of local failure (13%).[494] In contrast, Minsky and colleagues reported a general trend of increased local failure with more distal colon sites.[225] Patients with cecal cancer had a significantly lower incidence of local failure (3%) compared with those with cancer of the transverse (15%) or descending colon (25%). These data do not support the notion that bowel mobility is predictive of local failure.

Results of Local Radiation Therapy

Although all the series in local radiation therapy are retrospective (Table 30–11), the most comprehensive series examining the role of local radiation therapy in colon cancer is from the Massachusetts General Hospital.[500,501] After potentially curative surgery for stages T3N0–2M0 colon cancer,

TABLE 30–9. Cancer in Polyps: Risk for Lymph Node Metastases

Investigations	No. of Resected Patients	No. of Lymph Node Metastases
Sessile Polyps With Invasive Cancer		
Grinnell and Lane[690]		
Waye and Frankel[691]	13	3
	9	1
Wolff and Shinya[486]	5	2
Locke et al[692]	12	4
Kodaira et al[693]	34	2
Nivatvongs[694]	25	3
Percentage of lymph nodes with metastases = 15%		
Pedunculated Polyps With Invasive Cancer		
Grinnell and Lane[690]	39	3
Waye and Frankel[691]	8	0
Wolff and Shinya[486]	11	0
Shatney et al[695]	23	1
Locke et al[692]	15	1
Coutsoftides et al[696]	13	0
Colacchio et al[493]	24	6
Kodaira et al[693]	64	3
Nivatvongs[694]	16	3
Percentage of lymph nodes with metastases = 8%		
Pedunculated Polyps With Invasive Cancer Limited to Head of Polyp		
Grinnell and Lane[690]	28	0
Shatney et al[695]	14	0
Nivatvongs[694]	12	0
Colacchio et al[493]	11	2
Percentage of lymph nodes with metastases = 3%		

(Nivatvongs S. Management of polyps containing invasive carcinoma. In: Codner IJ, Fry RD, Roe JP, eds. Colon, rectal, and anal surgery 1985. St. Louis: CV Mosby, 1985:183–188)

133 patients received postoperative adjuvant local radiation therapy. Eligibility included patients with the following stages: T4N0–2M0 regardless of anatomic site, T3N1–2M0 excluding middle sigmoid and transverse colon, and selected high-risk T3N0M0 tumors with close margins. Patients received 4500 cGy to the primary tumor bed with a 5-cm margin and the primary draining lymph nodes. This was followed by a shrinking-field technique to 5040 to 5500 cGy depending on the volume of small bowel that could be excluded from the high-dose field. Twenty-two patients received bolus 5-FU in a variety of doses and schedules. The 5-year actuarial local control, disease-free survival, and overall survival were 82%, 61%, and 62%, respectively.

The results were compared with 395 historical surgical controls. For the total patient group, patients who received postoperative radiation therapy had a lower incidence of local failure (18% versus 26%). This improvement was limited to those with stages T4N0M0, T3N1–2M0, and T4N1–2M0. Patients with perforation or complete obstruction also had a lower incidence of local failure (16% versus 41%). For the total patient group, there was no impact of radiation therapy on 5-year survival compared with surgery alone (62% versus 58%).

Adjuvant Systemic Therapy of Colon Cancer Single-Agent Studies

As the natural history of colon cancer has been better defined, patient populations at increased risk for metastases after surgery have been identified. Systemic chemotherapy has been administered after primary resection for those with poor prognoses. The first generation of adjuvant trials was initiated in the late 1950s and is outlined in Table 30–12.[314,502–504] These were studies of heterogenous patient groups, often including patients with colon and rectal primaries, patients who had undergone curative and palliative resections, and patients at all Dukes' stages. Moreover, only thiotepa and the fluoropyrimidines, 5-FU and floxuridine (FUDR), were available, and usually they were used with suboptimal intensity.

Despite these flaws in study design and conduct, large patient cohorts were accrued and studied, establishing the clinical and scientific basis for subsequent adjuvant efforts. The

TABLE 30–10. Whole Abdominal Adjuvant Radiation Therapy for Colon Cancer

Investigations	No. of Patients	Stage	Chemotherapy	Dose (cGy)	In-Field Failure* (%)	Survival	Toxicity
Brenner et al[496]	21	T1–4N2	5-FU	2000	14	65% at 5 years (1 patient at risk)	10% SBO
Meek et al[495]	8	T3N0–2	None	3000 + a pelvic boost	50	50% NED at 10–35 months	38% unable to complete treatment
Wong et al[681]	30	T1–4N0–2	7 had 5-FU	1400–2250 ± a 1500–3000 boost	27	55% at 5 years	2% SBO, 5% severe diarrhea
Fabian et al[498]	38	T3N0 T1–4N1–2	5-FU	3000 + a 1600 boost	29	81% at 32 months	31% grade III–IV

In-field failure includes the tumor bed and the peritoneal cavity.
SBO, small bowel obstruction; NED, no evidence of diseease.

TABLE 30–11. Local Adjuvant Radiation Therapy in Colon Cancer

Investigations	Site	Stage	Locoregional Failure				5-Year Survival	
			No. of Patients	Surgery	No. of Patients	Surgery and Radiation Therapy	Surgery	Surgery and Radiation Therapy
Willett et al[500,501]	Colon	T3N0	163	10%	21	10%*	70%	77%
		T4N0	83	31%	37	8%	63%	81%
		T3N1–2	100	35%	47	21%	44%	47%
		T4N1–2	49	53%	28	31%	37%	51%
		Total	395	26%	133	18%	58%	62%
Shehata et al[680]	Cecum	T3N0			12	0%		
		T4N0			10	10%		
		T3N1–2			5	1/5		
		T4N1–2			4	2/4		
		Total			31	13%		
Wong et al[681]	Colon	T3N0				17%		
		T1–3N1–2				32%		
		Total			46	26%		
Loeffler[682]	Cecum	T3–4N0–2			10	0%		

* Actuarial component of total failure.

trials listed in Table 30–12 are conventionally considered negative studies, because dramatic benefits were not elicited. However, the third and fourth Veterans Administration Surgical Oncology Group (VASOG)[505] and the Central Oncology Group (COG)[504] studies demonstrated a 5% to 10% benefit in 5-year survival. For Dukes' C colon cancer, a significant disease-free survival benefit was noted ($p = 0.026$). Forty percent of adjuvantly treated patients had recurrence at 5 years, compared with 52% of patients not given systemic adjuvant treatment.[504] Moreover, an overall analysis of the fluoropyrimidine trials indicated a consistent therapeutic effect, confirmed by statistical pooling methodology.[506,507] Given the available drugs, existing pharmacologic understanding, size of patient groups studied, and dose intensity of therapy offered, it is not surprising that a major therapeutic impact was not observed. Rather, it is surprising that benefits were noted for any of the trials.

Combination Chemotherapy

The second generation of studies focused on combinations of agents and included chemotherapy and immunotherapy. Table 30–13 summarizes seven major trials initiated in the 1970s.[508–514] Six of the seven studies used a surgery-only control (the exception was the ECOG 2276 study). Six studies used a combination of methyl-CCNU and 5-FU with vincristine (MOF) or without (MF) vincristine. Combination chemotherapy—MOF or MF—was presumed to be more active than 5-FU alone in advanced disease. The empiric application of nonspecific immunotherapy with bacillus Calmette-Guérin (BCG), BCG-MER (BCG with methanol extraction residue of BCG), or levamisole was studied. A total of 4500 patients were evaluated in these seven studies. A trend favoring chemotherapy was noted in several studies, but statistically significant benefit was detected only in the NSABP C01 and the

TABLE 30–12. First-Generation Randomized Trials of Adjuvant Therapy for Large Bowel Cancer*

Investigations	Study Period	Treatment Regimen	Total Duration	Accrual
Dixon et al[502]	1957–1960	Thiotepa	2 d	695
Dwight et al[314]	1957–1961	Thiotepa	2 d	1064
Dwight et al[503]	1961–1964	FUDR	7 wk	548
Higgins et al[505]	1965–1969	5-FU	6 wk	308
	1969–1973	5-FU	18 mo	518
Grage and Moss[504]	1971–1976	5-FU	12 mo	233

* All studies had a surgery-only control group.
FUDR, floxuridine; 5-FU, 5-fluorouracil.

TABLE 30–13. Second-Generation Colon Cancer Adjuvant Trials

Investigations	Total Accrual	Chemotherapy	Immunotherapy	Chemoimmunotherapy	Results
VASOG 5[508]	654	5-FU, 9 mg/kg on d 1, + methyl-CCNU, 120 mg/m² on d 1, every 7 wk for 12 cycles			MF results in survival benefit for Dukes C1
GITSG 6175[511]	621	5-FU, 325 mg/m² on d 1–5, 375 mg/m² on d 36–40, + methyl-CCNU, 130 mg/m² on d 1, every 10 wk for 7 cycles	BCG-MER, 1 mg intradermally (ID) on d 1 and 0.5 mg ID once weekly at wk 1, 5, 10, 15, 20, 25, 40, 55, 70	MF + BCG-MER	Apparent overall improved survival compared with historical controls
ECOG 2276[514]	866	5-FU + methyl-CCNU, same as GTSG 6175, for 8 cycles or 5-FU, 450 mg/m²/d × 5 d, every 5 wk for 15 cycles			No significant differences in disease-free overall survival
NSABP C01[509]	1166	MF, same as in GTSG 6175 protocol, + VCR, 1 mg/m² on d 1 every 10 wk for 8 cycles	BCG, 6 × 10⁸ organisms by scarification weekly for 12 wk, then every other week for 33 wk		MOF results in 67% 5-year survival vs 58% for control
SWOG 7510[513]	626	5-FU, 400 mg/m² on d 1, 8, 15, + methyl-CCNU, 175 mg/m² on d 1, every 8 wk for 7 cycles		MF + BCG (6 × 10⁸ organisms po) every other wk for 26 wk	Superior disease-free survival benefit for MF with or without BCG
Cross Cancer Center[512]	253		BCG 120 mg po monthly × 5 yr	BCG + methyl-CCNU 130 mg/m² d 1 + 5-FU 325 mg/m²/d d 1–5 and 375 mg/m²/d d 36–40 for 8 cycles	No survival advantage for either treatment compared with untreated control
NCCTG 78-48-52[510]	398		Levamisole, 150 mg d 1, 2, 3, every 3 wk	Levamisole + 5-FU, 450 mg/m², weekly for 52 wk	5-FU with or without levamisole results in superior disease-free survival

MF, methyl-CCNU + 5-FU; VCR, vincristine; BCG, bacillus Calmette-Guérin; MER, methanol extraction residue of BCG; VASOG, Veterans Administration Surgical Oncology Group; GITSG, Gastrointestinal Tumor Study Group; ECOG, Eastern Cooperative Oncology Group; NSABP, National Surgical Adjuvant Breast and Bowel Project; SWOG, Southwest Oncology Group; NCCTG, North Central Cancer Treatment Group.

North Central Cancer Treatment Group (NCCTG 78-48-52) studies.

In the NSABP C01 study, conducted from 1977 to 1983, 1166 patients were randomly assigned to observation, chemotherapy, or immunotherapy. There was a statistically significant superiority in disease-free ($p = 0.02$) and overall survival ($p = 0.05$) for the MOF chemotherapy group compared with the control group. A patient who did not receive adjuvant chemotherapy had a 1.31 greater likelihood of dying than the counterpart who did, and an 8% survival improvement at the initial analysis.[509] Patients with right-sided colon tumors appeared to derive the most salutary benefits. Although a disease-free survival advantage was not demonstrated for BCG compared with control, an overall survival advantage was demonstrated (67% versus 59%; $p = 0.03$). Further analysis revealed that cardiovascular deaths in the BCG group were about half of those in the untreated control group. When overall survival was reassessed by excluding non–cancer-related deaths, there were no longer statistically significant differences between the control and BCG groups. This was the first prospective, randomized clinical trial to demonstrate a benefit in disease-free and overall survival for chemotherapy. With further follow-up the disease-free survival advantage has persisted, although the benefit in overall survival is of only borderline significance. Furthermore, the toxicity of this study included 5 patients randomized to receive MOF who developed myelodysplasia or acute leukemia. Overall, 19 of 2067 patients receiving methyl-CCNU in randomized trials developed myelodysplasia or acute leukemia at an estimated risk of 2.3 persons per 1000 persons per year.[515]

Levamisole Studies

Levamisole is a synthetic phenylimidothiazole that has been in use for many years as an antihelminthic agent. Interest in the use of levamisole in cancer therapy developed after the observation that it enhanced the immune response of mice vaccinated against *Brucella* bacteria. Subsequent studies have demonstrated that levamisole has a broad range of immunomodulatory properties including enhancement of specific immune responses in normal hosts and restoration of immunity in immune-deficient hosts.[516]

Levamisole has been evaluated alone and in combination with 5-FU as therapy for advanced colorectal cancer and as adjuvant therapy (Tables 30–14 and 30–15). Three randomized clinical trials involving more than 400 patients have evaluated the addition of levamisole to 5-FU chemotherapy for patients with metastatic disease. None of these studies demonstrated any improvement in response rate, time to progression, or survival in favor of the levamisole-containing treatment arms.[517–519]

The first study of single agent levamisole used as adjuvant therapy was initiated by Verhaegen in 1974.[520] Sixty patients were selected to receive levamisole or no further therapy after resection of Dukes' A, B, or C colon and rectal cancer. Five-year overall survival was 69% for patients receiving levamisole compared with 37% for patients in the control group. The greatest differences were noted for patients with Dukes' B2 and C colon cancer. Although this was a nonrandomized study in a few patients, the positive results stimulated further studies of levamisole used as adjuvant therapy. Two prospective, randomized, placebo-controlled trials have been completed and have failed to demonstrate a survival advantage for treatment with levamisole (Table 30–14).[521,522]

Based largely on the positive results reported by Verhaegen and colleagues,[520] several studies were performed in which levamisole was combined with 5-FU-based chemotherapy (see Table 30–15). Sertoli and colleagues randomly assigned 29 patients with Dukes' stage C colon cancer to receive methyl-CCNU and 5-FU with or without levamisole.[523] No benefit for levamisole was demonstrable during 8 years of follow-up. Bancewicz and colleagues compared oral 5-FU, oral 5-FU and levamisole, and no further treatment after surgery and failed to demonstrate any advantage for either treatment during a short period of follow-up.[524] Windle and colleagues randomized 131 patients with colon or rectal cancer to no further therapy, 5-FU alone, or the combination of 5-FU and levamisole.[525] In this study, 5-FU was administered intravenously on postoperative days 1 to 3 then orally for 6 months. Levamisole was given as 150 mg orally on postoperative days 1, 2, and 3. With a minimum follow-up of 5 years, the combined 5-FU and levamisole arm demonstrated a significant superiority to 5-FU alone in overall survival.

The most striking data on adjuvant chemotherapy with 5-FU and levamisole come from two recently reported studies. In 1989, the NCCTG and Mayo Clinic reported the results of a randomized study comparing levamisole alone to the combination of levamisole and 5-FU to no further therapy after surgery.[510] A total of 401 eligible patients were randomized, of which 21 had primary rectal cancer and the remainder colon cancer; 43% of patients had tumors invading through the bowel wall with spread to regional lymph nodes. With median follow-up in excess of 7 years, the levamisole and 5-FU combination demonstrated a significant improvement in disease-free survival compared with no further therapy (log rank, $p = 0.02$; Cox model, $p = 0.003$). Overall there was no improvement in survival. Subset analysis by stage demonstrated a significant disease-free survival advantage for 5-FU plus levamisole only in stage C patients. In this group, levamisole alone produced a modest disease-free survival advantage that did not reach statistical significance. The study did not reveal any treatment benefits for patients with stage B2 or B3 colon cancer. The results of this study were considered sufficiently promising to warrant a confirmatory national Intergroup study with participation by the NCCTG, the Eastern Cooperative Oncology Group, and the Southwest Oncology Group. This study differed from the NCCTG trial only in that patients with rectal cancer were excluded and those with stage B2 disease were randomized to observation only or to 5-FU and levamisole. The study was reported after enrollment of

TABLE 30–14. Adjuvant Studies of Single Agent Levamisole

Investigations	No. of Patients	Dukes' Stage	Treatment	Results
Verhaegen et al[520]	60	A–C	a) Levamisole 50 mg po tid ×3 d q 2wk × 2 y b) No further treatment	5-y survival 69% 5-yr survival 37% ($p = 0.028$)
Chlebowski et al[521]	78	B and C	a) Levamisole 30 mg/m² tid d 1–2 q wk × 18 mo b) Placebo	7-y survival B, 84% C, 46% B, 70%; C, 55%
Arnaud et al[522]	289	C	a) 100–250 mg d 1–2 q wk × 1 y b) Placebo	5-y survival 51% 5-y survival 39%

TABLE 30–15. Adjuvant Studies of Levamisole Plus 5-Fluorouracil

Investigations	No. of Patients	Dukes Stage	5-FU*	Levamisole	Survival	
Sertoli et al[523]	29	C	a) 325 mg/m²/d × 5 q 5 wk plus methyl-CCNU 150 mg/m² q 10 wk × 14 cycles	150 mg po × 3 d, wk 2 and 4 q 10 wk	8-y DFS 8-y OS	39% 60%
			b) As above	None	8-y DFS 8-y OS	50% 50%
Bancewicz et al[524]	52	B and C	a) None	200 mg po d 1–2 q wk × 1 y	2-y DFS 2-y OS	75% 81%
			b) 440 mg/m²/d × 5 d po q 4 wk	As above	2-y DFS 2-y OS	70% 76%
			c) None	None	2-y DFS 2-y OS	84% 89%
Windle et al[525]	131	B and C	a) 1000 mg d 1–3 then 1000 mg po q wk × 6 mo	50 mg tid po d 1–3	5-y OS ($p = 0.022$ and 0.046 vs B and C)	68%
			b) As above	None	5-y OS	48%
			c) None	None	5-y OS	56%
Laurie et al[510]	401	B and C	a) 450 mg/m²/d × 5 then q wk	50 mg tid p d 1–3 qow × 1 y	5-y DFS 5-y OS	60% 64%
			b) None	As above	5-y DFS 5-y OS	60% 60%
			c) None	None	5-y DFS 5-y OS	50% 58%
Moertel et al[526]	929	C	a) 450 mg/m²/d × 5 then q wk	50 mg tid p d 1–3 qow × 1 y	3-y DFS 3-y OS	63% 71%
			b) None	As above	3-y DFS 3-y OS	54% 65%
			c) None	None	3-y DFS 3-y OS	47% 55%

DFS, disease-free survival; OS, overall survival; po, by mouth; qow, every other week.
* Administered by intravenous push except when marked po.

1296 patients (929 stage C) and a median follow-up time of 3 years.[526] For stage C patients, levamisole alone produced no effect on recurrence rate or overall survival. The combination of levamisole and 5-FU resulted in a statistically significant reduction in tumor recurrence (disease-free survival 63% versus 47% for surgery only) and improved survival (3-year overall survival of 71% versus 55% for surgery only). The estimated reduction in death rate for 5-FU plus levamisole was 33% (95% confidence interval of 10–50%) compared with no further therapy. Of 318 patients with stage B2 cancer enrolled in the study, only 54 had recurrences and only 29 had died at the time of the initial report. At a median follow-up of 5 years in the Dukes' C study, a one-third reduction in cancer mortality can still be demonstrated.[526a]

Toxic effects attributable to the combination of 5-FU and levamisole are generally mild and reversible. Leukopenia, nausea, diarrhea, and stomatitis occur most commonly. Toxicities attributed primarily to levamisole have included nausea, diarrhea, dermatitis, metallic taste, fatigue, arthralgias, fever, seizures, tremors, agitation, and confusion.

The National Cancer Institute Consensus Development Conference convened in April 1990 recommended that stage C patients unable to participate in a clinical trial be offered adjuvant 5-FU and levamisole. However, many questions remain unanswered. The precise contribution of levamisole to the benefit observed in the NCCTG and Intergroup studies is difficult to determine. As a single agent, levamisole appears to have little utility in treatment of advanced colorectal cancer or as adjuvant therapy. In vitro, levamisole has no direct cytotoxic effects nor does it enhance 5-FU cytotoxicity at clinically achievable concentrations.[527] There are no data that levamisole, used in the doses and schedules in the NCCTG and Intergroup studies, produces immunomodulatory effects in humans. Whether the drug possesses biochemical or molecular effects remains to be determined.

Perhaps the greatest contribution of the NCCTG and Intergroup studies has been to stimulate additional clinical trials to evaluate adjuvant chemotherapy for colon cancer. Table 30–16 summarizes recently completed or ongoing studies for patients with stage B2 and C colon cancer. Accrual has been completed in NSABP studies CO3 and CO4 and the initial presentation of these results is eagerly awaited. The ongoing

TABLE 30–16. Ongoing or Recently Completed Adjuvant Colon Cancer Trials*

Investigations	Stage	Study Design
Recently Completed Studies		
NSABP CO3	B2, C	MOF vs 5-FU/LV
NSABP CO4	B2, C	5-FU/LV vs 5-FU/Lev vs 5-FU/LV/Lev
Ongoing Studies		
NCCTG 894641	B2, C	5-FU/Lev × 1 y vs 5-FU/Lev × 6 mo vs 5-FU/LV/Lev × 1 y vs 5-FU/LV/Lev × 6 mo
INT 0089 vs	B2, C	5-FU/Lev vs 5-FU/LV(hi) vs FU/LV/Lev vs 5-FU/LV(lo) vs 5-FU
NSABP CO5	B2, C	5-FU/LV vs 5-FU/LV/IFN
MAOP 5186A	C	5-FU/Lev vs infusional 5-FU/Lev
EST 1290	C	5-FU/Lev vs autologous vaccine + 5-FU
EST 5283	B2	Observation vs autologous vaccine
NCIC CO3	B2	Observation vs 5-FU/LV

* (p = 0.05) than 5-FU arm.
MOF, 5-FU + methyl-CCNU + vincristine; 5-FU, 5-fluorouracil; Lev, levamisole; LV, leucovorin; lo, low dose; hi, high dose LV.

Intergroup and NCCTG studies are evaluating the addition of leucovorin to combination 5-FU and levamisole, whereas the recently activated NSABP CO5 study seeks to determine the benefit of adding interferon to combination 5-FU and leucovorin. Another strategy being pursued is the use of autologous tumor vaccines. Between 1981 and 1988, Hoover and colleagues randomized 80 patients with stage B2 or C colorectal cancer to receive autologous tumor vaccine or no further therapy.[528] Autologous vaccine was administered as an intradermal injection weekly for 3 consecutive weeks. With a median follow-up of 68 months, there was a 75% reduction in the risk for recurrence in the treated arm compared with the control arm (p = 0.016). Although this approach is worthy of further study, the difficulty in harvesting adequate amounts of viable tissue for vaccine preparation has limited accrual to the ongoing randomized studies.

There has never before been so much documentation to support the contention that adjuvant systemic therapy is of value for Dukes' B and C colon cancer patients. It is not possible to specify precisely which regimen is optimal for each patient subgroup at this time. Nonetheless, the current generation of national trials presents an ideal opportunity to confirm the magnitude and character of the impact of adjuvant therapy, and patients and physicians should be encouraged to participate.

ADJUVANT PORTAL VEIN CHEMOTHERAPY

The rationale for adjuvant perioperative infusion of chemotherapy into the portal vein is based on the observation that cells embolize the portal venous system preoperatively and intraoperatively, seeding the liver.[302,529] Studies of portal vein infusion chemotherapy are summarized in Table 30–17. In 1955, Fisher and Turnbull demonstrated tumor cells in the portal circulation in 32% of patients at the time of colon carcinoma resection.[530] There is considerable clinical and autopsy evidence that the liver may be the most frequent and sometimes the only site of metastasis.[302,529] Although established metastases are fed primarily by the hepatic artery, micrometastases are still likely to depend on the portal venous blood.

In 1975, Taylor and colleagues began a randomized study of intraportal 5-FU using 1 g/day, with 5000 U heparin, infused continuously for 7 days immediately postoperatively for patients with Dukes' A, B, and C lesions. About 250 patients were studied; by 1985, with a median follow-up of greater

TABLE 30–17. Portal Vein Infusion Chemotherapy

Investigations	Patients	Treatment	No. of Patients	Decrease in Liver Metastases	Improved Survival
Taylor et al[531]	Dukes' A, B, and C, colon and rectal	5-FU/heparin vs control	127 117	Yes	Yes
Australia-New Zealand[532]	Dukes' B and C	5-FU (IP) vs 5-FU (I.V.) vs control	Total of 372	—	Yes
Dutch[535]	Dukes' A, B, and C, colon and rectal	5-FU/heparin vs urokinase vs control	99 103 102	Yes	No
SAKK5[533,534]	Dukes' A, B, and C colon and rectal	5-FU/mitomycin/ heparin vs control	236 233	No	Yes
NCCTG[536]	Dukes' B2 and C, colon and rectal	5-FU/heparin vs control	110 109	No	No
NSABP CO2[537]	Dukes' A, B, and C, colon	5-FU/heparin vs control	442 459	No	No

5-FU, 5-fluorouracil; I.V., intravenous; IP, intraportal.

than 50 months, 80 deaths had occurred. Patients with Dukes' B colon cancer and Dukes' C rectal cancer appeared to have a substantial survival benefit ($p = 0.002$ and 0.006 respectively) with intraportal venous 5-FU.[531] This preliminary study stimulated several randomized trials of similar design.

The Australia and New Zealand Trial evaluated 372 patients with colon cancer randomly allocated to observation alone or to immediate postoperative chemotherapy with 5-FU, 600 mg/m²/day for 7 days given intravenously or intraportally. Compared with the other two groups, portal vein 5-FU infusion resulted in a highly significant superior disease-free and overall survival in Dukes' C patients.[532] These data are not fully mature and require further follow-up to determine the magnitude and duration of benefits.

A second study of similar design was conducted by the Swiss Group for Clinical Cancer Research.[533,534] From 1981 to 1986, 469 eligible patients who had undergone resection for Dukes' A, B, or C lesions were randomly allocated to a control or to a chemotherapy group. The chemotherapy group received immediate postoperative intraportal 5-FU of 500 mg/m²/day, with 5000 U heparin, given by continuous infusion for 7 days. On the first day of therapy, a 10 mg/m² bolus of mitomycin C was also administered. After a median follow-up of 42 months, recurrences were detected in 36% of control patients, compared with 29% of infused patients ($p = 0.08$). The estimated 5-year survival rate was 71% for treated patients compared with 57% for untreated controls ($p = 0.03$). However, too few deaths have occurred in this trial to allow definitive conclusions regarding differences in survival, and further follow-up is required. An ongoing study by the Swiss group is comparing surgery alone, perioperative portal vein infusion of 5-FU and mitomycin, and systemic 5-FU and mitomycin to confirm their results and evaluate the importance of route of chemotherapy administration.

Wereldsma and colleagues have reported the results of a multiinstitutional Dutch study comparing portal vein infusion of 5-FU and heparin as administered by Taylor to portal vein infusion of urokinase (10,000 U over 24 hours) and to no further therapy.[535] Three hundred and seventeen patients were randomized intraoperatively. With a median follow-up of 44 months, a significant decrease in liver metastases was demonstrated in the patients receiving 5-FU with heparin (7% versus 23% in controls; $p = 0.01$). However, there was no improvement in overall survival after intraportal treatment.

Two recently reported randomized trials conducted in the United States evaluated perioperative portal venous infusion of 5-FU. The Mayo Clinic/NCCTG trial randomly assigned 219 patients with Dukes' B2 or C colorectal cancer to no further therapy after surgery or to receive portal vein infusion of 5-FU 500 mg/m²/day with 5000 U of heparin per day for 7 days.[536] Randomization was performed intraoperatively based on surgical findings and frozen-section pathology. With a median follow-up of 5.5 years, the incidence of hepatic metastases and estimated 5-year survival were essentially identical in the two arms of the study.

The largest randomized study conducted was reported by the NSABP in 1990.[537] Between 1984 and 1988, 1158 patients with Dukes' A, B, or C colon cancer were randomized to either no further treatment after surgery or to postoperative portal vein infusion of 5-FU 600 mg/m²/day with heparin 5000 U/day for 7 days. Randomization was conducted preoperatively;

almost 23% of patients were later declared ineligible, primarily due to documentation of metastatic disease at surgery. A total of 901 eligible patients were analyzed. A comparison between the two groups at 4 years revealed an improvement in disease-free survival (74% versus 64%; $p = 0.02$) and a trend toward improved survival (81% versus 73%; $p = 0.07$) in favor of the group receiving chemotherapy. However, there was no reduction in the incidence of liver metastases in the chemotherapy-treated group compared with the control group. The failure of portal vein infusion of chemotherapy to reduce the incidence of liver metastases while producing a modest survival advantage was attributed to a direct systemic effect of chemotherapy.

The use of portal vein infusion of chemotherapy in the immediate postoperative recovery period is attractive because of its convenience, modest toxicity, and relative lack of added expense. However, the clinical results are equivocal. Most studies have included small numbers of patients and heterogenous patient populations. Conflicting results have been reported, and the failure to demonstrate a consistent reduction in the incidence of liver metastases suggests that any benefit derived from this treatment approach is due to the systemic effects of chemotherapy.

SUMMARY OF ADJUVANT TREATMENT FOR COLON CANCER

Less than 1% of all patients with colorectal cancer are entered into randomized trials. To further define benefits of adjuvant treatment, patient participation in randomized trials is strongly encouraged. Recently completed clinical trials have demonstrated a survival benefit for Dukes' C patients treated with adjuvant 5-FU and levamisole. Ongoing studies will further define the optimal chemotherapy program for high-risk patients.

TREATMENT OF INITIALLY ADVANCED COLON CANCER

SYNCHRONOUS METASTATIC CANCER

About 10% to 15% of patients with primary colon cancers present with synchronous metastatic cancer. The treatment of patients with synchronous liver metastases is discussed in the section on treatment of recurrent and metastatic cancer. The operative finding of peritoneal seeding or extensive unresectable intraabdominal nodal metastases beyond the central nodal drainage should not deter surgical resection. An extended surgical lymphadenectomy in selected younger patients may be curative in a small subset despite gross involvement of high nodes, albeit probably at most in 10% to 15%.

LOCALLY UNRESECTABLE COLON CANCER

Tumors may be unresectable for cure whether or not distant metastases are present. Extensive direct extension into the retroperitoneum, pelvic sidewall, or duodenum or pancreas may be found. In the presence of concomitant metastatic disease, a bypass enterotoenterostomy is usually appropriate. In the absence of distant disease in otherwise healthy patients, an aggressive local surgical approach to these "unresectable" tumors should be taken.

FOLLOW-UP AFTER POTENTIALLY CURATIVE THERAPY

The goals of a follow-up strategy are to detect recurrent cancer at a potentially curable stage, to detect new primary colorectal neoplasia, to detect other cancers, to manage postoperative digestive and other symptoms, and to provide psychological benefit to the patient. An interval history and physical examination are straightforward. Colonoscopy is appropriate every year for several years, then every 2 to 3 years if adenomas have not been found. Breast examination, mammography, and pelvic examinations in women are appropriate. Although perhaps not cost-effective,[538] serial CEA assays detect asymptomatic recurrent cancer in many patients, particularly in those with hepatic metastases. Despite the absence of a clear benefit, we recommend postoperative serial assays every 2 to 4 months for 3 years in patients who are otherwise candidates for aggressive evaluation if the assay becomes elevated. Yearly chest x-ray films are reasonable. Routine CT scans in the general colon cancer patient population probably are not appropriate outside of clinical studies. Guidelines are listed in Table 30–18.

TREATMENT OF RECURRENT OR METASTATIC CANCER

TREATMENT INITIATED ON THE BASIS OF CEA ASSAY

Postoperative serial serum carcinoembryonic antigen levels may become elevated in an asymptomatic patient. After tran-sient CEA elevations, benign disorders, and laboratory error have been ruled out, most asymptomatic patients fall into one of three groups: they have a new primary cancer; they have a recurrent colorectal cancer, which can be ascertained by a more complete history, physical examination, or a panoply of tests and scans; or they have an entirely negative evaluation. This section discusses the management of the latter group.

Options in managing asymptomatic patients with elevated CEA levels and negative evaluations include continued observation and repeat examinations and tests, chemotherapy, and surgical exploration (second look surgery).

CHEMOTHERAPY

Because of the relative inefficacy of systemic chemotherapy, it is difficult to use this modality in asymptomatic patients without some way to monitor response to treatment. In a randomized trial of 5-FU and methyl-CCNU, a survival benefit could not be demonstrated in patients receiving early cytotoxic therapy rather than continued observation.[539]

SURGERY

In analyzing data relative to the usefulness of CEA-directed second look surgery, several issues are important (Table 30–19).

Sites Most Amenable to Curative Resection

In the various studies of CEA-directed second look operations, the term *curative resection* is used. This term is applied loosely to tumors amenable to complete surgical resection. It is unlikely that resection of paraaortic nodes, omental tumor, or other peritoneal nodules is truly curative. However, selected liver and lung metastases and some locally recurrent cancer may be resected for cure in a subset of patients.

TABLE 30–18. General Guidelines for Follow-up of Patients After Potentially Curative Surgery

Procedure/Test	Frequency	Comment
History/examination	Every 3–4 mo for 3 y then every 6 mo for 2 y	Detects one third of recurrences
Fecal occult blood	Same	
Sigmoidoscopy	Same	Only if anastomosis in pelvis
Colonoscopy	Preoperatively or 4–6 mo postoperatively, then every 6–36 mo	Every 3 years after free of polyps
Chest x-ray film	Yearly	
CEA	Every 2–4 mo for 3 y, then every 6 mo for 2 y	
Liver chemistries Chest CT scan Abdominal CT scan Pelvic CT scan Liver-spleen scan Liver US Bone scan	As indicated by findings on history, examination, or elevated CEA levels	

CEA, serum carcinoembryonic antigen; CT, computed tomography; US, ultrasound.

TABLE 30–19. Carcinoembryonic Antigen (CEA)-Initiated Second Look Surgery Issues

Is overall survival, as well as symptom-free survival, prolonged compared with that achieved with regular interval history and physical examination?

Optimal CEA assay frequency

Optimal definition of abnormal CEA

Optimal timing of second look surgery in patients with elevated CEA levels and negative evaluation for recurrent cancer

Value of adjuvant chemotherapy after second look surgery

Cost-benefit analysis

NEGATIVE EXPLORATION. Most groups have documented tumor recurrence in more than 90% of patients selected for second look surgery. At Ohio State University, tumor was confirmed in 139 of 146 surgical explorations.[540-542] The Memorial Sloan-Kettering group found recurrence in 33 of 37 patients explored.[543] Staab and associates reported tumor confirmation in 29 of 32 patients.[544] Most patients in whom surgical exploration is negative will ultimately develop clinical signs of recurrent cancer.

SURGICAL RESECTIONS. There has been great variability in the reports of second look operations in regard to the frequency of potentially curative resections. In a series of four reports from the Ohio State University group, a total of 146 patients underwent resection with curative intent.[540-542,545] Their resectability rate of 60% was ascribed to a policy of frequent CEA determinations (every 4–6 weeks) and early operation with CEA values less than 10 ng/ml. At Memorial Sloan–Kettering, 43% of patients had resectable tumors.[543] However, Steele and colleagues at Harvard University could resect only 27% of tumors,[546] Wilking and colleagues at Roswell Park Memorial Cancer Institute only 15%,[547] and Staab and colleagues in the Federal Republic of Germany only 12%.[544]

CURES. Despite considerable variability in long-term survival data, some patients who undergo second look operation based on CEA assay results have tumor resected and are alive and free of cancer at 5 years. Most reports refer to actuarial 5-year survival rates. However, in a recent publication from the Ohio State University group, the 5-year survival in the 45 patients who underwent curative resection and were at risk for 5 years was 31%.[540]

COST. The cost of CEA follow-up programs is considerable. When the expense of the assays, additional laboratory tests and scans, and exploratory surgery is tabulated, such programs cost $25,000 per patient found to have resectable cancer.[548] Actual costs are most likely far greater.[538]

OVERALL IMPACT ON SURVIVAL. August and colleagues have analyzed colorectal cancer from the perspective of the potential for surgical cure of recurrent cancer.[549] They estimate that 15% of patients have isolated local recurrence, with a cure rate of 20%. This results in a 3% incremental survival. About 25% of patients appear to have isolated hepatic metastases, with one fourth of these appropriate for resection.

With a 30% cure rate after liver resection, the overall incremental survival is an additional 2%. Therefore, it is likely that surgery, based on clinical criteria or on a CEA blood test, can improve overall survival only by 5% (3% and 2%, respectively) of the entire patient population undergoing potentially curative resection of colorectal cancer.

CURRENT STUDIES

The National Institutes of Health and the Medical Research Council are sponsoring a large cooperative trial in the United Kingdom to answer the following question: Does monthly CEA monitoring, added to quarterly routine histories and physical examinations, actually reduce the morbidity and mortality of colorectal cancer?[550] After resection of B2 or C colon or rectal cancer, patients undergo monthly CEA assays. The results of the tests are unknown to the patient and the physician. If recurrence is detected because of symptoms or physical examination, appropriate treatment is instituted. If the patient remains asymptomatic but has a rising CEA level (more than 10 ng/ml), the patient is randomized. In the standard follow-up arm, the physician and patient are not notified. In the intensive follow-up arm, the physician is notified, additional tests and scans are obtained, and second-look surgery is performed, if appropriate, based on the complete evaluation. At this time, no groups are studying the issue of the optimal timing of second look surgery in asymptomatic patients with a negative evaluation. Because most patients have no benefit from these explorations, a strategy of delayed surgery until tumor is detectable on a radiograph, scan, or examination or until symptoms develop may maximize symptom-free survival for the entire group.

One approach to focusing second-look surgery despite normal routine radiographs and scans is the use of isotope-labeled monoclonal antibodies to define recurrent tumor, with external scanning and with intraoperative γ detection. Iodine 131, iodine 125 and indium 111 isotopes with CEA antibody and monoclonal B72.3 have been studied.[551-557] The exact usefulness of these techniques is not known.

CHEMOTHERAPY FOR METASTATIC COLORECTAL CANCER

Single-Agent Chemotherapy

FLUOROPYRIMIDINES. The fluoropyrimidines remain the most widely used single chemotherapeutic agents for patients with colorectal cancer. Since the introduction of 5-FU in 1957,[558] tens of thousands of patients have been treated, and objective response rates of 8% to 85% have been reported.[559,560] The reasons for the wide range of response rates include various patient selection factors, such as performance status and comorbid conditions; disease factors, such as sites of metastases and previous therapy; and treatment-related factors. A particularly important treatment-related variable seems to be the intensity of 5-FU administration. Moertel found a 9% response rate for 5-FU therapy that induced no leukopenia, compared with a 23% response rate for 5-FU therapy that reduced the white blood cell count to between 1500 and 4500 cells/μL.[561] The Central Oncology Group compared four programs with different schedules, routes, and intensities of 5-FU.[562] They found that intravenous 5-FU, 12 mg/kg/day for 5 days, followed by 6 mg/kg every other day for 11 days, followed by 15 mg/kg/week resulted in a superior response rate (35%) and response duration ($p < 0.001$). Associated with this benefit was a higher incidence of drug toxicity, with 18% of patients experiencing severe or life-threatening leukopenia. This loading course schedule of 5-FU did not result in a significantly longer survival. It has been asserted that an objective response rate of about 20% is generally achievable with fluoropyrimidines.[559,561] Overall, 5-FU does not demonstrably affect survival for all patients treated; it is associated with a median survival of 6 or 8 months. For the few patients who have an objective response, the median survival may be in the 12- to 18-month range.[560] If 5-FU is administered with proper vigor, most patients experience mucositis, diarrhea, or leukopenia as dose-limiting effects of therapy.[560,563] Even after three decades of use, no single schedule or dose scheme has been shown to be ideal, but administration with proper intensity (to the point of definite but acceptable toxic effects) is appropriate.

Attempts to improve the therapeutic benefit of 5-FU have included modifications of route and schedule. Administering 5-FU by the oral rather than parenteral route has been abandoned because of erratic gastrointestinal absorption and poor response rates.[563–566] However, the use of prolonged or nearly continuous intravenous infusions of 5-FU has gained popularity. The advantages of ambulatory infusion 5-FU given over several days to months include the ability to deliver a higher dose per unit of time and the lack of myelotoxicity.[567–569]

CONTINUOUS INFUSION. For continuous intravenous infusion to be practical and economically feasible, dependable and affordable infusion devices were developed. The pump technology makes these devices easily available. Lokich and colleagues have demonstrated that for 5-FU the major toxic effect of 300 mg/m²/day given by continuous intravenous infusion for weeks to months is mucositis;[570] an additional 5% to 25% of patients experience a hand-foot syndrome of painful erythroderma.[571] The relative lack of hematologic toxicity makes this regimen attractive for combinations with myelotoxic drugs. Response rates ranging from 25% to 50% have been reported,[572–577] and some comparative studies suggest that infusion is more efficacious than bolus therapy. The Mid-Atlantic Oncology Program recently reported the results of a prospective randomized comparison of continuous infusion 5-FU with administration of the drug by intravenous bolus injection.[578] One hundred seventy-nine previously untreated patients with advanced, measurable colorectal cancer were randomly assigned to receive 5-FU by continuous venous infusion at 300 mg/m²/day or to receive 5-FU 500 mg/m²/day by bolus administration for 5 consecutive days every 5 weeks. The objective tumor response rate was 30% for those receiving infusional 5-FU compared with 7% ($p < 0.001$) for those receiving bolus 5-FU. Overall survival for the two groups was virtually identical. A similar study performed by the National Cancer Institute of Canada failed to demonstrate a survival advantage for infusional compared with bolus administration of 5-FU.[579] The major toxic effect in patients receiving intravenous bolus 5-FU is leukopenia, whereas hand-foot syndrome and mucositis occur most commonly in patients receiving 5-FU by infusion. The 30% response rate observed for infusional

5-FU is comparable to that found with the use of several biochemical modulation strategies, raising the possibility that the efficacy of infusional 5-FU might be enhanced further by the addition of leucovorin or other agents. Indeed, a 50% objective response rate has been reported recently in 42 patients with measurable colorectal cancer and no previous chemotherapy treated with continuous infusion 5-FU at 200 mg/m²/day for 7 days with a weekly intravenous bolus dose of leucovorin at 20 mg/m².[580] Treatment was administered for 3 consecutive weeks followed by 1 week of rest. The primary toxic effects were gastrointestinal and skin toxicities. This promising regimen currently is being compared with other combined 5-FU and leucovorin regimens in a phase III trial being conducted by the Southwest Oncology Group.

HEPATIC ARTERY INFUSION. Another special mode of administration of fluoropyrimidines is hepatic intraarterial therapy for patients with liver metastases. Because of the favorable pharmacodynamics of floxuridine (FUDR), there is high hepatic extraction and drug concentration with little systemic exposure. Moreover, preliminary phase II studies with continuous intrahepatic arterial infusion of FUDR at 0.2 to 0.4 mg/kg/day for 14 days out of 28 have reported objective response rates ranging from 30% to as high as 80%.[581–585] To confirm these findings, five randomized studies have been completed comparing intravenous with intraarterial FUDR or 5-FU (Table 30–20).[586–590] All of these trials have demonstrated significantly higher response rates (40–60%) for intrarterial therapy compared with systemic drug administration (10–20%), but none have revealed substantial survival benefits for intraarterial therapy. Toxicity of intraarterial treatment can be significant and include chemical hepatitis, biliary sclerosis, catheter thrombosis, and duodenal ulceration and hemorrhage.[591–596] Hepatic artery infusion chemotherapy should remain an investigational treatment program. The high regional response rate suggests that further study of this technique in combination with more effective systemic therapy should be considered.

OTHER AGENTS. Historically, the next most important family of compounds for colorectal cancer patients has been the nitrosoureas. Response rates of 10% to 15% have been reported for BCNU, CCNU, chlorozotocin, and methyl-CCNU.[559,597,598] Because of the convenience of oral administration and of single-agent activity equivalent to 5-FU demonstrated in one randomized trial, methyl-CCNU probably has been used the most frequently.[597] There are no firm data to support the contention of superiority for any particular nitrosourea.[599] The chlorethyl nitrosoureas have characteristic delayed and cumulative toxic effects on bone marrow, which often limit the ability to administer therapy for prolonged periods. In addition, patients receiving methyl-CCNU are at greater risk for myelodysplasia, preleukemia, and acute nonlymphatic leukemia. For 2067 patients retrospectively evaluated, the relative risk for such a hematologic syndrome was estimated to be 12.4 times greater than in those treated with other forms of chemotherapy. The chance of a leukemic syndrome was greater for those receiving higher total doses and living for a longer time. Patients receiving large total doses of methyl-CCNU as part of an adjuvant program are at the

TABLE 30–20. Hepatic Intraarterial Fluoropyrimidine Therapy for Liver Metastases in Colorectal Cancer

Investigations	Drug	Mode	No. of Patients	Dose	Objective Response Rate (%)	Survival (mo)
Kemeny et al[589]	FUDR	I.V.	51	0.125 mg/kg/d × 14 d q 28 d	20	12
		IA	48	0.3 mg/kg/d × 14 d q 28 d	50	17
Hohn et al[587]	FUDR	I.V.	72	0.075 mg/kg/d × 14 d q 28 d	10	16.1
		IA	64	0.20 mg/kg/d × 14 d q 28 d	42	16.7
Chang et al[586]	FUDR	I.V.	32	0.125 mg/kg/d × 14 d q 28 d	17	12
		IA	32	0.3 mg/kg/d × 14 d q 28 d	62	17
Martin et al[588]	5-FU	I.V.	33	500 mg/m²/d × 5 d q 5 wk	21	10.5
	FUDR	IA	36	0.3 mg/kg/d × 14 d q 28 d	48	12.6
Rougier et al[590]	5-FU	I.V.	82	500 mg/m²/d × 5 d q 4 wk	—	10
	FUDR	IA	81	0.3 mg/kg/d × 14 q 28 d	—	14

5-FU, 5-fluorouracil; FUDR, floxuridine; I.V., intranveous; IA, intraarterial.

greatest risk.[515] Preliminary analysis of two recently completed randomized studies has failed to demonstrate a significant benefit for the addition of methyl-CCNU to 5-FU in adjuvant therapy of colorectal cancer.[600,601] Therefore, use of this agent can no longer be recommended. Mitomycin has produced the same general quantitative and qualitative responses as the nitrosoureas.[563,599,602] Because both mitomycin and methyl-CCNU have the potential for substantial chronic hematologic and renal toxicity and yield median response durations of about 3 months, there is little to recommend one agent over the other.

Unfortunately, although dozens of new drugs have been screened, there is no convincing evidence of meaningful efficacy for any of them. Recently, taxol, a novel microtubule inhibitor, has produced minor responses in some patients with advanced colorectal cancer treated during phase I trials of the drug.[603] Due to limited drug supply, phase II studies to confirm taxol's efficacy have not been completed. Of greater interest is CPT-11, a novel topoisomerase I inhibitor, recently introduced into clinical trial. In preliminary studies conducted in Japan, a 46% response rate has been observed in 17 patients with advanced colorectal cancer.[604] These observations are particularly encouraging in view of preclinical data suggesting that colon tumors may be uniquely sensitive to inhibition of topoisomerase I.[605]

The modest responsiveness of colon adenocarcinoma to available chemotherapy has been the subject of intense basic science investigation. Adenocarcinoma of other organs (*e.g.*, breast, ovary, and stomach) is initially responsive to various alkylating and anthracycline agents, so histopathology is not an adequate explanation. One possible explanation for the poor response of colon adenocarcinoma to chemotherapy may lie in the observation of high expression of the *MDR1* gene in colon cancer cells de novo. This gene encodes a drug transport protein that modulates the access of cytotoxics to the interior of the cell. Other mechanisms of drug resistance, both acquired and arising de novo, are being explored.[606] Colon carcinoma cells evidence other aspects of the pleiotropic drug resistance phenomenon,[607] and characterization of the p170

glycoprotein, glutathione transferase and other biochemical marker activity is being pursued.

Combination Chemotherapy

Because of the limited number of chemotherapeutic options, most attempts to improve systemic treatment have consisted of empirically adding drugs to 5-FU.[559,599] One such popular regimen is based on the addition of methyl-CCNU to 5-FU. Enthusiasm for this combination arose from a small randomized comparison of MOF with 5-FU in metastatic bowel cancer patients at the Mayo Clinic. As reported initially, the objective response rate for MOF was twice that of 5-FU (43% versus 19%), but no significant survival advantage was observed.[608] Subsequent attempts to confirm this superiority have not been uniformly successful, and response rates for MOF or MF type regimens have ranged from 4% to 40%.[599,609–615] This observed heterogeneity should not be surprising, because the reported response rate for 5-FU alone varies tenfold. Perhaps MF combinations result in higher response rates than 5-FU alone, but most of the responses are partial and last less than 6 months. Nonetheless, the initial activity of MOF or MF combinations has influenced the design of adjuvant trials in colon and rectal cancer for more than a decade.

Simple attempts to substitute or add another alkylating-type agent, such as mitomycin, for the nitrosourea usually have not resulted in clinically meaningful differences.[616,617] There have been attempts to combine multiple alkylating-type agents such as 5-FU, methyl-CCNU, mitomycin or MOF, and streptozocin. Randomized trials with appropriate control groups have failed to demonstrate a significant survival superiority for any such combination.[615,618]

More recently, the addition of cisplatin to 5-FU has been evaluated based on preclinical studies demonstrating synergy between these agents. Although initial phase II studies produced response rates of 30% to 40%, several randomized trials (Table 30–21) subsequently have failed to demonstrate any advantage of the combination over 5-FU alone in response rate or survival.[619–624] In view of the increased toxicity that

TABLE 30–21. Randomized Studies of Combination 5-Fluorouracil (5-FU) + Cisplatin Compared With 5-FU Alone in Patients With Advanced Colorectal Cancer

Investigations	5-FU Dose	Cisplatin Dose	Response (%)	Survival (wk)
Poon et al[619]	a) 500 mg/m²/d × 5 q 5 wk	—	10	No difference
	b) 325 mg/m²/d × 5 q 5 wk	20 mg/m²/d × 5	15	
Kemeny et al[620]	a) 1000 mg/m²/d × 5 q 4 wk	—	3	52
	b) 1000 mg/m²/d × 5 q 4 wk	20 mg/m²/d × 5 q 4 wk	25	43
Lokich et al[621]	a) 300 mg/m²/d × 10 wk	—	33	42
	b) 300 mg/m²/d × 10 wk	20 mg/m²/wk	31	48
Loehrer et al[622]	a) 15 mg/kg/wk	—	19	39
	b) 15 mg/kg/wk	60 mg/m² q 3 wk	22	40
LaBianca et al[623]	a) 600 mg/m² wk	—	15	56
	b) 600 mg/m²/wk	60 mg/m² q 3 wk	20	43
Diaz-Rubio et al[624]	a) 1000 mg/m²/d × 5 d	—	23	39
	b) 1000 mg/m²/d × 5 d	100 mg/m² q 4 wk	21	51

results from addition of cisplatin, these regimens cannot be recommended for routine clinical use.

Fluorouracil Modulation

METHOTREXATE. Elucidation of the complex biochemical pathways followed by 5-FU intracellularly has led to the development of several biochemical modulation strategies designed to enhance the cytotoxic effects of the drug. These studies have concentrated on enhancing 5-FU activation by pretreatment with methotrexate (MTX), by depleting endogenous pyrimidine pools with phosphonacetyl-L-aspartate (PALA), or by expanding intracellular reduced folate pools with leucovorin. The sequential use of MTX and 5-FU enhances cell kill in various cell culture and animal tumor systems.[625–627] This effect is presumed to result from MTX inhibition of purine metabolism, causing accumulation of PRPP (5-phosphoribosyl-1-pyrophosphate) and increased conversion of 5-FU to its active metabolites 5-fluorouridine triphosphate (5-FUTP) and 5-fluoro-2'-deoxyuridylate (5-FdUMP).[626,627] Many MTX dosages (ranging from 40–800 mg/m²), intervals (1–24 hours before 5-FU), and schedules (bolus to infusion, weekly to monthly) have been reported. Mucositis and leukopenia have been the most notable toxic effects. Responses have been observed in untreated patients and in patients who have failed 5-FU regimens. Although there is no single regimen with a superior therapeutic index,[628–634,636,637] a recently reported randomized study has confirmed the importance of a 24-hour interval between administration of MTX and 5-FU. Marsh and colleagues randomly assigned 168 previously untreated patients with advanced measurable colorectal cancer to receive MTX 200 mg/m² followed by 5-FU 600 mg/m² either 24 hours or 1 hour after MTX.[635] Doses of leucovorin 10 mg/m² were administered by mouth every 6 hours for 6 doses beginning 24 hours after MTX administration. Compared with the 1-hour interval, the 24-hour scheduling interval resulted in a significantly better objective response rate (29% versus 14.5%; $p = 0.026$), median time to progression (9.9 versus 5.9 months; $p = 0.009$), and survival (median of 15.3 versus 11.4 months; $p = 0.003$). Interpretation of these results is confounded by the difference in leu-

covorin schedule in the two arms of the study. In one arm, leucovorin was administered concurrently with 5-FU, whereas in the other it was administered the day after 5-FU. Therefore, it is conceivable that the superiority of the 24-hour scheduling interval was related primarily to a combined 5-FU and leucovorin interaction.

LEUCOVORIN. The modulation of 5-FU by leucovorin is perhaps the most successful biochemical modulation strategy to be brought from the laboratory to the clinic. Considerable preclinical evidence indicates that intracellular reduced folate cofactor enhances 5-FU cytotoxicity by stabilizing the covalent ternary complex of thymidylate synthase and FdUMP.[638–640] Numerous phase II studies have been performed with varying doses of leucovorin (25 to 500 mg/m² per course) and 5-FU (150 to 600 mg/m² per course). Response rates of 10% to 60% have been reported in patients with and without previous 5-FU exposure.[641–644]

Seven prospective randomized trials comparing 5-FU to 5-FU with leucovorin have been reported (Table 30–22).[619,636,637,645–648] Six studies have demonstrated significantly higher response rates for the combination of 5-FU and leucovorin, and two studies have shown improved overall survival for it. The leucovorin doses used in these studies have ranged from 15 mg/m² to 500 mg/m². Higher doses have been used most often in an attempt to achieve plasma leucovorin concentrations of 1 to 10 μM, levels necessary for optimal synergy in vitro. The demonstration by Poon and colleagues that an leucovorin dose of 20 mg/m² could effectively enhance 5-FU efficacy and was equivalent to a dose of 200 mg/m² has generated considerable controversy regarding the optimal 5-FU/leucovorin doses and schedules.[619] In a recent update, Poon and colleagues reported on 457 patients with advanced colorectal cancer randomly assigned to treatment with 5-FU with low-dose leucovorin, 5-FU with high-dose leucovorin, or 5-FU with high-dose MTX and leucovorin rescue.[649] The combined 5-FU and leucovorin regimens were equivalent and superior to 5-FU with high-dose MTX for objective tumor response and time to progression. Moreover, 5-FU with low-dose leucovorin was found to confer a significant survival benefit ($p \leq 0.01$) compared with the combination of 5-FU

TABLE 30–22. Summary of Randomized Trials of 5-FU Plus Leucovorin Compared With 5-FU for the Treatment of Advanced Colorectal Cancer

Investigations	No. of Patients	Dose 5-Fluorouracil	Leucovorin	Comments
Roswell Park Memorial Institute[637]	74	a) 450 mg/m² IVP b) 600 mg/m² IVP c) 600 mg/m² IVP	— — 500 mg/m², 2-h infusion	No statistically significant survival difference; 44% PR and 4% CR with 5-FU and leucovorin, which was statistically superior to the other two arms ($p = 0.0009$).
GITSG[645]	343	a) 500 mg/m² IVP b) 600 mg/m² IVP c) 600 mg/m² IVP	— 500 mg/m², 2-h infusion 25 mg/m², 10-min infusion	A trend toward longer survival in arm b. High dose leucovorin (arm b) has a response rate of 30.3%, which is significantly greater than 5-FU alone ($p < 0.01$).
NCCTG/Mayo Clinic[619]	429	a) 500 mg/m² IVP b) 370 mg/m² IVP c) 370 mg/m² IVP	— 200 mg/m² IVP 20 mg/m² IVP	Significant survival advantage of the low- and high-dose leucovorin over 5-FU alone. Only 5-FU + low dose leucovorin was associated with benefit in quality of life parameters.
NORDIC[646]	249	a) 600 mg/m² IVP b) 500 mg/m² IVP	— 15 mg	Slight survival benefit in the combination treatment arm (8.5 mo vs 6 mo, $p < 0.02$). Objective responses were statistically significant.
Northern California Oncology Group[636]	249	a) 12 mg/kg/d IVP b) 400 mg/m², 15-min infusion c) 500 mg/m² IVP	— 200 mg/m² IVP 10 mg/m² po	No difference in response rates.
City of Hope[647]	79	a) 370 mg/m² IVP b) 370 mg/m² IVP	— 500 mg/m² continuous infusion	Superior response rates for combined treatment ($p = 0.0019$); no overall survival differences.
Princess Margaret Hospital[648]	130	a) 370 mg/m² IVP b) 370 mg/m² IVP	200 mg/m² IVP —	Statistically significant difference in response rates (33% vs 7%) in favor or 5-FU + leucovorin. Overall survival was longer in the 5-FU + leucovorin arm.

IVP, intravenous push.

and high-dose MTX. A final assessment regarding the optimal leucovorin dose awaits the results of ongoing randomized clinical trials. Compared with 5-FU alone, the 5-FU and low-dose-leucovorin combination regimen appears to provide enhanced efficacy, an improved quality of life, and an acceptable toxicity profile. The toxicity of 5-FU plus leucovorin therapy is noteworthy. If administered weekly, the combination results in mild leukopenia in about 10% of patients. The dose-limiting toxic effects are enteritis and diarrhea, which can be life-threatening but may be ameliorated by administration of somatostatin analogs.[650] In contrast, daily administration of the combination for 5 days produces oral mucositis in about 33% of all patients.

PALA. Other attempts to enhance the efficacy of 5-FU have used the pyrimidine synthesis inhibitor PALA to deplete intracellular pools of uridine triphosphate and thereby enhance formation of FUTP and its incorporation into RNA.[651,652] Initial clinical trials of PALA with 5-FU used high doses of the modulating agent, resulting in excessive toxicity requiring reductions in the administered dose of 5-FU.[651] These studies produced disappointingly low response rates and a loss of interest in the use of PALA as a modulating agent. More recent studies using lower doses of PALA have rekindled interest in this modulation strategy. Ardalan and colleagues performed a dose-finding study of PALA administered as an intravenous bolus

24 hours before beginning a 24-hour infusion of 5-FU.[653] Treatments were repeated on a weekly schedule. At a PALA dose of 250 mg/m², the maximally tolerated dose of 5-FU was 2600 mg/m². The dose-limiting toxicity of this regimen was ataxia, occurring in 4 of 8 patients treated at a 5-FU dose of 3400 mg/m². Other toxic effects included nausea, vomiting, stomatitis, diarrhea, and hand-foot syndrome. Eleven of 28 patients with advanced gastrointestinal cancer who received PALA with 5-FU had an objective tumor response. In a subsequent study, O'Dwyer and colleagues treated 39 patients with advanced, measurable colorectal cancer and no previous chemotherapy with PALA 250 mg/m² followed 24 hours later by a 24-hour infusion of 5-FU 2600 mg/m².[654] Among 37 evaluable patients, there were 3 complete and 13 partial remissions for an objective response rate of 43%. Mild to moderate gastrointestinal toxicity and neurotoxicity occurred in 30% to 40% of patients. The objective response rate observed in this study is comparable with that reported for many combination 5-FU and leucovorin regimens. Ardalan and colleagues have administered 5-FU 2600 mg/m² as a 24-hour infusion concurrently with leucovorin 500 mg/m² over 24 hours repeated weekly.[655] An objective response rate of 45% was observed among 22 patients with advanced colorectal cancer. These studies have led to the concept of double biochemical modulation using PALA before a 24-hour infusion of high-dose 5-FU and leucovorin.[656] Ongoing phase III clinical

trials are comparing combined PALA and 5-FU with combined 5-FU and leucovorin regimens in an attempt to define the optimal biochemical modulation strategy.

INTERFERON. Recent studies have focused attention on the use of interferon-α to modulate the cytotoxic effects of 5-FU. Preclinical studies have demonstrated synergistic cytotoxicity of these drugs on human colon cancer cell lines.[657,658] The mechanism of this effect is unknown, although interferon has been shown to enhance conversion of 5-FU to FdUMP,[659] to reduce cellular levels of thymidylate synthase,[660] and to inhibit thymidine salvage pathways—all of which would tend to enhance 5-FU effects. In addition to these biochemical interactions, some clinical trials have demonstrated reduced 5-FU clearance and increased pharmacologic area under the curve in the presence of interferon.[661]

A high response rate to the combination of 5-FU and interferon was initially reported by Wadler and colleagues (Table 30–23). Subsequent studies attempting to confirm the initial promising results have demonstrated response rates consistently in the range of 25% to 40% for previously untreated patients.[662-666] These results are comparable with those observed with other biochemical modulation strategies. The toxicity of treatment with 5-FU and interferon can be formidable. In addition to leukopenia, mucositis, and diarrhea, patients often experience fever, chills, and myalgias. Neurotoxicity manifests as somnolence, confusion, ataxia, or seizures in a small percentage of patients.

While ongoing phase III trials are attempting to define the efficacy of combination 5-FU and interferon compared with 5-FU alone, attempts to combine interferon with 5-FU plus leucovorin have begun. Grem and colleagues reported results of a pilot study conducted in 31 patients with metastatic adenocarcinoma of the gastrointestinal tract.[661] Patients received an initial cycle of 5-FU 370 or 425 mg/m²/day with leucovorin 500 mg/m²/day for 5 days. If tolerated, the patient received the same dose of combined 5-FU and leucovorin on cycle 2, with the addition of interferon on days 1 through 7 at doses ranging from 5 to 10 million U/m²/day. In 26 matched cycles, the addition of interferon was associated with an increased incidence of dose-limiting mucositis and diarrhea and greater thrombocytopenia. The recommended doses for subsequent study were 5-FU 370 mg/m²/day, leucovorin 500 mg/m²/day, and interferon 5×10^6 U/m²/day. Other phase I studies have demonstrated the feasibility of combining these three

agents.[667-670] Phase II and III studies are required to assess the efficacy of this double biochemical modulation strategy.

SUMMARY OF FLUOROURACIL MODULATION. Improved understanding of the biochemical pharmacology of 5-FU has led to the development of several biochemical modulation strategies now undergoing clinical trial. The combination of 5-FU with leucovorin, PALA, or interferon appears to produce response rates consistently in the range of 30% to 40%, although only the combination of 5-FU with leucovorin has been shown to be superior to 5-FU alone in prospective randomized trials. Two ongoing national cooperative group studies ultimately may define the optimal biochemical modulation strategy (Figure 30–11). Until the results from these studies are available, 5-FU with leucovorin must be considered standard therapy for previously untreated patients with metastatic colorectal cancer. Biochemical modulation strategies that use multiple modulating agents are worth pursuing until the discovery of effective new agents for treatment of colorectal cancer. Other drugs that have been combined with 5-FU include dipyridamole, a nucleoside transport inhibitor that inhibits thymidine salvage, and hydroxyurea, a ribonucleotide reductase inhibitor that depletes intracellular dUMP pools thereby enhancing the binding of FdUMP to thymidylate synthase.

Chemotherapy for Patients Not Benefitting From 5-FU Therapy

Most patients who receive 5-FU-based chemotherapy do not benefit from it and many patients are candidates for subsequent systemic therapy. Patients who fail to respond to an initial attempt at fluoropyrimidine therapy seldom respond to 5-FU administered on a different dose or schedule or with a different modulating agent. Regimens of combined 5-FU and leucovorin usually produce response rates of 10% or less in patients previously treated with 5-FU. In his initial report, Wadler observed no responses to 5-FU with interferon in patients previously treated with 5-FU, despite a high level of activity for this combination in previously untreated patients.[671] Variation of the method of administration of 5-FU is unlikely to produce clinically meaningful benefit once disease progression has occurred on chemotherapy. Outside of a formal research program, the options available for patients who do not improve with 5-FU-based therapy are limited. Oc-

TABLE 30–23. Phase II Studies of 5-FU Plus Interferon in Patients With Advanced Colorectal Cancer

Investigations	No. of Patients	5-FU Dose	Interferon Dose	Response Rate (%)	Survival
Wadler and Wiernik[662]	32	750 mg/m²/d × 5 then weekly	9 MU tiw	63	59% (at 1 year)
Pazdur et al[663]	52	750 mg/m²/d × 5 then weekly	9 MU tiw	35	16-month median
Kemeny et al[664]	35	750 mg/m²/d × 5 then weekly	9 MU tiw	26	Not reported
ECOG[665]	38	750 mg/m²/d × 5 then weekly	9 MU tiw	42	18-month median
Huberman et al[666]	42	750 mg/m²/d × 5 then weekly	9 MU tiw	39	Not reported

tiw, three times a week.

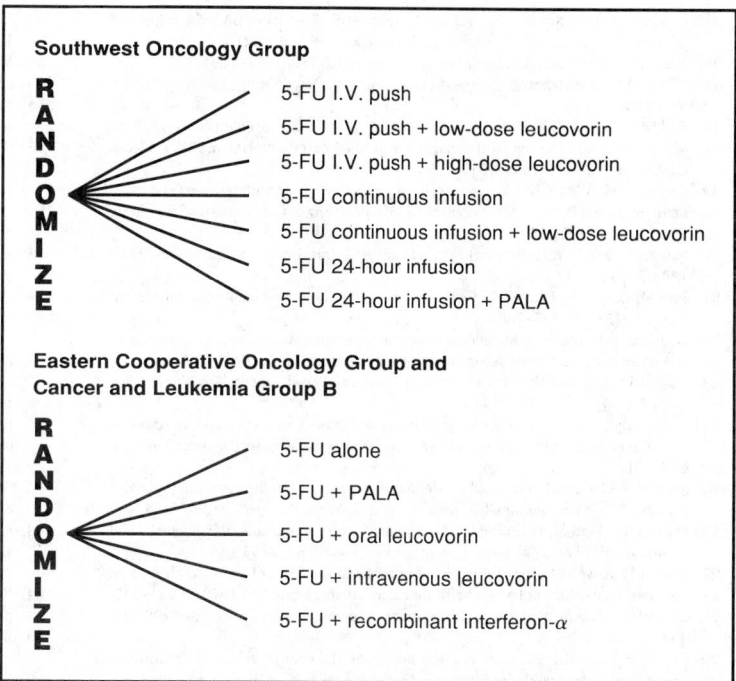

FIGURE 30–11. Ongoing phase III trials for previously untreated patients with metastatic colorectal cancer. 5-FU, 5-fluorouracil; PALA, phosphonacetyl-L-aspartate.

casional responses to nitrosoureas have been observed. Moertel and colleagues noted a 10% response rate in 112 patients treated with a chlorethyl nitrosourea as second-line therapy.[608] Likewise, two-drug combinations containing methyl-CCNU have proved to be effective in less than 10% of patients.[613] Patients with a good performance status should be considered for investigational chemotherapy protocols.

MISCELLANEOUS COLORECTAL TUMORS

CARCINOID TUMORS

Most alimentary tract carcinoids occur in the ileum and the appendix. The rectum is the next commonest site, with occasional tumors in the colon.[198] Almost all rectal carcinoids present as asymptomatic submucosal nodules less than 2 cm in size. In contrast to other sites, hematogenous and lymph node metastases are rare (<15%).[672] Malignant potential is seen almost exclusively in patients with tumors larger than 2 cm.[673–675] Transanal local excision suffices for tumors less than 2 cm, with radical surgery reserved only for larger tumors and those with histologic evidence of invasion of the muscularis propria.[674–676]

SARCOMA

Almost all smooth muscle tumors in the bowel occur in the stomach and small bowel. A few cases of rectal leiomyosarcoma have been reported.[199,677,678] The tumors may be small and asymptomatic or larger than 10 cm with typical rectal cancer symptomatology. The smaller submucosal tumors arise from the muscularis mucosa. Most are low grade and almost all are curable by local excision. Tumors arising in the muscularis propria are frequently high grade. Local recurrence is common with limited surgical approaches.[199,677] With high-

grade tumors, metastases to liver and lung occur in almost all patients despite radical surgery.[199,678]

LYMPHOMA

Primary rectal lymphoma is rare. It can be cured by surgery and postoperative irradiation.[679]

REFERENCES

1. National Institutes of Health. Annual cancer statistics review, including cancer trends: 1950–1985. 88th ed. Bethesda, MD: National Institutes of Health, 1988.
2. Schottenfeld D, Winawer SJ. Cancer, epidemiology and prevention. In: Schottenfeld D, Fraumeni JF Jr, eds. Philadelphia: WB Saunders, 1982:703–709.
3. Ziegler RG, Devesa SS, Fraumeni JF, et al. Epidemiology pattern of colorectal cancer. In: DeVita VT, Hellman S, Rosenberg SA, eds. Important advances in oncology. Philadelphia: JB Lippincott, 1986:209–232.
4. Waterhouse J, Carrea P, Muir C. Cancer incidence in five continents, IARC scientific publication 15. Lyon: International Agency for Research on Cancer, 1976.
5. Blot WJ, Fraumeni FJ, Stone BJ. Geographic patterns of large bowel cancer in the US. JNCI 1976;57:1225–1231.
6. Pickle LW, Greene MH, Ziegler RG. Colorectal cancer in rural Nebraska. Cancer Res 1984;44:363–369.
7. Burdette WJ. Carcinoma of the colon and antecedent epithelium. In: Burdette WJ, ed. Springfield, IL: Charles C. Thomas, 1970.
8. Phillips RL, Kuzma JW, Lotz TM. Cancer mortality among comparable members vs non-members of the Seventh Day Adventist Church. In: Cairns J, Lyon JL, Skolnick M, eds. Cancer incidence in defined populations. Cold Spring Harbor, NY: Cold Spring Harbor Laboratory, 1980:83–102.
9. Phillips RL, Garfinkel L, Kuzma JW. Mortality among California Seventh Day Adventists for selected cancer sites. JNCI 1980;65:1097–1107.
10. Enstrom JE. Health and dietary practices and cancer mortality among California Mormons. In: Lyon JL, Skolnick M, eds. Cancer incidence in defined populations. Cold Spring Harbor, NY: Cold Spring Harbor Laboratory, 1980:69–90.
11. Lyon JL, Sorenson AW. Colon cancer in a low-risk population. Am J Clin Nutr 1978;31:227–230.
12. Cady B, Persson AV, Monson DO. Changing patterns of colorectal cancer. Cancer 1974;33:433–436.
13. Axtell LM, Chiazze L. Changing relative frequency of cancer of the colon and rectum in the United States. Cancer 1966;19:750–754.
14. Rhodes JB, Holmes FF, Clark GM. Changing distribution of primary cancer in the large bowel. JAMA 1977;235:1641–1643.
15. Weisburger JH, Wynder EL. Etiology of colorectal cancer with emphasis on mechanism

In the figure:

Southwest Oncology Group

RANDOMIZE
- 5-FU I.V. push
- 5-FU I.V. push + low-dose leucovorin
- 5-FU I.V. push + high-dose leucovorin
- 5-FU continuous infusion
- 5-FU continuous infusion + low-dose leucovorin
- 5-FU 24-hour infusion
- 5-FU 24-hour infusion + PALA

Eastern Cooperative Oncology Group and Cancer and Leukemia Group B

RANDOMIZE
- 5-FU alone
- 5-FU + PALA
- 5-FU + oral leucovorin
- 5-FU + intravenous leucovorin
- 5-FU + recombinant interferon-α

of action and prevention. In: DeVita V, Hellman S, Rosenberg SA, eds. Important advances in oncology. Philadelphia: JB Lippincott, 1987:197–221.

16. Modan B. Dietary role in cancer etiology. Cancer 1977;40:1887–1891.
17. Willett NC, MacMahon B. Diet and cancer: An overview. N Engl J Med 1984;310:697–703.
18. Reddy B, Engle A, Katsifis S, et al. Biochemical epidemiology of colon cancer: Effects of types of dietary fiber on fecal mutagens, acid, and neutral sterols in healthy subjects. Cancer Res 1989;49:4629–4635.
19. Greenwald P, Witkin KM. Large bowel cancer: Policy, prevention research and treatment. In: Rozen P, Reich CB, Winawer SJ, eds. Frontiers of Gastrointestinal Research. Basel: Karger, 1991:25–37.
20. Palmer S, Bakshi K. Diet, nutrition and cancer: I. Interim dietary guidelines. JNCI 1983;70:1151–1170.
21. Jain M, Cook GM, Davis FG. A case-control study of diet and colorectal cancer. Int J Cancer 1980;26:757–768.
22. Haenszel WM, Kurihara M. Studies of Japanese immigrants: I. Mortality from cancer and other diseases among Japanese in the United States. JNCI 1968;40:43–47.
23. Correa P, Haenszel W. The epidemiology of large-bowel cancer. Adv Cancer Res 1978;26:1–141.
24. Armstrong B, Doll R. Environmental factors and cancer incidence and mortality in different countries with special reference to dietary practices. Int J Cancer 1975;15:617–631.
25. Ames BN, McCann J, Yamasaki E. Methods for detecting carcinogens and mutagens with the *Salmonella* mammalian microsome test. Mutat Res 1975;31:347–364.
26. Curren RD, Putman DL, Yang LL. Genotoxicity of fecapentaene-12 in bacterial and mammalian cell assay systems. Carcinogenesis 1987;8:349–353.
27. Ehrich M, Aswell JE, Van Tassell RL. Mutagens in the feces of three South African populations at different levels of risk for colon cancer. Mutat Res 1979;64:231–240.
28. Bruce WR. Recent hypotheses for the origin of colon cancer. Cancer Res 1987;47:4237–4242.
29. Correa P, Paschal J, Pizzolato P. Fecal mutagens and colorectal polyps:Preliminary report of an autopsy study. In: Bruce WR, Correa P, Lipkin M, et al, eds. Gastrointestinal cancer: Endogenous factors. New York: Cold Spring Harbor Laboratory, 1981:119–127.
30. Dion PW, Bright-See EB, Smith CC. The effect of dietary ascorbic acid and a-tocopherol on fecal mutagenicity. Mutat Res 1982;102:27–37.
31. Reddy BS, Sharma C, Simi B. Metabolic epidemiology of colon cancer: Effect of dietary fiber on fecal mutagens and bile acids in healthy subjects. Cancer Res 1987;47:644–648.
32. Susuki K, Bruce WR, Baptista J. Characterization of cytotoxic steroids in human feces and their putative role in the etiology of human colon cancer. Cancer Lett 1986;33:307–317.
33. Smith LL. Carcinogenic cholesterol products. In: Cholesterol autoxidation. New York: Plenum Press, 1981:432–446.
34. Lipkin M, Reddy BS, Weisburger J. Non-degradation of fecal cholesterol in subjects at high risk for cancer of the large intestines. J Clinical Invest 1981;67:304–307.
35. Bird RP, Bruce WR. Toxicity of dietary components to colonic mucosa in vivo. Proc Am Assoc Cancer Res 1983;24:89.
36. Bird RP. Effect of dietary components on the pathobiology of colonic epithelium: Possible relationship with colon tumorigenesis. Lipids 1986;21:289–291.
37. Sugimura T. Carcinogenicity of mutagenic heterocyclic amines formed during the cooking process. Mutat Res 1985;150:33–42.
38. Tanaka T, Barries WS, Weisburger JH. Multipotential carcinogenicity of the fried food mutagen 2-amino-emethylimudazo (4.b-f)quinoline (IQ) in rats. Jpn J Cancer Res (Gann) 1985;76:570–576.
39. Suzuki K, Bruce WR. Increase by deoxycholic acid of the colonic nuclear damage induced by known carcinogens in C57B1/6J mice. JNCI 1986;76:1129–1132.
40. Hill MJ, Drasar BS, Wiliams RED. Faecal bile-acid and clostridia in patients with cancer of the large bowel. Lancet 1975;1:535–539.
41. Linos DA, Beard CM, O'Fallon WM. Cholecystectomy and carcinoma of the colon. Lancet 1981;2:379–381.
42. Vernick LF, Kuller LH. Cholecystectomy and right-sided colon cancer: An epidemiological study. Lancet 1981;2:381–383.
43. Vernick LJ, Kuller LH, Lohsoonthorn P. Relationship between cholecystectomy and ascending colon cancer. Cancer 1980;45:392–395.
44. Bird RP, Medline A, Furrer R, Bruce WR. Toxicity of orally administered fat to the colonic epithelium of mice. Carcinogenesis 1985;6:1063–1066.
45. Caderni G, Stuart E, Bruce WR. Dietary factors affecting the proliferation of epithelial cells in the colon of the mouse. Gastroenterology 1987;92:1336.
46. Garland C, Shekelle RB, Barrett-Connor E. Dietary vitamin D and calcium and risk of colorectal cancer: A 19-year prospective study in men. Lancet 1985;1:307–309.
47. Thornton JR. High colonic PH promotes colorectal cancer. Lancet 1981;1:1081–1082.
48. Van Dokkum W, de Boer BCJ, van Faassen A. Diet, faecal pH and colorectal cancer. Br J Surg 1983;48:109–110.
49. Samelson SL, Nelson RL, Nyhus LM. Protective role of faecal pH in experimental colon carcinogenesis. J R Soc Med 1984;78:230–233.
50. Walker ARP, Walker AJ. Faecal pH, dietary fibre intake, and proneness to colon cancer in four South African populations. Br J Cancer 1986;53:489–495.
51. Pietroiusti A, Guliano M, Vita S. Faecal pH and cancer of the large bowel. Gastroenterology 1983;84:1273.
52. Winawer SJ. Diagnosis and prevention of gastrointestinal malignancies. Semin Oncol 1991;18:7–17.
53. Jensen OM, Mosbech J, Salaspuro M. A comparative study of the diagnostic basis for

cancer of the colon and cancer of the rectum in Denmark and Finland. Int J Epidemiol 1974;3:183–186.
54. Modan B, Barell V, Lubin F, et al. Low fiber intake as an etiologic factor in cancer of the colon. JNCI 1975;55:15–18.
55. Trock B, Lanza E, Greenwald P. Dietary fiber, vegetables, and colon cancer: Critical review and metaanalysis of the epidemiologic evidence. JNCI 1990;82:650–661.
56. Greenwald P, Lanza E. Role of dietary fiber in the prevention of cancer. In: DeVita VT Jr, Hellman S, Rosenberg SA, eds. Important advances in oncology. Philadelphia: JB Lippincott, 1986:37–54.
57. Glauert HP, Bennick MR, Sander CH. Enhanced 1,2-dimethylhydrazine-induced colon carcinogenesis in mice by dietary agar. Food Chem Toxicol 1981;19:281–286.
58. Freeman HJ, Spiller GA, Kim YS. A double blind study of the effect of purified cellulose dietary fiber on 1,2-dimethylhydrazine-induced rat colonic neoplasia. Cancer Res 1978;38:2912–2917.
59. Weisburger JH. Causes, relevant mechanisms, and prevention of large bowel cancer. Semin Oncol 1991;18:316–336.
60. Reddy BS. Molecular epidemiology of colon cancer. In: Rozen P, Reich CB, Winawer SJ, eds. Large bowel cancer: Policy, prevention, research, and treatment. Basel: Karger, 1991:88–98.
61. Reddy BS, Ekelund G, Bohe M, et al. Metabolic epidemiology of colon cancer: Dietary pattern and fecal sterol concentrations of three populations. Nutr Cancer [Abstract] 1978;5:34–40.
62. Garland CF, Garland F, Ko Shaw E, et al. Serum 25-hydroxyvitamin D and colon cancer: Eight-year prospective study. Lancet 1989;2:1176–1178.
63. Lipkin M, Friedman E, Winawer SJ, et al. Colonic epithelial proliferation in responders and nonresponders to supplemental dietary calcium. Cancer Res 1989;49:248–254.
64. Rozen P, Fireman E, Fine N, et al. Oral calcium suppresses increased rectal epithelial proliferation of persons at risk of colorectal cancer. Gut 1989;30:650–655.
65. Buset M, Lipkin M, Winawer S, et al. Inhibition of human colonic cell proliferation in vivo and in vitro by calcium. Cancer Res 1986;46:5426–5430.
66. Clark LC. The epidemiology of selenium and cancer. Fed Proc 1985;44:2584–2589.
67. Shamberger RJ. Nutrition and cancer. New York: Plenum Press, 1984.
68. Banner WP, DeCosse JJ, Tan QH, et al. Selective distribution of selenium in colon parallels its antitumor activity. Carcinogenesis 1984;5:1543–1546.
69. Bussey HJ, DeCosse JJ, Deschner EE. A randomized trial of ascorbic acid in polyposis coli. Cancer 1982;50:1434–1439.
70. McKeown-Eyssen GE, Bright-See E. Dietary prevention of recurrences of adenomatous polyps in the colon and rectum. In: UICC Cancer Congress, Budapest. Geneva: Union Internationale Contra le Cancer, 1986.
71. Lipkin M. Biomarkers of increased susceptibility to gastrointestinal cancer. Gastroenterology 1987;92:1083–1086.
72. McKusick VA. Genetics and large-bowel cancer. Am J Digest Dis 1974;19:954–957.
73. Lipkin M, Sherlock P, DeCosse JJ. Risk factors and preventative measures in the control of cancer of the large intestine. Curr Probl Cancer 1980;4:1057.
74. Bussey HJR. Gastrointestinal polyposis. Gut 1970;11:970–978.
75. Bussey AJR. Familial polyposis coli. Baltimore: Johns Hopkins University Press, 1975.
76. Erbe RW. Inherited gastrointestinal polyposis syndromes. N Engl J Med 1976;294:1101–1104.
77. DeCosse JJ, Adaurs MB, Condon RF. Familial polyposis. Cancer 1977;39:267–273.
78. Arvanitis ML, Jagelman DG, Fazio VW, et al. Mortality in patients with familial adenomatous polyposis. Dis Colon Rectum 1990;33:639–642.
79. Kelly PB, McKinnon DA. Familial multiple polyposis of the colon: Review and description of a large kindred. McGill Med J 1961;30:67–85.
80. Gardner EJ. Follow-up study of a family group exhibiting dominant inheritance for a syndrome including intestinal polyps, osteomas, fibromas and epidermal cysts. Am J Hum Genet 1962;14:376–390.
81. Oldfield MC. The association of familial polyposis of the colon with multiple sebaceous cysts. Br J Surg 1954;41:534–541.
82. Turcot J, Despres JP, St. Pierre F. Malignant tumors of the central nervous system associated with familial polyposis of the colon: Report of two cases. Dis Colon Rectum 1959;2:465–468.
83. Reid JD. Intestinal carcinoma in the Peutz-Jeghers syndrome. JAMA 1974;229:833–834.
84. Kussin SZ, Lipkin M, Winawer SJ. Inherited colon cancer: Clinical implications. Am J Gastroenterol 1979;72:443–457.
85. Lynch HT, Lynch PM. Heredity and gastrointestinal tract cancer. In: Lipkin M, Good RA, eds. Gastrointestinal tract cancer. New York: Plenum Press, 1978.
86. Lynch HT, Albano WA, Lynch JF, et al. Recognition of the cancer family syndrome. Gastroenterology 1983;84:672–673.
87. Law JP, Herberman RB, Oldham RL. Familial occurrence of colon, uterine and of lymphoproliferative malignancies: Clinical description. Cancer 1977;39:1224–1228.
88. Muto T, Kamiya J, Sawada T, et al. Small "flat adenoma" of the large bowel with special reference to its clinicopathologic features. Dis Colon Rectum 1985;28:847–851.
89. Lynch HT, Smyrk T, Lanspa SJ, et al. Flat adenomas in a colon cancer-prone kindred. JNCI 1988;80:278–282.
90. Muto T, Masaki T, Suzuki K. DNA ploidy pattern of flat adenomas of the large bowel. Dis Colon Rectum 1991;34:696–698.
91. Lynch HT, Smyrk T, Watson P, et al. Heriditary colorectal cancer. Semin Oncol 1991;18:337–366.
92. Lynch HT, Richardson JD, Amin M, et al. Variable gastrointestnal and urologic cancers in a Lynch syndrome II kindred. Dis Colon Rectum 1991;34:891–895.
93. Itoh H, Houlston RS, Harocopos C, et al. Risk of cancer death in first-degree relatives

of patients with hereditary non-polyposis cancer syndrome (Lynch type II): A study of 130 kindreds in the United Kingdom. Br J Surg 1990;77:1367–1371.

94. Macklin MT. Inheritance of cancer of the stomach and large intestine in man. JNCI 1960;24L:551–557.

95. Sherlock P. Heredity versus environment in colorectal cancer. In: Winawer SJ, Schottenfeld D, Sherlock P, eds. Colorectal cancer: Prevention, epidemiology and screening. New York: Raven Press, 1980:65–66.

96. Burt RW, Bishop DT, Cannon LA, et al. Dominant inheritance of adenomatous colonic polyps and colorectal cancer. N Engl J Med 1985;12:1540–1544.

97. Mulvihill JJ. Clinical ecogenetics: Cancer in families. N Engl J Med 1985;312:1569–1570.

98. Bodmer WF, Bailey CJ, Bodmer J, et al. Localization of the gene for familial adenomatous polyposis on chromosome 5. Nature 1987;328:2–4.

99. Kinzler KW, Nilbert MC, Su LK, et al. Identification of FAP locus genes from chromosome 5q21. Science 1991;253:661–664.

100. Groden J, Thliveris A, Samowitz W, et al. Identification and characterization of the familial adenomatous polyposis coli gene. Cell 1991;66:589–600.

101. Joslyn G, Carlson M, Thliveris A, et al. Identification of deletion mutations and three new genes at the familial polyposis locus. Cell 1991;66:601–613.

102. Vogelstein B, Fearon ER, Hamilton SR, et al. Genetic alterations during colorectal-tumor development. N Engl J Med 1988;319:525–532.

103. Forrester K, Almoguera C, Han K, et al. Detection of high incidence of K-ras oncogenes during human colon tumorigenesis. Nature 1987;327:298–303.

104. Bos JL, Fearon ER, Hamilton SR, et al. Prevalence of ras gene mutations in human colorectal cancers. Nature 1987;327:293–297.

105. Fearon ER, Cho KR, Nigro JM, et al. Identification of a chromosome 18q gene that is altered in colorectal cancers. Science 1990;247:49–56.

106. Kinzler KW, Mef CN, Vogelstein B, et al. Identification of a gene located at chromosome 5q21 that is mutated in colorectal cancers. Science 1991;251:1366–1370.

107. Edwards FC, Truelove SC. The course and prognosis of ulcerative colitis. Gut 1964;5:1–22.

108. Morson BC. Cancer and ulcerative colitis. Gut 1966;7:425–426.

109. Mir-Modjlessi SH, Farmer RG, Easley KA, et al. Colorectal and extracolonic malignancy in ulcerative colitis. Cancer 1986;58:1569–1574.

110. MacDougall PM. The cancer risk in ulcerative colitis. Lancet 1966;2:655–658.

111. Ekbom A, Helmick C, Zack M, et al. Ulcerative colitis and colorectal cancer: A population based study. N Engl J Med 1990;323:1228–1233.

112. Ohman U. Colorectal carcinoma in patients with ulcerative colitis. Am J Surg 1982;144:344–349.

113. Kewenter J, Ahlman H, Hulten L. Cancer risk in extensive ulcerative colitis. Ann Surg 1978;188:824–828.

114. Katzka I, Brody RS, Morris E, et al. Assessment of colorectal cancer risk in patients with ulcerative colitis: Experience from a private practice. Gastroenterology 1983;85:22–29.

115. Prior P, Gyde SN, Macartney JC, et al. Cancer morbidity in ulcerative colitis. Gut 1982;23:490–497.

116. Devroede GJ, Taylor WF, Sauer WG. Cancer risk and life expectancy of children with ulcerative colitis. N Engl J Med 1971;285:17–21.

117. Kirsner JB, Shorter RG. Inflammatory bowel disease of the large bowel and anal canal. In: Kirsner JB, Shorter RG, eds. Diseases of the colon, rectum and anal canal. Baltimore: Williams & Wilkins, 1987.

118. Biasco G, Paganelli GM, Migioloi M, et al. Rectal cell proliferation and colon cancer risk in ulcerative colitis. Cancer Res 1990;50:1156–1159.

119. Suzuki K, Muto T, Masaki T, et al. Microspectrophotometric DNA analysis in ulcerative colitis with special reference to its application in diagnosis of carcinoma and dysplasia. Gut 1990;31:1266–1270.

120. Hamilton SR. Colorectal carcinoma in patients with Crohn's disease. Gastroenterology 1989;89:398–407.

121. Heaton K. Crohn's disease and ulcerative colitis. In: Trowell H, Burkitt D, Heaton K, et al, eds. Dietary fibre, fibre-depleted foods and disease. New York: Academic Press, 1985:205–216.

122. Greenstein AJ, Sachar DB, Smith H, et al. Patterns of neoplasia in Crohn's disease and ulcerative colitis. Cancer 1980;46:403–407.

123. Weedon DD, Shorter RG, Ilstrup DM, et al. Crohn's disease and cancer. N Engl J Med 1973;289:1099–1104.

124. Morson BC. Genesis of colorectal cancer. Clin Gastroenterol 1976;5:505–525.

125. Heald RJ, Bussey HJR. Clinical experience at St. Mark's Hospital with multiple synchronous cancers of the colon and rectum. Dis Colon Rectum 1975;18:6.

126. Schottenfeld D, Berg JW, Vitsky B. Incidence of multiple primary cancers: II. Index cancers arising in the stomach and lower digestive system. JNCI 1969;43:77–86.

127. Burbank F. Patterns in cancer mortality in the United States: 1950–1967. Natl Cancer Inst Monogr 1971;33:127.

128. MacMahon CE, Rowe JW. Rectal reaction following radiation therapy of cervical carcinoma: Particular reference to subsequent occurrence of rectal carcinoma. Ann Surg 1971;173:264–269.

129. Castro EB, Rosen PP, Quan SH. Carcinoma of large intestine in patients irradiated for carcinoma of cervix and uterus. Cancer 1973;31:45–52.

130. McMichael AJ, Potter JD. Host factors in carcinogenesis: Certain bile-acid metabolic profiles that selectively increase the risk of proximal colon cancer. JNCI 1985;75:185–191.

131. Lowenfels AB, Domellof L, Lindstrom CG, et al. Cholelithiasis, cholecystectomy, and cancer: A case-control study in Sweden. Gastroenterology 1982;83:672–676.

132. Bristol JB, Williamson RCN. Ureterosigmoidostomy and colon carcinogenesis. Science 1981;214:351.

133. Appel MF, Spjut HJ, Estroda RG. The significance of villous component in colonic polyps. Am J Surg 1977;134:770–771.

134. Morson BC. Evolution of cancer of the colon and rectum. Cancer 1974;34:845–849.

135. Lipkin M. Phase 1 and phase 2 proliferative lesions of colonic epithelial cells in disease leading to cancer. Cancer 1974;34:878–888.

136. Muto T, Bussey HJR, Morson BC. The evolution of cancer of the colon and rectum. Cancer 1975;36:2251–2270.

137. McDermott FT, Hughes ESR, Pihl E, et al. Prognosis in relation to symptom duration in colon cancer. Br J Surg 1981;13:846–849.

138. Sherlock P, Lipkin M, Winawer SJ. The prevention of colon cancer. American J Med 1980;68:917–931.

139. Winawer SJ, Miller DG, Sherlock P. Risk and screening for colorectal cancer. Adv Intern Med 1984;30:471–496.

140. Devlin HB, Plant JA, Morris D. The significance of symptoms of carcinoma of the rectum. Surg Gynecol Obstet 1973;137:399–402.

141. Irvin TT, Greany MG. Duration of symptoms and prognosis of carcinoma of the colon and rectum. Surg Gynecol Obstet 1977;144:883–886.

142. Farrands PA, Hardcastle JD. Colorectal cancer by self completion questionnaire. Gut 1984;25:1445–4447.

143. Chapuis PH, Goulston KJ, Dent OF, et al. Predictive value of rectal bleeding in screening for rectal and sigmoid polyps. Br Med J Clin Res 1985;290:1546–1548.

144. Eddy DM, Nugent FW, Eddy JF, et al. Screening for colorectal cancer in a high-risk population: Results of a mathematical model. Gastroenterology 1987;92:682–692.

145. Winawer SJ, Schottenfeld D, Flehinger BJ. Colorectal cancer screening. JNCI 1991;83(4):243–253.

146. Ransohoff DF, Lang CA. Screening for colorectal cancer. N Engl J Med 1991;325:37–41.

147. Rozen P, Fireman Z, Figer A, et al. Family history of colorectal cancer as a marker of potential malignancy within a screening program. Cancer 1987;60:248–254.

148. Gryska PV, Cohen AM. Screening asymptomatic patients at high risk for colon cancer with full colonoscopy. Dis Colon Rectum 1987;30:18–20.

149. Winawer SJ, O'Brien MJ, Waye JD, et al. Risk and surveillance of individuals with colorectal polyps. Bull World Health Organ 1990;68:789–795.

150. Nava H, Pagana TJ. Postoperative surveillance of colorectal carcinoma. Cancer 1982;49:1043–1047.

151. Fantini GA, DeCosse JJ. Surveillance strategies after resection of carcinoma of the colon and rectum. Surg Gynecol Obstet 1990;171:267–273.

152. Winawer SJ, Ritchie M, Diaz B, et al. The National Polyp Study: Aims and Organization. In: Rozen P, Winawer SJ, eds. Frontiers of gastrointestinal research secondary prevention of colorectal cancer: An international perspective. Basel: Karger, 1986:216–225.

153. O'Brien MJ, Winawer SJ, Zauber AG, et al. The National Polyp Study: Patient and polyp characteristics associated with high-grade dysplasia in colorectal adenomas. Gastroenterology 1990;98:371–379.

154. Morson BC. Use of dysplasia as an indicator of risk for malignancy in patients with ulcerative colitis. In: Winawer SJ, Schottenfeld D, Sherlock P, eds. Colorectal cancer: Prevention, epidemiology and screening. New York: Raven Press, 1980:347–354.

155. Dobbins WO, Stock M, Ginsberg AL. Early detection and prevention of carcinoma of the colon in patients with ulcerative colitis. Cancer 1977;40:25–48.

156. Lofberg R, Brostrom O, Karlen P, et al. Colonoscopic surveillance in long-standing total ulcerative colitis: A 15-year follow-up study. Gastroenterology 1990;99:1021–1031.

157. Nugent FW, Haggitt RC, Gilpin PA. Cancer surveillance in ulcerative colitis. Gastroenterology 1991;100:1241–1248.

158. Winawer SJ, St.John D, Bond J, et al. Screening of average-risk individuals for colorectal cancer. Bull World Health Organ 1990;68:505–513.

159. Dales LG, Friedman GD, Collen MF. Evaluating periodic multiphase health check-ups: A controlled trial. J Chronic Dis 1979;32:385–404.

160. Hertz RE, Deddish MR, Day E. Value of periodic examination in detecting cancer of the rectum and colon. Postgrad Med 1960;27:290.

161. Winawer SJ, Cummins R, Baldwin MP, et al. A new flexible sigmoidoscope for the generalist. Gastrointest Endosc 1982;28:233–236.

162. Dubow RA, Katon RM, Benner KG, et al. Short (35 cm) versus long (60 cm) flexible sigmoidoscopy: A comparison of findings and tolerance in asymptomatic patients screened for colorectal neoplasia. Gastrointest Endosc 1985;31:305–308.

163. Wilking N, Petrelli NJ, Herrera L, et al. A comparison of the 25 cm rigid proctosigmoidoscope with the 65 cm flexible endoscope in the screening of patients for colorectal carcinoma. Cancer 1986;57:669–671.

164. Winnon G, Beri G, Parnish J. Superiority of the flexible to the rigid sigmoidoscope in routine proctosigmoidoscopy. N Engl J Med 1980;302:1011–1012.

165. Marks G, Boggs HW, Castro AF, et al. Sigmoidoscopic examinations with rigid and flexible fiberoptic sigmoidoscopes in the surgeon's office: A comparative prospective study of effectiveness in 1,012 cases. Dis Colon Rectum 1979;22:162–168.

166. Lipshutz GR, Katon RM, McCool MF, et al. Flexible sigmoidoscopy as a screening procedure for neoplasia of the colon. Surg Gynecol Obstet 1979;148:19–22.

167. Marks G, Gathright JB, Boggs HW, et al. Guidelines for use of the flexible sigmoidoscope in the management of the surgical patient. Dis Colon Rectum 1985;25:187–190.

168. Wherry DC. Screening for colorectal neoplasia in asymptomatic patients using flexible fiberoptic sigmoidoscopy. Dis Colon Rectum 1981;24:521–522.

169. Thomas WM, Pye G, Hardcastle JD, et al. Faecal occult blood screening for colorectal neoplasia: A randomized trial of three days or six days of tests. Br J Surg 1990;77:277–279.

170. Mandel JS, Bond JH, Bradley M, et al. Sensitivity, specificity and positive predictivity

of the hemoccult test in screening for colorectal cancers. Gastroenterology 1989;97: 597–600.

171. Knight KK, Fielding JE, Battista RN. Occult blood screening for colorectal cancer. JAMA 1989;261:587–593.

172. Morris JB, Stellato TA, Guy BB, et al. A critical analysis of the largest reported mass fecal occult blood screening program in the United States. Am J Surg 1991;161:101–106.

173. Ahlquist DA, McGill DB, Schwartz S, et al. Hemoquant, a new quantitative assay for fecal hemoglobin. Ann Intern Med 1984;101:297–302.

174. Ahlquist DA, McGill DB, Schwartz S, et al. Fecal blood levels in health and disease. N Engl J Med 1985;312:22–28.

175. Songster CL, Barrows GH, Jarrett DD. Immunochemical detection of fecal blood—the fecal smear pinch disc test. A new non-invasive screening test for colorectal cancer. Cancer 1980;45:1099–1102.

176. Saito H, Tsuchida S, Nakaji S, et al. An immunological test for fecal occult blood by counter immunoelectrophoresis. Cancer 1985;56:1549–1552.

177. Barry MJ, Mulley AG, Richter JM. Effect of workup strategy of the cost-effectiveness of fecal occult blood screening for colorectal cancer. Gastroenterology 1987;93:301–310.

178. Ahlquist DA, Beart RW Jr. Use of fecal occult blood test in the detection of colorectal neoplasia. Curr Problem Gen Surg 1985;2:200–210.

179. Winawer SJ, Fleisher M. Sensitivity and specificity of the fecal occult blood test for colorectal neoplasia. Gastroenterology 1982;82:986–991.

180. Griffith CDM, Turner DJ, Saunders JH. False-negative results of hemoccult test in colorectal cancer. Br J Med 1981;283:472.

181. Hardcastle JD, Armitage NC, Chamberlin J, et al. Fecal occult blood screening for colorectal cancer in the general population. Cancer 1986;58:397–403.

182. Feczko PJ, Halpert RD. Reassessing the role of radiology and hemoccult screening. Am J Radiol 1986;146:697–701.

183. Gilbertsen VA, Williams SE, Schuman L, et al. Colonoscopy in the detection of carcinoma of the intestine. Surgery,Gynecology & Obstetrics 1979;149:877–878.

184. Winawer SJ, Andrews M, Flehinger B, et al. Progress report on controlled trial of fecal occult blood testing for the detection of colorectal neoplasia. Cancer 1980;45: 2959–2964.

185. Winchester DP, Shull JH, Scanlon EF, et al. A mass screening program for colorectal cancer using chemical testing for occult blood in the stool. Cancer 1980;45:2955–2958.

186. Sontag SJ, Durczak C, Aranha GV, et al. Fecal occult blood screening for colorectal cancer in a Veterans' Administration hospital. Am J Surg 1983;145:89–94.

187. Hardcastle JD, Chamberland J, Sheffield J, et al. Randomized, controlled trial of faecal occult blood screening for colorectal cancer. Lancet 1989;II:1160–1164.

188. American Joint Committee on Cancer. Manual for staging of cancer. 2nd ed. Philadelphia: JB Lippincott, 1983.

189. Hermanek P. Evolution and pathology of rectal cancer. World J Surg 1982;6:502–509.

190. Spjut HJ. Pathology of neoplasms. In: Spratt JS, ed. Neoplasms of the colon, rectum, and anus: Mucosal and epithelial. Philadelphia: WB Saunders, 1984.

191. Morson BC, Sobin LH. Histological typing of intestinal tumours: WHO technical report 15. Geneva, World Health Organization, 1976.

192. Wood DA. Tumors of the intestines. In: Atlas of tumor pathology, section VI, fascicle 22. Washington, DC: Armed Forces Institute of Pathology, 1967.

193. Minsky BD. Clinicopathologic impact of colloid in colorectal carcinoma. Dis Colon Rectum 1990;33:714–719.

194. Mathews JL, Coyle D Jr, Little WP. Primary linitis plastica of the rectum: Report of a case. Dis Colon Rectum 1982;25:488–490.

195. Cooper HS. Carcinoma of the colon and rectum. In: Norris HT, ed. Pathology of the colon, small intestine, and anus. New York: Churchill Livingstone, 1983.

196. Black WA, Waugh JM. The intramural extension of carcinoma of the descending colon, sigmoid and rectosigmoid: A pathologic study. Surg Gynecol Obstet 1948;87: 457–464.

197. MacDonald RA. A study of 356 carcinoids of the gastrointestinal tract: Report of four new cases of the carcinoid syndrome. Am J Med 1956;21:867–878.

198. Orloff MJ. Carcinoid tumors of the rectum. Cancer 1971;28:175–180.

199. Evans HL. Smooth muscle tumors of the gastrointestinal tract: A study of 56 cases followed for a minimum of 10 years. Cancer 1985;56:2242–2250.

200. Akwari OE, Dozis RR, Weiland LH, et al. Leiomyosarcoma of the small and large bowel. Cancer 1978;42:1375–1384.

201. Lee WTN. Leiomyosarcoma of the gastrointestinal tract. General pattern of metastases in recurrence. Cancer Treat Rev 1983;10:91–101.

202. Broders AC. The grading of carcinoma. Minn Med 1925;8:726–730.

203. Dukes CE. The classification of cancer of the rectum. J Pathol 1932;35:323–332.

204. Qizilbash AH. Pathologic studies in colorectal cancer: A guide to the surgical pathology examination of colorectal specimens and review of features of prognostic significance. Pathol Annu 1982;17:1–46.

205. Jass JR, Atkin WS, Cuzick I, et al. The grading of rectal cancer: Histological perspectives and a multivariate analysis of 447 cases. Histopathology 1986;10:437–459.

206. Gordon-Watson C, Dukes C. The radium problem: III. The treatment of carcinoma of the rectum with radium. With an introduction on the spread of cancer of the rectum. Br J Surg 1930;17:643–669.

207. Dukes CE. Cancer of the rectum: An analysis of 1000 cases. J Pathol Bacteriol 1940;50: 527–539.

208. Dukes CE, Bussey HJR. The spread of rectal cancer and its effect on prognosis. Br J Cancer 1958;12:309–320.

209. Cole PP. The intramural spread of rectal carcinoma. Br Med J 1913;1:431–433.

210. Montessori GA, Donald JC. Invasion profile of colorectal carcinoma. Dis Colon Rectum 1978;21:26–28.

211. Templeton A. The value of whole mount sections in determining adequacy of surgical margins and in staging carcinoma of the colorectum. American Society of Therapeutic Radiology and Oncology abstract, 1991.

212. Seefeld P, Bargen JA. The spread of carcinoma of the rectum: Invasion of lymphatics, veins and nerves. Ann Surg 1943;118:76–90.

213. Astler VB, Coller FA. The prognostic significance of direct extension of carcinoma of the colon and rectum. Ann Surg 1954;139:846–851.

214. Gunderson LL, Sosin H. Areas of failure found at reoperation (second or symptomatic look) following "curative surgery" for adenocarcinoma of the rectum: Clinicopathologic correlation and implications for adjuvant therapy. Cancer 1974;34:1278–1292.

215. Gilbert SG. Symptomatic local tumor failure following abdomino-perineal resection. Int J Radiat Oncol Biol Phys 1978;4:801–807.

216. Cass AW, Million RR, Pfaff WW. Patterns of recurrence following surgery alone for adenocarcinoma of the colon and rectum. Cancer 1976;37:2861–2865.

217. Olson RM, Perencevich NP, Malcolm AW, et al. Patterns of recurrence following curative resection of adenocarcinoma of the colon and rectum. Cancer 1980;45:2969–2974.

218. Malcolm AW, Perencevich NP, Olson RM, et al. Analysis of recurrence patterns following curative resection for carcinoma of the colon and rectum. Surg Gynecol Obstet 1981;152:131–136.

219. Rao AR, Kagan AR, Chan PM, et al. Patterns of recurrence following curative resection alone for adenocarcinoma of the rectum and sigmoid colon. Cancer 1981;48:1492–1495.

220. Mendenhall WM, Million RR, Pfaff WW. Patterns of recurrence in adenocarcinoma of the rectum and rectosigmoid treated with surgery alone: Implications in treatment planning with adjuvant radiation therapy. Int J Radiat Oncol Biol Phys 1983;9:977–985.

221. Rich T, Gunderson LL, Lew R, et al. Patterns of recurrence of rectal cancer after potentially curative surgery. Cancer 1983;52:1317–1329.

222. Pilipshen SJ, Heilweil M, Quan SHQ, et al. Patterns of pelvic recurrence following definitive resections of rectal cancer. Cancer 1984;53:1354–1362.

223. Willett C, Tepper JE, Cohen A, et al. Obstructive and perforative colonic carcinoma: Patterns of failure. J Clin Oncol 1985;3:379–384.

224. Minsky BD, Mies C, Recht A, et al. Resectable adenocarcinoma of the rectosigmoid and rectum: 1. Patterns of failure and survival. Cancer 1988;61:1408–1416.

225. Minsky BD, Mies C, Rich TA, et al. Potentially curative surgery of colon cancer: 1. Patterns of failure and survival. J Clin Oncol 1988;6:106–118.

226. Gabriel WB, Dukes C, Bussey HJR. Lymphatic spread in cancer of the rectum. Br J Surg 1935;23:395–413.

227. Wood WQ, Wilkie DPD. Carcinoma of the rectum: An anatomico-pathologic study. Edinburgh Med J 1933;40:321–331.

228. Grinnell RS. The grading and prognosis of carcinoma of the colon and rectum. Ann Surg 1939;109:500–503.

229. Villemin F, Huard P, Montague M. Recherches anatomiques sur les lymphatiques du rectum et de l'anus. Rev Chir 1925;63:39–80.

230. Grinnell RS. Lymphatic block with atypical and retrograde lymphatic metastasis and spread in carcinoma of the colon and rectum. Ann Surg 1938;108:621–642.

231. Herter FP, Slanetz CA. Patterns and significance of lymphatic spread from cancer of the colon and rectum. In: Weiss L, Gilbert HA, Ballon SC, eds. Lymphatic system metastasis. Boston: GK Hall, 1980

232. Brown CE, Warren S. Visceral metastases from rectal carcinoma. Surg Gynecol Obstet 1938;66:611–621.

233. Grinnell RS. The lymphatic and venous spread of carcinoma of the rectum. Ann Surg 1942;116:200–215.

234. Weiss L, Grundmann E, Torhorst J, et al. Haematogenous metastatic patterns in colonic carcinoma: An analysis of 1541 necropsies. J Pathol 1986;150:195–203.

235. Batson OV. The function of the vertebral veins and their role in the spread of metastases. Ann Surg 1940;112:138–149.

236. Vider M, Maruyama Y, Narvaez R. Significance of the vertebral venous (Batson's) plexus in metastatic spread in colorectal carcinoma. Cancer 1977;40:67–71.

237. Umpleby HC, Williamson RCN. Anastomotic recurrence in large bowel cancer. Br J Surg 1987;74:873–878.

238. Beahrs OH, Phillips JW, Dockerty MB. Implantation of tumor cells as a factor in recurrence of carcinoma of the rectosigmoid: Report of four cases with implantation at dentate line. Cancer 1955;8:831–838.

239. LeQuesne LP, Thompson AD. Implantation recurrence of carcinoma of rectum and colon. N Engl J Med 1958;258:578–582.

240. Boreham P. Implantation metastases from cancer of the large bowel. Br J Surg 1958;46: 103–108.

241. Brodsky JT, Cohen AM. Peritoneal seeding following potentially curative resection of colonic carcinoma: Implications for adjuvant therapy. Dis Col Rect 1991;34:723–727.

242. Goligher JC. The Dukes' A, B and C categorization of the extent of spread of carcinomas of the rectum. Surg Gynecol Obstet 1976;143:793–794.

243. Krook JE, Moertel CG, Gunderson LL, et al. Effective surgical adjuvant therapy for high-risk rectal carcinoma. N Engl J Med 1991;324:709–715.

244. Stahle E, Glimelius B, Bergstrom R, et al. Preoperative prediction of outcome in patients with rectal and rectosigmoid cancer. Cancer 1989;63:1831–1837.

245. Minsky BD, Mies C, Rich TA, et al. Lymphatic vessel invasion is an independent prognostic factor for survival in colorectal cancer. Int J Radiat Oncol Biol Phys 1989;17: 311–318.

246. Chapuis PH, Dent OF, Fisher R, et al. A multivariate analysis of clinical and pathological

variables in prognosis after resection of large bowel cancer. Br J Surg 1985;72:698–702.

247. Moran K, Cooke T, Forster G, et al. Prognostic value of nucleolar organizer regions and ploidy values in advanced colorectal cancer. Br J Surg 1989;76:1152–1155.

248. Shepherd NA, Saraga EP, Love SB, et al. Prognostic factors in colonic cancer. Histopathol 1989;14:613–620.

249. Fisher ER, Pail SM, Rockette H, et al. Prognostic significance of eosinophils and mast cells in rectal cancer: Findings from the National Surgical Adjuvant Breast and Bowel Project (protocol R-01). Human Pathol 1989;20:159–163.

250. Mitmaker B, Begin LR, Gordon PH. Nuclear shape as a prognostic discriminant in colorectal carcinoma. Dis Colon Rectum 1991;34:249–259.

251. Hannisdal E, Thorsen G. Regression analysis of prognostic factors in colorectal cancer. J Surg Oncol 1988;37:109–112.

252. Steinberg SM, Barkin JS, Kaplan RS, et al. Prognostic indicators of colon tumors: The Gastrointestinal Tumor Group experience. Cancer 1986;57:1866–1870.

253. Jass JR, Love SB, Northover JM. A new prognostic classification of rectal cancer. Lancet 1987;1:1303–1306.

254. Quirke P, Durdey P, Dixon MF, et al. Local recurrence of rectal adenocarcinoma due to inadequate surgical resection. Histopathological study of lateral tumor spread and surgical excision. Lancet 1986;1:996–999.

255. Kokal WA, Gardine RL, Sheibani K, et al. Tumor DNA content in resectable, primary colorectal carcinoma. Ann Surg 1989;209:188–193.

256. Heimann TM, Miller F, Martinelli G, et al. Significance of DNA content abnormalities in small rectal cancer. Am J Surg 1989;159:525–528.

257. Jones DJ, Zaloudik J, James RD, et al. Predicting local recurrence of carcinoma of the rectum after preoperative radiotherapy and surgery. Br J Surg 1989;76:1172–1175.

258. Scivetti P, Riccardi A, Marsano B, et al. Flow cytometric DNA index in the prognosis of colorectal cancer. Cancer 1991;67:1921–1927.

259. Armitage NC, Ballantyne KC, Evans DF, et al. The influence of tumor cell DNA content of survival in colorectal cancer. Br J Cancer 1990;62:852–856.

260. Moertel CG, O'Fallon JR, Go VL, et al. The preoperative carcinoembryonic antigen test in the diagnosis, staging, and prognosis of colorectal cancer. Cancer 1986;58:603–610.

261. Lockhart-Mummery JP. Two hundred cases of cancer of the rectum treated by perineal excision. Br J Surg 1927;14:110–124.

262. Kirklin JW, Dockerty MB, Waugh JM. The role of the peritoneal reflection in the prognosis of carcinoma of the rectum and sigmoid colon. Surg Gynecol Obstet 1949;88:326–331.

263. Dukes CE. The surgical pathology of rectal cancer. J Clin Pathol 1949;2:95–99.

264. Turnbull RB Jr, Kyle K, Watson FR, et al. Cancer of the colon: The influence of the no-touch isolation technique on survival rates. Ann Surg 1967;166:420–427.

265. Wolmark N, Fisher B, Wieand HS. The prognostic value of the modifications of the Dukes' C class of colorectal cancer. Ann Surg 1986;203:115–122.

266. Phillips RKS, Hittinger R, Blesovsky L, et al. Large bowel cancer: Surgical pathology and its relationship to survival. Br J Surg 1984;71:604–610.

267. Gastrointestinal Tumor Study Group. Prolongation of the disease-free interval in surgically treated rectal carcinoma. N Engl J Med 1985;312:1465–1472.

268. International Union Against Cancer. TNM classification of malignant tumours. 4th ed. Berlin: Springer-Verlag, 1987.

269. Harmer MH, ed. TNM classification of malignant tumours. Geneva: International Union Against Cancer, 1978:69–76.

270. Chapuis PH, Dent OF, Newland RC, et al. An evaluation of the American Joint Committee (pTNM) staging method for cancer of the colon and rectum. Dis Colon Rectum 1986;29:6–10.

271. Enderlin F, Gloor F. Colorectal cancer: The relationship of staging to survival. A cancer registry study of 800 cases in St. Gallen-Appenzell. Prev Med 1986;31:85–88.

272. Hermanek P. Problems of pTNM classification of carcinoma of the stomach, colorectum and anal margin. Pathol Res Pract 1986;181:296–300

273. American Joint Committee on Cancer. Manual for staging of cancer. 3rd ed. Philadelphia: JB Lippincott, 1988.

274. Nathanson SD, Schultz L, Tilley B, et al. Carcinoma of the colon and rectum: A comparison of staging classifications. Am Surg 1986;52:428–433.

275. Newland RC, Chapuis PH, Smyth EJ. The prognostic value of substaging colorectal carcinoma: A prognostic study of 1117 cases with standardized pathology. Cancer 1987;60:852–857.

276. Fisher ER, Sass R, Palekar A, et al. Dukes's classification revisited: Findings from the national surgical adjuvant breast and bowel projects (protocol r-01). Cancer 1989;64:2354–2360.

277. Fisher ER, Robinsky B, Sass R, et al. Relative prognostic value of the Dukes and the Jass systems in rectal cancer: Findings from the National Surgical Adjuvant Breast and Bowel Projects (protocol R-01). Dis Colon Rectum 1989;32:944–949.

278. Hermanek P, Sobin LH, eds. TNM classification of malignant tumors (International Union Against Cancer). 4th ed. Berlin, Springer-Verlag, 1987:47–49.

279. American Joint Committee on Colon and Rectum Cancer. In: Beahrs OH, Henson DE, Hutter RV, et al. Manual for staging of cancer. 3rd ed. Philadelphia: JB Lippincott, 1988:75–80.

280. Cohen AM, Tremittera S, Candela F, et al. Prognosis of node-positive colon cancer. Cancer 1991;67:1859–1861.

281. Cawthorne SJ, Parmus DV, Gibbs NM, et al. Extent of mesorectal spread and involvement of lateral resection margin as prognostic factors after surgery for rectal cancer. Lancet 1990;335:1055–1059.

282. Hoerner MT. Carcinoma of the colon and rectum in persons under twenty years of age. Am J Surg 1958;96:47–53.

283. Recio P, Bussey HJR. The pathology and prognosis of carcinoma of the rectum in the young. Proc R Soc Lond 1965;58:789–790.

284. Coffey RJ, Cardenas F. Cancer of the bowel in the young adult. Dis Colon Rectum 1964;7:491–492.

285. Van Langenberg AV, Ong GB. Carcinoma of large bowel in the young. Br Med J 1972;3:374–376.

286. Odone V, Chang L, Caces J, et al. The natural history of colorectal carcinoma in adolescents. Cancer 1982;49:1716–1720.

287. Safford KL, Spebar MJ, Rosenthal D. Review of colorectal cancer in patients under age 40 years. Am J Surg 1981;142:767–769.

288. Simstein NL, Kovalcik PJ, Cross GH. Colorectal carcinoma in patients less than 40 years old. Dis Colon Rectum 1978;2:169–171.

289. Bulow S. Colorectal cancer in patients less than 40 years of age in Denmark, 1943–1967. Dis Colon Rectum 1980;23:327–336.

290. Umpleby HC, Williamson RCN. Carcinoma of the large bowel in the first four decades. Br J Surg 1984;71:272–277.

291. Welch CE, Burke JF. Carcinoma of the colon and rectum. N Engl J Med 1962;266:211–219.

292. McDermott FT, Hughes ESR, Pihl E, et al. Comparative results of surgical management of single carcinomas of the colon and rectum: A series of 1939 patients managed by one surgeon. Br J Surg 1981;68:850–855.

293. Spratt JS Jr, Spjut HJ. Prevalence and prognosis of individual clinical and pathologic variables associated with colorectal carcinoma. Cancer 1967;20:1976–1985.

294. Godwin JD, Brown CC. Some prognostic factors in survival of patients with cancer of the colon and rectum. J Chronic Dis 1975;28:441–454.

295. DeMello J, Struthers L, Turner R, et al. Multivariate analysis as aides to diagnosis and assessment of prognosis in gastrointestinal cancer. Br J Cancer 1983;48:341–348.

296. Eisenberg B, DeCosse JJ, Harford F, et al. Carcinoma of the colon and rectum: The natural history reviewed in 1704 patients. Cancer 1982;49:1131–1134.

297. Corman J, Arnoux R, Peloquin A, et al. Blood transfusions and survival after colectomy for colorectal cancer. Can J Surg 1986;29:325–329.

298. Fielding LP, Phillips RKS, Fry JS, et al. Prediction of outcome after curative resection for large bowel cancer. Lancet 1986;2:904–907.

299. Peter RK, Pike MC, Chang WWL, et al. Reproductive factors and colon cancers. Br J Cancer 1990;61:741–748.

300. Beahrs OH, Sanfelippo PM. Factors in the prognosis of colon and rectal cancer. Cancer 1971;28:213–217.

301. Pescatori M, Maria G, Beltrani B, et al. Site, emergency, and duration of symptoms in the prognosis of colorectal cancer. Dis Colon Rectum 1982;25:33–40.

302. Copeland EM, Miller LD, Jones RS, et al. Prognostic factors in carcinoma of the colon and rectum. Am J Surg 1968;116:875–881.

303. Ulin AW, Ehrlich EW. Current views related to management of large bowel obstruction caused by carcinoma of the colon. Am J Surg 1962;104:463–467.

304. Chang WYM, Burnett WE. Complete colonic obstruction due to adenocarcinoma. Surg Gynecol Obstet 1962;114:353–356.

305. Miller LD, Boruchow IB, Fitts WT. An analysis of 284 patients with perforative carcinoma of the colon. Surg Gynecol Obstet 1966;123:1212–1218.

306. Floyd CE, Cohn I. Obstruction in cancer of the colon. Ann Surg 1967;165:721–731.

307. Crowder VH, Cohn I. Perforation in cancer of the colon and rectum. Dis Colon Rectum 1967;10:415–420.

308. Glenn F, McSherry CK. Obstruction and perforation in colorectal cancer. Ann Surg 1971;173:983–992.

309. Welch JP, Donaldson GA. Management of severe obstruction of the large bowel due to malignant disease. Am J Surg 1974;127:492–499.

310. Welch JP, Donaldson GA. Perforative carcinoma of colon and rectum. Ann Surg 1974;180:734–740.

311. Wolmark N, Wieand HS, Rockette HE, et al. The prognostic significance of tumor and location and bowel obstruction in Dukes B and C colorectal cancer: Findings from the NSABP clinical trials. Ann Surg 1983;198:743–752.

312. Steinberg SM, Barwick KW, Stablein DM. Importance of tumor pathology and morphology in patients with surgically resected colon cancer: Findings from the Gastrointestinal Tumor Study Group. Cancer 1986;58:1340–1345.

313. Thomas WH, Larson RA, Wright HK, et al. An analysis of patients with carcinoma of the right colon. Surg Gynecol Obstet 1968;127:313–314.

314. Dwight RW, Higgins GA, Keehan RJ. Factors influencing survival after resection in cancer of the colon and rectum. Am J Surg 1969;117:512–522.

315. Freedman LS, Macaskill P, Smith AN. Multivariate analysis of prognostic factors for operable rectal cancer. Lancet 1984;2:733–736.

316. Gilchrist RK, David VC. A consideration of pathological factors influencing five year survival in radical resection of the large bowel and rectum for carcinoma. Ann Surg 1947;126:421–438.

317. Osnes S. Carcinoma of the colon and rectum: A study of 353 cases with special reference to prognosis. Acta Chir Scand 1956;110:378–388.

318. McSherry CK, Cornell GN, Glenn F. Carcinoma of the colon and rectum. Ann Surg 1969;169:502–512.

319. Cohen AM, Wood WC, Gunderson LL, et al. Pathological studies in rectal cancer. Cancer 1980;45:2965–2968.

320. Wolmark N, Fisher ER, Wieand HS, et al. The relationship of depth of penetration and tumor size to the number of positive nodes in Dukes C colorectal cancer. Cancer 1984;53:2707–2712.

321. Coller FA, Kay EB, MacIntyre RS. Regional lymphatic metastasis in carcinoma of the colon. Ann Surg 1941;114:56–63.

322. Burrows L, Tartter P. Effect of blood transfusions on colonic malignancy recurrence rate. Lancet 1982;2:662.

323. Agarwal M, Blumberg N. Colon cancer patients transfused perioperatively have an increased incidence of recurrence. Transfusion [Abstract] 1983;23:421.

324. Foster RS Jr, Costanza MC, Foster JC. Adverse relationship between blood transfusions and survival after colectomy for colon cancer. Cancer 1985;55:1195–1201.

325. Tartter PI. Perioperative blood transfusion and colorectal cancer recurrence: A review. J Surg Oncol 1988;39:197–200.

326. Beynon J, Davies PW, Billings PJ, et al. Perioperative blood transfusion increases the risk of recurrence in colorectal cancer. Dis Colon Rectum 1989;32:975–979.

327. Marsh J, Donnan PT, Hamer-Hodges DW. Association between transfusion with plasma and the recurrence of colorectal carcinoma. Br J Surg 1990;77:623–626.

328. Nathanson SD, Tilley BC, Schultz L, et al. Perioperative allogeneic blood transfusions: Survival in patients with resected carcinomas of the colon and rectum. Arch Surg 1985;120:734–738.

329. Eldar S, Kemeny MM, Terz JJ. Extended resections for carcinoma of the colon and rectum. Surg Gynecol Obstet 1985;161:319–322.

330. Kelley WE Jr, Brown PW, Lawrence W Jr, et al. Penetrating, obstructing, and perforating carcinomas of the colon and rectum. Arch Surg 1981;116:381–384.

331. Minsky BD, Rich T, Recht A, et al. Selection criteria for local excision with or without adjuvant radiation therapy for rectal cancer. Cancer 1989;63:1421–1429.

332. Riboli EB, Secco GB, Lapertosa G, et al. Colorectal cancer: Relationship of histologic grading to disease prognosis. Tumori 1983;69:581–584.

333. Godwin JD,II. Carcinoid tumors: An analysis of 2837 cases. Cancer 1975;36:560–569.

334. Symonds DA, Vickery AL Jr. Mucinous carcinoma of the colon and rectum. Cancer 1976;37:1891–1900.

335. Umpleby HC, Ranson DL, Williamson HC. Peculiarities of mucinous colorectal carcinoma. Br J Surg 1985;72:715–718.

336. Minsky BD, Mies C, Rich TA, et al. Colloid carcinoma of the colon and rectum. Cancer 1987;60:3103–3112.

337. Walton WW, Hagihara PF, Griffen WO. Colorectal adenocarcinoma in patients less than 40 years old. Dis Colon Rectum 1976;19:529–534.

338. Trimpi HD, Bacon HE. Mucoid carcinoma of the rectum. Cancer 1951;4:597–609.

339. Sundbald AS, Paz RA. Mucinous carcinomas of the colon and the rectum and their relation to polyps. Cancer 1982;50:2504–2509.

340. Minsky BD, Mies C, Rich TA, et al. Potentially curative surgery of colon cancer. The influence of blood vessel invasion. J Clin Oncol 1988;6:119–127.

341. Minsky BD, Mies C, Recht A, et al. Resectable adenocarcinoma of the rectosigmoid and rectum. 2) the influence of blood vessel invasion. Cancer 1988;61:1417–1424.

342. Krasna MJ, Flanobaum L, Cody RP, et al. Vascular and neural invasion in colorectal cancer. Cancer 1988;61:1018–1023.

343. Dukes CE, Bussey HJR. Venous spread in rectal cancer. Proc Royal Soc Med 1941;34:571–581.

344. Madison MS, Dockerty MB, Waugh JM. Venous invasion in carcinoma of the rectum as evidenced by venous radiography. Surg Gynecol Obstet 1954;99:170–178.

345. Khankhanian N, Maulight GM, Russel WO, et al. Prognostic significance of vascular invasion in colorectal cancer of Dukes' B class. Cancer 1977;39:1195–1200.

346. Heald RJ, Ryall RDH. Recurrence and survival after total meso-rectal excision for rectal cancer. Lancet 1986;1:1479–1482.

347. Talbot IC, Ritchie S, Leighton MH, et al. The clinical significance of invasion of veins by rectal cancer. Br J Surg 1980;67:439–442.

348. Horn A, Dahl O, Morild I. The role of venous and neural invasion on survival in rectal adenocarcinoma. Dis Colon Rectum 1990;33:598–601.

349. Horn A, Dahl O, Morild I. Venous and neural invasion as predictors of recurrence in rectal adenocarcinoma. Dis Colon Rectum 1991;34:798–804.

350. Wiggers T, Arends JW, Volovics A. Regression analysis of prognostic factors in colorectal cancer after curative resections. Dis Colon Rectum 1988;31:33–41.

351. Sunderland DA. The significance of vein invasion by cancer of the rectum and sigmoid: A microscopic study of 210 cases. Cancer 1949;2:429–437.

352. Swinton NW. Cancer of the colon and rectum: A statistical study of 608 patients. Surg Clin North Am 1959;39:745–753.

353. Michelassi F, Vannucci L, Ayala JJ, et al. Local recurrence after curative resection of colorectal adenocarcinoma. Surgery 1990;108:787–793.

354. Krasna MJ, Flancbaum L, Cody RP, et al. Vascular and neural invasion in colorectal carcinoma. Incidence and prognostic significance. Cancer 1988;61:1018–1023.

355. Murray D, Hreno A, Dutton J, et al. Prognosis in colon cancer: A pathologic reassessment. Arch Surg 1975;110:908–913.

356. Carlon CA, Fabris G, Arslan-Pagnini C, et al. Prognostic correlations of operable carcinoma of the rectum. Dis Colon Rectum 1985;28:47–50.

357. Svennevig JL, Lunde OC, Holter J, et al. Lymphoid infiltration and prognosis in colorectal carcinoma. Br J Cancer 1984;49:375–377.

358. Feil W, Wunderlich M, Neuhild N, et al. Rectal Cancer: Factors influencing the development of local recurrence after radical anterior resection. Int J Colorectal Dis 1988;3:195–200.

359. Fisher B, Wolmark N, Rockette H, et al. Postoperative adjuvant chemotherapy or radiation therapy for rectal cancer: Results from NSABP protocol R-01. JNCI 1988;80:21–29.

360. Patt DJ, Brynes RK, Vardiman JW, et al. Mesocolic lymph node histology is an important prognostic indicator for patients with carcinoma of the sigmoid colon: An immunomorphologic study. Cancer 1975;35:1388–1397.

361. Tsakraklides V, Wanebo HJ, Sternberg SS, et al. Prognostic evaluation of regional lymph node morphology in colorectal cancer. Am J Surg 1975;129:174–180.

362. Pihl E, Malahy MA, Khankhanian N, et al. Immunomorphological features of prognostic significance in Dukes' class B colorectal carcinoma. Cancer Res 1977;37:4145–4149.

363. LoGerfo P, Herter FP. Carcinoembryonic antigen and prognosis in patients with colon cancer. Ann Surg 1975;181:81–84.

364. Herrera MA, Chu TM, Holyoke ED. Carcinoembryonic antigen (CEA) as a prognostic and monitoring test in clinically complete resection of colorectal carcinoma. Ann Surg 1976;183:5–9.

365. Wanebo JH, Rao B, Pinsky CM, et al. Pre-operative carcinoembryonic antigen level as a prognostic indicator in colorectal cancer. N Engl J Med 1978;299:448–451.

366. Band PR, Beck IT, Dinner PJ, et al. Two year follow-up study of patients with known serum concentrations of carcinoembryonic antigen. Can Med Assoc J 1977;117:657–659.

367. Evans JT, Mittelman A, Chu M, et al. Pre- and post-operative uses of CEA. Cancer 1978;42:1419–1421.

368. Kohler JP, Simnonowitz D, Paloyan D. Pre-operative CEA level: A prognostic test in patients with colorectal carcinoma. Am Surg 1980;46:449–452.

369. Staab HJ, Anderer FA, Brummendorf T, et al. Prognostic value of pre-operative serum CEA level compared to clinical staging: I. Colorectal carcinoma. Br J Cancer 1981;44:652–662.

370. Szymendera J, Nowacki MP, Szalowski AW, et al. Predictive value of plasma CEA levels: Preoperative prognosis and postoperative monitoring of patients with colorectal carcinoma. Dis Colon Rectum 1982;25:46–52.

371. Onetto M, Paganuzzi M, Secco GB, et al. Preoperative carcinoembryonic antigen and prognosis in patients with colorectal cancer. Biomed Pharmacother 1985;39:392–395.

372. Aabo K, Pedersen H, Kjaer M. Carcinoembryonic antigen (CEA) and alkaline phosphatase in progressive colorectal cancer with special reference to patient survival. Eur J Cancer Clin Oncol 1986;22:211–217.

373. Goslin R, Steele G, MacIntyre J, et al. The use of pre-operative plasma CEA levels for the stratification of patients after curative resection of colorectal cancer. Ann Surg 1980;192:747–751.

374. Chapuis PH, Newland RC, Payne JE, et al. Preoperative carcinoembryonic antigen level and prognosis in colorectal cancer. Med J Aust 1980;2:140–143.

375. Blake KE, Dalbow MH, Concannon JP, et al. Clinical significance of preoperative plasma carcinoembryonic antigen (CEA) level in patients with carcinoma of the large bowel. Dis Colon Rectum 1982;25:24–32.

376. Lewi H, Blumgart LH, Carter DC, et al. Pre-operative carcinoembryonic antigen and survival in patients with colorectal cancer. Br J Surg 1984;71:206–208.

377. Steele G Jr, Ellenberg S, Ramming K, et al. CEA monitoring among patients in multi-institutional adjuvant G.I. therapy protocols. Ann Surg 1982;196:162–169.

378. Wobbes T, Hendriks T, DE Bower HHM. Collagen in colorectal cancer in relation to clinicopathologic stage and histologic grade. Dis Colon Rectum 1988;31:778–780.

379. Offerhaus GJ, Giardiello FM, Bruijn JA, et al. The value of immunohistochemistry for collagen IV expression in colorectal carcinomas. Cancer 1991;67:99–105.

380. Havenith MG, Arends JW, Simon R, et al. Type IV collagen immunoreactivity in colorectal cancer. Prognostic value of basement membrane deposition. Cancer 1988;62:2207–2211.

381. Heimann TM, Cohen RD, Szporn A, et al. Correlation of nuclear morphometry and DNA ploidy in rectal cancer. Dis Colon Rectum 1991;34:449–454.

382. Ambros RA, Pawel BR, Mescheryakov I, et al. Nuclear morphometry as a prognostic indicator in colorectal carcinoma resected for cure. Anal Quant Cytol Histol 1990;12:172–176.

383. Hiddemann W, von Bassewitz DB, Kleinemeier HJ, et al. DNA stemline heterogeneity in colorectal cancer. Cancer 1986;58:258–263.

384. Fischbach W, Mossner J, Seyschab H, et al. Tissue carcinoembryonic antigen and DNA aneuploidy in precancerous and cancerous colorectal lesions. Cancer 1990;65:1820–1824.

385. Giaretti W, Danova M, Geido E, et al. Flow cytometric DNA index in the prognosis of colorectal cancer. Cancer 1991;67:1921–1927.

386. Magnusson I, Falkmer UG, Nilsson R. Multiple primary colorectal adenocarcinomas: Cytometric DNA ploidy patterns and histopathologic features. Dis Colon Rectum 1991;34:810–815.

387. Heimann TM, Miller F, Martinelli G, et al. Significance of DNA content abnormalities in small rectal cancers. Am J Surg 1990;159:199–202.

388. Visscher DW, Zarbo RJ, Ma CK, et al. Flow cytometric DNA and clinicopathologic analysis of Dukes' A&B colonic adenocarcinomas: A retrospective study. Mod Pathol 1990;3:709–712.

389. Franssila K, Nordling S. The prognostic value of DNA-ploidy in colorectal carcinoma: A prospective study. Br J Cancer 1990;62:976–981.

390. Crissman JD, Zarbo RJ, Ma CK, et al. Histopathologic parameters and DNA analysis in colorectal adenocarcinomas 24. Pathol Annu 1989;24:103–147.

391. Goh HS, Jass JR, Atkin WS, et al. Value of flow cytometric determination of ploidy as a guide to prognosis in operable rectal cancer: A multivariate analysis. Int J Colorectal Dis 1987;2:17–21.

392. Emdin SO, Stenling R, Roos G. Prognostic value of DNA content in colorectal carcinoma:a flow cytometric study with some methodological aspects. Cancer 1987;60:1282–1287.

393. Quirke P, Dixon MF, Clayden AD, et al. Prognostic significance of DNA aneuploidy and cell proliferation in rectal c adenocarcinomas. J Pathol 1987;151:285–229.

394. Wirsching RP, Lamerz R, Wiebecke B, et al. Flow cytometric evaluation of colorectal carcinoma as completion of conventional tumor examination. J Exp Clin Cancer Res 1987;6:117–128.

395. Jones DJ, Moore M, Schofield PF. Refining the prognostic significance of DNA ploidy status in colorectal cancer: A prospective flow cytometric study. Int J Cancer 1988;41: 206–210.

396. Jass JR, Mukawa K, Goh HS, et al. Clinical importance of DNA content in rectal cancer measured by flow cytometry. J Clin Pathol 1989;42:254–259.

397. Scivetti P, Davona M, Riccardi A, et al. Prognostic significance of DNA content in large bowel carcinoma: A retrospective flow cytometric study. Cancer Lett 1989;46: 213–219.

398. Giaretti W, Sciallero S, Bruno S, Giaretti W. DNA flow cytometry of endoscopically examined colorectal adenocarcinomas. Pathol Res Pract 1989;185:589–593.

399. Halvorsen TB, Johannesen E. DNA ploidy, tumor site, and prognosis in colorectal cancer. Scand J Gastroenterol 1990;25:141–148.

400. Wolley RC, Schreiber K, Koss LG, et al. DNA distribution in human colon carcinomas and its relationship to clinical behavior. JNCI 1982;69:15–22.

401. Beauchamp RD, Townsend CM Jr, Singh P, et al. Proglumide, a gastrin receptor antagonist. Inhibits growth of colon cancer and enhances survival in mice. Ann Surg 1985;202:303–309.

402. Schillaci A, Tirindelli DD, Freei M, et al. Flow cytometric analysis in colorectal carcinoma: Prognostic significance of cellular DNA content. Int J Colorectal Dis 1990;5: 223–227.

403. Fisher ER, Siderits RH, Sass R, et al. Value of assessment of ploidy in rectal cancers. Archives Pathol Lab Med 1991;113:525–528.

404. Bauer KD, Lincon ST, Vera-Roman JM, et al. Prognostic implications of proliferative activity and DNA aneuploidy in colonic adenocarcinomas. Lab Invest 1987;57:329–335.

405. Rognum TO, Thorud E, Lund E. Survival of large bowel carcinoma patients with different DNA ploidy. Br J Cancer 1987;56:633–636.

406. Wiggers T, Arends JW, Schutte B, et al. A multivariate analysis of pathologic prognostic indicators in large bowel cancer. Cancer 1988;61:386–395.

407. Melamed MR, Enker WE, Banner P, et al. Flow cytometry of colorectal carcinoma with three-year follow-up. Dis Colon Rectum 1986;29:184–186.

408. Rognum TO, Lund E, Meling GI, et al. Near diploid large bowel carcinomas have better five-year survival than aneuploid ones. Cancer 1991;68:1077–1081.

409. Witzig TE, Loprinzi CL, Gonchoroff NJ, et al. DNA ploidy and cell kinetic measurements as predictors of recurrence and survival in stages B2 and colorectal adenocarcinoma. Cancer 1991;68:879–888.

410. Heerdt BG, Molinas S, Deitch D, et al. Aggressive subtypes of human colorectal tumors frequently exhibit amplification of the c-myc gene. Oncogene 1991;6:125–129.

411. Imaseki H, Hayashi H, Taira M, et al. Expression of c-myc oncogene in colorectal polyps as a biological marker for monitoring malignant potential. Cancer 1989;64: 704–709.

412. Michelassi F, Erroi F, Roncella M, et al. Ras oncogene and the acquisition of metastasizing properties by rectal adenocarcinoma. Dis Colon Rectum 1989;32:665–668.

413. Salhab N, Jones DJ, Bos JL, et al. Detection of ras gene alterations and ras proteins in colorectal cancer. Dis Colon Rectum 1989;32:659–664.

414. Mizoguchi T, Yamada K, Furukawa T, et al. Expression of the MDR1 gene in human gastric and colorectal carcinomas. JNCI 1990;82:1679–1683.

415. Murnane MJ, Sheahan K, Ozdemirli M, et al. Stage-specific increases in cathepsin B messenger RNA content in human colorectal carcinoma. Cancer Res 1991;51:1137–1142.

416. Kern SE, Fearon ER, Tersmette KWF, et al. Allelic loss in colorectal carcinoma. JAMA 1989;261:3099–3103.

417. Scott N, Sagar P, Stewart J, et al. p53 in colorectal cancer: Clinicopathological correlation and prognostic significance. Br J Cancer 1991;63:317–319.

418. Cohn KH, Wang F, DeSoto-LaPaiz F, et al. Association of nm23-H1 allelic deletions with distant metastases in colorectal carcinoma. Lancet 1991;338:722–724.

419. Liu C, Woo A, Tsao MS. Expression of transforming growth factor-alpha in primary human colon and lung carcinomas. Br J Cancer 1990;62:425–429.

420. Steele RJ, Kelly P, Ellul B, et al. Epidermal growth factor receptor expression in colorectal cancer. Br J Surg 1990;77:1352–1354.

421. Gold P, Freeman SO. Specific carcinoembryonic antigens of the human digestive system. J Exp Med 1965;122:467–481.

422. Ahnen DJ, Nakane PK, Brown WR. Ultrastructural localization of carcinoembryonic antigen in normal intestine and colon cancer: Abnormal distribution of CEA on the surface of colon cancer cells. Cancer 1982;49:2077–2090.

423. Primus FJ, Kuhns WJ, Goldenberg DM. Immunological heterogeneity or carcinoembryonic antigen: Immunohistochemical detection of carcinoembryonic determinants in colonic tumors with monoclonal antibodies. Cancer Res 1983;43:693–701.

424. Herlyn M, Blaszczyk M, Sears HF, et al. Detection of carcinoembryonic antigen and related antigens in sera of patients with gastrointestinal tumors using monoclonal antibodies in double-determinant radioimmunoassays. Hybridoma 1983;2:329–339.

425. Wiley EL, Murphy P, Mendelson D, et al. Distribution of blood group substances in normal human colon. Am J Clin Pathol 1981;76:806–809.

426. Ernst C, Thurin J, Atkinson B. Monoclonal antibody localization of A and B isoantigens in normal and malignant fixed human tissues. Am J Pathol 1984;117:451–461.

427. Schoentag R, Primus FJ, Kuhns W. ABH and Lewis blood group expression in colorectal carcinoma. Cancer Res 1987;47:1695–1700.

428. Compton C, Wyatt R, Konugres A, et al. Immunohistochemical studies of blood group substance H in colorectal tumors using a monoclonal antibody. Cancer 1987;59:118–127.

429. Itzkowitz SH, Yuan M, Ferrell LD, et al. Cancer-associated alterations of blood group antigen expression in human colorectal polyps. Cancer Res 1986;46:5976–5984.

430. Hakomori S. Blood group glycolipid antigens and their modifications as human cancer antigens. Am J Clin Pathol 1984;82:635–648.

431. Abe K, Hakomori S, Ohshiba S. Differential expression of difucosyl type II chain (Eey) defined by monoclonal antibody AH6 in different locations of colonic epithelia, various histological types of colonic polyps and adenocarcinomas. Cancer Res 1986;46: 2639–2644.

432. Sakamoto J, Furukawa K, Cordon-Cardo C, et al. Expression of Lewis A, Lewis B, X, Y blood group antigens in human colonic tumors and normal tissue in human tumor-derived cell lines. Cancer Res 1986;46:1553–1561.

433. Itzkowitz SH, Yuan M, Fukushi Y, et al. Lewis X- and sialylated Lewis X-related antigen expression in human malignant and non-malignant colonic tissues. Cancer Res 1986;46:2627–2632.

434. Koprowski H, Steplewski Z, Mitchell K, et al. Colorectal carcinoma antigens detected by hybridoma antibodies. Somatic Cell Mol Genet 1979;5:957–972.

435. Magnani JL, Nilsson B, Brockhaus M, et al. A monoclonal antibody-defined antigen associated with gastrointestinal cancer is a ganglioside containing sialylated lacto-N-fucopentose. J Biol Chem 1982;257:14365–14369.

436. Atkinson BF, Ernst CS, Herlyn M, et al. Gastrointestinal cancer-associated antigen in immunoperoxidase assay. Cancer Res 1982;42:4820–4823.

437. Herlyn D, Herlyn M, Steplewski Z, et al. Monoclonal antibodies in cell mediated cytotoxicity against human melanoma and colorectal carcinoma. Eur J Immunol 1979;9:657–659.

438. Herlyn D, Steplewski Z, Herlyn M, et al. Inhibition of growth of colorectal carcinoma in nude mice by monoclonal antibody. Cancer Res 1980;40:717–721.

439. Johnson VG, Schlom J, Patterson AJ, et al. Analysis of a human tumor associated glycoprotein (TAG-72) identified by monoclonal antibody B72-3. Cancer Res 1986;46: 850–857.

440. Lottich SC, Szpak CA, Johnston WW, et al. Phenotypic heterogeneity of a tumor-associated antigen in adenocarcinomas of the colon and their metastases as demonstrated by monoclonal antibody b72.3. Cancer Invest 1986;4(5):387–395.

441. Lambert R, Sobin LH, Waye JD, et al. The management of patients with colorectal adenomas. CA 1984;34:167–176.

442. Wegener M, Borsch G, Schmidt G. Colorectal adenomas: Distribution. Incidence of malignant transformation, and rate of recurrence. Dis Colon Rectum 1986;29:383–387.

443. Neugut AI, Johnsen CM, Forde KA, et al. Recurrence rates for colorectal polyps. Cancer 1985;55:1586–1589.

444. Nava H, Carlsson G, Petrelli NJ, et al. Follow-up colonoscopy in patients with colorectal adenomatous polyps. Dis Colon Rectum 1987;30:465–468.

445. Nivatvongs S, Nicholson JD, Rothenberger DA, et al. Villous adenomas of the rectum: The accuracy of clinical assessment. Surgery 1980;87:549–551.

446. Taylor EW, Thompson H, Oates GD, et al. Limitations of biopsy in reoperative assessment of villous papilloma. Dis Colon Rectum 1981;24:259–262.

447. Groff W, Rubin RJ, Salvati EP, et al. A method of management of a circumferential villous tumor of the rectum. Dis Colon Rectum 1981;24:151–154.

448. Pello MJ. Transanal excision of large sessile villous adenomas using an endorectal traction flap. Surg Gynecol Obstet 1987;164:281–279.

449. Corman ML, Prager ED, Hardy TG, et al. Comparison of the valtrac biofragmentable anastomosis ring with conventional suture and stapled anastomosis in colon surgery: Results of a prospective, randomized clinical trial. Dis Colon Rectum 1989;32:183–187.

450. Jagelman DG. Choice of operation in familial adenomatous polyposis. World J Surg 1991;15:47–49.

451. Bess MA, Adson MA, Elveback LR, et al. Rectal cancer following colectomy for polyposis. Arch Surg 1980;115:460–467.

452. Heimann TM, Gelernt I, Salky B, et al. Familial polyposis coli: Results of mucosal proctectomy with ileoanal anastomosis. Dis Colon Rectum 1987;30:424–427.

453. Herrera-Irbelas L. Familial polyposis coli. Seminars in Surgical Oncology 1987;3: 66–139.

454. Kewenter J, Hulten L, Ahren C. The occurrence of severe epithelial dysplasia and its bearing on treatment of longstanding ulcerative colitis. Ann Surg 1982;195:209–213.

455. Nugent FW, Haggitt RC, Colcher H, et al. Malignant potential of chronic ulcerative colitis. Gastroenterology 1979;76:1–5.

456. Lennard-Jones JE, Morson BC, Ritchie JK, et al. Cancer and colitis: Assessment of the individual risk by clinical and histological criteria. Gastroenterology 1977;73: 1280–1289.

457. Lennard-Jones JE. Cancer risk in ulcerative colitis: Surveillance or surgery? Br J Surg 1985;72:S84–S86.

458. Rosenstock E, Farmer RG, Petras R, et al. Surveillance for colonic carcinoma in ulcerative colitis. Gastroenterology 1985;89:1342–1346.

459. Wong WD, Rothenberger DA, Goldberg SA. Ileoanal pouch procedures. Curr Probl Surg 1985;22:1–78.

460. Taylor BA, Dozois RR. The J ileal pouch-anal anastomosis. World J Surg 1987;11: 727–734.

461. Enker WE, Laffer UT, Block GE. Enhanced survival of patients with colon and rectal cancer is based upon wide anatomic resection. Ann Surg 1979;190:350–360.

462. Grinnell RS. Results of ligation of inferior mesenteric artery at the aorta in resections of carcinoma of the descending and sigmoid colon and rectum. Surg Gynecol Obstet 1965;120:1031–1036.

463. Ault GW. A technique for cancer isolation and extended dissection for cancer of the distal colon and rectum. Surg Gynecol Obstet 1958;106:467–477.

464. Cole WH, Roberts SS, Strehl FW. Modern concepts of cancer of the colon and rectum. Cancer 1966;19:1347–1358.

465. Wiggers T, Jeekel J, Arends JW, et al. No-touch isolation technique in colon cancer: A controlled prospective trial. Br J Surg 1988;75:409–415.

466. Cohn I Jr, Gonzalez EA Jr, Atik M. Spillage and recurrence of colonic carcinoma. Surg Forum 1961;12:153–155.

467. Cohn I Jr, Floyd CE, Atik M. Control of tumor implantation during operations on the colon. Ann Surg 1963;157:825–838.

468. Cohn I Jr, Corley RG, Floyd CE. Iodized suture for control of tumor implantation in a colon anastomosis. Surg Gynecol Obstet 1963;116:366–370.

469. Douglass HO Jr, LeVeen HH. Tumor recurrence in colon anastomoses: Prevention by coagulation and fixation with formalin. Ann Surg 1971;173:201–205.

470. MacKeigan JM, Ferguson JA. Prophylactic oophorectomy in colorectal cancer in pre-menopausal patients. Dis Colon Rectum 1979;22:401–405.

471. Cutait R, Lesser ML, Enker WE. Prophylactic oophorectomy in surgery for large bowel cancer. Dis Colon Rectum 1983;26:6–11.

472. Graffner HOL, Alm POA, Oscarson JEA. Prophylactic oophorectomy in colorectal carcinoma. Am J Surg 1983;146:233–235.

473. O'Brien PH, Newton BB, Metcalf JS, et al. Oophorectomy in women with carcinoma of the colon and rectum. Surg Gynecol Obstet 1981;153:827–830.

474. Wolmark N, Gordon PH, Fisher B, et al. A comparison of stapled and hand-sewn anastomoses in patients undergoing resection of Duke's B and C colorectal cancer: An analysis of disease-free survival and survival from the NSABP prospective trials. Dis Colon Rectum 1986;29:344–350.

475. Gastrointestinal Tumor Study Group. Adjuvant therapy of colon cancer: Results of a prospectively randomized trial. Gastrointestinal tumor study group. N Engl J Med 1984;310:737–743.

476. Willett CG, Tepper JE, Cohen AM, et al. Failure patterns following curative resection of colonic carcinoma. Ann Surg 1984;200:685–690.

477. Russell AH, Pelton J, Reheis CE, et al. Adenocarcinoma of the colon: An autopsy study with implications for new therapeutic strategies. Cancer 1985;56:1446–1451.

478. Willett C, Tepper JE, Cohen AM, et al. Local failure following curative resection of colonic adenocarinoma. Int J Radiat Oncol Biol Phys 1984;10:645–651.

479. Welch JP, Donaldson GA. The clinical correlation of an autopsy study of recurrent colorectal cancer. Ann Surg 1979;189:496–502.

480. Enker WE, Dragacevic S. Multiple carcinomas of the large bowel. Ann Surg 1978;187:8–11.

481. Langevin JM, Nivatvongs S. The true incidence of synchronous cancer of the large bowel. Am J Surg 1984;147:330–333.

482. Isler JJ, Brown PC, Lewis FG. The role of preoperative colonoscopy in colorectal cancer. Dis Colon Rectum 1987;30:435–439.

483. Kelly WE Jr, Brown PW, Lawrence W, et al. Penetrating, obstructing, and perforating carcinomas of the colon and rectum. Arch Surg 1985;116:381–384.

484. Gall FP, Tonak J, Altendorf A. Multivisceral resections in colorectal cancer. Dis Colon Rectum 1987;30:337–341.

485. Hunter JA, Ryan JA Jr, Schultz P. En bloc resection of colon cancer adherent to other organs. Am J Surg 1987;154:67–71.

486. Wolff WI, Shinya H. Definitive treatment of "malignant" polyps of the colon. Ann Surg 1975;182:516–524.

487. Gordon MS, Cohen AM. Management of invasive carcinoma in pedunculated colorectal polyps. Oncology 1989;3:99–105.

488. Wilcox GM, Beck JR. Early invasive cancer in adenomatous colonic polyps: Evaluation of the therapeutic options by decision analysis. Gastroenterology 1987;92:1159–1168.

489. Cranley JP, Petras RE, Carey WD, et al. When is endoscopic polypectomy adequate therapy for colonic polyps containing invasive carcinoma? Gastroenterology 1987;91:419–427.

490. Wilcox JM, Anderson PB, Colacchio TA. Early invasive carcinoma in colonic polyps: A review of the literature with emphasis on the assessment of the risk of metastasis. Cancer 1986;57:160–171.

491. Haggitt RC, Glotzbach RE, Soffer EE, et al. Prognostic factors in colorectal carcinomas arising in adenomas: Implications for lesions removed by endoscopic polypectomy. Gastroenterology 1985;89:328–336.

492. Bartnik W, Burtuk E, Orlowska J. A conservative approach to adenomas containing invasive carcinoma removed colonoscopically. Dis Colon Rectum 1985;28:673–675.

493. Colacchio TA, Forde KA, Scantlebury VP. Endoscopic polypectomy: Inadequate treatment for invasive colorectal carcinoma. Ann Surg 1981;194:704–707.

494. Gunderson LL, Sosin H, Levitt S. Extrapelvic colon—areas of failure in a reoperation series: Implications for adjuvant therapy. Int J Radiat Oncol Biol Phys 1985;11:731–741.

495. Meek AG, Lam WC, Order SE. Carcinoma of the colon: Irradiation by delayed split whole-abdominal technique. Radiology 1983;148:845–849.

496. Brenner HJ, Bibi C, Chaitchik S. Adjuvant therapy for Dukes' C adenocarcinoma of the colon. Int J Radiat Oncol Biol Phys 1983;9:1789–1792.

497. Ghossein NA, Samala EC, Alpert S, et al. Elective postoperative radiotherapy after incomplete resection of colorectal cancer. Dis Colon Rectum 1981;24:252–256.

498. Fabian CJ, Reddy E, Jewell W, et al. Phase I-II pilot of AU whole abdomen radiation and concomitant 5-FU as an adjuvant in colon cancer: A Southwest Oncology Group Study. Int J Radiat Oncol Biol Phys 1988;15:885–892.

499. Patanaphan V, Salazar OM, Slawson RG, et al. A phase I/II trial of whole-abdominal plus pelvic irridation for Astler-Coller stage B2/C colorectal cancer. Am J Clin Oncol 1988;11:60–65.

500. Duttenhaver JR, Hoskins RB, Gunderson LL, et al. Adjuvant postoperative radiation therapy in the management of adenocarcinoma of the colon. Cancer 1986;57:955–963.

501. Willett CG, Tepper JE, Shellito PC, et al. Indications for adjuvant radiotherapy in extrapelvic colonic carcinoma. Oncology 1989;3:25–33.

502. Dixon WJ, Longmire WP Jr, Holden WD. Use of triethylenethiophosphomamide as adjuvant to the surgical treatment of gastric and colorectal cancer: Ten year follow-up. Ann Surg 1971;173:26–39.

503. Dwight RW, Humphrey EW, Higgins GA, et al. FUDR as an adjuvant to surgery in cancer of the large bowel. J Surg Oncol 1973;5:243–249.

504. Grage TB, Moss SE. Adjuvant chemotherapy in cancer of the colon and rectum: Demonstration of effectiveness of prolonged 5-FU chemotherapy in a prospectively controlled randomized trial. Surg Clin North Am 1981;61:1321–1329.

505. Higgins GA, Lee LE, Dwight RW, et al. The case for adjuvant 5-fluorouracil in colorectal cancer. Cancer Clin Trials 1978;1:35–41.

506. Rex DK, Lehman GA, Lappas JC, et al. Sensitivity of double contrast barium study for left colon polyps. Radiology 1986;158:69–72.

507. Macdonald JS. Adjuvant therapy of gastrointestinal cancer. In: Salmon SE, ed. Adjuvant therapy of cancer V. New York: Grune & Stratton, 1987:479–496.

508. Higgins GA, Amadeo JH, McElhinney J, et al. Efficacy of prolonged intermittent therapy with combined 5-fluorouracil and me-CCNU following resection for carcinoma of the large bowel. Cancer 1984;53:1–8.

509. Wolmark N, Fisher B, Rockette H, et al. Postoperative adjuvant chemotherapy or BCG for colon cancer: Results from NSABP protocol C-01. JNCI 1988;80:30–36.

510. Laurie JA, Moertel CG, Fleming TR, et al. Surgical adjuvant therapy of large-bowel carcinoma: An evaluation of levamisole and the combination of levamisole and fluorouracil. J Clin Oncol 1989;7:1447–1456.

511. Gastrointestinal Tumor Study Group. Adjuvant therapy of colon cancer: Results of a prospectively randomized trial. N Engl J Med 1984;310:737–743.

512. Abdi E, Harbora D, Hanson J, et al. Adjuvant chemoimmuno-and immunotherapy in stage B2 and C colorectal cancer. Proc Am Soc Clin Oncol 1987;6:93.

513. Panettiere FJ, Goodman PJ, Costanzi JJ, et al. Adjuvant therapy in large bowel adenocarcinoma: Long-term results of a Southwest Oncology Group study. J Clin Oncol 1988;6:947–954.

514. Mansour EG, MacIntyre JW, Johnson R, et al. Adjuvant studies in colorectal carcinoma: Experience of the Eastern Cooperative Oncology Group (ECOG)—preliminary report. In: Gerard A, ed. Progress and perspectives in the treatment of gastrointestinal tumors. New York: Pergamon Press, 1981.

515. Boice JD, Greene MH, Killen JY Jr, et al. Leukemia and pre-leukemia after adjuvant treatment of gastrointestinal cancer with semustine (methyl-CCNU). N Engl J Med 1983;309:1079–1083.

516. Stevenson HC, Green I, Hamilton JM, et al. Levamisole: known effects on the immune system, clinical results and future applications to the treatment of cancer. J Clin Oncol 1991;9:2052–2066.

517. Bedikian AY, Valdivieso M, Mavligit GM, et al. Sequential chemoimmunotherapy of colorectal cancer: Evaluation of methotrexate, Baker's antifol and levamisole. Cancer 1978;42:2169–2176.

518. Buroker TR, Moertel CG, Fleming TR, et al. A controlled evaluation of recent approaches to biochemical modulation of enhancement of 5-fluorouracil therapy in colorectal carcinoma. J Clin Oncol 1985;3:1624–1631.

519. Mansour EG, Cnaan A, Davis T, et al. Combined modality therapy following resection of colorectal carcinoma in patients with non-measurable intra-abdominal metastases. An ECOG study 3282. Proc Am Soc Clin Oncol 1990;9:107.

520. Verhaegen H, DeCree J, DeCock W, et al. Levamisole therapy in patients with colorectal cancer. In: Terry WD, Rosenberg SA, eds. Immunotherapy of human cancer. New York: Excerpta Medica, 1982:225–230.

521. Chlebowski RT, Nystrom S, Reynolds R, et al. Long-term survival following levamisole or placebo adjuvant treatment of colorectal cancer: A Western Oncology Group trial. Oncology 1988;45:141–143.

522. Arnaud JP, Buyse M, Nordlinger B, et al. Adjuvant therapy of poor prognosis colon cancer with levamisole: Results of an EORTC double-blind randomized clinical trial. Br J Surg 1989;76:284–289.

523. Sertoli MR, Guarneri D, Rubagotti A, et al. Adjuvant immunochemotherapy in colorectal cancer Dukes' C. Oncology 1987;44:78–81.

524. Bancewicz J, Macpherson SG, McVie JG, et al. Adjuvant chemotherapy and immunotherapy for colorectal cancer: Preliminary communication. J R Soc Med 1980;73:197–199.

525. Windle R, Bell PRF, Shaw D. Five year results of a randomized trial of adjuvant 5-fluorouracil and levamisole in colorectal cancer. Br J Surg 1987;74:569–572.

526. Moertel CG, Fleming TR, Macdonald JS, et al. Levamisole and fluorouracil for adjuvant therapy of resected colon carcinoma. N Engl J Med 1990;322:352–358.

526a. Moertel CG, Fleming TR, Macdonald J, Haller D. The Intergroup study of fluorouracil (5-FU) plus levamisole (LEV) and levamisole alone as adjuvant therapy for stage C colon cancer: A final report. Proc Am Soc Clin Oncol 1992;11:161.

527. Grem JL, Allegra CJ. Toxicity of levamisole and 5-fluorouracil in human colon carcinoma cells. JNCI 1989;81:1413–1417.

528. Hoover HC, Surdyke MG, Brandhorst JS, et al. Five year follow-up of a controlled trial of active specific immunotherapy in colorectal cancer. Proc Am Soc Clin Oncol 1990;9:106.

529. Pestana C, Reitemeyer RJ, Moertel CG, et al. The natural history of carcinoma of the colon and rectum. Am J Surg 1964;108:826–829.

530. Fisher ER, Turnbull RB Jr. The cytologic demonstration and significance of tumor cells in the mesenteric venous blood in patients with colorectal carcinoma. Surg Gynecol Obstet 1955;100:102–108.

531. Taylor I, Machin D, Mullee M, et al. A randomized controlled trial of adjuvant portal vein cytotoxic perfusion in colorectal cancer. Br J Surg 1985;72:359–362.

532. Gray BN, deZwart J, Fisher R, et al. The Australia and New Zealand Trial of adjuvant chemotherapy in colon cancer. In: Salmon SE, ed. Adjuvant therapy of cancer V. New York: Grune & Stratton, 1987:537–554.

533. Metzger U, Mermillod B, Aeberhard P, et al. Intraportal chemotherapy in colorectal carcinoma as an adjuvant modality. World J Surg 1987;11:452–458.

534. Metzger U, Laffer U, Castiglione M, et al. Adjuvant intraportal chemotherapy for colorectal cancer: 4 year results of the randomized Swiss study. Proc Am Soc Clin Oncol 1989;8:105.

535. Wereldsma JCJ, Bruggink ERM, Meijer WS, et al. Adjuvant portal liver infusion in colorectal cancer with 5-fluorouracil/heparin versus urokinase versus control: Results of a prospective randomized clinical trial (colorectal adenocarcinoma trial I). Cancer 1990;65:425–432.

536. Beart RW Jr, Moertel CG, Wieand HS, et al. Adjuvant therapy for resectable colorectal carcinoma with fluorouracil administered by portal vein infusion. Arch Surg 1990;125:897–901.

537. Wolmark N, Rockette H, Wickerham DL, et al. Adjuvant therapy of Dukes' A, B, and C adenocarcinoma of the colon with portal-vein fluorouracil hepatic infusion: Preliminary results of national surgical adjuvant breast and bowel project protocol C-02. J Clin Oncol 1990;8:1466–1475.

538. Kievit J, van de Velde CJH. Utility and cost of carcinoembryonic antigen monitoring in colon cancer follow-up evaluation: A Markov analysis. Cancer 1990;65:2580–2587.

539. Hine KR, Dykes PW. Prospective randomized trial of early cytotoxic therapy for recurrent colorectal carcinoma detected by serum CEA. Gut 1984;25:682–688.

540. Martin EW Jr, Minton JP, Carey LC. CEA-directed second-look surgery in the asymptomatic patient after primary resection of colorectal cancer. Ann Surg 1985;202:310–317.

541. Martin EW Jr, Cooperman M, King G, et al. A retrospective and prospective study of serial CEA determinations in the early detection of recurrent colorectal cancer. Am J Surg 1979;137:167–169.

542. Martin EW Jr, Cooperman M, Carey LC, et al. Sixty second-look procedures indicated primarily by rise in serial carcinoembryonic antigen. J Surg Res 1980;28:389–394.

543. Attiyeh FF, Stearns MW. Second-look laparotomy based on CEA elevations in colorectal cancer. Cancer 1981;47:2119–2125.

544. Staab HJ, Anderer FA, Stumpf E, et al. Eighty-four second look operations based on sequential carcinoembryonic antigen determinations and clinical investigations in patients with recurrent gastrointestinal cancer. Am J Surg 1985;179:198–204.

545. Minton JP, James KK, Hurtubise PE, et al. The use of serial carcinoembryonic antigen determinations to predict recurrence of carcinoma of the colon and the time for a second-look operation. Surg Gynecol Obstet 1978;147:208–210.

546. Steele G Jr, Zamcheck N, Mayer R, et al. Results of CEA-initiated second-look surgery for recurrent colorectal cancer. Am J Surg 1980;139:544–548.

547. Wilking N, Petrelli NJ, Herrera L, et al. Abdominal exploration for suspected recurrent carcinoma of the colon and rectum based upon elevated carcinoembryonic antigen alone or in combination with other methods. Surg Gynecol Obstet 1986;162:465–468.

548. Sandler RS, Freund DA, Herbst CA Jr, et al. Cost effectiveness of postoperative carcinoembryonic antigen monitoring in colorectal cancer. Cancer 1984;53:193–198.

549. August DA, Ottow RT, Surgarbaker PH. Clinical perspective of human colorectal cancer metastasis. Cancer Metastasis 1984;3:303–324.

550. Northover J, Slack WW. A randomized controlled trial of CEA-prompted second look surgery in recurrent colorectal cancer: A preliminary report. Dis Colon Rectum 1984;27:576.

551. Beatty JD, Duda RB, Williams LE, et al. Preoperative imaging of colorectal carcinoma with indium 111-labelled anticarcinoembryonic antigen monoclonal antibody. Cancer Res 1986;46:6494–6502.

552. Martin DT, Hinkel GH, Tuttle S, et al. Intraoperative radio immunodetection of colorectal tumor with a hand-held radiation detector. Am J Surg 1985;150:672–675.

553. Lyden MJ, Thompson CH, Liechtenstein M, et al. Visualization of metastases from colon carcinoma by an iodine 131-radio-labeled monoclonal antibody. Cancer 1986;57:1135–1139.

554. Begent RHJ, Keep PA, Searle F, et al. Radioimmunolocalization and selection for surgery in recurrent colorectal cancer. Br J Surg 1986;73:64–67.

555. Cohen AM, Martin EW, Lavery I, et al. Radioimmunoguided surgery using iodine 125 B72.3 in patients with colorectal cancer. Arch Surg 1991;126:349–352.

556. Dawson PM, Blair SD, Begent RHJ, et al. The value of radioimmunoguided surgery in first and second look laparotomy for colorectal cancer. Dis Colon Rectum 1991;34:217–222.

557. Doerr RJ, Abdel-Nabi H, Krag D, et al. Radiolabeled antibody imaging in the management of colorectal cancer: Results of a multicenter clinical study. Ann Surg 1991;214:118–124.

558. Heidelberger CG, Chandhari NK, Dannenberg P, et al. Fluorinated pyrimidines: A new class of tumor inhibitory compounds. Nature 1969;179:665–666.

559. Carter SK. Large bowel cancer: The current status of treatment. JNCI 1976;56:3–10.

560. Moertel CG, Reitemeyer RJ. In: Advanced gastrointestinal cancer: Clinical management and chemotherapy. New York: Harper & Row, 1969.

561. Moertel CG. Large bowel. In: Holland JF, Frei E, eds. Cancer medicine. Philadelphia: Lea & Febiger, 1973:1497–1626.

562. Ansfield F, Klotz J, Nealon T, et al. A phase III study comparing the clinical utility of four regimens of 5-fluorouracil. Cancer 1977;39:34–40.

563. Moertel CG. Clinical management of advanced gastrointestinal cancer. Cancer 1975;36:675.

564. Christophidis N, Vajda FJE, Lucas I, et al. Fluorouracil therapy in patients with carcinoma of the large bowel: A pharmacokinetic comparison of various rates and routes of administration. Clin Pharmacokinet 1978;3:330–336.

565. Bateman J, Irwin L, Pugh R, et al. Comparison of intravenous and oral administration of 5-fluorouracil for colorectal carcinoma. Proc Am Assoc Cancer Res 1975;16:242.

566. Hahn RG, Moertel CG, Shutt AJ, et al. A double-blind comparison of intensive course 5-FU by oral vs. intravenous route in the treatment of colon carcinoma. Cancer 1975;35:1031–1036.

567. Lokich J, Bothe A, Fine N, et al. Phase I study of protracted venous infusion of 5-fluorouracil. Cancer 1981;48:2565–2568.

568. Seifert P, Baker LH, Reed MD, et al. Comparison of continuously infused 5-fluorouracil with bolus injection in treatment of patients with colorectal adenocarcinoma. Cancer 1975;36:123–128.

569. Caballero GA, Ausman RK, Quebbeman EJ. Long-term, ambulatory, continuous intravenous infusion of 5-fluorouracil for treatment of advanced adenocarcinoma. Cancer Treat Rep 1985;69:13–15.

570. Lokich J, Gillings D, Gallo J, et al. Bolus versus infusion 5-fluorouracil (5-FU): A randomized clinical trial in advanced measurable colorectal cancer. Proc Am Soc Clin Oncol 1986;5:83.

571. Lokich JJ, Moor C. Chemotherapy associated palmar-plantar erythrodysesthesia syndrome. Ann Intern Med 1984;101:798–800.

572. Quebbeman E, Ausman R, Hansen R, et al. Long-term ambulatory treatment of metastatic colorectal adenocarcinoma by continuous intravenous infusion of 5-fluorouracil. J Surg Oncol 1985;30:60-65.

573. Wade JL, Herbst S, Greenburg A. Prolonged venous infusion (PVI) of 5-fluorouracil (5-FU) for metastatic colon cancer. Proc Am Soc Clin Oncol 1986;5:88.

574. Benedetto P, Davila E, Solomon J. Chronic continuous systemic infusion of 5-fluorouracil (CCI-5-FU) in the treatment of metastatic colorectal carcinoma (CCA). Proc Am Soc Clin Oncol 1984;3:142.

575. Hansen E, Quebbeman R, Ausman R, et al. Continuous 5-fluorouracil (5-FU) infusion in colorectal cancer: Update of the MCW experience. Proc Am Soc Clin Oncol 1987;6:80.

576. Belt RJ, Davidner ML, Myron MC, et al. Continuous low dose 5-fluorouracil (5-FU) for adenocarcinoma: Confirmation of activity. Proc Am Soc Clin Oncol 1985;4:90.

577. Leichman L, Seichman CG, Kinzie J, et al. Long term low dose 5-fluorouracil (5-FU) in advanced measurable colon cancer: No correlation between toxicity and efficacy. Proc Am Soc Clin Oncol 1985;4:86.

578. Lokich JJ, Ahlgren JD, Gullo JJ, et al. A prospective randomized comparison of continuous infusion fluorouracil with a conventional bolus schedule in metastatic colorectal carcinoma: A mid-Atlantic oncology program study. J Clin Oncol 1989;7:425-432.

579. Weinerman B, Shah A, Fields A, et al. A randomized trial of continuous systemic infusion versus bolus therapy with 5-fluorouracil in metastatic measurable colorectal cancer. Proc Am Soc Clin Oncol 1990;9:103.

580. Leichman CG, Leichman L, Spears CP, et al. Phase II study of prolonged infusion 5-fluorouracil with weekly leucovorin in disseminated colorectal cancer. Proc Am Soc Clin Oncol 1991;10:143.

581. Niederhuber JE, Ensminger W, Gyves J, et al. Regional chemotherapy of colorectal cancer metastatic to the liver. Cancer 1984;53:1336–1343.

582. Balch CM, Urist MM, Soong SJ, et al. A prospective phase II clinical trial of continuous FUDR regional chemotherapy colorectal metastases to the liver using a totally implantable pump. Ann Surg 1991;198(5):567–573.

583. Kemeny N, Daly J, Oderman P, et al. Hepatic artery pump infusion toxicity and results in patients with metastatic colorectal carcinoma. J Clin Oncol 1984;2:595–600.

584. Weiss GR, Barneck MB, Osteen RT, et al. Long-term hepatic arterial infusion of 5-fluorodeoxyuridine for liver metastases using an implantable infusion pump. J Clin Oncol 1983;1:337–344.

585. Shepard KV, Levin B, Karl RC, et al. Therapy for metastatic colorectal cancer with hepatic artery infusion chemotherapy using a subcutaneous implanted pump. J Clin Oncol 1985;3:161–169.

586. Chang AE, Schneider PD, Sugarbaker PH, et al. A prospective randomized trial of regional vs systemic continuous 5-FU chemotherapy in the treatment of colorectal metastases. Ann Surg 1987;206:685–693.

587. Hohn DC, Stagg RJ, Friedman MA, et al. A randomized trial of continuous intravenous versus hepatic intraarterial floxuridine in patients with colorectal cancer metastatic to the liver: The Northern California oncology group trial. J Clin Oncol 1989;7:1646–1654.

588. Martin JK, O'Connell MJ, Wieand HS, et al. Intra-arterial floxuridine vs systemic fluorouracil for hepatic metastases from colorectal cancer. Arch Surg 1990;125:1022–1027.

589. Kemeny N, Daly J, Reichman B, et al. Intrahepatic or systemic infusion of fluorodeoxyuridine in patients with liver metastases from colorectal carcinoma: A randomized trial. Ann Intern Med 1987;107:459–465.

590. Rougier P, Hay JM, Olivier JM, et al. A controlled multicentric trial of intrahepatic artery chemotherapy vs. standard palliative treatment for colorectal liver metastases. Proc Am Soc Clin Oncol 1990;9:104.

591. Hohn DC, Melnick J, Stagg R, et al. Biliary sclerosis in patients receiving hepatic arterial infusions of floxuridine. J Clin Oncol 1985;3:98–102.

592. Shepard KV, Levin B, Faintuch J, et al. Hepatitis in patients receiving intra-arterial chemotherapy for metastatic colorectal carcinoma. Am J Clin Oncol 1987;10:36–41.

593. Chuang VP, Wallace S, Stroehlein J, et al. Hepatic artery infusion chemotherapy: Gastroduodenal complications. Am J Radiol 1981;137:347–357.

594. Shike M, Scott-Gillin J, Kemeny N, et al. Severe gastroduodenal ulcerations complicating hepatic artery infusion chemotherapy for metastatic colon cancer. Am J Gastroenterol 1986;81:176–181.

595. Doria MI, Shepard KV, Levin B, et al. Liver pathology following hepatic arterial infusion chemotherapy. Cancer 1986;58:855–861.

596. Shea WJ, Demas BE, Goldberg HI, et al. Sclerosing cholangitis associated with hepatic

arterial FUDR chemotherapy: Radiographic-histologic correlation. AJR 1986;146: 717–724.

597. Moertel CG. Therapy of advanced gastrointestinal cancer with the nitrosoureas. Cancer Chemother 1973;3–4:27.

598. Macdonald JS, Neefe J. Chemotherapy in the management of gastrointestinal cancer. Abdom Surg 1979;21:126–131.

599. Moertel CG. Chemotherapy of gastrointestinal cancer. N Engl J Med 1978;299:1049–1052.

600. O'Connell M, Wieand H, Krook J, et al. Lack of value for methyl CCNU as a component of effective rectal cancer surgical adjuvant therapy. Interim analysis of intergroup protocol 86-47-51. Proc Am Soc Clin Oncol 1991;10:134.

601. Weaver D, Lindblad AS. Radiation therapy and 5-fluorouracil (5-FU) with or without MeCCNU for the treatment of patients with surgically adjuvant adenocarcinoma of the rectum. Proc Am Soc Clin Oncol [Abstract] 1990;9:409.

602. Wasserman TH, Comis RL, Goldsmith M, et al. Tabular analysis of clinical chemotherapy of solid tumors. Cancer Chemother Rep 1975;6:399.

603. Rowinsky EK, Cazenave LA, Donehower RC. Taxol: A novel investigational antimicrotubule agent. JNCI 1990;82:1247–1259.

604. Shimada Y, Yoshino M, Wakui A, et al. Phase II study of CPT-11: A new camptothecin derivative. Proc Am Soc Clin Oncol 1991;10:135.

605. Giovanella BC, Stehlin JS, Wall ME, et al. DNA topoisomerase I-targeted chemotherapy of human colon cancer in xenografts. Science 1989;246:1046–1048.

606. Pastan I, Gottesman M. Multiple-drug resistance in human cancer. N Engl J Med 1987;316:1388–1393.

607. Myers C, Cowan K, Sinha B, et al. The phenomenon of pleiotropic drug resistance. In: Devita VT, Hellman S, Rosenberg SA, eds. Important advances in oncology 1987. Philadelphia: JB Lippincott, 1987:27–37.

608. Moertel CG, Schutt AJ, Hahn RG, et al. Therapy of advanced colorectal cancer with a combination of 5-fluorouracil, methyl 3-cis (2-chloroethyl)-1-nitrosourea and vincristine. JNCI 1975;54:69–71.

609. Posey L, Morgan LR. Methyl CCNU versus methyl CCNU and 5-fluorouracil in carcinoma of the large bowel. Cancer Treat Rep 1977;61:1453–1458.

610. Baker LH, Talley RW, Matter R, et al. Phase III comparison of the treatment of advanced gastrointestinal cancer with bolus weekly 5-FU vs. methyl-CCNU plus bolus weekly 5-FU: A Southwest Oncology Group study. Cancer 1976;38:1–7.

611. Falkson G, Falkson HC. Fluorouracil, methyl-CCNU, and vincristine in cancer of the colon. Cancer 1976;38:1468–1470.

612. Macdonald JS, Kisner DF, Smythe T, et al. 5-Fluorouracil (5-FU), methyl-CCNU and vincristine in the treatment of advanced colorectal cancer: Phase II study utilizing weekly 5-FU. Cancer Treat Rep 1976;60:1597.

613. Kemeny N, Yagoda A, Braun D Jr, et al. Randomized study of 2 different schedules of methyl CCNU, 5-FU, and vincristine for metastatic colorectal carcinoma. Cancer 1979;43:78–82.

614. Engstrom P, MacIntyre J, Douglass H Jr, et al. Combination chemotherapy of advanced bowel cancer. Proc AACR-ASCO 1978;19:384.

615. Kemeny N, Yagoda A, Braun J. Metastatic colorectal carcinoma: A prospective trial of methyl CCNU, 5-fluorouracil (5-FU) and vincristine (MOF) versus MOF plus streptozotocin (MOF-Strep). Cancer 1983;51:20–25.

616. Buroker T, Kim PN, Groppe C, et al. 5-FU infusion with mitomycin C vs. 5-FU infusion with methyl CCNU in the treatment of advanced colon cancer. Cancer 1978;42:1228–1233.

617. Ramming KP, Tesler AS, Haskell CM. Gastrointestinal tract neoplasms. In: Haskell CM, ed. Cancer treatment. Philadelphia: WB Saunders, 1980:300–301.

618. Richards FD, Case LD, White DR, et al. Combination chemotherapy (5-fluorouracil, methyl-CCNU, mitomycin C) versus 5-fluorouracil alone for advanced previously untreated colorectal carcinoma: A phase III study of the Piedmont Oncology Association. J Clin Oncol 1986;4:565–570.

619. Poon MA, O'Connell MJ, Moertel CG, et al. Biochemical modulation of fluorouracil: Evidence of significant improvement of survival and quality of life in patients with advanced colorectal carcinoma. J Clin Oncol 1989;7:1407–1418.

620. Kemeny N, Israel K, Niedzwiecki D, et al. Randomized study of continuous infusion fluorouracil versus fluorouracil plus cis-platin in patients with metastatic colorectal cancer. J Clin Oncol 1990;8:313–318.

621. Lokich J, Cantrell J, Ahlgren J, et al. A phase III trial of protracted infusional 5-FU vs. PIF plus weekly bolus cis-platin in advanced measurable colon cancer. Proc Am Soc Clin Oncol 1989;8:104.

622. Loehrer PJ, Turner S, Kubilis P, et al. A prospective randomized trial of fluorouracil versus fluorouracil plus cis-platin in the treatment of metastatic colorectal cancer: A Hoosier Oncology Group trial. J Clin Oncol 1988;6:642–648.

623. Labianca R, Pancera G, Cesana B, et al. Cis-platin + 5-fluorouracil versus 5-fluorouracil alone in advanced colorectal cancer: A randomized study. Eur J Cancer Clin Oncol 1988;24:1579–1581.

624. Diaz-Rubio E, Milla A, et al. Lack of clinical synergism between cis-platin and 5-fluorouracil in advanced colorectal cancer: Results of a randomized study. Proc Am Soc Clin Oncol 1988;7:110.

625. Bertino JR, Sawicki WL, Lindquist A, et al. Schedule dependent antitumor effects of methotrexate and 5-fluorouracil. Cancer Rev 1977;37:327–328.

626. Cadman E, Heimer R, Davis L. Enhanced 5-fluorouracil nucleotide formation after methotrexate administration: Explanation for drug synergism. Science 1979;205:1135–1137.

627. Benz C, Cadman E. Modulation of 5-fluorouracil metabolism and cytoxicity by antimetabolite pretreatment in human colorectal adenocarcinoma HCT-8. Cancer Rev 1981;41:994–999.

628. Cantrell J, Hart R, Taylor R, et al. A phase II trial of continuous infusion (CI) 5-FU

and weekly low dose cis-platin (DDP) in colorectal carcinoma. Proc Am Soc Clin Oncol 1986;5:84.

629. Mehrotra S, Rosenthal CJ, Gardner B. Biochemical modulation of antineoplastic response in colorectal carcinoma: 5-fluorouracil (F), high dose methotrexate (M) with calcium leukovorin (L) rescue (FML) in two sequences of administration. Proc Am Soc Clin Oncol 1982;1:95.

630. Kemeny NE, Ahmed T, Michaelson RA, et al. Activity of sequential low dose methotrexate and fluorouracil in advanced colorectal carcinoma: Attempt at correlation with tissue and blood levels of phosphoribosylpyrophosphate. J Clin Oncol 1984;2:311–315.

631. Mahajan SL, Ajani JA, Kanoj A, et al. Comparison of two schedules of sequential high-dose methotrexate (MTX) and 5-fluorouracil (5-FU) for metastatic colorectal carcinoma. Proc Am Soc Clin Oncol 1983;2:122.

632. Rangineni RR, Ajani JA, Bedikian AY, et al. Sequential conventional dose methotrexate (MTX) and 5-fluorouracil (5-FU) in the primary therapy of metastatic colorectal carcinoma. Proc Am Soc Clin Oncol 1983;2:125.

633. Hansen R, Ritch P, Anderson T. Sequential methotrexate (MTX), 5-fluorouracil (5-FU), and leukovorin (LCV) in colorectal cancer. Proc Am Soc Clin Oncol 1983;2:117.

634. Drapkin R, McAloon E, Lyman G. Sequential methotrexate (MTX) and 5-fluorouracil in advanced measurable colorectal cancer. Proc Am Soc Clin Oncol 1983;2:118.

635. Marsh JC, Bertino JR, Katz KH, et al. The influence of drug interval on the effect of methotrexate and fluorouracil in the treatment of advanced colorectal cancer. J Clin Oncol 1991;9:371–380.

636. Valone FH, Friedman MA, Wittlinger PS, et al. Treatment of patients with advanced colorectal carcinomas with fluorouracil alone, high-dose leucovorin plus fluorouracil, or sequential methotrexate, fluorouracil and leucovorin: A randomized trial of the Northern California oncology group. J Clin Oncol 1989;7:1427–1436.

637. Petrelli N, Herrera L, Rustum Y, et al. A prospective randomized trial of 5-fluorouracil versus 5-fluorouracil and high dose leucovorin versus 5-fluorouracil and methotrexate in previously untreated patients with advanced colorectal carcinoma. J Clin Oncol 1987;5:1559–1565.

638. Ullman B, Lee M, Martin DW, et al. Cytotoxicity of 5-fluoro-2'-deoxyuridine: Requirement for reduced folate cofactors and antagonism of methotrexate. Proc Natl Acad Sci 1978;75:980–983.

639. Evans RM, Laskin JD, Hakala MT. Effect of excess folates and deoxyinosine on the activity and site of action of 5-fluorouracil. Cancer Res 1981;41:3283–3295.

640. Houghton JA, Maroda SJ Jr, Philips JO, et al. Biochemical determinants of responsiveness to 5-fluorouracil and its derivatives in xenografts of human colorectal adenocarcinomas in mice. Cancer Res 1981;41:144–149.

641. Machover D, Schwarzenberg L, Goldschmidt E, et al. Treatment of advanced colorectal and gastric adenocarcinomas with 5-FU combined with high-dose folinic acid: A pilot study. Cancer Treat Rep 1982;66:1803–1807.

642. Greene H, Desai A, Levick S, et al. Combined 5-fluorouracil infusion and high dose folinic acid in the treatment of metastatic gastrointestinal cancer. Proc Am Soc Clin Oncol 1986;5:89.

643. Lopez AR, Van Tiburg A, Bradley T, et al. Treatment of advanced malignancy with 5-fluorouracil combined with folinic acid. Proc Am Assoc Cancer Res 1984;25:178.

644. Schmoll HJ, LeBlanc S. Sequential high dose folinic acid and 5-fluorouracil in advanced colorectal cancer with measurable, progressive disease. Proc Am Soc Clin Oncol 1985;4:94.

645. Petrelli N, Douglass HO Jr, Herrera L, et al. The modulation of fluorouracil with leucovorin in metastatic colorectal carcinoma: A prospective randomized phase III trial. J Clin Oncol 1989;7:1419–1426.

646. Nordic Gastrointestinal Tumor Adjuvant Therapy Group. Superiority of sequential methotrexate, fluorouracil and leucovorin to fluorouracil alone in advanced symptomatic colorectal carcinoma: A randomized trial. J Clin Oncol 1989;7:1437–1446.

647. Doroshaw JH, Multhauf P, Leong L, et al. Prospective randomized comparison of fluorouracil versus fluorouracil and high dose continuous infusion leucovorin calcium for the treatment of advanced measurable colorectal cancer in patients previously unexposed to chemotherapy. J Clin Oncol 1990;8:491–501.

648. Erlichman C, Fine S, Wong A, et al. A randomized trial of fluorouracil and folinic acid in patients with metastatic colorectal cancer. J Clin Oncol 1988;6:469–475.

649. Poon MA, O'Connell MJ, Wieand HS, et al. Biochemical modulation of fluorouracil with leucovorin: Confirmatory evidence of improved therapeutic efficacy in advanced colorectal cancer. J Clin Oncol 1991;9:1967–1972.

650. Kennedy P, Presant CA, Blayney D, et al. Somatostatin therapy for chemotherapy and radiotherapy related diarrhea. Proc Am Soc Clin Oncol 1990;9:324.

651. Grem JL, King SA, O'Dwyer PJ, et al. Biochemistry and clinical activity of N-(phosphonacetyl)-L-aspartate: A review. Cancer Res 1988;48:4441–4454.

652. Martin DS, Stolfi RL, Sawyer RC. Therapeutic utility of utilizing low doses of N-(phosphonacetyl)-L-aspartic acid in combination with 5-fluorouracil: A murine study with clinical relevance. Cancer Res 1998;43:2317–2321.

653. Ardalan B, Singh G, Silberman H. A randomized phase I and II study of short-term infusion of high dose fluorouracil with or without N-(phosphonacetyl)-L-aspartic acid in patients with advanced pancreatic and colorectal cancers. J Clin Oncol 1988;6:1053–1058.

654. O'Dwyer PJ, Paul AR, Walczak J, et al. Phase II study of biochemical modulation of fluorouracil by low dose PALA in patients with colorectal cancer. J Clin Oncol 1990;8:1497–1503.

655. Ardalan B, Chua L, Tian E, et al. A phase II study of weekly 24 hour infusion with high dose fluorouracil with leucovorin in colorectal carcinoma. J Clin Oncol 1991;9:625–630.

656. Ardalan B, Sridhar KS, Hussein A, et al. Double biochemical modulation of 5-fluorouracil

with phosphonacetyl-L-aspartic acid and leucovorin: A phase I study. Proc Am Soc Oncol 1990;9:104.

657. Elias L, Crissman HA. Interferon effects upon the adenocarcinoma 38 and HL-60 cell lines: Antiproliferative responses and synergistic interactions with halogenated pyrimidine antimetabolites. Cancer Res 1988;48:4868–4873.

658. Wadler S, Wersto R, Weinberg V, et al. Interaction of fluorouracil and interferon in human colon cancer cell lines: Cytotoxic and cytokinetic effects. Cancer Res 1990;50:5735–5739.

659. Elias L, Sandoval JM. Interferon effects upon fluorouracil metabolism by HL-60 cells. Biochem Biophys Res Commun 1989;163:867–874.

660. Chu E, Zinn S, Boarman D, et al. The interaction of gamma interferon and 5-fluorouracil in the H630 human colon carcinoma cell line. Cancer Res 1990;50:5834–5840.

661. Grem JL, McAtee N, Murphy RF, et al. A pilot study of interferon alfa-2a in combination with fluorouracil plus high dose leucovorin in metastatic gastrointestinal carcinoma. J Clin Oncol 1991;9:1811–1820.

662. Wadler S, Wiernik PH. Clinical update on the role of fluorouracil and recombinant interferon alfa-2a in the treatment of colorectal carcinoma. Sem in Oncol 1990;17(Suppl 1):16–21.

663. Pazdur R, Ajani JA, Patt YZ, et al. Phase II study of fluorouracil and recombinant interferon alfa-2a in previously untreated advanced colorectal carcinoma. J Clin Oncol 1990;8:2027–2031.

664. Kemeny N, Younes A, Seiter K, et al. Interferon alfa-2a and 5-fluorouracil for advanced colorectal carcinoma: Assessment of activity and toxicity. Cancer 1990;66:2470–2475.

665. Wadler S, Lembersky B, Atkins M, et al. Phase II trial of fluorouracil and recombinant interferon alfa-2a in patients with advanced colorectal carcinoma: An Eastern Cooperative Oncology Group study. J Clin Oncol 1991;9:1806–1810.

666. Huberman M, McClay E, Atkins M, et al. Phase II trial of 5-fluorouracil and recombinant interferon alpha-2a in advanced colorectal cancer. Proc Am Soc Clin Oncol 1991;10:153.

667. Quan WDY, Madajewicz S, Skeel RT. Phase I trial of ALF: Alpha interferon, leucovorin and 5-fluorouracil in advanced cancer. Proc Am Soc Clin Oncol 1991;10:153.

668. Inoshita G, Yalavarthi P, Murthy S, et al. Phase I trial of 5-FU, leucovorin and rHu IFN-2a in metastatic colorectal cancer. Proc Am Soc Clin Oncol 1991;10:152.

669. Punt CJA, deMulder PHM, Burghouts JTM, et al. A phase I-II study of high dose 5-fluorouracil, leucovorin and α-interferon in patients with advanced colorectal cancer. Proc Am Soc Clin Oncol 1991;10:150.

670. Kreuser ED, Matthias M, Boewer C, et al. Double modulation of 5-fluorouracil with interferon α-2b and folinic acid in metastatic colorectal cancer. Proc Am Soc Clin Oncol 1991;10:150.

671. Wadler S, Schwartz EL, Goldman M, et al. 5-Fluorouracil and recombinant alpha-2a-interferon: An active regimen against advanced colorectal cancer. J Clin Oncol 1989;7:1769–1775.

672. Naunheim KS, Zeitels J, Kaplan EL, et al. Rectal carcinoid tumors: Treatment and prognosis. Surgery 1983;94:670–675.

673. Quan SHQ, Bader C, Berg JW. Carcinoid tumors of the rectum. Dis Colon Rectum 1964;7:197–206.

674. Federspiel BH, Burke AP, Sobin LH, et al. Rectal and Colonic Carcinoids: A clinicopathologic study of 84 cases. Cancer 1990;65:135–140.

675. Sauven P, Ridge JA, Quan SH, et al. Anorectal carcinoid tumors: Is aggressive surgery warranted? Ann Surg 1990;211:67–71.

676. Morgan JG, Marks C, Hearn D. Carcinoid tumors of the gastrointestinal tract. Ann Surg 1974;180:720–727.

677. Khalifa AA, Bong WL, Rao VK, et al. Leiomyosarcoma of the rectum: Report of a case and review of the literature. Dis Colon Rectum 1986;29:427–432.

678. Walsh TH, Mann CV. Smooth muscle neoplasms of the rectum and anal canal. Br J Surg 1984;71:597–599.

679. Devine RM, Beart RW Jr, Wolff BG. Malignant lymphoma of the rectum. Dis Colon Rectum 1986;29:821–824.

680. Shehata WM, Meyer RL, Jazy FK, et al. Regional adjuvant irradiation for adenocarcinoma of the cecum. Int J Radiat Oncol Biol Phys 1987;13:843–846.

681. Wong CS, Harwood AR, Cummings BJ, et al. Postoperative local abdominal irradiation for cancer of the colon above the peritoneal reflection. Int J Radiat Oncol Biol Phys 1985;11:2067–2071.

682. Loeffler RK. Postoperative radiation therapy for adenocarcinoma of the cecum using two fractions/day. Int J Radiat Oncol Biol Phys 1984;10:1881–1883.

683. Cummings KM, Michalek AJ, Tidings J, et al. Results of a public screening program for colorectal cancer. NY State Med 1986;86:68–72.

684. Bussey HJR, Eyers AA, Ritchie SM, et al. The rectum in adenomatous polyposis: The St. Mark's policy. Br J Surg 1985;72:S29–S35.

685. Moertel CG, Hill JR, Adson MA. Management of multiple polyposis of the large bowel. Cancer 1971;28:160–164.

686. Harvey JC, Quan SHQ, Stearns MW. Management of familial polyposis with preservation of the rectum. Surgery 1978;84:476–482.

687. Sarre RG, Jagelman DG, Beck GJ, et al. Colectomy with ileorectal anastomosis for familial adenomatous polyposis: The risk of rectal cancer. Surgery 1986;101:20–26.

688. Panettiere FJ, Chen TT. The SWOG large bowel study benefits from therapy. Proc Am Soc Clin Oncol [Abstract] 1985;4:76.

689. Laurie J, Moertel C, Flemming T, et al. Surgical adjuvant therapy of poor prognosis colorectal cancer with levamisole alone or combined levamisole and 5-fluorouracil: A North Central Cancer Treatment Group and Mayo Clinic study. Proc Am Soc Clin Oncol [Abstract] 1986;5:81.

690. Grinnell RS, Lane N. Benign and malignant adenomatous polyps and papillary adenomas of the colon and rectum: An analysis of 1,856 tumors in 1,335 patients. Int Abstr Surg 1958;106:519.

691. Waye JD, Frankel A. Treatment of early colon cancer. Gastroenterology 1974;66:796.

692. Locke MR, Cairns DW, Ritchie JK, et al. The treatment of early colorectal cancer by local excision. Br J Surg 1978;65:346–349.

693. Kodaira S, Teramoto T, Ono S, et al. Lymph node metastases from carcinomas developing in pedunculated and semi-pedunculated colorectal adenomas. Aust NZ J Surg 1981;51:429–433.

694. Nivatvongs S. Management of polyps containing invasive carcinoma. In: Codner IJ, Fry RD, Roe JP, eds. Colon, rectal, and anal surgery. St. Louis, CV Mosby, 1985:183–188.

695. Shatney CH, Lober PH, Gilbertsen VA, et al. The treatment of pedunculated adenomatous colorectal polyps with focal cancer. Surg Gynecol Obstet 1974;139:845–850.

696. Coutsoftides T, Lavery I, Benjamin SP, et al. Malignant polyps of the colon and rectum: A clinical pathological study. Dis Col Rect 1979;22:82–86.

Cancer: Principles & Practice of Oncology, Fourth Edition,
edited by Vincent T. DeVita, Jr., Samuel Hellman, Steven A. Rosenberg.
J.B. Lippincott Co., Philadelphia © 1993.

Alfred M. Cohen
Bruce D. Minsky
Michael A. Friedman

CHAPTER **31**

Rectal Cancer

The general issues of biology, diagnosis, and staging of colorectal cancer and the management of metastatic disease are discussed in Chapter 30. This chapter focuses on multidisciplinary approaches to the locoregional and systemic control of adenocarcinoma of the rectum. Treatment of rectal carcinoid, sarcoma, and lymphoma is discussed in Chapter 30.

ANATOMY

The rectum in the adult is approximately 15 cm long; for treatment purposes it is divided into 5-cm segments (Fig. 31–1). Actual rectal length and division into surgical segments reflect several patient features, such as height, body habitus, pelvic width (gynecoid or android), and curve of the sacral hollow, within which the rectum resides. The lowermost location of a rectal cancer is frequently defined in terms of distance from the anus. In reporting results, it should be stated whether the determination is made with a rigid or flexible endoscope and whether the reference point is the anal verge (*i.e.,* lowermost portion of the anal canal), the dentate line, or the anorectal ring.

LYMPHATIC DRAINAGE

The major portion of the lymphatic drainage of the rectum passes along the superior hemorrhoidal arterial trunk toward the inferior mesenteric artery. Only a few lymphatics pass along the inferior mesenteric vein. The pararectal nodes above the level of the middle rectal valve drain exclusively along the superior hemorrhoidal lymphatic chain. Below this level (*i.e.,* approximately 7 to 8 cm above the anal verge), some lymphatics pass to the lateral rectal pedicle. These lymphatics are associated with nodes along the middle hemorrhoidal artery, obturator fossa, and hypogastric and common iliac ar-

teries. There are extensive lymphatics in women contiguous with the rectovaginal septum and in men along Denonvilliers' fascia.[1,2] The entire extraperitoneal soft tissue (*i.e.,* mesorectum) is permeated with lymphatics.

NEUROMUSCULAR CONTROL MECHANISMS

Two muscular mechanisms are involved in maintaining fecal continence. The internal and external sphincter muscles control the anal canal lumen. The puborectalis sling system elevates the distal rectum when intraabdominal pressure increases, leading to kinking at the anorectal angle and enhanced continence, despite sneezing or coughing. This is the "flap-valve" theory of continence.[3] The intrarectal balloon proctogram defines the anorectal angle at rest and with straining.[4,5] Anorectal manometry and electromyography can be used to study subtle functional differences.[6]

Sphincter-saving treatment of rectal cancer may result in impaired bowel function. Frequency and urgency occur when the normal rectal reservoir is replaced with the less capacious proximal colon. Poor control of gas and fecal soilage, particularly with coughing, may lead to considerable embarrassment. Besides impairing motor function of the sphincter systems, surgery can cause sensory changes. Normal innervation is sensitive enough to differentiate gas, liquid, and solid feces, resulting in controlled differential release of these substances.

Sympathetic and parasympathetic nerve branches enter the rectum and anus. Preservation of the main branches to the bladder and prostate during rectal resection preserves potency, ejaculation, and bladder function.

DIAGNOSIS

Rectal and rectosigmoid cancer is much more likely to be symptomatic before diagnosis. Gross red blood (alone or mixed

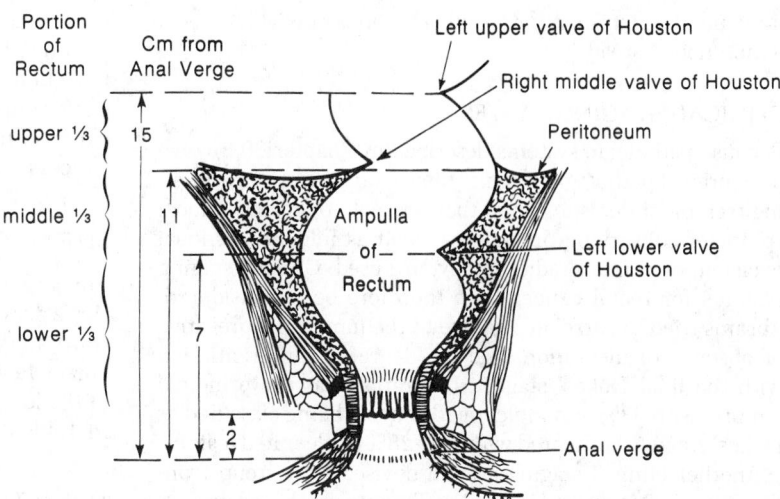

Portion of Rectum

Cm from Anal Verge

Left upper valve of Houston

Right middle valve of Houston

Peritoneum

upper ⅓ 15

middle ⅓ 11

Ampulla of Rectum

Left lower valve of Houston

lower ⅓ 7

2

Anal verge

FIGURE 31–1. Division of the rectum into upper, middle, and lower thirds.

with or covering stool) is frequently observed. Hemorrhoidal bleeding should always be a diagnosis of exclusion. All patients with rectal bleeding should be evaluated. If the blood is minimal and bright red, is located only on the toilet paper, and is associated with normal-colored stool, a sigmoidoscopy, preferably fiberoptic sigmoidoscopy with a 60- to 65-cm instrument, may suffice. All other patients should undergo sigmoidoscopy and barium enema examination or colonoscopy. Because a rectal cancer may be missed on barium enema, proctosigmoidoscopy complements the radiologic study. Small tumors may be missed on the cephalad portion of the rectal valves.

A change in bowel activity may occur with compromise of the rectal reservoir by tumor. Unexplained constipation or reduction in stool caliber should lead to evaluation. Obstructing rectal cancers frequently present with diarrhea, rather than constipation. Rigid sigmoidoscopy and barium enema examination or colonoscopy are the appropriate studies.

In cases of locally advanced rectal cancer with circumferential growth and extensive transmural penetration, urgency and inadequate emptying lead to tenesmus. This is usually a grave sign. Some degree of tenesmus may occur with less extensive distal rectal cancer as part of the normal rectal reflex. Urinary symptoms may occur with compression of the bladder, invasion of the prostate, or destruction of the high sacral nerve roots. Buttock or perineal pain from posterior extension also is a grave sign.

RADIOLOGIC EVALUATION

Pelvic Computed Tomography Scans

To evaluate the ureters and bladder, intravenous pyelography was traditionally obtained preoperatively. Data do not support its routine application.[7] Similar data is obtained with computed tomography (CT) scanning using intravenous contrast.

Initial reports of pelvic CT suggested an important role for this technique. A staging system was defined by Theoni and coworkers.[8] Koehler analyzed data from 23 patients, revealing unique information obtained from CT scans of 14.[9] Objective interpretation of these scans is not straightforward. A study of 91 patients revealed correlation with Dukes' staging for only 33% of cases. Interobserver agreement occurred for only 37%, and serial staging by the same radiologist was concordant only for 51%.[10]

Computed Tomography and Magnetic Resonance Imaging

A comparative trial of CT and 0.15-T magnetic resonance imaging (MRI) in 34 patients was reported by Hodgman and colleagues.[11] The overall accuracy of CT staging was 80%, but it was only 59% with MRI. In the detection of lymph node metastases, CT was more accurate than MRI (65% versus 39%). Specificity was 90% in both, but sensitivity 40% with CT and only 13% with MRI. Other studies using 0.6-T and 1.5-T coils suggest MRI does not add to the accuracy of CT scanning.[12,13]

Intrarectal Ultrasound

Intrarectal (IRUS) or transrectal ultrasound is excellent in detecting the degree of primary tumor penetration and fair to good in detecting lymph node metastases. An ultrasonic staging system (uT) of the tumor penetration has been proposed.[14] These stages correspond to the standard pathologic staging system. Practice is required to interpret these images.[15] In addition to image interpretation and scanner technical details, positioning the probe appropriately requires close interaction between surgeon and radiologist.

Saitoh and associates analyzed IRUS images of 99 rectal cancer patients.[16] If those with stages uT1 and uT2 were combined, transmural penetration was correctly determined in 79 of 88 patients. In 52 of the 71 patients with nodal metastases, IRUS made the correct preoperative assessment. Beynon and colleagues were able to predict transmural penetration of the primary tumor successfully for 97% of 51 patients.[17] Differentiating T1 from T2 is more problematic.[18] In all series, there is a tendency to overstate the extent of penetration.[15,19] Although in experienced hands the extent of tumor penetration is correctly assessed in more than 90% of patients, only recently have reports indicated lymph node spread correctly in 80%.[21] Several series have directly compared IRUS with pelvic CT. IRUS is as good or better than CT in determining transmural penetration.[22-26] Neither technique reliably detects lymph node spread.[22]

CLINICAL STAGING SYSTEMS

Because pathologic systems described in Chapter 30 involve postsurgical pathologic staging, they cannot be used for making treatment decisions, and they are not applicable if local sphincter-conserving procedures, such as fulguration, local excision, or contact radiotherapy, are used. Clinical staging systems for rectal cancer have therefore been considered. Abrams tried to correlate the size of the tumor, the presence or absence of ulceration, and the degree of differentiation with the final Dukes' stage.[27] Ulceration was the principal feature, with 63% of nonulcerated cancers being classified as Dukes' stage A, compared with only 28% of ulcerated lesions.

Another clinical staging system devised by a group from the Princess Margaret Hospital in Toronto was based on several prognostic variables: the presence or absence of metastases, whether the rectal tumor was fixed or mobile, whether it was annular, and whether the clinical symptoms of weight loss, anorexia, weakness, and anemia were present.[28] These variables were used to determine four clinical classes. In class I, none of the variables were present. Class II was characterized by annular rectal tumor or the systemic symptoms. Class III denoted a fixed rectal tumor, and in class IV, metastases existed. Patient survival correlated well with the breakdown into these classes and with the breakdown by Dukes' stages, but the correlation between clinical classes and Dukes' stages was not good. Univariate and multivariate analyses of prognostic features were performed for 824 rectal cancer patients in the Medical Research Council's preoperative radiation therapy trial in the United Kingdom.[29,30] Mobility of the tumor was the most important preoperative assessment related to curative resection.

An Australian clinicopathologic staging system combines features of both a pathologic staging system and a clinical system, based on local tumor characteristics alone.[31,32] York-Mason suggested the use of a clinical staging system based on mobility of the primary tumor. Clinical stage I represents a freely mobile tumor; stage II, a mobile tumor; stage III, tethered mobility; and stage IV, fixed tumor.[33] Clinical stages I and II encompass patients for whom local curative excision may be possible. Nicholls and colleagues tested the accuracy of the digital examination by comparing it with the final pathologic stage.[34] They assessed the morphology, number of quadrants involved, fixation, and presence of extrarectal involvement. For 70 tumors, there was 67% to 83% correlation with the final pathology by the consulting physicians, but the correlation was 44% to 68% if tumors were assessed by physicians with less experience. In a subsequent publication, Nicholls and coworkers reported that clinical determination of the local extent and penetration correlated positively with survival.[35]

TREATMENT OF RESECTABLE RECTAL CANCER

For patients, the treatment of rectal cancer is frequently associated with colostomy. This concern may lead to a delay in seeking medical care, but fewer than one third of patients with rectal cancer require a permanent colostomy. For most patients, the primary treatment modality is radical surgical resection. The results of these primarily surgical approaches can be improved with adjuvant therapy, and several techniques can maximize local and overall cure rates of resectable rectal cancers.

SITE-SPECIFIC TREATMENT OPTIONS

For surgical resections, the rectum is generally considered in three distinct sections in relation to the anal verge: the upper third, middle third, and lower third. These sections roughly correlate with 5-cm intervals. Treatment options for cancers of the lower two thirds (extraperitoneal rectum) are outlined in Table 31–1.

Upper Third

Treatment of cancers in the distal sigmoid or intraabdominal rectum (*i.e.*, rectosigmoid), cure rates, and patterns of recurrent cancer are similar to those of the more proximal colon. Tumors in the upper third of the rectum have their lowermost edge 11 to 12 cm from the anal verge. Extirpation is primarily by anterior or low anterior resection. In an anterior resection of the rectosigmoid, the rectum is mobilized from the sacral hollow. However, with a low anterior resection, the lateral rectal attachments (*e.g.*, middle hemorrhoidal arteries) are divided. Bowel continuity is always restorable, end to end or side to end. Single- or double-layer sutures or staples are suitable.

Middle Third

For cancers in the middle third of the rectum, abdominoperineal resection with permanent colostomy does not yield superior results to those achieved with sphincter-saving surgical treatment.[36] Every effort should be made to restore intestinal continuity in patients with cancers 6 to 11 cm from the anal verge. Overall surgical success depends on surgical expertise and on the patient's body habitus, pelvic width, and associated colonic disease like diverticulosis.

TABLE 31–1.   Primary Treatment of Cancers of the Extraperitoneal Rectum*

Abdominoperineal resection
Low anterior resection
   End-to-end versus side-to-end
   Sutures versus staples
Abdominosacral resection
Coloanal resection
   Endoanal versus pull-through
   Staples versus sutures
Localized procedures
   Local excision
   Fulguration
   Endocavitary irradiation or brachytherapy

* Less than 11 cm from the anal verge.

Lower Third

Most cancers in the lower 5 cm of the rectum require abdominoperineal resection. Abdominosacral resection or stapled low anterior resection may be feasible. Restorative proctectomy with a coloanal anastomosis can also be used in selected patients. Local procedures may be appropriate for selected patients with lower third rectal cancers.

EXTENT OF SURGERY

Before addressing the essential features of the approaches outlined in Table 31–1, it is important to understand the principles influencing the extent of radical extirpative surgery.

Distal Mucosal Margin

Sphincter-saving surgery for patients with distal rectal cancers requires an "adequate distal margin." A 5-cm distal margin is traditionally cited in surgical texts, but the data do not support this rule. Distal spread may occur by direct submucosal extension or intramural lymphatics. The spread may be continuous or discontinuous (*e.g.*, satellites). Histologic examination of the bowel wall distal to the gross tumor usually reveals a predominance of tumors without any distal spread, and only 2.5% of patients demonstrate disease spread greater than 2 cm.[36] The few patients with extensive distal spread usually have poorly differentiated, node-positive rectal cancers that disseminate rapidly.[37] Additional data suggest that a margin of 1.5 cm is adequate for potentially curable tumors.[38] There is no correlation between the risk of suture-line or local recurrences and the extent of distal margin in excess of 2 cm.[39,40]

Measured operative surgical margins always exceed pathologically measured margins because of shrinkage of the specimen. Because of the potential for miscalculation during surgery, we recommend a surgical margin of 3 cm. Exceptions are bulky, poorly differentiated, or anaplastic carcinomas, which may require a longer distal margin to maximize local control. Early nontransmural cancers may be resected with distal margins of 1 cm. It is unacceptable to intraoperatively transsect a rectal cancer in a desperate attempt to avoid a permanent colostomy.

Extent of Proximal Lymph Node Dissection

In patients with rectal cancer, the mesorectum should be removed at least to the level of the aortic bifurcation. This includes all nodes just distal to the origin of the left colic artery but not the periaortic nodes or those along the inferior mesenteric artery. A nonrandomized comparison of "high ligation" of the inferior mesenteric artery and resection distal to the left colic artery reported by the St. Mark's Hospital group did not elicit any survival benefit for the higher lymphadenectomy group.[41] The results in patients from whom pathologically positive nodes along the inferior mesenteric artery were surgically removed justify limiting routine resection to below the left colic origin. Hojo and colleagues had only a single 5-year survivor, and Grinnell had none.[42,43] However, it is frequently necessary to divide the inferior mesenteric artery and vein to mobilize an adequate length of proximal colon to reach the rectal remnant in sphincter-saving surgical procedures.

Distal and Lateral Extent of Pelvic Dissection

Although evidence justifies a more limited mucosal distal margin than was recommended in the past, the extent of surgical excision of distal lymphatics or lymph nodes may differ. These structures reside within the mesorectum. In a report by Williams and colleagues, only 3 of 50 patients who underwent abdominoperineal resection had positive lymph nodes caudad to the tumor within the mesorectum; these were poorly differentiated cancers.[37] Heald and associates strongly advocated complete excision of the mesorectum for distal rectal cancers, reporting a very low local recurrence rate with such an approach.[44,45]

Interest in formal pelvic lymph node dissection has been limited to a number of centers: Memorial Sloan-Kettering Cancer Center, the University of Chicago, St. Mark's Hospital, and the National Cancer Center Hospital in Tokyo. Elegant studies by Hojo and colleagues defined the incidence of metastasis to the various nodal groups.[42] An approximate 10% improvement in 5-year survival has been reported by several researchers from these centers.[46–49] The survival benefit was most notable among patients who underwent sphincter-saving procedures.[50] In a nonrandomized comparison conducted at St. Mark's Hospital, no survival advantage could be demonstrated with extended abdominopelvic nodal dissection.[51]

Data from Quirke and colleagues suggest that the lateral (*i.e.*, tangential or peripheral) margins are the major determinants of local recurrence.[52] In a series of 52 resected rectal cancers with negative lateral margins on routine pathologic review, serial step-sections demonstrated positive margins in 14. Disease recurred in 12 of these patients, compared with none who had truly negative margins. It is likely that some of the alleged local control benefits associated with hypogastric nodal dissection were obtained by the associated wide lateral dissection during surgery.

To maximize lateral margins, pelvic surgery should be performed by sharp dissection outside the mesorectum on the endopelvic fascia. This can be done while sparing the pelvic nerve plexus by using nerve-sparing pelvic side-wall dissection. Although a 2- to 3-cm distal mucosal margin is usually adequate, local cure of rectal cancer requires maximal extirpation of mesorectal and lateral pararectal tissues.

RADICAL TREATMENT OPTIONS

Abdominoperineal Resection

Abdominoperineal resection can be performed as a synchronous transabdominal and perineal procedure with two operative teams or performed sequentially. Surgery is greatly facilitated by placing the patient in the modified lithotomy position and using a single skin preparation and draping. The extent of the resection is illustrated in Figure 31–2.

An end sigmoid colostomy is brought out through the rectus sheath to minimize subsequent hernia. If postoperative radiation therapy is a possibility, clips should be placed around the tumor area to facilitate delivering the boost dose. Efforts to exclude the small bowel from the radiation field using the

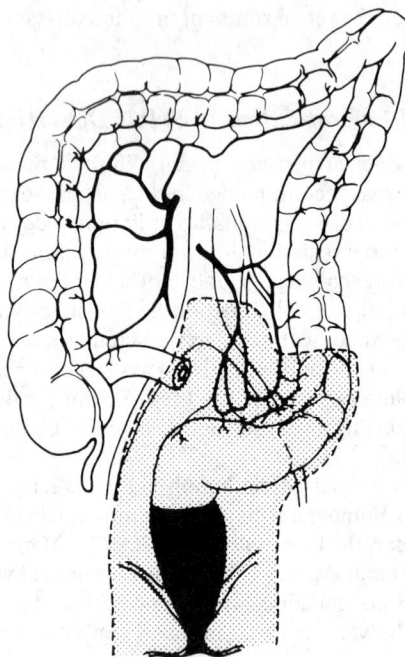

FIGURE 31–2.   Preferred extent of surgery in an abdominoperineal resection. (Modified from Enker WE. Surgical treatment of large bowel cancer. In: Enker WE, ed. Carcinoma of the colon and rectum. Chicago: Yearbook, 1978:73–106)

uterus, omentum, peritoneum, or absorbable mesh should be considered. The perineum was traditionally left open to heal by granulation, but in most patients the pelvic fat and skin can be closed primarily, with greatly improved recovery.

The surgical, nursing, and enterostomal team should work with the patient and family to relieve their anxiety concerning colostomy management. Preoperative visits by specially trained personnel or other patients can greatly reduce concerns about postoperative lifestyle for the patient with a new colostomy.

Sphincter-Saving Approaches

In all sphincter-saving surgical procedures, considerable tumor manipulation is required, resulting in intraluminal tumor-cell shedding. Although results of a randomized study are not available, it appears appropriate to irrigate the distal rectum with saline or water as part of most sphincter-saving procedures to minimize the risk of suture-line recurrences.

Low Anterior Resection

If transanal reconstruction with a stapler is contemplated, the patient is positioned in the modified lithotomy position. The initial stages of the operation with complete mobilization of the rectum to the level of the levators are identical to the initial stages of the abdominoperineal resection. Restorative options include end-to-end and side-to-end anastomoses constructed with sutures or staples. The most widely used approach uses the intraluminal circular stapler placed by a transanal approach (Fig 31–3). This approach allows the creation of very low anastomoses in the pelvis.[53–55] Temporary protective transverse colostomy is no longer a routine adjunct with low anterior resection.

Abdominosacral Resection

An operation pioneered by D'Allaines in the 1940s has been modified by several surgeons to allow direct anastomosis through a perineal incision.[56,57] The rectum is mobilized to the pelvic floor, as in the operations previously described. A second incision is made just above the anus, the coccyx is removed, and the pelvis is entered through the posterior fascia. An end-to-end anastomosis is performed through the perineal incision. To a great extent, this operation has been replaced by the use of the transanal stapling system. In expert hands, the operation can be combined with high-dose preoperative irradiation as a sphincter-saving approach to treating very low rectal cancers.[58,59]

Coloanal Resection

After complete mobilization of the rectum from an abdominal approach, the bowel continuity is restored by bringing the colon to the level of the anus and dentate line. With the pull-through approach, the anastomosis can be performed during the same procedure or delayed 10 days.[49] More commonly, a direct endoanal anastomosis is performed with staples or sutures (Fig 31–4).[60,61] Preoperative irradiation may be combined with coloanal reconstruction.[62,63]

Morbidity and Mortality From Radical Surgery

In addition to the usual potential postoperative complications of hemorrhage and infection, two additional areas of concern warrant comment. A neurogenic bladder with inability to void is common after extensive pelvic dissection. Catheter drainage of the bladder is used for 7 to 10 days, after which most patients are able to void spontaneously. If there is any mechanical obstructive component from urethral stricture or prostate enlargement, transurethral surgery may be required before voiding is possible. Bethanecol chloride (Urabeth) may be useful in improving bladder emptying. Intermittent or continuous catheterization for months may be necessary in some patients.

Sexual dysfunction, particularly in men, is common. Retrograde ejaculation is related to sympathetic nerve dysfunction. Erectile impotency results from damage to the pelvic parasympathetic plexus (*i.e.*, nervi erigentes).

The mortality from radical surgery for rectal cancer is 2% to 6%, with no difference between abdominoperineal resection or sphincter-saving procedures.[64–66]

TREATMENT OF INVASIVE RECTAL CANCER BY LOCAL APPROACHES

PATIENT SELECTION

Local treatment alone for rectal cancer was first applied to patients with medical contraindications to radical surgery. Severe cardiopulmonary disease may preclude extensive surgery because of high surgical mortality. Patient blindness has always been a concern if a colostomy is required, because it makes subsequent self-care difficult. However, a small subset of patients with early rectal cancers may be treated preferentially by more limited approaches. Exophytic, small (<3

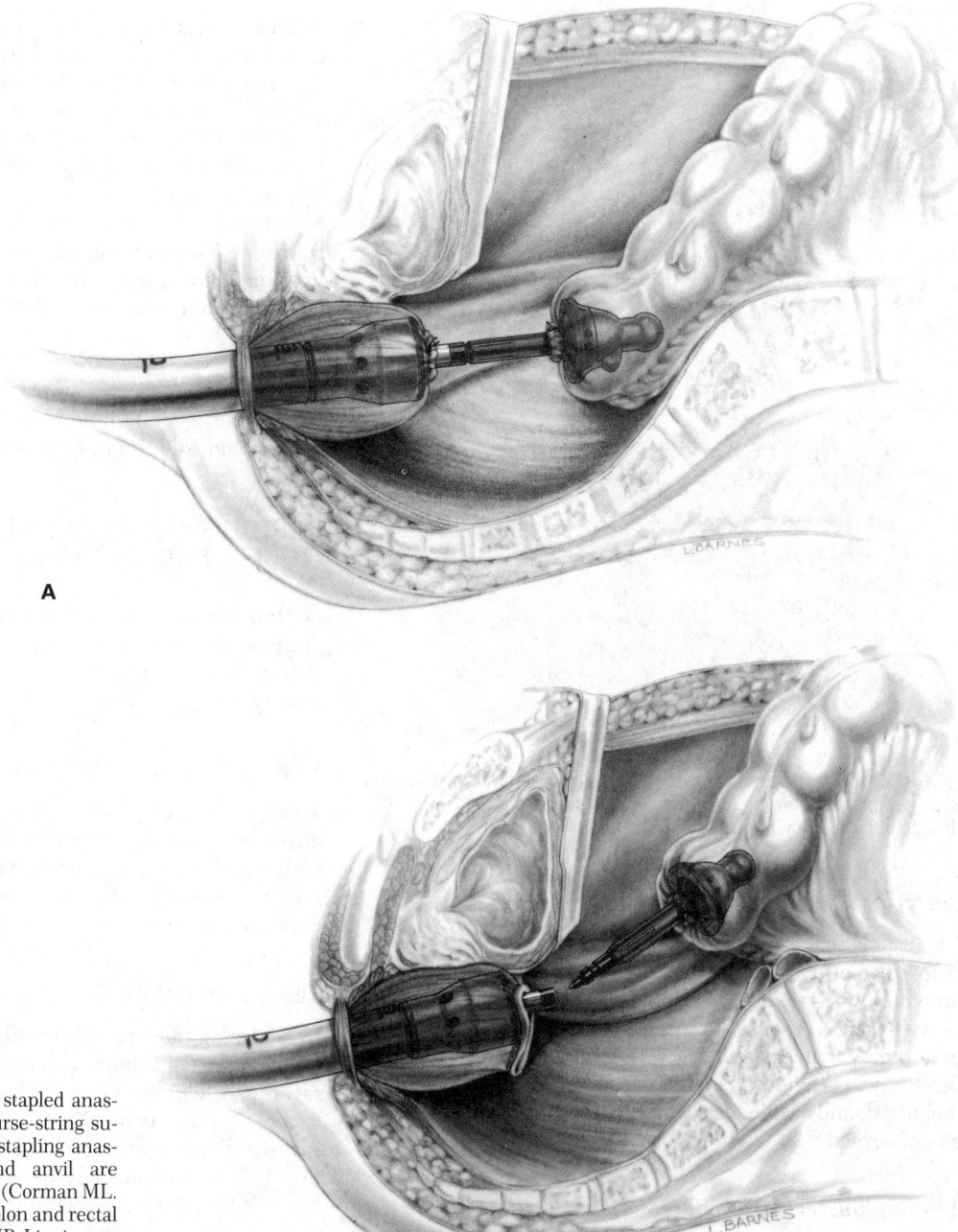

FIGURE 31–3. **(A)** Circular stapled anastomosis. Proximal and distal purse-string sutures are secured. **(B)** Double-stapling anastomosis. Detachable shaft and anvil are secured into the proximal colon. (Corman ML. Carcinoma of the rectum. In: Colon and rectal surgery. 2nd ed. Philadelphia: JB Lippincott, 1989:529)

cm), well-differentiated tumors, clinically limited to the submucosa, are ideal for a limited approach. However, tumors invading the muscle wall have been treated in limited fashion with good results. Improved clinical staging systems, combined with careful histologic and biologic analyses of various phenotypic markers, may enable us to define the appropriate subsets of rectal cancer patients for these treatment strategies.[35]

TREATMENT OPTIONS

A detailed analysis is beyond the scope of this chapter, but the various approaches are described to familiarize the reader with the therapeutic options. The results are presented in subsequent sections.

Transanal Local Excision

Transanal local excision is the most straightforward approach to removing rectal cancers. The deep plane of dissection should be a full-thickness excision in the perirectal fat. Adequate dilation of the anus and the use of special retractors, fiberoptic light, and traction sutures facilitate the procedure. Primary closure of the defect minimizes subsequent scarring.

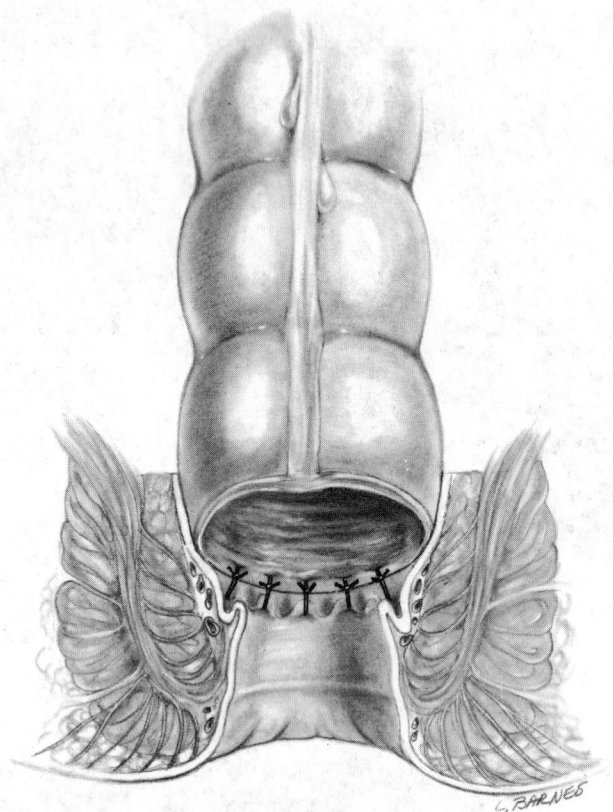

FIGURE 31–4.   Peranal hand-sewn coloanal anastomosis. (Corman ML. Carcinoma of the rectum. In: Colon and rectal surgery. 2nd ed. Philadelphia: JB Lippincott, 1989:551)

Posterior Proctotomy

For lesions too large or too proximal for transanal local excision, two other surgical approaches are available: posterior proctotomy (Kraske's procedure) and transsphincteric excision (Bevan's or York-Mason procedure). In the posterior proctotomy, a perineal incision is made just above the anus, the coccyx is removed, and the fascia divided. The rectum is mobilized, and a wide local excision or a sleeve resection can be performed.[67]

Transsphincteric Procedure

The transsphincteric approach is identical to the posterior proctotomy, except that the entire anal sphincter is divided posteriorly in the midline. As long as each portion of the sphincter mechanism is identified and marked, the anus can be reconstructed at the completion of the operation with minimal risk of functional impairment.[68]

Fulguration

Fulguration or cauterization has been used as an alternative to abdominoperineal resection by many surgeons.[69,70] The procedure is done in multiple stages under general or regional anesthesia. Tumor is charred, and then scraped with a curet. This approach is not without risk, primarily a delayed hemorrhage in 10% to 20% of patients from the slough of the scar at 7 to 10 days.

Endocavitary Irradiation

Irradiation has been used as a single-modality approach to early rectal cancer with curative intent. External-beam x-rays alone have been used, but most investigators have used intracavitary irradiation, alone or combined with temporary isotope implants.[71,72] The anus is dilated, and a 4-cm proctoscope is introduced. A low-energy x-ray unit is placed through the scope almost against the tumor. Generally, 50-kV x-rays, in doses of 3000 cGy per treatment, are given using this "contact" approach. Three or four sessions are required. Bulky tumors may require additional irradiation with iridium implants or external beam to reach the deeper pararectal tissues.

Other Local Options

Many other local treatment strategies have been used. Cryosurgery and Nd:YAG laser may play a role in future years.

RESULTS OF TREATMENT OF RECTAL CANCER

Overall cure rates for cancers in the lower third of the rectum are less than those for cancers in the upper two thirds.[73,74] Pelvic failure is reviewed in the discussion of patterns of recurrence.

CURE RATES FOR RECTAL CANCER

Three fourths of patients with node-negative rectal cancer are cured by radical surgical resection (Table 31–2).[64,75] Few patients whose rectal cancers have spread to regional lymph nodes are cured by surgery. Approximately one third of these patients achieve 5-year disease-free survival.

RESULTS WITH LOCAL TREATMENT OPTIONS

In analyzing the long-term results achieved with local treatment options, it is important to appreciate that case selection favors excellent results.[76] When in situ cancers were excluded, a local control rate of 82% was obtained for 378 patients with invasive cancer treated by local excision.[77–81] In a report from St. Mark's Hospital, treatment failed locally in 4 of 39 patients.[82] Hager and associates from Erlangen reported that 3

TABLE 31–2.   Cure Rates in Rectal Cancer

Investigations	Dukes Stage	5-Year Survival (%)
Wilson and Beahrs[214]	A, B	79
Eisenberg et al[215]	A	88
McDermott et al[216]	A	93
Eisenberg et al[215]	B	79
McDermott et al[216]	B	71
Wilson and Beahrs[214]	C	41
Eisenberg et al[215]	C	28
McDermott et al[216]	C	41

of 36 patients with T1 cancers and 3 of 18 with T2 cancers had local recurrences.[83] The largest series has been reported from the Mayo Clinic, with a local failure rate of 27% (38 of 141 patients).[84]

Local failure after fulguration occurs in 10% to 50% of patients.[78,79,85] Multiple sessions (average of 3.5) may be required to maximize local control.[78,85] A subset of these patients with recurrence are cured with subsequent radical surgery.[78,79,85–87]

Papillon and colleagues in Lyon, France, pioneered in the treatment of selected patients with rectal cancers using endocavitary irradiation. Exophytic superficial cancers exclusive of poorly differentiated or colloid histology and less than 4.5 cm in diameter were treated. If the tumor was thought to invade muscle, interstitial iridium 192 was added. In 245 patients, the 5-year disease-free survival rate was 76%. The local failure rate was only 5.3%.[81] Sischy and associates reported equally good results.[88] The local failure rate in 94 patients treated with endocavitary irradiation alone was 5%.

Five-year survival rates with local treatment options vary from 50% to 90%, with many deaths caused by illnesses other than cancer. In selected patients, a 10% cancer-related 5-year mortality can be expected with local excision, fulguration, or primary irradiation.

PATTERNS OF RECURRENCE AFTER RADICAL SURGERY

Despite radical surgery, locoregional failure occurs in 20% to 50% of patients with transmural or node-positive rectal cancers. The incidence of treatment failure in the pelvis is directly related to the extent of transmural penetration and the additive risks of lymph node metastases. Pelvic failure rates as a function of various pathologic parameters are listed in Table 31–

TABLE 31–3. Pelvic Recurrence Rates After Surgery Alone for Rectal Cancer

Investigations	Stage	Locoregional Recurrence (%)
McDermott et al[217]	Dukes' B	15
Phillips et al[218]	Dukes' B	15
Pilipshen et al[219]	Dukes' B	30
Pilipshen et al[219]	T2N0M0	14
Pilipshen et al[219]	T3N0M0	30
Rich et al[220]	T3$_m$ N0M0*	17
Rich et al[220]	T3$_g$ N0M0*	25
Rich et al[220]	T4N0M0	53
McDermott et al[217]	Dukes' C	32
Phillips et al[218]	Dukes' C	21
Pilipshen et al[219]	Dukes' C	39
Pilipshen et al[219]	T2N1M0	22
Pilipshen et al[219]	T3N1M0	49
Rich et al[220]	T3$_m$ N1M0*	28
Rich et al[220]	T3$_g$ N1M0*	52
Rich et al[220]	T4N1M0	67

* (m), microscopic transmural extension; (g), gross transmural extension.

3. Interpretation of local failure in rectal cancer is complex, with many reported variables: diagnosis by clinical surgical or autopsy criteria; first or cumulative site of failure; sole or component of failure.

Failure patterns determined at autopsy provide the most accurate insight into the relative risks of local and distant recurrence. In the series from the Massachusetts General Hospital, isolated pelvic recurrences were documented in 25% of patients, but a total of 75% of cancer-related deaths were associated with tumor in the pelvis. These data suggest that improved local control through multimodality treatment of the primary cancer may dramatically reduce cancer-related morbidity and may improve survival, particularly of node-negative patients.

MANAGEMENT PROBLEMS IN RECTAL CANCER

OBSTRUCTION

Subtotal obstruction from rectal cancers may manifest as increasing constipation or frank obstipation and more commonly as diarrhea and tenesmus. If dietary management with a minimal residue regimen is not effective in allowing an elective operation (perhaps including preoperative irradiation), a preliminary colostomy with intraoperative evaluation of the extent of disease should be considered.

CONTIGUOUS ORGAN INVOLVEMENT

In patients with rectal cancer, contiguous organ involvement usually entails direct invasion of the prostate and base of the bladder in men and invasion of the vagina in women. In women who have previously undergone a hysterectomy, a cancer of the upper third of the rectum may invade the base of the bladder. Management issues are discussed in a later section on unresectable, recurrent cancer and locally advanced rectal cancer.

RADIATION THERAPY ALONE FOR RESECTABLE CANCER

In most cases, radiation therapy is limited to patients who are medically inoperable. This section excludes discussion of patients amenable to a local and adjuvant therapy.

A variety of techniques have been used, including various combinations of external-beam irradiation, ^{192}Ir interstitial brachytherapy, and intracavitary irradiation. In an update from Papillon, 71 patients with clinical T2 or T3 rectal cancers received ten applications of 300 cGy to the pelvis.[89] Eight weeks later, an additional 2500 cGy was delivered by intracavitary irradiation and 2000 to 3000 cGy by ^{192}Ir interstitial brachytherapy. The 5-year disease-free survival was 65%, and 62% retained normal sphincter function. Although 7% developed anal necrosis, they all healed.

A similar approach was reported by Meyerson and coworkers.[90] Thirty patients received 4500 cGy followed 6 weeks later by 3000 to 9000 cGy with intracavitary irradiation. Their tumors were defined as larger than 3 cm, nonmobile, well or moderately well differentiated, and clinical stage T2 or pathologic stage T3. Deeply ulcerated or infiltrating tumors were excluded. With a median follow-up of 2 years, the local failure rate was 30%, and the 2-year disease-free survival rate was 42% (55% with salvage). Minor proctitis occurred in 17%.

SPHINCTER-SAVING ADJUVANT THERAPIES FOR RECTAL CANCER

Conservative management that preserves the sphincter has been used in several groups of distal rectal cancer patients as alternative to abdominoperineal resection. The first is patients with early localized tumors. These include small, exophytic, mobile tumors without adverse pathologic factors (*e.g.*, high grade, blood vessel invasion, lymphatic vessel invasion, colloid histology, penetration of tumor into or through the bowel wall).[91-93] These selected tumors comprise 3% to 5% of all rectal cancers and are adequately treated with a variety of local therapies alone. Adjuvant therapies have been applied to patients amenable to a local therapy but with adverse prognostic features. Another group of patients has tumors that are more locally advanced and resectable by a sphincter-saving approach but with inadequate margins.

LOCAL EXCISION AND POSTOPERATIVE RADIATION THERAPY

The use of local excision and postoperative radiation therapy is not a new concept. This organ-sparing technique has been used successfully in treating other tumors such as breast cancer, soft tissue sarcomas, and head and neck cancers. Only recently has this approach been applied to rectal cancer.

Local excision has been performed before and after radiation therapy. The advantage of performing a local excision before radiation therapy is that pathologic details such as margins, depth of bowel wall penetration, and histologic features can be characterized. Knowledge of these details is useful in the development of selection criteria.

Selection Criteria

To determine which tumors are likely to have a high enough incidence of local failure or positive pelvic lymph nodes to consider adjuvant irradiation, it first must be determined which tumors are adequately treated with local therapy alone. The selection of tumors for local therapy is based on clinical and pathologic factors. Clinical information such as tumor size, mobility, location, and circumference can be obtained at the time of physical examination. Accurate pathologic information is more difficult to obtain from a biopsy. Of the available local therapies, only a full-thickness local excision provides accurate pathologic information.

Results

Local excision followed by postoperative irradiation has been performed by a limited number of investigators (Table 31–4). In most series, patients had clinical T1 to T3 tumors and underwent a local excision followed in 4 to 6 weeks by 4500 to 5000 cGy in conventional fractionation to the whole pelvis. Some patients received external-beam or brachytherapy boosts.

In a limited series of 9 patients reported by Ellis and colleagues, there were no local failures and the disease-free survival rate was 89%.[94] The excellent results may be a result of

TABLE 31–4. Local Excision and Postoperative Pelvic Radiation Therapy

Investigations	No. of Patients	Median Follow-up (mo)	Size (cm)	T3 (%)	Margins	No. of Patients	Local Failure (%)	Survival	Sphincter Function*
Rich[95]	26	23	3.7 mean	19	Negative	17	6	88% DFS	N/A
					Positive	9	56	44% DFS	
Ellis[94]	9	65	2.0 median	0	Negative	8	0	89% DFS	100% rectal continence
					Positive	1	0		
McCready[97]	24	13	3.1 mean	33	Negative	24	0	92% DFS	Majority excellent
Willett[96]	26	26	4.0 mean	12	Negative	19	16	70% 5-y actuarial	Satisfactory
					Positive	6	0		
					Unevaluable	1	1/1		
Minsky[98]	14	29	2.5 median	29	Negative	14	21	88% 3-yr actuarial	82% satisfactory
Rosenthal[213]	16†	33	4.0 median	32%	Unevaluable	16	20‡	94% 3-yr actuarial	92% satisfactory

DFS, disease-free survival; N/A, not available from the manuscript.
* Sphincter function in locally controlled patients.
† Patients received 500-cGy pelvic radiation therapy preoperatively followed by local excision and postoperative radiation therapy.
‡ Crude incidence of cumulative local failure as a component of failure except the series by Rosenthal, which reports actuarial data.

the more favorable cancers that were treated (none had T3 cancers).

Rich and associates reported the results of treating 26 patients with T1, T2, or T3 rectal cancer.[95] The majority (81%) were located less than 5 cm from the anal verge. For the 17 patients with no gross residual tumor, the local failure rate was 6%, and the disease-free survival rate was 88%. Less satisfactory results were seen in the 9 patients with grossly positive margins. The incidence of local failure was 56%, and the disease-free survival rate was 44%.

At the Massachusetts General Hospital, Willett and colleagues treated 26 patients (T1:11; T2:11; T3:3; not evaluable, 1) with local excision followed by 4500 cGy plus 500- to 2250-cGy boosts.[96] The boost was limited to the 21 patients in whom the margins were positive, there was deep muscle invasion, or there was invasion into fat by tumor. Seven received 5-fluorouracil (5-FU) during the first and last 3 days of radiation therapy. The incidence of local failure was 15%, and the rate distant metastasis was 8%. In contrast to the series from Rich, there was no difference in the incidence of local failure in the 6 patients with microscopic positive margins and the 19 with negative margins.[95] All locally controlled patients maintained satisfactory sphincter function. Nineteen patients with T2 or T3 rectal cancer were treated by McCready and co-workers.[97] Their approach was limited to locally resected tumors which were mobile, involved more than 30% of the bowel circumference, were 4 cm or smaller, located 10 cm or less from the anal verge, well to moderately well differentiated, and had negative margins. Two to 6 weeks after a transsphincteric or transsacral excision, patients received 4500 cGy followed by a boost to a minimum of 5300 cGy. With a median follow-up of 13 months, no patients developed local failures. Survival data have not been reported.

Minsky and colleagues reported the results of 14 patients who underwent a full-thickness local excision followed by postoperative radiation therapy.[98] Patients received 4500 to 4680 cGy plus a boost to 5040 cGy. The 3-year actuarial disease-free survival rate was 66%, the overall survival rate was 88%, and the local failure rate was 21%. The incidence of local failure increased with T stage (T1:0/3, T2:1/7, T3:2/4) and tumor size (>3 cm, 33%; ≤3 cm, 0%). Of the 11 locally controlled patients, 82% had satisfactory sphincter function but did experience increased frequency of bowel movements, and 2 required diapers for incontinence of stool. None developed rectal stenosis.

The limited data suggest that the approach of local excision and postoperative radiation therapy should be limited to patients with T1 tumors with adverse pathologic factors and all T2 tumors. To address the issues of patient selection and results, a phase II intergroup trial of local excision and postoperative radiation and chemotherapy is ongoing.

PREOPERATIVE RADIATION THERAPY FOLLOWED BY SURGERY

One advantage of preoperative radiation therapy is to decrease the volume of the primary tumor. If the tumor is located in close proximity to the dentate line, the decreased tumor volume may allow the surgeon to perform a sphincter-conserving procedure that would not otherwise be possible. Two surgical approaches have been used after preoperative pelvic radiation: local excision or proctectomy and coloanal anastomosis.

Local Excision

Otmezguine and associates reported the results of 25 patients who received 3495 cGy in daily 233-cGy fractions to a partial pelvic field, followed in 6 to 8 weeks by transanal or transsphincteric local excision and a 2000- to 2500-cGy boost with afterloading [192]Ir.[99] The median tumor size was 4 cm, 80% were exophytic, 72% were well or moderately well differentiated, and all were mobile. With a mean follow-up of 41 months, the local failure rate was 20%, and 3 of the 5 failures were salvaged with abdominoperineal resections. Of the 6 patients with positive margins, 2 developed local failures. The 20 patients with local control had normal sphincter function.

In a report by Marks and colleagues, 14 patients who were medically unsuitable for a radical resection underwent a local excision after receiving 4000 to 4500 cGy.[100] With a minimum follow-up of 24 months and a median of 31 months, the 3-year actuarial incidence of local failure was 23%, and the overall survival rate was 61%.

Proctectomy and Coloanal Anastomosis

A total of 22 patients with resectable, primary adenocarcinoma of the rectum enrolled on a phase I–II trial of preoperative radiation therapy followed by proctectomy and coloanal anastomosis were reported from Memorial Sloan-Kettering Cancer Center.[62] The median tumor size was 4 cm (range, 1.5–6 cm), and the median distance from the anal verge was 4 cm (range, 3–7 cm). The whole pelvis received 4680 cGy followed by a 360-cGy boost to the primary tumor bed. The median follow-up was 23 months. Of the 21 patients who underwent resection, 10% had no tumor in the surgical specimen, and 90% were able to successfully undergo a coloanal anastomosis. The incidence of local failure as a component of failure was 14%. The overall 3-year actuarial survival rate was 83%.

Marks and coworkers reported the results of 43 patients who received preoperative radiation therapy followed by a variety of sphincter-preserving surgical techniques.[101] Of the 43, 14% of the tumors were clinically fixed, and 65% had unfavorable pathology (*e.g.*, deeply ulcerated, fixed, circumferential, obstruction, undifferentiated histology, palpable or indurated lymphatics). The sphincter-preservation rate in this series may be underestimated because some patients presented with unresectable disease. Patients received 4000 to 4500 cGy, and if the tumor was fixed, they received a boost to 6000 cGy. Surgical approaches included 31 combined abdominal transsacral procedures, eight transanal abdominal transanal proctosigmoidectomies and coloanal anastomoses, two low anterior resections, and two full-thickness wide local excisions. With a median follow-up of 51 months, the local failure rate was 16%. Of the 7 patients who developed local recurrences, 5 had fixed tumors. The 5-year actuarial survival rate was 72%, and 86% of patients retained a normal functioning sphincter. In an update limited to the 38 patients who underwent preoperative radiation followed by a transanal abdominal transanal proctosigmoidectomy and coloanal anastomosis, the local failure rate was 13%, and the 5-year actuarial survival rate was 91%.[102]

ADJUVANT RADIATION THERAPY FOR RESECTABLE RECTAL CANCER

The rationale of radiation therapy is based on the patterns of failure after potentially curative surgery. The incidence of local failure (as a component of failure) is less than 10% for T1–2N0M0 cancers, which increases 15% to 35% for stage T3N0M0 disease and is as high as 45% to 65% for T3–4N1–2M0 cancers. When local failure does occur, it is severely debilitating, and salvage has been of limited success. Even if it did not influence survival, the ability of radiation therapy to decrease local failure is an important endpoint. There are three major approaches for adjuvant treatment of resectable rectal cancer: postoperative, preoperative, and preoperative plus postoperative radiation therapy.

POSTOPERATIVE RADIATION THERAPY

The advantages of postoperative radiation therapy are that the stage is already known (*i.e.*, patients with stage T1–2N0M0–M1 may be spared treatment) and more accurate definition of the tumor bed for radiation planning is obtained by the placement of clips at the time of surgery. Disadvantages include an increased amount of small bowel in the radiation field, a potentially hypoxic postsurgical radiation field, and in the case of an abdominoperineal resection, the field must be extended inferiorly to include the perineal scar.

Nonrandomized Trials

Nonrandomized data from the Massachusetts General Hospital[103] and M.D. Anderson Cancer Center[104,105] reveal a local failure rate of 4% to 31% for patients with stage T3–4N0M0 disease and 8% to 53% for patients with stage T3–4N1–2M0 disease who received 4500 to 5500 cGy (Table 31–5). The Massachusetts General Hospital series is the larg-est reported experience from a single institution for which careful radiation techniques were used and long follow-up is available. Compared with a historic control group of 142 patients who underwent surgery only, there was an improvement in local control and survival among patients who received postoperative radiation therapy.

Randomized Trials

There are four randomized series examining the use of adjuvant postoperative radiation therapy for T3–4N1–2M0 rectal cancer (Table 31–6). The series from Odense University is a two-arm trial comparing postoperative radiation therapy with surgery alone.[106] In two of the series, one of the arms included radiation plus chemotherapy (Gastrointestinal Tumor Study Group [GITSG]) or chemotherapy alone (National Surgical Adjuvant Bowel and Breast Project [NSABP]).[107–109] In the Mayo Clinic/North Central Cancer Treatment Group (NCCTG) trial, there was no surgery-only control arm.[110] These trials are discussed at length in the section on combined-modality therapy of resectable rectal cancer. This discussion is limited to the comparison of the radiation therapy and surgical control arms.

Local failure rates depend on whether they are reported as first or cumulative failures. The four randomized trials express failure as first site of failure, and the nonrandomized trials express failure as cumulative failure. For example, in the Mayo Clinic/NCCTG trial, the incidence of local failure in node-positive patients was 25% if expressed as first failure but 63% if expressed as cumulative failure.[110] More favorable local failure results (local failure as the first site of failure) were reported from the GITSG (18%) and the NSABP (15%).[107–109]

In the GITSG series, there were no significant differences in local failure or survival rates with postoperative radiation.[107,108] There are many criticisms of the radiation therapy

TABLE 31–5. Adjuvant Postoperative Radiation Therapy for Resectable Rectal Cancer Selected by Nonrandomized Trials

| Investigation* | Stage | Local Failure (%)† | | | | 5-Year Survival (%) | |
		No. of Patients	S	No. of Patients	S + RT	S	S + RT
Massachusetts General Hospital[103]	T3N0	44	23	53	9	47	76 (NED)
	T4N0	15	53	7	0	27	69
	T1–2N1–2	4	50	10	20	25	69
	T3N1–2	34	17	77	21	27	34
	T4N1–2	6	67	15	53	0	13
M.D. Anderson Cancer Center[105]	T3N0		13	24	4		65
	T4N0		26	13	21		48
	T1–2N1–2			12	8		65
	T3N1–2		30	45	18		48
	T4N1–2		49	5	20		60

S, surgery alone; S + RT, surgery + postoperative radiation therapy; NED, no evidence of disease.
* MGH, 4500–5040 cGy + boost (14 patients had chemotherapy). M.D. Anderson, 4000–5000 cGy + boost.
† Cumulative failure as a component of failure.

TABLE 31–6. Randomized Trials of Postoperative Radiation Therapy for Rectal Cancer

Investigations	Dose (cGy)	No. of Patients		Stage	Local Failure (%)		Survival (%)		
		Surgery	RT		Surgery	RT	Surgery	RT	
GITSG[107,140]	4000–4800	58	50	T1–3N1–2M0	24	20	27	43	8-y actuarial
NSABP[141]	4600–4700	184	184	T1–3N1–2M0	25	16	43	41	5-y actuarial
Odense University[106]	4500–5000, split course	250	244	T2–3N0M0	6	6			
				T2-3N1-2M0	9	6	67	82	2-y actuarial LRS

RT, radiation therapy; LRS, local relapse-free survival.
* First failure.

techniques employed in the GTSG series. First, 39% of the patients treated with radiation therapy varied from the protocol specifications. Second, the radiation dose was chosen by the individual investigator (patients could receive 4000 or 4800 cGy). In the Mayo Clinic/NCCTG trial, patients in the radiation-alone arm who received 5040 cGy had a slightly lower local failure rate compared with those who received 4500 cGy (18% versus 24%).[110] Although there was no difference in overall survival, patients who received adjuvant radiation therapy in the NSABP series had a borderline significant decrease in local failure compared with surgery alone (16% versus 25%, $p = 0.06$).[109]

In the series from Odense University, 494 patients were randomized to postoperative radiation therapy (4500–5000 cGy) or to surgery alone.[106] Among patients with stage T2–3N0 disease, there was no difference in the incidence (6%) or mean time to local failure between the arms. In patients with stage T1–3N1–2M0 disease, there was no difference in local failure (6% versus 9%) however the mean time to local failure was significantly longer (19 versus 6 months, $p = 0.01$) in patients who received radiation therapy compared with the surgical control arm.

The retrospective data suggest that postoperative radiation therapy decreases local failure. The only randomized trial that confirms this finding (with borderline significance) is from the NSABP. Of the 3 randomized trials that compared radiation therapy with a surgical control arm, the NSABP was the only trial in which the radiation therapy was delivered with a continuous course, full doses, and with "modern" techniques.

PREOPERATIVE RADIATION THERAPY

There are biologic, physical, and functional advantages of preoperative irradiation for resectable rectal cancer: decreased tumor seeding at the time of surgery and increased radiosensitivity due to more oxygenated cells; no postsurgical small bowel fixation in the pelvis; and the ability to change the operation from an abdominoperineal resection to a sphincter-sparing low anterior resection and coloanal anastomosis.[111]

The major disadvantage of preoperative radiation therapy is possibly overtreating patients, such as patients with stages T1–2N0M0 disease who do not require adjuvant therapy or those with extensive distant metastases. With the use of CT and MRI, which increase the detection of unsuspected liver

metastasis, and intrarectal ultrasound, which increases the detection of transmural tumor penetration, the likelihood of patient overtreatment has been reduced.[9,12,14,112] There are also pathologic features that can help predict the presence of positive nodes.[91]

Nonrandomized Trials

Many nonrandomized trials of preoperative radiation therapy for patients with clinically resectable rectal cancer have been performed. Selected series are seen in Table 31–7. In the series from the University of Florida, there was a significant increase in 5-year absolute survival rate (70% versus 38%, $p = 0.001$) and decrease in local failure (8% versus 29%, $p = 0.015$).[113] Local failure was further decreased to 5% in patients who received more than 4000 cGy. Other series report local failure rates from 8% to 14% and a 5% to 10% pathologic complete response rate of the primary tumor.[89,102,114,115]

Retrospective data suggest that adequate doses of preoperative radiation therapy downstage pelvic lymph nodes, decrease local failure, and possibly improve survival.

Randomized Trials

There are eight modern randomized trials of preoperative radiation therapy for resectable rectal cancer (Table 31–8).[58,116–122] All use low to moderate doses of radiation. Some show a decrease in local failure, and in two of the series, this difference reached statistical significance.[116,117] The Stockholm trial[117] showed a significant advantage in disease-free survival, and the European Organization for Research on Treatment of Cancer (EORTC) combined radiation and 5-FU trial[120] revealed a borderline advantage in survival ($p = 0.06$). The most impressive improvement in results was reported from San Paulo Catholic University.[122]

There are significant flaws in the design of all of the randomized trials. First, none use adequate therapeutic radiation doses (>4500 cGy). Second, the interval between the completion of irradiation and surgery is inadequate. An interval of 4 to 6 weeks is recommended for maximal tumor downstaging and the recovery of normal tissues. Third, the radiation techniques employed were suboptimal and are known to be associated with an increased incidence of complications. For example, all used anteroposterior-posteroanterior (AP/PA) rather than multiple field techniques and made no attempt to

TABLE 31–7. Adjuvant Preoperative Radiation Therapy for Resectable Rectal Cancer: Selected Nonrandomized Trials

Investigations	No. of Patients	Clinical T Stage	Treatment	Local Failure (%)	Survival (%)
University of Florida[113]	74	T1–3	3500–5500 cGy, surgery	8	70 (5-y)
	135			29	38
Baystate[115]	40	T1–3	4000–4500 cGy surgery	9	71 (5-y)
	109			31	53
Lyon[89]	50	T2–3	300 cGy × 10	8	68 (DFS)
Thomas Jefferson[102]	143	T1–4	4500–6000 cGy	8	80 (5-y)*
Memorial Sloan-Kettering[114]	22	T2–3	5040 cGy	14	83 (3-y)

DFS, disease-free survival.
* Includes some patients with fixed cancers.

limit the dose to the small bowel. The superior border in most series was extended to L2 (rather than the more standard L5 or S1), further increasing the volume of small bowel in the radiation field. Moreover, the fraction sizes were unconventional and were as high as 510 cGy per day. These inferior radiation techniques contributed to the significant increase in complications, especially in the EORTC and Stockholm series.[116,117]

PREOPERATIVE VERSUS POSTOPERATIVE RADIATION THERAPY

It is difficult to compare, stage for stage, the results of preoperative and postoperative radiation trials because preoperative trials usually include a limited number of patients with T1–2N0 disease, full-dose preoperative radiation therapy downstages the T and N stage, and patients with pathologically confirmed M1 disease are excluded from adjuvant postoperative trials.[113]

The only randomized trial comparing preoperative with postoperative radiation therapy for resectable rectal cancer was reported by Pahlman and Glimelius.[123] In this multicenter randomized trial in Sweden, 471 patients were randomized to receive 2550 cGy preoperatively or 6000 cGy postoperatively. Postoperative irradiation was limited to patients with stages T3 and N1 or N2 disease. Those with stage T1–2N0 disease who were randomized to the postoperative radiation therapy arm did not receive radiation and were observed.

Patients who received preoperative irradiation had a decrease in local failure (12% versus 21%, $p = 0.02$), but there was no difference in 5-year survival rates (42% versus 38%). Although there was no increase in immediate radiation-related complications or postoperative mortality, there was a significant increase of perineal wound sepsis in the preoperative group (33% versus 18%, $p < 0.01$).

PREOPERATIVE PLUS POSTOPERATIVE RADIATION THERAPY

Preoperative plus postoperative radiation therapy, also known as the "sandwich technique" offers a short preoperative course of radiation therapy (500–1500 cGy), followed by surgery and, in patients with T3N1M0 disease, an additional 4140 cGy postoperatively. This approach was designed to employ the theoretical advantages of low-dose preoperative radiation (decreased tumor seeding) and reserve postoperative radiation therapy for those patients with T3N1–2M0 disease. The results of this approach has been reported in three series.[124–126] Local failure ranged from 0% to 13% and 3- to 5-year survival rates from 78% to 82%. Because of the short median follow-up (17–39 months), these data must be interpreted with caution. Because the randomized trials of combined radiation therapy and chemotherapy show a significant impact on survival and the benefits of preoperative radiation therapy (*i.e.*, downstaging and sphincter preservation) require full therapeutic doses rather than low or intermediate doses, there is limited interest in this approach for resectable rectal cancer.

FUTURE OF ADJUVANT RADIATION THERAPY

Given the increased morbidity and marginal benefits seen in the randomized trials of low- or moderate-dose adjuvant preoperative radiation, the limited interest in treating resectable rectal cancer with preoperative radiation therapy is understandable. The primary focus of clinical research in the adjuvant treatment of resectable rectal cancer for the past decade has involved the use of postoperative irradiation and chemotherapy. There are three reasons why the postoperative approach may not be the most innovative one: increased toxicity, less chance of sphincter preservation, and lower chemotherapy doses.

Despite the survival advantage of combined postoperative radiation therapy plus chemotherapy, it is associated with substantial toxicity. For example, the incidence of grade 3+ toxicity in patients who received combined radiation therapy plus chemotherapy in the GITSG trial was 26% for hematologic effects and 35% for nonhematologic effects.[108] In the Mayo Clinic/NCCTG trial, the most significant grade 3+ toxicities included diarrhea (41%) and leukopenia (33%).[110] The only grade 3+ toxic effect in patients receiving radiation therapy alone was diarrhea (5%). In the GITSG and Mayo Clinic/NCCTG trials, 35% of the patients never finished all the planned cycles of chemotherapy because of toxic reactions.

TABLE 31–8. Preoperative Radiation Therapy for Resectable Rectal Cancer: Randomized Trials

Investigations	No. of Patients	Treatment Arm	Fraction Size (cGy)	Irradiation-Surgery Interval	All Patients Local Failure (%)	All Patients 5-Year Survival (%)	Comments
Princess Margaret[118]	60	500 cGy	500	None‡	N/A§	35	Crude survival
	65	Surgery				35	
British MRC[121]	277	500 cGy	500	7 days	45	55	Includes 263 patients with partially fixed cancers
	272	2000 cGy	200	7 days	47	53	
	275	Surgery			43	57	
VASOG I[119]	302	2000–2500 cGy	200	14 days	29	43	Local failure included autopsy data
	311	Surgery			40	32	
VASOG II[58]	180	3150 cGy	175	None	N/A	50	
	181	Surgery			N/A	50	
EORTC[116]	231	3450 cGy	230	4–15 days	22*	60	% DFS Perineal Infection 66* 48%*
	228	Surgery			34	60	52* 29%*
EORTC[120]	124	3450 cGy + 5-FU	230	14 days	15	59†	5-FU = 375 mg/m²/d 1–4 of radiation therapy
	121	Surgery			15	46†	
Stockholm[117]	424	2500 cGy	500	1–7 days	17*	40	% DFS Morbidity Postop. Death 70* 26% 8%*
	425	Surgery			30*	43	59* 19% 2%*
Catholic Univ. San Paulo[122]	34	4000 cGy	200	7 days	15	80	
	34	Surgery			47	34	

* Statistically significant ($p \leq 0.05$).
† ($p = 0.06$).
‡ Interval is from completion of radiation therapy to surgery.
§ N/A, data not available.

In the Mayo/NCCTG trial, an additional 25% of patients did not finish due to patient refusal.

Preoperative radiation therapy increases the chance of sphincter preservation. By downstaging the primary tumor, preoperative irradiation allows the surgeon change the planned operation from an abdominoperineal resection to a low anterior resection and coloanal anastomosis.[111]

Higher initial doses of chemotherapy can be delivered with preoperative than with postoperative irradiation. This difference was observed in comparing two phase I trials of combined 5-FU, high-dose leucovorin, and radiation therapy (5040 cGy) reported from Memorial Sloan-Kettering.[114,127] Patients with unresectable disease received combined preoperative radiation therapy and two cycles of leucovorin and 5-FU followed by surgery and postoperative leucovorin and 5-FU.[127] Patients with resectable disease received the same leucovorin and 5-FU but postoperative radiation therapy.[114] The dose of leucovorin and radiation remained constant while the 5-FU dose was escalated. The maximal tolerated dose of 5-FU was higher with preoperative radiation therapy.

Based on its toxicity, increased chance of sphincter preservation, and higher chemotherapy doses, preoperative radiation therapy, if delivered with appropriate doses and techniques, is an attractive approach. Future trials with combined preoperative radiation therapy and chemotherapy for patients with resectable rectal cancer are warranted.

COMPLICATIONS OF PELVIC RADIATION THERAPY

Complications of pelvic radiation therapy are a function of the volume of the radiation field, overall treatment time, fraction size, radiation energy, total dose, and technique.[128,129] Large field sizes, a short overall treatment time, large fraction sizes (>200 cGy), orthovoltage or low-energy megavoltage radiation (cobalt 60), doses of more than 5000 cGy if there is small bowel in the high-dose field, the use of an AP/PA technique, treatment of only one field per day, the use of a direct perineal boost field, and the lack of computerized dosimetry all contribute to an increased incidence of radiation complications. Risk factors unrelated to irradiation techniques include pelvic inflammatory disease, hypertension, diabetes mellitus, obesity, prior pelvic surgery, or concomitant chemotherapy.[130]

Acute and delayed complications of pelvic radiation occur with distinct clinical courses and pathologic manifestations.[130]

The most frequent serious complication of pelvic radiation is damage of the small bowel.

Acute Complications

Acute complications are common during treatment and include thrombocytopenia, leukopenia, dysuria, and effects on the small bowel (*e.g.*, diarrhea, abdominal cramping, increased bowel frequency) and large bowel (*e.g.*, acute proctitis, tenesmus, bloody or mucus discharge). These are usually transient and resolve within a few weeks after the completion of radiation therapy. The symptoms appear to be a function of the dose rate and fraction size rather than the total dose. The management of bowel-related complications usually involves the use of diphenoxylate or narcotics. The bowel mucosa usually recovers in 1 to 3 months after the completion of therapy. Dysuria occurs in 10% to 15% of patients and is usually controlled with Pyridium. Skin erythema is common and is treated symptomatically with nonmetallic skin creams. If grade 3+ toxicity develops, a 1-week treatment break is commonly required.

Delayed Complications

Delayed complications occur less frequently than acute reactions, but they are substantially more serious. The initial symptoms commonly occur 6 to 18 months after completion of radiation therapy. Complications include persistent diarrhea, increased bowel frequency, proctitis, small bowel obstruction, perineal and scrotal tenderness, delayed perineal wound healing, urinary incontinence, and bladder atrophy or bleeding. Injury to the vascular and supporting stromal tissues of the bowel is the presumed pathophysiologic mechanism.[131]

The most common delayed complications are due to small bowel damage and include enteritis, adhesions, and small bowel obstruction requiring surgical intervention. The incidence of small bowel obstruction requiring surgery after postoperative pelvic irradiation for rectal cancer is 4% to 12% in recent series and as high as 17.5% in earlier series.[103–105] In patients treated with surgery only, 2% to 15% may develop similar complications. These late complications are directly proportional to the volume of small bowel in the radiation field.[128,132] Late radiation proctitis, similar to small bowel injury, is related to treatment volume and dose.

MINIMIZING TOXIC EFFECTS

Radiation Treatment Techniques

Several radiotherapeutic techniques can decrease radiation-related small bowel toxic effects (Table 31–9).[128,129] Contrast must be used to identify the location of the small bowel. The use of three or four fields allows a larger amount of small bowel to be blocked from the pelvis than with compared with an AP/PA (two-field) technique. The treatment of all radiation fields each day results in a lower integral dose and more homogenous dose distribution. Using lateral fields for the boost and positioning the patient prone with a distended bladder further decreases the volume of small bowel in the radiation fields. The treatment should be designed with the use of computerized dosimetry and be delivered by high-energy linear

TABLE 31–9. Techniques to Minimize Toxic Effect to Small Bowel With Pelvic Radiation Therapy

Surgical Techniques

Pelvic reconstruction to exclude small bowel from pelvis:
  Reperitonealize pelvic floor
  Retrovert the uterus
  Construct omental sling
  Insert absorbable mesh
Pelvic clips to delineate high-risk areas

Radiation Therapy Techniques

Use of preoperative radiation therapy during planning:
  Small bowel radiographs during simulation
  Liberal use of other diagnostic tools, such as US, CT, or MRI to
    delineate tumor-small bowel relation
  Place patient prone
  Use multiple fields for pelvic treatment with judicious blocking
  Use carefully planned boost fields
During treatment:
  Bladder distention (with patient prone)
  Use of external compression
  Use "false tabletop"
  Use standard fractions (180–200 cGy/day)
  Diet regulation
  Potential use of radioprotectors

US, ultrasound; CT, computed tomography; MRI, magnetic resonance imaging.

accelerators ($\geq$6 MV) that, by nature of their depth-dose characteristics, deliver a higher dose to the tumor volume while sparing the surrounding normal structures. If the perineal scar needs to be treated, it should be included in the pelvic radiation fields. The use of a separate perineal field is associated with an increased risk of field overlap and should be avoided.

The advantage of the combination of a four-field technique, high-energy photons, and computerized dosimetry is illustrated in Figure 31–5. With this combination, there is a homogenous dose distribution throughout the target volume, and prescribing to the 98% isodose line covers the volume at risk and gives only 62% of the dose to the small bowel. In contrast, when the same patient receives ^{60}Co AP/PA treatment, there is an heterogenous dose distribution throughout the target volume, and the radiologist must prescribe to the 90% isodose line to cover the volume at risk, giving 119% of the dose to the small bowel. Furthermore, if computerized treatment planning was not performed and the dose was prescribed to the midplane, parts of the tumor volume would be underdosed by 10%.

After pelvic surgery, the small bowel commonly fills the empty pelvis. Adhesions can result in fixed loops of small bowel in the radiation fields. In this situation, despite treatment of the patient in the prone position, the use of multiple fields may be of limited value (see Fig. 31–6). If radiation therapy is delivered preoperatively to a patient who has not undergone prior pelvic surgery, the small bowel is usually mobile. As illustrated in Figure 31–7, if there is no small bowel fixation, treatment in the prone position is successful

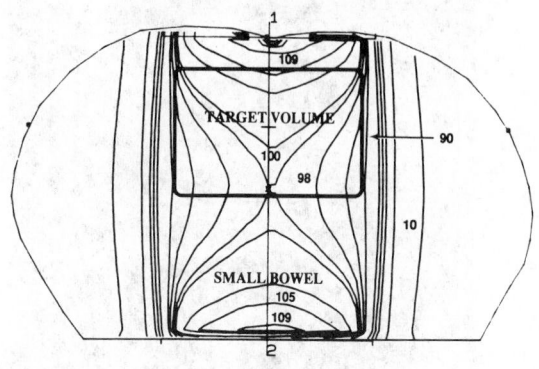

4-FIELDS 15 Mv

PRESCRIBE TO 98%

MAXIMUM SMALL BOWEL DOSE = 62%

AP/PA COBALT-60

PRESCRIBE TO 90%

MAXIMUM SMALL BOWEL DOSE = 119%

FIGURE 31–5. Isodose distribution of a 4-field technique compared with AP/PA cobalt 60 in a patient receiving radiation therapy for rectal cancer. The patient is prone, and the distribution is through the center of the field.

in excluding most of the small bowel from the AP/PA fields and completely from the lateral fields.

Immobilization Molds

The effectiveness of custom bowel immobilization molds (*i.e.*, belly board) for 30 patients with pelvic malignancies was analyzed by Shanahan and colleagues.[133] Using CT-based volumetric analysis, the combination of the prone position and immobilization molds decreased the mean small bowel volume in the radiation field by 66% compared with patients treated in the supine position without the immobilization mold.

Small Bowel Contrast

Small bowel contrast is essential to determine the position of small bowel during radiation simulation. It should be used

routinely during the simulation in patients receiving curative pelvic radiation therapy. For patients with endometrial and rectal cancer who had small bowel contrast used at the time of radiation simulation, there was a change in the treatment field and a lower incidence of overall and chronic complications.[134] Multivariate analysis revealed that the use of small bowel contrast and a lower superior border of the treatment field predicted decreased radiation toxicity. These data indicated that visualization of small bowel contributed to an adjustment in the radiation field, decreasing the incidence of toxicity.

Three-Dimensional Radiation Treatment Planning

Innovative techniques using three-dimensional treatment planning are being investigated. The Photon Treatment Plan-

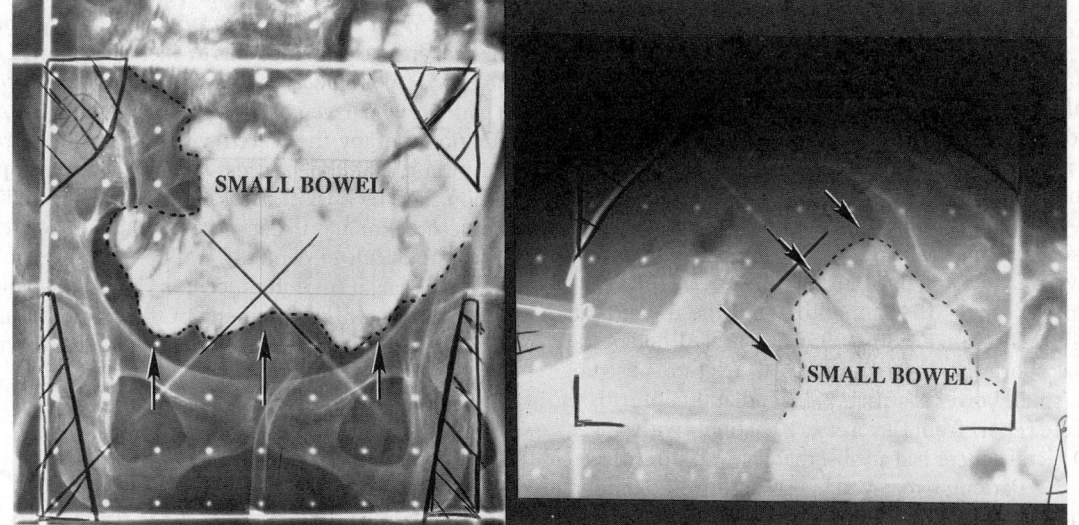

FIGURE 31–6. Radiation treatment fields in a patient in the prone position with a distended bladder receiving postoperative radiation therapy using a 4-field technique. Despite these maneuvers, the small bowel (*arrows*) remains fixed in the pelvis, and it cannot be excluded from the lateral fields.

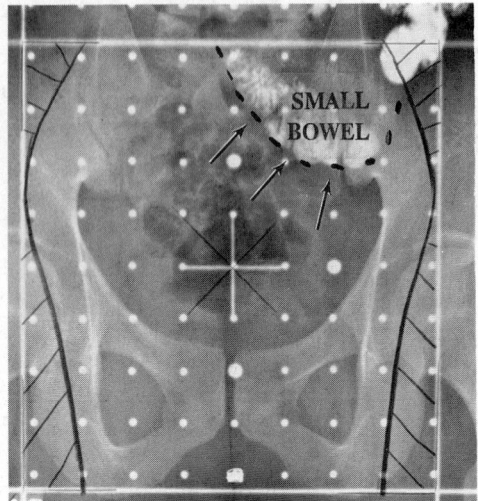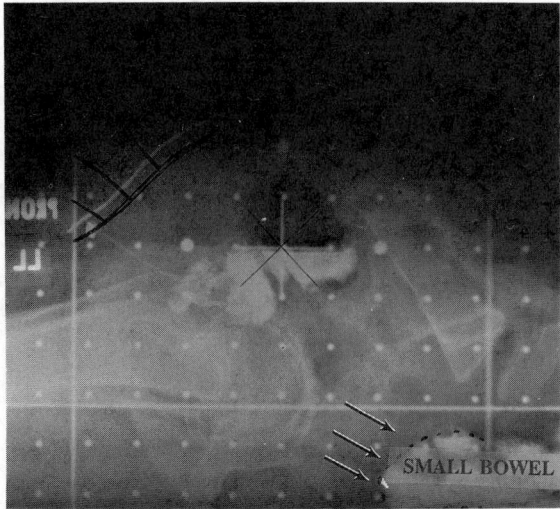

FIGURE 31–7.   Radiation treatment fields in a patient in the prone position with a distended bladder receiving preoperative radiation therapy using a 4-field technique.

ning Collaborative Working Group found that the most important contribution of three-dimensional treatment planing was the ability to plan and localize the target and normal tissues at all levels of the treatment volume, rather than using the traditional method of planning with only a single central transverse slice and simulation films.[135] There was also a slight improvement if there were no constraints on the type of plans (*e.g.,* if noncoplanar beams were used).

Radiation Therapy and Surgery Sequencing

The major disadvantage of delivering radiation therapy in the postoperative setting is the increased incidence of fixed loops of small bowel in the pelvis (see Fig. 31–6). The primary advantages of preoperative irradiation are decreased volume of small bowel in the radiation field and the absence of a perineal scar to be treated (Fig. 31–7).

Surgical Techniques

Surgical techniques to minimize small bowel injury include reperitonealization of the pelvic floor, construction of an omental pedicle flap, retroversion of the uterus, placing clips in the high risk areas to better define the tumor volume, and the use of absorbable mesh that temporarily removes the small bowel from the pelvis.[128] For 42 patients with rectal cancer who had absorbable mesh sling placed at surgery and received postoperative pelvic radiation therapy, the mean follow-up was 28 months (range, 10–57 months) and the mean total dose was 5450 cGy (range, 5300–5950 cGy).[136] Although the follow-up was short, there were no cases of stricture, obstruction, fistula, small bowel obstruction, or radiation enteritis.

In a separate report from Devereux, 19 patients with stages T4N1–2M0 rectal cancer had an absorbable mesh sling placed at surgery.[137] Patients received postoperative radiation therapy, but the details were not provided. With a mean follow-up of 33 months, no patient experienced obstruction, infection, nausea, vomiting, cramps, diarrhea, or acute radiation-associated small bowel injury.

Dietary Techniques

Elemental diets have been used to decrease the morbidity of pelvic irradiation. McArdle and colleagues compared the results of an elemental diet in 24 patients with bladder cancer who received five 400-cGy fractions before cystectomy with a similar historic group of 32 patients who received a regular diet or total parenteral nutrition with the same therapy.[138] There was a significant decrease in the incidence and severity of diarrhea, nausea and vomiting, and abdominal cramps and decreased time to the recovery of small bowel function in patients who received the elemental diet. The mechanism of protection of the mucosa by an elemental diet is unknown.

Recommendations

All cancer therapies have associated toxic effects. With pelvic radiation therapy, the exclusion of small bowel from the treatment field is the most important factor in decreasing the toxicity. With the use of careful radiation techniques and physical and surgical methods to exclude the small bowel from the pelvis, the toxicity can be reduced to an acceptable level. In patients who have not had prior pelvic surgery, preoperative radiation therapy (delivered with conventional fractionation and multiple fields) has less toxicity than postoperative radiation therapy.[114,127] Unless there is a contraindication, the simplest techniques to decrease radiation toxicity, such as the use of small bowel contrast, multiple field techniques, high energy linear accelerators, custom blocks, avoiding a direct perineal boost, and treatment in the prone position, should be part of the standard treatment of patients receiving curative adjuvant radiation therapy.

RADICAL SURGERY AND ADJUVANT CHEMOTHERAPY VERSUS CHEMORADIATION THERAPY

The anatomy and natural history of rectal adenocarcinoma require attention to issues of local and systemic tumor control.

Despite many clinical trials, until recently there was considerable controversy about whether additional therapy improved the survival rate of patients undergoing surgical resection of their primary tumors. Even a meta-analysis of the worldwide published experience, which demonstrated a statistically significant benefit for adjuvant chemotherapy in rectal cancer patients (38% decrease in the mortality rate), was not completely convincing for many physicians.[139] However, a Consensus Development Conference sponsored by the National Institutes of Health in 1990 concluded that effective adjuvant therapy exists for stage II and III (Dukes' stages B and C equivalent) rectal cancers. This conclusion was based on the clinical data derived over the past 20 years; especially important were five studies summarized in Table 31–10. Two of the studies included surgery-only groups, and three studies used surgery plus postoperative pelvic irradiation as the means for achieving definitive local control.[107,140-142]

GITSG study 7175 was initiated in 1975 and allocated patients with completely resected stage B2 or C disease to one of four treatment groups:[107,140]

1. Surgery only (control)
2. Methyl-CCNU (130 mg/m^2 on day 1) and 5-FU (325 mg/m^2 on days 1–5; 375 mg/m^2 on days 36–40), repeated every 10 weeks for 18 months
3. Radiation therapy employing 4000 to 4800 cGy to the pelvis
4. Radiation therapy using 4000 to 4400 cGy with concomitant 5-FU (500 mg/m^2) on the first three and last three days of radiation plus 5-FU and methyl-CCNU (doses as in the second group)

Although initially projected to accrue more than 500 patients, this trial was terminated after the entry of only 227 patients because of observed outcome differences between the regimens. At an 80-month median follow-up time, the control population had a 55% recurrence rate, but the rate was 33% for the radiation therapy plus chemotherapy group ($p < 0.009$). There were 14 local recurrences in the 32 control patients and 5 local recurrences in the 46 patients treated by combination therapy. A subsequent analysis at a median follow-up of 94 months showed an even larger margin of benefit for the combination therapy. In addition to a disease-free survival advantage, combination chemoradiation therapy was associated with a statistically significant overall survival benefit ($p = 0.005$). There was an approximate 20% superiority in survival rates at 6 years for the 96 patients at risk.[140]

Although these data support an aggressive multimodality approach to patients with rectal cancer, the morbidity of combined radiation therapy plus FU and methyl-CCNU must be considered.[143] Severe or life-threatening acute toxic effects occurred in 18% of patients in the chemoradiation therapy arm. Three late deaths occurred, two from enteritis in the combined treatment group and one from acute nonlymphocytic leukemia in a chemotherapy-alone patient.

Another major trial of adjuvant therapy for rectal cancer was initiated by the NCCTG (Study 79-47-51) in 1979.[110] A total of 204 eligible patients with Dukes' B2 and C rectal cancer were randomly assigned to postoperative radiation therapy only (4500 cGy with a 540-cGy boost) or to an integrated program of methyl-CCNU (130 mg/m^2 on day 1) plus 5-FU (350 mg/m^2/d on days 1–5; 400 mg/m^2/d on days 36–40), radiation therapy beginning on day 64 with concomitant 5-FU (500 mg/m^2) on the first three and last three days of radiation followed by one additional cycle of methyl-CCNU plus 5-FU (*i.e.*, sandwich therapy). At a median follow-up of more than 7 years, there were 62 recurrences in the group treated with radiation therapy alone and only 40 recurrences among those treated with combination therapy ($p < 0.0025$). Even after adjustment for known prognostic factors, the risk of relapse for patients receiving combination treatment was reduced by 47% compared with postoperative radiation therapy alone. The local failure rate in the combination treatment

TABLE 31–10. Rectal Cancer: Selected Completed Adjuvant Trials

Investigations	Total Accrual	Treatment (Arms)*	Results
GITSG 7175	227	Control MF RT → MF RT	RT + CT resulted in 59% 5-yr survival vs 43% in controls ($p < 0.01$)
NCCTG 79-47-51	204	MF → RT + FU → MF RT	RT + MF resulted in 63% 7-yr survival vs 48% for RT alone ($p = .04$)
NSABP R01	555	Control Pelvic RT MOF	MOF resulted in 52% 5-y survival vs 42% in controls (and RT) and significantly superior disease-free survival
GITSG 7180	210	RT + 5-FU → 5-FU RT + MF → MF	Interim analysis suggests 3-y probability of DFS is 45% for MF and 69% for 5-FU
NCCTG 86-47-51	453	MF → RT + 5-FU → MF 5-FU → RT + 5-FU → 5-FU (infusion vs bolus for 5-FU)	Interim analysis (16-mo median follow-up) suggests MF is not superior to 5-FU

MF, methyl-CCNU + 5-FU; MOF, methyl-CCNU + vincristine (Oncovin) + 5-FU; RT, pelvic radiation therapy; DFS, disease-free survival; →, sequential therapy.
* All patients undergo complete surgical resections.

group was 13.5% and 25% in those treated with postoperative irradiation only. The overall disease-free survival was superior with the combined treatment ($p = 0.0016$). An overall survival advantage was demonstrable for the combination therapy. The risk of cancer-related death was reduced by 36% ($p = 0.0071$) and overall death rate by 29% ($p = 0.025$). The therapy was well tolerated, and long-term toxicity was not apparent.

The largest study was performed by NSABP (R01) and required almost a decade to complete accrual.[109] A total of 555 patients with B2 or C lesions were randomized to one of three arms: postoperative observation; postoperative pelvic radiation therapy of 4700 cGy with a boost to 5300 cGy maximum; or MOF chemotherapy (methyl-CCNU, vincristine, 5-FU) as used in the NSABP C01 study (see Chap. 30). After a 64-month mean follow-up time, there was a statistically significant disease-free survival advantage for MOF chemotherapy ($p = 0.05$) and an overall survival improvement for selected subsets of patients receiving MOF, particularly men and patients younger than 65 years. Patients given only postoperative irradiation had no statistically demonstrable improvement in overall or relapse-free survival. There was, however, a reduction of locoregional recurrence rate from 25% without radiation therapy to 16% with radiation therapy. Despite 80 weeks of MOF chemotherapy, no leukemias have been observed; other toxic effects were predictable and tolerated.

These three studies permit the conclusion that combined radiation therapy and chemotherapy is superior to surgery alone, but the exact role of irradiation and the optimal protocol for chemotherapy are not defined. Two studies addressed the relative value of the addition of methyl-CCNU to 5-FU as part of a combined-modality irradiation plus chemotherapy treatment. The GITSG study 7180 evaluated 210 patients who successfully underwent surgical resection followed by 4140 cGy of pelvic irradiation and 5-FU (500 mg/m^2 given intravenously daily for 3 days at the beginning and end of irradiation). Patients were then assigned to receive 5-day courses of bolus 5-FU (300–500 mg/m^2/day) for 6 months or 5-FU (300–375 mg/m^2/day for 5 days each month) plus methyl-CCNU (100–130 mg/m^2 for 10 weeks) for a total of 12 months of treatment. With 3-year follow-up data, there was no superiority in recurrence or survival rates evident for the methyl-CCNU addition.[144]

The NCCTG study 86-47-51 used a 2×2 factorial statistical design to quantify the relative benefits of continuous infusion compared with bolus 5-FU and to determine the value of including methyl-CCNU in the chemotherapy regimen. All patients received pelvic radiation therapy and concomitant 5-FU in the sandwich sequence of chemotherapy-irradiation chemotherapy. Half the patients received methyl-CCNU and 5-FU chemotherapy as in the previous NCCTG trial (79-47-51), and the other half received 5-FU (500 mg/m^2 on days 1–5 and days 36–40. During the irradiation, patients received 5-FU (500 mg/m^2 on days 1–3 and days 36–39 as an intravenous bolus or 225 mg/m^2 as a continuous infusion each day for 5 weeks). The planned pelvic radiation therapy dose was 4500 cGy, with a boost to a total of 5400 to 5900 cGy. Patients received two more 5-day cyles of 5-FU, beginning 1 month after completing radiation.

A limited presentation of 453 patients with a median follow-up of 16 months, revealed no significant difference between 5-FU and methyl-CCNU plus 5-FU therapy in time to relapse or overall survival.[145] The reports of GITSG 7180 and NCCTG 86-47-51 are interim analyses, but neither study supports the addition of methyl-CCNU (in the setting of adequate surgery, irradiation, and 5-FU therapy).

The EORTC was unable to show a benefit with combined treatment.[120] This study of preoperative adjuvant therapies compared irradiation (3450 cGy in 230-cGy fractions) with the same radiation regimen combined with only an intravenous bolus of 5-FU (375 mg/m^2) on the first 4 days of irradiation. Among the 247 patients followed, overall survival was better with radiation therapy only. Because only minimal chemotherapy was employed, an overall advantage might not be detectable, but the incidence of liver metastases was reduced ($p = 0.07$) in the combined radiation therapy plus 5-FU group.

The integrated experience of five U.S. studies described indicate that meaningful survival benefits can be achieved with programs employing sufficient postoperative chemotherapy with or without pelvic irradiation. These data are supported by two earlier trials of adjuvant single-agent 5-FU in colorectal cancer patients. After the results in the rectal cancer patients were analyzed and reported separately, survival benefits with intensive 5-FU regimens were observed by Grage and coworkers[146] for the Central Oncology Group and by Higgins and colleagues for the Veterans Administration group.[147]

Although radiation therapy alone has had little impact on survival, an appropriately intensive combination of radiation therapy and chemotherapy may offer the greatest survival advantage.[148]

Several issues remain unresolved: the exact choice of chemotherapy agent(s) that can provide the most benefit with the least toxicity, the duration of chemotherapy, the scheduling and dosage of radiation therapy, and the integration of surgery, radiation therapy, and chemotherapy. In an attempt to address some of these therapeutic issues, two large cooperative group randomized effort are ongoing in the United States (Table 31–11).

The NSABP R02 study is summarized in Table 31–11. This protocol compares the standard NSABP MOF chemotherapy regimen with a 5-FU plus folinic acid program and is complementary to NSABP C03 for patients with colon cancer. Half the patients receive radiation therapy in conjunction with chemotherapy. Because of preliminary evidence of qualitative therapy interactions in specific subgroups, women receive 5-FU plus folinic acid, with or without radiation therapy, and men are randomly assigned among the four therapy options. The MOF chemotherapy doses are identical to those in NSABP C03. These two active studies address some of the most demanding questions in the treatment of rectal cancer. Programs employing pelvic irradiation and 5-FU plus methyl-CCNU have demonstrated benefits and toxicities. The new NSABP and NCCTG studies will help define the therapeutic advantage for methyl-CCNU and evaluate promising new ways of using 5-FU by infusion with folinic acid or levamisole modulation.

A large Intergroup Study (INT-0114) was initiated in 1990 to evaluate more than 1300 rectal cancer patients (Table 31–12). All patients undergo a complete resection and then receive one cycle of chemotherapy followed by 5000 to 5400 cGy of pelvic irradiation with chemotherapy and an additional cycle of therapy (*i.e.*, a treatment strategy similar to NCTTG-79-47-51 and 86-47-51). All patients receive 5-FU alone or with folinic acid or levamisole. Based on persuasive data for

TABLE 31–11. Rectal Cancer: National Cancer Institute Sponsored Randomized Adjuvant Trials

Investigation	Population	Target	Therapy	Comments
INT-0114	Stages B2, C	1378	5-FU → RT + 5-FU → 5-FU 5-FU + FA → RT + 5-FU + FA → 5-FU + FA 5-FU + LEV → RT + 5-FU → 5-FU + LEV 5-FU + LEV → RT + 5-FU + FA → 5-FU + FA + LEV	Completion of accrual anticipated by 11/1992
NASBP R02	Stages B2, C	750	MOF MOF → RT + 5-FU → MOF 5-FU + FA 5-FU + FA → RT + 5-FU → 5-FU + FA	Women are not randomized to MOF options; completion of accrual anticipated by 1/1993

RT, pelvic radiation therapy of 5040–5400 cGy; 5-FU, 5-fluorouracil; FA, folinic acid; MOF, methyl-CCNU + vincristine + 5-FU; LEV, levamisole; →, sequential therapy.

colon cancer patients with metastases that demonstrated higher response rates for 5-FU plus folinic acid (leucovorin) and for levamisole plus 5-FU for completely resected colon cancer patients, these combinations have been incorporated in adjuvant trials for colon and rectal cancer patients. A combination of all three agents is being evaluated. This high-priority clinical trial should reach its anticipated accrual goal by the end of 1992.

Until a complete analysis of all the previously cited studies becomes available, some form of adjuvant therapy should be considered for all patients and recommended for most patients with T3 or T4 and node-positive rectal cancer (stage II or III). Participation in a formal clinical trial should be encouraged. For those not entering a clinical study, the choice of adjuvant therapy depends on many medical, psychological, and financial factors. For many patients, the use of postoperative pelvic irradiation with postoperative 5-FU is entirely reasonable and justifiable.

CONTROL OF LOCALLY ADVANCED AND UNRESECTABLE RECTAL CANCER

A significant improvement in local control and survival can be achieved for patients with primary, resectable rectal cancer with the use of radiation therapy plus chemotherapy.[107,108,110] It is more difficult to obtain these results if the patient presents with locally advanced or unresectable cancer. For locally advanced rectal cancer, there is no uniform definition of resectability. Depending on the series, it can vary from a tethered or marginally resectable cancer to a fixed cancer with direct invasion of adjacent organs or structures. The definition also depends on whether the assessment of resectability is made clinically or at the time of surgery. For example, tumors thought to be unresectable at the time of clinical or radiographic examination may be found intraoperatively to be more mobile. There are also prognostic differences between primary

TABLE 31–12. Treatment Schema for Intergroup Protocol 0114

Treatment Arm		
Initial Chemotherapy →	*Chemoradiation →*	*Postradiation Chemotherapy†*
1. 5-FU (500 mg/m²/d, d 1–5, 29–33)*	RT (5040–5400 cGy) + 5-FU (500 mg/m²/d, d 57–59, 85–87)	5-FU (450 mg/m²/d, d 1–5, 29–33)
2. 5-FU (425 mg/m²/d, d 1–5, 29–33), leucovorin (20 mg/m²/d, d 1–5, 29–33)	RT (5040–5400 cGy) + 5-FU (400 mg/m²/d, d 57–60, 85–88) + leucovorin (20 mg/m²/d, d 57–60, 85–88)	5-FU (380 mg/m²/d, d 1–5, 29–33) + leucovorin (20 mg/m²/d, d 1–5, 29–33) (begin 28 days after end of RT)
3. 5-FU (450 mg/m²/d, d 1–5, 29–33) + levamisole (150 mg/d × 3, q 14 d × 4)	RT (5040–5400 cGy) + 5-FU (500 mg/m² d, 57–59, 85–87) (begin 28 days after end of RT)	5-FU (400 mg/m²/d, d 1–5, 29–33) + levamisole (150 mg/d × 3 q 14 d × 4)
4. 5-FU (425 mg/m²/d, d 1–5, 29–33) + leucovorin (20 mg/m²/d, d 1–5, 29–33) + levamisole (150 mg/d × 3 q 14 d × 4)	RT (5040–5400 cGy) + 5-FU (400 mg/m²/d, d 57–60, 85–88) +	5-FU (300 mg/m², d 1–5, 29–33) + leucovorin (20 mg/m²/d, d 1–5, 29–33) levamisole (150 mg/d, × 3 q 14 d × 4) (begin 28 days after end of RT)

* When given with RT, the duration of 5-FU therapy is 3 days for treatments 1 and 3, and 4 days for treatments 2 and 4.
† Postradiation chemotherapy begins 28 days after completing radiation (day 1 represents 29th day after radiation completion).

and recurrent tumors, but most series do not report the results separately. The heterogeneity of the disease and absence of a uniform definition may explain some of the variation in results seen among the series.

TUMORS AMENABLE TO POTENTIALLY CURATIVE RADICAL SURGERY

Some tumors can be cured with radical surgery. In this category are men with tumors invading the prostate or base of bladder and women with a prior hysterectomy and current invasion of the base of the bladder. In selected patients, abdominoperineal resection, pelvic exenteration, or wide perineal excision may be effective in eradicating the cancer.[149] Midline posterior tumors adherent or invading the distal sacrum may be resectable for cure with extended abdominoperineal resection that includes the sacrum. Occasionally, total pelvic exenteration including a portion of the sacrum is appropriate. Loss of nerves to the bladder is irrelevant in the last group, because the bladder is included in the specimen. We exclude anteriorly based cancers in women with rectovaginal septal invasion in whom a posterior vaginectomy or posterior exenteration renders them disease free.

Patient Selection

Physical examination, CT scan, MRI, and cystoscopy all play a role in staging these patients. Involvement of the sciatic notch indicated by symptoms or scans predicts a situation unlikely to be helped by surgery.

Surgery

Extended Lateral Dissection

Patients with bulky lateral extension as part of primary tumor growth may obtain an improved margin by a dissection lateral to the hypogastric vessels.[150]

Pelvic Exenteration

Reports from the Ellis Fischel State Cancer Center suggest that results with this radical approach in selected patients can be done with acceptable morbidity and mortality and with 5-year survival rates in excess of 40%.[151–153] Twenty-four patients have been treated, 17 at the time of initial surgery. In the node-negative patients, the 5-year survival rate was 60%. The group from Hong Kong obtained similar results in a large series of 49 patients, with a 5-year survival rate of 52% for node-negative patients and 27% for node-positive patients.[154] Ledesma and colleagues treated 30 patients with primary rectal cancers by total pelvic exenteration, and the mortality rate was 10%.[155] Eight of 17 node-negative patients and 2 of 8 node-positive patients were alive at 5 years.

RADIATION THERAPY

Preoperative Pelvic Radiation Therapy

Because surgery commonly leaves residual disease in the pelvis in patients with locally advanced or unresectable disease, a common strategy is preoperative pelvic radiation therapy. The goals of preoperative irradiation are to convert an un-

resectable cancer to a resectable status and decrease the incidence of local failure.

The optimal use of preoperative radiation therapy requires full dose ($\geq$4500 cGy) and, to achieve optimal downstaging, a 4- to 6-week delay between the completion of irradiation and surgery. This discussion is limited to the series that meet these criteria.

In an initial report from the Massachusetts General Hospital of 25 patients with recurrent or primary unresectable cancer, a complete resection with negative margins was possible in 64%.[156] Despite negative margins, the incidence of local failure was 38%. The 9 patients who were unable to undergo a complete resection were dead of disease within 28 months.

The results of the patients with primary cancers were more favorable than those with recurrent cancers. In an update of these results, the rate of complete resection with negative margins was 59% for patients with primary cancers compared with 44% of those with recurrent cancers.[157,158] Limiting the analysis to the most favorable group of patients with primary cancers and negative margins, the 5-year actuarial local failure rate was 29%, and the disease-free survival rate was 60%. Even in the most favorable group of patients (*i.e.*, primary cancer and negative margins), local failure with preoperative irradiation is still almost 30%.

In a separate report from the Massachusetts General Hospital, the results of 28 patients with tethered rectal cancers treated with preoperative radiation were presented.[159] Tethered was defined as the sensation by the examining finger of partial tumor mobility consistent with extensive perirectal spread and adherence but not fixation to unresectable structures. Tethered cancers represent the most favorable of all locally advanced or unresectable cancers. A complete resection with negative margins was possible in 93% of these patients, but the local failure rate for the total group was 24%.

A similar approach was reported from the University of Florida for 23 patients with fixed cancers.[113] In the 48% of patients who were able to undergo a complete resection, the local failure rate was 55%, and the 5-year determinate survival rate was 20%. Comparable data have been reported from Tufts University.[160] In the 59% of patients who were able to undergo a complete resection, the local failure rate was 35%. The mean survival of the patients with residual disease was 17 months, and all were dead of disease by 36 months. In an update by Kopelson, the 5 patients who did not undergo a resection all died with a component of local failure.[161] At Memorial Sloan-Kettering, 58% of patients underwent a complete resection with negative margins, and the local failure rate was 25%.[162]

After full-dose preoperative radiation therapy, most series report that 48% to 64% of patients are converted to a resectable status. Despite complete resection and negative margins, the local failure rate is still 24% to 55%, depending on the degree of tumor fixation.

Improving the Results of Preoperative Radiation Therapy

A major limitation of pelvic irradiation is that the dose required to achieve an adequate level of local control often exceeds the tolerance of the surrounding normal tissues. Several approaches have been used to improve the results of preoperative irradiation, including intraoperative radiation therapy (IORT) and the addition of systemic chemotherapy.

Intraoperative Radiation Therapy

The primary advantage of IORT is that the radiation can be delivered to the site with the highest risk of local failure (*i.e.*, tumor bed) while decreasing the dose to the surrounding normal tissues. IORT can be delivered by two techniques. The first is electron beam. With this technique, the electrons are delivered at the time of surgery by a linear accelerator and, with the use of a plastic cylinder, are directed to the tumor bed. The second technique is intraoperative brachytherapy. Brachytherapy techniques involve implantation of radioactive sources with removable afterloading catheters or permanent seeds. The permanent seeds (^{125}I or ^{103}Pd) can be sutured or implanted directly into the tissues or placed in an absorbable mesh that is then sutured to the tumor bed.[163] Most of the intraoperative brachytherapy experience has been in patients with gross residual disease, but it has recently been used as an alternative to electron-beam IORT in patients with negative margins.[127]

The largest experience with electron-beam IORT was reported from the Massachusetts General Hospital.[157,158] Patients received 5040 cGy preoperatively followed by attempted surgical resection 4 to 6 weeks later. A 1000- to 2000-cGy IORT boost (1000–1500 cGy for microscopic residual disease and 1500–2000 cGy for gross residual disease) to the tumor bed was performed at the time of surgery. The results were compared with a historic group of patients who received the same preoperative irradiation but did not receive IORT. Patients with primary cancer who underwent a complete resection with negative margins followed by IORT had a 5-year actuarial incidence of local failure of 12% compared historically with 29% of those who did not receive IORT.[157] Patients were selected to receive IORT if there was adherence or residual disease (*i.e.*, positive margins). The results were less satisfactory in the patients with positive margins. In this group, although all patients received IORT, the local failure rate was 40%. Patients with gross residual disease had a higher local failure rate compared with those with microscopic residual disease (50% versus 31%).

A similar approach was reported from the Mayo Clinic for 51 patients (15 primary unresectable, 36 recurrent) with colorectal cancers (39 rectal, 6 sigmoid, 6 extrapelvic).[164] Some patients received 3 days of bolus 5-FU (500 mg/m^2) during weeks 1 and 5 of radiation therapy. The 4-year actuarial survival rate was 57% for patients with primary cancer.

Complications of Electron-Beam Intraoperative Radiation Therapy

Initial reports of neuropathy, vasculitis, bone necrosis, and ureteral injury from IORT were reported in dogs by Gillette and associates.[165–168] As the IORT data have matured, similar morbidity have been reported in humans. The incidence of toxicity depends on whether the patient has primary or recurrent cancer. In the Massachusetts General Hospital IORT experience, the incidence of complications were higher in those with recurrent disease (*i.e.*, 10% soft tissue or sacral injury and 10% pelvic neuropathy) compared with primary disease (*i.e.*, 2% sacral necrosis or ureteral obstruction).[157,158]

Higher complication rates have been reported from the Mayo Clinic.[169] Among patients with primary or recurrent colorectal cancer, the incidence of peripheral neuropathy was 32%. Although the pain, numbness, and tingling resolved in 40% of patients, only 13% had resolution of weakness. Ureteral obstruction or hydronephrosis were seen in 63% of patients who did not have evidence of ureteral obstruction at presentation. The incidence of complications increased with the IORT dose.

The phase I–II nonrandomized trials suggest that the addition of electron-beam IORT to preoperative pelvic radiation improves local control compared with preoperative radiation therapy alone. The Radiation Therapy Oncology Group (RTOG) has an ongoing prospective phase III randomized trial to validate the phase I–II results.

Systemic Chemotherapy and Radiation Therapy

Given the advantage of chemotherapy for patients with resectable rectal cancer in the postoperative adjuvant trials and the in vitro and in vivo evidence of 5-FU sensitization to radiation, it is reasonable to combine 5-FU–based chemotherapy with radiation therapy in the preoperative setting.[107–110,170–172] A theoretical reason for adding systemic chemotherapy at the time of diagnosis rather than postoperatively is to deliver the chemotherapy when the metastatic burden is the smallest.[173]

There are major questions about using combined-modality therapy in patients with locally advanced or unresectable rectal cancer. Does the addition of chemotherapy increase the complete response, resectability, and local control rates? Does the addition of chemotherapy increase the survival rate?

There are limited, nonrandomized data from series in which patients received radiation therapy plus systemic chemotherapy. Frykholm and colleagues reported an enhanced resectability rate for 21 patients with unresectable rectal cancer who received 4000 cGy and concurrent 5-FU and methotrexate with leucovorin rescue compared with 38 patients who received radiation alone (71% versus 34%).[174] At Highland Hospital, 16 patients with unresectable rectal cancer received combined-modality therapy similar to that used for squamous cell carcinoma of the anus.[171] Patients received 4000 cGy and concurrent infusional 5-FU (1000 mg/m^2 for 96 hours) on days 2 and 28 and mitomycin C (10 mg/m^2) on day 2. The incidence of local failure was 13%. Neither trial used full doses (≥4500 cGy) of radiation.

In the Mayo Clinic IORT series, 11 patients received 3 days of bolus 5-FU during weeks 1 and 5 of radiation therapy.[164] The overall local failure rate was lower among the patients who received 5-FU plus radiation therapy than for those who received radiation therapy alone (9% versus 19%). Some patients in the Massachusetts General Hospital IORT series received 5-FU, but the data were not reported separately.[157,158]

Based on the Erlichman regimen[175] showing an advantage of bolus 5-FU plus high-dose (200 mg/m^2) leucovorin compared with 5-FU alone in patients with metastatic disease, the Memorial Sloan-Kettering group designed a phase I trial of combined preoperative 5-FU, high-dose leucovorin, and radiation therapy followed by surgery and postoperative leucovorin and 5-FU.[127] Some patients received intraoperative brachytherapy. Of the 20 patients enrolled, 13 had primary tumors, and 7 had recurrent disease. The dose of leucovorin and radiation remained constant while the 5-FU dose was escalated. Compared with a similar group of patients with unresectable cancer treated with the identical dose and technique of preoperative irradiation without leucovorin and 5-FU, those who received chemotherapy had a higher rate of complete resections with negative margins (89% versus 58%) and pathologically determined complete responses (21% versus 0%), and they had a lower incidence of positive nodes (30% versus 64%) compared with those who did not receive chemotherapy.[176] Based on the Mayo Clinic experience with low-dose leucovorin (20 mg/m^2), new trials are at Memorial Sloan-Kettering are determining the efficacy of low-dose leucovorin compared with high-dose leucovorin.

External-Beam Radiation Therapy Alone

Patients selected for radiation therapy alone are usually medically inoperable or have such advanced local disease that resection is not feasible for cure. In most series, patients received pelvic irradiation followed by a boost with external-beam or brachytherapy. The Princess Margaret Hospital reported a 2% 5-year actuarial survival rate and 91% local failure rate for 67 patients with primary unresectable cancer.[71] In a subgroup of patients without metastatic disease who received more than 4600 cGy, Overgaard and coworkers reported a 30% 2-year survival rate.[177] More favorable results for 37 patients were reported from Kaiser Permanente.[178] With 24 to 84 months of follow-up, 14% had no evidence of disease, and the local failure rate was 51%. A 30% 3-year survival rate was reported from Memorial Sloan-Kettering.[162] In other selected series, the incidence of local failure was 29% to 93%, and the 2- to 5-year survival rates ranged from 0% to 14%. Taylor and colleagues reported the results of 74 patients with recurrent, primary inoperable, or medically unfit patients with rectal cancer who received radiation therapy alone and 14 with gross or microscopic residual disease who received radiation therapy after surgery.[179] The actuarial 5-year survival rate was 4% for patients with residual disease after surgery; all others were dead of disease. Other series included patients with colon and rectal cancer, and the results were not reported separately.[180,181]

Postoperative Radiation Therapy and Chemotherapy

Two randomized trials compared postoperative irradiation plus chemotherapy with irradiation alone. In the RTOG trial, 129 patients with residual, primary unresectable, or recurrent rectal cancer were randomized to radiation therapy plus concurrent 5-FU followed by maintenance 5-FU and methyl-CCNU or to radiation therapy alone.[182] Some patients received IORT. There was no significant difference in the estimated actuarial 2-year survival rate for patients who received radiation therapy plus chemotherapy compared with radiation therapy alone (44% versus 36%). Of the patients with gross residual disease in either arm of the study, 25% had no evidence of disease, 6% were locally controlled, and 50% died with a component of local failure.

The ECOG randomized 30 patients with recurrent, residual, or primary inoperable rectal cancer to postoperative continuous-course radiation therapy or to split-course radiation therapy plus 5-FU followed by maintenance 5-FU and methyl-CCNU.[183] The median survival in both arms was 17 months. The 5 patients with primary inoperable cancer (considered gross residual) had the smallest 2-year survival rate (0%) compared with the 16 with recurrent (25%) or the 9 patients with residual disease (54%).

Chemotherapy plus postoperative radiation therapy, as delivered in these two randomized trials, did not significantly alter survival compared with postoperative radiation therapy alone. Other chemotherapeutic agents and schedules remain to be tested.

Investigational Radiation Therapy Approaches

Several investigational radiation therapy approaches have been employed to enhance the treatment results in patients with locally advanced rectal cancer or other pelvic malignancies. These include neutron-beam radiation, hyperthermia, and altered radiation fractionation schemes.

Neutron-Beam Radiation Therapy

The theoretical advantages of neutrons over more conventional radiation therapy include increased sensitivity of hypoxic cells and more advantageous radiation repair and sensitivity characteristics of the normal tissues. The results of two randomized trials that compared neutrons and photons for treating patients with unresectable and recurrent rectal cancers were reported by Duncan and associates.[184] A total of 35 patients received neutrons using a variety of techniques and doses. There were no significant differences in local control or survival, and patients who received neutrons experienced worse acute and late skin toxic effects (grades 3 and 4). The preferential absorption in fat of neutrons may have contributed to the complications seen in the skin and subcutaneous tissues. Similar severe and fatal complications were reported in a series of 25 patients with advanced rectal cancer treated by Batterman and colleagues.[185] Despite the theoretical advantages, there is little interest in the treatment of rectal cancer with neutrons because of these serious side effects.

Hyperthermia and Radiation Therapy

Hyperthermia has been used in conjunction with irradiation as a palliative modality in rectal cancer. Its use is based on an in vitro synergistic interaction of radiation and hyperthermia. The results of this combination in 41 patients with various pelvic malignancies has been reported in a phase I trial by the RTOG.[186] The preliminary acute and late toxicities were acceptable, but phase II data have not been reported. Goffinet and coworkers, using a hyperthermic interstitial radiofrequency technique with ^{192}Ir seeds, reported tolerable toxicity in 5 patients with recurrent rectal cancer.[187] Using regional hyperthermia to the whole pelvis, Feldmann and colleagues observed that there can be overheating of the perineal fat in eccentrically located presacral recurrences.[188]

Altered Radiation Fractionation Schemes

Various fractionation strategies have evolved with the goal of enhancing tumor-cell damage by radiation without augmenting normal tissue injury.[189] The repair of subcellular injury, regeneration, cell cycle redistribution, and reoxygenation are all factors at the cellular level contributing to how normal tissues and tumors respond to fractionated radiation therapy. The use of hyperfractionation and accelerated fractionation schemes take advantage of some of these factors. The major limitation of accelerated hyperfractionation is acute normal tissue toxicity, but late effects should be the same as or fewer than in conventional fractionation schemes.

There are limited data on the use of twice-daily irradiation of the pelvis. In a phase I–II trial from the RTOG, 54 patients with advanced bladder cancer received 120 cGy twice daily to a pelvic dose of 5040 followed by a boost to 6000 to 6900 cGy.[190] The actuarial incidence of grade III or IV complications was 11% at 2 years, which was that same as the incidence with conventional fractionation in prior RTOG protocols.

The RTOG is currently examining the use of twice-daily pelvic radiation therapy in adult patients with advanced pelvic malignancies. In this nonrandomized study, 370 cGy is delivered twice daily to the pelvis on 2 consecutive days every 3 to 6 weeks for a total dose of 5440 cGy. Results have not yet been reported.

FOLLOW-UP AFTER POTENTIALLY CURATIVE TREATMENT

The detection of asymptomatic recurrence is only one facet of patient follow-up. Maximizing the quality of life by management of treatment-related problems is extremely important in patients with colorectal disease.

Dietary modifications may be necessary for control of bowel function. A low-roughage diet may be helpful. After sphincter-saving rectal surgery, fecal urgency and frequency may be ameliorated with stool-bulking agents.

Small bowel obstruction, a late-occurring problem related to surgical scarring or radiation enteritis, necessitates surgery in 5% of patients.

The need for continued advice about colostomy management, irrigation techniques, and prevention of skin irritation may necessitate consultation with an enterostomal therapist.

Surgical castration or pelvic irradiation in premenopausal women leads to menopause with vaginal dryness with dyspareunia and general symptoms. Local and systemic estrogens may be helpful. Male impotence due to psychological and organic factors may require intervention. Papaverine injections and surgical implants can improve erectile impotence.

TREATMENT OF RECURRENCES

Recurrent disease can be treated with various combinations of surgery, irradiation, and chemotherapy. Systemic therapy for recurrent or metastatic cancer is discussed in Chapter 30.

RECURRENCE AFTER LIMITED LOCAL THERAPY

After treatment of rectal cancer by local excision, intracavitary radiation, or fulguration, some patients with limited local recurrences can be cured by radical surgery, perhaps combined with radiation therapy. Selected patients with superficial recurrences can be given additional local treatment before radical extirpative surgery, particularly if their medical conditions render radical surgery excessively risky. Although the data

are scant, low anterior resection or abdominoperineal resection can often be performed for patients without distant disease with a salvage rate of 25% to 50%.

SUTURE-LINE RECURRENCE

Limited suture-line recurrence in a patient with metastatic cancer may not require treatment. Radiation therapy may be useful for more advanced disease and to control bleeding. Prophylactic colostomy should be avoided, with partial obstruction managed by diet restriction and stool softeners. The Nd:YAG laser can be used to keep the lumen patent. In patients without distant metastases, long-term disease-free survival can be achieved with abdominoperineal resection, although cures are infrequent.[191-193]

RECURRENCE AFTER RADICAL SURGERY

Although isolated resectable local recurrences are encountered, most patients with pelvic failure have diffuse locoregional recurrences. Many of these patients also have distant metastatic disease. Patients with asymptomatic or minimally symptomatic pelvic recurrences and tumor outside the pelvis are usually treated with systemic chemotherapy. Regional chemotherapy of the pelvis is an experimental approach, with an encouraging initial report on the use of 5-FU and mitomycin C given by internal iliac artery infusion.[194] Results may be enhanced with hyperthermia.[195]

It is important to differentiate pelvic and perineal recurrences after abdominoperineal resection.[196] Isolated perineal recurrences can be palliated by wide local excision, but the disease is rarely cured.[197,198]

RADIATION THERAPY FOR PELVIC RECURRENCE

Unless there was prior pelvic irradiation, radiation therapy is the most useful palliative technique for patients with symptomatic pelvic recurrence. Although 80% to 90% of patients obtain initial pain relief, long-term symptom-free survival is uncommon with external-beam irradiation alone.[199,200] In patients with uncontrolled pelvic pain despite irradiation, symptomatic relief should be sought with pain control measures, not cancer treatment. Highly selected patients may be candidates for radical resection.

Patients with localized pelvic recurrences without prior irradiation have been treated at the Massachusetts General Hospital, Mayo Clinic, and Memorial Sloan-Kettering with an aggressive multimodality approach. Patients undergo high-dose external-beam irradiation and radical surgical resection with an intraoperative electron-beam boost. In the Massachusetts General series of 22 patients, an actuarial local control rate of 56% was obtained at 4 years in the subset of patients with tumors amenable to complete resection.[201] Thirty-six patients have been treated at the Mayo Clinic, with only a 17% local failure rate after a short follow-up.[158,202] Intraoperative brachytherapy yielded comparable results at Memorial Sloan-Kettering.[203,204]

As an alternative to intraoperative brachytherapy or electron-beam IORT, CT-guided transperineal implantation is available.[205] This technique can be performed under local anesthesia and offers an alternative, nonsurgical approach.

The technique is limited to tumors that are well delineated and, based on size and location, are technically implantable. Another nonsurgical technique is intraluminal brachytherapy.[206] With this technique, a remote afterloader is used to deliver a high-activity ^{192}Ir source. The source lies in the center of a rectal cylinder, and the dose is usually prescribed to 0.5 cm from the surface of the applicator. Its use is limited to patients with anastomotic recurrences whose tumors are 0.5 cm thick or smaller. It is difficult to draw conclusions because the series include patients with primary adjuvant and inoperable recurrent cancers and use various doses of external-beam radiation. Some include rectal and anal cancers, and most patients were treated in a palliative fashion.[205] If general anesthesia is not possible, these techniques may offer an alternative approach.

SURGERY FOR RECURRENT DISEASE

Abdominoperineal resection with in-continuity sacrectomy or pelvic exenteration with in-continuity sacrectomy (composite or abdominosacral exenteration) are useful for patients with extensive pelvic recurrent rectal cancer after low anterior resection or abdominoperineal resection combined with full-dose adjuvant irradiation. Multimodality options are limited for these patients. If the recurrence is primarily posterior without bladder involvement, sacrectomy up to the level of the S3 nerve roots may be performed without loss of bladder function.[207] If the bladder is involved and complete exenteration with in-continuity sacral resection is required, resection may be carried as high as S1.

The major experience with these extended operations for recurrent rectal cancer has been reported from three centers: Memorial Sloan-Kettering Cancer Center,[207,208] University of Virginia,[209,210] and the University of Colorado.[211,212] Wanebo and Marcove first reported the integration of the technique of primary sacral resection through the posterior approach with transabdominal visceral exenteration.[207,208]

The two-part approach begins with a thorough abdominal exploration to rule out extrapelvic cancer. The hypogastric vessels are preferentially ligated distal to the superior gluteal branch. The proximal line of sacral transection is determined, and the rectum or rectum and bladder are then mobilized. After complete anterior and partial lateral dissection, the abdomen is closed, and the surgery continues with the patient in the prone position. The sciatic nerves are identified and preserved, and the pelvis is entered. A laminectomy exposes and preserves the uppermost nerve roots, and the sacrum is transected with in-continuity removal of visceral contents, pelvic side-wall soft tissue, and the sacrum. Of the initial 7 patients who underwent potentially curative resection, only 2 patients had recurrences. Wanebo subsequently increased his series to 24 patients, and half underwent complete pelvic exenteration. Three patients died after surgery, and 5 patients were alive in excess of 4 years.[209,210]

Pearlman and associates resected 21 patients with recurrent rectal cancer, and 18 had prior radiation.[211,212] Twelve patients had complete abdominosacral exenteration. Of the 16 patients who had potentially curative surgery, 8 were free of recurrence at 6 to 48 months after the procedure.

All of these investigators attest to the excellent pain control associated with these operations, presumably related to the surgically induced hypesthesia and the tumor control.

REFERENCES

1. Enquist IF, Block IR. Rectal cancer in females: Selection of proper operation based upon anatomic studies of rectal lymphatics. Prog Clin Cancer 1966;2:73–85.
2. Reinhold P. Contribution a l'etude des facteurs de recidives postoperatoire du cancer rectal. Paris: These, 1924.
3. Bartolo DCC, AM R, Locke-Edmunds JC, et al. Flap-valve theory of anorectal continence. Br J Surg 1986;73:1012–1014.
4. Preston DM, Lennard-Jones JE, Thomas BM. The balloon proctogram. Br J Surg 1984;71:29–32.
5. Lahr CJ, Rothenberger DA, Jensen LL, et al. Balloon topography. Dis Colon Rectum 1986;29:1–5.
6. Read NW, Bartolo DCC, Read MG. Differences in anal function in patients with incontinence to solids and in patients with incontinence to liquids. Br J Surg 1984;71: 39–42.
7. Tartter PI, Steinberg BM. The role of preoperative intravenous pyelogram in operations performed for carcinoma of the colon and rectum. Surg Gynecol Obstet 1986;163: 65–69.
8. Thoeni RF, Moss AA, Schnyder P, et al. Detection and staging of primary rectal and rectosigmoid cancer by computed tomography. Radiology 1981;141:135–138.
9. Koehler PR, Feldberg MAM, van Waes PFGM. Preoperative staging of rectal cancer with computerized tomography: Accuracy, efficacy, and effect on patient management. Cancer 1984;54:512–516.
10. Shank B, Dershaw DD, Caravelli J, et al. A prospective study of the accuracy of preoperative computed tomographic staging of patients with biopsy-proven rectal carcinoma. Dis Colon Rectum 1990;33:285–290.
11. Hodgman CG, MacCarty RL, Wolff BG, et al. Preoperative staging of rectal carcinoma by computed tomography and 0.15 T magnetic resonance imaging: Preliminary report. Dis Colon Rectum 1986;29:446–450.
12. Butch RJ, Stark DD, Wittenberg J, et al. Staging rectal cancer by MR and CT. AJR 1986;146:1155–1160.
13. Guinet C, Buy JN, Ghossain MA, et al. Comparison of magnetic resonance imaging and computed tomography in the preoperative staging of rectal cancer. Arch Surg 1990;125:385–388.
14. Hildebrandt U, Feifel G. Preoperative staging of rectal cancer by intrarectal ultrasound. Dis Colon Rectum 1985;28:42–46.
15. Orrom WJ, Wong WD, Rothenberger DA, et al. Endorectal ultrasound in the preoperative staging of rectal tumors: A learning experience. Dis Colon Rectum 1990;33:654–659.
16. Saitoh N, Okui K, Sarashina H, et al. Evaluation of echographic diagnosis of rectal cancer using intrarectal ultrasonic examination. Dis Colon Rectum 1986;29:234–242.
17. Beynon J, Roe AM, Foy DM, et al. Preoperative staging of local invasion in rectal cancer using intraluminal ultrasound. J R Soc Med 1987;80:23–26.
18. Konishi F, Ugajin H, Ito K, et al. Endorectal ultrasonography with a 7.5 MHz linear array scanner for the assessment of invasion of rectal carcinoma. Int J Colorectal Dis 1990;5:15–20.
19. Dershaw DD, Warren EE, Cohen AM, et al. Transrectal ultrasonography of rectal carcinoma. Cancer 1990;66:2336–2340.
20. Glaser F, Schlag P, Herfarth C. Endorectal ultrasonography for the assessment of invasion of rectal tumours and lymph node involvement. Br J Surg 1990;77:883–887.
21. Hildebrandt U, Klein T, Feifel G, et al. Endosonography of pararectal lymph nodes—in vitro and in vivo evaluation. Dis Colon Rectum 1990;33:863–868.
22. Holdsworth PJ, Johnston D, Chalmers AG, et al. Endoluminal ultrasound and computed tomography in the staging of rectal cancer. Br J Surg 1988;75:1019–1022.
23. Waizer A, Zitron S, Ben-Baruch D, et al. Comparative study for preoperative staging of rectal cancer. Dis Colon Rectum 1989;32:53–56.
24. Rifkin MD, Ehrlich SM, Marks G. Staging of rectal carcinoma: Prospective comparison of endorectal US and CT. Radiology 1989;170:319–322.
25. Beynon J, Foy DMA, Roe AM, et al. Endoluminal ultrasound in the assessment of local invasion in rectal cancer. Br J Surg 1986;73:474–477.
26. Beynon J, McC.Mortensen NJ, Foy DMA, et al. Pre-operative assessment of local invasion in rectal cancer: Digital examination, endoluminal sonography or computed tomography? Br J Surg 1986;73:1015–1017.
27. Abrams JS. Clinical staging of colorectal cancer. Am J Surg 1980;139:539–543.
28. Zorzitto M, Germanson T, Cummings B, et al. A method of clinical prognostic staging for patients with rectal cancer. Dis Colon Rectum 1982;25:759–765.
29. Duncan W, Smith AN, Freedman LF, et al. Clinico-pathological features of prognostic significance in operable rectal cancer in 17 centres in the U.K. Br J Cancer 1984;50: 435–442.
30. Freedman LS, Macaskill P, Smith AN. Multivariate analysis of prognostic factors for operable rectal cancer. Lancet 1984;2:733–736.
31. Davis NC, Newland RC. The reporting of colorectal cancer: The Australian clinico-pathological staging system. Aust N Z J Surg 1982;52:395–397.
32. Davis NC, Evans EB, Cohen JR, et al. Clinicopathological staging of colorectal cancer: Has the time arrived? Br J Surg 1985;72:S47–S52.
33. York-Mason A. Rectal cancer: The spectrum of selective surgery. Proc R Soc Med 1976;69:237–244.

34. Nicholls RJ, York-Mason A, Morson BC, et al. The clinical staging of rectal cancer. Br J Surg 1982;69:404–409.

35. Nicholls RJ, Galloway DJ, Mason AY, et al. Clinical local staging of rectal cancer. Br J Surg 1985;72:S51–S52.

36. Williams NS. The rationale of preservation of the anal sphincter in patients with low rectal cancer. Br J Surg 1984;71:575–581.

37. Williams NS, Dixon MF, Johnston D. Reappraisal of the 5 centimetre rule of distal excision for carcinoma of the rectum: A study of distal intramural spread and of patient's survival. Br J Surg 1983;70:150–154.

38. Madsen PM, Christiansen J. Distal intramural spread of rectal carcinomas. Dis Colon Rectum 1986;29:279–282.

39. Hojo K. Anastomotic recurrence after sphincter-saving resection for rectal cancer: Length of distal clearance of the bowel. Dis Colon Rectum 1986;29:11–14.

40. Pollett WG, Nicholls RJ. The relationship between the extent of distal clearance and survival and local recurrence rates after curative anterior resection for carcinoma of the rectum. Ann Surg 1984;198:159–163.

41. Pezim ME, Nicholls RJ. Survival after high or low ligation of the inferior mesenteric artery during curative surgery for rectal cancer. Ann Surg 1984;200:729–733.

42. Hojo K, Koyama Y, Moriya Y. Lymphatic spread and its prognostic value in patients with rectal cancer. Am J Surg 1982;144:350–354.

43. Grinnell RS. Results of ligation of inferior mesenteric artery at the aorta in resections of carcinoma of the descending and sigmoid colon and rectum. Surg Gynecol Obstet 1965;120:1031–1036.

44. Heald RJ, Husband EM, Ryall RDH. The meso-rectum in rectal cancer surgery: The clue to pelvic recurrence. Br J Surg 1982;69:613–616.

45. Heald RJ, Ryall RDH. Recurrence and survival after total meso-rectal excision for rectal cancer. Lancet 1986;1:1479–1482.

46. Deddish MR. Surgical procedures for carcinoma of the left colon and rectum with five year end results following abdominopelvic dissection of lymph nodes. Am J Surg 1960;99:188–191.

47. Enker WE, Laffer UT, Block GE. Enhanced survival of patients with colon and rectal cancer is based upon wide anatomic resection. Ann Surg 1979;190:350–360.

48. Hojo K, Koyama Y. The effectiveness of wide anatomical resection and radical lymphadenectomy for patients with rectal cancer. Jpn J Surg 1982;12:111–116.

49. Koyama Y, Moriya Y, Hojo K. Effects of extended systemic lymphadenectomy for adenocarcinoma of the rectum: Significant improvement of survival rate and decrease of local recurrence. Jpn J Clin Oncol 1984;14:623–632.

50. Enker WE, Heilweil ML, Hertz REL, et al. En bloc pelvic lyphadenopathy and sphincter preservation in the surgical management of rectal cancer. Ann Surg 1986;203:426–433.

51. Glass RE, Ritchie JK, Thompson HR, et al. The results of surgical treatment of cancer of the rectum by radical resection and extended abdomino-iliac lymphadenectomy. Br J Surg 1985;72:599–601.

52. Quirke P, Durdey P, Dixon MF, et al. Local recurrence of rectal adenocarcinoma due to inadequate surgical resection. Histopathological study of lateral tumor spread and surgical excision. Lancet 1986;1:996–999.

53. Beart RW Jr, Kelly KA. Randomized prospective evaluation of the EEA stapler for colorectal anastomoses. Am J Surg 1981;141:143–147.

54. Griffen FD, Knight CD, Whitaker JM, et al. The double stapling technique for low anterior resection: Results, modifications, and observations. Ann Surg 1990;211:745–752.

55. Moritz E, Achleitner D, Holbling N, et al. Single vs. double stapling technique in colorectal surgery: A prospective randomized trial. Dis Colon Rectum 1991;34:495–497.

56. Donaldson GA, Rodkey GV, Behringer GE. Resection of the rectum with anal preservation. Surg Gynecol Obstet 1966;123:571–580.

57. Localio SA, Eng K, Coppa GF. Abdominosacral resection for mid-rectal cancer. Ann Surg 1983;198:320–324.

58. Higgins GA, Humphrey EW, Dwight RW, et al. Preoperative radiation and surgery for cancer of the rectum: Veterans Administration Surgical Oncology Group trial II. Cancer 1986;58:352–359.

59. Mohiuddin M, Yelovich RM, Komarnicky LT, et al. Preoperative radiation and surgery in unfavorable cancers of the rectum. Proc Am Soc Clin Oncol [Abstract] 1987;6:97.

60. Enker WE, Stearns MW Jr, Janov AJ. Peranal coloanal anastomosis following low anterior resection for rectal carcinoma. Dis Colon Rectum 1985;28:576–581.

61. Parks AG, Percy JP. Resection and sutured coloanal anastomosis for rectal carcinoma. Br J Surg 1982;69:301–304.

62. Cohen AM, Minsky BD. A phase I trial of preoperative radiation, proctectomy, and endoanal reconstruction. Arch Surg 1990;125:247–251.

63. O'Brien MJ, Winawer SJ, Zauber AG, et al. The National Polyp Study: Patient and polyp characteristics associated with high-grade dysplasia in colorectal adenomas. Gastroenterology 1990;98:371–379.

64. Welch JP, Donaldson GA. Recent experience in the management of cancer of the colon and rectum. Am J Surg 1974;127:258–266.

65. McDermott FT, Hughes ESR, Pihl EA, et al. Changing survival prospects in rectal carcinoma: A series of 1306 patients managed by one surgeon. Dis Colon Rectum 1986;29:798–803.

66. Slanetz CA Jr, Herter FP, Grinnell RS. Anterior resection versus abdominoperineal resection for cancer of the rectum and rectosigmoid. Am J Surg 1972;123:110–117.

67. Hargrove WC III, Gertner MH, Fitts WT Jr. The Kraske operation for carcinoma of the rectum. Surg Gynecol Obstet 1979;148:931–933.

68. Bevan AD. Carcinoma of the rectum: Treatment by local excision. Dis Colon Rectum 1986;29:906–910.

69. Madden JL, Kandalaft SI. Electrocoagulation as a primary curative method in the treatment of carcinoma of the rectum. Surg Gynecol Obstet 1983;157:164–179.

70. Crile G, Turnbull RB. Role of electrocoagulation in the treatment of carcinoma of the rectum. Surg Gynecol Obstet 1972;135:391–396.

71. Cummings BJ Jr, Rider WD, Harwood AR, et al. Radical external beam radiation therapy for adenocarcinoma of the rectum. Dis Colon Rectum 1983;26:30–36.

72. Papillon J. New prospects in the conservative treatment of rectal cancer. Dis Colon Rectum 1984;27:695–700.

73. Lockhart-Mummery HE, Ritchie JK, Hawley PR. The results of surgical treatment for carcinoma of the rectum at St. Marks Hospital from 1948 to 1972. Br J Surg 1976;63:673–677.

74. Whittaker M, Goligher JC. The prognosis after surgical treatment for carcinoma of the rectum. Br J Surg 1976;63:384–388.

75. Phillips RKS, Hittinger R, Blesovsky L, et al. Large bowel cancer: Surgical pathology and its relationship to survival. Br J Surg 1984;71:604–610.

76. Accarpio G, Scopinaro G, Claudiani F, et al. Experience with local rectal excision in light of two recent preoperative diagnostic methods. Dis Colon Rectum 1987;30:296–298.

77. Allgower M, Durig M, Hochstetter A, et al. The parasacral sphincter-splitting approach to the rectum. World J Surg 1982;6:539–548.

78. Killingback MJ. Indications for local excision of rectal cancer. Br J Surg 1985;72S:54–56.

79. Wilson E. Local treatment of cancer of the rectum. Dis Colon Rectum 1973;16:194–199.

80. Mason AY. Transsphincteric approach to rectal lesions. Surg Ann 1977;9:171–194.

81. Grigg M, McDermott FT, Pihl EA, et al. Curative local excision in the treatment of carcinoma of the rectum. Dis Colon Rectum 1984;27:81–83.

82. Whiteway J, Nicholls RJ, Morson BC. The role of surgical local excision in the treatment of rectal cancer. Br J Surg 1985;72:694–697.

83. Hager T, Gall FP, Hermanek P. Local excision of rectal cancer. Dis Colon Rectum 1983;26:149–151.

84. Biggers OR, Beart RW Jr, Ilstrup DM. Local excision of rectal cancer. Dis Colon Rectum 1986;29:374–377.

85. Salvati EP, Rubin RJ. Electrocoagulation as primary therapy for rectal carcinoma. Am J Surg 1976;132:583–586.

86. Wanebo HJ, Quan SHQ. Failures of electrocoagulation of primary carcinoma of the rectum. Surg Gynecol Obstet 1974;138:174–176.

87. Eisenstat TE, Deak ST, Rubin RJ, et al. Five-year survival in patients with carcinoma of the rectum treated by electrocoagulation. Am J Surg 1982;143:127–131.

88. Sischy B, Granez MJ, Hinson EJ. Endocavitary irradiation for adenocarcinoma of the rectum. Cancer 1984;34:333–339.

89. Papillon J. Present status of radiation therapy in the conservative management of rectal cancer. Radiother Oncol 1990;17:275–283.

90. Myerson RJ, Walz BJ, Kodner IJ, et al. Endocavitary radiation therapy for rectal cancer: Results with and without external beam. Endocurie Hypertherm Oncol 1989;5:195–200.

91. Minsky BD, Rich T, Recth A, et al. Selection criteria for local excision with or without adjuvant radiation therapy for rectal cancer. Cancer 1989;63:1421–1429.

92. Minsky BD, Cohen AM. Conservative management of invasive rectal cancer: Alternative to abdominoperineal resection. Oncology 1989;3:137–147.

93. Baker AR. Local procedures in the management of rectal cancer. Semin Oncol 1980;7:385–391.

94. Ellis LM, Mendenhall WM, Bland KI, et al. Local excision and radiation therapy for early rectal cancer. Am Surg 1988;54:217–220.

95. Rich TA, Weiss DR, Mies C, et al. Sphincter preservation in patients with low rectal cancer treated with radiation therapy with or without local excision or fulguration. Radiology 1985;156:527–531.

96. Willet CG, Tepper JE, Donnely S, et al. Patterns of failure following local excision and local excision and postoperative radiation therapy for invasive rectal adenocarcinoma. J Clin Oncol 1989;7:1003–1008.

97. McCready DR, Ota DM, Rich TA, et al. Prospective phase I trial of conservative management of low rectal lesions. Arch Surg 1989;124:67–70.

98. Minsky BD, Cohen AM, Enker WE, et al. Sphincter preservation in rectal cancer by local excision and postoperative radiation therapy. Cancer 1991;67:908–914.

99. Otmezguine Y, Grimard L, Calitchi E, et al. A new combined approach in the conservative management of rectal cancer. Int J Radiat Oncol Biol Phys 1989;17:539–545.

100. Marks G, Mohiuddin MM, Masoni L, et al. High-dose preoperative radiation and full-thickness local excision—a new option for patients with select cancers of the rectum. Dis Colon Rectum 1990;33:735–740.

101. Marks J, Mohiuddin M, Goldstein SD. Sphincter preservation for cancer of the distal rectum using high-dose preoperative radiation. Int J Radiat Oncol Biol Phys 1988;15:1065–1068.

102. Marks J, Mohiuddin M, Kakinic J. New hope and promise for sphincter preservation in the management of cancer of the rectum. Semin Oncol 1991;18:388–398.

103. Tepper JE, Cohen AM, Wood WC, et al. Postoperative radiation therapy of rectal cancer. Int J Radiat Oncol Biol Phys 1987;13:5–10.

104. Romsdahl MM, Withers HR. Radiotherapy combined with curative surgery: Its use as therapy for carcinomas of the sigmoid colon and rectum. Arch Surg 1978;113:446–453.

105. Vigliotti A, Rich TA, Romsdahl MM, et al. Postoperative adjuvant radiotherapy for adenocarcinoma of the rectum and rectosigmoid. Int J Radiat Oncol Biol Phys 1987;13:999–1006.

106. Balslev I, Pedersen M, Teglbjaerg PS, et al. Postoperative radiotherapy in Dukes' B and C carcinoma of the rectum and rectosigmoid: A randomized multicenter study. Cancer 1986;58:22–28.

107. Gastrointestinal Tumor Study Group. Prolongation of the disease-free interval in surgically treated rectal carcinoma. N Engl J Med 1985;312:1465–1472.

108. Gastrointestinal Tumor Study Group. Adjuvant therapy of colon cancer: Results of a prospectively randomized trial. N Engl J Med 1984;310:737–743.

109. Fisher B, Wolmark N, Rockette H, et al. Postoperative adjuvant chemotherapy or radiation therapy for rectal cancer: Results from NSABP protocol R01. JNCI 1988;80:21–29.

110. Krook JE, Moertel CG, Gunderson LL, et al. Effective surgical adjuvant therapy for high-risk rectal carcinoma. N Engl J Med 1991;324:709–715.

111. Minsky BD, Cohen AM, Enker WE, et al. Phase I/II trial of pre-operative radiation therapy and coloanal anastomosis in distal invasive resectable rectal cancer. Int J Radiat Oncol Biol Phys 1992;23:387–392.

112. Rifkin MD, Marks GJ. Transrectal US as an adjunct in the diagnosis of rectal and extrarectal tumors. Radiology 1985;157:499–502.

113. Mendenhall WM, Million RR, Bland KI, et al. Preoperative radiation therapy for clinically resectable adenocarcinoma of the rectum. Ann Surg 1985;202:215–222.

114. Minsky BD, Cohen AM, Kemeny N, et al. Phase I trial of postoperative 5-FU, radiation therapy, and high dose leucovorin for resectable rectal cancer. Int J Radiat Oncol Biol Phys 1991;22:139–145.

115. Reed WP, Garb JL, Park WC, et al. Long-term results and complications of preoperative radiation in the treatment of rectal cancer. Surgery 1988;103:161–167.

116. Gerard A, Buyse M, Nordlinger B, et al. Preoperative radiotherapy as adjuvant treatment in rectal cancer. Final results of a randomized study of the European Organization for research and treatment of cancer (EORTC). Ann Surg 1988;208:606–614.

117. Stockholm Rectal Cancer Study Group. Preoperative short-term preoperative radiation therapy in operable rectal cancer: A randomized trial. Cancer 1990;66:49–55.

118. Rider WD, Palmer JA, Mahoney LJ, et al. Preoperative irradiation in operable cancer of the rectum: Report of the Toronto Trial. Can J Surg 1977;20:335–338.

119. Roswit B, Higgins GA Jr, Keehn R. Preoperative irradiation for carcinoma of the rectum and rectosigmoid colon: Report of a national Veterans Administration randomized study. Cancer 1975;35:1597–1602.

120. Boulis-Wassif S, Gerard A, Loygue J, et al. Final results of a randomized trial on the treatment of rectal cancer with preoperative radiotherapy alone or in combination with 5-fluorouracil, followed by radical surgery. Cancer 1984;53:1811–1818.

121. Duncan W. Adjuvant radiotherapy in rectal cancer: The MRC trials. Br J Surg 1985;72:S59–S62.

122. Reis Neto JA, Quilici FA, Reis JA Jr. A comparison of nonoperative vs. preoperative radiotherapy in rectal carcinoma: A 10-year randomized trial. Dis Colon Rectum 1989;32:702–710.

123. Pahlman L, Glimelius B. Pre- or postoperative radiotherapy in rectal and rectosigmoid carcinoma: Report from a randomized multicenter trial. Ann Surg 1990;211:187–195.

124. Mohiuddin M, Derdel J, Marks G, et al. Results of adjuvant radiation therapy in cancer of the rectum: Thomas Jefferson University Hospital experience. Cancer 1985;55:350–353.

125. Gunderson LL, Dosoretz DE, Hedberg SE, et al. Low-dose preoperative irradiation, surgery, and elective postoperative radiation therapy for resectable rectum and rectosigmoid carcinoma. Cancer 1983;52:446–451.

126. Shank B, Enker WE, Santana J, et al. Local control with preoperative radiotherapy alone versus "sandwich" radiotherapy for rectal carcinoma. Int J Radiat Oncol Biol Phys 1987;13:111–115.

127. Minsky BD, Kemeny N, Cohen AM, et al. Preoperative high-dose leucovorin/5-fluorouracil and radiation therapy for unresectable rectal cancer. Cancer 1991;67:2859–2866.

128. Gunderson LL, Russell AH, Llewellyn HJ, et al. Treatment planning for colorectal cancer: Radiation and surgical techniques and value of small bowel films. Int J Radiat Oncol Biol Phys 1985;11:1379–1393.

129. Minsky BD, Cohen AM. Minimizing the toxicity of pelvic radiation therapy. Oncology 1988;2:21–25.

130. Kinsella TJ, Bloomer WD. Tolerance of the intestine to radiation therapy. Surg Gynecol Obstet 1980;151:273–284.

131. Rubin P, Casarett GW. Alimentary tract: Small and large intestine and rectum. In: Clinical radiation pathology. Philadelphia: WB Saunders, 1968.

132. Mameghan H, Fisher R, Mameghan J, et al. Bowel complications after radiotherapy for carcinoma of the prostate: The volume effect. Int J Radiat Oncol Biol Phys 1990;18:315–320.

133. Shanahan TG, Mehta MP, Bertelrud KL, et al. Minimization of small bowel volume within treatment fields utilizing customized "belly boards." Int J Radiat Oncol Biol Phys 1990;19:469–476.

134. Herbert SH, Curran WJ, Solin LJ, et al. Decreasing gastrointestinal morbidity with the use of small bowel contrast during treatment planning for pelvic radiation. Int J Radiat Oncol Biol Phys 1991;20:835–842.

135. Shank B, LoSasso T, Brewster L, et al. Three-dimensional treatment planning for postoperative treatment of rectal carcinoma. Int J Radiat Oncol Biol Phys 1991;21:253–265.

136. Devereux DF, Chandler JJ, Eisenstat T, et al. Efficacy of an absorbable mesh in keeping the small bowel out of the human pelvis following surgery. Dis Colon Rectum 1988;31:17–21.

137. Devereux DF, Eisenstat T, Zinkin L. The safe and effective use of postoperative radiation therapy in modified Astler-Coller stage C3 rectal cancer. Cancer 1989;63:2393–2396.

138. McArdle AH, Reid EC, Laplante MP, et al. Prophylaxis against radiation injury: The use of elemental diet prior and during radiotherapy for invasive bladder cancer and in early postoperative feeding following radical cystectomy and ileal conduit. Arch Surg 1986;121:879–885.

139. Buyse M, Zeleniunch-Jacquotte A, Chalmers T. Adjuvant therapy of colorectal cancer: Why we still don't know. JAMA 1988;259:3571–3578.

140. Douglass HO, Moertel CG, Mayer RJ, et al. Survival after postoperative combination treatment of rectal cancer. N Engl J Med 1986;315:1294–1295.

141. Fisher B, Wolmark N, Rockette HE, et al. Adjuvant chemotherapy or postoperative radiation for rectal cancer: Five-year results of NSABP R01. In: Salmon SE, ed. Adjuvant therapy of cancer. New York: Grune & Stratton, 1987:547–554.

142. Krook J, Moertel C, Wieand H, et al. Radiation vs sequential chemotherapy-radiation-chemotherapy: A study of the North Central Cancer Treatment Group, Duke University and the Mayo Clinic. Proc Am Soc Clin Oncol [Abstract] 1986;5:318.

143. Thomas PRM, Lindblad AS, Stablein DM, et al. Toxicity associated with adjuvant postoperative therapy for adenocarcinoma of the rectum. Cancer 1986;57:1130–1134.

144. Weaver D, Lindblad A for the Gastrointestinal Tumor Study Group (GITSG). Radiation therapy and 5-fluorouracil (5-FU) with or without MeCCNU for the treatment of patients with surgically adjuvant adenocarcinoma of the rectum. Proc Am Soc Clin Oncol [Abstract] 1990;9:106.

145. O'Connell M, Wieand H, Krook J, et al. Lack of value for methyl-CCNU (MeCCNU) as a component of effective rectal cancer surgical adjuvant therapy: Interim analysis of Intergroup Protocol 86-47-51. Proc Am Soc Clin Oncol [Abstract] 1991;10:134.

146. Grage TB, Moss SE. Adjuvant chemotherapy in cancer of the colon and rectum: Demonstration of effectiveness of prolonged 5-FU chemotherapy in a prospectively controlled randomized trial. Surg Clin North Am 1981;61:1321–1329.

147. Higgins GA, Lee LE, Dwight RW, et al. The case for adjuvant 5-fluorouracil in colorectal cancer. Cancer Clin Trials 1978;1:35–41.

148. Macdonald JS. Adjuvant therapy of gastrointestinal cancer. In: Salmon SE, ed. Adjuvant therapy of cancer, V. New York: Grune & Stratton, 1987:479–496.

149. Cohen AM, Minsky BD. Aggressive surgical management of locally advanced: Primary and recurrent rectal cancer. Dis Colon Rectum 1990;33:432–438.

150. Moriya Y, Hojo K, Sawada T, et al. Significance of lateral node dissection for advanced rectal carcinoma at or below the peritoneal reflection. Dis Colon Rectum 1989;32:307–315.

151. Kraybill WG, Lopez MJ, Bricker EM. Total pelvic exenteration as a therapeutic option in advanced malignant disease of the pelvis. Surg Gynecol Obstet 1988;166:259–263.

152. Lopez MJ, Kraybill WG, Downey RS, et al. Exenterative surgery for locally advanced rectosigmoid cancers. Is it worthwhile? Surgery 1987;102:644–651.

153. Eisenberg SB, Kraybill WG, Lopez MJ. Long-term results of surgical resection of locally advanced colorectal carcinoma. Surgery 1990;108:779–786.

154. Boey J, Wong J, Ong GB. Pelvic exenteration for locally advanced colorectal carcinoma. Ann Surg 1982;195:513–518.

155. Ledesma EJ, Bruno S, Mittelman A. Total pelvic exenteration in colorectal disease. Ann Surg 1981;194:701–703.

156. Dosoretz DE, Gunderson LL, Hedberg S, et al. Preoperative irradiation for unresectable rectal and rectosigmoid carcinomas. Cancer 1983;52:814–818.

157. Willet CG, Shellito PC, Tepper JE, et al. Intraoperative electron beam radiation therapy for primary locally advanced rectal and rectosigmoid carcinoma. J Clin Oncol 1991;9:843–849.

158. Willett CG, Shellito PC, Tepper JE, et al. Intraoperative electron beam radiation therapy for recurrent locally advanced rectal or rectosigmoid carcinoma. Cancer 1991;67:1504–1508.

159. Willett CG, Shellito PC, Rodkey GV, et al. Preoperative irradiation for tethered rectal carcinoma. Radiother Oncol 1991;21:141–142.

160. Emami B, Pilepich M, Willett C, et al. Effect of preoperative irradiation on resectability of colorectal carcinomas. Int J Radiat Oncol Biol Phys 1982;8:1295–1299.

161. Kopelson G. Long-term survivors after preoperative pelvic radiation therapy for locally unresectable rectal and sigmoid carcinoma. Dis Colon Rectum 1982;25:644–647.

162. Minsky BD, Cohen AM, Enker WE, et al. Radiation therapy for unresectable rectal cancer. Int J Radiat Oncol Biol Phys 1991;21:1283–1289.

163. Minsky BD, Cohen AM, Enker WE, et al. Intraoperative brachytherapy alone in incompletely resected recurrent rectal cancer. Radiother Oncol 1991;21:115–120.

164. Gunderson LL, Martin JK, Beart RW. Intraoperative and external beam irradiation for locally advanced colorectal cancer. Ann Surg 1988;207:52–60.

165. LeCouteur RA, Gilette EL, Powers BE, et al. Peripheral neuropathies following experimental intraoperative irradiation (IORT). Int J Radiat Oncol Bio Phys 1989;17:583–590.

166. Gilette EL, Powers BE, McChesney SL, et al. Response of aorta and branch arteries to experimental intraoperative irradiation. Int J Radiat Oncol Bio Phys 1989;17:1247–1255.

167. Powers BE, Gilette EL, McChesney SL, et al. Bone necrosis and tumor induction following experimental intraoperative irradiation. Int J Radiat Oncol Bio Phys 1989;17:559–567.

168. McChesney-Gilette SL, Gilette EL, Powers BE, et al. Ureteral injury following experimental intraoperative irradiation. Int J Radiat Oncol Bio Phys 1989;17:791–798.

169. Shaw EG, Gunderson LL, Martin JK, et al. Peripheral nerve and ureteral tolerance to intraoperative radiation therapy: Clinical and dose-response analysis. Radiother Oncol 1990;18:247–255.

170. Byfield JE, Frankel SS, Hoenback CL, et al. Phase I and pharmacological study of 72-hour infused and hyperfractionated cyclical radiation. Int J Radiat Oncol Biol Phys 1985;11:791–800.

171. Haghbin M, Sischy B, Hinson J. Combined modality therapy in poor prognostic rectal adenocarcinoma. Radiother Oncol 1988;13:75–81.

172. Rotman M, Aziz H. Concomitant continuous infusion chemotherapy and radiation. Cancer 1990;65:823–835.

173. Kelsen DP, Hilaris B, Martini N. Neoadjuvant chemotherapy and surgery of cancer of the esophagus. Semin Surg Oncol 1986;2:170–176.

174. Frykolm G, Glimelius B, Pahlman L. Preoperative irridation with and without chemotherapy (MFL) in the treatment of primarily nonresectable adenocarcinoma of the rectum. Results from two consecutive studies. Eur J Cancer Clin Oncol 1989;25:1535–1541.

175. Erlichman C, Fine S, Wong A, et al. A randomized trial of fluorouracil and folinic acid in patients with metastatic colorectal carcinoma. J Clin Oncol 1988;6:469–475.

176. Minsky BD, Cohen AM, Kemeny N, et al. Enhancement of radiation-induced downstaging of rectal cancer by fluorouracil and high-dose leucovorin chemotherapy. J Clin Oncol 1992;10:79–84.

177. Overgaard M, Overgaard J, Sell A. Dose-response relationship for radiation therapy of recurrent, residual, and primarily inoperable colorectal cancer. Radiother Oncol 1984;1:217–225.

178. Rao AR, Kagan AR, Chan PYM, et al. Effectiveness of local radiotherapy in colorectal carcinoma. Cancer 1978;42:1082–1086.

179. Taylor RE, Karr GR, Arnott SJ. External beam radiotherapy for rectal adenocarcinoma. Br J Surg 1987;74:455–459.

180. Ghossein NA, Samala EC, Alpert S, et al. Elective postoperative radiotherapy after incomplete resection of colorectal cancer. Dis Colon Rectum 1981;24:252–256.

181. Brizel HE, Tepperman BS. Postoperative adjuvant irradiation for adenocarcinoma of the rectum and sigmoid. Am J Clin Oncol 1984;7:679–685.

182. Rominger CJ, Gelber RD, Gunderson LL, et al. Radiation therapy alone or in combination with chemotherapy in the treatment of residual or inoperable carcinoma of the rectum and rectosigmoid or pelvic recurrence following colorectal surgery: Radiation Therapy Oncology Group study (76-16). Am J Clin Oncol 1985;8:118–127.

183. Danjoux CE, Gelber RD, Catton GE, et al. Combination chemo-radiotherapy for residual, recurrent, or inoperable carcinoma of the rectum: ECOG study (EST 3276). Int J Radiat Oncol Biol Phys 1985;11:765–771.

184. Duncan W, Arnott SJ, Jack WJL, et al. Results of two randomized trials of neutron therapy in rectal adenocarcinoma. Radiother Oncol 1987;8:191–198.

185. Battermann JJ. Results of d+T fast neutron irradiation on advanced tumors of the bladder and rectum. Int J Radiat Oncol Biol Phys 1982;8:2159–2164.

186. Meyerson RJ, Emani B, Perez CA, et al. Phase I/II study, combination of radiotherapy and hyperthermia in patients with deep-seated malignant tumors: Report of a pilot study. Int J Radiat Oncol Biol Phys 1989;17:204.

187. Goffinet DR, Prionas SD, Kapp DS, et al. Interstitial ^{192}Ir flexible catheter radiofrequency hyperthermia treatments of head and neck and recurrent pelvic carcinomas. Int J Radiat Oncol Biol Phys 1990;18:199–210.

188. Feldman HJ, Mollis M, Adler S, et al. Hyperthermia in eccentrically located pelvic tumors: Excessive heating of the perineal fat and normal tissue temperatures. Int J Radiat Oncol Biol Phys 1991;20:1017–1022.

189. Withers HR. Biological basis for altered fractionation schemes. Cancer 1985;55:2086–2095.

190. Cox JD, Guse C, Asbell S, et al. Tolerance of pelvic normal tissues to hyperfractionated radiation therapy: Results of protocol 83-08 of the Radiation Therapy Oncology Group. Int J Radiat Oncol Biol Phys 1988;15:1331–1336.

191. Sannella NA. Abdominoperineal resection following anterior resection. Cancer 1976;38:378–381.

192. Vassilopoulos PP, Yoon JM, Ledesma EJ, et al. Treatment of recurrence of adenocarcinoma of the colon and rectum at the anastomotic site. Surg Gynecol Obstet 1981;152:777–780.

193. Pihl E, Hughes ESR, McDermott FT, et al. Recurrence of carcinoma of the colon and rectum at the anastomotic suture line. Surg Gynecol Obstet 1981;153:495–496.

194. Patt YZ, Peters RE, Chuang VP, et al. Palliation of pelvic recurrence of colorectal cancer with intra-arterial 5-fluorouracil and mitomycin. Cancer 1985;56:2175–2180.

195. Estes NC, Morphis JG, Hornback NB, et al. Intraarterial chemotherapy and hyperthermia

196. Stearns MW Jr. Diagnosis and management of recurrent pelvic malignancy following combined abdominoperineal resection. Dis Colon Rectum 1980;23:359–361.

197. Polk HC Jr, Spratt JS Jr. The results of treatment of perineal recurrence of cancer of the rectum. Cancer 1979;43:952–955.

198. Wilking N, Herrera L, Petrelli NJ, et al. Pelvic and perineal recurrences after abdominoperineal resection for adenocarcinoma of the rectum. Am J Surg 1985;150:561–563.

199. Dobrowsky W, Schmid AP. Radiotherapy of presacral recurrence following radical surgery for rectal carcinoma. Dis Colon Rectum 1985;28:917–919.

200. Pacini P, Cionini L, Pirtoli L, et al. Symptomatic recurrence of carcinoma of the rectum and sigmoid: The influence of radiotherapy on the quality of life. Dis Colon Rectum 1986;29:865–868.

201. Cohen AM. Intraoperative radiation therapy for colorectal cancer. Probl Gen Surg 1987;4:76–82.

202. Beart RW Jr, Martin JK Jr, Gunderson LL. Management of recurrent rectal cancer. Mayo Clin Proc 1986;61:448–450.

203. Fourquet A, Enker WE, Shank B, et al. The value of interstitial radiation in advanced and recurrent colorectal cancer. Endocurie Hypertherm Oncol 1985;1:113–117.

204. Welch JP, Donaldson GA. The clinical correlation of an autopsy study of recurrent colorectal cancer. Ann Surg 1979;189:496–502.

205. Peretz T, Nori D, Hilaris B, et al. CT-guided transperineal implants in pelvic tumors. Proc Am Endocurie Soc [Abstract] 1988;4:13.

206. Kaufman N, Nori D, Shank B, et al. Remote afterloading intraluminal brachytherapy in the treatment of rectal, rectosigmoid, and anal cancer: A feasibility study. Int J Radiat Oncol Biol Phys 1989;17:663–668.

207. Wanebo HJ, Marcove RC. Abdominal sacral resection of locally recurrent rectal cancer. Ann Surg 1981;194:458–471.

208. Wanebo H. Resection of pelvic recurrence of rectal cancer. Contemp Surg 1982;21:21–33.

209. Wanebo HJ, Gaker DL, Whitehill R, et al. Pelvic recurrence of rectal cancer. Ann Surg 1987;205:482–495.

210. Wanebo HJ, Whitehill R, Gaker D, et al. Composite pelvic resection. Arch Surg 1987;122:1401–1406.

211. Pearlman NW, Donohue RE, Stiegmann GV, et al. Pelvic and sacropelvic exenteration for locally advanced or recurrent anorectal cancer. Arch Surg 1987;122:537–541.

212. Pearlman NW, Stiegmann GV, Donohue RE. Extended resection of fixed rectal cancer. Cancer 1989;63:2438–2441.

213. Rosenthal SA, Yeung RS, Weese JL, et al. Conservative management of extensive low-lying rectal carcinomas with transanal local excision and combined preoperative and postoperative radiation therapy: Report of a phase I/II trial. Cancer 1992;69:335–341.

214. Wilson SM, Beahrs OH. A curative treatment of carcinoma of the sigmoid, rectosigmoid and rectum. Ann Surg 1976;183:556–565.

215. Eisenberg B, DeCosse JJ, Harford F, et al. Carcinoma of the colon and rectum: The natural history reviewed in 1704 patients. Cancer 1982;49:1131–1134.

216. McDermott FT, Hughes ESR, Pihl E, et al. Prognosis in relation to symptom duration in colon cancer. Br J Surg 1981;13:846–849.

217. McDermott FT, Hughes ESR, Pihl E, et al. Local recurrence after potentially curative resection for rectal cancer in a series of 1008 patients. Br J Surg 1985;72:34–37.

218. Phillips RKS, Hittinger R, Blesovsky L, et al. Local recurrence following curative surgery for large bowel cancer. Br J Surg 1984;71:17–20.

219. Pilipshen SJ, Heilweil M, Quan SHQ, et al. Patterns of pelvic recurrence following definitive resections of rectal cancer. Cancer 1984;53:1354–1362.

220. Rich T, Gunderson LL, Lew R, et al. Patterns of recurrence of rectal cancer after potentially curative surgery. Cancer 1983;52:1317–1329.

Cancer: Principles & Practice of Oncology, Fourth Edition,
edited by Vincent T. DeVita, Jr., Samuel Hellman, Steven A. Rosenberg.
J.B. Lippincott Co., Philadelphia © 1993.

Brenda Shank
Alfred M. Cohen
David Kelsen

CHAPTER **32**

Cancer of the Anal Region

The treatment of epidermoid cancer of the anal region has undergone a major change. Twenty years ago, radical surgery in the form of abdominoperineal resection was the only possibility for cure. Combined modality treatment with irradiation and chemotherapy has resulted in increased survival and in sphincter preservation for most patients.[1-6] This approach serves as a model for successful combined modality therapy of other cancers.

EPIDEMIOLOGY AND ETIOLOGY

INCIDENCE, AGE, AND SEX

In the United States, cancer of the anal region accounts for 1% to 2% of all large bowel cancers and 3.9% of all anorectal carcinomas.[7-10] The figures are similar in the United Kingdom, where cancer of the anal region constitutes 3% to 3.5% of all anorectal tumors.[11,12] Most of these tumors are epidermoid carcinomas (Table 32–1).[13]

Epidermoid carcinoma of the anal region develops in persons between ages of 30 and 90 years, with the preponderance of cases occurring between 58 and 64 years, although an increased incidence has been observed in men younger than 45 years in the last decade.[7,8,10,13-16] This increase was not seen in men older than 45 years or in women of any age. McConnell correlated the site with age and found that 80% of anal *canal* carcinomas occurred in patients older than 60, but more than 50% of the anal *margin* carcinomas occurred in patients younger than 60 years of age.[12]

In the United States, anal carcinoma occurs more frequently in female than in male patients.[7,8,10,13,17] This is generally true for anal *canal* cancers in the Western world.[11,12,18-21] Anal *margin* cancers, however, are more frequent in men. Kapur

and colleagues reported a strong male preponderance for anal *canal* cancer in New Delhi, India.[22]

Several studies implicated male homosexuality in anal canal carcinoma, presumably from anal intercourse.[13,16,23-27] A case-control study reported by Daling and associates compared potential risk factors in 148 patients with anal cancer and 166 controls with colon cancer.[27] A history of anal-receptive intercourse in men (but not in women) was strongly associated with anal cancer (relative risk [RR]=33.1).

In a study by Peters and Mack of 970 Los Angeles County residents, the incidence of anal carcinoma was 6.0 times greater in single men than in married men (p<0.001).[13] The increased incidence was limited to squamous and transitional cell carcinomas in the anus; single women were not at an increased risk. In the group younger than 35 years of age, anal carcinoma was more common in men, which was the reverse of the sex ratio for patients older than 35, among whom there was a substantial female preponderance. Peters and Mack regarded these findings as consistent with the hypothesis that anal sexual activity is related to anal cancer. Mechanisms postulated were physical irritation of the anal canal, genital carcinogens (*e.g.*, lubricants), or the transmission of oncogenic viruses by sexual contact.

INFECTIOUS AGENTS

There is an association between papillomaviruses and the development of genital warts (condylomata acuminata), which can convert to squamous cell carcinomas after a latent period of 5 to 40 years.[28] Anal canal carcinoma has been associated with condylomata in the general population and in male homosexuals.[29-33] In the case-control study reported by Daling and colleagues, squamous cell carcinoma (but not transitional cell carcinoma) was strongly associated with a history of gen-

TABLE 32–1. Distribution of Histologic Types
in 970 Patients With Anal Carcinoma

Type	Patients (%)
Squamous cell carcinoma	63
Transitional (cloacogenic) carcinoma	23
Adenocarcinoma	7
Paget disease	2
Basal cell carcinoma	2
Melanoma	2

(Modified from Peters RK, Mack TM. Patterns of anal carcinoma by gender and marital status in Los Angeles County. Br J Cancer 1983;48: 629–636)

ital warts (RR=26.9 in men and 32.5 in women).[27] There is a sexual difference in susceptibility to development of anogenital malignancies in the presence of condylomata: in a study reported by Chuang and associates that spanned 28 years, 41 of 500 women with condylomata acuminata developed anogenital malignancies, but only 1 of 246 men developed anogenital malignancies.[34]

Nine (64%) of 14 patients with tumors positive for human papillomavirus (HPV) by in situ hybridization techniques had a history of warts. In an immunohistochemical study of anal cancers from 8 bisexual or homosexual men, HPV was identified in five specimens.[35]

In two studies, DNA of HPV type 16 was found most frequently in anal squamous cell carcinomas, but types 6 and 18 were also found, and type 11 was never found.[36,37] No HPV DNA was found in nonmalignant anal epithelium or in malignant rectal mucosa.

In a study by Scholefield and colleagues, 23 of 82 patients who had HPV infection by DNA hybridization performed on anal epithelial tissue also had a premalignant condition, anal intraepithelial neoplasia (AIN).[38] The incidence of AIN was significantly higher in homosexual men with HPV (17 of 28 patients) than in heterosexual men with HPV (1 of 26). AIN was not observed in women with anal HPV unless cervical intraepithelial neoplasia was present. In a study by Palevsky and associates, type 16 HPV was associated with high-grade AIN and invasive cancer, but types 6 and 11 were only associated with condylomata and low-grade AIN.[39]

In a 7-year cohort study of homosexual men, Goedert and colleagues found anal epithelial atypia in association with HPV detected by DNA hybridization but not by polymerase chain reaction; this suggested that atypia was related to a high level of replicative but not dormant HPV.[40] There also appeared to be an increased reactivation of HPV in the setting of human immunodeficiency virus (HIV)-induced immunodeficiency.

HPV RNA was investigated by Higgins and associates.[41] RNA transcripts were detected in 73% of 41 epidermoid carcinomas but in none of 6 anal and 11 rectal adenocarcinomas. Grade 3 AIN was not seen in the surrounding epithelium in any of the nine HPV RNA-negative tumors, but it was seen in 14 of 25 RNA-positive tumors. One explanation may be the loss of dependence on RNA expression for maintenance of the neoplastic state as the tumor develops. Despite all the evidence

linking homosexuality, HPV, and anal cancer, Oriel suggested caution in assuming a direct etiologic tie and stressed the need for more studies, including prospective cohort studies of men with anal HPV infection.[42]

In women without a history of genital warts, anal cancer was associated with seropositivity for herpes simplex virus type 1 (RR=4.1) and *Chlamydia trachomatis* (RR=2.3).[27] In men without a history of warts, there was an association with gonorrhea (RR=17.2). Although HIV infection has been questioned as a possible etiologic agent in homosexual men, Monfardini and colleagues showed that among 435 HIV-associated tumors in intravenous drug abusers in Italy, anal tumors were extremely rare.[43]

ASSOCIATED CONDITIONS

Anal canal carcinomas, especially mucinous adenocarcinomas, are associated with anal fistulas and other benign conditions, such as lymphogranuloma venereum and leukoplakia.[7,19,48–49] Brennan and Stewart reported the associations with condylomata acuminata, fistulas, fissures, abscesses, and hemorrhoids.[50] In one study, 41% of anal canal carcinomas were preceded by benign anorectal disease for at least 5 years.[51]

Prior radiation therapy may play a role in the development of anal carcinoma, as may immunosuppression.[19,52,53] Immunosuppressed renal transplant patients have a 100-fold increase in anogenital tumors compared with the rest of the population.[54] Many of these patients have a history of condylomata acuminata (29%) or herpes genitalis.

In the case-control study reported by Daling and associates, current cigarette smoking was a major risk factor in both sexes (RR=7.7 in women and 9.4 in men).[27] This substantiates the report by Daniell, who observed that 54% of 13 women with anal cancer were current smokers, compared with only 26% of 202 age-matched patients with colon cancer.[55] In a matched controlled study of 56 women with anal carcinoma, there were strong associations with herpes simplex virus titer, cigarette smoking, and increasing numbers of sexual partners. In a multivariate analysis, cigarette smoking was an independent variable ($p=0.0126$)[56] In murine studies, anal carcinomas may be induced by chemical carcinogens[57,58] and promoted by epidermal growth factor.[58]

Several general conclusions about causes of anal cancer can be made. Anal canal carcinoma is related to immunosuppression and correlates highly with HPV and condylomata acuminata. There is a clear-cut association with male homosexuality, which may be related to the presence of other viral diseases in these patients and to immunosuppression.

ANATOMIC CONSIDERATIONS

Squamous cell cancer of the anus can occur in the anal canal, the lower rectum, or the perianal skin.[59,60] Important gross anatomic landmarks associated with these locations are illustrated in Figure 32–1. Each level is associated with histologically distinct epithelium.

The lowest region lies caudad to the anal verge and is covered with keratinized stratified squamous epithelium, which is pigmented and has hair follicles. Anal cancers are defined

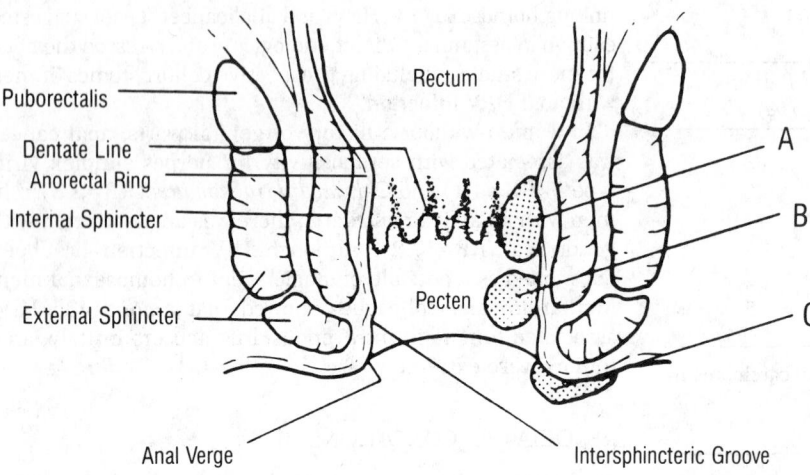

FIGURE 32–1.   Gross anatomy of the anal canal. A tumor in location *A* is always considered anal canal cancer; in location *C*, it is anal margin cancer; location *B* has been called anal canal or margin, depending on institutional preference, but it is now anal canal cancer by the AJCC-UICC definition.

distally as tumors that are within 5 cm of the anal verge, and they are referred to as perianal or anal margin cancers.[4]

Extending proximally from the anal verge to the pectinate or dentate line is the hairless stratified squamous epithelium of the anal canal. The rectal columns (*i.e.,* columns of Morgagni) extend for 1.0 to 1.5 cm proximal to the level of the anorectal ring. Proximal to the ring the mucosa is columnar. The mucosa over the rectal columns is cuboidal, giving rise to the transitional cell or cloacogenic anal cancers. Squamous epithelium can extend proximally to the pectinate line, which explains the finding of squamous cell cancers in the distal rectum. The anal crypts are located in the distal columns of Morgagni. From microscopic glandular components within these crypts the rare mucoepidermoid cancers arise.

The definition of the proximal extent of tumors referred to as anal margin has varied. The St. Mark's Hospital in London, Memorial Sloan-Kettering Cancer Center in New York, and the Melbourne, Australia, groups considered all tumors below the dentate line as *anal margin cancers.*[61–63] All tumors involving the dentate line were considered *anal canal cancers.* The Mayo Clinic and other groups defined *anal margin tumors* as those below the anal verge.[64] The American Joint Committee on Cancer (AJCC) and International Union Against Cancer (UICC) now define the *anal margin* as the hair-bearing skin beginning at the lower end of the anal canal mucous membrane (*i.e.,* below the anal verge).[65] The distinction is an important one, because squamous or basal cell cancers below the anal verge (perianal cancers) are skin cancers from a biologic and therapeutic perspective. Figure 32–1 demonstrates the various definitions of potential tumor sites within the anal region.

The *intersphincteric groove* is easily palpable during rectal examination. It represents the potential plane between the internal and external sphincter mechanism. The external sphincter surrounds the internal sphincter circumferentially and extends more caudad than the internal sphincter; therefore, the most superficial muscle beneath the anal verge is the superficial external sphincter. This is an important anatomic consideration when local excision is attempted. The superficial external and internal sphincter muscles can be resected without loss of continence in most patients. The entire sphincter mechanism caudad to the puborectalis sling

can be resected over a partial circumference with acceptable continence compared with a permanent colostomy.

The anal region is extremely well vascularized and has an extensive lymphatic system (Fig. 32–2). The lymphatics drain into the inguinal nodes, the lateral pelvic nodes, and the mesorectal nodes.[10] Tumors below the anal verge drain primarily into the inguinal nodal system. The distal 5 cm of rectum and the anal canal to the anal verge drain into the inguinal nodes, along the middle hemorrhoidal vessels to the pelvic side walls, and into the inferior mesenteric system. Lymph node metastases are the rule with advanced anal cancer. In a group of 29 patients undergoing primary abdominoperineal resection for anal squamous cell carcinoma at Roswell Park with pathologic "clearing" of all lymph nodes, widespread unpredictable patterns of spread to multiple nodal areas was detected.[66] Forty-four percent of the lymph node metastases were to nodes smaller than 5 mm in diameter.

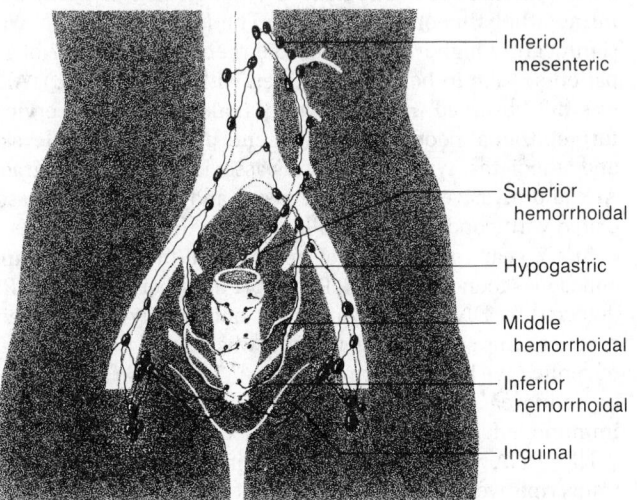

FIGURE 32–2.   Lymphatic drainage of the anus through three pathways: (1) inferiorly, from the margin and canal, across the perineum to the superficial inguinal lymph nodes; (2) from the upper canal and just superior to the dentate line, along the inferior and middle hemorrhoidal vessels to the hypogastric nodes; and (3) superiorly, from the rectum, along the superior hemorrhoidal vessels to the inferior mesenteric nodes.

PATHOLOGY

Many different histologic cell types may occur in the anal area.[67] In addition to the more common types (see Table 32–1), other rare histologic entities can arise, such as small-cell carcinomas similar to small-cell carcinoma of the lung,[68] lymphoma, basal cell carcinoma, Paget's disease,[69] and Bowen's disease. Melanomas constitute 1% to 2% of all anal cancers, and anal melanoma constitutes only 1.6% of all melanomas.[70] The importance of anal melanoma lies in its poor prognosis, with a 5-year survival rate of only 8% to 12%.[71,72]

Some pathologists divide anal canal tumors into those that exhibit keratinization and those that do not and further subdivide nonkeratinizing tumors into basosquamous, basaloid, and cloacogenic carcinomas.[61] Other investigators found no difference in clinical outcome with such subdivisions and assume that all histologic varieties are subsets of squamous cell carcinoma.[73,74] Most investigators currently think that prognosis depends more on stage than on histologic type.[75]

In one study, no HPV DNA was found in 14 cloacogenic carcinomas.[76] In another, there was no difference in the percentage of HPV RNA positivity (75%) between cloacogenic and squamous carcinomas.[41]

Chromosomal studies of eight anal canal cancers demonstrated abnormalities in chromosomes 11 and 3.[77] These alterations may be characteristic of anal canal carcinoma, but more cases should be studied to verify these findings.

In the anal margin, histologies other than squamous cell carcinoma include basal cell carcinoma identical with that in skin in other areas, Bowen's disease, and Paget's disease. Patients with Bowen's disease usually present with long-standing perianal pruritus. Patients with perineal Paget's disease also frequently present with pruritus, although they may be asymptomatic or have a bleeding erythematous or eczematoid plaque.[78] In the absence of an underlying anal canal cancer, the origin of the cells is probably from the apocrine glands. An associated anorectal carcinoma should be excluded.

Precancerous changes have been studied by several investigators. Fenger and Nielsen studied the incidence of precancerous changes in the anal canal epithelium.[79,80] In a group of 139 patients who underwent abdominoperineal resections (most with carcinomas of the rectum, but some with anal canal tumors), 15 (10.8%) had dysplasia that was thought to be precancerous or to represent carcinoma in situ. Severe dysplasia or carcinoma in situ was seen in 13 (81%) of the 16 patients with squamous cell carcinoma of the anal canal. They concluded that most anal canal tumors arising in the anal transition zone (ATZ) are preceded by multicentric areas of dysplasia.

Palefsky and colleagues studied the incidence of the premalignant condition, AIN, and its association to anal papillomavirus infection among homosexual males with group IV HIV disease.[81] Infection with multiple subtypes of human papillomavirus was detected in 12% of patients; these patients had a markedly increased risk for cytologic abnormalities (RR = 39.0). Patients with abnormal cytologies were significantly more likely to have lower median T4 cell counts. They concluded that immunosuppressed male homosexuals may be at significant risk for the development of anal canal neoplasia because of the presence of papillomavirus.

Flow cytometric analysis of normal epithelium along the ATZ and, in smaller groups of patients, of anal canal tumors was performed using fresh specimens by Fenger and Bichel.[82] Three patients with squamous cell carcinoma of the anal canal were studied; they had a high proliferative index but near-diploid peaks. In contrast, Goldman and associates found that most anal tumors had an aneuploid pattern.[83] Shepherd and colleagues studied flow cytometry in 235 patients with resected tumors of the anal canal and perianal skin.[84] In a multivariate analysis, depth of penetration, inguinal node involvement, and DNA ploidy were of independent prognostic significance.

EPIDERMOID CARCINOMA

NATURAL HISTORY

Squamous cell cancer of the anus and its variants spread by direct extension into contiguous soft tissues, with early dissemination through the lymphatics. Hematogenous spread is less common. The basaloid or cloacogenic subtypes have less biologic relevance than tumor location in considering the natural history of anal cancer.[75,85]

Anal margin cancers invade local tissues and cause clinically apparent local ulceration and spread. More proximal anal canal cancers frequently spread cephalad in the submucosal plane. If locally far advanced, the entire sphincter mechanism may be penetrated; there may also be direct invasion of the vagina, urethra, prostate, bladder, sacrum, or bone of the pelvic side walls.

Mesenteric lymph nodes are involved in one third to one half of patients with anal canal cancers treated by abdominoperineal resection.[9,19,63,73,86,87] The risk of mesenteric lymph node spread from anal margin cancers is less defined. In two small series of patients treated by abdominoperineal resection, mesenteric lymph node spread was identical to that in patients with anal canal cancers.[63,86] However, in two other series, the risk was almost zero.[9,88] Because the cure rate from local excision alone with anal margin cancers less than 5 cm in diameter is 90%, it appears that spread to mesenteric lymph nodes is infrequent, except in cases of massive disease.[62] In a series of 45 patients with anal cancer (primarily of the anal canal) treated at Memorial Sloan-Kettering Cancer Center with a surgical procedure that included excision of the obturator and hypogastric nodes, pelvic node metastases were found in one third.[73] However, case selection for such extensive surgery must result in overestimation of the risk of pelvic node spread.

The inguinal and external iliac nodes are the regional lymphatics considered in the TNM staging system. Patients may present with synchronous or metachronous inguinal lymph node metastases. Inguinal node metastases are extremely rare for T1 tumors or if the surface area of the primary tumor is less than 4 cm².[8,86] The overall risk of inguinal node metastases is approximately 30%.[73,86,89] This was equal to the incidence of pelvic node metastases in the Memorial Sloan-Kettering Cancer Center series.[10] If inguinal nodes originally negative on physical examination are destined to become clinically positive, they usually become so within 18 months of treatment of the primary tumor.[86]

Hematogenous metastases occur in few patients. Because of the dual venous drainage of the area, metastases occur equally to the liver and lung.[90]

Despite radical surgery, almost all recurrences of disease after surgery alone represent locoregional treatment failure. Most cancer-related deaths are secondary to uncontrolled pelvic and perineal disease.[64,68,87,91,92]

DIAGNOSIS

Because the initial symptoms of anal cancer are similar to those of common benign conditions, the patient often delays seeking a diagnosis. Because anal cancer is rare and examination may be painful and difficult if spasm occurs, physician-related delays also occur. Almost one third of the patients at Memorial Sloan-Kettering Cancer Center with squamous cell cancer of the anorectum were thought to have had benign disease until biopsies proved otherwise.[73] More than half of the patients in the Mayo Clinic study had associated benign anal abnormalities, such as fistula in ano, fissure, or hemorrhoids.[64]

Bleeding, pain, and a sensation of a mass are the most common symptoms. Pruritus is less frequent, except in patients with perianal cancer.[64] Physical examination should include digital anorectal examination, anoscopy and proctoscopy, and palpation of the inguinal lymph nodes. Associated Bowen's or Paget's disease of the perianal skin increases the likelihood of anal carcinoma. The differential diagnosis for bleeding, pain, or a mass sensation includes thrombosed hemorrhoid, fissure, fistula, perianal or crypt abscess, benign anal papilloma, and adenocarcinoma of the rectum. Patients with severe pain and spasm may be treated empirically with analgesics, stool softeners, warm baths, and topical ointments for 1 to 2 weeks. Persistent symptoms may require examination under sedation or general anesthesia to avoid missing the diagnosis of cancer or an inadequately treated infection.

An incisional biopsy is necessary to confirm the diagnosis. Excision should not be attempted, except for superficial lesions detected very early. Suspicious inguinal lymph nodes should be biopsied to differentiate inflammatory from metastatic lymphadenopathy. Formal groin dissection should be avoided. Needle aspiration of the groin nodes for cytology may be attempted first. If the results are negative, surgical biopsy should follow.

In addition to physical examination and surgical staging of a suspicious inguinal node site, an extent-of-disease staging includes chest radiography and liver function tests. Computed tomography (CT) and transanorectal sonography have been suggested as useful tools in evaluating primary anal tumors, but their value has not been rigorously assessed.[93,94] Marker studies have not been clinically useful, but a squamous cell carcinoma antigen can be monitored in serum and can reflect tumor status in some patients.[95]

STAGING

An early attempt at staging was made at the Mayo Clinic in 1962.[8] This anal canal staging was similar to the Dukes pathologic classification of rectal cancer, with stage A representing invasion into sphincter muscle, stage B representing invasion through the sphincter muscle, and stage C representing lymph node involvement. They also graded the tumors by the Broders system. This simple system was found to be prognostic for 5-year survival. Because the sphincter muscle

is thick, stage B was later subclassified further and stage D was added, representing unresectable regional tumor or distant metastases.[68] This classification was found to be prognostic for local and distant recurrence and for survival.

A similar surgical-pathologic staging classification developed at the Roswell Park Memorial Institute for application to the perianal area and the anal canal was found to be prognostic; major decrements in survival resulted from sphincter muscle or inguinal node involvement.[96]

The UICC established a dual staging system with a clinical staging and a pathologic staging after surgery, to be used only for carcinoma in the anal region.[97] Separate classifications were developed for the anal canal and for the anal margin; the anal margin staging system was analogous to that for other skin tumors. There were criticisms, and suggestions were incorporated into an illustrated guide of the UICC staging system.[98,99] Other variations of a TNM system have been used.[21,100]

In 1987, the UICC staging system was updated,[101] and the AJCC adopted the same staging system.[65] This unified AJCC/UICC system takes into account the fact that anal canal carcinoma is increasingly treated by nonsurgical methods, such as radiation therapy alone, or by multimodality therapy. T staging is determined by size and invasion into adjacent organs or tissues. The N classification for the anal canal subdivides the regional nodes, recognizing the poor prognosis of inguinal node involvement. Anal margin tumors are staged like skin cancers; the T staging is almost the same as for anal canal tumors. Grading is also stipulated. Grade 1 represents well-differentiated disease; grade 2, moderately differentiated disease; grade 3, poorly differentiated disease; and grade 4, undifferentiated disease.

In devising a staging system, it is important to ascertain which clinical features are the most prognostic. Survival correlates with size of the anal lesion and lymphadenopathy, both of which are considered in the current AJCC/UICC system. We recommend that this system be used routinely to facilitate comparison of results.

PROGNOSTIC FACTORS

Stage

Clinical stage, measured by 1978 UICC T stage, has been correlated with prognostic outcome. Goldman and coworkers retrospectively analyzed findings for a group of 43 patients from Sweden with anal canal cancers.[83] Clinical stage was highly statistically correlated with outcome: patients with T1 and T2 cancers had a greater than 80% 5-year survival rate, but those with T3 and T4 disease had survival rates less than 20%; few patients had T3 or T4 disease. This is not an independent association, because T stage is related to size. In a multivariate analysis of 242 cases, T stage was the only significant prognostic factor.[102] In an update that analyzed 286 cases by multivariate analysis, tumor size, clinically abnormal lymph nodes, and total irradiation dose influenced prognosis.[103] In another study, stage and radiation dose were the most important prognostic factors found by multivariate analysis, but gender was also important, with women faring better than men.[104]

Metastasis to inguinal lymph nodes is also an indicator of a poor prognosis.[75,105] However, Greenall and coworkers found a 55% 5-year survival rate despite the presence of inguinal lymph node metastases, if lymphadenectomy could be performed.[105] The use of multimodality therapy is also altering the historically poor prognosis associated with positive inguinal nodes.

Tumor Size

Tumor size (related to T stage) is of prognostic importance. Several investigators found that patients with lesions smaller than 2 cm in diameter have a markedly better prognosis than those with larger lesions.[68,86] Dillard and colleagues found a 75% 5-year survival rate for a group of 12 patients with tumors having a surface area less than 8 cm²; only 47% of patients with tumors greater than 8 cm² in surface area survived.[86] Boman and associates reported that, of a total of 108 patients with anal canal tumors, 13 had small (<2 cm in diameter), superficially invasive lesions.[68] All were treated with local excision, and although 1 patient later required abdominoperineal resection, all were cured. Kuehn and colleagues reported no survivors with tumors larger than 6 cm in diameter.[106] Even with aggressive therapy, Wanebo and associates found very poor survival among patients with lesions more than 10 cm in diameter.[107]

Salmon and colleagues also found that size was significantly related to survival in a study in which radiation therapy alone was the primary treatment.[75] In another radiation therapy series, size (≤4 cm or >4 cm in diameter) was prognostic for 5-year survival but not for tumor control.[108] In a large multivariate analysis with 235 cases, tumor thickness and anatomic infiltration (related to size) was an independent prognostic factor for survival, as was the presence of inguinal node involvement.[109] Because current initial therapy rarely involves abdominoperineal resection, it is difficult to accurately assess depth of penetration. If endoscopic ultrasonography continues to improve, depth of invasion measured by this technique may become a useful prognostic indicator.

Other Prognostic Features

Histologic cell type for squamous cancers of the anal canal (*i.e.*, epidermoid or cloacogenic) has no major prognostic relevance. The cloacogenic carcinomas were thought to have a slightly better prognosis in some series.[75,110] However, among 243 patients with resectable anal canal tumors, Papillon and Montbarbon found a worse prognosis for patients with nonkeratinizing and basaloid carcinoma than for patients with keratinizing lesions.[108] Small-cell carcinomas of the anus, like extrapulmonary small-cell cancers in other parts of the body, appear to have a worse prognosis, with a high propensity for systemic dissemination.[68,109]

Asymptomatic patients do better than symptomatic patients, but this may be directly related to the size of the tumor.[111]

Location may be of slight prognostic importance, with anal margin tumors having a better outcome than those in the anal canal. However, Paradis and associates found no difference in survival rates between patients with tumors within the anal canal and those with tumors in the perianal region.[96] No difference in survival according to sex was observed by Papillon and Montbarbon.[108]

Three studies looked at DNA content (*i.e.*, whether tumors were diploid or greater than diploid); two found no prognostic implications for this factor, but in one large multivariate analysis, DNA ploidy was an independent prognostic factor for the 184 patients whose tumors were analyzed for DNA.[83,84,109]

In one of the studies, grade was a significant prognostic factor, with low-grade tumors resulting in a 5-year survival of 75% compared with only 24% for high-grade tumors.[83]

TREATMENT

Anal Margin

Local Surgery

Superficial perianal skin carcinomas (*i.e.*, squamous and basal cell) outside the anal verge may be treated with wide local excision with good results. Excision with 1-cm margins, using primary closure, is usually appropriate. A skin graft can be placed if the surgical defect is large. Rarely are formal skin flaps necessary or desirable. A split-thickness skin graft will shrink with time, leaving a relatively small defect that will not interfere with the detection of local recurrence.

Treatment of Bowen's disease is by wide local excision, with frozen section control of the margins.[112] In the absence of invasive cancer, Paget's disease is treated by wide local excision, with or without skin grafting. Multiple biopsies from the margins are crucial.[113,114] For early noninvasive lesions, oral retinoids have been successful.[115] Primary abdominoperineal resection is almost never indicated as the initial treatment of margin lesions. The cure rate after local excision for superficial squamous cell tumors exceeds 80%.[61,62,64,89,116]

Local failure rates are higher if the anal margin includes cancers in the anal canal distal to (not involving) the dentate line.[62] In the Memorial Sloan-Kettering Cancer Center experience, disease recurred locally in 9 of 31 patients treated with local excision for anal margin cancers.[62] Eight of these tumors were amenable to second local excisions. In 4 patients, disease recurred in the inguinal nodes. There were only 3 cancer-related deaths among the 31 patients initially treated by local excision, and only 1 patient ultimately required abdominoperineal resection.

Deeply infiltrative anal margin carcinomas have been treated with abdominoperineal resection.[62,86] Although most patients were cured, the small number of reported cases of disease defined as anal margin cancers precludes detailed analysis of end results and patterns of failure. Patients with invasive Paget's disease or with an underlying associated anorectal carcinoma usually require abdominoperineal resection with wide excision of the perianal skin.

External Irradiation

Epidermoid carcinoma of the anal margin tends to be early or only moderately advanced at the time of diagnosis, with lymph nodes only rarely involved (0–15%), usually in larger tumors (≥5 cm in diameter).[117–120] Although these early cancers of the anal margin are successfully treated by local excision, radiation therapy should be considered for some patients. Papillon suggested that radiation therapy should be used for patients with anal margin carcinoma that is considered unresectable or patients who have extensive or recurrent lesions; patients who are medically inoperable can have radiation therapy.

Although some early studies of anal margin irradiation used interstitial radium needle implants, the high incidence of radionecrosis and the relatively poor geometry indicated that external-beam radiation therapy was a better modality.[100,117] Although photons are most frequently used for these treatments, electron-beam therapy may also be successfully used for early perianal epidermoid carcinomas.[121] Results of treating perianal lesions, stage for stage, are similar to results for anal canal lesions; more extensive lesions require more aggressive therapy.[118,122] Although some researchers recommended abdominoperineal resections for extensive lesions, radiation therapy appears to be an excellent alternative that yields cures with sphincter preservation.[118]

Two groups reported their results of treating anal margin carcinomas.[120,123–125] The Centre Leon Berard investigated the use of chemotherapy with mitomycin C and 5-fluorouracil (5-FU) concurrently with radiation therapy in a large proportion of the patients.[123–125] The investigators used direct perineal fields and cobalt 60 as the source to deliver a surface dose of 40 Gy in ten fractions. In a few patients with residual disease, iridium 192 implants were also used.[123–125] In the study from Princess Margaret Hospital, external-beam radiation therapy was used for treating most of the patients, who received a total of 50 Gy in 4 weeks or in 8 weeks as a split course.[120] At both institutions, local control was similar (80–85%). In the Centre Leon Berard study, the 5-year survival rate was 59%, and the cancer-specific survival rate was 80%.[125] Six of 7 local failures were controlled by local excision. Lymph node failures tended to occur later and were fatal in 8 of 9 patients. Prophylactic inguinal node irradiation is now recommended, because 6 of the 9 nodal failures occurred in patients who were N0 at presentation and did not receive groin irradiation. In the Princess Margaret Hospital study, local control was achieved in all 13 patients with a primary lesion smaller than 5 cm in diameter but in only 2 of 5 patients with a primary lesion larger than 10 cm.[120] Four patients had positive lymph nodes in this study, and disease in 2 patients was controlled by treatment. The investigators found that local necrosis developed in 3 of 11 patients treated with radiation therapy alone.

In another study, 5 patients with perianal tumors without nodal involvement were treated with radiation therapy (40–60 Gy) plus bleomycin; 2 with advanced disease (T4N0) also underwent abdominoperineal resection after chemotherapy and radiation therapy.[126] All 5 patients were alive and disease-free after 16 to 84 months of follow-up.

Most patients with anal margin tumors can be treated with excision alone, or with irradiation alone for more advanced or recurrent tumors. Concurrent irradiation and chemotherapy is an interesting but still investigational approach to advanced margin tumors.

Anal Canal

Local Disease
None of 10 patients initially treated at the Cleveland Clinic by local excision experienced recurrence of the disease.[127] Included were cancers of the anal margin and anal canal that extended less than one half the circumference; cancers involving the dentate line were excluded. Internal or full-thickness sphincter excision with skin-graft coverage resulted in acceptable continence. In a review from the Connecticut Cancer Registry reported by Kuehn and colleagues, 26 patients with anal cancer, including distal anal canal cancers, were treated by local excision, and 20 (77%) were cured.[59]

The Mayo Clinic experience with anal cancers between the dentate line and the anal verge includes 19 patients treated by local excision.[68] Treatment failed locally in 1 of 12 superficial tumors, which was subsequently cured with abdominoperineal resection. Seven patients with underlying sphincter muscle invasion refused radical surgery and were treated by wide local excision, some with adjuvant irradiation. Disease recurred locally in 3.[68] In a group of 5 patients (4 with T1 disease) treated at the Lahey Clinic by local excision, none had disease recurrence.[15] Of 144 patients treated at Memorial Sloan-Kettering Cancer Center for anal canal cancers (dentate line involvement), only 11 were suitable candidates for local excision. The 5-year survival rate was only 45% and most had local recurrence.[128] Fewer than 10% of the 91 anal canal tumors with dentate line involvement treated at St. Mark's Hospital with curative intent were amenable to local excision; of these patients, 75% were cured.[89] Klotz and associates compiled reports of anal canal "basaloid" cancers, 33 of which had been treated by local excision.[14] Most of the tumors had been found incidentally in hemorrhoidectomy specimens. The 5-year cure rate was 60%. Local excision should be considered only for T1 tumors with no evidence of nodal involvement and for patients who can be followed closely.

Hughes and colleagues treated 9 patients after local excision (*i.e.*, 1 Tis, 6 T1, 2 T2) with postoperative irradiation, using external irradiation only (3 patients), an ^{192}Ir implant only (3 patients), or both (3 patients).[129] All were locally controlled and free of disease after 16 to 93 months of follow-up.

Locoregional Disease
MULTIMODALITY THERAPY. Because integrated multimodality therapy improves overall survival and allows radical surgery to be avoided for most patients, the scope of initial diagnostic surgery should be limited to maximize the final functional result.

For anal margin cancers distal to the anal verge, a punch or surgical incisional biopsy performed in the office can suffice. For patients with considerable spasm and pain, examination and incisional biopsy under general anesthesia is appropriate. If a decision is made to proceed with local excision only (*i.e.*, small anal margin or T1 anal canal lesion), the bowel is prepared, and elective surgery is performed.

Grossly positive inguinal lymph nodes are studied initially by needle aspiration cytology; open biopsy is performed if the specimen is benign. Minimally suspicious nodes warrant an excisional biopsy of one or two lymph nodes, using great care to avoid a hematoma or lymphatic leak. A superficial groin dissection is not necessary or useful as part of the initial treatment strategy. It delays definitive chemotherapy and radiation treatment, and it may increase the risk of leg edema after combined treatment.

CHEMOTHERAPY AND IRRADIATION. In the past 15 to 20 years, increasing evidence amassed from single-arm phase II studies indicates that initial chemotherapy plus radiation therapy yields a very high rate of tumor regression, including a high rate of complete remission, and that surgery may not be required for many patients, or it may be limited to an excisional biopsy of residual scar. Even patients with relatively large anal epidermoid tumors may be spared a colostomy and have an excellent survival expectation.

Table 32–2 summarizes the results of therapy from several large series.[6,129-138] There are no results from prospective controlled randomized trials comparing multimodality therapy with irradiation alone or surgery alone. One retrospective study suggested a higher cure rate with multimodality therapy in patients with higher-stage disease.[139] Because phase II trials have been so impressive, with only modest morbidity, chemotherapy plus irradiation has been accepted as conventional treatment for most patients with anal canal disease. Some investigators still favor irradiation alone, but few support abdominoperineal resection as first line therapy.

The series in Table 32–2 followed a chemotherapy protocol similar to that pioneered by Nigro and coworkers. 5-FU was given by continuous 24-hour infusion for 4 to 5 days with a single bolus dose of mitomycin C.[140] Combined therapy has been given concurrently or sequentially. In the concurrent regimen, radiation therapy and chemotherapy are initiated on the same day. In the sequential regimen, chemotherapy is given before radiation therapy. In addition to differences in timing of administration, the dose of radiation therapy has also varied (see Table 32–2). In centers such as Wayne State University and the Memorial Sloan-Kettering Cancer Center, chemotherapy plus radiation therapy has been given before a planned surgical procedure—initially abdominoperineal resection and later local excision. At Highland Hospital in Rochester, New York, and the Princess Margaret Hospital, radiation therapy to higher total doses was definitive treatment; surgery was not part of the treatment plan. Despite these differences between trials, there is little evidence from these four studies that one schedule or dose level is markedly superior to another. Response and survival rates are similar, although fewer patients require an abdominoperineal resection after concurrent chemotherapy and radiation therapy to higher doses.

TABLE 32–2. Results of Multimodality Therapy for Locoregional Anal Canal Carcinoma

Investigations	Chemotherapy Regimen	Radiation Therapy Regimen	Patients Evaluable	Abdomino-perineal Resection Performed	Treatment-Related Deaths	5-Year Survival (%)
Wayne State[130]	5-FU: 1000 mg/m²/4 days 2 cycles* Mito: 15 mg/m² d 1	30 Gy/15 fx	104†	31	0	80
Memorial Sloan-Kettering[131]	5-FU: 750 mg/m²/5 days* Mito: 15 mg/m² d 1	30 Gy/15 fx	42	23	0	82
RTOG[132]	5-FU: 1000 mg/m²/4 days 2 cycles* Mito: 10 mg/m² d 2	40.8 Gy/24 fx	79	8	0	73 (3 y)
Highland Hospital[133]	5-FU: 1000 mg/m²/4 days 2 cycles* Mito: 10 mg/m² d 2	50–57.5 Gy/25–32 fx	33	4	0	
Fresno Community Hospital[134,135]	5-FU:1000 mg/m²/4 days 2 cycles* Mito: 10–15 mg/m² × 2	41–50 Gy/23–28 fx	30	1	0	90
Norwegian Radium Hospital[136]	5-FU: 1000 mg/m²/4 days* Mito: 10–15 mg/m²	50 Gy/25 fx	94	17	3 (3%)	72
Istituto Nazionale Tumori, Milano[137]	5-FU: 750 mg/m²/5 days 2–3 cycles* Mito: 15 mg/m² d 1	54 Gy/30 fx (split)	38	6	0	
Princess Margaret[138,139]	5-FU: 1000 mg/m²/4 days* Mito: 10 mg/m² d 1	48–50 Gy/24–20 fx (split or continuous)	69	10	0	65‡
	5-FU: 1000 mg/m²/4 days*	48–50 Gy/24–20 fx (split)	66	18	1 (2%)	64§
M.D. Anderson[140]	5-FU: 300 mg/m²/day for 32 days (median)*	45 Gy/25 fx	25	8	1 (4%)	

5-FU, 5-fluorouracil; Mito, mitomycin C; fx, fractions.
* Continuous 24-hour infusion.
† Wayne State had 44 of these patients, the other 60 were from elsewhere in the United States and analyzed through questionnaires.
‡ Cause-specific 5-year survival rate was 76%.
§ Cause-specific 5-year survival rate.

There are still major questions to be answered: How do we identify poor-risk patients for more aggressive chemotherapy plus concurrent radiation to further reduce the need for abdominoperineal resection? Is less treatment possible for lower-risk patients?

Long-term follow-up results are becoming available. These reports give a reasonable picture of the number of patients eventually requiring abdominoperineal resection and of the number of patients in whom a functional anal sphincter remained for a long period after nonoperative treatment with radiation therapy and chemotherapy. For example, Tanum and colleagues reviewed the experience in 106 Norwegian patients who received radiation plus concurrent mitomycin and 5-FU.[136] The radiation dose was 50 Gy given in 2-Gy fractions to most patients by anteroposterior and posteroanterior (AP/PA) parallel opposed fields. The complete response rate to chemotherapy was 84%; 16% of patients (*i.e.*, positive biopsy) underwent abdominoperineal resection. Of 89 patients who were followed for a minimum of 3 months after treatment, 14 (16%) had significant morbidity within 2 years of treatment, which eventually required surgery or seriously impaired normal social life.

When chemotherapy and irradiation are combined, AP/PA pelvic fields should probably not be treated to a dose higher than 40 Gy. Most investigators coned down to the primary site after 30 Gy. An update of the Memorial Sloan-Kettering Cancer Center experience by Miller and colleagues reported the results of 42 patients who received mitomycin and 5-FU followed by irradiation beginning 1 week after chemotherapy.[131] Twenty-three patients were initially treated with wide local excision. Two underwent abdominoperineal resection soon after local excision because of persistent cancer. Of 21 remaining patients, 3 patients later had abdominoperineal resections. Eighteen patients retained anal continence.

Some investigators found that any patient with a positive biopsy after initial treatment was certain to have recurrence of disease.[141] However, the Memorial Sloan-Kettering Cancer Center group has had long-term disease-free survival despite residual disease after induction therapy.[131,142,143] Of 44 patients in the original series, 18 (41%) had positive pathologic results after chemotherapy followed by irradiation.[142] At least half of these patients had no recurrent tumor detected at their most recent examinations.

Nigro made the point that combined therapy using chemotherapy plus irradiation can safely be given in a community setting.[144] This view is further strengthened by studies such as those of John and Flam (Fresno Community Hospital in Table 32–2)[134,135,145] and of Knecht.[146] In studies by Flam and associates, toxicity was tolerable, with no patient experiencing more than grade II toxicity on a modified scale.[134,147] Local failure rates and median disease-free survival rates appear similar to those of series from large cancer centers. A multiinstitutional Radiation Therapy Oncology Group single-arm study also demonstrated the feasibility and effectiveness of this regimen.[132] For 78 evaluable patients, the 3-year survival rate was 73%. Overall survival was significantly affected by protocol adherence: 92% survival for no or minor deviations and 45% survival for major deviations.

The best chemoradiation therapy regimen and the most appropriate radiation dose to use for patients with anal canal tumors limited to the primary site have not yet been defined.

Distant failure is not the major problem. Local recurrence is more common, especially if the radiation dose is low (30 Gy). 5-FU is probably a radiosensitizer, although there is some disagreement, but mitomycin is probably not synergistic.[148–150] Byfield and coworkers treated 11 patients with a 120-hour infusion of 5-FU (25 mg/kg/day) and concurrent irradiation, omitting mitomycin.[151] Radiation therapy was given in 4-day cycles (10 Gy/cycle), separated by at least 9 days, to a total dose of 30 Gy to 47.5 Gy. All patients had complete clinical regressions; only 1 patient had active disease histologically. There was only a single local recurrence.

Poorer local control was reported by the M.D. Anderson Cancer Center group when low-dose 5-FU (300 mg/m²/day) was used throughout the irradiation course (45–66 Gy).[129] Local control without an abdominoperineal resection was 67% in 24 patients, but 9 of 10 patients who received at least 55 Gy were controlled. Toxicity was considerable, with 6 of 25 patients experiencing grade 4 diarrhea, resulting in the death of 1 patient. In comparing two consecutive series of patients treated with 5-FU and irradiation, but with mitomycin omitted in the later series, Cummings and colleagues concluded that mitomycin is needed. The local control rate was only 60% for 58 patients after mitomycin was omitted, compared with 89% for 56 patients who received mitomycin.[138]

To better address this question, a Radiation Therapy Oncology Group study is currently underway comparing irradiation (45 Gy) and concurrent 5-FU to irradiation plus concurrent mitomycin and 5-FU. This trial, which is nearing its projected accrual, addresses the role of mitomycin. Patients with positive biopsies after initial treatment are eligible for cisplatin-based chemotherapy treatment, which addresses the issue of additional chemotherapy in poor-risk patients. Because the definitive results of this trial are not yet available, it is too early to conclude that mitomycin is not a necessary part of therapy, especially because the complications related to the use of this agent are quite small.

The chemotherapy regimen of mitomycin and 5-FU is quite active against anal canal tumors, but some patients do not respond or have less than a complete remission with this combination. The effectiveness of cisplatin-based treatment for patients with advanced disease has made use of this agent as part of multimodality therapy attractive. A few trials investigated the use of cisplatin with 5-FU and irradiation for initial therapy with promising results, especially for high-risk patients.[151–155]

RADICAL SURGERY. Before the widespread use of multimodality therapy, more than 90% of patients with potentially curable anal canal cancers required abdominoperineal resection. A wide perineal dissection in association with a posterior vaginectomy in women was recommended.[17,87] Despite initial enthusiasm of the oncology group at Memorial Sloan-Kettering Cancer Center for vaginectomy, a more recent analysis discounted its routine application.[10] Lateral pelvic lymphadenopathy was initially advocated by the same group on the basis of a 24% incidence of pathologically positive nodes.[73] Subsequent analysis could not define any therapeutic benefit for this extended abdominoperineal resection.[10] The overall cure rate with abdominoperineal resection is approximately 50%.[156]

The Mayo Clinic experience initially reported in 1976 by Beahrs and Wilson[64] was updated by Boman and associates.[68] Disease recurred in 40% of the 114 patients, with subsequent treatment resulting in a 71% 5-year survival rate. At the Ellis Fischel State Cancer Hospital in Columbia, Missouri, the 5-year survival rate in 46 patients was 58%.[86] The M.D. Anderson Hospital group reported a 62% 5-year survival rate for 109 patients treated with only abdominoperineal resection.[119] One sixth of the cases were anal margin cancers. A Memorial Sloan-Kettering Cancer Center update included 103 patients treated by radical surgery, with a 55% 5-year survival rate.[128] All of these tumors involved the dentate line. The 5-year survival rate for patients with tumors larger than 5 cm was only 40%. At St. Mark's Hospital, the 5-year survival rate among 83 patients with anal cancers involving the dentate line treated by radical surgery was 48%.[89]

Treatment failure despite radical surgery is locoregional and distant. In the Mayo Clinic experience, 84% of initial sites of failure included local and regional disease.[68] Most cancer-related deaths are secondary to uncontrolled locoregional tumor. One third to one half of patients with locally advanced anal cancers treated by abdominoperineal resection at the major centers known for their expertise in this disease still had local recurrence in the pelvis or perineum.[68,87,89,119,128]

With the success of combined modality therapy, abdominoperineal resection should be reserved for salvage of the few patients in whom multimodality treatment fails or for morbidity related to therapy, such as severe proctitis.

INTERSTITIAL RADIATION THERAPY. Interstitial radiation therapy was originally used because of the limitations of orthovoltage irradiation. It had the potential of curing only early lesions that were unlikely to spread to the lymph nodes. Radium needles have been used primarily, although interstitial implants with ^{192}Ir have also been used. Radium needles were used for many years at the Christie Hospital in Manchester, England, for early-stage anal cancers.[117,122] In an update from that institution, radium needles were the exclusive treatment modality for 74 patients, 43 with anal canal lesions and 31 with anal margin lesions.[122] Of the 68 evaluable patients with follow-up of 5 years, 33 (49%) were disease free at follow-up or at death and were considered to have been cured. Of the 35 locoregional failures, 7 were salvaged by a surgical procedure. Local control was achieved in 64% of tumors less than 5 cm in diameter but in only 23% of tumors 5 cm or larger. The investigators recommend only local excision or an implant for tumors smaller than 5 cm in diameter with clinically negative nodes and close follow-up and surgical resection for any recurrence.

Radium implantation was also used extensively by Papillon, but he abandoned this technique because of painful local reactions and an inability to achieve nodal control because of the small target volume.[100,108] Early studies with radium needles yielded a severe necrosis rate of about 25%.[117,157,158] Employing ^{192}Ir to a dose of 60 Gy, Keiling and coworkers observed no local failures in 12 patients but a 16% necrosis rate, although all healed with conservative treatment.[159] Disease recurred in regional lymph nodes in 2 patients, emphasizing the lack of control outside the very small target volume.

Combined multimodality techniques are yielding better local control, sphincter preservation, and survival rates and should be the treatment of choice for locoregional anal canal disease.

EXTERNAL IRRADIATION. External irradiation can be used with fields designed to cover the pelvic and inguinal node areas, which are at risk in anal canal cancer. CT may aid in the planning of treatment. For example, boost doses, whether given by external irradiation or by interstitial implant, may be better designed with the use of CT. A study reported from Duke University Medical Center found excellent definition of tumor extent (local spread, lymph node involvement, and distant metastases) with CT of the pelvis, and CT was also useful for follow-up for potential recurrence.[93]

The results of major studies using external irradiation alone are given in Table 32–3. Local control overall ranges from 60% to 80%, and overall survival ranges from 50% to 80%. The French studies show that 5-year survival is related to the extent of the primary tumor as determined from tumor size or the 1978 UICC T staging and is similar to or better than 5-year survival after abdominoperineal resection.[147,160,161] A study from San Francisco found that survival is better for patients with tumors smaller than 5 cm in diameter and with negative nodes.[16,162] In an update of the Institut Curie external irradiation data, the investigators expressed the belief that multimodality therapy is now the best approach for curative therapy.[163] Investigators at the Princess Margaret Hospital, who compared multimodality therapy with external irradiation, also concluded that multimodality therapy affords better local control and therefore a better colostomy-free survival rate.[164] In a study from Russia, in which the length of follow-up was unclear, similar results were obtained for 5-year survival rates by T stage.[165]

In all of the studies listed in Table 32–3, the rate of complications requiring surgery remains around 5% to 15%, probably reflecting the high doses (60–70 Gy) that must be delivered to the primary site to control this disease if radiation therapy is the sole treatment modality. The addition of bleomycin to external irradiation in 10 patients did not decrease the recurrence rate.[166] A British trial is comparing radiation therapy alone with radiation therapy plus mitomycin and 5-FU; 300 patients have been accrued, but no results are available yet.[167,168]

COMBINED INTERSTITIAL AND EXTERNAL IRRADIATION. Several studies using small numbers of patients have been done with external irradiation combined with implants (*i.e.*, ^{137}Cs, ^{192}Ir, radium needles).[119,121,161,167,169–172] Good local control was achieved, but there was still a relatively high rate of complications requiring surgery or leading to death. Delouche and colleagues, reporting the results of 22 patients followed for 5 to 13 years, found a 32% rate of moderate or severe complications with 30 to 40 Gy of external radiation therapy and 35 to 40 Gy administered by ^{192}Ir implant.[169] However, a 78% local control rate was achieved, with an overall survival of 45%.

The most extensive series is that from the Centre Leon Berard in which 221 patients with anal carcinoma were treated over a 15-year period with external radiation therapy (^{60}Co) to a dose of 35 Gy, followed 2 months later by an ^{192}Ir implant to deliver a dose of 15 to 20 Gy.[108,172] The investigators re-

TABLE 32–3. Treatment of Anal Canal Carcinoma With External Radiation Therapy Alone

Investigation	No. of Patients	Primary Site Dose (Gy)	Follow-up (y)	Complications Requiring Surgery (%)	5-Year Survival by Size or Stage*		Local Control (%)
Institut Curie[84]	158	65–70	3–14	8	T ≤ 4 cm	70	
					T > 4 but ≤6 cm	57	
					T > 6 cm	33	
					All	51	67
Institut Gustave Roussy[160]	64	60–65	2–13	14	T1, T2	72	91
					T3	} 35	76
					T4		67
					All	50	81
St. Francis Memorial Hospital[16,162]	39[16]	65	0.5–8.5	13	All	79	80
	35[162]	45–76		6	N0, <5 cm	92	77
Princess Margaret Hospital[164]	25	45–60	5–25	12	All	72	60
CRLC Val d'Aurelle[161]	28	60–65	5–14	4	T1–3	85	61
					T1	86	71
					T2	92	67
					T3	75	57

* UICC 1978 stage.

ported only a 3% rate of serious complications, 65% 5-year disease-free survival, and 79% locoregional control.

Another study from France confirmed a high 5-year survival rate (61%) and good local control (75%), but a 6% rate of complications requiring surgery.[171] The importance of treating the inguinal nodes prophylactically was shown in this study. In 28 N0 patients, there were 2 patients with inguinal recurrences, neither of which had received inguinal irradiation. Both developed metastases and died despite radiation treatment for recurrent disease. Combined brachytherapy and external irradiation may also be useful in treating extensive lesions.[173–175]

Combined interstitial and external radiation therapy may yield high local control rates but a significant complication rate. However, 5-year disease-free survival rates of 60% to 65% are excellent and compare favorably with results of surgically treated patients.

Locally Advanced, Residual, or Recurrent Cancer

Anal Margin Cancer

Recurrent anal margin cancer, after local excision, may require further local excision for salvage. In a study from Memorial Sloan-Kettering Cancer Center, 16 patients in whom disease recurred underwent additional surgical procedures; of these, 12 were alive at 5 years, and only 2 had died of disease.[105] One patient was unavailable for follow-up. Eleven of the 12 patients with local failure underwent local excision only for salvage. More advanced primary or recurrent anal margin lesions may be salvaged by external radiation therapy.[100]

Residual Anal Canal Cancer

Whether anal canal patients are treated by radiation therapy alone or chemoradiation therapy, histologic confirmation of complete remission should be obtained several weeks after irradiation is completed.[131] Patients with clinically complete remissions but microscopically residual superficial tumors should undergo sphincter-sparing wide local excisions. The deep margin may be increased by including a portion of the internal sphincter, with minimal impact on subsequent continence. If the margins are positive, an additional radiation boost may be used, if feasible, with external beam or an interstitial implant. The role of cisplatin-based chemotherapy in this setting is yet to be defined. If a radiation boost is not possible because maximal radiation has already been delivered, an abdominoperineal resection is probably required for cure.

Recurrent Anal Canal Cancer

Patients with recurrent anal canal cancer after surgery should be considered for multimodality therapy (described in the section on locoregional disease of the anal canal). Locoregional failures after initial multimodality therapy have been successfully treated with abdominoperineal resection[2] or with additional irradiation and chemotherapy.[134] The success rate of surgical salvage averaged about 60% for seven series.[102,129,132,138,162,171,176] Mitomycin plus 5-FU can also induce major remissions in previously treated patients who have locally recurrent disease.[177]

Locally Advanced Anal Canal Cancer

Multimodality therapy for locally advanced primary anal canal tumors may yield good palliation and, in some cases, cure. In a study reported from the University of Virginia, major regressions of disease were observed in 6 of 7 patients, 3 of whom were treated with chemotherapy alone and 3 with chemotherapy plus irradiation.[72] Abdominoperineal resections were performed on all patients, and all had delayed wound healing. Three of the 7 patients remained disease free for 24 to 26 months and 4 died, 2 of cancer and 2 of other causes. Another form of multimodality therapy, mitomycin and 5-FU with external irradiation and interstitial ^{192}Ir implant, was tried in 29 patients with advanced local disease.[178] After a follow-up of 5 to 54 months, 25 of 29 patients were alive and free of disease; only 2 patients required radical salvage surgery with loss of sphincter function. Papillon achieved a 90% local control rate in T3 tumors larger than 4 cm in diameter with a combination of mitomycin, 5-FU, external irradiation, and an ^{192}Ir implant.[175]

Brachytherapy combined with external irradiation has been used for advanced disease.[173–175] There was a 70% local control rate in Papillon's analysis of T3 tumors larger than 4 cm in diameter, which were treated with ^{60}Co external irradiation and an ^{192}Ir implant without combined chemotherapy.[175]

Inguinal Node Involvement

The initial experience from Memorial Sloan-Kettering Cancer Center suggested that patients with grossly positive inguinal lymph nodes *synchronous* with the primary tumor were incurable.[179] A subsequent report indicated that 2 of 13 patients survived 5 years after abdominoperineal resection, followed 6 weeks later by inguinal lymphadenectomy.[91] Other studies confirmed a small cure rate for surgical treatment of patients with synchronous unilateral inguinal nodes.[64,86] Table 32–4 shows that external irradiation[100] postoperatively may improve these results slightly, but radical external irradiation alone [100,102,171,180] can achieve a nodal control rate of about 65%, and external irradiation combined with chemotherapy[133,181,182] can achieve nodal control in approximately 90% of patients. Current recommendations are for limited surgical sampling, combined chemotherapy and radiation therapy with boost doses to the involved groin (45–50 Gy); surgical salvage may be done for isolated inguinal recurrence.

The development of unilateral *metachronous* inguinal lymph nodes usually does not carry such an ominous prognosis. After therapeutic groin dissection, the 5- to 7-year survival rate reported from Memorial Sloan-Kettering Cancer Center and St. Mark's Hospital exceeded 50%,[88,105] but it was zero in a small series reported from the Mayo Clinic.[64] Current strategies in patients with metachronous isolated inguinal node metastases

after multimodality therapy include a formal groin dissection followed by chemotherapy. The use of radiation under these circumstances depends on prior dose and fields.

Metastatic Disease

Because of its rarity and because many patients with anal canal tumors have locoregional disease that can be successfully treated by the methods described, data on the use of chemotherapy as a single modality in the treatment of advanced disease are scanty. Several anecdotal reports are available. Single-agent trials of doxorubicin (Adriamycin) and of cisplatin have been reported by several investigators. Fisher and associates reported response to doxorubicin as a single agent and, at another time, to cisplatin in an elderly man with advanced disease.[183] Salem and colleagues studied cisplatin as a single agent in 3 patients: 1 achieved complete remission, and the other 2 had partial regressions.[184] Earlier trials with 5-FU and vinblastine in small groups of patients were ineffective. Bleomycin and vincristine were used by Livingston and associates in a single patient, and a partial regression was observed.[185]

The results of combination chemotherapy with cisplatin plus 5-FU have now been reported from a few small series. Responses were seen with systemic and regional (hepatic arterial) routes. Of a total of 5 patients described in two reports, 2 complete and 3 partial remissions were observed.[186,187] In a study from France using this combination, which combined 7 patients who had local recurrences alone with 13 patients with metastases with or without local recurrences, there were 2 of 20 complete and 9 of 20 partial responses.[188]

One of the larger series of patients with advanced anal canal tumors treated with chemotherapy as primary management was reported by Wilking and colleagues.[189] They treated 15 patients with advanced disease with a combination of bleomycin, vincristine, and high-dose methotrexate (BOM regimen), with leucovorin rescue. Major objective regressions of disease occurred in 3 (25%) of 12 patients with measurable disease, but the duration of response ranged from only 1 to 5 months. The toxic effects were severe in one third of the patients, and 4 patients probably died as a result of toxicity. Wilking and associates concluded that although one fourth of

TABLE 32–4. Treatment of Synchronous Positive Inguinal Lymph Nodes in Epidermoid Anal Canal Carcinoma

Investigations	Treatment	Nodes Controlled/Nodes Treated	Controlled (%)
Greenall et al[91]	Surgery	2/13	~15
Papillon[100]	Surgery + postop. RT	3/12	~25
Cummings et al[180]	RT	8/11	
Papillon[100]	RT	4/10	
Kin et al[169]	RT	4/4	~65
Schlienger et al[102]	RT	17/24 (clin. +)	
Sischy[133]	RT + MITC/5-FU	3/3	
Cummings[181]	RT + MITC/5-FU	9/10	~90
Shank[182]	RT + MITC/5-FU	4/5	

RT, radiation therapy; MITC, mitomycin C; 5-FU, 5-fluorouracil; clin. +, clinically positive.

the patients had responses, these were of short duration and associated with severe toxicity.

Magill and colleagues treated a group of 24 patients (22 of whom had had prior chemotherapy) with a combination of cisplatin, bleomycin, and a vinca alkaloid (*i.e.*, vinblastine or vindesine). Six (29%) of 21 evaluable patients responded.[190]

Anal canal tumors are sensitive to several chemotherapeutic agents, including cisplatin and mitomycin or 5-FU. The optimal regimen remains to be defined. Complete remissions are possible, but relapse is the rule.

FOLLOW-UP

Patients with squamous cell cancer of the anus require careful follow-up. Those with local or regional recurrence can still be treated curatively, and those with systemic disease are eligible for effective chemotherapy. Follow-up examinations should include interval histories, physical examinations, and liver function tests every 2 to 3 months for the first 3 years and then semiannually for at least 10 years, because there can be recurrences after 5 years, although this is rare.[191] The detection of local and inguinal node recurrence requires follow-up by the same physicians to differentiate posttreatment scar and inflammatory lymphadenitis from progressive recurrent tumor. Annual chest radiography and abdominal or pelvic CT for the first 3 years is appropriate.

Management of patients with residual or recurrent local disease and those with metachronous regional lymph nodes was discussed in prior sections.

ANORECTAL MELANOMA

Melanomas in this region are rare (see Pathology section), and the etiology is unknown. They are rarely diagnosed at a curable stage, and most patients die within 1 year of diagnosis from systemic metastases. Ultraradical surgery involving an abdominoperineal resection with inguinal and pelvic lymphadenectomy was the recommended approach for many years.[192] The end results were poor, and current recommendations encourage a sphincter-saving local treatment if at all feasible.

CLINICAL AND PATHOLOGIC FEATURES

The diagnosis of anorectal melanoma is frequently delayed because the tumor is located deep within the anal canal and because symptoms are typically nonspecific "hemorrhoidal" complaints. Anal burning, pruritus, and minor, intermittent blood on the toilet paper are usual. A mass, frequently nonpigmented, seen at the dentate line is consistent with a thrombosed internal hemorrhoid. With progression, a prolapsing mass with increasing hemorrhage occurs, perhaps with palpable inguinal adenopathy. However, primary tumor progression is usually cephalad. Although most anal melanomas are pigmented on microscopic examination, few are grossly melanotic.[193] Asymptomatic anal melanoma is diagnosed as an incidental finding in hemorrhoidectomy specimens.

PATTERNS OF SPREAD

Extensive proximal submucosal spread of anorectal melanoma into the rectum occurs. Lymph node metastases are found in the mesorectal nodes in 50% of patients treated by radical surgery and in the inguinal nodes in 20%.[192,194] Hematogenous metastases occur early and spread widely, primarily to the liver and lungs.

TREATMENT AND END RESULTS

The Memorial Sloan-Kettering Cancer Center,[72,194–196] St. Mark's Hospital,[197] and Mayo Clinic[198] groups report the largest experience with these tumors, in addition to a composite experience from Israel.[199] In the initial reports from Memorial Sloan-Kettering Cancer Center, abdominoperineal resection, alone or combined with pelvic and inguinal lymphadenectomy, was recommended for all patients without distant disease, but there were only 3 5-year survivors of 50 patients so treated. In a smaller series at St. Mark's Hospital, there were no 5-year survivors. In the few patients treated by wide local excision (2-cm margins), all patients died of distant disease without local recurrence. The Mayo Clinic experience with abdominoperineal resection is equally grim. In a report from Israel, only 2 of 30 patients survived 5 years, both after local excision.

The dismal prognosis for patients with anal melanoma presenting with a palpable mass is confirmed in recent reports. Goldman combined cases from multiple institutions in Sweden.[200] One third of 49 patients presented with regional or distant metastases, and this group had a median survival of 5 months. Median survival of the remainder who underwent potentially curative wide local excision or abdominoperineal resection was only about 1 year, with only 2 long-term survivors. A comparable report from Duke University of 24 patients revealed median survivals of 1 to 2 years, and no survivors beyond 6 years.[201] Twenty-six patients underwent potentially curative local excision or abdominoperineal resection at the M.D. Anderson Cancer Center, with a median survival of approximately 1 year.[202] Patterns of failure reported by all of these investigators suggest local control of approximately 50% with wide local excision and 25% with abdominoperineal resection. However, local failure almost always occurs simultaneously with distant recurrence, raising doubt about the value of radical surgery for this rapidly progressive cancer.[202]

An analysis of the Memorial Sloan-Kettering Cancer Center experience includes some patients treated by local measures, such as local excision, fulguration, and cryosurgery.[72] The end results analyzed by tumor thickness provided the greatest insight into the far-advanced nature of these cancers when treatment is undertaken. All 3 patients with melanomas thinner than 2 mm were cured with abdominoperineal resection. No patient with a tumor thicker than 2 mm survived longer than 5 years, and 85% were dead in 2 years. It appears that only patients with "incidentally diagnosed" melanomas, usually as part of a hemorrhoidectomy specimen, are likely to be cured by surgery. Although the long-term survivors at Memorial Sloan-Kettering Cancer Center were treated with radical surgery, it does not preclude cure with a more limited approach.[203] More advanced lesions may be treated by local excision combined with external-beam radiation therapy at doses of at least 4 Gy per fraction.[204]

Patients with incidental anal melanomas less than 2 mm thick detected in hemorrhoidectomy specimens should undergo wide local excision. If the location of the tumor is unknown (multiple unmarked specimens sent to pathology), the patient may be observed closely for local recurrence or undergo abdominoperineal resection.

Intermediate tumors, those more than 2 mm thick but not overly bulky, may be palliated with a local procedure: wide local excision, fulguration, laser vaporization, or cryosurgery. External-beam or implant radiation therapy may play an adjuvant role.

Despite the incurability of bulky anal melanoma, if the lesion cannot be controlled with a local approach, abdominoperineal resection or radiation therapy may still be necessary to palliate symptoms of bleeding, tenesmus, or obstruction.

Patients with systemic disease should be considered for chemotherapy and immunotherapy regimens appropriate for skin melanoma.

ADENOCARCINOMA

Primary adenocarcinoma of the anal canal arising from the anal glands is a rare tumor.[205,206] Most adenocarcinomas in the canal represent rectal cancer with downward spread. With only a few cases reported, it appears reasonable to treat patients by abdominoperineal resection and, considering the vast lymphatics draining the anal canal, to use postoperative irradiation and 5-FU. As with squamous cell cancers, radiation fields should include the inguinal nodes. Schlienger and associates treated 21 patients with irradiation alone (16) or with irradiation combined with surgery (5) and obtained a 35% 5-year survival rate, despite the fact that 62% of the patients had early-stage disease: T1N0 and T2N0.[207]

FUTURE DIRECTIONS

Prevention of epidermoid carcinoma of the anal canal requires better knowledge of etiologic factors. Because accumulating evidence implicates papillomaviruses as causative factors and because the incidence of anal cancer appears to be increasing in the male homosexual community, it would be wise to direct further epidemiologic, virologic, and preventive studies along these lines. Increasing use of measures for "safe sex" initiated to stem the spread of acquired immunodeficiency syndrome (AIDS) may also affect the incidence of anal cancer. Early detection could result from increased awareness in high-risk persons; male homosexuals and immunosuppressed patients should be educated about the symptoms of anal cancer. Basic studies, such as the search for tumor markers or flow cytometric analyses for possible premalignant or diagnostic changes, may aid in detection and follow-up. Animal studies, such as those investigating epidermal growth factor, may offer etiologic insights and lead to means of prevention and new methods of treatment. Antiviral agents (*e.g.*, interferon) should be investigated further for treatment of condylomata before tumor development or after treatment of anal cancer if condylomata remain.

New approaches to treatment must be directed toward patients with late-stage disease, who are not as responsive to the multimodality regimen that has become well established. One potentially fruitful avenue is the addition of a biochemical modulator, such as a differentiation inducer, to therapy regimens.[130] Standard agents, such as cisplatin and 5-FU, should be explored further in conjunction with irradiation.

REFERENCES

1. Cummings BJ. The place of radiation therapy in the treatment of carcinoma of the anal canal. Cancer Treat Rev 1982;9:125–147.
2. Shank B. Treatment of anal canal carcinoma. Cancer 1985;55:2156–2162.
3. Papillon J. The responsibility of radiologists in the preservation of breast and rectum in cancer treatment. Clin Radiol 1986;37:303–309.
4. Cummings B. The treatment of anal cancer. Int J Radiat Oncol Biol Phys 1989;17:1359–1361.
5. Gordon PH. Current status—perianal and anal canal neoplasms. Dis Colon Rectum 1990;33:799–808.
6. Cummings BJ. Anal cancer. Int J Radiat Oncol Biol Phys 1990;19:1309–1315.
7. Grinnell RS. An analysis of forty-nine cases of squamous cell carcinoma of the anus. Surg Gynecol Obstet 1954;98:29–39.
8. Richards JC, Beahrs OH, Woolner LB. Squamous cell carcinoma of the anus, anal canal, and rectum in 109 patients. Surg Gynecol Obstet 1962;114:475–482.
9. Sawyers JL, Herrington JL Jr, Main FB. Surgical considerations in the treatment of epidermoid carcinoma of the anus. Ann Surg 1963;157:817–824.
10. Stearns MW Jr, Urmacher C, Sternberg SS, et al. Cancer of the anal canal. Curr Probl Cancer 1980;4:1–44.
11. Morson BC, Volkstadt H. Malignant melanoma of the anal canal. J Clin Pathol 1963;16:126–132.
12. McConnell EM. Squamous cell carcinoma of the anus: A review of 96 cases. Br J Surg 1970;57:89–92.
13. Peters RK, Mack TM. Patterns of anal carcinoma by gender and marital status in Los Angeles County. Br J Cancer 1983;48:629–636.
14. Klotz RG, Pamukcoglu T, Souilliard DH. Transitional cloacogenic carcinoma of the anal canal. Cancer 1967;20:1727–1745.
15. Corman ML, Haggitt RC. Carcinoma of the anal canal. Surg Gynecol Obstet 1977;145:674–676.
16. Cantril ST, Green JP, Schall GL, et al. Primary radiation therapy in the treatment of anal carcinoma. Int J Radiat Oncol Biol Phys 1983;9:1271–1278.
17. Welch JP, Malt RA. Appraisal of treatment of carcinoma of the anus and anal canal. Surg Gynecol Obstet 1977;145:837–841.
18. Gabriel WB. Discussion on squamous cell carcinoma of the anus and anal canal. Proc R Soc Med 1960;53:403–409.
19. Wolfe HRI, Bussey HJR. Squamous cell carcinoma of the anus. Br J Surg 1968;55:295–301.
20. Morson BC, Pang LSC. Pathology of anal cancer. Proc R Soc Med 1968;61:623–624.
21. Rousseau J, Mathieu G, Fenton J, et al. La telecobaltotherapie des cancers du canal anal. J Radiol Electrol Med Nucl 1973;54:622–626.
22. Kapur BML, Dhawan IK, Singhal KK. Epidermoid carcinoma of the anorectum: Review of 31 cases. Dis Colon Rectum 1977;20:252–254.
23. Cooper HS, Patchefsky AS, Marks G. Cloacogenic carcinoma of the anorectum in homosexual men: An observation of four cases. Dis Colon Rectum 1979;22:557–558.
24. Li FP, Osborn D, Cronin CM. Anorectal squamous carcinoma in two homosexual men. Lancet 1982;2:391.
25. Austin DF. Etiologic clues from descriptive epidemiology: Squamous carcinoma of the rectum or anus. NCI Monogr 1982;62:89–90.
26. Daling JR, Weiss NS, Klopfenstein LL, et al. Correlates of homosexual behavior and the incidence of anal canal cancer. JAMA 1982;247:1988–1990.
27. Daling JR, Weiss NS, Hislop G, et al. Sexual practices, sexually transmitted diseases, and the incidence of anal cancer. New Engl J Med 1987;317:973–977.
28. zur Hausen H. Human papillomaviruses and their possible role in squamous cell carcinomas. Curr Top Microbiol Immunol 1977;78:1–30.
29. Siegel A. Malignant transformation of condyloma acuminatum: Review of the literature and case report. Am J Surg 1962;103:613–617.
30. Friedberg MJ, Serlin O. Condyloma acuminatum: Its association with malignancy. Dis Colon Rectum 1963;6:352–355.
31. Oriel JD, Whimster IW. Carcinoma in situ associated with virus-containing anal warts. Br J Dermatol 1971;84:71–73.
32. Prasad ML, Abcarian H. Malignant potential of perianal condyloma acuminatum. Dis Colon Rectum 1980;23:191–197.
33. Croxson T, Chabon AB, Rorat E, et al. Intraepithelial carcinoma of the anus in homosexual men. Dis Colon Rectum 1984;27:325–330.
34. Chuang TY, Perry HO, Kurland LT, et al. Condyloma acuminatum in Rochester, Minnesota, 1950–1978. Arch Dermatol 1984;120:476–483.
35. Gal AA, Meyer PR, Taylor CR. Papillomavirus antigens in anorectal condyloma and carcinoma in homosexual men. JAMA 1987;257:337–340.
36. Beckmann AM, Daling JR, Sherman KJ, et al. Human papillomavirus infection and anal cancer. Int J Cancer 1989;43:1042–1049.
37. Palmer JG, Scholefield JH, Coates PJ, et al. Anal cancer and human papillomaviruses. Dis Colon Rectum 1989;32:1016–1022.
38. Scholefield JH, Sonnex C, Talbot IC, et al. Anal and cervical intraepithelial neoplasia: Possible parallel. Lancet 1989;2:765–769.

39. Palevsky JM, Holly EA, Gonzales J, et al. Detection of human papillomavirus DNA in anal intraepithelial neoplasia and anal cancer. Cancer Res 1991;51:1014–1019.

40. Goedert JJ, Causey D, Palefsky J, et al. Anal Pap smears and human papilloma viruses (HPV) in a 7-year cohort study of homosexual men. Proc Am Soc Clin Oncol 1990;9:3.

41. Higgins GD, Uzelin DM, Phillips GE, et al. Differing characteristics of human papillomavirus RNA-positive and RNA-negative anal carcinomas. Cancer 1991;68:561–567.

42. Oriel JD. Human papillomaviruses and anal cancer. Genitourin Med [Editorial] 1989;65:213–215.

43. Monfardini S, Vaccher E, Lazzarin A, et al. Characterization of AIDS-associated tumors in Italy: Report of 435 cases of an IVDA-based series. Cancer Detect Prev 1990;14:391–393.

44. McAnally AK, Dockerty MB. Carcinoma developing in chronic draining cutaneous sinuses and fistulas. Surg Gynecol Obstet 1949;88:87–96.

45. Winkelman J, Grosfeld J, Bigelow B. Colloid carcinoma of anal-gland origin: Report of a case and review of the literature. Am J Clin Pathol 1964;42:395–401.

46. Bretlau P. Carcinoma arising in anal fistula. Acta Chir Scand 1967;133:496–500.

47. Chaos A, Garrido H, Fernandez-Villoria JM. Carcinoma associated with fistula in ano. Int Surg 1973;58:497–499.

48. Binkley GE, Derrick WA. The association of squamous cancer with anal manifestations of lymphogranuloma venereum. Am J Dig Dis 1945;12:46–47.

49. Rainey R. The association of lymphogranuloma inguinale and cancer. Surgery 1954;35:221–235.

50. Brennan JT, Stewart CF. Epidermoid carcinoma of the anus. Ann Surg 1972;176:787–790.

51. Buckwalter JA, Jurayj MN. Relationship of chronic anorectal disease to carcinoma. Arch Surg 1957;75:352–361.

52. Cabrera A, Tsukada Y, Pickren JW, et al. Development of lower genital carcinomas in patients with anal carcinoma: A more than casual relationship. Cancer 1966;19:470–480.

53. Goligher JC. Surgery of the anus, rectum and colon. 3rd ed. London: Bailere, Tindell & Cassell, 1975:815.

54. Penn I. Cancers of the anogenital region in renal transplant recipients. Cancer 1986;58:611–616.

55. Daniell HW. Re: Causes of anal carcinoma. JAMA 1985;254:358.

56. Holmes F, Borek D, Owen-Kummer M, et al. Anal cancer in women. Gastroenterology 1988;95:107–111.

57. Kawaura A, Kumagai H, Shibata M, et al. Tumors of the anal region induced in mice painted with methylazoxymethanol acetate. Gann 1981;72:886–890.

58. Kingsnorth AN, Abu-Khalaf M, Ross JS, et al. Potentiation of 1,2-dimethylhydrazine-induced anal carcinoma by epidermal growth factor in mice. Surgery 1985;97:696–700.

59. Kuehn PG, Beckett R, Eisenberg H, et al. Epidermoid carcinoma of the perianal skin and anal canal. New Engl J Med 1964;270:614–617.

60. Adam YG, Efron G. Current concepts and controversies concerning the etiology, pathogenesis, diagnosis and treatment of malignant tumors of the anus. Surgery 1987;101:253–266.

61. Morson BC. The pathology and results of treatment of squamous cell carcinoma of the anal canal and anal margin. Proc R Soc Med 1960;53:414–420.

62. Greenall MJ, Quan SHQ, Stearns MW, et al. Epidermoid cancer of the anal margin. Am J Surg 1985;149:95–101.

63. Hardy KJ, Hughes ESR, Cuthbertson AM. Squamous cell carcinoma of the anal canal and anal margin. Aust N Z J Surg 1969;38:301–305.

64. Beahrs OH, Wilson SM. Carcinoma of the anus. Ann Surg 1976;184:422–428.

65. Beahrs OH, Henson DE, Hutter RVP, Myers MH. Manual for staging of cancer. 3rd ed. Philadelphia: JB Lippincott, 1987:81–83.

66. Wade DS, Herrera L, Castillo NB, et al. Metastases to the lymph nodes in epidermoid carcinoma of the anal canal studied by a clearing technique. Surg Gynecol Obstet 1989;169:238–242.

67. Wood DA. Tumors of the intestines. In: Atlas of tumor pathology. Washington, DC: Armed Forces Institute of Pathology, 1967:200–223.

68. Boman BM, Moertel CG, O'Connell MJ, et al. Carcinoma of the anal canal: A clinical and pathologic study of 188 cases. Cancer 1984;54:114–125.

69. Ordonez NG, Awalt H, Mackay B. Mammary and extramammary Paget's disease: An immunocytochemical and ultrastructural study. Cancer 1987;59:1173–1183.

70. Remigio PA, Der BK, Forsberg RT. Anorectal melanoma: Report of two cases. Dis Colon Rectum 1976;19:350–356.

71. Quinn D, Selah C. Malignant melanoma of the anus in a negro: Report of a case and review of the literature. Dis Colon Rectum 1991;20:627–631.

72. Wanebo HJ, Woodruff JM, Farr GH, et al. Anorectal melanoma. Cancer 1981;47:1891–1900.

73. Stearns MW, Quan SH. Epidermoid carcinoma of the anorectum. Surg Gynecol Obstet 1970;191:953–957.

74. Dougherty B, Evans H. Carcinoma of the anal canal: A study of 79 cases. Am J Clin Pathol 1985;83:159–164.

75. Salmon RJ, Zafrani B, Habib A, et al. Prognosis of cloacogenic and squamous cancers of the anal canal. Dis Colon Rectum 1986;29:336–340.

76. Wolber R, Dupuis B, Thiyagaratnam P, et al. Anal cloacogenic and squamous carcinomas. Comparative histologic analysis using in situ hybridization for human papillomavirus DNA. Am J Surg Pathol 1990;14:176–182.

77. Muleris M, Salmon R-J, Girodet J, et al. Recurrent deletions of chromosomes 11q and 3p in anal canal carcinoma. Int J Cancer 1987;39:595–598.

78. Tjandra J. Perianal Paget's disease: Report of three cases. Dis Colon Rectum 1988;31:462–466.

79. Fenger C, Nielsen VT. Precancerous changes in the anal canal epithelium in resection specimens. Acta Pathol Microbiol Immunobiol Scand [A] 1986;94:63–69.

80. Fenger C, Nielsen VT. Dysplastic changes in the anal canal epithelium in minor surgical specimens. Acta Pathol Microbiol Immunobiol Scand [A] 1981;89:463–465.

81. Palefsky J, Gonzalez J, Greenblatt R, et al. Anal intraepithelial neoplasia and anal papillomavirus infection among homosexual males with group IV HIV disease. JAMA 1990;263:1911–1916.

82. Fenger C, Bichel P. Flow cytometric DNA analysis of anal canal epithelium and anorectal tumours. Acta Pathol Microbiol Immunobiol Scand [A] 1981;89:351–355.

83. Goldman S, Auer G, Erhardt K, et al. Prognostic significance of clinical stage, histologic grade, and nuclear DNA content in squamous cell carcinoma of the anus. Dis Colon Rectum 1987;30:444–448.

84. Scott NA, Beart RW Jr, Weiland LH, et al. Carcinoma of the anal canal and flow cytometric DNA analysis. Br J Cancer 1989;60:56–58.

85. Singh R, Nime F, Mittelman A. Malignant epithelial tumors of the anal canal. Cancer 1981;48:411–415.

86. Dillard BM, Spratt JS Jr, Ackerman LV, et al. Epidermoid cancer of anal margin and canal. Arch Surg 1963;86:772–777.

87. Clark J, Petrelli N, Herrera L, et al. Epidermoid carcinoma of the anal canal. Cancer 1986;57:400–406.

88. Wolfe HRI. The management of metastatic inguinal adenitis in epidermoid cancer of the anus. Proc R Soc Med 1961;61:626–629.

89. Hardcastle JD, Bussey HJR. Results of surgical treatment of squamous cell carcinoma of the anal canal and anal margin seen at St. Mark's Hospital 1928–66. Proc R Soc Med 1968;61:629–630.

90. Kuehn PG, Beckett R, Eisenberg H, et al. Hematogenous metastases from epidermoid carcinoma of the anal canal. Am J Surg 1965;109:445–449.

91. Greenall MJ, Quan SHQ, DeCosse J. Epidermoid cancer of the anus. Br J Surg 1985;72:S97–S103.

92. Pyper PC, Parks TG. The results of surgery for epidermoid carcinoma of the anus. Br J Surg 1985;72:712–714.

93. Cohan RH, Silverman PM, Thompson WM, et al. Computed tomography of epithelial neoplasms of the anal canal. AJR 1985;145:569–573.

94. Goldman S, Glimelius B, Norming U, et al. Transanorectal ultrasonography in anal carcinoma: A prospective study of 21 patients. Acta Radiol 1988;29:337–341.

95. Petrelli NJ, Shaw N, Bhargava A, et al. Squamous cell carcinoma antigen as a marker for squamous cell carcinoma of the anal canal. J Clin Oncol 1988;6:782–785.

96. Paradis P, Douglass HO Jr, Holyoke ED. The clinical implications of a staging system for carcinoma of the anus. Surg Gynecol Obstet 1975;141:411–416.

97. Harmer MH, ed. TNM classification of malignant tumors. 3rd ed. Geneva: International Union Against Cancer (Union Internationale Contra le Cancer), 1978:77–81.

98. Hermanek P. Problems of pTNM classification of carcinoma of the stomach, colorectum and anal margin. Pathol Res Pract 1986;181:296–300.

99. Spiessl B, Hermanek P, Scheibe O, et al, eds. TNM atlas: Illustrated guide to the TNM/pTNM classification of malignant tumours. 2nd ed. New York: Springer-Verlag, 1982:114–123.

100. Papillon J. Rectal and anal cancers. New York: Springer-Verlag, 1982.

101. TNM Classification of malignant tumours. 4th ed. New York: Springer-Verlag, 1987.

102. Schlienger M, Krzisch C, Pene F, et al. Epidermoid carcinoma of the anal canal treatment results and prognostic variables in a series of 242 cases. Int J Radiat Oncol Biol Phys 1989;17:1141–1151.

103. Schlienger M, Touboul E, Mauban S, et al. Resultats du traitement de 286 cas de cancers epidermoides du canal anal dont 236 par irradiation a visee conservatrice. Lyon Chir 1991;87:61–69.

104. Goldman S, Glimelius B, Glas U, et al. Management of anal epidermoid carcinoma—an evaluation of treatment results in two population-based series. Int J Colorect Dis 1989;4:234–243.

105. Greenall M, Magill G, Quan S, et al. Recurrent epidermoid cancer of the anus. Cancer 1986;57:1437–1441.

106. Kuehn PG, Eisenberg H, Reed JF. Epidermoid carcinoma of the perianal skin and anal canal. Cancer 1968;22:932–938.

107. Wanebo H, Furrell W, Constable W. Multimodality approach to surgical management of locally advanced epidermoid carcinoma of the anorectum. Cancer 1981;47:2817–2826.

108. Papillon J, Montbarbon JF. Epidermoid carcinoma of the anal canal: A series of 276 cases. Dis Colon Rectum 1987;30:324–333.

109. Shepherd NA, Scholefield JH, Love SB, et al. Prognostic factors in anal squamous carcinoma: A multivariate analysis of clinical, pathological, and flow cytometric parameters in 235 cases. Histopathology 1990;16:545–555.

110. Serota AI, Weil M, Williams RA, et al. Anal cloacogenic carcinoma. Arch Surg 1981;116:456–459.

111. Grodsky L. Unsuspected anal cancer discovered after minor anorectal surgery. Dis Colon Rectum 1967;10:471–478.

112. Beck DE, Fazio VW, Jagelman DG, et al. Perianal Bowen's disease. Dis Colon Rectum 1988;31:419–422.

113. Beck DE, Fazio VW. Perianal Paget's disease. Dis Colon Rectum 1987;30:263–266.

114. Berardi R, Lee S, Chen HP. Perianal extramammary Paget's disease. Surg Gynecol Obstet 1988;167:359–366.

115. Emslie ES. Paget's disease of the anus. J R Soc Med [Letter] 1991;84:386.

116. Turell R. Epidermoid squamous cell cancer of the perianus and anal canal. Surg Clin North Am 1962;42:1235–1241.

117. Dalby JF, Pointon RS. The treatment of anal carcinoma by interstitial irradiation. AJR 1961;85:515–520.

118. Schraut WH, Wang C-H, Dawson PJ, et al. Depth of invasion, location, and size of cancer of the anus dictate operative treatment. Cancer 1983;51:1291–1296.

119. Frost DB, Richards PC, Montague ED, et al. Epidermoid cancer of the anorectum. Cancer 1984;53:1285–1293.

120. Cummings BJ, Keane TJ, Hawkins NV, et al. Treatment of perianal carcinoma by radiation (RT) or radiation plus chemotherapy (RTCT). Int J Radiat Oncol Biol Phys [Abstract] 1986;12:170.

121. Hintz BL, Charyulu KKN, Sudarsanam A. Anal carcinoma: Basic concepts and management. J Surg Oncol 1978;10:141–150.

122. James RD, Pointon RS, Martin S. Local radiotherapy in the management of squamous carcinoma of the anus. Br J Surg 1985;72:282–285.

123. Papillon J, Renard L, Pipard G. Le cancer de la marge de l'anus: Experience du Centre Leon Berard. J Eur Radiother 1985;6:29–34.

124. Papillon J, Chassard JL. Role respectif de la chirurgie et de la radiotherapie dans le traitement des cancers de la marge de l'anus: A propos de 59 cas. Lyon Chir 1991;87:85–87.

125. Papillon J, Chassard JL. Respective role of radiotherapy and surgery in the management of epidermoid carcinoma of the anal margin: A series of 57 patients. Dis Colon Rectum 1992;35:422–429.

126. Glimelius B, Pahlman L. Recurrent epidermoid cancer of the anus. Cancer 1986;57:1437–1441.

127. Al-Jurf AS, Turnbull RB, Fazio VW. Local treatment of squamous cell carcinoma of the anus. Surg Gynecol Obstet 1979;148:576–578.

128. Greenall MJ, Quan SHQ, Urmacher C, et al. Treatment of epidermoid carcinoma of the anal canal. Surg Gynecol Obstet 1985;161:509–517.

129. Hughes LL, Rich TA, Delclos L, et al. Radiotherapy for anal cancer: Experience from 1979–1987. Int J Radiat Oncol Biol Phys 1989;17:1153–1160.

130. Nigro ND, Vaitkeviceus VK, Herskovic AM. Preservation of function in the treatment of cancer of the anus. In: DeVita VT, Hellman S, Rosenberg SA, eds. Important advances in oncology. Philadelphia: JB Lippincott, 1989:161–177.

131. Miller EJ, Quan SH, Thaler T. Treatment of squamous cell carcinoma of the anal canal. Cancer 1991;67:2038–2041.

132. Sischy B, Doggett RLS, Krall JM, et al. Definitive irradiation and chemotherapy for radiosensitization in management of anal carcinoma: Interim report on radiation therapy oncology group study No. 8314. JNCI 1989;81:850–856.

133. Sischy B. The use of radiation therapy combined with chemotherapy in the management of squamous cell carcinoma of the anus and marginally resectable adenocarcinoma of the rectum. Int J Radiat Oncol Biol Phys 1985;11:1587–1593.

134. Flam MS, John M, Mowry P, et al. Definitive combined modality therapy of carcinoma of the anus: A report of 30 cases including results of salvage therapy in patients with residual disease. Dis Colon Rectum 1987;30:495–502.

135. John MJ, Flam MS, Mowry PA. Clinical potential of synchronous radiotherapy and chemotherapy for advanced squamous cell carcinoma. NCI Monogr 1988;6:375–378.

136. Tanum G, Tveit K, Karlsen KO, et al. Chemotherapy and radiation therapy for anal carcinoma. Cancer 1991;67:2462–2466.

137. Zucali R, Doci R, Bombelli L. Combined chemotherapy–radiotherapy of anal cancer. Int J Radiat Oncol Biol Phys 1990;19:1221–1223.

138. Cummings BJ, Keane TJ, O'Sullivan B, et al. Epidermoid anal cancer: Treatment by radiation alone or by radiation and 5-fluorouracil with and without mitomycin C. Int J Radiat Oncol Biol Phys 1991;21:1115–1125.

139. Ajlouni M, Mahrt D, Milad MP. Review of recent experience in the treatment of carcinoma of the anal canal. Am J Clin Oncol 1984;7:687–691.

140. Nigro ND, Vaitkeviceus VK, Considine B Jr. Combined therapy for cancer of the anal canal: A preliminary report. Dis Colon Rectum 1974;17:354–356.

141. Leichman L, Nigro N, Vaitkeviceus VK, et al. Cancer of the anal canal: Model for preoperative adjuvant combined modality therapy. Am J Med 1985;78:211–216.

142. Enker WE, Heilweil M, Janov AJ, et al. Improved survival in epidermoid carcinoma of the anus in association with pre-operative multi-disciplinary therapy. Arch Surg 1986;121:1386–1390.

143. Michaelson RA, Magill GB, Quan SHQ, et al. Pre-operative chemotherapy and radiation therapy in the management of anal epidermoid carcinoma. Cancer 1983;51:390–395.

144. Nigro ND. Multi-disciplinary management of cancer of the anus. World J Surg 1987;11:446–451.

145. John MJ, Flam M, Lovalvo L, et al. Feasibility of non-surgical definitive management of anal canal carcinoma. Int J Radiat Oncol Biol Phys 1987;13:299–303.

146. Knecht BH. Combined chemotherapy and radiotherapy for carcinomas of the anus. Am J Surg 1990;159:518–521.

147. Salmon RJ, Fenton J, Asselain B, et al. Treatment of epidermoid anal canal cancer. Am J Surg 1984;147:43–48.

148. Byfield JE, Calabro-Jones P, Klisak I, et al. Pharmacologic requirements for obtaining sensitization of human tumor cells in vitro to combined 5-fluorouracil or Ftorafur and x rays. Int J Radiat Oncol Biol Phys 1982;8:1923–1933.

149. Weinberg MJ, Rauth AM. 5-fluorouracil infusions and fractionated doses of radiation: Studies with a murine squamous cell carcinoma. Int J Radiat Oncol Biol Phys 1987;13:1691–1699.

150. Rockwell S, Sartorelli AC. Mitomycin C and radiation. In: Hill BT, Bellamy AS, eds. Antitumor drug-radiation interactions. Boca Raton: CRC Press, 1990:126–139.

151. Byfield JE, Barone RM, Sharp TR, et al. Conservative management without alkylating agents of squamous cell anal cancer using cyclical 5-FU alone and x-ray therapy. Cancer Treat Rep 1985;67:709–712.

152. Gerard JP, Romestaing P, Mahe M, et al. Cancer du canal anal: Role de l'association 5-FU/cisplatinum. Lyon Chir 1991;87:74–76.

153. Roca E, DeSimone G, Barugel M, et al. A phase II study of alternating chemoradiotherapy including cisplatin in anal canal carcinoma. Proc Am Soc Clin Oncol 1990;9:128.

154. Brunet R, Becouarn Y, Pigneux J, et al. Cisplatine (P) et fluorouracile (FU) en chimiotherapie neoadjuvante des carcinomes epidermoides du canal anal. Lyon Chir 1991;87:77–78.

155. Brunet R, Sadek H, Vignoud J, et al. Cisplatin (P) and 5-fluorouracil (5-FU) for the neoadjuvant treatment (Tt) of epidermoid anal canal carcinoma (EACC). Proc Am Soc Clin Oncol 1990;9:104.

156. Golden GT, Horsley JS III. Surgical management of epidermoid carcinoma of the anus. Am J Surg 1976;131:275–280.

157. Bond WH. . Proc R Soc Med 1960;53:411–414.

158. Devois A, Decker R. La curiepuncture du cancer de l'anus. Arch Fr Mal Appar Dig Malnutr 1960;49:54s–67s.

159. Keiling R, Grunewald JM, Achille E. Radiotherapie des cancers malpighiens de l'anus. J Radiol Electrol Med Nucl 1973;54:634–635.

160. Eschwege F, Lasser P, Chavy A, et al. Squamous cell carcinoma of the anal canal: Treatment by external beam irradiation. Radiother Oncol 1985;3:145–150.

161. Dubois JB, Garrigues JM, Pujol H. Cancer of the anal canal: Report on the experience of 61 patients. Int J Radiat Oncol Biol Phys 1991;20:575–580.

162. Doggett SW, Green JP, Cantril ST. Efficacy of radiation therapy alone for limited squamous carcinoma of the anal canal. Int J Radiat Oncol Biol Phys 1988;15:1069–1072.

163. Fenton J, Cutuli B, Rousseau J, et al. Anal canal carcinoma: Survival and sphincter preservation after radiotherapy (195 cases). Proceedings of the European Society for Therapeutic Radiology and Oncology [Abstract] 1986;54.

164. Cummings B, Keane T, Thomas G, et al. Results and toxicity of the treatment of anal canal carcinoma by radiation therapy or radiation therapy and chemotherapy. Cancer 1984;54:2062–2068.

165. Chruscov MM, Semakina EP, Raifel BA. Strahlentherapie des rektalen Epidermoidkarzinoms. Radiobiol Radiother (Berlin) 1978;19:683–689.

166. Glimelius B, Pahlman L. Radiation therapy of anal epidermoid carcinoma. Int J Radiat Oncol Biol Phys 1987;13:305–312.

167. Northover JMA. Anal cancer: A changing disease. Br J Hosp Med [Editorial] 1990;44:313.

168. Northover JMA. Personal communication, 1991.

169. Delouche G, Bachelot G, Cohen M, et al. La radiotherapie des cancers malpighiens de l'anus. J Radiol Electrol Med Nucl 1973;54:642–646.

170. Ager P, Samala E, Bosworth J, et al. The conservative management of anorectal cancer by radiotherapy. Am J Surg 1979;137:228–230.

171. Kin NYKNY, Pigneux J, Auvray H, et al. Our experience of conservative treatment of anal canal carcinoma combining external irradiation and interstitial implants: 32 cases treated between 1973 and 1982. Int J Radiat Oncol Biol Phys 1988;14:253–259.

172. Papillon J, Montbarbon JG, Gerard JP, et al. Interstitial curietherapy in the conservative treatment of anal and rectal cancers. Int J Radiat Oncol Biol Phys 1989;17:1161–1169.

173. Martinez A, Edmundson GK, Cox RS, et al. Combination of external beam irradiation and multiple-site perineal applicator (MUPIT) for treatment of locally advanced or recurrent prostatic, anorectal, and gynecologic malignancies. Int J Radiat Oncol Biol Phys 1985;11:391–398.

174. Puthawala AA, Syed N, Gates TC, et al. Definitive treatment of extensive anorectal carcinoma by external and interstitial irradiation. Cancer 1982;50:1746–1750.

175. Papillon J. Effectiveness of combined radio-chemotherapy in the management of epidermoid carcinoma of the anal canal. Int J Radiat Oncol Biol Phys 1990;19:1217–1218.

176. Habr-Gama A, da Silva e Sousa AH Jr, Nadalin W, et al. Epidermoid carcinoma of the anal canal: Results of treatment by combined chemotherapy and radiation therapy. Dis Colon Rectum 1989;32:773–777.

177. Barni S, Frigio F, Lissoni P, et al. Anal squamous cell carcinoma arising on radiodermatitis cured with chemotherapy alone: Case report. Tumori 1987;73:423–424.

178. Pipard G, Peytremann R, Marti MC. Conservative multidisciplinary treatment of locally advanced epidermoid and cloacogenic cancer of the anal canal. Proc Am Soc Clin Oncol [Abstract] 1986;5:268.

179. Stearns MW Jr. Epidermoid carcinoma of the anal region. Surg Gynecol Obstet 1958;106:92–96.

180. Cummings BJ, Thomas GM, Keane TJ, et al. Primary radiation therapy in the treatment of anal canal carcinoma. Dis Colon Rectum 1982;25:778–782.

181. Cummings BJ. Current management of epidermoid carcinoma of the anal canal. Gastroenterol Clin North Am 1987;16:125–142.

182. Shank B. Anal cancer: Primary radiation therapy. Cancer Res Clin Oncol 1990;116:852s.

183. Fisher W, Herbst K, Sims J, et al. Metastatic cloacogenic carcinoma of the anus: Sequential responses to Adriamycin and *cis*-dichlorodiamineplatinum (II). Cancer Treat Rep 1978;62:91–97.

184. Salem P, Habboubi N, Naanasissie E, et al. Effectiveness of cisplatin in the treatment of anal squamous cell carcinoma. Cancer Treat Rep 1985;69:891–893.

185. Livingston R, Bodey G, Gottlieb J, et al. Kinetic scheduling of vincristine and bleomycin in patients with lung cancer and other malignant tumors. Cancer Chemother Rep 1973;57:219–224.

186. Khater R, Frenay M, Bourry J, et al. Cisplatin plus 5-fluorouracil in the treatment of metastatic anal squamous cell carcinoma: A report of two cases. Cancer Treat Rep 1986;70:1345–1346.

187. Ajani J, Carrasco H, Jackson D, et al. Combination of cisplatin plus fluoropyrimidine chemotherapy effective against liver metastases from carcinoma of the anal canal. Am J Med 1989;87:221–224.

188. Mahjoubi M, Sadek H, Francois E, et al. Epidermoid anal canal carcinoma (EACC): Activity of cisplatin (P) and continuous 5-fluorouracil (5FU) in metastatic (M) and/or local recurrent (LR) disease. Proc Am Soc Clin Oncol 1990;9:114.

189. Wilking N, Petrelli N, Herrera L, et al. Phase II study of combination of bleomycin, vincristine and high-dose methotrexate (BOM) with leucovorin rescue in advanced squamous cell carcinoma of the anal canal. Cancer Chemother Pharmacol 1985;15:300–302.

190. Magill GB, Quan S. Salvage chemotherapy of anal epidermoid carcinoma with cisplatin-based protocols. Proc Am Soc Clin Oncol 1989;8:117.

191. Schlienger M. Radiotherapie des cancers epidermoides du canal anal. Ann Gastroenterol Hepatol 1991;27:125–131.

192. Pack GT, Martins FG. Treatment of anorectal malignant melanoma. Dis Colon Rectum 1960;3:15–24.

193. Morson BC, Volkstadt H. Malignant melanoma of the anal canal. J Clin Pathol 1963;16:126–132.

194. Quan SH, Deddish MR. Noncutaneous melanoma. CA 1966;16:111–114.

195. Quan SHQ, White JE, Deddish MR. Malignant melanoma of the anorectum. Dis Colon Rectum 1959;2:275–283.

196. Pack GT, Oropeza R. A comparative study of melanoma and epidermoid carcinoma of the anal canal: A review of 20 melanomas and 29 epidermoid carcinomas. Dis Colon Rectum 1967;10:161–176.

197. Ward MW, Romano G, Nicholls RJ. The surgical treatment of anorectal malignant melanoma. Br J Surg 1986;73:68–69.

198. Chiu YS, Unni KK, Beart RW. Malignant melanoma of the anorectum. Dis Colon Rectum 1980;23:122–124.

199. Siegel B, Cohen D, Jacob ET. Surgical treatment of anorectal melanomas. Am J Surg 1983;146:336–338.

200. Goldman S, Glimelius B, Pahlman L. Anorectal malignant melanoma in Sweden: Report of 49 patients. Dis Colon Rectum 1990;33:874–878.

201. Slingluff CL Jr, Vollmer RT, Seigler HF. Anorectal melanoma: Clinical characteristics and results of surgical management in twenty-four patients. Surgery 1990;107:1–9.

202. Ross M, Pezzi C, Pezzi T, et al. Patterns of failure in anorectal melanoma: A guide to surgical therapy. Arch Surg 1990;125:313–316.

203. Garnick M, Lokich JJ. Primary malignant melanoma of the rectum: Rationale for conservative surgical management. J Surg Oncol 1978;10:529–531.

204. Harwood AR, Cummings BJ. Radiotherapy for mucosal melanomas. Int J Radiat Oncol Biol Phys 1982;8:1121–1126.

205. Cabrera A, Tsukada Y, Pickren JW. Adenocarcinomas of the anal canal and peri-anal tissues. Ann Surg 1966;164:152–156.

206. Parks TG. Mucus-secreting adenocarcinoma of anal gland origin. Br J Surg 1970;57:434–436.

207. Schlienger M, Tiret E, Touboul E, et al. Cancer du canal anal diagnostic et traitement. Encyclopedie Medico Chirurgicale Vol. Pathol Digest (in press).

Cancer: Principles & Practice of Oncology, Fourth Edition,
edited by Vincent T. DeVita, Jr., Samuel Hellman, Steven A. Rosenberg.
J.B. Lippincott Co., Philadelphia © 1993.

W. Marston Linehan
William U. Shipley
David R. Parkinson

CHAPTER **33**

Cancer of the Kidney and Ureter

RENAL CELL CARCINOMA

Each year there are about 25,000 cases of kidney cancer in the United States, resulting in more than 10,600 deaths. This tumor accounts for about 3% of adult malignancies and occurs in a male to female ratio of 2 to 1. It is more common among urban than rural residents. Although most cases of renal cell carcinoma occur in persons aged 50 to 70 years, the disease has been observed in children as young as 6 months. Between 1973 and 1988, there was a modest increase of about 2% per year in the incidence of renal cell carcinoma.[1-8]

Renal cell carcinoma was first reported by Konig in 1826. As early as 1855, Robin concluded that the renal tubular epithelium was the most probable tissue of origin of the cancer, an observation that was confirmed by Waldeyer in 1867. In 1883, Grawitz noted that the fatty content of the cancer cells was similar to that of adrenal cells and he concluded that the tumors arose from adrenal rests within the kidney. He introduced the term stroma lipomatodes aberrata renis for these clear cell tumors. The term hypernephroid tumors was introduced in 1894 by Birch-Hirschfeld. Since that time, the conceptually incorrect term hypernephroma frequently has been applied to renal tumors.[9-12]

Renal cell carcinoma occurs in sporadic and familial forms. Familial renal cell carcinoma is a rare condition that is inherited in an autosomal dominant fashion. There is an increased incidence of renal cell carcinoma with von Hippel-Lindau (VHL) syndrome, and as many as 35% of patients with VHL syndrome develop renal cell carcinoma. In both familial syndromes, the kidney cancer often is bilateral and tends to occur at a younger age.[13-16] An increased incidence of renal cell carcinoma has been observed in patients with autosomal dominant polycystic kidney disease and tuberous sclerosis.[17,18]

ETIOLOGY

Environmental, hormonal, cellular, and genetic factors have been studied as possible causal factors in the development of renal cell carcinoma. Cigarette smoking has been found to be a definite risk factor.[17,19-22] A statistically significant dose-response relation has been observed in men and women for pack-years of cigarette use.[17,19-23] About 30% of renal cell carcinomas in men and 24% in women may be due directly to smoking.[17,19,24] Obesity is associated with an increased risk for development of renal cell carcinoma, particularly in women.[17,19,20] Analgesic abuse, which is known to be associated with renal pelvis cancer, is also associated with an increased incidence of kidney cancer. The increased risk for the development of renal cell carcinoma is observed primarily in patients who abuse phenacetin-containing analgesics and develop analgesic nephropathy.[17,19,20,25]

Environmental and occupational factors have been associated with the development of kidney cancer. There is an increased incidence of renal cell carcinoma among leather tanners, shoe workers, and workers exposed to asbestos.[26-28] Exposure to cadmium is associated with an increased incidence of kidney cancer, particularly in men who smoke.[29] Patients exposed to thorotrast, a 2.5% solution of thorium dioxide used in the 1920s as a contrast medium for renal and hepatic visualization, have an increased incidence of kidney cancer. Thorium dioxide is a radioactive agent that produces α-rays and γ-rays; it is thought that chronic exposure to radiation emitted by this agent is responsible for the development of renal cancer.[30] An association between gasoline exposure and kidney cancer has been observed in animal studies. Although the incidence of renal cell carcinoma increases with exposure to petroleum, tar, and pitch products, studies of oil refinery workers and petroleum products distribution workers do not identify a definite relation between gasoline exposure

1023

and renal cancer. There may be an increased risk for kidney cancer in older workers or in workers exposed to gasoline for prolonged periods.[31,32]

There is an increased incidence of renal cell carcinoma in patients with end-stage renal disease who develop acquired cystic disease of the kidney.[33–35] Acquired cystic disease is a recently described phenomenon in which patients on long-term dialysis for renal failure develop cysts in their native kidneys. Renal cell carcinoma has been found in association with the papillary hyperplasia observed in the cyst epithelium of these kidneys. The risk for developing kidney cancer has been estimated to be more than 30 times greater in dialysis patients with cystic changes in their kidney than in the general population.[36] It is estimated that 35% to 47% of patients on long-term dialysis develop acquired cystic disease, and that about 5.8% of the patients with acquired cystic disease develop renal cell cancer. Kidney cancer can develop at any time in patients with end-stage renal disease and can occur in kidney transplant recipients. Kidney cancer can occur in patients with end-stage renal disease who are undergoing hemodialysis or chronic ambulatory dialysis and has been reported to occur in patients with end-stage renal disease who are not being dialyzed.[33,34] Although many of these cancers are clinically insignificant and are found incidentally at autopsy or after bilateral nephrectomy, some have an aggressive course.[37–39] Careful surveillance of patients with end-stage renal disease with ultrasonography and computed tomography (CT) is recommended.

Growth Factors

Many patients with renal cell carcinoma have evidence of tumor-produced factors that have systemic effects. Pyrexia, cachexia, abnormal liver function, increased alkaline phosphatase levels, hypercalcemia, polycythemia, neuromyopathy, and amyloidosis have been reported in association with renal cell carcinoma.[40–43]

Humoral hypercalcemia of malignancy, frequently observed in patients with advanced renal cell carcinoma, is thought to be caused by a tumor-produced, systemically active bone-resorbing factor. Investigators have demonstrated that kidney cancer produces a factor with a bioactivity like that of parathyroid hormone (PTH).[44–49] A PTH-related protein that has been implicated in malignant hypercalcemia has been cloned from a human lung cancer cell line and is expressed in mammalian cells.[50] Thiede and colleagues demonstrated that human renal carcinoma expresses two messages encoding a PTH-like peptide with considerable similarity to PTH and to peptides isolated from human breast and lung carcinoma.[44] Whether the PTH-like factor induces paracrine and endocrine effects such as bone resorption or hypercalcemia of malignancy in patients with renal cell carcinoma is under study.

Molecular Genetics: Tumor Suppressor Genes in Familial and Sporadic Renal Cell Carcinoma

The first information with regard to the chromosomal location of the kidney cancer gene became available in 1979 when Cohen and colleagues described a pedigree with familial renal cell carcinoma in which the pattern of inheritance was consistent with an autosomal dominant gene.[51] Of particular interest was the association of renal cell carcinoma with a specific karyotypic abnormality, namely a balanced reciprocal translocation between the short arm of chromosome 3 and the long arm of chromosome 8. This abnormality was present in constitutional tissue and, therefore, presumably in tumor tissue of affected family members. All members of the family who developed renal cell carcinoma had a 3;8 translocation; no family member without a 3;8 translocation developed renal cell carcinoma. A second pedigree with renal cell carcinoma was described in 1982 by Pathak and colleagues.[52] In the propositus, the major karyotypic abnormality was a chromosome 3 to chromosome 11 translocation. This pedigree differed from the one described by Cohen and colleagues in that the karyotypic abnormality was limited to the tumor. Recently, chromosomal analysis performed on tumor cells from a patient with another familial form of kidney cancer associated with VHL disease revealed a proximal deletion in the short arm of chromosome 3 in the 3p14 region.[53]

Sporadic Kidney Cancer

The studies of chromosomal abnormalities in familial renal cell carcinoma focused attention on the possible role of alterations in the short arm of chromosome 3 in the genesis of nonfamilial renal cell carcinoma. Chromosomal analysis in four studies suggested that a structural change in chromosome 3 is linked to sporadic and hereditary renal cell carcinoma.[54–57] This information led to the use of restriction length fragment polymorphism (RFLP) analysis of chromosome 3 in constitutional and tumor tissue in patients with sporadic renal cell carcinoma.[58] The technique of RFLP analysis for detection of DNA sequence deletions in tumors described by Cavenee and colleagues in 1983 is significantly more sensitive than karyotype analysis for detecting DNA sequence deletions.[59] RFLP analysis has been used to detect DNA sequence deletions in human tumors such as Wilms' tumor,[60,61] retinoblastoma,[62–64] bladder cancer,[65,66] lung carcinoma,[67–69] and colorectal carcinoma.[70,71] In the initial study performed to use RFLP analysis to localize the kidney cancer disease gene, Zbar and colleagues evaluated normal and tumor tissue from 18 patients with renal cell carcinoma using three recombinant probes that have been mapped to the short arm of chromosome 3.[58] These investigators found evidence for a DNA sequence deletion (Fig. 33–1) in 11 of 11 evaluable patients with renal cell carcinoma. In a study performed to define more precisely the location of the renal cell carcinoma gene and to differentiate molecular changes occurring in early stages of renal neoplasia compared with those occurring later in malignant progression, Anglard and colleagues analyzed DNA from normal and tumor tissue from 60 patients with renal cell carcinoma for loss of alleles at different chromosomal loci.[72] In tumor tissue from 51 of 58 evaluable patients, these investigators determined loss of heterozygosity at one or more of 10 loci tested on the short arm of chromosome 3. Genotypic analysis identified the distal portion of 3p,3p21–26, as the region of the disease gene.[72–79] These investigators and others have reported abnormalities at loci of other tumor suppressor genes on chromosome 13, 11, and 17 in renal cell carcinoma.[72,77,80,81] The frequency of loss of 3p sequences in renal cell carcinoma is greater than that observed at other chromosomal loci in bladder carcinoma (42%), Wilms' tumor (55%), and other tumors and suggests that loss of heterozy-

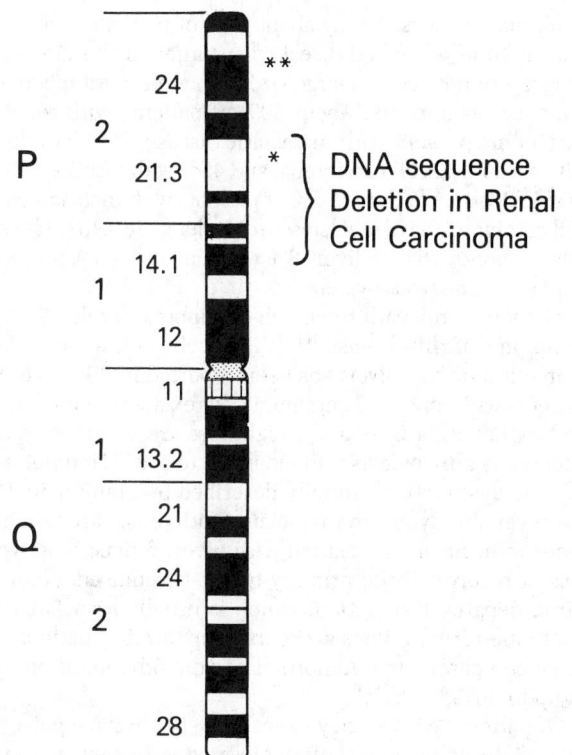

P
2
24
21.3
1
14.1
12
11
Q
1
13.2
1
21
24
2
28

** *
} DNA sequence Deletion in Renal Cell Carcinoma

FIGURE 33–1. A diagram of chromosome 3 shows the area of interstitial deletion in renal cell carcinoma at 3p14-26 locus. The asterisk denotes the site of the von Hippel-Lindau disease (VHL) gene locus.[92,347]

gosity in this region is a nonrandom alteration and that a functioning gene located on 3p may be involved in the origin or evolution of renal cell carcinoma.[58,71,82] Abnormalities at other tumor suppressor gene loci, such as retinoblastoma or p53, are thought to be involved in progression of this neoplasm.

Many of the biologic and genetic alterations in renal cell carcinoma are similar to those in retinoblastoma. Both neoplasms exist in hereditary and sporadic forms, and the hereditary form is associated with an earlier age at onset than is the sporadic form. The conceptual basis that seems to fit the genetic data on retinoblastoma is consistent with the molecular genetic data on renal cell carcinoma. The two-mutation theory of Knudson postulates that at least two mutations are necessary for the development of cancer.[83,84] The data generated by chromosomal and RFLP analysis of renal cell carcinoma suggest that a somatic mutation is a chromosome event that may involve the loss of the wild-type allele of a particular gene. In Wilms' tumor, which is associated with a DNA sequence deletion in the 13p region of chromosome 11, the introduction of a normal human chromosome 11 suppresses the tumorigenicity of Wilms' tumor cell lines.[85] Similarly, the introduction of a normal chromosome 3 back into a renal cell carcinoma cell line has been shown to suppress tumorigenicity, providing further support for the thesis that the sporadic kidney cancer disease gene is on chromosome 3.[86,87]

Familial Kidney Cancer

To identify the kidney cancer genes, investigators have initiated studies to localize the disease gene associated with a familial form of kidney cancer associated with VHL disease. VHL, an autosomal dominant disorder, is associated with the occurrence of tumors in organs such as the kidneys. Renal cell carcinoma is reported to occur in 28% to 45% of individuals affected with VHL.[88,89] Kidney involvement in patients with VHL is characterized by the occurrence of multiple, bilateral renal tumors and cysts.[88] Like familial (*i.e.*, non-VHL-associated) renal cell carcinoma, kidney tumors in VHL patients tend to be multifocal, bilateral, and occur at a younger age than those in patients with sporadic renal cell carcinoma. To determine whether there were abnormalities in kidney tumors from patients with this familial form of kidney cancer, Tory and colleagues evaluated loss of chromosome 3p alleles in tumors from patients with VHL disease.[90] These studies revealed a loss of alleles from chromosome 3p in 11 renal cell carcinomas that were tested. In each instance it was the wild-type allele from the nonaffected parent that was deleted.[90] These data suggested that an inherited disease gene on chromosome 3 was involved in the genesis of kidney cancer in VHL patients. To localize more precisely the *VHL* kidney cancer disease gene, linkage analysis has been performed in *VHL* kindreds. Seizinger and colleagues demonstrated linkage between the *VHL* gene and c-*RAF1*, a protooncogene that maps to 3p25.[91] Subsequently, Hosoe and colleagues used multipoint linkage analysis to determine that the location of VHL was in the interval between *RAF1* and an anonymous marker, D3S18, located telomeric to c-*RAF1* at 3p26.[92]

To determine if DNA-polymorphism analysis could be used to identify disease gene carriers for this familial form of kidney cancer, Glenn and colleagues conducted a prospective comparison of the results of DNA analysis with a comprehensive clinical screening examination in 16 families with VHL disease. After blood was collected from 182 members of these 16 kindred, 48 asymptomatic individuals who were at risk were examined for occult disease and tested by DNA polymorphism analysis. DNA polymorphism analysis predicted disease gene carrier status in 42 of 43 (98%) evaluable individuals.[93] This technique enables clinicians to focus their attention on those affected individuals who require periodic medical examination and it may help to alleviate the morbidity associated with this familial cancer syndrome.[93]

PATHOLOGY

For many years, renal cell carcinoma was thought to originate in adrenal rests within the kidney. However, immunohistologic and ultrastructural analysis has established that the proximal renal tubular epithelium is the true tissue of origin.[8,94] Renal cell tumors tend to be spheric, but may vary widely in size. The average diameter is about 7 cm, but renal tumors can often grow to fill the entire retroperitoneum. Previously, renal lesions 2 cm or less in diameter were considered to be renal adenomas, and lesions 2 cm or more in diameter were considered to be carcinomas. The distinction between benign and malignant tumors is no longer made on the basis of size but on the basis of classic histologic criteria.[94,95] Although renal cell carcinoma tends to arise in the cortex of the kidney, it can originate in the interior of the kidney. There is often a pseudocapsule formed around the tumor by compression of surrounding tissue. Hemorrhage and necrosis may be present, and frequently large areas of sclerosis and fibrosis are found within the tumor. Calcification and single or multiple fluid-filled cysts may be seen within the tumor. Sporadic renal cell carcinoma appears in either kidney with equal frequency; it is most often solitary and unilateral.

Renal cell carcinoma can occur in different cellular types: clear cell, granular cell, and spindle or sarcomatoid variant. Clear cell carcinomas contain lightly staining cells with vacuolated cytoplasm containing cholesterol-like substances, neutral lipids, phospholipids, and glycogen.[3,96] Granular cell carcinomas contain cells that have a ground-glass-appearing, eosinophilic-staining cytoplasm with abundant mitochondria. The large nuclei of granular cells stain darker than the nuclei of clear cells. In sarcomatoid renal cell carcinoma, there are spindle-type cells that may resemble fibroblasts, rhabdomyoblasts, lipoblasts, or pleomorphic mesenchymal cells.[3,96,97] Few tumors are purely clear or granular cell type; most are mixtures of clear and granular cells. Depending on the series, 1% to 6% of renal cell carcinomas are sarcomatoid variant.[98,99]

Some studies suggest that there is slightly better prognosis with clear cell variant than with granular or mixed renal cell carcinomas.[100] The sarcomatoid variant is associated with a significantly poorer prognosis than are carcinomas of the clear, granular, or mixed cell type.[99,101–103] Sella and colleagues recently reported a median survival of only 6.6 months in 44 patients with sarcomatoid-type renal cell carcinoma versus a 19.0-month median survival in 814 patients with nonsarcomatous renal cell carcinoma.[104] Although infrequently used in renal cell carcinoma, tumor grading may correlate with survival, particularly in patients with nonmetastatic cancer.[100,101,105]

CLINICAL PRESENTATION

Renal cell carcinoma may remain clinically occult for most of its course. The classic presentation of pain, hematuria, and flank mass occurs in only about 19% of patients and often is indicative of advanced disease.[3] A tumor in the kidney can progress unnoticed to a large size in the retroperitoneum until a metastasis appears. About 30% of patients with renal cell carcinoma present with metastatic disease, 25% with locally advanced renal cell carcinoma, and 45% with localized disease (Table 33–1).[8,106] Some 75% of patients with metastatic renal cell carcinoma have metastases to the lung, 36% to soft tissues, 20% to bone, 18% to liver, 8% to cutaneous sites, and 8% to the central nervous system.[107]

Many patients with renal cell carcinoma develop systemic symptoms of this disease.[108–111] Hypochromic anemia due to hematuria or hemolysis has been reported in 29% to 88% of patients with renal cell carcinoma. Pyrexia is observed in 20% and cachexia, fatigue, and weight loss are observed in 33%. Secondary amyloidosis is found in 3% to 5%.[40] Nonmetastatic hepatic dysfunction, initially described by Stauffer in 1961, is a reversible syndrome associated with renal carcinoma that tends to occur in association with fever, fatigue, and weight loss. It resolves if the primary tumor is removed. Nonmetastatic hepatic dysfunction, which is usually associated with poor long-term prognosis, occurs in up to 7% of patients with renal cell carcinoma. Abnormal hepatic function is observed in up to 40%.[102,112–114]

Of patients with kidney cancer, 1% to 5% have polycythemia.[115] Renin levels are often elevated in patients with renal cell carcinoma, but tend to return to normal after the kidney is removed. Whether the tumor itself produces renin or induces renin production by compression of adjacent tissue is unclear. Immunocytochemical studies suggest that renal cell carcinoma may produce renin, which, however, may be biologically inactive.[111,116,117] A recent report by Da Silva and colleagues demonstrated a strong erythropoietin signal by Northern analysis of tumor tissue from three patients with kidney cancer, showing that these malignant cells were able

TABLE 33–1. Presenting Symptoms, Laboratory Abnormality, or Abnormality on Physical Examination and Their Relation to Survival Rate in 309 Consecutive Patients Undergoing Nephrectomy for Renal Cell Carcinoma

Presenting Symptom, Abnormal Laboratory Findings, or Abnormality on Physical Examination	No. of Patients (% of Total)	No. of Patients Surviving 5 Years
Classic triad (gross hematuria, abnormal mass, pain)	29 (9)	9/29 (31)
Hematuria	183 (59)	74/183 (40)
Pain	127 (41)	56/127 (44)
Abdominal mass	139 (45)	49/139 (35)
Fever	21 (7)	8/21 (38)
Weight loss	85 (28)	29/85 (39)
Anemia	64 (21)	24/64 (38)
Erythrocytosis	10 (3)	4/10 (40)
Hypercalcemia	11 (3)	4/11 (35)
Acute varicocele	7 (2)	3/7 (43)
Tumor calcification on x-ray film	39 (13)	18/39 (46)
Symptoms of metastases	31 (10)	1/31 (3)
Cancer, incidental finding	20 (7)	13/20 (65)

(Modified from Skinner DG, Colvin RB, Vermillion CD, et al. Diagnosis and management of renal cell carcinoma: A clinical and pathologic study of 309 cases. Cancer 1971;28:1165–1177)

to produce erythropoietin constitutively.[115] Plasma fibrinogen levels are elevated in patients with renal cell carcinoma and may correlate with tumor stage, disease activity, and response to therapy.[118] Acquired dysfibrinogenemia has been associated with renal cell carcinoma and can be a sensitive plasma marker for the disease and for tumor progression.[119]

RADIOGRAPHIC EVALUATION

It is often difficult to determine whether a space-occupying renal mass lesion is benign or malignant. In a series of 940 asymptomatic space-occupying renal mass lesions reported by Lang, 515 (55%) were benign renal cysts, and only 52 (5.5%) were malignant neoplasms (Table 33–2).[120] Diagnostic modalities used to evaluate and stage renal mass lesions include excretory urography, CT, arteriography, venography, ultrasound, and magnetic resonance imaging (MRI). Excretory urography commonly is used in the initial evaluation of renal mass lesions, but because it is neither sensitive nor specific in renal cell carcinoma, a small- to medium-sized tumor may be present if the excretory urogram appears normal. Excretory urography provides important information about the location and function of the contralateral kidney, and this is particularly useful if surgery is being considered.

Ultrasound examination provides excellent staging and diagnostic information and can provide accurate anatomic detail of extrarenal extension of tumor, adrenal involvement, involvement of lymph nodes, and infiltration of adjacent viscera.[3,121–123] It can aid in the detection and delineation of renal vein or inferior vena caval involvement. Ultrasound examination is used frequently in the evaluation of renal cystic lesions that are detected on excretory urography or CT. If a cystic renal mass lesion appears potentially malignant on excretory urography, ultrasound, or CT, further evaluation by percutaneous cyst puncture under ultrasound or CT guidance may be performed. This procedure has two components: eval-

uation of cyst fluid and radiographic examination of the interior of the cyst. Cyst fluid aspirate is assessed for color, turbidity, and the presence of blood; fat, protein, lactic acid dehydrogenase (LDH), and glucose content are measured. If the cyst is benign, there is typically a clear, straw-colored fluid that is low in fat, protein, and LDH content. If a cystic or necrotic tumor is aspirated, the fluid may be bloody and may have a high fat, protein, or LDH content. After the fluid is removed, the cyst is filled with contrast medium and air and imaged radiographically. A benign cyst should appear as a homogenous sphere with a regular border, whereas a tumor may show up as a nodule or mass protruding into the cyst.[121] The combination of ultrasound and cyst puncture enables the clinician to make the correct diagnosis in most suspicious renal mass lesions.[3]

Renal arteriography historically has been a standard part of the evaluation of patients with a suspicious renal mass (Fig. 33–2). In a renal cell carcinoma, the arteriogram often shows neovascularity, arteriovenous fistulas, pooling of contrast medium, and accentuation of capsular vessels. Epinephrine may be used as an aid in the diagnosis of an equivocal renal mass lesion. If epinephrine is infused into a normal kidney during arteriography, the renal vessels constrict; the vessels in a renal cell carcinoma do not constrict due to lack of musculature in the tumor vessels.[3] A renal arteriogram is particularly useful in evaluating an indeterminant small renal mass lesion and as an aid to the surgeon in defining the vasculature during the surgical removal of a large tumor.[124,125] Although renal arteriography can be performed with minimal risk, false aneurysms, arterial emboli, hemorrhage, and decreased renal function secondary to contrast agent injection have been reported.[3] Digital subtraction arteriography can define the tumor vasculature without the morbidity associated with standard arteriography and can demonstrate the main renal arterial anatomy adequately in more than 80% of cases. The combination of CT and digital subtraction angiography yields satisfaction of CT and digital subtraction angiography yields satisfactory diagnostic and anatomic detail in most cases of renal cell carcinoma.[126]

CT is a useful imaging technique for renal cell carcinoma (Fig. 33–3).[7,123,124,127–132] In a study in which CT results were correlated with pathologic findings in 111 patients, perirenal extension was correctly identified in 79% of cases, lymph node involvement in 87%, renal vein involvement in 91%, and local advancement into adjacent viscera in 96%.[133]

Although arteriography and CT are equivalent in depicting renal vein involvement, CT is better for demonstrating local nodal involvement.[127] The use of contrast agent enhancement has greatly increased the sensitivity of CT for abnormal renal mass lesions.[130,131] Contrast-enhanced CT allows the clinician to detect small changes in the density of a renal lesion that might indicate the presence of an early neoplastic lesion. In a comparison study, dynamic CT was superior to standard CT arteriography, ultrasonography, and radionuclide scanning. Dynamic CT correctly demonstrated tumor involvement of the kidney, involvement of the renal fascia, or extension into adjacent organs in all the 22 patients studied.[123]

Inferior venacavography is performed if there is a large renal tumor or if there is uncertainty about tumor involvement of the vena cava. Ultrasound, CT, and MRI can provide information about tumor involvement of the vena cava (Fig.

TABLE 33–2. Underlying Pathologic Conditions in 940 Asymptomatic Space-Occupying Lesions of the Kidney

Type of Lesion	No. of Lesions	Percentage of Lesions
Cystic lesions		58
Benign cysts	515	
Benign hemorrhagic cysts	4	
Hydronephrosis	8	
Cystic dysplastic kidney	3	
Polycystic kidney	17	
Malignant neoplasms		5.5
Hypernephromas	21	
Other malignant neoplasms	31	
Benign neoplasms	40	4.2
Inflammatory lesions (pyelonephritis, abscess)	213	23
Intrarenal hematoma	7	0.7
Pseudotumors	81	8.6

(Modified from Lang EK. Diagnosis of renal and parenchymal tumors. In: Skinner DG, deKernion JB, eds. Genitourinary cancer. Philadelphia: WB Saunders, 1978:42)

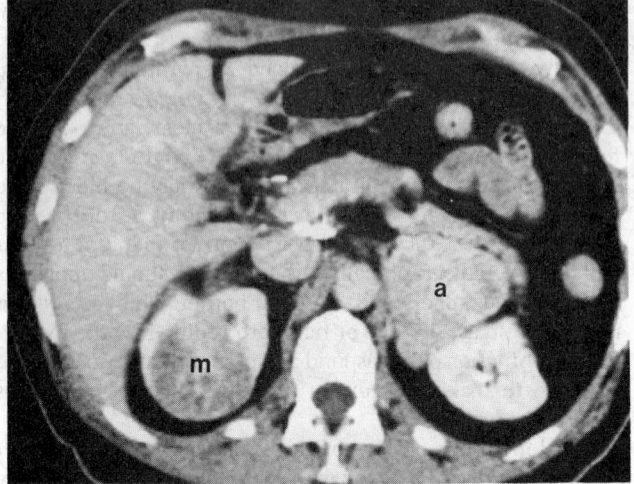

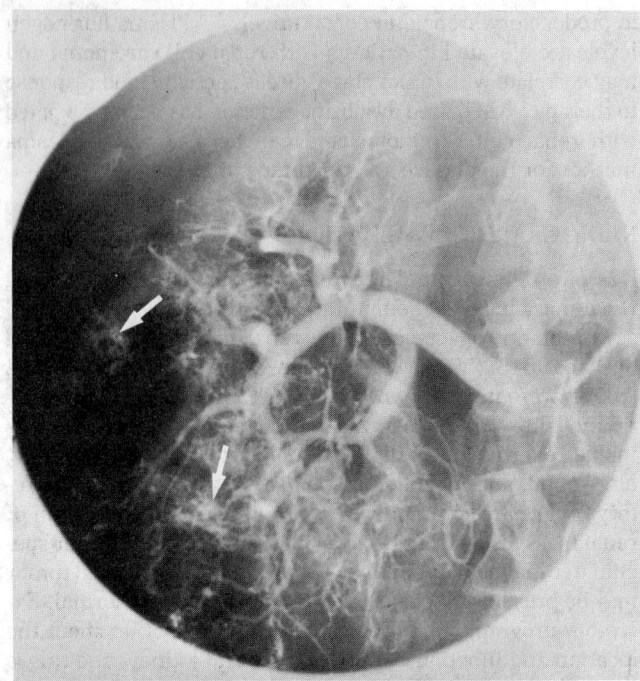

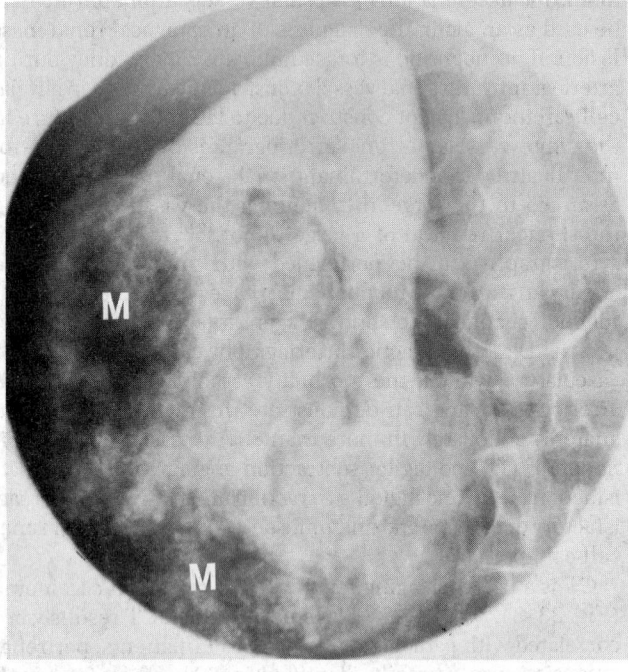

FIGURE 33–2.   Angiogram of a renal cell carcinoma. **(A)** CT demonstrates a right renal carcinoma (m) with a large contralateral adrenal metastasis (a). **(B)** Early phase of arteriogram demonstrates vascular changes indicative of a malignancy with puddling and tortuosity (*arrows*). **(C)** Late phase of the arteriogram demonstrates that the tumor (M) is relatively avascular despite its early appearance.

33–4)[134]; however, the inferior venacavogram is the most reliable means of accurately determining the precise extent of vena caval involvement by tumor. This information is important to the surgeon in planning the vascular aspect of the operative procedure. When Horan and colleagues prospectively compared the accuracy of venacavography and MRI, they found that venacavography and MRI offer equal diagnostic accuracy in the identification of venous extension of kidney cancer and that the combination of both tests results in higher diagnostic yield than use of either test alone.[135] MRI is useful for staging renal cell carcinoma.[136] MRI can produce a unique three-dimensional picture of the tumor which, in a large tumor, may be an invaluable aid to the surgeon in planning the operative approach. In patients with tumor involving the in-

ferior vena cava, transesophageal echocardiography has been shown to be an accurate diagnostic technique for tumor imaging to document the extent of involvement of the vena cava.[137]

There is no single imaging technique that is best for all patients with renal cell carcinoma. Depending on the size of the primary tumor and the extent of extrarenal disease, excretory urography, CT, ultrasound, arteriography, venography, and MRI each can provide unique information in an individual case. Because CT, MRI, and ultrasound are outpatient procedures and are less invasive than arteriography, arteriography is used less frequently. Multiple imaging modalities provide the most complete information, particularly if surgical removal of a large tumor is being considered.

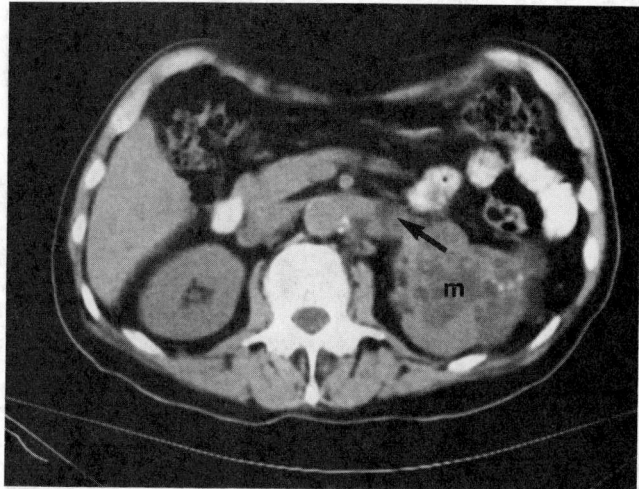

A

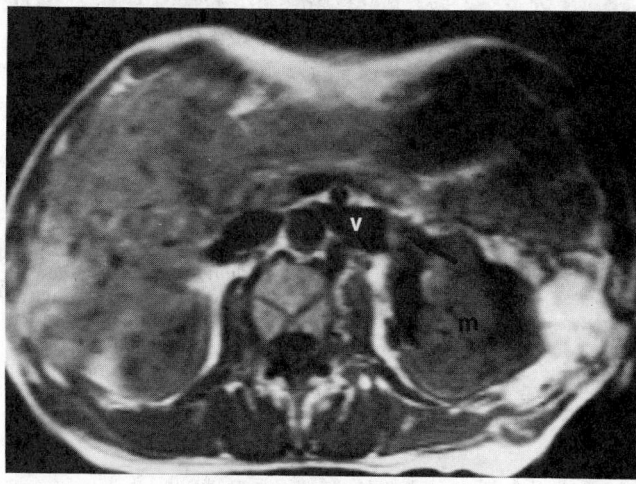

B

FIGURE 33–3.   Renal vein invasion by a renal carcinoma as shown by CT and MRI. **(A)** Nonenhanced CT shows large left renal mass with calcification (m) invading the left renal vein (*arrow*). **(B)** T1-weighted MRI demonstrates tumor (m) and vascular invasion (*arrow*). Flowing blood (v) in the left renal vein is black on this scan.

STAGING AND PROGNOSIS

The staging system used by most physicians in the United States is the Robson modification of the system of Flocks and Kadesky (Table 33–3).[138] In the Robson classification, stage I renal cell carcinoma is confined to the kidney. Stage II carcinoma extends through the renal capsule but is confined to Gerota's fascia, and stage III carcinoma involves the renal vein or inferior vena cava (stage IIIA) or the local hilar lymph nodes (stage IIIB). In stage IV renal cell carcinoma, the tumor has spread to local, adjacent organs (other than the adrenal gland) or to distant sites. The Robson staging system is uncomplicated and widely used. A disadvantage of this system is that it combines stages that may have significantly different survival prognoses. In this classification system, renal inferior vena caval involvement (stage IIIA) is considered the same stage as local lymph node metastasis (stage IIIB). Although

patients with stage IIIB renal cell carcinoma have a greatly decreased survival,[139,140] the prognosis for patients with stage IIIA renal cell carcinoma is not markedly different from that for patients with stage I or stage II renal cell carcinoma.[141] Patients who have disease that involves the inferior vena cava often have locally advanced or micrometastatic disease.[142-144] However, patients who are found to have no evidence of metastatic disease and who undergo a complete surgical excision have a reasonable chance for 5-year survival.

The TNM classification is a more accurate method for classifying extent of tumor involvement. In the TNM classification, T1 denotes a small tumor confined to the kidney, T2 denotes a large tumor that deforms the kidney or collecting system but is still confined to the kidney, T3 denotes tumor with perinephric or hilar extension, and T4 denotes tumor that has extended to neighboring organs (Table 33–4). N+ indicates local nodal involvement, and in M+ disease there are metastases.

The 5-year survival initially reported by Robson and colleagues in 1969 was 66% for stage I renal cell carcinoma, 64% for stage II, 42% for stage III, and only 11% for stage IV.[138] These survival statistics remained essentially the same for a number of years (Table 33–5).[100,112] Since then, it has been noted that whereas renal vein involvement does not have a markedly negative effect on prognosis, the 5-year survival for patients with stage IIIB renal cell carcinoma is only 18%.[8,100,101,112,145] Better survival is reported for patients with tumor confined to the kidney—about 95% 5-year survival for T1 renal cell carcinoma and 92% 5-year survival for T2 disease.[101,129] In patients with N0M0 tumors, studies have detected no markedly significant difference in survival in relation to the T stage of the disease.[146] The 5-year survival for patients with metastatic renal cell carcinoma continues to be low, ranging from no survival to 20%.[8,101,107,146,147] With the increased use of CT and ultrasonography, the rate of incidentally found carcinomas of the kidney has increased. The prognosis for patients whose tumor was diagnosed incidentally is more favorable than that of those who present with symptoms, because the former group consists of patients with smaller tumors that tend to be confined to the kidney.[148] Patients with metastatic renal cell carcinoma who present with humoral hypercalcemia of malignancy have a poor prognosis. Fahn and colleagues reported the median survival of patients with stage IV kidney cancer to be fewer than 50 days.[149]

Tumor DNA ploidy has been analyzed by flow cytometry in an effort to determine whether this technique will provide useful prognostic information about survival and, potentially, response to therapy. Ljungberg and colleagues recently reported that although nuclear grade, tumor cell type, and tumor size did not correlate with survival, there was a significant difference in survival between patients with diploid versus nondiploid kidney tumors.[150] In a study of DNA ploidy from primary renal cell carcinoma specimens from 106 patients, Currin and colleagues found a significant difference in the incidence of disease progression in patients with diploid tumors (13%) versus those with aneuploid tumors (35%).[151] If controlled for TNM stage, there was no clear survival advantage for evaluable patients with diploid versus aneuploid tumors.[151] Most studies show increased survival in patients diagnosed with metastatic disease under the following conditions: (1) there is a long disease-free interval between

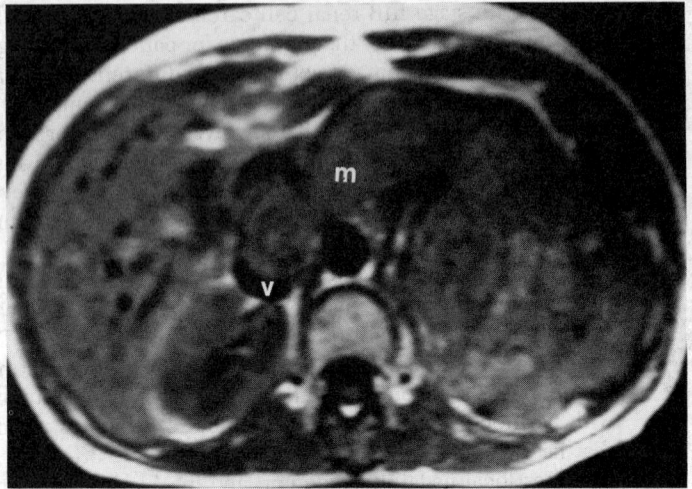

A

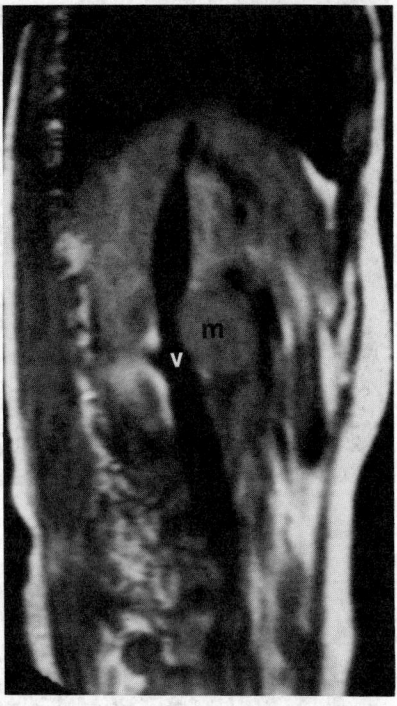

B

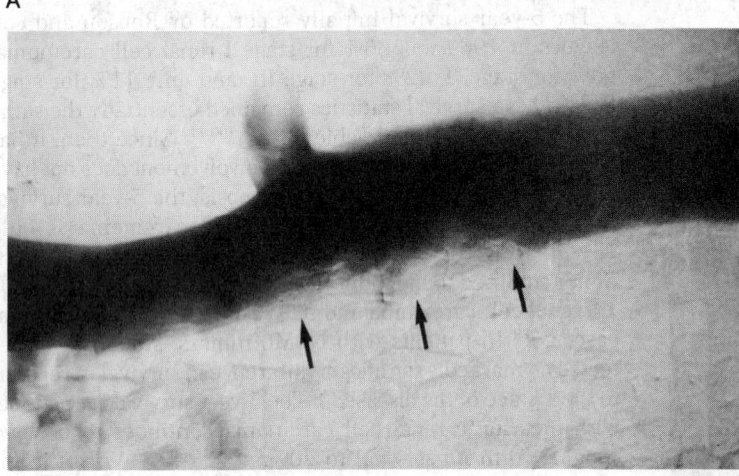

C

FIGURE 33–4. Invasion of inferior vena cava (IVC) by renal carcinoma demonstrated by MRI and venography. **(A)** Axial T₁-weighted image demonstrates a large left renal carcinoma with extension into the left renal vein (m) with protrusion into the IVC (v). **(B)** Sagittal T₁-weighted image shows the relation of the tumor thrombus (m) to the IVC (v) in the lateral projection. **(C)** An anteroposterior image of the inferior venacavagram demonstrates tumor in the medial aspect of the IVC.

initial nephrectomy and the appearance of metastases; (2) only pulmonary metastases are present; (3) there is a good performance status; and (4) the primary tumor has been removed.[107]

SURGICAL TREATMENT

Surgery is the only known effective therapy for localized renal cell carcinoma. The first nephrectomy was performed by Eratus B. Walcott in Milwaukee on June 4, 1861, on a 58-year-old man with a kidney tumor who died 15 days after surgery.[152] Professor Gustave Simon, after completing experimental nephrectomies on dogs, undertook the first deliberate, planned, and successful nephrectomy in Heidelberg on August 2, 1869, in a patient with a persistent ureteral fistula. The first successful nephrectomy in a patient with kidney cancer was performed in 1883 by Grawitz.[152] The standard procedure for treatment of localized renal cell carcinoma is radical nephrectomy (Fig. 33–5).[153] Radical nephrectomy includes complete removal of Gerota's fascia and its contents, including the kidney and the adrenal gland, and provides a better surgical margin than simple removal of the kidney.[154]

There are different surgical approaches to removal of a kidney cancer. Common approaches are the anterior transperi-

toneal approach, the flank approach, and the thoracoabdominal approach. The choice of surgical approach depends on the location and size of the tumor and the body habitus of the patient. The type of incision is chosen to ensure that the tumor may be removed safely. A flank incision, with or without removal of a portion of the 10th or 11th rib, is often used for

TABLE 33–3. Comparison of the Two Classification Systems for Staging of Renal Cell Carcinoma

	TNM (1978)	Robson
Small tumor, no enlargement of kidney	T1	A
Large tumor, cortex not broken	T2	A
Perinephric or hilar extension	T3	B
Extension to neighboring organs	T4	D
Nodal invasion	N+	C
Renal vein involved	V1	C
Vena cava involved	V2	C
Distant metastases	M+	D

(Selli C, Hinshaw WM, Woodard BH, Paulson DF. Stratification of risk factors in renal cell carcinoma. Cancer 1983;52:899)

TABLE 33–4. TNM Classification for Tumors
of the Kidney

Primary Tumor (T)

TX	Minimum requirements cannot be met
T0	No evidence of primary tumor
T1	Small tumor, minimal renal and caliceal distortion of deformity; circumscribed neovasculature surrounded by normal parenchyma
T2	Large tumor with deformity or enlargement of kidney or collecting system
T3A	Tumor involving perinephric tissues
T3B	Tumor involved renal vein
T3C	Tumor involving renal vein and infradiaphragmatic vena cava

Note: Under T3 tumor may extend into perinephric tissues, into renal vein, and into vena cava as shown on cavography. In these instances, the T classification may be shown as T3A, B, and C, or some appropriate combination, depending on extension, (*e.g.,* T3A–B is tumor in perinephric fat and extending into renal vein).

T4A	Tumor invasion of neighboring structures (*e.g.,* muscle, bowel)
T4B	Tumor involving supradiaphragmatic vena cava

Nodal Involvement (N)

The regional lymph nodes are the paraaortic and paracaval nodes. The juxtaregional lymph nodes are the pelvic nodes and the mediastinal nodes.

TX	Minimum requirements cannot be met
N0	No evidence of involvement of regional nodes
N1	Single, homolateral regional nodal involvement
N2	Involvement of multiple regional or contralateral or bilateral nodes
N3	Fixed regional nodes (assessable only at surgical exploration)
N4	Involvement of juxtaregional nodes

Note: If lymphography is course of staging, add *1* between *N* and designator number; if histologic proof is provided, + if positive, and − if negative. Thus, *N1*+ indicates multiple positive nodes seen on lymphography and proved at operation by biopsy.

Distant Metastasis (M)

MX	Not assessed
M0	No (known) distant metastasis
M1	Specify

Specify sites according to the following notations: Pulmonary, PUL; osseous, OSS; hepatic, HEP; brain, BRA; lymph nodes, LYM; bone marrow, MAR; pleura, PLE; skin, SKI; eye, EYE; other, OTH.

Note. Add "+" to the abbreviated notation to indicate that the pathology (p) is proved.

small tumors without venous involvement. A subcostal transabdominal incision may be used if there is a large tumor in the middle or lower aspect of the kidney or if vascular involvement is anticipated and access to the major vessels is essential. A thoracoabdominal incision often is required if there is a large middle or upper pole tumor. In a thoracoabdominal incision, a rib is removed, the thoracic cavity is opened, and the diaphragm is incised. The incision is then carried down transabdominally to allow maximal exposure of the upper abdominal region and the great vessels. In removal of a right-sided tumor, the hepatic flexure of the colon is mobilized toward the midline away from the kidney and duodenum. The duodenum is dissected up anteriorly and medially to the great vessels, and the renal artery and vein are iden-

tified. The renal vessels are divided and ligated early in the surgical procedure to decrease the vascularity of the tumor so that it may be removed with a minimum of blood loss. After ligation of the vessels, Gerota's fascia is incised away from the posterior abdominal wall, diaphragm, and liver (pancreas and spleen on a left-sided tumor; Fig. 33–6). Once Gerota's fascia and its contents have been dissected away from the surrounding structures and the vasculature has been ligated with nonabsorbable suture, the specimen can be lifted out of the retroperitoneum. If there is tumor in the renal vein, the renal vein can be ligated distal to the tumor thrombus. If there is tumor extension into the vena cava, the vena cava may need to be partially resected. If the tumor has grown into the side wall of the vena cava or if the vena caval involvement is too extensive for a simple partial wall resection, a portion of the vena cava itself may be resected. If the tumor is in the right kidney, the adjacent vena cava often can be resected safely.[142,144,155] If the tumors in the left kidney and the adjacent vena cava are resected, vascular reconstruction of the right renal vein may be needed to establish adequate venous drainage.[142,143,145,156] If the suprahepatic caval extension of a renal tumor thrombus extends up to the right atrium, cardiopulmonary bypass may be required for tumor removal.[143,157–160]

Regional lymphadenectomy often is performed at the time of radical nephrectomy, although its role in prolonging survival has not been demonstrated. In a regional lymphadenectomy, ipsilateral nodal tissue from the diaphragm to the bifurcation of the aorta and nodal tissue in the interaortacaval region at the hilum of the kidney is removed. Proponents of regional lymphadenectomy point out that 5-year survival in patients with nodal involvement is decreased greatly, and there is no known effective therapy for metastatic renal cell carcinoma. If local nodes were the first site of metastasis, resection of microscopic disease might be beneficial. Long-term survival in patients with nodal involvement who underwent lymphadenectomy has been reported. The ultimate role of regional lymphadenectomy remains to be determined in further randomized trials.[100,138–140,161–163]

Bilateral Renal Cell Carcinoma or Tumors in Solitary Kidneys

The treatment of patients with bilateral renal cell carcinoma or renal cell carcinoma in a solitary kidney is challenging. Patients with tumor in a solitary kidney may be treated by partial nephrectomy or nephrectomy followed by dialysis or transplantation or both.[164–172] A 5-year survival of 60% has been reported in patients with bilateral renal cell carcinoma or tumor in a solitary kidney treated by partial nephrectomy.[173] Some surgeons advocate surgical enucleation of a tumor in a patient with a solitary kidney. In one series, patients with bilateral renal cell carcinoma or tumor in a solitary kidney treated with enucleation had a 90% 3-year survival. There was excellent renal function in all patients: none required dialysis.[174] Others advocate caution in using surgical enucleation and favor partial nephrectomy instead. Marshall and colleagues evaluated standard nephrectomy specimens that were enucleated ex vivo and found positive margins, satellite tumor nodules, and occult metastatic disease in lymph nodes in a number of cases that were not appreciated fully in the operating room.[175] Most surgeons favor resection of a narrow

TABLE 33–5. Survival Rates in Renal Cell Carcinoma

Investigations	Length of Survival (y)	Survival by Stage (%)			
		I	II	III	IV
Robson et al, 1969[138]	5	66	64	42	11
	10	60	67	38	0
Skinner et al, 1971[100]	5	65	47	51	8
	10	56	20	37	7
Boxer et al, 1979[102]	5	56	100	50	8
	10	20	66	25	0
McNichols et al, 1981[105]	5	67	51	34	14
	10	56	28	20	3
Cherrie et al, 1982[145]	5	—	—	0–53	0
	10	—	—	—	—
Selli et al, 1983[101]	5	93	63	80	13
	10	—	—	—	—
Bassil et al, 1985[147]	5	91–100	—	—	18
	10	—	—	—	—
Golimbu et al, 1986[8]	5	88	67	40	2
	10	66	35	15	—

rim of normal tissue around the tumor in the kidney instead of simple enucleation.[176] Extracorporeal partial nephrectomy plus autotransplantation is a technique that allows the surgeon to remove large tumors in the center of a solitary kidney with accuracy.[173] This ex vivo procedure entails radical excision of the kidney and division of the ureter. The kidney is then placed on a table and is intermittently perfused with a chilled solution to enhance viability. Under optical magnification, the tumor is carefully dissected from the surrounding renal parenchyma. Care is taken to preserve the vasculature of the normal kidney, which has been defined by preoperative arteriography. A small rim of normal tissue is removed along with the tumor to provide a tumor-free margin of resection. After the kidney has been reconstructed surgically, it is autotransplanted back into the iliac space. Vascular anastomosis of the renal artery and vein to the iliac vessels and ureteroureterostomy are performed.[177,178] If multiple tumors are encountered in which small tumors are distributed throughout the parenchyma, autotransplantation is not indicated.[169]

Although familial renal cell carcinoma or renal cell carcinoma associated with VHL syndrome is often bilateral, sporadic renal cell carcinoma is only rarely bilateral.[179] Bilateral (synchronous or asynchronous) renal cell carcinoma has been reported to occur in 1.8% of 3.8% of cases.[153] Patients with synchronous bilateral renal cell carcinoma have a better prognosis than patients with asynchronous disease. Zincke and colleagues reported a 78% 5-year survival for patients seen initially with bilateral renal cell carcinoma compared with only a 38% 5-year survival for patients whose metastases in the contralateral kidney appeared after the primary had been removed.[179]

Radiation Therapy as an Adjuvant to Nephrectomy

The cure rates for patients with high pathologic stage renal cell carcinoma (*i.e.*, with nodal involvement or metastases) treated by nephrectomy are only fair and have improved little in the last two decades. Because patients with renal cell carcinoma can have variable and protracted courses, the benefit in survival from any adjunctive therapy to nephrectomy is difficult to demonstrate. No data clearly indicate that a combination of radical nephrectomy and lymph node dissection provides enhanced cure rate over treatment by nephrectomy alone.[147] Studies looking at the possible benefit of adjuvant irradiation combined with nephrectomy are few and inconclusive (Table 33–6). Reports of benefit with radiation therapy come from only one nonrandomized trial.[180] Two randomized studies found no benefit from postoperative irradiation. Any possible benefit from radiation therapy in the latter two studies was likely compromised by the radiation technique or the radiation dose. Four fatal liver complications occurred after postoperative irradiation of up to 5500 cGy in the 1973 study reported by Finney.[181] In a study in Denmark, reported in 1987, a high complication rate was noted.[182] In this series, the dose per fraction was 250 cGy, for a total dose of 5000 cGy delivered over about 4 weeks. Because of complications (44% severe, 19% fatal), mainly gastrointestinal, this trial was stopped.[182]

Two studies of preoperative radiation therapy given before partial nephrectomy have been reported. The first, reported by van der Werf-Messing,[183] found no benefit with a dose of 3000 cGy given before nephrectomy. However, 37% of the patients had tumors of low pathologic stage and would have been unlikely to benefit from the adjuvant treatment. Likewise, in the phase III trial reported from Finland of 3600 cGy given preoperatively, 70% of patients had tumors of low pathologic stage (pT1 and pT2). There are no wholly satisfactory analyses of the efficacy of well-tolerated model megavoltage preoperative or postoperative radiation therapy as an adjunct to radical nephrectomy in patients judged to be at high risk for local regional failure (*i.e.*, those with high pathologic stage tumors).

Patients with pathologic stage T1 or T2 tumors without lymph node metastases are not good candidates for adjunctive

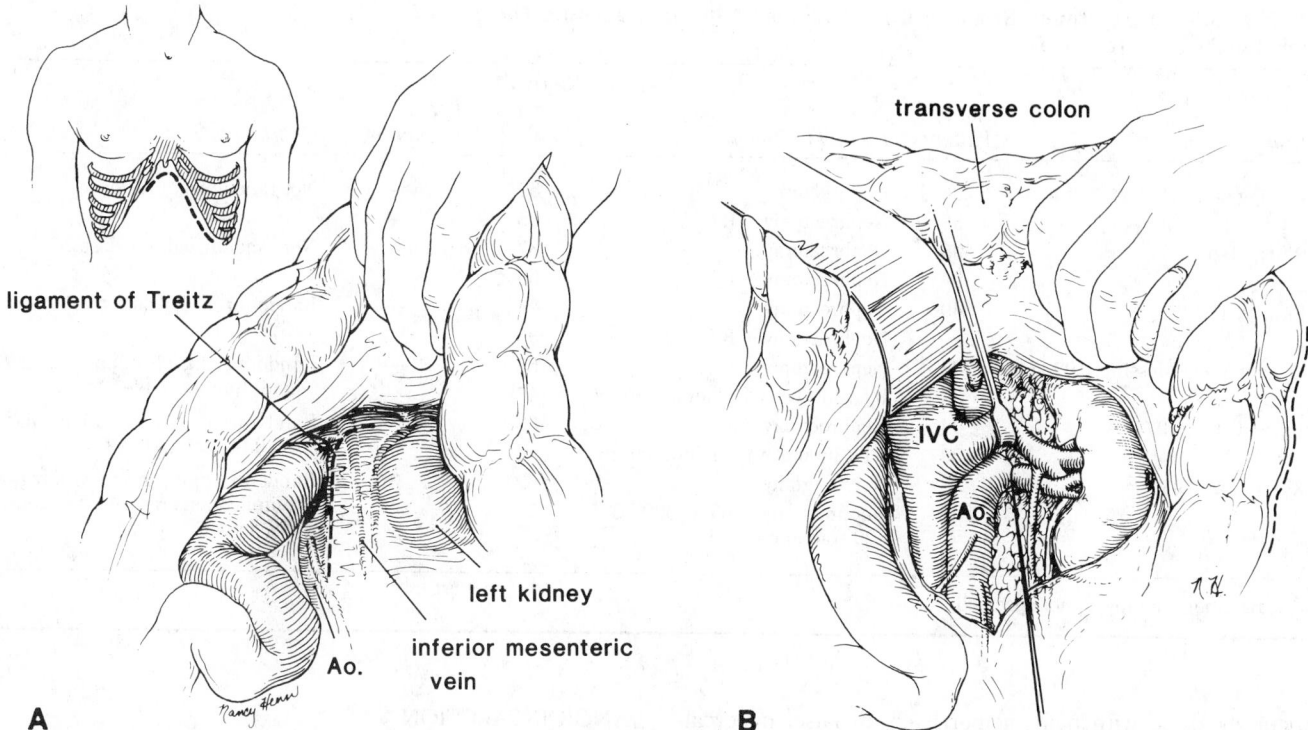

FIGURE 33–5. **(A)** Area of lymph node dissection for radical nephroureterectomy should be from the superior mesenteric artery to the level of the inferior mesenteric artery. The dotted line to the right of the descending colon indicates a line of incision on the left pericolic gutter that should extend superiorly to include division of the splenocolic attachments. **(B)** The left colon can be reflected from the anterior surface of Gerota's fascia with exposure of the renal artery before ligation and division. (Paulson DF, Perez CA, Anderson T. Cancer of the kidney and ureter. In: DeVita VT Jr, Hellman S, Rosenberg SA, eds: Cancer: Principles and practice of oncology. 2nd ed. Philadelphia: JB Lippincott, 1985:898)

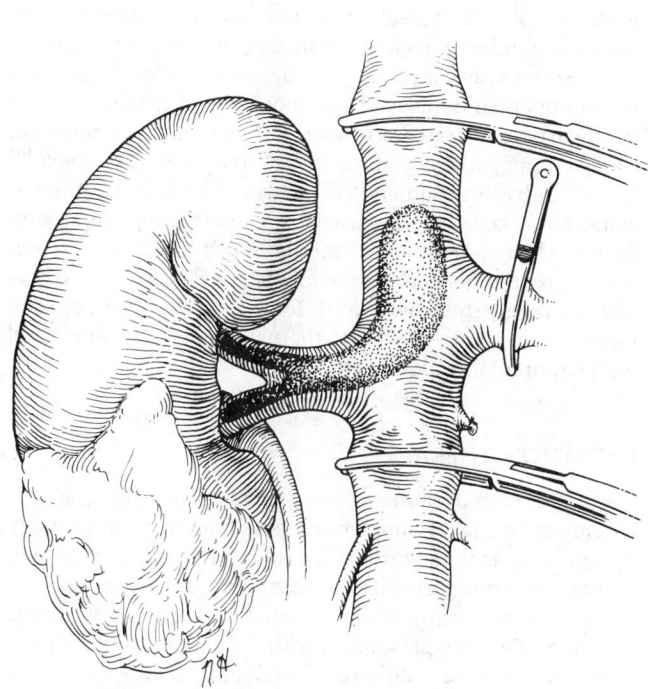

FIGURE 33–6. Surgical removal of a kidney tumor that has extended through the renal vein into the inferior vena cava.

therapy because they are likely to have a 5- to 10-year survival of 80% or more after radical nephrectomy alone.[140,147] Candidates for possible postoperative adjunctive radiation therapy include those with pathologic evidence of deep invasion of Gerota's fascia, adjacent organs, or regional lymph nodes and who have no known metastatic disease. Such patients are probably best treated with daily fractions of 180 to 200 cGy with 10- to 25-MV beams from linear accelerators to fields that include the renal fossa, tumor bed, and paraaortic paracaval lymph nodes, to a total dose of 4500 cGy in 5 weeks. The usual parallel-opposed anteroposterior isocentric fields are secondarily shaped with individual corner blocks. For right-sided tumors, the field often is reduced at the 3600 to 4600 cGy level to include only the tumor bed and the retroperitoneal lymph node regions, so that not more than 30% of the liver parenchyma receives a high dose. A postnephrectomy, preirradiation CT scan is useful as a baseline for subsequent comparison. Unless there is clear evidence of wound contamination by tumor spill at the time of nephrectomy, usually no effort is made to include the entire surgical incision in the treatment fields.

METASTATIC RENAL CELL CARCINOMA

NEPHRECTOMY AND RESECTION OF METASTASES

Adjuvant or palliative nephrectomy is not performed infrequently in patients with metastatic renal cell carcinoma, par-

TABLE 33–6. Treatment Results With and Without Adjuvant Radiation Therapy for Renal Cell Carcinoma

Investigations	No. of Patients	Local Treatment	5-Year Survival (%)	Local Recurrences	Comments
Peeling et al, 1969[338]	96	Nephrectomy	52	—	Not randomized; RT dose
	68	Nephrectomy + RT	25	—	
Rafla, 1970[180]	96	Nephrectomy	37	25	Not randomized; RT dose ?
	94	Nephrectomy + RT	56	7	
Finney, 1973[181]	49	Nephrectomy	44	—	Randomized; RT dose to 5500 cGy
		Nephrectomy + RT	36	—	
van der Werf-Messing, 1973[183]	85	Nephrectomy	63	—	Randomized; 37% of patients had small tumors (pT1–2)
	89	RT (3000 cGy) + nephrectomy	47		
Juusela et al, 1977[339]	44	Nephrectomy	63	—	Randomized; 70% of patients had small tumors (pT1–2)
	38	RT (3600 cGy) + nephrectomy			
Kjaer et al, 1987[182]	33	Nephrectomy	62	3	Randomized; RT group with high complications rate: 44% serious; 19% lethal
	32	Nephrectomy + RT (5000 cGy; 20 fractions)	38	0	

RT, radiation therapy; ?, not specified.

ticularly those with pain, hemorrhage, malaise, hypercalcemia, erythrocytosis, or hypertension. Removal of the primary tumor may alleviate some or all of these abnormalities.[184,185] Although there are isolated reports of regression of metastatic renal cell carcinoma after removal of the primary tumor, only 4 of 474 patients (0.8%) in nine series who underwent nephrectomy experienced an apparent regression of metastatic foci.[186] DeKernion and colleagues reported results in 26 patients with metastatic renal cell carcinoma who underwent palliative or adjuvant nephrectomy and found no increase in survival compared with survival in the entire group of 79 patients with metastatic renal cell carcinoma.[187] Middleton reported on 141 patients with metastatic renal cell carcinomas, 33 of whom underwent adjuvant nephrectomy; none of the 141 patients survived more than 24 months.[188] Adjuvant nephrectomy is not recommended for the purpose of inducing spontaneous regression; rather, it is performed to decrease symptoms or to decrease tumor burden in preparation for therapy in carefully controlled environments.

Of about 30% of patients with renal cell carcinoma who present with metastases, only 1.5% to 3.5% have solitary metastasis.[188,189] Patients with a solitary metastasis synchronous with a primary lesion have decreased survival compared with patients who develop metastasis after the primary tumor is removed.[180,187,190] Surgical resection is appropriate in selected patients with metastatic renal cell carcinoma. In one study, 59 patients with renal cell carcinoma who underwent surgical resection for a solitary metastasis had a 45% 3-year survival and a 34% 5-year survival.[188] O'Dea and colleagues reported on patients who presented with primary tumor in place and a solitary metastasis. Of the patients who underwent nephrectomy and later developed metastasis, 23% lived more than 5 years after removal of the metastatic lesions. Three of the 26 patients were alive 58, 94, and 245 months after resection of the metastatic lesions.[190] Nephrectomy and resection of metastases render few cures but frequently produce some long-term survivors.

ANGIOINFARCTION

Angioinfarction of the kidney is used with and without nephrectomy in the treatment of metastatic renal cell carcinoma. Techniques have been developed to occlude the renal artery for this purpose. Short-term embolization can be accomplished with alcohol, autologous blood clot, or gelatin sponge pads (Gelfoam). Other inert substances such as Silastic spheres, stainless pellets, or steel coils are used to embolize the renal artery.[191] Most patients develop a postinfarction syndrome consisting of pain, fever, and gastrointestinal complaints almost immediately after infarction.[184] Transcatheter arterial occlusion may decrease vascularity before nephrectomy in patients with large, locally advanced renal cell carcinoma or may lessen tumor bleeding, pain, or other systemic symptoms in patients with unresectable tumors.[191] Angioinfarction has not been demonstrated to be an effective method for inducing regression in patients with metastatic renal cell carcinoma.[192] In a study by Swanson and colleagues of patients with metastatic renal cell carcinoma who underwent angioinfarction followed by nephrectomy, a small number experienced complete or partial response of the metastatic disease to this therapy; however, there was no difference in survival between these patients (n = 100) and the patients who were treated with nephrectomy alone (n = 43).[193]

RADIATION THERAPY

The major sites of hematogenous metastases from renal cell carcinoma are bone, lung, and brain. Treatment in virtually all instances is noncurative. Therefore, the role of radiation therapy, neurosurgery, orthopedic surgery, or thoracic surgery in the local management of these metastases is nearly always palliative. Patients presenting with an initially solitary metastatic lesion have a 30% to 40% chance of surviving for 5 years. In these patients it is important to ensure as durable a palliative response as possible. In patients presenting with a solitary metastasis to the lung, spine, or brain, initial or de novo surgery should be considered, usually followed by postoperative irradiation. For a solitary metastasis to the spine, vertebral body resection by the anterior approach has proved satisfactory in carefully selected patients.[194,195] External-beam irradiation, the usual initial palliative approach for patients with symptomatic metastases, has been reported to yield a subjective or objective response in one half to two thirds of patients.[196,197] In a carefully selected and reviewed subset of patients irradiated for metastatic renal carcinoma, subjective improvement was noted in 16 of 19 analyzed patients, whereas objective evidence of regression, usually radiographic, was documented in only 13 of 26 treated patients. The external-beam irradiation doses were most commonly in the range of 4000 cGy.[196] Doses the equivalent of at least 5000 cGy in 5½ weeks are necessary to achieve a durable palliative response.[198] To deliver such high doses, multiple-field techniques are often necessary. Palliation of large renal bed recurrences by external-beam irradiation has been unsatisfactory. Some relief of pain has been achieved in about 50% of the patients, but it is usually of short duration.[197]

SYSTEMIC THERAPY

Appropriate management of the patient with metastatic renal cell carcinoma requires an appreciation of the unique natural history of this tumor, beyond the survival statistics described earlier in this chapter. Patients with metastatic renal cell carcinoma have a small but finite chance of undergoing spontaneous regression and can have stable disease for long periods of time; therefore, documentation of progressive metastatic disease is important before initiating systemic therapy. The natural history of this tumor in some patients is characterized by the development of solitary metastases, and surgical removal of these lesions can be associated with prolonged survival.[199] Therefore, surgical strategies to render a patient free of clinically evident disease may be appropriate in the management of selected patients with metastatic disease.

The results of systemic therapy in most patients with metastatic renal cell carcinoma continue to be unsatisfactory, and development of active therapy for metastatic renal cell carcinoma represents a significant challenge. Reproducible objective responses are being obtained with biologic agents, and there are new insights into the nature of the chemotherapy resistance of this tumor. Entry of patients into therapeutic clinical trials should remain a high priority for oncologists if therapeutic progress in renal cell carcinoma is to continue.

CHEMOTHERAPY

Renal cell carcinoma is a chemotherapy-resistant tumor. Review articles repeatedly conclude that commonly used cytotoxic agents exhibit only marginal response rates if modern objective response criteria are used, with no significant patient benefit.[199–201] Although weekly intravenous bolus vinblastine was once considered conventional therapy, this strategy is associated with only a 7% objective response rate,[200] activity that is not increased if the drug is administered by continuous infusion[202] or incorporated into a multidrug combination.[201]

There is no conventionally accepted, active cytotoxic chemotherapy for patients with this malignancy, and the search

for active new chemotherapeutic agents and treatment strategies remains an important goal. The conventional approach to testing new cytotoxic agents in phase II trials has had little success. A review of the results of 39 agents evaluated in phase II trials between 1983 and 1989 and involving 2120 patients revealed an objective response rate of less than 9%, usually of short duration.[203] A partial biologic explanation for this de novo drug refractoriness has emerged recently, with evidence suggesting that chemotherapy resistance reflects the expression on the renal carcinoma cell surface of the multidrug resistance (MDR) associated P-170 glycoprotein. Fojo and colleagues have described highly elevated *MDR1* mRNA levels in proximal tubule cells of normal kidney.[204] Furthermore, a series of studies confirm the strong *MDR1* gene expression in most renal cell adenocarcinomas.[205] These studies have demonstrated that the resistance of some renal cell carcinoma lines in vitro to doxorubicin can be reversed variably by inhibitors of P-170 function. Another P-170 independent cellular mechanism that may contribute to multidrug resistance in renal cell carcinoma, the glutathione redox cycle, has been demonstrated in studies on renal cell carcinoma cell lines and in fresh renal tumor specimens to contribute to the multidrug resistance of these tumors.[206,207] Successful strategies to overcome multidrug resistance may lead in the future to more effective cytotoxic chemotherapy-based treatment approaches in renal cell carcinoma.

Von Roemeling and Hrushesky have conducted preclinical and clinical studies to demonstrate that circadian rhythms predictably affect therapeutic indices of cytotoxic drugs such as floxuridine (FUDR).[208] They developed drug administration schedules for FUDR using implantation pumps that incorporate a circadian patterned variable rate infusion with a maximal flow rate in the late afternoon or early evening and a minimum flow rate during the early morning hours. Using this schedule, they demonstrated, first in mice and then in humans, less severe toxicities at similar daily dose intensity, and the ability to deliver as much as 1.45-fold more drug per unit time with minimal toxicity.[209] This treatment strategy was applied in patients with renal cell carcinoma using continuous infusion FUDR intravenously (61 patients with a starting dose of 0.15 mg/kg/day for 14 days) or intrahepatic arterially (7 patients with a starting dose of 0.25 mg/kg/day for 14 days).[210] Intravenous infusion was limited by diarrhea and nausea or vomiting, whereas intraarterial infusion was limited by abnormalities in hepatic function. Of 56 patients evaluable for response who were treated by intravenous infusion, 4 complete and 7 partial responses were observed, for a response rate of 19.6% and a median duration of response of 10.8 months. Of 7 patients evaluable for response who received intrahepatic arterial FUDR infusion, 1 complete response and 3 partial responses were observed. These results suggest that circadian-modified FUDR infusion may be beneficial in some patients with metastatic renal cell carcinoma. Preliminary results of confirmatory trials reported in abstract form have been positive[211–213] and negative.[214]

Hormonal Therapy

For decades, one approach to the therapy of patients with metastatic renal cell carcinoma was the use of medroxyprogesterone acetate. The rationale for this therapy was based on extensive preclinical studies of estrogen-induced renal cell cancer in the Syrian hamster.[215] Progesterone therapy inhibited the development of tumors in these animals, and high-dose progesterone therapy and adrenalectomy or orchiectomy inhibited tumor growth.[216] The higher incidence of renal cell carcinoma in men than women, the differential survival rates for men and women with this tumor, and the identification of hormonal receptors in renal cell tumors have been used to support hormonal approaches to therapy. The lack of effective alternative systemic therapies and the relatively low toxicity of progesterone therapy favored this approach. Three decades of experience with medroxyprogesterone acetate therapy and with testosterone or antiestrogens suggest that the animal models do not represent a valid model for human renal cell cancer.[200] The value of medroxyprogesterone therapy has been reviewed critically by Kjaer, who has concluded that irrespective of dose and schedule, human renal cell carcinoma is neither hormone-dependent nor, in general, hormone-responsive.[217] Using modern objective response criteria, responses are only occasional (1–2%) and are partial and of short duration with no clinical benefit if they do occur. There is no evidence to support a beneficial effect of adjuvant progesterone therapy and no evidence of a correlation between hormone receptor content and response.

Biologic Therapy

Interferons

After the first reports of objective responses to partially purified leukocyte interferon in patients with renal cell carcinoma,[218,219] extensive phase II experience has been accumulated with nonrecombinant interferon preparations and with recombinant interferon-α and -β.[220–223] Response rates with recombinant interferon-α are similar with different preparations and are in the 15% to 20% objective response range, with median response durations in different studies in the range of 6 to 10 months. An intermediate dose regimen (usually 5 to 10 million IU/m^2 given intramuscularly or subcutaneously daily or 3 to 5 times a week) has been used most often, although an optimal treatment regimen or duration of therapy has not been defined.[223] Objective responses have been reported with as little as 1 million U/day subcutaneously.[224] It does appear that chronic dosing is superior to intermittent higher doses with respect to tolerability and antitumor activity, and the development of response is often slow, taking months to develop. Responses correlate with good performance status, previous nephrectomy, and lung-predominant disease. Patients with nonresected primary tumors or bulky visceral metastatic disease are less likely to respond, although responses in all sites have been reported.[223]

The mechanisms of the interferon antitumor effect are not understood and may include direct tumor antiproliferative effects and immunostimulatory effects. In one study, the expression of a kidney-associated cell-surface differentiation antigen gp160 was associated with resistance to interferon growth-inhibitory effects in a series of renal cell carcinoma cell lines in vitro and during treatment after inoculation into mice.[225] The authors speculated that the absence of gp160 expression by a renal cell carcinoma might predict likelihood of response to interferon therapy in patients, and a clinical study to explore this question is underway. Similarly, the rea-

sons for loss of responsiveness to interferon therapy are not understood. There have been reports that the development of neutralizing antibodies in renal cell carcinoma patients was associated with loss of response,[226] but this phenomenon has not been studied extensively.

The reproducible objective response rates in favorable prognosis patients and the absence of major long-term toxicity with chronic interferon administration have led to the use of interferon-α in an ongoing adjuvant trial (EST 2886) conducted by the Eastern Cooperative Oncology Group (ECOG). In an attempt to improve the therapy of metastatic renal cell carcinoma, interferon has been combined with other antitumor agents. No advantage to the combination of interferon-α with vinblastine has been observed.[223] The combined use of interferon-α and IL-2 is discussed later. Preclinical data suggest a positive interaction of these two classes of agents, and phase II clinical trials are underway.

Reports of activity of interferon-γ in clinical trials of patients with renal cell carcinoma have appeared. In a multicenter Japanese study, 6 of 30 patients responded to 40 million U of interferon-γ administered on an intermittent schedule.[227] Aulitzky and colleagues used a low dose of interferon-γ (0.1 mg/week subcutaneously) and observed 2 complete and 4 partial responses in 20 evaluable treated patients.[228] Only 3 objective responses had been found in 32 patients treated on a continuous infusion schedule of interferon-γ,[229] and other smaller trials with single agent interferon-γ have been disappointing.

Interleukin-2-Based Therapies

The initial reports of the combination of IL-2 and lymphokine-activated killer (LAK) cell therapy included 4 complete and 8 partial responses in 36 patients with metastatic renal cell carcinoma.[230,231] Although objective responses already had been observed in this tumor with recombinant interferon-α, IL-2 differs from the interferons in that it is not known to have direct antiproliferative effects. IL-2 is a biologic agent that apparently mediates its antitumor effects entirely through the activation of host immune mechanisms. The reproducible complete and durable objective tumor responses it has achieved in a tumor refractory to standard therapeutic agents have served as a great stimulus to the investigation of biologic approaches to the therapy of renal cell cancer. The recent approvals in Europe and the United States of IL-2 for the treatment of patients with metastatic renal cell carcinoma makes available a treatment option that is capable of inducing durable objective responses in a reproducible subset of patients.

Preclinical studies showed that the antitumor efficacy of IL-2 was dose- and schedule-dependent (see Chap. 17). Furthermore, for any particular IL-2 treatment regimen, activity could be enhanced by the adoptive transfer of LAK cells or by the concomitant use of other cytokines such as interferon-α or tumor necrosis factor.[232,233] The initial clinical trials of IL-2 in renal cell carcinoma involved IL-2 administered at the maximally-tolerated dose and in combination with LAK cells. The dose-limiting toxicities in most patients treated in these high-dose IL-2 trials were principally hypotension and a vascular leak syndrome, although other serious toxicities were encountered. Vasopressor therapy and intensive care unit support allow the delivery of this high-dose therapy

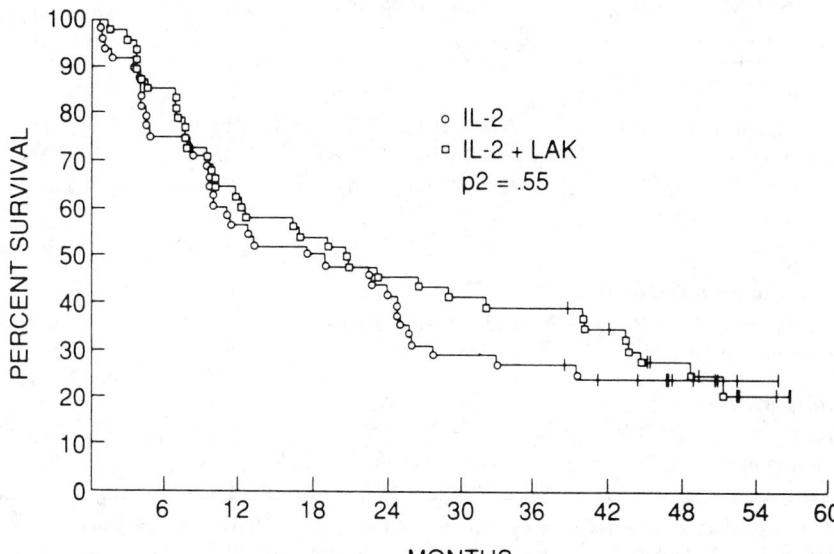

FIGURE 33-7. Survival of patients with metastatic kidney cancer treated at the National Cancer Institute with IL-2 or IL-2/LAK. The 18-month actuarial survival was 34% for patients who were treated with IL-2 and 46% for those treated with IL-2/LAK.[348] (Rosenberg SA. The immunotherapy and gene therapy of cancer. J Clin Oncol 1992;10:180–199)

safely in most patients. These cardiorespiratory toxicities and other renal, hepatic, gastrointestinal, and hematologic toxicities rapidly reverse in most patients after discontinuation of IL-2.[234–237]

The experience in early studies has led to the institution of more rigorous eligibility criteria for determination of patient suitability for IL-2 therapy. Patients considered for entry into high-dose IL-2 trials are screened carefully for the presence of underlying coronary artery disease or pulmonary impairment and must have an ECOG performance status of 0 or 1. Patients who are most safely treated are those who have relatively normal renal, hepatic, and hematologic values, an FEV_1 greater than 70% of predicted on pulmonary function testing, and no evidence of ischemic heart disease on stress treadmill or stress thallium study. Analysis of patients entered into these trials shows that most have had a previous nephrectomy and have been exposed to minimal pretreatment with chemotherapeutic, hormonal, or biologic agents. The influence of these latter factors on likelihood of response has not been defined. This attention to careful patient selection, a detailed knowledge of the pathophysiology of IL-2-related toxicities, and preferably experience with this form of treatment are important in minimizing the risks and maximizing the like-

lihood of benefit from high-dose IL-2 therapy. The results of the published IL-2 trials discussed later largely reflect the characteristics of treatment of this uniquely screened patient population. Understanding and consideration of these issues by physician and patient are necessary in making decisions about therapy with this biologic agent.

Results of Combined Interleukin-2 and LAK Cell Trials. The bulk of the initial therapeutic experience with high-dose IL-2 in renal cell carcinoma was with the combination IL-2 and LAK cell regimen developed in the Surgery Branch of the National Cancer Institute (NCI) and studied extensively by the NCI-sponsored Extramural IL-2 Working Group (Fig. 33–7 and Table 33–7).[230,231,238] In these trials, patients received high-dose intravenous bolus IL-2 (Cetus, Emeryville, CA; 600,000–720,000 IU/kg every 8 hours on days 1–5 and 11–15; Table 33–8).[239] The combined response rate of these published trials using high-dose IL-2 with LAK is 23.5% (43 of 183 patients, with 12 [6.5%] complete responses), and the median response duration of all responses is 11 months. At the time of analysis, 16 of the objective responders had been followed for more than 1 year; these responses were still ongoing at 19 to more than 55 months from entry to study. The

TABLE 33-7. Results of Immunotherapy for Renal Cell Carcinoma From the National Cancer Institute Surgery Branch

Total Evaluable Patients	No. of Patients (IL-2/LAK)	Response Duration (mo)	No. of Patients (IL-2 alone)	Response Duration (mo)
No. with complete response	72 8	20+, 17+, 15, 13+, 13, 11, 9, 6	52 4	24+, 18+, 17+, 15+
No. with partial response	17	26+, 17+, 13, 11, 10+, 10+, 10, 9, 7, 7, 6, 6, 6, 6, 3, 1, 1	7	17+, 17+, 15+, 11+, 11, 9+, 5+
Total responses	25 (35%)		11 (21%)	

TABLE 33–8. Collected Trials of Interleukin-2 in Renal Cell Carcinoma

Investigations	Regimen	No. of Evaluable Patients	Complete Response	Partial Response	Response Rate (%)
High-Dose Bolus IL-2					
Rosenberg et al, 1989[246]	720,000 IU/kg (C) q 8 h, d 1–5, 11–15	54	4	8	22
Atkins et al, 1991[247]	600,000 IU/kg (C) q 8 h, d 1–5, 15–19	30	1	7	27
Abrams et al, 1990[340]	600,000 IU/kg (C) q 8 h, d 1–5, 12–16	16	0	0	0
McCabe et al, 1991[341]	600,000 IU/kg (C) q 8 h, d 1–5, 11–15	37	1	2	8
Poo et al, 1991[342]	600,000 IU/kg (C) q 8 h, d 1–5, 11–15	15	0	4	27
Continuous Infusion IL-2					
Negrier et al, 1989[240]	18 mIU/m^2/d (C) d 1–5, 11–15	32	2	4	19
Bajorin et al, 1990[241]	9 mIU/m^2/d (HR) d 1–4, q wk × 4 wk	24	1	2	13
Outpatient IL-2					
Bukowski et al, 1990[244]	60 mIU/m^2 (C) I.V. tiw	41	1	4	12
Sleijfer et al, 1991[245]	9–18 mIU/d (C) d 1–5, q wk × 6 wk	21	2	4	19

C, IL-2 produced by Cetus Oncology Division of Chiron, Inc.; HR, IL-2 produced by Hoffman-LaRoche, Inc.; IL-2, interleukin-2; IU, international units; mIU, milli-international unit.
(Modified from Sznol M, Thurn A, Parkinson DR. Overview of interleukin-2 trials in patients with renal cell carcinoma. 1992 [in press])

response rate in trials using LAK cells administered with continuous infusion IL-2 was 17.9% (37 of 207 patients), with complete and durable responses observed (Table 33–9). Although attention originally was focused on this cellular therapy, it became clear that therapy with high-dose IL-2 alone, without the inconvenience and expense of LAK cell genera-tion, was capable of generating durable complete responses in patients with renal cell carcinoma (Figs. 33–7 to 33–10).

Results of Single-Agent Interleukin-2 Trials. In these trials, which formed the basis for the recent FDA approval of this agent for the treatment of renal cell carcinoma, IL-2 was ad-

TABLE 33–9. Collected Trials of Interleukin-2 in Combination With LAK Cells in Renal Cell Carcinoma

Investigations	Regimen	No. of Evaluable Patients	Complete Response	Partial Response	Response Rate (%)
Rosenberg et al, 1989[246]	720,000 IU/kg (C) I.V. q 8 h, d 1–5, 12–16	72	8	17	35
Fisher et al, 1988[343]	600,000 IU/kg (C) q 8 h, d 1–5, 12–16	35	2	3	14
Parkinson, 1990[251]	600,000 IU/kg (C) I.V. bolus q 8 h, d 1–3; 18 mIUm^2, CI, d 9–15	47	2	2	9
Gaynor et al, 1990[344]	18 mIU/m^2, CI, d 1–5 18–27 mIU/m^2, CI, d 11–15	25	2	2	16
Weiss et al, 1992[250]	600,000 IU/kg (C) I.V. q 8 h, d 1–5, 11–15	46	2	7	20
Weiss et al, 1992[250]	18 mIU/m^2, CI (C) d 1–5 22.5 mIU/m^2, CI, d 11–15	48	2	5	15
Dillman et al, 1991[345]	18 mIU/m^2, CI, d 1–5, 11–15	33	0	1	3
Negrier et al, 1989[240]	18 mIU/m^2/d, CI, d 1–5, 11–15	51	5	9	27
McCabe et al, 1991[341]	600,000 IU/kg (C) I.V. q 8 h, d 1–15, 11–15	30	0	4	12
Thompson et al, 1991[346]	18 mIU/m^2, CI (HR) d 1–5 6–18 mIU/m^2, CI, d 12–16 or d 10–19	29	4	5	31
Bajorin et al, 1990[241]	9 mIU/m^2, CI (HR), d 1–4 × 4 wk	21	1	1	10

C, IL-2 produced by Cetus Oncology Division of Chiron, Inc.; CI, continuous infusion; HR, IL-2 produced by Hoffman-LaRoche, Inc.; IL-2, interluekin-2; IU, international units; mIU, milli-international units.

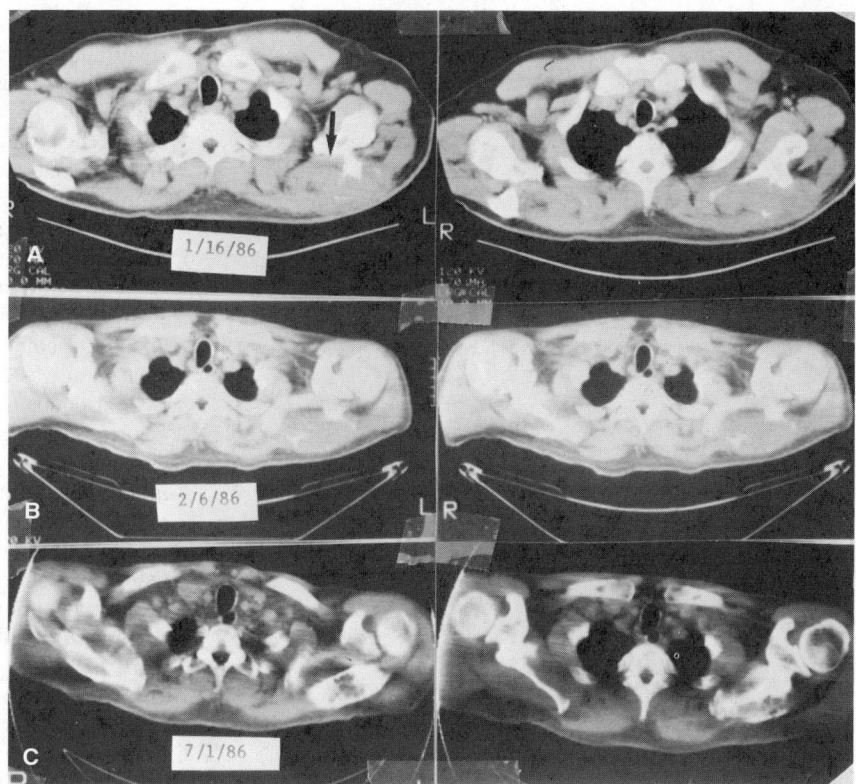

FIGURE 33–8. CT scan of a patient with renal cell carcinoma with a metastasis in the scapula (**A**) before treatment with IL-2 and LAK cells and (**B** and **C**) after treatment. All tumors regressed completely.

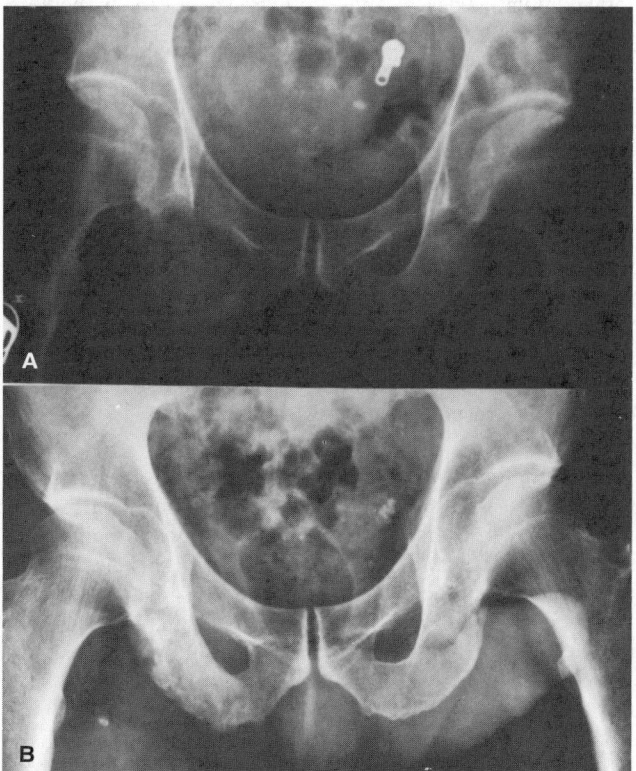

FIGURE 33–9. (**A**) Radiograph of the pelvis of a patient with metastatic renal cell carcinoma who had a large osseous metastasis before treatment with IL-2 and LAK cells. (**B**) After treatment, the osseous lesion regressed completely and the bone recalcified.

ministered in the same dose as in the IL-2/LAK trials and at the same schedule, except that the second 5-day course of IL-2 was sometimes administered from days 15 to 19 instead of days 11 to 15. Patients entered into these trials received a median of 15 to 20 doses of IL-2 (Cetus) over 3 weeks of treatment, and in the most recent analysis of this combined experience, an overall response rate of 17.8% objective response rate was observed (6 complete and 21 partial responses in 152 evaluable patients).[239] In general, responses were durable, ranging from 3 months to more than 50 months.

The complete therapeutic experience in patients with metastatic renal cell carcinoma treated with the high-dose bolus IL-2 regimen developed in the NCI Surgery Branch was the basis for the Product Licensing Application submitted to the FDA by the Cetus Oncology Division of Chiron Corporation. A recommendation for approval by the Biological Response Modifier Advisory Committee in January of 1992 was based on data including 255 patients treated using IL-2 (the regimen of bolus intravenous IL-2 [Cetus] every 8 hours) in seven clinical studies. These patients included almost all the patients listed in Table 33–8 and patients treated in other unpublished trials. In this experience, 9 complete (4%) and 28 partial (11%) responses were observed for an overall response rate of 15%; the median duration of response was projected to be 23.2 months. Although the response is low, the quality of these responses is further emphasized by the observation that 85% of responders were projected to remain in response at 12 months, and that even 79% of the PRs were projected to remain in response at 12 months. Although in this analysis a higher response rate (18%) and all the complete responses were observed in ECOG performance status 0 patients, and

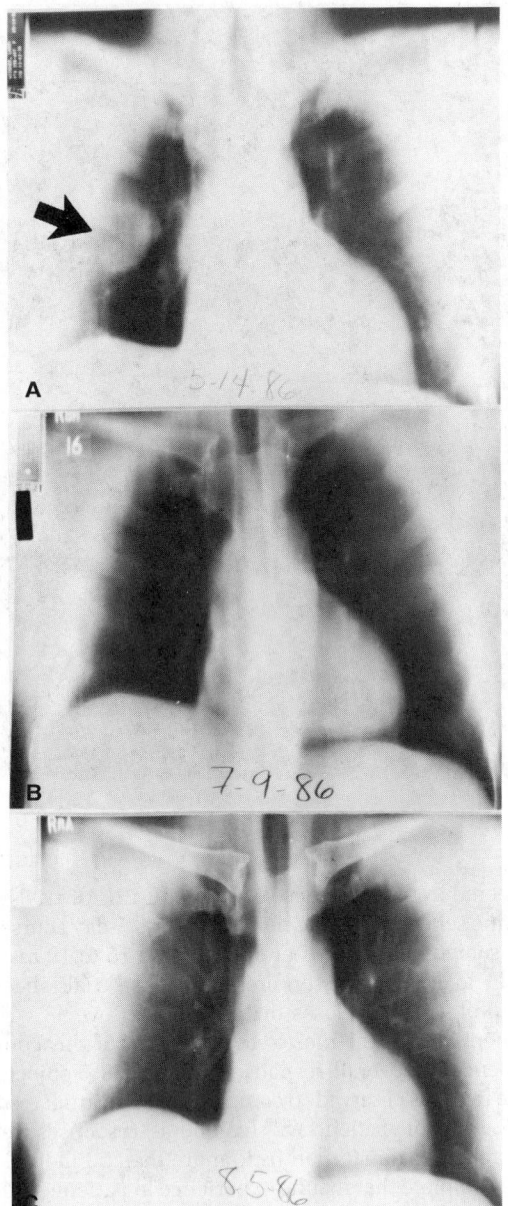

FIGURE 33–10. Lung tomograms of a patient with renal cell carcinoma and a large pulmonary metastasis (**A**) before IL-2 treatment and (**B** and **C**) after treatment. The pulmonary nodule regressed completely.

most responding patients had disease limited to lung or lymph nodes or both, responses were observed in these patients at most sites of metastatic involvement and in performance status 1 patients.

Consideration of the toxicities encountered during these therapeutic trials reveals the complexity of high-dose IL-2 therapy. Despite the careful attention to patient selection, a 4% on-study death rate was observed in this overall experience. More than half of the patients required vasopressors, and 7% required transient intubation secondary to treatment-associated respiratory failure. Somnolence or agitation during therapy occurred in 23% of patients, and more serious neurologic toxicities such as coma were observed. The most se-

rious gastrointestinal toxicities were gastrointestinal hemorrhage or perforation, which required surgical intervention. Although serious renal toxicities, principally severe oliguria and elevated serum creatinine, were observed in more than half of the patients, more long-lasting renal toxicity requiring dialysis occurred in only 4 patients. Sepsis, particularly with gram-positive organisms secondary to central lines, was common in these patients, although the use of prophylactic antibiotics has decreased this complication. Despite the severity of these acute toxicities occurring during high-dose bolus IL-2 therapy, most reverse rapidly after cessation of therapy, and the median time to discharge after completion of IL-2 treatment was 3 days.

Continuous infusion single-agent IL-2 has been studied in a series of trials (see Table 33–8). These studies were conducted primarily in Europe, in which IL-2 therapy using this method of administration has been approved by all members of the European Community. The studies used 19 million IU/m^2 for 120 hours separated by 1 week of rest. In a trial published by Negrier and colleagues, hypotension was managed by dose reduction rather than by the institution of vasopressor therapy, and no toxic death and only a 3% incidence of dyspnea were observed, whereas a response rate of 19% was obtained.[240] In a separate multicenter randomized trial comparing IL-2 (Roche) administered as a single agent (9 million IU/m^2/day for 4 days weekly for 4 weeks) with the same drug dose and schedule with LAK cells, 1 complete response and an overall 13% response rate were observed in the 24 patients in the IL-2 alone arm.[241] If IL-2 is administered by continuous infusion over 24 hours once or twice weekly, much higher total cumulative doses can be delivered over time without increased toxicity; responses have been observed with this approach.[242,243]

Outpatient single-agent IL-2 regimens have been studied in patients with renal cell carcinoma (see Table 33–8). In one trial, 41 evaluable patients, of whom only 56% had undergone previous nephrectomy and 50% had an ECOG performance status of 1 or 2, were treated with 60 million IU/m^2 of IL-2 (Cetus) by intravenous bolus administration 3 times weekly.[244] Dose reduction was necessary in most patients after a median of 4 doses, and an objective response rate of 12% was observed, with 4 of 19 (21%) ECOG performance status 0 patients responding. A study involving outpatient IL-2 (Cetus) administered subcutaneously at 18 million IU/m^2 produced a 29% response rate in 21 patients.[245]

Response Rates in Interleukin-2 and Interferon-α Combination Therapy. Rationales for the combination of IL-2 and interferon-α in therapy of renal cell carcinoma include the single-agent activity of each in patients with this disease and the results from preclinical models in which apparent synergy is present.[232] When interferon-α was added to high-dose IL-2 regimens, toxicities were similar or greater than those observed with high-dose IL-2 alone or with LAK cells. A 31% response rate, including 4 complete responses, was obtained among 35 patients with renal cell carcinoma treated in a phase I study at the NCI Surgery Branch.[246] However, phase II studies of IL-2 and interferon-α with and without LAK conducted by the NCI-sponsored Extramural IL-2/LAK Working Group did not suggest any improvement in antitumor activity associated with the addition of interferon-α to high-dose bolus IL-2.[247,248]

Preliminary response rates to outpatient IL-2/interferon-α combination regimens have been reported in the 17% to 32% range, involving a total of 150 patients treated in six trials in which 5 complete and 33 partial responses were observed (overall objective response rate of 25%).[239] Although more complete data are required for final assessment of this outpatient strategy, the results suggest that wider study of this approach is indicated. Phase III randomized outpatient trials of interferon-α versus the combination of IL-2 and interferon-α are necessary to define more fully the utility of these approaches. Such information is important in determining the nature of future adjuvant trials in renal cell carcinoma.

Summary of Interleukin-2 in the Treatment of Renal Cell Carcinoma. Response rates obtained in numerous trials with high-dose IL-2 in metastatic renal cell carcinoma, whether administered as a single agent by bolus or continuous infusion or in combination with LAK cells or interferon-α, are in the range of 15% to 20%. Response rates are higher in better performance status patients and have been defined in patients who have been selected carefully for adequate cardiopulmonary status and who in general have undergone previous nephrectomy. Comparison of results of different phase II trials in patients with metastatic renal cell carcinoma, given differences in source of IL-2, treatment regimens, and patient demographics, is difficult, and particular issues regarding optimal IL-2-based treatment approaches require comparative studies. The question of dose-response relation, for example, given all the other known and unknown influences on responsiveness to IL-2, is a phase III question which is the subject of an ongoing randomized trial at the NCI Surgery Branch. Similarly, the question of whether bolus or continuous infusion-based IL-2 regimens are more active in this malignancy is difficult to resolve. Although continuous infusion IL-2 produces greater biologic activity and toxicity on the basis of total dose per unit time,[249] the response data described earlier do not suggest that continuous infusion is more active in renal cancer. In a small randomized study in patients with renal cell carcinoma in which IL-2 was administered by bolus or by continuous infusion to equivalent toxicity, equivalent results were obtained.[250] Similarly, published data do not suggest that the addition of either LAK cells or interferon-α to high-dose IL-2 adds benefit, despite the predictions of the animals. In contrast, the initial results suggest that the addition of interferon-α to lower-dose IL-2 outpatient regimens results in a therapy that appears to be active and relatively nontoxic, although comparison with results obtained with either cytokine alone is a phase III question.

The question of net patient benefit in patients with metastatic renal carcinoma who are treated with IL-2 is difficult to answer with available data. No randomized phase III trials have been performed to compare survival in patients with renal cell carcinoma treated with IL-2 compared with non-IL-2-based therapy. Nevertheless, the durable complete and partial responses occurring in a subset of patients with this chemotherapy-refractory malignancy appear to represent a significant change in the natural history of this group of patients, and it was this information that led to the approval by the FDA of high-dose bolus IL-2 for metastatic renal carcinoma. Further characterization of the subset of patients most likely to respond to this therapeutic approach and the development of more active and toxic treatment strategies are clearly necessary for patients with renal cell carcinoma.[251,252] Efforts to develop a more effective adoptively transferred cell for use in the treatment of patients with advanced kidney cancer studies are underway, evaluating the use of IL-2 plus tumor-infiltrating lymphocytes (TIL). Preclinical studies have shown TIL to be more effective than LAK in treating established metastases in some murine models.[253] Clinical trials have demonstrated the efficacy of immunotherapy using TIL in patients with metastatic melanoma.[254] Studies evaluating the use of TIL in patients with advanced renal cell carcinoma are underway.

Other Immunobiologic Approaches

Autolymphocyte Therapy

Autolymphocyte therapy (ALT) involves the administration to patients of autologous peripheral blood lymphocytes (PBL) activated in vitro by supernatants of anti-CD3 activated autologous PBL. A randomized multicenter trial was conducted involving 90 patients with metastatic renal cell cancer who received ALT (about 10^9 cells administered monthly for 6 months with oral cimetidine 600 mg four times daily) or cimetidine alone at the same dose. The cellular therapy was administered on an outpatient basis with minimal toxicity. A statistically significant difference in median survival was observed in the ALT arm (>15 months compared with 9 months), with the significant survival benefit observed only in men, and particularly in those patients in whom the anti-CD3-activated supernatant contained high levels of IL-1.[255] Although the trial arms were balanced for conventional prognostic characteristics, the results are atypical for most cancer trials in that this highly significant survival benefit was observed in the setting of few objective tumor responses (no complete and 8 partial responses in 39 evaluable patients [21% objective response rate]). A confirmatory randomized trial of this therapy is being performed by the ECOG.

Coumarin

Based on preclinical studies suggesting favorable immunomodulatory properties to cimetidine and coumarin (a warfarin derivative), the combination of oral agents has been studied in patients with metastatic renal cell carcinoma. In both published studies, coumarin was administered at 100 mg/day and cimetidine at 300 mg four times a day. The initial optimistic report of a 33% response rate with 3 complete and 11 partial objective responses in a pilot study of 42 patients[256] was not confirmed in a phase II trial.[257] In the latter study, only partial responses in 50 patients were obtained, for an overall 6% response rate. Moreover, no evidence for immune stimulation was observed, based on studies of hypersensitivity skin testing, absolute numbers of circulating peripheral blood lymphocytes, phenotypic characterization of lymphocyte subsets, and in vitro lymphocyte blastogenesis. Similar negative results have been reported in abstract form by Herrmann and colleagues.[258]

Specific Immunotherapy

Future immunologic approaches will attempt to introduce more therapeutic specificity to the biologic therapy of melanoma. Although antibodies that recognize differentiation-related kidney antigens have been developed,[259] none have been applied in therapeutic trials in renal cell carcinoma. They may prove useful if used with immunostimulating agents such as IL-2 or as targeting ligands for cytotoxic drugs, toxins, or isotopes. The transfer of cytokine genes to autologous renal carcinoma cells may permit new vaccination strategies to induce specific antitumor immunity.[260]

CARCINOMA OF THE RENAL PELVIS

Carcinoma of the renal pelvis is a relatively rare tumor that accounts for 5% of all renal tumors. It occurs more frequently in men than in women (2–3:1). Upper urinary tract carcinoma is a multifocal process; patients with cancer at one site in the upper urinary tract are at greater risk for developing tumors elsewhere. The probability of multifocal occurrence is greater in patients with larger lesions and in those with carcinoma in situ. A patient with one upper tract urothelial tumor has a 30% to 50% chance of developing a bladder tumor as well. About 2% to 4% of patients with an upper tract urothelial tumor develop bilateral renal pelvic tumors. If a patient has a renal pelvic tumor and a ureteral tumor at the same time, there is a 75% chance that a bladder tumor will develop. Alternatively, a patient with a bladder tumor initially has a 2% to 3% chance of developing an upper tract tumor.[261–265]

ETIOLOGY

The major cause of cancer of the renal pelvis is smoking, and cessation of smoking can eliminate many of these tumors.[266] There is a significant increase in risk for upper genitourinary tract urothelial cancer in smokers; the risk is highest among the heaviest smokers.[28,265] In 1965, Hultengren and colleagues first identified a connection between epithelial tumors of the renal pelvis and abuse of compound analgesics.[267,268] Reports from Sweden,[269,270] Australia,[271–273] the Netherlands,[274] Denmark,[275,276] Italy,[277] Germany,[278] and the United States[28] demonstrated an association between analgesic abuse and renal pelvic tumors.[268,273] Most of the patients ingested a significant amount (5 kg) of compound analgesic, usually containing phenacetin, phenazone, and caffeine.[265,272] Typically, upper genitourinary tract tumors occur in patients in whom prolonged and heavy analgesic ingestion is followed by renal papillary necrosis.[272] Although the precise mechanism is not completely understood, studies have suggested a possible etiologic role of orthoaminophenols, the major phenacetin metabolites, in the development of renal pelvic tumors.[279] In a study of 192 patients with chronic pyelonephritis, 104 had pyelonephritis secondary to analgesic abuse. Of the 104 analgesic abusers, 8 developed transitional cell carcinoma of the renal pelvis. There were no tumors in the nonabusers.[269] In a case-control study of patients with renal pelvic transitional cell carcinoma, renal papillary necrosis and phenacetin abuse conferred relatively equal risks for the development of renal pelvic tumors. If these two conditions occurred together, the risk was 20 times that for nonconsumers of analgesics without renal papillary necrosis.[273]

Cancer of the renal pelvis is associated with Danubian endemic familial nephropathy (Balkan nephropathy). Balkan nephropathy is a slowly progressive inflammation of the interstitium of the kidney that ultimately results in renal failure. This disorder, which is prevalent in the Balkan countries (Yugoslavia, Rumania, Bulgaria, and Greece), is associated with multifocal, slow-growing, superficial, low-grade tumors of the renal pelvis.[265] The cause of Balkan nephropathy is unclear; however, potential etiologic agents such as fungal toxins, viruses, silicates, and heavy metals have been studied.[262]

An association has been observed between renal pelvic tumors and urban residence and occupation in the aniline dye, textiles, plastics, and rubber industries.[262,265] Chronic inflammation and irritation are associated with the development of renal pelvic tumors, particularly in patients who have upper urinary tract stones.

Studies of the molecular genetics of transitional cell carcinoma by RFLP analysis have identified abnormalities on chromosome 9, chromosome 17 near the p53 locus, chromosome 13 near the retinoblastoma locus, and chromosome 3 near the kidney cancer disease gene locus.[280–283] Although the transitional carcinoma disease gene has not been identified, it is thought to be located on chromosome 9, with abnormalities at other tumor suppressor gene loci involved in progression of disease.[280] There are reports of nine kindreds exhibiting a familial pattern in the development of transitional cell carcinoma of the urinary tract.[284,285] Of the affected family members, 22% had upper tract tumors, 59% had bladder cancer, and 18% had both upper and lower tract tumors.[284] One member of another cancer-prone family (Li-Fraumeni syndrome) developed bilateral upper tract urothelial carcinoma. A molecular defect, an activated c-*RAF1* gene, has been isolated from noncancerous cells from members of a family with Li-Fraumeni syndrome; however, material from affected family members with bladder or upper tract transitional cell carcinoma has not been analyzed for this abnormality.[286] Studies of the molecular and cellular aspects of urothelial transformation should provide further insight into the etiology and mechanisms of progression and metastasis of this disease.

PATHOLOGY

Transitional cell carcinoma accounts for 90% of the tumors of the renal pelvis and can be in situ, papillary, or planar. Squamous cell carcinoma, which is usually associated with chronic inflammation or infection of the renal pelvis, accounts for 7% of renal pelvic tumors. Squamous cell cancer of the renal pelvis is often deeply invasive and is associated with a worse prognosis than is transitional cell carcinoma.[287] Adenocarcinoma of the renal pelvis has been reported in few patients and occurs in association with inflammation, infection, or calculi.[262,265,288]

DIAGNOSTIC AND STAGING TECHNIQUES

The differential diagnosis of renal pelvic carcinoma is given in Table 33–10. Hematuria is the initial pelvic presenting symptom in most patients. Gross hematuria is present in 62% to 75% and microscopic hematuria in 10%. The triad of flank mass, pain, and hematuria is encountered in 20% of patients or less and is associated often with advanced disease.[262,265,289–292]

Excretory urography is used frequently to evaluate patients with renal pelvic tumors and often reveals a filling defect in

TABLE 33-10. Differential Diagnosis of Cancer of the Renal Pelvis

Intrinsic Lesions

Calculus
Blood clot
Cholesteatoma
Malacoplakia
Inflammatory lesions of urothelium (*e.g.*, pyelitis cystics)
Benign ureteropelvic junction obstruction
Benign (connective tissue) tumors of renal pelvis
Renal cell carcinoma
Suburothelial hemorrhage

Extrinsic Lesions

Vascular impressions
Parapelvic cyst

(Modified from Fraly EE. Cancer of the renal pelvis. In: Skinner DG, de Kernion JB, eds. Genitourinary cancer. Philadelphia; WB Saunders, 1978:141)

the collecting system. There may be a hydronephrotic or nonfunctional kidney due to obstruction by a blood clot or mass.[262,264] Retrograde pyelography, in which contrast medium is injected into the ureter through an endoscope, accurately delineates upper tract filling defects. If there is uncertainty about the nature of a renal pelvic lesion, CT performed before and after administration of intravenous contrast material differentiates a tumor from another radiolucent mass such as a stone. Angiography is not often used in the diagnostic evaluation of a suspected renal pelvic tumor; however, a renal mass lesion that lacks the characteristic neovascularity of a renal cell carcinoma may be the first indication of a renal pelvic tumor invading the renal parenchyma.[293-295]

Urine cytology is useful in evaluating a renal pelvis mass, and endoscopically obtained barbotage specimens allow an accurate diagnosis to be made in about 80% of cases.[296,297] Sidransky and colleagues have demonstrated recently that identification of p53 mutations in bladder cancers and urine samples by PCR is possible.[66] This technique could be potentially useful in the diagnosis and management of patients with upper tract urothelial lesions. Tissue can be obtained by introducing a biopsy brush into the ureter and removing a specimen for cytologic or histologic examination. Brush biopsy increases diagnostic accuracy to between 80% and 90%. Recently developed endoscopic ureteroscopy and percutaneous nephroscopy have dramatically improved the diagnosis of upper tract tumors. With available endoscopic instruments, the renal pelvis can be inspected visually in more than 90% of patients.[262,290,298,299]

STAGE AND GRADE

The most significant prognostic factors for survival of patients with renal pelvic carcinoma are stage and grade of tumor.[290,300] Renal pelvic cancer is divided into four stages. Stage I is papillary carcinoma without evidence of invasion, stage II denotes tumor that is superficially invasive but limited to the lamina propria, stage III denotes involvement of the muscularis, and

stage IV denotes extent to adjacent structures or metastatic disease (Table 33–11). Renal pelvic tumors are graded from I to III. The 5-year survival for patients with grade I transitional cell carcinoma of the renal pelvis approaches 100%; for grade II, it is 60% to 70%; and for grade III, it is 5%. Invasion of the renal hilum occurs in 95% of patients who ultimately develop metastases.[290,300,301]

TREATMENT

Carcinoma of the renal pelvis may be treated with a radical nephrectomy that includes removal of Gerota's fascia and its contents, total removal of the ipsilateral ureter, and removal of a cuff of bladder.[262,265,290,292,302-304] Simple intrafascial nephrectomy is associated with a decreased 5-year survival rate compared with that for radical nephrectomy, particularly in patients with stage III or IV tumors.[303] If transitional cell carcinoma of the renal pelvis invades the renal vein or vena cava, an extensive surgical procedure including thrombus extraction or partial vena cava resection may be required.[262,265,290,292,302,303,305,306]

A more conservative surgical excision is advocated by some researchers who note that renal pelvic carcinoma can be bilateral and that survival of patients with low-stage, low-grade renal pelvic carcinoma treated with a conservative surgical procedure is about the same as in patients treated with more radical surgery.[307-309] The incidence of low-grade, low-stage renal pelvic carcinoma is about 8% and that of bilateral disease is 2%. There is often a long latent period before recurrence.[262,291,304] In most studies reporting a low recurrence rate after local excision, the follow-up period is short. When even low-stage, low-grade tumors were resected from the renal pelvis, a 29% to 30% incidence of recurrence in the ipsilateral ureter was found during a 20-year follow-up.[262] Although the availability of new techniques such as intraoperative nephroscopy and brush cytology have made staging much more accurate, intraoperative pyeloscopy is not without risk. In a recent series of 18 patients with renal pelvic carcinoma who underwent intraoperative pyeloscopy for evaluation and staging, 2 experienced disease recurrence in the renal fossa.[310] Most clinicians consider local, partial excision appropriate for patients with a solitary kidney, with bilateral renal pelvic carcinoma, or with renal insufficiency. New treatment strat-

TABLE 33-11. Staging for Renal Pelvic Cancer

Stage I	Papillary or planar (nonpapillary) carcinoma with no evidence of invasion.
Stage II	Papillary or planar carcinoma. Superficially invasive but with invasion limited to the lamina propria.
Stage III	Papillary or planar carcinoma, extending to the level of the muscularis (may extend beyond the muscularis in intrarenal portions of the renal pelvis if confined to the kidney).
Stage IV	Papillary or planar carcinoma extending to the adventitial surface and involving adjuvant structures or metastatic structures or both.

(Modified from Bennington JL, Beckwith JB, eds. Tumors of the kidney, renal pelvis, and ureter. Fascicle 12. 2nd ed. Washington, DC: Armed Forces Institute of Pathology, 1975)

egies involving percutaneous or ureteroscopic resection of renal pelvic tumors followed by laser irradiation or supplemental intracavitary therapy with mitomycin C or bacillus Calmette-Guérin are being evaluated.[299,311-315]

FOLLOW-UP

Conscientious follow-up after surgery for renal pelvic carcinoma is essential. Urinalysis, urine cytology, and cystourethroscopy are performed every 3 months for 2 to 3 years, then less frequently. For patients who undergo a conservative upper tract procedure, periodic retrograde pyelography is performed.[262]

URETERAL CARCINOMA

Ureteral carcinoma is an uncommon neoplasm that accounts for only 1% of all malignancies of the upper genitourinary tract. Ureteral carcinoma was first reported by the French pathologist Rayer in 1841; the first ureteral carcinoma to be removed by nephroureterectomy was reported by Vorphl in 1905. Ureteral carcinoma tends to occur in the older age groups, predominantly in the sixth, seventh, and eighth decades of life. The male to female ratio is 2 to 1. The most common site for the occurrence of a ureteral tumor is in the lower third of the ureter, with a lesser incidence higher up.[316-321]

TABLE 33-12. Classification of Tumors of the Ureter

Primary Tumors

Epithelial
  Malignant
    Transitional cell carcinoma (71%)
    Transitional cell carcinoma with differentiation (20%)
      Squamous differentiation
      Glandular differentiation
      Mixed
    Squamous cell carcinoma (pure; 8%)
    Adenocarcinoma (1%)
    Undifferentiated carcinoma (1%)
  Benign
    Papilloma
Mesodermal
  Malignant
    Leiomyosarcoma
  Benign
    Fibroepithelial polyp
    Leiomyoma
    Neurilemmoma
    Angioma

Secondary Tumors (All Malignant)

Drop metastases
Metastases by way of blood or lymph
Direct extension

(Modified from Bennington JL, Beckwith JB, eds. Tumors of the kidney, renal pelvis, and ureter. Fascicle 12. 2nd ed. Washington, DC: Armed Forces Institute of Pathology, 1975)

Histology and Etiology

Ninety percent of malignant tumors of the ureter are transitional cell carcinomas; 20% have squamous or glandular differentiation. Eight percent of the tumors are pure squamous cell carcinomas and 1% are adenocarcinomas (Table 33-12). Tumors of the ureter share embryologic, morphologic, and etiologic characteristics with renal pelvic tumors. As with renal pelvic tumors, there is an increased incidence of ureteral carcinoma associated with Balkan nephropathy, prolonged exposure to phenacetin, or prolonged exposure to environmental agents such as aniline dyes.[322]

Clinical Presentation

Hematuria is the most common presenting symptom and is present in 75% of patients with ureteral carcinoma. The hematuria is usually painless; however, colicky pain due to obstruction by clot or by tumor occurs in up to 35% of these patients. Urinary frequency or dysuria, present in only 10% of patients with renal pelvic carcinoma, occurs in up to 50% of patients with ureteral carcinoma.[318,322]

Ureteral carcinoma is divided into five stages (Table 33-13). Stage 0 ureteral carcinoma is confined to the mucosa of the ureter; stage A disease involves the lamina propria. In stage B, the tumor involves the muscularis of the ureter, and in stage C, the tumor extends through the muscularis to the adventitia. Stage D is metastatic disease. Although up to 100% of grade I tumors and 85% of grade II tumors may be noninvasive, only 30% of grade II and 8% of grade IV tumors are noninvasive.[322]

Diagnosis

Excretory urography is an initial part of the evaluation of a suspected ureteral mass lesion. On excretory urography, the upper tract above the tumor may be completely normal or there may be hydronephrosis or complete nonfunction. Retrograde pyelography is performed to delineate accurately the precise location of the ureteral lesion.[322,323] Urine is collected for cytologic examination, and brush biopsy may be performed to obtain tissue for histologic examination. Flexible endoscopy has greatly improved the surgeon's ability to visualize and biopsy ureteral lesions, and its use is part of the standard management of this disease.[299,313-315] Abdominal CT also provides useful staging information, particularly with regard to extension of the tumor outside the ureter.

Treatment

Traditionally, carcinoma of the ureter has been treated by nephroureterectomy (Fig. 33-11) or partial ureterec-

TABLE 33-13. Staging of Ureteral Carcinoma

Stage 0	Limited to mucosa
Stage A	Lamina propria invasion
Stage B	Confined to muscularis
Stage C	Invasion through muscularis with involvement of adjacent structures of metastases
Stage D	Metastatic

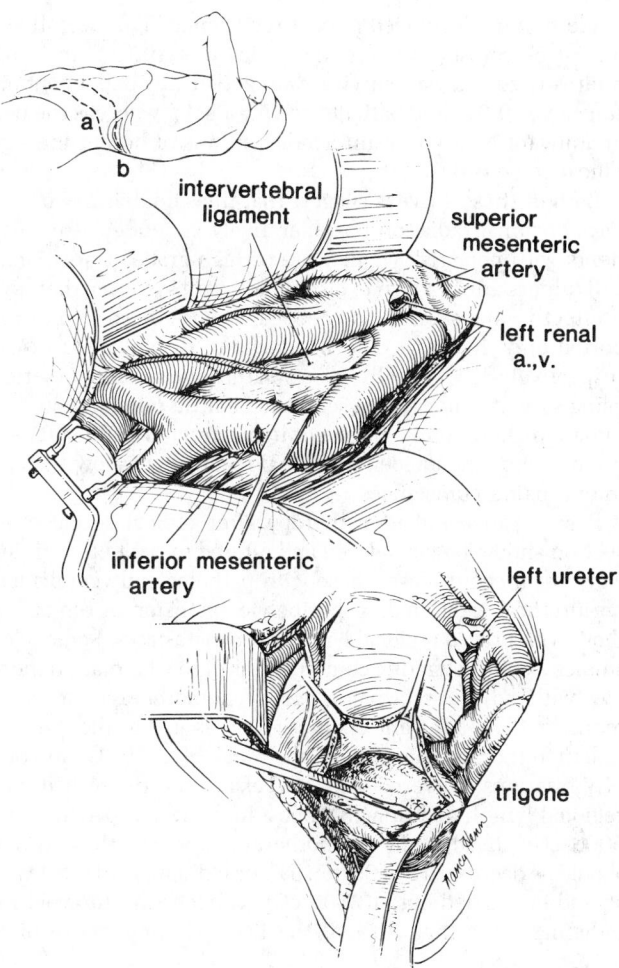

FIGURE 33–11. For a nephroureterectomy with lymph node dissection, the patient should be placed in a modified flank position and an incision made through line *a* or line *b*. The area of dissection is indicated in the middle panel, being divested from the superior mesenteric artery to the bifurcation. The ureter is removed by opening the bladder, circumscribing the orifice, and sharply dissecting the ureter from the surrounding detrusor muscle. The defect in the bladder is then closed appropriately. (Paulson DF, Perez CA, Anderson T. Cancer of the kidney and ureter. In: DeVita VT Jr, Hellman S, Rosenberg SA, eds: Cancer: Principles and practice of oncology. 2nd ed. Philadelphia: JB Lippincott, 1985:907)

TABLE 33–14. Correlation of Survival Rate With Pathologic Characteristics of Ureteral Cancer

	5-Year Survival Rate (%)	
	Bloom et al, 1970[325] *(54 Patients)*	*Batata et al, 1975*[321] *(41 Patients)*
Histologic Grade		
I	83.0	78.0
II	52.0	50.0
III	18.0	0
IV	12.0	0
Pathologic Stage		
0, A	62.0	91.0
B	50.0	43.0
C	33.3	23.0
D	0	

tomy.[264,317,318,324] The advantage of a partial ureterectomy is that the more conservative procedure preserves the kidney. However, mapping studies of the urothelium have demonstrated that carcinoma of the upper urinary tract is a multifocal disease. There is often atypia and carcinoma in situ in multiple areas of the urothelium, particularly in high-grade, high-stage carcinomas. Ureteral carcinoma treated by partial ureterectomy or by nephrectomy plus partial ureterectomy is associated with a 12% to 40% recurrence rate.[318,324] Those who advocate more conservative management of ureteral carcinoma note that in low-stage, low-grade carcinomas, distal ureterectomy with reimplantation of the distal ureter is associated with excellent survival[264,308] and that survival depends more on grade and stage of disease (Table 33–14) than on the type of operation performed.[291,325] In a study reported by Babaian and Johnson, there was a 100% 5-year survival rate

in patients with stage 0 or A distal ureteral carcinoma who were treated with distal ureterectomy plus reimplantation.[264] Distal ureterectomy plus reimplantation is recommended for patients with low-stage, low-grade disease that occurs in the distal third of the ureter. Nephroureterectomy is recommended for patients with high-grade or high-stage tumor and for those with disease at a location other than the distal third of the ureter.

Radical nephrectomy plus ureterectomy entails removal of the kidney and the entire contents of Gerota's fascia, the ureter, and a cuff of bladder including the ureteral orifice and intramural ureter. Regional lymph nodes may be removed, particularly if there is indication of involvement. This surgical procedure may be performed using one or two incisions, depending on the patient's body habitus and the surgeon's preference. When partial ureterectomy is performed, urinary tract continuity is reestablished with ureteroureterostomy or ureteroneocystostomy.

New strategies involving endoscopic resection, fulguration, and laser photocoagulation have been developed for treatment of patients with ureteral carcinoma.[326] Transurethral ureteropyeloscopy has become a standard diagnostic regimen for the investigation of upper tract filling defects.[315] Conservative endourologic techniques for management of upper tract urothelial tumors have been recommended for selected patients with low-grade transitional cell carcinoma.[299,315] Carcinoma in situ of the distal ureter has been treated with endoscopic fulguration, with encouraging preliminary results.[327] These new therapeutic strategies will be important in the future evaluation of the role of radical compared with local surgery for treatment of this disease.

Results of Therapy

The 5-year survival of patients with ureteral carcinoma is determined primarily by the grade and stage of the disease. Sex and age of the patient and multiplicity of tumor sites do not greatly influence survival. Patients with stage 0 or A ureteral carcinoma have a 90% to 100% 5-year survival rate. Patients with stage B disease have a 45% to 85% survival, and patients with stage C disease have a 25% to 30% 5-year survival rate. The 5-year survival for patients with stage D disease is 0% to 5%.

Adjuvant Radiation Therapy for Carcinoma of the Renal Pelvis and Ureter

The results of surgical resection alone by nephroureterectomy for patients with high-stage (C or III) or high-grade transitional cell carcinoma are poor, with less than 30% of the patients being cured by surgery alone.[319,328–330] Autopsy studies indicate that lymph node involvement occurs in 37% to 82% of patients with pelvic tumors related to initial tumor size and invasion.[289,331] In patients with ureteral transitional cell tumors, lymph node involvement has been reported in 22% to 41% of patients, depending on initial tumor size and grade.[320] The local recurrence rate has been reported to be higher after surgical resection for invasive pelvic transitional cell tumors (43%) than for invasive tumors of the ureter (14%). This is explained in part by the greater latency and diagnosis for patients with pelvic tumors.[288,318] Patients treated with radical surgery alone who have initial local recurrence often have the simultaneous or subsequent development of distant metastases. Distant metastases in many series are reported with much greater frequency than patients presenting with high-stage tumors. This rate is as high as that seen for patients presenting with invasive transitional cell carcinoma of the bladder. In a recent analysis, 14 of 26 patients with high-stage tumors (54%) developed distant metastases after radical surgery.[330] For patients with high-stage and high-grade transitional cell tumors, the need for successful therapies adjuvant to surgical removal clearly exists.

In the absence of data from randomized phase III trials, it is difficult to document benefit from adjuvant local and regional external-beam irradiation or from systemic chemotherapy. Nevertheless, two thorough retrospective reviews of patients with poor-risk (high-stage or high-grade) transitional cell carcinoma of the renal pelvis and ureter found that patients treated with postoperative radiation therapy had a lower incidence of local recurrence and a higher 5-year survival that was nearly statistically significant.[329,330] The first report, by Brookland and Richter, found that poor-risk patients receiving postoperative radiation therapy from 4000 to 5000 cGy had a lower incidence of local recurrence (1% versus 46%) and a higher 5-year survival (27% versus 17%) than patients treated with surgery alone.[329] The second thorough retrospective analysis, by Cozad and colleagues, involved 68 patients undergoing radical surgery for transitional cell carcinoma of the renal pelvis and ureter. Freedom from local recurrence and overall survival were improved in the subgroup (mostly with high-stage or high-grade tumors) who were selected for and treated with postoperative external-beam irradiation doses from 4500 to 5000 cGy.[330] Using multivariate analysis and considering sex, age, adjuvant radiation therapy, surgical procedure, grade, and tumor resection margins, the only significant predictors of local recurrence were high tumor grade and no administration of adjuvant external-beam irradiation. Four of 38 patients (11%) with low-grade tumors and 11 of 128 patients (61%) with high-grade tumors who did not undergo adjuvant radiation therapy developed local recurrence, whereas only 1 of 5 (20%) patients selected for and receiving adjuvant postoperative radiation therapy for high-

grade tumors developed a local recurrence. The overall actuarial 5-year survival for this series was 49%. Using Cox multivariate analysis, survival was statistically dependent on stage ($p = 0.01$) and patient age ($p = 0.01$), whereas the use of adjuvant external-beam irradiation was of borderline significance ($p = 0.07$).

Both of these surveys suggest that the safe delivery of external-beam irradiation postoperatively is beneficial for patients with poor-risk (high-stage or high-grade) transitional cell tumors after radical excision. Adjuvant systemic therapy, if effective and safe, is also needed because these studies reported only 45% and 54% incidence of distant metastases, respectively.[329,330] Finally, based on these series and on series using surgery alone, there seems to be little role for adjuvant radiation therapy for low-stage upper tract transitional cell tumors when the incidence of local recurrence is low, except in unusual circumstances.

Postoperative radiation therapy after radical surgical resection should be considered and offered to patients with locally advanced disease, those with pathologically confirmed periurethral, perirenal, or peripelvic extension of tumor, or those with proved regional lymph node metastases. Some pilot studies are investigating combinations of local radiation therapy with adjuvant cisplatin-based chemotherapeutic regimens.[332] If no adjuvant chemotherapy is given, the dose of radiation therapy should be in the range of 4500 cGy in 180-cGy fractions delivered over 5 weeks to the tumor bed and regional lymph nodes, with a boost to the tumor bed of up to 5000 cGy. If adjuvant chemotherapy is given, these doses should be decreased by 10% to 15%. In addition, field reduction should be carried out at 3600 cGy as necessary to avoid irradiating more than 30% of the liver parenchyma to high dose.

Chemotherapy for Metastatic Carcinomas of the Renal Pelvis and Ureter

Carcinomas arising in the ureters and renal pelvis are mainly transitional cell carcinomas.[264] They can be multiple (metachronously or synchronously),[333] occur with increased frequency in Balkan nephropathy (a toxic nephropathy indigenous to the Danube basin),[334] and give rise to metastases in about 40% of patients.[264] The histology, biology, and natural history make it appropriate for the medical oncologist to consider transitional cell carcinomas of the ureter and renal pelvis as pathologic entities indistinct from transitional cell carcinoma of the bladder. There are distinctive features to the surgical management of ureteral and renal pelvis tumors based on anatomic differences; however, the patterns of local recurrence and systemic spread and response to treatment are similar to histologically identical tumors arising in the bladder.[335]

The treatment of metastatic disease is the same as that for metastatic bladder cancer. The most active regimen is M-VAC, a four-drug regimen consisting of methotrexate, vincristine, doxorubicin, and cisplatin that was developed by Yagoda and colleagues at Memorial Sloan-Kettering Cancer Center.[336] M-VAC produces objective responses (complete and partial) in 69% of patients with metastatic transitional cell carcinoma of bladder, ureter, and renal pelvis.[336] The use of cyclophosphamide, doxorubicin, and cisplatin in varying doses; routes (intravenous and intraarterial); and schedules has produced a similar response rate.[337] Both regimens are being evaluated in neoadjuvant trials. Chapter 34 discusses the treatment options for metastatic carcinomas of the renal pelvis and ureter and the direction of treatment approaches in further detail.

REFERENCES

1. Ries LAG, Hankey BF, Miller BA, Hartman MA, Edwards BK, eds. Cancer statistics review. National Institutes of Health publication no. 91-2789. Bethesda: National Cancer Institute, 1991.
2. Silverberg E, Boring C, Squires T. Cancer statistics. CA 1991:9–26.
3. DeKernion JB. Renal tumors. In: Walsh PC, Gittes RF, Perlmutter AD, eds. Campbell's urology. Philadelphia: WB Saunders, 1986:1294–1342.
4. Goodman MT, Morgenstern H, Wynder EL. A case-control study of factors affecting the development of renal cell carcinoma. Am J Epidemiol 1986;124:926–941.
5. Goodman MT, Morgenstern H, Wynder EL. A case-control study of factors affecting the development of renal cell cancer. Am J Epidemiol 1986;124:926–941.
6. Lieber MM, Tomera FM, Taylor WF, Farrow GM. Renal adenocarcinoma in young adults: Survival and variables affecting prognosis. J Urol 1981;125:164–168.
7. Castellanos RD, Aron BS, Evans AT. Renal adenocarcinoma in children: Incidence, therapy and prognosis. J Urol 1974;111:534–536.
8. Golimbu M, Joshi P, Sperber A, Tessler A, Al-Askari S, Morles P. Renal cell carcinoma: Survival and prognostic factors. Urology 1986;27:291–301.
9. Carson WJ. Tumors of the kidney histologic study. In: Transactions of the Section on Urology of the American Medical Association, 1928.
10. Glenn JF. Renal tumors. In: Harrison JH, Gittes RF, Perlmutter AD, eds. Campbell's urology. Philadelphia: WB Saunders, 1979:967–1009.
11. Grawitz VP. Die sogenannten lipome der niere. Pathol Anat 1883;93:39–63.
12. Doderlein A, Birch-Hirschfeld FV. Embryonale drusengeschwulst der nierengegend im kindesalter. Sex Organe 1894;3:88–99.
13. Outzen HC, Maguire HC. The etiology of renal-cell carcinoma. Semin Oncol 1983;10:378–384.
14. Lauritsen JG. Lindau's disease: A study of one family through six generations. Acta Chir Scand 1973;139:482–486.
15. Green JS, Bowmer MI, Johnson GJ. Von Hippel-Lindau disease in a Newfoundland kindred. Can Med Assoc J 1986;134:133–146.
16. Malek RS, Omess PJ, Benson RC. Renal cell carcinoma in Von Hippel-Lindau syndrome. Am J Med 1987;82:236–238.
17. McLaughlin JK, Mandel JS, Blot WJ, Schuman LM, Mehl ES, Fraumeni JF. A population-based case control study of renal cell carcinoma. JNCI 1984;72:275–284.
18. Washecka R, Hanna M. Malignant renal tumors in tuberous sclerosis. Urology 1991;37:340–343.
19. Yu MC, Mack TM, Hanisch R, Cicioni C, Henderson BE. Cigarette smoking, obesity, diuretic use, and coffee consumption as risk factors for renal cell carcinoma. JNCI 1986;77:351–356.
20. Whittemore AS, Paffenbarger RS, Anderson K, Lee JE. Early precursors of urogenital cancers in former college men. J Urol 1984;132:1256–1260.
21. Talamini R, Baron AE, Barra S, et al. A case-control study of risk factor for renal cell cancer in northern Italy. Cancer Causes Control 1990;1:125–131.
22. La Vecchia C, Negri E, D'Avanzo B, Franceschi S. Smoking and renal cell carcinoma. Cancer Res 1990;50:5231–5233.
23. Maclure M, Willett W. A case-control study of diet and risk of renal adenocarcinoma. Epidemiology 1990;1:430–440.
24. Kantor AF. Current concepts in the epidemiology and etiology of primary renal cell carcinoma. J Urol 1977;117:415–417.
25. Lornoy W, Becaus I, De Vleeschouwer M. Renal cell carcinoma, a new complication of analgesic nephropathy. Lancet 1986;1:1271–1272.
26. Malker HR, Malker BK, McLaughlin JK, Blot WJ. Kidney cancer among leather workers. Lancet 1984;56–57.
27. Maclure M. Asbestos and renal adenocarcinoma: A case-control study. Environ Res 1987;42:353–361.
28. Ross RK, Paganini-Hill A, Landolph J, Gerkins V, Henderson BE. Analgesics, cigarette smoking, and other risk factors for cancer of the renal pelvis and ureter. Cancer Res 1989;49:1045–1048.
29. DeKernion JB, Smith RB. The kidney and adrenal glands. In: Paulson DF, ed. Genitourinary surgery. New York: Churchill Livingstone, 1984:1–153.
30. Kauzlaric D, Barmeir E, Binek J, Ramelli F, Petrovic M. Renal carcinoma after retrograde pyelography with thorotrast. AJR 1987;148:897–898.
31. Enterline PE, Viren J. Epidemiologic evidence for an association between gasoline and kidney cancer. Environ Health Perspect 1985;62:303–312.
32. McLaughlin JK, Blot WJ, Mehl ES, Stewart PA, Venable FS, Fraumeni JF. Petroleum-related employment and renal cell cancer. J Occup Med 1985;672–674.
33. Chung-Park M, Parveen T, Lam M. Acquired cystic disease of the kidneys and renal cell carcinoma in chronic renal insufficiency without dialysis treatment. Nephron 1989;53:157–161.
34. Matson MA, Cohen EP. Acquired cystic kidney disease: Occurrence, prevalence, and renal cancers. Medicine (Baltimore) 1990;69:217–226.
35. Bretan PN, Busch MP, Hricak H. Development of acquired renal cysts and renal cell carcinoma. Cancer 1986;57:1871–1879.
36. Brennan JF, Stilmant MM, Babayan RK, Siroky MB. Acquired renal cystic disease: Implications for the urologist. Br J Urol 1991;67:342–348.
37. Grantham JJ, Levin E. Acquired cystic disease: Replacing one kidney disease with another. Kidney Int 1985;28:99–105.
38. Hughson MD, Buchwald D, Fox M. Renal neoplasia and acquired cystic kidney disease in patients receiving long-term dialysis. Arch Pathol Lab Med 1986;110:592–600.
39. MacDougall ML, Welling LW, Wiegmann TB. Renal adenocarcinoma and acquired cystic disease in chronic hemodialysis patients. Am J Kidney Dis 1987;9:166–171.
40. Chisholm GD. Nephrogenic ridge tumors and their syndromes. Ann NY Acad Sci 1984;230:403–423.
41. Fan K, Smith DJ. Hypercalcemia associated with renal cell carcinoma: Probable role of neoplastic stromal cells. Hum Pathol 1983;14:168–173.
42. Evans BK, Fagan C, Arnold T, Dropcho EJ, Oh SJ. Paraneoplastic motor neuron disease and renal cell carcinoma: Improvement after nephrectomy [see comments]. Neurology 1990;40:960–962.
43. Sufrin G, Chasan S, Golio A, Murphy GP. Paraneoplastic and serologic syndromes of renal adenocarcinoma. Semin Urol 1989;7:158–171.
44. Thiede MA, Strewler GJ, Nissenson RA, Rosenblatt M, Rodan GA. Human renal carcinoma expresses two messages encoding a parathyroid hormone-like peptide: Evidence for the alternative splicing of a single-copy gene. Proc Natl Acad Sci USA 1988;85:4605–4609.
45. Klein RF, Strewler GJ, Leung SC, Nissenson RA. Parathyroid hormone-like adenylate cyclase-stimulating activity from a human carcinoma is associated with bone-resorbing activity. Endocrinology 1987;120:504–511.
46. Klein RF, Strewler GJ, Leung SC, Nissenson RA. Parathyroid hormone-like adenylate cyclase-stimulating activity from a human carcinoma is associated with bone-resorbing activity. Endocrinology 1987;120:504–511.
47. Nissenson RA, Strewler GJ, Williams RD, Leung SC. Activation of the parathyroid hormone receptor-adenylate cyclase system in osteosarcoma cells by a human renal carcinoma factor. Cancer Res 1985;45:5358–5363.
48. Strewler GJ, Williams RD, Nissenson RA. Human renal carcinoma cells produce hypercalcemia in the nude mouse and a novel protein recognized by parathyroid hormone receptors. J Clin Invest 1983;71:769–773.
49. Mehdizadeh S, Alaghband-Zadeh J, Gusterson B, Arlot M, Bradbeer JN, Loveridge N. Bone resorption and circulating PTH-like bioactivity in an animal model of hypercalcaemia of malignancy. Biochem Biophys Res Commun 1989;161:1166–1171.
50. Suva LJ, Winslow GA, Wettenhall REH, et al. A parathyroid hormone-related protein implicated in malignant hypercalcemia: Cloning and expression. Science 1987;237:893–896.
51. Cohen AJ, Li FP, Berg S, et al. Hereditary renal-cell carcinoma associated with a chromosomal translocation. N Engl J Med 1979;301:592–595.
52. Pathak S, Strong LC, Ferrell RE, Trindade A. Familial renal cell carcinoma with a 3:11 chromosome translocation limited to tumor cells. Science 1982;217:939–941.
53. King CR, Schimke RN, Arthur T, Davoren B, Collins D. Proximal 3p deletion in renal cell carcinoma cells from a patient with von Hippel-Lindau disease. Cancer Genet Cytogenet 1987;27:345–348.
54. Yoshida MA, Ohyashiki K, Ochi H, et al. Cytogenetic studies of tumor tissue from patients with nonfamilial renal cell carcinoma. Cancer Res 1986;46:2139–2147.
55. Yoshida MA, Ohyashiki K, Ochi H, et al. Rearrangement of chromosome 3 in renal cell carcinoma. Cancer Genet Cytogenet 1986;19:351–354.
56. Szucs S, Muller-Brechlin R, DeRiese W, Kovacs G. Deletion 3p: The only chromosome loss in a primary renal cell carcinoma. Cancer Genet Cytogenet 1987;26:369–373.
57. Carroll PR, Murty VVS, Reuter V, et al. Abnormalities of chromosome region 3p12-14 characterize clear cell renal carcinoma. Cancer Genet Cytogenet 1987;26:253–259.
58. Zbar B, Brauch H, Talmadge C, Linehan M. Loss of alleles of loci on the short arm of chromosome 3 in renal cell carcinoma. Nature 1987;327:721–724.
59. Cavenee WK, Dryja TP, Phillips RA, et al. Expression of recessive alleles by chromosomal mechanisms in retinoblastoma. Nature 1983;305:779–784.
60. Reeve A, Hiusiaux PJ, Gardner RJM. Loss of a Harvey ras allele in sporadic Wilms' tumor. Nature 1984;309:174–176.
61. Fearon ER, Vogelstein B, Feinberg AP. Somatic deletion and duplication of genes on chromosome 11 in Wilms' tumours. Nature 1984;309:176–178.
62. Xu H-J, Sumegi J, Hu S-X, et al. Intraocular tumor formation of RB reconstituted retinoblastoma cells. Cancer Res 1991;51:4481–4485.
63. Yandell DW, Campbell TA, Dayton SH, et al. Oncogenic point mutations in the human retinoblastoma gene: Their application to genetic counseling. N Engl J Med 1991;321:1689–1696.
64. Cavenee WK, Murphree AL, Shull MM, et al. Prediction of familial predisposition to retinoblastoma. N Engl J Med 1986;314:1201–1207.
65. Sklingelhutz AJ, Wu S-Q, Bookland EA, Reznikoff CA. Allelic 3p deletions in high-grade carcinomas after transformation in vitro of human uroepithelial cells. Genes Chromosom Cancer 1991;3:346–357.
66. Sidransky D, Von Eschenbach A, Tsai YC, et al. Identification of p53 gene mutations in bladder cancers and urine samples. Science 1991;252:706–709.
67. Brauch H, Johnson B, Hovis J, et al. Molecular analysis of the short arm of chromosome 3 in small-cell and non-small-cell carcinoma of the lung. N Engl J Med 1987;317:1109–1113.
68. Drabkin H, Kao FT, Hartz J, et al. Localization of human ERBA2 to the 3p22-3p24.1 region of chromosome 3 and variable deletion in small cell lung cancer. Proc Natl Acad Sci USA 1988;85:9258–9262.
69. Harbour JW, Lai SL, Whang-Peng J, Gazdar AF, Minna JD, Kaye FJ. Abnormalities

in structure and expression of the human retinoblastoma gene in SCLC. Science 1988;241:353–357.

70. Bodmer WF, Bailey CJ, Bodmer J, et al. Localization of the gene for familial adenomatous polyposis on chromosome 5. Nature 1987;328:614–616.

71. Solomon E, Voss R, Hall V, et al. Chromosome 5 allele loss in human colorectal carcinomas. Nature 1987;328:616–618.

72. Anglard P, Brauch TH, Weiss GH, et al. Molecular analysis of genetic changes in the origin and development of renal cell carcinoma. Cancer Res 1991;51:1071–1077.

73. Linehan M, Miller E, Anglard P, Merino M, Zbar B. Improved detection of allele loss in renal cell carcinomas after removal of leukocytes by immunologic selection. JNCI 1989;81:287–290.

74. Vogelstein B, Fearon ER, Kern SE, et al. Allelotype of colorectal carcinomas. Science 1989;244:207–211.

75. Kovacs G, Erlandsson R, Boldog F, et al. Consistent chromosome 3p deletion and loss of heterozygosity in renal cell carcinoma. Proc Natl Acad Sci USA 1988;85:1571–1575.

76. Ogawa O, Kakehi Y, Ogawa K, Koshiba M, Sugiyama T, Yoshida O. Allelic loss at chromosome 3p characterizes clear cell phenotype of renal cell carcinoma. Cancer Res 1991;51:949–953.

77. Presti JC, Rao PH, Chen Q, et al. Histopathological, cytogenetic, and molecular characterization of renal cortical tumors. Cancer Res 1991;51:1544–1552.

78. Van Der Hout A, Van Der Vlies P, Wijmenga C, Li FP, Oosterhuis JW, Buys CHCM. The region of common allelic losses in sporadic renal cell carcinoma is bordered by the loci D3S2 and THRB. Genomics 1991;11:537–542.

79. Yamakawa K, Morita R, Takahashi E, Hori T, Ishikawa J, Nakamura Y. A detailed deletion mapping of the short arm of chromosome 3 in sporadic renal cell carcinoma. Cancer Res 1991;51:4707–4711.

80. Leone A, McBride OW, Weston A, et al. Somatic allelic deletion of nm23 in human cancer. Cancer Res 1991;51:2490–2493.

81. Morita R, Ishikawa J, Tsutsumi M, et al. Allelotype of renal cell carcinoma. Cancer Res 1991;51:820–823.

82. Fearon ER, Feinberg AP, Hamilton SH, Vogelstein B. Loss of genes on the short arm of chromosome 11 in bladder cancer. Nature 1985;318:377–380.

83. Knudson AG. Genetics of human cancer. Annu Rev Genet 1986;20:231–251.

84. Moolgavkar SH, Knudson AG. Mutation and cancer: A model for human carcinogenesis. JNCI 1981;66:1037–1051.

85. Weissman BE, Saxon PJ, Pasquale SR, Jones GR, Geiser AG, Stanbridge EJ. Introduction of a normal human chromosome 11 into a Wilms' tumor cell line controls its tumorigenic expression. Science 1987;236:175–180.

86. Shimizu M, Yokota J, Mori N, et al. Introduction of normal chromosome 3p modulates the tumorigenicity of a human renal cell carcinoma cell line YCR. Oncogene 1990;5:185–194.

87. Oshimura M, Kugoh H, Koi M, et al. Transfer of a normal human chromosome 11 suppresses tumorigenicity of some but not all tumor cell lines. J Cell Biochem 1990;42:135–142.

88. Glenn GM, Choyke PL, Zbar B, Linehan WM. Von Hippel-Lindau disease: Clinical aspects and molecular genetics. In: Anderson EE, ed. Problems in urologic surgery: Benign and malignant tumors of the kidney. Philadelphia: JB Lippincott 1990:312–330.

89. Solomon D, Schwartz A. Renal pathology in von Hippel-Lindau disease. Hum Pathol 1988;19:1072–1079.

90. Tory K, Brauch H, Linehan M, et al. Specific genetic change in tumors associated with von Hippel-Lindau disease. JNCI 1989;81:1097–1101.

91. Seizinger BR, Rouleau GA, Ozelius LJ, et al. Von Hippel-Lindau disease maps to the region of chromosome 3 associated with renal cell carcinoma. Nature 1988;332:268–269.

92. Hosoe S, Brauch H, Latif F, et al. Localization of the von Hippel-Lindau disease gene to a small region of chromosome 3. Genomics 1990;8:634–640.

93. Glenn GM, Linehan WM, Hosoe S, et al. Screening for von Hippel-Lindau disease by DNA-polymorphism analysis. JAMA 1992;267:1226–1231.

94. Tannenbaum M. Ultrastructural pathology of human renal cell tumors. Pathol Annu 1971;6:249–277.

95. Fisher ER, Horvat B. Comparative ultrastructural study of so-called renal adenoma and carcinoma. J Urol 1972;108:382–386.

96. Mostofi FK, Davis CJ. Principles and management of urologic cancer. In: Javadpour N ed. Pathology of urologic cancer. Baltimore: Williams & Wilkins, 1983:54–126.

97. Bonsib SM, Fischer J, Plattner S, Fallon B. Sarcomatoid renal tumors: Clinicopathologic correlation of three cases. Cancer 1987;59:527–532.

98. Bertoni F, Ferri C, Benati A, Bacchini P, Corrado F. Sarcomatoid carcinoma of the kidney. J Urol 1987;137:25–28.

99. Ro JY, Ayala AG, Sella A, Samuels ML, Swanson DA. Sarcomatoid renal cell carcinoma: A clinicopathologic study of 42 cases. Cancer 1987;59:516–526.

100. Skinner DG, Calvin RB, Vermillion CD, Pfister RC, Leadbetter WF. Diagnosis and management of renal cell carcinoma. Cancer 1971;28:1165–1177.

101. Selli C, Hinshaw WM, Woodard BH, Paulson DF. Stratification of risk factors in renal cell carcinoma. Cancer 1983;52:899–903.

102. Boxer RJ, Waisman J, Lieber MM, Mampaso FM, Skinner DG. Renal carcinoma: Computer analysis of 96 patients treated by nephrectomy. J Urol 1979;122:598–601.

103. Sella A, Logothetis J, Ro JY, Swanson DA, Samuels ML. Sarcomatoid renal cell carcinoma: A treatable entity. Cancer 1987;60:1313–1318.

104. Antonarakis SE, Kazazian HH Jr, Orkin SH. DNA polymorphism and molecular pathology of the human globin gene clusters. Hum Genet 1985;69:1–14.

105. McNichols DW, Segura JW, Deweerd JH. Renal cell carcinoma: Long-term survival and late recurrence. J Urol 1981;126:17–23.

106. Silverberg E. Cancer statistics. Cancer 1981;31:13–28.

107. Maldazys JD, deKernion JB. Prognostic factors in metastatic renal carcinoma. J Urol 1986;136:376–379.

108. Samaan NA. Paraneoplastic syndromes associated with renal carcinoma: A pilot study. J Clin Oncol 1987;6:862.

109. Pinals RS, Krane SM. Medical aspects of renal carcinoma. Postgrad Med J 1962;38:507–529.

110. Cherukuri SV, Johenning PW, Ram MD. Systemic effects of hypernephroma. Urology 1977;X:93–97.

111. Sufrin G, Mirand A, Moore RH, Chu TM, Murphy GP. Hormones in renal cancer. J Urol 1977;117:433–438.

112. Utz DW, Warren MM, Gregg JA. Reversible hepatic dysfunction associated with hypernephroma. Mayo Clin Proc 1970;45:161.

113. Boxer RJ, Waisman J, Lieber MM, Mampaso FM, Skinner DG. Non-metastatic hepatic dysfunction associated with renal carcinoma. J Urol 1978;119:468–471.

114. Hanash KA, Utz DC, Ludwig J, Wakim KG, Ellefson RD, Kelalis PP. Syndrome of reversible hepatic dysfunction associated with hypernephroma: An experimental study. Invest Urol 1971;8:399–404.

115. Da Silva JL, Lacombe C, Bruneval P, et al. Tumor cells are the site of erythropoietin synthesis in human renal cancers associated with polycythemia. Blood 1990;75:577–582.

116. Lindop GB, Fleming S. Renin in renal cell carcinoma—an immunocytochemical study using an antibody to pure human renin. J Clin Pathol 1984;37:27–31.

117. Lindop GBM, Leckie B, Winearls CG. Malignant hypertension due to a renin-secreting renal cell carcinoma: An ultrastructural immunocytochemical study. Histopathology 1986;10:1077–1088.

118. Sufrin G, Mink I, Moore FR. Coagulation factors in renal adenocarcinoma. J Urol 1978;119:727–730.

119. Dawson NA, Barr CF, Alving BM. Acquired dysfibrinogenemia. Am J Med 1985;78:682–686.

120. Lang EK. Asymptomatic space-occupying lesions of the kidney: A programmed sequential approach and its impact on quality and cost of health care. South Med J 1977;70:277–285.

121. Frohmuller HGW, Grups JW, Heller V. Comparative value of ultrasonography, computerized tomography, angiography and exretory urography in the staging of renal cell carcinoma. J Urol 1987;138:482–484.

122. Juul N, Torp-Pedersen S, Gronvall S, Holm HH, Koch F, Larsen S. Ultrasonically guided fine needle aspiration biopsy of renal masses. J Urol 1985;133:579–581.

123. Lang EK. Comparison of dynamic and conventional computed tomography, angiography, and ultrasonography in the staging of renal cell carcinoma. Cancer 1984;54:2205–2214.

124. Karp W, Ekelung L, Olafsson G, Olsson A. Computed tomography, angiography and ultrasound in staging of renal carcinoma. Acta Radiol 1981;22:625–633.

125. Mauro MA, Wadsworth DE, Stanley RJ, McClenna BL. Renal cell carcinoma: Angiography in the CT Era. AJR 1982;139:1135–1138.

126. Zabbo A, Novick AC, Risius B, Montie JE. Digital subtraction angiography for evaluating patients with renal carcinoma. J Urol 1985;134:352–355.

127. Richie JP, Garnick MB, Seltzer S, Bettman MA. Computerized tomography scan for diagnosis and staging of renal cell carcinoma. J Urol 1983;129:1114–1116.

128. Stephenson TF, Iyengar S, Rashid HA. Comparison of computerized tomography and excretory urography in detection and evaluation of renal masses. J Urol 1984;131:11–13.

129. Jashke W, Kaick GV, Peter S. Accuracy of computed tomography in staging of kidney tumors. Acta Radiol 1982;23:593–598.

130. Kothari K, Segal AJ, Spitzer RM, Peartree RJ. Preoperative radiographic evaluation of hypernephroma. J Comput Assist Tomogr 1981;5:702–704.

131. Yokoyama M, Watanabe K, Inatsuki S. Computerized tomography of the kidney: Tissue-plasma ratio of contrast enhancement with bolus injection and renal function. J Urol 1982;127:721–723.

132. Lang EK. Angio-computed tomography and dynamic computed tomography in staging of renal cell carcinoma. Radiology 1984;151:149–155.

133. Medenica R, Slack N. Clinical results of leukocyte interferon-induced tumor regression in resistant human metastatic cancer resistant to chemotherapy and/or radiotherapy-pulse therapy schedule. Cancer Drug Deliv 1985;2:53–76.

134. Goldfarb DA, Novick AC, Lorig R, et al. Magnetic resonance imaging for assessment of vena caval tumor thrombi: A comparative study with venacavography and computerized tomography scanning. J Urol 1990;144:1100–1103.

135. Horan JJ, Robertson CN, Choyke PL, et al. The detection of renal carcinoma extension into the renal vein and inferior vena cava: A prospective comparison of venacavography and magnetic resonance imaging. J Urol 1989;142:943–948.

136. Karstaedt N, McCullough DL, Wolfman NT, Dyer RB. Magnetic resonance imaging of the renal mass. J Urol 1986;136:566–570.

137. Treiger BF, Humphrey LS, Peterson CV Jr, et al. Transesophageal echocardiography in renal cell carcinoma: An accurate diagnostic technique for intracaval neoplastic extension. J Urol 1991;145:1138–1140.

138. Robson CJ, Churchill BM, Anderson W. The results of radical nephrectomy for renal cell carcinoma. J Urol 1969;101:297–301.

139. Peters PC, Brown GL. The role of lymphadenectomy in the management of renal cell carcinoma. Urol Clin North Am 1991:705–709.

140. Siminovitch JMP, Montie JE, Straffon RA. Prognostic indicators in renal adenocarcinoma. J Urol 1983;130:20–23.

141. Ferrari P, Grassi D, Castagnetti G, Pollastri CA, Ferrari G. Neoplastic thrombosis in the renal cancer. Eur Urol 1990;17:27–29.

142. Kearney GP, Waters WB, Klein LA, Richie JP, Gittes RF. Results of inferior vena cava resection for renal cell carcinoma. J Urol 1981;125:769–773.

143. Sogani PC, Herr HW, Bains MS, Whitmore WF. Renal cell carcinoma extending into inferior vena cava. J Urol 1983;130:660–663.

144. Skinner DG, Pritchett TR, Lieskovsky G, Boyd SD, Stiles QR. Vena caval involvement by renal cell carcinoma. Surgical resection provides meaningful long-term survival. Ann Surg 1989;210:387–392.

145. Cherrie RJ, Goldman DG, Lindner A, deKernion JB. Prognostic implications of vena caval extension of renal cell carcinoma. J Urol 1982;128:910–912.

146. Giuliani L, Giberti C, Martorana G, Rovida S. Radical extensive surgery for renal cell carcinoma: long-term results and prognostic factors. J Urol 1990;143:468–473.

147. Bassil B, Dosoretz DE, Prout GR. Validation of the tumor, nodes and metastasis classification of renal cell carcinoma. J Urol 1985;134:450–454.

148. Tsukamoto T, Kumamoto Y, Yamazaki K, et al. Clinical analysis of incidentally found renal cell carcinomas. Eur Urol 1991;19:109–113.

149. Fahn HJ, Lee YH, Chen MT, Huang JK, Chen KK, Chang LS. The incidence and prognostic significance of humoral hypercalcemia in renal cell carcinoma. J Urol 1991;145:248–250.

150. Ljungberg B, Larsson P, Stenling R, Roos G. Flow cytometric deoxyribonucleic acid analysis in stage I renal cell carcinoma. J Urol 1991;146:697–699.

151. Currin SM, Lee SE, Walther PJ. Flow cytometric assessment of deoxyribonucleic acid content in renal adenocarcinoma: Does ploidy status enhance prognostic stratification over stage alone? J Urol 1990;143:458–463.

152. Gilbert JB. Diagnosis and treatment of malignant renal tumors. J Urol 1937;39:223–237.

153. McDonald MW. Current therapy for renal cell carcinoma. J Urol 1982;127:211–217.

154. Winter P, Miersch WD, Vogel J, Jaeger N. On the necessity of adrenal extirpation combined with radical nephrectomy. J Urol 1990;144:842–843.

155. Pritchett TR, Lieskovsky G, Skinner DG. Extension of renal cell carcinoma into the vena cava: Clinical review and surgical approach. J Urol 1986;135:460–464.

156. Linehan WM. Thoracoabdominal radical nephrectomy. In: Glenn JF, ed. Urologic surgery. Philadelphia: JB Lippincott, 1991:47–50.

157. Janosko EO, Powell CS, Spence PA, Hodges WE, Lust RM. Surgical management of renal cell carcinoma with extensive intracaval involvement using a venous bypass system suitable for rapid conversion to total cardiopulmonary bypass. J Urol 1991;145:555–557.

158. Stewart JR, Carey JA, McDougal WS, Merrill WH, Koch MO, Bender HW Jr. Cavoatrial tumor thrombectomy using cardiopulmonary bypass without circulatory arrest. Ann Thorac Surg 1991;51:717–721.

159. Belis JA, Pae WE Jr, Rohner TJ Jr, et al. Cardiovascular evaluation before circulatory arrest for removal of vena caval extension of renal carcinoma. J Urol 1989;141:1302–1307.

160. Marshall FF, Reitz BA, Diamond DA. A new technique for management of renal cell carcinoma involving the right atrium: Hypothermia and cardiac arrest. J Urol 1984;131:103–107.

161. DeKernion JB, Berry D. The diagnosis and treatment of renal cell carcinoma. Cancer 1980;45:1947–1956.

162. DeKernion JB. Lymphadenectomy for renal cell carcinoma: Therapeutic implications. Urol Clin North Am 1980:596–703.

163. Marshall FF, Powell KC. Lymphadenectomy for renal cell carcinoma: Anatomical and therapeutic considerations. J Urol 1982;128:677–681.

164. Novick AC, Gephardt G, Guz B, Steinmuller D, Tubbs RR. Long-term follow-up after partial removal of a solitary kidney [see comments]. N Engl J Med 1991;325:1058–1062.

165. Provet J, Tessler A, Brown J, Golimbu M, Bosniak M, Morales P. Partial nephrectomy for renal cell carcinoma: Indications, results and implications. J Urol 1991;145:472–476.

166. Angermeier KW, Novick AC, Streem SB, Montie JE. Nephron-sparing surgery for renal cell carcinoma with venous involvement. J Urol 1990;144:1352–1355.

167. Morgan WR, Zincke H. Progression and survival after renal-conserving surgery for renal cell carcinoma: experience in 104 patients and extended followup. J Urol 1990;144:852–857.

168. Palmer JM, Swanson DA. Conservative surgery in solitary and bilateral renal carcinoma: Indications and technical considerations. J Urol 1987;120:113–117.

169. Zincke H, Engen DE, Henning KM, McDonald MW. Treatment of renal cell carcinoma by in situ partial nephrectomy and extracorporeal operation with autotransplantation. Mayo Clin Proc 1985;60:651–662.

170. Mandel J, Kjellstrand CM. Long-term results of dialysis and transplantation in patients with end-stage renal failure from hypernephroma. Nephron 1986;44:111–114.

171. Smith RB, deKernion JB, Ehrlich RB, Skinner DG, Kaufman JJ. Bilateral renal cell carcinoma and renal cell carcinoma in the solitary kidney. J Urol 1984;132:450–454.

172. Jacobs SC, Berg SI, Lawson RK. Synchronous bilateral renal cell carcinoma: Total surgical excision. Cancer 1980;46:2341–2345.

173. Topley M, Novick AC, Montie JE. Long-term results following partial nephrectomy for localized renal adenocarcinoma. J Urol 1984;131:1050–1052.

174. Novick AC, Zincke H, Neves RJ, Topley HM. Surgical enucleation for renal cell carcinoma. J Urol 1986;135:235–238.

175. Marshall FF, Taxy JB, Fishman EK, Chang R. The feasibility of surgical enucleation for renal cell carcinoma. J Urol 1986;135:231–234.

176. DeKernion JB, Mukamel E. Selection of initial therapy for renal cell carcinoma. Cancer 1987;60:539–546.

177. Novick AC, Jackson CL, Straffon RA. The role of renal autotransplantation in complex urological reconstruction. J Urol 1990;143:452–457.

178. Clark RL, Brawer MK, Hunter GC, Pabst TS. Treatment of renal cell carcinoma by extracorporeal partial nephrectomy and autotransplantation using splenic vascular anastomosis. Surg Gynecol Obstet 1991;172:105–107.

179. Zincke H, Swanson SK. Bilateral renal cell carcinoma: Influence of synchronous and asynchronous occurrence on patient survival. J Urol 1982;128:913–915.

180. Rafla S. Renal cell carcinoma: Natural history and results of treatment. Cancer 1970;25:26–40.

181. Finney R. Radiotherapy in the treatment of hypernephroma: A clinical trial. Br J Urol 1973;45:26–40.

182. Kjaer M, Frederiksen PL, Engelholm SA. Postoperative radiotherapy in stage II and III renal adenocarcinoma: A randomized trial by the Cophenhagen renal cancer study group. Int J Radiation Oncology Biol Phys 1987;13:665–672.

183. van der Werf-Messing B. Carcinoma of the kidney. Cancer 1973;32:1056–1062.

184. DeKernion JB. Treatment of advanced renal cell carcinoma—traditional methods and innovative approaches. J Urol 1983;130:2–7.

185. Freed SZ. Nephrectomy for renal cell carcinoma with metastases. Urology 1977;9:613–175.

186. Montie JE, Stewart BH, Straffon RA, Banowsky LHW, Hewitt CB, Montague DK. The role of adjunctive nephrectomy in patients with metastatic renal cell carcinoma. J Urol 1977;117:272–275.

187. DeKernion JB, Ramming KP, Smith RB. The natural history of metastatic renal cell carcinoma: A computer analysis. J Urol 1978;120:148–152.

188. Middleton RG. Surgery for metastatic renal cell carcinoma. J Urol 1967;97:973–977.

189. Tolia BM, Whitmore WF. Solitary metastasis from renal cell carcinoma. J Urol 1975;114:836–838.

190. O'Dea MJ, Zincke H, Utz DC. The treatment of renal cell carcinoma with solitary metastasis. J Urol 1978;120:540–542.

191. Swanson DA, Wallace S, Johnson DE. The role of embolization and nephrectomy in the treatment of metastatic renal carcinoma. Urol Clin North Am 1980:719–730.

192. Flanigan RC. The failure of infarction and/or nephrectomy in stage IV renal cell cancer to influence survival or metastatic regression. Urol Clin North Am 1987:757–762.

193. Swanson DA, Johnson DE, von Eschenbach AC, Chung VP, Wallace S. Angioinfarction plus nephrectomy for metastatic renal cell carcinoma: An update. J Urol 1983;130:449–452.

194. Sundaresan N, Galicich JH, Baines MS. Vertebral body resection in the treatment of cancer involving the spine. Cancer 1984;53:1393–1396.

195. Sundaresan N, Scher H, Whitmore WF. Spinal cord compression in kidney cancer. Proc Am Soc Clin Oncol [Abstract] 1986;5:267.

196. Fossa SD, Kjolseth I, Lund G. Radiotherapy of metastasis from renal cancer. Eur Urol 1982;8:340–342.

197. Halperin EC, Harisiadis L. The role of radiation therapy in the management of metastatic renal cell carcinoma. Cancer 1983;51:614–617.

198. Onufrey V, Mohiuddin M. Radiation therapy in the treatment of metastatic renal cell carcinoma. Int J Radiat Oncol Biol Phys 1985;11:2007–2009.

199. Kjaer M. The treatment and prognosis of patients with renal adenocarcinoma with solitary metastasis: 10 year survival results. Int J Radiat Oncol Biol Phys 1987;13:619–621.

200. Harris DT. Hormonal therapy and chemotherapy of renal-cell carcinoma. Semin Oncol 1983;10:422–430.

201. Denis L, Van Oosterom A. Chemotherapy of metastatic renal cancer. Semin Surg Oncol 1988;4:91–94.

202. Yagoda A, Bander NH. Failure of cytotoxic chemotherapy, 1983–1988, and the emerging role of monoclonal antibodies for renal cancer. Urol Int 1989;44:338–345.

203. Yagoda A. Chemotherapy of renal cell carcinoma: 1983–1989. Semin Urol 1989;7:199–206.

204. Fojo AT, Ueda K, Slamon DJ, Poplack DG, Gottesman MM, Pastan I. Expression of a multidrug-resistance gene in human tumors and tissues. Proc Natl Acad Sci USA 1987;84:265–269.

205. Fojo AT, Shen DW, Mickley LA, Pastan I, Gottesman MM. Intrinsic drug resistance in kidney cancers is associated with expression of a human multidrug resistance gene. J Clin Oncol 1987;5:1922.

206. Mickisch G, Bier H, Bergler W, Bak M, Tschada R, Alken P. P-170 glycoprotein, glutathione and associated enzymes in relation to chemoresistance of primary human renal cell carcinomas. Urol Int 1990;45:170–176.

207. Mickisch GH, Roehrich K, Koessig J, Forster S, Tschada RK, Alken PM. Mechanisms and modulation of multidrug resistance in primary human renal cell carcinoma [see comments]. J Urol 1990;144:755–759.

208. Von Roemeling R, Hrushesky WJM. Determination of the therapeutic index of floxuridine by its circadian infusion pattern. JNCI 1990;82:386–393.

209. Von Roemeling R, Hrushesky WJM. Circadian patterning of continuous floxuridine infusion reduces toxicity and allows higher dose intensity in patients with widespread cancer. J Clin Oncol 1989;7:1710–1719.

210. Hrushesky WJ, von Roemeling R, Lanning RM, Rabatin JT. Circadian-shaped infusions of floxuridine for progressive metastatic renal cell carcinoma. J Clin Oncol 1990;8:1504–1513.

211. Huben RP, Dragone N, Wolf RM. Early results of a phase II study of continuous infusion FUDR in metastatic renal cell carcinoma. Proc Am Soc Clin Oncol [Abstract] 1989;8:131.

212. Damascelli B, Pizzocaro G, Spreadico C, et al. Improved survival in patients with continuous systemic infusion of FUDR. Proc Am Soc Clin Oncol [Abstract] 1989;30:259.

213. Geoffrois L, Conroy T, Hubert J, Krakowski I, Guillemin F, Volff D. Circadian modified FUDR infusion in patients with metastatic renal cell cancer: A confirmatory phase II study. Proc Am Soc Clin Oncol [Abstract] 1991;10:183.

214. Dexeus FH, Logothetis CJ, Sella A. Phase II study of continuous circadian infusion of

2-deoxy-5-fluorouridine (FURD) in metastatic renal cell carcinoma. Proc Am Assoc Cancer Res 1989;30:259.

215. Kirkman H, Bacon RL. Estrogen-induced tumors of the kidney. I. Incidence of renal tumors in intact and gonadectomized male golden hamsters treated with diethylstilbestrol. JNCI 1952;13:745–755.

216. Bloom HJG, Baker WH, Dukes CE, Mitchley BCV. Hormone-dependent tumours of the kidney: I. The oestrogen-induced renal tumor of the Syrian hamster—Hormone treatment and possible relationship to carcinoma of the kidney in man. Br J Cancer 1963;17:611–646.

217. Kjaer M. The role of medroxyprogesterone acetate (MPA) in the treatment of renal adenocarcinoma. Cancer Treat Rev 1988;15:195–209.

218. DeKernion JB, Sarna G, Figlin R. The treatment of renal cell carcinoma with human leukocyte alpha-interferon. J Urol 1983;130:1063.

219. Quesada JR, Swanson DA, Trindade A. Renal cell carcinoma: Antitumor effects of leukocyte interferon. Cancer Res 1983;43:940.

220. Krown SE. Interferon treatment of renal cell carcinoma: Current status and future prospects. Cancer 1987;59:647.

221. Quesada JR. Role of interferons in the therapy of metastatic renal cell carcinoma. Urology 1989;34:80–83.

222. Figlin RA, Abi-Aad AS, Belldegrun A, deKernion JB. The role of interferon and interleukin-2 in the immunotherapeutic approach to renal cell carcinoma. Semin Oncol 1991;18:102–107.

223. Muss MB. Renal cell carcinoma, in interferons clinical applications. In: DeVita VT, Hellman S, Rosenberg SA, eds. Biologic therapy of cancer. Philadelphia: JB Lippincott, 1991;298–310.

224. Marshall ME, Simpson W, Butler K, Fried A, Fer M. Treatment of renal cell carcinoma with daily low-dose alpha-interferon. J Biol Response Mod 1989;8:453–461.

225. Nanus DM, Pfeffer LM, Bander NH, Bahri S, Albino AP. Antiproliferative and antitumor effects of alpha-interferon in renal cell carcinomas: Correlation with the expression of a kidney-associated differentiation glycoprotein. Cancer Res 1990;50:4190–4194.

226. Quesada JR, Rios A, Swanson D. Antitumor activity of recombinant-derived interferon alpha in metastatic renal cell carcinoma. J Clin Oncol 1985;3:1522.

227. Recombinant human interferon gamma group: Phase II study of recombinant human interferon gamma (S6810 on renal cell carcinoma). Cancer 1992;60:929–930.

228. Aulitzky W, Gastl G, Aulitzky WE, et al. Successful treatment of metastatic renal cell carcinoma with a biologically active dose of recombinant interferon-gamma. J Clin Oncol 1989;7:1875–1884.

229. Garnick MB, Reich SD, Maxwell B. Phase I/II study of recombinant interferon gamma in advanced renal cell carcinoma. J Urol 1988;139:251–255.

230. Rosenberg SA, Lotze MT, Muul LM, et al. Observations on the systemic administration of autologous lymphokine-activated killer cells and recombinant interleukin-2 to patients with metastatic cancer. N Engl J Med 1985;313:1485–1492.

231. Rosenberg SA, Lotze MT, Muul LM, et al. A progress report on the treatment of 157 patients with advanced cancer using lymphokine-activated killer cells and interleukin-2 or high-dose interleukin-2 alone. N Engl J Med 1987;316:889–897.

232. Mule JJ, Rosenberg SA. Combination cytokine therapy: Experimental and clinical trials. In: DeVita VT, Hellman S, Rosenberg SA, eds. Biologic therapy of cancer. Philadelphia: JB Lippincott, 1991;393–416.

233. Yang JC, Rosenberg SA. Adoptive cellular therapy: preclinical studies. In: DeVita VT, Hellman S, Rosenberg JB, eds. Biologic therapy of cancer. Philadelphia: JB Lippincott, 1991;197–213.

234. Margolin KA, Raynor MJ, Hawkins MB, et al. Interleukin-2 and lymphokine-activated killer cell therapy of solid tumors: Analysis of toxicity and management guidelines. J Clin Oncol 1989;7:486.

235. Siegel JP, Puri RK. Interleukin-2 toxicity. J Clin Oncol 1991;9:694.

236. Lee RE, Lotze MT, Skibber JM, et al. Cardiorespiratory effects of immunotherapy with interleukin-2. J Clin Oncol 1989;7:7.

237. Belldegrun A, Webb DE, Austin HA III, et al. Effects of interleukin-2 on renal function in patients receiving immunotherapy for advanced cancer. Ann Intern Med 1987;106:817–822.

238. Rosenberg SA, Lotze MT, Yang JC, et al. Experience with the use of high-dose interleukin-2 in the treatment of 652 cancer patients. Ann Surg 1989;210:474–484.

239. Sznol M, Thurn A, Parkinson DR. Overview of interleukin-2 trials in patients with renal cell carcinoma. In: Bukowski RM, ed. Immunotherapy of renal cell carcinoma. New York: Marcel Dekker, 1992.

240. Negrier S, Philip T, Stoter G, et al. Interleukin-2 with or without LAK cells in metastatic renal cell carcinoma: A report of a European multicentre study. Eur J Cancer Clin Oncol 1989;25:S21.

241. Bajorin DF, Sell KW, Richards JM, et al. A randomized trial of interleukin-2 plus lymphokine-activated killer cells versus interleukin-2 alone in renal cell carcinoma. Proc Am Assoc Cancer Res 1990:1106.

242. Creekmore SP, Harris JE, Ellis TM, et al. A phase I clinical trial of recombinant interleukin-2 by periodic 24-hour intravenous infusions. J Clin Oncol 1989;7:276.

243. Perez EA, Schudder SA, Meyers FA, Tanaka MS, Paradise CH, Gandara DR. Weekly 24-hour continuous infusion interleukin-2 for metastatic melanoma and renal cell carcinoma: A phase I study. J Immunotherapy 1991;10:57.

244. Bukowski RM, Goodman P, Crawford ED, Sergi JS, Redman BGH, Whitehead RP. Phase II trial of high dose intermittent interleukin-2 in metastatic renal cell carcinoma: A southwest oncology group study. JNCI 1990;82:143–146.

245. Sleijfer D, Janssen R, Willemse P, et al. Subcutaneous interleukin-2 (Cetus) in patients with metastatic renal cell carcinoma. Proc Am Soc Clin Oncol 1991;163.

246. Rosenberg SA, Lotze MT, Yang JC, et al. Combination therapy with interleukin-2 and alpha-interferon for the treatment of patients with advanced cancer. J Clin Oncol 1989;7:1863–1874.

247. Atkins MB, Sparano J, Fisher RI, et al. Randomized phase II trial of high dose IL-2 either alone or in combination with interferon alpha 2B in advanced renal cell carcinoma. Proc Am Soc Clin Oncol 1991;166.

248. Aronson FR, Sznol M, Atkins MB, et al. A phase II trial of interleukin-2, interferon-alpha and lymphokine-activated killer cells for advanced renal cell carcinoma. Proc Am Soc Clin Oncol 1990;9:183.

249. Thompson JA, Lee DJ, Lindgren CG, et al. Influence of dose and duration of infusion of interleukin-2 on toxicity and immunodulation. J Clin Oncol 1988;6:669–678.

250. Weiss GR, Margolin KA, Aronson FR, et al. A randomized phase II trial of continuous infusion interleukin-2 or bolus injection IL-2 plus lymphokine-activated killer cells for advanced renal cell carcinoma. J Clin Oncol 1992;10:275–281.

251. Parkinson DR. Interleukin-2: Progress through further understanding. JNCI 1990;82:1374–1376.

252. Parkinson DR. Enhancement of the antineoplastic activity of interleukin-2. In: Atkins MB, Mier JW, eds. Therapeutic applications of interleukin-2. New York: Marcel Dekker, 1992 (in press).

253. Rosenberg SA, Spiess P, Lafreniere R. A new approach to the adoptive immunotherapy of cancer with tumor-infiltrating lymphocytes. Science 1986;233:1318–1321.

254. Rosenberg SA, Parckard B, Aebersold PM, Solomon D, Topalian SL. Immunotherapy of patients with metastatic melanoma using tumor infiltrating lymphocytes and interleukin-2: Preliminary report. N Engl J Med 1988;319:1676.

255. Osband ME, Lavin PT, Babayan RK, et al. Effect of autolymphocyte therapy on survival and quality of life in patients with metastatic renal-cell carcinoma. Lancet 1990;335:994–998.

256. Marshall ME, Mendelsohn L, Butler K. Treatment of metastatic renal cell carcinoma with coumarin (1.2-benzopyrone) and cimetidine: A pilot study. J Clin Oncol 1987;6:682.

257. Griffith KD, Read EJ, Carrasquillo JA, et al. In vivo distribution of adoptively transferred indium-111-labeled tumor infiltrating lymphocytes and peripheral blood lymphocytes in patients with metastatic melanoma. JNCI 1989;81:1709–1717.

258. Herrmann R, Egri T, Manegold C, et al. Coumarin and cimetidine in the treatment of metastatic renal cell carcinoma. Proc Am Soc Clin Oncol [Abstract] 1988;7:131.

259. Nanus DM, Pfeffer LM, Bander NH, Bahri S, Albino AP. Antiproliferative and antitumor effects of α-interferon in renal cell carcinomas: Correlation with the expression of a kidney-associated differentiation glycoprotein. Cancer Res 1990;50:4190–4194.

260. Gansbacher B, Zier K, Daniels. Interleukin-2 gene transfer into tumor cells abrogates tumorigenicity and induces protective immunity. J Exp Med 1990;172:1217–1224.

261. Oldbring J, Glifberg I, Mikulowski P, Hellsten S. Carcinoma of the renal pelvis and ureter following bladder carcinoma: Frequency, risk factors and clinicopathological findings. J Urol 1989;141:1311–1313.

262. Clayman RV, Lange PH, Fraley EE. Cancer of the upper urinary tract. In: Javadpour N, ed. Principles and management of urologic cancer. Baltimore: Williams & Wilkins, 1983;544–559.

263. Mahadevia PS, Karwa GL, Koss LG. Mapping of urothelium in carcinomas of the renal pelvis and ureter. Cancer 1983;51:890–897.

264. Babaian RJ, Johnson DE. Primary carcinoma of the ureter. J Urol 1980;123:357–359.

265. Droller MJ. Transitional cell cancer: Upper tracts and bladder. In: Walsh PC, Gittes RF, Perlmutter AD, Stamey TA, eds. Urology. Philadelphia: WB Saunders, 1986;1343–1440.

266. McLaughlin JK, Silverman DT, Hsing AW, et al. Cigarette smoking and cancers of the renal pelvis and ureter. Cancer Res 1992;52:254–257.

267. Hultengren N, Lagergren C, Ljungqvist A. Carcinoma of the renal pelvis in renal papillary necrosis. Acta Chir Scand 1985;130:314–320.

268. Palvio DHB, Andersen JC, Falk E. Transitional cell tumors of the renal pelvis and ureter associated with capillar sclerosis indicating analgesic abuse. Cancer 1987;59:972–976.

269. Bengtsson U, Angervall L, Ekman H, Lehmann L. Transitional cell tumors of the renal pelvis in analgesic abusers. Scand J Urol Nephrol 1968;2:145–150.

270. Bengtsson U, Johansson S, Angervall L. Malignancies of the urinary tract and their relation to analgesic abuse. Kidney Int 1978;13:107–113.

271. Adam WR, Dawborn JK, Price CG, Riddell J, Story H. Anaplastic transitional-cell carcinoma of the renal pelvis in association with analgesic abuse. Med J Aust 1970;1:1108–1109.

272. Mahony JF, Storey BG, Ibanez RC, Stewart JH. Analgesic abuse, renal parenchymal disease and carcinoma of the kidney or ureter. Aust N Z J Med 1977;7:463–469.

273. McCredie M, Stewart JH, Carter JJ, Turner J, Mahony JF. Phenacetin and papillary necrosis: Independent risk factors for renal pelvic cancer. Kidney Int 1986;30:81–84.

274. Gaakeer HA, Ruiter HJ. Carcinoma of the renal pelvis following the abuse of phenacetin-containing analgesic drugs. Br J Urol 1979;51:188–192.

275. Jensen OM, Knudsen JB, Tomasson H, Srensen BL. The Copenhagen case-control study of renal pelvis and ureter cancer: Role of analgesics. Int J Cancer 1989;44:965–968.

276. Hoybye G, Nielsen OE. Renal pelvic carcinoma in phenacetin abusers. Scand J Urol Nephrol 1971;5:190–192.

277. Campo B, Zanitzer L, Torelli T, et al. Renal cell carcinoma and transitional cell carcinomas of the pelvis and bladder in a patient affected by chronic renal failure due to abuse of phenacetin. Tumori 1986;72:215–217.

278. Rathert P, Melchior H, Lutzeyer W. Phenacetin: A carcinogen for the urinary tract? J Urol 1975;113:653–657.

279. Haber DA, Buckler AJ, Glaser T, et al. An internal deletion within an 11p13 zinc finger gene contributes to the development of Wilms' tumor. Cell 1990;61:1257–1269.

280. Tsai YC, Nichols PW, Hiti AL, Williams Z, Skinner DG, Jones PA. Allelic losses of chromosomes 9, 11, and 17 in human bladder cancer. Cancer Res 1990;50:44–47.

281. Presti JC, Reuter VE, Galan T, Fair WR, Cordon-Cardo C. Molecular genetic alterations

in superficial and locally advanced human bladder cancer. Cancer Res 1991;51:5405–5409.

282. Ishikawa J, Xu H, Hu S, et al. Inactivation of the retinoblastoma gene in human bladder and renal cell carcinomas. Cancer Res 1991;51:5736–5743.

283. Oka K, Ishikawa J, Bruner JM, Takahashi R, Saya H. Detection of loss of heterozygosity in the p53 gene in renal cell carcinoma and bladder cancer using the polymerase chain reaction. Mol Carcinogen 1991;4:10–13.

284. Orphali SLJ, Shols GW, Hagewood J, Tesluk H, Palmer JM. Familial transitional cell carcinoma of renal pelvis and upper ureter. Urology 1986;27:394–396.

285. Frischer Z, Waltzer WC, Gonder MJ. Bilateral transitional cell carcinoma of the renal pelvis in the cancer family syndrome. J Urol 1985;134:1197–1198.

286. Cahng EH, Pirollo KF, Zou ZQ. Oncogenes in radioresistant, noncancerous skin fibroblasts from a cancer-prone family. Science 1987;237:1036–1041.

287. Nativ O, Winkler HZ, Reiman HM Jr, Lieber MM. Squamous cell carcinoma of the renal pelvis: Nuclear deoxyribonucleic acid ploidy studied by flow cytometry. J Urol 1990;144:23–26.

288. Blacher EJ, Johnson DE, Abdul-Karim FW, Ayala AG. Squamous cell carcinoma of renal pelvis. Urology 1985;25:124–126.

289. Johansson S, Angervall L, Bengtsson U, Wahlqvist L. A clinicopathologic and prognostic study of epithelial tumors of the renal pelvis. Cancer 1976;37:1376–1383.

290. Grabstald H, Whitmore WF, Melamed MR. Renal pelvic tumors. JAMA 1971;218:845–853.

291. Murphy DM, Zincke H, Furlow WL. Management of high grade transitional cell cancer of the upper urinary tract. J Urol 1981;125:25–29.

292. Wagle DG, Moore RH, Murphy GP. Primary carcinoma of the renal pelvis. Cancer 1974;33:1642–1648.

293. Lang EK. The arteriographic diagnosis of primary and secondary tumors of the ureter or ureter and renal pelvis. Radiology 1969;93:799–805.

294. Pontes JE, Christensen LC, Pierce JM. Angiographic aspects of tumors of renal pelvis and ureter. Urology 1976;7:334–336.

295. Gatewood OMB, Goldman SM, Marshall FF, Siegelman SS. Computerized tomography in the diagnosis of transitional cell carcinoma of the kidney. J Urol 1982;127:876–887.

296. Cullen TH, Popham RR, Voss HJ. Urine cytology and primary carcinoma of the renal pelvis and ureter. Aust N Z J Surg 1972;41:230–236.

297. Highman WJ. Transitional carcinoma of the upper urinary tract: a histological and cytopathological study. J Clin Pathol 1986;39:297–305.

298. Smith AD, Orihuela E, Crowley AR. Percutaneous management of renal pelvic tumors: A treatment option in selected cases. J Urol 1987;137:852–855.

299. Bagley DH, Huffman JL, Lyon ES. Flexible ureteropyeloscopy: Diagnosis and treatment in the upper urinary tract. J Urol 1987;138:280–285.

300. Davis BW, Hough AJ, Gardner WA. Renal pelvic carcinoma: Morphological correlates of metastatic behavior. J Urol 1987;137:857–861.

301. Bennington JL, Beckwith JB, eds. Tumors of the kidney, renal pelvis, and ureter. 2nd ed. Washington, DC: Armed Forces Institute of Pathology, 1975;243–310.

302. Cummings KB. Nephroureterectomy: Rationale in the management of transitional cell carcinoma of the upper urinary tract. Urol Clin North Am 1991;569–578.

303. Johansson S, Wahlqvist L. A prognostic study of urothelial renal pelvic tumors: Comparison between the prognosis of patients treated with intrafascial nephrectomy and perifascial nephroureterectomy. Cancer 1979;43:2525–2531.

304. Johnson DE, DeBerardinis M, Ayala AG. Transitional cell carcinoma of the renal pelvis: Radical or conservative surgical treatment? South Med J 1974;67:1183–1186.

305. Geiger J, Fong Q, Fay R. Transitional cell carcinoma of renal pelvis with invasion of renal vein and thrombosis of subhepatic inferior vena cava. Urology 1986;28:52–54.

306. Jitsukawa S, Nakamura K, Nakayama M, Osawa A, Matsui K. Transitional cell carcinoma of kidney extending into renal vein and inferior vena cava. Urology 1985;25:310–312.

307. Gittes RF. Management of transitional cell carcinoma of the upper tract: Case for conservative local excision. Urol Clin North Am 1980;7:559–568.

308. Bazeed MA, Scharfe T, Becht E, Alken P, Thuroff JW. Local excision of urothelial cancer of the upper urinary tract. Eur Urol 1986;12:89–95.

309. Wallace DMA, Wallace DM, Whitfield HN, Hendry WF, Wickham JEA. The late results of conservative surgery for upper tract urothelial carcinomas. Br J Urol 1981;53:537–541.

310. Tomera KM, Leary FJ, Zincke H. Pyeloscopy in urothelial tumors. J Urol 1982;127:1088–1089.

311. Ramsey JC, Soloway MS. Instillation of bacillus Calmette-Guérin into the renal pelvis of a solitary kidney for the treatment of transitional cell carcinoma. J Urol 1990;143:1220–1222.

312. Schoenberg MP, Van Arsdalen KN, Wein AJ. The management of transitional cell carcinoma in solitary renal units. J Urol 1991;146:700–702.

313. Bagley DH, Rivas D. Upper urinary tract filling defects: Flexible ureteroscopic diagnosis. J Urol 1990;143:1196–1200.

314. Tasca A, Zattoni F. The case for a percutaneous approach to transitional cell carcinoma of the renal pelvis. J Urol 1990;143:902–904.

315. Blute ML, Segura JW, Patterson DE, Benson RC, Jr, Zincke H. Impact of endourology on diagnosis and management of upper urinary tract urothelial cancer [see comments]. J Urol 1989;141:1298–1301.

316. McIntyre D, Pyrah LN, Raper FP. Primary ureteric neoplasms. Br J Urol 1965;37:160–191.

317. Foord AG, Ferrier PA. Primary carcinoma of the ureter. JAMA 1939;112:596–601.

318. Abeshouse BS. Primary benign and malignant tumors of the ureter. Am J Surg 1956;91:237–271.

319. Heney NM, Nocks BN, Daley JJ. Prognostic factors in carcinoma of the ureter. J Urol 1981;125:632–636.

320. Hawtrey CE. Fifty-two cases of primary ureteral carcinoma: A clinical-pathologic study. J Urol 1971;105:188–193.

321. Batata MA, Whitmore WF, Hilaris BS, Tokita N, Grabstald H. Primary carcinoma of the ureter: A prognostic study. Cancer 1975;35:1626–1632.

322. Richie JP. Management of ureteral tumors. In: Skinner DG, deKernion JB, eds. Genitourinary cancer. Philadelphia: WB Saunders, 1978:150–165.

323. Bergman H, Friedenberg RM, Sayegh V. New roentgenologic signs of carcinoma of the ureter. Am Roentgen Ray 1961;86:707–717.

324. Strong DW, Pearse HD. Recurrent urothelial tumors following surgery for transitional cell carcinoma of the upper urinary tract. Cancer 1976;38:2178–2183.

325. Bloom NA, Vidone RA, Lytton B. Primary carcinoma of the ureter: A report of 102 new cases. J Urol 1970;103:590–598.

326. Carson CC. Endoscopic treatment of upper and lower urinary tract lesions using lasers. Semin Urol 1992 (in press).

327. Herr HW, Whitmore WF. Ureteral carcinoma in situ after successful intravesical therapy for superficial bladder tumors: Incidence, possible pathogenesis and management. J Urol 1987;138:292–294.

328. Johannson A, Angervall L, Bengtsson U. A clinicopathologic and prognostic study of epithelial tumors of the renal pelvis. Cancer 1976;37:1376–1381.

329. Brookland RK, Richter MP. Postoperative irradiation of transitional cell carcinoma of the renal pelvis and ureter. J Urol 1985;133:952–955.

330. Cozal SC, Smalley SR, Austenfeld M, et al. Transitional cell carcinoma of the renal pelvis or ureter: Patterns of failure. Am Radium Soc [Abstract] 1991:75.

331. Saitoh H, Hida N, Nakamura K. Distant metastases urothelial tumors of the renal pelvis and ureter. Tokai J Exp Clin Med 1985;7:355–361.

332. Shipley WU. Radiation therapy in the management of patients with genitourinary malignancies. In: Wang CC, ed. Clinical radiation oncology: Indications, techniques, and results. Boston: PSG Publishing, 1987:262–299.

333. Maruf NJ, Godec CJ, Kahn A. Synchronous tumors in both ureters and left renal pelvis. Urology 1983;21:305.

334. Edsmyr F, Eposti PL, Anderson L. Interferon therapy in disseminated renal cell carcinoma. Radiother Oncol 1985;4:21.

335. Trindade A, Samuels ML, Logothetis CJ. Chemotherapy of carcinoma of renal pelvis: Preliminary report. Urology 1981;18:54.

336. Sternberg C, Scher H. Current status of chemotherapy for urothelial tract tumors. Oncology 1987;1:41.

337. Logothetis CJ, Samuels ML, Selig DE. Combined intravenous and intraarterial cyclophosphamide, doxorubicin, and cisplatin (CISCA) in the management of select patients with invasive urothelial tumors. Cancer Treat Rep 1985;69:33.

338. Peeling WB, Mantell BS, Shepheard BCF. Postoperative irradiation in the treatment of renal cell carcinoma. Br J Urol 1969;41:23–31.

339. Juusela H, Malmio K, Alfthan D. Preoperative irradiation in the treatment of renal adenocarcinoma. Scand J Urol Nephrol 1977;11:277–281.

340. Abrams JS, Rayner AA, Wiernik PH, et al. High-dose recombinant interleukin-2 alone: A regimen with limited activity in the treatment of advanced renal cell carcinoma. JNCI 1990;82:1202–1206.

341. McCabe MS, Stablein D, Hawkins MJ. The modified group C experience: Phase III randomized trials of IL-2 vs IL-2/LAK in advanced renal cell carcinoma and advanced melanoma. Proc Am Soc Clin Oncol [Abstract] 1991;10:714.

342. Poo WJ, Fynan T, Davis C, Flynn S, Durivage H, Todd M. High-dose recombinant interleukin-2 alone in patients with metastatic renal cell carcinoma. Proc Am Assoc Cancer Res [Abstract] 1991;10:557.

343. Fisher RI, Coltman CA, Doroshow JH, et al. Metastatic renal cancer treated with interleukin-2 and lymphokine-activated killer cells. Ann Intern Med 1988;108:518.

344. Gaynor ER, Weiss GR, Margolin KA, et al. Phase I study of high-dose continuous-infusion recombinant interleukin-2 and autologous lymphokine-activated killer cells in patients with metastatic or unresectable malignant melanoma and renal cell carcinoma. JNCI 1990;82:1397.

345. Dillman RO, Oldham RK, Tauer KW, et al. Continuous interleukin-2 and lymphokine-activated killer cells for advanced cancer: A National Biotherapy Study Group trial. J Clin Oncol 1991;9:1233.

346. Thompson J, Benyunes L, Benz L, Lindgren C, Fefer A. Prolonged continuous intravenous infusion interleukin-2 and lymphokine-activated killer cell therapy for renal carcinoma. Proc Am Soc Clin Oncol [Abstract] 1991;10:179.

347. Latif F, Hosoe S, Brauch H, et al. A single recombinant event between the von Hippel-Lindau disease (VHL) gene and D3S18 (3p26) loci on human chromosome 3. Am J Hum Genet 1992 (in press).

348. Rosenberg SA. The immunotherapy and gene therapy of cancer. J Clin Oncol 1992;10:180–199.

Cancer: Principles & Practice of Oncology, Fourth Edition,
edited by Vincent T. DeVita, Jr., Samuel Hellman, Steven A. Rosenberg.
J.B. Lippincott Co., Philadelphia © 1993.

William R. Fair
Zvi Y. Fuks
Howard I. Scher

CHAPTER **34**

Cancer of the Bladder

Bladder cancer accounts for approximately 2% of all malignant tumors and approximately 7% of all urinary tract malignancies in U.S. men.[1] The American Cancer Society estimates that there will be more than 50,000 new bladder cancer cases in 1992, with an estimated 9500 deaths. On initial presentation, approximately 75% of all bladder cancers are limited to the mucosa, submucosa, or lamina propria. For these "superficial" tumors, recurrence rates are high (50–80%) after initial treatment, although progression to muscle-invading tumor occurs in only 10% to 25%.[2] In superficial disease, prevention of recurrence and progression are the two major considerations. In muscle-invading bladder cancers, the risk of distant metastases at the time of diagnosis is high and the clinician's main focus is on definitive treatment of the primary lesions plus distant disease.

EPIDEMIOLOGY

Like many solid tumors, bladder cancer is a disease of the older population, with a peak incidence in the seventh decade of life. In the United States, the male to female ratio of bladder cancer occurrence is approximately three to one, although this disparity narrows in populations in which cigarette smoking is common among women. The relative risk ratio of transitional cell carcinoma for whites and blacks is approximately 1.6. The elevated risk for whites compared with blacks was limited to disease confined to the mucosa and submucosa. For cancer extending to the bladder muscle or beyond, no increased risk for whites could be demonstrated.[3]

In 1895, Rehn was the first to suggest that occupational factors could be instrumental in development of bladder cancer.[4] He observed an increased risk for the disease in aniline dye workers. These observations have been confirmed and expanded to indicate a significant occupational hazard among people exposed to aryl amines, such as workers in the organic chemical, dye, rubber, and paint industries.

The strongest association is that observed between cigarette smoking and bladder cancer.[5-8] There is a consistent association between the amount and duration of cigarette smoking and the development of bladder cancer, although a latency period of 16 to 22 years has been observed. The association of bladder cancer and smoking appears to be true for transitional cell carcinoma and squamous cell carcinoma.[9] Other occupational and environmental factors, such as residence in urban areas and exposure to diesel fumes or automobile exhaust, have not been conclusively linked with bladder cancer. At least one epidemiologic study shows an increased incidence in bladder cancer for people living in rural areas.[6] An increased risk for transitional cell carcinoma of the urinary tract has been observed in persons who chronically abuse the analgesic phenacetin.[10]

The observation that dietary sweeteners such as cyclamate and saccharin function as potent bladder cancer-promoting agents in animals given methyl-nitrosourea followed by oral saccharin or cyclamates generated much concern about the safety of these agents for human use. Although it is not easy to separate dietary influences from factors like smoking and occupational exposure in epidemiologic studies, at least four case-control studies failed to show any significant relation between the use of dietary sweeteners and bladder cancer.[10-13]

Conditions leading to chronic bladder irritation are associated with the development of squamous cell carcinoma of the bladder. In addition to cigarette smoking, bilharziasis is a known etiologic factor, as is the effect of chronic urinary tract infections.[9] Although the mechanism action is unknown, urinary nitrites produced as a result of chronic infection with a subsequent production of nitrosourea may play a role in the development of squamous cell carcinoma of the bladder.

Few data are available on factors playing a protective role

against the development of bladder cancer, although there is a suggestion that milk and vitamin A ingestion may be inversely related to the development of bladder cancer.[14-16]

Recent data indicate that there may be a familial or genetic component to bladder cancer.[17-19] Kantor and colleagues found that a family history of urinary tract cancer significantly elevated the risk for bladder cancer (relative risk of 1.45), with higher risk observed among patients younger than 45.[18]

These epidemiologic observations are in keeping with cytogenetic and molecular genetic studies, which demonstrate deletions of several chromosomal arms, including 9q, 11p, and 17p, in bladder cancers.[20-23] Molecular genetic techniques have shown a significant correlation of tumor grade with deletions of 3p and 17p and tumor stage associated with deletions of 3p and 17p and altered expression of the *RB* (retinoblastoma) gene. Vascular invasion correlated with 17p deletions.[23] Centromeric copy number of chromosome 7 shows a strong correlation with tumor grade and labeling index in human bladder cancer.[24]

PATHOLOGY

HISTOLOGIC TYPES

In the United States, approximately 95% of malignant bladder lesions are transitional cell carcinomas. Of the remaining neoplasms, 3% are squamous cell carcinomas, and the remainder are adenocarcinomas. Some adenocarcinomas arise in the dome of the bladder from a primary site in the urachus. Primary adenocarcinoma of the bladder most commonly occurs on the trigone. One of the management problems is that carcinoma of the bladder is frequently multifocal. The entire bladder epithelium and the lining of the entire urothelial tract can undergo malignant change. After apparently successful treatment of a bladder lesion, new tumors may occur at the same site (*i.e.*, recurrence) or other urothelial cells in the bladder. Approximately 30% of bladder carcinomas appear as multiple lesions at the time of initial diagnosis.[25]

Most bladder tumors are papillary transitional cell carcinomas. In the World Health Organization (WHO) classification, three grades of urothelial carcinoma are recognized. Grade 1 represents well-differentiated papillary tumors with limited atypia and mitoses. At the other end of the spectrum, grade 3 lesions show a marked increase in the cell layers and cell size, and noticeable pleomorphism and mitoses are prominent. In some classifications, the tumors are graded on a scale of I to IV, although the behaviors of grade III and IV tumors are so similar that the approach used by WHO in combining these two into a single grade is clinically appropriate.

Tumor grade appears to correlate significantly with the natural history of transitional cell carcinoma. Gilbert and coworkers retrospectively analyzed the results of 365 patients with transitional cell carcinoma of the bladder treated conservatively.[26] The behavior of the tumors fell into three groups, based solely on the grading of the transurethral resection specimens. Five percent of the patients with grade I, 16% with grade II, 35% with grade III not involving muscle, and 83% with grade III disease involving muscle died from bladder cancer, with most deaths occurring within 2 years after initial diagnosis.

Tribukaite correlated tumor grade with the DNA ploidy, providing some objective evidence for the pathologic grading.[27]

A source of confusion for pathologists and clinicians has been differentiating benign papillomas from malignant epithelial lesions. In the WHO classification, the papilloma is designated as a grade 0 tumor and accounts for approximately 2% of all transitional cell carcinomas.[28] Although many pathologists continue to classify this as a grade 1 carcinoma, the studies by Lerman and colleagues[29] and Koss[30] provide convincing evidence that the papilloma is a benign lesion. The difficulty arises because a papilloma may signify an "unstable epithelium." Although the papilloma itself is not thought to undergo malignant change, the factors that give rise to a papilloma may, in other areas of the bladder, give rise to a more malignant growth. For this reason, patients with a papilloma of the bladder or those with low-grade epithelial lesions, although not requiring aggressive therapy, should be followed carefully.

PRENEOPLASTIC LESIONS

Damage to the urothelium caused by carcinogens, infection, stones, or catheters may result in permanent loss of the mature superficial cells and increase the rate of cell division in the basal layer, leading to the formation of hyperplastic urothelium of immature cells. The normal pattern of differentiation can easily be disturbed and give rise to various nonmalignant phenotypes, notably squamous or glandular metaplasia.

Most bladder carcinomas develop from a spectrum of preneoplastic and preinvasive urothelial disease. On the basis of multiple biopsies and mapping studies of cystectomy specimens, it is recognized that there may be a progression of normal urothelium to flat carcinoma in situ through possible early stages of tumor development: hyperplasia, atypical hyperplasia, or dysplasia. No unanimous agreement has been reached on the histopathologic limits between the various preneoplastic changes or of the terms preferred. Some investigators have recommended the term carcinoma in situ grade 1, 2, and 3 for similar lesions of the urothelium.[31]

Hyperplasia is defined as an increase in the number of cell layers without the loss of polarity and with differentiation and maturation from the base to the surface. Urothelial hyperplasia frequently accompanies tumors of the bladder and is the source of papillary neoplasia. However, it may occur as a benign reaction to injuries such as chronic inflammation.

Atypical hyperplasia is characterized by epithelial thickening with preservation of cell polarity, but nuclear crowding and various degrees of pleomorphism of the nuclei exist.

The term dysplasia of the urothelium has generated controversy. There is strong support for categorizing atypical hyperplasia in various degrees of severity. Others use the term dysplasia, which is characterized by the loss of cellular polarity. Nuclear crowding, granular chromatin, and small nucleoli are identified. Severe dysplasia should be regarded as carcinoma in situ and not merely as a preneoplastic lesion.

Preneoplastic changes in the bladder may be multifocal and may not be visualized cystoscopically. Most data about preneoplastic lesions have been accumulated for patients with known bladder tumors. Identification of dysplasia in an unselected population has not been feasible. Several reports have suggested that atypical hyperplasia or dysplasia is a risk factor for the development of recurrent or invasive bladder cancer. Althausen and coworkers reported that atypical cells at the margins of superficial tumors were associated with eventual progression to invasive cancer in 36% of patients, and if carcinoma in situ was reported, the frequency rose to 83%, compared with 7% if the epithelium was normal.[32] Murphy and associates prospectively studied selected urothelial biopsies from patients followed for urothelial cancer; 38% of patients with epithelial dysplasia had superficial recurrences after the appearance of premalignant lesions compared with only 16% of patients with normal urothelium at selected biopsy sites.[33] Wolf and Hojgaard found that approximately 50% of the patients with newly detected primary category T1 or T2 bladder tumors had concomitant widespread urothelial dysplasia or carcinoma in situ.[34] In a follow-up study of these patients treated with transurethral resection alone, it was found that new occurrences developed in 87% of patients with concomitant urothelial dysplasia, compared with 26% of those without dysplasia. Atypical hyperplasia and flat carcinoma in situ are probably the most common precursors to invasive bladder carcinoma.

CARCINOMA IN SITU

Carcinoma in situ is a flat, nonpapillary, noninvasive, histopathologically anaplastic epithelium closely resembling that seen in high-grade transitional cell carcinoma.[35] Carcinoma in situ has a spectrum of biologic potential. Most studies have suggested that urothelial carcinoma in situ is a biologically aggressive disease, while others point out cases of carcinoma in situ with a limited capacity to invade the bladder wall.

Carcinoma in situ may present in one of four different situations:

1. A localized lesion adjacent to a superficial papillary or an invasive tumor
2. As a diffuse urothelial disease concomitant with macroscopic tumors
3. A primary focal lesion in asymptomatic patients
4. Symptomatic, diffuse, or multifocal lesions of the urothelium, not associated with macroscopic tumors at the time of diagnosis

The most common form of carcinoma in situ is a small focus surrounding the base of a papillary or sessile tumor. The incidence of carcinoma in situ in areas adjacent to superficial papillary tumors ranges from 26% to 40% and is most prevalent adjacent to grade 4 transitional cell carcinoma, found in as many as 100% of the patients.[36] Carcinoma in situ adjacent to a superficial bladder tumor correlates strongly with the likelihood of muscle invasion. Althausen and coworkers demonstrated that 7% of patients with a normal mucosa surrounding papillary tumor and 83% of those with carcinoma in situ surrounding the papillary tumor developed invasive cancer within 5 years.[32]

Another presentation of carcinoma in situ is distant from the superficial tumor, sometimes diffused or multifocal. It may extend to one or both ureters, the prostatic urethra, or the prostatic ducts in approximately 20% of patients.

If a primary lesion of carcinoma in situ is localized and not accompanied by irritative symptoms, it is relatively innocuous and may not lead to infiltrating disease.[37]

In the fourth type of carcinoma in situ, there is extensive involvement of the urothelium at the time of initial diagnosis that is not associated with macroscopic tumors. Of these patients, 80% present with significant irritative bladder symptoms. If associated with total or near-total involvement of the urothelium and irritative symptoms, primary carcinoma in situ has been associated with a 50% to 80% incidence of infiltrating cancer. Farrow and associates followed 96 patients with biopsy-proven carcinoma in situ.[38] Invasive carcinoma developed in 37 patients within 5 years. Tannenbaum and associates reported a retrospective histologic study of 140 patients with primary carcinoma in situ who had been followed for 14 to 21 years; 40% developed muscle-invading lesions within 4 to 6 years, and 60% developed the lesions within 10 years.[39] At 15 to 21 years after initial documentation of carcinoma in situ, 40% had died from their disease, and the remaining 60% had invasive or metastatic bladder cancer. Although in both series there was a prolonged course of carcinoma in situ before invasion, carcinoma in situ is recognized as an aggressive malignancy with the potential for rapid progression and invasion.

CLINICAL PRESENTATION

SIGNS AND SYMPTOMS

Gross or microscopic hematuria is the most common presenting sign in patients with bladder cancer. Hematuria, with or without irritative symptoms, occurs in approximately 75% of patients with bladder cancer. Vesical irritation alone is the presenting symptom in approximately 30% of patients, and it often indicates carcinoma in situ. In women, the irritative symptoms may be mistaken for interstitial cystitis.

Patients with advanced bladder cancer may present with pelvic pain due to an enlarging tumor mass or a nerve root irritation. If ureteral obstruction occurs, flank pain may be the prominent symptom. With extensive local lesions, rectal obstruction with constipation may occur. Occasionally, lower extremity edema, secondary to lymphatic or venous obstruction, is the first presenting sign.

METHODS OF DIAGNOSIS

The standard method of diagnosis is through cystoscopy and biopsy. Urinary cytology with or without flow cytometry may detect malignant cells in the urinary tract, and it is useful in following patients with a history of bladder cancer. At the time of cystoscopy, bimanual examination enables the examiner to determine the presence of a mass, bladder wall thickening, and whether the bladder is freely mobile or fixed to the pelvic sidewall, which is important in planning definitive therapy. Adequate biopsies must include the muscle of the bladder wall in the specimen to enable the pathologist to ascertain muscle invasion. Selective mucosal biopsies at a site different from the tumor should be taken to detect concomitant carcinoma in situ. The "cold cup" punch biopsy is excellent for these purposes, because it provides a good sampling of the urothelium without cautery artifact.

STANDARD WORKUP

The standard workup required depends on the extent and grade of the primary tumor. Urinary cytology and flow cytometry are helpful in making an initial presumptive diagnosis and for follow-up. Because urothelial carcinoma may present anywhere along the lining of the genitourinary tract, some means should be employed to image the entire urothelial surface. Formerly, an intravenous pyelogram was the most commonly employed modality, but computed tomography (CT) scanning of the abdomen and pelvis enable visualization of the upper tracts and ureter and of the lymph node areas, which is important for proper staging. The CT scan often shows bladder wall thickening or an intraluminal filling defect. A bone scan and chest x-ray film completes the staging workup in patients with muscle-invading disease. The most common sites of distant spread in patients with invasive bladder tumor are the lymph nodes, lungs, or bone. These areas should be evaluated by means of a chest x-ray film, radioisotope bone scan, and CT scan of the abdomen and pelvis. In some centers, magnetic resonance imaging (MRI) may be preferable to a

CT scan for the staging evaluation. Ultrasonography of the bladder is useful for evaluating the bladder wall thickening, but it provides no information about lymph node status and is less informative than CT or MRI.

STAGING SYSTEMS

In 1946, Jewett and Strong were the first to relate the depth of penetration of the bladder wall to metastatic potential.[40] This system was subsequently modified by Marshall into the 0, A, B, C, D system based on the bimanual examination under anesthesia and the microscopic evaluation of the tissue removed at biopsy.[41] Although this system is adequate to address the depth of penetration to the muscle wall, it gives no information about the nodal or metastatic status and is not consistent with staging systems used in other anatomic sites or throughout much of the world. The International Union Against Cancer and the American Joint Committee adopted the tumor-node-metastasis (TNM) system illustrated in Figure 34–1, and it is the most appropriate system for accurate clin-

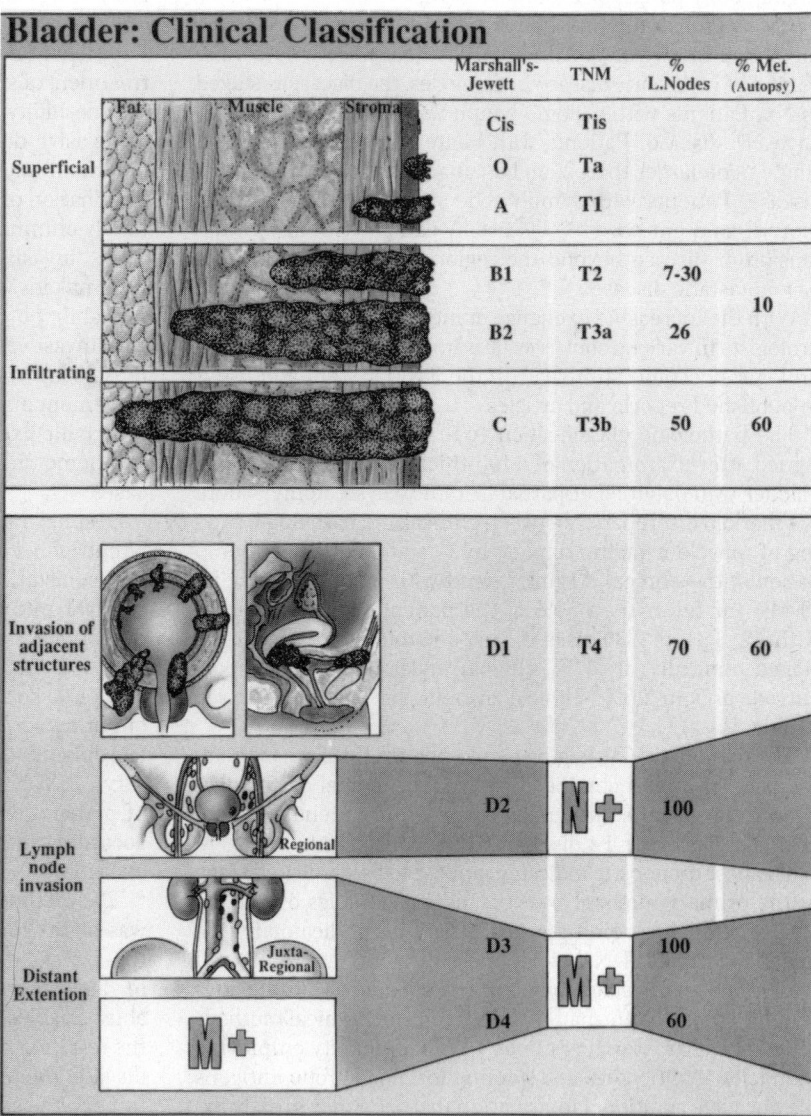

FIGURE 34–1. A comparison of the Marshall-Jewett and TNM system in the classification of bladder cancer.

ical staging. Carcinoma in situ, which is indicated by the term Cis in the Marshall-Jewett classification, is referred to as Tis in the TNM system. The stage 0 lesion in the older classification indicates a visible tumor limited to the mucosa (Ta) but not into the lamina propria (T1). Stage T2 through T4 lesions have invaded the muscle. T2 tumors are those muscle-invading tumors without a palpable mass or induration on bimanual examination after transurethral resection. A stage T3 tumor indicates a palpable mass or induration still remaining after transurethral resection (TUR). This represents a difference from the categorization of B1 and B2 lesions in the Marshall-Jewett classification, in which the B1 lesion represented invasion into less than one half of the muscle layer of the bladder wall, and B2 was more than halfway through the bladder wall without involving the perivesical fat. This difference between B1 and B2 is extremely difficult for the pathologist to make based on biopsy material only, and it represents another defect of the older system. T3a and stage B tumors do not have evidence of invasion beyond the bladder muscle, but T3b (stage C) indicates lesions that involve the perivesical fat. Clinical T4 tumors have evidence of extension into the surrounding organs, such as the prostate, rectum, vagina, bony pelvis, or abdominal wall.

The staging criteria for lymph node involvement presumes the actual biopsy of nodal tissue. Without histologic confirmation of metastatic disease in the nodes, the disease is staged as Nx. Patients with a single lymph node smaller than 2 cm have N1 disease. Patients with bilateral lymph nodes or a single node larger than 2 cm but smaller than 5 cm have N2 disease. Patients with lymph node involvement measuring more than 5 cm have N3 disease. A patient with distant extension of disease beyond the regional pelvic lymph nodes has metastatic disease.

With the increasing exchange of medical information from urologists in various countries, it is imperative that American urologists become familiar with the TNM system and use it in published reports and articles.

The pathologic classification (pT) refers to the stage assigned after examination of a full-thickness specimen of the bladder wall obtained at partial or radical cystectomy. There is a marked discrepancy between clinical and pathologic staging of muscle-invading tumors. In a combined series of 465 patients, the clinical staging agreed with pathologic staging (T=P) for fewer than 50% of the patients. In 341 patients with T2, T3a, or T3b disease, only one third were accurately staged clinically. In 41%, clinical understaging (T<P) occurred, and in 26%, clinical overstaging (T>P) occurred (Table 34–1).

The pathologic (P) staging employing a full-thickness bladder wall specimen obtained by partial or radical cystectomy is accurate in reflecting prognosis, even if patients with superficial disease or T4 disease are not considered.

The best prognostic indicators appear to be grade and stage of the primary tumor. However, the inaccuracies of clinical staging limit its usefulness as a prognostic indicator for individual patients. DNA ploidy measurements correlate well with grade and N stage, but as an independent variable adds little prognostic information. Immunohistochemical methods of further characterizing tumor T1 heterogeneity employing monoclonal antibodies and staining for blood group antigens may provide additional information that soon may greatly ex-

TABLE 34–1. T Versus P Staging for Radical Cystectomy Patients

T Stage	No. of Patients*	Patients for Whom T < P (%)	Patients for Whom T > P (%)
T1/Tis	124	23 (19)	18 (15)
T2	181	71 (39)	45 (25)
T3a	104	37 (36)	19 (18)
T3b	56	32 (57)	23 (45)
Total	465	163 (35)	105 (23)

* Combined series from Whitmore,[1977] Prout,[1977] Richie,[1975] and Skinner.[1982]

pand the prognostic information obtained from clinical staging alone.[42]

APPROACH TO TREATMENT

Urothelial tumors manifest heterogeneity in all stages. In the treatment of superficial tumors, the primary goal is to decrease the morbidity of recurrence. The overall risk of progression to invasive disease is low, but without infallible markers of potentially aggressive tumor behavior, careful follow-up, with elimination of all lesions as they occur, can minimize but not totally eliminate the risk for developing invasive disease. The term "invasive disease" encompasses papillary tumors with minimal invasion along a broad histologic front and a low probability of metastases; clinically more aggressive tumors, with invasion characterized by tentacular projections into the muscle layers, often demonstrating vascular or lymphatic involvement and a high probability of metastatic spread; or unresectable fixed lesions that produce severe pain, obstruction, and hemorrhage. The treatment goals vary for each of these cases.

Despite radical cystectomy (including bilateral pelvic lymphadenectomy) and high-dose local irradiation for treating nonmetastatic, locally invasive bladder cancer, the 5-year survival rate for patients presenting with muscle-invasive transitional cell carcinomas of the bladder is no better than 20% to 50%. Most patients who eventually succumb to bladder cancer do so as a result of distant disease, which was present but unrecognizable at the time of definitive local treatment. It is difficult to correlate the extent of local therapy with overall survival. Table 34–2 lists a compilation of 5-year survival rates of patients with transitional cell carcinomas of the bladder according to the stage of the tumor and the extent of local excision.[43–46]

The method of treatment employed for individual patients was highly selective, not based on T stage alone, and reflects the physician's judgment about the appropriateness of a bladder-conserving procedure based on several nonquantifiable variables. Because of the tremendous selectivity involved, the results cannot be strictly compared, but in muscle-invading disease, the overall failure rate is high. Except for TUR of T3 tumors, the specific method of treatment had little impact on

TABLE 34–2. Five-Year Survival After Surgery for Bladder Cancer

Treatment*	Tis, T1 (%)	T2 (%)	T3a (%)	T3b (%)
Transurethral resection	47–81	57–59	14–23	2–7
Segmental cystectomy	43–100	43–80	43–80	0–38
Simple cystectomy	27–88	45–52	16–40	2–31
Radical cystectomy	63–83	50–88	26–60	6–40

* Combined data from Whitmore.[43–46]

overall survival rates. The appeal of combining surgery or radiation therapy with chemotherapy is the hope of improving overall survival rates and permitting less extensive local resection that avoids total cystectomy and the resulting quality of life changes after bladder removal.

TREATMENT OF SUPERFICIAL BLADDER CANCER

The term superficial bladder cancer includes lesions of stage T0, Ta, T1, and Tis, and it encompasses a broad range of biologic implications, from tumors that may properly be considered benign lesions (*e.g.*, papilloma T0 grade 1) to those with a potential to be life threatening (*e.g.*, grade 3 T1 or Tis).

TUR of superficial bladder lesions is the primary modality of treatment, and more than 80% of lesions can be locally controlled by TUR. To be therapeutic, all tumors must be removed and only smooth bladder muscle should be visible at the completion of the resection. Although TUR is highly effective in eradicating an existing tumor, it has little impact on the development of additional lesions at sites removed from the initial surgery; recurrence rates of 30% to 85% after TUR have been recorded.[2,37]

Grade progression occurs in approximately 10% to 30% of cases, and stage progression occurs in 4% to 30%. Tumor multifocality and three or more episodes of recurrences seem to indicate patients with an increased risk for subsequent tumor, and these patients should be considered for intravesical therapy to minimize the rate of recurrence. The morbidity of repeated TUR or fulguration of superficial tumors is low and can often be carried out without the necessity of anesthesia. Close surveillance with endoscopic treatment of superficial lesions is appropriate for many patients. For patients with high-grade lesions, multiple recurrences, or endoscopically uncontrollable lesions, intravesical therapy may be considered.

The risk of progression is related to the stage and grade of the presenting tumor. In the U.S. collaborative bladder trials (NBCCGA), only 4% of patients with Ta tumors developed progressive disease, defined as bladder muscle involvement or metastases. In contrast, 30% of those with T1 tumors showed progression. Grade was a significant predictor of progression; only 2% of grade 1 lesions but 45% of grade 3 lesions progressed.[47,48] In patients with grade 3, stage T1 cancers,

Jakse and colleagues found only a 50% 10-year survival rate compared with a 95% survival rate for patients with Ta grade 1 lesions.[49]

The routine use of intravesical therapy in all patients, even those presenting with papillomas or low-grade lesions, is unnecessary; the morbidity of aggressive therapy can outweigh the morbidity of the natural course of the disease.

INTRAVESICAL THERAPY

Postoperative intravesical therapy is used to treat endoscopically unresectable lesions or after the complete resection of the initial lesion as adjuvant therapy designed to prevent recurrences. The most common agents used include thiotepa, doxorubicin (Adriamycin), mitomycin C, and Bacillus Calmette-Guérin (BCG). The use of intravesical chemotherapy is largely the result of empiric studies, and a lack of randomized studies confounds interpretation of the literature (Table 34–3). Nonetheless, the activities of these agents in reducing recurrence appears to be established, although the same cannot be said for the prevention grade or stage progression.[50]

The advantages of intravesical therapy include the ability to provide intimate contact of the drug with the tumor and the avoidance of systemic therapy. The agents are usually given diluted to an initial concentration of 1 mg/ml in sterile saline or water immediately after emptying the bladder with a catheter. The patient is asked to retain the chemotherapy for 2 hours. Chemotherapy doses employed are 30 to 60 mg for thiotepa, 20 to 80 mg for doxorubicin, and 20 to 60 mg for mitomycin C. BCG, the exact mechanism of action of which is unknown, is given in a dose of 120 mg in sterile saline.

TABLE 34–3. Effect of Intravesical Therapy on Recurrence and Progression

Agent	No. of Patients	Tumor Free ≥1 Year (%) Controls	Treated	Net Benefit (%)
Effect on Recurrence				
Thiotepa	757	48	56	8
Doxorubicin	860	59	69	10
Mitomycin C	880	46	58	12
Bacillus Calmette-Guérin	318	30	72	42
Effect on Progression Rate				
Thiotepa	513	6.0	4.5	NS
Doxorubicin	455	11.2	12.9	NS
Mitomycin C	455	5.0	2.4	NS
Bacillus Calmette-Guérin	329	28	14	14

NS, not significant.
(Data from Herr HW. Intravesical therapy. Hematol Oncol Clin North Am 1992; 6:1 and Lamm DL. Long-term results of intravesical therapy for superficial bladder cancer. Urol Clin North Am 1992;19:573–580)

Although few controlled studies have been done, it appears that thiotepa, doxorubicin, and mitomycin C are equally effective as prophylactic agents. Mitomycin C appears equivalent to doxorubicin and superior to thiotepa. BCG appears to be significantly superior to the chemotherapeutic agents for the prophylaxis of recurrence and retardation of progression.[50]

The key question concerning the use of any intravesical therapy is whether such treatment actually prevents disease progression or simply delays the inevitable. Recent data from Memorial Sloan-Kettering Cancer Center (MSKCC) suggests that BCG may confer durable protection. In this study, 61 patients initially presenting with Ta and T1 tumors with or without associated Tis were treated with intravesical BCG and followed from 10 to 13 years.[51] Nineteen (31%) patients remained tumor free during the follow-up period; another 17 (28%) had interval superficial recurrences, but no progression; and 41% had evidence of progression (*e.g.,* muscle involvement, prostatic urethra involvement, metastases). Of the 61 patients, 33 (54%) are alive and free of disease with an intact bladder; 13 (21%) are alive but subsequently required a cystectomy; 2 (3%) died from intercurrent disease; 1 (2%) is alive with metastases; and 12 (20%) died from metastatic disease. This study, which provides the longest BCG follow-up, suggests but does not prove that BCG significantly reduced tumor recurrence and the progression rate in this high-risk patient population. Overall, 75% of the patients were alive 10 years after therapy.

The toxic effects of intravesical chemotherapy include myelosuppression, bladder irritative symptoms, and allergic reactions. Due to its low molecular weight, thiotepa is easily absorbed, and mylosuppression is seen in 18% to 20% of patients treated.[52,189] Myelosuppression is rare in patients treated with mitomycin C because the larger molecular weight of mitomycin C retards absorption. Systemic toxicity of doxorubicin and mitomycin C is less than that observed with thiotepa, perhaps because of the molecular weight of these agents. The incidence of locally irritative symptoms with doxorubicin is significant. Fifty percent of patients complain of moderate or severe urgency, and another 25% have local irritative symptoms consistent with chemical cystitis. Symptoms of bladder irritation occur in 10% to 15% of patients treated with mitomycin C. Contact dermatitis occurs in 5% to 15% of patients. This can be avoided by washing the hands and perineum after treatment.

BCG produces an intense local inflammatory response in the bladder of most patients, although local symptoms do generally not require dose reduction or discontinuance of therapy if given for 6 weeks. With longer therapy, intolerance is a frequent occurrence. BCG has a cumulative effect, and toxicity escalates markedly with maintenance therapy. Maintenance therapy appears to be no more effective than a single 6-week course of treatment.[53]

Although local irritative symptoms are common, serious systemic complications are much less frequent and usually are a result of traumatic catheterization. Nonetheless, at least 7 deaths from BCG therapy have been recorded, and care must be exercised in its use. Other complications reported were fever, pneumonitis, hepatitis, arthritis, arthralgia, and skin rash. Because BCG vaccine contains viable bacteria, systemic BCGosis is rarely encountered but may require triple-drug antituberculosis treatment.[54]

CARCINOMA IN SITU

Therapy of carcinoma in situ of the bladder depends on the extent of the lesion, associated irritative symptoms, and its association with prior or concurrent bladder tumors. Patients presenting without irritative symptoms seem to have focal lesions characterized by a long latency period and clinical course. If all areas of Tis can be transurethrally resected or fulgurated, these patients can be safely followed with careful endoscopic surveillance.

Of greater concern are patients with carcinoma in situ associated with irritative bladder symptoms or bladder tumors. The initial Mayo Clinic series documented 73% of patients with a Tis developing subsequent bladder muscle invasion and 57% of patients dying of metastatic disease within 5 years.[55] Carcinoma in situ associated with prior or concurrent bladder tumor often produces severe symptoms of vesical irritability and has been associated with the subsequent development of infiltrating cancer in 50% to 80% of cases.

Although radical cystoprostatectomy may be required for endoscopically uncontrollable disease in the absence of involvement of extravesicle lesions or a severely contracted bladder, a trial of BCG therapy is warranted. A 6-week course of BCG usually is given, followed by a repeat cystoscopy and biopsy of the bladder and prostatic urethra 6 weeks after the completion of therapy to allow time for the inflammation accompanying BCG therapy to subside. Histologic evidence of persistence of carcinoma in situ in the bladder or presence of Tis in the prostatic ducts and invading stroma is an indication for radical cystectomy and urethrectomy.

Other modalities of treatment of superficial bladder cancer, such as laser therapy, have been used, but they appear to have no significant advantages over endoscopic management in terms of local control or likelihood of recurrence. Laser appears primarily useful in the treatment of small lesions, but resection of these lesions and histologic confirmation of the depth of invasion is preferable. Endoscopic photodynamic therapy using hematoporphyrin derivatives has also been used in association with laser therapy in an effort to treat the entire urothelium. Although this appears to be effective in some series, it is most active against small lesions. In uncontrolled studies, intracavitary irradiation has shown some effect, although external-beam therapy radiation therapy appears to be of little value in low-stage disease.[57]

TREATMENT OF INVASIVE DISEASE

SURGERY

For some patients with relatively small muscle-invading tumors, TUR provides an excellent means of control. In treating 43 patients, Miller and associates found a 55% 5-year survival rate for patients treated by TUR alone, a figure comparable to a nonrandomized group of patients treated at the same institution with preoperative irradiation and radical cystectomy.[58] At MSKCC, it is our policy to do a repeat TUR on all patients referred with a diagnosis of documented muscle-invading tumor. Approximately 20% of patients referred to our institution with muscle-invading disease documented elsewhere are found to be free of tumor (T0) after a restaging TUR. With a median follow-up of 5.1 years after initial diagnosis, 30 (67%) of 45 patients with a negative second TUR were tumor free and retained their bladders.[59] Overall, the survival rate was 82% (37 of 45 patients). For patients in whom endoscopic removal of all visible tumor is possible, the absence of residual tumor in a second TUR may suggest that conservative management is a feasible option.

Partial Cystectomy

The rationale of the partial cystectomy in the management of muscle-invading bladder cancer is consistent with the goal of providing the greatest possibility of local control with the least attendant morbidity. The application of partial cystectomy to clinical practice remains controversial. As indicated in Table 34–2, the results obtained in highly selected cases are comparable to those obtained with radical cystectomy. Partial cystectomy does not alter the underlying biologic potential for tumor formation in the remaining urothelium, and muscle-invading or superficial recurrent tumor may occur in approximately 50% of patients.

The ideal candidate for partial cystectomy is a patient with a muscle-invading tumor in an otherwise normal bladder confirmed by selected mucosal biopsies negative for carcinoma in situ or epithelial dysplasia. If there is concomitant Tis in other areas of the bladder, a partial cystectomy is not appropriate. The lesion should be small enough to allow adequate margins of resections, and confirmation of negative surgical margins should be obtained at the time of surgery. Ideally, the tumor should be in the dome or the posterior wall to allow the resection of the lesion with a 2 cm rim of uninvolved normal bladder mucosa. Although posterior wall tumors involving a ureteral orifice can technically be removed and the ureter reimplanted, this approach is rarely warranted because the lower ureter is also likely to be involved by tumor. Patients considered appropriate for partial cystectomy should have negative prostatic urethra biopsies before the contemplated procedure.

Before surgery, 900 to 1200 cGy of external-beam radiation therapy may be used to minimize the risk of bladder seeding. The overall 5-year survival rate for patients treated with partial cystectomy approximates those of total cystectomy. However, this procedure (*i.e.,* partial cystectomy plus radiation therapy) is appropriate for no more than 5% to 10% of patients with invasive bladder cancer.

Radical Cystectomy

In the United States and much of Western Europe, radical cystectomy is the most common treatment used for muscle-invading bladder tumors. In Great Britain and Canada, external-beam radiation therapy with salvage cystectomy in patients demonstrating persistent tumor has been used to identify tumors responsive to radiation therapy and spare some patients the morbidity of radical cystectomy. In an attempt to increase survival rates, Whitmore used 2000 to 4000 cGy preoperative irradiation, followed by cystectomy. In a nonrandomized study using historic controls, survival rates for T3 tumors doubled from approximately 20% to 40%, but no survival advantage was demonstrated in other stages.[60] Subsequent studies comparing radical cystectomy alone with pre-

operative radiation therapy plus cystectomy could not confirm a survival advantage.[61]

Radical cystectomy (Fig. 34–2) implies removal of the bladder and contiguous organs en bloc. In men, this includes the prostate and seminal vesicles, and in women, anterior exenteration includes the bladder, urethra, uterus, ovaries, and a segment of the anterior vaginal wall. At the time of radical cystectomy, a bilateral pelvic lymph node dissection is also performed. The margins of this dissection extend from approximately 2 cm above the bifurcation of the common iliac arteries superiorly, the genitofemoral nerve laterally, the inguinal ligament and node of Cloquet distally, the obturator nerve and vessels inferiorly, and the bladder wall medially. The technique used is described elsewhere.[62]

The data obtained from radical cystectomy series have emphasized the significant problems in clinical understaging (see Table 34–1) and provide further justification for the exploration of multimodal therapy. Most failures after radical cystectomy are due to distant disease, with fewer than 10% of patients demonstrating local failure.

Difficulties arise in attempting to compare the results of radical cystectomy in nonconcurrent series (Table 34–4). There has been a marked decrease in operative mortality resulting from improvements in surgical technique and preoperative management, and advances in staging modalities have identified patients with metastatic disease not appropriate for surgical treatment. The effect of this selection is apparent in an analysis of contemporary surgical results compared with older series.

The role of surgery as curative therapy for patients with nodal metastatic disease continues to evolve. Before the era of CT scanning, many patients with nodal disease were found to have large, bulky disease at surgery, but nodal disease in recent studies has more commonly been N1 disease, frequently microscopic, with normal-sized lymph nodes. Overall 5-year survival data of 4% to 35% have been recorded. Because a bilateral pelvic lymph node dissection at the time of cystectomy adds little to overall morbidity, improves staging accuracy, and may be curative in some patients with minimal nodal involvement, the procedure should be considered as standard in patients undergoing radical cystectomy.

In female patients, the entire urethra is removed with the specimen, but in male patients, the urethra beyond the prostate usually is left in place. Overall, the incidence of tumor recurrence in the retained urethra after cystectomy is 4% to 14%.[63] However, the incidence of Tis found in studies in which cystourethrectomies were routinely done is approximately twice that of the rate of urethral recurrence in patients in whom the urethra is left in place. What happens to the 50% of patients with urethral Tis who do not develop urethral cancer after cystectomy and how to identify these patients prospectively remain unanswered questions. The clinical data suggest that the urothelium left behind may benefit from the diversion of urine from the urethra. Although we cannot prospectively identify every patient who is at risk for developing a urethral recurrence after radical cystectomy, urethrectomy has been recommended for several clinical circumstances: multifocal papillary disease involving the bladder neck; diffuse carcinoma in situ of the bladder specimen, especially around the bladder neck; tumor in the prostatic urethra; and tumor involving the distal margin of the cystectomy specimen.

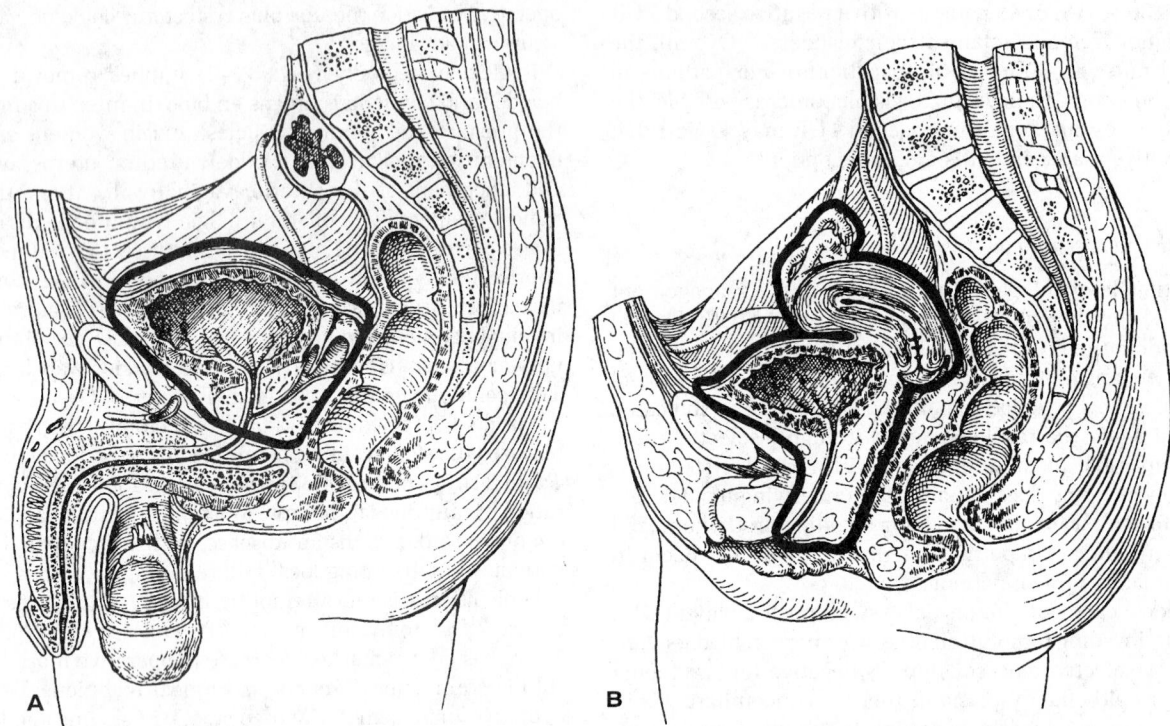

FIGURE 34–2. **(A)** Radical cystectomy in the male patient includes removal of the bladder, prostate, and seminal vesicles en bloc. **(B)** In women, the bladder, including the entire urethra, anterior vaginal wall, and uterus are excised. In postmenopausal women, the ovaries are included. At the time of radical cystectomy, a bilateral pelvic lymph node dissection is performed in men and women. Dissection is carried superiorly to the level of the common iliac artery just below the aortic bifurcation, laterally to the genitofemoral nerve, medially to the bladder wall, and caudally to the obturation fossa and the Cooper ligament.

The incidence of recurrent disease increases markedly in patients who had tumor involving the prostate. Hardeman and Soloway followed 86 patients after radical cystoprostatectomy to assess the incidence of urethral tumor recurrence. Of the 30 patients with tumor in the prostate, 11 (37%) had urethral recurrences. In 56 patients with other areas of the bladder involved but no prostatic involvement, only 2 (4%) had recurrences.[64] Levinson and colleagues, in a larger series of 124 men, found urethral recurrences in 17% of those who presented with disease extending into the prostate, including 3 (30%) of 10 with stromal invasion.[65] Among the patients whose tumor did not involve the bladder neck, the incidence of subsequent urethral cancer was 1.5%. Among patients with carcinoma in situ or multifocal tumors not involving the prostate, only 4.5% had recurrences, and among 9 patients with tumors at the bladder neck alone (without prostatic involvement), none had recurrences in this group followed for as long as 16 years.

In patients in whom the urethra is left in situ, the use of the urethral wash cytology should be routine; for a persistent positive cytology, urethrectomy should be performed. The overall survival rate is poor for patients presenting with symptomatic recurrences, usually manifested as the development of urethral bleeding or a mass. For patients in whom the diagnosis is made cytologically, the prognosis is much better.

TABLE 34–4. Cystectomy Alone for Invasive Transitional Cell Carcinoma

Investigations	No. of Patients	Study Period	5-Year Survival (%) by P Stage			Operative Mortality (%)
			P2	P3a	P3b	
Whitmore[60] (crude survival)	137	1949–1958	60	26	11	14.0
Montie[61] (cause-specific survival)	99	1960–1979	62	74	57	9.0
Mathur[168] (crude survival)	58	1967–1974	88	57	40	3.4
Skinner[47] (KM actuarial survival)	97	1971–1984	83	69	29	3.0
Pagano[139] (KM actuarial survival)	261	1979–1987	68	67	22	1.8

As we increasingly employ continent urinary diversion, especially involving an anastomosis directly between the bladder and the distal urethra, the eventual fate of the urethral remnant beyond the prostate assumes greater significance. Improved techniques of continent urinary diversions and preserving sexual function have revealed that routine performance of urethrectomy may be associated with poorer quality of life because of incontinence and impotency.

Our policy is to do a generous transurethral biopsy of the prostatic urethra in all patients being considered for continent urinary diversion. If the urethra is free of tumor, even if the bladder neck is involved, continent diversion may be considered.

Continent Urinary Diversion

During the past decade, a variety of innovative and challenging approaches to provide functional bladder substitutes for patients requiring radical cystectomy have been employed. The pioneering work of Koch,[66] Skinner and associates,[67] and Camay[68] have spawned a number of techniques of substitution enterocystoplasty.

The Koch pouch obviates the need for the patient to wear an external collecting device, but the difficulty of the operation, the short-term and long-term complications, the high reoperation rate, and the necessity for frequent catheterizations, with the risk of subsequent urinary tract infection and stone formation, have dimmed the enthusiasm for its routine performance in many centers. Other procedures employing the terminal ileum and right colon are at least theoretically less desirable because of the higher pressures within the colon, which may lead to a higher incontinence rate. Sacrifice of the terminal 15 to 20 cm of ileum is associated with impaired vitamin B_{12} and bile salt absorption, making resection of the terminal ileum physiologically equivalent to the removal of 70 to 100 cm of total ileum.

Although no alternative can be considered a normal bladder, the optimal bladder substitute should minimize the likelihood of incontinence and avoid repeat catheterization. To achieve these endpoints, a continent substitute should include the use of the small bowel, because the pressure in the ileum is lower than the pressure in the colon and may reduce the likelihood of incontinence. The detubularization of the intestinal segment eliminates "mass contraction," which can lead to sporadic loss of urine. If possible, the bladder substitute should be anastomosed directly to the urethra to approximate the normal bladder and to avoid the necessity for and the morbidity associated with repeat catheterization. Although a number of innovative approaches have been used, all based on the original ideas proposed by Camay, we have found the use of the ileal neobladder to be an extremely effective form of continent urinary diversion.[69] Hautmann and associates reported complete day and night continence in 78% of 145 patients.[70] Mild to moderate stress incontinence was reported in approximately 10% of patients, and 5% had severe stress incontinence. It appears that patients older than 70 are much more likely to have trouble with continence than younger patients. The rate of nocturnal continence depends on the instructions given to the patients and how the continence is reported. It is our practice to instruct all of the patients to set their alarm to rise and urinate one time during the night and empty the neobladder. Using this technique, none of our patients have required oral alkalinization to avoid hyperchloremic acidosis, and nocturnal enuresis has not been a problem.

RADIATION THERAPY

Treatment Techniques

The fact that radiation therapy can eradicate and permanently control urinary bladder tumors has been demonstrated in many studies. Duncan and Quilty reported that 46% of 963 patients with T1 through T4 disease treated with 5500 to 5750 cGy in 20 fractions over 4 weeks showed a complete response at first follow-up cystoscopy, although only approximately half of these patients had durable local control at 5 years.[71]

The level of the tumoricidal radiation dose is not clearly defined. The need to achieve maximal local control is stressed by the data demonstrating that patients succumb to local failure.[72,73] Davidson reported that 23% of bladder carcinoma patients who died after treatment with irradiation alone succumbed to local failure, 46% died with local and distant metastatic relapses, 13% with metastases only, and the other 18% from unrelated causes.[72] Although the tumor dose affected local control, several other clinical and pathologic parameters, such as T stage and grade, gross tumor morphology, ureteral obstruction, the hemoglobin level, and the size of the residual primary tumor after transurethral resection, also affected the likelihood of local control.[71,74-84] The problem is further complicated by the fact that disease recurs after years of apparent local control, with new tumors presumably reinduced by urinary carcinogens in genetically predisposed high-risk patients. Because most studies have not stratified patients by many of these covariates, the relative impact of dose on local control has frequently been obscured, and the tumoricidal dose level for a given set of clinical parameters is not well defined.

Edsmyr reported a prospective study of 168 patients with T2 through T4 disease who were randomized to receive 8400 cGy in 100-cGy fractions three times daily (4 hours apart) or to receive 6400 cGy in 200-cGy fractions once daily. Local eradication of the tumor at 6 months was observed in 65% of the patients receiving 8400 cGy but in only 36% of those receiving 6400 cGy ($p<0.001$).[85] Survival was also significantly improved in the high-dose group. However, a phase I–II RTOG protocol (83-08) of hyperfractionated radiation with two daily fractions of 120 cGy carried to 6000, 6490, or 6960 cGy failed to show an effect for the dose escalation.

Although the tumoricidal dose level is unknown, most recent series have recommended that a dose of 6500 cGy at daily single doses of 180 to 200 cGy should be given to the tumor region, although the dose to the whole bladder and perivesical dose should be restricted to 4750 to 5500 cGy.[71,72,86,87] When carefully planned, such treatments are considered safe, with acceptable acute and long-term toxic effects. The four-field box technique represents the most common approach, designed to include the entire bladder, the perivesical soft tissues, and the pelvic lymphatics, while minimizing the dose to the rectum and anus. Patients are simulated with radiopaque material in the bladder and rectum to delineate the tumor target volume. Treatment planning with CT is recommended to improve the delineation of extravesical tumor extensions. The pelvic fields extend from the level of L5–S1 to 1 cm below the obturator foramina (or to the bottom of the ischial tuberosities if inclusion of more distal urethral tissues is required) and laterally 1 to 2 cm beyond the bony pelvic brim. On the lateral portals, the posterior margin is set at least 3 cm behind the most posterior extent of the tumor as determined by palpation and CT scan. These fields are carried to a total dose of 4750 to 5500 cGy. An additional dose is delivered to the primary tumor volume to increase the tumor dose to approximately 6500 to 7000 cGy. This field should be designed based on tumor mapping produced with the aid of treatment planning cystoscopy and CT scans. Treatment is optimally delivered by opposed lateral fields or by arc rotation fields to decrease the dose to the rectum.

If treatment is delivered with radiation fractions of 200 cGy or less, it is well tolerated, with acute and self-limiting toxic effects such as dysuria, diarrhea, or urinary frequency occurring in 50% to 70% of the patients. These are usually treated symptomatically without requiring significant interruption in the treatment course. Long-term complications become clinically apparent within the first 3 years after completion of treatment. Shipley reported that only 4 of 35 patients treated with conventional daily doses of 180 to 200 cGy developed chronic frequency or hematuria causing incontinence or requiring surgery, and the RTOG 83-03 study reported that 10.5% of patients treated with hypofractionated radiotherapy (120 cGy twice daily) carried to 6000 to 6960 cGy developed grade 3 or 4 toxicities requiring medications or surgery at 18 to 36 months after completion of treatment.[82] Similarly, Mameghan reported that the 5-year actuarial complication rate with single daily fractions of 180 to 250 cGy was 9.4% for the bladder and 10.5% for the bowel.[88] A higher dose per fraction is not recommended, because hypofractionated regimens involve more serious acute complications that require interruptions during the course of treatment and because the rate of serious late complications increases to 20% to 25%.[71,89,90] Davidson and coworkers reported that split-course therapy (2–3-week interruptions) is associated with a statistically significant decrease in the overall 5-year survival rate, probably associated with tumor repopulation phenomena, as reported for other types of human tumors.[72]

Results of Treatment

RADIOTHERAPY ALONE. In many series, patients treated with radiotherapy alone were those regarded as poor candidates for cystectomy because of age or intercurrent medical contraindications for surgery, and they represented a group with a more limited potential for survival. The overall results of megavoltage radiotherapy when given alone have been disappointing, with 5-year survival ranging from 30% to 45% (Table 34–5). The probability of a curative success with radiotherapy alone depends on the ability to achieve a permanent eradication of the tumor in the bladder. Only 23% to 41% of patients with invasive tumors achieve a durable local control of the primary bladder tumor after radical radiotherapy (see Table 34–5), although survival critically depends on local control, with most locally relapsing patients succumbing to this condition with or without distant metastases.[72,91]

In a retrospective review from the Massachusetts General Hospital, the 5-year survival rate of patients with clinical stage T2 or T3 tumors who maintained permanent local control was 79%, compared with only 11% for patients who developed a local recurrence.[82] Because many patients succumb to locally recurring tumors, salvage cystectomy has become a common practice for patients relapsing locally after bladder irradiation, but such treatment can be deferred in completely responding patients until relapse occurs.[92–94] The 5-year survival rate after salvage cystectomy for patients selected as appropriate candidates for this procedure is 40% to 45%, but salvage cystectomy still carries significant risks because of difficulties in operating on heavily irradiated tissues and because many patients initially referred to radiation treatments are those regarded as poor candidates for surgery. Mortality rates associated with salvage cystectomy have been as high as 19%.[95,96]

Several clinical and histopathologic parameters have been identified as covariates that affect the local and metastatic outcome in carcinoma of the bladder. Although clinical staging has been recognized for its inaccuracies, it still represents the most significant factor affecting survival. Within each stage, the success of radiotherapy may be favorably influenced by low tumor grade, ploidy, a papillary rather than a sessile

TABLE 34–5. Five-Year Survival and Local Control Rates for Patients With Invasive Carcinoma of the Urinary Bladder Treated With Radical Radiation Therapy

Investigations	No. of Patients	Local Control (%)	Overall 5-Year Survival (%)	T1	T2	T3 (T3a/T3b)	T4 (T4a/T4b)
Goffinet, 1975[77]	384	24	40		46	35	
Rider, 1976[99]	554			56	50	18	20
Blandy, 1980[35]	704	30	29	70	27	38	9
Yu, 1985[36]	356	36		66	42	35/23	23
Duncan, 1986[71]	917	23	36	61	40	26	12
Jenkins, 1988[14]	182	41	40		46	35	
Gospodarowicz, 1989[84]	121	35	45		59	52/29	50/16
Davidson, 1990[72]	709		31	87	49	28	2
Greven, 1990[100]	116	27	34	39	59	10	0

tumor, the absence of ureteral obstruction, normal hemoglobin level, and the achievement of a visibly complete transurethral resection of the primary tumor.[82,83,97–100] In a recent multivariate Cox regression analysis of 121 patients with T2 through T4 bladder tumors, Gospodarowicz demonstrated that stage, grade, tumor size, configuration, and hemoglobin level were the independent covariates that significantly affected the outcome after radiotherapy.[84]

Because local control with external-beam radiotherapy has been frustratingly low, enhancement of the tumor dose has been recommended by intraoperative radiotherapy, involving external-beam tumor irradiation during open surgery with retraction of surrounding tissues, or temporary intratumoral implantation of radioactive sources. The rationale for these techniques is to facilitate the delivery of radiation to the tumor with concomitant exclusion of the surrounding normal tissues. The selection criteria for intraoperative radiotherapy is restricted by the need to perform surgery, and the technique is applicable to relatively few patients. Matsumoto and associates treated 116 patients with small, superficial (*e.g.*, Ta, T1, T2) tumors with 3.5- to 7.5-MeV electrons.[101] A single intraoperative dose of 2500 to 3000 cGy was delivered directly onto the tumor exposed during cystotomy by means of 4- to 6-cm cones. This was followed 3 to 4 weeks later by external-beam radiotherapy (3000–4000 cGy in 3 to 4 weeks). Among 28 patients treated for stage T2 tumors, there was freedom from recurrence in 82%, with an overall 62% 5-year survival rate.

Brachytherapy is also useful mainly in patients with small tumors (≤5 cm), because implantation of larger tumors requires large numbers of sources and high total activities, leading to severe complications. The largest experience with brachytherapy of bladder tumors has been reported by van der Werf-Messing at the Rotterdam Radiotherapy Institute. Implantation was initially carried out with radium needles and more recently with cesium 137 sources.[80] The sources were implanted into the tumor during cystotomy and left for several days until a dose of 3250 to 6500 cGy was delivered. Problems of wound seeding by tumor cells during cystotomy have been resolved by the use of preoperative irradiation with 1050 cGy in three fractions. The 5-year recurrence-free survival and overall survival rates for 328 patients with stage T2 disease were 77% and 56%, respectively. Mazeron, using modern afterloading techniques of iridium 192 after partial cystectomy of T2 tumors, reported similar favorable results, with 82% to 93% 5-year local control rates and 55% to 63% 5-year survival rates.[102] Van der Werf-Messing reported improved results with preimplant delivery of external-beam radiotherapy to a dose of 4000 cGy and radium implantation in T2 patients, producing a 5-year survival rate of 73%.[56] Although these data are impressive, they are biased by patient selection, and prospective trials comparing these techniques with conservative surgical treatments or with external-beam radiotherapy are necessary to establish the true role of intraoperative radiotherapy in the management of carcinoma of the bladder.

PREOPERATIVE IRRADIATION AND RADICAL CYSTECTOMY. The rationale for the use of preoperative irradiation is to sterilize microscopic tumor deposits that may be left behind in the pelvis after cystectomy and to prevent seeding of tumor cells caused by intraoperative tumor manipulation. The dose schedules commonly used are 2000 cGy in 1 week or 4000 to 5000 cGy in standard fractionation of 200 cGy per fraction over 4 to 5 weeks. Such treatment schedules have definite antitumor effects, because 14% to 43% of cystectomy specimens do not have identifiable tumor tissue after 4000 to 5000 cGy.[103–105] If pelvic lymphadenectomy is performed at the time of cystectomy in preirradiated stage B2 or C patients, the incidence of histologically positive lymph nodes decreases from the expected 37% to 53% to 10% to 25%.[38,41–43,103–106] A study by Whitmore and colleagues showed that the risk for recurrences was reduced from 37% (26 of 71 patients) after cystectomy alone to 14% (28 of 194) after 2000 to 4000 cGy to the pelvis plus cystectomy.[60]

Despite the definitive effects of preoperative irradiation on pelvic tumor tissues, its effects on survival are less clear. The data by Whitmore indicated an improved survival rate of 42% at 5 years for patients receiving 4000 cGy of preoperative irradiation and cystectomy compared with historic data that showed a survival rate of 37% for nonrandomized patients treated with cystectomy alone.[103] Parsons and Million summarized the published nonrandomized studies on the effects of preoperative irradiation in bladder tumors and showed that the calculated average for the 5-year survival rate after cystectomy in 784 patients with stage T3 disease who received preoperative irradiation was 48.3%, compared with 28.7% for 401 patients who did not receive irradiation.[107] However, such an analysis cannot be regarded as proof of benefit, which can only be provided by properly designed randomized studies.

There have been several randomized trials that compared cystectomy alone with preoperative irradiation and cystectomy, but the results are inconclusive. Two trials by the National Surgical Adjuvant Bowel and Breast Project suffered from major violations of the protocols, and the second protocol was terminated prematurely. Although the data suggest an advantage for the irradiated patients (44% versus 32% surviving at 5 years), these data cannot be regarded as conclusive.[108] Another study, carried out by eight Veterans Administration hospitals, suffered from poor accrual (total of 35 patients over 6 years) and failed to show a survival difference at 10 years.[109] The Southwest Oncology Group conducted a randomized study comparing 2000 cGy given in 1 week and cystectomy with cystectomy alone. Although the final results of this study are pending, the interim analysis showed no survival advantage to preoperative irradiation.[110] The current indications for preoperative irradiation are unclear, and its role in the routine management of carcinoma of the bladder remains controversial.

COMBINED RADIATION AND CHEMOTHERAPY. The demonstration that adjuvant chemotherapy can control metastatic disease and that neoadjuvant chemotherapy can completely or partially control primary bladder tumors and pelvic lymph node disease suggests that a combined-modality approach with neoadjuvant chemotherapy, limited surgery, and irradiation may lead to improved survival with bladder conservation.

CHEMOTHERAPY

The observation that most deaths from invasive bladder cancer are from metastases, and the development of effective combination programs led to the integration of chemotherapy in the management of invasive disease. This has been used in the preoperative or neoadjuvant setting, or as postoperative adjuvant treatment.[111] The approaches are contrasted in Table 34–6. Early use of chemotherapy exploits the inverse relationship between tumor burden and curability, and the higher

TABLE 34–6. Comparison of Adjuvant and Neoadjuvant Therapy

	Neoadjuvant	Adjuvant
A. Rationale: Early treatment of micrometastases		
1. Inverse relation of tumor burden and cure	+	+
2. Increased chemosensitivity of small volume high-growth-fraction tumors	+	+
3. Decreased chance of spontaneous resistance	+	+
B. Factors Favoring Neoadjuvant Therapy		
1. Chemosensitivity determined case by case		
a. Response assessment in vivo	+	−
b. Organ preservation possible	+	−
c. Endpoint of treatment more precise	+	−
2. "Downstaging" of the primary tumor		
a. Decrease the extent and need for additional therapy	+	−
b. Convert an "unresectable" to a "resectable" lesion	+	−
c. Drug delivery not compromised by previous surgery or radiation therapy	+	−
3. Prognostic significance of response in the primary	+	−
4. Potential for accelerated growth after surgery	+	−
5. Patient tolerance	+	±
C. Factors Favoring Adjuvant Therapy		
1. Case selection		
a. Staging error of T vs P	−	+
b. Need for therapy based on pathologic not clinical criteria	−	+
c. Exposure of patients "cured" by local therapies to cytotoxic agents	−	+
2. Timing of definitive local therapy		
a. Jeopardize curative therapy by prolonged treatment with ineffective agents	−	+
b. Refusal of potentially curative therapy	−	+

+, yes; −, no.
(Modified from Scher H. Chemotherapy for invasive bladder cancer. Neo-adjuvant vs. adjuvant. Semin Oncol 1990;17:555–564)

cure rate observed for patients with nodal as opposed to metastatic disease.[112–115]

Neoadjuvant Chemotherapy

Chemotherapy given in the neoadjuvant setting is directed at treating micrometastases, the cause of treatment failure, using response in the primary tumor as the marker of efficacy. That chemosensitivity is determined in vivo, allowing treatment of a patient to the point of maximal response, is the major advantage of the neoadjuvant approach. Response provides prognostic information and can be used as a guide for subsequent treatment of the primary tumor. Although "standard" therapy is radical cystectomy, several groups are investigating strategies of organ preservation using local radiation therapy with chemotherapy as treatment for the primary tumor.[116–122]

Most reported trials represent uncontrolled phase II studies, which vary in the criteria for treatment, staging and restaging techniques, response criteria, the specific chemotherapy program used, and whether the outcome measures are based on clinical (T; cystoscopic) or pathologic (P; laparotomy with cystectomy) grounds. In virtually all studies, P response proportions are inferior to T-based reporting. For example, using the combination of methotrexate, vincristine, doxorubicin (Adriamycin), and cisplatin (the MVAC regimen), 48% (13 of 27 patients; 95% confidence limits, 29–67%) of patients were T0 endoscopically after a median of three cycles of treatment, compared with 23% who were P0 (14 of 60, 95% confidence limits, 13–34%) after partial or radical cystectomy.[123]

Response varies inversely with the depth of tumor invasion. In our MVAC experience, pathologic complete response proportions (pCR) were observed in 46% (16 of 35, 95% confidence limits, 21–62%) of patients with T2 or T3a tumors, compared with 8.5% (3 of 35 patients, 95% confidence limits, 0–18%) of patients with more advanced T3b, T4a, or T4b lesions.[124] Nontransitional and mixed histology tumors and carcinoma in situ are generally less sensitive to chemotherapy, which is important if an attempt at bladder sparing is considered. Although a causal association cannot be implied, response in the primary does correlate with a good prognosis. In a summary series of 125 patients treated with cisplatin-based chemotherapy followed by radical surgery, 91% (53 of 58) of responders (≤P1 at cystectomy) but only 37% (25 of 67) of nonresponders (≥P2 at cystectomy) were alive and free of disease at a median follow-up of 25 months (range, 21.5–100).[25]

Cumulative data of 444 patients with residual disease in the bladder before the start of chemotherapy showed pathologic complete remissions (P0) in 30% of patients. Chemotherapy alone cannot replace definitive local therapy for most patients. Of equal concern is the inability to accurately predict by endoscopic and other noninvasive means which bladders that are clinically T0 will be pathologically P0. Summary data from several series show that as many as 50% of those with no tumor detected endoscopically harbor residual muscle infiltrating disease that is found at surgery.[111,123,126,127] For most patients, chemotherapy alone is inadequate as monotherapy for the primary tumor, and some form of definitive local treatment is required. Neoadjuvant chemotherapy has not yet been shown to improve survival, and randomized comparisons are needed.

Adjuvant Chemotherapy

Adjuvant therapy traditionally refers to the use of chemotherapy after surgery. The decision to recommend treatment is based on the pathologic findings at cystectomy. It also includes administration of chemotherapy in patients for whom all visible tumor has been resected endoscopically by TUR. The specific criteria for recommending chemotherapy have not been formalized, but many physicians offer therapy if there is nodal disease, extravesical tumor extension, or vascular or lymphatic invasion in the resected primary tumor specimen. Theoretically, the risks of delaying potentially curative surgery are diminished and the number of patients treated with cytotoxic drugs who may be cured by surgery alone is reduced. Removal of the bladder eliminates the risk of new tumor formation. The major limitation of adjuvant therapy is that response cannot be assessed, and the decision to continue therapy is largely empiric. However, as the techniques of internal urinary reservoirs become more refined, adjuvant treatment has become the preferred approach of many physicians.

Several studies using adjuvant therapy showed no benefit, partially because of the small number of patients treated and because the chemotherapy was suboptimal by 1990s' standards. Two trials using cisplatin, doxorubicin, and cyclophosphamide (CAP regimen) did show a benefit. At M.D. Anderson Cancer Center, 339 patients treated by radical cystectomy were categorized as high-risk (133 patients) or low-risk (206).[128] High risk included vascular or lymphatic invasion in the primary specimen (37), extravesical tumor spread (50), node-positive disease (24), or extension into the adjacent pelvic viscera (22). The survival distributions of the 71 high-risk patients who received chemotherapy were compared with the 62 high-risk and 206 low-risk patients who did not receive chemotherapy. A treatment benefit was suggested by a shift in the survival distributions for treated high-risk patients to those of the untreated low-risk group. Five-year survival rates for the untreated low-risk, treated high-risk, and untreated high-risk groups were 76%, 70%, and 35%, respectively. Patients in all risk groups appeared to benefit.

In a second trial at the University of Southern California, 91 patients with P3 or P4 with or without nodal disease after radical cystectomy and en bloc pelvic node dissection were randomized to receive four cycles of CAP or observation.[129] This group was derived from a total of 253 patients who met protocol criteria during the study period. The results showed a higher percentage of patients disease free at 3 years (70% versus 46%, $p=0.001$), longer median survival (4.25 versus 2.41 years), and lower risk of bladder cancer mortality for patients treated with adjuvant chemotherapy. In univariate analysis, the number of lymph nodes was the most important prognostic feature, but treatment benefit was only observed in patients with one or fewer nodes positive. Unfortunately, this trial was terminated before the planned accrual of 75 patients per arm, and the subgroup analyses were quite small. For example, only 7 patients with one positive lymph node were treated, which makes it difficult to extrapolate to a larger population of patients with nodal disease. Chemotherapy delivery was suboptimal, as 11 (25%) of the 44 patients randomized to chemotherapy never received it, and only 21 (48%) completed the full four chemotherapy cycles as intended. Therefore, the question whether adjuvant chemotherapy improves the survival of patients with P3 or P4 with or without nodal disease requires additional confirmation.

Chemotherapy and irradiation have been combined to reduce the incidence of metastatic disease. Several randomized comparisons of irradiation alone and irradiation plus single-agent systemic chemotherapy have been reported. No benefit has been shown for doxorubicin plus 5-fluorouracil, cisplatin, or methotrexate.[130-132] The outcome is not surprising considering the small response proportions observed in patients with metastatic disease.

Treatment and Cell Histologies of Nontransitional Cell Histologies

Nontransitional cell tumors are less sensitive to regimens employed for transitional cell carcinomas, although selected cases with small cell carcinoma have been reported to respond to MVAC, and one invasive adenocarcinoma was reported to respond to cisplatin, methotrexate, and vinblastine (CMV regimen). In our experience of treating invasive disease, 3 patients with mixed histology (*i.e.*, transitional plus squamous cell carcinoma or transitional cell plus adenocarcinoma) had only the nontransitional cell component left in the cystectomy specimen.

Most series reporting patients with adenocarcinomas include small numbers of patients treated with a variety of regimens, making generalizations about treatment policy difficult. Antitumor activity has been observed using a combination of 5-fluorouracil, doxorubicin and mitomycin C, and partial responses have been observed using the combination of 5-fluorouracil and cisplatin with or without mitomycin C. In these cases, elevations of CEA or CA 125 may be useful for monitoring outcome.

For squamous cell tumors, responses were reported using a combination of 5-fluorouracil, mitomycin C, and concurrent radiation therapy (NIGRO regimen), an approach similar to that used for squamous cell tumors of the anal canal.[167] Antitumor responses have been reported for squamous cell tumors of the bladder, urethra, and penis using 5-fluorouracil and cisplatin, which is the current approach used for tumors of squamous cell origin at MSKCC. Small cell tumors are treated with regimens similar to those used for primary small cell carcinomas of the lung, with similar dramatic, albeit short-lived, responses.

BLADDER PRESERVATION

Refinements in the techniques of urinary diversion, especially the availability of internal reservoirs and continent diversions, have lessened the interest in bladder preservation as a primary treatment goal. Although the relative quality of life of a patient treated with a radical cystectomy and ileal conduit, partial cystectomy, or ileal neobladder or who has received radiation therapy has not been adequately studied, it seems that retention of a functional "natural" bladder is preferable. Several series have reported that highly selected patients were able to safely retain their bladders by TUR alone, partial cystectomy, implantation, or laser therapy. However, these approaches are not appropriate for most patients with invasive disease.

Integrated Approaches

With radiation therapy alone, fewer than 50% of patients achieve a complete response to treatment, the prerequisite for bladder preservation. To improve local control rates and increase the proportion of patients who can retain their bladders, several groups have studied combinations of chemotherapy and radiation therapy. These two modalities can be integrated sequentially, in which the chemotherapy is given first and radiation therapy thereafter; as alternating chemotherapy and radiation therapy; or concurrently. Several chemotherapeutic agents have been studied, including cisplatin, 5-fluorouracil, mitomycin C, doxorubicin, methotrexate, or combinations of cisplatin and doxorubicin, MVAC, or CMV. The major limitations to the bladder-sparing approach are the potential for increased toxicities to the surrounding normal tissues, questions about the functional capability of the treated bladder, the continued risk of new superficial or invasive tumor formation in the bladder, the inability to predict which bladders are "tumor free" and safely left in place. Whether these approaches ultimately compromise survival is unknown. Although failure to control the disease locally can prevent cure, for patients with a high risk of metastases, inclusion of effective chemotherapy that treats the metastatic component is imperative if survival is to be improved.

It has been shown in several series that the probability of local control in the bladder with radiation therapy is improved if a visibly complete TUR is performed, rather than a simple biopsy or incomplete resection.[133] Recognizing the limitations of nonrandomized comparisons, the rates for these two groups were 68% and 11% for local control and 54% and 17% for 5-year survival, respectively. The probability of local control was higher for papillary than for solid tumors. To improve these results, the National Bladder Cancer Cooperative Group A study evaluated concomitant cisplatin (70 mg/m^2) at 3-week intervals with 180 cGy/day for 5 days a week for 5 weeks of radiation in patients who were not suitable for cystectomy. Of 57 patients with evaluable gross tumor who completed therapy, 45 (77%) were T0 after treatment. This included 88% of T2, 84% of T3, and 50% of T4 patients. Of those rendered tumor free, 73% were maintained at 4 years.[134]

To build on this experience and noting the results with MVAC in advanced disease, investigators at the Massachusetts General Hospital developed a protocol that evaluated the policy of a visibly complete endoscopic resection, followed by two cycles of MCV chemotherapy, followed by concurrent cisplatin and radiation therapy.[119,135] The relative contribution of each component of this combined modality approach is difficult to ascertain. After completion of treatment, the overall response in the primary is used to select patients for potential bladder preservation. Patients who were tumor free after 4500 cGy were continued to a total of 6500 cGy, and those with residual muscle infiltrating disease were referred for surgery. In the initial trial of 53 patients, 42 (81%) completed the protocol. Considering the entire group, 70% were free of metastases, 79% retained their bladders, but only 23% were tumor free, including recurrences in the bladder. An analysis of prognostic factors showed that increasing tumor size, increasing depth of invasion, and presence of carcinoma in situ adversely affected outcome.[136]

Case Selection

The results of these pilot investigations suggest that in a highly selected group of motivated patients, bladder preservation can be successfully accomplished. However, the risk of new tumor formation in the bladder remains, and careful follow-up is required for patients in whom the bladder is left. It is controversial whether the ability to visibly resect a tumor is in itself a favorable prognostic factor. Although preliminary data suggest that this approach does not compromise survival, a formal comparison with radical surgery has not been performed. It must therefore be considered investigational.

CLINICAL TRIALS

The heterogeneity of urothelial tract tumors in all stages and the differences in patient demographics with respect to extent of disease, performance status, and intercurrent illness makes it difficult to extrapolate a standard treatment policy that can be applied to all patients. Within the different stages—superficial, invasive, regionally advanced, and metastatic—many clinical trials have attempted to define standards of care. For patients with metastatic disease, combination chemotherapy is now standard or first-line treatment. For those with invasive disease, controversy continues about whether preoperative radiation therapy improves survival. Despite the recognized risk of metastatic disease for those with invasive lesions, the question of using chemotherapy as neoadjuvant or adjuvant therapy remains unanswered.

The routine application of chemotherapy for all patients with invasive bladder cannot be considered standard. Combining the results of single-arm phase II trials or comparison of contemporary chemotherapy-treated patients with historic surgical results does not permit definitive conclusions.[137] Surgical results have improved. Operative mortality has decreased to less than 2%, and careful pathologic examination of the lymph nodes removed at surgery results in a higher frequency of discovery of microscopic nodal disease. This resultant upstaging of patients with minimal tumor burdens produces a "stage migration" and an apparent improvement in survival for all stages of patients.[138] As a result, 5-year survival rates for patients with microscopic N2 disease, previously thought to be incurable, have recently been reported in the range of 15% to 20%.[139,140]

Although the design of a trial to demonstrate a survival benefit for patients with invasive bladder tumors seems straightforward, application of this methodology to this patient population has been limited.[141] This may reflect the elderly population treated, the problem administering aggressive therapies, and the recognized reluctance of physicians and patients to participate in randomized trials. The results in advanced-disease patients provide a basis for estimating the number of patients required to demonstrate a survival benefit. These estimates are crucial to ensure that the appropriate patients are considered and that the trial is completed on a timely basis. Relative risk also affects the number of patients needed. Fewer patients would be required if the risk of the event were 90% instead of 10%. Many randomized trials accrued too few patients to answer the question they were designed to address. For example, a West Midlands trial and a separate Australian trial designed to assess the benefit of neoadjuvant cisplatin before definitive local radiation therapy fell short of planned accrual; only 155 of 300 and 87 of 250, respectively, were entered.[131] Hall estimated that a 10% to 15% improvement in survival would be clinically meaningful and have the potential to change clinical practice.[142] This aim is realistic based on currently available therapies. However, sample size estimates show that to improve the 2-year survival rate of 50% in a control group to 65% in an experimental group would require 400 patients.[143]

Ongoing clinical trials for patients with invasive disease are listed in Table 34–7. The trials differ on the basis of the patient populations under study, the proportion that are surgically resectable at the start of therapy, and metastatic risk. Two trials designed to assess survival are the Intergroup study comparing three cycles of MVAC followed by cystectomy with cystectomy alone and an international study comparing CMV chemotherapy, followed by radical cystectomy or radiation therapy.[144] For the latter, an accrual of 800 to 1000 patients is planned. The RTOG is comparing their previous standard, cisplatin plus radiation therapy, with two cycles of MCV plus cisplatin and radiation therapy, with an endpoint of bladder preservation. Survival will be evaluated, but the results cannot be compared with radical surgery. Investigators at M.D. Anderson Cancer Center are comparing the policy of adjuvant and neoadjuvant therapies in a high-risk population. The effect on downstaging, drug delivery, and patient tolerance will be assessed. Data from these trials are awaited to refine the role of chemotherapy for invasive disease.

MANAGING ADVANCED DISEASE

Left untreated, patients with metastatic urothelial tract tumors die from their disease.[145] Before the development of effective chemotherapy, median survivals rarely exceeded 3 to 6 months. For these patients, the aim is palliation, although long-term survival was reported using aggressive combination regimens in selected patients. The choice of a particular chemotherapy program depends on the patient and tumor-related factors that may affect tolerance to treatment. Histology can also affect outcome, because the regimens commonly in use have limited efficacy against nontransitional cell histologies such as adenocarcinomas and squamous cell tumors.

Urothelial tract tumors are sensitive to several single agents with different mechanisms (Table 34–8).[145–147] In general, responses to single agents are partial, with virtually no complete remissions, and they last a median of 3 to 4 months. Cisplatin is thought to be the most active agent, followed by methotrexate. Response occurs rapidly, and the drug can be discontinued if no response is seen in one or two cycles. The standard schedule is 70 mg/m² every 3 weeks; higher doses (100–120 mg/m²) have not improved outcome. The primary limitations are the inability to administer the adequate doses in patients with compromised renal function and the fluid load required to maintain hydration in patients with cardiac disease. In some cases, divided doses (20–35 mg/m²/day) have been used, but it is unclear whether this strategy results in equivalent therapeutic efficacy. Cumulative data suggest a higher response proportion for localized than for metastatic disease.

Methotrexate is usually given on a weekly or biweekly basis in a dose range of 30 to 40 mg/m². The overall (*i.e.*, complete plus partial) response proportion is 30% (95% confidence limits, 25–35%). Administration of higher doses with or without leucovorin rescue has not improved outcome, despite the suggestion from cumulative phase II trials.[148] Several investigational analogs have shown activity, including 10-deazaaminopterin, trimetrexate, and dichloromethotrexate, but none has replaced the parent compound in combination regimens. Other agents with significant activity include doxo-

TABLE 34–7. Selected Randomized Trials

Investigations	Experimental Arm	Control Arm	Eligible	Endpoint(s)	No. of Patients
Intergroup	MVAC × 3 → cystectomy	Cystectomy	T2–4N0M0	Downstaging, time to metastases, survival	300
MRC/EORTC	CMV × 3 → local therapy (Cystectomy or radiation)	Local therapy (Cystectomy or radiation)	T2–4N0M0	Survival	800–1000
MDAH	Both arms experimental: MVAC × 2 → cystectomy → MVAC × 3 vs cystectomy → MVAC × 5		T3b–4N0M0	Policy of adjuvant vs neoadjuvant	150
RTOG	Local therapy based on response in primary MCV × 2 → DDP/RT	DDP/RT	T2–4N0M0	Bladder preservation, survival	250

MVAC, methotrexate, vincristine, doxorubicin (Adriamycin), cisplatin; C, cisplatin; RT, radiation therapy; MRC, Medical Research Council; EORTC, European Organization for the Research and Treatment of Cancer; MDAH, M.D. Anderson Cancer Center; RTOG, Radiation Therapy Oncology Group.
(Scher HI, Norton L. Chemotherapy for urothelial tract malignancies. Semin Surg Oncol 1992;88: 316–341)

TABLE 34–8.   Single Agents for Urothelial Tract Tumors

Agent	No. of CR + PR/ No. Entered	CR + PR (%)	95% Confidence Interval (%)
Cisplatin			
Single institution	70/206	34	28–40
Randomized trials	55/316	17	37–55
Neoadjuvant	75/184	40	34–48
Overall	200/706	28	26–32
Carboplatin	21/186	15	11–19
CHIP	7/39	18	6–30
Methotrexate			
"Low" dose	68/236	29	23–35
"High" dose	16/57	45	37–50
Doxorubicin	47/274	17	13–22
Vinblastine	6/38	16	4–28
Cyclophosphamide	30/98	31*	22–40
5-Fluorouracil	22/141	17*	11–25
Mitomycin C	5/42	13*	2–22
Gallium nitrate	9/29	29	13–45

CR, complete response; PR, partial response.

* Reflects early trials using varied doses, schedules and response criteria.

(Modified from Arap W, Scher HI. The value of cytotoxic chemotherapy in locally invasive and metastatic bladder cancer. In: Williams G, Waxman J, eds. Urological cancer: A consensus. London: Edward Arnold, 1991:185–199)

(Scher HI, Norton L. Chemotherapy for urothelial tract malignancies. Semin Surg Oncol. 1992;8:316–341)

rubicin, vinblastine, 5-fluorouracil, and gallium nitrate (see Table 34–8).

Several multidrug programs (Table 34–9) have been developed from carefully designed and executed phase II studies showing the independent activity of each component. In general, combinations of cisplatin and methotrexate (CM) with or without vinblastine (CMV) and with or without doxorubicin (MVAC) or the combination of cisplatin, doxorubicin, and cyclophosphamide (CISCA or CAP) have been the most extensively studied. This may in part explain the dramatic in-

crease in the overall and complete response proportions reported in these trials. For example, using MVAC, a four-drug regimen developed at MSKCC in 1983, in 121 evaluable patients, complete clinical (cCR) and pathologic (pCR) responses were observed in 25% of patients, and an additional 12% were rendered disease free with chemotherapy followed by resection of residual disease (overall CR proportion of 37%), and 36% obtained partial remissions after treatment.[114] With a 6-year follow-up, the median survival for patients with advanced nodal and metastatic disease was 32.9 and 12 months, respectively, with a 6-year survival rate of 32% and 17%, respectively.[149] Durable complete remissions have also been reported using CAP and CMV, with 19% of 92 patients alive beyond 200 weeks with the former and 9% of 62 patients alive at 3.9 years using the latter program.[150,151] A change in the natural history of the disease is also suggested by the increasing proportion of responding patients who develop central nervous system relapse as the first site of failure.

Several randomized trials comparing multidrug regimens to single agents have been reported. Only one showed the superiority of a combination with respect to response proportion, response duration, and survival.[152] This was due to the limited efficacy of previously available regimens and the inadequate number of patients treated to exclude a large β-error. In a seminal study, MVAC was compared with single-agent cisplatin. With 224 evaluable patients, MVAC was superior with respect to the complete response proportion (13% versus 3%), overall response proportion (34% versus 9%, $p=0.01$), and survival (12.6 versus 8.7 months, $p=0.02$).[152] In a second trial, MVAC was superior to CISCA with respect to overall response proportion (65% versus 46%) and median survival (18.4 versus 9.3 months, $p=0.0003$).[115] The relative superiority, if any, of MVAC over CMV, differs by the inclusion of doxorubicin in MVAC and a higher dose of cisplatin (100 versus 70 mg/m²) in CMV. No randomized trial has been performed, and the median survivals are similar. However, the median survivals for completely responding patients is longer for MVAC than for CMV-treated patients (38 versus 14 months, respectively) . Combination chemotherapy with three or four agents should be considered standard first-line therapy.

Other investigators have observed lower response proportions and shorter durations of response using MVAC. The toxic

TABLE 34–9.   Combination Chemotherapy Programs

Regimen	Drugs	No. of Trials	Evaluable Patients	Complete Responses (%)	Complete and Partial Responses (%)	95% Confidence Interval (%)
MTX/DDP	Methotrexate, cisplatin	9	293	41 (14)	135 (46)	(17–34)
CMV	Cisplatin, methotrexate, vinblastine	4	157	35 (22)	82 (52)	(29–39)
CAP/CISCA	Cyclophosphamide, doxorubicin, cisplatin	10	293	65 (22)	166 (57)	(13–31)
MVAC	Methotrexate, vinblastine, doxorubicin, cisplatin	12	526	106 (20)	281 (53)	(22–34)

(Scher HI, Norton L. Chemotherapy for urothelial tract malignancies. Semin Surg Oncol. 1992;8: 316–341)

effects include myelosuppression, sepsis, mucositis, nephrotoxicity, and peripheral neuropathy. Deaths have also been reported.[114,153-155] Therefore, before starting treatment, careful consideration must be given to pretreatment factors that may influence an individual patient's tolerance to the planned chemotherapy program. Patients with metastatic disease include those who present de novo and those with recurrence after primary therapies. The ability to deliver chemotherapy varies for each group. For example, long ileal conduits or internal reservoirs can alter the kinetics of methotrexate, which can predispose a patient to mucositis at presumably nontoxic levels. The intensive hydration required for cisplatin administration risks severe distension of these low-pressure reservoirs. Prior radiation therapy predisposes the patient to more severe myelosuppression. Consideration must also be given to any intercurrent medical conditions that may affect the tolerance to the components of a particular regimen. For example, underlying cardiac dysfunction may make the administration of doxorubicin contraindicated; ascites or edema preclude full doses of methotrexate; and severe renal dysfunction precludes cisplatin. Pretreatment prognostic factors can also affect outcome. Positive factors include high initial performance status, nodal versus metastatic disease, absence of bone or liver metastases, and no history of weight loss. Age per se has not been shown to inhibit outcome.[156,157]

The potential difficulties that can occur when using aggressive high-dose chemotherapy programs in an elderly population have led to several modifications of the standard programs. Some researchers advocate deletion of the day 15 or day 22 doses of methotrexate and vinblastine in MVAC. Epiadriamycin (MVEC) has been substituted for doxorubicin (MVAC) with the aim of reduced cardiac toxicity and myelosuppression, and carboplatin has been substituted for cisplatin in patients with compromised renal function. In two trials of carboplatin and methotrexate, overall response proportions of 50% and 53% and complete responses in 6% and 12%, respectively, were reported.[158,159]

A regimen of methotrexate, vinplastine, mitoxantrone, and carboplatin may be useful for elderly patients with intercurrent disease who cannot tolerate full doses of MVAC. A formal comparison with MVAC has not been undertaken. Therefore, routine substitution of carboplatin for cisplatin cannot be recommended, because a review of the single-agent experience with this compound shows a lower response proportion (see Table 34–8).

Toxicities can be reduced and drug delivery improved by coadministration of hematopoietic growth factors, such as granulocyte colony-stimulating factor (G-CSF). One study compared treatment cycles with MVAC plus G-CSF and treatment cycles with MVAC alone in an individual patient. It showed that a higher percentage of patients were eligible to receive full doses of chemotherapy on day 14 and 21 as planned (100% versus 29%, $p=0.0015$), that there were significantly fewer days (3 versus 32) with an absolute neutrophil count less than 1000 cells/mm^3 ($p=0.0039$), and that there was less mucositis (11% versus 44%, $p=0.041$) during cycles that included the growth factor.[160] This may permit safer treatment of patients with adverse prognostic features.

Unfortunately, most patients with advanced disease relapse after an initial response or are resistant de novo. In these cases, effective salvage therapies are required. Investigators

at M.D. Anderson Cancer Center observed partial responses in 9 (30%) of 30 patients who had progressed on MVAC (95% confidence interval, 15–47%) with 5-fluorouracil and interferon.[161] After an initial report showing activity using a weekly schedule, two recent studies showed the activity of gallium nitrate given by continuous infusion.[162,163] Three (2 CR, 1 PR) of 5 patients who had progressed on cisplatin as a single agent responded. An investigational antifolate, pirotrexim, effected partial responses in 3 of 4 patients who had progressed on MVAC, and short-term responses were reported with high-dose methotrexate and cisplatin after MVAC.[164,165] In a fifth study, escalated doses of MVAC with granulocyte-macrophage colony stimulating factor showed 7 complete and 5 partial responses (40%) in 30 patients who had progressed after MVAC and CAP, a population generally refractory to therapy.[166]

Several phase I studies using escalated doses of the components of the MVAC regimen are ongoing, but randomized comparisons of high-dose and conventional-dose programs have not been completed. At this point, it is not proven whether the addition of hematopoietic growth factors can significantly increase complete response proportions, a prerequisite for cure.[169]

REFERENCES

1. Boring CC, Squires TS, Tong T. Cancer Statistics 1991. CA 1991;41:19.
2. Heney NM, Nocks BN, Daly JJ, et al. TA and T1 bladder cancer: Occassion, recurrence and progression. Br J Urol 1982;54:152.
3. Schairer C, Hartge P, Hoover RN. Racial differences in bladder cancer risk: A case-control study. Am J Epidemiol 1988;125:1027.
4. Rehn L. Blasen Geschwülte bei Fuchsin-Arbeitern. Arch Klin Chir 1895;50:588.
5. Iyer V, Harris RE, Wynder EL. Diesel exhaust exposure and bladder cancer risk. Eur J Urol Epidemiol 1990;6:49.
6. Mills PK, Beeson WL, Phillips, RL, et al. Bladder cancer in a low risk population: Results from the adventists health study. Am J Epidemiol 1991;133:230.
7. Gonzalez CA, Lopez-Abente G, Errezola M, et al. Occupation and bladder cancer in Spain: A multi-center case-control study. Int J Epidemiol 1989;18:569.
8. Clavel J, Cordier S, Baccon-Jibod L, et al. Tobacco and bladder cancer in males: Increased risk for inhalers and smokers of black tobacco. Int J Cancer 1989;44:605.
9. Kantor AF, Hartge P, Hoover RN, et al. Epidemiological characteristics of squamous cell carcinoma and adenocarcinoma of the bladder. Cancer Res 1988;48:3853.
10. Piper JN, Matanoski GM, Tonascia J. Bladder cancer in young women. Am J Epidemiol 1986;123:1033.
11. Risch HA, Burch JD, Miller AB. Dietary factors and the incidence of cancer of the urinary bladder. Am J Epidemiol 1988;126:1179.
12. Sullivan JW. Epidemiological survey of bladder cancer in Greater New Orleans. J Urol 1982;128:281.
13. Morrison AS, Verhoek WG, Leck I, et al. Artificial sweeteners and bladder cancer in Manchester, UK, and Nagoya, Japan. Br J Cancer 1982;45:332.
14. Slattery ML, West DW, Robinson LM. Fluid intake and bladder cancer in Utah. Int J Cancer 1988;42:17.
15. Kolonel LN, Hinds MW, Nomura AM, et al. Relationship of dietary vitamin A and ascorbic acid intake to the risk for cancers of the lung, bladder and prostate in Hawaii. NCI Monogr 1985;69:137.
16. Mettlin, Graham S. Dietary risk factors in human bladder cancer. Am J Epidemiol 1979;110:255.
17. Lynch HT, Kimberling WJ, Lynch JF, et al. Familial bladder cancer in an oncology clinic. Cancer Genet Cytogenet 1987;27:161.
18. Kantor AF, Hartge P, Hoover RN, et al. Familial and environmental interactions in bladder cancer risk. Int J Cancer 1985;35:703.
19. Thompson IN Jr, Fair WR. Occupational and environmental factors in bladder cancer. In: Chisholm JD, Fair WR, eds. Scientific foundations of urology. 3rd ed. Oxford: Heineman, 1990.
20. Fearon ER, Feinberg, Hamilton SH, et al. Loss of genes on the short arm of chromosome-11 in bladder cancer. Nature 1985;318:377.
21. Tsai YC, Nichols PW, Hiti AL, et al. Allelic loss of chromosomes 9, 11 and 17 in human bladder cancer. Cancer Res 1990;50:44.
22. Olumi AF, Tsai YC, Nichols PW, et al. Allelic loss of chromosome 17p distinguishes high grade from low grade transitional cell carcinomas of the bladder. Cancer Res 1990;50:7081.
23. Presti JC Jr, Reuter VE, Galin T, et al. Molecular genetic alterations in superficial and locally advanced human bladder cancer. Cancer Res 1991;51:405.
24. Waldman FM, Carroll PR, Kerschmann R, Cohen MB, Field FG, Mayall BH. Centromeric

copy number of chromosome 7 is strongly correlated with tumor grade and labeling index in human bladder cancer. Cancer Res 1991;51:3807–3813.

25. Pode D, Fair WR. The development of bladder cancer. AUA Update, vol 7, lesson 40. Bellaire, Texas: American Urological Associates Office of Education, 1987.

26. Gilbert HA, Logan JL, Kagan AR, et al. The natural history of papillary transitional cell carcinoma of the bladder and its treatment in an unselected population on the basis of histologic grading. J Urol 1978;119:488.

27. Tribukaite B, Gustafson H, Esposti P. Ploidy and proliferation in human bladder tumors as measured by flow cyto-fluorometric DNA analysis and its relation to histopathology and cytology. Cancer 1979;43:1742.

28. Friedel GH, Bell JR, Burney SW, et al. Histopathology and classification of urinary bladder carcinomas. Urol Clin North Am 1976;3:53.

29. Lerman RJ, Hutter RVP, Whitmore WF Jr. Papilloma of the urinary bladder. Cancer 1970;25:333.

30. Koss LG. Mapping of the urinary bladder: Its impact on the concepts of bladder cancer. Human Pathol 1979;10:533.

31. Mostofi FK, Davis DC Jr, Cesterhenn IA. Pathology of tumors of the urinary tract. In: Skinner DG, Lieskovsky G, eds. Genitourinary cancer. Philadelphia: WB Saunders, 1988.

32. Althausen AF, Prout GR Jr, Daly JJ. Noninvasive papillary carcinima of the bladder associated with carcinoma in situ. J Urol 1976;116:575.

33. Murphy WM, Nagy GT, Rao MK, et al. "Normal" urothelium in patients with bladder cancer: A preliminary report from the National Bladder Cancer Collaborative Group A. Cancer 1979;44:1050.

34. Wolf H, Hojgaard K. Urothelial displasia concomitant with bladder tumors as a determinant factor for future new occurrences. Lancet 1983;2:134.

35. Friedell GH, Soloway MS, Hilgar AG, et al. Summary of workshop on carcinoma in situ of the bladder. J Urol 1986;136:1047.

36. Cooper PH, Waisman J, Johanston, et al. Severe atypia of transitional epithelium and carcinoma of the urinary bladder. Cancer 1973;31:1055.

37. Riddle TR, Chisholm GD, Trott PA. Flat carcinoma in situ of the bladder. Br J Urol 1975;47:829.

38. Farrow GM, Utz DC, Rife CC, et al. Clinical observations on 69 cases of carcinoma in situ of the urinary bladder. Cancer Res 1977;37:2794.

39. Tannenbaum M, Romas NA, Droller MJ. The pathobiology of early urothelial cancer. In: Skinner DG, Lefskovsky G, ed. Genitourinary cancer. Philadelphia: WB Saunders, 1988.

40. Jewett HJ, Strong GH. Infiltrating carcinoma of the bladder: Relation of depth of penetration of the bladder wall to incidence of local extension in metastases. J Urol 1946;55:366.

41. Marshall VF. The relation of the preoperative estimate to the pathologic demonstration of the extent of vesicle neoplasms. J Urol 1952;68:714.

42. Fradet Y, Cordon-Cardo C, Whitmore WF Jr, et al. Cell surface antigens of human bladder tumors: Definition of tumor subsets by monoclonal antibodies and correlation with growth characteristics. Cancer Res 1986;46:5183.

43. Whitmore WF Jr. Bladder cancer: Future directions in management. Proceedings of a symposium, Marco Island, FL, John Wiley and Sons Medical Group, 1986.

44. Whitmore WF Jr. Surgical management of low stage bladder cancer. Semin Oncol 1973;6:207.

45. Whitmore WF Jr. Management of invasive bladder neoplasms. Semin Urol 1983;1:34.

46. Smith JA, Whitmore WF Jr. Regional lymph node metastases from bladder cancer. J Urol 1981;126:591.

47. Skinner DG. Current perspectives in the management of high grade invasive bladder cancer. Cancer 1980;45:1866.

48. Prout GR Jr, Griffin PP, Shipley WU. Bladder carcinoma as a systemic disease. Cancer 1979;43:2532.

49. Jakse G, Loidl W, Seeber G, et al. Stage T1, grade 3 transitional cell carcinoma of the bladder: An unfavorable tumor? J Urol 1987;137:39.

50. Herr HW, Ludone VP. Intravesical therapy for superficial bladder cancer. AUA Update Series, vol 8, lesson 12. Bellaire, Texas: American Urological Associates Office of Education, 1989.

51. Herr HW, Wartinger DD, Fair WR, et al. Bacillus Calmette-Guerin therapy for superficial bladder cancer: A 10-year follow-up. J Urol 147:1020–1023, 1992.

52. Hollister D, Coleman M. Hematologic effects of intravesical thiotepa therapy for bladder cancer. JAMA 1980;224:2065.

53. Badalament RA, Herr HW, Wong GY. A prospective randomized trial of maintenance vs. non-maintenance intravesical BCG therapy of superficial bladder cancer. J Clin Oncol 1987;5:441.

54. Rawls WH, Lamm DL, Lowe BA, et al. Fatal sepsis following intravesical bacillus calmette-guerin administration for bladder cancer. J Urol 1990;144:1328.

55. Utz CD, Hansh KA, Farrow GM. The plight of the patient with carcinoma in situ of the bladder. J Urol 1970;103:160.

56. van der Werf-Messing BHP, Hop WCJ. Carcinoma of the urinary bladder treated either by radium implant or by transurethral resection only. Int J Radiat Oncol Biol Phys 1981;7:299.

57. Whitmore WF, Prout GR. Discouraging results for high dose external beam radiation therapy in low stage (O and A) bladder cancer. J Urol 1982;127:902.

58. Miller J. TUR promising in stage B bladder cancer. Urol Times 1989.

59. Herr HW. Conservative management of muscle-infiltraing bladder cancer: Prospective experience. J Urol 1987;138:1162.

60. Whitmore WF Jr, Batata MA, Ghonein MA, et al. Radical cystectomy with or without prior radiation in the treatment of bladder cancer. J Urol 1977;118:184.

61. Montie JE, Straffon RA, Stewart BA. Radical cystectomy with and without radiation therapy for carcinoma of the bladder. J Urol 1984;131:477.

62. Fair WR, Atlas I. Radical cystectomy. In: Surgical management of urologic disease: An anatomic approach. St. Louis: Mosby Year Book, 1992.

63. Kaver I, Koontz WW Jr. The fate of the remaining uroepithelium following total cystectomy for bladder cancer. AUA Update Series, vol 8, lesson 30, 1989.

64. Hardeman SW, Soloway MS. Urethral recurrence following radical cystectomy. J Urol 1990;144:666.

65. Levinson AK, Johnson DE, Wishnow KI. Indications for urethrectomy in an era of continent urinary diversion. J Urol 1990;144:73.

66. Koch NG. Ileostomy without external appliances: A survey of 25 patients provided with intra-abdominal intestinal reservoir. Ann Surg 1971;173:545.

67. Skinner DG, Lieskovsky G, Boyd SD. Continuing experience with the continent ileal reservoir (Kock pouch) as an alternative to cutaneous urinary diversion: An update after 250 cases. J Urol 1987;137:1140.

68. Camay M, Le Duc A. L'entero-cystoplastie avec cystoprostatectomie totale pour cancer de la vessie. Indications, techniques operatoire, surveillance et resultats sur quatre-vingt-sept cas. Ann Urol 1979;13:114.

69. Hautmann RE, Egghart G, Frohneberg D, Miller K. The ileal neobladder. J Urol 1988;139:39.

70. Fair WR. The ileal neobladder. Urol Clin North Am 1991;18:3:555–559.

71. Duncan W, Quilty PM. The results of a series of 963 patients with transitional cell carcinoma of the urinary bladder primarily treated by radical megavoltage x-ray therapy. Radiother Oncol 1986;7:299.

72. Davidson SE, Symonds RP, Snee MP, et al. Assessment of factors influencing the outcome of radiotherapy for bladder cancer. Br J Urol 1990;66:288.

73. Quilty PM, Duncan W, Kerr GR. Results of a randomised study to evaluate influence of dose on morbidity in radiotherapy for bladder cancer. Clin Radiol 1985;36:615.

74. Miller LS. Bladder cancer: Superiority of preoperative irradiation and cystectomy in clinical stages B2 and C. Cancer 1977;39:973.

75. Morrison R. The results of treatment of cancer of the bladder: A clinical contribution to radiobiology. Clin Radiol 1975;26:67.

76. Parsons JT, Thar TL, Bova FJ, et al. An evaluation of split-course irradiation for pelvic malignancies. Int J Radiat Oncol Biol Phys 1980;6:175.

77. Goffinet DR, Schneider MJ, Glatstein EJ, et al. Bladder cancer results of radiation therapy in 384 patients. Radiology 1975;117:149.

78. Hoppe-Stone HF, Oliver RTD, England HR, et al. T3 bladder cancer: Salvage rather than elective cystectomy after radiotherapy. Urology 1984;24:315.

79. Abratt RP, Tucker RD, Barnes DR. Radical irradiation of T2 grade III and T3 bladder cancer-tumor response and prognosis. Int J Radiat Oncol Biol Phys 1983;9:1213.

80. van der Werf-Messing B, Menon RS, Hop WC. Carcinoma of the urinary bladder T3NXM0 treated by combination radium implant and external beam irradiation: Second report. Int J Radiat Oncol Biol Phys 1983;9:177.

81. Shipley WU, Rose MA, Perrone TL, et al. Full-dose irradiation for patients with invasive bladder carcinoma: Clinical and histological factors prognostic of improved survival. J Urol 1985;134:679.

82. Shipley WU, Rose MA, Perrone TL, et al. Full-dose irradiation for patients with invasive bladder carcinoma: Clinical and histological factors prognostic of improved survival. J Urol 1985;134:679.

83. Quilty PM, Duncan W. The influence of hemoglobin level on the regression and long term local control of transitional cell carcinoma of the bladder following photon irradiation. Int J Radiat Oncol Biol Phys 1986;12:1735.

84. Gospodarowicz MK, Hawkins NV, Rawlings GA, et al. Radical radiotherapy for the muscle invasive transitional cell carcinoma of the bladder: Failure analysis. J Urol 1989;142:1448.

85. Edsmyr F, Andersson L, Esposti PL, et al. Radiother Oncol 1985;4:197.

86. Marks LB, Kaufman SD, Prout Jr GR, et al. Invasive bladder carcinoma: Preliminary report of selective bladder conservation by transurethral surgery, upfront MCV (methotrexate, cisplatin, and vinblastine) chemotherapy and pelvic irradiation plus cisplatin. Int J Radiat Oncol Biol Phys 1988;15:877.

87. Parsons JT, Million RR. The role of radiation therapy alone or as an adjunct to surgery in bladder carcinoma. Semin Oncol 1990;17:566.

88. Mameghan H, Fisher R. Invasive bladder cancer. Prognostic factors and results of radiotherapy with and without cystectomy. Br J Urol 1989;63:251.

89. Goodman GB, Hislop TG, Ekwiidm JM, et al. Conservation of bladder function in patients with invasive bladder cancer treated by definitive irradiation and selective cystectomy. Int J Radiat Oncol Biol Phys 1981;7:569.

90. Gospodarowicz MK, Rider WD, Keen CW. Bladder cancer: Long-term follow-up results of patients treated with radical radiation. Clin Oncol 1991;3:155.

91. Shipley WU, Prout GR Jr, Kaufman SD, Perrone TL. Invasive bladder carcinoma. The importance of initial transurethral surgery and other significant prognostic factors for improved survival with full-dose irradiation. Cancer 1987;160:514.

92. Freiha FS, Faysal MH. Salvage cystectomy. Urology 1983;22:496.

93. Swanson DA, von Eschenbach AC, Bracken RB, et al. Salvage cystectomy for bladder carcinoma. Cancer 1981;47:2275.

94. Smith JA Jr, Whitmore WF Jr. Salvage cystectomy for bladder cancer after failure of definitive irradiation. J Urol 1981;125:643.

95. Timmer PR, Hartlief HA, Hooijkaas JAP. Bladder cancer: Pattern of recurrence in 142 patients. Int J Radiat Oncol Biol Phys 1984;11:899.

96. Osborn DE, Honon RP, Palmer MK, et al. Factors influencing salvage cystectomy results. Br J Urol 1982;54:122.

97. Jenkins BJ, Martin JE, Baithun SI, et al. Prediction of response to radiotherapy in invasive bladder cancer. Br J Urol 1990;65:345.

98. van der Werf-Messing B. Preoperative irradiation followed by cystectomy to treat carcinoma of the urinary bladder category T3NX,0–4M0. Int J Radiat Oncol Biol Phys 1979;5:394.

99. Rider WD, Evans DH. Radiotherapy in the treatment of recurrent bladder cancer. Br J Urol 1976;48:595.

100. Greven KM, Solin LJ, Hanks GE. Prognostic factors in patients with bladder carcinoma treated with definitive irradiation. Cancer 1990;65:908.

101. Matsumoto K, Kakizoe T, Mikuriya S, et al. Clinical evaluation of intraoperative radiotherapy for carcinoma of the urinary bladder. Cancer 1981;47:509.

102. Mazeron J-H, Crook J, Chopin D, et al. Conservative treatment of bladder carcinoma by partial cystectomy and interstitial iridium 192. Int J Radiat Oncol Biol Phys 1988;15:1323.

103. Whitmore WF Jr, Batata M. Status of integrated irradiation and cystectomy for bladder cancer. Urol Clin North Am 1984;1:681.

104. Bloom HJG, Hendry WF, Wallace DM, Skeet RG. Treatment of T3 bladder cancer: Controlled trial of preoperative radiotherapy and radical cystectomy versus radical radiotherapy: Second report and review (for the Clinical Trials Group, Institute of Urology). Br J Urol 1982;54:136.

105. Scanlon PW, Scott M, Segura JW. A comparison of short-course low-dose and long-course high-dose preoperative radiation for carcinoma of the bladder. Cancer 1983;52:1153.

106. Marshal VF. The relation of the preoperative estimate to the pathologic demonstration of the extent of vesical neoplasma. J Urol 1952;68:714.

107. Parsons, JT, Million RR. Planned preoperative irradiation in the management of clinical stage B2-C (T3) bladder carcinoma. Int J Radiat Oncol Biol Phys 1988;14:797.

108. Slack NH, Bross IDJ, Prout GR Jr. Five-year follow-up results of a collaborative study of therapies for carcinoma of the bladder. J Surg Oncol 1977;9:393.

109. Madsen PO, Hoyme UB, Byar DP, VA Cooperative Research Group. Paper presented to the North Central Section of the AUA. (No differences reported in 10-year survival rates in three bladder cancer groups). Urol Times 1980;:20.

110. Smith JA Jr, Crawford ED, Blumenstein B, et al. A randomized prospective trial of pre-operative irradiation plus radical cystectomy versus surgery alone for transitional cell carcinoma of the bladder: A Southwest Oncology Group study. J Urol 1988;139:266A.

111. Scher HI. Chemotherapy for invasive bladder cancer: Neoadjuvant versus adjuvant. Semin Oncol 1990;17:555–565.

112. Goldin A, Venditti JM, Humphreys SR, et al. Influence of the concentration of leukemic inoculum on the effectiveness of treatment. Science 1956;840.

113. Skipper HE, Schabel FM, Wilcox WS. Experimental evaluation of potential anticancer agents. XII. On the criteria and kinetics associated with curability of experimental leukemia. Cancer Chemother Rep 1964;35:1–9.

114. Sternberg CN, Yagoda A, Scher HI, et al. M-VAC for advanced transitional cell carcinoma of the urothelium: Efficacy, and patterns of response and relapse. Cancer 1989;64:2448–2458.

115. Logothetis CJ, Dexeus F, Sella A, et al. A prospective randomized trial comparing CISCA to MVAC chemotherapy in advanced metastastic urothelial tumors. J Clin Oncol 1990;8:1050–1055.

116. Venturini M, Merlano M, Michelotti A, et al. Neoadjuvant or definitive alternating chemotherapy and radiotherapy for infiltrating bladder cancer. Am J Clin Oncol 1989;12:63–67.

117. Shipley WU, Kaufman DS, Heney NM. Can chemo-radiotherapy plus transurethral tumor resection make cystectomy unnecessary for invasive bladder cancer? Oncology 1990;4:25–32.

118. Russell KJ, Boileau MA, Higano C, et al. Combined 5-fluorouracil and irradiation for transitional cell carcinoma of the urinary bladder. Int J Radiat Oncol Biol Phys 1990;19:693–699.

119. Prout GR Jr, Shipley WU, Kaufman DS, et al. Preliminary results in invasive bladder cancer with transurethral resection, neoadjuvant chemotherapy and combined pelvic irradiation plus cisplatin chemotherapy. J Urol 1990;144:1128–1134.

120. Rotman M, Aziz H, Porrazzo M, et al. Treatment of advanced transitional cell carcinoma of the bladder with irradiation and concomitant 5-fluorouracil infusion. Int J Radiat Oncol Biol Phys 1990;18:1131–1137.

121. Sauer R, Dunst J, Altendorf-Hofmann A, et al. Radiotherapy with and without cisplatin in bladder cancer. Int J Radiat Oncol Biol Phys 1990;19:687–691.

122. Moore M, Tannock I. How expert physicians would wish to be treated if they developed genitourinary malignancies. J Clin Oncol 1991;6:1736–1745.

123. Scher H, Herr H, Sternberg C, et al. Neo-adjuvant chemotherapy for invasive bladder cancer: Experience with the M-VAC regimen. Br J Urol 1989;64:250–256.

124. Seidman A, Scher HI, Herr H, et al. Survival of patients (pts) with invasive (T2-4N0M0) bladder cancer treated with neoadjuvant methotrexate, vinblastine, adriamycin and cisplatin (MVAC). 3rd Intl Cong Neo-Adjuvant [Abstract] Chemotherapy 1991;35.

125. Splinter TA, Scher HI, Denis L, et al. The prognostic value of pathological response to combination chemotherapy before cystectomy in patients with invasive bladder cancer. J Urol 1992;147:606–608.

126. Simon SD, Srougi M. Neoadjuvant M-VAC chemotherapy and partial cystectomy for treatment of locally invasive transitional cell carcinoma of the bladder. Prog Clin Biol Res 1990;353:169–174.

127. McCullough DL, Cooper RM, Yeaman LD, et al. Neoadjuvant treatment of stages T2 to T4 bladder cancer with cis-platinum, cyclophosphamide and doxorubicin. J Urol 1989;141:849–852.

128. Logothetis CJ, Johnson DE, Chong C, et al. Adjuvant cyclophosphamide, doxorubicin, and cisplatin chemotherapy for bladder cancer: An update. J Clin Oncol 1988;6:1590–1596.

129. Skinner DG, Daniels JR, Russell CA, et al. The role of adjuvant chemotherapy following cystectomy for invasive bladder cancer: A prospective comparative trial. J Urol 1991;145:459–464.

130. Schaeffer A, Grayhack JT, Merrill JM, et al. Treatment of stage D bladder cancer with adjuvant doxorubicin hydrochloride and radiation. Urology 1982;20:393–399.

131. Wallace DM, Raghavan D, Kelly KA, et al. Neo-adjuvant (preemptive) cisplatin therapy in invasive transitional cell carcinoma of the bladder. Br J Urol 1991;67:608.

132. Shearer RJ, Chilvers CF, Bloom HJ, et al. Adjuvant chemotherapy in T3 carcinoma of the bladder. A prospective trial: Preliminary report. Br J Urol 1988;62:558–564.

133. Shipley WU, Prout GR Jr, Kaufman SD, et al. Invasive bladder carcinoma. The importance of initial transurethral surgery and other significant prognostic factors for improved survival with full-dose irradiation. Cancer 1987;60:514–520.

134. Shipley WU, Prout GR Jr, Einstein AB, et al. Treatment of invasive bladder cancer by cisplatin and radiation in patients unsuited for surgery. JAMA 1987;258:931–935.

135. Marks LB, Kaufman SD, Prout GR Jr, et al. Invasive bladder carcinoma: Preliminary report of selective bladder conservation by transurethral surgery, upfront MCV (methotrexate, cisplatin, and vinblastine) chemotherapy and pelvic irradiation plus cisplatin. Int J Radiat Oncol Biol Phys 1988;15:877–883.

136. Fung CY, Shipley WU, Young RH, et al. Prognostic factors in invasive bladder carcinoma in a prospective trial of preoperative adjuvant chemotherapy and radiotherapy. J Clin Oncol 1991;9:1533–1542.

137. Geller NL, Scher HI, Parmar MK, et al. The effects of neoadjuvant chemotherapy for invasive bladder cancer? Semin Oncol 1990;17:628–634.

138. Feinstein AR, Sossin DM, Wells CR. The Will Rogers phenomenon: Stage migration and new diagnostic techniques as a source of misleading statistics for survival in cancer. N Engl J Med 1985;312:1604–1608.

139. Pagano F, Bassi P, Galetti TP, et al. Results of contemporary radical cystectomy for invasive bladder cancer: A clinicopathological study with an emphasis on the inadequacy of the tumor, nodes and metastases classification. J Urol 1991;145:45–50.

140. Bosl GJ, Scher HI, Fair WR, et al. Carcinoma of the bladder. In: ASCO Annual Meeting. Chicago: American Society of Clinical Oncology, 1991:123–139.

141. Tannock IF. Endpoints of clinical trials in invasive bladder cancer. Semin Oncol 1990;17:619–627.

142. Hall RR, Parmar MK. Randomised intercontinental trial of locoregional therapy with or without neoadjuvant chemotherapy. Prog Clin Biol Res 1990;353:105–109.

143. Dalesio O. Neoadjuvant chemotherapy in invasive bladder cancer. Trial design and statistics. Prog Clin Biol Res 1990;353:57–64.

144. Crawford ED, Natale RB, Burton H, Southwest Oncology Group study (8710): Trial of cystectomy alone versus neo-adjuvant M-VAC and cystectomy in patients with locally advanced bladder cancer (Intergroup trial 0080). Prog Clin Biol Res 1991;353:111–114.

145. Yagoda A. Chemotherapy for advanced urothelial cancer. Semin Urol 1983;1:60–74.

146. Yagoda A. Chemotherapy of metastatic bladder cancer. Cancer 1980;45:1879–1888.

147. Sternberg CN, Scher HI. Current status of chemotherapy for urothelial tract tumors. Oncology 1987;1:41–50.

148. Yagoda A. Chemotherapy of urothelial tract tumors. Cancer 1987;60:574–585.

149. Arap W, Scher HI. The value of cytotoxic chemotherapy in locally invasive and metastatic bladder cancer. In: Williams G, Waxman J, eds. Urological cancer: A consensus. London: Edward Arnold, 1991:185–199.

150. Logothetis CJ, Dexeus FH, Chong C, et al. Cisplatin, cyclophosphamide and doxorubicin chemotherapy for unresectable urothelial tumors: The M.D. Anderson experience. J Urol 1989;141:33–37.

151. Lo R, Freiha FS, Torti FM. CMV for metastatic urothelial tumors. In: Johnson DE, Logothetis CJ, von Eschenbach AC, eds. Systmeic therapy for genitourinary cancers. Chicago, Year Book Medical Publishers, 1989:59–63.

152. Loehrer PJ, Elson P, Kuebler JP, et al. Advanced bladder cancer: A prospective Intergroup trial comparing single agent cisplatin (CDDP) versus M-VAC combination therapy (INT 0078). Proc Am Soc Clin Oncol [Abstract] 1990;10:112.

153. Connor JP, Olsson CA, Benson MC, et al. Long-term follow-up in patients treated with methotrexate, vinblastine, doxorubicin, and cisplatin (M-VAC) for transitional cell carcinoma of the urinary bladder: Cause for concern. Urology 1989;34:353–356.

154. Tannock I, Gospodarowicz M, Connolly J, et al. M-VAC (meth otrexate, vinblastine, doxorubicin and cisplatin) chemotherapy for transitional cell carcinoma: The Princess Margaret Hospital experience. J Urol 1989;142:289–292.

155. Igawa M, Ohkucki T, Ueki T, et al. Usefulness and limitations of methotrexate, vinblastine, doxorubicin and cisplatin for the treatment of advanced urothelial cancer. J Urol 1990;144:662–665.

156. Geller NL, Sternberg CN, Penenberg D, et al. Prognostic factors for survival of patients with advanced urothelial tumors treated with methotrexate, vinblastine, doxorubicin, and cisplatin chemotherapy. Cancer 1991;67:1525–1531.

157. Dreicer R, Messing EM, Loehrer PJ, et al. Perioperative methotrexate, vinblastine, doxorubicin and cisplatin (M-VAC) for poor risk transitional cell carcinoma of the bladder: An Eastern Cooperative Oncology Group pilot study. J Urol 1990;144:1123–1126.

158. Stalder M, Leyvraz S, Bauer J, et al. An outpatient treatment for advanced urothelial tract cancer including patients with impaired renal function. Proc Am Soc Clin Oncol [Abstract] 1990;9:A576.

159. Dogliotti L, Bertetto O, Berruti A, et al. Carboplatin (CBDCA) and methotrexate (MTX) combination chemotherapy in advanced urothelial cancer (UC). A phase II study. J Cancer Res Clin Oncol 1992 (in press).

160. Gabrilove JL, Jakubowski A, Scher H, et al. Effect of granulocyte colony-stimulating factor on neutropenia and associated morbidity due to chemotherapy for transitional-cell carcinoma of the urothelium. N Engl J Med 1988;318:1414–1422.

161. Logothetis CJ, Hossan E, Sella A, et al. Fluorouracil and recombinant human interferon alfa-2a in the treatment of metastatic chemotherapy-refractory urothelial tumors. JNCI 1991;83:285–288.

162. Crawford ED, Saiers JH, Baker LH. Treatment of metastatic bladder cancer with gallium nitrate. 13th Intl Cong Chemother 1983;240:12.1.7.

163. Seidman AD, Scher HI, Bajorin DF, et al. Gallium nitrate: An active agent in advanced refractory transitional cell carcinoma of the bladder. Cancer 1991;68:2651–2655.

164. Clendeninn NA, Savaraj N, Benedetto P, et al. Compassionate use of oral piritrexim in advanced bladder cancer: An effective drug after progression on MVAC chemotherapy. Proc Am Assoc Cancer Res [Abstract] 1991;32:186.

165. Pizzocaro G, Gederico M, Berri G, et al. Methotrexate, vinblastine, adriamycin and cisplatin versus methotrexate and cisplatin in advanced urothelial cancer. A randomized study. Eur Urol 1991;20:89–92.

166. Logothetis CJ, Dexeus FH, Sella A, et al. Escalated therapy for refractory urothelial tumors: Methotrexate-vinblastine-doxorubicin-cisplatin plus unglycosylated recombinant human granulocyte-macrophage colony-stimulating factor. JNCI 1990;82:667–672.

167. Patterson JM, Ray EH Jr, Mendiondo OA, et al. A new treatment for invasive squamous cell bladder cancer: The Nigro regimen: Preoperative chemotherapy and radiation therapy. J Urol 1988;140:379–380.

168. Mathur UK, Krahn HP, Ramsey EW. Total cystectomy for bladder cancer. J Urol 1981;125:784–786.

169. Scher HI, Norton LN. Chemotherapy for urothelial tract malignancies. Breaking the deadlock. Semin Surg Oncol 1992;8:316–341.

Cancer: Principles & Practice of Oncology, Fourth Edition,
edited by Vincent T. DeVita, Jr., Samuel Hellman, Steven A. Rosenberg.
J.B. Lippincott Co., Philadelphia © 1993.

Gerald E. Hanks

Charles E. Myers

Peter T. Scardino

CHAPTER **35**

Cancer of the Prostate

Second only to lung cancer as a cause of cancer deaths, prostate cancer has become the most common cancer among American men.[1] The age-specific mortality rate, which in black American men is nearly double that in whites, has increased slowly over the past 50 years.[2] Prostate cancer is responsible for almost 3% of all deaths in men older than 55 years.[1] Because the incidence of prostate cancer increases more rapidly with age than the incidence of any other cancer, and the average age of American men is rising, the number of patients with prostate cancer is expected to increase steadily over the next decade.[2] The widespread use of more efficient diagnostic tests, including measurement of prostate-specific antigen (PSA) levels and transrectal ultrasonography (TRUS), will further increase the number of cases detected.[3-5] It was estimated that in 1992 more than 134,000 men in the United States would be diagnosed with prostate cancer and 32,000 would die from the disease.[6] More than half of the patients diagnosed with prostate cancer die from the disease within 10 years (Table 35–1), and more than two-thirds suffer local or systemic progression of the disease despite therapy.[7-9] In autopsies, 30% of men older than 50 years harbor foci of cancer within the prostate.[10-12] This remarkably high prevalence of cancer, unmatched in any other organ, makes prostate cancer the most common malignancy in humans. Nevertheless, only 1% of these men will be diagnosed with prostate cancer each year, and only 0.3% will die from the disease. This enormous discrepancy between the high prevalence of the disease at autopsy and the low incidence of the disease clinically has confounded our understanding of its clinical significance and has stymied efforts to detect and treat prostate cancer.[2,8,11,13,14]

Over the past decade, our understanding of the pathogenesis and natural history of prostate cancer has improved substantially, as have techniques for diagnosis and staging, such as monitoring of PSA levels and TRUS. Refinements in treatment have reduced the morbidity of the therapy substantially. However, we do not understand the etiology of prostate cancer, and we have no means of preventing the disease. Treatment still threatens the sexual and urinary function of patients, and the prognosis for those with advanced disease remains dismal. The challenge of the next decade is to understand the molecular mechanisms of progression of prostate cancer and to intervene more effectively in the course of the disease with treatment that is appropriate to the risk of the cancer.

EPIDEMIOLOGY

Incidence and mortality from prostate cancer have climbed steadily since 1970. The prostate cancer death rate was projected to exceed that for colorectal cancer by 1992, and become second only to carcinoma of the lung. In part, the increased incidence may result from more efficient screening tools such as the use of TRUS and measurement of PSA levels. In addition, the increased use of transurethral resection for benign prostatic hypertrophy has led to the discovery of localized prostate cancer with increased frequency. Even taking these changes into consideration, there appears to be an increased incidence of carcinoma of the prostate. This has led to increased interest in the epidemiology of prostate carcinoma in an attempt to find avoidable risk factors and to identify high-risk populations.

The incidence of latent carcinoma of the prostate increases with age, but shows little geographic, racial, or ethnic variation.[13,15–17] Clinically evident carcinoma of the prostate, on the other hand, shows a more than 10-fold difference in incidence according to geography, race, or ethnicity. In portions of the United States and Europe, the incidence is more than 200 persons per 100,000, whereas in Thailand it is less than 50 persons per 100,000. In the United States, race is associated

TABLE 35–1. Prostate Cancer: Diagnosis, Risk of Death, and Cure Rate by Clinical Stage

Percentage of Patients	Stage*	Prognosis	10-Year Cancer-Specific Survival Rate (%)	Estimated Cure Rate† (%)
30	M+	Incurable	10	<1
20	N+	Rarely curable	40	<5
10	T3–4 N0M0	Occasionally curable	60	25
30	T0B2N0M0	Often curable	80	65
10	T0AN0M0	Treatment unnecessary	95	85
100	All stages		51	32
	Excluding T0A (stage A1)		45	25

* Based on clinical stage, pelvic lymph node dissection, bone scan, and acid phosphatase.
† Cure rate is the approximate percentage of patients with lifelong freedom from prostate cancer.
(Scardino PT, Weaver R, Hudson MA. Early detection of prostate cancer. Hum Pathol 1992;23:211–222)

strongly with the incidence and mortality of prostatic carcinoma. Prostate cancer is more common in American blacks, is more often of later stage and less well differentiated at diagnosis, and survival time is shorter than that seen in whites.[18-25] In contrast, black Africans have a low incidence of carcinoma of the prostate. The incidence of prostate cancer usually is low in Asia, but rises rapidly in Asian immigrants to the United States (Table 35–2).[20,26,27] There are a number of possible explanations for this effect. Prostate cancer is a tumor whose growth is promoted by androgens, and American blacks have been found to have higher testosterone levels than white or black Africans. The risk of carcinoma of the prostate also is associated with dietary factors, including fat, selenium,[28-30] carotene or vitamin A,[22,25,31,32] and protein.[22,25,28,30] Of these, fat intake has received the greatest attention, although the evidence in general is not as persuasive or consistent as it is for colon carcinoma.[22,23,25,26,28,30,33,34] For example, Eskimos, who have a high-fat diet, are at much less risk for prostate cancer than are whites in Canada or the United States and other Native American groups.[35] A potential clue to this puzzle is the observation by Prentice and Sheppard that monounsaturated fat intake is associated with a higher risk than that of saturated fat.[26] Because few epidemiologic studies contain information about the composition of the fat in the diet, it is difficult to verify this finding. However, recent laboratory findings are consistent with these observations. The growth of human prostate cancer cells in tissue culture and in nude mice is stimulated by the availability of the unsaturated fatty acid, arachidonic acid, or its precursors, and suppressed by the omega-3 fatty acids found in marine lipid.[34,36,37] This provides an attractive explanation for the low incidence of prostate cancer in Eskimos, because they subsist on a diet of cold-water marine lipid rich in omega-3 fatty acids.

Chemical carcinogens often require metabolic activation. This process is commonly mediated by aryl hydrocarbon hydroxylase or prostaglandin H synthetase. Prostatic epithelium is rich in both enzyme activities, and prostatic homogenates have been shown to be effective in activating chemical carcinogens.[38-40] The risk for prostate cancer has been reported to be higher in workers in agricultural,[41] nitrate fertilizer,[42] or ferrochromium industries,[43] but otherwise does not show a strong correlation with industrial exposure to potential chemical carcinogens.

In animals, cadmium toxicity has been shown to include an increased risk for carcinoma of the prostate.[23,24,30,44,45] In humans, exposure to cadmium has been shown to be associated with an increased risk for carcinoma of the prostate, and patients with carcinoma of the prostate often have elevated cadmium levels.[45a] A comparison of cadmium levels in serum and prostate tissue of high-risk and low-risk populations showed similar levels among controls and patients with benign

TABLE 35–2. Geographic Variations in the Incidence and Mortality Rates of Prostate Cancer*

	Clinical Cancer				Latent Cancer	
	Incidence		Mortality		Prevalence	
	%	Ratio	%	Ratio	%	Ratio
Singapore	3.6	1.0	—		13.2	1.0
Hong Kong			2.2	1.0	15.8	1.2
Uganda	4.4	1.2	—		19.5	1.5
Israel	14.3	4.9	7.9	3.6	22.0	1.7
Jamaica	20.7	5.8	13.9	6.3	29.8	2.3
German Federal Republic	21.1	5.9	13.9	6.3	28.4	2.2
Sweden	38.8	10.8	18.4	8.4	31.6	2.4

* Geographic variations (8.4-fold to 10.8-fold) in the incidence and mortality rates of clinical prostate cancer (per 100,000 men/y) are much greater than variations in the prevalence of latent cancer (2.4-fold). This discrepancy strongly supports the multistep concept that clinical cancer differs from latent or histologic cancer.[28] *Ratio* refers to the ratio between the lowest incidence or prevalence rate and each higher rate.
(Data from Breslow N, Chan CW, Dhom G, et al. Latent carcinoma of the prostate at autopsy in seven areas. Int J Cancer 1977;20:680–688)

prostatic hypertrophy and carcinoma. This suggests that elevated serum cadmium levels may well be a marker of, rather than a risk factor for, carcinoma of the prostate.

In addition to these environmental factors, there is evidence to support the existence of a genetic predisposition to develop carcinoma of the prostate.[33,46-48] In relatives of patients with prostate cancer, the risk for developing carcinoma of the prostate is more than twice that in controls. Familial clusters have been documented. One common genetic mechanism found in cancer families is the loss of tumor suppressor genes such as *RB* and p53. Prostate cancer cell lines have been reported to contain altered or defective *RB* and p53.[4,49-52] Transfection with wild-type p53 or *RB* has been reported to suppress the growth of human prostate cancer cells in vitro.[4,51-54] There is an extensive body of literature on the role of positive oncogenes in carcinoma of the prostate. Early studies suggested a firm association between aggressive behavior and the expression of c-*MYC*[54-56] and activated *RAS*[57] such as Ha-*RAS*. Models of rodents with prostate cancer were established by double transfection with c-*MYC* and activated *RAS*.[58,59]

More recently, it has become apparent that activated *RAS* or c-*MYC* plays a minor role in clinical prostate cancer.[60-64] Expression of v-*RAS* in a hormone-sensitive prostate cancer cell line has been reported to be sufficient to establish hormone independence.[65]

NATURAL HISTORY

CLINICAL CANCER

Anecdotal reports suggest a benign behavior of prostate cancer. However, recent reports of unselected, properly staged, carefully followed patients with clinically detected prostate cancer who received no treatment until progression was documented or symptoms appeared, indicate that, if detected clinically, prostate cancer progresses slowly but relentlessly in the absence of treatment and threatens the life of the host.[66-75]

Handley and colleagues reported a large series of patients managed by deferred treatment.[66] Although 75% of the patients had clinically localized disease at the time of diagnosis, only 30% survived 5 years compared with the expected survival rate of 65% for an age-matched population. Two thirds of all deaths within 5 years were due to prostate cancer. Although the policy was to defer treatment until the patients became symptomatic, only 11% survived 5 years without requiring any further treatment, and 17% of the patients died from cancer without ever having received hormonal therapy. Handley concluded that a deferred treatment policy was temporary, that most patients became symptomatic soon after diagnosis, and that some suffered death as their first symptomatic event.

George and associates reported an apparently favorable outcome of a no treatment policy in 120 patients.[68] Only 19% required treatment for symptomatic local progression. Distant progression occurred in 11% and death from prostate cancer in 4%, whereas 40% died from other causes in this elderly group of patients (mean age 74.8 years). Nevertheless, 84% of the patients developed evidence of local progression measured by palpation. The actuarial rate of distant metastases

was about 45% and the actuarial cancer-specific mortality rate was about 35% at 5 years. George concluded that "the progression of localized prostatic cancer is indeed predictable—growth will be slow and regular and the patient is unlikely to die of metastatic disease. The potential for full expression of the disease in older men will . . . always be limited by the likelihood of death from other causes." Although these conclusions are applicable to the population studied, the high rate of local progression over a short period belies the benign nature of clinically detected localized prostate cancer even in elderly patients.

Whitmore and colleagues reported the outcome of expectant management of 75 patients with predominantly well-differentiated clinical stage B tumors.[70] Each patient apparently was followed without treatment for up to 21 years from the time of diagnosis with no apparent change in the tumor.[76] Nearly all patients showed local progression within 15 years, although fewer developed distant metastases. Within the period of follow-up (24-298 months), prostate cancer accounted for 39% of all deaths.

Johansson and colleagues emphasized the slow rate of progression and low rate of death from prostate cancer observed in 223 patients with very early stage disease.[69] During a mean of 78 months, only 29% of the patients showed evidence of progression (9% distant, 20% local only). Overall, 19% of the deaths were due to prostate cancer. These patients had very early-stage disease (one third were stage A1) and well differentiated tumors. The progression rate at 5 years was 36% to 38% for stages A2 and B.

In summary, small, clinically detectable prostate cancers have a slow doubling time, over 2 years in published reports.[73,74] But all studies that have followed untreated patients for long periods show that progression is inexorable, with local recurrence often preceding distant metastases.[66,68,70] Clinically localized prostate cancer is not a benign disease; it has a slow but steadily progressive natural history.

LATENT CANCER

About 30% of men older than 50 years with no clinical evidence of prostate cancer have foci of cancer within the prostate that can be detected at autopsy (Table 35-3).[14,77,78] Such a high prevalence is seen in no other organ and makes prostate cancer the most common malignancy in human beings.[10] Yet the number of men diagnosed with clinical prostate cancers in 1990 was about 100,000, only 1% of the estimated 10 million men with cancer present in the prostate (Fig. 35-1).[13] There were about 30,000 deaths from prostate cancer that year, or 0.3% of men with cancer. This enormous discrepancy between the high prevalence of the disease at autopsy and the low incidence of the disease clinically has provided a theoretical basis for a so-called no-treatment policy and has stymied efforts at early detection.[11,79-81]

This discrepancy has been exaggerated by the failure to consider the effect of time. Although the clinical incidence of prostate cancer is low (about 0.31% per year for men older than 50 years), the lifetime risk for developing prostate cancer for a man older than 50 years is 9.51% (Table 35-4).[82] Similarly, the annual mortality rate for men older than 50 years in 1985 was only 0.09%, but the lifetime risk for dying from prostate cancer was 2.89%. A 50-year-old man is expected to

TABLE 35–3. More Than Thirty Percent of Men Over Age 50 With No Clinical Evidence of Prostate Cancer Have Foci of Cancer Within the Prostate That Can Be Detected at Autopsy in Contrast to No Breast Cancer in Women at Autopsy

	Autopsy Incidence of Cancer in 173 Breasts* (Wellings, 1980)			Autopsy Incidence of Cancer in 220 Prostates (Franks, 1954)	
Age	No. of Patients Examined	Percent With Cancer	Age	No. of Patients Examined	Percent With Cancer
20–29	16	0	20–29	4	0
30–39	16	0	30–39	8	0
40–49	15	0	40–49	18	0
50–59	40	0	50–59	38	29
60–69	29	0	60–69	53	30
70–79	31	0	70–79	70	40
80–89	32	0	80–89	17	67
90+	4	0	90+	2	100

* 14 breasts had DCIS.
(Stamey TA. Cancer of the prostate. Monographs in Urology 1982;3:67–94)

live to the age of 75. Autopsy data confirm that prostate cancer is not found in every 75-year-old man but in only about 42%.[13] For a 50-year-old man, therefore, it can be estimated that the lifetime risk for developing cancer in the prostate is about 42%; the risk for developing the disease clinically is about 9.5%; and the risk for dying from the disease is about 2.9% (see Table 35–4).[13] Over their lifetimes, then, 23% of men with cancer in the prostate develop the disease clinically and 7% die from prostate cancer. Most histologic (autopsy) cancers do not progress within the lifespan of the host, but some do. Latent cancers appear cytologically and architecturally similar to cancers detected clinically. One of the greatest challenges to effective control of this disease is to find objective criteria to differentiate between these two forms of prostate cancer.[10,14,77,78,83–86]

There are important differences between autopsy cancers and clinically detected cancers in the volume, grade, and invasiveness of the tumor.[10,14,78,83,85] Most cancers found at autopsy are small, well differentiated, and show no tendency to invade normal structures such as the prostatic capsule or the seminal vesicles.[10] The proportion that are large and invasive is greater in men with a higher mortality rate from prostate cancer,[85] as reviewed in Dhom[10] and Scardino[13] (see Table 35–2). These observations strongly support the concept of a multistep process in the pathogenesis of prostate cancer, in which latent cancers have progressed through some of the steps necessary for full malignant expression.[87]

CLINICALLY IMPORTANT AND UNIMPORTANT CANCERS

Because some cancers found at autopsy have the features of clinical cancers[10,14,85,86] and some cancers detected clinically have the features of autopsy or latent cancers (for example, stage A1 or T0A),[88–90] we find it more helpful to describe prostate cancers as *clinically important*, that is, threatening the life or well-being of the host within his remaining life expectancy, or as *clinically unimportant*, that is, a latent cancer of no threat to the host.[13] At the light microscope level,

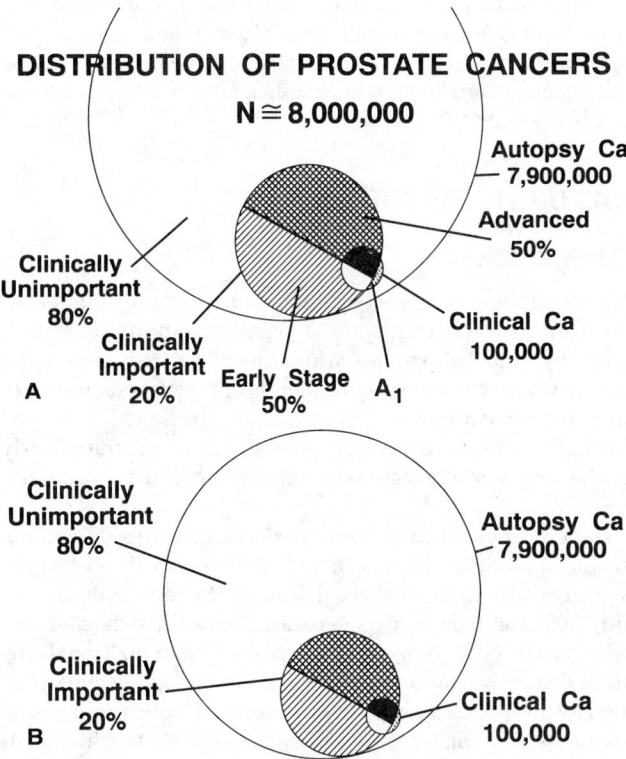

FIGURE 35–1. **(A)** If the prevalence of adenocarcinoma among men older than 50 years is 30%, then about 8 million American men harbor foci of cancer in their prostate. In 1990 only about 100,000 men were diagnosed with the disease (*i.e.*, clinical cancer) and the other 7.9 million were considered to have incidental or autopsy cancer. Based on the pathologic features of prostate cancer found at autopsy and the lifetime risk of developing prostate cancer, we estimate that 20% of these cancers are clinically important, that is, they will threaten the life or well being of the host if not treated effectively, and 80% are truly latent cancer (clinically unimportant). **(B)** Of the clinically detected cancers, nearly half are advanced. About 40% are early stage and may be curable, and 10% are focal, well-differentiated stage A1 (T0A) and may be clinically unimportant. Of the large pool of undetected but clinically important cancers, similar proportions are estimated to apply. (Scardino PT, Weaver R, Hudson MA. Early detection of prostate cancer. Hum Pathol 1992;23:211–222)

TABLE 35-4. Lifetime Risk of Developing or Dying From Prostate Cancer for a 50-year-old Man in 1985*

	Lifetime Risk (%)	Ratio
Lifetime risk of developing autospy cancer: Scardino, 1989[13]	42.0	14.5
Lifetime risk of developing clinical cancer: Seidman et al, 1985[82]	9.51	3.3
Lifetime risk of dying from prostate cancer: Seidman et al, 1985[82]	2.89	1.0

* The ratio indicates that for every death from prostate cancer, 3.3 men are diagnosed with the clinical disease and 14.5 develop histologic evidence of cancer in the prostate during their lifetime.

TABLE 35-5. Features That Help Distinguish Clinically Important From Unimportant Prostate Cancers

	Clinically Important	Clinically Unimportant
Volume	Large	Small
Grade	Moderate/poor (Gleason grade 3, 4, 5)	Well-differentiated (Gleason grade 1 or 2)
Pattern of growth	Invasive, proliferative	Noninvasive
Ploidy	Nondiploid	Diploid
Serum PSA*	Elevated	Normal
Zone of Origin	Peripheral zone	Transition zone

Note: Most features can be clinically detected. Approximately 20% of autopsy cancer cases have two or more of the features of clinically important cancers.
* Elevated indicates ≥10 ng/ml (Hybritech monoclonal assay).
(Scardino PT, Weaver R, Hudson MA. Early detection of prostate cancer. Hum Pathol 1992;23:211–223)

tumor volume, grade, and invasiveness are some of the features that help to differentiate clinically important from unimportant cancers (Table 35-5). Unfortunately, no objective markers of progression or prognosis in human cancer have been developed,[91] and other features that seem to be associated strongly with the biologic behavior of prostate cancer are the DNA ploidy status of the tumor, the degree of PSA production (serum PSA level), and, possibly, the zone of origin of the tumor within the prostate (see Table 35-5).

Among men older than 50 years, the proportion of prostate cancers that are clinically important is difficult to determine precisely. Data from detailed morphometric studies of prostate cancers found at autopsy and in cystoprostatectomy specimens suggest that about 20% of undetected cancers are clinically important on the basis of the features listed in Table 35-5 (see Fig. 35-1).[10,13,14,78,83,85,86]

ANATOMY AND PATHOLOGY

Prostatic cancers are commonly subdivided by site of origin as illustrated in Table 35-6.[92] The regional anatomy of the pelvis and prostate is illustrated in Figures 35-2 and 35-3. The acinar structure or proximal ducts of the prostate give rise to 98% of prostate cancers that prove to be adenocarcinomas. This adenocarcinoma group contains the recognizable histologic subdivisions outlined in Table 35-6. The other cancers of acinar or ductal origin are rare, as are all of the group arising from the distal ducts. The latter groups are at least as aggressive as the common adenocarcinoma and are usually less responsive to hormone manipulation.[93] Radiation therapy and cystoprostatectomy are recommended for management of localized nonacinar carcinomas, whereas radiation therapy is preferred for locally extensive disease.[94] In a study of the results of radical prostatectomy in 15 patients with ductal cancer most of whom had clinical stage B (T2) disease, Christensen and colleagues found the pathologic stage of disease to be more extensive than is typical of stage B (T2) adenocarcinomas with 93% capsular invasion, 47% positive margins, 40% seminal vesicle involvement, and 27% positive nodes.[95] Of these patients, 54% were noted to have cancers that were diploid on DNA analysis, and short-term follow-up (generally less than 2 years) showed that 47% had persisting disease.

GRADING SYSTEMS

The histologic grade of prostate cancer is the strongest independent clinical variable predictive of outcome.[96] Of the systems separating patients into 3 or 4 groups, including those proposed by Broders,[97] and Mostofi,[98] the Brawn (M.D. Anderson Cancer Center) system[99] has been particularly successful in discriminating outcome. The system described by Gleason[100] has been widely accepted as increasing numbers of studies have confirmed its reproducibility and predictive value.[101-103] The Gleason system recognizes five histologic patterns, which are assigned grade numbers, and combines the dominant and secondary pattern number into a histologic sum (Table 35-7). As originally proposed, a numeric representation of anatomic stage was combined with the histologic score to produce a final Gleason combined score that was most predictive of outcome. The numeric staging system has not gained wide acceptance.

DNA PLOIDY: CORRELATION WITH GRADE AND PROGNOSTIC SIGNIFICANCE

Nuclear shape has been used by Diamond to segregate patients treated by radical prostatectomy into good and bad outcome groups[104] and by Shaeffer and colleagues to correlate shape with outcome of radiation therapy.[105] In a computer-assisted image analysis of roundness, Diamond and colleagues observed that nuclear roundness was highly discriminatory in separating long-term survivors from those who developed metastasis in a group of 17 clinical stage B2 patients ($p = 0.005$).[104] They observed no overlap of roundness values between these two groups. Shaeffer and colleagues compared 23 patients with local failure to 23 matched patients who showed no evidence of disease after treatment.[105] They observed a highly significant difference in nuclear roundness of tumor cells in the two groups of patients when the tumors were well differentiated. They believe that this identifies a subset of well-differentiated tumors with an increased risk of local failure.

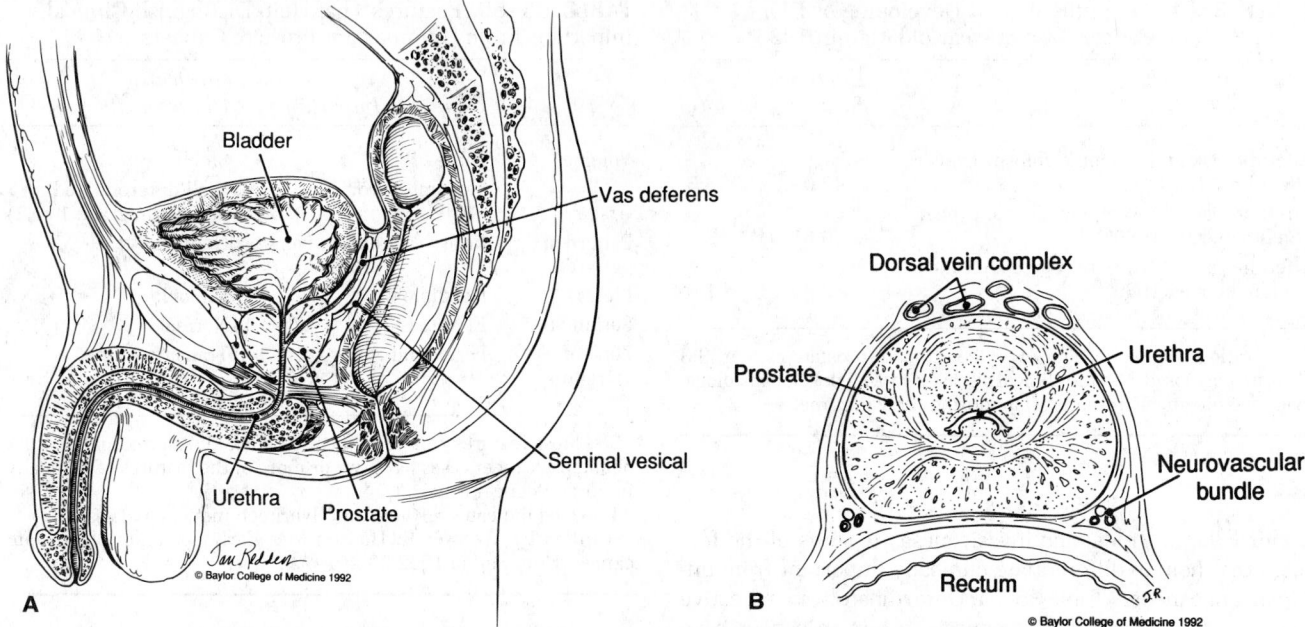

FIGURE 35–2. **(A)** Regional anatomy of the pelvis. The prostate is located at the outlet of the urinary bladder and is accessible to palpation through the rectum. **(B)** A transverse section through the midportion of the prostate gland shows the proximity to the rectum and the relation of the neurovascular bundles to the prostate. The cavernous nerves, responsible for penile erections, accompany small vessels in the groove between the rectum and the posterolateral peripheral zone of the prostate, where most prostate cancers arise.

DNA Analysis

Nuclear DNA content can be measured by image cytometry or by flow cytometry. These measurements correlate with pathologic stage and survival in prostate cancer. Frankfurt and colleagues examined 45 patients with prostate cancer and noted that all 11 patients with organ-confined cancer had diploid tumors.[106] Of a total of 25 diploid tumors, 8 invaded the capsule and 6 had nodal or other metastasis. *None* of the aneuploid tumors were organ confined. Patients with stage A and B prostate cancer treated by radical prostatectomy show a strong correlation of ploidy and outcome. Blute and colleagues reported that in their radical prostatectomy series, 63% of 38 patients showing tumor progression had nondiploid tumors

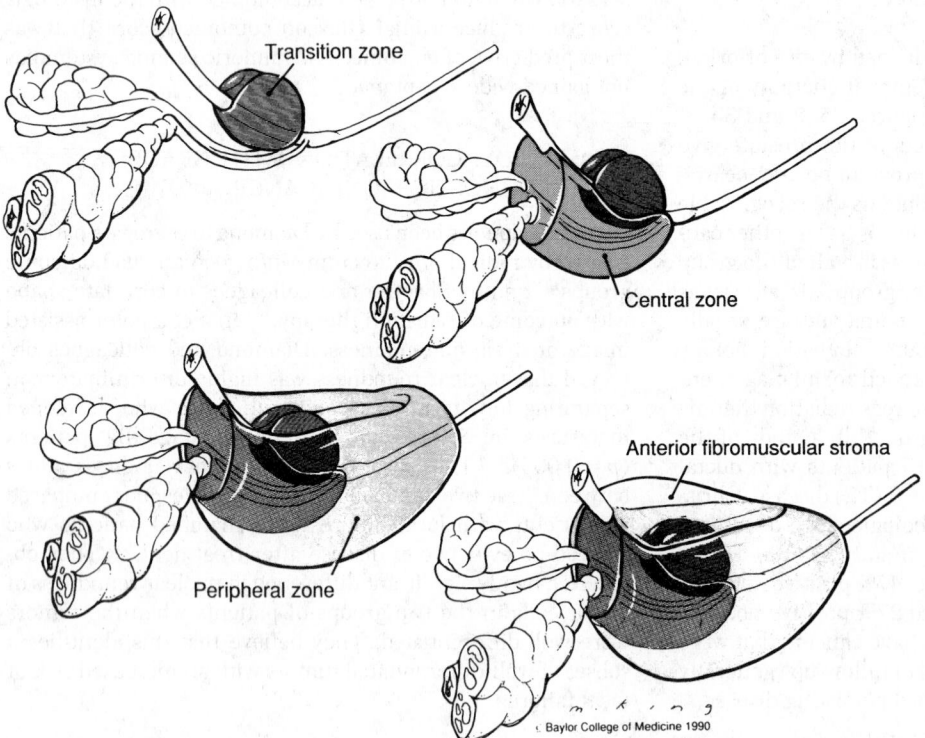

FIGURE 35–3. Zonal anatomy of the prostate. There are three glandular zones and the anterior fibromuscular stroma. In the young adult prostate, the transition zone is composed of 10% of the glandular tissue, the central zone 25%, and the peripheral zone 65%.

TABLE 35–6. Classification of Prostatic Carcinoma

Acinar and Proximal Duct Origin (98%)
Adenocarcinoma (papillary, cribriform, comedo, acinar)
Mucinous carcinoma
Adenoid cystic carcinoma
Carcinoid tumor
Undifferentiated carcinoma, small cell type

Distal Duct Origin (2%)
Transitional cell carcinoma
Squamous cell carcinoma
Papillary carcinoma
Ductal carcinoma with endometroid features

(Modified from Petersen RO. Urologic pathology. Philadelphia: JB Lippincott, 1986:617)

TABLE 35–7. Gleason Scoring System

Pattern 1	Closely packed, single, separate, round, uniform glands; well-defined tumor margin
Pattern 2	Single, separate, round, less uniform glands separated by stroma up to one gland diameter; tumor margin less well defined
Pattern 3	Single, separate, irregular glands of variable size; enlarged masses with cribriform or papillary pattern; poorly defined tumor margin
Pattern 4	Fused glands in mass with infiltrating cords, small glands with papillary, cribriform, or solid patterns; cells small, dark, or hypernephroid (clear cells)
Pattern 5	Few or no glands in background of masses with comedo pattern; cords or sheets of tumor cells infiltrating stroma

* Gleason tumor grade = dominant pattern + secondary pattern.
(Modified from Petersen RO. Urologic pathology. Philadelphia: JB Lippincott, 1986)

and 37% had diploid tumors.[88] In an age-matched control group of 38 patients with nonrecurrent tumors, there were no aneuploid tumors. In the Mayo Clinic prostatectomy series, ploidy was the only significant predictive factor found in a multivariate analysis of tumor characteristics. Patients with tumors of all stages that were still operable were used by Nativ and colleagues to compare ploidy and PSA values.[107] They observed that all nondiploid tumors were associated with elevated PSA levels. Although all normal PSA values occurred in patients with diploid tumors, only 35% of diploid tumors were not associated with an elevation of the PSA. Miller and colleagues studied 103 D2 patients, including 66 who died within 1 year (the "bad" group), and compared them with 37 patients, all of whom survived 5 years (the "good" group).[101] Of the "bad" outcome group, 76% had poorly differentiated tumors and 88% were nondiploid. In the "good" group, 65% had well-differentiated tumors and 64% were diploid tumors. DNA analysis added little to histologic differentiation in this series because the two were highly correlated. Stephenson and associates examined the ploidy value of cancer found in pelvic lymph node metastases and observed a strong correlation between mean survival time and ploidy status.[108] This correlation remained true even when they compared only patients with tumors of intermediate histologic grade. This suggests that DNA analysis contributes prognostic information beyond differentiation, at least in the intermediate differentiation group.

Robertson and Paulson observed a similarly enhanced usefulness of DNA analysis in intermediate differentiation of surgical patients.[109] Peters and colleagues correlated grade and ploidy in 44 patients including 33 with small palpable tumors treated by iodine 125 implantation (Table 35–8).[110] Progression was noted in 21% (5/24) of tumors with Gleason grades 5 through 7 and 25% (2/8) of tumors with grades 8 through 10, whereas only 10% of diploid tumors (3/29) and 100% of aneuploid tumors (4/4) progressed. In this small series, ploidy was more predictive than grade. Patients with external-beam irradiation are not reported but would be expected to have similar results. The correlation of nondiploid tumors with increased progression rates and decreased mean survival times is shown in all stages of prostate cancer. The correlation is not sufficiently accurate for exclusion of patients from one form of therapy or another.

MARKERS OF PROSTATE CANCER

The two tumor markers of proved clinical utility in the diagnosis and management of carcinoma of the prostate are the measurement of levels of prostatic acid phosphatase (PAP) and PSA. Although measurement of PAP levels have been widely used in the past, it is rapidly being replaced by measurement of PSA levels for most indications. There appear to be only three areas in which the use of PAP is justified. First, monoclonal antibodies to PAP provide an immunohistochemical reagent of value equivalent to that provided by antibodies

TABLE 35–8. Progression After ^{125}I Implantation Related to DNA Content and Grade

Stage	No. of Patients	Fraction Progressing		Stage	No. of Patients	Fraction Progressing	
		Diploid	Aneuploid			GL 5–7	GL 8–10
A2	4	0/2	1/2	A2	4	0/3	1/1
B1	33	3/29	4/4	B1	32	5/24 (21%)	2/8 (25%)
B2	7	1/4	3/3	B2	7	4/6 (67%)	0/1
Total	44	4/35 (11%)	8/9 (89%)	Total	43	9/33 (27%)	3/10 (30%)

(Modifed from Peters JM, Miles BJ, Kubus JJ, Crissman JD. Prognostic significance of the nuclear DNA content in localized prostatic carcinoma. Anal Quant Cytol Histol 1990;12:359–365)

to PSA.[111] Second, radioimmunoscintigraphy with anti-PAP antibodies has proved superior to similar studies with anti-PSA reagents.[112] Third, although levels of PSA tend to increase in proportion to the total mass of normal and malignant prostatic tissue, PAP levels are much more likely to become elevated only in the presence of metastatic disease.[113–115] PAP exhibits greater specificity but less sensitivity than PSA in the detection of metastatic disease.

PAP and PSA are subject to the general constraints of all tumor markers. First, no tumor marker is expressed consistently. PAP and PSA are expressed less in poorly differentiated than in well-differentiated tumors.[111,116] Histochemical studies typically reveal considerable variation in the expression of both markers from cell to cell within a tumor mass. Treatment can alter the expression of markers by tumor cells. For example, androgen removal lessens PSA expression in the surviving prostate cancer.[117] In addition, drug-induced sublethal injury may lessen marker expression. All the factors listed above lead to considerable patient-to-patient variability in marker elevation associated with any given clinical stage and render markers inaccurate staging tools.[113–115] Finally, the correlation between shrinkage of tumor mass and the decline of a marker is not straightforward. An ideal marker would reflect changes in tumor volume. However, objective responses usually are expressed in terms of an alteration in the products of the perpendicular diameters of measurable disease. The latter is proportional to area, not volume. Figure 35–4 shows the relation between area and volume for a sphere. A 50% decline in area correlates with a change in volume of nearly 70%. Because treatment may result in decreased marker expression in sublethally injured cells, a partial remission should be expected not to correlate with a 50% decline in a marker, but with alterations of more than 70% to 80%.

CHROMOSOMAL LOCATION, GENE STRUCTURE, AND BIOCHEMISTRY

PAP is a protein phosphatase that can dephosphorylate tyrosine and serine-threonine phosphates.[118–121] In prostate tissue, its preferred substrate appears to be an 83-kd phosphoprotein. The enzyme is composed of dimers assembled from α, β, or γ monomers, each about 50 kd in size.[122] The major component of PAP, PAP-A, is composed of two α monomers, whereas the minor isozyme, PAP-B, is composed of equal amounts of the α-β and α-γ dimers. The chromosomal location of PAP is 3q21.[123] The amino acid sequence of PAP shows a 45% to 49% homology with lysosomal acid phosphatase.[124–126] The major difference between these two proteins is that the membrane-anchoring domain of lysosomal acid phosphatase is lacking in PAP, in keeping with the secretory nature of PAP. Although the biologic function of PAP in normal prostate epithelial cell function remains obscure, it has been shown to stimulate directly the collagen and alkaline phosphatase content of isolated bone cells and may play a role in the development of osteoblastic lesions.[127]

PSA is a serine protease secreted into the seminal fluid. Its normal role appears to be the liquefaction of the seminal coagulum.[128] As a protease, it is a member of a subclass of glandular or tissue kallikreins.[117,128,129] All members of this family are characterized by posttranslational processing of polypeptide precursors to their biologically active forms. Other members of the kallikrein gene family include human glandular kallikrein 1 through 3, the α and γ subunits of nerve growth factor, γ renin, and the epidermal growth factor binding protein. The *PSA* gene is located at 19q13 in close association with human glandular kallikrein 1 and renal kallikrein. The *PSA* gene exhibits an 82% homology with H-*GK1* and has a similar structure.[117,130] In the normal prostate and benign prostatic hypertrophy, but not in cancer, *PSA* and H-*GK1* expression correlate. Expression of the *PSA* gene contains an androgen response element and is regulated by the presence of androgen and other unidentified tissue-specific elements. As a result, *PSA* gene expression increases with puberty and decreases after androgen removal. In blood, most *PSA* is bound to α_1-antichymotrypsin and is enzymatically inactive. Because circulating PSA has a 2- to 4-day terminal half life, circulating levels rapidly reflect the rate of production.

PSA has been called a specific marker for prostatic epithelium, normal or malignant. PSA and PAP are repressed in a selected range of other normal tissues and tumors. The prostate develops from the cloacogenic glandular epithelium, and other products of this fetal tissue may be found in the anal and urethral glands. The epithelia of these tissues exhibit expression of both markers.[131,132] In addition, cells from the cloacogenic epithelium may be found scattered within the bladder and rectal wall. Tumors arising from these cells can

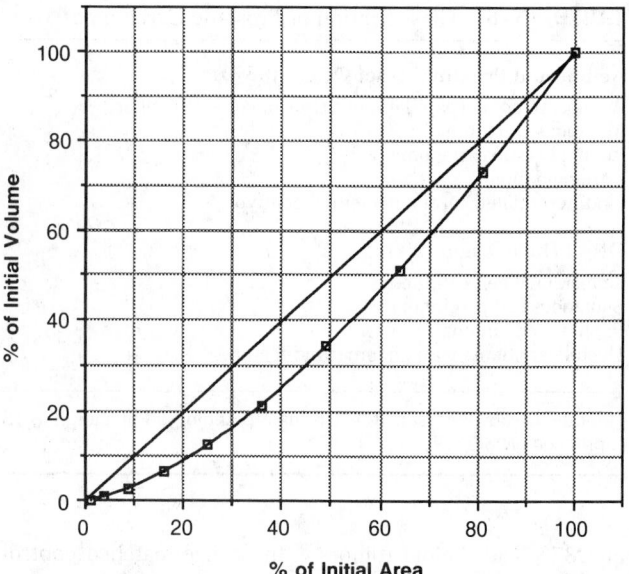

FIGURE 35–4.   The relation between partial remission and changes in tumor volume. The conventional definition of a partial response is a decline of 50% or more in the sum of the products of the perpendicular diameters of measurable tumor masses (the formula for the area of a quadrilateral). However, tumor shape is better represented by a sphere, the volume of which is π times the radius cubed. This figure shows the relation between the product of the diameters and volume of a spherical tumor mass as open boxes connected by a curved line. The straight line shows the relation that would be found if these two parameters were equivalent. A 50% decline in the product of the diameters correlates with a 65% decline in volume. On the other hand, a 50% decline in volume correlates with a 37% change in the product of the diameters. Because markers correlate with tumor volume and not area, a decline in pretreatment marker levels of 65% to 70% would be equivalent to a partial response as determined by traditional techniques.

manifest as PSA- and PAP-positive bladder tumors and PSA-negative PAP-positive rectal carcinoids.[133] In addition, normal axillary and perineal apocrine sweat glands, some apocrine foci in fibrocystic breast disease, and apocrine sweat gland carcinomas may stain positive with polyclonal, but not monoclonal, anti-PSA antibody. There is a single report of a PSA-producing small cell carcinoma of unknown primary.[134]

FOLLOWING RESPONSE TO TREATMENT

PSA has proved to be superior to PAP as a marker to follow the course of treatment with surgery, radiation therapy, and hormonal therapy. Levels of PSA also have proved more sensitive than the bone scan in detecting recurrent disease and may begin to rise 6 to 12 months before the bone scan shows recurrent disease.[135-137] The cost of a PSA evaluation is much less than that of the bone scan. The only real disadvantage to using PSA in place of the bone scan to follow patients is that occasionally progress occurs without an elevation in circulating PSA levels.[138] Detailed information is available on the use of PSA to follow the results of radical prostatectomy.[74,139-144] The mass of prostate tissue removed correlates well with the difference between presurgical and postsurgical PSA levels. After successful radical prostatectomy, the PSA level should decline to that found in females (<0.4 ng/ml). Levels in excess of this value indicate residual disease and predict early recurrence. The appropriate management of patients with elevated PSA levels after radical prostatectomy is controversial. Some of these patients experience a decline or normalization of PSA after radiation therapy to the pelvis.[145-147] There is no evidence that this alters the time to clinical recurrence or survival. Stamey and colleagues found that these responses usually were not durable.[146] Similarly there is no convincing evidence that adjuvant hormonal therapy in such patients alters eventual outcome. In a second group of patients, PSA levels initially exhibit a rapid decline to the female range, but subsequently begin to rise. A subset of these patients are reported to experience a lasting response to pelvic irradiation.[146]

PSA levels have been used to monitor the response of early-stage prostate carcinoma to radiation therapy.[148-153] Although PSA may begin to decline during the course of radiation therapy, a nadir typically is not reached until 6 months after treatment and may take as long as 12 months. The PSA decline generally follows an exponential function, and deviations from that pattern may provide an early indication of progressive disease.

The use of PSA to follow response to hormonal therapy is complicated by the fact that expression of PSA is stimulated by the presence of androgen. A portion of the decline in PSA seen after androgen ablation is due not to tumor cell death but to diminished expression. Nevertheless, with appropriate safeguards, it is possible to use PSA levels to monitor response of patients to hormonal therapy.[117,128,154-158] The speed and magnitude of the PSA decline have proved to be important. The most durable responses are seen in patients who experience at least an 80% decline in PSA within the first 4 weeks. On the other hand, there is no evidence that a decrease of 50% or less in PSA levels is of prognostic significance. For the patient with bone involvement alone, the evaluation of PSA levels has several advantages over other methods available to detect response. First, with a terminal half life of 2 to

4 days, PSA is a much more rapid indicator of healing than the bone scan or radiographic measurement of osteoblastic lesions. In addition, PSA has been shown to be more sensitive than the bone scan. In patients who experience a hormonal response, monitoring PSA becomes a valuable means of follow-up, with elevations in PSA levels preceding other indicators of disease progression by 6 to 12 months.

There is little information on the use of PSA levels to follow the course of chemotherapy. Scher and colleagues evaluated the use of PSA to monitor the course of patients treated with methotrexate.[159] The drug was not sufficiently active for proper assessment of the role of PSA in monitoring response or duration of response, but it showed that there is enough day-to-day variation in PSA so that multiple determinations are needed for optimal accuracy. Suramin has shown a high enough response rate to provide information relating PSA decline to treatment outcome.[160] In a pattern similar to that observed with hormonal therapy, a decline of 75% or greater over the first 8 weeks correlated with a prolongation in survival, with 80% of these patients alive at 1 year and more than 60% alive at 2.5 years. On the other hand, declines of 50% or less in PSA levels had no clinical significance. As with hormonal therapy, sublethal concentrations of suramin suppress expression of PSA by prostate cancer cells. These results suggest that PSA may prove valuable in evaluating the results of phase II drug trials in metastatic prostatic carcinoma.

SCREENING

Over the last 40 years, physicians have concerned themselves with finding ways to ensure that manipulations of a cancer during examination, biopsy, or resection do not contribute to the spread of that cancer.[161,162] In the past, this concern was expressed in the limitation of the number of examiners of patients with bulky pediatric and adult tumors and by the development of no-touch surgical techniques with control of blood vessels and lymphatics before the cancer is manipulated.[163,164]

Transurethral resection of the prostate (TURP) has been shown to be accompanied by the entrance of large amounts of irrigating fluid into the blood stream and the associated appearance in the blood stream of what appear to be prostate tumor cells.[165] There has been no direct proof that these cells are capable of establishing metastasis, but the possibility that TURP could increase in the role of distant metastasis gives rise to caution that this operation be used sparingly on patients with clinically localized prostate cancer. An adverse effect of TURP on the course of prostate cancer was first suggested by McGowan,[166] and other retrospective studies support and extend his observation that patients who undergo TURP have a lower survival rate than similarly staged patients undergoing a needle biopsy for diagnosis.[167-172] The subgroup most frequently affected has been patients with stage C or T3T4 cancers of poor and intermediate differentiation.[167,172] The severity of the effect is illustrated in Table 35–9, in which the frequency of metastasis is increased threefold at 5 years and the frequency of deaths is increased 2.5-fold after TURP in the Patterns of Care data.[96,167] The data from the Radiation Therapy Oncology Group (RTOG), analyzed by Sandler and Hanks, illustrate an apparent "wave" of metastasis appearing

TABLE 35–9.   Possible Adverse Effect of Transurethral Resection of the Prostate in Selected Patients (T3–4, Moderate and Poorly Differentiated, N0 or X, Normal Serum Acid Phosphatase)

		5-Year		10-Year	
Method of Diagnosis	*No. of Patients*	*Frequency of Metastasis*	*Dead*	*Frequency of Metastasis*	*Dead*
Transurethral resection of the prostate	87	38%	59%	56%	87%
Needle biopsy	52	13%	24%	22%	48%

(Modified from Hanks GE. Optomizing the radiation treatment and outcome of prostate cancer. Int J Radiat Biol Oncol Phys 1985;11:1235–1245)

after TURP that is less evident after needle biopsy, suggesting a pattern consistent with the dissemination of disease by the procedure (Fig. 35–5).[172] These reports are summarized in Table 35–10 along with other reports that failed to show an adverse effect of TURP.[173–176] Nevertheless, a review of the RTOG patients who were staged by lymph node dissection shows no significant increase in nodal metastasis in the group of patients requiring TURP (Table 35–11).

Hammarsten and Johansson in Sweden demonstrated prospectively a significant decrease in metastasis and death for prostate cancer patients who underwent TURP with low-pressure irrigation rather than the usual higher pressure irrigation.[177] They found significantly less intravascular absorption of irrigating fluid by the low-pressure method. This

correlation of the amount of intravascular fluid absorption with frequency of metastasis strongly suggests that the processes are causally related and that the TURP effect is real.

Strategies have been suggested to avoid the need for TURP in patients with a clinical stage C intermediate or poorly differentiated cancer. A single 500-cGy dose of irradiation given shortly before TURP would be expected to decrease the chance of viability of any cells forced into the blood stream by a factor of 10.[96] It must be emphasized that tumors in patients who do not fit into the affected subset do not appear to be disseminated by the TURP. Nevertheless, Meacham and colleagues did not observe an adverse effect of TURP and suggested that the apparent effect of TURP on the rate of development of distant metastases was a reflection of the poor prognosis of

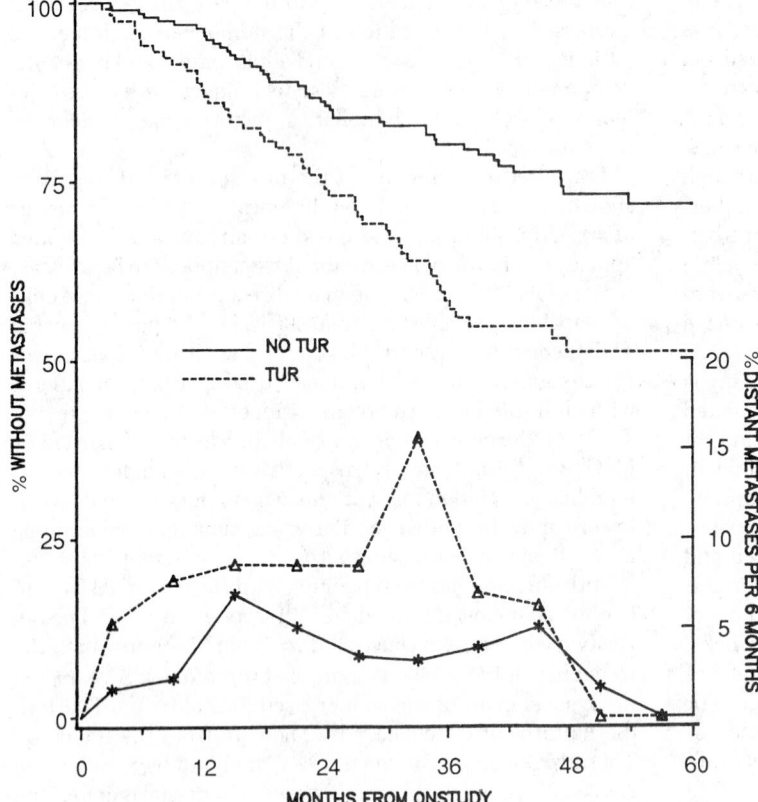

FIGURE 35–5. The data from the Radiation Therapy Oncology Group illustrate an apparent "wave" of metastasis appearing after transurethral resection that is less evident after needle biopsy, a pattern consistent with the dissemination of disease by the procedure. (Sandler HM, Hanks GE. Analysis of the possibility that transurethral resection promotes metastasis in prostate cancer. Cancer 1988;62:2622–2627)

TABLE 35–10. Effect of Transurethral Resection of the Prostate: Stage C

Investigations	No. of patients
Effect Observed	
PCS	195*
RTOG	433*
Stanford	353†
Mallinckrodt	263*
Mason Clinic	224*
Johns Hopkins	127†
Cross Cancer Institute	56†
Total	1651
Effect Not Observed	
Baylor	71†
E. Virginia	55†
Memorial	43†
Total	169

* Intermediate and poor differentiation.
† All.

TABLE 35–11. Frequency of Nodal Involvement by Method of Diagnosis (RTOG 75-06)

	Positive Nodes	
Stage B		
TURP	17/43 (28%)	NS
No TURP	21/55 (23%)	
Stage C		
TURP	24/40 (60%)	NS
No TURP	24/55 (44%)	

NS, no significant difference; TURP, transurethral resection of the prostate.

patients with severe obstructive voiding symptoms.[173] They showed that the presence of such symptoms was associated with a poorer prognosis and a greater frequency of pelvic lymph node metastases. Because TURP is recommended for relief of obstructive voiding symptoms and is not an appropriate technique for the diagnosis of cancer in men with a palpable tumor,[67,178,179] it was expected that patients with stage B or C prostate cancer who had a TURP would have a more extensive cancer, contributing to the outlet obstruction, and a higher incidence of positive nodes. The risks of metastases after TURP and after needle biopsy were compared, controlling for the degree of obstructive voiding symptoms on the status of the pelvic lymph nodes. No difference in time to distant metastasis was observed (Fig. 35–6).

Nevertheless, TURP is a major operation associated with important complications (*e.g.*, retrograde ejaculation, erectile impotence, and urinary incontinence) and even death in 0.5% to 1.2% of patients.[180] This procedure is not indicated for the diagnosis of cancer, which should be made by needle biopsy whenever feasible. Patients with prostate cancer who have severe obstructive voiding symptoms should proceed immediately to definitive therapy (radical prostatectomy, irradiation therapy, or hormonal therapy) and the TURP should be delayed or avoided if possible.

Because PAP usually is not elevated in early stage patients, it is of little use in screening patients for early stage prostate cancer. On the other hand, PSA is sensitive and frequently abnormal in early-stage disease; patients with A2 disease may have PSA values above 10 ng/ml.[148] However, benign prostatic hypertrophy, prostatitis, and prostatic trauma can result in levels that overlap with those of early-stage prostate cancer, so that the PSA test lacks specificity.[181] Nevertheless, several large studies attempt to assess the role of PSA as a screening tool.[5,182–186] A PSA level above 10 ng/ml has a positive predictive value of 65% for carcinoma of the prostate. With a

PSA level between 4 and 10 ng/ml (Hybritech assay) in association with rectal examination, PSA increases the detection rate of prostate cancer compared with rectal examination alone.[5]

Controversy surrounds the concept of screening for prostate cancer. First, there is no consensus as to the optimum management of early stage prostate cancer and no unequivocal evidence that treatment affects survival, especially within the first 10 years. Second, the cost of mounting a national screening effort for men over 50 years of age would be high and might not be cost effective. Currently, an NCI-funded randomized trial is underway to determine the survival advantage of screening.

ROUTES OF SPREAD

Cancer of the prostate regularly spreads by direct extension and lymphatic and vascular routes.

LYMPHATIC SPREAD

True lymphatic and lymph node metastases are common, and their frequency correlates with stage, tumor volume, and histologic grade, as demonstrated in the classic work of Barzell and colleagues (Table 35–12).[187] This information can be used to identify patients whose risk for nodal metastasis is low and to identify groups of patients whose risk for nodal and other metastasis is so great that nonsurgical therapy is indicated and lymph node dissection may not be needed. Fowler and Whitmore[188] and Donahue and colleagues[189] identified in greater detail the frequency of nodal metastasis by stage and grade (Table 35–13). Perineural lymphatic invasion commonly is described in the prostate but probably represents the infiltration of least resistance tissue spaces rather than of lymphatics. The problem of penetration of the prostatic capsule through these paths is greatest at the apex of the gland, where the capsule is anatomically susceptible to penetration. This was shown by Stamey and colleagues, who noted that in 39 of 78 patients with stage B cancer and capsular extension, direct extension along perineural spaces exited from the gland at the point of penetration of the capsule by the nerve.[190]

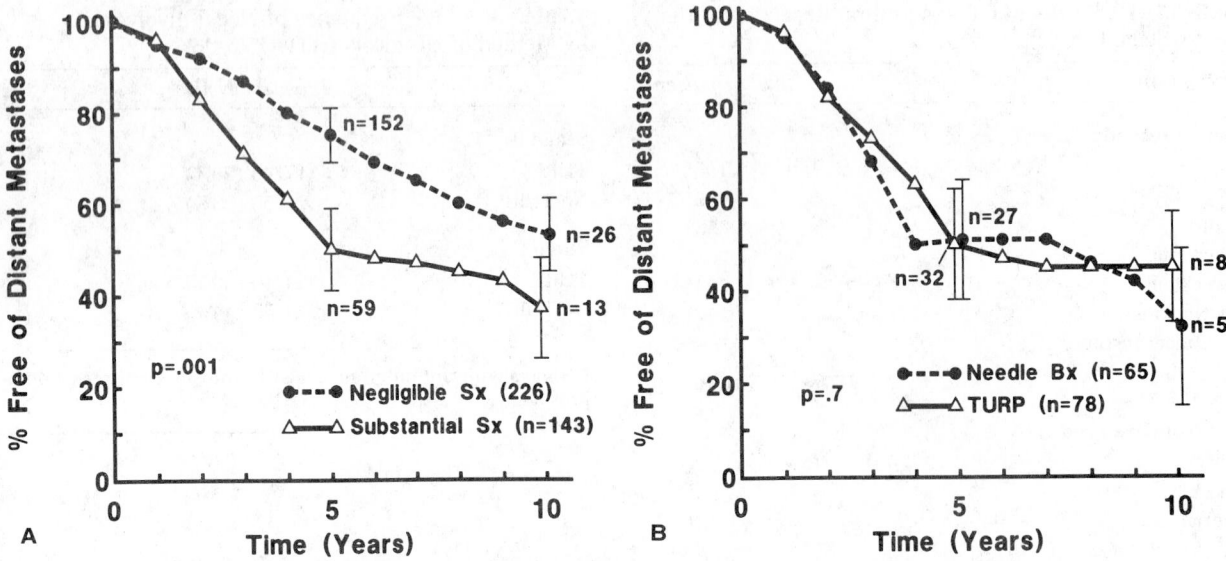

FIGURE 35–6. **(A)** Actuarial rate of development of distant metastases based on degree of obstructive voiding symptoms (Sx). Presence of such symptoms at diagnosis was a significant prognostic feature. **(B)** When analysis was restricted to patients with substantial obstructive voiding symptoms (all stages), there was no longer a significant difference between transurethral prostatic resection (TURP) and needle biopsy (Bx) groups. Brackets at 5 and 10 years indicate a 95% confidence interval. n, number of patients still alive and being followed without distant metastases. (From Meacham RB, Scardino PT. The role of transurethral resection of the prostate in the dissemination of prostatic carcinoma. In: Fitzpatrick JM, Crane RJ, eds. The prostate. London: Churchill Livingstone, 1989:315–318)

DIRECT EXTENSION

Direct extension is a common route of spread beyond the capsule and is difficult to detect by digital rectal examination. The risk of extracapsular extension is strongly correlated with clinical stage and differentiation. Patients with clinical stage B2 (T2B) prostate cancers of tumors of any anatomic extent that are poorly differentiated have at least a 66% rate of positive surgical margins or extensive extracapsular tumor,[191,192] whereas the rate in differentiated B1 (T1A) tumors is 15% to 30%.

TABLE 35–12. Correlation of Stage, Grade, and Volume With Nodal Metastasis

Factor	No. of Positive Regional Nodes/Total	Percentage	p Value
Stage			
Stage B	15/59	25	<0.01
Stage C	26/41	63	
Grade			
Well-differentiated	3/19	16	
Differentiated	18/46	39	
Poorly differentiated	9/15	60	<0.01
Size			
<0.25	1/18	5	
2.5–7.9	17/50	34	<0.01
8.0–18.0 cm³	23/32	72	

(Modified from Barzell W, Beam JA, Hilaris BS, Whitmore WF. Prostatic adenocarcinoma: Relationship of grade and local extent to the pattern of metastases. J Urol 1977;11:278–282)

VASCULAR SPREAD

Metastases to bone have been observed in up to 80% of patients with prostate cancer as a result of direct invasion of the venous system and systemic dissemination. The cells can gain access to Batson's veins but do not show a pattern that suggests preferential spread by that venous system.[193,194]

IMAGING STUDIES OF THE PROSTATE AND LYMPH NODES

There is a crucial need for a diagnostic test to determine before the initiation of treatment whether the cancer substantially penetrates the prostatic capsule or involves the seminal vesicles or pelvic lymph nodes. This would enable the surgeon to identify for operation the one third of patients with clinical stage B2 disease who do not have these adverse pathologic features and thereby avoid surgery in the two thirds for whom there is no demonstrated long-term benefit.[195] Similarly, the radiation oncologist could restrict the volume treated in patients with truly localized disease, a program associated with fewer side effects, while treating an appropriately larger volume in those with extracapsular extension. Patients with seminal vesicle and lymph node involvement could be directed to appropriate clinical trials.

LYMPH NODE EVALUATION

Imaging studies of the lymph nodes have advocates in institutions in which experience or expertise leads them to have confidence in the results of lymphangiography (LAG)[196–198] or computed tomographic (CT) scans. The single prospective trial of magnetic resonance imaging (MRI) in evaluating lymph node metastasis in early A–B (T1B–T2) prostate cancer

TABLE 35–13. Frequency of Positive Nodes Related to Clinical Stage and Grade

| | *Differentiation* | | | | | |
| | *Well* | | *Moderate* | | *Poor* | |
Stage	Donahue[189]	Fowler[188]	Donahue[189]	Fowler[188]	Donahue[189]	Fowler[188]
A1	2%	—	—	—	—	—
A2	5%	—	23%	—	50%	—
B1	5%	6%	20%	7%	27%	—
B2	28%	31%	27%	47%	38%	80%
C	18%	64%	42%	62%	68%	60%

(Data from Donahue RE, Man JH, Whitsel JA, et al. Pelvic lymph node dissection: Guide to patient management in clinically locally confined adenocarcinoma of the prostate. Urology 1982;20:559–565; and from Fowler JE, Whitmore WF. The incidence and extent of pelvic lymph node metastases in apparently localized prostatic cancer. Cancer 1981;47:2941–2945)

showed poor results, with only 1 of 23 true-positive results identified correctly (Table 35–14). Therefore, MRI is not recommended for identifying nodal metastasis. Hanks and colleagues reviewed in great detail two RTOG prospective clinical trials in which lymph node status was evaluated by LAG, CT, or biopsy.[199] Results of various methods of determining nodal status are shown in Table 35–15. Imaging studies in patients with and without positive lymph nodes were not able to show differences in survival, in survival with no evidence of disease, or in frequency of metastasis. In contrast, biopsy determination of positive lymph nodes was highly discriminating and all differences were significant. In this broad-based experience in more than 20 clinical research institutions, the imaging tests were of no prognostic value. For patients who will receive radiation therapy, it is recommended that MRI or CT be delayed until it can be done as part of the treatment planning process in which it has value and does not require a costly repetition of the examination.[199,200]

EVALUATION OF THE PROSTATE

The Radiological Diagnostic Oncology Group (RDOG) has reported a prospective trial comparing the accuracy of TRUS with that of MRI (body surface) in identifying extraprostatic extension and seminal vesicle involvement.[201] In 187 patients who had both examinations, the tests did not differ significantly in their ability to detect extraprostatic extension or seminal vesicle involvement; however, the level of accuracy was poor. For extraprostatic extension, pathologic data agreed with imaging in 46 of 65 cases.

TABLE 35–14. MRI Detection of Nodal Metastasis

| *Pathologic Nodal Status* | *MRI Results* | |
	Negative	*Positive*
Negative		
162	155	7
Positive		
23	22	1

(Data from references 198, 199, and 201)

Ultrasound identified 14 of 65 patients who had seminal vesicle involvement, and MRI identified 18 of 65. When TRUS or MRI correctly identified seminal vesicle invasion or extracapsular extension, the result correlated with the pathologic data in only 31% of patients. The crucial preoperative determination of the extent of disease can be made with a positive ultrasound or surface MRI, and unnecessary surgery can be avoided. Many instances of extracapsular extension and seminal vesicle invasion are missed. More controlled prospective studies with pathologic correlation are needed to settle these issues.

To summarize, LAG, CT, and body coil MRI are not accurate in determining nodal involvement. If they are used and a positive node is reported and that finding alters the patient's treatment, then the status of the node must be proved by fine-needle aspiration or by open biopsy.

ENDORECTAL SURFACE COIL

MRI, adapted for endorectal examination by Schnall and associates[201a] at the University of Pennsylvania, may be superior to body coil image examination in their hands. They noted an overall accuracy of 82% in differentiating pathologic stage B cancers from stage C, whereas the accuracy of three examiners at their institution with the body coil was an average of 16% lower. Unfortunately, only 22 patients are included in this first report[201a] and there has not been a proper prospective comparison of endorectal and surface MRI. Table 35–16 contains a summary of accuracy in identifying stage C disease by ultrasound, surface MRI, and endorectal MRI, with data pooled from several sources.

TREATMENT OF CLINICALLY LOCALIZED PROSTATE CANCER

1987 CONSENSUS CONFERENCE ON THE MANAGEMENT OF CLINICALLY LOCALIZED PROSTATE CANCER

The National Cancer Institute and the Office of Medical Application of Research convened a Consensus Development Conference on the management of clinically localized prostate cancer in 1987. The Consensus Committee considered the data presented by experts and agreed on answers to five ques-

TABLE 35–15. Outcome at 5 Years* by Stage and Method of Lymph Node Assessment (RTOG 7506/7706; n = 805)

| | | Pathologic Nodal Status | | | | | | Clinical Nodal Status | | | | |
| | | Negative | | | Positive | | | Negative | | Positive | |
Outcome	Stage	N†	5-Year (%)		N†	5-Year (%)		N†	5-Year (%)	N†	5-Year (%)
Survival											
	B	97	84	S‡	38	61	S‡	249	77	23	80
	C	47	82	S	48	66	S	199	65	21	60
Survival With No Evidence of Disease											
	B	97	72	S	38	32	S	249	63	23	55
	C	47	64	S	48	32	S	199	44	21	38
Free From Metastases											
	B	97	85	S	38	46	S	249	84	23	85
	C	47	75	S	48	44	S	199	60	21	55

* Actuarial estimates.
† Sample sizes shown (N) are initial sample sizes.
‡ S, differences between pathologically negative and positive nodes are significant for stages B and C.
(Modified from Hanks GE, Asbell S, Krall JM, et al. Outcome for lymph node dissection negative T-1b, T-2 (A-2, B) prostate cancer treated with external beam radiation therapy in RTOG 77-06. Int J Radiat Oncol Biol Phys 1991;21:1099–1103)

tions.[202] The reader is encouraged to review the Consensus Development Statement, the conclusion of which is reproduced here in its entirety.[203]

Radical prostatectomy and radiation therapy are clearly effective forms of treatment in the attempt to cure tumors limited to the prostate for appropriately selected patients. Comparisons across studies suggest comparable 10-year survival rates with either form of management. What remains unclear is the relative merit of each in producing lifelong freedom from cancer recurrence. It is known that traditional radical prostatectomy can provide 15-year cancer-free survival, in appropriately selected patients, equivalent to that of a comparably aged control population. On the other hand, sufficient long-term followup does not exist to permit a conclusion about the ability of radiation therapy to eradicate such cancer in an equivalent proportion of patients. After appropriate primary irradiation, the long-term complication rate is now well defined and appears acceptable. The new approach to prostatectomy is clearly associated with a reduction in postoperative impotence. The true comparative incidence of impotence over time, however, awaits prospective evaluation. While impotence may result from the alteration of normal anatomy, the psychological considerations should not be overlooked. Sexual rehabilitation should address both medical and psychological needs.

TABLE 35–16. Accuracy of Various Methods of Identifying Stage C Disease

	Correct Identification of Stage C	Incorrect Identification of Stage C
Body coil[201]	86/121 (71%)	31/82 (38%)
Surface coil[201a]	5/6 (83%)	1/6 (17%)
Ultrasound[201]	84/134 (63%)	50/92 (54%)

Information that should be available to a patient considering with his physician the choice of treatment includes:

1. Probability of cure, mortality, complications, and other side effects of radical prostatectomy and radiation therapy.
2. Risk of impotence and incontinence for either treatment.
3. Psychosocial consequences of either choice.
4. Extent and risk of pretreatment staging assessment tests.
5. Economic consequences of each form of treatment.

As competing, noncancer-related causes of death (*e.g.,* cardiovascular disease) may be expected to decrease for men over the age of 50, the issue of cure will become more important in low stage disease. Properly designed and completed randomized trials that evaluate both disease control and quality of life after modern radiation therapy compared with radical prostatectomy are essential.[203]

In addition to concerns about management and decision making in treatment of localized prostate cancer, the panel reviewed and recommended appropriate directions for future basic and clinical research.

The Consensus Conference report was not received with unparalleled enthusiasm by urologic surgeons or radiation oncologists, probably an indication that the committee had achieved a fair consensus. Since the conference, there has been a tremendous increase in the number of clinical trials in all aspects of prostate cancer care and an infusion of funds to support more laboratory and clinical investigations. It appears that prostate cancer will be a major focus of research in the 1990s, initiated in part by the 1987 consensus.

STAGING

Every patient's disease must be staged before definitive treatment. Staging requires a minimal workup described elsewhere in this chapter. The most commonly used staging system is the American Urological Association system which is based on the original system proposed by Whitmore and modified by Jewett.[11] Recently, the American Joint Committee on Cancer (AJCC) and the Union Internationale Contra le Cancer (UICC) agreed on a joint TNM classification that includes histopathologic grade to determine final stage grouping.[204] These two systems are shown in Table 35–17.

A major problem with both of these systems is a lack of sufficient subdivision of stage B or T2 tumors.[205,206] The current systems only separate small tumors (<1.5 cm) from those that may involve all of both palpable lobes. Although concerned about adding another system, the Organ Systems Program developed a primary staging classification that divides stage B (T2) tumors into three subcategories and similarly divides stage C (T3–4) into three different categories based on extent of tumor (Table 35–18). Recently, the AJCC and UICC updated their system so that there is one internationally accepted staging system.[201b]

CLINICAL TRIALS

The 1987 Consensus Conference along with federal and investigator initiatives of the last 4 years stimulated an important series of prospective random trials in prostate cancer.[202] Additional initiatives stimulated pilot studies of new modalities such as hypoxic sensitizers in combination with radiation therapy and cytoreduction before radiation or radical surgery. In the absence of a prospective random trial, the variation in natural history associated with different prostate cancers allows one to demonstrate any desired end result by careful case selection.

A prospective randomized clinical trial is difficult to organize, complete, and analyze so that the results will be accepted by treating physicians. A series of reasonable criteria are listed in Table 35–19. Studies exhibiting poor compliance with these criteria are illustrated in Table 35–20, which lists six trials that were widely reported. Table 35–21 lists two RTOG trials

TABLE 35–18. Organ Systems Program Staging Classification (OSS) for Primary Tumor

TA	Digitally unrecognizable neoplasm, proved histologically
TA1	Five percent or less of the total surgical specimen, and of low or medium grade
TA2	Five percent or more of specimen, and/or of high grade
TB	Palpable tumor, not beyond the prostatic capsule
TB1	No more than one half of one lobe
TB2	More than one half of one lobe, but no more than one lobe
TB3	More than one lobe or more than one palpable tumor
TC	Palpable tumor extending beyond the prostatic capsule
TC1	Beyond margin of gland unilaterally
TC2	Beyond margin of gland bilaterally
TC3	Involvement of seminal vesicles, base of bladder and/or rectum and/or levator muscle(s) and/or pelvic side wall(s)

testing the value of elective nodal irradiation by using imaging studies (*e.g.*, CT, LAG) to determine lymph node status, studies that subsequently have been demonstrated to be inaccurate. *The trials could not be expected to prove the point in question favorably or not.*[199] These trials have been cited widely to show that elective nodal irradiation has no value when it is not possible to make *any statement* about the value of nodal irradiation.

Table 35–22 lists clinical trials that were completed in early 1992 but were not analyzed and reported. They illustrate the recent interest in combining radiation treatment with androgen manipulation. Table 35–23 lists prospective random trials under case accession in 1992, limited to national clinical research groups. The Southwest Oncology Group (SWOG) comparison of surgery and radiation was discontinued because of poor patient accrual. The SWOG trial of adjuvant radiation is slow in accessing patients, as is the ECOG study, but renewed investigator interest may salvage these studies.

Johansson and colleagues in Sweden recently completed a trial of androgen deprivation with radiation therapy and are continuing trials comparing radical prostatectomy with observation and comparing radiation therapy with observation.[207] These studies are important because irradiation and radical surgery are destructive procedures that should be used only if needed, and it will be helpful to have clinical trials that demonstrate their primary value. Adjuvant hormone alteration is an equally serious problem because there are physical and psychological objections to eliminating androgens by surgical or chemical suppression. The high cost of using luteinizing hormone-releasing hormone agonists and antiandrogen in large numbers of patients will burden an already troubled

TABLE 35–17. Comparison of the American Urologic Association (AUA) and TNM Classification Systems for Prostate Cancer

	TNM	AUA
Tumor is incidental histologic finding	T1	A
Three or fewer microscopic foci	T1A	A1
More than three microscopic foci	T1B	A2
Tumor is present clinically or grossly and limited to the prostate	T2	B
Tumor <1.5 cm, with normal tissue on at least three sides	T2A	B1
Tumor >1.5 cm or in more than one lobe	T2B	B2
Tumor invades the prostatic apex or into or beyond the prostatic capsule, bladder neck, or seminal vesicle, but is not fixed	T3	C
No invasion of seminal vesicles	T3	C1
Invasion of seminal vesicles	T3	C2
Pelvic wall fixation	T4	C2
Lymph node metastasis	N	D
Distant metastasis	M	D

TABLE 35–19. Clinical Trials in Prostate Cancer: Reasonable Criteria for a Clinical Trial

- Selection of a valid question
- Randomization process eliminating bias
- Accession of adequate numbers of patients
- Appropriate stratification
- Complete case accession in 3–4 years
- Acceptable fraction with major deviations
- Careful quality control
- Data analysis independent of investigators

TABLE 35–20. Clinical Trials in Prostate Cancer not Meeting Reasonable Criteria of Adequacy

Stage	Group	Question	Published Outcome
A1, A2, B	VACURG[365]	Prostatectomy vs placebo	No difference in survival
A1, A2	VACURG[366]	Orchiectomy ± estrogen	No difference in survival
A1, A2	VACURG[366]	Prostatectomy vs hormonal therapy	No difference in survival
A2, B	Uro-Oncology[367]	Prostatectomy vs radiation	Prostatectomy superior
T3, N0	Uro-Oncology[368]	Radiation vs delayed hormone	1. Radiation superior 2. No difference
N+	Uro-Oncology[368]	Radiation vs delayed hormone	Radiation superior

health care financing system, and the value of these agents must be understood clearly. For these reasons, there is a pressing need for further clinical trials in prostate cancer.

INDICATIONS FOR RADIATION TREATMENT AND SPECIAL POINTS

EARLY PROSTATE CANCER

All patients with early (T1, T2A, B unilobar) prostate cancer should participate in two decisions relative to their cancers. The first decision is whether treatment is required or careful observation is sufficient, a decision greatly influenced by tumor volume, histologic differentiation, patient age, and patient comorbidities.[208] Attitudes about the advisability of observation vary greatly between the United States and parts of Europe, but the strongly held opinions on both sides are largely conjectural because there has not been a prospective trial of treatment versus observation in appropriately selected patients. A recent report describes a trial of observation alone,[69] and appropriate clinical trials prospectively randomizing patients between radical prostatectomy and observation and between radiation therapy and observation have been initiated in Sweden.

The second decision in which the patient should participate is the choice of therapy for early cancer, assuming he is medically fit for either. By default, the less healthy and the older patients with poorly differentiated tumors are properly treated with radiation therapy. Data show that when similarly staged

TABLE 35–21. Clinical Trials in Prostate Cancer Studies of Elective Nodal Irradiation in Which Criteria of Nodal Evaluation Are Inaccurate

Stage	Group	Question	Published Result*
A2, B, C	RTOG 7506	Elective nodal irradiation	No value demonstrated
A2, B	RTOG 7706	Elective nodal irradiation	No value demonstrated

* Studies did not prove or disprove value of elective irradiation.

patients are treated with prostatectomy or irradiation and carefully compared at 10-year endpoints, there is no difference in outcome.[209] In addition, there is no basis in fact for the frequently made statements that younger patients should be treated with surgery because they will live longer, that radiation shows late failure, and that the patient sacrifices a survival advantage when he selects radiation treatment.[210] For patients with B1 nodules, a historical comparison of the survival rates found by Elder and colleagues,[211] Gibbons and colleagues,[212] and Bagshaw[213] is interesting but of little help in choosing treatment. Figure 35–7 shows the same 15-year survival for all three series, although they have never been matched with regard to prognostic indicators and similarity of patients; both surgical series were screened carefully for ability to tolerate the surgery. Using these old data to make decisions is unwise, because lymph node status was unknown, the operation performed (perineal prostatectomy) is not a common procedure, the radiation techniques currently are not considered optimal, and the patient's age and the histologic differentiation of cancer in each patient in each series were not known.

In theory, radioactive implant has the potential to be as successful as radical prostatectomy or external-beam irradiation for treatment of some early stages of disease, but data are limited.[214] Late local recurrences associated with technical misapplication of ^{125}I implants and observed after 5 years have discouraged its use.[215–217] Use of implants remains an optional treatment, but one that is perhaps best applied as part of a controlled clinical trial designed to compare their effectiveness with that of external-beam irradiation and radical prostatectomy, which are the existing standards.

If the patient understands that there is an equal chance for cure by radiation or surgery, he must understand the side effects of treatment by these two methods. The presentation of complications of treatment should reflect the results of management of the 1980s rather than that of 15 and 20 years ago, which makes either method of treatment seem inappropriately morbid. To participate intelligently in the decision-making process and to receive objective counseling, the patient should consult with a knowledgeable proponent of both treatments. Finally, the patient may have legitimate concerns about the quality and safety of treatment he will receive in his community compared with that received in a major urologic or radiation oncology center, and he should feel free to discuss

TABLE 35–22. Clinical Trials in Prostate Cancer Recently Completed and Not Yet Reported

Stage	Group	Question	Completed
B2, C (T2B, 3, 4)	RTOG 8610	Preirradiation cytoreduction	Fall 1991
(T1B, T2, N+), T3–4	RTOG 8531	Adjuvant goserelin acetate	Spring 1992

frankly the physician's personal experience and results with the procedure proposed.

A recent 15-year follow-up study indicates the long-term outcome of radiation therapy across the entire United States is good.[96] In contrast, the only published results of radical prostatectomy come from a few centers of surgical excellence, and there is concern as to whether the urologist who performs an occasional radical prostatectomy can do it with the same success and safety as the surgeon who performs the procedure every week.[191,192,218,219] Similarly, there are a limited number of radiation oncology facilities that have access to the most advanced and developmental technology.[205,220–225] Surgeons or radiation oncologists who obtain poor results do not report them, and community practitioners of both specialities usually do not analyze their personal treatment results to help the patient make his decision.

LOCALLY EXTENSIVE PROSTATE CANCER

The need for treatment of locally advanced (T2B bilobar, T3–4) prostate cancer is usually clear and the choice of treatment is limited. There is a long history of published success with thousands of patients treated with external-beam irradiation.[96,191,220–222,96,224–228] New methods of conformal therapy have been developed to provide the opportunity to increase the dose to the prostate, which may further improve local control with appropriate clinical testing. External-beam irradiation is the standard of treatment of extensive local disease. New methods (whether they involve surgery, radiation sensitizers, or interstitial implants) must be compared with external-beam irradiation in formal clinical trials to demonstrate that they are superior.[229] Without structured trials, use of new procedures or technology is experimentation without the patient's real understanding and true informed consent, and the failure of a method may not become evident for 5 to 10 years, as observed with ^{125}I implants.[191,192,215–217,219,230] Worse, the true failure of a new method may not be observed

at all because of patient selection and inadequate long-term follow-up.

THE ROLE OF PELVIC LYMPHADENECTOMY

Knowing the status of the pelvic lymph nodes would be a helpful addition to the radiation management of many patients. A judgment based on tumor volume and histologic differentiation may identify patients whose chances of a positive lymph node dissection are predictably low and in whom the risk of the procedure is not warranted. In other groups of patients, the predicted chance of positive nodes or other spread are so high that it is not worth the risk of a surgical procedure to prove it (see Tables 35–12 and 35–13).

When recommending lymphadenectomy to patients who are candidates for medical treatment, we must remember that lymph node dissection is a less than perfect procedure. If positive nodes are used to assign the patient to a different treatment, then the procedure can be useful. If treatment is the same for positive and negative node patients, nothing has been accomplished. A negative lymph node dissection, however, is only a reasonably accurate assurance that lymph nodes are not involved. Data reported by Fowler and Whitmore show that 12% of all positive node patients or 5% of all patients subjected to lymphadenectomy have positive nodes missed because they are isolated metastases to the external iliac chain and are not included in the modern modified node dissection.[188] Golimbu, who has done the only superextensive dissections, obtained 30 total dissections and showed that isolated nodal metastasis to the external iliac, presciatic and presacral lymph nodes occurred in 5 of 15 node positive patients.[231] The chance of missing an isolated metastasis appears to be at least 12% (Whitmore) and may be as high as 33% (Golimbu) of those that are truly positive.[188,231] This equates to 5% to 17% of all patients submitting to lymph node dissection. The lymph node sampling procedure done by some urologists is inadequate and further increases the rate of error in as-

TABLE 35–23. Randomized Clinical Trials in Prostate Cancer Active in 1992

Stage	Group	Question	Comment
T2B, T3, T4	RTOG 1050	Cytoreduction and irradiation vs cytoreduction, androgen suppression	Beginning Fall, 1992
T3†	SWOG 8794	Adjuvant radiation after prostatectomy	Slow case accrual*
T1B, T2	SWOG 8890	Radical prostatectomy vs external-beam irradiation	Closed
N+	ECOG 3886	Androgen suppression vs observation	Poor case accrual*

* These trials will close if case accession does not improve.
† Pathologic stage.

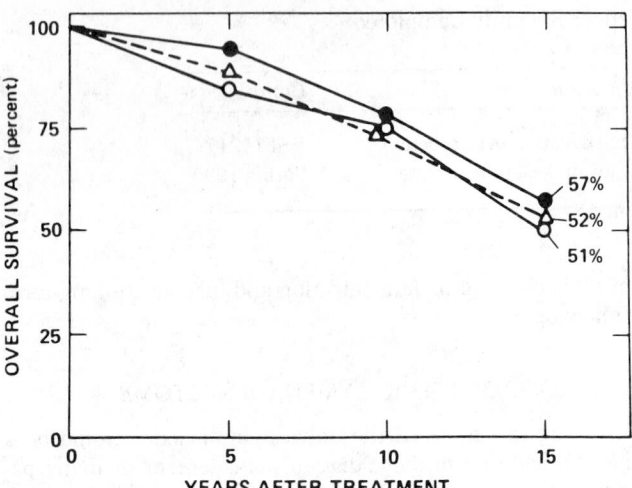

FIGURE 35–7.   Long-term survival of patients with B1 (T2A) prostate cancer treated at Stanford (131 patients) with irradiation (*triangles*), at Johns Hopkins (51 patients) with surgery (*open circles*), and at Virginia Mason Medical Center (195 patients) with surgery (*solid circles*).

sessing lymph node involvement, resulting in incorrect clinical decisions and treatment.

If finding a positive node assigns a patient to a different treatment strategy and the predicted risk for nodal disease is between about 15% as a lower limit and 70% as an upper limit, then lymph node dissection may be useful in otherwise healthy patients. Again, the patient should participate in the decision to perform this procedure and must understand there is no proved benefit from the procedure or knowledge obtained.

The recent interest in replacing the modified lymphadenectomy with a procedure performed through a laparoscope seems likely to decrease further the accuracy of the procedure and can probably be considered only a rough screen except in the most expert hands.[232]

The patient with a positive node proved by lymph node dissection presents a dilemma for subsequent management. If radiation is delivered to the external iliac and common iliac nodes after a lymph node dissection, leg and genital edema increases, and that risk may not be considered warranted.[168] One is then committed to treat patients with positive nodes with a radiation program that excludes likely sites of disease. At Fox Chase Cancer Center, we commonly use local radiation to the prostate in these positive-node patients. The stated goal is to control or minimize subsequent problems with urinary function that develop as the cancer in the prostate grows. There are few data to support this approach, but Tomlinson and colleagues observed major local symptoms, increased hospital stay, increased transfusions, and infections when bulky prostate cancer was treated with hormone therapy only.[233]

EXTERNAL-BEAM IRRADIATION

External-beam irradiation has been the gold standard for the treatment of prostate cancer over the last 30 years.[205] There are several basic technical principles that must be understood.

1. Day-to-day reproducibility of treatment is crucial to the delivery of a homogenous dose to the intended target volume. At Fox Chase Cancer Center, this day-to-day variation is significantly reduced by using a posterior body cast that extends from the middle thighs to the middle thorax, providing rigid day-to-day positioning and immobilization (Fig. 35–8). The cast eliminates variations of more than 7 mm in location of the treatment field, which will occur in 25% of daily setups without the immobilizing cast (Table 35–24).[224] The materials for this cast cost little, add only a few minutes to the simulation procedure, and must be used to position the patient for the treatment planning CT scan.

2. The CT-assisted three-dimensional reconstruction of the prostate and seminal vesicles is a major aid in determining the correct location and contour of the prostate, seminal vesicles, and normal structures.

3. The retrograde urethrogram is the most accurate means of identifying the inferior margin of the prostate, which cannot be accurately identified on the planning CT scan. This simple procedure should be adopted if possible. This triad of rigid immobilization, localization of the prostate by CT, and urethrogram identification of the inferior prostate margin is necessary for the most accurate determination of treatment fields, and treatment planned in this manner for early prostate cancer is associated with reduced morbidity.[200,224,227]

Table 35–25 illustrates two important technical factors in treatment.[96] Multiple fields or moving beam treatment should be used, unless photons over 20 MeV are used. If anteroposterior and posteroanterior fields are used with common photon energies, complications are increased without the justification of improved cancer control. All fields should be treated each day so that some portions of the target volume do not receive less than the prescribed daily dose and so that normal tissues do not receive excessive daily doses. Complications can in-

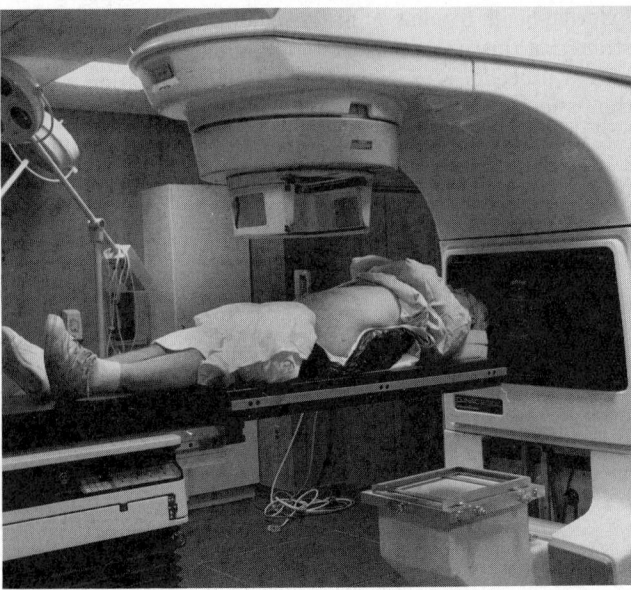

FIGURE 35–8.   Example of posterior half cast used to immobilize patients during treatment. Cast extends from midthigh to midthorax.

TABLE 35–24. Comparison of Portal Films With Patients Casted and Not Casted

	Cast*	No Cast†
Average range daily error (mm)	3.3	8.0
Median daily error (mm)	1	3
Exact agreement with simulation (%)	43	22
Greatest error (mm)		
Superoinferior	6	10
Anteroposterior	6	15
Lateral	7	13

* Total number of observations = 280.
† Total number of observations = 216.
(Modified from Soffen EM, Hanks GE, Hwang CC, Chu JCH. Conformal static field therapy for low-volume, low-grade prostate cancer with rigid immobilization. Int J Radiat Biol Oncol Phys 1991;20:141–146)

crease if one field is treated each day. High-energy photons (≥6 MeV) are associated with an improved local control rate and are recommended for all patients with prostate cancer.[234,235] Radiation dose should be increased with increasing tumor volume.[236,237] Short-term (4-year) local control is not different for T1 and T2 tumors treated with a dose between 6000 and 6999 cGy, but long-term evaluation may show a difference. At 4 years, that local control is improved for bulky stage T3–4 tumors at or above 7000 cGy. The common practice of treating all stages of prostate cancer with the same dosage of radiation is not logical.

Treatment is most accurately planned with rigid immobilization. The diagnostic CT scan commonly obtained before radiation for evaluation of the extent of primary disease and status of nodes *cannot* be used to localize the prostate at the time of treatment planning, because in 25% of patients it will be inaccurate by more than 1 cm.[238] The study is better delayed so that it can be performed as part of the treatment planning procedure.

Figure 35–9 illustrates standard radiation fields in use in the United States and the type of widely used fields that produced all the long-term results. They were not the state of the art in 1992.

CONFORMAL TREATMENT TECHNIQUES

The logical extension of an attempt to identify accurately the location of the prostate in the carefully immobilized patient is to locate the target volume by three-dimensional computer reconstruction of the prostate and seminal vesicles. This is achieved by integrating the results of the treatment planning CT scan with the planning computer. One can then determine a beam configuration for early prostate cancer that conforms precisely to the shape of each individual prostate rather than forcing all prostates to fit into similar size boxes. Examples of anterior and lateral conformal treatment portals used in early prostate cancer are given in Figure 35–10A and B, which illustrate a 1.5-cm margin of normal tissue around the prostate, *a margin that is safe only with the described technology.* Anterior and lateral conformal coned-down fields are used to treat the prostate and seminal vesicles with a margin of 1.5

TABLE 35–25. Complication Rate and Local Recurrence Rate Associated With Radiotherapeutic Techniques

Treatment Fields		Complications
AP and PA fields only		18/373 6.0%
All other techniques		10/320 3.0%
		p = 0.08

Energy Source	n	Local Recurrence Rate
Cobalt	309	20% ⎫
4 MeV	305	18% ⎬ p = 0.01
≥6 MeV	246	10% ⎭

n, number of patients.

to 2.0 cm (see Fig. 35–10C and D). Conformal techniques are associated with about 50% fewer side effects during treatment, and only one serious complication has been observed in more than 100 patients followed for 6 to 30 months.[200,224,227] These technologies should be adopted by most practicing radiation oncologists over the next few years. There is considerable variation in size, shape, and position of the prostate and seminal vesicles (Fig. 35–11).

REAL-TIME PORTAL IMAGES

Real-time portal images are available and have the potential for improving the technical execution of radiation therapy. These devices replace the time and trouble of taking an x-ray portal film by recording a digital portal image during a portion of the actual radiation treatment. The recording is, therefore, a more accurate reflection of what was actually treated and can be checked on a daily basis if necessary. The true usefulness of these imaging devices is realized as the digital image is entered, stored, and reviewed as part of our local area network with personal computers.[239,240]

SPECIAL TYPES OF RADIATIONS

A pilot study of mixed-beam (neutrons and photons) treatment compared with photon treatment of prostate cancer was published by the RTOG.[241] It showed that 93% local control was achieved with mixed-beam irradiation, compared with 78% with photons. That observation encouraged the members of the neutron research group to proceed with a prospective random trial, but problems with the neutron program make it unlikely that this trial will be completed. We probably will not learn whether the biologic advantage of neutrons would prove useful in treating prostate cancer patients. The Massachusetts General Hospital has been conducting a prospective trial of proton-boost irradiation in prostate cancer.[242] The main advantage of using protons is a greater ability to focus the radiation, in what was probably the first conformal treatment program. It has allowed an increase in the local dose to the prostate. This study has not been completed.

INTERSTITIAL RADIATION THERAPY

Over the last 20 years, prostate cancer has been treated with some frequency by three general techniques involving the interstitial placement of sealed isotopes. The oldest and most

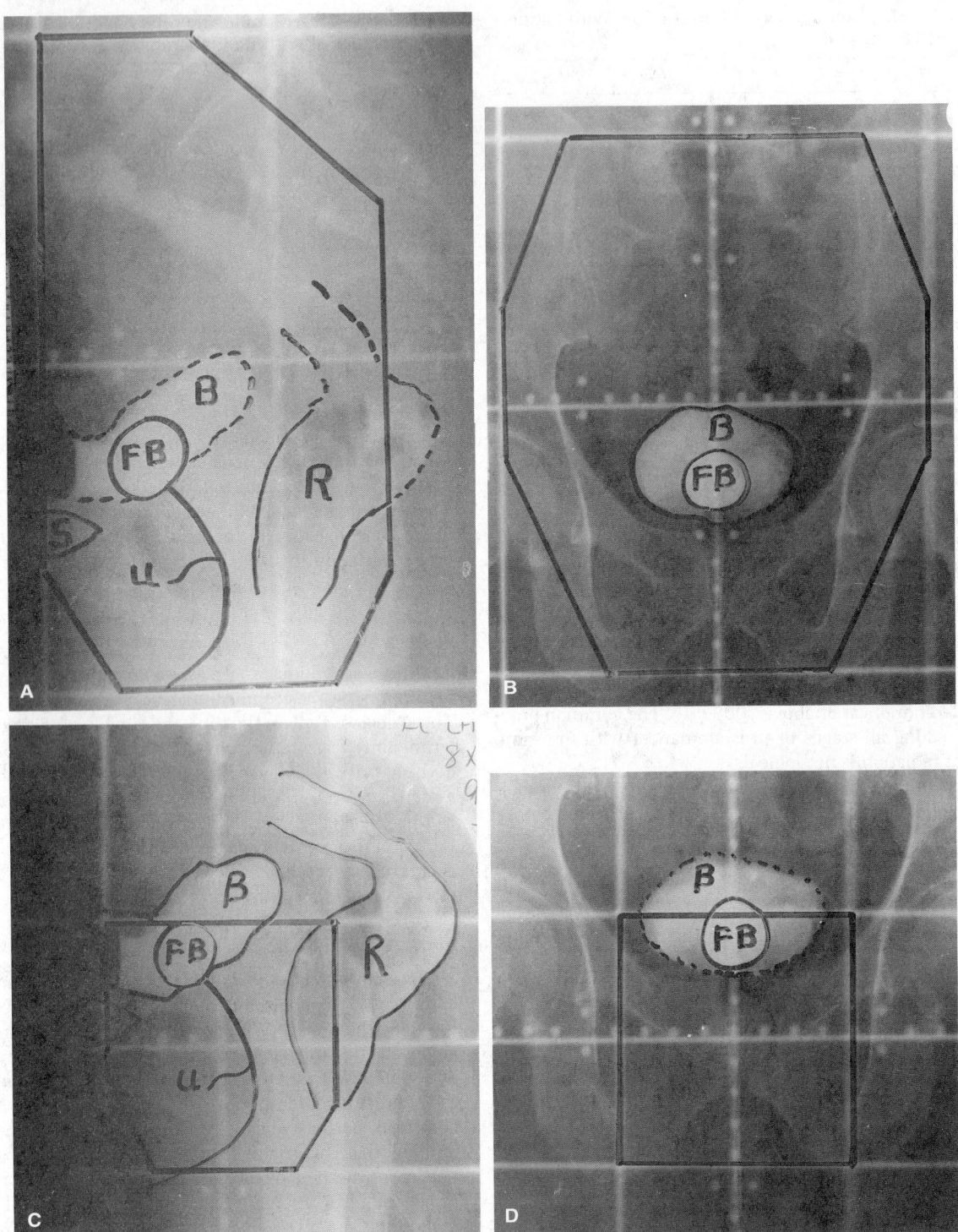

FIGURE 35–9. **(A)** Anteroposterior simulation film with whole pelvis field outlined. **(B)** Lateral simulation film with whole pelvis field outlined. **(C)** Anteroposterior simulation film with prostate boost field outlined. **(D)** Lateral simulation film with prostate boost field outlined.

commonly used method has been the freehand placement at laparotomy of ^{125}I or gold (^{198}Au) seeds. Recently, palladium seeds have been placed by similar techniques.[243–245] The major technical problem of this freehand implant technique is difficulty in obtaining the homogenous distribution of radioactive materials throughout the target volume necessary to obtain a homogenous radiation dose.

A second technique involves positioning of hollow needles in the tumor with guidance through a perforated template designed to encompass the prostate. The needles or catheters are subsequently loaded with radioactive materials to provide the interstitial radiation. Following the guide provided by the template directs the sources to an improved distribution of radiation throughout the target volume. This technique usually

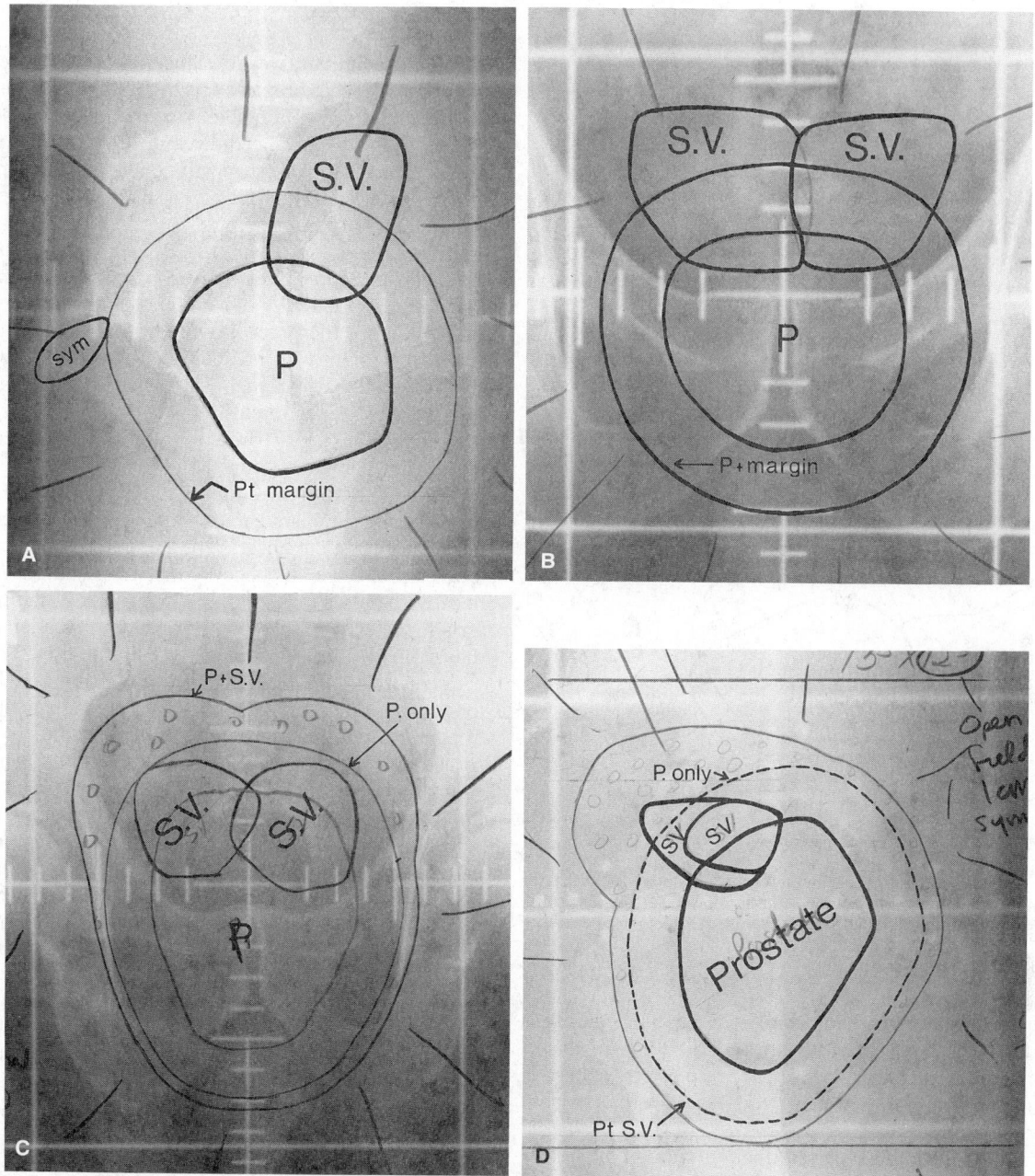

FIGURE 35–10. Examples of treatment volumes with beam's eye view after CT-assisted reconstruction of the prostate. The urethrogram was used in all patients. **(A)** Anteroposterior conformal field at simulation with 1.5 cm margin around the prostate. **(B)** Lateral conformal field at simulation with 1.5 cm margin. **(C)** Anteroposterior conformal field including prostate and seminal vesicles. **(D)** Lateral conformal field including prostate and seminal vesicles.

uses iridium, frequently is combined with external-beam irradiation, and the sources remain in place in the tumor for 3 to 7 days.

The third and most recent technique uses TRUS to direct the freehand placement of ^{125}I or palladium seeds in the prostate. Again, the goal is to improve the distribution of dose.

FREEHAND TECHNIQUES

The technique of freehand ^{125}I seed implants has been shown by Kuban and colleagues[215] and by Fuks and colleagues[216] to be associated with an increase in local failures, particularly

during the second 5-year interval after treatment. In Kuban's experience, 43% of all failures appeared after 5 years of follow-up. Local failure was associated with an 83% rate of subsequent development of metastasis compared with an 18% rate of metastasis in patients in whom local control was achieved by the implant, strongly suggesting the importance of achieving local control. Fuks reported that 328 of 679 patients (48%) treated with ^{125}I developed local failure with grades II and III histology and that B2 and B3 stage tumors all exceeded 50% local failure rates, confirming the association of local failure with an increase in distant metastasis. In the group of patients in whom local failure was achieved with the

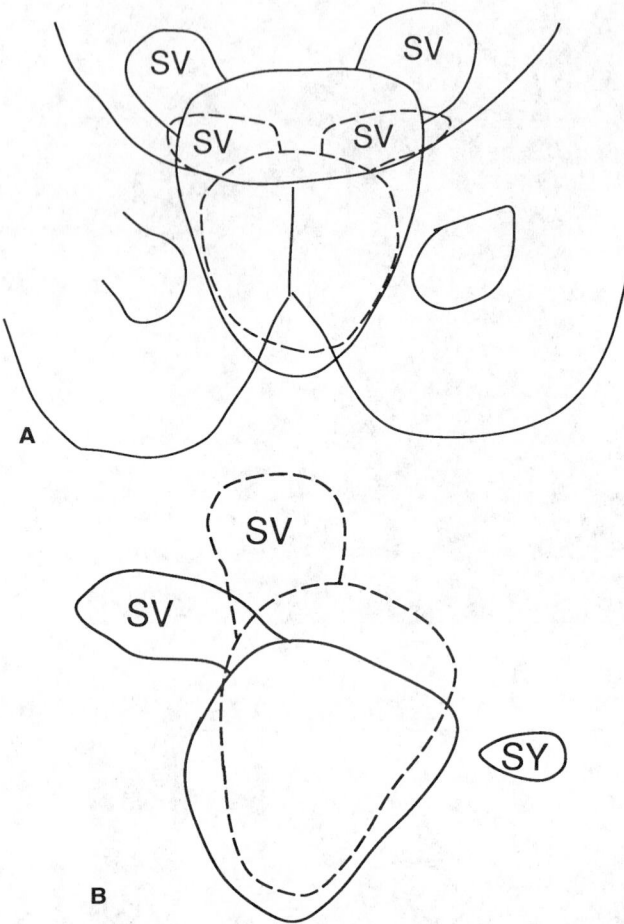

FIGURE 35–11. Composite diagram of the location of the prostate and seminal vesicles in 3 patients selected to show observed variations that warrant conformal field shaping.

^{125}I implant, the tumors were small volume and well differentiated in both series. In patients with larger, intermediate, and poorly differentiated cancers, better results were achieved in Kuban's institution when they were treated with external-beam irradiation.

Carlton and Scardino reported the treatment of all stages of prostate cancer with lymphadenectomy, gold grain insertion, and supplemental external-beam irradiation.[244] Fifteen-year survival for stages A and B was 28% and for stage C 17%. They reported that more than 55% of patients were free of local recurrence at 10 years. Koprowski and colleagues reported the results of treating 101 patients with ^{125}I and compared them with results in 175 treated with external-beam irradiation.[217] These two groups were selected for analysis from 983 patients. Survival at 5 years was similar for the two groups, but survival with no evidence of disease differed markedly, from 80% for external-beam irradiation to 55% for implant treatment. By 9 years, the implant group showed less than 20% survival with no evidence of disease. Clinical local failure was equally dramatic: at 5 years, 95% of patients treated with external-beam irradiation and 62% of patients treated with implants were free of local recurrence. The freehand technology used in these studies has been replaced by methods that allow more accurate distribution of sources.

TEMPLATE TECHNIQUES

Template techniques were designed to provide more accurate placement of seeds or linear sources within the target volume, and this method is often combined with external-beam irradiation in locally advanced disease. There are no published 10-year results to compare with results of radical prostatectomy or external-beam irradiation, so results of these methods must remain preliminary.

In the largest series reported, 8- and 9-year results of operative, temporary, interstitial iridium implants in 200 patients are described.[214,246] Lymph node dissections were performed before the procedure, and 3000 to 3500 cGy were given by implant with no additional radiation or with 3000 cGy of additional external-beam irradiation, depending on stage, given by small fields (7 × 7 or 8 × 8). Survival was more than 85% at 9 years for well-differentiated and moderately differentiated tumors. However, survival fell steeply for poorly differentiated tumors to about 35% at 7 years, illustrating that implants are of limited value in less well-differentiated prostate cancers. The authors do not report clinical local control or the frequency of metastasis, but they do report negative biopsies in 61 of 74 patients without stating the criteria for selection for biopsy. Serious complications (not further defined) were substantial, 11% in the first 100 patients but reduced to 4% with changes in treatment technique in the second 100 patients. About 25% of potent patients became impotent after treatment. This favorable outcome was observed in a highly selected group of patients. There was no comparison with standard methods of management, and some important details are not included in the report.

Brindel and colleagues reported results of treatment of 51 patients with stages B2 or C prostate cancer treated with lymphadenectomy, prostate implant, and external-beam irradiation.[247] Five-year actuarial disease-free survival is reported as 89%, with a 20% incidence of serious rectal problems.

The template interstitial treatment method awaits further developmental use, critical reporting, and direct long-term comparison with standard treatment results in comparable patients. Complicated template technology is proceeding at Memorial Sloan-Kettering Cancer Center, and the template is described as the Wallner Interstitial prostate implanter.[248] This device allows integration of computed tomography for source distribution planning and TRUS for confirmation of needle placement through a specially drilled perineal implant guide essentially fixed to the patient. Short-term results are available in 20 patients.

TRANSRECTAL ULTRASOUND-AIDED IMPLANT

Implant methods using ultrasound-guided seed positioning have been developed to the greatest extent by Blasko and associates in the Northwest United States.[248a] They are accumulating treatment data from several regional institutions that are treating early disease with interstitial implants alone and more advanced and less well-differentiated tumors with a combination of implant and external-beam irradiation. More than 500 patients have been treated in 5 years, and the first 5-year data should be available soon. Again, there is no comparison with results with standard management.

IMPLANTS AND RADICAL PROSTATECTOMY

Kwon and colleagues have followed lymphadenectomy and radical prostatectomy with the insertion of gold seeds into the surrounding undissected tissues.[245] The results presented are not different from those recently reported with radical prostatectomy alone except that there is a 15% complication rate that seems unacceptably high. The report does not present convincing support for this procedure.

SUMMARY

Local implants with even distributions of adequate doses through the entire target volume should be an effective treatment of early differentiated prostate cancer. These techniques fail when applied to tumors of larger volume and poorer differentiation or when distributions are not homogenous, but this failure may not be observed for many years.

Various implants should be suitable for providing an alternate form of boost to increase the local dose and thereby improving local control of large-volume prostate cancers if used in combination with external-beam irradiation. However, because of co-morbidities, many patients with locally advanced prostate cancer that requires treatment are not candidates for the more invasive techniques represented by interstitial radiation. Few radiation oncologists have mastered the technology needed to use the various interstitial treatments, and these treatments are not available to all patients.

RESULTS OF EXTERNAL-BEAM IRRADIATION

It is difficult to compare the results of surgery and radiation in early prostate cancer because of differences in the patients and their cancers that are treated by the two methods (see Table 35–26).[191,192,209] The main categories of difference are as follows:

Age. Surgical patients are younger, with mean ages ranging from less than 60 to 64 years, whereas in radiation series, ages range from 65 to more than 70 years.

General Health. Surgical patients are selected for better health, with fewer significant comorbidities and less likelihood of dying from intercurrent disease.

Size of Cancer Within Stage. Surgical patients are appropriately selected for tumors of small size, reaching 72% B1 (1.5 cm) and 17% B2 tumors in Walsh's experience compared with a reversal of those percentages in radiation series (Table 35–26). The results of equally effective treatment of T2 (B) cancers in the three series noted in Table 35–26 would not be expected to

produce equal results because of differences in cancer volume within the one stage.

Differentiation. Surgical series are appropriately selected for well-differentiated and intermediately differentiated tumors, whereas radiation series do not exclude poorly differentiated tumors with their worse prognosis.

Nodal Status. Modern surgical patients have pathologically proved negative nodes and improved outcome, whereas most patients in radiation series have unknown nodal status and about 40% of patients have positive nodes (25% in T1A–2 group).[6] An understanding of these difficulties makes it possible to examine the success of radiation in a limited number of patients of known nodal status and to attempt to compare results with surgical series, despite differences in patient and tumor status (*e.g.,* patients in the radiation series are older and have larger and less well-differentiated tumors).

UNITED STATES NATIONAL AVERAGES
(UNKNOWN NODAL STATUS)

The favorable long-term results of radiation in the treatment of prostate cancer in the United States are well illustrated by the results reported in the Patterns of Care National Surveys describing the results of treatment delivered in 1973, 1978, and 1983.[96,202,229] Figure 35–12 illustrates by stage the survival to 15 years for patients treated in 1973, and Figure 35–13 shows similar results to 10 years for the series of patients treated in 1978. Figure 35–14 shows the 5-year results of treatment given in 1983.[238] The expected survival of age-matched controls is also shown. In these two large series at 10 years, 63% and 57% of stage A, 47% and 45% of stage B, and 33% and 35% of stage C patients are alive. At 15 years, the survival rates are 40% for stage A, 25% for stage B, and 23% for stage C. Table 35–27 includes tabular results, with the added endpoints of free of any failure and free of clinical local recurrence. Two thirds of stage A patients, and one third of stage B and C patients are free of any failure at 15 years, whereas at 10 years 70% to 80% of stage A, 40% to 50% of stage B, and 30% to 40% of stage C patients are free of any failure. These data are true United States national averages, and there are no comparable data for patients treated with surgery.[235,249]

SELECTED SINGLE INSTITUTIONS
(UNKNOWN NODAL STATUS)

Table 35–27 includes selected long-term data by stage from Stanford,[220] Washington University,[222] and the M.D. Anderson Cancer Center[223,250] as examples of single-institution centers of excellence. The tabular results of the Patterns of Care survey are also listed. These single-institution data are accu-

TABLE 35–26. Tumor and Patient Characteristics for Contemporary Series of Prostate Cancer Patients

				Stage				
Investigations	*No. of Patients*	*Mean Age (y)*	*Older Than 70 Years*	*T1A (A1)*	*T1B (A2)*	*T2A (B1)*	*T2B (B2)*	*D0*
Hanks et al.[209]	104	67	32%	0%	15%	24%	61%	0%
Catalona and Bigg[369]	250	64	11%	5%	16%	33%	45%	0%
Walsh[192]	206	<60	3%	2%	8%	72%	17%	1%

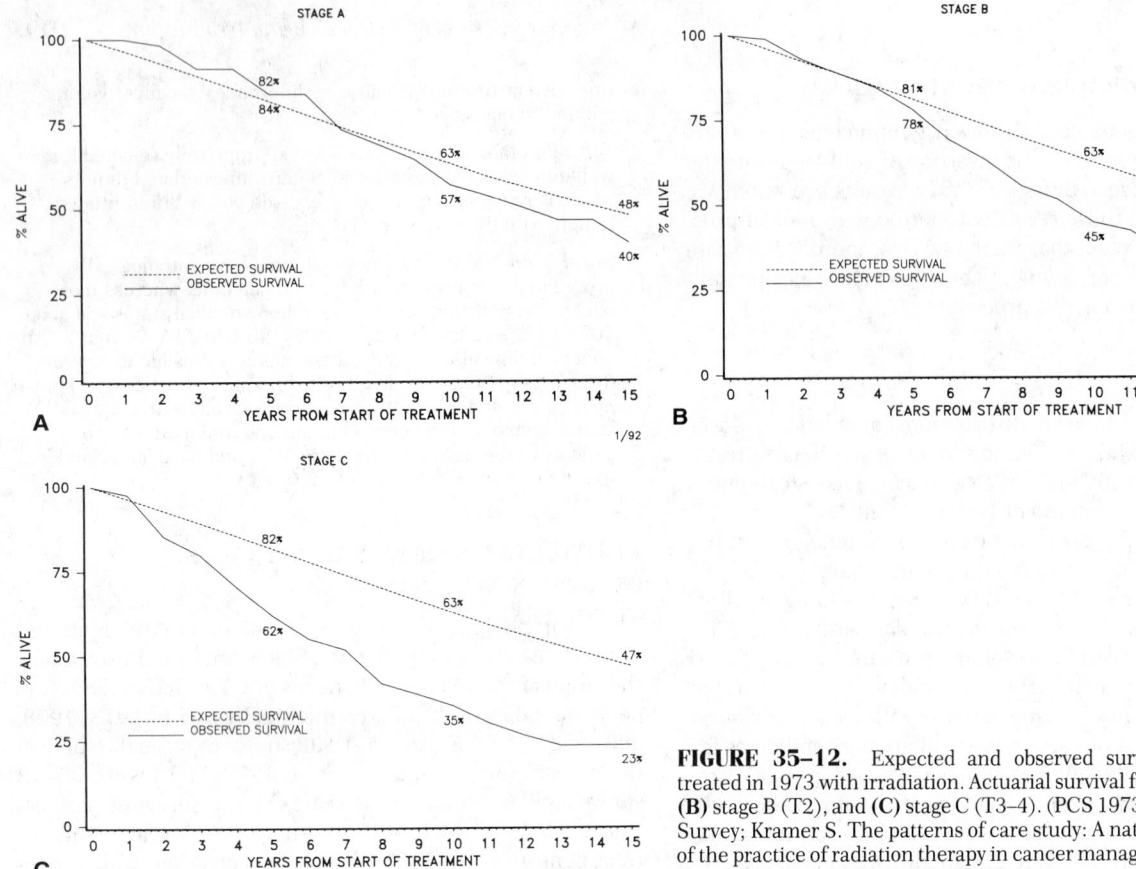

FIGURE 35–12. Expected and observed survivals for patients treated in 1973 with irradiation. Actuarial survival for **(A)** stage A (T1), **(B)** stage B (T2), and **(C)** stage C (T3–4). (PCS 1973 Prostate Outcome Survey; Kramer S. The patterns of care study: A nationwide evaluation of the practice of radiation therapy in cancer management. Int J Radiat Oncol Biol Phys 1976;1:1231–1236)

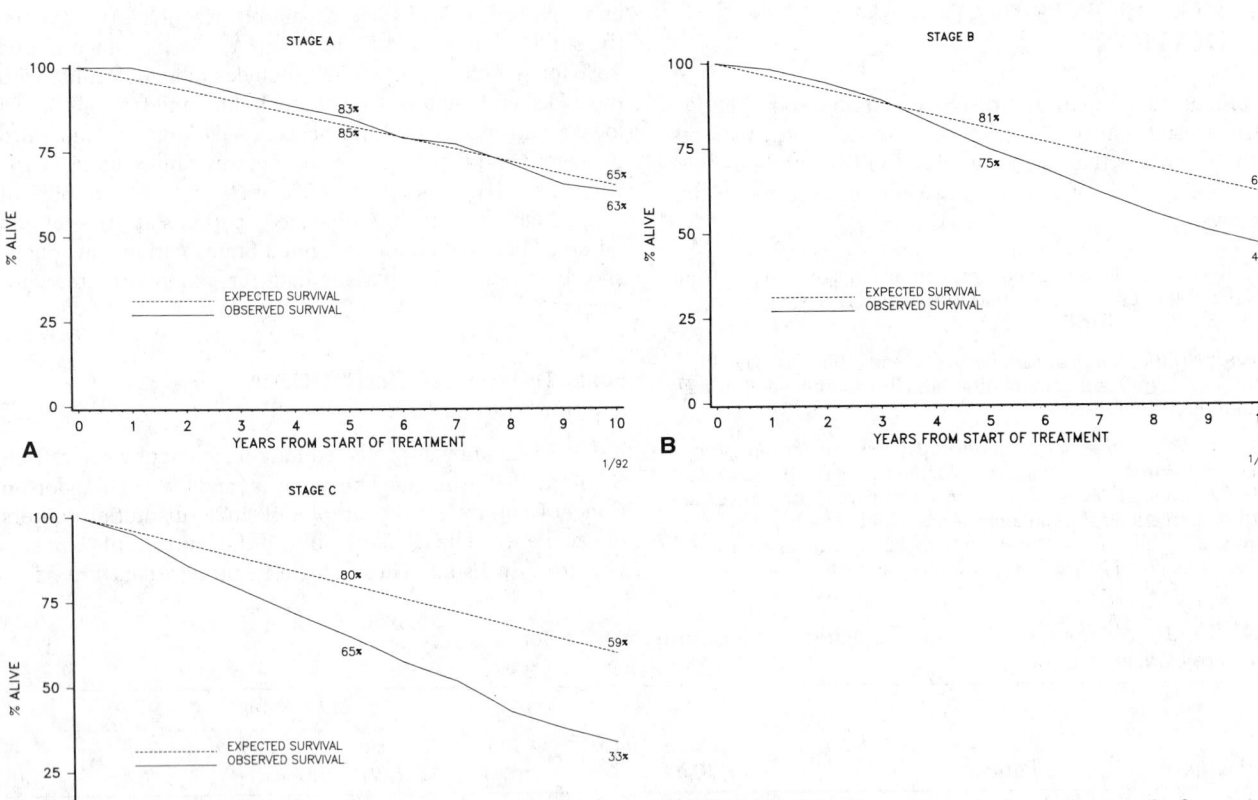

FIGURE 35–13. Expected and observed survivals for patients treated in 1978 with irradiation. Actuarial survival for **(A)** stage A (T1), **(B)** stage B (T2), and **(C)** stage C (T3–4). (PCS 1978 Prostate Outcome Survey; Hanks GE. External beam radiation for prostate cancer: Patterns of Care studies in the United States. NCI Monogr 1988;7:85–94)

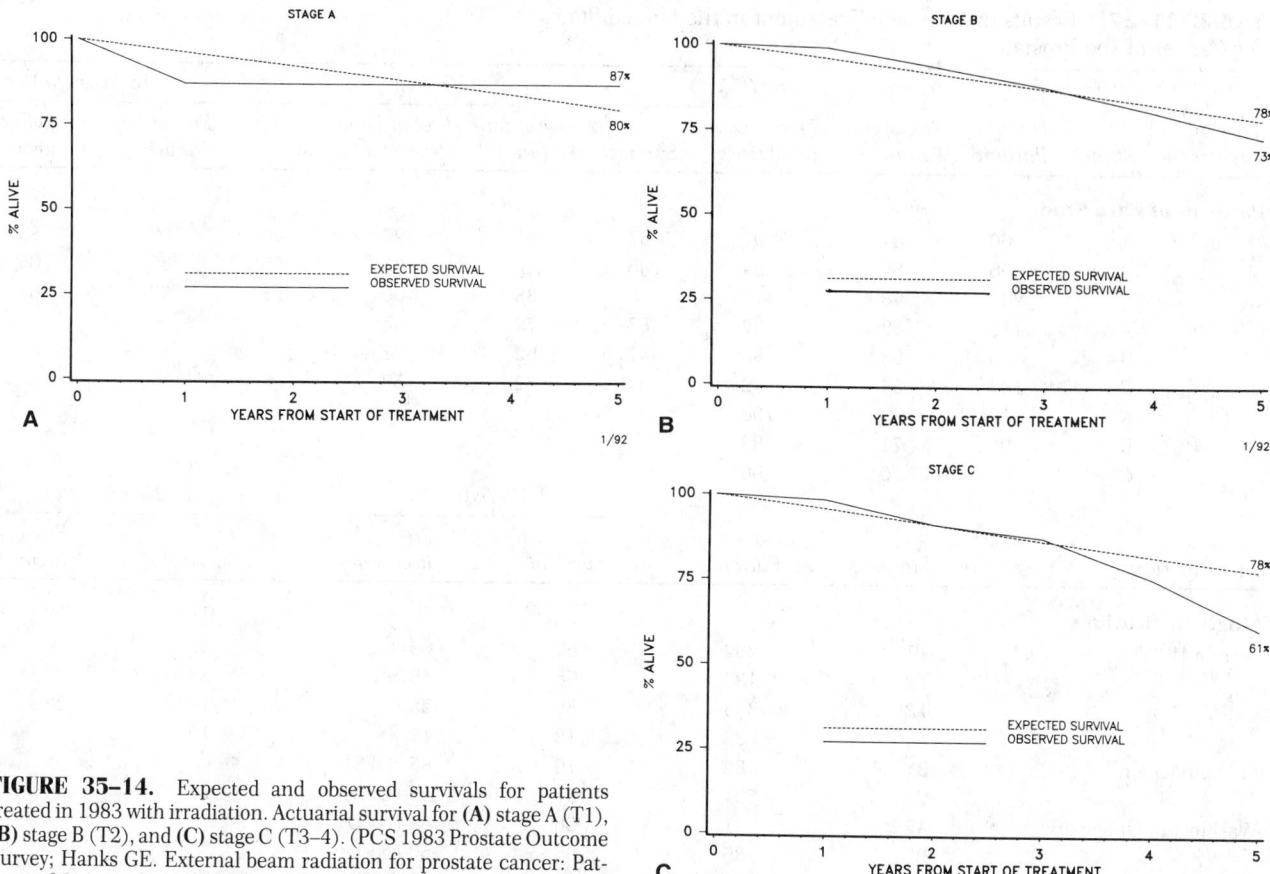

FIGURE 35–14. Expected and observed survivals for patients treated in 1983 with irradiation. Actuarial survival for **(A)** stage A (T1), **(B)** stage B (T2), and **(C)** stage C (T3–4). (PCS 1983 Prostate Outcome Survey; Hanks GE. External beam radiation for prostate cancer: Patterns of Care studies in the United States. NCI Monogr 1988;7:85–94)

mulated over a long time and are susceptible to stage migration and time-based changes in adjuvant treatment policies.[96] The results are not greatly different from the United States national average, indicating that excellent outcome is available throughout the United States. In thousands of cases treated over the last 20 years and treated for all extents and degrees of differentiation of prostate cancer, the 10- and 15-year outcome is excellent.

RESULTS OF THE EXTERNAL-BEAM IRRADIATION TREATMENT OF SURGICAL CANDIDATES: LYMPH NODE DISSECTION NEGATIVE STAGES A2 AND B (T1B–2)

There are three reports describing 10-year results of radiation treatment of clinical stage A2 and B patients who have had a negative lymph node dissection.[209,220] These reports offer the best basis for comparison with the results of radical prostatectomy, even though the patients treated with radiation were not always similar. Figure 35–15 shows rates of survival, freedom from local recurrence, and freedom from cancer death for the 104 patients from the RTOG prostate trial. This trial included studies of elective nodal irradiation, and patients were subjected to lymph node dissection to establish nodal status before irradiation. The study benefited from the rigid quality control of the RTOG group, and survival at 10 years exceeded the expected survival; 85% of patients were free of clinical local recurrence and only 15% of patients died from cancer.

Table 35–28 lists important 10-year endpoints of the RTOG series, the Stanford series, and the Patterns of Care series. All three series show the same excellent outcome, with 6% to 15% cancer deaths and 85% local control for these early patients with disease treated with irradiation.

In two recent surgical reports of 10-year data with radical prostatectomy, none of the endpoints are different from those obtained with radiation, and the difference observed in overall survival is due to patient age selection (Table 35–29). The 10-year results of Middleton and colleagues[219] and of Paulson and colleagues[230] for radical prostatectomy are identical to the results of Hanks' and colleagues'[209] analysis of RTOG data for radiation and similar to Bagshaw's Stanford series[220] and Hanks' Patterns of Care series (see Table 35–28). Five-year results are preliminary at best, but they are included to show the first report of the nerve-sparing radical prostatectomy[251] and the anomaly of the Uro-Oncology trial reported by Paulson (Table 35–30). In this trial, no local recurrences were reported after surgery or irradiation, and 41% of radiation-treated patients developed metastasis in 5 years. Survival, cause-specific survival, and complications are not reported, and further problems of this study are discussed elsewhere.[252] Walsh makes the important observation of elevated PSA levels in 11% without clinical signs of recurrence, and the other authors do not report PSA data.[251]

SUMMARY

The available 10-year follow-up in roughly similar patients with T1B–2 prostate cancers treated with modern methods

TABLE 35–27. Results of Radiation Treatment in the United States for Cancer of the Prostate

Year of Treatment	Stage*	No. of Patients	5-Year (%)			10-Year (%)			15-Year (%)	
			Free of Any Failure	Free of Local Recurrence	Survival	Free of Any Failure	Free of Local Recurrence	Survival	Free of Any Failure	Free of Local Recurrence
Patterns of Care Study										
1973	A	60	84	97	57	81	97	40	64	83
	B	306	66	94	45	42	71	25	35	65
	C	287	48	73	35	38	66	23	33	61
1978	A	116	82	92	63	72	85			
	B	415	63	80	47	52	71			
	C	197	54	72	33	32	58			
1983	A	16	92	100						
	B	96	71	88						
	C	61	70	90						

Investigations	Stage	No. of Patients	10-Year (%)		15-Year (%)	
			Survival	Free of Recurrence	Survival	Free of Recurrence
Single Institutions						
Stanford† [78]	T1	282	60	63	35	50
	T2	183	55	45	33	37
	T3	348	35	28	18	23
	T4	32	12	17	10	
M.D. Anderson [223,250]	B	82	70	85 (DFS)		
	C	551	57	45 (DFS)	27	40 (DFS)
Washington University [222]	A2	41	66	68 (NED)		
	B	185	55	50 (NED)		
	C	328	35	32 (NED)		

DFS, disease-free survival; NED, no evidence of disease.
* See Table 35–17 for stage definitions.
† Stanford staging system.

shows that the results of radical prostatectomy and external-beam irradiation therapy are similar. Patients should have the opportunity to choose between the available effective modalities through informed consent.

The 10- and 15-year results of treatment of stage B and C disease show that many 10-year and most 15-year survivors after radiation are without evidence of cancer and are presumed cured. No other treatment has demonstrated long-term benefit in patients with these extensive cancers. Problems needing clinical solutions are evident. The fact that local failure occurs in 30% to 50% of patients with bulky disease and metastasis develops in 30% to 50% of patients illustrates a need for more effective local treatment and more effective screening for metastasis.

COMPLICATIONS OF TREATMENT

The undesirable side effects or sequelae of treatment are a necessary by-product of aggressive treatment focusing on the goal of eliminating the cancer. Advances in knowledge of the disease process and the technology of treatment have given us the opportunity to reduce morbidity at current radiation dose and local control rates and to attempt to increase dose and related local control without increasing undesired side effects.[200,224,225,227,253-255] Patients at increased risk for major complications after treatment include patients with multiple transurethral resections or recurring bladder infections or stones, patients with collagen, vascular, or autoimmune diseases such as lupus, and patients with ulcerative colitis, regional enteritis, or multiple prior abdominal surgical procedures. These individuals should be aware of their increased risk for morbidity and usually should receive high-dose radiation only if there are no equally effective alternatives and if they fully understand the potential sequelae.

The method of reporting complication rates influences the numeric value. If these are expressed as absolute percentages, they are always lower than if expressed as actuarial values for any treatment method.

GENERAL COMMENTS

There is more variability in technique, dose, and equipment across the United States than is observed in a single institution.[256,257] The report of Patterns of Care does not reflect side effects of the most aggressive or of the least aggressive treat-

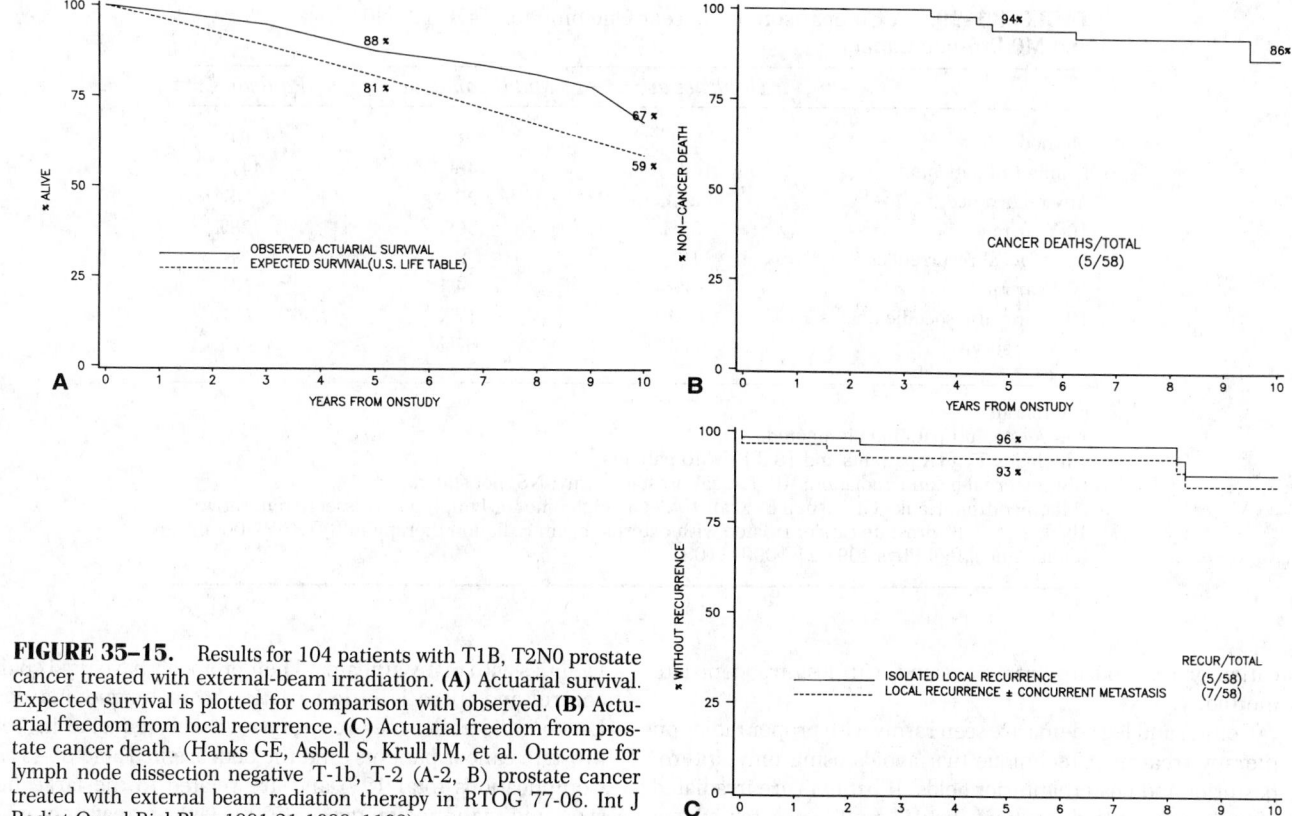

FIGURE 35–15. Results for 104 patients with T1B, T2N0 prostate cancer treated with external-beam irradiation. **(A)** Actuarial survival. Expected survival is plotted for comparison with observed. **(B)** Actuarial freedom from local recurrence. **(C)** Actuarial freedom from prostate cancer death. (Hanks GE, Asbell S, Krull JM, et al. Outcome for lymph node dissection negative T-1b, T-2 (A-2, B) prostate cancer treated with external beam radiation therapy in RTOG 77-06. Int J Radiat Oncol Biol Phys 1991;21:1099–1103)

ment, but an average, and it describes results for treatment given 18 years, 13 years, and 8 years ago, respectively.[236] It shows that, as was previously known, serious side effects appear most commonly between 6 and 30 months after treatment and sporadically thereafter and that they may decrease over time.[220] Appropriate management of these patients can usually preclude the need for hospitalization for treatment and surgery for resolution. Mortality from radiation complications is rare and less frequent than surgical mortality. Our experience is similar to observations reported in the Patterns of Care Study. We have observed 1 death due to complications in 1633 patients surveyed.[229]

The most common gastrointestinal side effect is rectal bleeding due to ulceration on the anterior rectal wall, where the full dose unavoidably is received. This ulceration usually can be treated successfully with enemas containing steroids

or by laser fulguration. In rare cases, a diverting colostomy is necessary to allow time and rest for healing. Small bowel injury is rare, may present as partial bowel obstruction, and usually responds to conservative treatment. In some cases, the affected segment must be resected to resolve symptoms.

Severe bladder symptoms are more common than severe gastrointestinal symptoms and are aggravated by the presence of increased risk factors. Careful management of infection and symptomatic management of frequency and dysuria help during treatment. Attention to dose, field size, and volume of bladder irradiated reduces symptoms. One of the more common bladder complications requires transurethral surgery for relief of stenosis after radiation, and this need for transurethral surgery is considered a major complication. Careful immobilization, CT-assisted treatment planning, and conformal fields are associated with fewer side effects requiring medi-

TABLE 35–28. Stage A2 and B Lymph Node Dissection Negative

Investigations	No. of Patients	10-Year Survival (%)	10-Year Free of Local Recurrence (%)	Cancer Death (%)
Hanks et al[209]	104	63	85	15
Bagshaw[220]	51	78	?	14
Hanks*	37	63	87	6

* Hanks GE. Unpublished data, January 1992.

TABLE 35–29.   A Comparison of 10-Year Outcome for T1B, T2, N0, and M0 Prostate Cancer

	Hanks et al[209] *	Middleton et al[219]†	Paulson[230] *‡
Method	EBI	RP	RP
Number of patients	104	46	441
Any recurrence	24	23	NS
10-Year rate	33%	50%	28%
No. of local recurrences	10	2	NS
10-Year rate	14%	4%	NS
10-Year cause-specific deaths	14%	17%	NS
10-Year survival	63%	67%	88%

* Actuarial.
† Absolute, lost patients eliminated.
‡ Includes 27 T1A patients and 18 T12NM0 patients.
EBI, external-beam irradiation; RP, radical prostatectomy; NS, not stated.
(Modified from Hanks GE, Asbell S, Krall JM, et al. Outcome for lymph node dissection negative T-1b, T-2 (A-2, B) prostate cancer treated with external beam radiation therapy in RTOG 77-06. Int J Radiat Oncol Biol Phys 1991;21:1099–1103)

cation or rests during treatment and with less frequent late morbidity.

Genital and leg edema are seen rarely with proper radiation therapy treatment technique that avoids using only anteroposterior and posteroanterior fields. If patients are irradiated after lymph node dissection, the 1% to 2% risk for edema may increase to 10% when the whole pelvis is treated.[168] That frequency of sequelae usually is not warranted if lymph nodes are positive, nor is the whole pelvis treatment indicated if nodes are negative.

SELECTED RESULTS

Data on complications have been drawn from three sources. The RTOG is a nationwide consortium of about 20 committed facilities with many affiliates. Their protocols have rigid quality control and there is little variation in technique and dose. Lawton and colleagues recently reviewed sequelae in 1020 prostate cancer patients, and the data are in Table 35–31.[254] Complications total 12% and are related to the large field sizes and high median doses (7000 cGy) of treatment given in the late 1970s. A dose of more than 7000 cGy was the only significant factor in a multivariate analysis. There were only 2 deaths, and only 1.8% of patients required surgery beyond cystoscopy.

Sequelae observed in the Patterns of Care surveys are presented in Table 35–31. In three surveys of a total of 1633 patients, the average number of serious complications was 4.3%.[238] These are true national averages. Radiation dose was lower than in the RTOG studies and more broadly spread,

TABLE 35–30.   Patterns of Failure After Radiation or Surgery for T1B, T2, N0, and M0 Prostate Cancer (5-Year Results)

	Hanks et al[209] *	Middleton[219] †	Paulson[230] *		Walsh[251]
Method	XRT	RP	XRT	RP	RP
Number	104	153	56	45	586
Any recurrence	24	14	17	4	40
5-Year rate	15%	10%	41%	14%	11%
Local recurrence	10	9	0	0	11
5-Year rate	4%	7%	0%	0%	4%
Cause-specific mortality	4%	3%	NS		3%
Survival	87%	94%†	NS		93%
Isolated PSA elevation	NS	NS	NS		10%
5-Year rate	NS	NS	NS		NS

* Actuarial analysis.
† Absolute with lost patients eliminated 17/153.
NS, not stated; RP, radical prostatectomy; XRT, radiation therapy.
(Modified from Hanks GE, Asbell S, Krall JM, et al. Outcome for lymph node dissection negative T-1b, T-2 (A-2, B) prostate cancer treated with external beam radiation therapy in RTOG 77-06. Int J Radiat Oncol Biol Phys 1991;21:1099–1103)

TABLE 35–31.   Complications of External-Beam Irradiation

| No. of Patients | RTOG* | | | |
	GI†	GU	Other	Total‡
1020	3.3%	7.7%	1.6%	12.6%

Patterns of Care[205]§

Year RX Administered	No. of Patients	No. of Deaths	No. Requiring Surgery¶	No. Hospitalized	Total No.	Percentage
1973	682	0‖	12	8	20	3
1978	769	0	18	28	46	6
1983	182	0	3	1	4	2
	1633				70	4.3

Fox Chase Cancer Center[206,229]#

Year RX Administered	No. of Patients	GI	GU	Other	No. of Deaths	Total	Percentage
1985–1989	177	1**	2††	0	0	3	1.7

GI, gastrointestinal; GU, genitourinary; RX, radiation therapy.
* Grades III, IV, and V RTOG Scale. Seven-year follow-up of large fields. Median dosage to pelvis was 5400 cGy, and median dosage to prostate was 7000 cGy.
† Includes two deaths.
‡ Only 1.8% required surgery other than cytoscopy.
§ Grades III, IV, and V PCS Scale. Five-year follow-up of variable fields. Median dosage to prostate was 6600 cGy.
‖ One death after 5 years.
¶ Includes transurethral resection.
# Small fields 35%; large fields 65%. Median dosage to prostate was more than 7000 cGy (6600–7500 cGy).
** Transfusion for rectal bleeding.
†† Hemorrhagic cystitis and urethral stricture.

and the field sizes were smaller. There was only 1 death in 1633 patients that was related to complications.

Bagshaw and colleagues have reported a decrease in sequelae with adjustments in dose and technique.[220] Data from Fox Chase Cancer Center[209] are included to represent sequelae observed in a carefully managed individual practice. The principles of immobilization and three-dimensional planning for conformal therapy have been in use since 1989, and careful field shaping has allowed the delivery of median doses above 7000 cGy with less than 2% serious morbidity. Our studies of conformal treatment show side effects during treatment that we believe are reflected in decreased long-term morbidity.[224,227] The patient who is eligible for both treatments must understand the complications of radiation therapy and surgery when considering which treatment he desires.[257]

POSTRADIATION BIOPSIES

Over the last 15 years, interest has increased in evaluating the postirradiation prostate by biopsy. The goal has been to understand better prostate cancer and its response to radiation rather than to provide a specific diagnosis that leads to an effective intervention. Some of these reports of biopsy results

have not included correlation with subsequent clinical course and therefore have been incomplete. All the reported studies have sampled only a fraction of the total number of patients treated, so that case selection and the absence of a complete denominator are a concern in interpreting results of the biopsy.

The initial report of Sewall and colleagues[258] demonstrating that 87% of 15 irradiated patients were positive after radiation therapy was followed by Cox's and Staffel's[259] report demonstrating that a decreasing fraction of positive biopsies are obtained as the time after treatment increases to 18 months or 2 years.[258,259] The implication was that this slow-growing tumor regressed slowly and that biopsy data within 18 to 24 months of treatment were unreliable in reflecting the true result of treatment. It is generally believed that the results of biopsies obtained before 18 months may be unreliable and should be avoided.

BIOPSIES AFTER INTERSTITIAL AND EXTERNAL-BEAM IRRADIATION

Scardino performed biopsies in 124 of 803 patients treated at Baylor with lymph node dissection, radioactive gold seed implantation, and external-beam irradiation.[260] The patients were followed a mean of 64 months after treatment biopsy without therapy. Forty-three patients had a positive biopsy ranging from 22% for B1 nodules to 50% for C1 lesions. Clinical local recurrences developed within 5 years in 58% of patients with positive biopsies and within 10 years in 82% of patients with positive biopsies. In patients with negative biopsies, there was local recurrence in 18% by 5 years and in 32% by 10 years. When the biopsy was abnormal, it was positive 71% of the time. This study suggests an extremely slow progression of the appearance of clinical disease after a positive biopsy, with 42% not progressing within 5 years. The question has been raised about whether this method of treatment would have been expected to result in optimal local control because of dose inhomogeneity throughout the prostate with a limited implant volume. As with all sampling studies, one wonders how the 123 were selected from the 803 and whether the same result would be observed in the other 580 patients.

Schellhammer and colleagues reported the results of biopsies obtained more than 18 months after treatment by ^{125}I implant or external-beam irradiation.[261] No difference in percent of positive biopsies was observed between the two treatment groups, with positive biopsies in 25% of 71 patients treated with ^{125}I (35%) and 16 of 55 treated with external-beam irradiation (29%). Of the 26 patients with positive biopsies, 46% had a local recurrence. Of the 77 patients whose biopsies were negative, 9% developed local recurrence. Surprisingly, in this series, a positive biopsy was associated with clinical local recurrence less than half the time, and a patient with a negative biopsy developed local recurrence only 9% of the time.

Schellhammer's group demonstrated that their ^{125}I implant was unsatisfactory in achieving adequate local control in the patients with bulkier stage B tumors and in those with intermediate or poorly differentiated histology, and that local control by external-beam irradiation in those patients was superior to that obtained by ^{125}I.[174,215]

BIOPSY AFTER EXTERNAL-BEAM IRRADIATION

Freiha and Bagshaw reported biopsies in 72 patients treated with external-beam irradiation.[262] Sixty-one percent had positive biopsies. Of the 61%, 85% had clinically abnormal prostates and 31% had clinically normal prostates. Of the patients with positive biopsies, 71% subsequently developed metastasis, and 24% of patients with negative biopsies developed metastasis. A more recent report from the urologists at Stanford illustrates the problems of patient selection and interpretation of this posttreatment biopsy data.[263] Kabalin and colleagues reported 22 positive biopsies from 23 patients treated with external-beam irradiation 1.5 to 12 years before biopsy. There was no correlation with PSA levels or ultrasound findings. The selection criteria for the 23 patients chosen from a large cohort of survivors after irradiation were not explained, and on the basis of these biopsies 5 patients were said to have poorly differentiated prostate cancer in their glands without clinical abnormality.

Except for learning about the biology of prostate cancer after treatment, there seems to be no reason to recommend systematic biopsy after irradiation or after radical prostatectomy. There is no clear course of action if the biopsy is positive, and not all patients with positive biopsy progress. Some physicians no longer perform biopsies routinely.[264] Resolving this question requires a thorough examination of an entire radiation-treated population and a similar investigation of a complete group of radical prostatectomy patients.

ADJUVANT OR SALVAGE TREATMENT AFTER RADICAL PROSTATECTOMY

The increasing use of radical prostatectomy for treating prostate cancer has stimulated interest in developing data and criteria that indicate which patients with adverse pathologic features may benefit from adjuvant radiation therapy and illustrate the value of irradiation for patients who develop signs of recurrence after radical prostatectomy.[179] Many of the patients who are likely to develop these adverse features can be identified in advance and excluded from candidacy for radical prostatectomy. For example, patients with poorly differentiated tumors and bilobar B2 tumors have a more than 70% likelihood of demonstrating positive nodes, positive seminal vesicles, or positive surgical margins.[195] Under any of those three circumstances, surgery is not advisable and has not been demonstrated to have long-term benefit for the patient.[179,211] Despite these well-documented observations, such patients are still submitted to radical prostatectomy and we are faced with the problem of many patients who have positive surgical margins, positive seminal vesicles, poorly differentiated tumors, or signs of local recurrence.

PATIENT SELECTION FOR ADJUVANT TREATMENT

The initial reports of Bagshaw and colleagues showed that good local control could be obtained with radiation therapy but that their use of 7000 cGy was associated with a 16% rate of serious complications.[220] Gibbons and colleagues confirmed the association of a high complication rate with a high radiation dose and with the use of cobalt treatment equipment.[212] Hanks and Dawson showed that when adjuvant therapy was given shortly after surgery, a high rate of local control was obtained (94%).[265] If this treatment was delayed until there was a clinical recurrence, local control was achieved in only 70% of patients with the added disadvantage of an increased complication rate associated with the necessarily higher doses of radiation.

Pathologic indications for postoperative adjuvant radiation are not completely clear because of limited information about local recurrence rates after surgery and the admixture of androgen deprivation for patients with adverse pathologic features who are followed without more specific local treatment.[265] It is generally agreed that patients with positive margins or extensive extracapsular disease have a 30% to 40% risk for local recurrence, a level of risk that may warrant adjuvant treatment. However, simple capsular penetration is not associated with a local failure rate in excess of 10% and those patients are not likely to benefit from treatment. It is sometimes argued that all patients with seminal vesicle involvement ultimately fail systemically and that these patients do not benefit from postoperative radiation treatment,[219] but there are few cases and no proper study has been conducted. The most sophisticated analysis of the risk of local recurrence in relation to pathologic features found at radical prostatectomy has been reported by Anscher and Prosnitz.[266] The results in their multivariate analysis included in Table 35–32 show that poorly differentiated histology, positive seminal vesicles, positive surgical margins, and elevated levels of acid phosphatase are significantly correlated with local failure. The variable of positive seminal vesicles was positive only on univariate analysis and not on multivariate analysis. In their series, there were 40 patients with local relapse, 15 (38%) of whom have developed distant metastasis. In a more positive light, 62% of these patients with local failure have not developed distant metastasis. Table 35–32 illustrates that local failures range from 36% to 58% in the subgroups listed at 10 years and from 19% to 39% at 5 years.

LOCAL CONTROL WITH IRRADIATION

The likelihood of achieving local control is better if radiation is given soon after recovery from surgery. In a review of three studies, local control was achieved in 150 of 157 patients (96%) who were treated before recurrence compared with 45 of 65 patients (70%) who were treated after local recurrence developed.[265-267]

If one favors early treatment, an appropriate radiation dose should be selected. Because an excessive complication rate of more than 10% is associated with radiation doses greater than 6500 cGy, radiation doses should be between 5500 and 6500 cGy. Radiation should not be started until the patient has stable urinary function because continued improvement in function is unusual after radiation therapy is begun. In patients with high-grade tumors, there is concern about delaying treatment more than 6 months after surgery because of the risk for local tumor proliferation, although this concern is based on theory alone.

The goal of treatment should be to treat the entire prostate-seminal vesicle surgical bed with a generous margin. Four-field or other multiple-field techniques should be used. The treatment volume is best determined with the aid of a presurgical CT or MRI. Without this examination, one guesses at the location of the organs, and the fields of treatment are not optimal.

TABLE 35–32. Risk Factors for Local Failure After Radical Prostatectomy

	No. of Patients		Actuarial Rate of Local Failure	
	Total	Local		
Factors	No.	Failure	*5-Year*	*10-Year*
Multivariate Analysis				
Poorly differentiated histology	72	20	19%	44%
Positive surgical margins	102	28	26%	58%
Elevated acid phosphatase	47	12	31%	36%
Univariate Analysis				
Positive seminal vesicles	45	17	39%	50%

(Modified from Anscher MS, Prosnitz LR. Multivariate analysis of factors predicting local relapse after radical prostatectomy—possible indications for postoperative radiotherapy. Int J Radiat Oncol Biol Phys 1991;21:941–947)

SURVIVAL BENEFIT

There is no demonstrated survival benefit associated with adjuvant radiation after radical prostatectomy, and it is unrealistic to expect confirmation of benefit from single-institution retrospective data. However, such a relation is suggested by recent reports of increased metastases in patients with local failure compared with patients with local control.[174,216]

A major benefit of radiation can be decreased symptoms as a result of achieving local control. Unfortunately, the severity of problems presented by uncontrolled local tumor in the absence of such treatment is unknown. Tomlinson and colleagues have shown that there are major local problems in patients with stage C cancer when no specific local treatment is given in addition to androgen deprivation, and they prefer aggressive local treatment.[233] Table 35–33 illustrates the impressive problems that developed in these patients. Past experience supports local treatment, but new and modern data are needed on this issue. Under any circumstance, the largest series includes fewer than 75 treated patients, so that it is unrealistic to expect these limited retrospective reviews to show a survival advantage. The ongoing SWOG prospective trial should provide some data about the adjuvant treatment of the surgical patient with adverse pathologic features.

IRRADIATION FOR ELEVATIONS OF PSA AFTER RADICAL PROSTATECTOMY

Patients treated primarily by radical prostatectomy may show an elevation of PSA levels after a period of return to undetectable levels. This usually signals recurrence but does not define the site, which remains unknown in the absence of a positive bone scan, palpable abnormality, or other clinical sign. Most of these patients have had adverse pathologic features, suggesting that the prostate-seminal vesicle bed is suspect. Lange and colleagues obtained positive needle biopsies from the area of anastomosis in 42% of 57 patients with elevated PSA levels and no other clinical signs of disease, and there was no positive biopsy found in 30 patients with normal PSA levels.[139] In Walsh's recent series of 580 patients, 10% had elevated PSA levels without other evidence of disease.

Patients with a rising PSA level after surgery should be considered for regional radiation to the area of the prostate bed

TABLE 35–33. What Happens When Stage C Cancer Receives No Local Treatment Except Antiandrogen Management (20 Patients)

Problem	*Incidence*
Urethral obstruction	75.0
Ureteral obstruction	40.0
Infection	80.0
Hematuria	45.0
Hospital admission	2.4 per patient
Hospital days	23.0 per patient
Surgical procedure	28 total in 20 patients

(Data from Tomlinson RL, Currie DP, Boyce WH. Radical prostatectomy: Palliation for stage C carcinoma of the prostate. J Urol 1977;117:85-87)

and seminal vesicle. There usually is a preoperative CT or MRI to aid localization. Irradiation of the regional nodes is not recommended because problems may result from irradiating areas of lymph node dissection. Link and colleagues have noted a durable PSA response in 7 of 13 patients who were irradiated after a delayed elevation of PSA, but only in 1 of 2 who were treated for detectable elevations immediately after surgery.[146] Substantially more data of long duration are needed to clarify the response of these two groups of patients.

THERAPY FOR ADVANCED DISEASE

Clinically apparent distant metastatic spread of prostate carcinoma (stage D2) is limited to the bone in about 80% to 85% of patients. This bony involvement is unusual in that it most commonly appears as a mixture of blastic and lytic elements. However, individual patients can have pure blastic lesions radiographically identical to Paget's disease of the bone or pure lytic lesions similar to those seen with carcinoma of the breast.[268] Microscopic examination of the areas of bone involvement does not show normal trabecular bone, but bone with an abnormal woven appearance.[269] In patients with prostate cancer, unlike patients with breast cancer, hypercalcemia is uncommon and patients more commonly exhibit circulating calcium levels in the low normal to mildly hypocalcemic range.[270] Areas of uninvolved bone typically exhibit erosion of the bone cortex and osteomalacia.[268,269,271,272] As a result of these changes, patients with osteoblastic lesions are at increased risk for fractures in involved and uninvolved sites.

These observations point to an unusual and interesting association of prostate cancer with bone. Prostate carcinoma cells have been shown to release products that stimulate osteoblasts and, in turn, bone fibroblasts have been shown to stimulate the growth of prostate carcinoma cells.[273]

Bone pain represents one of the most difficult problems in the management of carcinoma of the prostate. However, individuals vary considerably in this regard and often have extensive, but painless, bone involvement. These observations suggest that the pain is not simply a result of bone involvement but is the consequence of another process. Carcinoma of the prostate has been shown to produce prostaglandins, well-known mediators of pain and inflammation.[274–282] In addition, prostaglandin synthetase inhibitors such as indomethacin may be effective in providing pain relief.

About 10% to 15% of patients with prostate carcinoma are found to have soft tissue lesions. This typically occurs in two clinical settings: late in the course of patients who initially presented with bone involvement alone or at the initial evaluation of patients with poorly differentiated, rapidly growing, aggressive tumors. Lymph node involvement is probably the most common site of soft tissue spread. This is not limited to contiguous spread to the paraaortic lymph nodes from the pelvic lymph nodes but can be found as generalized adenopathy involving axillary, supraclavicular, and cervical lymph node chains. Liver and lung are the other two common sites of soft tissue metastatic spread.

Death from metastatic prostate carcinoma may result from several processes. Thrombophlebitis with fatal pulmonary embolism is a common problem even in patients not treated with estrogens. As with other malignancies, carcinoma of the prostate can cause diffuse intravascular coagulation that results in lethal hemorrhage.[283–291] If the patient has not had hormonal therapy, use of heparin or fresh frozen plasma is warranted to protect the patient until a hormonal response has occurred. As with pancreatic carcinoma, carcinoma of the prostate can cause severe cachexia and the resulting debilitation can contribute to the patient's demise.[292] Myelophthisic replacement of the bone marrow can result in pancytopenia with increased risk of infection, anemia, and thrombocytopenia. Death due to replacement of liver or lung, two of the frequent sites of extraosseous spread, is uncommon.

EVALUATION OF RESPONSE

Evaluation of response in patients with bone involvement alone has been problematic. Blastic lesions heal slowly and have been shown to persist even when biopsy documents absence of disease.[293] Although the bone scan is a useful indicator of bone involvement, it has proved to be a less than adequate indicator of response. Perhaps because bone lesions in this disease are most commonly a mixture of lytic and blastic elements, the bone scan can increase in intensity in the initial phase of a response. Because bone remodeling is slow in elderly men, the bone scan can take more than 6 months to reflect a response. Soft tissue disease is evaluable using the standard criteria of medical oncology. Soft tissue disease is not always representative of events in the bone lesions. The acid phosphatase test has proved to be a poor indicator of clinical course in patients undergoing surgery, x-ray therapy, hormonal treatment, or chemotherapy. Measurement of PSA levels has proved uniformly superior to the prostatic acid phosphatase as a marker in following patient response to radical prostatectomy and radiation therapy. Recently, several investigators have shown that this marker is useful in following response to hormonal therapy and chemotherapy.[293a] PSA has several important advantages over other indicators of response. First, because the half life of this marker is 2 to 4 days, it provides a much more rapid indication of tumor status than does bone scan or radiographic evidence of tumor healing. Second, compared with these imaging techniques, it is inherently more quantitative, reproducible, and objective. Third, it is much less expensive and demonstrably more sensitive.

Because of the problematic nature of the tools available to assess response, quality of life and survival have been advocated as alternate methods of judging the effectiveness of hormonal and chemotherapeutic agents.[294–298] This approach has much to recommend it. Survival is an unambiguous endpoint and has proved to be reproducible. Improved survival and relief from suffering accurately match the goals of patients seeking treatment. This approach has several disadvantages. For a single agent to alter survival, response rates usually must exceed 50%. It is unusual for single agents to reach such response levels in any carcinoma of adult life. There is considerable interest in quality of life assessment tools but no widely accepted method to measure this endpoint.

PRINCIPLES OF ENDOCRINE THERAPY

ANDROGEN PHYSIOLOGY

Normal and malignant prostatic epithelial cells are composed of three populations: hormone dependent, hormone sensitive, and hormone independent.[299,300] Hormone-dependent cells die when androgen is withdrawn, and hormone-sensitive cells stop dividing until resupplied with androgen.[301-303] The process of cell death seen after androgen withdrawal has been termed programmed cell death or apoptosis and is characterized by a series of biochemical and morphologic changes. The earliest well-characterized event is a sudden increase in intracellular free calcium. This is followed by activation of a calcium-dependent endonuclease, which digests the cellular DNA predominantly in the linker regions joining DNA segments that are wrapped around nucleosomes and protected. The result is DNA fragmentation in which DNA chains are shortened in a step-wise fashion as each nucleosomal unit is freed from the chain. The process is an active one and can be slowed by calcium-channel blockers or inhibitors of protein synthesis, such as cyclohexamide. This results in a characteristic and diagnostic ladder appearance on polyacrylamide gel. This process, which may be recognized pathologically by the destruction of the nucleus and preservation of cytoplasm, is distinct from necrosis, in which nuclear detail is preserved and cytoplasmic structure is lost.

Although the androgen receptor has an affinity for testosterone, the androgen with the highest affinity is 5-dihydrotestosterone (DHT), which plays the dominant role in androgen response in prostatic epithelium. Most of the DHT active within the prostate gland is formed peripherally within the prostate gland by the action of a 5-α reductase. Fenasteride, an inhibitor of this reductase, causes a marked drop in prostatic DHT and a dramatic increase in prostatic testosterone.[304] Under these circumstances, sufficient testosterone is available to bind to and activate the androgen receptor.

The cloning of the androgen receptor has shed new and provocative light on mechanisms by which cells might escape traditional methods of hormonal therapy. A single-point mutation has been shown to result in a receptor currently able to bind well to estrogen, progesterone, and the antiandrogen flutamide.[305] In the human hormone-sensitive prostatic carcinoma cell line, LNCaP, which expresses this receptor, flutamide can replace testosterone as a growth stimulus.

Synthesis of androgen begins with the conversion of 17-hydroxyprogesterone to dehydroepiandrosterone (DHEA) followed by the formation of dehydroepiandrosterone sulfate (DHEAS), androstenedione, and testosterone (Fig 35-16). Although the complete pathway to testosterone is present only in the testes, in humans the adrenal gland releases DHEA, DHEAS, and androstenedione.[306-308] Enzymes for subsequent conversion of DHEA, DHEAS, and androstenedione to testosterone are present in many peripheral tissues, including the prostate gland. Harper and colleagues[306] and Geller and colleagues[307] have shown that in humans, infusion of radiolabeled DHEA or DHEAS results in the formation of prostatic DHT. As a result, although about 90% of circulating testosterone is of testicular origin, only about 60% of prostatic testosterone is from this source. The results published by Geller and colleagues show considerable patient to patient variability in the source of prostatic DHT; in about 20% of patients, prostatic DHT levels after castration overlap with those seen in the prostate gland before castration.[307] This suggests that in some patients the adrenal gland represents an important alternate source of androgenic stimulation. As a consequence, adrenal blockade of androgen production can be shown to decrease the levels of prostatic DHT further.

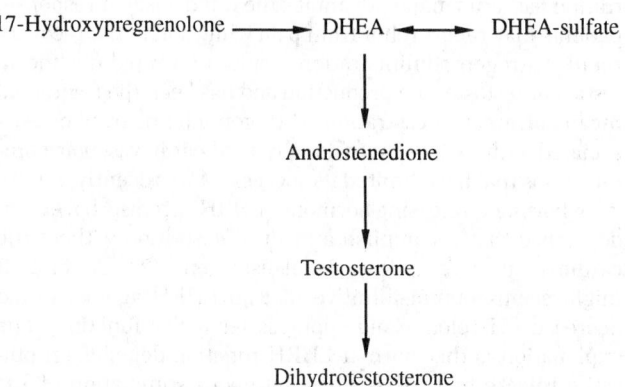

FIGURE 35-16. Androgen synthesis. In humans, dihydroepiandrosterone (DHEA), dihydroepiandrosterone sulfate (DHEA-sulfate), and androstenedione are produced in the adrenal gland and released into the circulation. Within prostate tissue, all three androgen precursors may be converted to testosterone and dihydrotestosterone. The latter represents the dominant active androgen in prostate tissue and for male pattern hair loss, whereas testosterone is responsible for muscle mass and sex drive.

Not all prostatic cells, normal or malignant, die on androgen withdrawal. Castration of normal animals results in a dramatic reduction of prostate size in the adult male. On administration of exogenous androgen, the gland rapidly resumes its normal size and function. There must be prostatic epithelial cells able to survive androgen withdrawal and respond to subsequent androgen administration by proliferation and differentiation into androgen-sensitive and dependent-cell populations. Isaacs and colleagues have shown through classic genetic techniques that androgen-responsive tumors contain an androgen-independent population before the initiation of hormone therapy and that this population emerges as a result of selection when androgen is withdrawn.[299,300,309] Human trials confirm the presence of androgen-independent tumor cells: even after surgical castration and adrenalectomy, patients with metastatic carcinoma of the prostate always progress and ultimately die from metastatic prostate cancer.

The physiology described defines the limits of hormonal therapy for metastatic prostate carcinoma and prevents this therapy from ever resulting in cure of metastatic prostate cancer. The success of surgical or medical castration is limited by the presence of an adrenal androgen source and by the presence of androgen-independent cells, but the importance of adrenal androgens and the proportion of the tumor population initially hormone-independent show considerable variation among patients. Secondary hormonal treatment results in clinical responses, but they are often of short duration and occur in less than 20% of patients. Combined testicular and adrenal blockade are limited by the presence of hormone-independent tumor cells.

INITIAL HORMONE THERAPY

Monotherapy

After the landmark observation in 1941 by Huggins and Hodges that androgen ablation caused regression of prostate carcinoma,[310,311] the standard method of management of metastatic prostate cancer became medical or surgical castration. Until recently, this was typically accomplished by surgical castration or estrogen administration. Surgical castration has as its major advantage the rapid onset of response; patients may report relief from pain while still in the recovery room. Estrogen administration results in a rapid decline in testicular testosterone production and has been the traditional means of medical castration. Estrogen administration is associated with serious, occasionally fatal cardiovascular complications that have limited its success. More recently, luteinizing hormone-releasing hormone (LHRH) agonists have been developed that accomplish a medical castration without the cardiovascular complications of estrogen.[312–314] At first, it might seem counter-intuitive that an LHRH agonist would decrease LH release and suppress testicular function. The explanation is that normal LHRH function depends on pulsatile release of LHRH. The continuous stimulation of LH release caused by LHRH agonists causes an initial increase in LH release and, therefore, testosterone synthesis followed by down-regulation of the LHRH receptors and a decline in LH release. As a result, LH release peaks on day 2 or 3 after initiation of LHRH agonist administration and testosterone levels peak on days 3 through 5. Thereafter, LH release and testosterone production gradually decline to castrate levels about 3 to 4 weeks after initiation of LHRH agonist administration. As a result of this initial increase in testosterone production, patients may experience an increase in tumor activity during the initial week of treatment. For this reason, patients with lesions that threaten key organ functions should not receive LHRH agonist monotherapy. An example would be the patient with symptoms of cord compression. The LHRH agonists approved by the FDA for marketing in the United States include leuprolide and goserelin acetate. Both are available in time-release formulations that permit once a month administration. There are no significant differences in efficacy between these two compounds.

The advent of antiandrogens has offered another therapeutic option. Antiandrogens may be steroidal or nonsteroidal.[315–323] Steroidal antiandrogens (*e.g.*, megestrol acetate [Megace] and cyproterone acetate) have antiandrogen action and variable progestin and glucocorticoid action. In some experimental systems, these drugs show androgen rather than antiandrogen action. The nonsteroidal antiandrogens include pure antiandrogens such as flutamide, Casodex, or nilutamide. These compounds act peripherally rather than at the testes or adrenal gland. Flutamide, the only member of this class approved by the FDA, has been shown to block androgen uptake and receptor binding or processing. Although flutamide appears to cause an initial drop in prostatic DHT, it can induce a compensatory increase in LH release, resulting in a gradual increase in testosterone levels that ultimately reverses androgen blockade. Flutamide can cause gynecomastia, gastrointestinal complications, and a chemical hepatitis that is occasionally severe.

There is no convincing evidence that monotherapy, given early or late, alters the survival of patients with metastatic disease. Therefore, it is regarded reasonable to delay monotherapy until the patient requires palliation.

Combined Blockade of Testicular and Adrenal Androgen

This approach is based on the role of adrenal androgens in the formation of prostatic DHT.[308,324–328] This approach is further supported by the fact that responses are seen when patients failing medical or surgical castration are subjected to medical or surgical adrenalectomy. Labrie and colleagues have argued forcefully in favor of the combination of an LHRH agonist, such as leuprolide or surgical castration, with flutamide.[308] Additional advantages of the combination include blockade of the LHRH agonist flare by flutamide and blockade of flutamide gynecomastia by LHRH agonist. Although Labrie and colleagues initially reported outstanding results,[308] recent large cooperative group randomized clinical trials have better defined the benefit of combined androgen blockade.[309,327,328] For patients with widespread bone or soft tissue involvement and a poor performance status, responses are typically short, and combined androgen blockade offers no significant advantage over LHRH agonist alone or orchiectomy alone. At the other extreme, in patients without symptoms and with minimal bone metastasis, combined androgen blockade gave results superior to that of LHRH alone or orchiectomy alone in terms of duration of response and overall survival. The overall survival advantage for combined androgen blockade in such patients is about 2 years. Unfortunately, most patients are diagnosed with disease intermediate in severity between these two extremes and have widespread bone disease but good performance status. For such patients, the advantage of combined androgen blockade results in an increase in overall duration of response and survival of about 6 months.

These results strongly support the concept of early aggressive rather than late palliative use of combined androgen blockade. Although the Intergroup trial reported by Crawford and colleagues[309,327,328] identified the patients likely to benefit from combined androgen blockade as having a high performance status and disease limited to pelvis and spine, others are rapidly identifying additional prognostic factors that can be used to identify patients with a good prognosis. For example, having fewer than 5 bone lesions, a testosterone level of less than 300 ng/ml, a PSA value of less than 100 ng/ml, and absence of anemia are all associated with a better prognosis.[329] The major disadvantage of combined androgen blockade is that available LHRH agonists and pure antiandrogens such as flutamide are expensive and beyond the means of many elderly patients. Surgical castration can replace LHRH agonist in such treatment and may result in significant savings in patients with minimal metastatic disease, when overall survival is projected to be greater than 4 years.

The appropriate management of patients with advanced metastatic disease is less defined. None of the therapeutic options result in a meaningful prolongation of life, and duration of response to hormonal therapy is typically less than 1 year. Combined adrenal androgen blockade does not add significantly to the treatment of these patients but does add to the cost.

Therapy for Patients in Whom Initial Hormonal Therapy Fails

After initial hormonal therapy, secondary hormonal treatment has been studied extensively. Most approaches have been based on blockade of adrenal androgens. Responses have been noted in as many as 20% of such patients but usually are less than 6 months in duration and do not significantly alter survival. Flutamide may be used in patients who have failed monotherapy with estrogen, surgical castration, or LHRH agonist. Hydrocortisone alone, given at replacement doses, can provide significant relief of pain to patients with metastatic disease, and an occasional patient has shown objective evidence of antitumor activity.[330-332] Aminoglutethimide and hydrocortisone are widely used and responses have been reported. Aminoglutethimide is usually started at a dose of 125 mg four times daily for several days and then escalated to a dose of 250 mg four times a day. However, randomized trials indicate that most of the hormonal effects and responses are due to the hydrocortisone alone.[331,332] The side effects of aminoglutethimide are significant and include skin rash, fever, lethargy, and weakness. Ketoconazole inhibits adrenal androgen synthesis and in vitro it exhibits antitumor activity against hormone-independent human tumor cell lines. Ketoconazole alone or in combination with hydrocortisone has been used and can result in a response in up to 25% of all patients.[333] Administration of ketoconazole usually is initiated at a total daily dose of 600 to 800 mg in three divided doses. Thereafter, the dose may be increased to a total dose of up to 1200 mg/day according to patient tolerance. Nausea and vomiting are common at this dose range and often limit therapy. This drug may cause significant liver injury. In addition to its hormonal effects, ketoconazole has shown some activity in hormone refractory carcinoma of the prostate.[334]

As with most epithelial cells, prostatic epithelial cells exhibit growth hormone receptors.[335,336] Growth hormone causes the release of insulin-like growth factor-I (IGF-I) by the liver, and this cytokine supports the proliferation of many epithelial cells and carcinomas. It is not surprising that prostatic epithelia have been shown to exhibit IGF-I receptors.[337] Somatostatin blocks growth hormone action and prevents IGF-I release by the liver.[338] Unfortunately, somatostatin itself is short-lived and therefore is not useful as a drug. Somatostatin agonists have been developed that are potent and long-lived. Two agents, octreotide acetate (commercially available as Sandostatin) and Somatulin, have shown activity in preclinical models and have been given to small numbers of patients with prostate cancer who have had relief of pain and a decrease in PSA levels.[339-344] Objective responses were not well documented and the overall response rate remains to be defined. The major side effects of somatostatin agonists are abdominal pain and diarrhea that tend to subside with continued use.

PALLIATIVE RADIATION THERAPY

External-beam irradiation therapy provides an effective, well-tolerated, and reliable means of controlling individual bone lesions in patients with hormone refractory prostate cancer. It can result in relief of pain and lessening of the risk of fracture. In addition, it is the standard method of treating impending cord compression. Hemibody irradiation has been reported to provide relief of pain when lesions are too numerous or widespread to respond to conventional radiation therapy.[174,345-347]

There are several radioactive isotopes, such as phosphorus 32, strontium, samarium 53, and rhenium 186, which are handled in biologic systems in a fashion similar to calcium.[348-357] As a result, they accumulate selectively within the blastic bone lesions that are characteristic of carcinoma of the prostate. These agents have proved effective in the management of bone pain but are experimental.

CYTOTOXIC CHEMOTHERAPY

Eisenberger and colleagues have effectively reviewed the problems associated with the evaluation of chemotherapeutic agents in carcinoma of the prostate.[295-298] For any given agent, response rates vary over a wide range from center to center. Response rates for doxorubicin, for example, range from no response to more than 50% response. Median survival, on the other hand, has been remarkably similar from study to study at 30 to 40 weeks with no agent consistently altering overall survival. Since this review was written, there have been two important developments that may simplify evaluation of new agents. The first development has been the rapid development of PSA as a reliable marker to follow the clinical course of carcinoma of the prostate after radical prostatectomy, radiation therapy, and hormonal therapy. There are already two reports of its use to evaluate response to chemotherapy. This marker has proved itself in other settings to be a more sensitive and rapidly responding indicator of disease status than other measures of tumor mass. Should additional experience establish its use as an indicator of response to chemotherapy, evaluation of drug activity would be markedly simplified. The second development has been the recent focus on improved quality of life as a criteron for drug approval by the FDA. Because pain and debilitation are such a prominent part of hormone refractory prostate cancer, agents that improve quality of life should be easy to identify. The only major barrier is the lack of a universally accepted instrument to assess quality of life.

Despite early optimistic reports, doxorubicin and other DNA intercalators that operate by a topoisomerase-2-dependent mechanism exhibit objective response rates of less than 15%. Standard alkylating agents such as cyclophosphamide and the antimetabolites 5-fluorouracil and methotrexate have exhibited minimal antitumor activity with objective response rates of less than 20%. The tubulin-binding agents, vinblastine and vindesine, exhibit greater single-agent activity with response rates between 15% and 30%. Estramustine, which binds to the tubulin-associated proteins, exhibits useful activity with objective response rates in the 15% to 30% range. The reductive alkylator, mitomycin C, exhibits activity within this same range.

SURAMIN

Suramin has elicited interest because of its unique mechanism of action and initial reports of its activity in hormone refractory carcinoma of the prostate. Suramin was originally synthesized in 1917 as part of the search for a drug active against African trypanosomiasis. In 1984, it was shown to be effective in inhibiting the action of the cytokine platelet-derived growth factor (PDGF). Malignant transformation due to the PDGF-like peptide product of the v-*SIS* oncogene was reversed by addition of suramin.[358,359] Subsequent studies have shown that suramin is able to block the action of a wide range of heparin-binding cytokines including the fibroblast growth factors, transforming growth factor-β, interleukin-2, and IGF-I and IGF-II. Because several of these cytokines, including fibroblast growth factor,[360] transforming growth factor-β,[361-363] and IGF-I[363,364] are involved in growth regulation of prostatic epithelium, suramin was tested as an agent in the treatment of carcinoma of the prostate. The initial phase II trial of suramin in prostate carcinoma yielded a response rate of 33% in patients with hormone refractory carcinoma of the prostate.[160] Two subsequent phase II trials have confirmed activity and report response rates of greater than 40%. In the initial trial, the incidence of severe side effects exceeded 80%. In subsequent studies, careful monitoring of plasma drug levels has reduced the incidence of serious side effects to less than 20%. Although these early results are promising, the drug is still investigational and its final role in the treatment of carcinoma of the prostate remains to be defined.

REFERENCES

1. Boring CC, Squires TS, Tong T. Cancer statistics, 1991. Bol Asoc Med PR 1991;41:225–242.
2. Carter HB, Coffey DS. The prostate: An increasing medical problem. Prostate 1990;16:39–48.
3. Cooner WH, Mosley BR, Rutherford CL, et al. Prostate cancer detection in a clinical urological practice by ultrasonography, digital rectal examination, and prostate specific antigen. J Urol 1990;143:1146–1154.
4. Lee WH. The molecular basis of cancer suppression by the retinoblastoma gene. Int Symp Princess Takamatsu Cancer Res Fund 1989;20:159–170.
5. Catalona WJ, Smith DS, Ratliff TL, et al. Measurement of prostate-specific antigen in serum as a screening test for prostate cancer [published erratum appears in N Engl J Med 1991;325(18):1324]. N Engl J Med 1991;324:1156–1161.
6. Harrison SH, Seale-Hawkins C, Schum CW, Dunn JK, Scardino PT. Correlation between side of palpable tumor and side of pelvic lymph node metastasis in clinically localized prostate cancer. Cancer 1992;69:750–754.
7. Williams RD, ed. Controversies in prostate cancer management. Philadelphia: JB Lippincott, 1990:408–419.
8. Scardino PT, Weaver R, Hudson MA. Early detection of prostate cancer. Hum Pathol 1992;23:211–222.
9. National Cancer Institute. Roundtable on prostate cancer: Future research directions. Cancer Res 1991;51:2498–2505.
10. Dhom G. Epidemiologic aspects of latent and clinically manifest carcinoma of the prostate. J Cancer Res Clin Oncol 1983;106:210–218.
11. Whitmore WF. Natural history and staging of prostate cancer. Urol Clin North Am 1984;11:205–220.
12. Chiquet-Ehrismann R, Kalla P, Pearson CA. Participation of tenascin and transforming growth factor-b in reciprocal epithelial-mesenchymal interactions of MCF7 cells and fibroblasts. Cancer Res 1989;49:4322–4325.
13. Scardino PT, Weaver R, Hudson MA. Early detection of prostate cancer. Hum Pathol 1992;23:211–222.
14. McNeal JE, Kindrachuk RA, Freiha FS, Bostwick DG, Redwine EA, Stamey TA. Patterns of progression in prostate cancer. Lancet 1986;11:60–63.
15. Tulinius H. Latent malignancies at autopsy: A little-used source of information on cancer biology. IARC Sci Publ 1991:253–261.
16. Whittemore AS, Keller JB, Betensky R. Low-grade, latent prostate cancer volume: Predictor of clinical cancer incidence? [see comments]. JNCI 1991;83:1231–1235.
17. Yatani R, Kusano I, Shiraishi T, Hayashi T, Stemmermann GN. Latent prostatic carcinoma: Pathological and epidemiological aspects. Jpn J Clin Oncol 1989;19:319–326.
18. Austin JP, Aziz H, Potters L, et al. Diminished survival of young blacks with adenocarcinoma of the prostate. Am J Clin Oncol 1990;13:465–469.
19. Mebane C, Gibbs T, Horm J. Current status of prostate cancer in North American black males. J Natl Med Assoc 1990;82:782–788.
20. Muir CS, Nectoux J, Staszewski J. The epidemiology of prostatic cancer: Geographical distribution and time-trends. Acta Oncol 1991;30:133–140.
21. Ross R, Bernstein L, Judd H, Hanisch R, Pike M, Henderson B. Serum testosterone levels in healthy young black and white men. JNCI 1986;76:45–48.
22. Ross RK, Shimizu H, Paganini HA, Honda G, Henderson BE. Case-control studies of prostate cancer in blacks and whites in southern California. JNCI 1987;78:869–874.
23. Ross RK, Paganini HA, Henderson BE. The etiology of prostate cancer: What does the epidemiology suggest? Prostate 1983;4:333–344.
24. Ogunlewe JO, Osegbe DN. Zinc and cadmium concentrations in indigenous blacks with normal, hypertrophic and malignant prostate. Cancer 1989;63:1388–1392.
25. Heshmat MY, Kaul L, Kovi J, et al. Nutrition and prostate cancer: A case-control study. Prostate 1985;6:7–17.
26. Prentice RL, Sheppard L. Dietary fat and cancer: Consistency of the epidemiologic data, and disease prevention that may follow from a practical reduction in fat consumption [published erratum appears in Cancer Causes Control 1990;1(3):253]. Cancer Causes Control 1990;1:81–97.
27. Shimizu H, Ross RK, Bernstein L, Yatani R, Henderson BE, Mack TM. Cancers of the prostate and breast among Japanese and white immigrants in Los Angeles County. Br J Cancer 1991;63:963–966.
28. Palmer S. Diet, nutrition, and cancer. Prog Food Nutr Sci 1985;9:283–341.
29. Willett WC, Polk BF, Morris JS, et al. Prediagnostic serum selenium and risk of cancer. Lancet 1983;2:130–134.
30. West DW, Slattery ML, Robison LM, French TK, Mahoney AW. Adult dietary intake and prostate cancer risk in Utah: A case-control study with special emphasis on aggressive tumors. Cancer Causes Control 1991;2:85–94.
31. Reichman ME, Hayes RB, Ziegler RG, et al. Serum vitamin A and subsequent development of prostate cancer in the first National Health and Nutrition Examination Survey Epidemiologic Follow-up Study. Cancer Res 1990;50:2311–2315.
32. Kolonel LN, Hinds MW, Nomura AM, Hankin JH, Lee J. Relationship of dietary vitamin A and ascorbic acid intake to the risk for cancers of the lung, bladder, and prostate in Hawaii. Natl Cancer Inst Monogr 1985;69:137–142.
33. Meikle AW, Smith JJ. Epidemiology of prostate cancer. Urol Clin North Am 1990;17:709–718.
34. Rose DP, Connolly JM. Effects of fatty acids and eicosanoid synthesis inhibitors on the growth of two human prostate cancer cell lines. Prostate 1991;18:243–254.
35. Lanier AP, Bulkow LR, Ireland B. Cancer in Alaskan Indians, Eskimos, and Aleuts, 1969–83: Implications for etiology and control. Public Health Rep 1989;104:658–664.
36. Drago JR, Al MH. The effect of prostaglandin modulators on prostate tumor growth and metastasis. Anticancer Res 1984;4:391–394.
37. Anderson KM, Wygodny JB, Ondrey F, Harris J. Human PC-3 prostate cell line DNA synthesis is suppressed by eicosatetraynoic acid, an in vitro inhibitor of arachidonic acid metabolism. Prostate 1988;12:3–12.
38. Flammang TJ, Yamazoe Y, Benson RW, et al. Arachidonic acid-dependent peroxidative activation of carcinogenic arylamines by extrahepatic human tissue microsomes. Cancer Res 1989;49:1977–1982.
39. Kahng MW, Smith MW, Trump BF. Aryl hydrocarbon hydroxylase induction and binding of dimethylbenz(a)anthracene in human prostate. Prog Clin Biol Res 1981;75B:183–190.
40. Sirigu P, Cossu M, Perra MT. Histochemical localization of prostaglandin synthetase in human exocrine glands. Anat Rec 1982;204:101–104.
41. Pearce N, Reif JS. Epidemiologic studies of cancer in agricultural workers. Am J Ind Med 1990;18:133–148.
42. Hagmar L, Bellander T, Andersson C, Linden K, Attewell R, Moller T. Cancer morbidity in nitrate fertilizer workers. Int Arch Occup Environ Health 1991;63:63–67.
43. Langard S, Andersen A, Ravnestad J. Incidence of cancer among ferrochromium and ferrosilicon workers: An extended observation period. Br J Ind Med 1990;47:14–19.
44. Kazantzis G. Cadmium: Sources, exposure and possible carcinogenicity. IARC Sci Publ 1986;76:93–101.
45. Lee JS, White KL. A review of the health effects of cadmium. Am J Ind Med 1980;1:307–317.
45a. Greenwald P. The prostate. In: Scottenfeld D, Fraumeni JF. Cancer epidemiology and prevention. Philadelphia: WB Saunders, 1982:944.
46. Ghadirian P, Cadotte M, Lacroix A, Perret C. Family aggregation of cancer of the prostate in Quebec: The tip of the iceberg. Prostate 1991;19:43–52.
47. Pottern LM, Linet M, Blair A, et al. Familial cancers associated with subtypes of leukemia and non-Hodgkin's lymphoma. Leuk Res 1991;15:305–314.
48. Spitz MR, Currier RD, Fueger JJ, Babaian RJ, Newell GR. Familial patterns of prostate cancer: A case-control analysis. J Urol 1991;146:1305–1307.
49. Bookstein R, Lee WH. Molecular genetics of the retinoblastoma suppressor gene. Crit Rev Oncol 1991;2:211–227.
50. Szekely L, Uzvolgyi E, Jiang WQ, et al. Subcellular localization of the retinoblastoma protein. Cell Growth Differ 1991;2:287–295.
51. Rubin SJ, Hallahan DE, Ashman CR, et al. Two prostate carcinoma cell lines demonstrate abnormalities in tumor suppressor genes. J Surg Oncol 1991;46:31–36.
52. Bookstein R, Rio P, Madreperla SA, et al. Promoter deletion and loss of retinoblastoma gene expression in human prostate carcinoma. Proc Natl Acad Sci U S A 1990;87:7762–7766.
53. Bookstein R, Shew JY, Chen PL, Scully P, Lee WH. Suppression of tumorigenicity of human prostate carcinoma cells by replacing a mutated RB gene. Science 1990;247:712–715.
54. Fleming WH, Hamel A, MacDonald R, et al. Expression of the c-myc protooncogene in human prostatic carcinoma and benign prostatic hyperplasia. Cancer Res 1986;46:1535–1538.
55. Matusik RJ, Fleming WH, Hamel A, et al. Expression of the c-myc proto-oncogene in prostatic tissue. Prog Clin Biol Res 1987;239:91–112.
56. Nag A, Smith RG. Amplification, rearrangement, and elevated expression of c-myc in the human prostatic carcinoma cell line LNCaP. Prostate 1989;15:115–122.
57. Viola MV, Fromowitz F, Oravez S, et al. Expression of ras oncogene p21 in prostate cancer. N Engl J Med 1986;314:133–137.
58. Merz VW, Miller GJ, Krebs T, et al. Elevated transforming growth factor-beta 1 and beta 3 mRNA levels are associated with ras + myc-induced carcinomas in reconstituted mouse prostate: Evidence for a paracrine role during progression. Mol Endocrinol 1991;5:503–513.
59. Thompson TC, Southgate J, Kitchener G, Land H. Multistage carcinogenesis induced by ras and myc oncogenes in a reconstituted organ. Cell 1989;56:917–930.
60. Gumerlock PH, Poonamallee UR, Meyers FJ, de Vere WR. Activated ras alleles in human carcinoma of the prostate are rare. Cancer Res 1991;51:1632–1637.
61. Varma VA, Austin GE, O'Connell AC. Antibodies to ras oncogene p21 proteins lack immunohistochemical specificity for neoplastic epithelium in human prostate tissue. Arch Pathol Lab Med 1989;113:16–19.
62. Carter BS, Epstein JI, Isaacs WB. Ras gene mutations in human prostate cancer. Cancer Res 1990;50:6830–6832.
63. Sumiya H, Masai M, Akimoto S, Yatani R, Shimazaki J. Histochemical examination of expression of ras p21 protein and R 1881-binding protein in human prostatic cancers. Eur J Cancer 1990;26:786–789.

64. Funa K, Nordgren H, Nilsson S. In situ expression of mRNA for proto-oncogenes in benign prostatic hyperplasia and in prostatic carcinoma. Scand J Urol Nephrol 1991;25: 95–100.
65. Voeller HJ, Wilding G, Gelmann EP. v-rasH expression confers hormone-independent in vitro growth to LNCaP prostate carcinoma cells. Mol Endocrinol 1991;5:209–216.
66. Handley R, Carr TW, Travis D, Powell PH, Hall RR. Deferred treatment of prostate cancer. Br J Urol 1988;62:249–253.
67. Catalona WJ. Prostate cancer. New York: Grune & Stratton, 1984.
68. George NJR. Natural history of localized prostatic cancer managed by conservative therapy alone. Lancet 1988:494–497.
69. Johansson J-E, Adami H-O, Andersson S-O, Bergstrom R, Krusemo UB, Kraaz W. Natural history of localized prostatic cancer: A population-based study in 223 untreated patients. Lancet 1989:799–803.
70. Whitmore WF, Warner JA, Thompson IM. Expectant management of localized prostatic cancer. Cancer 1991;67:1091–1096.
71. Norlen BJ. Epidemiology: Is prostatic cancer mostly a "benign" tumour? Scand J Urol Nephrol 1988;110(Suppl):71–75.
72. Larson A, Norlen BJ. Five-year follow-up of patients with localized prostatic carcinoma initially referred for expectant treatment. Scand J Urol Nephrol 1985;93(Suppl): 19–30.
73. Schroeder FH, Carpentier PJ, Maksimovic PA, Bentvelsen FMJ. Transrectal ultra-sonography (TRUS) volumetric applications to prostatic carcinoma. In: Resnick M, WH Karr JP, eds. Diagnostic ultrasound of the prostate. New York: Elsevier, 1989: 124–128.
74. Stamey TA, Kabalin JN, McNeal JE, et al. Prostate specific antigen in the diagnosis and treatment of adenocarcinoma of the prostate. II. Radical prostatectomy treated patients. J Urol 1989;141:1076–1083.
75. Barnes R, Hadley H, Axford P, Kronholm S. Conservative treatment of early carcinoma of prostate. Urology 1979;14:359–362.
76. Whitmore W. Natural history of low-stage prostatic cancer and the impact of early detection. Urol Clin North Am 1990;17:689–697.
77. Franks LM. Latency and progression in tumors: The natural history of prostatic cancer. Lancet 1956;2:1037–1039.
78. Scott RJ, Mutchnik DL, Laskowski TZ. Carcinoma of the prostate in elderly men: Incidence, growth characteristics and clinical significance. J Urol 1969;101:602–607.
79. Hinman F. Screening for prostatic carcinoma. J Urol 1991;145:126–130.
80. Chodak GW, Schoenberg HW. Progress and problems in screening for carcinoma of the prostate. World J Surg 1989;13:60–64.
81. Thompson IM, Fair WR. Screening for carcinoma of the prostate: Efficacy of available screening tests. World J Surg 1989;13:65–70.
82. Seidman H, Mushinski MH, Geib SK. Probabilities of eventually developing or dying of cancer—United States 1985. Cancer 1985;35:35–56.
83. Kabalin JN, McNeal JE, Price HM, Freiha FS, Stamey TA. Unsuspected adenocar-cinoma of the prostate in patients undergoing cystoprostatectomy for other causes: Incidence, histology and morphometric observations. J Urol 1989;141:1091–1094.
84. Montie JE, Wood DP, Pontes JE, Levin HS, Boyett J. Adenocarcinoma of the prostate identified by serial sectioning of the prostate after cystoprostatectomy for carcinoma of the bladder: A prospective study. J Urol [Abstract 611] 1988;139:315.
85. Breslow N, Chan CW, Dhom G, et al. Latent carcinoma of the prostate at autopsy in seven areas. Int J Cancer 1977;20:680–688.
86. McNeal JE. Origin and development of carcinoma in the prostate. Cancer 1969;23: 24.
87. Carter HB, Piantodosi S, Isaacs JT. Clinical evidence for and implications of the multistep development of prostate cancer. J Urol 1990;143:742–746.
88. Blute ML, Nafir O, Lincke H, Farrow G, Thermen T, Lieber M. Pattern of failure after radical retropubic prostatectomy for clinically and pathologically localized ad-enocarcinoma of the prostate: Influence of tumor deoxyribonucleic acid ploidy. J Urol 1989;142:1262.
89. Shinohara K, Scardino PT, Carter SSC, Wheeler TM. Pathologic basis of the sono-graphic appearance of the normal and malignant prostate. Urol Clin North Am 1989;16: 675–691.
90. McClennan BL. Transrectal ultrasound: Is the technology leading the science? Ra-diology 1988;168:571–577.
91. Thompson TC, Kadmon D, Timme TL, et al. Experimental oncogene-induced prostate cancer. Cancer Surveys 1991;11:55–71.
92. Petersen RO. Urologic pathology. Philadelphia: JB Lippincott, 1986:617–620.
93. Dube VE, Garrow GM, Greene LF. Prostatic adenocarcinoma of ductal origin. Cancer 1973;32:402–409.
94. Kopelson G, Harisiadis L, Romas NA, Veenema RJ, Tannenbaum M. Periurethal prostatic duct carcinoma: Clinical features and treatment results. Cancer 1978;42: 2894–2902.
95. Christensen WN, Steinberg G, Walsh PC, Epstein JI. Prostatic duct adenocarcinoma: Findings at radical prostatectomy. Cancer 1991;67:2118–2124.
96. Hanks GE. Optimizing the radiation treatment and outcome of prostate cancer. Int J Radiat Oncol Biol Phys 1985;11:1235–1245.
97. Broders AC. Epithelioma of the genitourinary organs. Anal Surg 1922;75:574.
98. Mostofi FK. Grading of prostatic carcinoma. Cancer Chemother Rep 1975;59:111.
99. Brawn PN, Ayala AG, Von Eschenbach AC. Histologic grading study of prostate ad-enocarcinoma: The development of a new system and comparison with other meth-ods—a preliminary study. Cancer 1982;49:525.
100. Gleason DF. Classification of prostatic carcinomas. Cancer Chemother Rep 1966;50: 125.
101. Miller GJ, Shikes JL. Nuclear roundness as a predictor of response to hormonal

therapy of patients with stage D$_2$ prostatic cancer. In: Karr JP, Coffey DS, Gardner W, eds. Prognostic cytometry and cytopathology of prostate cancer. New York: Elsevier, 1988:349–353.
102. Guileyardo JM, Sama DP, Johnson WD. Incidental prostatic carcinoma: Tumor extent versus histologic grade. Urology 1982;20:40.
103. Harada M, Mostofi FK, Carle DK. Preliminary studies of histologic prognosis in cancer of the prostate. Cancer Treat Rep 1977;61:223.
104. Diamond DA, Berry SF, Jewett HJ, Eggleston JC, Coffey DS. A new method to assess metastatic potential of human prostate cancer: Relative nuclear roundness. J Urol 1982;128:729–734.
105. Shaeffer J, Tegeler JA, Kuban DA, Philput CB, El-Mahdi AM. Nuclear roundness factor and local failure from definitive radiation therapy for prostatic carcinoma. Int J Radiat Oncol Biol Phys (in press).
106. Frankfurt OS, Chin JL, Englander LS. Relationship between DNA ploidy, glandular differentiation and tumor spread in human prostate cancer. Cancer Res 1985;45: 1418–1423.
107. Nativ O, Winkler HZ, Raz Y, et al. Stage C prostatic adenocarcinoma: Flow cytometric nuclear DNA ploidy analysis. Mayo Clin Proc 1989;64:911–919.
108. Stephenson RA, James BC, Gay U. Flow cytometry of prostate cancer: Relationship of DNA content to survival. Cancer Res 1987;47:2504–2509.
109. Robertson CN, Paulson DF. DNA in radical prostatectomy specimens: Prognostic value of tumor ploidy. Acta Oncol 1991;30:205–207.
110. Peters JM, Miles BJ, Kubus JJ, Crissman JD. Prognostic significance of the nuclear DNA content in localized prostatic adenocarcinoma. Anal Quant Cytol Histol 1990;12: 359–364.
111. Abrahamsson PA, Lilja H. Three predominant prostatic proteins. Andrologia 1990;1: 122–131.
112. Babaian RJ, Lamki LM. Radioimmunoscintigraphy of prostate cancer. Semin Nucl Med 1989;19:309–321.
113. Seamonds B, Yang N, Anderson K, Whitaker B, Shaw LM, Bollinger JR. Evaluation of prostate-specific antigen and prostatic acid phosphatase as prostate cancer markers. Urology 1986;28:472–479.
114. Stamey TA, Yang N, Hay AR, McNeal JE, Freiha FS, Redwine E. Prostate-specific antigen as a serum marker for adenocarcinoma of the prostate. N Engl J Med 1987;317: 909–916.
115. Leitenberger A, Altwein JE. Efficacy and discriminative ability of prostate-specific antigen as a tumor marker. Eur Urol 1990;17:12–16.
116. Gallee MP, Visser de JE, van der Korput Ja, et al. Variation of prostate-specific antigen expression in different tumour growth patterns present in prostatectomy specimens. Urol Res 1990;18:181–187.
117. Young CY, Montgomery BT, Andrews PE, Qui SD, Bilhartz DL, Tindall DJ. Hormonal regulation of prostate-specific antigen messenger RNA in human prostatic adeno-carcinoma cell line LNCaP. Cancer Res 1991;51:3748–3752.
118. Lee H, Chu TM, Lee CL. Endogenous protein substrates for prostatic acid phosphatase in human prostate. Prostate 1991;19:251–263.
119. Lin MF, Li SS, Chu TM, Lee CL. Comparison of prostate acid phosphatase with acid phosphatase isoenzymes from the lung and spleen. J Clin Lab Anal 1990;4:420–425.
120. Nguyen L, Chapdelaine A, Chevalier S. Prostatic acid phosphatase in serum of patients with prostatic cancer is a specific phosphotyrosine acid phosphatase. Clin Chem 1990;36:1440–1455.
121. Van ER, Davidson R, Stevis PE, MacArthur H, Moore DL. Covalent structure, disulfide bonding, and identification of reactive surface and active site residues of human prostatic acid phosphatase. J Biol Chem 1991;266:2313–2319.
122. Lee H, Chu TM, Li SS, Lee CL. Homodimer and heterodimer subunits of human prostate acid phosphatase. Biochem J 1991;277:759–765.
123. Winqvist R, Virkkunen P, Grzeschik KH, Vihko P. Chromosomal localization to 3q21-qter and two TaqI RFLPs of the human prostate-specific acid phosphatase gene (ACPP). Cytogenet Cell Genet 1989;52:68–71.
124. Peters C, Geier C, Pohlmann R, et al. High degree of homology between primary structure of human lysosomal acid phosphatase and human prostatic acid phosphatase. Biol Chem Hoppe Seyler 1989;370:177–181.
125. Solin T, Kontturi M, Pohlmann R, Vihko P. Gene expression and prostate specificity of human prostatic acid phosphatase (PAP): Evaluation by RNA blot analyses. Biochim Biophys Acta 1990;1048:72–77.
126. Roiko K, Janne OA, Vihko P. Primary structure of rat secretory acid phosphatase and comparison to other acid phosphatases. Gene 1990;89:223–229.
127. Ishibe M, Rosier RN, Puzas JE. Human prostatic acid phosphatase directly stimulates collagen synthesis and alkaline phosphatase content of isolated bone cells. J Clin Endocrinol Metab 1991;73:785–792.
128. Oesterling JE. Prostate specific antigen: A critical assessment of the most useful tumor marker for adenocarcinoma of the prostate. J Urol 1991;145:907–923.
129. Bilhartz DL, Tindall DJ, Oesterling JE. Prostate-specific antigen and prostatic acid phosphatase: Biomolecular and physiologic characteristics. Urology 1991;38:95–102.
130. Henttu P, Vihko P. cDNA coding for the entire human prostate specific antigen shows high homologies to the human tissue kallikrein genes. Biochem Biophys Res Commun 1989;160:903–910.
131. Fernandez P.L, Gomez M, Caballero T, Alfaro P, Aguilar D. Prostatic acid phosphatase in cloacogenic carcinoma. Acta Oncol 1990;29:776–777.
132. Kamoshida S, Tsutsumi Y. Extraprostatic localization of prostatic acid phosphatase and prostate-specific antigen: Distribution in cloacogenic glandular epithelium and sex-dependent expression in human anal gland. Hum Pathol 1990;21:1108–1111.
133. Azumi N, Traweek ST, Battifora H. Prostatic acid phosphatase in carcinoid tumors: Immunohistochemical and immunoblot studies. Am J Surg Pathol 1991;15:785–790.

134. Freeman NJ, Doolittle C. Elevated prostate markers in metastatic small cell carcinoma of unknown primary. Cancer 1991;68:1118–1120.

135. Amico S, Liehn JC, Desoize B, Larbre H, Deltour G, Valeyre J. Comparison of phosphatase isoenzymes PAP and PSA with bone scan in patients with prostate carcinoma. Clin Nucl Med 1991;16:643–648.

136. Gerber G, Chodak GW. Assessment of value of routine bone scans in patients with newly diagnosed prostate cancer. Urology 1991;37:418–422.

137. Hetherington JW, Siddall JK, Cooper EH. Contribution of bone scintigraphy, prostatic acid phosphatase and prostate-specific antigen to the monitoring of prostatic cancer. Eur Urol 1988;14:1–5.

138. Goldrath DE, Messing EM. Prostate specific antigen: Not detectable despite tumor progression after radical prostatectomy. J Urol 1989;142:1082–1084.

139. Lange PH, Ercole CJ, Lightner DJ, Fraley EE, Vassella R. The value of serum prostate specific antigen determinations before and after radical prostatectomy. J Urol 1989;141:873–879.

140. Pontes JE. New developments in biological markers in prostate cancer. Recent Results Cancer Res 1990;118:186–189.

141. Lange PH. Prostate-specific antigen for staging prior to surgery and for early detection of recurrence after surgery. Urol Clin North Am 1990;17:813–817.

142. Meek AG, Park TL, Oberman E, Wielopolski L. A prospective study of prostate specific antigen levels in patients receiving radiotherapy for localized carcinoma of the prostate. Int J Radiat Oncol Biol Phys 1990;19:733–741.

143. Walsh PC, Oesterling JE, Epstein JI, Bruzek DJ, Rock RC, Chan DW. The value of prostate-specific antigen in the management of localized prostatic cancer. Prog Clin Biol Res 1989;303:27–33.

144. Oesterling JE, Chan DW, Epstein JI, et al. Prostate specific antigen in the preoperative and postoperative evaluation of localized prostatic cancer treated with radical prostatectomy. J Urol 1988;139:766–772.

145. Morgan WR, Zincke H, Rainwater LM, Myers RP, Klee GG. Prostate specific antigen values after radical retropubic prostatectomy for adenocarcinoma of the prostate: Impact of adjuvant treatment (hormonal and radiation). J Urol 1991;145:319–323.

146. Link P, Freiha FS, Stamey TA. Adjuvant radiation therapy in patients with detectable prostate specific antigen following radical prostatectomy. J Urol 1991;145:532–534.

147. Lange PH. Controversies in management of apparently localized carcinoma of prostate. Urology 1989;34(Suppl):13–17.

148. Zagars GK, Sherman NE, Babaian RJ. Prostate-specific antigen and external beam radiation therapy in prostate cancer. Cancer 1991;67:412–420.

149. van Eijkeren M, van Haelst JP. Monitoring of prostate-specific antigen during external beam radiotherapy for carcinoma of the prostate. Strahlenther Onkol 1990;166:557–561.

150. Schellhammer PF, Schlossberg SM, el MA, Wright GL, Brassil DN. Prostate specific antigen levels after definitive irradiation for carcinoma of the prostate. J Urol 1991;145:1008–1010.

151. Landmann C, Hunig R. Prostatic specific antigen as an indicator of response to radiotherapy in prostate cancer. Int J Radiat Oncol Biol Phys 1989;17:1073–1076.

152. Kaplan ID, Cox RS, Bagshaw MA. A model of prostatic carcinoma tumor kinetics based on prostate specific antigen levels after radiation therapy. Cancer 1991;68:400–405.

153. Chodak GW, Neumann J, Blix G, Sutton H, Farah R. Effect of external beam radiation therapy on serum prostate-specific antigen. Urology 1990;35:288–294.

154. Arai Y, Yoshiki T, Yoshida O. Prognostic significance of prostate specific antigen in endocrine treatment for prostatic cancer. J Urol 1990;144:1415–1419.

155. Dupont A, Cusan L, Gomez JL, Thibeault MM, Labrie F. Prostate specific antigen and prostatic acid phosphatase for monitoring therapy of carcinoma of the prostate. J Urol 1991;146:1064–1067.

156. Leo ME, Bilhartz DL, Bergstralh EJ, Oesterling JE. Prostate specific antigen in hormonally treated stage D2 prostate cancer: Is it always an accurate indicator of disease status? J Urol 1991;145:802–806.

157. Matzkin H, Lewyshon O, Ayalon D, Braf Z. Changes in prostate-specific markers under chronic gonadotrophin-releasing hormone analogue treatment of state D prostatic cancer. Cancer 1989;63:1287–1291.

158. Mecz Y, Barak M, Lurie A, Gruener N. Prognostic importance of the rate of decrease in prostate specific antigen levels after treatment of patients with carcinoma of the prostate. J Tumor Marker Oncol 1989;4:323–328.

159. Scher HI, Curley T, Geller N, et al. Trimetrexate in prostatic cancer: Preliminary observations on the use of prostate-specific antigen and acid phosphatase as a marker in measurable hormone-refractory disease. J Clin Oncol 1990;8:1830–1838.

160. Myers C, Cooper M, Stein C, et al. Suramin: A novel growth factor antagonist with activity in hormone-refractory metastatic prostate cancer. J Clin Oncol 1992;10:881–889.

161. Gerster AG. On surgical dissemination of cancer. NY Med J 1885;41:233–236.

162. Roberts S, Jonasson O, Long L, McGrew EA, McGrath R, Cole WH. Relationship of cancer cells in circulating blood to operation. Cancer 1962;15:332–340.

163. Cole WH, McDonald GO, Roberts SS, Southwick HW. Dissemination of cancer: Prevention and therapy. New York: Appleton-Century-Crofts, 1961.

164. Turnbull RB, Kyle K, Watson FR, Spratt J. Cancer of the colon: The influence of the no-touch isolation technique on survival rates. Ann Surg 1967;166:420–427.

165. Jonasson O, Long L, Roberts S, McGrew E, McDonald JH. Cancer cells in the circulating blood during operative management of genitourinary tumors. J Urol 1961;85:1–12.

166. McGowan DH. The adverse influence of prior transurethral resection on prognosis in carcinoma of prostate treated by radiation therapy. Int J Radiat Oncol Biol Phys 1980;6:1121–1126.

167. Hanks GE, Leibel S, Kramer S. The dissemination of cancer by transurethral resection of locally advanced prostate cancer. J Urol 1983;129:309–311.

168. Forman JD, Zinreich E, Lee D, Wharam MD, Baumgardner RA, Order SE. Improving the therapeutic ratio of external beam irradiation for carcinoma of the prostate. Int J Radiat Oncol Biol Phys 1985;11:2072–2080.

169. Perez CA. Carcinoma of the prostate, a vexing biological and clinical enigma. Int J Radiat Oncol Biol Phys 1983;9:1427–1438.

170. Elder JS, Haferman MD. Does transurethral resection disseminate prostatic cancer? Radiology 1984;153:156.

171. Pilepich MV, Krall JM. Correlation of pretreatment transurethral resection and prognosis in patients with stage C carcinoma of the prostate treated with definitive radiotherapy—RTOG experience. Int J Radiat Oncol Biol Phys 1987;13:195–199.

172. Sandler HM, Hanks GE. Analysis of the possibility that transurethral resection promotes metastasis in prostate cancer. Cancer 1988;62:2622–2627.

173. Meacham RB, Scardino PT, Hoffman GS, Easley JD, Wilbanks JH, Carlton CEJ. The risk of distant metastases after transurethral resection of the prostate versus needle biopsy in patients with localized prostate cancer. J Urol 1989;142:320–325.

174. Kuban DA, El-Mahdi AM, Schellhammer PF, Babb TJ. The effect of transurethral prostatic resection on the incidence of osseous prostatic metastasis. Cancer 1985;56:961–964.

175. Fowler JE, Fisher HAG, Kaiser DL, Whitmore WF. Relationship of pretreatment transurethral resection of the prostate to survival without distant metastases in patients treated with 125-I implantation for localized prostatic cancer. Cancer 1984;53:1857–1863.

176. Paulson DF, Cox EB. Does transurethral resection of the prostate promote metastatic disease? J Urol 1987;138:90–91.

177. Hammarsten, Johansson JE. Personal communication. November, 1991.

178. Catalona WJ, Scott WW. Carcinoma of the prostate. In: Walsh PC, Gittes RF, Perlmutter AD, Stamey TA. Campbell's urology. Philadelphia: WB Saunders, 1986:1463–1534.

179. Catalona WJ, Miller DR, Kavoussi LR. Intermediate-term survival results in clinically understaged prostate cancer patients following radical prostatectomy. J Urol 1988;140:540–543.

180. McConnell JD. Medical management of benign prostatic hyperplasia with androgen suppression. Prostate 1990;3(Suppl):49–59.

181. Bernstein LH, Rudolph RA, Pinto MM, Viner N, Zuckerman H. Medically significant concentrations of prostate-specific antigen in serum assessed. Clin Chem 1990;36:515–518.

182. Moon TD, Clejan S. Prostate cancer screening in younger men: Prostate-specific antigen and public awareness. Urology 1991;38:216–219.

183. Littrup PJ, Kane RA, Williams CR, et al. Determination of prostate volume with transrectal US for cancer screening. I. Comparison with prostate-specific antigen assays. Radiology 1991;178:537–542.

184. Chadwick DJ, Kemple T, Astley JP, et al. Pilot study of screening for prostate cancer in general practice. Lancet 1991;338:613–616.

185. Babaian RJ, Miyashita H, Evans RB, von EA, Ramirez EI. Early detection program for prostate cancer: Results and identification of high-risk patient population. Urology 1991;37:193–197.

186. Perrin P, Maquet JH, Bringeon G, Devonec M. Screening for prostate cancer. Comparison of transrectal ultrasound, prostate specific antigen and rectal examination. Br J Urol 1991;68:263–265.

187. Barzell W, Beam MA, Hilaris BS, Whitmore WF. Prostatic adenocarcinoma: Relationship of grade and local extent to the pattern of metastases. J Urol 1977;118:278–282.

188. Fowler JE, Whitmore WF. The incidence and extent of pelvic lymph node metastases in apparently localized prostatic cancer. Cancer 1981;47:2941–2945.

189. Donahue RE, Man JH, Whitesel JA, et al. Pelvic lymph node dissection: Guide to patient management in clinically locally confined adenocarcinoma of the prostate. Urology 1982;20:559–565.

190. Stamey TA, Villers AA, McNeal JE, Link PC, Freiha FS. Positive surgical margins at radical prostatectomy: Importance of the apical dissection. J Urol 1990;143:1166–1173.

191. Catalona WJ, Bigg SW. Nerve-sparing radical prostatectomy: Evaluation of results after 250 patients. J Urol 1990;143:538.

192. Walsh PC. Radical prostatectomy, preservation of sexual function, cancer control: The controversy. Urol Clin North Am 1987;14:663.

193. Batson OV. The function of the vertebral veins and their role in the spread of metastases. Ann Surg 1940;112:138–149.

194. Dodds PR, Caride VJ, Lytton B. The role of vertebral veins in the dissemination of prostatic carcinoma. J Urol 1981;126:753–755.

195. Hanks GE. Radiotherapy or surgery for prostate cancer: Ten and fifteen-year results of external beam therapy. Acta Oncol 1991;30:231–237.

196. Bagshaw MA. Radiotherapeutic treatment of prostatic carcinoma with pelvic node involvement. Urol Clin North Am 1984;11:297–304.

197. Spellman MC, Castellino RA, Ray GR. An evaluation of lymphography in localized carcinoma of the prostate. Radiology 1977;25:637.

198. Hricak H. Noninvasive imaging for staging of prostate cancer: Magnetic resonance imaging, computed tomography, and ultrasound. NCI Monogr 1988;7:31–36.

199. Hanks GE, Krall JM, Pilepich MV. Comparison of pathologic and clinical evaluation of lymph nodes in prostate cancer: Implications of RTOG data for patient management and trial design and stratification. Int J Radiat Oncol Biol Phys 1992;23:293–298.

200. Hanks GE, Soffen EM, Chu JC, Stafford PM. Conformal static field radiation therapy treatment of low volume low grade prostate cancer: Immobilization, dose volume histograms, and acute morbidity. Proc Euro Soc Therap Radiol Oncol 1990:27–40.

201. Rifkin MD, Zerhouni EA, Gatsonis CA, et al. Comparison of magnetic resonance imaging and ultrasonography in staging early prostate cancer. N Engl J Med 1990;323: 621–626.

201a. Schnall MD, Imai Y, Tomaszewski J, et al. Prostate cancer: Local staging with endorectal surface coil MR imaging. Radiology 1991;178:797–802.

201b. Schroeder FH, Hermanke P, Denis L, Fair WR, Gospodarowicz MK, Pavone-Macaluso M. The TNM classification of prostate cancer. Prostate 1992;4(Suppl):129–138.

202. U.S. Dept of Health and Human Sciences. Consensus development conference on the management of clinically localized prostate cancer. NCI Monogr 1988;7:1–185.

203. National Institutes of Health. Consensus development conference statement. U.S. Government Printing Office 1987:6.

204. Beahrs OH, Henson DE, Hutter RV, Myers MH. Manual for staging of cancer. Philadelphia: JB Lippincott, 1988:177–182.

205. Hanks GE. External beam radiation for prostate cancer: Patterns of Care studies in the United States. NCI Monogr 1988;7:85–94.

206. Epstein BE, Hanks GE. Prostate cancer: Definitive treatment in the 1990's. Cancer (in press).

207. Johansson JE. Personal communication.

208. Markiewicz D, Hanks GE. Therapeutic options in the management of incidental carcinoma of the prostate. Int J Radiat Oncol Biol Phys 1991;20:153–167.

209. Hanks GE, Asbell S, Krall JM, et al. Outcome for lymph node dissection negative T-1b, T-2 (A-2, B) prostate cancer treated with external beam radiation therapy in RTOG 77-06. Int J Radiat Oncol Biol Phys 1991;21:1099–1103.

210. Mulholland G. A second look at prostate cancer. Am Cancer Soc News 1988;III.

211. Elder JS, Jewett MJ, Walsh PC. Radical perineal prostatectomy for clinical stage B2 carcinoma of the prostate. J Urol 1986;127:704–706.

212. Gibbons RP, Correa RJ, Brannen E. Total prostatectomy for localized prostatic cancer. J Urol 1984;131:73–76.

213. Bagshaw MA. Potential for radiotherapy alone in prostatic cancer. Cancer 1985;55: 2079–2085.

214. Syed AMN, Puthawala A, Austin P, et al. Temporary iridium-192 implant in the management of carcinoma of the prostate. Cancer 1992;69:2515–2524.

215. Kuban D, El-Mahdi A, Schellhammer P. I-125 interstitial implantation for prostate cancer. Cancer 1989;63:2415–2420.

216. Fuks Z, Leibel S, Wallner K, et al. The effect of local control on metastatic dissemination in carcinoma of the prostate: Long term results in patients treated with I-125 implantation. Int J Radiat Oncol Biol Phys 1991;21:537–547.

217. Koprowski CD, Berkenstock KG, Borofski AM, Ziegler JC, Lightfoot dA, Brady LW. External beam irradiation versus 125 iodine implant in the definitive treatment of prostate carcinoma. Int J Radiat Oncol Biol Phys 1991;21:955–960.

218. Paulson DF, Lin GH, Hinshaw W. Radical surgery versus radiotherapy for adenocarcinoma of the prostate. J Urol 1982;128:502–504.

219. Middleton RG, Smith JA, Melzer RB. Patient survival and local recurrence rate following radical prostatectomy for prostatic carcinoma. J Urol 1986;136:422–424.

220. Bagshaw MA, Cox RS, Ray GR. Status of radiation treatment of prostate cancer at Stanford University. NCI Monogr 1988;7:47–60.

221. Shipley WU, Prout GR, Coachman NM, et al. Radiation therapy for localized prostate carcinoma: Experience at the Massachusetts General Hospital (1973–1981). NCI Monogr 1988;7:85–94.

222. Perez CA, Pilepich MW, Garcia D, Simpson JR, Zivnuska F, Hederman MA. Definitive radiation therapy in carcinoma of the prostate localized to the pelvis: Experience at the Mallinckrodt Institute of Radiology. NCI Monogr 1988;7:85–94.

223. Zagars GK, von Eschenbach AC, Johnson DE, Oswald MJ. Stage C adenocarcinoma of the prostate: An analysis of 551 patients treated with external beam radiation. Cancer 1987;60:1489–1499.

224. Soffen EM, Epstein BE, Hunt MA, Hanks GE. Decreased acute morbidity with conformal static field radiation therapy treatment of early prostate cancer as compared to non-conformal techniques. Int J Radiat Oncol Biol Phys (in press).

225. Ten Haken RK, Perez-Tamayo C, Tesser RJ, McShan DL, Fraass BA, Lichter AS. Boost treatment of the prostate using shaped, fixed fields. Int J Radiat Oncol Biol Phys 1989;16:193–200.

226. Hanks GE. The prostate. Moss WT, Cox JD, eds. Radiation oncology rationale, technique, results. St. Louis: CV Mosby, 1989:487–511.

227. Soffen EM, Hanks GE, Hwang CC, Chu JCH. Conformal static field therapy for low volume low grade prostate cancer with rigid immobilization. Int J Radiat Oncol Biol Phys 1991;20:142–146.

228. Biggs PJ, Shipley WU. A beam width improving device for a 25 MV x-ray beam. Int J Radiat Oncol Biol Phys 1986;12:131–135.

229. Hanks GE. External beam radiation for prostate cancer: The gold standard of treatment for 30 years. Oncology 1992;6:79–86.

230. Paulson DF, Moul JW, Walther PJ. Radical prostatectomy for clinical stage T1-2N0M0 prostatic adenocarcinoma: Long term results. J Urol 1990;144:1180–1184.

231. Golimbu M, Morales P, Al-Askari S, Brown J. Extended pelvic lymphadenectomy in prostate cancer. J Urol 1979;121:617–620.

232. Schuessler WW, Vancaillie TG, Raich H, Griffith DP. Transperitoneal endosurgical lymphadenectomy in patients with localized prostate cancer. J Urol 1991;145:988–991.

233. Tomlinson RL, Currie DP, Boyce WH. Radical prostatectomy: Palliation for stage C carcinoma of the prostate. J Urol 1977;117:85–87.

234. Hanks GE, Diamond JJ, Kramer S. The need for complex technology in radiation oncology: Correlations of facility characteristics and structure with outcome. Cancer 1985;55:2198–2201.

235. Kramer S. The patterns of care study: A nationwide evaluation of the practice of radiation therapy in cancer management. Int J Radiat Oncol Biol Phys 1976;1:1231–1236.

236. Hanks GE, Martz KL, Diamond JJ. The effect of dose on local control of prostate cancer [see comments]. Int J Radiat Oncol Biol Phys 1988;15:1299–1305.

237. Perez CA, Walz BJ, Zivnuska FR. Irradiation of carcinoma of the prostate localized to the pelvis: Analysis of tumor response and prognosis. Int J Radiat Oncol Biol Phys 1980;6:555–565.

238. Hanks GE. Unpublished data.

239. Stafford PM, Martin EE, Chu JCH, Davidson BA, Hanks GE. Digital imaging in the radiation oncology environment: A personal computer local area network solution. J Digit Imaging 1991;4:177–184.

240. Stafford PM, Chakraborty DP, Martin E, Wong J, Hanks GE. A characterization of two commercially available real-time portal imaging systems. Int J Radiat Oncol Biol Phys 1991;21:124–125.

241. Laramore GE, Krall JM, Thomas FJH, Griffin TW, Maor MH, Hendrickson FR. Fast neutron radiotherapy for locally advanced prostate cancer: Results of an RTOG randomized study. Int J Radiat Oncol Biol Phys 1985;11:1261–1267.

242. Dutenhaver JR, Shipley WU, Perrone TL. Protons or megavoltage x-rays as boost therapy for patients irradiated for localized prostatic carcinoma. Cancer 1983;51: 1599–1604.

243. Whitmore WF. Interstitial radiation therapy for carcinoma of the prostate. Prostate 1980;1:157.

244. Carlton CE, Scardino PT. Long-term results after combined radioactive gold seed implantation and external beam radiotherapy for localized prostate cancer. In: Coffey DS, Resnick MI, Dorr FA, Karr JP, eds. A multidisciplinary analysis of controversies in the management of prostate cancer. New York: Plenum, 1988:109–121.

245. Kwon ED, Loening SA, Hawtrey CE. Radical prostatectomy and adjuvant radioactive gold seed placement: Results of treatment at 5 and 10 years for clinical stages A2, B1 and B2 cancer of the prostate. J Urol 1991;145:524–531.

246. Syed AMN, Puthawala A, Austin P, Cherlow J, Shanberg A, Tansey L. Role of temporary iridium-192 implant in the treatment of carcinoma of the prostate. Int J Radiat Oncol Biol Phys 1990;19:190-.

247. Brindel JS, Martinez A, Schray M, et al. Pelvic lymphadenectomy and transperineal interstitial implantation of IR-192 combined with external beam radiotherapy for bulky stage C prostatic carcinoma. Int J Radiat Oncol Biol Phys 1989;17:1063–1066.

248. Wallner K, Chiu-Tsao S, Roy J, et al. An improved method for computerized tomography-planned transperineal 125-iodine prostate implants. J Urol 1991;146:90–95.

248a. Blasko JC, Radge H, Grimm PD. Transperineal ultrasound-guided implantation of the prostate: Morbidity and complications. Scand J Urol Nephrol 1991;137(Suppl): 113–118.

249. Sedransk N, Sedransk J. Distinguishing among distributions using data from complex designs. J Am Stat Assoc 1979;74:754–760.

250. Zagars GK, von Eschenbach AC, Johnson DE, Oswald MJ. The role of radiation therapy in stages A2 and B adenocarcinoma of the prostate. Int J Radiat Oncol Biol Phys 1988;14:701–709.

251. Morton RA, Steiner MS, Walsh PC. Cancer control following anatomical radical prostatectomy: An interim report. J Urol 1991;145:1197–1200.

252. Hanks GE. More on the Uro-Oncology Research Group report of radical surgery vs. radiotherapy for adenocarcinoma of the prostate 'letter.' Int J Radiat Oncol Biol Phys 1988;14:1053–1054.

253. Rounsaville MC, Green JP, Vaeth JM, Purdon RP, Heltzel MM. Prostatic carcinoma: Limited field irradiation. Int J Radiat Oncol Biol Phys 1987;13:1013–1020.

254. Lawton CA, Won M, Pilepich MV, et al. Long-term treatment sequelae following external beam irradiation for adenocarcinoma of the prostate: Analysis of RTOG studies 7506 and 7706. Int J Radiat Oncol Biol Phys 1991;21:935–939.

255. Pilepich MV, Krall JM, Johnson RJ, et al. Extended field (peri-aortic) irradiation in carcinoma of the prostate: Analysis of RTOG 75-06. Int J Radiat Oncol Biol Phys 1986;12:345–351.

256. Hanks GE, Edland RW, Diamond JJ. Variation in the technical support of radiation oncology in different practice settings. Am J Surg Pathol 1989;16:1583–1586.

257. Hanks GE. Radical prostatectomy or radiation therapy for early prostate cancer: Two roads to the same end. Cancer 1988;61:2153–2160.

258. Sewell RA, Braren V, Wilson SK. Extended biopsy followup after full course radiation for resectable prostatic carcinoma. J Urol 1975;113:371–373.

259. Cox JD, Staffel TJ. The significance of needle biopsy after irradiation for stage C adenocarcinoma of the prostate. Cancer 1977;40:156–160.

260. Scardino PT. The prognostic significance of biopsies after radiotherapy for prostatic cancer. Sem Urol 1983;1:243–251.

261. Schellhammer PF, Lagada LE, El-Mahdi A. Histologic characteristics of prostatic biopsies after iodine-125 implantation. J Urol 1980;123:700–705.

262. Freiha FS, Bagshaw MA. Carcinoma of the prostate: Results of post-irradiation biopsy. Prostate 1984;5:19–25.

263. Kabalin JN, Hodge KK, McNeal JE, Freiha FS, Stamey TA. Identification of residual cancer in the prostate following radiation therapy: Role of transrectal ultrasound guided biopsy and prostate specific antigen. J Urol 1989;142:326–331.

264. Kuban DA, El-Mahdi AM, Schellhammer PF, Lagada LE. The significance of post-irradiation prostate biopsy with long-term follow-up. Int J Radiat Oncol Biol Phys 1991;21(Suppl 1):191.

265. Hanks GE, Dawson AK. The role of external beam radiation therapy after prostatectomy for prostate cancer. Cancer 1986;58:2406–2410.

266. Anscher MS, Prosnitz LR. Multivariate analysis of factors predicting local relapse after radical prostatectomy—possible indications for postoperative radiotherapy. Int J Radiat Oncol Biol Phys 1991;21:941–947.

267. Robey EL, Schellhammer PF. Local failure after definitive therapy for prostatic cancer. J Urol 1987;137:613–619.

268. Percival RC, Urwin GH, Harris S, et al. Biochemical and histological evidence that carcinoma of the prostate is associated with increased bone resorption. Eur J Surg Oncol 1987;13:41–49.

269. Clarke NW, McClure J, George NJ. Morphometric evidence for bone resorption and replacement in prostate cancer. Br J Urol 1991;68:74–80.

270. Riancho JA, Arjona R, Valle R, Sanz J, Gonz:alez MJ. The clinical spectrum of hypocalcaemia associated with bone metastases. J Intern Med 1989;226:449–452.

271. Burki F, Coindre JM, Mauriac L. Sclerotic bone metastases of prostatic origin and osteomalacia: Importance of a histomorphometry study. Prog Clin Biol Res 1987;243: 569–571.

272. Minisola S, Perugia G, Scarda A, et al. Biochemical picture accompanying sclerotic bone metastases of prostatic origin. Br J Urol 1987;60:443–446.

273. Chackal RM, Niemeyer C, Moore M, Zetter BR. Stimulation of human prostatic carcinoma cell growth by factors present in human bone marrow. J Clin Invest 1989;84: 43–50.

274. Bennett A. The role of biochemical mediators in peripheral nociception and bone pain. Cancer Surv 1988;7:55–67.

275. Davies P, Bailey PJ, Goldenberg MM, Ford HA. The role of arachidonic acid oxygenation products in pain and inflammation. Annu Rev Immunol 1984;2:335–357.

276. Drago JR, Rohner TJ, Demers LM. The synthesis of prostaglandins by the Nb rat prostate tumor. Anticancer Res 1985;5:393–395.

277. Dunzendorfer U, Zahradnik HP, Gerster K. 13,14-Dihydro-15-keto-prostaglandin F2 alpha in patients with urogenital tumors. Urol Int 1980;35:171–175.

278. Hensby CN, Khan QM, Williams G, Dollery CT. The possible role of circulating 6-oxo-PGF1 alpha in monitoring the growth and spread of malignant disease of the prostate. Prog Lipid Res 1981;20:681–683.

279. Karmali RA, Reichel P, Cohen LA, et al. The effects of dietary omega-3 fatty acids on the DU-145 transplantable human prostatic tumor. Anticancer Res 1987;7:1173–1179.

280. Khan O, Hensby CN, Williams G. Prostacyclin in prostatic cancer: A better marker than bone scan or serum acid phosphatase? Br J Urol 1982;54:26–31.

281. Norrdin RW, Jee WS, High WB. The role of prostaglandins in bone in vivo. Prostaglandins Leukot Essent Fatty Acids 1990;41:139–149.

282. Urwin GH, Percival RC, Yates AJ, et al. Biochemical markers and skeletal metabolism in carcinoma of the prostate: Use of decision matrix theory and ROC analysis. Br J Urol 1985;57:711–714.

283. Al MH, Drago J, Bartholomew MJ. The fibrinolytic system in experimental prostate tumor. Thromb Haemost 1986;56:133–136.

284. Al MH, Manni A, Owen J, Gordon R. Hemostatic effects of hormonal stimulation in patients with metastatic prostate cancer. Am J Hematol 1988;28:141–145.

285. Bhadoria DP, Mukhopadhyay DK, Mehta S, Mittal D, Rao YV, Malhotra KK. Emergency treatment with ketoconazole in disseminated intravascular coagulation due to metastatic prostatic carcinoma [published erratum appears in J Assoc Physicians India 1990;38(3): 205]. J Assoc Physicians India 1989;37:792–793.

286. Blomback M, Hedlund PO, Sawe U. Changes in blood coagulation and fibrinolysis in patients on different treatment regimens for prostatic cancer: Predictors for cardio-vascular complications? Thromb Res 1988;49:111–121.

287. Goldenberg SL, Fenster HN, Perler Z, McLoughlin MG. Disseminated intravascular coagulation in carcinoma of prostate: Role of estrogen therapy. Urology 1983;22: 130–132.

288. Henriksson P, Blomback M, Bratt G, Edhag O, Eriksson A. Activators and inhibitors of coagulation and fibrinolysis in patients with prostatic cancer treated with oestrogen or orchidectomy. Thromb Res 1986;44:783–791.

289. Koller A, Kirchheimer J, Pfluger H, Binder BR. Tissue plasminogen activator activity in prostatic cancer. Eur Urol 1984;10:389–394.

290. Martinez JF, Tabernero RM, Alberca SI, Lopez BA. Disseminated intravascular coagulation in prostatic carcinoma reversed by antiandrogenic therapy. JAMA [Letter] 1988;260:2507.

291. Shepherd SM, Lyon WK. Gingival bleeding: Initial presentation of prostate cancer. J Fam Pract 1990;30:98–100.

292. Schacter L, Rozencweig M, Canetta R, Kelley S, Nicaise C, Smaldone L. Megestrol acetate: Clinical experience. Cancer Treat Rev 1989;16:49–63.

293. Scher HI, Yagoda A. Bone metastases: Pathogenesis, treatment, and rationale for use of resorption inhibitors. Am J Med 1987;82:6–28.

293a. Miller JI, Ahmann FR, Drach GW, et al. The clinical usefulness of serum prostate specific antigen after hormonal therapy of metastatic prostate cancer. J Urol 1992;147: 956–961.

294. Eisenberger MA. Chemotherapy for endocrine resistant cancer of the prostate. Prog Clin Biol Res 1990;359:155–164.

295. Eisenberger MA., Kennedy P, Abrams J. How effective is cytotoxic chemotherapy for disseminated prostatic carcinoma? Oncology (Williston Park) 1987;1:59–71.

296. Eisenberger MA, Simon R, O'Dwyer PJ, Wittes RE, Friedman MA. A reevaluation of nonhormonal cytotoxic chemotherapy in the treatment of prostatic carcinoma. J Clin Oncol 1985;3:827–841.

297. Eisenberger MA, Bezerdjian L, Kalash S. A critical assessment of the role of chemotherapy for endocrine-resistant prostatic carcinoma. Urol Clin North Am 1987;14: 695–706.

298. Eisenberger MA, Abrams JS. Chemotherapy for prostatic carcinoma. Semin Urol 1988;6:303–310.

299. Isaacs JT, Schulze H, Coffey DS. Development of androgen resistance in prostatic cancer. Prog Clin Biol Res 1987;243:21–31.

300. Schulze H, Isaacs JT, Coffey DS. A critical review of the concept of total androgen ablation in the treatment of prostate cancer. Prog Clin Biol Res 1987;243:1–19.

301. Martikainen P, Kyprianou N, Tucker RW, Isaacs JT. Programmed death of nonproliferating androgen-independent prostatic cancer cells. Cancer Res 1991;51:4693–4700.

302. Martikainen P, Isaacs J. Role of calcium in the programmed death of rat prostatic glandular cells. Prostate 1990;17:175–187.

303. Kyprianou N, English HF, Isaacs JT. Programmed cell death during regression of PC-82 human prostate cancer following androgen ablation. Cancer Res 1990;50: 3748–3753.

304. Rittmaster RS, Magor KE, Manning AP, Norman RW, Lazier CB. Differential effect of 5 alpha-reductase inhibition and castration on androgen-regulated gene expression in rat prostate. Mol Endocrinol 1991;5:1023–1029.

305. Brinkmann AO, Kuiper GG, Ris SC, et al. Androgen receptor abnormalities. J Steroid Biochem Mol Biol 1991;40:349–352.

306. Harper M, Pike A, Peeling W, Griffiths K. Steroids of adrenal origin metabolized by human prostatic tissue both in vivo and in vitro. J Endocr 1974;60:117–122.

307. Geller J, Albert J, Vik A. Advantages of total androgen blockade in the treatment of advanced prostate cancer. Semin Oncol 1988;15:53–61.

308. Labrie F, Luthy I, Veilleux R, Simard J, Belanger A, Dupont A. New concepts on the androgen sensitivity of prostate cancer. Prog Clin Biol Res 1987;243:145–172.

309. Carter HB, Isaacs JT. Experimental and theoretical basis for hormonal treatment of prostatic cancer. Semin Urol 1988;6:262–268.

310. Huggins C. The effect of castration, of estrogen and of androgen injections on serum phosphatases in metastatic carcinoma of the prostate: Studies on prostatic cancer. Cancer Res 1941;1:293–297.

311. Huggins C, Stevens R, Hodges C. The effect of castration on advanced carcinoma of the prostate gland: Studies on prostatic cancer. Arch Surg 1941;43:209–223.

312. Swanson LJ, Seely JH, Garnick MB. Gonadotropin-releasing hormone analogs and prostatic cancer. Crit Rev Oncol Hematol 1988;8:1–26.

313. Smith JA. Luteinizing hormone-releasing hormone (LH-RH) analogs in treatment of prostatic cancer: Clinical perspective. Urology 1986;27(Suppl):9–15.

314. Garnick MB. Leuprolide versus diethylstilbestrol for previously untreated stage D2 prostate cancer: Results of a prospectively randomized trial. Urology 1986;27(Suppl): 21–28.

315. Namer M. Clinical applications of antiandrogens. J Steroid Biochem 1988;31:719–729.

316. De Voogt HJ. Cyproterone acetate as monotherapy in prospective randomized trials. Prog Clin Biol Res 1990;359:85–91.

317. Gaillard MM. Pharmacology of antiandrogens and value of combining androgen suppression with antiandrogen therapy. Urology 1991.

318. Goldenberg SL, Bruchovsky N. Use of cyproterone acetate in prostate cancer. Urol Clin North Am 1991;18:111–122.

319. Habenicht UF, Schroder H, el EM, Neumann F. Advantages and disadvantages of pure antiandrogens and of antiandrogens of the cyproterone acetate-type in the treatment of prostatic cancer. Prog Clin Biol Res 1988;260:63–75.

320. Kennealey GT, Furr BJ. Use of the nonsteroidal anti-androgen Casodex in advanced prostatic carcinoma. Urol Clin North Am 1991;18:99–110.

321. Schroder FH. Antiandrogenic substances in the management of prostatic cancer. Recent Results Cancer Res 1990;118:163–173.

322. Schroder FH. Pure antiandrogens as monotherapy in prospective studies of prostatic carcinoma. Prog Clin Biol Res 1990;359:93–103.

323. Tunn UW. Cyproterone acetate in the management of prostatic cancer. Prog Clin Biol Res 1989;303:105–110.

324. Nicholson RI, Walker KJ, Davies P. Hormone agonists and antagonists in the treatment of hormone sensitive breast and prostate cancer. Cancer Surv 1986;5:463–486.

325. Labrie F, Dupont A, Giguere M, et al. Combination therapy with flutamide and castration (orchiectomy or LHRH agonist): The minimal endocrine therapy in both untreated and previously treated patients. J Steroid Biochem 1987;27:525–532.

326. Kung TT, Mingo GG, Siegel MI, Watnick AS. Effect of adrenalectomy, flutamide, and leuprolide on the growth of the Dunning rat R-3327 prostatic carcinoma. Prostate 1988;12:357–363.

327. Crawford ED, Eisenberger MA, McLeod DG, et al. A controlled trial of leuprolide with and without flutamide in prostatic carcinoma [published erratum appears in N Engl J Med 1989 Nov 16;321(20):1420]. N Engl J Med 1989;321:419–424.

328. Crawford ED, Blumenstein BA, Goodman PJ, et al. Leuprolide with and without flutamide in advanced prostate cancer. Cancer 1990.

329. Soloway MS. The importance of pretreatment testosterone and other prognostic variables in the response to androgen deprivation therapy. Prog Clin Biol Res 1990;350: 141–148.

330. Tannock I, Gospodarowicz M, Meakin W, Panzarella T, Stewart L, Rider W. Treatment of metastatic prostatic cancer with low-dose prednisone: Evaluation of pain and quality of life as pragmatic indices of response. J Clin Oncol 1989;7:590–597.

331. Dowsett M, Shearer RJ, Ponder BAJ, Malone P, Jeffcoate SL. The effects of aminoglutethimide and hydrocortisone, alone and combined, on androgen levels in post-orchiectomy prostatic cancer patients. Br J Cancer 1988;57:190–192.

332. Plowman PN, Perry LA, Chard T. Androgen suppression by hydrocortisone without aminoglutethimide in orchidectomised men with prostatic cancer. Br J Urol 1987;59: 255–257.

333. Shaw M, Nicholls P, Smith H. Aminoglutethamide and ketoconazole: Historical perspectives and future prospects. J Biochem 1988;31:137–146.

334. Eichenberger T, Trachtenberg J. Effects of high-dose ketoconazole in patients with androgen-independent prostatic cancer. Am J Clin Oncol 1988;11:104S–107S.

335. Lobie PE, Breipohl W, Aragon JG, Waters MJ. Cellular localization of the growth hormone receptor/binding protein in the male and female reproductive systems. Endocrinology 1990;126:2214–2221.

336. Prieto JC, Carmena MJ. Growth hormone binding and stimulation of amino acid uptake in epithelial cells of rat ventral prostate. Cell Biochem Funct 1987;5:63–68.

337. Davies P, Eaton CL, France TD, Phillips ME. Growth factor receptors and oncogene expression in prostate cells. Am J Clin Oncol 1988.

338. Ho KY, Weissberger AJ, Marbach P, Lazarus L. Therapeutic efficacy of the somatostatin analog SMS 201-995 (octreotide) in acromegaly: Effects of dose and frequency and long-term safety [see comments]. Ann Intern Med 1990;112:173–181.

339. Bogden AE, Taylor JE, Moreau JP, Coy DH. Treatment of R-3327 prostate tumors with a somatostatin analogue (somatuline) as adjuvant therapy following surgical castration. Cancer Res 1990;50:2646–2650.

340. Manni A, Boucher AE, Demers LM, et al. Somatostatin analogues in the treatment of breast and prostate cancer. J Steroid Biochem Mol Biol 1990;37:1083–1087.

341. Zalatnai A, Paz BJ, Redding TW, Schally AV. Histologic changes in the rat prostate cancer model after treatment with somatostatin analogs and D-Trp-6-LH-RH. Prostate 1988;12:85–98.

342. Schally AV, Redding TW, Paz-Bourza JI, Comaru-Schally AM, Mathe G. Current concept for improving treatment of prostate cancer based on combination of LH-RH agonists with other agents. Prog Clin Biol Res 1987;243:173–197.

343. Murphy WA, Lance VA, Moreau S, Moreau JP, Coy DH. Inhibition of rat prostate tumor growth by an octapeptide analog of somatostatin. Life Sci 1987;40:2515–2522.

344. Siegel RA, Tolcsvai L, Rudin M. Partial inhibition of the growth of transplanted dunning rat prostate tumors with the long-acting somatostatin analogue sandostatin (SMS 201–995). Cancer Res 1988;48:4651–4655.

345. Aziz H, Choi K, Sohn C, Yaes R, Rotman M. Comparison of 32P therapy and sequential hemibody irradiation (HBI) for bony metastases as methods of whole body irradiation. Am J Clin Oncol 1986;9:264–268.

346. Hoskin PJ, Ford HT, Harmer CL. Hemibody irradiation (HBI) for metastatic bone pain in two histologically distinct groups of patients. Clin Oncol (R Coll Radiol) 1989;1:67–69.

347. Nseyo UO, Fontanesi J, Naftulin BN. Palliative hemibody irradiation in hormonally refractory metastatic prostate cancer. Urology 1989;34:76–79.

348. Burnet NG, Williams G, Howard N. Phosphorus-32 for intractable bony pain from carcinoma of the prostate. Clin Oncol (R Coll Radiol) 1990;2:220–223.

349. Laing AH, Ackery DM, Bayly RJ, et al. Strontium-89 chloride for pain palliation in prostatic skeletal malignancy. Br J Radiol 1991;64:816–822.

350. Maxon HR, Schroder LE, Hertzberg VS, et al. Rhenium-186(Sn)HEDP for treatment of painful osseous metastases: Results of a double-blind crossover comparison with placebo. J Nucl Med 1991;32:1877–1881.

351. Blake GM, Zivanovic MA, McEwan AJ, Ackery DM. Sr-89 therapy: Strontium kinetics in disseminated carcinoma of the prostate. Eur J Nucl Med 1986;12:447–454.

352. Kim SI, Chen DC, Muggia FM. A new look at radionuclides therapy in metastatic disease of bone (review and prospects). Anticancer Res 1988;8:681–684.

353. Lewington VJ, McEwan AJ, Ackery DM, et al. A prospective randomised double-blind crossover study to examine the efficacy of strontium-89 in pain palliation in patients with advanced prostate cancer metastatic to bone. Eur J Cancer 1991;27:954–958.

354. Maxon HR, Schroder LE, Thomas SR, et al. Re-186(Sn) HEDP for treatment of painful osseous metastases: Initial clinical experience in 20 patients with hormone-resistant prostate cancer. Radiology 1990;176:155–159.

355. Robinson RG, Spicer JA, Preston DF, Wegst AV, Martin NL. Treatment of metastatic bone pain with strontium-89. Int J Rad Appl Instrum [b] 1987;14:219–222.

356. Robinson MR. Carcinoma of the prostate. Objective criteria of response. Am J Clin Oncol 1988;11(Suppl):S48–S52.

357. Turner JH, Claringbold PG, Hetherington EL, Sorby P, Martindale AA. A phase I study of samarium-153 ethylenediaminetetramethylene phosphonate therapy for disseminated skeletal metastases [see comments]. J Clin Oncol 1989;7:1926–1931.

358. Garrett JS, Coughlin SR, Niman HL, Tremble PM, Giels GM, Williams LT. Blockade of autocrine stimulation in simian sarcoma virus-transformed cells reverses downregulation of platelet-derived growth factor receptors. Proc Natl Acad Sci USA 1984;81:7466–7470.

359. Williams LT, Tremble PM, Lavin MF, Sunday ME. Platelet-derived growth factor receptors form a high affinity state in membrane preparations. Kinetics and affinity cross-linking studies. J Biol Chem 1984;259:5287–5294.

360. Coffey RJ, Leof EB, Shipley GD, Moses HL. Suramin inhibition of growth factor receptor binding and mitogenicity in AKR-2B cells. J Cell Physiol 1987;132:143–148.

361. McCaffrey TA, Falcone DJ, Brayton CF, Agarwal LA, Welt F, Weksler BB. TGF-β activity is potentiated by heparin via dissociation of TGF-β-alpha 2 macroglobulin inactive complex. J Cell Biol 1988;109:441–448.

362. Coffey RJ, Goustin AS, Soderquist AM, et al. Transforming growth factor alpha and beta expression in human colon cancer lines: Implications for an autocrine model. Cancer Res 1987;47:4590–4594.

363. Pollak M, Richard M. Suramin blockade of insulinlike growth factor I-stimulated proliferation of human osteosarcoma cells [published erratum appears in JNCI 1990;82:1349–1352.

364. Mohan S, Jennings JC, Linkhart TA, et al. Primary structure of human skeletal growth factor, homology with IGF-II. Biochim Biophys Acta 1988;966:44–55.

365. Madsdeu PO, Graveson PH, Gasser TC, et al. Treatment of localized prostatic cancer: Radical prostatectomy versus placebo. A 15-year follow up. Scand J Urol Nephrol 1988;110(Suppl):95–100.

366. Byar DP, Corle DK, Veterans Administration Cooperative Urological Research Group. VACURG randomized trial of radical prostatectomy for stages I and II prostate cancer. Urology 1981;17:7.

367. Paulson DF. Randomized series of treatment with surgery versus radiation for prostate adenocarcinoma. Monographs NCI 1988;7:127–131.

368. Paulson DF. Carcinoma of the prostate: The therapeutic dilemma. Annu Rev Med 1984;35:341–372.

369. Catalona WJ, Biggs SW. Nerve sparing radical prostatectomy: Evaluation of results of 250 patients. J Urol 1990;143:538–544.

Cancer: Principles & Practice of Oncology, Fourth Edition,
edited by Vincent T. DeVita, Jr., Samuel Hellman, Steven A. Rosenberg.
J.B. Lippincott Co., Philadelphia © 1993.

William R. Fair
Zvi Y. Fuks
Howard I. Scher

CHAPTER **36**

Cancer of the Urethra and Penis

Primary cancer of the urethra and penis is uncommon. The relative rarity of urethral and penile malignancies has contributed to the controversies surrounding their management. No single institution has sufficient patient treatment and follow-up data to define the natural history and establish categorical recommendations for therapy. Most articles dealing with urethral and bladder cancer reflect empiric management strategies and remain essentially anecdotal.

Squamous cell carcinoma is the most common cancer in the penis and urethra. The pattern of spread is primarily a reflection of the area of the organ affected. Likewise, the treatment approach and overall prognosis are related to the region of the urethra or penis involved by tumor.

CARCINOMA OF THE MALE URETHRA

Carcinoma of the male urethra is extremely rare. Approximately 600 cases have been reported in the world literature.[1] Urethral carcinoma has been reported for boys as young as 13 years of age and men in their nineties, although most patients are older than 50 years of age, and the peak incidence occurs at 58 years.[2] Significant etiologic factors have not been identified, but chronic inflammation is thought to play a role in the initiation of the disease on the basis of the observation that many patients relate a history of prior venereal disease, urethritis, or urethral stricture. The incidence of urethral stricture in men with carcinoma of the male urethra ranges from 24% to 76%, and the most frequent site of stricture (*i.e.,* bulbomembranous urethra) is the most frequent site of malignancy.[3–6] No racial predisposition has been recorded.

As with bladder cancer, a high percentage of males with carcinoma of the urethra give a history of smoking or occupational exposure to known carcinogens. However, no epidemiologic studies have unequivocally linked these factors to the development of urethral carcinoma.

SYMPTOMS

The lesion is often insidious at onset, with the symptoms attributed to benign stricture disease rather than to malignancy. Urethral stricture or bleeding in a patient without a history of trauma or venereal disease or the onset of a perineal abscess or fistula in an elderly man should suggest the possibility of urethral carcinoma. Because of the nonspecific nature of the symptoms, the interval between the initiation of symptoms and the diagnosis is as long as 15 years, with an average of 5 months.[7] The most common presenting symptoms are listed in Table 36–1; most reflect local involvement by the lesion.

PATHOLOGY

Tumors of the male urethra can be categorized according to the histology of the cells lining the anatomic region of origin (Fig. 36–1). The epithelium of the prostatic urethra gives rise to transitional cell malignancy that is histologically and clinically distinct from the adenocarcinoma commonly associated with prostatic malignancy, but that is identical to the bladder urothelium. Tumors originating in the area of the trigone or bladder neck with direct extension into the prostatic urethra may be mistakenly diagnosed as primary urethral carcinoma unless careful examination and biopsy excludes the vesical neck area as the site of origin. Benign lesions of condyloma acuminatum, benign papillomas, and urethral caruncles are found within the distal penile urethra and meatus. In published reports, 59% of malignant tumors occurred in the bulbomembranous urethra, 34% in the penile urethra, and 7% in the prostatic urethra. Histologically, 78% of male urethral car-

TABLE 36–1. Cancer of the Urethra and Penis

Symptoms*	No. of Patients (%)
Palpable urethral mass	34 (72)
Obstructive symptoms (with or without retention)	32 (65)
Pain	12 (26)
Urethral fistula or periurethral abscess	10 (21)
Hematuria	10 (21)
Palpable inguinal mass	9 (19)

* Presenting symptoms of 47 patients.
(Fair WR, Yang CR. Urethral carcinoma in males. In: Resnick M, Kursch E, eds. Current therapy in surgery. Toronto: BC Decker, 1987)

TABLE 36–2. Staging System for Carcinoma of the Male Urethra

Stage	Criteria
O	Confined to mucosa only (in situ)
A	Into but not beyond lamina propria
B	Into but not beyond substance of corpus spongiosum or into but not beyond prostate
C	Direct extension into tissues beyond corpus spongiosum (corpora cavernosa, muscle, fat, fascia, skin, direct skeletal involvement), or beyond prostatic capsule
D1	Regional metastasis including inguinal and/or pelvic lymph nodes (with any primary tumor)
D2	Distant metastasis (with any primary tumor)

(Modified from Ray B, Canto AR, Whitmore W. Experience with primary carcinoma of the male urethra. J Urol 1977;117:591–594)

cinomas were squamous cell carcinoma, 15% were transitional carcinoma, 6% were adenocarcinoma, and 1% were undifferentiated carcinoma.[2]

Male urethral carcinoma tends to spread by direct extension to adjacent structures and usually involves the vascular spaces of the corpus spongiosum and the periurethral tissues. Carcinoma of the bulbomembranous urethra often extends to the urogenital diaphragm, prostate, perineum, and scrotal skin. Hematogenous spread is uncommon except in advanced disease. Metastasis occurs by lymphatic embolization to regional lymph nodes. The lymphatics from the anterior urethra drain into the superficial and deep inguinal nodes and occasionally to the external iliac nodes, and the lymphatics from the posterior urethra drain into the external iliac, obturator, and hypogastric nodes. Tumors of the anterior urethra usually metastasize to the inguinal nodes, and tumors of the posterior urethra most commonly spread to pelvic nodes, although exceptions occur.[8]

EVALUATION AND STAGING

The diagnosis is made by transurethral or needle biopsy. The extent of local involvement can be determined by careful inspection and palpation of the external genitalia and perineum at the time of cystourethroscopy and by bimanual examination with the patient under anesthesia. Cytologic studies of voided urine may be helpful for diagnosing some patients.[1] Computed tomography (CT) or magnetic resonance imaging (MRI) may help to evaluate the pelvic and paraaortic nodes. A lymphangiogram may be of value if the CT scan is equivocal, but it is not required routinely.

A commonly used staging system is listed in Table 36–2. A system proposed by the American Joint Committee on Cancer

TABLE 36–3. American Joint Committee on Cancer Staging System for Urethral Cancer

T—Primary Tumor (Male)

Tx	Primary tumor cannot be assessed
T0	No evidence of primary tumor
Tis	Carcinoma in situ
Ta	Noninvasive papillary, polypoid, or verrucous carcinoma
T1	Tumor invades subepithelial connective tissue
T2	Tumor invades corpus spongiosum or prostate or periurethral muscle
T3	Tumor invades corpus cavernosum or beyond prostatic capsule or bladder neck
T4	Tumor invades other adjacent organs

N—Regional Lymph Nodes

Nx	Regional lymph nodes cannot be assessed
N0	No regional lymph node metastasis
N1	Metastasis in a single lymph node, 2 cm or less in greatest dimension
N2	Metastasis in a single lymph node, more than 2 cm but no more than 5 cm in greatest dimension, or multiple lymph nodes, none more than 5 cm in greatest dimension
N3	Metastasis in a lymph node(s) more than 5 cm in greatest dimension

M—Distant Metastasis

Mx	Presence of distant metastasis cannot be assessed
M0	No distant metastasis
M1	Distant metastasis

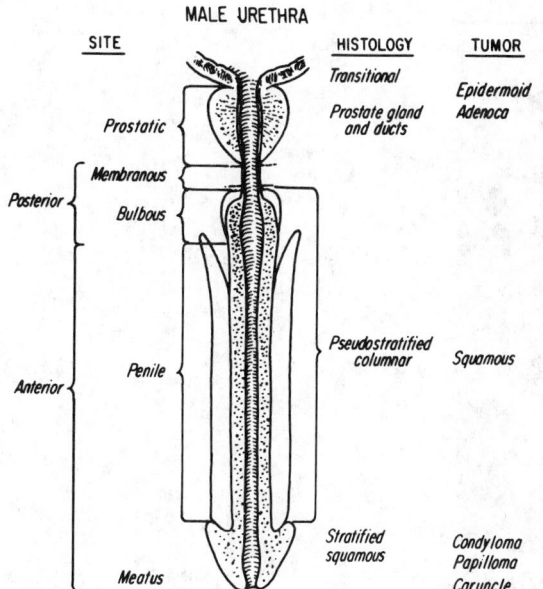

FIGURE 36–1. Anatomy and pathology of urethral carcinoma.

(AJCC) based on the depth of invasion of the primary tumor and the presence or absence of regional lymph node involvement or distant metastases is given in Table 36–3. The TNM staging system is much more valuable and should be the preferred method of describing tumor extent (Fig. 36–2).

TREATMENT

The primary mode of therapy for carcinoma of the male urethra is surgical excision, and its extent depends on the location and stage of the tumor. In general, anterior urethral carcinoma is more amenable to surgical control than posterior urethral carcinoma. Perhaps as a consequence, the prognosis for patients with lesions originating in the anterior urethra is better than that of those with tumors situated posteriorly.

A comparison of the results of surgical excision and radiation therapy is difficult because of the low incidence of the disease and no controlled study comparing the two modalities has been done. As with surgery, the results of radiation therapy depend on the site of the tumor. Anterior urethral lesions respond better than posterior tumors.[2] The main problem with the radiation approach is the high incidence of locoregional reoccurrences.

Modern combinations of chemotherapy are capable of producing meaningful objective regression of regionally advanced or metastatic urothelial carcinomas. The MVAC regimen (methotrexate, vinblastine, doxorubicin [Adriamycin], and cisplatin) has produced significant tumor regression in most patients with transitional cell carcinoma of the urinary tract.[9-11] Tumors of nontransitional histology appear to be resistant to this combination. The MVAC regimen causes significant myelosuppression, and the potential for nephrotoxicity and cardiotoxicity necessitates careful attention to detail in drug administration. However, on the basis of the response to MVAC chemotherapy in bladder and upper tract urothelial tumors, investigation into its use in transitional cell carcinoma of the urethra is warranted.

Untreated patients with carcinoma of the urethra can anticipate a median survival of 3 months (range, 1 week to 15 months). Only 16% of these patients survive more than 5 years.[12]

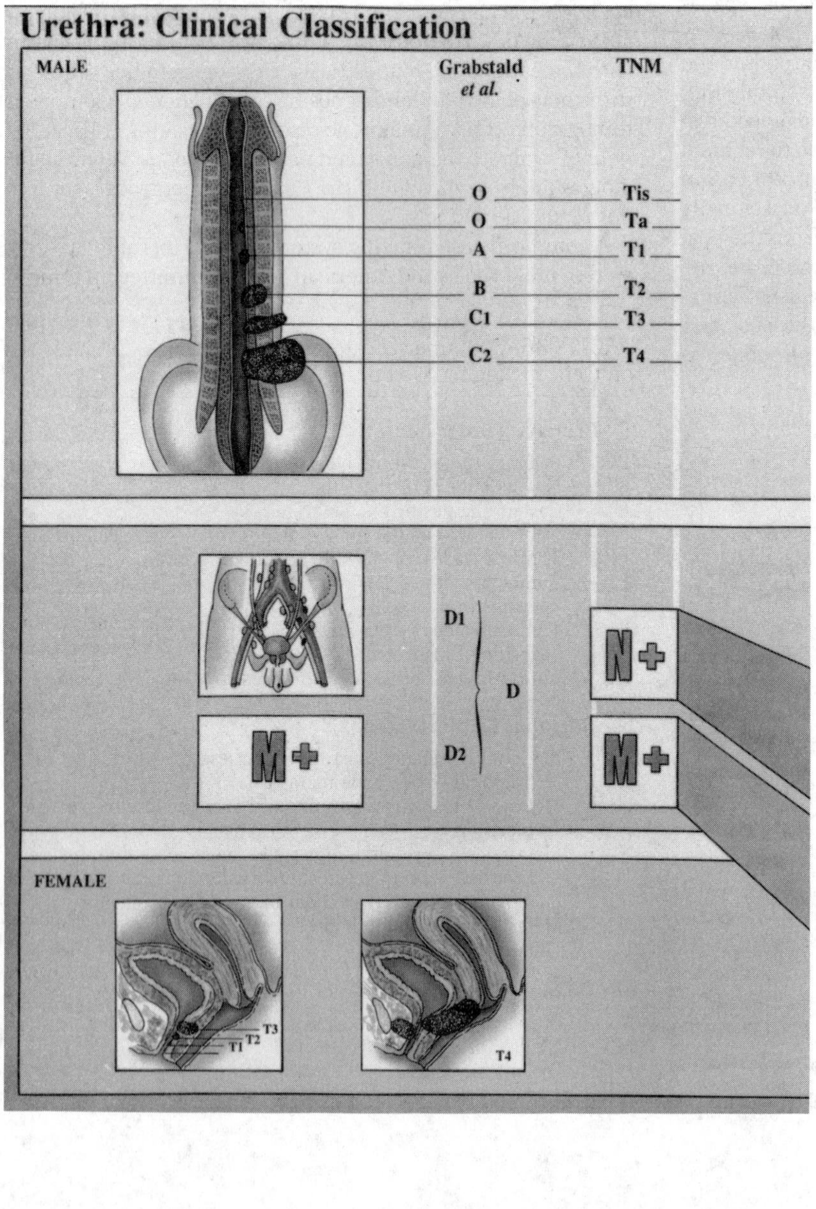

FIGURE 36–2. Clinical classification of urethral cancer.

Surgery

CARCINOMA OF THE DISTAL URETHRA. Carcinoma of the penile urethra can be treated by transurethral resection, local excision, partial amputation, or radical amputation with or without emasculation. For superficial, papillary, or in situ tumors, transurethral resection may be sufficient. For tumor infiltrating the corpus and localized to the distal half of the penis, a partial amputation with a 2-cm margin proximal to any visible or palpable lesion is the accepted treatment. If the infiltrating tumor is located in the proximal penile urethra or involves the entire penile urethra, radical amputation should be done. Emasculation is indicated only if the scrotal skin is involved.

Unlike the situation that exists in carcinoma of the penis, clinically palpable adenopathy in the groin of patients with urethral carcinoma usually represents metastases and is not often the result of reactive inflammation. Ilioinguinal node dissection is indicated only if the inguinal nodes are palpable; there is no evidence of benefit from prophylactic groin dissection. After excision of the primary tumor, the patient should be followed with careful examinations of the inguinal areas for evidence of lymphadenopathy, and a groin dissection should be done if metastatic disease is detected.[1,3,5,7,13] The 5-year survival rates usually correlate with the location and type of lesion, and overall rates are poor (Table 36–4).

CARCINOMA OF THE BULBOMEMBRANOUS URETHRA. Early lesions of the bulbomembranous urethra have been treated successfully by transurethral resection or by resection of the involved urethral segment with end-to-end anastomosis, but cases appropriate for limited resection are rare.[13,14] Poor survival figures have been recorded for all forms of treatment, but it appears that radical excision offers the best opportunity for long-term disease control and the lowest incidence of local recurrence. Unfortunately, most patients with bulbomembranous urethral carcinoma present with locally advanced disease.

In-continuity resection of the pubic rami has been suggested as a means of improving local control, but the small number of patients treated in this manner prevents definitive conclusions.[15] Patients with carcinoma of the posterior urethra should have simultaneous deep pelvic node dissection to ascertain nodal metastatic disease. There is no evidence that cure can be effected for patients with gross pelvic disease by surgical excision or radiation therapy alone.

PRIMARY CARCINOMA OF THE PROSTATIC URETHRA. Carcinoma arising from the prostatic urethra is rare. There are no characteristic symptoms of this lesion, and the serum acid phosphatase or prostatic-specific antigen (PSA) concentration is not elevated. Superficial lesions of the prostatic urethra have been managed successfully by transurethral resection in some patients, but such tumors are uncommon.[1] In many instances, the tumor involves the bulk of the prostate with extension to the bulbomembranous urethra or the bladder neck and trigone. In this situation, radical prostatectomy alone may not provide a tumor-free margin, and anterior exenteration is the treatment of choice. As with other carcinomas in the posterior urethra, the overall 5-year survival rates for invasive prostatic urethral carcinoma are poor.[5] There are anecdotal reports of successful treatment of primary carcinoma of the prostatic urethral stroma with combination chemotherapy (*i.e.*, MVAC) plus extensive transurethral resection of the prostate or radical prostatectomy.[16] Although these cases are few, if successful, this multimodal approach has the advantage of retaining the patient's bladder. The use of systemic therapy to address the problem of unrecognized, distant, micrometastatic disease is conceptually appealing. Long-term survivors have been recorded, and use of this approach is likely to increase in the future.

RADIATION THERAPY

The results of radiation therapy for carcinoma of the male urethra are difficult to evaluate because only a few reports are available for patients treated with this modality. The most common approach has been external-beam radiotherapy, using a variety of techniques to deliver 5000 to 6000 cGy in 5 to 9 weeks.[8,17–19] A few cases of interstitial implantation of radioactive sources have been reported, mostly with bulbomembranous or prostatic lesions in which brachytherapy was used preoperatively or to control recurrences.[8,17,19,20] The long-term results of radiotherapy have been mixed, with the best results reported for patients with distal lesions, for whom the outcome seems to be similar to that reported with surgery.[18]

CARCINOMA OF THE FEMALE URETHRA

Carcinoma of the urethra is unusual among genitourinary tract neoplasms in that it occurs more often in women than in men. The tumors most commonly present in older and postmenopausal women, with 75% of patients older than 50 years of age. The disease is more prevalent among whites than other races.

ETIOLOGY

The cause of urethral carcinoma in women has not been established, although a causal relation is reported between chronic irritation and malignancy. Proliferative lesions, such as caruncles, papillomas, adenomas, and polyps, have been associated with subsequent malignancy. Leukoplakia of the urethra should be considered a premalignant lesion and treated accordingly.

TABLE 36–4. Five-Year Survival in Carcinoma of Male Urethra

Histologic Type	No. of Surviving Patients (%)/ Total No. of Patients		
	Penile	Bulbomembranous	Prostatic
Squamous	12/27 (44)	4/40 (10)	0/1 (0)
Transitional	1/3 (33)	0/4 (0)	4/13 (31)
Adenocarcinoma		1/4 (25)	
Undifferentiated		0/1 (0)	
Total	13/30 (43)	5/49 (10)	4/14 (29)

(Modified from Ray B, Canto AR, Whitmore WF. Experience with primary carcinoma of the male urethra. J Urol 1977;117:591–594)

SYMPTOMS

The tumor usually presents as a papillary growth and later becomes a soft, fungating mass that bleeds easily. Ulcerative lesions may produce a foul-smelling discharge. Spread from the primary lesion is by local extension and infiltration with subsequent involvement of the bladder neck and vulva. It may be difficult on initial physical examination to differentiate malignant tumors of the urethra from those of the vulva.

The lymphatic drainage of the various segments of the female urethra is poorly defined. It is generally accepted that the lymphatics of the distal urethra drain into the inguinal region, and the drainage from the more proximal urethra is to the obturator and iliac nodes. Between 25% and 50% of patients have inguinal node involvement at the time of initial diagnosis, and an additional 15% of patients develop metastatic nodal disease during follow-up.[2,21–23] As with urethral carcinoma in males, inguinal lymphadenopathy usually indicates malignant involvement.

PATHOLOGY

Stratified squamous epithelium lines the distal two thirds of the female urethra, and transitional epithelium lines the proximal one third (Fig. 36–3). Tumor histology is a reflection of the site, and the predominant tumor is squamous cell carcinoma, usually presenting in the proximal two thirds. In general, carcinomas of the anterior urethra are low grade, and carcinomas of the proximal or entire urethra are of higher grade. However, histologic characteristics do not significantly affect the prognosis. For practical purposes, transitional cell carcinoma, squamous cell carcinoma, and adenocarcinoma are treated in a similar fashion, although for metastatic transitional cell carcinoma, combination chemotherapy may be considered.[9,10]

TREATMENT

The most significant prognostic factor is the anatomic location of the tumor. For example, meatal tumors, if diagnosed early, are associated with an excellent 5-year survival rate.[24,25] The treatment is based primarily on the tumor stage at the time of presentation.

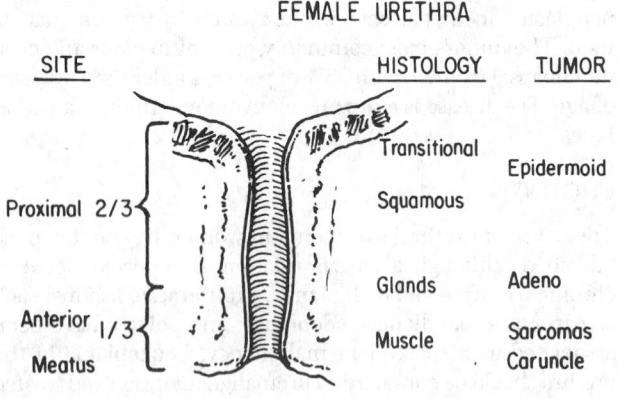

FEMALE URETHRA

SITE · HISTOLOGY · TUMOR

Transitional · Epidermoid
Proximal 2/3 · Squamous
Glands · Adeno
Anterior 1/3
Meatus · Muscle · Sarcomas · Caruncle

FIGURE 36–3.   Anatomy and pathology of the female urethra.

Surgery

Local excision is often sufficient in selected patients with carcinoma of the distal urethra, because the incidence of lymph node metastasis with distal urethral carcinoma is low.

For tumors involving the proximal urethra or with extension beyond the urethra into the adjacent structures, more aggressive therapy is required. When surgery is considered, extensive resection is necessary, including total urethrectomy, cystectomy with pelvic node dissection, and in cases of palpable inguinal lymph nodes, inguinal lymphadenectomy. Removal of the vulva and vagina have also been advocated as part of an anterior exenteration.[13,26]

Although there has been some success with radiation therapy alone in advanced-stage disease, the cure rates have been low. Bracken and coworkers reported 81 cases of carcinoma of the female urethra, and the overall 5-year survival rate for the entire group was 32%.[25] There is a high incidence of local recurrence, ranging from 46% to 64%, for all forms of single-modality therapy, suggesting the need to explore combination treatment.

Radiation Therapy

The potential advantage of radiotherapy is that it can control the tumor while preserving the function of the urethra. Small meatal tumors are best treated with interstitial implantation of radioactive sources, and larger tumors, especially those invading the labia, vagina, or the urinary bladder, require the addition of external-beam therapy. Combined modality approaches with surgery and brachytherapy or external-beam radiotherapy have also been used to improve the local outcome of treatment in advanced-stage disease.[27]

Advanced technology with iridium 192 interstitial implantation was introduced to optimize the dose distributions throughout the tumor, using specialized templates to guide the placements of the radioactive sources within and around the urethra.[28,29] The template consists of a 1- to 2-cm-thick plastic plate that is placed in apposition with the urethral meatus and is usually stabilized by a perpendicular vaginal cylinder or by a central urethral stainless steel catheter.[28,29] One or two circles of equally spaced holes are drilled in the plastic plate to guide the insertion and placement of 17-gauge stainless steel implant needles around the urethra, as required by the specific tumor size and its anatomic configuration. Afterloading of the ^{192}Ir sources is carried out according to individualized computer-aided treatment planning to ensure a homogenous dose distribution throughout the tumor with minimal irradiation of the surrounding normal tissues. Usually, an implant dose of 4000 to 4500 cGy is delivered to the tumor, and external irradiation is added to increase the total tumor dose to 6500 to 7000 cGy. This technique enables the delivery of tumoricidal doses to the tumor with concomitant elective irradiation of presumed sites of microscopic involvement and nontoxic doses to the bowel, rectum, and bladder.

The rates of 5-year survival for meatal tumors are 60% to 90%.[13,25,30–34] Neoplasms involving the entire urethra are more difficult to treat, and the overall control rates for these tumors have been 20% to 40%, with chronic complications (*e.g.*, strictures, vesicovaginal fistulas, urethral necrosis) occurring in 15% to 40% of treated patients.[13,24,25,30–34] Several studies have recommended combined-modality approaches of preoperative irradiation and radical cystourethrectomy or concomitant external-beam radiotherapy and low-dose 5-fluorouracil plus mitomycin C according to protocols used in carcinoma of the anus, with excellent preliminary results.[33–37]

Urethral strictures develop in some patients, necessitating dilation. More severe complications are necrosis secondary to overdosage and fistula, primarily vesicovaginal or urethrovaginal.[25,38] In advanced neoplasms, fistula formation is unavoidable because of tumor erosion of the organ and subsequent tumor necrosis.[39] Less common complications include osteomyelitis of the symphysis pubis, radiation cystitis, urinary incontinence or stress incontinence, radiation enteritis, and small-bowel obstruction. Johnson and O'Connell[32] encountered a 42% complication rate in patients treated by radiotherapy, and in the series treated by Prempree and colleagues,[39] 2 of 10 patients treated definitively by radiotherapy developed strictures. Bracken and associates[25] reported a complication rate of 45% among their patients who were treated with radiation, and Taggart and colleagues[38] encountered severe complications in 5 of 37 patients.

CANCER OF THE PENIS

Carcinoma of the penis represents 2% to 5% of all urogenital cancers.[40,41] Although rare in North America, tumors of the penis are a significant clinical problem in populations in which circumcision is not a common practice and proper hygiene is lacking. In some populations, squamous cell carcinoma of the penis accounts for 10% to 12% of all malignancies in males.

Penile cancer is the most common genitourinary cancer in Paraguay, representing 45% to 76% of all genitourinary malignancies. In Uganda, where circumcision is usually not performed, penile cancer is the most commonly diagnosed cancer in males.[42,43] Although malignant penile lesions have been found in young men, most patients are older than 50 years of age.

ETIOLOGY

The occurrence of penile carcinoma correlates strongly with the existence of a foreskin and the irritative effects of smegma combined with the products of poor hygiene within the pre-putial sac. Carcinoma is rare among men who were circumcised in the neonatal period, but circumcision performed at puberty or in adulthood does not have the same protective potential as neonatal circumcision.[44–47] In one series, 15 patients circumcised as adolescents developed carcinoma of the penis.[48] Although the annual age-adjusted incidence of carcinoma of the penis for males in the United States is only 1.0 per 100,000, the lifetime risk of penile cancer developing in uncircumcised males may be as high as 1 in 600.[49] Smegma, the product of bacterial action or desquamated epithelial cells, has been identified as carcinogenic in animal systems, although the specific component responsible for malignant degeneration in human males has not been identified.

Conflicting reports support and deny the association of penile carcinoma with cervical carcinoma in sexual partners or with herpetic infection.[50,51] There are no compelling data to support the assertion that penile cancer is a sexually transmitted disease.[52] No persistent etiologic relation has been documented between carcinoma of the penis and the venereal diseases of syphilis, granuloma inguinale, or chancroid. Evidence that human papillomavirus (HPV) may be causative is scanty, although HPV type 16 transfection alters human epithelial cell differentiation in vitro.[53–55]

SYMPTOMS

The most common presenting manifestation of penile cancer is a mass or a persistent sore or ulcer of the glans or foreskin.[41,56,57] Most penile carcinomas are painless, and there may be significant ulceration and bleeding without patient concern. Less commonly, the initial symptoms are related to inguinal lymphadenopathy.

It has been estimated that more than half of patients delay more than 1 year in seeking treatment after the appearance of the lesion.[12,47,57–59]

PATHOLOGY

Penile carcinoma is most often squamous cell in origin, although malignant melanoma, basal cell carcinoma, Bowen's disease (carcinoma in situ), mesenchymal tumors (including Kaposi's sarcoma), metastatic lesions, and leukemic or lymphomatous infiltrates may involve the penis.[60] Several premalignant lesions have been identified (Table 36–5).

TABLE 36–5. Premalignant Lesions of the Penis

Lesion	Characteristic	Treatment
Leukoplakia	White plaque	Local excision
Erythroplasia of Queyrat	Raised, red, velvet lesion; cellular disorientation with multiple mitoses; identical to carcinoma in situ of skin; 10–20% may develop areas of squamous cell carcinoma. May be painful	Local excision; topical 5-fluorouracil; radiation therapy
Bowen's disease	Red plaque	Local excision
Balanitis xerotica obliterans	Scaly, atrophic with fissure or ulceration; meatus often involved	Local exicision; topical steroids (?)
Buschke-Lowenstein tumor	Large verrucous lesion, histologically benign; may undergo malignant degeneration	Local excision with negative margins; topical therapy doubtful; radiation therapy has limited effectiveness

STAGING

The initial diagnosis must be made by incisional or, preferably, excisional biopsy. Careful physical examination to determine the extent of local invasion and the status of the inguinal lymph nodes is essential to proper staging (Fig. 36–4). A CT or MRI scan to evaluate the pelvic and abdominal lymph nodes is also required. Lymphangiography is rarely required, but it can be combined with fine-needle aspiration biopsy of suspicious nodes to improve staging accuracy.[61]

Table 36–6 shows the Jackson staging system for penile carcinoma.[62] Although widely used, this system suffers to the extent that inguinal nodal involvement is not subcategorized; all patients with tumorous nodes are grouped together.[63]

Table 36–6 provides a summary of five large series encompassing 526 patients for whom Jackson stage is available.[57,64–67] Of patients with stage I, II, or III disease, approximately half are grouped in stage I, with one third of the remainder in stage II. Because patients' survivals were not reported in a uniform manner and the pathologic staging of lymph nodes was not always provided, the "poor prognosis" grouping in the table includes patients dying of their disease or subsequently developing positive lymph nodes. As the table illustrates, although the risk of nodal disease or death from cancer is significant in stages II and III, mere classification of patients into stage I does not deny the development of metastatic disease. One patient in 10 subsequently develops nodal disease. Although this method of patient selection offers some assistance to the clinician in deciding on the necessity of a lymphadenectomy, it is not completely reliable.

The tumor-node-metastasis (TNM) classification, outlined in Figure 36–4, is an attempt to quantify more precisely the nodal and metastatic disease.

TREATMENT

Adequate therapy implies an accurate assessment of the extent of the disease with particular reference to the status of the

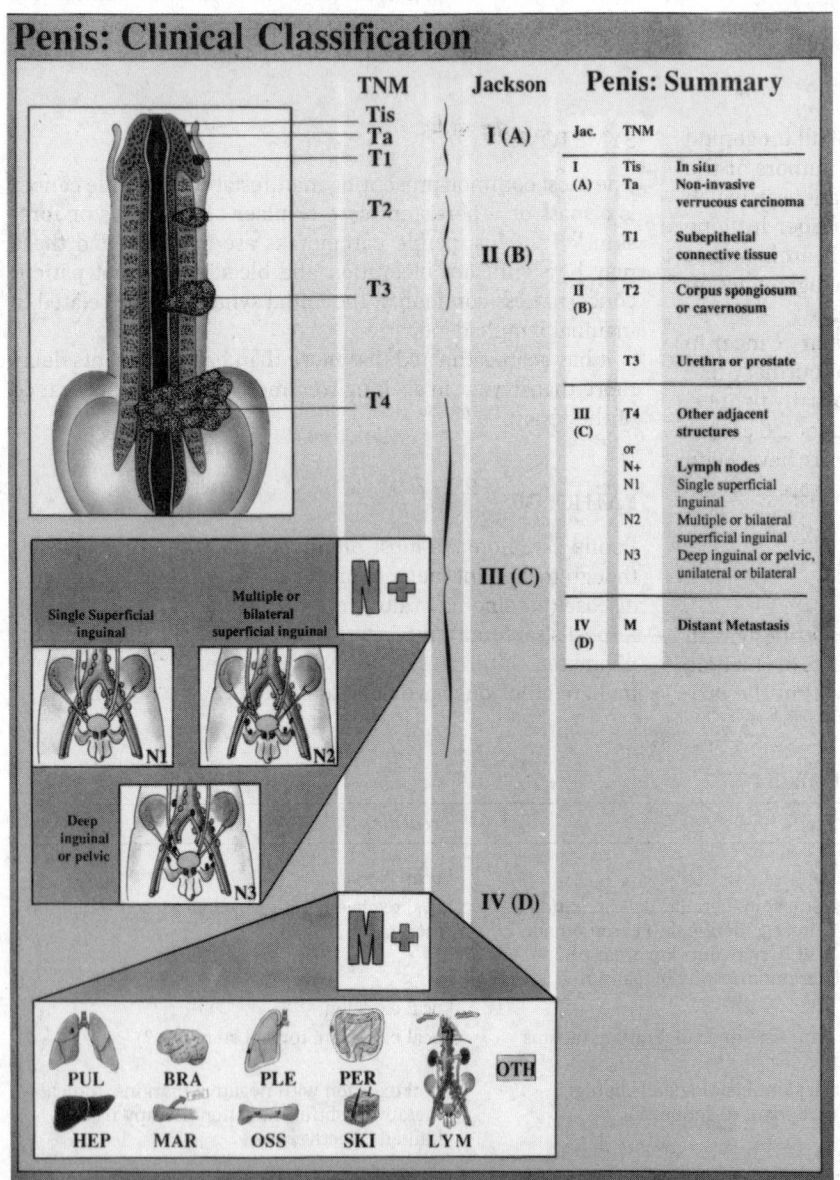

FIGURE 36–4. Clinical classification of penile cancer.

TABLE 36–6. Prognostic Value of Jackson Stage

Jackson Stage	No. of Patients*	No. of Patients With Positive Nodes or Dying From Cancer (%)
I	278	33 (12)
II	80	27 (34)
III	168	94 (57)
Total	526	154 (29)

* The 526 patients were accumulated from five series.[57,64–67]

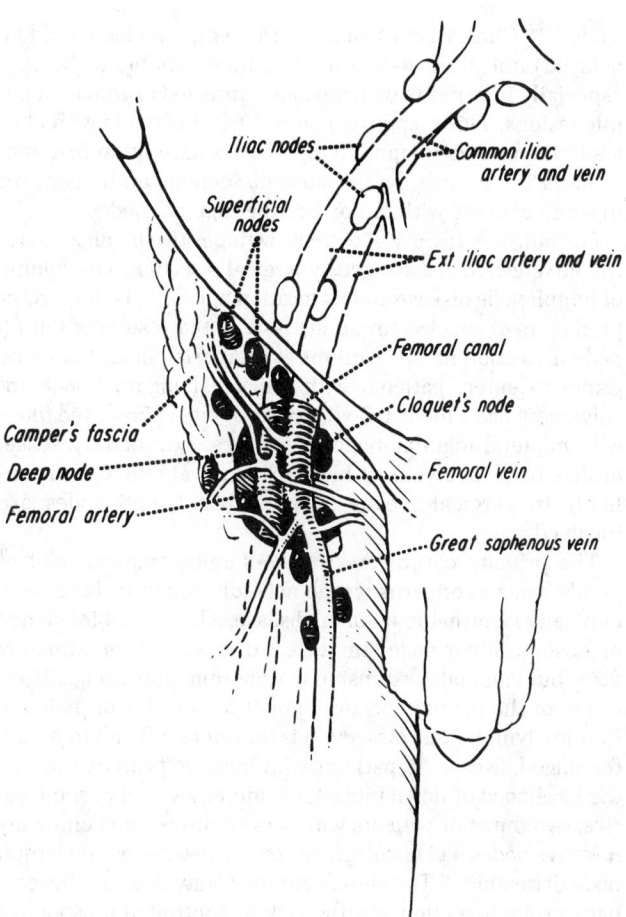

FIGURE 36–5. Lymphatic drainage of the penis.

regional lymph nodes. Controversies exist about the best management of the primary lesion, resulting mainly from the lack of controlled clinical studies in this rare disease. Wide excision or partial penectomy with or without inguinal lymph node dissection is the most commonly accepted treatment for small and well-localized tumors.[66,68–69] For larger tumors, partial or total penectomy with or without inguinal and pelvic lymph node dissection is generally necessary, although some researchers have demonstrated that organ-preserving techniques of radiotherapy may be effective for some patients and may avoid the functional sacrifice associated with penectomy.[68–71] Proponents of the surgical approach have argued that radiation is associated with severe complications, such as necrosis or urethral stenosis, but the techniques and dose schedules used in some of the older series that are commonly quoted may not be considered optimal according to current standards.[57,65,70] Several investigators have demonstrated that local relapses after radiotherapy can be salvaged by a partial or total amputation of the penis without apparently affecting the prognosis.[70,72]

Paramount in any treatment philosophy is a consideration of the lymphatic drainage of the penis as a prelude to rational therapeutic planning (Fig. 36–5). The skin of the penis and the lymphatics of the prepuce drain primarily into the superficial inguinal nodes. Bilateral drainage occurs as a result of a freely anastomosing system and crossover at the base of the penis.[65] The glans is drained by the superficial inguinal nodes, but along with those of the corpora, the lymphatics of the glans penis empty into the deep inguinal and iliac nodes. The superficial nodes are located in the deep portion of Camper's fascia superficial to the deep fascia of the thigh, the fascia lata. Subsequently, the superficial lymphatics drain into the deep inguinal lymphatics surrounding the femoral vessels and then to the external iliac, common iliac, and periaortic lymphatic channels. Tumor invasion of the corpora cavernosa or the posterior urethra is consistent with involvement of the deep pelvic lymphatic structures of the internal iliac and obturator regions.

Surgery

Two areas of surgical concern in disease management are the selection of the appropriate treatment for the primary lesion and the role of surgery in the evaluation and therapy of nodal disease.

TREATMENT OF PRIMARY LESION. Adequate control of the primary tumor must be accomplished for a cure to be expected. Surgical therapy involves removal of the lesion with adequate margins to minimize the risk of local recurrence. Small tumors that are limited to the prepuce are treated by circumcision alone. Lesions that on physical examination involve only the skin, not the underlying structures, may be controllable by excisional biopsy. Partial or total penectomy is indicated for lesions that, because of their size, invasiveness, or location on the shaft, are not amenable to more conservative treatment. Partial penectomy requires that a 2-cm margin of grossly normal shaft be available proximal to the primary lesion. For extensive lesions approaching the base of the shaft, total penectomy should be accomplished with excision of both corpora and creation of a perineal urethrostomy.[66]

MANAGEMENT OF REGIONAL LYMPH NODES. Several factors determine the role of regional lymphadenectomy in patients with penile cancer. First, between 35% and 60% of patients with squamous cell penile cancer present with palpable inguinal lymph nodes.[66,73,74] Second, the incidence of false-positive lymph nodes on clinical examination averages 40%, with series reporting figures between 13% and 82%, because of the well-known association of inflammatory inguinal lymphadenopathy with ulcerated or infected penile lesions.[63,66] Clinical assessment of the lymph nodes should be delayed until after a 4- to 6-week course of antibiotic therapy, especially in patients with obviously infected or inflamed penile lesions. Third, approximately 20% of patients with clinically tumor-free inguinal lymph nodes have lymphatic metastases.[66,73] Fourth, lymph node dissection can be curative in some patients with tumor-bearing inguinal nodes.

Overall, 40% to 50% of patients with positive inguinal nodes can be rendered disease free by surgical resection. The volume of lymph node disease and its location appear to be important predictors of success. In an analysis of the results of lymph node dissection in 119 patients at Memorial Sloan-Kettering Cancer Center, patients with unilateral inguinal-node involvement had a median 5-year survival rate of 56%, and those with bilateral inguinal-node metastases, extranodal disease, or iliac node involvement had a 9% survival rate. Cure is unlikely by surgical means if the pelvic lymph nodes are involved.[63]

The primary controversy in the surgical management of penile cancer concerns lymph node dissection if there is no clinically identifiable inguinal disease. The overall incidence of false-negative nodes in stage I disease is approximately 20%, but late nodal extension to the groin after adequate excision of the primary occurs in only 5% to 11% of patients. Routine lymph node dissection is therefore difficult to justify for stage I disease. In patients with invasive primary tumors, the likelihood of nodal metastases increases, and in some series, two thirds of patients with stage II disease and clinically negative nodes had histologically confirmed disease on lymph node dissection.[64] The significant morbidity that may accompany groin dissection and the lack of controlled prospective studies to document the benefit of early "prophylactic" versus late "therapeutic" groin dissection has led many surgeons and centers to delay lymphadenectomy until clinical evidence of lymph node involvement exists.[50,74]

Ekstron and Edsmyr identified a 50% disease control rate among patients who had node dissection delayed until adenopathy was evident.[75] Frew and colleagues could identify no cancer deaths among patients in whom lymph node excision was deferred until clinical node disease was found.[76] Beggs and Spratt reported no significant adverse effect on survival in patients with delayed groin dissection; the 1% mortality rate from lymphadenectomy was essentially the same as the percentage of patients who died from cancer as a result of therapeutic delay.[74] However, others have reported a significant decrease in 5-year survival rates in patients with therapeutic rather than prophylactic groin dissection and have suggested that delayed surgery is inappropriate.[64,77]

Cabanas described a technique of "sentinel node" biopsy followed by formal node dissection if metastatic disease is found.[78] The sentinel lymph node is found radiographically, on the anteroposterior view, at the junction of the femoral head and the ascending pubic ramus. Anatomically, the sentinel node is part of the lymphatic system around the superficial epigastric vein located medial to and above the superficial epigastric-saphenous junction. In Cabanas' series, inguinal-femoral-iliac node involvement was not demonstrated without a positive sentinel node biopsy. However, Perinetti and coworkers reported a patient with a negative sentinel node biopsy who had unresectable bilateral groin disease 3 months later.[79]

It seems appropriate that patients with noninvasive tumor and clinically negative nodes (stage I) should be followed carefully and groin dissection considered only if lymphadenopathy occurs. In patients with stage II disease, the sentinel node biopsy is appealing as a means of increasing diagnostic and prognostic accuracy without significant morbidity, although proponents of prophylactic and therapeutic groin dissection exist. In patients with clinically positive nodes (stage II), initial bilateral dissection should be performed because of the high incidence (60%) of bilateral inguinal node involvement.[75] Unilateral node dissection in patients managed by delayed lymphadenectomy is reasonable because the incidence of contralateral involvement in these patients is less than 10%.[12] Controversy also exists over the benefit obtained by pelvic node dissection if there are pelvic nodal metastases. Although positive pelvic nodes appear to be an indicator of incurable disease, some physicians report a 20% to 29% cure rate with surgery in these patients. Whether this apparent long-term survival reflects a beneficial impact of surgery or represents a subset of patients with apparently indolent disease is undetermined.[78]

Technical Aspects of Lymphadenectomy. The operation is performed essentially as described by Whitmore and Vagaiwala.[80] The patient is placed in the supine position with the thighs slightly flexed, abducted, and externally rotated and with support under the knees. The incision for the bilateral pelvic node dissection, which may be performed before (usually) or after the inguinal dissection, is a midline incision from the umbilicus to the pubis. The dissection limits are defined by the genitofemoral nerve laterally, the bladder medially, the bifurcation of the common iliac artery superiorly, and the fascia covering the obturator internus and levator ani muscles inferiorly (Fig. 36–6). Cloquet's node can usually be removed through the pelvic incision as the vessels are cleaned as they enter the femoral canal.

The inguinal incision is planned to provide adequate margins surrounding lymph nodes containing obvious tumor and simultaneously to remove the area of skin at greatest risk of devitalization and necrosis. An elliptical incision is made over the inguinal ligament from the anterosuperior iliac spine toward, but lateral to, the pubic tubercle. The borders of the ellipse parallel the inguinal ligament and extend 4 to 6 cm in a vertical diameter at the widest point. The incision is beveled outward from the skin and down, describing a pyramidal wedge of tissue truncated by the skin surface. Because penile cancers appear to involve the inguinal lymph nodes by tumor embolization rather than through permeation of lymphatic channels, wide, thin skin flaps and a thorough dissection, as is required for malignant melanoma, are not indicated. The surgeon's goal should be to remove completely the nodes in the superficial and deep inguinal areas; this can be done without widely undermining the skin flaps. With this technique, the incidence of postoperative wound necrosis is markedly reduced.

Complications. The most common complication is skin flap necrosis. Particular attention to operative detail, especially with regard to skin flap thickness, infection control, perioperative antibiotic coverage, protection of femoral vessels by sartorius transfer, appropriate drainage, and postoperative immobilization, appears to lessen this most disturbing complication. Other problems include lymphedema (19–45%),

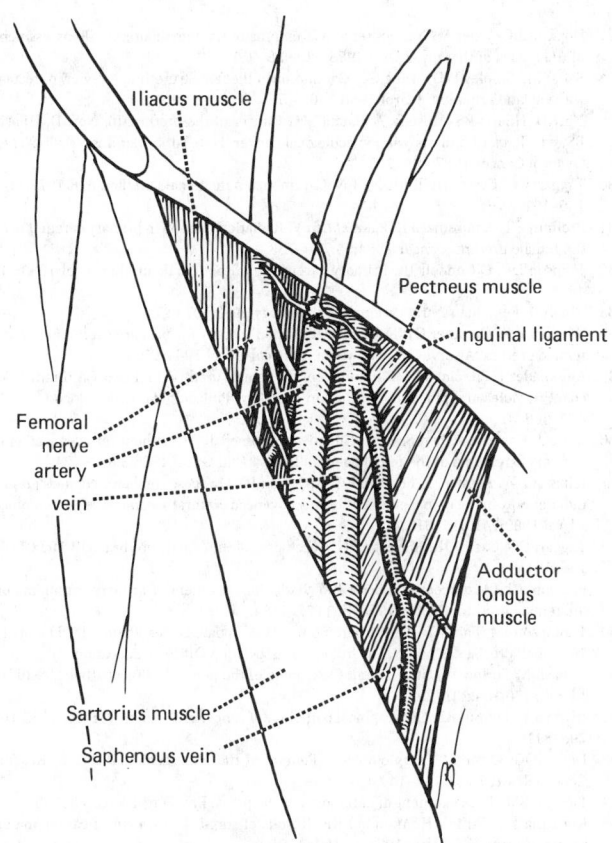

FIGURE 36–6. Anatomic limits of deep groin dissection.

Labels on figure: Iliacus muscle; Pectneus muscle; Inguinal ligament; Femoral nerve artery vein; Adductor longus muscle; Sartorius muscle; Saphenous vein

wound infection (10%), and rarely, hemorrhage, hernia, or death. Persistent lymphedema can be a problem. Meticulous ligation of lymphatic channels during the dissection by cautery, metal clips, or fine ligatures appears to reduce the likelihood of severe, persistent lymphedema. The use of preoperatively fitted compression stockings, elevation, and immobilization also appears to be important in reducing the incidence of this problem.

Radiation Therapy

The main advantage for radiation therapy in penile tumors is that it provides an option of functional preservation of the penis. However, for radiation to represent an alternative to surgery, it must yield comparable local control rates with minimal toxic effects. Grabstald and Kelley showed that 9 of 10 irradiated patients with small superficial tumors remained free of disease at 6 years, but several developed urethral stenosis.[81] Other series reported initial rates of local control in 80% to 90% of patients treated with radiotherapy, but 10% to 20% eventually relapsed and required surgical salvage.[67,69–71,82,83] Although this may represent a distinct advantage over the categorical approach with partial or total penectomy, it indicates that all aspects of treatment planning are critical in the management of this disease to minimize toxicities and the likelihood of local relapse.

Treatment techniques have included interstitial implantation of radium needles, ^{192}Ir sources, or external-beam radiotherapy. The use of brachytherapy has been limited to small

tumors. Results from a series of 50 patients implanted with ^{192}Ir wires showed that the tumor was controlled in 95% of the patients with noninfiltrating tumors of 4 cm or less, with the penis conserved in 80% without major impairments of function.[84] When external-beam radiotherapy is used, treatment is usually delivered with custom-made plastic or wax molds to ensure a uniform dose distribution and to overcome the skin-sparing effects of supervoltage beams.[69–71] Circumcision is usually recommended before radiotherapy to minimize radiation morbidity associated with cellulitis of the prepuce and the adjacent structures, which frequently exists in patients with carcinoma of the penis.[71] The whole shaft of the penis is treated to 4000 cGy in 20 fractions in 4 weeks, and the primary lesion is then boosted to a total dose of 6000 cGy. Superficial small lesions can be treated with localized fields using superficial x-rays or electron beams carried to a similar dose.

External-beam radiotherapy of stage I to III tumors usually produces 70% to 80% local success rates, and most local failures that appear in 10% to 20% of the patients can be salvaged with surgery.[69–71,83] If prophylactic or therapeutic lymph node dissection cannot be performed, external-beam radiotherapy to the inguinal and pelvic lymph nodes carried to 5000 cGy can provide permanent control in a substantial percentage of the patients.[69–71] Meatal-urethral stricture represents the most common late effect, and its incidence can be decreased with protracted fractionation schemes.[57–65,71] Mucosal changes and telangiectasia are frequent long-term sequelae.

Chemotherapy

Chemotherapy for urethral and penile carcinomas varies with the histology of the lesion. For patients with pure transitional tumors, the regimens that have been used for bladder primary tumors have shown efficacy. Difficulties arise in the limited ability to document response.

Malignancies of the penis are squamous cell tumors, which do not respond to the regimens used for transitional cell tumors of bladder origin. The results with chemotherapy vary according to the extent of disease, with higher rates of response for locoregional (inguinal) than metastatic (pelvic and beyond) disease. Antitumor activity has been demonstrated with single-agent bleomycin, methotrexate, or cisplatin. Using bleomycin as a single agent, response was observed in 12 of 24, 3 of 14, and in cumulative results of 41 (46%) of 93 patients.[85–87] With cisplatin, cumulative data showed partial responses in 8 of 29 patients and no complete remissions, and methotrexate produced partial responses in 12 of 17, which suggests that this may be the most active single agent.[86–90]

In combination, cyclophosphamide, bleomycin, and cisplatin produced partial responses in 31% of 13 patients, and sequential treatment with bleomycin and methotrexate followed by radiation therapy produced complete responses lasting 30 and 44 months in two separate reports.[90–92] Investigators at the M.D. Anderson Cancer Center evaluated intravenous methotrexate with mitomycin and cisplatin given intraarterially, determined by angiography. Twelve patients with squamous cell carcinomas, including 10 penile, 1 scrotal, and 1 prostate tumor, had 10 responses, including 2 complete responses (72%; 95% confidence interval, 57–92%) for a median duration of 5.9 months. Three patients with unresectable disease received treatment in the neoadjuvant setting, but all had residual unresectable disease at surgery despite preoperative tumor regression.[93] At Memorial Sloan-Kettering Cancer Center, 2 patients treated with MVAC did not respond.

Two reports showed activity of cisplatin and 5-fluorouracil, a combination that has been extensively evaluated in head and neck tumors. Hussein and colleagues treated 6 men with recurrent (4) or unresectable (2) squamous cell carcinomas (*i.e.*, 1 urethral and 5 penile) with cisplatin (100 mg/m^2 on day one) plus 5-fluorouracil (960 mg/m^2/day) for 4 days.[87] Overall, 1 complete response and 5 partial responses were documented, including 2 patients with unresectable disease who were rendered disease free by surgery. Fisher and coworkers treated 5 patients with biopsy-proven unresectable disease and reported major responses in 4 patients, including 2 men who were pathologically free of disease at surgery.[94] Additional confirmatory data are awaited.

REFERENCES

1. Fair WR, Yang CR. Urethral carcinoma in males. In: Resnick M, Kursh E, eds. Current therapy in surgery. Toronto: BC Decker, 1987.
2. Grabstald H. Tumors of the urethra in men and women. Cancer 1973;32:1236–1255.
3. Kaplan GW, Bulkey GJ, Grayhack JT. Carcinoma of the male urethra. J Urol 1967;96:365–371.
4. King LR. Carcinoma of the urethra in male patients. J Urol 1964;92:555–559.
5. Ray B, Canto AK, Whitmore WF Jr. Experience with primary carcinoma of the male urethra. J Urol 1977;117:591–594.
6. Zaslow J, Priestly JT. Primary carcinoma of the male urethra. J Urol 1947;58:207–211.
7. Mandler JT, Pool TL. Primary carcinoma of the male urethra. J Urol 1966;96:67–72.
8. Hopkins SC, Nag SK, Soloway MS. Primary carcinoma of male urethra. Urol 1984;23:128.
9. Sternberg CN, Yagoda A, Scher HI, et al. Preliminary results of MVAC (methotrexate, vinblastine, Adriamycin and cisplatin) for transitional cell carcinoma of the urothelium. J Urol 1985;33:403–407.
10. Scher HI, Yagoda A. Herr HW, et al. Neoadjuvant M-VAC (methotrexate, vinblastine, Adriamycin and cisplatin) for extravesical urinary tract tumors. J Urol 1988;139:470–474.
11. Scher HI, Yagoda A, Herr HW, et al. Neoadjuvant M-VAC (methotrexate, vinblastine, Adriamycin and cisplatin): Effect on the primary bladder lesion. J Urol 1988;139:475–477.
12. Paulson DF, Perez CA, Anderson T. Cancer of the urethra and penis. In: DeVita VT Jr, Hellman S, Rosenberg SA, eds. Principles and practice of oncology, vol 1. Philadelphia: JB Lippincott, 1985:965–977.
13. Pointon RCS, Poole-Wilson DS. Primary carcinoma of the urethra. Br J Urol 1968;40:682–685.
14. Lower WE, Hausfeld KF. Primary carcinoma of the male urethra: Report of 10 cases. J Urol 1947;58:192–206.
15. Klein FA, Whitmore WF Jr, Herr HW, et al. Inferior pubic rami resection with en bloc radical excision for invasive urethral carcinoma. Cancer 1983;51:1238–1242.
16. Davis BE, Fair WR. Management of primary transitional cell carcinoma of the prostatic urethra with bladder preservation. [Abstract] American Urological Association, Annual Meeting, Washington, DC, 1992.
17. Bracken RB, Henry R, Ordonez N. Primary carcinoma of the male urethra. South Med J 1980;73:1003.
18. Heysek RV, Parsons JR, Drylie DM, et al. Carcinoma of the male urethra. J Urol 1985;134:753.
19. Ticho BH, Perez-Tamayo C, Konnak JW. Primary carcinoma of the distal male urethra: A case treated with lymphadenectomy and interstitial radiation therapy. J Urol 1987;139:1302–1303.
20. Kaplan GW, Bulkley GJ, Grayhack JT. Carcinoma of the male urethra. J Urol 1967;98:365.
21. Desai S, Libertino JA, Zinman L. Primary carcinoma of the female urethra. J Urol 1973;110:693–695.
22. Staubitz WJ, Carden LM, Oberkircher OJ, et al. Management of urethral carcinoma in the female. J Urol 1955;73:1045–1053.
23. Ritter DW. Primary malignancy of the female urethra. West J Surg Obstet Gynecol 1953;51:420–429.
24. Antoniades J. Radiation therapy in carcinoma of the female urethra. Cancer 1969;24:70–76.
25. Bracken RB, Johnson DE, Miller LS, et al. Primary carcinoma of the female urethra. J Urol 1976;116:188–192.
26. Grabstald H, Hilaris B, Henschike U, Whitmore WF Jr. Cancer of the female urethra. JAMA 1966;197:835–837.
27. Hopkins SC, Vider M, Nag SK, et al. Carcinoma of the female urethra: Reassessment of the modes of therapy. J Urol 1983;129:958–961.
28. Sailer SL, Shipley WU, Wang CC. Carcinoma of the female urethra: A review of results with radiation therapy. J Urol 1988;140:1–5.
29. Nori D, Hilaris BS, Mostafa A, Batata MA. Cancer of the urethra. In: Nori D, Hilaris BS, eds. Radiation therapy in gynecological cancer. New York: Alan Liss. Radiat Ther Gynecol Cancer 1987:199–205.
30. Taggart CG, Castro JR, Rutledge FN. Carcinoma of the female urethra. AJR 1972;114:145–151.
31. Prempree T, Amoremarn R, Patanaphan V. Radiation therapy in primary carcinoma of the female urethra. Cancer 1984;54:729–733.
32. Johnson DE, O'Connell JR. Primary carcinoma of the female urethra. Urol 1983;21:42.
33. Chu AM. Female urethral carcinoma. Radiology 1973;107:627.
34. Weghaupt K, Gerstner GJ, Kucera H. Radiation therapy for primary carcinoma of the female urethra: A survey over 25 years. Gynecol Oncol 1984;17:58.
35. Antoniades J, Pilepich MV. Carcinoma of the female urethra. In: Perez CA, Brady LW, eds. Principles and practice of radiation oncology. Philadelphia: JB Lippincott, 1987:863–866.
36. Kalra J, Cortes E, Chen S, et al. Effective multimodality treatment for advanced epidermoid carcinoma of the female genital tract. J Clin Oncol 1985;3:917–924.
37. Johnson DW, Kessler JF, Ferrigni RG, Anderson JD. Low dose combined chemotherapy/radiotherapy in the management of locally advanced urethral squamous cell carcinoma. J Urol 1989;141:615–616.
38. Taggart CG, Castro JR, Rutledge FN. Carcinoma of the female urethra. AJR 1972;114:145–151.
39. Prempree T, Wizenberg MJ, Scott RM. Radiation treatment of primary carcinoma of the female urethra. Cancer 1978;42:1177–1184.
40. Thompson IM, Fair WR. Penile carcinoma. AUA Update Series Volume IX, Lesson 1, 1990, Bellaire, Texas American Urological Association Office of Education.
41. Hanash K, Furlow W, Utz D, et al. Carcinoma of the penis: A clinicopathologic study. J Urol 1970;104:291–297.
42. Riveros M, Lebron RF. Geographical pathology of cancer of the penis. Cancer 1963;16:798–811.
43. Dodge OG, Owor R, Templeton AC. Tumors of the male genitalia. Recent Results Cancer Res 1973;41:132–144.
44. Jackson SM. The treatment of carcinoma of the penis. Br J Surg 1966;53:33–35.
45. Kuruvilla JT, Garlic RH, Mamnen KE. Results of surgical treatment of carcinoma of the penis. Aust N Z J Urol 1971;41:157–159.
46. Schellhammer PF, Spaulding JP. Carcinoma of the penis. In: Paulson DF, ed. Genitourinary surgery. New York: Churchill Livingstone, 1983:629.
47. Thomas JA, Small CS. Carcinoma of the penis in southern India. J Urol 1963;160:520–524.
48. Bissada NK, Morcos RR, El-Senoussi M. Post-circumcision carcinoma of the penis. I. Clinical aspects. J Urol 1986;135:283–284.
49. Koenen, M, McCurdy S. Circumcision and the risk of cancer of the penis: A life-table analysis. Am J Dis Child 1980;134:484–486.
50. Gursel EO, Georgountzod C, Uson AC, et al. Penile cancer. Urology 1973;1:569–578.
51. Schrek L, Lenowitz H. Etiologic factors in carcinoma of the penis. Cancer Res 1947;7:180–184.
52. Hellberg D, Valentin J, Eklund T, Nilsson S. Penile cancer: Is there an epidemiological role for smoking and sexual behavior? Br Med J 1987;295:1306–1308.
53. Moriyama N, Hagase Y, Ueki T, et al. In situ hybridization study of human papillomavirus from the penile cancer. Jpn J Urol 1990;81:1706–1710.
54. Iwasawa A, Kumamoto Y, Fukushima M, Fujinaga K. Studies of human papillomavirus (HPV) in urological tumors. Jpn J Urol 1990;81:1626–1632.
55. McCance DJ, Kopan R, Fuchs E, Laimins LA. Human papillomavirus type 16 alters human epithelial cell differentiation in vitro. Proc Natl Acad Sci USA 1988;85:7169–7173.
56. Paymaster JC, Gangadharin P. Cancer of the penis in India. J Urol 1967;97:110–113.
57. Hardner GJ, Bhanalaph T, Murphy GP, et al. Carcinoma of the penis: Analysis of therapy in 100 consecutive cases. J Urol 1972;108:428–430.
58. Buddington WT, Kickham CJ, Smithy WE. An assessment of malignant disease of the penis. J Urol 1963;89:442–446.
59. Dean AL. Epithelioma of the penis. J Urol 1935;33:252–254.
60. Fair WR, Perez CA, Anderson T. Cancer of the urethra and penis. In: DeVita VT Jr, Hellman S, Rosenberg SA, eds. Cancer: Principles and practice of oncology. 3rd ed. Philadelphia: JB Lippincott, 1989:1059–1063.
61. Wajsman Z, Gamarra M, Park JJ, et al. Fine needle aspiration of metastatic lesions and regional lymph nodes in genitourinary cancer. Urology 1982;19:356–360.
62. Jackson SM. The treatment of carcinoma of the penis. Br J Surg 1966;53:33–35.
63. Srinivas V, Morse MJ, Herr HW, et al. Penile cancer: Relation of extent of nodal metastasis to survival. J Urol 1987;137:880–882.
64. McDougal WS, Kirchner FK, Edwards RH, et al. Treatment of carcinoma of the penis: The case of primary lymphadenectomy. J Urol 1986;136:38–41.
65. Skinner DG, Ledbetter WR, Kelley SP. The surgical management of squamous cell carcinoma of the penis. J Urol 1972;107:273–277.
66. Persky L, deKernion JB. Carcinoma of the penis. CA 1986;36:258–272.
67. Narayana AS, Olney LE, Leoning SA, et al. Carcinoma of the penis. Cancer 1982;49:2185–2192.
68. Fraley EE, Zhang G, Sazama R, Lange PH. Cancer of the penis: Prognosis and treatment plans. Cancer 1985;55:1618–1624.
69. Jones WG, Fossa SD, Hamers H, van den Bogaert WV. Penis cancer: A review by the joint radiotherapy committee of the European Organization for Research and Treatment

of Cancer (EORTC) genitourinary and radiotherapy groups. J Surg Oncol 1989;40: 227–231.

70. Sagerman RH, Yu WS, Chung CT, Puranik A. External beam irradiation of carcinoma of the penis. Radiology 1984;152:183–185.

71. Kaushal V, Sharma SC. Carcinoma of the penis. Acta Oncol 1987;26:413–417.

72. Krieg RM, Luk KH. Carcinoma of the penis: Review of cases treated by surgery and radiation therapy, 1960–1977. Urol 1981;16:145–154.

73. deKernion JB, Tynberg P, Persky L, et al. Carcinoma of the penis. Cancer 1973;32: 1256–1262.

74. Beggs JH, Spratt JS Jr. Epidermoid carcinoma of the penis. J Urol 1964;91:166–172.

75. Ekstrom T, Edsmyr F. Cancer of the penis: A clinical study of 29 cases. Acta Chir Scand 1958;115:25–45.

76. Frew ID, Jefferies JD, Swinney J. Carcinoma of the penis. Br J Urol 1967;39:398–401.

77. Johnson DE, Lo RK. Management of regional lymph nodes in penile carcinoma: Five-year results following therapeutic groin dissections. Urology 1984;24:308–311.

78. Cabanas RM. An approach for the treatment of penile carcinoma. Cancer 1977;39: 456–466.

79. Perinetti EP, Crane DD, Catalona WJ. Unreliability of sentinel lymph node biopsy for staging penile carcinoma. J Urol 1980;124:734–735.

80. Whitmore WF Jr, Vagaiwala MR. A technique of ilioinguinal lymph-node dissection of carcinoma of the penis. Surg Gynecol Obstet 1984;159:573–578.

81. Grabstald H, Kelley CD. Radiation therapy of penile cancer: Six to ten years' follow-up. Urol 1980;15:575–576.

82. Haile K, Delclos L. The place of radiation therapy in the treatment of carcinoma of the distal end of the penis. Cancer 1987;45:1980–1984.

83. Salaverria JC, Hope-Stone HF, Paris AMI, et al. Conservative treatment of carcinoma of the penis. Br J Urol 1979;51:32–37.

84. Mazeron JJ, Langlois D, Lobo PA, et al. Interstitial radiation therapy for carcinoma of the penis using iridium 192 wires: The Henri Mondor Experience (1970–1979). J Radiat Oncol Biol Phys 1984;10:1891–1893.

85. Ichikawa T. Chemotherapy of penis carcinoma. Recent Results Cancer Res 1977;60: 140–156.

86. Ahmed T, Sklaroff R, Yagoda A. Sequential trials of methotrexate, cisplatin and bleomycin for penile cancer. Cancer 1984;132:465–468.

87. Hussein AM, Benedetto P, Sridhar KS. Chemotherapy with cisplatin and 5-fluorouracil for penile and urethral squamous cell carcinomas. Cancer 1990;65:433–438.

88. Gagliano R, Blumenstein BA, Crawford ED, et al. cis-Diamminedichloroplatinum in the treatment of advanced epidermoid carcinoma of the penis: A Southwest Oncology Group study. J Urol 1989;141:66–67.

89. Garnick MB, Skarin AT, Steele GD. Metastatic carcinoma of the penis: complete remission after high dose methotrexate chemotherapy. J Urol 1979;122:265–266.

90. Edsmyr F, Andersson L, Esposti P. Combined bleomycin and radiation therapy in carcinoma of the penis. Cancer 1985;56:1257–1263.

91. Palmieri G, Gridelli C, Vitale A, Bianco R. Contemporary chemotherapy and radiotherapy for inguinal metastases of carcinoma of the penis: A case report. Tumori 1988;74:585–586.

92. Abratt RP, Barnes RD, Pontin AR. The treatment of clinically fixed inguinal lymph node metastases from carcinoma of the penis by chemotherapy and surgery. Eur J Surg Oncol 1989;155:285–286.

93. Dexeus FH, Logothetics CJ, Sipahi H. Chemotherapy for advanced squamous carcinoma of the male external genital tract and urethra. In: Johnson DE, Logothetics CJ, von Eschenbach AC, eds. Systemic therapy for genitourinary cancers. Chicago: Year Book Medical Publishers, 1989:255–259.

94. Fisher HAG, Barada JH, Horton J, Von Roemeling R. Neoadjuvant therapy with cisplatin and 5-fluorouracil for stage III squamous cell carcinoma of the penis. J Urol [Abstract] 1990;143:352A.

Cancer: Principles & Practice of Oncology, Fourth Edition,
edited by Vincent T. DeVita, Jr., Samuel Hellman, Steven A. Rosenberg.
J.B. Lippincott Co., Philadelphia © 1993.

Lawrence H. Einhorn
Jerome P. Richie
William U. Shipley

CHAPTER **37**

Cancer of the Testis

With an incidence of approximately 3 in 100,000 men per year, testicular cancer represents the most common malignancy in men from the ages of 15 to 35 years. In the 1990s, testicular cancer has become one of the most curable solid neoplasms, and it can serve as a paradigm for the multimodal treatment of solid malignancies. Dramatic improvements in survival, with an almost total reversal from a 10% survival rate in the 1970s to a 90% survival rate in the 1990s, has resulted from the combination of effective diagnostic techniques, improvement in serum tumor markers, effective multidrug chemotherapeutic regimens, and modifications of surgical technique. All of these advances have led to a decrease in morbidity and mortality rates. In the 1990s, overall survival for all stages of testicular cancer should be well above 80% and should approach 100% for patients with low-stage disease.

Survival advances have resulted from a better understanding of accurate serum tumor markers, which allow careful follow-up with intervention earlier in the course of disease, and additional characteristics of testicular tumors that favor successful therapy. These characteristics include an origin from germ cells that generally are more sensitive to radiation therapy, various chemotherapeutic agents, and a capacity for differentiation, rapid rate of growth, predictable and systematic patterns of spread, and occurrence in young people without comorbid disease.

Approximately 5500 new cases related to testicular cancer are seen annually in the United States. Estimates of lifetime probability of American white men developing testicular cancer are approximately 0.2%.[1] The average age-adjusted rate for American men from 1969 to 1971 was 3.7 in 100,000, nearly twice the rate of 2 in 100,000 seen in the 1930s. Among American black men, the rate is 0.9 in 100,000, which has not changed in 40 years. Similar trends have been noted in Denmark, with an almost doubled age-adjusted incidence between 1945 and 1970.[2]

The peak incidence of testicular tumor occurs in men between the ages of 20 and 40 and again in late adulthood (men older than 60 years of age). Seminoma is rare in patients younger than 10 years of age and older than 60, but it is the most common histologic type overall. Approximately 2% to 3% of testicular cancers are bilateral, occurring either simultaneously or successively. A history of cryptorchidism in nearly half the men with bilateral tumors is consistent with observations that bilateral dysgenesis occurs frequently even in patients with unilateral maldescent.

CRYPTORCHIDISM

LeComete in 1851 was credited with the initial observation of a relation between cryptorchidism and subsequent tumor formation.[3] Approximately 10% of patients with testicular tumors have a prior history of cryptorchidism. Based on the observed incidence of cryptorchidism in military inductees, Gilbert and Hamilton in 1940 calculated estimated risks of tumorogenesis in a man with a history of cryptorchidism to be 48 times that of a man with normally descended testes.[4] More recent studies have reported the relative risk to be lower, some 3 to 14 times the normal expected incidence.[5] Approximately 5% to 10% of patients with a history of cryptorchidism develop malignancy in the contralateral normally descended gonad. This observation may be representative of carcinoma in situ or some hormonal dysfunction in patients predisposed to the development of subsequent malignancy.

CLINICAL SYMPTOMS

SIGNS AND SYMPTOMS

Survival in patients with germ cell tumors usually is related to the stage at presentation and, therefore, the amount of tumor burden. Delay in diagnosis of 1 to 2 months or longer is common in most patients and seems to be related directly to patient factors, such as ignorance, denial, and fear, and physician factors, such as misdiagnosis. *The need clearly exists for patient education through programs such as Advocation of Testicular Self-Examination.* Only through these widespread public health techniques will the knowledge of testicular tumors be promulgated so the diagnosis can be achieved in an earlier fashion. Physician-related causes remain major factors in delay of treatment, emphasizing the need for continuing education.

The usual presentation is a painless swelling or nodule in one gonad, noted incidentally by the patient or his sexual partner. Classically, this finding is described as a lump or hardness of the testis, with occasional heaviness or a dull, aching sensation in the lower abdomen or scrotum. In approximately 10% of patients, acute pain is the presenting symptom. Rarely, infertility may be the presenting complaint. In approximately 10% of patients, presenting symptoms may result from metastases, such as a neck mass, respiratory symptoms, gastrointestinal disturbance, or lumbar back pain. Gynecomastia is seen in approximately 5% of patients with testicular germ cell tumors.

Physical Examination

Physical examination of the testis should be performed by bimanual examination, beginning with the normal contralateral testis. This examination provides a baseline to appreciate the relative size, the contour, and the consistency of the normal testis and the suspected gonad. Careful palpation of the testis is performed between the thumb and first two fingers of the examining hand. The normal testis is homogenous in consistency, freely movable, and separable from the epididymis. Any firm, hard, or fixed area within the substance of the tunica albuginea should be considered suspicious.

Testicular tumors tend to remain ovoid, being limited by the tough investing tunica albuginea. Spread to the epididymis may occur in 10% to 15% of patients. A hydrocele may be present and increase the difficulty of appreciation of a testicular mass. Ultrasonography of the scrotum is a rapid and reliable technique to exclude hydrocele or epididymitis and should be used in patients if there is any suspicion of tumor.

Differential Diagnosis

Differential diagnosis should include testicular torsion, epididymitis, or epididymal orchitis. Less commonly, hydrocele, hernia, hematoma, or spermatocele may mimic testicular tumor. In any patient with a solid, firm intratesticular mass within the tunica albuginea, testicular cancer must be the considered diagnosis until proved otherwise.

IMAGING STUDIES

High-resolution ultrasonography may aid in the clinical evaluation of scrotal masses.[6] Ultrasonography reliably demonstrates whether a mass is intratesticular or extratesticular. In patients with intratesticular masses, testicular cancer must be the diagnosis until proved otherwise. In patients with extratesticular involvement without involvement of the tunica albuginea, conservative treatment may be elected. Ultrasonography is also useful to identify occult testicular neoplasms in patients with palpably normal genitalia and evidence of extragonadal germ cell malignancy.[7]

HISTOLOGY

The seminiferous tubules contain two cell populations: supporting, or Sertoli's, cells and spermatogenic cells known as *spermatogonia.* The Sertoli cells line the basement membrane of the tubules and envelop germ cells as they pass through various stages of spermatogenesis. The stroma that connects the seminiferous tubules is connected to tissue in which interstitial Leydig's cells (androgen-producing cells) are arranged in clusters. These cells are the androgen-producing cells that are necessary for spermatogenesis.

Most primary neoplasms of the testis arise from germinal elements, accounting for 95% of all testicular neoplasms. Nongerminal elements, Sertoli's and Leydig's cells, account for roughly 5% of primary testicular neoplasms. Metastatic tumors to the testis are distinctly uncommon, although involvement by lymphoma may occur in older patients.

Histologic classifications have traditionally provided a major clinical basis for therapeutic decisions. Germinal neoplasms are traditionally divided into seminomas and a variety of other types of germinal neoplasms, known collectively as *nonseminomatous germ cell tumors.* Table 37–1 presents the histology of primary neoplasms of the testis. Although histologic systems play an important role in treatment selection, grading schema have not been employed uniformly. Since 1940 there have been at least six major attempts to classify germinal tumors with a clinical basis. A major distinction exists between British and American systems, with the British referring to all nonseminomatous germ cell tumors as malignant teratomas of one cell type or another. In the United States, classification

TABLE 37–1. Histologic Classification of Primary Neoplasms

A. Germinal neoplasms (demonstrating one or more of the following components)
  1. Seminoma
    a. Classic (typical) seminoma
    b. Anaplastic seminoma
    c. Spermatocytic seminoma
  2. Embryonal carcinoma
  3. Teratoma (with or without malignant transformation)
    a. Mature
    b. Immature
  4. Choriocarcinoma
  5. Yolk sac tumor (endodermal sinus tumor; embryonal adenocarcinoma of the prepubertal testis)
B. Nongerminal neoplasms
  1. Specialized gonadal stromal neoplasms
    a. Leydig cell tumor
    b. Other gonadal stromal tumor
  2. Gonadoblastoma
  3. Miscellaneous neoplasms
    a. Adenocarcinoma of the rete testis
    b. Mesenchymal neoplasms
    c. Carcinoid
    d. Adrenal rest "tumor"

is based on the initial work of Friedman and Moore in 1946.[8] This system, with modifications by Mostofi and Sobin, has generally become the North American standard classification (Table 37–2).[9]

Preneoplastic changes in the testis, so-called carcinoma in situ, have been described by many investigators. Controversy exists, however, concerning the premalignant alteration of intratubular germ cell neoplasia with the development of frank malignancy. Skakkebaek and associates have described the occurrence of intratubular germ cell clusters that are atypical when seen on testicular biopsies in men who presented with infertility.[10] Precancerous changes have been described in adjacent uninvolved areas of the testis in patients with germinal tumors.[11] These findings raise the difficult question of how to deal with the opposite gonad, particularly because there is a known tendency for patients to develop contralateral tumor in approximately 1% of cases. The rate of intratubular germ cell neoplasia has been well defined. The problem that remains in the 1990s is identifying how to deal with this intratubular germ cell neoplasia and what percentage of patients will develop clinically apparent testicular tumors.

FREQUENCY OF HISTOLOGIC TYPES

Seminoma is the most common single germinal cell tumor, accounting for 40% of tumors, with embryonal carcinoma accounting for 20% to 25%, teratocarcinoma accounting for 25% to 30%, teratoma accounting for 5% to 10%, and pure choriocarcinoma accounting for 1%. When combined histologic patterns are considered as a separate entity, the frequency approximates seminoma 30%, embryonal carcinoma 30%, teratoma 10%, teratocarcinoma 25%, choriocarcinoma 1%, and other combined patterns 15%.[12]

SEMINOMA

TYPICAL SEMINOMA

Typical, or classic, seminoma accounts for 85% of all seminomas and occurs most commonly in the fourth decade. Histologically, classic seminoma is composed of sheets of relatively large cells with clear cytoplasm and densely staining nuclei. Synctiotrophoblastic elements may be noted in 10%

TABLE 37–2.   Germ Cell Nomenclature

Serminoma
  Spermatocytic
Teratoma
  Mature
  Immature
  With malignant transformation
Embryonal carcinoma and teratoma
Embryonal carcinoma (adult type)
Choriocarcinoma with or without embryonal carcinoma and/or
  teratoma
Yolk sac tumor (endodermal sinus tumor)

(Mostofi FK, Sobin LH. International histological classification of tumors of testes [No. 16]. Geneva: World Health Organization, 1977)

to 15% of cases, and lymphocytic infiltration is seen in approximately 20%. Synctiotrophoblastic elements correspond to the frequency of production of the tumor marker, β-human chorionic gonadotropin (β-HCG).

ANAPLASTIC SEMINOMA

Anaplastic seminoma accounts for approximately 10% of all seminomas. Anaplastic seminomas are noteworthy because as many as 30% of patients who die with seminoma are found to have anaplastic morphology. Various features suggest that anaplastic seminoma may be more aggressive than is the variant of typical seminoma, including greater mitotic activity, higher rate of local invasion, and higher rate of tumor marker production.

Anaplastic seminoma is typified by increased mitotic activity, with three or more mitoses per high-power field, nuclear pleomorphism, and cellular anaplasia. Anaplastic seminomas tend to have a greater metastatic potential. There is no difference between anaplastic and classic seminoma in terms of survival when patients are treated appropriately and compared stage for stage.

SPERMATOCYTIC SEMINOMA

Spermatocytic seminoma is composed of cells with deeply pigmented cytoplasm and rounded nuclei containing chromatin. Cells closely resemble those of different phases of the maturing spermatogonia. Spermatocytic seminoma accounts for approximately 10% of all seminomas, nearly half occurring in men older than the age of 50 years. The metastatic potential of spermatocytic seminoma is minimal, and the prognosis is extremely favorable.

NONSEMINOMATOUS GERM CELL TUMORS

EMBRYONAL CARCINOMA

Embryonal carcinoma shows a histologic appearance of malignant epithelioid cells arranged in glands or tubules. Cell borders are indistinct, cytoplasm vacuolated, and nuclei rounded with chromatin and large nucleoli. Pleomorphism, mitotic figures, and giant cells are common to these highly malignant tumors.

CHORIOCARCINOMA

Microscopically, choriocarcinoma consists of two distinct and oriented cell types, syncytiotrophoblasts and cytotrophoblasts, that must be present to satisfy the histologic diagnosis. Syncytiotrophoblasts are large, multinucleated cells usually vacuolated with large hyperchromatic nuclei. Cytotrophoblasts are closely packed, intermediate-sized uniform cells with a distinct cell border and a single nucleus.

CLINICAL STAGING

Once the diagnosis of germ cell neoplasm has been established by radical inguinal orchiectomy, with early clamping of the cord, clinical staging is necessary to define treatment modal-

TABLE 37–3. Clinical Staging Systems for Seminoma

Boden-Gibb Stage	MSKCC	American Joint Committee
A (I)—Tumor confined to testis	A	I (A)—Negative
		II (B)—Positive
		N1—Microscopic involvement
B (II)—Spread to regional nodes	B1 < 5 cm	N2—Nodes grossly involved
		A (B1)—<5 Nodes involved with none >2-cm diameter
	B2 > 5 cm	B (B2)—>5 nodes involved and/or nodes >2 cm diameter
		N3—Extranodal extension (gross or microscopic), resectable
	B3 > 10 cm ("bulky")	N4(B3)—Incompletely resected/unresectable disease
C (III)—Spread beyond retroperitoneal nodes	C	

MSKCC, Memorial Sloan-Kettering Cancer Center.

ities further. Staging should take into account the pathologic examination of the primary specimen, history, physical findings, and other diagnostic modalities. Clinical staging attempts to define the extent of disease at the time of diagnosis. The accuracy of clinical assessment is imperative if the physician is to be able to make a logical decision about therapy. The importance of clinical staging cannot be overemphasized; such knowledge allows the orderly decision of algorithms for appropriate treatment and reasonable expectations for prognosis. With the advent of alternative treatment protocols (surveillance) for patients with clinical low-stage testicular cancer, the impact of staging and its accuracy assumes greater importance.

STAGING SYSTEMS

The predictable mode of metastases, along with advances in imaging and biochemical markers, has improved the accuracy of initial clinical evaluations, although they remain far from perfect. A variety of clinical staging systems have been advocated.

For seminoma, the system proposed by Boden and Gibb in 1951 has remained the mainstay of clinical staging (Table 37–3).[13] These investigators separated the extent of disease into the following three stages:

Stage I Tumor limited to the testis with no spread through the capsule or the spermatic cord.

Stage II Clinical or radiologic evidence of tumor extension beyond the testicle but contained within the regional lymph nodes.

Stage III Disseminated disease above the diaphragm or visceral disease.

The system of Boden and Gibb has been modified as clinical staging procedures have become more precise. The Memorial Sloan-Kettering Cancer Center group has subdivided stage B patients into B1 (<5 cm in diameter), B2 (>5 cm in diameter),

and B3 (bulky retroperitoneal disease). The American Joint Committee on Cancer has described the tumor, node, metastasis (TNM) system. All of these systems are detailed in Table 37–3.

For nonseminomatous germ cell tumors, accurate clinical staging is desirable. The principal differences among staging systems for seminomas and nonseminomas relate to the roles of surgical lymph node sampling and serum tumor markers. Pathologic staging systems for nonseminomatous germ cell tumors are detailed in Table 37–4, including the University of Southern California (USC) system, the Walter Reed system, and the TNM system.[14,15]

STAGING EVALUATION

Findings at Orchiectomy

Radical orchiectomy with early clamping of the spermatic cord removes a primary tumor and allows effective local staging. The orchiectomy specimen should be processed carefully to evaluate all tumor elements so that the histologic diagnosis

TABLE 37–4. Pathologic Staging Systems for Nonseminomatous Germ Cell Tumors

Skinner[14]	Walter Reed[15]	TNM
A—Confined to testis	I	N0
B—Spread to retroperitoneum		
B1—<6 positive nodes; no node >2 cm; no extranodal extension	IIA	N1, N2A
B2—>6 positive nodes; any node >2 cm	IIB	N2B
B3—Massive retroperitoneal disease	IIC	N3
C—Metastatic	III	M+

TNM, tumor node metastasis.

can be secure. Equally important is local extent of tumor. Pathologists should record whether tumor is confined within the body of the testis (T1), extends beyond the tunica albuginea (T2), involves the rete testis or epididymis (T3), or invades the spermatic cord (T4A) or scrotal wall (T4B). The histologic report should also determine whether lymphatic or vascular invasion exists and the percentage of subtypes of tumor present.

The extent of staging is determined somewhat by decisions for therapy; for example, if surveillance protocols are to be elected, every effort should be made to exclude patients with any evidence of retroperitoneal disease. If retroperitoneal lymphadenectomy is likely to be elected, then efforts should be directed toward delineation of regional nodal versus distant metastases.

Chest X-Ray Films

Posteroanterior and lateral chest x-ray films provide the initial radiographic procedure. These x-ray films provide minimal assessment of lung parencyma and mediastinal structures. Chest computed tomography (CT) provides more sensitive evaluations of the thorax and may increase the detection of pulmonary metastases. Chest CT, however, delineates lesions as small as 2 mm in size. Approximately 70% of these small lesions are benign.

Computed Tomography Scan

Abdominal CT scans are the most effective means to identify retroperitoneal lymph node involvement. CT scanning has replaced intravenous urography and pedal lymphangiography. Abdominal CT scans, especially with third- and fourth-generation scanners, can identify lymph node deposits smaller than 2 cm in diameter in the upper paraaortic regions. CT scanning generally provides a three-dimensional estimate of tumor size and involvement of soft-tissue structures, but it has significant limitations. In thin patients, with absence of intraperitoneal versus retroperitoneal fat plains, retroperitoneal metastases may often be missed even when they are 2 to 3 cm in diameter. CT scanning is not sufficiently accurate to distinguish fibrosis, teratoma, or malignancy. There is an estimated 25% underestimation of regional nodal involvement with negative CT scans.[16] A positive CT scan is likely to identify metastatic disease accurately. The converse, however, is not necessarily true. As many as an estimated 25% to 30% of patients with documented retroperitoneal metastases have apparently negative CT scans.

Tumor Markers

Germinal testicular tumors produce marker proteins that are relatively specific and measurable in minute quantities using radioimmunoassay technology. These markers may be capable of detecting small tumor burdens that are not detectable by currently available imaging techniques. Two tumor markers, α-fetoprotein (AFP) and the β-subunit of β-HCG, are clinically useful in diagnosis, staging, and monitoring of treatment response in patients with germ cell neoplasms. An additional nontumor marker, lactic acid dehydrogenase (LDH), is associated with bulk disease.

α-Fetoprotein

AFP is a single-chain glycoprotein with a molecular weight of approximately 7 kd that was initially described as an embryonic protein produced by fetal yolk sac, liver, and gastrointestinal tract. Highest concentrations are detected during the 12th to 14th weeks of gestation. AFP levels decline gradually, so that by 1 year after birth, the glycoprotein is detectable at low levels.

Postnatally, AFP may be detected in association with a number of malignancies, including testis, liver, pancreas, stomach, and lung. AFP may be produced by pure embryonal carcinoma, teratocarcinoma, yolk sac tumor, or combined tumors *but should not be produced by pure seminoma*. One of the major importances of AFP is to reclassify an apparently pure seminoma as a nonseminomatous germ cell tumor. The half-life of AFP is approximately 5 to 7 days, a fact useful in evaluation of treatment response.

Human Chorionic Gonadotropin

HCG is composed of α- and β-chains and is normally produced by trophoblastic tissue. β-HCG is structurally distinct from that of pituitary hormones, although there is marked homology between the α-subunits of HCG and luteinizing hormone. β-HCG may be demonstrated in various malignancies, including liver, pancreas, stomach, lung, breast, kidney, and bladder. In germ cell tumors, syncytiotrophoblastic cells have been found responsible for the production of β-HCG.

The serum half-life of β-HCG is between 24 and 36 hours. β-HCG levels are increased in patients with choriocarcinoma and in approximately 50% of patients with embryonal carcinoma. Five percent to 10% of patients with pure seminoma have detectable levels of β-HCG, apparently produced by syncytiotrophoblast-like giant cells.

Clinical Staging Accuracy

After orchiectomy, persistent elevation of one or both tumor markers suggests residual tumor. Rapid normalization of previously elevated markers conceivably represents elimination of tumor, although this is not necessarily the case. In patients with disease clinically confined to the testis, approximately 30% develop metastatic disease while under surveillance, despite negative tumor markers immediately postorchiectomy. Tumor markers, when elevated, are helpful in predicting residual disease. The converse, however, is not necessarily true. Approximately 40% of patients with documented disease in the retroperitoneum have negative tumor markers.

Lactic Acid Dehydrogenase

LDH is an enzyme with a molecular weight of 134 kd, with levels detectable in smooth, cardiac, and skeletal muscles and numerous other organs. Elevations of serum LDH levels have been useful in monitoring germ cell tumors. Because of its low specificity, serum LDH must be correlated with other clinical findings in the making of therapeutic decisions.

TREATMENT

STAGE I: NONSEMINOMATOUS GERM CELL TUMORS

Removal of the testis by an inguinal approach remains the definitive procedure for pathologic diagnosis and local treatment of nonseminomatous germ cell tumors (Fig. 37–1). Morbidity is minimal, and mortality should be virtually zero while allowing 100% local control. Transscrotal biopsy should be condemned. The inguinal approach has the advantages of early control of the vascular and lymphatic supply and en bloc removal of the testis with its surrounding tunics.

In patients with nonseminomatous germ cell tumor, the accuracy of clinical staging is critical as a determinant for further treatment selection after inguinal orchiectomy. Because of the inexactitude of clinical staging, retroperitoneal lymphadenectomy remains the mainstay of surgical therapy in patients with nonseminomatous germ cell tumors. Two- to 5-year survival rates in patients after orchiectomy and retroperitoneal lymph node dissection in pathologic stage I germ cell tumors average higher than 90% in more than 300 patients from collected series in the literature (Table 37–5).[17–19]

Thorough excision of retroperitoneal lymph nodes remains the gold standard of staging. Noninvasive staging techniques are somewhat accurate, but 20% to 25% of patients with clinical stage I disease are understaged by all available modalities of nonsurgical staging. The cure rate for patients with pathologically confirmed stage I disease is roughly 96% with surgery alone. The 5% to 10% of patients who relapse after negative retroperitoneal lymph node dissection, usually within 2 years, have a high cure rate with salvage chemotherapy. Careful follow-up studies are necessary for the first 2 years, generally with monthly chest x-ray films and tumor markers (AFP and β-HCG) for the first year and every other month for the second year.

Modified Retroperitoneal Lymph Node Dissection

Although retroperitoneal lymph node dissection remains the gold standard, there was a high incidence of infertility before 1980 in patients who had experienced retroperitoneal lymph node dissection for testicular cancer. This infertility, either failure of seminal emission or retrograde ejaculation, resulted from the disruption of postganglionic sympathetic nerve fibers that coursed over the aortic bifurcation to form the hypogastric

TABLE 37–5. Two- to Five-Year Survival After Orchiectomy and RPLND in Pathologic Stage I NSGCT

Investigations	NED	Follow-Up (y)
Staubitz et al, 1974[17]	42/45 (93%)	3
Fraley et al, 1979[18]	28/28 (100%)	2
McLeod et al, 1991[19]	259/264 (98%)	5
Total	329/337 (Average 97.6%)	

NSGCT, nonseminomatous germ cell tumor; RPLND, retroperitoneal lymph node dissection; NED, no evidence of disease.

plexus. In the 1980s, Narayan and associates published an important article concerning ejaculation after extended retroperitoneal lymph node dissection.[20] This study showed that modification of surgical boundaries could allow the return of ejaculation in approximately 50% of patients.

In 1990, Richie reported an 8-year prospective study of modified retroperitoneal lymph node dissection in 85 patients with clinical stage I nonseminomatous germ cell tumor.[21] The technique involves a thoracoabdominal approach through the ipsilateral side with mobilization of the peritoneal envelope.

For a right-sided tumor, the dissection would encompass the renal hilar area bilaterally to the level of the left ureter or gonadal vein (Fig. 37–2). Dissection on the left side is carried down to the level of the inferior mesenteric artery, then across to and down the right side of the aorta, encompassing the right common iliac artery. All nodal-bearing tissue in the interaortal caval area is removed, with the posterior margin of the anterior spinous ligament. Both sympathetic chains are preserved. On the right side, the dissection is carried along the right renal hilar area to the level of the right ureter and down to the area where the ureter crosses the common iliac artery. The ipsilateral spermatic vessels are removed to the level of the deep inguinal ring. For a left-sided dissection, a similar dissection is performed, with the exception of the right lateral margin. Because nodal spread tends to be from right to left, dissection is carried only to the lateral margin of the inferior vena cava. Dissection is bilateral above the inferior mesenteric artery and unilateral below the inferior mesenteric artery.

In 85 patients who underwent modified retroperitoneal lymph node dissection, 64 were pathologic stage A and 21 stage B1. Patients have been followed for a median of 38 months. Seven patients relapsed, all with pulmonary metastases; all were cured with chemotherapy.

Ejaculatory function was preserved in 75 of 85 patients, usually within 1 month postoperatively. An additional 5 patients were converted to antegrade ejaculation with imipramine. Eighty of 85 patients (94%) have recovered antegrade ejaculation. Sperm counts range from a low of 2×10^6/ml to a high of 120×10^6/ml. To date, there have been 11 pregnancies in this group of patients' sexual partners.

The template or boundary method of retroperitoneal lymph node dissection has significant advantages. A complete dissection can be performed, but this modification is less likely to cause ejaculatory consequences. Donohue and associates

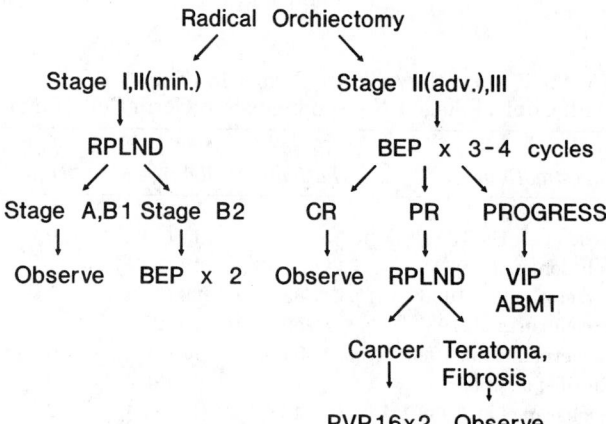

FIGURE 37–1. Treatment algorithm for patients with nonseminomatous germ cell testicular tumors. RPLND, retroperitoneal lymph node dissection; BEP, bleomycin, etoposide, and cisplatin; VIP, vinblastine, ifosfamide and cisplatin; ABMT, autologous bone marrow transplantation.

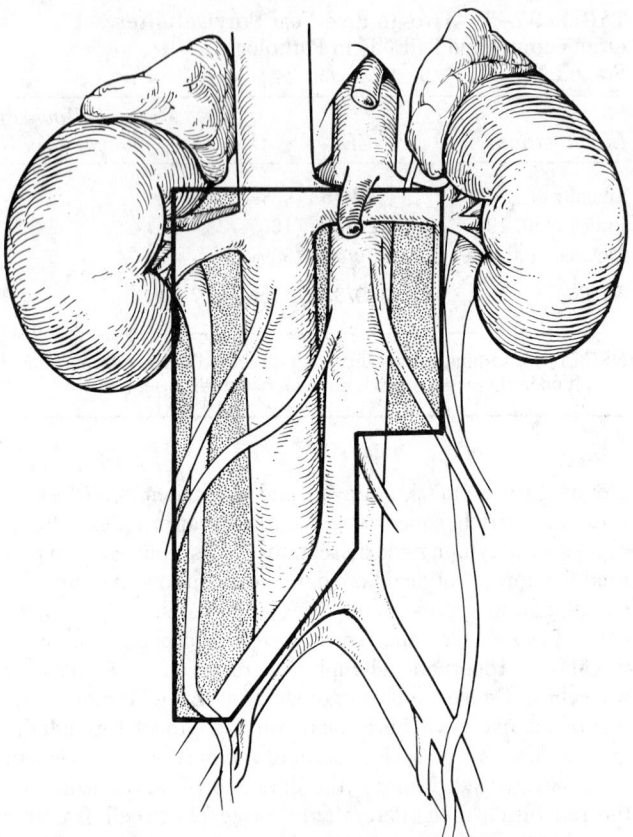

FIGURE 37–2. Modified right-sided retroperitoneal lymph node dissection template. The dissection is complete above the level of the inferior mesenteric artery, but limited to the unilateral-ipsilateral side below the level of the inferior mesenteric artery.

reported modifications with prospective nerve identification with excellent return of ejaculation.[22] These techniques involve removal of nodal-bearing tissue from around the postganglionic fibers. The techniques are somewhat more time consuming and may require a steeper learning curve.

Surveillance

If staging modalities were sufficiently accurate to identify patients whose disease is truly confined to the testis, orchiectomy alone should yield survival results equal to therapeutic strategies that incorporate treatment of the regional lymph nodes. With the inaccuracies of staging, however, retroperitoneal lymph node dissection remains the only modality that can accurately delineate pathologic stage I from pathologic stage II testicular cancer. Clinical understaging approximates 25% even in the best of series. Nonetheless, approximately 70% of patients who undergo retroperitoneal lymph node dissection are found to have pathologic stage I disease and, therefore, receive no therapeutic benefit from the operation. Additionally, 5% to 10% of patients relapse outside of the field of the retroperitoneal node dissection.

With the advent of effective chemotherapy, coupled with concerns about the need for retroperitoneal lymph node dissection in all patients with clinical stage I testicular cancer

and the complications of loss of ejaculation and infertility, postorchiectomy observation or surveillance has a certain appeal. Several large surveillance programs have been undertaken throughout the world. In several of the largest series, detailed in Table 37–6, the relapse rate is approximately 30%. Unfortunately, the death rate in those patients who relapse has been 7%, or 1.8% of the entire series. Even with monitoring, 80% of relapses are detected at a more advanced stage compared with those patients who undergo retroperitoneal lymph node dissection and who tend to relapse with pulmonary metastases at a lower stage of advanced disease.[32] Considering that most of these patients have favorable factors to enter a surveillance protocol, death rates should be exceedingly rare in this subset of patients.

As more experience has been generated, patient selection should identify those persons at low risk for metastases in whom close observation could be elected. These patients require meticulous evaluation before entering a well-designed and well-managed surveillance protocol. Staging should be carried out compulsively in selected patients with no evidence of suspicious nodes or pulmonary masses.

Several series have evaluated prognostic factors associated with relapse.[33,34] Patients with a significant percentage of embryonal carcinoma in the primary are believed to be at high risk of relapse. The local T stage, or extent of involvement of the tumor, is also an important prognostic factor. Patients with invasion of the epididymis or tunica albuginea (T2 or greater) have a higher rate of relapse. Finally, and most importantly, the presence of vascular or lymphatic invasion is significantly associated with relapse.

In patients for whom surveillance therapy is elected, this should be considered an active form of treatment, with careful follow-up studies being mandatory. Physical examination, chest x-ray films, and tumor markers are performed monthly for the first year, every 2 months for the second year, and every 3 to 6 months thereafter. Because of the difficulty with assessment of the retroperitoneum, CT scan should be performed approximately every 2 to 3 months for the first 2 years and at least every 6 months thereafter. Surveillance is necessary for a minimum of 5 years and possibly 10 years after orchiectomy.

TABLE 37–6. Surveillance Studies in Patients With Clinical Stage I Nonseminomatous Germ Cell Tumor

Investigations	No. of Patients	No. Relapsed	No. Dead
Read et al, 1983[23]	45	11 (24%)	0
Johnson et al, 1984[24]	36	12 (33%)	2
Pizzocaro et al, 1986[25]	85	23 (27%)	1
Freedman et al, 1987[26]	259	70 (27%)	3
Gelderman et al, 1987[27]	54	11 (20%)	0
Rørth et al, 1987[28]	79	24 (30%)	2
Raghavan et al, 1988[29]	46	13 (8%)	2
Sogani et al, 1988[30]	45	10 (22%)	2
Thompson et al, 1988[31]	36	12 (33%)	2
Total	680	179 (26%)	12 (7%)

STAGE II:
SPREAD TO RETROPERITONEAL LYMPH NODES

Surgical Treatment

The potential advantages of retroperitoneal lymph node dissection for testicular cancer stem from the fact that retroperitoneal deposits are usually the first and, often, the only evidence of spread beyond the testis. Therefore, retroperitoneal lymph node dissection should be capable of eradicating all disease in more than half of patients with stage II tumors. A variety of surgical approaches has been used, including the thoracoabdominal or midline transperitoneal exposure. Clinical experience has shown that surgical exploration alone is more than 90% accurate in assessing the presence or the absence of lymph node metastases. When suspicious lymph nodes are encountered at operation, a complete bilateral retroperitoneal lymphadenectomy is recommended. Suprarenal nodal metastases occur infrequently in the absence of advanced infrarenal disease. Retrocrural metastases must be evaluated carefully.

Retroperitoneal lymph node dissection is capable of controlling regional nodal metastases in selective patients. For those patients with metastases larger than 3 cm in diameter, chemotherapy is often necessary, and these patients are usually recommended for primary chemotherapy. In patients with clinical metastases smaller than 3 cm in diameter, retroperitoneal lymph node dissection often suffices without the need for additional chemotherapy.

TREATMENT OF SEMINOMA

The treatment of testicular seminoma is one of the most gratifying endeavors in all of oncologic clinical practice. With the advent of effective multidrug chemotherapy, which allows the cure of men with disseminated disease, the overall cure rate for all stages is now higher than 90% in most treatment centers. Because these tumors occur in a young population, and because surgical resection, external-beam irradiation, and multidrug chemotherapy are all effective (either alone or in combination) modes of treating patients with metastatic deposits, consideration of cure *with* maintenance of fertility *and* the avoidance of potential harmful sequelae are important.

Seminoma is exquisitely sensitive to radiation therapy and usually presents at an early stage. Postorchiectomy external-beam irradiation therapy to the retroperitoneal lymph nodes achieves high cure rates for patients presenting with early-stage tumors. The optimum treatment (*i.e.*, chemotherapy, radiation therapy, or both) for patients presenting with large retroperitoneal nodal metastases or more distant metastases (both uncommon presentations) remains undecided.

After orchiectomy, the clinical evaluation for possible extragonadal metastatic disease should include quantitative postorchiectomy serum radioimmunoassays of HCG and AFP, chest x-ray films, and abdominal CT scan. If the abdominal CT scan shows nodal metastases, then a mediastinal and chest CT is necessary. If the abdominal CT scan is negative for nodal masses, then a bipedal lymphangiogram (LAG) is indicated. Recent studies have shown that the LAG detects abnormal paraaortic lymph nodes in 13% to 22% of seminoma patients with negative abdominal CT scans.[35-37] The absolute incidence of occult retroperitoneal lymph nodal disease in

stage I seminoma (both the abdominal CT and LAG are normal) is not known, because for the last three decades, patients have been treated by regional radiation therapy. The accepted incidence of radiographically occult retroperitoneal lymph node metastases is approximately 15%.[38-40] Specific histopathologic characteristics of the primary tumors have been evaluated with regard to their influence on metastatic potential in men with pure seminoma, but no useful significant predictors have been identified.[41-43] In a histopathologic study, there was no significant difference in the incidence of either vascular invasion by tumor or invasion of the epididymis or spermatic cord structures by tumor in patients who were radiographically staged as I compared with those staged as II.[43]

STAGES I AND IIA:
POSTORCHIECTOMY RADIATION TECHNIQUE

The schematic of a typical radiation therapy field for stage I patients is shown in Figure 37–3.

The contralateral testis can be optimally and conveniently shielded using the three additional shields outside the primary

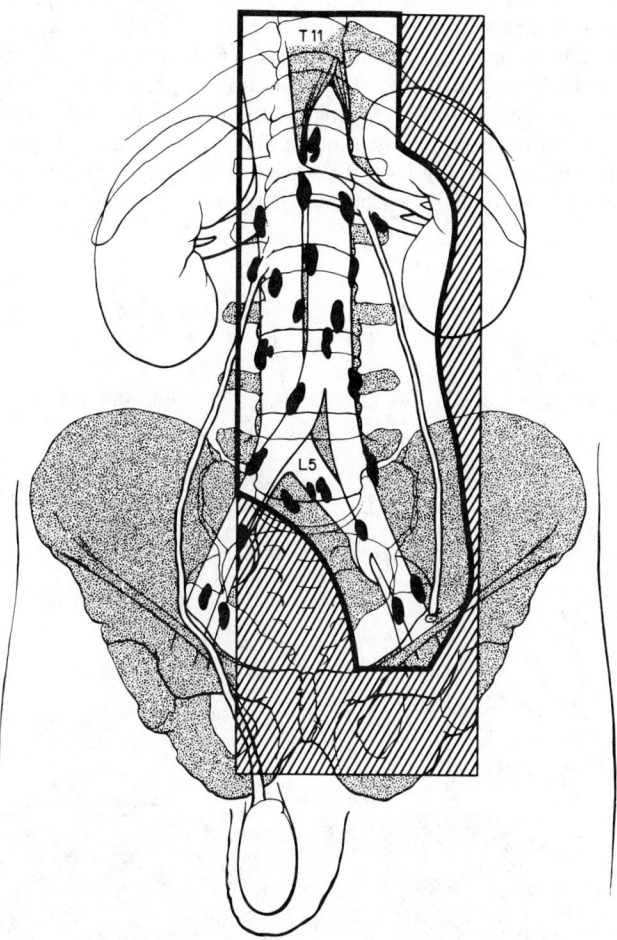

FIGURE 37–3. Contoured anterior and posterior radiation treatment fields for men with clinical stage I or IIA left testicular cancer. The diagonally shaded area and individually made, 8-cm-thick cerrobend block. (Kudo HD, Shipley WU. Reduction of the scatter dose to the testicle outside the radiation treatment fields. Int J Radiat Oncol Biol Phys 1982;8:1741–1745)

radiation beam. As shown in Figure 37–4, these three shields are a 10-cm-thick lead shield immediately above the contralateral testicle; an extention of the cerrobend block for an additional 5 cm below the inferior border of the field; and a more comprehensive gonadal shielding device preventing most internally scattered photons from reaching the remaining testicle. This combination of shields limits the contralateral testicle dose to approximately 0.1% of the treatment dose or to approximately 3 cGy over 20 treatment fractions in 4 weeks.[44] These fields are treated with conventional fractionation (150 cGy/day, 5 sessions per week) using 6- to 10-MeV linear accelerator beams to a total dose of 3000 cGy for stage I patients. For stage IIA patients, a boost dose to the involved nodes with a 5-cm margin of 3600 cGy is recommended. Both the anterior and the posterior fields are treated each day. Elective radiation of the mediastinum is no longer necessary.[45] Adequate coverage of the renal hilum is most important for left-sided tumors, because the testicular lymphatics often drain directly into the renal hilum, as does the testicular vein. From right-sided tumors, the lymphatic drainage is usually to a first-echelon lymph node at the level of L4 adjacent to the inferior vena cava. Radiation therapy fields are adjusted in some special situations. If the primary tumor invades the epididymis, the ipsilateral internal iliac (hypogastric) lymph nodes should be included within the treatment field, because they are in lymphatic drainage of the epididymis and cord structures. If the patients had a scrotal orchiectomy (a procedure that is not recommended), the ipsilateral hemiscrotum needs to be treated only if there was tumor spill or for a microscopic positive margin. In the past, if the patient had a prior ipsilateral orchiopexy or inguinal herniorrhaphy, the contralateral inguinal lymph nodal region was irradiated. More recently, many clinicians find this is no longer necessary.[45–47]

If the patient had a massive primary tumor invading into part of the scrotum but not requiring a hemiscrotectomy, or if microscopic seminoma cells are judged to remain in this scrotum after a removal of the seminoma through a scrotal incision, then the ipsilateral hemiscrotum is best treated by 12- to 15-MeV electron-beam field matched to the lower border of the photon field. The ipsilateral hemiscrotum is held to the involved side with a soft clamp while the patient holds his remaining testicle high in the (contralateral) inguinal canal under a 2-cm-thick lead cup. With this technique, the contralateral testicle can usually be moved more than 4 cm from the electron beam edge and has consistently been measured to receive less than 3% of the given electron dose by scatter.

STAGES I AND IIA: TREATMENT RESULTS

The results from many series for patients with clinically stage I seminoma who received radiation therapy after orchiectomy are shown in Table 37–7. The 3- and 5-year disease-free survival rates are near the absolute cure rates in these patients, because there are few late relapses in the series. With effective chemotherapy against disseminated disease, cure is currently possible in nearly all of the few patients who relapse with distant disease. These excellent results shown in Table 37–7 (the cure rate is approaching 100%) were often *without* elective mediastinal radiation therapy.[54] Therefore, prophylactic mediastinal irradiation has been discontinued by most treatment centers for at least 5 years. Postorchiectomy irradiation for seminoma patients with minimal (<5 cm in diameter)

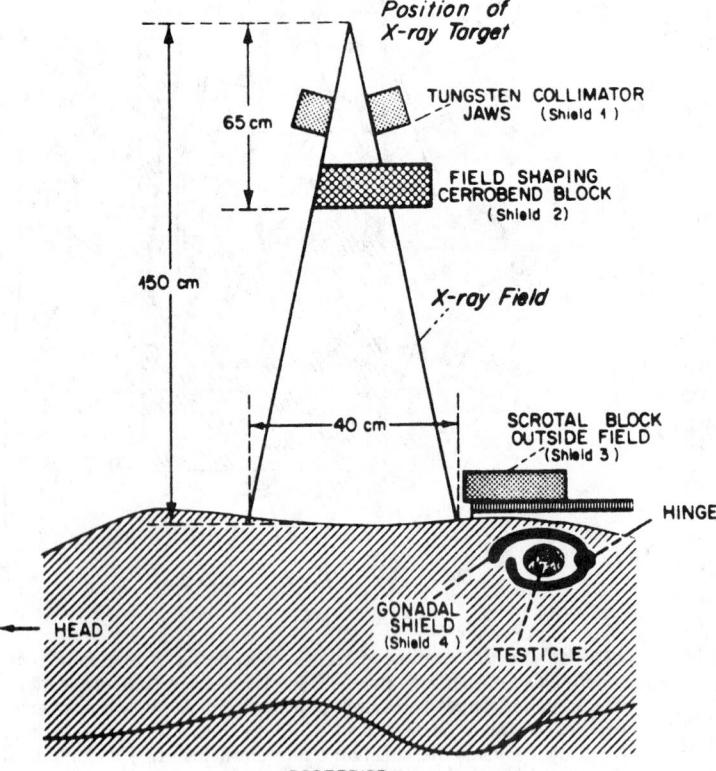

FIGURE 37–4. A schematic sagittal diagram of the treatment setup and shielding for the treatment of a patient with a testicular seminoma after radical orchiectomy. Patient is supine, and the contralateral testis is shown diagrammatically. Field size is 40 cm in the longitudinal direction, and the treatment distance from source to skin is 150 cm. Four shielding devices are illustrated: the collimator jaws of the linear accelerator, cerrobend field-shaping blocks, a lead scrotal block, and a gonadal shield whose front or cephalad wall separates the testicle from the horizontal internal scatter. (Kubo HD, Shipley WU: Reduction of the scatter dose to the testicle outside the radiation treatment fields. Int J Radiat Oncol Biol Phys 1982;8:1741–1745)

TABLE 37–7. Results of Postorchiectomy Radiation Therapy in Stage I Seminoma Testis

Investigations	No. of Patients	5-Year Survival (%)
Walter Reed Army Hospital[48]	284	97
Royal Marsden Hospital[46]	232	98
M. D. Anderson Cancer Center[42]	161	98
Princess Margaret Hospital[45]	150	99
Massachusetts General Hospital[49]	135	98
U. S. Patterns of Care Study[50]	229	98
Cross Cancer Institute[51]	147	98
Harvard Joint Center[52]	79	97
Norwegian Radium Center[53]	365	99
Johns Hopkins Hospital[36]	42	100
Total	1824	98

TABLE 37–8. Results of Postorchiectomy Radiation Therapy in Minimal or ≤5 cm Stage IIA Seminoma Testis

Investigations	No. of Patients	5-Year Survival (%)
Royal Marsden Hospital[55]	39	95
M. D. Anderson Cancer Center[56]	37	95
Princess Margaret Hospital[57]	16	94
Massachusetts General Hospital[49]	18	100
Cross Cancer Institute[51]	20	85
Harvard Joint Center[52]	25	96
Queensland Radium Center[53]	25	96
Johns Hopkins Hospital[36]	16	100
Total	196	95

lymph node masses (stage IIA) results in an 85% to 100% survival rate (Table 37–8). Patients irradiated (usually to doses of 3600 cGy with conventional fractionation) for stage IIA seminoma have a low incidence of distant metastases developing, whether or not they are treated with elective medastinal irradiation.[45,56]

Infradiaphragmatic radiation therapy usually is well tolerated. Because the irradiated volume includes a portion of the stomach, intestine, and bone marrow, some patients may have transient nausea, diarrhea, or a decline in their platelet or leukocyte counts, or both. Moderate or severe acute complications are extremely uncommon. The most frequently seen long-term sequela is dyspepsia or ulcer disease, which has been reported in approximately 5% of patients.[46] The issue of fertility after radiation therapy is important. With the shielding of the contralateral testicle as described previously, there is usually no associated azoospermia or even oligospermia.[44] Because some of these men present with oligospermia at the time of diagnosis of tumor,[58] thorough evaluation of the influence of scattered irradiation on spermatogenesis requires a pretreatment and a posttreatment sperm analysis.

The excellent results achievable with infradiaphragmatic radiation therapy represent the standard against which all other therapeutic approaches should be compared. Because approximately 85% of these patients will not have retroperitoneal lymph node metastases, the use of a comprehensive surveillance program recently has been suggested as an alternative approach in men with clinically stage I seminoma. The Royal Marsden Hospital has carried out such a surveillance program in 113 patients with a median follow-up period of 30 months.[59] These patients were followed closely with serial markers, chest and abdominal x-ray films, and, less frequently, abdominal CT scans. Thirteen patients under observation have had relapses, for a cumulative incidence at 3 years of 16%. Only 4 of these 13 patients had small-volume abdominal disease at the time of relapse. No patient has died yet of seminoma, although the follow-up period is relatively short. The Princess Margaret Hospital has reported an early experience with 81 men with clinically stage I seminoma under a careful surveillance protocol with the mean observation time of 19 months.[47] Only 3 patients have relapsed to date.

Were it possible to identify a subset of clinical stage I patients who are at low risk for having occult paraaortic metastases, these men might be treated safely with careful observation. However, it has not been possible to identify any histopathologic characteristics of the primary tumor that define such a subset.[43,60] Therefore, we and most specialists in urologic oncology recommend infradiaphragmatic irradiation for men with clinical stage I seminoma. The only exception is the patient who develops a second contralateral testis tumor in whom reirradiation of the paraaortic lymph node is likely to be associated with an increased risk for normal tissue injury (such as small bowel obstruction); therefore, reirradiation is not usually recommended.

From observations made more than two decades ago that patients with testicular seminoma either with anaplastic histology or elevated urinary gonadotropin titers did relatively poorly, additional therapy was suggested. However, updated reviews from several large institutions have documented that patients with stages I and IIA disease who have the anaplastic histology have as high an overall success rate as do patients with well-differentiated seminoma when they are treated with conventional radiation therapy.[61,62] Also, recent reviews have documented that stages I and IIA patients with elevated serum HCG titers have all remained in complete remission after conventional treatment with radiation therapy.[63,64] Patients with stages I and IIA pure seminoma with elevated serum HCG levels and anaplastic histology should be treated with conventional external-beam irradiation, with dosages that are usual for the patient's clinical stage.

BULKY STAGES II AND III: TREATMENT OF ADVANCED SEMINOMA

Nearly all series reporting on patterns of failure after irradiation alone for patients with bulky retroperitoneal lymph nodal mass (stage IIB) find that the disease-free survival is low (approximately 60%) and that the incidence of the subsequent development of distant metastases is high (about 30%) when compared with patients with minimal lymph nodal metastases (Table 37–9). The reported cure rate for stage IIB patients treated with radiation alone in older series in which there was no opportunity for salvage with modern chemotherapy is approximately 60%,[45,49,56] which is significantly

TABLE 37–9. Results of Postorchiectomy Radiation Therapy in Bulky Stage IIB Abdominal Seminoma

Treatment Center	No. of Patients	Disease-Free Survival	Patterns of Failure		
			L	L + D	D
Princess Margaret Hospital[45]	46	22/46	10	0	14
Royal Marsden Hospital[65]	23	14/23	2	4	3
Massachusetts General Hospital[49]	7	3/7	1	2	1
M. D. Anderson Cancer Center[56]	11	7/11	2	0	2
Queensland Radium Center[53]	24	18/24	0	1	5
Harvard Joint Center[36]	9	3/9	2	0	4
Mayo Clinic Hospital[66]	20	16/20	—	—	—
Cross Cancer Institute[51]	14	8/14	0	0	6
Total	154	91/154 (59%)	17/134 (13%)	7/134 (5%)	35/134 (26%)

L, local; D, distant.

lower compared with a current cure rate of more than 90% with effective modern cisplatin combination chemotherapy.

Controversial Aspects of Seminoma

Before the advent of cisplatin combination chemotherapy, seminoma represented a noncontroversial topic. This histology represented a markedly radiosensitive and radiocurable tumor. Even occasional patients who presented with both supradiaphragmatic and infradiaphragmatic metastases were potentially curable with radiation therapy alone.

There is no debate about therapeutic strategy for current patients who present with stage III disease (tumor above diaphragm—nodal or visceral). All patients are treated with platinum-based chemotherapy,[165,166] usually with similar regimens and results as for nonseminomatous disease. Horwich and colleagues have evaluated single-agent carboplatin in this patient population and achieved excellent results. Twenty-seven of 34 patients (80%) are found continuously with no evidence of disease (NED) for 12+ to 40+ months. Of six relapses from complete remission, five are currently NED (9+–18+ months) with cisplatin combination chemotherapy.[167] A national multicenter study by Clemm in Munich, Germany, is currently randomizing bulky seminoma patients to single-agent carboplatin compared with cisplatin plus etoposide (VP-16) plus ifosfamide.[168]

There is debate about the proper treatment for bulky but localized seminoma (*e.g.*, primary extragonadal or testicular seminoma with >5 cm retroperitoneal mass). Most of these patients are treated with cisplatin combination chemotherapy, with a greater than 90% cure rate. However, it is equally logical to treat them with initial radiation therapy, unless the retroperitoneal mass is larger than 10 cm or the primary mediastinal seminoma is associated with a superior vena caval (SVC) syndrome or the presence of supraclavicular or axillary adenopathy. Data are scarce, especially in the modern era of

serum markers such as AFP, to exclude obvious nonseminomatous elements. However, the cure rate with radiation therapy alone is probably 70% to 90%, and most failures are salvaged with subsequent chemotherapy.

A final area of controversy involves the proper management of patients who present with bulky seminoma and have persistent radiographic abnormalities after chemotherapy. A certain subset of these patients have persistent seminoma, and it is controversial as to which (if any) of these patients should undergo a postchemotherapy retroperitoneal lymph node dissection. Investigators at Memorial Sloan-Kettering Cancer Center recommend further therapy if the diameter of the residual mass is 3 cm or larger. They recommend surgery and, if viable seminoma is found, then further chemotherapy or radiation therapy should follow. If surgery is not done in such patients, they recommend postchemotherapy abdominal irradiation.[169] These recommendations are based on their careful retrospective evaluation of patients with metastatic seminoma. They culled 14 postchemotherapy patients with persistent retroperitoneal masses larger than 3 cm in diameter. These patients underwent subsequent surgery, and 6 of 14 had viable residual tumor.[170] The opposite viewpoint has been expressed by investigators at Indiana University. Regardless of the size of the residual postchemotherapy mass, none of their patients receive any form of subsequent therapy (surgery, radiation therapy, or chemotherapy), unless there is radiologic or serologic evidence of progressive disease. At Indiana University, 8 of 9 patients with residual masses larger than 3 cm in diameter remain continuously NED after chemotherapy with follow-up of 24+ to 122+ months. One of these patients had a persistent 10-cm mass after chemotherapy and remains without progression for 83+ months.[171]

A cooperative study currently in progress at Indiana University and Memorial Sloan-Kettering Cancer Center may possibly solve this controversy. Patients with bulky seminoma are imaged before and after chemotherapy with gallium scans.

Gallium scans have been used in staging germ cell tumors for 20 years. The results in nonseminomatous germ cell tumors have been disappointing. However, similar to lymphoma, results in seminoma have been excellent.[172,173] Willan and colleagues evaluated 77 consecutive testicular seminomas and reported gallium scan sensitivity and specificity of 83% and 95%, respectively.[173] Data are prospectively collected to see if patients who retain gallium avidity after completion of chemotherapy represent those patients who have persistent seminoma at resection.

CHEMOTHERAPY FOR DISSEMINATED TESTIS CANCER

Historical Perspectives: Pre-Cisplatin Era

Germ cell tumors were known to be chemosensitive and even occasionally chemocurable before the advent of "modern chemotherapy." Therapy was based on dactinomycin, either as a single agent or a component of combination chemotherapy.[69,70] The objective response rate was 50%, including a 10% complete remission and a 5% cure rate. These results were obtained in an era when tumor markers and CT scans were not routinely available, and it was not surprising that at least half of these patients who had clinical complete remissions subsequently relapsed and died. During the 1960s, several other single agents were used, such as mithramycin, vinblastine, and bleomycin, with similar activity compared with dactinomycin.[71–73] Mithramycin has a particularly interesting history, because this drug demonstrated little, if any, activity in preclinical systems, but actually cured a small cohort of patients with metastatic embryonal cell carcinoma.

Combination chemotherapy with vinblastine plus bleomycin was pioneered by Samuels and colleagues at M.D. Anderson Cancer Center.[74] This regimen represented a major improvement over contemporary dactinomycin studies. However, the major advance was the discovery of cisplatin, the first heavy metal to be evaluated in human oncology. Cisplatin is one of a group of coordination compounds of platinum identified by Rosenberg and colleagues that inhibits *Escherichia coli* replication.[75] Phase I and early phase II studies demonstrated remarkable activity in refractory advanced testicular cancer, with complete and partial remissions achieved.[76] Cisplatin is widely recognized currently as the single most active agent in testicular cancer and the most effective cytolytic drug in any neoplasm. The incorporation of cisplatin in the management of disseminated germ cell tumors revolutionized the cure rate in this previously highly lethal tumor.

VAB Programs at Memorial Sloan-Kettering Cancer Center

In the early 1970s, the Memorial Sloan-Kettering Cancer Center group began their vinblastine, dactinomycin, and bleomycin (VAB) studies. VAB-I tested this three-drug combination in 71 evaluable patients treated from 1972 to 1974.[77] A modest 36% objective response rate was attained, including 14% complete remissions. VAB-II switched to continuous-infusion bleomycin and added cisplatin (administered only every 3–4 months) to the original VAB regimen. Fifty evaluable patients were treated with the VAB-II regimen from 1974 to 1976, with a 50% complete remission rate and 24% long-term remissions.[78] Slight modifications were made in the protocol from July 1975 through September 1976, creating VAB-III. In September 1976, another modification resulted in VAB-IV.[79]

Between January 1979 and November 1982, 166 patients were treated with the last VAB regimen (VAB-VI). This differed markedly from earlier VAB regimens in that the cisplatin dosage was 120 mg/m² and was given with each course (every 4 weeks) for three courses (Table 37–10). The complete remission rate was 78%, and this time the remissions were usually durable.[83]

PVB Studies at Indiana University

In August 1974, we began studies at Indiana University in disseminated testicular cancer with the already-established two-drug regimen of vinblastine plus bleomycin and added to this the then-experimental drug, cisplatin (the combination is known as PVB).[80] The original regimen is depicted in Table 37–11. The cisplatin was dissolved in 50 ml of normal saline and given at a rate of 1 mg/minute. Saline hydration at a rate of 100 ml/hour was given continuously during all 5 days of cisplatin administration. Mannitol diuresis was not employed and has never been believed to be necessary in any of the subsequent studies. In this trial, 33 of 47 patients (70%) achieved a complete remission, and an additional 5 patients (11%) were rendered disease free by post-PVB resection of teratoma or carcinoma. Thirty patients (64%) survived 5 years, and 28 (60%) survived 10 years.

After four courses of PVB, if the markers were normal and there were persistent radiographic abnormalities, we resected residual disease 4 to 6 weeks after the final cisplatin chemotherapy, if anatomically feasible. Surgery consists of retroperitoneal lymph node dissection, lateral thoracotomy, median sternotomy with wedge resection of bilateral pulmonary metastases, or a combined thoracoabdominal procedure. If carcinoma was found in the completely resected specimen

TABLE 37–10. VAB-VI Regimen

Agent	Dosage
Vinblastine	4 mg/m²
Cyclophosphamide	600 mg/m²
Dactinomycin	1 mg/m²
Bleomycin	30 U I.V. push day 1 and then 20 U/m² continuous infusion days 1–3
Cisplatin	120 mg/m² day 4

TABLE 37–11. Original PVB Regimen

Agent	Dosage
Cisplatin	20 mg/m² for 5 consecutive days every 3 wk × 4
Vinblastine	0.2 mg/kg day 1 and 2 every 3 wk × 4
Bleomycin	30 U I.V. push weekly × 12
Maintenance vinblastine	0.3 mg/kg monthly × 21 months

TABLE 37–12.   Results of PVB Study No. 2

	PVB 0.4 mg/kg (n = 26)	PVB 0.3 mg/kg (n = 27)	PVB Plus Doxorubicin (n = 25)
NED	23 (88%)	21 (78%)	20 (80%)
Relapses	5 (19%)	2 (10%)	3 (15%)
Currently NED	20 (77%)	19 (70%)	18 (72%)

NED, no evidence of disease.

and the markers remained normal, two postoperative courses of the original induction regimen (fifth and sixth courses of cisplatin combination chemotherapy) were given, with deletion of bleomycin. This strategy resulted in a 67% long-term disease-free survival rate in such patients.[82] Similar results have been obtained with post-VAB-VI resection at Memorial Sloan-Kettering Cancer Center.[83]

The principal serious toxicity of the original PVB protocol was related to the high-dose (0.4 mg/kg) vinblastine. Myalgias, constipation, neuropathy, and paralytic ileus all were troublesome, but severe granulocytopenia with potential sepsis was the most worrisome toxicity. In 1976, we started a randomized, prospective trial comparing our original PVB with the same regimen but with a 25% reduction in the vinblastine dosage (to 0.3 mg/kg). A third arm, adding doxorubicin to PVB with vinblastine at 0.2 mg/kg, was also studied. Again, maintenance vinblastine was employed for a total of 2 years.

Seventy-eight patients were entered in this study. The 25% reduction in the vinblastine dosage resulted in the expected decrease in hematologic and neuromuscular toxicity. There was no significant difference in the efficacy of the three induction arms (Table 37–12).[84] Fifty-eight patients (73%) currently are alive and disease free.

Based on the results of this study, we abandoned our original PVB regimen in 1978 in favor of the equally effective but less toxic program involving the reduced dosage of vinblastine. A similar but larger study was conducted by the European Organization for Research on Treatment of Cancer in 214 patients randomized to receive vinblastine 0.4 or 0.3 mg/kg in combination with cisplatin and bleomycin.[85] This study also showed no benefit for the higher dose of vinblastine; the complete remission rates were 68% for the regimen using vinblastine at 0.4 mg/kg versus 71% with 0.3 mg/kg. There was no significant difference in the disease-free or overall survival rates, but there was a significant increase in hematologic

($p=0.01$) and nonhematologic toxicity with the higher dose of vinblastine.

We began a third-generation study in 1978 in conjunction with the Southeastern Cancer Study Group. We randomized patients achieving a complete remission or disease-free status after resection of teratoma to maintenance vinblastine, as in the first two studies, versus no maintenance therapy (just four courses of PVB over 12 weeks). This study confirmed the facts that optimal cure rates were achieved with induction PVB and that maintenance vinblastine was unnecessary.[81] One hundred forty-seven patients from Indiana University entered this study, and 117 (80%) are alive and disease free with a minimum follow-up of 5 years. The Memorial Sloan-Kettering Cancer Center group also evaluated maintenance therapy (vinblastine plus dactinomycin) with VAB-VI and, likewise, found no value.[83]

The results of these three PVB studies are depicted in Table 37–13. Two hundred one of 272 (74%) patients with disseminated testicular cancer are alive and presumably cured of their disease. Similar results with PVB have been published by numerous other investigators and cooperative groups around the world.

PVB Versus Cisplatin Plus VP-16 Plus Bleomycin

VP-16 is an epipodophyllotoxin derivative with definite single-agent activity in refractory testicular cancer.[86] In preclinical systems, there is marked synergy with VP-16 plus cisplatin.[87] In 1978, we began our initial salvage chemotherapy studies with cisplatin plus VP-16 in patients who were not cured with PVB or similar induction therapy. VP-16, unlike vinblastine, is essentially devoid of neuromuscular toxicity.

The three-drug combination of cisplatin, VP-16, and bleomycin (PVP-16B) was initially used as first-line induction chemotherapy at the Royal Marsden Hospital.[88] Thirty-seven of 43 patients (86%) achieved disease-free status.

From 1981 through 1984, the Southeastern Cancer Study Group conducted a randomized, prospective study comparing PVB and PVP-16B as initial induction chemotherapy (Table 37–14).[89] No maintenance therapy was given in either arm, and if the markers were normal after chemotherapy but there were persistent radiographic abnormalities, appropriate surgery was done. If carcinoma was found, two more courses of the original induction regimen were given.

A total of 244 patients from 24 institutions entered this trial. Of 121 patients treated with PVB, 74 (61%) had a complete remission, and another 15 (13%) became disease free after resection of teratoma (10 patients) or carcinoma (5 pa-

TABLE 37–13.   Summary of PVB Studies at Indiana University

Study No.	Period	No. of Patients	CR	NED With Surgery	Currently NED
1	1974–1976	47	33 (70%)	5 (11%)	27 (57%)
2	1976–1978	78	53 (68%)	13 (17%)	57 (73%)
3	1978–1981	147	92 (63%)	31 (21%)	117 (80%)

CR, complete response; NED, no evidence of disease.

tients). Among the 123 patients given PVP-16B, 74 (60%) had a complete remission, and 28 (23%) became free of disease after resection of teratoma (22 patients) or carcinoma (6 patients). Therefore, 74% became disease free after treatment with PVB and 83% after PVP-16B. Nine patients receiving PVB and 6 receiving PVP-16B subsequently had recurrences. The 2-year survival rate was approximately 80% in both arms with a slight, but not statistically significant, survival advantage for PVP-16B. However, in the subgroup of advanced disseminated disease, there was a clear survival advantage for this combination ($p=0.02$).

Granulocytopenic toxicity, including granulocytopenic fever, was similar in the two arms. Severe thrombocytopenia was more common with PVP-16B, because 14% had a platelet count lower than $50,000/mm^3$ at some time during treatment compared with 5% of the patients given PVB. Hemorrhage was seen in 2 patients given PVB and in 1 given PVP-16B. There was a major reduction in neuromuscular toxicity as manifested by paresthesias, abdominal cramps and ileus, and myalgias. This was significant statistically and clinically (Table 37–15). On the basis of this study, which demonstrated a reduction in morbidity and an equivalent (if not superior) survival, we now use PVP-16B as first-line therapy for disseminated testicular cancer.

PROGNOSTIC FACTORS IN DISSEMINATED GERM CELL TUMORS

Prognostic factors in metastatic germ cell tumors have been analyzed by many authors. There is only minimal disagreement on what constitutes good prognosis ("favorable") disease, because this is a relatively homogenous patient population. Most published series achieve a higher than 90% disease-free status in patients with "good-risk" disease. However, there is considerable debate over what constitutes "poor-risk" disease. This is clearly a more heterogenous group with known and unknown prognostic variables. Tumor volume, multiplicity of anatomic sites, and primary mediastinal nonseminomatous germ cell tumors are independent prognostic variables in virtually all staging systems. Serum markers are usually of independent value, although individual markers (HCG, AFP, and LDH) are given different importance in separate staging systems. The presence of bulky teratoma is not often mentioned or appreciated. For example, if a patient has pure embryonal cell carcinoma in the orchiectomy specimen

TABLE 37–14. Treatment Arms of Southeastern Cancer Study Group Comparison of PVB and PVP-16B

Agent	Dosage
PVB	
Cisplatin	20 mg/m^2 × 5 every 3 wk × 4
Vinblastine	0.15 mg/kg days 1 and 2 every 3 wk × 4
Bleomycin	30 U weekly × 12
PVP-16B	
Cisplatin	20 mg/m^2 × 5 every 3 wk × 4
VP-16	100 mg/m^2 × 5 every 3 wk × 4
Bleomycin	30 U weekly × 12

TABLE 37–15. Neuromuscular Toxicity (% of Patients)

	PVB (n = 114)	PVP-16B (n = 110)
Paresthesias*		
None	62	77
Mild	27	19
Moderate	11	4
Abdominal Cramps†		
None	80	95
Mild	12	3
Moderate	8	2
Myalgias‡		
None	81	99
Mild	5	1
Moderate	14	0

* $p = 0.0003$.
† $p = 0.0008$.
‡ $p = 0.0002$.

with a palpable abdominal mass, mediastinal and left supraclavicular adenopathy, and multiple bilateral pulmonary metastases, his curability is directly predicated by the effectiveness of his cisplatin combination chemotherapy. However, if this same presentation is associated with an orchiectomy histology revealing predominantly teratoma (with or without nongerm cell elements, such as sarcoma) with elements of embryonal cell carcinoma, the patient's curability is determined by both the chemosensitivity of his embryonal cell carcinoma and whether the chemoresistant persistent teratoma is capable of total surgical extirpation.[91]

Arguments about proper categories for inclusion in the advanced group have practical importance due to different chemotherapy strategies for good- versus poor-risk presentations. It has not been demonstrated that more aggressive chemotherapy is superior; therefore, the different therapeutic strategies are less dissimilar (*e.g.*, three versus four courses of PVP-16B).

At Indiana University, we have developed a relatively simple and easily reproducible staging system that places patients into good-risk ("minimal" or "moderate") or poor-risk ("advanced") disease categories.[92] We have modified this system so that *all* patients with primary mediastinal nonseminomatous germ cell tumors are in the advanced category, as are patients with a palpable abdominal mass and any supradiaphragmatic disease. This system is depicted in Table 37–16.

The British system also categorizes patients into three subgroups, with 91%, 72%, and 47% 3-year survival.[93] Other European authors have performed meticulous retrospective analyses of their patients with germ cell tumors.[94,95]

Investigators at Memorial Sloan-Kettering Cancer Center have used a mathematic model incorporating the sites of disease and the pretreatment values of the LDH and HCG levels.[96]

Obviously, no staging system is flawless. Future staging systems will probably evaluate laboratory parameters such as

TABLE 37–16. Indiana University Staging System
for Disseminated Testicular Cancer

Minimal Extent

1. Elevated markers only
2. Cervical nodes (± nonpalpable retroperitoneal nodes)
3. Unresectable, nonpalpable retroperitoneal disease
4. Fewer than five pulmonary metastases per lung field *and* largest
   <2 cm (± nonpalpable retroperitoneal nodes)

Moderate Extent

1. Palpable abdominal mass only (no supradiaphragmatic disease)
2. Moderate pulmonary metastases: 5–10 metastases per lung field
   and largest <3 cm *or* solitary pulmonary metastasis of any size
   >2 cm (± nonpalpable retroperitoneal disease)

Advanced Extent

1. Advanced pulmonary metastases: primary mediastinal
   nonseminomatous germ cell tumor *or* >10 pulmonary
   metastases per lung field, *or* multiple pulmonary metastases
   with largest >3 cm (± nonpalpable retroperitoneal disease)
2. Palpable abdominal mass plus supradiaphragmatic disease
3. Liver, bone, or CNS metastases

flow cytometry, oncogene expression, serum markers, and
anatomic extent of disease.

MANAGEMENT OF GOOD-RISK DISEASE

Regardless of which staging system is used, patients in the
good-risk disease category have a higher than 90% probability
of achieving a disease-free status with standard chemotherapy
and an 80% to 90% expectation for cure. The goal is to achieve
these excellent results with the least morbidity to the host.
The success rate is so high that it would be statistically impossible to prove that any new regimen produced superior
therapeutic results. Although reduction of toxicity is important, it cannot be done at any sacrifice in the cure rate in this
young patient population.

At Indiana University, we have performed consecutive phase
III studies in both good- and poor-risk patient populations and
have supported the following findings:

1. A 25% reduction in the dosage of vinblastine reduced
   toxicity while maintaining therapeutic efficacy.[84]
2. Maintenance vinblastine is unnecessary.[81]
3. VP-16 could be substituted for vinblastine with a reduction in toxicity and a concomitant improvement in therapeutic results, especially in patients with poor-risk
   disease.[89]

From 1984 through 1987, Indiana University, in conjunction with the Southeastern Cancer Study Group, conducted a
phase III study in the cohort of patients previously defined as
good risk (minimal or moderate disease).

One hundred eighty-four patients were randomized to four
courses of PVP-16B as a control arm versus an experimental
arm of identical chemotherapy, but the fourth course (last 3
weeks) of therapy was deleted.[97] This was not simply elimination of *a* course of therapy, but represented deletion of the
most toxic course due to cumulative anorexia, nausea, vomiting, neurotoxicity (cisplatin), and pulmonary fibrosis. The

TABLE 37–17. Comparison of Three and Four Courses
of PVP-16B

	PVP-16B × 3	*PVP-16B × 4*
No. entered	88	96
NED status	86 (98%)	93 (97%)
Continuously NED	81 (92%)	88 (92%)

NED, no evidence of disease.

therapeutic results are demonstrated in Table 37–17. This
random, prospective study confirmed the high cure rate in
favorable-prognosis disease and documented that optimal cure
rates in this patient population could be attained with merely
9 weeks (three courses) of cisplatin combination chemotherapy. There was only one drug-related death (secondary to
sepsis) in these 184 patients with good-risk disease. Further,
there were no episodes of clinically significant bleomycin-
induced pulmonary fibrosis in any of the 88 patients randomized to three courses.

The next study in minimal-moderate extent (good-risk)
disease was performed by Indiana University under the aegis
of the Eastern Cooperative Oncology Group (ECOG). Based
on the previous study, three courses of PVP-16B were accepted
as the standard arm. In this phase III trial, the experimental
arm was the identical chemotherapy, but with the deletion of
bleomycin. At the onset of this study, there was a growing
opinion that bleomycin was not necessary in this patient population. However, bleomycin had a single-agent response rate
of 30% to 50% and exhibited little or no myelosuppression,
permitting a full dosage of all three agents in the regimen.
Although pulmonary fibrosis is a well-recognized cumulative
side effect of bleomycin, as discussed earlier, this toxicity is
essentially negligible in good-risk patients receiving only 9
weeks (270 U) of bleomycin. In November 1987, this ECOG
phase III study commenced. One hundred seventy-eight patients were entered and were stratified in their randomization
according to minimal versus moderate category. Overall, 95%
of patients receiving all three drugs achieved a disease-free
status compared with 90% on the nonbleomycin regimen. This
group included only 2 patients with the three-drug regimen
compared with 8 with the two-drug treatment who had persistent carcinoma in the postchemotherapy-resected specimen. These patients were, therefore, at higher risk for subsequent relapse and death and required two postoperative
treatments (fourth and fifth courses) with cisplatin plus VP-
16. The most striking difference was in the relapse rate, as 8
of 82 NED patients with the three-drug regimen relapsed
compared with 18 of 78 in the two-drug regimen ($p=0.01$).[98]
The overall results are depicted in Table 37–18. Toxicity was
similar in both arms, with one early death from sepsis on the
three-drug regimen and no clinically significant pulmonary
toxicity. Based on this large multiinstitution phase III study,
bleomycin was shown to be an essential component of therapy
in this highly curable patient population. It is possible that
bleomycin could be deleted if *four* courses are given.[99] However, because the toxicity of 9 weeks of bleomycin was negligible, this additional course of cisplatin plus VP-16 would

TABLE 37–18. Cisplatin + VP-16 ± Bleomycin

	PVP-16B	PVP-16
No. patients entered	86	86
Complete remission	67 (78%)	62 (72%)
NED—teratoma	13 (15%)	8 (9%)
NED—carcinoma	2 (2%)	8 (9%)
Relapse	8 (9%)	18 (23%)
Continuously NED	74 (86%)	60 (70%)

NED, no evidence of disease.

add to the overall toxicity in an attempt to eliminate a less toxic component (bleomycin).

Important phase III studies in good-risk patients have been performed by other institutions as well, most notably Memorial Sloan-Kettering Cancer Center. Between November 1982 and July 1986, 164 eligible patients were randomized to the five-drug VAB-VI regimen compared with a two-drug regimen consisting of cisplatin (20 mg/m² for 5 consecutive days) plus VP-16 (100 mg/m² for 5 consecutive days). One hundred sixty-four eligible patients were treated. Ninety-six percent of VAB-VI and 93% of cisplatin plus VP-16 patients achieved a disease-free status and relapse rate was similar in both arms. However, there was considerably more toxicity with VAB-VI with more emesis ($p=0.05$), lower leukocyte count nadir ($p=0.06$), platelet nadir ($p=0.01$), more hypomagnesemia ($p=0.0001$), and more mucositis ($p=0.09$).[100] The authors concluded that cisplatin plus VP-16 is equally effective but considerably less toxic than the five-drug VAB-VI regimen.

The Memorial Sloan-Kettering Cancer Center group, in conjunction with the Southwest Oncology Group (SWOG), conducted a study in good-risk patients comparing four courses of cisplatin plus VP-16 with four courses of carboplatin plus VP-16. The purpose of this study was to determine if a "less toxic" platinum compound (carboplatin) could produce equivalent results when substituted for cisplatin. At the start of this study, highly effective 5-hydroxytryptamine antagonists, such as ondansetron, were not commercially available to mitigate cisplatin-induced nausea and vomiting. Two hundred sixty-three patients were randomized. The VP-16 dosage was identical in both arms (100 mg/m² for 5 consecutive days), but courses were given every 3 weeks with cisplatin (20 mg/m² for 5 consecutive days) compared with every 4 weeks with carboplatin. The carboplatin dosage was initially 350 mg/m² in the first 25 patients and subsequently increased to 500 mg/m² in the remaining large patient population.[101] At the time of the presentation of this trial, the carboplatin arm had statistically significant more hematologic toxicity. In addition, there were fewer patients continuously NED with carboplatin.

Other successful regimens have been evaluated in phase II trials. At Royal Marsden, 76 patients were treated with variable doses of carboplatin in combination with VP-16 and bleomycin.[102] Follow-up was 6 to 54 months. Sixty-nine of 76 (91%) are alive and continuously NED.

In conclusion, the following statements can be made about chemotherapy for good-risk disease:

1. Three courses of PVP-16B is equivalent to four courses of the same therapy.
2. When only three courses of cisplatin combination chemotherapy are given, bleomycin must be included (with cisplatin plus VP-16) to achieve optimal cure rates. There is little or no clinically significant pulmonary fibrosis in this relatively healthy patient population.
3. Four courses of cisplatin plus VP-16 is superior to four courses of carboplatin plus VP-16.

We believe that standard therapy should consist of three courses of PVP-16B. It is unlikely that any further modification could ever statistically improve the cure rate or clinically lessen patient morbity.

MANAGEMENT OF POOR-RISK (ADVANCED) DISEASE

The definition of what constitutes poor-risk disease varies among authors in different staging systems. However, one constant is the relation of bulk disease and multiplicity of anatomic sites to an inferior cure rate with standard chemotherapy compared with good-risk patients. Depending on the definition, the potential cure rate has varied from 35% to 65%. This is a more complicated and heterogenous patient population than is the good-risk patient group, with an 80% to 95% cure rate with standard chemotherapy.

The Southeastern Cancer Study Group protocol comparing PVB with PVP-16B randomized both good- and poor-risk patients.[89] This study, conducted from 1981 through 1984, clearly demonstrated superior continuous disease-free survival and overall survival for the VP-16 arm in the cohort of patients with advanced disease. It would seem logical to incorporate VP-16 as an essential ingredient in any platinum combination chemotherapy regimen in advanced disseminated germ cell tumors.

A phase III National Cancer Institute study in advanced disease started in 1981 before results of the study just discussed were available. Standard therapy consisted of PVB, and this was compared with double-dose (40 mg/m² for 5 consecutive days) cisplatin in combination with vinblastine, bleomycin, and VP-16. There were two variables in this study: the dosage of cisplatin and the inclusion of VP-16 in the high-dose cisplatin regimen. Randomization was in a 2 to 1 ratio. Thirty-four patients were assigned to high-dose therapy, and 30 (88%) obtained an NED status. In contrast, only 12 of 18 (67%) PVB patients attained disease-free status ($p=0.14$). Sixty-eight percent (23 of 34) of high dose and only 33% (6 of 18) of PVB patients are continuously disease free ($p=0.02$).[103]

Based on this study design (and the lack of information about the value of VP-16 at study inception), it was impossible to determine whether these superior results were the result of double-dose cisplatin, the inclusion of VP-16, or a combination of both of these factors. Therefore, from October 1984 through August 1989, a phase III study was designed for poor-risk patients in which the *only* variable was the cisplatin dosage (Fig. 37–5). This study was conducted by Indiana University, the Southeastern Cancer Study Group, and SWOG. One hundred fifty-three patients were evaluable. Patients receiving

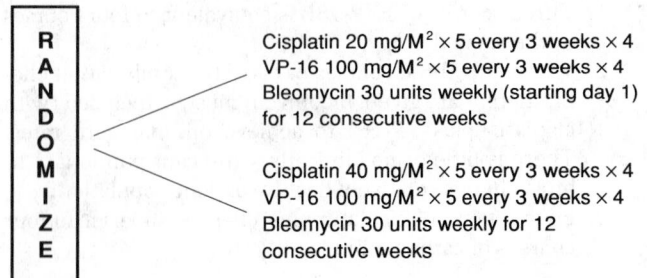

Cisplatin 20 mg/M² × 5 every 3 weeks × 4
VP-16 100 mg/M² × 5 every 3 weeks × 4
Bleomycin 30 units weekly (starting day 1)
for 12 consecutive weeks

Cisplatin 40 mg/M² × 5 every 3 weeks × 4
VP-16 100 mg/M² × 5 every 3 weeks × 4
Bleomycin 30 units weekly for 12
consecutive weeks

FIGURE 37–5.   PVP-16B versus P-2VP-16B in advanced disease.

TABLE 37–20.   Therapeutic Results

	PVP-16B	P2VP-16B
No. patients evaluable	77	76
Complete remission	36 (47%)	35 (46%)
NED—teratoma	15 (19%)	16 (21%)
NED—cancer	5 (6%)	1 (1%)
Continuously NED	47 (61%)	48 (63%)

P2, double dose cisplatin; NED, no evidence of disease.

the high-dose cisplatin regimen experienced significantly more toxicity (Table 37–19). Despite the toxicity encountered, there was no evidence for any therapeutic superiority of double-dose cisplatin (Table 37–20). This large phase III intergroup study failed to demonstrate value for doubling the dosage of the most active single agent in the treatment of germ cell tumors.[104]

A successor study in the same advanced disease patient population was recently completed. This study was being conducted by Indiana University, ECOG, SWOG, and Cancer and Leukemia Group B. The standard arm was four courses of cisplatin (20 mg/m²×5) plus VP-16 plus bleomycin and was compared with the salvage chemotherapy regimen of VP-16 plus ifosfamide plus cisplatin (VIP). The VP-16 dosage in the VIP regimen was attenuated 25% (75 mg/m²×5) because of inclusion of the other myelosuppressive drug, ifosfamide. This study completed accrual in 1992.

An innovative and dynamic approach is being tested currently in advanced disease patients at Memorial Sloan-Kettering Cancer Center. Retrospective analysis of prior Memorial Sloan-Kettering Cancer Center studies revealed that the lack of appropriate decay of serum tumor markers allowed early identification of patients unlikely to be cured with standard therapy.[105] A current phase II study is evaluating this diagnostic approach to identify patients needing an early change in therapy. Patients with advanced disease are treated with VAB-6 initially. If after two cycles there is not an appropriate decrease in serum HCG and AFP levels, patients are immediately switched to high-dose chemotherapy with carboplatin plus VP-16 with autologous bone marrow rescue.[106]

TABLE 37–19.   Toxicity

	PVP-16B	P2VP-16B
No. patients evaluable	77	76
Grade 3–4 ototoxicity*	0	24 (32%)
Grade 3–4 neurotoxicity*	1 (1%)	20 (26%)
Grade 3–4 gastrointestinal toxicity*	3 (4%)	20 (26%)
Leukocytes <1 × 10⁹/L*	12 (16%)	27 (36%)
Granulocytopenic fevers*	12 (16%)	38 (50%)
Platelets <100 × 10⁹/L*	8 (10%)	44 (58%)

P2, double dose cisplatin.
* $p < 0.001$.

EXTRAGONADAL GERM CELL TUMORS

Primary extragonadal germ cell tumors may arise in midline structures such as the mediastinum and the retroperitoneum or in the pineal gland, the prostate, the stomach, or the thymus. During early embryogenesis, germinal epithelium arises in the yolk sac and undergoes a midline migration (from the level of C6 to S2) down the dorsal mesentery of the hind gut to the urogenital ridge and eventually forms aggregates of testicular tissue in the scrotum. During the migration, germinal epithelium may be sequestered along the route and ultimately undergoes malignant transformation.

Patients with presumed primary retroperitoneal germ cell tumors must have a careful search for an occult testicular primary. This is critically important, because the testis is a relative sanctuary site from the effects of chemotherapy, and a missed small primary there is not necessarily eradicated with chemotherapy.[90] Patients with a normal testis on palpation should have bilateral testicular ultrasound performed. If physical examination or ultrasound is abnormal, an orchiectomy should be performed, usually after completion of chemotherapy. Also, a primary retroperitoneal germ cell tumor should be a midline mass. If the abdominal CT scan reveals predominantly right- or left-sided adenopathy, this is compatible with an occult primary site of origin in the ipsilateral testis, and strong consideration should be given to removal of the suspected testis.

The treatment philosophy for a primary retroperitoneal germ cell tumor should parallel that for the testicular tumors in general, and the prognosis for cure is similar to that of testicular primaries with similar amounts of disease and marker elevation.

There is a paucity of literature guidelines for the management of suprasellar germ cell tumors (pinealomas). Most of these are seminoma, but anatomic location often precludes accurate histologic diagnosis. An area of significant controversy is whether cranial irradiation alone is adequate or whether the entire neuroaxis should be irradiated. The incidence of positive spinal fluid cytology ranges from 6% to 55% in various series, and about 35% of patients relapse in the spine. However, the routine use of craniospinal radiation therapy makes the subsequent delivery of myelosuppressive chemotherapy difficult should the patient relapse. The Harvard Joint Center for Radiation therapy recently detailed their results in 25 suprasellar germ cell tumors.[107] Nineteen of the patients (76%) are continuously disease free, and most of these received radiation to the entire neuraxis.

Primary mediastinal germ cell tumors represent a challenging and fascinating subject for oncologists, pathologists, and developmental biologists. A recent review by Nichols details the clinical features and biologic correlates of these rare tumors.[108] There is a definite association between primary mediastinal nonseminomatous germ cell tumor and Klinefelter's syndrome. The Indiana group has prospectively performed chromosomal analyses on 22 consecutive patients, and 5 (22%) had karyotypic or pathologic evidence of Klinefelter's syndrome.[109] Data from M.D. Anderson confirm that approximately 20% of patients with mediastinal nonseminomatous germ cell tumors have Klinefelter's syndrome.[110]

Primary mediastinal nonseminomatous germ cell tumors have been associated with hematologic disorders. Nichols and colleagues reported 16 cases of this linkage.[111] These cases included 5 patients who developed a hematologic malignancy among the 31 patients receiving initial chemotherapy at Indiana University from 1976 to 1989. The most common disorder was acute megakaryocytic leukemia (French-American-British [FAB] M7) with 6 cases. This is a remarkable association, because the incidence of this rare leukemia in the general population is 1 in 500,000, and there have been no cases seen in association with mediastinal seminoma, primary retroperitoneal germ cell tumors, or testicular primary. The median time to the development of the hematologic malignancy in these 16 patients was 6 months.

There is a unique and definite linkage between hematologic disorders and primary mediastinal nonseminomatous germ cell tumors. One possible explanation for this association is that the hematologic malignancy is a consequence of multipotential differentiation of the malignant germ cell tumors in a proper microenvironment (*e.g.*, sternal marrow) with development of hematopoietic cells. Recently, Bosl and coworkers reported that the finding of the isochromosome of chromosome 12 (i[12p]) was a marker chromosome for germ cell tumors.[112] The Memorial Sloan-Kettering Cancer Center group subsequently reported the finding of i(12p) in the cytogenetic analysis of bone marrow in a patient with primary mediastinal nonseminomatous germ cell tumor and leukemia. Cytogenetic analysis was identical for the mediastinal germ cell tumor and the leukemia.[113]

Extragonadal germ cell tumors must always be considered in the diagnosis of "carcinoma, primary unknown," especially in young patients with mediastinal or retroperitoneal masses. Assays for HCG and AFP should be performed. The investigators at Vanderbilt University accumulated data on 119 patients with poorly differentiated carcinoma, primary unknown.[114] Reviewing pathologists found features suggestive of germinal neoplasm in only 6 patients, and only 2 of these achieved complete remission with cisplatin combination chemotherapy. Overall, 27 of 96 patients (28%) who received at least one course of chemotherapy attained a complete remission and an additional 42 (44%) a partial remission. Sixteen patients (17%) are currently without evidence of disease 16 to 133 months (median 65 months) after completion of chemotherapy. Only 3 of the 27 achieving a complete remission were HCG or AFP positive. This study points out that neither light microscopy nor marker elevation can differentiate curable from incurable patients.

The results of PVB in extragonadal germ cell tumors at Indiana and Vanderbilt Universities have been published.[115] Approximately 50% of these patients were cured. Similar results were observed with PVB by the Southeastern Cancer Study Group[116] and with VAB-VI at Memorial Sloan-Kettering Cancer Center.[117] Investigators at M.D. Anderson used a complicated five-drug regimen and also achieved similar results, with 16 of 19 patients with seminoma and 12 of 30 with nonseminomatous tumors without evidence of disease at the time of publication.[118]

Primary mediastinal nonseminomatous germ cell tumors are associated with an inferior survival compared with other germ cell tumors with similar bulk disease. Part of the reason for this is associated with the biologic correlates listed earlier. However, another major factor is related to the difficulty in surgically extirpating residual teratoma after chemotherapy because of anatomic constraints within the anterior mediastinal. Nevertheless, a recent review of the Indiana experience in 31 patients with primary mediastinal nonseminomatous germ cell tumors revealed that 18 (58%) achieved a disease-free status. However, only 10 of these 18 patients are continuously NED. Two patients had a relapse with teratoma that was resected successfully. Three patients relapsed with recurrent germ cell tumors, and 3 patients in complete remission developed a hematologic malignancy at 13, 39, and 105 months.[119] Overall, 13 of 31 patients (42%) are currently alive and NED with minimal follow-up of 2 years. These results contrast dramatically with published series just a decade ago. Economou and colleagues summarized the experience of many groups before 1978.[120] Of 63 patients with mediastinal nonseminomatous germ cell tumors, only 2 patients (3%) survived after 16 months.[120]

SALVAGE CHEMOTHERAPY

First-line cisplatin combination chemotherapy cures 70% of patients with disseminated germ cell tumors. By definition, then, 30% become candidates for salvage chemotherapy.

It is our philosophy to resect residual disease after a maximum of four courses of induction therapy, if the serum markers are normal, and if it is anatomically feasible to extirpate the persistent disease. Traditionally, we do not administer more than four courses of induction therapy, even if there is continued serologic and radiographic regression. Most patients with persistently elevated markers at this time demonstrate a plateau in their marker decline, allowing the physician to realize that a fifth or sixth course will be incapable of normalizing the markers. Further, by continuing the same "ineffective" induction regimen beyond four courses, there is a risk that the disease will worsen, thereby depriving the patient of the opportunity to enroll in a potentially curative cisplatin salvage regimen. A patient who progresses *during* cisplatin combination chemotherapy is not a candidate for cisplatin salvage chemotherapy regimen, whereas a patient progressing while no longer receiving cisplatin is still potentially curable with agents to which his tumor has not been exposed, in combination with a platinum compound.

The marker results of a hypothetical patient of this type are shown in Table 37–21. This patient had his maximal marker regression with his first course of chemotherapy. He still had a greater than 1 log reduction with his second course; however, he had a clear plateau in his HCG decline subsequently. It should be obvious that giving a fifth and sixth course

TABLE 37–21. Results of Exceeding Four Courses

Cisplatin + VP-16 + Bleomycin Course No.	*HCG Level*
1	100,000
2	4000
3	380
4	190
5	130
6	120
7	500

HCG, human chorionic gonadotropin.

of the identical induction regimen would never normalize his HCG. Instead, because of continuation of a noncurative regimen, he eventually developed marker-evidenced progression and is no longer a candidate for a cisplatin-based salvage regimen, because his disease has progressed during cisplatin chemotherapy.

If a patient has a partial remission with anatomically unresectable disease but has normal serum markers, he is observed monthly (receiving no therapy) until he develops serologic or radiographic evidence of progressive disease. This practice is followed because some patients with an "unresectable partial remission" have no remaining tumor; that is, they have persistent necrotic fibrous tissue with or without teratoma. Some of these patients become radiographically free of disease later as their necrotic fibrous deposits spontaneously dissipate.

Candidates for salvage chemotherapy are patients who progress after achieving a complete remission or patients with progression after an unresectable partial remission (either anatomically unresectable or elevated HCG or AFP level, or both, after four courses of induction chemotherapy). However, if a patient progresses with normal markers, the investigator must be aware that this may represent growing teratoma and require surgery rather than salvage chemotherapy. Likewise, progression documented as an elevated marker but with normal radiographic studies must be studied carefully. Among the pitfalls are laboratory error, cross-reactivity of leutinizing hormone with HCG, or a second primary in the contralateral testis. Once the need for salvage chemotherapy is determined, a different platinum recipe (*i.e.*, cisplatin plus other active drugs not previously employed) may be curative if there was not progression during cisplatin combination chemotherapy (*i.e.*, within 4 weeks of the last course).

The two-drug combination of cisplatin and VP-16 is highly synergistic in preclinical systems.[87] Single-agent VP-16 is an active, albeit noncurative, drug in refractory testicular cancer. We first began PVP-16 salvage chemotherapy in 1978 and documented a 30% cure rate.[121] These results have been confirmed subsequently by other single institutions and by the Southeastern Cancer Study Group.[122] This represented the first curative salvage regimen for an adult solid tumor.

Another active drug in refractory testicular cancer is ifosfamide, with a 22% single-agent response rate after PVB and PVP-16.[123] We have evaluated cisplatin plus ifosfamide in refractory testicular cancer.[124] Perhaps the most impressive results are with this therapy as a third-line or later regimen in

patients previously given PVB or PVP-16 combinations: 20 of 56 patients (36%) achieved disease-free status, and 9 (18%) are continuously disease free. Our current first-line regimen is PVP-16B. Therefore, our present initial salvage regimen is cisplatin plus vinblastine plus ifosfamide (VeIP; Table 37–22). The uroprotector mesna, in a dosage of 120 mg/m^2 by intravenous push, is given just before starting ifosfamide and then continued for all 5 days of each ifosfamide course.

Einhorn and colleagues from Indiana University recently reported their results with VeIP as second-line therapy.[125] One hundred twenty-four patients were treated, with a minimal follow-up of 27 months from initiation of VeIP. All patients had prior first-line chemotherapy with PVP-16B. Hematologic toxicity was significant, with 48% requiring erythrocyte transfusion and 28% platelet transfusion, and 73% of patients developed granulocytopenic fever. In addition, 11 patients (7%) had treatment-related azotemia (usually reversible) with serum creatinine levels higher than 4 mg/dl. There were three drug-related deaths. Therapeutically, 56 patients (45%) achieved NED status, and 29 (23%) are alive and continuously disease free. Although only 10% of patients attaining a disease-free status with first-line chemotherapy relapse, the relapse rate for salvage chemotherapy is usually 50%. Only 1 of 31 patients with extragonadal germ cell tumors are continuously NED compared with 28 of 93 (30%) patients with a testicular primary.

Similar results with ifosfamide-based salvage therapy were reported by Motzer and colleagues from Memorial Sloan-Kettering Cancer Center.[126] Ten of 42 patients (25%) achieved a disease-free status, and 6 of 42 (15%) remain NED.

The second course of salvage chemotherapy always begins on day 22, regardless of the blood cell count. We try to give courses three and four on time also, and if therapy is delayed, we never delay it by more than 7 days. We believe it is safe and effective to start subsequent courses even in the presence of unrecovered myelosuppression; however, if on day 5 of a course of salvage chemotherapy there is no obvious hematologic recovery, we delete the fifth day of ifosfamide. Drug dosages are never lowered based on nadir blood counts or day-of-treatment counts. However, if granulocytopenic fever or thrombocytopenic bleeding occurs, subsequent ifosfamide and vinblastine are reduced by 25%. Cisplatin dosages are never reduced. If the serum creatinine level is higher than 2 mg/dl, ifosfamide (alone) is reduced by 25%, and if hematuria (more than 10 erythrocytes per high-power field) is found during daily urinalysis, ifosfamide is not administered that particular day but the regular dose is resumed after hematuria clears.

Because of the high incidence (40%) of granulocytopenic fevers requiring antibiotics with salvage chemotherapy, cur-

TABLE 37–22. Initial Salvage Chemotherapy at Indiana University*

Agent	*Dosage*
Cisplatin	20 mg/m^2 × 5
Vinblastine	0.11 mg/kg on days 1 and 2
Ifosfamide	1.2 g/m^2 × 5

* Drugs are given every 3 wk for 4 courses.

rently we routinely employ a hematologic growth factor with each course. We currently use granulocyte-colony stimulating factor (G-CSF), 5 μg/kg subcutaneously, usually for 10 consecutive days on day 6 through 15.

RADIATION THERAPY FOR RESIDUAL MASSES OF METASTATIC NONSEMINOMATOUS GERM CELL CANCER

Many medical oncologists do not appreciate the marked radiation sensitivity of embryonal carcinoma and teratocarcinoma, which is similar to that of non-Hodgkin's lymphoma. Therefore, patients who have residual masses after first-line chemotherapy who are surgically unresectable frequently are offered for second-line chemotherapy without the addition of local irradiation. Like non-Hodgkin's lymphoma, radiation therapy is excellent at sterilizing minimal disease and lymph nodal disease that is not bulky. For instance, in the Royal Marsden Hospital experience, only 2 of 84 men with clinical stage I cancer who were irradiated developed a retroperitoneal recurrence—1 in 44 patients with primary teratocarcinoma and in 1 in 40 patients with primary embryonal carcinoma.[67] In this setting, based on surveillance studies, 15% to 20% of men without treatment would have recurred in the retroperitoneum. The radiosensitivity of nonseminoma testis cancer recently has been highlighted further by the results of the randomized trial involving radiation therapy by the Danish Testicular Cancer Study Group.[68] In this study, 150 evaluable patients were randomized to receive either retroperitoneal radiation therapy or surveillance for clinical stage I disease. A significant reduction in retroperitoneal lymph nodal relapses was seen in the radiation therapy group (0 of 73 compared with 14 of 77 in the surveillance group). The Royal Marsden Hospital also reported that radiation therapy sterilized more than 90% of patients treated primarily with radiation whose lymph node metastases were no larger than 2 cm in greatest diameter by lymphangiographic evaluation. However, unlike non-Hodgkin's lymphoma, the ability of radiation to sterilize bulky lymph node masses in the retroperitoneum was reduced to 31% when used as initial therapy.[67]

AUTOLOGOUS BONE MARROW TRANSPLANTATION

We are also evaluating high-dose chemotherapy with autologous bone marrow transplantation (ABMT) in patients who are otherwise incurable (progression during cisplatin or prior PVB, VP-16, and ifosfamide). Results with this approach in the past have been disappointing, with virtually no remissions longer than 1 year. However, most preparative regimens used chemotherapy regimens without a platinum compound (*e.g.*, cyclophosphamide, VP-16, BCNU). Carboplatin (CBDCA) has activity similar to cisplatin, with myelosuppression as its dose-limiting toxicity, making it ideal for high-dose therapy with ABMT in refractory testicular cancer. Further, in preclinical systems, the drug is highly synergistic with VP-16. At Indiana University, we began a phase I–II regimen in 1986 in heavily pretreated patients with high-dose CBDCA plus VP-16 with

BMT. Eligible patients were believed to be incurable with any other therapeutic strategy. All patients either progressed during cisplatin combination chemotherapy or had prior exposure to cisplatin, vinblastine, bleomycin, VP-16, and ifosfamide. Bone marrow was harvested for two courses of high-dose therapy (double transplant), because it was hypothesized that in a rapidly growing tumor incapable of pretransplant cytoreduction it would be unlikely that a single course of therapy, regardless of the dosage, could eradicate 100% of tumor cells. Unlike allogeneic transplants, there would be no graft versus tumor response. Likewise, total body irradiation, as used in lymphoma transplants, was impractical, especially in lieu of prior bleomycin and the propensity for pulmonary fibrosis.

Testis cancer is an ideal disease for ABMT. It is a remarkably chemosensitive tumor, marrow involvement is exceedingly rare, and most of these patients with testis cancer are young and healthy with normal organ function. Platinum compounds and VP-16 are two of the most active (if not *the* most active) drugs and are particularly suited for dose escalation with ABMT. The primary dose-limiting toxicity for VP-16 is myelosuppression. Cisplatin is not practical (at four times the recommended dose) for ABMT because of nonmarrow neurotoxicity, ototoxicity, and nephrotoxicity. However, CBDCA, like VP-16, only rarely exhibits extramedullary toxicity.

Between 1986 and 1988, 33 consecutive patients were entered on this ABMT protocol. Twenty-two had progressed during prior cisplatin therapy. The VP-16 dosage was fixed at 1200 mg/m^2, and the CBDCA dosage started at 900 mg/m^2 and ranged as high as 2000 mg/m^2. As expected, hematologic toxicity was substantial, and each course was associated with granulocytopenic fever; 7 (21%) patients died from therapy. A larger experience in more selected patients has been associated with a reduced treatment-related mortality of 10% to 15%. Hematopoietic growth factors currently are routinely employed. Overall,[14] (42%) responses were seen, including 8 (24%) complete remissions.[127] This was a phase I and a phase II study, and several patients with poor pulmonary function were treated, with a high mortality rate—such patients would be excluded now. A follow-up on this study was reported recently for the first 40 patients. Twenty-four of 40 (60%) received both courses of high-dose CBDCA plus VP-16 with ABMT. Reasons for not giving the second course were drug-related mortality, unacceptable morbidity, or inadequate response to the first course. Twelve of 40 (30%) were in complete remission, and 8 of 40 (20%) were continuously NED with minimal follow-up of 24 months. Unfortunately, 1 of these 8 patients died from acute myelogenous leukemia 28 months after transplant while still in complete remission from germ cell tumor.[128]

SALVAGE SURGERY

An unusual form of salvage therapy not often appreciated is surgery. There are occasional patients with rising markers (HCG or AFP, or both) who are deemed to be incurable with any chemotherapy strategy but have anatomically localized disease. Such patients may be candidates for salvage surgery with curative intent, especially if the disease is confined to the retroperitoneum.[129]

Finally, despite all the potential tools of salvage therapy, approximately 15% to 20% of all patients with disseminated germ cell tumors eventually succumb from their malignancy. It is often difficult to discern when the direction of salvage therapy should change from an aggressive potentially curative strategy to a palliative philosophy. When that does occur, older drugs such as mithramycin, dactinomycin, cyclophosphamide, vincristine, and methotrexate have no significant activity alone or in combination. The most appropriate approach in this setting is either a phase I or II agent or daily oral VP-16. VP-16 has been shown to be a schedule-dependent drug in several preclinical models.[130] Results of a clinical trial in previously untreated extensive small cell lung cancer confirmed these early preclinical observations. Slevin and colleagues conducted a phase III study of single-agent VP-16 in which the only variable was schedule.[131] Patients were randomized to 500 mg/m^2 as a 24-hour infusion compared with 100 mg/m^2 for 5 consecutive days every 3 weeks. The response rates were 10% compared with 78% ($p < 0.0001$) and median survival 6 compared with 10 months ($p = 0.03$), respectively, favoring the 5-day course. Because of the schedule dependency of VP-16, it was hypothesized that daily exposure for 21 consecutive days might offer further benefit over the standard 5-day regimen. The availability of the oral capsules facilitated this approach. Because part of the cytotoxicity of VP-16 is related to its inhibition of topoisomerase II, it is possible that prolonged inhibition with daily oral VP-16 also might be advantageous. The standard VP-16 dose (100 mg/m^2 for 5 consecutive days) is probably equivalent to 200 mg/m$^2 \times 5$ (1000 mg/m^2) when the oral capsules are used. This amount translates to approximately 50 mg/m^2/day for 21 consecutive days. Therefore, patients with refractory germ cell tumors deemed to be incurable were entered on this phase II trial of 50 mg/m^2 orally for 21 consecutive days, with courses repeated every 4 weeks. Therapy was well tolerated. The median number of prior chemotherapy regimens was three. Of 21 evaluable patients, there were three objective responses. All 3 of these patients had a greater than 90% decline in their markers and a greater than 50% radiographic improvement. One of these patients had progressed during intravenous cisplatin plus VP-16 plus ifosfamide, implying that VP-16-refractory patients can be made sensitive to VP-16 with this schedule. In addition, three other patients had more than a 90% decrease in markers but with stable radiographic disease.[132] Similar results were reported in a small series of patients in Newcastle by Cantwell and colleagues.[133]

ADJUVANT CHEMOTHERAPY FOR STAGE II DISEASE

The criteria for successful application of adjuvant chemotherapy are poor prognosis for cure with primary therapy alone and evidence that the proposed adjuvant therapy is effective in metastatic disease. However, in nonseminomatous germ cell tumors, there is a third consideration, namely, whether similar cure rates can be achieved by using chemotherapy when a patient relapses after a retroperitoneal lymph node dissection.

An intergroup study has been completed in patients with pathologic stage II nonseminomatous germ cell tumors. Patient entry was from 1979 to 1987, and there were 197 evaluable patients.[134] Median time on study was in excess of 7

years. Patients were randomized to two postoperative courses of cisplatin combination chemotherapy versus observation, which consisted of history and physical examination, HCG and AFP assays, and posteroanterior and lateral chest x-ray films monthly the first postoperative year, every 2 months during the second year, and, subsequently, every 6 months. Ninety-seven patients entered the adjuvant arm, and only 2 patients have relapsed. One of these 2 patients subsequently died of metastatic testicular cancer. Forty-eight of 98 patients on the observation arm have relapsed. However, with this close follow-up, relapse was detected in a favorable setting: only 3 of these patients have died from recurrent testicular cancer, and the remaining 95 continue to be disease free. There was no independent risk factor for relapse that would mandate adjuvant chemotherapy in any subtype (*e.g.*, marker-negative patients and vascular invasion). Two courses of cisplatin-based adjuvant chemotherapy almost always prevent relapse; however, when surgery, follow-up, and chemotherapy are optimal, either approach produces excellent cure rates.

LATE CONSEQUENCES OF CISPLATIN COMBINATION CHEMOTHERAPY

Approximately 80% of patients with disseminated germ cell tumors are cured with their initial chemotherapy or with some form of salvage therapy. The most dire "late consequence" is a late relapse (after 2 years). Fortunately, this is uncommon (<3%) and usually is associated with prior advanced disease, often with bulky teratoma. Some of these patients relapse with only teratoma and are surgically curable. However, those who recur with elevated markers (usually AFP) do extremely poorly with any form of chemotherapy. The complete remission rate is low, further relapse rate high, and cure rate much lower than 20%. A partial explanation is that in these rare cases, slow-growing clones develop that are not uniquely sensitive to cisplatin combination chemotherapy.

A retrospective study of the first 229 cases (1974–1980) treated with PVB at Indiana University revealed that 146 are NED with a minimum follow-up of 6 years and median follow-up of 8.5 years at the time of publication.[135]

At 12 years, the probability of survival was 65% and for complete responders, 84%. Similar long-term survival results with PVB have been reported from Australia[136] and England.[137] Long-term organ toxicity or therapy-related second malignancies were not seen. More than 95% of patients returned to their pretherapy functional status, and approximately 90% are fully employed.

FERTILITY

Drasga and associates have evaluated with serial semen analyses 69 patients with disseminated germ cell tumors who did not undergo a retroperitoneal lymph node dissection.[138] Before any chemotherapy was administered, 77% of patients were severely oligospermic, and 17% were azoospermic. After four courses of PVB, 96% were azoospermic. However, 2 years after initiation of chemotherapy, 50% had recovered a normal sperm count and motility, and approximately half of the patients who had attempted to impregnate their partners had been successful, with the infants having no congenital abnormalities. Fossa and colleagues reported similar results, with

50% to 60% of patients having active spermatogenesis 1 to 3 years after PVB.[139] In contrast, Nijman and associates recently reported that 2 years after PVB, only 28% of patients had a sperm count greater than 60 million/ml; however, unlike the previous two studies, these patients all received maintenance cisplatin for 12 months.[140]

The fertility data with more contemporary chemotherapy is relatively meager. We have retrospectively evaluated a single semen analysis for 21 patients who received three to four courses of PVP-16B. None of these patients had undergone a retroperitoneal lymph node dissection. The minimal follow-up from initiation of chemotherapy was 2 years.

Six patients (29%) were azoospermic, and 7 (33%) had sperm counts lower than 40 million/ml.[141] These results indicate that patients with germ cell tumors cured with contemporary chemotherapy remain at substantial risk for diminished reproductive capacity.

The exact incidence of chemotherapy-induced infertility is impossible to define accurately, because a certain percentage of cured patients remain permanently oligospermic as a result of dysgenetic abnormalities in the contralateral testis caused by the effects from the cancer itself.[142] Approximately 10% to 15% of all patients with testis cancer probably will be infertile due to nontreatment-related abnormalities.

VASCULAR COMPLICATIONS

Vogelzang and colleagues first identified and clarified the relation between Raynaud's phenomenon and chemotherapy for testicular cancer.[143] Narrowing of the terminal digital arterioles was described. Twenty-two of 60 men (37%) in their series developed Raynaud's phenomenon, which was seen with the two-drug combination of vinblastine plus bleomycin and with PVB. Other authors have reported Raynaud's phenomenon with just vinblastine plus bleomycin.[144]

The incidence of Raynaud's phenomenon with distal arteriolar narrowing raises the specter of generalized vascular disease with acute myocardial infarction secondary to coronary artery disease, deep venous thrombosis, and cerebrovascular accident. Bleomycin and vinca alkaloids, such as vinblastine, have been anecdotally associated with myocardial ischemia.[145,146]

Two reports have raised concern about vascular complications of cisplatin combination chemotherapy. Samuels and colleagues described 5 patients with both acute and long-term vascular toxicity,[147] and 3 of these patients had no evidence of cancer at autopsy. These cases were culled from 65 patients treated at the University of Minnesota from 1978 to 1982. However, 1 of these patients came from the University of Chicago, and the denominator at that institution is unknown. The frequency of these problems cannot be determined currently.

These 5 patients are not proof of PVB-based toxicity. One patient may have had clostridial sepsis as the causative agent of his vascular toxicity, namely rectal infarction. Another patient had sepsis and hypotension during high-dose cytarabine and a questionable myocardial infarction. A third patient received doxorubicin, a known cardiotoxic drug, and other agents. Finally, in an additional patient, Koch's postulates were not fulfilled, because rechallenge with five more courses of PVB produced no immediate further problems.

Doll and associates described four additional cases of vascular complications after cisplatin combination chemotherapy in 23 patients treated from 1983 to 1985.[148] None of these patients had known risk factors, such as prior mediastinal radiation therapy, family history of cardiac disease, history of heavy smoking, hypertension, diabetes, or hyperlipedemia.

There are several plausible explanations for vascular toxicity, including the previously mentioned Raynaud's phenomenon progressing to generalized vascular disease. Also, bleomycin can cause endothelial changes cumulatively in capillaries and arterioles.[149] Cisplatin-induced hypomagnesemia can cause ventricular irritability and coronary artery spasm. High levels of circulating von Willebrand's factor antigen, which have been associated with Raynaud's phenomenon, may be a marker for endothelial damage[150] and may lead to thrombosis.[151]

The following conclusions and statements about vascular complications can be made:

1. The incidence of vascular complications is low (less than 5%).
2. Vascular complications vary temporally and anatomically.
3. Some patients with complications can be retreated with the same chemotherapy without apparent problems.
4. It is not possible to know whether these vascular complications are secondary to treatment or to the disease process (*e.g.*, tumor emboli or deep venous thrombosis in association with large pelvic mass). If treatment is implicated, which drug or drug combination is the culprit remains unknown.

The recently completed adjuvant intergroup stage I–II study provided a unique forum to address these important concerns. Questionnaires concerning deep venous thrombosis, pulmonary embolus, myocardial infarction, and cerebrovascular accident were sent to 459 patients, and 270 were returned. Median follow-up was more than 5 years. The results are depicted in Table 37–23. This large retrospective analysis of an intergroup trial failed to implicate chemotherapy as the cause of vascular abnormalities.[152]

BLEOMYCIN-RELATED COMPLICATIONS

Barneveld and colleagues evaluated 93 patients treated with PVB, of whom 8 had clinical evidence of bleomycin pneumonitis.[153] One of these patients died from bleomycin toxicity; the other 7 were fully recovered with a minimum follow-up of 2 years. Chest films normalized at a median of 9 months (range 6–13 months), and all symptoms abated in 4 to 5 months.

The risk factors for the development of bleomycin-induced pulmonary fibrosis are age of more than 45 years, prior mediastinal radiation therapy, total cumulative dose of bleomycin, and advanced pulmonary disease. The incidence of clinically significant bleomycin pulmonary fibrosis for patients with good-risk disease receiving 9 weeks (270 U) of bleomycin is less than 1%.

A different bleomycin-related complication relates to radiographic abnormalities that can simulate metastatic pulmonary nodules.[154,155]

TABLE 37–23. Cardiovascular Complications: Intergroup Trial

Event	Observation Arm* (n = 168)	Adjuvant Chemotherapy (n = 49)	Metastatic Chemotherapy (n = 53)
Smoking history	72 (43%)	26 (53%)	31 (58%)
Antihyerptensive use	7 (4%)	1 (2%)	6 (11%)
Hypertension	14 (8%)	6 (12%)	4 (8%)
Heart disease	2 (1%)	1 (2%)	0
Stroke	0	0	0
Blood clot	3 (2%)	0	1 (2%)

* Pathologic stage I or II patients who never received any chemotherapy for adjuvant or metastasic disease.

Subclinical bleomycin pulmonary fibrosis can produce a coalescence of fibrous tissue that, on chest film or CT, has the appearance of metastatic nodules. If such nodules are seen after chemotherapy in areas different from those of the original pulmonary metastases, they are assumed to be secondary to bleomycin, and it is not necessary to biopsy these areas by fine-needle aspiration or thoracotomy.

LEUKEMIA

Perhaps the most worrisome late complication of cytolytic chemotherapy is the development of secondary malignancies, such as acute nonlymphocytic leukemia. This complication is relatively rare in cured patients with germ cell tumors compared with Hodgkin's disease, presumably because the former patients are immunologically intact and receive short-duration chemotherapy. However, if longer duration chemotherapy is employed, secondary leukemia can be a late consequence of curative therapy.[156]

There have been several articles concerning epipodophyllotoxin derivatives, such as VP-16, causing an increased risk for myelodysplasia or acute leukemia, or both.[157,158] Whitlock and colleagues described 37 patients with a variety of malignancies treated with VM-26 (teniposide) or VP-16 combination chemotherapy.[157] These patients frequently had a cytogenetic abnormality involving 11q23. Pedersen-Bjergaard and colleagues retrospectively evaluated 212 patients with germ cell tumors treated with PVP-16B.[158] There were four cases of acute myeloid leukemia and one case of myelodysplasia. Three of these leukemias involved balanced chromosome translocations affecting bands 11q23 and 21q22. However, all 5 of these patients with leukemic complications were among the 82 who had received a cumulative dose of more than 2000 mg/m² of VP-16. It is questionable whether there is any increased risk with standard therapy consisting of cisplatin plus bleomycin plus VP-16 (100 mg/m² for 5 consecutive days for three to four courses), because no cases of leukemia were observed among the 130 patients in this series who received 2000 mg/m² or less of VP-16.

A retrospective review of all patients with germ cell tumors entering clinical trails using conventional-dose VP-16 was completed recently at Indiana University. Dosages of VP-16 ranged from 1500 (three courses) to 2000 mg/M² (four courses). Five hundred thirty-six patients were entered, with median follow-up of 5 years. One patient developed acute undifferentiated leukemia with a t(4:11)(q21;q23) abnormality at 27 months, and another patient developed acute myelomonocytic leukemia with normal cytogenetics 2 years after starting chemotherapy.[159] Leukemia associated with conventional-dose VP-16 is rare and probably not substantially different from the incidence in the general population.

ADDITIONAL TOPICS

THE TESTIS AS A SANCTUARY SITE

Testicular relapse can terminate a complete remission in childhood acute lymphoblastic leukemia in the absence of marrow or meningeal relapse, implying that the testis is a sanctuary site. In germ cell tumors, the testis is affected by chemotherapy, with resultant testicular atrophy and impaired spermatogenesis. Nevertheless, the primary tumor in the testis is not always eradicated by systemic chemotherapy. Greist and coworkers described 20 patients with occult testicular primaries who underwent a delayed orchiectomy after cisplatin combination chemotherapy.[90] These patients were initially believed to have a primary retroperitoneal germ cell tumor, but subsequently were found to have a testicular primary on careful palpation or bilateral testicular ultrasound demonstrating a characteristic hypoechogenic mass. Three of these patients had embryonal cell carcinoma in the testis after cisplatin chemotherapy, and an additional 6 had teratoma. None of the 20 patients had persistent carcinoma in the original areas of bulky retroperitoneal disease. Similar results have been reported by other investigators.[160,161]

An orchiectomy, therefore, must be performed initially or after chemotherapy in any patient with a known or suspected testicular primary, because it is erroneous to assume that the chemotherapy will eradicate the primary. If carcinoma is found in the orchiectomy specimen, we recommend two postoperative courses of cisplatin combination induction chemotherapy. This same therapy is recommended if carcinoma is found in the retroperitoneum or chest after chemotherapy. However, this view is controversial,[160] and there is not enough information to permit a firm recommendation based on hard data.

CENTRAL NERVOUS SYSTEM METASTASES

Metastasis in the central nervous system (CNS) is an uncommon initial presentation, occurring in fewer than 5% of all patients with stage III disease. Most of these patients have concomitant advanced pulmonary metastases. CNS metastases are more common in patients with pure choriocarcinoma and in patients with primary mediastinal nonseminomatous germ cell tumors. The presence of CNS metastases does not preclude cure, and such patients should be treated aggressively.

At M.D. Anderson, 12 patients with disseminated testicular cancer and CNS metastases were treated from 1977 to 1979 with chemotherapy plus whole-brain irradiation therapy.[162] Although none of the 6 patients with multiple CNS metastases were cured, 4 of the 6 with single CNS metastases were disease free at 13+ to 41+ months.

A unique approach for CNS metastases has been advocated by investigators at Charing Cross Hospital in London, England.[163]Ten patients with germ cell tumors and CNS metastases were treated from 1977 to 1984 with no CNS irradiation. A complicated chemotherapy regimen, platinum-oncovin - methotrexate - bleomycin / doxorubicin - cyclophosphamide-etoposide or etoposide-platinum/oncovin-methotrexate-bleomycin (POMB/ACE or EP/OMB), was employed in conjunction with high-dose (1 g/m²) methotrexate and intrathecal methotrexate. Eight patients were disease free at 3+ to 54+ months.

Recently, we have reviewed our results of therapy for patients with germ cell tumors and brain metastases.[164] A retrospective review of patients treated from 1975 to 1988 uncovered 24 patients. Ten of these patients presented initially with CNS metastases. All 10 of these patients also had extensive intrathoracic disease. Chemotherapy consisted of four courses of PVB, PVB plus doxorubicin, or PVP-16B. Most of these patients received concurrent CNS irradiation therapy, 5000 cGy in 25 fractions over 5 weeks, starting with the first day of chemotherapy. Three of 10 patients (30%) are continuously NED with a minimum follow-up of 5 years (67+, 77+, and 142+ months). Two additional patients survived more than 5 years (74+ and 122+ months), but eventually died from progressive generalized testicular cancer. A second group of patients (n=4) consisted of those patients who achieved an initial complete remission with cisplatin combination chemotherapy, but developed a relapse confined to the brain. Three of these 4 patients had a solitary CNS lesion and were treated with craniotomy with metastatectomy followed by whole-brain irradiation therapy (4000 cGy in 20 fractions in 4 weeks) with concurrent cisplatin combination chemotherapy for two courses. The reason for the latter modality was our concern that a CNS-only relapse could herald a systemic relapse; therefore, two "consolidation" courses of chemotherapy were used. The fourth patient in this group relapsed with multiple CNS metastases with no other anatomic site of involvement. He received 5000 cGy in 25 fractions plus two courses of PVB and is continuously NED for more than 13 years. Two of the 3 resected patients also remain disease free for 6+ and 7+ years. Therefore, overall, 6 of 14 patients with potentially curable disease are continuously NED in this series. None of these 6 patients have any evidence of treatment-related neuropsychological sequelae. Finally, a separate group of 10 patients who were treated with palliative intent were also included in this review. These patients had multiple anatomic sites of disease in the CNS and elsewhere, and most were refractory to cisplatin at the time they developed their

brain metastases. As expected, survival was brief in this refractory and advanced patient population. The median survival from initiation of CNS irradiation therapy was only 3 months (with a range of 1–56 weeks), and all 10 patients have died from progressive disease.

REFERENCES

1. Silverberg E. Cancer statistics. CA 1991;40:9.
2. Clemmesen J. Statistical studies in malignancy. Microbiol Scand 1974;247(Suppl):1.
3. LeComete (1851). quoted by Grove JS. The cryptorchid problem. J Urol 1954;71:735.
4. Gilbert JB, Hamilton JB. Studies in malignant testis tumors: Incidence and nature of tumors in ectopic testis. Surg Gynecol Obstet 1940;71:731.
5. Farrer JH, Walker AH, Rajfer J. Management of the postpubertal cryptorchid testis: A statistical review. J Urol 1985;134:1071.
6. Richie JP, Birnholz J, Garnick MB. Ultrasonography as a diagnostic adjunct for the evaluation of masses in the scrotum. Surg Gynecol Obstet 1982;154:695.
7. Glazer HS, Lee JKT, Melson GL, McClennan BC. Sonographic detection of occult testicular neoplasms. AJR 1982;138:67.
8. Friedman NB, Moore RA. Tumor of the testis: A report on 922 cases. Milit Surg 1946;99:57.
9. Mostofi FK, Sobin LH. International histological classification of tumors of testes (No 16). Geneva: World Health Organization, 1977.
10. Skakkebaek NE. Possible carcinoma in situ of the testis. Lancet 1972;2:516.
11. Skakkebaek NE. Atypical germ cells in the adjacent "normal" tissue of testicular tumors. Acta Pathol Microbiol Scand 1975;84:127.
12. Mostofi FK. Testicular tumors: Epidemiologic, etiologic and pathologic features. Cancer 1973;32:1186.
13. Boden JP, Gibb R. Radiotherapy and testicular neoplasms. Lancet 1951;2:119.
14. Skinner DG. Non-seminomatous testis tumors: A plan of management based on 96 patients to improve survival in all stages by combined therapeutic modalities. J Urol 1976;115:65.
15. Maier JG, Sulak MH. Radiation therapy in malignant testis tumors: II. Non-seminoma. Cancer 1973;32:1212.
16. Stomper PC, Kalish LA, Garnick MB, Richie JP, Kantoff PW. CT and pathologic predictive features of residual mass histologic findings after chemotherapy for non-seminomatous germ cell tumors: Can residual malignancy or teratoma be excluded? Radiology 1991;180:711–714.
17. Staubitz WJ, Early KS, Magoss IV, Murphy GP. Surgical management of testis tumors. J Urol 1974;111:205.
18. Fraley EE, Lange PH, Kennedy BJ. Germ-cell testicular cancer in adults. N Engl J Med 1979;301:1370, 1420.
19. McLeod DG, Weiss RB, Stablein DM, et al. Staging relationships and outcome in early stage testicular cancer: A report from the testicular cancer intergroup study. J Urol 1991;146:1178.
20. Narayan P, Lange PH, Fraley EE. Ejaculation and fertility after extended retroperitoneal lymph node dissection for testicular cancer. J Urol 1982;127:685.
21. Richie JP. Clinical stage I testicular cancer: The role of modified retroperitoneal lymphadenectomy. J Urol 1990;144:1160–1163.
22. Donohue JP, Foster RS, Rowland RG, Bihrle R, Jones J, Grier G. Nerve-sparing retroperitoneal lymphadenectomy with preservation of ejaculation: I. J Urol 1990;144:287, 291.
23. Read G, Johnson RJ, Wilkinson PM, et al. Prospective study on follow-up alone in stage I teratoma of the testis. Br Med J 1983;287:1503.
24. Johnson DE, Lo RK, von Eschenbach AC, et al. Surveillance alone for patients with clinical stage I nonseminomatous germ cell tumors of the testis: Preliminary results. J Urol 1984;131:491.
25. Pizzocaro G, Zanoni F, Milani A, et al. Orchiectomy alone in clinical stage I nonseminomatous testis cancer: A critical appraisal. J Clin Oncol 1986;4:35.
26. Freedman LS, Jones WG, Peckham MJ, et al. Histopathology in the prediction of relapse of patients with stage I testicular teratoma treated by orchidectomy alone. Lancet 1987;2:294.
27. Gelderman WAH, Koops HS, Sleijfer DF, et al. Orchidectomy alone in stage I non-seminomatous testicular germ cell tumor. Cancer 1987;59:578.
28. Rørth M, von der Maase H, Nielsen ES, et al. Orchidectomy alone versus orchidectomy plus radiotherapy in stage I nonseminomatous testicular cancer: A randomized study by the Danish Carcinoma Study Group. Int J Androl 1987;10:255.
29. Raghavan D, Colls B, Levi J, et al. Surveillance for stage I nonseminomatous germ cell tumors of the testis: The optimal protocol has not yet been defined. Br J Urol 1988;61:522.
30. Sogani PC, Whitmore WF Jr, Herr HW, et al. Long-term experience with orchiectomy alone in treatment of clinical stage I non-seminomatous germ cell tumor of the testis. J Urol 1988;133:246A.
31. Thompson PI, Nixon J, Harvey VJ. Disease relapse in patients with stage I non-seminomatous germ cell tumor of the testis on active surveillance. J Clin Oncol 1988;6:1597.
32. Rowland RG, Weisman D, Williams S, Einhorn L, Donohue JP. Accuracy of preoperative staging in stage A and B non-seminomatous germ cell testis tumors. J Urol 1982;127:718.
33. Dunphy CH, Ayala AG, Swanson DA, et al. Clinical stage I nonseminomatous and

mixed germ cell tumors of the testis: A clinicopathologic study of 93 patients on a surveillance protocol after orchiectomy alone. Lancet 1988;62:1202.

34. Fung CY, Kalish LA, Brodsky GL, et al. Stage I nonseminomatous germ cell testicular tumor: Prediction of metastatic potential by primary histology. J Clin Oncol 1988;6:1467.

35. Taylor RE, Duncan W, Best JJ. Influence of computed tomography scanning and lymphography on the management of testicular germ cell tumors. Clin Radiol 1986;37:539–543.

36. Epstein BE, Order SE, Zinreich ES. Staging, treatment and results in testicular seminoma: A 12-year report. Cancer 1990;65:405–411.

37. Marks LB, Walker TG, Shipley WU, et al. The role of lymphangiography in staging testicular seminoma. Urology 1991;38:264–266.

38. Barzell W, Whitmore WF. Neoplasms of the testis. In: Campbell's Urology. Vol 2. Philadelphia: WB Saunders, 1979:1141.

39. Maier JG, Sulak MH, Mittemeyer BT. Seminoma of the testis: Analysis of treatment success and failure. AJR 1968;102:596–602.

40. Heiken JP, Balfe DM, McClennan BL. Testicular tumors: Oncologic imaging and diagnosis. Int J Radiat Oncol Biol Phys 1984;10:275–287.

41. Hoeltl W, Kosak D, Pont J, et al. Testicular cancer: Prognostic implications of vascular invasion. J Urol 1987;137:683–685.

42. Zagars GK, Babaian RJ. Stage I testicular seminoma: Rationale for post-orchiectomy radiation therapy. Int J Radiat Oncol Biol Phys 1987;13:155–162.

43. Marks LB, Rutgers JL, Shipley WU, et al. Testicular seminoma: Clinical and pathological features that may predict para-aortic lymph node metastases. J Urol 1990;143:524–527.

44. Kubo HD, Shipley WU. Reduction of the scatter dose to the testicle outside the radiation treatment fields. Int J Radiat Oncol Biol Phys 1982;8:1741–1745.

45. Thomas GM, Rider WD, Dembo AJ, et al. Seminoma of the testis: Results of treatment and patterns of failure after radiation therapy. Int J Radiat Oncol Biol Phys 1982;8:165–174.

46. Hamilton C, Horwich A, Easton D, et al. Radiotherapy for stage I seminoma testis: Results of treatment and complications. Radiother Oncol 1986;6:115–120.

47. Thomas GM, Sturgeon JF, Alison R, et al. A study of post-orchiectomy surveillance in stage I testicular seminoma. J Urol 1989;142:313–316.

48. Maier JG, Sulak MH. Radiation therapy in malignant testis tumors: I. Seminoma. Cancer 1973;32:1212–1216.

49. Dosoretz DE, Shipley WU, Blitzer PH, et al. Megavoltage irradiation for pure testicular seminoma: Results and patterns of failure. Cancer 1981;48:2184–2190.

50. Hanks GE, Herring DF, Kramer S. Patterns of care outcome studies results of the national practice in seminoma of the testis. Int J Radiat Oncol Biol Phys 1981;7:1413–1417.

51. Willan BD, McGowan DG. Seminoma of the testis: A 22-year experience with radiation therapy. Int J Radiat Oncol Biol Phys 1985;11:1769–1775.

52. Lederman GS, Sheldon TA, Chaffey JT, et al. Cardiac disease after mediastinal irradiation for seminoma. Cancer 1987;60:772–776.

53. Fossa SD, Aass N, Kaalhus O. Radiotherapy for testicular seminoma stage I: Treatment results and long-term post-irradiation morbidity in 365 patients. Int J Rad Oncol Biol Phys 1989;16:383–388.

54. Lester SG, Morphis JG II, Hornback NB. Testicular seminoma: Analysis of treatment results and failures. Int J Rad Oncol Biol Phys 1986;12:353–358.

55. Gregory C, Peckham MJ. Results of radiotherapy for stage II testicular seminoma. Radiother Oncol 1986;6:285–292.

56. Zagars GK, Babaian RJ. The role of radiation therapy in stage II testicular seminoma. Int J Radiat Oncol Biol Phys 1987;13:163–170.

57. Thomas GM. Controversies in the management of testicular seminoma. Cancer 1985;55:2296–2302.

58. Fossa SD, Abyholm T, Normann N, et al. Post-treatment fertility in patients with testicular cancer: Influence of radiotherapy in seminoma patients. Br J Urol 1986;58:315–319.

59. Duchesne GM, Horwich A, Dearnaley DP, et al. Orchiectomy alone for stage I seminoma of the testis. Cancer 1990;65:1115–1118.

60. Zagars GK, Babaian RJ. Stage I testicular seminoma: Rationale for post-orchiectomy radiation therapy. Int J Rad Oncol Biol Phys 1987;13:155–162.

61. Percarpio B, Clements JC, McLeod DG, et al. Anaplastic seminoma: An analysis of 77 patients. Cancer 1979;43:2510–2513.

62. Cockburn AG, Vugrin D, Batata M, et al. Poorly differentiated (anaplastic) seminoma of the testis. Cancer 1984;53:1991–1994.

63. Mauch P, Weichselbaum R, Botnick L. The significance of positive chorionic gonadotropins in apparently pure seminoma of the testis. Int J Radiat Oncol Biol Phys 1979;5:887–889.

64. Mirimanoff RO, Shipley WU, Dosoretz DE, et al. Pure seminoma of the testis: The results of radiation therapy in patients with elevated human chorionic gonadotropins titers. J Urol 1985;134:1124–1126.

65. Ball D, Barrett A, Peckham MJ. The management of metastatic seminoma of the testis. Cancer 1982;50:2289–2294.

66. Smalley SR, Earle JD, Evans RG, et al. Modern radiotherapy results with bulky stages II and III seminoma. J Urol 1990;144:684–689.

67. Tyrrell CJ, Peckham MJ. The response of lymph node metastases of testicular teratoma to radiation therapy. Br J Urol 1976;48:363–370.

68. Rorth M, Jacobson GK, von der Maase H, Danish Testicular Cancer Study Group. Surveillance alone versus radiotherapy after orchiectomy for clinical stage I nonseminomatous testicular cancer. J Clin Oncol 1991;9:1543–1548.

69. Li MC, Whitmore WF, Golbey R, et al. Effects of combined drug therapy on metastatic cancer of the testis. JAMA 1960;174:145–153.

70. MacKenzie AR. Chemotherapy of metastatic testis cancer: Results in 154 patients. Cancer 1966;19:1369–1376.

71. Kennedy BJ. Mithramycin therapy in advanced testicular neoplasms. Cancer 1970;26:755–766.

72. Blum RH, Carter S, Agre K. A clinical review of bleomycin: A new anti-neoplastic agent. Cancer 1973;31:903–914.

73. Samuels ML, Howe CD. Vinblastine in the management of testicular cancer. Cancer 1970;25:1009–1017.

74. Samuels ML, Johnson DE, Holoye PY. Continuous intravenous bleomycin therapy with vinblastine in stage III testicular neoplasia. Cancer Chemother Rep 1975;59:563–570.

75. Rosenberg B, VanCamp L, Krigas T. Inhibition of cell division in E. coli by electrolysis products from a platinum electrode. Nature 1965;205:678–699.

76. Higby DJ, Wallace HJ, Albert DJ, et al. Diamminedichloroplatinum: A phase I study showing responses in testicular and other tumors. Cancer 1974;33:1219–1225.

77. Wittes RE, Yagoda A, Silvay O, et al. Chemotherapy of germ cell tumors of the testis. Cancer 1976;37:637–645.

78. Cheng E, Cvitkovic E, Wittes RE, et al. Germ cell tumors: VAB II in metastatic testicular cancer. Cancer 1978;42:2162–2168.

79. Cvitkovic E, Wittes R, Golbey R, et al. Primary combination chemotherapy for metastatic or unresectable germ cell tumors. Proc Am Assoc Cancer Res [Abstract] 1978;19:174.

80. Einhorn LH, Donohue JP. Cis-diamminedichloroplatinum, vinblastine, and bleomycin combination chemotherapy in disseminated testicular cancer. Ann Intern Med 1977;87:293–298.

81. Einhorn LH, Williams SD, Troner M, et al. The role of maintenance therapy in disseminated testicular cancer. N Engl J Med 1987;305:727–731.

82. Fox EP, Einhorn LH, Weathers T, Williams SD, Donohue JP. Outcome analysis for patients with persistent germ cell carcinoma in post-chemotherapy retroperitoneal lymph node dissections. Proc Am Soc Clin Oncol [Abstract] 1992;11:198.

83. Bosl GJ, Gluckman R, Geller NL, et al. VAB-6: An effective chemotherapy regimen for patients with germ cell tumors. J Clin Oncol 1986;4:1493–1499.

84. Einhorn LH, Williams SD. Chemotherapy of disseminated testicular cancer. Cancer 1980;46:1339–1344.

85. Stoter G, Sleyfer DT, Bokkel Huinink WW, et al. High-dose versus low-dose vinblastine in cisplatin-vinblastine-bleomycin combination chemotherapy of non-seminomatous testicular cancer: A randomized study of the EORTC Genitourinary Tract Cancer Cooperative Group. J Clin Oncol 1986;4:1199–1206.

86. Fitzharris BM, Kaye SB, Saverymuttu S, et al. VP-16-213 as single agent in advanced testicular tumors. Eur J Cancer 1980;16:1193–1197.

87. Schabel FM Jr, Trader MW, Laster WR Jr, et al. Cis-dichlorodiammine-platinum: Combination chemotherapy and cross-resistance studies with tumors of mice. Cancer Treat Rep 1979;63:1459–1473.

88. Peckham MJ, Barrett A, Liew KH, et al. The treatment of metastatic germ cell testicular tumors with bleomycin, etoposide, and cisplatin (BEP). Br J Cancer 1983;47:613–619.

89. Williams SD, Birch R, Einhorn LH, et al. Treatment of disseminated germ cell tumors with cisplatin, bleomycin, and either vinblastine and etoposide. N Engl J Med 1987;316:1435–1440.

90. Greist A, Einhorn LH, Williams SD, et al. Pathologic findings at orchiectomy following chemotherapy for disseminated testicular cancer. J Clin Oncol 1984;2:1025–1027.

91. Loehrer PJ, Sledge GW, Einhorn LH. Heterogeneity among germ cell tumors of the testis. Semin Oncol 1985;12:304–316.

92. Birch R, Williams SD, Cone A, et al. Prognostic factors for favorable outcome in disseminated germ cell tumors. J Clin Oncol 1986;4:400–407.

93. Peckham MJ, Oliver RTD, Bagshawe KD, et al. Prognostic factors in advanced nonseminomatous germ cell testicular tumors: Results of a multicentre study. Lancet 1985;1:8–11.

94. Stoter G, Denis L. The chemotherapy of disseminated testicular non-seminomatous germ cell tumors and the clinical research of the EORTC Genitourinary Group. Acta Urol Belg 1985;53:428–435.

95. Aass N, Klepp O, Cavallin-Stahl E, et al. Prognostic factors in a multicenter experience. J Clin Oncol 1991;9:818–826.

96. Bajorin D, Katz A, Chan E, et al. Comparison of criteria for assigning germ cell tumor patients to "good risk" and "poor risk" studies. J Clin Oncol 1988;6:786–792.

97. Einhorn LH, Williams SD, Loehrer PJ, et al. Evaluation of optimal duration chemotherapy in favorable prognosis disseminated germ cell tumors: A Southeastern Cancer Study Group Protocol. J Clin Oncol 1989;7:387–391.

98. Loehrer PJ, Elsen P, Johnson DH, et al. A randomized trial of cisplatin plus etoposide with or without bleomycin in favorable prognosis disseminated germ cell tumors: An ECOG study. Proc Am Soc Clin Oncol [Abstract] 1991;10:169.

99. Bajorin DF, Geller NL, Weisen SF, Bosl GJ. Two-drug therapy in patients with metastatic germ cell tumors. Cancer 1991;67:28–32.

100. Bosl GJ, Geller NL, Bajorin D, et al. A randomized trial of etoposide plus cisplatin versus vinblastine, bleomycin, cisplatin, cyclophosphamide, and dactinomycin in patients with good-prognosis germ cell tumors. J Clin Oncol 1988;6:1231–1238.

101. Bajorin DF, Sarosdy MF, Bosl GJ, et al. A randomized trial of etoposide plus carboplatin versus etoposide plus cisplatin in patients with metastatic germ cell tumors. Proc Am Soc Clin Oncol [Abstract] 1991;10:168.

102. Horwich A, Dearnaley DP, Nicholls J, et al. Effectiveness of carboplatin, etoposide and bleomycin combination chemotherapy in good-prognosis metastatic testicular nonseminomatous germ cell tumors. J Clin Oncol 1991;9:62–69.

103. Ozols RF, Ihde DC, Linehan M, et al. A randomized trial of standard chemotherapy versus a high-dose chemotherapy regimen in the treatment of poor prognosis nonseminomatous germ cell tumors. J Clin Oncol 1988;6:1031–1040.

104. Nichols CR, Williams SD, Loehrer PJ, et al. Randomized study of cisplatin dose intensity in advanced germ cell tumors: A Southeastern Cancer Study Group and Southwest Oncology Group protocol. J Clin Oncol 1991;9:1163–1172.

105. Toner GC, Geller NL, Tan C, Nisselbaum J, Bosl GJ. Serum tumor marker half-life during chemotherapy allows early prediction of complete resposne and survival in nonseminomatous germ cell tumors. Cancer Res 1990;50:5904–5910.

106. Motzer RJ, Gulati SC, Crown J, et al. High-dose carboplatin plus etoposide with autologous bone marrow rescue in poor-risk nonseminomatous germ cell tumor patients with slow serum tumor markers decline during induction with VAB-6. Proc Am Soc Clin Oncol [Abstract] 1991;10:164.

107. Rich TA, Cassady JR, Strand RD, et al. Radiotherapy for pineal and suprasellar germ cell tumors. Cancer 1985;55:932–940.

108. Nichols CR. Mediastinal germ cell tumors. Chest 1991;99:472–479.

109. Nichols CR, Heerema NA, Palmer C, et al. Klinefelter's syndrome associated with mediastinal germ cell neoplasms. J Clin Oncol 1987;5:1290–1294.

110. Dexeus FH, Logothetis CJ, Chong C, et al. Genetic abnormalities in men with germ cell tumors. J Urol 1988;140:80–84.

111. Nichols CR, Roth BJ, Heerema N, et al. Hematologic neoplasms associated with primary mediastinal germ cell tumors. N Engl J Med 1990;322:1425–1429.

112. Bosl GJ, Dmitrosky E, Reuter V, et al. Isochromosome of chromosome 12: Clinically useful marker for male germ cell cancer. JNCI 1989;81:1874–1878.

113. Ladanyi M, Sammaniego F, Reuter VE, et al. Cytogenetic and immunohistochemical evidence for the germ cell origin of a subset of acute leukemia associated with mediastinal germ cell tumors. JNCI 1990;82:221–227.

114. Hainsworth JD, Wright EP, Gray GF, Greco FA. Poorly differentiated carcinoma of unknown primary: Correlation of light microscopic findings with response to cisplatin-based combination chemotherapy. J Clin Oncol 1987;5:1275–1280.

115. Hainsworth JD, Einhorn LH, Williams SD, et al. Advanced extragonadal germ cell tumors. Ann Intern Med 1982;97:7–11.

116. Vugrin D, Einhorn LH, Williams SD, et al. A multi-institutional experience in extragonadal germ cell tumors: An SECSG study. Proc Am Assoc Cancer Res [Abstract] 1985;26:172.

117. Israel A, Bosl GJ, Golbey RB, et al. The results of chemotherapy for extragonadal germ cell tumors in the cisplatin era: The MSKCC experience (1975–1982). J Clin Oncol 1985;3:1073–1078.

118. Logothetis CJ, Samuels ML, Selig DE, et al. Chemotherapy of extragonadal germ cell tumors. J Clin Oncol 1985;3:316–325.

119. Nichols CR, Saxman S, Williams SD, et al. Primary mediastinal nonseminomatous germ cell tumors. Cancer 1990;65:1641–1646.

120. Economou JS, Trump DL, Holmes EC, Eggleston JE. Management of primary germ cell tumors of the mediastinum. J Thorac Cardiovasc Surg 1982;83:643–649.

121. Williams SD, Einhorn LH, Greco FA, et al. VP-16-213 salvage therapy for refractory germinal neoplasms. Cancer 1980;46:2154–2158.

122. Hainsworth JD, Williams SD, Einhorn LH, et al. Successful treatment of resistant germinal neoplasms with VP-16 and cisplatin: Results of a Southeastern Cancer Study Group trial. J Clin Oncol 1985;3:666–671.

123. Wheeler BM, Loehrer PJ, Williams SD, Einhorn LH. Ifosfamide in refractory germ cell tumors. J Clin Oncol 1986;4:28–34.

124. Loehrer PJ, Einhorn LH, Williams SD. Salvage therapy for refractory germ cell tumors with VP-16 plus ifosfamide plus cisplatin. J Clin Oncol 1986;4:528–536.

125. Einhorn LH, Weathers T, Loehrer PJ. Second-line chemotherapy with vinblastine, ifosfamide and cisplatin after initial chemotherapy with cisplatin, VP-16 and bleomycin in disseminated germ cell tumors: Long-term followup. Proc Am Soc Clin Oncol [Abstract] 1992;11:

126. Motzer RJ, Cooper K, Geller NC, et al. The role of ifosfamide plus cisplatin-based chemotherapy as salvage therapy for patients with refractory germ cell tumors. Cancer 1990;66:2476–2481.

127. Nichols CR, Tricot G, Williams SD, et al. Dose-intensive chemotherapy in refractory germ cell cancer—a phase I–II trial of high-dose carboplatin and etoposide with autologous bone marrow transplantation. J Clin Oncol 1989;7:932–939.

128. Broun ER, Tricot G, Fox E, et al. Long-term follow of salvage chemotherapy in relapsed and refractory germ cell tumors using high-dose carboplatin and etoposide with autologous bone marrow rescue. Proc Am Soc Clin Oncol [Abstract] 1991;10:167.

129. Murphy B, Breeden E, Donohue J, et al. Surgical salvage of chemorefractory germ cell tumors. Proc Am Soc Clin Oncol [Abstract] 1992;11:198.

130. Vendetti JM. Treatment-schedule dependency of experimentally active anti-leukemic (L-1210) drugs. Cancer Chemother Rep 1971;2:35–39.

131. Slevin ML, Clark PI, Joel SP, et al. A randomized trial to evaluate the effect of schedule on the activity of etoposide in small cell lung cancer. J Clin Oncol 1989;7:1333–1340.

132. Miller JC, Einhorn LH. Phase II study of daily oral etoposide in refractory germ cell tumors. Semin Oncol 1990;17:36–39.

133. Cantwell BMJ, Millnard MJ, Lind MJ, Calvert AH. Twenty-one day cycles of oral etoposide in heavily pre-treated metastatic germ cell cancer. Lancet 1990;336:1011.

134. Williams SD, Stablein DM, Einhorn LH, et al. Pathologic stage II testis cancer: Immediate adjuvant chemotherapy versus observation with treatment relapse—a report from the Testicular Cancer Intergroup Study. N Engl J Med 1987;317:1433–1438.

135. Roth BJ, Greist A, Kubilis PS, et al. Cisplatin-based combination chemotherapy for disseminated germ cell tumors: Long-term followup. J Clin Oncol 1988;6:1239–1247.

136. Levi JA, Thomson D, Bishop J, et al. Dose intensity and outcome with combination chemotherapy for germ cell carcinoma. Eur J Cancer Clin Oncol 1989;25:1073–1077.

137. Peckham MJ, Horwich A, Easton DF, Hendry WF. The management of advanced testicular teratoma. Br J Urol 1988;62:63–68.

138. Drasga RE, Einhorn LH, Williams SD, et al. Fertility after chemotherapy for testicular cancer. J Clin Oncol 1983;1:179–183.

139. Fossa SD, Ous S, Abyholm T, et al. Post-treatment fertility in patients with testicular cancer. Br J Urol 1985;57:210–214.

140. Nijman JM, Koops HS, Kremer J, et al. Gonadal function after surgery and chemotherapy in men with stages II and III non-seminomatous testicular tumors. J Clin Oncol 1987;5:651–656.

141. Poirier S, Einhorn, LH, Rubin L. Evaluation of reproductive capacity in germ cell tumor patients following chemotherapy with cisplatin, VP-16 and bleomycin. Proc Am Soc Clin Oncol [Abstract] 1992;11:379.

142. Schlsky RL. Infertility in patients with testicular cancer. Testis, tumor, or treatment? JNCI 1989;81:1204–1205.

143. Vogelzang NJ, Bosl GJ, Johnson K, et al. Raynaud's phenomenon: A common toxicity after combination chemotherapy for testicular cancer. Ann Intern Med 1981;95:288–292.

144. Teutsch C, Lipton A, Harvey HA. Raynaud's phenomenon as a side effect of chemotherapy with vinblastine plus bleomycin for testicular cancer. Cancer Treat Rep 1977;61:925–926.

145. Subar M, Muggia FM. Apparent myocardial ischemia associated with vinblastine administration. Cancer Treat Rep 1986;70:690–691.

146. Vogelzang NJ, Freming DH, Kennedy BJ. Coronary artery disease after treatment with bleomycin and vinblastine. Cancer Treat Rep 1989;64:1159–1160.

147. Samuels BL, Vogelzang NJ, Kennedy BJ. Severe vascular toxicity associated with vinblastine, bleomycin, and cisplatin chemotherapy. Cancer Chemother Pharmacol 1987;19:253–256.

148. Doll DC, List AF, Greco FA, et al. Acute vascular ischemic events after cisplatin-based combination chemotherapy for germ cell tumors of the testis. Ann Intern Med 1986;105:48–51.

149. Burkhardt A, Haltje WJ, Gebbens JO, et al. Vascular lesions following perfusion with bleomycin: Electron microscopic observations. Virchows Arch [A] 1976;372:227–236.

150. Kahaleh MD, Osborn I, LeRoy EC. Increased factor VIII antigen in scleroderma and Raynaud's phenomenon. Ann Intern Med 1981;94:842–845.

151. Pui Ch, Chesney CM, Weed J, et al. Altered von Willebrand factor molecule in children with thrombus following asparaginase-prednisone-vincristine therapy for leukemia. J Clin Oncol 1985;3:1266–1271.

152. Nichols CR, Roth B, Williams SD, et al. Cardiovascular complications of chemotherapy for testicular cancer. Proc Am Soc Clin Oncol [Abstract] 1990;9:132.

153. Barneveld PW, Sleijfer DT, van der Mark TW, et al. Natural course of bleomycin induced pneumonitis. Am Rev Respir Dis 1987;135:48–51.

154. Nachman JB, Baum ES, White H, et al. Bleomycin-induced pulmonary fibrosis mimicking recurrent metastatic disease in a patient with testicular cancer. Cancer 1981;47:236–239.

155. McCrea ES, Diaconis JN, Wade JC, et al. Bleomycin toxicity simulating metastatic nodules to the lungs. Cancer 1981;48:1096–1100.

156. Redman JR, Vugrin D, Arlin ZA, et al. Leukemia following treatment of germ cell tumors in men. J Clin Oncol 1984;2:1080–1087.

157. Whitlock JA, Greer JP, Lukens JN. Epipodophyllotoxin-related leukemia. Cancer 1991;68:600–604.

158. Pedersen-Bjergaard J, Daugaard G, Hansen SW, et al. Increased risk of myelodysplasia and leukemia after etoposide, cisplatin, and bleomycin for germ cell tumors. Lancet 1991;338:359–363.

159. Nichols C, Breeden E, Loehrer P, Williams S, Einhorn LH. Secondary leukemia associated with standard dose etoposide: Review of germ cell tumor protocols. Proc Am Soc Clin Oncol [Abstract] 1992;11:2000.

160. Chong C, Logothetis CJ, von Eschenbach A, et al. Orchiectomy in advanced germ cell carcinoma following intensive chemotherapy: A comparison of systemic to testicular response. J Urol 1986;136:1221–1223.

161. Fowler JE Jr, Whitmore WF Jr. Intratesticular germ cell tumors: Observations on the effect of chemotherapy. J Urol 1981;126:412–415.

162. Logothetis CJ, Samuels ML, Trindode A. The management of brain metastases in germ cell tumors. Cancer 1982;49:1278–1281.

163. Bustin GJS, Newlands ES, Bagshawe KE, et al. Successful management of metastatis and primary germ cell tumors in the brain. Cancer 1986;57:2108–2113.

164. Spears WT, Morphis JG, Lester SG, Williams SD, Einhorn LH. Brain metastases and testicular tumors: Long-term survival. Int J Radiat Biol Phys 1991;22:17–22.

165. Stanton GF, Bosl GJ, Whitmore WF, et al. VAB-6 as initial treatment of patients with advanced seminoma. J Clin Oncol 1985;33:336–339.

166. Loehrer PJ, Birch R, Williams SD, et al. Chemotherapy of metastatic seminoma: The Southeastern Cancer Study Group experience. J Clin Oncol 1987;5:1212–1220.

167. Horwich A, Dearnaley DP, Duchesne GM, et al. Simple non-toxic treatment of advanced metastatic seminoma with carboplatin. J Clin Oncol 1989;7:1150–1156.

168. Hartenstein RC, Mair W, Gerl A, Wilmanns W. VIP combination chemotherapy in bulky seminoma. Proc Am Soc Clin Oncol 1991;10:178.

169. Motzer RJ, Bosl GJ, Geller N, et al. Advanced seminoma: The role of chemotherapy and adjunctive surgery. Ann Intern Med 1988;108:513–518.

170. Motzer R, Bosl G, Heelan R, et al. Residual mass: An indication for further therapy in patients with advanced seminoma following systemic chemotherapy. J Clin Oncol 1987;5:1064–1070.

171. Schultz SM, Einhorn LH, Conces DJ, Williams SD, Loehrer PJ. Management of post-chemotherapy residual mass in patients with advanced seminoma: Indiana University experience. J Clin Oncol 1989;7:1497–1503.

172. Patterson AHG, Peckham MJ, McCready VR. Value of gallium scanning in seminoma of the testis. Br Med J 1976;1:1118–1121.

173. Willan BD, Penney H, Castor WR, et al. The usefulness of gallium-67 citrate scanning in testicular seminoma. Clin Nucl Med 1987;10:813–815.

Cancer: Principles & Practice of Oncology, Fourth Edition,
edited by Vincent T. DeVita, Jr., Samuel Hellman, Steven A. Rosenberg.
J.B. Lippincott Co., Philadelphia © 1993.

William J. Hoskins
Carlos A. Perez
Robert C. Young

CHAPTER **38**

Gynecologic Tumors

Gynecologic cancer represents 12.7% of all cancers that occur in women and accounts for 9.8% of all cancer deaths.[1] Table 38–1 lists the estimated number of new cases and deaths from gynecologic malignancies in 1992.

The physician who diagnoses and treats patients with cancer of the female genital tract must have a thorough understanding of the pathophysiology of the disease and the various therapeutic options that are available. In this chapter, we provide current information on all the female genital cancers except ovarian cancer, which is discussed separately in Chapter 39. We describe the epidemiology, natural history, routes of spread, and pathologic characteristics that affect treatment planning. We emphasize methods of diagnosis and current therapeutic options.

CARCINOMA OF THE VULVA

Carcinoma of the vulva accounts for 3% to 4% of all female genital cancers, and squamous cell cancer accounts for 90% of vulvar cancers. Other cell types that can be found in the vulva include malignant melanoma, basal cell carcinoma, and adenocarcinoma of the Bartholin's and Skene's glands. Primary vulvar sarcoma and verrucous carcinoma occur infrequently. Paget's disease can be associated with invasive adenocarcinoma of the sweat glands.

Vulvar cancers tend to develop slowly. They spread by direct continuity to adjacent tissues or by the lymphatics to the inguinal lymph nodes. Treatment is usually surgical, which in the past resulted in physical disfigurement and sexual dysfunction.[2] However, clinical studies of this disease report alternative methods of therapy that modify treatment to reduce disfigurement while improving survival.

EPIDEMIOLOGY

Carcinoma of the vulva accounts for 3% to 4% of all primary genital cancers in women. The median age for patients with carcinoma in situ of the vulva is 44.[3-7] For those with microinvasive carcinoma, the median age is 58.[7,8] Patients with frankly invasive carcinoma have a median age of 61.[9,10] Some researchers suggest that carcinoma in situ and microinvasive carcinoma are being seen more frequently and are occurring in younger women, but that impression remains to be verified by large studies. The age-incidence associations for invasive cancer do not appear to have changed.

Japaze and colleagues reported no increase in the incidence of vulvar cancer in any ethnic group.[5] However, Mack and Casagrande reported that women of the lowest socioeconomic class had three times the incidence that was seen in women of the highest socioeconomic class.[11]

Medical illnesses associated with vulvar cancer are hypertension, cardiovascular disease, obesity, and diabetes.[8,12,13] A variety of sexually transmitted diseases, including granulomatous venereal disease, syphilis, herpes hominis type II, and condylomata acuminata, have been associated with vulvar carcinoma.[7,14] Recent evidence suggests an association between the human papillomavirus or the herpes simplex virus and vulvar neoplasia.[15-19] Other associations, such as leukoplakia of the vulva, genitourinary cancer, and an occupational history in the laundry and cleaning industries, were observed.[20] Patients with vulvar cancer have an increased incidence of anogenital carcinomas, especially cervical cancer.[21,22]

NATURAL HISTORY AND PATTERNS OF SPREAD

The association of carcinoma in situ, microinvasive carcinoma, and invasive vulvar carcinoma indicates a continuum

TABLE 38-1. Estimated New Cases and Deaths From Cancer in 1992

Site	Estimated New Cases	Estimated Deaths
Corpus	32,000	5,600
Ovary	21,000	13,000
Cervix	13,500	4,400
Other	5,000	1,000
Total	71,500	24,000

(Adapted from Boring CC, Squires TS, Tong T. Cancer statistics. CA 1992;42:19)

from preinvasive to invasive disease. However, this process occurs more slowly in the vulva than in the vagina or cervix, and although most cervical cancers are associated with an intraepithelial lesion, this holds true for only a third of vulvar carcinomas.[23]

A difference of almost 20 years exists between the peak incidence of vulvar carcinoma in situ and the peak incidence of invasive vulvar carcinoma. Some researchers suggest that the multifocal carcinoma in situ of women in their thirties or forties is less likely to progress to invasive cancer than is the localized carcinoma in situ of older women. However, proof does not yet exist for this theory, and therapy for young women should not be delayed.

Plentl and Friedman reported that the labia are the most common sites of primary vulvar lesions, followed by the clitoris.[24] Labial lesions occur three times more frequently on the labia majora than on the labia minora. Metastatic lesions spread predictably to the inguinal lymph nodes, followed by spread to the pelvic nodes. With the possible exception of vulvar melanoma, vulvar cancer does not usually spread by the blood stream.

The embryologic derivation of the lymphatics of vulvar skin is similar to that of abdominal skin, and primary drainage is logically to the superficial and deep inguinal lymph nodes.[24] Direct drainage to the pelvic lymph nodes occurs infrequently. The labia minora are characterized by a fine network of lymphatics that extends to the folds between the labia minora and labia majora. At these folds, the lymphatic vessels coalesce and extend cephalad. The lymphatics of the labia majora are more coarse than those of the labia minora. They run laterally to the crural fold, where they turn cephalad. The clitoral vessels drain into the connecting trunks of the labia minora. All of these channels eventually drain into the superficial inguinal nodes that lie beneath Camper's fascia and anterior to the cribriform fascia. Connecting lymphatics lead to the deep inguinal nodes that surround the femoral vessels and drain into the iliac nodal system. Although the clitoral lymphatics may drain directly into the pelvic lymphatics, metastases to pelvic nodes without inguinal involvement are rare.[24] Way found involvement of pelvic lymph nodes without inguinal lymph node involvement in only 3% of his patients.[25]

Iversen and Aas further clarified lymphatic drainage from the vulva.[26] The investigators injected ^{99m}Tc colloid in 54 patients who were undergoing radical hysterectomy and pelvic lymphadenectomy for carcinoma of the cervix. Radioactivity was measured in vivo with a scintillation camera and in the removed lymph nodes with a well counter. Although most radioactivity from the vulva was emitted by the ipsilateral inguinal lymph nodes, a small but detectable contralateral flow occurred. Bilateral flow from the clitoris and the perineum was confirmed, and a significant amount of contralateral flow in the anterior labia minora was found. The investigators were unable to document direct flow of lymphatics from the clitoris to the pelvic lymph nodes. They did find that 13% of lymph flow bypassed Cloquet's node in traveling to the pelvic lymph nodes.

In a literature review by Plentl and Friedman, the overall incidence of positive lymph nodes (inguinal and pelvic) was 46% in more than 1100 patients with vulvar cancer.[24] Because the incidence of pelvic node metastases is 5% to 10%, inguinal node metastases can be expected to occur in 35% to 40% of patients. Plentl and Friedman also reported a 62% incidence of metastases in clinically palpable lymph nodes and a 35% incidence of metastases in nonpalpable lymph nodes. The incidence of positive lymph nodes increases with the size of the lesion, with the depth of invasion, and by location. Midline lesions have a higher incidence of bilateral positive lymph nodes.

PATHOLOGY

Intraepithelial neoplasia of the vulva exhibits a variety of gross and microscopic patterns. Grossly, the lesions can be flat and raised (maculopapular) or verrucous. They can be brown (hyperpigmented), red (erythroplastic), or white (leukoplakia). This variety of gross and microscopic patterns led to the use of terms such as Bowen's disease, erythroplasia of Queyrat, carcinoma simplex, and Paget's disease to differentiate the types of neoplasia.[27]

In 1976, to standardize nomenclature, the International Society for the Study of Vulvar Disease published a classification that is widely accepted throughout the world.[28] A summary is shown in Table 38-2. In this classification system, only two types of true intraepithelial neoplasia are accepted: carcinoma in situ and Paget's disease.

Histologically, carcinoma in situ is characterized by disordered orientation and maturation of the epithelial cells that extend for the full thickness of the epithelium. Giant cells, multinucleated cells, dyskeratosis, parakeratosis, and increased density of cells are seen. The morphologically abnormal nucleus has irregular borders and clumped chromatin.[28]

TABLE 38-2. International Society for the Study of Vulvar Disease: Abbreviated Classification of Vulvar Diseases

A. Hyperplastic dystrophy
   1. Without atypia
   2. With atypia
B. Lichen sclerosis
C. Mixed dystrophy
   1. Without atypia
   2. With atypia
D. Paget's disease of the vulva
E. Carcinoma in situ

Paget's disease is characterized microscopically by Paget's cells, which are large and round or oval with pale, vacuolated cytoplasm. These cells appear singly and in nests surrounded by small hyperchromatic basaloid cells. Helwig and Graham reported that one third of their cases of Paget's disease of the vulva were associated with underlying adenocarcinomas of an adnexal structure.[29] Associated carcinomas of the breast and Bartholin's gland and squamous cell carcinomas of the cervix have been reported.[30-32]

Invasive squamous cell cancer is the most common vulvar malignancy and accounts for more than 90% of all cases. Grossly, the lesions are ulcerated and endophytic in one third of the patients and exophytic in the remainder.[28] Histologically, squamous cell cancers tend to be well differentiated, with whorls and nests of keratin. Gosling and colleagues[33] and Way[34] report that 5% to 10% of these cancers are anaplastic.

Squamous cell cancers that are less than 2 cm in diameter and invade less than 5 mm are often called microinvasive carcinoma.[35] However, the International Society for the Study of Vulvar Disease concluded that "microinvasive" should not be used in vulvar cancer because of its ambiguity. They proposed that the International Federation of Gynecology and Obstetrics (FIGO) designate a stage IA vulvar carcinoma to be defined as solitary squamous cell cancer of the vulva with a lesion of 2 cm or less that invades 1 mm or less.[36] The metastatic potential of these lesions and the proper management of patients who exhibit them are currently being evaluated.

Two rare varieties of squamous cell cancer are adenoid squamous cancer and verrucous carcinoma.[37,38] Verrucous carcinoma is well differentiated and resembles extensive condylomata acuminata. It invades locally but seldom metastasizes.[39]

Melanoma accounts for 2% to 9% of vulvar cancers.[28] Two varieties of melanoma are the nodular melanoma and the superficial spreading melanoma.[28] Depth of invasion is directly related to the incidence of nodal metastases and survival.[40]

Although basal cell carcinomas are common in other parts of the body, they seldom occur in the vulva.[41] Rarely, sarcomas arise in the vulvar connective tissue. Leiomyosarcoma is the most common, but neurofibrosarcomas, rhabdomyosarcomas, fibrosarcomas, and angiosarcomas were reported.[42] Adenocarcinomas occasionally arise from the periurethral Skene's glands, but most are from the Bartholin's gland or from vulvar adnexal structures associated with Paget's disease.

Bartholin's carcinomas are squamous if they originate near the orifice of the duct, papillary if they arise from the transitional epithelium of the duct, or adenocarcinoma if they arise from the gland itself. The adenoid cystic variety of Bartholin's gland carcinoma is similar to the adenoid cystic tumor of the salivary gland and tends to invade locally, with metastases occurring late, if at all.[28]

CLINICAL PRESENTATION AND STAGING

The most common complaint of the patient with vulvar cancer is a growth or mass on the vulva.[13] Pruritus vulvae, bleeding, and pain are also seen, although up to 20% of patients are asymptomatic.[12,43] Physician and patient delay have resulted in delays in diagnosis, but improved education appears to have reduced delays in treatment. Most recent series report smaller

lesions, and the available literature on early invasive cancer is increasing.

The best way of diagnosing vulvar cancer is to maintain a high index of suspicion and to perform an early biopsy. A wedge biopsy with a knife or a circular biopsy with a Keye's or Baker's dermal punch under local infiltration anesthesia provides an excellent specimen. The punch biopsy instruments are especially useful because hemostasis can usually be obtained by silver nitrate application without sutures. Colposcopy is often helpful in defining the limits of the lesion, but it is too time consuming to be used as a standard screening procedure. Toluidine blue staining of the vulva was advocated as a method of identifying areas for biopsy, but it has a 20% false-positive rate.

If invasive carcinoma is found on biopsy, the patient should undergo a metastatic evaluation. The vagina and cervix should be carefully inspected, and a Papanicolaou (Pap) smear of the cervix must be obtained. A careful bimanual examination, cystoscopy, proctoscopy, chest radiograph, computed tomography (CT) scan, and biochemical profile are required. If indicated, barium enema or other diagnostic studies may be employed. Because most patients with vulvar carcinoma are elderly, a thorough medical evaluation is often indicated before treatment.

Radiographic evaluation of regional lymphatics in carcinoma of the vulva is of limited value and is rarely used. Preoperative lymphography was evaluated at the Mallinckrodt Institute of Radiology in 32 patients with vulvar carcinoma. Correlations with surgical specimens revealed an overall accuracy of 54.5% with a sensitivity of 15.7% and a specificity of 66.1%.[44] Computed tomography or magnetic resonance imaging (MRI) may aid in outlining the extent of tumor and in evaluating the inguinal and pelvic/periaortic lymph nodes. The standard workup for these patients is described in Table 38–3.[45]

In 1989, FIGO approved a new staging system for vulvar cancer. Based on surgical findings, the new system uses a surgical-pathologic staging classification (Table 38–4).[46] For malignant melanoma, the Clark[47] or Breslow[48] classifications of depth of invasion should also be provided. Bartholin's gland carcinomas are staged by the FIGO system, and metastatic tumors are not staged. Because the FIGO system does not include a subdivision for microinvasive vulvar cancer, the depth of invasion for stage I tumors must be described accurately. The presence or absence of lymphovascular invasion should be documented for later determining the prognosis.

TREATMENT

Historically, vulvar carcinoma was thought to be most effectively managed by radical surgery, with minimal response to radiation therapy, chemotherapy, or conservative surgery. The slow growth of the disease, with its orderly progression of metastases to regional lymph nodes, argues for en bloc surgical resection, and survival rates of 85% to 98% for patients with negative lymph nodes and 30% to 70% for those with positive inguinal nodes were consistently reported after radical surgery. Table 38–5[49] shows 5-year survival rates for patients with carcinoma of the vulva.

Radical vulvectomy, inguinal node dissection, and pelvic node dissection significantly disrupt normal anatomy. These

TABLE 38–3. Diagnostic Workup for Vulvar Tumors

General

History

Physical examination, including careful bimanual pelvic
  examination

Special Studies

Exfoliative cytology of cervix and vagina

Colposcopy and directed biopsies (including Schiller's test)

Biopsies and examination under anesthesia to determine tumor
  extent

Cytoscopy

Proctosigmoidoscopy (as indicated)

Radiographic Studies

Standard

  Chest radiographs

  Intravenous pyelogram

Complementary

  Barium enema

  Lymphangiogram

  Computed tomography or magnetic resonance imaging scans
  of pelvis and abdomen

Laboratory Studies

Complete blood count

Blood chemistry

Urinalysis

(Perez CA, Grigsby PW. Vulva. In: Perez CA, Brady LW, eds. Principles
and practice of radiation oncology. 2nd ed. Philadelphia: JB Lippincott,
1992:1273–1289)

treatments are often complicated by wound breakdown,
lymphedema, and sexual dysfunction. A more conservative
approach to vulvar cancer is currently in use, and innovative
approaches that decrease short-term and long-term morbidity
are being evaluated. In the past 5 years, significant changes
have come about in the management of vulvar cancer, and
additional changes are likely to occur in the next decade.

Carcinoma in Situ

In the 1960s, Collins and coworkers advocated radical vulvectomy for carcinoma in situ of the vulva because 4 of their
41 patients had unsuspected invasive cancer in the final specimen.[3] Boutselis reported almost 100% survival with simple
vulvectomy.[4] Rutledge and Sinclair described the skinning
vulvectomy, which removed the skin of the vulva but preserved
the fat, muscles, and glandular structures.[50] Better cosmesis
was obtained if this incision was covered with a split-thickness
skin graft from the thigh or buttock. Forney and colleagues
used this procedure in 8 patients and reported only 1 recurrence.[6] In 1983, Barnhill and colleagues described the rhomboid flap technique for vulvar reconstruction after wide local
excision of carcinoma in situ.[51]

Current treatment for carcinoma in situ of the vulva is wide
local excision followed by primary closure, skin flaps, or skin
graft to restore normal anatomy. Many researchers reported
successful control of the disease, with recurrence rates of only
9% to 12%.[6,7,52,53] Considering the improved function and
cosmesis with wide local excision, this method of therapy and
close follow-up appears to provide optimal management for
carcinoma in situ of the vulva. Most patients, even if they
require repeat excisions for recurrence, can be managed by
wide local excisions, providing they obtain frequent follow-
up examinations.

Other methods of treatment for carcinoma in situ of the
vulva include topical 5-fluorouracil, cryosurgery, dinitrochlo-
robenzene-induced hypersensitivity, and laser vaporization.
Of these methods, none provide a pathologic specimen for
histologic review, and only laser vaporization is significantly
useful. Extensive laser vaporization is painful, and most authorities use it only for small lesions.

Paget's disease of the vulva extends subepithelially and requires wide excision to achieve free margins. Frozen section
of the margins in the operating room may assist the surgeon
to ensure complete removal. Although some authorities recommend simple vulvectomy for Paget's disease, this lesion is
like carcinoma in situ and can usually be managed by less
radical excision. A slightly deeper excision than is used for
carcinoma in situ is necessary for Paget's disease in order to
remove the epidermis and corium down to the level of the
underlying fat to ensure removal of the adnexal skin structures. Gregori and colleagues reported a 12.4% recurrence
rate after surgical excision (many patients initially underwent
simple vulvectomy).[54]

Some researchers reported success with topical chemotherapy for recurrent Paget's disease, but this treatment should
not be used as primary therapy because of the possibility of
overlooking an underlying adenocarcinoma.[55] If an invasive
adenocarcinoma is found, the patient should be managed according to the extent of invasion.

Stage I

Stage I vulvar cancer encompasses all tumors that show any
degree of invasion, providing they are less than 2 cm in diameter, do not involve the anus, vagina, or urethra, and have
not metastasized to lymph nodes. However, a growing body
of literature indicates that certain early lesions should be separated into a category of limited invasion. In 1974, Wharton
and colleagues described a series of patients with vulvar tumors that were less than 2 cm in diameter and exhibited less
than 5 mm of stromal invasion.[35] They performed lymphadenectomies in 10 of 25 patients and found no positive lymph
nodes. Since these reports, several researchers reported small
series of patients with an average incidence of inguinal node
metastases of 5% to 10%.[8,56,57] Hacker and colleagues reviewed the literature and described the incidence of inguinal
nodal metastases by depth of invasion.[58] They reported no
nodal metastases in patients with less than 1 mm of invasion,
but invasion of 1 to 2 mm was associated with nodal metastases
in 6.6% of patients. Metastases in 8.2% to 25% were reported
with invasion of 3 to 5 mm, and metastases of 27.5% were
reported with invasion of more than 5 mm. Other factors that
may influence the incidence of nodal metastases are anaplastic
tumors, confluency of invading foci, and lymphovascular
invasion.[8,57]

There is disagreement about the management of patients
with early invasive carcinoma. No clear-cut evidence exists

TABLE 38–4.   FIGO Staging for Carcinoma of the Vulva

Stage 0

Tis — Carcinoma in situ; intraepithelial carcinoma

Stage I

T1N0M0 — Tumor confined to the vulva and/or perineum—2 cm or less in greatest dimension, nodes are not palpable

Stage II

T2N0M0 — Tumor confined to the vulva and/or perineum—more than 2 cm in greatest dimension, nodes are not palpable

Stage III

T3N0M0 — Tumor of any size with. . .

T3N1M0 — 1) Adjacent spread to the lower urethra and/or the vagina, or the anus, and/or. . .

T1N1M0 — 2) Unilateral regional lymph node metastasis

T2N1M0

Stage IVA

T1N2M0 — Tumor invades any of the following:

T2N2M0 — Upper urethra, bladder mucosa, rectal mucosa, pelvic bone, and/or bilateral regional node metastasis

T3N2M0

T4 any NM0

Stage IVB

Any T — Any distant metastasis including pelvic lymph

Any N, M1 — nodes

Rules for Clinical Staging

The rules for staging are similar to those for carcinoma of the cervix.

TNM Classification of Carcinoma of the Vulva (FIGO)

T	*Primary tumor*
Tis	Preinvasive carcinoma (carcinoma in situ)
T1	Tumor confined to the vulva and/or perineum—≤2 cm in greatest dimension
T2	Tumor confined to the vulva and/or perineum—>2 cm in greatest dimension
T3	Tumor of any size with adjacent spread to the urethra and/or vagina and/or to the anus
T4	Tumor of any size infiltrating the bladder mucosa and/or the rectal mucosa, including the upper part of the urethral mucosa and/or fixed to the bone
N	*Regional lymph nodes*
N0	No lymph node metastasis
N1	Unilateral regional lymph node metastasis
N2	Bilateral regional lymph node metastasis
M	*Distant metastasis*
M0	No clinical metastasis
M1	Distant metastasis (including pelvic lymph node metastasis)

(International Federation of Gynecology and Obstetrics. Annual report on the results of treatment in gynecological cancer. Int J Gynecol Obstet 1989;28:189–190)

in the literature to enable us to establish firm guidelines. Di Saia and colleagues recommended an operative procedure in which the superficial inguinal lymph nodes are removed and sent for frozen section.[59] If positive nodes are found, bilateral complete groin dissections and radical vulvectomy are performed. If the nodes are negative, wide local excision of the primary cancer is performed. This therapeutic option appears to offer an acceptable treatment plan based on the meager information available. However, no large prospective trial of this therapy was conducted. A major concern is whether su-

TABLE 38–5.   Survival Rates for Carcinoma of the Vulva Using the 1988 FIGO Staging Classification

Stage	*Five-Year Survival Rate (%)*
I	98
II	85
III	74
IV	31

(Adapted from Homesley HD, Bundy BN, Sedlis A, et al. Assessment of current International Federation of Gynecology and Obstetrics staging of vulvar carcinoma relative to prognostic factors for survival [a Gynecologic Onolcogy Group study]. Am J Obstet Gynecol 1991;164:997)

perficial inguinal node dissection is as accurate an assessment of nodal status as a full inguinofemoral node dissection.

The Gynecologic Oncology Group (GOG) is prospectively evaluating patients with tumor diameter of less than 2 cm and tumor invasion of less than 5 mm. In this protocol, patients are managed by modified radical hemivulvectomy and ipsilateral node dissection.

Most authorities manage stage I carcinomas of the vulva (*i.e.*, invasion >5 mm) by modified radical vulvectomy or hemivulvectomy with ipsilateral inguinofemoral lymphadenectomy. For patients with midline lesions, bilateral node dissections are performed. Analysis of the literature indicates that the incidence of local recurrence after wide local excision of stage I tumors is no higher than after radical vulvectomy.[58] Heaps and colleagues published a report indicating that the lateral and deep margins of resection should clear the lesion by at least 1 cm.[60]

Stage II

The lesion in stage II vulvar carcinoma is greater than 2 cm in diameter and confined to the vulva or perineum (*i.e.*, no nodal metastases). The traditional treatment for stage II carcinoma of the vulva is radical vulvectomy and bilateral inguinal lymphadenectomy. Three basic surgical approaches can be employed. The so-called "butterfly" incision removes the skin over the mons, from the level of the iliac crest and the vulva, and a wedge of skin over the inguinal dissection. An alternative to the butterfly incision is to mobilize a skin flap over the inguinal dissection without excising this skin. Some researchers advocated separate groin incisions for the inguinal dissections coupled with a radical excision of the vulva. The incidence of local recurrence appears to be similar for each technique, and most gynecologic oncologists use separate groin incisions (Fig. 38–1A,B).[61]

Some researchers recommend conservative resection of more advanced lesions. Burrell and colleagues reported the use of modified radical vulvectomy for 14 patients with lesions greater than 2 cm.[62] They also performed bilateral inguinofemoral lymphadenectomy (see Fig. 38–1C).[61] Although 5 of 14 patients had positive lymph nodes, none developed local recurrence. Burke and coworkers reported 32 patients with invasion greater than 1 mm managed by wide local excision.[63] Seventeen patients had tumors less than 2 cm in diameter, and 15 patients had tumors larger than 2 cm. The diameters

of the tumors ranged from 5 to 65 mm, and the depth of invasion ranged from 1.5 to 13 mm. Only 2 patients developed local recurrences, and both were salvaged by reexcision. Heaps and colleagues found no local recurrences in patients treated with radical vulvectomy if the margins were larger than 8 mm, but the recurrence rate was 48% if the margins were less than 8 mm.[60]

Although radical vulvectomy and bilateral inguinofemoral lymphadenectomy remain the standard therapy for stage II lesions, many surgeons manage these patients by modified radical vulvectomy. Preliminary evidence indicates that this treatment may be acceptable if the margins of resection are at least 1 cm.

Many surgeons perform only an ipsilateral lymphadenectomy for unilateral lesions. Bilateral lymphadenectomy, however, is necessary in treating midline lesions and if the ipsilateral lymph nodes contain metastases.

Although most researchers previously recommended rou-

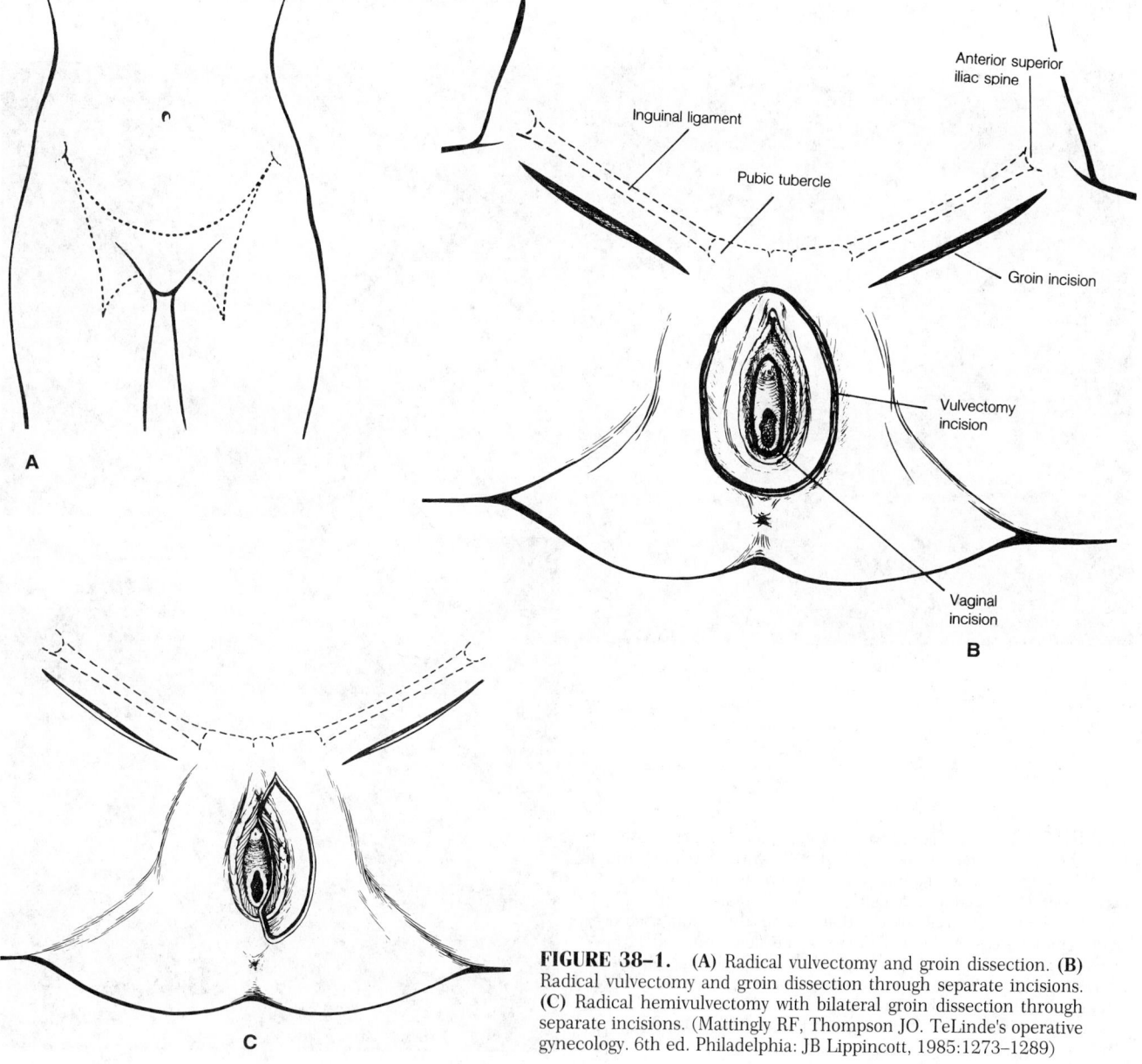

FIGURE 38–1. **(A)** Radical vulvectomy and groin dissection. **(B)** Radical vulvectomy and groin dissection through separate incisions. **(C)** Radical hemivulvectomy with bilateral groin dissection through separate incisions. (Mattingly RF, Thompson JO. TeLinde's operative gynecology. 6th ed. Philadelphia: JB Lippincott, 1985:1273–1289)

tine performance of pelvic lymphadenectomy if the inguinal lymph nodes were positive, current evidence indicates that these patients are best managed by pelvic irradiation. Homesley and colleagues reported a randomized trial of pelvic irradiation or pelvic lymphadenectomy in patients with positive inguinal nodes.[64] The investigators demonstrated statistically significant improved survival and no increased morbidity in the group receiving pelvic irradiation.

Because of the morbidity associated with radical vulvectomy, an attempt is being made to combine a wide local excision or simple vulvectomy to remove the primary tumor (plus an inguinofemoral lymph node dissection in patients with clinically positive nodes) with moderate doses of radiation therapy (5000 cGy for subclinical disease with a boost of 1000 to 1500 cGy through reduced portals for microscopically involved areas) to the remaining vulva and regional lymph node-bearing areas (Fig. 38-2). The biologic and therapeutic principles that are the basis for this method have already been validated in the treatment of head and neck, breast, and soft tissue sarcomas.

The role of radiation therapy alone in the primary management of carcinoma of the vulva remains controversial, mainly because of a lack of data on the results of treatment with modern techniques and because of the traditional belief that vulvar tissues cannot tolerate high doses of radiation (>6000 cGy). Historically, the reported rate of control was low, and the rate of complications was substantial. Radiation therapy is most often used for palliation or for treatment of disease not amenable to surgical resection.

Stages III and IV

Stage III vulvar carcinoma is a tumor of any size that has spread to the urethra, vagina, anus, or to the lymph nodes in the inguinal area. For these patients, radical vulvectomy often involves removal of a portion of the distal urethra or vagina and may require excision of a portion of the anus. Exenteration is rarely required. Based on the GOG study by Homesley and colleagues, these patients should undergo postoperative pelvic irradiation if the inguinal lymph nodes contain cancer.[64]

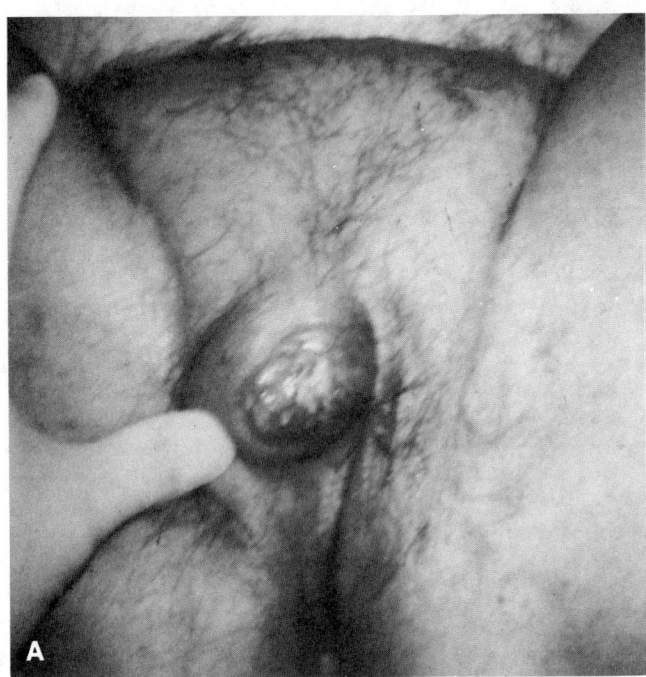

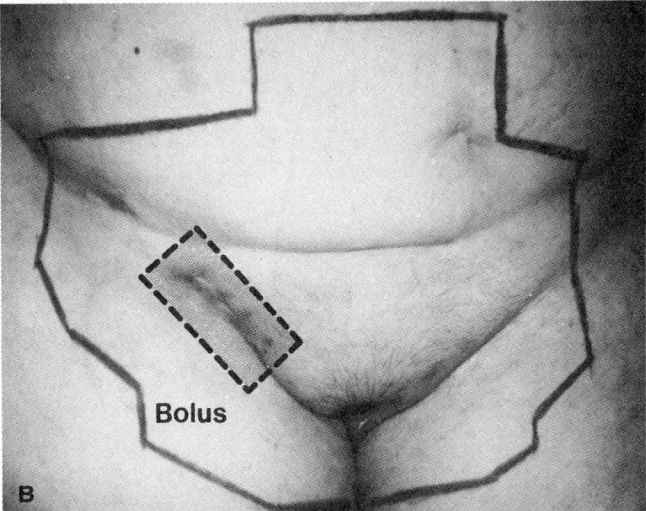

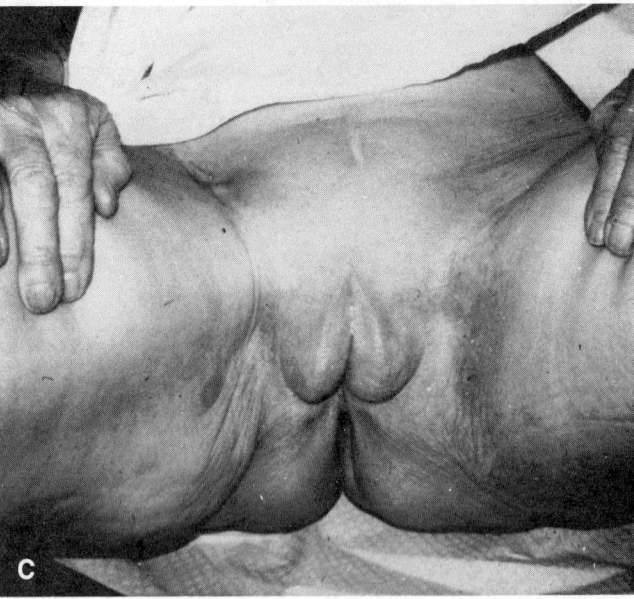

FIGURE 38-2. **(A)** Patient with a 4-cm epidermoid carcinoma in the right labia and clitoris and a 4 × 4 × 3 cm right inguinal lymph node. Wide local excision of the primary tumor and lymph nodes was carried out. **(B)** Portal used to deliver external irradiation to treat pelvic and vulvar areas to 5000 cGy. Bolus (2 cm thick) was used over right inguinal areas. Additional 1500 cGy was delivered with 12 MeV electrons to right tumor volume. **(C)** Posttreatment photograph 3 years later, showing excellent cosmetic results. Patient is tumor free. (Perez CA, Grigsby PW. Vulva. In: Perez CA, Brady LW, eds. Principles and practice of radiation oncology. 2nd ed. Philadelphia: JB Lippincott, 1992:1277)

Stage IVA vulvar cancer involves the upper one third of the urethra or involves the bladder or rectum. Stage IV disease also indicates bilateral positive inguinal lymph nodes or fixation of tumor to bone. Distant metastases are classified as stage IVB disease.

Treatment of tumors involving the bladder or upper urethra may require anterior exenteration in addition to radical vulvectomy and inguinal node dissections. Posterior exenteration may be used if the lesion involves the rectum.

Boronow and colleagues reported 37 primary cases of advanced vulvar cancer and 11 cases of recurrent vulvar cancer managed by preoperative radiation.[65] The 5-year survival rate for the patients with primary disease was 75.6%, and the 5-year survival rate for those with recurrent disease was 62.6%. Seventeen of 40 patients had no residual cancer in the final specimen. The investigators reported 8 patients with local recurrences and 5 with fistulae, but only 2 of 48 patients eventually required exenteration.

If the tumor is fixed to bone or distant metastases have occurred, treatment is usually palliative and consists of combinations of irradiation and chemotherapy. These therapies are discussed in more detail later in this chapter.

Treatment of Other Vulvar Tumors

MALIGNANT MELANOMA OF THE VULVA. Chung and colleagues found no lymph node metastases in patients with Clark's level I or II malignant melanoma.[40] Positive lymph nodes were associated with deeper levels of invasion. Current recommendations for treatment are wide local excision for all malignant melanomas. Ipsilateral lymph node dissection should be considered for melanomas that are deeper than Clark's level II.

Some authorities question the value of routine lymph node dissection in any case of malignant melanoma. The GOG prospectively evaluated wide local excision and inguinal lymphadenectomy for all cases of vulvar melanoma. The study reached its accrual goal, but the follow-up time is still too short for complete evaluation of the data.

Woolcott and associates reported results for 50 patients with primary melanoma of the vulva, 42 of whom were treated with definitive therapy (*i.e.*, 16 with wide local excision, 2 with unilateral inguinofemoral lymphadenectomy, 2 with bilateral inguinofemoral lymphadenectomy, 2 with hemivulvectomy and inguinofemoral lymph node dissection, 1 with simple vulvectomy alone).[66] Twenty-three patients were treated with radical vulvectomy, and all but one of these procedures were combined with bilateral inguinofemoral lymphadenectomy. Two patients also had pelvic lymphadenectomy. Three of the 42 patients treated with curative intent received adjuvant radiation therapy. Seventeen of the 50 patients were alive and free of disease at the last follow-up examination. The 5-year survival rate for 32 eligible patients was 43.8%. Eighty percent (12 of 15) of patients treated with wide local excision were alive at 2 years, and 50% (5 of 10) were alive at 5 years. Seventy-four percent (14 of 19) of the patients treated with radical vulvectomy and bilateral inguinofemoral lymphadenectomy were alive at 2 years and 50% (7 of 14) were alive at 5 years. The depth of melanocytic penetration was the main prognostic factor. Seven of 23 patients treated with radical vulvectomy developed local recurrence; 4 had

inguinofemoral nodal recurrences, and 8 developed distant metastases. Of the 16 patients treated with wide local excision, 3 developed local recurrence, 4 had inguinofemoral recurrences, and 2 had distant metastases.

BARTHOLIN'S GLAND CARCINOMA. Bartholin's gland carcinoma is usually managed by radical vulvectomy and bilateral inguinal node dissection. Copeland and colleagues reported 36 patients with Bartholin's gland carcinoma, of whom 12 were managed by wide local excision or hemivulvectomy.[67] The recurrence rate was 17% in the group managed by local excision and 21% in the group managed by radical vulvectomy.

Resection of the local tumor must be extensive due to its deep location. Although some researchers recommend pelvic node dissection for all Bartholin's gland carcinomas, current evidence suggests that pelvic irradiation may be an acceptable treatment option. Adenoid cystic carcinoma of the Bartholin's gland should be treated by wide local excision. Lymph node metastases are rare.

OTHER VULVAR CANCERS. Basal cell carcinoma and verrucous carcinoma are managed by wide local excision. Lymph node dissection is not indicated for these patients. Metastatic tumors of the vulva should be excised, if possible, to control local symptoms. Further treatment depends on the site of the primary cancer. All soft tissue sarcomas should be locally excised, if possible. After excision, treatment should include combinations of systemic chemotherapy and local and regional irradiation.

Radiation Therapy

The role of radiation therapy in the management of carcinoma of the vulva continues to be actively explored. The traditional belief that vulvar tissues cannot tolerate therapeutic doses of radiation has for many years limited the use of radiation therapy to palliation or treatment of unresectable disease.

RADIATION THERAPY TECHNIQUES FOR UNRESECTABLE PRIMARY TUMORS. For patients who are not candidates for surgical resection, the primary tumor site needs to be irradiated to the customary tumoricidal dose of 6500 to 7000 cGy over 35 to 40 treatments. Small lesions may be controlled with somewhat lower doses (6000 cGy). It is important to use a daily fraction size of 180 cGy or less. Usually, parallel opposed anteroposterior-posteroanterior (AP/PA) portals are used, preferably loaded anteriorly (or a high-energy single anterior beam with bolus). These portals cover the vulva and the inguinofemoral lymphatics. An electron beam (9–12 MeV) or low-energy photon beam supplement (4–6 MV) aimed directly at the vulva is needed at the end of the course to bring the dose to full tumoricidal level. An interstitial implant may also be considered as a means of providing the "boost" to the primary tumor site. Use of appropriate bolus material over the areas of the skin at risk for tumor involvement is essential. Interruption of therapy is sometimes necessary in the third or fourth week of treatment to prevent severe moist desquamation and maceration of tissues.

RADIATION THERAPY TECHNIQUES FOR THE REGIONAL LYMPHATICS. In patients with no clinical indications of regional lymphatic involvement, the inguinal lymph

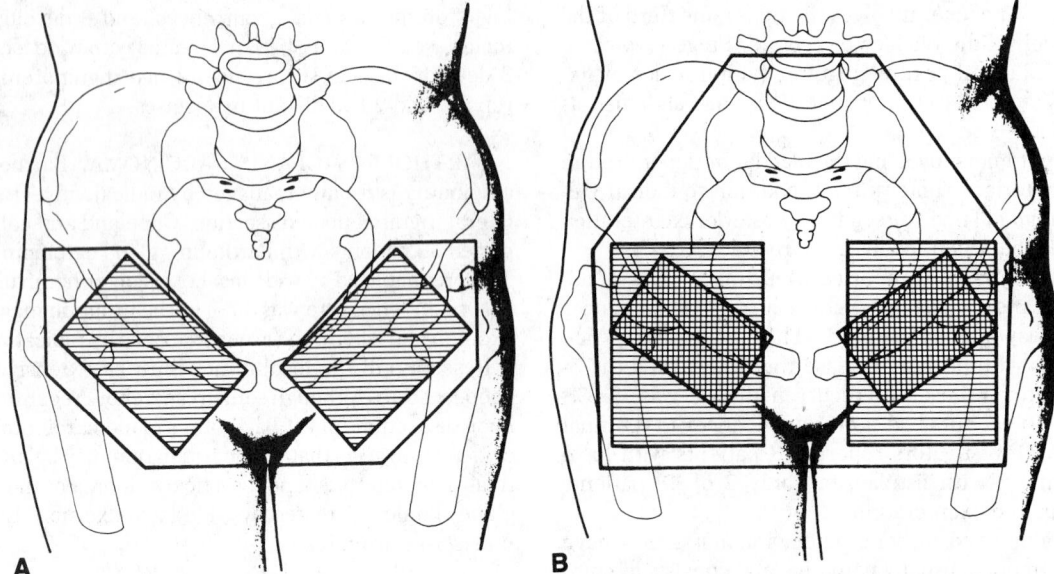

A **B**

FIGURE 38–3. **(A)** Portals for elective irradiation of regional lymphatics in patients with no clinical evidence of inguinal lymph node involvement. **(B)** Setup for patients with positive inguinal lymph nodes. The entire pelvis is treated to a dose of 4500 to 5000 cGy. This is followed by a boost to the inguinal-femoral areas and distal iliac chain to bring the total dose to that area to 5500 to 6000 cGy and a final boost to the positive inguinal lymph nodes consisting of 500 to 1000 cGy, bringing the total dose to that area to approximately 6500 cGy (calculated at 3–4 cm). (Perez CA, Grigsby PW. Vulva. In: Perez CA, Brady LW, eds. Principles and practice of radiation oncology. 2nd ed. Philadelphia: JB Lippincott, 1992)

nodes are treated electively (prophylactically) to a dose of 5000 cGy (180–200 cGy/day). Depending on the available equipment, an anteroposterior beam, differentially loaded parallel opposed AP/PA beams, or an electron beam (for part of the treatment) can be used. Care should be taken to deliver adequate doses to the superficial inguinal nodes and to the femoral nodes and the first echelon of deep pelvic nodes if indicated (Fig. 38–3).[45]

For patients with regional lymph node involvement, the dose must be in the range of 6500 to 7000 cGy, depending on the size of the nodes. For patients with evidence of involved inguinal lymph nodes, the pelvis should be treated with elective (prophylactic) irradiation of 4500 to 5000 cGy. For patients with evidence of involvement of the pelvic nodes, the dose may be boosted to 5500 to 6000 cGy (Fig. 38–4).[45] Because some of the patients with involved pelvic lymph nodes are curable, irradiation of the lower paraaortic chain in the presence of pelvic lymph node involvement may be appropriate.

POSTOPERATIVE RADIATION THERAPY. Radiation therapy is being used more often in combination with surgery. For a patient who has undergone resection of the primary lesion and is considered at high risk for recurrence because of inadequate resection margins, postoperative irradiation is indicated and should consist of at least 4500 cGy, preferably 5000 cGy (180–200 cGy/day). If the resection margins are clearly involved or there is known gross residual tumor, higher doses of irradiation (6000–7000 cGy) are required.

PREOPERATIVE RADIATION THERAPY. Patients with advanced primary lesions involving surrounding structures that are of questionable resectability or are clearly unresect-

able can be treated with preoperative radiation therapy. If moderately high doses of 4500 to 5500 cGy are delivered preoperatively, an increase in the resectability rate can be expected, and mutilating procedures such as exenteration may be avoided.[68]

IRRADIATION OF RECURRENT LESIONS. Recurrences after surgical resection are potentially curable and need to be treated aggressively in the manner described previously, with

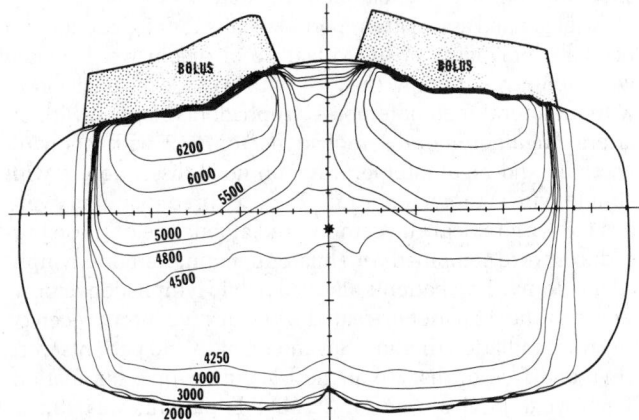

FIGURE 38–4. Representative treatment plan for irradiation of regional lymphatics in patients with carcinoma of the vulva or the vagina. Parallel opposed 18 MV photon beams are preferentially loaded anteriorly (2700 cGy anteriorly, 1800 cGy posteriorly), and a bolus is added over the inguinal areas to improve dose distribution in subcutaneous tissues in that area. A boost of 1500 cGy using 16-MeV electrons (without bolus) is added to the groin. (Perez CA, Grigsby PW. Vulva. In: Perez CA, Brady LW, eds. Principles and practice of radiation oncology. 2nd ed. Philadelphia: JB Lippincott, 1992:1273–1289)

doses in the range of 6500 to 7000 cGy (daily fractions of 180 cGy).

Prempree and Amornmarn described results of 21 patients with recurrent carcinoma of the vulva treated with irradiation alone (*i.e.*, external-beam irradiation and interstitial brachytherapy).[69] Most of these patients received doses ranging from 5500 to 8000 cGy. Patients with recurrent tumor limited to the introitus or adjacent vagina had the best prognosis, with all 6 exhibiting tumor control and surviving longer than 5 years. Two of 4 patients with small inguinal lymph nodes were cured. None of the patients with extensive recurrences survived, although a few had transient tumor responses.

Buchler and colleagues reported 73% tumor control in 18 patients presenting with recurrences after radical vulvectomy (8) or local excision.[6,70] Most of these recurrences involved only the perineum. Seven of the patients were treated with irradiation, and 11 were treated surgically (*i.e.*, wide local excision, radical vulvectomy, or posterior exenteration). Two patients survived for 4 and 13 years, respectively.

RESULTS OF RADIATION THERAPY. Numerous attempts were made to combine radiation therapy and surgery to improve therapeutic results.[65,71–76] Frankendal and colleagues reported 55 patients, 22 of whom had palpable lymph nodes that were considered tumorous.[71] Nodal involvement was histologically confirmed in 19 patients. Primary lesions were electrocoagulated, resected, or irradiated, and the regional nodes were dissected if clinically involved. Clinically negative nodes were observed without treatment unless the primary tumor was quite large or poorly differentiated. In these situations, the groins were irradiated to a dose of 3000 to 6000 cGy over 15 to 55 days. Of the 12 patients who were irradiated prophylactically to the inguinal areas because of unfavorable primary lesions, none developed inguinal metastasis. Of the 7 patients with clinically negative nodes and early lesions who were observed only, 3 developed regional lymph node metastases.

Kucera treated the primary lesion with electrocoagulation, and the inguinal areas were irradiated to a total dose of 6000 cGy (orthovoltage or cobalt 60).[75] For patients with stages III and IV disease (*i.e.*, positive lymph nodes), the inguinal nodes were dissected; this was performed in fewer than 20% of the patients. Eighty-three percent of the stage I patients, 69% of the stage II patients, 58% of the stage III patients, and 10% of the stage IV patients survived 5 years.

Daly and Million tested a combination of radical vulvectomy followed by elective nodal irradiation of 4500 cGy in 5 weeks.[73] In their small series of 6 patients, treatment was well tolerated, with no nodal failures and no radiation complications. There was no delay in healing of the surgical site. The value of elective irradiation of the pelvic lymph nodes was further demonstrated by Homesley and colleagues in a report of 114 patients with invasive carcinoma of the vulva and positive inguinal nodes who were randomized after radical vulvectomy and bilateral groin lymphadenectomy to receive postoperative radiation therapy to the pelvic and groin lymph nodes (4500–5000 cGy in 5 to 6 weeks).[64] The irradiated patients had a recurrence rate of 32.3% and a 2-year survival rate of 68%, in contrast to a recurrence rate of 45.5% and a 2-year survival rate of 54% in the nonirradiated group. The incidence of recurrence at the primary site was similar in both groups: 8.5%

in the irradiated group and 9.1% in the pelvic lymph node dissection group. Surgical morbidity was comparable, and late effects of irradiation and surgery were similar in both groups.

The rationale for a combination of radiation therapy and conservative surgery in advanced tumors that would ordinarily require exenteration was discussed by Boronow.[68] In a series of 9 patients, only 1 had a local recurrence. The incidence of operative morbidity was minimal, and 5 patients remained disease free for 11 months to 4.5 years. This experience has been updated, and the results indicate a 75% to 80% 5-year salvage probability for advanced primary and recurrent cancer.[65] Hacker and colleagues treated 8 patients with locally advanced vulvar cancer, who would ordinarily have required an exenteration, with 4400 to 5400 cGy before resection (*i.e.*, vulvectomy).[74] Significant tumor regression was observed in 7 patients, and there was no viable tumor in the surgical specimens of 4 patients. Five (62.5%) of 8 patients remained alive without evidence of disease from 15 months to 10 years. Acosta and collaborators found no macroscopic residual tumor in 13 patients who underwent surgery after receiving 3500 to 5500 cGy.[72]

Kucera and Weghaupt analyzed 607 patients treated with electrocoagulation of the primary lesions and 4500 cGy (300 cGy fractions) to inguinal nodes smaller than 2 cm or 6000 cGy and local excision for inguinal nodes larger than 2 cm.[77] The primary excision site was not irradiated. The 5-year overall survival rates were 78%, 71%, 57%, and 12% for stages I to IV, respectively.

Miyazawa and associates reported results in 18 patients treated with combined irradiation and surgery and 15 patients treated with irradiation alone.[78] Of the patients treated surgically, 5 had a local excision or simple vulvectomy, and 12 had a radical vulvectomy with or without lymph node dissection. Ten of these patients presented with local recurrences, with 60% occurring in the first 2 years after initial surgery. Seven patients were referred for irradiation because of positive lymph nodes in the surgical specimen. Of the 10 patients treated for local recurrences, only 2 survived longer than 5 years. Seven patients were referred for irradiation of positive lymph nodes; only 1 survived 1 year. The second group consisted of 15 patients treated with irradiation alone because of associated medical problems or extensive local disease. Six had stage III tumors, and 9 had stage IV tumors. Thirteen of these patients were followed for up to 5 years. Four were alive at 1 year, 2 were alive at 2 years, and 1 was alive at 3 years. Severe moist desquamation, ulceration, and pain were observed in 4 of 6 patients treated with orthovoltage x-rays compared with 2 of 27 patients treated with megavoltage irradiation, 1 of whom developed an ileocutaneous fistula.

Pao and colleagues reported 40 patients with histologically confirmed primary or recurrent vulvar carcinoma treated with radiation therapy for locoregional disease at Washington University Medical Center.[79] Nineteen of the patients with primary tumors received postoperative radiation therapy (5000 cGy in 6 weeks) after wide local excision or simple vulvectomy (9 patients) or radical vulvectomy (10 patients). Fifteen of the 19 patients exhibited local tumor control. Five patients with stage III or IV disease were managed with radiation therapy alone. Four had a complete response, and 2 currently have no evidence of disease. Two patients who received preoperative radiation therapy with local excision are also free of disease. The 4-year disease-free survival rates for the study population are 100%, 28%, 50%, 0%, and 10% for stages I, II, III, IV, and recurrent tumors, respectively. The poor results obtained in stage II tumors are probably due to selection, because 4 of 7 patients developed distant metastases. Two of 14 patients treated for recurrent disease remain disease free after local excision of their tumors and irradiation. No dose response for subclinical disease could be found between 4500 and 7000 cGy. Treatment morbidity was acceptable; only 2 patients developed severe long-term complications requiring surgical intervention.

The wide range of techniques, doses, and fractionation patterns complicates any attempt to evaluate the side effects of radiation therapy using modern techniques and treatment schemes. A tumor located at the skin or mucosal surface requires that the peak dose be at the surface, and these patients are likely to experience significant acute cutaneous and mucosal irritation. However, the incidence of late sequelae is often of even greater concern, and some of these can be attributed to the fractionation schemes. Schulz and colleagues reported a high incidence of late sequelae for patients who were treated with 500-cGy fractions.[80] The complication rate was consistently low in patients treated with the conventional 200 cGy per day or similar schemes. Prospective, large-scale, multidimensional studies are needed to assess the side effects of radiation therapy and the optimal indications for it in vulvar carcinoma.

Chemotherapy

TOPICAL CHEMOTHERAPY. Topical chemotherapy was used to treat selected patients with vulvar or vaginal intraepithelial neoplasia. Topical 5-fluorouracil (5-FU) is the most commonly used agent.[81] Three 7-day courses of 5% 5-FU cream are usually given 2 weeks apart. A study of 27 patients treated in this way demonstrated that, although 3 patients required retreatment at 3, 9, and 11 months, all 25 evaluable patients were free of disease for 3+ to 40+ months after treatment.[82]

Stillman and colleagues combined topical 5-FU pretreatment and colposcopically directed surgical excision to manage 16 patients with lower genital tract intraepithelial neoplasia.[83] This approach was based on the researchers' observation that neoplastic epithelium is more easily dissected from the underlying stroma after local 5-FU application. Before surgery, the patient applies 4 ml of 5% topical 5-FU to the lesions every night for 1 week. On the eighth day, colposcopically directed excisional biopsies are performed. All 16 patients in this series had remissions, and although 2 required retreatment, no patient had a recurrence of severe dysplasia.

SYSTEMIC CHEMOTHERAPY. Very limited data exist on the activity of chemotherapeutic agents in the various malignancies of the vulva. A variety of drugs were tested in phase II trials, but only doxorubicin (Adriamycin) and bleomycin demonstrated activity in squamous cell carcinoma of the vulva.[84,85] Cisplatin, active in most gynecologic tumors, has little activity in vulvar carcinoma. Combination chemotherapy was tried, usually in patients with inoperable disease, before definitive surgery or radiation. One study, using bleomycin, vincristine, mitomycin C, and cisplatin, produced 6 responses (2 complete responses [CR], 4 partial responses [PR]) in 22 patients (27%).[86] Another trial with bleomycin, methotrexate, and CCNU had 18 responders (3 CR, 15 PR) in 28 patients (64%).[87] Approaches using more active agents may warrant further study, although toxicity (primarily mucositis, fever, and infections) is often significant in this elderly population.

Other investigators used combination chemotherapy shortly before or concomitantly with irradiation therapy in advanced and inoperable disease. Levin and colleagues used preoperative chemotherapy (mitomycin C and 5-FU) followed by pelvic irradiation before surgery for advanced carcinoma of the vulva.[88] On day 1, mitomycin C (10 mg/m^2) was given intravenously, followed 30 minutes later by a 24-hour infusion of 5-FU (1000 mg/m^2). 5-FU was repeated for 3 additional days at a similar dose and schedule, followed by 10 days of equal fractions of radiation therapy. Courses of chemotherapy and radiation therapy lasted 2 weeks. After adequate response had been achieved, usually with one to two cycles, surgery was performed. Marked local tumor shrinkage in 6 patients allowed more definitive surgery after chemotherapy.

Thomas and associates reported the use of chemotherapy with irradiation in 33 patients with stages II, III, or IV disease. Infusional 5-FU with or without mitomycin C was used. Seven of 9 patients treated with neoadjuvant therapy remain disease free 5 to 45 months after treatment. Of the 9 patients treated with combined modality therapy for cure, 6 are alive and free of disease at 5 to 45 months. Of the 15 patients treated with chemotherapy as salvage, 7 are alive and free of disease 5 to 45 months after therapy.[89] Despite these interesting results, further studies are required to establish the role of chemotherapy in the therapy of squamous cell carcinoma of the vulva.

No significant activity of chemotherapy was reported for melanoma or Bartholin's gland carcinomas of the vulva.

TRENDS IN TREATING CARCINOMA OF THE VULVA

Future studies in vulvar cancer should attempt to define microinvasive carcinoma and should continue searching for ways to reduce the radical nature of therapy. Further investigations of surgical reconstruction of the vulva should focus on restoring normal anatomy and function.[90,91]

Radiation therapy may come to play a significant role in the management of patients with carcinoma of the vulva. The current data on the primary therapy of vulvar cancer with modern radiation therapy techniques are inconclusive. However, for patients with advanced, inoperable carcinoma of the vulva, radiation therapy combined with chemotherapy may prove useful.

None of these new approaches to the therapy of vulvar cancer have been widely used, and careful, prospective trials are necessary. The potential efficacy of irradiation and chemotherapy in the management of carcinoma of the vulva is promising.

CARCINOMA OF THE VAGINA

Carcinoma of the vagina is a primary carcinoma arising in the vagina that does not involve the cervix or vulva. Primary vaginal cancer is uncommon; it accounts for only 1% to 2% of all gynecologic cancers.[24,92,93] More commonly, tumors involve the vagina by direct extension or are metastases from other genital areas, particularly the cervix. The vagina can also be involved by tumors of the rectum. If primary carcinomas of the vagina occur, they are usually squamous cell cancers, with the exception of diethylstilbestrol (DES)-related clear cell carcinomas. Primary sarcomas and melanomas of the vagina are rare.

EPIDEMIOLOGY

The median age for patients with carcinoma in situ of the vagina is the early fifth decade, and the median age for patients with invasive cancer is the middle of the sixth decade.[24,92–97] One percent to 3% of patients who develop squamous cell carcinoma of the vagina have had squamous neoplasia of the cervix. Hummer and colleagues reported that carcinoma in situ of the vagina can follow carcinoma in situ of the cervix up to 17 years later, but that one third of the cases were diagnosed within 2 years.[95]

Brinton and colleagues identified low socioeconomic level, a history of human papillomavirus infection, early hysterectomy, and a previous abnormal Pap test as significant risk factors for vaginal carcinoma in situ or invasive carcinoma.[96] A history of vaginal trauma had less significance as a risk factor.

Prior radiation therapy may also be a predisposing factor in primary vaginal carcinoma.[92,97,98] Pride and associates observed that 9 (20.9%) of 43 patients with invasive cancer of the vagina had prior radiation therapy.[97] The interval from previous irradiation to development of the primary squamous cell cancer was 7 to 20 years. However, an analysis of 1200 patients at Washington University failed to demonstrate an increase in the incidence of second pelvic malignancies after prior radiation therapy.[99]

In 1971, Herbst and colleagues related an increase in the number of clear cell carcinomas of the vagina to maternal ingestion of DES during pregnancy.[100] The youngest DES-exposed patient who developed clear cell adenocarcinoma was 7 years old, and the peak incidence occurred at age 19.[101,102] The actual risk that an exposed woman will develop clear cell adenocarcinoma is 0.14 to 1.4 per 1000 women through 24 years of age.[101] A plateau of patients was reached in the middle of the 1970s, with a gradual decline in the number of patients each year since then. It is unknown whether these women remain at risk for the development of other cancers of the genital tract.

Primary sarcomas of the vagina account for approximately 2% of all vaginal cancers.[103,104] Leiomyosarcoma is the most frequent, but reticulum cell and stromal sarcomas have also been reported. Age at diagnosis is the fifth and sixth decades.[103] Sarcoma botryoides, although rare, is the most common tumor of the genital tract in female children.[105] The mean age for the appearance of these tumors is between 2 and 3 years.

Malignant melanoma rarely occurs in the vagina as a primary neoplasm. In the vagina, as in other parts of the genital tract, melanoma spreads locally by direct extension and through the lymphatics and blood stream.[106]

NATURAL HISTORY AND PATTERNS OF SPREAD

The location of primary vaginal carcinoma was evaluated in an extensive literature review of more than 1200 cases by Plentl and Friedman.[24] They found that 26.9% occurred on the anterior wall, 57.2% on the posterior wall, and 15.9% on the lateral walls. Of 743 cases reviewed for axial location, they found that 50.7% occurred in the upper third of the vagina, 18.8% in the middle third, and 30.4% in the lower third. Clear cell adenocarcinoma of the vagina associated with maternal DES ingestion occurs most commonly on the anterior vagina and is usually seen in the upper third of the vaginal canal.

Vaginal carcinomas spread to adjacent structures by direct extension or by lymphatics. By convention, tumors that involve the cervix or vulva are considered primary in those sites because they are more common. The close proximity of the urethra, bladder, and rectum results in early involvement of these structures and has a major effect on treatment planning. If spreading laterally, vaginal tumors may invade the paracolpial, parametrial, and pararectal tissues, with extension to the pelvic sidewalls.

The lymphatic drainage of the vagina begins with the fine capillary meshwork in the mucosa and submucosa.[24] Both of these systems flow into collecting trunks near the lateral aspect of the vagina. The ventral portion of the vagina drains primarily to lateral pelvic lymph nodes, and the posterior portion drains into the rectal and paraaortic lymph nodes. Significant overlap occurs in these patterns of drainage. The upper third of the vagina drains primarily, like the cervix, but the middle third tends to spread into the pelvic nodes and into the inferior gluteal nodes near the ischial spine. The lower third of the vagina drains laterally, posteriorly, and to the femoral nodes.

In addition to this distribution of lymphatics, a rich interconnection exists between the lymphatics of the vagina and those of the bladder and rectum. In their review of the literature, Plentl and Friedman reported an overall positive node rate of 20.8% for vaginal carcinoma.[24] These results were obtained from surgical series and autopsy reports. Patients with clear cell carcinoma have distant spread to supraclavicular nodes or lungs more frequently than would be expected for a similar group of patients with squamous cell carcinoma of the vagina or cervix.[102]

PATHOLOGY

Squamous cell carcinomas of the vagina may appear grossly as ulcerated and endophytic tumors or as exophytic tumors that protrude into the vaginal canal. Microscopically, most of them are keratinizing epidermoid carcinomas with pleomorphic squamous cells that display a lack of organization and a loss of cellular cohesion.[107] The lesions may exhibit patterns of dysplasia, carcinoma in situ, and invasion, and premalignant lesions can be multifocal. For squamous cell carcinoma, a grade is assigned based on a combination of cytologic and histologic features, but there is little demonstrated correlation between grade and survival.[108,109]

Verrucous carcinoma, a distinctive variant of well-differentiated squamous cell carcinoma, rarely occurs in the vagina.[110] This tumor is a relatively large, well-circumscribed, soft, cauliflower-like mass. Microscopically, it exhibits a papillary growth pattern, with marked hyperkeratosis and broad, bulbous pegs of acanthotic epithelium that push into the underlying stroma. Because of the well-differentiated character of verrucous carcinoma, microscopic diagnosis can be difficult, especially if the biopsy is superficial. Verrucous carcinoma can recur locally after surgery, but it rarely metastasizes.

Small cell carcinoma can occur in the vagina, in pure form or associated with squamous or glandular elements. Many show ultrastructural or immunohistochemical evidence of neuroendocrine differentiation.

Vaginal adenosis is a condition in which müllerian-type glandular epithelium is present after vaginal development is complete. Much attention was focused on this lesion because it was discovered in women exposed to DES in utero. Although adenosis is the most common histologic abnormality in women exposed to DES in utero, it is not strictly confined to this population.[111,112] In the DES cohort, adenosis most commonly involves the anterior wall and upper third of the vagina, but it may also extend into the middle and lower thirds of the vagina. The classic gross appearance of adenosis is red, velvety, grape-like clusters in the vagina. The surface epithelium or the glands in the superficial stroma may be involved.[113,114] The glandular epithelium may be composed of any of the müllerian epithelial cell types.

Malignant melanoma is the second most common cancer of the vagina, accounting for 2.8% to 5% of all vaginal neoplasms.[115,116] Melanoma can occur in any portion of the vagina, but it is most frequently seen in the lower third. These tumors show considerable variation in size, color, and growth pattern.[117] Microscopically, they are similar to melanomas that occur at other sites. The tumor may be composed of spindle-shaped, epithelioid, or small, lymphocyte-like cells. The cells may or may not be pigmented. Junctional activity, if present, is an important observation because it helps exclude the possibility of metastasis. Poorly differentiated lesions that are difficult to differentiate from sarcomas or squamous cell carcinomas can be identified by their distinctive ultrastructural features or immunoperoxidase staining pattern.[118] Tumor depth should be assessed according to the method of Breslow, because depth of tumor invasion is the best predictor of survival.[116,119]

Benign pigmented lesions are extremely rare in the vagina. The blue nevus has been reported.[120]

Nonepithelial tumors of the vagina include leiomyosarcomas and rhabdomyosarcomas. *Leiomyosarcomas,* although rare, are reported to be the most common benign and malignant mesenchymal tumors in adult women.[121] Although they can originate in any part of the vagina, most are submucosal. Their gross appearance depends on cellularity, the type and extent of degenerative change, and the amount of necrosis and hemorrhage.[122,123] Microscopically, smooth muscle tumors are composed of interlacing bundles of spindle-shaped cells with blunt-ended nuclei and fibrillar cytoplasm. An epithelioid pattern and extensive myxoid change were reported in a few vaginal smooth muscle tumors.[122]

Predicting the behavior of some smooth muscle tumors based on histologic appearance can be difficult. Factors considered important in predicting outcome include status of the tumor border (infiltrating versus circumscribed), mitotic rate, and degree of cytologic atypicality. Based on a small number of patients, Tavassoli and Norris concluded that smooth muscle tumors with 5 or more mitoses per 10 high-power fields, significant cellular atypia, a diameter of 3 cm or more, and infiltrating margins are most likely to recur or metastasize.[122]

The botryoid variant of embryonal *rhabdomyosarcoma* is the most common malignant tumor of the vagina in infants and children.[123] Ninety percent occur in children younger than 5 years of age. Although rhabdomyosarcomas vary in size and location, they have a characteristic gross appearance that consists of multiple, gray-red, translucent, edematous, grape-like masses that fill and protrude from the vagina. Microscopically, a continuous zone of condensed round or spindle cells (*i.e.,* cambium layer) can be seen immediately beneath the intact vaginal epithelium. Elsewhere, the tumor is composed of small, dark cells sparsely distributed in a myxoid stroma.

Rare reports of *other primary sarcomas* involving the vagina include endometrial stromal sarcoma (arising in endometriosis), alveolar soft-part sarcoma, malignant fibrous histiocytoma, synovial-like sarcoma, malignant mixed tumor, angiosarcoma, and hemangiopericytoma.[124–129]

Malignant lymphoma can be localized to the female genital tract or can occur there as part of a widespread disease process.[130] Most primary malignant lymphomas involving the vagina are the diffuse, large cell type, but nodular lymphomas also occur. Characteristically, the mucosa is intact. An important clinical correlate is the presence of a mass. Marker studies are useful in differentiating difficult or equivocal cases from lymphoma-like lesions. Leukemic infiltration, especially granulocytic sarcoma, may be impossible to differentiate from malignant lymphoma. A chloroacetate esterase stain is helpful in some cases.

CLINICAL PRESENTATION, DIAGNOSIS, AND STAGING

Preinvasive lesions of the vagina are asymptomatic, and diagnosis is usually made during evaluation of an abnormal Pap smear. Examination of the vagina by colposcopy should be conducted in all patients with abnormal cytologic results, even if a cervical lesion appears to explain the abnormality. Although vaginal biopsies are not totally painless, local anesthesia is usually not required. A skin hook, used to tent and stabilize the vaginal mucosa, can help in obtaining an adequate biopsy.

Abnormal vaginal bleeding is the most common symptom of invasive vaginal carcinoma.[103,131] The bleeding is often postmenopausal, because that population is most likely to develop the disease, but bleeding may be postcoital or, in younger patients, intermenstrual. Vaginal discharge is common. Pain or symptoms referable to the bladder or rectum usually occur with more advanced disease. Brady reported that the average duration of symptoms before diagnosis is 7.4 months.[132]

Detection of invasive vaginal carcinoma is made by inspection, palpation, and biopsy. In performing a speculum examination, the physician must rotate the speculum or remove it slowly to visualize the entire vagina. Lesions that arise on the posterior vaginal wall are particularly likely to be missed because they can be obscured by the posterior blade of the speculum. Any lesions found during examination should be biopsied. Wharton and colleagues published data from M.D. Anderson Cancer Center showing that 67.5% of patients seen at that institution had lesions larger than 2 cm when the initial diagnoses were made.[131]

The staging workup of the patient with vaginal cancer includes careful inspection of the vagina and cervix, with biopsies as needed and a careful bimanual examination. Chest radiograph, biochemical profile, CT scan (with contrast) of the abdomen and pelvis, barium enema, cystoscopy, and proctoscopy are necessary. MRI may be helpful in certain situations. Chang and coworkers found the use of MRI in vaginal carcinoma to be reliable.[615] The FIGO classification of vaginal carcinoma is listed in Table 38–6.

TREATMENT

The anatomic position of the vagina, located between the urethra and bladder anteriorly and the rectum posteriorly, is the predominant factor in treatment planning. The vaginal tube is thin-walled, and the thickness of the vesicovaginal and rectovaginal septa is usually measured in millimeters.

Surgical extirpation of carcinoma of the vagina is often unfeasible because the proximity of the bladder and rectum require exenterative procedures to allow adequate surgical margins. With the exception of clear cell adenocarcinoma of the vagina occurring in young women and localized to the upper third of the vaginal canal, the primary treatment for vaginal carcinoma, especially squamous cell carcinoma, is radiation therapy. Chau pointed out the need for careful radiation therapy techniques, which resulted in survival similar to that for carcinoma of the uterine cervix.[133] Perez and colleagues correlated the doses of radiation given to various tumor stages and the probability of local tumor control.[134]

Carcinoma In Situ

A wide range of therapeutic options are available for carcinoma in situ of the vagina, and the best option depends on the location of the lesion, the size of the lesion, and whether it has a single focus or multiple foci. Local excision is ideal therapy for patients with single lesions or several lesions located in a single portion of the vagina, especially patients who develop recurrence in the vaginal cuff after hysterectomy. Total vaginectomy is a difficult procedure and requires split-thickness grafts for repair. Multiple lesions can often be treated in stages, with multiple excisions and primary closure.

Cryotherapy has had limited usefulness in the treatment of vaginal carcinoma in situ, because it usually requires anesthesia and multiple applications. It can easily damage the urethra, bladder, or rectum because of difficulty controlling the

TABLE 38–6. International Federation of Gynecology and Obstetrics Classification for Carcinoma of the Vagina

Stage 0	Carcinoma in situ: intraepithelial carcinoma
Stage I	Carcinoma limited to the vaginal wall
Stage II	Carcinoma has invaded the subvaginal tissue but has not extended to the pelvic wall
Stage III	Carcinoma has extended to the pelvic wall
Stage IV	Carcinoma has extended beyond the true pelvis or has involved the mucosa of the bladder or rectum. Bullous edema as such does not permit a case to be allotted to Stage IV
Stage IVA	Spread of the growth to adjacent organs
Stage IVB	Spread to distant organs

depth of the freeze. CO_2 laser has become popular and has the advantage of being able to be tailored to the depth and extent of disease. Additional studies with long-term follow-up are needed to define the extent of its usefulness in this disease.

Woodruff and colleagues reported the use of topical 5-FU in preinvasive vaginal carcinoma and observed complete eradication of lesions in 8 of 9 patients.[135] Townsend recommends 5 g of 5-FU cream instilled in the vagina every night for 5 days.[136] He repeats these courses of therapy every 6 to 12 weeks until eradication of the lesion is documented. Contamination of the vulva must be prevented, because 5-FU cream can produce an intense chemical reaction.

Radiation therapy of carcinoma in situ is rarely indicated. However, for some patients who were poor operative risks, irradiation of the vagina using intracavitary and interstitial sources alone produced excellent cure rates.[137,138] Radiation therapy may also be considered if extensive surgical resection is necessary because of multifocal involvement of the entire vagina.

Stage I

Stage I lesions of the vagina that are located in the upper third of the vagina can be managed by radical hysterectomy, partial vaginectomy and pelvic lymphadenectomy, or radical radiation therapy. The proximity of the bladder and rectum often dictates that vaginal carcinoma would be best managed by irradiation. Irradiation appears to allow considerably more flexibility than surgery, and good functional results are obtained with adequate radiation therapy. Surgical procedures are often reserved for the treatment of irradiation failures. However, some researchers recommended a surgical approach for stage I lesions.[93,138,139] Lesions of the middle or lower vagina, unless they are superficial and do not lie in the rectovaginal or vesicovaginal septa, often require anterior or posterior exenteration as primary surgical therapy.

Brown and associates[137] and Perez and associates[134] reported excellent tumor control and survival in patients with stage I vaginal carcinoma. These researchers warned against overly aggressive therapy in early lesions because of the possibility of mucosal injury and interference with sexual function. Most patients with stage I superficial tumors can be treated adequately with intracavitary and interstitial sources alone. If the carcinoma is less than 0.5 cm thick, intracavitary irradiation with a vaginal cylinder to deliver 8000 cGy to the mucosa yields excellent results (>90% tumor control). If the lesion is thicker or localized to one of the walls of the vagina, the addition of an interstitial single-plane implant delivers an adequate dose of irradiation to the tumor, limiting exposure to uninvolved normal tissues.

In patients with more extensive stage I lesions, external irradiation, in addition to intracavitary and interstitial therapy, should be administered to treat paravaginal tissues and regional lymph nodes.

Stage II

Patients with stage II carcinoma of the vagina require a comprehensive approach to treatment that should include external-beam irradiation and brachytherapy. Survival was shown by Perez and colleagues to improve with the addition of ex-

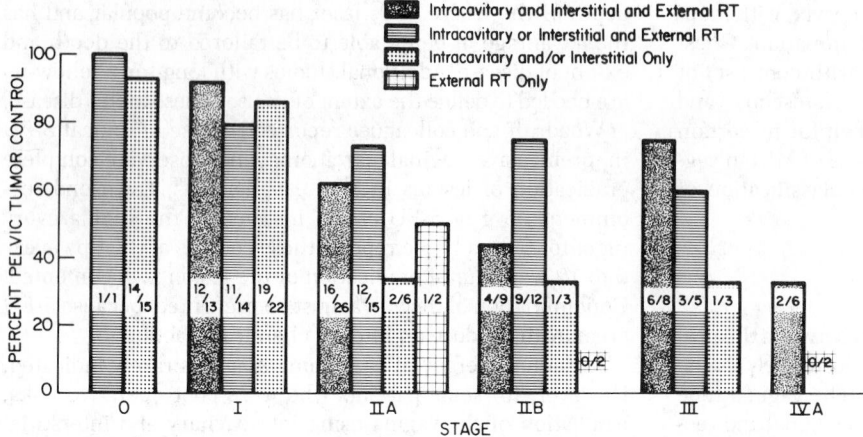

FIGURE 38–5. Tumor control in the vagina and the pelvis (MIR 1950–1984) as a function of the type of treatment used and the anatomic stage of the disease. In patients with tumor beyond stage I, there is a critical need for the addition of external-beam irradiation to improve tumor control. (Perez CA, Camel HM, Galakatos AE, et al. Definitive irradiation in carcinoma of the vagina: Long-term evaluation of results. Int J Radiat Oncol Biol Phys 1988;15:1283–1290)

ternal irradiation compared with brachytherapy alone (Fig. 38–5).[134] The investigators reported a survival rate of 65% with brachytherapy plus external irradiation but only 40% with brachytherapy alone. In general, doses of 2000 cGy to the whole pelvis are followed by a supplemental dose (3000 cGy) to the parametria with a midline shielding block. This is combined with interstitial and intracavitary therapy for a minimum of 6500 to 7000 cGy to the base of the tumor and 5000 cGy to the pelvic lymph nodes.

Stages III and IV

In more advanced lesions (stages III and IVA), results with irradiation were less than satisfactory. Only 25% to 30% pelvic tumor control and survival rates were reported. Therefore, higher irradiation doses with a greater contribution from external irradiation are used. Table 38–7 summarizes the results of 165 patients with carcinoma of the vagina treated at the Mallinckrodt Institute of Radiology at the Washington University School of Medicine.[134]

Hopkins and associates reported 3 patients with small cell tumors, containing neuroendocrine granules, who were treated with a combination of irradiation and chemotherapy.[140] As in the lung counterpart, local tumor control was good, but distant metastases to the brain, bones, and other organs were frequent.

Treatment by Tumor Type

CLEAR CELL CARCINOMA OF THE VAGINA. Stage I lesions of the cervix or vagina can be treated with surgery or radiation therapy.[102,148] All other stages should be treated with radiation therapy. Surgery for stage I clear cell carcinoma may have the advantage of ovarian preservation and better vaginal function after skin graft, although Wharton and colleagues advocated intracavitary or transvaginal irradiation for the treatment of small tumors.[148] They describe excellent tumor control, with maintenance of functional vagina and preservation of ovarian function.

If surgery is to be performed, a radical hysterectomy and vaginectomy with radical lymph node dissection are necessary for vaginal clear cell carcinoma. Paraaortic nodes should be sampled before the procedure to determine whether there is lymphatic disease beyond the pelvis.

Fletcher reported results of 19 young women treated with irradiation alone (2 were treated with irradiation combined with surgery).[149] Fifteen of the women were followed for more than 2 years. Eighteen of the patients are alive, and 17 of 18 are tumor free. One patient with an extensive lesion has a vaginal recurrence, and 1 patient died from a pulmonary embolus after removal of radium needles.

NONEPITHELIAL TUMORS OF THE VAGINA. The treatment of embryonal rhabdomyosarcoma of the vagina re-

TABLE 38–7. Carcinoma of the Vagina, Mallinckrodt Institute of Radiology: Anatomic Sites of Failure

Stage	No. of Patients	Local/Parametrial Only	Local/Parametrial Plus Distant Metastases	Distant Metastases Only	Dead From Intercurrent Disease
0	16	1 (6.3%)	0	0	6 (37.5%)
I	50	4 (8%)	3 (6%)	5 (10%)	20 (40%)
IIA	49	10 (20.4%)	9 (18.4%)	6 (12.2%)	15 (30.6%)
IIB	26	5 (19.2%)	7 (26.9%)	5 (19.2%)	6 (23.1%)
III	16	0	6 (37.5%)	4 (25%)	1 (6.3%)
IVA	8	2 (25%)	4 (50%)	0	1 (12.5%)

(Perez CA, Camel HM, Galakatos AE, et al. Definitive irradiation in carcinoma of the vagina: Long-term evaluation of results. Int J Radiat Oncol Biol Phys 1988;15:1283–1290)

quires combined treatment with chemotherapy, irradiation, and surgery. This therapy allows children to be treated without pelvic exenteration.[150,151] Survival rates of 46% to 63% were reported after combined therapy. Sordillo and colleagues[152] and Kinsella and Glatstein[153] reported the use of combinations of chemotherapy or radiation sensitizer and irradiation in adult soft tissue sarcomas. These same principles may be applicable to adult sarcomas of the vagina.

The results of surgical or irradiation therapy or both for vaginal melanoma are poor. Morrow and Di Saia reported only 21% survival after radical surgery.[117] These researchers reported an 80% recurrence rate in patients managed by excision with or without irradiation. Further studies are needed to determine optimal methods of therapy for these patients.

Radiation Therapy

The pelvic portals should encompass the entire vagina down to the introitus and should encompass the pelvic lymph nodes to the upper portion of the common iliac chain. Portals of 15 × 15 cm or 15 × 18 cm (at patient's surface) are usually adequate. In lesions of the lower two thirds of the vagina, the inguinal lymph nodes should be electively included in the irradiated field even if there are no palpable lymph nodes.

Intracavitary therapy is carried out with vaginal cylinders of various diameters, such as the Burnett, Bloedorn, or Delclos applicators. The largest possible diameter should be used to improve the dose ratio of mucosa to tumor (Fig. 38–6).[141,142] A new afterloading vaginal applicator retaining the charac-

teristics of the Bloedorn applicator was designed at Washington University Medical Center by Perez and colleagues.[143] Interstitial therapy with ^{137}Cs, ^{226}Ra needles, or afterloading ^{192}Ir needles was employed. Single-plane, double-plane, or volume implants should be planned, depending on the extent and thickness of the tumor.

If the lesion is in the upper third of the vagina, radiation oncologists recommend treating the upper vagina with the same intracavitary arrangement used for carcinoma of the uterine cervix, including an intrauterine tandem and vaginal colpostats. The middle and distal vagina are treated with a vaginal cylinder. For carcinoma in situ and stage I lesions, a dose of 6000 cGy at 0.5 cm under the mucosa is adequate. For larger lesions, doses in the range of 7000 to 8000 cGy are necessary. The vaginal mucosa receives an estimated 9000 to 10,000 cGy, which is usually well tolerated. The pelvic lymph nodes receive 5000 to 6000 cGy with application to the whole pelvis and split fields.

The importance of combined external irradiation and interstitial implants was emphasized by Perez and colleagues, who observed better tumor control (65%) in stage I and II disease with the addition of external irradiation than with brachytherapy only (40%).[134] MacNaught and colleagues, in an analysis of 78 patients of primary vaginal carcinomas (61 of which were squamous cell carcinomas), reported better tumor control and survival with combination external-beam and interstitial treatment than with brachytherapy alone.[144]

In stage II and stage IVA vaginal carcinoma, irradiation resulted in rates of only 25% to 50% for pelvic tumor control,

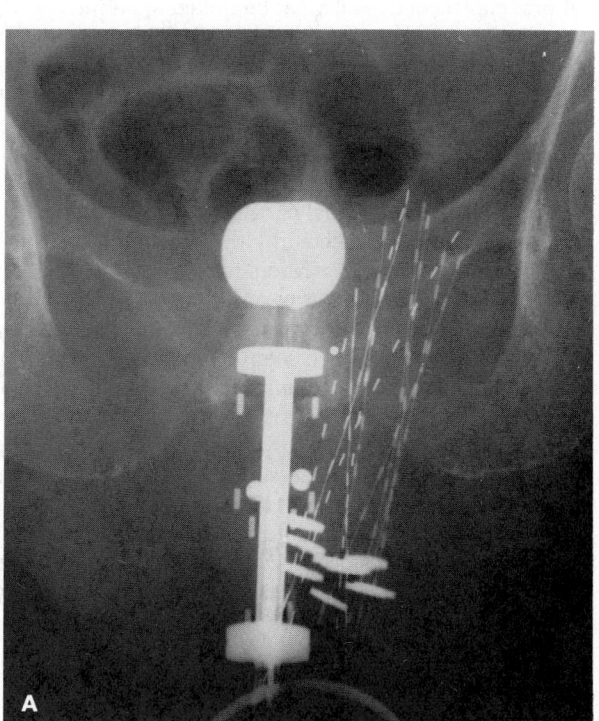
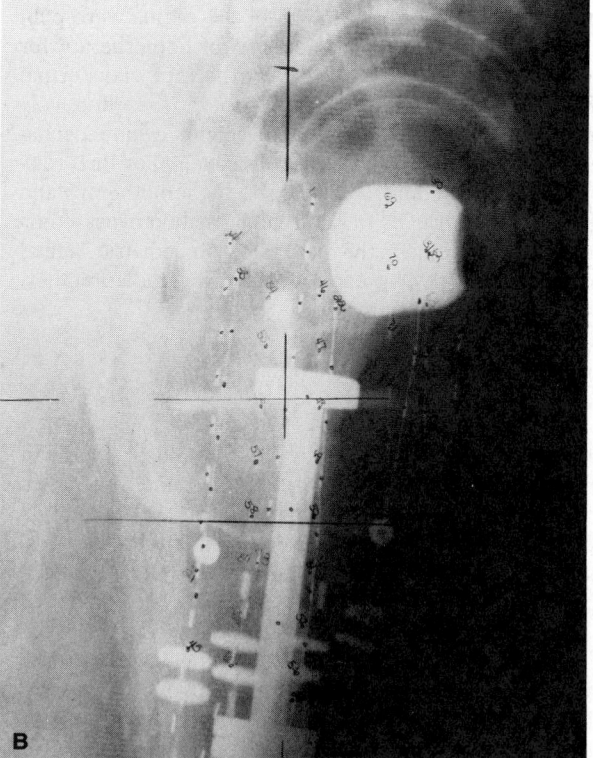

FIGURE 38–6. **(A)** Anteroposterior and **(B)** lateral view of intracavitary single-plane interstitial implant used to treat a stage IIA (left paravaginal extension) carcinoma of the vagina. This was combined with external-beam 18-MV photon irradiation (4000 cGy whole pelvis and additional 2000 cGy parametrial dose).

and therefore higher doses with a greater contribution from external irradiation are being used.

Prempree and Amornmarn[145] and Puthawala and co-workers[146] described tumor control rates in the pelvis ranging from 65% to 80% with a combination of external irradiation and, if appropriate, paravaginal or parametrial interstitial implant in addition to intracavitary brachytherapy.

Dancuart and colleagues reported results in 167 patients with primary squamous cell carcinoma of the vagina treated with irradiation alone at M.D. Anderson Cancer Center.[147] The central failure rate was 18% for 71 patients with stage I disease, 14% for 42 patients with stage II, 24% for 38 patients with stage III, and 30% for 11 patients with stage IVA disease. A few pelvic or central failures combined with distant metastases occurred in each stage. No significant difference was seen in the failure rate if brachytherapy or external irradiation or a combination of both was used. The investigators advocate treating subclinical disease in the inguinal lymph nodes with 4000 or 5000 cGy.

CHEMOTHERAPY

Most patients with vulvar carcinoma do not require chemotherapy, because they present with local disease and are managed with surgery or radiation therapy. Because these tumors are rare, few institutions have significant experience with salvage chemotherapy, and data are therefore sparse.

Squamous cell carcinomas of the vagina were included in a variety of phase II trials, but only doxorubicin appears to have significant activity.[154] Drug combinations and combined radiation and chemotherapy were tried in patients with locally advanced disease.[155] No studies of chemotherapy for adenocarcinomas or clear cell carcinoma of the vagina were published, and poor results were achieved with chemotherapy for melanoma of the vagina.[156] However, the rare endodermal sinus tumors that present in the vagina can be effectively treated with VAC (vincristine, doxorubicin, cyclophosphamide), PVB (cisplatin, vinblastine, bleomycin), or PEB (cisplatin, etoposide, bleomycin) regimens of chemotherapy and conservative surgery.[157,158] Embryonal rhabdomyosarcoma (*i.e.,* sarcoma botryoides), the most common pediatric vaginal tumor, can be effectively treated with surgery, radiation therapy, and VAC chemotherapy.[159]

CARCINOMA OF THE CERVIX

Carcinoma of the uterine cervix is the third most frequent of the female genital cancers.[160] Thirteen thousand cases of invasive cervical cancer were estimated for 1992, in addition to more than 50,000 cases of carcinoma in situ and several times that number of cases of preinvasive dysplasia of the cervix.[160]

Of all the female genital cancers, only cervical cancer can be reliably prevented by an effective, inexpensive screening technique that allows detection and treatment of precancerous conditions. Most deaths due to cervical cancer each year could be prevented if women would avail themselves of routine screening with cervical cytologic analysis. Unfortunately, screening for cervical cancer is less frequent in the underserved population.

EPIDEMIOLOGY

The peak age incidence for carcinoma of the cervix is between 48 and 55 years, with a mean of 53.8 years and a median of 51.5 years.[161,162] The peak incidence for carcinoma in situ occurs between the ages of 25 and 40.[162] Barber reviewed data from the State of Connecticut and the Third National Cancer Survey and found that only 9% of women with invasive cancer younger than 35 years of age and 53% of women with carcinoma in situ were younger than 35.[163]

Cervical cancer is most frequent in women of low socio-economic status, women who began sexual intercourse at a young age, women with a large number of sexual partners, women who became pregnant at a young age, multiparous women, and prostitutes.[163–166] In contrast, the disease is infrequent in nulliparous women, in women with inactive sexual lives (such as nuns), and in women who have a mutually monogamous relationship and no children.[163,166,167]

Cancer of the cervix is infrequent in Jewish and Moslem women, and circumcision of Jewish and Moslem men was postulated as a cause.[168] Abou-Daoud questioned the role of circumcision as a protective factor after he found an equal incidence of cervical cancer in Lebanese Moslems and Christians.[169] Ackerman and del Regato postulated genetic factors as a cause of the low incidence of cervical cancer in Jewish women.[170] Kessler demonstrated that the risk for cervical cancer may be increased in the wives of men who have previously been married to women who developed cervical cancer.[171]

Chemical irritants have not been linked with increased incidence of cervical carcinoma in women, although cervical carcinoma was induced in animals by direct application of chemical carcinogens.[172] Hormonal compounds in the form of oral contraceptives cannot be linked to an increased incidence of cervical cancer, but use of DES in pregnant women resulted in an increased incidence of clear cell carcinoma of the cervix and vagina in their offspring.[173,174]

Infectious agents may play a role in the development of cervical cancer. Cervical cancer has many characteristics of a sexually transmitted disease. The disease is associated with the total number of sexual partners a woman had in her lifetime, and it is also affected by the number of partners her male sexual partner or partners had.

The identification of herpesvirus type 2 (HSV-2) and the finding of higher antibody titers against this virus in cervical cancer patients than were seen in controls suggests a cause and effect relation.[175] Hollinshead and colleagues reported that the sera of 88% of patients with invasive cervical cancer contained antibodies to herpesvirus tumor-associated antigens, compared with 11% of the sera of controls.[176] Several researchers demonstrated that HSV-2 viruses can transform animal cells or human embryonic cells into malignant cells.[177,178] Wentz and associates produced in situ an invasive carcinoma of the cervix and vagina of mice inoculated with inactivated HSV-2.[179] However, only one report of transcription of the HSV genome was detected in cervical cancer, and it is now thought that HSV is not important in the development of cervical neoplasia, except perhaps as a cofactor.[180,181]

In a similar interpretation, other sexually transmitted diseases such as chlamydial and trichomonal infections are not considered etiologic in cervical cancer. They are probably only related in that they are associated with sexual promiscuity.[182,183]

Human papillomavirus (HPV) does appear to be associated with the development of cervical neoplasia. Meisels and Fortin first demonstrated the high frequency of HPV infection in 1976 and observed its association with dysplasia of the cervix.[184] Kurman and associates studied 322 cases of cervical dysplasia and carcinoma in situ for the presence of papilloma antigen and found these proteins in over 20% of patients.[185] Current studies indicate that almost 50% of intraepithelial neoplasias show evidence of HPV infection.[186,187] Viral particles were demonstrated in invasive cervical cancer.[187] HPV types 6 and 11 are common in nonneoplastic condylomata acuminata, and HPV types 16 and 18 (and, less often, types 31 and 33–35) are common in cervical intraepithelial neoplasia and invasive cervical cancer. Currently, 22 different types of HPV may infect the human anogenital tract. Using the polymerase chain reaction, HPV was detected in as many as 33% of college-aged women.[188] In studies of penile swabs from healthy blood donors, HPV was detected in approximately 8% of men between the ages of 16 and 35.[189,190] At least 12.5 million men and women in the United States between the ages of 15 and 49 years are estimated to have HPV infections.[191]

Although the exact mechanism for cervical cancer development has not been explained, considerable insight has been obtained in the past few years. High-risk populations and cofactors such as cigarette smoking were identified. Infection with HPV appears to play an important role in the transformation process.

NATURAL HISTORY AND PATTERNS OF SPREAD

Squamous cell carcinoma usually arises from the squamocolumnar junction of the cervix and is preceded by cervical dysplasia and carcinoma in situ.[192] Petersen reported 127 patients with untreated carcinoma in situ of the cervix and described invasive carcinoma in 30% of patients by the tenth year after diagnosis.[193] Clemmesen and Poulsen reported a progression rate of 40% from carcinoma in situ to invasive cancer.[194] Kottmeier reported that of 31 patients with carcinoma in situ, 71% developed invasive cancer within 12 years and 80% within 30 years.[195]

Although most authorities agree that dysplasias and carcinoma in situ proceed to invasive cancer, less agreement exists about the time scale of progression. Richart and Barron followed 557 women with abnormal Pap smears and reported mean progression rates to carcinoma in situ of 85 months for mild dysplasia, 58 months for moderate dysplasia, and 12 months for severe dysplasia.[196] The Walton Report describes intervals of 1 to 20 years for progression from carcinoma in situ to invasive cancer, although most investigators accept the figure of 10 years as reported by Patton and others.[197–200]

Invasive carcinoma occurs when the malignant epithelial cells break through the basement membrane and enter the stroma. Continued growth results in a visible lesion that involves progressively more of the cervical tissue. Cervical cancer spreads by direct extension into the paracervical tissue, the vagina, or the endometrium. Continued local growth involves the pelvic side walls laterally, the bladder anteriorly, or the rectum posteriorly. Metastases usually occur by means of the lymphatics, although blood-borne metastases do occur.

The cervix has a rich lymphatic network. Microscopic lymphatics lie beneath the squamous mucosa and surround the endocervical glands.[24] In the outer third of the cervix, the lymphatics turn cephalad. In these lateral channels, the cervical lymphatics are joined by vaginal lymphatics. Plentl and Friedman comment on the interconnection of all the lymphatics from the various levels of the cervix with those of the uterus and upper vagina.[24] The lateral collecting trunks are relatively large and leave the cervix with the uterine artery and veins. The upper branches of these collecting lymphatics drain into the interiliac lymph nodes, and the middle branches drain into the obturator and deep hypogastric lymph nodes. The lower branches drain into the inferior gluteal and sacral lymph nodes and then into the lower aortic nodes. The interiliac, obturator, and hypogastric nodes drain into the common iliac and aortic lymph nodes.

In a review of 31 reports (>6000 patients), Plentl and Friedman found that the average incidence of positive lymph nodes was 15.4% in stage I disease and 28.6% in stage II disease.[24] Fuller and colleagues reported a series from Memorial Sloan-Kettering Cancer Center that evaluated 431 patients, finding a 15% rate of positive lymph nodes in stage IB cervical cancer and 22% in stage IIA cervical cancer.[201] Table 38–8 shows the distribution of paraaortic nodal metastases reported

TABLE 38–8. Metastases to Paraaortic Lymph Nodes in Carcinoma of the Uterine Cervix

Investigations	*Stage IB (%)*	*Stage IIA (%)*	*Stage IIB (%)*	*Stage IIIA (%)*	*Stage IIIB (%)*	*Stage IV (%)*
Sudarsanam et al[202]	11/155 (7)	3/21 (14)	4/22 (18)	0/3 (0)	3/16 (19)	0/3 (0)
Nelson et al[203]			5/31 (16)		13/28 (46)	
Piver et al[204]			6/46 (13)		18/49 (36)	4/7 (57)
Wharton et al[205]	0/21 (0)	0/10 (0)	10/47 (21)		14/42 (33)	
Lagasse et al[206]	8/143 (5)	4/22 (18)	19/58 (33)	0/3 (0)	19/61 (31)	1/4 (25)
Buchsbaum[207]	0/23 (0)	1/12 (7)			7/20 (35)	1/2 (50)
Averette et al[208]	3/40 (8)	2/9 (8)	2/9 (22)		2/20 (10)	1/2 (50)
Welander et al[209]			8/41 (20)	2/6 (33)	8/32 (25)	4/12 (33)
Berman et al[210]	8/158 (5)	3/25 (12)	40/240 (17)	1/3 (33)	44/177 (25)	3/17 (18)
Total	30/540 (6)	13/99 (13)	94/494 (19)	3/15 (20)	128/445 (29)	14/47 (30)

by several researchers.[202-210] The incidence of positive para-aortic nodes is 6% in stage IB disease, 12% in stage IIA, 19% in stage IIB, and 29% in stage IIIB.

Spread by hematogenous dissemination is relatively unusual in the early stages of cervical cancer, but the risk increases with more advanced stages. Carlson and colleagues reported distant metastases in 4.7% of patients with stage IB disease and 9.2% of stage IIA.[211] In stage IIB disease through stage IV, the average incidence of distant metastases was 20.4%, ranging from 16.2% in stage IIB to 24% in stage IV.

PATHOLOGIC CHARACTERISTICS

Gross Characteristics

In situ and microinvasive cervical cancers are usually diagnosed by exfoliative cytology and colposcopy, and they do not present with gross abnormalities. The term "occult" carcinoma refers to an invasive cancer that is not clinically apparent and tends to be the result of an endophytic carcinoma that develops high in the endocervix.

Visible lesions are usually divided into endophytic and exophytic lesions. A variant of the endophytic type of tumor extends into and expands the endocervix so that the diameters of the corpus and cervix appear to be equal, resembling a barrel. These barrel-shaped carcinomas are usually described as having transverse diameters of 6 cm or more, and they present special treatment problems. Just as endophytic tumors can have a misleading appearance and be more extensive than they appear at first examination, exophytic tumors can appear more extensive than they are. An exophytic tumor may appear to fill the upper vagina and be connected to the cervix by a relatively small stalk with only moderate invasion or enlargement of the cervix.

Microscopic Characteristics

Preinvasive cervical carcinoma was traditionally described by one of two different classifications, both of which are in common usage. The first system divides lesions into dysplasias (*i.e.*, mild, moderate, and severe) and carcinoma in situ. The second system uses three divisions of cervical intraepithelial neoplasia (*i.e.*, CIN-1, CIN-2, CIN-3). The precursor stage of cervical carcinoma begins with minimal morphologic changes (CIN-1 or mild dysplasia) and progresses until the entire epithelium from the basement membrane to the surface is composed of malignant cells (CIN-3 or carcinoma in situ).

Richart proposed a terminology that follows the cytologic descriptions of the Bethesda System, in which all preinvasive cervical lesions are divided into two groups: squamous cell intraepithelial lesion 1 (SIL-1), which includes HPV-related changes and CIN-1 (mild dysplasia); and squamous intraepithelial lesion 2 (SIL-2), which includes CIN-2 and CIN-3 (moderate dysplasia, severe dysplasia, and carcinoma in situ).[212]

Most carcinomas of the cervix are squamous cell carcinomas. Although many researchers state that these carcinomas represent 90% or more of all cervical cancer, Regan and Ng pointed out that if rigid histologic criteria are used, only 75% to 80% are of the squamous cell type.[213] They proposed that squamous cell carcinomas be classified as large cell nonkera-

tinizing, large cell keratinizing, and small cell nonkeratinizing. There was a survival rate of 68.3% for patients with large cell nonkeratinizing carcinomas, 41.7% for large cell keratinizing carcinomas, and 20% for small cell nonkeratinizing carcinomas. Other researchers used different types of histologic grading. Wentz divided these cancers into well-differentiated, moderately differentiated, and poorly differentiated carcinomas and reported differences in survival by grade.[214] Many other terms were used, including high grade and low grade, anaplastic, and grades 1 through 4. This lack of uniformity has inhibited comparison of results and hampered the development of useful clinical protocols based on differentiation of the carcinomas.

Adenocarcinomas of the cervix arise from the endocervical columnar cells. They are thought to account for 10% to 15% of cervical carcinomas, although some researchers reported incidences of 16% to 34%.[213-216] This apparent increase in incidence may be due to improved detection and treatment of squamous cell cancers during their relatively prolonged preinvasive stage.[216] Histologically, endocervical adenocarcinoma is composed of glands that are composed of malignant columnar cells with enlarged, bizarre nuclei and increased mitoses. As these adenocarcinomas become less differentiated, they can lose their glandular appearance and become more solid.

Adenosquamous cell carcinomas of the cervix represent 2% to 5% of all cervical carcinomas.[213] They are a mixture of malignant adenocarcinoma and malignant squamous cell carcinoma. These tumors are poorly differentiated and are associated with decreased survival.[213]

Clear cell carcinoma, glassy cell carcinoma, adenoid cystic carcinoma, and mucoepidermoid carcinoma are rarely seen, but they usually behave like poorly differentiated carcinomas.[213,217-219] Other rare primary carcinomas of the cervix are malignant melanoma, carcinoid tumors, sarcomas, malignant lymphoma, Hodgkin's disease, and verrucous carcinoma.[220-224] Verrucous carcinoma is a well-differentiated squamous cell carcinoma that invades locally but rarely metastasizes.

CLINICAL MANIFESTATIONS

Preinvasive cervical carcinoma is detected by Pap smear at the time of routine periodic examination and is not associated with symptoms. Any symptoms the patient has, such as vaginal discharge, represent coexisting problems. Early invasive carcinoma can produce a vaginal discharge or vaginal bleeding; the most common type of vaginal bleeding is postcoital spotting. As the tumor becomes more extensive, serosanguineous or purulent discharge becomes more pronounced. Bleeding may occur intermenstrually and be of greater volume.

Pain is a late symptom in cervical carcinoma, as are symptoms relating to the urinary tract or rectum. Dull, aching pain low in the pelvis may be associated with chronic inflammation, tumor necrosis, or a combination of both. Low back pain or leg pain may result from compression of lumbosacral nerves, direct involvement of lumbosacral nerve roots, pressure from a large tumor mass, or ureteral obstruction. In advanced disease, urinary frequency or urgency, hematuria, rectal tenesmus, and rectal bleeding can result from direct invasion of the bladder or rectum.

DIAGNOSIS

The purpose of periodic cytologic screening with the Pap smear is to prevent the development of invasive cervical cancer. Although the early detection of microinvasive and early invasive cervical cancer is valuable in decreasing the death rate, all cervical abnormalities should ideally be detected in the premalignant stage to prevent invasion.

Pap smears are performed at the time of routine pelvic examination. Screening with Pap smears has reduced mortality from cervical cancer.[225] How often this routine screening examination should be performed is the subject of considerable debate. In 1976, a task force was appointed by the Conference of Deputy Ministers of Health of Canada.[197] Their report, the Walton Report, identified two major categories of risk. The low-risk group is made up of women who never had a period of sexual activity during their lives, who had a hysterectomy for nonmalignant disease, or who reached the age of 60 after regular participation in a screening program without having had an abnormal cytologic smear. The at-risk group is made up of women who reached the age of 18, are sexually active, and do not otherwise fall into the low-risk group. Within the at-risk group is a high-risk subgroup made up of women who had an early onset of sexual activity with multiple partners. Mainly as a result of this report, the American Cancer Society recommended that asymptomatic women 20 years of age and older and those under 20 years of age who are sexually active have cytologic screening for 2 consecutive years and at least one screening every 3 years until age 65. They further recommended that women who are at high risk for developing cervical carcinoma because of early age at first coitus, multiple sexual partners, and multiparity should have a yearly cytologic screening.

A complete gynecologic examination should be performed when the Pap smear is obtained.[226] The American College of Obstetricians and Gynecologists recommends that cervical cytologic screening take place at the time of an annual gynecologic examination.[227] In 1988, The American College of Obstetricians and Gynecologists and the American Cancer Society concurred on the following recommendation: "All women who are, or have been, sexually active, or have reached the age of 18 years, should have an annual Pap test and pelvic examination. After a woman has had three or more consecutive satisfactory normal annual examinations, the Pap test may be performed less frequently at the discretion of her physician."[228]

Although the distribution of women into risk groups seems reasonable, it is difficult in practice. To effectively establish risk categories, the physician must have a detailed and reliable sexual history. Even then, the woman's risk status may be influenced by the sexual history of her partner, which can be even more difficult to determine accurately. Other issues are whether the value of annual screening is influenced by the bimanual examination and the breast examination and whether that annual examination by the gynecologist is the only periodic health screening that many women receive.

For many years, the Papanicolaou System of terminology was used to describe Pap smears. This system divided exfoliated cells into five groups or classes.[229] Because different laboratories often modified the system and reported the results of Pap tests differently, the World Health Organization established guidelines in 1973 for accepted terminology for reporting Pap tests: normal, atypical, dysplasia, carcinoma in situ, invasive squamous cell carcinoma, and adenocarcinoma.[230]

In 1988, a National Institute of Health consensus panel was formed to develop a uniform terminology for reporting the results of Pap tests.[231] This new terminology, called the Bethesda System, is illustrated in Table 38–9.[232] The three major features of the Bethesda System include an estimation of the adequacy of the smear, a characterization of the smear as normal or abnormal, and a descriptive diagnosis. This system uses two categories to describe preinvasive lesions of the vagina and cervix that are labeled squamous intraepithelial lesion 1 (HPV changes and mild dysplasia) or squamous intraepithelial lesion 2 (moderate dysplasia, severe dysplasia, and carcinoma in situ). The three systems for reporting Pap tests are compared in Table 38–9.

The adequacy of Pap tests has been questioned. Most authorities agree that, despite their accuracy for detecting high-

TABLE 38–9. Nomenclature in Cervical Cytology

Pap Smear	WHO System	Bethesda System
Class I	Normal	Within normal limits
Class II	Atypical	Reactive or reparative change
Class III	Dysplasia	Squamous epithelial cell abnormality; atypical squamous cells of undetermined significance; squamous intraepithelial lesion
	Mild dysplasia	Low grade (includes human papillomavirus)
	Moderate dysplasia	High grade
	Severe dysplasia	High grade
Class IV	Carcinoma in situ	High grade
Class V	Invasive squamous cell carcinoma	Squamous cell carcinoma
	Adenocarcinoma	Glandular cell abnormalities: adenocarcinoma or nonepithelial malignant neoplasm

(Wright TC, Richart RM. Preinvasive lesion of the lower genital tract. In: Hoskins WJ, Perez CA, Young RC, eds. Principles and practice of gynecologic oncology. Philadelphia: JB Lippincott, 1992: 528)

grade preinvasive disease and invasive cancer, Pap tests are not very sensitive. False-negative rates run from 8% to 50%.[233,234] This is usually not a problem if the Pap test is repeated annually, because a woman is unlikely to be in a false-negative group each year.

One of the most important steps that can be taken to minimize false negatives is to perform a proper smear of the cervix. To obtain an optimal Pap smear, the transformation zone must be sampled. This is relatively easy in women with a visible transformation zone, and it can be performed with a moistened cotton applicator or a plastic or wooden spatula. For women without a visible transformation zone, a moistened cotton applicator, a glass pipette, or a cytobrush should be used. The smear must be fixated immediately to prevent drying of the specimen.

Colposcopy is the recommended method for evaluating an abnormal Pap smear. A bright light with a green filter enhances vascular patterns, and 10 to 15 power magnification allows abnormal areas to be visualized and identified for biopsy with considerable accuracy. Most obstetrics and gynecology programs in the United States provide thorough experience in this technique, and colposcopes are a relatively inexpensive piece of office equipment. Colposcopy is designed to allow properly directed biopsies; it is not a substitute for cervical biopsy and endocervical curettage. If colposcopy is inadequate in the patient with dysplastic or malignant cells on Pap smear, cervical conization is mandatory.

Cervical conization is the removal of a cone-shaped portion of tissue from the cervix, including most or all of the transformation zone. This procedure is indicated for any patient with dysplastic or malignant cells on cervical cytology, inadequate colposcopy, and no grossly visible lesion on the cervix. It is also indicated for patients with microinvasive cancer and patients in whom the depth of invasion cannot be determined by biopsy. A cone biopsy should not be performed on a patient with a visible lesion of the cervix unless a cervical biopsy of the area fails to make the diagnosis of invasive cancer.

Any grossly visible cervical lesion should be biopsied. Pap smears and colposcopic examination are not substitutes for cervical biopsy. The inflammation that accompanies many cervical carcinomas can be misleading on the colposcopic examination and the Pap smear, resulting in a false-negative evaluation.

CLINICAL EVALUATION AND STAGING

The standard clinical evaluation for patients with cervical carcinoma includes examination by inspection and palpation (under anesthesia, if necessary), a biochemical profile that includes evaluation of liver and renal functions, a chest radiograph, cystoscopy, proctosigmoidoscopy, and a CT scan. In patients with advanced-stage disease or patients in whom there is suspicion of involvement based on examination, results from a barium enema should be obtained.

CT scan is being used more frequently, and at some institutions, attempts were made to replace lymphangiography with this procedure.[235] Performed with intravenous contrast, CT can be a substitute for intravenous pyelography. The diagnostic accuracy of the CT scan is under evaluation, particularly in assessing the status of extrapelvic lymph nodes. Camilien reported 61 patients with carcinoma of the cervix who had preoperative CT scans and exploratory laparotomy.[236] The radiographic and surgical-pathologic findings were correlated, showing that 75% of the enlarged pelvic lymph nodes on CT scan contained metastases, and 97% of the patients with negative nodes on CT scan were pathologically negative (*i.e.,* specificity of 97%). However, histologically positive pelvic nodes were often missed on CT scan (*i.e.,* sensitivity of 25%). The CT scan was more valuable in the evaluation of paraaortic lymph nodes (*i.e.,* specificity of 100% and sensitivity of 67%) (Table 38–10).[236–239] The reliability of CT scan was reported for evaluating lymph nodes of nonsurgically staged patients and for patients who underwent surgical staging by the GOG.[235]

Lymphangiograms were used in the nonsurgical evaluation of cervical cancer and may be helpful if clearly positive. Piver and Chung reported 98% accuracy by biopsy or laparotomy in patients with a positive lymphangiogram but a 20% false-negative rate in studies reported as negative.[240] Piver and associates reported 102 patients for whom lymphangiograms were correlated with operative findings.[241] Of 41 abnormal lymphangiograms, 40 were subsequently confirmed by biopsy and laparotomy (*i.e.,* 98% accuracy). In contrast, in 12 of 61

TABLE 38–10. CT Scan in the Evaluation of Paraaortic Nodes

Investigations	No. of Cases	FIGO Stage	Sensitivity (%)	Specificity (%)	Accuracy (%)
Kilcheski et al[237]	36	I–IV, rec			80
Brenner et al[238]	42	I–IV, rec	77	86	83
Bandy et al[239]	44	I–IV, rec	75	91	86
DMC, 1986[236]	10	IIB–IV	67	100	90
	61	I–IV	67	100	98
Camilien et al[236]	51	IB–IIA	67	100	100
Camilien et al[236]	10	IIB–IV	67	100	90

rec, recurrent.
(Modified from Camilien L, Gordon D, Fruchter RG, Maiman M, Boyce JG. Predictive value of computerized tomography in the presurgical evaluation of primary carcinoma of the cervix. Gynecol Oncol 1988;30:209–215)

patients in whom lymphangiograms were interpreted as normal, the patients had metastases in the lymph nodes found at laparotomy (about a 20% false-negative rate). The initial enthusiasm for the use of the lymphangiogram has been replaced with more realistic expectations. De Muylder and coworkers reported 100 patients with stage IB carcinoma of the uterine cervix for whom lymphangiography was done before radical hysterectomy with lymphadenectomy.[242] The lymphangiograms of 5 patients were classified as abnormal, 15 were suspicious, and 80 were normal. Surgical-pathologic findings demonstrated pelvic lymph node metastasis in 18 patients (*i.e.*, 5 with abnormal, 3 with suspicious, and 10 with normal findings on the lymphangiogram). The specificity of this test was 100%, but the sensitivity to detect metastases was only 28%. Others, including Lagasse and coworkers, found lymphangiogram an unreliable basis for modifying treatment.[243]

Heller and coworkers reported a prospective evaluation of 320 patients with stage IIB, III, or IVA carcinoma of the cervix entered into a GOG protocol on whom preoperative CT scan, lymphangiogram, and ultrasound of the aortic area were performed.[244] Paraaortic node dissection was performed in patients with negative staging studies. Positive paraaortic nodes were seen in 21% of patients with stage IIB disease, 31% with stage III, and 13% with stage IVA. The lymphangiogram, CT scan, and ultrasound had false-negative frequencies for pelvic lymph node evaluation of 14.2%, 25%, and 30%, respectively, for 111 patients who had sampling of pelvic lymph nodes. The sensitivity of the lymphangiogram was 79%, CT scan was 34%, and ultrasound was 19%. The specificity of these tests was 73%, 96%, and 99%, respectively. These findings suggest that a negative lymphangiogram may be adequate to eliminate surgical staging in subgroups at low risk for metastases to the paraaortic lymph nodes. The lymphangiogram definitely is of value in outlining abnormal lymph nodes that can be included in the irradiated fields or, in the case of surgical management, those that should be removed by the surgeon for pathologic examination. Hammond and coworkers correlated lymphangiographic findings and prognosis in 215 patients with stage IB through IIIB treated with definitive irradiation.[245]

MRI is being evaluated and may prove to be helpful. It is being used more frequently for assessment of extracervical extension.[246] Parametrial tumor was easily identified on T2-weighted images from the low-signal-intensity cervix and uterine ligaments.[247] Ebner and associates reported that, in comparing MRI findings in 12 women with recurrent pelvic tumors and 10 with fibrotic masses (confirmed by laparotomy or biopsy in 21 of the patients), they were able to differentiate the two processes accurately in most instances.[248] However, no reliable evaluation supports the accuracy of this procedure or the contributions that it can make to staging or therapeutic decisions. It is highly desirable to confirm abnormal or suspicious lymph node radiographic findings with CT-guided thin-needle aspiration biopsies.[249]

Ultrasound has limited value in the evaluation of extrauterine tumor involvement, but it may be used to detect uterine perforation, which can occur during intracavitary insertion.[250]

Griffin and colleagues emphasized that routine radiographic procedures may have a low yield of positive findings.[251] However, these examinations must be selectively carried out, depending on the stage of the tumor. Even if normal, these assessments have value as a baseline for evaluation after therapy.

Other symptoms may require evaluation with appropriate studies, such as bone scans or specialized x-ray procedures.

Clinical Staging

The clinical staging of cervical carcinoma consists of physical examination (*i.e.*, inspection, palpation, biopsy), laboratory studies, and radiographic evaluation as outlined previously. Surgical staging, if performed, does not alter the official stage of the patient for the purpose of reporting treatment results. If possible, cervical cancer should be staged as part of a multidisciplinary effort involving the gynecologist, radiation oncologist, and medical oncologist. The staging examination can usually be performed adequately in an outpatient setting, but if the adequacy of the examination is questionable, examination under anesthesia should be performed.

In 1985, the Oncology Committee of FIGO made changes in the FIGO classification of cervical carcinoma, which were published in 1987.[252] The new FIGO classification is listed in Table 38–11.[253] The changes in the staging system are limited to stage I. Stage IA, which in the 1985 report was described as "microinvasive carcinoma (early stromal invasion)," is now divided into two categories. Stage IA1 is defined as "preclinical carcinomas of the cervix; that is, those diagnosed only by microscopy" and should be limited to the earliest forms of microinvasion, including patients in whom invasion can be seen but the area of invasion is too small for measurement. Stage IA2 is defined as "lesions detected microscopically that can be measured." The upper limit of the depth of invasion should be less than 5 mm, taken from the base of the epithelium (surface or glandular) from which it originates, and a second dimension, the horizontal spread, should not exceed 7 mm. Larger lesions should be staged as IB. Stage IB is now defined as "lesions of greater dimensions than stage IA2, whether seen clinically or not." Preformed space involvement should not alter the staging but should be recorded to determine whether it affects treatment decisions in the future. The remainder of the staging classification is unchanged.

The impact of these changes on the staging system is not clear at this time, because most authorities in the United States still use "less than 3 mm of invasion without lymphovascular invasion" as the definition for stage IA cervical carcinoma. The Society of Gynecologic Oncologists (SGO) officially opposed the new FIGO staging classification and recommended that the definition of IA carcinoma be "less than 3 mm of invasion with no lymphovascular invasion." Current clinical practice patterns are unlikely to be changed by this new classification, and the effect it has on the reporting of results has not yet been determined.

Kolstad reviewed the results of therapy in 643 patients with microinvasive carcinoma reclassified as stage IA1 or IA2.[254] Three of the 232 patients with stage IA1 disease (1.3%) and 12 of 411 stage IA2 patients (2.9%) had local recurrences in addition to four pelvic recurrences, confirming the validity of the staging modification. Similar conclusions were reached by Tsukamoto and coworkers.[255]

Surgical Staging

In the early 1970s, Averette and associates[208] and Nelson and associates[203] introduced the concept of pretreatment surgical

TABLE 38–11.   Staging of Carcinoma
of the Uterine Cervix

AJC	FIGO	

Primary Tumor (T)

TX		Primary tumor cannot be assessed
T0		No evidence of primary tumor
Tis	0	Carcinoma in situ
T1	I	Cervical carcinoma confined to uterus (extension to corpus should be disregarded)
T1A	IA	Preclinical invasive carcinoma, diagnosed by microscopy only
T1A1	IA1	Minimal microscopic stromal invasion
T1A2	IA2	Tumor with invasive component 5 mm or less in depth taken from the base of the epithelium and 7 mm or less in horizontal spread
T1B	IB	Tumor larger than T1A2
T2	II	Cervical carcinoma invades beyond uterus but not to pelvic wall or to the lower third of vagina
T2A	IIA	Without parametrial invasion
T2B	IIB	With parametrial invasion
T3	III	Cervical carcinoma extends to the pelvic wall and/or involves lower third of vagina and/or causes hydronephrosis or nonfunctioning kidney
T3A	IIIA	Tumor involves lower third of the vagina, no extension to pelvic wall
T3B	IIIB	Tumor extends to pelvic wall and/or causes hydronephrosis or nonfunctioning kidney
T4*	IVA	Tumor invades mucosa of bladder or rectum and/or extends beyond true pelvis

Regional Lymph Nodes (N)

Regional lymph nodes include paracervical, parametrial, hypogastric (obturator), common internal and external illiac, presacral and sacral

NX		Regional lymph nodes cannot be assessed
N0		No regional lymph node metastasis
N1		Regional lymph node metastasis

Distant Metatasis (M)

MX		Presence of distant metastasis cannot be assessed
M0		No distant metastasis
M1	IVB	Distant metastasis

* Presence of bullous edema is not sufficient evidence to classify a tumor as T4.
(Beahrs OH, Henson DE, Hutter, RVP, Myers MH, eds. Manual for staging of cancer. 3rd ed. Philadelphia; JB Lippincott, 1988:151–153)

staging of cervical carcinoma. Averette and colleagues reported a lack of correlation between clinical staging and the results of surgical exploration, with reported errors of 26% for stage IB, 45% for stage IIA, 60% for stage IIB, 66% for stage IIIA, and 95% for stage IIIB disease.[208] Both researchers demonstrated the relatively high frequency of paraaortic nodal metastases in cervical carcinoma, particularly in more advanced stages. Table 38–8 summarizes the results of several reports of positive paraaortic lymph nodes in cervical cancer.

Wharton and colleagues[205] and Piver and Barlow[204] reported the treatment of patients with positive paraaortic nodes with extended-field radiation therapy. Wharton and colleagues gave 5500 cGy to the paraaortic area and reported a 27% serious complication rate, with a 13% treatment-related mortality rate.[205] Piver and Barlow used 6000 cGy and found a similarly high complication rate.[204] Berman and coworkers reported fewer intestinal complications after using a retroperitoneal approach to the paraaortic lymph nodes.[256] Welander and colleagues, using a transperitoneal approach to the paraaortic lymph nodes, reported that a 4400 cGy dose to the paraaortic nodes was not associated with a high complication rate.[209]

Survival of patients with positive paraaortic lymph nodes was addressed by several researchers.[203–205,207,209,210] The average disease-free survival rate was approximately 18%. Welander and colleagues pointed out that because the maximal tolerated dose of paraaortic irradiation was in the range of 4400 to 4500 cGy, patients with more than microscopic disease were unlikely to be cured by extended-field irradiation.[209] If patients with positive paraaortic lymph nodes have bulky local disease, control of paraaortic disease cannot improve survival if the local disease cannot be controlled. Moreover, spread to paraaortic lymph nodes may be a sign of systemic disease. Buchsbaum reported that 34.8% of patients with positive paraaortic lymph nodes have metastatic cancer in the scalene lymph nodes.[207] Welander and colleagues found that 54.8% of patients with positive paraaortic lymph nodes developed distant metastases, compared with 25% of a similar group of patients with negative paraaortic lymph nodes.[209] Berman and colleagues, in a collective multivariate analysis of 626 patients by the GOG, found the relative risk of recurrence to be 11.0 for positive paraaortic lymph nodes.[210] The decrement in survival time had a relative risk of 6.2. These researchers also reported an increased likelihood of extrapelvic failure with positive paraaortic lymph nodes.

The role of pretreatment surgical staging in carcinoma of the cervix remains unclear. Several large institutions across the United States routinely perform prospective protocols, and the GOG used pretreatment laparotomy as an integral part of many of their advanced cervix protocols. The operation has a place in the research setting, but whether the data that are being accumulated in these studies can provide enough survival benefit to recommend the procedure routinely remains to be seen. It is likely that an improvement in survival based on surgical staging will require an effective systemic therapy.

PROGNOSTIC FACTORS

Prognosis in cervical cancer is worse with advancing stage of disease, which represents increasing tumor bulk or increasing extent of tumor involvement of adjacent or distant organs. In the early stage of disease, survival is influenced by multiple factors.

Patients with stage IB and IIA carcinoma treated by radical hysterectomy and pelvic lymphadenectomy have survival rates of 82% to 92% if there are no metastases to pelvic lymph nodes, compared with survival rates of 45% to 61% for patients with positive lymph nodes.[240,257–259] The incidence of positive lymph nodes in patients has been related to tumor diameters of greater than 4 cm, lymphovascular invasion, deep invasion into the cervical stroma, and histologic grade.[240,257,260–263]

Two researchers looked at recurrence in patients who had

negative lymph nodes.[257,263] Fuller and colleagues found that, after stratifying for nodal metastases, the size of the primary tumor, the depth of invasion into the cervix, and the histologic grade were associated with an increased incidence of recurrence.[257] The investigators observed an increased incidence of recurrence in patients who had adenocarcinoma compared with those with squamous histology, even though patients with adenocarcinoma did not have an increased incidence of positive lymph nodes. Burke and colleagues found that adenomatous cell type and lymphovascular invasion placed patients with negative lymph nodes at an increased risk.[263] Figge and Tamimi found an increased recurrence rate in patients with adenocarcinoma, but this was only in association with lymphovascular space involvement and positive lymph nodes.[264] Several researchers reported increased recurrence rates and decreased survival as the number of metastatic lymph nodes or the number of metastases in lymph node groups increases.[201,240]

Delgado and coworkers described 3-year disease-free survival rates of 94.8%, 88.1%, and 67.6%, respectively, for occult, smaller than 3 cm, and larger than 3 cm invasive squamous cell carcinoma of the cervix at stage I treated with radical surgery.[265] Survival also strongly correlated with depth of tumor invasion of the stroma: 86% to 94% for less than 10 mm, 71% to 75% for 11 to 20 mm, and 60% for 21 mm or larger. For patients without parametrial involvement, the survival rate was 84.9%, and it was 69.6% for those with parametrial tumor extension. Similar observations were reported by Rotman and associates in surgically treated patients.[266] Podczaski and associates found that patients with tumors larger than 5 cm fared worse than those with smaller tumors.[267]

Alvarez and colleagues, reporting on 185 patients with stage IB or IIA carcinoma of the cervix with nodal metastasis at the time of radical hysterectomy and pelvic lymphadenectomy, described several groups closely associated with prognosis.[268] Patients with small primary tumors (<1 cm in diameter) and no more than two positive lymph nodes had a survival rate of 90%. Those with lesions smaller than 4 cm and two positive nodes had a 50% to 70% survival rate, and those with tumors larger than 4 cm or more than two positive nodes had a 10% 5-year survival rate.

Several researchers described a greater incidence of lymphatic and distant metastasis in patients with bulky stage IB and IIA tumors treated by radical hysterectomy (Table 38–12).[240,261,269] Similar findings after treatment with irradiation were reported by Fletcher[149] and by Perez and associates.[270] Metastasis correlated with decreased survival.

The effects of other factors on outcome are less clear. Age at the time of diagnosis was reported to have no effect by Kyriakos and colleagues.[271] Other researchers observed a decrease in survival for young patients or for older patients.[266,272-274]

Some studies suggested a decrease in survival and an increased incidence of distant metastases in patients with endometrial extension of a primary cervical carcinoma (*i.e.*, endometrial stromal invasion or replacement of the endometrium by tumor only). Grimard and associates confirmed these findings only in patients with stage IB tumors but not with more advanced disease.[275] Similar findings were reported by Noguchi and colleagues in 301 patients treated with radical hysterectomy (*i.e.*, uterine body invasion in 7.8% of stage IB patients, 25.5% of IIA and 38.2% of IIB patients).[276] Extension of cervical cancer in the uterine body was associated with a higher incidence of peritoneal carcinomatosis and distant metastases. Patients without uterine body invasion had a 5-year survival rate of 92.4% compared with 53.8% for patients with invasion.

Several researchers reported lower survival and an increased incidence of pelvic recurrences in patients with anemia who were managed by radiation therapy.[277] Jenkin and Stryker found more pelvic recurrences and complications in patients with hypertension.[278] Van Herik[279] and Kapp and Lawrence[280] found decreased survival if patients had oral temperatures over 100°F. Although some patients with ele-

TABLE 38–12. Nodal Metastases and Parametrial Extension Related to the Maximal Depth of Tumor Invasion

Depth of Invasion (mm)	No. of Patients	Nodal Metastases		Parametrial Extension	
		No.	Percent	No.	Percent
0–4.9	97	1	1.0*	0	0.0
5–9.9	153	19	12.4†	5	3.3¶
10–14.9	169	44	26.0‡	29	17.2#
15–19.9	96	31	32.3 ⎫	27	28.1**
20–24.9	58	21	36.2 ⎬ 34.4§	20	34.5††
25–29.9	29	11	37.9 ⎭	16	55.2 ⎫ 56.4‡‡
≥30	26	16	61.5‖	15	57.7 ⎭
Total	628	143	22.8	112	17.8

Significant differences between * and † (*p* < 0.005), † and ‡ (*p* < 0.005), § and ‖ (*p* < 0.01), ¶ and # (*p* < 0.001), # and ** (*p* < 0.05), and †† and ‡‡ (*p* < 0.05).
(Inoue T. Prognostic significance of the depth of invasion relating to nodal metastases, parametrial extension, and cell types. A study of 628 cases with stage IB, IIA, and IIB cervical carcinoma. Cancer 1984;54:3035–3042)

vated temperatures had pelvic infections, more than half of the patients had no specific etiologic factor for the temperature elevation.

Attempts were made to correlate the distribution of peridiploid and aneuploid tumors by flow cytometry with prognosis. Some researchers found no significant difference in recurrence rates between patients with diploid or aneuploid tumors, but others observed a less favorable prognosis for those with tumors with a diploid or tetraploid DNA content compared with the nondiploid or nontetraploid tumors if the parameters were combined with age (<51 years) and degree of differentiation of the tumor.[281-283] However, the difference is not statistically significant.

DNA content of cancer cells was evaluated in 12 cases of cervical carcinoma and 2 cases of vaginal carcinoma treated with radiation therapy.[284] Nuclear extinction, mean nuclear area, and 5N-exceeding rate (5 NER) were analyzed after different doses of radiation. The values increased gradually after various doses. Cancer cells disappeared in patients exhibiting good responses before 3000 cGy. Low mean nuclear areas and low 5 NER were observed in two patients who died with poor response to irradiation.[284]

Strang and associates found more relapses of tumors with an S-phase rate of 20% or greater.[282] Kelland and Steel, analyzing the response to irradiation of five established carcinomas of the cervix cell lines exposed to various dose rates (1.6, 3.2, or 150 cGy/minute), observed a significant difference in radiosensitivity of various cell lines.[285] The data were well fitted by the incomplete repair model.[286]

Kenter and associates reported a 49% (44 of 89) rate of DNA aneuploidy in patients with stage IB or IIA squamous cell carcinoma of the cervix.[287] There was no difference in survival between these patients and those with no DNA diploid index (81% and 79%, respectively).

TREATMENT

The primary method of therapy for preinvasive (stage 0) and microinvasive (stages IA1 and IA2) carcinoma of the cervix is surgery. Only rarely does radiation therapy have a place in the management of early disease.

Stage IB and IIA carcinoma of the cervix can be managed effectively by radical surgery or irradiation therapy.[288] Some patients are better managed surgically, but others benefit most from primary therapy with irradiation. The optimal situation is for all patients to be treated in institutions that have personnel and equipment suitable for either type of therapy and for selection of therapy to be a joint decision of the surgeon, the radiation oncologist, and the patient. Only in this setting can the best results be obtained for all patients.

Patients with stage IIB through stage IVA disease are usually managed by radiation therapy, with the exception a few patients with stage IVA who are candidates for primary pelvic exenteration. Patients with IVB cervical carcinoma are usually managed by a combination of chemotherapy and irradiation. Phase I and II trials of concomitant chemotherapy and irradiation were performed using patients with locally advanced disease. Although this is an intriguing concept, its usefulness is unproved.

Selected types of cervical carcinoma may be managed by combinations of surgery and irradiation. These situations are discussed later in this chapter.

Carcinoma In Situ

Although the definitive therapy for cervical intraepithelial neoplasia (CIN), grade 3 (severe dysplasia and carcinoma in situ), is conization of the cervix, selected patients can be managed by outpatient therapy with cryotherapy or laser ablation. These lesions should be entirely visible by colposcopy, the squamocolumnar junction must be visible, the endocervical curettage must be negative, and the colposcopically directed biopsy must be at least as severe as the cytologic smear. Some physicians also require that the lesion occupy no more than one quadrant of the cervix and that there be no gland involvement. To be a candidate for outpatient therapy, the patient must be reliable and must agree to long-term follow-up. Townsend and colleagues, in a review of patients in whom invasive carcinoma developed after outpatient therapy, found obvious deviation from these criteria in most of the patients.[289] Similar findings were reported by Sevin and associates.[290]

A new technique for diagnosis and therapy of preinvasive lesions of the cervix employs a thin wire loop electrode to excise the lesions and the transformation zone.[291,292] This technique is called the loop electrosurgical excision procedure, and it appears to be bringing rapid changes to the management of preinvasive disease. As with any new method, additional reports are needed to establish its proper role.

In the past, abdominal or vaginal hysterectomy was the treatment for CIN-3. However, based on current evidence, this treatment choice is no longer justified. In an extensive review of the literature, Coppleson found that only 18 (0.3%) of 5442 women treated for carcinoma in situ by conization of the cervix subsequently developed overt invasive cancer.[293] This result can be compared with 38 (0.4%) of 8995 women who developed invasive carcinoma of the vagina after hysterectomy for carcinoma in situ. Based on these findings, routine hysterectomy for CIN-3 cannot be recommended.

Patients who do not desire further childbearing and have intraepithelial neoplasia involving the margins of the cone biopsy may be treated by hysterectomy. Hysterectomy may also be indicated in patients with other gynecologic disorders that require removal of the uterus. However, only rarely does a patient who desires further childbearing require a hysterectomy for preinvasive cancer.

Stage IA

In the 1987 classification of cervical carcinoma by FIGO, microinvasive carcinoma is divided into IA1 and IA2 (see Table 38-11).[253] Stage IA1 microinvasive carcinoma is so small that it cannot be measured. It should be treated by abdominal or vaginal hysterectomy in the healthy patient who does not desire further childbearing. Women who desire to preserve fertility or who are poor surgical risks can be managed by conization and followed closely, if the cone margins are free of disease. Kolstad stated that invasion of less than 1 mm, with negative margins of resection, can be managed by cone biopsy and careful follow-up.[254]

The proper management of stage IA2 cervical carcinoma is less clear. Averette and associates found no patients with positive lymph nodes if invasion was less than 1 mm without lymphovascular invasion, but they reported a 3.5% incidence of positive nodes if invasion extended to 5 mm.[294] Simon and colleagues found no metastasis to lymph nodes in 43 patients with invasion of less than 3 mm, but they reported a rate of 3.9% positive lymph nodes in 26 patients with invasion of 3.1 to 5 mm.[295] Their review of the literature revealed a rate of 8% nodal metastasis in patients with invasion of 3 to 5 mm.

In addition to depth of invasion, several researchers reported an increased incidence of nodal metastases if there was lymphovascular space invasion.[296,297] Based on these results, most authorities in the United States recommend abdominal or vaginal hysterectomy for stage IA cervical cancer if invasion is less than 3 mm and there is no lymphovascular space involvement. Cervical carcinoma with invasion of over 3 mm or in which there is lymphovascular invasion is managed like stage IB disease.

Greer and associates reported histologically positive margins in 66% of patients with stage IA2 carcinoma of the cervix who had undergone conization.[298] They found residual carcinoma in 24% of patients who had negative cone margins. Two of 50 patients had positive lymph nodes. The influence of volume of invasive cancer as a criteria for planning therapy was recommended by Burghardt.[296] Because such measurements are part of the new FIGO classification, additional data may be available in the future.

Patients with stage IA can be treated with intracavitary irradiation. In 34 patients with stage IA carcinoma treated at Washington University, 13 of whom received intracavitary therapy alone, no local or regional failures occurred.[299] The corrected 5-year survival rate for intercurrent disease was 100%.

Hamberger and associates reported 151 patients with stages IA or IB lesions smaller than 1 cm in diameter treated with intracavitary therapy alone.[300] No failures occurred in 41 patients with stage IA carcinoma, and there were only 4 (4%) failures in 93 patients with small-volume stage IB carcinoma. However, of 17 patients with more advanced stage IB lesions, 3 patients (18%) treated with intracavitary therapy alone had regional failures.

Stages IB and IIA

Stages IB and IIA cervical carcinoma can be managed equally well by radical hysterectomy and pelvic lymphadenectomy or definitive irradiation.[288] Surgical therapy is sometimes preferred because ovarian function can be preserved. In young women, the vagina is usually more pliable after surgery than if irradiation is used. Overall treatment time is shorter, and long-term radiation complications in pelvic tissues are avoided. Other reasons to select surgery include concomitant inflammatory gastrointestinal disease, pelvic inflammatory disease, presence of an adnexal mass, and pregnancy. Radiation therapy avoids major intraoperative and postoperative surgical complications. Most of the therapy can be given on an outpatient basis, and it is suitable for virtually any patient. Some noncontrolled studies demonstrated that radical surgery and definitive irradiation are equally effective therapies for stage IB and IIA cervical cancer.[301,302] Newton[303] and Roddick and Greenlow[304] reported comparable survival and complication rates for stages IB and IIA cervical cancer if patients were prospectively randomized to radiation therapy or radical hysterectomy. The results of a literature review that compared the two modalities is presented in Table 38–13 and Table 38–14.[216,257,258,288,303,305–331]

Some caution in interpreting surgical data is warranted because surgical findings can modify the treatment plan. In a GOG trial, 80 of 1125 patients were found to have less than 3 mm of invasion, and an additional 129 patients did not undergo radical hysterectomy because of intraoperative complications (49 patients) or because more advanced disease was found (80 patients).[265] Failure to account for these patients could bias the results.

Volterrani and Lombardi reported a 5-year survival of 82.6% in 23 patients with occult stage IB carcinoma of the cervix treated with intracavitary radium only (^{226}Ra application using a derivation from the Paris method to deliver 7500 mgh).[332] However, in stage IB, the 5-year survival rate was only 65.8%; in stage II, the 5-year survival rate was 50%; and in stage III, the 5-year survival rate was 29.8%. These results are substantially inferior to those obtained with a combination of intracavitary and external irradiation. Intracavitary therapy alone is grossly inadequate for treating large primary tumors, including the barrel-shaped lesions and any parametrial extension. Unfortunately, the sites of the failures were not reported.

Van Nagell and associates found that the recurrence rate after radical hysterectomy or irradiation for stage IB disease was 5% for tumors smaller than 2 cm in diameter treated with either modality.[319] For lesions that were 2 to 5 cm in diameter, the failure rate was 24% for surgery but 11% for radiation. Keilbinska and colleagues, in a long-term follow-up of 792 women treated by irradiation and 789 women treated with hysterectomy and irradiation for stage I cervical carcinoma, found no difference in survival, general health, incidence of recurrent carcinoma, or appearances of second primary malignancies.[333] Perez and associates reported comparable results from a randomized trial of preoperative irradiation and radical hysterectomy compared with irradiation alone for stage IB and IIA cervical cancers (Fig. 38–7).[334]

Patients with bulky endocervical carcinoma (*i.e.*, barrel-shaped cervix) had higher incidences of central recurrence, pelvic and paraaortic node metastases, and distant metastases.[335] Because of the difficulty of obtaining central control of these large lesions, higher doses of irradiation to the central pelvis, a surgical procedure that removes the uterus, and both treatments together were advocated.[336] Durrance and coworkers[337] and Nelson and colleagues[338] recommended an extrafascial, conservative hysterectomy 6 weeks after completion of high-dose preoperative irradiation (2000 cGy to the whole pelvis, an additional 3000 cGy to the parametria with midline shielding, and one intracavitary insertion for 6000 mgh, delivering about 7500 cGy to point A). Several nonrandomized studies,[142,339] as well as several small randomized trials,[142,340] failed to show a survival advantage for the combination of radiation and surgery. The GOG is evaluating the benefits of postirradiation hysterectomy in a prospective, randomized trial. Although the trial is near closure, results will not be available for several months.

The use of irradiation for patients with positive lymph nodes after radical hysterectomy is controversial. In a panel report summarizing the experience at several institutions in the United States, Morrow found no consistent practice and no evidence of benefit from such therapy.[340] Investigators from

TABLE 38–13. Five-Year Survival Rates for Stage I and II Carcinoma of the Uterine Cervix Treated by Radical Hysterectomy and Pelvic Lymphadenectomy

Investigations	Stage	No. of Patients	Survivors*	Percent Survival
Allen[305]	IB	116		88.0
Artman[216]	IB	153	129	84.3
Benedet[306] ± node dissection	IB	43	33	76.7
	IIA	3	2	66.7
Blaikley et al[307]	IB	98	64	65.5
	IB and IIA	161	96	50.8
Brunschwig and Barber[308]	IB (A)†	173	141	81.5
	IB and IIA (B)†	308	231	76.0
Burghardt[258]	IB			82.0
	IIA			76.9
Christensen et al[309]	IB	168	137	82.7
	IB and IIA	219	168	77.0
Delgado[310]	IB	645	Actuarial	80.0
Fuller[257]	IB	295	Actuarial	86.0
	IIA	136	Actuarial	72.0
Hoskins[288]	IB	56		84.0
Ketcham et al[311]	IB	28	Actuarial	86.0
	IB and IIA	42		87.0
Lee[312]	IB	237	204	86.1
	IIA	106	76	71.7
Liu and Meigs[313]	IB	116	91	78.4
	IB and IIA	165	119	72.1
Masterson[314]	IB	120	105	87.5
	IB and IIA	150	124	82.5
Newton[303]	IB	58	46	81.0
Park et al[315]	IB	126	Actuarial	91.0
Piver[316]	IB	55	50	92.0
Symmonds[317]	IB	48	46	95.8
	IIA	16	14	87.5
Underwood[318]	IB	139	119	85.6
Van Nagell[319]	IB	190	164	86.0
	IIA	43	34	79.0

* Patients dead from intercurrent disease were included with survivors when data were available.
† Surgical and pathologic classification.
(Modified from Hoskins WJ, Ford JJ, Lutz MH, Averette HE. Radical hysterectomy and pelvic lymphadenectomy for the management of early invasive cancer of the cervix. Gynecol Oncol 1976;4:278–290)

the Memorial Sloan-Kettering Cancer Center reported improved survival of patients with nodal metastases at radical hysterectomy if treated postoperatively with a combination of whole-pelvis irradiation and chemotherapy.[341]

Fuller and coworkers found pelvic lymph node metastases in 71 of 431 patients with stage IB or IIA carcinoma of the uterine cervix treated with radical hysterectomy.[201] Postoperative irradiation (4000 cGy in 4 weeks) was given. In 32 patients with one or two positive nodes, the 5-year survival rate in the irradiated group was slightly higher than in the nonirradiated group (about 60% and 40%, respectively).

Hogan and associates evaluated 31 patients with positive pelvic nodes, 22 with parametrial extension and 14 with a positive margin of resection.[342] Adjuvant postoperative irradiation was given to 21 patients. The reduction in local recurrence in the treated group approached statistical significance.

Gonzalez and associates reported 89 patients with stage IB or IIA disease with positive lymph nodes who received postoperative irradiation.[343] The 5-year and 10-year survival rates were 60% and 51%, respectively. By comparison, 43 patients with negative lymph nodes had a survival rate of 85%. In the 89 patients with metastatic disease in lymph nodes, 37 (41.5%) developed recurrences, 21 (23.6%) in the pelvis, alone or combined with distant metastasis. In the 43 patients with negative lymph nodes, only 3 (7%) had pelvic failures, 2 of which were combined with distant metastasis. In the surviving patients, 4 had gastrointestinal and 7 had genitourinary complications severe enough to require surgical correction. In 4 patients, asymptomatic stenosis of the ureters was detected by annual intravenous pyelogram.

Kim and associates reported 38 patients (selected from 240 with stage IB disease) who received postoperative pelvic irradiation after radical hysterectomy because of close surgical

TABLE 38–14. Five-Year Survival Rates of Patients With Stage I and II Carcinoma of the Uterine Cervix Treated by Radiation Therapy

Investigations	Stage	No. of Patients	Survivors*	Percent Survival
Blaikley et al[307]	I	183	123	67.2
	I and II	551	296	53.7
Dickson[320]	IB	348	249	71.6
	IB and IIA	983	589	60.0
Fletcher[321]	IB	549	Actuarial	91.5
	IB and IIA	973		83.5
Hanks[322]	IB			87.0
	II, NOS			66.0
Haie[323]	IB	299	Actuarial	85.0
	IIA	315	Actuarial	76.0
Kim[324]	IB	169	Actuarial	82.0
	IIA	83	Actuarial	76.0
Kline et al[325]	IB	45	37	81.4
	IB and IIA	64	47	70.5
Kottmeier[326]	IB	611	547	89.5
	IB and IIA	1576	1244	78.9
Lanciano[327]	IB	618	Actuarial	79.0
Montana[328]	IB	177	Actuarial	83.0
	II			
Muirhead and Green[329]	I	194	152	78.0
	I and II	306	208	68.0
Perez et al[330]	IB	312	Actuarial	85.0
	IIA	98	NED	70.0
Piver[316]	IB	48	44	91.0
Wall et al[331]	I	101	87	86.4
	I and II	208	153	73.5

* Patients dead from intercurrent disease included with survivors when data available.
(Modified from Hoskins WJ, Ford JJ, Lutz MH, Averette HE. Radical hysterectomy and pelvic lymphadenectomy for the management of early invasive cancer of the cervix. Gynecol Oncol 1976;4:278–290)

margins or metastatic pelvic lymph nodes.[344] Patients with close surgical margins were treated with intracavitary vaginal ovoid insertions (5000 cGy at 1 cm above and between the two ovoids). Patients with positive margins and pelvic lymph nodes received external whole-pelvis irradiation only (5000–6000 cGy in 6 weeks delivered through AP/PA portals). The overall recurrence rate was 45% (17 of 38). In the total group, 9 of the recurrences were in the pelvis, and 4 were associated with distant metastasis. Five (15%) of 33 patients treated with whole-pelvis irradiation with or without vaginal intracavitary therapy had major bowel complications that required surgical intervention (*i.e.*, 4 small bowel obstructions, 1 enterovesical fistula). Five patients treated only with intravaginal ovoids had no major complications.

For 60 patients receiving external irradiation for pelvic node metastasis after radical hysterectomy, Bianchi and colleagues observed a 65% 5-year survival rate.[345] Among 15 patients who refused postoperative irradiation, only 3 (20%) survived 5 years. The improvement in survival was particularly notable in the stage II patients. After pelvic irradiation was given after radical hysterectomy, the major complication rate was 21.1%, compared with 19.8% if hysterectomy was preceded by an intracavitary radium application or 10.5% with surgery alone.

Kinney and colleagues compared the results of therapy in 82 patients with stage IB or IIA carcinoma of the cervix who had pelvic lymph node metastases at Wertheim hysterectomy and bilateral lymphadenectomy and did not receive additional adjuvant therapy with a group of 103 similar patients who received 5000 cGy to the pelvis postoperatively.[346] Of these 185 patients, 60 pairs matched for stage, tumor size, and number and location of positive nodes were analyzed. The 5-year survival rate was 72% for the surgery-only group and 64% for the group receiving adjuvant irradiation. The incidence of pelvic recurrences was 67% in the surgery-only group and 27% in the patients receiving adjuvant irradiation. The lack of impact on overall survival was probably related to the higher incidence of distant metastases in the irradiated patients, which may be a reflection of longer survival.

Stages IIB, III, and IV

The treatment for cervical cancer more advanced than stage IIA is irradiation. In stage IIB, practically all patients are treated with irradiation alone, and the 5-year survival rate is 60% to 65%. Occasionally, a conservative hysterectomy is performed after high-dose preoperative irradiation in patients with a

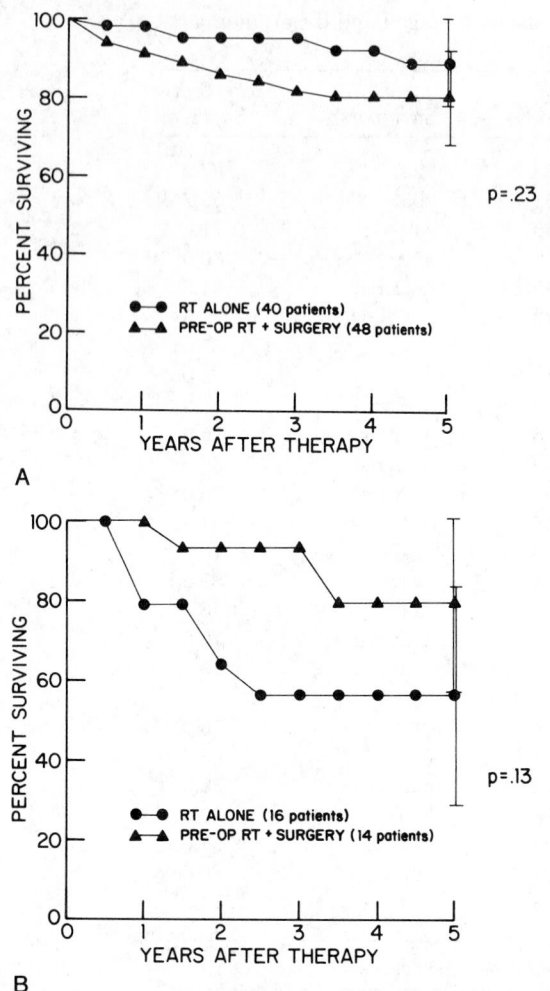

FIGURE 38–7. Actuarial survival without evidence of disease in patients with **(A)** stage IB or **(B)** IIA carcinoma of the uterine cervix treated with irradiation alone (*solid circles*) or a combination of low-dose preoperative irradiation and surgery (*solid triangles*). Randomized study, 1966–1979. Difference in survival is not statistically significant. (Perez CA, Camel HM, Kao MS, et al. Randomized study of preoperative radiation and surgery or irradiation alone in the treatment of stage IB and IIA carcinoma of the uterine cervix: Final report. Gynecol Oncol 1987;27:129)

barrel-shaped cervix and limited medial parametrial infiltration, which regresses completely 4 to 6 weeks after completion of irradiation.

In stage IIIB, the 5-year survival rates range from 25% to 48%. This variation may be related to the socioeconomic status of the patients, the extent of the disease, the techniques of irradiation, and the doses delivered to the parametria. Johns reported better pelvic tumor control and survival and fewer complications in a group of 65 patients with stages IIB or III cervical carcinoma treated with 23-MV photons compared with 61 patients treated with ^{60}Co external irradiation and intracavitary insertions.[347]

Isolated cases of stage IVA cervical cancer with involvement of the bladder or rectum without pelvic sidewall involvement can be treated by primary pelvic exenteration, but the best choice of therapy is primary irradiation.

Million and associates reported 16 (30%) of 53 patients

surviving 5 years after irradiation alone or combined with a surgical procedure for stage IVA carcinoma of the uterine cervix involving the bladder.[348] Most of these patients received 6000 cGy in 6 to 7 weeks to the whole pelvis supplemented with individualized doses of intracavitary radium. Six major complications were reported: 1 rectovaginal fistula, 2 vesicovaginal fistulae, 1 sigmoid perforation, and 2 skin necroses.

Kramer and associates reported 48 patients with stage IVA carcinoma of the cervix treated with definitive radiation therapy of 3000 to 4500 cGy to the whole pelvis with additional parametrial doses to complete 4000 to 6000 cGy combined with one or two intracavitary insertions for approximately 3000 to 5000 mgh, delivering 7000 to 8000 cGy or more to point A.[349] Fifteen of these patients also received 4000 to 4500 cGy of periaortic irradiation. Nine patients survived without recurrence; the 5-year actuarial survival rate was 18%. The rate of major complications was 22%, consisting mainly of vesicovaginal fistulae in 5 patients and severe radiation enteritis in 1 patient. The degree of parametrial involvement had a significant impact on prognosis. Patients with minimal disease had a 5-year survival rate of 46% compared with 5% for those with extensive parametrial tumor.

Interstitial parametrial implants were used to supplement standard external and intracavitary techniques. Prempree reported a 96% local tumor control rate and a 61% 5-year disease-free survival rate for 23 patients with intact uteri and stage IIIB carcinoma of the cervix treated with a combination of external irradiation and intracavitary and interstitial implants to the parametrium.[350] Prempree described a 23% local failure rate and a 69% 5-year survival rate for 26 patients with a similar stage carcinoma of the cervix treated in the same manner but for whom the uterine cavity could not be probed or was absent. Overall, major complications were observed in 8% of the 49 patients.

Aristizabal and colleagues described the treatment of 21 patients with locally advanced invasive carcinoma of the uterine cervix treated with transperineal interstitial implants using a specially designed plastic template.[351] With a mean follow-up of 26 months, local tumor control was reported in 18 (85%) of the patients. Seven patients (33%) developed grade 2 or 3 complications, which included vesicovaginal fistula (1 patient), rectovaginal fistula (1), or both fistula (1). Three patients developed severe radiation proctitis, cystitis, or both.

Martinez and associates, using a special applicator consisting of two acrylic cylinders, a template with an array of holes that serve as guides to localize the trocars, and a cover plate, treated 37 patients with advanced or recurrent carcinoma of the cervix and 26 patients with vaginal-urethral tumors.[352] The investigators reported 6 local failures in the patients with cervical lesions and 5 in the group with vaginal-urethral tumors. The overall complication rate was 5.1%.

Pierquin and associates described locoregional recurrences in 6% of 53 patients with T1, 11% of 47 patients with T2, and 42% of 19 patients with T3 primary tumors of the uterine cervix treated with a combination of external-beam irradiation and interstitial implantation of ^{192}Ir sources in a plastic cervical-vaginal moulage and a uterine tandem.[353]

Maruyama and Muir used californium 252 (^{252}Cf) neutron brachytherapy in conjunction with fractionated external irradiation to treat carcinoma of the uterine cervix.[354] They reported 41 patients with stage IB treated with 4000 to 5000 cGy to the whole pelvis followed by a 500- to 1500-cGy boost dose to the lateral pelvic wall. The ^{252}Cf neutron therapy was usually delivered in a single intracavitary insertion in approximately 8 hours. Near-total tumor clearance was achieved in more than 90% of the patients. Only a small group exhibited a slow clearance pattern.

Maruyama and associates reported 80 patients treated with ^{137}Cs brachytherapy and 544 treated with ^{252}Cf (combined with external pelvic irradiation), followed by extrafascial hysterectomy for bulky cervical carcinoma.[355] There were 37.5% positive specimens after ^{137}Cs and 22% after ^{252}Cf. The 5-year survival rate was 95%, and the pelvic failure rate was 5% in the negative-specimen group, and the 5-year survival rate was 58% with a 19% pelvic recurrence rate after ^{252}Cf and positive specimens. With ^{137}Cs, the 5-year survival rates were 89% with negative and 76% with positive specimens.

Maor and colleagues reported results in 156 patients with locally advanced cervical carcinoma (*i.e.*, stages IIB, III, IVA) treated at five institutions and randomized to receive external photons only to the pelvis (5000 cGy in 25 fractions in 5 weeks) or photon and neutron mixed-beam external irradiation (three fractions of photons per week) to a total relative biologic effectiveness adjusted dose of 5000 cGy over 5 weeks.[356] All patients were scheduled to receive intracavitary brachytherapy. Of 146 evaluable patients, 80 were treated with mixed beam and 66 were treated with photons. Only 50% of the patients in the mixed-beam group and 75% in the photon group underwent brachytherapy applications. Local control rates at 2 years were 45% in the mixed-beam group and 52% in the photon group. Median survival was 1.9 years and 2.3 years, respectively. Severe complications occurred in 19% of the mixed-beam group and 11% of the photon-beam group ($p < 0.13$). The inferior outcome with neutrons may have resulted from the use of horizontal beams of various energies and penetrations. A new randomized trial using high-energy hospital-based cyclotrons with gantry-mounted beam-delivery systems was activated.

If brachytherapy procedures cannot be performed for medical reasons or because of an unusual anatomic configuration of the pelvis or the tumor (*e.g.*, extensive lesion, inability to identify the cervical canal), higher doses of external irradiation may be used. Castro and colleagues reported results of 118 patients with invasive cervical carcinoma treated with 5000 to 6000 cGy to the whole pelvis (four-field box technique) and additional doses to residual tumor with reduced AP/PA portals to complete a 7000 cGy tumor dose.[357] With doses below 5000 cGy, no pelvic tumor control was obtained in 32 patients. However, disease control and survival were significantly enhanced with higher doses. Complications increased with higher doses.

Coia and coworkers, in an analysis of 565 patients with various stages of cervical carcinoma treated in the Patterns of Care Study, reported better survival (67%) and pelvic tumor control (78%) compared with patients who had no intracavitary brachytherapy applications (36% 4-year survival and 47% in-field failure).[358] Patients treated with two intracavitary applications had a higher 4-year survival rate (73%) and in-field tumor control (83%) than those receiving only one application (60% 4-year survival rate and 71% in-field tumor control).

Hanks and associates[322] and Montana and colleagues[328] reported a higher incidence of central-pelvic recurrences for patients with stage III cervical carcinoma treated with external beam alone than for patients receiving brachytherapy in addition to external-beam irradiation (Table 38–15).[322,328,358,359] The incidence of major complications was similar in both groups.

Combined Irradiation and Surgery

The results of several series that used combined irradiation and surgery are comparable with those obtained with irradiation alone. Perez and associates reported a randomized study of 118 selected patients with stages IB or IIA carcinoma of the uterine cervix.[334] Patients were treated with irradiation alone (as described previously) or with irradiation and surgery (2000 cGy to the whole pelvis and one intracavitary insertion for 5000 to 6000 mgh followed by a radical hysterectomy with pelvic lymphadenectomy 4 to 6 weeks later). The tumor-free actuarial 5-year survival rate for 40 stage IB patients treated with irradiation alone was 80%, and for 48 patients treated with preoperative irradiation and surgery, it was 82% ($p = 0.23$). For 16 patients with stage IIA carcinoma, the actuarial tumor-free survival rate was 56% with irradiation alone and 79% for 14 patients treated with irradiation and

TABLE 38–15. Carcinoma of the Uterine Cervix: Incidence of Central and Pelvic Recurrences According to Method of Therapy

| | | Incidence of Pelvic Failures | | |
| | | *External Beam Only (%)* | *External Beam and Intracavitary (%)* | *P Value* |
Investigations	*Stage*			
Hanks et al[322]	III	33/38 (86)	55/109 (50)	0.0002
Montana et al[328]	III	14/35 (40)	12/37 (32)	0.6725
Coia et al[358]	I, II, III	(53)	(22)	<0.01

(Perez CA, Kurman RJ, Stehman FB, Thigpen JT. Carcinoma of the uterine cervix. In: Hoskins WJ, Perez CA, Young RC, eds. Principles and practice of gynecologic oncology. Philadelphia: JB Lippincott, 1992:632)

surgery ($p = 0.13$). For patients with stage IB disease treated with irradiation alone, the pelvic failure rate was 2.5%, and the rate of distant metastases was 7.5%. For the preoperative irradiation and surgery group, the pelvic failure rate was 12.5%, and the rate of distant metastases was 4.2%. For stage IIA carcinoma, patients who received radiation therapy alone had a pelvic failure rate of 6.3%, a rate of 18.8% for combined pelvic recurrence with distant metastases, and a 12.5% rate for distant metastases alone. The incidence of grade 2 to 3 complications in patients receiving radiation therapy alone was 13.8% (*i.e.*, two vesicovaginal fistulae, one rectovaginal fistula, one rectal stricture). For patients treated with preoperative irradiation and surgery, 11% developed grade 2 to 3 complications (*i.e.*, one rectal stricture, one severe proctitis, one small bowel obstruction, three ureteral strictures).

Einhorn and colleagues, in a nonrandomized study, reported better survival in 49 patients with stage IB carcinoma treated with a combination of surgery and irradiation (100% at 5 years) than for 64 patients treated with irradiation alone (81% at 5 years).[360] No difference was observed for 25 patients with stage IIA cervical carcinoma treated with combined therapy and 40 patients treated with irradiation alone; both groups had a 5-year survival rate of approximately 75%. Patients with metastases to lymph nodes had survival rates that were approximately 50% of those with negative nodes.

The dose of irradiation delivered to the lymph nodes, the time of the operation, and the pathologic examination of the specimens are critical in determining the presence of post-irradiation residual tumor (Table 38–16).[309,361–371] Rampone and associates reported a 15% incidence of metastatic lymph nodes in 537 patients with stage IB cervical carcinoma treated with two preoperative intracavitary insertions (total of 6000 mgh), which delivered 1500 cGy to the pelvic lymph nodes.[364] All patients with positive nodes in the operative specimen were given postoperative external radiation to the pelvis. The 5-year survival rate was 92.9% for 456 patients with negative nodes and 52% for 81 patients with positive nodes.

Rutledge and coworkers reported a 3.3% rate of metastatic lymph nodes in 30 patients with stage I carcinoma and 10.3% in 39 patients with stage IIA carcinoma of the uterine cervix who underwent a bilateral pelvic lymphadenectomy 6 weeks after completing definitive radiation therapy.[370] The dose of irradiation to the lymph nodes was in the range of 5000 cGy, delivered with megavoltage external photon beam and two intracavitary radium insertions. The survival rates for the patients treated with irradiation alone or irradiation combined with lymphadenectomy were the same (Fig. 38–8).[372] The rate of complications was somewhat higher for patients treated with combinations of the two modalities.

For patients with large endocervical lesions (barrel-shaped) or with endometrial extension of cervical carcinoma, Durrance and associates recommend an extrafascial conservative hysterectomy 6 weeks after completing high-dose preoperative radiation consisting of 2000 cGy to the whole pelvis, 3000 cGy in split fields, and one intracavitary insertion of 6000 mgh.[337]

In an analysis of 128 patients with barrel-shaped stage IB or IIA carcinoma of the cervix, Perez and colleagues reported similar results with the combined treatment or with higher intracavitary doses (7500 cGy to point A) in addition to external irradiation consisting of 2000 cGy to whole pelvis and 3000 cGy to parametria with midline block.[270] The major cause of treatment failure with either approach was distant metastases.

Weems and associates, in comparing 123 patients with stage IB, IIA, or IIB carcinoma of the cervix of 6 cm or larger in diameter treated with irradiation alone and 44 patients treated with irradiation combined with hysterectomy, found no significant difference in the pelvic tumor control or survival with either treatment modality.[339]

TABLE 38–16. Carcinoma of the Uterine Cervix, Stages IB and IIA: Percentage of Metastatic Pelvic Lymph Nodes and Dose of Irradiation Delivered to Lymph Nodes

	Stage IB		*Stage IIA*		
Investigations	*Surgery Alone*	*Preoperative XRT*	*Surgery Alone*	*Preoperative XRT*	*Estimated Dose (cGy) to Nodes*
Christensen[309]	29/167 (17.4%)		27/104 (26%)		0
Morley[361]	18/143 (12.6%)				0
Morton[362]	9/38 (23.7%)	4/32 (12.5%)			1800
Sweeney and Douglas[363]		5/39 (13%)		9/54 (17%)	3500
Rampone[364]		81/137 (15%)			2000
Decker[365]		5/38 (13.2%)		11/45 (24.4%)	4000
Quigley[366]		13/136 (9.6%)			1800
Parker[367]	15/95 (16%)	6/73 (8%)	7/16 (44%)	20/71 (28%)	Not stated
Gray[368]	5/44 (11.4%)	3/58 (5.2%)	6/17 (35.3%)	Inc. with I	4500
Perez[369]		2/43 (4.6%)		2/24 (8.3%)	3000–4000
Perez[369]	0/32 (0)				4001–5000
Rutledge[370]		1/30 (3.3%)		4/39 (10.3%)	5000

(Modified from Perez CA, Breaux S, Askin F, et al. Irradiation alone or in combination with surgery in stage IB and IIA carcinoma of the uterine cervix. A non-randomized comparison. Cancer 1979;43: 1062)

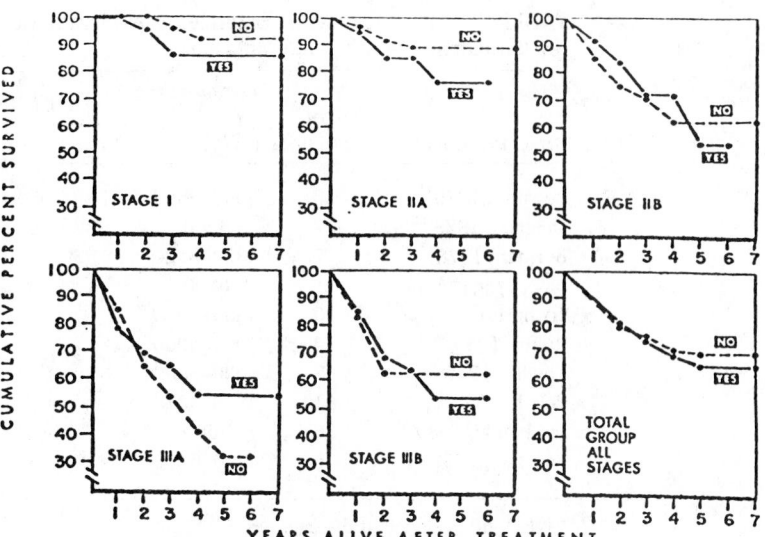

FIGURE 38–8. Survival curves of patients treated for squamous cell carcinoma of the cervix: stages I, IIA, IIB, IIIA, IIIB, and all stages combined. Patients who had lymphadenectomy after definitive irradiation to their treatment are represented by solid lines. The broken lines are for patients who had radiation treatment only. (Rutledge FM, Fletcher GM, Macdonald EJ. Pelvic lymphadenectomy as an adjunct to radiation therapy in treatment for cancer of the cervix. Am J Roentgenol Radium Ther Nucl Med 1969;106:831)

Thomas and coworkers reported 363 patients with bulky endocervical carcinoma treated with curative intent (*i.e.*, 246 with irradiation alone and 117 with irradiation and surgery).[373] Patients treated with radiation therapy alone had a 10-year survival rate of 45% compared with a survival rate of 64% with radiation therapy and surgery. However, the more bulky lesions were treated with radiation therapy alone. In a subset of 48 patients treated with radiation therapy alone and 45 patients treated with radiation therapy and surgery, the 10-year survival rates were comparable, and pelvic tumor control was 90% and 87%, respectively.

For patients with primary carcinoma of the uterine cervix who had endometrial stromal invasion of tumor in the curettings only, the addition of hysterectomy did not improve survival, and most of the patients failed because of distant dissemination.[371] Stage IVB cancer is managed by combinations of irradiation and chemotherapy.

RESULTS OF TREATING DISEASE METASTATIC TO PARAAORTIC LYMPH NODES. Paraaortic lymph node metastases are often an indication of distant dissemination, but they are clinically apparent in only 10% to 20% of the patients who have recurrences.

Nelson and associates reported 104 patients with stage II and III cervical carcinoma who underwent exploratory laparotomy and paraaortic lymph node biopsies.[374] Metastatic paraaortic lymph nodes were found in 12.5% of the patients with stage IIA disease, 14.9% with stage IIB disease, and 38.4% with stage III disease. These patients were treated with 6000 cGy to the paraaortic region. Within 4 years, 50% of these patients had distant metastases. Only 1 of 13 patients with positive paraaortic nodes was alive at the end of 4 years. Thirty-nine percent of the patients treated with paraaortic lymph node irradiation had grade 2 or 3 complications, compared with 32% of the patients who received radiation therapy to the pelvis only. No significant increase in intraperitoneal complications was observed among the patients who received paraaortic irradiation. However, the researchers did not recommend that 6000 cGy be given to the paraaortic area. They concluded that the main goal of exploratory laparotomy and paraaortic lymph node biopsy is to define the extent of the disease; extended dissection of the paraaortic lymph nodes is not, in itself, therapeutic.

Lovecchio and associates reported a 50% 5-year survival rate for 36 patients with stage IB or IIA cervical carcinoma identified before therapy at surgical staging laparotomy as having histologically confirmed paraaortic lymph node metastases.[375] These patients were treated with radiation therapy, including 4500 cGy to the paraaortic lymph nodes. Fourteen of 31 evaluable patients developed pelvic recurrence (12 combined with distant metastases). Unfortunately, the researchers did not specify how many patients had paraaortic recurrences, although they reported 4 with abdominal failures. Podczaski and associates reported 5 of 35 patients with surgically documented paraaortic metastasis treated with extended-field and pelvic irradiation (in 7 with concurrent chemotherapy).[376] Actuarial survival rates at 2 and 5 years were 32% and 29%, respectively. Twenty-three patients died from cervical cancer, and 4 patients died from intercurrent disease.

Goodman and associates compiled survival statistics on patients with paraaortic lymph node metastases and found an average 5-year survival rate of about 40% (Table 38–17).[265,375–383]

RESULTS OF ELECTIVE PARAAORTIC LYMPH NODE IRRADIATION. Rotman reported for the Radiation Therapy Oncology Group (RTOG) a randomized study of 335 patients with stages IB, IIA, or IIB carcinoma of the uterine cervix, with no clinical or radiographic evidence of paraaortic lymphadenopathy, who were randomized to electively receive or not receive 4500 cGy to the paraaortic region in addition to standard pelvic irradiation.[384] No significant difference was seen between the two groups ($p = 0.21$) in the rate of pelvic tumor control. The 5-year survival rate was 66% for the patients receiving elective paraaortic irradiation and 55% for those treated to the pelvis ($p = 0.043$). Although not statistically significant, the tumor control rate was better among the patients electively irradiated to the paraaortic area (75% versus 66% for the pelvic irradiated group) (Fig. 38–9).[385] Fourteen (8%) severe and 6 (4%) life-threatening complications occurred in the patients treated with pelvic irradiation

TABLE 38–17.   Results of Extended-Field Irradiation
for Paraaortic Lymph Node Metastases

Investigations	No. of Patients	Paraaortic Dose (cGy)	NED Survival*		Incidence of Severe Complications (%)
			2 Years	5 Years	
Lepanto, 1975[378]	36	5000–5500	11/26 (42%)	4/8 (50%)	19.5
Delgado, 1978[265]	13	4500	38%†		46.0
Berman, 1978[379]	7	4320–5120	57%‡		
Piver, 1981[380] (two cohorts)	21	6000		9.6%	61.9
	10	4400–5000		43.0%	10.0
Rubin, 1984[381]	14	4000–5000			36.0
Tewfik, 1982[382]	23	5000–5500	22.6§		35.0
Potish, 1983[383]	81	4350–5075		40.0%	2.4
Lovecchio, 1989[375]	36	4500	70%	50%	
Podczaski, 1990[376]	35	4250–5100	38	39%	9.0

* NED, no evidence of disease.
† Follow-up of 13 to 36 months.
‡ Follow-up of 4 to 25 months.
§ Follow-up of 45 months.
(Modified from Goodman HM, Bowling MC, Nelson JH Jr. Cervical malignancies. In: Knapp RC, Berkowitz RS, eds. Gynecologic oncology. New York, Macmillan, 1986:225–273)

only, and 13 (8%) severe and 11 (7%) life-threatening complications occurred in patients irradiated to the paraaortic lymph nodes.

A similar randomized study of 441 patients with cervical carcinoma who had an increased risk for lymph node metastasis but no clinical, radiographic, or surgical evidence of paraaortic lymph node involvement was reported by Haie and EORTC.[323] The paraaortic area received 4500 cGy with external-beam irradiation. No statistically significant difference was observed between the two treatment arms for local control, distant metastases, or survival. However, the incidence of paraaortic and distant metastases without pelvic failure was significantly higher among patients who received pelvic irradiation alone. The incidence of small bowel injury is 0.9%

in the pelvic irradiation group and 2.3% in the pelvic and paraaortic irradiation groups. A severe complication rate of 9% was observed among patients who received paraaortic irradiation, compared with 4.8% for those treated to the pelvis only.

Occult involvement of the paraaortic lymph nodes is a significant cause of treatment failure in some patients with carcinoma of the cervix. Treating the paraaortic region electively avoids the morbidity of treatment after surgical staging. Extended-field irradiation still has greater morbidity than pelvic therapy alone, even without surgical staging. Unfortunately, 37% of patients entered on the RTOG study had no radiographic evaluation of the paraaortic nodes before study entry. The reason the extended-field group had improved pelvic disease control (75% versus 66%) is unclear, but these studies provide a provocative alternative to surgical staging or systemic therapy.

Radiation Therapy

The application of radium therapy in the treatment of carcinoma of the cervix was first presented in 1913 at the Congress at Halle. Despite a slower regression after irradiation, reflecting cellular kinetics and slow growth, no difference in tumor control or survival was observed for adenocarcinomas compared with epidermoid carcinoma.[386] Because the endocervix is often involved in adenocarcinoma, a combination of irradiation and conservative hysterectomy was advocated.[302,338]

EXTERNAL IRRADIATION.   External irradiation is used to treat the whole pelvis and the parametria, including the common iliac lymph nodes, but central disease (*i.e.*, cervix, vagina, and medial parametria) is primarily irradiated with intracavitary sources. External pelvic irradiation is delivered before intracavitary insertions in patients with these indications:

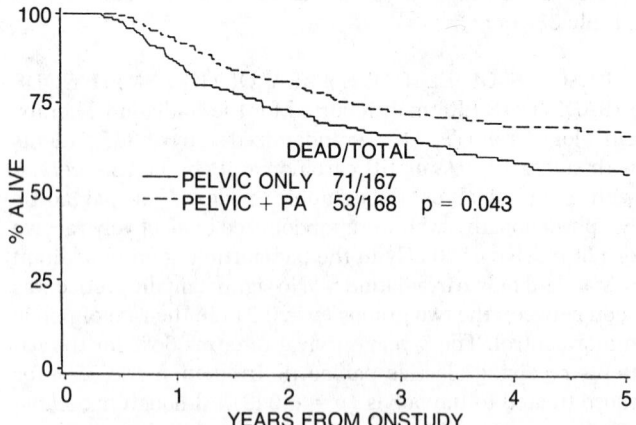

FIGURE 38–9.   Survival by assigned treatment for patients treated on Radiation Therapy Oncology Group protocol 79-20. (Rotman M, Choi K, Guse C, et al. Survival by assigned treatment (Kaplan-Meier) for patients treated on RTOG protocol 79-20. Int J Radiat Oncol Biol Phys 1990;19:513)

1. Bulky cervical lesions, to improve the geometry of the intracavitary application
2. Exophytic, easily bleeding tumors
3. Tumors with necrosis or infection
4. Parametrial involvement

VOLUME. In treating invasive carcinoma of the uterine cervix, it is critical to deliver adequate doses of irradiation to the pelvic lymph nodes. For stage IB carcinoma, 15×15 cm portals (at the surface of the patient) are sufficient. For patients with IIA, IIB, III, or IVA carcinoma, somewhat larger portals of 18×15 cm are required to cover all the common iliac nodes in addition to the cephalad half of the vagina (Fig. 38–10). A 2-cm margin lateral to the bony pelvis is sufficient. If no vaginal extension is present, the lower margin of the port is at the inferior border of the obturator foramen. If the vagina is involved, its entire length should be treated down to the introitus.

If metastatic periaortic lymph nodes are suspected or confirmed, the retroperitoneal tissues should be irradiated through a separate portal or with a field that includes the periaortic nodes and the pelvic tissues (*i.e.*, anterior and posterior, occasionally lateral portals).

BEAM ENERGIES. Because of the thickness of the pelvis, high-energy photon beams are especially suited for this treatment. They decrease the dose of radiation delivered to the peripheral normal tissues and provide a more homogenous dose distribution in the central pelvis. With lower-energy megavoltage beams (^{60}Co, 4–6-MV photons), higher maximal doses must be given, and a more complex portal arrangement is needed (*i.e.*, three fields or pelvic box technique) to minimize the dose to the bladder and the rectum while delivering an adequate dose in the cervix and the parametria.

BRACHYTHERAPY. Brachytherapy can be delivered with intracavitary techniques using applicators that consist of an

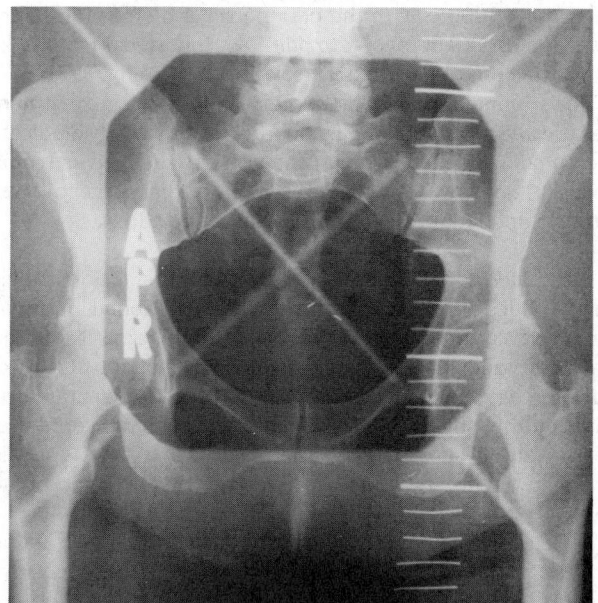

FIGURE 38–10. Simulation anteroposterior film of the pelvis, showing the volume treated with external irradiation that includes uterus, upper vagina, parametria, and pelvic lymph nodes.

intrauterine tandem and vaginal colpostats or, if necessary, with vaginal cylinders. Interstitial implants with needles or catheters, in which the radioisotopes (usually ^{192}Ir seeds in nylon strands) are implanted in limited tumor volumes, can be helpful in specific clinical situations (*e.g.*, localized residual tumor).

Intracavitary therapy, with its rapid dose fall-off as a function of distance, yields a high dose to the uterus and paracervical tissues (Fig. 38–11).[387] However, as the only modality used for treating pelvic lymph nodes, it is inadequate. Several isotopes are available, including ^{226}Ra, ^{60}Co, and ^{137}Cs. Currently, ^{137}Cs is the most popular.

Various applicators are used for intracavitary therapy. Remote control afterloading applicators allow better application, because the operators are not concerned about radiation exposure. The technique can be exploited to achieve an optimal dose distribution, with replacement or removal of sources in the tandem or the vaginal ovoids at different times. Radiographs of the application are always obtained with dummy sources; the active sources are inserted after the films are reviewed and the applicators are in a satisfactory position.

The first intracavitary insertion is scheduled after 1000 to 2000 cGy of external irradiation if an adequate geometry exists in the pelvis. Otherwise, 2000 to 4000 cGy are delivered before the first application to decrease the size of the lesion and to improve the relation of the applicators to the cervix and vagina. The second application is performed 1 to 3 weeks after the first insertion.

DOSES OF IRRADIATION. The optimal dose of irradiation for invasive carcinoma of the cervix is delivered with a combination of whole-pelvis, intracavitary, and sometimes interstitial therapy. Some institutions use lower doses of whole-pelvis external irradiation (*e.g.*, 1000 cGy for stage IB and 2000 cGy for stages IIA, IIB, III, and IVA) in addition to parametrial doses to complete 5000 cGy for stages IB, IIA, and IIB and 6000 cGy in more advanced stages. An assortment of step wedges, designed in accordance with the isodose curves of the intracavitary applications, or a 3-cm-wide rectangular 5 half value layer block is used to shield the midline. In addition, two intracavitary insertions deliver 7000 to 8000 mgh (6500–7200 cGy to point A).

This technique affords a high central dose to the cervix, paracervical tissues, and parametria and a moderate, homogenous dose to the external iliac lymph nodes, without exceeding the bladder and rectal tolerance doses (Fig. 38–12).[387] Other institutions prefer higher doses of whole-pelvis external irradiation (usually 4000 cGy) with an additional parametrial dose to complete 5000 cGy in patients with stages IB or IIA tumors and 6000 cGy for patients with IIB, III, or IVA tumors. This treatment is usually combined with one or two intracavitary insertions, for approximately 5000 to 6000 mgh (4500–5500 cGy to point A). If residual tumor is palpated at the completion of the prescribed course of therapy, an additional 1000 cGy through a small field of 8×12 cm to one parametrium or 12×12 cm to both parametria may be used to deliver an additional 1000 cGy. The midline block is left in place.

PREOPERATIVE IRRADIATION. At some institutions, the combination of preoperative irradiation and hysterectomy was used to treat patients with stages IB or IIA cervical cancer.[270]

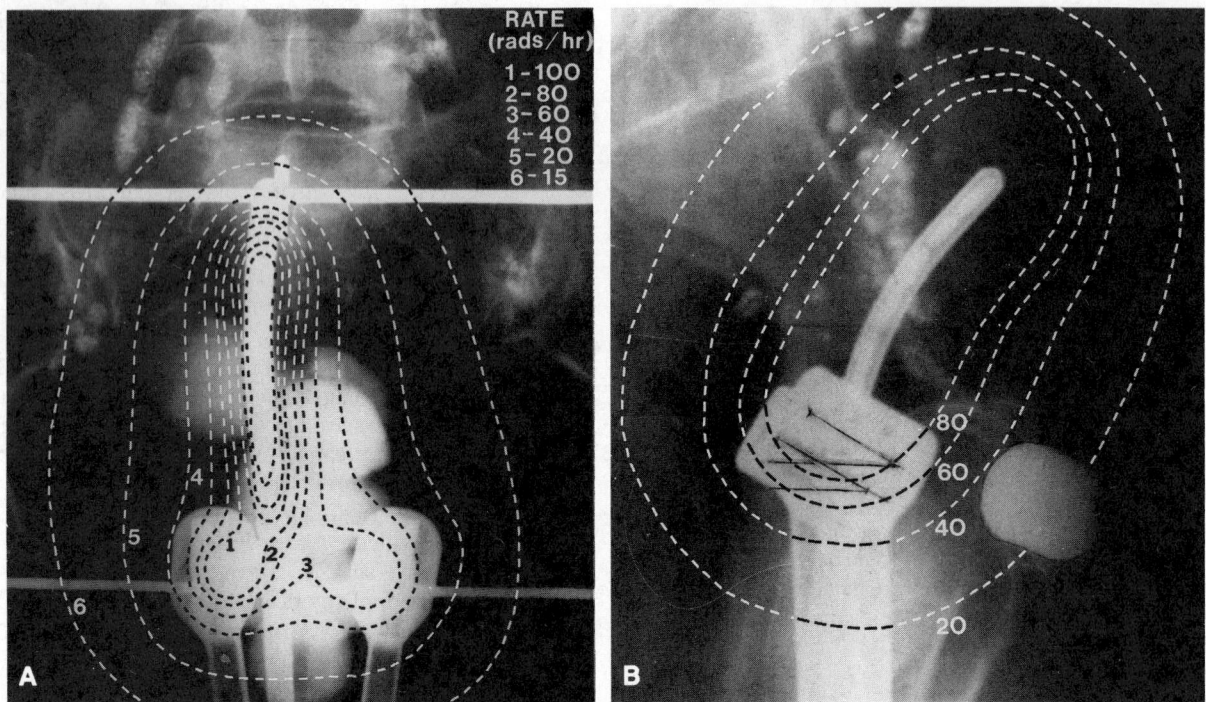

FIGURE 38–11.   (A) Anteroposterior and (B) lateral radiographs of a standard intracavitary insertion with afterloading Fletcher-Suit tandem and ovoids. Slight deviation of the tandem to the left is apparent. However, there is good symmetry between the tandem and the ovoids. On the lateral projection, the tandem is crossing the ovoids near the center of the long axis. Radiopaque marker is placed on the anterior lip of the cervix. A Foley balloon with Hypaque outlines the bladder neck. (Perez CA. Uterine cervix. In: Perez CA, Brady LW, eds. Principles and practice of radiation oncology. 2nd ed. Philadelphia: JB Lippincott, 1992:1169)

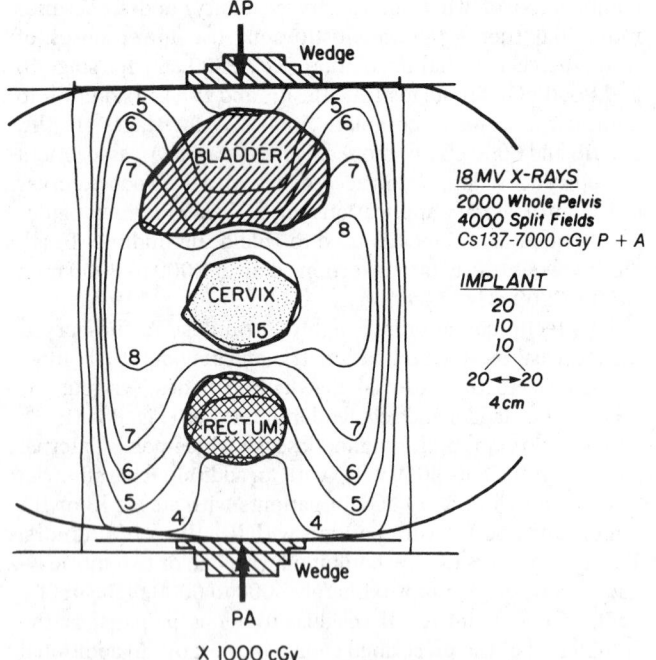

FIGURE 38–12.   Composite isodose curves through point A for patient with stage IIB carcinoma of the uterine cervix treated with external irradiation and two intracavitary insertions. Doses and source arrangement are shown. High doses can be delivered to the cervix and parametrial tissues with relative sparing of the bladder and rectum. (Perez CA. Uterine cervix. In: Perez CA, Brady LW, eds. Principles and practice of radiation oncology. 2nd ed. Philadelphia: JB Lippincott, 1992:1167)

Sometimes, an intracavitary insertion alone is used (5000–6000 mgh) before radical hysterectomy with pelvic lymphadenectomy. Brachytherapy can be combined with external irradiation (2000 cGy to the whole pelvis), in which case a radical hysterectomy and pelvic lymphadenectomy are performed. In other patients, 2000 cGy is delivered to the whole pelvis plus 3000 cGy to the parametria and an intracavitary insertion (5000–6000 cGy to point A), followed 4 to 6 weeks later by a conservative extrafascial hysterectomy.[270]

The rationale for adding surgery to irradiation treatment was the alleged inability of irradiation to completely eradicate the tumor at bulky primary sites or in the pelvic lymph nodes.[388] Some gynecologists also believe that surgery leaves a more functional vagina in sexually active patients.

POSTOPERATIVE IRRADIATION. If metastatic pelvic lymph nodes or positive surgical margins are found after hysterectomy, postoperative irradiation is delivered. If only intracavitary therapy was given preoperatively, 2000 cGy is administered to the whole pelvis and 3000 cGy to the parametria with midline shielding. If external therapy is delivered preoperatively, an additional parametrial dose of 5500 cGy should be given again, shielding the midline with an appropriate block.

For patients who were not irradiated preoperatively and in whom postoperative irradiation is indicated because of positive (central) surgical margins, we administer a combination of external irradiation consisting of 2000 cGy to the whole pelvis and 3000 cGy to the parametria with a small midline block, combined with an intracavitary insertion for 6000 cGy to the vaginal mucosa (1800 mgh) with two colpostats. For patients with positive pelvic or periaortic lymph nodes, external irradiation alone (5000 cGy to the midplane of the pelvis) is administered.

For patients receiving postoperative irradiation, extreme care should be taken in designing treatment techniques that include intracavitary insertions. Because of the surgical extirpation of the uterus, the bladder and the rectosigmoid may lie closer to the radioactive sources than in a patient with an intact uterus.[389] The vascular supply may have been affected by the surgical procedure, and adhesions can prevent mobilization of the small bowel loops that are occasionally fixed in the pelvis, increasing the risk of complications.

HYPERBARIC OXYGEN, HYPOXIC SENSITIZERS, AND HYPERTHERMIA COMBINED WITH IRRADIATION. Several reports were published on clinical trials evaluating the efficacy of hyperbaric oxygen combined with irradiation in the treatment of a variety of human tumors, including carcinoma of the uterine cervix.[390] Watson and colleagues, in a randomized clinical trial of 320 patients (stages III and IVA disease) who were treated at four institutions, reported a 5-year survival rate of 33% in the oxygen-treated group and 27% in the control group treated in air ($p = 0.08$).[391] The greatest improvement in survival was observed in women younger than 55, in whom the 5-year survival rate for those treated with oxygen was 50%, compared with 30% for the control group treated in air. The local recurrence rate was 33% for the 161 patients treated with oxygen and 53% for the 159 patients treated in air. The difference is statistically significant ($p = 0.001$). Morbidity among the patients treated with oxygen was greater (20 severe and 13 moderate complications) than in those treated in air (6 severe and 8 moderate). The difference was particularly striking for complications of the bowel (13 versus 2 severe complications).

Fletcher and colleagues reported that 233 patients with stages IIB, III, or IV cervical disease randomized to conventional irradiation in air or with hyperbaric oxygen demonstrated no significant benefit in survival or tumor control; 20 of 109 patients treated with oxygen failed in the pelvis in contrast to 29 of 124 treated in air.[392] The morbidity was greater (26 complications) in patients treated with hyperbaric oxygen than in the control group (15 complications). A smaller series reported by Glassburn and associates showed no benefit in survival but showed an increased morbidity with hyperbaric oxygen.[393] Hyperbaric oxygen, administered with fewer high-dose fractions, may be more efficacious than if combined with conventional dose and fractionation schemes.[394] The reported trials did not show an increased incidence of distant metastasis, which was reported in a clinical study and in some animal experiments.[395]

Thomas and colleagues described a phase I study of metronidazole in 80 patients with various stages of carcinoma of the uterine cervix.[396] The researchers suggested that a daily dose of 1.3 g/m² was well tolerated, but no tumor response data were reported. Phase III clinical trials were recommended.

Dische reported preliminary observations on the use of misonidazole in 10 patients with advanced carcinoma of the cervix.[397] The morbidity of this therapy is similar to that observed with irradiation alone, except for some misonidazole neurotoxicity. All 10 patients had more than 50% tumor regression, which was thought to be promising.

Leibel and the RTOG reported a randomized study of 119 patients with FIGO stage IIIB or IVA squamous cell carcinoma of the cervix who received radiation therapy alone (4600 cGy to the pelvis plus a 1000 cGy parametrium boost) followed by intracavitary or external boost to the primary tumor with or without misonidazole (400 mg/m² daily 2 to 4 hours before radiation therapy).[398] With a median follow-up of 33 months, 64% of the patients treated with radiation therapy alone and 54% receiving irradiation plus misonidazole were alive at 18 months. The median survivals were 1.9 years and 1.6 years, respectively. Grades 3 and 4 toxicity were observed in 5 patients receiving radiation therapy alone and in 3 patients in the irradiation plus misonidazole group.

These findings are similar to those reported by Overgaard and associates, who, in a randomized study of 331 patients with stage IIB, III, or IVA carcinoma of the uterine cervix treated with misonidazole or a placebo and irradiation, found no significant difference in local tumor control (50% versus 54%), disease-free survival (47% versus 46%), or crude survival (39% versus 45%).[399] Patients with hemoglobin levels below 7 mmol/L had significantly lower local tumor control (24% versus 47%).

The GOG has developed a protocol to compare misonidazole or hydroxyurea in combination with definitive irradiation in patients with stages IIB, III, or IV carcinoma of the uterine cervix.

HYPERTHERMIA AND IRRADIATION. Because of technologic limitations in attempting to deliver adequate heat to large parts of the body such as the pelvis, the evaluation of hyperthermia in the treatment of carcinoma of the uterine cervix was sparse. Hornback and associates reported a nonrandomized study indicating that the combination of microwave hyperthermia and irradiation (433 mgh) resulted in improved tumor control in a group of 79 patients with stage IIIB (72% local tumor control) compared with previously irradiated controls (35% and 53% tumor control).[400] However, 5-year survival rates were similar in all groups (22% to 30%).

Sharma and associates reported a 70% disease-free survival rate at 18 months in 20 patients with stage IIB or III carcinoma of the uterine cervix treated with a combination of irradiation and hyperthermia (*i.e.*, 13.5 MHz, 42°C to 43°C, 30 minutes before irradiation) compared with a 50% disease-free survival rate for 22 patients treated with irradiation alone.[401] The grade 3 complication rate (8%) was similar in both groups.

SEQUELAE OF IRRADIATION. Major complications of radiation therapy for stages I and IIA carcinoma of the cervix range from 3% to 5%, and for stages IIB and III, they range from 10% to 15%. The most frequent major complications for the various stages are listed in Table 38–18 and Table 38–19.[334,387] Perez and associates,[402] Kottmeier,[403] Pourquier and associates,[404] and others demonstrated a greater incidence of complications after high doses of irradiation. High doses of external irradiation to the whole pelvis were associated with a greater number of complications (Fig. 38–13).[402] Injury to the gastrointestinal tract usually is evident within the first 2

TABLE 38–18. Carcinoma of the Uterine Cervix: Grade 2 Complications
(MIR 1959–1986)

	Stage				
	IB	*IIA*	*IIB*	*III*	*IVA*
Total no. of patients treated	374	124	314	271	18
Number of complications	46 (12.3%)	16 (12.9%)	40 (12.7%)	25 (9.2%)	1 (5.6%)
Intestinal Complications					
Proctitis	6	1	10	4	
Rectal ulcer	1			2	
Sigmoid stricture		2	1	1	
Diverticulitis			1		
Small bowel obstruction	2		2	3	
Small bowel perforation				1	
Malabsorption	3		1	1	
Urinary Complications					
Chronic cystitis	2	2	6	3	
Bladder ulcer	2	1	1		
Ureteral stricture		1			
Incontinence			1		
Urethral stricture			1		
Extensive cystocele	1				
Other Complications					
Pelvic abscess				1	
Pulmonary embolus			1		
Subcutaneous fibrosis	1				
Vault necrosis	6	3	1	3	
Leg edema			1		
Hemorrhage			1		
Vaginal stenosis	21	4	6	6	1
Thrombophlebitis		1	2		
Arteriosclerosis	1		3		
Thrombosis of pelvic blood vessels		1			
Neuropathy			1		

(Perez CA. Uterine cervix. In: Perez CA, Brady LW, eds. Principles and practice of radiation oncology. 2nd ed. Philadelphia: JB Lippincott, 1992:1143–1202)

years after radiation therapy, but complications of the urinary tract are not likely to be seen until 3 to 4 years after treatment.

If preoperative radiation is combined with surgery, the complication rate tends to be somewhat higher (5–10%) because of the potential injury to the ureters or bladder (*e.g.,* ureteral stricture, ureterovaginal or vesicovaginal fistula). The dose and technique of irradiation and the type of surgical procedures that are performed are important in determining the morbidity of combined therapy.

The pretherapy staging laparotomy can lead to a significant increase in the rate of complications, particularly if irradiation (5000–5500 cGy) is given, because of metastases to paraaortic lymph nodes. The most common operative complications include pneumonia, thrombophlebitis, cardiovascular accident, hepatitis, and evisceration. Late sequelae resulting from combined surgery and irradiation in the abdomen and pelvis include small bowel obstruction, stricture and fibrosis of the

intestine, and rectosigmoid, rectovaginal, or vesicovaginal fistulae.

Improvements in anesthesia, surgical technique, and antibiotic therapy have reduced the mortality from radical hysterectomy with pelvic lymphadenectomy to 1% or less.[288] Complications of this procedure include ureterovaginal fistula, the incidence of which has decreased to less than 3%.

The overall incidence of complications is between 5% and 20%, depending on the extent of periaortic lymph node dissection, the choice of transperitoneal or retroperitoneal approach, and the dose of irradiation.[405] Tewfik and colleagues reported a 27.8% complication rate for a group of 23 patients (most of whom had stage IIIB carcinoma of the cervix) who were treated with laparotomy and pelvic or periaortic nodal irradiation.[382] Komaki and colleagues reported 3 patients (14%) with small bowel obstructions in a group of 22 patients who received 5000 to 5500 cGy to the periaortic areas for

TABLE 38–19. Carcinoma of the Uterine Cervix, MIR 1966–1979, Stages IB and IIA: Major Complications of Treatment

| | Stage IB | | | | Stage IIA | | | |
| | Radiation Therapy Alone (40 Patients) | | Preoperative Radiation Therapy + Surgery (48 Patients) | | Radiation Therapy Alone (16 Patients) | | Preoperative Radiation Therapy + Surgery (14 Patients) | |
Complications	Grade 2	Grade 3	Grade 2	Grade 3	Grade 2	Grade 3	Grade 2	Grade 3
Rectovaginal fistula		1 (2.5%)						
Vesicovaginal fistula		2 (5%)						
Ureteral stricture		1 (2.5%)		1 (2.1%)				2 (14.3%)
Wound infection			1 (2.1%)					
Subcutaneous fibrosis	1 (2.5%)							
Vault necrosis	1 (2.5%)		1 (2.1%)		1 (6.3%)		1 (7.1%)	
Pelvic infection		1 (2.5%)						
Vaginal stenosis	6 (15%)		1 (2.1%)		2 (12.5%)			
Thrombophlebitis			2 (4.2%)					
Pelvic arteriosclerosis	1 (2.5%)							
Proctitis								1 (7.1%)
Rectal stricture						1 (6.3%)		1 (7.1%)
Acute pelvic cellulitis							1 (7.1%)	
Small bowel stricture								1 (7.1%)
Lymphocyst							1 (7.1%)	

(Perez CA, Camel HM, Kao MS, et al. Randomized study of preoperative radiation and surgery or irradiation alone in the treatment of stage IB and IIA carcinoma of the uterine cervix: Final report. Gynecol Oncol 1987;27:129)

histologically proved nodal metastases from carcinoma of the cervix or endometrium.[405] Potish and associates described only 2 patients with small bowel obstructions and 3 patients with large bowel complications among 81 patients with cervical carcinoma treated with radiation therapy alone (including periaortic lymph nodes) and no surgical exploration.[383]

The risks of paraaortic nodal irradiation should be compared with its effect on survival. Several researchers reported survival rates of 30% to 40%, but others reported lower rates.[382,405,406]

Surgical Techniques

From Freund's first hysterectomy for cervical cancer in 1878 to the description of total pelvic exenteration by Brunschwig in 1948, surgical treatment played a vital role in the management of this disease.[407,408] The following sections of this chapter discuss the major surgical procedures that are used, but we do not provide detailed descriptions or illustrations of these procedures. The interested reader is referred to *Telinde's Operative Gynecology*.[409]

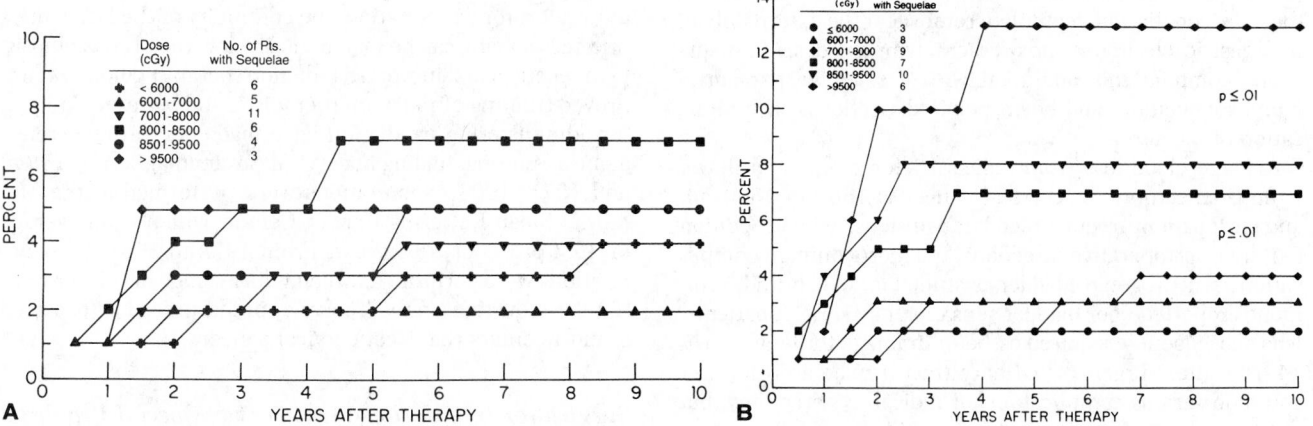

FIGURE 38–13. Carcinoma of the uterine cervix between 1959 and 1986. **(A)** Actuarial rate of severe urinary sequelae correlated with total dose to the bladder. **(B)** Actuarial rate of severe rectal or rectosigmoid sequelae correlated with total dose to the rectum. (Perez CA, Fox S, Lockett MA, et al. Impact of dose in outcome of irradiation alone in carcinoma of the uterine cervix: Analysis of two different methods. Int J Radiat Oncol Biol Phys 1991;21:885–898)

CERVICAL CONIZATION. Conization of the cervix may be diagnostic or therapeutic. It is used for the diagnostic evaluation of patients with cervical intraepithelial neoplasia or microinvasive carcinoma and is the standard therapeutic option for patients with CIN-3. Complications associated with cervical conization include hemorrhage, cervical stenosis, and uterine perforation.

TOTAL EXTRAFASCIAL ABDOMINAL HYSTERECTOMY. Total abdominal hysterectomy for the treatment of cervical carcinoma involves the removal of the uterus and the cervix. The plane of excision lies just outside the pubocervical fascia and does not require unroofing of the ureters as they pass through the cardinal ligaments. A small vaginal cuff can easily be excised. Hysterectomy is indicated in selected cases of CIN-3 and of microinvasive cervical carcinoma of less than 3 mm invasion if there is no lymphovascular invasion. Extrafascial hysterectomy is also used by some physicians after irradiation for barrel-shaped stages IA and IB cervical carcinoma and after irradiation in early stage disease if the endometrium is involved.

MODIFIED RADICAL HYSTERECTOMY. In the modified radical hysterectomy, the ureter is unroofed from its canal, but the lateral attachments with their blood supply are preserved. Parametrial and paracervical tissues medial to the ureter are removed, and a larger vaginal cuff is taken. This operation is rarely used today, although some authorities recommended it for microinvasive carcinoma of the cervix.

RADICAL ABDOMINAL HYSTERECTOMY WITH BILATERAL PELVIC LYMPHADENECTOMY. In the radical hysterectomy, the ureters are dissected completely free from their tunnels through the paracervical tissues, and the bladder is dissected free of the upper third of the vagina. The uterosacral ligaments are severed posteriorly near their point of origin, and the cardinal ligaments are severed at the lateral pelvic sidewall. This allows complete removal of the parametrial, paracervical, and upper paravaginal tissues and removal of the upper one fourth to one third of the vagina.

The lymphadenectomy begins at the middle of the common iliac vessels and consists of removal of the distal one half of the common iliac and complete removal of the external iliac, hypogastric, obturator, and presacral lymph nodes. Many surgeons combine this operation with a selective paraaortic lymphadenectomy and begin pelvic dissection at the bifurcation of the aorta.[288]

Average blood loss from radical hysterectomy and pelvic lymphadenectomy for cervical cancer is 1500 to 1800 ml, and most patients require blood transfusions.[216,288] In addition to minor postoperative infections, the most common complication is neurogenic bladder dysfunction. Webb and Symmonds reported poor bladder sensation in 31.5% of patients, who subsequently required catheter drainage for longer than 14 days after surgery.[410] Urinary tract fistulae are the most common serious complications of radical hysterectomy, but most modern series report an incidence of less than 2%.[216,288,317] Pelvic lymphocysts and pelvic abscess are infrequent problems that result from the use of closed suction drainage of the pelvis.

Radical hysterectomy is used for stages IB and IIA cervical carcinoma. Its advantages and disadvantages were cited previously. In the hands of well-trained, experienced surgeons, this procedure has an acceptable complication rate that is comparable with the complication rate for full pelvic irradiation. Symmonds pointed out that the complications of radical hysterectomy are more often amenable to correction than are the late complications of irradiation.[317]

SELECTIVE PARAAORTIC LYMPHADENECTOMY. Selective paraaortic lymphadenectomy or paraaortic lymph node biopsy is an integral part of the management of patients with cervical carcinoma. Its use in pretreatment surgical staging has been discussed. Many surgeons perform this procedure before radical hysterectomy, believing that the patient is better treated by extended-field irradiation if the lymph nodes contain metastatic cancer. Enlarged or suspicious lymph nodes seen on CT scan or lymphangiography can sometimes be sampled by fine-needle aspiration guided by CT scan or fluoroscopy. If the sampling procedure is inadequate, paraaortic node biopsy is indicated.

PELVIC EXENTERATION. The use of pelvic exenteration for recurrent cervical cancer after irradiation therapy was introduced at the Memorial Sloan-Kettering Cancer Center by Brunschwig in 1948.[408] In 1960, Brunschwig and Daniel reported 592 exenterations with a 5-year survival rate of 17% and an operative mortality of 23%.[411] In 1987, Lawhead and associates reviewed the Memorial Sloan-Kettering Cancer Center experience with pelvic exenteration for the years 1972 to 1981 and reported an operative mortality of 9.8% and a 5-year survival rate of 23%.[412] As of December 1981, 1129 pelvic exenterations had been performed on the Gynecology Service at the Memorial Sloan-Kettering Cancer Center.

Total pelvic exenteration includes removal of the bladder, urethra, uterus, cervix, vagina, rectum, and all lateral supporting tissues. Most surgeons differentiate between supralevator exenterations that stop at the floor of the pelvis and infralevator exenterations that excise part or all of the pelvic floor and include removal of the vulva. Posterior exenteration allows preservation of the urinary tract, and anterior exenteration preserves the rectum. The urinary conduit can be constructed from the ileum, sigmoid, or transverse colon. In a supralevator exenteration, the continuity of the large intestine occasionally can be maintained by low rectal anastomosis.

In recent years, improved radiation therapy equipment, improved training of radiation therapists, and better techniques for administering irradiation have made central recurrence alone an unusual finding in cervical carcinoma. Between 1948 and 1971, 1064 exenterations were performed at the Memorial Sloan-Kettering Cancer Center, which is an average of 46.3 procedures per year. From 1972 to 1981, 65 exenterations were performed, which is an average of 6.5 per year. Similar reductions in the frequency of this procedure occurred at most centers that treat cervical cancer.

Surgical or Irradiation Treatment of Special Problems

PALLIATION OF LOCALLY ADVANCED CARCINOMA OF THE CERVIX. Irradiation can be effective for palliation of pelvic pain or bleeding. It can also be useful for patients with advanced tumors whose general condition does not warrant a prolonged course of external irradiation with conventional fractionation. If vaginal bleeding is the main concern, a single intracavitary insertion with tandem and colpostats for about 6000 mgh (5500 cGy to point A) suffices. If previous irradiation was delivered, lower intracavitary doses are prescribed (4500 to 5000 mgh).

Several high-dose fractionation schedules were used, and Meoz and colleagues described satisfactory palliation with single doses of 1000 cGy combined with misonidazole, delivered every 3 to 6 weeks for a total of 3000 cGy.[413] The rate of complications in the long-term survivors was 15%, which is relatively high.

Spanos and associates reported a phase II study of daily multifraction split-course irradiation in 142 patients; half had recurrent or metastatic disease in the pelvis only, and the other half had associated extrapelvic metastases.[414] Irradiation consisted of 370 cGy per fraction given twice daily for two consecutive days, repeated at 3- to 6-week intervals for a total of three courses and a total tumor dose of 4440 cGy. The dose was based on linear quadratic equation considerations of acute and late effects, assuming an α/β ratio of 10 for acute and 4 for late effects. Occasionally, this regimen was combined with an intracavitary insertion (4500 mgh), blocking the midline for the last 1440 cGy external dose. Eighty-three (59%) of the 142 evaluable patients received three courses of irradiation; 29 (20%) received two courses, and an additional 29 (20%) received one course. Complete responses were observed in 15 patients (10.5%), and partial responses occurred in 32 (22.5%). For patients who completed three courses of irradiation, the complete plus partial response rate was 45%. Twenty-seven patients survived more than 1 year; only two cases of grade 3 toxicity (lower gastrointestinal) were reported.

These results show a significant decrease from the 11% incidence of grade 3 and 19% incidence of grade 4 complications (mostly intestinal) previously reported by Spanos and associates for 46 patients treated with 1000-cGy fractions given every 4 weeks for a total of 3000 cGy combined with misonidazole (4 g/m² administered 4 to 6 hours before irradiation).[413,415] Multiple daily fractionation appears to be a safe way to deliver palliative irradiation. The RTOG study was expanded to a phase III protocol, randomizing between a 2-week or 4-week rest period between the split courses of irradiation.

TREATMENT OF RECURRENT CARCINOMA OF THE CERVIX AFTER DEFINITIVE IRRADIATION. Irradiation of previously irradiated patients must be undertaken with extreme caution. The techniques used in the initial treatment (*e.g.,* beam energy, volume, external or intracavitary irradiation) must be analyzed, and the period of time between the two treatments must be taken into account.

We usually give external irradiation to limited volumes (*i.e.,* 4000–4500 cGy, 180 cGy/fraction, preferentially using lateral portals). Intracavitary or interstitial irradiation occasionally can be used to treat relatively circumscribed recurrences. In some patients, this treatment is combined with weekly regional hyperthermia.[210]

Sommers and colleagues described the results of retreatment of 376 patients with recurrent carcinoma of the uterine cervix.[416] Ninety-one patients received irradiation, mostly external (86.8%) and occasionally combined with brachytherapy

(7.7%), to control bleeding of central recurrences; brachytherapy alone was administered in 5.5% of the patients. The mean pelvic dose was 4130 cGy. Significant morbidity was observed in only 1 of 4 patients. The usual dose for paraaortic lymph node metastases was 4500 to 5000 cGy in 5 weeks. Other metastatic sites were treated with approximately 3500 to 4000 cGy over 3 to 4 weeks. Pelvic exenteration was attempted in 23 patients, only 10 of whom were deemed inoperable (43.5%), but it was completed in only 7. Chemotherapy was administered to 22 patients, frequently alone, but occasionally combined with surgery or irradiation. Multiple cytotoxic agent combinations were employed, mostly cisplatin (50–75 mg/m²) or 5-FU (750–1000 mg/m²) in continuous infusion over 4 days.

The probability of 5-year survival after treatment for recurrence was 30% for patients treated with combined surgery and external irradiation, 12% for patients treated with surgery, and 4% for patients who received external irradiation (Fig. 38–14).[417] The 5-year survival rate for the 10 patients who underwent pelvic exenteration was 16%. Patients who had failed only in the pelvis and were reirradiated with a secondary curative aim had a 40% (2 of 5) 5-year survival rate. Only 1% of the untreated patients survived 5 years. Six (4.3%) of 140 patients experienced grade 2 or 3 complications. Four of these complications (*i.e.,* cystitis, urethral constricture, malabsorption, leg edema, each in one patient) were thought to be related to irradiation and two to surgery (*i.e.,* pulmonary embolism, small bowel perforation, each in one patient). These results indicate that, although patients who fail after initial treatment have a poor prognosis, some patients with limited pelvic disease and particularly with central recurrences can be salvaged by additional aggressive therapy.

Contrary to this report, Thomas and colleagues found a median survival of only 7 months for 242 patients with recurrent carcinoma of the uterine cervix of all stages who were primarily treated with irradiation.[396] All the patients died within

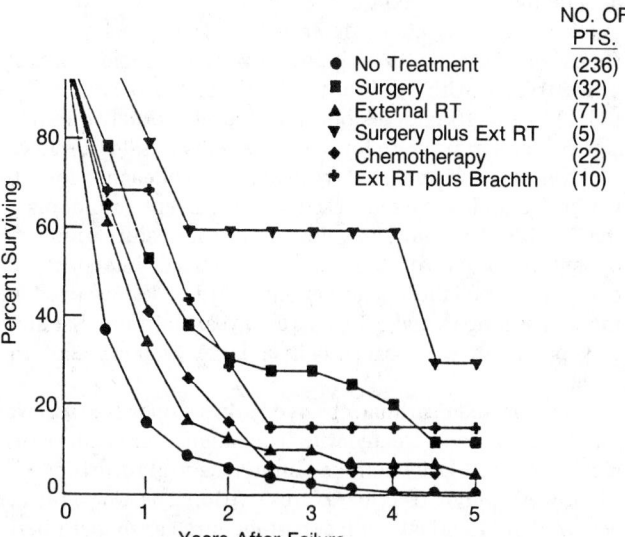

FIGURE 38–14. Actuarial survival after treatment of recurrent disease by type of therapy. (Sommers GM, Grigsby PW, Perez CA, et al. Actuarial survival after treatment of recurrent disease by type of therapy. Gynecol Oncol 1989;35:150)

24 months of treatment for recurrence, with the exception of 1 patient who was salvaged by hysterectomy for a central failure.

Puthawala and associates used interstitial implants to treat 14 patients with pelvic recurrences who had received definitive radiation therapy at the time of initial treatment for carcinoma of the uterine cervix.[418] Seven (50%) of the 14 patients exhibited tumor control. Palliation of symptoms after reirradiation was obtained in about 80% of the patients. No postoperative mortality was reported. Severe complications occurred in 15% of the patients, including soft tissue necrosis and one instance each of rectovaginal fistula, vesicovaginal fistula, enterovaginal fistula, and rectal stricture.

Prasasvinichai and associates reported a 17.6% 5-year survival rate for 51 patients with recurrent tumors limited to the pelvis who were treated with irradiation alone (31 patients), pelvic exenteration (10), or a combination of exploratory laparotomy, debulking, and irradiation (10).[419] Prempree and colleagues treated 8 patients with late invasive cervical carcinoma who had recurrences after primary irradiation.[420] Three survived tumor free for more than 5 years after retreatment.

After Previous Surgery. Recurrences can be more easily treated with irradiation after surgery than after initial irradiation. We recommend a combination of external irradiation of 2000 to 4000 cGy total dose, depending on tumor volume, and an additional parametrial dose with midline shielding, for a total of 5000 to 6000 cGy. An intracavitary insertion, covering the vaginal vault or the entire vagina, depending on tumor volume, should also be delivered. The total mucosal dose from external and intracavitary therapy can approach 14,000 cGy in the upper vagina and 9800 cGy in the distal vagina without high risk. This treatment can be combined with interstitial irradiation to boost the dose to the vaginal vault, the parametrium, or the paravaginal tissues, as indicated by the volume of disease. Doses in the range of 2000 to 3000 cGy are administered with single, double, or volume implants, depending on the extent of the tumor.

Jobsen and associates described 16 (88%) complete responses in 18 patients with postsurgical locoregional recurrence treated with 5000 to 6000 cGy to the pelvis.[421] Five (31%) of the 16 patients developed a second pelvic failure. The 5-year survival rate for the 18 patients was 44%. A lower survival rate was reported by Evans and colleagues for 114 patients found to have unresectable recurrent carcinoma of the cervix after primary irradiation or surgical treatment.[422] Seventy patients were treated with external, interstitial, or combined irradiation. Ten percent of the patients lived 15 months or longer, and 5% survived 5 years or more. Satisfactory palliation was observed in a large proportion of the patients.

Friedman and Pearlman observed a 42% tumor-free survival rate for 38 patients treated with irradiation after primary surgical therapy, 14 of whom had limited central recurrence.[423] Eight were tumor free for 3.5 to 9 years. The worst results occurred in 11 patients with persistent or recurrent peripheral pelvic tumor, 3 of whom survived tumor free for more than 5 years, and in 6 patients with massive pelvic recurrences, in whom only palliation was attained.

Krebs and associates, in 312 patients with carcinoma of the cervix that had been treated surgically, reported 40 recurrences (13%).[424] Eleven were limited to the central pelvis. The 5-year salvage rate for the 40 patients with recurrences was 13%. Webb and colleagues analyzed 104 recurrences after initial surgical treatment (predominantly for stage IB tumors) and found a 5.7% 5-year survival rate after treatment for recurrence.[425]

Larson and associates reported 27 (11%) recurrences in 249 patients treated with radical hysterectomy and pelvic lymphadenectomy for stage IB of the cervix.[426] Seventeen patients had recurrences in the pelvis or vulva; the other 10 patients developed recurrences outside the pelvis. Eight (53%) of 15 patients treated with irradiation for an isolated recurrence in the pelvis or vulva were tumor free at 10 to 126 months after treatment of the recurrence (median, 48 months).

Nori and colleagues reported 75 patients with recurrent cervical cancer treated with external, intracavitary, or interstitial irradiation, and some were treated with surgery.[427] Relief was obtained in 70% of the patients with symptoms. Ten percent of the patients survived 5 years. Early complications were observed in 10 patients, and 5 patients developed late complications that required surgical intervention.

CARCINOMA OF THE CERVICAL STUMP. Subtotal hysterectomy, which was a relatively popular procedure for benign conditions of the uterus in past years, is rarely performed today. Patients who undergo this procedure are at risk for carcinoma of the uterine cervix.

Patients with carcinoma of the cervical stump are divided into two groups: *true*, if the first symptom occurs 3 or more years after subtotal hysterectomy, or *coincidental*, if the symptoms are noticed before the third postoperative year. Moss and colleagues recommend 2 elapsed years after hysterectomy as the time for classification of these lesions.[428] This distribution is important because the prognosis for carcinoma of the true stump is significantly better than for coincidental lesions that probably indicate that carcinoma was present when the hysterectomy was performed.

The natural history and patterns of spread for carcinoma of the cervical stump are similar to those for cervical cancer in the intact uterus. The diagnostic workup, clinical staging, and basic principles of therapy are the same. If surgery is performed for stage I tumors, it is somewhat more difficult because of the previous surgery and adhesions in the pelvis. Nevertheless, radical trachelectomy and bilateral pelvic lymphadenectomy is excellent therapy for selected patients.

The lack of a uterine cavity in which to insert a tandem with three or more sources makes intracavitary therapy difficult. If possible, sources should be inserted into the remaining cervical canal. Transvaginal irradiation may be used to boost the dose delivered to central disease in the stump. More whole-pelvis irradiation should be delivered.

Patients with stage I disease usually are treated with a combination of 2000 cGy to the whole pelvis and 3000 cGy to the parametria, with midline shielding, combined with two intracavitary insertions. The dose of intracavitary therapy depends on the number of sources that can be placed in the cervical canal (*e.g.*, 1000–3000 mgh for 1–3 sources). The vaginal vault should receive about 7000 cGy mucosal dose (approximately 2000 mgh).

More advanced stages of disease should be treated with a dose of 4000 cGy to the whole pelvis and 2000 cGy to the parametria with midline shielding, combined with the same intracavitary doses. For bulky disease in the cervix, parametrium, or vagina, interstitial therapy with needles is advisable. If sources cannot be inserted into the cervical canal, the whole-pelvis dose must be increased to 6000 cGy. If using intravaginal irradiation, a 3000- to 5000-cGy air dose is delivered over 2 to 4 weeks in three to five weekly fractions. Moss and colleagues limit the transvaginal irradiation dose to the vaginal vault to 3000 cGy over 10 days.[428]

The 5-year survival rate for carcinoma of the cervical stump treated with irradiation is similar to that reported for patients with carcinoma of the intact uterus.[429] Creadnick reported results of 83 patients, 25 of whom were treated with radical trachelectomy and pelvic lymphadenectomy.[430] The salvage rate was 85.7% for squamous cell carcinoma and 50% for adenocarcinoma (stages I and II). The anatomic sites of failure and the incidence of recurrences were similar to those seen with an intact uterus. Distant metastases also follow the same distribution.

For 253 patients with carcinoma of the cervical stump treated at the M.D. Anderson Cancer Center, the median survival was 203, 140, and 32 months for stages I, II, and III, respectively.[431] Goodman and coworkers described pelvic recurrences in 4 of 7 patients with stage I adenocarcinoma of the cervical stump treated with external irradiation (4500–5500 cGy) to the whole pelvis and intracavitary insertions.[432] Only 1 patient was alive tumor free, and 2 died from intercurrent disease at 28 and 63 months. Six (66%) of 9 patients with stage IIA to IIIB tumors developed pelvic failures, and only 1 patient survived 5 years. Although 3 patients with adenoacanthoma survived, none of 5 with adenosquamous cell carcinoma survived.

Kovalic and colleagues reported 70 patients with carcinoma of the surgical stump treated with various irradiation techniques; 16 of these patients also underwent a surgical procedure.[433] The 10-year disease-free survival rates were 100% for stage IA, 79% for stage IB, 66% for stage IIB, and 39% for stage IIIB disease. The pelvic failure rates were 10% in stage IB (2 of 19), 9% in stage II (2 of 12), and 50% in stage IIIB disease (3 of 6). Major gastrointestinal complications were observed in 9% of the patients, and urinary complications occurred in 3.8%. These results are comparable to those seen in patients treated for invasive carcinoma of the cervix with an intact uterus.

Because of the proximity of the bladder, rectum, and small intestine to the intracavitary sources and the higher doses of whole-pelvis external-beam irradiation that are often given, complications are somewhat more frequent in carcinoma of the cervical stump than in carcinoma of the cervix with an intact uterus. Wimbush and Fletcher reported 5 patients with fistulae, 6 with severe proctosigmoiditis, and 12 with vault necrosis among 238 patients treated with definitive radiation therapy.[429]

CARCINOMA OF THE CERVIX DURING PREGNANCY. Preinvasive and invasive cervical carcinomas that occur during pregnancy require the combined expertise of the gynecologic oncologist, maternal-fetal medicine specialist, and sometimes the radiation oncologist. An abnormal Pap smear in a pregnant patient should be evaluated by colposcopy and biopsy.[434] Endocervical curettage should not be performed, but the physiologic eversion of the cervix in pregnancy usually allows easy visualization of the squamocolumnar junction. Biopsy of the cervix requires a well-equipped treatment room because of the likelihood of profuse bleeding. Conization of the cervix should be performed in patients with biopsies or Pap smears indicating invasion, but less severe lesions can usually be followed by colposcopy and Pap smears with biopsy as needed until the postpartum period. Several researchers reported the use of cervical conization in pregnancy with small to significant increases in morbidity and pregnancy wastage.[435,436]

If invasive cancer of the cervix is encountered, the patient must be evaluated by an oncologist and a specialist in maternal-fetal medicine. The patient should be informed of all therapeutic options and the possible effects on her and the fetus.

A tertiary care level intensive care nursery can reliably obtain survival rates of about 80% for fetuses delivered at 28 weeks of gestation (1000-g fetus).[437] For fewer than 24 weeks of gestation, the pregnancy should be disregarded. Patients who are 28 weeks pregnant or more should deliver the fetus by cesarean section. Between 24 and 28 weeks, the patient and her physician must weigh the advantages and disadvantages of all courses of action, because even though fetal survival rates at 28 weeks' gestation are excellent, significant morbidity is associated with the small-birth-weight infant. Greer and colleagues reviewed 600 infants without congenital abnormalities and found that, in cases of stage IB cervical carcinoma during pregnancy, neonatal mortality decreased from 30% at 26 to 28 weeks to 2.7% if the fetus was allowed to mature to 34 to 35 weeks.[438] The investigators could not define any adverse maternal outcomes with delays of up to 17 weeks. The actual treatment of the cancer depends on the stage of disease and the usual considerations in selecting therapy. Radical hysterectomy can be performed with the fetus in situ or, in the case of a viable fetus, immediately after delivery by cesarean section. If radiation is used, the patient usually aborts during the course of pelvic irradiation; if this does not occur, the uterus must be evacuated before insertion of intracavitary irradiation.[439,440] Survival was similar in pregnant and nonpregnant patients matched by stage of disease, regardless of the gestational age of the pregnancy.[439]

Common practice is to avoid vaginal delivery in pregnancy because of the fear that delivery through a cancerous cervix may cause the disease to spread more rapidly. However, Creasman and colleagues were unable to document a decrease in survival for stage I patients who delivered vaginally before definitive treatment.[439]

Chemotherapy

Because effective therapy using surgery and irradiation is available for most patients with cervical carcinoma, chemotherapy has not been extensively studied.[441] However, chemotherapy could play an important role if effective regimens were identified. Patients who would be good candidates for chemotherapy include those with stages III or IV disease, those with recurrent disease after surgery and radiation therapy, and those with pelvic and periaortic nodal metastasis. These patients have a low chance of cure with standard treatment modalities.

TABLE 38–20. Single-Agent Chemotherapy in Cervical Cancer

Drugs	No. of Responders/Total Treated
Alkylating Agents	
Cyclophosphamide	38/251 (15%)
Chlorambucil	11/44 (25%)
Dibromodulcitol	16/55 (29%)
Dianhydrogalacitol	7/36 (19%)
Ifosfamide	25/84 (29%)
Antimetabolites	
5-Fluorouracil	65/348 (20%)
Methotrexate	17/96 (18%)
Mitotic Inhibiters	
Vincristine	10/55 (18%)
Antitumor Antibiotics	
Doxorubicin	33/205 (16%)
Bleomycin	17/172 (10%)
Other Agents	
Cisplatin	182/785 (23%)
Iproplatin	19/177 (11%)
Carboplatin	27/175 (15%)
Piprazinedione	5/38 (13%)
Hexamethylmelamine	12/64 (19%)

Several novel approaches using chemotherapy were studied in cervical cancer. The location of cervical carcinoma and the regional vascularization of the pelvis provide a rationale for the study of regional perfusion of chemotherapy using intraarterial infusion. Chemotherapy was studied as a sensitizer to enhance conventional irradiation treatment, and neoadjuvant chemotherapy is being used with concomitant radiation therapy.

Factors that complicate the effective use of chemotherapy in cervical carcinoma include decreased pelvic vascular perfusion, limited bone marrow reserve, and poor renal function related to ureteral obstruction from tumor or fibrosis.

SINGLE-AGENT CHEMOTHERAPY. Table 38–20 lists the single agents with suggested activity against cervical carci-

noma. These data were collected from the literature in which variable criteria for response were used. Activity in well-designed studies with adequate patient numbers was documented for cisplatin, dibromoducitol, and ifosfamide.[442–444]

Cisplatin is the single agent with the best-documented activity against cervical cancer.[442] The GOG evaluated 782 patients on a variety of dose schedules. Objective responses occurred in 23% of patients, with little evidence for better responses with increased doses.[445] Twenty-four-hour infusions were associated with significantly less nausea and vomiting than bolus administration.[446]

Ifosfamide, an alkylating agent, produced a 29% response rate in 84 patients in European trials, although lower overall response rates (14%) were seen in GOG studies.[447,448]

Dibromoducitol produced 16 (29%) responses in 55 patients in GOG trials.[449]

COMBINATION CHEMOTHERAPY. Because several classes of cytotoxic agents with different mechanisms of action showed activity in carcinoma of the cervix, a number of combinations were used. Several studies demonstrated 10% to 29% complete remission rates that suggest some enhancement of effect. Table 38–21 lists combination chemotherapy studies in which reasonable numbers of evaluable patients were studied. The response rates appear to exceed those of single agents, but most studies did not compare combination chemotherapy regimens to standard single agents, and the toxicity of the combination regimens is substantial. None of these combinations was definitely superior to single-agent cisplatin in duration of response or survival, particularly in patients with recurrent disease after primary therapy.

INTRAARTERIAL CHEMOTHERAPY. Intraarterial infusion of chemotherapeutic agents for cervical carcinoma was of interest because of the distinct arterial supply to the tumor-bearing area. Unfortunately, responses were limited, and the toxicity was significant. Morrow and colleagues[450] and Swenerton and colleagues[451] each studied 20 patients treated with bleomycin or a combination of bleomycin, mitomycin C, and vincristine. Morrow's group observed only 2 of 26 objective regressions; Swenerton's group reported 3 of 20.

The intraarterial approach continues to be evaluated, using injections of single drugs or combinations into the internal iliac arteries. A few studies reported a reduction in compli-

TABLE 38–21. Combination Chemotherapy in Cervical Carcinoma

Regimen	Evaluable Patients	No. of Responses (%)	Complete Responses (%)
Doxorubicin (Adriamycin) and methotrexate	59	39 (66)	13 (22)
Doxorubicin and methotrexate	24	7 (28)	0 (0)
Doxorubicin and methyl-CCNU	13	14 (45)	9 (29)
Doxorubicin and cisplatin	19	6 (31)	2 (10)
Mitomycin C and bleomycin	33	12 (36)	5 (15)
Mitomycin C, vincristine, and bleomycin	91	46 (51)	14 (15)
Mitomycin C, vincristine, bleomycin, and cisplatin	14	6 (43)	4 (29)
Cisplatin, bleomycin, and velban	33	22 (66)	6 (18)
Cisplatin, bleomycin, vincristine, and methotrexate	15	10 (66)	3 (20)

cations and some responses.[452–455] However, randomized comparisons are necessary to establish any benefits of intraarterial chemotherapy infusions.

CHEMOTHERAPY AS A RADIOSENSITIZER. Continued interest in the use of chemotherapeutic agents as radiation sensitizers was stimulated by the initial positive results with hydroxyurea. Piver and associates studied 130 patients with stages IIB to IIIB cervical carcinoma in a prospective, randomized study in which patients received split-course radiation therapy with or without hydroxyurea.[456] In clinical stage IIB patients, a significant improvement in 2-year survival rates was achieved for the group who received hydroxyurea (74%) compared with the control group who were treated with radiation therapy and a placebo (43.5%). In clinically staged IIIB patients, 52% of those receiving hydroxyurea were alive at 2 years, compared with 33% of those receiving placebo with irradiation ($p = 0.22$). Increased toxicity was observed in the hydroxyurea arm.

Hreshchyshyn and colleagues[457] and Piver and colleagues[458] compared treatment with hydroxyurea to treatment with a placebo combined with irradiation in stages IIIB and IV cervical cancer. In 104 evaluable patients randomized to two treatment regimens, the complete response rate was 68% for the hydroxyurea-treated group and 48% for the placebo group; p intervals and survival were significantly better for the patients who received hydroxyurea. However, hematologic toxicity was more common and more severe in these patients. The results of these studies continue to be controversial because the patients were not all surgically staged, and substantial numbers of randomized patients were not evaluable. Moreover, with effective radiation therapy alone, Fletcher[321] and Perez and colleagues[459] demonstrated survival and tumor control similar to those observed with the addition of hydroxyurea in these two adjuvant trials.

The most recent GOG trial compared hydroxyurea with misonidazole in patients with stage IIB through IVA disease and negative paraaortic nodes.[460] The progression-free interval was marginally better for the hydroxyurea treatment ($p = 0.08$), but survival was not significantly different between hydroxyurea-treated (34% mortality) and misonidazole-treated patients (39% mortality). Isolated pelvic relapse was more common in patients treated with misonidazole (24%) than with hydroxyurea (18%). The current GOG trial is comparing adjuvant hydroxyurea with cisplatin and 5-FU.

NEOADJUVANT CHEMOTHERAPY IN LOCALLY ADVANCED DISEASE. Many recent trials used chemotherapy (most commonly cisplatin or cisplatin and 5-FU) with irradiation to treat patients with locally advanced or recurrent cervical cancer.

Studies from the Princess Margaret Hospital included 200 patients treated with neoadjuvant chemotherapy (mitomycin C and 5-FU) and pelvic irradiation.[461] Local control at 3 years for stage IB and II patients was 85%, and 50% for stage III and IV patients, compared with 58% for all stages treated previously with irradiation alone. The toxic effects of these approaches is significant, especially bladder and bowel toxicity.

Other investigators used cisplatin with or without 5-FU in nonrandomized neoadjuvant trials and reported encouraging results.[462–464]

One randomized trial compared irradiation alone (25 patients) with irradiation and weekly cisplatin (22) with irradiation and twice-weekly cisplatin (17).[465] Complete responses were similar in the three groups, as was the 5-year survival rate (45%). Whether neoadjuvant chemotherapy can produce a significant improvement in long-term survivals is still unclear.

TRENDS IN TREATING CERVICAL CANCER

Conservative therapy (*i.e.,* less than hysterectomy) is well established for stage 0 carcinoma (CIN-3) of the cervix. Prospective studies may show that conization of the cervix with negative margins and close follow-up is sufficient for most patients with microinvasive cervical cancer (<3 mm and no lymphovascular invasion). For patients with stage IB or IIA cervical cancer, the identification of high-risk subgroups may allow early use of adjunctive therapy with further improvements in survival. Combination therapy using irradiation and chemotherapy may be able to improve survival in advanced disease. Preliminary results of neoadjuvant chemotherapy followed by surgery or irradiation should be followed with larger, prospective randomized studies. Every effort should be expended to develop chemotherapeutic agents effective in the therapy of squamous cell carcinoma and adenocarcinoma of the cervix. All patients with advanced and recurrent cervical cancer should be considered for entry in clinical trials.

CARCINOMA OF THE ENDOMETRIUM

Carcinoma of the endometrium is the most common female genital cancer. There were approximately 33,000 new patients in 1992, which represented 46% of all female genital cancers and 11% of all malignancies occurring in women.[160] Although carcinoma of the endometrium accounts for almost half of all new cases of female genital cancer, it causes only 23% of all gynecologic cancer deaths.[160] This low death rate is primarily due to early diagnosis. Approximately 85% to 90% of all uterine cancer is diagnosed while it is still confined to the uterus.

EPIDEMIOLOGY

The largest number of cases of endometrial cancer occur in women between the ages of 55 and 60, although 75% to 80% of cases occur after menopause and a significant number of cases are reported in each decade after age 50. Only 5% of cases occur in women younger than 40, and the median age is 61.1 years.[466,467] Obesity, nulliparity, late menopause, polycystic ovarian disease, estrogen-secreting tumors of the ovary, and exogenous estrogen are associated with an increased incidence of endometrial cancer.[468–471] Nachtigall and colleagues[472] and Gambrel[473] showed that if progesterone is given with exogenous estrogen, there is no increased risk of endometrial cancer. Medical disorders that are associated with the development of endometrial cancer include diabetes, hypertension, arthritis, and hypothyroidism. Of these, hypertension and diabetes mellitus are most frequently observed.[468] Sommers and colleagues reported an increased susceptibility to endometrial cancer in some families, but the familial association does not appear to be strong.[474]

NATURAL HISTORY, ROUTES OF SPREAD, AND CLINICAL MANIFESTATIONS

The association of hyperplasia of the endometrium with endometrial carcinoma is well documented.[475] Cystic and adenomatous hyperplasias may be physiologic if they occur in an anovulatory hormonal environment before menopause but are of more concern in a postmenopausal woman. Atypical adenomatous hyperplasia is a cause of concern in any woman, regardless of menstrual status.

Carcinoma of the endometrium may spread along the uterine cavity to the cervix, penetrate the uterine wall, or spread through the fallopian tubes. The carcinoma can spread by local extension to the ovary, broad ligament, vagina, or other pelvic organs. Malignant cells may spread by way of the lymphatics or less frequently through the blood stream. The endometrial lymphatics begin beneath the glandular lining cells of the endometrium and drain into lymphatic vessels in the myometrium. Myometrial lymphatics drain into the subserosal network that coalesces into larger channels before exiting the uterus. Lymph flow from the fundus travels toward the adnexa and infundibulopelvic ligaments, and flow from the lower and middle thirds tend to spread in the base of the broad ligament toward the lateral pelvic sidewall.[24] There are four drainage channels from the uterus, according to Plentl and Friedman: from the fundus with the ovarian vessels; in the folds of the broad ligament; along the mesosalpinx and fallopian tubes; and along the round ligaments to the femoral nodes.[24]

In a review of the literature, Plentl and Friedman found nodal metastases in 202 (10%) of 1978 patients undergoing lymphadenectomy at the time of surgical therapy for endometrial carcinoma.[24] In an autopsy series, these same researchers reported an incidence of 65%. Creasman and colleagues, analyzing a GOG study in which patients with stage I and stage II adenocarcinoma had selective pelvic and para-aortic lymph node sampling, reported an incidence of positive pelvic lymph nodes of 1% to 25% and of aortic nodes of 1% to 18%, depending on histology, grade, and depth of invasion (Table 38–22).[476]

Metastases or extension of endometrial cancer to the fallopian tubes or the ovaries occurs in 5% to 10% of patients.[477] Cervical involvement occurs with the same frequency.[478] Extension to the vagina occurs in about 7% of patients.[24] Metastases to the peritoneal cavity and the omentum are occasionally seen. Creasman and colleagues reported a recurrence rate of 34% for patients with positive peritoneal cytology, compared with a 10% recurrence rate in patients with negative results.[479] Other researchers have not confirmed this high recurrence rate.[480] Creasman later reported a 25% rate of metastases to pelvic nodes and 19% rate of metastases to para-aortic nodes for patients with positive peritoneal cytology, compared with rates of 7% and 4%, respectively, if the results of peritoneal cytology were negative.[476] Morrow and colleagues reported an 18.8% recurrence rate for patients with positive peritoneal cytology as their only risk factor, compared with a 10.5% recurrence rate in similar patients without positive

TABLE 38–22. Frequency of Nodal Metastasis Among Risk Factors

Risk Factor	No. of Patients	Pelvic Metastases (%)	Aortic Metastases (%)
Histology			
Endometrioid			
Adenocarcinoma	599	56 (9)	30 (5)
Others	22	2 (9)	4 (18)
Grade			
1 Well	180	5 (3)	3 (2)
2 Moderate	288	25 (9)	14 (5)
3 Poor	153	28 (18)	17 (11)
Myometrial invasion			
Endometrial	87	1 (1)	1 (1)
Superficial	279	15 (5)	8 (3)
Middle	116	7 (6)	1 (1)
Deep	139	35 (25)	24 (17)
Site of tumor			
Fundus	524	42 (8)	20 (4)
Isthmus-cervix	97	16 (16)	14 (14)
Capillary-like space involvement			
Negative	528	37 (7)	19 (9)
Positive	93	21 (27)	15 (19)
Adnexal involvement			
Negative	587	47 (8)6	27 (5)
Positive	34	11 (32)	7 (20)
Other extrauterine metastasis			
Negative	586	40 (7)	26 (4)
Positive	35	18 (51)	8 (23)
Peritoneal cytology*			
Negative	537	38 (7)	20 (4)
Positive	75	19 (25)	14 (19)

* Nine patients did not have cytology reported.
(Modified from Creasman WT, Morrow CP, Bundy BN, Homesley HD, Graham JE, Heller PB. Surgical pathologic spread patterns of endometrial cancer. A Gynecologic Oncology Group study. Cancer 1987;60:2035–2041)

peritoneal cytology. The increase included distant recurrences and regional or distant recurrences.[481]

Almost all women with endometrial cancer report abnormal vaginal bleeding. Because 70% to 75% of women who develop the disease are postmenopausal, this symptom should be easily identified. The character of the abnormal bleeding varies from a serosanguineous discharge to frank bleeding. Pyometria and hematometra may be seen in patients with stenosis of the cervical canal. The finding of pyometria in a postmenstrual woman should suggest endometrial cancer. Pain is usually a symptom of advanced disease.

PATHOLOGY

The gross appearance of endometrial hyperplasia is not distinctive. The major distinction is usually the thickness of the endometrium, which is not necessarily characteristic, because normal endometrium and malignant endometrium can be thickened. Microscopically, this condition is described on the basis of two distinct features: architectural pattern and cytologic atypia. The classification of endometrial hyperplasia is shown in Table 38–23.[482] This classification was accepted by the International Association of Gynecological Pathologists. Any proliferation that has cytologic atypia is considered atypical, regardless of architectural pattern, and lesions with and without atypia are classified as simple or complex depending on the architectural abnormalities of glandular complexity or crowding.

Endometrial carcinoma is a polypoid growth that arises most often in the fundus of the uterus. The tumor may be small and focal or diffusely involve the uterine cavity. The diffuse lesions often show extensive hemorrhage and necrosis. The posterior wall is more likely to be involved than the anterior wall.

Histologically, most endometrial carcinomas are adenocarcinomas.[483] There is no evidence that adenoacanthoma behaves differently from pure adenocarcinoma. Several pathologists began using the term "adenocarcinoma with squamous metaplasia" to describe an adenoacanthoma. Adenosquamous carcinoma of the endometrium contains malignant adenocarcinoma and malignant squamous cell carcinoma. Ng and associates[484] and Silverberg and colleagues[485] described these lesions and reported a worse prognosis for them than for pure adenocarcinomas. Silverberg and colleagues[485] and Salazar and colleagues[486] correlated prognosis for these tumors to the differentiation of the adenocarcinoma portion of the tumor.

Uncommon carcinomas of the endometrium include clear cell carcinoma, secretory carcinoma, and squamous cell carcinoma.[487–489] The two varieties of papillary endometrial carcinoma are endometrioid papillary carcinoma and serous papillary carcinoma. Although both were reported to behave as poorly differentiated tumors, the serous papillary variety appears to carry the worse prognosis.[490]

The histologic grading of endometrial carcinoma is divided by FIGO into well-differentiated (grade 1), moderately differentiated (grade 2), and poorly differentiated (grade 3). A GOG pilot study of 222 patients found the distribution of cases to be 42% for grade 1, 40% for grade 2, and 18% for grade 3.[491] These researchers were able to correlate increasing grade with an increased frequency of nodal metastases.

TABLE 38–23. Classification of Endometrial Hyperplasia

Types of Hyperplasia	Progressing to Cancer (%)
Simple (cystic without atypia)	1
Complex (adenomatous without atypia)	3
Atypical	
Simple (cystic with atypia)	8
Complex (adenomatous with atypia)	29

(Park RC, Grigsby PW, Muss HB, Norris HJ. Corpus: Epithelial tumors. In: Hoskins WJ, Perez CA, Young RC, eds. Principles and practice of gynecologic oncology. Philadelphia: JB Lippincott, 1992:664–665)

DIAGNOSIS, CLINICAL EVALUATION, AND STAGING

The diagnosis of endometrial carcinoma is made on the basis of a fractional dilatation and curettage. The endocervical curettage should be performed before sounding or dilating the cervix to prevent contamination of the cervical sample by endometrial tissue that may be dislodged by the sound or dilator. If there is a visible lesion or a suspicious area on the cervix, biopsies should be obtained. If the diagnosis was made by office biopsy, a separate endocervical curettage should be obtained. Some authorities recommend that dilatation and curettage be performed if carcinoma is diagnosed on office biopsy to be sure that the worst lesion is sampled, but because most patients are managed primarily by surgery, most physicians would not perform a dilatation and curettage in patients with a diagnosis of endometrial cancer made on endometrial biopsy. The Pap smear is not a reliable method of detecting endometrial cancer, even though malignant endometrial cells may occasionally be found in the Pap smears of asymptomatic patients with endometrial cancer. In these cases, an endometrial biopsy or dilatation and curettage is indicated.

Patients diagnosed as having endometrial carcinoma should undergo a thorough history and physical examination, a careful pelvic examination, a chest radiograph, and a CT scan. Barium enema is an optional procedure, and most authorities would not obtain an intravenous pyelogram. Cystoscopy and proctosigmoidoscopy are advisable. Laboratory studies should include a complete blood count and biochemical profile to include renal and liver function tests. MRI and lymphangiography may be helpful but are rarely indicated. Although there are no tumor markers specific for endometrial carcinoma, serum CA 125 was elevated in some patients with endometrial cancer.[492,493] It may be wise to obtain a baseline CA 125 level in patients with endometrial cancer, because those with elevated levels may benefit from following the levels during and after therapy.

The FIGO staging classification was changed from a clinical staging system to a surgical staging system in 1988.[494] They are listed in Table 38–24. Patients who are considered medically inoperable are staged by the old clinical staging system.

The 1988 FIGO system requires evaluation of operative findings, such as histologic grade, depth of myometrial invasion, peritoneal cytology, pelvic and paraaortic nodal status, and evaluation for extrauterine spread. This presents some problems and has been grounds for some controversy. The major area of contention in this staging system is the requirement for evaluation of pelvic and paraaortic lymph nodes. Some authorities argued that, because the incidence of pelvic and paraaortic lymph node metastases is low in patients with grade 1 tumors that do not invade deeply (most cases), it is not proper to sample nodes in these patients. At Memorial Sloan-Kettering Cancer Center, we routinely obtain a frozen section analysis of depth of invasion in grade 1 tumors and perform nodal sampling only in those with invasion into the outer half of the myometrium. Many oncologists argue that sampling pelvic nodes does not add beneficial information and may cause increased morbidity, because patients with grade 3 lesions or deep invasion should have postoperative pelvic irradiation. Despite these limitations, it seems likely that surgical staging does provide a better evaluation of prognosis and probably provides valuable information for planning postoperative adjunctive therapy.

TABLE 38–24. FIGO Corpus Cancer Staging

Old Staging

I	The carcinoma is confined to the corpus
IA	The length of the uterine cavity is 8 cm or less
IB	The length of the uterine cavity is 8 cm or more

Stage I cases should be subgrouped by histologic type of the adenocarcinoma as follows:

> G1—Highly differentiated carcinomas
> G2—Differentiated adenocarcinomas with partly solid areas
> G3—Predominantly solid or entirely undifferentiated carcinomas

II	The carcinoma involves the corpus and the cervix
III	The carcinoma extends outside the corpus, but not outside the true pelvis (it may involve the vaginal wall or the parametrium but not the bladder or rectum)
IV	The carcinoma involves the bladder or rectum or extends outside the pelvis

New Staging

IA G123	Tumor limited to endometrium
IB G123	Invasion to $<\frac{1}{2}$ myometrium
IC G123	Invasion to $>\frac{1}{2}$ myometrium
IIA G123	Endocervical glandular involvement only
IIB G123	Cervical stromal invasion
IIIA G123	Tumor invades serosa and/or adnexae and/or positive peritoneal cytology
IIIB G123	Vaginal metastases
IIIC G123	Metastases to pelvic and/or paraaortic lymph nodes
IVA G123	Invasion of bladder and/or bowel mucosa
IVB	Distant metastases, including intraabdominal and/or inguinal lymph node

PROGNOSTIC FACTORS

Age at the diagnosis of endometrial carcinoma is a prognostic factor. Jones attributed improved survival to an increased incidence of less extensive, better-differentiated lesions in younger women.[495]

Stage at diagnosis is also related to survival. Creasman and Weed reviewed three large series and reported average survivals of 79% for stage I, 50% for stage II, 27% for stage III, and 9% for stage IV.[496] Cervical involvement was associated with a worse prognosis in most series. Surwit and colleagues reviewed 117 patients with histologic involvement of the cervix.[497] The overall survival rate for the entire group was 58%. However, if divided into those with stromal invasion and those with involvement of endocervical glands only, the survival rates were 47% and 74%, respectively.

Perhaps the most significant prognostic factors for planning therapy in patients with early disease are histologic grade, depth of myometrial penetration, and lymph node metastases. Plentl and Friedman, in an extensive review of the literature, found decreased survival was directly related to histologic grade and depth of tumor penetration of the myometrium.[24] These same researchers found that vaginal recurrence was also directly related to histologic grade. They reported a 4.3% rate of vaginal recurrence with grade 1 tumors, 9.2% with grade 2, and 24.4% with grade 3. A large prospective protocol by the GOG evaluated prognostic factors in carcinoma of the endometrium as determined by operative staging. The findings are presented in Table 38–25.[476,481,482] The uterine risk factors are histologic cell type, histologic grade, depth of myometrial invasion, extension of the tumor to the cervix, and vascular

TABLE 38–25. Risk Factors in Endometrial Carcinoma

Uterine Factors	Extrauterine Factors
Histologic type	Adnexal metastasis
Grade	Intraperitoneal spread
Myometrial invasion	Positive peritoneal cytology
Isthmus-cervix extension	Pelvic node metastasis
Vascular space invasion	Aortic node metastasis

(Park RC, Grigsby PW, Muss HB, Norris HJ. Corpus: Epithelial tumors. In: Hoskins WJ, Perez CA, Young RC, eds. Principles and practice of gynecologic oncology. Philadelphia: JB Lippincott, 1992:671)

space invasion. The extrauterine factors are adnexal metastases, status of peritoneal cytology, pelvic and paraaortic lymph node metastases, and other extrauterine spread.

The importance of uterine risk factors is their influence on the likelihood of lymph node metastases and ultimate survival, and the extrauterine risk factors directly influenced survival. Cell type (regardless of histologic grade) influences lymph node metastases and survival, with serous papillary carcinomas, clear cell carcinomas, and undifferentiated and squamous cell carcinomas carrying a worse prognosis (in that order) than endometrioid adenocarcinoma. For the endometrioid carcinomas, histologic grade of the tumor is an important prognostic factor. As the histologic grade becomes less differentiated, the incidence of deep myometrial invasion and lymph node metastases increases. The greater the depth of myometrial invasion, the greater is the likelihood of extrauterine spread and lymph node metastases. Involvement of the cervix increases the percentage of lymph node metastases, as does vascular space involvement. Extrauterine spread manifested by adnexal involvement, intraperitoneal spread, and positive peritoneal cytology is a poor prognostic sign, indicating lymph node metastasis and decreased rates of survival.

TREATMENT

The lower rate of deaths from endometrial carcinoma than ovarian carcinoma is due to the large percentage of patients diagnosed in stage I. In a literature review, Morrow and colleagues reported survival rates of 76% for stage I, 51% for stage II, 26% for stage III, and 9% for stage IV.[498] Boronow found that survival in endometrial cancer was similar to cervical cancer if corrected for stage distribution.[499] In other series, the 5-year survival rate of surgery alone or combined with preoperative or postoperative radiation therapy varied from 80% to 95%.[500–502]

The therapeutic approach for endometrial cancer is determined by FIGO stage, histologic type and grade, depth of myometrial penetration, and the medical condition of the patient.[501,502] Hysterectomy is the central feature of the management of most patients. The place of radiation therapy is in the adjunctive therapy of high-risk early stage disease, in the management of advanced disease, and for patients with early disease who are medically unsuitable for hysterectomy.[503]

Stages I and II

Patients with stage I (A, B, C) and stage II (A, B) endometrial carcinoma should undergo total abdominal hysterectomy and bilateral salpingo-oophorectomy with appropriate surgical staging. Sampling of pelvic and paraaortic lymph nodes is required by the 1987 FIGO staging system, although there is controversy about whether nodal sampling is always indicated. Some authorities recommend frozen section analysis of the depth of myometrial invasion, with nodal sampling performed only for grade 1 tumors with invasion greater than 50% or for cervical involvement. Most physicians recommend nodal sampling for grade 2 and 3 tumors or for cervical involvement (stages IIA and IIB). Some recommend only paraaortic nodal sampling. Most recommend the addition of whole-pelvis radiation therapy for patients with grade 3 tumors or those with invasion greater than 50% of the myometrium. Pelvic irradiation is added for patients with metastases to pelvic lymph nodes or adnexal spread. There is evidence that the addition of pelvic radiation in these patients improves local control, but little evidence of improved overall survival.[504] Whether postoperative vaginal irradiation should be added in grade 1 patients with minimal myometrial invasion is controversial. The incidence of vaginal metastases is less than 5% for grade 1 carcinomas.[24,505] However, most oncologists recommend vaginal irradiation in grade 2 carcinomas with less than 50% myometrial invasion. Paraaortic irradiation is added for patients with metastases to paraaortic lymph nodes.

Patients with histologic grade 2 or 3 carcinomas have a 15% and 39% incidence, respectively, of deep myometrial invasion.[491] The incidence of metastases to pelvic lymph nodes is 10% for grade 2 and 36% for grade 3, and aortic lymph nodes are involved in 4% of grade 2 tumors and 28% of grade 3 tumors.[506] Because of these factors, preoperative intracavitary or whole-pelvis irradiation may be used, and paraaortic nodal sampling is performed at the time of hysterectomy.

In preoperative insertions (^{137}Cs) for stage I tumors, Perez used 3500 to 4000 mgh in the endometrial cavity. A dose of 6000 to 6500 cGy is delivered to the surface of the vaginal fornices (1800–2000 mgh). Surgery is usually scheduled 3 days to 1 week after removal of the brachytherapy insertion to ensure that the true pathologic extent of the tumor can be adequately evaluated histologically. Although a higher degree of tumor sterilization is observed if surgery is performed 4 to 6 weeks after the brachytherapy placement, the pathologic features that can be helpful in determining if further treatment is necessary, such as depth of myometrial invasion, are more difficult to evaluate.[500,507] Preoperative brachytherapy delivers an inadequate radiation dose to the pelvic lymph nodes. If tumor extension greater than 50% of the thickness of the myometrium or tumor extension beyond the uterus is demonstrated at the time of surgery, external-beam irradiation should be added postoperatively (with midline shielding block as required). In patients treated with total abdominal hysterectomy and bilateral salpingo-oophorectomy, the irradiation fields are the same as those used for preoperative irradiation. Whole-pelvis fields are used for this boost, using a midline shield at some point during the treatment course as determined by calculating the bladder and rectal doses from the intracavitary insertion. A dose of 2000 cGy is delivered to the whole pelvis with 3000 cGy to the parametria with a midline

block. If the patient has residual tumor left in the pelvis, a boost to the area of residual tumor is indicated. The indications for postoperative radiation therapy by the Washington University group are deep myometrial invasion, transection of tumor, unsuspected advanced stage (*i.e.*, ovary, tube, or node involvement), and unsuspected poorly differentiated tumors.

The initial surgical management of FIGO stages IIA and IIB is not different from that of stage I cancers, except that these patients always require lymph node evaluation and postoperative irradiation. Gross cervical involvement, which is not categorized separately in the 1987 FIGO staging system, differs from occult cervical involvement and requires a different treatment regimen. These patients require radical hysterectomy and pelvic lymphadenectomy or combination therapy with preoperative whole-pelvis irradiation, an intracavitary brachytherapy application, and subsequent total abdominal hysterectomy and bilateral salpingo-oophorectomy with paraaortic lymph node sampling. Most researchers report decreased survival for these patients.[24,485,507] Homesley and colleagues, in a review from Memorial Sloan-Kettering Cancer Center, reported survival rates of 61% if cervical involvement was occult and 48% if there was gross involvement of the cervix.[507] Larson and associates from M.D. Anderson Cancer Center divided patients into three groups: gross cervical involvement, occult stromal invasion, and no evidence of stromal invasion.[508] They reported survival rates of 70%, 65%, and 67%, respectively, and they concluded that there is no prognostic significance in the extent of cervical involvement.

At Washington University, based on experience reported by Grigsby and associates, patients with stage II endometrial carcinoma who have only microscopic involvement of the endocervix are treated with a preoperative intracavitary insertion followed by an extrafascial hysterectomy and bilateral salpingo-oophorectomy.[509] The dose delivered usually is 3500 to 4000 mgh to the body of the uterus and 6000 cGy to the vaginal vault (1800 to 2000 mgh) with 2-cm colpostats. If there is gross or multiple-quadrant microscopic involvement of the exocervix, in addition to the intracavitary insertion, the patient receives external irradiation of 2000 cGy to the whole pelvis and 3000 cGy additional dose to the parametria with midline shield, followed by an extrafascial hysterectomy approximately 4 weeks later. Radiation alone is used for the inoperable patient or if surgery is refused.

Stages III and IV

The therapy for patients with stage III or IV endometrial carcinoma must be individualized. By the 1987 FIGO staging classification, patients with stage III disease on the basis of serosal involvement, adnexal spread, or pelvic nodal metastases are usually treated by postoperative pelvic radiation therapy. Patients with paraaortic nodal metastases usually receive pelvic and paraaortic radiation therapy. Patients with vaginal metastases (stage IVA) are usually treated primarily with irradiation. Because the distribution of tumor within the pelvis may vary, no single technique is applicable to all patients. External-beam irradiation is the mainstay of treatment; whole-pelvis irradiation is given for a dose of 2000 to 4000 cGy, with an additional boost to the parametria given with midline shield to complete 5000 to 6000 cGy in 5 to 7 weeks. The central dose is supplemented with at least two brachytherapy applications for approximately 6000 to 8000 mgh, depending on whole-pelvis external irradiation dose. Afterloading Simon-Heyman capsules and the Fletcher-Suit applicators provide the differential loading necessary to achieve the best possible dose distribution. If there is lower-third vaginal extension, volume interstitial implantation with brachytherapy sources is indicated. Stage IIIB endometrial carcinoma with involvement of only the upper vagina may be managed by preoperative whole-pelvis and intracavitary irradiation and total abdominal or modified radical hysterectomy and a wide vaginal cuff.

There is no standard therapy for patients with positive peritoneal cytologic examinations (stage IIIA). Heath and associates[510] and Soper and colleagues[511] recommended intraperitoneal ^{32}P in these patients, and Piver and colleagues[512] recommended medroxyprogesterone (Provera) for 1 year.

Surgery

The usual surgical procedure for adenocarcinoma of the endometrium is abdominal hysterectomy and bilateral salpingo-oophorectomy with sampling of the pelvic and paraaortic lymph nodes. In removing the uterus, tubes, and ovaries, an extrafascial hysterectomy is performed with the plane of excision lying outside the pubocervical fascia and does not require unroofing of the ureters. A small vaginal cuff is usually excised. Paraaortic nodal sampling can be performed through a midline peritoneal incision over the common iliac arteries and lower aorta or by mobilizing the right and left colon medially to allow access to the retroperitoneum. In either case, a sample of right and left paraaortic lymph nodes are removed from the lower aorta and vena cava. On the left side, the lymphatics lie slightly posterior to the aorta, and on the right side, they lie primarily in the fat pad over the vena cava. Pelvic lymph node sampling consists of a sample of nodes from the distal common iliacs on either side and a second sample from the external iliac chain. A third sample is then taken from the obturator-hypogastric chain, although some surgeons separate these nodes into two samples. The procedure is performed on both sides of the pelvis and should provide a representative sample. It is not a complete lymphadenectomy.

Most surgeons do not recommend that the cervix be sutured closed before abdominal hysterectomy for endometrial carcinoma, although this was common practice in the past. Neither do most surgeons tie the fimbriated ends of the fallopian tubes on opening the abdomen, although most recommend placing clamps across the cornual region to occlude the fallopian tubes and provide traction during the procedure.

Pelvic exenteration was used for central recurrence after irradiation, but the utility of this procedure in endometrial carcinoma is limited.[554]

Radiation Therapy

Statistically valid data are not available to support the impact of adjuvant radiation therapy on survival, but in a randomized study, Graham reported better 5-year survival rates with combination therapy than for hysterectomy alone, although the difference between the preoperative and postoperative irradiation groups was not statistically significant.[513]

There was a significantly decreased incidence of vaginal recurrences in patients treated with irradiation (1% to 3%) compared with those treated with hysterectomy alone (15%). A review of 858 patients treated at the Mallinckrodt Institute of Radiology, using preoperative intracavitary therapy alone in 538 patients, additional external irradiation (usually 2000–3000 cGy to the whole pelvis) in 82 patients, and postoperative irradiation in 218 patients, demonstrated an overall pelvic recurrence rate of 4% for grade 1, 3% for grade 2, and 9% for grade 3 lesions.[514] Survival is shown in Figure 38–15, and Table 38–26 shows 5-year survival figures for patients with stage I disease.[330,500,505,513–520]

Several researchers reported a greater incidence of vaginal and pelvic recurrences and distant metastases in patients with poorly differentiated (grade 3) tumors or in those with advanced stage disease. However, radiation therapy was shown to decrease the incidence of pelvic recurrences. Bedwinek and colleagues reported a 71% overall 5-year disease-free survival rate, 9.6% incidence of pelvic recurrences, and 15.6% distant failures for 83 patients with stage I grade 3 endometrial carcinoma treated with intracavitary irradiation alone or combined with pelvic external radiation therapy.[521]

Uterine size in stage I disease was found to correlate with prognosis only if the enlargement is related to tumor infiltra-

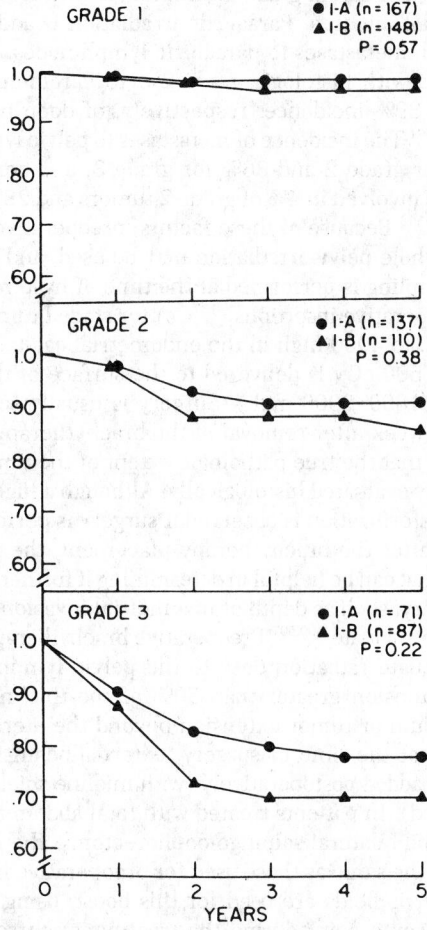

FIGURE 38–15. Progression-free survival by FIGO (1971) clinical stage and tumor grade. (Grigsby PW, Perez CA, Kuten A, et al. Clinical stage I endometrial cancer: Results of adjuvant irradiation and patterns of failure. Int J Radiat Oncol Biol Phys 1991;21:379–385)

TABLE 38–26. Stage I Endometrial Carcinoma Survival at 5 Years

Investigations	No. of Patients	Survival at 5 Years (%)
Beiler et al[515]	282	64 crude
Wharam et al[505]	269	81 without disease
Graham[513]	123	74 crude
Malkasian et al[516]	409	82 actuarial
Underwood et al[500]	220	91 actuarial
Frick et al[517]	239	78 crude
Salazar et al[518]	307	84 actuarial
Brady et al[519]	99	88 crude
Stokes et al[330]	304	87 actuarial

(Modified from Glassburn JR, Brady LW. Carcinoma of the endometrium. In Perez CA, Brady LW, eds. Principles and practice of radiation oncology. Philadelphia: JB Lippincott, 1987:966–987)

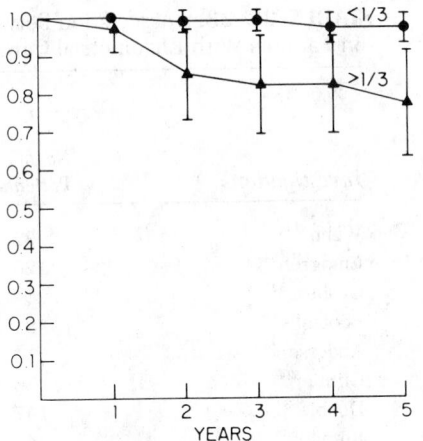

● No tumor, superficial–no invasion or invasion <1/3 (69)
▲ Invasion >1/3 (33)
Error Bars: 90% Confidence Limits

FIGURE 38–16. Survival without evidence of disease by depth of myometrial invasion (quick or postoperative radiotherapy) for endometrial carcinoma patients. (Stokes S, Bedwinek JM, Kao M-S, et al. Treatment of stage I adenocarcinoma of the endometrium by hysterectomy and adjuvant irradiation: A retrospective analysis of 304 patients. Int J Radiat Oncol Biol Phys 1986;12:339)

tion in the myometrium (Table 38–27).[495,517,522–531] Wade and associates[532] and Javert[533] observed that benign conditions such as myomas and adenomyosis often contribute to uterine enlargement and have no significant impact on prognosis. Stokes and colleagues observed similar survival rates in stage IA and IB patients, regardless of the tumor differentiation.[330] Myometrial invasion decreases the 5-year survival rate from 85% to 90% for no involvement to 60% to 79% if involvement is more than half way through the myometrium (Fig. 38–16).[330] Similar results are correlated with the degree of differentiation of the tumor (Table 38–28).[495,515,517,522–526,529,531,532,534–538]

A few reports compared the effectiveness of external irradiation or intracavitary radium without conclusive results. Sala and del Regato compared survival after 4000 cGy external irradiation to the pelvis (70 patients) or a radium implant for 6000 cGy (48 patients).[539] The 3-year survival rates were 87% and 77%, respectively. No vaginal recurrences were documented in either group. The survival rate was similar whether residual tumor was present in the surgical specimen or not.

TABLE 38–27. Five-Year Survival Rates Correlated With Depth of Myometrial Invasion

Investigations	No Invasion		Superficial Invasion		Deep Invasion	
	No. of Patients	5-Year Survival Rate (%)	No. of Patients	5-Year Survival Rate (%)	No. of Patients	5-Year Survival Rate (%)
Anderson[522]	12	100	22	86	7	42
Gusberg[523]	245	67	96	70	94	34
Climie[524]	56	87	20	80	23	56
Austin[525]	133	91	239	95	163	81
Cheon[526]	181	81	91	77	73	42
Nilson[527]			205	89	131	76
Lewis[528]	16	93	41	88	22	54
Ng[529]	129	88	48	72	22	27
Sall[530]			75	92	16	75
Nahhas[531]	75	85	33	82	28	56
Frick[517]	63	79	101	77	42	45
Total patients	910		971		621	
Total survivors	736		827		376	
Average 5-year survival rate		80		85		50

(Adapted from Jones HW III. Treatment of adenocarcinoma of the endometrium. Obstet Gynecol Surv 1975;30:147)

TABLE 38–28. Association Between Tumor Differentiation and 5-Year Survival Rates in Patients With Endometrial Carcinoma

	Grade I		Grade II		Grade III	
Investigations	No. of Patients	5-Year Survival Rate (%)	No. of Patients	5-Year Survival Rate (%)	No. of Patients	5-Year Survival Rate (%)
Webb[534]	32	84	155	52	37	30
Lindgren[535]	120	88	153	82	56	80
Gusberg[523]	204	62	85	53	65	32
Boutselis[536]	81	75	42	64	49	14
Anderson[522]	14	100	51	82	26	65
Climie[524]	56	93	24	75	18	44
Dobbie[537]	147	81	74	78	45	73
Roman[538]	47	87	105	78	113	51
Wade[532]	65	84	150	78	50	42
Austin[525]	126	96	239	96	163	75
Cheon[526]	196	81	72	78	77	44
Ng[529]	91	86	101	75	62	37
Nahhas[531]	106	84	57	75	35	48
Beiler[515]	54	83	130	65	67	40
Frick[517]	218	79	76	54	54	30
Total patients	1558		1515		917	
Total survivors	1267		1124		462	
Average 5-year survival rate		81		74		50

(Adapted from Jones HW III. Treatment of adenocarcinoma of the endometrium. Obstet Gynecol Surv 1975;30:147)

Similar findings were reported by Silverberg and DeGiorgi in 76 patients treated with preoperative irradiation and hysterectomy.[540] Weigensberg, in a randomized study involving small groups of patients in two community hospitals, observed a 5-year actuarial disease-free survival rate of 75% for 53 patients treated with intracavitary irradiation and hysterectomy and 48% for 38 patients treated with external-beam irradiation.[541] Patients treated with intracavitary radium received 5400 cGy, and those treated with external-beam irradiation received 4000 cGy. Two of the intracavitary therapy patients and 9 in the external-beam group had pelvic recurrences. Uterine size or degree of tumor differentiation was similar in both groups. Aalders and colleagues,[504] in a ran-

domized trial, and Bedwinek and colleagues,[521] in a nonrandomized retrospective review, reported similar survival with intracavitary therapy alone or combined with external irradiation. However, pelvic recurrences can be decreased with external irradiation in patients with less differentiated tumors from about 20% to 5%.

In 19 patients with stage II endometrial carcinoma treated by an intracavitary insertion and external-beam irradiation to the whole pelvis, a 63% 5-year survival rate was obtained.[542] A report by Grigsby and associates from the Mallinckrodt Institute of Radiology disclosed 8 (10%) pelvic recurrences in 79 patients with stage II endometrial carcinoma treated by a combination of preoperative or postoperative intracavitary

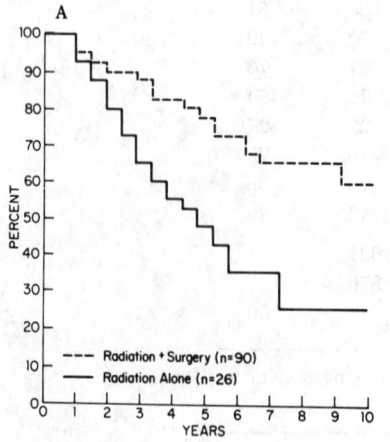
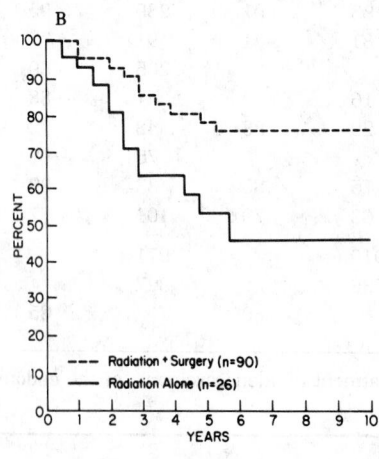

FIGURE 38–17. **(A)** Overall survival and **(B)** disease-free survival in 116 patients with stage II carcinoma of the endometrium. MIR, 1960–1981. (Grigsby PW, Perez CA, Camel HM, et al. Stage II carcinoma of the endometrium: Results of therapy and prognostic factors. Int J Radiat Oncol Biol Phys 1985;11:1915)

insertion and external irradiation.[509] Eleven patients with microscopic endocervical involvement treated only with a preoperative intracavitary insertion had no pelvic or vaginal recurrence. For a small group of 26 patients with stage II endometrial carcinoma treated with irradiation alone, the overall incidence of pelvic failure was 34.6%, compared with an incidence of only 8.9% among those treated with a combination of irradiation and surgery. The survival and disease-free survival rates are illustrated in Figure 38–17.[509]

It is known that gross involvement of the cervix carries a worse prognosis than microscopic involvement. Grigsby and associates reported lower survival rates for patients with ectocervical tumor invasion, even if it was microscopic only.[509] Numbers and sites of recurrence for radiation therapy plus surgery versus radiation alone reported by various researchers for patients with stage II endometrial carcinoma are summarized in Table 38–29.[503,518,543–546]

The results of treatment for stage III disease are poor. A 25% 5-year survival rate can be expected with aggressive therapy, with somewhat better results for patients who had ovarian involvement only (Table 38–30).[507,529,547–553] Patients with stage IV disease are rarely cured, and most researchers report 5% alive at 5 years.

COMBINATIONS OF IRRADIATION AND SURGERY. A variety of techniques were used in combining irradiation and surgery in the treatment of stage I endometrial cancer, including external beam, brachytherapy, or combinations of both. Irradiation was administered preoperatively, postoperatively, or as a combination of both.

Preoperative irradiation aims to decrease the opportunity of viable tumor cells seeded in the operative field to develop into a local recurrence, to render the tumor cells nonviable and decrease the possibility of distant dissemination of the tumor, and to irradiate the areas of frequent nodal involvement that are not removed at the time of surgery. The techniques

TABLE 38–29. Carcinoma of the Endometrium: Treatment Outcome of Stage II Disease

Investigations	No. of Patients	Survival (%)	Vagina	Pelvis	Vagina Plus Pelvis	Pelvis Plus DM	DM
Stage II—Radiation Therapy and Surgery							
Gagnon et al[543]	20	44.8*		1 (5)			2 (10)
Onsrud et al[544]	44†	85			1 (2.3)		4 (9.1)
	40‡	85	2 (5)	2 (5)	3 (7.5)		4 (10)
Salazar et al[518]	20			1 (5)			3 (15)
Spanos et al[545]	61				12 (19.7)§		Not reported
Total‖	124		2 (1.6)	4 (3.2)	4 (3.2)	0	13 (10.5)
				Total pelvis 8%		Total DM 10.5%	
Stage II—Radiation Therapy Alone							
Landgren et al[503]	38	65¶		3 (7.9)		4 (10.5)	9 (23.7)
Salazar et al[518]	8			3 (37.5)			2 (25)
Spanos et al[545]	21				4 (19)**		Not reported
Total‖	46			6 (13)		4 (8.7)	11 (23.9)
				Total pelvis 21.7%		Total DM 32.6%	

* Five years.
† Radium only.
‡ Radium plus external.
§ Value is the combined total of recurrences in pelvis, vagina and pelvis, and pelvis plus distant metastases (DM) in the study by Spanos et al.[545]
‖ Excluding Spanos et al.
¶ Actuarial, 5 years.
** Value is the combined total of recurrences in pelvis and pelvis plus DM in the study by Spanos et al.[545]
(Perez CA, Bedwinek JM, Breaux SR. Patterns of failure after treatment of gynecological tumors. Cancer Treat Symp 1983;2:217)

TABLE 38–30. Stage III Endometrial Carcinoma:
Survival Rates at 5 Years

Investigations	No. of Patients	Survival at 5 Years (%)
Antoniades et al[547]	37	25
Rutledge and Ehrlich[548]		21
Buchler et al[549]	32	22
Kottmeier[550]	136	30
Homesley et al[507]	23	4
Boronow[551]	49	18
Geisler and Gibbs[552]	19	5.3
Ng and Reagan[529]	14	13.6
Danoff et al[553]	17	11.7

(Danoff BF, McDay J, Louka M, et al. Stage III endometrial carcinoma: Analysis of patterns of failure and therapeutic implications. Int J Radiat Oncol Biol Phys 1980;6:1491)

of external-beam irradiation, volume to be treated, and portals used are similar to those used in the treatment of carcinoma of the uterine cervix.

For the intracavitary insertions, in addition to afterloading tandem and vaginal ovoids, it is common practice to pack the uterine cavity with Heyman or afterloading Heyman-Simon capsules (Fig. 38–18).[142] This technique allows the placement of sources in the body of the uterus around the tumor. Some pressure can be exerted on the uterine wall to try to reduce its thickness. These two effects may result in higher doses of radiation delivered to the serosa of the uterus and immediately adjacent paracervical tissues. The lower segment of the uterus and the endocervical canal can be treated with capsules or

with a tandem. The vaginal vault is always irradiated with vaginal colpostats. If there is tumor extension into the vagina, the entire length of this organ should be treated with a cylinder or special applicator (*e.g.*, Burnett, Bloedorn, Delclos) to include the suburethral regions and introitus because of the propensity of advanced endometrial adenocarcinoma to metastasize to this site through submucosal venous and lymphatic plexuses.

RADIATION THERAPY ALONE. A significant proportion of medically inoperable patients with stage I or II disease can be cured with a combination of external-beam therapy and brachytherapy. Usually, two intracavitary insertions are carried out, 2 weeks apart, to deliver 4500 to 5000 mgh to the uterine cavity and an additional 3000 mgh to the vaginal vault. This is combined with external-beam therapy for an additional 2000 to 4000 cGy to the whole pelvis and subsequent boosting of the lateral pelvic dose to a total of 5000 cGy with a midline pelvic shield to protect the bladder and bowel. Survival rates of 74% to 78% at 5 years were reported.[503]

Complications of Therapy

Surgical or combined treatment by surgery and adjuvant irradiation of endometrial carcinoma is well tolerated. Major complications, as reported by Stokes and colleagues, with a preoperative implant and hysterectomy occurred in 1% of 199 patients.[555] However, if the intracavitary insertion was given postoperatively, 12% of the patients (3 of 26) had significant complications. With adjuvant external whole-pelvis irradiation, the complication rate was 2% (5 of 264) but increased to 18% (7 of 40) if the whole-pelvis dose exceeded 3000 cGy. Eight major gastrointestinal and four urinary com-

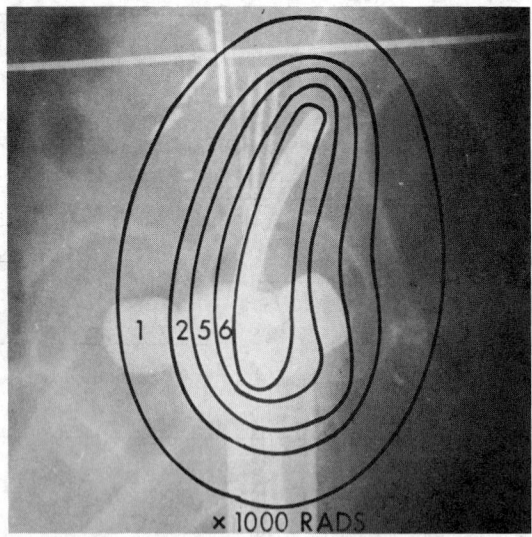

A

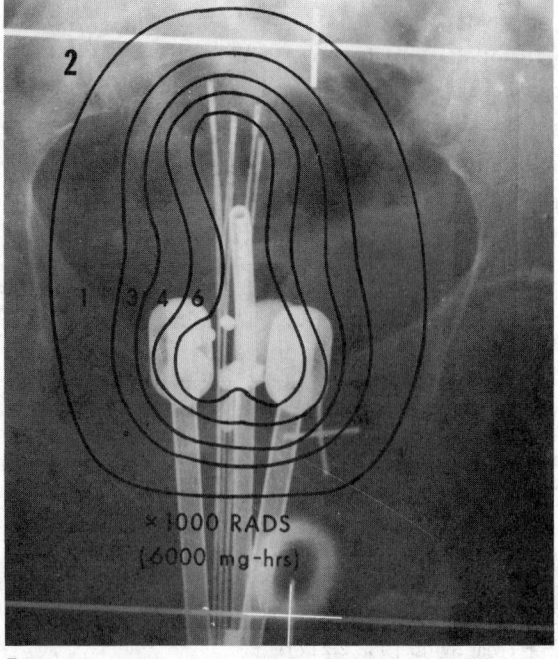

B

FIGURE 38–18. (A) Frontal and (B) lateral radiographs of intracavitary insertion in a patient with carcinoma of the endometrium, showing a Heyman-Simon afterloading capsule in the uterine fundus, tandem in the lower uterine segment, and ovoids in the vaginal vault. (Perez CA, DiSaia PJ, Knapp RC. Gynecologic tumors. In: DeVita VT Jr, Hellman S, Rosenberg SA, eds. Cancer: Principles and practice of oncology. 2nd ed. Philadelphia: JB Lippincott, 1985:1013–1081)

plications occurred in 304 patients, and the most frequent complications were bowel obstruction, ureterovaginal fistula, urethral stricture, hemorrhagic cystitis, and rectal ulcer.

Chemotherapy

HORMONAL THERAPY. The most commonly used systemic treatment in recurrent endometrial carcinoma was synthetic progestational agents. The response rates range from 15% to 29%.[556,557] Responses were associated with prolonged survival. Median survival for patients responding to progesterone therapy was 23 to 29 months compared with 6 months for patients without an objective response.[558] Response to hormonal therapy is related to the histologic grade of the tumor, and well-differentiated tumors respond more frequently than those with poorly differentiated histologies. Other factors that influence response to hormonal therapy include disease-free interval and receptor status. Responses are more common in vaginal or lung metastases and lymph nodes and less common in pelvic recurrences.

The progesterone receptor content of endometrial tumors correlates well with subsequent response to progesterone therapy.[556,559,560] Even though well-differentiated tumors tend to have the highest progesterone receptor positivity, receptor positivity appears to be a better correlate than grade.

In studies on 114 endometrial adenocarcinomas, the mean progesterone-binding capacity was inversely related to tumor grade.[559] Although more data are needed to establish the value of progesterone receptor analysis, this study reported that 88% (30 of 34) of progesterone-responsive lesions were receptor positive and that 94% (34 of 36) of unresponsive lesions were receptor negative.

Hormonal therapy with progestogens was well established as first-line systemic therapy for patients with recurrent or disseminated disease. The most commonly used progestogens were hydroxyprogesterone (Delalutin) or medroxyprogesterone (Depo-Provera, 400 mg intramuscularly weekly). Oral megestrol acetate (Megace, 160 mg/day), produces similar results. These progestogens should be continued indefinitely until recurrence or distant metastases develop.

Studies using alternative endocrine therapy for advanced endometrial cancer, including the antiestrogen tamoxifen and the synthetic 17-ethinyl testosterone derivative danazol, suggested some activity.[561,562] Data from several studies with tamoxifen suggest an overall response rate of approximately 18%, with well-differentiated tumors more likely to respond.[563-565] Attempts were made to enhance the activity of hormonal therapy by sequential therapy with tamoxifen, which induces progesterone receptors.[566] Although an increase in progesterone receptors was documented, the overall response rate was 33%, which is not significantly different from progesterone alone.

Other combination hormonal therapies, including medroxyprogesterone with tamoxifen, estradiol, or aminoglutethimide, have not enhanced response over that of progesterone alone.[567-569]

The use of progestogen therapy as prophylaxis in early stage endometrial carcinoma remains controversial. In one large adjuvant trial, stage I patients received adjuvant Depo-Provera or a placebo.[570] Despite unbalanced stratification with regard to prognostic factors and lack of evaluable patients, there was

no difference in 5-year survival rates. Another study of 35 stage IA and IB patients treated with surgery with or without subsequent treatment with 6-methyl-17-hydroxyprogesterone reported no benefit.[571] Despite these results, several investigators advocated the use of prophylactic progestational agents in high-risk patients.[572,573] The worth, if any, of adjuvant progesterone therapy in early stage endometrial carcinoma must be considered unproved. Ongoing trials in Australia and Italy that include only high-risk patients suggest some beneficial effect, but longer follow-up is needed in this important subgroup of patients.[558,574]

SINGLE-AGENT CHEMOTHERAPY. Nonhormonal chemotherapy was studied to a limited degree. Table 38–31 lists single agents with some activity against advanced endometrial cancer.[550,575-577] These data can only be used to suggest activity because of the small numbers of patients studied and the variability of prognostic factors. Of these agents, only doxorubicin, hexamethylmelamine, and cisplatin appear to have unambiguous activity, with response rates in the range of 15% to 30%.[578,579]

Of all single agents, doxorubicin was most extensively evaluated and appears to be the standard single agent to which new agents or combinations should be compared. Thigpen and colleagues treated 43 patients with advanced or recurrent disease using 60 mg/m² intravenous doxorubicin every 3 weeks.[580] They reported a 37% response rate (16 of 43), and 26% (11 of 43) had clinically complete regression of disease. Median survival was 14 months for patients achieving complete responses, 6.8 months for those with partial regressions, and 3.5 months for patients with progressive disease. Age, time to first recurrence, histologic grade of primary site of metastasis, and previous therapy had no effect on probability of response. Toxicity was similar to other studies in which doxorubicin was used as a single agent.

Conflicting reports on the activity of cisplatin in this disease may relate to its low activity (4%) when used as second-line treatment and its reasonable response rate (46%) when used at higher doses (100 mg/m²) in patients who have not been previously treated with chemotherapy.[467,576]

Although the response rates to doxorubicin and cisplatin

TABLE 38–31. Results of Single-Agent Chemotherapy for Endometrial Carcinoma

Drug	Patients Responding/ Total Treated	Response Rate (%)
Alkylating agents Cyclophosphamide	4/37	11
Antimetabolites 5-Fluorouracil	10/43	23
Antitumor antibiotics Doxorubicin	42/161	26
Mitoxantrone	2/46	4
Miscellaneous agents	9/54	17
Hexamethylmelamine Cisplatin	29/127	23
Carboplatin	7/26	27
Cytembena	10/30	33

are significant, the duration of single-agent responses are short, and the median survival of treated patients is only 4 to 8 months. The benefit is therefore modest.

COMBINATION THERAPY. Combination chemotherapy for advanced endometrial carcinoma has not been studied extensively. The relatively few studies that were published include small patient numbers.[578,579] Recent studies employing doxorubicin and cisplatin report higher response rates (30–90%), but only a few patients were treated. Comparison of this two-drug regimen with doxorubicin alone demonstrates a 45% response rate for the combination compared with 20% for the single agent.[580-583] Cisplatin, doxorubicin, and cyclophosphamide (PAC regimen) demonstrated a 45% overall response rate in 209 patients at a cost of moderate to severe toxicity.[584] Another study of the three-drug regimen CAP, including cisplatin (50 mg/m^2), cyclophosphamide (500 mg/m^2), and doxorubicin (50 mg/m^2) intravenously every 4 weeks, produced a 58% response rate, including 28% complete remissions in 18 patients with advanced disease.[585] Both the AP and CAP regimens appear to have some enhanced activity and should be compared with doxorubicin alone in larger trials.

Other studies included combination chemotherapy with progestogens, but the independent contribution of the drugs and the hormone cannot be assessed in these single-arm studies.[586-589]

The combination of megestrol, cyclophosphamide, and doxorubicin with or without 5-FU was given to 126 patients in the cooperative group study.[590] The response rate (22%) and the median survival (27 weeks) were the same in both arms and represent only a marginal improvement over the 19% response rate achieved by the same group with doxorubicin alone.

Ayoub and colleagues did a randomized comparison of combination chemotherapy (cyclophosphamide, doxorubicin, and 5-FU) with or without medroxyprogesterone alternating with tamoxifen.[591] Responses were higher (43% versus 15%) for the hormone-containing combination, but there was no difference in median survival (14 versus 11 months). Two other randomized trials compared different chemotherapy regimens, with all patients receiving hormone therapy (Megace).[589,590] Neither produced enhanced survival.

Whether the use of combinations of hormones with single-agent chemotherapy or combinations substantially enhance the antitumor effect remains unresolved and should be subjected to well-controlled clinical trials.

TRENDS IN TREATING ENDOMETRIAL CARCINOMA

Prospective studies should be undertaken to improve therapeutic results in high-risk groups of patients with early disease. Publication of the extensive surgical staging data from the GOG should allow selection of high-risk groups for which to attempt better adjunctive therapeutic regimens.

It is imperative that chemotherapeutic agents useful in endometrial cancer be developed. This provides hope for recurrent disease, and it allows the development of useful neoadjuvant regimens. The evaluation of whole-abdominal irradiation and new radiation therapy techniques such as hyperfractionation should be continued in this patient population. At this time, all patients with advanced and recurrent disease should be considered candidates for investigational protocols.

UTERINE SARCOMAS

Uterine sarcomas account for 1% to 6% of all cancers of the corpus uteri.[592-598] These variations in reported incidence depend on the criteria used to classify these cancers and the nature of the series on which the reports are based. Table 38–32 lists a classification of uterine sarcomas. It is based on Kempson's[593] simplification of the classification by Ober.[594] A new system of classification was adopted by the International Society of Gynecologic Pathologists for pure nonepithelial uterine sarcomas (Table 38–33) and mixed epithelial-nonepithelial uterine tumors (Table 38–34). Clinically, the most important tumors are, in order of frequency, carcinosarcoma, leiomyosarcoma, endometrial stromal sarcoma, and müllerian adenosarcoma.

Although there is no FIGO staging classification for uterine sarcomas, most researchers use a modification of the 1971 FIGO classification for endometrial carcinoma. This classification is listed in Table 38–35. It is a surgical classification based on the findings at initial surgical treatment of the sarcoma.

CARCINOSARCOMA

Carcinosarcomas (*i.e.*, malignant mixed mesodermal tumor, malignant mixed müllerian tumors) are composed of two types of cells: an adenocarcinoma of the endometrium and a sarcomatous element. They are called homologous if the sarcomatous element is from a cell type found in the uterus and heterologous if the sarcomatous element is from cell types not found in the uterus (*e.g.*, rhabdomyosarcoma, chondro-

---

TABLE 38–32. Classification of Uterine Sarcomas

I. Pure sarcomas
  A. Pure homologous
    1. Leiomyosarcoma
    2. Stromal sarcoma
    3. Angiosarcoma
    4. Fibrosarcoma
  B. Pure heterologous
    1. Rhabdomyosarcoma
    2. Chondrosarcoma
    3. Osteogenic sarcoma
    4. Liposarcoma
II. Mixed sarcomas
  A. Mixed homologous
  B. Mixed heterologous
  C. Mixed homologous and heterologous
III. Malignant mixed müllerian tumors
  A. Malignant mixed müllerian tumor, homologous type; carcinoma plus one or more of the homologous sarcomas listed under IA above
  B. Malignant mixed müllerian tumor, heterologous type; carcinoma plus one or more of the heterologous sarcomas listed under IB; homologous sarcoma(s) may also be present
IV. Sarcoma, unclassified
V. Malignant lymphoma

TABLE 38–33. Pure Nonepithelial Tumors

I. Endometrial stromal tumors
   A. Stromal nodule
   B. Low-grade stromal sarcoma
   C. High-grade stromal sarcoma
II. Smooth muscle tumors
   A. Leiomyoma
      1. Cellular
      2. Epithelioid
      3. Bizarre (symplastic, pleomorphic)
      4. Lipoleiomyoma
   B. Smooth muscle tumor of uncertain malignant potential
   C. Leiomyosarcoma
      1. Epithelioid
      2. Myxoid
   D. Other smooth muscle tumors
      1. Metastasizing leiomyoma
      2. Intravenous leiomyomatosis
      3. Diffuse leiomyomatosis
III. Mixed endometrial stromal and smooth muscle tumors
IV. Adenomatoid tumor
V. Other soft tissue tumors (benign and malignant)
   A. Homologous
   B. Heterologous

sarcoma, osteosarcoma, liposarcoma). The reported peak age of incidence for carcinosarcomas is between 55 and 65 years.[592] Vaginal bleeding is the most common presenting symptom.[595,596] A history of prior irradiation is reported in 5% to 30% of patients.[595,596] Diagnosis is made by dilatation and curettage. Spread of disease is usually by local extension in the pelvis, to lymph nodes, and to the lungs. This pattern is similar to that seen in endometrial adenocarcinoma, although carcinosarcomas are more aggressive than most endometrial adenocarcinomas, with early lymphatic or hematogenous spread. Major and colleagues reported a 15.5% incidence of positive lymph nodes in 174 patients with carcinosarcomas and correlated these metastases with depth of myometrial penetration, lymphovascular invasion, and cervical involvement.[597]

The primary treatment for carcinosarcomas is surgical removal of the uterus, fallopian tubes, and ovaries. Perez and associates reported a group of 54 patients with carcinosarcoma of the uterus who received combined radiation therapy and surgery.[598] In stage I disease, a preoperative uterine packing

TABLE 38–34. Mixed Epithelial and Nonepithelial Tumors

I. Benign
   A. Adenofibroma
   B. Adenomyoma
      1. Atypical polypoid adenomyoma
II. Malignant
   A. Adenosarcoma
      1. Homologous
      2. Heterologous
   B. Carcinosarcoma (malignant mixed mesodermal tumor; malignant mixed müllerian tumor)
      1. Homologous
      2. Heterologous
   C. Carcinofibroma

TABLE 38–35. Modified Staging Classification for Endometrial Carcinomas Used for Staging of Uterine Sarcomas

Stage I	Sarcoma is confined to the corpus
Stage II	Sarcoma is confined to the corpus and cervix
Stage III	Sarcoma has spread outside the uterus but is confined to the true pelvis
Stage IV	Sarcoma has spread outside the true pelvis

for 6000 mgh was recommended. Treatment for patients with stage II disease consisted of an intracavitary insertion for 5000 to 6000 mgh, combined with external-beam irradiation of 2000 cGy to the whole pelvis and a 3000-cGy boost to the parametrium with a midline shield. They found that local failures decreased compared with other series in which surgery alone was the only local treatment. This increase in local control with radiation was confirmed by others, and there is a tendency in the combined radiation and surgery group toward improved survival.[599,600] However, the patient numbers in most series are quite small, the reports are unrandomized, and it is difficult to make a definite statement about treatment efficacy.

Belgrad and colleagues, in reviewing patients treated at four institutions, found improved 2-year survival rates for patients treated by combined radiation and surgery for endometrial stromal sarcomas and carcinosarcomas.[600] In the carcinosarcoma category, 35% survived 2 years after combined-modality therapy, and 20% survived after surgery only. Salazar and associates found that in patients who received local radiation therapy as part of their program of management, local failures decreased but survival was not changed.[601]

In a GOG randomized trial of chemotherapy for advanced uterine sarcomas, responses to doxorubicin alone or doxorubicin plus DTIC were observed in 10% to 23% of patients.[602] This same group was unable to demonstrate a statistically significant survival advantage with the adjunctive use of doxorubicin in stage I or II disease.[603] In a phase II trial, ifosfamide, given at a dose of 1.5 g/m^2/day for 5 days every 4 weeks produced five complete responses and four partial responses in 28 patients who had not received prior chemotherapy.[448] Ifosfamide appears to hold promise for the treatment of carcinosarcomas of the uterus.

The GOG evaluated single-agent cisplatin in previously treated and untreated carcinosarcomas, reporting response rates of 18% and 19%, respectively.[604] A study from M.D. Anderson Cancer Center also reported activity.[605]

The prognosis of carcinosarcoma tumors is directly related to the extent of disease at the time of diagnosis. Kempson and Bari reported that all of their patients with disease extending into the outer half of the myometrium died.[593] Piver and Lurain reviewed 610 patients and reported an overall survival rate of 21%.[606] Most reports in their review indicated survival rates of 15% to 30%.

LEIOMYOSARCOMA

Leiomyosarcomas are tumors of the smooth muscle and arise in the myometrium. The distinction between cellular leiomyomas and leiomyosarcoma is not clear. Kempson and Bari reported death from tumor or metastases in all of their patients if the tumors had 5 to 9 mitoses per 10 high-power fields.[593] Silverberg reported death or metastases in one half of his patients if the tumor had 5 to 9 mitoses per 10 high-power fields.[607] Other factors that seem to influence prognosis are cellular atypia, vascular invasion, and infiltrating tumor margins.[607] It appears clear that most tumors with fewer than 5 mitoses per 10 high-power fields are benign, all with greater than 10 mitoses per 10 high-power fields are malignant, and those with 5 to 9 mitoses per 10 high-power fields are of uncertain malignant potential. Piver and Lurain, in a review of 265 patients, reported 99% survival for 0 to 4 mitoses per 10 high-power fields, 30% survival for 5 to 9 mitoses per 10 high-power fields, and 16% survival for tumors with 7 to 10 mitoses per 10 high-power fields.[606] Silverberg contends that mitosis counting alone is not the ideal method for determining which leiomyosarcomas are more malignant and stresses the need to consider other microscopic features.[607] He also points out the lack of uniformity in the counting of mitoses among different pathologists.

The median age for patients who develop leiomyosarcoma is between 43 and 56 years.[608] The presenting symptoms are abnormal vaginal bleeding, an enlarging pelvic mass, and pain or pressure in the pelvis. Dilatation and curettage produce a correct diagnosis for fewer than one third of the patients.[609] Spread of disease is by direct extension to other pelvic viscera, through the lymphatics, and by invasion of blood vessels and hematogenous spread, especially to the lungs.

Treatment consists of removal of the uterus and adnexa. Adjuvant radiation therapy did not benefit patients with leiomyosarcoma.[592] Adjuvant chemotherapy with doxorubicin for stages I and II disease was evaluated by the GOG.[603] The recurrence rate was 40% among patients receiving doxorubicin and 57% in the no-therapy group. The difference was not significant. Responses of 25% and 30% were seen in advanced disease by the GOG using doxorubicin alone compared with doxorubicin and DTIC.[602] The GOG found that ifosfamide produced four partial responses among 28 patients with leiomyosarcoma.[610] The prognosis for uterine leiomyosarcoma varies from essentially no survival in patients with advanced disease to 20% to 30% for disease confined to the uterus at initial diagnosis.[592]

ENDOMETRIAL STROMAL SARCOMA

Endometrial stromal sarcoma is a uterine tumor of pure endometrial stromal type. This tumor was best characterized by Norris and Taylor in 1966.[611] These researchers categorized three tumor types by behavior: stromal nodule, a benign tumor; low-grade endometrial stromal sarcoma (*i.e.*, endolymphatic stromal myosis); and high-grade endometrial stromal sarcoma. Evans proposed the addition of a fourth diagnostic group called poorly differentiated endometrial stromal sarcoma.[612]

Stromal nodule is a well-circumscribed proliferation of uniform cells that resemble endometrial stromal cells with "pushing" margins. Despite occasionally growing to 4 to 5 cm, these lesions are uniformly benign. Low-grade stromal sarcomas are composed of cells identical to those found in stromal nodules, but the margins of the low-grade stromal sarcoma are infiltrative, and extrauterine extension occurs in as many as one third of patients.[612] Low-grade stromal sar-

comas spread by direct extension and by contiguous lymphatic channels. Local recurrence is a problem, but these tumors are less likely to metastasize. In their original paper, Norris and Taylor used mitotic count to distinguish endometrial stromal sarcoma from low-grade stromal sarcoma, labeling tumors with 10 or more mitoses per 10 high-power fields as endometrial stromal sarcoma and those with fewer than 10 mitoses per 10 high-power fields as low-grade stromal sarcoma.[611] Others questioned this definition and suggested that the appearance of the cellular component of the tumors is equally or more important.[613,614] Evans[612] and Chang and associates[615] described poorly differentiated stromal sarcomas that had an anaplastic appearance and aggressive behavior.

Stromal tumors are seen most frequently in patients between the ages of 45 and 50 years, and the most common symptoms are vaginal bleeding and an enlarged, boggy uterus. Diagnosis is made by dilatation and curettage or as an unexpected finding at hysterectomy for leiomyomas. Endolymphatic stromal myosis spreads by direct extension and by the lymphatics. It extends beyond the uterus by the time of diagnosis in one third of the patients, although two thirds of the patients have disease confined to the pelvis.[606] Recurrence rates of 50% are reported, but spreading outside the pelvis is rare.[616] Endometrial stromal sarcomas are highly malignant neoplasias with tumor-free survival rates of 0% to 33%.[593,603,617] Distant metastases are more frequent in this group of patients.

The treatment of low-grade stromal sarcomas and endometrial stromal sarcoma is removal of the uterus and adnexa. More radical local resection was recommended for low-grade stromal sarcoma, but no large series supports this recommendation. Adjunctive irradiation for stromal sarcoma is probably effective in obtaining local control and preventing pelvic recurrences, and Belgrad and colleagues reported modest improvements in survival.[600] In their report, the 2-year survival rate in patients with endometrial stromal sarcoma treated by radiation therapy and surgery was 57%, and for those treated by surgery alone it was 37%.

Norris and Taylor reported a beneficial effect of irradiation on residual disease in low-grade stromal sarcoma.[611] Koss and colleagues recommended pelvic irradiation for recurrences and postsurgical residual disease.[618] There are few data on chemotherapy for stromal sarcomas, although Baggish and Woodruff reported responses with high-dose progestins.[619] Low-grade stromal sarcomas have a large number of estrogen and progesterone receptors and may respond to progesterone therapy.[629,621,622]

ADENOSARCOMA

Adenosarcoma was first described in 1974.[623] Several hundred cases were reported; the larger series had 25 to 100 patients.[624–626] This tumor is composed of a benign epithelial component and a malignant nonepithelial (stromal) component. The tumor is usually limited to the endometrium, but myometrial invasion does occur. Extrauterine spread was reported in 6 of 31 patients by Kaku and colleagues.[625]

These tumors appear in a slightly younger age group than the carcinosarcomas, with a peak incidence in the patients between 55 and 60 years. They have a more favorable prognosis than carcinosarcomas unless there is sarcomatous overgrowth. Recurrences were reported in 44% to 70% of patients with sarcomatous overgrowth but only 14% to 25% of patients without sarcomatous overgrowth.

Treatment of adenosarcomas is surgical, with total abdominal hysterectomy and bilateral salpingo-oophorectomy. There is little experience with radiation therapy or chemotherapy in this disease.

TRENDS IN TREATING UTERINE SARCOMAS

Surgery remains the treatment of choice for all sarcomas arising in the uterus. A total abdominal hysterectomy and bilateral salpingo-oophorectomy constitute the preferred treatment, although there are advocates of a more radical surgical approach for the low-grade endometrial stromal sarcomas. Lymph node dissections or lymph node sampling, although adding information for determining prognosis, have not improved survival. Although local failures are common, most patients fail because of hematogenous dissemination of their tumors. The role of radiation therapy in the treatment of uterine sarcomas remains controversial, with no clear evidence that its preoperative or postoperative use improves survival. In patients with stage III or IV disease who are not operative candidates, some palliation and control of local symptoms can be achieved by the judicious use of external-beam therapy and brachytherapy placements.

Because the major pattern of failure is that of disseminated tumor, alone or in combination with local failure, an effective systemic means of therapy must be devised to improve survival significantly. Because of the rarity of sarcomas arising in the uterus, multiinstitutional studies are necessary to evaluate new treatment approaches.

CARCINOMA OF THE FALLOPIAN TUBE

The fallopian tube gives rise to the smallest number of primary malignant tumors of the female genital tract. These tumors comprise 0.5% to 1.1% of all gynecologic malignancies.[627,628] Because of its anatomic association with the uterus and ovary (the two most common sites of gynecologic cancers), rigid criteria were recommended to label a tumor as being a primary cancer of the fallopian tube.[628] To be considered a primary carcinoma of the fallopian tube, the tumor must be located within the fallopian tube, and the uterus and ovary must not contain carcinoma, or if they contain carcinoma, it must be clearly different from the fallopian tube carcinoma. The tubal carcinoma must involve the tubal mucosa with transition from benign to malignant epithelium, except in the case of sarcomas arising from nonmucosal structures. The most common malignant tumors involving the fallopian tube are metastatic from other genital organs.[629]

EPIDEMIOLOGY

Benedet and White reviewed eight studies of fallopian tube carcinomas reported between 1961 and 1979 and found a mean age incidence of 55 years among 393 patients.[630] Although the disease had developed in patients 18 and 87 years of age, most occurred in women between the ages of 40 and 65. The most commonly associated conditions in patients who develop fallopian tube cancer are infertility and chronic salpingitis. However, the common association of infertility and salpingitis and the high frequency in which salpingitis is found, compared with the rarity of fallopian tube carcinoma, renders chronic infection an unlikely etiologic factor. Some researchers found an increased incidence of tuberculous salpingitis in association with tubal carcinoma, but there was no definite etiologic link.

PATHOLOGY

The most common malignant tumors of the fallopian tube are adenocarcinomas. The tumor presents as a swollen, dilated fallopian tube that, when opened, is filled with papillary and solid tumor. Areas of degeneration with hemorrhage and necrosis are commonly seen.[628] The fimbriated end of the tube is closed in approximately one half of the patients, and before opening the tube, it is difficult to differentiate tubal carcinoma from a hydrosalpinx or tuboovarian abscess.[631] Microscopically, alveolar, papillary, and medullary patterns of tumor growth have been described, with abrupt transitions from normal to neoplastic epithelium.[632] Ninety percent of primary fallopian tube cancers are papillary serous carcinomas.[633] Grading of fallopian tube carcinomas has not been of prognostic significance, but this may be due to the relatively small numbers in most series.[634]

Pure sarcomas of the fallopian tube such as leiomyosarcoma and chondrosarcomas are exceedingly rare.[635] Mixed mesodermal tumors of the fallopian tube contain mixtures of adenocarcinoma and sarcoma and are homologous if they contain sarcomas of tubal elements such as smooth muscle or heterologous if they contain tissues not found in the tube, such as cartilage or bone.[636] The presence of heterologous elements does not appear to affect the behavior of the carcinoma.

Other rare tumors of the fallopian tube are lymphomas and choriocarcinoma.[637,638] They are probably associated with tubal pregnancies. A primary adenosquamous carcinoma was reported.[639]

PATTERNS OF SPREAD, CLINICAL MANIFESTATION, AND STAGING

Malignant tumors of the fallopian tube spread by exfoliation of clonogenic cells into the lumen of the fallopian tube that then migrate into the pelvic and abdominal cavity or, in the case of tumors that penetrate the serosa, shed cells directly into the pelvic and abdominal cavity. Although many tubal carcinomas exhibit occlusion of the fimbriated end of the tube, the potential for transtubal migration may have existed earlier in the course of the disease. After the entry of cells into the abdominal cavity, spread is similar to that of ovarian carcinoma. Fallopian tube cancer also spreads by contiguous invasion of adjacent structures and through lymphatics. Hematogenous spread appears to occur less frequently. Commonly involved organs are the pelvic peritoneum, broad ligament, omentum, diaphragm, and surfaces of the intestines.[24]

Plentl and Friedman described the lymphatics of the fallopian tube.[24] Efferent lymphatics travel in the mesosalpinx to join efferent channels from the ovary and uterus and follow the ovarian vessels to the paraaortic lymph nodes. Lymphatics also course within the broad ligament to the iliac lymph nodes and superior gluteal lymph nodes. Metastatic disease to pelvic and paraaortic nodes is most common, although inguinal node metastases are occasionally seen.[24]

Bilateral tubal involvement was reported in one half of their patients by Novak and Woodruff.[640] Benedet and White, after reviewing more than 400 cases from the literature, reported the incidence of tumors to be roughly equal in the right and left fallopian tubes and found bilateralism in 21%.[630] Bilateralism may be due to multicentric involvement of paired organs or to metastases.

Schiller and Silverberg reported 76 published cases of fallopian tube cancer and documented the association of depth of invasion of tumor and survival.[641] They found a 91% survival rate for lesions confined to the mucosa, 53% for tumors with mucosal wall invasion, and 25% for tumors that penetrated the tubal serosa.

Frick stated that the diagnosis of fallopian tube cancer is made preoperatively in only 5% of patients.[642] The most common symptoms are abnormal vaginal bleeding and abdominal pain. Benedet and White reviewed eight series of patients and found that 101 (50%) of 203 patients reported abnormal vaginal bleeding or discharge, 62 (30%) described abdominal pain, and in 25 (12%), a mass was the presenting symptom.[630] Pain may be intermittent and colicky or dull and aching and probably results from tubal distension similar to that seen with a tubal pregnancy. Rarely, an asymptomatic patient may present with adenocarcinoma cells on Pap smear.[628] The symptom complex of *hydrops tubae profluens* consists of the triad of a profuse vaginal discharge, abdominal pain, and an adnexal mass. This triad is said to be pathognomonic for tubal carcinoma but is uncommon in most series.

Staging of carcinoma of the fallopian tube is determined at surgical exploration, as in ovarian carcinoma. The preoperative diagnostic evaluation is the same as for ovarian carcinoma, because most patients undergoing surgery do so with the diagnosis of a pelvic mass. Only rarely is fallopian tube cancer high on the list of differential diagnoses. There is no FIGO staging classification for fallopian tube carcinoma. In 1970, Dodson and colleagues adapted the staging for ovarian carcinoma to tubal carcinoma by substituting fallopian tube for ovary and vice versa.[643] In 1971, Schiller and Silverberg developed a different system that is more like the Dukes' classification for colon cancer.[641] Benedet and White[630] modified the staging system reported by Erez and associates[644] in 1967 and reported survival in 142 patients staged by their "modified Erez" classification. They found 5-year survival rates of 60% in stage I, 30% in stage II, 16% in stage III, and 19% in stage IV. Table 38–36 compares the three staging systems.[630,641,643] The most widely accepted method of staging of fallopian tube cancers is that described by Dodson, which uses a modification of the FIGO staging for ovarian carcinoma.

Fallopian tube cancer tends to present at an early stage. Although two thirds of patients with ovarian carcinoma present with advanced disease, most patients with fallopian tube cancer are diagnosed at an early stage of disease. Among 558 patients from eight studies, 33% were stage I, 33% were stage II, and only 34% were stage III or IV.[645]

TREATMENT

Because of the relative rarity of fallopian tube carcinoma and because its histology and patterns of spread are similar to those of ovarian carcinoma, most researchers recommended treatment plans of surgery, radiation therapy, and chemotherapy similar to those used for carcinoma of the ovary.

Surgery

The recommended surgical approach for tubal carcinoma is total abdominal hysterectomy, bilateral salpingo-oophorectomy, omentectomy, and resection of as much gross disease as possible. If the disease is limited to the pelvis or if all gross disease is resectable, a full surgical staging operation including multiple peritoneal biopsies, diaphragmatic biopsy, and sampling of the pelvic and paraaortic nodes is required. The importance of evaluation of the lymph nodes was pointed out by many

TABLE 38–36. Three Suggested Classifications for Fallopian Tube Carcinoma

Stage	FIGO Type[643]	Dukes' Type[641]	Modified Erez[630]
0		Carcinoma in situ	
I	Growth limited to tube	Tumor extends into submucosa or muscularis, not serosa	Tumor limited to the tube (mucosa or muscularis)
IA	One tube, no ascites		
IB	Both tubes, no ascites		
IC	One or both tubes with ascites with malignant cells		
II	Growth limited to the true pelvis	Tumor extends to serosa	
IIA	Extension to uterus or ovary		Tumor has extended through the serosa but not to contiguous organs
IIB	Extension to other pelvic tissues		Tumor directly invading surrounding organs in pelvis or abdomen or metastases to pelvic organs
III	Growth involving one or both ovaries with intraperitoneal metastases	Tumor extends to ovary or endometrium	True metastatic lesions outside the pelvis but confined to the abdomen
IV	Growth involving one or both tubes with distant metastases outside the peritoneal cavity	Tumor extends beyond reproductive organs	Metastatic disease outside the abdomen

researchers.[646,647] Tamimi and Figge[647] reported a 53% incidence of lymph node metastases for 15 patients, and Schray and associates[646] reported a 35% incidence for 34 patients.

Because of the potential for early exfoliation of malignant cells by the tubal lumen, no recommendation for conservative surgery in the young patient can be made. This same potential for early dissemination of malignant cells led most oncologists to recommend that all patients with tubal cancer be treated adjunctively with irradiation or chemotherapy. MacMurray and colleagues suggested that all patients with disease more advanced than stage I be treated with aggressive postoperative therapy.[648] In their series of 30 patients, 50% of failures were in the upper abdomen, and 44% failed in extraperitoneal sites.

The role of second-look surgery in fallopian tube cancer is not defined. Barakat and associates reported a lower recurrence rate among patients with a negative second-look operation than among similar patients with ovarian cancer.[645] He reported similar findings after a review of the literature.

Radiation Therapy

Postoperative radiation therapy in patients with fallopian tube carcinoma was recommended by some investigators and questioned by others.[627,634,649] Radiation therapy techniques currently used include 5000 cGy external-beam irradiation to the whole pelvis for the more aggressive stage I and II tumors. For stage III disease, whole-pelvis and abdominal irradiation are required. Techniques resemble those used for ovarian tumors. Instillation of radioactive colloidal gold (^{198}Au) and chromic phosphate (^{32}P) was recommended in cases without macroscopic disease in the peritoneal cavity.

Several studies suggested benefits from postoperative radiation therapy. In 1957, Engstrom reported significant improvement in patients with fallopian tube carcinoma treated with postoperative radium and deep external-beam irradiation; patients treated with postoperative radiation therapy had a 38% 5-year survival rate, and those treated with surgery only had a 5-year survival rate of 15%.[650] Green and Scully reported an average survival of 2 years with postoperative radiation and no survivors 1 year after surgery without radiation therapy.[628]

Phelps and Chapman reported good results for patients with stage I or II disease treated with megavoltage irradiation.[651] Nine patients with stage I or II disease received 2500 to 5000 cGy to the pelvis or abdomen. Six also received intraperitoneal radioactive colloidal gold or phosphate. Eight of the 9 patients were alive at the time of publication of the study, and 6 patients were 5-year survivors. Six patients with stage III disease were treated with postoperative radiation therapy; none survived. In a study of 34 patients, Amendola and colleagues reported 1 of 4 patients alive 5 years after therapy consisting of less than 3000 to 5000 cGy.[652] However, 5 of 14 patients who received more than 5000 cGy were alive and disease free.

MacMurray and associates reported 30 patients with adenocarcinoma of the fallopian tube treated at Washington University.[648] Nine had stage I disease, 11 had stage II, 7 had stage III, and 3 had stage IV. Primary surgical treatment consisted of total abdominal hysterectomy and bilateral salpingo-oophorectomy in 70% of patients; 23% had more extensive surgery than this, and 13% had incomplete extirpation of the female genitalia. Three patients with stage I tumors were treated with surgery alone, and the remainder received postoperative radiation, chemotherapy, or both. Survival was unrelated to grade but highly dependent on stage. Disease-free survival at 3 years was 86% for stage I, 27% for stage II, 29% for stage III, and 0% for stage IV. Four of 5 patients treated after surgery with a combination of cisplatin, doxorubicin, and cyclophosphamide survived at least 3 years. Patterns of initial treatment failure showed 56% with a component of pelvic failure, 50% with a component of upper abdominal failure, and 44% with extraperitoneal metastases as a component of failure. The results according to method of treatment suggest that aggressive postoperative adjuvant therapy targeted at upper abdominal and distant sites for metastases of all lesions beyond stage I can improve survival and tumor control (Table 38–37).[653]

Chemotherapy

Because of the paucity of data about the chemosensitivity of this tumor and because its histology and pattern of spread resemble those of epithelial ovarian tumors, it was common practice to treat these rare carcinomas with chemotherapeutic regimens active in epithelial ovarian cancer. However, one study of 30 patients suggests that, although the tumors behave like ovarian cancer, they present at earlier stages and there is an increased frequency of failure due to distant metastases.[648] These observations coupled with the generally poor

TABLE 38–37. Survival According to Treatment and Stage for Patients Surviving 3 Years or More

Stage	S	S + RT	S + CT	S + PAC	S + CT + RT	Total
I	3/3	1/2	3/3*		1/1	8/9
II		2/5	0/2	3/3†	0/1	5/11
III			0/3	1/2	1/2*	2/7
IV			0/1		0/2	0/3

S, surgery; RT, radiation therapy; CT, chemotherapy; PAC, cisplatin, doxorubicin (Adriamycin), and cyclophosphamide (Cytoxan).
* Two patients received RT.
† One patient alive with disease.
(Jacobs AJ, MacMurray EH, Parham J, et al. Treatment of carcinoma of the fallopian tube using cisplatin, doxorubicin, and cyclophosphamide. Am J Clin Oncol 1986;9:436–439)

prognosis suggest a potential role for adjuvant postoperative chemotherapy, but few adjuvant studies were done. Adjuvant chlorambucil used with pelvic irradiation produced some long-term survivors, but the independent contribution of the adjuvant chemotherapy is difficult to assess.[654]

Several single agents have activity against fallopian tube carcinoma, including the alkylating agents (*e.g.,* melphalan, thiotepa, cyclophosphamide, chlorambucil), doxorubicin, and cisplatin.[655,656]

Combination chemotherapy was more commonly used in recent years, and the CAP regimen (*i.e.,* cyclophosphamide, doxorubicin and cisplatin) used in 9 patients produced four complete remissions with 3 of the 4 patients surviving without evidence of disease at 18 to 56 months.[653] This small study suggests significant activity for this combination, and it should be further investigated.

More than 50 patients were treated with cisplatin-based combinations, with overall response rates and survivals similar to patients with similar stages of epithelial ovarian cancer.[657,658] In a summary of the Roswell Park experience, Rose and colleagues treated 14 patients with cisplatin-based chemotherapy. There were three responses (21%), two complete and one partial.[659]

Hormonal therapy, particularly progestational agents, used in a few small studies was not successful.[655,660]

GESTATIONAL TROPHOBLASTIC DISEASE

Gestational trophoblastic disease is actually a spectrum of neoplasia that encompasses benign hydatidiform mole, locally invasive mole, and choriocarcinoma. Although the disorder is uncommon in the United States and makes up less than 1% of female gynecologic malignancies, it is extremely important because of the high degree of curability with appropriate treatment. Because of the rarity of the disease, most patients should be treated at trophoblastic disease centers, where sufficient expertise exists to deal with the complex and life-threatening nature of this disorder. Because of adherence to these principles, death from this disease is now rare.

EPIDEMIOLOGY

Although rare in the United States, the disease is much more common in other areas of the world, particularly in Asia and in South America, where incidences as high as 1 in 120 pregnancies were reported. Although the precise explanation for this increase is unknown, many investigators suggested nutritional or dietary factors. Studies in Philippine populations revealed a lower incidence among the meat-eating, wealthy populations than in the poorer populations, whose diets were heavily based on fish and rice and whose incidence of molar pregnancy was as high as 1 in 200.[661] The incidence is approximately 1 in 1200 pregnancies in the United States. In most series, increasing age, particularly above the age of 40, increases the risk. This is true in all countries but is most dramatic in countries in which a high baseline risk is already existent. Studies in Singapore demonstrate a 12-fold increase in risk for women older than 45.[662] Although risk increases with pregnancies after age 40, there appears to be no increasing risk with advancing parity. The patient's age or the parity does not affect the outcome of a molar pregnancy.

CLASSIFICATION AND PATHOLOGY

Approximately half of all trophoblastic tumors develop after a molar pregnancy, but they can develop after an abortion, an ectopic pregnancy, or an apparently normal term pregnancy. If the disease occurs after a molar pregnancy, the tumor can be a hydatidiform mole or choriocarcinoma. If the disease develops in any of the other settings, virtually all the tumors are choriocarcinoma. The trophoblastic neoplasias can be classified morphologically as hydatidiform mole, invasive mole, and choriocarcinoma.

Hydatidiform moles have clusters of hydropic villi, absence of fetal vessels, and trophoblastic hyperplasia. Invasive moles have similar histologic findings but display a greater tendency to invade surrounding tissues. These tumors are locally invasive in about 15% of patients after a molar pregnancy. Locally invasive moles are sometimes called chorioadenoma destruens if they follow a molar pregnancy. Trophoblastic disease can undergo spontaneous regression or local invasion or can metastasize hematogenously. Choriocarcinomas consist of anaplastic trophoblastic tissue with cytotrophoblastic and syncytiotrophoblastic elements and no identifiable villi.

Several attempts were made to develop pathologic classifications that would correlate with clinical outcome.[663,664] Although classifications that include patterns of growth, extent of stromal invasion, nuclear grade, and lymphocytic infiltration have broadly correlated, the management and outcome have been based on staging and clinical definitions of low-, moderate-, and high-risk patients.

TUMOR MARKERS

A major reason for the successful management of this tumor was the availability of a marker that is invariably present with the disease. All types of trophoblastic disease produce human chorionic gonadotropin (hCG), and the quantity produced is proportional to the volume of the disease.[665] The hCG titers can be used as an accurate monitor of response to therapy. Diagnosis and management depend on careful radioimmunoassay of this substance. Pregnancy tests or biologic assays have no place in the management of the disease.

HCG consists of α and β chains. Because the α chain is cross-reactive with leutinizing hormone (LH), it was the source of some confusion in diagnosis and subsequent management. An assay for the β subunit was developed that selectively assays hCG in the presence of normal LH.[666] Use of this specific radioimmunoassay is required for monitoring all patients with trophoblastic disease. After evacuation of a molar pregnancy, the elevated hCG titers disappear in 8 to 10 weeks, although clearance may be delayed as long as 14 to 16 weeks in about 25% of patients.[667]

CLINICAL EVALUATION AND STAGING

Molar pregnancies are associated with first-trimester bleeding, ectopic pregnancies, or threatened abortions. The uterus is often large for the estimated length of the gestation, and the hCG titers are elevated in excess of a normal pregnancy. Fetal heart sounds are absent, and obviously fetal parts are not palpable. Early toxemia of pregnancy may occur. Expulsion of grape-like villi often provides the most common presenting finding for invasive mole or choriocarcinoma. Occasionally, patients present with metastatic disease as the first manifestation of their illness.

Ultrasound evaluation is increasingly used to evaluate molar pregnancies, and the characteristic findings can be diagnostic. These techniques may also define extrauterine extension but are not always diagnostic.[668] Amniography produces a typical moth-eaten appearance that is also characteristic. Neither amniography or angiography is used frequently because of the current sophistication of ultrasonography. The diagnosis is based on the clinical findings, hCG titer, ultrasound, and pathologic confirmation. Patients with molar pregnancy should be further evaluated with chest radiographs, careful pelvic examinations, and weekly serial monitoring of the hCG titers. Patients who have evidence of persistent disease and those found to have choriocarcinoma should have chest radiographs and brain and liver scans to define the extent of metastatic spread.

Distant metastases are found in about 5% of patients who have molar pregnancies. Choriocarcinoma spreads hematogenously, and the common metastatic sites are the lungs (80%), vagina (30%), pelvis (20%), liver (10%), brain (10%), and bowel, kidney, and spleen (5%).[669]

No uniform staging classification has received widespread adoption. Many investigators classify patients according to whether disease is metastatic or nonmetastatic, and those with metastatic disease are further divided into low-risk and high-risk groups.[670] Several staging schemes have been used, including those of Bagshawe,[670] the Dutch Working Group for trophoblastic tumors,[671] and the New England Trophoblastic Disease Center.[670] Comparisons of all three staging classifications documented similar degrees of specificity and prognostic value.[671] The latter two classifications are easier to apply because they are based on data that are readily available and do not require information about the husband's blood group, lymphocytic infiltration of the tumor, or the patient's immune status. None of these retrospective comparisons identify a particular staging classification as superior, but the staging classification used by the New England Trophoblastic Disease Center is straightforward and useful (Table 38–38).[669] Patients are divided into high-risk and low-risk molar pregnancies, patients with disease confined to the corpus of the uterus (stage I), patients with local pelvic spread (stage II), and patients with more advanced disease (stages III and IV). Patients thought to have low-risk molar pregnancies include those with

TABLE 38–38. Staging of Gestational Trophoblastic Neoplasms

Stage 0	Molar pregnancy
	A. Low risk
	B. High risk
Stage I	Confined to uterine corpus
Stage II	Metastases to pelvis and vagina
Stage III	Metastasis to lung
Stage IV	Distant metastases

(Goldstein DP, Berkowitz RS. The management of gestational trophoblastic neoplasms. Curr Probl Obstet Gynecol 1980;4:1)

hCG titers less than 100,000 IU/ml, small uterine size, ovarian enlargement less than 6 cm, and no other poor-prognosis metabolic or epidemiologic factors.[672] Patients at high risk include those with hCG titers greater than 100,000 IU/ml, uterine size greater than normal for date of gestation, enlarged ovaries, and any of the poor-prognosis metabolic or epidemiologic factors, including maternal age over 40, toxemia, coagulopathy, trophoblastic tumor with or without embolization, and hyperthyroidism.

Seventy-five percent of patients with stage I disease have classic invasive mole, and the remaining 25% have locally invasive choriocarcinoma. Stages 0 to 3 have good prognoses if treated with currently available therapies. Stage IV patients include those with poor prognostic findings. All have choriocarcinoma and include those with initial hCG titers more than 100,000 IU/ml, persistence of disease longer than 4 months after initial therapy, and those with brain or liver metastasis.

TREATMENT

Patients with hydatidiform mole require evacuation of the uterus by suction curettage and oxytocin. After evacuation, patients usually have dilatation and curettage. In 80% of patients, no additional therapy is needed. Subsequent follow-up requires weekly hCG assay until the titer returns to normal.

The mainstay of treatment for the other gestational trophoblastic neoplasias is chemotherapy. Before chemotherapy, only 40% of patients could be cured with hysterectomy alone, even if the disease appeared localized. If there was evidence of metastatic spread, fewer than 10% of those patients survived, despite aggressive surgery and irradiation. The classic reports of Li and colleagues[673] of the activity of methotrexate in the 1950s and the subsequent documentation of the curative capacity of chemotherapy by Hertz and associates[674] represent milestones in cancer treatment and ushered in the era of modern chemotherapy.

Chemotherapy is now commonly used to manage many patients with gestational trophoblastic neoplasia. Patients with hydatidiform mole receive chemotherapy if there is a persistent plateau in the weekly hCG level, a rise in the hCG titer, or the development of metastases. Patients with invasive mole or choriocarcinoma or any patient who presents with metastatic disease requires immediate chemotherapy.

Patients requiring chemotherapy are divided into good-risk patients who can be cured with single-agent chemotherapy and poor-risk patients who require initial combination chemotherapy for best results. Poor-risk features include stage IV disease, cerebral or hepatic metastases, hCG levels of greater than 100,000 IU/ml, previous unsuccessful treatment, persistence of symptoms for longer than 4 months, or disease after a full-term pregnancy. Using these criteria, treatment selection can be based on risk factors and stage.

Treatment of Low-Risk Patients

Historically, single-agent chemotherapy was most commonly used for low-risk patients (*i.e.*, stages I and II and low-risk metastatic disease). Intramuscular methotrexate or dactinomycin were the standard single-agent therapies, with methotrexate given intramuscularly (0.4 mg/kg/day) for 5 days every 2 weeks or dactinomycin (10–12 μg/kg/day) given for 5 days every 2 weeks. Although this therapy is extremely effective for low-risk trophoblastic disease, both regimens have significant toxic effects. Moderate-dose methotrexate with leucovorin rescue achieved similar results with less toxicity. The New England Trophoblastic Disease Center (NETDC) published their 10-year experience with this regimen.[675] For 185 patients treated, complete remissions were achieved in 88% of patients, including 90% of the 163 patients with non-metastatic disease and 68% of those with low-risk metastatic disease. In 82% of these patients, complete remission was achieved with a single course of methotrexate and leucovorin. The regimen includes methotrexate (1 mg/kg) given intramuscularly every other day for four doses, followed by leucovorin (0.1 mg/kg) given intramuscularly 24 hours after each methotrexate dose.

After the initial course of chemotherapy, the response to therapy is monitored by hCG regression curves.[674] One log or greater fall in hCG titer over the subsequent 18 days allows the physician to withhold further therapy. If the hCG titer does not fall to this degree, reaches a plateau, or begins rising, a second course of therapy is administered. Therapy continues until the hCG titer normalizes for 3 weeks. Patients are monitored at monthly intervals for 1 year. If hCG titers remain normal for a year, pregnancy may be allowed.

Toxicity was modest in the NETDC study. Granulocytopenia occurred in 6% of patients and thrombocytopenia in fewer than 2%. There was no alopecia, and nausea and vomiting were rare. Although 14% of patients developed enzyme evidence of hepatic toxicity, this resolved within 2 weeks after completing therapy. All of the patients in this series who failed initial induction therapy with methotrexate-leucovorin achieved complete remissions with subsequent combination chemotherapy. On the basis of this extensive experience, this regimen appears to be the treatment of choice for low-risk gestational trophoblastic disease.

Treatment of High-Risk Patients

All high-risk patients should receive initial combination chemotherapy. One of the most commonly used regimens was methotrexate (0.3 mg/kg) given intramuscularly, dactinomycin (10 μg/kg) given intravenously, and chlorambucil (10 mg) given orally daily for 5 days, with courses repeated as required until 3 successive weeks of normal hCG levels are achieved.[676] Other effective regimens include CHAMOCA, MAC, or PVB.[677–680] Using these regimens, complete responses are usually achieved in approximately 80% of patients, although lower responses (60–70%) are seen in patients with hepatic or cerebral metastases.[681]

Newlands from Bagshawe's group reported 10-year results of 148 patients with high-risk disease treated with etoposide, methotrexate, dactinomycin, cyclophosphamide (Cytoxan), Oncovin (EMA/CO).[683] Of the 76 patients who had not had prior therapy, 82% had sustained complete remissions. Some of the partial remissions and relapses were salvaged with cisplatin or surgery. Relapse after complete remission was uncommon (5.4%). Toxicity was primarily expressed as myelosuppression. Overall survival for all 148 patients was 85%. He concluded that EMA/CO is the treatment of choice for high-risk patients.

Salvage chemotherapy for patients failing initial induction therapy for high-risk disease employs six to seven drugs in combination.[677,682] One salvage regimen using high-dose cisplatin, vincristine, and methotrexate with leucovorin achieved durable complete remissions in 35% of previous failures.[683] With the identification of VP-16 and cisplatin as active agents in a salvage setting, several investigators used these drugs in new regimens.[682–685]

PVB, after failure of conventional triple therapy, produced complete remissions in 50% of patients, although only 20% (2 of 11) had sustained complete remissions.

In the EMA/CO study, 72 patients with high-risk disease had been previously treated with chemotherapy. Fifty-seven (79%) achieved a complete remission, but an additional 10% were salvaged with surgery or cisplatin, and 89% of these salvaged patients were alive at mean follow-up of 50 months.[686]

Patients with brain or liver metastasis are generally treated with local irradiation to the sites. Patients with proved brain metastasis or elevations of cerebrospinal fluid hCG are treated with 3000 cGy of whole-brain irradiation. Surgery is rarely required. Patients with hepatic metastasis are often treated with 2500 cGy before initiating chemotherapy to reduce the risk of intrahepatic hemorrhage during chemotherapy.

Long-Term Complications of Chemotherapy

Several studies of the long-term consequences of successful therapy for gestational trophoblastic disease were published, and there is no evidence of increased risk of maternal complications or fetal abnormalities associated with these treatments.[687,688]

POSTIRRADIATION GYNECOLOGIC MALIGNANCIES

Several reports were published on the incidence of malignant tumors of the endometrium or other pelvic organs in patients treated with irradiation for benign or malignant pelvic conditions. Smith and Doll reported an increased incidence of leukemia (7 deaths observed versus 2.3 expected) and cancers of the heavily irradiated sites (59 observed versus 40.1 expected) 5 or more years after irradiation to the pelvis for benign metropathia hemorrhagica.[689] The mean dose of radiation to the bone marrow was estimated to correlate with the projected excess rate of leukemia, which is about 1.2 case/million/women/year/cGy. However, researchers like Hutchinson did not observe this increased incidence (3 cases observed versus 16 expected).[690] Dickson reported 2 deaths from leukemia, but only 1.1 were expected.[691] Wagoner observed no excess leukemia among 7835 women treated with radium and roentgen rays for primary uterine cancer.[692] Others observed no significant increase of malignancy in patients treated with irradiation for carcinoma of the uterine cervix.[693,694]

Storm carried out a comprehensive analysis of the Danish Cancer Registry data for 24,970 women with invasive cervical cancer and 19,470 with in situ carcinoma of the cervix treated between 1943 and 1982.[695] There was a small overall excess of second primary cancers in the lung, stomach, pancreas, rectum, and bladder and acute connective tissue sarcomas, although there was a decreased incidence of breast cancer in the irradiated patients compared with nonirradiated patients. The significant decreased incidence of breast cancer observed may be attributable to the effect of ovarian ablation by radiation therapy. In the patients irradiated for invasive carcinoma, there was an excess of 64 cases per 10,000 women per year of tumors in organs close to or at intermediate distance from the cervix, reaching the maximum after 30 or more years of follow-up. A high risk for development of acute nonlymphatic leukemia was observed in irradiated patients with carcinoma in situ, but not in those with invasive lesions. This could be explained by the lower doses of irradiation delivered to the bone marrow in the in situ tumors treated with brachytherapy alone. Lower doses of irradiation, with greater induction of mutations and less cell killing, may be responsible for the leukemogenic effect.

Decreased risk was also observed for tumors of the brain, myeloma of the skin, and tumors of the colon other than rectal. Storm recommended follow-up for life of the irradiated patients to evaluate the long-term carcinogenic effects of irradiation.[695]

Wagoner studied 1803 patients treated for benign gynecologic disorders with radium and observed 10 deaths from leukemia against 3.6 expected; in a similar series in Connecticut, 9 cases of leukemia were seen against 2.8 expected.[692] A decreased death rate from carcinoma of the breast was observed with an artificial inducement of menopause.[696,697,689] Among patients treated for carcinoma of the cervix at Washington University, a similar lower mortality from breast cancer was observed. It is possible that the castration induced by irradiation in younger women may influence the subsequent development of carcinoma of the breast. Villasanta and Rubel reported 15 cases of pelvic malignancy in 174 patients irradiated for benign uterine bleeding in contrast to 3 cases of malignant tumors in 147 nonrandomized control patients who were not irradiated.[698] Most of the tumors developed in the endometrium or the ovary. The dose of irradiation was relatively small (2000–2400 mgh). The same researchers observed only 19 patients developing a second pelvic malignancy among 569 women with malignant tumors of the gynecologic tract treated with doses of irradiation above 5000 cGy and followed for 4 years or longer. Dickson pointed out that the incidence of malignancy after irradiation for benign uterine bleeding was significantly less in patients treated with external irradiation than in those treated with intracavitary radium.[691] Most postirradiation malignancies of the uterus are adenocarcinomas of the endometrium, followed by mixed müllerian tumors and sarcomas of the uterine cervix.[699] The prognosis of these patients after treatment was similar to that of patients who had not had irradiation.[699]

The principles of management for these patients are similar to those for patients who received no previous irradiation. Most researchers agree that the primary treatment of these patients is surgical. There is some controversy about whether preoperative or postoperative irradiation should be delivered. However, the number of patients is small, and no definite conclusions can be drawn.

REFERENCES

1. Boring CC, Squires TS, Tong T. Cancer statistics. CA 1992;42:19.
2. Andersen BL, Hacker NF. Psychosexual adjustment after vulvar surgery. Obstet Gynecol 1983;62:457–462.
3. Collins CG, Roman-Lopez JJ, Lee FYL. Intraepithelial carcinoma of the vulva. Am J Obstet Gynecol 1987;108:1187.
4. Boutselis JG. Intraepithelial carcinoma of the vulva. Am J Obstet Gynecol 1972;113:733–738.
5. Japaze H, Garcia BR, Woodruff JD. Primary vulvar neoplasia: A review of in situ and invasive carcinoma, 1935–1972. Obstet Gynecol 1977;49:404–411.
6. Forney JP, Morrow CP, Townsend DE, Di Saia PJ. Management of carcinoma in situ of the vulva. Am J Obstet Gynecol 1977;127:801–806.
7. Friedrich EJ, Wilkinson EJ, Fu YS. Carcinoma in situ of the vulva: A continuing challenge. Am J Obstet Gynecol 1980;136:830–843.
8. Magrina JF, Webb MJ, Gaffey TA, Symmonds RE. Stage I squamous cell cancer of the vulva. Am J Obstet Gynecol 1979;134:453–459.
9. Podratz KC, Symmonds RE, Taylor WF, Williams TJ. Carcinoma of the vulva: Analysis of treatment and survival. Obstet Gynecol 1983;61:63–74.
10. Hacker NF, Leuchter RS, Berek JS, Castaldo TW, Lagasse LD. Radical vulvectomy and bilateral inguinal lymphadenectomy through separate groin incisions. Obstet Gynecol 1981;58:574–579.
11. Mack T, Casagrande JT. Epidemiology of gynecologic cancer: II. Endometrium, ovary, vagina, and vulva. In: Coppleson MC, ed. Gynecologic oncology: Fundamental principles and clinical practice. New York: Churchill Livingstone, 1981:28–30.
12. Green TJ. Carcinoma of the vulva. A reassessment. Obstet Gynecol 1978;52:462–469.
13. Morley GW. Infiltrative carcinoma of the vulva: Results of surgical treatment. Am J Obstet Gynecol 1976;124:874–888.
14. Josey WE, Nahmias AJ, Naib ZM. Viruses and cancer of the lower genital tract. Cancer 1976;38:526–533.
15. Bornstein J, Kaufman RH, Adam E, Adler SK. Multicentric intraepithelial neoplasia involving the vulva. Clinical features and association with human papillomavirus and herpes simplex virus. Cancer 1988;62:1601–1604.
16. Carson LF, Twiggs LB, Okagaki T, Clark BA, Ostrow RS, Faras AJ. Human papillomavirus DNA in adenosquamous carcinoma and squamous cell carcinoma of the vulva. Obstet Gynecol 1988;72:63–67.
17. Downey GO, Okagaki T, Ostrow RS, Clark BA, Twiggs LB, Faras AJ. Condylomatous carcinoma of the vulva with special reference to human papillomavirus DNA. Obstet Gynecol 1988;72:68–73.
18. Gupta J, Pilotti S, Rilke F, Shah K. Association of human papillomavirus type 16 with neoplastic lesions of the vulva and other genital sites by in situ hybridization. Am J Pathol 1987;127:206–215.
19. Kaufman RH, Bornstein J, Adam E, Burek J, Tessin B, Adler SK. Human papillomavirus and herpes simplex virus in vulvar squamous cell carcinoma in situ. Am J Obstet Gynecol 1988;158:862–871.
20. Mabuchi K, Bross DS, Kessler II. Epidemiology of cancer of the vulva. A case-control study. Cancer 1985;55:1843–1848.
21. Deligdisch L, Szulman AE. Multiple and multifocal carcinomas in female genital organs and breast. Gynecol Oncol 1975;3:181–190.
22. Stern BD, Kaplan L. Multicentric foci of carcinomas arising in structures of cloacal origin. Am J Obstet Gynecol 1969;104:255–266.
23. Buscema J. The significance of the histological alterations adjacent to invasive vulvar carcinoma. Am J Obstet Gynecol 1987;156:212–222.
24. Plentl AA, Friedman EA. Lymphatic system of the female genitalia: The morphologic basis of oncologic diagnosis and therapy. Philadelphia: WB Saunders, 1971.
25. Way S. Carcinoma of the vulva. In: Meigs JV, Sturgis SH, ed. Progress in gynecology. New York: Grune & Stratton, 1957.
26. Iversen T, Aas M. Lymph drainage from the vulva. Gynecol Oncol 1983;16:179–189.
27. Kaufman RH, Gardner HL. Intraepithelial carcinoma of the vulva. Clin Obstet Gynecol 1965;8:1035–1050.
28. Friedrich EG Jr, Wilkinson EJ. The vulva. In: Blaustein A, ed. Pathology of the female genital tract. New York: Springer-Verlag, 1977.
29. Helwig EB, Graham JH. Anogenital (extramammary) Paget's disease. Cancer 1963;16:387.
30. Friedrich EJ, Wilkinson EJ, Steingraeber PH, Lewis JD. Paget's disease of the vulva and carcinoma of the breast. Obstet Gynecol 1975;46:130–134.
31. Tchang F, Okagaki T, Richart RM. Adenocarcinoma of Bartholin's gland associated with Paget's disease of vulvar area. Cancer 1973;31:221–225.
32. Woodruff JD, Richardson EH. Malignant vulvar Paget's disease. Obstet Gynecol 1957;10:10.
33. Gosling JRH, Abell MR, Drolette BM, et al. Infiltrative squamous cell carcinoma of the vulva. Cancer 1961;14:330.
34. Way S. Carcinoma of the vulva. Am J Obstet Gynecol 1960;79:692.
35. Wharton JT, Gallager S, Rutledge FN. Microinvasive carcinoma of the vulva. Am J Obstet Gynecol 1974;118:159–162.
36. Kneale BL. Microinvasive cancer of the vulva: Report of the International Society for the Study of Vulvar Disease Task Force, VIIth Congress. J Reprod Med 1984;29:454.
37. Lasser A, Cornog JL, Morris JM. Adenoid squamous cell carcinoma of the vulva. Cancer 1974;33:224–227.
38. Gallousis S. Verrucous carcinoma. Report of three vulvar cases and review of the literature. Obstet Gynecol 1972;40:502–507.
39. Lucas WE, Benirschke K, Lebherz TB. Verrucous carcinoma of the female genital tract. Am J Obstet Gynecol 1974;119:435–440.
40. Chung AF, Woodruff JM, Lewis JL Jr. Malignant melanoma of the vulva. Obstet Gynecol 1975;345:638.
41. Breen JL, Neubecker RD, Greenwald E, et al. Basal cell carcinomas of the vulva. Obstet Gynecol 1975;46:122.
42. Tavassoli FA, Norris HJ. Smooth muscle tumors of the vulva. Obstet Gynecol 1979;53:213–217.

43. Buscema J, Woodruff JD, Parmley TH, Genadry R. Carcinoma in situ of the vulva. Obstet Gynecol 1980;55:225–230.
44. Weiner SA, Lee JKT, Kao MS, Moon TE. The role of lymphangiography in vulvar carcinoma. Am J Obstet Gynecol 1986;5:1073.
45. Perez CA, Grigsby PW. Carcinoma of the vulva. In: Perez CA, Brady LW, eds. Principles and practice of radiation oncology. 2nd ed. Philadelphia: JB Lippincott, 1992.
46. International Federation of Gynecology and Obstetrics. Annual report on the results of treatment in gynecological cancer. Int J Gynecol Obstet 1989;28:189–190.
47. Clark WH Jr. A classification of malignant melanoma in men correlated with histogenesis and biologic behavior. In: Montagna W, Hu F, eds. Advances in biology of skin and pigmentary system. London: Pergamon Press, 1967.
48. Breslow A. Thickness, cross-sectional areas and depth of invasion in the prognosis of cutaneous melanoma. Ann Surg 1970;172:902–908.
49. Homesley HD, Bundy BN, Sedlis A, et al. Assessment of current International Federation of Gynecology and Obstetrics staging of vulvar carcinoma relative to prognostic factors for survival (a Gynecologic Oncology Group study). Am J Obstet Gynecol 1991;164:997–1003.
50. Rutledge FN, Sinclair M. Treatment of intraepithelial carcinoma of the vulva by skin excision and graft. Am J Obstet Gynecol 1986;102:806.
51. Barnhill DR, Hoskins WJ, Metz P. Use of the rhomboid flap after partial vulvectomy. Obstet Gynecol 1983;52:444.
52. Woodruff JD, Julian C, Puray T, Mermut S, Katayama P. The contemporary challenge of carcinoma in situ of the vulva. Am J Obstet Gynecol 1973;115:677–686.
53. Dean RE, Taylor ES, Weisbrod DM, Martin JW. The treatment of premalignant and malignant lesions of the vulva. Am J Obstet Gynecol 1974;119:59–68.
54. Gregori CA, Smith CI, Breen JL. Extramammary Paget's disease. Clin Obstet Gynecol 1978;21:1107–1115.
55. Watring WG, Roberts JA, Lagasse LD, et al. Treatment of recurrent Paget's disease of the vulva with topical bleomycin. Cancer 1978;41:10–11.
56. Di Paola GR, Gomez RN, Arrighi L. Relevance of microinvasion in carcinoma of the vulva. Obstet Gynecol 1975;45:647–649.
57. Kneale BLG, Elliott PM, McDonald IA. Microinvasive carcinoma of the vulva: Clinical features and management. In: Coppleson M, ed. Gynecologic oncology: Fundamental principles and clinical practice. New York: Churchill Livingstone, 1981:320–328.
58. Hacker NF. Vulvar cancer. In: Berek JS, Hacker NF, eds. Practical gynecologic oncology. Baltimore: Williams & Wilkins, 1989:391–407.
59. Di Saia PJ, Creasman WT, Rich WM. An alternate approach to early cancer of the vulva. Am J Obstet Gynecol 1979;133:825–832.
60. Heaps JM, Fu YS, Montz FJ, Hacker NF, Berek JS. Surgical-pathologic variables predictive of local recurrence in squamous cell carcinoma of the vulva. Gynecol Oncol 1990;38:309–314.
61. Mattingly RF, Thompson JO. Telinde's operative gynecology. 6th ed. Philadelphia: JB Lippincott, 1985.
62. Burrell MO, Franklin E, Campion MJ, Crozier MA, Stacy DW. The modified radical vulvectomy with groin dissection: An eight-year experience. Am J Obstet Gynecol 1988;159:715–722.
63. Burke TW, Stringer CA, Gershenson DM, Edwards CL, Morris M, Wharton JT. Radical wide excision and selective inguinal node dissection for squamous cell carcinoma of the vulva. Gynecol Oncol 1990;38:328–332.
64. Homesley HD, Bundy BN, Sedlis A, Adcock L. Radiation therapy versus pelvic node resection for carcinoma of the vulva with positive groin nodes. Obstet Gynecol 1986;68:733–740.
65. Boronow RC. Combined therapy as an alternative to exenteration for locally advanced vulvo-vaginal cancer: Rationale and results. Cancer 1982;49:1085–1091.
66. Woolcott RJ, Henry RJ, Houghton CR. Malignant melanoma of the vulva. Australian experience. J Reprod Med 1988;33:699–702.
67. Copeland LJ, Sneige N, Gershenson DM, McGuffee VB, Abdul KF, Rutledge FN. Bartholin gland carcinoma. Obstet Gynecol 1986;67:794–801.
68. Boronow RC, Hickman BT, Reagan MT, Smith RA, Steadham RE. Combined therapy as an alternative to exenteration for locally advanced vulvovaginal cancer. II. Results, complications, and dosimetric surgical considerations. Am J Clin Oncol 1987;10:171–181.
69. Prempree T, Amornmarn R. Radiation treatment of recurrent carcinoma of the vulva. Cancer 1984;54:1943–1949.
70. Buchler DA, Kline JC, Tunca JC, Carr WF. Treatment of recurrent carcinoma of the vulva. Gynecol Oncol 1979;8:180–184.
71. Frankendal B, Larsson LG, Westling P. Carcinoma of the vulva. Results of an individualized treatment schedule. Acta Radiol Ther Phys Biol 1973;12:165–174.
72. Acosta AA, Given FT, Frazier AB, Cordoba RB, Luminari A. Preoperative radiation therapy in the management of squamous cell carcinoma of the vulva: Preliminary report. Am J Obstet Gynecol 1978;132:198–206.
73. Daly JW, Million RR. Radical vulvectomy combined with elective node irradiation for TXN0 squamous carcinoma of the vulva. Cancer 1974;34:161–165.
74. Hacker NF, Berek JS, Juillard GJ, Lagasse LD. Preoperative radiation therapy for locally advanced vulvar cancer. Cancer 1984;54:2056–2061.
75. Kucera H. Treatment of the carcinoma of the vulva at the first University-Clinic of Gynecology in Vienna (386 cases). [Author's translation]. Strahlentherapie 1980;156:598–600.
76. Simonsen E, Nordberg UB, Johnsson JE, Lamm IL, Trope C. Radiation therapy and surgery in the treatment of regional lymph nodes in squamous cell carcinoma of the vulva. Acta Radiol Oncol 1984;23:433–442.
77. Kucera H, Weghaupt K. The electrosurgical operation of vulvar carcinoma with postoperative irradiation of inguinal lymph nodes. Gynecol Oncol 1988;29:158–167.
78. Miyazawa K, Nori D, Hilaris BS, Lewis JJ. Role of radiation therapy in the treatment of advanced vulvar carcinoma. J Reprod Med 1983;28:539–541.
79. Pao WM, Perez CA, Kuske RR, Sommers GM, Camel HM, Galakatos AE. Radiation therapy and conservation surgery for primary and recurrent carcinoma of the vulva: Report of 40 patients and a review of the literature. Int J Radiat Oncol Biol Phys 1988;14:1123–1132.
80. Schulz U, Callies R, Kruger KG. Efficiency of postoperative electron therapy for localized cancer of the vulva. [Author's translation]. Strahlentherapie 1980;156:326–330.
81. Stillman FH, Sedlis A, Boyce JG. A review of lower genital intraepithelial neoplasia and the use of topical 5-fluorouracil. Obstet Gynecol Surv 1985;40:190–220.
82. Caglar H, Hertzog RW, Hreshchyshyn MM. Topical 5-fluorouracil treatment of vaginal intraepithelial neoplasia. Obstet Gynecol 1981;58:580–583.
83. Stillman FH, Boyce JG, Macasaet MA, Nicastri AD. 5-Fluorouracil/chemosurgery for intraepithelial neoplasia of the lower genital tract. Obstet Gynecol 1981;58:356–360.
84. Deppe G, Bruckner HW, Cohen CJ. Adriamycin treatment of advanced vulvar carcinoma. Obstet Gynecol 1977;50:13–14.
85. Trope C, Johnsson JE, Larsson G, et al. Bleomycin alone or combined with mitomycin-C in treatment of advanced or recurrent squamous cell carcinoma of the vulva. Cancer Treat Rep 1980;64:639–642.
86. Belinson JL, Stewart JA, Richards A, et al. Bleomycin, vincristine, mitomycin-C, and cisplatin in the management of gynecologic squamous cell cancer. Gynecol Oncol 1985;120:387–393.
87. Durrant KR, Mangione C, Lacave AJ, et al. Bleomycin, methotrexate, and CCNU in advanced inoperable squamous carcinoma of the vulva: A phase II study of the EORTC Gynaecological Cancer Cooperative Group (GCCG). Gynecol Oncol 1990;37:359–362.
88. Levin W, Goldberg G, Altaras M, Bloch B, Shelton MG. The use of concomitant chemotherapy and radiotherapy prior to surgery in advanced stage carcinoma of the vulva. Gynecol Oncol 1986;25:20–25.
89. Thomas G, Dembo A, DePetrillo A, et al. Concurrent radiation and chemotherapy in vulvar carcinoma. Gynecol Oncol 1989;34:263.
90. Hoskins WJ, Burke TW, Weiser EB, et al. Take advantage of rotational flaps for vulvar and vaginal surgery. Contemp Obstet Gynecol 1986;28:159.
91. Julian CG, Callison J, Woodruff JD. Plastic management of extensive vulvar defects. Obstet Gynecol 1971;38:193–198.
92. Rutledge F. Cancer of the vagina. Am J Obstet Gynecol 1967;97:635–655.
93. Herbst AL, Green TJ, Ulfelder H. Primary carcinoma of the vagina. An analysis of 68 cases. Am J Obstet Gynecol 1970;106:210–218.
94. Gallup DG, Morley GW. Carcinoma in situ of the vagina. A study and review. Obstet Gynecol 1975;46:334–340.
95. Hummer WK, Massey E, Decker DG, et al. Primary invasive squamous carcinoma of the vagina. Obstet Gynecol 1959;53:218.
96. Brinton LA, Nasca PC, Mallin K, et al. Case-control study of in situ and invasive carcinoma of the vagina. Gynecol Oncol 1990;38:49–54.
97. Pride GL, Schultz AE, Chuprevich TW, et al. Primary invasive squamous carcinoma of the vagina. Obstet Gynecol 1959;53:218.
98. Novak ER, Woodruff JD. Postirradiation malignancies of the pelvic organs. Am J Obstet Gynecol 1959;77:667.
99. Lee JY, Perez CA, Ettinger N, Fineberg BB. The risk of second primaries subsequent to irradiation for cervix cancer. Int J Radiat Oncol Biol Phys 1982;8:207–211.
100. Herbst AL, Ulfelder H, Poskanzer DC. Adenocarcinoma of the vagina: Association of maternal stilbesterol therapy with tumor appearance in young women. N Engl J Med 1971;11:284.
101. Herbst AL, Cole P, Colton T, et al. Age-incidence and risk of diethylstilbestrol-related clear cell adenocarcinoma of the vagina and cervix. Am J Obstet Gynecol 1977;128:48.
102. Herbst AL, Robboy SJ, Scully RE, Poskanzer DC. Clear-cell adenocarcinoma of the vagina and cervix in girls: Analysis of 170 registry cases. Am J Obstet Gynecol 1974;119:713–724.
103. Park RC, Parmley TH. Vaginal cancer. In: McGowan L, ed. Gynecologic oncology. New York: Appleton-Century-Crofts, 1978:174–184.
104. Perez CA, Arneson AN, Galakatos A, Samanth HK. Malignant tumors of the vagina. Cancer 1973;31:36–44.
105. Smith J. Malignant gynecologic tumors in children. Obstet Gynecol 1973;116:201.
106. Norris JH, Taylor HB. Melanomas of the vagina. Am J Clin Pathol 1966;46:420.
107. Blaustein A. Diseases of the vagina. In: Blaustein A, ed. Pathology of the female genital tract. New York: Springer-Verlag, 1977:59–86.
108. Cavanagh D, Praphat H, Ruffolo EH. Cancer of the vagina. Obstet Gynecol Annu 1980;9:311–325.
109. Perez CA, Arneson AN, Dehner LP, Galakatos A. Radiation therapy in carcinoma of the vagina. Obstet Gynecol 1974;44:862–872.
110. Vayrynen M, Romppanen T, Koskela E, Castren O, Syrjanen K. Verrucous squamous cell carcinoma of the female genital tract. Report of three cases and survey of the literature. Int J Gynaecol Obstet 1981;19:351–356.
111. Kurman RJ, Scully RE. The incidence and histogenesis of vaginal adenosis. An autopsy study. Hum Pathol 1974;5:265–276.
112. Robboy SJ, Herbst AL, Scully RE. Clear-cell adenocarcinoma of the vagina and cervix in young females: Analysis of 37 tumors that persisted or recurred after primary therapy. Cancer 1974;34:606–614.
113. Robboy SJ, Kaufman RH, Prat J, et al. Pathologic findings in young women enrolled in the National Cooperative Diethylstilbestrol Adenosis (DESAD) project. Obstet Gynecol 1979;53:309–317.
114. Robboy SJ, Scully RE, Welch WR, Herbst AL. Intrauterine diethylstilbestrol exposure

and its consequences: Pathologic characteristics of vaginal adenosis, clear cell adenocarcinoma, and related lesions. Arch Pathol Lab Med 1977;101:1–5.

115. Chung AF, Casey MJ, Flannery JT, Woodruff JM, Lewis JJ. Malignant melanoma of the vagina—report of 19 cases. Obstet Gynecol 1980;55:720–727.

116. Iversen K, Robins RE. Mucosal malignant melanomas. Am J Surg 1980;139:660–664.

117. Morrow CP, Di Saia PJ. Malignant melanoma of the female genitalia: A clinical analysis. Obstet Gynecol Surv 1976;31:233–271.

118. Berman ML, Tobon H, Surti U. Primary malignant melanoma of the vagina: Clinical, light and electron microscopic observations. Am J Obstet Gynecol 1981;139:963–965.

119. Bonner JA, Perez TC, Reid GC, Roberts JA, Morley GW. The management of vaginal melanoma. Cancer 1988;62:2066–2072.

120. Tobon H, Murphy AI. Benign blue nevus of the vagina. Cancer 1977;40:3174–3176.

121. Peters W, Kumar NB, Andersen WA, Morley GW. Primary sarcoma of the adult vagina: A clinicopathologic study. Obstet Gynecol 1985;65:699–704.

122. Tavassoli FA, Norris HJ. Smooth muscle tumors of the vagina. Obstet Gynecol 1979;53:689–693.

123. Copeland LJ, Gershenson DM, Saul PB, Sneige N, Stringer CA, Edwards CL. Sarcoma botryoides of the female genital tract. Obstet Gynecol 1985;66:262–266.

124. Ulbright TM, Kraus FT. Endometrial stomal tumors of extra-uterine tissue. Am J Clin Pathol 1981;76:371–377.

125. Chapman GW, Genda J, Williams T. Alveolar soft-part sarcoma of the vagina. Gynecol Oncol 1984;18:125.

126. Webb MJ, Symmonds RE, Weiland LH. Malignant fibrous histiocytoma of the vagina. Am J Obstet Gynecol 1974;119:190–192.

127. Okagaki T, Ishida T, Hilgers RD. A malignant tumor of the vagina resembling synovial sarcoma: A light and electron microscopic study. Cancer 1976;37:2306–2320.

128. Prempree T, Tang CK, Hatef A, Forster S. Angiosarcoma of the vagina: A clinicopathologic report. A reappraisal of the radiation treatment of angiosarcomas of the female genital tract. Cancer 1983;51:618–622.

129. Buscema J, Rosenshein NB, Taqi F, Woodruff JD. Vaginal hemangiopericytoma: A histopathologic and ultrastructural evaluation. Obstet Gynecol 1985;66:82S–85S.

130. Harris NL, Scully RE. Malignant lymphoma and granulocytic sarcoma of the uterus and vagina. A clinicopathologic analysis of 27 cases. Cancer 1984;53:2530–2545.

131. Wharton JT, Fletcher GH, Declos L. Invasive tumors of the vagina: Clinical features and management. In: Coppleson M, ed. Gynecologic oncology: Fundamental principles and clinical practice. New York: Churchill Livingstone, 1981:345–359.

132. Brady LW. Radiation therapy for carcinoma of the vagina. In: McGowan L, ed. Gynecologic oncology. New York: Appleton-Century-Crofts, 1978:185–190.

133. Chau PM. Radiotherapeutic management of malignant tumors of the vagina. Am J Roentgenol Radium Ther Nucl Med 1963;89:502.

134. Perez CA, Camel HM, Galakatos AE, et al. Definitive irradiation in carcinoma of the vagina: Long-term evaluation of results. Int J Radiat Oncol Biol Phys 1988;15:1283–1290.

135. Woodruff JD, Parmley TH, Julian CG. Topical 5-fluorouracil in the treatment of vaginal carcinoma-in-situ. Gynecol Oncol 1975;3:124–132.

136. Townsend DE. Intraepithelial neoplasia of the vagina. In: Coppleson M, ed. Gynecologic oncology: Fundamental principles and clinical practice. New York: Churchill Livingstone, 1981:339–344.

137. Brown GR, Fletcher GH, Rutledge FN. Irradiation of in situ and invasive squamous cell carcinomas of the vagina. Cancer 1971;28:1278–1283.

138. Perez CA, Camel HM. Long-term follow-up in radiation therapy of carcinoma of the vagina. Cancer 1982;49:1308–1315.

139. Underwood PJ, Smith RT. Carcinoma of the vagina. JAMA 1971;217:46–52.

140. Hopkins MP, Kumar NB, Lichter AS, Peters W, Morley GW. Small cell carcinoma of the vagina with neuroendocrine features. A report of three cases. J Reprod Med 1989;34:486–491.

141. Perez CA, Korba A, Sharma S. Dosimetric considerations in irradiation of carcinoma of the vagina. Int J Radiat Oncol Biol Phys 1977;2:639–649.

142. Perez CA, Di Saia PJ, Knapp RC. Gynecologic tumors. In: DeVita VT, Hellman S, Rosenberg SA, eds. Cancer: Principles and practice of oncology. Philadelphia: JB Lippincott, 1985:1013–1081.

143. Perez CA, Slessinger E, Grigsby PW. Design of an afterloading vaginal applicator (MIRALVA). Int J Radiat Oncol Biol Phys 1990;18:1503–1508.

144. MacNaught R, Symmonds RP, Hole D, Watson ER. Improved control of primary vaginal tumors by combined external beam and interstitial radiotherapy. Clin Radiol 1986;37:29.

145. Prempree T, Amornmarn R. Radiation treatment of primary carcinoma of the vagina. Patterns of failures after definitive therapy. Acta Radiol Oncol 1985;24:51–56.

146. Puthawala A, Syed AM, Nalick R, McNamara C, Di Saia PJ. Integrated external and interstitial radiation therapy for primary carcinoma of the vagina. Obstet Gynecol 1983;62:367–372.

147. Dancuart F, Delclos L, Wharton JT, Silva EG. Primary squamous cell carcinoma of the vagina treated by radiotherapy: A failures analysis—the M. D. Anderson Hospital experience 1955–1982. Int J Radiat Oncol Biol Phys 1988;14:745–749.

148. Wharton JT, Rutledge FN, Gallager HS, Fletcher G. Treatment of clear cell adenocarcinoma in young females. Obstet Gynecol 1975;45:365–368.

149. Fletcher GH. Textbook of radiotherapy. 3rd ed. Philadelphia: Lea and Febiger, 1980.

150. Grosfeld JL, Smith JP. Pelvic rhabdomyosarcoma in infants and children. J Urol 1973;107:673.

151. Ghavimi F, Exelby PR, D'Angio GJ, et al. Proceedings: Combination therapy of urogenital embryonal rhabdomyosarcoma in children. Cancer 1973;32:1178–1185.

152. Sordillo PP, Magill GB, Schauer PK, Vikram B, Kim JH, Hilaris BS. Preliminary trial of combination therapy with Adriamycin and radiation in sarcomas and other malignant tumors. J Surg Oncol 1982;21:23–26.

153. Kinsella TJ, Glatstein E. Clinical experience with intravenous radiosensitizers in unresectable sarcomas. Cancer 1987;59:908–915.

154. Piver MS, Barlow JJ, Xynos FP. Adriamycin alone or in combination in 100 patients with carcinoma of the cervix or vagina. Am J Obstet Gynecol 1978;131:311.

155. Evans LS, Kersh CR, Constable WC, et al. Concomitant 5-Fluorouracil, mitomycin-C, and radiotherapy for advanced gynecologic cancer. Int J Radiat Oncol Biol Phys 1988;15:901.

156. Brand E, Fu YS, Lagasse LD, et al. Vulvovaginal melanoma: Report of seven cases and literature review. Gynecol Oncol 1989;33:54.

157. Anderson WA, Sabio H, Durso N, et al. Endodermal sinus tumor of the vagina: The role of primary chemotherapy. Cancer 1985;56:1025.

158. Collins HS, Burke TW, Heller PB, et al. Endodermal sinus tumor of the infant vagina treated exclusively by chemotherapy. Obstet Gynecol 1989;73:507.

159. Hays DM, Shimada H, Rancy RB, et al. Sarcomas of the vagina and uterus: The Intergroup Rhabdomyosarcoma Study. J Pediatr Surg 1985;20:718.

160. Boring CC, Squires TS, Tong T. Cancer statistics. CA 1991;41:19–36.

161. Barber HRK. Incidence, prevalence, and median survival rates of gynecologic cancer. In: Van Nagell JR, Barber HRK, eds. Modern concepts of gynecologic oncology. Boston: John Wright PSG, 1982:1–19.

162. Cramer DW, Cutler SJ. Incidence and histopathology of malignancies of the female genital organs in the United States. Am J Obstet Gynecol 1974;118:443–460.

163. Barber HRK. Cervical cancer. In: McGowan L, ed. Gynecologic oncology. New York: Appleton-Century-Crofts, 1975:206–216.

164. Christopherson WM, Parker JE. Relation of cervical cancer to early marriage and childbearing. N Engl J Med 1965;273:235.

165. Keighley E. Carcinoma of the cervix among prostitutes in a women's prison. Br J Vener Dis 1968;44:254–255.

166. Rotkin ID. Epidemiology of cancer of the cervix. III. Sexual characteristics of a cervical cancer population. Am J Public Health Nations Health 1967;57:815–829.

167. Taylor RS, Carroll BE, Lloyd JW. Mortality among women in 3 Catholic religious orders with special references to cancer. Cancer 1959;12:1207.

168. Terris M, Wilson F, Nelson JJ. Relation of circumcision to cancer of the cervix. Am J Obstet Gynecol 1973;117:1056–1066.

169. Abou-Daud KT. Epidemiology of carcinoma of the cervix uteri in Lebanese Christians and Moslems. Cancer 1967;20:1706–1714.

170. Ackerman LV, del Regato JA. Cancer diagnosis, treatment, and prognosis. St. Louis: CV Mosby, 1977.

171. Kessler II. Human cervical cancer as a venereal disease. Cancer Res 1976;36:783–791.

172. Joneja MG, Coulson DB. Histopathology and cytogenetics of tumors induced by the application of 7,12-dimethybenz(a)anthracene (DMBA) in mouse cervix. Eur J Cancer 1973;9:367–374.

173. Herbst AL, Cole P, Norusis MJ, Welch WR, Scully RE. Epidemiologic aspects and factors related to survival in 384 Registry cases of clear cell adenocarcinoma of the vagina and cervix. Am J Obstet Gynecol 1979;135:876–886.

174. Boyce JG, Lu T, Nelson JJ, Joyce D. Cervical carcinoma and oral contraception. Obstet Gynecol 1972;40:139–146.

175. Melnick JL, Adams E, Rawls WE. The causative role of herpes virus 2 in cervical cancer. Cancer 1974;34:1376.

176. Hollinshead AC, Chretien PB, Lee OB, et al. In vivo and in vitro measurements of the relationship of human squamous carcinomas to herpes simplex virus tumor-associated antigens. Cancer Res 1976;36:821–828.

177. Rapp F, Duff R. Oncogenic conversion of normal cells by inactivated herpes simplex virus. Cancer 1974;34:1353.

178. Darai G, Munk K. Human embryonic lung cells abortively infected with herpes virus hominis type 2 show some properties of cell transformation. Nature New Biol 1973;241:268–269.

179. Wentz WB, Reagan JW, Heggie AD. Cervical carcinogenesis with herpes simplex virus, type 2. Obstet Gynecol 1975;46:117–121.

180. McDougall JK, Crum CP, Fenoglio CM, Goldstein LC, Galloway DA. Herpesvirus-specific RNA and protein in carcinoma of the uterine cervix. Proc Natl Acad Sci USA 1982;79:3853–3857.

181. Zur Hausen H. Human genital cancer: Synergism between two virus infections of synergism between a virus infections of synergism between a virus infection and initiative agents. Lancet 1982;2:489.

182. Hulka BS. Risk factors for cervical cancer. J Chronic Dis 1982;35:3–11.

183. Schacter J, Hill EC, King EB, et al. *Chlamydia trachomatis* and cervical neoplasia. JAMA 1982;248:2134.

184. Meisels A, Fortin R. Condylomatous lesions of the cervix and vagina. I. Cytologic patterns. Acta Cytol 1976;20:505–509.

185. Kurman RJ, Jenson AB, Lancaster WD. Papillomavirus infection of the cervix. II. Relationship to intraepithelial neoplasia based on the presence of specific viral structural proteins. Am J Surg Pathol 1983;7:39–52.

186. Reid R, Crum CP, Herschman BR, et al. Genital warts and cervical cancer. III. Subclinical papillomaviral infection and cervical neoplasia are linked by a spectrum of continuous morphologic and biologic change. Cancer 1984;53:943–953.

187. Crum CP, Levine RU. Human papillomavirus infection and cervical neoplasia: New perspectives. Int J Gynecol Pathol 1984;3:376–388.

188. van den Brule AJ, Claas EC, du MM, et al. Use of anticontamination primers in the polymerase chain reaction for the detection of human papilloma virus genotypes in cervical scrapes and biopsies. J Med Virol 1989;29:20–27.

189. Grussendorf-Conen EI, de Villiers EM, Gissmann L. Human papillomavirus genomes in penile smears of healthy men. Lancet [Letter] 1986;2:1092.

190. Schneider A. HPV infection in women and their male partners. Contemp Obstet Gynecol 1988;32:131.

191. Koutsky LA, Galloway DA, Holmes KK. Epidemiology of genital human papillomavirus infection. Epidemiol Rev 1988;10:122–163.

192. Richart RM. Natural history of cervical intraepithelial neoplasia. Clin Obstet Gynecol 1967;110:748.

193. Petersen O. Spontaneous course of cervical pre-cancerous conditions. Am J Obstet Gynecol 1956;72:1063.

194. Clemmesen J, Poulsen H. Report of the Ministry of the Interior, Document 3. Copenhagen: , 1971.

195. Kottmeier HL. Evolution et traitment des epitheliomas. Rev Fr Gynecol Obstet 1961;56:821.

196. Richart RM, Barron BA. A follow-up study of patients with cervical dysplasia. Am J Obstet Gynecol 1969;105:386–393.

197. Walton R. Cervical cancer screening program, epidemiological and natural history of cancer of the cervix. Can Med Assoc J 1976;114:1003.

198. Patton SF. Diagnostic cytology of the uterine cervix—Monograph. Baltimore: Williams & Wilkins, 1969.

199. Barron BA, Richart RM. A statistical model of the natural history of cervical carcinoma based on a prospective study of 557 cases. JNCI 1968;41:1343–1353.

200. Barron BA, Richart RM. A statistical model of the natural history of cervical carcinoma. II. Estimates of the transition time from dysplasia to carcinoma in situ. JNCI 1970;45:1025.

201. Fuller AJ, Elliott N, Kosloff C, Lewis JJ. Lymph node metastases from carcinoma of the cervix, stages IB and IIA. implications for prognosis and treatment. Gynecol Oncol 1982;13:165–174.

202. Sudarsanam A, Charyulu K, Belinson J, et al. Influence of exploratory celiotomy on the management of carcinoma of the cervix. A preliminary report. Cancer 1978;41:1049–1053.

203. Nelson JH, Macasaet MA, Lu T, et al. The incidence and significance of para-aortic lymph node metastases in late invasive carcinoma of the cervix. Am J Obstet Gynecol 1974;118:749–756.

204. Piver MS, Barlow JJ. High dose irradiation to biopsy confirmed aortic node metastases from carcinoma of the uterine cervix. Cancer 1977;39:1243–1246.

205. Wharton JT, Jones H, Day TJ, Rutledge FN, Fletcher GH. Preirradiation celiotomy and extended field irradiation for invasive carcinoma of the cervix. Obstet Gynecol 1977;49:333–338.

206. Lagasse LD, Creasman WT, Shingleton HM, Ford JH, Blessing JA. Results and complications of operative staging in cervical cancer: Experience of the Gynecologic Oncology Group. Gynecol Oncol 1980;9:90–98.

207. Buchsbaum HJ. Extrapelvic lymph node metastases in cervical carcinoma. Am J Obstet Gynecol 1979;133:814–824.

208. Averette HE, Ford JJ, Dudan RC, Girtanner RE, Hoskins WJ, Lutz MH. Staging of cervical cancer. Clin Obstet Gynecol 1975;18:215–232.

209. Welander CE, Pierce VK, Nori D, et al. Pretreatment laparotomy in carcinoma of the cervix. Gynecol Oncol 1981;12:336–347.

210. Berman ML, Keys H, Creasman W, Di Saia P, Bundy B, Blessing J. Survival and patterns of recurrence in cervical cancer metastatic to periaortic lymph nodes (a Gynecologic Oncology Group study). Gynecol Oncol 1984;19:8–16.

211. Carlson V, Delclos L, Fletcher GH. Distant metastases in squamous-cell carcinoma of the uterine cervix. Radiology 1987;88:961.

212. Richart RM. A modified terminology for cervical intraepithelial neoplasia. Obstet Gynecol 1990;75:131–133.

213. Regan JW, Ng ABP. The cellular manifestations of uterine carcinomas. In: Norris HJ, Hertig AT, Abell MR, eds. The uterus: International Academy of Pathology, monographs in pathology. Baltimore: Williams & Wilkins, 1973.

214. Wentz WB. Histological grade and survival in cervical cancer with respect to cell type. Cancer 1961;18:412.

215. Davis JR, Moon LB. Increased incidence of adenocarcinoma of uterine cervix. Obstet Gynecol 1975;45:79–83.

216. Artman LE, Hoskins WJ, Bibro MC, et al. Radical hysterectomy and pelvic lymphadenectomy for stage IB carcinoma of the cervix: 21 years' experience. Gynecol Oncol 1987;28:8–13.

217. Hart WR, Norris HJ. Mesonephric adenocarcinomas of the cervix. Cancer 1972;29:106–113.

218. Ulbright TM, Gersell DJ. Glassy cell carcinoma of the uterine cervix. A light and electron microscopic study of five cases. Cancer 1983;51:2255–2263.

219. Hoskins WJ, Averette HE, Ng AB, Yon JL. Adenoid cystic carcinoma of the cervix uteri: Report of six cases and review of the literature. Gynecol Oncol 1979;7:371–384.

220. Abell MR. Primary melanoblastoma of the uterine cervix. Am J Clin Pathol 1961;36:248.

221. Warner TFCS. Carcinoid tumor of the uterine cervix. J Clin Pathol 1978;31:990.

222. Abell MR, Ramirez JA. Sarcomas and carcinosarcomas of the uterine cervix. Cancer 1973;31:1176–1192.

223. Chorlton I, Karnei RF, King FM, et al. Primary malignant reticuloendothelial disease involving the vagina, cervix, and corpus uteri. Obstet Gynecol 1974;44:735.

224. Jennings RH, Barclay DL. Verrucous carcinoma of the cervix. Cancer 1972;30:430–434.

225. Fidler HK, Boyes DA, Worth AJ. Cervical cancer detection in British Columbia. A progress report. J Obstet Gynaecol Br Commonw 1968;75:392–404.

226. American CS. ACS report of the cancer-related health check-up. Cancer 1980;30:194.

227. American College of Obstetricians and Gynecologists. Statement of policy: Periodic cancer screening; ACOG, 1980.

228. American College of Obstetricians and Gynecologists. Report; ACOG, 1988.

229. Papanicolaou G. Atlas of exfoliative cytology. Boston: Massachusetts Commonwealth Fund and Boston University Press, 1954.

230. Riottan G, Christopherson WM. Cytology of the female genital tract: International histological classification of tumors, No. 8. Geneva: World Health Organization, 1973.

231. National Cancer Institute. The 1988 Bethesda System for reporting cervical/vaginal cytologic diagnoses. JAMA 1989;262:931.

232. Wright TC, Richart RM. Preinvasive lesions of the lower genital tract. In: Hoskins WJ, Perez CA, Young RC, eds. Principles and practice of gynecologic oncology. Philadelphia: JB Lippincott, 1992.

233. Coppleson LW, Brown B. Estimation of the screening error rate from the observed detection rates in repeated cervical cytology. Am J Obstet Gynecol 1974;119:953–958.

234. Vooijs GP, Elias A, van der Graaf Y, et al. The influence of sample takers on the cellular composition of cervical smears. Acta Cytol 1986;30:251–257.

235. Walsh JW, Amendola MA, Konerding KF, Tisnado J, Hazra TA. Computed tomographic detection of pelvic and inguinal lymph-node metastases from primary and recurrent pelvic malignant disease. Radiology 1980;137:157–166.

236. Camilien L, Gordon D, Fruchter RG, Maiman M, Boyce JG. Predictive value of computerized tomography in the presurgical evaluation of primary carcinoma of the cervix. Gynecol Oncol 1988;30:209–215.

237. Kilcheski TS, Arger PH, Mulhern CJ, Coleman BG, Kressel HY, Mikuta JI. Role of computed tomography in the presurgical evaluation of carcinoma of the cervix. J Comput Assist Tomogr 1981;5:378–383.

238. Brenner DE, Whitley NO, Prempree T, Villasanta U. An evaluation of the computed tomographic scanner for the staging of carcinoma of the cervix. Cancer 1982;50:2323–2328.

239. Bandy LC, Clarke PD, Silverman PM, Creasman WT. Computed tomography in evaluation of extrapelvic lymphadenopathy in carcinoma of the cervix. Obstet Gynecol 1985;65:73–76.

240. Piver MS, Chung WS. Prognostic significance of cervical lesion size and pelvic node metastases in cervical carcinoma. Obstet Gynecol 1975;46:507–510.

241. Piver MS, Wallace S, Castro JR. The accuracy of lymphangiography in carcinoma of the uterine cervix. Am J Roentgenol Radium Ther Nucl Med 1971;111:278–283.

242. de Muylder X, Belanger R, Vauclair R, Audet LP, Cormier A, Methot Y. Value of lymphography in stage IB cancer of the uterine cervix. Am J Obstet Gynecol 1984;148:610–613.

243. Lagasse LD, Ballon SC, Berman ML, Watring WG. Pretreatment lymphangiography and operative evaluation in carcinoma of the cervix. Am J Obstet Gynecol 1979;134:219–224.

244. Heller PB, Maletano JH, Bundy BN, Barnhill DR, Okagaki T. Clinical-pathologic study of stage IIB, III, and IVA carcinoma of the cervix: Extended diagnostic evaluation for paraaortic node metastasis—A Gynecologic Oncology Group study. Gynecol Oncol 1990;38:425–430.

245. Hammond JA, Herson J, Freedman RS, et al. The impact of lymph node status on survival in cervical carcinoma. Int J Radiat Oncol Biol Phys 1981;7:1713–1718.

246. Hricak H, Lacey CG, Sandles LG, Chang YC, Winkler ML, Stern JL. Invasive cervical carcinoma: Comparison of MR imaging and surgical findings. Radiology 1988;166:623–631.

247. Worthington JL, Balfe DM, Lee JK, et al. Uterine neoplasms: MR imaging. Radiology 1986;159:725–730.

248. Ebner F, Kressel HY, Mintz MC et al. Tumor recurrence versus fibrosis in the female pelvis: Differentiation with MR imaging at 1.5 T. Radiology 1980;166:333.

249. Zornoza J, Lukeman JM, Jing BS, Wharton JT, Wallace S. Percutaneous retroperitoneal lymph node biopsy in carcinoma of the cervix. Gynecol Oncol 1977;5:43–51.

250. Wong F, Bhimji S. The usefulness of ultrasonography in intracavitary radiotherapy using Selectron applicators. Int J Radiat Oncol Biol Phys 1990;19:477–482.

251. Griffin TW, Parker RG, Taylor WJ. An evaluation of procedures used in staging carcinoma of the cervix. AJR 1976;127:825–827.

252. International Federation of Gynecology and Obstetrics. Change in definitions of clinical staging for carcinoma of the cervix and ovary. Am J Obstet Gynecol 1987;156:263–264.

253. Beahrs OH, Henson DE, Hutter RVP, Myers MH. Manual for staging of cancer. 3rd ed. Philadelphia: JB Lippincott, 1988.

254. Kolstad P. Follow-up study of 232 patients with stage IA1 and 411 patients with stage IA2 squamous cell carcinoma of the cervix (microinvasive carcinoma). Gynecol Oncol 1989;33:265–272.

255. Tsukamoto N, Kaku T, Matsukuma K, et al. The problem of stage IA (FIGO, 1985) carcinoma of the uterine cervix. Gynecol Oncol 1989;34:1–6.

256. Berman ML, Lagasse LD, Watring WG, et al. The operative evaluation of patients with cervical carcinoma by an extraperitoneal approach. Obstet Gynecol 1977;50:658–664.

257. Fuller AJ, Elliott N, Kosloff C, Hoskins WJ, Lewis JJ. Determinants of increased risk for recurrence in patients undergoing radical hysterectomy for stage IB and IIA carcinoma of the cervix. Gynecol Oncol 1989;33:34–39.

258. Burghardt E, Pickel H, Hass J, Lahousen M. Prognostic factors and operative treatment of stages IB to IIB cervical cancer. Am J Obstet Gynecol 1987;156:988–996.

259. Martimbeau PW, Kjorstad KE, Iversen T. Stage IB carcinoma of the cervix, the Norwegian Radium Hospital. II. Results when pelvic nodes are involved. Obstet Gynecol 1982;60:215–218.

260. Chung CK, Nahhas WA, Stryker JA, Curry SL, Abt AB, Mortel R. Analysis of factors contributing to treatment failures in stages IB and IIA carcinoma of the cervix. Am J Obstet Gynecol 1980;138:550–556.

261. van Nagell JR Jr, Donaldson ES, Wood EG, Parker JC Jr. The significance of vascular

invasion and lymphocytic infiltration in invasive cervical cancer. Cancer 1978;41: 228–234.

262. Boyce J, Fruchter RG, Nicastri AD, Ambiavagar PC, Reinis MS, Nelson JJ. Prognostic factors in stage I carcinoma of the cervix. Gynecol Oncol 1981;12:154–165.

263. Burke TW, Hoskins WJ, Heller PB, Bibro MC, Weiser EB, Park RC. Prognostic factors associated with radical hysterectomy failure. Gynecol Oncol 1987;26:153–159.

264. Figge DC, Tamimi HK. Patterns of recurrence of carcinoma following radical hysterectomy. Am J Obstet Gynecol 1981;140:213–220.

265. Delgado G, Bundy BN, Fowler WJ, et al. A prospective surgical pathological study of stage I squamous carcinoma of the cervix: A Gynecologic Oncology Group Study. Gynecol Oncol 1989;35:314–320.

266. Rotman M, John M, Boyce J. Prognostic factors in cervical carcinoma: Implications in staging and management. Cancer 1981;48:560–567.

267. Podczaski ES, Palombo C, Manetta A, et al. Assessment of pretreatment laparotomy in patients with cervical carcinoma prior to radiotherapy. Gynecol Oncol 1989;33:71–75.

268. Alvarez RD, Soong SJ, Kinney WK, et al. Identification of prognostic factors and risk groups in patients found to have nodal metastasis at the time of radical hysterectomy for early-stage squamous carcinoma of the cervix. Gynecol Oncol 1989;35:130–135.

269. Inoue T. Prognostic significance of the depth of invasion relating to nodal metastases, parametrial extension, and cell types. A study of 628 cases with stage IB, IIA, and IIB cervical carcinoma. Cancer 1984;54:3035–3042.

270. Perez CA, Kao MS. Radiation therapy alone or combined with surgery in the treatment of barrel-shaped carcinoma of the uterine cervix (stages IB, IIA, IIB). Int J Radiat Oncol Biol Phys 1985;11:1903–1909.

271. Kyriakos M, Kempson RL, Perez CA. Carcinoma of the cervix in young women. I. Invasive carcinoma. Obstet Gynecol 1971;38:930–944.

272. Prempree T, Patanaphan V, Sewchand W, Scott RM. The influence of patients' age and tumor grade on the prognosis of carcinoma of the cervix. Cancer 1983;51:1764–1771.

273. Meanwell CA, Kelly KA, Wilson S, et al. Young age as a prognostic factor in cervical cancer: Analysis of population based on data from 10,022 cases. Br Med J 1988;296:391.

274. van der Graaf Y, Peer PG, Zielhuis GA, Vooijs PG. Cervical cancer survival in Nijmegen region, The Netherlands, 1970–1985. Gynecol Oncol 1988;30:51–56.

275. Grimard L, Genest P, Girard A, et al. Prognostic significance of endometrial extension in carcinoma of the cervix. Gynecol Oncol 1988;31:301–309.

276. Noguchi H, Shiozawa I, Kitahara T, Yamazaki T, Fukuta T. Uterine body invasion of carcinoma of the uterine cervix as seen from surgical specimens. Gynecol Oncol 1988;30:173–182.

277. Bush RS, Jenkin RD, Allt WE, et al. Definitive evidence for hypoxic cells influencing cure in cancer therapy. Br J Cancer Suppl 1978;37:302–306.

278. Jenkin RD, Stryker JA. The influence of the blood pressure on survival in cancer of the cervix. Br J Radiol 1968;41:913–920.

279. Van Herik M. Fever as a complication of radiation therapy for carcinoma of the cervix. Am J Roentgenol Radium Ther Nucl Med 1965;43:104.

280. Kapp DS, Lawrence R. Temperature elevation during brachytherapy for carcinoma of the uterine cervix: Adverse effect on survival and enhancement of distant metastasis. Int J Radiat Oncol Biol Phys 1984;10:2281–2292.

281. Dyson JE, Joslin CA, Rothwell RI, Quirke P, Khoury GG, Bird CC. Flow cytofluorometric evidence for the differential radioresponsiveness of aneuploid and diploid cervix tumours. Radiother Oncol 1987;8:263–272.

282. Strang P, Eklund G, Stendahl U, Frankendal B. S-phase rate as a predictor of early recurrences in carcinoma of the uterine cervix. Anticancer Res 1987;7:807–810.

283. Rutgers DH, van der Linden PM, van Peperzeel HA. DNA flow cytometry of squamous cell carcinomas from the human uterine cervix: The identification of prognostically different subgroups. Radiother Oncol 1986;7:249–268.

284. Izutsu T, Kagabu T, Nishiya I, Wied GL. DNA analysis cervical and vaginal cancer cells during radiotherapy by rapid high-resolution cytometry. Nippon Sanka Fujinka Gakkai Zasshi 1988;40:621–626.

285. Kelland LR, Steel GG. Differences in radiation response among human cervix carcinoma cell lines. Radiother Oncol 1988;13:225–232.

286. Thames HD. An "incomplete-repair" model for survival after fractionated and continuous irradiations. Int J Radiat Biol Rel Stud Phys Chem Med 1985;47:319–339.

287. Kenter GG, Cornelisse CJ, Aartsen EJ, et al. DNA ploidy level as prognostic factor in low stage carcinoma of the cervix. Gynecol Oncol 1990;39:181–185.

288. Hoskins WJ, Ford JJ, Lutz MH, Averette HE. Radical hysterectomy and pelvic lymphadenectomy for the management of early invasive cancer of the cervix. Gynecol Oncol 1976;4:278–290.

289. Townsend DE. Invasive carcinoma following outpatient evaluation and therapy for cervical disease. Obstet Gynecol 1971;57:145.

290. Sevin BU, Ford JH, Girtanner RD, et al. Invasive cancer of the cervix after cryosurgery. Pitfalls of conservative management. Obstet Gynecol 1979;53:465–471.

291. Cartier R. Practical colposcopy. 2nd ed. Paris: Laboratoire Cartier, 1984.

292. Wright TC, Gagnon S, Ferenczy A, Richart RM. Excising CIN lesions by loop electrosurgical procedure. Contemp Obstet Gynecol 1991;36:56.

293. Coppleson M. Cervical intraepithelial neoplasia: Clinical features and management. In: Coppleson M, ed. Gynecologic oncology: Fundamental principles and clinical practice. New York: Churchill Livingstone, 1981:451–464.

294. Averette HE, Nelson JJ, Ng AB, Hoskins WJ, Boyce JG, Ford JJ. Diagnosis and management of microinvasive (stage IA) carcinoma of the uterine cervix. Cancer 1976;38:414–425.

295. Simon NL, Gore H, Shingleton HM, et al. Study of superficially invasive carcinoma of the cervix. Obstet Gynecol 1986;69:19.

296. Burghardt E. Microinvasive carcinoma. Obstet Gynecol Surv 1979;34:836–838.

297. van Nagell JR Jr, Greenwell N, Powell DF, Donaldson ES, Hanson MB, Gay EC. Microinvasive carcinoma of the cervix. Am J Obstet Gynecol 1983;145:981–991.

298. Greer BE, Figge DC, Tamimi HK, Cain JM, Lee RB. Stage IA2 squamous carcinoma of the cervix: Difficult diagnosis and therapeutic dilemma. Am J Obstet Gynecol 1990;162:1406–1409.

299. Grigsby PW, Perez CA. Radiotherapy alone for medically inoperable carcinoma of the cervix: Stage IA and carcinoma in situ. Int J Radiat Oncol Biol Phys 1991;21:375–378.

300. Hamberger AD, Fletcher GH, Wharton JT. Results of treatment of early stage I carcinoma of the uterine cervix with intracavitary radium alone. Cancer 1978;41:980–985.

301. Pilleron JP, Durand JC, Lenoble JC. Carcinoma of the uterine cervix, stages I and II, treated by radiation therapy and extensive surgery (1000 cases). Cancer 1972;29:593–596.

302. Sall S, Pineda AA, Cananoq A, et al. Surgical treatment of stages IB and IIA invasive carcinoma of the cervix by radical abdominal hysterectomy. Am J Obstet Gynecol 1979;135:422.

303. Newton M. Radical hysterectomy or radiotherapy for stage I cervical cancer. A prospective comparison with 5 and 10 years' follow-up. Am J Obstet Gynecol 1975;123:535–542.

304. Roddick JW Jr, Greenlow RH. Treatment of cervical cancer. Am J Obstet Gynecol 1971;19:754.

305. Allen HH, Collins JA. Surgical management of carcinoma of the cervix. Am J Obstet Gynecol 1977;127:741–744.

306. Benedet JL, Turko M, Boyes DA, et al. Radical hysterectomy in the treatment of cervical cancer. Am J Obstet Gynecol 1980;137:254.

307. Blaikley JB, Lederman M, Pollard W. Carcinoma of the cervix at Chelsea Hospital for Women, 1933–65. Five-year and ten-year results of treatment. J Obstet Gynaecol Br Commonw 1969;76:729–740.

308. Brunschwig A, Barber HR. Surgical treatment of carcinoma of the cervix. Obstet Gynecol 1966;27:21–29.

309. Christensen A, Lange P, Neilsen E. Surgery and radiotherapy for invasive cancer of the cervix: Surgical treatment. Acta Obstet Gynecol 1964;43:59.

310. Delgado G, Coglar H, Walker P. Survival and complications in cervical cancer treated by pelvic and extended field radiation after para-aortic lymphadenectomy. AJR 1978;130:141.

311. Ketcham AS, Hoye RC, Taylor PT, Deckers PJ, Thomas LB, Chretien PB. Radical hysterectomy and pelvic lymphadenectomy for carcinoma of the uterine cervix. Cancer 1971;28:1272–1277.

312. Lee YN, Wang KL, Lin MH, et al. Radical hysterectomy with pelvic lymph node dissection for treatment of cervical cancer: A clinical review of 954 cases. Gynecol Oncol 1989;32:135–142.

313. Liu W, Meigs JV. Radical hysterectomy and pelvic lymphadenectomy: A review of 473 cases, including 244 for primary invasive carcinoma of the cervix. Am J Obstet Gynecol 1955;69:1–32.

314. Masterson JG. The role of surgery in the treatment of early carcinoma of the cervix. Clin Obstet Gynecol 1967;10:922–939.

315. Park RC, Patow WE, Rogers RE, Zimmerman EA. Treatment of stage I carcinoma of the cervix. Obstet Gynecol 1973;41:117–122.

316. Piver MS, Marchetti DL, Patton T, Halpern J, Blumenson L, Driscoll DL. Radical hysterectomy and pelvic lymphadenectomy versus radiation therapy for small (less than or equal to 3 cm) stage IB cervical carcinoma. Am J Clin Oncol 1988;11:21–24.

317. Symmonds RE. Morbidity and complications of radical hysterectomy with pelvic lymph node dissection. Am J Obstet Gynecol 1966;94:663–678.

318. Underwood PJ, Wilson WC, Kreutner A, Miller M, Murphy E. Radical hysterectomy: A critical review of twenty-two years' experience. Am J Obstet Gynecol 1979;134:889–898.

319. van Nagell JR Jr, Rayburn W, Donaldson ES, et al. Therapeutic implications of patterns of recurrence in cancer of the uterine cervix. Cancer 1979;44:2354–2361.

320. Dickson RJ. Late results of radium treatment of carcinoma of the cervix. Clin Radiol 1972;23:528–535.

321. Fletcher GH. Cancer of the uterine cervix: Janeway lecture. Am J Roentgenol Radium Ther Nucl Med 1971;111:225.

322. Hanks GE, Herring DF, Kramer S. Patterns of care outcome studies. Results of the national practice in cancer of the cervix. Cancer 1983;51:959–967.

323. Haie C, Pejovic MH, Gerbaulet A, et al. Is prophylactic para-aortic irradiation worthwhile in the treatment of advanced cervical carcinoma? Results of a controlled clinical trial of the EORTC radiotherapy group. Radiother Oncol 1988;11:101–112.

324. Kim RY, Trotti A, Wu CJ, Soong SJ, Salter MM. Radiation alone in the treatment of cancer of the uterine cervix: Analysis of pelvic failure and dose response relationship. Int J Radiat Oncol Biol Phys 1989;17:973–978.

325. Kline JC, Schultz AE, Vermund H, Peckham BM. High-dose radiotherapy for carcinoma of the cervix. Method and results. Am J Obstet Gynecol 1969;104:479–484.

326. Kottmeier HL. Annual report on the results of treatment in carcinoma of the uterus, vagina, and ovary. : FIGO, 1973; 15.

327. Lanciano RM, Won M, Coia LR, et al. Pretreatment and treatment factors associated with improved outcome in squamous cell carcinoma of the uterine cervix: A final report of the 1973 and 1978 Patterns of Care Studies. Int J Radiat Oncol Biol Phys 1990;19:126.

328. Montana GS, Fowler WC, Varia MA, Walton LA, Mack Y, Shemanski L. Carcinoma of the cervix, stage III. Results of radiation therapy. Cancer 1986;57:148–154.

329. Muirhead W, Green LS. Carcinoma of the cervix. Five-year results and sequelae of treatment. Am J Obstet Gynecol 1968;101:744–749.

330. Stokes S, Bedwinek J, Kao MS, Camel HM, Perez CA. Treatment of stage I adenocarcinoma of the endometrium by hysterectomy and adjuvant irradiation: A retrospective analysis of 304 patients. Int J Radiat Oncol Biol Phys 1986;12:339–344.

331. Wall JA, Collins VP, Hudgins PT, Kaplan AL, Adams RM. Carcinoma of the cervix. Review of clinical experience during a 20 year period (1946–1965). Am J Obstet Gynecol 1966;96:57–63.

332. Volterrani F, Lombardi F. Long-term results of radium therapy in cervical cancer. Int J Radiat Oncol Biol Phys 1980;6:565–570.

333. Keilbinska S, Ludwika , Tarlowska L, Fraczek O. Studies of mortality and health status in women cured of cancer of the cervix uteri. Comparison of long-term results of radiotherapy and combined surgery and radiotherapy. Cancer 1973;32:245–252.

334. Perez CA, Camel HM, Kao MS, Hederman MA. Randomized study of preoperative radiation and surgery or irradiation alone in the treatment of stage IB and IIA cancer of the uterine cervix: Final report. Gynecol Oncol 1987;27:129–140.

335. Lu T, Macasaet MA, Nelson JJ. The barrel-shaped cervical carcinoma. Am J Obstet Gynecol 1976;124:596–600.

336. O'Quinn AG, Fletcher GH, Wharton JT. Guidelines for conservative hysterectomy after irradiation. Gynecol Oncol 1980;9:68–79.

337. Durrance FY, Fletcher GH, Rutledge FN. Analysis of central recurrent disease in stages I and II squamous cell carcinomas of the cervix on intact uterus. Am J Roentgenol Radium Ther Nucl Med 1969;106:831–838.

338. Nelson A, Fletcher GH, Wharton JT. Indications for adjunctive conservative extrafascial hysterectomy in selected cases of carcinoma of the uterine cervix. Am J Roentgenol Radium Ther Nucl Med 1975;123:91–99.

339. Weems DH, Mendenhall WM, Bova FJ, Marcus RJ, Morgan LS, Million RR. Carcinoma of the intact uterine cervix, stage IB-IIA-B, greater than or equal to 6 cm in diameter: Irradiation alone vs preoperative irradiation and surgery. Int J Radiat Oncol Biol Phys 1985;11:1911–1914.

340. Morrow CP. Panel report: Is pelvic radiation beneficial in the postoperative management of stage IB squamous cell carcinoma of the cervix with pelvic node metastases managed by radical hysterectomy and pelvic lymphadenectomy? Gynecol Oncol 1980;10:105.

341. Wertheim MS, Hakes TB, Daghestani AN, Nori D, Smith DH, Lewis JJ. A pilot study of adjuvant therapy in patients with cervical cancer at high risk of recurrence after radical hysterectomy and pelvic lymphadenectomy. J Clin Oncol 1985;3:912–916.

342. Hogan WM, Littman P, Griner L, Miller CL, Mikuta JJ. Results of radiation therapy given after radical hysterectomy. Cancer 1982;49:1278–1285.

343. Gonzalez GD, Ketting BW, van BB, van DJ. Carcinoma of the uterine cervix stage IB and IIA. Results of postoperative irradiation in patients with microscopic infiltration in the parametrium and/or lymph node metastasis. Int J Radiat Oncol Biol Phys 1989;16:389–395.

344. Kim RY, Salter MM, Shingleton HM. Adjuvant postoperative radiation therapy following radical hysterectomy in stage IB CA of the cervix—analysis of treatment failure. Int J Radiat Oncol Biol Phys 1988;14:445–449.

345. Bianchi UA, Sartori E, Pecorelli S, et al. Treatment of primary invasive cervical cancer. Considerations on 997 consecutive cases. Eur J Gynaecol Oncol 1988;9:47–53.

346. Kinney WK, Alvarez RD, Reid GC, et al. Value of adjuvant whole-pelvis irradiation after Wertheim hysterectomy for early-stage squamous carcinoma of the cervix with pelvic nodal metastasis: A matched-control study. Gynecol Oncol 1989;34:258–262.

347. Johns HE. Optimization of energy and equipment. In: Kramer S, Suntharalingam N, Zinneger GF, eds. High energy photons and electrons: Clinical applications in cancer management. New York: John Wiley & Sons, 1976:333.

348. Million RR, Rutledge F, Fletcher GH. Stage IV carcinoma of the cervix with bladder invasion. Am J Obstet Gynecol 1972;113:239–246.

349. Kramer C, Peschel RE, Goldberg N, et al. Radiation treatment of FIGO stage IVA carcinoma of the cervix. Gynecol Oncol 1989;32:323–326.

350. Prempree T. Parametrial implant in stage IIIB cancer of the cervix. III. A five-year study. Cancer 1983;52:748–750.

351. Aristizabal SA, Surwit EA, Hevezi JM, Heusinkveld RS. Treatment of advanced cancer of the cervix with transperineal interstitial irradiation. Int J Radiat Oncol Biol Phys 1983;9:1013–1017.

352. Martinez A, Edmundson GK, Cox RS, Gunderson LL, Howes AE. Combination of external beam irradiation and multiple-site perineal applicator (MUPIT) for treatment of locally advanced or recurrent prostatic, anorectal, and gynecologic malignancies. Int J Radiat Oncol Biol Phys 1985;11:391–398.

353. Pierquin B, Marinello G, Mege JP, Crook J. Intracavitary irradiation of carcinomas of the uterus and cervix: The Creteil method. Int J Radiat Oncol Biol Phys 1988;15:1465–1473.

354. Maruyama Y, Muir W. Human cervical cancer clearance after ^{252}Cf neutron brachytherapy versus conventional photon brachytherapy. Am J Clin Oncol 1984;7:347–352.

355. Maruyama Y, van Nagell J, Yoneda J, et al. Dose-response and failure pattern for bulky or barrel-shaped stage IB cervical cancer treated by combined photon irradiation and extrafascial hysterectomy. Cancer 1989;63:70–76.

356. Maor MH, Gillespie BW, Peters LJ, et al. Neutron therapy in cervical cancer: Results of a phase III RTOG study. Int J Radiat Oncol Biol Phys 1988;14:883.

357. Castro JR, Issa P, Fletcher GH. Carcinoma of the cervix treated by external irradiation alone. Radiology 1970;95:163–166.

358. Coia L, Won M, Lanciano R, Marcial VA, Martz K, Hanks G. The Patterns of Care outcome study for cancer of the uterine cervix. Results of the Second National Practice Survey. Cancer 1990;66:2451–2456.

359. Perez CA, Kurman RJ, Stehman FB, Thigpen JT. Carcinoma of the uterine cervix. In: Hoskins WJ, Perez CA, Young RC, eds. Principles and practice of gynecologic oncology. Philadelphia: JB Lippincott, 1992.

360. Einhorn N, Bygdeman M, Sjoberg B. Combined radiation and surgical treatment for carcinoma of the uterine cervix. Tumors 1980;45:720–723.

361. Morley GW, Seski JC. Radical pelvic surgery versus radiation therapy for stage I carcinoma of the cervix (exclusive of microinvasion). Am J Obstet Gynecol 1976;126:785–798.

362. Morton DG, Lagasse LD, Moore JG. Pelvic lymphadenectomy following radiation in cervical carcinoma. Am J Obstet Gynecol 1964;88:932.

363. Sweeney WJ, Douglas RG. Treatment of carcinoma of the cervix with combined radiation and extensive surgery. Am J Obstet Gynecol 1962;84:981.

364. Rampone JF, Klem V, Kolstad P. Combined treatment of stage IB carcinoma of the cervix. Obstet Gynecol 1973;41:163–167.

365. Decker DG, Aaro LA, Hunt AG, et al. Sequential radiation and operation in carcinoma of the uterine cervix. Am J Obstet Gynecol 1965;92:35.

366. Quigley MM, Knab DR, MacMahon EB. Carcinoma of the cervix: A third treatment. Obstet Gynecol 1975;45:650–655.

367. Parker RT, Wilbanks GD, Yowell RK. Radical hysterectomy with and without preoperative radiotherapy for cervical cancer. Am J Obstet Gynecol 1967;99:993.

368. Gray MJ, Gusberg SB, Guttman R. Pelvic lymph node dissection following radiotherapy. Am J Obstet Gynecol 1958;76:629.

369. Perez CA, Camel HM, Kao MS, et al. Randomized study of preoperative radiation and surgery or irradiation alone in the treatment of stage IB and IIA carcinoma of the uterine cervix: Preliminary analysis of failure and complications. Cancer 1980;45:2759.

370. Rutledge FN, Fletcher GH, MacDonald EJ. Pelvic lymphadenectomy as an adjunct to radiation therapy in treatment for cancer of the cervix. Am J Roentgenol Radium Ther Nucl Med 1965;93:607.

371. Perez CA, Breaux S, Askin F, Camel HM, Powers WE. Irradiation alone or in combination with surgery in stage IB and IIA carcinoma of the uterine cervix: A nonrandomized comparison. Cancer 1979;43:1062–1072.

372. Rutledge RM, Fletcher GM, MacDonald EJ. Pelvic lymphadenectomy as an adjunct to radiation therapy in treatment for cancer of the cervix. Am J Roentgenol Radium Ther Nucl Med 1969;106:831.

373. Thomas WW, Eifel PJ, Delclos L, et al. Bulky endocervical carcinomas of the uterine cervix: A 23-year experience at the M.D. Anderson Cancer Center. Int J Radiat Oncol Biol Phys 1990;19:127.

374. Nelson JJ, Boyce J, Macasaet M, et al. Incidence, significance, and follow-up of para-aortic lymph node metastases in late invasive carcinoma of the cervix. Am J Obstet Gynecol 1977;128:336–340.

375. Lovecchio JL, Averette HE, Donato D, Bell J. 5-Year survival of patients with periaortic nodal metastases in clinical stage IB and IIA cervical carcinoma. Gynecol Oncol 1989;34:43–45.

376. Podczaski E, Stryker JA, Kaminski P, et al. Extended-field radiation therapy for carcinoma of the cervix. Cancer 1990;66:251–258.

377. Goodman HM, Bowling MC, Nelson JH. Cervical malignancies. In: Knapp RC, Berkowitz RS, eds. Gynecologic Oncology. New York: Macmillan, 1986:225–273.

378. Lepanto P, Littman P, Mikuta J, Davis L, Celebre J. Treatment of para-aortic nodes in carcinoma of the cervix. Cancer 1975;35:1510–1513.

379. Berman ML, Lagasse LD, Ballon SC, Watring WG, Tesler A. Modification of radiation therapy following operative evaluation of patients with cervical carcinoma. Gynecol Oncol 1978;6:328–332.

380. Piver MS, Barlow JJ, Krishnamsetty R. Five-year survival (with no evidence of disease) in patients with biopsy-confirmed aortic node metastasis from cervical carcinoma. Am J Obstet Gynecol 1981;139:575–578.

381. Rubin SC, Brookland R, Mikuta JJ, Mangan C, Sutton G, Danoff B. Para-aortic nodal metastases in early cervical carcinoma: Long-term survival following extended-field radiotherapy. Gynecol Oncol 1984;18:213–217.

382. Tewfik HH, Buchsbaum HJ, Latourette HB, Lifshitz SG, Tewfik FA. Para-aortic lymph node irradiation in carcinoma of the cervix after exploratory laparotomy and biopsy-proven positive aortic nodes. Int J Radiat Oncol Biol Phys 1982;8:13–18.

383. Potish R, Adcock L, Jones TJ, et al. The morbidity and utility of periaortic radiotherapy in cervical carcinoma. Gynecol Oncol 1983;15:1–9.

384. Rotman M, Choi K, Guse C, et al. Prophylactic irradiation of the para-aortic lymph node chain in stage IIB and bulky stage IB carcinoma of the cervix, initial treatment results of RTOG 79-20 [published erratum appears in Int J Radiat Oncol Biol Phys 1991;20:193. Int J Radiat Oncol Biol Phys 1990;19:513–521.

385. Rotman M, Choi K, Guse C, et al. Survival by assigned treatment (Kaplan-Meier) for patients treated on RTOG protocol 79-20. Int J Radiat Oncol Biol Phys 1990;19:513.

386. Cuccia CA, Bloedorn FG, Onal M. Treatment of primary adenocarcinoma of the cervix. Am J Roentgenol Radium Ther Nucl Med 1967;99:371–375.

387. Perez CA. Uterine cervix. In: Perez CA, Brady LW, eds. Principles and practice of radiation oncology. Philadelphia: JB Lippincott, 1992.

388. Taussig FJ. Iliac lymphadenectomy with irradiation in the treatment of cancer of the cervix. Am J Obstet Gynecol 1934;28:650.

389. Perez CA. Carcinoma of the uterine cervix. In: Perez CA, Brady LW, eds. Principles and practice of radiation oncology. Philadelphia: JB Lippincott, 1987:919.

390. Fowler JF. Radiobiological considerations from the hyperbaric oxygen trials. Br J Radiol 1978;51:68.

391. Watson ER, Halnan KE, Dische S, et al. Hyperbaric oxygen and radiotherapy: A Medical Research Council trial in carcinoma of the cervix. Br J Radiol 1978;51:879–887.

392. Fletcher GH, Lindberg RD, Caderao JB, Wharton JT. Hyperbaric oxygen as a radiotherapeutic adjuvant in advanced cancer of the uterine cervix: Preliminary results of a randomized trial. Cancer 1977;39:617–623.

393. Glassburn JR, Damsker JI, Brady LW, et al. Hyperbaric oxygen and radiation in the treatment of advanced cervical carcinoma. In: Fifth International Hyperbaric Congress Proceedings. : Simon Fraser University, 1974;2:813–819.

394. Dische S. Hyperbaric oxygen: The Medical Research Council trials and their clinical significance. Br J Radiol 1979;51:888.
395. Johnson RJR, Walton RF. Sequential study on the effect of the addition of hyperbaric oxygen on the 5-year survival rates of carcinoma of the cervix treated with conventional fractional irradiations. Am J Roentgenol Radium Ther Nucl Med 1974;120:111.
396. Thomas GM, Rauth AM, Bush RS, Black BE, Cummings BJ. A toxicity study of daily dose metronidazole with pelvic irradiation. Cancer Clin Trials 1980;3:223–230.
397. Dische S. Misonidazole in the clinical at Mount Vernon. Cancer Clin Trials 1986;3:175.
398. Leibel S, Bauer M, Wasserman T, et al. Radiotherapy with or without misonidazole for patients with stage IIIB or stage IVA squamous cell carcinoma of the uterine cervix: Preliminary report of a Radiation Therapy Oncology Group randomized trial. Int J Radiat Oncol Biol Phys 1987;13:541–549.
399. Overgaard J, Bentzen SM, Kolstad P, et al. Misonidazole combined with radiotherapy in the treatment of carcinoma of the uterine cervix. Int J Radiat Oncol Biol Phys 1989;16:1069–1072.
400. Hornback NB, Shupe RE, Shidnia H, Marshall CU, Lauer T. Advanced stage IIIB cancer of the cervix treatment by hyperthermia and radiation. Gynecol Oncol 1986;23:160–167.
401. Sharma S, Patel FD, Sandhu APS, et al. A prospective randomized study of local hyperthermia as a supplement and radiosensitizer in the treatment of carcinoma of the cervix with radiotherapy. Endocur Hyperther Oncol 1989;5:151.
402. Perez CA, Fox S, Lockett MA, et al. Impact of dose in outcome of irradiation alone in carcinoma of the uterine cervix: Analysis of two different methods. Int J Radiat Oncol Biol Phys 1991;21:885–898.
403. Kottmeier HL. Complications following radiation therapy in carcinoma of the cervix and their treatment. Am J Obstet Gynecol 1964;88:854.
404. Pourquier H, Dubois JB, Delard R. Cancer of the uterine cervix: Dosimetric guidelines for prevention of late rectal and rectosigmoid complications as a result of radiotherapeutic treatment. Int J Radiat Oncol Biol Phys 1982;8:1887–1895.
405. Komaki R, Mattingly RF, Hoffman RG, Barber SW, Satre R, Greenberg M. Irradiation of para-aortic lymph node metastases from carcinoma of the cervix or endometrium. Preliminary results. Radiology 1983;147:245–248.
406. Rotman M, John M. Current concepts in cancer: Updated cervix cancer III. Stages III and IV. Para-aortic irradiation in cervical carcinoma. Int J Radiat Oncol Biol Phys 1979;5:2139–2141.
407. Freund AW. Zu meiner methods des totalen uterus-extripation. Zentralbl Gynak 1978;2:265.
408. Brunschwig A. Complete excision of pelvic viscera for advanced carcinoma: A one-step abdominoperineal operation with end colostomy and bilateral ureteral implantation into the colon above the colostomy. Cancer 1948;1:177.
409. Thompson JD, Rock JA. Telinde's operative gynecology. 7th ed. Philadelphia: JB Lippincott, 1992.
410. Webb MJ, Symmonds RE. Wertheim hysterectomy: A reappraisal. Obstet Gynecol 1979;54:140–145.
411. Brunschwig A, Daniel WW. Pelvic exenteration operations. Ann Surg 1960;151:71.
412. Lawhead RJ, Clark DG, Smith DH, Pierce VK, Lewis JJ. Pelvic exenteration for recurrent or persistent gynecologic malignancies: A 10-year review of the Memorial Sloan-Kettering Cancer Center experience (1972–1981). Gynecol Oncol 1989;33:279–282.
413. Meoz RT, Spanos WJ, Doss L, Johnson R, Wasserman TH. Misonidazole combined with large-fraction pelvic irradiation in the treatment of patients with advanced pelvic malignancies. Preliminary report of an ongoing RTOG phase I–II study. Am J Clin Oncol 1983;6:417–422.
414. Spanos WJ, Guse C, Perez C, Grigsby P, Doggett RL, Poulter C. Phase II study of multiple daily fractionations in the palliation of advanced pelvic malignancies: Preliminary report of RTOG 8502. Int J Radiat Oncol Biol Phys 1989;17:659–661.
415. Spanos WJ, Wasserman T, Meoz R, Sala J, Kong J, Stetz J. Palliation of advanced pelvic malignant disease with large fraction pelvic radiation and misonidazole: Final report of RTOG phase I/II study. Int J Radiat Oncol Biol Phys 1987;13:1479–1482.
416. Sommers GM, Grigsby PW, Perez CA, et al. Outcome of recurrent cervical carcinoma following definitive irradiation. Gynecol Oncol 1989;35:150–155.
417. Sommers GM, Grigsby PW, Perez CA, et al. Actuarial survival after treatment of recurrent disease by type of therapy. Gynecol Oncol 1989;35:150.
418. Puthawala AA, Syed AM, Fleming PA, Di Saia PJ. Re-irradiation with interstitial implant for recurrent pelvic malignancies. Cancer 1982;50:2810–2814.
419. Prasasvinichai S, Glassburn JR, Brady LW, Lewis GC. Treatment of recurrent carcinoma of the cervix. Int J Radiat Oncol Biol Phys 1978;4:957–961.
420. Prempree T, Kwon T, VillaSanta U, Scott RM. Management of late second or late recurrent squamous cell carcinoma of the cervix uteri after successful initial radiation treatment. Int J Radiat Oncol Biol Phys 1979;5:2053–2057.
421. Jobsen JJ, Lee JW, Cleton FJ, Hermans J. Treatment of locoregional recurrence of carcinoma of the cervix by radiotherapy after primary surgery. Gynecol Oncol 1989;33:368–371.
422. Evans SJ, Hilaris BS, Barber HR. External vs. interstitial irradiation in unresectable recurrent cancer of the cervix. Cancer 1971;28:1284–1288.
423. Friedman M, Pearlman AW. Carcinoma of the cervix: Radiation salvage of surgical failures. Radiology 1965;84:801.
424. Krebs HB, Helmkamp BF, Sevin BU, Poliakoff SR, Nadji M, Averette HE. Recurrent cancer of the cervix following radical hysterectomy and pelvic node dissection. Obstet Gynecol 1982;59:422–427.
425. Webb MJ, Symmonds RE. Site of recurrence of cervical cancer after radical hysterectomy. Am J Obstet Gynecol 1980;138:813–817.
426. Larson DM, Copeland LJ, Stringer CA, Gershenson DM, Malone JJ, Edwards CL.

427. Nori D, Hilaris BS, Kim HS, et al. Interstitial irradiation in recurrent gynecological cancer. Int J Radiat Oncol Biol Phys 1981;7:1513–1517.
428. Moss WT, Brand WN, Battifor H. Radiation oncology: Rationale, technique, results. St. Louis: CV Mosby, 1973.
429. Wimbush PR, Fletcher GH. Radiation therapy of carcinoma of the cervical stump. Radiology 1969;93:665.
430. Creadnick RN. Carcinoma of the cervical stump. Am J Obstet Gynecol 1958;75:5465.
431. Miller BE, Copeland LJ, Hamberger AD, et al. Carcinoma of the cervical stump. Gynecol Oncol 1984;18:100–108.
432. Goodman HM, Niloff JM, Buttlar CA, et al. Adenocarcinoma of the cervical stump. Gynecol Oncol 1989;35:188–192.
433. Kovalic JJ, Grigsby PW, Perez CA, Lockett MA. Cervical stump carcinoma. Int J Radiat Oncol Biol Phys 1991;20:933–938.
434. De Petrillo AD, Townsend DE, Morrow CP, Lickrish GM, Di Saia PJ, Roy M. Colposcopic evaluation of the abnormal Papanicolaou test in pregnancy. Am J Obstet Gynecol 1975;121:441–445.
435. Averette HE, Nasser N, Yankow SL, Little WA. Cervical conization in pregnancy. Analysis of 180 operations. Am J Obstet Gynecol 1970;106:543–549.
436. Mikuta JJ, Enterline HT, Braun TJ. Carcinoma in situ of the cervix associated with pregnancy. A clinical-pathological review. JAMA 1968;204:763–766.
437. Boyle MH, Torrance GW, Sinclair JC, Horwood SP. Economic evaluation of neonatal intensive care of very-low-birth-weight infants. N Engl J Med 1983;308:1330–1337.
438. Greer BE, Easterling TR, McLennan DA, et al. Fetal and maternal considerations in the management of stage I-B cervical cancer during pregnancy. Gynecol Oncol 1989;34:61–65.
439. Creasman WT, Rutledge FN, Fletcher GH. Carcinoma of the cervix associated with pregnancy. Obstet Gynecol 1970;36:495–501.
440. Sablinska R, Tarlowska L, Stelmachar J. Invasive carcinoma of the cervix associated with pregnancy: Correlation between age, advancement of cancer and gestation, and results of treatment. Gynecol Oncol 1979;5:383.
441. Bonomi PD, Yordan EL. Chemotherapy of cervical carcinoma. In: Deppe G, ed. Chemotherapy of gynecologic cancer. New York: Alan R Liss, 1984:103.
442. Thigpen T, Shingleton H, Homesley H, Lagasse L, Blessing J. Cis-platinum in treatment of advanced or recurrent squamous cell carcinoma of the cervix: A phase II study of the Gynecologic Oncology Group. Cancer 1981;48:899–903.
443. Lira-Puerta V, Tenovio F, Wernz J, et al. Phase II study of cisplatin or dibromoducitol for carcinoma of the cervix. Proc Am Soc Clin Oncol 1982;1:111.
444. Stehman FB, Blom J, Blessing JA, Ehrlich CE, Mangan C. Phase II trial of galactitol-1,2:5,6-dianhydro-(NSC 132313) in the treatment of advanced gynecologic malignancies: A Gynecologic Oncology Group study. Gynecol Oncol 1983;15:381–390.
445. Bonomi P, Blessing J. Randomized trial of three cisplatin dose schedules in squamous-cell carcinoma of the cervix: A Gynecologic Oncology Group study. J Clin Oncol 1985;3:1079–1085.
446. Thigpen JT, Blessing JA, Di Saia PJ, et al. A randomized comparison of a rapid versus prolonged (24 hr) infusion of cisplatin in therapy of squamous cell carcinoma of the uterine cervix: A Gynecologic Oncology Group study. Gynecol Oncol 1989;32:198–202.
447. Thigpen T, Lambuth B, Vance R. Ifosamide in the management of gynecologic cancers. Semin Oncol 1990;17:11–18.
448. Sutton GP, Blessing JA, Rosenshein N, Photopulos G, Di Saia PJ. Phase II trial of ifosfamide and mesna in mixed mesodermal tumors of the uterus (a Gynecologic Oncology Group study). Am J Obstet Gynecol 1989;161:309–312.
449. Stehman FB, Blessing JA, McGehee R, Barrett RJ. A phase II evaluation of mitolactol in patients with advanced squamous cell carcinoma of the cervix: A Gynecologic Oncology Group study. J Clin Oncol 1989;7:1892–1895.
450. Morrow CP, Di Saia PJ, Mangan CF, Lagasse LD. Continuous pelvic arterial infusion with bleomycin for squamous carcinoma of the cervix recurrent after irradiation therapy. Cancer Treat Rep 1977;61:1403–1405.
451. Swenerton KD, Evers JA, White GW, Boyes DA. Intermittent pelvic infusion with vincristine, bleomycin, and mitomycin C for advanced recurrent carcinoma of the cervix. Cancer Treat Rep 1979;63:1379–1381.
452. Ohta A. Basic and clinical studies on the simultaneous combination treatment of cervical cancer (especially advanced cases) with a carcinostatic agent and radiation. J Tokyo Med Coll 1978;36:529.
453. Oku T, Iwasaki M, Toto S. Study on surgical chemotherapy for advanced cancer of the uterine cervix—particularly on the problem of clinical effect and drug concentration. Acta Obstet Gynaecol Jpn 1979;31:1833.
454. Kavanagh JJ, Rutledge F, Wharton JT, et al. Palliation of advanced recurrent pelvic malignancies by selective intra-arterial combination chemotherapy. Proc Am Soc Clin Oncol 1982;1:109.
455. Carlson JJ, Freedman RS, Wallace S, Chuang VP, Wharton JT, Rutledge FN. Intraarterial cis-platinum in the management of squamous cell carcinoma of the uterine cervix. Gynecol Oncol 1981;12:92–98.
456. Piver MS, Barlow JJ, Vongtama V, Webester J. Hydroxyurea and radiation therapy in advanced cervical cancer. Am J Obstet Gynecol 1974;120:969–972.
457. Hreshchyshyn MM, Aron BS, Boronow RC, Franklin E, Shingleton HM, Blessing JA. Hydroxyurea or placebo combined with radiation to treat stages IIIB and IV cervical cancer confined to the pelvis. Int J Radiat Oncol Biol Phys 1979;5:317–322.
458. Piver MS, Barlow JJ, Vongtama V, Blumenson L. Hydroxyurea as a radiation sensitizer in women with carcinoma of the uterine cervix. Am J Obstet Gynecol 1977;129:379–383.
459. Perez CA, Breaux S, Madoc JH, et al. Radiation therapy alone in the treatment of

Recurrent cervical carcinoma after radical hysterectomy. Gynecol Oncol 1988;30:381–387.

carcinoma of uterine cervix. I. Analysis of tumor recurrence. Cancer 1983;51:1393–1402.

460. Stehman F, Bundy B, Keys H, et al. A randomized trial of hydroxyurea versus misonidazole adjunct to radiation therapy in carcinoma of the cervix. Am J Obstet Gynecol 1988;159:87–94.

461. Thomas G, Dembo P, Fyles A, et al. Concurrent chemoradiation in advanced cervical cancer. Gynecol Oncol 1990;38:446–451.

462. Kuske RR, Perez CA, Grigsby PN, et al. Phase I/II study of definitive radiotherapy and chemotherapy (cisplatin and 5-fluorouracil) for advanced or recurrent gynecologic malignancies. Am J Clin Oncol 1989;12:467–473.

463. Choo YC, Choy TK, Wong LC, Ma HK. Potentiation of radiotherapy by *cis*-dichlorodiammine platinum (II) in advanced cervical carcinoma. Gynecol Oncol 1986;23:94–100.

464. Monyak DJ, Twiggs LB, Potish RA, et al. Tolerance and preliminary results of simultaneous therapy with radiation and cisplatin for advanced cervical cancer. NCI Monogr 1988;6:369–373.

465. Wong LC, Choo YC, Choy D, et al. Long-term follow-up of potentiation of radiotherapy by *cis*-platinum in advanced cervical cancer. Gynecol Oncol 1989;35:159–163.

466. Gallup DG, Stock RJ. Adenocarcinoma of the endometrium in women 40 years of age or younger. Obstet Gynecol 1984;64:417–420.

467. Whitaker GK, Lee RB, Benson WL. Carcinoma of the endometrium in young women. Milit Med 1986;151:25–31.

468. MacMahon B. Risk factors for endometrial cancer. Gynecol Oncol 1974;2:122.

469. McDonald TW, Malkasian GD, Gaffey TA. Endometrial cancer associated with feminizing ovarian tumor and polycystic ovarian disease. Obstet Gynecol 1977;49:654–658.

470. Smith DC, Prentice R, Thompson DJ, Herrmann WL. Association of exogenous estrogen and endometrial carcinoma. N Engl J Med 1975;293:1164–1167.

471. Amtunes CMF, Stolley PD, Rosensheim NB, et al. Endometrial cancer and estrogen use (report of a large case-control study). N Engl J Med 1979;300:9.

472. Nachtigall LE, Nachtigall RH, Nachtigall RD, Beckman EM. Estrogen replacement therapy II: A prospective study in the relationship to carcinoma and cardiovascular and metabolic problems. Obstet Gynecol 1979;54:74–79.

473. Gambrel DR Jr. Role of hormones in the etiology and prevention of endometrial and breast cancer. Acta Obstet Gynecol Scand 1982;106:337.

474. Sommers SC, Hertig AT, Beugloff H. Genesis of endometrial carcinoma: 11 cases, 19 to 35 years old. Cancer 1949;2:957.

475. Gore H, Hertig AT. Premalignant lesions of the endometrium. Clin Obstet Gynecol 1962;5:1148.

476. Creasman WT, Morrow CP, Bundy BN, Homesley HD, Graham JE, Heller PB. Surgical pathologic spread patterns of endometrial cancer. A Gynecologic Oncology Group study. Cancer 1987;60:2035–2041.

477. Berman ML, Ballon SC, Lagasse LD, Watring WG. Prognosis and treatment of endometrial cancer. Am J Obstet Gynecol 1980;136:679–688.

478. Tak WK. Carcinoma of the endometrium, with cervical involvement (stage II). Cancer 1979;43:2504.

479. Creasman WT, Di Saia PJ, Blessing J, et al. Prognostic significance of peritoneal cytology in patients with endometrial cancer and preliminary data concerning therapy and intraperitoneal pharmaceuticals. Am J Obstet Gynecol 1981;141:931.

480. Kennedy AW, Peterson GL, Becker SN, Nunez C, Webster KD. Experience with pelvic washings in stage I and II endometrial carcinoma. Gynecol Oncol 1987;28:50–60.

481. Morrow CP, Bundy BN, Kurman RJ, et al. Relationship between surgical-pathological risk factors and outcome in clinical stage I and II carcinoma of the endometrium: A Gynecologic Oncology Group study. Gynecol Oncol 1991;40:55–65.

482. Park RC, Grigsby PW, Muss HB, Norris HJ. Corpus: Epithelial tumors. In: Hoskins WJ, Perez CA, Young RC, eds. Principles and practice of gynecologic oncology. Philadelphia: JB Lippincott, 1992.

483. Reagan JW, Fu YS. Pathology of endometrial carcinoma. In: Coppleson M, ed. Gynecologic oncology: Fundamental principles and clinical practice. New York: Churchill Livingstone, 1981:546–561.

484. Ng AB, Reagan JW, Storaasli JP, Wentz WB. Mixed adenosquamous carcinoma of the endometrium. Am J Clin Pathol 1973;59:765–781.

485. Silverberg SG, Bolin MG, DeGiorgi LS. Adenoacanthoma and mixed adenosquamous carcinoma of the endometrium. A clinicopathologic study. Cancer 1972;30:1307–1314.

486. Salazar OM, DePapp EW, Bonfiglio TA, Feldstein ML, Rubin P, Rudolph JH. Adenosquamous carcinoma of the endometrium. An entity with an inherent poor prognosis? Cancer 1977;40:119–130.

487. Kurman RJ, Scully RE. Clear cell carcinoma of the endometrium: An analysis of 21 cases. Cancer 1976;37:872–882.

488. Hertig AT, Gore H. Tumors of the female sex organs: Part 2. Tumors of the vulva, vagina, and uterus. Washington, DC: Armed Forces Institute of Pathology, 1960.

489. Fluhman CF. Squamous epithelium in benign and malignant conditions. Surg Gynecol Obstet 1928;46:309.

490. Hendrickson M, Ross J, Eifel P, Martinez A, Kempson R. Uterine papillary serous carcinoma: A highly malignant form of endometrial adenocarcinoma. Am J Surg Pathol 1982;6:93–108.

491. Boronow RC, Morrow CP, Creasman WT, et al. Surgical staging in endometrial cancer: Clinical-pathologic findings of a prospective study. Obstet Gynecol 1984;63:825.

492. Berchuck A, Soisson AP, Clarke PD, et al. Immunohistochemical expression of CA 125 in endometrial adenocarcinoma: Correlation of antigen expression with metastatic potential. Cancer Res 1989;49:2091–2095.

493. Niloff JM, Klug TL, Schaetzl E, Zurawski VJ, Knapp RC, Bast RJ. Elevation of serum CA 125 in carcinomas of the fallopian tube, endometrium, and endocervix. Am J Obstet Gynecol 1984;148:1057–1058.

494. International Federation of Gynecology and Obstetrics. Classification and staging of malignant tumors in the female pelvis. Int J Gynaecol Obstet 1971;9:172.

495. Jones HW. Treatment of adenocarcinoma of the endometrium. Obstet Gynecol Surv 1975;30:147.

496. Creasman WT, Weed JC Jr. Carcinoma of the endometrium (FIGO stages I and II): Clinical features and management. In: Coppleson M, ed. Gynecologic oncology: Fundamental principles and clinical practice. New York: Churchill Livingstone, 1985:562–574.

497. Surwit EA, Fowler WC Jr, Rogoff EE, et al. Stage II carcinoma of the endometrium. Int J Radiat Oncol Biol Phys 1979;5:323.

498. Morrow CP, Disaia SP, Townsend DE. Current management of endometrial carcinoma. Obstet Gynecol 1973;42:399–406.

499. Boronow RC. Endometrial cancer: Not a benign disease. Obstet Gynecol 1976;47:630–634.

500. Underwood PJ, Lutz MH, Kreutner A, Miller M, Johnson RJ. Carcinoma of the endometrium: Radiation followed immediately by operation. Am J Obstet Gynecol 1977;128:86–98.

501. Gusberg SB, Chen SY, Cohen CJ. Endometrial cancer: Factors influencing the choice of treatment. Gynecol Oncol 1974;2:308–313.

502. Malkasian GJ. Carcinoma of the endometrium: Effect of stage and grade on survival. Cancer 1978;41:996–1001.

503. Landgren RC, Fletcher GH, Delclos L, Wharton JT. Irradiation of endometrial cancer in patients with medical contraindication to surgery or with unresectable lesions. AJR 1976;126:148–154.

504. Aalders J, Abeler V, Kolstad P, Onsrud M. Postoperative external irradiation and prognostic parameters in stage I endometrial carcinoma: Clinical and histopathologic study of 540 patients. Obstet Gynecol 1980;56:419–427.

505. Wharam MD, Phillips TL, Bagshaw MA. The role of radiation therapy in clinical stage I carcinoma of the endometrium. Int J Radiat Oncol Biol Phys 1976;1:1081–1089.

506. Creasman WT, Boronow RC, Morrow CP, et al. Adenocarcinoma of the endometrium: Its metastatic lymph node potential. Gynecol Oncol 1976;4:239.

507. Homesley HD, Boronow RC, Lewis JJ. Stage II endometrial adenocarcinoma. Memorial Hospital for Cancer, 1949–1965. Obstet Gynecol 1977;49:604–608.

508. Larson DM, Copeland LJ, Gallagher HS, et al. Nature of cervical involvement in endometrial carcinoma. Cancer 1987;59:959.

509. Grigsby PW, Perez CA, Camel HM, Kao MS, Galakatos AE. Stage II carcinoma of the endometrium: Results of therapy and prognostic factors. Int J Radiat Oncol Biol Phys 1985;11:1915–1923.

510. Heath R, Rosenman J, Varia M, Walton L. Peritoneal fluid cytology in endometrial cancer: Its significance and the role of chromic phosphate (^{32}P) therapy. Int J Radiat Oncol Biol Phys 1988;15:815–822.

511. Soper JT, Creasman WT, Clarke-Pearson DL, Sullivan DC, Vergadoro F, Johnston WW. Intraperitoneal chromic phosphate ^{32}P suspension therapy of malignant peritoneal cytology in endometrial carcinoma. Am J Obstet Gynecol 1985;153:101.

512. Piver MS, Lele SB, Gamarra M. Malignant peritoneal cytology in stage I endometrial adenocarcinoma: The effect of progesterone therapy (a preliminary report). Eur J Gynaecol Oncol 1988;9:187.

513. Graham H. The value of preoperative or postoperative treatment by radium for carcinoma of the uterine body. Surg Gynecol Obstet 1971;1323:855.

514. Grigsby PW, Perez CA, Kuten A, et al. Clinical stage I endometrial cancer: Results of adjuvant irradiation and patterns of failure. Int J Radiat Oncol Biol Phys 1991;21:379–385.

515. Beiler DD, Schumtz DA, O'Rourke TL. Carcinoma of the endometrium: Radiation and surgery versus surgery alone. Radiology 1972;102:159–164.

516. Malkasian GDJ, McDonald TW, Pratt JH. Carcinoma of the endometrium: Mayo Clinic experience. Mayo Clinic Proc 1977;51:175.

517. Frick H, Munnell EW, Richart RM, Berger AP, Lawry MF. Carcinoma of the endometrium. Am J Obstet Gynecol 1973;115:663–676.

518. Salazar OM, Feldstein ML, DePapp EW, et al. Endometrial carcinoma: Analysis of failures with special emphasis on the use of initial preoperative external pelvic radiation. Int J Radiat Oncol Biol Phys 1977;2:1101–1107.

519. Brady LW, Lewis GJ, Antoniades J, et al. Evolution of radiotherapeutic techniques. Gynecol Oncol 1974;2:314–323.

520. Glassburn JR, Brady LW. Carcinoma of the endometrium. In: Perez CA, Brady LW, eds. Principles and practice of radiation oncology. Philadelphia: JB Lippincott, 1987.

521. Bedwinek J, Galakatos A, Camel M, Kao MS, Stokes S, Perez C. Stage I, grade III adenocarcinoma of the endometrium treated with surgery and irradiation. Sites of failure and correlation of failure rate with irradiation technique. Cancer 1984;54:40–47.

522. Anderson JC, Meltzer HD, Scarborough JE, et al. Adenocarcinoma of the endometrium. Cancer 1965;1:955.

523. Gusberg SB, Yannopoulos D. Therapeutic decisions in corpus cancer. Am J Obstet Gynecol 1964;120:73.

524. Climie ARW, Rachmaninoff N. A ten-year experience with endometrial carcinoma. Surg Gynecol Obstet 1965;120:73.

525. Austin JH, MacMahon B. Indicators of prognosis in carcinoma of the corpus uteri. Surg Gynecol Obstet 1969;128:1247.

526. Cheon HK. Prognosis of endometrial carcinoma. Obstet Gynecol 1969;34:680–684.

527. Nilsen PA, Koller O. Carcinoma of the endometrium in Norway 1957–1960 with special reference to treatment results. Am J Obstet Gynecol 1969;105:1099–1109.

528. Lewis BV, Stallworthy JA, Cowdell R. Adenocarcinoma of the body of the uterus. J Obstet Gynaecol Br Commonw 1970;77:343–348.

529. Ng AB, Reagan JW. Incidence and prognosis of endometrial carcinoma by histologic grade and extent. Obstet Gynecol 1970;35:437–443.

530. Sall S, Sonnenblick B, Stone ML. Factors affecting survival of patients with endometrial adenocarcinoma. Am J Obstet Gynecol 1970;107:116–123.

531. Nahhas WA. Prognostic factors in endometrial carcinoma. 1971; (personal communication).

532. Wade ME, Kohorn EI, Morris JM. Adenocarcinoma of the endometrium. Am J Obstet Gynecol 1967;99:869–876.

533. Javert CT. The spread of benign and malignant endometrium in the lymphatic system with a note on coexisting vascular involvement. Am J Obstet Gynecol 1952;64:780.

534. Webb GA, Margolis AJ, Traut HF. Adenocarcinoma of the endometrium: An evaluation of factors influencing prognosis and an outline of a plan of therapy based on these factors. West J Surg Obstet Gynecol 1955;63:407.

535. Lindgren L. The prognosis of carcinoma of the endometrium in its different stages treated by surgery combined with postoperative radiotherapy. Acta Obstet Gynecol Scand 1957;36:426.

536. Boutselis JG, Bair JR, Nichols V, et al. Carcinoma of the uterine corpus: A study of 269 cases. Am J Obstet Gynecol 1963;85:994.

537. Dobbie BMW, Taylor CW, Waterhouse JAH. A study of carcinoma of the endometrium. J Obstet Gynaecol Br Commonw 1965;72:659.

538. Roman TN, Beck RP, Latour JP. Correlation of histologic grading with 5-year survival rates in endometrial carcinoma. Am J Obstet Gynecol 1967;97:117–119.

539. Sala JM, del Regato JA. The treatment of carcinoma of the endometrium. Radiology 1969;79:12.

540. Silverberg SG, DeGiorgi LS. Histopathologic analysis of preoperative radiation therapy in endometrial carcinoma. Am J Obstet Gynecol 1974;119:698–704.

541. Weigensberg IJ. Preoperative radiation therapy in endometrial carcinoma: Preliminary report of a clinical trial. Am J Roentgenol Radium Ther Nucl Med 1976;127:391.

542. Greenberg SB, Glassburn JR, Antoniades J, Brady LW. Management of carcinoma of the uterus stage II. Cancer Clin Trials 1981;4:183–186.

543. Gagnon JD, Moss WT, Gabourel LS, Stevens KJ. External irradiation in the management of stage II endometrial carcinoma. Cancer 1979;44:1247–1251.

544. Onsrud M, Aalders J, Abeler V, Taylor P. Endometrial carcinoma with cervical involvement (stage II): Prognostic factors and value of combined radiological-surgical treatment. Gynecol Oncol 1982;13:76–86.

545. Spanos WJ, Fletcher GH, Wharton JT, Gallager HS. Patterns of pelvic recurrence in endometrial carcinoma. Gynecol Oncol 1978;6:495–502.

546. Perez CA, Bedwinek JM, Breaux SR. Patterns of failure after treatment of gynecological tumors. Cancer Treat Symp 1983;2:217.

547. Antoniades J, Brady LW, Lewis GC. The management of stage III carcinoma of the endometrium. Cancer 1967;38:1838.

548. Rutledge F, Ehrlich C. Adenocarcinoma of the endometrium. In: Gray LAS, ed. Endometrial carcinoma and its treatment: The role of irradiation, extent of surgery, and approach to chemotherapy. Springfield, IL: Charles C Thomas, 1977:128–137.

549. Buchler DA, Peckham BM, Carr WF. Treatment and results of endometrial carcinoma from 1956–1974. In: Gray LAS, ed. Endometrial carcinoma and its treatment: The role of irradiation, extent of surgery, and approach to chemotherapy. Springfield, IL: Charles C Thomas, 1977:146–150.

550. Kottmeier HL. Endometrial carcinoma and its treatment: Recent experience of the Radiumhemmet, Stockholm. In: Gray LAS, ed. Endometrial carcinoma and its treatment: The role of irradiation, extent of surgery, and approach to chemotherapy. Springfield, IL: Charles C Thomas, 1977:118–126.

551. Homesley HD, Lewis JLJ. Treatment of endometrial adenocarcinoma at Memorial Hospital, New York, 1884–1976. In: Gray LAS, ed. Endometrial carcinoma and its treatment: The role of irradiation, extent of surgery, and approach to chemotherapy. Springfield, IL: Charles C Thomas, 1977:99–117.

552. Geisler HE, Gibbs CP. Invasive carcinoma of the endometrium. A 5 to 16 year follow-up of 183 patients. Am J Obstet Gynecol 1968;102:516–520.

553. Danoff BF, McDay J, Louka M, Lewis GC, Lee J, Kramer S. Stage III endometrial carcinoma: Analysis of patterns of failure and therapeutic implications. Int J Radiat Oncol Biol Phys 1980;6:1491–1495.

554. Barber HR, Brunschwig A. Treatment and results of recurrent cancer of corpus uteri in patients receiving anterior and total pelvic exenteration 1947–1963. Cancer 1968;22:949–955.

555. Stokes S, Bedwinek J, Breaux S, Kao MS, Camel M, Perez CA. Treatment of stage I adenocarcinoma of the endometrium by hysterectomy and irradiation: Analysis of complications. Obstet Gynecol 1985;65:86–92.

556. Podratz KC, O'Brien PC, Malkasian GJ, Decker DG, Jefferies JA, Edmonson JH. Effects of progestational agents in treatment of endometrial carcinoma. Obstet Gynecol 1985;66:106–110.

557. Thigpen JT, Blessing J, Di Saia P. Oral medroxyprogesterone acetate in advanced or recurrent endometrial carcinoma: Results of therapy and correlation with estrogen and progesterone levels. In: Baulieu EE, Iacobelli S, McGuire WL, eds. Endocrinology and malignancy: Basic and clinical issues. Proceedings of the First International Congress on Cancer and Hormones, Rome. NJ: Parthenon Publishing Group. 1986:446.

558. Kneale BL. Adjunctive and therapeutic progestins in endometrial cancer. Clin Obstet Gynaecol 1986;13:789–809.

559. Ehrlich CE, Young PC, Cleary RE. Cytoplasmic progesterone and estradiol receptors in normal, hyperplastic, and carcinomatous endometria: Therapeutic implications. Am J Obstet Gynecol 1981;141:539–546.

560. Quinn MA, Cauchi M, Fortune D. Endometrial carcinoma: Steroid receptors and response to medroxyprogesterone acetate. Gynecol Oncol 1985;21:314–319.

561. Swenerton KD. Treatment of advanced endometrial adenocarcinoma with tamoxifen. Cancer Treat Rep 1980;64:805–811.

562. Bonte J. Recente aanwinten in de behandeling van endometriaal adenocarcinoma. Voor Geneeskind 1981;37:1377.

563. Slavik M, Petty WM, Blessing JA, Creasman WT, Homesley HD. Phase II clinical study of tamoxifen in advanced endometrial adenocarcinoma: A Gynecologic Oncology Group study. Cancer Treat Rep 1984;68:809–811.

564. Hald I, Salimtschik M, Mouridsen HT. Tamoxifen treatment of advanced endometrial carcinoma. A phase II study. Eur J Gynaecol Oncol 1983;4:83–87.

565. Edmonson JH, Krook JE, Hilton JF, et al. Ineffectiveness of tamoxifen in advanced endometrial carcinoma after failure of progestin treatment. Cancer Treat Rep 1986;70:1019.

566. Carlson JJ, Allegra JC, Day TJ, Wittliff JL. Tamoxifen and endometrial carcinoma: Alterations in estrogen and progesterone receptors in untreated patients and combination hormonal therapy in advanced neoplasia. Am J Obstet Gynecol 1984;149:149–153.

567. Zaino RJ, Satyaswaroop PG, Mortel R. Hormonal therapy of human endometrial adenocarcinoma in a nude mouse model. Cancer Research 1985;45:539.

568. Kline RC, Freedman RS, Jones LA, Atkinson EN. Treatment of recurrent or metastatic poorly differentiated adenocarcinoma of the endometrium with tamoxifen and medroxyprogesterone acetate. Cancer Treat Rep 1987;71:327.

569. Tatman JL, Freedman RS, Scot W, Atkinson EN. Treatment of advanced endometrial adenocarcinoma with cyclic sequential ethinyl estradiol and medroxyprogesterone acetate. Eur J Cancer Clin Oncol 1989;25:1619.

570. Lewis GJ, Slack NH, Mortel R, Bross ID. Adjuvant progestogen therapy in the primary definitive treatment of endometrial cancer. Gynecol Oncol 1974;2:368–376.

571. Malkasian GJ, Decker DG. Adjuvant progesterone therapy for stage I endometrial carcinoma. Int J Gynaecol Obstet 1978;16:48–49.

572. Gusberg SB. Current concepts in cancer: The changing nature of endometrial cancer. N Engl J Med 1980;302:729–731.

573. Bochman YV, Chepik OF, Volkova AT, et al. Can primary endometrial carcinoma stage I be cured without surgery and radiation therapy? Vopr Onkel 1982;28:42.

574. De Palo G, Spatti GB, Bandieramonte G, Luciani L. Pilot study with adjuvant hormone therapy in FIGO stage I endometrial carcinoma with myometrial invasion. Tumori 1983;69:65–67.

575. Lagasse L, Thigpen T, Morrison F. Phase II trial of piperazinedione in treatment of advanced endometrial carcinoma, uterine sarcoma, and vulvar carcinoma. Proc Am Assoc Cancer Res 1970;20:388.

576. Seski JC, Edwards CL, Herson J, Rutledge FN. Cisplatin chemotherapy for disseminated endometrial cancer. Obstet Gynecol 1982;59:225–228.

577. Seski JC, Edwards CL, Copeland LJ, Gershenson DM. Hexamethylmelamine chemotherapy for disseminated endometrial cancer. Obstet Gynecol 1981;58:361–363.

578. Deppe G, Malviya VK, Zbella E. Nonhormonal chemotherapy in endometrial cancer—a review. Wien Klin Wochenschr 1984;96:747–756.

579. Cohen CJ. Cytotoxic chemotherapy for patients with endometrial carcinoma. Clin Obstet Gynecol 1986;13:811.

580. Thigpen JT, Buchsbaum HJ, Mangan C, Blessing JA. Phase II trial of Adriamycin in the treatment of advanced or recurrent endometrial carcinoma: A Gynecologic Oncology Group study. Cancer Treat Rep 1979;63:21–27.

581. Pasmantier MW, Coleman M, Silver RT, Mamaril AP, Quiguyan CC, Galindo AJ. Treatment of advanced endometrial carcinoma with doxorubicin and cisplatin: Effects on both untreated and previously treated patients. Cancer Treat Rep 1985;69:539–542.

582. Seltzer V, Vogl SE, Kaplan BH. Adriamycin and cis-diamminedichloroplatinum in the treatment of metastatic endometrial adenocarcinoma. Gynecol Oncol 1984;19:308–313.

583. Chauvergne J, Granger C, Mage P, Pigneux J, David M. Palliative chemotherapy of endometrial cancer. Value of combinations with doxorubicin and cisplatin. Rev Fr Gynecol Obstet 1986;81:547–551.

584. Turbow MM, Thornton J, Ballon S, et al. Chemotherapy of advanced endometrial carcinoma with platinum, Adriamycin, and cyclophosphamide. Proc Am Soc Clin Oncol 1982;1:108.

585. Hancock KC, Freedman RS, Edwards CL, Rutledge FN. Use of cisplatin, doxorubicin, and cyclophosphamide to treat advanced and recurrent adenocarcinoma of the endometrium. Cancer Treat Rep 1986;70:789–791.

586. Bruckner HW, Deppe G. Combination chemotherapy of advanced endometrial adenocarcinma with Adriamycin, cyclophosphamide, 5-fluorouracil, and medroxyprogesterone acetate. Obstet Gynecol 1977;50:415.

587. Cohen CJ, Deppe G, Bruckner HW. Treatment of advanced adenocarcinoma of the endometrium with melphalan, 5-fluorouracil, and medroxyprogesterone acetate: A preliminary study. Obstet Gynecol 1977;50:415–417.

588. Lovecchio JL, Averette HE, Lichtinger M, Townsend PA, Girtanner RW, Fenton AN. Treatment of advanced or recurrent endometrial adenocarcinoma with cyclophosphamide, doxorubicin, cis-platinum, and megestrol acetate. Obstet Gynecol 1984;63:557–560.

589. Piver MS, Lele SB, Patsner B, Emrich LJ. Melphalan, 5-fluorouracil, and medroxyprogesterone acetate in metastatic endometrial carcinoma. Obstet Gynecol 1986;67:261–264.

590. Horton J, Elson P, Gordon P, Hahn R, Creech R. Combination chemotherapy for advanced endometrial cancer. An evaluation of three regimens. Cancer 1982;49:2441–2445.

591. Ayoub J, Audet-Lapointe P, Methot Y, et al. Efficacy of sequential cyclical hormonal therapy in endometrial cancer and its correlation with steroid hormone receptor status. Gynecol Oncol 1988;31:327.

592. Berchuck A, Rubin SC, Hoskins WJ, et al. Treatment of uterine leiomyosarcoma. Obstet Gynecol 1988;71:845.

593. Kempson RL, Bari W. Uterine sarcomas. Classification, diagnosis, and prognosis. Hum Pathol 1970;1:331–349.

594. Ober WB. Uterine sarcomas: Histogenesis and taxonomy. Ann NY Acad Sci 1959;75: 568.

595. Norris HJ, Roth E, Taylor HB. Mesenchymal tumors of the uterus. II. A clinical and pathological study of 31 mixed mesodermal tumors. Obstet Gynecol 1966;28:57.

596. Salazar OM, Bonfiglio TA, Patten SF, et al. Uterine sarcomas: Natural history, treatment and prognosis. Cancer 1978;42:1152–1160.

597. Major F, Silverberg S, Morrow P, et al. A preliminary analysis of prognostic factors in uterine sarcomas. Gynecol Oncol 1987;26:411.

598. Perez CA, Askin F, Baglan RJ, et al. Effects of irradiation on mixed mullerian tumors of the uterus. Cancer 1979;43:1274–1284.

599. Vongtama V, Karlen JR, Piver SM, Tsukada Y, Moore RH. Treatment, results and prognostic factors in stage I and II sarcomas of the corpus uteri. AJR 1976;126:139–147.

600. Belgrad R, Elbadawi N, Rubin P. Uterine sarcoma. Radiology 1975;114:181–188.

601. Salazar OM, Bonfiglio TA, Patten SF, et al. Uterine sarcomas: Analysis of failures with special emphasis on the use of adjuvant radiation therapy. Cancer 1978;42:1161–1170.

602. Omura GA, Major FJ, Blessing JA, et al. A randomized study of Adriamycin with and without dimethyl triazenoimidazole carboxamide in advanced uterine sarcomas. Cancer 1983;52:626–632.

603. Omura GA, Blessing JA, Major F, et al. A randomized clinical trial of adjuvant Adriamycin in uterine sarcomas: A Gynecologic Oncology Group study. J Clin Oncol 1985;3:1240–1245.

604. Thigpen JT, Blessing JA, Orr JJ, Di Saia PJ. Phase II trial of cisplatin in the treatment of patients with advanced or recurrent mixed mesodermal sarcomas of the uterus: A Gynecologic Oncology Group study. Cancer Treat Rep 1986;70:271–274.

605. Gershenson DM, Kavanagh JJ, Copeland LJ, Edwards CL, Stringer CA, Wharton JT. Cisplatin therapy for disseminated mixed mesodermal sarcoma of the uterus. J Clin Oncol 1987;5:618–621.

606. Piver MS, Lurain JR. Uterine sarcomas: Clinical features and management. In: Coppleson M, ed. Gynecologic oncology: Fundamental principles and clinical practice. New York: Churchill Livingstone, 1981:608–618.

607. Silverberg SG. Leiomyosarcoma of the uterus. A clinicopathologic study. Obstet Gynecol 1971;38:613–628.

608. Christopherson WM, Williamson EO, Gray LA. Leiomyosarcoma of the uterus. Cancer 1972;29:1512–1517.

609. Giarratano RC, Slate TA. Sarcomas of the uterus. Obstet Gynecol 1971;38:472–477.

610. Sutton G, Blessing J, McGuire W, Photopoulos G, Di Saia P. Phase II trial of ifosfamide and mesna in leiomyosarcomas of the uterus. Gynecol Oncol 1990;36:295.

611. Norris HJ, Taylor HB. Mesenchymal tumors of the uterus. I. A clinical and pathologic study of 53 endometrial stromal tumors. Cancer 1966;19:755.

612. Evans HJ. Endometrial stromal sarcoma and poorly differentiated endometrial sarcoma. Cancer 1982;50:2170.

613. Tavassoli FA, Norris HJ. Mesenchymal tumours of the uterus. VII. A clinicopathological study of 60 endometrial stromal nodules. Histopathology 1981;5:1–10.

614. Fekete PS, Vellios F. The clinical and histologic spectrum of endometrial stromal neoplasms: A report of 41 cases. Int J Gynecol Pathol 1984;3:198–212.

615. Chang KL, Crabtree GS, Lim TS, Kempson RL, Hendrickson MR. Primary uterine endometrial stromal neoplasms. A clinicopathologic study of 117 cases. Am J Surg Pathol 1990;14:415–438.

616. Newlands ES. New chemotherapeutic agents in the management of gestational trophoblastic disease. Semin Oncol 1982;9:239–243.

617. Wong LC, Choo YC, Ma HK. Etoposide, methotrexate, and bleomycin in drug-resistant gestational trophoblastic disease. Gynecol Oncol 1986;24:51–57.

618. Koss LG, Spiro RH, Brunschwig A. Endometrial stromal sarcoma. Surg Gynecol Obstet 1965;121:531.

619. Baggish MS, Woodruff JD. Uterine stromatosis. Clinicopathologic features and hormone dependency. Obstet Gynecol 1972;40:487–498.

620. Katz L, Merino MJ, Sakamoto H, Schwartz PE. Endometrial stromal sarcoma: A clinicopathologic study of 11 cases with determination of estrogen and progestin receptor levels in three tumors. Gynecol Oncol 1987;26:87–97.

621. Tosi P, Sforza V, Santopietro R. Estrogen receptor content, immunohistochemically determined by monoclonal antibodies, in endometrial stromal sarcoma. Obstet Gynecol 1989;73:75–78.

622. Sutton GP, Stehman FB, Michael H, Young PC, Ehrlich CE. Estrogen and progesterone receptors in uterine sarcomas. Obstet Gynecol 1986;68:709–714.

623. Clement PB, Scully RE. Mullerian adenosarcoma of the uterus. A clinicopathologic analysis of ten cases of a distinctive type of mullerian mixed tumor. Cancer 1974;34:1138–1149.

624. Clement PB, Scully RE. Mullerian adenosarcoma of the uterus: A clinicopathologic analysis of 100 cases with a review of the literature. Hum Pathol 1990;21:363–381.

625. Kaku T, Silverberg SG, Major FJ, et al. Adenosarcoma of the uterus: A Gynecologic Oncology Group clinicopathologic study of 31 cases. Int J Gynecol Pathol 1992;11:75–88.

626. Zaloudek CJ, Norris HJ. Adenofibroma and adenosarcoma of the uterus: A clinicopathologic study of 35 cases. Cancer 1981;48:354–366.

627. Roberts JA, Lifshitz S. Primary adenocarcinoma of the fallopian tube. Gynecol Oncol 1982;13:301–308.

628. Green TH, Scully RE. Tumors of the fallopian tube. Clin Obstet Gynecol 1962;5:886.

629. Woodruff JD, Julian CG. Multiple malignancy in the upper genital canal. Am J Obstet Gynecol 1969;103:810–822.

630. Benedet JL, White GW. Malignant tumors of the fallopian tube. In: Coppleson M, ed. Gynecologic oncology: Fundamental principles and clinical practice. New York: Churchill Livingstone, 1981:621–629.

631. Woodruff JD, Pauerstein CJ. The fallopian tube. Baltimore: Williams & Wilkins, 1969.

632. Wheeler JE, Mastroianni L Jr. Pathology of the fallopian tube. In: Blaustein A, ed. Pathology of the female genital tract. New York: Springer-Verlag, 1977:359–362.

633. Berg JW, Lampe JG. High-risk factors in gynecologic cancer. Cancer 1981;48:429–441.

634. Hanton EM, Malkasian GJ, Dahlin DC, Pratt JH. Primary carcinoma of the fallopian tube. Am J Obstet Gynecol 1966;94:832–839.

635. Scheffey LC, Lang WR, Nugent FB. Clinical and pathologic aspects of primary sarcoma of the uterine tube. Am J Obstet Gynecol 1941;52:904.

636. Wu JP, Tanner WS, Fardal PM. Malignant mixed mullerian tumor of the uterine tube. Obstet Gynecol 1973;41:707–712.

637. Hertig AT, Gore H. Tumors of the female sex organs: Part 3. Tumors of the ovary and fallopian tubes. Washington, DC: Armed Forces Institute of Pathology, 1961.

638. Patton GJ, Goldstein DP. Gestational choriocarcinoma of the tube and ovary. Surg Gynecol Obstet 1973;137:608–612.

639. Weiss PD, MacDougall MK, Regan JW, et al. Primary adenosquamous carcinoma of the fallopian tube. Obstet Gynecol 1980;55:885.

640. Novak ER, Woodruff JD. Novak's gynecologic and obstetric pathology. Philadelphia: WB Saunders, 1971.

641. Schiller HM, Silverberg SG. Staging and prognosis in primary carcinoma of the fallopian tube. Cancer 1971;28:389–395.

642. Frick MC. Cancer of the fallopian tube. In: Gusberg SG, Frick MC, eds. Corscaden's gynecologic cancer. Baltimore: Williams & Wilkins, 1978.

643. Dodson MG, Ford JJ, Averette HE. Clinical aspects of fallopian tube carcinoma. Obstet Gynecol 1970;36:935–939.

644. Erez S, Kaplan AL, Wall JA. Clinical staging of carcinoma of the uterine tube. Obstet Gynecol 1967;30:547–550.

645. Barakat RR, Rubin SC, Hoskins WJ, et al. Cisplatin-based combination chemotherapy in carcinoma of the fallopian tube. Gynecol Oncol 1991;42:156–160.

646. Schray MF, Podratz KC, Malkasian GD. Fallopian tube cancer: The role of radiation therapy. Radiother Oncol 1987;10:267–275.

647. Tamimi HK, Figge DC. Adenocarcinoma of the uterine tube: Potential for lymph node metastases. Am J Obstet Gynecol 1981;141:132–137.

648. MacMurray EH, Jacobs AJ, Perez CA, Camel HM, Kao MS, Galakatos A. Carcinoma of the fallopian tube. Management and sites of failure. Cancer 1986;58:2070–2075.

649. Raju KS, Barker GH, Wiltshaw E. Primary carcinoma of the fallopian tube. Report of 22 cases. Br J Obstet Gynaecol 1981;88:1124–1129.

650. Engstrom L. Primary carcinoma of the fallopian tube. Acta Obstet Gynecol Scand 1957;36:289.

651. Phelps HM, Chapman KE. Role of radiation therapy in treatment of primary carcinoma of the uterine tube. Obstet Gynecol 1974;43:669–673.

652. Amendola BE, La Rouere J, Amendola MA, et al. Adenocarcinoma of the fallopian tube. Surg Gynecol Obstet 1983;158:223.

653. Jacobs AJ, MacMurray EH, Parham J, et al. Treatment of carcinoma of the fallopian tube using cisplatin, doxorubicin, and cyclophosphamide. Am J Clin Oncol 1986;9:436–439.

654. Griffiths CT. Ovary and the fallopian tube. In: Holland JF, Frei E III, eds. Cancer medicine. Philadelphia: Lea and Febiger, 1972:1718.

655. Boronow RC. Chemotherapy for disseminated tubal cancer. Obstet Gynecol 1973;42:62.

656. Yoonessi M. Carcinoma of the fallopian tube. Obstet Gynecol Survey 1979;34:257.

657. Deppe G, Bruckner HW, Cohen CJ. Combination chemotherapy for advanced carcinoma of the fallopian tube. Obstet Gynecol 1980;56:530.

658. Peters WA, Anderson WA, Hopkins MP. Results of chemotherapy in advanced carcinoma of the fallopian tube. Cancer 1987;63:836.

659. Rose PG, Piver MS, Tsukada Y. Fallopian tube cancer: The Roswell Park experience. Cancer 1990;66:2661–2667.

660. Yoonessi M, Leberer JP, Crickard K. Primary fallopian tube carcinoma: Treatment and spread pattern. J Surg Oncol 1988;38:97.

661. Acosta-Sison H. Statistical study of chorionephithelioma in the Philippine General Hospital. Am J Obstet Gynecol 1949;58:125.

662. Teoh ES, Dawood MY, Ratnam SS. Epidemiology of hydatidiform mole in Singapore. Am J Obstet Gynecol 1947;110:53.

663. Hertig AT, Sheldon WH. Hydatidiform mole—A pathologicoclinical correlation of 200 cases. Am J Obstet Gynecol 1947;53:1.

664. Deligdisch L, Driscoll SG, Goldstein DP. Gestational trophoblastic neoplasms: Morphologic correlates of therapeutic response. Am J Obstet Gynecol 1978;130:801–806.

665. Goldstein DP. Endocrine assay in chorionic tumors. Clin Obstet Gynecol 1978;18:41.

666. Vaitukaitis JL, Braunstein GD, Ross GT. A radioimmunoassay which specifically measures human chorionic gonadotropin in the presence of human luteinizing hormone. Am J Obstet Gynecol 1976;38:453.

667. Goldstein DP. Chorionic gonadotropin. Cancer 1976;38:453.

668. Woo JSK, Ngan HYS, Ma HK. Non-resolution of pelvic sonographic abnormality after chemotherapy for persistent trophoblastic disease—A word of caution. Eur J Obstet Gynecol Reprod Biol 1983;22:153.

669. Goldstein DP, Berkowitz RS. The management of gestational trophoblastic neoplasms. Curr Probl Obstet Gynecol 1980;4:1.

670. Bagshawe KD. Risk and prognostic factors in trophoblastic neoplasia. Cancer 1976;38:1373–1385.

671. Dijkema HE, Aalders JG, de Bruijn HW, Laurini RN, Willemse PH. Risk factors in gestational trophoblastic disease, and consequences for primary treatment. Eur J Obstet Gynaecol Reprod Biol 1986;22:145–152.

672. Goldstein DP, Berkowitz RS, Cohen SM. The current management of molar pregnancy. Curr Probl Obstet Gynecol 1978;3:1.

673. Li MC, Hertz R, Spence DB. Effect of methotrexate therapy upon choriocarcinoma and chorioadenoma. Proc Soc Exp Biol Med 1956;93:361.

674. Hertz R, Lewis JL Jr, Lipsett MB. Five years' experience with the chemotherapy of metastatic choriocarcinoma and related trophoblastic disease. Gynecol Oncol 1986;23:111.

675. Berkowitz RS, Goldstein DP, Bernstein MR. Ten years' experience with methotrexate and folinic acid as primary therapy for gestational trophoblastic disease. Gynecol Oncol 1986;23:111–118.

676. Surwit EA, Hammond CB. Treatment of metastatic trophoblastic disease with poor prognosis. Obstet Gynecol 1979;53:207.

677. Bagshawe KD. Treatment of trophoblastic tumors. Ann Acad Med 1976;5:273.

678. Weed JJ, Barnard DE, Currie JL, Clayton LA, Hammond CB. Chemotherapy with the modified Bagshawe protocol for poor prognosis metastatic trophoblastic disease. Obstet Gynecol 1982;59:377–380.

679. Berkowitz RS, Goldstein DP, Bernstein MR. Modified triple chemotherapy in the management of high-risk metastatic gestational trophoblastic tumors. Gynecol Oncol 1984;19:173–181.

680. Hansen LA, Clayton BD. Treatment of gestational trophoblastic tumors. Drug Intell Clin Pharm 1984;18:569–576.

681. Ballon SC, Berman ML, Lagasse LD, et al. The unique aspects of gestational trophoblastic disease. Obstet Gynecol 1977;32:405.

682. Surwit EA, Sucia TN, Schmidt HJ, Hammond CB. A new combination chemotherapy for resistant trophoblastic disease. Gynecol Oncol 1979;8:110–118.

683. Newlands ES, Bagshawe KD. Activity of high-dose cis-platinum (NCI 119875) in combination with vincristine and methotrexate in drug-resistant gestational choriocarcinoma. A report of 17 cases. Br J Cancer 1979;40:943–945.

684. Newlands ES, Bagshawe, KD. The role of VP16-213 (etoposide; NSC-141540) in gestational choriocarcinoma. Cancer Chemother Pharmacol 1982;7:211–214.

685. Amiel JL, Droz JP, Tursz T. Placental tumors resistant to usual chemotherapy: Treatment with cis-diaminedichloroplatinum (2 case reports). Nouv Presse Med 1978;7:1933–1935.

686. Newlands FS, Bagshawe KD, Begent RHJ, et al. Results with the EMA/CO regimen in high-risk gestational trophoblastic tumors. Br J Obstet Gynecol 1991;98:550–557.

687. Ross GT. Congenital anomalies among children born to mothers receiving chemotherapy for gestational trophoblastic neoplasms. Cancer 1976;37:1043.

688. Kuten A, Cohen Y, Tatcher M, Kobrin I, Robinson E. Pregnancy and delivery after successful treatment of epidural metastatic choriocarcinoma. Gynecol Oncol 1978;6:464–466.

689. Smith PG, Doll R. Late effects of x-irradiation in patients treated for metropathia haemorrhagica. Br J Radiol 1976;49:224–232.

690. Hutchinson GB. Leukemia in patients with cancer of the cervix uteri treated with radiation: A report covering the first five years of an international study. JNCI 1968;40:9591.

691. Dickson RJ. The late results of radium treatment for benign uterine haemorrhage. Br J Radiol 1969;42:582.

692. Wagoner JK. Leukemia and other malignancies following radiation therapy for gynecological disorders. In: Boice JD, Fraumeni JF Jr, eds. Radiation carcinogenesis: Epidemiology and biological significance. New York: Raven Press, 1984:153–159.

693. Arneson AN, Schellhas HF. Multiple primary cancers in patients treated for carcinoma of the cervix. Am J Obstet Gynecol 1970;106:1155–1170.

694. Spratt JJ, Hoag MG. Incidence of multiple primary cancers per man-year of follow up: 20-year review from the Ellis Fischel State Cancer Hospital. Ann Surg 1966;164:775–784.

695. Storm HH. Second primary cancer after treatment for cervical cancer. Late effects after radiotherapy. Cancer 1988;61:679–688.

696. Wagoner JK. American Public Health Association Meeting, 1969.

697. Feinleib M. Breast cancer and artificial menopause: A cohort study. JNCI 1968;41:315–329.

698. Villasanta U, Rubel H. Radium treatment of benign uterine bleeding. Long-term follow-up. Obstet Gynecol 1969;33:813–817.

699. Thomas WJ, Harris HH, Enden JA. Postirradiation malignant neoplasms of the uterine fundus. Am J Obstet Gynecol 1969;104:209–219.

Cancer: Principles & Practice of Oncology, Fourth Edition,
edited by Vincent T. DeVita, Jr., Samuel Hellman, Steven A. Rosenberg.
J.B. Lippincott Co., Philadelphia © 1993.

Robert C. Young
Carlos A. Perez
William J. Hoskins

CHAPTER **39**

Cancer of the Ovary

Ovarian cancer is the fourth most common cause of cancer death in women and the leading cause of gynecologic cancer death in the United States. More women die from ovarian cancer each year than from cervical and endometrial carcinoma combined. Incidence and mortality estimates for 1992 indicate that 21,000 new patients are diagnosed yearly, and 13,000 women die from this disease.[1] A steady increase in the age-adjusted cancer death rates in the United States has occurred during the past 25 years, and similar increases have occurred in other industrialized nations.[2] Approximately 1 in every 70 women will develop ovarian cancer, and approximately 1% of all female deaths result from this disease.

EPIDEMIOLOGY

The highest ovarian cancer rates are reported in highly industrialized countries. The notable exception is Japan, where rates of death from ovarian cancer are among the lowest in the world. Studies of migrant populations strongly suggest environmental influences. Japanese migrants to Hawaii and their first-generation offspring in the United States have a significantly higher incidence of ovarian cancer than Japanese women in Japan, but the incidence is still lower than that observed in the indigenous white population of the United States.[3,4]

In the United States, the common epithelial neoplasms usually develop in adult white populations. They rarely occur before menarche, but the rate of occurrence tends to increase significantly thereafter. Incidences range from 15.7 of 100,000 women in the 40 to 44 age group to 54 of 100,000 women in the 75 to 79 age group. In contrast, germ cell ovarian tumors are primarily seen in children and young women, and they occur frequently in nonwhite populations.

Several epidemiologic studies suggest that disordered endocrine function may contribute to the development of ovarian cancer. A higher incidence of epithelial tumors is seen in women with a lower mean number of pregnancies, in nulliparous women, and in women with a history of infertility.[5-7] Compared with a relative risk of 1.0 for nulliparous women, women who have had one to two pregnancies have a risk of 0.49 to 0.97, and women with three or more pregnancies have a relative risk of 0.35 to 0.76.[8] Each additional pregnancy appears to lower the risk by about 10%. No clear association between ovarian cancer and the administration of synthetic estrogens has been established, but oral contraceptives reduce ovarian cancer risk.[9-13] In a World Health Organization study, 368 women with ovarian cancer were compared with 2397 matched controls. The relative risk for women who had used oral contraceptives was 0.75.[13] Oral contraceptives are estimated to have prevented over 1700 cases of ovarian cancer in the United States.[12] Risk appears to fall after several months of contraceptive use, but the reduction is greatest for long-term users.

An increased frequency of ovarian thecomas has been described in patients who undergo long-term anticonvulsant therapy. This increase is probably related to variations in the patients' ability to metabolize anticonvulsant drugs.[14]

No association with a viral infection has been identified, but a lower than expected frequency of mumps and other viral exanthems has been reported for women with ovarian cancer.[15]

Cancers of the ovary and breast appear to share some common etiologic factors. For example, women with breast cancer have twice the expected risk for ovarian carcinoma. Women with ovarian cancer have a threefold to fourfold increase in the incidence of subsequent breast cancer. Most studies that have evaluated breast feeding have not found it to be a risk factor.

Familial and genetic associations have been reported but are uncommon. Cases of familial ovarian cancer may constitute 5% to 10% of the total cases. Ovarian cancer has been reported in multiple members of the same or succeeding generations.[16] Case-control studies have been done in an effort to estimate the increased risk in cancer-prone families. Relative risks of 3.6 for first-degree relatives and 2.9 for second-degree relatives were reported.[17,18] Families with two or more first-degree relatives with the disease are at high risk but occur rarely and comprise only 0.5% of all ovarian cancer patients.

There are three types of hereditary ovarian cancer: site-specific ovarian cancer; breast-ovarian cancer syndrome; and Lynch II syndrome, which is a combination of Lynch I hereditary colon cancer and the frequent occurrence of ovarian, breast, and uterine cancers.[19-22] All these syndromes appear to be the result of autosomal dominant genes with incomplete penetrance. All but the site-specific syndromes exhibit variable expressivity. Relative risks of families with the site-specific pattern have been estimated to be increased 20-fold (RR=20). In the breast-ovarian syndrome, relative risks have been estimated at 13, compared with 10 for the Lynch type II families.

Several unusual genetic disorders seem to cause a predisposition to ovarian neoplasms, although the tumors that develop are usually benign and stromal in origin. Females with Peutz-Jeghers syndrome (*i.e.*, mucocutaneous pigmentation and intestinal polyps) have a 5% to 14% chance of developing ovarian tumors. Women with inherited basal cell nevus syndrome develop benign fibromas or, rarely, other tumors. Patients with gonadal dysgenesis (*i.e.*, 46 XY genotype or mosaic) are prone to the development of gonadoblastomas. Patients with Turner's syndrome (*i.e.*, 45 X0) and undeveloped gonads have no such tendency.

Although epidemiologic evidence strongly suggests that ovarian cancer may be caused primarily by environmental factors, these associations have not been firmly established. Diagnostic or therapeutic irradiation does not seem to increase the frequency of this malignancy. No association with known chemical carcinogens has been proved, although a study implicated exposure to triazine herbicides.[23] Ovarian cancer is not found with increased frequency among women with industrial exposures to dyes, tars, or anthracene-containing compounds.[24] However, exposure to asbestos and talc appears to be associated with an increased risk for ovarian carcinoma in humans.[25] Studies indicate a higher than expected frequency of ovarian and peritoneal neoplasms in asbestos workers. Passage of these materials through the bowel wall or retrograde through the female reproductive tract has been described and may explain how they arrive at the ovarian epithelium.[25,26] However, other studies have failed to demonstrate an association between talc use for diaphragm storage and ovarian cancer. The risk, if any, may lessen as talc products are progressively cleared of asbestos contamination.[27]

Cramer and associates evaluated the relation of lactose consumption (usually yogurt) and ovarian cancer and implicated lactose and transferase abnormalities as etiologic factors.[28] Another multinational study correlated lactose persistence and ovarian cancer.[29] These observations need additional study. Use of coffee and tobacco do not seem to increase the risk for ovarian cancer, but a slight increase has been seen with alcohol consumption.[8,30]

PATHOGENESIS

Epithelial carcinomas of the ovary account for 80% to 90% of ovarian malignancies. The remaining 10% to 20% of ovarian tumors arise from germ or stromal cells. Epithelial tumors arise from the serosal mesothelial layer of the gonads. In the embryo, the ovary develops from the genital ridge of thickened celomic epithelium. Germ cells originate in the primitive streak, migrate to the gonad, and proliferate to form the bulk of the cortex. The mesenchyma of the medulla gives rise to the ovarian stroma. All three cell types (*i.e.*, celomic epithelial, germ, and stromal cells) can give rise to malignant neoplasms.[31] Celomic epithelium has the capability to differentiate into endometrioid, mucinous, or serous epithelium, and the common epithelial tumors of the ovary have these characteristic cell types.[32]

Epithelial tumors disseminate primarily by surface shedding, lymphatic spread, or less commonly, by hematogenous metastasis. Most of the errors committed by surgeons in the operative management of this disease can be related to a lack of understanding about the patterns of spread. Figure 39–1 illustrates the typical spread of this disease. Commonly, tumors spread by continuity and intraperitoneal dissemination.[33] Spread to the opposite ovary occurs in 6% to 13% of patients with disease that is otherwise stage IA.[34,35] Transperitoneal tumor implantation and lymphatic spread to the uterus and fallopian tubes occur in approximately 5% of patients otherwise thought to have stage IA disease.[34] In more advanced stages, the uterus is involved in 25% of patients, sometimes with demonstrable retrograde lymphatic tumor emboli.[33] Direct spread can also involve the peritoneal surfaces of the bladder, rectosigmoid, or pelvic peritoneum.

The most common type of extraovarian spread is transperitoneal dissemination, in which free tumor cells shed from gross or microscopic tumor excrescences on the surface of

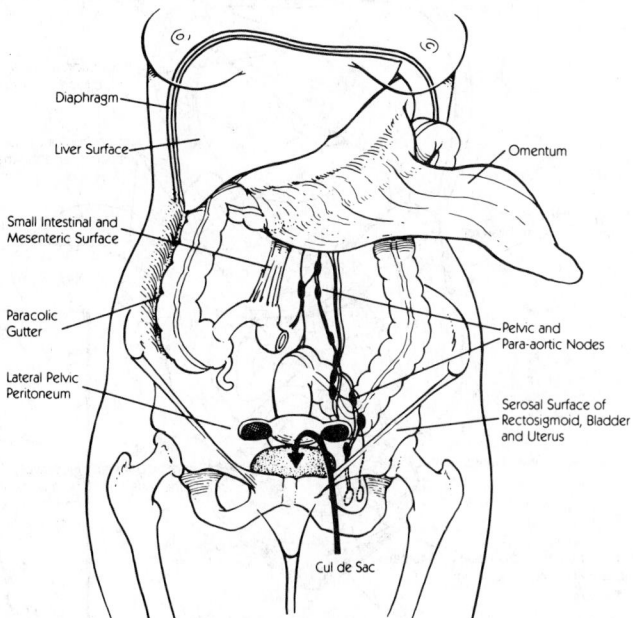

FIGURE 39–1. Spread of disease in ovarian cancer.

the primary tumor. Malignant cells in the peritoneal cavity despite an apparently intact capsule indicates that cancers can exfoliate cells even before the capsule is disrupted.[36] Exfoliated clonogenic cells attach to the peritoneal surfaces and form micrometastases that continue to exfoliate clonogenic cells. These free-floating cells are removed from the peritoneal cavity through lymphatic channels in the diaphragm.[37,38] Clearance does not take place evenly over the whole diaphragm surface; it is more extensive on the right side overlying the liver, where respiratory movements create a flow of peritoneal fluid along the abdominal gutters that travel predominately to the right hemidiaphragm.[39,40] Drainage occurs into submesothelial lymphatic capillaries of the diaphragm that intercommunicate with the pleural surface and subsequently communicate with the anterior mediastinal lymph nodes.[37,41,42] This pathway accounts for 80% of peritoneal clearance. Peritoneoscopic studies have shown that a significant fraction of stage I and II patients have involvement of the undersurface of the diaphragm, which accounts for the failure to cure some of these patients.[43-45] Partial or complete obstruction of the diaphragmatic lymphatics by tumor cells allows implantation on the omentum and at various other sites on the serosal surface of the peritoneum. It also causes accumulation of carcinomatous ascites.[46] The force of gravity in the upright adult leads to early implantation in the cul-de-sac and along the surface of the rectum.

Autopsy studies almost invariably demonstrate omental involvement in patients who die from ovarian carcinoma. Occult omental metastases have been found in 3% to 11% of untreated patients thought to have stage I or II disease at initial surgical exploration.[45,47] Steinberg reported that 22% of 55 grossly negative omenta had histologically proved tumor.[48] In one half of these patients, the omentum was the only demonstrable site of stage III disease.

The ovarian lymphatic system is an important pathway of dissemination (Fig. 39–2).[49] The lymphatic vessels of the ovarian parenchyma drain into the ovarian hilus to form the subovarian plexus. From this plexus, three routes of lymphatic drainage emerge. The main pathway ascends bilaterally among the ovarian blood vessels and terminates in the paraaortic group of lymph nodes between the bifurcation of the aorta and the renal arteries. The second route passes within the broad ligaments toward the lateral and posterior pelvic wall and terminates in the uppermost external iliac and hypogastric nodes. The third group of efferent lymphatics runs along the round ligaments and drains into the external iliac and inguinal nodes, accounting for the occasional spread of ovarian carcinoma to the inguinal nodes.

The use of lymphangiography in early and advanced stages of the disease demonstrates dissemination in about 15% of patients with stage I ovarian carcinoma, 17% with stage II, 31% with stage III, and 64% with stage IV.[50,51] At autopsy, the frequency of involved pelvic and aortic lymph nodes is approximately 80%.[52] Burghardt and colleagues performed complete pelvic and paraaortic lymphadenectomies in 48 patients with untreated ovarian cancer.[53] They found a 14% rate of positive lymph nodes in stages I and II and 63% in stages III and IV. Pelvic nodes were involved more frequently than paraaortic nodes, which were never involved unless pelvic nodes were involved. Similar results were reported by Wu and associates.[54] Data from a Gynecologic Oncology Group (GOG) surgical staging study indicated that patients with stages I, II and optimal III disease, defined in this study as less than 3 cm of abdominal disease before debulking, had an 8% incidence of positive paraaortic lymph nodes.[55] The paraaortic nodes were only sampled, unlike the studies of Burghart and Wu, in which full paraaortic lymphadenectomy was performed.

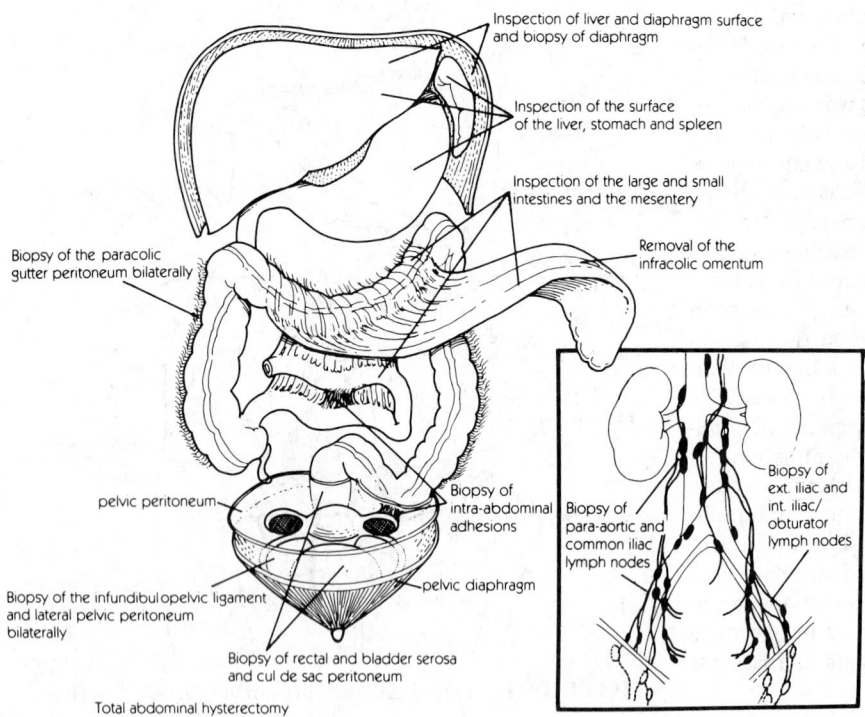

FIGURE 39–2. Staging laparotomy for the patient with ovarian cancer. (Hoskins WJ. The role of cytoreductive surgery in ovarian cancer. PPO Updates 1987;1[2])

Although peritoneum, omentum, bowel surfaces, and retroperitoneal lymph nodes are the most frequent sites of spread in ovarian cancer, other organs are also at risk. The distant organs that may be involved include, in order of decreasing frequency, the liver, lungs, pleura, kidneys, bone, adrenal glands, bladder, and spleen.[33] The major pathways of spread are shown in Figure 39–2. Studies of recurrence after negative second-look laparotomy found disease outside the abdominal cavity in as many as 50% of patients.[56]

HISTOLOGY

Several comprehensive reviews of ovarian cancer pathology provide detailed pathologic descriptions for each type.[57-61] The World Health Organization (WHO) and the International Federation of Gynecology and Obstetrics (FIGO) adopted a unified classification of the common epithelial tumors, the sex cord and stromal tumors, and the germ cell tumors (Table 39–1). Eighty-five percent to 90% of malignant ovarian tumors seen in the United States are epithelial, and their approximate overall frequency varies: serous cystadenocarcinoma, 42%; mucinous cystadenocarcinoma, 12%; endometrioid carcinoma, 15%; undifferentiated carcinoma, 17%; and clear cell carcinoma, 6%. The remaining 8% of primary tumors are sex cord, stromal, and germ cell tumors.

EPITHELIAL OVARIAN CARCINOMAS

Epithelial tumors are classified as benign, malignant (*i.e.*, invasive), or of low malignant potential (*i.e.*, borderline malignancy). The latter group contains neoplastic epithelial cells, detached cellular clusters from sites of origin, increased mitotic activity, and nuclear abnormalities. However, they lack obvious invasion of the supporting stroma. The incidence of borderline epithelial tumors varies but may approach 15% of all epithelial tumors.

Tumors of borderline malignancy possess a different natural history from benign and malignant tumors. They progress and metastasize slowly. Five-year survival rates for patients with serous and mucinous epithelial tumors with low malignant potential range from 74% to 98%.[62] The 5-year and 10-

TABLE 39–1. World Health Organization Classification of Malignant Ovarian Tumors

Common Epithelial Tumors	**Sex Cord-Stromal Tumors** (*continued*)
Malignant serous tumors	Tubular androblastoma, Sertoli cell tumor (tubular adenoma of Pick)
Adenocarcinoma, papillary adenocarcinoma, papillary cystadenocarcinoma	Tubular androblastoma with lipid storage, Sertoli cell tumor with lipid storage (folliculome lipidique of Lecene)
Surface papillary carcinoma	Sertoli-Leydig cell tumor (tubular adenoma with Leydig cells)
Malignant adenofibroma, cystadenofibroma	Leydig cell tumor, hilus cell tumor
Malignant mucinous tumors	Of intermediate differentiation
Adenocarcinoma, cystadenocarcinoma	Poorly differentiated (sarcomatoid)
Malignant adenofibroma, cystadenofibroma	With heterologous elements
Malignant endometrioid tumors	Gynandroblastoma
Carcinoma	Unclassified
Adenocarcinoma	
Adenoacanthoma	**Lipid (Lipoid) Cell Tumors**
Malignant adenofibroma, cystadenofibroma	Germ cell tumors
Endometrioid stromal sarcomas	Dysgerminoma
Mesodermal (müllerian) mixed tumors: homologous and heterologous	Endodermal sinus tumor
Clear cell (mesonephroid) tumors, malignant	Embryonal carcinoma
Carcinoma and adenocarcinoma	Polyembryoma
Brenner tumors, malignant	Choriocarcinoma
Mixed epithelial tumors, malignant	Teratomas
Undifferentiated carcinoma	Immature
Unclassified	Mature dermoid cyst with malignant transformation
	Monodermal and highly specialized
Sex Cord-Stromal Tumors	Struma ovarii
Granulosa-stromal cell tumors	Carcinoid
Granulosa cell tumor	Struma ovarii and carcinoid
Tumors in the thecoma-fibroma group	Others
Fibroma	Mixed forms
Unclassified	Gonadoblastoma
Androblastomas: Sertoli-Leydig cell tumors	Pure
Well-differentiated	Mixed with dysgerminoma or other form of germ cell tumor

(Modified from Serov SF, Scully RE, Solvin LH. International Histological Classification of Tumors, No. 9. Histological Typing of Ovarian Tumors. Geneva: World Health Organization, 1973)

year survival rates of patients with borderline tumors in one study were 93% and 91%, respectively, compared with 34% and 29% for patients with invasive epithelial carcinomas.[63] Patients with borderline tumors must be considered separately from patients with invasive ovarian carcinoma in planning treatment.

Proper therapy for borderline tumors is unsettled. In stage I and II disease, surgical resection alone usually produces excellent results. In more advanced stages, some investigators advocate therapeutic approaches similar to those used for more invasive tumors. Despite the fact that tumors of low malignant potential grow slowly, approximately 10% to 15% of patients die from disease within the first 5 to 10 years.

Fort and associates reported a series of patients with borderline tumors of the ovary who were left with residual disease and had negative second-look operations after chemotherapy.[64] This study seems to indicate that some patients with residual disease can be rendered disease free by systemic chemotherapy. Some authorities differentiate borderline tumors that have invasive metastatic implants from those that have noninvasive implants and suggest that patients with invasive implants should be treated aggressively.[65] However, other studies do not demonstrate survival differences, and the issue remains controversial.[66,67] Other studies used DNA content and ploidy analysis to differentiate indolent from aggressive tumors, but this also produced inconsistent results.[68] The GOG is prospectively evaluating borderline ovarian tumors. The slow progression of disease in these patients requires a long-term study.

For invasive epithelial carcinomas, survival has not consistently correlated with histologic type.[69-72] The current consensus is that the histologic type of malignant epithelial ovarian cancer has limited prognostic significance independent of clinical stage, extent of residual disease, and histologic grade. The apparently better survival rates for mucinous and endometrioid carcinomas are related to the less frequent occurrence of poorly differentiated tumors. Poorly differentiated mucinous tumors have a poor prognosis, and poorly differentiated endometrioid carcinomas are often misdiagnosed as undifferentiated adenocarcinomas. Although several studies suggest that clear cell carcinomas have a worse prognosis, others do not.[73,74] The matter remains unsettled.

The degree of cellular differentiation of epithelial cancers (*i.e.*, histologic grade) is an important independent prognostic factor that helps predict survival and response to treatment.[75-78] Studies from the Mayo Clinic, using Broders' classification of stage II serous cystadenocarcinoma, demonstrated a survival rate of 80% for patients with grade 1 tumors, 47% for grade 2, and 10% for grades 3 and 4.[76] Day and colleagues made similar observations with the pattern system of grading.[77] In stages I and II serous carcinoma of the ovary, patients with grade 1 tumors had a 78% 7-year survival rate compared with a 35% 7-year survival rate for grade 2 and a 0% 7-year survival rate for grade 3 tumors.

Initial studies emphasized the effect of grade on prognosis in early stage disease, but some studies also suggest its prognostic importance in more advanced disease. Using grading systems based on cytologic detail (*i.e.*, Broders') or the pattern-grading classification based on the degree to which the tumor forms papillary structures or glands versus solid tumor (*i.e.*, FIGO classification), investigators showed grade to affect the outcome of patients with advanced disease treated with chemotherapy.[78]

A study by Dembo and Bush suggests a more complex interaction between grade and histologic type.[79] In patients with serous tumors, the effect of grade was highly significant, but grade was not significant in the prognosis of patients with mucinous, endometrioid, or clear cell tumors. When the two variables of grade and histologic type were combined, significant survival differences were seen between patients with "favorable" pathologies (*i.e.*, serous, well-differentiated and mucinous, endometrioid, and clear cell types of all grades). The 5-year survival rate was 59% compared with a five-year survival rate of 19% in patients with "unfavorable" pathologies (*i.e.*, serous, moderately and poorly differentiated, and the unclassified type).

Histologic grading of ovarian tumors has not been accepted enthusiastically by pathologists, primarily because no standardized, easily reproducible, and objective classification exists. Despite the different classifications, virtually every published study demonstrates the prognostic significance of grade. Grading of epithelial ovarian tumors should be required in every carefully designed clinical study.

STROMAL TUMORS

Fewer than 10% of all ovarian tumors are of stromal origin. These tumors contain granulosa, theca, Sertoli, Leydig, and collagen-producing stromal cells or their embryonic precursors.[61,80-82] Of the many stromal tumors listed in Table 39-1, only the granulosa cell tumor is seen with significant frequency. This tumor is composed of granulosa cells with or without an admixture of theca cells, and it may contain folliculoid structures known as Call-Exner bodies. The granulosa cell tumor can be associated with feminizing effects and precocious puberty resulting from tumor-related estrogen secretion.

Presenting signs and symptoms are similar to those seen in epithelial ovarian tumors, with the exception of those related to hyperestrogenism. These tumors tend to be discovered at earlier stages, and they have a more indolent course than epithelial tumors. Late recurrences can sometimes be effectively treated with repeated cytoreductive surgery. There is no convincing evidence that granulosa cell tumors are particularly sensitive to radiation therapy or chemotherapy, but some responses to alkylating agents and doxorubicin (Adriamycin) have been published. One small study of 11 patients treated with a combination of cisplatin, bleomycin, and vinblastine reported pathologically documented complete remissions in 6 patients.[83] However, follow-up in this study was short, and toxicity was significant.

Sertoli-Leydig cell tumors are characterized by differentiation toward testicular structures. The tumors contain various mixtures of Sertoli and Leydig cells and tissues similar to the fetal testis. The clinical behavior of these tumors is directly related to their differentiation, and poorly differentiated tumors behave in a malignant fashion.[84] Because these tumors are rare, little is known about their response to therapy.

Gonadal stromal tumors occasionally contain granulosa cell elements combined with tubules and Leydig cells characteristic of the arrhenoblastoma. They are called gynandroblastomas.

GERM CELL TUMORS

Although germ cell tumors comprise fewer than 5% of all ovarian malignancies, they are important because they occur in young women, display an unusual natural history, and require different treatment from the common epithelial ovarian cancers. Most of these patients can now be cured with combination chemotherapy and limited surgery. Of these tumors, dysgerminoma, endodermal sinus tumor, and embryonal carcinoma are most often encountered.

The dysgerminomas comprise fewer than 2% of all ovarian malignancies. They are cytologically similar to seminoma of the testis and have a similar natural history. These tumors are frequently unilateral (90%) and tend to be localized. Secondary spread occurs by way of the lymphatics to the paraaortic nodes. The tumor is very radiosensitive, and dysgerminomas are also effectively treated by multidrug chemotherapy.[85] Chemotherapy preserves reproductive capacity and ovarian function, and it is currently the treatment of choice.

The terms "endodermal sinus tumor" and "embryonal carcinoma" have been used interchangeably to describe highly malignant germ cell tumors of the ovary, but evidence indicates that the two disorders are distinct.[80] Embryonal carcinoma, with patterns typical of embryonal carcinoma of the testis, is associated with elevations of human chorionic gonadotropin or α-fetoprotein. It is rarely seen in the ovary. Endodermal sinus tumors are more common, and they are similar morphologically to the infantile orchioblastoma of the testis. The endodermal sinus tumor, also called a yolk sac tumor, is characterized by reticular patterns, papillary formations known as Schiller-Duval bodies, and intracellular and extracellular hyaline droplets. This tumor is derived from extraembryonic rather than embryonic tissues.

Endodermal sinus tumors and embryonal carcinomas are highly aggressive, and they metastasize hematogenously. Chemotherapy for these tumors is highly effective and is discussed later.

DIAGNOSIS AND STAGING

Ovarian cancer has no specific signs or symptoms, particularly in early stage disease. Symptoms can include nausea, dyspepsia, and lower abdominal discomfort, but these vague signs are often ignored by the patient or her doctor. When more obvious problems appear, they are usually manifestations of advanced disease. Cancer in 75% of patients has spread beyond the ovary at diagnosis, and 60% have disease that has spread beyond the pelvis. Sall and Stone found that 37% of patients had abdominal discomfort or pain, 35% had abdominal swelling or masses, and 15% experienced vaginal bleeding.[86] Gastrointestinal symptoms occurred in 10%, and urinary tract symptoms were present in 1.5%. In two other large series, the main presenting symptoms were pain (57%), abdominal distention (51%), and vaginal bleeding (25%).[87,88]

The ovary lies in the rather spacious pelvic cavity and is suspended loosely by the ovarian and infundibulopelvic ligaments. An ovarian mass can become quite large without producing symptoms of pain or pressure. When pain does occur, it is probably the result of stretching of the supporting ligaments, and it is often nonspecific and intermittent. Discomfort caused by compression of the bladder or rectum is also nonspecific. All women, particularly perimenopausal or postmenopausal women with pelvic or abdominal symptoms, should have a thorough physical and pelvic examination, with careful evaluation of the adnexal area. These women often are subjected to several weeks or months of expensive diagnostic x-ray studies, although an office pelvic examination would have revealed a large pelvic mass almost immediately. An even more serious delay in diagnosis can occur if physicians attempt to treat symptoms with various therapies without performing a pelvic examination.

An adnexal mass in a premenarchal girl or postmenopausal woman is usually an indication for exploratory laparotomy. Functional ovarian cysts should not occur in these age groups, and a mass often indicates neoplastic growth. The incidence of malignancy is difficult to determine, but the high mortality rate of ovarian cancer that has spread beyond the ovary usually mandates early surgical exploration. Barber and Graber pointed out that a normal ovary during reproductive years is approximately $3.5 \times 2.0 \times 1.5$ cm, but in the postmenopausal patient, it should be $2.0 \times 1.0 \times 0.5$ cm or smaller.[89] Palpation of an ovary in a postmenopausal woman may indicate ovarian enlargement, and pelvic or vaginal probe ultrasound is indicated. A complex mass on ultrasound is usually an indication for surgery. A simple cyst smaller than 4 cm can often be observed by serial ultrasound examinations. Any growth, even a cyst, is an indication for surgical exploration in this age group. Barber and Graber originally suggested surgical exploration for any palpable ovary, but improvement in ultrasound techniques and additional experience allows the surgeon to be more discriminatory. Flynt and Gallup performed exploratory laparotomy on 11 patients with a palpable postmenopausal ovary and found only one malignancy, a colon carcinoma.[90]

Ovarian enlargement in a woman during reproductive years is usually benign. Most of these enlargements are caused by follicular or corpus luteum cysts (*i.e.,* functional cysts). Most enlargements regress in one to three menstrual cycles. Patients should be followed by repeat pelvic examination and pelvic or vaginal probe ultrasound at 4- to 6-week intervals. Some gynecologists recommend oral contraceptives to prevent stimulation of the ovary by pituitary hormones, but no data establish this practice. Table 39–2 outlines the suggested management of patients with an adnexal mass. Patients who are older than 40 years of age, although still of reproductive age, are at a greater risk for ovarian cancer. Fortunately, retention of reproductive function is usually of less concern in these patients.

Conventional Papanicolaou (Pap) smears are rarely positive for ovarian cancer and only in advanced disease. However, a patient with adenocarcinoma cells on a Pap smear and a negative evaluation of the vulva, vagina, cervix, and endometrium should be considered to have carcinoma of the ovary, fallopian tube, or other intraabdominal organs until proved otherwise. If a metastatic evaluation is negative, the patient should be considered for surgical exploration. Some investigators have attempted mass screenings of asymptomatic patients by peritoneal lavage with culdocentesis.[91] However, poor patient acceptance and high false-negative results make this approach unacceptable.

TABLE 39–2. Management Approach to the Patient With an Adnexal Mass

Observe and Repeat Examination in 4–6 Weeks	Surgical Exploration
Reproductive age	Premenarchal
	Postmenarchal*
Mass <8 cm	Mass >8 cm
Simple cysts on ultrasound	Complex cysts on ultrasound
Decreasing size	Increase in size or persistence through 2–3 menstrual cycles
Cystic and smooth	Solid and irregular
Mobile	Fixed
Unilateral	Bilateral
Asymptomatic	Pain or other symptoms of acute intraabdominal process
No ascites	Ascites

* Simple cysts smaller than 3 cm may be followed closely with ultrasound.

Laparoscopy should be discouraged as a diagnostic tool for ovarian carcinoma. Although it can occasionally differentiate uterine leiomyomas or endometriosis from ovarian cancer, these cases are infrequent. Laparoscopic biopsy or needle aspiration of an unruptured ovarian mass can spill malignant cells into the peritoneal cavity, and aspiration of cyst fluid for cytologic examination is not a reliable method of diagnosing ovarian cancer. Rubin and associates evaluated cell washings in patients with gross intraabdominal disease at second-look surgery and found only a 66% rate of positive cytology.[92] A similar false-negative rate in the evaluation of cyst fluid would make the technique of little value.

Ultrasound is a safe, noninvasive procedure that can be used to define intrapelvic disease. Solid elements and prominent papillary projections with involvement of adjacent viscera suggest a malignant neoplasm. Ultrasound can also be used to differentiate ascites from a large ovarian cyst. A mass separate from the uterus and associated with internal echoes suggests ovarian cancer. Ultrasound can also be used to guide direct percutaneous needle aspirations of suspected metastasis and aspiration biopsies of aortic nodes.[93,94] The recent refinement of the technique of vaginal probe ultrasound allows improved evaluation of the pelvic viscera. Vaginal probe ultrasound does not require a full bladder and is usually a more comfortable procedure for the patient. Preliminary evidence suggests that transvaginal ultrasound is more effective in evaluating adnexal abnormalities than is transabdominal ultrasound.[95,96] Studies at the University of Kentucky on 1000 asymptomatic women (≥40 years) found 31 (3.1%) abnormal transvaginal sonograms. Twenty-four of these women had a laparotomy, and 17 ovarian tumors were detected, although only 1 was malignant. Doppler color flow imaging may enhance the accuracy of sonography and reduce the high false-positive rate seen with transvaginal ultrasound alone.[97] It is not obvious what role either of these techniques has in screening for early ovarian cancer.

Lymphangiography may be useful in evaluating patients with ovarian carcinoma and is positive in about 30%.[51,98] Among patients with positive lymphangiograms, 32% have disease in pelvic nodes only, and 46% have diffuse retroperitoneal involvement of pelvic and paraaortic nodes.[34] Lymphangiography is accurate when aortic lymph nodes are enlarged or replaced by tumor and the radiologist has sufficient expertise. In one study of patients with positive preoperative lymphangiograms, histologic confirmation was obtained in 100%. In 63 patients with negative preoperative lymphangiograms, the lymphographic-histologic correlation was 87.3%. Eight (12.7%) of these 63 patients had microscopic nodal involvement at surgery. The overall accuracy of bipedal lymphangiography in this study was 91.7%.[51]

Computed tomography (CT) adds useful diagnostic and staging information to the results of ultrasound, lymphangiography, and surgery. CT can delineate liver and pulmonary nodules, large abdominal and pelvic masses, and retroperitoneal nodal involvement. However, CT is costly, and it cannot reliably detect masses smaller than 2 cm in diameter. CT has been useful in ovarian carcinoma if bowel gas makes an ultrasonogram difficult to interpret.[99]

Preoperative evaluation of a patient with suspected ovarian cancer is outlined in Table 39–3. The extent of evaluation requires that the physician use clinical judgment. An apparently healthy young woman with a persistent, unilateral, cystic mass requires only basic preoperative studies, but a postmenopausal woman with a large, irregular mass should undergo more extensive evaluation.

TUMOR MARKERS

Tumor markers capable of detecting early ovarian cancer would be valuable, because most patients are not diagnosed until the disease is advanced. Although markers are helpful in detecting and monitoring germ cell and some epithelial malignancies, they have not been reliable in detecting early epithelial ovarian tumors.

The serial measurement of α-fetoprotein has facilitated the postsurgical evaluation of therapy for patients with endodermal sinus tumors.[100] After surgical resection, serum α-fetoprotein levels progressively decline and, with recurrence, become elevated before clinically palpable disease. The levels

TABLE 39–3. Evaluation of Patients With Suspected Ovarian Carcinoma

Careful history and physical examination to include breast and pelvic examination and Papanicolaou smear

Complete blood count, biochemical profile, and CA 125 assay

Chest radiograph

Intravenous urogram

Cystoscopy

Proctoscopy

Barium enema

CT, MRI, or ultrasound*

Upper gastrointestinal series with small bowel follow-through in patients with upper gastrointestinal symptoms or symptoms of partial bowel obstruction

* As indicated by clinical evaluation.

may be helpful in diagnosing an endodermal sinus tumor in a woman with a rapidly enlarging, solid ovarian mass.

Human chorionic gonadotropin, or its beta subunit, has been a valuable tumor marker in the postsurgical evaluation of patients with ovarian choriocarcinoma or embryonal carcinoma and in evaluating germ cell tumors with choriocarcinomatous elements.[101]

Carcinoembryonic antigen (CEA) is elevated in approximately 58% of patients with stage III epithelial ovarian cancer.[102] The frequency of elevated CEA levels progressively increases with advancing stage and bulk of tumor. It is most likely to be elevated in patients with mucinous tumors. Because serum levels of CEA can also be elevated in patients with cirrhosis, chronic pulmonary disease, inflammatory bowel disease, and a history of heavy cigarette smoking, its diagnostic use in ovarian cancer is limited. For patients with ovarian cancer who have elevated CEA levels before therapy, serial CEA measurements may be valuable for monitoring subclinical disease.

Numerous investigators have tried to isolate tumor-specific antigens for use in serologic diagnosis and monitoring of patient therapy. The monoclonal antibody (OC-125) directed against the antigen (CA 125) common to most nonmucinous epithelial ovarian tumors appears to be the most useful.[103] The OC-125 antibody recognizes multiple antigen determinants on a high-molecular-weight (>500,000 d) glycoprotein. These determinants are found in celomic epithelium during embryonic development and can be detected on fetal tissues, müllerian duct remnants, amnion, and amnionic fluid. The antigen is not found in normal ovarian tissue, but it is found in nonmucinous epithelial ovarian carcinomas. Eighty-two percent of ovarian cancer patients react positively, and rising or falling titers correlate with disease in 93% of patients. Approximately 25% of patients with nongynecologic malignancies, 5% of patients with benign disease, and 1% of apparently healthy persons have elevated antigen levels (>35 U of CA 125/ml of serum).

Several studies explored the use of serum CA 125 levels in the early detection of ovarian carcinoma. Zurawski and associates studied 915 nonhospitalized Roman Catholic nuns in whom CA 125 levels ranged from 0 to 574 U/ml.[104] Thirty-six women (3.9%) had CA 125 levels greater than 35 U/ml, and 7 women had levels greater than 65 U/ml. Of the 7 women with CA 125 levels over 65 U/ml, 5 had benign or malignant neoplasms, including 1 colon carcinoma, 1 uterine leiomyoma, 1 endometrioma, 1 fibroadenoma of the breast, and 1 sclerosing adenosis of the breast. None of the 36 patients with levels of greater than 35 U/ml had ovarian cancer. Einhorn and colleagues measured CA 125 levels in 100 women undergoing diagnostic laparotomy for a palpable adnexal mass.[105] CA 125 levels were greater than 35 U/ml in 11 (61%) of 18 patients with some form of ovarian cancer and greater than 65 U/ml in 9 of these 11.

Two large studies of CA 125 for screening for ovarian cancer have been published. Jacobs and associates evaluated 1010 asymptomatic postmenopausal women.[106] Serum CA 125 had a specificity of 0.970 and, when combined with ultrasound, a specificity of 0.998. Einhorn and colleagues screened 5550 apparently healthy women and found elevations of more than 30 U/ml in 175 women.[105] After further evaluation, laparotomies were performed on 12 women, and 6 were found to

have ovarian cancer. However, only 2 of these 6 patients had stage I disease. One significant problem with CA 125 as a screening test is that only 50% of patients with clinically detectable ovarian cancer have elevated CA 125 levels.[107]

Persistent elevation of CA 125 in patients after surgery has almost invariably been associated with residual disease at second-look surgery, but even after the level falls into the normal range, residual disease often remains. Bast and co-workers performed second-look surgery on 15 women whose CA 125 levels had fallen into the normal range and, in 11 of the 15 women, residual disease was detected.[103] Since that report, several researchers demonstrated the lack of specificity of serum CA 125 levels in predicting which patients are disease free after primary chemotherapy.[108-116] These reports are summarized in Table 39–4. Several researchers tried to use CA 125 to predict response to initial chemotherapy. Most studies show that failure of CA 125 levels to return to normal by the fourth treatment course is a bad prognostic sign. Investigators from the GOG evaluated 400 patients with monthly CA 125 levels obtained during therapy. They calculated a 2.8 relative risk for every one log (10-fold) elevation of the CA 125 above baseline, with the greatest specificity at course four. They also found a 2.2 relative risk for every rise or fall of the CA 125 over each unit of time (3 weeks in their study).[117]

The elevation of CA 125 levels may antedate the appearance of disease or recurrence. Levels can be elevated several months before clinical detection of recurrent disease. Patients who have completed primary therapy and are being followed should have serial CA 125 levels obtained at frequent intervals, usually every 2 to 3 months. Doubling of the CA 125 level over 35 U/ml or an absolute value of over 100 U/ml usually indicates recurrence. Patients with high initial levels of CA 125 whose values return to normal during therapy often show early and significant CA 125 elevation when they develop recurrent disease.

TABLE 39–4. CA 125 Levels and Findings at Second-Look Laparotomy

Investigations	Normal CA 125 Second Look –	+	Elevated CA 125 Second Look –	+	Total
Niloff et al, 1985[108]	14	22	1	19*	56
Berek et al, 1986[109]	24	18	0	12	54
Atack et al, 1986[110]	8	6	0	3	17
Khoo et al, 1986[111]	19	11	1	11	42
Mogensen et al, 1986[112]	44	19	0	18	81
Vergote et al, 1987[113]	16	3	0	2*	21
Rome et al, 1987[114]	18	15	0	16	49
Rubin et al, 1989[115]	11	18	0	67*	96
Podczaski et al, 1989[116]	19	19	0	7	45
Total	173	131	2	155	461
Percent accurate	57%		99%		

* One recurrence after negative second-look laparotomy.

SURGERY

Initial Surgical Staging

Staging of ovarian cancer is based on the extent and location of disease found at surgical exploration. The FIGO classification was revised in 1985.[118] The new classification is listed in Table 39–5. Major changes have been made in stages I, II, and III. In stages I and II, the subdivisions "Ai and Aii" and "Bi and Bii" that identified tumor rupture or surface spread were made part of subdivision C. Malignant cells must be identified in cell washings or ascites to assign a patient to stages IC or IIC. Ascites alone (without malignant cells), regardless of the volume, are insufficient. In stage III, subdivi-

sions A, B, and C designate the size of tumor found at initial surgical exploration. Any lymph node metastasis, including inguinal lymph nodes, places the patient in stage IIIC. The staging classification is based on findings after opening the abdomen but not after surgical debulking. A patient with disease (>2 cm) confined to the omentum who is cytoreduced to no residual disease is still stage IIIC. The surgeon must define the amount of disease after opening the abdomen.

An accurate and complete initial surgical procedure is crucial for proper management of ovarian carcinoma. Although only a few patients with ovarian cancer can be managed by surgery alone, the success of subsequent therapy is in large part determined by the initial surgical procedure. Proper selection of appropriate adjuvant therapy depends on accurate assessment of the extent of residual disease at the conclusion of the initial operation. The chance of achieving a complete pathologic response (negative second-look laparotomy) is directly related to the extent of residual disease left after initial surgery.

For best results, the surgeon must understand the pathogenesis of the disease and must be appropriately aggressive in performing the surgical procedure. Most surgeons prefer a vertical midline incision for patients with suspected ovarian cancer. This incision provides excellent access to the pelvis and can be extended as far as needed into the upper abdomen. Patients with apparent early stage disease often require different therapy from those with microscopic metastases to the upper abdomen, and proper evaluation of the upper abdomen is rarely possible through a lower abdominal incision. If there is gross disease in the upper abdomen, proper resection requires adequate exposure. Unfortunately, it is still common to see patients who have had two or more operations for ovarian cancer and have no abdominal scar above the umbilicus.

In a young patient with a nonsuspicious pelvic mass, a low transverse incision may be appropriate but should be large enough to remove the mass without danger of rupture. An ovarian mass must never be aspirated to fit the incision. When carcinoma is found after a Pfannenstiel's incision has been used, the incision should be converted to a true transverse incision by dividing the rectus muscles and making a second, upper abdominal midline incision. The patient should be told of this possibility preoperatively by her surgeon.

Initial exploration of the abdomen must be thorough and methodical. Figure 39–2 illustrates the essentials of the staging laparotomy. The presence, amount, and character of any ascitic fluid should be noted and the fluid submitted in toto for cytology. In the absence of ascitic fluid, cell washings should be obtained from the pelvis, each abdominal gutter, and each subdiaphragmatic surface.

If a unilateral mass is found, the surgeon must decide whether to perform a cystectomy or to remove the tube and ovary. A cystectomy is indicated only in young (<40) patients. If cystectomy is performed, the abdomen should be protected from rupture and spillage by the use of laparotomy tapes. If frozen section indicates a malignancy, the fallopian tube and ovary must be removed, and a full abdominal exploration is necessary. In a patient not concerned about future childbearing, a total abdominal hysterectomy and bilateral salpingo-oophorectomy should be performed. Unilateral salpingo-oophorectomy is only indicated in the young patient desiring additional children in whom careful inspection reveals no ev-

TABLE 39–5. FIGO Stage Grouping
for Primary Carcinoma of the Ovary (1987)

Stage I	Growth limited to the ovaries	
	IA	Growth limited to one ovary; no ascites. No tumor on the external surface; capsule intact
	IB	Growth limited to both ovaries; no ascites. No tumor on the external surfaces; capsules intact
	IC*	Tumor either stage IA or IB but with tumor on the surface of one or both ovaries, or with capsule ruptured, or with ascites present containing malignant cells, or with positive peritoneal washings
Stage II	Growth involving one or both ovaries with pelvic extension	
	IIA	Growth involving one or both ovaries with pelvic extension
	IIB	Extension and/or metastases to the uterus and/or tubes
	IIC*	Tumor either stage IIA or IIB but with tumor on the surface of one or both ovaries, or with capsule(s) ruptured, or with ascites present containing malignant cells, or with positive peritoneal washings
Stage III	Tumor involving one or both ovaries with peritoneal implants outside the pelvis and/or positive retroperitoneal or inguinal nodes. Superficial liver metastases equal stage III. Tumor is limited to the true pelvis but with histologically verified malignant extension to small bowel or omentum	
	IIIA	Tumor grossly limited to the true pelvis with negative nodes but with histologically confirmed microscopic seeding of abdominal peritoneal surfaces
	IIIB	Tumor of one or both ovaries with histologically confirmed implants of abdominal peritoneal surfaces, none exceeding 2 cm in diameter. Nodes negative
	IIIC	Abdominal implants greater than 2 cm in diameter and/or positive retroperitoneal or inguinal nodes
Stage IV	Growth involving one or both ovaries with distant metastasis. If pleural effusion is present, there must be positive cytologic test results to allot a case to stage IV. Parenchymal liver metastasis equals stage IV.	

* To evaluate the impact on prognosis of the different criteria for alloting cases to stage IC or IIC, it would be of value to know if rupture of the capsule was spontaneous or caused by the surgeon and if the source of malignant cells detected was peritoneal washings or ascites.

idence of disease other than in one ovary. If careful and methodical inspection of the entire abdomen is negative, biopsies as outlined in Table 39–6 are performed.

A set sequence should be established for inspecting the abdomen and obtaining biopsies so that nothing is omitted. Table 39–6 outlines the recommended exploration and biopsy procedure. It is reasonable to maintain the written procedure in the operating room to ensure accuracy.

Postsurgical Staging

If the appropriate surgical staging procedure is performed at initial surgery, little additional evaluation is required for clinical evaluation. However, if the upper abdomen was not properly evaluated at the initial operation, postoperative reevaluation by laparotomy or laparoscopy may be necessary before initial treatment is begun. Unfortunately, understaging as a result of inadequate initial surgery is common. Several studies that used laparoscopy to evaluate patients who did not have full surgical staging documented upper abdominal spread in 30% to 40% of patients with apparently early (FIGO stage I

TABLE 39–6. Operative Procedure for Proper Surgical Staging of the Patient With Ovarian Cancer

Step 1. If ascites is present, remove as much as possible for cytology. If no ascites is present, obtain cell washings from the pelvis, both abdominal gutters, and both subdiaphragmatic areas.

Step 2. Determine whether the mass is malignant; if malignant, perform appropriate pelvic procedure (total abdominal hysterectomy and bilateral salpingo-oophorectomy unless patient desires additional childbearing, and there is no evidence of spread beyond the ovary).

Step 3. Carefully examine pelvic peritoneum; if lesions are present, remove as much as possible and biopsy any lesion that cannot be removed. If no lesions are seen, sample at a minimum the peritoneum of the lateral pelvic sidewalls, the bladder, the rectosigmoid, and the cul-de-sac.

Step 4. Examine the paracolic gutters, and remove any lesions seen. If no lesions are seen, obtain a 1 × 3-cm strip of peritoneum on either side.

Step 5. Examine the omentum, and remove any that contains visible tumor (including the supracolic omentum if involved by tumor). If no lesions are seen, remove the infracolic omentum.

Step 6. Examine and palpate both diaphragms and the surface of the spleen and liver. If lesions are present, remove as much as possible; biopsy if they cannot be removed. If no lesions are seen, a strip of peritoneum 1 × 2 cm should be carefully excised from the right hemidiaphragm. (*Note:* only peritoneum is needed, and care should be taken not to create a pneumothorax.)

Step 7. Beginning at either the rectum or cecum, carefully inspect the entire large colon and remove and/or biopsy any suspicious lesion of the intestine or mesentery.*

Step 8. Beginning at either the ileocecal valve or ligament of Treitz, carefully inspect the entire small bowel and mesentery, removing and/or biopsing any lesions.*

Step 9. If, after all of the above procedures, no gross disease larger than 1 or 2 cm is left, the pelvic and paraaortic lymph nodes should be sampled.

* If resection of intestine is necessary to cytoreduce the tumor optimally or to relieve obstruction, it should be performed.

or II) disease.[43–45] Piver and coworkers found diaphragmatic metastases in 11% and aortic lymph node metastases in 13% of patients otherwise felt to have stage I disease.[45] The use of laparoscopy in patients with ovarian carcinoma has been of value as an adjunct to initial staging and as a means of surveillance to assess therapeutic response.[43,44] In the National Cancer Institute (NCI) experience, laparoscopy documented new involved sites that had gone undetected during conventional radiologic and isotopic procedures in 42% of patients.[134] This technique provided the only evidence of disease in 38% of patients. Twenty percent to 30% of patients who were referred with stages I and II disease were reclassified as having stage III disease based on diaphragmatic metastases detected at laparoscopy.

The procedure was found to be safe and feasible even after prior laparotomies. In 6% of patients, technical problems precluded complete evaluation. Of 159 procedures performed, there were few serious complications; only 2.5% of the patients required medical therapy to manage a complication. Complications included pneumothorax (1), bleeding requiring transfusion (1), wound infection (1), and hypotension (2). Other complications that did not require therapy were pneumomediastinum and subcutaneous or mesenteric emphysema. There were no deaths or viscous perforations, and no patient required surgical exploration because of a complication of laparoscopy. Other institutions have had similar experiences. Berek, Griffiths, and Leventhal reviewed 112 laparoscopies performed in 57 patients without clinical evidence of disease.[135] In 80 (71%) of procedures, the entire peritoneal cavity was visualized; visualization was totally inadequate in only 16 procedures. Complications were similar to those previously listed, but none were serious.

CYTOREDUCTIVE SURGERY

Cytoreductive surgery is an integral part of initial patient management, and it demands substantial skill and judgment. Technically difficult cytoreductive surgery requires detailed knowledge of gynecologic surgery, and the surgeon must be prepared for complicated abdominal and urologic surgery as well. Formal residency programs in obstetrics and gynecology and general surgery do not usually provide the depth of knowledge and experience needed for the surgical management of ovarian cancer. If possible, patients with ovarian cancer should be referred to physicians with special training in surgical or gynecologic oncology.

The surgeon faces a formidable task if ovarian carcinoma has spread throughout the abdomen and pelvis. The tumor fills the pelvis and leaves little room for visualization of vital structures such as the iliac vessels and the ureters. All peritoneal surfaces may be involved, including the lateral pelvic walls, the bladder peritoneum, and the serosa of the rectosigmoid. The optimal approach to the pelvis is through the retroperitoneum, as illustrated in Figure 39–2. By opening the peritoneum lateral to the iliac vessels (and, if necessary, the colon), the surgeon gains access to the pararectal and paravesical spaces, allowing identification of the major blood vessels and ureter. Ligation of the infundibulopelvic ligament and round ligament allows the surgeon to mobilize the pelvic viscera and tumor masses. The ureter can be dissected free of the medial flap of peritoneum, and the uterine artery can be identified and ligated.

If the tumor is large or has extended into the obturator foramen, the obturator nerve should be identified and preserved. When the ureter, obturator nerve, and major blood vessels are identified and the uterine artery and infundibulopelvic ligament are ligated, the surgeon can remove the uterus, adnexa, and pelvic tumor. In some cases, the tumor peels away from the peritoneum, and in other cases, the peritoneum must be removed with the tumor. Occasionally, a portion of the bladder or rectosigmoid colon must be removed. Primary reanastomosis of the rectum is usually feasible, although a colostomy may be necessary. In some patients, pelvic involvement of the cecum or terminal ileum may require resection of these structures with reconstruction of intestinal continuity by ileo-ascending or ileo-transverse colostomy. Although the ureter usually can be separated from the pelvic tumor, resection and reimplantation into the bladder may be necessary to achieve complete cytoreduction. If disease involves the infracolic omentum, it can be removed below the transverse colon. If disease involves the supracolic omentum, it should be detached from the transverse colon and resected along the greater curvature of the stomach, as shown in Figure 39–3. The dissection should be carried up toward the spleen to remove all gross tumor. The spleen must sometimes be removed. Tumor implants in the paracolic gutters and on the surface of the intestine can usually be separated from underlying structures, although it may be necessary to resect portions of the intestine. Bulky disease on the liver surface and undersurface of the diaphragm can often be partially debulked, and venous oozing can usually be controlled with pressure from a laparotomy pack. Some surgeons recommend using the CUSA in the dissection of ovarian cancer.

The surgeon must often make difficult decisions about how extensive the resection of gross tumor should be in relation to possible benefit. Leaving a patient with a colostomy or resecting large segments of small intestine if bulk disease cannot be removed from other sites probably provides little benefit. However, the resection may be feasible if it leaves the patient with minimal residual disease. As with any surgical procedure for cancer, the experienced cancer surgeon must weigh the benefits of an extended operation against the potential morbidity. Optimal cytoreduction is not possible in all patients.

IMPACT OF PRIMARY CYTOREDUCTIVE SURGERY

In 1968, Munnell reported improved survival in stage III and IV ovarian carcinoma after omentectomy.[119] He also demonstrated improved survival in patients undergoing definitive operations rather than "partial removal" or "laparotomy and biopsy." A year later, Delclos and Quinlan reported that patients with "nonpalpable" disease survived longer than patients with "palpable" disease when treated with radiation therapy.[120] For nonpalpable disease, the 4-year survival rate for stages II and III was 72% and 25%, respectively, and for palpable disease, it was 33% and 9%, respectively.

In the mid-1970s, Griffiths used chemotherapy after cytoreductive surgery and compared survival in patients grouped by the amount of residual disease.[121] He demonstrated that duration of survival was directly related to the amount of residual disease after initial cytoreductive surgery. Patients with no residual disease had a mean survival of 39 months compared with 29 months for residual disease of less than 0.5 cm and 18 months for residual disease of 0.6 to 1.5 cm. Patients whose tumors were not cytoreduced below 1.5 cm had a mean survival of 11 months, and none of the suboptimally cytoreduced patients survived beyond 26 months.

Table 39–7 summarizes nine reports in which median survival is based on primary cytoreductive surgery to less than or greater than 2 cm of residual disease. Most of these patients received postoperative multidrug chemotherapy. Mean survival was 29.4 months in the optimally cytoreduced group and 13.4 months in the group in whom cytoreductive surgery was suboptimal. In a GOG study that evaluated cisplatin and cyclophosphamide with or without doxorubicin in patients with residual disease of less than 1 cm, a marked difference was seen in progression-free interval and survival in patients with no gross residual disease compared with those with gross residual disease of less than 1 cm.[127] The median progression-free interval for patients with no gross residual disease was 20 months, compared with 42 months for patients with gross residual disease of less than 1 cm. Improvement in survival is much more pronounced for patients with no gross residual and less than 1 cm of residual disease than for groups of patients with large residual disease. Figure 39–4 shows survival in a prospective randomized trial of the Netherlands Cancer Group and demonstrates that differences in survival based on the volume of residual disease become less pronounced when patients with residual greater than 1 cm are considered.[128]

Fuks and associates described two radiation therapy series in which the median survival was 24 months for "small residual" or "no residual" disease compared with 6 to 11 months for "large residual" disease.[129] Dembo reported a 43% 5-year survival rate for stage III patients with less than 2 cm of residual disease treated with whole-abdominal irradiation, compared with an 18% 5-year survival rate for a group of patients with more than than 2 cm of disease.[130]

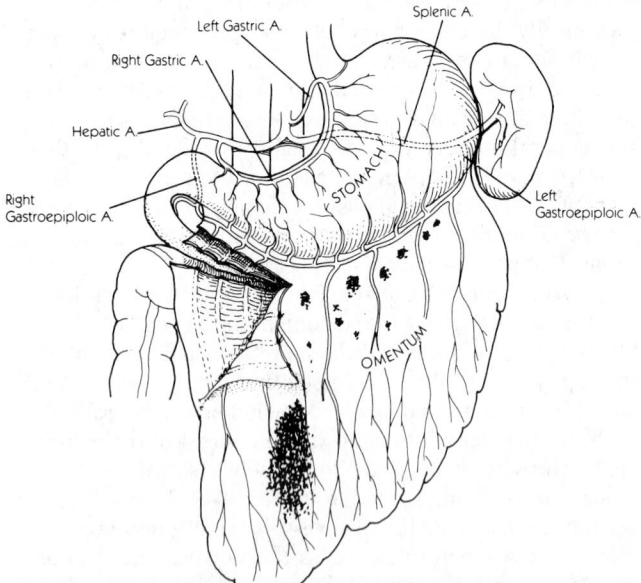

FIGURE 39–3.   Omentectomy in patients with metastatic ovarian cancer. (Hoskins WJ. The role of cytoreductive surgery in ovarian cancer. PPO Updates 1987;1[2])

TABLE 39–7.   The Effect of Residual Disease at the Conclusion of Primary Cytoreductive Surgery on Survival

Investigations	Treatment	Residual Disease	No. of Patients	Survival (mo)
Griffiths, 1975[121]	L-PAM	0	29	39
		0–0.5	28	29
		0.6–1.5	16	18
		>1.5	29	11
Hacker, 1983[122]	Varied	<0.5	7	40
		0.6–1.5	24	18
		>1.5	16	6
Vogl, 1983[123]	CHAP	<2 cm	32	>40
		>2 cm	68	16
Pohl, 1984[124]	Varied	<2 cm	37	45
		>2 cm	57	16
Delgado, 1984[125]	Varied	<2 cm	21	45
		>2 cm	54	16
Redman, 1986[400]	CAP	<3 cm	34	38
		>3 cm	51	26
Conte, 1986[277]	CAP or CP	<2 cm	37	>40
		>2 cm	38	16
Neijt, 1987[128]	CHAP or CP	<1 CM	88	40
		>1 CM	219	21
Piver, 1988[126]	PAC	<2 cm	35	48
		>2 cm	5	21
		Optimal	388*	36.7†
		Suboptimal	537*	16.6†

* Total number of patients.
† Mean survival.

To evaluate the operative morbidity and quality of life of primary cytoreductive surgery, Chen and colleagues reviewed 60 patients who underwent optimal primary cytoreductive surgery.[131] They reported a mean operating time of 3.6 hours, a mean blood loss of 1644 ml, and a mean hospital stay of 16 days (with most patients receiving their first course of chemotherapy before discharge). The rate of operative morbidity was 5%. Blythe and Wahl compared the survival of 19 patients whose tumors were cytoreduced to less than 2 cm (i.e., optimal) by an extensive surgical procedure to 17 patients whose disease could not be debulked (i.e., suboptimal).[132] Mean survival was 14.3 months in the optimal group and 10.2 months in the suboptimal group. Quality of life was judged to be "good" or "good to fair" for 75% of the optimal group but for only 18% of the suboptimal group.

Some researchers have argued that patients who can be optimally cytoreduced represent a different population of patients, whose improved survival may be related to factors other than the primary cytoreduction. This is a difficult argument to refute or to study prospectively. Hoskins and associates reanalyzed a GOG study and attempted to evaluate the role of primary cytoreductive surgery.[133] Patients entered on a trial of cisplatin-based multidrug therapy were divided into patients who, after the abdomen was opened, had abdominal disease of less than 1 cm and those who were found to have larger tumors but were cytoreduced to 1 cm. These investigators found a statistically significant difference in survival in favor of the patients who were found to have optimal disease compared with those rendered optimal by surgery. They concluded that, although cytoreductive surgery may impact survival, the status of disease found when the patient undergoes surgical exploration has important prognostic significance. Survival is affected by the biology of the disease and by the degree of success of the surgery.

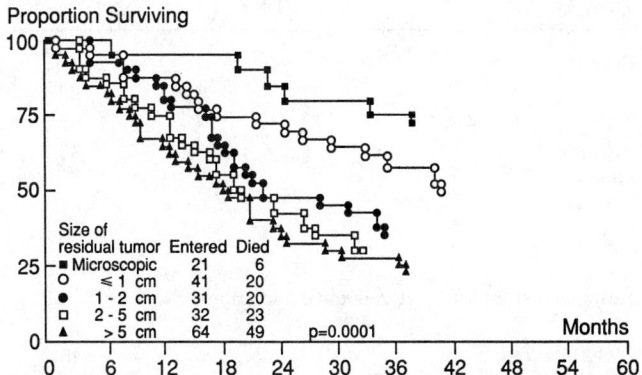

FIGURE 39–4.   Survival of patients in relation to the largest cross-sectional tumor diameter before the initiation of chemotherapy. (Neijt JP, ten Bokkel Huinink WW, van der Burg MEL, et al. Randomized trial comparing two combination chemotherapy regimens (CHAP-5 v CP) in advanced ovarian carcinoma. J Clin Oncol 1987;5:1157)

SECOND-LOOK SURGICAL REASSESSMENT

The term "second-look surgical reassessment" should be restricted to a systematic surgical reexploration of patients who have completed a planned course of treatment after initial surgical staging and cytoreductive surgery. Patients should be clinically without evidence of disease by physical examination and routine diagnostic studies such as chest radiographs, liver function tests, CA 125 levels, and CT scans. The fact that approximately 50% of patients who are clinically without evidence of disease still have residual disease illustrates the limitations of nonsurgical evaluation in this disease.

Wangenstein[136] introduced the concept of second-look surgery, and a series of studies from the M.D. Anderson Cancer Center defined its application to ovarian cancer.[137,138] The technique of second-look surgical reassessment requires considerable care, because most patients with negative second-look operations do not receive additional therapy. The abdomen should be entered through a generous midline incision extending from the symphysis pubis to well above the umbilicus. If no disease is found or if upper abdominal disease is to be cytoreduced, the incision should probably be extended to near the xyphoid. All adhesions in the abdomen and pelvis should be lysed, and portions of these adhesions should be submitted for pathologic analysis. A thorough examination of the abdomen and pelvis is then performed. The same procedures are followed as for the primary staging of ovarian cancer (see Table 39–6). Washings of the pelvis, paracolic gutters, and subdiaphragmatic areas are essential. If no gross disease is found, pelvic and paraaortic lymph nodes should be biopsied. A second-look operation usually results in 20 to 40 pathologic specimens. Residual disease should be resected if possible, and any disease that cannot be resected should be documented in the operative report.

Table 39–8 summarizes the effects of initial residual disease on the outcome of second-look surgical reassessment in epithelial ovarian cancer. The likelihood of a complete pathologic response (negative second-look surgical reassessment) is 82% if no residual disease remains after initial surgery, 53% if initial residual remains, and only 23% if suboptimal residual disease is present.

The timing of second-look surgical reassessment has varied since the concept was introduced. Patients treated with single alkylating agents were usually treated for 12 to 18 months. Smith and associates indicated that patients treated with at least 10 courses of melphalan had better survival than those who had shorter courses of therapy before second-look surgery.[138] With the introduction of multidrug regimens, toxicity was greater, and 10 to 12 months of such chemotherapy was difficult to administer without significant dose reduction or prolongation of chemotherapy intervals. Greco and associates[139] and Berek and colleagues[140] used second-look laparotomy after 6 courses of therapy. In a prospective randomized trial at Memorial Sloan-Kettering Cancer Center, five courses of cisplatin, doxorubicin, and cyclophosphamide were compared with 10 courses of the same regimen. There was no difference in the frequency of negative second-look surgical reassessment or in survival between the two arms.[141] A similar study from the Netherlands cancer group found the same results.[142] Based on these studies, it would appear that five to six courses of cisplatin-based multidrug therapy is optimal before second-look surgical reassessment. Rubin and associates found that, although short-course cisplatin-based chemotherapy produced a high complete response rate, there was a high recurrence rate after negative second-look surgical reassessment.[56]

Second-look surgical reassessment is summarized in Table 39–9.[143] The chances of a patient having a negative second-look surgical reassessment is directly related to stage of disease, grade of tumor, and the amount of residual disease at the conclusion of the initial cytoreductive operation. Of 1255 patients included in the 16 reports reviewed by Rubin and Lewis, 53.9% had residual disease detected at second-look surgery.[143] Persistent disease at second-look surgical reassessment has been described in the pelvis, on the surfaces of the intestine, on the diaphragm, in the omentum, and in retroperitoneal lymph nodes.[144-147] Berek and colleagues[148] and Creasman[149] reported retroperitoneal lymph node spread as the sole positive finding at second-look surgical reassessment.

Second-look surgical reassessment is a significantly invasive

TABLE 39–8. Effect of Residual Disease at End of Initial Cytoreductive Operation on Extent of Disease at Second-Look Surgical Reassessment

	Percentage With Negative Second Look		
Investigations	No Residual	Optimal Residual	Suboptimal Residual
Feldman[46]	67	61	14
Greco[139]	76	50	28
Berek[140]		40	11
Rubin[143]	75		25
Smirz[144]	95	36	20
Podratz[145]	82	44	33
Ballon[146]		49	13
Schwartz[147]	79	45	22
Berek[148]	100	100	40
	82 (mean)	53 (mean)	23 (mean)

TABLE 39–9. Results of Second-Look Surgery in Ovarian Carcinoma (Collected Series)*

Disease	Negative (%)
Stage	
I	80
II	68
III	35
Grade	
1	61
2	50
3	41
Residual disease after cytoreductive operation	
None	77
Optimal	45
Suboptimal	25

(Rubin SR, Lewis JLJ. Second look surgery in ovarian carcinoma. Crit Rev Oncol Hemat 1988;8:75–78)

procedure that involves the expense and discomfort of a major abdominal operation and results in disruption of the patient's normal activities. Nevertheless, published reports have documented acceptable morbidity. In the review by Rubin and Lewis, there were no deaths in 682 operations, and the overall rate of morbidity, including minor complications, was 19%.[143] Most of these complications were infections involving the surgical incision, the urinary tract, or lungs.

Recurrent ovarian carcinoma after negative second-look surgery occurs in 15% to 20% of all patients in the multiple studies previously cited. However, in certain groups of patients, the recurrence rate is much higher. The Memorial Sloan-Kettering Cancer Center group reported recurrence rates of approximately 50% among stage III and IV, grade 2 and 3 patients after treatment with cisplatin-based chemotherapy.[56] It is possible that patients in these high-risk categories should receive additional therapy rather than second-look surgical reassessment.

Several investigators have questioned the value of second-look surgery because of the poor survival of patients with positive second looks and the high recurrence rates of patients with negative second-look results. However, as new second-line therapeutic options become available, their effectiveness must be evaluated with second-look laparotomy. Patients most likely to respond to these second-line therapies are those with small amounts of residual disease. If second-line therapeutic options are not available, the patient should be referred to centers where active investigational treatment is ongoing.

Other techniques for monitoring response to therapy can be used under some circumstances. The NCI group has used peritoneoscopy.[134] In 66 restaging peritoneoscopies, residual disease was found in 33 patients (50%), and peritoneoscopic findings provided the only evidence of disease in 24 patients (36%). These patients were spared an unnecessary second-look laparotomy, but patients with negative results on peritoneoscopy underwent laparotomy. Residual ovarian cancer was found in 55%, mainly in the pelvis and mesentery. A negative peritoneoscopy must be followed by laparotomy before a patient with ovarian cancer can be considered disease free.

SECONDARY CYTOREDUCTIVE SURGERY

Although the role of primary cytoreductive surgery has been well defined, the value of secondary cytoreduction is controversial. The recent availability of cisplatin analogs, intraperitoneal chemotherapy, and new drugs such as taxol have expanded our second-line treatment capabilities, and because these agents are most effective in minimal residual disease, secondary cytoreduction may be important.

Table 39–10 summarizes the frequency with which secondary cytoreduction can be accomplished. Berek and associates performed secondary cytoreduction on 32 patients and found that 12 (38%) had their tumors reduced to optimal (<1.5 cm) residual disease.[150] Median survival for that group was 20 months, compared with 5 months for the 20 patients with disease that could not be optimally cytoreduced. Factors that were associated with a greater likelihood of optimal secondary cytoreduction were previous optimal primary cytoreduction, less than 1000 ml of ascites, tumor size less than 5 cm at second operation, and interval from primary to secondary surgery longer than 12 months. Age, tumor grade, type of subsequent chemotherapy, and presence or absence of bowel obstruction did not influence survival after secondary cytoreductive surgery.

TABLE 39–10. Frequency of Successful Secondary Cytoreductive Operations in Patients With Advanced or Recurrent Epithelial Ovarian Cancer

Investigations	No. of Patients	Patients Optimally Cytoreduced (%)
Lippman[152]	32	12 (37.5)
Podratz[153]	13	11 (84.6)
Eymer[156]	29	13 (44.7)
Young[157]	26	15 (57.7)
Berek[135]	38	9 (24.0)
Raju[388]	207 (total)	89 (43.0%)

In one study, Hoskins and associates evaluated 67 patients who had disease at second-look laparotomy.[151] Seventeen patients had microscopic disease, and another 16 patients had disease that was cytoreduced to microscopic disease. The 5-year survival rate for both of these groups of patients exceeded 50%. The investigators concluded that secondary cytoreduction to microscopic disease provides survival benefit. Lippman and coworkers reported a survival benefit with secondary cytoreduction at second-look laparotomy.[152] Podratz and associates reported a 55% 4-year survival rate for patients with microscopic residual disease and 19% for patients with macroscopic disease.[153] They found no difference in survival between those with microscopic disease and those with tumors cytoreduced to microscopic disease.

Others have not found a survival benefit for secondary cytoreduction. Chambers and colleagues reported no survival benefit for 23 patients with microscopic disease compared with 6 patients with macroscopic disease.[154] Luesley and coworkers found no survival benefit for secondary cytoreduction.[155]

The role of secondary cytoreduction surgery remains controversial. However, the increased availability of second-line therapy probably increases the importance of these surgical procedures. It appears that about one third of patients can have their tumors cytoreduced to microscopic disease at second-look surgery, and this may be the optimal population of patients in which to use aggressive second-line therapy.

RADIATION THERAPY

EXTERNAL IRRADIATION

Radiation therapy has been traditionally used as an adjuvant after maximal surgical cytoreduction; for treating patients with inoperable tumors not responding to chemotherapy; and for salvaging patients with persistent disease after primary treatment, including chemotherapy and second-look operation. Radiation therapy also has a useful palliative role in incurable patients with symptomatic pelvic masses or metastatic deposits.

Radiation therapy for ovarian carcinoma was first used in 1912 by Eymer, who reported durable remissions in 8 patients treated with low-dose whole-abdominal irradiation.[156] The low-energy radiation from the early orthovoltage machines had poor penetration and produced significant skin toxicity, which compromised the delivery of high-dose radiation to peritoneal tumors. As a result, radiation was used for palliation, but its curative value was not established. The megavoltage radiation therapy of the 1950s was more penetrating and skin sparing, and it allowed large and shaped fields with higher radiation doses. However, the radiation sensitivities of many important normal tissues (*i.e.*, kidneys, liver) limited the use of irradiation as a curative modality in many patients, especially in those with advanced disease. Nonetheless, when appropriate techniques are used, radiation therapy does represent an effective curative modality for certain patients with ovarian carcinoma.[157]

IRRADIATION OF EARLY DISEASE

The impact of radiation therapy or chemotherapy on the survival of patients with limited-stage disease has been evaluated in several clinical trials. Two randomized studies that included external-beam pelvic irradiation for patients with stage I tumors have been reported.[158,159] In a GOG study, stage I patients were randomized postoperatively to observation, pelvic radiation therapy, or melphalan administration.[159] The elimination of almost half of the entered patients from the analysis and the absence of meticulous staging make it difficult to draw conclusions from this study. The Princess Margaret Hospital study randomized stage IA patients between postoperative pelvic irradiation or observation, but the study did not require comprehensive staging.[158] Both studies suggested that pelvic irradiation reduced the rate of pelvic relapses, but because relapses occurred throughout the peritoneal cavity, there was no impact on the overall relapse or survival rates.

Abdominopelvic irradiation has not been the subject of a phase III trial with patients with stage I disease only, but it has been retrospectively compared with pelvic irradiation or no treatment.[160] No benefit was found for patients with grade I tumors, for whom the risk of relapse was under 5% overall; for grade II and II lesions, a statistically nonsignificant reduction in relapses was observed. In patients whose tumors were densely adherent, a significant reduction in relapse risk was associated with the use of abdominopelvic irradiation, but these tumors are more correctly classified as stage II.

The volume treated with irradiation and the dose and fractionation schemes used represent a compromise between the tumoricidal doses required to eradicate tumor deposits and the danger of clinically significant injury to normal tissues. Although the tumoricidal dose levels for ovarian tumors have not been established, there is evidence that irradiation can permanently eradicate tumor deposits in patients with residual ovarian cancer.

Fuks and Bagshaw reported an actuarial 5-year disease-free survival rate of 46% among 16 stage IIB patients with residual pelvic disease treated with 5000 to 6000 cGy.[161] Schray treated 26 patients with minimal residual tumors (<2 cm in diameter) with similar radiation doses.[162] Only 4 (16%) relapsed in the pelvis compared with 9 (45%) of 20 patients who had more extensive tumors. Dembo treated stage I, II, and III patients

with 4500 cGy to the pelvis and 2250 cGy to the upper abdomen.[130,163] The 5-year survival rate for 50 patients with small or no residual tumors was 78%, compared with 19% for 26 patients with larger residual.

These data suggest that tumoricidal dose levels are a function of tumor size. For tumors larger than 2 cm, the required dose probably exceeds 5000 to 6000 cGy, but for tumors smaller than 2 cm in diameter, it is probably 5000 cGy. For microscopic tumor deposits, the tumoricidal dose levels may be even lower. The Princess Margaret Hospital study randomized patients with no residual tumor after surgery to 4500 cGy to the pelvis or 4500 cGy to the pelvis and 2250 cGy to the upper abdomen.[158,163,164] The 5-year survival rate for patients receiving abdominopelvic radiation therapy was 78%, compared with 51% for patients receiving only pelvic irradiation. There was a 30% better control rate of occult upper abdominal metastases in the patients receiving abdominopelvic radiation. This study suggests that 2250 cGy given to microscopic upper abdominal tumor deposits was tumoricidal.

Fuller and associates reported a 71% 10-year actuarial relapse-free survival rate for 42 women with stage I through IIIA with less than 2 cm pelvic residual disease treated with total abdominopelvic irradiation, compared with 40% for a similar group of women treated by subtotal abdominopelvic techniques.[165] Delclos and Smith showed that stage II patients treated with 5550 cGy to the pelvis and 2600 to 2800 cGy to the upper abdomen by the moving-strip technique had a higher survival at 5 years (56%) than the patients treated to the pelvis only (17%).[166] Similarly, Perez and associates reported a 5-year survival rate of 56% for stage II patients treated with a similar technique to the whole abdomen and 16% for patients receiving pelvic irradiation only.[167]

These reports have been criticized, particularly because the patients were not surgically staged, and in the randomized series from the Princess Margaret Hospital and M.D. Anderson Cancer Center, it is possible that the groups were not truly comparable. The M.D. Anderson Cancer Center study was criticized for the use of irradiation techniques that failed to encompass the entire subdiaphragmatic area.[163] This was substantiated by the Princess Margaret study, which reported that the 5-year survival rate was 75% for patients treated with optimal radiation fields but only 33% if technical violations were identified in a retrospective review of the portal films.

No current trials are in progress to compare the efficacy of cisplatin-based multiagent chemotherapy with abdominopelvic irradiation. Several cooperative groups, including RTOG and GOG, attempted such a study, but because of the great difference in the treatment approaches and strong investigator bias, the small patient accrual led to the demise of these important studies, leaving the question unanswered.[168]

Because abdominopelvic irradiation encompasses only the peritoneal cavity and retroperitoneum, its use as primary adjuvant treatment is restricted to patients with stage I, II, or III disease who have no macroscopic tumor in the upper abdomen and small macroscopic (<2 cm) or no macroscopic residual disease in the pelvis.[130,163] Multivariate analysis of prognostic factors demonstrated that, in addition to age, stage, and amount of residual disease, histopathology is an important factor.[160,163,169]

Several studies compared abdominopelvic or pelvic irradiation alone with single-agent alkylating chemotherapy in patients with minimal residual disease after primary surgery (Table 39–11).[165,170–172] These studies demonstrate a superior outcome with abdominopelvic irradiation. The Princess Margaret Hospital study was the only one of the four that was randomized; it compared pelvic irradiation, alone or with chlorambucil, and abdominopelvic irradiation in patients with stage I, II, or III tumors.[170] With minimum follow-up of 7 years, the survival difference for the 76 patients treated with abdominopelvic radiation therapy was significantly superior to that of the 71 patients treated with pelvic irradiation and chlorambucil (46% versus 31%, *p* = 0.05). This survival benefit was seen only in patients with small macroscopic residuum or no tumor residuum (64% versus 40%, *p* = 0.0007). The long-term survival benefit of approximately 25% was thought to be related to the 25% reduction in abdominal tumor relapse in patients treated with abdominopelvic irradiation. With extensive residual tumor, there was no advantage to abdominopelvic irradiation over the other two methods (12% versus 10%). Because the patients in all three treatment arms were comparable with respect to age, stage, grade, histology, and presence or absence of gross tumor residuum, the most likely explanation for the outcome observed was that it was due to the whole-abdominal irradiation. The other three studies were not randomized but show similar confirmatory results; the Salt Lake City report is the most recent and supportive.[165,171,172]

Patterns of spread indicate that the entire peritoneal cavity is at risk. Two radiation therapy extended-field techniques have been used in ovarian carcinoma: open field and moving strip.[173–175] The open field employs anterior and posterior large portals shaped to encompass the entire peritoneal cavity. In some patients with stage I or stage II disease, radiation portals have been restricted to the lower half of the peritoneal cavity. However, in view of the frequent involvement of the retroperitoneal paraaortic lymph nodes in early stage ovarian carcinoma, Hanks and Bagshaw suggested that treatment should encompass these nodes.[173] Because many of these patients also have metastatic deposits on the undersurface of the diaphragms, Fuks[50] and Glatstein and colleagues[176] suggested further modifications to encompass large portions of the diaphragms in addition to the paraaortic region.[43]

When the open-field techniques are used, radiation is delivered at a rate of 800 to 1000 cGy/week. The total dose to the lower abdomen usually is 5500 cGy delivered in 27 fractions over 37 days. The total dose to the pelvis is 89, expressed in time-dose-fractionation (TDF) value.[177] When the upper abdomen is treated, the dose is usually 3000 to 4000 cGy delivered in 15 to 20 fractions over 21 to 33 days (TDF value of 64). Shielding the kidneys and liver (including the right hemidiaphragm) to protect these organs from radiation damage limits the effective dose to the underlying organs to approximately 2000 to 3000 cGy, respectively.

Another open-field technique was described by Martinez and colleagues (Fig. 39–5).[178,179] It involves a special field design and dose fractionation scheme to reduce the toxicity of the open-field technique. Using this approach, treatment is delivered by a series of anteroposterior-posteroanterior opposed fields. Beginning with radiation to the true pelvis, the field extends from the lower border of the obturator foramina up to the level of L5. Five fractions of 180 cGy each are given in 1 week. The field is then opened to include the entire abdominal and pelvic peritoneum, extending to 1 cm above the diaphragms. Twenty fractions of 150 cGy each are given to this volume in 4 weeks. A full-thickness posterior block is introduced after 1000 cGy to shield the kidneys, and a 50% transmission block is introduced anteriorly and posteriorly to shield the liver after 1500 cGy. The third and last field is a continuous pelvic, paraaortic, and partial diaphragmatic T-shaped field. Eight fractions of 150 cGy each are given in 10 days. The whole peritoneal cavity receives 3000 cGy in 20 fractions in 4 weeks, the pelvis receives 5100 cGy in 33 fractions in 6 to 7 weeks, and the paraaortic region with the medial part of the diaphragm receives 4200 cGy in 28 fractions in 5 to 6 weeks. The total dose to the liver is 2250 cGy and to the kidneys is 2000 cGy, given in 20 fractions in 4 weeks. This technique has been well tolerated.[162,178]

The moving-strip technique divides the peritoneal cavity into equal horizontal segments (2.5-cm-wide strips).[174] Treatment begins with irradiation to the lowest pelvic segments. At each radiation therapy session, four adjacent segments are treated simultaneously. On consecutive days, the irradiated volume is moved cephalad one segment to encom-

TABLE 39–11.   Radiation Therapy in Ovarian Cancer

Invesigations	Study Design	No. of Patients	Stage	Results
Dembo[158]	Pelvic RT vs pelvic RT and chlorambucil vs pelvic + whole-abdominal RT	43 76 76	I–III	5-y survival and relapse improved by whole-abdominal RT
Delclos[171]	Pelvic RT vs pelvic + whole-abdominal RT	47 148	I–IV	Improved survival for whole-abdominal RT (43% vs 31%)
Dubois[172]	Pelvic RT ± chemotherapy vs pelvic + whole-abdominal RT	58 52	II–III	Whole-abdominal RT superior only in stage II
Fuller[401]	Modified-abdominal RT vs abdominal RT ± pelvic RT	64 42	I–III	Survival improved by 30% with abdominal RT

* RT, radiation therapy.
(Ozols RF, Rubin SC, Dembo AJ, Robboy S. Epithelial ovarian cancer. In: Hoskins WJ, Perez CA, Young RC, eds. Principles and practice of gynecologic oncology. Philadelphia: JB Lippincott, 1992)

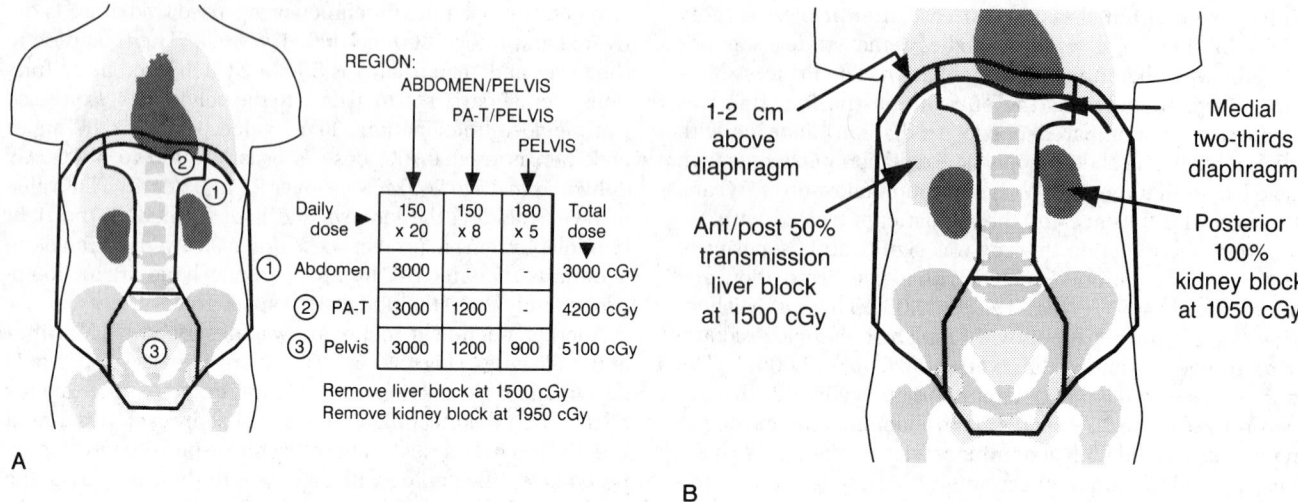

FIGURE 39–5. Martinez technique and dose schedule. Field boundaries and blocks for treatment of gynecologic malignancies by whole-abdomen irradiation with diaphragmatic, paraaortic, and pelvic boost. PA-T, paraaortic nodes T-shaped part. (Martinez A, Schray MF, Howes AE, et al. Postoperative radiation therapy for epithelial ovarian cancer: The curative role based on a 24-year experience. J Clin Oncol 1985;3:901–922)

pass the four adjacent segments in an orderly fashion until the entire abdomen has been treated. The dose to each point in the abdominal cavity usually is 3000 cGy delivered in 10 fractions over 12 days (TDF value of 62). The kidneys and liver are usually shielded by partial-thickness lead blocks designed to allow the delivery of 50% of the dose. An additional dose of 2000 cGy in 10 fractions over 12 days usually is delivered to the pelvis by an open-field technique to increase the pelvic dose. The total pelvic dose by the TDF method is 1713 rets (TDF value 95).

Studies comparing the open-field and moving-strip techniques have shown that the rates of acute morbidity, chronic complications, and survival are similar.[130,180] In the two randomized studies that compared the techniques, the difference in 5-year survival was less than 1% between the two treatment approaches.[180,181] A detailed analysis of the Princess Margaret Hospital study showed the two techniques to be comparable in all patient subgroups, regardless of stage, histology, grade, or disease residuum.[181] Acute toxicity was similar in the two treatment arms. Significant late toxic effects occurred infrequently with either technique, but toxicity was less commonly encountered using the open-field technique. Because of the shorter duration, simplicity, reduced toxicity, and equal efficacy, the open-field technique (or variant) has become the standard in most centers (Fig. 39–6).

RADIATION THERAPY FOR ADVANCED DISEASE

Calkins and colleagues reported 58 patients with advanced ovarian malignancy treated with a delayed, split-course whole-abdomen irradiation technique delivering 200 cGy per fraction for a total dose of 4000 cGy to the lower hemiabdomen and, after 2 to 6 hours delay, 150 cGy to the upper hemiabdomen for a total dose of 3000 cGy.[182] Fifty-three of the patients completed the prescribed course of therapy, 3 (5%) experienced a grade III or greater acute gastrointestinal toxicity, and 14 (24%) required treatment breaks because of thrombocytopenia. Twenty-five percent of stage III optimally cytoreduced

patients were disease free at 5 years, with a median survival of 45 months. Seven patients (12%) developed delayed small bowel obstruction in the absence of documented or suspected intraabdominal recurrence. Five of these patients required surgical resection of the obstruction, and 2 patients had diffusely matted bowel loops. All 5 patients received ^{32}P in ad-

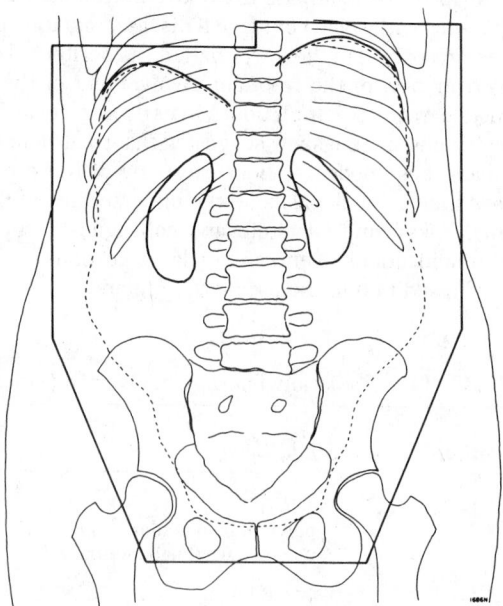

FIGURE 39–6. Treatment volume for abdominopelvic radiation therapy in patients with ovarian cancer. The entire peritoneal cavity must be encompassed. Liver shielding is not used. The kidneys are shielded to keep the renal dose at 1800 to 2000 cGy. The true pelvis is given a boost dose in 180- to 220-cGy fractions to a total dose of 4500 to 5000 cGy. Parallel opposing portals are used with beam energy sufficient to ensure dosage variation of less than 5%. (With permission from Dembo J. Cancer 1985;55:2285; from Ozols RF, Rubin SC, Dembo AJ, Robboy S. Epithelial ovarian cancer. In: Hoskins WJ, Perez CA, Young RC, eds. Principles and practice of gynecologic oncology. Philadelphia: JB Lippincott, 1992)

dition to the external abdominopelvic irradiation. Two patients developed hepatitis; 1 died. Both patients had received ^{32}P in addition to the external whole-abdominal irradiation. Two patients developed acute myelogenous leukemia at 13 and 44 months after completion of treatment. Both patients had been treated with melphalan after irradiation.

RADIATION THERAPY AFTER SURGERY AND CHEMOTHERAPY

In an attempt to reduce toxicity of abdominopelvic irradiation, several hyperfractionation schedules have been tried. The delivery of two doses of irradiation (120–150 cGy/fraction) with 5- to 6-hour intervals between fractions theoretically results in a greater killing of tumor cells with significant repair of the radiation effects on normal tissues.[183] Morgan and coworkers treated stage III patients with residual tumor after induction therapy with cisplatin-based regimens to deliver 2600 to 3060 cGy to the whole abdomen with 80-cGy fractions twice daily and an additional 1500 to 1920 cGy to the pelvis.[184] All patients completed therapy, and only 2 required a treatment break for thrombocytopenia. No patients developed small bowel obstruction requiring surgery. With a follow-up of 8 to 48 months, 6 (40%) of the patients were alive without disease.

Kong and colleagues treated 23 patients with advanced ovarian carcinoma after multiagent chemotherapy with 3000 cGy to the whole abdomen (100 cGy/fraction twice daily) with a rest period of 3 weeks after 1500 cGy.[185] Six patients with gross residual disease also received a boost of 1500 cGy to limited fields, without achieving tumor control. Five of the patients required surgery for intestinal obstruction with pathologic evidence of radiation bowel injury. Nine of 23 patients were without tumor at the time of the report, with follow-up ranging from 4 to 30 months (median, 13.5 months). A subsequent report from the same institution by Eifel and colleagues updated their experience with 34 patients.[186] All patients received the same dose of abdominopelvic irradiation with hyperfractionation and a split-course schedule. Eleven patients had a boost of 900 to 2000 cGy for gross residual disease. Only 1 patient did not complete therapy, and 2 had a 1-week interruption of treatment because of hematologic toxicity. Three patients with grade 1 tumors have no evidence of disease 20 to 50 months after irradiation. Patients with grade 2 and 3 tumors who had microscopic residual disease had relapse-free survival rates at 3 years of 10% and 14%, respectively. None of 12 patients with gross residual disease had significant response to therapy. Of the patients treated, 14 (38%) experienced small bowel obstructions, all associated with recurrent tumors. None of 5 patients currently believed to be free of tumor has experienced small bowel obstruction.

Hacker and associates treated 30 patients found to have residual epithelial ovarian cancer at second-look laparotomy with 3000 cGy to the whole abdomen (120 cGy/day) with a boost to the pelvis to complete 5000 cGy at 180-cGy fractions per day.[187] Fourteen patients (47%) completed therapy without interruption, and 7 (23%) had interruptions ranging from 1 to 4 weeks due to myelosuppression. Therapy was never completed in 9 patients (30%). Four (25%) of 16 patients with only microscopic residual disease remained disease free at 22 to 41 months. Two (33%) of 6 patients with minimal

(≤5 mm) residual disease were disease free at 19 to 40 months after radiation therapy. Patients with larger residual disease did poorly. Those who progressed on primary chemotherapy had a median survival of 7 months compared with more than 38 months for those who had responded to chemotherapy. The major morbid effect was late small bowel obstruction, requiring surgery in 8 (30%) of 24 patients who survived at least 4 months after completion of therapy. Two patients developed severe radiation enteritis. Five of the 8 patients undergoing laparotomy had no evidence of disease in multiple peritoneal biopsy specimens or washings. Eventually, 24 of the 30 patients developed recurrent disease; in 22, the initial site of recurrence was in the irradiated field. This therapy may be of limited value in patients with minimal or microscopic residual disease at second-look laparotomy, but morbidity is substantial.

Intraperitoneal ^{32}P has been used in patients with residual tumor at second-look laparotomy, with conflicting reports about efficacy.[188,189] No randomized trials have been conducted to assess the value of this therapy in patients with residual disease. The limited penetration (3–4 mm) of the β particles of the radioisotope restricts its application to minimal residual disease. In patients who have been previously operated and developed adhesions, it is extremely difficult to ensure an adequate distribution of the radioisotope throughout the entire peritoneal cavity.

RADIATION THERAPY INTEGRATED WITH SURGERY AND CHEMOTHERAPY

In patients with advanced or recurrent disease, there may be an advantage in combining adjuvant irradiation and chemotherapy. Fuks and associates studied sequential administration of cisplatin-based chemotherapy and reexploration with cytoreductive surgery, followed by abdominopelvic irradiation.[129] Several single-arm studies have reported encouraging, equivocal, or negative results.[185,187,189–198] Three randomized studies compared whole-abdominal and pelvic irradiation with chemotherapy after cisplatin induction.[199–201] One of the reports suggests that irradiation is inferior to continued chemotherapy if persistent disease is found at second-look surgery.[200] The other two studies indicated that abdominopelvic irradiation and chemotherapy, with carboplatin or chlorambucil, yields equivalent results.[199,201] Reports of abdominopelvic irradiation after initial therapy and second-look operation have described a higher incidence of complications, particularly small intestinal obstruction. One study correlated this morbidity with pelvic irradiation doses above 4500 cGy or whole-abdominal doses above 2500 cGy in patients who had second-look laparotomy.[202]

Franchin and associates treated 42 patients with advanced ovarian carcinoma with aggressive surgery, three courses of intraperitoneal cisplatin-based chemotherapy, followed by alternating combination chemotherapy, second-look laparotomy, and abdominopelvic irradiation (2200 cGy in 20 fractions to the abdomen and 1800 cGy in 10 fractions to the pelvis).[203] All except 2 patients relapsed within the abdominopelvic cavity. Three patients developed small bowel obstructions requiring surgery, and 1 died from surgical complications without evidence of tumor. Only 8 patients were alive and disease free at 5 years. They concluded that this type of therapy should be discontinued for patients with advanced ovarian cancer.

ACUTE MORBIDITY AND LONG-TERM SEQUELAE

The most common sequelae of radiation therapy for ovarian carcinoma is enteritis.[50,70,180] The incidence and severity are directly related to the volume irradiated and the radiation dose. Acute morbidity, including diarrhea, nausea, vomiting, and weight loss, was reported in 78% of the 167 patients treated with high-dose radiation therapy (4500–6000 cGy) to the lower abdomen.[204] In most patients, gastrointestinal symptoms subsided within a few weeks after completion of treatment. In 29% of the patients, diarrhea with or without gastrointestinal bleeding persisted for months to years after treatment. In 24 (14%) of the 167 patients, severe bowel stenosis and bleeding developed requiring surgery. Similar rates of acute and chronic radiation enteritis have been reported with the moving-strip technique.[205,206] Although acceptable, this frequency of morbidity and complications is regarded as high, despite the fact that the treatment is considered potentially curative for some patients.

Four studies summarize the frequency of major complications with abdominopelvic irradiation.[163,172,207,208] Of 1098 patients, 61 (5.6%) required bowel surgery for treatment complications (1.4–14%). However, only 4 (0.36%) died as a result of bowel damage. The frequency and severity of fatal bowel damage is related to the total dose of radiation, the dose per fraction, the extent of previous surgery, and results of lymph node sampling.[209]

Some hematopoietic toxicity usually accompanies irradiation.[50] Blood counts usually return to normal shortly after cessation of treatment, but there is evidence that the irradiated bone marrow remains somewhat impaired for extended periods after radiation therapy.[210]

Radiation-induced nephritis is a well-known complication of irradiation doses exceeding 2300 cGy.[211] Biochemical evidence of liver dysfunction, with elevation of the alkaline phosphatase, serum glutamic-pyruvic transaminase, serum glutamic-oxaloacetic transaminase, and lactic dehydrogenase, are observed in 25% to 50% of the patients, but clinical jaundice and ascites are rare (<1%).[163] Between 10% and 15% of patients experience persistent bloating or diarrhea, which is usually related to particular foods. Frank malabsorption is extremely rare if appropriate attention is paid to dose and technique. If careful portal design and shielding are not performed, these syndromes are common.[70,174,212] Hepatitis and nephritis are reported less frequently with careful application of appropriate shielding of the liver and kidneys.

Postirradiation chest radiographs show basal pneumonitis or fibrosis in 15% to 20% of patients, but few patients are symptomatic. The process is usually self-limiting.[168]

RADIOISOTOPES

Intraperitoneal installation of radioactive colloidal ^{196}Au or ^{32}P to irradiate the peritoneal cavity was once widely used.[213,188] Radioactive ^{196}Au is no longer available for therapy. Data show that radiation dose distribution on the peritoneal surface was quite variable and unpredictable and that the dose to lymph nodes and the retroperitoneum was usually negligible.[214] A multivariate, retrospective analysis of Norwegian Radium Hospital patients with stage I and II tumors showed a nonsignificant excess of relapses in patients who received ^{32}P or ^{196}Au compared with pelvic irradiation or no treatment.[160] Unacceptably high bowel toxicity was reported for radioisotopes given with pelvic irradiation.[215] The colloidal particles increase isotope uptake by the mesothelial peritoneal cells and lymph nodes and decrease systemic radioisotope elution. Radioactive phosphorus (chromic phosphate) has a half-life of 14.2 days and emits only β particles (1.7 MeV maximum energy). The range of β particles in tissue is only 3 to 5 mm; radioisotopes like ^{32}P may sterilize microscopic peritoneal implants, but they are inadequate to treat large masses because of the limited range of the β particle. Because of adhesions or loculation, poor distribution within the peritoneal cavity may occur. Adequate distribution within the peritoneal cavity can be defined by injecting diluted Hypaque or by instilling technetium 99m in the peritoneal cavity. Follow-up abdominal radiographs or scans are obtained before the therapeutic dose is administered.

After radioisotope therapy, subsequent surgical management may be more difficult because of fibrosis, although with ^{32}P, this problem has been infrequent. The usual dose of intraperitoneal radiophosphorus (as chromic phosphate) is 15 to 20 mCi diluted in sterile saline (1500–2000 ml) and properly distributed throughout the entire peritoneal cavity. If the average peritoneal surface is estimated at 30,000 cm^2, the dose of irradiation delivered to the peritoneum is 6000 cGy, and the dose to the omentum is 7000 cGy.[216]

The limited toxicity of intraperitoneal ^{32}P (particularly no known leukemia risk) and the absence of a therapeutic difference between patients receiving the radiocolloid and those receiving oral melphalan have led to the acceptance of ^{32}P by the GOG as the standard form of treatment for subsequent clinical trials recruiting patients with stage I tumors.[73] On the basis of studies of patients with advanced ovarian cancer demonstrating the effectiveness of platinum-based chemotherapy, the GOG has initiated a replacement trial comparing intraperitoneal ^{32}P with three cycles of cisplatin and cyclophosphamide in patients with unfavorable early stage disease.[168]

Intraperitoneal colloidal radioisotopes may be complicated by small bowel obstruction and stenosis. Pezner and coworkers, reporting on 104 patients treated with intraperitoneal radioisotopes, observed that 11% required surgery for adhesions or fibrosis of the small intestine.[217] Among patients treated with radioactive colloidal gold, only 1 (2.2%) of 45 developed small bowel complications, although 12 (24%) of 50 treated with radioisotopes and pelvic external radiation therapy developed complications. The frequency of small bowel complications appears to be lower with ^{32}P than with ^{196}Au. Complication rates tend to be slightly higher among patients who have uneven distribution of the radioactive material in the peritoneal cavity.

PALLIATIVE RADIATION THERAPY

Radiation therapy has been effectively used to relieve symptoms of patients with advanced inoperable or recurrent tumors. One of the most common applications is treatment of a large pelvic mass that may produce pressure on the urinary tract or rectosigmoid or of metastasis to the uterus or the vagina with ulceration and bleeding. Doses in the range of 5000 cGy with various fractionation schedules, depending on the condition of the patient, may be of value. A similar approach may be used in patients with localized abdominal or extraabdominal masses, including lymph nodes. Novel fractionation schedules have included 1000 cGy in a single weekly fraction for 2 or 3 weeks (2000–3000 cGy). However, the major complication rate of approximately 15% was difficult to justify in a palliative situation. Spanos and associates observed better tolerance and good palliative results in patients with large pelvic masses treated with a twice-daily fractionation schedule of 370 cGy per fraction (fractions separated by 5–6 hours), with the same treatment delivered every 3 to 4 weeks for a total of 4440 cGy.[218]

Patients with brain metastases may be palliated with doses of 3000 to 4000 cGy to the whole brain, delivered at daily doses of 250 to 300 cGy for five fractions per week. Although radiation therapy has no significant role in treating patients with pulmonary parenchyma metastasis or pleural effusion, mediastinal irradiation may palliate symptoms secondary to mediastinal or hilar metastatic lymph nodes.

Symptomatic liver metastasis can be treated with doses of approximately 3000 cGy delivered in 200- to 300-cGy fractions, five times per week. Radiation therapy has not produced satisfactory palliative results for patients with ascites.

Patients with painful bone metastasis or asymptomatic lesions in weight-bearing bones (*e.g.*, vertebral bodies, pelvis, femur) may benefit from a palliative course of radiation therapy delivering 3000 to 4000 cGy with 250- to 300-cGy fractions for four or five weekly fractions.

CHEMOTHERAPY

SINGLE AGENTS

Chemotherapy has been commonly employed as initial treatment in patients with advanced disease (*i.e.*, FIGO stages III and IV).[219] With the discovery of more active chemotherapeutic agents, chemotherapy has become the most common form of therapy for patients with advanced disease.

Alkylating agents have been used more extensively than any other class of chemotherapeutic agents. Melphalan, chlorambucil, cyclophosphamide, and thiotepa have produced similar objective response rates (33–65%).[71] The median survival of treated patients is approximately 10 to 14 months; the median survival of those responding to alkylating agents is 17 to 20 months; and for those not responding, the median survival is 6 to 13 months. The 5-year survival rate of treated patients ranges from 0% to 9% (mean, 7%). The 5-year survival rate for the largest single series of patients treated with melphalan was 9%; approximately 20% of the responders in that series were alive at 5 years, with some patients alive and free of disease for longer than 10 years. Second-look studies indicate that patients with no residual tumor at second-look laparotomy have a 5-year survival rate of 60% to 80% without additional therapy.[147,220] Approximately 5% to 10% of women with advanced ovarian cancer can be cured with single alkylating agent therapy alone.

Other drugs including carboplatin, cisplatin, doxorubicin, hexamethylmelamine, and taxol have been well studied and have response rates in the range of 20% to 35%.[221-224]

Cisplatin is one of the most active agents in ovarian cancer. Overall response rates of 25% to 40% have been reported in single-agent trials.[225] In a randomized trial of cisplatin versus cyclophosphamide, a longer duration of response (18 versus 8 months) and significantly better survival (19 versus 12 months; $p = 0.009$) was seen with cisplatin.[226] Toxicities include nausea and vomiting, ototoxicity, peripheral neuropathy, nephrotoxicity, and bone marrow suppression. Techniques are now available using hydration and chloruresis, which markedly reduce the nephrotoxicity of the agent.[227] Several studies have suggested a clinically important dose-response relation with cisplatin.[228,229] Hryniuk and colleagues have demonstrated an association between dose intensity and outcome in 33 chemotherapy trials in ovarian cancer.[230] The overall response rate and median survival correlated with the dose intensity (measured as mg/m^2/week) for combinations of drugs, particularly those containing cisplatin. When analyzed as single drugs, the dose intensity effect was seen primarily for cisplatin. Although hydration programs have modified or largely eliminated the nephropathy, the bone marrow toxicity, peripheral neuropathy, and ototoxicity remain significant problems when higher doses of cisplatin (>100 mg/m^2) are used.

Doxorubicin is a first-line agent active against advanced ovarian cancer. Collected experience indicates a response rate of approximately 30%.[231] Two metaanalyses, which pooled data from doxorubicin-containing combination chemotherapy trials, demonstrated a modest survival benefit of 5% to 7% at 6 years for patients treated with doxorubicin-containing regimens.[232,233] Unfortunately, several studies indicate that the drug has little activity when used as a second- or third-line agent, with only 3 (5%) of 56 patients responding to the drug after failing initial chemotherapy.[222,234]

One study of hexamethylmelamine in 54 previously untreated patients documented an overall response rate of 32%.[235] The drug was given orally on a daily schedule continuously in this study, and there was significant gastrointestinal, hematologic, and neurologic toxicity. Recent studies suggest reduced toxicity with intermittent schedules of 14 day per month. Updated information on hexamethylmelamine indicates definite single-agent activity against ovarian cancer.[236]

Cisplatin derivatives, particularly carboplatin, have been studied extensively in ovarian cancer and have significant activity.[224,237] Carboplatin (400 mg/m^2) appears to be roughly equivalent to 100 mg/m^2 of cisplatin. Carboplatin produces bone marrow suppression with little or no nephrotoxicity, ototoxicity, or peripheral neuropathy.

Taxol is a relatively new drug with a unique mechanism of action. It binds preferentially to microtubules and results in their polymerization and stabilization. Pharmacokinetics indicate that the drug is extensively protein bound, and metabolism, biliary excretion, and extensive tissue binding account for its systemic clearance. Renal clearance is minimal (<5%).

Initial phase II trials in 40 drug-refractory patients explored doses of taxol from 110 to 250 mg/m^2 given in 24-hour infusions and established doses of 110 to 150/m^2 for previously treated patients and 200 to 250 mg/m^2 for untreated patients. Response rates of 30%, including a response rate of 24% for platinum-refractory patients, were reported.[223] The durations of response ranged from 1 to 15 months (median, 6 months). Due to some hypersensitivity reactions apparently related to the Cremophor vehicle, the infusions were given with intravenous dexamethasone (20 mg), intravenous diphenhydramine (50 mg), and intravenous cimetidine (300 mg) 30 minutes before taxol.

A follow-up trial of taxol by the GOG in 41 previously treated patients produced a 36% response rate (*i.e.*, 24% partial, 12% complete). Overall responses of 30% were seen in platinum-refractory patients.[238] Nevertheless, the median duration of these responses was 6 months, and few long-term survivals have been reported from the salvage taxol trials.

The toxic effects of taxol include bone marrow suppression, alopecia, myalgias, arthralgias, and hypersensitivity reactions. The dose-limiting toxicity is most commonly neutropenia, which can be partially ameliorated by administering granulocyte colony-stimulating factor (G-CSF). It allows doses of taxol up to 250 mg/m² to be administered with safety. Nevertheless, there is no evidence of a significant dose-response effect with taxol. Results of preliminary trials using previously untreated patients and administering taxol (250 mg/m²) followed by cisplatin (75 mg/m²) with G-CSF appear to be appropriate for subsequent phase II combination trials.

Taxol is now available as a salvage agent through NCI-designated comprehensive cancer centers. It is given in doses of 135 mg/m² every 3 weeks for advanced ovarian cancer patients who meet eligibility criteria.

Other single agents that have received adequate testing and appear to have some activity in advanced ovarian cancer include ifosfamide, AZQ (aziridinylbenzoquinone), VP-16, and low-dose mitomycin C.[224,237,239,240]

Table 39–12 provides a summary of the activity of potentially important single agents in ovarian cancer.

HORMONE THERAPY

Although the ovary is the major source of estrogen in women, the extent to which hormones regulate the ovarian epithelium is unclear. After the demonstration of estrogen and progesterone receptors in approximately half of all ovarian carcinomas, the use of hormone treatment in the disease was actively investigated.[241,242] Clinical trials of various hormonal manipulations, including antiandrogens, gonadotropin-releasing hormone analogs, and antiestrogens, have been reported.[243–245] Overall response rates to progestational agents have been 5% to 15% in most studies.[224] Similar response rates have been achieved with leuprolide acetate (17%) and cyproterone acetate (7%).[243,244] Initial reports of activity for Megace, medroxyprogesterone, and tamoxifen have been followed by larger studies demonstrating less impressive activity. One trial of medroxyprogesterone in 41 patients resulted in one partial response.[245–250] Two trials of tamoxifen demonstrated no responses in 22 and 23 patients, respectively.[251,252] One study attempted to induce progesterone receptors by sequencing estradiol with medroxyprogesterone. Sixty-five patients were treated in two different dose schedules. The overall response was 14%.[253]

One prospective randomized trial of chemohormonal therapy has been published.[254] One hundred patients with previously untreated advanced disease were entered, and all received cisplatin and doxorubicin, with half of the patients

TABLE 39–12. Single Agents Active in Advanced Ovarian Adenocarcinoma

Drugs	No. of Patients	Percent Response (% Complete Response)
Alkylating Agents		
Melphalan	494	47 (20)
Chlorambucil	280	50
Thiotepa	144	65
Cyclophosphamide	126	49
Mechlorethamnine	81	35
Ifosfamide	41	20
AZQ	26	15
Antimetabolites		
5-Fluorouracil	81	32 (18–20)
	21	33
Methotrexate	16	25
	23	13
Antitumor Antibiotics		
Doxorubicin (Adriamycin)	18	28
	33	36
Mitomycin C	43	23
Plant Alkaloids		
Vinblastine	16	13
VP-16	22	32
Taxol	81	30 (12)
Miscellaneous		
Hexamethylmelamine	53	41
Cisplatin	34	27
Carboplatin	22	50 (17)
Dianhydrogalacticol	39	15
Peptichemio	47	24 (14)

randomized to concomitant tamoxifen. There was no difference in disease-free or overall survival rates between the two groups. Although the toxicity of these agents is low, the activity appears to be extremely modest.

In Vitro Clonogenic Assays in Ovarian Cancer

For many years, attempts have been made to define the activity of potentially useful chemotherapeutic agents using a variety of in vitro screening techniques. These have not been particularly successful. An in vitro tumor colony assay that evaluates clonogenic potential after exposure to chemotherapy has been used for a variety of tumors and has been studied in ovarian carcinoma.[255] Unfortunately, subsequent larger studies with ovarian cancer and other solid tumors have highlighted serious shortcomings of the human tumor clonogenic assay.[256]

The technical limitations of the clonogenic assay include difficulty in preparation of single cell suspensions, lack of optimal growth conditions for specific tumor types, and persistence of nonclonogenic clumps of tumor cells. It is unclear whether the assay predicts successful drugs or merely identifies patients who are more generally responsive to chemotherapy. These technical limitations, coupled with the absence of sufficient numbers of active drugs for relapsed ovarian cancer patients and the short duration of response in relapsed patients, make the assay an experimental tool and not a clinically proved means for selection of chemotherapy.

COMBINATION CHEMOTHERAPY

Combination chemotherapy in advanced ovarian cancer has been extensively studied during the past decade. From these studies, important prognostic factors, such as stage, histologic grade, and extent of residual disease, have been well defined, and most trials now stratify for important prognostic factors or at least analyze trial results by these factors.[231] Nevertheless, response rates have varied from 20% to 90%, with complete response rates varying from 10% to 65%, depending on the types of patients included and the criteria used for assessing response. There is still great variation in patient selection, prognostic factors, and response criteria in many trials of combination chemotherapy. These differences in patient characteristics may have a more important influence on survival than the therapies being reported. The published studies on previously untreated patients can be divided into three major groups: studies comparing single agents with combinations; randomized comparisons of different combination regimens; and experimental combination regimens.

Single Agents Versus Combination Chemotherapy

The first prospective study to demonstrate significantly improved survival for any combination compared with a standard alkylating agent was published in 1978.[257] Eighty previously untreated patients were randomized to receive melphalan in conventional doses or hexamethylmelamine, cyclophosphamide, methotrexate, and 5-fluorouracil (Hexa-CAF regimen).

Treatment with the four-drug combination achieved a significantly higher overall response rate (75% versus 54%; $p < 0.05$), more complete remissions (33% versus 16%; $p = 0.06$), and significantly longer median survival (29 versus 17 months; $p < 0.02$). However, Hexa-CAF was most effective in patients with minimal residual disease (overall response, 84% versus 53%; $p < 0.05$). Important stratification factors, such as extent of residual disease and histologic grade, and age, stage, and histologic type were well balanced. The toxicity of the combination was greater than that of the single agent. Dutch investigators confirmed the activity of the Hexa-CAF combination in previously untreated patients (overall response rate 57%, with 30% complete response rate), they but also demonstrated that Hexa-CAF in previously treated patients had a much lower overall response rate (3 of 13, 25%), produced no complete remissions, and had increased toxicity.[258] Their study emphasized the marked reduction of activity of any combination regimen used as second-line therapy in advanced ovarian cancer.

A series of trials randomly comparing single-agent chemotherapy (usually alkylating agents) with combination chemotherapy show improved response rates, improved disease-free survival, improved overall survival, or all three.[259-264] A summary of trials demonstrating improved response rates or disease-free survival and those demonstrating improved survival are shown in Table 39–13. These trials provide substantial evidence for the increased effectiveness of combinations compared with single agents in treating this disease. Other studies have not shown such benefit, but patient compliance and substantial dose modifications may have played a major role in the negative results of these studies.[265,266] One example is a large cooperative trial that compared oral chlorambucil with cisplatin at relapse with the combination of chlorambucil and cisplatin.[267] Response rates (53% versus 51%) and median

TABLE 39–13. Combination Chemotherapy Versus Single Agents in Advanced Previously Untreated Ovarian Carcinoma

Investigations	Regimen	Results
Clinical Trials Demonstrating Increased CR Rates and/or Disease-Free Survival		
Vogl[259]	CHAD vs LPAM	38% CR vs 21% CR: progression-free survival increased for CHAD
Delgado[260]	CHF vs LPAM	85% RR vs 57% RR; 50% CR vs 17% CR
Edmonson[261]	AC vs C	Improved progression-free survival with AC in patients with minimal residual disease
Williams[262]	PAC vs CLB	RR: 68% vs 26%, $p = 0.0004$ PCR: 26% vs 15%
Clinical Trials Demonstrating Improved Survival		
Young[257]	Hexa-CAF vs LPAM	75% RR vs 43%; 33% CR vs 16%; median survival, 29 mo vs 17 mo
Trope[263]	A + LPAM vs LPAM	67% RR vs 40%; 23+ mo vs 8.1 mo for duration of response; median survival, 17 mo vs 11 mo
Decker[264]	CP vs C	2-year disease-free interval: 52% vs 10%; 2-year survival: 62% vs 19%

CHAD, cyclophosphamide, hexamethylmelamine, doxorubicin (Adriamycin), cisplatin; LPAM, melphalan; CHF, cyclophosphamide, hexamethylmelamine, 5-fluorouracil; AC, doxorubicin, cyclophosphamide; C, cyclophosphamide; PAC, cisplatin, doxorubicin, cyclophosphamide; CLB, chlorambucil; Hexa-CAF, hexamethylmelamine, cyclophosphamide, methotrexate, 5-fluorouracil; CP, cyclophosphamide, cisplatin; RR, response rate; CR, complete response.

survival (16 versus 17 months) were similar, but only 57% of patients on combination chemotherapy had significant myelosuppression, and even fewer (25%) had bone marrow suppression during sequential treatment. Despite the minimal myelosuppression, the investigators demonstrated that myelosuppression had an important and favorable effect on survival. The relatively poor survival for both arms of the trial (similar to that achieved with single alkylating agents alone) coupled with the demonstrated positive effect of myelosuppression on subsequent survival illustrate the problem with this and similar trials. It is common to demonstrate equivalence of single agents and combinations if the trial is designed without full doses of the drugs used in combination.

A metaanalysis addressed the survival of 8139 patients with advanced disease treated with cisplatin and other single agents and combinations. The analysis indicated that platinum-based treatment was better than nonplatinum regimens and that platinum in combination was better than single-agent platinum at the same dose. It also demonstrated that cisplatin and carboplatin were equally effective.[268]

Several earlier trials used alkylating agents as maintenance therapy for several years after induction chemotherapy.[262,267] These trials failed to show any survival benefit for maintenance, and they reported leukemias.[269,270] Maintenance therapy for this disease should be abandoned.

Several conclusions can be drawn from the prospective, randomized trials and metaanalyses. Platinum-based combination chemotherapy produces higher overall response rates and higher complete response rates than single agents, although survival is not altered significantly in some studies. Long-term disease-free survivals, although uncommon, are more frequent with combinations, particularly if full doses of the most active drugs are included. The best chance for achieving a complete remission in advanced ovarian carcinoma exists when initial therapy is begun with an effective platinum-based combination regimen of full therapeutic doses.

Randomized Comparisons of Combination Regimens

Many studies using combination chemotherapy as initial treatment in advanced disease have now been published. Earlier trials were often single-arm studies, but recent randomized trials have compared two or more combinations. Most of these studies contain sufficient information about prognostic factors, response duration, and survival to allow realistic comparisons with currently established regimens of combination chemotherapy or single agents.

Several groups reported results of two-, three-, and four-drug combinations in nonrandomized studies in previously untreated stage III and stage IV disease. Most of these trials used combinations of cisplatin, doxorubicin, cyclophosphamide, hexamethylmelamine, methotrexate, or 5-FU.[139,257,271,272] The overall response rates have been 60% to 80%, with clinical complete remissions in approximately 40% to 50% of patients. Careful restaging demonstrates that approximately half of those clinically free of disease actually have residual disease at second-look laparotomy. Approximately 25% to 30% of all patients treated with combination chemotherapy are free of disease at restaging, and it is this subset of patients who experience prolonged disease-free survival. Using data from early, nonrandomized trials, there did not seem to be a striking difference between one combination regimen and another.

Several well-designed trials have been performed testing various combination regimens. Several of the more significant studies are summarized in Table 39–14.

Dutch investigators compared cyclophosphamide, hexamethylmelamine, doxorubicin, and cisplatin (CHAP-5) with Hexa-CAF, and they demonstrated a statistically greater response rate (79% versus 50%) and complete remission rate (30% versus 17%), improved disease-free survival (19.5 versus 6.8 months), and improved overall survival (30.7 versus 19.6 months) for the CHAP-5 combination.[273] The Nether-

TABLE 39–14. Randomized Comparisons of Combination Chemotherapy in Advanced Ovarian Adenocarcinoma

Investigations	Regimen*	Results
Neijt[258]	CHAP-5 vs Hexa-CAF	79% RR vs 50%; 30% CR vs 17%; median survival, 31 vs 20 mo
Omura[275]	PAC vs AC	51% CR vs 26% in patients with measurable disease. Response duration (15 vs 19 mo), progression-free interval (13 vs 7 mo), and overall survival (20 vs 16 mo) all statistically significant
Neijt[274]	CHAP-5 vs CP	78% RR vs 76%. PCR 34% vs 37% and no differences in survival
Edmonson[279]	HCAP vs CP	Survival at 30 mo equivalent for the two regimens (24.6 mo)
Conte[277]	PAC vs PC	41% clinical CR vs 20% CR; in those patients going to second-look, significant increase in PCR for PAC (62% vs 40%, $p < 0.05$). No difference in overall survival
Jakobsen[278]	PAC vs CP	CR 24% vs 11% ($p < 0.05$); at 3 years more PAC survivors (48% vs 20%)

* Abbreviations: see footnote of Table 39–13.

lands Cancer Institute subsequently performed a large trial comparing CHAP-5 with cyclophosphamide and cisplatin (CP). The overall response rate (78% versus 76%) and the pathologically documented complete response rate (34% versus 37%) were identical for the two regimens.[274]

The 10-year follow-up results of these important trials has been published.[128] At 10 years, 9% of patients treated with Hexa-CAF and 21% of patients treated with CHAP-5 were alive. Sixty percent of all the patients who achieved complete remission were alive at 5 years, and 40% were alive at 10 years. Results with CP were statistically similar to those achieved with CHAP-5 and better than those with Hexa-CAF.

The GOG compared doxorubicin and cyclophosphamide (AC) with cisplatin, doxorubicin, and cyclophosphamide (PAC) in 227 patients with measurable disease.[275] The progression-free interval (13 versus 7.7 months) and overall survival (19.7 versus 15.7 months) were statistically better for the platinum-containing combination. These trials provide substantial evidence for the importance of platinum in any ovarian cancer regimen. It is not clear that the addition of other agents to regimens that include full dose intensities of cyclophosphamide and cisplatin is necessary or beneficial.

The impact of additional agents, particularly doxorubicin, used in cisplatin-containing combinations has been the focus of several trials. The GOG compared CP with the PAC combination in 349 patients with advanced disease.[276] Complete remission rates were similar (30% versus 33%). Progression-free intervals (22.7 versus 24.6 months) and overall survivals (31.2 versus 38.9 months) were similar in these optimal (<1 cm of residual disease) stage III patients.

Two studies comparing CP with CAP have come to somewhat different conclusions. A study by Conte and colleagues compared CP and PAC in 125 patients who had localized and advanced disease.[277] The objective response rates were similar for the two groups (54% versus 56%), but the PAC regimen induced a higher percentage of complete remissions (41% versus 20%) in patients with measurable disease, and there were more surgically documented complete remissions (62% versus 40%). Progression-free interval and survival were not statistically different. The second trial compared CP and PAC in 154 patients with advanced disease.[278] The complete remission rate favored PAC (24% versus 11%), and at 3 years follow-up, there was improved survival for the PAC-treated group (48% versus 20%). These somewhat conflicting results probably account for the small contribution that doxorubicin made to the outcome of the metaanalyses mentioned previously.[232,233]

The potential contribution of hexamethylmelamine to combination regimens is controversial. A study from the Mayo Clinic compared CP with hexamethylmelamine, cyclophosphamide, doxorubicin, and cisplatin (H-CAP) in 181 patients.[279] An early publication at a median follow-up of 30 months reported identical survivals (24.6 months). However, longer follow-up of this trial and results of two others suggested some effect for hexamethylmelamine. In the Mayo Clinic trial, the 5-year survival rates were 22% for the CP-treated group and 33% for the H-CAP group (two-sided $p = 0.14$).[279] The Vanderbilt group also studied H-CAP. Nineteen (35%) of 54 patients had a complete response, and 10 (18%) remain disease free 108 months after treatment.[280] In an NCI study of cyclophosphamide, hexamethylmelamine, 5-fluorouracil, and cisplatin (CHex-UP), the complete response rate was only 19%. However, the median survival of the complete responder group exceeds 7.5 years.[220]

Interpretation of these trials is hampered by the variation of the dose intensities of the drugs included. The ultimate contribution of doxorubicin and hexamethylmelamine will be clarified when equitoxic regimens of CP, CAP, and H-CAP are compared prospectively. Current evidence suggests that no combination regimen produces significantly better results than the two-drug CP regimen used in full therapeutic doses.

Experimental Combinations

Because of the activity of taxol and ifosfamide, attention has focused on trials incorporating these drugs into platinum-based combinations.[281,282] Trials have also substituted carboplatin for cisplatin in standard combinations and other trials have studied combinations containing both carboplatin and cisplatin.[283–286]

Attempts are being made to reduce the dose-limiting myelotoxicity of these combinations by using granulocyte-macrophage colony-stimulating factor, G-CSF, or WR-2721.[287,288] High-dose chemotherapy with stem cell support is another experimental approach that is being increasingly used in advanced ovarian cancer.

Shae and colleagues treated relapsed ovarian cancer patients with high-dose carboplatin and bone marrow transplantation. There were 7 responders among 11 heavily pretreated patients.[289]

Shpall and associates used high-dose cyclophosphamide, thiotepa, and cisplatin followed by transplantation. Among 8 evaluable patients, there were 6 partial remissions (median duration, 6 months), but 3 (35%) died of toxic side effects.[290]

Stoppa and coworkers used high-dose melphalan and autologous bone marrow transplantation in a more favorable group of patients with advanced disease. Of the 12 patients with evaluable disease, 9 (75%) responded, and 4 (33%) had complete responses. There was a 9% treatment-related mortality rate.[291]

These pilot studies suggest significant activity but serious toxicity when the experimental regimens were given to heavily pretreated patients. These approaches are now being applied to patients with small volume residual disease where the benefits may be greater.[292]

Combination Chemotherapy After Single-Drug Failure

In the past, many attempts were made to use combination chemotherapy after patients had failed initial single-agent therapy. Details of these regimens are presented in the original publications and in reviews.[157] None of these trials really establish any combination regimen as particularly useful in managing chemotherapy failures. High overall response rates have been reported, but the number of patients is small, and most responses are partial and of short duration (4–6 months). The reported toxicity appears to be substantial.

INTRAPERITONEAL CHEMOTHERAPY

Techniques for delivering chemotherapy to patients with minimal residual peritoneal disease have been extensively

TABLE 39–15. Intraperitoneal Chemotherapy in Ovarian Cancer

Investigations	Drug	Pharmacologic Advantage*
Brenner[393]	Cytosine arabinoside	300–1000
Speyer[342]	5-Fluorouracil	111–898
Gyves[394]		550–7852
Ozols[343]	Doxorubicin	474
Howell[395]	Melphalan	63–93
Jones[341]	Methotrexate	18–36
Howell[396]		7–303
Howell[397]	Cisplatin	21
Pretorius[398]		47–72
Casper[399]		50–100

* Ratio of peak peritoneal level to plasma level or ratio of area under curve (AUC).

studied. The clinical rationale and pharmacologic basis for high-volume intraperitoneal chemotherapy ("belly bath") in ovarian cancer are based on several observations. The disease remains confined to the intraperitoneal space throughout most of its natural history, and currently available combination chemotherapy produces clinically complete responses in approximately 40% of patients, but at least half or more of these patients have minimal residual disease. The pharmacologic rationale depends on the differences in peritoneal clearance and clearance from the systemic circulation.[338–340] The slower the peritoneal clearance of a drug, the greater is the potential pharmacologic advantage. High-molecular-weight compounds with a low lipid solubility have slow peritoneal clearance and have an increased pharmacologic advantage.

Intraperitoneal chemotherapy has been used for many years to control malignant ascites. The major differences between previous methods of intraperitoneal chemotherapy and current techniques are the use of a semipermanent Tenckhoff dialysis catheter or Portacath system and the delivery of the antineoplastic agents in a large volume (2 L of dialysate) instead of 50 to 100 ml of saline. The use of a large volume of dialysate for drug administration is based partially on theoretical pharmacokinetic modeling studies.[338] Initial trials of methotrexate, 5-fluorouracil, doxorubicin, and other drugs documented a marked pharmacologic advantage with intra-

peritoneal chemotherapy (Table 39–15).[341–343] These studies indicated that intraperitoneal therapy was possible in about 80% of patients. In 20%, adhesions or maldistribution of fluid prevented proper drug delivery.[344–346]

Although the pharmacologic success of intraperitoneal chemotherapy has been established, the therapeutic benefit remains less clear. The early trials established that patients with minimal residual disease are most likely to respond and that responses of patients with bulky disease are uncommon.[347] Two studies using intraperitoneal cisplatin established the drug as the current intraperitoneal drug of choice.[348,349] A summary of the study design and results are listed in Table 39–16.

In an intraperitoneal chemotherapy study where survival was reported, for patients with bulky residual disease treated with intraperitoneal cisplatin, the median survival was 6.5 months. For those with minimal residual disease before therapy, the 2-year actuarial survival rate was 74%.[350] The survival rates for patients with microscopic residual, positive washings, or minimal residual disease have varied in several studies.[128,273,274] There is still no evidence that the intraperitoneal administration of any single agent or combination prolongs survival.[351] There is a European study underway in which patients in complete remission are randomized to receive intraperitoneal chemotherapy or no additional treatment.[352] Other studies are exploring the role of intraperitoneal therapy as a part of initial therapy. An intergroup study of patients with previously untreated small-volume disease is comparing intravenous and intraperitoneal cisplatin, with all patients receiving systemic cyclophosphamide.[353] Studies are also underway using sequential intravenous and intraperitoneal cisplatin during induction.[354]

Taxol has been used intraperitoneally because of its high molecular weight and complex chemical structure. Markman and colleagues studied intraperitoneal taxol (25–200 mg/m² every 3–4 weeks) in 25 previously treated patients.[387] Severe abdominal pain was the dose-limiting toxic effect for doses of 125 mg/m² or more. At 125 mg/m², satisfactory drug levels were reached and maintained for several days with a single dose. Pharmacokinetic studies showed that plasma taxol levels reached therapeutic range with this intraperitoneal dose. The area-under-the-curve ratio for taxol in these studies was 1000. Additional studies of intraperitoneal taxol are warranted.

The current use of intraperitoneal therapy remains experimental. Cisplatin appears to be the current drug of choice, and there is no evidence of substantial activity for any intra-

TABLE 39–16. Intraperitoneal Cisplatin in Small-Volume Residual-Disease Ovarian Cancer After Induction Chemotherapy

Variables	Mount Sinai[346]	Netherlands Cancer Institute[348]
No. of patients	23	21
Cisplatin dose	50 mg/m² in 2 L every 3 wk	60–150 mg/m² in 2 L every 2–3 wk
No. of cycles	6	6–10
Sodium thiosulfate	Not used	If toxicity developed in previous cycle
Catheter	Temporary in 75% of patients	Tenckhoff
Results	6/19 (32%) negative laparotomy	7/21 (33%) negative laparotomy

peritoneal therapy in patients with bulky residual disease. Combination chemotherapy administered intraperitoneally has not improved survival over results achieved with single agents. Whether intraperitoneal chemotherapy in any phase of ovarian cancer management can play an important role is unknown.[355,356]

LATE COMPLICATIONS OF CHEMOTHERAPY

As therapy for advanced ovarian cancer improves, a variety of late complications are being observed that are related to the treatment or the altered natural history of the disease. Late relapse with unusual lesions, such as bone metastases or central nervous system involvement, have been reported. Acute leukemia as a late complication of ovarian cancer therapy has been reported in several studies. A published survey of 70 institutions with 5455 patients revealed 13 patients who developed leukemia, representing a 21-fold increase in risk.[269] Risks were highest in patients who had alkylating-agent chemotherapy in excess of 2 years, and approximately two thirds of the patients had received irradiation as well. A prolonged period of pancytopenia often antedated frank leukemic transformation. Two thirds of the leukemic patients who died showed no evidence of ovarian cancer at autopsy.

Similar results have been published in an analysis of 1399 women in five randomized trials, for whom the cumulative risk of acute nonlymphocytic leukemia was 9.6% at 7 years.[270] Nevertheless, the overall risk of acute leukemia in ovarian cancer is quite small (0.3%).[269] Techniques for minimizing the risk, such as cyclic intermittent chemotherapy rather than continuous treatment with alkylating agents, avoidance of combined irradiation and chemotherapy, and better techniques for defining the complete remissions so that therapy can be discontinued, can undoubtedly minimize this risk.

OTHER EXPERIMENTAL APPROACHES

Immunotherapy

Immunotherapy has been investigated in a few studies. A good experimental basis for immunotherapy exists, including the existence of tumor-associated antigens demonstrated in ovarian cancer; circulating lymphocytes that are reactive to the patient's tumor cells; defects in B-cell function demonstrated in patients with advanced ovarian cancer, although T-cell function appears intact; and animal models of ovarian cancer demonstrate enhanced tumoricidal activity with chemotherapy and nonspecific immunotherapy or specific antibodies generated against ovarian tumor cells.[293,294] Most studies have used nonspecific immunotherapy with chemotherapy. However, trials with intraperitoneal *C. parvum*, interferon, and melphalan with levamisole have been reported.[295–298] Nonspecific immunotherapy in conjunction with chemotherapy has shown activity against ovarian cancer in two randomized studies, but the independent contribution of immunotherapy to the therapeutic result is ambiguous.[299,300] Randomized trials of melphalan with or without *C. parvum* and CAP with or without bacillus Calmette-Guérin immunization failed to show improvement in survival for patients on the immunotherapy arms.[301]

Studies have used intraperitoneal interleukin-2 with or without lymphokine-activated killer cells.[302] Some reduction in the systemic toxicity was achieved by intraperitoneal administration, and objective regressions were reported, but the local peritoneal toxicity was severe.[302]

Several murine monoclonal antibodies have been generated against ovarian cancer specifically or are cross-reactive to ovarian cancer cell lines. Because most murine antibodies lack intrinsic cytotoxicity, they have been coupled to toxic moieties, such as radioisotopes, chemotherapeutic agents, or natural toxins like ricin or *Pseudomonas aeruginosa* exotoxin.[303,304] In early phase I and II trials, radioisotope conjugates and immunotoxins have been associated with serious toxicity, including central nervous system toxicity, neuropathy, and pancytopenia.[305,306]

Drug Resistance in Ovarian Cancer

The effectiveness of drug therapy in this disease is limited by the development of acquired drug resistance. This resistance is drug specific and frequently associated with a broad cross-resistance to structurally dissimilar drugs. This pleiotropic drug resistance may be due to the *MDR1* gene with its protein product, the P170 glycoprotein, which enables the drug-resistant tumor to limit drug accumulation of structurally unrelated agents.[307–310] This cross-resistance is most frequently seen with natural products, such as the vinca alkaloids, doxorubicin, and VP-16. Although this mechanism appears to be important in certain other tumors, it does not seem to be the primary mechanism of broad cross-resistance in ovarian cancer. Other mechanisms of resistance include the elevation of intracellular glutathione and increased DNA repair in drug-resistant human ovarian cancer.[311,312]

Approaches to overcome these mechanisms of drug resistance are being explored. Certain calcium channel blockers can overcome drug resistance associated with decreased drug accumulation. Verapamil can reverse doxorubicin resistance in ovarian carcinoma cell lines by blocking drug efflux.[313] A pilot clinical trial has been completed, but adequate levels of verapamil to produce clinical effectiveness could not be achieved without unacceptable cardiac toxicity.[314] Other calcium channel blockers are currently under study.

Glutathione is a tripeptide thiol found ubiquitously in human cells. Drug resistance in ovarian cancer cells is associated with a marked increase in intracellular glutathione.[315,316] Buthionine sulfoximine (BSO), a synthetic amino acid analog, inhibits the synthesis of glutathione and markedly reduces intracellular glutathione in vitro and in vivo.[317,318] This is associated with a restoration of drug sensitivity in cell lines and prolongation of survival in a nude mice model of ovarian cancer.

A phase I trial of melphalan and BSO is underway. Preliminary results indicate that BSO can be safely given to patients at doses that lower intracellular gluthione to 20% of normal, the level at which the antitumor effect was restored in animals.[319] Ethacrynic acid can restore sensitivity to alkylating agents in experimental tumors, and a clinical trial using drug-refractory patients is underway.[321,322]

It has also been demonstrated that drug resistance in ovarian cancer is associated with increased DNA repair.[320] Aphidicolin, a potent inhibitor of polymerase, can block DNA repair and partially restore drug sensitivity in these resistant cell lines.[312] Clinical trials with aphidicolin have shown it to be nontoxic in phase I trials.

Drug resistance in ovarian cancer is an interaction of multiple factors, and a single explanation of drug resistance is not likely. Nevertheless, there are clinical trials underway to test a variety of ways in which resistance can be overcome.

RESULTS OF TREATMENT

Historically, the treatment of ovarian cancer has been discussed by separating early disease (FIGO stages I and II) from advanced disease (FIGO stages III and IV). Other important prognostic variables are tumor residuum, grade, histologic subtype, and the age of the patient at diagnosis.[63,79,178] A multivariate analysis of these variables in 430 ovarian carcinoma patients revealed residual disease and tumor grade to be the most important variables ($p < 0.001$), followed by stage ($p = 0.002$), age ($p = 0.004$), and histologic type ($p = 0.058$).[79] Tumor residuum is significantly more powerful in predicting the therapeutic outcome than FIGO stage, and this is reflected in the change in the FIGO stage classification for advanced disease (see Table 39–4).

The extent of residual disease after surgery affects outcome.[79,323] There are three prognostically distinct subgroups based on early disease (stages I and II) and the presence or absence of large postsurgical residual disease (usually >2 cm). Patients with minimal residual disease stand a good chance of disease eradication by postoperative therapy and have the highest probability of long-term survival.

We discuss the treatment of these three groups of patients separately: patients with early (FIGO stages I and II) ovarian cancer and microscopic or no residual disease; patients with advanced disease but minimal residual (<2 cm) after initial surgery; and patients with bulky residual tumor and advanced stage III or IV disease.

EARLY OVARIAN CANCER WITH MICROSCOPIC OR NO RESIDUAL DISEASE

The surgical management of stage I ovarian cancer is influenced by the cell type and grade of the tumor and the reproductive desires of the patient. Although certain types of epithelial ovarian cancer may present more frequently at an early stage than other cell types, there is probably little difference in survival or recommended surgical management of these carcinomas when matched for stage and grade. Scully summarized three series in which cancer was confined to a single ovary and reported a survival rate of 78% for conservative surgical treatment and 79% for radical therapy.[57,61] Munnell reported a survival rate of 75% for two similar groups of patients.[35] Webb and coworkers reported a survival rate of 90% for stage I patients with intact capsules and 57% if the tumor had penetrated the capsule or ruptured.[324]

These studies suggest that patients with epithelial ovarian cancer confined to one ovary with otherwise negative comprehensive surgical exploration results can be managed by unilateral salpingo-oophorectomy and no additional therapy if the tumor is grade 1 or 2 and the patient wants to have children. For patients who undergo conservative surgery (i.e.,

unilateral salpingo-oophorectomy), the opposite ovary should be biopsied. For patients with grade 3 tumors or those who do not desire to have children, a total abdominal hysterectomy and bilateral salpingo-oophorectomy should be performed.

A series of studies attempted to define whether well-staged patients with IA and IB, well-differentiated or moderately differentiated tumors require additional therapy. Dembo studied a group of 54 stage IA patients randomized between observation or pelvic radiation therapy after initial surgery.[170] There were relapses among 30 patients with moderately or poorly differentiated tumors, compared with no relapses among 24 patients with well-differentiated tumors, regardless of whether pelvic irradiation was given or not. Similarly, the GOG reported 1 relapse among 56 stage IA or IB patients with well-differentiated or moderately differentiated tumors.[73,159] In the GOG study, patients in this favorable-prognosis group were randomized to receive oral melphalan (48 patients) or no additional therapy (38 patients). With a median follow-up in excess of 6 years, there were only 6 deaths. The 5-year disease-free survival rates (91% and 98%) and the overall survival rates (94% versus 98%) are similar in the two groups.[73] Based on these studies, stage I patients with well-differentiated tumors and without positive peritoneal cytology, densely adherent tumors, or cyst rupture do not require postoperative therapy.[73,159,164]

For patients with stage II disease or with stage I disease with incomplete surgical staging or poor prognostic findings, more aggressive management is required. Stage II epithelial ovarian carcinoma always requires total abdominal hysterectomy, bilateral salpingo-oophorectomy, and a full staging operation. Particular care must be exercised to ensure that the carcinoma has not spread to the upper abdomen. Every effort should be made to remove all visible tumor in the pelvis, using retroperitoneal surgical approaches if necessary.

If microscopic or small macroscopic residual disease remains, adjuvant therapy is employed, and the choice of management is similar to that used for patients with advanced stages and minimal residual disease.

The GOG in an early trial studied patients with stage IA and IB epithelial ovarian cancer (staged in a conventional manner) and compared no additional therapy, pelvic irradiation, or intermittent oral melphalan.[159] Forty-nine percent of patients were not evaluable, and the three treatment arms were not well balanced for prognostic variables. The frequency of relapse was greatest after pelvic irradiation (7 of 23, 30%) compared with observation (5 of 29, 17%) and intermittent oral melphalan (2 of 34, 6%), although there were no significant differences in overall survival.

In trials that required careful surgical staging before entry, the Ovarian Cancer Study Group and GOG studied two groups of patients with early disease.[73] The first studied good-prognosis stage I patients, and the second included patients with IC, IIA, IIB, or IIC disease and poor-prognosis stage I patients and compared melphalan with intraperitoneal ^{32}P.[306] In the second trial, 141 patients were randomized to oral melphalan or intraperitoneal ^{32}P. With a follow-up in excess of 6 years, the disease-free survival rates (80% versus 80%) and overall survival rates (81% versus 78%) are similar ($p = 0.48$). A replacement trial is underway, using the same patient population and comparing intraperitoneal ^{32}P with three courses of cyclophosphamide and cisplatin. Because radiocolloids are transported to the diaphragm and concentrated there, this treatment technique delivers high-dose radiation to the diaphragm, which may explain the good survival observed in patients receiving intraperitoneal radioactive colloids.[214,217]

POOR-PROGNOSIS STAGE I DISEASE AND STAGES II, III, OR IV WITH MINIMAL OR NO RESIDUAL DISEASE POSTOPERATIVELY

Patients in the second category include most of the patients with poor-prognosis stage I and II disease and 20% to 30% of stage III patients who are left without gross tumor after initial surgery (stage IIIA). Current evidence indicates that these patients require postoperative therapy, although it is not clear what form of therapy is optimal.

One commonly used approach has been postoperative irradiation with doses of 4500 to 5000 cGy given to the pelvis and 2250 to 3000 cGy delivered to the upper abdomen. Previous studies indicated that whole-abdominal irradiation is necessary. Bush showed that 4500 cGy given to the pelvis reduced the number of pelvic recurrences in stage I patients, but the overall risk of relapse did not decrease, because most of the irradiated patients relapsed in the upper abdomen.[325] Similarly, Schray reported that 14 of 19 stage I and II patients treated with high-dose lower abdominal irradiation relapsed in the upper abdomen.[162] Irradiation of the upper abdomen decreases the risk of upper abdominal relapse, and improves survival.

The Princess Margaret Hospital group studied patients with stage IB, II, and IIIA ovarian carcinoma, randomized to receive pelvic irradiation, pelvic irradiation plus oral chlorambucil for 2 years, or pelvic and upper abdominal irradiation.[158,325] In 8 of 31 patients treated with irradiation of the pelvis only, upper abdominal relapses without concomitant pelvic relapses occurred, compared with no relapses among 51 in patients receiving whole-abdominal irradiation.[158] The 5-year survival rate for patients with whole-abdominal irradiation was 78%, compared with 51% for the patients receiving pelvic irradiation with or without chlorambucil.[325] Similarly, Delclos and Smith reported that only 17% of 18 stage II patients treated with pelvic irradiation alone survived at 5 years, compared with 49% of 71 patients treated with whole-abdominal irradiation.[166] Based on these data, it is generally accepted that whole-abdominal radiation therapy is the optimal radiation technique for this group of patients.

Chemotherapy has been used in this group of patients, and data suggest that results are similar to that observed with external-beam radiation therapy. The M.D. Anderson Cancer Center group studied patients with stages I through IIIA disease with minimal residual disease. They compared single-agent melphalan with total-abdominal irradiation by moving strip in a slightly different dose and port design from that used by the Princess Margaret Hospital group.[326] The 2- and 5-year survival rates for the groups were 86.5% and 71.5%, respectively, for radiation and 90% and 78% for melphalan. At 10 years follow-up, there were still no differences in survival between the two groups.[327] The M.D. Anderson Cancer Center group concluded that chemotherapy is as effective as irradiation, has fewer serious side effects, and is less expensive.

The Radiumhemmet Group randomized stage I and stage IIA patients with seropapillary ovarian carcinoma to adjuvant postsurgical treatment with lower abdominal radiation, single alkylating agent chemotherapy, or to radiation therapy followed by chemotherapy. Analysis showed that the lowest 5-year survival rate was observed for patients treated with chemotherapy alone (68%), compared with 88% for the radiation alone group and 91% for the combined radiation and chemotherapy group.[328]

Many of these early studies did not require comprehensive surgical staging before therapy. When systematic restaging is performed prospectively, 31% of these patients are found to have a more advanced stage of disease, and 77% actually have stage III disease. A major reason why local treatment fails in many patients with apparent localized disease is because they have unsuspected extrapelvic metastases that are not being treated by surgery or pelvic irradiation.

Although radiation and chemotherapy are effective against small ovarian tumors (<2 cm in diameter), resulting in high rates of clinical and pathologic complete responses, the cure rates for patients with residual tumor after initial surgery have been less favorable than those in patients with no residual tumor.[164,178] Whole-abdominal irradiation with doses of 5000 to 6000 cGy given to the lower abdomen and 3000 to 4000 cGy delivered to the upper abdomen has frequently been employed in such patients. Using radiation therapy, Dembo reported a 5-year survival rate of 58% for 36 stage II patients and 43% for 55 stage III patients left with minimal residual tumor after initial surgery.[164] Martinez and associates reported a 54% 5-year survival rate for 42 similar stage II and III patients.[178]

Combination chemotherapy has been used in similar groups of patients. The initial response rates are high, and the pathologically confirmed complete remissions are about 56% (Table 39–17). These patients usually experience long survival. The M.D. Anderson Cancer Center group reported a 34% 4-year survival rate for 83 patients treated with a variety of single-agent chemotherapies (*e.g.*, melphalan, 5-fluorouracil, doxorubicin, cisplatin, hexamethylmelamine) and a rate of 51% for patients treated with various combinations.[329,330] Belinson reported a 53% survival rate for 21 patients treated with CAP chemotherapy.[329] These survival rates are similar to those observed with total-abdominal irradiation.

The frequency of surgically confirmed complete remissions is approximately half the clinically observed complete response rate, but it depends on the volume of disease at initial therapy. The effect of the extent of residual disease on the frequency of a pathologic complete remission is shown in Table 39–17.

Patients who have negative second-look laparotomies after combination chemotherapy usually have long survival periods, although this varies from institution to institution. Greco and colleagues reported a 74% 4-year disease-free survival rate for patients with negative second-look surgical results after chemotherapy.[191,331] The NCI experience is similar, and long-term follow-up of patients treated with CHex-UP indicate that 63% of the patients with pathologically documented complete remissions are alive without relapse at 5 years.[220] Studies from Memorial Sloan-Kettering Cancer Center on survival after negative second-look surgery project a 65% relapse rate by 48 months.[332] In a 7-year follow-up of patients treated with PAC, only 3 (38%) of 8 patients were alive without recurrence at 7 to 8 years after treatment.[271] Recent evidence indicates

TABLE 39–17. Effect of Residual Disease on Pathologic Complete Remission Rate

Investigations	Chemotherapy*	Surgically Confirmed Complete Remissions (%)	
		<3-cm Residua	>3-cm Residua
Young[257]	Hexa-CAF	8/8 (100)	5/32 (16)
Louie[220]	CHEX-UP	5/14 (36)	5/37 (14)
Edmonson[279]	H-CAP	18/21 (86)	3/29 (11)
Parker[389]	AC	11/12 (92)	1/24 (4)
Erlich[271]	PAC	5/17 (30)	5/39 (13)
Hacker[390]	PAC/Hexa-CAF	6/22 (27)	1/17 (6)
	Total	53/94 (56)	20/178 (11)

* Abbreviations: see footnote of Table 39–13.

STAGES II, III, AND IV AND BULKY RESIDUAL DISEASE

Most stage III patients and some stage II patients are left with extensive residual disease after initial diagnosis and surgery. These patients respond poorly to conventional therapies of all types. The major challenge for the future lies in identifying successful therapy for this large group of women. In recent years, the mainstay of therapy for this group has been systemic chemotherapy, but some patients with unique presentations may be appropriately treated with radiation therapy. It is worthwhile to separate patients with gross abdominal tumors from those with only retroperitoneal lymph node metastases, because the latter group may have a different prognosis if treated with appropriate irradiation therapy. Hintz and colleagues observed that patients with retroperitoneal lymph nodes as the only site of extrapelvic disease have a survival rate of about 55% at 5 years, compared with 10% for patients with peritoneal spread.[212]

The prognosis of patients with gross abdominal tumors exceeding 2 cm in diameter has been poor after treatment with whole-abdominal irradiation. Even after aggressive radiotherapeutic approaches were used with radiation to the whole peritoneal cavity at maximal tolerable doses, the 5-year survival rates were 9% to 12%.[69,119,333] The tolerance of treatment by these patients has been extremely poor. Attempts to improve survival by additional treatment with single alkylating agent chemotherapy given before or after irradiation usually failed to improve survival and were even less well tolerated.[120,175,334–336] Postoperative whole-abdominal irradiation given as the primary modality with curative intent is not indicated for patients with large (>2 cm) abdominal tumors, unless effective cytoreductive surgery can be performed before radiation therapy, leaving the peritoneal cavity without gross disease or with minimal residual disease (<2 cm).

The lack of a satisfactory cure rate with irradiation or combination chemotherapy in patients with bulky disease and the frequent inability to cytoreduce the tumor at the initial laparotomy led to the introduction of combined-modality therapy. Combination chemotherapy is highly effective in debulking such tumors, resulting in significant clinical responses in 80% to 90% of patients. If second-look surgery is performed, the residual tumors found are often small, and their complete or near-complete resection can frequently be achieved. The elimination of minimal residual disease after induction therapy is being studied.[129]

Fuks and coworkers treated 38 patients with initial induction therapy, using 3 to 14 courses of CHAD combination chemotherapy for tumor mass reduction, and a second laparotomy for resection of residual tumors, followed by a consolidation phase with curative doses of whole-abdominal irradiation.[198] The initial rate of complete and partial clinical responses to CHAD was 91%. After second-look surgery, 76% of patients were without residual disease. Whole-abdominal irradiation, using the Martinez technique, was then given. The actuarial 5-year survival and disease-free survival rates for the irradiated group were 27% and 17%, respectively. These survival data are similar to those for patients treated with CHAP-5 combination chemotherapy without subsequent whole-abdominal irradiation.[128] These data suggest that the consolidation radiation therapy had little additional effect on long-term survival.

This observation is consistent with other reports. Hacker and associates treated 30 patients with a variety of combination protocols, followed by a second surgical tumor reduction and whole-abdominal radiation therapy.[187] Only 4 of 16 patients with completely resected tumors during the second laparotomy survived 22 to 41 months after radiation therapy. Hainsworth, using a similar approach after H-CAP or H-FAP combination chemotherapy, showed that 14 of 17 patients relapsed between 2 and 20 months after completion of radiation therapy.[337] Coltart and colleagues reported a 30% 3-year survival rate for 10 stage III patients treated with CP chemotherapy, second debulking surgery, and whole-abdominal irradiation.[197] Survival was poor, and by 37 months only 2 patients were disease free.

The probability of achieving a prolonged (>2 year) disease-free survival using postchemotherapy total-abdominal irradiation is low. The influence of the extent of residual disease is shown in Table 39–18.

TABLE 39–18. Patients Surviving 2 Years or Longer After Salvage Abdominal Irradiation for Disease Found at Second-Look Surgery

Investigations	Microscopic Disease	Residual Disease	
		<1 cm	>1 cm
Piver[194]	1/4	0/3	0/1
Hainsworth[191]	3/11	0/5	0/1
Kucera[391]	2/10	0/4	0/2
Hacker[187]	4/16	2/6	0/18
Hoskins[195]	0/1	0/6	0/1
Peters[196]	2/9	0/7	0/6
Menczer[392]	0/4		0/4
	12/55 (22%)*	2/31 (7%)*	0/33 (0%)*

* Total.

Other attempts to control the minimal residual disease remaining after initial induction chemotherapy have included intraperitoneal radioisotopes (primarily ^{32}P) and intraperitoneal chemotherapy.

MANAGEMENT OF STROMAL AND GERM CELL OVARIAN TUMORS

Although germ cell and stromal tumors of the ovary only make up about 5% to 10% of all ovarian tumors, they require separate discussion because of their unusual natural history and clinical manifestations. Different therapies are required for the various tumor types. These tumors are particularly important, because some of the most aggressive lesions are now curable with combination chemotherapy and conservative surgery. These tumors can be separated into three groups:

1. Tumors with ovarian stromal components, such as the granulosa cell and Sertoli-Leydig cell tumors
2. Tumors derived from germ cell elements, such as malignant teratoma embryonal carcinoma, endodermal sinus tumor, and dysgerminoma
3. Choriocarcinoma

OVARIAN STROMAL TUMORS

Ovarian stromal tumors comprise approximately 5% of all ovarian tumors, generally have an indolent natural history, and sometimes recur many years after initial therapy. They are sometimes associated with precocious feminization, and their association with unopposed estrogen secretion and an increased incidence of concomitant endometrial carcinoma (7.8%) has been well documented.[357] In a review of 51 patients, 43% of the tumors were theca, 24% were pure granulosa cell tumors, and 33% were mixed granulosa and theca cell tumors.[358] None of the patients with thecomas died as a result of their disease; deaths occurred only among patients having granulosa cell tumors with metastases.

Stromal tumors can be managed by unilateral salpingo-oophorectomy in young patients and rarely require additional therapy. The incidence of bilaterality is low. There are too few reported cases of stage II stromal tumors to make definitive recommendations, but the lack of effective adjuvant therapy makes more extensive surgery necessary for these patients. Factors such as tumor size, degree of differentiation, histologic patterns of the tumor, and tumor spillage are of prognostic importance. Because of their protracted natural history, it is difficult to document the value of postoperative irradiation. However, for tumors that are not completely resected, a dose of 5000 to 6000 cGy to the pelvis has been advocated. Experience with 37 patients at M.D. Anderson Cancer Center resulted in a 5-year survival rate of 75% for stage I and 50% to 60% for stages II and III.[138] Retrospective analyses of studies of stage I disease discerned no difference in survival between patients treated with irradiation or surgery alone.[359]

The role of chemotherapy in treating the granulosa-theca cell tumors has been poorly defined because so few patients have been studied. There are anecdotal reports of responses to alkylating agents and doxorubicin.[138,360,361] The polypeptide hormone inhibin may be a useful marker in granulosa cell tumors.[362]

Experience with 9 patients with Sertoli-Leydig cell tumors was reported from the M.D. Anderson Cancer Center. Two patients with recurrent lesions had a complete response after a combination of vincristine, dactinomycin, and cyclophosphamide.[138] The largest published study described 11 patients with granulosa cell tumors who were treated with cisplatin, vinblastine, and bleomycin (PVB regimen).[83] Six of the 11 had surgically confirmed complete remissions. Substantial drug toxicity was seen, but this combination merits additional study for treating stromal tumors in light of the paucity of activity seen with other regimens or with radiation therapy.

Recurrent stromal tumors are treated with surgical resection and postoperative irradiation if the residual tumor can be encompassed by external irradiation or by chemotherapy if the disease is extensive.

OVARIAN GERM CELL TUMORS

Ovarian germ cell tumors are rare, accounting for 2% to 3% of all ovarian cancers. These tumors may have a mixed histologic pattern, and treatment should be designed to address the most malignant component of the tumor. Before modern combination chemotherapy, malignant embryonal carcinoma, endodermal sinus tumors, and malignant teratomas had extremely poor prognoses with surgery alone, and long-term survival was achieved by only a small percentage of patients, even those with stage I disease.[363] The Ovarian Tumor Registry of the American Gynecological Society reported that 31 of 34 patients with endodermal sinus tumor were dead of disease after surgery alone, and the only 3 survivors had stage IA disease.[364] Gallion and coworkers reviewed the literature on 150 cases of pure endodermal sinus tumors.[365] Before the use of chemotherapy, the overall 2-year survival rate for patients with stage I disease was 27%, which did not differ from patients presenting with more advanced disease. Surgery alone was ineffective, producing a 16% 2-year survival rate. Even total abdominal hysterectomy and bilateral salpingo-oophorectomy for stage IA disease in one study produced only a 13% 2-year survival rate. Pelvic or total-abdominal irradiation added little to these 2-year survival figures.

Improved survival rates followed the observation that germ cell tumors are highly curable with combination chemotherapy. Surgery is now more limited.

For germ cell tumors confined to one ovary, unilateral salpingo-oophorectomy is the surgery of choice for the young patient. For germ cell tumors that have spread to pelvic structures other than the opposite ovary, fallopian tube, or uterus, complete tumor removal without total abdominal hysterectomy or removal of the uninvolved adnexa is appropriate. These patients can usually be cured with combination chemotherapy and preserve reproductive function.

ENDODERMAL SINUS TUMORS

Endodermal sinus tumors are unusual and aggressive tumors of germ cell origin. They reproduce the extraembryonic structures of the early embryo. The tumor is rarely bilateral. Before the use of combination chemotherapy, the tumor was almost invariably fatal.

The general consensus is that all patients, regardless of stage, should receive chemotherapy. The earliest effective regimen reported was vincristine, dactinomycin, and cyclophosphamide (VAC). Cangir and coworkers described 21 patients (*i.e.*, 8 malignant teratomas, 6 endodermal sinus tumors, 6 mixed germ cell tumors, and 1 Sertoli-Leydig tumor).[366] Fourteen of the 21 patients who had a second-look operation after chemotherapy showed no evidence of disease. They concluded that surgical resection followed by adjuvant VAC was the therapy of choice. They felt that irradiation had no role in the initial management of these patients. Slayton and colleagues summarized the GOG with VAC in aggressive germ cell tumors.[367] Seventy-six patients were treated with VAC postoperatively, including 54 who were disease free after surgery. Thirty-nine (72%) of 54 patients remain disease free. The best results were seen in patients with immature (*i.e.*, grade II and III) teratomas; 19 of 20 remained disease free. Results were not as good for patients with significant residual disease; 7 (32%) of 22 were disease free after VAC chemotherapy.

Reports indicate that PVB is at least as good and may be better than VAC. Collected experience from published series indicate that 53 (87%) of 61 PVB-treated patients are alive without evidence of disease.[368-370] A combination of cisplatin, VP-16, and bleomycin (PEB) was used by the Royal Marsden group for treating 9 patients (6 with stage III or IV disease).[369] Eight of the 9 are disease free at 6 to 62+ months. Although no randomized trials exist comparing VAC with PVB or PEB, it is likely that the latter two regimens are preferred therapy for endodermal sinus tumors.

MALIGNANT TERATOMA

Malignant teratoma of the ovary is a rare but lethal germ cell tumor. Over half of the presenting patients are younger than 20. The tumor is rarely bilateral. Prognosis seems to be related to the histologic grade of the tumor.[371] Before the use of combination chemotherapy, patients were managed with aggressive surgery followed by irradiation or single-agent chemotherapy, but few survived. Combination chemotherapy with VAC or one of the other regimens previously mentioned is now the therapy of choice for these tumors. Preliminary re-

sults from a GOG trial indicate that 50 of 52 stage I, II, and III patients with completely resected disease are disease free after three cycles of BEP.[372]

DYSGERMINOMA

Dysgerminomas comprise about 2% of all ovarian malignancies, and they are unique among the germ cell tumors because of the high cure rate and sensitivity to radiation therapy. They are the only ovarian germ cell malignancy that occurs bilaterally with significant frequency. Although these tumors are the counterpart of testicular seminoma in males, they are much rarer. They are bilateral in approximately 10% of patients. If confined to the ovary, these tumors can be cured with limited surgery. Although sensitive to modest doses of radiation, many are now managed with combination chemotherapy.

At initial surgery, the contralateral ovary should be carefully examined. If there is any question of disease, the ovary should be bivalved, and wedge biopsies should be obtained for frozen section. If the tumor is localized to one ovary, a unilateral salpingo-oophorectomy should be performed, but a full staging operation should be done, and the pelvic and paraaortic nodes should be sampled. If the tumor is localized to one ovary, there is no disruption of the capsule, and there are no elements of other malignant germ cell types, no postoperative therapy is indicated. If dysgerminoma involves both ovaries, bilateral salpingo-oophorectomy and a full staging operation should be carried out. Unless involved by cancer, the uterus should not be removed because in vitro fertilization with a donor ovum may allow the woman to carry a pregnancy. Metastatic disease demands complete cytoreductive surgery.

Typical early results for 36 patients with pure dysgerminoma were reported.[373] Sixty-one percent of the patients had stage I disease, and 34% had advanced disease (*i.e.*, FIGO stages III and IV). In 5 patients with stage IA disease treated only with unilateral salpingo-oophorectomy, there were no recurrences. All patients are alive 3 to 20 years after initial treatment, and 3 have had children. Management of the other patients was with aggressive debulking surgery followed by total-abdominal irradiation. Lymphangiography was used to assess disease in the paraaortic nodes. The overall survival rate for the entire group of patients was 86%.

De Palo and associates recommend radiation therapy for all patients with stages I, II, or III disease.[374] For stage IA lesions, irradiation is given as adjuvant therapy; for stages I and II, they recommend radiation therapy to the ipsilateral hemipelvis (with shielding of the contralateral ovary and head of the femur) and paraaortic nodes to doses of 2500 to 3000 cGy. The upper limit of the field is at T10–T11 (Fig. 39–7). For stage III retroperitoneal disease found at surgery, they recommend radiation therapy as for stage I and additional elective treatment to the mediastinal and supraclavicular lymph nodes. If there is peritoneal involvement, the whole abdomen and pelvic, mediastinal, and supraclavicular nodes are irradiated to a dose of 2500 to 3000 cGy (750–900 cGy/week). In curative irradiation, 3500 to 4000 cGy is given; a boost of 1000 cGy is delivered to involved nodes. When irradiating above the diaphragm, 3000 cGy in 3 to 4 weeks is administered after completion of irradiation below the diaphragm. When the entire abdominal cavity is irradiated, the

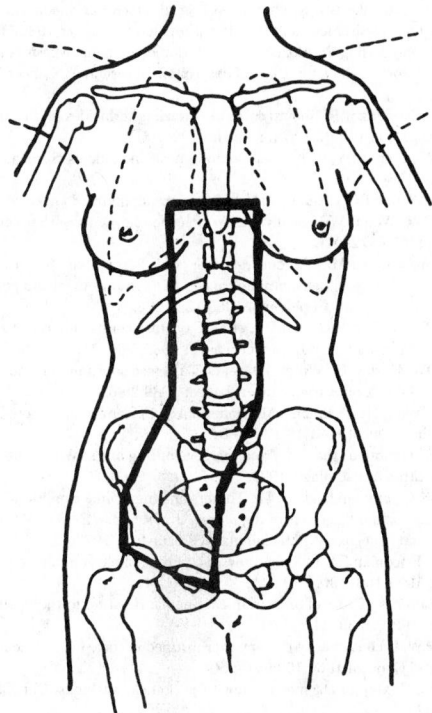

FIGURE 39–7. Ipsilateral and hemipelvic field for irradiation of dysgerminoma. (Horowitz CJ, Brady LW. Ovary. In: Perez CA, Brady LW, eds. Principles and practice of radiation oncology. 2nd ed. Philadelphia: JB Lippincott, 1992)

fields are similar to those used for epithelial tumors.[375] The kidneys are shielded after 1800 cGy. Lawson and Adler reported giving 3000 cGy (1000 cGy/week) to pelvic and paraaortic fields.[376] Only 2 patients were treated with whole-abdomen irradiation, one with the moving-strip technique and 1 with open fields. The patient treated with the moving-strip technique received 2250 cGy to the whole abdomen and 4500 cGy to the pelvis.

De Palo and associates reported 100% overall 5-year survival and 90% recurrence-free 5-year survival rates for 31 patients with stages IA, IB, and IC disease.[374] At 4 years, the overall survival rate was 80%, and the recurrence-free survival rate was 57% for stage III patients. Lawson and Adler reported 10 of 14 stage I through III patients alive with a median follow-up of 54 months.[376] In this small series, there was no correlation between survival and the stage of the disease at presentation or the size of the primary tumor found at laparotomy. Similar results have been reported from the Radiumhemmet Institute.[378] Of 56 patients treated with radiation therapy, the overall 5-year survival rate was 75%, with 36% of the patients developing recurrences. The extent of the tumor was a critical factor in determining survival and recurrences. In 40 patients treated at the Radiumhemmet, there were 13 recurrences, and 8 of these patients survived for 5 years or more after the beginning of therapy.

Asadourian and Taylor reported recurrences or metastasis in 23 (24%) of 105 patients; additional therapy resulted in the cure of 10 of these patients.[379] There was a 96% 5-year actuarial survival rate for 78 patients with tumor localized to one or both ovaries, compared with a rate of 63% for 17 pa-

tients with extraovarian extension. There were 18 pregnancies after treatment in 10 patients. Fifteen of the babies were normal, and 1 was malformed. There were 2 abortions, 1 therapeutic and 1 spontaneous.

Recurrent disease can be surgically resected and subsequently treated with radiation therapy or chemotherapy. Eighty percent of recurrences appear within 2 years of the initial surgery, and 75% occur within the first year. The abdomen and pelvis are the most frequent sites of failure, followed by the paraaortic and supraclavicular nodes.[377]

Although there is no question that dysgerminomas are quite sensitive to radiation therapy and that cure rates are high with this type of therapy, these young patients are almost always rendered sterile and lose ovarian function after abdominal irradiation. This fact and the excellent results with chemotherapy in male seminomas led investigators to evaluate chemotherapy in women with dysgerminomas. Williams and co-workers reported the GOG experience with chemotherapy for dysgerminomas.[380] They reported 18 patients with stage III or IV tumors, all of whom had more than 2 cm of residual disease. Using vinblastine, bleomycin, and cisplatin or etoposide, bleomycin, and cisplatin, 17 of 18 of the high-risk patients were free of disease 9 to 66 months after therapy. The GOG is evaluating carboplatin and etoposide as primary therapy in patients with stages II, III, or IV dysgerminoma. The Royal Marsden group treated 7 patients with stages III or IV dysgerminoma using cisplatin, vinblastine, and bleomycin (4 had failed irradiation). All 7 had complete responses, and 6 of the 7 were free of disease for more than 1 year.

Chemotherapy with a platinum-based regimen is the treatment of choice for dysgerminoma. Radiation therapy should be reserved for those rare patients with persistent disease after chemotherapy.

OVARIAN CHORIOCARCINOMA

Ovarian choriocarcinoma is extremely rare, accounting for fewer than 1% of ovarian tumors. Chemotherapy, as for trophoblastic lesions, has been the treatment of choice.[381] The prognosis, however, is extremely poor. Rutledge reported a few patients responding to a combination of methotrexate, dactinomycin, and cyclophosphamide (MAC regimen).[382] Fanning and associates reported successful treatment of patients with stage III mixed germ cell tumor with pure choriocarcinoma in the paraaortic nodes.[383] The patient was treated with alternating sequences of VAC and PVB, and at 30 months, she was free of disease. The researchers stated that this is the first reported long-term survival of a patient with pure choriocarcinoma metastases.

OVARIAN CARCINOMA
ASSOCIATED WITH PREGNANCY

Although unusual, ovarian carcinoma does occur during pregnancy.[384] Palpation of an adnexal mass during the first trimester of pregnancy without other evidence of malignancy should be managed by close follow-up with pelvic examinations and ultrasound. A persistent corpus luteum cyst usually resolves spontaneously, and surgical exploration for an asymptomatic mass is best carried out during the second trimester. Although most adnexal masses in pregnancy are benign, a persistent mass should be removed. Creasman and colleagues reported 17 patients with ovarian carcinoma managed at M.D. Anderson Cancer Center who were pregnant or were within 6 months of delivery at the time of diagnosis.[385] One third of the patients were diagnosed at delivery.

Hess and associates reported 54 patients who underwent surgical exploration during pregnancy because of an adnexal mass.[386] The incidence of adnexal masses that require surgery during pregnancy is 1 per 1300 live births. In this report, the masses were malignant ovarian tumors in 5.9% of patients. The investigators reported an increased incidence of premature delivery or abortion among patients who had emergency operations because of torsion or rupture of the mass. They recommended elective surgical removal of the mass during the second trimester of pregnancy.

Unless there is spread outside of the ovary, unilateral salpingo-oophorectomy and a full staging operation constitute recommended treatment. If the carcinoma has spread beyond the ovary, a full staging and debulking operation should be performed, although hysterectomy with sacrifice of the fetus should be undertaken only if necessary to debulk the tumor. Postoperative chemotherapy should be administered as indicated by the stage, cell type, and grade of the tumor, because most chemotherapeutic agents useful in ovarian cancer can be administered during pregnancy without known adverse effects on the fetus.

REFERENCES

1. Boring CC, Squires TS, Tong T. Cancer statistics, 1992. CA 1992;42:19–38.
2. Doll R, Muir C, Waterhouse J. International Union Against Cancer. Cancer incidence in five continents. Berlin: Springer-Verlag, 1970.
3. Buell P, Dunn JE. Cancer mortality among Japanese Issei and Nisei of California. Cancer 1965;18:656–664.
4. Haenszel W, Kurihara M. Studies of Japanese migrants. I. Mortality from cancer and other diseases among Japanese in the United States. JNCI 1968;40:43–68.
5. Joly DJ, Lilienfeld AM, Diamond EL, Bross ID. An epidemiologic study of the relationship of reproductive experience to cancer of the ovary. Am J Epidemiol 1974;99:190–209.
6. Beral V, Fraser P, Chilvers C. Does pregnancy protect against ovarian cancer? Lancet 1978;1:1083–1087.
7. Lingeman CH. Etiology of cancer of the human ovary: A review. JNCI 1974;53:1603–1618.
8. Greene MH, Clark JW, Blayney DW. The epidemiology of ovarian cancer. Semin Oncol 1984;11:209–226.
9. Hoover R, Gray LA, Fraumeni JF. Stilbestrol and the risk of ovarian cancer. Lancet 1977;2:1083–1086.
10. Cancer and Steroid Hormone Study of the Centers for Disease Control and the National Institute of Child Health and Development. The reduction in risk of ovarian cancer associated with oral contraceptive use. N Engl J Med 1987;316:650–655.
11. Hartge P, Schiffman MH, Hoover R, McGowan L, Lesher L, Norris HJ. A case-controlled study of epithelial ovarian cancer. Am J Obstet Gynecol 1989;161:10–16.
12. Cramer DW, Hutchinson GE, Welch WR, Scully RE, Knapp RC. Factors affecting the association of oral contraceptives and ovarian cancer. N Engl J Med 1982;307:1047–1051.
13. World Health Organization. The World Health Organization collaborative study of neoplasia and steroid contraceptives: Epithelial ovarian cancer and combined oral contraceptives. Int J Epidemiol 1989;18:538–545.
14. Schweisguth O, Gerard MR, Plainfosse B, Lemerle J, Watchi JM, Seringe P. Bilateral nonfunctioning thecoma of the ovary in epileptic children under anticonvulsant therapy. Acta Paediatr Scand 1971;60:6–10.
15. West RO. Epidemiologic study of malignancies of the ovaries. Cancer 1966;19:1001–1007.
16. Fraumeni JJ, Grundy GW, Creagan ET, Everson RB. Six families prone to ovarian cancer. Cancer 1975;36:364–369.
17. Koch M, Gaedke H, Jenkins H. Family history of ovarian cancer patients: A case-control study. Int J Epidemiol 1989;18:782.
18. Schildkraut JM, Thompson WD. Familial ovarian cancer: A population-based case-control study. Am J Epidemiol 1988;128:456.
19. Lynch HT, Bewtra C, Lynch JF. Familial ovarian carcinoma. Am J Med 1986;81:1073–1076.
20. Lynch HT, Fitzscommons ML, Conway TA, Bewtra C, Lynch J. Hereditary carcinoma of the ovary and associated cancers: A study of two families. Gynecol Oncol 1990;36:48–55.
21. Lynch HT, Scheulke GS, Kimberlins WJ, et al. Hereditary neopolyposis colorectal cancer (Lynch syndromes I and II): Biomarker studies. Cancer 1985;56:939–951.
22. Lynch HT, Kimberling W, Albano WA, et al. Hereditary nonpolyposis colorectal cancer (Lynch syndrome I and II): I. Clinical description of resources. Cancer 1985;56:934–938.
23. Donna A, Crosignani P, Robutti F, et al. Triazine herbicides and ovarian epithelial neoplasms. Scand J Work Environ Health 1989;15:47.
24. Hueper WC, Conway WD. Chemical carcinogenesis and cancers. Springfield, IL: Charles C Thomas, 1964.
25. Longo DL, Young RC. Cosmetic talc and ovarian carcinoma. Lancet 1979;2:349–351.
26. Cramer DW, Welch WR, Scully RE, Wojciechowski CA. Ovarian cancer and talc. Cancer 1982;50:372–376.
27. Whittemore AS, Wu ML, Paffenbarger RS, et al. Personal and environmental characteristics related to epithelial ovarian cancer. II. Exposures to talcum powder, tobacco, alcohol and coffee. Am J Epidemiol 1988;128:1228.
28. Cramer DW, Willett WC, Bell DA, et al. Galactose consumption and metabolism in relation to the risk of ovarian cancer. Lancet 1989;2:66–71.
29. Cramer DW, Harlow BI, Willett WC, et al. Galactose consumption and metabolism in relation to the risk of ovarian cancer. Lancet 1989;2:66.
30. Piver MS, Baker TR, Piedmonte M, Sandecki AM. Epidemiology and etiology of ovarian cancer. Semin Oncol 1991;18:177–185.
31. Scully RE. Tumors of the ovary and maldeveloped gonads. Washington, DC: Armed Forces Institute of Pathology, 1979.
32. Janovski NA, Paramandandhan TL. Tumors and tumor-like conditions of the ovaries, fallopian tubes, and ligaments of the uterus. In: Friedman EA, ed. Major problems in obstetrics and gynecology. Philadelphia: WB Saunders, 1973:12.
33. Plentl AA, Friedman EA. Lymphatic system of the female genitalia. Philadelphia: WB Saunders, 1973:168–180.
34. Fuks Z. Patterns of spread of ovarian carcinoma: Relation to therapeutic strategies. Adv Biosci 1980;26:39–51.
35. Munnell EW. Is conservative therapy ever justified in stage I (Ia) cancer of the ovary? Am J Obstet Gynecol 1969;103:641–650.
36. Keettel WC, Pixley E. Diagnostic value of peritoneal washings. Clin Obstet Gynecol 1958;1:592.
37. Joffey JM, Courtice FC. Lymphatics, lymph and lymphoid complexes. New York: Academic Press, 1970:295–305.
38. Feldman GB, Knapp RC. Lymphatic drainage of the peritoneal cavity and its significance in ovarian cancer. Am J Obstet Gynecol 1974;119:991–994.
39. Meyers MA. The spread and localization of acute intraperitoneal effusions. Radiology 1970;95:547–554.
40. Dyre JC. Intraperitoneal pressure in the human. Surg Gynecol Obstet 1948;87:472.
41. French JE, Florey HW, Morris BL. The absorption of particles by the lymphatics of the diaphragm. Q J Exp Biol 1960;45:88–103.
42. Coates G, Bush RS, Aspin N. A study of ascites using lymphoscintigraphy with ^{99m}Tc-sulfur colloid. Radiology 1973;107:577–583.
43. Bagley CM, Young RC, Schein PS, Chabner BA, DeVita VT. Ovarian carcinoma metastatic to the diaphragm: Frequently undiagnosed at laparotomy. J Obstet Gynecol 1973;116:397–400.
44. Rosenoff SH, DeVita VT, Hubbard S, Young RC. Peritoneoscopy in the staging and follow-up of ovarian cancer. Semin Oncol 1975;2:223–228.
45. Piver MS, Barlow JJ, Lele SB. Incidence of subclinical metastasis in stage I and II ovarian carcinoma. Obstet Gynecol 1978;52:100–104.
46. Feldman GB, Knapp RC, Order SE, Hellman S. The role of lymphatic obstruction in the formation of ascites in a murine ovarian carcinoma. Cancer Res 1972;32:1663–1666.
47. Fisher RI, Young RC. Advances in the staging and treatment of ovarian cancer. Cancer 1977;39:967.
48. Steinberg JJ, Demopoulos RI, Bigelow B. The evaluation of the omentum in ovarian cancer. Gynecol Oncol 1975;2:253.
49. Eichner E, Bove ER. In vivo studies on the lymphatic drainage of the human ovary. Obstet Gynecol 1954;3:287–297.
50. Fuks Z. External radiotherapy of ovarian cancer: Standard approaches and new frontiers. Semin Oncol 1975;2:253–266.
51. Musumeci R, De Palo G, Kenda R, Tesoro-Tess JD, et al. Retroperitoneal metastases from ovarian carcinoma: Reassessment of 365 patients studied with lymphography. AJR 1980;134:449–452.
52. Fuks Z. Patterns of spread of ovarian carcinoma: Relation to therapeutic strategies. In: Newman CE, Ford CH, Jordan JA, eds. Ovarian cancer. Oxford: Pergamon Press, 1980.
53. Burghardt E, Pickel H, Stettner H. Management of advanced ovarian cancer. Eur J Gynaecol Oncol 1984;3:155.
54. Wu PC, Lang JH, Huang RL, et al. Lymph node metastasis and retroperitoneal lymphadenectomy in ovarian cancer. Baillieres Clin Obstet Gynaecol 1989;3:143–155.
55. Buchsbaum HJ, Delgado G, Blessing J, et al. Surgical staging of ovarian carcinoma. Gynecol Oncol 1986;23:253.
56. Rubin SC, Hoskins WJ, Hakes TB, et al. Recurrence following negative second-look laparotomy for ovarian cancer: Analysis of risk factors. Am J Obstet Gynecol 1988;159:1094.
57. Scully RE. Recent progress in ovarian cancer. Hum Pathol 1970;1:73–98.
58. Novak ER, Woodruff JD. Novak's gynecologic and obstetric pathology. Philadelphia: WB Saunders, 1974.
59. Serov SF, Scully RE, Solvin LH. International histologic classification of tumors. Geneva: World Health Organization, 1973.

60. FIGO. Classification and staging of malignant tumors in the female pelvis. Acta Obstet Gynaecol Scand 1971;50:1–7.

61. Scully RE. Ovarian tumors. Am J Pathol 1977;87:686–720.

62. Nikrui N. Survey of clinical behavior of patients with borderline tumors of the ovary. Gynecol Oncol 1981;12:107–119.

63. Bjorkholm E, Petterson F, Einhorn N, et al. Long term follow-up and prognostic factors in ovarian carcinoma: The Radiumhemmet series, 1953–1973. Acta Rad Oncol 1982;21: 413–419.

64. Fort MG, Pierce VK, Saigo PE, Hoskins WJ, Lewis JLJ. Evidence for the efficacy of adjuvant therapy in epithelial ovarian tumors of low malignant potential. Gynecol Oncol 1989;32:269.

65. Bell DA, Weinstock MA, Scully RE. Peritoneal implants of ovarian serous borderline tumors: Histologic features and prognosis. Cancer 1988;62:2212–2222.

66. Gershenson DM, Silva FG. Serous ovarian tumors of low malignant potential with peritoneal implants. Cancer 1990;65:578–585.

67. Michael H, Roth LM. Invasive and noninvasive implants in ovarian serous tumors of low malignant potential. Cancer 1986;57:1240–1247.

68. Brescia RJ, Barakat RA, Beller U, et al. The prognostic significance of nuclear DNA content in malignant epithelial tumors of the ovary. Cancer 1990;65:141.

69. Aure JC, Hoeg K, Kolstad P. Clinical and histologic studies of ovarian carcinoma: Long-term follow-up of 900 cases. Obstet Gynecol 1971;37:1–9.

70. Perez CA, Walz BZ, Jacobson PL. Radiation therapy in the management of carcinoma of the ovary. NCI Monogr 1975;42:119–125.

71. Young RC, Hubbard SP, DeVita VT. The chemotherapy of ovarian carcinoma. Cancer Treat Rev 1974;1:99–110.

72. Smith JP, Rutledge F, Wharton JT. Chemotherapy of ovarian cancer: New approaches to treatment. Cancer 1972;30:1565–1571.

73. Young RC, Walton LA, Ellenberg SS, et al. Adjuvant therapy in stage I and stage II epithelial ovarian cancer: Results of two prospective randomized trials. N Engl J Med 1990;322:1021–1027.

74. Jenison EL, Montag AG, Griffiths CT, et al. Clear cell adenocarcinoma of the ovary: A clinical analysis and comparison with serous carcinoma. Gynecol Oncol 1989;32: 65.

75. Munnell EW, Taylor HC. Ovarian carcinoma: A review of 200 primary and 51 secondary cases. Am J Obstet 1949;58:943.

76. Decker DG, Mussey E, Williams TJ. Grading of gynecologic malignancy. Philadelphia: JB Lippincott, 1972:223–231.

77. Day TG, Gallager HS, Rutledge F. Epithelial carcinoma of the ovary: Prognostic importance of histologic grade. NCI Monogr 1975;42:15–18.

78. Ozols RF, Garvin WJ, Costa J, et al. Advanced ovarian cancer: Correlation of histologic grade with response to therapy and survival. Cancer 1980;45:572–581.

79. Dembo AJ, Bush RS. Choice of postoperative therapy based on prognostic factors. Int J Radiat Oncol Biol Phys 1982;8:893–897.

80. Scully RE. World Health Organization classification and nomenclature of ovarian cancer. NCI Monogr 1975;42:5–7.

81. Young RH, Clement PB, Scully RD. The ovary. In Sternberg SS, Antonioli DA, Carter D, et al, eds. Diagnostic surgical pathology. New York: Raven Press, 1989:1655.

82. Clement PB. Histology of the ovary. Am J Surg Pathol 1987;11:277.

83. Colombo N, Sessa C, Landoni F, et al. Cisplatin, vinblastine, and bleomycin combination chemotherapy in metastatic granulosa cell tumor of the ovary. Obstet Gynecol 1986;67: 265.

84. Hoskins WJ, Rubin SC. Malignant gonadal stromal tumors of the ovary: Clinical features and management. In: Coppleson M, Monaghan JM, Morrow CP, Tattersall MHN, eds. Gynecologic oncology. London: Churchill Livingstone, 1991.

85. Williams SD, Blessing JA, Hatch KD, Homesley HD. Chemotherapy of advanced dysgerminoma: Trials of the Gynecologic Oncology Group. J Clin Oncol 1991;9:1950–1955.

86. Sall S, Stone ML. The treatment of ovarian cancer. Prog Clin Cancer 1973;5:249.

87. Kent SN, McKay DG. Primary cancer of the ovary. Am J Obstet Gynecol 1960;80: 430–438.

88. Pearse WH, Behrman SJ. Carcinoma of the ovary. Obstet Gynecol 1954;3:32–45.

89. Barber HRK, Graber EA. The PMPO syndrome. Obstet Gynecol 1971;38:921.

90. Flynt JR, Gallup DG. The postmenopausal palpable ovary syndrome: A 14-year review. Milit Med 1981;146:666–686.

91. Bolandgray A, Mehellati KA, Ardekany MS. Early detection of ovarian malignancy by culdocentesis. J Reprod Med 1971;9:32.

92. Rubin SC, Dulaney ED, Markman M, Hoskins WJ, Saigo PE, Lewis JL Jr. Peritoneal cytology as an indicator of disease in patients with residual ovarian carcinoma. Obstet Gynecol 1988;71:851.

93. Samuels BI. Usefulness of ultrasound in patients with ovarian cancer. Semin Oncol 1975;2:229–233.

94. Berkowitz RS, Leavitt, TJ, Knapp RC. Ultrasound directed percutaneous aspiration biopsy of periaortic lymph nodes in cervical carcinoma recurrence. Am J Obstet Gynecol 1978;131:906–908.

95. Higgins RV, van Nagell JR, Donaldson ES, et al. Transvaginal sonography as a screening method for ovarian cancer. Gynecol Oncol 1989;34:402.

96. Van Nagell JR, Higgins RV, Donaldson ES, et al. Transvaginal sonography as a screening method for ovarian cancer. A report of the first 1000 cases screened. Cancer 1990;65: 573.

97. Bourne T, Campbell S, Steer C, et al. Transvaginal colour flow imaging: A possible new screening technique for ovarian cancer. Br Med J 1989;299:1367.

98. Parker BR, Castellina RA, Fuks ZY, Bagshaw MA. The role of lymphography in patients with ovarian cancer. Cancer 1974;34:100–105.

99. Schaner EG, Head GL, Kalman MA, et al. Whole body computed tomography in the diagnosis of abdominal and thoracic malignancy: Review of 600 cases. Cancer Treat Rep 1977;61:1537–1560.

100. Kurman RJ, Norris HJ. Endodermal sinus tumor of the ovary: A clinical and pathologic analysis of 71 cases. Cancer 1976;38:2404–2419.

101. Goldstein DP, Piro AJ. Combination chemotherapy in the treatment of germ cell tumors containing choriocarcinoma in males and females. Surg Gynecol Obstet 1971;134: 61–66.

102. Di Saia PJ, Morrow CP, Haverback BJ, Dyce BJ. Carcinoembryonic antigen in cancer of the female reproductive system: Serial plasma values correlated with disease state. Cancer 1977;39:2365–2370.

103. Bast RC, Klug TL, St. John E, et al. A radioimmunoassay using a monoclonal antibody to monitor the course of epithelial ovarian cancer. N Engl J Med 1983;309:883–887.

104. Zurawski VR, Broderick SF, Pickens P, et al. Serum CA-125 levels in a group of non-hospitalized women. Relevance for the early detection of ovarian cancer. Obstet Gynecol 1987;69:606.

105. Einhorn N, Sjovall K, Schoenfeld DA, et al. Prospective evaluation of the specificity of serum CA-125 levels for detection of ovarian cancer in a normal population. Am Soc Clin Oncol 1990;9:157.

106. Jacobs I, Bridges J, Reynolds C, et al. Multimodal approach to screening for ovarian cancer. Lancet 1988;2:268–271.

107. Van Nagell JR, De Priest PD. Early diagnosis of ovarian cancer. In: Markman M, Hoskins WJ, eds. Cancer of the ovary. New York: Raven Press, (in press).

108. Niloff JS, Bast RC Jr, Schaetzl EM, Knapp RC. Predictive values of CA-125 antigen levels in second-look procedures for ovarian cancer. Am J Obstet Gynecol 1985;151: 981.

109. Berek JS, Knapp RC, Malkasian GD, et al. CA-125 levels correlated with second-look operations among ovarian cancer patients. Obstet Gynecol 1986;67:685.

110. Atack DB, Nisker JA, Allen HH, Tustanoff ER, Levin L. CA-125 surveillance and second-look laparotomy in ovarian cancer. Am J Obstet Gynecol 1986;154:287.

111. Khoo SK, Hurst T, Webb MJ, Dickie GJ, Kemsky JH, Mackay EV. Predictive value of serial CA-125 antigen levels in ovarian cancer evaluated by second-look laparotomy. Eur J Cancer Clin Oncol 1987;23:765.

112. Mogensen O, Mogensen B, Jakobsen A, SE11: Measurement of the ovarian cancer-associated antigen CA-125 prior to second-look operation. Eur J Cancer Clin Oncol 1988;24:1835.

113. Vergote IB, Bormer OP, Abeler VM. Evaluation of serum CA 125 levels in the monitoring of ovarian cancer. Am J Obstet Gynecol 1987;157:88.

114. Rome RM, Koh H, Fortune D, Cauchi M. CA 125 serum levels and secondary laparotomy in epithelial ovarian tumors. Aust N Z J Obstet Gynaecol 1987;27:142.

115. Rubin SC, Hoskins WJ, Hakes TB, Markman M, Reichman BS, Chapman D, Lewis JL Jr. Serum CA 125 levels and surgical findings in patients undergoing secondary operations for epithelial ovarian cancer. Am J Obstet Gynecol 1989;160:667.

116. Podczaski E, Whitney C, Manetta A, Larson JE, Kirk J, Stevens CW, Lytes J, Mortel R. Use of CA 125 to monitor patients with ovarian epithelial carcinomas. Gynecol Oncol 1989;33:193.

117. Hoskins WJ, McGuire WP, Brady MS, Homesley HD, Clarke-Pearson DL. Serum CA 125 for prediction of progression in advanced epithelial ovarian carcinoma (AOC). Cairnes, Australia: International Gynecologic Cancer Society, 1991.

118. FIGO. Changes in definitions of clinical staging for carcinoma of the cervix and ovary. Am J Obstet Gynecol 1987;156:236.

119. Munnell EW. The changing prognosis and treatment in cancer of the ovary: A report of 235 patients with primary ovarian carcinoma 1952–1961. Am J Obstet Gynecol 1968;100:790.

120. Delclos L, Quinlan EJ. Malignant tumors of the ovary managed with postoperative megavoltage irradiation. Radiology 1969;93:659.

121. Griffiths CT. Surgical resection of tumor bulk in the primary treatment of ovarian carcinoma. NCI Monogr 1975;42:101.

122. Hacker NF, Berek, JS, Lagasse LD, et al. Primary cytoreductive surgery for epithelial ovarian cancer. Obstet Gynecol 1983;61:413.

123. Vogl SE, Pagano M, Kaplan BH, et al. Cisplatin based combination chemotherapy for advanced ovarian cancer: High overall response rate with curative potential only in women with small tumor burdens. Cancer 1983;51:2024.

124. Pohl R, Dallenback-Hellweg G, Plugge T, et al. Prognostic parameters in patients with advanced malignant ovarian tumors. Eur J Gynaecol Oncol 1984;3:160.

125. Delgado G, Oram DH, Petrilli ES. Stage III ovarian cancer: The role of maximal surgical reduction. Gynecol Oncol 1984;18:293.

126. Piver MS, Lele SB, Marchetti DL, et al. The impact of aggressive debulking surgery and cisplatin chemotherapy on progression-free survival in stage III and IV ovarian carcinoma. J Clin Obstet Gynecol 1988;6:983.

127. Omura GA, Bundy RN, Berek JS, Curry S, Delgado G, Mortel R. Randomized trial of cyclophosphamide plus cisplatin with or without doxorubicin in ovarian carcinoma: A Gynecologic Oncology Group study. J Clin Oncol 1989;7:457.

128. Neijt JP, Huinink TB, van der Burg MEL, et al. Long-term survival in ovarian cancer. Eur J Cancer 1991;27:1367–1372.

129. Fuks Z, Rizel S, Anteby SO, et al. The multimodal approach to the treatment of stage IV ovarian carcinoma. Int J Radiat Oncol Biol Phys 1982;8:903.

130. Dembo AJ. Radiotherapeutic management of ovarian cancer. Semin Oncol 1984;2: 238–250.

131. Chen SS, Bochner R. Assessment of morbidity and mortality in primary cytoreductive surgery for advanced ovarian cancer. Gynecol Oncol 1985;20:190.

132. Blythe JG, Wahl TP. Debulking surgery: Does it increase the quality of survival? Gynecol Oncol 1982;14:396.

133. Hoskins WJ, Bundy BN, Thigpen JT, Omura GA. The influence of initial surgery on

progression-free interval (PFI) and survival (S) in optimal (<1cm) stage III epithelial ovarian cancer (EOC). Gynecol Oncol (in press).

134. Ozols RF, Fisher RI, Anderson T, Makuch R, Young RC. Peritoneoscopy in the management of ovarian cancer. Am J Obstet Gynecol 1981;140:611–619.

135. Berek JS, Griffiths CT, Leventhal JM. Laparoscopy for second-look evaluation in ovarian cancer. Obstet Gynecol 1981;58:192–198.

136. Wangenstein OH, Lewis FJ, Tongen L. The "second look" in cancer surgery. Lancet 1951;71:303.

137. Smith JP, Rutledge F. Chemotherapy in the treatment of cancer of the ovary. Obstet Gynecol 1970;107:691.

138. Smith JP, Delgado G, Rutledge F. Second look operation in ovarian cancer. Cancer 1976;38:1438.

139. Greco FA, Julian CG, Richardson RL, et al. Advanced ovarian cancer: Brief intensive combination chemotherapy and second look operation. Obstet Gynecol 1981;58:199.

140. Berek JS, Hocha NF, Lagasse LD, et al. Second look laparotomy in stage III epithelial ovarian cancer: Clinical variables associated with disease status. Obstet Gynecol 1981;64:14.

141. Hakes T, Hoskins W, Jones W, Markman M, et al. Randomized prospective trial of 5 versus 10 cycles of cyclophosphamide, doxorubicin and cisplatin (CAP) in stage III and IV ovarian carcinoma. Proc Am Soc Clin Oncol 1990;9:156.

142. Bertelsen K, Jakobsen A, Kern M, et al. A randomized trial of six cycles versus twelve cycles of cyclophosphamide, Adriamycin and cisplatin (CAP) in advanced ovarian cancer. Proc Am Soc Clin Oncol 1989;8:150.

143. Rubin SR, Lewis JLJ. Second look surgery in ovarian carcinoma. Crit Rev Oncol Hemat 1988;8:75.

144. Smirz LR, Stehman FB, Ulbright TM, et al. Second look laparotomy after chemotherapy in the management of ovarian malignancy. Am J Obstet Gynecol 1985;152:661.

145. Podratz KC, Malkasian GDJ, Hilton JF, et al. Second look laparotomy in ovarian cancer: Evaluation of pathologic variables. Am J Obstet Gynecol 1983;192:230.

146. Ballon SC, Protnuf JC, Sikic BI, et al. Second look laparotomy in ovarian carcinoma: Precise definition, sensitivity, and specificity of the operative procedure. Gynecol Oncol 1984;17:154.

147. Schwartz PE, Smith JP. Second-look operations in ovarian cancer. Am J Obstet Gynecol 1980;138:1124–1130.

148. Berek JS, Hacker NF, Lagasse LD, et al. Second look laparotomy in stage III epithelial ovarian cancer: Clinical variables associated with disease status. Obstet Gynecol 1984;64:207.

149. Creasman WT, Aba-Ghazaleh S, Schmidt HJ. Retroperitoneal metastatic spread of ovarian carcinoma. Gynecol Oncol 1978;6:447.

150. Berek JS, Hacker NF, Lagasse LD, et al. Survival of patients following secondary cytoreductive surgery in ovarian cancer. Obstet Gynecol 1983;61:189.

151. Hoskins WJ, Rubin SC, Dulaney E, et al. Influence of secondary cytoreduction at the time of second-look laparotomy on the survival of patients with epithelial ovarian carcinoma. Gynecol Oncol 1989;34:365–371.

152. Lippman SM, Alberts DS, Slymen DJ, et al. Second-look laparotomy in epithelial ovarian carcinoma: Prognostic factors associated with survival duration. Cancer 1988;51:2571–2577.

153. Podratz KC, Schray MF, Wiegand HS, et al. Evaluation of treatment and survival after positive second-look laparotomy. Gynecol Oncol 1988;31:9–24.

154. Chambers SK, Chambers JT, Kohorn EI, Lawrence R, Schwartz PE. Evaluation of the role of second-look surgery in ovarian cancer. Obstet Gynecol 1988;72:404–408.

155. Luesley DM, Chan KK, Fielding JW, Hurlow R, Blackledge GR, Jordon JA. Second-look laparotomy in the management of epithelial ovarian carcinoma: An evaluation of fifty cases. Obstet Gynecol 1984;64:421–426.

156. Eymer H. Beeinflussung von proliferenden ovarialtumoren durch roetgen strahlen. Strahlen 1912;1:358–361.

157. Young RC, Fuks Z, Hoskins WJ. Cancer of the ovary. In: DeVita VTJ, Hellman S, Rosenberg SA, eds. Principles and practice of oncology. Philadelphia: JB Lippincott, 1989.

158. Dembo AJ, Bush RS, Beale FA, et al. The Princess Margaret study of ovarian carcinoma stages I, II, and asymptomatic III presentations. Cancer Treat Rep 1979;63:249–254.

159. Hreshchyshyn MM, Park RC, Blessing JA, et al. The role of adjuvant therapy in stage I ovarian cancer. Am J Obstet Gynecol 1980;138:139–145.

160. Dembo AJ, Davy S, Stenwig AE, Berle EJ, Bush RS, Kjorstad K. Prognostic factors in patients with stage I epithelial ovarian cancer. Obstet Gynecol 1990;75:263–273.

161. Fuks Z, Bagshaw MA. The rationale for curative radiotherapy for ovarian carcinoma. Int J Radiat Oncol Biol Phys 1975;1:21–32.

162. Schray M, Martinez A, Cox R, Ballon S. Radiotherapy in epithelial ovarian cancer: Analysis of prognostic factors on long-term experience. Obstet Gynecol 1983;62:373–382.

163. Dembo AJ. Abdominopelvic radiotherapy in ovarian cancer. A 10-year experience. Cancer 1985;55:2285–2290.

164. Dembo AJ. The sequential multiple modality treatment of ovarian cancer. Radiol Oncol 1985;3:187–192.

165. Fuller DB, Sause WT, Plenk HP, Menlove RL. Analysis of postoperative radiation therapy in stage I through III epithelial ovarian carcinoma. J Clin Oncol 1987;5:897–905.

166. Delclos L, Smith JP. Tumors of the ovary. In: Fletcher G, ed. Textbook of radiotherapy. Philadelphia: Lea & Febiger, 1973:690–702.

167. Perez CA, Korba A, Zivnusk F, et al. Cobalt 60 moving strip technique in the management of carcinoma of the ovary: Analysis of tumor control and morbidity. Int J Radiat Oncol Biol Phys 1978;4:379–388.

168. Ozols RF, Rubin SC, Dembo AJ, Robboy S. Epithelial ovarian cancer. In: Hoskins WJ,

169. Leers WH, Kock HCLV. The evaluation of postoperative irradiation in patients with early-stage ovarian cancer. Gynecol Oncol 1989;28:41–49.

170. Dembo AJ, Bush RS, Beale FA. Ovarian carcinoma: Improved survival following abdominopelvic irradiation in patients with a completed pelvic operation. Am J Obstet Gynecol 1979;134:793–800.

171. Delclos L, Smith JP. Ovarian cancer, with special regard to types of radiotherapy. NCI Monogr 1975;42:129–135.

172. Dubois JB, Joyeux H, Solassol CL, Pourquier H, Pujol H. Les tumeurs epithelialées de l'ovaire. Resultats therapeutiques a propos de 165 stades II et III. J Gynecol Obstet Biol Reprod 1985;14:627–632.

173. Hanks G, Bagshaw MA. Megavoltage radiation therapy and lymphangiography in ovarian cancer. Radiology 1969;93:649–654.

174. Delclos L, Barun EJ, Herrera JR Jr, et al. Whole abdominal irradiation by cobalt-60 moving strip technique. Radiology 1963;81:632–641.

175. Perez CA, Korba A, Zivnuska F, et al. ^{60}Co moving strip technique in the management of carcinoma of the ovary: Analysis of tumor control and morbidity. Int J Radiat Oncol Biol Phys 1978;4:379–388.

176. Glatstein E, Fuks Z, Bagshaw MA. Diaphragmatic treatment in ovarian carcinoma: A new radiotherapeutic technique. Int J Radiat Oncol Biol Phys 1977;2:357–362.

177. Orton CG, Ellis F. A simplification in the use of the NSD concept in practical radiotherapy. Br J Radiol 1973;46:529–537.

178. Martinez A, Schray MF, Hoes AE, Bagshaw MA. Postoperative radiation therapy for epithelial ovarian cancer: The curative role based on a 24-year experience. J Clin Oncol 1985;3:901–922.

179. Martinez A. Perspective: The role of radiation therapy in the treatment of epithelial ovarian cancer. In: Ballon SC, ed. Gynecologic oncology: Controversies in cancer treatment. Boston: Hall, 1981:300–310.

180. Fazekas JT, Maier JF. Irradiation of ovarian carcinomas: A prospective comparison of the open-field and moving-strip techniques. Am J Roentgenol Radium Ther Nucl Med 1974;120:118–123.

181. Dembo AJ, Bush RS, Beale FA, et al. A randomized clinical trial of moving strip versus open field whole abdominal irradiation in patients with invasive epithelial cancer of the ovary. Int J Radiat Oncol Biol Phys 1983;9:97.

182. Calkins AR, Rosenshein NB, Fox MG, Order SE. Delayed split whole abdominal irradiation in the combined modality treatment of ovarian cancer. Int J Radiat Oncol Biol Phys 1991;20:661–665.

183. Withers HR, Peters LJ, Thames HD, Fletcher GH. Hyperfractionation. Int J Radiat Oncol Biol Phys 1982;8:1807–1809.

184. Morgan L, Chafe W, Mendenhall W, Marcus R. Hyperfractionation of whole-abdomen radiation therapy: Salvage treatment of persistent ovarian carcinoma following chemotherapy. Gynecol Oncol 1988;31:122–134.

185. Kong JS, Peters LJ, Wharton JT, et al. Hyperfractionated split-course whole abdominal radiotherapy for ovarian carcinoma: Tolerance and toxicity. Int J Radiat Oncol Biol Phys 1988;14:737–743.

186. Eifel PJ, Gershenson DM, Delclos L, Wharton JT, Peters LJ. Twice-daily, split-course abdominopelvic radiation therapy after chemotherapy and positive second-look laparotomy for epithelial ovarian carcinoma. Int J Radiat Oncol Biol Phys 1991;21:1013–1018.

187. Hacker NF, Berek JS, Brunison CM, Heintz APM, Juillard GJF, Lagasse LD. Whole abdominal radiation as salvage therapy for epithelial ovarian cancer. Obstet Gynecol 1985;65:60–66.

188. Potter ME, Partridge EE, Shingleton HM, et al. Intraperitoneal chromic phosphate in ovarian cancer: Risks and benefits. Gynecol Oncol 1989;32:314–318.

189. Schray M, Martinez A, Howes A, et al. Advanced epithelial cancer: Salvage whole abdominal irradiation for patients with recurrent or persistent disease after combination chemotherapy. J Clin Oncol 1988;6:1433–1439.

190. Cain JM, Russell AH, Greer BE, Tamimi HK, Figge DC. Whole abdomen radiation for minimal residual epithelial ovarian carcinoma after surgical resection and maximal first-line chemotherapy. Gynecol Oncol 1988;29:168–175.

191. Hainsworth JD, Malcolm A, Johnson DH, Burnett LS, Jones HW, Greco FA. Advanced minimal residual ovarian carcinoma: Abdominopelvic irradiation following combination chemotherapy. Obstet Gynecol 1983;61:619.

192. King LA, Downey GO, Potish RA, Adcock LL, Carson LF, Twiggs LB. Concomitant whole-abdominal and intraperitoneal chemotherapy in advanced ovarian carcinoma. Cancer 1991;67:2867–2871.

193. Rustin GJS, Minton M, Southcott B, et al. Surgery, chemotherapy and whole abdominal radiotherapy in the management of advanced ovarian carcinoma. Clin Radiol 1987;38:269–272.

194. Piver MS, Barlow JJ, Lee FT, Vongtama V. Sequential therapy for advanced ovarian adenocarcinoma: Operation, chemotherapy, second-look laparotomy, and radiation therapy. Am J Obstet Gynecol 1975;122:355–357.

195. Hoskins WJ, Lichter AS, Whittington R, Artman LE, Bibro MC, Park RC. Whole abdominal and pelvic irradiation in patients with minimal disease at second-look surgical reassessment for ovarian cancer. Gynecol Oncol 1985;20:271–280.

196. Peters WA, Blasko JC, Bagley CMJ, Rudolph RH, Smith MR, Rivkin SE. Salvage therapy with whole-abdominal irradiation in patients with advanced carcinoma of the ovary previously treated with combination chemotherapy. Cancer 1986;58:880–882.

197. Coltart RS, Nethersell BW, Brown CH. A pilot study of high dose abdominopelvic radiotherapy following surgery and chemotherapy for stage III epithelial carcinoma of the ovary. Gynecol Oncol 1986;23:105–110.

198. Fuks Z, Rizel S, Biran S. Chemotherapeutic and surgical induction of pathological

complete remission and whole abdominal irradiation for consolidation does not enhance the cure of stage III ovarian carcinoma. J Clin Oncol 1988;6:509–516.

199. Lawton F, Luesley D, Blackledge G, et al. A randomized trial comparing whole abdominal radiotherapy with chemotherapy following cisplatinum cytoreduction in epithelial ovarian cancer: West Midlands Ovarian Cancer Group Trial II. Clin Oncol 1990; 2:4–9.

200. Mangioni C, Elpis A, Vassena L, et al. Radiotherapy versus chemotherapy as second-line treatment of minimal residual disease (MRD) in advanced epithelial ovarian cancer (EOC). Amsterdam: International Gynecologic Cancer Society, 1987.

201. Lambert JE. Advanced carcinoma of the ovary: A comparative trial between carboplatin versus radiotherapy as maintenance therapy. Toronto: North Thames Ovary Group, 1989.

202. Whelan TJ, Dembo AJ, Bush RS, et al. Complications of whole abdominal and pelvic radiotherapy following chemotherapy for advanced ovarian cancer. Int J Radiat Oncol Biol Phys (in press).

203. Franchin G, Tumolo S, Scarabelli C, et al. Whole abdomen radiation therapy after a short chemotherapy course and second-look laparotomy in advanced ovarian cancer. Gynecol Oncol 1991;41:206–211.

204. Fuks Z. The role of radiation therapy in the management of ovarian carcinoma. Isr J Med Sci 1977;8:815–828.

205. Smith JP, Rutledge FN, Delclos L. Postoperative treatment of early cancer of the ovary: A random trial between postoperative irradiation and chemotherapy. NCI Monogr 1975;42:149–153.

206. Brady LW. Advances in the management of gynecologic cancer: Radiation therapy. Cancer 1975;36:661–668.

207. Weiser EB, Burke TW, Heller PB, Woodward J, Hoskins WJ, Park RC. Determinants of survival of patients with epithelial ovarian carcinoma following whole abdominal irradiation (WAR). Gynecol Oncol 1988;30:201–208.

208. Goldberg N, Peschel RE. Postoperative abdominopelvic radiation therapy for ovarian cancer. Int J Radiat Oncol Biol Phys 1988;14:425–429.

209. Van Bunnigen B, Bouma J, Kooijman C, Warlam-Rodenhuis CC, Heintz APM, van Lindert A. Total abdominal irradiation in stage I and II carcinoma of the ovary. Radiother Oncol 1988;11:305–310.

210. Kjellgren O, Johnsson L. Bone marrow depression in the pelvis after megavoltage irradiation for ovarian carcinoma. Obstet Gynecol 1969;105:849–855.

211. Luxton R. Radiation nephritis. Q J Med 1953;22:215–242.

212. Hintz BL, Fuks Z, Kempson RL, et al. Results of postoperative megavoltage radiotherapy of malignant surface epithelial tumors of the ovary. Radiology 1975;114:695–700.

213. Aure JC, Hoeg K, Kolstad P. Radioactive colloidal gold in the treatment of ovarian carcinoma. Acta Radiol Ther (Stockh) 1971;10:399–407.

214. Rosenshein NB. Radioisotopes in the treatment of ovarian cancer. Clin Obstet Gynecol 1983;10:279–295.

215. Klassen D, Starreveld A, Shelly W, et al. External beam pelvic radiotherapy plus intraperitoneal radioactive chromic phosphate in early stage ovarian cancer: A toxic combination. A National Cancer Institute of Canada Clinical Trials Group Report. Int J Radiat Oncol Biol Phys 1985;11:1801–1804.

216. Moore DW, Langley II. Routine use of radiogold following operation for ovarian cancer. Am J Obstet Gynecol 1967;98:624–630.

217. Pezner RD, Stevens KRJ, Tong D, et al. Limited epithelial carcinoma of the ovary treated with curative intent by intraperitoneal installation of radiocolloids. Cancer 1978;42:2563–2671.

218. Spanos WJ, Guse C, Perez CA, et al. Phase II study of multiple daily fractionation in the palliations of advanced pelvic malignancies. Int J Radiat Oncol Biol Phys 1989;17: 659–661.

219. Bagley CMJ, Young RC, Canellos GP, et al. Treatment of ovarian carcinoma. Possibilities for progress. N Engl J Med 1972;287:856–862.

220. Louie KG, Ozols RF, Myers CE, et al. Long-term results of a cisplatin-containing combination chemotherapy regimen for the treatment of advanced ovarian carcinoma. J Clin Oncol 1986;4:1579.

221. Johnson BL, Fisher RI, Bender RA, et al. Hexamethylmelamine in alkylating agent resistant ovarian carcinoma. Cancer 1978;42:2157.

222. Hubbard SM, Barkes P, Young RC. Adriamycin therapy for advanced ovarian carcinoma after chemotherapy. Cancer Treat Rep 1978;62:1375.

223. McGuire WP, Rowinski EK, Rosenshein NB, et al. Taxol: A unique antineoplastic agent with significant activity in advanced ovarian epithelial neoplasms. Ann Intern Med 1989;111:273.

224. Thigpen JT, Vance RB, Balducci I, et al. New drugs and experimental approaches in ovarian cancer treatment. Semin Oncol 1984;11:314.

225. Young RC, Von Hoff DD, Gormley P, et al. Cis-dichlorodiammineplatinum (II) for the treatment of advanced ovarian cancer. Cancer Treat Rep 1979;63:1539–1544.

226. Lambert HE, Berry RJ. High dose cisplatin compared with high dose cyclophosphamide in the management of advanced epithelial ovarian cancer (FIGO stages III and IV): Report from the North Thames Cooperative Group. Br Med J 1985;290:889–892.

227. Ozols RF, Young RC. High-dose cisplatin therapy in ovarian cancer. Semin Oncol 1985;12:21–30.

228. Bruckner HW, Wallach R. High-dose cisplatinum for the treatment of refractory ovarian cancer. Gynecol Oncol 1984;12:64–67.

229. Barker GH, Wiltshaw E. Use of high dose cis-dichlorodiammine platinum-II following failure on previous chemotherapy for advanced carcinoma of the ovary. Br J Obstet Med 1981;88:1192–1199.

230. Levin L, Hryniuk WM. Dose intensity analysis of chemotherapy regimens in ovarian carcinoma. J Clin Oncol 1987;5:756–767.

231. Ozols RF, Young RC. Chemotherapy of ovarian cancer. Semin Oncol 1984;11:251–263.

232. Gruppo Intergionale Cooperativo Oncologico Ginecologia. Randomized comparisons of cisplatin with cyclophosphamide/cisplatin and with cyclophosphamide/doxorubicin/cisplatin in advanced ovarian cancer. Lancet 1987;2:353.

233. Omura GA, Buyse M, Marsoni S, et al. CP versus CAP chemotherapy of ovarian carcinoma: A meta-analysis. J Clin Oncol 1991;9:1668.

234. Bolis G, D'Incalci M, Gramellini F, et al. Adriamycin in ovarian cancer patients resistant to cyclophosphamide. Eur J Cancer 1978;14:1401.

235. Wharton JT, Rutledge F, Smith JP, et al. Hexamethylmelamine: An evaluation of its role in the treatment of ovarian cancer. Am J Obstet Gynecol 1979;133:833.

236. Foster BJ, Clagett-Carr K, Marsoni S, et al. Role of hexamethylmelamine in the treatment of ovarian cancer. Where is the needle in the haystack? Cancer Treat Rep 1986;70: 1003.

237. Canetta R, Carter SK. Developing new drugs for ovarian cancer: A challenging task in a changing reality. J Cancer Res Clin Oncol 1984;107:111.

238. Thigpen T, Blessing J, Ball H, et al. Phase II trial of taxol as second-line therapy for ovarian carcinoma: A Gynecologic Oncology Group study. Proc Am Soc Clin Oncol 1990;9:156.

239. Hillcoat BL, Campbell JJ, Pepperell R, et al. Phase II trial of VP-16-213 in advanced ovarian cancer. Gynecol Oncol 1985;22:162.

240. Creech RH, Shah MK, Catalano RB, et al. Phase II study of low-dose mitomycin in patients with ovarian cancer previously treated with chemotherapy. Cancer Treat Rep 1985;69:1271.

241. Willocks D, Toppila M, Hudson CN, et al. Estrogen and progesterone receptors in human ovarian tumors. Gynecol Oncol 1983;16:246.

242. Ford LC, Berek JS, Lagasse LD, et al. Estrogen and progesterone receptors in ovarian neoplasms. Gynecol Oncol 1983;15:299.

243. Thompson P, Osborne R, Slevin M, et al. A phase II study of cyproterone acetate in advanced ovarian cancer. London Gynecology Oncology Group. Proc Am Assoc Clin Oncol 1990;9:160.

244. Kavanagh JJ, Roberts W, Townsend P, Hewitt S. Leuprolide acetate in the treatment of refractory or persistent epithelial ovarian cancer. J Clin Oncol 1989;7:115.

245. Schwartz PE, Keating G, MacLusky N, et al. Tamoxifen therapy for advanced ovarian cancer. Obstet Gynecol 1982;59:583.

246. Geisler H. Megestrol acetate for the palliation of advanced ovarian carcinoma. Obstet Gynecol 1983;61:95.

247. Aabo K, Pedersen AG, Haid I, et al. High-dose medroxyprogesterone acetate (MPA) in advanced chemotherapy-resistant ovarian carcinoma: A phase II study. Cancer Treat Rep 1982;66:407–408.

248. Trope C, Johnsson JE, Sigurdsson K, et al. High-dose medroxyprogesterone acetate for the treatment of advanced ovarian carcinoma. Cancer Treat Rep 1982;66:1441–1443.

249. Myers M, Moore GE, Major FJ. Advanced ovarian carcinoma: Response to antiestrogen therapy. Cancer 1981;48:2368–2370.

250. Hamerlynck JVTH, Maskens AP, Mangioni C, et al. Phase II trial of medroxyprogesterone acetate in advanced ovarian cancer: An EORTC gynecological cancer cooperative group study. Gynecol Oncol 1985;22:313.

251. Slevin ML, Harvey VJ, Osborne RJ, et al. A phase II study of tamoxifen in ovarian cancer. Eur J Cancer Clin Oncol 1986;22:309.

252. Shirey DR, Kavanagh JJ, Gershenson DM, et al. Tamoxifen therapy of epithelial ovarian cancer. Obstet Gynecol 1985;66:575.

253. Freedman RS, Saul PB, Edwards CL, et al. Ethinylestradiol and medroxyprogesterone in patients with epithelial ovarian carcinoma: A phase II study. Cancer Treat Rep 1986;70:369.

254. Schwartz PE, Chambers JP, Kohorn EI, et al. Tamoxifen in combination with cytotoxic chemotherapy in advanced epithelial ovarian cancer. Cancer 1989;63:1074.

255. Hamburger AW, Salmon SE, Kim MB, et al. Direct cloning of human ovarian carcinoma cells in agar. Cancer Res 1978;38:3438–3444.

256. Hanauske AR, Von Hoff DD. The value of the human tumor cloning assay in ovarian cancer. Clin Obstet Gynecol 1986;29:638.

257. Young RC, Chabner BA, Hubbard SP, et al. Prospective trial of melphalan (L-PAM) versus combination chemotherapy (hexa-CAF) in ovarian adenocarcinoma. N Engl J Med 1978;299:1261–1266.

258. Neijt JP, Vanlindert ACM, Vendrijk CPJ, et al. Hexa-CAF combination chemotherapy and other multiple drug regimens in advanced ovarian carcinoma. Present and future. Neth J Med 1979;22:28.

259. Vogl SE, Pagano M, Davis T, et al. Platinum based combination chemotherapy versus melphalan for advanced ovarian carcinoma. Proc Int Congr Chemother 1983;207:9–13.

260. Delgado G, Smith FP, McLaughlin EF, et al. Single agent vs. combination chemotherapy for ovarian cancer. Am J Clin Oncol 1985;8:33–37.

261. Edmonson JH, Fleming TR, Decker DG, et al. Different chemotherapeutic sensitivities and host factors affecting prognosis in advanced ovarian carcinoma versus minimal residual disease. Cancer Treat Rep 1979;63:241–247.

262. Williams CJ, Mead GM, Macbeth FR, et al. Cisplatin combination chemotherapy versus chlorambucil in advanced ovarian carcinoma: Mature results of a randomized trial. J Clin Oncol 1985;3:1455.

263. Trope C. A prospective randomized trial comparison of melphalan vs. melphalan-Adriamycin in advanced ovarian carcinoma. Proc Am Clin Oncol 1981;22:469.

264. Decker DG, Fleming TR, Malkasian GD, et al. Cyclophosphamide plus cisplatinum in combination: Treatment program for stage III or IV ovarian carcinoma. Obstet Gynecol 1982;60:481–486.

265. Medical Research Council. MRC Working Party on Ovarian Cancer: Medical Research Council study on chemotherapy in advanced ovarian cancer. Br J Obstet Gynecol 1981;88:1174.

266. Carmo-Pereira J, Costa FO, Henriques E, et al. Advanced ovarian carcinoma. A prospective and randomized clinical trial of cyclophosphamide versus combination cytotoxic chemotherapy (hexa-CAF). Cancer 1981;48:1947–1951.

267. Gynecological Group, Clinical Oncological Society of Australia, and the Sydney Branch, Ludwig Institute for Cancer Research. Chemotherapy of advanced ovarian adenocarcinoma: A randomized comparison of combination versus sequential therapy using chlorambucil and cisplatin. Gynecol Oncol 1986;23:1–13.

268. Chemotherapy in advanced ovarian cancer: An overview of randomised clinical trials: Advanced Ovarian Cancer Trials Group. Br Med J 1991;303:884–893.

269. Reimer RR, Hoover R, Fraumeni JF, Young RC. Acute leukemia after alkylating agent therapy in ovarian cancer. N Engl J Med 1977;297:117.

270. Greene MH, Boice JD, Greer BE, et al. Acute non-lymphocytic leukemia after therapy with alkylating agents for ovarian cancer. N Engl J Med 1982;307:1416.

271. Ehrlich CE, Einhorn L, Williams SD, et al. Chemotherapy for stage III–IV epithelial ovarian cancer with *cis*-dichlorodiammineplatinum (II), adriamycin, and cyclophosphamide: A preliminary report. Cancer Treat Rep 1979;63:281–288.

272. Wiltshaw E, Eavans B, Rustin G, et al. A prospective randomized trial comparing high-dose cisplatin with low-dose cisplatin and chlorambucil in advanced ovarian carcinoma. J Clin Oncol 1986;4:722.

273. Neijt JP, van der Burg MEL, Vriesendorp R, et al. Randomized trial comparing two combination chemotherapy regimens (hexa-CAF vs. CHAP-5) in advanced ovarian carcinoma. Lancet 1984;2:594–598.

274. Neijt JP, ten Bokkel Huinink WW, van der Burg, et al. Randomized trial comparing two combination chemotherapy regimens (CHAP-5 v CP) in advanced ovarian carcinoma. J Clin Oncol 1987;5:1157.

275. Omura G, Blessing JA, Ehrlich CE, et al. A randomized trial of cyclophosphamide and doxorubicin with or without cisplatin in advanced ovarian carcinoma. Cancer 1986;57:1725–1730.

276. Omura G, Bundy B, Berek J, et al. Randomized trial of cyclophosphamide plus cisplatin with or without doxorubicin in ovarian carcinoma: A Gynecologic Oncology Group study. J Clin Oncol 1989;7:457.

277. Conte PF, Bruzzone M, Chiara S, et al. A randomized trial comparing cisplatin plus cyclophosphamide versus cisplatin, doxorubicin, and cyclophosphamide in advanced ovarian cancer. J Clin Oncol 1986;4:965–971.

278. Jakobsen A, Bertelsen K, Sell A, et al. Advantage of CAP over CP in terms of survival in advanced ovarian carcinoma. Proc Am Soc Clin Oncol 1985;4:113.

279. Edmonson JH, McCormack GW, Fleming TR, et al. Comparison of cyclophosphamide plus cisplatin versus hexamethylmelamine, cyclophosphamide, doxorubicin, and cisplatin in combination as initial chemotherapy for stage III and IV ovarian carcinomas. Cancer Treat Rep 1985;69:1243–1246.

280. Hainsworth J, Grosh W, Burnett L, et al. Advanced ovarian cancer: Long-term results of treatment with intensive cisplatin-based chemotherapy of brief duration. Ann Intern Med 1988;108:165.

281. Gynecologic Oncology Group. GOG Protocol: Phase III randomized study of cyclophosphamide and cisplatin versus taxol and cisplatin in patients with suboptimal stage III and stage IV epithelial ovarian carcinoma.

282. Green JA, Slater AJ. A study of cisplatinum and ifosfamide in alkylating agent-resistant ovarian cancer. Gynecol Oncol 1989;32:233.

283. Sutton GP. Pilot study of hexamethylmelamine, cyclophosphamide and carboplatin in previously untreated patients with advanced ovarian cancer. Hoosier Oncology Group protocol.

284. Lund B, Hansen M, Hansen OP, Hansen H. High-dose platinum consisting of combined carboplatin and cisplatin in previously untreated ovarian cancer patients with residual disease. J Clin Oncol 1989;7:1469.

285. Fox Chase Cancer Center Protocol: A pilot study of carboplatin, cisplatin and cyclophosphamide in patients with advanced epithelial ovarian cancer.

286. Muggia F, Christian M, Parker R, et al. Phase I study of carboplatin (CB) day 1 and cisplatin (CP) day 3. Proc Am Soc Clin Oncol 1990;9:286.

287. Kemp GM, Glover DJ, Schein PS. The role of WR-2721 in the reduction of combined cisplatin and cyclophosphamide toxicity. Proc Am Soc Clin Oncol 1990;9:76.

288. Reed E, Janik J, Bookman M, et al. High-dose carboplatin and rGM-CSF in refractory ovarian cancer. Proc Am Soc Clin Oncol 1990;9:609.

289. Shae TC, Flaherty M, Elias A, et al. A phase I clinical and pharmacokinetic study of carboplatin and autologous bone marrow support. J Clin Oncol 1989;7:651.

290. Shpall EJ, Clarke-Pearson D, Soper JT, et al. High-dose alkylating agent chemotherapy with autologous bone marrow support in patients with stage III/IV epithelial ovarian cancer. Gynecol Oncol 1990;38:386.

291. Stoppa A, Maraninchi D, Viens P, et al. High doses of melphalan and autologous marrow rescue in advanced common epithelial ovarian carcinomas: A retrospective analysis in 35 patients. Proceedings of the Fourth International Symposium. University of Texas Cancer Center, M.D. Anderson Hospital, Houston, 1989;125.

292. Shpall E. Autologous bone marrow transplantation in ovarian cancer patients with small volume residual disease: Trial in progress. (personal communication).

293. Bast RC, Knapp RC. Immunologic approaches to the management of ovarian carcinoma. Semin Oncol 1984;11:264–274.

294. Hamilton TC, Ozols RF, Longo DL. Biologic therapy for the treatment of malignant common epithelial tumors of the ovary. Cancer 1987;60:2054–2063.

295. Mantovani A, Sessa C, Peri G, et al. Intraperitoneal administration of Corynebacterium parvum in patients with ascitic ovarian tumors resistant to chemotherapy. Effects on cytotoxicity of tumor-associated macrophages and NK cells. Int J Cancer 1981;27:437–446.

296. Bast RC, Berek JS, Obrist E, et al. Intraperitoneal immunotherapy of human ovarian carcinoma with *Corynebactyerium parvum*. Cancer Res 1983;43:1395.

297. Berek JS, Hacker NF, Lichtenstein A, et al. Intraperitoneal recombinant alpha interferon for "salvage" immunotherapy in stage III epithelial ovarian cancer: A GOG study. Cancer Res 1985;45:4447.

298. Gudson JP, Homesley HD, Muss HB, et al. Chemotherapy of advanced ovarian epithelial carcinoma with melphalan and levamisole: A pilot study of the Gynecologic Oncology Group. Am J Obstet Gynecol 1981;141:65–70.

299. Creasman WT, Yale SA, Blessing JA, et al. Chemoimmunotherapy in the management of primary stage III ovarian cancer. Cancer Treat Rep 1979;63:319.

300. Alberts DS, Moon TE, Stephens RA, et al. Randomized study of chemoimmunotherapy for advanced ovarian carcinoma. Cancer Treat Rep 1982;63:325.

301. Creasman WT, Omura GA, Brady MF, et al. A randomized trial of cyclophosphamide, doxorubicin, and cisplatin with or without *Bacillus Calmette-Guerin* in patients with suboptimal stage III and IV ovarian cancer: A Gynecologic Oncology Group study. Gynecol Oncol 1990;39:239.

302. Steis R, Bookman M, Clark J, et al. Intraperitoneal lymphokine activated killer (LAK) cell and interleukin-2 (IL-2) therapy for peritoneal carcinomatosis: Toxicity, efficacy, and laboratory results. Proc Am Soc Clin Oncol [Abstract 984] 1987.

303. Pirker R, Fitzgerald DJP, Hamilton TC, et al. Anti-transferrin receptor antibody linked to pseudomonas exotoxin as a model immunotoxin in human ovarian carcinoma cell lines. Cancer Res 1985;45:751–757.

304. Pirker R, Fitzgerald DJP, Hamilton TC, et al. Characterization of immunotoxins active against ovarian cancer cell lines. J Clin Invest 1985;76:1261–1267.

305. Bookman M, Godfrey S, Padavic K, et al. Anti-transferrin receptor immunotoxin therapy: Phase I intraperitoneal trial. Proc Am Soc Clin Oncol 1990;9:772.

306. Epenetos AA, Hooker G, Krausz T, et al. Antibody-guided irradiation of advanced ovarian cancer with intraperitoneally administered radiolabeled monoclonal antibodies. J Clin Oncol 1987;5:1890.

307. Shen DW, Fojo A, Chin JE, et al. Human multidrug-resistant cell lines: Increased *mdr-1* expression can preceded gene amplification. Science 1986;232:643–645.

308. Fojo A, Hamilton TC, Young RC, et al. Multidrug resistance in ovarian cancer. Cancer 1987;60:2075–2080.

309. Juliano RL, Ling V. A surface glycoprotein modulating drug permeability in Chinese hamster ovary cell mutants. Biochem Biophys Acta 1976;455:152–162.

310. Riordan JR, Deuchars K, Kartner N, et al. Amplification of P-glycoprotein genes in multidrug-resistant mammalian cell lines. Nature 1985;316:817–819.

311. Louie KG, Hamilton TC, Winker MA, et al. Adriamycin accumulation and metabolism in Adriamycin-sensitive and resistant human ovarian cancer cell lines. Biochem Pharmacol 1986;35:467–472.

312. Hamilton TC, Masuda H, Young RC, Ozols RF. Modulation of cisplatin cytotoxicity by inhibition of DNA repair in a cisplatin-resistant human ovarian cancer cell line 2780-cp. Proc Am Soc Cancer Res 1987;28:291.

313. Rogan AM, Hamilton TC, Young RC, et al. Reversal of Adriamycin resistance by verapamil in human ovarian cancer. Science 1984;224:994–998.

314. Ozols RF, Cunnion RE, Klecker RW, et al. Verapamil and Adriamycin in the treatment of drug resistant ovarian cancer patients. J Clin Oncol 1987;5:641–647.

315. Meister A. Selective modification of glutathione metabolism. Science 1983;220:472–477.

316. Green JA, Vistica DT, Young RC, et al. Potentiation of melphalan cytotoxicity in human ovarian cancer cell lines by glutathione depletion. Cancer Res 1984;44:5427–5431.

317. Ozols RF, Louie KG, Plowman J, et al. Enhanced alkylating agent cytotoxicity in human ovarian cancer in vitro and in tumor-bearing nude mice by buthionine sulfoximine depletion of glutathione. Biochem Pharmacol 1987;36:147–153.

318. Ozols RF, Hamilton TC, Masuda H, Young RC. The role of thiols in drug resistance. In: Woolley PVI, Tew KD, eds. Mechanisms of drug resistance in neoplastic cells. New York: Academic Press 1988:289–306.

319. Hamilton TC, O'Dwyer PJ, Young RC, et al. Phase I trial of buthionine sulfoximine plus melphalan in patients with advanced cancer. Proc Am Soc Clin Oncol 1990;9:291.

320. Behrens BC, Hamilton TC, Masuda H, et al. Characterization of a *cis*-diamminedichloroplatinum (II)-resistant human ovarian cancer cell line and its use in evaluation of platinum analogs. Cancer Res 1987;47:414–418.

321. Tew KD, Clapper ML.L Glutatione S-transferases and anticancer drug resistance. In Wooley PV, Tew KD, eds. Bristol-Myers cancer symposia. New York: Academic Press, 1988.

322. O'Dwyer P. Phase I trial of ethacrynic acid and thiotepa. Philadelphia: Fox Chase Cancer Center, 1990.

323. Smith JP, Day TG. Review of ovarian cancer at the University of Texas Center, M.D. Anderson Hospital and Tumor Institute. Am J Obstet Gynecol 1979;135:984–993.

324. Webb MJ, Decker DG, Massey, et al. Factors influencing survival in stage I ovarian cancer. Am J Obstet Gynecol 1973;166:222.

325. Bush RS. Radiotherapy for patients with ovarian cancer. Strahlentherapie 1983;159:131–137.

326. Drouin P, Rutledge FN, Delclos L, et al. Comparison of external radiotherapy and chemotherapy in ovarian cancer. Ann R Coll Phys Surg Can 1979;12:61.

327. Delclos L. International Symposium on Combined Modalities Approach on Gynecologic Cancer, Mexico City, 1983:61.

328. Einhorn N. The place of adjuvant chemotherapy in early stages. Int J Radiat Oncol Biol Phys 1982;8:257–258.

329. Belinson JT, McClure M, Ashikaga T, Karakoff IH. Treatment of advanced and recurrent ovarian carcinoma with cyclophosphamide, doxorubicin, and cisplatin. Cancer 1984;54:1983–1990.

330. Wharton JT, Edwards CL, Rutledge FN. Long-term survival after chemotherapy for advanced epithelial ovarian carcinoma. Am J Obstet Gynecol 1984;148:997–1005.

331. Greco FA, Hande KR, Jones HW, et al. Advanced ovarian cancer: Long-term follow-up after brief intensive chemotherapy. Proc Am Soc Clin Oncol 1984;3:166.

332. Dougherty J, Hakes T, Cain J, et al. Recurrence pattern of advanced ovarian carcinoma after negative laparotomy. Proc Am Soc Clin Oncol 1985;4:122.

333. Sigurdson K, Johnsson JE, Trope C. Carcinoma of the ovary in stage III. Effects of postoperative chemotherapy, radiation therapy, and repeat laparotomy. Acta Rad Oncol 1982;21:181–189.

334. Potish R, Adcock L, Brooker D, et al. Sequential surgery, radiation therapy, and alkeran in the management of epithelial carcinoma of the ovary. Cancer 1980;45:2754–2758.

335. Nevin JE, Pinzon G, Baggerly TJ, et al. The use of intravenous phenylalanine mustard followed by supervoltage irradiation in the treatment of carcinoma of the ovary. Cancer 1984;51:1273–1283.

336. Griffiths CT, Grogan RH, Hall TC. Advanced ovarian cancer: Primary treatment with surgery, radiotherapy, and chemotherapy. Cancer 1972;29:1–7.

337. Hainsworth JD, Malcolm A, Johnson DH. Treatment of minimal residual ovarian carcinoma: Abdominopelvic irradiation following incomplete response to combination chemotherapy. Obstet Gynecol 1983;61:619–623.

338. Dedrick RL, Myers CE, Bungay PM, et al. Pharmacokinetic rationale for peritoneal drug administration in the treatment of ovarian cancer. Cancer Treat Rep 1978;62:1.

339. Dedrick RL. Theoretical and experimental bases of intraperitoneal chemotherapy. Semin Oncol 1985;12:1–6.

340. Myers C. The use of intraperitoneal chemotherapy in the treatment of ovarian cancer. Semin Oncol 1984;11:275–284.

341. Jones RB, Myers CE, Guarino AM, et al. High volume intraperitoneal chemotherapy ("Belly Bath") for ovarian cancer. Cancer Chemother Pharmacol 1978;1:161–166.

342. Speyer JL, Collins JM, Dedrick RL, et al. Phase I and pharmacologic studies of 5-fluorouracil administered intraperitoneally. Cancer Res 1980;40:567.

343. Ozols RF. Intraperitoneal chemotherapy in the management of ovarian cancer. Semin Oncol 1985;12:75–80.

344. Pfeifle CE, Howell SM, Markman M, Lucas WE. Totally implantable system for peritoneal access. J Clin Oncol 1984;2:1277.

345. Piccart MJ, Speyer JL, Markman M, et al. Intraperitoneal chemotherapy: Technical experience at five institutions. Semin Oncol 1985;12:90.

346. Cohen CJ. Therapeutic staging. In Brucker HW, Cohen CJ, eds. Ovarian cancer: New approaches with curative intent. Morristown, NJ: Sieher & McIntyre, 1984:37–50.

347. Ozols RF, Speyer JL, Jenkins J, et al. Phase II trial of 5-FU administered IP to patients with refractory ovarian cancer. Cancer Treat Rep 1984;68:1229–1232.

348. ten Bokkel Huinink WW, Dubbelman R, Aartsen E, et al. Experimental and clinical results with intraperitoneal cisplatin. Semin Oncol 1985;12:43–46.

349. Cohen CV. Surgical considerations in ovarian cancer. Semin Oncol 1985;12:53–56.

350. Markman M, Howell S, Cleary S, et al. Survival following cisplatin (DDP)-based intraperitoneal chemotherapy for refractory ovarian carcinoma. Proc Am Soc Clin Oncol 1986;5:113.

351. Ozols RF. Intraperitoneal therapy in ovarian cancer: Time's up. J Clin Oncol 1991;2:197.

352. EORTG Trial of intraperitoneal cisplatin in patients with a complete remission.

353. Alberts DS. Clinical trial of intraperitoneal cisplatin vs intravenous cisplatin with all patients receiving intravenous cyclophosphamide in previously untreated patients with optimal disease. (personal communication).

354. Hakes T, Hoskins W, Jones W, et al. Randomized prospective trial of 5 versus 10 cycles of cyclophosphamide, doxorubicin and cisplatin (ACP) in stage III and IV ovarian cancer. Proc Am Soc Clin Oncol 1990;9:156.

355. Markman M, Howell SB, et al. Intraperitoneal chemotherapy with high dose cisplatin and cytarabine for refractory ovarian carcinoma and other malignancies principally involving the peritoneal cavity. J Clin Oncol 1985;3:925.

356. Zimm S, Cleary S, Lucas W, et al. Phase I/pharmacokinetic study of intraperitoneal (IP) cisplatin and etoposide. Proc Am Soc Clin Oncol 1986;5:49.

357. Stage AH, Grafton WD. Thecomas and granulosa-theca cell tumors of the ovary: An analysis of 51 tumors. Obstet Gynecol 1977;50:21.

358. Diddle AW. Granulosa and theca-cell ovarian tumors: Prognosis. Cancer 1952;5:215–228.

359. Stenwit JT, Hazekamp JT, Beecham JB. Granulosa cell tumors of the ovary. A clinicopathological study of 118 cases with long-term follow-up. Gynecol Oncol 1979;7:136–162.

360. Lusch CJ, Mercurio RM, Runyeon WK. Delayed recurrence and chemotherapy of a granulosa cell tumor. Obstet Gynecol 1978;51:505.

361. Di Saia PJ, Saltz A, Kagan AR, et al. A temporary response of recurrent granulosa cell tumors to Adriamycin. Obstet Gynecol 1978;52:355.

362. Lapoohn RE, Burger HG, Bouma J, et al. Inhibin as a marker for granulosa cell tumors. N Engl J Med 1989;321:790–793.

363. Woodruff JD, Protos P, Peterson WF. Ovarian teratomas. Am J Obstet Gynecol 1968;102:702–715.

364. Jimerson GK, Woodruff JD. Ovarian extraembryoneal teratoma I. Endodermal sinus tumor. Am J Obstet Gynecol 1977;127:78–79.

365. Gallion H, van Nagell JR, Powell DR, et al. Therapy of endodermal sinus tumor of the ovary. Am J Obstet Gynecol 1979;135:447.

366. Cangir A, Smith J, Van Eys J. Improved prognosis in children with ovarian cancers following modified VAC (vincristine sulfate, dactinomycin and cyclophosphamide) chemotherapy. Cancer 1978;42:1234.

367. Slayton RE, Park RC, Silverberg SG, et al. VAC treatment of malignant germ cell tumors of the ovary. Cancer 1985;56:243–248.

368. Williams S, Blessing J, Adcock L, et al. Treatment of malignant ovarian germ cell tumors with PVB. Proc Am Soc Clin Oncol 1984;3:175.

369. Smales E, Peckham MJ. Chemotherapy of germ cell ovarian tumors. Eur J Cancer Clin Oncol 1987;23:469–473.

370. Carlson RW, Sikic BI, Turbow MM, Ballon SC. Combination PVB for malignant germ cell tumors of the ovary. J Clin Oncol 1983;1:546–651.

371. Curry SL, Smith JP, Gallagher HS. Malignant teratoma of the ovary: Prognostic factors and treatment. Am J Obstet Gynecol 1978;131:845.

372. Williams SD, Blessing J, Slayton R, et al. Ovarian germ cell tumors: Adjuvant trials of the Gynecologic Oncology Group. Proc Am Soc Clin Oncol 1989;8:150.

373. Krepart G, Smith JP, Rutledge F, Delclos L. The treatment for dysgerminoma of the ovary. Cancer 1978;41:986–990.

374. De Palo G, Pilotti S, Kendra R, et al. Natural history of dysgerminoma. Am J Obstet Gynecol 1982;143:799–807.

375. Horowitz CJ, Brady LW. Ovary. In: Perez CA, Brady LW, eds. Principles and practice of radiation oncology. Phildelphia: JB Lippincott, 1992.

376. Lawson AP, Adler GF. Radiotherapy in the treatment of ovarian dysgerminomas. Int J Radiat Oncol Biol Phys 1988;14:431–434.

377. Slayton RE. Management of germ cell and stromal tumors of the ovary. Semin Oncol 1984;11:299–313.

378. Brody S. Clinical aspects of dysgerminoma of the ovary. Acta Radiol Ther Stockh 1961;56:209–230.

379. Asadourian LA, Taylor HB. Dysgerminoma: An analysis of 105 cases. Obstet Gynecol 1969;33:370–379.

380. Williams SD, Blessing J, Hatch K, et al. Chemotherapy of advanced ovarian dysgerminoma: Trials of the Gynecologic Oncology Group. Proc Am Soc Clin Oncol 1990;9:155.

381. Goldstein DP, Piro AJ. Combination chemotherapy in the treatment of germ cell tumors containing choriocarcinoma in males and females. Surg Gynecol Obstet 1972;134:61–66.

382. Rutledge FN, Fletcher GH, Smith JP, et al. In: Clark RL, Howe CD, eds. Cancer patient care at M.D. Anderson Hospital and Tumor Institute. Chicago Year Book Medical Publishers, 1976:263–308.

383. Fanning J, Walker RLA, Shah NR. Mixed germ cell tumor of the ovary with pure choriocarcinoma metastasis. Obstet Gynecol 1986;58:84.

384. Munnell EW. Primary ovarian cancer associated with pregnancy. Clin Obstet Gynecol 1963;6:983–993.

385. Creasman WT, Rutledge F, Smith JP. Carcinoma of the ovary associated with pregnancy. Obstet Gynecol 1971;38:111.

386. Hess LW, Peaceman A, O'Brien WF, Winkel CA, Cruikshnk DP, Morrison JC. Adnexal mass occurring with intrauterine pregnancy: Report of fifty-four patients requiring laparotomy for definitive management. Am J Obstet Gynecol 1988;158:1029.

387. Markman M, Rowinsky E, Hakes T, et al. Phase I study of taxol administered by the intraperitoneal route. Proc Am Soc Clin Oncol 1991;10:601.

388. Raju KS, McKinna JA, Barker GH, et al. Second look operations in the planned management of advanced ovarian carcinoma. Am J Obstet Gynecol 1982;144:650–654.

389. Parker LM, Griffiths CT, Yankee RA, et al. Combination chemotherapy with Adriamycin-cyclophosphamide for advanced ovarian carcinoma. Cancer 1980;46:669–674.

390. Hacker NF, Berek JS, Burnison CM, et al. Whole abdominal radiation salvage therapy for epithelial ovarian cancer. Obstet Gynecol 1985;65:619–623.

391. Kucera RP, Sheets EE, Micha JP, et al. Whole abdominal radiotherapy for patients with minimal residual epithelial ovarian cancer. Presented at the Thirteenth Annual Meeting of the Western Association of Gynecologic Oncologists. San Diego, California, June, 1985.

392. Menczer J, Moda M, Brenner DE, et al. Abdominopelvic irradiation for stage II-IV ovarian carcinoma patients with limited or no residual disease at second-look laparotomy after completion of cisplatin-based combination chemotherapy. Gynecol Oncol 1986;24:149–153.

393. Brenner DE. Intraperitoneal chemotherapy: A review. J Clin Oncol 1986;4:1135–1147.

394. Gyves JW, Ensminger WD, Stetson P, et al. Constant intraperitoneal 5-fluorouracil infusion through a totally implanted system. Clin Pharmacol Ther 1984;35:83–89.

395. Howell SB, Pfeifle CL, Wung WE, et al. Intraperitoneal chemotherapy with melphalan. Ann Intern Med 1984;101:14–18.

396. Howell SB, Chu BB, Wung WE, et al. Long-duration intracavitary infusion of methotrexate with systemic leucovorin protection in patients with malignant effusions. J Clin Invest 1981;67:1161–1170.

397. Howell S, Pfeifle C, Wung W, et al. Intraperitoneal cisplatin with systemic thiosulfate protection. Ann Intern Med 1982;97:845–851.

398. Pretorius RG, Hacker NF, Berek JS, et al. Pharmacokinetics of IP cisplatin in refractory ovarian carcinoma. Cancer Treat Rep 1983;67:1085–1092.

399. Casper ES, Kelsen DP, Alcock NW, et al. IP cisplatin in patients with malignant ascites: Pharmacokinetic evaluation and comparison with the IV route. Cancer Treat Rep 1983;67:235–238.

400. Redman JR, Petrini GR, Saigo PE, et al. Prognostic factors in advanced ovarian carcinoma. J Clin Oncol 1986;4:515–520.

401. Fuller DB, Sause WT, Plenk HP, et al. Analysis of post-operative radiation therapy in stage I through III epithelial ovarian carcinoma. J Clin Oncol 1987;5:897–902.

Cancer: Principles & Practice of Oncology, Fourth Edition,
edited by Vincent T. DeVita, Jr., Samuel Hellman, Steven A. Rosenberg.
J.B. Lippincott Co., Philadelphia © 1993.

Jay R. Harris
Monica Morrow
Gianni Bonadonna

CHAPTER **40**

Cancer of the Breast

In North America, breast cancer is the most common malignancy among women and accounts for 27% of their cancers. Eighteen percent of the female cancer deaths are due to breast cancer, but since 1985, lung cancer has equaled or exceeded breast cancer as a cause of cancer death in women. Among women in the United States between the ages of 40 and 55 years, breast cancer is the leading cause of death. In 1992, approximately 181,000 new cases of breast cancer will be diagnosed in the United States, and 46,000 women will die from breast cancer.[1] Between 1940 and 1982, the age-standardized incidence rose by an average of 1.2% per year, and between 1982 and 1986, the incidence rose more sharply at 4% per year. Age-adjusted breast cancer mortality rates have been remarkably stable in the United States. The relatively constant mortality despite increases in incidence may be the result of increases in a more benign form of the disease, earlier detection, or advances in treatment.

The natural history of breast cancer is characterized by a long duration and marked heterogeneity within and among patients. Breast cancer is among the more slow-growing tumors, and the preclinical period before diagnosis and the clinical phases after initial treatment and even after the appearance of metastasis are measured in years and decades. Nevertheless, some patients have aggressive forms of the disease and do poorly. Other patients have such indolent forms of the disease that it is difficult to demonstrate that therapy has any effect on survival. During the long clinical phase, there is ample opportunity for clonal mutation and evolution, and it seems probable that individual patients may have multiple tumor clones, each with its own growth rate, propensity to metastasize, and sensitivity to drugs. Advances in molecular biology during the next decade should enable a more precise estimate of a patient's clinical course than is now possible based on clinical criteria.

In this chapter, we describe the salient features of the disease, stressing practical information of importance to clinicians and findings that are new since the last edition of this book. Readers interested in a more comprehensive source should consult another book in this series.[2]

ONCOGENES AND GROWTH FACTORS IN BREAST CANCER

Advances in molecular biology have enabled researchers to examine the mechanisms of neoplastic growth at the level of gene expression. Delineation of the genetic, molecular, and biochemical events that are responsible for the initiation and transformation of mammary epithelial cells are crucial for understanding the cause, pathogenesis, and prognosis of this disease and for developing new methods of treatment and prevention.[3-8] Two important examples are presented here.

It is hoped that identification of oncogenes in breast tumors can help in assessing prognosis. Some of the oncogenes linked to human mammary carcinoma are *ERBB2* (*i.e.,* human homolog of the gene originally called *NEU* in rat neuroblastomas), *HRAS* (Ha-*ras*), *MYC*, and WNT2 (*i.e.,* updated name of INT2), of which *ERBB2* has been the most studied. The ERBB2 (or NEU) protein is a member of the tyrosine kinase family, and because of the similarity of its transmembrane topology to the epidermal growth factor receptor, it is thought to be a growth factor receptor, although the putative ligand has not been identified. In more than 1500 human breast carcinomas, amplification of the *ERBB2* oncogene or its overexpression at the level of mRNA transcription were found in 21% of the tumor specimens, showing increased gene copy number ranging from twofold to more than a 100-fold greater than normal.[9] In 1987, Slamon and colleagues published findings of a strong association between the oncogene's amplification and nodal status but not with other previously defined prognostic factors, including progesterone receptor status, tumor size, or patient age. For the patients with histologically positive lymph nodes, a significant correlation was found between the degree of gene amplification and both the time to relapse and survival. These findings have been confirmed by some but not all investigators.[10,11] Some of the conflicting findings may be a result of small sample sizes, nonconsecutive case series, differences in study design, or the use of different techniques to demonstrate *ERBB2* gene amplification. Only prospective studies involving large numbers of patients can clarify its usefulness and that of other oncogenes in assessing prognosis.

An improved understanding of the biology of breast cancer may provide new avenues of therapy. During the past 2 decades, a new model of the growth regulation of human breast cancer was developed (Fig. 40–1).[12–15] Breast tumors have the capacity to make growth factors that stimulate their own growth in an autocrine fashion, such as the transforming growth factor-α (TGF-α) and insulin growth factors (IGFs), or that affect stromal tissues or tumor invasiveness by paracrine mechanisms, such as TGF-β and platelet-derived growth factor.[3,13,14] The synthesis and secretion of several of these growth factors are regulated by estrogen in some estrogen receptor (ER)-positive breast cancer cell lines, and they are produced constitutively by certain ER-negative cell lines.[12,13]

This new model of breast cancer growth regulation proposes that stromal tissues such as fibroblasts, mononuclear cells, or endothelial cells play an important role in the development and growth of mammary carcinoma by producing diffusible products that enhance the growth of the breast cancer cells. There appear to be important communications in the form of secreted polypeptide messengers among the various cellular elements of a breast tumor.[14] This new model of breast cancer regulatory mechanisms provides exciting opportunities for new therapies to inhibit tumor growth by interfering specifically with the actions of these growth factors. Such therapies are currently being investigated in phase I–II studies.

SCREENING FOR BREAST CANCER

Screening for cancer represents an important advance in the management of the disease and is described in detail elsewhere in this book. The main methods for earlier detection of breast cancer have been mammography and physical examination performed by a trained health professional. The ability of mammography to detect cancers well before they are apparent on physical examination has been established. The usefulness of mammography has been enhanced by technical improvements that provide better visualization of the breast parenchyma with less exposure to radiation, improvements in film quality and processing, improved techniques for imaging (*e.g.,* compression, focal spot size reduction, magnification, ancillary use of ultrasonography), better guidelines for the diagnosis of cancer, and greater availability of well-trained mammographers. Using these newer techniques, a large percentage of cancers detected are 2 cm or smaller with uninvolved axillary nodes or at the noninvasive

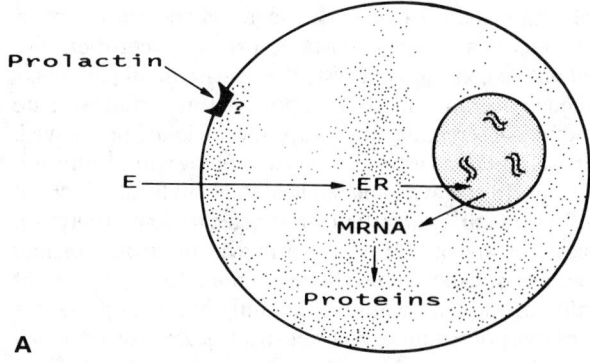

A

Breast Cancer Cell

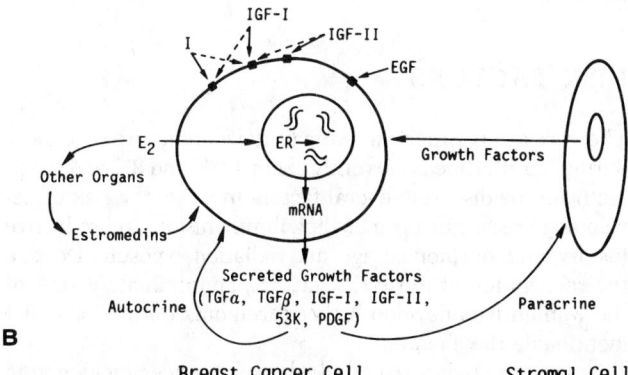

B

Breast Cancer Cell   **Stromal Cell**

FIGURE 40–1. **(A)** Simplified mechanisms of breast cancer growth regulation based on data from the early 1970s. Prolactin was considered important, mainly because it has a pivotal role in rodent mammary carcinoma. The importance of this hormone in human breast cancer development and growth remains questionable. Estrogen (E) stimulation of cells involves the binding of E to estrogen receptor (ER) protein, followed by the tight coupling of the receptor-hormone complex to DNA, resulting in alterations of specific gene transcription and protein synthesis. **(B)** Schema depicting possible growth regulatory pathways in human breast cancer based on recent experimental data. The model preserves the estrogen response pathway mediated through cellular ER, and there is considerable evidence to suggest that E can directly affect cell proliferation. E may also indirectly influence tumor growth through the secretion of growth factors (estromedins) produced at distant sites. In addition to steroid hormones, a host of polypeptide hormones and growth factors may play a role in the regulation of breast cancer growth. (With permission from Osborne CK, Artega CL. Autocrine and paracrine growth regulation in breast cancer: Clinical implications. Breast Cancer Res Treat 1990;15:3–11)

stage (*i.e.,* ductal carcinoma in situ). The use of randomized trials to assess the effect of screening on breast cancer mortality eliminates potential sources of bias, and the trials have demonstrated that screening reduces breast cancer mortality by approximately 25%.[16–22]

The finding that screening reduces breast cancer mortality has important implications for the natural history of the disease. Some evidence suggests that metastases occur very early in the course of the disease and that breast cancer should be considered a systemic disease from its onset.[23] However, the reduction in breast cancer mortality by screening provides compelling evidence that early diagnosis and treatment of breast cancer can avert metastasis. Breast cancer therefore should not be considered a systemic disease in all patients.

Although the randomized trials provided an overall estimate of the effect of screening, they leave several issues unresolved. One important issue is the effect of screening within different age groups. In the available studies, the beneficial effects of screening are fairly consistently restricted to women between the ages of 50 and 69. There is no firm evidence that screening reduces breast cancer mortality in women 40 to 49 years of age, although it can be argued that only in recent years has the sensitivity of mammography been adequate to detect small lesions reliably in this age group. The available results from trials provide little information on the value of mammography in women 70 years or older and have not defined the optimal periodicity of screening or the relative effects of mammography and physical examination in reducing breast cancer mortality.

RISK FACTORS

The risk of an American woman developing breast cancer during her lifetime is currently about 11%, and 3% to 4% will die from the disease. Several factors increase the risk of developing breast cancer, including family history, reproductive history, diet, hormone usage, and radiation exposure. Despite the recognition of these risk factors, approximately 70% of the women who develop breast carcinoma do not have any identifiable risk factors.

Numerous studies have linked breast cancer incidence to the age of menarche, menopause, and first pregnancy. Age at menarche and the establishment of regular ovulatory cycles seem to be strongly associated with breast cancer risk.[24,25] A review of case-control studies suggests that a 20% decrease in breast cancer risk exists for each year that menarche is delayed.[24] The late onset of menarche is associated with a delay in the establishment of regular ovulatory cycles, which is thought to have an additional protective effect by some investigators, although there is dispute on this point.[25–27] A woman's level of physical activity, even if moderate, can have an impact on the likelihood of ovulatory cycles and may alter breast cancer risk.[28] The age-specific incidence of breast cancer rises at a steep rate with age up to the time of menopause and then slows to a rate one sixth of that seen in the premenopausal period. It has been suggested that this age-specific incidence curve is shaped largely by the effects of ovarian activity.[29]

Age at menopause is another factor in breast cancer risk. The relative risk of developing breast cancer for a woman with natural menopause before age 45 is 0.73 compared with a woman with natural menopause between the ages of 45 and 54.[30] Oophorectomy before age 50 decreases breast cancer risk, with an increasing magnitude of risk reduction as the age at oophorectomy decreases.[31] From these data, it seems likely that the total duration of menstrual life is an important factor in breast cancer risk, although the mechanisms through which risk is altered remain uncertain.

Parity and age at first birth are other endogenous hormonal factors that influence breast cancer risk. Nulliparous women are at greater risk for the development of breast cancer than parous women, with a relative risk of about 1.4.[32] It has become increasingly apparent that the effect of term pregnancy on breast cancer risk varies with the age at first birth, with women whose first term pregnancy occurs after age 30 having a twofold to fivefold increase in breast cancer risk compared with women having a first term pregnancy before age 18 or 19.[33,34] Abortion, whether spontaneous or induced, before full-term pregnancy has no protective effect, and in several studies, it has been shown to increase breast cancer risk. The apparently contradictory effects of pregnancy on risk are explained in a variety of ways.[32,35,36] Breast tissue may undergo differentiation as a result of the hormonal changes of pregnancy, and these differentiated cells are less likely to undergo malignant transformation, or the persisting changes in hormone levels after pregnancy may alter the proliferative rate of the breast epithelium.[29,37,38] In incomplete pregnancy, the breast is exposed only to the high estrogen levels of early pregnancy, and this may be responsible for the increased risk seen in these women.

The associations between the use of oral contraceptives or postmenopausal estrogen replacement and breast cancer were reviewed by Henderson.[39] Of 27 reported studies of oral contraceptive use, only two showed an overall increase in risk for all patients in the study population. One of these studies found a twofold increase in breast cancer risk with any use of oral contraceptives.[40] These data suggest that if oral contraceptives increase overall breast cancer risk, the magnitude of the increase is small. Despite this, there is continuing concern about the potential risks in a variety of subgroups. Several studies have demonstrated an increased risk of breast cancer in long-term users of oral contraceptives.[40–43] Risk estimates range from 1.7 for use longer than 8 years to 4.1 for use for 10 or more years.[40,41] However, the Centers for Disease Control's Cancer and Steroid Hormone study failed to find any increase in risk related to duration of oral contraceptive use or in users with a family history of breast cancer or a personal history of benign breast disease.[44] Currently, there is no compelling evidence to avoid the use of oral contraceptives for any subgroup of patients. Most studies of oral contraceptives involve women treated with higher estrogen doses than those currently used. Since 1960, the average estrogen content of contraceptive pills has dropped from 150 to 35 mg, and currently available contraceptives may have even less of an effect than that previously observed. Due to uncertainties regarding the latent interval between oral contraceptive use and the onset of cancer and their recent widespread use by very young women, firm conclusions about the safety of oral contraceptives must await further follow-up.

The use of postmenopausal estrogen replacement therapy may be associated with a small increase in breast cancer risk in the range of 1.5 to 2.0 for moderate-dose conjugated estrogen therapy for periods of 10 to 20 years.[39] The use of estrogen replacement for short periods of time appears safe, and little information is available about the effect of long-term, low-dose therapy. In evaluating the potential risk of estrogen replacement therapy, its proven benefits in reducing osteoporosis and subsequent fracture and lowering the risk of coronary artery disease should be kept in mind.[45]

A possible relation between breast cancer and diet has been suggested by the large variation in international breast cancer incidence rates. National per capita fat consumption correlates with incidence and mortality from breast cancer (Fig. 40–

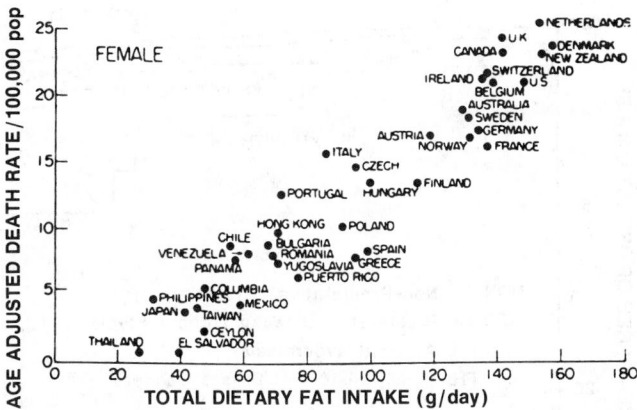

FIGURE 40–2. The relation between total dietary fat intake by country and the death rate from breast cancer. (With permission from Carroll K. Experimental evidence of dietary factors and hormone dependent cancers. Cancer Res 1975;35:3374–3383)

2).[46] That these differences are not solely due to genetics is suggested by studies of migrants. Japanese women immigrating to the United States and first-generation American-born Japanese were found to have an incidence of breast cancer almost equal to that of whites in the same area and considerably higher than that of women in Japan.[47] Although this suggests that environmental factors are important in breast cancer incidence, it does not implicate diet as the sole cause of the observed differences.

Epidemiologic studies of diet and studies of populations with special diets have produced inconclusive results. Kinlen compared breast cancer rates between nuns who were vegetarians or ate only small amounts of meat and single British women who ate regular diets and observed no differences.[48] Breast cancer mortality among Seventh Day Adventists, a group that eats a diet low in animal fats, is not significantly lower than expected.[49] In the largest prospective study of dietary fat, 89,538 nurses between the ages of 34 and 59 were studied.[50] No relation between breast cancer risk and total fat, saturated fat, linoleic acid, or cholesterol intake was found. The difference in fat intake between women at the lowest and highest extremes of fat intake was only 25%. This suggests that dietary fat reduction in the context of the usual American diet is unlikely to reduce breast cancer risk. In another prospective study with more than 10 years of follow-up, breast cancer risk was actually lower in women with the highest total fat intake, although this difference was not statistically significant after adjustments for total caloric intake were made.[51] Currently, there is no conclusive evidence that dietary modification reduces breast cancer incidence or alters prognosis after a diagnosis of breast cancer.[52]

A positive but modest association between alcohol use and breast cancer risk is seen in most studies. A metaanalysis of 16 case-control and cohort studies found a relative risk of breast cancer of 1.4 for women with an alcohol intake of two drinks per day.[53] A clear-cut dose-response association was observed. The largest cohort study of alcohol and breast cancer, based on data from the American Cancer Society, found no increase in risk in occasional users of alcohol, but risk was elevated in all other categories of alcohol use.[54] Several studies have found that alcohol has its greatest effect on breast cancer risk in women under the age of 30.[55,56]

Women with a family history of breast cancer in a first- or second-degree relative are at increased risk for developing the disease. The risk of developing breast cancer is increased 1.5 to 3.0 times if a mother or sister has the disease, and risk may be greater if a sibling is affected than if a mother is affected.[57,58] For women whose relatives have unilateral breast carcinoma, its occurrence premenopausally or postmenopausally does not seem to significantly affect risk.[57] In some studies, risk increases with the number of cancer-affected first-degree relatives, but this is an inconsistent finding.[59,60] Bilateral premenopausal breast cancer in a relative has been associated with the highest risk of breast cancer development.[57,61] For most persons with a family history of breast cancer, the lifetime probability of developing breast cancer is rarely greater than 30%, and the magnitude of risk conferred by a positive family history is similar to that seen with many other risk factors. Only 5% of carefully studied breast cancer patients are thought to have a pedigree consistent with hereditary breast cancer.[62] Breast cancer is observed as part of cancer family syndromes in association with other tumors. These are listed in Table 40–1.

Epidemiologic studies have shown that women exposed to ionizing radiation due to nuclear war or medical diagnostic and therapeutic procedures are at increased risk for the development of breast carcinoma.[63–66] Multiple chest fluoroscopies, breast irradiation for mastitis, and thymic irradiation increase breast cancer risk.[64–66] There is a long latent period for radiation-induced breast cancer, and the risk of developing the disease is related to the age at radiation exposure. Radiation exposure after age 40 results in a minimal increase in risk, and radiation in adolescence is associated with the greatest risk of breast cancer development.[64] Girls irradiated during infancy for thymic enlargement had a linear dose-response risk for subsequent breast cancer development.[66]

An assessment of the breast cancer risk associated with benign breast disease cannot be made without specific knowledge of the histologic features of the biopsy. Fibrocystic disease includes a heterogeneous group of pathologic changes associated with various degrees of breast cancer risk. A useful system for classifying benign breast diseases was proposed by Dupont and Page,[67] and subsequently adopted at a consensus meeting of the American College of Pathologists.[68] Benign breast conditions were classified as nonproliferative or proliferative, and on the basis of a review of more than 10,000 breast biopsies, relative risks of breast cancer were determined.[67] Women with proliferative disease were found to have

TABLE 40–1. Breast Cancer in Hereditary Syndromes

Syndrome	Sites of Other Tumors
Li-Fraumeni syndrome	Sarcomas (*e.g.*, soft tissue, bone), brain tumors, leukemia, adrenocortical carcinoma
Cowden's disease	Facial trichilemmomas, papillomatosis of lips and oral mucosa, acral keratoses, gastrointestinal polyps, uterine leiomyomata
Muir syndrome	Basal cell carcinoma, benign and malignant gastrointestinal tumors

a relative risk of 1.9, and the subcategory of women with atypical hyperplasia were found to have a relative risk of 4.4. Nonproliferative breast disease was associated with no excess risk of breast cancer. Sixty-nine percent of the reviewed biopsies were found to have nonproliferative breast disease, and of the biopsies demonstrating proliferative changes, only 3.6% were atypical.[67] The histologic diagnoses grouped under the headings of proliferative and nonproliferative disease are shown in Table 40–2.

The risk of breast cancer development after a diagnosis of proliferative breast disease with or without atypia is greatest in the first 10 years after the biopsy, with the relative risk associated with atypical hyperplasia halved after this interval and the relative risk for women with proliferative disease without atypia returning to the level of the index population.[69] A marked interaction between atypia and a family history of a first-degree relative with breast cancer was also found by Dupont and Page.[67] This subgroup of patients had a risk 11 times that of women with nonproliferative disease. The effect of a family history of breast carcinoma in conjunction with atypical hyperplasia on the incidence of cancer for a 25-year period is shown in Figure 40–3. The absolute risk of breast cancer development in women with a positive family history and atypical hyperplasia was 20% at 15 years, compared with 8% in women with atypical hyperplasia and a negative family history of breast carcinoma. No increased risk of breast cancer development was observed in women with a diagnosis of proliferative disease who used estrogens after their breast biopsies.[70]

Risk factor assessment for the individual patient is poorly understood by many clinicians. Risk may be expressed as absolute risk or relative risk. Relative risk cannot be multiplied by lifetime risk to determine the risk status of an individual patient. Many believe that risk is most meaningfully discussed with a patient as the risk over a given time interval. Although the lifetime risk of breast cancer development for an American woman is about 11%, more than half of this risk is expressed after age 65. Moreover, the risk of dying from breast cancer is one third the risk of developing the disease. Risk figures by age interval are shown in Table 40–3. For most women with identified risk factors, the lifetime absolute risk of developing breast cancer is in the range of 20% to 40%. Gail and colleagues developed a model that incorporates age at menarche, age at first live birth, number of previous biopsies, and number of first-degree relatives with breast cancer to provide an in-

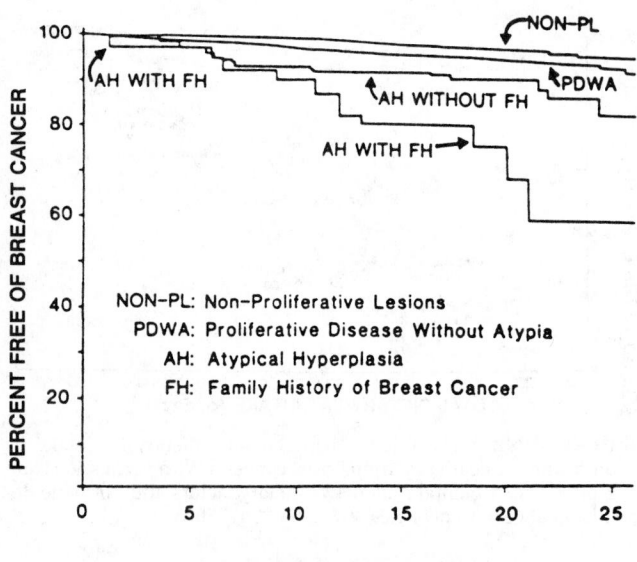

FIGURE 40–3. Freedom from breast cancer in relation to types of benign breast lesions and family history. (With permission from Dupont W, Page D. Risk factors for breast cancer in women with proliferative breast disease. N Engl J Med 1985;312:146–151)

dividualized risk estimate for breast cancer development at different ages over various time intervals.[71] For example, a 30-year-old nulliparous female with menarche at age 12, a history of one benign breast biopsy and one relative with breast cancer is estimated to have a 2.3% risk of developing breast cancer in the next 10 years. A 50-year-old with the same risk factors has a 7.6% risk of developing breast cancer in the next 10 years. The 30-year risk for the 30-year-old woman is 14.9%, and the corresponding risk for the 50-year-old woman is 19.9%. A precise estimate of an individual patient's risk is often helpful, because the extensive publicity about breast cancer causes many women at increased risk to feel that they are doomed to die from the disease.

There are no interventions proven to decrease risk. The data on the use of exogenous hormones are controversial enough that a firm recommendation to avoid their use cannot be made. Similarly, the link between dietary fat and breast cancer is weak, and there is little evidence to suggest that altering diet or alcohol consumption in adult life changes breast cancer risk. Patient education with instruction in breast self-examination, regular physical examinations every 4 to 6 months, and mammography in accordance with standard guidelines are appropriate surveillance techniques.

PREVENTION OF BREAST CANCER

Prevention of breast cancer is possible only by bilateral prophylactic mastectomy. This is a radical approach, particularly because breast-conserving therapy is increasingly employed for the treatment of established cancer. Research is now directed toward developing agents for the primary chemoprevention of breast cancer, an approach that, if successful, will be more applicable to the general population.

TABLE 40–2. Classification of Benign Breast Diseases

Nonproliferative	*Proliferative*
Adenosis	Moderate or florid hyperplasia
Cysts, macro or micro	Papilloma with fibrovascular core
Duct ectasia	Atypical hyperplasia, ductal or lobular
Fibroadenoma	
Fibrosis	
Mastitis	
Metaplasia, apocrine or squamous	
Mild hyperplasia	

TABLE 40–3. Probability of Developing and Dying From Breast Cancer

Age (y)	Risk of Developing Breast Cancer (%)	Risk of Developing Invasive Breast Cancer (%)	Risk of Dying From Breast Cancer (%)
Birth to 110	10.2	9.8	3.6
20 to 30	0.04	0.04	0.000
20 to 40	0.49	0.42	0.09
35 to 45	0.88	0.83	0.14
35 to 55	2.53	2.37	0.56
35 to 110	10.27	9.82	3.56
50 to 60	1.95	1.86	0.33
50 to 70	4.67	4.48	1.04
50 to 110	8.96	8.66	2.75
65 to 75	3.17	3.08	0.43
65 to 85	5.48	5.29	1.01
65 to 110	6.53	6.29	1.53

(Seidman H, Mushinski M, Gelb SEA. Probabilities of eventually developing or dying of cancer: United States, 1985. CA 1985;35:36–56). The data are derived from white females.

PROPHYLACTIC MASTECTOMY

Little agreement exists on the indications for prophylactic breast removal. Some have suggested the use of prophylactic mastectomy for women with a family history of breast cancer, carcinoma of the contralateral breast, high-risk benign histologies, lumpy breasts, or a high degree of anxiety.[72–75] This list includes women with true hereditary breast cancer who may have a risk of developing breast cancer that is as high as 50% and women with lumpy breasts due to nonproliferative fibrocystic disease who have no increased risk of developing breast cancer.[76] There are currently no absolute indications for prophylactic mastectomy. Decisions about surgery should be made only after a detailed discussion with the woman of her relative and absolute risk of developing breast cancer.

Another problem with prophylactic mastectomy is that the efficacy of the procedure is difficult to assess due to inadequate follow-up and poor definition of the risk classification of women who have undergone the surgery. In the Mayo Clinic series of 1500 women treated with prophylactic subcutaneous mastectomy, only 5 (0.0033%) were identified who subsequently developed breast carcinoma at a maximal follow-up of 22 years.[77] However, many of these women were at relatively low risk for the development of breast carcinoma, and not all patients were systematically followed. Prophylactic mastectomy does not offer 100% protection against breast cancer. Pennisi followed 1244 women for 7 years after prophylactic subcutaneous mastectomy and found a cancer incidence of 0.5%.[78] Subcutaneous mastectomy is an unsatisfactory operation for breast cancer prophylaxis because glandular breast tissue is left behind beneath the nipple and often on the skin flaps and in the tail of the breast.[75,79] In animals, a reduction in the volume of breast tissue is not associated with a proportionate reduction in breast cancer risk.[80] If prophylactic surgery is undertaken, the operative procedure should be a total mastectomy with sacrifice of the nipple-areolar complex. Even with this procedure, breast tissue may be left behind on the flaps or in the axilla unless great care is taken with operative technique.[81] In considering prophylactic mastectomy, it should be kept in mind that for nearly all women, their chances of not having breast cancer exceed their risk of developing the disease, and even bilateral mastectomy is not an absolute guarantee that breast cancer will not develop.

CHEMOPREVENTION

One of the most important new strategies to address the breast cancer problem is the use of agents for the chemoprevention or the chemosuppression of the disease. The two main agents being evaluated are tamoxifen and retinoids. Much of the impetus for the use of tamoxifen as a chemopreventive agent comes from the trials of its use as an adjuvant systemic agent, which demonstrated a reduction of approximately 40% in the number of contralateral breast cancers in tamoxifen-treated women compared with controls. A trial to test the value of tamoxifen as a prevention for breast cancer is currently underway in the United Kingdom and will be underway soon in the United States by the National Surgical Adjuvant Breast and Bowel Project (NSABP). Retinoids have been shown to be effective in preventing or reducing the incidence of breast cancer in several animal studies.[82–84] A clinical trial of the synthetic retinoid N-(4-hydroxyphenyl) retanamide (HPR) has been undertaken by the National Cancer Institute in Milan. Three thousand women previously treated for a unilateral T1 or T2, node-negative breast carcinoma have been randomized to HPR or no treatment, and the incidence of contralateral breast cancer will be assessed. No data are currently available from this trial. There is no indication for the use of tamoxifen or the retinoids as chemopreventive agents outside of a clinical trial.

BREAST BIOPSY

INDICATIONS FOR BIOPSY: CLINICAL ABNORMALITIES

The most common clinical indications for breast biopsy are a dominant breast mass or a pathologic nipple discharge. Although this seems straightforward, the determination of what constitutes a dominant breast mass is frequently difficult, particularly in the premenopausal woman. Normal breasts are a mixture of fat and glandular tissue. The glandular tissue, most of which is located in the upper outer quadrant, changes throughout the menstrual cycle, and this type of physiologic nodularity should not be considered an indication for a breast biopsy. Dominant masses are characterized by their persistence throughout the menstrual cycle. Breast pain, in the absence of a dominant mass, should not be an indication for a breast biopsy. Breast pain is an uncommon presenting symptom of breast carcinoma, seen in only 7% of cases reported by Preece, and if it is not accompanied by clinical or mammographic evidence of a breast mass, medical management, rather than surgical intervention, is appropriate.[85]

If a dominant breast mass is detected in a premenopausal woman, it should be aspirated to determine if it is a cyst. Cysts require biopsy only if the aspirated fluid is bloody, the palpable abnormality does not completely resolve after the aspiration of fluid, or the same cyst recurs multiple times. This policy can be safely followed because intracystic carcinoma accounts for fewer than 1% of all breast cancers.[86] Routine cytologic examination of breast cyst fluid is not indicated because of the low likelihood of carcinoma in the absence of bloody fluid or recurrent cysts.[87,88] Noncystic masses in premenopausal women that are clearly different from the surrounding breast tissue should be biopsied using one of the techniques described later. Observation for one to two menstrual cycles is only appropriate for vague asymmetry or nodularity if it is uncertain that a dominant mass exists. In women older than 35, a mammogram is an essential part of the prebiopsy workup of a breast mass. Communication with the radiologist allows a complete radiographic evaluation, which may include compression and magnification views to define the extent of associated microcalcifications, or ultrasound if a cyst is suspected.

In postmenopausal women, clinical examination of the breasts is frequently easier due to atrophy of the nodular glandular elements. Without exogenous estrogen, cysts are uncommon after the perimenopausal years, and the masses should be regarded with a higher degree of suspicion than those in premenopausal women. Benign breast conditions causing palpable masses are less frequent, and small areas of nodularity that might be observed in premenopausal women should be considered for prompt biopsy in the postmenopausal patient.

Although nipple discharge is a common complaint, it is an uncommon sign of breast carcinoma. Three percent to 11% of women with malignant disease have an associated nipple discharge.[89–91] The likelihood of a nipple discharge being secondary to malignancy increases as patient age increases. A 32% incidence of carcinoma was found for women older than 60 presenting with a discharge and no mass, compared with a 7% incidence in women younger than 60.[91] Discharges are considered pathologic if they are unilateral, spontaneous, and localized to one duct. Discharges secondary to carcinoma may be bloody or serous. Bloody discharges are reported in 70% to 85% of the cancers that present with nipple discharge.[89,90,92] If a discharge occurs, it should be tested for occult blood and localized to one quadrant of the breast. A mammogram should be obtained to look for dilated ducts or occult masses. Galactography cannot reliably differentiate benign from malig-

nant causes of discharge and is not usually helpful in cases where clinical indications for surgery are present.[93] A persistent pathologic discharge is an indication for duct exploration. In a review of 1956 cases of pathologic discharge, 44% were due to papilloma or papillomatosis, 23% to duct ectasia, 16% to fibrocystic disease, and only 11% were associated with malignancy.[94] Terminal duct excision is the procedure of choice for the diagnosis and treatment of nipple discharge in the absence of a breast mass. If a mass is associated with the discharge, the mass should be biopsied.

BIOPSY TECHNIQUES

Palpable Masses

Four techniques are available for the diagnosis of breast masses. They are fine-needle aspiration, core-cutting needle biopsy, incisional biopsy, and excisional biopsy. Fine-needle aspiration and core-cutting needle biopsy are office procedures. Excisional biopsy, with rare exceptions, is an outpatient procedure that can be done using local anesthesia.

Fine-needle aspiration is becoming increasingly popular for the diagnosis of dominant breast masses. The procedure has the advantages of being quick, relatively painless, and inexpensive to perform. The main drawbacks of the procedure are the need for an experienced cytopathologist to interpret smears and the risk of false-negative results. Strawbridge, reviewing 890 lesions with histologic confirmation of cytologic results, found a 9.6% false-negative rate.[88] Bell and coworkers reported a 4% false-negative rate in their series of 1680 aspirates.[87] Kline and colleagues, in a review of 3545 breast aspirates, reported a 9.6% incidence of false negatives.[95] In half of Kline's cases, the needle tract did not extend into the tumor, most of which were smaller than 1 cm in diameter. Extremely fibrotic tumors were found to be a source of false-negative results, and invasive lobular carcinoma was more likely to be a source of false-negative results than infiltrating ductal carcinoma.[95] In addition to false-negative aspirates, specimens with material insufficient for diagnosis are reported in 1% to 10% of aspirates.[88,95,96] Barrows found that the experience of the physician performing the aspirate was the factor that most strongly predicted a successful aspirate. False-positive aspirates are extremely uncommon, reported in fewer than 1% of cases in most large series.[88,95,96] However, fine-needle aspiration cannot identify cases of gross ductal carcinoma in situ as noninvasive tumors, potentially leading to overtreatment.

Fine-needle aspiration is an excellent technique for establishing a diagnosis of breast cancer before placing an incision in the breast. A treatment option can then be selected by the patient, and only a single operative procedure is needed. Because of the false-negative rate of up to 10% seen with fine-needle aspiration, dominant masses for which a malignant diagnosis is not obtained should be excised. Several physicians have suggested that patients with benign cytologic results and a mammogram and physical examination suggesting benign breast disease can be followed expectantly, with a rate of missed breast cancer of less than 1%. In view of the low morbidity of breast biopsy, this seems unnecessarily risky if a dominant breast mass is present.[97–99]

Core-cutting needle biopsy has many of the advantages of

fine-needle aspiration. It is a rapid, relatively painless office procedure. Because a core of tissue is obtained for histologic examination, more details of tumor structure are available, and ductal carcinoma in situ can be identified. Fentiman reported a 79% accuracy rate for core-cutting needle biopsy, and no false-positive results were seen.[100] Minkowitz found an 89% sensitivity for the technique, which increased to 94% for lesions larger than 2.5 cm.[101] Aspiration cytology and core-cutting needle biopsy were prospectively compared for 81 women by Shabot and coworkers. The accuracy of fine-needle aspiration was 96.2%, compared with 78.9% for core-cutting needle biopsy.[102] The choice of core-cutting needle biopsy or fine-needle aspiration depends on the availability of an experienced cytopathologist.

Excisional biopsy has been the standard technique for the diagnosis of breast masses. It has the advantage of allowing a complete evaluation of the tumor size and its histologic characteristics before instituting definitive therapy. When an excisional biopsy is done for the diagnosis of a breast mass, it should be done as a definitive lumpectomy, with the mass excised with a surrounding margin of normal breast tissue. The biopsy incision should be placed directly over the mass in a curvilinear fashion. The exception to this rule is the young woman with a clinical diagnosis of fibroadenoma; the mass can be shelled out without removing additional breast tissue. Breast tissue should not usually be reapproximated after biopsy to avoid distortion of the breast contour, and drains should be avoided for the same reason. Proper handling of the specimen is crucial to the success of the biopsy. The specimen should be excised as a single piece of tissue and orienting sutures placed for the pathologist. The tissue should not be placed in formalin and should be promptly sent to the pathology department to allow inking for evaluation of the margins and sampling for hormone receptors. Most excisional biopsies are done as outpatient procedures. There is no evidence that a one-step procedure (*i.e.*, biopsy under general anesthesia followed by definitive surgery if positive) is associated with any survival benefit compared with biopsy followed later by definitive surgery, and outpatient breast biopsy is more cost effective.[23,103–105]

Incisional biopsy is used to establish a diagnosis of breast cancer in masses too large to excise completely. It is frequently employed in women with metastatic disease or those with locally advanced breast cancer who will be receiving systemic therapy as an initial treatment approach. The problems of poor wound healing, which can occasionally occur in this setting, can be avoided by the use of fine-needle aspiration with immunohistochemical hormone receptor determination rather than incisional biopsy.

Mammographic Abnormalities

The classic mammographic signs of clinically occult malignancy are clustered microcalcifications and a stellate mass. A review of 5500 biopsies from 17 reports of 100 or more cases identified microcalcifications as the indication for biopsy in 45% of cases, masses in 43%, masses containing microcalcifications in 6%, and asymmetric density in 5%.[106] The incidence of positive biopsies done for mammographic findings ranges from 9% to 65%, with most investigators reporting a 15% to 30% positive biopsy rate.[107–110] Moskowitz found

that the predictive value of microcalcifications for the presence of cancer was 11.5±1.7%, based on his review of 40,431 screening mammograms.[111] The predictive value of masses that were thought to be definitely malignant was 74%, but masses thought to be possibly malignant yielded carcinoma in only 5.4% of cases. Because the predictive value of any mammographic sign depends on the skill of the observer and the quality of the mammograms, positive biopsy yields in some institutions may be lower than those reported in the literature.

Special mammographic views are frequently helpful in the evaluation of equivocal findings on two-view mammography. Tabar found that 62% of abnormalities identified on a single-view screening examination were shown to be of no concern with additional views.[110] Sickles evaluated 302 women with indeterminate microcalcifications with magnification views and demonstrated 61% of the lesions to be benign and 11% to have previously unsuspected malignant characteristics.[112] Even if biopsy is clearly indicated on the basis of the initial mammogram, magnification views are useful in delineating the extent of microcalcifications in women considering breast-conserving therapy.

Magnification views of mass lesions are helpful in equivocal cases. Magnification mammography increased diagnostic accuracy from 29% to 69% in 216 cases with indeterminate masses or microcalcifications on initial studies.[113] Other radiologic techniques are not particularly helpful in the evaluation of occult breast masses, although sonography is useful for determining if mass lesions are cysts. Transillumination light scanning, computerized tomography (CT), and magnetic resonance imaging (MRI) have not been shown to be superior to mammography.

Nonpalpable Masses

Because only 15% to 30% of mammographic abnormalities are shown to be cancer, a biopsy technique that reliably excises the lesion with a good cosmetic result is essential. Blind excisions of large amounts of breast tissue or the use of skin marking as a localization technique are unsatisfactory, with failure to excise the mammographic abnormality reported in 17% of cases, even with the removal of large amounts of breast tissue.[114] Localization can be done using straight needles, hook wires, or dye injection along a needle tract. The most important factor in the success of localization is how close the wire is placed to the mammographic abnormality. Gallagher reported wire placement to within 2 mm of the target in 96% of cases, with 96% of the lesions being successfully removed on the first attempt.[115] The average specimen size was 6 cm³. Communication between the mammographer and the surgeon is important to ensure that the incision for the needle localization biopsy is placed over the termination of the wire rather than at the entry of the wire into the skin to avoid tunneling to the lesion. Specimen radiography should be carried out in all biopsies done for microcalcifications to confirm the presence of the calcifications in the biopsy specimen. Compression and magnification views are useful for specimen evaluation. Although nonpalpable masses can frequently be identified grossly at the time of biopsy, it is still useful to obtain x-ray films of the specimen to ensure that the gross lesion corresponds to the mammographic abnormality. The specimen should be marked with orienting sutures and inked to allow evaluation of margins.

Frozen section is reliable in the diagnosis of palpable breast masses, but indications for its use in the evaluation of non-palpable breast abnormalities are limited. If a definite mass is palpable intraoperatively, a frozen section may be done and tissue saved for estrogen receptors if the frozen-section specimen is positive. Tinnemans evaluated the reliability of frozen-section diagnoses in 297 clinically occult lesions.[116] Diagnosis was deferred to permanent section in 12% of cases, and if a definitive diagnosis was made, there was a 3% incidence of false-negative results and two instances of false-positive results. Because the abnormalities being sought by needle localization are usually small and often represent histologically borderline lesions, they may be difficult to diagnose on frozen section. Because needle localization is rarely undertaken with a plan to proceed to definitive therapy at the same operation, a careful examination of all the available pathologic material in paraffin sections would seem to be the most prudent course. Failure to remove the mammographic abnormality occurs in 2% to 8% of localizations.[106] In these cases, persistence of the lesion on mammogram should be confirmed and repeat biopsy undertaken.

Aspiration cytology, using a stereotactic device for needle positioning, has been employed for the diagnosis of nonpalpable breast abnormalities. Azavedo and coworkers aspirated 2594 mammographic abnormalities.[117] Seventy-seven percent of the patients had benign aspirates and received no further therapy if the mammographic finding was thought to be of low suspicion. One of these 2005 women developed a carcinoma 14 months later. Overall, only 21.9% of the mammographic abnormalities were biopsied, and 76% of those biopsied were carcinoma. Diagnostic sensitivities and specificities over 90% are reported from several centers using this procedure.[117-119] The major use of aspiration cytology of non-palpable breast masses has been to avoid biopsy of minimally suspicious lesions unless cytologic evidence of atypia is found.[120] Stereotactic fine-needle aspiration is unlikely to be of major use in the management of highly suspicious mammographic abnormalities, because it does not reliably differentiate invasive and in situ disease. The availability of stereotactically directed core biopsies may partially resolve this problem, but only complete excision of the mammographic abnormality allows a reliable assessment of invasion to be made.

CLASSIFICATION OF TUMOR TYPES

Histopathologic examination of breast cancer makes available information that establishes the diagnosis of the lesion, aids in determining patient prognosis, and leads to a better understanding of the nature of breast cancer.

Several pathologic classifications of mammary carcinomas are in use. The most commonly used are those presented by the Armed Forces Institute of Pathology (AFIP)[121] and the World Health Organization.[122] Breast carcinomas are classified as ductal or lobular, corresponding to the ducts and lobules of the normal breast. However, there is evidence that most tumors arise in the terminal duct section of the breast, regardless of pathologic type.[123] A comparison of the histologic types of infiltrating breast carcinomas from the AFIP is given in Table 40–4.[121]

CARCINOMA IN SITU

Tumors arising from duct epithelium that are confined within the lumen of the ducts or lobules of the breast are referred to as carcinoma in situ. Carcinoma in situ has been classified as ductal or lobular, depending on the cytologic features and pattern of growth. Ductal carcinoma in situ (DCIS), also known as intraductal carcinoma or noninvasive ductal carcinoma, and lobular carcinoma in situ (LCIS) are characterized by a proliferation of malignant epithelial cells confined to the mammary ducts or lobules, without light-microscopic evidence of invasion through the basement membrane into the surrounding stroma. The distinction between DCIS and LCIS is usually not difficult, but overlaps exist. The natural history and management of these lesions are discussed later.

INFILTRATING DUCTAL CARCINOMAS

A variety of histologic types of invasive (infiltrating) carcinomas of the breast have been described. Infiltrating ductal carcinomas in which no special histologic features are recognized are designated NOS (not otherwise specified) and

TABLE 40–4. Comparison of Histologic Types of Infiltrating Breast Carcinoma

Characteristic	Ductal	Lobular	Medullary	Colloid	Comedo	Papillary
Percent*	78.1%	8.7%	4.3%	2.6%	4.6%	1.2%
Average age (y)	50.7	53.8	49.0	49.7	48.6	51.9
Average size (cm)	3.1	3.5	3.4	3.8	3.9	3.4
Involved nodes	60%	60%	44%	32%	32%	17%
Survival						
At 5 years	59%	57%	69%	76%	84%	89%
At 10 years	47%	42%	68%	72%	77%	65%
At 15 years	38%	34%	62%	62%	74%	65%

* Percent of all infiltrating carcinomas.
(McDivitt R, Stewart F, Berg J. Tumors of the breast. In: Atlas of tumor pathology. Bethesda, MD: Armed Forces Institute of Pathology, 1967)

account for almost 70% of breast cancers. They are characterized by their stony hardness to palpation. When transected, a gritty resistance is typically encountered, and the tumor retracts below the cut surface. Histologically, various degrees of fibrotic response and associated DCIS are present. These tumors commonly metastasize to the axillary lymph nodes, and their prognosis is the poorest of the various ductal types.

MEDULLARY CARCINOMA

Medullary carcinomas are circumscribed lesions that can attain large dimensions, but they demonstrate only low-grade infiltrative properties. They constitute 5% to 7% of all mammary carcinomas and are characterized by a well-circumscribed border, poorly differentiated nuclei, syncytial growth pattern, and an intense infiltration with small lymphocytes and plasma cells. The 5-year survival rate after treatment for medullary carcinoma is better than for NOS ductal carcinomas. The more favorable prognosis requires the presence of *all* of these characteristics; tumors with some of these features (*i.e.*, atypical medullary tumors) do not have a more favorable prognosis.[124]

TUBULAR CARCINOMA

A tumor in which tubule formation is conspicuous is known as tubular or well-differentiated carcinoma. This diagnosis is made only if 75% or more of the tumor is composed of these elements. Axillary metastases are uncommon, and the prognosis is considerably better than for NOS ductal carcinoma.

MUCINOUS CARCINOMA

Another ductal type, the mucinous or colloid carcinoma, comprises about 3% of all mammary carcinoma. It is slow growing and can reach bulky proportions. When the tumor is predominantly mucinous, the prognosis tends to be good.

Rarer types of ductal carcinomas include papillary, adenocystic, apocrine, secretory, squamous, and carcinosarcoma or metaplastic duct carcinoma. In many cases, NOS ductal carcinomas contain small areas of these special types.

INFILTRATING LOBULAR CARCINOMA

Another histologic type of breast cancer is infiltrating lobular carcinoma. It is relatively uncommon, accounting for only 5% to 10% of breast tumors in most series. The clinical presentation is often an area of ill-defined thickening in the breast, unlike the dominant lump characteristic of ductal carcinoma. Microscopically, lobular carcinomas typically are composed of small cells in a linear arrangement ("Indian filing") with a tendency to grow around ducts and lobules (*i.e.*, targetoid growth). Lobular carcinomas are characterized by a greater proportion of multicentric tumors in the same or the opposite breast than are found in NOS ductal carcinoma. Overall, infiltrating lobular carcinoma has a similar likelihood of axillary nodal involvement and prognosis as infiltrating duct carcinoma. However, the sites of metastases for these two types tend to differ. Ductal carcinomas more characteristically metastasize to bone or to intraparenchymal sites within lung,

liver, or brain, and lobular carcinomas more often show a predilection for meningeal and serosal surfaces.[125]

INFILTRATING COMEDOCARCINOMA

Infiltrating comedocarcinoma is a type of infiltrating ductal carcinoma. It is composed primarily of the comedo type of ductal carcinoma in situ, which is characterized by large poorly differentiated nuclei with frequent mitoses and central necrosis with areas of invasion. This term has not been used recently because of possible confusion with pure comedo DCIS. Tumors with an extensive intraductal component appear to have important implications in breast-conserving treatment and are discussed in the section on local treatment.

PAGET'S DISEASE

Paget's disease of the breast occurs in 1% of all patients with breast cancer. Clinically, the patient presents with a relatively long history of eczematous changes in the nipple with itching, burning, oozing, bleeding, or some combination of these. The nipple changes are associated with an underlying carcinoma in the breast that can be palpated in one half to two thirds of the patients. The subadjacent tumor may be the intraductal or invasive duct type. The prognosis is related to the histologic type of the associated tumor. Histologically, the nipple epidermis contains tumor cells singly and in nests. Treatment of Paget's disease is discussed later in this chapter.

INFLAMMATORY BREAST CARCINOMA

Inflammatory breast cancer is characterized clinically by prominent skin edema, redness and warmth, a visible erysipeloid margin, and induration of the underlying tissue. In approximately half of these patients, a mass is not palpated. These criteria in the past were sufficient for the diagnosis, but currently, pathologic corroboration must be obtained by a skin biopsy demonstrating involvement of the dermal lymphatics with cancer cells. Inflammatory cells rarely are present. The prognosis of patients with inflammatory breast cancer is poor, even if the disease is apparently localized. The management of inflammatory cancer is discussed later in this chapter.

LOCAL AND REGIONAL SPREAD OF BREAST CANCER

The features of breast cancer related to its local and regional involvement provide the basis for local treatment, which is discussed later in this chapter.

LOCAL INVOLVEMENT

The primary site of breast cancer is described by the quadrant of the breast in which it is found. In one series of 696 patients, 48% of the tumors were located in the upper outer quadrant, 15% in the upper inner quadrant, 11% in the lower outer quadrant, 6% in the lower inner quadrant, and 17% in the central region (*i.e.*, within 1 cm of the areola).[126] An additional 3% were called diffuse because of multifocal origin or involvement of the entire breast. The higher frequency of breast cancer in the upper outer quadrant is thought to be attributable simply to the greater amount of breast tissue in that quadrant. In this series of patients, no differences in survival based on quadrant location were found. The relation between the location of the primary tumor and prognosis was examined in another large NSABP series. Relapse and ultimate survival were related to the pathologic status of the axillary nodes, and there were no significant differences in prognosis by primary tumor location (Table 40–5).[127]

The spread of cancer through the breast was summarized by Haagensen.[128] This spread occurs by direct infiltration into the breast parenchyma, along mammary ducts, and through breast lymphatics. Direct infiltration tends to occur by ramifying projections that have a characteristic stellate appearance on gross examination. If untreated, direct involvement of overlying skin or deep pectoral fascia is common. Involvement along ducts is observed frequently and may include wide segments of the breast. It is unclear whether this intraductal involvement represents true spread of a primary cancer along previously uninvolved ducts or a "field cancerization" that results in simultaneous transformation along entire lengths of ducts. Spread can occur by the extensive network of breast lymphatics. Investigators have emphasized lymphatic spread vertically down to the lymphatic plexus in the deep pectoral fascia underlying the breast, and spread to the central subareolar region has been described. These multiple mechanisms of spread emphasize the likelihood of cancer being present in the breast well beyond the palpable primary mass.

A detailed study of the sites of cancer in a breast containing a primary tumor has been performed by Holland and associates.[129] They examined 264 mastectomy specimens from patients with clinically unifocal breast cancer measuring 4 cm or less. In only 40% of cases was the cancer in the breast restricted to the primary tumor (Fig. 40–4). The probability of finding additional foci of cancer decreased as a function of the distance from the primary tumor: 41% of the specimens had additional foci of cancer 2 cm or more from the primary tumor, and 11% had additional foci 4 cm or more from the primary tumor. Of the cases with additional foci beyond 2 cm, the additional foci were intraductal in approximately two thirds of the patients.

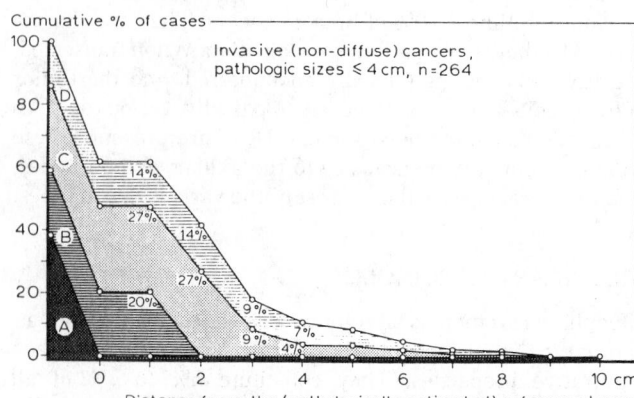

FIGURE 40–4. Distribution of tumor foci at different distances from the reference tumor. **(A)** Cases without tumor foci outside the reference tumor. **(B)** Cases with tumor foci within 2 cm. **(C)** Cases with noninvasive tumor foci at a distance greater than 2 cm. **(D)** Cases with invasive tumor foci at a distance greater than 2 cm. (With permission from Holland R, Veling S, Mravunac M, Hendriks J. Histologic multifocality of T1S, T1–2 breast carcinomas. Implications for clinical trials of breast-conserving surgery. Cancer 1985;56:979–990)

REGIONAL NODAL INVOLVEMENT

The most common sites of regional lymph node involvement in breast cancer are the axillary, internal mammary, and supraclavicular lymph node regions. A knowledge of the likelihood of involvement of these areas and their significance is critical for planning treatment. The axillary lymph node region is the principal site of regional metastases from carcinoma of the breast, and approximately 40% of patients have evidence of spread to the axillary nodes. The likelihood of axillary nodal involvement appears to be related directly to the size of the primary tumor.[130]

To some extent, the incidence of histologic involvement of axillary nodes depends on the extent of the pathologic analysis of the specimen. Pickren was the first to show that a more thorough clearing and sectioning of the axillary specimen resulted in a greater yield of positive nodes.[131] Of 51 specimens analyzed in routine fashion and found to be negative, 11 (22%) showed evidence of involvement on more careful analysis in that study.

Detection of axillary involvement by physical examination has high false-positive and high false-negative rates (Table 40–6).[132–135] If axillary lymph nodes are palpable, histologic evidence of metastatic disease is not found in approximately 25% of patients. Conversely, if axillary nodes are not palpable, histologic involvement is detected in approximately 30% of patients. These shortcomings of clinical evaluation are of particular importance because histologic involvement of ax-

TABLE 40–5. Five-Year Relapse Rate According to the Location of the Primary Tumor and Nodal Status

Location*	Negative Nodes†	Positive Nodes†
UOQ	17 (208)	63 (239)
UIQ	25 (75)	59 (37)
LIQ	22 (23)	55 (22)
LOQ	26 (46)	70 (44)

* U, upper; O, outer; Q, quadrant; I, inner; L, lower.
† Five-year relapse rate, with the number of patients in the subgroup in parentheses.)
(Fisher B, Slack N, Ausman R. Location of breast carcinoma and prognosis. Surg Gynecol Obstet 1969;129:705–716)

TABLE 40–6. Accuracy of Physical Examination in Predicting Histologic Involvement of Axillary Nodes

Accuracy of Prediction	Series 1[132]	Series 2[133]	Series 3[134]	Series 4[135]
False-positive rate (%)	25	31	26	29
False-negative rate (%)	32	28	27	29

TABLE 40–7. Ten-Year Survival by Axillary Node Status for Patients Treated With Radical Mastectomy

Investigations	Negative Nodes (%)	Positive Nodes (%)	1–3 Positive Nodes (%)	4 or More Positive Nodes (%)
Valagussa[136]	80	38	50	24
Haagensen[137]	76	48	63	27
Schottenfeld[135]	72	43		
Fisher[138]	65	25	38	13
Spratt and Donegan[139]	68	27		
Payne[140]	76	35		
Ferguson[141]	72	39	52	27

illary nodes has a high correlation with prognosis. Table 40–7 shows 10-year survival figures according to axillary involvement from seven separate series of patients treated with radical mastectomy.[135–141] Patients with histologically negative axillary nodes have a markedly greater likelihood of survival than patients with histologic involvement. The prognosis is inversely related to the number of involved nodes.[142] The combination of the presence and extent of metastases to the axilla represents the single most important prognostic factor for patients with breast cancer.

The axilla is a triangle bounded by the axillary vein superiorly, the latissimus dorsi laterally, and the serratus anterior medially (Fig. 40–5). For the purposes of analysis, the axilla is commonly divided into three levels: proximal, which is tissue inferior to the lower border of the pectoralis minor muscle (level I); middle, which is tissue directly beneath the pectoralis minor (level II); and distal, which is tissue superior to the pectoralis minor (level III). Prognosis is related to the level of axillary involvement (Table 40–8).[135] Involvement of the upper level nodes carries a worse prognosis than involvement of proximal level nodes alone. In a series of 182 mastectomy specimens examined by clearing, involvement of nodes at the apex of the axilla was found in 15, and all 15 patients relapsed, indicating the grave prognosis associated with involvement high in the axilla.[128] Involvement of upper-level nodes usually is associated with a high total number of lymph nodes involved; in this group of 15 patients, the mean number of involved nodes was 16.2 (range, 4–37). In another study, axillary node involvement and survival were examined in 385 patients to determine whether the total number of involved nodes or the level of axillary involvement was the better indicator of prognosis.[143] For any given number of involved nodes, survival was independent of the level of involvement, and the investigators concluded that prognosis was related more directly to the total number of nodes involved than to the level of involvement.

The distribution of axillary node involvement by level has been studied in two large series, with nearly identical re-

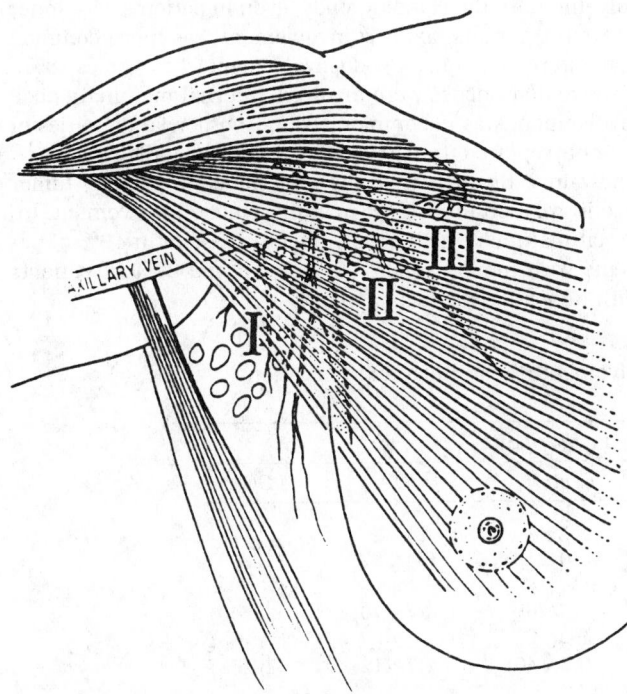

FIGURE 40–5. Anatomy of the axilla. The levels are defined in relation to the pectoralis minor muscle. (Kinne DW. Primary treatment of breast cancer. In: Harris JR, Hellman S, Henderson IC, Kinne DW, eds. Breast diseases. 2nd ed. Philadelphia: JB Lippincott, 1991)

TABLE 40–8. Ten-Year Survival Related to Primary Tumor Size and Level of Axillary Involvement

| Axillary Status | Size of Primary Tumor (cm) | | | |
	<2	2–5	>5	Total
Negative	82	65	44	72
Positive				
Proximal only	73	74	39	65
Middle or distal	—*	28	37	31
All	68	51	37	

* Insufficient data.
(Schottenfeld D, Nash A, Robbins G, Beattie E. Ten-year results of the treatment of primary operable breast cancer. Cancer 1976;38: 1001–1007)

TABLE 40–9. Five-Year Relapse Rate (%) According to Size of Primary and Axillary Node Involvement

Axillary Status	Size of Primary Tumor (cm)		
	<2	2–5	>5
Negative Axillary Nodes			
Fisher et al[146]	12	24	27
Nemoto et al[142]	13	19	25
Valagussa et al[136]	8	24	19
Positive Axillary Nodes			
Fisher et al[146]	50	60	79
Nemoto et al[142]	39	50	65
Valagussa et al[136]	37	64	74

sults.[144,145] Involvement of level I alone was seen in 54% to 58% of patients and level I and II in 20% of patients. Involvement of levels II or III without involvement of level I (*i.e.*, skip metastases) was seen in only 2% to 4% of patients with nodal involvement. These results indicate that involvement of the axilla is usually sequential. A level I dissection is highly effective for determining nodal involvement but frequently underestimates the extent of involvement.

Prognosis is related to the size of the primary tumor and to axillary node involvement. Whether these two factors independently predict the outcome is addressed in Table 40–9. If axillary nodes are involved, the size of the tumor still has prognostic value. For example, in the data from Valagussa and colleagues, the 5-year relapse rate was 37% for patients with positive nodes and small (≤2 cm) tumors and 79% for patients with positive nodes and large (>5 cm) tumors.[136] In the data from Fisher and coworkers, this correlation was analyzed further according to the number of positive axillary nodes (*i.e.*, 1 to 3 or 4 or more).[146] Within each subgroup with positive axillary nodes, the size of the primary tumor was still an independent prognostic factor. However, if axillary nodes are negative, the relation is less clear. The prognosis for patients with small tumors and negative nodes is exceptionally good, with a 5-year relapse rate of approximately 10%. For tumors larger than 2 cm, the prognosis is not as good.

However, the prognosis for patients with large tumors and negative nodes is not significantly worse than that of patients with 2- to 5-cm tumors and negative nodes. These data imply that the results of an axillary sampling are of value for prognostic purposes in patients with large primary tumors, because patients with histologically negative axillary nodes do relatively well even without adjuvant therapy. The 30-year survival rate was 61% if the primary tumor was no larger than 2 cm, 46% if it was 2 to 5 cm, and 50% if it was larger than 5 cm.[147] For patients with involvement of level I axillary nodes, the 30-year survival rate was 40% if the tumor was no larger than 2 cm, 31% if it was 2 cm to 5 cm, and only 14% if it was larger than 5 cm.

The axillary nodal region is the principal drainage site for carcinoma of the breast, and a histologic analysis of the axilla provides a useful guide to prognosis. The more practical issue of what treatment is required for the axillary region is discussed in later sections.

The second major site of regional metastases for carcinoma of the breast is the internal mammary lymph node chain, which lies at the anterior ends of the intercostal spaces by the side of the internal thoracic artery. Because of their intrathoracic location and their uncommon clinical presentation, the frequency of internal mammary node involvement was not appreciated as early as was axillary node involvement. One of the first to document this second route of spread was Sampson Handley, who reported his results of internal mammary node biopsy in 1000 patients in 1975 (Table 40–10).[148] These results illustrate that internal mammary node involvement is more common for inner quadrant or central tumors than for outer quadrant tumors and that axillary lymph node involvement is more likely than internal mammary node involvement. In the Handley study, even in patients with inner or central tumors, axillary involvement was more common than internal mammary node involvement (42% versus 28%). If the axillary nodes were involved, internal mammary node involvement was uncommon (8%). Another larger series of patients reported from Italy confirmed the Handley results.[132] These investigators stress the importance of primary tumor size in relation to internal mammary node involvement. Internal mammary node involvement was seen in 19% of patients with tumors smaller than 5 cm and 37% of patients with tumors larger than 5 cm.

TABLE 40–10. Internal Mammary Node Involvement (%) in Relation to Location of the Primary and Axillary Node Involvement

Node Involvement	Primary Site				
	UIQ*	LIQ	Central	UOQ	LOQ
Total†	27% (67/248)‡	33% (20/61)	32% (70/216)	14% (54/382)	13% (12/93)
Axilla not involved	14% (20/143)	6% (2/36)	7% (5/76)	4% (7/170)	5% (2/40)
Axilla involved	45% (47/105)	72% (18/25)	46% (65/140)	22% (47/212)	19% (10/53)

* U, upper; I, inner; Q, quadrant; L, lower, O, outer.
† All patients regardless of axillary status.
‡ Numbers in parentheses are crude results.
(Handley R. Carcinoma of the breast. Ann R Coll Surg Engl 1975;57:59–66)

The significance of internal mammary node involvement is similar to that of axillary node involvement. In a large series reported by Veronesi and coworkers, the 10-year rate of disease-free survival was 73% if the axillary nodes and the internal mammary nodes were negative, 47% if axillary nodes alone were positive, 52% if the internal mammary nodes alone were positive, and only 25% if both areas were positive.[149] In practice, biopsy of the internal mammary nodes is associated with a greater likelihood of morbidity than biopsy of axillary nodes and is rarely performed.

The principal route of spread to the supraclavicular lymph node areas is through the axillary node chain. In one series of patients undergoing routine supraclavicular dissection, involvement of the region was found in 23 (18%) of the 125 patients who had involvement of axillary nodes but in none of the 149 patients who did not have involvement of axillary nodes.[145] The significance of supraclavicular node involvement was first shown by Halsted, who performed a supraclavicular dissection in 119 patients. Forty-four (37%) women were found to have involvement of these nodes, and only two were free of cancer at 5 years.[150] Supraclavicular node involvement represents a late stage of axillary nodal involvement and carries a grave prognosis.

DISTANT METASTASES

Metastatic spread from carcinoma of the breast can involve a variety of organs. The likelihood of organ involvement has been studied in several autopsy series, and the results are shown in Table 40–11.[128,151,152]

TABLE 40–11. Percentage of Patients With Metastatic Breast Cancer at Various Sites in Three Collected Series

Site	Series 1[151] (n = 160)	Series 2[152] (n = 43)	Series 3[128] (n = 100)
Lung	59	65	69
Liver	58	56	65
Bone	44		71
Pleura	37	23	51
Adrenals	31	41	49
Kidneys	NR*	14	17
Spleen	14	23	17
Pancreas		11	17
Ovaries	9	16	20
Brain		9	22
Thyroid			24
Heart			11
Diaphragm			11
Pericardium	5	21	19
Intestine			18
Peritoneum	12	9	13
Uterus			15
Lymph nodes	72		76
Skin	34	7	30

* NR, not recorded.

PRETREATMENT EVALUATION

The pretreatment evaluation of the breast cancer patient is directed at identifying the clinical stage of the patient's disease and disease sites that would alter the treatment plan. A complete history and physical examination is the first step in this evaluation. The components of the breast-directed history and physical examination are listed in Table 40–12. A chest roentgenogram (posteroanterior and lateral views), complete blood count, and liver chemistries should be obtained for all patients. The likelihood of identifying metastases by the routine use of scans in the asymptomatic patient is greatly influenced by the clinical stage of disease. Bone scans are fre-

TABLE 40–12.
Breast-Directed History and Physical Examination

History
Breast and axillary symptoms: first observed and evolution
    Breast mass
    Nipple discharge: spontaneous or induced, color
    Nipple and skin retraction
    Axillary mass
    Arm swelling or pain
History of prior breast biopsies, cyst aspirations
Reproductive history
    Age at onset of menses
    Date of last menstrual period, regularity of cycles
    Number of pregnancies, children, abortions
    Age at first birth
    Age at menopause
    History of hormone use
Family history: relationship, age at diagnosis of breast cancer
Date of last mammogram
Review of systems directed toward evidence of metastases

Physical Examination
Breast mass
    Size (measured)
    Location (clock position and distance from areola)
    Consistency
    Fixation to skin, pectoral muscle, chest wall
Skin changes
    Erythema
    Edema
    Dimpling
    Satellite nodules
    Ulceration
Nipple changes
    Retraction
    Discoloration
    Erosion
    Discharge: color, location
Nodes
    Axillary size, number, fixation
    Supraclavicular
    Infraclavicular
    Arm edema

quently used as a preoperative screening test, but Khansur and coworkers found positive scans in only 2.1% of 187 women with stage I and II disease.[153] Baker reported a similar low incidence of occult bony metastases detected by scanning, with disease demonstrated for only 1.8% of stage I and II patients.[154] An incidence of bony metastases of less than 5% for patients with stage I and II disease has been reported in several other studies, including a review of 1118 patients by Lee.[155-158] False-positive scans are obtained frequently, particularly for older patients. In contrast, positive bone scans are obtained for 20% to 25% of asymptomatic women with stage III breast cancer, making this a worthwhile screening procedure in locally advanced breast cancer.[153,154,156]

The yield of screening liver scans is even lower than that seen with bone scanning, and the test is of little benefit in the preoperative evaluation of stage I and II breast cancer. Nomura and colleagues reviewed 129 patients with stage I, II, and III breast carcinoma and had a 0% yield from liver scanning.[159] Abnormal liver scans secondary to causes other than metastatic disease are common. Weiner found 12 abnormal scans in 234 patients, but only 4 (1%) were due to metastatic disease.[160] Sears and associates reviewed 100 patients with five abnormal liver scans, only one of which was a true positive finding.[161] Liver scans should be reserved for patients with abnormal liver chemistries, hepatomegaly, or significant weight loss suggesting hepatic metastases. Because false-positive scans are common, histologic confirmation of metastases should be considered before abandoning definitive primary therapy on the basis of an abnormal liver scan.

Bilateral mammography is an essential part of the preoperative workup. Ideally, a mammogram should be obtained before a breast biopsy is done to allow adequate evaluation of the index breast for breast-conserving therapy. In these patients, the use of magnification views is recommended to assess the presence and extent of the microcalcifications suggestive of associated DCIS. In patients who will undergo mastectomy, complete visualization of the contralateral breast to exclude an occult synchronous tumor is necessary. In a report from Guy's Hospital, the use of routine preoperative mammography resulted in a synchronous breast cancer incidence of 2.4%, a fivefold increase over prior clinical detection rates.[162]

The evaluation of serum tumor markers has not been shown to be of benefit preoperatively. Although carcinoembryonic antigen (CEA) may be useful in monitoring response to therapy, it is infrequently elevated in primary breast cancer. Lee found that only 3% of patients with stage I breast carcinoma and 6% with stage II disease had CEA levels greater than 5 mg/ml.[163] Other markers, such as assays to identify sialomucin (*e.g.*, CA 15-3, CA 549), are more commonly elevated in primary breast cancer, with abnormalities seen in 20% to 50% of patients.[164-166] However, 20% of patients with benign breast disease have elevated CA 15-3 levels, and elevated levels are seen in benign gastrointestinal disease, diminishing the usefulness of this marker as a screening test.[166] The value of tumor markers in primary breast cancer has not been clearly established. The available markers have no real utility in the preoperative evaluation of the patient. The identification of a highly specific and sensitive marker, such as a shed tumor product, is currently an active area of research.

STAGING

Staging refers to the grouping of patients according to the extent of their disease. It is useful in choosing treatment for individual patients, estimating prognosis, and comparing the results of different treatment programs. Staging of breast cancer is performed initially on a clinical basis, according to the physical examination and laboratory radiologic evaluation. The most widely used clinical staging system is the one adopted by the International Union against Cancer (UICC) and the American Joint Committee on Cancer (AJCC) Staging and End Results Reporting. It is based on the tumor-nodes-metastases (TNM) system as detailed in the 1988 *Manual for Staging of Cancer:*

T	*PRIMARY TUMORS*
TX	Primary tumor cannot be assessed
T0	No evidence of primary tumor
Tis	Carcinoma in situ: intraductal carcinoma, lobular carcinoma, or Paget's disease with no tumor
T1	Tumor 2 cm or less in its greatest dimension

    a. 0.5 cm or less in greatest dimension

    b. Larger than 0.5 cm, but not larger than 1 cm in greatest dimension

    c. Larger than 1 cm, but not larger than 2 cm in greatest dimension

T2	Tumor more than 2 cm but not more than 5 cm in its greatest dimension
T3	Tumor more than 5 cm in its greatest dimension
T4	Tumor of any size with direct extension to chest wall or to skin. Chest wall includes ribs, intercostal muscles, and serratus anterior muscle, but not pectoral muscle.

    a. Extension to chest wall

    b. Edema (including peau d'orange), ulceration of the skin of the breast, or satellite skin nodules confined to the same breast

    c. Both of the above

    d. Inflammatory carcinoma

Dimpling of the skin, nipple retraction, or any other skin changes except those in T4b may occur in T1, T2, or T3 without affecting the classification.

N	*REGIONAL LYMPH NODES*
NX	Regional lymph nodes cannot be assessed (*e.g.*, previously removed)
N0	No regional lymph node metastases
N1	Metastasis to movable ipsilateral axillary node(s)
N2	Metastases to ipsilateral axillary nodes fixed to one another or to other structures
N3	Metastases to ipsilateral internal mammary lymph node(s)

M	*DISTANT METASTASIS*
M0	No evidence of distant metastasis
M1	Distant metastases (including metastases to ipsilateral supraclavicular lymph nodes)

Another clinical staging system, the Columbia Clinical Classification, is less widely used but is of historic importance. Like the UICC-AJCC system, patients are grouped according to the extent of disease in the primary tumor site, nodal areas, and distant metastases:

Stage A — No skin edema, ulceration, or solid fixation of the tumor to the chest wall. Axillary nodes are not involved clinically.

Stage B — No skin edema, ulceration, or solid fixation of the tumor to the chest wall. Clinically involved nodes, but less than 2.5 cm in transverse diameter and not fixed to overlying skin or deeper structures of the axilla.

Stage C — Any one of the five grave signs of advanced breast carcinoma:
1. Edema of the skin of limited extent (involving less than one third of the skin over the breast)
2. Skin ulceration
3. Solid fixation of the tumor to the chest wall
4. Extensive involvement of axillary lymph nodes (measuring 2.5 cm or more in transverse diameter)
5. Fixation of the axillary nodes to overlying skin or deeper structures of the axilla

Stage D — All other patients with more advanced breast carcinoma:
1. A combination of any two or more of the five grave signs listed under stage C
2. Extensive edema of the skin (involving more than one third of the skin over the breast
3. Satellite skin nodules
4. Inflammatory type of carcinoma
5. Clinically involved supraclavicular lymph nodes
6. Internal mammary metastases as evidenced by a parasternal tumor
7. Edema of the arm
8. Distant metastases

Clinical evaluation of spread to the axilla has high false-positive and false-negative rates. For this reason, pathologic staging based on histologic study of the axillary specimen is preferable. For the individual patient, prognosis is better determined by pathologic staging than by clinical staging (Table 40–13). For patients who have clinical indications of spread of tumor but negative histologic evaluations, the survival rate (72%) is similar to that of the entire group of patients with histologically negative nodes (76%), not to that of the group with histologically positive nodes (48%).[137] Similarly, if a patient does not have clinical evidence of axillary involvement but microscopic involvement is detected pathologically, the survival rate (57%) is similar to that of the entire group of patients with microscopic involvement (48%).

Pathologic stage is commonly given as stage I (*i.e.*, axillary nodes not involved) or stage II (*i.e.*, axillary nodes involved). Refinements of this simple staging format have been made, such as subdividing stage II according to the number of positive axillary nodes. Because prognosis is clearly related to the ex-

TABLE 40–13. Ten-Year Survival (%) According to Clinical and Pathologic Assessment of Axillary Nodes

	Pathologic Assessment		
Clinical Assessment	*Node Negative*	*Node Positive*	*All Patients*
N0	77	57	71
N1	72	34	44
All patients	76	48	

(Haagensen C. Treatment of curable carcinoma of the breast. Int J Radiat Oncol Biol Phys 1977;2:975–980)

tent of axillary involvement (see Table 40–7), it has become convention to subdivide axillary involvement into one to three nodes positive or more than four nodes positive. Another refinement is based on the recognition that micrometastatic involvement of axillary lymph nodes is not associated with the poor prognosis seen with macrometastatic involvement. A comparison of the significance of these two types of axillary metastases has been the object of recent pathologic study. In one study, occult metastases were demonstrated in the regional lymph nodes by an extended histopathologic technique in 24% of 78 cases of invasive breast cancer that would have been regarded as pathologic stage I (*i.e.*, no nodal metastases) after routine pathologic examination. Patients in whom the largest nodal metastases measured 2 mm or less in the greatest diameter (*i.e.*, micrometastases) were compared with those in whom the lesions were larger than 2 mm (*i.e.*, macrometastases). Life table analysis revealed no significant difference in survival rates between patients with micrometastases and those without nodal metastases, and both of these groups exhibited a significantly greater likelihood of survival than patients with macrometastases. In another study, by Huvos and coworkers from Memorial Hospital in New York City, prognosis was related to pathologic extent of axillary nodal involvement.[167] For the 62 patients with no involvement of the axillary nodes, the 8-year survival rate was 82% (51 of 62 patients). When micrometastatic involvement (<2 mm) of level I axillary nodes was found, the 8-year survival rate was 94% (17 of 18). The survival rate was 62% (28 of 45) for patients with macrometastatic involvement of level I axillary nodes. Other refinements of the pathologic staging scheme are based on the recognition that extension of metastatic disease beyond the lymph node capsule or involvement of an axillary node larger than 2 cm has been associated with a worse prognosis, independent of the number of nodes involved.

The Postsurgical Treatment Pathologic Classification was developed by the UICC-AJCC in 1988:

PRIMARY TUMOR (pT)

pTx — Criteria to assess the primary tumor can not be met

pT0 — No evidence of primary tumor

pT1–4 — Same as UICC-AJCC classification

NODAL INVOLVEMENT (pN)

pNX	Regional lymph node metastasis cannot be assessed
pN0	No regional lymph node metastasis
pN1	Metastasis to movable ipsilateral axillary node(s)
pN1a	Only micrometastasis (none larger than 0.2 cm)
pN1b	Metastasis to lymph node(s), any larger than 0.2 cm

    i. Metastasis in one to three lymph nodes, any larger than 0.2 cm and all smaller than 2 cm in greatest dimension

    ii. Metastasis to four or more lymph nodes, any larger than 0.2 cm and all smaller than 2 cm in greatest dimension

    iii. Extension of tumor beyond the capsule of a lymph node metastasis smaller than 2 cm in greatest dimension

    iv. Metastasis to a lymph node 2 cm or more in greatest dimension

pN2–3	Same as clinical UICC-AJCC classification

LOCAL TREATMENT OF BREAST CARCINOMA

The modern era of breast cancer surgery began with Halsted's description of the radical mastectomy in 1894.[168] At that time, breast cancer was thought to begin with a tumor in the breast and to spread in an orderly fashion through lymphatics from the low axillary nodes to the high axillary nodes and then to distant sites. The radical mastectomy incorporated this concept of tumor biology by extirpating the tumor and its draining lymphatics en bloc with a wide margin of normal tissue. Halsted contended that the histologic tumor type, degree of local spread, patient age, and thoroughness of the operative procedure all influenced survival after surgery.[150] Although our understanding of tumor biology has changed considerably since Halsted's time, the surgical treatment of breast cancer that he popularized remained unchallenged dogma for the next 70 years.

Radical mastectomy is the en bloc removal of the breast, the skin overlying the tumor (usually with a 5-cm margin), the pectoralis major and minor muscles and all of the axillary contents (Fig. 40–6). Skin graft closure of the operative defect is not uniformly required but was advocated by Haagensen to allow more radical skin excision.[134] The radical mastectomy is technically feasible in virtually all women with breast cancer. Of 1640 women seen at Memorial Hospital from 1940 to 1943, 88.9% were thought to have tumors resectable for cure by this technique.[147] In 1974, Adair and Berg reported the 30-year follow-up of the 1458 women in this series who underwent surgical resection.[147] Fifty-seven percent of the patients died from breast cancer, 24% died from other causes, and only 13% survived 30 years free of cancer. Six percent of the total group were lost to follow-up.

Although radical mastectomy does not cure most women with breast carcinoma, it is an effective means of maintaining local control of the primary tumor. Local recurrence on the chest wall or in the axilla is relatively rare after the procedure, occurring in only 6% of 935 patients reported by Haagensen[169] and 17% of 704 women in Donegan's series.[170] It is possible that complete local control of the primary tumor in the breast and axilla may play a role in long-term survival for a small number of women as indicated by the observation of Adair and coworkers that 33% of their 30-year survivors treated with surgery alone had positive axillary nodes.[147] Similar observations were made by Brinkley and Haybittle,[171] Fentiman,[172] and Rosen and colleagues,[173] who found that about 25% of 20-year survivors had positive axillary nodes.

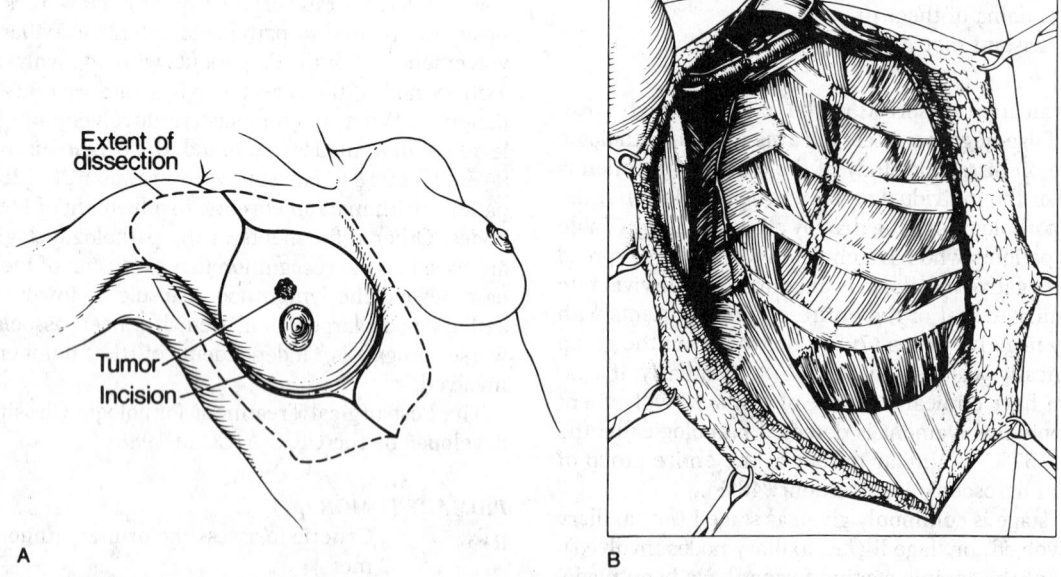

FIGURE 40–6. Radical mastectomy. **(A)** Extent of dissection. Notice the vertical orientation of the incision. **(B)** Postresection anatomy. Notice the absence of the pectoralis major and minor muscles. (Kinne DW. Primary treatment of breast cancer. In: Harris JR, Hellman S, Henderson IC, Kinne DW, eds. Breast diseases. 2nd ed. Philadelphia: JB Lippincott, 1991)

Radical mastectomy, in addition to failing to cure a large number of women, is associated with significant long-term morbidity. Limitation of arm elevation and chronic lymphedema are seen in 25% to 53% of women after this procedure, and removal of the pectoralis major muscle leaves a noticeable cosmetic defect on the patient's chest wall.[174,175] Breast reconstruction after radical mastectomy usually requires tissue flaps to provide adequate skin and muscle coverage.

The failure of radical mastectomy to cure many women with breast cancer was thought by some surgeons to be due to its failure to extirpate all of the draining lymphatics of the breast. It was recognized in the 1950s that approximately one quarter of the lymphatic drainage of the breast is through the ipsilateral internal mammary nodes, and this drainage occurs from all quadrants of the breast.[176] In an attempt to address this, the extended radical mastectomy was developed. This operation is a radical mastectomy with en bloc removal of the internal mammary nodes. Nonrandomized reports suggested that survival might be improved in selected patients by this more radical procedure.[177,178] However, a prospective randomized trial reported by Veronesi and Valagussa failed to show a survival difference between women treated with radical and those treated with extended radical mastectomy.[179] Isolated internal mammary node metastases are uncommon, occurring in 4.9% of 7070 patients in whom axillary and internal mammary nodes were sampled. Metastases to this node group seem to have the same prognostic significance as axillary node metastases.[136,180] The extended radical mastectomy is an operation of historic interest, demonstrating that extension of the Halstedian principles of breast cancer surgery does not result in improved survival.

Modified radical mastectomy is now the standard operative treatment for patients with invasive breast cancer in the United States. Surveys by the American College of Surgeons indicate that only 28% of women were treated with modified radical mastectomy in 1972, but by 1981, this figure rose to 72%.[181] A survey of breast cancer treatment in New Mexico through 1985 found that 72% of node-negative women and 79% of node-positive women continued to be treated with modified radical mastectomy.[182] A concomitant decrease in the number of radical mastectomies performed has been observed, with this procedure accounting for only 3.2% of breast cancer operations in 1981.[181]

A modified radical mastectomy (*i.e.*, total mastectomy and axillary dissection) includes removal of the entire breast and some or all of the axillary lymph nodes. The pectoralis minor muscle may be removed or transected, but it is usually preserved (Fig. 40–7). Although it still involves removal of the entire breast, the modified radical mastectomy is less morbid than the radical mastectomy. The incidence of arm edema and shoulder dysfunction is decreased, and the cosmetic defect is less noticeable in a variety of types of clothing (Fig. 40–8).[183] Breast reconstruction is more easily performed after modified radical mastectomy.

Although the modified radical mastectomy may not seem to differ significantly from the radical mastectomy, it represented a major departure from Halstedian principles of cancer surgery, because it is not an en bloc procedure. The switch to modified radical mastectomy occurred as it became increasingly apparent that treatment failure after breast cancer surgery is usually due to systemic tumor dissemination before

surgery rather than an inadequate operative procedure. Several retrospective studies showed similar survival rates for women treated with the radical or modified radical mastectomy.[184,185] These findings were confirmed in two prospective randomized trials. Between 1969 and 1981, 606 women with stage I or II breast carcinoma were randomized to treatment with radical mastectomy or modified radical mastectomy in Manchester, England.[186] No differences in disease-free survival, overall survival, or local recurrence rates were seen between the groups. In a smaller trial involving 311 women, Maddox and associates failed to demonstrate any significant benefit in survival or local control for women undergoing radical mastectomy.[187] The NSABP provided further evidence that radical en bloc surgery did not prolong survival with a trial (B-04) in which patients with clinically node-negative breast cancer were randomized to three treatment groups: radical mastectomy; total mastectomy with observation of the untreated axillary nodes, and a delayed dissection if positive nodes appeared; or total mastectomy with radiation therapy to the regional lymph nodes.[188] No survival differences were found among the groups, despite the fact that approximately 40% of patients in the axillary observation arm were presumed to have histologically positive nodes (as seen in the group undergoing axillary dissection) that were untreated. Although this trial did not directly compare radical mastectomy and modified radical mastectomy, it provided further support for the use of modified radical mastectomy, by demonstrating the limitations in the Halsted notion of cancer spread.

There are few, if any, indications for radical mastectomy. If the pectoral fascia has been violated at the time of biopsy or the tumor seems to abut the fascia or invade a portion of the pectoral muscle, a small portion of the muscle directly beneath the tumor can be excised to obtain a negative deep margin of resection.[189] Large tumors that involve greater amounts of the pectoral muscle are best treated with chemotherapy or radiation therapy as the initial therapeutic modality. In these situations, this multimodal approach frequently allows a standard modified radical mastectomy to be done after a response to the initial therapy.

Total mastectomy, referred to as simple mastectomy, involves removal of the entire breast, including the nipple areola complex, with preservation of the pectoral muscles and the axillary nodes. Because of the importance of axillary dissection as a staging procedure, total mastectomy is not considered a standard surgical approach for the management of infiltrating carcinomas. The indications for total mastectomy include patients with ductal carcinoma in situ who elect mastectomy (among whom the incidence of axillary node metastases is less than 1%); women undergoing prophylactic surgery to prevent the development of breast cancer; patients who develop a recurrence in the breast after breast-conserving surgery that had included an axillary dissection, and patients who require mastectomy for local control of tumor in whom information about axillary node status does not influence therapy. This includes women with metastatic disease undergoing "toilet mastectomy" or elderly women with significant comorbidities.

OPTIONS IN LOCAL TREATMENT

The major options for local treatment are modified radical mastectomy and breast-conserving treatment consisting of

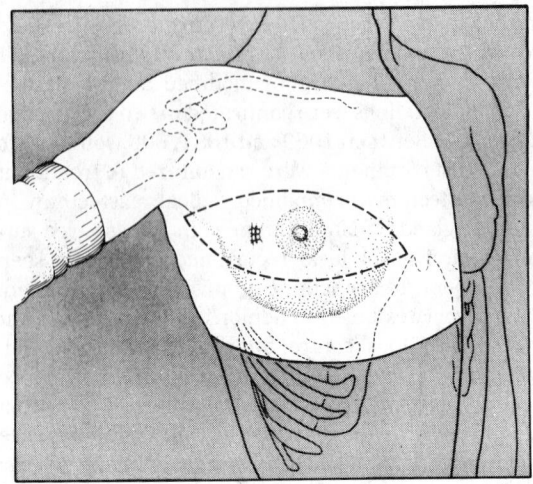

FIGURE 40–7.   Modified radical mastectomy. **(A)** Extent of dissection. Notice the horizontal orientation of the incision. **(B)** The clavipectoral fascia is incised and reflected caudad. The pectoralis minor muscle is divided near the coracoid process. **(C)** Postresection anatomy. The pectoralis muscles are retracted, not resected. (Kinne DW, DeCosse JJ. Modified radical mastectomy for carcinoma of the breast. Am Surg 1982;48:543–556)

A

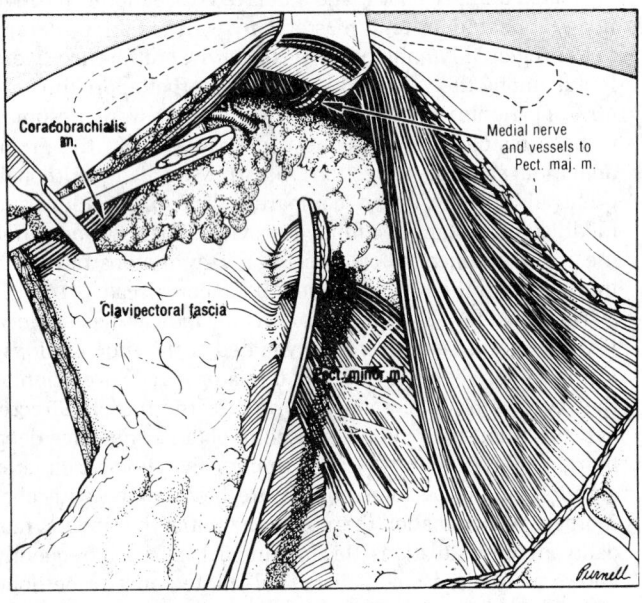

B

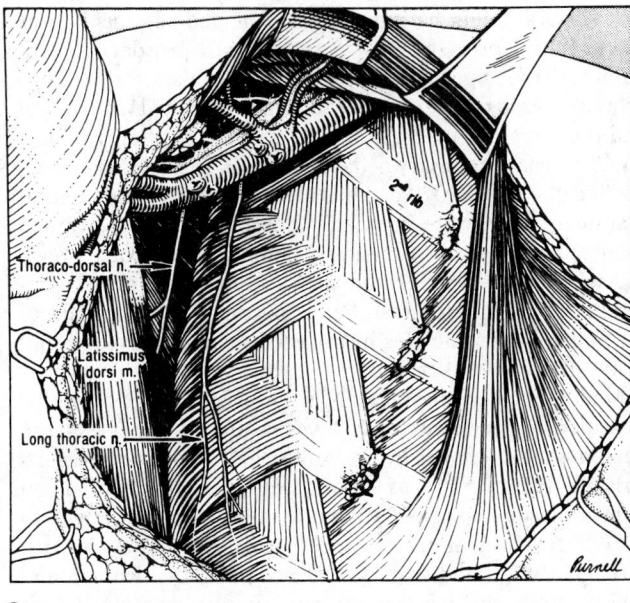

C

conservative surgery and irradiation. Breast-conserving surgery involves removal of the primary tumor and a variable margin of surrounding normal breast tissue, usually accompanied by an axillary dissection. A variety of terms, imprecisely defined, are used to describe this approach to the surgical therapy of breast cancer. They include lumpectomy, tumorectomy, segmental mastectomy, and local excision, which imply the removal of a relatively small amount of normal breast tissue, and partial mastectomy and quadrantectomy, which usually imply the excision of a larger amount of breast tissue.

In the past, excision of less than the entire breast was thought to be contraindicated due to the multicentricity of breast carcinoma. The actual frequency of multicentricity is debatable, with reported incidences in mastectomy specimens ranging from 9% to 75%.[190] The large discrepancy in the reported incidence of multicentricity is related to a variety of factors: differences in the definition of multicentricity, quantitation of invasive and noninvasive carcinoma, variations in

the extent of tissue sampling, and different techniques of pathologic examination. It is important to differentiate foci of cancer in the vicinity of the tumor (*i.e.*, multifocality) and totally independent foci of cancer (*i.e.*, true multicentricity). The work of Holland and coworkers described earlier was instrumental in demonstrating that breast cancer is commonly multifocal, but uncommonly multicentric.[129] The clinical importance of multifocal tumor is readily apparent in reviewing the local failure rates of women treated only with excision of the primary tumor. The NSABP found a 39% incidence at 8 years of recurrent tumor in the breast in patients treated with an excision of the primary tumor in which the margins of resection were histologically negative.[191] Lagios observed a 19% local failure rate at a mean follow-up of only 24 months in women treated with gross tumor excision without consideration of margin status.[192] Several additional experiences with local excision alone confirm local failure rates in the range of 25% to 35%.[193–196] In all these series, the site of recurrence in the breast is at or near the site of the primary

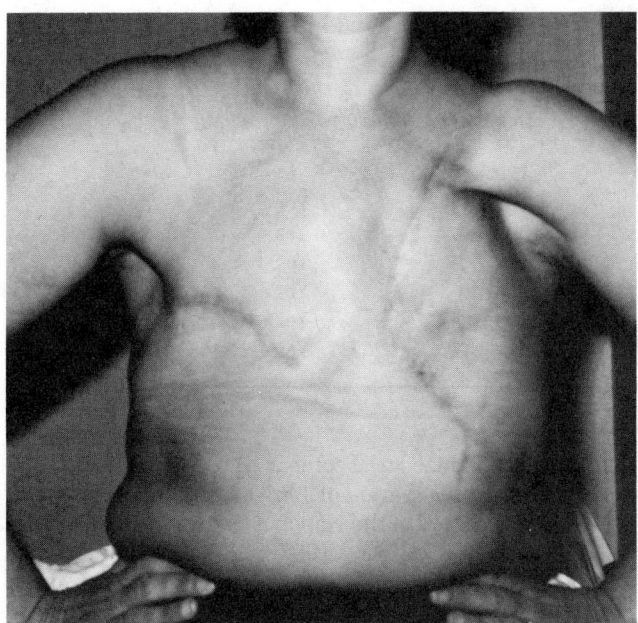

FIGURE 40–8. Cosmetic results of a radical mastectomy on the patient's left and a modified radical mastectomy on the right.

tumor in most cases. These data emphasize that multifocal breast cancer commonly remains after an excision, even if the margins of resection are histologically negative.

Although it is clear from the preceding data that breast conservation using excision of the primary tumor alone provides inadequate local control, there is now ample data from retrospective and prospective studies indicating that the addition of radiation therapy to tumor excision reduces breast failure rates to the range of 4.4% to 16% at 10 years, and survival does not differ from that seen after mastectomy.[191,197–205]

Since 1970, there have been seven prospective randomized trials using modern radiation therapy techniques in which breast-conserving surgery and radiation therapy has been compared with mastectomy. At the National Cancer Institute of Italy in Milan, 701 women with clinical stage I breast carcinoma (<2 cm, negative axillary nodes) were randomized to treatment with conservative surgery or radical mastectomy.[199,200] Conservative surgery consisted of a quadrantectomy and complete axillary dissection. Radiation therapy was administered to the breast alone through two opposing tangential fields, giving a dose of 5000 cGy in 5 weeks. Another 1000 cGy was given to the tumor site by orthovoltage radiation. After 1975, all patients with histologically positive axillary lymph nodes were treated with 12 cycles of cyclophosphamide, methotrexate, and 5-fluorouracil (CMF regimen). Microscopically involved axillary nodes were found in 25% of the radical mastectomy group and 27% of the conservatively treated group. The latest report of the Milan trial was published in 1990.[200] No differences in relapse-free and overall survival rates were observed. This was true for node-positive and node-negative patients. Recurrence in the ipsilateral breast occurred in 3% of the quadrantectomy patients. There were 19 cases of contralateral breast carcinoma in the quadrantectomy group and 20 in the mastectomy group.

The NSABP began a three-arm trial (protocol B-06) in 1976 comparing mastectomy with lumpectomy with or without radiation therapy.[191] A total of 1843 evaluable patients with clinical stage I or II carcinoma whose primary tumors clinically measured no more than 4 cm were entered, but 174 patients refused their assigned treatment and were excluded from analysis. All patients underwent axillary dissection. Those with involved lymph nodes received adjuvant chemotherapy. In contrast to the Milan trial, in which an entire quadrant of the breast was removed, a lumpectomy was performed in the NSABP trial that involved resection of the tumor with only enough normal tissue around it to ensure that the microscopic margins of the specimen were tumor free. It was considered impossible to obtain tumor-free margins in 10% of the patients randomly assigned to lumpectomy, and total mastectomy was carried out in these patients. Radiation therapy was delivered to the breast alone with supervoltage equipment using opposed tangential fields, often without wedge filters to compensate for the slope of the breast, to a dose of 5000 to 5300 cGy in 5 to 6 weeks. The regional lymph nodes were not treated, and no boost was given to the tumor site. After 8 years of follow-up, no differences in distant disease-free survival or overall survival rates were observed between patients undergoing mastectomy and those undergoing lumpectomy with or without radiation therapy. Although the use of radiation therapy did not effect survival, it significantly reduced the incidence of local recurrence in the breast. The probability of a local recurrence 8 years after surgery was only 10% for women who received radiation and 39% for those who did not. The benefit of radiation was seen in patients with positive or negative nodes.

Additional smaller and more recent trials have been performed by the Institut Gustave-Roussy in Paris,[201] the National Cancer Institute of the United States,[202] Guy's Hospital in London,[203] the European Organization for Research on Treatment of Cancer,[204] and the Danish Breast Cancer Group.[205] All of these trials show comparable results for conservative surgery and radiation therapy and mastectomy. The randomized trials comparing these treatments are summarized in Table 40–14.

Based on the information obtained in these randomized trials and from nonrandomized series with long-term follow-up, a panel of experts at a Consensus Development Conference on the Treatment of Early Stage Breast Cancer convened by the National Cancer Institute and held in June 1990 concluded: "Breast conservation treatment (excision of the primary tumor and adjacent breast tissue followed by radiation therapy) is an appropriate method of primary therapy for the majority of women with stage I and II breast cancer and is preferable because it provides survival equivalent to total mastectomy and axillary dissection while preserving the breast."[206]

BREAST-CONSERVING SURGERY AND AXILLARY DISSECTION

The goal of breast-conserving surgery is to maintain local tumor control in the breast while preserving a good cosmetic appearance. The surgical techniques used for breast-conserving surgery differ from those employed for mastec-

TABLE 40–14.   Modern Randomized Trials of Conservative Surgery and Irradiation Compared With Mastectomy

Investigations	Dates of Trial	No. of Patients	Survival Equivalent
Gustave-Roussy[201]	1972–1979	179	Yes
NCI Milan[200]	1973–1980	701	Yes
NSABP B-06[191]	1976–1984	1843	Yes
NCI Bethesda[202]	1980–1986	112	Yes
EORTC[204]	1980–1986	903	Yes
Guy's Hospital[203]	1981–1986	399	Yes
Danish Breast Cancer Group[205]	1983–1987	619	Yes

tomy. Breast-conserving surgery should be done through an incision directly over the tumor. Incisions that are transverse or curvilinear usually give the best cosmetic results (Fig. 40–9). The use of circumareolar incisions, with tunneling through the breast tissue to the carcinoma, should be avoided, because this approach makes control of margins more difficult and increases the amount of tissue that must be treated with a boost of radiation therapy. A crucial step in breast-conserving surgery is avoidance of thin skin flaps.[207] Preservation of the subcutaneous fat beneath the incision and the breast tissue superficial to the tumor helps maintain normal breast contour. Attempts to obliterate the lumpectomy cavity with sutures and the use of breast drains worsen the cosmetic result by altering breast contour.

The extent of breast tissue that should be excised is the subject of some debate. The NSABP reported a 10% incidence of recurrence in the breast 8 years after excision with histologically negative margins.[191] Margins were considered negative if tumor cells were not directly at inked resection margins, regardless of how close to the margins the cells were. The lowest rates of local failure are reported by Veronesi and colleagues, who observed a 2.8% incidence of recurrence at the primary tumor site and a 1.6% incidence of new tumors elsewhere in the breast after treatment with quadrantec-

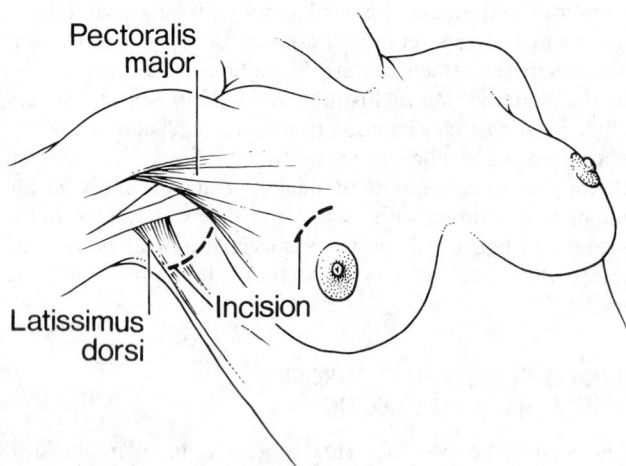

FIGURE 40–9.   Breast-conserving surgery and axillary dissection. Notice the use of separate incisions. (Kinne DW. Primary treatment of breast cancer. In: Harris JR, Hellman S, Henderson IC, Kinne DW, eds. Breast diseases. 2nd ed. Philadelphia: JB Lippincott, 1991)

tomy.[197] A randomized trial comparing quadrantectomy to tumor excision with a margin of 1 cm of grossly normal breast tissue was conducted at the National Cancer Institute of Italy in Milan between 1985 and 1987.[208] After quadrantectomy, patients received external-beam irradiation alone, but women randomized to tumorectomy received an iridium 192 implant and external-beam therapy. Local recurrence was less common in patients treated with quadrantectomy (2.5%) than patients treated with more limited excision (7.2%). A significant cosmetic advantage was observed for patients treated with lumpectomy, even though quadrantectomy was performed by surgeons with extensive experience in the technique. At the time of latest follow-up, survival was the same in the patients treated with quadrantectomy and with excision. These results are consistent with the findings of Holland and associates.[129] Because the probability of finding additional microscopic foci of cancer decreases as a function of distance from the primary tumor, the removal of larger amounts of breast tissue would be expected to decrease local failure rates.

The extent of breast resection appears to be only one of several variables that influence the likelihood of local recurrence after breast-conserving surgery and radiation therapy. The most important of these appear to be the presence of an extensive intraductal component (EIC), patient age at diagnosis, and the use of adjuvant systemic therapy. An EIC is defined for an infiltrating ductal carcinoma in which DCIS is prominently present within the tumor (typically greater than 25%) and present in grossly normal adjacent breast tissue *or* in which the tumor is composed primarily of DCIS with areas of focal invasion. Data from the Joint Center for Radiation Therapy (JCRT) series indicate that 28% of patients with infiltrating ductal carcinoma have an EIC. Local recurrence occurred in 27% of EIC-positive tumors but only 8% of EIC-negative tumors.[209] The effect of an EIC on local recurrence decreases as the extent of breast resection increases. One study reported a decrease of local recurrence rates in EIC-positive tumors from 36% to 9% as the volume of breast tissue resected increased from 35 to 74 cm[3].[210] This result is consistent with a pathologic study of mastectomy specimens by Holland and coworkers, in which an EIC predicted the likelihood of finding extensive multifocal involvement beyond the edge of the tumor.[211] Age less than 35 to 40 years has been associated with a substantially increased risk of local failure in several series.[197,209,212,213] In part, this is explained by an association between young patient age and the presence of an EIC.[198,214]

The use of adjuvant chemotherapy or hormonal therapy in conjunction with radiation therapy appears to reduce the incidence of local failure in the breast. In the NSABP trial (B-13) testing the value of methotrexate and fluorouracil in node-negative, ER-negative women, patients randomized to the treatment arm had a 0.9% rate of recurrence in the ipsilateral breast after 4 years of follow-up, compared with 3.7% for women who did not receive cytotoxic therapy.[215] Similar results were seen in a trial (B-14) testing the value of tamoxifen in node-negative, ER-positive patients treated with tamoxifen had a 0% recurrence rate in the ipsilateral breast, compared with 2.2% in the control group.[216] This finding is supported by the data from NSABP trial B-06, in which node-positive women, all of whom received chemotherapy, had a 6% rate of failure in the breast after lumpectomy and irradiation, compared with 12% for node-negative women undergoing the same local treatment with no systemic chemotherapy.[191]

The value of obtaining histologically negative margins of resection in preventing local recurrence is unclear. The lack of a universally accepted definition of what constitutes an involved margin, problems with sampling breast specimens, and the presence of additional foci of cancer in the breast, even if margins are negative, limit the reliability of margin status as a predictor of local failure.[217,218] Veronesi was unable to correlate margin status and local failure in his tumorectomy patients.[208] The 10% incidence of local recurrence in NSABP trial B-06, in which tumor-free margins were required, indicates that negative margins alone do not ensure local control after conservative surgery and radiation therapy.[191]

The available data suggest that the amount of breast tissue that must be excised in breast-conserving procedures needs to be individualized. Although the lowest local failure rate is obtained with quadrantectomy, it is at the expense of a lesser cosmetic result. For most women, excision of the primary tumor with a 1- to 2-cm margin reduces the tumor burden to a point where it can be controlled with radiation therapy. Important factors in determining the adequacy of surgical resection are the presence and extent of tumor at the inked resection margins, the presence or absence of an EIC, and the patient's relative concerns about cosmetic outcome and local recurrence.

Until recently, axillary dissection was considered an essential aspect of local treatment, whether by mastectomy or by a breast-conserving approach. The principal purpose of axillary dissection is to provide prognostic information that can direct further therapy. Axillary dissection is effective in obtaining local control in the axilla and simplifies the technique of irradiation in patients treated with breast-conserving treatment. However, because of the widespread use of adjuvant systemic therapy, even if axillary nodes are histologically negative, the role and the conduct of axillary dissection are being questioned.

If an axillary dissection is to be performed, it can be the classic axillary dissection in which nodal tissue at all three levels is removed or a more limited dissection of levels I and II. As nodal dissection has come to be regarded as a staging procedure, rather than a therapeutic one, a more limited dissection has become increasingly popular in the United States. Many surgeons think that a complete three-level axillary dissection should be carried out if the axillary nodes are grossly positive or if knowledge of the exact number of positive nodes influences treatment, because there is a 20% to 30% chance that additional positive nodes will be identified at level III if metastases are present in the low axillary nodes.[144,145,219,220]

Major complications of axillary dissection are infrequent and include injury or thrombosis of the axillary vein and injury to the motor nerves of the axilla. Minor complications are reported in 8% to 13% of patients and include wound infection, seroma formation, mild shoulder dysfunction, loss of sensation in the distribution of the intercostobrachial nerve, and edema of the breast and arm.[221,222] The extent of axillary dissection correlates with the degree of breast edema seen after breast-preserving surgery and the risk of arm edema. Clark and coworkers found a 6% incidence of breast edema if no axillary surgery was done, compared with a 25% incidence after axillary sampling and a 79% incidence after complete dissection.[233] The incidence of lymphedema of the arm after axillary dissection varies with the definition of lymphedema, but an incidence of 6% to 8% is commonly reported.[183,224–226] Factors that contribute to the development of lymphedema are radiation therapy to the dissected axilla, postoperative wound complications, subsequent cellulitis of the arm, obesity, the extent of axillary dissection, and advanced age.[174,224,227,228] The morbidity of axillary dissection can be minimized by the use of appropriate surgical techniques. Avoiding unnecessary dissection superior to the axillary vein and preservation of the fat and lymphatic tissue surrounding the vein decreases edema of the arm and breast. The identification of the long thoracic nerve minimizes the risk of injury to this structure. In the clinically negative axilla, it is reasonable to preserve the thoracodorsal neurovascular bundle and the intercostobrachial nerve.

The appropriateness of eliminating axillary dissection depends on the institutional approach to the use of adjuvant systemic therapy. Women who would not be candidates for adjuvant therapy unless positive nodes were identified, such as those with invasive tumor less than 1 cm in diameter and those participating in clinical trials, continue to require axillary dissection. If different chemotherapy is given depending on the presence and extent of nodal involvement, axillary dissection continues to be necessary. If decisions regarding adjuvant therapy are being made independent of nodal status, the purposes of axillary dissection are for local control and to provide prognostic information. In the woman who is undergoing breast-conserving treatment, radiation therapy to the axilla is an equally effective method of maintaining local control. In women undergoing mastectomy, axillary dissection remains the preferred method of achieving local control.

IRRADIATION IN BREAST-CONSERVING TREATMENT

The technical details of irradiation are important in obtaining satisfactory results using breast-conserving treatment. It is important that the techniques of surgery and irradiation be coordinated. In general, the larger the surgical resection, the less intensive the irradiation needs to be. The optimal combination of surgery and irradiation to achieve the dual objectives of local tumor control and preservation of the cosmetic appearance is controversial and varies from patient to patient, depending on the extent, nature, and location of the tumor, the patient's breast size, and the patient's relative concerns about local recurrence and preservation of the cosmetic appearance.

There is a consensus about some elements in the technique of irradiation. It is considered standard to require patient immobilization, treatment simulation, treatment planning with the use of tissue compensators to improve dose homogeneity, and supervoltage equipment (*i.e.*, 4, 6, or 8 MV or ^{60}Co with 6 MV preferred for dose homogeneity and skin sparing). More sophisticated treatment planning is now available to assess three-dimensional dose distributions and to account for the lower density of lung tissue in the treatment field, but the impact of these developments on patient outcome has not been demonstrated, and they are not considered standard at this time.[229] (In standard treatment planning, the lung is considered to have unit density; the use of actual lung density results in a small alteration in the dose distribution.) Each field should be treated daily, and bolus should not be used. To minimize the risk of radiation pneumonitis, not more than 3 cm of lung (as projected on the beam radiograph at isocenter) should be treated.[230] The dose to the breast should be in the range of 4500 to 5000 cGy given at 180 to 200 cGy per day for 5 days each week.

There is controversy about the need for delivering additional dose to the primary site (*i.e.*, boost) and for treating nodal areas in addition to the breast. The rationales for using a boost are that histologic studies show that residual cancer after resection of the primary tumor is typically in the vicinity of the primary site, recurrences after treatment are most commonly seen at or near the primary site, and boost treatment can be delivered without significant morbidity. Although boost irradiation is usually employed in this country, it is likely that patients treated with more extensive breast resections in whom the margins of resection are clearly negative do not benefit greatly from the use of a boost. It is generally agreed that a boost should be employed in patients with focally positive margins of resection. Boost irradiation is typically delivered using an electron beam or interstitial implantation, and the dose to the primary site is increased to approximately 6000 cGy. There is not a consensus about the advisability of treating nodal areas with irradiation, and this needs to be considered in relation to the use and extent of axillary dissection. In patients who do not undergo axillary dissection, the axillary and supraclavicular regions are usually treated with irradiation. There is general agreement that axillary irradiation should not be given after a complete axillary dissection, that overlap between adjacent fields (if used) should be avoided, and that a photon-only "hockey stick" (used to treat the internal mammary nodes) should be avoided. The use of supraclavicular irradiation in patients with positive axillary nodes is reasonable to decrease the risk of recurrence in this area, but it must be balanced against the small increase in complications.[231] The major trials providing the justification for breast-conserving treatment (*i.e.*, NSABP B-06 and Milan trials) were conducted using breast irradiation alone, establishing this technique as a reasonable option in all patients (after axillary dissection).

PATIENT SELECTION FOR LOCAL TREATMENT

Patient selection is based on the results of patient evaluation. Critical elements in patient evaluation are history and physical examination, mammography, histologic assessment of the resected breast specimen, and assessment of the patient's wishes. There appears to be a consensus about the guidelines for an adequate mammographic evaluation.[232] This includes dedicated mammography in an approved unit, ideally with magnification views of the primary site to determine the presence and extent of associated microcalcifications. In patients with mammographic microcalcifications, if there is any doubt about the adequacy of the resection after review of the original and specimen mammograms, a follow-up mammogram with magnification views is recommended. The use of high-quality mammograms can identify about two thirds of patients with EIC-positive tumors.[233]

The surgeon should orient the resected breast specimen by the use of sutures or other means, and the pathologist should evaluate the margins of resection for tumor involvement by the use of inking or some other method. A careful gross description is essential to detail the size of the specimen, the size of the tumor, and the proximity of the tumor to the margin. The pathology report should mention the presence of microscopic and gross involvement of the margins, although no established definition of "involved margins" has been demonstrated to predict local recurrence after breast-conserving treatment.

Perhaps the most difficult aspect of patient evaluation is the assessment of the patient's wishes about breast preservation in the face of having just been diagnosed with a potentially lethal disease. The patient and her physician need to discuss the implications of the options of mastectomy and breast-conserving treatment with regard to long-term survival, the possibility and consequences of local recurrence, the treatment options if local recurrence occurs, psychological adjustment, cosmetic outcome, sexual adaptation, and functional competence, and the guidelines, effectiveness, and cost of follow-up procedures. For most patients, this decision does not have an impact on the likelihood of survival, but it may influence the quality of life.

Randomized clinical trials have demonstrated equivalent survival for patients treated with mastectomy and breast-conserving treatment, but there are some absolute and some relative contraindications to breast-conserving treatment. An ongoing pregnancy is an absolute contraindication to the use of breast irradiation. It is feasible in many cases to perform breast-conserving surgery in the third trimester and deliver breast irradiation after delivery. Women with two or more gross cancers situated in separate quadrants of the breast or those with diffuse malignant-appearing microcalcifications are not considered candidates for breast-conserving treatment. Another absolute contraindication is a history of prior therapeutic irradiation to the breast region that would necessitate retreatment to an excessively high total radiation dose to a significant volume. For example, breast-conserving treatment is not feasible in a woman with a history of Hodgkin's disease treated with mantle irradiation. A history of collagen vascular disease is considered a contraindication to breast-conserving treatment because of the reports indicating that these patients tolerate irradiation poorly.

Tumor size is not an absolute contraindication to breast-conserving treatment, although there is little published experience in treating patients with tumors larger than 4 to 4.5 cm. A relative contraindication is a large tumor in a small breast, for which adequate resection would result in significant cosmetic alteration. Breast size can be a relative contraindication. Treatment of women with large or pendulous breasts is feasible if there is sufficient expertise to ensure reproducibility of patient set-up and the availability of 6 to 10 MeV radiation to obtain adequate dose homogeneity. The location of the tumor in the breast may be a consideration in the choice of local treatment. In a patient with a tumor beneath the nipple, an adequate resection usually involves removal of all or part of the nipple-areola complex. Whether this is preferable to mastectomy needs to be assessed by the patient and her physicians. The use of breast-conserving treatment in an elderly patient, especially with impaired performance, is generally contraindicated because of poor tolerance of the treatment.

There is still some controversy about whether certain pathologic and clinical features influence the likelihood of recurrence after breast-conserving treatment and therefore should affect the choice of local therapy. These include young patient age (<35 years), focal involvement of the margins of resection, and an extensive intraductal component. It is controversial whether a breast that is difficult to evaluate by mammography and physical examination should influence the choice of local therapy. Further research is required to evaluate the significance of these factors in the selection of patients.

There are certain clinical and pathologic features that should not mitigate against the use of breast-conserving treatment. These include the presence of clinically suspicious (and mobile) axillary lymph nodes or microscopic tumor involvement in axillary nodes. The changes in the breast after conservative surgery and irradiation do allow for the detection of local recurrence at an early stage using physical examination and mammography, and the use of irradiation in this setting has not been shown to result in a significant risk of second tumors in the treated area.

BREAST RECONSTRUCTION AFTER MASTECTOMY

Breast reconstruction is an important option for women undergoing mastectomy for the treatment of breast cancer. Reconstruction may be done at the time of mastectomy or as a secondary procedure, but the possibility of reconstruction should be discussed with the patient before definitive surgery. Reconstruction should be offered to all women who are not candidates for or do not desire breast-conserving surgery with radiation therapy. The indication for breast reconstruction is the patient's desire for the operative procedure. The only true contraindications are significant comorbid conditions that would interfere with the patient's ability to tolerate a longer operative procedure in the case of immediate reconstruction or additional procedures in the case of delayed reconstruction. Patient age, the need for adjuvant chemotherapy, or a poor long-term prognosis are not contraindications to reconstruction. In the past, there were major concerns that the performance of breast reconstruction would obscure local recurrence after mastectomy, and the procedure was restricted to women with early stage carcinoma, usually after a delay of 2 or more years from the time of extirpative surgery.

As our knowledge of the pathophysiology of breast cancer has increased and as more women are diagnosed with early stage breast cancer, there has been an increasing trend toward performing breast reconstruction at the time of mastectomy. Several nonrandomized studies of immediate reconstruction have demonstrated that the incidence of local recurrence after the procedure is similar to that after mastectomy alone.[234-237] Local recurrences after reconstruction were detected at an early stage and, in many cases, treated without loss of the reconstructed breast. The advantages of an immediate reconstruction include avoidance of an additional operative procedure, decreased psychological trauma, and improved coordination of the efforts of the oncologic and reconstructive surgeons to produce an optimal cosmetic result without compromising the oncologic aspects of the surgery.[238] The potential disadvantages of immediate reconstruction are a possible increase in the number of surgical complications and a delay in the institution of adjuvant therapy. Vinton and colleagues compared the incidences of infection, hematoma, seroma, and epidermolysis among 305 women who underwent modified radical mastectomy and 90 who underwent modified radical mastectomy with immediate reconstruction during the same time period.[239] No increase in the frequency of complications was found in the reconstruction group. Eberlein and colleagues reported 199 consecutive patients treated with immediate reconstruction, including 109 with flaps and 90 with implants.[240] Thirty percent of the reconstruction patients underwent chemotherapy, and no delays in initiating treatment were found, a finding similar to that of Frazier.[234]

The two techniques of reconstruction involve the use of implants and the use of tissue from elsewhere in the body (Table 40–15). In January of 1992, the Food and Drug Administration (FDA) declared that silicone gel-filled implants could not be used until more information is available about their long-term safety. This moratorium does not apply to saline-filled implants. In February, a panel of experts appointed by the FDA recommended that silicone gel-filled implants be allowed in breast cancer patients pending the results of further study, and this was approved by the FDA in April of 1992. The complications associated with implants are discussed later. The availability of adequate skin coverage, the size and shape of the patient's contralateral breast, and the patient's cosmetic expectations influence the choice of reconstructive technique.

Until recently, the most commonly used technique for reconstruction was the placement of a silicone gel implant beneath the pectoralis major muscle. This approach is best suited for women with small or moderate-size breasts with minimal ptosis, and requires adequate skin to cover an implant of a size similar to the contralateral breast. The use of limited skin excision, with operative exposure gained by the incision, usually leaves enough skin to cover an implant. Oncologic surgeons agree that the only skin that it is necessary to excise for reasons of cancer control is the nipple-areola complex and the biopsy scar. If insufficient skin is available to achieve symmetry with the contralateral breast or for larger or ptotic breasts, a tissue expander may be employed. This technique involves placement of a prosthesis that is only partially inflated beneath the pectoral muscle. Using a subcutaneous injection port, the prosthesis is gradually filled with saline over a period of weeks to months until the desired breast size and shape are achieved.

Many questions have been raised about the safety of silicone

TABLE 40-15. Types of Reconstruction After Mastectomy

Type	Advantages	Disadvantages
Local Tissue (plus implant)		
Submuscular implant	Simple, single stage	Lack of projection, little natural ptosis
Tissue expansion	Gradual recruitment and stretching of skin, improved projection	Many postoperative visits, complications, time, second-stage surgery to place permanent implant
Permanent expander	Expander is also permanent prosthesis, second stage minor	Many postoperative visits, complications, time
Distant Tissue (with or without implants)		
Myocutaneous latissimus dorsi	Dependable, nice contour axillary fold	Donor site scar, turn patient during surgery
Transverse rectus abdominis myocutaneous (TRAM) flap	Excellent bulk Rarely need implant Abdominoplasty	Big operation (doubles mastectomy time), wound-healing problems, vascularity, hernias
Microvascular free flaps	Bulk depends on donor site	5% failure rate, long and complicated surgery (2 teams), donor site deformity comparable to myocutaneous flaps

breast implants. Silicone implants have been available for the past 30 years, and approximately 2 million women have had implants for reconstruction or augmentation.[241] The major recognized complication of this procedure is fibrous encapsulation or capsular contracture, which is the formation of excessive scar tissue around the implant, possibly leading to deformation of the appearance and pain. There is no convincing data to substantiate the idea that silicone breast implants increase breast cancer risk in humans, although it is true that women with breast implants have not been systematically followed.[241-244] Two epidemiologic studies did not demonstrate an increased incidence of breast carcinoma in women with silicone implants.[242,243] Review of the Surveillance, Epidemiology, and End Results program (SEER) data from 1973 to 1986 did not reveal an increase in the number of breast sarcomas, a neoplasm that can be induced in rats with silicone implants.[244]

There is concern that leakage of silicone from implants may lead to collagen-vascular conditions. Over the past 26 years, there have been more than 100 cases reported of women who developed connective tissue disease in conjunction with the use of free silicone injections or silicone breast prostheses.[245-248] However, only one third of the reported cases have occurred in women with silicone breast implants, and it is uncertain whether the observed number of cases of connective tissue diseases in women with breast implants exceeds the number expected by chance. Based on the lack of good long-term information on the safety of silicone implants, the FDA concluded that the implants should not be used outside of a clinical trial until there is better documentation of their safety. Women with these implants have been advised that there is no information to indicate that implants should be removed, but that they should be monitored for any problems. Further research is needed to clarify this issue.

Another technique of reconstruction is the use of myocutaneous flaps to transfer skin, fat, and muscle from distant parts of the body. The most commonly used flaps are the latissimus dorsi and transverse rectus abdominis (TRAM) myocutaneous flaps. The use of a flap for reconstruction requires a more lengthy operative procedure than the implant method, and postoperative recovery is somewhat longer because of two separate incision sites. The latissimus flap is often used in conjunction with a prosthesis because the flap alone provides insufficient bulk to achieve symmetry in most cases. The survival rate for this flap is high, with only a 1% incidence of complete flap loss reported in most series.[249] The TRAM flap usually allows an adequate breast mound to be fashioned without the use of a prosthesis, but its blood supply is more tenuous than that of the latissimus flap, with major necrosis reported in 5% of patients and partial necrosis in as many as 31% of patients.[250,251] If these myocutaneous flaps are not available or not suitable for use, it is possible to transfer composite tissues from distant sites and to perform a microvascular anastomosis to nearby vessels.[252] This technique, known as a free flap, requires a skilled microsurgeon and prolonged operating time and is only occasionally chosen for primary reconstruction.[249] The potential benefits and complications of the various reconstructive procedures are listed in Table 40–15.

Regardless of the technique of reconstruction chosen, the creation of a breast mound is the chief goal in breast reconstruction. Surgery on the contralateral breast, such as reduction or mastopexy, may be required to achieve symmetry. Reconstruction of a nipple-areolar complex is another secondary procedure that some patients elect to improve the cosmetic appearance. The patient's own nipple should not be used for this purpose, because recurrent carcinoma due to persistence of breast tissue on the nipple has been reported.[253-255] Microscopic involvement of the nipple is seen in 30% of mastectomy specimens but is frequently not apparent at the time of gross pathologic examination.[256-258] The nipple can be reconstructed using a variety of local flap techniques or by the use of full-thickness skin grafts.[249] Tattooing of the grafts produces a color match to the patient's own areola, and allows any site to be used as the donor.[259] Tissue from the contralateral nipple should not be used for nipple reconstruction because of the concern of transferring breast tissue to the reconstruction site.

POSTOPERATIVE IRRADIATION

The first major use of radiation therapy in the primary management of patients with breast cancer was as an adjuvant to radical mastectomy. There were two rationales for prophylactic radiation therapy. The first was that prophylactic radiation therapy could be used to reduce the risk of locoregional tumor recurrence. The overall risk of local recurrence after mastectomy is 10% to 15% and is related to whether axillary nodes are negative or positive. One purpose of postoperative radiation therapy is to decrease this risk of local recurrence. It has been argued that prevention of local recurrence is important because these recurrences are often distressing for patients and because clinically manifested recurrences can be treated effectively in only approximately 50% of patients. The second rationale for postoperative radiation therapy is to improve the likelihood of survival.

Postoperative radiation therapy markedly decreases the risk of locoregional recurrence, but the effect of adjuvant radiation therapy on survival remains uncertain. The survival value of postoperative radiation therapy ideally would be determined by large, properly conducted, prospective, randomized clinical trials. The trials testing the value of postoperative radiation therapy are shown in Table 40–16. It should be stressed that the number of patients entered into these trials is relatively small (*i.e.*, small or moderate benefits may be missed) and that the trials before the late 1960s used techniques of irradiation that did not adequately treat the target volume (*i.e.*, the chest wall and regional nodal areas) and gave excessive doses to critical structures, such as the heart. In the Stockholm trial, the most modern of the trials using patients without adjuvant systemic therapy, there was a long-term improvement in relapse-free survival after postoperative irradiation, but the improvement in survival was only marginal (*p* = 0.09) and restricted to the subset of node-positive patients. In node-negative patients, there was no benefit.

It is possible that postoperative irradiation may be detrimental to survival. An overview of postoperative radiation therapy by Cuzick and associates published in 1987 included the results from the Manchester trials, the Oslo trials, the Stockholm trial, and an unpublished small trial from Heidelberg.[260] No difference was seen in mortality comparing patients treated with or without radiation therapy over the first 10 years after surgery. After 10 years, there was a lower rate of survival associated with the use of radiation therapy (*p* = 0.005). This decrease in survival was primarily due to an increase in late cardiac deaths and was evident in patients treated for left-sided breast cancer in the trials that gave large doses of radiation to the heart. In a recent retrospective analysis of cause-specific mortality in the Stockholm trial, in which cardiac doses were calculated in relation to the patient's lat-

erality and the technique employed, a clear relation between cardiac dose and late cardiac death was demonstrated. With a mean follow-up time of 16 years, patients who received low or intermediate cardiac doses had a 20% reduction in breast cancer deaths and no increase in cardiac deaths. This study provides good evidence that late cardiac mortality can be avoided using proper techniques of irradiation.

The use of postoperative radiation therapy needs to be reconsidered in patients who receive adjuvant chemotherapy. It is possible that the chest wall and regional nodes are the sites of greatest tumor burden after mastectomy in certain subgroups, such as patients with larger primary tumors or positive axillary nodes. According to the Goldie-Coldman hypothesis, spontaneous mutations of tumor cells to drug resistance accounts for failures of chemotherapy, and the likelihood that drug-resistant cells will emerge is directly related to the tumor burden. In theory, by decreasing the local tumor burden, adjuvant radiation therapy may decrease the probability of drug resistance and increase the probability of cure. The use of adjuvant chemotherapy by itself decreases the rate of local recurrence, but to a lesser degree than after irradiation. In a randomized trial from Sweden that compared the adjuvant use of CMF chemotherapy and irradiation, the local recurrence rate for patients treated with irradiation was approximately one half that of patients treated with chemotherapy.[261] Table 40–16 shows the results of trials in which patients were randomized to receive irradiation or to not receive irradiation in conjunction with adjuvant systemic therapy. The largest of these is from the Danish Breast Cancer Cooperative Group, in which patients with high-risk breast cancer (*i.e.*, T3 or T4 or with positive nodes) were randomized to various adjuvant therapies. In an abstract of the results at 7 years, the local recurrence rate was 32% among the 737 premenopausal patients treated with CMF and only 9% among the 736 premenopausal patients treated with irradiation (*p* < 0.0001), and the corresponding survival rates were 61% for CMF and 57% for irradiation (*p* < 0.05).[262]

The role of postoperative irradiation is not established. The modern trials suggest that the treatment can be given safely and is associated with a modest benefit in the survival of node-positive patients, particularly if used in conjunction with adjuvant chemotherapy. Further research is required to substantiate these observations, but many physicians favor the use of postoperative irradiation to prevent locoregional recurrence, particularly in patients with four or more positive nodes. In patients to be treated with chemotherapy and irradiation, the optimal sequencing of these modalities is not determined. The results of the Dana-Farber Cancer Institute/JCRT trial indicate that radiation therapy can effectively be added at the completion of adjuvant chemotherapy, avoiding any possible interference with the administration of the chemotherapy.[263]

TREATMENT OF SPECIFIC PROBLEMS IN BREAST CANCER

AXILLARY METASTASES WITH AN OCCULT BREAST PRIMARY

Breast carcinoma presenting as an axillary metastasis with no apparent primary tumor is an uncommon problem that was described by Halsted in 1907, and it remains a treatment

TABLE 40-16. Randomized Trials Testing the Value of Radiation Therapy After Radical or Modified Radical Mastectomy

Investigations	Treatment Arms*	No. of Patients	Years	Type of Irradiation	Follow-up	Survival
Without Systemic Therapy						
Manchester[563]	RM	752	1949–1955	Orthovoltage	34 y	Decreased survival in RT pts seen after 15 y
	RM + RT	709				
NSABP B-02	RM	632	1961–1968	Super- and orthovoltage	5 yr	No significant difference
	RM + RT	470				
Oslo I[564]	RM	264	1964–1967	Orthovoltage	10 y	No significant difference
	RM + RT	282				
Oslo II[564]	RM	277	1968–1972	Supervoltage	10 y	No significant difference
	RM + RT	265				
Stockholm	MRM	321	1971–1976	Supervoltage	13.5 y	No significant difference (for node-pos. pts, RT slightly better)
	MRM + RT	323				
Compared With Systemic Therapy						
Stockholm II[565]	MRM + RT	311	1976–1984	Supervoltage	6.5 y	No significant difference (RT slightly better in postmenopausal pts)
	MRM + CMF	345				
In Conjunction With Systemic Therapy						
DFCI/JCRT[263]	MRM + CT	84	1974–1984	Supervoltage	44 mo	No significant difference
	MRM + CT + RT	76				
SECSG[566]	MRM + CMF × 6	133	1976–1983	Supervoltage	10 y	No significant difference, but combined treatment favored
	MRM + CMF × 12	61				
	MRM + RT + CMF × 6	137				
Danish Breast Cancer Coop Group[567]	MRM + CMF	737	1982–1989	Supervoltage	5 y (2 y median)	63% vs 68%; $p = 0.03$ (combined treatment favored)
	MRM + RT + CMF (premenop pts only)	736				
Danish Breast Cancer Coop Group[567]	MRM + Tam	600	1982–1989	Supervoltage	5 y (2 y median)	No significant difference
	MRM + RT + TAM (postmenop pts only)	602				
Mayo Clinic[568]	MRM + L-PAM	81	1974–?	Supervoltage	5 y	No significant difference
	MRM + CFP	104				
	MRM + RT + CFP	108				
POA[569]	MRM + CT	86	1977–?	Supervoltage	11 y	No significant difference
	MRM + RT + CT (CT = L-PAM or CMF)	72				
Glasgow[570]	RT	103	1976–1982	Orthovoltage	63 mo	No significant difference
	RT + CMF	111				
	CMF	108				
British Columbia	CMF + RT	161	1979–1985	Supervoltage	10 y	DFS better for CMF + RT Survival for CMF + RT 63% vs CMF 58%; $p = 0.01$
	CMF	155				

* RT, radiation therapy; RM, radical mastectomy; MRM, modified radical mastectomy; CT, chemotherapy; CMF, cyclophosphamide, methotrexate, and 5-fluorouracil; Tam, tamoxifen; CFP, cyclophosphamide, 5-fluorouracil, and prednisone.

dilemma today. This entity accounted for 0.35% of 10,014 patients treated for primary breast carcinoma at Memorial Sloan-Kettering Cancer Center from 1975 to 1988.[264] A similar incidence of 0.4% of 12,000 breast cancers treated over a 20-year period at the National Cancer Institute in Milan was reported by Vezzoni and associates.[265] The mean age of women with occult primary tumors is between 50 and 54 years, which does not differ significantly from that of women with clinically detectable primary carcinomas.[265–267]

Axillary adenopathy due to metastatic adenocarcinoma may be secondary to a variety of primary tumors, but in women, the breast is by far the most common primary site. After a diagnosis of adenocarcinoma is obtained, the radiologic evaluation should be confined to high-quality bilateral mammography, a chest radiograph, and a bone scan to exclude metastases before definitive therapy. There is uniform agreement that additional radiologic studies looking for another primary tumor site are unrewarding if there are no symptoms and should not be done.[264–269]

The sensitivity of mammography in the identification of the occult primary lesion is low. Of 36 women undergoing mammography in Vezzoni's series, only 36% had tumors detected.[265] In the M.D. Anderson Cancer Center experience, only three possible mammographic abnormalities were identified in 40 women with axillary adenopathy due to a presumed occult breast primary.[266] Of 24 patients reviewed by Kemeny,[268] only 1 woman had a mammogram suggesting carcinoma, and Baron and coworkers[264] reported a 29% sensitivity for mammography in detecting occult primary tumors. These reports, using modern mammographic techniques and equipment, suggest that although abnormalities on mammogram should be aggressively pursued, the absence of a mammographic abnormality does not exclude the presence of a primary breast tumor.

When an axillary node biopsy of an occult primary tumor is done in the clinical setting, the pathologist should be alerted to this fact so that appropriate diagnostic studies can be obtained. Tissue should be sent in a fresh, nonpreserved state to the pathology laboratory and portions retained for hormone receptor determination, immunohistochemistry, and routine light microscopy. Iglehart and coworkers reported the utility of using electron microscopy in a study of 5 patients.[269] However, no features that clearly established the breast as the primary tumor site were identified. Bhatia and coworkers obtained hormone receptor studies for the axillary nodes of 11 women with occult primary breast carcinoma and identified positive estrogen or progesterone receptors in 7 patients, unequivocally establishing the breast as the site of the primary lesion.[270] Others have reported receptor positivity in 62%, 50%, and 40% of patients.[264,268,271] A negative receptor analysis does not rule out the breast as the site of the primary.

Most women with axillary node metastases secondary to a presumed breast primary have been treated with mastectomy. Table 40–17 summarizes the results of mastectomy in 228 patients, and a primary tumor was identified in 64%. The highest rates of primary tumor identification were seen in some of the older reports from a time when high-quality mammography was not routinely available. Kemeny[268] and Ellerbroek,[266] reviewing case material in which virtually all patients had mammography, found 45% and 8%, respectively, of mastectomy specimens to contain a primary.

TABLE 40-17. Identification of Primary Tumors in Mastectomy Specimens From Patients With Occult Breast Cancer

Investigations	No. of Patients	No. of Cancers/ No. of Mastectomies		Five-Year Survivors (%)
Ashikari[272]	42	22/34	(65%)	79
Baron[264]	35	22/33	(67%)	75
Ellerbroek[266]	42	1/13	(8%)	72
Fitts[275]	13	11/13	(85%)	71
Haagensen[128]	18	13/14	(93%)	57
Kemeny[268]	20	5/11	(46%)	Not stated
Owen[571]	25	15/25	(60%)	50
Patel[267]	29	16/29	(55%)	28
Vezzoni[265]	49	33/44	(75%)	84
Westbrook[273]	18	9/12	(75%)	61
Total		147/228	(64%)	

The size of the carcinomas identified in the mastectomy specimen varies widely. DCIS was the only histologic evidence of malignancy in several cases.[264,267,268,272,273] This finding may be secondary to sampling error with failure to identify a small invasive carcinoma or invasion through the basement membrane identifiable only by electron microscopy.[274] Vezzoni found that 30% of pathologically identified carcinomas were 1 to 2 cm in diameter.[265] Forty-five percent of the 22 cancers reported by Baron and colleagues[264] were multifocal, and Rosen[271] reported a median tumor size of 1.5 cm (range, 0.1–6.5 cm) in his series. Infiltrating ductal carcinoma is the most common histologic tumor type seen.[128,272,273,275]

With the increasing use of breast preservation in the management of breast carcinoma, several groups have applied these techniques to occult breast cancer.[266,268,276,277] Theoretical objections to this approach include the fact that the tumor burden in the breast may be extensive, even if the disease is clinically occult, and that it is not feasible to deliver a boost dose of radiation therapy to the primary tumor site. Thirty patients were treated at the Institut Curie with radiation therapy to the breast and axillary, supraclavicular, and internal mammary fields to a mean midbreast dose of 6200 cGy.[277] Eleven (37%) women developed breast recurrences. Local recurrence occurred as an isolated event in 4 women, in conjunction with nodal recurrence in 4, and as part of systemic failure in 3. The mean time to breast recurrence was 9.3 years, and in another report from this group, only 1 of 3 patients alive at 15 years after treatment retained her breast.[276] Ellerbroek reported 29 patients in which a breast-preserving approach was employed.[266] Sixteen patients had radiation therapy using a mean breast dose of 5170 cGy, producing a 17% 5-year actuarial breast failure rate. An additional 13 woman had an axillary biopsy with irradiation of the axilla only. Seven of the 13 developed clinical primary breast tumors at a mean follow-up of 27 months, and the 5-year actuarial risk of breast failure in this group was 57%. No apparent survival differences between patients treated with mastectomy and breast preservation were observed in these studies, a finding supported by the reports of Kemeny[268] and Baron[264] for small numbers of women treated with a breast-preserving approach.

Overall, survival for women with occult primary tumors does not differ greatly from the survival of patients with the same extent of axillary involvement and a known primary. This is shown in Figure 40–10. A difference in survival is not observed between patients in whom the histologic tumor is identified in the breast and those in whom tumor can not be documented, suggesting that the breast is the primary tumor site in both cases. Adjuvant chemotherapy should be given postoperatively to these patients, using the same indications and therapeutic selection criteria employed for any stage II breast cancer patients.

LOCALLY ADVANCED BREAST CANCER

The designation of locally advanced breast carcinoma (LABC) encompasses a heterogeneous group of tumors ranging from neglected, relatively slow-growing, large primary tumors to small breast tumors presenting with extensive nodal metastases. Locally advanced breast cancer corresponds to stage III as defined by the UICC-AJCC system. Patients may be stage III by virtue of a T3 or T4 tumor or N2 or N3 disease. Inflammatory carcinoma, characterized clinically by a diffuse edema and erythema of the breast, frequently without a palpable breast mass, and defined pathologically by the presence of tumor emboli in the subdermal lymphatics, is a particularly virulent form of locally advanced breast cancer. The biologic diversity seen in locally advanced tumors makes a comparison of different treatment results or the formation of a single treatment recommendation for all women difficult.

Despite increasing recognition by physicians and the public of the importance of screening and early detection to decrease breast cancer mortality, 10% to 20% of women with breast cancer have locally advanced disease at diagnosis.[278,279] Although clinical features at presentation and prognosis among women with locally advanced cancer may vary, there are two common problems in the treatment of these patients: obtaining local control and prolonging survival by preventing or delaying distant metastases.

Historically, treatment of LABC was surgical. By 1942,

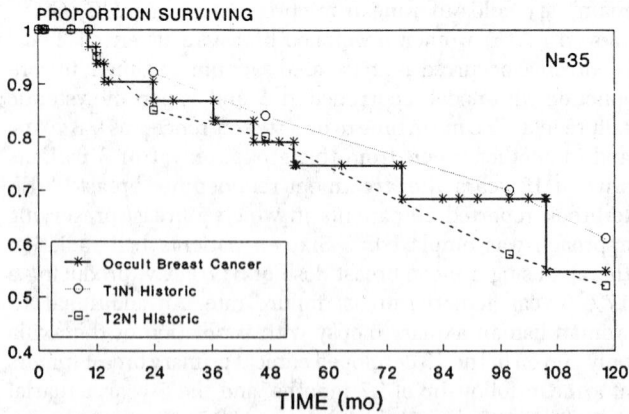

FIGURE 40–10. Survival among patients with occult breast cancer compared with patients with an identified breast primary. (Baron P, Moore M, Kinne D. Occult primary cancer presenting with axillary metastases. Arch Surg 1990;125:210–214)

Haagensen and Stout developed the Columbia Clinical Classification of breast cancer based on 1135 carcinomas treated at Columbia Presbyterian Hospital from 1915 through 1942.[280] This classification identified clinical features associated with a high local recurrence rate and poor survival after surgery. These are listed in the earlier section on staging. Radical mastectomy in these patients was associated with a 53% local failure rate and a 0% 5-year disease-free survival.

Haagensen identified five grave signs, including edema of less than one third of the skin of the breast, skin ulceration, fixation of the tumor to the chest wall, fixed axillary lymph nodes, or an axillary node larger than 2.5 cm in diameter, that were associated with a high likelihood of local recurrence, although a single grave sign was not thought to connote inoperability.

The poor results seen with radical surgery resulted in the use of radiation therapy as local treatment in women with locally advanced breast cancer. Early studies demonstrated that the ability of radiation therapy to control LABC depends on dose. Fletcher and Montague reviewed the M.D. Anderson Hospital experience from 1948 to 1962 with the treatment of locally advanced breast cancer by radiation alone.[281] Forty-four (28%) of 159 women with tumors larger than 7 cm and 19 (17%) of 114 patients with tumors smaller than 7 cm failed locally after radiation therapy. Fletcher emphasized the concept that, although microscopic disease can be sterilized by 4500 cGy in 5 weeks in 90% of all instances, large tumors require large doses (7500–8000 cGy) to control gross disease. Sheldon and associates corroborated the importance of dose in a report of 192 stage III patients.[282] At 5 years, women receiving 6000 cGy or higher doses to the primary site had an 83% local control rate, compared with 70% for those who received less than 6000 cGy. However, local control rates over 70% are not reported in all groups of stage III patients treated with radiation therapy. A 5-year actuarial risk of local recurrence of 59% was found in a review of patients with inflammatory cancer treated from 1968 to 1986 at the JCRT.[283] Two thirds of the local failures occurred before the appearance of distant metastases, and 26% were associated with moderate to severe symptoms. Bedwinek observed that 65% of 43 women with noninflammatory T4 lesions failed locally after treatment doses of 4000 to 7000 cGy.[284]

Increasing the dose of radiation therapy may increase the likelihood of local tumor control and increase the risk of complications. Spanos and associates reviewed treatment sequelae in patients at the M.D. Anderson Cancer Center and found that the most severe consequences of high-dose radiation were fibrosis and necrosis.[285] The incidence of severe complications ranged from 17% at 5100 to 6000 cGy to 28% at 8100 cGy, but all patients were reported to have some component of fibrosis. Bedwinek and colleagues reported 4 cases of severe breast fibrosis among 83 patients.[284] Twenty moderately severe complications were reported, including breast fibrosis, breast and arm edema, stiff shoulder, and one brachial plexus injury. Sheldon and coworkers observed 18 severe or moderate complications in 15 of 192 patients (197 breasts treated).[282] These included moderate or severe arm edema in 6 patients and brachial plexopathy in 4 patients. A cosmetic evaluation of these patients revealed that satisfactory cosmetic results were obtained in only 56% of patients, and 19% of the patients had poor cosmetic results.

The poor results using local treatment in patients with LABC led to use of initial treatment with chemotherapy. It was actually in these stage III noninflammatory breast cancer patients that primary or neoadjuvant chemotherapy containing doxorubicin (Adriamycin) was first tested. These early results demonstrated prompt tumor shrinkage in many patients that facilitated subsequent radiation therapy or mastectomy.[286] Treating the tumor with primary chemotherapy allows the clinician to assess the efficacy of a particular drug regimen using the local disease as a marker. This approach may help in the design of systemic adjuvant treatment.[279,287-289] The use of primary chemotherapy in patients with LABC is discussed later.

Two randomized trials examined whether mastectomy or radiation therapy is the more effective local treatment modality if combined with chemotherapy.[290,291] De Lena and colleagues randomized 132 women to mastectomy or radiation therapy after three cycles of doxorubicin and vincristine.[290] Additional chemotherapy was given after local treatment. No significant differences in duration of response, relapse-free survival, or overall survival were observed. Similar findings were reported by the Cancer and Leukemia Group B in a study of radiation therapy versus surgery after three cycles of cyclophosphamide, doxorubicin, fluorouracil, vincristine, and prednisone.[291] In the 87 patients eligible for randomization after induction, no differences in relapse rates or survival were found.

In an attempt to improve local control rates and to avoid the complications of high-dose radiation therapy, several institutions combined preoperative or postoperative radiation therapy with mastectomy. Although excellent local control rates were reported with the combination therapy, it is difficult to compare the results in patients who were able to undergo surgery with those in patients who are technically inoperable, frequently due to more diffuse disease, and receive radiation alone.[284,292-294] High-dose radiation therapy or combinations of surgery and radiation therapy may result in excellent local tumor control in stage III breast carcinoma, but survival remains poor because of frequent distant recurrences. Bedwinek and associates observed that, although women treated with surgery and radiation therapy had a local failure rate of only 13% compared with 61% after radiation therapy alone, a high frequency of distant metastases was seen after either treatment approach.[284]

Few randomized studies have been performed to evaluate the addition of chemotherapy to local treatment in locally advanced breast cancer. These trials can be criticized because the chemotherapy used was not sufficiently aggressive. In a study from Finland, 120 patients with stage III cancer underwent modified radical mastectomy and were randomized to receive radiation therapy alone, chemotherapy alone, or both treatments.[295] Disease-free survival after combined chemotherapy and radiation therapy was significantly better than after either modality alone, but a significant benefit in overall survival for the combined-treatment group was seen only in comparison with the radiation therapy group. Schaake-Koning and coworkers reported a randomized study of 118 patients with locally advanced breast cancer, including inflammatory cancer, comparing radiation therapy alone, radiation therapy followed by CMF chemotherapy, and radiation therapy preceded and followed by alternating cycles of CMF and doxo-

rubicin plus vincristine.[261] Although there were trends toward improved relapse-free survival in the chemotherapy arms, these differences were not statistically significant. The projected 5-year survival rate was 37%, with no differences observed between treatment groups. The negative results of this study should be viewed in light of problems with its design. The technique of radiation therapy differed in the third arm of the study, and 6 of the 8 patients with T1 tumors were assigned to the radiation therapy-alone arm.

A European Organization for Research and Treatment of Cancer randomized study assigned 363 evaluable patients (13% with inflammatory cancer) to receive radiation therapy alone, radiation therapy plus endocrine therapy, radiation therapy plus CMF, or radiation therapy plus endocrine therapy plus CMF.[296] The systemic treatments prolonged the disease-free interval if compared with radiation therapy alone, and the prolongation of disease-free survival was most notable for the combined endocrine and chemotherapy group. However, this improvement was accounted for primarily by a delay in locoregional relapse and no significant improvement in distant disease-free survival was found. Differences in overall survival, although appearing to favor the combined modality therapy, did not reach statistical significance.

There has been an increasing trend toward the use of induction chemotherapy before undertaking local treatment in the management of LABC. This approach has several potential benefits, including the prompt treatment of presumed systemic disease, the reduction of tumor burden before definitive local therapy, and the use of the response of the primary tumor as an in vivo chemosensitivity assay. Clinical response rates of 70% to 90% have been reported for a variety of induction therapies.[297-300] Pathologic studies, however, indicate that the clinical assessment of response is relatively inaccurate. Feldman[300] and Morrow[299] each observed a 60% error rate in the clinical assessment of response compared with the pathologic findings at mastectomy. The amount of residual tumor (microscopic versus gross) in the mastectomy after induction therapy was found to be the most significant predictor of disease-free and overall survival in the experience of Feldman and coworkers.[300] No increase in surgical morbidity has been reported for patients undergoing mastectomy after induction chemotherapy.[301]

Representative results of combined-modality treatment are those reported from the M.D. Anderson Cancer Center.[302] Of 174 patients with LABC treated with three cycles of fluorouracil, doxorubicin, and cyclophosphamide followed by surgery, radiation therapy, or both and additional chemotherapy, disease-free and overall survivals at 5 years were 71% and 84% for stage IIIA patients and 33% and 44% for IIIB patients. Seventy percent of treatment failures in this study occurred at distant sites. The results appear related to tumor size and clinical nodal status, as shown in the experience from the National Cancer Institute of Italy in Milan. In their 10-year analysis of 277 patients with stage IIIB disease treated with a combined-modality approach, the survival rate was 48% for patients with primary tumors smaller than 5 cm, 20% for 5 to 10 cm, and 4% for tumors larger than 10 cm.[303] The relation between nodal status and survival followed a similar pattern (N0, 27%; N1, 28%; N2, 12%). Premenopausal or postmenopausal status had no prognostic influence (24% versus 23%). In a review of trials using a multidisciplinary approach, a benefit in survival was observed when compared with historic controls.[289]

In most institutions, it is standard to treat patients with LABC with combined-modality treatment consisting of induction or primary chemotherapy and a combination of mastectomy and radiation therapy. Typically, primary chemotherapy is started using a doxorubicin-containing regimen (*e.g.*, FAC or AC regimens) and given at full dose for four to six cycles, depending on the magnitude of response. After maximal tumor shrinkage has been obtained, it is still uncertain whether the next step should be surgery followed by radiation therapy or the opposite sequence. Usually, surgery is performed first if the local disease has become technically operable, and postoperative irradiation to the chest wall and appropriate nodal areas is reserved until the completion of all chemotherapy. The experiences at the National Cancer Institute of Italy and M.D. Anderson Cancer Center strongly suggest maintenance chemotherapy is useful after induction chemotherapy and surgery to improve treatment outcome.[289,303] Based on the results from the National Cancer Institute of Italy, six cycles of CMF is a reasonable approach to adjuvant therapy.[304,305] In steroid receptor-positive tumors, tamoxifen (20 mg/day given orally) can be added for 3 or more years after adjuvant chemotherapy is completed.

The trials using combined-modality treatment appear to show an improvement in outcome, but this approach is still associated with a high rate of distant metastases. Further progress in treating women with LABC awaits improvements in systemic therapy.

INFLAMMATORY BREAST CANCER

Inflammatory breast cancer is a rare type of breast cancer accounting for only 1% to 4% of all mammary carcinomas.[279] Inflammatory breast cancer carries an invariably poor prognosis if treated with radiation therapy or surgery alone. Almost 20 years ago, a combined-modality approach with primary chemotherapy (doxorubicin plus vincristine [AV]) was first attempted.[306] Currently, treatment consists of primary chemotherapy followed by local treatment and additional chemotherapy, as for patients with LABC. Using four to six cycles of a doxorubicin-containing regimen (*e.g.*, FAC, AVCMF) as induction chemotherapy, the objective response rate is about 70% with a 10% to 15% complete tumor response.[306–311] In patients with inflammatory breast cancer, radiation therapy rather than mastectomy follows chemotherapy at many institutions because of concerns about "cutting through" dermal lymphatic involvement. Later, if feasible, mastectomy is performed.[312]

The use of combined modality treatment in patients with inflammatory breast cancer has resulted in a large improvement in the 5-year survival rate compared with the results in historic series in which local therapy alone was used. As for patients with LABC, there continues to be a high rate of metastatic disease with time, and improvements in systemic therapy are required for this patient subset.

PAGET'S DISEASE OF THE NIPPLE

Paget's disease of the nipple is a rare form of breast cancer that is characterized clinically by eczematoid changes of the nipple. Associated symptoms include itching, erythema, and nipple discharge.[313–315] Histologically, Paget's disease is diagnosed by the presence of large cells with pale cytoplasm and prominent nucleoli known as Paget's cells. Sir James Paget found that this condition was invariably followed by cancer of the breast, which usually occurred within 1 year of diagnosis.[316] In approximately 54% of women with Paget's disease, a breast mass is detected at presentation, and in most of the remainder, infiltrating or intraductal carcinoma is identified in the mastectomy specimen.[317] The average age of women with Paget's disease does not differ from that of women with other forms of breast cancer, but symptoms are frequently present for 6 months or more before diagnosis.[313,318]

The relation between the changes observed in the nipple and the underlying breast cancer remains a matter of controversy. One theory suggests that the nipple involvement represents the migration of malignant cells from the underlying breast tumor. This view is based primarily on older histologic studies in which ducts containing malignant cells were connected to the overlying nipple containing Paget's cells.[319,320] The alternative hypothesis proposes that the Paget's cells are a separate disease process and in fact are not neoplastic.[315,321] If changes indicate Paget's disease, a mammogram may be helpful in identifying nonpalpable masses or microcalcifications indicating intraductal carcinoma. Regardless of the findings of the mammogram, all suspicious lesions of the nipple should be promptly biopsied.

Paget's disease has traditionally been treated with mastectomy. The rationales for this approach are the need to sacrifice the nipple-areola complex, the fact that the subareolar ducts may be diffusely involved with tumor, and the observation that carcinoma may be found at a considerable distance from the nipple.[315] The prognosis in Paget's disease is related to the stage of the disease and appears to be similar to that of women with other types of breast carcinoma. A limited experience with breast-conserving procedures in the management of Paget's disease has been analyzed. Paone reported 5 patients who underwent excision of the nipple with a wedge resection of underlying breast tissue who remained free of disease at 10-year follow-up.[315] Lagios and coworkers reported 5 patients with no palpable breast mass and negative mammograms treated by excision of the nipple-areola complex.[322] One patient, treated with only partial nipple excision, developed recurrent Paget's disease at 12 months, which was resected. At a mean follow-up of 36 months, no patient had developed parenchymal breast recurrence. Twenty selected patients with Paget's disease without clinical or radiologic evidence of tumor were treated with radiation therapy alone or excision plus radiation therapy at the Institut Curie from 1960 to 1984.[323] At a median follow-up of 7.5 years, 3 patients had recurrent disease in the nipple-areolar region and were treated with mastectomy. The 7-year actuarial probability of survival with the breast preserved was 81%. Osteen collected a total of 79 patients treated by local excision with or without radiation therapy, with 9 local recurrences.[317]

When considering therapeutic options in Paget's disease, it is helpful to think of the condition as an intraductal carcinoma involving the nipple that usually is associated with additional intraductal or invasive carcinoma in the underlying breast parenchyma. Mastectomy is considered the standard therapy. In patients with apparently localized Paget's disease after clinical and radiographic evaluation, breast-conserving therapy can be considered. The selection criteria and treatment techniques applied to other women with breast cancer should be applied in this setting, with the understanding that the nipple-areola complex must be sacrificed and the risk of local recurrence may be higher than after mastectomy.

MALE BREAST CANCER

Cancer of the male breast is an uncommon disease, with an estimated 900 cases diagnosed in the United States in 1991 and 300 deaths in the same period.[324] Rare families have been reported with more than one man with breast cancer, and in some reports, as many as 60% of men with the disease have affected female relatives.[325] Other factors that increase the risk of male breast cancer include Klinefelter's syndrome, schistosomiasis, and radiation exposure.[326-328] The presence of gynecomastia does not seem to be associated with an increased risk of male breast carcinoma, although the microscopic changes of gynecomastia were associated with male breast cancer in 40% of patients reported from Memorial Hospital.[329-331]

Clinically, male breast cancer presents as a mass beneath the nipple-areolar complex in most cases.[329,330,332,333] Ulceration of the nipple is a frequent sign, although isolated nipple discharge is uncommon.[334] The mean age of men with breast carcinoma is between 60 and 70, approximately 10 years older than that of women with the disease.[327,330,335] Infiltrating ductal carcinoma is the most common tumor type, but Paget's disease of the nipple and inflammatory carcinoma have been reported in men. Lobular carcinoma in situ is not seen in the male breast.[335,336] As many as 80% of male breast carcinomas are ER positive.[337,338] An inverse correlation exists between receptor positivity and age, similar to that seen in women.[338]

The standard treatment for male breast carcinoma has been mastectomy. If the tumor is not fixed to the pectoral muscle, a modified radical mastectomy can be done, or if muscle involvement is limited, a portion of this structure can be removed. For patients with extensive involvement of the pectoral muscle, a radical mastectomy may be required.[339] Postoperative radiation is considered in patients with close surgical margins or extensive nodal involvement. Reports of primary radiation therapy for male breast carcinoma are scarce, but Ramantanis' series included 22 men treated by tumor excision and radiation therapy, producing a 35% 5-year survival rate.[329]

There is some controversy about the prognosis of male breast cancer. Most oncologists think that, after accounting for differences in stage between male and female breast cancer, survival rates do not differ.[331,335] Axillary node involvement has the same prognostic significance in men as it does in women. Heller and associates found a 90% 5-year survival rate for node-negative men and a 59% survival rate for node-positive men, which was similar to the survival of women with breast cancer treated in the same time period.[331]

Systemic therapy of metastatic male breast cancer has usually involved hormonal manipulations to eliminate sources of androgen. Response rates of 50% to 80% are reported, and responses to second-line therapy are commonly seen.[338-340] The traditional method of hormonal manipulation has been

orchiectomy. A recent literature review found a 53% response rate to this treatment.[339] Tamoxifen has a similar response rate and has become increasingly popular as a first-line hormonal manipulation, with orchiectomy reserved for patients who have failed multiple other therapies.[339,340] Responses to progestins, antiandrogens, luteinizing hormone-releasing hormone analogs, and aminoglutethimide have been reported.[339]

The available data on the use of chemotherapy in metastatic male breast cancer is limited. The drugs reported are those used to treat women, and the approach to chemotherapy for these patients should be the same as that employed for women.[339,341,342] Two small studies of adjuvant chemotherapy in node-positive men project 5-year survivals greater than 80%, suggesting that adjuvant chemotherapy may be of benefit.[343,344] Without definitive data, the guidelines for the use of adjuvant therapy in male breast cancer commonly follow those used in female breast cancer.

BREAST CANCER DURING PREGNANCY

Breast cancer occurring during pregnancy is relatively uncommon, accounting for 2.8% of 45,881 patients reviewed by White.[345] If only breast cancer patients in their childbearing years are considered, 7% to 14% have breast cancer during pregnancy.[346,347] A review of 416,441 pregnancies found an incidence of 2.2 breast cancers per 10,000 pregnancies.[348]

The clinical presentation of breast cancer during pregnancy is the same as in the nonpregnant patient, and a palpable mass is the most common symptom. Nipple discharge, including a thin, bloody discharge from multiple ducts, may be a physiologic accompaniment of pregnancy. However, a persistent, pathologic, unilateral, bloody discharge during pregnancy requires surgical investigation. Mammography is not particularly helpful in the pregnant woman due to the increased density of the breast during pregnancy. Decisions about the need for breast biopsy should be made on the basis of clinical examination. Delays in the diagnosis of breast masses in pregnant women are common, and most of this delay is due to physicians.[346,347,349] Breast biopsy under local anesthesia is safe at any time during pregnancy and should be done for any suspicious mass.

The options for the local treatment of breast cancer during pregnancy are limited for the woman who wishes to continue her pregnancy. The use of radiation therapy is contraindicated, due to the inability to shield the fetus from the internal scatter of radiation. If cancer is diagnosed in the third trimester, lumpectomy and axillary dissection can be performed and radiation therapy delayed until after delivery. Delays for longer periods to allow breast preservation may be detrimental.

Immediate reconstruction is contraindicated during pregnancy. It would be extremely difficult to obtain symmetry with the postpartum breast, and the risk to the fetus of a more prolonged anesthesia and increased blood loss is not warranted. Therapeutic abortion does not play a role in the treatment of nonmetastatic breast carcinoma. Donegan, reviewing the literature, found a 5-year survival rate of 62% for women undergoing therapeutic abortion compared with 54% for those whose pregnancy was completed.[350] King and colleagues found no survival differences between women whose pregnancies were interrupted and those who delivered after stratification for stage of disease.[351]

Breast cancer during pregnancy was thought to be a particularly virulent disease. Haagensen and Stout originally thought that breast cancer during pregnancy was categorically incurable.[280] Much of the poor prognosis seems to be due to advanced stage of disease at diagnosis in pregnant women. Nugent[352] found that 74% of women in his series had positive axillary nodes, a figure similar to the 65% reported by King,[351] and 72% reported by Holleb.[353] Petrek compared 56 pregnant breast cancer patients treated at Memorial Hospital from 1960 to 1980 with 166 nonpregnant women of the same age treated in the same period and found that 61% of the pregnant women and 38% of the nonpregnant women had positive lymph nodes ($p < 0.05$) and that 31% of the pregnant women and 50% of their counterparts had T1 tumors ($p < 0.05$).[354]

After correction for tumor stage, survival in women treated during pregnancy is similar to that seen in nonpregnant women. Ribeiro and Palmer compared the survival of 40 pregnant patients with 120 controls matched for age, stage, and year of treatment and found no differences between groups.[355] Petrek reported a 77% 10-year survival rate for node-negative women treated during pregnancy and a rate of 75% for nonpregnant women with negative nodes.[354] King observed a 71% 10-year survival rate for node-negative pregnant patients.[351] It appears that delay in diagnosis and treatment, rather than pregnancy itself, is responsible for the poor prognosis observed in some series of women treated for breast cancer during pregnancy. Subsequent pregnancy does not seem to have a detrimental effect on prognosis.[352,354,356]

The use of chemotherapeutic agents in pregnant women is controversial. The effect of chemotherapy on the fetus is influenced by gestational age, the drugs used, and drug dosage. Schapira reviewed 71 patients treated with chemotherapeutic agents during the first trimester and found a 12.7% fetal malformation rate.[357] Another review found a low incidence of fetal malformations in women receiving antineoplastic drugs during pregnancy, although 40% of resulting offspring had low birth weights.[358] The decision to treat an individual patient with chemotherapy during pregnancy depends on the strength of the indication for treatment and the woman's desire to continue her pregnancy after being informed of the potential risks and benefits of treatment. In the third trimester, chemotherapy can usually be postponed until fetal maturity, when delivery can be induced.

LOCAL RECURRENCE AFTER MASTECTOMY OR CONSERVATIVE SURGERY AND RADIATION THERAPY

Local recurrence refers to the reappearance of breast cancer in the surgical or radiation field. The term local recurrence includes tumor in the chest wall, the overlying skin, residual breast tissue, ipsilateral axillary lymph nodes, supraclavicular nodes, or internal mammary lymph nodes. Local failure after mastectomy differs from local failure after conservative surgery in its time course, treatment, and prognosis.

The axillary node status is the best predictor of local recurrence after mastectomy. Local recurrences are seen in fewer than 10% of women with negative axillary nodes, but 12% to 27% of node-positive women fail locally.[136,169,359] The greater the number of involved axillary nodes, the higher is the risk of local failure. High local recurrence rates are also seen in women with locally advanced breast cancer treated with surgery alone. Sixty percent to 80% of local failures after mastectomy occur in the first 2 years after surgery, and failures are uncommon after 5 years.[136,360,361] The mechanism of local recurrence is uncertain. Although the number of involved axillary nodes is highly predictive of local failure, relapse in the axilla alone is uncommon. The chest wall and the overlying skin are the sole sites of local recurrence in more than 50% of patients.[360,361]

Approximately one third of patients with local recurrences after mastectomy have concurrent metastatic disease, and another 25% develop metastases shortly after the diagnosis of local failure.[361-363] The median survival for patients with isolated local recurrence is 2 to 3 years.[364] A review of patients treated for local recurrence at the JCRT revealed that only 7% were free of metastases at 10 years.[365]

Surgery and radiation therapy have been used as treatment modalities for local recurrence. Local excision is applicable only for patients with limited amounts of disease. Simple excision is a relatively poor way of maintaining long-term local control, with fewer than 30% of women treated by this method remaining free of further local relapses.[170,366,367] Radical chest wall resection has been employed for highly selected women with locally recurrent breast carcinoma. Local control has been achieved in approximately 90% of patients with this technique, and 5-year survivors are reported.[368,369] This may be secondary to the selection of women with long disease-free intervals and relatively limited disease for this procedure. Hospitalization ranges from 14 to 21 days, and operative mortality is less than 5%.

Radiation therapy has been employed more frequently than surgery in the management of local failure after mastectomy. Initial complete tumor regression is seen in most patients, with reported complete remission rates ranging from 63% to 97%.[365-367,370] Unfortunately, additional local relapses occur in 36% to 61% of women. The removal of all gross disease before radiation is associated with more favorable long-term local control rates in some series.[365]

The routine use of systemic therapy after local relapse remains controversial. Although it is recognized that most of these patients fail distantly, the optimal timing of systemic therapy is unknown.

Local failure after breast-conserving therapy is defined as recurrence in the breast parenchyma, skin of the breast, or nodal areas. About 95% of local recurrences involve the breast parenchyma alone, and most local recurrences occur at or near the primary tumor site.[371-374] However, as the interval from initial therapy to local recurrence increases, more recurrences are seen elsewhere in the breast, and these recurrences probably represent new primary tumors. Kurtz and associates, reviewing 178 local recurrences in 1593 patients, found that only 21% were distant from the primary tumor site, but 64% of recurrences seen after 10 years were in other quadrants of the breast.[374] Recht and coworkers observed that the hazard rate for local failure at or near the primary site increases over the first 2.5 postoperative years to a rate of 2% per year until year 5 and then decreases to about 0.5% per year by 8 years after treatment.[198] In contrast, the risk of failure elsewhere in the breast is about 1% per year at 5 years, with little change after further follow-up. The time course of local recurrence after breast-preserving therapy is much more protracted than that after mastectomy.

Approximately one third of breast recurrences are detected solely by mammography, one third by physical examination alone, and one third by both modalities.[375,376] Most recurrences are of the same histologic type as the primary cancer, although recurrences detected solely by mammography have a higher likelihood of being purely intraductal.[375,376]

Unlike local recurrence after mastectomy, distant metastases are rarely seen in conjunction with local recurrence after breast-preserving therapy. Ninety-five percent of recurrences are described as operable, and the main reason for unresectability is diffuse skin involvement (*i.e.*, inflammatory recurrence).[372,374] Total mastectomy has been the mainstay of surgical therapy. Five-year survival rates after salvage surgery for breast recurrence range from 48% to 84%.[373,374,377] If reconstruction is performed with salvage mastectomy, autogenous tissue should be used. A small experience with wide excision as a treatment for selected breast recurrences has been reported.[214,378] At a median follow-up of 5 years, 23% of patients had further local failure in the breast, suggesting that mastectomy is the treatment of choice. The role of systemic therapy after breast recurrence is controversial.

IN SITU CARCINOMA

In 1932, Broders defined carcinoma in situ as a condition in which malignant epithelial cells and their progeny are found in or bear positions occupied by their ancestors before the ancestors underwent malignant transformation. In the breast, carcinoma in situ has traditionally been categorized as lobular or ductal, depending on the cytologic features and the pattern of growth.

DUCTAL CARCINOMA IN SITU

DCIS (*i.e.*, noninfiltrating or intraductal carcinoma) is a proliferation of presumably malignant epithelial cells confined to the mammary ducts and lobules without demonstrable evidence of invasion through the basement membrane into the surrounding stroma. The management of ductal carcinoma in situ has become one of the most important and controversial topics in breast diseases. In this section, we review the available information about the incidence, diagnosis, pathologic and mammographic features, natural history, workup, and treatment options for patients with DCIS.

The incidence of DCIS has increased dramatically since approximately 1983. In the period between 1983 and 1985, the incidence of DCIS *doubled* for premenopausal and postmenopausal women. The reasons for this increase are not certain, but a major factor is believed to be the increased used of high-quality screening mammography combined with biopsy for suspicious lesions. However, the incidence of breast cancer has been increasing at about 1% per year for several decades before the use of screening mammography, and the incidence of breast cancer has increased approximately 2% per year since 1970 in women younger than 35 in whom screening mammography is rarely used. If the recent in-

creased incidence of DCIS is primarily due to earlier detection, the mortality due to breast cancer should decrease with time.

The clinical spectrum of DCIS is broad and includes lesions discovered incidentally during microscopic examination of breast tissue removed because of another abnormality (*e.g.*, fibroadenoma or an area of fibrocystic change); small foci detected by mammography; nipple discharge with or without an associated mass; localized, sometimes large, palpable tumors; and large areas of abnormality found on mammography. The frequency with which these various patterns of presentation are observed depends on the population under study. In series reported before the advent of screening mammography, most patients with DCIS presented with a palpable mass, nipple discharge, or both. With the use of mammographic screening, most in situ cancers are detected exclusively by mammography.

The most common mammographic abnormality associated with DCIS is clustered microcalcifications. The probability of finding malignant disease is related to the number of clustered microcalcifications, and with their appearance. Of particular concern are branching, irregularly shaped calcifications. However, mammographically detected calcifications, even if clustered, are not specific, and pathologic examination reveals carcinoma, most often DCIS, for only approximately 25% of patients for whom the mammogram shows suspicious calcifications. Less frequently, DCIS may have the mammographic appearance of a soft tissue mass with or without calcifications. In one series of 100 consecutive cases of DCIS seen at the Brigham and Women's Hospital and Dana-Farber Cancer Institute, 10% presented on mammography with only soft tissue abnormality and another 12% with soft tissue abnormality and microcalcifications.[379] The soft tissue abnormality was associated with gross involvement and dilation of ducts or lobules or periductal fibrosis on pathologic correlation of these lesions.

There are three histopathologic entities that can be confused with DCIS: atypical ductal hyperplasia, lobular carcinoma in situ, and ductal carcinoma in situ with minimal stromal invasion.

Atypical ductal hyperplasia is a nonmalignant intraductal epithelial proliferation closely resembling DCIS, although not completely fulfilling its histologic criteria. No special techniques are available that enable a clear and objective differentiation of the two lesions. Atypical ductal hyperplasia carries a risk of the development of a subsequent cancer and is believed to be the precursor of noncomedo DCIS.[69] In most cases, the distinction between DCIS and atypical ductal hyperplasia is obvious. In a few borderline lesions, particularly if small, differentiation may be difficult. In a recent study of concordance among a group of five experts in breast cancer pathology, little agreement was seen in the diagnosis of borderline lesions.[380]

Lobular carcinoma in situ is often difficult to differentiate from the solid type of the noncomedo subtype of DCIS. In some instances, both may be present in the same lesion, and it has been conjectured that this type of DCIS may be a manifestation of lobular carcinoma in situ in ductal structures.[381]

The ability to identify small clusters of tumor cells close to the intraductal foci as evidence of minimal stromal invasion may be difficult for several reasons. Sampling error may hamper the detection of microinvasion. DCIS may extend to involve adjacent lobular units and mimic the appearance of invasive cancer. In cases of DCIS with severe periductal fibrosis, a distorted small duct may be mistaken for invasion. Because of these difficulties and the clinical implication of diagnosing invasive cancer, most experts in breast pathology restrict the diagnosis of minimal stromal invasion to cases in which invasion is straightforward. Muscle-specific antibody to actin or one of the components of the basement membrane, which would be expected to be positive in the myoepithelial cells around in situ lesions and lacking in the invasive foci, may help in this differential diagnosis, but is not used in routine cases.[382]

DCIS is heterogeneous in terms of its histopathologic growth pattern, cell type, extent, and biologic behavior. Based on the growth pattern and cell type (*e.g.*, cribriform, micropapillary, clinging, solid), DCIS can be classified into comedo and noncomedo subtypes, and there may be a combination of these types. The comedo type is characterized by nuclear polymorphism, numerous mitoses, and significant necrosis. The noncomedo subtype is characterized by monomorphic nuclei, few or no mitoses, and the absence of significant necrosis. Many investigators believe that it is useful to divide DCIS into the comedo and noncomedo types, because the comedo type appears more malignant cytologically, has a higher proliferative rate as determined by thymidine-labeling studies, more frequently expresses the *ERBB2* oncogene, and is more likely to be associated with areas of microinvasion than the other types.[383,384] The mammographic presentation of the two types of DCIS is different.[211] The comedo type is associated with the so-called casting (*i.e.*, linear) or coarse granular microcalcifications that usually develop in the necrotic debris of the tumor. The noncomedo type is associated with the fine granular microcalcifications that appear to develop in the secretion produced by the lesion. In most cases, the mammographic detection of the comedo DCIS is straightforward, because few benign lesions have a similar type and pattern of microcalcifications. Benign lesions often have microcalcifications similar to those of the noncomedo DCIS. There is a difference in the reliability of mammography in predicting the histologically assessed size of the two types of DCIS. Mammographic estimates of the comedo type closely approximate the histologic size of the tumor, and the estimates of size of the noncomedo type based on the extent of microcalcifications may be considerably smaller than the histologic size.[211] The distinction between the comedo and noncomedo subtypes is limited by the lack of a clear and reproducible definition, the fact that many lesions contain both subtypes, and the lack of a clear association between subtype and clinical behavior.

DCIS has been considered by some to be a multicentric process with separate areas of involved ducts. This concept is based on studies using the standard pathologic examination of surgical biopsies and subsequent mastectomy specimens. Residual tumor foci in the latter were considered as separate foci and therefore evidence of multicentricity. However, in a study using a correlated radiologic-pathologic technique in combination with a subgross sectioning and extensive sampling of a series of 82 mastectomies harboring DCIS, only one was found to have a multicentric distribution.[211] The tumor foci are more likely to be evenly distributed within a given region (typically corresponding to a breast segment) without intervening areas of uninvolved breast tissue. This concept is supported by clinical data showing that local tumor recurrence after breast-conserving treatment of DCIS typically appears in the vicinity of the biopsy site. The finding that most DCIS has a unicentric distribution is important in allowing the possibility of a complete resection of the lesion and implies that the extent of the lesion is the main factor influencing the feasibility of breast-conserving treatment.

Reports on the size distribution of DCIS are conflicting. In a series of 115 patients, Lagios and colleagues reported 52% of patients to have tumors that were 25 mm or smaller.[385] In this series, 79 patients with mammographically detected DCIS with a reported average size of 7 mm were treated by excision alone. The resection margins were carefully assessed for completeness and considered negative. In the series of Silverstein and associates, only about 20% of lesions were smaller than 2 cm.[386] In about half of the patients with small lesions who were selected for breast-conserving treatment, the margins of the initial biopsy were considered involved, suggesting that the extent of the lesion was even larger than originally assessed. In the series reported by Holland, only 15% of the DCIS lesions were smaller than 2 cm and 51% were larger than 5 cm.[211] The size distribution was not affected by the mode of detection, with a similar distribution found for tumors detected by mammography and by clinical examination. Sixty-six percent of the lesions were confined to one breast quadrant, 23% extended over more than one quadrant, and 11% were centrally located. There was a 52% rate of occult involvement in the nipple-subareolar region. For many cases of DCIS, adequate resection requires wide excision and may be feasible in only a few patients.

The chief issue in treating DCIS is its risk of progression to invasive cancer. The available information on this subject is extremely limited, because most patients with DCIS have been treated by mastectomy. The only long-term studies to address this issue are those in which patients with DCIS were inadvertently treated by biopsy alone. Two studies have identified patients with DCIS during histologic review of biopsies originally categorized as benign. However, in both of these studies, a complete excision of the lesion was not attempted and the status of the resection margins was unknown. In one of these studies, Page and coworkers found subsequent invasive carcinoma in the ipsilateral breast in 7 (28%) of 25 patients at intervals of 3 to 10 years (mean, 6.1 years) after the initial biopsy.[387] All seven invasive cancers occurred in the vicinity of the original biopsy. In the other study by Rosen and colleagues, 8 (53%) of 15 patients with follow-up data or 8 (27%) of 30 total patients subsequently developed an invasive carcinoma in the same breast an average of 9.7 years after the initial biopsy showing DCIS.[388] In most of these patients, the invasive tumor occurred at or near the original biopsy site. In both series, the cases of DCIS were all micropapillary or cribriform (noncomedo) types. These studies suggest that some patients with noncomedo DCIS treated by biopsy alone develop invasive cancer in the ipsilateral breast, usually in the region of the initial lesion. The invasive carcinoma commonly occurs a long time after the initial biopsy.

Insight into the biologic significance of DCIS can be obtained from studies that indicate that foci of DCIS are frequently detected in the contralateral breast of women with invasive breast cancer. However, there is a discrepancy between this incidence of contralateral DCIS and the risk of developing a subsequent, clinically evident, opposite breast cancer. Alpers and Wellings found DCIS in 48% of breasts contralateral to cancer-containing breasts, yet the cumulative 20-year risk of opposite breast cancer in patients with an ipsilateral breast cancer is only about 10%.[389] These data suggest that not all examples of histologically detectable DCIS progress to clinically significant cancers.

It may be possible to discern the biologic significance of DCIS based on its frequency in autopsy series. Unfortunately, there are few studies, because routine systematic examination of breast tissue at autopsy is not performed, and the available studies are not consistent. Alpers and Wellings reported 185 randomly selected breasts from autopsies in 101 patients.[389] Each breast was examined in toto by a subgross sampling technique. Of these 185 breasts, one or more foci of DCIS were found in 11 (6%). The average number of foci per involved breast was 1.5. The likelihood of finding DCIS was not directly related to age. DCIS was found in 3 (5%) of 56 patients 49 years of age or younger, in 7 (10%) of 70 patients between the ages of 50 and 69, and in 1 of 59 patients older than 70. Bartow and associates studied the breasts from autopsies of 519 female patients who were 14 years or older.[390] All breasts were studied by examination in toto by subgross sampling technique. Only 1 (0.2%) patient (40 years old) was found to have DCIS, and 5 patients were found to have invasive cancers. These studies from the United States indicate that DCIS is uncommonly found on routine autopsy which suggests that the presence of DCIS is of potential significance. A study from Denmark reported by Anderson and coworkers suggested a higher incidence of DCIS in autopsies.[381] They examined 83 patients and found DCIS (with or without lobular carcinoma in situ [LCIS]) in 11 (13%). It is possible that variations in diagnostic criteria may account for these differences.

It is not possible by routine pathologic examination to differentiate examples of DCIS that are likely to progress to invasive cancer from lesions that are biologically innocuous. The various histologic subtypes may have different likelihoods of progression to invasive disease, but the differences are incompletely understood, because most clinical series have not differentiated subtypes in reporting outcome. It is possible

that recently developed techniques for studying oncogenes and their products, growth factors, and markers of cell proliferation and DNA content may ultimately determine the effects of the types of DCIS. In one study of 69 patients with DCIS treated by excision, only 1 of 31 diploid noncomedo lesions recurred, compared with about 40% of the other 38 lesions ($p < 0.05$).[391]

The results of treatment with mastectomy indicate that about 99% of patients with DCIS are cured.[386,392] However, patients with an initial biopsy that showed DCIS but who later had invasive cancer in the mastectomy specimen were generally excluded from the series. In the study by Silverstein and colleagues of 75 patients with DCIS (average tumor size of 4.1 cm) treated by mastectomy, 51 (68%) had residual disease at the time of mastectomy, including 10 (13%) with microinvasive disease.[386] For this reason, it may be difficult to compare outcome after mastectomy with outcome in series of patients treated by breast-conserving approaches.

The results of the use of excision alone for DCIS (listed in ascending order of follow-up time) are given in Table 40–18.[393-398] Local recurrence rates after excision alone tend to increase with time of follow-up; in those studies with longer follow-up, the local recurrence rates are close to 50%. This most likely reflects the propensity of this lesion for late recurrences, although it is possible that patients in the series with longer follow-up had less adequate excisions. Approximately half of local recurrences contain invasive cancer. Although these recurrences have generally been detected at an early stage, the salvage of patients with these recurrences as determined by 5- and 10-year relapse-free and overall survival rates has not yet been established.

Results of the use of excision combined with breast irradiation are given in Table 40–19.[396,399-404] Local recurrence rates after excision and breast irradiation appear to be lower than those after excision alone (by at least 50%), although the results in some of the series are less favorable than in others, and as in the studies using excision alone, approximately half of local recurrences contain invasive cancer.[399,402] Only short-term information is available about the salvage of recurrences after excision combined with breast irradiation.

Several trials comparing excision with and without breast

TABLE 40-18. Results of Treatment With Excision Alone for Ductal Carcinoma In Situ

Investigations	No. of Patients	Median Follow-up (mo)	Percent With Recurrence	No. With Invasion
Carpenter, 1979–86[393]	28	38*	18	1/5
Arnesson, 1978–84[394]	38	60	13	2/5
Lagios, 1972–87[395]	79	68	13	5/10
Fisher, 1976–84[396]	22	85*	43	5/9
Graham, 1969–88[397]	53	97	38	7/14
Gallagher, 1944–81[398]	13	100	38	3/5
Price, 1972–82[572]	35	108	63	12/22
Total				35/70 (50%)

* Mean follow-up (mo).

TABLE 40-19. Results of Excision Combined With Radiation Therapy for Ductal Carcinoma In Situ

Investigations	No. of Patients	Median Follow-up (mo)	Percent With Recurrence	No. With Invasion
McCormick, 1977–88[399]	54	35	18%	3/10
Kurtz, 1975–85[400]	44	61	7%	3/3
Solin, 1978–85[401]	51	68	10%	2/5
Bornstein, 1976–85[402]	38	81	21%	5/8
Fisher, 1976–84[396]	29	85	7%	1/2
Stotter, 1958–87[403]	42	92	9%	4/4
Fourquet, 1967–85[404]	67	104	10%	5/7
Total				25/42 (60%)

irradiation for patients with DCIS have been undertaken, but published results from these trials are not yet available. There were a few patients with DCIS inadvertently entered onto the NSABP trial B-06, suggesting that irradiation is useful in avoiding recurrence, but this number is too small to provide meaningful conclusions (see Fisher in Tables 40–18 and 40–19).[396] There are no firm guidelines for the use of irradiation after breast-conserving surgery for DCIS. Breast irradiation is commonly recommended in patients electing breast conservation if the lesion is greater than 1 to 2 cm or if the lesion approaches the margins of resection.

Careful mammographic and pathologic evaluations are essential for patients with DCIS considered for breast-conserving treatment. A careful mammographic evaluation consists of the standard mammographic views, but it is extended by magnification views for better evaluation of the form, distribution, and extent of the microcalcifications. The area between the lesion and the nipple should receive special attention. Larger lesions should preferably be localized at their margins using two hook-wires to ensure an adequate excision. A postoperative mammogram may be required to confirm the completeness of resection if there is any doubt based on review of the specimen mammogram. A careful pathologic evaluation requires a proper orientation of the specimen. The surgeon should label the specimen at two points: for example, at the closest point to the nipple and at 12 o'clock. The entire surface of the specimen should be inked to facilitate recognition of the surgical edges on microscopy. Radiographs should be obtained of the specimen while it is intact to permit comparison of the lesion with that of the preoperative mammograms and again after sectioning at 4- to 5-mm intervals to allow recognition of the exact site of the microcalcifications.

Generous sampling of the area of microcalcifications and the margins is recommended to facilitate the detection of possible microinvasion and the assessment of the margins. Adequate orientation and sampling of the specimen are essential to assess the extent of the lesion and the adequacy of the resection. A portion of the lesion should *not* be sent for biochemical assay of hormone receptors or other assays, because of the concern that the portion sent might contain an undiagnosed area of invasive cancer. A recent consensus committee on DCIS recommended that the following should be described routinely: tumor size; margin involvement; nuclear features including size, pleomorphism, and mitoses; necrosis; and architecture.[405] It is useful for the pathology report to include a statement about the type of the microcalcifications and their relation to the malignant ducts.

The histologic evaluation of the surgical margins is considered an important part of the assessment in any patient being considered for breast-conserving treatment. Unfortunately, there is no established definition of what constitutes a negative margin. The minimal definition of an negative margin is the absence of foci of DCIS at the surgical edge. It is not known if a certain distance is required between any foci of DCIS and the margin to be certain about the adequacy of the resection. It has been suggested that a negative margin should include uninvolved glandular structures beyond the lesion at the margin of the specimen.[405a]

With the increased risk for local recurrence with breast-conserving treatment, the frequency of invasive cancer in these recurrences, and the uncertain effectiveness of salvage for recurrence, mastectomy is viewed as the safest option. This is always true for a patient with a locally extensive lesion. The greater difficulty arises in treating a patient with an apparently localized lesion that has been adequately resected and for whom breast conservation is an important issue. It is useful to attempt to estimate for the patient the degree of risk associated with breast conservation. With the information currently available and after a careful mammographic and pathologic assessment, breast conservation may be associated with a 15% to 20% risk of a recurrence over a 10-year period. Because approximately half of these contain invasive cancer, there is a 7% to 10% risk of an invasive cancer over a 10-year period. If approximately 50% of invasive cancers can be cured, the breast cancer mortality associated with breast conservation is in the range of 3% to 5%. (These estimates are given to illustrate the level of risk and may need to be modified as additional information is obtained.) Patients show a wide variety of reactions to a discussion of these estimates of risk. For some patients, this level of risk is unacceptable, but for others, it is viewed as a reasonable risk to assume to avoid breast amputation.

Is it reasonable to allow a patient to assume this level of risk? There is not a consistent policy of prophylactic mastectomy for high-risk patients. Because DCIS is, strictly speaking, not a cancer, it is of interest to view the policy for DCIS in relation to the policy for other high-risk conditions. The risk of developing an invasive breast cancer over a 10-year period for a 50-year-old woman in the United States is approximately 1.8%. For a 50-year-old woman identified as high risk on the basis of family history, hormonal and reproductive factors, or a prior breast biopsy revealing atypical epithelial hyperplasia, the risk is in the range of 2% to 10% or even greater. For a woman with a diagnosis of lobular carcinoma in situ (discussed later), the risk is approximately 1% per year or 10% over a 10-year period. Prophylactic mastectomy is not routinely recommended for patients with these high-risk conditions. The 10-year risk of an invasive cancer for a woman with DCIS is in the range of 7% to 10% or similar to that for other high-risk conditions for which prophylactic mastectomy is not recommended. Based on all these considerations, the option of breast conservation is reasonable assuming that the lesion is apparently localized, has been adequately resected, and that the patient comprehends and accepts the risk assumed by breast-conserving treatment.

DCIS represents a challenge and an opportunity for the 1990s. Because DCIS probably represents breast cancer at its earliest stage, it is an opportunity to identify the earliest genetic abnormalities associated with the disease. It is important to determine whether the real incidence of the lesion is increasing and what factors (*e.g.*, dietary and hormonal) may be responsible for this. The identification of markers for progression to invasive breast cancer would greatly improve the management of patients with DCIS. Given the importance of breast conservation for many women, it is important to develop rules for the successful use of breast-conserving treatment. Clinical trials currently in progress may help to define guidelines for the use of breast irradiation. It may be useful to consider some patients with DCIS (especially those with the noncomedo type) as being at high risk for invasive cancer and candidates for trials testing the value of prevention (*e.g.*, tamoxifen). The use of tamoxifen is being tested in the current NSABP trial for DCIS in which patients are randomized after excision and irradiation.

LOBULAR CARCINOMA IN SITU

In 1941, Foote and Stewart described a noninvasive form of mammary carcinoma arising from the lobules and terminal ducts that they called lobular carcinoma in situ (LCIS).[406] Their initial report included three important features of LCIS. The lesion is an incidental microscopic finding that cannot be identified clinically or by gross pathologic examination, invasive cancers that develop after LCIS may be infiltrating ductal or infiltrating lobular tumors, and the lesion is multifocal in the breast. These observations led Foote and Stewart to conclude that simple mastectomy was the appropriate treatment for LCIS. Additional information about LCIS has been accrued since the report of Foote and Stewart, but the appropriate clinical management of this lesion remains controversial.

The true incidence of LCIS in the general population is unknown because it lacks clinical or mammographic signs. LCIS is found in from 0.8% to 8.0% of breast biopsies.[407–409] In all reports, LCIS is more frequent in premenopausal women, with a mean age of 44 years in one series of 98 patients.[408–410] This age distribution may reflect the fact that the benign breast abnormalities that require biopsy are primarily seen in premenopausal women. The frequency with which LCIS is diagnosed appears to be increasing, with a 15% rise in the number of cases seen from 1973 to 1988 reported in one series.[411] This increase in the incidence of LCIS may be due to the increased number of breast biopsies done for mammographic abnormalities. Although LCIS lacks mammographic signs, it accounted for 14% of mammographically detected cancers in one large series.[412,413]

The major issue in the management of LCIS is whether the LCIS is a premalignant lesion or a marker of increased risk for the development of breast carcinoma. Support for the idea that LCIS is a premalignant lesion came from the report of McDivitt and associates,[414] which was subsequently updated by Rosen.[415] Of 40 women with LCIS treated with biopsy alone, a cumulative risk of ipsilateral breast cancer of 10% at 5 years, 15% at 10 years, and 30% at 15 years was found. The risk of contralateral breast cancer was 15% at 15 years. Rosen and coworkers found a similar degree of risk that continued to increase with the length of follow-up through 24 years.[415] Rosen recommended ipsilateral mastectomy with a large contralateral biopsy as the appropriate treatment for LCIS. However, a significant body of data supports the idea that LCIS is a marker of increased risk for the development of cancer in either breast rather than a precancerous lesion.[408,410,416] Anderson found a 19.5% incidence of ipsilateral breast cancer and an 8.5% incidence of contralateral carcinoma in 52 women followed after a biopsy demonstrating LCIS.[417] Haagensen followed 211 women and found a 17% incidence of invasive carcinoma that was equally distributed between the index breast and the contralateral breast.[410] In a review of 228 published cases of LCIS treated by biopsy alone, 15.5% developed invasive carcinoma of the ipsilateral breast and 9.3% had a contralateral carcinoma.[416]

It appears that most women with LCIS do not develop breast cancer, and the risk of breast cancer development is approximately equal in both breasts. Treatment strategies addressing one breast, such as unilateral mastectomy with contralateral biopsy, appear to be illogical, because the risk of LCIS is bilateral regardless of the findings of the contralateral biopsy. One treatment option for the woman with LCIS is careful observation, as would be carried out for any woman known to be at increased risk for the development of breast cancer due to a positive family history or prior history of breast cancer. In women unwilling to accept the 20% to 30% risk of the development of breast cancer associated with this policy, bilateral simple mastectomy, usually with immediate breast reconstruction, is another therapeutic option. Radiation therapy has no role in the management of LCIS. It is unnecessary to obtain histologically negative margins in women who will be followed expectantly, because LCIS is known to be a diffuse lesion. If observation is elected, it must last for the patient's lifetime, because the increased risk of breast cancer persists indefinitely.[415] Efforts to identify features of LCIS associated with a higher likelihood of the development of malignancy have been largely unsuccessful. Haagensen found that the ratio of observed to expected cases of breast cancer increased from 5.7 for women with LCIS alone to 8.5 in women with a positive family history and LCIS.[418] Histologic features, including the amount of LCIS, have not predicted the subsequent development of invasive carcinoma.[415]

SYSTEMIC ADJUVANT THERAPY

SCIENTIFIC BACKGROUND

Many of the experimental foundations of systemic adjuvant therapy were derived from laboratory studies performed more than 25 years ago by investigators in North America, and these are summarized in Table 40–20.[304,419–423] This evidence indicated that the lymphatic and blood vascular systems were so interrelated that it was impractical to consider them as independent routes of neoplastic cell dissemination. This meant that the regional lymph nodes were of prognostic, rather than anatomic, importance in cancer survival. This provided a basis on which an alternative hypothesis (*i.e.*, biologic, rather than the anatomic and mechanistic one proposed by Halsted) could be formulated. Observations on the survival of mice with transplantable solid tumors of various sizes subjected to resection revealed that the surgical cure rates correlated with tumor size, although there was great variability in survival and the metastatic tumor burden at the time of surgery among the animals. There were breakpoints in the survival curves, after which time no further recurrences were found. These breakpoints appeared at similar times after surgery, although the percentage of survival in the various groups was different. This observation suggested that the biology of the tumor was similar in the various animals but that the extent of the tumor cell burden determined the cure rates. A corollary to this observation is that definitive conclusions about curative effects of any treatment must be withheld until this breakpoint is reached.

Empiric and practical considerations were used in the selection of chemotherapeutic agents, the treatment schedule, and the duration of treatment. The selection of drugs and the treatment schedule (typically given in cycles) must achieve a net reduction in the cell burden by the time to deliver the next cycle, and the optimal treatment intensity must be at least as intense as that which yields the optimal results in advanced disease. In mice bearing mammary tumors, survival was invariably superior after a combination of drugs compared

TABLE 40-20. Laboratory Findings, Clinical Observations, and Biologic Hypotheses Influencing the Beginning of Modern Adjuvant Chemotherapy for High-Risk Operable Breast Cancer

- By the time cancer becomes clinically detectable, it is advanced (about 30 doublings) and has had ample opportunity to establish distant micrometastases.
- There is no orderly pattern of tumor cell dissemination, and the blood stream is of considerable importance in tumor spread.
- The likelihood of metastatic disease is directly related to the size of the tumor mass; surgical "cure" rates drop as tumor volume at surgery increases.
- Tumor growth fraction is inversely related to population size.
- In homogenous tumor cell populations, effective drug kill follows first-order reaction kinetics.
- The use of a combination of drugs is superior to the use of a single agent and can eradicate 10 to 100 times as many cells.
- In transplantable tumors, surgical adjuvant chemotherapy increases the long-term cure rates.
- The optimal kinetic conditions to achieve cure exist if microscopic foci of disease are present after curative surgery and/or radiation therapy.
- The efficacy of chemotherapy is dose dependent, related to the tumor cell burden at the time of drug treatment and to the presence of primary resistant tumor cells.
- Operable breast cancer is often a systemic disease and variations in local-regional therapy are unlikely to substantially affect survival. Only by control of distant disease can there be an improvement in the outcome of breast cancer patients.

with single-agent chemotherapy. The animal models showed that the emergence of drug resistance increases with the extent of the disease and that this constitutes a major element in the failure of adjuvant therapy. The experimental systems demonstrated that surgery followed by adjuvant chemotherapy yielded superior survival results to either modality alone.

It was the evaluation of two surgical trials that challenged the principles of the Halstedian hypothesis and supported the laboratory investigations.[136,138] The high recurrence rate, especially during the first 3 years after the Halsted radical and extended radical mastectomy, could have only one reasonable explanation: micrometastases may exist at the time of surgery, and they are unaffected by local treatment. This observation helped to challenge the old anatomic and mechanistic dogma, opened the pathway to biologic hypotheses, and paved the way for breast-conserving treatment and adjuvant chemotherapy. During the mid-1970s, hormones began to receive renewed attention as potential adjuvant treatments.[424] In a carcinogen-induced mammary tumor model in rats, it was demonstrated that the antiestrogen compound, tamoxifen, could delay the appearance of tumors and decrease their overall frequency. This was of great interest because of its relevance in the adjuvant treatment of breast cancer and because of its possible inhibition of a carcinogenic process.

ADJUVANT CHEMOTHERAPY

The first randomized trials based on the modern concepts of adjuvant chemotherapy were performed by the NSABP and by the National Cancer Institute of Italy, using patients with positive axillary nodes.[425,426] The first NSABP study used single-agent chemotherapy (melphalan or L-phenylalanine mustard [L-PAM]), and the Milan trial used a multidrug regimen that included cyclophosphamide, methotrexate, and fluorouracil (CMF). Eventually, the strategy of using combination chemotherapy proved superior in the adjuvant situation as it had in animals, and it became the standard approach. The long-term results of these trials established the effectiveness of adjuvant chemotherapy in node-positive breast cancer and provided evidence or confirmation of important biologic and pharmacologic concepts: the prognostic importance of the tumor burden in the ipsilateral axilla, the dose-response relation for adjuvant chemotherapy, and the clinical relevance of drug resistance.[286,427]

Long-term results are now available from the initial Milan trial.[304] Figure 40–11 displays the 15-year results of CMF administered for 12 monthly cycles starting within 4 weeks after surgery and compared with a no-treatment control group. The benefit of adjuvant chemotherapy occurred during the first 3 years after radical mastectomy, and the difference between controls and CMF patients remained about the same for the subsequent 12 years. This observation suggests that early findings can predict the late outcome with sufficient accuracy and that, in some patients, micrometastases include aggressive tumor clones that are resistant to chemotherapy. The results of the CMF trial confirmed the prognostic importance of the extent of nodal involvement in the axilla; there was a consistent inverse relation between the number of histologically involved lymph nodes and the treatment outcome (Table 40–21). In the first CMF trial, the significant survival benefit observed in premenopausal women (Fig. 40–

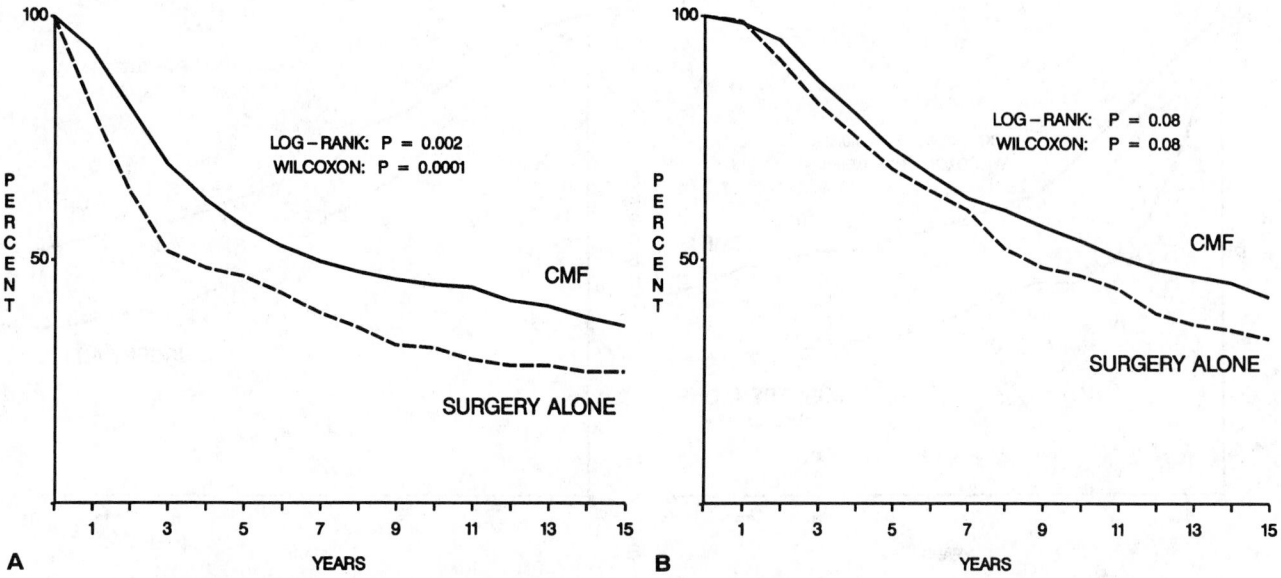

FIGURE 40–11. First Milan trial comparing adjuvant cyclophosphamide, methotrexate, and 5-fluorouracil (CMF) with surgery alone (control). 15-year results. **(A)** Comparative relapse-free survival. **(B)** Comparative total survival. (Bonadonna G. Evolving concepts in the systemic adjuvant treatment of breast cancer. Cancer Res 1992;52[8]:2127–2137)

12) was not duplicated in postmenopausal patients. However, as a consequence of trial design and protocol deviations, the drug doses employed in postmenopausal patients were initially low and were often arbitrarily further reduced during most cycles.[427,428]

The second CMF adjuvant program attempted to determine whether six cycles of combination chemotherapy was as effective as 12 cycles.[286,304,427] After 14 years, relapse-free (Fig. 40–13) and total survival rates are equal in the two treatment groups. In this trial in which full doses of drug were frequently used, there was equal benefit for premenopausal and postmenopausal patients. Comparable findings with the same theoretical and practical considerations were recently reported

TABLE 40-21. Fifteen-Year Results of the First CMF Program Carried Out at the Milan Cancer Institute

Patient Group	Control (%)	CMF (%)	p
Relapse-Free Survival			
All patients	26	36	0.002
Premenopausal	28	42	0.002
Postmenopausal	25	31	0.22
1–3 nodes positive	31	42	0.009
>3 nodes positive	15	24	0.05
Total Survival			
All patients	33	42	0.08
Premenopausal	35	51	0.02
Postmenopausal	32	35	0.85
1–3 nodes positive	37	48	0.08
>3 nodes positive	24	31	0.31

by the Dana-Farber Cancer Institute[429] and the NSABP group[430] using doxorubicin-containing regimens. Although the optimal treatment duration has not been firmly established, six cycles of full-dose CMF or one of the other effective poly-drug regimens (Table 40–22) are currently recommended in the adjuvant treatment of node-positive breast cancer if given outside the context of a clinical trial. Although other effective polydrug regimens are delivered in various centers of the world, those reported in the table have been exhaustively tested through large prospective trials and found to be reproducible in terms of benefit and toxicity. If chemotherapy is indicated, these regimens can be administered in an adjuvant situation as primary (neoadjuvant) treatment or in the management of locally advanced or clinically metastatic disease.

The first CMF schedule is the so-called standard regimen and includes oral cyclophosphamide. Whether the addition of prednisone improves treatment outcome remains unsettled. The schedules with intravenous cyclophosphamide were devised at the Milan Cancer Institute to improve patients' compliance. Although the intravenous administration on days 1 and 8 of all three drugs provides a greater dose intensity, a recent trial of administration every 3 weeks in women with one to three positive nodes indicated that the 5-year results are equivalent to those achieved with standard CMF.[431] In clinical practice, the well-known CMFVP (cyclophosphamide, methotrexate, fluorouracil, vincristine, prednisone) regimen has been used less frequently during the past few years because of severe myelosuppression and neurotoxicity without clear-cut evidence of a superior long-term benefit. Other drug regimens, including cisplatin, paraplatin, mitomycin C, mitoxantrone, vinorelbine (Navelbine), taxol, growth factor-supported, high-dose chemotherapy with or without autologous bone marrow or cryopreserved circulating hematopoietic progenitor cells, are effective, but they are still considered experimental.

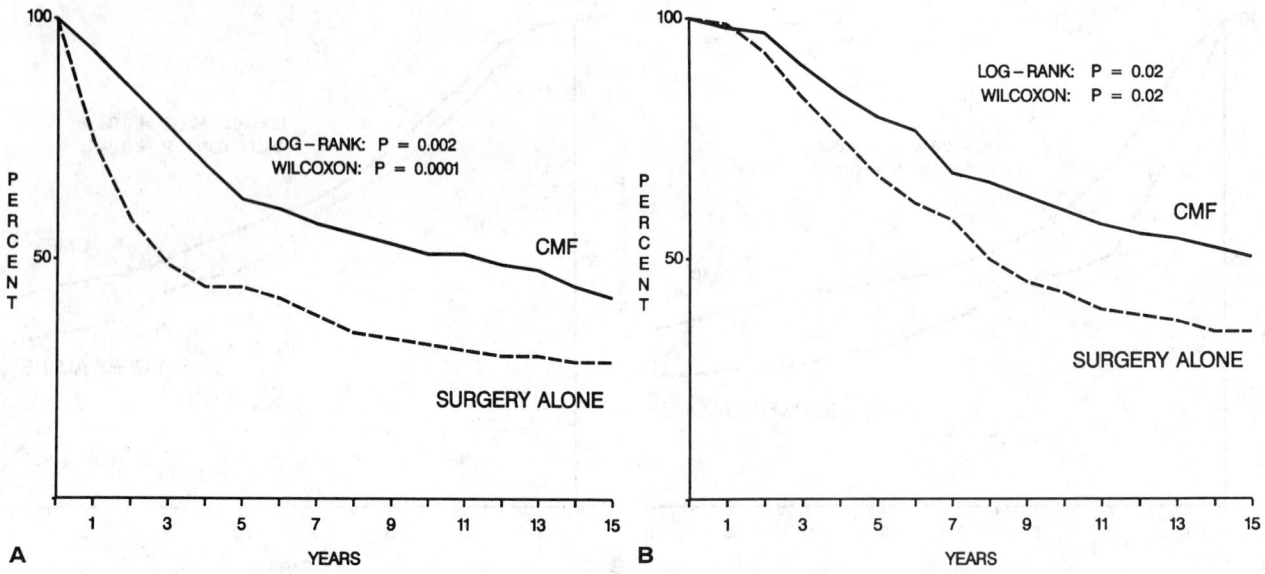

FIGURE 40–12.   First Milan trial comparing adjuvant chemotherapy (CMF) with surgery alone (control): 15-year results in premenopausal women. **(A)** Comparative relapse-free survival. **(B)** Comparative total survival. (Bonadonna G. Evolving concepts in the systemic adjuvant treatment of breast cancer. Cancer Res 1992;52[8]:2127–2137)

DOXORUBICIN COMBINATIONS

Twenty years after its first reported clinical use, the anthracycline doxorubicin remains the single most effective drug in the treatment of advanced breast cancer.[432] Combination chemotherapy regimens that include doxorubicin or its analog epirubicin have repeatedly been shown to induce a higher response rate in patients with locally advanced or clinically disseminated breast carcinoma than regimens that do not contain an anthracycline. However, the median duration of response and survival have not been unquestionably superior using an anthracycline. The initial reluctance to include

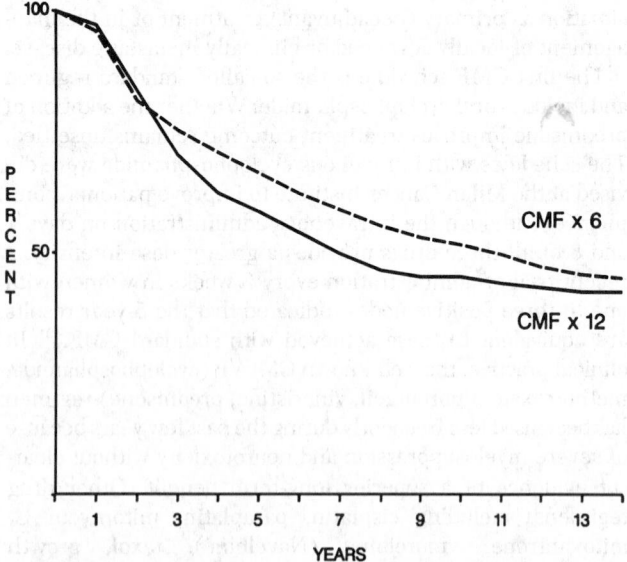

FIGURE 40–13.   Second Milan trial comparing adjuvant chemotherapy (CMF) for 6 and 12 cycles: comparative relapse-free survival at 14 years. (Bonadonna G. Evolving concepts in the systemic adjuvant treatment of breast cancer. Cancer Res 1992;52[8]:2127–2137)

doxorubicin in an adjuvant situation was due to its potential for myocardial damage after prolonged treatment.

The M.D. Anderson Cancer Center and the University of Arizona tested the potential efficacy of adjuvant doxorubicin in nonrandomized studies but did not document a clear superiority for doxorubicin-containing regimens over CMF or CMFP.[433,434] After it became clear that adjuvant chemotherapy could be limited to about 6 months, randomized trials with doxorubicin-containing regimens were started in Europe and in the United States.[286,305,427,429–431,435] Possibly due to the low dose (30 mg/m² every 3 weeks) of doxorubicin administered in combination with PF (L-PAM and fluorouracil) by the NSABP group, patients treated with this anthracycline showed only a marginal advantage at 5 years compared with patients given PF alone and similar outcome if adjuvant tamoxifen was added to both drug combinations.[435] In a subsequent NSABP trial (B-15) consisting of tamoxifen-nonresponsive tumors, node-positive patients were randomized to one of three arms: doxorubicin (60 mg/m²) plus cyclophosphamide (600 mg/m²) given every 3 weeks for four cycles (AC regimen); AC followed 6 months later by three monthly cycles of a slightly modified intravenous CMF; or standard CMF for six monthly cycles. The 3-year results did not reveal any significant difference in outcome among the three arms; the relapse-free survival rate was 62% for AC; 68% for AC followed by CMF; and 63% for CMF. The investigators concluded that AC chemotherapy should be preferred to CMF because of the shorter treatment duration and lesser toxicity.[430] In node-positive patients with a median of seven positive nodes treated at the Dana-Farber Cancer Institute, 15 and 30 weeks of the AC regimen consisting of doxorubicin (45 mg/m²) plus cyclophosphamide (500 mg/m²) given intravenously every 3 weeks were compared. At the 8-year analysis, the disease-free survival rate was comparable in the two arms, indicating that there was no significant advantage for the use of longer durations of AC.[429]

TABLE 40-22. Effective Combination Chemotherapy Regimens Commonly Used to Treat Breast Cancer

Regimen	Dose (mg/m²)	Route	Day(s) of Treatment	Recycle
CMF (P)				
Cyclophosphamide	100	PO	1 to 14	
Methotrexate	40 (60)	I.V.	1 and 8	4 wk
Fluorouracil	600 (700)	I.V.	1 and 8	
Prednisone	(40)	(PO)	(1 to 14)	
CMF				
Cyclophosphamide	600	I.V.	1	
Methotrexate	40	I.V.	1	3 wk
Fluorouracil	600	I.V.	1	
CMF				
Cyclophosphamide	600	I.V.	1 and 8	
Methotrexate	40	I.V.	1 and 8	4 wk
Fluorouracil	600	I.V.	1 and 8	
CA				
Cyclophosphamide	200	PO	3 to 6	3–4 wk
Doxorubicin	40	I.V.	1	
AC				
Doxorubicin	45	I.V.	1	3 wk
Cyclophosphamide	500	I.V.	1	
FAC				
Fluorouracil	500	I.V.	1 and 8	
Doxorubicin	50	I.V.	1	4 wk
Cyclophosphamide	500	I.V.	1	

Recent results on the use of adjuvant doxorubicin are available from the Milan Cancer Institute.[304,305,431] Patients with one to three positive nodes were randomized to receive 12 courses of intravenous CMF every 3 weeks (see Table 40–22) or intravenous CMF for eight courses followed by four courses of doxorubicin (75 mg/m²) given every 3 weeks. The 5-year results did not show improved outcome with the use of doxorubicin compared with CMF alone (relapse-free survival rates: 72% versus 74%). In another trial involving patients with more than three positive nodes, sequential administration of doxorubicin (as previously described) followed by eight courses of CMF (as described) yielded significantly improved treatment outcome at 5 years (relapse-free survival rates: 61% versus 38%) in both menopausal groups compared with the alternating administration of the same drug regimens. The superiority of the sequential to the alternating chemotherapy is still observed at the 6-year analysis in this subset of patients (Fig. 40–14).[304] These findings suggest that the use of doxorubicin and this scheduling are responsible for this improved outcome. If the Milan data with doxorubicin followed by CMF are confirmed by other research groups, this sequence (*i.e.*, four cycles of doxorubicin followed by four cycles of intravenous CMF on days 1 and 8; see Table 40–22) could replace CMF as the standard adjuvant treatment in patients with node-positive breast cancer, regardless of menopausal status.

PERIOPERATIVE CHEMOTHERAPY

Perioperative chemotherapy refers to the administration of a single course of chemotherapy (single agent or drug combination) within a few days after surgery. Studies testing the value of a single dose of perioperative chemotherapy in node-positive and node-negative breast cancer patients have not shown any consistent benefit. The Ludwig Trial V, testing the value of a single cycle of chemotherapy given perioperatively, included a total of 2504 evaluable patients. In 1229 node-positive patients, the study demonstrated that one course of CMF was inferior to the same perioperative chemotherapy followed by six monthly cycles of standard adjuvant combination chemotherapy or standard combination chemotherapy without perioperative treatment.[436] In 1275 node-negative patients, the use of perioperative CMF was associated with a marginal benefit at 5 years compared with no treatment (74% versus 68% for controls).[437] This benefit was significant in ER-negative tumors, particularly in the postmenopausal subset (79% for CMF, 56% for controls).

Investigators at the Cancer Institute in Genoa designed a study protocol using randomization to one course of CEF (cyclophosphamide, epidoxorubicin, and fluorouracil) or to no perioperative treatment.[438] Node-negative patients did not receive further therapy, and node-positive women were given CEF alternating with CMF for a total of 12 cycles given every 3 weeks. This trial, which included 467 patients, failed to reveal any significant difference in treatment outcome at 5 years. The findings do not support the hypothesis that perioperative chemotherapy is an important strategy in the management of breast cancer. These clinical findings are in agreement with the experimental studies that demonstrated that tumor cell killing by drugs follows first-order reaction kinetics. Unless perioperative chemotherapy involves the use of very high doses, one treatment cycle is insufficient to yield a consistent benefit.

DRUG DOSE INTENSITY AND HIGH-DOSE CHEMOTHERAPY

Except for the initial studies with polydrug regimens in acute leukemia and Hodgkin's disease, it was only during the past decade that clinicians began to appreciate that treatment failure could be the consequence of insufficient dose intensity.[439] In the area of adjuvant therapy of breast cancer, the Milan CMF program was the first to provide retrospective evidence that the outcome at 5 and 10 years was related to the use of full doses of drugs.[427,428] Despite the intrinsic limitations of retrospective evaluations, these findings generated the initial interest in the subject of dose intensity.

Dose intensity is a concept developed in 1984 by Hryniuk and coworkers, who emphasized received dose rate, rather than total dose received.[440] The concept is complex, because it is a mathematical combination of the total amount of drug received and the amount of drug received per unit time (*e.g.*, mg/m²/week). Hryniuk and colleagues evaluated the relation between relapse-free survival and the dose intensity of CMF adjuvant chemotherapy in node-positive breast cancer (Fig. 40–15).[441] This analysis showed a highly significant relation between projected dose intensity and the 3-year relapse-free survival within all four subsets of patients: one to three positive

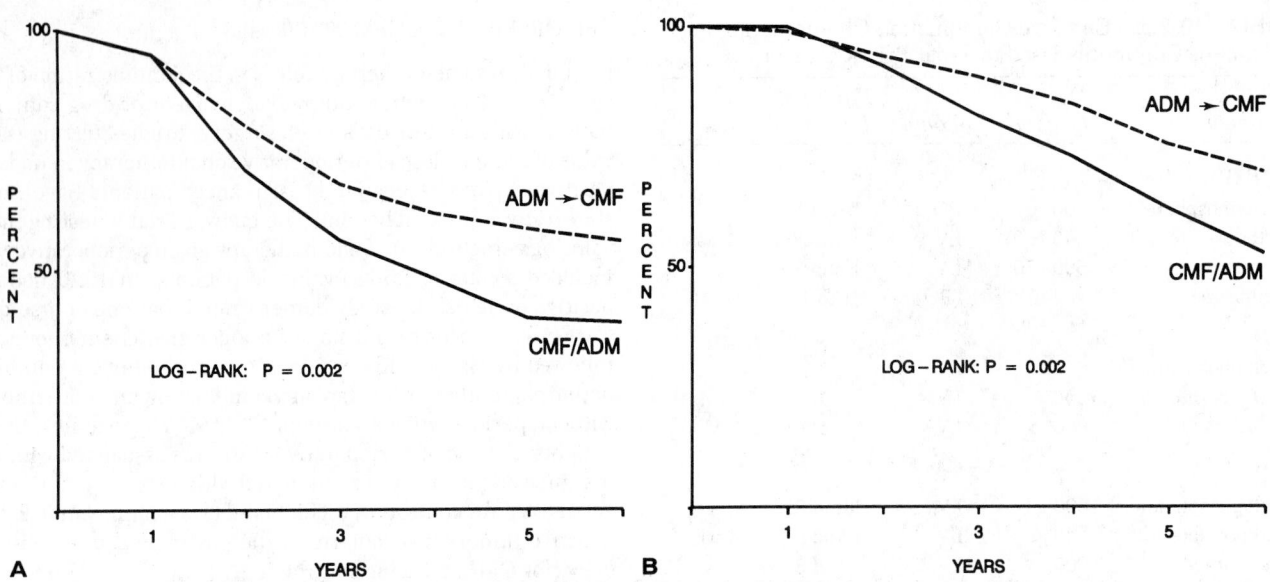

FIGURE 40–14. Milan trial comparing doxorubicin-containing regimens: 6-year results in patients with more than 3 positive axillary lymph nodes. **(A)** Comparative relapse-free survival. **(B)** Comparative total survival. (Bonadonna G. Evolving concepts in the systemic adjuvant treatment of breast cancer. Cancer Res 1992;52[8]:2127–2137)

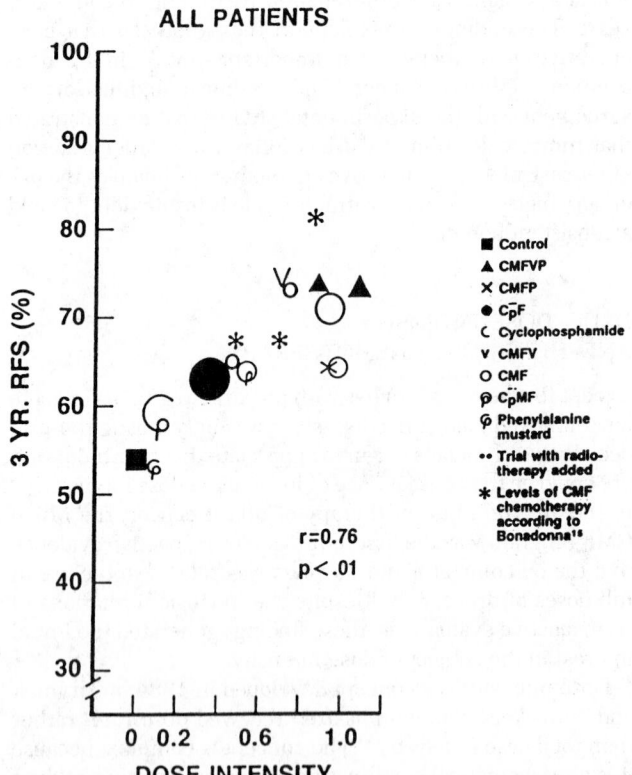

FIGURE 40–15. Three-year relapse-free survival in stage II breast cancer related to the average relative dose intensity of the adjuvant chemotherapy used. The size of the symbols is proportional to the number of cases at each dose intensity. (Hryniuk WM, Bonadonna G, Valagussa P. The effect of dose intensity in adjuvant chemotherapy. In: Salmon SE, ed. Adjuvant therapy of cancer V. Philadelphia: Grune & Stratton, 1987:13–23)

nodes or more than three positive nodes in premenopausal and postmenopausal women. Henderson and associates summarized the results of retrospective analyses of chemotherapy dose and treatment outcome in adjuvant chemotherapy trials.[442] Although conclusions from data-derived results may be biased, it appears that the trials refuting the dose-response hypothesis mostly employed single-agent or low-dose combination chemotherapy. Recent prospective randomized trials carried out using patients with advanced breast cancer have shown that the use of higher doses of CMF is superior to lower doses.[443,444] Medical oncologists must be aware that frequent dose reductions or treatment delays may compromise treatment results. It is considered preferable to delay treatment for a few days for myelosuppression rather than to reduce the drug dose by 50%.

Dose-intensive adjuvant chemotherapy is being evaluated in patients with 10 or more positive axillary nodes. The Johns Hopkins Cancer Center devised a five-drug regimen using weekly chemotherapy, sequential administration of antimetabolites, and continuous infusion of fluorouracil to minimize dose reduction and treatment delay.[445] At a median follow-up of 17 months, only 8 of the 53 treated patients relapsed. This encouraging preliminary outcome, the manageable side effects of the regimen, and the demonstrated ability to deliver more than 90% of the planned doses provide the rationale for a phase III comparison of this new dose-intense regimen to standard chemotherapy.

During the 1980s, the use of high-dose chemotherapy and autologous bone marrow transplantation was shown to produce rapid and complete responses in patients with advanced breast cancer.[446] With the exception of a few women presenting with small tumor burdens, sustained complete remissions were limited. The limited success can be attributed to drug-resistant tumor cells in these relapsed patients, who usually had large tumor burdens. The current strategy of bone marrow transplantation focuses on the adjuvant setting for patients with 10 or more positive axillary nodes. Without absolute drug resistance, increasing the dose intensity should increase the log kill and improve the results.

Table 40–23 presents the treatment program of the Milan Cancer Institute, which consists of the sequential administration of cyclophosphamide, vincristine, methotrexate plus folinic acid, cisplatin, and melphalan.[304] It is important to point out that patients were also treated with recombinant human granulocyte-macrophage colony-stimulating factor (rhGM-CSF) or interleukin-3 (rhIL-3) as a means of harvesting by leukapheresis large quantities of peripheral blood precursors capable of accelerating hematopoietic recovery after subsequent myeloablative chemotherapy (Fig. 40–16).[447] To minimize hematologic toxicity after high-dose melphalan, cryopreserved circulating hematopoietic cells, harvested during the leukocyte rebound phase after the postcyclophosphamide nadir, were autotransplanted in combination with bone marrow cells. Although clinical data are still premature (*i.e.*, only 48 patients were treated, with a median follow-up period of 21 months at the end of 1991), the 2-year relapse-free survival was 93%.[448] Patient tolerance of this therapy was excellent, and there were no life-threatening complications. These findings, which compare favorably with those from Duke University (*i.e.*, 53 patients, 80% 3-year relapse-free survival rate), appear superior to those achieved with the best available adjuvant therapy (*i.e.*, doxorubicin followed by CMF), for which the 2-year relapse-free survival rate for the subset with more than 10 positive nodes is only 60%.[305,446] A longer follow-up is necessary to demonstrate that the approach using growth factor-supported high-dose sequential adjuvant chemotherapy is superior and can be used effectively in properly selected patients outside a research center.

TABLE 40-23. The Milan High-Dose Chemotherapy Regimen for the Adjuvant Treatment of Patients Having More Than 10 Positive Axillary Nodes

Regimen	Intravenous Dose (mg/m²)	Approximate Scheduled Day
Surgery		−30 to −45
Cyclophosphamide	7000	0
rhGM-CSF (µg/kg/day)*	5	1 to 14–16
Leukphereses (CPC harvest)		13–16
Bone marrow harvest		17
Vincristine	1.4	18
Methotrexate plus rescue	8000	18
Cisplatin	60	23 and 30
Melphalan	200	40
Marrow plus CPC autoinfusion		41
Radiation therapy (4500 cGy)		60

* rhGM-CSF, recombinant human granulocyte-macrophage colony-stimulating factor; CPC, circulating progenitor cells.

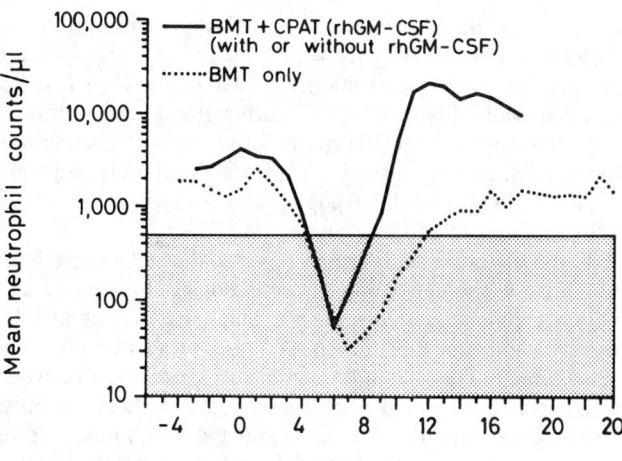

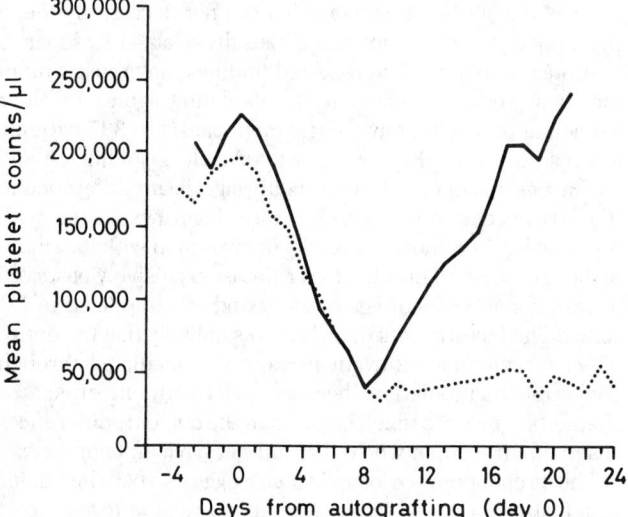

FIGURE 40–16. Effect of rhGM-CSF–mobilized hematopoietic progenitor cells on granulocyte (*upper panel*) and platelet (*lower panel*) recovery after high-dose melphalan (200 mg/m²) treatment and bone marrow transplant (BMT). Compared with the 15 controls receiving BMT only, the 14 breast cancer patients who received circulating progenitor autotransfusion (CPAT) experienced a much faster median recovery, which was particularly striking for platelets. (Modified from Gianni AM, Bregni M, Siena S. Recombinant human granulocyte-macrophage colony-stimulating factor reduces hematologic toxicity and widens clinical applicability of high-dose cyclophosphamide treatment in breast cancer and non-Hodgkin's lymphoma. J Clin Oncol 1990;8:768–778)

DRUG-INDUCED AMENORRHEA AND TREATMENT OUTCOME

Based on adjuvant trial results indicating the treatment benefit was better for premenopausal than for postmenopausal patients and the relatively high frequency of drug-induced amenorrhea, many clinicians hypothesized that the mechanism of action of adjuvant chemotherapy (which included alkylating agents) was chemical castration.[425,427,449] However, the results of trials carried out by the NSABP and Milan groups indicated that women who developed amenorrhea as a result of adjuvant treatment failed to show a longer disease-free interval or increased overall survival than patients who did not develop amenorrhea.[450,451] In the Milan series, premenopausal women who relapsed were equally likely to respond to subsequent ovarian castration whether or not they had developed prior amenorrhea.[286,452] Although some investigators reported that the effect of drug-induced amenorrhea was documented almost exclusively in ER-positive tumors, adjuvant cytotoxic therapy has been equally efficacious in patients with ER-negative and ER-positive tumors.[453,454]

Two cooperative study groups reported the endocrine effects of adjuvant chemotherapy in premenopausal breast cancer patients. Bianco and coworkers evaluated 221 patients who received adjuvant CMF for six or nine cycles with or without tamoxifen.[455] They found a significant correlation between drug-induced amenorrhea and subsequent treatment outcome. Drug-induced amenorrhea was age related, with women closer to menopause more likely to develop amenorrhea. The existence of a statistical association does not necessarily mean that drug-induced amenorrhea is causally related to a superior treatment outcome. The reported findings may represent an increasing ovarian sensitivity to alkylating agents in older women approaching physiologic menopause. In 387 patients given adjuvant CMFP for at least six cycles, Goldhirsch and colleagues documented a marginally significant difference in the 4-year relapse-free survival rate, favoring women with drug-induced amenorrhea (68%) over women without amenorrhea (61%).[456] This effect was almost exclusively observed in patients 40 years of age or older and was unrelated to ER status. The investigators thought it was unlikely that the entire effect of cytotoxic adjuvant therapy was mediated through endocrine manipulation, because the treatment effects of chemotherapy were much larger than the outcome differences observed for women who did or did not have amenorrhea.[456]

The preponderance of evidence suggests that the major benefit from adjuvant chemotherapy is related to its direct cytotoxic effect on micrometastatic breast cancer, but a possible treatment effect on the female endocrine axis cannot be excluded.

ADJUVANT ENDOCRINE THERAPY

The concept that at least a fraction of breast tumors are hormone dependent and therefore responsive to various endocrine manipulations is an old one, supported by innumerable laboratory and clinical observations.[424,457] The discovery of steroid receptors in the mid-1970s provided the rationale for a more selective application of endocrine treatment. In advanced disease, endocrine ablative (*e.g.*, surgical castration, ovarian irradiation) or additive endocrine therapies have a response rate of 30% in unselected patients, of about 50% in ER-positive patients, and of 70% to 80% if ER and progesterone receptors (PGR) are positive. Only 5% to 10% of patients with receptor-negative tumors respond to hormonal manipulations. The response rates are proportional to the level of hormone receptor measured by the dextran-coated charcoal method, and the receptor status in the primary tumor appears to correspond largely to that of metastases.

Since the initial proposal of Schnitzinger in 1889 to use adjuvant oophorectomy in breast cancer patients, there have been more than 20 trials of various types of ovarian ablation. The earliest endocrine studies were limited by the same de-

fects as the studies using adjuvant chemotherapy performed before 1972: use of historic, nonmatched, or nonrandomized controls and insufficient information on nodal status. An analysis of the results was further hampered by the absence of adequate statistical methodology.[424,457] Several recent trials with ovarian ablation, including several prospective randomized studies, have shown improvement in recurrence-free and overall survival rates in premenopausal women.[424,457-459] The trial that was instrumental in reviving interest in the use of adjuvant ovarian ablation was the Toronto study.[460] In this trial, patients 45 years or older were randomized, after a radical mastectomy, into one of three groups: radiation-induced menopause, radiation-induced menopause followed by 5 years of prednisone (7.5 mg daily), or no adjuvant systemic therapy. Although postmenopausal patients showed no survival gain from either of the adjuvant regimens, patients who were premenopausal at entry and given prednisone and castration had a significantly increased survival rate at 10 years compared with the group given no adjuvant therapy. In this trial, patients younger than 45 years were not included in the prednisone therapy arm, and the use of ovarian ablation alone in this group was not associated with a statistically significant survival advantage compared with the no-treatment group.

Adjuvant chemotherapy is being compared with adjuvant castration in premenopausal patients in Scotland in a trial initiated in March of 1980. By May 1990, 332 premenopausal patients with node-positive operable breast cancer regardless of ER status were randomized to receive intravenous CMF or to undergo ovarian ablation, each with or without prednisolone for 5 years. The low rate of accrual is a function of the relatively small number of premenopausal patients with breast cancer, the reluctance of surgeons to disregard ER status (known for 80%) in assigning adjuvant therapy, and the reluctance of patients to be entered onto the trial. The initial local treatment was by mastectomy or local excision and sampling or clearance of the axilla, with immediate postoperative radiation therapy if indicated. Although the preliminary reported findings suggest no difference in the recurrence rate between CMF and ovarian ablation, the trial is still open, and formal analysis is not yet available.[458]

Another form of adjuvant hormonal treatment is the use of the antiestrogen tamoxifen. Two characteristics of tamoxifen encouraged research clinicians to assess its role as an adjuvant therapy. It is known to be effective in postmenopausal receptor-positive breast cancer patients with metastatic disease, especially those with limited disease and a disease-free interval in excess of 2 years, and there are fewer side effects compared with chemotherapeutic agents.

In 1977, the Nolvadex Adjuvant Trial Organization designed the first modern adjuvant trial with randomization to tamoxifen or to a no-treatment control arm. In a series of 1131 patients with node-positive or node-negative breast cancer, the 5- and 10-year results provided evidence that overall survival was moderately, but significantly, improved with the use of adjuvant tamoxifen.[461] Based on the preliminary results of this trial, additional trials testing the value of adjuvant tamoxifen were initiated among major research centers. The results of large randomized studies, activated in Europe during the late 1970s, confirmed the benefit of adjuvant tamoxifen, especially in patients presenting with strongly ER-positive tumors.[462-464] Based on these results, tamoxifen has become widely used in clinical practice during the past decade, primarily in postmenopausal patients with ER-positive tumors and with one to three positive nodes. The recommended dose is 20 mg per day for a minimum of three consecutive years.[465,466] However, based on the available results, many oncologists believe that treatment with adjuvant tamoxifen should be given for 5 or more years, if not indefinitely, in patients remaining disease free. The benefits of prolonged administration of tamoxifen need to be balanced against potential long-term toxicity, and this is being addressed in current trials.

CHEMOTHERAPY WITH ENDOCRINE THERAPY

With the results achieved using adjuvant chemotherapy and adjuvant tamoxifen, it is logical to ask whether the combined use of cytotoxic and endocrine modalities results in an additive or synergistic effect. The biologic rationale for combining these two treatment modalities is tumor cell heterogeneity. It is likely that breast tumors consist of various populations of cells with different sensitivities to cytotoxic and hormonal agents, and these two modalities may be effective in killing different tumor populations. During the past decade, a few research groups have tested adjuvant chemoendocrine treatment, particularly in postmenopausal patients. The only large study that yielded a positive result, favoring chemoendocrine treatment (PF plus tamoxifen) over chemotherapy (PF) alone, is that of the NSABP. The investigators observed that the benefit was almost entirely restricted to the subset of patients older than 50 years of age with more than four involved axillary nodes and with positive estrogen and progesterone receptors.[467] Trials from the Eastern Cooperative Oncology Group[468] and the Mayo Clinic[469] failed to show a significant advantage for the addition of tamoxifen to combination chemotherapy. There is not yet clear evidence from individual trials that the addition of tamoxifen to effective chemotherapy (CMF or CMF-like regimens) has improved treatment outcome over chemotherapy alone. However, the addition of chemotherapy to tamoxifen has consistently resulted in superior treatment outcome compared with adjuvant tamoxifen alone (given for 3 to 5 years) in postmenopausal patients with ER-positive tumors.[470-472]

The pharmacologic reasons for these disparate clinical findings are unknown. In vitro studies demonstrated that endocrine therapies may decrease the cytotoxic effect of chemotherapeutic drugs by unfavorably altering tumor cell kinetics, and this effect may occur clinically if chemotherapy and hormonal treatments are delivered concurrently.[473] It is important to compare sequential and concurrent administration of the two modalities in properly designed clinical trials. It may be determined that relatively short intensive chemotherapy should be given first to kill rapidly proliferating tumor cells and that tamoxifen should be given after chemotherapy to kill or retard the growth of slowly proliferating cells. Although the potential benefit of giving tamoxifen after cessation of chemotherapy was suggested by studies of the NSABP[465] and ECOG,[466] this important issue remains unsettled. Additional studies are required to develop effective combined chemotherapy and endocrine therapy regimens.

ADJUVANT THERAPY IN NODE-NEGATIVE PATIENTS

For many decades, it was believed that histologically node-negative breast cancer represented an almost invariably curable disease. This was a logical consequence of the Halstedian hypothesis of cancer spread. About 20 years ago, however, the evaluation of large surgical series indicated that the overall 10-year relapse-free survival rate after radical mastectomy in this patient subgroup was only about 70% to 75%.[136,138] As in patients with node-positive tumors (regardless of tumor size and menopausal status), about half of all recurrences manifest within the first 3 years after locoregional treatment.[474] Research efforts using new prognostic variables indicate that, in given subsets of node-negative patients, the distant recurrence rate is as high as 50%. These clinical findings are in agreement with the modern hypothesis that stresses the importance of early hematogenous dissemination of cancer cells.

During the late 1980s, the reports of a few randomized trials using node-negative patients with ER-negative tumors supported the strategy of using adjuvant systemic therapy in high-risk subsets of node-negative patients. A Clinical Alert released in May 1988 by the National Cancer Institute, in which the results of these trials were described before their publication, informed physicians and women about the need to reconsider the overall prognosis of node-negative breast cancer and encouraged their participation in clinical trials in an attempt to refine patient subsets and treatment outcome.

The results of combination chemotherapy in node-negative and receptor-negative tumors are summarized in Table 40–24.[215,304,475,476] Although the three series have some dissimilarities, the use of adjuvant treatment yielded comparable results at follow-up of 5 or more years. Combination chemotherapy reduced the annual odds of recurrence by at least 30% in patients with node-negative breast cancer. In the Milan trial, the 8-year total survival was significantly improved using adjuvant chemotherapy, with no difference in benefit between premenopausal and postmenopausal patients.[304,475] Based on these results, CMF(P) for six monthly cycles is recommended for node-negative patients who are selected to receive adjuvant chemotherapy. As for node-positive patients, chemotherapy should be started within 4 weeks after surgery and administered at full dose with minimal dose reductions for myelosuppression.

Should all node-negative patients be treated with adjuvant chemotherapy? Currently, the answer is no. Although there is no established method to integrate the various morphologic and biologic indicators of prognosis, it is possible to identify patients with a low (<15%) risk of recurrence.[477] This includes patients with tumors characterized by tumor size less than 1 cm in diameter, grade I malignancy, with positive steroid receptors, particularly if ER and PGR are highly positive, or with a low proliferative rate measured by flow cytometric DNA analysis (S phase). Most of these patients can be spared chemotherapy. The converse is true for patients having tumors larger than 3 cm in the largest diameter, grade III tumors, negative steroid receptors (particularly if both types are negative), or high S-phase components. These patients have a risk of recurrence that is greater than 30%. If two or more of these unfavorable prognostic factors are present (*e.g.*, large tumor size and high S-phase component), adjuvant chemo-

TABLE 40-24.   Chemotherapy in Node-Negative Breast Cancer: Results of Modern Adjuvant Trials in Receptor-Negative Tumors

Study Factors	Milan[304,475]	NSABP[215]	Intergroup[476]
Selection Criteria			
Menopausal status	Pre and post	Pre and post	Pre and post
Tumor size	T1–T3a	Any	Any
Estrogen receptor status	Negative	Negative	Negative: all T
			Positive: T > 3 cm
Regimen	Intravenous CMF	M → F	CMFP
Number of patients	90	737	425
Median follow-up	8 y	5 y	5 y
Relapse-Free Survival (%)			
Control group	39	66	61
Chemotherapy	80	78	83
p value	0.0002	0.0007	<0.0001

C, cylophosphamide; M, methotrexate; F, fluorouracil; P, prednisone.

therapy is strongly advised. Additional research into the identification of prognostic factors should simplify this process.

The current indications for adjuvant endocrine therapy in node-negative tumors are not well defined. Although relapse-free survival has been significantly improved by the use of prolonged tamoxifen in a large series of patients with ER-positive tumors, the advantage in terms of total survival remains somewhat questionable.[216] However, the use of tamoxifen has been associated with favorable effects on bone and blood lipids and is relatively nontoxic.

The 1990 Consensus Development Conference suggested that the oncologist have a thorough discussion with the patient in arriving at a final decision.[206] The clinician should first estimate the risk of recurrence for that individual patient after locoregional therapy alone and then should explain the potential benefits and risks of endocrine and cytotoxic treatments.

INDICATORS FOR SELECTING ADJUVANT TREATMENT IN NODE-NEGATIVE PATIENTS

Laboratory studies and clinical experience have demonstrated that breast cancer is a highly heterogenous disease in its pathologic and clinical behavior. It is not surprising that the clinical course of this malignancy—the risk of recurrence and the response to systemic therapy—often varies. The major determinants of prognosis are tumor cell burden and drug resistance. During the 1970s, the criteria defining high-risk patients were the presence and number of histologically involved axillary nodes, tumor size, and tumor grade. These firmly established prognostic features were later followed by steroid receptor values and assessments of tumor cell proliferative activity (*e.g.,* thymidine labeling index, DNA ploidy, and S-phase fraction by DNA flow cytometry). Because even these indicators are not absolute, clinicians need additional information to better define tumors associated with poor or good prognoses.

A variety of biochemical and immunocytochemical variables have been the subjects of numerous studies (Table 40–25).

There is abundant literature on the putative utility of these individual prognostic indicators, which does not enable the clinician to compare one factor with the others and to select the most useful ones among them. The sharpness of *p* values in any given series is not enough to provide complete information. Provisional data from many research groups conflict about the additional predictive potential of these newer prognostic factors compared with conventional prognostic factors. The constellation of newly proposed variables, such as *ERBB2* oncogene amplification, epidermal growth factor receptor, protease cathepsin D, stress-response proteins, monoclonal antibodies for detecting peritumoral lymphatic and blood vessel invasion, high-molecular-weight mucin-like antigens, a variety of serum tumor markers, and timing of breast cancer surgery during the menstrual cycle, have been claimed to influence treatment outcome and to help in the treatment de-

TABLE 40-25.   Risk Factors for Relapse in Node-Negative Breast Cancer

Established
Primary tumor size
Histologic tumor grade
Steroid receptor status
Tumor cell proliferative activity

Requiring Additional Investigation
DNA ploidy
Oncogene amplification (*e.g., ERBB2*)
Protease cathepsin D
Epidermal growth factor receptor
Stress-response proteins
Haptoglobin-related protein
Laminine receptor expression
Serum tumor markers (*e.g.,* CA 15-3)
Detection of occult bone marrow micrometastases by monoclonal antibodies

cision, but they have left the average clinician confused. What is required to resolve this issue is a sufficiently large series of consecutive patients who have been uniformly staged, managed, and evaluated using the established and the newer prognostic factors.[477,478] It is less critical to determine the underlying biologic principles or laboratory evidence supporting these various factors than to determine their utility in making treatment decisions. The search for new biologic indicators of prognosis remains important for clinicians, but the novel markers should be "handled with care" in the selection of high-risk patients.

THE INTERNATIONAL OVERVIEW

In 1984, an international overview (*i.e.*, metaanalysis) of the effect on mortality of the various adjuvant systemic treatments (*e.g.*, chemotherapy, endocrine therapy, immunotherapy) was organized by the Early Breast Cancer Trialists' Collaborative Group with the cooperation of several individual investigators who contributed their data. Performing a metaanalysis requires the use of proper statistical procedures, which includes obtaining treatment results in *all* trials, published and not published, and evaluating the effects from each trial individually before combining them. The major advantage of metaanalysis is the ability to demonstrate a moderate, but clinically relevant, reduction in mortality in a disease that is common. Such a reduction in mortality may not be demonstrated in individual randomized studies because of insufficient patient numbers, even in trials accruing 300 to 400 patients.

The first metaanalysis was conducted in 1987 for a total of about 30,000 patients and evaluated the 5-year results of adjuvant treatment. When all drug treatments (*e.g.*, single agents and various combinations) were considered, the analysis demonstrated a significant overall reduction in the annual odds of death for patients treated with chemotherapy, compared with no-treatment controls.[449] When only CMF-type regimens were analyzed, the reduction for all patients was 23%, with a 37% reduction for patients younger than 50 years old and a 9% reduction for older patients. The use of tamoxifen was associated with an overall reduction in the odds of death of

16%, and among women older than 50 years, the reduction was 20%.

The updated metaanalysis at 10 years was conducted in 1991 for a total of 75,000 women enrolled in 133 randomized trials involving 31,000 (41%) recurrences and 24,000 (32%) deaths. Thirty thousand women were included in tamoxifen trials, 11,000 in polychemotherapy trials, 15,000 in other chemotherapy comparisons, 3000 in ovarian ablation trials, and 6000 in immunotherapy trials.[479] Table 40–26 summarizes the essential data and demonstrates the following points:

1. The long-term (10-year) results essentially confirmed the intermediate (5-year) results.
2. The cumulative difference in total survival was *larger* at 10 than at 5 years. Tamoxifen produced a highly significant mortality reduction during the first 5 years and an additional mortality reduction during the next 5 years. For polychemotherapy, the absolute mortality difference at 5 years was about doubled by 10 years.
3. Longer courses of chemotherapy (*e.g.*, 12 months) were no more effective than shorter courses (*e.g.*, 6 months).
4. At the 10-year analysis, polychemotherapy was documented to reduce the annual odds of mortality, even in women 50 years of age or older (relative reduction = 14±5%).
5. For the ER-poor (<10 fmol/mg cytosol total protein) subset, the 10-year mortality reduction after adjuvant tamoxifen was only 11%, compared with 21% for the ER-positive subset.
6. Among the 1746 women younger than 50 years, ovarian ablation was associated with a highly significant reduction in the annual odds of recurring (26%) and of dying (25%).
7. The proportional annual odds reductions were similar for node-positive and node-negative patients, but the absolute improvement in 10-year survival was about twice as great for the former as for the latter group.
8. The use of adjuvant immunotherapy was not associated with a significant improvement in recurrence-free survival or in mortality.

TABLE 40-26. Main Results of the Updated International Overview

Types of Systemic Adjuvant Therapy Compared	*Age <50 Years**		*Age ≥50 Years**	
	Recurrence (% ± SD)	*Death (% ± SD)*	*Recurrence (% ± SD)*	*Death (% ± SD)*
Polychemotherapy alone vs no treatment	37 ± 5	27 ± 6	22 ± 4	14 ± 5
Chemotherapy plus tamoxifen vs chemotherapy	7 ± 4	3 ± 5	28 ± 3	20 ± 4
Tamoxifen for about 2 years vs no treatment	27 ± 7	[17 ± 10]†	30 ± 2	19 ± 3
Chemotherapy plus tamoxifen vs tamoxifen	[32 ± 16]‡	[−6 ± 23]‡	26 ± 5	10 ± 7

* Data are expressed as a relative reduction in the annual odds of recurrence or death from any cause at 10 years.
† Brackets denote statistically unstable results with SD ≥ 9.
‡ Only 383 patients (Early Breast Cancer Trialists' Collaborative Group, 1992).[407]

The updated results of the International Overview should have a major impact on clinical practice, because they confirm the results from the individual trials and indicate that the benefit is greater at 10 years than at 5 years. The validation of the benefit from adjuvant systemic treatments reemphasizes the importance of the biologic concepts that are the basis of this treatment. The highest recurrence rates in treated patients were documented to be within the first 3 to 4 years, implying that a considerable fraction of patients have resistant tumor cells and that they do not benefit from the prolonged administration of the same polychemotherapy. Despite the considerable amount of information contained in the Overview, the results do not necessarily reflect the evolving state of the art, nor should they be expected to provide a detailed guide for physicians in the choice of treatment outside the context of clinical trials. For example, the most recent metaanalysis did not evaluate the use of full- and intensive-dose chemotherapy, sequential drug regimens, or the role of anthracyclines. The updated International Overview provides evidence for the long-term benefit of adjuvant systemic therapy and a measure of what a practicing physician can reasonably expect from "standard" adjuvant therapy. This is particularly true for the use of tamoxifen, because most patients were treated with 20 mg/day for a minimum of 2 years.

Polychemotherapy includes a heterogenous group of treatments delivered by means of various drugs, doses, and intensities. It is possible that the results of the metaanalysis may underestimate the benefit seen using full-dose standard therapy. This also applies to patients treated with CMF, the most widely tested drug combination, although this drug regimen was "the only one which separately demonstrated survival advantage in the present overview."[479]

TOXICITY OF ADJUVANT THERAPY

Treatment-related morbidity is still a major concern in the use of adjuvant chemotherapy. Table 40–27 summarizes the early toxic effects and their average frequency for the four most commonly used polydrug regimens. Marked alopecia (requiring the patient to wear a wig) occurs in fewer than 10% of patients after CMF, but it is more frequently observed in women receiving CMFVP and is even more common if using an doxorubicin-containing regimen, such as FAC or AC. After CMFVP administration, paresthesias can be documented in about half of women. About a third of patients undergoing treatment complain of anticipatory vomiting, which obviously reflects the patient's psychological distress. Weight gain during adjuvant chemotherapy has been consistently documented in at least half of women, with an average gain of 3 to 4 kg. This has occurred irrespective of menopausal status or whether drug-induced amenorrhea occurs in premenopausal patients. Although none of 3000 women treated at the National Cancer Institute of Italy with adjuvant CMF alone or combined with doxorubicin required supportive therapy for life-threatening toxic effects, other trial reports indicate that toxic deaths may occur in fewer than 0.5% of patients.

Thromboembolic complications after adjuvant chemotherapy were recently described by several research groups, but the actual incidence of these complications remains unknown.[468,480,481] They are probably uncommon. In the Milan 15-year experience with CMF chemotherapy, these episodes

TABLE 40-27. Acute and Late Toxicity From Commonly Used Adjuvant Chemotherapy Combinations

Toxicity	CMF (%)	CMFVP (%)	FAC or AC (%)
Acute			
Vomiting	>90	>90	>90
Oral mucositis	<10	25	
Marked alopecia	≤10	40	>90
Leukopenia*	≤10	<12	≤25
Thrombocytopenia†	<10	<15	<5
Conjunctivitis	≤30		
Cystitis	≤15	≤15	<5
Delayed			
Amenorrhea	70	70	80
Congestive heart failure	0	0	1–2
Late			
Acute leukemia	<1	<1	<1

* <2500/mm^3.
† <75,000/mm^3.
(Data are averages derived from the published literature)

were almost never documented. It is possible that the type of drugs used and the duration of chemotherapy are partially responsible for these events. In a survey of ECOG studies, thromboembolic complications were more than doubled when prednisone (1.5%) and prednisone plus tamoxifen (3.5%) were added to CMF (0.5%).[468]

The major delayed toxicity of adjuvant chemotherapy is irreversible amenorrhea, which is secondary to the administration of alkylating agents, such as cyclophosphamide. The incidence of amenorrhea is age related (<40 years: 40%, >40 years: 95%), and it is reversible in about 40% of women younger than 40 years of age. The available results suggest that the current adjuvant treatments have not been followed by a high incidence of chronic organ failure. After FAC or AC chemotherapy, the incidence of congestive heart failure is only 1% to 2% if the cumulative dose of doxorubicin does not exceed 300 to 350 mg/m^2. The Dana-Farber Cancer Institute reported that the frequency of congestive heart failure increased from 1.6% to 6% when the duration of AC chemotherapy was prolonged from 15 to 30 weeks.[429] The increase in the frequency of laboratory-proven and symptomatic myocardial damage in patients treated with conservative surgery and irradiation to the left breast combined with doxorubicin-containing regimens partially depended on the technique of irradiation used.

The primary toxic effects associated with high-dose chemotherapy and autologous bone marrow support are myelosuppression-associated infections, thrombocytopenia, and therapy-related organ system toxicity.[446] Use of hematopoietic growth factors (*e.g.*, rhGM-CSF, rhG-CSF, rhIL-3) has shortened the period of absolute granulocytopenia to a few days. With rhGM-CSF, the number of platelet transfusions required by the patient has been drastically reduced (see Fig. 40–16). Growth factor-supported high-dose sequential adjuvant chemotherapy is becoming more tolerable and practically devoid of iatrogenic mortality.[446-448]

The major late toxic effect of adjuvant chemotherapy is the risk of secondary neoplasms, mainly acute nonlymphocytic leukemia (Table 40–28). There may be a slightly increased risk of myeloproliferative disease in patients treated with melphalan-containing regimens (1.3%), but induced acute leukemias after adjuvant CMF have been reported only occasionally.[482,483] There is no apparent increase in the incidence of solid tumors, although longer follow-up is required to assess this possibility.[483,484]

The major toxicities of adjuvant tamoxifen are menopausal-like symptoms, atrophic vaginitis, occasional uterine bleeding, and thrombophlebitis. The estrogenic effect of tamoxifen may decrease circulating levels of antithrombin III, predisposing to thromboembolic disorders.[457,485]

There are insufficient data on the long-term consequences of prolonged tamoxifen use, but there is evidence that tamoxifen does not have deleterious effect on bone density after prolonged administration, and this drug produces a beneficial blood lipid profile in women. It has been reported that in athymic mice transplanted with both hormone-dependent breast and endometrial tumors and treated with tamoxifen, the estrogen-stimulated growth of the breast tumor is controlled, but the growth of the endometrial tumor is not.[486] Physicians should be aware of the possibility that an occult endometrial carcinoma may not be controlled during prolonged adjuvant tamoxifen therapy for breast cancer.[487,488] The cumulative frequency of infiltrating endometrial cancer in women receiving tamoxifen is 0.5%, compared with 0.1% in the control group.[489] When the Stockholm trial (in which higher doses of tamoxifen were used) is excluded, the differences in the frequency of endometrial cancer using tamoxifen doses of 20 mg daily are not dramatic. This twofold increase in risk of endometrial cancer is similar in magnitude to that associated with postmenopausal estrogen-replacement therapy.

PRACTICAL GUIDELINES FOR ADJUVANT THERAPY

Despite 20 years of progress in the development of adjuvant therapy, many issues remain unsettled. Physicians are still encouraged to enter patients into prospective studies. Treatment guidelines provide recommendations for patients who are treated outside the context of clinical trials. The Consensus Development Conferences held in Bethesda in 1985 and 1990 provided guidelines for the use of adjuvant chemotherapy and tamoxifen.[206,490] During the past few years, additional information has become available from recent studies, particularly from the Overview report and studies of node-negative breast cancer.

Node-Positive Tumors

The available data indicate that patients with node-positive tumors benefit from adjuvant treatment. Regardless of hormone receptor status, an established combination chemotherapy (*e.g.,* full-dose CMF for six monthly cycles) is now the standard of care for a premenopausal patient. For a postmenopausal patient, the hormone receptor status determines the approach. In patients with receptor-positive tumors, tamoxifen is given for a minimum of 3 years, and in patients with receptor-negative tumors, chemotherapy (*e.g.,* CMF) is given. If there are other unfavorable prognostic indicators (*e.g.,* undifferentiated tumors, aneuploidy, high tumor cell proliferative activity), it is reasonable to use chemotherapy in addition to tamoxifen in receptor-positive patients. In patients presenting with more than three positive nodes (especially those having ≥10 nodes) full-dose doxorubicin, given every 3 weeks for four cycles, followed by intravenous CMF for four

TABLE 40-28. Frequency of Second Primary Malignancies After Adjuvant Systemic Treatment

Investigations	Total No. of Patients	Median Follow-up (y)	Second Malignancies	Postsurgical Treatment	Actuarial Risk (%)
Milan[286,483]	845	14	Acute leukemia	Control	0
				CMF	0
			Solid tumors*	Control	8.1
				CMF	4.7
NSABP[482]	8013	10	Acute leukemia or Myeloproliferative disease	Control	0.1
				Radiation therapy	1.4
				L-PAM ± other drugs	1.3
Danish[487]	1710	9	Endometrial ca.	Radiation therapy	0.27
				Radiation therapy plus TAM 30 mg/day × 1 y	1.01
Stockholm[488]	1846	4.5	Endometrial ca.	Control	<0.5
				TAM 40 mg/day × 2 y	1.0
				TAM 40 mg/day × 5 y	5.5

* Contralateral breast cancer and cutaneous basal cell carcinomas excluded; L-PAM, L-phenylalanine mustard (melphalan); TAM, tamoxifen.

monthly cycles should be considered, regardless of menopausal and receptor status. In this high-risk subset, tamoxifen can be administered after chemotherapy is completed if the tumor is receptor positive.

Node-Negative Tumors

The available data do not clearly indicate which patients in this subset should be routinely treated with adjuvant therapy. There is consistent evidence that, regardless of menopausal status, receptor-negative tumors benefit from adjuvant chemotherapy (*e.g.*, full-dose CMF for six monthly cycles). Other high-risk subsets, including patients with tumors larger than 3 cm, undifferentiated tumors, and tumors with a high proliferative activity, should be treated with adjuvant therapy. Conversely, patients with favorable tumors (*e.g.*, size <1 cm, well differentiated, low proliferative activity) do not routinely require adjuvant therapy, particularly if all three favorable indicators are present. In women who have tumors with positive hormone receptors, there is evidence that adjuvant tamoxifen prolongs relapse-free and overall survival, although the fraction of patients who benefit from this systemic treatment remains to be defined.

PRIMARY CHEMOTHERAPY

Primary (*i.e.*, neoadjuvant) chemotherapy is a somewhat novel treatment approach in women presenting with resectable tumors. This strategy is based in part on the experience achieved in the treatment of stage III breast cancer. Two clinical developments have helped to bring about the use of chemotherapy as initial treatment in earlier disease stages: the similarity of treatment outcome between breast-conserving procedures and radical mastectomy in small tumors and the demonstrated efficacy and safety of adjuvant postoperative chemotherapy.[191,491]

In an attempt to reduce the frequency of mutilating surgery for tumors larger than 3 cm, the Milan Cancer Institute in 1988 initiated a prospective study using neoadjuvant chemotherapy in patients with operable breast cancers larger than 3 cm.[304,478,492] It was hoped that the use of chemotherapy before surgery would improve long-term results compared with the classic strategy of surgery followed by chemotherapy. The updated results of the Milan Cancer Institute for 227 evaluable

patients presenting with operable breast cancer 3 cm or larger are summarized in Table 40–29. The degree of tumor response was inversely proportional to the initial tumor size, and pathologic complete remission was documented in 8 (4%) of 220 patients subjected to surgery. Conservative surgery (*i.e.*, quadrantectomy or tumorectomy with ample free margins plus full axillary dissection) was performed in a total of 201 (91%) of 220 patients.

There was additional important information from this prospective study. Tumor response was similar for the four drug combinations (CMF, FAC, FEC with epirubicin substituting for doxorubicin, FNC with mitoxantrone substituting for anthracycline), and there was no difference in response rates for three and four cycles of CMF or FAC. Three cycles of single-agent doxorubicin (75 mg/m^2 every 3 weeks) yielded an objective tumor response (79%) comparable to that of combination chemotherapy (78%). Age, menopausal status, tumor proliferative activity, and DNA ploidy did not influence the degree of tumor reduction, but the frequency of response was greater in receptor-negative tumors. With a median follow-up of 18 months after surgery, local recurrences were detected in fewer than 2% of the 201 patients treated with conservative surgery and postoperative breast irradiation. In this protocol, high-energy radiation therapy was started 4 to 6 weeks after surgery, the breast was irradiated with two opposing tangential fields, and treatment consisted of five fractions each week to a total dose of 6000 cGy in 6 weeks. There is insufficient follow-up to evaluate relapse-free and total survival rates in this trial.

A French study initiated by Jacquillat and others attempted to avoid surgery altogether by the use of primary chemotherapy followed by irradiation and further systemic therapy.[287] For 192 patients with stage I through IIIA breast cancers, they reported a 5-year relapse-free survival of 100% for stage I, 82% for stage IIA, 61% for stage IIB, and 46% for stage IIIA. The overall rate of breast preservation at 5 years was 94%. They concluded that most women with breast cancer should be given the option of breast-preserving treatment. A more recent French study included 272 patients with operable breast cancers measuring greater than 3 cm, who were prospectively randomized to primary chemotherapy followed by locoregional treatment or to mastectomy with postoperative adjuvant chemotherapy given to high-risk patients (*i.e.*, node-positive and node-negative ER-negative tumors).[493] Conservative treatment was feasible for 63% of women treated with

TABLE 40-29. Operable Breast Cancer Candidates for Mastectomy Treated With Primary Chemotherapy (Milan)

Initial T (cm)	Patients Subjected to Surgery	T at Surgery (cm)*			Conservative Surgery
		<3	0	pCR†	
3.0–4.0	110	102	11	5	107
4.1–5.0	73	58	10	3	67
>5	37	23	5		27

* Initial clinical size compared with size at surgery after three or four cycles of primary chemotherapy.
† pCR, pathologic complete remission.

primary chemotherapy. At a median follow-up of 34 months, overall survival, but not relapse-free survival, favored the group of patients treated with primary chemotherapy. This interesting study requires longer follow-up to draw meaningful conclusions, particularly about the adequacy of locoregional treatment and patterns of disease recurrence.

Other research groups are conducting randomized clinical trials comparing primary chemotherapy and postoperative chemotherapy. For example, the NSABP is evaluating the use of four cycles of doxorubicin and cyclophosphamide (AC regimen) given before or after local regional therapy. Additional studies are required to determine the optimal integration of primary and adjuvant chemotherapy. What can firmly be stated today is that the delivery of short-term full-dose primary chemotherapy in large but resectable breast cancers can result in downstaging of the primary tumor to less than 3 cm in diameter in most patients, allowing breast-conserving treatment. These results challenge the classic indication for primary mastectomy and offer the possibility of an effective and safe alternative for women concerned about preservation of body integrity. Currently in the United States, the use of primary chemotherapy in operable breast cancer should be restricted to patients entered onto clinical trials.

FOLLOW-UP EXAMINATIONS AFTER PRIMARY THERAPY

The follow-up of patients after primary therapy should ideally be carried out in a simple, regular, and uncostly manner. An important objective is the early detection of persistent or recurrent disease in the ipsilateral breast and new cancers in the contralateral breast or in other high-risk organs, such as the uterus, large intestine, and lung. For patients treated using breast-conserving treatment, periodic mammography of both breasts is recommended. The optimal periodicity of performing mammography of the treated breast has not been established, but annual mammography would be considered a minimum. Some clinicians favor performing mammography of the treated breast every 6 months for the first 5 years, especially in patients whose cancer was detected only on mammography.

The benefit of early detection of distant metastases has not been established, and the periodicity of screening tests for metastases (*e.g.*, bone scans, chest radiographs, serum markers, liver function tests) should be individualized, based on the needs of the patient. One reasonable program is to obtain a chest radiograph and radionuclide bone scan every 6 months during the first 3 years and then annually. The routine use of circulating tumor markers deserves a word of caution.[494] CEA and CA 15-3 are elevated at presentation in approximately 20% of patients with stage I or II breast cancer. CA 15-3 appears to be a more sensitive marker than CEA. If the marker(s) persist(s) at the same level after surgery, this should not be considered tantamount to signaling micrometastatic disease. Only if the abnormal values progressively increase over time is there a high likelihood of metastatic disease. Isolated abnormal laboratory findings usually create considerable anxiety for the patient and the physician, but they should not be used as a basis to alter therapy.

TREATMENT OF OVERT METASTATIC BREAST CANCER

The treatment of clinically overt metastatic breast cancer is currently in a static phase. Despite innumerable trials using the available cytotoxic drugs, hormonal agents, biologic response modifiers, and various combinations of these three modalities, the survival of patients with metastatic disease has not consistently and substantially improved over that of the previous decade. Overall, the frequency of durable complete remissions has not dramatically changed, even if high-dose chemotherapy is combined with autologous bone marrow reinfusion. With the exception of taxol, there are few promising new drugs or innovative strategies on the immediate horizon. The clinical situation is somewhat complicated by the fact that many patients with widespread disease have relapsed after prior adjuvant chemotherapy, and their tumors may be resistant to most effective drugs. Current medical treatment in this large patient subset is palliative, and recurrent breast cancer remains incurable. However, the judicious application of available treatment can control the disease for several months or years in some patients.

In treating patients with metastatic disease with hormonal or chemotherapy, it is important for the clinician to document carefully the patient's response to treatment. The rules for assessing a response have been established by the UICC and are shown in Table 40–30.

ENDOCRINE THERAPY

Manipulation of the endocrine system is the oldest form of systemic therapy for breast cancer. Overall, approximately one third of unselected patients with metastatic disease respond to endocrine therapies (Table 40–31). The discovery of steroid receptors contributed considerably to the selection of patients for endocrine therapy. In advanced disease, the objective response rate is 50% to 60% in patients with ER-positive tumors and 65% to 75% if the tumor is also PGR positive.[495] Only 5% to 10% of patients with receptor-negative tumors respond to hormonal manipulation.

Receptor levels measured in the primary tumor, in the absence of intervening hormonal therapy, are remarkably similar to levels measured in recurrent disease. In a multivariate analysis of ER, PGR, age, site, and number of metastases, the quantitation of the ER level was shown to be the most important predictor of hormone response to tamoxifen, with response rates increasing from approximately 20% for women with ER values of 3 to 10 fmol/mg of protein to approximately 75% response for women with tumors having ER values greater than 30 fmol/mg of protein. Patients with PR levels greater than 10 fmol/mg of protein have a significantly higher response rate (55%) than those with values less than 10 fmol/mg of protein (25%). In general, neither the level of ER nor the presence of PR correlates with the duration of response.[496]

Ablative Procedures

Oophorectomy commonly induces an almost immediate subjective response in menstruating women whose tumors are ER-positive. The median duration of response is longer than 8 months, and 20% to 30% of patients achieve complete re-

TABLE 40-30. Assessment of Response to Medical Therapy in Clinically Advanced Breast Cancer: Recommendations of UICC, 1979

A. Recording of lesions
This should be done by anatomic site. Dimensions should be stated when applicable and the method of evaluation stated (*e.g.*, direct measurement, photograph, radiograph). Pleural effusion, ascites, hepatomegaly, pulmonary shadows, etc., may be the result of nonmalignant processes. When possible, histologic proof of involvement should be obtained if these abnormalities are to be used for evaluation of response or stratification in a clinical trial
 1. Soft tissue. Breast: ipsilateral or contralateral.
    Skin: intracutaneous or subcutaneous or both.
    Lymphedema.
 2. Bone. Sites recorded (state whether lytic and/or blastic).
 3. Visceral. Lung (nodular or diffuse), pleura (nodular and/or malignant effusion), ascites, abdominal or pelvic masses, central nervous system.

B. Menopausal Status
There are three physiologic categories of menopausal status which may be classified in various ways. The following is suggested:
 1. Premenopausal—a menstrual period has occurred within the previous year.
 2. Early postmenopausal—last period: 1–5 years.
 3. Late postmenopausal—last period: >5 years.
Women who have had a hysterectomy with one or both ovaries left in place may be considered premenopausal if <50 years of age and postmenopausal if >55 years of age: those 50–55 years are classified as early postmenopausal. Vaginal cytology or hormone studies may clarify the true menopausal status. Younger women who have had an artificial menopause should be considered separately.

C. Disease-Free Interval
This is the time from treatment of the primary tumor by surgery or radiation therapy or adjuvant systemic therapy to the time of the first recurrence.
 1. No free interval (*e.g.*, stage IV or M1)
 2. <2 years
 3. >2 years

D. Definition of Response
 1. Measurable lesions. Ideally, all lesions should be measured at each assessment. When multiple lesions are present, this may not be possible and, under such circumstances, a representative number of eight or more lesions may be selected for measurement. For bidimensional lesions, regression is defined as when all lesions disappear, or the sum of the products of the diameters of each individual lesion, or those selected for study, decreases by 50% or more, with no lesion increasing in size. In each case, no new lesions should appear. Progression is defined as when (i) new lesions appear, (ii) there is a 25% or more increase in the sum of the products of the diameters of each lesion measured. If an increase of less than 25% makes additional treatment necessary, this is also regarded as progression.
 2. For unidimensional lesions, in the case of regression, the same rules apply as for bidimensional lesions, except that regression is taken as a decrease of 50% or more in one measurement. In situations such as infiltration of the breast, liver involvement, and mediastinal enlargement, objective regression is a 50% or greater decrease in that measurement which is regarded as being in excess of that usual for the site under consideration.
 3. Evaluable, but nonmeasurable lesions (*e.g.*, osseous metastases, pulmonary infiltration, pleural effusion, skin infiltration). Serial evidence of appreciable change documented by radiography or photography must be obtained and be available for subsequent review. The assessment must always be objective. Pathologic fractures or collapse of bones are not necessarily evidence of progressive disease. Neither the development nor healing of skin ulcers should be taken as sole evidence of change.

E. Categories of Response
Objective regression applies to 1 and 2.
 1. Complete response: disappearance of all known disease. In case of lytic bone metastases, these must be shown radiologically to have calcified.
 2. Partial response: ≥50% decrease in measurable lesions and objective improvement in evaluable, but nonmeasurable lesions. No new lesions. It is not necessary for every lesion to have regressed to qualify for partial response, but no lesion should have progressed.
 3. No change: lesions unchanged (*i.e.*, <50% decrease or <25% increase in the size of measurable lesions).
    Note: if nonmeasurable but evaluable lesions represent the bulk of disease and these clearly do not respond, even though measurable lesions have improved, this is considered as "no change," not "objective regression."
 4. Progressive disease: Mixed—some lesions regress while others progress or new lesions appear. Failure—progression of some or all lesions or appearance of new lesions. No lesions regress.

F. Duration of Response
In a patient who has an objective regression, this is to be dated from the start of therapy until new lesions appear or any one existing lesion increases by 25% or more above its smallest size recorded.
It is essential to categorize a patient as having a regression at a stated time. It is also essential that all baseline studies should have been repeated at this time.

G. Survival
Survival is dated from time of commencement of treatment to death.

(Adapted from Hayward JL, Carbone PP, Heuson JC. Assessment of response to therapy in advanced breast cancer. A project of the Programme on Clinical Oncology of the International Union against Cancer, Geneva, Switzerland. Eur J Cancer 1977;13:89–94)

TABLE 40-31. Endocrine Therapies in Clinically Metastatic Breast Cancer: Response Rates in Unselected Patients

Therapy	No. of Patients	Response Rate (%)	Range (%)	Effective in
Tamoxifen	1269	32	16–52	Pre- and postmenopause
Oophorectomy	3380	33	21–41	Premenopause or within 1 year from last menstrual period
Progestins	3479	31	9–67	Pre- and postmenopause
Aminoglutethimide	1153	32	16–43	Postmenopause
LHRH analogs	293	40	32–45	Premenopause
Estrogens	1683	26	15–38	Postmenopause
Androgens	2250	21	10–38	Pre- and postmenopause
Adrenalectomy	3739	32	23–46	Pre- and postmenopause
Hypophysectomy	1174	36	22–58	Pre- and postmenopause

(Harris JR, Hellman S, Henderson IC, Kinne DW. Breast diseases. 2nd edition. Philadelphia: JB Lippincott, 1991)

missions that can last for years for some women. Although the frequency and duration of objective response is about the same after radiation castration (2000 cGy), the benefit from radiation therapy becomes evident only after the second to the tenth week. In the absence of steroid receptor values, ovarian ablation or other endocrine manipulations (see Table 40–31) are indicated in premenopausal women with slow-growing metastatic disease, a long disease-free interval, and age over 35 years. The response rate to oophorectomy in premenopausal women younger than 35 is lower than the response rate in older premenopausal women. In one study, an objective response to castration occurred in about 20% of amenorrheic women who relapsed after CMF adjuvant chemotherapy.[452] This observation supports the concept that the benefit from chemotherapy is not necessarily related to ovarian suppression and that drug-induced amenorrhea is not tantamount to castration. There are no data indicating that maintenance therapy with tamoxifen can improve the treatment outcome of patients who respond to ovarian ablation.

Other endocrine ablative procedures, such as adrenalectomy and hypophysectomy, are considered obsolete forms of treatment for patients with metastatic breast cancer because of the availability of newer endocrine treatments, such as antiestrogens, progestins, aminoglutethimide, and luteinizing hormone-releasing hormone analogs.

Antiestrogens

During the past 20 years, the nonsteroidal antiestrogen tamoxifen has replaced diethylstilbestrol and androgens and has become the most widely used hormonal therapy for patients with metastatic breast cancer. Tamoxifen appears to exert its main antiproliferative effect by competing with estrogen for binding to ER proteins. Presumably, the drug-ER complex inhibits gene transcription and protein synthesis of factors important to tumor growth. The degree of tumor-cell inhibition correlates with the affinity of tamoxifen and its active metabolites for the ER. After binding to the ER, tamoxifen antagonizes many of the cellular events affected by estrogen.[457,497-499] Other cellular mechanisms of tamoxifen may augment tumor inhibition. The precise subcellular actions for tumor inhibition by tamoxifen remain uncertain. In model systems, this compound slows estrogen-induced growth and leads to a cell-cycle blockade. Tumor cells are prevented from entering late phases of the cell cycle and accumulate in the early G_1 phase. In vitro and in vivo data suggest that the predominant effect of tamoxifen is cytostatic.[500] At low concentrations, the inhibitory effects of tamoxifen, mediated through ER, can be completely reversed by the addition of estradiol, but at very high concentration, the inhibitory effects are not reversible and are probably not mediated through the ER. Although tamoxifen behaves primarily as an estrogen antagonist, it may act as a partial agonist for some organs; in fact, the drug shows weak estrogenic properties.[499]

Acquired tamoxifen resistance represents a major cause of treatment failure in all stages of breast cancer. It has been reported that tamoxifen resistance in MCF-7 human breast cancer cell lines is associated with changes in tamoxifen metabolism and the accumulation and retention of the drug by the breast cancer cells.[501]

Tamoxifen has complex endocrine effects that depend on treatment duration and dose, menopausal status, and the target organ. In postmenopausal women, the normally elevated gonadotropins, follicle-stimulating hormone (FSH) and luteinizing hormone (LH), decrease with tamoxifen therapy (although levels remain in the normal range), but serum estradiol and progesterone levels are unaffected. In premenopausal women, estradiol and progesterone levels show a striking elevation of up to three times normal, and FSH and LH levels remain unchanged or only slightly increased from pretherapy levels. The antiestrogenic properties of tamoxifen usually are not sufficient to suppress ovarian function. Recent data from the University of Wisconsin have demonstrated that long-term adjuvant tamoxifen for stage I or II breast cancer continues to result in an increase in steroidogenesis in premenopausal women.[502] Because ovulation continues, there is a risk for pregnancy, and patients should be advised to use contraception. Approximately half of patients on long-term tamoxifen therapy continue to have regular ovulatory menstrual cycles. In women developing oligomenorrhea or amenorrhea while on treatment, menses return to normal in more than 90%.

The standard therapeutic dose is 20 mg/day orally and treatment is continued until there is documented evidence of disease progression. The use of doses higher than 20 mg/day is associated with a greater increase in menstrual irregularities but not an increase in the objective response rate. Tamoxifen is currently recommended for postmenopausal patients with metastatic disease and ER-positive tumors. The frequency of response is related to the level of the ER protein. Tamoxifen is an active agent for premenopausal patients with metastatic disease, although its value is less well documented. The response rates appear to be comparable to those reported for ovarian ablation, although there are no firm data indicating that they are equivalent.[499,503,504] This drug can be offered as a reasonable alternative to women who wish to avoid surgical or radiation castration. It is not yet clear whether the response to tamoxifen can predict response to subsequent ovarian ablation.[499]

The toxicity from tamoxifen is minimal and transient.[505] The frequency of nausea and vomiting, weight gain, vaginal bleeding, skin rash, edema, leukopenia, thrombophlebitis, and abnormal liver function tests is less than 3%. Transient ocular disturbances of the lens, retina, and optic nerve are rare (<1%).[506] Thrombocytopenia, flare, and hypercalcemia may occur in about 5% of patients and hot flashes in 7% to 10%. The main side effects from prolonged tamoxifen therapy were described in the section on adjuvant endocrine therapy.

Other antiestrogens have been studied to identify compounds with less estrogenic effect or no cross-resistance to tamoxifen. Trioxifene, droloxifene, zindoxifene, toremifene, and ICI 164384 have been studied, but they have not been proven to be more active or less toxic than tamoxifen. The results of randomized multicenter trials comparing toremifene and tamoxifen are not yet available, and toremifene therefore remains experimental. The antiestrogens clomiphene and nafoxidine have no role in the current treatment of breast cancer.

Progestins

The semisynthetic progestins medroxyprogesterone acetate and megestrol acetate are the two most active compounds of this class of hormones available for the treatment of metastatic breast cancer.[507] The other effective compounds, norethistrone and hydroxyprogesterone caproate, are rarely used in the current treatment of breast cancer. The mechanism of action of the progestins is not well understood. Several potential mechanisms have been suggested, and it is probable that the predominant effects vary with drug dosage.[508] Studies with the MCF-7 hormone-sensitive cell line suggest that at low concentrations megestrol acetate causes direct cytotoxicity mediated by the hormone receptors. Other investigators have shown that there is dose-dependent inhibition of the hypothalamic-pituitary-adrenal axis that results in suppression of adrenal steroid production. A third potential mechanism for this class of hormones is through their effects on the autocrine growth factors and their receptors. The presence and levels of ER predict response to the progestins, but there is

no evidence that patients whose tumors contain high PGR levels are more likely to respond than those with low levels.

Medroxyprogesterone acetate has been evaluated, mostly in Europe, in a variety of doses and schedules.[509–511] At the end of several trials, it was concluded that very high doses (>1000 mg/day) were not required to influence the response rate, duration of response, or survival. The most frequently used dose schedule is 1000 mg/day given orally or intramuscularly for the first month, followed by 500 mg/day once or twice each week. The drug is almost exclusively administered in postmenopausal patients, for whom the overall response rate is 33% (range, 10–67%). The objective response is higher in women who have not received prior endocrine therapy (40–45%) compared with those who have been treated with tamoxifen (5–10%). In patients presenting with considerable liver involvement, the tumor response is practically nil.

Megestrol acetate has been widely evaluated, primarily in the United States, and has shown an overall response rate of 28% (range, 14–56%).[512–514] The therapeutic dosage commonly used is 160 mg/day in divided oral doses. It remains to be confirmed through the ongoing randomized studies conducted by Cancer and Leukemia Group B that higher doses (800–1600 mg/day) yield superior objective response and survival compared with lower doses. Randomized trials have confirmed that, for patients without prior endocrine therapy, megestrol acetate is therapeutically equivalent to tamoxifen and that the response rate is low (<10%) if megestrol acetate is used after two or three other hormone treatments.[515]

Prolonged high doses (≥1000 mg/day) of medroxyprogesterone acetate are associated with an increased incidence of side effects, including gluteal abscesses after intramuscular administration (15%), facies lunaris (10%), increased sweating (6%), fine tremors and leg cramps (20%), weight gain (>50%), fluid retention (≤10%), hypertension (≤10%), worsening of diabetes mellitus, hypertrichosis (≤50%), skin rash, and hypercalcemia. Unlike the experience with medroxyprogesterone acetate, toxicity at the highest dose of megestrol acetate is milder and transient and includes fluid retention, hypertension, hyperglycemia, and mild congestive heart failure.[514] Because of superior oral bioavailability and ease of administration, megestrol acetate is becoming the progestin of choice in the United States. The considerable increase in appetite and body weight associated with the use of medroxyprogesterone acetate and megestrol acetate at high doses is being used in the management of cachexia.

Aminoglutethimide and Aromatase Inhibitors

Aminoglutethimide was developed to effect a medical adrenalectomy and function as an antiestrogen. The major source of estrogen in postmenopausal women is from the adrenal gland, which produces androstenedione. Androstenedione is converted by an aromatase reaction in peripheral tissues to estrone and estradiol. Aminoglutethimide blocks several steroid hydroxylations and cleavage enzymes. It is capable of inhibiting the conversion of cholesterol to D-5-pregnenolone, blocking all adrenal steroid synthesis. The drug can inhibit the aromatase reaction responsible for conversion of androstenedione to estrone in peripheral tissue.

Adrenal suppression with aminoglutethimide results in

negative feedback to the pituitary, increased levels of ACTH, and further stimulation of the adrenal gland to overcome the block. Patients treated with aminoglutethimide are usually given glucocorticoid replacement to prevent addisonian symptoms.[516] When aminoglutethimide is given orally at the dose of 1000 mg/day, the recommended glucocorticoid is hydrocortisone (20 mg twice daily or in a more physiologic schedule of 10 mg in the morning, 10 mg in the afternoon, and 10 mg before bed time). Clinical trials demonstrated that low doses of aminoglutethimide (250–500 mg/day) can suppress circulating estrogens to the same level as full doses without compromising treatment efficacy.[517-519] The standard dose in clinical practice is 250 mg twice daily combined with 40 mg/day of hydrocortisone, although the deletion of glucocorticoid replacement has been shown to be safe and effective.

In patients with previously untreated metastatic breast cancer, aminoglutethimide has replaced surgical adrenalectomy and has been shown to be as effective as any other form of endocrine therapy in postmenopausal patients.[520] The overall response rate is about 35% (range, 25–53%). When used as second-line endocrine treatment, the overall response rate is approximately 25%. Compared with tamoxifen, it appears that aminoglutethimide is more likely to induce objective response in sites of bone metastases.

Most of the side effects induced by aminoglutethimide can be documented during the first 6 weeks of treatment and include lethargy (35–45%), skin rash (≤30%), orthostatic dizziness (20%), ataxia (10%), and mild hypertension (5%). In fewer than 1% of patients, thrombocytopenia or leukopenia may be observed, and in a few cases, fatal pancytopenia has occurred. To avoid or diminish lethargy and pruritic skin rash, it is advisable to start treatment for a few days with hydrocortisone only. If pruritus develops, aminoglutethimide should not be discontinued, because this symptom can be easily alleviated by doubling the dose of hydrocortisone for about 1 week.

The development of new aromatase inhibitors and adrenal suppressants is an active area of drug development, with several promising agents, including 4-hydroxyandrostenedione and CGS 16949A, on the horizon.[521-524] Both drugs are effective in postmenopausal patients, with response rates of approximately 30%. Neither has been shown to be superior to aminoglutethimide, but several clinical studies are ongoing, and these drugs remain experimental.

Trilostane is not an aromatase inhibitor, but it does inhibit the 3β-hydroxysteroid dehydrogenase system and therefore the conversion of pregnenolone to progesterone, of 17α-hydroxypregnenolone to 17α-hydroxyprogesterone, and dehydroepiandrosterone to androstenedione. Trilostane is effective in about 25% of postmenopausal patients with metastatic breast cancer, and its administration must be supplemented with glucocorticoids.[525] Side effects include diarrhea (≥30%), anorexia, lethargy, dizziness, and headache. This compound is experimental.

Inhibitors of Pituitary Function

Based on the observation that interruption of pituitary function by hypophysectomy has a beneficial effect in patients with metastatic breast cancer, medical inhibitors of pituitary function are being evaluated. Few objective responses have been documented after the use of prolactin inhibitors, such as levodopa or bromocriptine. Danazol, a synthetic steroid whose primary effect is to inhibit pituitary function, has been shown in small trials to have some efficacy in postmenopausal women with metastatic breast cancer.[525] All of these drugs appear inferior to the well-established endocrine manipulations, such as castration, tamoxifen, progestins, and aminoglutethimide.

Luteinizing Hormone-Releasing Hormone Analogs

Luteinizing hormone-releasing hormone (LHRH) agonists or antagonists are promising new areas of research and treatment for breast cancer. The agonist drugs, including buserelin, leuprolide (Leupron), and goserelin (Zoladex) decrease FSH and LH excretion, decrease prolactin excretion, and decrease the levels of sex hormones. The mechanism of action usually ascribed to this group of compounds is a medical oophorectomy.[526] However, it is possible that these agents have a direct effect on breast cancer.

Several phase II studies have provided convincing evidence that LHRH agonists are effective in the treatment of premenopausal women with metastatic disease and have shown a total response rate of 40% (range, 32–50%). Some postmenopausal women may respond to these agents.[527-529] Goserelin is easy to administer through a depot preparation injected monthly as a single subcutaneous injection of 3.6 mg. Toxicity is minimal and consists mainly of hot flashes. Cessation of menses persists only as long as the patient continues taking the drug. Prospective randomized trials ongoing in Europe and North America are comparing LHRH agonists (with or without tamoxifen) with oophorectomy in premenopausal women who have metastatic disease and with adjuvant chemotherapy.

COMBINED ENDOCRINE THERAPY

Theoretically, combining two or three endocrine therapies may provide therapeutic advantages, because different endocrine therapies can inhibit tumor growth through different mechanisms. However, it is possible that combinations of hormones may produce an antagonistic interaction. To investigate this, several trials were activated during the past decade.[530] The most frequently tested combinations have been tamoxifen with fluoxymesterone, glucocorticosteroids, medroxyprogesterone acetate, or goserelin, and the results are intriguing. The response rate after polyhormonal treatment often is superior to the use of a single endocrine therapy. However, this superiority in the response rate has not been associated with a significant and reproducible improvement in the duration of response or survival.[531] This is probably due to the fact that patients who respond to a single endocrine therapy subsequently respond to other hormonal treatments, and women treated with combinations of hormones lose this sequential response. Patients treated with a combination of hormonal therapies experience the combined toxicities as well. Combinations of hormones are not recommended outside of a clinical trial.

GUIDELINES FOR ENDOCRINE THERAPY

Considering that the probability of responding to an endocrine therapy in an unselected patient is only about 30%, hormonal therapy is only indicated for patients whose tumors are receptor-positive. The ER protein is a good predictor of response to all forms of endocrine therapy and helps to exclude women who are not likely to benefit from hormonal treatment. The response rate to hormonal treatment is related to the dominant site of disease and is highest in women with disease in soft tissue, lower in those with bone metastases, and still lower in those with limited nodular pulmonary metastases. Physicians should remember that the predictive value of a response to one endocrine therapy for a subsequent response to the second appears to be independent of the type of endocrine therapy used and that the level of ER protein is a more powerful predictor of response to endocrine therapy than prior response to therapy. The median duration of response to a single course of endocrine therapy is between 1 and 2 years, and this appears to be independent of the type of hormonal therapy. For patients with negative-receptors, the response rate is consistently less than 10%, regardless of clinical presentation. If receptors are not available and a biopsy is not feasible, medical oncologists should follow the established clinical guidelines outlined in Table 40–32.

Premenopausal Patients

For women older than 35 years of age and regularly menstruating, surgical castration is generally recommended as the first endocrine treatment. A good (not necessarily equivalent) alternative is the use of tamoxifen. Goserelin may prove to be an even better treatment than oophorectomy or tamoxifen, but it is still being evaluated.

If a patient who responded to oophorectomy relapses, tamoxifen is the treatment of choice. Second-line endocrine treatment is associated with about a 50% response rate in patients who are ER-positive and who respond to a first course of endocrine therapy. Fewer than 25% of patients with receptor-positive tumors who fail to respond to a first course of endocrine therapy respond to a subsequent endocrine therapy. In patients who respond to tamoxifen, third-line treatment is a progestational agent (medroxyprogesterone acetate or me-

gestrol acetate) or aminoglutethimide. The latter drug is preferred in patients with disease predominantly in bone. If a patient with a receptor-positive tumor progresses after surgical castration, combination chemotherapy is indicated.

Postmenopausal Patients

The treatment of choice is tamoxifen for postmenopausal women, unless the patient has rapidly growing visceral (*e.g.*, liver, lymphangitic lung) involvement. In case of a favorable response, second- or third-line endocrine treatment is indicated, and the sequence is usually the same as outlined for premenopausal patients. It is rare for a patient to respond to a fourth endocrine manipulation, and after the third hormonal treatment, patients are usually treated with combination chemotherapy.

CHEMOTHERAPY

General Principles

In the treatment of clinically disseminated breast cancer, the aim of conventional chemotherapy is to palliate symptoms and improve the quality of life. Because the selection of patients for chemotherapy is largely a process of exclusion, clinicians should carefully evaluate the general indications outlined in Table 40–32 before deciding to start chemotherapy.[532] Because the administration of chemotherapy always involves the principle of dose intensity, physicians should carefully evaluate patients to rule out certain organ dysfunctions (*e.g.*, high blood urea nitrogen for methotrexate, high serum bilirubin or cardiac insufficiency for doxorubicin, poor bone marrow reserve due to prior extensive irradiation of the spine and pelvis) that may preclude delivering full doses of drugs.[440] Age is not a substantial impediment to the use of chemotherapy, unless increased age is associated with one or more organ dysfunctions.

During treatment, measurable lesions should be objectively evaluated to avoid prolongation of ineffective but toxic treatment. The criteria of response for endocrine therapy and chemotherapy are shown in Table 40–30.

For most patients, chemotherapy is delivered using a polydrug regimen, because combinations of drugs are superior to the use of a single agent. The one exception is the use of single-agent doxorubicin, which is as effective as several standard combination regimens.[533,534] As in the adjuvant setting, treatment should be applied according to the principles of dose intensity whenever safety allows. If the patient has moderate leukopenia (<3000 peripheral leukocytes/mm^3), it is usually preferable to delay the subsequent treatment for a few days rather than reduce the drug dose by 50%.

In considering the indications for systemic therapy, medical oncologists should not neglect the contribution of local treatment in certain clinical situations. The most common events are listed in Table 40–33. For example, a patient with a single chest wall lesion appearing 4 or 5 years after mastectomy can easily and effectively be treated with excision and irradiation, if restaging excludes distant metastases. A similar strategy can be applied in a patient with a long disease-free interval (>2 years) and a small supraclavicular recurrence or an isolated bony metastasis. The decision to add endocrine therapy,

TABLE 40-32. General Criteria to Select Patients for Endocrine Manipulations or Chemotherapy

Endocrine Therapy	Chemotherapy
Slow-growing disease particularly in soft tissue* or skeleton	Rapidly growing disease, massive liver involvement, lung or skin involvement with lymphangitic metastases
Free interval > 2 years	Free interval < 2 years
Age > 35 years	Any age group
Objective response to prior endocrine manipulations	Negative response to first endocrine manipulations

* Inflammatory carcinoma excluded.

TABLE 40-33. Clinical Situations in Which Surgery or Radiation Therapy are used in Addition to or Instead of Systemic Therapy

Limited recurrence (*e.g.*, chest wall, supraclavicular adenopathy, a single vertebra) after a free interval > 2 years
Impending fracture in a long bone
Persistent localized bone pain
Spinal cord compression
Brain or choroidal metastases
Pleural or pericardial effusion

TABLE 40-34. Response After Combination Chemotherapy in Patients Previously Untreated With Cytotoxic Drugs

Total with PR or CR (%)	45–80% of all patients
Total with CR (%)	5–25% of all patients
Time to initial response (median)	4–8 wk
Duration of response (median)	5–13 mo
Survival of responders (median)	15–33 mo

PR, partial response; CR, complete response.

such as tamoxifen, to local treatment depends on the patient's hormone receptor status, but the use of chemotherapy usually can be delayed because survival is not improved by earlier use. Patients with a single site of recurrence and a short disease-free interval should preferentially be treated with systemic therapy, using the isolated lesion as a means of measuring response.

Combination Regimens

The most common drug regimens currently used in the treatment of advanced breast cancer are shown in Table 40–22. Doxorubicin-containing regimens yield a 10% to 20% higher response rate than polydrug regimens without doxorubicin. However, it has not been demonstrated that the use of doxorubicin or its analog epirubicin can improve overall survival in this setting. The same applies to CMFP when compared with CMF, for which the magnitude of the advantage provided by prednisone is minimal. The role of vincristine remains undefined, because there is no difference in the response rate between CAFVP and CAF.[532,535,536]

Table 40–34 presents the average therapeutic results that can be expected after adequate delivery of an effective combination regimen. The reported differences reflect differences in patient selection, response criteria, frequency of assessment, and total tumor volume. The response rate is higher among patients who present with disease predominantly in soft tissues than those with visceral and osseous metastases. The initial signs of response are usually measurable within the first 2 months after starting treatment, but in the case of osteolytic metastases, it may take a few months to detect partial bone recalcification. Patients who do not show signs of tumor shrinkage within the first 6 months of chemotherapy usually do not show an objective response using additional treatment with the same drug regimen. Because it is difficult to determine the optimal second-line treatment for a patient who no longer responds to doxorubicin, we usually prefer CMF as initial chemotherapy, and use doxorubicin, alone or in combination, when the disease progresses. An additional reason for choosing this sequence is that CMF and doxorubicin are not cross-resistant and are roughly equivalent in efficacy.[537]

The optimal duration of chemotherapy in patients with metastatic breast cancer is controversial. The results of recent trials indicate that the continuous use of chemotherapy results in a twofold to threefold longer median time to progression than a six-course induction regimen followed by observation.[538,539] However, total survival is essentially the same in the two treatment groups. The physician should carefully assess whether the patient is more concerned about the discontinuation of treatment without a complete remission or about the continuing symptoms of treatment, including nausea, vomiting, mucositis, and hair loss. In the few patients who achieve a complete remission, chemotherapy is discontinued and resumed after detection of tumor recurrence. Occasionally, patients who have complete responses may live in unmaintained remissions for as long as 5 years after the completion of their chemotherapy.[535]

Other important strategies in the treatment of advanced breast cancer using drug combinations are the use of alternating noncross-resistant regimens, the sequencing of endocrine therapy and chemotherapy, and the use of combinations of chemotherapy and endocrine therapy. The common rationale for all of these strategies is that breast tumors are characterized by multiple clones, and the patient may benefit from the use of multiple different treatments. It is possible that some clones are sensitive to chemotherapy and resistant to endocrine manipulations and that other clones manifest the opposite behavior. Several trials carried out over the past 15 years have shown some improvement in the response rate and the frequency of complete remission, but they have not demonstrated a consistent increase in the duration of response or in survival.[2,540–542] These strategies have not been established as standard practice in the treatment of disseminated breast cancer.

Salvage Chemotherapy

Salvage chemotherapy is increasingly used for women who develop clinically disseminated breast cancer after adjuvant systemic therapy. Patients who fail after adjuvant tamoxifen can be treated with one of the standard drug combinations (see Table 40–22). There is no evidence that the response rate, the duration of response, or total survival are inferior compared with previously untreated patients with similar disease extent. If the disease-free interval from the completion of adjuvant chemotherapy is longer than 12 months, retreatment with the same drug regimen can yield a complete and partial remission rate of about 50%, with a median duration of response of 22 months. In women who had recurrences within the first 12 months after starting adjuvant CMF, retreatment with CMF was totally ineffective, and full-dose doxorubicin (75 mg/m^2 every 3 weeks) yielded a 38% response rate, with a median response of 17 months.[452] As in malignant lymphomas, the disease-free interval can differentiate patients who require noncross-resistant therapy and those who can be retreated with the same regimen.

Patients with metastatic breast cancer who are refractory to first-line chemotherapy generally do not respond to second- and third-line drug regimens. The most common situation is for a patient with metastatic disease to develop progressive disease after treatment with CMF. As in women who develop recurrences after adjuvant CMF chemotherapy, doxorubicin (or epirubicin) represents the treatment of choice, and it can induce a second response in 25% to 40% of patients. The use of full-dose doxorubicin alone appears to yield results superior to its administration with other drugs. If there is an objective response, treatment can be continued, but not to a cumulative dose exceeding 450 to 500 mg/m^2 to avoid the risk of congestive heart failure. In patients with a poor performance status or bone marrow reserve, massive liver involvement, or lymphangitic pulmonary metastases, weekly administration of 15 to 20 mg/m^2 of doxorubicin is associated with fewer cardiac and noncardiac complications without a reduction in its effectiveness compared with a dose of 50 to 75 mg/m^2 every 3 weeks.[543]

There is no third-line treatment of choice for patients who have become refractory to doxorubicin. Among the several regimens tested, a combination of mitomycin C and vinblastine is probably the most effective, yielding a response rate between 25% and 35%.[544–547] Various dose regimens of this combination have been attempted to avoid excessive bone marrow toxicity. The regimen using mitomycin (10 mg/m^2) on day 1 and vinblastine (5 mg/m^2) on days 1 and 15, recycled every 4 weeks, yielded a response rate of about 30% with less hematologic toxicity than regimens using mitomycin at the dose of 20 mg/m^2 every 6 weeks.[546] Single-agent treatments with nitrosourea derivatives (BCNU or CCNU), vinorelbine, platinum derivatives, or mitoxantrone are associated with lower response rates.[2]

NEW DRUGS AND TREATMENTS

Taxol

Taxol is the single new drug that holds promise in the treatment of breast cancer. Taxol is a complex molecule derived from the needles and bark of the Pacific yew tree, *Taxus brevifolia*. It functions as a mitotic spindle poison by interfering with the formation of the structural apparatus used by dividing cells to partition chromosomes between daughter cells. Although other plant-derived drugs (*e.g.*, colchicine, podophyllotoxin, vinblastine, vincristine) interfere with cell division by inhibiting assembly of the microtubules that make up the spindle, taxol instead promotes assembly of microtubules and stabilizes those already formed. This prototype of a novel class of antimicrotubule agents that induces excessive polymerization of tubulin has demonstrated significant activity in advanced refractory ovarian epithelial neoplasms and objective responses in various malignancies including breast cancer.[548]

The administration of taxol is associated with several nonprohibitive side effects (*e.g.*, neutropenia, neurotoxicity, myalgias, alopecia, vomiting, diarrhea, bradycardia, asymptomatic ventricular tachycardia). To avoid hypersensitivity reactions (probably due to the cremophor vehicle), the time span of intravenous infusion was prolonged, and routine premedication was implemented. Using a 6-hour intravenous infusion, the recommended phase II starting dose is 225 mg/

m^2 every 3 weeks.[549] Sequences of taxol and cisplatin have yielded only mild to modest neurotoxicity in 27% of patients.[548] Taxol appears to merit broad investigation at the phase II level. Because of the scarcity of taxol, research is being directed toward identifying active taxol analogs synthesized from the abundant but inactive taxol-like natural chemicals, taxanes.

Biochemical Modulation

Biochemical modulation refers to strategies that favorably alter the interaction of conventional therapeutic agents with their target end points in malignant and nonmalignant cells. The development of clinically useful modulatory strategies requires a solid knowledge of the mechanism of action of chemotherapeutic agents and the means by which malignant cells become insensitive to their cytotoxic effects. Several investigations illustrated the value of modulating the cytotoxicity of fluorouracil with leucovorin and demonstrated that the addition of leucovorin in the treatment of patients with advanced colorectal carcinoma is associated with a significant survival advantage compared with patients given fluorouracil alone.

Therapeutic trials using a combination of fluorouracil and leucovorin in patients with refractory breast cancer and as initial therapy in patients with previously untreated advanced disease have shown encouraging results in the past few years.[550,551] Phase II trials from Vanderbilt and Baylor Universities using a combination of mitoxantrone with leucovorin-modulated fluorouracil in previously treated advanced breast carcinoma suggest that this may be an effective second-line chemotherapy regimen.[552,553]

The anthracenedione mitoxantrone is considered a substitute for doxorubicin because it is less toxic. Randomized trials comparing mitoxantrone (14 mg/m^2) and doxorubicin as second-line treatment of metastatic breast cancer demonstrated comparable activity but less alopecia, vomiting, mucositis, and cardiotoxicity in the mitoxantrone-treated group.[554] The combination of mitoxantrone, methotrexate, and mitomycin (MMM regimen) was as effective as CMF.[555] The results from the Vanderbilt and Baylor groups, using a 21-day cycle of mitoxantrone on day 1 and 3 days of fluorouracil and leucovorin, showed impressive 65% and 42% response rates, respectively, with a median duration of 6 months. It is likely that the reported findings in these previously treated populations may underestimate its effect in previously untreated patients. The combination of mitoxantrone, fluorouracil, and high-dose leucovorin appears to be active and well tolerated, and comparison with other standard combinations as first- or second-line treatment for breast cancer is indicated.

Bone Marrow Transplantation

Dose-intensity analyses provided the impetus to study a variety of high-dose regimens using autologous bone marrow support.[440,441] In patients with stage IV disease, this approach has produced high complete remission rates (35–50%), but they are insufficient to conclude that this form of therapy is superior to conventional drug treatments.[446,556–558] The duration of response in these series has not yet been convincingly demonstrated to be prolonged compared with more conventional treatments. The results have been achieved in highly selected series of previously untreated patients, and the median follow-up time is still short. For clinically advanced disease, it is possible that the major obstacle to curative high-dose chemotherapy is the high frequency of drug-resistant tumor cells. If this is the case, high-dose treatment is unlikely to work in these patients, and future trials should instead concentrate on the adjuvant treatment of high-risk women (≥ 10 positive axillary lymph nodes).

New techniques, including the administration of hematopoietic growth factors, have considerably decreased the toxicity and mortality associated with dose-intensive regimens and reduced the hospital costs of the procedure.[446–448] Additional follow-up of the current studies and randomized studies using high-dose chemotherapy with autologous bone marrow transplantation are required to assess the impact of this approach.

Biologic Response Modifiers

Lymphokines, cytokines, and monoclonal antibodies, all products of biotechnology, were devised to enable the immune system to inhibit the growth of human malignancy.[559] Several of the biologic response modifiers (*e.g.*, interferon-α, lymphokine-activated killer cells, recombinant human tumor necrosis factor) have been investigated in phase I trials as treatment of metastatic breast cancer. The results achieved so far are disappointing or controversial. The interferons may be used as modulatory agents, because they represent a new class of biochemical modulators that appear capable of circumventing mechanisms by which malignant cells became resistant to the fluoropyrimidines.

TREATMENT OF METASTATIC COMPLICATIONS

Metastases to the Central Nervous System

Approximately 25% of patients with metastatic breast cancer eventually develop a nervous system problem: brain metastases, epidural spinal cord compression syndrome, carcinomatous meningeal infiltration, choroidal metastases, brachial plexus syndrome, or paraneoplastic syndrome. Brain metastases are often multiple, and they usually become symptomatic late in the course of patients with disseminated disease. After diagnosis by MRI or CT scans, standard therapy is prompt administration of dexamethasone (16–24 mg/day) followed by whole-brain irradiation. About two thirds of patients improve, and some patients remain free of symptoms for many months or years. Resection before radiation therapy is indicated if the diagnosis is in doubt or if there is a single accessible metastasis. Small-field or gamma knife irradiation has been used in conjunction with standard external-beam irradiation in patients with limited metastases. The impact of systemic treatment on brain metastases has not been fully evaluated. Single-agent (*e.g.*, lomustine, fluorouracil, high-dose methotrexate) chemotherapy, combinations of drugs, or tamoxifen may produce objective responses in 25% to 50% of patients.

Carcinomatous meningeal infiltration is a disease complication that is associated with a poor prognosis. Fewer than 10% of patients survive 12 months. The treatment involves intrathecal administration of methotrexate, thiotepa, and cytosine arabinoside in single-drug or combination regimens.

Treatment is optimally administered through an Ommaya reservoir and is usually started with methotrexate (10 mg/m²) given twice weekly until the cerebrospinal fluid cytology becomes negative. The frequency of methotrexate administration can be gradually decreased, first to a weekly course and eventually to a single administration every 2 months. Radiation therapy is generally not recommended because treatment would involve more than 40% of the bone marrow, and it cannot be delivered concomitantly with intrathecal chemotherapy. In patients with symptomatic cranial nerve palsies, whole-brain irradiation is usually given. Choroidal metastases are rare ($\leq 5\%$ of all patients) and may be bilateral. The treatment of choice is radiation therapy, which can improve visual acuity in most patients.

Epidural spinal cord compression syndrome is one of the most serious disease complications. After localizing the exact level of compression by MRI or CT scans, dexamethasone and radiation therapy should be promptly instituted. In the presence of rapid development of paralysis and sphincter dysfunction, laminectomy should be considered. However, the results of surgery followed by radiation therapy have not been demonstrated to be superior to the results achieved by irradiation alone. Brachial plexopathy can be caused by tumor infiltration or radiation damage, if prior irradiation has been given to that area. Early diagnosis of brachial plexopathy secondary to tumor and prompt administration of radiation therapy (and systemic treatment if the patient has not been previously receiving treatment) can alleviate neurologic symptoms in most patients. If symptoms are longstanding, the likelihood of alleviating them is considerably decreased.

Bone Metastases and Hypercalcemia

Pathologic bone fractures can be devastating, and it is preferable to attempt to prevent them. A femoral fracture may result in marked limitation of mobility, and a vertebral body compression fracture may result in severe pain or profound neurologic dysfunction due to spinal cord injury. In patients with known metastatic disease, attention must be paid to areas of bony involvement and suspicion maintained for areas where pathologic fractures can occur. If recognized promptly, fracture can be prevented in most areas of bony destruction by the early use of radiation therapy or by orthopedic stabilization. The choice of treatment depends on the site and extent of involvement and the degree of pain; in patients with painful lesions with significant (>33%) destruction of the cortex in the peritrochanteric region, the treatment is usually surgery.

Hypercalcemia is the most common life-threatening metabolic abnormality in patients with breast cancer and osseous metastases. This complication is associated with significant morbidity and mortality, especially in patients in the latter stages of their disease (see Chap. 60). Besides the use of systemic anticancer therapy, the bisphosphonates and gallium nitrate are new agents for the treatment of hypercalcemia that work as potent inhibitors of bone resorption.[560] To directly compare therapeutic effectiveness, a randomized, double-blind, multicenter study of gallium nitrate compared with etidronate was recently conducted using patients with cancer-related hypercalcemia.[561] Both drugs were given daily for 5 consecutive days. Gallium nitrate was given by continuous intravenous infusion (200 mg/m²/day), and etidronate was given as a 4-hour intravenous infusion (7.5 mg/kg). In 71 randomized patients, normocalcemia was achieved in 82% of patients given gallium nitrate and in 43% of those treated with etidronate. The conclusion of the study is that gallium nitrate is highly effective and superior to etidronate for acute control of moderate to severe cancer-related hypercalcemia.

REFERENCES

1. American Cancer Society. Cancer statistics. CA 1992;42:30–31.
2. Harris JR, Hellman S, Henderson IC, Kinne DW. Breast diseases. 2nd ed. Philadelphia: JB Lippincott, 1991.
3. Lippman ME, Dickson RB. Regulatory mechanisms in breast cancer. Boston: Kluwer Academic Publishers, 1990.
4. McGuire WL, Johnson BE, Seeger RC. Oncogenes in clinical cancer: A panel discussion. Breast Cancer Res Treat 1987;10:217–227.
5. Lee EY-H. Tumor suppressor genes: A new era for molecular genetic studies of cancer. Breast Cancer Res Treat 1991;19:3–13.
6. Liotta LA. Gene products which play a role in cancer invasion and metastasis. Breast Cancer Res Treat 1988;11:113–124.
7. O'Malley BW. Steroid hormone receptors as transactivators of gene expression. Breast Cancer Res Treat 1991;18:67–71.
8. Clarke R, Dickson RB, Brunne R. The process of malignant progression in human breast cancer. Ann Oncol 1990;1:401–407.
9. Slamon DJ, Clark GM, Wong SG. Human breast cancer: Correlation of relapse and survival with amplification of the *HER-2/neu* oncogene. Science 1987;235:177–182.
10. Tandon AD, Clark GM, Chamness GC. *HER-2/neu* oncogene protein and prognosis in breast cancer. J Clin Oncol 1989;7:1120–1128.
11. Paik S, Hazan R, Fisher ES. Pathologic findings from the National Surgical Adjuvant Breast and Bowel Project: Prognostic significance of erbB-2 protein overexpression in primary breast cancer. J Clin Oncol 1990;8:103–112.
12. Lippman ME, Dickson RB, Bate S. Autocrine and paracrine growth regulation of human breast cancer. Breast Cancer Res Treat 1986;7:59–70.
13. Lippman ME, Dickson RB, Gelmann EP. Growth regulation of human breast carcinoma occurs through regulated growth factor secretion. J Cell Biochem 1987;35:1–16.
14. Osborne CK, Arteaga CL. Autocrine and paracrine growth regulation in breast cancer: Clinical implications. Breast Cancer Res Treat 1990;15:3–11.
15. Yee D, Favoni RE, Lippman ME. Identification of insulin-like growth factor binding proteins in breast cancer cells. Breast Cancer Res Treat 1991;18:3–10.
16. Andersson I, Aspegren K, Janson L. Mammographic screening and mortality from breast cancer: The Malmo mammographic screening trial. Br Med J 1988;297:943–948.
17. Chu K, Smart C, Tarone R. Analysis of breast cancer mortality and stage distribution by age for the Health Insurance Plan clinical trial. JNCI 1988;80:1125–1132.
18. UK Trial of Early Detection of Breast Cancer Group. First results on mortality reduction in the UK trial of early detection of breast cancer. Lancet 1988;2:411–416.
19. Roberts M, Alexander FE, Anderson T, et al. Edinburgh trial of screening for breast cancer: Mortality at seven years. Lancet 1990;335(8684):241–246.
20. Rutqvist L, Miller A, Andersson I, et al. Reduced breast-cancer mortality with mammography screening—an assessment of currently available data. Int J Cancer 1990;5:76–84.
21. Tabar L, Fagerberg C, South M, Day N, Duffy S. Update of the Swedish two-country trial of mammographic screening for breast cancer. Radiol Clin North Am 1992;30:187–210.
22. Wald N, Cuckle H, Frost C. Breast cancer screening: The current position. Br Med J 1991;302:845–846.
23. Fisher E, Sass R, Fisher B. Biologic considerations regarding the one and two-step procedures in the management of patients with invasive carcinoma of the breast. Surg Gynecol Obstet 1985;161:245–249.
24. MacMahon B, Cole P, Brown J. Etiology of human breast cancer: A review. JNCI 1973;50:21–42.
25. Henderson B, Ross R, Ludd H. Do regular ovulatory cycles increase breast cancer risk? Cancer 1985;56:1206–1208.
26. MacMahon B, Trichopoulos D, Brown J. Age at menarche, probability of ovulation and breast cancer risk. Int J Cancer 1982;29:12–16.
27. Trichopoulos D, Yen S, Brown J. The effect of westernization on urine estrogens, frequency of ovulation, and breast cancer risk. Cancer 1984;53:187–192.
28. Bernstein L, Ross R, Lobo R. The effects of moderate physical activity on menstrual cycle patterns in adolescence: Implications for breast cancer prevention. Br J Cancer 1987;55:681–685.
29. Henderson B, Ross R, Bernstein L. Estrogens as a cause of human cancer: The Richard and Hinda Rosenthal Foundation Award Lecture. Cancer Res 1988;48:246–253.
30. Thomas D, Lilienfeld A. Geographic, reproductive and sociobiological factors. In: Stoll BA, ed. Risk factors in breast cancer. Chicago: Heinemann Medical Books, 1976:25–53.
31. Trichopoulos D, MacMahon B, Cole P. Menopause and breast cancer risk. JNCI 1972;48:605–613.
32. MacMahon B, Cole P, Lin T. Age at first birth and breast cancer risk. Bull WHO 1970;43:209–221.
33. Trichopoulos P, Hsieh C, MacMahon B. Age at any birth and breast cancer risk. Int J Cancer 1983;31:701–704.
34. Brinton L, Hoover R, Fraumeni J. Reproductive factors in aetiology of breast cancer. Br J Cancer 1983;47:757–762.
35. Pike M, Henderson B, Casagrande J. Oral contraceptive use and early abortion as risk factors for breast cancer in young women. Br J Cancer 1981;43:720–776.
36. Hadjimichael O, Boyle C, Meigs J. Abortion before first live birth and risk of breast cancer. Br J Cancer 1986;53:281–284.
37. Moolgavkar S, Day N, Stevens R. Two stage model for carcinogenesis: Epidemiology of breast cancer in females. JNCI 1980;65:559–569.
38. Anderson T, Ferguson D, Raab G. Cell turnover in the "resting" human breast: Influence of parity, contraceptive pill, age and laterality. Br J Cancer 1982;46:376–382.
39. Henderson I. What can a woman do about her risk of dying of breast cancer? Curr Probl Cancer 1990;14:166–230.
40. Miller D, Rosenberg L, Kaufman D. Breast cancer before age 45 and oral contraceptive use: New findings. Am J Epidemiol 1989;129:269–280.
41. Bernstein L, Pike M, Krailo M, Henderson B. Update of the Los Angeles study of oral contraceptives and breast cancer. In: Mann R, ed. Oral contraceptives and breast cancer. London: Parthenon Publishing Group, 1990:169.
42. Meirik O, Lund E, Adami H. Oral contraceptive use and breast cancer in young women. Lancet 1986;2:650–653.
43. McPherson K, Vessey M, Neil A. Early oral contraceptive use and breast cancer. Results of another case-control study. Br J Cancer 1987;56:653–660.
44. The Centers for Disease Control Cancer and Steroid Hormone Study. Long-term oral contraceptive use and the risk of breast cancer. JAMA 1983;259:1591–1595.
45. Paganini-Hill A, Ross R, Gerkins V. Menopausal estrogen therapy and hip fractures. Ann Intern Med 1981;95:28–31.
46. Carroll K. Experimental evidence of dietary factors and hormone dependent cancers. Cancer Res 1975;35:3374–3383.
47. Buell P. Changing incidence of breast cancer in Japanese-American women. JNCI 1973;51:1479–1483.
48. Kinlen L. Meat and fat consumption and cancer mortality. A study of strict religious orders in Britain. Lancet 1982;1:946–949.
49. Phillips R, Garfinkel L, Kuzma J. Mortality among California Seventh Day Adventists for selected cancer sites. JNCI 1980;65:1097–1107.
50. Willett W, Stampfer M, Colditz G. Dietary fat and risk of breast cancer. N Engl J Med 1987;316:22–28.
51. Jones G, Schatzkin A, Green S. Dietary fat and breast cancer in the National Health and Nutrition Examination Survey I epidemiologic follow-up study. JNCI 1987;79:465–471.
52. Zollinger T, Phillips R, Kuzma J. Breast cancer survival rates among Seventh-Day Adventists and non-Seventh Day Adventists. Am J Epidemiol 1984;119:503–509.
53. Longnecker P, Berlin J, Orz M. A metaanalysis of alcohol consumption in relation to breast cancer risk. JAMA 1988;206:652–656.
54. Garfinkel L, Boffetta P, Stellman S. Alcohol and breast cancer: A cohort study. Prev Med 1988;17:686–693.
55. Harvey E, Schairer C, Brinton L. Alcohol consumption and breast cancer. JNCI 1987;78:657–661.
56. Veer P, Kok F, Hermus R, Sturmans F. Alcohol dose, frequency and age at first exposure in relation to the risk of breast cancer. Int J Epidemiol 1989;18:511–517.
57. Ottman R, King M, Pike M, Henderson B. Practical guide for estimating risk for familial breast cancer. Lancet 1983;2:556–558.
58. Anderson D. Genetic study of breast cancer: Identification of a high risk group. Cancer 1974;34:1090–1097.
59. Sattin R, Rubin G, Webster L. Family history and the risk of breast cancer. JAMA 1985;253:1908–1913.
60. Baak J, Van Dop H, Kurver P, Hermans J. The value of morphometry to classic prognosticators in breast cancer. Cancer 1985;56:374–382.
61. Anderson D, Badzioch M. Bilaterality in familial breast cancer patients. Cancer 1985;56:2092–2098.
62. Lynch H, Guingis M, Brodkey F. Genetic heterogenicity and familial carcinoma of the breast. Surg Gynecol Obstet 1976;142:693–699.
63. Tokunaga M, Land C, Yamamoto T, et al. Incidence of female breast cancer among atomic bomb survivors, Hiroshima and Nagasaki, 1950–1980. Radiat Res 1987;112:243–272.
64. Miller A, Howe G, Sherman G. Mortality from breast cancer after irradiation during fluoroscopic examinations in patients being treated for tuberculosis. N Engl J Med 1989;321:1285–1289.
65. Shore R, Hildreth N. Breast cancer among women given x-ray therapy for acute postpartum mastitis. JNCI 1986;77:689–696.
66. Hildreth N, Shore L, Dvoretsky P. The risk of breast cancer after irradiation of the thymus in infancy. N Engl J Med 1989;321:146–151.
67. Dupont W, Page D. Risk factors for breast cancer in women with proliferative breast disease. N Engl J Med 1985;312:146–151.
68. Cancer Committee of the College of American Pathologists. Is "fibrocystic disease" of the breast precancerous? Arch Pathol Lab Med 1986;110:171–173.
69. Dupont W, Page D. Relative risk of breast cancer varies with time since diagnosis of atypical hyperplasia. Hum Pathol 1989;20:723–725.
70. Dupont W, Page D, Rogers L, Parl F. Influence of exogenous estrogens, proliferative breast disease, and other variables on breast cancer risk. Cancer 1989;63:948–951.
71. Gail M, Brinton L, Byar D, et al. Projecting individualized probabilities of developing

breast cancer for white females who are being examined annually. JNCI 1989;81:1879–1886.

72. Schechter M. Breast cancer risk factors: Can we select women for prophylactic mastectomy? Can J Surg 1985;28:242–244.

73. Ariyan S. Prophylactic mastectomy for precancerous and high risk lesions of the breast. Can J Surg 1985;28:262–267.

74. Snyderman R. Cancer. Prophylactic mastectomy: Pros and cons. Cancer 1984;53:803–808.

75. Eldar S, Mequid M, Beatty J. Cancer of the breast after prophylactic subcutaneous mastectomy. Am J Surg 1984;148:692–693.

76. Lynch M, Watson P, Conway T. Breast cancer family history as a risk factor for early onset breast cancer. Br Cancer Res Treat 1988;11:263–267.

77. Woods J, Meland N. Conservative management of full thickness nipple areolar necrosis after subcutaneous mastectomy. Plast Reconstr Surg 1989;84:258–254.

78. Pennisi V. Total mammary adenectomy with histologic evaluation and immediate reconstruction. Plast Reconstr Surg 1981;68:510–518.

79. Goodnight J, Quagliana J, Morton D. Failure of subcutaneous mastectomy to prevent the development of breast cancer. J Surg Oncol 1984;26:198–201.

80. Jackson C, Palmquist M, Swanson J. The effectiveness of prophylactic subcutaneous mastectomy in Sprague Dawley rats induced with 7,12-dimethylbenzanthracene. Plast Reconstr Surg 1984;73:249–260.

81. Temple W, Lindsay R, Magi E, Urbanski S. Technical considerations for prophylactic mastectomy in patients at high risk for breast cancer. Am J Surg 1991;161:413–415.

82. Moon R, Thompson H, Becci P. N-(4-hydroxyphenyl) retinamide, a new retinoid for prevention of breast cancer in the rat. Cancer Res 1979;39:1229–1346.

83. Silverman J, Katayama S, Radok R. Effect of short-term administration of N-(4-hydroxyphenyl)-all *trans*-retinamide on chemically induced mammary tumors. Nutr Cancer 1983;4:186–191.

84. McCormick D, Menta R, Thompson C. Enhanced inhibition of mammary carcinogenesis by combined treatment with N-(4-hydroxyphenyl) retinamide and ovariectomy. Cancer Res 1982;42:508–512.

85. Preece P, Baum M, Mansel R. Importance of mastalgia in operable breast cancer. Br Med J 1982;284:1299.

86. Divitt J, Barr J. The clinical recognition of cystic carcinoma of the breast. Surg Gynecol Obstet 1984;159:130–132.

87. Bell D, Hajdu S, Urban J. The role of aspiration cytology in the diagnosis and management of mammary lesions in office practice. Cancer 1983;51:1182–1189.

88. Strawbridge H, Bassett A, Foldes I. Role of cytology in management of lesions of the breast. Surg Gynecol Obstet 1981;152:1–7.

89. Urban J, Egeli R. Non-lactational nipple discharge. Cancer 1978;28:3.

90. McLaughlin C, Coe J. A study of nipple discharge in the non-lactating breast. Ann Surg 1963;157:810.

91. Seltzer M, Perloff L, Kelley R, Fitts W. The significance of age in patients with nipple discharge. Surg Gynecol Obstet 1970;131:519.

92. Murad T, Contesso G, Mouriesse H. Nipple discharge from the breast. Ann Surg 1982;195:259.

93. Di Petro S, Coopmans de Yoldi G, Bergorzi S. Nipple discharge as a sign of preneoplastic lesion and occult carcinoma of the breast: Clinical and galactographic study in 103 consecutive patients. Tumori 1979;65:317–324.

94. Morrow M. Nipple discharge in breast diseases. In: Harris J, Hellman S, Henderson IC Kinne D, eds. Breast diseases. 2nd ed. Philadelphia: JB Lippincott, 1991:73–76.

95. Kline T, Joshi L, Neal H. Fine needle aspiration of the breast: Diagnoses and pitfalls. Cancer 1979;44:1458–1464.

96. Barrows G, Anderson T, Lamb J. Fine needle aspiration of breast cancer. Relationship of clinical factors to cytology results in 689 primary malignancies. Cancer 1986;58:1493–1498.

97. Dixon J, Anderson T, Lamb J. Fine needle aspiration cytology, in relationship to clinical examination and mammography in the diagnosis of a solid breast mass. Br J Surg 1984;71:593–596.

98. Bicker T, Schandorf H, Naujoks H. Long-term follow-up in patients with mammary gland changes found unsuspicious by aspiration cytology. Cancer Detect Prev 1988;11:319–322.

99. Goodson W, Mailman R, Miller T. Three year follow-up of benign fine-needle aspiration biopsies of the breast. Am J Surg 1987;154:58–61.

100. Fentiman I, Millis R, Hayward J. Value of needle biopsy in outpatient diagnosis of breast cancer. Arch Surg 1980;115:652–653.

101. Minkowitz S, Moskowitz R, Khafif R, Alderete M. Tru-cut needle biopsy of the breast. An analysis of its specificity and sensitivity. Cancer 1986;57:320–323.

102. Shabot M, Goldbert I, Schick P. Aspiration cytology is superior to Tru-cut needle biopsy in establishing the diagnosis of clinically suspicious breast masses. Ann Surg 1982;196:122–126.

103. Bertario L, Reduzzi D, Piromalli D. Outpatient biopsy of breast cancer. Influence on survival. Ann Surg 1985;201:64–67.

104. Walker G, Foster R, McKegney C, McKegney F. Breast biopsy. A comparison of outpatient and inpatient experience. Arch Surg 1978;113:942–946.

105. Doberneck R. A study of cost effectiveness. Ann Surg 1980;192:152–156.

106. Morrow M. Management of nonpalpable breast lesions. PPO Updates 1990;4:1–11.

107. Schwartz G, Feig S, Patchefsy A. Significance and staging of nonpalpable carcinomas of the breast. Surg Gynecol Obstet 1988;166:6.

108. Ciatto S, Cataliotti L, Distante V. Nonpalpable lesions detected with mammography. Review of 512 consecutive cases. Radiology 1987;165:99.

109. Choucair R, Holcomb M, Matthews R, Hughes T. Biopsy of nonpalpable breast lesions. Am J Surg 1988;156:453.

110. Tabar L, Gad A. Screening for breast cancer. The Swedish trial. Radiology 1981;138:219–222.

111. Moskowitz M. The predictive value of certain mammographic signs in screening for breast cancer. Cancer 1983;51:1007–1011.

112. Sickles E. Further experience with microfocal spot magnification mammography in the assessment of clustered microcalcifications. Radiology 1980;137:9.

113. Sickles E. Microfocal spot magnification mammography using xeroradiographic and screen film recording systems. Radiology 1979;131:599.

114. Powell R, McSweeney M, Wilson C. X-ray calcifications as the only basis for breast biopsy. Ann Surg 1983;197:555–559.

115. Gallagher W, Cardenosa G, Rubens J. Minimal volume excision of nonpalpable breast lesions. AJR 1989;153:957–961.

116. Tinnemans J, Wobbes T, Holland R. Mammographic and histopathologic correlation of nonpalpable lesions of the breast and the reliability of frozen section diagnosis. Surg Gynecol Obstet 1987;165:523.

117. Azavedo E, Auer G, Svane G. Stereotactic fine needle biopsy in 2594 mammographically detected nonpalpable lesions. Lancet 1989;1:1033.

118. Dowlatshai K, Gent H, Schmidt R. Nonpalpable breast tumors: Diagnosis with stereotaxic localization and fine-needle aspiration. Radiology 1989;1770:427–433.

119. Gent H, Springer E, Dowlatshahi K. Stereotaxic needle localization and cytological diagnosis of occult breast lesions. Ann Surg 1986;204:580.

120. Schmidt R, Morrow M, Bibbo M, Cox S. Mammographic screening: Potential cost benefits of stereotactic aspiration cytology. Administr Radiol 1990;9:35.

121. McDivitt R, Stewart F, Berg J. Tumors of the breast. In: Atlas of tumor pathology. Bethesda, MD: Armed Forces Institute of Pathology, 1967.

122. World Health Organization. Histologic typing of breast tumors. Tumori 1982;68:181.

123. Wellings S, Jensen H. On the origin and progression of ductal carcinoma in the human breast. JNCI 1973;50:1111–1118.

124. Fisher E, Kenny J, Sass R, et al. Medullary cancer of the breast revisited. Breast Cancer Res Treat 1990;16:215–229.

125. Harris M, Howell A, Chrissohou M, Swindell R, Hudson M, Sellwood R. A comparison of metastatic pattern of infiltrating lobular and infiltrating ductal carcinoma of the breast. Br J Cancer 1984;50:23–30.

126. Spratt J, Donegan W. Cancer of the breast. Philadelphia: WB Saunders, 1967.

127. Fisher B, Slack N, Ausman R. Location of breast carcinoma and prognosis. Surg Gynecol Obstet 1969;129:705–716.

128. Haagensen C. Diseases of the breast. Philadelphia: WB Saunders, 1971:486–491.

129. Holland R, Veling S, Mravunac M, Hendriks J. Histologic multifocality of Tis, T1–2 breast carcinomas. Implications for clinical trials of breast-conserving surgery. Cancer 1985;56:979–990.

130. Carter C, Allen C, Henson D. Relation of tumor size, lymph node status, and survival in 24,740 breast cancer cases. Cancer 1989;63:181–187.

131. Pickren J. Significance of occult metastases. Cancer 1961;14:1266–1271.

132. Bucalossi P, Veronesi U, Zingo L, Conti C. Enlarged mastectomy for breast cancer: Review of 1,213 cases. Am J Roentgenol Radium Ther Nucl Med 1971;111:119–122.

133. Butcher H. Radical mastectomy for mammary carcinoma. Ann Surg 1969;170:883–884.

134. Haagensen C. Diseases of the breast. 3rd ed. Philadelphia: WB Saunders, 1986:872.

135. Schottenfeld D, Nash A, Robbins G, Beattie E. Ten-year results of the treatment of primary operable breast cancer. Cancer 1976;38:1001–1007.

136. Valagussa P, Bonadonna G, Veronesi U. Patterns of relapse and survival following radical mastectomy: Analysis of 716 consecutive patients. Cancer 1978;41:1170–1178.

137. Haagensen C. Treatment of curable carcinoma of the breast. Int J Radiat Oncol Biol Phys 1977;2:975–980.

138. Fisher B, Slack N, Katrych D, Wolmar N. Ten-year follow-up results of patients with carcinoma of the breast in a co-operative clinical trial evaluating surgical adjuvant chemotherapy. Surg Gynecol Obstet 1975;140:528–534.

139. Spratt J, Donegan W. Carcinoma of the breast. Philadelphia: WB Saunders, 1971:136.

140. Payne W, Taylor W, Knonsari S. Surgical treatment of breast cancer: Trends and factors affecting survival. Arch Surg 1970;101:105–113.

141. Ferguson D, Meier P, Karrison T, et al. Staging of breast cancer and survival rates: An assessment based on 50 years of experience with radical mastectomy. JAMA 1970;248:1337–1341.

142. Nemoto T, Vana J, Bedwani R. Management and survival of female breast cancer. Cancer 1980;45:2917–2924.

143. Smith J, Gamez-Araujo J, Gallager H, White E, McBride C. Carcinoma of the breast. Cancer 1977;39:527–532.

144. Veronesi U, Rilke F, Luini R. Distribution of axillary node metastases by level of invasion. An analysis of 539 cases. Cancer 1987;59:682–687.

145. Rosen P, Lesser M, Kinne D. Discontinuous or "skip" metastases in breast carcinoma: Analysis of 1228 axillary dissections. Ann Surg 1983;187:276–283.

146. Fisher B, Slack N, Bross ID. Cancer of the breast: Size of neoplasm and prognosis. Cancer 1969;24:1071–1080.

147. Adair F, Berg J, Joubert L, Robbins G. Long-term follow-up of breast cancer patients: The 30 year report. Cancer 1974;33:1145–1150.

148. Handley R. Carcinoma of the breast. Ann R Coll Surg Engl 1975;57:59–66.

149. Veronesi U, Cascinelli N, Greco M. Prognosis of breast cancer patients after mastectomy and dissection of internal mammary nodes. Ann Surg 1985;202:702–707.

150. Halsted W. The results of radical operations for the cure of carcinoma of the breast. Ann Surg 1907;46:1–19.

151. Warren S, Witman E. Studies on tumor metastases: The distribution of metastases in cancer of the breast. Surg Gynecol Obstet 1937;57:1018.

152. Saphillo O, Parker M. Metastases from primary carcinoma of the breast with special reference to spleen, adrenal glands and ovaries. Arch Surg 1941;42:1003.

153. Khansur T, Haick A, Patel B. Evaluation of bone scan as a screening work-up in primary and local-regional recurrence of breast cancer. Am J Clin Oncol 1987;10:167–170.

154. Baker R. Preoperative assessment of the patient with breast cancer. Surg Clin 1984;64:1039–1050.

155. Butzelaar R, Van Dongen J, Van Der Schoot J. Evaluation of routine preoperative bone scintigraphy in patients with breast cancer. Eur J Cancer Clin Oncol 1977;13:19.

156. Gerber F, Goddreau J, Kirchner P. Efficacy of preoperative and postoperative bone scanning in the management of breast carcinoma. N Engl J Med 1977;297:300.

157. Green D, Jeremy R, Towson J. The role of fluorine 18 scanning in the detection of skeletal metastases. Aust N Z J Surg 1973;43:251.

158. Lee Y. Bone scanning in patients with early breast carcinoma: Should it be a routine staging procedure? Cancer 1981;47:486.

159. Nomura Y, Kondo H, Yamagata J. Evaluation of liver and bone scanning in patients with early breast cancer, based on results obtained from more advanced cancer patients. Eur J Cancer 1978;14:1129.

160. Weiner S, Sachs S. An assessment of routine liver scanning in patients with breast cancer. Arch Surg 1978;113:126.

161. Sears H, Gerber F, Sturtz D. Liver scan and carcinoma of the breast. Surg Gynecol Obstet 1975;140:409.

162. Chaudry M, Millis R, Hoskins E. Bilateral primary breast cancer: A prospective study of disease incidence. Br J Surg 1984;71:711–714.

163. Lee Y. Carcinoembryonic antigen as a monitor of recurrent breast cancer. J Surg Oncol 1982;20:109.

164. Colomer R, Ruibal A, Navarro M. Circulating CA 15-3 levels in breast cancer. Our present experience. Int J Biol Markers 1986;1:89.

165. Gion M, Mione R, Dittadi R. Evaluation of CA 15-3 serum levels in breast cancer patients. J Nucl Med Allied Sci 1986;30:29.

166. Hayes D, Zurawski V, Kufe D. Comparison of circulating CA 15-3 and carcinoembryonic antigen levels in patients with breast cancer. J Clin Oncol 1986;4:1542.

167. Huvos A, Hutter V, Berg J. Significance of axillary macrometastases and micrometastases in mammary cancer. Ann Surg 1971;1:44–46.

168. Halsted W. The results of operations cure of cancer of the breast performed at Johns Hopkins Hospital. Johns Hopkins Hosp Bull 1984;4:497–555.

169. Haagensen C, Bodian C. A personal experience with Halsted's radical mastectomy. Ann Surg 1984;199:143–150.

170. Donegan W, Perez-Mesa C, Watson F. A biostatistical study of locally recurrent breast carcinoma. Surg Gynecol Obstet 1966;122:529–540.

171. Brinkley D, Haybittle J. The curability of breast cancer. Lancet 1975;2:95–97.

172. Fentiman I, Cuzick J, Millis R. Which patients are cured of breast cancer? Br Med J 1984;289:1108–1111.

173. Rosen P, Groshen S, Saigo P, Kinne D, Hellman S. A long-term follow-up study of survival in stage I and stage II breast carcinoma. J Clin Oncol 1989;7:355–366.

174. Say C, Donegan W. A biostatistical evaluation of complications from mastectomy. Surg Gynecol Obstet 1974;138:370–376.

175. Forrest A, Roberts M, Cant E. Simple mastectomy and pectoral node biopsy: The Cardiff–St. Mary's Trial. World J Surg 1977;1:320–323.

176. Turner-Warwick R. Lymphatics of the breast. Br J Surg 1958;46:574–582.

177. Urban J. Management of operable breast cancer. The surgeon's view. Cancer 1978;42:2066–2077.

178. Meir P, Ferguson D, Harrison T. A controlled trial of extended radical mastectomy. Cancer 1985;55:880–891.

179. Veronesi U, Valagussa P. Inefficacy of internal mammary node dissection in breast cancer surgery. Cancer 1981;47:170–175.

180. Morrow M, Foster R. Staging a breast cancer. A new rationale for internal mammary node biopsy. Arch Surg 1981;116:748–751.

181. Wilson R, Donegan W, Mettlin C. The 1982 national survey of carcinoma of the breast in the United States by the American College of Surgeons. Surg Gynecol Obstet 1984;159:309–318.

182. Mann B, Samet J, Hunt W. Changing treatment of breast cancer in New Mexico from 1969 through 1985. JAMA 1988;259:3413–3417.

183. Aitken D, Minton J. Complications associated with mastectomy. Surg Clin North Am 1983;63:1331–1352.

184. Robinson G, Van Heerden J, Payne WEA. The primary surgical treatment of carcinoma of the breast. A changing trend toward modified radical mastectomy. Mayo Clin Proc 1976;51:433–442.

185. Baker R, Montague A, Childs J. A comparison of modified radical mastectomy to radical mastectomy in the treatment of operable breast cancer. Ann Surg 1979;189:553–559.

186. Turner L, Swindell R, Bell W. Radical versus modified radical mastectomy for breast cancer. Ann R Coll Surg Engl 1981;63:239–243.

187. Maddox W, Carpenter J, Laws H. A randomized prospective trial of radical mastectomy versus modified radical mastectomy in 311 breast cancer patients. Ann Surg 1983;198:207–212.

188. Fisher B, Redmond C, Fisher E. Ten year results of a randomized clinical trial comparing radical mastectomy and total mastectomy with or without radiation. N Engl J Med 1985;312:674–681.

189. Kinne D, De Cosse J. Modified radical mastectomy for carcinoma of the breast. Ann Surg 1982;48:543–556.

190. Lagios M, Westdahl P, Rose M. The concept and implications of multicentricity in breast carcinoma. Pathol Annu 1981;16:83–102.

191. Fisher B, Redmond C, Poisson R, et al. Eight year results of a randomized clinical trial comparing total mastectomy and lumpectomy with or without irradiation in the treatment of breast cancer. N Engl J Med 1989;320:822–828.

192. Lagios M, Richards V, Rose M, Yee E. Segmental mastectomy without radiotherapy. Short-term follow-up. Cancer 1983;52:2173–2179.

193. Clark R, Wilkinson R, Mahoney L. Breast cancer: A 21-year experience with conservative surgery and radiation. Int J Radiat Oncol Biol Phys 1982;8:967–975.

194. Montgomery A, Greening W, Levene A. Clinical study of recurrence rate and survival time of patients with carcinoma of the breast treated by biopsy excision without any other therapy. J R Soc Med 1978;71:339–342.

195. Tagart R. Partial mastectomy for breast cancer. Br Med J 1978;2:1268.

196. Freeman C, Belliveau N, Kim T. Limited surgery with or without radiotherapy for early breast carcinoma. J Can Assoc Radiol 1981;32:125–128.

197. Veronesi W, Salvadori B, Luini A. Conservative treatment of early breast cancer. Long-term results of 1232 cases treated with quadrantectomy, axillary dissection, and radiotherapy. Ann Surg 1990;211:250–259.

198. Recht A, Silen W, Schnitt S, et al. Time course of local recurrence following conservative surgery and radiotherapy for early stage breast cancer. Int J Radiat Oncol Biol Phys 1988;15:255–261.

199. Veronesi U, Saccozzi R, Del Vecchio M. Comparing radical mastectomy with quadrantectomy, axillary dissection, and radiotherapy in patients with small cancers of the breast. N Engl J Med 1981;305:6–11.

200. Veronesi U, Banfi A, Salvadori B. Breast conservation is the treatment of choice in small breast cancer: Long-term results of a randomized trial. Eur J Cancer 1990;26:668–670.

201. Sarrazin D, Le M, Arriagada R, et al. Ten-year results of a randomized trial comparing a conservative treatment of mastectomy in early breast cancer. Radiother Oncol 1989;14:177–184.

202. Straus K, Lichter A, Lippmann M, et al. Results of the National Cancer Institute early breast cancer trial. JNCI Monographs 1992; 11:27–32.

203. Habibollahi F, Fentiman I, Chandry M. Conservation treatment of operable breast cancer. Proc Am Soc Clin Oncol 1987;6:59.

204. van Dongen JA, Bartelink H, Fentiman IS, et al. Randomized clinical trial to assess the value of breast-conserving therapy in stage I and II breast cancer, EORTC 10801 trial. JNCI Monographs 1992;11:15–18.

205. Blichert-Toft M, Rose C, Andersen JA, et al. Danish randomized trial comparing breast conservation therapy with mastectomy: Six years of life table analysis. JNCI Monographs 1992;11:19–26.

206. National Institute for Health Consensus Conference. Treatment of early stage breast cancer. JAMA 1991;265:391–395.

207. Margolese R, Poisson R, Shibata H. The technique of segmental mastectomy (lumpectomy) and axillary dissection: A syllabus from the National Surgical Adjuvant Breast Project workshops. Surgery 1987;102:828–834.

208. Veronesi U, Volterrani F, Luini A. Quadrantectomy versus lumpectomy for small size breast cancer. Eur J Cancer 1990;26:671–673.

209. Harris J, Recht A. Conservative surgery and radiotherapy. In: Harris J, Hellman S, Henderson IC, Kinne D, eds. Breast diseases. 2nd ed. Philadelphia: JB Lippincott, 1991:399–404.

210. Vicini F, Eberlein T, Connolly J, et al. The optimal extent of resection for patients with stages I or II breast cancer treated with conservative surgery and radiotherapy. Ann Surg 1991;214:200–205.

211. Holland R, Connolly JL, Gelman R, et al. The presence of an extensive intraductal component following a limited excision correlates with prominant residual disease in the remainder of the breast. J Clin Oncol 1990;8(1):113–118.

212. Fourquet A, Campana F, Zafrani B. Prognostic factors of breast recurrence in the conservative management of early breast cancer: A 25-year follow-up. Int J Radiat Oncol Biol Phys 1989;17:719–725.

213. Delouche G, Bachelot F, Premont M, Kurtz J. Conservation treatment of early breast cancer: Long-term results and complications. Int J Radiat Oncol Biol Phys 1987;13:29–34.

214. Kurtz J, Jacquemier J, Amalric R, et al. Why are local recurrences after breast-conserving therapy more frequent in younger patients? J Clin Oncol 1990;8(4):591–598.

215. Fisher B, Redmond C, Dimitrov N, et al. A randomized clinical trial evaluating sequential methotrexate and fluorouracil in the treatment of patients with node negative breast cancer who have estrogen receptor negative tumors. N Engl J Med 1989;320:473–478.

216. Fisher B, Costantino J, Redmond C, et al. A randomized clinical trial evaluating tamoxifen in the treatment of patients with node negative breast cancer who have estrogen receptor positive tumors. N Engl J Med 1989;320:479–484.

217. Frazier T, Wong R, Rose D. Implications of accurate pathologic margins in the treatment of primary breast cancer. Arch Surg 1989;124:37–38.

218. Carter D. Margins of "lumpectomy" for breast cancer. Hum Pathol 1986;17:330–332.

219. Danforth D, Findlay P, McDonald H. Complete axillary lymph node dissection for stage I–II carcinoma of the breast. J Clin Oncol 1986;4:655–662.

220. Chevinsky A, Ferrara J, James A. Prospective evaluation of clinical and pathologic detection of axillary metastases in patients with carcinoma of the breast. Surgery 1990;108:612–618.

221. Schwartz G, Rosenberg A, Danoff B. Lumpectomy and level I axillary dissection prior to irradiation for operable breast cancer. Ann Surg 1984;200:554–560.

222. Siegel B, Mayzel K, Love S. Level I and II axillary dissection in the treatment of early stage breast cancer. Arch Surg 1990;125:1144–1147.

223. Clark D, Martinez A, Cox R. Breast edema following staging axillary node dissection in patients with breast carcinoma treated by radical radiotherapy. Cancer 1982;49:2295–2299.

224. Brismar B, Ljungdahl I. Postoperative lymphoedema after treatment of breast cancer. Acta Chir Scand 1983;149:687–689.

225. Feigenberg Z, Zer M, Dintsman M. Comparison of postoperative complications following radical and modified radical mastectomy. World J Surg 1977;1:207–211.

226. Budd D, Cochran R, Stutz D. Surgical morbidity after mastectomy operations. Am J Surg 1978;135:218–220.

227. Larson D, Weinstein M, Goldberg I, et al. Edema of the arm as a function of the extent of axillary surgery in patients with stage I–II carcinoma of the breast treated with primary radiotherapy. Int J Radiat Oncol Biol Phys 1986;12:1575–1582.

228. Pezner R, Patterson M, Hill L. Arm edema in patients treated conservatively for breast cancer: Relationship to patient age and axillary node dissection technique. Int J Radiat Oncol Biol Phys 1986;12:2079–2083.

229. Chin L, Cheng C, Siddon R, Rice R, Mijnheer B, Harris J. Three dimensional photon dose distributions with and without lung corrections for tangential breast intact treatments. Int J Radiat Oncol Biol Phys 1989;17:1327–1335.

230. Bornstein B, Cheng C, Rhodes LM, et al. Can simulation measurements be used to predict the irradiated lung volume in the tangential fields in patients treated for breast cancer? Int J Radiat Oncol Biol Phys 1990;18:181–187.

231. Pierce SM, Recht A, Lingos TI, et al. Long-term radiation complications following conservative surgery and radiation therapy in patients with early stage breast cancer. Int J Radiat Oncol Biol Phys 1992;23:915–923.

232. Sadowsky N, Semine A, Harris H. Breast imaging: A critical aspect of breast conserving treatment. Cancer 1989;65:2113–2118.

233. Healey E, Osteen R, Schnitt S, et al. Can the clinical and mammographic findings at presentation predict the presence of an extensive intraductal component in early stage breast cancer? Int J Radiat Oncol Biol Phys. 1989;17:1217–1221.

234. Frazier T, Noone R. An objective analysis of immediate simultaneous reconstruction in the treatment of primary carcinoma of the breast. Cancer 1985;55:1202–1205.

235. Kroll S, Ames F, Singletary S, Schusterman M. The oncologic risks of skin preservation at mastectomy combined with immediate reconstruction of the breast. Surg Gyn Obstet 1991;172:17–20.

236. Johnson C, Van Heerden J, Donohue J. Oncological aspects of immediate breast reconstruction following mastectomy for malignancy. Arch Surg 1989;124:819–824.

237. Webster D, Mansel R, Hughes L. Immediate reconstruction of the breast after mastectomy. Is it safe? Cancer 1984;53:1416–1419.

238. Stevens L, McGrath M, Durss R. The psychological impact of immediate breast reconstruction for women with early breast cancer. Plast Reconst Surg 1984;73:619–626.

239. Vinton A, Traverso W, Zehring R. Immediate breast reconstruction following mastectomy is as safe as mastectomy alone. Arch Surg 1990;125:1303–1308.

240. Eberlein T, Cresop L, Smith B. Prospective evaluation of immediate reconstruction following mastectomy. Paper Session, Clinical Congress of the American College of Surgeons, 1991.

241. Kessler DA. The basis of the FDA's decision on breast implants. N Engl J Med 1992;326:713–715.

242. Deapen D, Pike M, Casagrande J, Brody G. The relationship between breast cancer and augmentation mammoplasty: An epidemiologic study. Plast Reconstr Surg 1986;77:361–367.

243. Glasser J, Lee N, Wingo P. Does breast augmentation increase the risk of breast cancer? [Abstract] Epidemic Intelligence Service Conference. Atlanta: Centers for Disease Control, 1989.

244. May D, Stroup N. The incidence of sarcomas of the breast among women in the United States, 1973–1986. Plast Reconstr Surg 1991;87:193–194.

245. Weissman M, Vecchione D, Albert L, Moore M. Connective tissue disease following breast augmentation: A preliminary test of the human adjuvant disease hypothesis. Plast Reconstr Surg 1988;82:626–630.

246. Van Nunen S, Gatenby P, Basten A. Post-mammoplasty connective tissue disease. Arthritis Rheum 1982;25:694.

247. Kumagai Y, Shiokawa Y, Medsger T, Rodnan G. Clinical spectrum of connective tissue disease after cosmetic surgery. Arthritis Rheum 1984;27:1.

248. Byron M, Venning V, Mowat A. Post-mammoplasty human adjuvant disease. Br J Rheumatol 1984;23:227.

249. Krizek T. Breast reconstruction after mastectomy. In: Harris J, Hellman S, Henderson IC, Kinne D, eds. Breast diseases. 2nd ed. Philadelphia: JB Lippincott, 1991:491–495.

250. Hartrampf C. Breast reconstruction with a transverse abdominal island flap. A retrospective evaluation of 335 patients. Perspect Plast Surg 1987;1:123.

251. Bunkis J, Walton R, Mathes S. Experience with the transverse lower rectus abdominis operation for breast reconstruction. Plast Reconstr Surg 1983;72:819–827.

252. Shaw W. Microvascular free flap breast reconstruction. Clin Plast Surg 1984;11:333–341.

253. Allison A, Howorth M. Carcinoma in a nipple preserved by heterotopic auto implantation. N Engl J Med 1978;298:1132.

254. Parry R, Cochran T, Wolfort F. When is there nipple involvement in carcinoma of the breast? Plast Reconstr Surg 1977;59:535–537.

255. Smith J, Payne W, Carney J. Involvement of the nipple and areola in carcinoma of the breast. Surg Gynecol Obstet 1976;143:546–548.

256. Andersen J, Pallesen R. Spread to the nipple and areola in carcinoma of the breast. Ann Surg 1979;189:367–372.

257. Lagios M, Gates E, Westdahl P. A guide to the frequency of nipple involvement in breast cancer. A study of 149 consecutive mastectomies using a serial subgross and correlated radiographic technique. Am J Surg 1979;138:135–142.

258. McCarty K, Barton T, Georgiade N. Selection of patients for heterotopic implantation of the areola and nipple. Surg Gynecol Obstet 1980;150:545–547.

259. Becker H. The use of intradermal tattoo to enhance the final result of nipple-areola reconstruction. Plast Recontr Surg 1986;77:673–675.

260. Cuzick J, Stewart H, Peto R, et al. Overview of randomized trials of postoperative adjuvant radiotherapy in breast cancer. Cancer Treat Rep 1987;71:15–29.

261. Schaake-Koning C, Van der Linden E, Hart G. Adjuvant chemo- and hormonal therapy in locally advanced breast cancer: A randomized clinical study. Int J Radiat Oncol Biol Phys 1985;11:1759–1763.

262. Overgaard M, Christensen J, Rose C, et al. Importance of loco-regional tumour control in high-risk breat cancer patients given adjuvant systemic treatment with or without radiotherapy. Presented at the Fifth EORTC Breast Cancer Working Conference, 1991.

263. Griem K, Henderson I, Gelman R, et al. The 5-year results of a randomized trial of adjuvant radiation therapy after chemotherapy in breast cancer patients treated with mastectomy. J Clin Oncol 1987;5:1546.

264. Baron P, Moore M, Kinne D. Occult primary cancer presenting with axillary metastases. Arch Surg 1990;125:210–214.

265. Vezzoni P, Balestrazzi A, Bignami P. Axillary lymph node metastases from occult carcinoma of the breast. Tumori 1979;65:87–91.

266. Ellerbroek N, Holmes F, Singletary E. Treatment of patients with isolated axillary nodal metastases from an occult primary carcinoma consistent with breast origin. Cancer 1990;66:1461–1467.

267. Patel J, Nemoto T, Rozner D, Dao T, Pickren J. Axillary lymph node metastasis from an occult breast cancer. Cancer 1981;47:2923–2927.

268. Kemeny M, Rivera D, Terz J, Benfield J. Occult primary adenocarcinoma with axillary metastases. Am J Surg 1986;152:43–47.

269. Iglehart J, Ferguson B, Shingleton W. An ultrastructural analysis of breast carcinoma presenting as isolated axillary adenopathy. Ann Surg 1982;196:8–13.

270. Bhatia S, Saclarides T, Witt T. Hormone receptor studies in axillary metastases from occult breast cancer. Cancer 1987;59:1170–1172.

271. Rosen P, Kimmel M. Occult breast carcinoma presenting with axillary lumph node metastases: A follow-up study of 48 patients. Hum Pathol 1990;21:518–523.

272. Ashikari R, Rosen P, Urban J, Senoo T. Breast cancer presenting as an axillary mass. Ann Surg. 1976;183:415–417.

273. Westbrook K, Gallager H. Breast carcinoma presenting as an axillary mass. Am J Surg 1971;122:607–611.

274. Ozzello L, Sanpitak P. Epithelial-stromal junction of intraductal carcinoma of the breast. Cancer 1970;26:1186–1198.

275. Fitts W, Steiner G, Enterline H. Prognosis of occult carcinoma of the breast. Am J Surg 1963;106:460–463.

276. Vilcoq J, Calle R, Ferme F, Veith F. Conservative treatment of axillary adenopathy due to probable subclinical breast cancer. Arch Surg 1982;117:1136–1138.

277. Campana F, Forquet A, Ashby M. Presentation of axillary lymphadenopathy without detectable breast primary (T0N1B breast cancer): Experience at Institut Curie. Radiol Oncol 1989;15:321–325.

278. Donegan W. Cancer of the breast. 3rd ed. Philadelphia: WB Saunders, 1988:389.

279. Swain MS. Selection of therapy for stage III breast cancer. Surg Clin North Am 1990;70:1061–1080.

280. Haagensen C, Stout A. Carcinoma of the breast. Criteria of operability. Ann Surg 1943;118:859–870.

281. Fletcher G, Montague E. Carcinoma of the breast; criteria of operability. Am J Roentgenol Radium Ther Nucl Med 1965;93:573–584.

282. Sheldon T, Hayes D, Cady B, et al. Primary radiation for locally advanced breast cancer. Cancer 1987;60:1219–1225.

283. Parker L, Boyages J, Eberlein T, et al. Inflammatory carcinoma of the breast. In: Harris J, Hellman S, Henderson IC, Kinne D, eds. Breast diseases. 2nd ed. Philadelphia: JB Lippincott, 1991:775–782.

284. Bedwinek J, Rao D, Perez C. Stage III and localized stage IV breast cancer: Irradiation alone vs. irradiation plus surgery. Int J Radiat Oncol Biol Phys 1982;8:31–36.

285. Spanos W, Montague E, Fletcher G. Late complications of radiation only for advanced breast cancer. Int J Radiat Oncol Biol Phys 1980;6:1473–1476.

286. Bonadonna G. Conceptual and practical advances in the management of breast cancer. Karnofsky Memorial Lecture. J Clin Oncol 1989;7:1380–1397.

287. Jacquillat C, Weil M, Baillet F. Results of neoadjuvant chemotherapy and radiation therapy in the breast-conserving treatment of 250 patients with all stages of infiltrative breast cancer. Cancer 1990;66:119–129.

288. Ragaz K. Emerging modalities for adjuvant therapy of breast cancer: Neoadjuvant chemotherapy. NCI Monogr 1986;1:145–152.

289. Hortobagyi GN. Comprehensive management of locally advanced breast cancer. Cancer 1990;66:1387–1391.

290. DeLena M, Varini M, Zucali R. Multinodal treatment for locally advanced breast cancer. Cancer Clin Trials 1981;4:229–236.

291. Perloff M, Lesnick G, Korzun A. Combination chemotherapy with mastectomy or radiotherapy for stage III breast carcinoma: A Cancer and Leukemia Group B study. J Clin Oncol 1988;6:261–269.

292. Terz J, Romeroo C, Kay S. Preoperative radiotherapy for stage III carcinoma of the breast. Surg Gynecol Obstet 1978;147:497–502.

293. Zucali R, Uslenghi C, Kenda R, Bonadonna G. Natural history and survival of inoperable breast cancer treated with radiotherapy and radiotherapy followed by radical mastectomy. Cancer 1976;37:1422–1431.

294. Balawajder I, Antich P, Boland J. An analysis of the role of radiotherapy alone and in combination with chemotherapy and surgery in the management of advanced breast carcinoma. Cancer 1983;51:574–580.

295. Gohn P, Heinonen E, Klefstrom P. Adjuvant postoperative radiotherapy, chemotherapy, and immunotherapy in stage III breast cancer. Cancer 1984;54:670–674.

296. Rubens R, Bartelink H, Englesman E. Locally advanced breast cancer: The contribution of cytotoxic and endocrine treatment of radiotherapy. An EORTC Breast Cancer Cooperative Group trial (10792). Eur J Cancer Clin Oncol 1989;25:667–678.

297. Israel L, Breau J, Morere J. Two years of high dose cyclophosphamide and 5-fluorouracil followed by surgery after 3 months for acute inflammatory breast carcinomas. Cancer 1986;57:24–28.

298. Awain S, Sorace R, Bagley C. Neoadjuvant chemotherapy in the combined modality approach of locally advanced nonmetastatic breast cancer. Cancer Res 1987;47:3889–3894.

299. Morrow M, Braverman A, Thelmo W. Multimodal therapy for locally advanced breast cancer. Arch Surg 1986;121:1291–1296.

300. Feldman L, Hortobagyi G, Buzdar A. Pathological assessment of response to induction chemotherapy in breast cancer. Cancer Res 1986;46:2578–2581.

301. Broadwater J, Edwards M, Kuglen C. Mastectomy following preoperative chemotherapy. Ann Surg 1991;213:126–129.

302. Hortobagyi GN, Ames FC, Buzdar AU. Management of stage III primary breast cancer with primary chemotherapy, surgery and radiation therapy. Cancer 1988;62:2507–2516.

303. Valagussa P, Zambetti M, Bonadonna G. Prognostic factors in locally advanced non inflammatory breast cancer. Long-term results following primary chemotherapy. Breast Cancer Res Treat 1990;15:137–147.

304. Bonadonna G. Evolving concepts in the systemic adjuvant treatment of breast cancer. Cancer Res 1992;52(8):2127–2137.

305. Buzzoni R, Bonadonna G, Valagussa P. Adjuvant chemotherapy with doxorubicin plus cyclophosphamide, methotrexate, and fluorouracil in the treatment of resectable breast cancer with more than three positive axillary nodes. J Clin Oncol 1991;9:2134–2140.

306. De Lena M, Zucali R, Viganotti G. Combined chemotherapy and radiotherapy approach in locally advanced breast cancer. Cancer Chemother Pharmacol 1978;1:53–59.

307. Fastenberg NA, Buzdar AU, Montague ED. Management of inflammatory carcinoma of the breast. A combined modality approach. Am J Clin Oncol 1985;8:134–141.

308. Perez CA, Fields NC. Role of radiation therapy for locally advanced and inflammatory carcinoma of the breast. Oncology 1987;1:81–93.

309. Fowble BF, Glover D, Rosato ER. Combined modality treatment of inflammatory breast cancer. Int J Radiat Oncol Biol Phys 1986;12:11–12.

310. Rouesse J, Sarrazin D, Mouriesse H. Primary chemotherapy in the treatment of inflammatory breast carcinoma: A study of 230 cases from the Institut Gustave-Roussy. J Clin Oncol 1986;4:1765–1771.

311. Rouesse J, Friedman S, Mouriesse H. Therapeutic strategies in inflammatory breast carcinoma based on prognostic factors. Breast Cancer Res Treat 1990;16:15–22.

312. Fields JN, Kuske RR, Perez CA. Prognostic factors in inflammatory breast cancer. Univariate and multivariate analysis. Cancer 1989;63:1225–1232.

313. Nance F, De Loach D, Welsh R, Becker W. Paget's disease of the breast. Ann Surg 1970;171:684–874.

314. Ashikari R, Park K, Huvos AU J. Paget's disease of the breast. Cancer 1970;26:680–685.

315. Paone J, Baker R. Pathogenesis and treatment of Paget's disease of the breast. Cancer 1981;48:825–829.

316. Paget J. Disease of the mammary areola preceding cancer of the mammary gland. St Bart Hosp Rep 1874;10:79–89.

317. Osteen R. Paget's disease of the nipple. In: Harris J, Hellman S, Henderson IC, Kinne D, eds. Breast diseases. 2nd ed. Philadelphia: JB Lippincott, 1991:797–803.

318. Maier W, Rosemond G, Harasym E. Paget's disease in the female breast. Surg Gynecol Obstet 1969;128:1253–1263.

319. Inglis K. Paget's disease of the nipple. London: Oxford University Press, 1936:10.

320. Muir R. Pathogenesis of Paget's disease of the nipple and associated lesions. Br J Surg 1935;22:728–737.

321. Orr J, Parish D. The nature of the nipple changes in Paget's disease. J Pathol Bacteriol 1962;84:201–208.

322. Lagios M, Westdahl P, Rose M, Concannon S. Paget's disease of the nipple. Alternative management in cases without or with minimal extent of underlying breast carcinoma. Cancer 1984;54:545–551.

323. Fourquet A, Campana F, Vielh P. Paget's disease of the nipple without detectable breast tumor: Conservative management with radiation therapy. Int J Radiat Oncol Biol Phys 1987;13:1463–1465.

324. Boring C, Squires T, Tong T. Cancer Statistics, 1991. CA 1991;41:19–51.

325. Kozak F, Hall J, Band P. Familial breast cancer in males. A case report and review of the literature. Cancer 1986;58:2736–2739.

326. Jackson A, Muldal S, Ockey C, O'Connor P. Carcinoma of the male breast in association with Klinefelter syndrome. Br Med J 1965;1:223–225.

327. El-Gazarerli M, Abdul-Aziz A. On bilharziasis and male breast cancer in Egypt: A preliminary report and review of the literature. Br J Cancer 1963;17:566–571.

328. Eldar S, Nash E, Abrahamson J. Radiation carcinogenesis in the male breast. Eur J Surg Oncol 1989;15:274–287.

329. Ramantanis G, Besbeas S, Garas J. Breast cancer in the male: A report of 138 cases. World J Surg 1980;4:621–624.

330. Axelsson J, Andersson A. Male breast cancer. World J Surg 1983;7:281–287.

331. Heller K, Rosen P, Schottenfeld D. Male breast cancer: A clinicopathologic study of 97 cases. Ann Surg 1978;188:60–65.

332. Treves N, Holleb A. Cancer of the male breast. A report of 146 cases. Cancer 1955;8:1239–1250.

333. Langlands A, Maclean N, Ken G. Cancer of the male breast: Report of a series of 88 cases. Clin Radiol 1976;27:21–25.

334. Donegan W, Perez-Mesa C. Carcinoma of the male breast. A 30-year review of 28 cases. Arch Surg 1973;106:273–279.

335. Gupta S, Khanna N, Khanna S. Paget's disease of the male breast: A clinicopathologic study and a collective review. J Surg Oncol 1983;22:151–156.

336. Treves N. Inflammatory carcinoma of the breast in the male patient. Surgery 1953;34:810–820.

337. Friedman M, Hoffman P, Dandolos E. Estrogen receptors in male breast cancer: Clinical and pathologic correlations. Cancer 1981;47:134–137.

338. Everson R, Lippman M, Thompson E. Clinical correlations of steroid receptors and male breast cancer. Cancer Res 1980;40:991–997.

339. Kinne D, Hakes T. Male breast cancer. In: Harris J, Hellman S, Henderson IC, Kinne D, eds. Breast diseases. 2nd ed. Philadelphia: JB Lippincott, 1991:782–790.

340. Bezwoda W, Hesdorffer C, Dansey R. Breast cancer in men. Clinical features, hormone receptor status, and response to therapy. Cancer 1987;60:1337–1340.

341. Kraybill W, Kaufman R, Kinne D. Treatment of advanced male breast cancer. Cancer 1981;47:2185–2189.

342. Yap H, Toshima C, Blumenschein G. Chemotherapy for advanced male breast cancer. JAMA 1980;243:1739–1741.

343. Patel H, Buzdar A, Hortobagyi G. Role of adjuvant chemotherapy in male breast cancer. Cancer 1989;64:1583–1585.

344. Bagley C, Wesley M, Young R. Adjuvant chemotherapy in males with cancer of the breast. Am J Clin Oncol 1987;10:55–60.

345. White T. Prognosis of breast cancer for pregnant and nursing women; analysis of 1413 cases. Surg Gynecol Obstet 1955;100:661.

346. Applewhite R, Smith L, Divicenti F. Carcinoma of the breast with pregnancy and lactation. Am Surg 1973;39:101–104.

347. Treves N, Holleb A. A report of 549 cases of breast cancer in women 35 years of age or younger. Surg Gynecol Obstet 1958;107:271–283.

348. Torres J, Mickal A. Carcinoma of the breast in pregnancy. Clin Obstet Gynecol 1975;18:219–225.

349. Byrd B, Bayer D, Robertson J. Treatment of breast tumors associated with pregnancy and lactation. Ann Surg 1962;155:940–947.

350. Donegan W. Breast cancer and pregnancy. Obstet Gynecol 1977;60:244–252.

351. King R, Welch J, Martin J, Coulam C. Carcinoma of the breast associated with pregnancy. Surg Gynecol Obstet 1985;160:228–32.

352. Nugent P, O'Connell T. Breast cancer and pregnancy. Arch Surg 1985;120:1221–1224.

353. Holleb A, Farrow J. The relation of carcinoma of the breast and pregnancy in 283 patients. Surg Gynecol Obstet 1962;115:65–71.

354. Petrek J. Breast cancer and pregnancy. In: Harris J, Hellman S, Henderson IC, Kinne D, eds. Breast diseases. 2nd ed. Philadelphia: JB Lippincott, 1991:809–816.

355. Ribeiro G, Palmer M. Breast carcinoma associated with pregnancy: A clinician's dilemma. Br Med J 1977;2:1524–1527.

356. Bunker M, Peters V. Breast cancer associated with pregnancy or lactation. Am J Obstet & Gynecol 1963;85:312–319.

357. Schapira D, Chudley A. Successful pregnancy following continuous treatment with combination chemotherapy before conception and throughout pregnancy. Cancer 1984;54:800–803.

358. Sweet D, Kinzie J. Consequences of radiotherapy and antineoplastic therapy for the fetus. J Reprod Med 1976;17:241–246.

359. Fisher B. Ten-year results of a randomized trial comparing radical mastectomy and total mastectomy with or without radiation. N Engl J Med 1985;312(11):674–681.

360. Zimmerman K, Montague E, Fletcher G. Frequency, anatomical distribution and management of local recurrences after definitive therapy for breast cancer. Cancer 1966;19:67–74.

361. Gilliland M, Barton R, Copeland E. The implications of local recurrence of breast cancer as the first site of therapeutic failure. Ann Surg 1983;197:284–287.

362. Marshall K, Redfern A, Cady B. Local recurrences of carcinoma of the breast. Surg Gynecol Obstet 1974;139:406–408.

363. Fentiman I, Matthews P, Davison O. Survival following local skin recurrence after mastectomy. Br J Surg 1985;72:14–16.

364. Recht A, Hayes D. Local recurrence following mastectomy. In: Harris J, Hellman S, Henderson IC, Kinne D, eds. Breast diseases. 2nd ed. Philadelphia: JB Lippincott, 1991:527–540.

365. Aberizk W, Silver B, Henderson I, et al. The use of radiotherapy for treatment of isolated locoregional recurrence of breast cancer after mastectomy. Cancer 1986;58:1214–1218.

366. Beck T, Hart N, Woodard D, Smith C. Local or regionally recurrent carcinoma of the breast: Results of therapy in 121 cases. J Clin Oncol 1983;1:400–405.

367. Bedwinek J, Fineberg B, Lee J. Analysis of failures following local treatment of isolated local-regional recurrence of breast cancer. Int J Radiat Oncol Biol Phys 1981;7:581–585.

368. McKenna R, McMurtrey M, Larson D, Mountain C. A perspective on chest wall resection in patients with breast cancer. Ann Thorac Surg 1984;38:482–487.

369. McCormick P, Bains M, Burt M. Local recurrent mammary carcinoma failing multimodality therapy: A solution. Arch Surg 1989;124:158–161.

370. Chen K, Montague E, Oswald M. Results of irradiation in the treatment of locoregional breast cancer recurrence. Cancer 1985;56:1269–1273.

371. Fisher E, Sass R, Fisher B. Pathologic findings from the National Surgical Adjuvant Breast Project II. Relation of local recurrence to multicentricity. Cancer 1986;57: 1717–1724.

372. Fowble B, Solin L, Schultz D. Breast recurrence following conservative surgery and radiation: Patterns of failure, prognosis, and pathologic findings from mastectomy specimens with implications for treatment. Int J Radiat Oncol Biol Phys 1990;19: 833–842.

373. Recht A, Silver B, Schnitt S, et al. Breast relapse following primary radiation therapy for early breast cancer. I. Classification, frequency and salvage. Int J Radiat Oncol Biol Phys 1985;11:1271–1276.

374. Kurtz J, Amalric R, Brandone M. Local recurrence after breast conserving surgery and radiotherapy. Frequency, time course and prognosis. Cancer 1989;63:1912–1917.

375. Solin L, Fowble B, Schultz D. The detection of local recurrence after definitive irradiation for early stage carcinoma of the breast. Cancer 1990;65:2497–2502.

376. Stomper P, Recht A, Berenberg A, et al. Mammographic detection of recurrent cancer in the irradiated breast. AJR 1987;148:39–43.

377. Haffty B, Goldberg N, Fischer D. Conservative surgery and radiation therapy in breast carcinoma: Local recurrence and prognostic implications. Int J Radiat Oncol Biol Phys 1989;17:727–732.

378. Kurtz J, Amalric R, Brandone H. Results of wide excision for mammary recurrence after breast conserving therapy. Cancer 1988;61;1969–1972.

379. Stomper P, Connolly J, Meyer J, Harris J. Clinically occult ductal carcinoma in situ detected with mammography: Analysis of 100 cases with radiologic-pathologic correlations. Radiology 1989;172:235–241.

380. Rosai J. Borderline epithelial lesions of the breast. Am J Surg Pathol 1991;15:209–221.

381. Andersen J, Nielsen M, Christensen L. New aspects of the natural history of in situ and invasive carcinoma in the female breast: Results from autopsy investigations. Verh Dtsch Ges Pathol 1985;69:88–95.

382. Wetzels R, Holland R, van Haelst U, Lane E, Leigh I, Ramaekers F. Detection of basement membrane components and basal cell keratin 14 in noninvasive and invasive carcinomas of the breast. Am J Pathol 1989;134:571–579.

383. Meyer J. Cell kinetics of histologic variants of in situ breast carcinoma. Breast Cancer Res Treat 1986;7:171–180.

384. van de Vijver M, Peterse J, Mooi W, et al. Neu protein overexpression in breast cancer: Association with comedo-type ductal carcinoma in situ and limited prognostic value in stage II breast cancer. N Engl J Med 1988;319:1239–1245.

385. Lagios M, Margolin F, Westdahl P, Rose M. Mammographically detected duct carcinoma in situ: Frequency of local recurrence following tylectomy and prognostic effect of nuclear grade on local recurrence. Cancer 1989;63:618–624.

386. Silverstein M, Waisman J, Gierson E, Colburn W, Gamagami P, Lewinsky B. Radiation therapy for intraductal carcinoma: Is it an equal alternative? Arch Surg 1991;126: 424–427.

387. Page D, Dupont W, Rogers L, Landenberger M. Intraductal carcinoma of the breast: Follow-up after biopsy only. Cancer 1982;49:751–758.

388. Rosen P, Braun D, Kinne D. The clinical significance of pre-invasive breast carcinoma. Cancer 1980;46:919–925.

389. Alpers C, Wellings S. The prevalence of carcinoma in situ in normal and cancer-associated breasts. Hum Pathol 1985;16:796–807.

390. Bartow S, Pathak D, Black W, Key C, Teaf S. Prevalence of benign, atypical, and malignant breast lesions in populations at different risk for breast cancer. Cancer 1987;60:2751–2760.

391. Aasmundstad T, Haugen O. Recurrence-free survival in patients with intraductal carcinomas grouped according to combinations of DNA ploidy and histopathological classification. Eur J Cancer 1990;26:956–959.

392. Kinne D, Petrek J, Osborne M, Fracchia A, De Palo A, Rosen PP. Breast carcinoma in situ. Arch Surg 1989;124:33–36.

393. Carpenter R, Boulter PS, Cooke T, Gibbs MN. Management of screen detected ductal carcinoma in situ of the female breast. Br J Surg 1989;76:564–567.

394. Arnesson L, Smeds S, Fagerberg G. Follow-up of two treatment modalities for ductal cancer in situ of the breast. Br J Surg 1989;76:672–675.

395. Lagios M. Ductal carcinoma in situ: Pathology and treatment. Surg Clin North Am 1990;70:853–871.

396. Fisher E, Leeming R, Anderson S, Redmond C, Fisher B. Conservative management of intraductal carcinoma (DCIS) of the breast. J Surg Oncol 1991;47:139–147.

397. Graham M, Lakhani S, Gazet J. Breast conserving surgery in the management of in situ breast carcinoma. Eur J Surg Oncol 1991;17:258–264.

398. Gallagher W, Koerner F, Wood W. Treatment of intraductal carcinoma with limited surgery: Long-term follow-up. J Clin Oncol 1989;7:376–380.

399. McCormick B, Rosen P, Kinne D, Cox L, Yahalom J. Ductal carcinoma in situ of the breast: Does conservation surgery and radiotherapy provide acceptable local control? Int J Radiat Oncol Biol Phys [Abstract] 1990;19:132.

400. Kurtz J, Jacquemier J, Torhorst J, et al. Conservation therapy for breast cancers other than infiltrating ductal carcinoma. Cancer 1989;63:1630–1635.

401. Solin L, Fowble B, Schultz D, et al. Definitive irradiation for intraductal carcinoma of the breast. Int J Radiat Oncol Biol Phys 1990;19:843–850.

402. Bornstein B, Recht A, Connolly J, Harris J. Results of treating ductal carcinoma in situ of the breast with conservative surgery and radiation therapy. Cancer 1991;67: 7–13.

403. Stotter AT, McNeese M, Oswald MJ, Ames FC, Romsdahl MM. The role of limited surgery with irradiation in primary treatment of ductal in situ breast cancer. Int J Radiat Oncol Biol Phys 1990;18:283–287.

404. Fourquet A, Zafrani B, Campana F, Durand J, Vilcoq J. Breast conserving treatment of ductal carcinoma in situ. Semin Radiat Oncol 1992;2:116–124.

405. Van Dongen J, Holland R, Peterse J, et al. Ductal carcinoma in situ of the breast: Second EORTC consensus meeting. Eur J Cancer 1992;28(2-3):626–629.

405a. Roland Holland, personal communication.

406. Foote F, Stewart F. Lobular carcinoma in situ: A rare form of mammary cancer. Am J Pathol 1941;17:491–496.

407. Schwartz G, Feig S, Rosenberg A. Staging and treatment of clinically occult breast cancer. Cancer 1984;53:1379.

408. Wheeler J, Enterline H, Roseman J. Lobular carcinoma in situ of the breast. Long-term follow-up. Cancer 1974;34:554–563.

409. Frykberg E, Santiago F, Betsill W, O'Brien P. Lobular carcinoma in situ of the breast. Surg Gynecol Obstet 1987;164:285–301.

410. Haagensen C, Lane N, Lattes R, Bodian C. Lobular neoplasia of the breast. Cancer 1978;421:737–769.

411. Lemanne D, Simone M, Martino S, Swanson M. Breast carcinoma in situ: Greater rise in ductal carcinoma in situ vs lobular carcinoma in situ. Proc Am Soc Clin Oncol 1991;10:45.

412. Pope T, Fechner R, Wilhem M. Lobular carcinoma in situ of the breast: Mammographic features. Radiology 1988;168:63–66.

413. Silverstein M, Gamagami P, Colburn W. Nonpalpable breast lesions: Diagnoses with slightly overpenetrated screen film mammography and hook wire-directed biopsy in 1014 cases. Radiology 1989;171:632–638.

414. McDivitt R, Hutter R, Foote F, Stewart F. In situ lobular carcinoma. A prospective followup study indicating cumulative patient risks. JAMA 1967;201:82–86.

415. Rosen P, Lieberman P, Braun D. Lobular carcinoma in situ of the breast. Am J Surg Pathol 1978;2:225–251.

416. Andersen J. Lobular carcinoma in situ of the breast. An approach to rational treatment. Cancer 1977;39:2597–2602.

417. Andersen J. Lobular carcinoma in situ. A long-term follow-up in 52 cases. Acta Pathol Microbiol Scand 1974;82:519–533.

418. Haagensen C, Bodian C, Haagensen D. Breast carcinoma, risk and detection. Philadelphia: WB Saunders, 1981:238.

419. Fisher B, Fisher ER. The interrelationship of hematogenous and lymphatic tumor cell dissemination. Surg Gynecol Obstet 1966;122:791–798.

420. Martin DS, Fugman RA. A role of chemotherapy as an adjuvant to surgery. Cancer Res 1957;17:1098–1101.

421. Skipper HE, Schabel FMJ. Tumor stem cell heterogeneity: Implication with respect to the classification of cancers by chemotherapeutic effect. Cancer Treat Rep 1984;68: 43–61.

422. Schabel FM, Griswold DP, Corbett TH. Increasing the therapeutic response rates to anticancer drugs by applying the basic principles of pharmacology. Cancer 1984;54: 1160–1167.

423. Bonadonna G, Valagussa P. The contribution of medicine to the primary treatment of breast cancer. Cancer Res 1988;48:2314–2324.

424. Pritchard Kl. Current status of adjuvant endocrine therapy for resectable breast cancer. Semin Oncol 1987;14:23–33.

425. Fisher B, Carbone P, Economou SG. L-Phenylalanine mustard (L-PAM) in the management of primary breast cancer: A report of early findings. N Engl J Med 1975;292: 117–122.

426. Bonadonna G, Brusamolino E, Valagussa P. Combination chemotherapy as an adjuvant treatment in operable breast cancer. N Engl J Med 1976;294:405–410.

427. Bonadonna G, Valaguss AP, Rossi A. Ten-year results with CMF-based adjuvant chemotherapy in resectable breast cancer. Breast Cancer Res Treat 1985;5:95–115.

428. Bonadonna G, Valagussa P. Dose-response effect of adjuvant chemotherapy in breast cancer. N Engl J Med 1981;304:10–15.

429. Shapiro CL, Henderson IC, Gelman RS. A randomized trial of 15 vs. 30 weeks of adjuvant chemotherapy in high risk breast cancer patients: Results after a median follow-up of 9.1 years. Proc Am Soc Clin Oncol [Abstract] 1991;10:44.

430. Fisher B, Brown AM, Dimitrov NV, et al. Two months of doxorubicin-cyclophosphamide with and without interval reinduction therapy compared with 6 months of cyclophosphamide, methotrexate and fluorouracil in positive-node breast cancer patients with tamoxifen nonresponsive tumor: Results from the National Surgical Adjuvant Breast and Bowel Project B-15. J Clin Oncol 1990;8:2483–2496.

431. Moliterni A, Bonadonna G, Valagussa P. Cyclophosphamide, methotrexate, and fluorouracil with and without doxorubicin in the adjuvant treatment of resectable breast cancer with one to three positive axillary nodes. J Clin Oncol 1991;9:1124–1130.

432. Bonadonna G, Monfardini S, De Lena M. Phase I and preliminary phase II evaluation of Adriamycin (NSC-123127). Cancer Res 1970;30:2572–2582.

433. Buzdar AU, Hortobagyi GN, Kau SW. Doxorubicin-containing adjuvant therapy for patients with stage II breast cancer: M.D. Anderson Cancer Center experience. In: Salmon SE, ed. Adjuvant therapy of cancer VI. Philadelphia: WB Saunders, 1990: 210–215.

434. Dalton W, Brooks R, Jones S. Breast cancer adjuvant therapy trials at Arizona Cancer Center using Adriamycin and cyclophosphamide. In: Salmon SE, ed. Adjuvant therapy of cancer V. Philadelphia: Grune & Stratton, 1987:263–269.

435. Fisher B, Redmond C, Wicherham DL. Doxorubicin-containing regimens for the treatment of stage II breast cancer: The National Surgical Adjuvant Breast and Bowel Project experience. J Clin Oncol 1989;7:572–582.

436. The Ludwig Breast Cancer Study Group. Combination chemotherapy for node-positive breast cancer: Inadequacy of a single perioperative cycle. N Engl J Med 1988;319: 677–683.

437. The Ludwig Breast Cancer Study Group. Prolonged disease-free survival after one course of perioperative adjuvant chemotherapy for node-negative breast cancer. N Engl J Med 1989;320:491–496.

438. Sertoli M, Pronzato P, Rubagotti A. A randomized study of perioperative chemotherapy in primary breast cancer. In: Salmon SE, ed. Adjuvant therapy of cancer VI. Philadelphia: WB Saunders, 1990:196–203.

439. Frei EL, Canellos GP. Dose: A critical factor in cancer chemotherapy. Am J Med 1980;69:585–593.

440. Hryniuk W, Bush H. The importance of dose intensity in chemotherapy of metastatic breast cancer. J Clin Oncol 1984;2:1281–1288.

441. Hryniuk WM, Bonadonna G, Valagussa P. The effect of dose intensity in adjuvant chemotherapy. In: Salmon SE, ed. Adjuvant therapy of cancer V. Philadelphia: Grune & Stratton, 1987:13–23.

442. Henderson IC, Hayes DF, Gelman R. Dose-response in the treatment of breast cancer: A critical review. J Clin Oncol 1986;6:1501–1515.

443. Tannock IF, Boyd NF, De Boer G. A randomized trial of two dose levels of cyclo-phosphamide, methotrexate, and fluorouracil chemotherapy for patients with metastatic breast cancer. J Clin Oncol 1986;6:1377–1387.

444. Engelsman E, Klijn JCM, Rubens RD. "Classical" CMF versus a 3-weekly intravenous CMF schedule in postmenopausal patients with advanced breast cancer. An EORTC Breast Cancer Co-operative Group phase III trail (10808). Eur J Cancer 1991;27: 966–970.

445. Abeloff M, Beveridge RA, Donehower RC. Sixteen-week dose-intense chemotherapy in the adjuvant treatment of breast cancer. JNCI 1990;82:570–574.

446. Peters WP. High-dose chemotherapy and autologous bone marrow support for breast cancer. In: DeVita VT Jr, Hellman S, Rosenberg SA, eds. Important advances in oncology, 1991. Philadelphia: JB Lippincott, 1991:135–156.

447. Gianni AM, Bregni M, Siena S. Recombinant human granulocyte-macrophage colony-stimulating factor reduces hematologic toxicity and widens clinical applicability of high-dose cyclophosphamide treatment in breast cancer and non-Hodgkin's lymphoma. J Clin Oncol 1990;8:768–778.

448. Gianni AM, Siena S, Bregni M. Growth factor-supported high-dose sequential adjuvant chemotherapy in breast cancer with ≥10 positive nodes. Proc Am Soc Clin Oncol [Abstract] 1992;11 (in press).

449. Early Breast Cancer Trialists' Collaborative Group. Effects of adjuvant tamoxifen and of cytotoxic therapy on mortality in early breast cancer. An overview of 61 ran-domized trials among 28,896 women. N Engl J Med 1988;319:1681–1692.

450. Fisher B, Sherman B, Roakcette H. L-Phenylalanine mustard (L-PAM) in the man-agement of premenopausal patients with primary breast cancer. Lack of association of disease-free survival with depression of ovarian function. Cancer 1979;44:847–857.

451. Bonadonna G, Valagussa P, De Palo G. The results of adjuvant chemotherapy are predominantly caused by the hormonal changes such therapy induces. Opposed. In: Van Scoy-Mosher MB, ed. Medical oncology. Controversies in cancer treatment. Boston: GK Hall, 1981:100–109, 112–115.

452. Valagussa P, Brambilla C, Zambetti M. Salvage treatments in relapsing resectable breast cancer. Recent Results Cancer Res 1989;115:69–76.

453. Padmanabhan N, Howell A, Rubens RD. Mechanism of action of adjuvant chemo-therapy in early breast cancer. Lancet 1986;2:411–414.

454. Valagussa P, Bonadonna G. Mechanism of action of adjuvant chemotherapy in early breast cancer. Letter to the editor. Lancet 1986;2:1035–1036.

455. Bianco AR, Del Mastro L, Gallo C. Prognostic role of amenorrhea induced by adjuvant chemotherapy in premenopausal patients with early breast cancer. Br J Cancer 1991;63:799–803.

456. Goldhirsch A, Gelber RD, Castiglione M. The magnitude of endocrine effects of ad-juvant chemotherapy for premenopausal breast cancer patients. Ann Oncol 1990;1: 183–188.

457. Gibson DFC, Jordan VC. Adjuvant antiestrogen therapy for breast cancer. Past, present, and future. Surg Clin North Am 1990;70:1103–1113.

458. Stewart HJ. Adjuvant endocrine therapy for operable breast cancer. Bull Cancer 1991;78:379–384.

459. Goldhirsch A, Valagussa P. Old and new trends in the adjuvant treatment of early breast cancer. Ann Oncol [Editorial] 1991;2:320–322.

460. Meakin JW, Allt WEC, Beale FA. Ovarian irradiation and prednisone following surgery and radiotherapy for carcinoma of the breast. Breast Cancer Res Treat 1983;3(suppl 1):45–48.

461. Baum M, Ebb S, Brooks M. Biological fall out from trials of adjuvant tamoxifen in early breast cancer. In: Salmon SE, ed. Adjuvant therapy of cancer VI. Philadelphia: WB Saunders, 1990:269–274.

462. Breast Cancer Trials Committee. Adjuvant tamoxifen in the management of operable breast cancer: The Scottish trial. Lancet 1987;2:171–175.

463. Rose C, Thorpe SM, Anderson KW. Beneficial effect of adjuvant tamoxifen therapy in primary breast cancer patients with high estrogen receptor values. Lancet 1985;1: 16–19.

464. Rutqvist LE, Cedermark B, Glas U. The Stockholm trial on adjuvant tamoxifen in early breast cancer. Correlation between estrogen receptor level and treatment effect. Breast Cancer Res Treat 1987;10:255–266.

465. Fisher B, Brown A, Wolmark N. Prolonging tamoxifen therapy for primary breast cancer. Findings from the National Surgical Adjuvant Breast and Bowel Project clinical trial. Ann Intern Med 1987;106:694–754.

466. Tormey DC, Rasmussen P, Jordan VC. Long-term adjuvant tamoxifen study: Clinical update. Breast Cancer Res Treat 1987;9:157–158.

467. Fisher B, Redmond C, Brown A. Adjuvant chemotherapy with and without tamoxifen in the treatment of primary breast cancer: 5-year results from the NSABP trial. J Clin Oncol 1986;4:459–471.

468. Tormey DC, Gray R, Taylor SGI. Postoperative chemotherapy and chemohormonal therapy in women with node-positive breast cancer. NCI Monogr 1986;1:75–80.

469. Ingle JN, Everson LK, Wieand HS. Randomized trial of observation versus adjuvant therapy with cyclophosphamide, fluorouracil, prednisone with or without tamoxifen following mastectomy in postmenopausal women with node-positive breast cancer. J Clin Oncol 1988;6:1388–1396.

470. Fisher B, Redmond C, Legault-Poisson S. Postoperative chemotherapy and tamoxifen compared with tamoxifen alone in the treatment of positive-node breast cancer patients aged 50 years and older with tumors responsive to tamoxifen: Results from the National Surgical Adjuvant Breast and Bowel Project B-16. J Clin Oncol 1990;8:1005–1018.

471. Pearson OH, Hubay CA, Gordon NH. Endocrine versus endocrine plus five-drug che-motherapy in postmenopausal women with stage II estrogen receptor-positive breast cancer. Cancer 1989;64:1819–1823.

472. Goldhirsch A, Gelber RD. Adjuvant chemo-endocrine therapy or endocrine therapy alone for postmenopausal patients: Ludwig studies III and IV. Recent Results Cancer Res 1989;115:153–162.

473. Osborne CK, Kitten L, Arteaga CL. Antagonism of chemotherapy-induced cytotoxicity for human breast cancer cells by antiestrogens. J Clin Oncol 1989;7:710–717.

474. Henderson IC, Hayes DF, Parker LM. Adjuvant systemic therapy for patients with node-negative tumors. Cancer 1990;65:2132–2147.

475. Zambetti M, Bonadonna G, Valagussa P. CMF for node-negative and estrogen receptor-negative breast cancer. JNCI Monogr 1992;11:77–83.

476. Mansour EG, Eudey L, Shatila AH. Adjuvant therapy in node-negative breast cancer. Is it necessary for all patients? An Intergroup study. In: Salmon SE, ed. Adjuvant therapy of cancer VI. Philadelphia: WB Saunders, 1990:174–189.

477. McGuire WL, Clark GM. Prognostic factors and treatment decisions in axillary-node-negative breast cancer. N Engl J Med 1992;326:1756–1761.

478. Bonadonna G, Valagussa P, Brambilla C. Adjuvant and neoadjuvant treatment of breast cancer with chemotherapy and/or endocrine therapy. Semin Oncol 1991;18:515–524.

479. Early Breast Cancer Trialists' Collaborative Group. Systemic treatment of early breast cancer by hormonal, cytotoxic or immune therapy: 133 randomised trials involving 31,000 recurrences and 24,000 deaths among 75,000 women. Lancet 1992;339:1–15, 71–85.

480. Levine MN, Gent M, Hirsh J. The thrombogenic effects of anticancer drug therapy in women with stage II breast cancer. N Engl J Med 1988;318:404–407.

481. Weiss RB, Tormey DC, Holland JF. Venous thrombosis during multimodal treatment of primary breast carcinoma. Cancer Treat Rep 1981;65:677–679.

482. Fisher B, Rockette H, Fisher ER. Leukemia in breast cancer patients following adjuvant chemotherapy or postoperative therapy: The NSABP experience. J Clin Oncol 1985;3: 1640–1658.

483. Valagussa P, Tancini G, Bonadonna G. Second malignancies after CMF for resectable breast cancer. J Clin Oncol 1987;5:1138–1142.

484. Arriagada R, Rutqvist LE. Adjuvant chemotherapy in early breast cancer and incidence of new primary malignancies. Lancet 1991;338:535–8.

485. Jordan VC, 1991. Are we giving tamoxifen for too long? Eur J Cancer 1991;27:1072–1074.

486. Jordan VC. Tamoxifen and endometrial cancer. Letter to the editor. Lancet 1988;2: 1019.

487. Andersson M, Storm HH, Mouridsen HT. Incidence of new primary cancers after tamoxifen therapy and radiotherapy for early breast cancer. JNCI 1991;83:1013–1017.

488. Fornander T, Rutqvist LE, Cedermark B. Adjuvant tamoxifen in early breast cancer: Occurrence of new primary cancers. Lancet 1989;1:117–120.

489. Nayfield SG, Karp JE, Ford LG. Potential role of tamoxifen in prevention of breast cancer. JNCI 1991;83:1450–1459.

490. Consensus Conference: Adjuvant chemotherapy for breast cancer. JAMA 1985;254: 3461–3463.

491. Veronesi U, Banfi A, Del Vecchio M. Comparison of Halsted mastectomy with quad-rantectomy, axillary dissection, and radiotherapy in early breast cancer. Long-term results. Eur J Cancer Clin Oncol 22:1085.

492. Bonadonna G, Veronesi U, Brambilla C. Primary chemotherapy to avoid mastectomy in tumors with diameters of three centimeters or more. JNCI 1990;82:1539–1545.

493. Mauriac L, Durnad M, Avril A. Effects of primary chemotherapy in conservative treatment of breast cancer patients with operable tumors larger than 3 cm. Results of a randomized trial in a single centre. Ann Oncol 1991;2:347–354.

494. Bates C. Clinical applications of serum tumor markers. Ann Intern Med 1991;115: 623–638.

495. Osborne CK, Yochnowitz MG, Knight WA. The value of estrogen and progesterone receptors in the treatment of breast cancer. Cancer 1980;46:2884–2888.

496. Bezwuoda WR, Esser JD, Kansey R. The value of estrogen and progesterone receptor determination in advanced breast cancer: Estrogen receptor level but not progesterone receptor level correlates with response to tamoxifen. Cancer 1991;68:867–872.

497. Jordan VC. Biochemical pharmacology of antiestrogen action. Pharmacol Rev 1984;36: 245–276.

498. Furr BJA, Jordan VC. The pharmacology and clinical uses of tamoxifen. Pharmacol Ther 1984;35:127–205.

499. Sunderland MD, Osborne CK. Tamoxifen in premenopausal patients with metastatic breast cancer: A review. J Clin Oncol 1991;9:1283–1297.

500. Osborne CK, Boldt DH, Clark GM. Effects of tamoxifen on human breast cancer cell cycle kinetics: Accumulation of cells in early G_1 phase. Cancer Res 1983;43:3583–3585.

501. Osborne CK, Coronado E, Allred DC. Acquired tamoxifen resistance: Correlation with reduced breast tumor levels of tamoxifen and isomerization of *trans*-4-hydroxytamoxifen. JNCI 1991;83:1477–1482.

502. Jordan VC, Fritz NF, Langan-Fahey S. Alteration of endocrine parameters in premenopausal women with breast cancer during long-term adjuvant therapy with tamoxifen as single agent. JNCI 1991;83:1488–1491.

503. Ingle JN, Krook JE, Green SJ. Randomized trial of bilateral oophorectomy versus tamoxifen in premenopausal women with metastatic breast cancer. J Clin Oncol 1986;4:178–185.

504. Buchanan RB, Blamey RW, Durrant KR. A randomized comparison of tamoxifen with surgical oophorectomy in premenopausal patients with advanced breast cancer. J Clin Oncol 1986;4:1326–1330.

505. Mouridsen H, Palshof T, Patterson J. Tamoxifen in advanced breast cancer. Cancer Treat Rev 1978;5:131–141.

506. Ashford AR, Donev HA, Hamilton RW. Reversible ocular toxicity related to tamoxifen therapy. Cancer 1988;61:33–35.

507. Haller DG, Glick JH. Progestational agents in advanced breast cancer: An overview. Semin Oncol 1986;13:2–8.

508. Allegra JC, Kiefer SM. Mechanisms of action of progestational agents. Semin Oncol 1985;12:3–5.

509. Pannuti F, Martoni A, Di Marco AR. Prospective randomized clinical trial of two different high dosages of medroxyprogesterone acetate (MPA) in the treatment of metastatic breast cancer. Eur J Cancer 1979;15:593–601.

510. Cavalli F, Goldhirsch A, Jungi F. Randomized trial of low-versus high-dose medroxyprogesterone acetate in the induction treatment of postmenopausal patients with breast cancer. J Clin Oncol 1978;2:414–419.

511. Davila E, Vogel CL, East D. Clinical trial of high dose oral medroxyprogesterone acetate in the treatment of breast cancer and review of the literature. Cancer 1988;61:2161–2167.

512. Gregory EJ, Cohen SC, Oines DW. Megestrol acetate therapy for advanced breast cancer. J Clin Oncol 1985;3:155–160.

513. Muss HB, Wells HB, Paschold EH, et al. Megestrol acetate versus tamoxifen in advanced breast cancer: 5-year analysis—a phase III trial of the Piedmont Oncology Association. J Clin Oncol 1988;6:1098–1106.

514. Parnes HL, Abrams JS, Tchekmedyian S. A phase I/II study of high-dose megestrol acetate in the treatment of metastatic breast cancer. Breast Cancer Res 1991;18:171–177.

515. Muss HB, Well HB, Paschold EH. Megestrol acetate versus tamoxifen in advanced breast cancer: 5-year analysis—a phase III trial of the Piedmont Oncology Association. J Clin Oncol 1985;12:40–42.

516. Santen RJ, Henderson IC. A comprehensive guide to the therapeutic use or aminoglutethimide. Berlin: Karger, 1982.

517. Murray R, Pitt P. Low-dose aminoglutethimide without steroid replacement in the postemenopausal women with advanced breast cancer. Eur J Cancer Clin Oncol 1985;21:19–22.

518. Harris AL, Cantwell BMJ, Sainsbury JR. Low dose aminoglutethimide (125 mg twice daily) with hydrocortisone for the treatment of advanced postemnopausal breast cancer. Breast Cancer Res Treat 1986;7:1–44.

519. Bruning PF, Bonfrer JMG, Hart AAM. Low dose aminoglutethimide without hydrocortisone for the treatment of advanced postmenopausal breast cancer. Eur J Cancer Clin Oncol 1989;25:369–376.

520. Santen RJ, Worgul TJ, Samojlik E. A randomized trial comparing surgical adrenalectomy with aminoglutethimide plus hydrocortisone in women with advanced breast cancer. N Engl J Med 1981;305:545–551.

521. Gross PE, Powles TJ, Dowsett M. Treatment of advanced postmenopausal breast cancer with an aromatase inhibitor, 4-hydroxyandrostenedione. Phase II report. Cancer Res 1986;46:823–826.

522. Dowsett M, Metha H, Smith IE. Endocrine pharmacology of the aromatase inhibitor 4-hydroxyandrostenedione (4-HA) in orally treated breast cancer. Breast Cancer Res Treat 1989;14:151–155.

523. Lipton A, Harvey HA, Demers LM. A phase I trial of CGS 16949A: A new aromatase inhibitor. Cancer 1990;65:1279–1285.

524. Stein RC, Dowsett M, Davenport J. Preliminary study of the treatment of advanced breast cancer in postmenopausal women with the aromatase inhibitor CGS 16949A. Cancer Res 1990;50:1381–1384.

525. Ingle JN, Krook JE, Schaid DJ. Evaluation of trilostane plus hydrocortisone in women with metastatic breast cancer and prior hormonal therapy exposure. Am J Clin Oncol 1990;13:93–97.

526. Santen RJ, Manni A, Harvey H. Gonadotropin releasing hormone (GnRH) analogs for the treatment of breast cancer and prostatic carcinoma. Breast Cancer Res Treat 1986;7:129–145.

527. Harvey HA, Lipton A, Max DT. Medical castration produced by the GnRH analogue leuprolide to treat metastatic breast cancer. J Clin Oncol 1985;3:1068–1072.

528. Jackson IM, Matthews MJ, Diver JMJ. LH-RH analogues in the treatment of cancer. Cancer Treat Rev 1989;16:161–175.

529. Dixon AR, Jackson L, Nicholson RI. The use of goserelin (Zoladex) in premenopausal advanced breast cancer. Br J Cancer 1990;62:32–39.

530. Stoll BA. Combination endocrine therapy in breast cancer. Eur J Cancer Clin Oncol 1985;21:413–416.

531. Powles TJ, Ford HT, Nash AG. Treatment of disseminated breast cancer with tamoxifen, aminoglutethimide, hydrocortisone, and danazol, used in combination or sequentially. Lancet 1984;1:1369–1373.

532. Henderson IC, Garber JE, Breitmeyer JB. Comprehensive management of disseminated breast cancer. Cancer 1990;66:1439–1448.

533. Jones RB, Holland JF, Bhardway S. A phase I-II study of intensive-dose Adraiamycin for advanced breast cancer. J Clin Oncol 1987;5:172–177.

534. Ahman DL, Schaid D, Bisel HF. The effect on survival of initiating chemotherapy in advanced breast cancer: Polychemotherapy versus single drug. J Clin Oncol 1987;5:1928–1932.

535. Garber JE, Henderson IC. The use of chemotherapy in metastatic breast cancer. Hematol Oncol Clin North Am 1989;3:807–821.

536. Tranum BL, McDonald B, Thigpen T. Adriamycin combinations in advanced breast cancer: A Southwest Oncology Group study. Cancer 1982;49:835–839.

537. Brambilla C, De Lena M, Rossi A. Response and survival in advanced breast cancer after two non-cross resistant combinations. Br Med J 1976;1:801–804.

538. Coates A, Gebski V, Bishop JF. Improving the quality of life during chemotherapy for advanced breast cancer: A comparison of intermittent and continuous treatment strategies. N Engl J Med 1987;317:1490–1495.

539. Muss HB, Case LD, Richards F. Interrupted versus continuous chemotherapy in patients with metastatic breast cancer. N Engl J Med 1991;325:1342–1348.

540. Henderson IC, Hayes DF, Come S. New agents and new medical treatments for advanced breast cancer. Semin Oncol 1987;14:34–64.

541. Brambilla C, Valagussa P, Bonadonna G. Sequential combination chemotherapy in advanced breast cancer. Cancer Chemother Pharmacol 1978;1:35–39.

542. Lippman ME, Cassidy J, Wesley M. A randomized attempt to increase the efficacy of cytotoxic chemotherapy in metastatic breast cancer by hormonal synchronization. J Clin Oncol 1984;2:28–36.

543. Scheithauer W, Zielinski C, Ludwig. Weekly low dose doxorubicin therapy in metastatic breast cancer resistant to previous hormonal and cytostatic treatment. Breast Cancer Res Treat 1985;6:89–93.

544. Konits P, Aisner J, Van Echo D. Mitomycin C and vinblastine chemotherapy in advanced breast cancer. Cancer 1981;48:1295–1298.

545. Kardinal C, Perry M, Korzum A. Responses to chemotherapy or chemohormonal therapy in advanced breast cancer patients treated previously with adjuvant chemotherapy. A subset analysis of CALGB study 8081. Cancer 1988;61:415–419.

546. Brambilla C, Zambetti M, Ferrari L. Mitomycin and vinblastine in advanced refractory breast cancer. Tumori 1989;75:141–144.

547. Buckner JC, Ingle JN, Everson LK. Results of salvage hormonal therapy and salvage chemotherapy in women failing adjuvant chemotherapy after mastectomy for breast cancer. Breast Cancer Res Treat 1989;13:135–142.

548. Rowinsky EK, Cazenae LA, Donehower RC. Taxol: A novel investigational antineoplastic agent. JNCI 1990;82:1247–1259.

549. Brown T, Havlin K, Weiss G. A phase I trial of taxol given by a 6-hour intravenous infusion. J Clin Oncol 1991;9:1261–1267.

550. Doroshow JH, Leong L, Margolin K. Refractory metastatic breast cancer: Salvage therapy with fluorouracil and high-dose continuous infusion leucovorin calcium. J Clin Oncol 1989;7:439–444.

551. Swain SM, Lippman ME, Egan EF. 5-Fluorouracil and high-dose leucovorin in previously treated patients with metastatic breast cancer. J Clin Oncol 1989;7:890–899.

552. Hainsworth JD, Andrews MB, Johnston DH. Mitoxantrone, fluorouracil, and high-dose leucovorin: An effective, well-tolerated regimen for metastatic breast cancer. J Clin Oncol 1991;9:1731–1735.

553. Jones SE, Mennel RG, Brookes B. Phase II study of mitoxantrone, leucovorin, and infusional fluorouracil for treatment of metastatic breast cancer. J Clin Oncol 1991;9:1736–1739.

554. Henderson IC, Alegra JC, Woodcock T. Randomized clinical trial comparing mitoxantrone with doxorubicin in previously treated patients with metastatic breast cancer. J Clin Oncol 1989;7:560–571.

555. Jodrell DI, Smith IE, Mansi JL. A randomized comparative trial of mitozantrone/methotrexate/mitomycin C (MMM) and cyclophosphamide/methotrexate/5FU (CMF) in the treatment of advanced breast cancer. Br J Cancer 1991;63:794–798.

556. Shpall EJ, Jones RB, Bast RCJ. 4-Hydroxyperoxycyclophosphamide purging of breast from the mononuclear cell fraction of bone marrow in patients receiving high dose chemotherapy and autologous marrow support: A phase I trial. J Clin Oncol 1991;9:85–93.

557. Kennedy MJ, Beveridge RA, Rowley SD. High-dose chemotherapy with reinfusion of purged autologous bone marrow following dose-intense induction as initial therapy for metastatic breast cancer. JNCI 1991;83:920–926.

558. Williams SF, Mick R, Desser R. High-dose consolidation therapy with autologous stem cell rescue in stage IV breast cancer. J Clin Oncol 1989;7:1824–1830.

559. Borden EC, Sondel PM. Lymphokines and cytokines as cancer treatment: Immunotherapy realized. Cancer 1990;65:800–814.

560. Muggia F. Therapeutic approaches to management of metabolic complications of cancer. Semin Oncol 1991;18:1–31.

561. Warrell RPJ, Murphy WK, Shulman P. A randomized double-blind study of gallium nitrate compared with etidronate for acute control of cancer—related hypercalcemia. J Clin Oncol 1991;9:1467–1475.

562. Seidman H, Mushinski M, Gelb SEA. Probabilities of eventually developing or dying of cancer: United States, 1985. CA 1985;35:36–56.

563. Jones J, Ribeiro G. Mortality patterns over 34 years of breast cancer patients in a clinical trial of post-operative radiotherapy. Clin Radiol 1989;40:24–28.

564. Host H, Brennhoud I, Loeb M. Post-operative radiotherapy in breast cancer—Long-term results from the Oslo study. Int J Radiat Oncol Biol Phys 1986;12:727–732.

565. Rutqvist L, Cedermark B, Glas U, et al. Radiotherapy, chemotherapy, and tamoxifen as adjuncts to surgery in early breast cancer: A summary of three randomized trials. Int J Radiat Oncol Biol Phys 1989;16:629–639.

566. Vélez-Garcia E, Carpenter JT, Moore M, et al. Comparison of adjuvant chemotherapy versus loco-regional radiotherapy followed by adjuvant chemotherapy in breast cancer patients with 4 or more positive axillary nodes: A Southeastern Cancer Study Group study. Eur J Cancer 1992;28A:1833–1837.

567. Overgaard M, Christensen J, Johansen H, et al. Evaluation of radiotherapy in high-risk breast cancer patients. Int J Radiat Oncol Biol Phys 1990;19:1121–1124.

568. Ahmann D, O'Fallon J, Scanlon PW, et al. A preliminary assessment of factors associated with recurrent disease in a surgical adjuvant clinical trial for patients with breast cancer with special emphasis on aggressiveness of therapy. Am J Clin Oncol 1982;5:371–381.

569. Muss H, Cooper R, Brockschmidt J, et al. A randomized trial of adjuvant chemotherapy (CT) without radiation therapy (RT) for stage II breast cancer: 11-year follow-up of Piedmont Oncology Association protocol 74176. Breast Cancer Res Treat 1989;14:185.

570. McArdle C, Crawford D, Dykes EH, et al. Adjuvant radiotherapy and chemotherapy in breast cancer. Br J Surg 1980;73:264–266.

571. Owen H, Dockerty M, Gray H. Occult carcinoma of the breast. Surg Gynecol Obstet 1954;98:302–307.

572. Price P, Sinnett HD, Gusterson B, Walsh G, A'Hern RP, McKinna JA. Duct carcinoma in situ: Predictors of local recurrence and progression in patients treated by surgery alone. Br J Cancer 1990;61:869–872.

573. Hayward JL, Carbone PP, Heuson JC. Assessment of response to therapy in advanced breast cancer. A project of the Programme on Clinical Oncology of the International Union against Cancer, Geneva, Switzerland. Eur J Cancer 1977;13:89–94.

Cancer: Principles & Practice of Oncology, Fourth Edition,
edited by Vincent T. DeVita, Jr., Samuel Hellman, Steven A. Rosenberg.
J.B. Lippincott Co., Philadelphia © 1993.

Jeffrey A. Norton
Bernard Levin
Robert T. Jensen

CHAPTER **41**

Cancer of the Endocrine System

THE THYROID GLAND

Malignant disease of the thyroid gland is a heterogenous disorder that affects all age groups but is more serious in the elderly. No single treatment plan is preferred because of the high long-term survival in most patients with differentiated thyroid cancers regardless of the type of treatment and even with no treatment.[1] The thyroid gland is the most common site of endocrine tumor. Occult thyroid cancer is found in 3% of individuals who die from other causes and microscopic cancer in 10% of individuals who die from other causes.[2] Because some thyroid cancers are malignant and potentially lethal, a thorough attempt to provide definitive diagnosis of all lesions of the thyroid gland is indicated and will suggest the appropriate therapy. Mortality from thyroid cancer equals or exceeds mortality from all other endocrine glands combined excluding the ovary.[2]

EPIDEMIOLOGY

The estimated number of new cases of thyroid cancer in the United States during 1990 was 12,100, with 8900 of these cases in women (Table 41-1).[3] The estimated number of deaths from thyroid cancer in 1990 was 1025, about 9% of the total number of new cases (see Table 41-1). The incidence of thyroid cancer in females was 5.8 persons per 100,000 in 1986, whereas the incidence in males was only 2.4 persons per 100,000 population.[4] Thyroid neoplasms are the most common endocrine cancers, accounting for 89% of endocrine malignancies and for 59% of deaths related to endocrine cancer (see Table 41-1).

Between 1973 and 1987, the estimated incidence of thyroid cancer increased by 14.6%, whereas the estimated death rate caused by thyroid cancer decreased by 20.6%.[4] Most cases occur in patients between 25 and 65 years of age, but thyroid cancer also occurs in the very young and the elderly. For well-differentiated thyroid cancers, age at diagnosis is an important prognostic variable[5-13] and some reports indicate that it is the most important prognostic variable.[6,7,13] The recurrence and survival rates of patients in the low-risk group (men younger than 40 years and women younger than 50 years) are strikingly different from patients in the high-risk group (all older patients). The high-risk age for well-differentiated thyroid cancer is the fourth or fifth decade.[5-14]

Since the report in 1969 by Sampson and associates on the prevalence of thyroid carcinoma in the autopsy population of Hiroshima and Nagasaki, there have been similar studies of the prevalence of thyroid cancer at autopsy in patients dying of other diseases.[15,16] The more carefully the gland is examined, the more occult and minute cancers are found. Most series report a prevalence of thyroid cancer at autopsy between 5% and 10%,[17] except in Japan and Hawaii, where the incidence can be as high as 28%.[18] These small, occult (almost always papillary) cancers are of minimal clinical significance even if lymph node spread is present.[19] However, other investigators suggest that some occult, small papillary carcinomas of the thyroid may be locally invasive and have a propensity for local recurrence and spread to cervical nodes.[20] The prevalence of thyroid cancer in autopsy series does not correlate with increased clinical incidence, recurrence, or mortality from thyroid cancer.[21]

The prevalence of clinical thyroid cancer increases with solitary nodular or multinodular thyroid disease. The evaluation of nodular thyroid disease is an integral part of the clinical evaluation of thyroid cancer. The prevalence of thyroid nodules depends on the population studied. In children not exposed to radiation, the prevalence is between 0.22% and 1.5%.[22] Prevalence increases linearly with age, with sponta-

TABLE 41-1. Estimated New Cases of and Deaths From Thyroid Cancer in the United States in 1990

Gland	Estimated New Cases			Estimate Deaths		
	Both Sexes (%)	Male (%)	Female (%)	Both Sexes (%)	Male (%)	Female (%)
Thyroid	12,100 (89)	3200 (80)	8900 (93)	1025 (59)	375 (48)	650 (67)
Other*	1500 (11)	800 (20)	700 (7)	725 (41)	400 (52)	325 (33)
Total	13,600	4000	9600	1750	775	975

* Other sites include the endocrine glands except the thyroid but exclude the reproductive organs.
(Data from Silverberg E, Boring CC, Squires TS. Cancer statistics. CA 1990;40:9)

neous nodules occurring at a rate of 0.08% per year through the eighth decade. In the United States, clinical nodules are present in 4% to 7% of the adult population and are more common in women than men.[23] The absolute prevalence of thyroid cancer in solitary and multinodular glands is about 10% to 20%.[24-27] Thyroid irradiation increases the incidence of thyroid nodules and the likelihood that a thyroid nodule will be malignant, and after radiation exposure as many as 30% of thyroid nodules are found to be malignant.[28]

PATHOLOGY

Most malignant tumors of the thyroid gland are of glandular epithelial origin and are carcinomas (Table 41-2). Some well-differentiated thyroid cancers grow slowly,[1] so that the diagnosis of malignancy depends on blood vessel or capsular invasion rather than on histopathologic appearance.[21] Because lesions with vascular invasion and distant spread may have a benign clinical course, some investigators argue that aggressive therapy is not warranted.[1]

TABLE 41-2. Incidence and Classification of Malignant Tumors of the Thyroid Glands

Incidence (%)	Tumor Type
	I. Well-Differentiated Thyroid Carcinoma
	A. Papillary or Mixed Papillary-Follicular Carcinoma
70	1. Good-prognosis variants of papillary Micropapillary Encapsulated Solid Follicular
5	2. Poor-prognosis variants of papillary Tall cell Columnar Diffuse sclerosing Insular
15	B. Follicular Carcinoma Hürthle cell
5	II. Carcinoma of the Parafollicular C Cells (Medullary)
<5	III. Undifferentiated (Anaplastic)
Rare	IV. Other A. Sarcoma B. Lymphoma C. Metastatic Tumor

Primary tissue given to the pathologist must be adequate and include the thyroid nodule and the adjacent ipsilateral thyroid lobe. This resection allows the pathologist to evaluate carefully the margin of the nodule or tumor and the thyroid. Examination of the junction of the neoplasm and the thyroid allows determination of capsular invasion. Malignant papillary neoplasms of the thyroid may be multifocal, a finding with adverse prognostic importance.[29] Multifocality has been documented in up to 80% of patients with papillary cancer.[30] A recent prospective analysis of the totally resected thyroid gland from 44 patients with papillary thyroid carcinoma found an incidence of bilateral disease (both lobes involved) of 32% and an incidence of multicentric disease (multiple tumor loci in one lobe) of 50%.[31] An important prognostic feature is the age of the patient at diagnosis,[6-14] which is also an important criterion in staging.[29] An important clinicopathologic observation is the presence or absence of direct extension into contiguous structures in the neck or of extracapsular invasion which affect subsequent recurrence rates.[2,29,32] There is controversy about the prognostic significance of lymph node metastases in patients with papillary thyroid cancer. Some investigators suggest that lymph node metastases are associated with a favorable prognosis,[13,33] whereas others suggest that they are linked to a less favorable prognosis.[7,9,10] In patients with medullary thyroid cancer, lymph node metastasis is associated with a poorer prognosis.

The diagnosis of undifferentiated or anaplastic thyroid cancer has a uniformly poor prognosis regardless of stage at presentation or method of treatment.[34] Because of the problems posed by staging of thyroid carcinoma, a uniform staging system has not been applied routinely. An acceptable staging system based on the TNM classification has been developed recently by the American Joint Committee on Cancer (Table 41-3).[29] Prognosis depends on the type of thyroid cancer, the extent of disease, and, for papillary or follicular histologies, the age of the patient.

Papillary Adenocarcinoma

In the United States, papillary cancer of the thyroid represents the most common type of thyroid malignancy (about 75%). It is the most common thyroid cancer in patients older than 45 years.[35,36] Papillary cancer is characterized by an infiltrative pattern of growth, multicentricity, and spread to regional lymph nodes.[36] The nuclear membrane of the papillary cancer cells is delicate and has an opaque, ground-glass appearance

TABLE 41–3. Staging Malignant Tumors of the Thyroid Gland

Definition of TNM

Primary Tumor (T)

TX	Primary tumor cannot be assessed
T0	No evidence of primary tumor
T1	Tumor 1 cm or less
T2	Tumor > 1 cm and < 4 cm
T3	Tumor > 4 cm
T4	Tumor extending beyond thyroid capsule

Lymph Nodes (N)

NX	Regional nodes cannot be assessed
N0	No metastasis
N1	Regional nodal metastasis
	N1a ipsilateral node
	N1b contralateral or bilateral or mediastinal node(s)

Distant Metastasis (M)

MX	Distant metastasis cannot be assessed
M0	No distant metastasis
M1	Distant metastasis

Staging

Papillary or Follicular

	Patients Under 45 Years	Patients Older Than 45 Years
Stage I	Any T, any N, M0	T1, N0, M0
Stage II	Any T, any N, M1	T2, N0, M0
Stage III		T4, N0, M0
Stage IV		Any T, any N, M1

Medullary

Stage I	T1	N0	M0
Stage II	T2	N0	M0
	T3	N0	M0
	T4	N0	M0
Stage III	Any T	N1	M0
Stage IV	Any T	Any N	M1
Undifferentiated	All cases stage IV		

(Data from American Joint Committee on Cancer. Manual for staging of cancer. Philadelphia: JB Lippincott, 1988)

(the so-called Orphan Annie appearance).[36] Mixed papillary and follicular carcinomas are classified as papillary carcinomas because they have similar biologic behaviors and prognoses. Most papillary cancers are slow growing, and few prognostic differences have been detected.

The variants of papillary thyroid cancer associated with a good prognosis include the micropapillary, encapsulated, solid, and follicular variants.[36] Micropapillary tumors may be called *occult* or *small* and usually are less than 1.5 cm in diameter and detected incidentally. Encapsulated tumors have a well-defined fibrous demarcation between the neoplastic cells and the adjacent thyroid tissue, although capsular infiltration without vascular invasion is often found. Solid variants of papillary thyroid cancer consist primarily (at least 50% or more) of solid elements. The follicular variant is composed of follicles lined by the characteristic clear or ground-glass nuclei.[36]

Papillary thyroid carcinoma varies in necrosis and gross appearance depending on size. Occult thyroid papillary can-

cers usually are small (less than 1.0 or 1.5 cm in diameter) and often are minute. They are sometimes multiple and have no clinical significance. There is a high incidence of occult thyroid cancer in autopsy studies, but most patients (517 of 518 in one study)[37] reach the end of normal lifespan without clinical manifestations or awareness of a tumor. Even if occult papillary cancers metastasize to lymph nodes, the prognosis is still excellent and it is important not to overtreat these occult tumors. Only a rare case of a metastasis to bone from an occult cancer has been reported.[38] The larger tumors usually are poorly defined, although some may show attempts at encapsulation. Associated fibrosis is common, and calcium may be deposited in fibrotic areas. The classic appearance is one of papillary projections formed by a fibrovascular pedicle with its covering epithelium. Mitoses are uncommon. Squamous metaplasia, psammoma bodies, multifocality (30–40%), and lymphatic invasion are common. Whether the multifocality is multicentricity of primary papillary tumors or lymphatic spread through the thyroid has been debated. Extension of the tumor into adjacent neck structures worsens the prognosis, as does the presence of distant metastasis.

Just as there are types of papillary thyroid cancer associated with good prognosis (about 90%), there are types that appear to be associated with poor prognosis. These include the tall cell, columnar cell, and diffuse sclerosing types.[36] The tall cell variant is composed of tall columnar cells lining the glandular and papillary structures. These tumors tend to occur in older patients, to have extrathyroidal and vascular invasion, and to be associated with distant metastases to lung and bone.[39,40] The columnar cell variant is associated with poor prognosis, and patients may die of the disease. Histologically, it is similar to the tall cell variant.[41] Each of these tumor types appears to be more aggressive than typical papillary thyroid cancer.

Follicular Carcinoma

Follicular carcinoma of the thyroid gland occurs less frequently than does papillary carcinoma of the thyroid gland.[2,35,42] Although the incidence of papillary thyroid cancer is nearly seven times the incidence of follicular cancer, patients with follicular cancer account for more deaths from disease than do patients with papillary thyroid cancer (Table 41–4). Follicular adenomas and carcinomas usually have a uniform, microfollicular pattern. The detection of papillae or

TABLE 41–4. The Incidence and Deaths From Papillary and Follicular Thyroid Cancer Among 961 Cases of Differentiated Thyroid Cancer*

	No. of Patients (%)	Deaths From Thyroid Cancer No. (% of Cases) (% of Deaths)
Papillary thyroid cancer	842 (87)	17 (2) (35)
Follicular thyroid cancer	119 (13)	31 (26) (65)

* Data are a tabulation of three recently reported series.[2,35,42]

cytologic characteristics of papillary carcinoma (*e.g.*, Orphan Annie nucleus, psammoma bodies) are not consistent with follicular carcinoma. The distinction between follicular adenomas and carcinomas is based on the presence or absence of invasion of vessels or the tumor capsule. The term *atypical adenoma* denotes a follicular tumor without invasion but with sufficient cellular and nuclear atypia to suggest cancer. *Encapsulated follicular carcinoma* is a follicular tumor that appears encapsulated but has microscopic invasion of the capsule or vessels or both. Nineteen patients with this diagnosis treated with surgical resection and thyroid replacement had a 10-year survival rate of 78%. Primary lesions larger than 3.5 cm were associated with recurrent or metastatic disease.[43]

Multivariate analyses of populations of patients with follicular thyroid cancer emphasize the slow growth and good prognosis of these tumors if the tumor is small ($\leq$4.0 cm), occurs in a person younger than 50 years, and is localized without marked vascular invasion.[42] Compared with papillary thyroid carcinoma, lymph node metastases are infrequent. The prognosis is poorer in patients older than 50 years, in males, in cancer that extends into contiguous neck structures, and in cancer that develops distant metastases.[42] The most important diagnostic distinction with regard to prognosis is between minimally invasive (encapsulated) and extensively invasive carcinomas.[42,44] The growth rate of distant metastases may be slow and they may respond, at least temporarily, to radioiodine therapy if the thyroid gland has been ablated.

Hürthle cell (or oxyphil cell) tumors, when studied by electron microscopy or biochemistry, have been shown to be derived from the follicular cell. Tumors show occasional formation of colloid and thyroglobulin and may have enzymes to synthesize thyroid hormone. Hürthle cell neoplasms usually are composed of sheets of Hürthle cells and not just an occasional Hürthle cell. Malignant criteria for these tumors are similar to those for other follicular neoplasms, namely capsular or vascular invasion. Thompson and colleagues started a controversy in 1974 when they described 25 patients with Hürthle cell tumor, most of whom died, including 3 of 4 in whom the diagnosis of adenoma had been made.[45] They concluded that the diagnosis of oxyphil or Hürthle cell adenoma should not be used. A follow-up study from the same institution indicated that total thyroidectomy for malignant Hürthle cell neoplasms or benign neoplasms larger than 2 cm resulted in a lower recurrence rate than in historical controls (21% versus 59%).[46] However, studies done at other institutions disagree and the pathologist can reliably distinguish a benign from a malignant Hürthle cell neoplasm based on capsular or vascular invasion. The chance of a benign Hürthle cell adenoma demonstrating malignant behavior is low (1.5–2.5%).[47,48] In general, the pathologist's diagnosis of Hürthle cell adenoma or carcinoma corresponds to the clinical behavior of the tumor.

Medullary Thyroid Carcinoma

Medullary thyroid carcinoma (MTC) makes up about 5% of all thyroid cancers (see Table 41–2). MTC is slightly more common in women. It may occur at any age with the highest incidence in the fifth and sixth decades. MTC is a tumor of calcitonin-secreting cells (C cells) of the thyroid gland. These tumors secrete a variety of other hormone products, and plasma levels of calcitonin gene-related peptide recently have

been used to identify patients with MTC.[49–51] Although plasma levels of calcitonin remain the circulating marker of choice, plasma levels of calcitonin gene-related peptide may help predict more malignant tumors and the presence of metastases.[49] MTC can serve as an important model for the study of human epithelial cell transformation. About 20% of patients acquire this neoplasm through an autosomal dominant inheritance pattern, and considerable progress has been made in identifying chromosomal abnormalities associated with MTC. Investigators first proposed that a constitutional deletion of part of the short arm of chromosome 20 was a predisposing factor in some families with hereditary MTC.[52] Other investigators have not been able to detect this deletion in most families with the tumor or in MTC cells grown in tissue culture.[53] Germ line abnormalities on chromosome 10 are linked to three different familial forms of MTC: multiple endocrine neoplasia type IIa (MEN-IIa), MEN-IIb, and familial non-MEN MTC.[54–58] The genetic abnormality associated with each of the familial forms of MTC maps to the pericentromeric region of chromosome 10. This finding suggests that each abnormality is an allelic mutation at the same locus or represents a cluster of genes involved in the regulation of neuroendocrine tissue development.[54–58]

In patients with MEN-IIa, the earliest thyroid abnormality is referred to as C-cell hyperplasia and is characterized by multicentric patches of C cells. These lesions progress to become foci of microscopic carcinoma as cells break out of the C cell hyperplasia cluster and grow. Ultimately, macroscopic foci of MTC are evident. In the future, hybridization histochemistry by Northern gel analysis of mRNA for calcitonin and calcitonin gene-related peptide may help differentiate C-cell hyperplasia from MTC in situ.[59] This diagnosis has been difficult to make pathologically and some investigators have relied on sensitive preoperative elevations in plasma levels of calcitonin in response to calcium or pentagastrin stimulation.[60] These agents are especially useful in establishing the diagnosis of MTC at an early stage. Two recent studies demonstrated that of 41 patients who were from kindreds with MEN-IIa and had MTC diagnosed by an abnormal plasma calcitonin response to pentagastrin or calcium, each had MTC within the resected thyroid gland and 38 (93%) were biochemically cured.[51,61] Furthermore, because familial MTC is inherited most commonly as an autosomal dominant trait in patients from families with MEN-IIa, it is possible to determine who is at risk for the development of MTC and who is not. Using specific genetic markers linked to the pericentromeric region of chromosome 10, it is possible to predict individuals from kindreds with MEN-IIa who are at risk for developing clinical evidence of the disease (MTC) and who, therefore, should be screened periodically for pentagastrin-stimulated or calcium-stimulated plasma levels of calcitonin. Conversely, it is possible to determine who does not need to be screened.[62,63]

In patients with familial MTC or MEN-II, the neoplasm is present in both thyroid lobes.[64] In sporadic (nonfamilial) MTC, the neoplasm occurs unilaterally.[65] The solid, firm tumor is usually gray-white, and the cut surface shows areas of hemorrhage, necrosis, fibrosis, and calcification. The tumors usually are located at the junction of the upper and middle portion of each lobe, the area with the highest concentration of C cells. The tumor cells commonly are arranged in solid, irregular cords and clusters. The anaplastic variant can be recognized only by argyrophilic and calcitonin immunoreactivity. The tumor stroma is hyaline and variable in amount, and amyloid is almost always demonstrated by amyloid stains such as congo red or by electron microscopy. Calcitonin determination in tumor tissue by immunoperoxidase technique has been diagnostic.

The tumor metastasizes by way of the lymphatics and the blood stream. The growth rate of MTC compared with anaplastic carcinoma is slow and variable, yet the ultimate prognosis is not good, with about 50% 10-year survival. With earlier diagnosis and treatment, that is, with needle aspiration of thyroid mass lesions for sporadic patients and provocative testing of plasma calcitonin levels for familial patients, the survival appears to be better than 50%. In recent analyses, the 10-year survival of patients with sporadic MTC is 80%.[51] With MTC in the setting of MEN-IIa, survival is about 90%.[51,66] The prognosis is worse for older patients, patients with MEN-IIb,[67] and patients with large tumor size, lymph node metastases, or distant metastases.[66,68] There is considerable evidence that hyperplasia of the C cells precedes neoplasia. Basal and pentagastrin stimulated plasma levels of calcitonin are elevated in hyperplasia, and thyroidectomy is recommended. In familial settings, the cure rate is high (nearly 100%) if calcitonin levels are elevated and the tumor is not palpable but low if the tumor is palpable (17%).[69]

Anaplastic Thyroid Cancer

The relative frequency of undifferentiated or anaplastic thyroid cancer has been decreasing steadily for several decades to about 5% or less of all thyroid cancers (see Table 41–2).[70,71] The decreasing incidence of anaplastic thyroid tumors may mean that newer diagnostic techniques are better able to differentiate two confusing diagnoses, MTC and lymphoma. In one study, 9 of 14 undifferentiated thyroid cancers were reviewed with immunoperoxidase staining for calcitonin and electron microscopy and found to be MTC.[72] Newer monoclonal antibody methods specific for lymphoma can detect lymphomas masquerading as small cell anaplastic thyroid carcinoma.[73] Electron microscopy studies have shown that anaplastic cancers have cells with features such as lysosomal bodies and microvilli that resemble normal follicular cells.[74] Studies to determine the frequency of hormonal, epithelial, and sarcoma markers in anaplastic thyroid carcinoma indicate that 27% stain for thyroglobulin, 48% for α-antichymotrypsin, and 47% for vimentin. Thirty percent were not positive for any marker, indicating a total lack of differentiation.[70] Keratin and vimentin antibodies are generally found in anaplastic thyroid tumors. Of 32 different anaplastic thyroid cancers, between 70% and 80% stained positive with antibodies to keratin and 94% were positive for vimentin.[34] These findings are nonspecific and markers are of limited value in differentiating anaplastic from other thyroid tumors.

The prognosis of anaplastic thyroid cancer is dismal. All tumors of this type are placed in stage IV (see Table 41–3), regardless of extent of disease. Most studies show almost no 2-year survival. The mean survival in a recent series from the M. D. Anderson Hospital was only 7 months.[71] Aldinger found a 7% 5-year survival in 84 patients treated with combination therapy.[75] About 35% of anaplastic thyroid cancer arises in preexisting differentiated thyroid cancer in the elderly. There may be a greater incidence in countries with endemic goiter.[21]

ETIOLOGY

Radiation

The treatment of thymic enlargement in infancy with external irradiation was first reported in 1907. Subsequently, x-irradiation was used to treat enlarged tonsils and adenoids, mastoiditis, sinusitis, hemangiomas, lymphadenopathy, and acne. Thousands of patients in this country have received neck irradiation for these indications. In 1950, thyroid carcinoma was reported in 9 of 28 children who had previously received thymic irradiation.[76] Many subsequent studies have confirmed the association between therapeutic irradiation of the head and neck region and the development of thyroid carcinoma, salivary, neural, and parathyroid tumors 20 to 35 years later.[77] The risk for developing thyroid cancer is dose-dependent and the risk increases with doses as small as 6.5 to 80 cGy. At more than 2000 cGy, the risk declines. Risk is inversely related to age at the time of irradiation and is highest among children exposed before the age of 10.[78] The incidence of radiation-induced thyroid cancer has been increasing but appears to be reaching a plateau. The incidence of death from radiation-induced thyroid cancer appears to be decreasing.[79]

Marshall Islanders, who received about 1200 cGy from the atomic bomb fallout, showed an increased incidence of thyroid neoplasia, especially among children. There was a linear dose-response relation between distance from bomb blast site and chance of development of thyroid nodules.[80] Treatment of Graves' disease with radioactive iodine does not cause thyroid cancer because the gland receives a dose in excess of 5000 cGy.[81] It seems likely that lower doses of irradiation damage thyroid tissue and lead to mutational changes. However, lower doses of ^{131}I exposure have not been linked to increased cancer rates.[79] These studies of ^{131}I exposure are relevant to nuclear accidents, such as the Chernobyl incident in 1986, which appear likely to increase the rate of thyroid cancer.[82] Studies of people in China exposed to continuous chronic low-dose background radiation for years (330 mR/year, which is three times the normal background radiation) found no evidence of increased risk for thyroid cancer.[83] The incidence of thyroid neoplasia appears to be a function of the radiation dose, with the dose-response curve being linear, initially at 3 per 200 person-years at risk per 1000 cGy. Risk factors include sex (women have increased risk), age (the younger the patient at the time of radiation the greater the risk for subsequent cancer), interval (the more years since radiation the greater chance of cancer), and dose (risk is linear from 300–1200 cGy). Radiation increases the risk for thyroid cancer and thyroid nodules.[80,84] Furthermore, increased secretion of thyroid-stimulating hormone (TSH) as a result of impaired thyroid hormone secretion may play a cancer-promoting role in this condition.[85]

Iodine

Papillary carcinoma of the thyroid may be more common in areas with iodination of salt (United States) or a high-iodine diet (Sweden).[86] In contrast to papillary carcinoma, follicular carcinoma is much more common in iodine-deficient goitrous areas (Switzerland). The high incidence of follicular neoplasia in goitrous areas may be related to the prolonged stimulatory effect of TSH.[87]

Goiters

In the rat, prolonged exposure of the thyroid gland to TSH stimulation induced by antithyroid drugs causes a high yield of malignant tumors including rat MTC. Some series have indicated that a higher proportion of anaplastic and follicular carcinomas of the thyroid gland occur in endemic goiter regions.[21,88] Many studies suggest that anaplastic carcinoma may originate within long-standing abnormal thyroid glands. A history of nodular goiter is obtained in a high proportion of patients affected with anaplastic carcinoma.[70] The preexisting abnormality may represent an adenomatous goiter, an adenoma, or a well-differentiated carcinoma. This striking association and its frequency by history and histology has led several investigators to infer transformation of a low-grade or benign lesion into a highly malignant one.[21,70,89] Some researchers suggest that external radiation may enhance the potential for this transformation.[89] However, most radiation-induced thyroid cancers are well differentiated and behave biologically exactly like excellent prognosis papillary cancer.[90,91]

Familial

The carcinoma of the thyroid that is most influenced by genetic factors is MTC. Although the exact genetic abnormality remains unclear, recent research has pinpointed it to the centromere of chromosome 10.[54–58] This tumor is inherited as an autosomal dominant trait in 20% of cases.[64,92] It occurs in three distinct familial settings: familial MTC,[93] MEN-IIa,[65] and MEN-IIb.[51,67] Papillary thyroid carcinoma usually does not show a familial disposition, but two groups have suggested that it occurs in families and one group has suggested an association with familial polyposis of the colon and Gardner's syndrome (benign adenomatous colonic polyps, lipomas, fibromas, and mandibular osteomas).[94,95]

Oncogenes

Models for tumorigenesis suggest that a series of genetic alterations occur during progression from the normal cell to the malignant phenotype. Mutations in each of the 3 RAS genes (K-RAS, H-RAS, and N-RAS) have been identified in many human tumors including thyroid cancer. In one recent study, normal thyroid tissue did not contain point mutations in codons 12, 13, and 61 of these RAS oncogenes. However, 4 of 19 nodules from benign goiter (21%), 6 of 24 from benign tumors (25%), and 3 of 14 papillary carcinomas (21%) contained RAS point mutations, whereas none of 3 follicular carcinomas had these changes.[96] Similarly, another study demonstrated that RAS gene activation was found in a similar proportion of benign and malignant tumors of the thyroid.[97] Together, these two studies suggest that RAS gene activation is equally prevalent in benign and malignant thyroid neo-plasms. The mutation of these oncogenes may be an early event in the tumoral process.

Thyroid tumors, benign and malignant, have been screened for a variety of gene rearrangements of the protooncogenes, including C-MYC, C-MYB, C-FOS, c-ERBB1, c-ERBB2, c-ERBA, N-RAS, K-RAS, and H-RAS. Only mutations of H-RAS were observed. Of 18 malignant thyroid tumors studied, 4 (22%) had H-RAS gene rearrangement.[98] Some suggest that RAS gene activation correlates with the metastatic potential of thyroid tumors, because 80% of follicular cancers in one study had activated RAS oncogenes, whereas only 20% of papillary tumors had this finding.[99] This finding was confirmed in a more recent study in which 2 of 14 patients with follicular carcinomas had N-RAS oncogene mutations and both of these patients had bone metastases.[100] In animal studies, H-RAS activation has been associated with chemically induced thyroid tumors, whereas K-RAS activation has been associated with ionizing radiation-induced tumors. Another recent study found a significantly greater rate (10-fold) of K-RAS mutation in radiation-associated follicular carcinomas than in nonradiation-associated follicular carcinomas. These findings suggest that radiation may preferentially activate K-RAS gene expression in human tumors as it does in animal tumors.[101]

Using DNA transfection analysis on NIH 3T3 cells, a new oncogene was identified from 5 separate papillary thyroid cancer specimens and 2 of the respective human lymph node metastases.[102] That the same oncogene is active in 5 thyroid papillary carcinomas suggests a tissue-specific activation for the oncogene. The transforming oncogene was called PTC for papillary thyroid cancer and was detected in about 15% of papillary thyroid carcinoma specimens.[103] Later it was determined that PTC is a novel rearrangement of the RET protooncogene and displays tyrosine protein kinase activity.[103] The gene has been cloned.[104] The gene appears to be specific for papillary thyroid carcinoma and has been detected in 19% of a large number of papillary thyroid cancer specimens. It has not been detected in other benign and malignant thyroid tumors including follicular, anaplastic, and medullary thyroid cancers.

Summary of Etiologic Factors

Chronic TSH stimulation appears to play a permissive but not initiative role in the etiology of well-differentiated thyroid cancer. Iodine deficiency may lead to follicular cancer, and iodine abundance is associated with papillary thyroid cancer. Low-dose radiation leads to thyroid nodules and papillary thyroid cancer. Preliminary experimental data suggest that the K-RAS oncogene is associated with radiation-induced thyroid cancer.[101] The RAS and PTC oncogenes appear to play a role in the pathogenesis, with the former activated in various well-differentiated forms (especially follicular forms) and the latter primarily in papillary carcinomas.[54–57,105] Genetic factors are most important in the genesis of MTC and related syndromes. The defect in familial MTC appears to be near the centromere of chromosome 10.[54–58] Thyroiditis does not appear to predispose patients to carcinoma; however, the prevalence of lymphoma of the thyroid gland may increase in patients with severe Hashimoto thyroiditis.[106]

DIAGNOSIS

Clinical Presentation

The manner of evaluating and treating a thyroid nodule is evolving. The incidence of thyroid nodules is relatively high (4–7% of the adult population and 20–30% of the radiation-exposed adult population).[28] Cancer occurs relatively infrequently, however, with a 10% to 20% incidence of cancer in nodules without radiation exposure[23] and a 30% to 50% incidence of cancer in radiation-exposed nodules.[28] For these reasons, the workup of a thyroid nodule should suggest surgical resection for nodules that are malignant and should avoid unnecessary surgery for nodules that are benign. The problem is that no preoperative test can perfectly differentiate malignant from benign nodular disease.

History and Physical Examination

The history may suggest the likelihood of cancer in a thyroid nodule. Exposure to ionizing radiation is a well-documented risk factor for the later development of thyroid cancer.[107] Whether patient age affects the likelihood of a nodule being cancerous is not clear. Local symptoms such as airway obstruction, hoarseness, and dysphagia may be associated with extensive thyroid cancer or goiter. The appearance of a new nodule or rapid growth of a nodule are associated with malignancy but are nonspecific. Because thyroid cancer is usually slow growing, a dominant nodule of long duration needs the same diagnostic attention as a new nodule. The risk for malignant disease in a multinodular goiter is significantly lower than the risk in a solitary nodule.[23] The neck must be examined for jugular or central lymph nodes, which increase the likelihood of a thyroid nodule being malignant; however, physical examination characteristics of the nodule are poor predictors of a malignant lesion. It is important to be able to palpate the thyroid nodule, because workup and evaluation of a nodule are based on the presence of the nodule on physical examination.

Laboratory Tests

Laboratory tests are minimally helpful in the evaluation of a patient with a thyroid nodule. Thyroid function studies, including measurement of serum levels of TSH, triiodothyronine (T_3), thyroxine (T_4), and free T_4, are done first. Most patients with malignant thyroid nodules have normal serum levels of these hormones. If the patient has elevated serum levels of T_3 and T_4 with low TSH levels, a thyroid scan is indicated to determine if the palpable thyroid nodule is hot (*i.e.*, hyperfunctional compared with the remainder of the thyroid). Hot nodules should be removed surgically but are seldom malignant.

Serum levels of thyroglobulin may be of use in the management of patients with well-differentiated thyroid cancer and nodular disease of the thyroid secondary to previous neck irradiation. Serum levels of thyroglobulin are elevated in patients with differentiated thyroid tumors that arise from follicular epithelium and are normal or low in patients with anaplastic or medullary tumors. The levels of thyroglobulin cannot predict whether a given nodule is benign or malignant, nor can they predict whether a cancer is present in a multi-

nodular goiter. After total thyroidectomy for differentiated thyroid cancer with follicular elements, serum thyroglobulin levels return to normal and may become elevated with recurrent or metastatic disease.[108] Serum thyroglobulin levels have been used to follow patient populations at risk for developing thyroid cancer after radiation treatment in childhood. Increasing levels of serial serum thyroglobulin determinations in this patient population were associated with individuals who subsequently developed thyroid nodules and cancer.[109] An increment of serum level of thyroglobulin greater than 18 ng/ml in this specific patient population was predictive for the development of cancer.[109] Thyroglobulin levels are elevated in noncancerous thyroid diseases such as Graves' disease, nontoxic goiter, and thyroiditis. Because of lack of specificity and sensitivity, only sequential thyroglobulin determinations are useful in an individual patient (*e.g.*, follow-up of patients with metastatic or recurrent thyroid cancer and serial evaluation of patients with a history of radiation).

Serum levels of carcinoembryonic antigen (CEA) are elevated in many patients with MTC,[110] but serum calcitonin elevations are specific for MTC and are the most specific marker available in oncology. Combined with provocative agents such as calcium or pentagastrin, calcitonin levels become the most sensitive marker available in clinical oncology.[111] Although MTC is a rare form of thyroid cancer, these tests are useful if there is a family history of the cancer.

Thyroid Gland Suppression

A thyroid nodule is suppressed by administering thyroid hormone exogenously for several months. Supposedly, benign nodules will suppress in size but malignant nodules will not. TSH receptors are present and binding occurs on normal and malignant thyroid tissue.[112,113] Indirect evidence for the TSH dependence of thyroid cancer includes lower recurrence rates for patients receiving thyroid hormone postoperatively than for those who do not receive it.[107] The success rate of suppression therapy for solitary nodules has ranged from 0 to 60%, with 0 to 38% of patients having a complete response and 10 to 60% a partial response.[23] A prospective double-blind placebo-controlled study of the ability to suppress solitary nodules of the thyroid demonstrated that none of 28 patients randomized to receive TSH-suppressive doses of synthroid had evidence of a decrease in nodule size by repetitive ultrasonography.[114] This study failed to demonstrate any efficacy of levothyroxine sodium (Synthroid) therapy for thyroid nodules. Furthermore, the incidence of malignant disease that suppresses is completely unknown. Successful suppression of thyroid nodules does not exclude malignant disease, and confirmed carcinomas have been reported that responded to suppression.[115,116] The lack of suppression to thyroid hormone is not specific for malignant disease; most benign nodules will not suppress.[114] In two small studies in which nonresponders to suppression underwent thyroid resection, the incidence of thyroid cancer was 20% and 40%.[117,118] We use suppression for selected small nodules that have a benign cellular appearance on aspiration cytology. If an aspiration indicates malignant cytology, we proceed to surgery without suppression. When trying to suppress a nodule, measure TSH levels and make certain that circulating levels are actually suppressed on a given dose of levothyroxine sodium. If the nodule increases on suppression, a surgical resection should be done. At the end of 6 months of suppression, reevaluate the nodule with another aspiration if it is smaller but has not disappeared. If it remains unchanged, surgical resection may be necessary. With careful follow-up, delay in definitive treatment of well-differentiated thyroid cancer does not appear to translate into morbidity or mortality.

Radionuclide Imaging

The three common isotopes used in thyroid scanning are iodine 123, iodine 131, and sodium pertechnetate Tc 99m. These isotopes image nodules and thyroid tissue because these tissues trap iodine.[119] [123]I has advantages over ^{131}I for imaging studies because ^{123}I does not have the high β-emission of [131]I. Although the β-emission is useful therapeutically, it does not contribute diagnostic information and adds to the patient's dose of radiation.[119] A survey indicated that ^{99m}Tc and ^{123}I accounted for 54% and 35%, respectively, of the thyroid imaging done in the United States.[120] [131]I remains indicated for uptake studies, for evaluation of metastatic thyroid carcinoma, and for treatment. Malignant thyroid tissue either does not incorporate iodine or incorporates less iodine than normal thyroid tissue, so that a malignant lesion appears as a cold area on the scan.[121]

Thyroid scanning cannot differentiate benign from malignant nodules and can be used only to assign a probability of malignancy based on the functional status of a nodule. Ashcraft and Van Herle reviewed 22 series in which radioiodine scans were obtained and all patients underwent operation regardless of the functional status of a nodule. They reported that 84% of nodules were cold, 10.5% were warm (same as normal thyroid), and 5.5% were hot.[122,123] Malignant thyroid disease was documented in 16% of cold nodules, 9% of warm nodules, and 4% of hot nodules. These results indicate that thyroid scanning does not successfully differentiate benign from malignant thyroid nodules. Cold nodules are more likely to be malignant, but hot and warm nodules also may be malignant.[123] Another group takes strong exception to the claim that hot nodules may be malignant because they have found no evidence for any malignant hot nodules.[124,125] Whether hot thyroid nodules can be malignant is not crucial because hot nodules comprise only 5.5% of all nodules and only 4% are malignant. The problem is that the likelihood of cold nodules (85% of all nodules) being malignant is also small (10–20%), so that the nuclide scan cannot reliably differentiate benign from malignant thyroid nodules. Therefore, we have not used thyroid scanning as part of the initial workup of a thyroid nodule unless the patient has serum levels of thyroid hormones that suggest hyperthyroidism.

MTC that recurs locally in the neck after thyroidectomy and in metastatic locations has been imaged using thallium ^{99m}Tc scintigraphy.[126] This study may help image recurrent or metastatic disease in patients who develop elevation of plasma calcitonin levels after thyroid resection.[126] Thallium is a blood pool marker. Because MTC and thyroid are vascular,[126] thallium is concentrated in the tumor and thyroid, whereas ^{99m}Tc is concentrated only in thyroid. A computer is used to subtract the technetium scan from the thallium scan to image MTC. This technique has been used to image parathyroid adenomas and is not specific for MTC.[127]

Meta-iodobenzylguanidine (MIBG) labeled with ^{131}I has imaged primary[128] and metastatic[129] MTC successfully. ^{131}I-MIBG also has been used to image pheochromocytomas. In one patient with MEN-IIa who had pheochromocytomas and MTC, it also imaged the MTC.[128] Subsequently, it has been used to image metastatic MTC to bone and liver. Because the isotope is taken up and incorporated into the MTC cell, it has been suggested that metastatic MTC can be treated with doses of ^{131}I-MIBG. In our experience, locally recurrent or metastatic MTC generally is not imaged by labeled MIBG and has not been useful for this tumor type. Two recent approaches appear to have developed a more efficacious method. First, anti-CEA monoclonal antibodies labeled with indium or iodine may image metastatic MTC in selected patients (2 have been reported).[130,131] Imaging by this method may have treatment implications, but treatment efficacy has not been demonstrated. Second, pentavalent ^{99m}Tc dimercaptosuccinic acid (DMSA) scintigraphy has been used to image 10 patients with suspected primary, recurrent, or metastatic MTC. It was helpful in 9 of 10 patients, including 7 of 8 asymptomatic patients with elevated peak plasma levels of calcitonin.[132,133] These findings are by a single group and are preliminary; however, if the findings are confirmed by others, noninvasive DMSA scintigraphy may be the method of choice to localize recurrent and metastatic disease in patients with MTC and hypercalcitonemia.

Ultrasonography

Ultrasound examination of the thyroid gland accurately measures the size of a given nodule, determines whether it is solid or cystic, and detects the exact number of nodules. Conventional B-mode ultrasound classifies nodules as solid, cystic, or mixed solid-cystic, with more than 90% accuracy. In one large review of 16 series in which conventional techniques were used, 21% of the solid lesions, 12% of the mixed lesions, and only 7% of the cystic lesions were malignant.[122] A solid mass within the thyroid most often is benign, but it has the highest chance of being malignant. Conversely, a cystic mass is not always benign, but it has a higher likelihood of being benign than a solid mass.

In patients with previous radiation exposure who are at risk for developing radiation-induced thyroid carcinoma, the results of two different groups support conservative management (close observation or aspiration and not surgical resection) of small nodules that are not palpable or are barely palpable and are detected by ultrasonography. The chance of this type of nodule becoming clinically significant thyroid cancer, even in patients with previous radiation, is low.[134]

Ultrasound cannot differentiate benign from malignant lesions. High-resolution real-time scanning depicts most malignant thyroid tumors as sonolucent compared with the surrounding echogenic thyroid. No ultrasound appearance is unequivocal for malignant or benign tumors. The *halo sign* is a thin sonolucent rim that supposedly occurs around a benign tumor[135] and has been observed around papillary and follicular carcinomas.[136] Lymph node metastases from a thyroid neoplasm can be detected and have the sonolucent characteristics of the primary. Nonspecific lymph node enlargement also may appear sonolucent. Ultrasound is observer-dependent and requires a dedicated ultrasonographer. It is noninvasive and sensitive but not specific. It is the most accurate method to measure and follow the exact size of a lesion in a patient on thyroid suppression. It can be used to guide aspiration or biopsy of large lesions (1–3 cm) in the posterior part of the thyroid, which may be clinically significant but not readily palpable. In patients from kindreds with MEN-II and in patients with elevated calcitonin levels, it can detect small foci of MTC that appear sonolucent with calcification.[137] It is more sensitive than physical examination in detecting locally recurrent thyroid carcinoma in high-risk individuals after thyroidectomy.[136] Because of its safety, flexibility, and sensitivity as a real-time extension of the physical examination, high-resolution ultrasound has a role in the evaluation and follow-up of thyroid neoplasms.

Biopsy

Fine-needle aspiration biopsy has emerged as the most valuable aid in the diagnosis and management of thyroid nodular disease because it is safe and inexpensive and has resulted in better selection of patients for operation.[23] The diagnostic accuracy of cytologic analysis with aspiration biopsy has been low in some centers (71%) and high in other centers (96%; Table 41–5).[123,138] The experience and technique of physicians performing the biopsy and of cytopathologists reading the slides appear to be the major reasons why one institution has excellent results and another poor results. We use local anesthesia, a syringe holder, and a 21- or 22-gauge needle in most instances. The lesion should be fixed between two fingers and the needle placed in the center of the nodule for small lesions (1–2 cm) and at the periphery for larger lesions (2–4 cm). We advise taking at least 6 good samples because most false-negative results are caused by inadequate sampling. For a detailed description of the preferred method for aspiration cytology, the reader is referred to the discussion by Hamburger and Hamburger.[139] The difficulty of obtaining adequate cytologic specimens decreases with physician experience and number of aspirations,[138] so that satisfactory specimens can be obtained in about 95% of nodules.[118,140] Large rapidly growing lesions (greater than 4 cm) in which there is a concern about lymphoma or anaplastic thyroid carcinoma may be better assessed by cutting-needle biopsy.[141,142] In lymphoma of the thyroid, fine-needle aspiration may give a diagnosis of thyroiditis, whereas cutting-needle biopsy usually provides the correct diagnosis.[142] This differentiation is important because surgery is not part of the usual treatment for lymphoma. The

fine-needle aspiration cytology and the large-needle biopsy are complementary. In studies analyzing both in the same patient,[141] biopsy has given fewer false-negative diagnoses than aspiration.[143] Reported false-negative rates for fine-needle aspiration range from 2.2% to 10%.[144] The sensitivity and specificity of fine-needle aspiration is about 80% (see Table 41–5).[145] The addition of large-needle biopsy can decrease the false-negative rate to 1% and increase the sensitivity and specificity.[146] The problem with large-needle cutting biopsy is that small nodules (<4 cm) are not easily amenable to this technique. Large-needle cutting biopsy has more side effects than fine-needle aspiration[134] and, in general, has similar or better accuracy rates.[141] Nevertheless, large-needle cutting biopsy of lesions that are indeterminant on fine-needle aspiration may occasionally provide a definitive diagnosis.[141,147] We reserve fine-needle aspiration cytology for most thyroid nodules, but we use cutting-needle biopsy for larger nodules (>4 cm) that are more consistent with anaplastic carcinoma or lymphoma.

When a satisfactory fine-needle aspirate has been obtained, three cytologic results are possible: benign, suspicious, or malignant.[145] Reviewing results from four series with a total of 848 patients, 78% of the patients had benign aspirates, 20% had suspicious aspirates, and 12% had malignant aspirates.[148–151] These data indicate improvement in fine-needle aspiration results with more experience, because previous studies included about 35% of patients in the suspicious or indeterminant group.[147,152,153] In studies in which all patients with suspicious lesions underwent operation, the incidence of thyroid cancer ranged from 11% to 71%, with an overall rate of 36% (Table 41–6). If a fine-needle aspiration indicates a benign diagnosis, the probability of a malignant lesion is low (3%). Conversely, if the aspirate is diagnostic for cancer, there is a high probability that the lesion is malignant (85%; see Table 41–6). The predictive value of fine-needle aspiration biopsy is affected by whether suspicious lesions are considered positive. If a suspicious nodule is not included in the positive group, the procedure has few false-positive results but is not sensitive enough and misses too many cancers in the suspicious group (overall 36% chance of a suspicious aspirate having cancer). If the suspicious aspirate is included in the positive group, the aspiration cytology can diagnose about 97% of thyroid cancers but the specificity decreases to about 70% (see Table 41–6).

The difficulty in evaluating suspicious lesions reflects the inability to differentiate benign Hürthle cell and follicular tu-

TABLE 41–5. Analysis of Accuracy of Fine-Needle Aspiration in the Evaluation of Patients With Nodular Thyroid Disease

No. of Studies	Total No. of Patients	Mean Sensitivity % (Range)	Mean Specificity % (Range)	Mean Accuracy % (Range)	Mean Negative Predictive Value % (Range)	Mean Positive Predictive Value % (Range)
10	1553	79 (46–93)	78 (44–94)	80 (71–96)	72 (50–96)	86 (72–91)

(Data from Cusick EL, MacIntosh CA, Krukowski VMM, et al. Management of isolated thyroid swellings: a prospective six year study of fine needle aspiration cytology in diagnosis. Br Med J 1990;301: 318)

TABLE 41–6.   Accuracy of Preoperative Fine-Needle Aspiration (FNA) Cytology

Investigations	Group	FNA (No.)	Pathology		
			Benign (No.)	Malignant (No.)	Malignant (%)
Hawkins et al, 1987[153]	Benign	336	326	10	3
	Suspicious	28	13	15	54
	Malignant	51	3	47	92
Harsoulis et al, 1986[1094]	Benign	150	146	4	3
	Suspicious	14	4	10	71
	Malignant	26	3	23	88
Abu-Nema et al, 1987[1095]	Benign	89	88	1	1
	Suspicious	28	28	0	0
	Malignant	7	0	7	100
Ramacciotti et al, 1984[1096]	Benign	87	79	8	9
	Suspicious	15	12	3	20
	Malignant	17	4	13	76
Hamburger and Hamburger, 1986[139]	Benign	—	—	—	—
	Suspicious	149	133	16	11
	Malignant	284	66	218	77
Mayo[139]	Benign	—	—	—	—
	Suspicious	233	173	60	26
	Malignant	98	0	98	100
Cusick et al, 1990[145]	Benign	115	115	0	0
	Suspicious	165	39	126	76
	Malignant	21	0	21	100
Cumulative Experience	Benign	777	754	23	3
	Suspicious	632	402	230	36
	Malignant	504	76	427	85

mors from their malignant counterparts.[154] Papillary carcinoma is less of a cytologic problem except when the cellularity of a sample is poor or diagnostic features of cancer such as psammoma bodies are not present. Repeat aspiration or cutting-needle biopsy may be helpful. However, with follicular neoplasms no preoperative evaluation has been able to differentiate benign from malignant tumors consistently. The diagnosis does not depend on cell features but on invasion of the capsule or blood vessels. This distinction is poorly evaluated on frozen section tissue examination and may require permanent histologic examination. Attempts have been made to use DNA content, nuclear size, and nuclear ploidy to differentiate malignant from benign follicular neoplasms, but conflicting results have been reported.[155–157] In general, the potential value of DNA aneuploidy in differentiating benign from malignant follicular thyroid neoplasms is limited, and definitive diagnosis requires histologic examination.[158] Surgical excision of all suspicious thyroid nodules is recommended, because the complications of surgery are infrequent ($\leq$1%), the chance of malignancy is 20% to 40%, and there is no way to identify only malignant nodules.

The real benefit of fine-needle aspiration cytology is for the benign aspiration group and the malignant aspiration group. Benign aspiration results may be present in about 78% of patients.[148–151] Only about 3% of patients with benign aspiration results have thyroid cancer, and the development of thyroid cancer can be detected by repeat aspiration cytology.[148] When 246 patients who initially had a benign aspirate were

followed for 6 months, and underwent repeat fine-needle aspiration, changes in diagnosis from benign to suspicious occurred in 12 patients. Changes in diagnosis from benign to malignant occurred in 6 patients, and only 6 cancers were detected (2%).[159] Another recent study demonstrated that the risk of cancer developing in 641 patients with a benign fine-needle aspiration diagnosis was only 0.7% with a median follow-up of 6.1 years.[160] Therefore, surgical resection is not necessary for patients with benign aspirations. These patients can undergo suppression and careful follow-up evaluations with repeat aspiration cytology. Patients with malignant aspiration cytologies should undergo immediate surgical resection, and they have about an 85% chance of a true malignant lesion. Some investigators advocate definitive surgical resection based on aspiration cytology rather than on frozen section.[149] Most studies demonstrate that this strategy results in occasional incorrect diagnoses and that operative frozen section determination or postoperative permanent section determination is necessary before proceeding with a definitive cancer-type operation.[161,162]

Fine-needle aspiration cytology has had a substantial impact on the management of thyroid nodules and provides far more diagnostic information than any other diagnostic technique. Workup of nodules with history, physical examination, thyroid scan, and ultrasound yielded only 10% to 20% malignancy rates in surgically resected nodules. Fine-needle aspiration cytology has halved the number of patients who undergo operations and has doubled the incidence (40%) of malignant disease found at surgical resection.[23] This effect has been estimated to eliminate significant health care costs in the management of patients with a thyroid nodule.[150,151]

Standard Workup

The initial step in patient evaluation is a careful history of childhood irradiation, including the dose and the interval from treatment to presentation with a thyroid nodule. Physical examination determines the size and location of the nodule or nodules. Careful palpation is required to detect jugular, supraclavicular, and submandibular lymph nodes. Hoarseness, difficulty swallowing liquids, or dyspnea with exertion may necessitate indirect laryngoscopy. Fine-needle aspiration cytology is the primary diagnostic procedure for smaller lesions (≤4 cm). Ultrasound is used to measure exact lesion size before suppression and to ensure that no larger thyroid masses or suspicious lymph nodes have been missed. If the lesion appears totally cystic on ultrasound, aspiration may completely eliminate it. If the thyroid mass is large (>4 cm), cutting-needle biopsy is the preferred diagnostic maneuver. Therapeutic intervention is based on biopsy results.

If the fine-needle aspiration cytology or biopsy is benign, ultrasound is used to measure the mass and thyroid suppression is started. It the results are suspicious or malignant, surgical resection is indicated. During TSH suppression therapy for benign tumors, the responsible physician must be certain that TSH levels are actually suppressed by the dose of levothyroxine sodium. If the nodule remains unchanged or decreases without resolution after 6 months, repeat aspiration cytology is indicated. If the nodule increases in size, surgical resection is indicated. Nodule size can be accurately reevaluated by physical examination and ultrasound as necessary. The entire scheme is outlined in Figure 41-1.

TREATMENT

Thyroid Nodules: Surgical Approach

Once the decision is made to operate, surgical resection is performed on the assumption that the nodule represents a carcinoma. Nodule excision is not performed. Thyroid lobectomy of the ipsilateral thyroid lobe is the procedure of choice. For isthmus lesions, the isthmus is resected along with the lobe in closer propinquity to the nodule. The pathologist needs the relation of the nodule to the adjacent normal thyroid to make the diagnosis. In addition, in the event that a given nodule is malignant and a simple nodulectomy is performed, any reoperation in the same lobe is technically difficult and increases the risk for recurrent laryngeal nerve injury sixfold. The local recurrence rate of a simple nodulectomy compared with a lobectomy may be higher because some well-differentiated carcinomas are multifocal or multicentric (about 20–40%).[152]

Most studies that have considered the extent of thyroid resection for primary well-differential thyroid carcinoma (*i.e.*, total thyroidectomy versus subtotal or partial thyroidectomy) have concluded that subtotal resection is preferred, especially in patients with small tumors (about 1 cm) and younger than 45 years.[163,164] The reasons are that there is no difference in survival or recurrence rates between the two groups and that total thyroidectomy is associated with greater morbidity. In older patients with larger, locally aggressive, or metastatic well-differentiated tumors, near-total

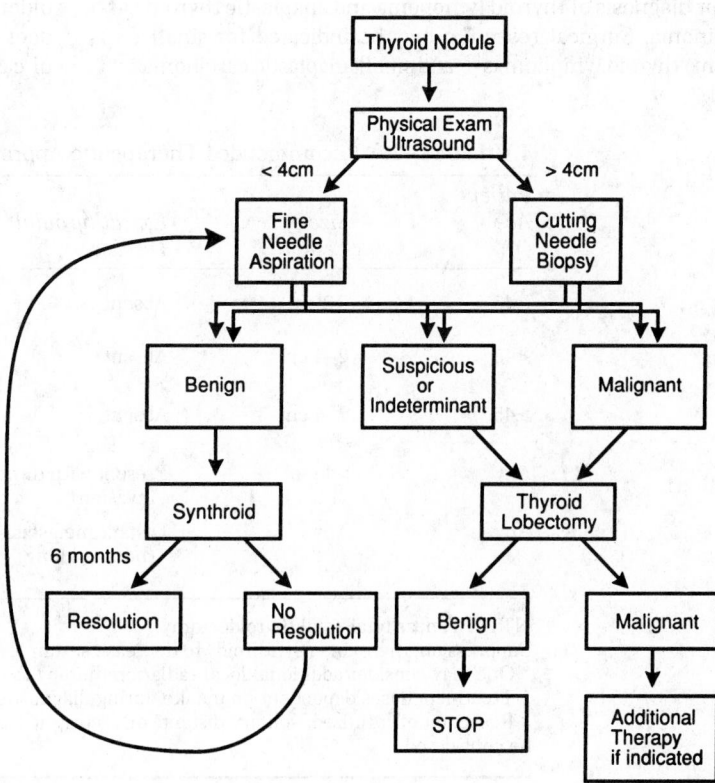

FIGURE 41-1. Flow diagram for evaluation of a thyroid nodule.

or total thyroidectomy is preferred because the tumors may be bilateral or multifocal, and tumor treatment with ^{131}I is facilitated. Prospective randomized trials regarding the extent of resection for thyroid carcinoma have not been done and may be impossible because of the slow-growing benign nature of the neoplasm in most patients. Thyroid carcinoma can behave like cancer in older patients with large tumors and extracapsular invasion.[5–13,32,165,166]

If the nodule is benign on frozen section, malignant, and small, or if the pathologist cannot be certain of malignancy, the operative procedure may be terminated with one lobe removed. The contralateral lobe is exposed and carefully palpated to make certain that no obvious tumors or suspicious nodules are present in it. If permanent pathology results indicate that the removed nodule is malignant, we use the same criteria used intraoperatively to remove the contralateral lobe. Indications for completion of near-total thyroidectomy include large lesions (>2 cm), older patients, and poor-prognosis variants of papillary thyroid cancer including tall cell, columnar, diffuse sclerosing, and follicular cancers. This point is controversial and some surgeons would not reoperate.[167] The risk of a reoperation on the contralateral lobe done before 1 week postoperatively is no greater than the same procedure performed at the initial operation. The risk would increase if the lobe was extensively dissected and about 1 month had passed.

Management of Well-Differentiated Thyroid Cancer

Surgery

Surgical resection is the method of choice for exact diagnosis and initial treatment of well-differentiated thyroid carcinoma and MTC. Large-needle biopsy is the preferred method for diagnosis of thyroid lymphoma and anaplastic thyroid carcinoma. Surgical resection may be indicated for small (<3 cm) thyroid lymphomas[168] and small anaplastic carcinomas,[169] but most of these malignancies present with large bulky lesions and surgery has no role in treatment. The extent of surgical resection and adjuvant treatment for well-differentiated thyroid carcinoma is given in Table 41–7. In general, the use of near-total or total thyroidectomy is advocated except in younger patients with tumors less than 2 cm and no evidence of lymph nodes or extrathyroidal disease. In patients undergoing near-total or total thyroidectomy for well-differentiated thyroid carcinoma, the incidence of disease in the contralateral lobe ranges from 20% to 87%.[152,170]

Tumors recur in the neck more than twice as often in patients who have had subtotal thyroidectomy than in patients who have had total thyroidectomy, although these recurrences are not associated with decreased survival. Another argument for total thyroidectomy is the ease of subsequent documentation of recurrent or metastatic disease by serum thyroglobulin determination and ^{131}I uptake. [131]I ablation doses are reduced so that treatment doses can be administered within a safer range. Studies report no postoperative mortality after total thyroidectomy for differentiated thyroid carcinomas. The incidence of permanent recurrent laryngeal nerve damage is 2% to 2.5%, and there is a 1% to 2.7% incidence of permanent hypoparathyroidism.[171] Experienced thyroid surgeons can perform total thyroidectomy safely. In patients with papillary and follicular thyroid carcinoma, TSH-suppressive doses of thyroid hormone and ^{131}I ablation after thyroidectomy have been demonstrated to decrease recurrence rates, but neither treatment has been shown to improve survival.[107,172] The presence of lymph node metastases at diagnosis is not associated with decreased survival rates but is associated with increased local recurrence rates. The correlation of younger age with frequent nodal metastases and older age with less frequent nodal metastases suggests a biologic difference between risk groups with thyroid cancer. Even in poor-prognosis older patients with thyroid cancer, lymph node involvement does not appear to influence survival as seen in other types of cancer.[6]

TABLE 41–7. Recommended Therapeutic Approach to Well-Differentiated Thyroid

Patient Age (y)	Size of Lesion	Extrathyroidal Disease	Recommended Therapy
<45	<2 cm	Absent	Thyroid lobectomy or NTT with suppression
<45	2–4 cm	Absent	NTT/TT with suppression ^{131}I ablation and treatment†
≥45	2–4 cm	Absent	NTT/TT with suppression ^{131}I ablation and treatment
Any	>4 cm*	Present with direct invasion†	NTT/TT with suppression ^{131}I ablation and treatment
Any	Any	Distant metastasis‡ (bone on lung)	NTT/TT with suppression ^{131}I ablation and treatment

NTT/TT, near total/total thyroidectomy.
Suppression, thyroxine (Synthroid) to decrease serum levels of TSH.
* One may consider additional local radiation therapy (see text).
† Treatment doses dependent on uptake during diagnostic whole-body scan.
‡ Resection of localized, solitary distant, or recurrent local well-differentiated thyroid cancer may be considered.

In general, the prognosis of well-differentiated thyroid cancer is excellent as long as some type of thyroid resection is performed. In certain risk groups, ^{131}I is added, along with levothyroxine sodium (Synthroid) to suppress serum levels of TSH. A suggested treatment strategy is outlined in Table 41–7. Certain factors indicate more aggressive disease and may dictate more aggressive treatment. The higher risk factors include distant metastases at presentation, older age (>45 years), males, direct invasion into adjacent structures from large primary lesions, and poor-prognosis variants of papillary including those with tall cell, columnar, diffuse sclerosing, and follicular histology.[5,7,10,32,44,162,165,173] Contrary to previous reports, radiation-induced thyroid carcinoma does not worsen prognosis[91] but behaves exactly like well-differentiated thyroid carcinoma. Regardless of the type of treatment, the survival of patients with papillary or follicular thyroid carcinoma is excellent as long as surgical resection is performed with or without levothyroxine sodium or [131]I (Table 41–8). The major morbidity and mortality appear to occur in elderly patients (5%) who present with locally advanced or distant disease. The use of more aggressive treatment strategies may be indicated in this subgroup.

Management of Hürthle Cell Neoplasia

Hürthle cell neoplasms of the thyroid, also called *oxyphil cell tumors*, are really a subgroup of follicular carcinomas of the thyroid gland.[21,174] The histologic appearance is not merely an occasional oxyphil or Hürthle cell, but rather sheets of uniform Hürthle cells. The controversy regarding these tumors comes from a single institution's experience in which the authors describe Hürthle cell neoplasms larger than 2 cm that resulted in metastatic or locally recurrent disease and death of the patient, even in the absence of vascular or capsular invasion.[45,46] This study indicates that total thyroidectomy for all histologically malignant tumors and for tumors greater than 2 cm in size results in a lower recurrence rate (21% versus 59%) than a historical control group.[46] Rosen and colleagues reported that 9% of patients with Hürthle cell malignancies had carcinoma in the contralateral lobe after total thyroidectomy and that 12% of patients developed contralateral lobe tumors after lobectomy.[175] Therefore, the incidence of bilateral malignant Hürthle cell neoplasms was about 10%.[175]

The first question that must be answered about Hürthle cell neoplasms of the thyroid gland is whether they usually appear benign or malignant. A review of nine series indicates that most of these neoplasms appear benign pathologically; that is, they do not have vascular or capsular invasion (Table 41–9). The recurrence rate in tumors that are diagnosed as malignant pathologically ranges from 25% to 53%. Malignant Hürthle cell carcinomas have been found to have a greater proportion of aneuploidy on flow cytometry studies, but the hallmark pathologic finding of malignancy remains capsular or vascular invasion.[176,177] The 10-year survival for malignant Hürthle cell carcinoma ranges from 65% to 95%, with a median survival of 80%.[176] The recurrence rate in tumors that are diagnosed as benign ranges from no recurrence to 12%, with a mean rate of 2% (see Table 41–9). This review indicates that most Hürthle cell neoplasms are benign and act benign after thyroid lobectomy. If the pathologist diagnoses a malignant Hürthle cell carcinoma, there is a higher incidence of recurrent disease. Total or near-total thyroidectomy is advocated for Hürthle cell carcinomas proved pathologically. Total thyroidectomy should not be performed for all Hürthle cell neoplasms. Recent updated reviews corroborate this approach.[174,176-178]

TABLE 41–8. Survival of Well-Differentiated Thyroid Carcinoma After Treatment

Investigations	No. of Patients	5-Year Survival (%)	10-Year Survival (%)	20-Year Survival (%)
Papillary				
Schroder et al, 1986[1097]	104	97	—	—
McConahey et al, 1986[152]	859	—	—	93
Mazzaferri et al, 1977[107]	576	—	92.4	—
Joensuu et al, 1986[5]	121	92	74	—
Akslen et al, 1991[7]	1528	93	—	—
Simpson et al, 1987[10]	1074	90	87	—
Radiation-Induced Papillary Carcinoma				
Schneider et al, 1985[77]	296	—	99	—
Follicular Carcinoma				
Schroder et al, 1986[1097]	23	96	—	—
Lang et al, 1986[44]	170	—	94	—
Harness et al, 1984[173]	37	—	84	—
Crile et al, 1985[1098]	84	73	43	—
Joensuu et al, 1986[5]	46	87	66	—
Akslen et al, 1991[7]	459	83	—	—
Simpson et al, 1987[10]	504	75	65	—

TABLE 41–9. Incidence of Hürthle Cell Carcinoma, Recurrence Rates, and Late Metastases in Patients With Hürthle Cell Neoplasm of the Thyroid Gland

Investigations	No. of Patients With Hürthle Cell Tumors (Benign and Malignant)	No. of Patients With Benign Tumors (%)	Recurrence Rate in Malignant Tumors (%)	Recurrence Rate in Benign Tumors (%)
Thompson et al, 1974[45]	62	26 (42)	29	12
Heppe et al, 1985[47]	20	10 (50)	—	0
Savino et al, 1981[1099]	42	27 (64)	53	0
Rosen et al, 1985[175]	34	25 (73)	—	0
Bondeson et al, 1981[183]	42	34 (81)	25	0
Arganini et al, 1986[48]	47	40 (85)	43	2.5
Caplan et al, 1984[1100]	27	24 (88)	33	0
Gosain and Clark, 1984[1101]	75	71 (95)	25	0
Bronner and LiVolis, 1988[174]	50	34 (68)	31	0
Total	399	291 (73)	34	2

(Modified from Arganini M, Behar R, Wu C, et al. Hürthle cell tumors: a twenty-five year experience. Surgery 1986;100:1108)

Management of Radiation-Induced Thyroid Carcinoma

There is considerable evidence that clinically inapparent thyroid cancer, even radiation-induced occult thyroid cancer, runs an indolent course and does not result in morbidity or mortality. Autopsy studies demonstrate that there is increased papillary cancer in patients exposed to previous radiation, that the clinical course of that cancer was benign, and that the patients died of other causes.[2,15,17] Experience with radiation-induced thyroid carcinoma compared with thyroid carcinoma in patients with no history of head and neck irradiation demonstrates that patients with previous thyroid irradiation more often present with cancer not limited to the thyroid gland and bilateral thyroid lobe involvement.[179] The prognosis of well-differentiated thyroid cancer in patients with a history of irradiation was similar to the prognosis of patients with the same disease extent but without such a history.[179] These data underline the importance of careful follow-up with physical examination and serial serum thyroglobulin levels as a predictor of new malignancy.[109] If a patient has a history of head and neck irradiation, other risk factors can make the patient likely to develop cancer, including higher doses, being female, and younger age at the time of irradiation. Some groups recommend total thyroidectomy for all radiation-induced thyroid carcinomas because the incidence of bilaterality is high (54–75%).[180] However, a prospective study indicated that although thyroid lobectomy may leave occult malignancies in unresected thyroid tissue, there was no significant difference in outcome between patients with limited resection and total thyroidectomy after a 12-year follow-up.[181]

The administration of thyroid hormone to suppress TSH levels has reduced the number of postresection recurrences in radiation-induced papillary and follicular carcinoma.[91] No reduction in recurrence rate could be demonstrated with a greater extent of surgical resection or with the administration of postoperative radioactive iodine,[91] which has been advocated in all radiation-induced carcinomas by some researchers.[182] The clinical course of radiation-induced thyroid carcinoma appears to be similar to neoplasms without a history

of radiation (Table 41–8), and therapy should be similar to that of other well-differentiated thyroid carcinomas (see Table 41–7). Furthermore, some investigators estimate that the incidence of radiation-induced thyroid cancer is decreasing.[178]

Postoperative Therapy and Follow-up of Well-Differentiated Thyroid Cancers

There is good evidence that all patients with well-differentiated thyroid cancer should take thyroid hormone (Synthroid) postoperatively to suppress TSH levels.[107,172] This treatment can decrease the recurrence rate of radiation-induced thyroid carcinoma,[91] although reduced recurrence rates do not appear to translate into any difference in survival with the use of levothyroxine sodium postoperatively.[10,107,172] We recommend the postoperative administration of levothyroxine sodium to suppress TSH levels in all patients with thyroid carcinoma (see Table 41–7). The use of postoperative ^{131}I therapy has provided similar data; that is, decreased recurrence rates but no prolongation of survival.[10,112,183] Ablative doses of [131]I (30 mCi) should be administered postoperatively to the following patients with primary well-differentiated thyroid cancers: patients older than 45 years, patients with multiple or locally invasive tumors or tumors larger than 2.5 cm, and patients with local or distant metastases, provided adequate uptake of the radionuclide can be demonstrated on scan (see Table 41–7).[182]

Locally recurrent disease in the neck that is detected by physical examination or ultrasound should be surgically excised if the procedure can be performed with low morbidity. Radical neck dissections are not indicated for differentiated thyroid carcinoma. Localized distant metastases that do not take up radioiodine may be resected.[2] External-beam irradiation may be of benefit for less differentiated recurrent or locally advanced lesions (see the section on treatment of anaplastic carcinoma). Metastatic thyroid carcinoma confined to lung has been treated successfully by radioactive iodine, and 54% of patients were alive and without disease 20 years after ^{131}I treatment.[184] In contrast, patients with bony involvement treated by radioactive iodine seldom survive 10 years after treatment.[184] Some patients who have localized bony metastases that take up iodine on whole-body scan and who are treated with radioactive iodine plus aggressive surgery may be rendered disease free, and 30% of patients are still alive at 86 months.[185] After a successful ablative dose of ^{131}I and failure to find extrathyroidal uptake, a patient should be given thyroid hormone replacement (levothyroxine sodium) and TSH levels should be measured to ensure suppression. If the ablation is successful, the patient is not scanned again unless serum thyroglobulin levels are persistently elevated or become elevated, suggesting recurrent or persistent disease.[186]

In a recent study of 98 patients, a serum thyroglobulin level of more than 23 ng/ml correlated 100% with recurrent disease in patients with well-differentiated thyroid cancer who had undergone a total thyroidectomy and received an ablative dose of [131]I. The converse was also true; if the serum thyroglobulin level was less than 23 ng/ml, the patient did not have recurrent tumor.[187] Some patients with thyroid cancer may develop antithyroglobulin antibodies that interfere with the ability to measure serum levels of thyroglobulin. This appears to be more common in patients with progressive metastatic disease.[188] As useful and sensitive as serum levels of thyroglobulin are in the follow-up of patients with well-differentiated thyroid cancer, they are inadequate alone and should be coupled with diagnostic whole-body scan for maximal determination of recurrent disease.[189]

Although the use of radioactive iodine to treat metastatic or persistent well-differentiated thyroid cancer is efficacious and generally safe, it can be associated with complications. The side effects of ^{131}I therapy in order of frequency include temporary bone marrow suppression, nausea, sialoadenitis, pain in metastatic deposits, vomiting, pulmonary fibrosis, and leukemia.[186] Patients who have had less extensive surgery (*e.g.*, lobectomy) for the primary tumor often have more neck pain with radioactive iodine.[190] Most authorities use a therapeutic dose of 100 to 200 mCi to treat recurrent or metastatic disease and may repeat the dose several times.[2] A reasonable limiting factor is 200 cGy to blood. One mCi of ^{131}I gives 0.67 cGy to blood, so 300 mCi would be the maximum tolerable dose. If bulk disease or distant metastatic disease exists, dosimetry is required to allow maximal dose with minimal risk. Hematologic complications such as hypoplasia and leukemia may occur when the total dose exceeds 800 mCi.[184,191] Women have had normal pregnancies and deliveries after a total dose of 500 to 600 mCi.

Survival rates from time of discovery of lung and bone metastases from differentiated thyroid carcinoma are less favorable than rates for localized disease. One analysis of 283 patients indicates that 53% were alive at 5 years, 38% at 10 years, and 30% at 15 years.[191] A more recent analysis suggests that the 1-year survival is 50%.[8] Survival after the development of pulmonary metastases from well-differentiated thyroid cancer depends on whether the tumor takes up radioactive iodine. Fortunately, 63% to 80% of metastases from well-differentiated thyroid cancer avidly take up [131]I. Metastases that take up ^{131}I are usually treatable with ^{131}I therapy.[192] Six variables have an independent prognostic significance for survival in these patients: extensive metastases, older age at discovery of metastases, advanced local disease, male sex, absence of radioactive iodine uptake by metastases, and fol-

licular cell type.[8,191] These variables were documented in another study, in which pulmonary metastases occurred less often in patients treated initially by total thyroidectomy than in those treated with less than total thyroidectomy.[193]

The aim of management of patients with differentiated thyroid carcinoma after surgery should be to detect and treat metastases with radioactive iodine as early as possible. The incidence of pulmonary metastases is lowest in patients with papillary carcinoma (9%), intermediate with follicular carcinoma (13%), and highest with Hürthle cell carcinoma (25%).[176,178,193] Surgical resection of distant metastases from differentiated thyroid carcinoma has been advocated by some researchers.[2] Indications for resection include reduced administration of radioiodine, pain, and pathologic fracture. Estimated cumulative survival rates from the time of resection of distant disease were 45% for 5 years and 33% for 20 years after removal of a solitary metastasis.[2] This heroic treatment may be indicated for solitary metastases to bone or lung that do not take up radioiodine.

Chemotherapy for metastatic well-differentiated thyroid cancer has not been effective. The best regimen has been high-dose single-drug therapy with doxorubicin. Doses in the range of 60 to 150 mg/m^2 given every 3 weeks have resulted in a 33% to 39% partial response rate. Combination regimens have not had better results than monotherapy doxorubicin (see the section on chemotherapy in the treatment of anaplastic thyroid cancer).[194]

Management of Medullary Thyroid Carcinoma

In 1959, Hazard and colleagues described MTC as a distinct clinical and pathologic entity. This neoplasm presents in sporadic form (nonfamilial) and is associated with three clinical syndromes: MEN-IIa, MEN-IIb, and familial non-MEN MTC, a disease characterized by hereditary MTC without associated endocrinopathies.[51,65,93,178] In the three familial presentations of MTC, the disease is almost always bilateral and requires a total thyroidectomy combined with central lymph node dissection.[51,178,195] MTC that presents sporadically is usually unilateral, but it still requires the same operation because the familial disease cannot be ruled out by history alone. In MEN-IIa and MEN-IIb, MTC is associated with pheochromocytoma, a potentially life-threatening situation if an unprepared patient undergoes anesthetic stress for thyroidectomy. For this reason, if the diagnosis of MTC is known preoperatively by abnormal plasma level of calcitonin or by needle biopsy, pheochromocytoma must be ruled out by measurement of 24-hour urine for vanillylmandelic acid (VMA), metanephrines, and catecholamines or by measurement of serum levels of norepinephrine and epinephrine.[51,65] In the familial setting, individuals from kindreds who are at risk for the development of MTC can be identified accurately by specific genetic probes.[62,63] These individuals can then be screened at yearly intervals for the early diagnosis of MTC (Fig. 41–2). The early diagnosis of C-cell hyperplasia, C-cell carcinoma in situ, or MTC confined to the thyroid gland can be made by provocative testing with calcium and pentagastrin. An abnormal response is a rise in plasma calcitonin levels after use of these agents (see Fig. 41–2). This abnormal response to pentagastrin or calcium is diagnostic for MTC or MTC in situ or premalignant C-cell hyperplasia (see Fig. 41–2). Individuals

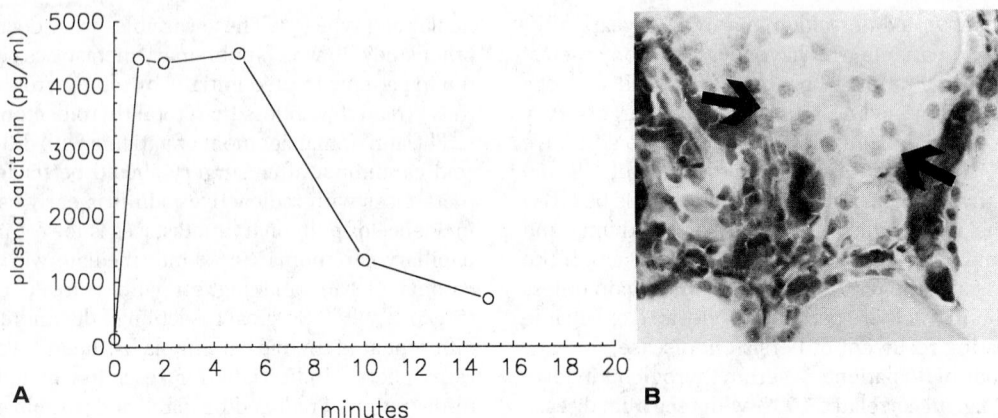

FIGURE 41–2.   The results of a screening pentagastrin stimulation test and a photomicrograph from a 21-year-old man whose family has multiple endocrine neoplasia. **(A)** Although the patient's basal calcitonin level was normal (<200 pg/ml), his peripheral plasma level was abnormally elevated at 1, 2, 5, 10, and 20 minutes after the intravenous administration of pentagastrin (0.5 µg/kg body weight). **(B)** A thyroidectomy specimen showing C-cell hyperplasia (*arrows*). A similar focus was found in both thyroid lobes. The patient had no evidence of extrathyroidal metastases and was cured by total thyroidectomy (H & E, original magnification × 250). (Alexander HR, Norton JA. Biology and management of medullary thyroid carcinoma of the parafollicular cells. Ann Intern Med 1991;115:133)

diagnosed in this fashion have a high probability of cure (Table 41–10).

Plasma calcitonin levels (basal and stimulated) increase with an increase in the extent of disease. In a study of patients from kindreds with MTC who had undetectable basal calcitonin levels and who had levels less than 100 pg/ml after pentagastrin-calcium stimulation, 24 of 25 patients had MTC localized to the thyroid gland and were cured after total thyroidectomy.[111] Telander and colleagues demonstrated that MTC is present in children from kindreds at a mean age of 7 years (range, 1.5–12 years).[196] A total thyroidectomy cured 14 of 17 children at this early age, and the 3 children with persistent disease had MEN-IIb. Provocative testing helps in the management of patients from kindreds with MEN-IIa and familial non-MEN MTC. Furthermore, recent reports contradict past dogma[67] and suggest that children with MTC in the setting of MEN-IIb may be cured. Investigators at Washington University School of Medicine performed total thyroidectomy and central node dissection in 7 children (age 3–10 years) with a family history of MEN-IIb based on increased plasma concentrations of calcitonin (either basal or pentagastrin stimulated). Five of 7 children treated in this manner had no evidence of MTC 3 to 10 years after thyroidectomy.[197] In older studies, most patients with MEN-IIb had spread of MTC outside the thyroid gland at presentation. These patients were not cured by thyroid surgery.[67]

Sporadic MTC usually presents with a neck mass, and the diagnosis can be obtained by aspiration cytology, cutting-needle biopsy, or measurement of serum calcitonin levels. Serum calcitonin is a specific, sensitive circulating marker for MTC but usually is not measured as part of the workup of a thyroid nodule. Patients with sporadic MTC may present with lymph node metastases or extrathyroidal disease, and surgery may not be curable in this setting. However, in a study of 12 patients with sporadic MTC who were treated at the National Institutes of Health, 5 were cured after total thyroidectomy and central lymph node dissection (see Table 41–10).[51] High-resolution real-time ultrasound can be used to stage accurately the extent of disease in the neck. MTC appears bright and echogenic and may be detected in the thyroid or lymph nodes.[198] The only significant predictor of survival after resection of primary MTC is tumor invasion beyond the

TABLE 41–10.   Outcome of Patients With Medullary Thyroid Carcinoma According to Method of Diagnosis

Investigations	Disease and Method of Diagnosis	No. of Patients	Follow-Up (y)	No. of Cured Patients (%)	No. of Patients Dead From Disease (%)
Alexander and Norton, 1991[51]	MEN-IIa* by screening	19	13	19 (100)	0
Gagel et al, 1988[61]	MEN-IIa by screening	22	11	19 (86)	0
Alexander and Norton, 1991[51]	MEN-IIa by palpation of mass	17	19	5 (29)†	2 (12)
Alexander and Norton, 1991[51]	Sporadic MTC by palpation of mass	12	12	5 (42)†	2 (17)

* MEN-IIa, multiple endocrine neoplasia type IIa.
† Significantly less than MEN-IIa by screening (*p* < 0.01, Fisher's exact test).

thyroid capsule or metastases to cervical lymph nodes. The overall survival after surgical resection of sporadic MTC varies; the historical 10-year survival was 40% to 60%.[21,199] With meticulous surgery and earlier diagnosis, the 10-year survival may be better (about 80%).[51]

Several studies have attempted to localize and resect lymph nodes containing microscopic or macroscopic MTC after thyroidectomy. One study used selective venous catheterization and pentagastrin stimulation to detect regions draining calcitonin in patients with recurrent and MTC.[200] Another study used additional extensive neck dissections after thyroidectomy to remove tumor in lymph nodes.[201] Both studies were able to remove MTC in clinically normal-appearing lymph nodes, and both were able to normalize postoperative basal calcitonin levels in some patients. The impact of these techniques on survival has not been demonstrated.[200,201] Most recent analyses of larger groups of patients with MTC suggest that this strategy can normalize plasma levels of calcitonin in 50% of patients and may render some patients free of disease.[202] Several groups have used thallium and technetium scanning or pentavalent ^{99m}Tc-DMSA to detect recurrent MTC and advocate resection of recurrent or persistent macroscopic disease.[126,132,133,203] Surgery alone seldom has been able to cure patients with MTC spread outside the thyroid gland. Whether resection of local or distant metastases from MTC impacts on survival is not clear because of the indolent course of this neoplasm.

The tragedy of not detecting MTC confined to the thyroid gland when it is surgically curable can be appreciated if one considers the ineffectiveness of nonoperative treatment of recurrent or metastatic disease.[65] Chemotherapy has been of little use for metastatic MTC. Gottlieb and Hill reported remissions in 3 of 5 patients with metastatic MTC,[204] but these results have not been confirmed by others.[205] Cisplatin, streptozocin, carmustine (BCNU), methotrexate, and 5-fluorouracil (5-FU) have been used without benefit.[65] One recent case report demonstrated some efficacy of low-dose doxorubicin at 15 mg/m^2 intravenously each week for 20 weeks for a total dose of 300 mg/m^2. The patient had a complete response that has lasted 18 months.[206] Another patient had a partial response to a combination of dacarbazine and 5-FU that lasted 10 months.[207] Because ^{131}I-MIBG is taken up by metastatic and recurrent MTC,[128,129] it may be of use in the treatment of metastatic MTC, although no studies have been reported. We have attempted to image several patients with metastatic MTC with iodinated MIBG without success. This strategy does not appear useful. Monoclonal antibodies to CEA have been used to image metastatic MTC and may have potential in experimental treatment of metastatic MTC.[130,131]

Radiation therapy for localized inaccessible tumor deposits may be useful in patients with MTC.[208] Work with sensitizers may increase radiation efficacy in MTC, but the data are limited (see the section on anaplastic thyroid carcinoma). In general, MTC is not very sensitive to radiation. Potential benefits from radiation therapy must be weighed against complications.

Patients with metastatic MTC may be asymptomatic even with substantial tumor burdens. The most troubling symptom is severe voluminous secretory diarrhea, which generally develops when plasma calcitonin levels exceed 20 ng/ml. The etiology of this diarrhea is unknown. It may be due to calcitonin[209] or to other tumor hormone products, because C

cells in MTC can secrete many different hormones.[65] This symptom is especially bothersome because it is not well controlled by medical regimens. In some cases, debulking of grossly evident tumor ameliorates the diarrhea. One patient with metastatic MTC, elevated pancreatic polypeptide levels, and severe refractory diarrhea has been reported to respond with complete resolution of diarrhea to the long-acting somatostatin analog octreotide.[210] Three other patients with metastatic MTC have had their diarrhea controlled with octreotide in a similar protocol, in which octreotide was administered by continuous pump at a dose of 0.6 to 1.0 mg/day.[211] Octreotide does not appear to have antitumor effects in these studies. It does lower circulating levels of calcitonin and other hormones and appears to derive its beneficial effects on the diarrhea by inhibiting secretion of diarrhea-producing peptides. Tachyphylaxis may develop and requires increasing the administered dose.[211] Low-dose use of interferon-α (3 million units) three times per week subcutaneously ameliorated the diarrhea in 2 patients with metastatic MTC.[212] This immune stimulatory agent appears to decrease plasma levels of calcitonin without any change in tumor size.[212]

Management of Anaplastic Thyroid Carcinoma

Treatment of anaplastic thyroid carcinoma is poor, and most patients with this diagnosis are dead within 1 year with a median survival of 4 months.[213] The clinical manifestations of thyroid carcinoma present a true paradox; it is a cancer that in its differentiated form may be one of the most benign types of cancer[1] and in its undifferentiated form may be one of the most malignant forms.[213] Surgical resection is indicated for small tumors or tumors in which it is technically feasible;[169] however, most tumors are unresectable at presentation. If the tumor is large and apparently unresectable, cutting-needle biopsy is recommended to establish the diagnosis. Radiation therapy alone has not been useful for anaplastic thyroid carcinoma; however, the combination of doxorubicin as a sensitizer and 5760 cGy delivered over 40 days has had dramatic local control rates for anaplastic giant and spindle cell carcinoma of the thyroid gland.[214] The regimen consists of once weekly low-dose doxorubicin (10 mg/m^2) and hyperfractionated radiation therapy. The radiation therapy is carried out with fractional doses of 160 cGy per treatment twice a day for 3 days each week to a total dose of 5760 cGy in 40 days. Using this protocol, 16 of 19 patients (84%) achieved complete tumor regression in the primary area and 13 (68%) remained disease free in the neck until death.[214,215] The same group has treated 22 patients with locally advanced differentiated thyroid carcinoma with a similar treatment regimen, and 91% of patients achieved complete tumor regression in the neck.[215,216] The regimen did not disproportionately enhance normal tissue morbidity and appears to be a breakthrough for the treatment of locally advanced anaplastic or differentiated thyroid carcinoma. External-beam irradiation has been shown to reduce massive mediastinal disease from follicular thyroid carcinoma, resolving superior vena caval syndrome.[217] Most patients with anaplastic cancer develop distant metastases and die within 1 year, and systemic therapies need to be developed.

Drug therapies for advanced thyroid carcinoma and anaplastic thyroid carcinoma have been disappointing. Regimens with doxorubicin have shown the highest response rates, and doxorubicin itself is the best single agent (Table 41–11). Some researchers suggest that doxorubicin-only therapy is better than multidrug therapy.[194] Cisplatin and bleomycin have had some activity, although two trials using these active agents in advanced thyroid carcinoma had conflicting results. The combination of doxorubicin (60 mg/m²) and cisplatin (60 mg/m²) had only 2 (9%) partial remissions in 22 evaluable patients with advanced thyroid cancer.[218] These results were inconsistent with a previous study that showed that doxorubicin plus cisplatin was significantly better than doxorubicin alone in a similar group of patients with advanced thyroid carcinoma.[219] Eighty-four evaluable patients were stratified by histologic type and randomized to doxorubicin alone (60 mg/m² intravenously every 3 weeks) or to a combination of doxorubicin (60 mg/m²) and cisplatin (40 mg/m²) intravenously every 3 weeks. The total dose of doxorubicin was 550 mg/m². Forty-one patients received doxorubicin alone and 7 had partial responses (17%). Forty-three patients received the combination of drugs, and there were 5 complete and 6 partial responses (26%). The finding of 5 complete responses in the combination group was significantly better than no complete responses in the doxorubicin alone group. The 5 CRs in the combination group included 3 complete responders of 18 with anaplastic carcinoma, and an overall response rate in anaplastic carcinoma of 33%. Four of 5 complete responders survived for more than 2 years. The toxicity was similar in the two-drug regimens and indicated that doxorubicin plus cisplatin had a better response rate than doxorubicin alone.[219] Bukowski and colleagues treated 11 patients with advanced thyroid carcinoma with a combination of doxorubicin, bleomycin, vincristine and melphalan.[220] They reported a response in 4 of 11 patients (36%), with one durable complete response in a patient with anaplastic carcinoma.[220]

The findings of durable complete response in patients with anaplastic carcinoma are provocative. One potential diagnostic error is thyroid lymphoma, which may mimic anaplastic carcinoma. However, there may be subsets of patients with advanced or anaplastic thyroid carcinoma that will respond to combination chemotherapy. A recent phase II study of 15 patients in Germany with anaplastic thyroid carcinoma showed more potential efficacy with a different regimen. Drugs included cisplatin (100 mg/m²), mitoxantrone (20 mg/m²), and vincristine (1.5 mg/m²). Ten of 15 patients (67%) responded to chemotherapy, with 4 patients (27%) having a compete response. Responders demonstrated a longer survival than nonresponders (mean 21 months versus 4 months).[105] Patients with anaplastic thyroid carcinoma are rare, and it will take cooperative trials to answer questions about certain regimens. The treatment of anaplastic thyroid carcinoma should include doxorubicin, fractionated radiation therapy to control primary tumors, and combination chemotherapy using either doxorubicin with cisplatin or the combination of Bukowski and colleagues.[214,219,220]

THE PARATHYROID GLAND

Primary hyperparathyroidism is a common disease, with an incidence between 1 and 5 persons per 1000. An increased incidence of hyperparathyroidism has been reported in persons who have been exposed previously to irradiation of the head and neck.[221] The parathyroid tumor associated with previous radiation has been adenoma and not carcinoma. Patients usually present with symptoms related to increased urinary excretion of calcium (urinary calculi and nephrocalcinosis) or demineralization of bony skeleton (bone pain and elevated serum alkaline phosphatase) or both. The diagnosis of primary hyperparathyroidism is established biochemically by concomitant serial elevations of serum calcium levels and inappropriately elevated serum parathyroid hormone levels. Elevated urinary cyclic adenosine monophosphate (UcAMP) levels are present in 92% of patients with primary hyperparathyroidism.[222] Once the diagnosis is established, surgical exploration generally is recommended. The extent of surgery depends on the etiology of the hyperparathyroidism. The three possible etiologies of primary hyperparathyroidism and incidences are adenoma (83%), hyperplasia (15%), and car-

TABLE 41–11.   Chemotherapy for Thyroid Carcinoma

Investigations	Drugs	No. of Evaluable Patients	No. of Responders (%)	No. of Complete Responders (%)
Gottlieb and Hill, 1974[204]	Doxorubicin alone	43	15 (35)	0
Shimaoka et al, 1985[219]	Doxorubicin alone	41	7 (17)	0
Ahuja and Ernst, 1987[194]	Doxorubicin alone	248	95 (38)	8 (3)
Shimaoka et al, 1985[219]	Doxorubicin + cisplatin	43	11 (26)	5 (12)
Williams et al, 1986[218]	Doxorubicin + cisplatin	22	2 (9)	0
Bukowski et al, 1983[220]	Doxorubicin + bleomycin + vincristine + melphalan	11	4 (36)	1 (19)
Sokal and Harmar, 1978[1102]	Doxorubicin + vincristine + bleomycin	14	9 (64)	0
Kober et al, 1990[105]	Cisplatin, mitoxantrone, vincristine	15	10 (67)	4 (27)

cinoma (1–2%; Table 41–12). Parathyroid hyperplasia means multiple gland involvement and can be inherited as part of two familial syndromes (MEN-I and MEN-IIa). Parathyroid adenomas are the most common cause of primary hyperparathyroidism and require identification and simple excision of the tumor. Parathyroid carcinomas are rare and require identification and resection of the tumor along with the ipsilateral lobe of the thyroid and abnormal central nodal tissue. The diagnosis of parathyroid carcinoma can be confusing and it is the purpose of this section to help the clinician and the pathologist differentiate parathyroid carcinoma from parathyroid adenoma.

The diagnosis of parathyroid carcinoma may be suspected at the time of clinical presentation. Parathyroid carcinoma

has been reported in 3 patients from different families with familial hyperparathyroidism. This finding is rare and implies transformation of hyperplastic parathyroid tissue into carcinoma.[223,224] Parathyroid carcinoma usually presents in the fourth decade. The hallmark preoperative signs are severe hypercalcemia (serum calcium >15 mg/dl), palpable neck mass, and bone and renal disease.[225] Parathyroid adenomas rarely present with palpable tumors, and serum levels of calcium are usually significantly lower, although similar hypercalcemia can be seen with parathyroid adenomas.[226] The principal histologic features of parathyroid carcinoma that distinguish it from adenoma include a trabecular pattern, mitotic figures, thick fibrous bands, and capsular and blood vessel invasion.[225] The major problem with parathyroid carcinoma

TABLE 41–12. Differential Causes of Primary Hyperparathyroidism: Etiology, Incidence, Diagnostic Features, and Long-Term Results

Diagnosis	Etiology	Relative Frequency	Palpable Neck Mass or Vocal Cord Paralysis	Serum Calcium Level (mg/dl)	Parathyroid Hormone	Gross Pathology	Surgical Procedure	Microscopic Pathology	Recurrent Hyperparathyroidism*
Hyperplasia	Familial pattern	14%	Absent	12	Elevated	Multiple gland enlargement; soft reddish brown appearance	Either 3½ gland resection or 4 gland resection with autograft	Decreased fat content and increased gland cellularity in multiple glands	Intermediate (10–30%)
Adenoma	Associated with previous irradiation	85%	Absent	12	Elevated	Single gland enlargement; soft reddish brown appearance	Excision of abnormal gland	Decreased fat content and increased cellularity; occasionally attached normal parathyroid gland	Low (<1%)
Carcinoma	? Familial pattern	1%	Usually	>14	Markedly elevated	Single enlarged gland that is firm, whitish gray	Resection of abnormal gland in continuity with ipsilateral thyroid lobe and suspicious central lymph nodes	Trabecular pattern; mitotic figures; thick fibrous bands; capsular and blood vessel invasion	High (>50%)

* Recurrent means that patient initially has normal serum levels of calcium postoperatively and more than 6 months later develops recurrent hypercalcemia.

is intraoperative recognition of the malignancy and performance of an appropriate resection procedure including ipsilateral thyroid lobectomy and dissection of the central lymph node region.[227] In two large series of patients, the 5-year survival rates were 44% and 29% and the 10-year survival rates were 22% and 15%, respectively.[228,229] This is in marked contrast to a more recent series in which 8 of 9 patients were alive with a median follow-up of 6 years.[227] Distant metastases develop to lung, bone, and liver in order of highest frequency.[229,230] Radiation therapy has been unsuccessful at controlling primary and metastatic lesions.[229,230] Bukowski and colleagues reported a single patient with metastatic lesions who had a complete remission of 5 months' duration with a combination of 5-fluorouracil (500 mg/m^2), cyclophosphamide (500 mg/m^2), and dacarbazine (200 mg/m^2).[231] Another group also documented a dramatic response of metastatic parathyroid cancer to dacarbazine.[232] Based on these two reports, dacarbazine appears active and may be useful in the treatment of parathyroid carcinoma.

The major morbidity of recurrent or metastatic parathyroid carcinoma is due to severe hypercalcemia, which is difficult to control medically and results in death. Aggressive surgical resection of bulk recurrent or metastatic disease has been advocated by some surgeons because of the indolent, slow-growing nature of the tumor and the potential to control hypercalcemia.[233] Unfortunately, surgery is not always possible or successful, especially if the carcinoma has metastasized widely. Attempts to inhibit the actions of parathyroid hormone with calcitonin, mithramycin, or diphosphonates have been disappointing. Recent evidence suggests that gallium nitrate is effective for cancer-related hypercalcemia and may be useful to manage the hypercalcemia of patients with parathyroid cancer.[234] Intravenous etidronate may be helpful in the acute setting with severe hypercalcemia.[235] Unfortunately, the hypercalcemia associated with parathyroid cancer is a chronic problem and needs better antitumor therapy to control. Proper intraoperative identification of malignancy and appropriate initial surgery is crucial to therapy of parathyroid carcinoma. The characteristics that distinguish patients at risk preoperatively and the intraoperative malignant tumor characteristics that allow the surgeon and pathologist to make the correct diagnosis are listed in Table 41–12. If malignant parathyroid neoplasms are recognized and proper initial resections performed, a greater number of patients will be cured.

THE ADRENAL GLAND

PATHOLOGY OF THE ADRENAL CORTEX

Hyperplasia

The term hyperplasia is defined as an increased number of cells in an organ.[236] It is a pathologic change associated with increased function or compensatory change. In pituitary-based hypercortisolism (Cushing's disease), which is the most common endogenous form of hypercortisolism, the gross adrenal enlargement is not impressive. The adrenal gland is about twice the normal size. The weight of each adrenal ranges from 6 to 8 g, although occasionally the adrenal weighs 12 g (a normal adrenal weighs from 3–6 g). Microscopically, there is a widened inner zone of the compact zona reticularis and

a sharply demarcated outer zone of clear cells. The appearance of adrenal glands in ectopic ACTH syndrome is similar except that the glands are usually larger, weighing at least 12 g and as much as 30 g. Macronodular adrenal hyperplasia (3-cm nodules of adrenal cortex weighing 30–50 g and as much as 100 g) usually is a secondary response of the adrenal gland to adrenocorticotropic hormone (ACTH), whereas pigmented micronodular adrenal hyperplasia (1- to 5-mm nodules with pigmented appearance and normal glandular weight) is more likely to be autonomous and to occur in children including infants.[237] ACTH levels are low or undetectable. This histology is rare and can occur in a familial pattern.[238]

Adrenocortical Adenoma

Adrenal adenoma is a benign neoplasm of adrenocortical cells that resembles normal adrenal cells histologically but may possess functional autonomy.[236] An adenoma usually does not exceed 5 cm, although benign tumors exceeding 10 cm have been reported. One suggested cut-off for benign adenomas is a weight of 100 g. Cellular pleomorphism and tumor necrosis may be present but are rare. The exact functional type of neoplasm cannot be described based solely on histology, although there are consistent differences. Adenomas produce syndromes of hypercortisolism and hyperaldosteronism but seldom produce adrenogenital syndromes. Larger tumors producing adrenogenital syndromes are consistent with carcinoma,[239] as are pleomorphism, tumor necrosis, and mitotic activity.[239] The prognosis of adrenocortical adenomas producing Cushing's syndrome is excellent, and successful resection invariably produces cure. The prognosis of adrenocortical adenomas producing hyperaldosteronism may not be as favorable. Resection is followed by a response in blood pressure and correction of hypokalemia; however, 30% of patients with resected aldosteronomas develop recurrent hypertension but not recurrent hypokalemia. If the preoperative diagnosis was incorrect and the patient had hyperaldosteronism secondary to hyperplasia, unilateral adrenalectomy does not improve the syndrome. Adenomas that produce the adrenogenital syndrome have the least favorable outcome. Many of these tumors are really misdiagnosed carcinomas that develop local recurrence or metastases.[239]

Adrenocortical Carcinoma

Adrenocortical carcinoma is a malignant neoplasm of adrenocortical cells demonstrating partial or complete histologic and functional differentiation. Adrenocortical carcinomas are rare neoplasms and comprise only 0.05% to 0.2% of all cancers.[240] This incidence translates to a rate of only 2 persons per million in the world population.[241] Women appear to develop functional adrenocortical carcinomas more commonly than men, and men develop nonfunctioning malignant adrenal tumors more commonly than women. There is a bimodal occurrence by age with a peak incidence at less than 5 years of age and a second peak in the fourth and fifth decade. Adrenocortical carcinoma has been described as part of a complex hereditary syndrome including sarcoma and breast and lung cancer.[242] Cytogenetic analysis of primary adrenocortical carcinoma revealed clonal rearrangements of several autosomes and sex chromosomes. In all metaphases, the following marker chromosomes were present: 4 pt, t(3;12) (p14;p3), 14q+,t(15;20)(p11;q11), t(5;18)(p13.3;p11.2), psu dic (18) t(18;3) (p11.39;p12), and psu dic (20)t(20;9) (q11.2;p11).[243] Two recent studies suggest that loss of heterozygosity at loci on the short arm of chromosome 11 (11p) may be important in the pathogenesis of malignant adrenocortical tumors.[244,245]

Adrenocortical carcinomas weigh between 100 and 5000 g. Areas of necrosis and hemorrhage are common and are consistent with malignancy. Invasion and metastases are common. Microscopically, their appearance varies with the functional syndrome but also varies within the same tumor. The presence of cells with big nuclei, hyperchromatism, and enlarged nucleoli are all consistent with malignancy.[236] Nuclear changes are more common in tumors larger than 500 g. Vascular invasion and mitoses are diagnostic of adrenocortical malignancy. Broad desmoplastic bands are associated with metastatic potential of tumors.

The diagnosis of malignancy in adrenocortical neoplasms is difficult, especially in tumors that weigh between 50 and 100 g. Differentiating between adrenal carcinoma and renal carcinoma also may be difficult. Immunostaining for vimentin, epithelial membrane antigen, cytokeratin, and blood group antigens can separate the two diagnoses. Adrenal carcinoma and adenoma stain positive for vimentin, whereas renal carcinoma is negative for vimentin but positive for the others.[246] Table 41–13 attempts to differentiate benign from malignant adrenal tumors based on criteria suggested by Page and colleagues.[236] Immunostaining profiles of adrenocortical carcinoma and adenoma are similar, so that the pathologist must rely on clinical and morphologic criteria.[246] Although the difference in natural history between benign and malignant adrenocortical neoplasms is clear, it is not always possible to histologically separate one from the other. The only reliable criterion is the presence of nodal or distant metastases. The data used to differentiate benign from malignant adrenocortical neoplasms include whether hormone is produced and what type, the amount of tumor necrosis, fibrosis, vascular invasion, number of mitoses, and tumor weight. In a series that analyzed 43 adrenocortical tumors histologically, mitotic activity and venous invasion correlated best with metastasizing or recurring tumors (*i.e*, carcinoma).[247] Another more recent analysis demonstrated that number of mitoses is the most important predictor of outcome. Patients who had more than

20 mitoses per 50 high-power fields had a median survival of 14 months, whereas patients with fewer than 20 had a median survival of 58 months.[248] Nuclear DNA ploidy may predict survival because patients with aneuploid tumors appear to have shortened survival.[249] A final criterion is based on the observation that cells from carcinomas produce abnormal amounts of androgens and 11-deoxysteroids.[250] Only 10% of malignant tumors are associated with masculinization and only 12% with feminization; the rest usually produce a combination of hormones including aldosterone.

CLINICAL PRESENTATIONS OF ADRENOCORTICAL NEOPLASMS

Cushing's Syndrome or Hypercortisolism

Signs

Hypercortisolism results in the signs and symptoms of Cushing's syndrome. The signs and symptoms are widespread and diverse, affecting nearly every organ in the body.[251,252] However, no single symptom or sign is common to every patient with endogenous hypercortisolism. Although hypercortisolism is the most common presentation for adrenocortical neoplasms, Cushing's syndrome is rare with an estimated incidence of only 10 persons per million population.[251] The most common cause of hypercortisolism is iatrogenic administration of steroids to treat other diseases. Hypercortisolism usually is not associated with MEN-I, although it can be present in this familial syndrome.[253] It has been reported in 5% of patients with sporadic Zollinger-Ellison syndrome (ZES) and in 19% of patients with both ZES and MEN-I.[251,254]

Progressive weight gain is the most universal symptom of patients with hypercortisolism. Obesity is usually truncal, and patients demonstrate thin extremities due to muscle wasting. Increased fat in the dorsal neck region combined with dorsal kyphosis secondary to osteoporosis gives the appearance of a buffalo hump. Serial photographs demonstrate a rounding of the face. Increased blood pressure in Cushing's syndrome is usually mild and is caused primarily by excess mineralocorticoid secretion. Hypertension is less frequent in iatrogenic Cushing's syndrome because physicians prescribe pure glucocorticoids. Striae are reliable clinical signs of Cushing's. Hirsutism consists of excessive fine hair on the face, upper

TABLE 41–13. Diagnosis of Malignancy in Adrenocortical Neoplasms

Reliability	Clinical Criteria	Pathologic Criteria
Diagnostic of malignancy	Weight loss, feminization, nodal or distant metastases	Tumor weight >100 g, tumor necrosis, fibrous bands, vascular invasion, mitosis
Consistent with malignancy	Virilism, Cushing's virilism, no hormone production	Nuclear pleomorphism
Suggestive of malignancy	Elevated urinary 17-ketosteroids	Capsular invasion
Unreliable	Hypercortisolism, hyperaldosteronism	Tumor giant cells, cytoplasmic size variation, ratio between compact and clear cells

(Adapted from Page DL, DeLillis RA, Hough AJ. Tumors of the adrenal. In: Atlas of tumor pathology. Washington DC: Armed Forces Institute of Pathology, 1986)

back, and arms. Virilization including clitoromegaly, deep voice, and balding suggest adrenocortical carcinoma. Glucose intolerance with hyperglycemia is common, and patients may present with diabetes mellitus. Weakness secondary to muscle atrophy is a common complaint and is especially common in ectopic ACTH syndrome with hypokalemia. Menstrual irregularity or amenorrhea is common in women with Cushing's syndrome, whereas men with Cushing's syndrome have loss of libido or impotency. Dilatation of blood vessels and thinning of the subcutaneous tissue give the face a ruddy appearance. Mental changes in Cushing's syndrome vary from mild depression to severe psychosis and appear to correlate directly with serum levels of cortisol and ACTH. Hypokalemia worsens the weakness associated with Cushing's syndrome and suggests the etiology of adrenocortical carcinoma or ectopic ACTH syndrome. Impaired immune surveillance is an important part of the morbidity associated with Cushing's syndrome. Opportunistic infections including cryptococcosis, aspergillosis, nocardiosis, and *Pneumocystis carinii* pneumonia are more common in patients with Cushing's syndrome and may be lethal.[255-257] In children with Cushing's syndrome, the most common presenting sign is obesity or an arrest of normal

growth with short stature.[258] The early diagnosis of Cushing's syndrome depends primarily on a knowledge of the many different signs and symptoms of the disorder and a high clinical index of suspicion.

Workup and Diagnosis of Cushing's Syndrome

The initial step in the workup of a patient with presumptive hypercortisolism is to establish biochemically whether hypercortisolism is present. The second step is to determine whether the hypercortisolism is considered pituitary-dependent or pituitary-independent, and the final step is to determine the exact etiology of the hypercortisolism (Fig. 41–3). Laboratory testing allows the correct diagnosis of the presence and the cause of the hypercortisolism in nearly every case.[251]

Establish Hypercortisolism. Urinary excretion of unmetabolized (free) cortisol is directly proportional to the amount of free cortisol in the plasma. As the cortisol-binding globulin becomes saturated (at plasma cortisol levels of 20 μg/dl), small increases in cortisol secretion produce exponential increases in urinary free cortisol. This amplification effect makes 24-hour urinary free cortisol the single best measurement to dif-

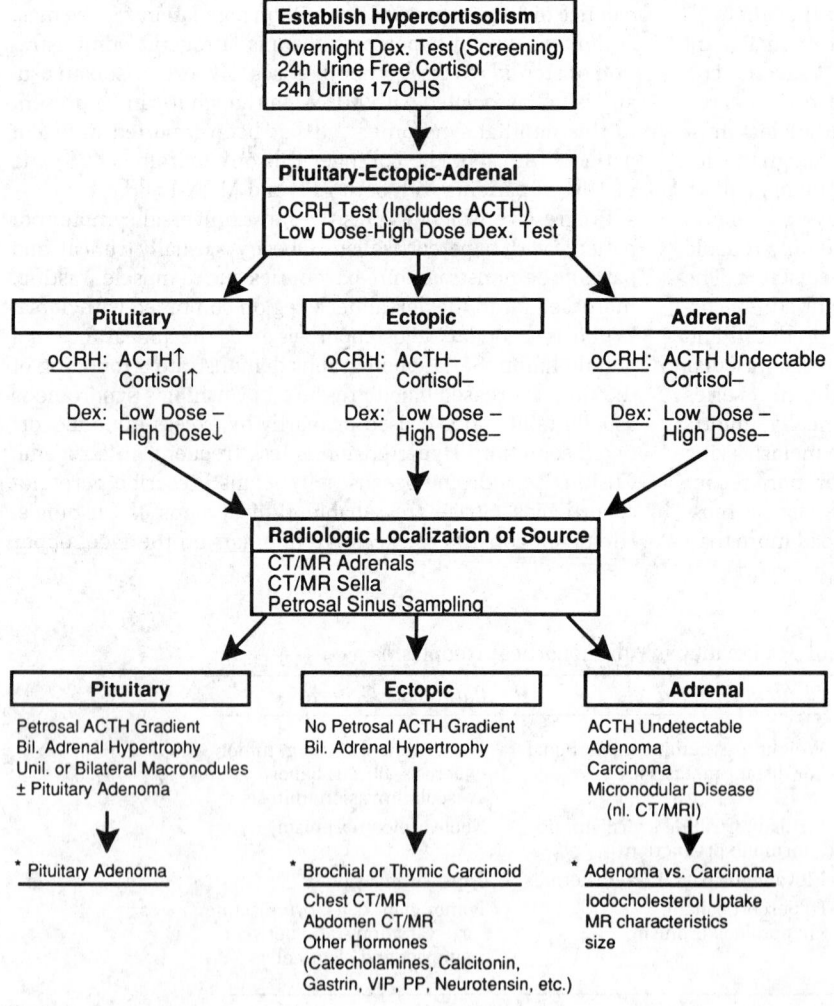

FIGURE 41–3. Flow diagram for evaluation of a patient with suspected hypercortisolism or Cushing's syndrome.

* Most probable diagnosis

ferentiate normal from hypercortisolemic states (see Fig. 41–3). The overnight single-dose dexamethasone test works because of the lack of normal feedback that occurs in all forms of hypercortisolism (Fig. 41–4).[259] Normal subjects given 1 mg of dexamethasone orally at 11:00 P.M. have plasma cortisol levels less than 5 μg/dl at 8:00 A.M. the next day. Patients with endogenous hypercortisolism do not suppress and have cortisol levels greater than 5 μg/dl. The major advantage of this test is a 3% incidence of false-negative results (patients with Cushing's syndrome whose cortisol levels suppress). This test may have false-positive results (30%) including depression, alcoholism, stress, and primary cortisol resistance.[260–262] A normal-single dose dexamethasone test and urinary free cortisol (less than 100 μg/day in most laboratories) virtually exclude the diagnosis of hypercortisolism.[251] Another study that can be used to discriminate hypercortisolism is the 24-hour urine test for 17-hydroxysteroids corrected for gram creatinine. This study is older but has results similar to urinary measurement of free cortisol levels.

Etiology of Hypercortisolism. Patients with pituitary Cushing's syndrome respond to 1 μg/kg of corticotropin-releasing hormone (CRH) by increasing plasma ACTH and cortisol levels, and patients with depression have a blunted ACTH response to CRH.[263] A CRH test can differentiate pituitary Cushing's syndrome (Cushing's disease) from ectopic secretion of ACTH. Twenty-nine of 33 patients with Cushing's disease had increased plasma ACTH and cortisol levels after CRH, whereas none of 8 patients with ectopic ACTH responded. The CRH test worked as well as the standard dexamethasone test, and the diagnostic power was enhanced when the two tests were combined.[264] Patients with Cushing's syndrome have abnormalities in the diurnal rhythm of plasma cortisol and ACTH levels. Serial samples taken over several days are necessary because patients with Cushing's disease can have episodic secretion of cortisol. Nevertheless, a low midnight cortisol level (<2 μg/dl) excludes the diagnosis of

endogenous hypercortisolism. Determination of simultaneous plasma ACTH levels are helpful. Primary adrenal tumors or hyperplasia cause very low plasma ACTH levels. Pituitary-dependent hypercortisolism causes intermediate levels of plasma ACTH, and ectopic ACTH-producing tumors have very high levels of plasma ACTH (about 60% of these patients have ACTH levels of more than 300 pg/ml). Radioimmunoassays for ACTH in plasma have been difficult to perform reliably and to interpret because of platelet-associated proteases that degrade ACTH. Samples must be collected using recommended procedures including pre-chilled tubes on ice. Urinary 17-ketosteroids can help the differential diagnosis of hypercortisolism. Low levels (<10 mg/day) suggest an adrenal adenoma and very high levels (>60 mg/day) occur more commonly in patients with adrenal cancer and ectopic ACTH. Hypokalemia is seen in most patients with ectopic ACTH (16/16 in one series) and in only 10% of patients with Cushing's disease.[265]

The standard dexamethasone suppression test remains one of the most useful tests in establishing the cause of hypercortisolism (see Fig. 41–3). The expected results are that urinary 17-hydroxysteroid levels will be less than 2.5 mg/day when normal subjects receive 2 mg of dexamethasone per day, but this dose has no effect on patients with endogenous hypercortisolism. High-dose dexamethasone (8 mg/day) suppresses urinary 17-hydroxysteroids to less than 50% of baseline levels in patients with pituitary-dependent hypercortisolism (Cushing's disease), but has no effect on hypercortisolism from other causes. This single test differentiates hypercortisolism from normal and pituitary-dependent hypercortisolism, the most common cause, from all other causes with about 95% accuracy.[266]

Radiologic Evaluation of Hypercortisolism. Sellar computed tomography (CT) scans detect abnormal sellar enlargement in up to 15% of patients with pituitary-dependent Cushing's disease and can detect more subtle abnormalities in 23% to 60% of these patients.[267] Sellar CT scans may detect ACTH-secreting tumors whose greatest diameter is between 5 and 10 mm, but this study cannot reliably detect the more common microadenoma (less than 5 mm). Pituitary magnetic resonance imaging (MRI) studies have similar resolution capabilities, even those done with gadolinium.[268] In patients with pituitary-dependent hypercortisolism, CT and MRI may be normal, but simultaneous bilateral petrosal sinus sampling for ACTH concentrations produces a hormone gradient in most cases. Resection of the ipsilateral half of the pituitary with the ACTH gradient is followed by biochemical and clinical remission, and pathologic analysis demonstrates microadenomas in most patients.[269] Recent data in 281 patients indicate that petrosal sinus sampling is the single best method to differentiate a pituitary source of hypercortisolism (Cushing's disease) from an ectopic ACTH-producing tumor.[268] Petrosal sinus sampling worked best when combined with the administration of ovine corticotropin-releasing hormone and requires bilateral sampling of the inferior petrosal sinus and peripheral sampling for plasma ACTH levels before and after CRH. A peak inferior petrosal sinus to peripheral plasma ACTH level greater than 3.0 after CRH administration correctly identified all 203 patients with Cushing's disease (sensitivity, 100%) with no false-positive results (specificity,

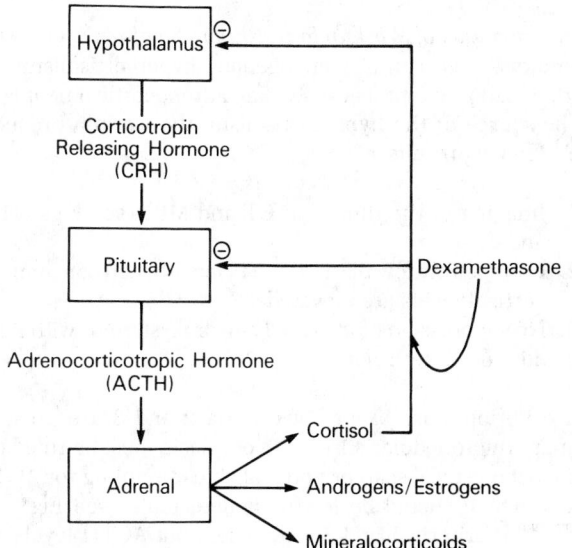

FIGURE 41–4. Model of cortisol secretion indicates the mechanism of dexamethasone suppression and CRH stimulation of normal cortisol secretion.

100%). Furthermore, petrosal sinus sampling predicted correct localization of the ACTH-producing microadenoma in about 70% of patients.[268] Although this new study is invasive and requires a significant degree of experience and expertise by the radiologist, it is the study of choice to diagnose and localize pituitary tumors in patients with Cushing's disease, the most common form of endogenous hypercortisolism.

Adrenal CT and MRI have been able to detect small adrenal abnormalities with certainty (Fig. 41–5). CT scans can detect

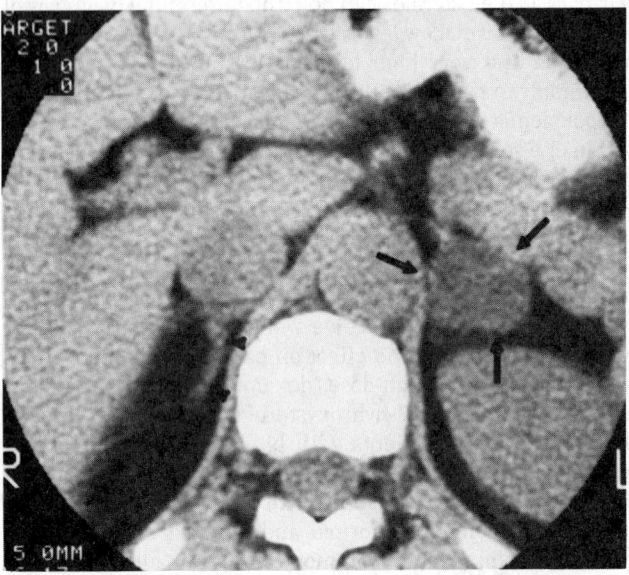

A

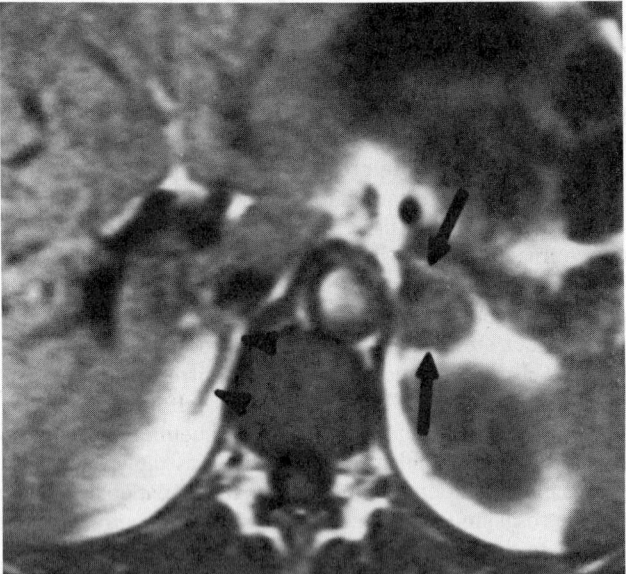

B

FIGURE 41–5. Left adrenal adenoma in a patient with Cushing's syndrome. **(A)** CT scan of the left adrenal (*arrows*) shows a mass and a normal contralateral adrenal gland (*arrowheads*). **(B)** T2-weighted MRI of the same tumor (*arrows*) and normal contralateral adrenal gland (*arrowheads*). Because the tumor has less density than the liver (darker) on T2 image, the image suggested a benign adrenal adenoma, which was removed subsequently for resolution of the hypercortisolism.

normal adrenal glands in about 97% of patients.[270] CT scans can differentiate cortical hyperplasia from tumor.[271–274] Although CT scanning has great sensitivity (>95%), it lacks specificity. In a patient with Cushing's syndrome, early detection of an adrenal neoplasm by CT scan simplifies the workup. About 15% of patients with Cushing's syndrome have a primary adrenal neoplasm as the source of the hypercortisolism. Unilateral adrenal tumors require the detection of a normal adrenal gland on the contralateral side (Figure 41–5A). Adrenal hyperplasia may be detected if both glands appear enlarged. MRI may be able to add specificity to the sensitivity of CT scanning and to differentiate adrenal adenoma (Fig. 41–5B) from carcinoma or from a pheochromocytoma by the brightness of the lesion on the T2-weighted image.[272,275] Functional adenoma and nonfunctional adenoma appear darker than the liver on the T2-weighted MRI. Carcinomas, whether primary adrenocortical or metastatic, appear as bright as or slightly brighter than the liver on T2-weighted image (Fig. 41–6). Pheochromocytomas appear about three times brighter than the liver on T2-weighted MRI.[275]

Radioisotope imaging of adrenals using labeled iodocholesterol such as ^{131}I-6-β-iodomethyl norcholesterol can be useful in differentiating unilateral adrenal adenoma with suppression of the contralateral gland from bilateral hyperplasia.[276] It can help differentiate a benign cortical neoplasm (adenoma), which usually takes up iodocholesterol (images), from a malignant cortical neoplasm (carcinoma), which usually does not take up the tracer.[277] A recent study demonstrated that labeled iodocholesterol correctly imaged 14 of 14 benign functional adenomas, only 1 of 4 carcinomas, and 4 of 4 adrenal pairs in primary nodular adrenocortical hyperplasia.[278] Radioisotope imaging is helpful in micronodular hyperplasia, in which uptake in both adrenal glands confirms the diagnosis, and can be useful in instances of recurrent hypercortisolism after bilateral adrenalectomy, in which ectopic rests of tissue enlarge with chronic ACTH stimulation. The limitations of radioiodocholesterol scans are the magnitude of the radiation dose, limited availability of the scan and isotope, and poor imaging of malignant adrenal neoplasms.

Interpretation of Workup for Cushing's Syndrome. Once the laboratory tests confirm endogenous hypercortisolism, the workup can pinpoint its cause. If an adrenocortical neoplasm is the source of the hypercortisolism, the workup produces the following results:

1. Imaging of the tumor on CT and MRI (see Figs. 41–5 and 41–6)
2. Consistently low plasma ACTH levels when concomitant cortisol levels are elevated
3. No suppression of urinary 17-hydroxysteroids with high-dose dexamethasone.

If criterion 1 is absent but criteria 2 and 3 are present, primary micronodular adrenal hyperplasia must be ruled out by iodocholesterol scan or petrosal sinus sampling for ACTH levels, which should be low or undetectable (see Fig. 41–3).[279,280] If criteria 1 and 3 are present but ACTH levels are consistently elevated, urinary catecholamines, VMA, and metanephrines should be measured because the patient may have an ACTH-producing pheochromocytoma.[281]

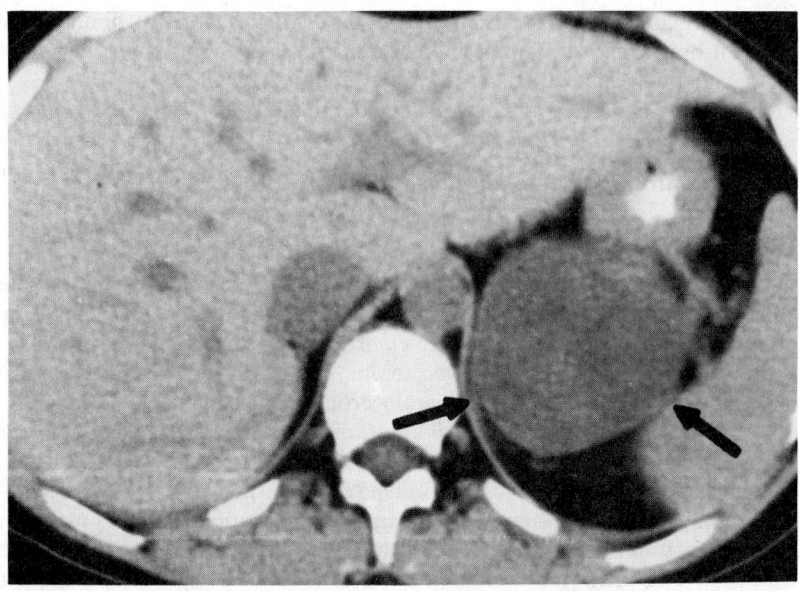

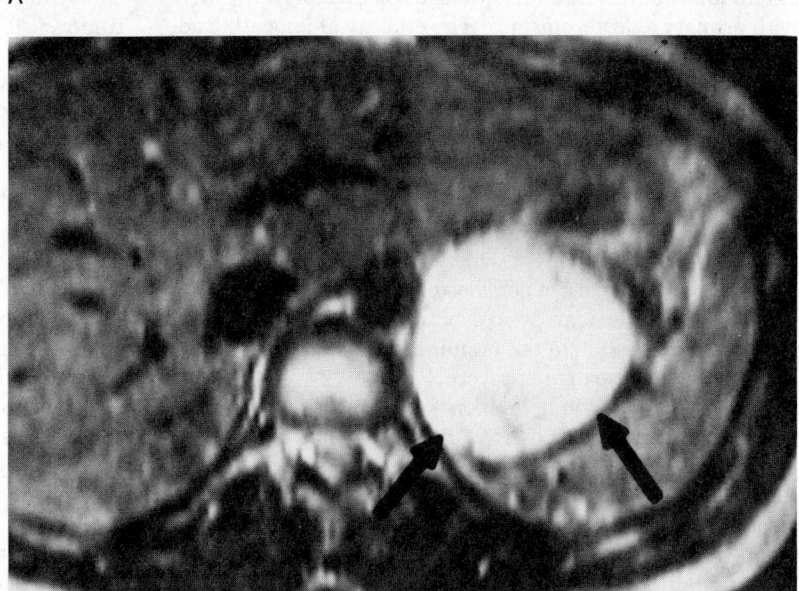

FIGURE 41–6. Adrenocortical carcinoma of the left adrenal. **(A)** CT scan of mass in left adrenal gland (*arrows*) in a patient with Cushing's syndrome. **(B)** T2-weighted MRI demonstrates that the mass (*arrows*) is brighter than the liver, consistent with adrenal cortical carcinoma. After surgical resection, pathologic analysis diagnosed adrenocortical carcinoma.

In patients with ectopic ACTH syndrome, one would expect to find the following:

1. Normal or bilateral hyperplasia of adrenals on CT
2. Normal or greatly elevated ACTH levels in plasma
3. No suppression with high-dose dexamethasone
4. No evidence of lateralization of ACTH plasma levels on petrosal sinus sampling with CRH.

Some bronchial ACTH-producing carcinoid tumors may suppress with dexamethasone, but the false suppression of ectopic ACTH-producing tumors is rare.[251] If the results are inconsistent, rely on petrosal sinus sampling for ACTH levels[268,269] and on CRH test results. More than 95% of patients with ectopic ACTH have no ACTH or cortisol increase after CRH.[264]

If the patient has pituitary-dependent hypercortisolism or Cushing's disease, the most common cause of endogenous hypercortisolism, one expects to find the following:

1. Normal or bilateral hyperplasia of the adrenal glands
2. Normal or mildly elevated plasma ACTH levels
3. No suppression with low-dose dexamethasone but greater than 50% suppression with high-dose dexamethasone
4. Lateralization with petrosal sinus sampling and a petrosal sinus to peripheral gradient of 3 or more after CRH.

More than 90% of patients with Cushing's disease have increased plasma levels of ACTH and cortisol after CRH,[264] and all patients have a gradient on petrosal sinus sampling with CRH.[268,269] In less than 5% of instances, results may be confusing and ectopic ACTH syndrome may not be distinguishable from Cushing's disease. This problem fortunately is not common,[282] and new data with petrosal sinus sampling with CRH suggest that diagnostic ambiguity may be eliminated.[268]

Conn's Syndrome (Primary Aldosteronism)

Diagnosis

Aldosterone overproduction with elevated plasma levels is the cause of hypertension in patients with primary aldosteronism or Conn's syndrome. Elevated urinary or serum levels of deoxycorticosterone, 18-hydroxycorticosterone, 18-hydroxydeoxycorticosterone, corticosterone, 18-hydroxycortisol, 18-oxocortisol, and other mineralocorticoids have been detected in patients with primary aldosteronism.[283,284] These mineralocorticoid metabolites contribute to the hypertension detected clinically.[285] The most common cause of primary aldosteronism is an aldosterone-producing adenoma, and the second most common cause is idiopathic hyperaldosteronism.[286,287] The third most common cause is adrenocortical carcinoma, but it is rare for adrenal cancers to present solely with primary aldosteronism.[288] The etiology of idiopathic adrenal hyperplasia is not clear, but some studies have suggested that a pituitary factor stimulates proliferation of the adrenal cortex.[289]

Hypertension, hypokalemia, hyperaldosteronism, and decreased plasma renin levels are essential for the diagnosis of primary aldosteronism. Secondary aldosteronism that occurs with renal artery stenosis, cirrhosis, and conditions of decreased kidney perfusion is diagnosed by an increase in plasma renin activity. Primary hyperaldosteronism is associated with weakness, muscle cramps, polyuria, and polydipsia. These clinical signs are due to the prominent hypokalemia.[285] The hypertension is usually not severe.

The serum potassium level in primary aldosteronism is usually less than 3.9 mEq/L.[290] Another possible diagnosis is essential hypertension that has been treated with diuretics. Although patients with the later diagnosis seldom have potassium levels of less than 3.9 mEq/L, the diuretic should be stopped and 24-hour urinary potassium excretion should be measured. In most patients with primary aldosteronism, 24-hour urinary excretion of potassium is greater than 30 mEq. Patients who are taking antihypertensive medications including diuretics and spironolactone should have all medications stopped for 1 month before measurement of plasma aldosterone levels and concomitant plasma renin activity. Patients with primary hyperaldosteronism are expected to have elevated plasma aldosterone levels and low renin activity. The plasma aldosterone to renin ratio is usually greater than 30. The final proof of the diagnosis of primary hyperaldosteronism relies on an inability to lower plasma aldosterone levels and a similar inability to raise plasma renin activity. A suppression test that simplifies the evaluation of primary aldosteronism uses captopril.[291] The patient takes 25 mg of captopril orally in the morning. Two hours later, plasma levels of aldosterone and renin activity are obtained. In normal subjects and in patients with essential hypertension, plasma aldosterone levels decrease and plasma renin activity increases after captopril administration. In patients with primary aldosteronism, plasma levels of aldosterone and renin activity do not change. A postcaptopril plasma aldosterone level greater than 15 ng/dl and an aldosterone to renin ratio greater than 50 are diagnostic of primary aldosteronism (Table 41–14).

Etiology: Adenoma Versus Hyperplasia

Once the diagnosis of primary aldosteronism is established, the next important consideration is whether the patient has idiopathic adrenocortical hyperplasia (IAH) or a tumor that produces aldosterone (see Table 41–14). Determining the exact cause of primary aldosteronism is crucial because treatment is primarily medical for IAH and primarily surgical for a neoplasm. Patients with neoplasm generally have serum 18-hydroxycorticosterone levels greater than 100 ng/dl, whereas patients with IAH have levels less than 90 ng/dl; however, there is some overlap and these measurements do not always discriminate between the two diagnoses.[283]

About 75% to 90% of aldosteronomas can be imaged preoperatively on CT scans; however, tumors smaller than 7 to 10 mm may not be imaged.[292–294] CT scanning does not accurately identify IAH because these glands appear normal and small tumors may be missed. CT scan evidence of a tumor does not predict the functional significance of the tumor.[292–294]

Iodocholesterol scans are able to image 64% of aldosteronomas, and the agent ^{131}I-β-iodomethyl-19-norcholesterol combined with adrenal suppression with dexamethasone can image 88% of tumors.[292] The advantage of these nuclear studies over CT scans is that they provide functional information about the neoplasm. Generally, CT scanning is more sensitive, more available, and uses less radiation per study than iodocholesterol scans. However, in some patients with equivocal studies, iodocholesterol scans may be helpful. In patients with IAH as a cause of hyperaldosteronism, the adrenal scan shows symmetrical uptake in both adrenal glands; and in patients with adrenal carcinoma causing hyperaldosteronism, the study may show no uptake by the tumor, whereas in adenomas tumor uptake is usually evident.[292]

The study of choice for determining whether hyperaldosteronism is caused by a tumor or by hyperplasia is sampling of the adrenal veins for aldosterone.[294] The procedure is performed by simultaneous selective catheterization of the veins and a peripheral vein. Serum levels of aldosterone and cortisol are measured at each site. A unilateral elevation of the aldosterone level or of the aldosterone to cortisol ratio indicates the presence of an aldosterone-secreting adenoma. Bilateral levels of aldosterone that are similar and are greater than peripheral levels are consistent with IAH. Adrenal venous sampling for aldosterone (96%) has been more sensitive than CT scans (75%) and adrenal venography (78%) in prospective comparisons.[287,294] Venous sampling is invasive and expensive, but it is the best study to confirm a functioning aldosteronoma.

The clinical response to spironolactone appears to be useful in predicting the subsequent outcome of surgical resection of an aldosteronoma. In one series before a trial of spironolactone, only 66% of patients were cured after surgical resection. When the guideline of a good response to the preoperative administration of spironolactone was used, the cure rate was increased to 92%.[295]

Treatment of Hyperaldosteronism

The treatment of primary aldosteronism depends on the diagnosis. IAH is best managed medically with spironolactone

TABLE 41–14. Evaluation of Patient With Hyperaldosteronism

Diagnosis of Primary Aldosteronism

Measure	Result
Blood pressure	Hypertension
Serum potassium levels	Hypokalemia (serum K^+ < 3.9 mEq/L)
Urinary potassium levels	Elevated urinary K^+ excretion (>25–30 mEq/day)
Plasma aldosterone and plasma renin activity	Ratio > 30 (elevated aldosterone and low renin)
Captopril suppression test (25 mg orally)	After captopril aldosterone > 15 ng/ml
	Aldosterone/renin ratio > 50

Etiology of Primary Aldosteronism: Idiopathic Adrenal Hyperplasia (IAH) Versus Neoplasm

Measurement	IAH	Neoplasm
Serum 18-hydroxycorticosterone	<90 ng/dl	>100 ng/dl
High-resolution CT scan	Normal adrenals	Tumor (tumors < 7–10 mm may be missed)
Iodocholesterol scan	Symmetric uptake bilaterally	Uptake or tracer by benign adenoma (malignant tumors may not take up tracer)
Spironolactone	Fair response	Good repsonse
Adrenal vein sampling	Aldosterone levels elevated from both adrenal veins and greater than simultaneous peripheral sample	Aldosterone levels elevated on side with tumor, contralateral side equal to simultaneous peripheral samples

or amiloride, in conjunction with other antihypertensive drugs. Another drug with potential for managing the hypokalemia and hypertension associated with primary aldosteronism (IAH and adenoma) is the calcium-channel blocker nifedipine. In a 4-week study of 10 patients (5 with aldosteronoma and 5 with IAH), nifedipine controlled blood pressure and normalized potassium and aldosterone levels in every patient.[296] These drugs usually allow effective blood pressure control.[285,297] There may be subsets of patients with primary adrenal hyperplasia who respond favorably to subtotal (75%) adrenalectomy.[298] However, most patients with hyperplasia (IAH) should be treated medically. Because of adrenal venous aldosterone levels and the ability to localize a small aldosteronoma to one adrenal gland, it is preferable to use a posterior approach for unilateral adrenalectomy in patients with a localized adrenocortical adenoma.

Results for resection of an aldosteronoma have not been entirely satisfactory. A high percentage of patients become normotensive and normokalemic postoperatively (about 95%, dependent on accurate diagnosis), and 20% to 30% of patients develop recurrent hypertension within 2 to 3 years.[297] This hypertension may not be associated with recurrent hypokalemia. Prolonged preoperative hypertension from an aldosteronoma may alter renal function and lead to renal impairment and persistent postoperative hypertension despite successful resection of the tumor.[299] Aldosterone-producing adrenocortical carcinomas are rare (2% of all carcinomas).[300] Patients with primary aldosteronism due to adrenocortical carcinoma usually have higher levels of deoxycorticosterone and aldosterone than patients with benign adenomas.[301] In addition, their hypokalemia and weakness are usually more severe than in the typical patient with Conn's syndrome.[301]

Treatment is similar to that for other patients with adrenal carcinoma and is discussed later in this chapter.

Asymptomatic Adrenal Mass

With the availability of high-resolution CT scanners, a new diagnostic problem has arisen—the evaluation of a patient with an asymptomatic adrenal mass seen or detected by CT scan. Unexpected adrenal masses have been detected on 0.6% of abdominal CT scans.[302,303] Most adrenal masses detected in this manner are benign, silent adrenocortical adenomas, which occur in 8.7% of autopsy series (incidentalomas may appear similar to the tumors shown in Fig. 41–5).[304] Adrenal carcinomas are rare. Metastases to the adrenal gland from a known or occult primary tumor, a pheochromocytoma, or an early adrenal carcinoma cannot be diagnosed based on CT scan morphology. When managing these masses, one must remember that most are benign and nonfunctional. Percutaneous aspiration biopsy of occult unsuspected pheochromocytomas identified in this manner has resulted in severe morbidity including hypertensive crises, hemorrhage, and even sudden death.[305] The suggested procedure for evaluating an incidental adrenal mass (incidentaloma) is given in Figure 41–7.

In the evaluation of an adrenal incidentaloma, two questions arise: is the tumor functional, and is it cancer?[304] Attempting to answer these questions is the basis for the diagnostic evaluation. One difficulty is that nonfunctioning adrenocortical carcinomas may occur.[306,307] With earlier diagnosis and measurement of urinary 17-ketosteroids, most nonfunctional adrenocortical carcinomas are secreting increased amounts of some steroid.[308]

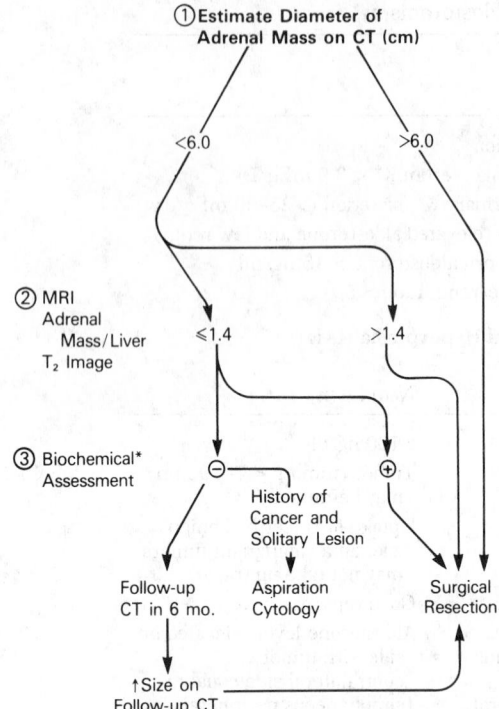

①Estimate Diameter of
Adrenal Mass on CT (cm)

<6.0   >6.0

②MRI
Adrenal
Mass/Liver
T₂ Image

≤1.4   >1.4

③Biochemical*
Assessment   ⊖   ⊕

History of
Cancer and
Solitary Lesion

Follow-up   Aspiration   Surgical
CT in 6 mo.   Cytology   Resection

↑Size on
Follow-up CT

FIGURE 41–7. Flow diagram for evaluation of an incidentally discovered adrenal mass. All three studies are performed on each patient. *Biochemical assessment includes 24-hour urine for VMA, metanephrine, catecholamines, and serum levels of potassium. Biochemical assessment for hypercortisolism or virilization is reserved for patients with clinical signs of the disease.

The first step in evaluation of an asymptomatic adrenal mass is a careful history and physical examination including blood pressure. The clinician should examine for evidence of the following: weight change, weakness, or hypokalemia; Cushing's syndrome; hypertension; virilization or feminization; change in menstruation; and evidence of occult malignancy (stool guaiac, pap smear, anemia).

The laboratory evaluation of an asymptomatic adrenal mass should consist of measurement of a 24-hour urine for VMA, metanephrines, and catecholamines. If urinary levels of catecholamines are elevated, see the section on management of pheochromocytoma. If the patient is hypertensive, the serum potassium concentration should be measured. Hormonal screening for an excess of glucocorticoids or androgens to detect functional adrenocortical tumors that have a low prevalence, such as glucocorticoid-producing adenoma, should be limited to patients with clinical features suggestive of these disorders.[309] Therefore, plasma testosterone levels should be measured if a woman or child has clinical evidence of hirsutism or virilization. Elevated serum testosterone levels are usually associated with elevated urinary levels of 17-ketosteroids, but serum testosterone levels may be elevated in some patients with normal urinary levels of 17-ketosteroids.[310] Serum estrogen levels should be measured if there is a clinical suspicion of feminization. Although urinary levels of 17-ketosteroids are usually elevated in patients with feminization, levels may be normal, so that measurement of serum estrogen levels may be indicated.[304] Serum levels of aldosterone should be measured in any patient

with an adrenal mass accompanied by hypertension or hypokalemia.

The size of the adrenal mass on CT scan is probably the most helpful determinant of the nature of a biochemically silent lesion.[304] Most adrenocortical carcinomas are greater than 6 cm in diameter, and most benign lesions are less than 6 cm. A smaller lesion should not be ignored. Early diagnosis may lead to discovery of smaller adrenocortical carcinomas, which lead to better prognosis and survival. In three series, all 5 patients with nonmetastatic adrenocortical carcinoma and primary tumors less than 5 cm were alive 5 years postoperatively, whereas only about 10% of patients with larger tumors or metastases survived longer than 5 years.[311–313] CT scans can accurately image normal glands, hyperplastic adrenal glands, and neoplasms but cannot differentiate benign from malignant neoplasms by criteria other than size, direct invasion, or distant metastases. More recent studies confirm earlier reports that CT scanning cannot differentiate benign from malignant adrenal masses.[314] MRI of the adrenal gland is a new modality but already has resolution similar to that of CT. Small tumors (<1 cm) can be imaged accurately by MRI.[315] Some studies suggest that MRI can reliably differentiate adrenal cancer or metastases from pheochromocytoma and adenoma based on appearance on T2-weighted spin echo scans.[275,315] Adenomas appear dark, carcinomas intermediate (1.4 times as bright as liver), and pheochromocytomas bright (3 times as bright as liver) when T2-weighted images are compared with the adjacent liver.[316–318]

Fine-needle aspiration biopsy of an adrenal mass is of limited use in differentiating benign from malignant adrenal lesions. Because fine-needle aspiration cytology may be catastrophic if the patient has an unsuspected pheochromocytoma, MRI or measurement of urinary catecholamine levels is indicated before needle biopsy.[305,319] In patients with suspected metastatic disease to the adrenal gland and inconclusive MRI, needle aspiration may be helpful. In a study of 16 patients with known primary cancers, 7 patients had adrenal metastases confirmed by aspiration cytology.[320] Because aspiration cytology usually cannot differentiate benign from malignant adrenal neoplasms and may be life-threatening if the patient has an unsuspected pheochromocytoma, it should not be performed routinely in the evaluation of asymptomatic adrenal masses.

The suggested approach to an asymptomatic adrenal mass is outlined in Figure 41–7. All three suggested tests—CT, MRI, and biochemical assessment—should be performed on each patient because each provides information important to management. Initially, the adrenal mass diameter is carefully measured by CT scans, with a size greater than 6 cm an indication for surgical resection. Because the incidence of cancer in solid adrenal masses larger than 6 cm ranges from about 35% to 98%, most experts recommend excision of these adrenal mass lesions.[309] Ultrasound may be useful in the evaluation of large masses to determine if the mass is solid or cystic. Cystic masses are rare but should be aspirated with ultrasound guidance. Lesions smaller than 3.5 to 4 cm on CT scan are usually benign adenomas,[318] but aldosteronoma, pheochromocytoma, and early carcinomas must be considered. MRI and measurement of urinary catecholamine levels can rule out the presence of pheochromocytoma. Density of fat as determined by CT scan may raise the diagnostic possibility of myolipoma. An increase in MRI signal intensity (>1.4 compared with liver) on T2-weighted image for an intermediate-size adrenal lesion may suggest surgical resection for possible cancer. If a surgical resection is not done, a follow-up CT scan examination in 3 months is indicated to determine whether the mass has enlarged. If it has increased in size, surgical excision is recommended.[309] Finally, clinical evidence of hypercortisolism or Conn's syndrome and a positive biochemical assessment also mandate surgical resection. This schema provides early surgical intervention for functional and malignant adrenal masses, and it is hoped that it will limit surgical resection of nonfunctional benign adrenal adenomas.

Sex Hormone Excess

The final way adrenocortical carcinoma may present is with excessive sex hormone secretion. This presentation may consist primarily of excessive levels of estrogen or testosterone or may be combined with excessive levels of cortisol or aldosterone or both. In children, the clinical signs of increased androgen production include increased growth, premature development of pubic and facial hair and acne, genital enlargement, increased muscle mass, and deepening voice. In women, the clinical signs of excess androgen production include hirsutism, acne, amenorrhea, infertility, increased muscle mass, deep voice, and temporal balding. In children, the clinical signs of increased estrogen production include gynecomastia in boys and precocious breast enlargement or vaginal bleeding in girls. In men, hyperestrogenism presents with gynecomastia, decreased sexual drive, impotence, and infertility. In women, hyperestrogenism presents primarily with irregular menses in premenopausal women and dysfunctional uterine bleeding or vaginal bleeding in postmenopausal women.[251] The workup requires measurement of 24-hour urinary 17-ketosteroids, 17-hydroxysteroids, and urinary free cortisol levels and, depending on virilization or feminization, serum levels of testosterone or estrogen.

Virilization secondary to an adrenal neoplasm may accompany Cushing's syndrome and usually indicates adrenocortical carcinoma. Adrenal-induced virilization in the absence of Cushing's syndrome may occur due to adrenocortical adenoma[310] or carcinoma.[321] Although many other disorders can cause virilization in women and children, in working up a patient with virilization, an imaging study of both adrenals (either CT or MRI) is indicated to rule out an adrenal neoplasm. Hyperestrogenism of adrenal origin is usually caused by an adrenal adenoma or carcinoma and may be associated with hypercortisolism. An imaging study of both adrenal glands (either CT or MRI) is indicated to rule out a neoplasm before proceeding with the differential diagnosis of hyperestrogenism.

TREATMENT OF ADRENOCORTICAL NEOPLASM

Adenomas of the Adrenal Cortex

The definitive treatment of benign adenomas is surgical resection of the adrenal gland with the adenoma. MRI can help characterize the biology of a tumor, and if the tumor appears malignant on MRI (adrenal mass to liver ratio of >0.4:<3.0 on T2-weighted image), the anterior approach is preferred.[275]

Baker and colleagues reported 2 patients who had benign adrenal adenomas with increased adrenal mass to liver ratio on T2-weighted MRI, but they agree with the general ability of the MRI signal intensity to differentiate malignant neoplasms from pheochromocytomas.[322] In patients who are undergoing resection of an adrenal tumor that causes Cushing's syndrome, steroid replacement during and after surgery is necessary. Mineralocorticoid replacement is not required. Postoperative glucocorticoid replacement is necessary until the patient has complete recovery of the hypothalamic-pituitary-adrenal axis. In most cases, glucocorticoid replacement is necessary for about 2 years.[323] Surgical resection of an adenoma is curative.[323] Larger lesions that weigh between 50 to 100 g and appear benign histologically (no mitoses and no vascular invasion) may need careful follow-up including detection of hormonal abnormalities and CT or MRI.

Carcinoma of the Adrenal Cortex

The mainstay of treatment of adrenocortical carcinoma is complete resection of all gross tumor. If the carcinoma is intimately associated with the kidney, liver, or diaphragm on the right, or with the pancreas on the left, it may be necessary to resect part or all of the contiguous structures at the time of definitive resection. The best time for potentially curative surgery is at the initial surgery. The surgeon needs adequate imaging of the mass including CT and MRI.[275,322] CT and MRI should include the chest to rule out metastatic disease above the diaphragm. If the right adrenal is involved and the inferior vena cava is compressed, an inferior vena caval contrast study or caval ultrasound is useful to assess blood flow through the cava. If resection of one kidney is planned along with resection of the primary tumor, an intravenous pyelogram or an intravenous contrast CT scan is indicated to be sure that the contralateral kidney is functioning. A bone scan is necessary to rule out bony metastases. A complete bowel preparation is helpful in case the tumor invades bowel.

In children, adrenocortical carcinoma usually occurs before age 6, with a higher incidence in girls than in boys. Twice as many girls as boys develop childhood adrenal cancer. The median age in children with adrenal cancer is 4 years. Virilization is the most common presenting feature (93%), although children may present with precocious puberty or Cushing's syndrome.[324-328] Some children with adrenal cancer can be cured primarily by complete surgical resection. In one recent report, 17 of 26 (65%) children with completely resected adrenal cancer remained in continuous complete remissions.[327] In a multivariate analysis of predictors of outcome, only primary tumor size greater than 200 cm³ independently identified a poor-prognosis group of children who may require more aggressive adjuvant therapy after surgery.[327]

The second peak age of occurrence of adrenal cancer is between 40 and 50 years, and about 70% of these patients present with hormonal syndromes.[300] The surgical staging of adrenal carcinoma is outlined as follows (Table 41–15):

Stage I	Tumor less than 5 cm without local invasion of nodal or distant metastases
Stage II	Same as stage I except the tumor is greater than 5 cm

TABLE 41–15. Staging Criteria
for Adrenocortical Carcinoma*

Stage	Criteria
	Tumor ≤ 5 cm, invasion absent
T1	Tumor > 5 cm, invasion absent
T2	Tumor outside adrenal in fat
T3	Tumor invading adjacent
T4	organs
N0	No positive lymph nodes
N1	Positive lymph nodes
M0	No distant metastases
M1	Distant metastases
	TNM Criteria
I	T1, N0, M0
II	T2, N0, M0
III	T1 or T2N1M0, T3N0M0
IV	Any T, any NM1, T3T4N1

* Staging criteria from references 312, 329, and 1103.

Stage III	Tumor with local invasion or positive lymph nodes
Stage IV	Tumor with local invasion and lymph nodes or distant metastases

Most patients (70%) present with stage III or IV disease.[300,329]

The definitive initial treatment for all stage disease including locally aggressive stage III disease is en bloc resection, which may include the adjacent kidney. This procedure usually requires a combined thoracoabdominal approach. Surgical resection of localized disease can be curative.[300,312,329] However, in a recent analysis of 105 patients with adrenal cancer, only 80 patients were able to undergo surgery for possible cure and the median disease-free interval postoperatively was 12 months.[330] The overall 5-year survival was 22%.[330] Age of more than 40 years and the presence of metastases at the time of diagnosis were predictive of a poor prognosis.[330]

If complete resection of tumor cannot be achieved, remove as much of the primary tumor as possible to decrease the amount of cortisol-secreting tissue and to minimize complications due to tumor mass. Patients who undergo definitive resection should be monitored for appropriate steroid hormone levels postoperatively. The steroid levels depend on the secretion of the neoplasm before resection and at the time of diagnosis. If hypercortisolism was present, urinary free cortisol levels should be measured. If levels of urinary 17-ketosteroids were elevated preoperatively, postoperative levels are most helpful. Plasma measurements of 11-deoxycortisol, dehydroepiandrosterone, deoxycorticosterone, or other steroids may help detect recurrences in an individual patient.[251] CT and MRI can help detect local recurrences and pulmonary metastases. If a solitary recurrence is detected, it should be removed surgically if possible with acceptable morbidity. Prolonged remissions have been reported after resection of hepatic, pulmonary, and cerebral metastases from adrenocortical

carcinoma.[331–335] If complete resection of tumor metastases is not possible, near-total resection may still be helpful in some hormonally productive, slow-growing adrenocortical cancers.[306,335] A recent nonrandomized retrospective study of patients with locally recurrent or metastatic adrenal cancer compared treatment by surgery plus mitotane chemotherapy with treatment by mitotane alone.[335] The benefit of aggressive re-resection of adrenal cancer appeared greatest in one third of patients who were able to survive more than 5 years from the time of first recurrence with an improvement in the symptoms and signs of hypercortisolism. However, aggressive surgical therapy was not able to cure any patient with recurrent adrenal cancer.[335] Palliation of bony metastases may be achieved by radiation therapy.[300] Percapto and Knowlton reported that abdominal radiation therapy was palliative in two thirds of patients with local recurrences and that it even relieved one bowel obstruction.[334] However, it did not improve the length of survival.[300,334]

Chemotherapy of Adrenocortical Carcinoma

Once a patient has recurrent or metastatic adrenocortical carcinoma, chemotherapy with o,p-DDD (mitotane) is usually started.[336] Therapy is initiated at a dose of 2 to 6 g daily in two or three divided doses and increased until adverse reactions occur. Adverse reactions include gastrointestinal toxicity (anorexia, nausea, vomiting, and diarrhea), neuromuscular toxicity (depression, dizziness, tremors, headache, confusion, and weakness) and skin rash. Of patients treated with mitotane, 79% suffer from gastrointestinal toxicity, 50% from neuromuscular toxicity, and 15% from skin rash.[336] Mitotane is associated with prolonged bleeding time and abnormal platelet aggregation responses consistent with an aspirin-like defect. It may cause a significant defect in platelet function.[337] A decrease in levels of urinary 17-hydroxysteroids and 17-ketosteroids occurs in 67% of patients treated with mitotane, due to its direct effect on steroid metabolism,[338,339] and a partial response occurs in about 33% of patients. It is important to measure blood levels of o,p-DDD and to achieve serum levels higher than 14 μg/ml. In one study, patients who had blood levels less than 10 μg/ml had no demonstrable therapeutic effects, whereas 7 of 8 patients who had levels greater than 14 μg/ml had objective responses and significantly longer survival rates.[340] Unfortunately, the difference between efficacy and toxicity is small, and levels greater than 20 μg/ml are associated with symptoms of neuromuscular toxicity.[340]

Tumor responses usually occur in the first 6 weeks after the initiation of mitotane treatment. Although most patients who demonstrate an objective response to o,p-DDD subsequently relapse, there have been a few long-term survivors with metastatic adrenocortical carcinoma.[341] Mitotane can be an unpleasant drug, and if clinical toxicity is present, the dose must be adjusted to minimize side effects. Because patients with adrenocortical carcinoma are rare, there have been no controlled studies to establish that mitotane can significantly alter the natural course of adrenocortical carcinoma. Some suggest that adjuvant o,p-DDD improves survival after initial surgery for adrenocortical carcinoma.[342] although most experts do not recommend it as an adjuvant drug after total resection of primary adrenocortical cancer. In a recent report of 59 patients with adrenal cancer who received mitotane therapy at a dose between 7 and 10 g/day, 37 patients were evaluable for tumor response.[330] Of the 37 patients, only 8 (22%) had a documented partial response. These findings are similar to three other recent reports, none of which recommends mitotane for the management of patients with adrenocortical cancer.[335,343–345] Other researchers argue that the dose of mitotane is critical and must be pushed to toxicity to see the higher response rates described in some studies.[346] At best, the response rate with mitotane alone is 60%, and few complete responses have been seen. Mitotane appears to be of use in controlling hypercortisolism but of limited use as an antitumor agent. We do not recommend mitotane because the dose of drug must be pushed to toxicity to see modest efficacy. A potential use of mitotane in patients with adrenal cancer is to block the decreased chemotherapy drug accumulation mediated by the multidrug resistance gene (*MDR1/* p-glycoprotein). It appears that adrenocortical cancers have high levels of expression of this gene and that treatment with mitotane blocks gene expression and increases chemotherapeutic drug accumulation within the cancer.[347] This in vitro finding suggests a rationale for combining chemotherapy and mitotane in the treatment of adrenocortical cancer, but human trials have not been done.

Chemotherapy regimens besides o,p-DDD have been ineffective against adrenocortical carcinoma. Partial responses have been reported with regimens based on doxorubicin[345,348,349] and alkylating agents.[349] Promising regimens include cisplatin and etoposide. In two different studies using cisplatin and etoposide in patients with metastatic adrenocortical carcinomas for whom mitotane therapy had not been effective, there were 5 responses in 6 patients, including 1 patient with a complete response that lasted only 1 year.[350,351] In another study, an active regimen that included 5-FU, doxorubicin, and cisplatin produced a response in all 3 patients treated, and 1 patient had a complete response that lasted for 42 months.[352,353] Suramin is known to inhibit the binding of growth factors (*e.g.*, epidermal growth factor, platelet-derived growth factor, and transforming growth factor-β) to tumor receptors and may reduce tumor growth by antagonizing the ability of these factors to stimulate tumor growth.[354] Suramin was used as a phase I agent in 21 patients with metastatic adrenocortical cancer in whom other therapy had failed. It produced 3 partial responses (14%) but no complete responses.[354–356] It has toxicity related to blood coagulation, and some patients have had thrombocytopenia and hemorrhage.[357] In one recent retrospective review, 2 inoperable patients were treated preoperatively with mitotane and streptozocin and each had a 50% reduction in primary tumor size. One patient also had complete regression of pulmonary metastases. Tumor was resected in both patients and both were treated with more chemotherapy postoperatively. Both patients have remained completely free of disease for 9 and 5 years postoperatively.[358] Gossypol has been shown to inhibit adrenal cancer growth and prolong survival in in vitro studies with adrenocortical carcinoma cells and in nude mice studies.[359] In phase I human studies with metastatic cancer, it has only had a partial response rate of about 20%. There is no consistently active cytotoxic drug or drug combination in the treatment of adrenocortical carcinoma. Steroid hormone receptors have been detected in vitro in adrenocortical carcinomas, indicating a dependence on pro-

gesterone and glucocorticoid.[360] In vivo studies of therapy related to manipulation of receptors have not been done. The available chemotherapy agents and results are summarized in Table 41–16.

Survival of Patients With Adrenocortical Carcinoma

Adrenocortical carcinoma is a rare but very malignant tumor. Some have categorized it into two subpopulations, anaplastic and differentiated, with different prognoses and survival. The anaplastic variant of adrenocortical carcinoma occurred more commonly in males, produced more frequent cutaneous metastases, and was associated with a lack of clinical or laboratory evidence of hormone production. Median survival of patients with anaplastic adrenocortical cancer was only 5 months. Differentiated adrenocortical cancer usually occurred in women, produced clinical or laboratory evidence of hormonal excess, and had a median survival of 40 months.[306]

Most patients present with stage III and stage IV tumors (see Table 41–15). The metastatic sites of adrenal cancer are lymph nodes (68%), lung (71%), liver (42%), and bone (26%).[307] Surgical cure is possible only in stage I or II tumors (tumors confined to the adrenal gland).[361]

In patients with invasion of contiguous structures at presentation, median survival was 2.3 years.[300] In one large series from the Mayo Clinic, 39% of patients presented with stage I or stage II adrenocortical carcinoma.[329] Mean survival for patients presenting with stage I and stage II tumors was only 25 and 24 months, respectively, compared with 28 and 12 months for stages III and IV. Only patients with stage IV tumors had a significantly shortened survival.[329] In a recent study from the Cleveland Clinic, patients who presented with stage I disease had a 50% 5-year survival, whereas patients who presented with stage II or III disease had a 10% 5-year survival.[343] In another study, most patients presented with functional tumors, abdominal mass, and distant or nodal metastases (stage IV). In those patients with tumors confined to the adrenal gland, the mean duration of survival was 5 years.[300] For all patients, the 6-year survival is only about 10% to 20%, indicating that most patients present with locally advanced or distant disease.[330] Most clinicians recommend aggressive surgical resection of locally recurrent or metastatic cancer in these patients, but a recent study demonstrates that even with this aggressive intervention the 5-year survival is about 10% to 20%.[335] These data indicate the poor prognosis of all patients with adrenocortical carcinoma and support the use of adjuvant systemic chemotherapy for resectable lesions (stages I, II, and III). However, chemotherapy is not recommended except as part of a study because effective regimens have not been developed.

Future challenges for the treatment of adrenocortical carcinoma include facilitating earlier diagnosis and finding better adjuvants than o,p-DDD. Earlier diagnosis can be facilitated by an index of suspicion for hormonal excess during history and physical examinations. Changes in body appearance and menstrual history are important clues to earlier diagnosis. The use of MRI to differentiate benign from malignant incidentalomas of the adrenal may help clinicians find early resectable adrenocortical cancers. Drugs such as cisplatin and etoposide or mitotane combined with mitotane[347] may be useful in the management of this difficult disease.

TABLE 41–16. Chemotherapy Agents Used to Treat Adrenocortical Carcinoma

Investigations	Drug	Dose	Frequency	No. of Patients	Efficacy
Gutierrez and Crooke, 1980[336] Fukishima et al., 1971[338] Hellman et al, 1973[339] Luton et al, 1990[330] Van Slooten et al, 1984[340] Jarabak and Rice, 1981[341]	o,p-DDD (mitotane)	1–12 g/d	bid or tid	37	22–33% PR 0 CR
Venkatesh et al, 1989[344]		7–10 g/d not given	bid	72	29% PR 0 CR
Decker et al, 1991[345]		6 g/d	—	36	22% PR
Stein et al, 1989[354] Allolio et al, 1989[355] LaRocca et al, 1990[356]	Suramin	1–1.5 mg/m²	q wk	21	3 PR
Stein et al, 1989[345]	Doxorubicin	60 mg/m²	q 3 wk	16	19% PR
Hag et al, 1980[349]		40 mg/m²	q 4 wk	8	1 PR
Chun et al, 1983[1104]	Cisplatin	120 mg/m²	q 4 wk	5	0 PR 0 CR
Johnson and Creco, 1986[350]	Cisplatin + etoposide (VP-16)	40 mg/m²/d 100 mg/m²/d	Daily for 3 d	2	2 PR 0 CR
Van Slooten and van Oosterom[348]	Cyclophosphamide + doxorubicin + cisplatin	600 mg/m² 40 mg/m² 50 mg/²	q 3 wk	11	2 PR 0 CR
Hag et al, 1980[349]	Cyclophosphamide + vincristine + methyl-CCNU + bleomycin	Not given	Not stated	2	1 PR 0 CR
Hag et al, 1980[349]	Cyclophosphamide + melphalan or peptichermio	Not given		12	2 PR 0 CR
Heskel et al, 1987[351]	Cisplatin + etoposide + bleomycin	40 mg/m² 100 mg/m² 30 U	q 4 wk	4	1 CR 2 PR
Schlumberger et al, 1991[352]	5-Fluorouracil + doxorubicin + cisplatin	500 mg/m² on days 1, 2, 3 60 mg/m² on day 2 120 mg/m² on day 2	q 4 wk	13	1 CR 2 PR

PR, partial remission; CR, complete remission.

Ectopic ACTH Syndrome

The first report of a patient who exhibited features of Cushing's syndrome described an oat cell carcinoma of the bronchus secreting a peptide now called corticotropin or ACTH.[362] Similar patients who had adrenal hyperplasia without pituitary tumors were reported over the next 30 years, but it was Christy[363] and Liddle[364] who established the presence of ACTH-like material in tumors other than pituitary tumors and in the blood, and the presence of subnormal quantities in the pituitary itself.[363,364] The term *ectopic ACTH syndrome* was introduced in 1962.[364]

The diagnosis of ectopic ACTH syndrome is based on the metabolic evaluation of the patient who presents with hypercortisolism. An early clue to the diagnosis is the presence of Cushing's syndrome and severe hypokalemia (potassium <3.3 mEq/L). The diagnosis is based primarily on high plasma ACTH and cortisol levels, which do not change with high-dose dexamethasone or administration of CRH,[264] and on results of petrosal sinus sampling, which demonstrate low levels of ACTH draining the pituitary gland that do not change with CRH.[252,268,269] The simultaneous bilateral inferior petrosal sinus venous and peripheral determination of ACTH levels with and without CRH stimulation always differentiates ectopic ACTH syndrome from pituitary Cushing's disease.[268] Once the diagnosis is established, the primary therapeutic goal is to find and eradicate the neoplasm that is secreting ACTH. When this is accomplished by surgery, chemotherapy, or radiation therapy, long-term cures can be achieved.[251] The main clinical problems have been finding the source of ectopic ACTH in some patients and treating the aggressive, underlying tumor in others.

The causative tumors, in approximate order of frequency, are as follows:

1. Oat cell carcinoma of the bronchus
2. Carcinoid tumor of the bronchus
3. Epithelial carcinoma of the thymus or thymic carcinoids
4. Pancreatic endocrine tumor
5. Medullary carcinoma of the thyroid gland
6. Pheochromocytoma

7. Gut carcinoids
8. Ovarian adenocarcinoma
9. Pancreatic cystadenoma
10. Adenocarcinoma of unknown site[365-367]

Other than small cell carcinoma of the lung, the most common cause of ectopic ACTH syndrome is a bronchial or thymic carcinoid tumor that secretes ACTH. The recommended radiographic procedures to localize ACTH producing tumors include the following:

Chest and abdominal CT
Chest and abdominal MRI
Urinary catecholamines to screen for pheochromocytomas
Plasma level of calcitonin to rule out MTC
Inferior petrosal sinus sampling with CRH in any patients in whom the differential diagnosis of Cushing's disease (pituitary) is unclear

Any suspicious finding in chest or abdomen can be unequivocally confirmed by fine-needle aspiration and radioimmunoassay for ACTH in the aspirate.[368]

The goal of therapy for patients with ectopic ACTH production is to find and treat (usually by resection except in oat cell carcinoma) the neoplasm that is the source of ACTH. Cancer resection is indicated for patients with bronchial carcinoid tumors (lobectomy with lymph nodes) because 50% have positive lymph node metastases. Despite this malignant potential, about 75% of patients are cured by surgical resection.[369] The proper therapy for ACTH-producing neoplasms depends on the diagnosis (exact tumor that produces ACTH) and extent of disease.

Any of these tumors may be malignant and may metastasize. Therefore, in some patients with ectopic ACTH production the primary disease cannot be eradicated and therapy must be directed toward correcting the life-threatening metabolic and hormonal abnormalities. Hypokalemia and excess mineralocorticoid activity may be managed with potassium supplementation and spironolactone. Hypercortisolism may be managed with metyrapone,[370] aminoglutethimide,[371] or mitotane. Bilateral adrenalectomy is recommended for patients who have ectopic ACTH secondary to tumors that cannot be localized despite diligent radiographic efforts and for patients who have stable but unresectable metastatic disease.[367]

Pheochromocytoma

Pheochromocytomas are rare tumors that rise from chromaffin cells in the adrenal medulla and elsewhere. Pheochromocytomas secrete catecholamines and cause intermittent, episodic, or sustained hypertension. In autopsy series, only 0.005% to 0.1% of persons have unsuspected pheochromocytomas.[236] When urinary catecholamines are measured as a screening test for pheochromocytoma in hypertensive patient populations, the tumor is present in only 0.1% of the patients.[372] Although these tumors are rare, it is important to diagnose and localize pheochromocytomas for several reasons.[373] Sustained hypertension caused by a pheochromocytoma may be curable with tumor resection. Sudden death has been described in patients with pheochromocytoma secondary to paroxysmal hypertensive crisis. Pheochromocytomas can be malignant. Earlier diagnosis and therapy may lessen the

probability of death from malignancy and improve the prognosis. Incidence of malignancy in pheochromocytomas has been reported to be as low as 5%[373] and as high as 46%.[374] Extraadrenal tumors are more commonly cancerous.[375] The presence of pheochromocytomas can be part of associated endocrine or nonendocrine inherited disorders.

Bilateral adrenal medullary pheochromocytomas are components of MEN-IIa and MEN-IIb. MEN-IIa includes MTC, parathyroid hyperplasia, and pheochromocytomas. MEN-IIb includes a characteristic body and facial appearance, bony abnormalities, MTC, and pheochromocytomas. The presence of pheochromocytomas must be excluded before operating on patients with MTC because an unexpected pheochromocytoma can result in hypertensive crisis and death during general anesthesia. Familial pheochromocytoma also has been described. Affected individuals have bilateral adrenal pheochromocytomas and no other manifestation of MEN syndromes.[376] In other families without evidence of MEN, extraadrenal pheochromocytomas have been reported usually in the same extraadrenal location (*e.g.*, bladder) in all affected individuals from one kindred.[377] Pheochromocytomas occur in about 25% of patients with von Hippel-Lindau disease[378] and have been reported in less than 1% of patients with neurofibromatosis and von Recklinghausen's disease.[379]

Pheochromocytomas produce catecholamines, which can cause the clinical symptoms of anxiety attacks and marked or sustained hypertension. Pheochromocytomas produce other hormones, including ACTH, and patients may have concomitant Cushing's syndrome.[252,281] Pheochromocytomas contain other peptide hormones, including somatostatin,[380] calcitonin,[381] oxytocin, and vasopressin,[382] that are seldom of clinical significance.

Oncogene

Pheochromocytomas originate from the neural crest and may develop by arrest at various points during normal differentiation.[383] The *RAS* oncogene does not appear to be involved in the tumoral process of pheochromocytoma because one recent study failed to detect any abnormality of *RAS* gene sequence in 10 pheochromocytomas.[384] Loss of heterozygosity at specific loci may help localize tumor suppressor genes involved in the formation of various familial and sporadic pheochromocytomas. Of 41 tumors tested, significant allelic losses were found on chromosome 1p (42%), 3p (16%), 17p (24%) and 22q (31%). Furthermore, there appeared to be a correlation between loss of heterozygosity on chromosome 1p with urinary excretion of metanephrine and loss of heterozygosity on chromosomes 1p, 3p, and 17p with tumor volume.[385]

Pathology

Pheochromocytomas arise from chromaffin cells,[373] which are widespread and are associated with sympathetic ganglia during fetal life. After birth, most chromaffin cells degenerate but many remain in the adrenal medulla.[373] This may explain why about 90% of pheochromocytomas are in the adrenal medulla. Extraadrenal pheochromocytomas may arise anywhere including in the carotid body, within the heart,[386] along the aorta (thoracic and abdominal), and within the urinary bladder. The most common extraadrenal location is the organ of Zuckerkandl, which is near the origin of the inferior mesenteric artery to the left of the aortic bifurcation. Bilateral adrenal pheochromocytomas occur in familial syndromes including MEN-IIa and MEN-IIb. Some researchers believe that unilateral adrenal medullary tumors can occur in these patients, but with resection both adrenals usually have neoplasms or medullary hyperplasia. In patients with MEN-IIa who undergo unilateral adrenalectomy for pheochromocytoma, recurrent biochemical disease and imageable pheochromocytomas may develop in the contralateral adrenal gland with a long follow-up period.[387] Sturge-Weber syndrome is associated with cavernous hemangiomas of the trigeminal nerve and pheochromocytoma.

Data from series of patients with sporadic pheochromocytomas indicate that the right adrenal gland harbors a tumor more commonly than the left gland does.[372,388] Pheochromocytomas resected from hypertensive patients usually measure between 3 and 5 cm in diameter and weigh about 100 g.[389] These tumors appear tan or gray and have a soft, smooth consistency. Larger tumors may be cystic or have necrotic areas and often have calcification. Microscopically, pheochromocytomas resemble the cell of origin. Tumors are usually arranged in cords or alveolar patterns[236] and may be composed of cords of cells lining vascular structures and having an angiomatous appearance.[390] Tumors generally are separated clearly from the adrenal cortex by a thin band of fibrous tissue. Extension of the pheochromocytoma into the cortex or vascular invasion may occur in benign neoplasms.[236]

The pathologic distinction between benign and malignant pheochromocytomas is not clear, and pathologists have relied on the reported benign natural history of most pheochromocytomas. However, pheochromocytomas may be malignant more often than expected.[374] In one large series, the tumor recurrence rate was 10% and most recurrences occurred within 5 years.[388] In another series, tumors recurred in 16 of 69 (23%).[391] In another experience, tumors recurred in 46%

of 176 patients studied.[374] These results partly reflect the referral pattern of tertiary institutions, but they may also reflect a higher malignancy rate than originally predicted. Malignant tumors tend to be larger and weigh more than benign pheochromocytomas, although this is not an absolute criterion.[236] The only absolute criteria for malignancy are secondary tumors in sites where chromaffin cells are not usually present and visceral metastases.[392] Paradoxically, benign pheochromocytomas may demonstrate marked nuclear pleomorphism, whereas malignant ones may demonstrate less.[236] Malignant pheochromocytomas usually have many more mitoses than benign tumors, but capsular and vascular invasion occurs with equal frequency in both.[236] Nuclear DNA ploidy may indicate malignant potential.[393–395] Flow cytometry has been used to define a subgroup of patients with pheochromocytoma who have malignant tumor. Tumors in which DNA ploidy studies demonstrated tetraploidy, polyploidy, or aneuploidy had a significantly higher chance of a malignant course compared with most other tumors, which were normally diploid.[394] It has been suggested that neuropeptide Y gene expression by tumors may be used to differentiate benign from malignant pheochromocytomas. In one study, neuropeptide Y mRNA was expressed in 9 of 9 benign tumors and in only 4 of 11 malignant tumors, suggesting that expression of this gene is seen more often in benign pheochromocytomas.[396] Other investigators have attempted to differentiate benign pheochromocytomas from malignant pheochromocytomas by measuring serum levels of neuron-specific enolase and neuropeptide Y, but observed differences were not significantly different.[397] Finally, a study by Medeiros and colleagues indicates that the malignant potential of a tumor correlates best with tumor weight and amount of necrosis (Table 41–17).[398] The prospective distinction between benign and malignant pheochromocytoma based on pathologic criteria remains a chal-

TABLE 41–17.   Differentiation of Benign Versus Malignant Pheochromocytomas

Investigations	Characteristic	Benign	Malignant
Sherwin, 1964[392]	Metastases	−	+
Medeiros et al, 1985[398]	Weight (g)	156	759
Beierwaltes et al, 1986[374]	Occurrence (%)	50–90	10–50
Remine et al, 1974[388]			
Page et al, 1986[236]	Vascular invasion	+	+
Page et al, 1986[236]	Capsular invasion	+	+
Page et al, 1986[236]	Mitoses	±	++++
Page et al, 1986[236]	Nuclear pleomorphism	+	−
Sherwin, 1964[392]	Ploidy	Diploid	Hyperdiploid, triploid
Lewis, 1971[393]			
Hosaka et al, 1986[394]			
Sheps et al, 1990[395]			
Medeiros et al, 1985[398]	Necrosis	±	++
Helman et al, 1989[396]	Tumors with neuropeptide Y gene expression (%)	100	36
Grouzmann et al, 1990[397]	Proportion of patients with elevated serum levels of neuron-specific enolase (%)	0	50

+, extent present; −, extent absent.

lenge. This distinction is increasingly important because recent studies indicate that more patients have malignant recurrent tumors than originally believed.

Clinical Manifestations and Diagnosis

Patients with pheochromocytomas may present with symptoms such as mild labile hypertension or may experience sudden death secondary to a hypertensive crisis, myocardial infarction, or cerebral vascular accident. The classic symptoms described by patients are spells of paroxysmal headaches, pallor, palpitations, hypertension and diaphoresis. In 50% of patients, the hypertension is intermittent, whereas in the other 50% it is sustained. In 90% of children with pheochromocytomas, the hypertension is sustained.[399] Patients may have signs of chronic hypovolemia such as orthostatic hypotension secondary to excessive α-catecholaminergic stimulation and vasoconstriction. Most patients have mild weight loss, but obesity does not rule out pheochromocytoma.

The diagnosis of pheochromocytoma is based on measuring catecholamines in the urine and blood and on the clonidine suppression test (Fig. 41–8). There is no single best screening test for pheochromocytoma. Some clinicians prefer measurement of a spot urine for metanephrines. The false-negative rate is about 5%. Another recommended screening method is the separate measurement of norepinephrine and epinephrine and their metabolites in the urine or serum.[400] Measuring urinary free catecholamines by ion-pair high pressure liquid chromatography (HPLC) is another sensitive screening test.[401]

If a pheochromocytoma is suspected clinically or if a patient has a family history of MEN-IIa or MEN-IIb, the best study is a measurement of 24-hour urine for catecholamine, metanephrine, and VMA. In a recent report testing 64 patients, 30 of whom had pheochromocytomas, 24-hour urine collections for VMA, dopamine, epinephrine, and norepinephrine were analyzed. The measurement of 24-hour urine for levels of VMA and norepinephrine had the greatest sensitivity (97%), whereas the measurement for levels of VMA had the best specificity (91%).[402] Another recent study reports that urinary measurement of catecholamine, VMA, and metanephrine levels was the most sensitive screening test.[403] When patients with MTC are screened for pheochromocytomas by these urinary studies in the MEN-II setting, false-negative results can occur. Radioenzymatic assays for plasma catcholamines can provide a more direct measurement of catecholamine excess, but there have been conflicting reports comparing the value of urinary or plasma catecholamines in the diagnosis of pheochromocytoma. As the plasma assay becomes more reliable, it may be a more sensitive and specific method than the urinary assay, especially when combined with the clonidine suppression test.[400] This depends on the laboratory and the method, because recent studies still report that 24-hour urinary measurement of levels of free norepinephrine are more sensitive (sensitivity 100%) than plasma assays (sensitivity 82%). Urinary assay may be more specific if 24-hour levels of 3,4-dihydroxyphenyl glycol are also measured (specificity, 99%).[404]

Plasma levels of chromogranin A may be used as a confirmatory but not diagnostic circulating marker for pheochromocytomas. Levels are not specific for patients with pheochromocytoma but are elevated in any condition in which excessive catecholamine secretion occurs (*e.g.*, cardiac arrest).[405] The clonidine suppression test has become the test of choice to determine whether a patient with borderline urinary or plasma catecholamine level has a pheochromocytoma.[406–410] It may be the most definitive test for pheochromocytoma. In this test, the patient rests supine in a quiet room while a venous catheter for blood drawing is inserted. Blood samples are obtained for plasma epinephrine, norepinephrine, and total catecholamines after a 30-minute period. Clonidine (300 μg) is then administered orally, and 3 hours later another blood sample is obtained. In normal subjects and in patients with idiopathic hypertension, clonidine suppresses plasma levels of epinephrine and norepinephrine into the normal or less than normal range. In patients with pheochromocytomas, clonidine did not suppress these plasma levels. Combing two studies from different groups, plasma levels of epinephrine and norepinephrine after clonidine were found to be suppressed in 14 normal subjects and in 51 essential hypertensive patients without pheochromocytomas but were not suppressed in the 16 patients with proved pheochromocytomas.[408,409] Only 2 patients were diagnosed incorrectly using the clonidine suppression test; 1 patient had a false-positive result and 1 patient had a false-negative result.[411]

The clonidine suppression test remains the study of choice to diagnose pheochromocytomas in patients with plasma catecholamine concentrations between 500 and 2000 pg/ml.[412] An overnight method of this test is based on the measurement of urinary levels of norepinephrine and epinephrine that do not suppress in patients with pheochromocytoma but do suppress in other forms of hypertension.[410] This test may be more valuable because urinary determinations of catechol-

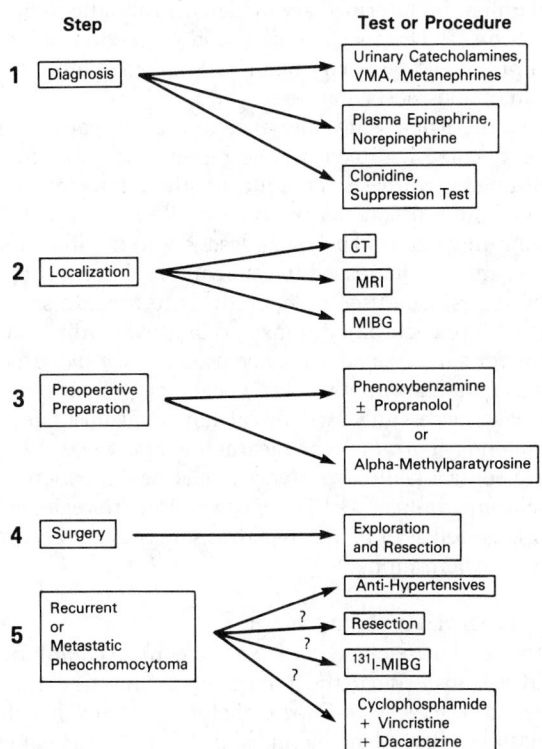

FIGURE 41–8. Flow diagram for diagnosis, localization, preoperative preparation, treatment, and follow-up of a patient with a pheochromocytoma.

amines may be more sensitive and specific than plasma determinations.[404]

Localization Studies

CT and MRI are the two radiologic (non-nuclear medicine) procedures of choice to localize pheochromocytomas preoperatively (see Fig. 41–8).[318,413] Both are noninvasive and sensitive, being able to detect tumors about 1 cm in diameter. MRI is specific because of the signal intensity on the T2-weighted image. Pheochromocytomas appear more than three times as bright as liver and few if any other adrenal tumors have a similar MRI appearance.[316] CT has a greater resolution and availability than MRI does, but MRI is rapidly improving in both areas. In a Mayo Clinic study of 52 patients with pheochromocytoma, CT scans detected 51 of 52 tumors, including 9 of 10 bilateral tumors.[414] In another study, unenhanced high-resolution CT scans detected pheochromocytomas in 6 of 6 patients who had tumors found at surgery, including 2 extraadrenal retroperitoneal tumors.[415] MRI of pheochromocytomas has remarkable resolution without any radiation. In 7 patients with pheochromocytomas demonstrated on CT, MRI imaged all primary lesions and metastases to the chest, retroperitoneum, and liver.[316] Because it has no radiation exposure, it has been used to image successfully a life-threatening pheochromocytoma during pregnancy in a patient with severe hypertension.[416] In a recent study, CT scans imaged 16 of 19 pheochromocytomas (84%), whereas MRI imaged 12 of 15 (75%) for comparable sensitivity.[417] In addition, MRI successfully imaged an intrapericardial pheochromocytoma and differentiated it from the cardiac chambers and surrounding great vessels, which could not be determined by CT.[418] Adrenal arteriography and venography, formerly the best studies to localize pheochromocytomas, are no longer indicated.

Another important technique for the localization of pheochromocytomas is nuclear scanning after the administration of labeled MIBG. The compound is similar to norepinephrine and is taken up and concentrated in adrenergic tissue. ^{131}I-MIBG has been studied in 400 patients to localize suspected pheochromocytoma.[419] The results were rated as true positive, false positive, true negative, and false negative based on a combination of other imaging studies, venous sampling, and surgical pathologic results after exploration. The sensitivity of MIBG scanning was 78% in sporadic pheochromocytoma, 91% in malignant pheochromocytoma, and 94% in familial pheochromocytoma. The overall sensitivity was 87%. The specificity was nearly 100% in each category and overall. ^{131}I-MIBG used in 48 patients at another institution demonstrated a sensitivity of 77% and a specificity of 96%,[420] and two other institutions reported similar findings.[421,422] Recent data confirm previous studies and demonstrate that labeled MIBG is a useful diagnostic and imaging study for the detection and localization of pheochromocytoma.[402] In three recent studies from different institutions, it had a sensitivity of 86% and correctly diagnosed and imaged tumor in 71 of 83 patients.[402,417] It appears that MIBG scanning is safe, noninvasive, and efficacious for the localization of pheochromocytomas, including those that arise in nonadrenal sites, and malignant disease. Metastatic bone involvement of pheochromocytoma can be imaged by ^{131}I-MIBG, but standard bone scintigraphy may be more sensitive.[423,424] In summary, MIBG scanning images catecholamine-producing tumors with a high specificity and sensitivity. Whereas CT scans and MRI reflect changes in morphology, scintigraphic imaging relies on tissue function.[422] False-positive results with MIBG scintigraphy are rare, although tumors such as MTC and neuroblastoma can image, accounting for the high specificity (98% to 100%) of the study. False-negative results can occur and have an incidence of about 13% to 20%, which lowers sensitivity.[402,417,425,426] It appears that these false-negative results may be more common with multiple tumors and with metastatic disease in the same patient.[427]

Preoperative Preparation

Once the diagnosis is established and the tumor localized, preoperative preparation includes α-adrenergic blockade. Patients are started on phenoxybenzamine 10 mg orally two or three times daily (see Fig. 41–8). If tachycardia develops (heart rate of more than 100 beats/minute), β-adrenergic blocking agents (*e.g.*, propranolol) are added 1 week before surgery. Propranolol should never be started before α-blockade because unopposed vasoconstriction may worsen hypertension. One problem with intraoperative management of patients with pheochromocytomas is decreased blood volume and plasma volume secondary to tumor production of excess α-adrenergic hormones. Phenoxybenzamine blocks this excessive α-adrenergic activity and after 14 days increases the total blood volume and plasma volume to normal levels in patients with pheochromocytoma.[428] This standard regimen has been used by many and has been a marked improvement over historical unprepared patients with pheochromocytoma.[402,403,429] In addition, lactic acidosis is often present in patients with pheochromocytoma related to the effect of catecholamines on intermediary metabolism and the peripheral circulation.[430] The measurement and correction of arterial blood pH should be performed in all patients before the induction of anesthesia and surgery.[430]

Alpha-methyltyrosine (metyrosine) is a competitive inhibitor of tyrosine hydroxylase, the rate-limiting step in catecholamine biosynthesis. Treatment with metyrosine reduces catecholamine production by 50% to 80% in patients with pheochromocytoma. The usual dose is 250 mg four times a day and may be increased to a maximum dose of 3 to 4 g/day.[431] It has been used preoperatively to prepare some patients with pheochromocytoma and unusual cardiac complications for surgery, and it may be used to treat hypertensive crisis in patients with pheochromocytoma.[431,432] Other clinicians have successfully used the calcium-antagonist nifedipine with phenoxybenzamine or nicardipine alone (60–120 mg/day) to control labile hypertensive episodes in patients with pheochromocytoma.[433,434] These newer drug strategies appear to work as well as or better than the more traditional strategy of phenoxybenzamine.

Intraoperative Management

Patients who are elderly or have had cardiac complications should be transferred to the intensive care unit the day before surgery to have a Swan-Ganz catheter inserted. This allows correction of hemodynamic imbalances and optimization of cardiac performance. The morning of the operation, an arterial catheter and peripheral intravenous catheters should be inserted. Arterial blood gas should be measured to rule out acidosis. During surgery, especially during manipulation of the tumor, marked increased in blood pressure may occur, and hypertensive episodes should be controlled with α-adrenergic blocking agents such as regitine or with agents that directly relax arterial and venous smooth muscle such as sodium nitroprusside. Nitroprusside is the preferred drug because of its rapid onset and short duration. It is administered by continuous intravenous infusion with a pump, and the blood pressure is continuously titrated to acceptable levels. The use of preoperative preparation with oral α-adrenergic blocking agents and intraoperative adjustment and regulation of blood pressure with nitroprusside has greatly facilitated the surgical resection of pheochromocytomas and has reduced operative morbidity and mortality.

The operation is performed using a transabdominal incision that is either a bilateral subcostal or long midline incision. Preoperative localization studies such as CT, MRI, and ^{131}I-MIBG guide the exploration, but the entire abdomen must be carefully visualized and palpated. Others argue that localization procedures are so sensitive and specific that more direct approaches may be preferred.[435] Most pheochromocytomas can be well localized. In instances of malignant pheochromocytomas or multiple pheochromocytomas in known or unsuspected MEN syndromes, some tumors may be missed. Extraadrenal pheochromocytomas may be difficult to find. The most common locations of intraabdominal extraadrenal pheochromocytoma are the hilar region of the kidneys and the chromaffin tissue along the aorta from the celiac axis to the aortic bifurcation. The organ of Zuckerkandl at the aortic bifurcation is the most common extraadrenal location for a pheochromocytoma. Pheochromocytomas have even been described within the bladder.[436] Multiple locations, metastatic potential, and multiple tumors all support the necessity for a complete exploration of the entire abdominal cavity, which includes Kocherization of the duodenum and exploration of the lesser sac. The *rule of ten* may be of value in the management of pheochromocytomas and states that 10% are malignant, 10% are extraadrenal, and 10% are bilateral in the adrenal medulla.[407] Some researchers suggest that nearly 100% of patients with MEN-II have or will develop bilateral benign adrenal medullary pheochromocytomas,[437] whereas others suggest that the incidence of bilaterality, although high, may be significantly less (70%).[65]

Malignant Pheochromocytomas

It is generally believed that malignant pheochromocytomas do not occur in MEN syndromes and are present in about 10% of patients with pheochromocytoma.[407] However, two reports indicate that substantially more than 10% of sporadic pheochromocytoma may be malignant.[374,391] In one study, 25 of 69 patients (36%) had malignant pheochromocytomas diagnosed by recurrent or metastatic disease.[391] In another study using the same criteria, 81 of 176 patients (46%) with pheochromocytomas had malignant disease.[374] In the latter study, original histologic review by blinded pathologists failed to discriminate malignant versus benign neoplasms with accuracy. Pathologic analysis was not helpful in predicting which tumors were malignant.[374] Patients who developed metastases did not develop them until 0.2 to 28.7 years after their initial surgery. Incidence of detection for the first 9 years was 5% per year. Males were more likely to develop metastatic pheochromo-

cytoma. Imaging with ^{131}I-MIBG was usually able to detect recurrent or metastatic pheochromocytoma. Some surgeons recommend yearly ^{131}I-MIBG scans to detect recurrent disease in all patients after resection of pheochromocytoma.[374] Others recommend lifetime follow-up with measurement of blood pressure and urinary levels of catecholamines.[391] The detection of recurrent or metastatic pheochromocytoma should be based on the same methods as detection of primary or initial pheochromocytoma. These methods include measurement of urinary and serum catecholamines, clonidine suppression test, CT, MRI, and ^{131}I-MIBG scan. Careful follow-up requires some of these studies on a yearly basis (see Fig. 41–8). With careful follow-up, the incidence of malignant pheochromocytoma may be more than 10% and may approach 30% to 50%.

Treatment of Malignant Pheochromocytoma. The basic principles in the treatment of malignant pheochromocytomas have been surgical resection of recurrences or metastases if possible and treatment of hypertensive symptoms by catecholamine blockade.[438,439] Painful bony metastases, which may be diagnosed by ^{131}I-MIBG scans or by standard bone nuclide scans,[424] respond well to radiation therapy.[440] Soft tissue masses or bony masses generally respond well to radiation therapy, if doses of 4000 cGy or more can be administered.[395] Localized or solitary soft tissue masses may be successfully resected surgically, even when metastatic to the liver or lung.[441] Standard chemotherapy regimens including doxorubicin plus streptozocin[438] and BCNU plus doxorubicin have not been effective in the treatment of malignant pheochromocytomas.

Survival data of patients with malignant pheochromocytoma are difficult to obtain because of the rarity and indolence of the tumor.[441] In a large series from the Mayo clinic, the 5-year survival rate was 36%.[439] Other investigators reported a 5-year survival rate of 60% in 15 patients with malignant pheochromocytoma.[442] In this study, patients were treated primarily by aggressive surgery and medical blood pressure control. In a final series, patients who succumbed from malignant pheochromocytoma did so within 3 years of the appearance of metastases.[443]

The early success with streptozocin in the treatment of neuroendocrine tumors of the gastrointestinal tract[444] suggested that it might be useful in the treatment of malignant pheochromocytomas. Streptozocin has had mixed responses in patients with malignant pheochromocytoma. Initial work with streptozocin was disappointing and suggested no role for it in the treatment of malignant pheochromocytoma.[438,443] However, Feldman treated one patient with a good response and suggested that the dosage schedule might be important in obtaining a beneficial result.[445] Three-year follow-up data on that patient showed that the patient maintained an 85% reduction in urinary homovanillic acid levels and a 73% reduction in urinary VMA levels with normal renal function despite 66 g of streptozocin.[446] Other investigators have tried this regimen and found no response and deterioration of renal function.[447] Some patients with malignant pheochromocytoma may respond to streptozocin chemotherapy, but many do not and it does not appear to play a major role in the treatment of patients with these rare tumors.

Because of the high sensitivity (85%) and specificity (100%) of ^{131}I-MIBG in the imaging of pheochromocytomas, its use in higher doses to treat recurrent or metastatic pheochromocytomas is a logical progression. Imaging of pheochromocytoma permits accurate dosimetry to the tumor on the basis of the diagnostic dose of ^{131}I-MIBG administered. If uptake by the primary tumor or metastases is high, it is possible to deliver radiation doses on the order of several thousand cGy by increasing the administered activity. Specific activity of ^{131}I-MIBG of 200 mCi in 5 mg has been achieved.[448] With the remarkable ability of MIBG to image tumors, one would expect its ability to treat metastatic or recurrent tumors to be equally effective; unfortunately, it has not been dramatic. Treatment response in patients with pheochromocytomas can be measured by catecholamine secretion and standard tumor size measurements. Blood pressure control of a few patients with malignant pheochromocytoma has been facilitated by ^{131}I-MIBG therapy.[442] A recent trial reports the use of ^{131}I-MIBG therapy in 15 patients with malignant pheochromocytoma. Patients were treated with ^{131}I-MIBG (specific activity 740 MBq/mg) every 3 months. The typical patients received 3 doses, with an absorbed cumulative tumor dose of 1200 to 15,500 cGy. A beneficial response to treatment was observed in 9 of the 15 patients (60%). Four patients did not respond, and the others had a slight response. No complete responses were observed. Five patients had measurable partial responses to treatment and 7 had hormonal responses. Toxicity included pancytopenia in 1 patient that resolved after discontinuation of therapy.[449] In another study of 12 patients treated with ^{131}I-MIBG, 5 (42%) had reduced catecholamine levels and 2 had decreased tumor size (17%).[450] Vetter and colleagues reported that 2 patients with malignant pheochromocytomas treated with ^{131}I-MIBG had minor reductions in tumor size but no change in catecholamine secretion.[451] There have been no complete responses.[448–451]

For a malignant pheochromocytoma to concentrate and retain ^{131}I-MIBG, the tumor must have an active neuronal pump mechanism.[451] Keiser and colleagues found that only 1 of 5 patients with metastatic pheochromocytoma had an appreciable uptake of ^{131}I-MIBG into the tumor.[452] When ^{131}I-MIBG was administered to 9 patients with metastatic pheochromocytoma, 40% to 55% of the administered radioactivity appeared in the urine as ^{131}I-MIBG in 24 hours and 70% to 90% appeared in the urine within 4 days.[453] This study suggests that the agent is stable and rapidly excreted by the kidneys and that malignant pheochromocytomas do not take up much of the administered dose. This inability of malignant pheochromocytoma to absorb ^{131}I-MIBG may be partially explained by a study in which plasma levels of dopa and catecholamines from patients with benign pheochromocytoma were compared with levels from patients with malignant pheochromocytomas and neuroblastoma.[454] Neuroblastomas are aggressive tumors of neural-crest origin that occur in children and have no association with hypertension. All the patients with neuroblastoma had high plasma levels of dopa. Patients with benign pheochromocytomas had elevated plasma levels of norepinephrine or epinephrine, and none had elevated plasma levels of dopa. In contrast, 60% of patients with malignant pheochromocytomas had elevated plasma levels of dopa. These observations suggest that patients with benign pheochromocytomas have well-differentiated tumor cells that function as normal chromaffin tissue. These cells synthesize and store norepinephrine and

epinephrine, leading to hypertension. Malignant pheochromocytomas that are composed of less differentiated cells grow more rapidly and have deficient mechanisms for catecholamine synthesis or storage, explaining why malignant tumors do not take up as much ^{131}I-MIBG and why dopa is detected in the plasma of 60% of patients with malignant pheochromocytoma and in no patients with benign pheochromocytoma.[454] The similarity between malignant pheochromocytoma and neuroblastoma is further supported by the astonishing responsiveness of malignant pheochromocytomas to therapy effective in treating neuroblastomas.[452,455,456]

There are many similarities between pheochromocytoma and neuroblastoma. Both tumors arise from neuroectoderm, for example, and both contain neuron-specific enolase. Dopa is found to circulate in the plasma of patients who have either of these tumors.[452,454] Because of these similarities and because a combination of cyclophosphamide, vincristine, and dacarbazine has an 80% response rate for metastatic neuroblastoma,[457] this regimen has been used in patients with metastatic pheochromocytoma.[452] The chemotherapy regimen consisted of cyclophosphamide 750 mg/m^2 given intravenously on day 1, vincristine 1.4 mg/m^2 intravenously on day 1, and dacarbazine 600 mg/m^2 intravenously on days 1 and 2, repeated every 21 days. Doses of cyclophosphamide and dacarbazine were increased or decreased on the basis of neurotoxicity. Each of the 3 patients treated had decreased levels of catecholamines, decreased blood pressure, and a documented partial response on imaging studies. Each patient had either progressed on ^{131}I-MIBG therapy or failed to image tumor on ^{131}I-MIBG scan.[452] In a study of this regimen in 14 patients with metastatic pheochromocytoma, the ability to respond to the chemotherapy regimen correlated with plasma norepinephrine level before therapy.[456] One patient had a complete response (biochemical and imageable) that lasted for 9 months. One other patient had a biochemically complete response, and a total of 8 patients (57%) had decreases in 24-hour levels of urinary catecholamines. Seven patients (50%) had at least a 50% decrease in measurable size of tumor. Biochemical response (urinary catecholamines) correlated well with response evaluated on imaging studies. The median duration of response was more than 18 months. All responding patients have had dramatic improvement in hypertension control and performance status. The regimen has been well tolerated and toxicity has been mild.[456] Malaise, nausea, and vomiting have been limited to the 48 hours after chemotherapy. Reversible granulocytopenia has been controlled by dose reductions of cyclophosphamide and dacarbazine. Hypertensive crisis after cytotoxic drug therapy in patients with unsuspected pheochromocytomas has been reported,[458] but this potentially life-threatening complication is not a problem as long as the patients are treated with adequate α-adrenergic blockade.[452] Table 41–18 lists possible treatment regimens for metastatic pheochromocytoma.

In summary, malignant pheochromocytomas are difficult to diagnose accurately based on pathology alone. They are indolent tumors, and the overall 5-year survival rates are between 34% and 60%. These malignant tumors may be more common than previously reported, mandating diligent lifelong follow-up of all patients who undergo resection of a primary pheochromocytoma. In patients with malignant pheochro-

TABLE 41–18. Treatment of Metastatic Malignant Pheochromocytoma

Investigations	*Compound*	*No. of Patients*	*No. With Change in Catecholamine Secretion*	*Result of Imaging in Urine Levels of Catecholamine*
McEwan et al, 1985[448]	^{131}I-MIBG	12	5 partial decrease (40%)	2 decrease (16%)
Feldman et al, 1984[450]	^{131}I-MIBG	3	No change	Questionable decrease
Krempf et al, 1991[449]	^{131}I-MIBG	15	7 partial decrease (47%) 4 normal	5 decrease (33%)
Feldman, 1983[445]	High-dose streptozocin	1	Marked decrease	Marked decrease
Gross et al, 1985[447]	High-dose streptozocin	1	No change	No change
Keiser et al, 1985[452]	Cyclophosphamide + vincristine + darcarbazine	3	3 Marked decrease	3 Marked decrease
Averbuch et al, 1988[456]	Cyclophosphamide + vincristine + darcarbazine	14	2 normal 6 partial decrease (57%)	1 CR 6 PR (50%)

CR, complete remission; PR, partial remission.

mocytoma, hypertension should be controlled medically with α-adrenergic blocking agents or other antihypertensive agents. Recurrent or metastatic tumors that are solitary and well localized should be resected surgically. Bony metastases that are painful should be treated with radiation therapy. ^{131}I-MIBG scans can localize recurrent or metastatic tumor and may be used to treat malignant disease if the isotope localizes to the tumor on scan. Treatment with combination chemotherapy cyclophosphamide, vincristine, and dacarbazine may be more efficacious than ^{131}I-MIBG.

CARCINOID TUMORS

Carcinoid tumors are believed to arise from enterochromaffin (EC) cells, which are scattered throughout the body but occur primarily in the submucosa of the intestine and main bronchi. In the intestine, these cells are present at the base of the crypts and are sometimes called Kultchitzky's cells.[459,460] Some EC cells can take up and reduce silver and are called argentaffin cells. Others take up silver but do not reduce it and are called argyrophilic cells.

PATHOLOGY AND TUMOR HISTOLOGY

Carcinoids are neuroendocrine tumors and have been proposed to derive from the diffuse neuroendocrine cell system.[461,462] They have been classified as APUDomas (amine precursor uptake and decarboxylation) and share cytochemical features with melanomas, pheochromocytomas, MTC, and pancreatic endocrine tumors.[461,462] The APUDomas all share histologic, ultrastructural, and biochemical features. Histologically, they are similar to pancreatic endocrine tumors.[463,464] Both are composed of monotonous sheets of small round cells with uniform nuclei and cytoplasm. Mitotic figures are rare.[463,464] Pathologists cannot differentiate benign from malignant carcinoids based on histology, nor can they differentiate pancreatic endocrine tumors from carcinoids histologically. Malignancy can be determined unequivocally only

if there is lymph node invasion or distant metastases. Ultrastructurally, carcinoid tumors possess electron-dense neurosecretory granules.[465] Studies using immunoperoxidase staining have shown that carcinoid tumors synthesize numerous bioactive amines, peptides such as neuron-specific enolase, 5-hydroxytryptamine, 5-hydroxytryptophan, synaptophysin, and chromogranin A and C, other peptides such as insulin, growth hormone, neurotensin, ACTH, melanocyte stimulating hormone (B-MSH), gastrin, pancreatic polypeptide, calcitonin, substance P and other tachykinins (*e.g.*, neuropeptide K), growth hormone-releasing hormone, and bombesin.[466–472] Shared biochemical characteristics include increased activity of tissue enzymes such as diamine oxidase, L-dopa decarboxylase, cholinesterase, and nonspecific esterase.[462] APUDomas originally were proposed to be of neural crest origin.[461,462] Later studies suggest that some of these tumors are of endodermal origin.[468] The numerous similarities of these tumors to carcinoid tumors make the concept of the APUDoma useful.

Most carcinoid tumors can be identified tentatively on routine histology.[469,472] Diagnostic problems can arise because adenocarcinomas occasionally have carcinoid-like features, in that both produce mucus, express carcinoembryonic antigen, and produce various cytokeratins.[473–476] For this reason, general endocrine tumor markers such as the argyrophil reaction of Grimelius and the immunocytochemical localization of chromogranin, synaptophysin, and neuron-specific enolase generally have been used.[469,472] The chromogranins (A, B, and C) are a family of acidic polypeptides that are the major components of the secretory granules of many neuroendocrine cell types.[469,471,472] There usually is a close correspondence between neuroendocrine cells sharing chromogranin A immunoreactivity and an argyrophil reaction, which may be partially explained by argyrophilic nature of pure chromogranin A.[472] Generally, chromogranin A immunoreactivity is more specific than the argyrophil reaction because the latter identifies other intracellular proteins such as melanin.[472] Neuron-specific enolase is a glycolytic enzyme that occurs in the cytoplasm of most neuroendocrine cells and is positive in most carcinoid tumors and other APUDomas.[469,472,477] NSE occasionally can be misleading because some tumors not considered to be neuroendocrine (*e.g.,* breast tumors) may show considerable neuron-specific enolase activity.[472] Synaptophysin is a calcium-binding vesicle membrane glycoprotein that is synthesized independently of other neuroendocrine proteins.[478] In a recent study of 12 patients with carcinoid tumors, special staining for neuron-specific enolase was positive in 100%, chromogranin A in 92%, synaptophysin in 50%, and the Grimelius reaction in 75%.[479]

In addition to the general histologic neuroendocrine tumor markers discussed above, specific markers for carcinoid tumors may help identify the tumor as a carcinoid tumor. Serotonin can be identified by various methods including the argentaffin reaction of Masson or the use of antibodies to serotonin.[469,472,480] In midgut carcinoids, the argentaffin reaction of Masson generally is positive and the serotonin antibody localization weak or negative, whereas in foregut and hindgut carcinoids, serotonin immunoreactivity is detected more often than is the argentaffin reaction.[472,480]

Numerous biogenic amines and peptide hormones are secreted by carcinoid tumors and can be detected in the plasma (Table 41–19). Many of these cause symptomatic syndromes such as the carcinoid syndrome, Cushing's syndrome, and the classic syndromes caused by pancreatic endocrine tumors (*e.g.,* ZES, acromegaly due to release of growth-hormone releasing factors [GRFoma], and somatostatinoma syndrome). Measurement of the plasma levels of these secreted products (*e.g.,* biogenic amines, serotonin and its precursors or metabolites, chromogranins, or subunits of human chorionic gonadotropin [HCG]) are used to diagnosis and assess malignancy and are discussed in later sections.

Williams and Sanders originally proposed a classification of carcinoids by their site of origin. This classification is useful because carcinoid tumors from different areas have different functional manifestations, histochemistry, and secretory products (see Table 41–19).[481] Foregut carcinoids generally have a low serotonin (5-HT) content, are argentaffin negative but argyrophilic, occasionally secrete 5-hydroxytryptophan (5-HTP) and ACTH, are associated with the typical carcinoid syndrome, are often multihormonal, and may metastasize to bone (see Table 41–19). Although many foregut carcinoids contain peptides, clinical syndromes rarely are produced, and elevated levels of hormones in the plasma generally are not detected. Midgut carcinoids are argentaffin positive, have a high serotonin content, have smaller number of endocrine cells than foregut tumors, cause the classical carcinoid syndrome when they metastasize, release serotonin and tachykinins (substance P, neuropeptide K, substance K), rarely secrete 5-HTP or ACTH, and rarely metastasize to bone. Hindgut carcinoid tumors are argentaffin negative, often argyrophilic, rarely contain 5-HT, rarely cause carcinoid syndrome, contain numerous gastrointestinal hormones, rarely secrete 5-HTP or ACTH, and may metastasize to bone.

Carcinoid tumors can be ubiquitous, but most arise from four sites: the bronchus, appendix, rectum, and jejunoileum.[482] Carcinoid tumors most frequently occur in the appendix (about 40%; Table 41–20). The most common extraappendiceal sites are the small intestine (27%), rectum (13%), and bronchus (11.5%). The distribution of carcinoid tumors found

TABLE 41–19. Classification of Carcinoid Tumors

	Origin		
	Foregut (Respiratory Tract, Pancreas, Stomach, Proximal Duodenum)	*Midgut (Jejunum, Ileum, Appendix, Meckel's Diverticulum, Ascending Colon)*	*Hindgut (Transverse and Descending Colon, Rectum)*
Histochemistry			
Silver staining	Argentaffin negative, argyrophilic or negative	Argentaffin positive	Argentaffin negative (75%) or occasional argyrophilic (55%)
Neuron-specific enolase	Positive	Positive	Positive
Chromogranin A staining	Positive	Positive	Positive (42%)
Cytoplasmic granules (Electron microscopy)	Round, variable density, 180 nm in size	Pleomorphic, uniform density 230 nm in size	Round, variable density, about 190 nm in size
Products			
Tumor	Low 5-HT content, multihormonal*	High 5-HT content, multihormonal*	Rarely 5-HT multihormonal*
Blood	5-HTP, histamine, multihormonal,* occ ACTH	5-HT, multihormonal,* rarely secrete ACTH	Rarely release 5-HTP or ACTH
Urine	5-HTP, 5-HT, 5-HIAA, histamine and others	5-HT, 5-HIAA	Negative
Carcinoid syndrome	Occurs but is atypical	Occurs frequently (with metastases)	Rarely occurs
Metastasize to bone	Common	Rarely	Common

* Multihormonal tumors include tachykinins (substance P, substance K, neuropeptide K), neurotensin, insulin, glucagon, pastrin, glicentin, VIP, somatostatin, pancreatic polypeptide, ACTH, and α subunit of human chorionic gonadotropin.
(Data from references 467, 472, 481, 483, 521–524, 532, and 554)

TABLE 41–20. Carcinoid Tumors: Location, Incidence of Metastases, and Incidence of Carcinoid Syndrome by Location

	Location of Tumors (%)	Incidence of Metastases by Site (%)	Incidence of Carcinoid Syndrome by Site (%)
Foregut			
Esophagus	<1	—	—
Stomach	2	22	9.5
Duodenum	2.6	20	3.4
Pancreas	<1	20	20
Gallbladder	<1	33	5
Bile duct	<1	—	—
Ampulla	<1	14	—
Larynx	<1	50	—
Bronchus	11.5	20	13
Thymus	2	25	—
Midgut			
Jejunum	1.3	35	9
Ileum	23	35	9
Meckel's diverticulum	1	18	13
Appendix	38	2	<1
Colon	2	60	5
Liver	<1	—	—
Ovary	<1	6	50
Testis	<1	—	50
Cervix	<1	24	3
Hindgut			
Rectum	13	3	—

Percentages from review of 4349 carcinoid tumors.
(Godwin JD. Carcinoid tumors: an analysis of 2837 cases. Cancer 1975;36:560)

in surgical or clinical series differs markedly from that found at autopsy.[483,484] At autopsy, as many as 76% of all carcinoid tumors are found in the jejunoileum, whereas these make up about 25% of tumors found in clinical and surgical series, demonstrating that most small intestinal carcinoid tumors are clinically silent. The anatomic origin of carcinoid tumors has presented a changing clinical pattern over the last 10 years.[483] There has been an approximate doubling in the percentage of all carcinoid tumors of foregut origin, primarily due to an increase in occurrence of carcinoids of the bronchus from 10% (1961–1980) to 30% (1981–1989). There was a marked decrease from 65% to 25% in the occurrence of tumors of the jejunoileum, and the occurrence of tumors of the rectum decreased from 15% to 6%.[483] The percentage of tumors in the colon, stomach, liver, pancreas, and lymph nodes remained about the same. Although the reasons for this change in distribution are not clear, the authors speculate that it is due to improved diagnostic histologic methods such as the increased use of staining with neuron-specific enolase and chromogranin, which have identified some cases originally

thought to be small cell lung cancer or adenocarcinoma as carcinoid tumors.[483] The exact clinical incidence of carcinoid tumors varies in different studies. In Ireland between 1920 and 1985, they were reported to occur at an annual incidence of 13 per million population per year and were 11 times as common as insulinomas and 26 times as common as gastrinomas.[485] In a series from Scandinavia, the annual incidence of clinically significant tumors was 7 per million population per year, a rate twice that for all pancreatic endocrine tumors, 7 times that of gastrinomas, and 8 times that of insulinomas.[486–489] The clinical presentation of carcinoids underestimates their occurrence, because many are asymptomatic. This is demonstrated by recent data from the Surveillance, Epidemiology, and End Results program reporting an annual incidence of 2.8 per million population for small intestinal carcinoids.[490] An autopsy study at the Mayo Clinic found 6500 cases per million.[463] In another study, the annual incidence of malignant carcinoid tumors at autopsy was 21 per million population per year.[491]

About 1 in every 200 to 300 appendectomies has a carcinoid tumor in the resected appendix.[463] Most tumors occur in the tip of the appendix and most (about 90%) are less than 1 cm in diameter without metastases.[463,492] About 50% of those tumors between 1 and 2 cm metastasize to lymph nodes.[493]

Small intestinal carcinoids may be multiple; 87% present within the ileum and 40% present within 2 feet of the ileocecal valve.[463] Primary tumors tend to remain small. If they spread to local lymph nodes, a marked fibrotic reaction can distort the gut or mesentery and present clinically as a small bowel obstruction or mesenteric infarction. Further spread generally occurs to the liver and possibly bone. Only about 20% to 35% of small intestinal carcinoids are malignant and metastasize (see Table 41–20). About 20% to 30% of patients with ileal carcinoid have one or more additional ileal primary carcinoid tumors.[494] The incidence of metastases from small intestinal carcinoid tumors depends on the size of the primary lesion. If the tumor is less than 1 cm, metastases occur in less than 15% of cases.[463] If the tumor is between 1 and 2 cm in size, metastases occur in 60% to 80% of cases.[463] If the tumor is larger than 2 cm, metastases nearly always occur.[463] In contrast to jejunoileal carcinoids, duodenal carcinoids often are discovered by endoscopy.[495] In a recent study of 99 patients with duodenal carcinoid tumors, 21% had metastases.[495] Invasion into the muscularis propria, size, and mitotic activity all correlated with metastatic spread, with invasion being the strongest predictor. No duodenal carcinoid smaller than 1 cm metastasized, whereas 33% of the tumors larger than 2 cm or 35% of tumors invading the muscularis mucosa metastasized. In this series, 25% of the tumors stained positively for somatostatin, 20% for gastrin, and 3% for both.[495] Only 5% of patients had clinical ZES, and no patient had the somatostatinoma syndrome.

In about 1 in every 2500 proctoscopies, a small gray-yellow nodule is seen and is diagnosed as a carcinoid tumor on pathologic examination.[463] Nearly all rectal carcinoids occur submucosally on the anterior or lateral walls between 4 and 13 cm above the dentate line.[463] About 80% are smaller than 1 cm in diameter and never metastasize. Tumors between 1 and 2 cm can metastasize, and tumors larger than 2 cm (which are rare) almost always metastasize.[463,493] Colorectal carcinoids not detected at autopsy are almost entirely limited to the sigmoid colon and rectum, with most occurring in the rectum.[496] Metastatic disease occurs in about 10% of colorectal carcinoids, and in all patients with metastatic disease the tumor was larger than 2 cm in diameter and invaded the muscularis propria. Greater invasiveness correlates with increased numbers of mitoses.[496] The frequency or intensity of immunohistochemical or silver positivity does not differ between metastasizing and nonmetastasizing colorectal carcinoid tumors.[496]

As recently as 1981, bronchial carcinoids were reported to be rare, accounting for only 1% to 6% of primary lung tumors.[497] However, in a study for the years 1981 to 1989, they accounted for 30% of all carcinoid tumors.[483] Pathologic features indicating a poor prognosis for bronchial carcinoid tumors include increased mitotic count, nuclear pleomorphism, vascular invasion, undifferentiated growth pattern, and lymphatic invasion. The bronchus is the site of the primary carcinoid tumor in about 2% of cases.[497,498]

Gastric carcinoids account for 3 of every 1000 gastric neoplasms, and all gastric carcinoid tumors may not be similar.[499,500] In older studies, these tumors frequently were reported to be multifocal and metastatic (36–55% of cases) and were associated with a high mortality rate of 80%.[501,502] Muscularis propria invasion was associated with tumors larger than 2 cm. Recently, gastrin-producing argyrophil carcinoids have been found with increased frequency in patients with various causes of hypergastrinemia such as pernicious anemia, atrophic gastritis, and ZES.[466,500,503] These carcinoids have been shown to be tumors of the gastric enterochromaffin-like (ECL) cell.[499,504,505] These tumors characteristically react with argyrophil stains and chromogranin A antibodies and are negative for staining with gastrin, somatostatin, or chromogranin B.[499] Only 9% of these tumors show metastases, mostly to local lymph nodes, and only 2% show distant metastases.[499] These tumors appear to have a markedly different growth behavior from gastric carcinoids, which arise independently from hypergastrinemic states and are usually solitary.[499]

Carcinoid tumors are classified by their histologic growth patterns: insular, trabecular, glandular, undifferentiated, or mixed.[472,473] The midgut carcinoid tumors frequently possess the most typical morphology, with an insular formation of regular tumor cells, surrounded by fibrotic stroma.[472] Most foregut carcinoids show a more mixed growth pattern, with a solid, ribbon-like, trabecular, or acinar pattern. Hindgut carcinoids frequently are solid or trabecular.[472,473] The histologic types have prognostic significance.[506,507] Glandular and undifferentiated carcinoids have a worse prognosis, whereas midgut carcinoids have a better prognosis than foregut or hindgut carcinoids.[506] One study demonstrated that 27% of midgut carcinoids, which have the best prognosis, were in the favorable histologic group (insular structure), whereas there were no foregut or hindgut carcinoids, which have a worse prognosis, in the insular histologic group.[507] Multivariate analysis demonstrated that histologic type and primary site have independent prognostic significance.[507]

Neither the stimulus for malignant growth nor the factors that promote the growth of carcinoid tumors are known. For some gastric carcinoids, recent data have led most[503–505] but not all[508] investigators to conclude that gastrin may be an important growth factor. Studies have shown an increased occurrence of gastric carcinoids in disease states that result in

high fasting gastrin concentrations.[499,503] In pernicious anemia and atrophic gastritis, basal hypergastrinemia develops as achlorhydria develops, and the development of endocrine cell hyperplasia, nodules of mucosal argyrophilic cells and carcinoid tumors have been reported.[466,503,505,509,510] Gastric carcinoids have been reported in some patients with ZES.[466,499,503] Rats treated for prolonged periods with omeprazole, a potent long-acting inhibitor of the gastric H^+-K^+-ATPase, or rats and other animals treated by other patent gastric antisecretory agents or by partial fundectomy, develop prolonged achlorhydria and basal hypergastrinemia that result in EC hyperplasia and gastric carcinoids.[499,503,505,511] These experimental changes occur more frequently in female rats, suggesting other hormonal factors may be involved in the development of gastric carcinoids.[499,505]

CLINICAL FEATURES

The age of patients with carcinoid tumors ranges from 10 to 93 years, with a mean of 55 years and a median age of 57.[484] In most series, the most frequent age is between 50 and 70 years.[483,484] However, in one series, 17% of patients were younger than 40 years at the time of diagnosis.[484]

Carcinoid Tumors Without Systemic Features

The presentation of carcinoid tumors that do not cause the carcinoid syndrome is diverse and related to the site of origin of the tumor and the malignant spread of the tumor. In the most common site of occurrence, the appendix, carcinoid tumors are almost always found incidentally during surgery for suspected appendicitis.[492] Small intestinal carcinoids in the jejunoileum are the most common location for carcinoid tumors of clinical significance.[463,483,484,494] Most small intestinal carcinoids do not cause symptoms, but these tumors can cause fibrosis of the mesentery, which results in kinking of the bowel, intestinal obstruction, obstruction of blood supply, and gut infarction or intussusception either secondary to the tumor itself or to direct spread of the tumor. The most common clinical presentation for small intestinal carcinoid is periodic abdominal pain that is consistent with a diagnosis of intermittent small bowel obstruction.[463,484,494] Gastrointestinal bleeding is uncommon, and small intestinal carcinoids rarely ulcerate.[463] Only 24 patients with small intestinal carcinoids have been described as presenting with bleeding.[512] Because of the vagueness of the symptoms, the diagnosis of small intestinal carcinoid is frequently delayed, with the median time of onset from symptoms to diagnosis being 2 years in one study,[463,494] with a range up to 20 years. Except for an abdominal mass with or without hepatomegaly, there are no physical signs to suggest small intestinal carcinoid tumors.[463] Duodenal and gastric carcinoids are usually found incidentally during endoscopy.[484,495,500] Rectal carcinoids are usually found incidentally during endoscopy but can occasionally be large and cause obstruction.[459,496] Rectal carcinoid tumors seldom cause bleeding. Bronchial carcinoids are usually discovered as a lesion on chest x-ray films (43% in one series).[484] Patients may present with pneumonitis (11%) or cough (7%).[484] Thymic carcinoids usually present as anterior mediastinal masses on chest x-ray films or CT scans. Ovarian and testicular carcinoids may present as masses that can be reliably detected by physical examination or ultrasound. Most carcinoids present as an isolated disease; however, foregut carcinoids are associated with MEN-I,[499,513-515] gastric carcinoids with diseases causing hypergastrinemia,[466,499,503,509,510,514-517] ampullary somatostatin-rich carcinoids with von Recklinghausen's disease,[518-520] and duodenal carcinoids with tumors causing ZES.[484,503] Metastatic carcinoid tumors frequently present in fully active and productive patients with a grossly enlarged liver, minimal symptoms, and normal or near-normal liver function test results.[463]

Carcinoid Tumors With Systemic Features

The most common systemic syndrome caused by carcinoids is the malignant carcinoid syndrome, which is discussed in the following section. Carcinoid tumors have been demonstrated to contain and occasionally secrete gastrointestinal peptides. Immunocytochemical studies have identified ACTH, gastrin, somatostatin, insulin, motilin, growth hormone, calcitonin, neurotensin, B-MSH, pancreatic polypeptide (PP), vasoactive intestinal peptide (VIP), and other peptides thought to be involved in the pathogenesis of the carcinoid syndrome.[467,470,471,521-525] Because all APUDomas are carcinoid tumors and it cannot be determined which of the gastrointestinal hormones demonstrated by immunocytochemistry or histology are released in amounts sufficient to cause symptoms, carcinoids that are found in a patient with a given clinical syndrome due to excess release of a peptide are classified by that clinical syndrome (*e.g.*, carcinoid syndrome, gastrinoma, insulinoma, somatostatinoma, GRFoma, and so forth). In studies of patients with carcinoid tumors, elevated serum concentrations of PP have been reported in 43%,[467,486] motilin in 14%,[467] and subunits of HCG in 12%.[486] A slightly elevated

level of gastrin was reported in 15% of these patients,[486] and no patient had an elevated level of VIP[467] or plasma gastrin-releasing peptide.[467] Even though these gastrointestinal peptides were present in the serum, they did not appear to contribute to any clinical symptoms.

Foregut carcinoids have been reported to be more likely to produce gastrointestinal peptides than midgut carcinoids.[521] Ectopic ACTH production with Cushing's syndrome is increasingly seen with carcinoid tumors.[484] In one recent study, carcinoid tumors were the most common cause of the ectopic ACTH syndrome and accounted for 54% of all patients.[526] Foregut carcinoids are reported to be more likely than midgut carcinoids to release ACTH and cause Cushing's syndrome, whereas hindgut carcinoids are not reported to cause Cushing's syndrome.[483,521,527] Acromegaly due to growth-hormone releasing factors (GRFoma) has been reported with carcinoid tumors.[520,527,528]

The Carcinoid Syndrome

Clinical Features

Even though carcinoid tumors have been known for more than 80 years, the endocrine manifestations of these tumors were not described until 1954.[529,530] The principal clinical endocrine manifestations are cutaneous flushing, diarrhea, valvular heart disease, asthma or wheezing, and facial telangiectasia. The relative percentages of patients who have these clinical features are summarized in Table 41–21.

The cardinal feature of the carcinoid syndrome is flushing attacks, which occur in 25% to 73% of patients initially and in 63% to 94% at some time during the course of the disease (see Table 41–21). The typical flush appears as a sudden deep-

TABLE 41–21. Clinical Characteristics in Patients With Malignant Carcinoid Syndrome

	At Presentation		During Course of Disease		
	Davis et al, 1973[531]	Norheim et al, 1987[486]	Thornson, 1958[540]	Feldman, 1987[538]	Norheim et al, 1987[486]
No. of patients	91	91	79	111	91
Symptom (%)					
Diarrhea	73	32	68	73	84
Flushing	65	23	74	63	75
Pain	NR	10	NR	NR	NR
Asthma/wheezing	8	4	18	3	15
Pellagra	2	NR	5	NR	NR
None	12	NR	NR	22	NR
Carcinoid heart disease present	11	NR	41	14	33
Sex (% males)	59	46	61	NR	46
Mean age (y)	57	59	52	NR	NR
(Range)	(25–79)	(ND)	(18–80)		
Tumor Location (%)					
Foregut	5	9	2	NR	9
Midgut	78	87	75	NR	87
Hindgut	5	1	8	NR	1
Unknown	11	2	15	NR	2

NR, not reported.

red or violaceous erythema of the upper part of the body, primarily the face and neck. Flushes often are associated with an unpleasant feeling of warmth, occasionally with lacrimation, itching, palpitations, facial or conjunctival edema, and diarrhea. Flushes may be spontaneous or precipitated by stress, alcohol, foods such as cheese, exercise, or pharmacologically by injections of agents such as catecholamines (adrenaline, noradrenaline, isoproterenol), calcium, pentagastrin, or the COOH-terminal octapeptide of cholecystokinin.[483,484,531–537] Initially, flushing attacks may be brief, lasting only 2 to 5 minutes, although they may be prolonged for hours, especially later in syndrome. These flushes usually are seen with carcinoid tumors of midgut origin but can occur in some patients with foregut tumors.[484] Although flushing has been classified into four characteristic types,[532] the most distinctive types are those associated with bronchial carcinoids or gastric carcinoids. With bronchial carcinoids, the flushes are more frequently prolonged, last for hours to days, are reddish in color, and are associated with salivation, lacrimation, diaphoresis, facial swelling, palpitations, deep furrowing of the forehead, diarrhea, and hypotension.[484,532] The flushing with bronchial carcinoids has a greater tendency to cause diffuse body involvement, and after repeated flushing of this type, patients may develop a constant red or cyanotic coloration.[463] The flush associated with gastric carcinoids is reddish and distributed in patches over the neck and face. It is frequently provoked by food intake or pentagastrin, with erythema associated with blotches and wheals with central clearing. It frequently occurs around the root of the neck and on the arms, and the lesions frequently are associated with pruritus.[463,484,532,533,537]

Diarrhea initially is present in 32% to 78% of patients with the carcinoid syndrome and in 68% to 84% at some time during the course of the disease (see Table 41–21). If diarrhea is present, it usually occurs with flushing (85% of cases) but may occur alone (15% of cases).[484,538] Typically, the patient describes the stools as watery and less commonly as frothy or as the pale bulky stool of steatorrhea, with the stool number ranging from 2 to 30 per day.[484,531,532] Steatorrhea can occur but is unusual and much less common than diarrhea.[532,539] Abdominal pain may be present with the diarrhea or independently, and the frequency of its occurrence in carcinoid syndrome ranges from 10% to 50% in different series (see Table 41–21). In one series, 55% of patients with diarrhea had abdominal cramps at the time of the diarrhea.[540]

Cardiac manifestations have been reported in 11% to 53% of patients (see Table 41–21). The cardiac disease is due to a unique form of fibrosis involving the endocardium, primarily of the right side of the heart, although left-side lesions can occur.[532,541,542] The fibrous deposits are diffuse and are found most commonly on the ventricular aspect of the tricuspid valve and the associated chordae and less commonly on the pulmonary valve cusps. These fibrous deposits tend to constrict the tricuspid and pulmonic valves. At the pulmonic valve, stenosis is usually predominant, whereas at the tricuspid valve, where the constriction results in the valve being fixed open, tricuspid regurgitation is usually predominant, although some degree of clinical tricuspid stenosis can occur.[532,541–543] In two studies, 80% of patients with cardiac lesions had evidence of heart failure.[531,540] Simultaneous appearance of the lesions on the right and left sides of the heart occurs in 30% of autopsy

cases.[542] Lesions on the left side are much less extensive than those on the right side and most frequently occur on the mitral valve.[542]

Other clinical manifestations of carcinoid syndrome are wheezing or asthma-like symptoms in 8% to 25% of patients and pellagra-like skin lesions with hyperkeratosis and pigmentation in 2% to 6% of patients (see Table 41–21). Symptoms rarely reported to occur in carcinoid syndrome are rheumatoid arthritis,[540] arthralgias,[540] changes in mental state or confusion, and ophthalmic changes during flushing leading to vessel occlusion.[540,544] Noncardiac problems secondary to increased fibrous tissue have been reported, including retroperitoneal fibrosis leading to ureteral obstruction, Peyronie's disease of the penis, intraabdominal fibrosis, and occlusion of mesenteric arteries or veins.[484,532] Sexual dysfunction is a common complaint of men with carcinoid syndrome and may be related to the vascular effects of serotonin on pelvic blood vessels.[484]

Pathobiology

The carcinoid syndrome occurs only when sufficient concentrations of the hormonal products released by the tumor reach the systemic circulation. The occurrence and severity of the carcinoid syndrome are related directly to tumor size in an area that drains into the systemic circulation.[463] In almost all cases, especially with midgut carcinoids, this only occurs after distant metastases (especially to the liver). In one study, the carcinoid syndrome was associated with the presence of hepatic metastases in 95% of patients with gastrointestinal carcinoids,[545] and with distant metastases in 100% of these patients in another study.[531] In rare cases, primary gut tumors with nodal metastases, with peritoneal metastases that are extensively invasive retroperitoneally or into the ovarian veins, or with direct access to the systemic circulation can produce the carcinoid syndrome without hepatic metastases.[531,546] Ovarian carcinoids in the absence of hepatic metastases have produced the carcinoid syndrome due to the direct venous drainage of these tumors into the systemic circulation.[546] Bronchial tumors can give rise to the carcinoid syndrome without metastatic disease; however, metastases are present in most cases.[547–549] Tumors of thyroid C cells and oat cell tumors rarely have been reported to cause the carcinoid syndrome.[532,548] All carcinoid tumors do not have the same propensity to metastasize and to produce the carcinoid syndrome (see Table 41–20). Because midgut tumors are the most common tumors and frequently metastasize, they account for 75% to 87% of the carcinoids causing the carcinoid syndrome. In most series, foregut tumors account for 2% to 9% of these carcinoids, hindgut tumors for 1% to 8%, and unknown primary locations for 2% to 15% (see Table 41–21).

In the original description of the complete carcinoid syndrome, symptoms were attributed to secretion of serotonin by the tumor.[529,530] In three reports, the carcinoid syndrome with overproduction of serotonin was estimated to occur in 6%, 10%, and 18% of patients with carcinoid tumors.[494,531,550] However, it was assumed in these reports that patients with carcinoid syndrome had overproduction of serotonin, so that serotonin production was not systematically examined in all patients with carcinoid tumors.[538] In one study of 380 patients with carcinoid tumors, 56% had evidence of serotonin overproduction.[484] Eighteen percent of 500 patients in a second study[531] and 88% of 103 patients with carcinoid tumors in a third study had elevated levels of urinary 5-hydroxyindolacetic acid (5-HIAA), the major metabolite of serotonin (Fig. 41–9).[486] In one of the above series, many patients were assessed only for serotonin overproduction after resection of the tumor, so the incidence of serotonin overproduction may be underestimated.[484] When 44 consecutive cases were studied before any resection, 84% of the patients had serotonin overproduction.[484] In two of these studies, 12% to 22% of all patients with evidence of serotonin overproduction had no symptoms, and in one study only 44% of the patients with serotonin overproduction had flushing and diarrhea.[484] Serotonin overproduction was associated with 70% of carcinoid tumors arising from the cecum, jejunum, pancreas, ileum, or an unknown site, with 25% to 40% of tumors arising from the stomach, bronchus, or thymus, with 10% to 16% of tumors arising from the duodenum and rectum, with 8% of tumors arising from the appendix, and with no tumors arising from the left colon.[484]

Patients may develop typical or atypical carcinoid syndromes (see Fig. 41–9). In patients with the typical carcinoid syndrome, the conversion of tryptophan to 5-HTP is the rate-limiting step. Once formed, the 5-HTP is rapidly converted to 5-HT in the tumor by L-dopa decarboxylase and stored in the neurosecretory tumor granules or released into vascular compartments. Most 5-HT is taken up and stored in the granules of platelets. A small amount remains in the plasma, but most 5-HT in the circulation is converted by monoamine oxidase and aldehyde dehydrogenase to 5-HIAA, which appears in large amounts in the urine (see Fig. 41–9).[538,551] Characteristically, patients with carcinoid syndrome have expansion of the serotonin pool size, increase in blood and platelet concentrations of serotonin, and elevated levels of 5-HIAA in the urine.[551] This is the typical pattern in argentaffin-positive and argyrophil-positive tumors such as midgut carcinoids, which characteristically secrete large amounts of serotonin and make up 75% to 87% of all cases of carcinoid syndrome (see Table 41–21). Some carcinoid tumors cause an atypical carcinoid syndrome[484,521,543,552,553] and are thought to be deficient in the enzyme L-dopa decarboxylase; therefore, they cannot convert 5-HTP to 5-HT, and 5-HTP is secreted into the blood stream (see Fig. 41–9). Serotonin plasma levels are normal in these patients, but urinary levels usually are elevated because some of the 5-HTP is decarboxylated at the kidney and excreted as 5-HT. Patients with this type of carcinoid tumor may have a marked increase in urinary 5-HT and 5-HTP levels but normal or only slightly elevated 5-HIAA levels (see Fig. 41–9).[484,538] Foregut carcinoid tumors are more likely to excrete high levels of 5-HT and 5-HTP in the urine and give the atypical carcinoid syndrome.[484]

Flushing is not thought to be due to serotonin overproduction, because serotonin antagonists such as methysergide, cyproheptadine, and ketanserin generally have no effect on the flushing.[554–557] It has been proposed that serotonin has a role in provoking flushing attacks.[484,538] Early studies demonstrated that kinins, which are vasoactive substances, are released from carcinoids. Carcinoids contain kallikrein, an enzyme capable of converting plasma kininogen to lysylbradykinin, which is converted to bradykinin.[558–560] Not all patients have increased levels of bradykinin during flushing.[536,558] Moreover, a study demonstrated that plasma kallikrein levels were no different in patients with carcinoids than in normal patients and did not increase after alcohol administration, despite the fact that some patients developed a flush; these findings suggest that kallikrein levels did not cause the flush in these patients.[561] The exact etiology of the flushing in patients with carcinoid syndrome may differ depending on the tumor type. In patients with gastric carcinoids, the red, patchy, pruritic flush is thought to be caused by histamine, because this type of flushing can be prevented by the use of histamine 1 and 2 (H_1 and H_2) receptor antagonists.[534,562] Candidates for mediators of flushing seen with midgut carcinoids, which comprise 75% to 87% of all tumors causing the carcinoid syndrome (see Table 41–21), include the tachykinins (substance P, neuropeptide K) and gastrointestinal peptides or prostaglandins.[538,556,557,563] Prostaglandins E and F and other unidentified prostaglandins have been extracted from carcinoid tumors.[564] In one study, plasma prostaglandin concentrations have been shown to correlate with the severity of flushing in 1 patient, whereas in other studies there no correlation between clinical symptoms and prostaglandin blood levels.[564–566] In a review of numerous reports of prostaglandin measurements in the carcinoid syndrome and of studies generally showing a lack of effect of prostaglandin synthesis inhibitors on flushing or diarrhea in the carcinoid syndrome, the investigators concluded that prostaglandins are unlikely to be major mediators of the flushing or diarrhea in carcinoid syndrome.[567] A more recent study reached the same conclusion.[538] Studies demonstrate

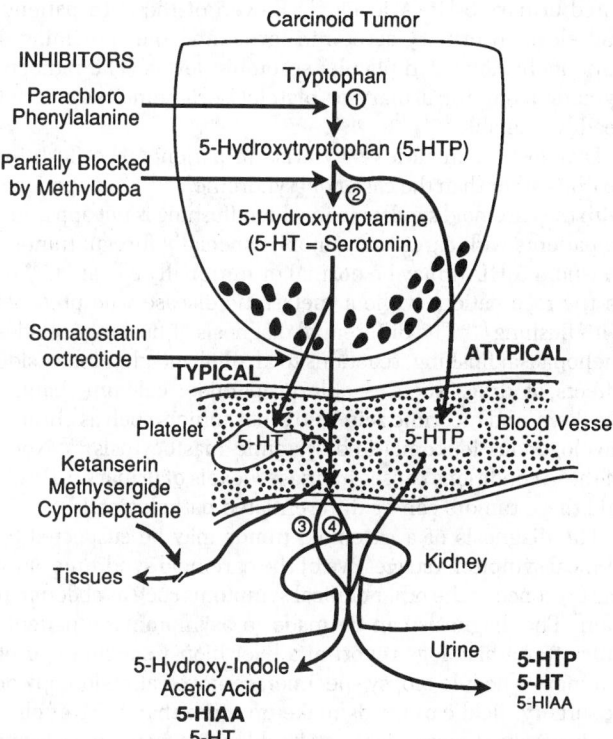

FIGURE 41–9. Synthesis, secretion, and metabolism of serotonin (5-HT) and 5-hydroxytryptophan (5-HTP) in patients with typical and atypical carcinoid syndrome. (1) Tryptophan hydroxylase; (2) Aromatic 1-amino acid decarboxylase (dopa decarboxylase); (3) Monoamine oxidase; and (4) Aldehyde dehydrogenase. Arrows indicate the sites of action of therapeutic agents used in the treatment of the carcinoid syndrome.

that numerous tachykinins are stored in carcinoid tumor and released during flushing.[467,486,557,563,568–571] One study reported that plasma levels of neuropeptide K increased during spontaneous and pentagastrin-stimulated flush.[572] Although flushing can be produced by infusion of substance P,[573] some researchers found that changes in plasma levels of substance P or neuropeptide K did not correlate with the occurrence of flushing, leading them to conclude that circulating tachykinins have a minor role or no role in flushing.[538,556,563] A recent study demonstrated that 8 of 8 patients with midgut carcinoids had elevated plasma substance P levels (*i.e.*, >10 pg/ml).[557] In addition, 88% of patients with pancreatic endocrine tumors and 71% of patients with idiopathic flushing had elevated plasma levels of substance P. With pentagastrin stimulation, plasma levels of substance P increased to more than 150 pg/ml in 50% of patients with carcinoid tumors and in 38% of patients with pancreatic endocrine tumors.[557] In this study, octreotide acutely relieved pentagastrin-induced flushing in all patients without necessarily altering the substance P response. Furthermore, pentagastrin caused flushing in some patients without rises in plasma levels of substance P, suggesting that mediators other than substance P must be important in inducing the flushing.[557] Although gastrointestinal peptides have been proposed to be involved in the flush, no changes in gastric inhibitory peptide, neurotensin, VIP, PP, motilin, insulin, glucagon, or enteroglucagon occurred with provocation of the flush.[561] The exact etiology of flushing in the carcinoid syndrome remains unexplained.

Serotonin is thought to be responsible for the diarrhea by means of its effects on gut motility.[538,574,575] It may cause fat malabsorption and probably induces a secretory state in the small intestine.[538,575,576] Furthermore, serotonin receptor antagonists (methysergide, cyproheptadine, and ketanserin) have been shown to relieve diarrhea but not flushing.[554–556,577,578] In combination with histamine, serotonin may be responsible for producing asthma[579] and may be involved in the fibrotic reactions that contribute to heart disease, Peyronie's disease, and ureteral obstruction.[521,532,556] The pathogenetic link between the carcinoid tumor and the characteristic heart disease remains a subject of debate.[484] No correlation has been established between the severity of the heart disease and other common manifestations such as flushing, diarrhea, or duration of disease.[484,580] Patients with heart disease have higher levels of urinary 5-HIAA excretion and higher plasma levels of neurokinin A and substance P than those without heart disease.[580]

Diagnosis

Diagnosis of the carcinoid syndrome relies on the measurement of levels of serotonin or its metabolites in the urine. The most commonly used test is measurement of 5-HIAA levels in a 24-hour urine sample. False-positive results may occur if the patient is eating serotonin-rich foods such as bananas, plantains, pineapple, kiwi fruit, walnuts, hickory nuts, pecans, and avocados, which elevate urinary levels of 5-HIAA.[581] Medications that contain guaifenesin, acetaminophen, salicylates, and L-dopa (*e.g.*, cough medicine) should be avoided because they may affect urinary 5-HIAA levels.[483,582]

Although a simple and inexpensive qualitative test can be used to measure increased excretion of 5-HIAA in the urine, the test is only positive if patients excrete more than 30 mg of 5-HIAA daily.[484,583] If the urine collection bottle is not re-

frigerated, the addition of acid before the urine collection is necessary to prevent oxidation.[484] With properly controlled dietary and medicinal intake, the normal range for urinary 5-HIAA excretion is between 2 and 8 mg every 24 hours.[484] Many patients with serotonin-secreting carcinoid tumors have an increase in urinary 5-HIAA excretion in the range of 8 to 30 mg/24 hours, making the quantitative test measuring urinary 5-HIAA levels the preferred method for diagnosing carcinoid syndrome.[584] Determination of 5-HIAA levels alone has a 73% sensitivity and a 100% specificity for the carcinoid syndrome.[538]

Most physicians rely on the measurement of urinary 5-HIAA for diagnosis; however, urinary and platelet measurement of serotonin levels may give additional information and it has been recommended recently that serotonin levels should be measured.[484,538,584] Elevated levels of 5-HIAA can occur in malabsorption states.[532,577] Foregut carcinoids tend to produce an atypical carcinoid syndrome with increases in plasma 5-HTP levels but not in serotonin levels because they lack the appropriate decarboxylase (see Fig. 41–9), with the result that urinary 5-HIAA is usually not markedly increased.[484] Patients with a normal or minimally elevated 5-HIAA should be screened for other urinary metabolites of tryptophan if there is a strong suspicion of the carcinoid syndrome.[584] Usually this is not necessary because some of the 5-HTP is decarboxylated in the intestine and other tissues and many of these patients have elevated levels of urinary 5-HT or 5-HIAA (see Fig. 41–9).[537,584] In an evaluation of 75 patients with known carcinoid tumors, 15 patients had normal or borderline elevated urinary 5-HIAA levels.[584] Eleven of these 15 patients had elevated urinary serotonin levels and the remaining 4 patients had elevated platelet serotonin levels. The radioenzymatic assay for urinary or platelet serotonin levels is not readily available.[584–586]

Diagnostic difficulties may arise in patients who flush for reasons other than the carcinoid syndrome,[483,484,587] in patients with the carcinoid syndrome in whom flushing is not apparent, in patients with carcinoid tumors, especially foregut tumors, in whom 5-HIAA may be normal or minimally elevated,[584] or in the rare patient without metastatic disease who presents with flushing.[546] The differential diagnosis of flushing includes menopausal flushing, reactions to alcohol and glutamate, side effects of drugs such as chlorpropamide, calcium-channel blockers, and nicotinic acid, and other tumors such as chronic myelogenous leukemia and systemic mastocytosis.[587] None of these conditions causes increased levels of urinary 5-HIAA, and these tumors can be differentiated pathologically.

The diagnosis of a carcinoid tumor may be suspected by clinical symptoms suggestive of the carcinoid syndrome or by the presence of the other clinical symptoms such as abdominal pain. The diagnosis can be made in asymptomatic patients only after a histology report of a liver biopsy specimen or of a tumor or nodule biopsy specimen removed at endoscopy or at surgery. Ileal carcinoids make up more than 25% of clinically detected carcinoids and should be suspected if a patient presents with bowel obstruction, abdominal pain, flushing, or diarrhea.[484] In a study of 154 consecutive patients with gastrointestinal carcinoid tumors, 60% of those tumors found at surgery were asymptomatic and 40% were symptomatic.[493] In patients with symptomatic carcinoid tumors, the time from the onset of symptoms until the diagnosis is frequently delayed, varying from 1 to 2 years in different studies.[463,486] Attempts are being made to identify specific and sensitive serum markers for carcinoid tumors that allow earlier diagnosis.[467,470,471,484,486,538,557] In one study, measurement of levels of urinary 5-HIAA had a sensitivity of 73% and a specificity of 100%, levels of plasma substance P had a sensitivity of 32% and a specificity of 85%, and levels of plasma neurotensin had a sensitivity of 41% and a specificity of 60%.[467] In another study, 88% of patients with carcinoid tumors (93% with hepatic metastases) had elevated levels of 5-HIAA, 66% has elevated levels of plasma neuropeptide K, and 43% has elevated plasma PP concentrations.[486] In a recent study, plasma levels of substance P were reported to be elevated in 100% of patients with carcinoid tumors, and in 88% of patients with pancreatic endocrine tumors, demonstrating a low specificity.[557] When a value of 50 pg/ml was used as the cutoff (normal <10 pg/ml), 63% of patients with carcinoid tumors were positive, whereas none of the noncarcinoid tumors was positive.[557] Plasma elevations of substance P were reported in 100% of 47 patients with carcinoid tumors, of whom 13 patients had midgut carcinoids and 3 had foregut carcinoids.[557] In another study of 30 patients with limited disease carcinoid tumors, all patients had an elevated plasma chromogranin levels using an antibody that recognizes chromogranin A and B, whereas only 3 patients had increased urinary 5-HIAA levels.[470] These results suggest that plasma chromogranin A and B levels may be useful in recognizing carcinoid tumors. The α-HCG or β-HCG subunits of human chorionic gonadotropin are reported to be present in carcinoid tumors as determined by immunocytochemistry,[588] and elevated plasma levels of HCG are reported in 28% of carcinoid tumors.[540,589] In a review of an ongoing prospective study, it was pointed out that HCG levels are elevated in the plasma in a much lower percentage of cases than the literature suggests; therefore, it is unlikely to be useful in diagnosis.[484] Although CEA antigen is elevated in some neuroendocrine tumors, it is usually normal or minimally elevated in patients with metastatic carcinoid tumors.[590] Markedly elevated levels suggest the presence of a second tumor.[484]

Because measurements of urinary 5-HIAA levels and plasma assays of amines or peptides are unable to identify all patients with carcinoid tumors, various provocative tests have been proposed. Adrenergic agents[535,591] and pentagastrin can stimulate flushing attacks.[533,557] Pentagastrin has been used as a provocative test in patients with carcinoid tumors,[533,538,557] and caused flushing in 100% of patients in two series.[555,557] In one study, more than 75% of patients demonstrated enhanced release of substance P after pentagastrin stimulation,[557] whereas in another study none of the patients demonstrated increased levels after pentagastrin.[555] In one study, 50% of patients demonstrated an increase of more than 150 pg/ml in plasma levels of substance P; however, 38% of patients with pancreatic endocrine tumors also demonstrated an increase, suggesting this test may be of limited usefulness.[557] Provocative tests have been used in too few patients to assess their potential usefulness.

Localization

Many techniques have been used to determine the location of the primary tumor and the tumor extent, including gastrointestinal endoscopy, gastrointestinal barium x-ray films, chest x-ray films, imaging studies (ultrasound, CT scan, MRI, angiography), selective venous sampling for hormones, and radionuclide scanning (radiolabeled octreotide, iodinated MIBG).[483,484]

Bronchial carcinoids usually are detected by chest x-ray film, MRI, and CT and occasionally are detected by bronchoscopy.[484,526,549] The bronchial carcinoid tumors appear most frequently (37%) as opacities with sharp or notched margins.[592] They were slow growing and often induced airway compression with resultant atelectasis, and enlarged hilar lymph nodes from metastasis were rare.[592] Rectal, colonic, and gastric carcinoids almost always are detected by gastrointestinal endoscopy, with barium x-ray films generally having negative results.[493,500] In one study, positive barium x-ray studies showed dilated loops of small bowel or extrinsic filling defects but rarely detected a mucosal lesion,[493] whereas ileal, cecal, and right colon tumors were diagnosed or suggested on x-ray studies by others.[483,593,594]

The main problem is in localizing small bowel carcinoids, which may be small and frequently are missed by barium studies,[594] and small carcinoids in other gastrointestinal tissues.[483] Some of these tumors can be localized by angiography[595,596] or CT scanning[596–598] but many are not seen with these modalities. Liver metastases usually are detected by CT scanning, however, and angiography remains the most sensitive method for detecting liver metastases.[484,596,597,599,600] CT scanning is the primary diagnostic modality for tumor staging. Liver lesions appear as focal hypodense lesions on nonenhanced CT scans.[600]

Recently, scanning with ^{123}I-MIBG or ^{131}I-MIBG either alone or with CT scanning has been recommended for carcinoid tumors.[483,484,601,602] ^{125}I-MIBG, which is concentrated by a sodium-dependent neuronal pump in pheochromocytomas, is also concentrated by carcinoid tumors. In a recent review of a number of series, the overall sensitivity was reported as 55% with a specificity of 95%.[483] In a study of 82 patients with carcinoid tumors, ^{131}I-MIBG identified 59% of the primary or distant metastatic sites, localized 68% of ileal carcinoids, and localized 64% of patients with an unknown carcinoid site. In only 38% of patients did ^{131}I-MIBG localize foregut tumors.[601] ^{131}I-MIBG was more likely to accumulate in patients with elevated urinary 5-HIAA levels (70%), elevated urinary serotonin levels (70%), and elevated serum serotonin levels (80%), than in patients with normal 5-HIAA levels (23%), urinary serotonin levels (44%), or plasma serotonin levels (12%).[601] However, the likelihood of the ^{131}I-MIBG scan being positive did not correlate with the presence of absence of the carcinoid syndrome (68% versus 44%).[601] In general, ^{131}I-MIBG was more useful for visualizing metastatic tumors than for identifying the primary tumor.[484,601] Because the liver concentrates a small amount of ^{131}I-MIBG, the combination of a ^{99m}Tc-liver-spleen scan and ^{131}I-MIBG scan is recommended to detect liver involvement.[484]

Carcinoid tumors possess high-affinity receptors for the hormone somatostatin in 87% of cases.[603] The somatostatin receptors were present in the primary tumor and in the metastases.[603] Recently, ^{123}I-labeled octreotide, a synthetic somatostatin analog that has a high affinity for somatostatin receptors and is only slowly degraded, has been used to localize carcinoid tumors and pancreatic endocrine tumors.[604–606] In one study, primary tumors or metastases, often previously unrecognized, were identified in 12 of 13 patients with carcinoid tumors.[606] Metastatic tumor in the liver was detected in 85% of cases, and primary tumor in the ileum was detected in all 6 cases.[606] In more than 50% of patients, extensive metastatic disease that had not been appreciated by other modalities was detected.[606] However, only a small number of patients have been assessed with iodinated MIBG or octreotide and compared with patients assessed by widely used imaging modalities such as CT with or without contrast or MRI. Therefore, the roles of these two new methods have not been defined clearly.

Bone metastases are increasingly being recognized in patients with metastatic carcinoid and pancreatic endocrine tumors.[606–608] In one recent study of 12 patients with carcinoid tumors, of which 11 had liver metastases, bony metastases were found in 8 patients (75%) using ^{125}I-radiolabeled octreotide.[606] In general, ^{99m}Tc bone scanning is more sensitive than conventional radiographs for detecting metastases to bone.[484,607]

Prognosis

The carcinoid syndrome is generally a manifestation of advanced disease. Two of every 3 patients with the carcinoid syndrome have physical signs of cancer such as an abdominal mass or hepatomegaly.[463] In the remaining patients, the disease is easy to identify on imaging studies. A positive correlation between tumor mass and urinary 5-HIAA levels makes this laboratory test a good marker for extent of disease.[463,506,531] Flushing alone does not indicate an extremely poor prognosis or the need for immediate aggressive intervention. Patients with elevated levels of urinary 5-HIAA may have only minimal symptoms such as occasional flushing or mild diarrhea for many years.

Survival rates depend on the site and the extent of the carcinoid tumors.[482] For patients with local disease only, the 5-year survival was found to be 94%, ranging from 75% for carcinoids of the small intestine and ileum to 99% for carcinoids of the appendix (Table 41–22). In patients with regional involvement, 5-year survival was 64% overall, ranging from 23% for the stomach to 100% for the appendix. For patients with distant metastases, the overall 5-year survival was 18%, ranging from no survival with carcinoids of the stomach to 19% for carcinoids of the small intestine. Five-year survival rates were highest for carcinoids of the appendix (92%–99%),[463,482] followed by lung (87%),[482] rectum (76%–100%),[482,493,609,610] small intestine (42%–71%),[463,482,494,611,612] and colon and stomach (52%; see Table 41–22).[482] The chance of finding regional invasion or metastatic disease is directly proportional to the size of the primary tumors.[463,612–615] If carcinoid tumors are smaller than 1 cm in diameter, less than 15% to 18% of patients with small bowel primaries have metastases, up to 20% with rectal primaries have metastases, and up to 2% with appendiceal primaries have metastases.[463,486,492,610] Of patients with carcinoid tumors larger than 2 cm in diameter, 86% to 95% with small bowel primaries have metastases, almost all with rectal primaries have metastases, and 33% with appendiceal primaries have metastases.[463,494,610] For all patients with carcinoid tumors, the reported 5-year survivals range from 65% to 82%.[482,486] Race, age, and sex have no influence on survival.[482]

The histologic stage of the carcinoid tumor has been shown to correlate with disease-specific survival and the risk of metastases.[493,495,496,612,613] In one recent study, carcinoid tumors were staged according to Dukes' classification and demonstrated a 10-year disease-specific survival of 100% for Dukes' A (n=3 patients), 80% for Dukes' B (n=12 patients), 55% for Dukes' C (n=22 patients), and 10% for Dukes' D classification.[612] Recently, flow cytometry has been used to define the malignant potential for gastrointestinal and bronchial carcinoids.[616–621] In two studies of gastrointestinal carcinoids, aneuploidy was found in 5% and 45% of patients and tetraploidy in 5% and 6% of patients.[616,619] The presence of metastases or decreased survival correlated with the presence of aneuploidy. In bronchial carcinoids, aneuploidy was reported to occur in 50% to 79% in two studies.[621,622] In some studies[621–623] but not others,[624] flow cytometry was able to predict the presence of metastasis or decreased survival. In one study, aneuploidy was seen significantly more frequently in atypical tumors (74% of cases) than in typical bronchial carcinoid tumors (18%; $p<0.001$).[622]

The median survivals reported for patients with carcinoid syndrome from the time of the onset of symptoms range from 3.5 to 8.5 years, and the presence of the carcinoid syndrome is associated with decreased survival.[486,531] The mean survival

TABLE 41–22. Prognosis of Carcinoid Tumors

Site	No. of Patients	Patients With Metastases (%)	5-Year Survival (%)			
			Local	Regional Metastasis	Distant Metastasis	All Stages
Appendix	820	5	99	100	27	99
Rectum	295	15	92	44	7	83
Lung and bronchus	190	21	96	71	11	87
Small intestine and ileocecum	366	60	75	59	19	54
Colon	112	71	77	65	17	52
Stomach	41	54	93	23	0	52
All sites	1824	23	94	64	18	82

(Modified from Godwin JD. Carcinoid tumors: an analysis of 2837 cases. Cancer 1975;36:560)

after recognition of abnormal excretion of 5-HIAA was 23 months,[531] and the 5-year survivals after onset of symptoms in two studies were 30% and 67%.[486,531] Although an occasional patient lives for 30 years with carcinoid syndrome,[463] and some may live for many years excreting 300 to 400 mg of 5-HIAA per day,[531] the level of urinary 5-HIAA excretion generally correlates with survival.[531] In one study, patients who excreted 10 to 49 mg of 5-HIAA daily had a mean survival of 29 months; those with daily 5-HIAA excretions of 50 to 149 mg had a mean survival of 24 months; and those excreting more than 150 mg of 5-HIAA daily had a mean survival of 13 months.[531]

The most immediate life-threatening complication of the carcinoid syndrome, the carcinoid crisis, is observed more frequently in patients who have intense symptoms from foregut carcinoids or who have greatly elevated urinary 5-HIAA levels (>200 mg/day).[625] The carcinoid crisis may occur spontaneously or may be associated with stress, anesthesia, chemotherapy, or even biopsy of hepatic metastases.[463,626–629] Patients usually develop an intense flush, diarrhea, and abdominal pain. Mentation is altered, ranging from lightheadedness to coma. Cardiac abnormalities may occur, including tachycardia, hypertension, or profound hypotension. This crisis can be treated successfully but in many patients may be a terminal event.[463,625,626] Recent treatment strategies using the somatostatin analog octreotide have improved the treatment of carcinoid crises greatly, and these methods are discussed in the next section.

Treatment of the Carcinoid Syndrome

Many patients can have hepatic metastases from carcinoid tumor and remain active and well except for occasional episodes of flushing or diarrhea. Management of these patients includes avoiding stress and conditions or substances that precipitate flushing and dietary supplementation with nicotinamide (Fig. 41–10).[521] Heart failure may require diuretics, wheezing may require oral bronchodilators (*e.g.*, salbutamol, a bronchodilator that interacts with β-adrenergic receptors and does not induce flushing, or aminophylline), and mild diarrhea may respond to antidiarrheal agents (*e.g.*, loperamide or diphenoxylate; see Fig. 41–10). If patients still have carcinoid syndrome symptoms, agents that may help relieve the flushing, diarrhea, or wheezing should be used on a trial-and-error basis. These agents act in various ways: they inhibit the synthesis of serotonin, act as serotonin receptor antagonists, block the action of serotonin on target tissues, or inhibit the release of vasoactive substances. Parachlorophenylalanine blocks the hydroxylase enzyme that converts tryptophan to 5-HTP (see Fig. 41–9) and has been shown to relieve diarrhea and improve flushing in some patients and to reduce urinary levels of 5-HIAA.[625,630] The side effects of this agent, including hypersensitivity reactions and psychiatric disturbances, make it intolerable for long-term clinical use.[625,630] Alpha-methyldopa partially blocks the conversion of 5-HTP to serotonin (see Fig. 41–9), but its effect is partial.[537] It occasionally relieves flushing, which may be secondary to inhibiting catecholamine-stimulated release of vasoactive substances, and has little effect on gastrointestinal symptoms.[521,532] Phenoxybenzamine, an α-adrenergic antagonist, and phenothiazines, possibly acting as α-adrenergic antagonists, may block flushing provoked by alcohol or other agents, although patients frequently become refractory.[521,532,554,577] The serotonin receptor antagonists methylsergide,[554] cyproheptadine,[577,578,631–633] and,

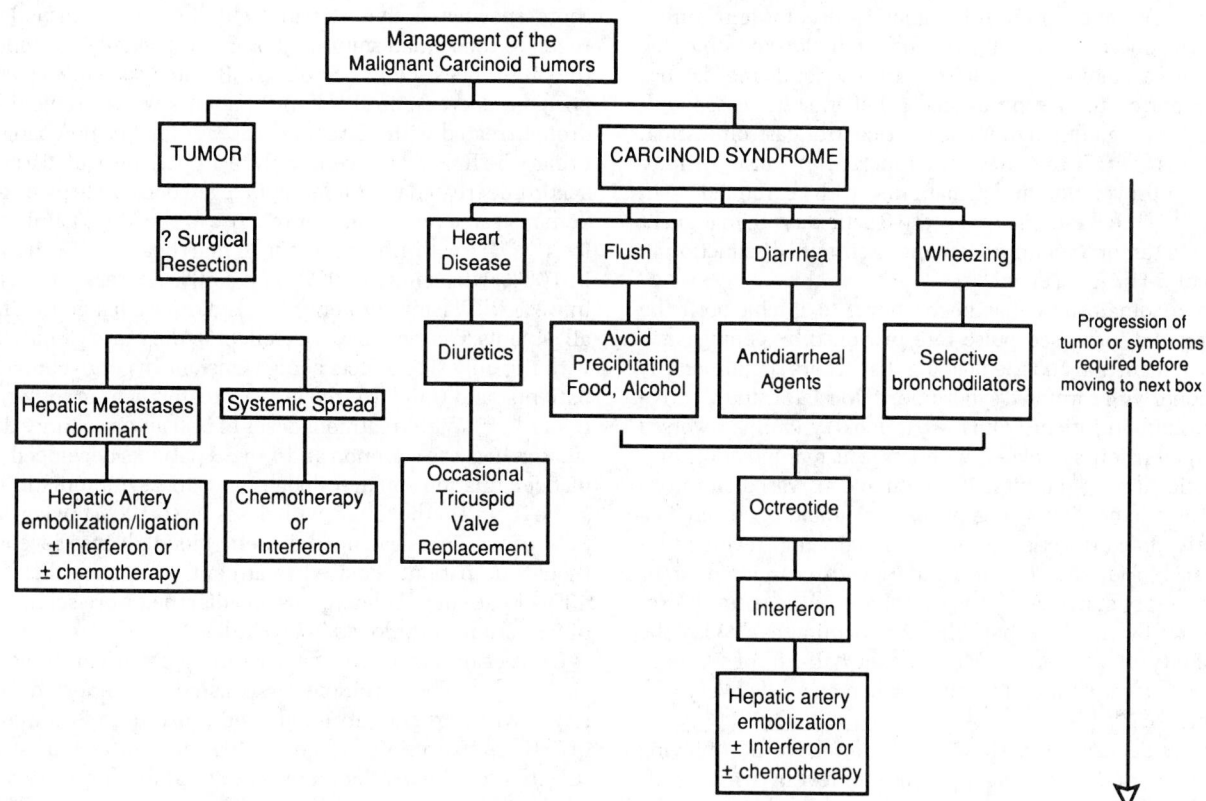

FIGURE 41–10. Flow diagram for the treatment of malignant carcinoid tumors.

more recently, ketanserin[634,635] have been used with success to treat gastrointestinal symptoms such as diarrhea but usually do not decrease flushing. In one study, cyproheptadine used at a dose of 3 to 8 mg three times daily reduced diarrhea in 50% of patients, with minimal or no effect on flushing or excretion of 5-HIAA.[463] In a study of 16 patients with carcinoid syndrome who were given up to 48 mg of cyproheptadine daily, diarrhea decreased by 50% or more in 58%, flushing decreased more than 50% in 17%, and levels of 5-HIAA did not decrease more than 50% in any patient.[578] Cyproheptadine was discontinued in 19% of patients because of side effects.[578] The recommended starting dose is 0.4 mg/kg/day given in divided portions and then reduced to a level that produces only minimal side effects.[578] If no benefit is seen in 1 week, the drug should be discontinued. Cyproheptadine is reported to have antitumor activity.[578,633] The use of methysergide is limited because it can cause or enhance retroperitoneal fibrosis. Ketanserin, like cyproheptadine, is a selective serotonin type II (S_2) receptor antagonist and has weak α-blocking and H_1 receptor blocking properties.[635] In one placebo-controlled study, a daily dose of 40 to 160 mg of ketanserin diminished the frequency and severity of flushing in 70% of patients and of diarrhea in 30% of patients.[635] In another study, ketanserin controlled pentagastrin-provoked flushing, dyspnea, and diarrhea in all patients (n=6).[634] Ketanserin decreased pentagastrin-provoked gastrointestinal symptoms in 93% of patients in another study, whereas flushing was controlled in only 6% of patients.[655] In open trials, ketanserin decreased the severity and frequency of flushing in 68% of 31 patients and lessened diarrhea in 75% of 29 patients.[634,636] An antagonist of the S_3 receptor recently has been reported to decrease diarrhea in patients with the carcinoid syndrome.[637] A combination of H_1- and H_2-receptor antagonists has been reported to be effective in carcinoid syndrome due to gastric carcinoids.[534] Prednisone in doses of 20 mg/day has been reported to give occasional relief in some cases with severe flushing, although it does not control gastrointestinal symptoms.[521,532] Tamoxifen was reported to cause symptomatic improvement in 2 patients with carcinoid syndrome.[638,639] However, in a study of 16 patients with malignant carcinoid tumors, no improvement or sustained reduction in levels of 5-HIAA occurred.[640]

Native somatostatin has been shown to inhibit both the flushing and increased pulse rate provoked by pentagastrin and food ingestion and the flushing that occurs spontaneously in patients with carcinoid syndrome.[533] In a later study, native somatostatin in patients with the carcinoid syndrome reversed the hypotension associated with surgical manipulation of a carcinoid tumor,[641] inhibited the cutaneous vasodilation induced by ethanol or norepinephrine,[642] inhibited the diarrhea and bronchoconstriction in one patient,[643] and reversed intestinal chloride secretion in a patient with a carcinoid tumor and secretory diarrhea.[644] The usefulness of the natural form is limited by its short half-life (2.5–3 minutes). With the availability of octreotide, which has a half-life of 90 minutes,[645,646] treatment can be given subcutaneously every 6 to 12 hours.[645-647]

Octreotide has been shown to be effective at relieving symptoms and decreasing hormone levels when self-administered every 6 to 12 hours subcutaneously in patients with carcinoid syndrome[463,648-652] and pancreatic endocrine tumors, which are discussed in a later section (see Pancreatic Endocrine Tumors). Octreotide recently has been shown to decrease serotonin and neuropeptide K release from midgut carcinoids by a direct action on tumor cells.[653] Octreotide inhibited release of serotonin and neuropeptide K from tumor cell cultures prepared from 4 midgut carcinoids and the synthesis of these substances by the tumor cells.[653] In Mayo Clinic studies of 53 patients with carcinoid syndrome, octreotide caused complete improvement in flushing in 53% and a 50% or more decrease in an additional 32%.[463,650,654] Diarrhea was completely improved in 25% of patients and partially improved in an additional 49%.[463,650] Levels of 5-HIAA excretion decreased by 50% or more in 68% of all patients and were reduced to normal in 5%.[463,650,654] Only 7% failed to respond in any way.[463] Forty percent of patients escaped from control after a median time of 4 months, with the remaining patients having sustained control for up to 2.5 years with all responding for more than 1 year and 33% for more than 2 years.[463] The recommended starting dose is 150 μg subcutaneously three times a day.[655] Results with octreotide vary. In one study of 23 patients, in which an objective response was defined as more than a 50% decrease in 5-HIAA levels, plasma neuropeptide K levels or tumor size were reported to decrease significantly in only 28% of patients,[652] whereas in the earlier studies,[463,650,654] 68% of patients showed such a response. In the recent study, 50% of patients showed a subjective response with less diarrhea or flushing.[652] The octreotide dose had to be increased to maintain this response in all patients. The difference between these two studies is that in the latter study patients were started on a low dose (50 μg twice daily ×6 months) then increased, whereas in the earlier study patients were treated with 150 μg three times daily.[463,650,654] The authors speculated that starting with low doses may downregulate the somatostatin receptor and partially account for the differences seen.[652] Similarly, Richter and colleagues reported a decrease in 5-HT in 8 patients with carcinoid syndrome treated with octreotide 150 μg/day but no change in urinary 5-HIAA.[656] A recent study of 14 patients with carcinoid syndrome treated with at least 100 μg of octreotide twice daily demonstrated results similar to those of the Mayo Clinic studies,[463,650,654] with improvement in diarrhea in 83%, flushing in 100%, wheezing in 100%, and a 50% decrease in 5-HIAA in 62%.[651] Plasma serotonin levels did not change in almost all patients. Octreotide was excellent in the Mayo Clinic study, with the only side effects being transient hyperglycemia in 2 patients and mild to moderate steatorrhea in other patients.[463,650] With treatment doses of 500 μg three times daily, steatorrhea was common and 1 of 28 patients developed gallbladder dilation, biliary sludge, and an asymptomatic gallstone.[655] In another study with doses up to 100 μg twice daily, 36% of patients developed diabetic blood glucose levels, although no patient required treatment other than diet.[652] In 43% of patients, borborygmus and diarrhea were seen, and 1 of 23 patients developed bradycardia.

Octreotide has been effective in cases of carcinoid crisis.[629,655,657] The carcinoid crisis usually is reported in patients with foregut carcinoids and more than 250 mg/day of 5-HIAA excretion. It frequently is precipitated by stressful situations such as chemotherapy, tumor biopsy, or anesthesia and may result in death. The use of octreotide may be life-saving.[463,626-629,655,657]

Interferon-α is reported to be effective in the carcinoid syndrome either alone[658-662] or with hepatic artery embolization.[662,663] In one study, patients improved significantly and there was a reduction in 5-HIAA excretion in 12 of 36 patients (42%).[658] In another study, flushing and diarrhea improved in 75% of patients, but the positive effect for diarrhea disappeared by 1 year of treatment.[661] In a study in which 24 patients with malignant carcinoid syndrome were treated with 24 million units/m² body surface area (24 mU/m²), 39% had a decrease in 5-HIAA excretion, flushing improved in 65%, and diarrhea improved in 33%.[662] These responses were transient, lasting a median of only 7 weeks. Human interferon-2b has been combined with hepatic embolization in 7 patients and compared with interferon given alone in 12 patients (5 mU/daily) with the carcinoid syndrome.[663] Evaluation after 1 year of treatment showed that a 50% decrease in urinary levels of 5-HIAA with interferon alone in 50% of patients; when combined with embolization, 71% of patients had such a decrease. With interferon alone, 58% of patients had decreased flushing and 67% had decreased diarrhea, whereas with embolization 86% had decreased flushing and 43% decreased diarrhea.[663]

For a patient with severe carcinoid syndrome who does not respond to other measures, hepatic artery embolization or ligation either alone or combined with interferon or chemotherapy may be effective (see Fig. 41–10).[463,662-669] In two recent studies involving 32 patients with metastatic liver disease and the carcinoid syndrome, hepatic artery embolization or ligation resulted in 50% decrease in urinary 5-HIAA levels in 63% of patients.[668,669] In the largest study, diarrhea and flushing disappeared in all patients immediately after the procedure, and 61% were free of symptoms at 1 year later.[669] Chemoembolization with gelfoam embolization and simultaneous chemotherapy (doxorubicin, mitomycin, cisplatin) was reported to result in symptomatic improvement in a significant number of patients with carcinoid syndrome.[463,666,667] Hepatic artery occlusion can have significant side effects, however, including septicemia. In one study, 5% of patients died of a complication of hepatic artery occlusion.[666] The mortality is reported as less than 3%, pain occurs in 100%, pyrexia and leukocytosis occur in 50%, and there can be occasional acute gangrenous cholecystitis from obstruction of the cystic artery, hepatic abscess, paralytic ileus, and renal failure.[668]

The approach to treatment of the carcinoid syndrome is summarized in Figure 41–10. After symptomatic treatment, patients should avoid precipitating food and alcohol. Oral antidiarrheal agents are given for mild diarrhea and oral selective bronchodilators for wheezing. Octreotide in a dose of 100 to 150 μg three times daily subcutaneously is the drug of choice, self-administered by the patient. If tachyphylaxis develops, the dose can be increased. If symptoms recur, are severe, and do not respond to an increased octreotide dose, serotonin receptor antagonists such as cyproheptadine or ketanserin should be considered. If these agents are ineffective, interferon should be considered.

TREATMENT OF THE CARCINOID TUMOR

Surgery should be considered as the only potentially curative therapy in patients with carcinoids (see Fig. 41–10). Resection

of local disease or resection of local and regional nodal metastatic disease can result in cure in some patients. Because the probability of metastatic disease is directly related to primary tumor size in most carcinoid tumors, the extent of surgical resection for possible cure should be determined accordingly. In the case of appendiceal tumors smaller than 1 cm in diameter without gross metastases (more than 98% of cases encountered in the appendix), a simple appendectomy is sufficient.[463] Of 103 such patients treated with simple appendectomy, of whom 103 were followed for 5 years and 83 for 10 to 35 years, no patient developed a local recurrence or metastatic disease.[463,492] With rectal carcinoids smaller than 1 cm, local resection is adequate and results in cure.[463,496,670,671] There is no agreement about treatment of intestinal carcinoids smaller than 1 cm. In two series, 15% and 18% of tumors less than 1 cm had metastases; in other series, 69% of tumors smaller than 0.5 cm had metastases.[672] One group concluded that with midgut carcinoids malignancy is independent of size.[672] This had led one group to recommend a wide resection with en bloc resection of the adjacent lymph node-bearing mesentery for all small intestinal carcinoids.[493] If the carcinoid tumor is 2 cm or larger, which is uncommon in the case of carcinoids of the rectum or appendix but occurs in 40% of small bowel carcinoids, a full-scale cancer operation should be done.[463] In the case of a carcinoid tumor of the appendix that is 2 cm or larger, a right hemicolectomy is the operation of choice.[463,492,493] In such a tumor in the rectum, an abdominoperineal resection or a low anterior resection with primary anastomosis is recommended.[493] In one recent study, all 13 cases of patients with rectal carcinoid tumors greater than 2 cm died of metastatic complications with a median survival of 10 months after abdominal perineal or low anterior resection.[671] The investigators concluded that radical surgery is inappropriate if anorectal carcinoids can be removed by local excision. In the case of a small intestinal carcinoid 2 cm or larger, a wide resection is recommended with en bloc resection of the adjacent lymph node-bearing mesentery.[493] For carcinoids of the appendix between 1 and 2 cm, some surgeons recommend simple appendectomy,[463,492] whereas others favor partial cecectomy for those lesions located at the base of the appendix to ensure clear margins[493] or formal right hemicolectomy. For carcinoids of the rectum between 1 and 2 cm, it is estimated that only 11% have metastases.[673] It is recommended that these tumors be locally resected with a wide local full-thickness excision[671] and that tumors found to invade the muscularis propria undergo abdominoperineal or low anterior resection.[463,493,674] For gastric and duodenal carcinoids, lesions smaller than 1 cm can be locally excised[493,674] or removed endoscopically.[500,675] With larger gastric tumors, there is no agreement about the best course of treatment. If the tumor is greater than 2 cm or there is local invasion, some recommend total gastrectomy.[493,674] Another study recommends that larger tumors (2 cm or more in diameter) without muscle invasion be resected locally.[500] It is not clear whether gastric carcinoids arising in patients with atrophic gastritis or pernicious anemia should be treated differently.[675] Of 137 cases arising in patients with hypergastrinemic states, only 9% developed metastases, whereas of those arising outside of these hypergastrinemia states, 55% had metastases.[499]

Resection of isolated hepatic metastases may be markedly beneficial or curative in selected patients.[625] In one series, 10 patients who apparently had isolated areas of hepatic metastases in a surgically accessible region of the liver were chosen for possible resection.[463,625] All patients with carcinoid syndrome had symptomatic relief, and 5-HIAA levels were reduced to normal. Although only one patient was cured, the mean survival was 5 years and extended to 13.5 years in 1 patient.[463] In the presence of extensive metastases, partial hepatic resection is not indicated. One study has recommended debulking mesenteric metastases and removal of compromised intestinal segments even in the presence of liver metastases.[672] In this study of 138 patients with midgut carcinoids of whom 51 patients were subjected to surgery with the principal aim of removing the primary and debulking mesenteric metastases, the researchers concluded that surgery provided considerable symptomatic relief.[672] A similar approach involving a aggressive surgical debulking combined with transarterial embolization of hepatic arteries has been used recently in patients with carcinoid syndrome.[676]

Although a study reported that radiation therapy induced a prolonged disease-free remission for carcinoid tumors with metastases,[677] a follow-up study from the same group showed no benefit.[678] In general, radiation therapy has not been useful in the treatment of metastatic carcinoid tumors, except for treatment of symptomatic bone and skin metastases.[521] In one recent study, radiation therapy was used in 44 patients with symptomatic metastatic carcinoid tumors.[679] Survival was not prolonged, although substantial palliation was achieved in most cases. Of 8 patients with intracranial lesions, none demonstrated progression of these lesions (median dose of 3300 cGy). Local control of osseus or epidural metastases was achieved in 78% and 77% of sites respectively, and local control was obtained in 62% of patients with intraabdominal disease.[679] It is recommended that nonhepatic sites be treated with 4500 to 5000 cGy over 4 to 5 weeks.[679]

Because MIBG frequently is taken up by carcinoid tumors and concentrated, the possibility of using radiolabeled MIBG therapeutically has been evaluated recently in a small number of patients.[483,680–683] In three studies involving 10 patients with metastatic carcinoid tumors, 3 patients had decreased urinary excretion of 5-HIAA.[680–683] In one study, 20% of patients had a decrease of 50% or more.[680]

There is no general agreement on when, or even if, chemotherapy should be started in patients with malignant carcinoid tumors. One group with considerable experience suggests that only patients suffering from significant symptoms or disability due to malignant disease or syndromes or those who have a poor prognosis should undergo chemotherapy.[463] The signs of poor prognosis include impaired liver function, high levels of 5-HIAA (150 mg/day or more), or clinical evidence of carcinoid heart disease.[463] Chemotherapy for metastatic carcinoid tumors has, in general, been disappointing. With single agents such as 5-FU, doxorubicin, actinomycin, cisplatin, etoposide, cyclophosphamide, or streptozocin, responses ranged from no response to a 30% response rate (Table 41–23).[521,625,655,684–686] Combination chemotherapy for metastatic carcinoid has not been shown to have any advantage compared with single-agent chemotherapy.[687] For streptozocin with 5-FU,[506,655,688] with cyclophosphamide,[506] or with doxorubicin,[689,690] response rates varied from 11% to 40%. There was no response to the combination of ectoposide and cisplatin (see Table 41–23).[691] A three-drug regimen of

streptozocin, doxorubicin, and cyclophosphamide,[692] or a four-drug regimen of streptozocin, doxorubicin, cyclophosphamide, and 5-FU, offered no additional therapeutic advantage (see Table 41–23).[655,692,693] Remissions have been short-lived with an average duration of 4 to 7 months.[463,625,655,694] Given the indolent nature of the tumor, poor efficacy, undisputed toxicity of chemotherapy, and availability of excellent symptomatic therapy (octreotide), chemotherapy usually is reserved for advanced tumors with radiologic evidence of progression.

The long-acting somatostatin analog octreotide has an antitumor effect in addition to controlling symptoms and reducing secretion of 5-HIAA or various peptides (see Table 41–23).[632,695,696] In 25 patients with carcinoid syndrome who underwent octreotide treatment (150 μg three times daily), tumor size increased in 3, remained unchanged in 22, and was reduced in 4 (a 16% response rate).[650] To determine whether an increased dose of octreotide was more effective, the effect of octreotide (500 μg three times daily) on tumor size was evaluated in 23 patients with metastatic carcinoid syndrome.[696] Of the 23 patients, 4 (17%) demonstrated a decrease of more than 50% in the diameter of the tumor, a response similar to that seen with the lower dose.[650] In more recent studies of patients with metastatic carcinoid tumors, octreotide decreased tumor size in 0 to 9% of patients (see Table 41–23).[652,695] The antitumor effects of octreotide have not been impressive in all studies.

Human leukocyte interferon or recombinant interferon-α can decrease tumor size in a significant number of patients with metastatic tumors (see Table 41–23). In early studies with human leukocyte interferon in 36 patients with malignant carcinoid tumors treated with doses of 3 to 6 million units/day, decreases in tumor size were seen in 11%.[658,697] Nineteen patients previously had failed standard chemotherapy. The median duration of response was 34 months. Adverse side effects were surmountable and less severe than with cytotoxic chemotherapy.[658,698] In a recent study using 24 million units of recombinant interferon-α three times weekly, 4 of 20 patients (20%) with metastatic carcinoid tumors had measurable regression of tumor metastases (20%); the regression was always partial.[699] The mean duration of the regression was 7 weeks from the onset of therapy, with a range of 4 to 26 weeks.[699] In a large prospective study of 111 patients with metastatic disease, 16 patients (14%) demonstrated more than a 50% reduction in tumor size, with 66% demonstrating a stabilization of the disease, and only 19% a progressive disease.[660] In this study, the mean survival of patients treated with interferon was prolonged compared with the median survival with chemotherapy with streptozocin plus 5-FU. In patients treated with interferon alone, the mean survival was more than 80 months; with chemotherapy first and then interferon, it was 64 months.[660] In this large study, interferon treatment (3–9 million units three times weekly) was associated with tolerable but significant side effects including flu-like symptoms (89% of patients), fatigue (70%), weight loss (57%), reduction of blood counts or anemia (31%), leukopenia (3%), thrombocytopenia (14%), and increased serum levels of tryglycerides (32%), liver enzymes (31%), and antibodies (5%).[660] Clinical thyroid disease developed in 76% of patients with thyroid antibodies.[700] In 22 patients, induction of the enzyme 2′,5′-oligoadenylate synthetase with interferon treatment was correlated with the development of a clinical re-

TABLE 41–23. Drug Therapy of Carcinoid Tumors

Investigations	Agent	No. of Patients	Objective Response* Number (%)
Single Drug			
Moertel, 1983[625]	DOX	33	7 (21)
Moertel, 1983[625]	5-FU	19	5 (26)
Kvols, 1989[655]	DTIC	18	3 (17)
Van Hazel et al, 1983[684]			
Van Hazel et al, 1983[684]	Dactinomycin	17	1 (6)
Moertel et al, 1986[685]	Cisplatin	15	1 (6)
Maton and Hodgson, 1984[521]	Alkylating agents	39	9 (23)
Kelsen et al, 1987[686]	ETOP	17	0 (0)
Maton and Hodgson, 1984[521]	STZ	23	7 (30)
	Interferon		
Oberg et al, 1986[658]	Human leukocyte	36	4 (11)
Norbin et al, 1989[661]		13	2 (15)
Valimaki et al, 1991[1106]		7	1 (14)
Moertel et al, 1989[699]	Interferon-α	20	4 (20)
Norbin et al, 1989[661]		10	1 (10)
Doberanr et al, 1987[690]		7	0 (0)
Creutzfeldt et al, 1991[695]		10	0 (0)
Kvols et al, 1986[650]	Octreotide	25	4 (16)
Creutzfeldt et al, 1991[695]		10	0 (0)
Oberg et al, 1991[652]		23	2 (9)
Kvols et al, 1987[696]		23	4 (17)
Norbin et al, 1989[669]	Hepatic artery occlusion or embolization	27	10 (37)
Marlink et al, 1991[668]		4	3 (75)
Combination			
Oberg and Erickson, 1991[660]	STZ + 5-FU	19	2 (11)
Moertel and Hanley, 1979[506]		42	14 (33)
Kvols, 1989[655]			
Engstrom et al, 1984[688]		80	18 (22)
Moertel and Hanley, 1979[506]	STZ + CTX	47	12 (26)
Kelsen et al, 1982[689]	STZ + DOX	10	4 (40)
Doberaur et al, 1987[690]		9	2 (22)
Moertel et al, 1991[1024]	ETOP + Cisplatin	13	0 (0)
Bukowski et al, 1987[692]	STZ + CTX + 5-FU	9	2 (21)
Bukowski et al, 1987[692]	STZ + DOX + CTX + 5-FU	56	17 (31)
Bukowski et al, 1983[1107]			
Moertel, 1987[463]	Hepatic artery occlusion + DTIC + DOX + 5-FU + STZ	21 / 10	18 (86) / 9 (90)
Hanssen, 1989[663]	Hepatic artery occlusion + inteferon-α, 2β	7	5 (71)

DOX, doxorubicin; 5-FU, 5-fluorouracil; ETOP, etoposide; STZ, streptozocin; DTIC, dacarbazine; CTX, cyclophosphamide.
* Objective response is defined as a decrease in tumor size using the investigator's criteria. Changes in tumor markers or functional improvement was not included as an objective response.

sponse.[701] It is not known whether it is predictive of changes in tumor size with interferon treatment.

Selective hepatic artery infusion of 5-FU had a response rate similar to that reported for systemic 5-FU.[521] Hepatic artery ligation surgically or embolization by interventional radiology has been reported to reduce hepatic tumor bulk.[463,662,663,665,667,669] In one series of 14 patients with metastatic carcinoid to the liver after hepatic artery occlusion either surgically or percutaneously, 7% showed complete improvement, 43% showed 75% to 100% improvement, and 43% showed a 50% to 75%[463] improvement in endocrine responses and in regression of hepatic metastases. The duration of response was short, with a mean of 5 months.[463] In two recent studies involving 31 patients, 19 patients had temporary liver dearterialization and 12 patients were treated by liver embolization.[668,669] After temporary liver dearterialization, 41% had a decrease in metastatic hepatic tumor size, whereas with embolization 50% showed a decrease and in almost all cases the reduction lasted more than 12 months. The combination of hepatic artery ligation and combination chemotherapy with dacarbazine, doxorubicin, 5-FU, and streptozocin has led to dramatic response rates in patients with carcinoid and hepatic metastases.[463,649,666,667] Of 21 patients with carcinoid tumors treated with sequential hepatic artery occlusion and cytotoxic drugs (doxorubicin, dacarbazine, streptozocin, and 5-FU), 19% had complete improvement, 57% had 75% to 100% improvement, and 10% a 50% to 75% improvement, for an 80% overall response rate that lasted a median of 24 months.[463] In a recent study of 15 patients with liver metastases from carcinoid (n=7) or pancreatic endocrine tumors (n=8) who were treated with chemoembolization (gelfoam occlusion with doxorubicin, mitomycin, and cisplatin), 4 patients (33%) demonstrated a 75% decrease in tumor size, 17% (2 patients) stable disease, and 4 patients (33%) progressive disease.[667] The median survival was 6 months (range, 0–55 months). Hepatic artery embolization has been combined with treatment with human interferon 2b (see Table 41–23).[662,663] One year after the chemoembolization, 5 of 7 patients (71%) continued to demonstrate a decrease in tumor size within the liver, whereas with interferon alone (n=10) only 10% demonstrated a decrease in tumor size.

The therapeutic potential of the uptake of MIBG by carcinoid tumors has been investigated recently.[680] In 5 patients with progressive metastatic disease who were given 5.2 to 29.5 GBq of ^{131}I-MIBG cumulatively, no decrease in tumor size was seen in any patient even though symptomatic improvement was seen.

PANCREATIC ENDOCRINE TUMORS

Pancreatic endocrine tumors share a number of features with carcinoid tumors, and their histologic features cannot be differentiated from those of carcinoid tumors.[702] Both carcinoid and pancreatic endocrine tumors can be classified as an APUDomas by histologic criteria (see the earlier section on pathology) and, except for insulinoma, both are malignant in most cases (more than 60%; Table 41–24). Both are vascular tumors with similar radiographic appearances and metastatic patterns (primarily to regional lymph nodes and the liver).

Pancreatic endocrine tumors are classified as functional if they are associated with a clinical syndrome due to ectopic hormone release of a functional tumor. They are considered nonfunctional if they are not associated with a clinical symptom due to hormone release. This latter category includes tumors releasing PP (PPomas) or neurotensin (neurotensinomas) and tumors are not associated with elevated plasma hormone levels, even though they are histologically indistinguishable from functional tumors.[702] Despite elevated plasma levels of PP or neurotensin, these tumors are classified as nonfunctional because no specific symptoms occur in most studies due to elevated plasma levels of these hormones.[702,703]

TABLE 41–24.   Characteristics of Gastropancreatic and Endocrine Tumors

Tumor Name	Syndrome Name	Hormone Producing Symptoms	Malignant (%)	Location (%)
Symptoms Not Due to Released Hormones				
PPoma	PPoma	None	>60	Pancreas
Nonfunctioning	Nonfunctioning Pancreatic Endocrine Tumor	None	>60	Pancreas
Symptoms Due to Released Hormones				
Gastrinoma	Zollinger-Ellison syndrome	Gastrin	60–90	Pancreas (30–60%) Duodenum (30–43%) Other (10–20%)
Insulinoma	Insulinoma	Insulin	10–15	Pancreas (>99%)
VIPoma	Pancreatic cholera Verner-Morrison syndrome WDHA	Vasoactive intestinal peptide	80	Pancreas (90%) Adrenal (10%)
Glucagonoma	Glucagonoma	Glucagon	60	Pancreas (>99%)
Somatostatinoma	Somatostatinoma	Somatostatin		Pancreas (56%) Upper small intestine (44%)
GRFoma	GRFoma	Growth hormone-releasing peptide	30	Pancreas (33%) Lung (53%) Small intestine (10%) Other (7%)

PPoma, pancreatic endocrine tumor releasing pancreatic polypeptide; VIPoma, vasoactive intestinal peptide; GRFoma, growth hormone-releasing factor tumor; WDHA, watery diarrhea hypokalemia achlorhydria.

In general, these tumors are uncommon. Functional pancreatic endocrine tumors are reported to have a prevalence of 10 persons per million population.[704] The prevalence in unselected autopsy studies is 0.5% to 1.5%.[704-707] It is not apparent why the autopsy detection rate is so much higher than the clinical detection rate.[520] It may be because most tumors are nonfunctional, symptoms frequently are missed, or peptides are released in quantities too small to cause symptoms. The incidence of clinically significant pancreatic endocrine tumors is 3.6 to 4 persons per million population per year.[488,708] Nonfunctional pancreatic endocrine tumors or PPomas are reported to account for 15% to 30% of all pancreatic endocrine tumors.[488,709-711] Gastrinomas and PPomas are the most common malignant pancreatic endocrine tumors. Gastrinomas due to ZES usually are clinically recognized and have been studied extensively; they are discussed in detail.[712] The localization, surgical approach, and the approach to advanced disease are similar to approaches used for the more rare pancreatic tumors. Other syndromes are discussed in separate sections. The treatment of metastatic disease is similar for all metastatic pancreatic endocrine tumors and is discussed at the end of this chapter.

ZOLLINGER-ELLISON SYNDROME

In 1955, Zollinger and Ellison described 2 patients with severe peptic ulcer disease treatable only by total gastrectomy. The disease was characterized by extreme hypersecretion of gastric acid and a non-β islet cell tumor of the pancreas.[713] Extracts of tumors from patients with ZES were demonstrated to contain a potent acid secretagogue that was gastrin-like.[714] Amino acid analysis and enzymatic degradation of purified tumor extracts demonstrated that the secretagogue in the tumor was identical to human antral gastrin.[715,716] Because these tumors synthesize and release large amounts of gastrin, they have been called gastrinomas.

Recent studies estimate that ZES occurs in 1 person per 100,000 population in Denmark,[717] in 0.5 persons per million population in Ireland,[708] and in 1 to 3 persons per million per year in Sweden.[488] The prevalence of ZES varies from half

as common[708] to 1.2 times as common as insulinomas.[488] Gastrinomas occur less frequently than the original estimate of 0.1% of all persons in the United States with duodenal ulcer disease.[718] In one series, gastrinomas were the most common pancreatic endocrine tumor, making up 30% of all such tumors.[488]

Pathogenesis, Pathology, and Tumor Biology

Almost all clinical manifestations, except for those late in the course of the disease, are due to gastric acid hypersecretion secondary to hypergastrinemia.[691] Effective control of the gastric hypersecretion medically or surgically abolishes all clinical manifestations, including peptic ulcer disease and diarrhea (Table 41–25).[691,719-722] In patients late in the course of their disease with metastatic gastrinoma or large primaries, symptoms such as pain or cachexia can arise due to the tumor itself. Besides basal gastric acid hypersecretion, hypergastrinemia causes trophic changes in the gastric mucosa,[723] with the result that patients with ZES have increased numbers of parietal cells and an increased maximal acid secretory capacity.[719,724,725]

Many patients with ZES have diarrhea and in some patients it is the sole presenting manifestation (see Table 41–25). The diarrhea is due to the consequences of gastric acid hypersecretion including direct injury to the small intestinal mucosa, inactivation of pancreatic lipase at low pH, and precipitation of bile acids at low pH.[719] Hypergastrinemia itself has been proposed to contribute to the diarrhea by increasing intestinal secretion.[726] This hypothesis is not supportable because diarrhea disappears and patients remain asymptomatic when the gastric acid hypersecretion is controlled, even though the hypergastrinemia remains unchanged.[503,719]

Gastrin in normal subjects and in patients with ZES has been found in different molecular sizes. In gastrinomas, gastrin-17 (G-17) is the major gastrin component, comprising 74% to 80% of the total immunoreactivity, with so-called big gastrin or gastrin-34 (G-34) comprising most of the remainder.[719,727,728] In contrast, in sera from normal subjects and patients with gastrinoma, G-34 comprises more than 60% of

TABLE 41–25. Clinical Features of Patients With Zollinger-Ellison Syndrome

Characteristic	Ellison et al, 1964[757]	Regan et al, 1978[791]	Stage et al, 1979[717]	Mignon et al, 1986[822]	Jensen et al, 1991[712]
No. of patients	260	40	34	144	165
MEN-I (%)	21	23	24	24	18
Mean duration of symptoms before diagnosis (y)	ND (53% = 1–4) (27% = >4)	6.5	6.4	ND	6.4
First symptoms (%)					
Abdominal pain	93	98	85	26	24
Pain and diarrhea	30	28	56	49	55
Diarrhea only	7	2	9	15	18
Dysphagia/pyrosis	0	0	6	ND	31
Mean age at onset (y)	ND	50.5	50.4	47	45
Sex (% male)	60	60	62	68	58

MEN-I, multiple endocrine neoplasia type I; ND, no data.

the total gastrin immunoreactivity.[702,719,727] In addition to G-17 and G-34, smaller and larger forms of gastrin have been described in sera and in gastrinomas from patients with ZES. Each of the gastrins can exist in two different forms (sulfated or nonsulfated), which are reported to be equipotent.[719] Early studies reported that G-17 was five times more potent than G-34,[729] but a recent study using synthetic peptides found G-34 and G-17 to be equally potent.[730] In ZES, plasma gastrin immunoreactivity includes a high-molecular-weight gastrin (big, big gastrin), an uncategorized gastrin slightly larger than G-34 (component I gastrin), and small amounts of amino-terminal, carboxyl-terminal, and carboxyl-terminal-extended fragments of gastrin.[728,731-737] Altered posttranslational processing of gastrin may occur in gastrinoma, leading to altered ratios of various fragments of gastrin and precursors.[734,738,739] In a recent study, less than 50% of the total progastrin in tumors was processed to α-amidated gastrins, whereas in normal subjects only small amounts of unprocessed, nonamidated gastrins were found.[738] In patients with ZES, large amounts of glycine-extended forms of G-17, G-34, and component I have been described in the plasma.[735,738] In addition, a high-molecular-weight progastrin has been described in plasma and tumors of patients with gastrinomas.[734,737,738,740] Elevated levels of progastrin have been found in patients with gastrinoma metastatic to liver, whereas the smaller glycine-extended gastrins predominated in benign disease.[738] Furthermore, a significantly lower percentage of α-amidated gastrin was found in patients with metastatic disease to the liver compared with patients without metastases.[738] These results suggest that a low degree of processing of progastrin predicts a malignant clinical course.[738] Some researchers reported that the relative amounts of G-17 and amino-terminal fragments and the ratio of G-17 amino-terminal immunoreactivity to G-17 carboxyl-terminal immunoreactivity was predictive of the extent of gastrinoma.[733,734,741] Others did not confirm these findings.[738] These results are preliminary and appear to vary considerably from patient to patient. It is unclear whether analysis of gastrin fragments and precursors will provide useful clinical information to help establish the presence of malignancy.

Initially, gastrinomas were thought to occur most commonly in the pancreas (Table 41–26). In early studies, gastrinomas were reported to occur in a frequency of 4:1:4 for the pancreatic head:body:tail, and 14% of all gastrinomas were found in the duodenum.[720,742] Gastrinomas in the duodenum and in lymph nodes in the pancreatic head area have been reported increasingly[741,743-745] and have been found recently in 60% of all patients in whom a tumor is found at surgery (Table 41–27).[745] Of all gastrinomas found at surgery, 65% to 90% are in the pancreatic head and duodenal area (see Table 41–27).[741,743,745,746] Occasionally, gastrinomas have been found in the liver, stomach, jejunum, mesentery, and spleen. In women, there are numerous reports of ovarian gastrinomas that are functionally indistinguishable from other gastrinomas.[747-751]

Because gastrin-containing cells (G cells) normally are not present in the adult pancreas, it has been proposed that pancreatic gastrinomas be considered ectopic, whereas gastrinomas in areas that normally contain G cells (*e.g.*, duodenum, stomach, jejunum) be considered entopic.[510,752-754] Earlier studies found a lower incidence of malignant change (38%) for gastrinomas in entopic locations and a higher incidence for ectopic gastrinomas (60–70%).[752] In recent prospective studies, duodenal gastrinomas have been found to be malignant with metastatic spread in 54% to 75% of patients.[745,755,756] The disease-free interval was shortest in patients who had resected duodenal gastrinomas and normal serum levels of gastrin and provocative tests immediately postoperatively, suggesting the presence of metastases (Fig. 41–11).[745] These data suggest that the malignant potential of ectopic and entopic gastrinomas does not differ as suggested originally and that both groups are malignant in more than 60% of cases. In early studies, 60% to more than 90% of patients with ZES had metastatic gastrinoma at the time of diagnosis.[727,757-759] In recent studies, only 34% have had metastatic disease at the time of diagnosis (see Table 41–26). Metastases usually are to the peripancreatic lymph nodes and the liver.[712] Recently, bony metastases have been reported in 12% of patients with metastatic gastrinoma in the liver.[608]

The cell of origin of gastrinomas remains obscure. Duodenal gastrinoma usually contains many well-differentiated antral G cells, in contrast to pancreatic gastrinoma, and is believed to originate from gastrin cells in the duodenal crypts and

TABLE 41–26. Pathology, Tumor Location, and Extent in Patients With Zollinger-Ellison Syndrome in Various Series

*Extent of Tumor** (% of All Patients)	*Tumor Location** (% of All Patients)	*Pathology Found*
No tumor found in 30% (8–48%)	Pancreatic in 42% (21–65%)	Gastrinoma in 90% (87–94%)†
Tumor present in 70% (52–92%)	Duodenal in 15% (6–31%)	Malignant in 61–90%‡
Metastatic in 34% (13–52%)	Other, 11% (1–26%)	Benign in 10–39%‡
Localized in 36% (23–51%)	Metastases only in 2% (0–11%)	Islet cell hyperplasia only in 10% (6–13%)†

* Mean percentages and ranges are calculated from references 722, 741–743, 745, 746, 757–759, 762, 766, 767, 799, and 823.
† Percentages from references 722, 741, 745, 757, 758, and 822.
‡ Percentages from references 727, 757, 759, and 822.

TABLE 41–27. Location of Primary Gastrinomas in a Recent Prospective 10-Year Surgical Study

	Location of Primary Gastrinoma Number (%)				
Surgical Group*	Duodenum	Pancreatic	Lymph Nodes Only	Other†	No Tumor Found
Group 1 (n = 36)	4 (11)	12§ (33)	6 (17)	1 (3)	13 (36)
Group 2 (n = 37)	16‡ (43)	11 (30)	7 (19)	—	3 (8)
Both groups (n = 73)	20 (27)	23 (32)	13 (18)	1 (1)	16 (22)

* Group 1 and Group 2 differed in that patients in Group 2 underwent additional procedures to search for duodenal gastrinomas (duodenotomy, endoscopy at surgery).
† One patient had an ovarian gastrinoma.
‡ Proportion of duodenal gastrinomas found was significantly greater in group 2 versus group 1 patients ($p < 0.01$).
§ Proportion of pancreatic gastrinomas found in group 1 was greater than that of duodenal gastrinomas found in group 1 ($p < 0.05$).
(Data from Norton JA, Doppman JL, Jensen RT. Curative resection in Zollinger-Ellison syndrome: Results of a ten year prospective study. Ann Surg 1992;215:8)

Brunner's glands.[510,754] Because G cells are not seen in human pancreas and because pancreatic gastrinomas are pleomorphic with heterogenous cell types, they have been proposed to originate from a multipotential, endocrine-programmed stem cell that undergoes somewhat inappropriate and incomplete differentiation toward the G cell.[510,754] An argyrophilic cell with atypical granules has been described in islet cell tumors and may well be the precursor or stem cell for these tumors.[727]

In early studies, in which patients presented late in the course of their disease, gastrinomas were found at surgery in most patients with ZES (81–94%).[727,757,758] In subsequent studies, gastrinomas were found in only 70% of the patients with ZES (see Table 41–26).[712] In one-half of the patients, the tumor is nonmetastatic (36% of all patients), and in about one-half of these patients the tumors are multiple.[715,758] Therefore, in only 20% of all patients with ZES was a single, nonmetastatic gastrinoma found. In a recent large prospective study, when attention was directed to finding duodenal gastrinomas, tumors were found in 93% of patients.[745] Forty-three percent were duodenal, 30% were pancreatic, and 20% were in the lymph nodes (see Table 41–27). Islet cell hyperplasia and nesidioblastosis have been suggested as causes of

FIGURE 41–11. (A) Typical secretin and (B) calcium provocative test results in a patient with Zollinger-Ellison syndrome (ZES). Secretin (2 U/kg intravenous bolus) was given (*arrow*), and serum levels of gastrin increased more than 200 pg/ml consistent with ZES. This response is seen in 87% of patients with ZES. Calcium gluconate (54 mg/kg/h) is infused over 3 hours and serum levels of gastrin increase greater than 395 pg/ml. This response is seen in 56% of patients with ZES. Percentage data is based on responses in 96 patients with ZES.

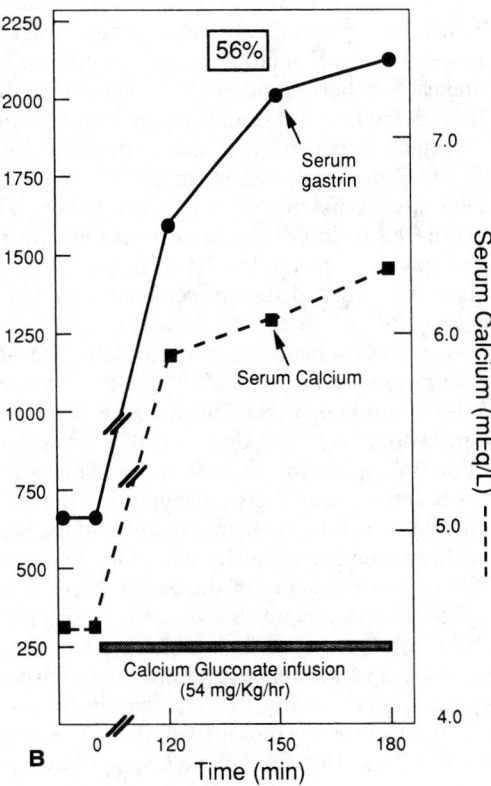

ZES in some cases in which no gastrinoma is found.[757,758,760] Most authorities do not accept islet cell hyperplasia or nesidioblastosis as a cause of ZES for three reasons. First, islet cell hyperplasia or nesidioblastosis is common in patients with ZES who have a gastrinoma located. Second, the hyperplastic islets do not contain gastrin. Third, the possibility of a small gastrinoma that was not detected at surgery cannot be excluded. Islet cell hyperplasia or nesidioblastosis is regarded not as a cause but as a consequence of the disease.[707,727,754,761]

The percentage of gastrinomas that are actually malignant is unclear. In early studies, 60% to more than 90% of patients with ZES had a malignant gastrinoma.[727,757–759] In recent studies, only 50% of patients have had a malignant gastrinoma at the time of diagnosis (see Table 41–26). Whether this change represents earlier diagnosis or inclusion of a spectrum of the disease not previously appreciated is unclear. The diagnosis of malignancy is complicated by the fact that no histologic criteria predicts malignancy; therefore, malignancy can be established only by the presence of metastases. Even metastatic disease can be difficult to establish, because a number of extrapancreatic gastrinomas localized in lymph nodes have been described with no evidence of primary tumor. Some of these patients apparently have been cured by excision of lymph nodes, which suggests that the gastrinoma was not metastatic but originated in the lymph node.[707,746,762–764]

About 20% of patients with ZES (see Table 41–25) have a familial form of the disease with evidence of MEN-I (Wermer's syndrome). MEN-I is an autosomal dominant trait characterized by hyperplasia or tumors of multiple endocrine organs, with hyperparathyroidism the most common abnormality.[513,514] Islet cell tumors of the pancreas are the second most common characteristic, occurring in 82% of MEN-I patients, with 57% having ZES and 25% having insulinomas.[513] Pituitary and adrenal adenomas are less common. Patients with MEN-I and ZES differ from sporadic cases in that they frequently present at a younger age. Their tumors almost always are multiple and frequently are small. In some studies[762,765] but not others,[766,767] patients with MEN-I have an increased survival rate compared with sporadic cases.

Immunocytochemical studies of tumors from patients with ZES have demonstrated gastrin in 90% to 100% of tumors in some studies and in 56% to 78% in others.[691] This difference may be due to differences in tissue fixation, the type of gastrin antibody used, or the low levels of gastrin in small tumors. More than 50% of tumors demonstrate other peptides, including PP in 17% to 50%, insulin in 20% to 33%, glucagon in 0 to 33%, somatostatin in 0 to 33%, and ACTH-like immunoreactivity in 0 to 30%.[691,727,768–770] A review of seven different immunocytochemical studies of tumors from 75 patients with ZES found gastrin in 80%, insulin in 30%, human PP in 35%, glucagon in 29%, and somatostatin in 21%.[703] It has become increasingly difficult, if not impossible, to determine by immunocytochemistry which of the hormones found in the tumor are clinically important in a given patient.[691] The endocrine nature of the tumor is not always apparent, and to obtain a precise classification, a combination of clinical and biochemical data and immunocytochemical studies for peptides and for chromogranins, neuron-specific enolase, synaptophysin, and PCP 7.5 frequently are needed.[712,768]

It is not clear why most patients with ZES or other gastrointestinal endocrine tumors have symptoms characteristic of hypersecretion of only one peptide, even though their tumors contain multiple peptide hormones. It may be that only one of the peptides is released in quantities sufficient to cause symptoms, that only one of the peptides is biologically active, or that all the peptides are released and biologically active but have antagonistic physiologic actions. Early studies involving small numbers of cases reported elevated plasma concentrations of various gastrointestinal peptides in patients with ZES.[691,718,771–775] A recent prospective study of 45 consecutive cases of patients with ZES demonstrated increased plasma concentrations of a peptide besides gastrin in 62% of patients.[703] Forty-four percent had one additional peptide in abnormal amounts and 18% had two additional peptides. No patient had abnormal levels of three additional peptides. Motilin was the peptide most often present at abnormally high levels (29%). Human PP plasma levels were elevated in 27% of patients, compared with plasma PP elevations of 10% to 60% described previously.[772,773,776] Some investigators[774] but not others[777] have proposed that elevations in plasma PP levels might be a useful marker for identifying patients with ZES and metastatic liver disease. Elevated levels of neurotensin occurred in 20% of patients in one study[703] and in no patients in another study.[771] Plasma levels of gastrin-releasing peptide were elevated in 10% of patients in one study.[703] Although there have been frequent reports of finding insulin, glucagon, or somatostatin by immunocytochemical studies, and of occasional patients having ZES with a concomitant insulinoma[778] or glucagonoma,[712] the prospective study of 45 patients with ZES found no patient with increased plasma levels of these peptides.[703] The presence or absence of abnormal plasma levels of a particular peptide or extent of elevation did not correlate with location of tumor, extent of tumor, or the presence or absence of a particular symptom.[703]

Elevated concentrations of HCG subunits (α or β chains) in sera, or the presence of HCG in the tumor as determined by immunocytochemistry, have been found in some patients with gastrinoma and may be predictive of a malignant tumor.[779–782] In a recent study of 30 patients with ZES, 57% of patients with malignant disease and 45% of those with benign disease had elevated concentrations of α-HCG in plasma.[781] Seven patients had elevated levels of β-HCG in plasma. Of these 7 patients, 4 had malignant disease. The usefulness of elevated plasma concentrations of α-HCG or β-HCG or their presence in the tumor in predicting malignancy is not established.[712,764,783]

Chromogranin A is a 48-kd protein that is co-stored and co-released with peptide hormones from gut endocrine cells and tumors.[782,784–787] Chromogranin A is not produced by nonendocrine cells. Immunocytochemical staining for chromogranin A has shown its presence in gastrinomas, carcinoids, antral G cells, and fundic ECL cells of the stomach.[784–788] The latter location is particularly important because conditions that elevate the fasting gastrin concentration (*e.g.*, ZES, chronic atrophic gastritis, pernicious anemia, and antral exclusion or pharmacologic inhibition of gastric acid hypersecretion) can lead to gastric ECL hyperplasia and in some cases to the development of multiple gastric carcinoid tumors (see the discussion of omeprazole under Medical Treatment of Gastric Hypersecretion). In a study of patients with ZES, abnormal levels of chromogranin A correlated best with plasma pepsinogen levels, not with tumor characteristics.[789] The researchers speculated that the chromogranin A-producing cells in the stomach, not the gastrinoma, could be the principal source of plasma chromogranin A due to long-term hypergastrinemia with resultant hyperplasia of ECL cells.[789] This study measured plasma chromogranin A levels in 10 patients with ZES and found that the mean value was 5 times that in normal patients.[789] There was no correlation between the plasma level of chromogranin A and the amount of tumor, presence or absence of metastatic disease, or presence or absence of MEN-I.[789]

Histologic studies have demonstrated that tumors from patients with ZES are similar to other carcinoid tumors.[691,770] Different histologic classifications have been proposed based on growth patterns, including classifying tumors into a glandular pattern, solid nests of cells (solid pattern), a trabecular or ribbon-like structure (gyriform pattern), and an unclassified pattern.[691,712,754,768,770,790] Similar patterns have been demonstrated in tumors from patients with other endocrine tumors, and the type of histologic pattern does not correlate with the type of hormone produced, clinical symptoms, or malignancy. Ultrastructural classifications have been based on the type of granules seen, but this does not correlate with malignancy or clinical features.[510,691,727,754,768,783]

Clinical Features

The clinical features of ZES as reported in several studies are summarized in Table 41–25. ZES is slightly more common in males (60%) than in females (40%); the mean age is 45 to 50 years old, and about 20% have MEN-I. Abdominal pain remains the most common initial symptom, with 90% to 95% of patients developing peptic ulcer disease at some time during the course of the disease. The abdominal pain cannot be differentiated from that which occurs in patients with idiopathic peptic esophagitis or peptic ulcer disease. Diarrhea and esophageal disease are increasingly the first symptoms (see Table 41–25). Esophageal symptoms were only reported in 3% of 355 patients with ZES in early studies.[757,787,791] However, in two later small series in which esophageal disease was specifically sought, 33% of 32 patients had symptoms or endoscopic evidence of esophagitis.[792,793] In a study of 122 patients with ZES, esophageal symptoms, endoscopic abnormalities, or both were present in 61%.[794]

The change in presenting symptoms is reflected in changes in radiologic and endoscopic findings. In early studies, up to 93% of patients had a peptic ulcer, and in 36% of patients the ulcers were multiple or in unusual locations.[719,757] Although atypical ulcers, when present, strongly suggest the diagnosis, most patients with ZES have typical duodenal ulcers, and 18% to 25% of patients have no ulcer at the time of diagnosis.[719] This change in presenting symptoms and severity of peptic disease suggests that patients with ZES are being diagnosed earlier. Nevertheless, in almost all series there is a delay of 3 to 6 years between the onset of symptoms and diagnosis (see Table 41–25). Intestinal perforation, especially of the jejunum, is a presenting event, even today, in as many as 7% of patients with ZES.[795]

Diagnosis

None of the original triad of symptoms described by Zollinger and Ellison is required for the diagnosis of ZES. At time of diagnosis, 38% to 68% of patients have a solitary peptic ulcer and 14% to 25% have no peptic ulcer.[719] Although gastric acid hypersecretion remains an essential criterion of ZES, it may not be extreme, and in 8% to 48% of patients, gastrinomas are not located at the time of diagnosis (see Table 41–26). ZES is suspected on the basis of the clinical presentation and established in almost all patients by demonstrating elevated basal gastric acid secretion (basal acid output [BAO]) and fasting hypergastrinemia.

ZES should be suspected clinically in any of the clinical settings of ulcer with diarrhea, familial ulcer, ulcer in unusual locations, and recurrent or resistant ulcer. One of the most common clinical presentations is a patient whose peptic ulcer fails to heal on conventional doses of H_2 receptor antagonists.[712] Most patients present with symptoms that are similar to those in patients with idiopathic peptic disease.[717,719] Therefore, at least one preoperative fasting serum gastrin should be done for all patients who have peptic ulcer disease severe enough to require gastric surgery.

To make the diagnosis of ZES it is necessary to demonstrate fasting hypergastrinemia and an elevated BAO.[796] The fasting gastrin concentration is usually done first, and although occasional normal values have been reported in patients with ZES, this is a rare occurrence.[707,796] Disorders other than ZES are known to elevate the fasting serum level of gastrin.[719] These disorders fit into two categories—those associated with gastric acid hypersecretion (Table 41–28) and those associated with hypochlorhydria or achlorhydria including chronic gastritis, gastric cancer, pernicious anemia, or postvagotomy.[719] No absolute level of elevation of serum gastrin concentration distinguishes these two categories causing hypergastrinemias, and they can be differentiated only by measuring the BAO. If facilities are not available to measure the basal output, the pH of the gastric contents should be determined while the patient is not taking antisecretory medications. A pH of 3 or higher virtually excludes the diagnosis of ZES.[796]

The most commonly used secretory criteria for diagnosing ZES are a BAO of 15 mEq/hour or more in patients without previous acid-reducing operations and 5 mEq/hour or more in patients with previous acid-reducing operations.[712,719,798] The mean BAO in five series ranged from 34 to 53 mEq/hour in patients without previous gastric surgery and from 6 to 20 mEq/hour for patients with previous acid-reducing surgery.[691,721,791,798,799] In early studies, 33% of patients with ZES without previous gastric surgery were reported to have a BAO of less than 15 mEq/hour.[721,791,798] In recent studies, only 1 of 77 patients without previous gastric surgery had a BAO of less than 15 mEq/hour.[691,799,800] Requiring a BAO of at least 15 mEq/hour will include 66% to 99% of all patients with ZES and exclude 90% of patients with routine duodenal ulcer.[719] In patients with previous acid-reducing surgery, the mean BAO exceeded 5 mEq/hour in most studies, but in three studies, 6%, 33%, and 45% of patients had a BAO of less than 5 mEq/hour.[503,773,801] Patients with ZES have an elevated maximal acid output (MAO) and an elevated BAO/MAO ratio that often exceeds 0.6.[802] In some series, the BAO/MAO ratio is less than 0.6 in a significant proportion of patients.[721,791,798,799] Criteria based on the MAO or BAO/MAO ratio have not been shown to offer an advantage over the BAO alone.[712,719]

TABLE 41–28. Differential Diagnosis of Increased Fasting Gastrin Level and Basal Acid Output

Diagnosis	Secretion Injection	Calcium Infusion	Meal Test	Other Discriminating Features
Zollinger-Ellison syndrome	Increase > 200 pg/ml over basal	Increase > 395 pg/ml over basal	NC or increase < 100% over basal (70%)	About 50% of patients have tumor on imaging studies
Retained gastric antrum	NC or increase < 200 pg/ml	NC or small increase	NC, decrease or increase < 50% over basal	History of Billroth II operation. Positive ^{99m}Tc scan
Chronic gastric outlet obstruction	NC or increase < 200 pg/ml	NC or small increase	ND	Decreased gastric emptying; with nasogastric suction serum gastrin levels return to normal
Antral G-cell hyperplasia	NC or decrease or increase < 200 pg/ml	NC or small increase	Increase > 100% over basal	Increased numbers of G cells may be seen by immunocytochemical staining
Antral G-cell hyperfunction	NC or decrease or increase < 200 pg/ml	NC or small increase	Increase > 100% over basal	Normal number of G cells; frequently familial; may be associated with hyperpepsinogenemia I
After small bowel resection	NC or increase < 200 pg/ml	NC or small increase	ND	History of extensive small bowel resection

NC, no change; ND, not determined.

If a patient has a fasting gastrin concentration of 1000 pg/ml or more with basal acid hypersecretion, the diagnosis of ZES generally is established.[691,796] The only other disorder that can mimic ZES and cause similar elevations of acid secretion and fasting gastrin concentration is the retained gastric antrum syndrome, a rare condition that occurs in patients who underwent a Billroth II gastroenterostomy in which part of the antrum was left attached to the excluded proximal duodenal stump.[803,804] This diagnosis can be excluded if there is no history of gastric surgery. If there is such a history, the diagnosis can be excluded using the secretin test and gastric ^{99m}Tc scanning as outlined in Table 41–28.[804,805]

In a recent study, 32% of patients with ZES had a fasting gastrin concentration of 1000 pg/ml or greater.[806] In the remaining 68%, the fasting gastrin concentration was elevated but less than 1000 pg/ml, a range that overlaps with other conditions that can cause similar elevations of fasting gastrin and BAO.[719,806] These conditions are listed in Table 41–28. To differentiate them from ZES, various gastrin provocative tests frequently are necessary (Table 41–29). Provocative tests including the secretin test,[712,729,800,806–809] calcium infusion test,[800,806,807,809] and meal test[809] have been developed, and each measures the serum gastrin response. Recently, the secretin, calcium, and meal provocative tests were evaluated prospectively.[806,810] In terms of sensitivity to the three proposed criteria of positivity, gastrin levels increased by 110 pg/ml in 93%, 200 pg/ml or more in 87%,[808] and more than 50% in 85% of patients with ZES (see Table 41–29).[809] There was no significant difference in results in patients with or without MEN-I, and fasting serum gastrin levels above or below 1000 pg/ml did not correlate with extent, size, or location of tumor. The study concluded that an increase of 200 pg/ml after injection of secretin is the diagnostic criteria of choice.[806]

This study analyzed different gastrin sampling times and found that 6% of patients had a positive secretin test only at 2 minutes and that no secretin test was positive at more than 20 minutes that was not positive previously. It was therefore recommended that serum gastrin levels be sampled at −15, 0, +2, +5, +10, and +20 minutes only. A typical result is shown in Figure 41–11.

During the calcium infusion test, calcium gluconate is infused at a rate of 54 mg/kg/hour for 3 hours, and serum levels of calcium and gastrin are measured.[800,806] It has been suggested that serum samples be obtained at −15, 0, +120, and +180 minutes.[806] A typical result is shown in Figure 41–11. The calcium infusion test was evaluated using the proposed criteria of at least a 395 pg/ml[800] or 50% increase[806] and compared with the secretin test results. The 395 pg/ml criteria was less sensitive (see Table 41–29). Although the 50% increase criteria had equal sensitivity to secretin, it can be seen in patients with ordinary peptic ulcer disease without ZES.[503,806]

Because of its ease, lack of side effects, high sensitivity, and low number of false-positive results, the secretin test is the provocative test of choice.[719,806,808] The calcium infusion test should be reserved for the rare patient in whom ZES is strongly suspected but the secretin test is negative.[796,808] In 33% of such patients, the calcium test is positive.[806]

To separate ZES from antral G-cell hyperfunction or hyperplasia, serum gastrin response as determined after a standard meal is reported to be useful.[809,810] After a standard meal, serum gastrin is measured at -15, 0, +30, +60, and +90 minutes.[809,810] Patients with ZES are reported to have less than 50% increase over basal values (see Fig. 41–11), whereas patients with antral G-cell hyperfunction or hyperplasia have an exaggerated response (Table 41–28).[809,810] In a recent re-

TABLE 41-29. Results of Provocative Tests Using Secretin, Calcium, and a Standard Meal Test in Patients With Zollinger-Ellison Syndrome: Proposed Criteria for a Positive Test

	Serum Gastrin Increase*								
	After Secretin			After Calcium		After Meal			
	≥110 pg/ml	≥200 pg/ml	≥50%	≥395 pg/ml	≥50%	<50%	50-99%	≥100%	≥150%
Tumor demonstrated	93%	84%	78%	43%	74%	46%	36%	18%	9%
Tumor not demonstrated	93%	89%	93%	70%	100%	43%	14%	43%	10%

* Results are the percentage of patients with the indicated tumor status who demonstrated the indicated change in serum gastrin after receiving a secretin bolus (2 U/kg), calcium infusion (54 mg calcium gluconate/h for 3 h) or a standard meal.[809] Results are for patients with Zollinger-Ellison syndrome with fasting serum gastrin concentration < 1000 pg/ml (secretin, 54 patients; calcium 46 patients; meal, 53 patients).
(Data from Lamers CBH, van Tongeren JHM. Comparative study of the value of calcium, secretin, and meal stimulated increase in serum gastrin in the diagnosis of Zollinger-Ellison syndrome. Gut 1979;18:128; and from Frucht HJ, Howard JM, Stark HA, et al. Prospective study of meal provocative gastrin testing in patients with Zollinger-Ellison syndrome. Am J Med 1989;87:528)

view of 52 patients with antral G-cell disease, 98% of patients had an increase of 100% or more and 92% had an increase of 150% or more postmeal.[810] In a recent prospective study of patients with ZES, only 46% of patients had an increase of 50% or less, 26% had an increase of 50% to 99%, 30% had an increase of less than 100%, and 10% had a greater than 150% increase (see Table 41-28).[810] It was therefore concluded that the meal test frequently is positive in patients with ZES and does not reliably differentiate ZES from antral syndromes.[810] Antral G-cell hyperplasia is reported to mimic ZES clinically with elevated fasting serum levels of gastrin and BAO, to occur frequently in patients postvagotomy, to be due to increased numbers of antral G cells, to be curable by antrectomy, and to be differentiated from ZES by a negative secretin test and a postmeal increase of 100% or more in serum gastrin levels (see Table 41-28).[712,719,811-814] Antral G-cell hyperfunction is similar to antral G-cell hyperplasia except that normal numbers of G cells are found, the syndrome frequently is familial with autosomal dominant inheritance, and the syndrome is associated with hyperpepsinogenemia I.[712,815,816] This syndrome also was reported to be differentiated from ZES by having a negative secretin test and exaggerated increase in serum gastrin postmeal.[719,815,816] Thirty percent of patients with ZES have a positive meal test (see Tables 41-28 and 41-29).[810]

Chronic gastric outlet obstruction can be difficult to differentiate from ZES because the obstruction can be caused by ZES or can mimic ZES and be secondary to other causes of duodenal obstruction (see Table 41-28).[719,817] ZES can be differentiated from the other causes of obstruction by a secretin test and prolonged gastric suction.[719,818] In ZES, the secretin test is positive (more than 200 pg/ml increase) and prolonged nasogastric suction does not change the serum gastrin concentrations. In the other conditions, the secretin test is negative and serum gastrins decrease with nasogastric suction.[817] Massive small bowel resection has been reported to cause a transient hypergastrinemia and an elevation of BAO that can be differentiated from ZES by the history and the secretin test (see Table 41-28).[719]

Tumor Localization

Precise localization of the gastrinoma has become an increasingly important factor in evaluating patients with ZES.[764,796,819] With the increased ability to control gastric acid hypersecretion with H_2 receptor antagonists, emergency total gastrectomy is rarely necessary, allowing time to determine the location and extent of the gastrinoma.[719,820] With the increased ability to control gastric acid hypersecretion long-term medically or surgically, the growth and possible metastatic spread of the gastrinoma has become an increasingly important determinant of long-term survival.[691,712,720,759,821] In previous studies, 13% to 52% of all patients at surgery had metastatic disease (usually to the liver), and identification of these patients preoperatively can prevent unnecessary surgery (see Table 41-26).[746,762,822] Gastrinomas frequently are multiple and extrapancreatic (see Tables 41-26 and 41-27).[757,762,823,824] In as many as 40% to 60% of patients in some series (see Table 41-26), no gastrinoma is found at surgery.[823-825] Therefore, careful imaging studies should be used to assist the surgeon in localizing the tumor. A recent study using careful imaging studies was able to identify 15% of patients with metastatic disease to the liver in whom the gastrinoma was resectable.[826]

A number of techniques are helpful in localizing gastrinomas, including abdominal ultrasound, CT scans, selective abdominal angiography, MRI, selective venous sampling for gastrin from portal venous tributaries, intraarterial secretin with hepatic venous gastrin sampling, intraoperative ultrasonography (IOUS), and transillumination of the duodenum at surgery (Table 41-30). Although ultrasound has a low sensitivity for localizing primary and metastatic tumors, a recent prospective study recommended that it continue to be used because it is highly specific, noninvasive, and on occasion localizes gastrinomas not found by other modalities.[827] The CT scan detects on average 50% of all primaries and patients with metastatic liver disease (see Table 41-30). Its ability to detect primary tumors has been shown to be directly related to tumor size, detecting no tumor smaller than 1 cm, 30% of

TABLE 41–30. Ability of Various Modalities to Localize Primary and Metastatic Gastrinoma in Patients With Zollinger-Ellison Syndrome

	Sensitivity (%) Mean (Range)	Specificity (%) Mean (Range)
Primary Tumor		
Ultrasound	23 (21–28)	92 (92–92)
CT scan	50 (35–59)	90 (83–100)
Angiography	68 (35–68)	89 (84–94)
IOUS	83	NE
MRI	21	33
PVS	73	33
Intraarterial secretin test	78 (55–100)	100
Transillumination of duodenum*	83	88
Metastatic Tumor		
Ultrasound	14 (14–63)	100
CT scan	54 (35–72)	99 (98–100)
Angiography	62 (33–86)	98 (96–100)
IOUS	NE	NE
MRI	67	100
PVS	NE	NE

IOUS, intraoperative ultrasound; PVS, selective gastrin sampling from portal venous tributaries; NE, not evaluated.
* Data are for duodenal gastrinomas only.
(Data from Jensen RT, Gardner JD. Zollinger-Ellison syndrome: Clinical presentation, pathology, diagnosis, and treatment. In: Dannenberg A, Zakim D, eds. Peptic ulcer and other acid-related diseases. New York: Academic Research Association, 1991:117)

tumors between 1 and 3 cm, and 95% of tumors larger than 3 cm.[828] Primary tumors smaller than 1 cm, which increasingly are being found in the duodenum, usually are missed by CT.[743,745,783,829] Furthermore, CT is less sensitive for detecting extrahepatic and extrapancreatic tumors than pancreatic gastrinomas.[828] A typical CT scan showing gastrinoma metastatic to the liver is shown in Figure 41–12. Selective angiography was able to detect 68% of primary tumors and 86% of hepatic metastases in a recent large prospective study (see Table 41–30).[830] The ability to detect tumors depended on their location, with the study finding 90% of gastrinomas in the pancreatic head, 80% in the body, 45% in the tail, 34% in the duodenum, and 50% in extrapancreatic, extrahepatic, and extraduodenal locations.[830] A typical angiogram of a primary gastrinoma in the pancreatic head area is shown in Figure 41–13. In a comparative study, angiography detected 68% of hepatic metastases, 17% more than CT scans did, and the combination detected 98% of all patients with liver metastases.[830]

MRI was reported in early studies to be useful in localizing gastrinoma in a small number of cases (see Table 41–30).[831,832] A typical positive imaging study identifying metastatic disease in the liver is shown in Figure 41–13. A prospective study from 1986 to 1987 reported that MRI was less sensitive than CT or angiography.[833] A recent preliminary study suggests that contrast agents such as gadolinium may increase the sensitivity of MRI.[834] In this study, in which gadolinium was given by continuous intravenous infusion, MRI was found to be as sensitive as CT for detecting hepatic metastases in 4 of 15 patients with metastatic gastrinomas. In another recent study of 16 patients with ZES, gadolinium did not enhance the ability to find the primary or metastatic tumor.[835] MRI is rapidly improving, and in a study using MRI that corrects for motion by respiratory gating, signal averaging, and fast image analysis, MRI was more sensitive than angiography or CT for metastatic disease.[835] MRI may be the initial imaging study of choice for metastatic disease, although MRI studies remain less sensitive than angiography for primary tumor.[835]

Even though gastrinomas frequently occur in the duodenum (see Tables 41–26 and 41–27), they rarely are seen by routine upper gastrointestinal endoscopy because they are small and submucosal.[712] Endoscopic transillumination of the duodenum at surgery has been attempted and was useful in localizing small gastrinomas not found by other modalities (see Table 41–30).[836] In a recent prospective study of 26 patients, 12

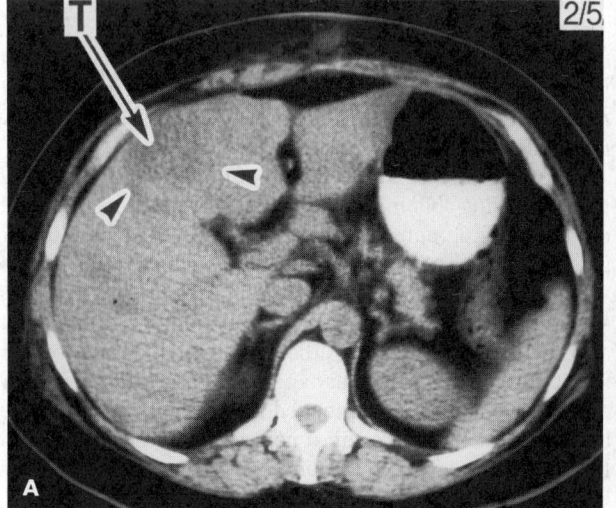
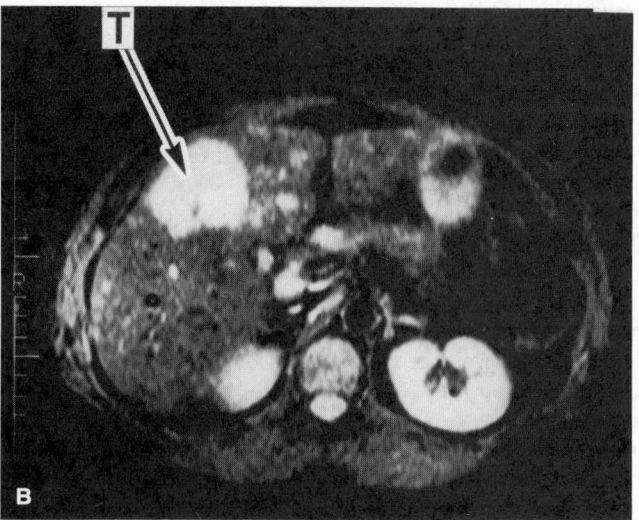

FIGURE 41–12. CT and MRI scans in a patient with metastatic gastrinoma. **(A)** The CT scan shows a large metastatic tumor (T) deposit in the left lobe of the liver (*arrowheads*). **(B)** The MRI STIR sequence more clearly demonstrates the metastatic tumor (T).

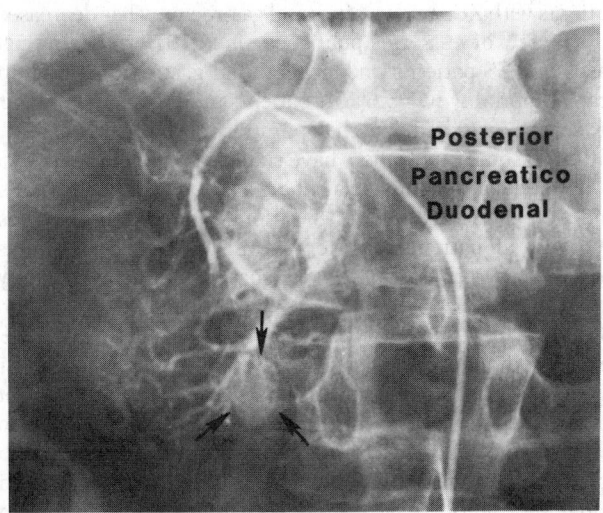

FIGURE 41–13. Selective injection of the posterior pancreatico-duodenal artery shows a small gastrinoma (*arrows*) in the postero-inferior portion of the pancreatic head in a patient with Zollinger-Ellison syndrome.

duodenal gastrinomas were found at surgery in 10 patients.[836] Operative endoscopic transillumination detected 10 of the 12 (83% sensitivity), a sensitivity significantly greater than that of preoperative imaging, which detected 3 duodenal gastrinomas (25% sensitivity), or of IOUS and palpation, which detected 5 (42% sensitivity). It is not known whether this procedure is as sensitive as duodenotomy or has less morbidity. A preliminary report suggests that endoscopic ultrasound should be helpful for preoperatively localizing duodenal tumors.[837] In this study, endoscopic ultrasound localized tumor in 8 of 13 patients (61%), including a primary pancreatic gastrinoma or gastrinoma in lymph nodes not seen on CT scan; however, it failed to localize 3 duodenal gastrinomas. Future prospective studies are needed to evaluate its potential fully.

Early studies in a small number of patients with ZES suggested that selective venous sampling for gastrin from portal venous tributaries (PVS) would be helpful (see Table 41–30).[838–840] In a recent prospective study, a combination of PVS and imaging yielded results only marginally better than imaging alone in identifying gastrinomas.[808] In this study, neither the magnitude of the gastrin gradient nor its presence or absence correlated with finding a gastrinoma at surgery. A typical result localizing a gastrinoma to the pancreatic head area is shown in Figure 41–14. A gradient of more than 50% is reported to occur in 74% of all patients with ZES.[808,841] PVS requires expertise, is time consuming, and has some morbidity, primarily abdominal pain at the catheter insertion site.[808,841] These drawbacks, combined with its limited availability and the fact that 70% to 80% of gastrinomas are in the pancreatic head, have led most investigators[796,808] but not all[842] to conclude that this procedure has limited usefulness in ZES. PVS, although occasionally helpful, is not recommended for gastrinomas. PVS has proved valuable in localizing insulinomas, which can occur throughout the pancreas.[843,844]

Most gastrinomas (91%) demonstrate a paradoxical release of gastrin with intravenous injection of secretin (see Fig. 41–11).[806–808] This characteristic has been used to localize gas-

PORTAL VENOUS GASTRIN SAMPLING

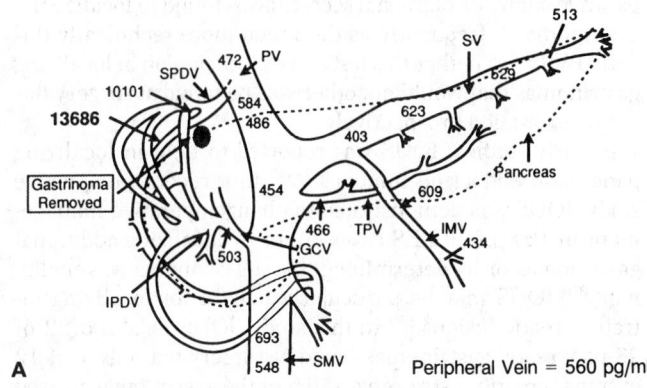

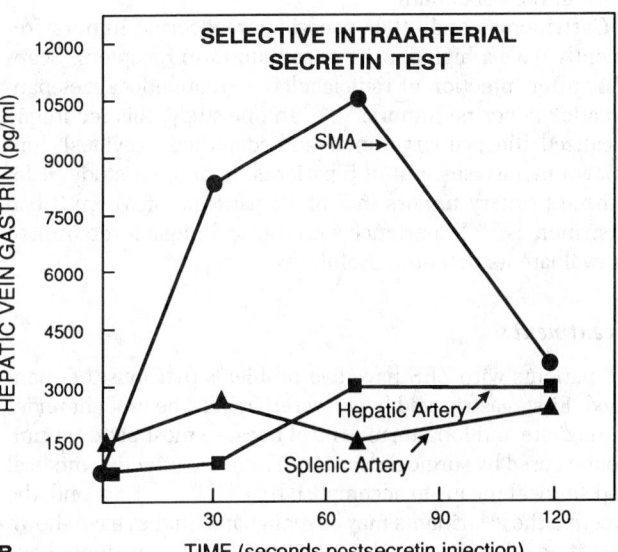

FIGURE 41–14. Selective portal venous sampling and intraarterial secretin injection to localize gastrinoma in a patient with ZES. **(A)** The selective venous gastrin concentration at different locations with a simultaneous peripheral gastrin of 560 pg/ml. This patient had a marked gradient of 2343% in the pancreatic head. The solid dot indicates the location of the 1-cm gastrinoma found subsequently in the pancreatic head at surgery. **(B)** The serum gastrin concentration (from the same patient) in the hepatic vein after secretin injection (30 units) sequentially into the hepatic, superior or mesenteric (SMA), and splenic arteries. Hepatic venous samples were collected before injection and at 0.5, 1 and 2 minutes after injection. A rapid rise from 520 pg/ml to 10,500 pg/ml at 30 seconds occurred with the SMA injection, whereas the increase with injection in the other arteries occurred later and was of less magnitude. These results localized the gastrinoma to the pancreatic head area supplied by the SMA, which was the area in which a 1-cm gastrinoma was found subsequently **(A)**. GCV, gastrocolic vein; TPA, tranverse pancreatic vein; IMV, inferior mesenteric vein; SMV, superior mesenteric vein; SPDV, superior pancreaticoduodenal vein; IPDV, inferior pancreaticoduodenal vein; PV, portal vein.

trinomas selectively by injecting secretin intraarterially into various abdominal arteries and collecting venous samples from the hepatic veins for assays of gastrin.[843,845,846] Figure 41–14 (lower panel) demonstrates a rapid increase in hepatic vein gastrin concentration after injection of secretin into the superior mesenteric artery. The other vessels demonstrated smaller increases that occurred at later times. A gastrinoma was found in this patient in the pancreatic head, which is supplied by the superior mesenteric artery. In a recent comparative study, intraarterial secretin was found to localize the gastrinoma as frequently as the much more technically difficult PVS.[846] Whether this test assists the surgeon in localizing gastrinomas that would not otherwise be found at surgery has not been studied prospectively.

In early studies, IOUS was reported to help in localizing pancreatic endocrine tumors.[847–849] In a recent prospective study, IOUS was demonstrated to change operative management in 10% of all ZES cases either by localizing additional gastrinomas or by determining that a gastrinoma was malignant.[850] IOUS may be particularly helpful for localizing intrapancreatic lesions.[850] In this study, IOUS localized 22 of 23 pancreatic gastrinomas found at surgery but only 7 of 12 extrapancreatic gastrinomas. All 5 of the gastrinomas missed were in the duodenum.[850]

Gastrinomas and other pancreatic endocrine tumors frequently have a high density of somatostatin receptors. Scanning after injection of radiolabeled octreotide localizes pancreatic endocrine tumors.[604–606] In one study, this technique localized the primary tumor and identified previously unknown metastases in 4 of 5 patients. In another study, it localized primary tumors in 7 of 12 patients, of whom 3 had gastrinomas.[606] Experience with this technique is too limited to evaluate its potential usefulness.

Treatment

All patients with ZES have two problems that must be managed. First, gastric acid hypersecretion must be brought under immediate and long-term control because most patients cannot be cured by surgical excision. There are effective medical and surgical means to accomplish this.[691,712,715,719] Second, the fact that the gastrinoma may be malignant. Studies have shown that if acid hypersecretion is controlled, these patients have an excellent quality of life. Long-term prognosis increasingly is being determined by the malignant nature of the gastrinoma.[712] Although in recent studies only about 30% patients at diagnosis have metastatic disease, in previous studies 60% to 90% of patients had metastatic disease (see Table 41–26). The exact percentage of gastrinomas that are malignant is not clear. However, in contrast to insulinomas, of which only 15% are malignant, as many as 60% to 90% of gastrinomas may be malignant (see Table 41–26).[520,702,851] Therefore, it is important to consider therapy directed at the gastrinoma itself, including therapies for metastatic disease and surgical excision of nonmetastatic gastrinoma.

Treatment of Acid Secretion

Surgical Treatment of Gastric Hypersecretion. Until recently, all patients with ZES required total gastrectomy to control gastric acid hypersecretion. In early studies, patients at the time of surgery were debilitated with complicated ulcer disease, had electrolyte abnormalities, and were malnourished. The operation frequently had to be done as an emergency, leading to a mortality rate of 15% in the postoperative period.[757,758] Operative results were unsatisfactory for patients who had less than total gastrectomy, with most patients developing recurrent ulcer disease, often with lethal complications, within days of surgery.[757,758] With the development of increasingly effective medical therapy, the mortality for

patients with ZES undergoing total gastrectomy has decreased. In a review of 10 series published since 1978 involving 248 cases of ZES patients undergoing total gastrectomy, the operative mortality was 5.6%. If patients undergoing emergency procedures are excluded, the operative mortality was 2.4%.[762] Although some researchers have stated that the morbidity rate is low, adequate follow-up is not always apparent.[762] In at least one well-studied series of 18 patients undergoing total gastrectomy, all patients experienced one or several side effects, including symptoms of esophageal reflux, early satiety, cramping, or diarrhea.[766] These side effects were moderate to severe in 50% of the patients, and in 3 patients (27%) serious additional complications developed, including stenosis of the esophageal anastomosis in 2 patients, and recurrent, severe vomiting in the third patient.[766] The morbidity associated with total gastrectomy may be significant and is probably underestimated in many series.[691] Furthermore, a nutritional morbidity is associated with total gastrectomy that includes weight loss and anemia. Although one early study claimed that total gastrectomy could lead to regression of the gastrinoma in some patients,[852] recent studies have failed to substantiate this claim.[759,799,821] There is no evidence that medical therapy of gastric hypersecretion or total gastrectomy affects the growth rate of the gastrinoma.[503]

The development of increasingly effective medical therapy has led to a considerable debate over the role of total gastrectomy in controlling gastric acid hypersecretion.[691,719,762,853] Some groups continue to advocate total gastrectomy, citing high failure rates with medical therapy and improved morbidity and mortality now that total gastrectomy can be performed electively after correcting malnutrition.[722,762,853] Gastric acid hypersecretion can be controlled medically long-term in every patient who takes oral medication, using the H^+-K^+-ATPase inhibitor omeprazole.[854–861] The availability of omeprazole and its long duration of action has greatly simplified management because it can be taken once or twice per day. Therefore, most authorities recommend that total gastrectomy be reserved for patients who do not have access to routine medical follow-up or who cannot or will not take oral medication.[764,796] In all other patients, medical therapy is the treatment of choice.

A combination of anticholinergic agents and H_2 receptor antagonists has a greater effect than either drug alone.[862–864] The use of anticholinergic agents frequently is associated with side effects that limit patient acceptance.[865] Richardson and colleagues reported that parietal cell vagotomy in patients with ZES in whom no tumor was found at surgery decreased the BAO by 66% and decreased the antisecretory drug requirement by 95% in all patients.[825] Even though it is likely that the antisecretory drug dose requirement will increase slowly as the gastrinoma progresses, use of a parietal cell vagotomy will delay high-dose requirements for years in most patients.[825] Because of the availability of potent antisecretory agents such as omeprazole, parietal cell vagotomy should not be performed routinely.[796] Rather, it should be reserved for the occasional patient who has a high-dose antisecretory medication requirement and an unresectable tumor or tumor not found (Fig. 41–15).

In patients with ZES and the MEN-I syndrome, medical control of gastric hypersecretion can be facilitated greatly by correction of the hyperparathyroidism, which almost always

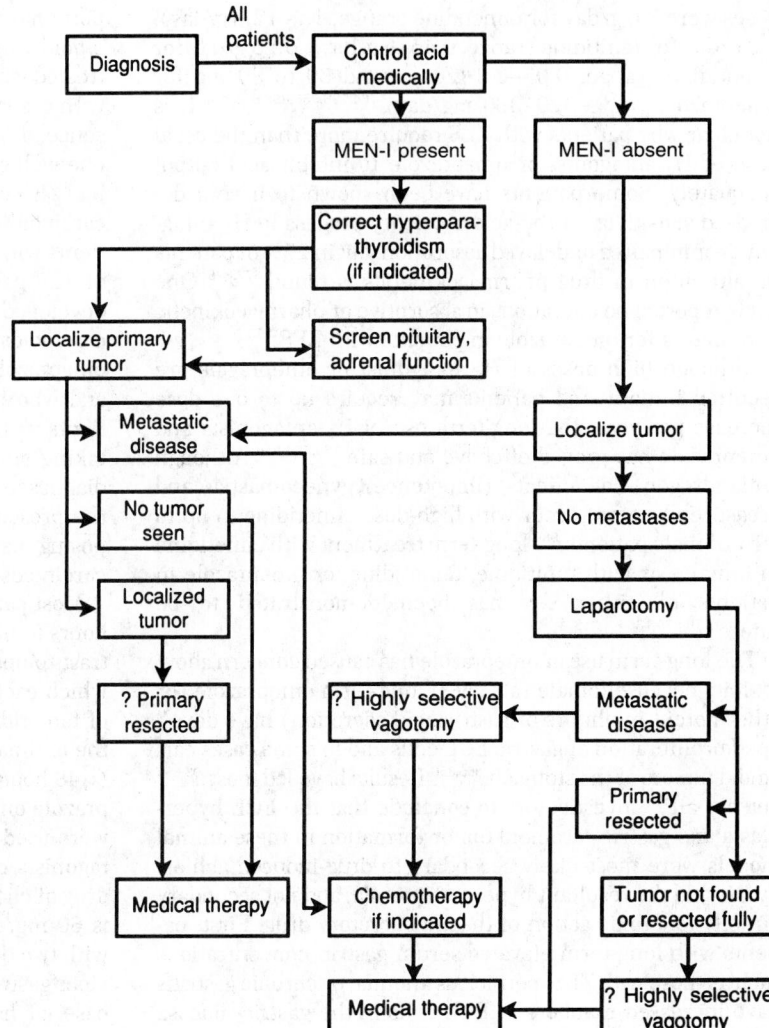

FIGURE 41–15. Flow diagram for the management of patients with Zollinger-Ellison syndrome. It is unclear whether a highly selective vagotomy should be performed in a patient in whom metastatic disease is found at the time of surgery. With the availability of omeprazole, gastric acid hypersecretion can be controlled in all such patients so that parietal cell vagotomy is indicated less frequently. If a primary tumor is seen on imaging studies in patients with MEN-I, there is no general agreement as to whether patients should undergo surgery because resection of a pancreatic tumor does not result in cure.

is present by the time ZES develops.[514] Correction of hyperparathyroidism may reduce the fasting serum gastrin concentration, increase the responsiveness to a given dose of antisecretory medication, and decrease the BAO.[866–868] Therefore, in patients with MEN-I and hyperparathyroidism, parathyroidectomy should be performed before any other surgical procedure to control acid hypersecretion.

Medical Treatment of Gastric Hypersecretion. The results of medical treatment of gastric acid hypersecretion have been reviewed extensively.[691,764,796,820,856,865,869] H_2 antagonists (*e.g.,* cimetidine, ranitidine, famotidine) alone or in combination with anticholinergic agents probanthine (*e.g.,* propantheline bromide and isopropamide) and more recently omeprazole, the substituted benzimidazole that functions as a H^+-K^+-ATPase inhibitor, have been used successfully in the long-term treatment of gastric hypersecretion in ZES. The number of patients failing medical therapy varies greatly in different series,[691,719,796,869] with failure rates ranging from 0 to 65% for cimetidine,[691,704,766,870–872] from 0 to 40% for ranitidine,[691,757,873] no reported failure for famotidine,[862,874] and from 0 to 7.5% for omeprazole.[854–861] An analysis of these series concluded that the principal factors contributing to

failure of H_2 receptor antagonists to control acid hypersecretion were inadequate doses of antisecretory medication and the failure to use reliable criteria for assessing the ability of these agents to suppress BAO.[869] In general, relief of symptoms does not reflect adequately the effectiveness of antisecretory therapy.[871,872,875] To assess the adequacy of antisecretory therapy, gastric acid secretion must be measured while the patient is taking medication.[691,719,876]

The amount of antisecretory medication required varies widely from patient to patient and increases slowly with time. The optimal dose of medication must be determined for each patient initially and periodically reevaluated.[691,764,820,856] If enough antisecretory drug is used to decrease gastric acid secretion to less than 10 mEq/hour for the hour before the next dose of medications in patients without previous gastric surgery and to less than 5 mEq/hour in patients with previous acid-reducing procedures or severe esophageal disease, peptic ulcers will heal and complications of peptic ulcer disease will be prevented.[721,764,794,854,873,875] To reduce acid output to these levels before the next dose of medication, patients usually require more than twice the usual dose of H_2 antagonist or three times the usual dose of omeprazole recommended for idiopathic peptic ulcer disease. In recent studies, the median doses were 3.6 g/day for cimetidine (range, 1.2–12.6 g/day), 1.2 g/day for ranitidine (range, 0.45–6 g/day), 0.25 g/day for famotidine (range, 0.05–0.8 g/day), and 60 to 80 mg for omeprazole (range, 20–360 mg/day).[764,796,856,862,873,874] It is not clear why patients with ZES require more than the usual dose of H$_2$ antagonist or omeprazole to inhibit acid output adequately. Some patients have been shown to have a decreased sensitivity of the acid secretory process to H$_2$ antagonists or impaired or delayed absorption, but in 25% of patients no alteration in drug pharmacokinetics is found.[877,878] One study reported no alterations in absorptive or pharmacokinetic parameters for omeprazole in patients with ZES.[879]

Although high doses of H$_2$ antagonist or omeprazole are required initially and patients may require up to one dose increase per year, the long-term use of H$_2$ antagonists and omeprazole has proved effective and safe.[764,796,856] Although antiandrogen side effects (impotence, gynecomastia, and breast tenderness) occur with high-dose cimetidine in up to 60% of male patients,[880] long-term treatment with cimetidine in females or with ranitidine, famotidine, or omeprazole in patients of either sex has been demonstrated to be safe.[691,764,796,865]

The long-term use of omeprazole has caused concern about toxicity because female rats given long-term omeprazole (or other potent inhibitors of gastric acid secretion) have developed proliferation of gastric ECL cells and in some cases carcinoid tumors of the stomach.[505,856] Results have led most[505,856] but not all[508] investigators to conclude that the ECL hyperplasia and gastric carcinoid tumor formation in these animal models were most likely secondary to drug-induced achlorhydria and the resultant hypergastrinemia, and not secondary directly to a toxic action of the antisecretory drug. First, patients with long-term elevated serum gastrin concentrations such as those with ZES, pernicious anemia, or chronic gastritis have increased numbers of ECL cells in the gastric mucosa and have been reported to develop gastric carcinoid tumors.[505,856] Second, gastrin has been shown to be trophic to the gastric mucosa in animals and to cause ECL hyperplasia.[503,505,723,856] Third, ECL hyperplasia is caused not only by omeprazole or unsurmountable inhibitors of gastric acid secretion but also by large doses of H$_2$ receptor antagonists such as ranitidine, loxtidine, SKF9378, BL-6431, ICI 162,846, or sodium bicarbonate.[503,505,508,856] Fourth, in animal studies, hyperplasia of the ECL cells was proportional to the hypergastrinemia produced by various means and was prevented by antrectomy.[503,505,856] Fifth, other means of inducing hypergastrinemia such as gastric antral exclusion and fundectomy can increase the number of ECL cells and in some cases cause the development of carcinoid tumors.[511,881]

Hyperplasia of gastric endocrine cells occurs in patients with ZES. Quantitative studies indicate that gastric ECL cells are increased about twofold, independent of administration of antisecretory agents.[499,503,856,882–884] Of the six types of gastric endocrine cells, only the ECL cells were increased and underwent neoplastic changes in patients with ZES.[884] In two studies in which omeprazole treatment was prolonged for up to 4 years, there was no statistical increase in gastric ECL cells due to this drug.[882,883] The lack of effect of omeprazole on ECL-cell hyperplasia in patients with ZES appears to conflict with reports of gastric carcinoids in patients with ZES, some of whom were taking omeprazole.[503,856,884] Recent reports have described patients with ZES who developed carcinoid tumors of the stomach, some of whom were being treated with omeprazole.[503,856,884] In 15 of 16 patients reported with gastric carcinoids and ZES in whom the presence or absence of MEN-I could be determined, 14 had MEN-I.[503,856] In one well-studied series of 170 patients, 24% of the patients had ZES with MEN-I.[822] Both patients who developed gastric carcinoid tumors had MEN-I.[883] Therefore, about 2 of 41 patients with MEN-I and ZES developed gastric carcinoids, but of 129 patients with the sporadic form of ZES, no patient developed gastric carcinoids. Two of the 16 cases of gastric carcinoids occurred in patients with ZES who were taking omeprazole when the gastric carcinoid tumors were diagnosed and who had ZES with MEN-I.[856] Therefore, 14 of the patients with ZES reported to have gastric carcinoids were not taking omeprazole when the gastric carcinoid tumors were diagnosed, and almost all had MEN-I. These data suggest that the presence of MEN-I may be an important factor predisposing patients with ZES to the development of gastric carcinoids.[499,856]

Most patients with ZES require H$_2$ antagonists every 4 to 8 hours to inhibit gastric secretion adequately.[796,820,865] In contrast to optimally effective doses of cimetidine or ranitidine, which each have a duration of action of 6 to 8 hours,[862] and of famotidine, which has a duration of action of 10 hours,[720] the optimal dose of omeprazole has a long duration of action (>48 hours),[854–856,879] allowing most patients to require omeprazole only once or twice a day. Anticholinergic agents that were used extensively in the past[865] are rarely used. H$_2$ antagonists continue to be useful, although omeprazole is the drug of choice.[503,820,856] The usual starting dose of omeprazole is 60 mg/day, although some patients are better controlled with two doses daily.[856] Patients with ZES who have had previous gastric surgery, have moderate to severe esophageal disease, or have MEN-I usually require a higher dose and are best treated by starting with 40 mg twice a day.[794,856,885]

If the patient presents with a complication and cannot take oral antisecretory medication, or if during surgery it is important to control secretion, continuous infusions of cimetidine (median dose 3 mg/kg/hour) or ranitidine (median dose 1 mg/kg/hour) or bolus doses of omeprazole (injectable, 60 mg every 12 hours; not available in the United States) are all effective.[876,886–889] These drugs should be continued until oral antisecretory agents can be restarted.[503,876,888,889]

Treatment of Gastrinoma

The 5-year survival rate for patients with ZES ranges from 62% to 75%, and the 10-year survival ranges from 47% to 53% (Table 41–31). Although the growth of a gastrinoma generally is slow, long-term studies of patients originally treated by total gastrectomy found that in 57% of patients, death was due to tumor progression.[758,759] Therefore, with the ability to control gastric acid hypersecretion, the malignant potential of the tumor is an increasingly important determinant of long-term prognosis. Various factors that contribute to long-term survival have been identified. The extent of the tumor and whether MEN-I is present or absent have been reported to determine survival rates (see Table 41–31). In patients with no tumor found at laparotomy or in whom tumor is completely resectable, 5-year and 10-year survival rates are 90% to 100% (see Table 41–31).

TABLE 41–31. Prognosis in Patients With Zollinger-Ellison Syndrome

Investigations	No. of Patients	5-Year Survival (%)	10-Year Survival (%)
All Patients			
Thompson et al, 1983[762]	27	75	52
Zollinger et al, 1984[765]	40	62	47
Mignon et al, 1986[822]	144	62	53
Ellison et al, 1987[891]	60	63	52
Related to Tumor Resectability			
No tumor found			
Malagelada et al, 1983[766]	13	100	100
Zollinger et al, 1984[765]	6	100	—
Stabile and Passaro, 1984[767]	10	90	90
Zollinger, 1985[890]	8	ND	63
Norton et al, 1992[745]	16	90	ND
Tumor resected			
Malagelada et al, 1983[766]	7	100	100
Zollinger et al, 1984[765]	22	76	—
Stabile and Passaro, 1984[767]	10	90	90
Ellison et al, 1987[891]	33	69	62
Norton et al, 1992[745]	42	95	ND
Tumor incompletely resected or recurrence			
Malagelada et al, 1983[766]	10	75	20
Zollinger et al, 1984[765]	7	14	—
Norton et al, 1992[745]	15	95	ND
Unresectable			
Malagelada et al, 1983[766]	13	80	—
Zollinger et al, 1984[765]	7	30	—
Stabile and Passaro, 1984[767]	14	40	30
Hancke, 1979[1108]	15	20	—
Norton et al, 1992[745]	18	18	ND
Related to MEN-I Status			
MEN-I present			
Malagelada et al, 1983[766]	14	—	80
Thompson et al, 1983[762]	11	85	85
Zollinger et al, 1984[765]	13	85	62
Stabile and Passaro, 1984[767]	23	80	75
Zollinger, 1985[890]	7	ND	71
Ellison et al, 1987[891]	16	75	70
Podevin et al, 1990[892]	45	70	63
MEN-I absent			
Malagelada et al, 1983[766]	36	—	64
Thompson et al, 1983[762]	26	70	50
Zollinger et al, 1984[765]	27	52	40
Stabile and Passaro, 1984[767]	42	70	65
Zollinger, 1985[890]	7	ND	71
Ellison et al, 1987[891]	44	70	65
Podevin et al, 1990[892]	135	66	55

MEN-I, multiple endocrine neoplasia type I; ND, not determined.

Survival curves from a recent large prospective study of curative resection in ZES are shown in Figure 41–16, demonstrating excellent long-term survival in patients with resected disease or tumors so small they cannot be detected at surgery, whereas patients who develop advanced metastatic disease have a poor survival.[745] In contrast, patients with tumor incompletely resected or unresectable have 5-year survival averaging 50% and an average 10-year survival of 25%. In two studies, patients with MEN-I are reported to have a better 5-year and 10-year survival than patients without MEN-I,[762,765] whereas in other studies[766,767,890–892] the difference was not significant (see Table 41–31). The presence of Cushing's syndrome is associated with a poor prognosis.[893] It has not been proved a poor prognostic factor, because it usually occurs in patients with ZES without MEN-I when extensive metastases are present, a condition that already has a poor prognosis.[893]

Because of the excellent prognosis of patients with gastrinoma who are resected and the increased importance of the malignancy in determining survival, surgical resection of the gastrinoma should be considered in all patients with ZES. The general approach to the gastrinoma is summarized in the flow diagram in Figure 41–15. The first step is to control gastric acid hypersecretion medically. It must then be determined whether the patient has sporadic ZES (ZES without MEN-I) or whether ZES is present with MEN-I.[691] The role of surgery is controversial in patients with MEN-I (see the sections on MEN-I and on pancreatic endocrine tumors in MEN-I).

Treatment of Nonmetastatic Gastrinoma. The role of surgery in the treatment of the gastrinoma is becoming better defined.[745,783] All physicians agree that the ideal treatment of ZES is the surgical excision of the gastrinoma, but in early studies this was possible in only 8 of 157 patients.[717,719–721,799] Even this figure was probably an overestimation of the cure rate because in many cases follow-up was less than 1 year and in no cases were multiple secretin provocative tests performed postoperatively.[503,691] In series reported since 1986, the cure rate is higher, averaging about 40% and ranging from 17% to 100% (Table 41–32).

Surgical cure rates may continue to increase. With the development of effective antisecretory agents, all patients can undergo extensive preoperative investigational studies, surgery can be done electively, and the surgery can emphasize gastrinoma localization and removal rather than control of gastric acid hypersecretion.[503,745,783] The preoperative localization and clinical distinction between patients with and without MEN-I identifies groups of patients with different potential for cure. More than 90% of patients with gastrinoma metastatic to the liver can be identified with imaging studies, obviating unnecessary attempts at curative surgery in these patients.[745,783,828,830] Because gastrinomas occur more frequently in the duodenum than previously thought (see Tables 41–26 and 41–27), preoperative localization studies frequently do not identify extrapancreatic gastrinomas.[691,741,745,783,828–830] Even when the gastrinoma is localized, potential resectability cannot be predicted if hepatic metastases are not present.

In a recent large prospective study, the overall percentage of patients with no evidence of disease immediately postoperatively was 58%.[745] At 5 years, 30% of all patients remained

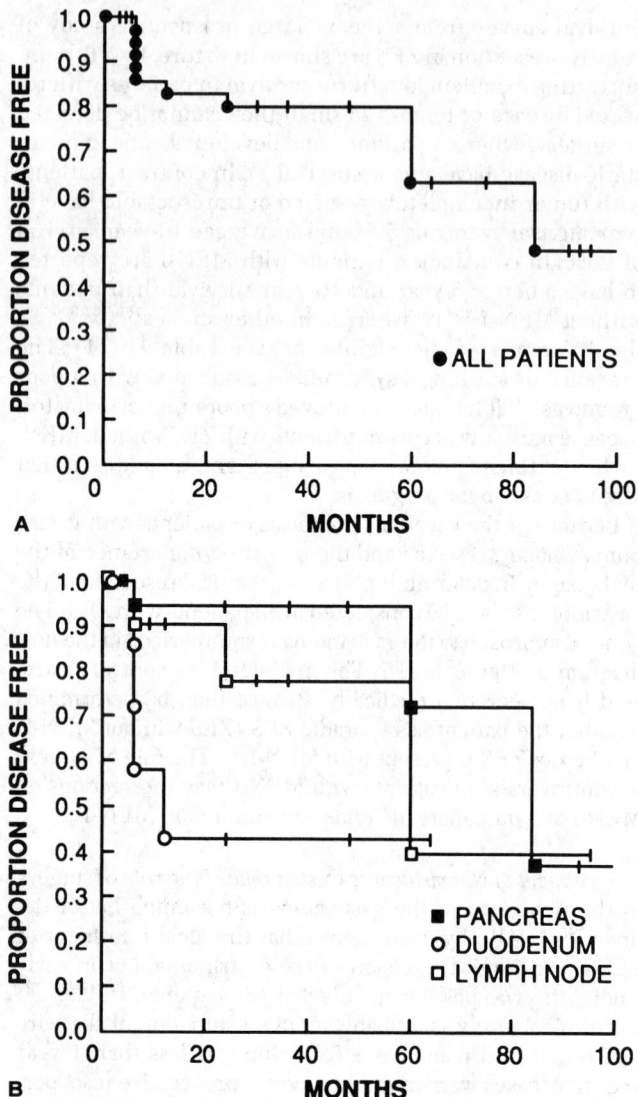

A

B

FIGURE 41–16.   Time to recurrence of Zollinger-Ellison syndrome in patients initially disease-free by surgery. **(A)** The Kaplan-Meier plot of the time to recurrence for all patients (n = 42) who were disease free of Zollinger-Ellison syndrome at the initial (3- or 6-month) postoperative follow-up. *Disease-free* is defined as no evidence of gastrinoma on imaging studies, normal fasting gastrin concentration, and negative secretin and calcium provocative tests. **(B)** Kaplan-Meier plot of the time to recurrence of Zollinger-Ellison syndrome of patients who were rendered disease-free of Zollinger-Ellison syndrome at the initial postoperative follow-up divided by primary disease site: duodenum (n = 12), pancreas (n = 19), and lymph node (n = 10). One patient with the primary ovarian gastrinoma is excluded. Patients with primary duodenal gastrinomas had a significantly shorter disease-free interval than patients with pancreatic gastrinomas (*p* <0.01). The difference between patients with duodenal gastrinomas and those with lymph node only gastrinomas was not significant (*p* = 0.1). The median disease-free survival for patients with duodenal, pancreatic, or lymph node primary gastrinomas was 12, 84, and 60 months, respectively. (Modified from Norton JA, Doppman JL, Jensen RT. Curative resection in Zollinger-Ellison syndrome: results of a 10 year prospective study. Ann Surg 1992;215:8)

TABLE 41–32. Long-Term Results of Attempts at Complete Surgical Resection of Gastrinoma

Investigations	No. of Patients Operated*	Patients With Normal Gastrin Postresection Number (%)
Stage and Stadil, 1979[717]	25	1 (4)
Zollinger et al, 1980[720] †	42	2 (5)
Bonfils et al, 1981[722] †	32	6 (6.5)
Friesen, 1982[853] †	23	9 (39)
Wilson, 1982[1109] †	28	6 (22)
Wolfe et al, 1982[744] †	18	4 (22)
Thompson et al, 1983[762] †	26	3 (12)
Deveney et al, 1983[823] †	52	6 (12)
Malagelada et al, 1983[766]	44	7 (16)
Stabile et al, 1984[746] †	45	5 (11)
Richardson et al, 1985[825]	22	4 (18)
Norton et al, 1986[743]	29	12 (43 postop) (30; 6 mo–4 y)
Mignon et al, 1986[822]	125	32 (26)
Vogel et al, 1987[1110] †	20	5 (25)
Ellison et al, 1987[891]	60	10 (17)
Howard et al, 1990[748]	11	8 (73)
Delcore et al, 1989[1111]	43	12 (27)
Thompson et al, 1989[829]	5	5 (100)
Norton et al, 1992[745]	73	42 (58; 3 mo) 22 (30; 5 y)

* The total number of patients reported to have undergone exploratory laparotomy in each series.
† Series in which total gastrectomy was performed in most cases.

cured (see Fig. 41–16). The recurrence rate varied markedly for different groups of patients at different times, depending on where the primary tumor was found (see Fig. 41–16). The recurrence rate was significantly greater in patients with duodenal primaries.[745] Furthermore, 55% of duodenal tumors and only 25% of pancreatic tumors were associated with metastases, suggesting that duodenal primaries are much more malignant than previously believed.[503,755,894] The long-term survival in this study for all patients was excellent, with more than 90% surviving for all the nonmetastatic groups (Fig. 41–17).[745] Survival was similar for patients cured, patients resected but not cured, and patients in whom a small gastrinoma was not found. It might be concluded that surgery is not helpful because patients with no gastrinoma found or those cured had equal 5-year survival rates (see Fig. 41–17). It is known that if patients have a gastrinoma so small it cannot be found on a detailed exploratory laparotomy, they have an excellent prognosis.[766] Preliminary evidence suggests this group is not representative of patients with gastrinomas, including the patients who had gastrinomas found and resected. In preliminary long-term studies at the National Institutes of Health, a number of patients who did not undergo surgical resection developed metastatic disease to the liver. There is no way to predict which patients will develop metastatic disease. Therefore, all patients with sporadic gastrinoma (*i.e.,* ZES that is not associated with MEN-I) and with no serious contraindication to surgery should undergo localization studies (selective hepatic and pancreatic angiography, CT, MRI, ultrasound), preferably

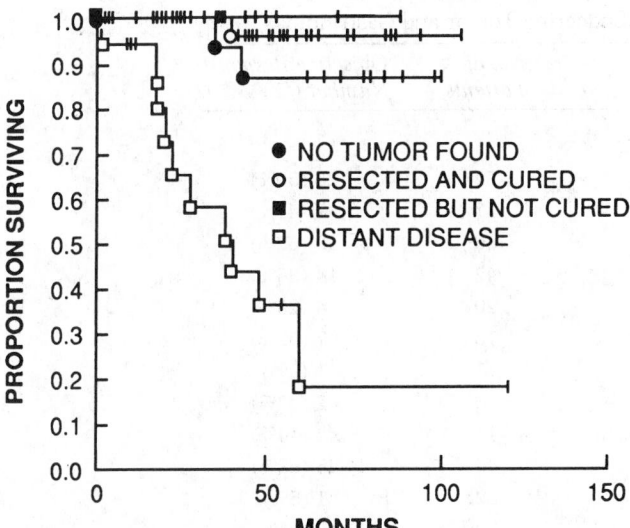

FIGURE 41–17. Survival of patients with Zollinger-Ellison syndrome from the day of diagnosis. Patients were divided into four groups based on preoperative evaluation, operative findings, and initial postoperative evaluation: (1) patients who had biopsy confirmation of bulky metastatic gastrinoma on initial evaluation (n = 18, open squares); (2) patients who had all tumor resected and were functionally disease-free (cured) at initial postoperative evaluation (n = 42, open circles); (3) patients who had all tumor resected but were functionally not disease-free (cured) (n = 15, closed squares); and (4) patients with no tumor found (closed circles). There were no significant differences seen among the three groups who did not have metastatic gastrinoma. However, the group with distant disease survived for a significantly shorter time than all other patient groups (p <0.001). (Modified from Norton JA, Doppman JL, Jensen RT. Curative resection in Zollinger-Ellison syndrome: results of a 10 year prospective study. Ann Surg 1992; 215:8)

in a center with considerable experience with these patients.[691,764,796,843] If no metastases are found, the patient should undergo surgical exploration (Fig. 41–15).

In our experience, the single most important factor in achieving good surgical results is the expertise of the surgeon. Even very experienced pancreatic surgeons have almost no experience with islet cell tumors and no appreciation of the difficulty in identifying the extrapancreatic gastrinomas or the technique of enucleating lesions within the pancreas. A gastrinoma found at laparotomy as a solitary lesion in the liver should be removed, provided the resection can be performed safely. If gastrinoma is found in the pancreatic head, it should be enucleated.[743,745,796,895] If unresectable gastrinoma is found in the pancreatic head area, a pancreaticoduodenectomy (Whipple's operation) is not indicated. No studies have demonstrated an increased survival overall in patients with ZES after pancreaticoduodenectomy. Furthermore, because of the marked morbidity and mortality associated with this operation (up to 37% in one study)[783,838] and the excellent long-term prognosis of these patients, it is not established that the adverse consequences of a pancreaticoduodenectomy might not outweigh the adverse consequences of an unresected solitary gastrinoma. If no gastrinoma is found at surgery, as occurs in 7% to 30% of cases overall but in 60% of cases in one series,[825] a blind distal pancreatectomy should not be performed, because 65% to 90% of gastrinomas are found in the

pancreatic head or duodenum (gastrinoma triangle[743,745,746,783] and because such an approach has not improved cure rates.[796] The use of IOUS to localize additional lesions and to confirm the significance of a palpated mass is recommended.[847–850] This allows identification of some masses as malignant and can help determine the extent of resection that may be needed.[850]

Special attention needs to be paid to finding duodenal gastrinomas. In a recent prospective study, gastrinomas were found in 64% of patients using the above described procedures, of which 11% were in the duodenum and 33% in the pancreas (see Table 41–27).[745] When transillumination of the duodenum at surgery[836] and a duodenotomy were used, gastrinomas were found in 92% of patients,[745] 43% in the pancreas and 30% in the duodenum (see Table 41–27). The increase was entirely due to the detection of additional duodenal gastrinomas, which frequently are small. A 3-cm duodenotomy is recommended along the antimesenteric aspect of the duodenum and entering on the second portion of the duodenum with the option to extend in either direction.[745] The duodenal wall should be palpated carefully, with the index finger inside the duodenum and the thumb on the outside, and the distal third and fourth parts of the duodenum examined by everting them into the incision. If no tumor is found at laparotomy, or if the gastrinoma is unresectable or metastatic to the liver and the patient had a high antisecretory drug requirement before surgery (>4.8 g/day cimetidine), a highly selective vagotomy may be considered (see Fig. 41–15).

The role of surgery in the treatment of patients with ZES with MEN-I is unclear (see Fig. 41–15).[712,719,783,896] Surgery is discussed later in this chapter in the section on pancreatic endocrine tumors in MEN-I.

Treatment of Metastatic Gastrinoma. Because patients with metastatic gastrinomas have a markedly decreased survival (Table 41–31 and Fig. 41–17) and because the malignant nature of the gastrinoma is becoming an increasingly important determinant of survival, there is an increasing need for effective treatment of metastatic gastrinoma and other metastatic pancreatic endocrine tumors. Chemotherapy, hepatic embolization, systematic removal of all resectable tumor, hormonal therapy with a somatostatin analog, and treatment with interferon (Table 41–33) have been advocated, but the role of each remains unclear.

Chemotherapy using streptozocin alone or in combination with 5-FU or 5-FU plus doxorubicin has been reported to be effective at reducing tumor size in 5% to 63% of patients with islet cell tumors (see Table 41–33). In one study, the combination of streptozocin plus 5-FU was more effective than streptozocin alone.[897] Dacarbazine and doxorubicin have given poor response rates alone (9–20%), and chlorozotocin has given about the same response rate (50%; see Table 41–33) as streptozocin alone. Almost all single studies that include significant numbers of patients and investigate the effects of chemotherapeutic agents on pancreatic endocrine tumors have been combined series that include all pancreatic endocrine tumors often compared with carcinoids. Whether these results can be extrapolated to include metastatic gastrinoma is not clear. Two studies have demonstrated no difference in response rates of various islet cell tumors to streptozocin;[897,898] however, there were only small numbers of patients with the

TABLE 41–33.   Drug Therapy of Pancreatic Endocrine Tumor and Gastrinomas

Investigations	Agent	No. of Patients	Objective Response Number (%)
All Pancreatic Endocrine Tumors			
Broder and Carter 1973[444]	STZ	52	26 (50%)
Kvols and Buck, 1987[1019]		17	7 (41%)
Buchanan et al, 1986[898]		16	10 (62%)
Moertel et al, 1980[897]		42	14 (36%)
Moertel et al, 1982[1112]	DOX	20	4 (20%)
Bukowski et al, 1983[1113]	CZT	13	7 (53%)
Manger et al, 1986[463]	DTIC	11	1 (9%)
Manger et al, 1986[463]	Tubercidin	6	2 (33%)
Moertel et al, 1991[1024]	Etoposide + cisplatin	14	2 (14%)
Moertel et al, 1982[897]	STZ + 5-FU	40	25 (63%)
Maton, 1989[905]		22	1 (5%)
Oberg and Erikson, 1989[489]		30	19 (68%)
Kelsen et al, 1982[689]	STZ + DOX	5	1 (20%)
Frame et al, 1988[1114]		14	3 (21%)
Bonfils et al, 1986[1115]	STZ or STZ + 5-FU	45	19 (42%)
Von Schrenk et al, 1988[899]	STZ + 5-FU + DOX	10	4 (40%)
Maton et al, 1989[903]	Octreotide	46	8 (17%)
Maton 1989[905]		66	8 (11%)
Erikson et al, 1986[909]	Interferon	22	6 (27%)
Gastrinomas Only			
Jensen et al, 1983[719]	STZ	24	12 (50%)
Moertel et al, 1980[897]			
NIH 1987 (unpub. data)	DTIC	5	0 (0%)
Moertel et al, 1980[897]	STZ + 5-FU	3	1 (33%)
Mignon et al, 1986[822]		10	8 (80%)
Hofman et al, 1973[742]		5	1 (20%)
Ruszniewski et al, 1989[900]		22	1 (5%)
Bonfils et al, 1986[1115]	STZ + 5-FU	28	(42%)
Bonfils et al, 1986[1115]	STZ	17	(42%)
Von Schrenk et al, 1988[899]	STZ + 5-FU + DOX	10	4 (40%)
Kvols et al, 1987[1116]	Octreotide	9	1 (11%)
Maton et al, 1989[903]		16	3 (19%)
Maton, 1989[905]		22	3 (14%)
Erikson et al, 1986[909]	Interferon	4	2 (50%)
Slimak et al, 1991[910]		9	3 (33%)

STZ, streptozotocin; DOX, doxorubicin; CZT, chlorozotocin; 5-FU, 5-fluorouracil; DTIC, dacarbazine.

different type of pancreatic endocrine tumor. Other studies have suggested differential responses of gastrinomas, glucagonomas, and VIPomas to chemotherapeutic agents such as dacarbazine or streptozocin. When results from a number of small series are combined, streptozocin alone appears to cause an objective response in 50% of patients with metastatic gastrinoma (see Table 41–33). Streptozocin combined with 5-FU or 5-FU plus doxorubicin causes an objective response in 5% to 80% of patients with metastatic gastrinoma (see Table 41–33). For all pancreatic endocrine tumors, the combination of streptozocin and 5-FU gave a response rate of 63%, which was significantly better than the 40% response rate with streptozocin alone.[897] In a prospective study of 10 patients

with metastatic gastrinoma to the liver that had increased in size over the 6 months before the patient entered the study, chemotherapy with streptozocin, 5-FU, and doxorubicin resulted in only a 40% objective response rate, no complete remissions, and no statistical difference in survival in responders versus nonresponders.[899] In another recent study of a similar group of 22 patients, only 5% of patients demonstrated an objective decrease in tumor size.[900] Therefore, the precise role and efficacy of chemotherapy in patients with metastatic gastrinoma has not been established, and it is not clear when chemotherapy should be considered in a given patient. Some patients have been followed for 20 years with stable metastatic disease,[759] whereas most die within 5 years, with a mean survival of 3 to 5 years.[720,722,762,799,826] Of the two groups with considerable experience with metastatic gastrinoma, one group proposed that patients be treated with chemotherapy when they become symptomatic.[897] If gastric acid hypersecretion is controlled adequately, symptoms due to the tumor will arise only late in the course of the disease. The other group proposed that after the initial evaluation patients be reassessed in 3 to 6 months and that those patients with evidence of increasing size of hepatic metastases should be treated with chemotherapy.[719,899] No studies have recommended chemotherapy in patients with metastases only to regional lymph nodes.

For tumors metastatic to the liver, hepatic arterial embolization has been recommended in patients with gastrinoma and other gastrointestinal endocrine tumors.[665,668,901,902] Only small numbers of gastrinomas have been treated by this technique and its effect on long-term survival is not known. Furthermore, distant metastases to bone recently have been reported to occur in 12% of all patients with hepatic metastases,[608] suggesting that procedures directed only at the disease in the liver, such as embolization, may be of limited value in many patients with extensive disease.

The data of Zollinger and colleagues suggest that removal of all resectable tumor or *debulking surgery* prolongs life expectancy.[720] There are no studies that have systematically evaluated debulking surgery. Norton and colleagues reported the successful resection of all metastatic disease in 5 of 20 patients with extensive disease, 2 of whom have maintained normal gastrin levels postoperatively.[826] Although debulking surgery requires systematic evaluation before it can be routinely recommended, these results raise the possibility that a small percentage of patients with extensive disease can be identified in whom removal of all resectable tumor may provide prolonged remission.

Hormonal therapy with octreotide is effective in controlling the symptoms of pancreatic endocrine or carcinoid-like tumors, including VIPomas, glucagonomas, GRFomas, insulinomas, gastrinomas, and carcinoids (see Table 41–33).[903-905] Octreotide has been reported to decrease the size of metastases or tumor growth of pancreatic endocrine tumors in animals[906] and humans.[905] Studies have reported a decrease in hepatic metastases in 3 patients of 22 with gastrinoma (see Table 41–33).[903,905,907,908] Another recent study of 9 patients with metastatic gastrinoma who were treated with octreotide for 1 to 11 months reported no effect.[904] Until controlled trials are done, treatment with octreotide cannot be recommended for routine use in patients with metastatic gastrinoma.

Human leukocyte interferon may be helpful in patients with metastatic pancreatic endocrine tumors including gastrinoma (see Table 41–33). In one study using interferon, 17 of 22 patients, most of whom had previously failed chemotherapy, demonstrated an objective response (defined as a decrease of more than 50% in tumor size or in tumor markers).[909] In a more recent study of 9 patients with metastatic gastrinoma to the liver that was increasing in size, interferon-α (5 million units/day) did not decrease tumor bulk but did slow tumor growth in 3 patients.[910] Because of the small numbers of cases and limited follow-up, it is unclear whether interferon can provide long-term benefit for patients with metastatic gastrinoma.

INSULINOMA

Insulin-secreting islet cell tumors encompass a broad range of diagnostic and therapeutic features. Insulinomas were first recognized by Whipple, who had seen 30 patients with hypoglycemia and pancreatic adenomas by 1935.[911] Whipple's triad, which consisted of the characteristic symptoms of hypoglycemia, blood sugars below 50 mg/dl, and immediate relief after ingestion of glucose, remained for many years the major diagnostic criteria for insulinoma.[911]

Insulinomas usually occur in patients between the ages of 20 and 75 years. The average age of presentation is between 44 and 46 years.[702,851,912,913] There is a preponderance of women in most series (60%),[702,851,914] and the reported incidence of insulinomas ranges from 0.8 to 0.9 persons per million population per year.[488,708] In these studies, the prevalence of insulinomas varied from twice as common as gastrinomas[708] to slightly less common than gastrinomas,[488] and insulinomas made up 27% of the pancreatic endocrine tumors in one series.[488]

Symptoms

The clinical symptoms of insulinomas are due to hypoglycemia in almost all instances. Most symptoms are neuroglycopenic, that is, provoked by insufficient availability to the CNS of glucose, which is the main source of energy to the brain.[482,914-917] The most common symptoms are visual disturbances (59%), confusion (51%), altered consciousness (38%), and weakness (32%). Seizures occur but are less common (23%).[482,914-917] Symptoms can occur due to catecholamine release (adrenergic symptoms)[482,915,916] such as sweating (43%) and tremulousness (23%). In one study of the initial presenting symptoms, 49% of patients had both neuroglycopenic symptoms and adrenergic symptoms, 38% had neuroglycopenic symptoms only, and 12% had adrenergic symptoms only.[915] Symptoms characteristically are associated with fasting, as when a meal is delayed or missed or with exercise.[482,851,914-916] There are numerous reports of erroneous psychiatric or neurologic diagnoses for patients with insulinomas.[918] These reports highlight the need for blood glucose measurements during any transient neuropsychiatric incident, particularly if it is recurrent. The duration of neuroglycopenic symptoms before diagnosis is usually longer than 3 years. Some patients present with a history of self-treatment by consuming frequent small meals.[919] Most patients with insulinomas are overweight and many are obese.

Diagnosis

Although there are useful clues to diagnosis of insulinoma, such as symptoms after a fast, symptoms often are nonspecific and the diagnosis can only be established by fasting with concomitant laboratory examination.[702,914,915] Investigation of patients with neuroglycopenic episodes begins with the documentation of hypoglycemia during these symptoms provoked by a fast. Organic hypoglycemia is usually defined as a blood sugar level of less than 40 mg/dl in the fasting state.[482,851,915] In healthy individuals, the blood glucose value usually does not decrease to less than 70 mg/dl after an overnight fast.[915]

In a study of patients with insulinomas, blood glucose levels after an overnight fast were less than 60 mg/dl in 53% of patients and less than 50 mg/dl in 39% of patients.[482] If this test is combined with measurement of plasma insulin levels, plasma insulin levels will be inappropriately elevated in 65% of people.[482,915] Because a single overnight fast, even when combined with a measurement of plasma insulin levels, does not establish the diagnosis of insulinoma in more than 55% of patients, a 72-hour fast usually is done with measurement of blood glucose and insulin levels at 2- to 4-hour intervals and more frequently if blood glucose levels decrease to less than 50 mg/dl.[851,914,915,917] If at any point the patient becomes symptomatic during the fast, plasma insulin and glucose values should be obtained before intravenous glucose is given and the test stopped. Within 24 hours of starting the fast, 75% of patients with an insulinoma have symptoms and a blood sugar level of less than 40 mg/dl. By 48 hours, 92% to 98% are hypoglycemic, and by 72 hours virtually all patients with insulinomas are hypoglycemic.[482,915,917,920] The test is considered positive for insulinoma if the plasma insulin to glucose ratio is greater than 0.3.[851] In some normal obese subjects, the fasting plasma insulin to glucose ratio may be elevated because hyperinsulinemia due to insulin resistance mimics the pattern in insulinoma.[915] In these patients, the fasting glucose is normal, and even with prolonged fasting blood glucose levels do not decrease to less than 55 mg/dl; therefore, during fasting they can be easily differentiated.[915]

The presence of hypoglycemia or an elevated fasting blood insulin to blood glucose ratio during fasting is consistent with but may not be caused by insulinoma. Other conditions can cause a similar result, including organic hyperinsulinism due to pancreatic islet diseases, factitious use of insulin or hypoglycemic agents, or autoantibodies against the insulin receptor or insulin.[851,920–922] To differentiate insulinoma from these other conditions, additional tests are required, including plasma determinations of proinsulin, C peptide, antibodies to insulin, and plasma sulfonylurea levels.[482,851,922] Plasma proinsulin levels are elevated in 80% to 90% of patients with insulinoma to more than 22% of the plasma insulin level.[851,915,922] In patients with surreptitious use of insulin or oral hypoglycemic agents, the proinsulin level is normal or decreased.[922] The measurement of C peptide has proved useful in differentiating organic hypersecretion of insulin such as in patients with insulinoma from patients surreptitiously using insulin, because commercial insulin preparations contain no C peptide.[922] In insulinoma, the characteristic finding is an elevated or normal C peptide plasma concentration,[922] whereas in patients surreptitiously using insulin the plasma insulin level is high and the C peptide level low.[920,922] The C peptide level does not differentiate patients surreptitiously taking oral hypoglycemic agents from patients with insulinomas in that both have low blood sugars and elevated levels of insulin and C peptide,[702,920,922] but most oral hypoglycemia drugs do produce elevated plasma levels of sulfonylurea.

Pathology

As with other APUDomas, malignancy is only defined by the presence of metastases at the time of surgery or metastases documented by other investigations.[923] Insulinomas are the opposite of gastrinomas in that 60% to 90% of gastrinomas

are malignant but only 5% to 16% of insulinomas are malignant.[482,851,915,916] The pattern of metastatic spread of insulinomas is local invasion followed by spread to peripancreatic and portal nodes and then to the liver. Most insulinomas are found to be solitary benign pancreatic nodules, often encapsulated; only 2% to 10% of patients have multiple tumors.[482,920] In patients with multiple insulinomas, MEN-I should be suspected.[513] Insulinomas are uniformly distributed throughout the entire pancreas, and most are smaller than 1.5 cm in diameter.[482,915,916]

Localization

After a firm diagnosis of insulinoma is established, an attempt should be made to localize the tumor (Table 41–34 and Fig. 41–18). Radiographic investigations are concentrated on the pancreas because most insulinomas (unlike gastrinomas) are within the pancreas.[851,915,924] Preoperative localization is essential because insulinomas frequently are small (90% are less than 2 cm in diameter) and unnecessary surgery may be prevented if metastatic spread is present. CT scanning local-

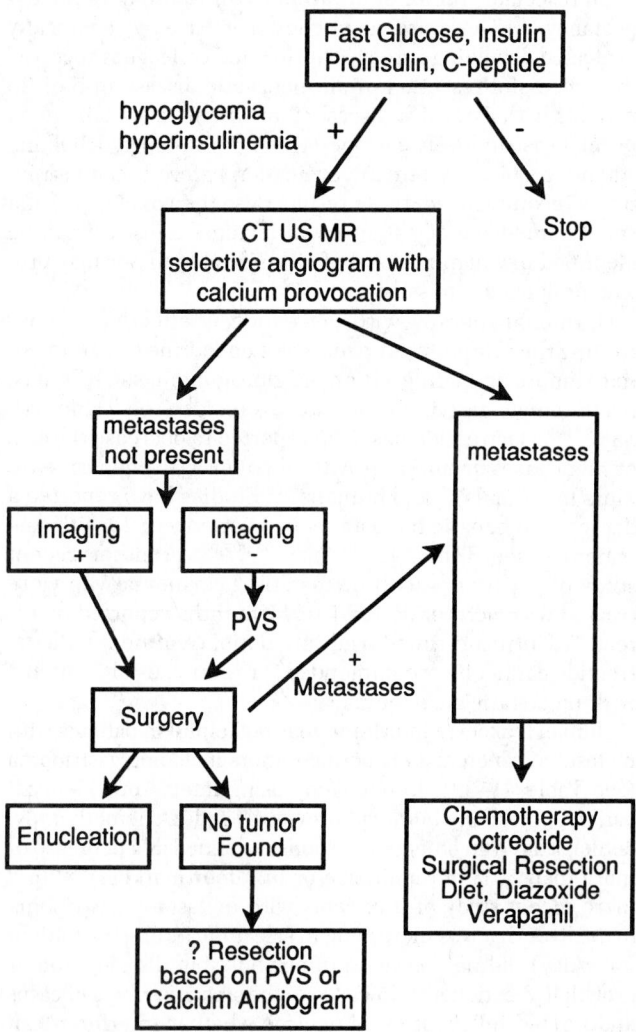

FIGURE 41–18. Flow diagram for the evaluation and management of patients with hypoglycemia.

TABLE 41–34. Localization Procedures for Insulinoma

Procedure	Successful Localization Mean (Range)	References
Ultrasound	33% (0–66%)	482, 927, 928, 1117
CT scan	35% (11–50%)	482, 927, 928, 1117
Dynamic CT scan	66%	925
Selective arteriography	63% (17–100%)	482, 927, 928, 1117
All imaging studies	80% (50–90%)	482, 927
Transhepatic portal venous sampling	92% (89–96%)	844, 926, 927, 929, 1117–1119
Operative ultrasound	83–90%	844, 850, 930

izes 35% of cases. Dynamic CT scanning is reported to be more sensitive, localizing 66% of insulinomas.[925] Selective arteriography localizes the greatest proportion of insulinomas (see Table 41–34). An average of 40% of patients do not have insulinomas localized by these imaging procedures (see Table 41–34).[482,844,926–928] Most large series report an even distribution of insulinomas within the pancreas,[915,924,928] so that a blind distal pancreatectomy has only a one in three chance of finding tumor. Therefore, additional localization procedures may be needed in some patients. PVS for insulin can localize an insulinoma to the exact region of the pancreas (head, body,

or tail) in nearly all patients (see Table 41–34). A typical result localizing tumor in the pancreatic tail is shown in Figure 41–19. Four groups have reported successful localizations by PVS in the subgroup of patients not visualized by angiography, identifying 10 of 10 in one series and 6 of 7 in another.[844,851,926,928,929] In a recent study of 12 patients with insulinomas with negative imaging studies, selective venous sampling correctly localized the tumor in 75% of cases.[844] In another recent study of 35 patients with insulinoma in whom imaging studies localized the tumors in 46%, PVS localized the tumor in 100%.[926] Because PVS only localizes tumors to

PORTAL VENOUS INSULIN SAMPLING

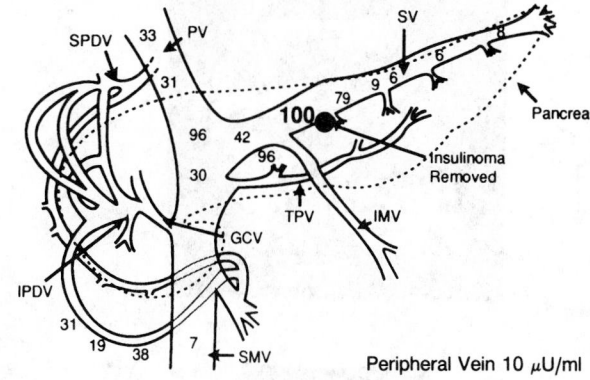

FIGURE 41–19. Selective venous sampling for insulin from portal venous tributaries (**A**) and a selective intraarterial calcium provocative test in a patient with insulinoma (**B**). (**A**) Numbers are the plasma insulin concentrations at different locations. The simultaneous peripheral value was 10 μU/ml. A significant gradient of 900% (increase to 100 μU/ml) is seen in the proximal splenic vein. The closed circle indicates the location of a 1-cm insulioma found at surgery. (**B**) Results of calcium (0.01–0.25 mEq/kg) injected into the splenic, gastroduodenal hepatic, and superior mesenteric arteries (SMA) and of venous blood obtained from the hepatic veins. A rapid increase in plasma insulin levels was seen with injection of the splenic artery, which supplies the area where the tumor was found.

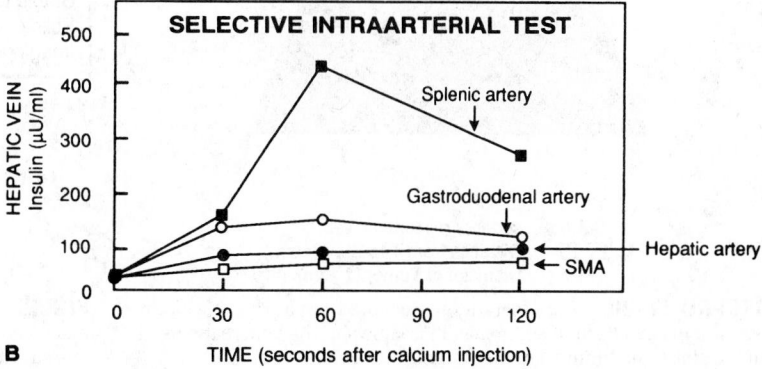

a general area of the pancreas and insulinomas may be so small that they cannot be localized by palpation at surgery within this area, IOUS has been useful in localizing insulinomas.[844,848,850,930] A typical IOUS result is shown in Figure 41–20, in which a 1.1-cm insulinoma is localized in the pancreatic head area. In one recent study of 12 patients with negative imaging studies of which 75% had a PVS gradient localizing the insulinoma to the appropriate pancreatic area, insulinomas could be localized by palpation at surgery in only 41%.[844] IOUS identified insulinomas in 5 additional patients and was the single best modality in locating the insulinoma at surgery.[844]

A new study that may be helpful in the future and may replace selective sampling for insulin from portal venous tributaries is the use of selective intraarterial injection of calcium with hepatic venous insulin sampling.[927] Small amounts of calcium (0.01–0.25 mEq Ca^{2+}/kg) are infused directly into the branches of the celiac plexus (gastroduodenal, splenic, hepatic) and superior mesenteric artery, and simultaneous blood samples are taken from the right and left hepatic artery for measurement of plasma insulin concentrations (see Fig. 41–19B). In all 4 patients, insulin increased in one of the hepatic veins after the calcium injection into one of the arteries, correctly localizing the insulinoma.[927] A typical result is shown in Figure 41–19 and compared with the PVS. In this patient, PVS demonstrated a positive gradient (900% increase; Fig. 41–19A) in the proximal pancreatic tail, and intraarterial calcium into the splenic artery demonstrated an increase in plasma insulin (Fig. 41–19B). A 1-cm insulinoma was resected from the proximal pancreatic tail. If the usefulness of this test is confirmed, it will likely obviate the need for PVS because it can be done in most centers and requires less expertise.

Many pancreatic endocrine tumors possess somatostatin receptors,[604–606,850,931] and radiolabeled somatostatin is reported to localize some tumors not localized by other modalities. The experience with this technique in patients with insulinomas is limited, with too few patients with insulinoma studied to determine whether this technique will localize tumors not found by any other modalities.

In our experience, more than 70% of insulinomas are visualized by arteriography, and 75% of the unidentified lesions are localized by PVS.[844,851] If all preoperative localization studies are negative, the patient should undergo surgical exploration by a group with experience in the use of IOUS (Fig. 41–21). Previously, the decision for surgical exploration patients with negative localization studies rested on whether the patient's symptoms could be effectively controlled medically.[932] The recent results with IOUS in these patients indicate that the insulinoma can be found and resected successfully at surgery.

Surgery

All insulinomas without evidence of metastases should be surgically removed, regardless of the severity of symptoms. Of

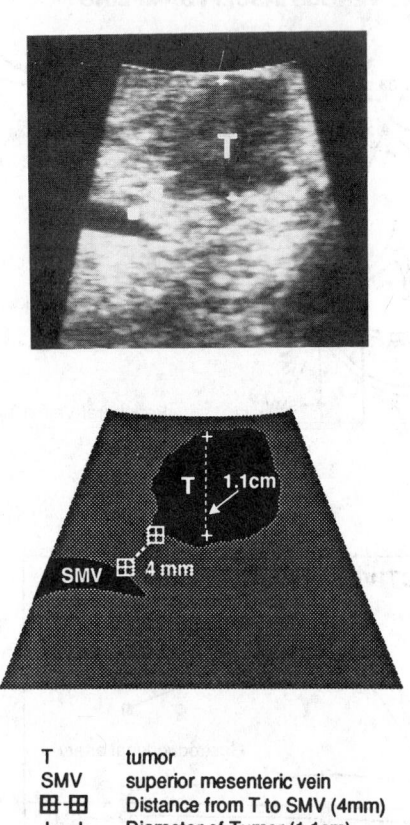

T	tumor
SMV	superior mesenteric vein
⊞-⊞	Distance from T to SMV (4mm)
+--+	Diameter of Tumor (1.1cm)

FIGURE 41–20. Intraoperative ultrasound from a patient with an insulinoma. A 1.1-cm insulinoma (T) is shown in the pancreatic head at a distance of 4 mm from the superior mesenteric vein (SMV).

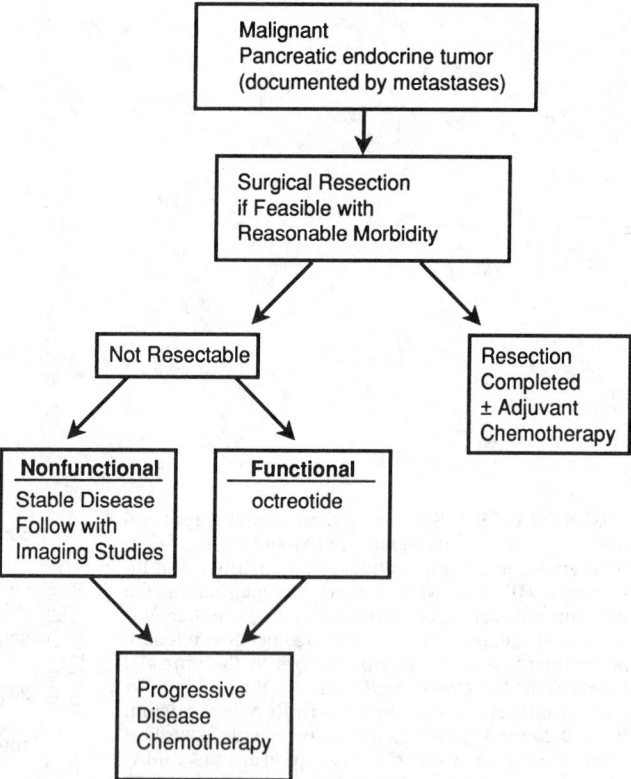

FIGURE 41–21. Flow diagram for management of patients with malignant pancreatic endocrine tumors. Chemotherapy may be required with progressive disease.

all insulinomas, 80% are benign isolated lesions whose surgical removal is curative.[915,921] The liver always must be explored for evidence of metastatic disease and the entire abdomen explored to rule out rare extrapancreatic tumors. The entire pancreas must be explored for other tumors, because multifocal tumors occur in at least 10% of patients.[844,851] Isolated lesions of the tail may be enucleated or removed en bloc by distal pancreatectomy. Body and head lesions require enucleation with careful dissection to avoid damage to the main pancreatic duct and its attendant morbidity. Division of the peritoneum lateral to the duodenum (Kocher's maneuver) is necessary to palpate the pancreatic head, and division of the peritoneum along the inferior border of the pancreas is required to palpate the body and the tail adequately. Distal pancreatectomy usually requires concomitant splenectomy. Pneumococcal vaccine (Pneumovax) should be administered preoperatively to lower the risk of catastrophic postsplenectomy sepsis.

Anecdotal reports of hypoglycemia during manipulation of the pancreas have focused attention on glucose monitoring during surgery. Use of the artificial pancreas (Biostator) has documented an increased glucose requirement during removal of insulinomas.[851] A number of centers have used the artificial pancreas or frequent glucose measurements to monitor patients for hypoglycemia and to document successful removal of the tumor by noting a *rebound hyperglycemia* or sudden decreased glucose requirement. A large retrospective study at the Mayo Clinic showed that the rebound hyperglycemia did not occur in 23% of patients who had successful extirpation of insulinoma.[933] This technique may be of more limited use in aiding the localization of insulinomas occult to preoperative studies. Kudlow and colleagues showed sensitive detection of an unlocalized tumor using a noncrushing clamp to isolate regions of the pancreas from the circulation while monitoring blood glucose with an artificial pancreas programmed to amplify small increases in blood glucose concentrations.[934] We do not use intraoperative monitoring of insulin or glucose to guide tumor localization or removal.

Even in cases of documented metastatic disease, refractory debilitating symptoms may be an indication for debulking the pancreatic lesion. Metastases are not always secretory. Removal of peripancreatic lymph nodes may be curative for malignant insulinoma if no liver metastases are present.[851,914]

Medical Therapy

The simplest form of nonsurgical treatment for insulinoma is dietary management.[851,915] Many insulinoma patients begin frequent small meals to alleviate symptoms before seeking medical evaluation, and a significant percentage report weight gain in the year before diagnosis. Slowly absorbed oral nutrients such as cornstarch, bread, potatoes, and rice are recommended.[851,926] In unusually severe cases, intravenous glucose may be required to prevent neuroglycopenic attacks. Hypertonic solutions, such as 10% dextrose, should be avoided because of electrolyte imbalances generated by combining high levels of glucose and hyperinsulinemia simultaneously. During a hypoglycemia episode, rapidly absorbable forms of carbohydrates such as fruit juice with glucose or sucrose are preferable.

A number of drugs have been reported to control the hyperinsulinemia. Diazoxide, a benzothiazide analog, directly inhibits insulin release from β cells through stimulation of α-adrenergic receptors. It has an extrapancreatic, hyperglycemic effect, possibly by inhibiting cyclic AMP phosphodiesterase, which enhances glycogenolysis.[915,920] The major side effects of diazoxide are sodium retention, gastrointestinal symptoms such as nausea, and occasional hirsutism.[851,915,920] Edema can result from the sodium retention and the addition of a diuretic such as trichlormethiazide, a benzothiadiazine derivative, can correct the edema and augment the hyperglycemia effect.[702,851,915,920] Diazoxide should be initiated with 150 to 200 mg given in two to three divided doses a day and, if not effective, increased to a maximum of 600 to 800 mg/day.[851,920] About 60% of patients respond to the diazoxide.[851,914] The calcium-channel inhibitor verapamil has been used alone and in combination with other drugs to help control hypoglycemia in a small number of patients,[935-937] as has propanolol.[915,938] Phenytoin (Dilantin) inhibits the release of insulin from β cells and has been used successfully to treat a small number of patients with refractory hypoglycemia.[915,939] Maintenance doses of 300 to 600 mg/day are used, and only in less than 33% of patients is the hypoglycemia effect of phenytoin of any clinical significance.[915] Glucocorticoids (prednisone, 1 mg/kg) and glucagon either alone or with diazoxide have been used in a few patients.[915]

The most promising results are with octreotide, which has been reported to control symptoms and hypoglycemia in 40% to 60% of patients.[903,905,940-942] Octreotide generally is well tolerated and usually is given in starting doses of 50 μg two or three times daily, which can be increased to 1500 μg/day.[905] The main side effects are gastrointestinal (*e.g.*, bloating and abdominal cramping), and long-term side effects include malabsorption and cholelithiasis.[713,905,940-942] Besides improving symptoms, octreotide decreases plasma insulin levels in 65% of patients.[905] Most patients were treated for less than 1 week before surgery, so that the long-term efficacy is not known in a significant number of patients.

Malignant Insulinoma

The documentation of metastatic disease, either at the time of surgery or by imaging studies, is the only accurate means of diagnosing malignant insulinoma. Unlike all other islet cell tumors, malignant insulinomas are uncommon, occurring in only 10% to 15% of cases (see Table 41-24). Malignant primary insulinomas usually are not occult and have a mean size of 6 cm, which is more than twice the mean size of benign insulinomas.[702,914,915,923] The median disease-free survival after curative resection of malignant insulinomas was 5 years in one recent series.[923] The recurrence rate was 63%, with the median interval to recurrence 2.8 years. The median survival with recurrent tumor was 19 months. Palliative re-resection was associated with a median survival of 4 years, and biopsy only with a survival of 11 months.[923] Surgical resection of primary and metastatic insulinomas is preferred when possible (see Fig. 41-21).[923] Malignant insulinomas, like other pancreatic endocrine tumors, may respond to chemotherapy and treatment with octreotide.[905,940-942] The use of these agents for all malignant pancreatic endocrine neoplasms is described at the end of this section (see Chemotherapy).

NONFUNCTIONAL PANCREATIC ENDOCRINE TUMORS AND PPOMAS

Nonfunctional pancreatic endocrine tumors and PPomas present in the fourth and fifth decade of life.[943–945] PPomas release the hormone PP.[702,944,945] Nonfunctioning pancreatic endocrine tumors are not associated with elevated plasma levels of any peptide.[520,943] Because no active hormone is secreted by these tumors, symptoms arise from mechanical or mass effects of the neoplasm; therefore, they present late and the tumors are usually large and locally invasive at diagnosis. In one series, 72% were greater than 5 cm in diameter.[943]

These tumors usually are solitary except in patients with MEN-I, in whom multiple microadenomata can be seen.[711,770] The tumors are distributed throughout the pancreas with a ratio of 14:2:3 for pancreatic head:body:tail in one study.[943] The malignancy rate varied from 64% to 92% in different series (see Table 41–24).[488,711,943–945] Histologically, PPomas and nonfunctioning tumors are similar and cannot be differentiated from other pancreatic endocrine tumors even by immunocytochemistry. Nonfunctioning tumors are only differentiated from PPomas by the detection of an elevated level of plasma PP.[702] Increasingly, what in the past were thought to be nonfunctioning pancreatic endocrine tumors are found to have elevated plasma PP levels.[945] In one study of those pancreatic endocrine tumors not associated with any clinical syndrome and classified as nonfunctioning in the past, 50% to 75% were PPomas.[944] That elevated plasma PP levels are specific for endocrine pancreatic tumors is suggested by a study of 53 patients with adenocarcinoma of the pancreas, in which no patient had an elevated plasma PP level.[944] There are no data to suggest that nonfunctioning pancreatic endocrine tumors and PPomas differ in biologic behavior or presentation.[702] Immunocytochemically, nonfunctioning tumors and PPomas can contain numerous other gastrointestinal peptides. In one series of 30 nonfunctioning tumors, 50% had insulin-like immunoreactivity, 30% had glucagon immunoreactivity, 43% had PP immunoreactivity, 13% had somatostatin immunoreactivity, and only 13% produced none of these peptides.[770]

Infusions of PP into animals and humans have shown this peptide to have numerous biologic effects including the following: a net secretory effect on water and electrolytes in the small intestine; inhibitory effects of fluid, electrolyte, and enzyme secretion by the pancreas; effects on esophageal, gastric, intestinal, and gallbladder motility; and metabolic effects such as decreasing somatostatin or insulin release.[946] Patients with PPomas have been reported to have symptoms that were attributed to elevated plasma levels of PP,[944] although most patients have no such symptoms.[702,947] In one study, 36% of patients presented with abdominal pain and 28% with jaundice.[948] In 16% of patients, the tumors were found incidentally at surgery, and the remaining patients had a variety of symptoms due to the tumor mass. In this series, no patient was diagnosed preoperatively. In the future, it is likely that the histologic diagnosis will be established by cytologic analysis after fine-needle aspiration. This technique has been used extensively to diagnose pancreatic cancer and increasingly is being used to diagnose pancreatic endocrine tumors.[949–952] In a recent study of 10 patients with pancreatic endocrine tumors using fine-needle aspiration combined with immunocyto-

chemical analysis, cytologic studies showed the typical pattern of monotonous cytologic features with few mitoses.[949] Positive staining for chromogranin was seen in 5 patients, with a 78% concordance between cytochemical studies and final histology studies.

Elevated plasma levels of PP do not establish the diagnosis of a PPoma, even when a pancreatic mass is present. Plasma PP levels are reported to be elevated in 22% to 71% of patients with functional pancreatic endocrine tumors and nonpancreatic carcinoid tumors.[702,776,945,947] Furthermore, elevated plasma levels of PP can occur in other situations such as old age, bowel resection, alcohol abuse, infection, chronic noninfective inflammatory disorders, acute diarrhea, chronic renal failure, diabetes, chronic relapsing pancreatitis, hypoglycemia, or even after eating.[947] Therefore, an elevated plasma level of PP is not diagnostic of a PPoma. To increase the specificity of an elevated plasma level for a pancreatic tumor, an atropine suppression test has been proposed.[776,953] In one study of 48 patients with elevated plasma PP levels, atropine (1 mg intramuscularly) did not suppress the levels in any of the 18 patients with pancreatic endocrine tumors but did suppress the level by 50% in all patients without tumors.[776] Others have proposed a secretin provocative test.[947] A response of more than a 5000 pg/ml/minute increase is more than two standard deviations greater than seen in normal subjects. The usefulness of the atropine suppression or secretin provocative test for PP has not been investigated extensively and cannot be recommended as a routine procedure.[520]

The treatment of these tumors is surgical if possible. In more than 60% of patients, metastases are present at the time of diagnosis. Of 25 patients in one series, a Whipple procedure was done in 20%, a partial or total pancreatectomy in 25%, and a tumor excision in 10%.[948] The remaining patients had a biopsy only. The survival rates were 60% at 3 years and 44% at 5 years in this series. The cure rate of these tumors is low because of their late recognition.

LESS FREQUENT PANCREATIC ENDOCRINE TUMORS

Other pancreatic endocrine tumors occur less frequently and include VIPomas, glucagonomas, ACTHomas, somatostatinomas, and GRFomas (see Table 41–24). Each of these pancreatic endocrine tumors is usually malignant.

VIPomas

The VIPoma syndrome was first described by Verner and Morrison in 1958 and is commonly called the Verner-Morrison syndrome (see Table 41–24).[954] Because of the resemblance of the diarrheal fluid to that seen in patients with cholera, the term pancreatic cholera was proposed in 1967[955] and the acronym WDHA (watery diarrhea, hypokalemic, and achlorhydric) proposed in 1967.[954,956,957]

In adults, more than 80% to 90% of VIPomas are pancreatic in location,[958,959] with rare cases caused by VIP-producing intestinal carcinoids or pheochromocytomas.[959] VIPomas are usually large solitary tumors.[711,958,959] In one series, only 2% of tumors were multiple.[959] Seventy-five percent were reported in the pancreatic tail in one review.[941] In various series,

37% to 68% of the VIPomas have metastases at the time of diagnosis or surgery.[944,956,958-960] In one detailed pathology study, 61% of VIPomas were identified as malignant by the occurrence of metastases.[958] Characteristically in children younger than 10 years and rarely in adults (5% of cases), the VIPoma syndrome is due to a ganglioneuroma or ganglioneuroblastoma.[959] In one series, 16% of all cases were due to this tumor.[959] These tumors are extrapancreatic and are less often malignant than pancreatic VIPomas, being malignant in only 10% of cases.[959]

By immunocytochemistry, VIP was detected in 86%[958] and 57%[770] of VIPomas. Using immunocytochemical studies, 34% to 38% of VIPomas possess PP, 19% glucagon, 10% somatostatin, 5% insulin, and none gastrin.[770,958] VIPomas elaborate the peptide histidine methionine (PHM-27), a 27 amino acid peptide that shares with VIP a common precursor peptide (prepro VIP/PHM-27), and PHM-27-like immunoreactivity has been found in the plasma and tumors of patients with VIPomas.[702,957,961] On conventional microscopy, VIPomas show the typical microscopic features of endocrine tumors.[958] Mitoses were uncommon, seen in only 12%.[958] On electron microscopy, a mixture of cells were seen, usually in the same tumor.[958] The secretory granules were small (120–180 nm) and resembled those of the so-called D cells of normal gut.[958] The histologic and electron microscopic studies do not allow VIPomas to be differentiated clearly from some other pancreatic endocrine tumors; however, the presence of immunoreactive VIP is strongly suggestive for VIPoma because it is found uncommonly in other pancreatic endocrine tumors (10 of 104 pancreatic endocrine tumors in one study).[946,958]

The pathophysiology of the VIPoma syndrome is clear in that VIP is the major mediator.[958,962] For a number of years there was considerable controversy about the mediator.[962,963] In early studies, levels of substances other than VIP were reported to be elevated in the plasma of patients.[702,957,962] In early studies, plasma VIP infusions in humans did not produce the syndrome.[702,962,963] Plasma levels of VIP are consistently elevated in patients with the VIPoma syndrome.[702,957,959,962] A continuous infusion of VIP for 10 hours in normal human subjects to achieve plasma levels similar to that seen in patients with the VIPoma syndrome produced watery diarrhea in 6 to 7 hours.[964] The ability of VIP to produce diarrhea is consistent with its known actions in the intestine.[965] Receptors for VIP have been identified on intestinal epithelial cells. VIP stimulates intestinal electrolyte and fluid secretion in animals, stimulates chloride secretion with increased short circuit current, and activates adenylate cyclase and cyclic AMP in intestinal cells, which leads to intestinal secretion.[965] PHM-27-like immunoreactivity was found in 92% of VIPomas.[961] PHM was 32-fold less potent than VIP at causing intestinal secretion.[702,966] Because VIP is always present, it is likely to be the important peptide in most cases.

In two large series, the mean age for adults at the time of diagnosis was 49 and 50 years, with a range of 32 to 81 years.[959,967] There was a slight female predominance. The mean age in children was 4 years[959] and 2 years[967] in these studies, with a range from 10 months to 9 years.

The principal features of the VIPoma syndrome are the presence of severe, secretory diarrhea (100%) associated with hypokalemia (100%) and dehydration (100%).[702,957,959,967] The diarrhea is large volume with all patients with VIPomas, having

more than 1 L in a number of studies and in most more than 3 L/day.[959,962] A volume of less than 700 g/day has been proposed to rule out the diagnosis of VIPoma.[962] The diarrhea fluid is described as having the appearance of weak tea and persisting during fasting.[955,962] Although abdominal cramping pain and colic were reported to be absent in earlier studies, more recent studies report these characteristics in 63% of patients.[959,968] Gross steatorrhea usually is not present, and in one study none of 52 patients with VIPomas had 24-hour fecal fat of more than 15 g/day.[959] Weight loss is almost universally present.[959] Flushing is reported in 21% of patients, is usually present in the head or trunk area, and is characteristically erythematous.[957] The clinical laboratory studies invariably demonstrate hypokalemia (100%) and, to a lesser degree, hypercalcemia (41%), hypochlorhydria (70%), and hyperglycemia (18%).[702,957,959,967] The hypokalemia is often severe, being less than 2.5 mmol/L. At some time, 93% of patients will have serum levels of potassium less than 3 mmol/L (normal 3.5-5 mmol/L).[959] The hyperglycemia is mild.[959]

The diagnosis of a VIPoma requires the demonstration of an elevated plasma concentration of VIP and the establishment of the presence of a large volume secretory diarrhea. The possibility that VIPoma is responsible for the secretory diarrhea is strongly suggested by the volume of the diarrhea.[702,956,957] In 80% to 85% of patients, the diarrhea volume is more than 3 L/day and never less than 700 ml/day.[959,962] Many possible causes for the diarrhea can be excluded by fasting the patient, because in patients with VIPomas the diarrhea persists during fasting.[702,957,962] The diarrheal fluid should be characteristic of a secretory diarrhea,[962] in which the stool electrolytes can account for all the stool water osmolality ([sodium+potassium]×2=measured osmolality]).[962] Other diseases can give a chronic secretory diarrhea with large volume and be confused with a possible VIPoma; one such syndrome is called the pseudoVIPoma syndrome.[962] Other causes include ZES[712,962] and chronic laxative abuse.[969] In some cases, the secretory diarrhea is of unknown origin.[969–971] The diagnosis of ZES can be excluded by measuring fasting serum gastrin and gastric acid secretory rate.[712,764]

To differentiate VIPomas from these other conditions, a reliable measurement of plasma VIP concentrations is required. The fasting plasma VIP level ranges in most laboratories is 0 to 170 pg/ml.[959,962,967] In one study of patients with VIPomas, the mean value was 965 pg/ml, with the lowest value at 225 pg/ml (normal less than 170 pg/ml).[967] In another large study, the mean value in patients with VIPomas was 675 pg/ml, with the highest normal value (being 53 pg/ml) seen in normal patients and the lowest value seen in a VIPoma patient was 160 pg/ml.[959] Originally, plasma VIP levels were not found to increase in some patients with VIPomas or were increased in patients without VIPomas, including patients with laxative abuse. In most recent studies, this is not the case if a reliable assay is used.[702,957,959,962]

The first objective in these patients even before considering the diagnosis is the replenishment of fluid and electrolyte losses to correct the profound hypokalemia, dehydration, and acidosis that is usually present. The patients may require 5 L/day or more of fluid[957] and more than 350 mEq/day of potassium.[957,972] In the past, numerous drugs have been used in small numbers of VIPoma patients to control, to varying degrees, the diarrheal output. These drugs include prednisone

(60 to 100 mg/day), clonidine, indomethacin, phenothiazines, lithium carbonate, propranolol, metoclopramide, loperamide, lidamidine, angiotensin II, and norepinephrine.[702,957,967] Octreotide provides short-term and long-term control of the diarrhea in 87% of patients with VIPoma and is the agent of choice.[903,905,940–942,957] In two recent reviews of 20 and 25 patients with VIPomas treated with octreotide, the drug completely abolished diarrhea in 10% of patients in one study and in 65% in the other; diarrhea improved in 90% of patients in one study and in 95% in the other.[903,905,941] In one study, octreotide continued to be effective for all patients (n=13) at 6 months.[941] Some patients have short-lived responses or may respond initially to a low dose (50–100 μg three times daily) but subsequently require a larger dose to control the diarrhea, and some symptoms may become refractory even with doses up to 1200 μg/day.[905] In a small number of nonresponsive patients or patients whose symptoms recur, the administration of glucocorticoids concomitant with octreotide has proved effective.[905] With octreotide, plasma VIP concentrations decreased in 80% to 88% of patients.[905,941]

After imaging studies to localize the primary VIPoma and determine the extent of the tumor, possible surgical cure should be considered for all patients without metastatic disease. In one series, surgical resection of a pancreatic VIPoma relieved all symptoms in 17 patients (33% of patients).[959] In another series, 30% were cured.[960] Surgical removal with complete control of all symptoms was possible in 78% of all patients with VIP-producing ganglioneuroblastomas.[959]

Glucagonoma

In 1974, Mallinson and colleagues established the association of a cutaneous rash with glucagon-producing tumors of the pancreas when they reported 9 patients with the full clinical syndrome and a glucagon-releasing tumor of the pancreas.[973] The disease was described earlier by others, but the association with elevated plasma levels of glucagon had not been established.[702,914] In 1942, the association of a pancreatic tumor with a skin rash was first described.[974] In 1966, McGavran and colleagues reported a patient with an elevated fasting glucagon level, dermatitis, diabetes, and a pancreatic endocrine tumor.[975] Wilkinson and associates in 1973 described the rash associated with endocrine tumor as necrolytic migratory erythema.[976]

Most glucagonomas are large at the time of diagnosis, with the average size between 5 and 10 cm and a range from 0.4 to 35 cm.[977] Fifty percent of glucagonomas occurred in the tail in one study[978] and 80% in another study,[979] whereas in the largest study 22% were in the head, 14% in the body, and 51% in the pancreatic tail.[977] Between 50% and 80% had evidence of metastatic spread or invasion establishing malignancy.[977–979] The most common site of metastatic spread was to the liver (43% to 82%), with metastasis to lymph nodes, bone, and mesentery less common. In most cases, glucagonomas are within the pancreas; however, a glucagonoma associated with the typical clinical syndrome was found in the proximal duodenum.[979] Glucagonomas usually occur as a single tumor, although in one series multiple tumors or diffuse involvement by a single mass were found in 10% of patients.[979]

The pathophysiology of the glucagonoma syndrome is related to the known actions of glucagon.[980] Glucagon stimulates glycogenolysis, gluconeogenesis, ketogenesis, lipolysis, and insulin secretion. Glucagon affects gut secretion, inhibits pancreatic and gastric secretion, inhibits gut motility, and increases heart rate and force of contraction. Hyperglycemia in the glucagonoma syndrome results from the increased hepatic glycogenolysis and glyconeogenesis. The weight loss has been attributed to the known catabolic effects of glucagon.[974] It is not clearly established that the skin rash is due to the hyperglucagonemia per se, because numerous patients have been given large doses of glucagon over extended periods and the skin rash did not develop.[702,974] The glucagon-induced hypoaminoacidemia that develops in 80% to 90% of patients[977–979] may be involved in causing the skin rash, because correction of the hypoaminoacidemia has been shown to correct the dermatitis without changing plasma glucagon concentrations in some patients.[702,822,974,981] The similarity of the lesions to those seen in patients with zinc deficiencies have resulted in trials of zinc in some patients with some responses.[974]

Immunocytochemical and histologic studies of glucagonomas show results typical of pancreatic endocrine tumors. Glucagon is one of the most frequently seen peptides in immunocytochemical studies of pancreatic endocrine tumors, although in many cases it is not associated with any syndrome. In one series of 1366 autopsy cases, a 0.8% frequency of adenomas was reported, and all contained glucagon-producing cells.[711,770,974] The morphology of most glucagon-producing tumors demonstrate no general features that distinguish them from other pancreatic endocrine tumors.[702,770,974,979]

Glucagonomas usually occur in middle to late age with only 16% occurring in persons younger than 40 years and most occurring in persons between 50 and 70 years.[977–979] The typical dermatitis, called necrolytic migratory erythema, occurs in 64% to 90% of patients. Diabetes mellitus or glucose intolerance occurs in 83% to 90% of patients, weight loss in 56% to 90%, diarrhea in 14% to 15%, abdominal pain in 12%, thromboembolic disease with venous thrombosis in 24%, pulmonary emboli in 11%, and psychiatric disturbances in a few patients.[520,974,977–979] Laboratory abnormalities include anemia in 44% to 85% of patients, hypoaminoacidemia in 26% to 100%, hypocholesterolemia in 80%, and renal glycosuria.[520,974,977,978]

The presence of cutaneous lesions often precedes the diagnosis of the syndrome for long periods, with a mean of 6 to 8 years in one study and a maximum of 18 years.[977] The skin lesions may wax and wane, and because of their variable nature have been misdiagnosed in various studies as pemphigus foliaceus, pemphigoid, vasculitis, acrodermatitis enteropathica, psoriasis, herpes, seborrheic or contact dermatitis, eczema, pellagra, or even a chemical burn.[979] Numerous excellent descriptions of necrolytic migratory erythema associated with glucagonoma have been published.[973,974,977–979] Typically, the rash starts as an erythematous area, usually at periorifacial or intertriginous areas such as the groin, buttocks, thighs, or perineum, and then spreads laterally. The lesions later become raised with superficial central blistering. The top of the bullae frequently detach or rupture, leaving eroded areas that crust. The lesions tend to heal in the center, while the edges continue to spread with a well-defined crusting edge. Lesions may become confluent. Healing is associated with hyperpigmentation. This entire sequence characteristically takes 1 to 2 weeks. While some new lesions are developing, others are healing; therefore, a mixed pattern of erythema, bullous formation with epidermal separation, crusting, and hyperpigmentation can occur together with normal skin. The histopathology can be as varied as the clinical presentation.[979] In their classical form, early lesions demonstrate a superficial spongiosis and necrosis with subcorneal and midepidermal bullae.[973,974,976] Fusiform keratinocytes with pyknotic nuclei are often seen, as are mononuclear inflammatory infiltrates.[973,974,976] This characteristic histologic pattern is best seen in an early lesion. Glossitis or angular stomatitis is reported to occur in 34% to 68% of patients.[977,978]

Once the diagnosis is suspected, it can be confirmed by establishing the presence of a marked elevation in plasma glucagon concentration. In most laboratories, the upper limit of normal for fasting glucagon concentration is 150 to 200 pg/ml.[977] In one large review of glucagonomas, only 2 patients had a plasma glucagon level of 200 to 500 pg/ml, 4 patients had levels between 500 and 1000 pg/ml, and 52 patients had levels of more than 1000 pg/ml.[977] These results agree with another study, in which the mean plasma glucagon concentration in 73 patients with glucagonoma was 2110±334 pg/ml, with a range of 550 to 6600 pg/ml.[979] In this study, no patient had a level less than 500 pg/ml, 30% of patients had levels between 500 and 1000 pg/ml, and the remaining patients had levels of more than 1000 pg/ml. Hyperglucagonemia is reported to occur in chronic renal insufficiency, diabetic ketoacidosis, prolonged starvation, acute pancreatitis, acromegaly, hypercortisolism, septicemia, severe burns, severe stress (trauma, exercise), familial hyperglucagonemia, and hepatic insufficiency.[974,977–979] Plasma glucagon levels in these conditions have not been reported to exceed 500 pg/ml.[974,977]

In terms of medical therapy, the rash improved with octreotide in 54% to 90% of patients and disappeared completely in up to 30%.[903,905,941] In 5 patients in whom the time course was described, the rash disappeared in 2 patients within 1 week, and within 1 month in three other patients.[905] In one study, diarrhea improved in 4 of 6 patients and resolved in the other 2 patients.[941] Diabetes mellitus was not improved with octreotide treatment.[905,941] The diabetes mellitus was severe enough to require oral hypoglycemic agents in 42% of patients and insulin in 27%.[977] With octreotide treatment, plasma glucagon levels decreased in 80% to 90% of patients but only decreased in the normal range in 10% to 20% of patients.[903,905,941]

In 50% to 80% of patients, metastases are present at the time of diagnosis.[974,977,979] In patients with resectable disease, surgical resection has been successful in many cases.[702,974,977] The exact percentage of cases that can be cured is not known. In one large review involving 92 cases of glucagonoma, only 16 of the malignant cases were treated by surgical resection only.[977] Only 7 patients had normal plasma glucagon levels after resection, and of the 5 patients that had no evidence of metastatic spread, plasma glucagon levels postoperatively were normal in 2. Even if a patient eventually develops a recurrence, an extended disease-free interval may be attained.[974] Some studies have reported a benefit to patients even if only surgical debulking is done.[974,977–979] In patients with widely metastatic disease in which surgical debulking is not possible, chemotherapeutic agents frequently are used and are described later in this chapter (see Chemotherapy).

Somatostatinoma

Somatostatin is a hormone that inhibits numerous endocrine and exocrine functions.[982] Somatostatin inhibits the release of almost all gut hormones, including insulin, glucagon, gastrin, secretin, cholecystokinin, and motilin. Somatostatin has direct effects on target organs (*e.g.*, inhibition of gastric acid secretion), increases intestinal motility, and reduces the absorption of fat.[982]

The first two cases of somatostatinoma were described in 1977 by Ganda and colleagues[983] and Larsson and colleagues.[984] Somatostatinomas are the least common of the pancreatic endocrine tumors, and fewer than 50 cases have been described.[947] Patients characteristically have diabetes mellitus, gallbladder disease, diarrhea, weight loss, steatorrhea, and hypochlorhydria.[702,944,947,983,985,986]

Somatostatinomas occur in the pancreas in 56% to 75% of cases, and the remainder occur in the upper small intestine.[944,986] The distribution of the tumors within the pancreatic head:body:tail was 11:0:3.[986] and 14:2:5.[944] In 90% of patients, the tumors were solitary and varied from 1.5 to 10 cm in diameter (mean 4.9 cm).[986] In one series, 84% of all tumors had evidence of metastatic spread.[986] However, in another study, 92% of pancreatic tumors were associated with metastases, whereas metastases were seen in only 69% of those originating in the intestine.[944] Metastases occur to the liver in about 75% of patients with metastases and less frequently to the regional lymph nodes (31%) and to bone.[944,986]

With light microscopic studies, most tumors appear as well-differentiated tumors within varying degrees of fibrous septa. In 89% of the tumors examined, the secretory granules are typical of those in D cells.[944,986] Immunocytochemical analysis of 15 cases demonstrated somatostatin-like immunoreactive material in all tumors, and 33% contained insulin, 27% calcitonin, and 13% gastrin.[986] The mean age of patients was 51 to 53 years.[944,986] Of patients with intestinal somatostatinomas, 43% were females and 66% had with pancreatic tumors.[986] Diabetes mellitus was present in 95% of patients with pancreatic tumors and in 21% of those with intestinal tumors.[944,947] Gallbladder disease was seen in 94% of pancreatic tumors and in 36% of intestinal tumors, whereas weight loss was seen in 90% of pancreatic and in 44% of intestinal cases.[944,947] Steatorrhea and hypochlorhydria occurred in 83% to 86% of pancreatic cases but in only 12% to 17% of intestinal tumors.[520,944,947] Somatostatinomas generally are found by accident.[944,986] The symptoms produced by somatostatinomas are less pronounced than those seen with other pancreatic endocrine tumors and often are not detected until patients develop high somatostatin blood levels, usually late in the course of the disease when the tumor is large. In most cases, somatostatinomas are found at the time of laparotomy for cholecystectomy or during gastrointestinal imaging studies for various nonspecific complaints such as abdominal pain or diarrhea.[944,986]

Surgery was performed in 83% of patients in one series[987] and in 60% of patients in another series.[986] In one study, 65% of patients were reported to have successful resection, but the percentage actually cured was not stated.[987] Although an occasional patient might be cured,[987] this is not possible in most series because of the late diagnosis. In patients in whom a combination of surgical resection and cytotoxic therapy was used, 60% were alive 6 months to 5 years after diagnosis.[944,986,988] Because of the malignant nature of these tumors, patients benefit from surgical resection if imaging studies demonstrate possible resectable tumor.

GRFomas

GRFomas are the most recently described pancreatic endocrine tumor syndrome and are due to excessive release of growth hormone-releasing factor (GRF).[989-991] In one recent review of 30 cases of GRFomas,[528] 30% originated in the pancreas, 53% in the lung, 10% from small intestinal tumors, and 1 case from the adrenal gland.

Multiple pancreatic tumors have been reported,[992,993] occurring in 30% of the pancreatic GRFomas in one series.[528] All occurred in patients with MEN-I. Tumors were generally large (>6 cm), varying from 1 to 25 cm in diameter.[528] Metastases were present in 30% of patients with pancreatic GRFomas and in 2 of the 3 patients with intestinal GRFomas.[528] Metastases were to regional lymph nodes and less frequently to the liver. In one series, there were no relations among tumor size, GRF levels, and the presence of metastases, and the three largest tumors were not associated with metastatic disease or invasion.[528] About 40% of all GRFomas occur in patients with ZES, and in 40% of patients Cushing's syndrome was also present.[528,702]

On light microscopic studies, the typical features of a pancreatic endocrine tumor are seen: trabecular or solid nests and sheets of uniform tumor cells.[528] In electron microscopic studies, tumor cells containing 100- to 250-nm secretory granules are seen.[528,992,994,995] Immunochemical studies demonstrated GRF-immunoreactive material in all tumors examined, with 10% to 80% of cells possessing GRF.[528] GRF-immunoreactive material was seen in 31% of all pancreatic endocrine tumors in one study[996] and in 0 to 100% in other pathology studies,[528,997,998] although few of these patients had acromegaly. The known actions of GRF as a stimulant of growth hormone release account for the clinical presentation with acromegaly.[528,989,990,999]

Patients are from 15 to 63 years old with an average age of 38.[528] The patients with intestinal GRFomas were younger, with 2 of the 3 patients younger than 20 years.[528] A female predominance (73%) is seen for all GRFomas and for patients with pancreatic GRFomas (78%). Acromegalic features were indistinguishable from patients with classical acromegaly and included enlargement of hands and feet, facial changes, skin changes, headache, and peripheral nerve entrapment.[528,999] The average time from the onset of the acromegalic changes to diagnosis was 5.3 years in patients with pancreatic GRFomas.[528] The syndromes due to other hormones were due to the presence of ZES, Cushing's syndrome, or to hyperinsulinemia and hypoglycemia.[528,702]

Patients without metastatic disease should undergo surgical resection of the GRFoma. Before surgery and in those patients with nonresectable lesions, various agents may reduce plasma growth hormone (GH) levels. Dopamine agonists such as bromocriptine are widely used in patients with classical acromegaly, having more than a 50% response rate in some series.[999] However, they rarely are able to normalize plasma GH levels in patients with GRFomas.[991] Octreotide is the agent of choice because it always significantly suppresses or nor-

malizes growth hormone levels[905,999-1002] and in some cases is associated with pituitary shrinkage.[1000,1002] The suppression of GH secretion is mainly due to suppression at the pituitary level.[999] Surgical resection resulted in regression of the GRFoma syndrome in a small number of cases.[528,989,993,1003] The actual number of patients with long-term cure is unknown.

Other Pancreatic Endocrine Tumors

In a few studies in patients with pancreatic endocrine tumors secreting the peptide neurotensin, a neurotensinoma syndrome has been proposed.[771,944,1004-1009] Neurotensin is a 13 amino acid peptide originally isolated from bovine brain[1010] and later from human intestine and has biologic effects including tachycardia, hypotension, and cyanosis. It affects intestinal motility, stimulates jejunal and ileal fluid and electrolyte secretion, and stimulates pancreatic protein and bicarbonate secretion.[1010] Clinical features of patients with possible neurotensinomas include hypokalemia, weight loss, diabetes mellitus, cyanosis, hypotension, and flushing in a patient with a pancreatic endocrine tumor.[944] In a review of 6 patients, 50% were cured by resection of the pancreatic endocrine tumor and the remaining 50% improved with chemotherapy.[771,944,1004-1009] Recent studies question the existence of a specific neurotensinoma syndrome.[702,703,771] Of 180 patients with functional pancreatic endocrine tumors, elevated plasma neurotensin levels were found in 6 patients with VIPomas and their symptoms did not differ from patients with normal levels.[771] In another study, a similar result was found in patients with gastrinomas.[703]

Patients with pancreatic endocrine tumors with Cushing's syndrome (ACTHoma) have been reported.[893,947] In a recent study, Cushing's syndrome was reported in 19% of patients with both ZES and MEN-I.[893] In these patients, the disease was of pituitary origin and was mild. Cushing's syndrome occurs in sporadic cases of ZES[893] and in one recent prospective study was found in 5% of all cases.[702,893,1011] In these patients, the Cushing's syndrome was severe, due to ectopic ACTH production, occurred with metastatic pancreatic endocrine tumors that responded poorly to chemotherapy, and was associated with a poor prognosis.[893] Cushing's syndrome as the only manifestation of pancreatic endocrine tumors occurs and may precede any other hormonal syndrome.[1011]

Hypercalcemia has been reported to be due to a pancreatic endocrine tumor secreting a peptide similar to parathyroid hormone (PTH) or to an unknown substance that mimics the action of PTH and causes hyperparathyroidism.[1012-1017] The tumor generally has been metastatic to the liver by the time of diagnosis,[1012-1014] although in one recent case, radical resection of a pancreatic tail tumor with subsequent treatment with chemotherapy resulted in a total remission for 5 years.[1017]

Treatment

Most pancreatic endocrine tumors including VIPomas, glucagonomas, nonfunctional tumors or PPomas, somatostatinomas, and GRFomas resemble gastrinomas and are malignant with diligent follow-up. The exception is insulinoma, which has a low incidence of malignancy (10–15%; see Table 41–24). The malignant nature of these tumors cannot be detected accurately by pathology, so they require careful follow-up with imaging studies and appropriate plasma markers. The principles and treatment of malignant insulinomas, VIPomas, glucagonomas, somatostatinomas, nonfunctioning islet cell tumors, PPomas, and GRFomas are similar to that discussed previously in detail for gastrinomas. Although these tumors frequently may metastasize, many patients live comfortably and productively for many years with metastatic disease if symptoms can be controlled.

Chemotherapy alone has yielded few, if any, complete remissions in patients with metastatic disease.[520,563,702,1018,1019] Chemotherapy combined with aggressive surgical resection of all visible disease may be helpful, especially in patients with functional tumors in which medical therapy is not controlling the symptoms.[702,947,957,974] Because of the indolent growth pattern of these tumors and the fact that chemotherapy has not cured any patients with metastatic disease, chemotherapy has usually been withheld until a patient demonstrates progression of disease during follow-up or demonstrates refractory symptoms due either to the tumor or to the secreted hormone. Progression usually means increase in size or number of metastatic lesions on an imaging study. In some studies, an increase in plasma hormone marker for a given tumor has been used to assess disease activity. The former documentation is more reliable. A recent study has shown no relation between tumor growth and plasma levels of gastrin in patients with ZES treated with chemotherapy.[899]

Treatment of metastatic and primary tumors requires control of bulk disease and control of symptoms secondary to the hormonal excess in patients with functional tumors. The initial consideration and the only potentially curative treatment of malignant pancreatic endocrine tumors is surgical resection (see Fig. 41–21). This should be considered (if feasible with a reasonable operative risk) for any patient with a pancreatic endocrine tumor whether primary or metastatic. The goal of surgery is to locate and remove all gross disease. Resection must be performed with acceptable morbidity and mortality because often the disease is slow-growing and some patients may live for years with documented metastases.

Therapy for malignant pancreatic endocrine tumors consists of controlling the symptoms with octreotide or other medical therapies in patients with functional tumors. This therapy is used alone or coupled with debulking surgery in some cases and various cytotoxic therapies in others (see Table 41–33). Treatment with octreotide, with other medical therapies, and with surgical resection is discussed under the functional tumor syndromes. The remainder of this section considers cytotoxic therapies directed at the tumor itself in patients with metastatic disease.

MANAGEMENT OF METASTATIC DISEASE

The treatment of all metastatic pancreatic endocrine tumors is considered together because in most aspects it is similar for each tumor. Cytotoxic protocols and surgical approaches generally are the same. The long-term natural history of most functional pancreatic endocrine tumors (malignant insulinomas, VIPomas, glucagonomas, GRFomas, somatostatinomas) is not known because, until recently, effective treatment for the functional syndrome did not exist. Patients died of com-

plications of the hormonal excess rather than of the tumor itself.[702] This may change with the recent availability of agents such as octreotide. In contrast to PPomas, nonfunctional pancreatic endocrine tumors, and gastrinomas, for which effective therapy for the gastric hypersecretion has existed for more than 30 years, the natural history of the malignant tumor itself can be assessed. Because of the similar biologic behavior of all endocrine tumors, the assessment of the latter tumors will likely provide insights into the natural history of all malignant pancreatic endocrine tumors.[702,948,1018] As shown in Table 41–31, the overall 5-year survival rate with gastrinomas is 63% to 75%, and survival is influenced primarily by the extent of the tumor. If the tumor is thought to be completely resected at the time of surgery, 5-year survival is 69% to 100%. If the tumor is resected incompletely or recurs, 5-year survival rates are 14% to 95%. If the tumor is unresectable, 5-year survival rates are 18% to 75%. There are no data to suggest that other pancreatic endocrine tumors differ in behavior. Limited data from PPomas, of which most were metastatic, report a 5-year survival rate of 44%, which is similar to that with metastatic gastrinomas.[948] Most authorities would therefore agree that treatment directed at the metastatic disease is indicated. There is no agreement about what type of therapy is most appropriate, when therapy should be started, and even the efficacy of various therapies because of the small numbers of patients treated with various protocols. Chemotherapy either alone or with debulking surgery, hepatic arterial embolization either alone or with chemotherapy, hormonal therapy with octreotide, and interferon all have been reported useful in small numbers of cases (see Table 41–33).

CHEMOTHERAPY

Chemotherapy for insulinomas and the less common islet cell tumors is similar to that discussed previously for gastrinomas and summarized in Table 41–33. Because of the rarity of these tumors, in most studies of chemotherapy for pancreatic endocrine tumors, chemotherapy of all pancreatic endocrine tumors is considered together. Although two series reported no difference in responsiveness to chemotherapeutic agents in different tumors, the numbers of individual tumors studied were small and it is not established that each tumor responds equally to chemotherapy.[702,897] As with gastrinomas, chemotherapy is reserved for patients with metastatic disease that is increasing in size on imaging studies or with refractory symptoms. The recommended choice for metastatic pancreatic endocrine tumors is the combination of streptozocin and 5-FU.[702,1019] Streptozocin is a glycocyamine nitrosourea compound originally derived from a *Streptomyces* species and has been in clinical use since 1967.[1020,1021] In preclinical studies, it was found to have cytotoxic effects on pancreatic islets.[1022] In 1968, streptozocin was found to have clinical effectiveness against a pancreatic endocrine tumor[1023] and since then has been used as the initial agent either alone or in combination with other agents for treating metastatic pancreatic endocrine tumors (see Table 41–33). Streptozocin alone gives an objective tumor response in 36% to 62% of patients. In contrast, other single agents such as doxorubicin, dacarbazine, or tubercidin have had a lower response rate of 6% to 33% (see Table 41–33). In various series, streptozocin treatment has caused nausea and vomiting in almost all patients

(100%),[899] transient dose-related renal dysfunction including proteinuria (40% to 50%),[899,1018] decreased creatinine clearance (26%),[1018] abnormalities in hepatic function (27%),[1018] and leukopenia and thrombocytopenia (6%).[1018] In one study, 5 patients died of renal failure, and the use of streptozocin must be carefully monitored.[444]

Etoposide, dactinomycin, or cisplatin alone have been used in a few cases but generally are not effective.[1019] Recently, a combination of etoposide and cisplatin was evaluated in 14 patients with metastatic pancreatic endocrine tumors and the results compared with metastatic carcinoid tumors (13 patients) or anaplastic neuroendocrine tumors (18 patients: 6 with tumors in the pancreas, 8 with tumors in the stomach and intestine, 1 with tumor of the lung, and 3 with tumors in unknown locations).[1024] This study was performed because recent studies demonstrate that these two agents are effective in small cell lung cancer, which has neuroendocrine features histologically similar to those seen in pancreatic endocrine tumors.[1024] Sixty-seven percent of the anaplastic neuroendocrine tumors, 14% of the pancreatic endocrine tumors, and none of the metastatic carcinoid tumors demonstrated partial to complete regression.[1024]

The combination of streptozocin and 5-FU was found to be more effective than streptozocin alone.[897] In this study, streptozocin gave a 36% response rate with 12% showing a complete response, whereas with streptozocin plus 5-FU, 63% demonstrated a response with 33% having a complete response. Response rates for different functional tumors or between functional and nonfunctional tumors did not differ.[897] In two more recent prospective studies, the response rate with streptozocin plus 5-FU was significantly lower in patients with metastatic gastrinomas to the liver (5% and 40%).[899,900] In neither study did any patient have a complete response, and in one study there was no difference in survival for responders and nonresponders.[899] The difference in response rate in the early study and the more recent ones remains unexplained. Streptozocin has been used in combination with other agents such as doxorubicin or tubercidin in small numbers of patients with response rates ranging from 20% to 100% (see Table 41–33).

Glucagonomas are reported to respond to dacarbazine.[694,1025–1031] Some patients have complete remissions with dacarbazine, whereas in other pancreatic endocrine tumors the response rate is low. In one study, 90% of VIPomas were reported to respond to streptozocin, a percentage higher than that seen in series of all pancreatic endocrine tumors (see Table 41–33).[967] Only small numbers of patients are reported with the different pancreatic endocrine tumors, and these possible differences have not been established.

SURGICAL TREATMENT

If possible, systematic removal of all resectable tumor (debulking surgery) is recommended for VIPomas,[957,967] glucagonomas,[920,974] and somatostatinomas.[1032] The survival of patients with gastrinomas was reported to improve with this approach.[720,759] Whether such an approach actually increases survival is not clear. This approach may be required in patients with symptomatic tumors in whom octreotide or the use of chemotherapy alone is not reducing plasma hormone levels and symptoms are not controlled sufficiently.

HEPATIC ARTERY EMBOLIZATION

Hepatic artery embolization with or without postocclusion chemotherapy has been used successfully in small numbers of patients with metastatic pancreatic endocrine tumors to the liver.[463,666,668,901,902,1033] Because the liver derives only 20% to 25% of its blood supply from the hepatic artery and 75% to 80% from the portal vein,[1033] and because most pancreatic islet cell tumors are vascular with an arterial supply, hepatic artery embolization has been used if the portal vein is patent. In some studies, 80% to 90% of patients demonstrate symptomatic improvement.[1033] In one study, only 14% had symptomatic improvement.[901] In a study combining hepatic arterial occlusion with chemotherapy, 64% of patients had complete symptomatic remission, 18% had a 75% to 100% improvement, and 9% had a 50% to 75% improvement.[463,666] The symptomatic improvement lasts longer with the addition of chemotherapy than without it.[463,666] This procedure is not without side effects, and almost all patients report abdominal pain, nausea, vomiting, and fever, usually lasting 3 to 10 days.[1033] Severe complications occur in 10% to 15%, including hepatic failure, infection, and death.[901,1033] Even more important than the possible side effects is the recent report that metastases to bone occur in 12% of patients with gastrinoma metastatic to liver.[608] This raises the likelihood in some cases that treatment directed only at the liver may be of limited value. Hepatic artery embolization should be considered in a patient with a symptomatic pancreatic endocrine tumor who has diffusely metastatic disease to the liver, minimal or no bone metastases, and hormone symptoms that cannot be controlled by octreotide, chemotherapy, or other medical treatment.

HORMONAL THERAPY WITH SOMATOSTATIN ANALOGS

In animal studies, somatostatin analogs can inhibit tumor growth[1034] and the growth of transplantable insulinomas and chondrosarcomas.[906] Pancreatic endocrine tumors frequently possess somatostatin receptors, which may mediate the action of somatostatin on these tumors.[605,931,1035] In one recent study, all 15 pancreatic endocrine tumors examined had somatostatin receptors.[603] Hormonal treatment with octreotide was reported to decrease tumor size in 8 of 66 patients (see Table 41–33). This included 3 of 29 patients with gastrinomas, 4 of 10 patients with VIPomas, 1 of 3 patients with GRFomas, and none of 5 patients with insulinomas, 10 patients with glucagonomas, 4 with Cushing's syndrome secondary to a pancreatic endocrine tumor, and 5 with nonfunctioning tumors. In no case did the metastases disappear.[905] Therefore, the antitumor effects of octreotide are small, at least at the doses of less than 1000 μg/day used in most of these studies.

INTERFERON

Interferon has been reported to effective at controlling symptoms in many patients with pancreatic endocrine tumors.[489,698,909,1036,1037] In one study of 22 patients with advanced pancreatic endocrine tumors, treatment with 3 to 6 million U/day of human leukocyte interferon resulted in responses in 77% of patients, with a mean duration of 8.5 months (2–

36 months).[909] In this study, 7 of 7 patients (100%) with VI-Pomas and 6 of 9 patients (66%) with PPomas or nonfunctioning tumors responded, whereas patients with somatostatinoma and insulinoma did not. Only 6 of 22 patients (27%) demonstrated an actual decrease in tumor size, although each patient had failed chemotherapy. One study demonstrated no effect of recombinant interferon-α in 2 patients with VIPomas.[1037] In another study of 16 patients with neuroendocrine tumors treated with doxorubicin plus interferon, 3 (18%) partial responses were reported.[1018] The exact percentage of patients who will respond with tumor reduction is unknown but appears to be low.[1038]

MULTIPLE ENDOCRINE NEOPLASIA TYPE I

In 1954, Wermer described the familial occurrence of tumors involving the pituitary gland, parathyroid glands, and the endocrine pancreas.[1039] Of the 5 affected patients, 4 had pituitary tumors, 3 had hyperparathyroidism, and 3 had pancreatic tumors. The syndrome was initially called Wermer's syndrome and then multiple endocrine adenomatosis type I. It is now termed multiple endocrine neoplasia type I (MEN-I) because the parathyroid disease is hyperplasia and some of the pancreatic endocrine tumors in affected individuals can be malignant.[513,514,1040]

MEN-I is inherited as an autosomal dominant trait.[514,1040,1041] Recent chromosomal linkage studies have localized the genetic defect to the long arm of chromosome 11 (q12,q13 locus), which is closely linked to the skeletal muscle glycogen phosphorylase locus that is altered in McArdle's disease (Table 41–35).[1041–1044] In 2 insulinomas from patients with MEN-I, there was a loss of one constitutional allele on chromosome 11 and hyperplastic pancreatic tissue showed a similar alteration.[1043] This suggests that the oncogenesis of MEN-I follows the two-hit theory of neoplasia of Knudsen,[1045] in which an inherited mutation in one chromosome is unmasked by a somatic deletion or mutation on the other normal chromosome, thereby removing the suppressor effect of the normal gene. These results are in contrast to patients without MEN-I who develop pancreatic endocrine tumors, in whom the pancreatic neoplasms even when malignant do not develop homozygous inactivation of the MEN-I gene.[1046] Recent work concerning the etiology of primary hyperparathyroidism in patients with MEN-I suggests that a circulating factor in the serum stimulates bovine parathyroid cells to proliferate.[1047,1048] Subsequent analyses of the mitogenic activity in the plasma of MEN-I patients demonstrated that basic fibroblast growth or a closely related growth factor was present in this plasma.[1048,1049] A monoclonal abnormality has been found in the hyperplastic parathyroid glands of patients with MEN-I, suggesting that the hyperplastic process in these glands may develop by inactivation of the MEN-I gene in a precursor cell.[1050]

CLINICAL PRESENTATION

The peak incidence of symptoms in women with MEN-I is during the third decade of life, whereas the peak incidence in men is during the fourth decade. More than half of patients

TABLE 41–35. Multiple Endocrine Neoplasia Syndromes and Familial Medullary Thyroid Cancer

Characterstic	MEN-II	MEN-IIa	MEN-IIb	Familial Non-MEN MTC
Genetic defect location	Chromosome 11q 12–13 near PYGM locus	Chromosome 10 near centrosome	Chromosome 10 near centrosome	—
MTC present	No	Bilateral	Bilateral	Bilateral
Pheochromocytoma present	No	70% bilateral	70% bilateral	No
Parathyroid disease	Hyperplasia	Hyperplasia	Rare	No
Specific phenotype	No	No	Bony abnormalities, multiple mucosal neuromas, marfanoid habitus, bumpy lips	No
Familial, autosomal dominant trait	Yes	Yes	Yes, but may be nonfamilial	Yes
Course of MTC	No MTC	Variable, frequently indolent	Generally more virulent	Indolent
Pancreatic endocrine tumors	PPomas (80–100%) Gastrinomas (54%) Insulinomas (21%) Glucagonomas (3%) GRFomas, VIPomas (uncommon)	No	No	No

MEN, multiple endocrine neoplasia; MTC, medullary thyroid carcinoma; PYGM locus, skeletal muscle glycogen phosphorylase locus; PPoma, pancreatic endocrine tumor releasing pancreatic polypeptide; VIPoma, vasoactive intestinal peptide; GRFoma, growth hormone-releasing factor tumor.

with MEN-I have adenomas of more than one gland, and about 20% have 3 affected glands. The frequency of glandular involvement, in descending order, is parathyroid, pancreas, pituitary, adrenal cortex, and thyroid. The frequency of clinical symptoms, in descending order, is hypercalcemia, nephrolithiasis, peptic ulcer disease, hypoglycemia, headache, visual-field loss, hypopituitarism, acromegaly, galactorrhea-amenorrhea, and Cushing's syndrome.[514,1040,1051]

PARATHYROID GLAND INVOLVEMENT

Hyperparathyroidism is the most common clinically detected abnormality in patients with MEN-I, occurring in 88% to 97% of all patients in different series.[513,514,1042,1052] The pathology associated with primary hyperparathyroidism is always hyperplasia or multiple gland disease (see Table 41–35).[513,1052] The surgical management requires removal of 3½ or 4 parathyroid glands to control the hypercalcemia. If 4 glands are removed, immediate autograft of some of the parathyroid tissue into the musculature of the nondominant forearm is recommended.[1053] Unfortunately, the incidence of recurrent or persistent hyperparathyroidism after surgery for hyperparathyroidism in MEN-I patients varies from 16% to 54% and the incidence of hypoparathyroidism from 10% to 25%.[1054,1055] Primary hyperparathyroidism adversely affects the medical management of the gastric acid hypersecretion in MEN-I patients with hyperparathyroidism and ZES. A recent study indicates that successful parathyroidectomy in these patients greatly facilitates the management of the gastric acid hypersecretion.[868]

PANCREATIC ENDOCRINE TUMORS

Pathologic examination of the resected pancreas in patients with MEN-I demonstrated multiple tumors producing multiple different hormones.[1056,1057] These pathologic studies suggest that PPomas are the most common pancreatic endocrine tumor, occurring in 80% to 100% of these patients.[520] These tumors cause symptoms only due to the tumor itself and often present when tumor growth is advanced. Furthermore, because patients with MEN-I have not been able to survive until late adulthood, the frequency with which this tumor will be clinically significant is unknown. In two large series, 81% to 82% of patients with MEN-I developed functional pancreatic endocrine tumors—54% had gastrinomas, 21% insulinomas, 3% glucagonomas, and 1% VIPomas (see Table 41–35).[513,514] Up to 33% of patients with GRFomas have MEN-I, and this tumor may occur much more frequently in patients with MEN-I than previously suspected.[702] The diagnosis and management of each of these syndromes are described earlier in this chapter.

The ideal treatment of ZES is surgical excision of the gastrinoma; however, in patients with MEN-I, excision of gastrinomas rarely results in normal serum gastrin levels.[712,719,896] In early studies in six different surgical series, no patient with MEN-I was cured by resection of gastrinoma, indicating that the probability of curing these patients in this manner is remote.[719] Therefore, the role of pancreatic surgery in the treatment of the gastrinoma in patients with ZES with MEN-I is unclear.[712,719,783,896] The possibility of surgical cure is much lower in patients with ZES and MEN-I than in patients with

sporadic disease.[712,783,796,1058] Because of the low possibility of cure and the recent suggestion that the gastrinoma may be less malignant in MEN-I, some groups recommend that patients with MEN-I do not undergo explorative laparotomy.[758,766] Others recommend laparotomy only if a localized lesion is predicted by a localized gastrin gradient from selective venous sampling for gastrin,[1058] if the fasting serum PP concentration is more than three times normal,[1059] or if a localized tumor is identified by imaging studies and there is a family history suggesting early metastatic disease.[712,778] The best approach is unclear because all the above criteria are flawed. It is not established clearly that familial gastrinoma has a less malignant course.[712] In a recent study, an elevated or normal level of PP had no predictive value.[778] Selective gastrin sampling from portal venous tributaries in patients with MEN-I with ZES was not helpful.[777]

Many gastrinomas in patients with ZES with MEN-I are reported to appear in the duodenum[756,783] and not in the pancreas, as earlier studies suggested.[1056] No study has examined prospectively whether such tumors can be found routinely at surgery and what the long-term cure rate will be. These patients often have multiple duodenal nodularities with more than one endocrine tumor in the duodenum. It is not clear how the gastrinoma can be identified without radical surgery. Therefore, it is not known whether these patients will benefit by routine exploration with duodenotomy to the same extent as patients with sporadic disease.[783] In particular kindreds in which patients' parents died of metastatic gastrinoma and presentation occurs at a relatively young age with a large pancreatic tumor, a surgical approach similar to the one used in patients with sporadic disease may be warranted.[712,764,778,783] Therefore, we recommend that all patients with ZES and MEN-I have extensive localization studies but that only patients with unequivocally positive imaging studies undergo surgical exploration (see Fig. 41–15). At surgery, tumors identified in the pancreatic head are enucleated, the duodenum is carefully explored and any identified tumor is resected, and tumors in the pancreatic body or tail are resected. In a recent study, almost 50% of the patients treated in this manner had evidence of lymph nodes metastases.[778] Using this approach, cure of ZES is almost never seen; however, it is hoped that such surgery reduces the risk of later metastatic disease. No data demonstrate that this approach increases survival.

MEN-I is reported to be present in 20% of all patients with ZES and in 4% of patients with insulinomas.[520,764] The exact percentage of patients with VIPoma, glucagonomas, or somatostatinoma with MEN-I is not known but is estimated to be low (<5%).[520] The management of insulinomas and VIPomas is different from gastrinoma in patients with MEN-I.[702] Medical management of VIPomas and insulinomas is not as reliable as medical management of gastric acid hypersecretion in ZES patients. Diazoxide and octreotide are available and may be useful for short-term treatment, but they are not as reliable as surgical resection for long-term treatment (see the sections on these tumors). Unlike gastrinomas, insulinomas or VIPomas in patients with MEN-I frequently are solitary tumors, and resection may prove helpful in symptomatic management and may result in cure.[778,1056,1058,1060] Preoperative PVS for insulin or VIP can help identify the tumor or region of the pancreas from which the abnormal hormone source originates.[778,1058]

PITUITARY TUMORS

Pituitary tumors occur in 54% to 80% of patients with MEN-I.[513,514,1051] Symptoms caused by pituitary adenomas in MEN-I are usually due to local encroachment of tumor including headache and visual-field defects. In early studies, most tumors were described as nonfunctioning chromophobe adenomas, with 15% of patients having eosinophilic tumors often with acromegaly and 5% having basophilic tumors with Cushing's disease.[1051] It is likely that many of these nonfunctioning tumors are prolactinomas because serum prolactin levels were not routinely measured in these early cases.[1051] Prolactinomas are now thought to have a prevalence of 15%.[1051] Of the functional tumors, prolactinomas comprise 70%. The second most common hormone secreted is GH (25%), with resulting acromegaly.[1051] Cushing's syndrome may be more common in some patients with MEN-I than previously thought. In one recent study of patients with MEN-I and gastrinoma, 20% of patients had Cushing's syndrome.[893] In this series, Cushing's syndrome was always of pituitary origin and was mild.[893] Cushing's syndrome can result from release of ACTH-like material from the pancreatic tumor itself,[520,893,1061] although in patients with MEN-I this appears to be much less common than in patients with sporadic pancreatic endocrine tumors such as gastrinomas.[893] Transsphenoidal pituitary surgery is indicated to control any detectable pituitary mass lesion in patients with MEN-I. Incompletely resected patients can be managed with bromocriptine.

ADRENAL AND THYROID TUMORS

Adrenal abnormalities occur in 27% to 36% of patients with MEN-I.[513,514] The most common abnormality is a benign, nonfunctional cortical adenoma, although adrenocortical carcinomas and hyperplasia may occur.[513,514] Adrenocortical hyperfunction may be found secondary to a pituitary tumor[893] or rarely to a pancreatic endocrine tumor.[1061] Adrenocortical neoplasms usually are nonfunctional in patients with MEN-I. Thyroid adenomas occur in about 5% to 30% of patients with MEN-I involving diffuse or nodular hyperplasia and have little clinical significance.[513]

FAMILIAL MEDULLARY THYROID CARCINOMA AND MULTIPLE ENDOCRINE NEOPLASIA TYPES IIa AND IIb

HISTORY AND PATHOLOGY

The coexistence of thyroid cancer and pheochromocytoma was first described in 1932 by Eisenberg and Wallerstein.[1062] In 1959, Hazard and colleagues first described MTC and its striking histologic characteristics of cellular argentaffin staining and amyloid production.[1063] MTC is associated with three distinct familial syndromes: MEN-IIa, MEN-IIb, and familial non-MEN MTC, a disease characterized by hereditary MTC without associated endocrinopathies (see Table 41–35).[1064] In 1970, a radioimmunoassay was developed for calcitonin and a kindred with MEN-IIa was described with elevated serum calcitonin levels.[1065] Subsequently, patients with increased serum calcitonin levels were identified whose resected thyroid glands were normal macroscopically but on microscopic examination showed C-cell hyperplasia.[1066,1067]

In 1961, Sipple reported the unusually high incidence of bilateral pheochromocytomas in patients with thyroid malignancy.[1068] These patients were later found to have MTC, and the familial disease was inherited as a mendelian autosomal dominant trait with high gene penetrance (see Table 41–35).[1069,1070] Hyperparathyroidism later was identified as part of the syndrome.[1071] In 1968, this syndrome of MTC, pheochromocytomas, and hyperparathyroidism was termed MEN-II. It is now called MEN-IIa (see Table 41–35).

In 1966, Williams and Pollock called attention to the finding that some patients with MTC and pheochromocytomas had multiple mucosal neuromas, with or without marfanoid habitus, puffy lips, prominent jaw, pes cavus, and medullated corneal nerves (Fig. 41–22).[1072] For this group of patients, the terms MEN-IIb and MEN-II were suggested.[92] Patients with MEN-IIb do not have parathyroid disease (see Table 41–35). Recent chromosomal linkage studies have localized the genetic defects of MEN-IIa and MEN-IIb to chromosome 10 (see

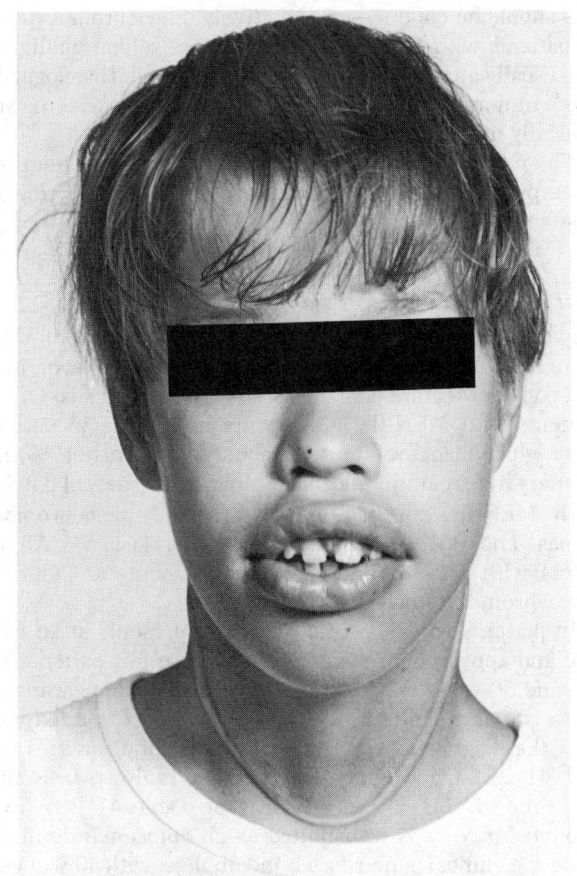

FIGURE 41–22. Characteristic appearance of a patient with multiple endocrine neoplasia type IIb. Note the mucosal neuromas, pronounced lips, poor dentition, and prominent jaw. (Norton JA, Fromme LC, Farrell RE, Wells SA Jr. Multiple endocrine neoplasia type IIb: the most aggressive form of medullary thyroid carcinoma. Surg Clin North Am 1979;59:109)

Table 41–35).[1073] In MEN-IIa, the defect has been localized to near *RBP3*, D10S5, *FNRB*, D10S15, and D10ZI near the centrosome of chromosome 10.[1074–1077] Recent linkage studies have localized the defect in MEN-IIb to chromosome 10 near *FNRB*, D10Z1.[1077–1079]

Histologically, MTC in patients with familial MTC, MEN-IIa and MEN-IIb appears identical to the MTC occurring sporadically. In each syndrome, there is bilateral involvement and the MTC usually occupies a position in the superior-lateral part of the thyroid lobe and may be multicentric, whereas in the sporadic setting it is usually unilateral. MTC is a malignant tumor of the parafollicular cells or the calcitonin-secreting cells (C cells). MTC comprises 5% to 12% of all thyroid cancers, and only 10% of all MTC is familial.[1080]

The pheochromocytomas in patients with MEN-IIa or MEN-IIb usually present in the second or third decades of life and are usually bilateral (70%).[437,1080] Tumors in patients with MEN-IIa usually are smaller than 2 to 3 cm and usually are larger in patients with MEN-IIb. Even in MEN-IIa patients with apparent unilateral pheochromocytomas, the contralateral adrenal gland almost always demonstrates medullary hyperplasia on pathologic analysis.[437] Patients with medullary hyperplasia rarely have symptoms of pheochromocytoma. ^{131}I-MIBG scans in patients with MEN-IIa may be useful to predict the presence of a clinically significant pheochromocytoma and should be obtained preoperatively. Pheochromocytomas in patients with MEN-IIa or MEN-IIb are seldom malignant and usually are found within the adrenal gland. Histologically, these tumors are indistinguishable from those occurring sporadically in a nonfamilial setting.

The parathyroid lesions in MEN-IIa consist of generalized hyperplasia[1052] and must be managed like the parathyroid disease in MEN-I (see Table 41–35).[1053]

CLINICAL PRESENTATION

Any of the neoplasms that make up the syndromes of MEN-IIa or MEN-IIb may be the presenting problem; however, MTC is a constant feature and affects 100% of individuals. Of 164 patients with MEN-IIa, all patients had MTC, 35 patients (21%) had pheochromocytomas, and 28 patients (17%) had primary hyperparathyroidism.[1080] In another study of patients with MEN-IIa, all had MTC, 40% had pheochromocytomas, and 60% had parathyroid hyperplasia.[1081] All patients with MEN-IIb have MTC and about 60% develop pheochromocytomas.[1082]

In patients with MEN-IIb, the MTC presents at an early age and appears more aggressive because few patients live beyond 30 years of age.[67] The characteristic appearance of these patients is often the first sign of disease and may suggest the diagnosis before other clinical abnormalities (see Fig. 41–22). On investigation, the MTC is always present at the time of clinical recognition (see Table 41–33). Even though MEN-IIa is transmitted as an autosomal dominant trait, the clinical penetrance is incomplete, with 40% of gene carriers not presenting with symptoms even by the age of 70 years.[1083]

Patients initially may seek medical advance because of episodic spells with headache, dizziness, or symptoms suggestive of hypertension. It is unusual for patients with MEN-IIa to present with symptoms related to parathyroid disease.[1064]

PREOPERATIVE EVALUATION AND SCREENING

When the presence of MEN-IIa or MEN-IIb is suspected, precise diagnosis depends on hormonal changes consistent with MTC, hyperparathyroidism, and pheochromocytoma. For MTC, the production of calcitonin by the tumor cells holds the key for diagnosis. Most investigators believe that the upper normal limit of plasma calcitonin levels is 300 pg/ml. Virtually all patients with MTC have elevated basal levels or stimulated plasma levels of calcitonin. Patients who present with clinically apparent disease usually have basal plasma calcitonin levels exceeding 1 ng/ml.[1084] Generally, there is a direct correlation between the tumoral mass of MTC and plasma calcitonin levels.[1084]

Minimal plasma elevations of plasma calcitonin are indicative of MTC in patients who have no other clinical evidence of the neoplasm.[1085] Some patients with normal basal plasma calcitonin levels have an increase to abnormal levels after calcium infusion (15 mg/kg over 4 hours), or pentagastrin injection (see Fig. 41–2). Short bolus calcium injection (2 mg calcium gluconate/kg over 1 minute) provokes elevated plasma calcitonin levels in MTC patients. The peak plasma calcitonin levels in patients with MTC were higher with the combination test of calcium and pentagastrin injection than with calcium chloride alone, calcium gluconate alone, or pentagastrin alone.[1086] Patients with MTC and undetectable basal calcitonin levels (<300 pg/ml) all had peak calcitonin responses above 300 pg/ml after pentagastrin and calcium injection. Three of 12 patients with MTC had peak calcitonin levels below 300 pg/ml with pentagastrin alone and with calcium gluconate alone, and would not have been diagnosed if these two provocative agents had been used separately. The combination test provides a higher diagnostic accuracy than any other provocative test and may be the most efficacious method of screening for MTC.[1086] The pentagastrin test alone is usually diagnostic (see Fig. 41–2), and patients diagnosed with MTC using this test almost always have been cured (see Table 41–12). In kindred members at risk who have borderline elevated plasma calcitonin levels (200–600 pg/ml), selective inferior thyroid venous catheterization and sampling during provocative testing is recommended.[1087] Patients with MTC have strikingly increased plasma calcitonin levels in the inferior thyroid vein effluent after provocative testing, whereas normal subjects do not. Furthermore, such subjects with MTC and minimally elevated plasma CT levels after stimulation have minimal MTC and are usually cured by thyroidectomy.[1084]

Patients and members of kindreds with MEN-IIa or MEN-IIb have been screened using various DNA markers from the pericentromeric region of chromosome 10.[1074,1077,1078] In one study,[1078] family members with a negative pentagastrin-stimulated calcitonin test were screened and the linkage study resulted in substantial changes in carrier risk for various family members. In another study of a 5-year-old child, the pentagastrin provocative test was negative but DNA linkage studies suggested a 96% chance of carrying the MEN-IIa gene.[1074] A repeat provocative test at a later time was positive for MTC. Studies combining calcitonin and restriction fragment length polymorphism tests have identified up to 99% of MEN-IIa carriers age 25.[1076] This is an apparent improvement over pentagastrin-stimulated calcitonin screening, which detects

90% by age 30.[1078] Patients with MEN-IIa or MEN-IIb must have a pheochromocytoma excluded before undergoing surgery for MTC. Pheochromocytomas usually can be excluded by measuring normal urinary levels of epinephrine, norepinephrine, VMA, and metanephrines. If levels are elevated, tumor localization studies should be done. Abdominal CT and MRI are helpful in localizing the pheochromocytoma, but more sensitive studies may be needed.[1088,1089] MIBG is concentrated into pheochromocytoma cells and provides a means to localize these tumors functionally using scintigraphy.[1089] The sensitivity of this method varies from 79% to 91%, with a specificity of 94% to 99%.[1089]

SURGICAL MANAGEMENT

The ability to diagnose MTC in patients at risk for familial MTC allows the physician to diagnose and treat this malignancy in an early preclinical stage. If MTC is diagnosed in a patient from a MEN-IIa kindred, it is essential to screen the remainder of the family members at risk. It is in this situation that calcium gluconate and pentagastrin provocative test and DNA linkage studies are of greatest use. Most patients diagnosed with only biochemically evident MTC have surgically curable C-cell hyperplasia or carcinoma confined to the thyroid gland (see Fig. 41–3).[1090] Provocative testing is usually done in family members at risk beginning at 5 years of age and continuing at yearly intervals through the fifth decade. DNA linkage studies require only a blood sample and can be done even earlier with ease.

MEN-II patients with pheochromocytoma merit abdominal exploration and evaluation of both adrenal glands. Before surgical exploration, all patients need effective α-adrenergic receptor blockade.[1082,1089] Phenoxybenzamine should be administered 1 to 2 weeks before surgery, starting with a dose of 10 mg twice daily and increasing every second day to a usual dose of 20 to 30 mg three times daily.[1089] The end point is normotension with mild to moderate asymptomatic posterial hypotension (15 mm Hg) accompanied by symptoms of blockade including nasal stuffiness. β-Adrenergic blockade is not required[1091] except in patients with persistent sinus tachycardia.[1082,1089] The β blocker should never be administered before the institution of α-adrenergic blockage because this may result in unopposed agonism with hypertensive crises.[1089]

If a solitary pheochromocytoma is present at surgery, it should be resected. Some advocate resecting only abnormal adrenal glands confirmed by palpation,[1092] whereas others recommend routinely resecting both adrenal glands because bilateral pathology is present in most patients.[437] However, some patients have undergone only unilateral adrenalectomy and remained asymptomatic with normal urinary catecholamines for a mean follow-up of 8 years.[1092] A preoperative MIBG scan can determine unilateral versus bilateral adrenalectomy in these patients. Patients with MEN-IIa undergoing unilateral adrenalectomy should be followed carefully at 6-month or 1-year intervals because a second adrenal tumor may be diagnosed biochemically before it is clinically apparent.

The surgical management of familial MTC is total thyroidectomy with a central lymph node dissection. A total thyroidectomy must be performed because the MTC is always bilateral.

POSTOPERATIVE FOLLOW-UP

In patients with MEN-IIa and MEN-IIb, the disease that is most frequently lethal is MTC. The MTC in patients with MEN-IIb seems to be more virulent than in patients with MEN-IIa.[67] However, a recent group of children with MTC in the setting of MEN-IIb have been reported, some of whom appear to be cured of MTC.[197] Survival of patients with MTC and MEN-IIa is difficult to predict because some patients die at a young age, whereas others live a normal life expectancy. However, survival of patients with MEN-IIa depends on the extent of MTC at initial surgical resection (see Table 41-10).[1084] The survival of patients with MTC in the presence of MEN-IIa is excellent.

In a familial setting, MTC must be diagnosed at an early stage when it is confined to the thyroid gland.[1090] The prognostic significance of the stimulated plasma calcitonin level was demonstrated in a study of 92 patients with hereditary MTC.[1090] The patients were divided into four groups according to their preoperative stimulated plasma calcitonin level (group 1, 1000–1250 pg/ml; group 2, 1000–5000 pg/ml; group 3, 5000–10,000 pg/ml; and group 4, more than 10,000 pg/ml). In the 25 patients in group 1, the MTC was clinically occult and evident only on biochemical testing. Only 1 of these patients had regional lymph node metastases and only 1 patient had an elevated stimulated plasma calcitonin level postoperatively, indicating residual disease. None of the patients had distant metastases and none died during the period of observation. In the group 4 patients, 13 of the 23 had metastases to regional lymph nodes and 14 had biochemical evidence of residual disease.[1090] The only patients who had distant metastatic disease and succumbed to disease were in group 4.[1090]

With the widespread availability of reliable radioimmunoassays for calcitonin, a patient can be easily followed postoperatively. Detection of an elevated basal plasma calcitonin level, or the finding of an abnormal response to calcium and pentagastrin, indicates recurrent or persistent disease. The best strategy for patients with metastatic MTC is unclear. Radioactive iodine ablation, thyroid suppression, and radiation therapy have not been helpful. MTC is relatively insensitive to chemotherapy. Because of the indolent nature of the tumor, most physicians do not treat metastatic disease aggressively.

The 10-year survival of MTC is about 80% to 90%. Aggressive surgical resection has been used to control recurrent MTC locally because it is the only known effective therapy. In patients with MEN-IIa, the MTC may be well tolerated. The average life expectancy of patients with MTC and MEN-IIa is more than 50 years.[1093] The best therapy for familial MTC is early diagnosis and complete resection of intrathyroidal disease at initial surgery. Ablation of extrathyroidal disease when detected as persistent or current elevations of plasma calcitonin levels after total thyroidectomy requires the development of effective systemic adjuvant treatment (see Management of Medullary Thyroid Carcinoma).

REFERENCES

1. Schwartz TB. Benign metastases from thyroid malignancies. Lancet 1986;733.
2. Robbins J, Merino MJ, Boice JD Jr, et al. Thyroid cancer: A lethal endocrine neoplasm. Ann Intern Med 1991;115:133.
3. Silverberg E, Boring CC, Squires TS. Cancer Statistics. CA 1990;40:9.

4. Cancer Statistics Review. A report on the status of cancer control: 1973–1986. Cancer Statistics Review I-45, 1989.

5. Joensuu H, Klemi PJ, Paul R, Tuominen J. Survival and prognostic factors in thyroid carcinoma. Acta Radiol Oncol 1986;25:243.

6. Cady B, Rossi R, Silverman M, Wool M. Further evidence of the validity of risk group definition in differentiated thyroid carcinoma. Surgery 1985;98:1171.

7. Akslen LA, Haldorsen T, Thoresen SO, Glattre A. Survival and causes of death in thyroid cancer: A population-based study of 2479 cases from Norway. Cancer Res 1991;51:1234.

8. Hoie J, Stenwig AE, Kullmann G, Lindegaard N. Distant metastases in papillary thyroid cancer. Cancer 1988;61:1.

9. Schelfhont LJDM, Creutzberg CL, Hamming JF, et al. Multivariate analysis of survival in differentiated thyroid cancer: The prognostic significance of the age factor. Eur J Cancer Clin Oncol 1988;24:331.

10. Simpson WJ, McKinney SE, Carruthers JS, Gospodarowicz MK, Sutcliffe SB, Panzarella T. Papillary and follicular thyroid cancer. Am J Med 1987;83:479.

11. Rossi RL, Cady B, Silverman ML, et al. Surgically incurable well-differentiated thyroid carcinoma. Arch Surg 1988;123:569.

12. Schindler AM, van Melle G, Evequoz B, Scazziga B. Prognostic factors in papillary carcinoma of the thyroid. Cancer 1991;68:324.

13. Cady B. Papillary carcinoma of the thyroid. Semin Surg Oncol 1991;7:81.

14. Mueller-Gaertner HW, Grzac HT, Rehpenning W. Prognostic indices for tumor relapse and tumor mortality in follicular thyroid carcinoma. Cancer 1991;67:1903.

15. Sampson RJ, Key CF, Buncher CR, Lijima S. Thyroid carcinoma in Hiroshima and Nagasaki: Prevalence of thyhroid carcinoma at autopsy. JAMA 1969;209:65.

16. Bondeson L, Ljungberg O. Occult thyroid carcinoma at autopsy in Malmo, Sweden. Cancer 1981;47:319.

17. Sampson RJ, Woolner LB, Bahn RC, et al. Occult thyroid carcinoma in Olmsted County, Minnesota: Prevalence at autopsy compared with that in Hiroshima and Nagasaki. Cancer 1975;36:1095.

18. Fukunaga FH, Yatani R. Geographic pathology of occult thyroid carcinoma. Cancer 1975;366:1095.

19. McConahey WM, Hay ID, Woolner LB, van Heerden JA, Taylor WF. Papillary thyroid cancer treated at the Mayo Clinic 1946 through 1970: Initial manifestations, pathologic findings, therapy and outcome. Mayo Clin Proc 1986;61:968.

20. Allo MD, Christianson W, Koivunen D. Not all "occult" papillary carcinomas are "minimal." Surgery 1988;104:971.

21. Meisner WA. Tumors of the thyroid gland. In: Atlas of tumor pathology. Washington, DC: Armed Forces Institute of Pathology, 1984 (monograph).

22. Rallison ML, Dobyns BM, Keating FR, et al. Thyroid nodularity in children. JAMA 1975;233:1069.

23. Rojeski MT, Gharib H. Nodular thyroid disease. N Engl J Med 1985;313:428.

24. Shimaoka K, Sokal JE. Differentiation of benign and malignant thyroid nodules by scintiscan. Arch Intern Med 1974;114:36.

25. Groesbeck HP. Evaluation of routine scintiscanning of nontoxic thyroid nodules 1: The preoperative diagnosis of thyroid carcinoma. Cancer 1959;12:1.

26. Liechty RD, Stoffel PT, Zimmerman DE, Silverberg SG. Solitary thyroid nodules. Arch Surg 1977;112:59.

27. Messaris G, Kyriakou K, Vasilopoulos P, Tountas C. The single thyroid nodule and carcinoma. Br J Surg 1974;661:943.

28. DeGroot LJ, Reilly M, Pinnameneni K, Refetoff S. Retrospective and prospective study of radiation-induced thyroid disease. Am J Med 1983;74:852.

29. American Joint Committee on Cancer. Manual for staging of cancer. Philadelphia: JB Lippincott, 1988.

30. Clark RL, White EC, Russell WO. Total thyroidectomy for cancer of the thyroid: Significance of intraglandular dissemination. Ann Surg 1959;149:858.

31. LoGerfo P, Chabot J, Gazetas P. The intraoperative incidence of detectable bilateral and multicentric disease in papillary cancer of the thyroid. Surgery 1990;108:958.

32. Torres J, Volpato RD, Power EG, et al. Thyroid cancer survival in 148 cases followed for 10 years or more. Cancer 1985;566:2298.

33. Cady B, Sedgwick E, Meisner WA, et al. Changing clinical pathologic therapeutic and surgical patterns in differentiated thyroid carcinoma. Ann Surg 1980;192:701.

34. Ordonez NG, El-Naggar AK, Hickey RC, Samaan NA. Anaplastic thyroid carcinoma. Am J Clin Pathol 1991;96:15.

35. Mazzaferi FL. Papillary thyroid carcinoma: Factors influencing prognosis and current therapy. Semin Oncol 1987;14:315.

36. Merino MJ. Variant forms of thyroid carcinoma. In: Robbins J, moderator. Thyroid cancer: A lethal endocrine neoplasm. Ann Intern Med 1991;115:133.

37. Sampson RJ. Thyroid carcinoma. Arch Pathol Lab Med 1978;102:270.

38. Patchefsky AS, Keller IB, Mansfield CM. Solitary vertebral column metastasis from occult sclerosing carcinoma of the thyroid gland. Am J Clin Path 1970;53:596.

39. Merino MJ, Kennedy SM, Norton JA, Robbins J. Pleural involvement by metastatic thyroid carcinoma "tall cell variant": An unusual occurrence. Surg Pathol 1990;3:59.

40. Johnson TL, Lloyd RV, Thompson NW, Beierwaltes WH, Sisson JC. Prognostic implications of the tall cell variant of papillary thyroid carcinoma. Am J Surg Pathol 1988;12:22.

41. Sobrinho-Simoes MA, Nesland JM, Johannessen JV. Columnar-cell carcinoma: Another variant of poorly differentiated carcinoma of the thyroid. Am J Clin Pathol 1988;89:264.

42. Brennan MD, Bergstralh EJ, van Heerden JA, McConahey WM. Follicular thyroid cancer treated at the Mayo Clinic: 1946 through 1970. Initial manifestations, pathologic findings, therapy and outcome. Mayo Clin Proc 1991;66:11.

43. Schmidt RJ, Wang CA. Encapsulated follicular carcinoma of the thyroid: Diagnosis, treatment and results. Surgery 1986;100:1068.

44. Lang W, Choritz H, Hundeshagen H. Risk factors in follicular thyroid carcinoma. Am J Surg Pathol 1986;10:246.

45. Thompson NW, Dunn EL, Batsakis JG, Nishiyama RH. Hurthle cell lesions of the thyroid gland. Surg Gynecol Obstet 1974;139:555.

46. Gundry SR, Burney RE, Thompson NW, Lloyd R. Total thyroidectomy for Hurthle Cell Neoplasm of the thyroid. Arch Surg 1983;118:529.

47. Heppe H, Armin A, Calandra DB, et al. Hurthle cell tumors of the thyroid gland. Surgery 1985;98:1162.

48. Arganini M, Behar R, Wu TC, et al. Hurthle cell tumors: A twenty-five year experience. Surgery 1986;100:1108.

49. Carter WB, Taylor RL, Kao PC, Heath H. Determination of plasma calcitonin-gene related peptide concentrations by a new immunochemiluminometric assay in normal persons and patients with medullary thyroid carcinoma and other neuroendocrine tumors. J Clin Endocrinol Met 1991;72:327.

50. Poston GJ, Seitz PK, Townsend CM Jr, et al. Calcitonin gene-related peptide: Possible tumor marker for medullary thyroid cancer. Surgery 1987;102:1–49.

51. Alexander HR, Norton JA. Biology and management of medullary thyroid carcinoma of the parafollicular cells. In: Robbins J, moderator. Thyroid cancer: A lethal endocrine neoplasm. Ann Intern Med 1991;115:133.

52. Babu VR, Van Dyke DL, Jackson CE. Chromosome 20 deletion in human multiple endocrine neoplasias types 2A and 2B: A double blind study. Proc Natl Acad Sci USA 1985;84:2525.

53. Tanaka K, Baylin SB, Nelkin BD, Testa JR. Cytogenetic studies of a human medullary thyroid carcinoma cell line. Cancer Genet Cytogenet 1987;25:27.

54. Nelkin BD, deBustros AC, Mabry M, Baylin SB. The molecular biology of medullary thyroid carcinoma. JAMA 1989;261:3130.

55. Lairmore TC, Howe JR, Korte JA, et al. Familial medullary thyroid carcinoma and multiple endocrine neoplasia type 2B map to the same region of chromosome 10 as multiple endocrine neoplasia type 2A. Genomics 1991;9:181.

56. Mathew GGP, Chin KS, Easton DF, et al. A linked genetic marker for multiple endocrine neoplasia type 2A on chromosome 10. Nature 1987;328:527.

57. Simpson NE, Kidd KK, Goodfellow PJ, et al. Assignment of multiple endocrine neoplasia type 2A to chromosome 10 by linkage. Nature 1987;328:528.

58. Jackson CE, Norum RA, O'Neal LW, Nikolai TF, DeLaney JP. Linkage between MEN 2B and chromosome 10 markers linked to MEN 2A. Am J Hum Genet [Abstract] 1988;43:147.

59. Zajac JD, Penschow J, Mason T, et al. Identification of calcitonin and calcitonin gene-related peptide messenger ribonucleic acid in medullary thyroid carcinomas by hybridization histochemistry. J Clin Endocrinol Metab 1986;62:1037.

60. Wells SA Jr, Ontjes DA, Cooper CW, et al. The early diagnosis of medullary carcinoma of the thyroid gland in patients with multiple endocrine neoplasia type II. Ann Surg 1975;182:362.

61. Gagel RF, Tashjian AH Jr, Cummings T, et al. The clinical outcome of prospective screening for multiple endocrine neoplasia type 2a. N Engl J Med 1988;318:478.

62. Matthew CGP, Easton DF, Nakamura Y, Ponder BAJ. MEN2a International Collaborative Group. Presymptomatic screening for multiple endocrine neoplasia type 2A with linked DNA markers. Lancet 1991;337:7.

63. Sobol H, Narod SA, Assouline D, Lenon GM (GETC). Genetic screening of endocrine tumour syndromes with DNA probes: The example of medullary thyroid carcinoma. Horm Res 1989;32:34.

64. Wells SA Jr. Multiple endocrine neoplasia type II. Recent Results Cancer Res 1990;118:70.

65. Cance WG, Wells SA Jr. Multiple endocrine neoplasia type IIa. Curr Probl Surg 1985;22:1.

66. Van Heerden JA, Grant CS, Gharib H, Hay ID, Ilstrup DM. Long-term course of patients with persistent hypercalcitonemia after apparent curative primary surgery for medullary thyroid carcinoma. Ann Surg 1990;212:395.

67. Norton JA, Fromme LC, Farrell RE, Wells SA Jr. Multiple endocrine neoplasia type 2b: The most aggressive form of medullary thyroid carcinoma. Surg Clin North Am 1979;59:109.

68. Rossi R, Cady B, Meissner WA, et al. Nonfamilial medullary thyroid carcinoma. Am J Surg 1980;139:554.

69. Block MA, Jackson CE, Greenawald KA, et al. Clinical characteristics distinguishing hereditary from sporadic medullary thyroid carcinoma. Arch Surg 1980;115:142.

70. LiVolsi VA, Brooks JJ, Arendash-Durand B. Anaplastic thyroid tumors immunohistology. Am J Clin Pathol 1987;87:434.

71. Venkatesh YSS, Ordonez NG, Schultz PN, Hickey RC, Goepfert H, Samoan NA. Anaplastic carcinoma of the thyroid. Cancer 1990;66:321.

72. Kruseman ACN, Bosman FT, Henegouw JCV, et al. Medullary differentiation of anaplastic thyroid carcinoma. Am J Clin Pathol 1982;77:541.

73. Carcangiu ML, Steeper T, Zampi G, Rosai J. Anaplastic thyroid carcinoma. Am J Clin Pathol 1985;83:135.

74. Krisch K, Holzner JH, Kokoschkar J. Hemangioendothelioma of the thyroid gland: True endothelioma or anaplastic carcinoma? Pathol Res Pract 1980;170:230.

75. Aldinger KA, Samaan NA, Ibanez M, Hill CS. Anaplastic carcinoma of the thyroid. Cancer 1978;41:2267.

76. Duffy BJ Jr, Fitzgerald PJ. Cancer of the thyroid in children: A report of 28 cases. J Clin Endocrinol Metab 1950;10:1296.

77. Schneider AB, Shore-Freedman E, Ryo UY, et al. Radiation-induced tumors of the head and neck following childhood irradiation. Medicine 1985;64:1.

78. Ron E, Kleinerman RA, Boice JD Jr, LiVolsi VA, Flannery JT, Fraumeni JF Jr. A population-based case-control study of thyroid cancer. JNCI 1987;79:1.

79. Boice JD Jr, Ron E. Epidemiology of radiation-induced thyroid cancer. Ann Intern Med 1991;115:135.

80. Hamilton TE, van Belle G, LoGerfo JP. Thyroid neoplasia in Marshall islanders exposed to nuclear fallout. JAMA 1987;258:629.

81. Holm LE, Dahlquist I, Israelsson A, et al. Malignant thyroid tumors after [131]iodine therapy. N Engl J Med 1980;303:188.

82. Anspaugh LR, Catlin RJ, Goldman M. The global impact of Chernobyl Reactor Accident. Science 1988;242:1513.

83. Wang Z, Boice JD Jr, Wei L, et al. Thyroid nodularity and chromosome aberrations among women in areas of high background radiation in China. JNCI 1990;82:478.

84. Pottern LM, Kaplan MM, Larsen PR, et al. Thyroid nodularity after childhood irradiation for lymphoid hyperplasia: A comparison of questionnaire and clinical findings. J Clin Epidemiol 1990;43:449.

85. Larsen PR, Conrad RA, Knudsen KD, et al. Thyroid hypofunction after exposure to fallout from a hydrogen bomb explosion. JAMA 1982;247:1571.

86. Harach HR, Escalant DA, Onatavia A, et al. Thyroid cancer and thyroiditis in an endemic goiter region before and after iodine prophylaxis. Acta Endocrinol 1985;108:55.

87. William ED. The aetiology of thyroid tumours. Clin Endocrinol Metab 1979;8:193.

88. Heitz P, Moser H, Staub JJ. Thyroid cancer. Cancer 1976;37:2329.

89. Kapp DS, Li Volsi VA, Sanders MM. Anaplastic carcinoma following well-differentiated thyroid cancer: Etiological considerations. Yale J Biol Med 1982;55:521.

90. Deaconson TF, Wilson SD, Cerletty JM, Komorowski RA. Total or near total thyroidectomy versus limited resection for radiation-associated thyroid nodules: A twelve-year follow-up of patients in a thyroid screening program. Surgery 1986;100:1116.

91. Schneider AB, Recant W, Pinsky SM, et al. Radiation-induced thyroid cancer. Ann Intern Med 1986;105:405.

92. Chong GC, Beahrs OH, Sizemore GW, Woolner LH. Medullary carcinoma of the thyroid gland. Cancer 1975;35:695.

93. Farndon JR, Leight GS, Dilley WG, et al. Familial medullary thyroid carcinoma without associated endocrinopathies: A distinct clinical entity. Br J Surg 1986;73:278.

94. Phade V. R, Lawrence WR, Max MH. Familial papillary carcinoma of the thyroid. Arch Surg 1981;116:836.

95. Lote K, Andersen A, Nordal E, Brennhovd IO. Familial occurrence of papillary thyroid carcinoma. Cancer 1980;46:1291.

96. Namba H, Rubin SA, Fagis JA. Point mutations of ras oncogenes are an early event in thyroid tumorigenesis. Mol Endocrinol 1990;4:1474.

97. Lemoine NR, Mayall ES, Wyllie FS, et al. High frequency of ras oncogene activation in all stages of human thyroid tumorigenesis. Oncogene 1989;4:159.

98. Namba H, Gutman RA, Matsuo K, Alvarez A, Fagin JA. H-ras protooncogene mutations in human thyroid neoplasms. J Clin Endocrinol Metab 1988;48:4459.

99. Lemoine NR, Mayall ES, Wyllie FS, et al. Activated ras oncogenes in human thyroid cancers. Cancer Res 1988;48:4459.

100. Karga H, Lee JK, Vickery AL Jr, Thor A, Guz RD, Jameson JL. Ras oncogene mutations in benign and malignant thyroid neoplasms. J Clin Endocrinol Metab 1991;73:832.

101. Wright PA, Williams ED, Lemoine NR, Wynford-Thomas D. Radiation-associated and spontaneous human thyroid carcinomas show a different pattern of ras oncogene mutation. Oncogene 1991;6:471.

102. Fusco A, Grieco M, Santoro M, et al. A new oncogene in human thyroid papillary carcinomas and their lymph-nodal metastases. Nature 1987;328:170.

103. Bongarzone I, Pierotti MA, Monzini N, et al. High frequency of activation of tyrosine kinase oncogenes in human papillary thyroid carcinoma. Oncogene 1989;4:1457.

104. Grieco M, Santoro M, Berlingieri MT, et al. PTC is a novel rearranged form of the ret proto-oncogene and is frequently detected in vivo in human papillary thyroid carcinoids. Cell 1990;60:557.

105. Kober F, Heiss A, Keminger K, Depisch D. Chemotherapy of highly malignant thyroid tumors. Wien Klin Wochenschr 1990;102:274.

106. Jackson IMD, Cobb WE. Disorders of the thyroid. In: Kohler PO, ed. Clinical endocrinology. New York: John Wiley, 1986;73–165.

107. Mazzaferri EL, Young RL, Oertel JE. Papillary thyroid carcinoma: The impact of therapy in 576 patients. Medicine 1977;56:171.

108. Van Herle AJ, Uller RP. Elevated serum thyroglobulin: A marker of metastases in differentiated thyroid carcinoma. J Clin Invest 1975;56:272.

109. Schneider AB, Shore-Freedman E, Ryo UY, et al. Prospective serum thyroglobulin measurements in assessing the risk of developing thyroid nodules in patients exposed to childhood neck irradiation. J Clin Endocrinol Metab 1985;661:547.

110. Wells SA Jr, Haagensen DE Jr, Linehan WM, et al. The detection of elevated plasma levels of carcinoembryonic antigen in patients with suspected or established medullary thyroid carcinoma. Cancer 1978;42:1498.

111. Wells SA Jr, Dilley WG, Farndon JA, et al. Early diagnosis and treatment of medullary thyroid carcinoma. Arch Intern Med 1985;145:1248.

112. Clark OH. TSH suppression in the management of thyroid nodules and thyroid cancer. World J Surg 1981;5:39.

113. Field JB, Bloom G, Chou MCY, et al. Effects of thyroid-stimulating hormone on human thyroid carcinoma and adjacent normal tissue. J Clin Endocrinol Metab 1978;47:1052.

114. Gharib H, James FM, Charkmeau JW, Naessens JM, Offord KP, Gorman CA. Suppressive therapy with levothyroxine for solitary thyroid nodules. N Engl J Med 1987;317:70.

115. Getaz EP, Shimaoka K, Razack M, et al. Suppressive therapy for post-irradiation thyroid nodules. Can J Surg 1980;23:558.

116. Hill LD, Beebe HG, Hipp R, Jones HW. Thyroid suppression. Arch Surg 1974;108:403.

117. Blum M, Rothschild M. Improved nonoperative diagnosis of the solitary "cold" thyroid nodule: Surgical selection based on risk factors and three months of suppression. JAMA 1980;243:242.

118. Gershengorn MC, McClung MR, Chu EW, et al. Fine needle aspiration cytology in the preoperative diagnosis of thyroid nodules. Ann Intern Med 1977;87:265.

119. Schick RM. Thyroid nodules. N Engl J Med [Letter] 1986;314:452.

120. Parker TW, Mettler FA Jr, Christie JH, Williams AG. Radionuclide thyroid studies: A survey of practice in the United States in 1981. Radiology 1984;150:547.

121. Dobyns BM, Maloof F. The study and treatment of 119 cases of carcinoma of thyroid with radioactive iodine. J Clin Endocrinol Metab 1951;11:1323.

122. Ashcraft MW, Van Herle AJ. Management of thyroid nodules I. History, physical examination, blood tests, x-ray tests and ultrasonograph. Head Neck Surg 1981;3:216.

123. Ashcraft MW, Van Herle AJ. Management of thyroid nodules II. Scanning techniques, thyroid suppressive therapy, and fine needle aspiration. Head Neck Surg 1981;3:297.

124. Hamburger JI. Thyroid nodules. N Engl J Med [Letter] 1986;314:452.

125. Miller JM, Hamburger JI. The thyroid scintigram. One hot nodule. Radiology 1965;84:66.

126. Arnstein NB, Juni JE, Sisson JC, et al. Recurrent medullary carcinoma of the thyroid demonstrated by thallium-201 scintigraphy. J Nucl Med 1986;27:1564.

127. Skibber JM, Reynolds JC, Spiegel AM, et al. Computerized technetium/thallium scan and parathyroid reoperation. Surgery 1985;98:1077.

128. Asari AN, Siegel ME, DeQuattro V, Gazarian LH. Imaging of medullary thyroid carcinoma and hyperfunctioning adrenal medulla using Iodine-131 metaiodobenzylguanidine. J Nucl Med 1986;27:1858.

129. Sone T, Fukunaga M, Otsuka N, et al. Metastatic medullary thyroid cancer: Localization with iodine-131 metaiodobenzylguanidine. J Nucl Med 1985;26:604.

130. Zanin DFA, van Dongen A, Hoefnagel CA, Bruning PF. Radioimmunoscintigraphy using iodine-131-anti-CEA monoclonal antibodies and thallium-201 scintigraphy in medullary thyroid carcinoma: A case report. J Nucl Med 1990;31:1854.

131. Edington HD, Watson CG, Levine G, Tauxe WN, Yousem SA, Unger M, Kowal CD. Radioimmunoimaging of metastatic medullary carcinoma of the thyroid gland using an indium-111-labelled monoclonal antibody to CEA. Surgery 1988;104:1004.

132. Mojiminyi OA, Udelsman R, Soper ND, Shepstone BJ, Dudley NE. Pentavalent Tc99m DMSA scintigraphy: Prospective evaluation of its role in the management of patients with medullary carcinoma of the thyroid. Clin Nucl Med 1991;16:259.

133. Udelsman R, Mojiminyi OA, Soper ND, Buley ID, et al. Medullary carcinoma of the thyroid: Management of persistent hypercalcitonemia utilizing ^{99m}Tc dimercaptosuccinic acid scintigraphy. Br J Surg 1989;76:1278.

134. Stockwell R, Davidoff F. Radiation-induced thyroid carcinoma. Ann Intern Med [Letter] 1987;106:637.

135. Nassani SN, Bard R. Evaluation of solid thyroid neoplasms by gray scale and real-time ultrasonography: The halo sign. Ultrasound Med Biol 1978;4:323.

136. Simeone JF, Daniels GH, Hall DA, et al. Sonography in the follow-up of 100 patients with thyroid carcinoma. AJR 1987;148:45.

137. Schwerk WB, Grun R, Wahl R. Ultrasound diagnosis of c-cell carcinoma of the thyroid. Cancer 1985;55:624.

138. Van Herle AJ, Rich P, Ljung BME, et al. The thyroid nodule. Ann Intern Med 1982;966:221.

139. Hamburger JI, Hamburger SW. Fine needle biopsy of thyroid nodules: Avoiding the pitfalls. New York State J Med 1986;86:241.

140. Walfish PG, Hazani E, Strawbridge HTG, et al. Combined ultrasound and needle aspiration cytology in the assessment and management of hypofunctioning thyroid nodule. Ann Intern Med 1977;87:270.

141. Nishiyama RH, Bigos ST, Goldfarb WB, et al. The efficacy of simultaneous fine-needle aspiration and large-needle biopsy of the thyroid gland. Surgery 1986;100:1133.

142. Hamburger JI, Miller JM, Kini SR. Lymphoma of the thyroid. Ann Intern Med 1983;99:685.

143. Broughan TA, Esselstyn CB. Large-needle biopsy: Still necessary. Surgery 1986;100:1138.

144. Schwartz AE, Nieburgs HE, Davies TF, et al. The place of fine needle biopsy in the diagnosis of nodules of the thyroid. Surg Gynecol Obstet 1982;155:54.

145. Cusick EL, MacIntosh CA, Krukowski Z, Williams VMM, Ewen SWB, Matheson NA. Management of isolated thyroid swellings: A prospective six year study of fine needle aspiration cytology in diagnosis. Br Med J 1990;301:318.

146. Boey J, Hsu C, Collins RJ. False-negative errors in fine-needle biopsy of dominant thyroid nodules: A prospective follow-up study. World J Surg 1986;10:623.

147. Block M. A, Dailey GE, Robb JA. Thyroid nodules indeterminant by needle biopsy. Am J Surg 1983;146:72.

148. Hamburger JI. Consistency of sequential needle biopsy findings for thyroid nodules, management implications. Arch Intern Med 1987;147:97.

149. Hamburger JI, Hamburger SW. Declining role of frozen section in surgical planning for thyroid nodules. Surgery 1985;98:307.

150. Miller JM, Hamburger JI, Kini SR. The impact of needle biopsy on the preoperative diagnosis of thyroid nodules. Henry Ford Hosp Med J 1980;28:145.

151. Hamburger B, Gharib H, Melton LJ III. Fine needle aspiration biopsy of thyroid nodules: Impact on thyroid practice and cost of care. Am J Med 1982;73:381.

152. McConahey WM, Hay ID, Woolner LB, et al. Papillary thyroid cancer treated at the Mayo Clinic, 1946 through 1970: Initial manifestations, pathologic findings, therapy and outcome. Mayo Clin Proc 1986;61:978.

153. Hawkins F, Bellido D, Bernal C, et al. Fine needle aspiration biopsy in the diagnosis of thyroid cancer and thyroid disease. Cancer 1987;59:1206.

154. Gharib H, Boellner JR, Zinsmeister AR, et al. Fine needle aspiration biopsy of the thyroid: The problem of suspicious cytologic findings. Ann Intern Med 1984;101:25.

155. Boon ME, Lowhagen T, Cardozo PL, et al. Computation of preoperative diagnosis probability for follicular adenoma and carcinoma of the thyroid on aspiration smears. Anal Quant Cytol 1982;4:1.

156. Luck JB, Mumaw VR, Frable WJ. Fine needle aspiration biopsy of the thyroid: Differential diagnosis by videoplan image analysis. Acta Cytol 1982;26:793.

157. Sprenger E, Lawhagen T, Vogt-Schaden M. Differential diagnosis between follicular adenoma and follicular carcinoma of the thyroid by nuclear DNA determination. Acta Cytol 1977;21:528.

158. Cusick EL, Ewen SWB, Krukowski ZH, Matheson NA. DNA aneuploidy in follicular thyroid neoplasia. Br J Surg 1991;78:94.

159. Hamburger JI. Consistency of sequential needle biopsy findings for thyroid nodules. Arch Intern Med 1987;147:97.

160. Grant CS, Hay ID, Gough IR, McCarthy PM, Goellner JR. Long-term follow-up of patients with benign thyroid fine-needle aspiration cytologic diagnoses. Surgery 1989;106:980.

161. Layfield LJ, Mohrmann RL, Kopald KH, Guiliano AE. Use of aspiration cytology and frozen section examination for management of benign and malignant thyroid nodules. Cancer 1991;68:130.

162. Shaha AR, DiMaio T, Webber C, Jaffe BMJ. Intraoperative decision making during thyroid surgery based on the results of preoperative needle biopsy and frozen section. Surgery 1990;108:964.

163. Rossi R, Cady B, Silverman ML, et al. Current results of conservative surgery for differentiated thyroid carcinoma. World J Surg 1986;10:612.

164. Cohn KH, Backdahl M, Forsslund G, et al. Biologic considerations and operative strategy in papillary thyroid carcinoma: Arguments against the routine performance of total thyroidectomy. Surgery 1984;96:957.

165. Tubiana M, Schlumberger M, Rougier P, et al. Long-term results and prognostic factors in patients with differentiated thyroid carcinoma. Cancer 1985;55:794.

166. Hannequin P, Liehn JC, Delisle MJ. Multifactorial analysis of survival in thyroid cancer. Cancer 1986;58:1749.

167. Brennan MF. Cancer of the endocrine system. In: DeVita VT, Hellman S, Rosenberg SA, eds. Cancer principles and practice of oncology. Philadelphia: JB Lippincott, 1985:1179–1241.

168. Tupchong L, Phil D, Hughes F, Harmer CL. Primary lymphoma of the thyroid: Clinical features, prognostic factors and results of treatment. Int J Radiat Oncol Biol Phys 1986;12:1813.

169. Goldman JM, Goren EN, Cohen MH, et al. Anaplastic thyroid carcinoma: Long-term survival after radical surgery. J Surg Oncol 1980;14:389.

170. Tollefson HR, DeCosse JJ. Papillary carcinoma of the thyroid: Recurrence in the thyroid gland after initial treatment. Am J Surg 1983;1066:728.

171. Van Heerden JA, Groh MA, Grant CS. Early postoperative morbidity after surgical treatment of thyroid carcinoma. Surgery 1986;101:224.

172. Young RL, Mazzaferri EL, Rahe AJ, et al. Pure follicular thyroid carcinoma: Impact of therapy in 214 patients. J Nucl Med 1980;21:735.

173. Harness JK, Thompson NW, McLeod MK, et al. Follicular carcinoma of the thyroid gland: Trends and treatment. Surgery 1984;966:972.

174. Bronner MP, LiVolsi VA. Oxyphilic (Askanazy/Hurthle cell) tumors of the thyroid: Microscopic features predict biologic behavior. Surg Pathol 1988;1:137.

175. Rosen IB, Luk S, Katz I. Hurthle cell tumor behavior: Dilemma and resolution. Surgery 1985;98:777.

176. Cooper DS, Schneyer CR. Follicular and Hurthle cell carcinoma of the thyroid. Endocrinol. Metab Clin North Am 1990;19:577.

177. Flint J, Lloyd RV. Hurthle-cell neoplasms of the thyroid gland. Pathol Annu 1990;577.

178. Kramer JB, Wells SA Jr. Thyroid carcinoma. Adv Surg 1989;22:195.

179. Schneider AB, Shore-Freedman E, Weinstein RA. Radiation-induced thyroid and other head and neck tumors: Occurrence of multiple tumors and analysis of risk factors. J Clin Endocrinol Metab 1986;63:107.

180. Calandra DB, Shah KH, Lawrence A, Paloyan E. Total-thyroidectomy in irradiated patients. Ann Surg 1985;202:356.

181. Deaconess TF, Wilson SD, Cerletty JM, Komorowski RA. Total or near total thyroidectomy versus limited resection for radiation-associated thyroid nodules: A twelve-year follow-up of patients in a thyroid screening program. Surgery 1986;100:1116.

182. DeGroot LJ, Reilly M. Comparison of 30- and 50- mCi doses of Iodine-131 for thyroid ablation. Ann Intern Med 1982;96:51.

183. Bondeson L, Bondeson AG, Ljungberg O, Tibblin S. Oxyphil tumors of the thyroid. Follow-up of 42 cases. Ann Surg 1981;194:677.

184. Brown AP, Greening WP, McCready VR, et al. Radioiodine treatment of metastatic thyroid carcinoma: The Royal Marsden experience. Br J Radiol 1984;57:323.

185. Marocci C, Pacini F, Elisei R, et al. Clinical and biological behavior of bone metastases from differentiated thyroid carcinoma. Surgery 1989;106:960.

186. Leeper RD. Thyroid cancer. Med Clin North Am 1985;669:1079.

187. Ruiz-Garcia J, Ruiz de Almodovar JM, Olea N, Pedraza V. Thyroglobulin as a predictive factor of tumoral recurrence in differentiated thyroid cancer. J Nucl Med 1991;32:395.

188. Rubello D, Girelli ME, Casara D, Piccolo M, Perin A, Busnardo B. Usefulness of the combined antithyroglobulin antibodies and thyroglobulin assay in the follow-up of patients with differentiated thyroid cancer. J Endocrinol Invest 1990;13:737.

189. Robnga G, Fiorentino A, Paserio E, Signore A, Todino V, Tummarello MA, Filesi M, Baschierri I. Can iodine-131 whole-body scan be replaced by thyroglobulin measurement in the post-surgical follow-up of differentiated thyroid carcinoma? J Nucl Med 1990;31:1766.

190. Burmeister LA, deCret RP, Mariash CN. Local reactions to radioiodine in the treatment of thyroid cancer. Am J Med 1991;906:217.

191. Schlumberger M, Tubiana M, De Vathaire F, et al. Long-term results of treatment of 283 patients with lung and bone metastases from differentiated thyroid carcinoma. J Clin Endocrinol Metab 1986;63:9660.

192. Maxon MR, Smith HS. Radioactive ^{131}I in the diagnosis and treatment of metastatic well differentiated thyroid cancer. Endocrinol Metab Clin North Am 1990;19:685.

193. Samaan NA, Schultz PN, Haynie TP, Ordonez NG. Pulmonary metastasis of differentiated thyroid carcinoma: Treatment results in 101 patients. J Clin Endocrinol Metab 1985;665:376.

194. Ahuja S, Ernst H. Chemotherapy of thyroid cancer. J Endocrinol Invest 1987;10:303.

195. Duh QY, Sancho JJ, Greenspan FS, et al. Medullary thyroid carcinoma. Arch Surg 1989;124:1206.

196. Telander RL, Zimmerman D, van Heerden JA, Sizemore GW. Results of early thyroidectomy for medullary thyroid carcinoma in children with multiple endocrine neoplasia type 2. J Pediatr Surg 1986;21:1190.

197. Decker RA, Toyama WM, O'Neal LW, Telander RL, Wells SA Jr. Evaluation of children with multiple endocrine neoplasia type IIb following thyroidectomy. J Pediatr Surg 1990;25:939.

198. Gorman B, Charboneau JW, James EM, et al. Medullary thyroid carcinoma: Role of high-resolution. Ultrasound Radiology 1987;162:147.

199. Tennvall J, Biorklund A, Moller T, et al. Prognostic factors of papillary, follicular and medullary carcinoma of the thyroid gland. Acta Radiologica Oncol 1985;24:17.

200. Norton JA, Doppman JL, Brennan MF. Localization and resection of clinically inapparent medullary carcinoma of the thyroid. Surgery 1980;87:616.

201. Tisell LE, Hansson G, Jansson S, Salander H. Reoperation in the treatment of asymptomatic metastasizing medullary thyroid carcinoma. Surgery 1986;99:60.

202. Tisell LE, Hansson S. Recent results of reoperative surgery in medullary carcinoma of the thyroid. Wien Klin Wochenschr 1988;100:347.

203. Talpos GB, Jackson CB, Froelich JW, et al. Localization of residual medullary thyroid cancer by thallium/technetium scintigraphy. Surgery 1985;98:1189.

204. Gottlieb JA, Hill CS Jr. Chemotherapy of thyroid cancer with adriamycin: Experience with 30 patients. N Engl J Med 1974;290:193.

205. Stepanas AV, Samaan NA, Hill CS Jr, Hickey RC. Medullary thyroid carinoma: Importance of serial serum calcitonin measurement. Cancer 1979;43:825.

206. Porter AT, Ostrowski MJ. Medullary carcinoma of the thyroid treated by low-dose adriamycin. Brit J of Clin Pract 1990;44:517.

207. Petursson SR. Metastatic medullary thyroid carcinoma, complete response to combination chemotherapy with dacarbazine and 5-fluorouracil. Cancer 1988;62:1899.

208. Tubiana M, Haddad E, Schlumberger M, et al. External radiotherapy in thyroid cancers. Cancer 1985;55:2062.

209. Cox TM, Fagan EA, Hillward CJ, et al. Role of calcitonin in diarrhea associated with medullary carcinoma of the thyroid. Gut 1979;20:629.

210. Jerkins TW, Sacks HS, O'Dorisio TM, et al. Medullary carcinoma of the thyroid, pancreatic nesidioblastosis and microadenosis, and pancreatic polypeptide hypersecretion: A new association and clinical and hormonal responses to long-acting somatostatin analog SMS 201-995. J Clin Endocrinol Metab 1987;64:1313.

211. Mahler C, Verhelst J, DeLonueville M, Harris A. Long-term treatment of metastatic medullary thyroid carcinoma with the somatostatin analogue octreotide. Clin Endocrinol 1990;33:261.

212. Gröhn P, Kumpulainen E, Jakobsson M. Response of medullary thyroid cancer to low-dose alpha-interferon therapy. Acta Oncol 1990;29:950.

213. Nel CJC, van Heerden JA, Goellner JR, et al. Anaplastic carcinoma of the thyroid: A clinicopathologic study of 82 cases. Mayo Clin Proc 1985;60:51.

214. Kim JH, Leeper RD. Treatment of anaplastic giant and spindle cell carcinoma of the thyroid gland with combination adriamycin and radiation therapy a new approach. Cancer 1983;52:954.

215. Kim JH, Leeper RD. Treatment of locally advanced thyroid carcinoma with combination doxorubicin and radiation therapy. Cancer 1987;60:2372.

216. Kim JH, Leeper RD. Combination adriamycin and radiation therapy for locally advanced carcinoma of the thyroid gland. Int J Radiat Oncol Biol Phys 1983;9:565.

217. Wilford MR, Chertow BS, Lepanto PB, Leidy JW Jr. Dramatic response of follicular thyroid carcinoma with superior vena cava syndrome and tracheal obstruction to external beam radiotherapy. Am J Med 1991;90:753.

218. Williams SD, Birch R, Einhorn D. Phase II evaluation of doxorubicin plus cisplatin in advanced thyroid cancer: A Southeastern Cancer Study Group trial. Cancer Treat Rep 1986;70:405.

219. Shimaoka K, Schoenfeld DA, DeWys WD, et al. A randomized trial of doxorubicin versus doxorubicin plus cisplatin in patients with advanced thyroid carcinoma. Cancer 1985;566:2155.

220. Bukowski RM, Brown L, Weick JK, et al. Combination chemotherapy of metastatic thyroid cancer. Am J Clin Oncol 1983;6:579.

221. Christensson T. Hyperparathyroidism and radiation therapy. Ann Intern Med 1978;89:216.

222. Norton JA, Brennan MF, Saxe AW, et al. Intraoperative urinary cyclic adenosine monophosphate as a guide to successful reoperative parathyroidectomy. Ann Surg 1984;200:389.

223. Mallette LE, Bilizikian JP, Ketcham AS, Aurbach GD. Parathyroid carcinoma in familial hyperparathyroidism. Am J Med 1974;57:642.

224. Dinnen JS, Greenwood RH, Jones JH, et al. Parathyroid carcinoma in familial hyperparathyroidism. J Clin Pathol 1977;30:966.

225. Schantz A, Castleman B. Parathyroid carcinoma a study of 70 cases. Cancer 1973;31:6600.

226. Levin KE, Galante M, Clark OH. Parathyroid carcinoma versus parathyroid adenoma in patients with profound hypercalcemia. Surgery 1987;101:649.

227. Cohn K, Silverman M, Corrado J, Sedgewick C. Parathyroid carcinoma: The Lahey Clinic experience. Surgery 1985;98:1095.

228. Wang C, Gaz RD. Natural history of parathyroid carcinoma. Diagnosis, treatment, and results. Am J Surg 1985;149:522.

229. Shane E, Bilezikian JP. Parathyroid carcinoma: A review of 62 patients. Endocr Rev 1982;3:218.

230. Gutter RD, Maier H. Carcinoma of the parathyroid. Arch Intern Med 1972;130:413.

231. Bukowski RM, Sheeler L, Cunningham J, Esselstyn C. Successful combination chemotherapy for metastatic parathyroid carcinoma. Arch Intern Med 1984;144:399.

232. Calandra DB, Chejfec G, Foy BK, et al. Parathyroid carcinoma: Biochemical and pathologic response to DTIC. Surgery 1984;96:1132.

233. Flye MW, Brennan MF. Surgical resection of metastatic parathyroid carcinoma. Ann Surg 1981;193:425.

234. Warrell RP Jr, Israel R, Frisone M, Snyder T, Gaynor JJ, Bockman RS. Gallium nitrate for acute treatment of cancer-related hypercalcemia a randomized, double-blind comparison to calcitonin. Ann Intern Med 1988;108:669.

235. Singer FR, Ritch PS, Lad TE, Ringenberg QS, et al. Treatment of hypercalcemia of malignancy with intravenous etidronate. Arch Intern Med 1991;151:471.

236. Page DL, DeLellis RA, Hough AJ. Tumors of the adrenal. In: Atlas of tumor pathology. Washington, DC: Armed Forces Institute of Pathology, 1986 (monograph).

237. Travis WD, Tsokos M, Doppman JL, et al. Primary pigmented nodular adrenocortical disease. Am J Surg Pathol 1989;13:921.

238. Schweizer-Cagrianut M, Salomon F, Hedinger E. Primary adrenocortical nodular dysplasia with cardiac myxomas. Virchows Arch [A] 1982;397:183.

239. Hough AJ, Hollifield JW, Page DL, Hartmann WH. Diagnostic factors in adrenal cortical tumors. Am J Clin Pathol 1979;72:390.

240. Hutter AM Jr, Kayhoe DE. Adrenal cortical carcinoma. Am J Med 1966;4:572.

241. National Cancer Institute Monograph. Third national cancer surgery: incidence data (DHEW publication NIH75-787). Bethesda, MD: National Cancer Institute, 1975:41.

242. Lynch HT, Katz DA, Bogard PJ, Lynch JF. The sarcoma, breast cancer, lung cancer, and adrenocortical carcinoma syndrome revisited. Am J Dis Child 1985;139:134.

243. Limon J, Dal Cin P, Kakati S, et al. Cytogenetic findings in a primary adrenocortical carcinoma. Cancer Genet Cytogenet 1987;266:271.

244. Yano T, Linehan M, Anglard P, et al. Genetic changes in human adrenocortical carcinomas. JNCI 1989;81:518.

245. Henry I, Grandjovans S, Couillin P, et al. Tumor-specific loss of 11 p 15.5 alleles in del 11 p 13 Wilms tumor and in familial adrenocortical carcinoma. Proc Natl Acad Sci USA 1989;86:3247.

246. Wick MR, Cherwitz DL, McGlennen RC, Dehner LP. Adrenocortical carcinoma, an immunohistochemical comparison with renal cell carcinoma. Am J Pathol 1986;122:343.

247. Weiss LM. Comparative histologic study of 43 metastasizing and nonmetastasizing adrenocortical tumors. Am J Surg Pathol 1984;8:163.

248. Weiss LM, Medeiros LJ, Vickery AL. Pathologic features of prognostic significance in adrenocortical carcinoma. Am J Surg Pathol 1989;13:202.

249. Hosaka Y, Rainwater LM, Grant CS, et al. Adrenocortical carcinoma: Nuclear deoxyribonucleic acid ploidy studied by flow cytometry. Surgery 1987;102:1027.

250. O'Hare MJ, Monaghan P, Neville AM. The pathology of adrenocortical neoplasia: A correlated structural and functional approach to the diagnosis of malignant disease. Hum Pathol 1979;10:137.

251. Loriaux DL, Cutler GB. Diseases of the adrenal glands. In: Kohler PO, ed. Clinical endocrinology. New York: John Wiley and Sons, 1986:167–238.

252. Perry RR, Nieman LK, Cutler GB, et al. Primary adrenal causes of Cushing's syndrome: Diagnosis and surgical management. Ann Surg 1989;210:59.

253. Raker JW, Henneman PH, Graf WS. Coexisting primary hyperparathyroidism and Cushing's syndrome. J Clin Endocrinol Metab 1962;22:273.

254. Maton PN, Gardner JD, Jensen RT. Cushing's syndrome in patients with the Zollinger-Ellison Syndrome. N Engl J Med 1986;315:1.

255. Kramer M, Corrado ML, Bacci V, et al. Pulmonary cryptococcosis and Cushing's syndrome. Arch Intern Med 1983;143:2179.

256. Fulkerson WJ, Newman JH. Endogenous Cushing's syndrome complicated by pneumocystis carinii pneumonia. Am Rev Respir Dis 1984;129:188.

257. Graham BS, Tucker WS Jr. Opportunistic infections in endogenous Cushing's syndrome. Ann Intern Med 1984;101:334.

258. Thomas CG Jr, Smith AT, Griffith JM, et al. Hyperadrenalism in childhood and adolescence. Ann Surg 1984;199:538.

259. Pavlatos FC, Smilo RP, Forsham PH. A rapid screening test for Cushing's syndrome. JAMA 1965;193:720.

260. Willenbring M. L, Morley JE, Niewoeher CB, et al. Adrenocortical hyperactivity in newly admitted alcoholics: Prevalence, course and associated variables. Psychoneuroendocrinology 1984;9:415.

261. Chrousos GP, Vingerhoeds A, Brandon D, et al. Primary cortisol resistance in man: A glucocorticoid receptor-mediated disease. J Clin Invest 1982;69:1261.

262. Chrousos GP, Schuermeyer TH, Doppman J, et al. Primary cortisol resistance: A family study. J Clin Endocrinol Metab 1983;56:1243.

263. Chrousos GP, Schuermeyer TH, Doppman J, et al. Clinical applications of corticotropin-releasing factor. Ann Intern Med 1985;102:344.

264. Nieman LK, Chrousos GP, Oldfield EH, et al. The ovine corticotropin-releasing hormone stimulation test and the dexamethesone suppression test in the differential diagnosis of Cushing's syndrome. Ann Intern Med 1986;105:862.

265. Howlett TA, Drury PL, Perry L, et al. Diagnosis and management of ACTH-dependent Cushing's syndrome: Comparison of the features in ectopic and pituitary ACTH production. Clin Endocrinol 1986;24:699.

266. Weiss E. R, Rayjis SS, Nelson DH, et al. Evaluation of stimulation and suppression tests in the etiological diagnosis of Cushing's syndrome. Ann Intern Med 1969;71:941.

267. Tyrrell JB, Brooks RM, Fitzgerald PA, et al. Cushing's disease: Selective transphenoidal resection of pituitary microadenomas. N Engl J Med 1978;298:753.

268. Oldfield EH, Doppman JL, Nieman LK, et al. Petrosal sinus sampling with and without corticotropin-releasing hormone for the differential diagnosis of Cushing's syndrome. N Engl J Med 1991;325:897.

269. Oldfield EH, Chrousos GP, Shulte HM. Preoperative lateralization of ACTH-secreting pituitary microadenomas by bilateral and simultaneous inferior petrosal sinus sampling. N Engl J Med 1985;312:100.

270. Epstein AJ, Patel SK, Petasnick JP. Computerized tomography of the adrenal gland. JAMA 1979;242:2791.

271. Doppman JL, Nieman LK, Travis WD, et al. CT or MR imaging of massive macronodular adrenocortical disease: A rare cause of autonomous primary adrenal hypercortisolism. J Comput Assist Tomogr 1991;15:773.

272. Roubidoux M, Dunnick NR. Adrenal cortical tumors. Bull N Y Acad Med 1991;67:119.

273. Remer EM, Weinfeld RM, Glazer GM, Quint LE, Francis IR, Gross MD, Bookstein FL. Hyperfunctioning and nonhyperfunctioning benign adrenal cortical lesions: Characterization and comparison with MR imaging. Radiology 1989;171:681.

274. Doppman JL, Travis WD, Nieman L, et al. Cushing syndrome due to primary pigmented nodular adrenocortical disease: Findings at CR and MR imaging. Radiology 1989;172:415.

275. Doppman JL, Reinig JW, Dwyer AJ, et al. Differentiation of adrenal masses by magnetic resonance imaging. Surgery 1987;102:1018.

276. Bierwaltes WH, Sisson JC, Shapiro JC, Shapiro B. Diagnosis of adrenal tumors with radionuclide imaging. Spec Top Endocrinol Metab 1984;6:1.

277. Schteingart DE, Seabold JE, Gross MD, Swanson DP. Iodocholesterol adrenal tissue uptake and imaging in adrenal neoplasms. J Clin Endocrinol Metab 1981;52:1156.

278. Fig LM, Gross MD, Shapiro B, Ehrmann DA, Freitas JE, Schteingart DE, Galzer GM, Francis IR. Adrenal localization in the adrenocorticotropic hormone-independent Cushing syndrome. Ann Intern Med 1988;109:547.

279. McArthur RB, Bahn RC, Hayles AB. Primary adrenocortical nodular dysplasia as a cause of Cushing's syndrome in infants and children. Mayo Clin Proc 1982;57:58.

280. Donaldson MDC, Grant DB, O'hare MJ, et al. Familial congenital Cushing's syndrome due to bilateral nodular adrenal hyperplasia. Clin Endocrinol 1981;14:519.

281. Spark RF, Connolly PB, Gluckin DS, et al. ACTH secretion from a functioning pheochromocytoma. N Engl J Med 1979;301:416.

282. Boggan JE, Tyrrell JB, Wilson CB. Transsphenoidal microsurgical management of Cushing's disease: Report of 100 cases. J Neurosurg 1983;59:195.

283. Kern DC, Tang K, Hanson CS, et al. The prediction of anatomical morphology of primary aldosteronism using serum 18-hydroxycorticosterone levels. J Clin Endocrinol Metab 1985;60:67.

284. Gomez-Sanchez CE, Montgomery M, Ganguly A, et al. Elevated urinary excretion of 18-oxocortisol in glucocorticoid-suppressible aldosteronism. J Clin Endocrinol Metab 1984;59:1022.

285. Brown RD, Hollifield JW. Endocrine hypertension. In: Kohler PO, ed. Clinical endocrinology. New York: John Wiley & Sons, 1986:239–262.

286. Conn JW. Presidential address. Part I. Painting background. II. Primary aldosteronism, a new clinical syndrome. J Lab Clin Med 1972;264:9.

287. McLeod MK, Thompson NW, Gross MD, Grekin RJ. Idiopathic aldosteronism masquerading as discrete aldosterone-secreting adrenal cortical neoplasms among patients with primary aldosteronism. Surgery 1989;106:1161.

288. Tenschert W, Maurer R, Vetter H, Vetter W. Primary aldosteronism by carcinoma of the adrenal cortex. Klin Wochenschr 1987;65:428.

289. Carey RM, Sen S, Dolan LM, et al. Idiopathic hyperaldosteronism: A possible role for aldosterone-stimulating factor. N Engl J Med 1984;311:94.

290. Weinberger MH, Grim CE, Hollifield JW, et al. Primary aldosteronism: Diagnosis, localization and treatment. Ann Intern Med 1979;90:386.

291. Lyons DG, Kern DC, Brown RD, et al. Single dose captopril as a diagnostic test for primary aldosteronism. J Clin Endocrinol Metab 1983;57:892.

292. Guerin CK, Wahner HW, Gorman CA, et al. Computed tomographic scanning versus radioisotope imaging in adrenocortical diagnosis. Am J Med 1983;75:653.

293. Falke THM, Strake L, Shaff MI, et al. MR imaging of the adrenals: Correlation with computed tomography. J Comput Assist Tomogr 1986;10:242.

294. Geisinger MA, Zelch M, Bravo E, et al. Primary hyperaldosteronism: Comparison of CT, adrenal venography, and venous sampling. AJR 1983;141:299.

295. Auda SP, Brennan MF, Gill JR. Evolution of the surgical management of primary aldosteronism. Ann Surg 1980;191:1.

296. Nadler JL, Hsueh W, Horton R. Therapeutic effect of calcium channel blockade in primary aldosteronism. J Clin Endocrinol Metab 1985;60:896.

297. Alder GK, Williams GH. Primary aldosteronism. In: Krieger DT, Bardin CW, eds. Current therapy in endocrinology and metabolism. Toronto: BC Decker, 1985:116–121.

298. Banks WA, Kastin AJ, Biglieri EG, Ruiz AE. Primary adrenal hyperplasia: A new subset of primary hyperaldosteronism. J Clin Endocrinol Metab 1984;58:783.

299. Biglieri EG, Schambelan M, Slaton PE, et al. The intercurrent hypertension of primary aldosteronism. Circ Res 1970;26:1.

300. Cohn K, Gottesman L, Brennan M. Adrenocortical carcinoma. Surgery 1986;100:1170.

301. Arteaga E, Biglieri EG, Kater C, et al. Aldosterone-producing adrenocortical carcinoma, preoperative recognition and course in three cases. Ann Intern Med 1984;101:316.

302. Glazer HS, Weyman PJ, Sagel SS, et al. Nonfunctioning adrenal masses: Incidental discovery on computed tomography. AJR 1982;139:81.

303. Prinz RA, Brooks MH, Churchill R, et al. Incidental asymptomatic adrenal masses detected by computed tomographic scanning: Is operation required? JAMA 1982;248:701.

304. Copeland PM. The incidentally discovered adrenal mass, diagnosis and treatment. Ann Intern Med 1983;98:940.

305. McCorkell SJ, Miles NL. Fine-needle aspiration of catecholamine-producing adrenal masses: A possibly fatal mistake. AJR 1985;145:113.

306. Hogan TF, Gilchrist KW, Westring DW, Citrin DL. A clinical and pathological study of adrenocortical carcinoma. Cancer 1980;45:2880.

307. Didolkar MS, Bescher RA, Elias EG, Moore RH. Natural history of adrenal cortical carcinoma: A clinicopathologic study of 42 patients. Cancer 1981;47:2153.

308. Bertagna C, Orth DN. Clinical and laboratory findings and results of therapy in 58 patients with adrenocortical tumors admitted to a single medical center 1951 to 1978: Am J Med 1981;71:855.

309. Ross NS, Aron DC. Hormonal evaluation of the patient with an incidentally discovered adrenal mass. N Engl J Med 1990;323:1401.

310. Gabrilove JL, Seman AT, Sabet R, et al. Virilizing adrenal adenoma with studies on the steroid content of the adrenal venous effluent and a review of the literature. Endocr Rev 1981;2:462.

311. Tang CK, Gray GF. Adrenocortical neoplasms: Prognosis and morphology. Urology 1975;5:691.

312. Sullivan M, Boileau M, Hodges CV. Adrenal cortical carcinoma. J Urol 1978;120:660.

313. Bradley EL. Primary and adjunctive therapy in carcinoma of the adrenal cortex. Surg Gynecol Obstet 1975;141:507.

314. Hussain S, Belldegrun A, Seltzer SE, et al. Differentiation of malignant from benign adrenal masses: Predictive indices on computed tomography. AJR 1985;144:61.

315. Reinig JW, Doppman JL, Dwyer AJ, et al. Distinction between adrenal adenomas and metastases using MR imaging. J Comput Assist Tomogr 1985;9:898.

316. Fink IJ, Reinig JW, Dwyer AJ, et al. MR imaging of pheochromocytomas. J Comput Assist Tomogr 1985;9:454.

317. Reinig JW, Doppman JL, Dwyer AJ, Frank J. MRI of indeterminate adrenal masses. AJR 1986;147:493.

318. Reinig JW, Doppman JL. Magnetic resonance imaging of the adrenal. Radiologe 1986;26:186.

319. Casola G, Nicolet V, Van Sonnenberg E, et al. Unsuspected pheochromocytomas: Risk of blood pressure alterations during percutaneous adrenal biopsy. Radiology 1986;159:733.

320. Katz RL, Shirkhoda A. Diagnostic approach to incidental adrenal nodules in the cancer patient. Cancer 1985;55:1995.

321. Gabrilove JL, Frieberg EK, Nicolis GL. Peripheral blood steroid levels in Cushing's syndrome due to adrenocortical carcinoma or adenoma. Urology 1983;22:576.

322. Baker ME, Spritzer C, Blinder R, et al. Benign adrenal lesions mimicking malignancy on MR imaging: Report of two cases. Radiology 1987;163:669.

323. Doherty GM, Nieman LK, Cutler GB Jr, Chrousos GP, Norton JA. Time to recovery of the hypothalamic-pituitary-adrenal axis after curative resection of adrenal tumors in patients with Cushing's syndrome. Surgery 1990;108:1085.

324. Jones GS, Shah KJ, Mann JR. Adreno-cortical carcinoma in infancy and childhood: A radiological report of ten cases. Clin Radiol 1985;36:257.

325. Daneman A, Chan HSL, Martin J. Adrenal carcinoma and adenoma in children: A review of 17 patients. Pediatr Radiol 1983;13:11.

326. Neblett W, Frexes-Steed M, Scott HW. Experience with adrenocortical neoplasia in childhood. Am J Surg 1987;53:117.

327. Ribeiro RC, Sandrini NR, Schell MJ, Lacerda L, Sambaio GA, Cat I. Adrenocortical carcinoma in children: A study of 40 cases. J Clin Oncol 1990;8:67.

328. Chudler RM, Kay R. Adrenocortical carcinoma in children. Urol Clin North Am 1989;16:469.

329. Henley DJ, van Heerden JA, Grant CS, Carney JA, Carpenter PC. Adrenal cortical carcinoma—A continuing challenge. Surgery 1983;94:226.

330. Luton JP, Cerdas S, Billaud L, et al. Clinical features of adrenocortical carcinoma, prognostic factors and the effect of mitotane therapy. N Engl J Med 1990;322:1195.

331. Hajjar RA, Hickey RC, Samaan NA. Adrenal cortical carcinoma: A study of 32 patients. Cancer 1975;35:549.

332. Appelqvist P, Kostiainen S. Multiple thoracotomy combined with chemotherapy in metastatic adrenal cortical carcinoma: A case report and review of the literature. J Surg Oncol 1983;24:1.

333. Potter DA, Strott CA, Javadpour N, Roth JA. Prolonged survival following six pulmonary resections for metastatic adrenal cortical carcinoma: A case report. J Surg Oncol 1984;25:273.

334. Percarpio B, Knowlton AH. Radiation therapy of adrenal cortical carcinoma. Acta Rad Ther Phys Biol 1976;15:288.

335. Jensen JC, Pass HI, Sindelar WF, Norton JA. Recurrent or metastatic disease in select patients with adrenocortical carcinoma. Arch Surg 1991;126:457.

336. Gutierrez ML, Crooke ST. Mitotane (o,p-DDD). Cancer Treat Rev 1980;7:49.

337. Haak HR, Caekibcke-Peerlinck KMH, Van Seters AP, Briet E. Prolonged bleeding time due to mitotane therapy. Eur J Cancer 1991;27:638.

338. Fukushima DK, Bradlow HL, Hellman L. Effects of o, p-DDD on cortisol and 66-B-hydroxycortisol secretion and metabolism in man. J Clin Endocrinol Metab 1971;32:192.

339. Hellman L, Bradlow HL, Zumoff B. Decreased conversion of androgens to normal 17-ketosteroid metabolites as a result of treatment with o,p-DDD. J Clin Endocrinol Metab 1973;36:801.

340. Van Slooten H, Moolenaar AJ, Van Seters AP, Smeek D. The treatment of adrenocortical carcinoma with o,p-DDD: Prognostic implications of serum levels monitoring. Eur J Clin Oncol 1984;20:47.

341. Jarabak J, Rice K. Metastatic adrenal cortical carcinoma, prolonged regression with mitotane therapy. JAMA 1981;246:1706.

342. Thompson NW. Adrenocortical carcinoma. In: Thompson NW, Vinik AI, eds. Endocrine surgery update. New York: Grune & Stratton, 1983:119–128.

343. Bodie B, Novick AC, Pontes JE, Straffon RA, et al. The Cleveland Clinic experience with adrenal cortical carcinoma. J Urol 1989;141:257.

344. Venkatesh S, Hickey RC, Sellin RV, Fernandez JF, Samoan NA. Adrenal cortical carcinoma. Cancer 1989;64:765.

345. Decker RA, Elson P, Hogan TF, et al. Eastern Cooperative Oncology Group Study 1989: Mitotane and adriamycin in patients with advanced adrenocortical carcinoma. Surgery 1991;110:1006.

346. Haak HR, Van Seters AP, Moolenaar AJ. Mitotane therapy of adrenocortical carcinoma. N Engl J Med 1990;322:758.

347. Bates SE, Shieh CY, Mickley LA, Dichek HL, Gazdar A, Loriaux DL, Fojo AT. Mitotane enhances cytotoxicity of chemotherapy in cell lines expressing a multidrug resistance gene (mdr-1/P-glycoprotein) which is also expressed by adrenocortical carcinomas. J Clin Endocrinol Metab 1991;73:18.

348. Van Slooten H, van Oosterom AT. CAP (cyclophosphamide, doxorubicin and cisplatin) regimen in adrenal cortical carcinoma. Cancer Treat Rep 1983;67:377.

349. Hag MM, Legha SS, Samaan NA, et al. Cytotoxic chemotherapy in adrenal cortical carcinoma. Cancer Treat Rep 1980;64:909.

350. Johnson DH, Creco A. Treatment of metastatic adrenal cortical carcinoma with cisplatin and etoposide (VP-16). Cancer 1986;58:2198.

351. Hesketh PJ, McCaffrey RP, Finkel HE, et al. Cisplatin-based treatment of adrenocortical carcinoma. Cancer Treat Rep 1987;71:222.

352. Schlumberger M, Brugieres L, Gicquel C, Travagli JP, Droz JP, Parmentier C. 5-fluorouracil, doxorubicin, and cisplatin as treatment for adrenal cortical carcinoma. Cancer 1991;67:2997.

353. Schlumberger M, Ostronoff M, Bellaiche M, Rougier P, Driz JP, Parmentier C. 5-fluorouracil, doxorubicin and cisplatin regimen in adrenal cortical carcinoma. Cancer 1988;61:1492.

354. Stein CA, LaRocca RV, Thomas R, McAtee N, Myers CE. Suramin: An anticancer drug with a unique mechanism of action. J Clin Oncol 1989;7:499.

355. Allolio B, Reincke M, Arlt W, Deuss U, Winkelmann W, Siekmann L. Suramin for treatment of adrenocortical carcinoma. Lancet 1989;1:277.

356. LaRocca RV, Stein CA, Danesi R, Jamis Dow CA, Weiss GH, Myers CE. Suramin in adrenal cancer: Modulation of steroid hormone production, cytotoxicity in vitro and clinical antitumor effect. J Clin Endocrinol Metab 1990;71:497.

357. Stein CA, LaRocca R, Myers CE. A phase II trial of suramin in metastatic adrenocortical cancer, 1991 (personal communication).

358. Grondal S, Cedermark B, Eriksson B, Grimelius L, Harach R, Kristoffersson A, Rastad J, Uden P, Akerstrom G. Adrenocortical carcinoma. A retrospective study of a rare tumor with a poor prognosis. Eur J Surg Oncol 1990;16:500.

359. Wu YW, Chek CL, Knazck RA. An in vitro study of antitumor effects of gossypol in human SW-13 adrenocortical carcinoma. Cancer Res 1989;49:3754.

360. Sanfilippo JS, Wittliff JL. Steroid hormone receptors in adrenal cortical carcinoma. Am J Obstet Gynecol 1984;150:326.

361. Richie JP, Gittes RF. Carcinoma of the adrenal cortex. Cancer 1980;45:1957.

362. Brown WH. A case of pluriglandular syndrome. Lancet 1928;2:1022.

363. Christy NP. Adrenocorticotrophic activity in plasma of patients with Cushing's syndrome associated with pulmonary neoplasms. Lancet 1961;1:85.

364. Liddle GW, Island D, Meador CK. Normal and abnormal regulation of corticotropin secretion in man. Recent Prog Horm Res 1962;18:125.

365. Imura H. Ectopic hormone syndrome. Clin Endocrinol Metab 1980;9:235.

366. Davies CJ, Hoplin GF, Welbourn RB. Surgical management of the ectopic ACTH syndrome. Ann Surg 1982;196:246.

367. Jex RK, van Heerden JA, Carpenter PC, Grant CS. Ectopic ACTH syndrome. Am J Surg 1985;149:276.

368. Doppman JL, Loughlin T, Miller DL, et al. Identification of ACTH-producing intra-thoracic tumors by measuring ACTH levels in aspirated specimens. Radiology 1987;163:501.

369. Pass HI, Doppman JL, Nieman L, et al. Management of the ectopic ACTH syndrome due to thoracic carcinoids. Ann Thorac Surg 1990;50:52.

370. Liddle GW, Nicholson WE, Island DP, et al. Clinical and laboratory studies of ectopic humoral syndromes. Recent Prog Horm Res 1969;25:283.

371. Misbin RI, Canary J, Williard D. Aminoglutethimide in the treatment of Cushing's syndrome. J Clin Pharmacol 1976;16:645.

372. Beard CM, Sheps SG, Kurland L. T, et al. Occurrence of pheochromocytoma in Rochester, Minnesota, 1950 through 1979. Mayo Clin Proc 1983;58:802.

373. Cryer PE. Phaeochromocytoma. Clin Endocrinol Metab 1985;14:203.

374. Beierwaltes WH, Sisson JC, Shapiro B, et al. Malignant potential of pheochromocytoma. Proc Am Assoc Cancer Res 1986;27:617.

375. Melicow MM. One hundred cases of pheochromocytoma (107 tumors) at the Columbia Presbyterian Medical Center, 1926–1976. Cancer 1977;40:1987.

376. Irvin GL, Fishman LM, Sher JA. Familial pheochromocytoma. Surgery 1983;94:938.

377. Glowniak JV, Shapiro B, Sisson JC, et al. Familial extra-adrenal pheochromocytoma. Arch Intern Med 1985;145:257.

378. Loughlin KR, Gittes RF. Urological management of patients with von Hippel-Lindau's disease. J Urol 1986;136:789.

379. Nakagawara A. Malignant pheochromocytoma with ganglioneuroblastomatous elements in a patient with von Ricklinghausen's disease. Cancer 1985;55:2794.

380. Berelowitz M, Szabo M, Barowsky HW, et al. Somatostatin-like immunoactivity and biological activity is present in human pheochromocytoma. J Clin Endocrinol Metab 1983;56:134.

381. Weinstein RS, Ide LF. Immunoreactive calcitonin in pheochromocytomas. Proc Soc Exp Biol Med 1980;165:215.

382. Ang VTY, Jenkins JS. Neurohypophysical hormones in the adrenal medulla. J Clin Endocrinol Metab 1984;58:688.

383. Cooper MJ, Helman LJ, Israel MA. Molecular biology and the pathogenesis of neuroblastoma and pheochromocytoma. Cancer Cells 1989;7:95.

384. Moley JF, Brother MB, Wells SA, Spengler BA, Bredler JL, Brodeur GM. Low frequency of ras gene mutations in neuroblastomas, pheochromocytomas and medullary thyroid cancers. Cancer Res 1991;51:1596.

385. Khosia S, Patel VM, Hay ID, Schaid DJ, Grant CS, van Heerden JA, Thibodeau SN. Loss of heterozygosity suggests multiple genetic alterations in pheochromocytomas and medullary thyroid carcinomas. J Clin Invest 1991;87:1691.

386. Orringer MB, Sisson JC, Glazer G, et al. Surgical treatment of cardiac pheochromocytomas. J Thorac Cardiovasc Surg 1985;89:753.

387. Lips KJM, Veer JVDS, Struyvenberg A, et al. Bilateral occurrence of pheochromocytoma in patients with multiple endocrine neoplasia syndrome type 2a (Sipple's syndrome). Am J Med 1981;70:1051.

388. Remine WH, Chang GC, van Heerden JA, et al. Current management of pheochromocytoma. Ann Surg 1974;179:740.

389. Sutton MGS, Sheps SG, Lie JT. Prevalence of clinically unsuspected pheochromocytoma: Review of a 50 year autopsy series. Mayo Clin Proc 1981;56:354.

390. Shin WY, Groman CS, Berkman JI. Pheochromocytoma with angiomatous features. Cancer 1977;40:275.

391. Scott HW, Halter SA. Oncologic aspects of pheochromocytoma: The importance of follow-up. Surgery 1984;96:1061.

392. Sherwin RP. Present status of the pathology of the adrenal gland in hypertension. Am J Surg 1964;107:136.

393. Lewis PD. A cytophotometric study of benign and malignant pheochromocytomas. Virchows Arch 1971;9:371.

394. Hosaka Y, Rainwater LM, Grant CS, et al. Pheochromocytoma: Nuclear deoxyribonucleic acid patterns studied by flow cytometry. Surgery 1986;100:1003.

395. Sheps SG, Jiang NS, Klec GG, van Heerden JA. Recent developments in the diagnosis and management of pheochromocytoma. Mayo Clin Proc 1990;65:88.

396. Helman LJ, Cohen PS, Averbuch SD, Cooper MJ, Keiser HR, Israel MA. Neuropeptide y expression distinguishes malignant from benign pheochromocytoma. J Clin Oncol 1989;7:1720.

397. Grouzmann E, Gicquel C, Pluin PF, Schlumberger M, Conroy E, Bohuon C. Neuropeptide Y and neuron specific enolase levels in benign and malignant pheochromocytomas. Cancer 1990;66:1833.

398. Medeiros LJ, Wolf BC, Balogh K, Federman M. Adrenal pheochromocytoma: A clinicopathologic review of 60 cases. Hum Pathol 1985;16:580.

399. Manger WM, Gifford RW. Pheochromocytoma. New York: Springer-Verlag, 1977.

400. Hengstmann JH. Evaluation of screening tests for pheochromocytoma. Cardiology 1985;72:153.

401. Kremer R, Crawhall JC, Kolanitch R. Rapid and reliable estimation of urinary free catecholamines in patients with pheochromocytoma. J Chromatogr 1985;344:313.

402. Hanson MW, Feldman JM, Beam CA, Leight GS, Coleman E. Iodine ¹³¹-labelled metaiodobenzylguanidine scintigraphy and biochemical analyses in suspected pheochromocytoma. Arch Intern Med 1991;151:1397.

403. Samaan NA, Hickey RC, Shutts PE. Diagnosis, localization and management of pheochromocytoma. Cancer 1988;62:2451.

404. Duncan MW, Compton P, Lazarus L, Smythe GA. Measurement of norepinephrine and 3,4-dihydroxyphenylglycol in urine and plasma for the diagnosis of pheochromocytoma. N Engl J Med 1988;319:136.

405. Cryer PE, Wortsman J, Shah SD, Nowak RM, Deftos LJ. Plasma chromogranin A as a marker of sympathochromaffin activity in humans. Am J Physiol 1991;260:E243.

406. Karlberg BE, Hedman L. Value of the clonidine suppression test in the diagnosis of pheochromocytoma. Acta Med Scand 1986;714:15.

407. Gifford RW, Bravo EL, Manger WM. Diagnosis and management of pheochromocytoma. Cardiology 1985;72:186.

408. Brandstetter K, Krause U, Beyer W. Preliminary results with the clonidine suppression test in the diagnosis of pheochromocytoma. Cardiology 1985;72:157.

409. Karlberg BE, Hedman L, Lennquist S, Pollace T. The value of the clonidine-suppression test in the diagnosis of pheochromocytoma. World J Surg 1986;10:753.

410. MacDougall IC, Isles CG, Stewart H, et al. Overnight clonidine suppression test in the diagnosis and exclusion of pheochromocytoma. Am J Med 1988;84:993.

411. Taylor HC, Mayes D, Anton AH. Clonidine suppression test for pheochromocytoma: Examples of misleading results. J Clin Endocrinol Metab 1986;63:238.

412. Bravo EL, Tarazi RC, Fouad FM, et al. Clonidine suppression test: A useful aid in the diagnosis of pheochromocytoma. N Engl J Med 1981;305:623.

413. Dunnick NR, Doppman JL, Gill JR, et al. Localization of functional adrenal tumors by computed tomography and venous sampling. Radiology 1982;142:429.

414. Welch TJ, Sheedy PF, van Heerden JA, et al. Pheochromocytoma: Value of computed tomography. Radiology 1983;148:501.

415. Radin DR, Ralls PW, Boswell WD, et al. Pheochromocytoma: Detection by unenhanced CT. AJR 1986;146:741.

416. Greenberg M, Moawad AH, Wieties BM, et al. Extraadrenal pheochromocytoma: Detection during pregnancy using MR imaging. Radiology 1986;161:475.

417. Velchik MG, Alavi A, Kressel HY, Engelman K. Localization of pheochromocytoma: MIBG, CT and MRI correlation. J Nucl Med 1989;30:328.

418. Fisher MR, Higgins CB, Andereck W. MR imaging of an intrapericardial pheochromocytoma. J Comput Assist Tomogr 1985;9:1103.

419. Shapiro B, Copp JE, Sisson JC, et al. Iodine-131 metaiodobenzylguanidine for the locating of suspected pheochromocytoma: Experience in 400 cases. J Nucl Med 1985;26:576.

420. Swenson SJ, Brown MJ, Sheps SG, et al. Use of ¹³¹I-MIBG scintigraphy in the evaluation of suspected pheochromocytoma. Mayo Clin Proc 1985;60:299.

421. Koizumi M, Endo K, Sakahara H, et al. Computed tomography and ¹³¹I-MIBG scintigraphy in the diagnosis of pheochromocytoma. Acta Radiologica Diagn 1986;27:305.

422. Fischer M, Galanski M, Winterberg B, Vetter H. Localization procedures in pheochromocytoma and neuroblastoma. Cardiology 1985;72:143.

423. Shulkin B. L, Shen SW, Sisson JC, Shapiro B. Iodine 131 MIBG scintigraphy of the extremities in metastatic pheochromocytoma and neuroblastoma. J Nucl Med 1987;28:315.

424. Lynn MD, Braunstein EM, Wohl RL, et al. Bone metastases in pheochromocytoma: Comparative studies of efficacy of imaging. Radiology 1986;160:701.

425. Lynn MD, Shapiro B, Sisson JC, et al. Pheochromocytoma and the normal adrenal medulla: Improved visualization with I-123 MIBG scintigraphy. Radiology 1985;156:851.

426. Cheung PSY, Thompson NW, Dmuchowski CF, Sisson JC. Spectrum of pheochromocytoma in the ¹³¹I-MIBG era. World J Surg 1988;12:546.

427. Gouch IR, Thompson NW, Shapiro B, Sisson JC. Limitations of ¹³¹I-MIBG scintigraphy in locating pheochromocytomas. Surgery 1985;98:115.

428. Stenstrom G, Kutti J. The blood volume in pheochromocytoma patients before and during treatment with phenoxybenzamine. Acta Med Scand 1985;218:381.

429. Stenstrom G, Haljamae H, Tisell LE. Influence of pre-operative treatment with phenoxybenzamine on the incidence of adverse cardiovascular reactions during anaesthesia and surgery for phaeochromocytoma. Acta Anaesthesiol Scand 1985;29:797.

430. Bornemann M, Hill SC, Kidd GS. Lactic acidosis in pheochromocytoma. Ann Intern Med 1986;105:880.

431. Perry RR, Keiser HR, Norton JA, et al. Surgical management of pheochromocytoma with the use of metyrosine. Ann Surg 1990;212:621.

432. Imperato-McGinley J, Gautier T, Ehlers K, et al. Reversibility of catecholamine-induced dilated cardiomyopathy in a child with a pheochromocytoma. N Engl J Med 1987;316:793.

433. Chimori K, Miyazaki S, Nakajima T, Muira D. Preoperative management of pheochromocytoma with the calcium-antagonist nifedipine. Clin Ther 1985;7:372.

434. Proye C, Thevenin D, Cecat P, et al. Exclusive use of calcium channel blockers in preoperative and intraoperative control of pheochromocytomas: Hemodynamics and free catecholamine assays in ten consecutive patients. Surgery 1989;106:1149.

435. Irvin GL, Fishman LM, Sher JA, Yeung LK, Irane H. Pheochromocytoma lateral vs anterior operative approach. Ann Surg 1989;209:774.

436. Zimmerman ID, Biron RE, MacMahon HE. Pheochromocytoma of the urinary bladder. N Engl J Med 1953;249:25.

437. Carney JA, Sizemore GW, Sheps SG. Adrenal medullary disease in multiple endocrine neoplasia, type 2. Am J Clin Pathol 1976;66:279.

438. Brennan MF, Keiser HR. Persistent and recurrent pheochromocytoma: The role of surgery. World J Surg 1982;6:397.

439. Van Heerden JA, Sheps SG, Hamberger B, et al. Pheochromocytoma: Current status and changing trends. Surgery 1982;91:367.

440. James RE, Baker HL, Scanlon PW. The roentgenological aspects of metastatic pheochromocytoma. AJR 1972;115:783.

441. Lewi HJE, Reid R, Mucci B, et al. Malignant phaeochromocytoma. Br J Urol 1985;57:394.

442. Guo JZ, Gong LS, Chen SX, Luo BY, Xu MY. Malignant pheochromocytoma: Diagnosis and treatment in fifteen cases. J Hypertens 1989;7:261.

443. Scott WH, Reynolds V, Green N, et al. Clinical experience with malignant pheochromocytoma. Surg Gynecol Obstet 1982;154:801.

444. Broder LE, Carter SK. Pancreatic islet cell carcinoma II Results of therapy with streptozotocin in 52 patients. Ann Intern Med 1973;79:108.

445. Feldman JM. Treatment of metastatic pheochromocytoma with streptozotocin. Arch Intern Med 1983;143:1799.

446. Feldman JM. In reply to a letter to the editor by Gross DJ, Schlank E, Ipp E. Arch Intern Med 1985;145:368.

447. Gross DJ, Schlank E, Ipp E. Streptozotocin therapy for malignant pheochromocytoma. Arch Intern Med [Letter] 1985;145:368.

448. McEwan A, Shapiro B, Sisson JC, et al. Radio-iodobenzylguanidine for the scintigraphic location and therapy of adrenergic tumors. Semin Nucl Med 1985;15:132.

449. Krempf M, Lumbroso J, Mornex R, et al. Use of ¹³¹Im iodobenzylguanidine in the treatment of malignant pheochromocytoma. J Clin Endocrinol Metab 1991;72:455.

450. Feldman JM, Frankel N, Coleman RE. Platelet uptake of the pheochromocytoma-scanning agent ¹³¹I-meta-iodobenzylguanidine. Metabolism 1984;33:397.

451. Vetter H, Fischer M, Muller-Rensing R, et al. [¹³¹I]-meta-iodobenzylguanidine in treatment of malignant pheochromocytomas. Lancet 1983;2(8341):107.

452. Keiser H. R, Goldstein DS, Wade JL, et al. Treatment of malignant pheochromocytoma with combination chemotherapy. Hypertension 1985;7:1-18.

453. Manger TJ, Tobes MC, Wieland DW, et al. Metabolism of Iodine-131 metaiodobenzylguanidine in patients with metastatic pheochromocytoma. J Nucl Med 1986;27:37.

454. Goldstein DS, Stull R, Eisenhofer G, et al. Plasma 3,4-dihydroxyphenylalanine (Dopa) and catecholamines in neuroblastoma or pheochromocytoma. Ann Intern Med 1986;105:887.

455. Averbuch S, Steakley C, Gelmann E, et al. Malignant pheochromocytoma: Treatment

with a combination of cyclophosphamide, vincristine and darcarbazine. Proc American Society of Clinical Oncology 1987;6:241.

456. Averbuch SD, Steakley CS, Young RC, et al. Malignant pheochromocytoma: Effective treatment with a combination of cyclophosphamide, vincristine and dacarbazine. Ann Intern Med 1988;109:267.

457. Finklestein JZ, Klemperer MR, Evans A, et al. Multiagent chemotherapy for children with metaststic neuroblastoma: A report from children's cancer study group. Med Pediatr Oncol 1979;6:179.

458. Taub MA, Osburne RC, Georges LP, Sode J. Malignant pheochromocytoma: Severe clinical exacerbation and release of stored catecholamines during lymphoma chemotherapy. Cancer 1982;50:1739.

459. Masson P. Carcinoid (argentaffin-cell tumours) and nerve hyperplasia of appendicular mucosa. Am J Pathol 1982;4:181.

460. Kultschitzky N. Zur frage ueber den bau des darmkanals. Arch Mikrosk Anat 1987;49:7.

461. Bolande RP. The neurocrestopathies: A unifying concept of disease arising from neural crest maldevelopment. Hum Pathol 1974;5:409.

462. Pearse HGE. The APUD concept and hormone production. Clin Endocrinol Metab 1980;9:211.

463. Moertel CG. An odyssey in the land of small tumors. J Clin Oncol 1987;5:1502.

464. Kloppel G, Heitz PU. Pancreatic endocrine tumors. Pathol Res Pract 1988;183:155.

465. Black WC III. Enterochromaffin cell types and corresponding carcinoid tumors. Lab Invest 1968;19:473.

466. Carney JA, Go VLW, Fairbanks JF, Moore SB, Alport EC, Nora EE. The syndrome of gastric argyrophil carcinoid tumors and nonantral gastric atrophy. Ann Intern Med 1983;99:761.

467. Feldman JM, O'Dorisio TM. The role of neuropeptides and serotonin in the diagnosis of carcinoid tumors. Am J Med 1986;81:41.

468. Pearse AGE, Tabor TT. Embryology of the diffuse neuroendocrine system and its relationship to the common peptides. Fed Proc 1979;38:2288.

469. Wilander E, Scheibenpflug L, Eriksson B, Oberg K. Diagnostic criteria of classical carcinoids. Acta Oncol 1991;30:469.

470. Eriksson B, Oberg K. Peptide hormones as tumor markers in neuroendocrine gastrointestinal tumors. Acta Oncol 1991;30:477.

471. Eriksson B, Arnberg H, Oberg K, et al. Chromogranins: A new sensitive marker for neuroendocrine tumors. Acta Oncol 1989;28:325.

472. Wilander E. Diagnostic pathology of gastrointestinal and pancreatic neuroendocrine tumors. Acta Oncol 1989;28:363.

473. Soga J, Tazawa K. Pathologic analysis of carcinoids. Histologic reevaluation of 62 cases. Cancer 1971;28:990.

474. Nash SV, Said JW. Gastroenteropancreatic neuroendocrine tumors. A histochemical and immunohistochemical study of epithelial (keratin proteins, carcinoembryonic antigen) and neuroendocrine (neuron-specific enolase, bombesin and chromogranin) markers in foregut, midgut and hindgut tumors. J Clin Pathol 1986;86:415.

475. Moll R, Franke WW. Cytoskeletal differences between human neuroendocrine tumors: A cytoskeletal protein of molecular weight 46,000 distinguishes cutaneous from pulmonary neuroendocrine neoplasms. Differentiation 1985;30:165.

476. Pinkus GS, Etheridge CL, O'Connor EM. Are keratin proteins a better tumor marker than epithelial membrane antigen? A comparative immunohistochemical study of various paraffin-embedded neoplasms using monoclonal and polyclonal antibodies. Am J Clin Pathol 1986;85:269.

477. Marangos PJ, Polak JM, Pearse AGE. Neuron-specific enolase. A prove for neurons and neuroendocrine cells. TINS 1982;5:193.

478. Wiedenmann B, Franke WW, Kuhn C, Moll R, Gould VE. Synaptophysin: A marker protein for neuroendocrine cells and neoplasms. Proc Natl Acad Sci USA 1986;83:3500.

479. Vyberg M, Horn T, Francis D, Askaa J. Immunohistochemical identification of neuron-specific enolase, synaptophysin, chromogranin and endocrine granule constituent in neuroendocrine tumors. Acta Histochem 1990;38:S179.

480. Wilander E, Lundquist M, El-Salhy M. Serotonin in foregut carcinoids: A survey of 60 cases with regard to silver stains, formalin-induced fluorescence and serotonin immunocytochemistry. J Pathol 1985;145:251.

481. Williams ED, Sanders M. The classification of carcinoid tumors. Lancet 1963;1:238.

482. Godwin JD. Carcinoid tumors: An analysis of 2837 cases. Cancer 1975;36:560.

483. Vinik AI, McLeod MK, Fig LM, Shapiro B, Lloyd RV, Cho K. Clinical features, diagnosis, and localization of carcinoid tumors and their management. Gastroenterol Clin North Am 1989;18:865.

484. Feldman JM. Carcinoid tumors and the carcinoid syndrome. Curr Probl Surg 1989;26:835.

485. Watson RGP, Johnston CF, et al. The frequency of gastrointestinal endocrine tumors in a well-defined population: Northern Ireland 1970–1985. Q J Med 1989;72:647.

486. Norheim I, Oberg K, Theodorsson-Norheim E, et al. Malignant carcinoid tumors. Ann Surg 1987;206:115.

487. Eriksson B. Recent advances in the diagnosis and management of endocrine pancreatic tumors. Acta Universitatis Upsaliensis 1988:160:28.

488. Eriksson B, Oberg K, Skogseid B. Neuroendocrine pancreatic tumors. Acta Oncol 1989;28:373.

489. Oberg K, Eriksson B. Medical treatment of neuroendocrine gut and pancreatic tumors. Acta Oncol 1989;28:425.

490. Weiss NS, Yang CP. Incidence of histologic types of cancer of the small intestine. JNCI 1987;78:653.

491. Berge T, Linell F. Carcinoid tumors. Acta Pathol Microbiol Immunol Scand 1976;84:322.

492. Moertel CG, Dockerty MB, Judd ES. Carcinoid tumors of the vermiform appendix. Cancer 1968;21:270.

493. Thompson GB, van Heerden JA, Martin JK, et al. Carcinoid tumors of the gastrointestinal tract: Presentation, management and prognosis. Surgery 1985;98:1054.

494. Moertel CG, Suer WG, Doherty MG, et al. Life history of the carcinoid tumor of the small intestine. Cancer 1961;14:901.

495. Burke AO, Sobin LH, Federspiel BH, Shekitka KM, Helwig EB. Carcinoid tumors of the duodenum. Arch Pathol Lab Med 1990;114:700.

496. Federspiel BH, Burke AP, Sokin LH, Shekitka KM. Rectal and colonic carcinoids. Cancer 1990;65:135.

497. Bronchial adenomas. Br Med J [Editorial] 1981;282:252.

498. Hasleton PS, Gomm S, Blair V, Thatcher N. Pulmonary carcinoid tumours: A clinico-pathological study of 35 cases. Br J Cancer 1986;54:963.

499. Solcia E, Capella C, Fiocca R, Cornaggia M, Bosi F. The gastroenteropancreatic endocrine system and related tumors. Gastroenterol Clin North Am 1989;18:671.

500. Davies MG, O'Dowd GO, McEntree GP, Hennessey TPJ. Primary gastric carcinoid tumors: A view on management. Br J Surg 1990;77:1013.

501. Hasdu SI, Winawer SJ, Myer WP. Surgical management of carcinoid tumors of the gastrointestinal tract. Ann Surg 1980;41:429.

502. Sanders RJ. Carcinoids of the gastrointestinal tract. Springfield, IL: Charles L. Thomas, 1973.

503. Jensen RT, Gardner JD. Gastrinoma. In: Go VLW, Brooks FA, DiMagno EP, Gardner JD, Lebenthal E, Scheele GA, eds. The exocrine pancreas: Biology, pathobiology and disease. New York: Raven Press, 1992 (in press).

504. Solcia E, Capella C, Sessa F, et al. Gastric carcinoids and related endocrine growths. Digestion 1986;35:3.

505. Ekman L, Hansson E, Havu N, et al. Toxicological studies on omeprazole. Scand J Gastroenterol 1985;20:53.

506. Moertel CG, Hanley JA. Combination chemotherapy trials in metastatic carcinoid and malignant carcinoid syndrome. Cancer Clin Trials 1979;2:327.

507. Johnson LA, Lavin PT, Moertel CG, et al. Carcinoids: The prognostic effect of primary site histologic type variations. J Surg Oncol 1986;33:81.

508. Penston J, Wormsley KG. Achlorhydria-hypergastrinaemia: Carcinoids—a flawed hypothesis. Gut 1987;28:488.

509. Borch K, Renvall H, Liedberg G. Gastric endocrine cell hyperplasia and carcinoid tumors in pernicious anemia. Gastroenterology 1985;88:638.

510. Solcia E, Capella C, Buffa R, et al. Endocrine cells of the gastrointestinal tract and related tumors. Pathol Annu 1979;9:163.

511. Mattson H, Havu N, Brautigam J, Carlsson K, Lundell L, Carlsson E. Partial fundectomy results in hypergastrinemia and development of gastric enterochromaffin-like cell carcinoids in rats. Gastroenterology 1991;100:311.

512. Krets DJ, Guerra JJ, Saltz M, et al. Gastrointestinal hemorrhage due to carcinoid tumors of the small intestine. JAMA 1986;255:234.

513. Eberle F, Grun R. Multiple endocrine neoplasia type I. Adv Intern Med Pediatr 1981;5:76.

514. Ballard HS, Frame B, Hartsock RT. Familial multiple endocrine adenoma: Peptic ulcer complex. Medicine 1964;43:481.

515. Creutzfeldt W. The achlorhydria—carcinoid sequence: Role of gastrin. Digestion 1988;39:61.

516. Wilander E. Achylia and the development of gastric carcinoids. Virchows Arch Anat Pathol 1981;394:151.

517. Hodges JR, Isaacson P, Wright R. Diffuse enterochromaffin-like (ECL) cell hyperplasia and multiple gastric carcinoids: A complication of pernicious anemia. Gut 1981;22:237.

518. Johnson L, Weaver M. Von Recklinghausen's disease and gastrointestinal carcinoids. JAMA 1981;245:2496.

519. Wheeler MH, Curley IR, Williams ED. The association of neurofibrometasis, pheochromocytoma, and somatostatin rich duodenal carcinoid tumor. Surgery 1986;100:1163.

520. Jensen RT, Norton JA. Pancreatic endocrine tumors. In: Fordtran JS, Sleisinger MH, Feldman M, Scharschmidt B, eds. Gastrointestinal diseases: Pathophysiology, diagnosis and management. Philadelphia: WB Saunders, 1992 (in press).

521. Maton PN, Hodgson HJF. Carcinoid tumors and the carcinoid syndrome. In: Bouchier IAD, Allan RN, Hodgson HJF, Keighly MRB, eds. Textbook of gastroenterology. London: Bailliere-Tindall, 1984:620.

522. Falkner S, Martensson H, Nobin A, Sundler F. Peptide hormones in various types of gastro-entero-pancreatic tumors: immunohistochemical patterns and evolutionary background. In: Bresciani F, King RJB, Lippman ME, Namers M, Raynaud JP, eds. Progress in cancer research and therapy. New York: Raven Press, 1984:597.

523. Dayal Y. Endocrine cells in the gut and their neoplasms. In: Norris HT, ed. Contemporary issues in surgical pathology. New York: Churchill Livingstone, 1983:267.

524. Dayal Y, Wolfe HJ. Regulatory substances in clinically nonfunctioning gastrointestinal carcinoids. In: Falkmers W, Hakanson R, Sundler F, eds. Evolution and tumor pathology of the neuroendocrine system. Amsterdam: Elsevier Science Publishers, 1984:497.

525. Wilander E, Ed-Salhy M, Lundquist M. Argyrophilic reaction in rectal carcinoids. Path Microbiol Scand 1983;91:84.

526. Doppman JL, Nieman L, Miller DL, et al. Ectopic adreno-corticotropic hormone syndrome: Localization studies in 28 patients. Radiology 1989;172:115.

527. Leveston SA, McKeel DW Jr, Buckley PG, et al. Acromegaly and Cushing's syndrome associated with a foregut carcinoid. J Clin Endocrinol Met 1981;53:682.

528. Sano T, Asa SL, Kovacs K. Growth hormone releasing-producing tumors: Clinical, biochemical and morphological manifestations. Endocr Rev 1988;9:357.

529. Thorson A, Bjork G, Bjorkman G, Waldenstrom J. Malignant carcinoid of the small intestine with metastases to the liver, valvular disease of the right heart (pulmonary stenosis and tricuspid regurgitation without septal defect), peripheral vasomotor symptoms, bronchoconstriction and an unusual type of cyanosis. Am Heart J 1954;47:795.

530. Pernow B, Waldenstrom J. Paroxysmal flushing and other symptoms caused by 5-hydroxytryptamine and histamine in patients with malignant tumors. Lancet 1954;2:951.

531. Davis Z, Moertel CG, McIlrath DC. The malignant carcinoid syndrome. Surg Gynecol Obstet 1973;137:637.

532. Grahame-Smith DG. The carcinoid syndrome. London: William Heineman Medical Books, 1972.

533. Frolich JC, Bloomgarden ZT, Oates JA, et al. The carcinoid flush: Provocation by pentagastrin and inhibition by somatostatin. N Engl J Med 1978;19:1055.

534. Roberts LJ, Marney SR, Oates JA. Blockade of the flush associated with metastatic gastric carcinoid by combined H_1 and H_2 receptor antagonists: Evidence for an important role of H_2 receptors in human vasculature. N Engl J Med 1979;300:236.

535. Peart WS, Robertson JS, Andrews TM. Facial flushing produced in patients with carcinoid syndrome by intravenous adrenaline and noradrenaline. Lancet 1959;2:715.

536. Adamson AR, Grahame-Smith DG, Peart WS, et al. Pharmacological blockade of carcinoid flushing provoked by catecholamines and alcohol. Lancet 1967;2:293.

537. Oates JA, Sjoerdsma A. A unique syndrome associated with secretion of 5-hydroxytryptophan by metastatic gastric carcinoids. Am J Med 1962;32:333.

538. Feldman JM. Carcinoid tumors and syndrome. Semin Oncol 1987;14:237.

539. Knowlessar OD, Law DH, Sleisenger MH. Malabsorption syndrome associated with carcinoid tumors. Am J Med 1959;27:673.

540. Thorson AH. Studies on carcinoid disease. Acta Med Scand 1958;334:81.

541. Roberts WC, Sjoerdsma A. The cardiac disease associated with carcinoid syndrome (carcinoid heart disease). Am J Med 1964;36:5.

542. Lundin L. Carcinoid heart disease. Acta Oncol 1991;30:499.

543. Schiller VL, Fishbein MC, Siegel RJ. Unusual cardiac involvement in carcinoid syndrome. Am Heart J 1986;112:1322.

544. Wong VW, Melman KL. Ophthalmic manifestations of the carcinoid flush. N Engl J Med 1967;277:406.

545. Waldenstrom J. Clinical picture of carcinoidosis. Gastroenterology 1958;35:565.

546. Feldman JM, Jones RS. Carcinoid syndrome from gastrointestinal carcinoids without liver metastases. Ann Surg 1982;196:33.

547. Ricci C, Patrassi N, Massa R, et al. Carcinoid syndrome in bronchial adenoma. Am J Surg 1973;126:671.

548. Moertel CG, Beahrs O, Woolmer LB, Tyce GM. Malignant carcinoid syndrome associated with noncarcinoid tumors. N Engl J Med 1965;273:244.

549. McCaughan BC, Martini H, Bains MS. Bronchial carcinoids: review of 124 cases. J Thorac Cardiovasc Surg 1985;89:8.

550. Cheek RC, Wilson H. Carcinoid tumors. Curr Probl Surg 1970;11:4.

551. Sjoerdsma A. Serotonin. N Engl J Med 1959;261:181.

552. Campbell ACP, Gowenlock AH, Platt DS, et al. A 5-hydroxytryptophan-secreting carcinoid tumor. Gut 1963;4:61.

553. Feldman JM. Serotonin metabolism in carcinoid tumors: Incidence of 5-hydroxytryptophan secreting tumors. Gastroenterology 1978;75:1109.

554. Grahame-Smith DG. Natural history and diagnosis of the carcinoid syndrome. Clin Gastroenterol 1974;3:575.

555. Ahlman H, Dahlstrom A, Gronstadt K, et al. The pentagastrin test in the diagnosis of carcinoid syndrome: Blockage of gastrointestinal symptoms by ketanserin. Ann Surg 1985;201:81.

556. Creutzfeldt W, Stockman F. The carcinoid syndrome. Am J Med 1987;82(Suppl 5B):4.

557. Vinik AI, Gonin J, England BG, Jackson T, McLeod MK, Cho K. Plasma substance-P in neuroendocrine tumors and idiopathic flushing: The value of pentagastrin stimulation tests and the effects of the somatostatin analog. J Clin Endocrinol Metab 1990;70:1702.

558. Oates JA, Melman K, Sjoersdma M, Gillespie L, Mason DT. Release of a kinin peptide in the carcinoid syndrome. Lancet 1964;2:514.

559. Oates JA, Pettinger WA, Doctor RB. Evidence for the release of bradykinin in the carcinoid syndrome. J Clin Invest 1966;45:173.

560. Melman K, Lovenberg W, Sjoerdsma A. Identification of lysylbradykinin as the peptide formed in vitro by carcinoid tumor kallikrein. Clin Chim Acta 1965;12:292.

561. Lucas KJ, Feldman JM. Flushing in the carcinoid syndrome and plasma kallikrein. Cancer 1986;58:2290.

562. Wilkin JK, Roundtree CB. Blockade of the carcinoid flush with cimetidine and clonidine. Arch Dermatol 1982;118:109.

563. Oates JA. The carcinoid syndrome. N Engl J Med 1986;315:702.

564. Sandler M, Karim SM, Williams ED. Prostaglandins in amine-peptide-secreting tumors. Lancet 1968;2:1053.

565. Smith AG, Greaves MW. Blood prostaglandin activity associated with noradrenaline-provoked flush in the carcinoid syndrome. Br J Dermatol 1974;90:547.

566. Jaffe BM, Landon C. Prostaglandin E and F in endocrine diarrheagenic syndromes. Ann Surg 1976;84:516.

567. Metz SA, McRae JR, Robertson PR. Prostaglandins as mediators of paraneoplastic syndromes: Review and update. Metabolism 1981;30:299.

568. Hakanson R, Bengmark S, Brondin E, et al. Substance P like immunoreactivity in intestinal carcinoid tumors. In: Van Euler US (Pernow B, ed). New York: Raven Press, 1977:55.

569. Theodorsson-Norheim E, Norheim I, Oberg K, et al. Neuropeptide K: A major tachykinin in plasma and tumor tissues from carcinoid patients. Biochem Biophys Res Comm 1985;131:77.

570. Conlon JM, Deacon CF, Richter G, Schmidt WE, Stockmann F, Creutzfeldt W. Measurement and partial characterization of the multiple forms of neurokinin A-like immunoreactivity in carcinoid tumors. Regul Pept 1985;131:77.

571. Emson PC, Gilbert RFT, Martensson H, Nobin A. Elevated concentrations of substance P and 5-HT in patients with carcinoid tumors. Cancer 1984;54:715.

572. Norheim I, Theodorsson-Norheim E, Brondin E, Oberg K. Tachykinins in carcinoid tumors: Their use as a tumor marker and possible role in carcinoid flush. J Clin Endocrinol Metab 1986;63:605.

573. Schaffalitsky de Muckadell OB, Aggestrup S, Stentoft P. Flushing and plasma substance P concentration during infusion of synthetic substance P in normal man. Scand J Gastroenterol 1986;21:498.

574. Hendrix TR, Arkinson M, Clifton JA, Ingelfinger FJ. The effect of 5-hydroxytryptamine on intestinal motor function in man. Am J Med 1957;23:886.

575. Feldman JM, Plank JW. Gastrointestinal and metabolic function in patients with the carcinoid syndrome. Am J Med Sci 1977;273:43.

576. Donowitz M, Binder JH. Jejunal fluid and electrolyte secretion in carcinoid syndrome. Am J Dig Dis 1975;20:1115.

577. Warner RRP. Carcinoid tumor. In: Berk JE, Haubrich WS, Kalser MH, Roth JLA, Schnaffner F, eds. Bockus: Gastroenterology. Philadelphia: WB Saunders, 1985:1074.

578. Moertel CG, Kvols LK, Rubin J. A study of cyproheptadine in the treatment of metastatic carcinoid tumor and the malignant carcinoid syndrome. Cancer 1991;67:33.

579. Herxheimer H. Influence of 5-hydroxytryptamine on bronchial function. J Physiol (Lond) 1953;122:49.

580. Lundin L, Norheim I, Landelius J, Oberg K, Theodorsson-Norheim E. Carcinoid heart disease: relationship of circulating vasoactive substances to ultrasound detectable cardiac abnormalities. Circulation 1988;77:264.

581. Feldman JM, Lee EM. Serotonin content of foods: Effect on urinary excretion of 5-hydroxyindoleacetic acid. Am J Clin Nutr 1985;42:639.

582. Feldman JM, Butler SS, Chapman BA. Interference with measurement of 3-methoxy-4-hydroxymandelic acid and 5-hydroxyindoleacetic acid by reducing metabolites. Clin Chem 1974;20:607.

583. Sjoerdsma A, Weissbach H, Udenfriend H. Simple test for diagnosis of metastatic carcinoid (argentaffinoma). JAMA 1955;159:397.

584. Feldman JM. Urinary serotonin in the diagnosis of carcinoid tumors. Clin Chem 1986;32:840.

585. Hussain MN, Sole MJ. A simple, specific radioenzymatic assay for picogram quantities of serotonin or acetylserotonin in biological fluids of tissues. Anal Biochem 1981;111:105.

586. Feldman JM, Davis JA. Radioenzymatic assay of platelet serotonin, dopamine and norepinephrine in subjects with normal and increased serotonin production. Clin Chim Acta 1981;109:275.

587. Wilkin JK. Flushing reactions: Consequences and mechanisms. Ann Intern Med 1981;95:468.

588. Fukayama M, Hayashi Y, Shiozawa Y, Okabe S, Koike M. Human chorionic gonadotropin alpha subunit in rectal carcinoids. Am J Pathol 1989;135:1065.

589. Oberg K, Wide L. HLG and HCG subunits as tumor markers in patients with endocrine pancreatic tumors and carcinoid tumors. Acta Endocrinol 1981;98:256.

590. Feldman JM, Plonk JW. Carcinoembryonic antigen and carcinoid tumors. Ann Intern Med 1975;83:82.

591. Robertson JIS, Peart WS, Andrews TM. The mechanism of facial flushes in the carcinoid syndrome. Q J Med 1961;31:103.

592. Nessi R, Ricci D, Ricci SB, Bosco M, Blanc M. Bronchial carcinoid tumors: Radiologic observations in 49 cases. J Thorac Imaging 1991;6:47.

593. Jeffree MA, Barter SJ, Hemingway AP, Nolan DJ. Primary carcinoid tumors of the ileum: The radiological appearances. Clin Radiol 1985;35:451.

594. Banks NH, Goldstein MH, Dodd G. The roentgenologic spectrum of small intestinal carcinoid tumors. AJR 1975;123:274.

595. Goldstein HM, Miller M. Angiographic evaluation of carcinoid tumors in the small intestine: The value of epinephrine. Radiology 1975;115:23.

596. Sako M, Lunderquist A, Owman T, Martensson H, Norbin A. Angiographic and computed tomographic appearance of secondary carcinoid tumor of the liver. Cardiovasc Intervent Radiol 1982;5:90.

597. McCarthy SM, Stark DD, Moss AA, Goldberg HI. Computed tomography of malignant carcinoid disease. J Comput Assist Tomogr 1984;8:846.

598. Lackey BM, Fishman EK, Jones B, Siegelman SS. Computed tomography of abdominal carcinoid tumors. J Comput Assist Tomogr 1985;9:38.

599. Collatz L, Stage JG, Henriksen FW. Angiography in the diagnosis of carcinoid syndrome. Scand J Gastroenterol 1979;53:111.

600. Gould M, Johnson RJ. Computed tomography of abdominal carcinoid tumour. Br J Radiol 1986;59:881.

601. Hanson MW, Feldman JM, Blinder RH, Moore JO, Coleman RE. Carcinoid tumors: Iodine ^{131}I MIBG scintigraphy. Radiology 1989;172:699.

602. Adolph JMG, Kimmig BN, Georgi P, et al. Carcinoid tumors: CT and ^{131}I-meta-iododobenzylguanidine scintigraphy. Radiology 1976;164:199.

603. Reubi JC, Kvols LK, Waser B, et al. Detection of somatostatin receptors in surgical and percutaneous needle biopsy samples of carcinoids and islet cell tumors. Cancer Res 1990;50:5969.

604. Bakker WH, Krenning EP, Breeman WA, et al. Receptor scintigraphy with radiolabelled somatostatin analogue: Radiolabelling, purification, biologic activity and in vivo application. J Nucl Med 1990;31:501.

605. Lamberts SW, Hofland LJ, van Koetsveld PM, et al. Parallel in vivo and in vitro detection of functional somatostatin receptors in human endocrine tumors: Consequences with regard to diagnosis, localization and therapy. J Clin Endocrinol Metab 1990;31:566.

606. Lamberts SW, Bakker WH, Reubi JC, Krenning EP. Somatostatin receptor imaging in the localization of endocrine tumors. N Engl J Med 1990;323:1246.

607. Feldman JM, Plunk JW. 99mTc-pyrophosphate bone scans in patients with metastatic carcinoid tumors. J Med 1977;8:71.
608. Barton JC, Hirschowitz BI, Maton PN, Jensen RT. Bone metastases in malignant gastrinoma. Gastroenterology 1986;91:915.
609. Orloff MJ. Carcinoid tumors of the rectum. Cancer 1971;28:175.
610. Caldarola VT, Jackman RJ, Moertel CG, et al. Carcinoid tumors of the rectum. Am J Surg 1964;107:844.
611. Brookes VS, Waterhouse JAH, Pawel DJ. Malignant carcinoids of the small intestine: A ten year survey. Br J Surg 1968;55:405.
612. Agranovich AL, Anderson GH, Manji M, Acker BD, MacDonald WC, Threlfall WJ. Carcinoid tumor of the gastrointestinal tract: Prognostic factors and disease outcome. J Surg. Oncol 1991;47:45.
613. Eller R, Frazee R, Roberts J. Gastrointestinal carcinoid tumors. Am Surg 1991;57:434.
614. MacGillivary DG, Snyder DA, Druker W, Remine SR. Carcinoid tumors: The relationship between clinical presentation and the extent of disease. Surgery 1991;110:68.
615. Martensson H, Norbin A, Sundler F. Carcinoid tumors in the gastrointestinal tract: An analysis of 156 cases. Acta Chir Scand 1983;149:607.
616. Tsushima K, Nagorney DM, Weiland LH, Lieber MM. The relationship of low cytometry DNA analysis and clinicopathology in small-intestinal carcinoids. Surgery 1989;105:366.
617. Tsioulias G, Muto T, Kubota Y, et al. DNA ploidy pattern of rectal carcinoid tumors. Dis Colon Rectum 1991;34:31.
618. Von Herbay A, Sieg B, Schurmann G, Betzler M, Otto HF. Proliferative activity of neuroendocrine tumors of the gastroenteropancreatic endocrine system: DNA flow cytometric and immunohistochemical investigations. Gut 1991;32:949.
619. Kujari H, Joensuu H, Klemi P, Asola R, Nordman E. A flow cytometric analysis of 23 carcinoid tumors. Cancer 1988;61:2517.
620. Wilander E, Bjelkenkrantz K, Risberg B. Nuclear DNA recordings in gastric carcinoids. A cytofluorometric study in single tumor cells. Pathol Res Pract 1987;182:331.
621. Jones DJ, Hasleton PS, Moore PN. DNA ploidy in bronchopulmonary carcinoid tumors. Thorax 1988;43:195.
622. El Nugger AK, Pallance W, Karim FW, et al. Typical and atypical bronchopulmonary carcinoids. A clinicopathologic and flow cytometry study. Am J Clin Pathol 1991;95:828.
623. Thunnissen FB, Van Eijk J, Book JP, et al. Bronchopulmonary carcinoids and regional lymph node metastases: A quantitative pathologic investigation. Am J Pathol 1988;132:119.
624. Travis WD, Linnoila RI, Tsokos MG, et al. Neuroendocrine tumors of the lung with proposed criteria for large-cell neuroendocrine carcinoma: An ultrastructural immunohistochemical and flow cytometry study of 35 bases. Am J Surg Pathol 1991;15:529.
625. Moertel CG. Treatment of the carcinoid tumor and the malignant carcinoid syndrome. J Clin Oncol 1983;1:727.
626. Bissonette RT, Gibney RG, Berry BR, Buckley AR. Fatal carcinoid crisis after percutaneous fine-needle biopsy of hepatic metastasis: Case report and literature review. Radiology 1990;174:751.
627. Sukamaran M, Wilkinson ZS, Christainson L. Acute carcinoid syndrome: A complication of flexible fiberoptic bronchoscopy. Ann Thorac Surg 1982;34:702.
628. Miller R, Patel AV, Warner RPR, Parres IH. Anaesthesia for the carcinoid syndrome: A report of nine cases. Can Anaesth Soc J 1978;25:240.
629. Kvols LK, Martin JK, Marsh HM, Moertel CG. Rapid reversal of carcinoid crises with a somatostatin analogue. N Engl J Med 1985;313:1229.
630. Sjoerdsma H, Loyenberg W, Engelman K, Carpenter WT Jr, Wyatt RJ, Gessa GL. Serotonin now: Clinical implications of inhibiting its synthesis with parachlorophenylalanine. Ann Intern Med 1970;73:607.
631. Berry EM, Maunder C, Wilson M. Carcinoid myopathy and treatment with cyproheptadine (Periactin). Gut 1974;15:34.
632. Ureles AL, Murray M, Wolf R. Results of pharmacologic treatment in the malignant carcinoid syndrome. N Engl J Med 1962;267:435.
633. Harris AL, Smith IL. Regression of carcinoid tumor with cyproheptadine. Br Med J 1982;285:475.
634. Robertson JIS. Carcinoid syndrome and serotonin: Therapeutic effects of ketanserin. Cardiovasc Drug Therapy 1990;4:53.
635. Gustafsen J, Lendorf A, Raskov H, Boesby S. Ketanserin versus placebo in carcinoid syndrome. Scand J Gastroenterol 1985;21:816.
636. Sullivan PA, O'Donovan M. Ketanserin as the antagonist in symptomatic treatment of carcinoid syndrome. Irish J Med Sci 1985;155:436.
637. Coupe MO, Anderson JV, Morris JH, Alstead EM, Bloom SR, Hodgson HJF. The effect of the 5-hydroxytryptamine (5HT) receptor antagonist ICS 205-930 in the carcinoid syndrome. Aliment Pharmacol Ther 1988;2:167.
638. Stathopoulous GR, Karvountzis GG, Yiotis J. Tamoxifen in carcinoid syndrome. N J Med 1981;305:52.
639. Myers CF, Ershler WB, Tannenbaum MA, et al. Tamoxifen and carcinoid tumor. Ann Intern Med 1982;96:383.
640. Moertel CG, Engstrom PF, Schutt AJ. Tamoxifen therapy for metastatic carcinoid tumor: A negative study. Ann Intern Med 1984;100:531.
641. Thulin L, Samnegard H, Tyden G, Long DH, Efendic S. Efficacy of somatostatin in a patient with carcinoid tumor. Lancet 1978;2:43.
642. Long RG, Peters JR, Bloom SR, et al. Somatostatin, gastrointestinal peptides and the carcinoid syndrome. Gut 1981;22:549.
643. Dharmsathaphorn K, Sherwin RS, Calaland S, Jaffe B, Dobbins J. Somatostatin inhibits diarrhea in the carcinoid syndrome. Ann Intern Med 1980;92:68.
644. Davis GR, Camp RG, Raskin P, Krejs GJ. Effect of somatostatin infusion on jejunal

water and electrolyte transport in a patient with secretory diarrhea due to malignant carcinoid syndrome. Gastroenterology 1980;78:346.
645. Bauer W, Briner U, Doefner W, et al. SMS-201-995 a very potent and selective octapeptide of somatostatin with prolonged actions. Life Sci 1982;31:1183.
646. Pless J, Bauer W, Briner U, et al. Chemistry and pharmacology of SMS-201-995, a long-acting octapeptide of somatostatin. Scand J Gastroenterol 1986;21(Suppl 119):54.
647. Kutz K, Nuesch J, Rosenthaler J. Pharmacokinetics of SMS-201-995 in healthy subjects. Scand J Gastroenterol 1986;21:65.
648. Vinik AI, Tsai ST, Moattari AR, Cheung P, Eckhauser FE, Cho K. Somatostatin analogue (SMS-201-995) in the management of gastroentero-pancreatic tumors and diarrhea syndromes. Am J Med 1986;81:23.
649. Kvols LK. Metastatic carcinoid tumors and the carcinoid syndrome. Am J Med 1986;81:49.
650. Kvols LK, Moertel CG, O'Connell MJ, Schutt AJ, Rubin J, Hahn RG. Treatment of the malignant carcinoid syndrome: Evaluation of a long-acting somatostatin analogue. N Engl J Med 1986;315:663.
651. Vinik AI, Moattari AR. Use of somatostatin analogue in management of carcinoid syndrome. Dig Dis Sci 1989;34:14S.
652. Oberg K, Norheim I, Theodorsson E. Treatment of malignant carcinoid tumors with a long-acting somatostatin analogue octreotide. Acta Oncol 1991;30:503.
653. Wangberg B, Nilsson O, Theodorsson E, Dahlstrom A, Ahlman H. The effect of somatostatin analogue on the release of hormones from human midgut carcinoid tumor cells. Br J Cancer 1991;64:23.
654. Kvols LK. Therapeutic considerations for the malignant carcinoid syndrome. Acta Oncol 1989;28:433.
655. Kvols LK. Therapy of malignant carcinoid syndrome. Endocrinol Metab Clin North Am 1989;18:557.
656. Richter G, Stockmann F, Lembeke B, Conlon JM, Creutzfeldt W. Short-term administration of somatostatin analogue SMS-201-995 in patients with carcinoid tumor. Scand J Gastroenterol 1986;21:193.
657. Roy RC, Carter RF, Wright KD. Somatostatin, anesthesia and the carcinoid syndrome: Perioperative administration of a somatostatin analogue to suppress carcinoid tumor activity. Anaesthesia 1987;42:627.
658. Oberg K, Norheim I, Lind E, et al. Treatment of malignant carcinoid tumors with human leukocyte interferon: Long term results. Cancer Treat Rev 1986;70:1297.
659. Oberg IL, Funa K, Alma GV. Effects of leukocyte interferon on clinical symptoms and hormone levels in patients with mid gut carcinoid tumors and carcinoid syndrome. N Engl J Med 1983;309:129.
660. Oberg K, Erickson B. The role of interferons in the management of carcinoid tumors. Acta Oncol 1991;30:519.
661. Norbin A, Lindblom A, Mansson B, Sundberg M. Interferon treatment in patients with malignant carcinoids. Acta Oncol 1989;28:445.
662. Hanssen LE, Schrompf E, Jacobsen MB, Kolbenstredt AN, Kolmannskug F, Bergan A, Dulva LO. Extended experience with recombinant 2b interferon with or without hepatic artery embolization in the treatment of midcut carcinoid tumors: A preliminary report. Acta Oncol 1991;30:523.
663. Hanssen LE, Schrumpt E, Kalbenstvedt AN, Tausjo J, Dowa LO. treatment of malignant metastatic midgut carcinoid tumors with recombinant human 2b interferon with or without prior hepatic artery embolization. Scand J Gastroenterol 1989;24:787.
664. Stockman F, von Tomatowski HJ, Reimold WV, Schuster R, Creutzfeldt W. Hepatic artery embolization for treatment of endocrine gastrointestinal tumors with liver metastases. Z Gastroenterol 1984;22:652.
665. Maton PN, Camilleri M, Friggin G, et al. The role of hepatic arterial embolization in the carcinoid syndrome. Br Med J 1983;287:932.
666. Moertel CG, May GR, Martin JK, et al. Sequential hepatic artery occlusion and chemotherapy for metastatic carcinoid tumor and islet cell carcinoma. Proc Amer Soc Clin Oncol 1985;4:80.
667. Venook A, Stagg R, Frye J, Gorden R, Ring E. Chemoembolization of patients with liver metastases from carcinoid and islet cell tumors. Proc Amer Soc Clin Oncol [Abstract] 1991;10:386.
668. Marlink RG, Lakich JJ, Robins JR, Clouse ME. Hepatic arterial embolization for metastatic hormone secreting tumors. Cancer 1991;65:2227.
669. Norbin A, Mansson B, Lunderquist A. Evaluation of temporary liver dearterialization and embolization in patients with metastatic carcinoid tumors. Acta Oncol 1989;28:419.
670. Andaker L, Lamke LO, Smeds S. Follow-up of 102 patients operated for gastrointestinal carcinoid. Acta Chir Scand 1985;151:469.
671. Sauven P, Ridge JE, Quan SH, Siguardson ER. Anorectal carcinoid tumors: Is aggressive surgery warranted? Ann Surg 1990;211:67.
672. Makridis C, Oberg K, Juhlin C, et al. Surgical treatment of midgut carcinoid tumors. World J Surg 1990;14:377.
673. Naunheim KS, Zeitel J, Kaplan EL, et al. Rectal carcinoid tumors - treatment and prognosis. Surgery 1983;94:670.
674. Arunha G. U, Greenlee HB. Surgical management of carcinoid tumors of the gastrointestinal tract. Ann Surg 1980;41:429.
675. Stuart RC. Primary gastric carcinoids. Br J Surg 1991;78:122.
676. Ahlman H, Schensten T, Tisell L-E. Surgical treatment of patients with carcinoid syndrome. Acta Oncol 1989;28:403.
677. Gaitan-Gaitan A, Riden WD, Rush RS. Carcinoid tumor: Cured by radiation. Int J Radiat Oncol Biol Phys 1975;1:9.
678. Keane TS, Rider WP, Harwood HR, et al. Whole body radiation in the management of the metastatic carcinoid tumor. Int J Radiat Oncol Biol Phys 1981;7:1519.
679. Shupak KP, Wallner KE. The role of radiation therapy in the treatment of locally unresectable or metastatic carcinoid tumors. Int J Radiat Oncol Biol Phys 1991;20:489.

680. Shapiro B, Fig LM. Management of pheochromocytomas. Endocrinol Metab Clin North Am 1989;18:443.

681. Bauer P, van de Fierdt E, Stettmeier H, Langhammer HR, Pabst HW. ^{125}I-MIBG therapy of carcinoid tumor of intestinal origin. Eur J Nucl Med 1988;14:234.

682. Hoefnagel LA, der van Hartog Jaeger FC, Tool GB, Abeling NG, Engelsman EE. The role of ^{125}I-MIBG in the diagnosis and therapy of carcinoids. Eur J Nucl Med 1987;13: 187.

683. Hoefnagel CA, der van Hartog Jaeger FC, van Gennig AM, et al. Diagnosis and therapy of carcinoid tumor using ^{131}I metaiodobenzylguanidine. Clin Nucl Med 1986;11:150.

684. Van Hazel GA, Rubin J, Moertel CG. Treatment of metastatic carcinoid tumor with dactinomycin or dacarbazine. Cancer Treat Rep 1983;67:583.

685. Moertel CG, Rubin J, O'Connell MJ. Phase II study of cisplatin therapy in patients with metastatic carcinoid tumor and the malignant carcinoid syndrome. Cancer Treat Rep 1986;70:1459.

686. Kelsen D, Fiore J, Heelar R, et al. Phase II trial of ectoposide in APUD tumors. Cancer Treat Rep 1987;71:305.

687. Kvols LK, Buck M. Chemotherapy of endocrine malignancies. Semin Oncol 1987;14: 343.

688. Engstrom PF, Lavin PT, Folsch E, Moertel CG, Douglas HO. Streptozotocin plus fluorouracil versus doxorubicin therapy for metastatic carcinoid tumors. J Clin Oncol 1984;2:1255.

689. Kelsen DG, Cheng E, Kemeny N, Magill GB, Yagoda A. Streptozotocin and adriamycin in the treatment of APUD tumors (carcinoid, islet cell and medullary thyroid). Proc Amer Assoc Cancer Res 1982;23:433.

690. Doberauer C, Niecterle N, Klobe O, Kurschel E, Schmidt GS. Zur behandlung des metastatasserten karzoids van ileum und cecum mit arkombinatem interferon alpha-2b. Oncologie 1987;10:340.

691. Jensen RT, Doppman JL, Gardner JD. Gastrinoma. In: Go VLW, Brooks FA, DiMagno EP, Gardner JD, Lebenthal E, Scheele GA, eds. The exocrine pancreas: Biology, pathobiology and disease. New York: Raven Press, 1986:727–744.

692. Bukowski RM, Johnson KG, Peterson RF, et al. A Phase II trial combination chemotherapy in patients with metastatic carcinoid tumors: A Southwest Oncology Group study. Cancer 1987;60:2891.

693. Boddie AW Jr, McMurtrey MJ, Diacco GG, McBride CM. Palliative total gastrectomy and esophagogastrectomy. Cancer 1983;51:1195.

694. Kvols LK, Buck M. Chemotherapy of endocrine malignancies: A review. Semin Oncol 1987;14:343.

695. Creutzfeldt W, Bartsch HH, Jacubaschke U, Stockmann F. Treatment of gastrointestinal endocrine tumors with interferon-α and octreotide. Acta Oncol 1991;30:529.

696. Kvols LK, Moertel CG, Schutt AJ, Rubin J. Treatment of the malignant carcinoid syndrome with a long acting somatostatin analogue (SMS 201-995): Preliminary evidence that more is not better. Proc Amer Soc Clin Oncol 1987;6:95.

697. Oberg K, Norheim I, Alm G, et al. Long-term treatment of malignant carcinoid tumors with human leukocyte interferon. In: Stewart WE, et al, eds. Biology of the interferon system. New York: Elsevier Science Publisher, 1985:433.

698. Oberg K, Eriksson B, Norheim I. Interferon treatment of neuroendocrine gut tumors. J Clin Oncol 1987;6:80.

699. Moertel CG, Rubin J, Kvols LK. Therapy of metastatic carcinoid tumor and the malignant carcinoid syndrome with recombinant leukocyte A interferon. J Clin Oncol 1989;7:865.

700. Ronnblom LE, Alm GV, Oberg KE. Autoimmunity after alpha-interferon therapy for malignant carcinoid tumors. Ann Intern Med 1991;115:178.

701. Grander D, Oberg K, Lundquist M-L, Jansun ET, Eriksson B, Einhorn S. Interferon-induced enhancement of 2',5'-oligoadenylate synthetase in mid-gut carcinoid tumors. Lancet 1990;336:337.

702. Jensen RT, Norton JA. Pancreatic endocrine tumors. In: Yamada T, Alpers DH, Owyang C, Powell DW, Silverstein FE, eds. Textbook of gastroenterology. Philadelphia: JB Lippincott, 1991:1912.

703. Chiang HC, O'Dorisio TM, Huang SC, et al. Multiple hormone elevations in patients with Zollinger-Ellison syndrome: Prospective study of clinical significance and of development of a second symptomatic pancreatic endocrine tumor syndrome. Gastroenterology 1990;99:1565.

704. Schein PS, DeLellis RA, Kahn CR, Gorden P, Kraft AR. Islet cell tumors: Current concepts and management. Ann Intern Med 1973;79:239.

705. Becker V. Pathologisch-anatomische aspekte bei endokrin wirksamon. Tumoren Langenbecks Arch 1971;88:426.

706. Grimelius L, Hultquist D, Stenkvist B. Cytological differentiation of asymptomatic pancreatic endocrine tumors in autopsy material. Virchows Arch A Pathol Anat Histopathol 1975;365:275.

707. Weil C. Gastroenteropancreatic endocrine tumors. Klin Wochenschr 1985;63:433.

708. Buchanan KD, Johnston CF, O'Hare MMT, et al. Neuroendocrine tumors: A European view. Am J Med 1986;81(Suppl 68):14.

709. Dent RB, van Heerden JA, Weiland LH. Nonfunctioning islet cell tumors. Ann Surg 1981;193:185.

710. Broder LE, Carter SK. Pancreatic islet cell carcinoma: Clinical features of 52 patients. Ann Intern Med 1973;79:101.

711. Koppel G, Heitz PU. Pancreatic endocrine tumors. Pathol Res Pract 1988;183:155.

712. Jensen RT, Gardner JD. Zollinger-Ellison syndrome: Clinical presentation, pathology, diagnosis and treatment. In: Dannenberg A, Zakim D, eds. Peptic ulcer and other acid-related diseases. New York: Academic Research Association, 1991:117.

713. Zollinger RM, Ellison EH. Primary peptic ulceration of the jejunum associated with islet cell tumors of the pancreas. Ann Surg 1955;142:709.

714. Gregory RA, Tracy HJ, French JM, Sircus W. Extraction of a gastrin-like substance

715. from a pancreatic tumor in a case of Zollinger-Ellison syndrome. Lancet 1960;1: 1045.

715. Gregory RA, Grossman MI, Tracy HJ, Bentley PH. Nature of the gastric secretogue in Zollinger-Ellison tumors. Lancet 1967;2:543.

716. Gregory RA, Tracy JH, Agarwal KL. Amino acid constitution of two gastrins isolated from Zollinger-Ellison tumor tissue. Gut 1969;10:603.

717. Stage JG, Stadil F. The clinical diagnosis of the Zollinger-Ellison syndrome. Scand J Gastroenterol 1979;14:79.

718. Grossman MI, ed. Peptic ulcer. Chicago: Yearbook Medical Publishers, 1981:141–151.

719. Jensen RT, Gardner JD, Raufman JP. Zollinger-Ellison syndrome. NIH combined clinical staff conference. Ann Intern Med 1983;98:59.

720. Zollinger RM, Ellison EC, Fabri PJ, et al. Primary peptic ulceration of the jejunum associated with islet cell tumors: Twenty-five year appraisal. Ann Surg 1980;192: 422.

721. Thompson JC, Reeder DD, Villar HV, et al. Natural history and experience with diagnosis and treatment of the Zollinger-Ellison syndrome. Surg Gynecol Obstet 1975;140:721.

722. Bonfils S, Landor SH, Mignon M, Hervoir P, et al. Results of surgical management in 92 consecutive patients with Zollinger-Ellison syndrome. Ann Surg 1981;194:692.

723. Johnson LR. Gut hormones on growth of gastrointestinal mucosa. In: Chey WY, Brooks FP, eds. Endocrinology of the gut. Thorofare, NJ: Charles B. Slack, 1974:163.

724. Neurburger PH, Lewin M, Bonfils S. Parietal and chief cell populations in 4 cases of the Zollinger-Ellison syndrome. Gastroenterology 1972;937.

725. Sum P, Perey BJ. Parietal cell mass (PCM) in a man with Zollinger-Ellison syndrome. Can J Surg 1969;12:285.

726. Wright HK, Hersh T, Floch MH, Weinstein LD. Impaired intestinal absorption in the Zollinger-Ellison syndrome independent of gastric hypersecretion. Am J Surg 1970;119:150.

727. Creutzfeldt W, Arnold R, Creutzfeld C, et al. Pathomorphological, biochemical and diagnostic aspects of gastrinomas (Zollinger-Ellison syndrome). Hum Pathol 1975;6: 47.

728. Dockray GJ, Walsh JH, Passaro E Jr. Relative abundance of big and little gastrins in the tumors and blood of patients with Zollinger-Ellison syndrome. Gut 1975;16:353.

729. Walsh JH, Grossman MI. Gastrin. N Engl J Med 1975;292:1324.

730. Eysselein VE, Maxwell V, Peedy T, Wunsch E, Walsh JH. Similar and stimulatory potencies of synthetic human big and little gastrins in man. JNCI 1984;73:1284.

731. Dockray GJ, Walsh JH. Amino terminal gastrin fragment in serum of Zollinger-Ellison syndrome patients. Gastroenterology 1975;68:222.

732. Rehfeld JF, Stadil F. Gel filtration studies on immunoreactive gastrin in serum from Zollinger-Ellison patients. Gut 1973;14:369.

733. Kothary PC, Fabri PJ, Gower W, O'Dorisio TM, Ellis J, Vinik A. Evaluation of NH2-terminus gastrins in gastrinoma syndrome. J Endocrinol Metab 1986;62:970.

734. Kothary PC, Mahoney WC, Vinik AI. Identification of gastrin molecular variants in gastrinoma syndrome. Regul Pept 1987;17:71.

735. Hilsted L, Bardram LC. Terminally glycine extended gastrins in serum and tumors from patients with Zollinger-Ellison syndrome. Can J Physiol Pharmacol 1986:136.

736. Desmond H, Parcevelo S, Varro A, Gregory H, Yaund J, Dockray GJ. Isolation and characterization of the intact gastrin precursor from a gastrinoma. FEBS Lett 1987;210: 185.

737. Pauwels S, Desmond H, Dimaline R, Dockray GJ. Identification of progastrin in gastrinoma, antrum and duodenum by a novel radioimmunoassay. J Clin Invest 1986;77:376.

738. Bardram L. Progastrin in serum from Zollinger-Ellison patients: An indicator of malignancy? Gastroenterology 1990;98:1420.

739. Del Valle G, Sugano K, Yamada T. Progastrin and its glycine-extended posttranslational processing intermediates in human gastrointestinal tissues. Gastroenterology 1987;87: 1908.

740. Dockray GJ, Varro A, Desmond H, Young J, Gregory H, Gregory RA. Posttransitional processing of the porcine gastrin precursor by phosphorylation of the COOH-terminal fragment. J Biol Chem 1987;262:8643.

741. Johnson JA, Fabri PJ, Lott JA. Serum gastrins in Zollinger-Ellison syndrome: Identification of localized disease. Clin Chem 1980;26:867.

742. Hofman JW, Fox PS, Wilson SD. Duodenal wall tumors and the Zollinger-Ellison syndrome. Arch Surg 1973;107:334.

743. Norton JA, Doppman JL, Collen MJ, Harmon JW, Maton PN, Gardner JD, Jensen RT. Prospective study of gastrinoma localization and resection in patients with Zollinger-Ellison syndrome. Ann Surg 1986;204:468.

744. Wolfe MM, Alexander RW, McGuigan JE. Extrapancreatic, extraintestinal gastrinoma: Effective treatment by surgery. N Engl J Med 1982;306:1533.

745. Norton JA, Doppman JL, Jensen RT. Curative resection in Zollinger-Ellison syndrome: Results of a 10 year prospective study. Ann Surg 1992;215:8.

746. Stabile BE, Morrow DJ, Passaro E. The gastrinoma triangle: Operative implications. Am J Surg 1984;147:25.

747. Maton PN, Macken SM, Norton JA, Gardner JD, O'Dorisio TM, Jensen RT. Ovarian carcinoma as a cause of Zollinger-Ellison syndrome. Gastroenterology 1989;97:464.

748. Howard TJ, Zinner MJ, Stabile BE, Passaro E Jr. Gastrinoma excision for cure. Ann Surg 1990;211:9.

749. Primrose JN, Maloney M, Wells M, Bulgin O, Johnston D. Gastrin-producing ovarian mucinous cystadenomas: A cause of Zollinger-Ellison syndrome. Surgery 1988;104: 830.

750. Bollen ECM, Lamers CBHW, Jansen JBMJ, Larsson LI, Joosten HJ. Zollinger-Ellison syndrome due to a gastrin-producing ovarian cystadenoma. Br J Surg 1981;68:776.

751. Cocco AE, Conway SJ. Zollinger-Ellison syndrome associated with ovarian mucinous cystadenocarcinomas. N Engl J Med 1975;293:485.

752. Friesen SR. Tumors of the endocrine pancreas. N Engl J Med 1982;306:580.

753. Larsson LI, Rehfeld JR, Goltermann N. Gastrin in the human fetus. Distribution and molecular forms of gastrin in the antro-pyloric gland area, duodenum, and pancreas. Scand J Gastroenterol 1977;12:869.

754. Solcia E, Capella C, Buffa R, Frigerio G, Fiocca R. Pathology of the Zollinger-Ellison syndrome. In: Fengolio LM, Wolff M, eds. Progress in surgical pathology. 1980;119.

755. Thom AK, Norton JA, Axiotix CA, Jensen RT. Location, incidence and malignant potential of duodenal gastrinomas. Surgery 1991;110:1086.

756. Pipeleers-Marichal M, Somers G, Willems G, Foulis A, Imrie C, Bishop AE, et al. Gastrinomas in the duodenums of patients with multiple endocrine neoplasic type 1 and the Zollinger-Ellison syndrome. N Engl J Med 1990;322:723.

757. Ellison EC, Wilson SD. The Zollinger-Ellison syndrome: Re-appraisal and evaluation of 260 registered cases. Ann Surg 1964;160:512.

758. Fox PS, Hofmann JW, Wilson SD, DeCosse JJ. Surgical management of the Zollinger-Ellison syndrome. Surg Clin North Am 1974;54:394.

759. Zollinger RM, Martin EW, Carey LC. Observations on the post-operative tumor growth of certain islet cell tumors. Ann Surg 1976;184:525.

760. Friesen SR. The development of endocrinopathies in the prospective screening of two families with MEN-1. World J Surg 1979;3:753.

761. Larsson LI, Ljungberg O, Sundler F, et al. Antropyloric gastrinoma associated with pancreatic nesidioblastosis and proliferation of islets. Virchows Arch [A] 1973;360:305.

762. Thompson JC, Lewis BG, Wiener I, Townsend CM Jr. The role of surgery in the Zollinger-Ellison Syndrome. Ann Surg 1983;197:594.

763. Harmon JW, Norton JA, Collen MJ. Removal of gastrinomas for control of Zollinger-Ellison syndrome. Ann Surg 1984;200:396.

764. Jensen RT, Maton PN. Zollinger-Ellison syndrome. In: Gustavsson S, Kumar D, Graham DY, eds. The stomach. London: Churchill Livingstone, 1991:341.

765. Zollinger RM, Ellison EC, O'Dorisio T, Sparks J. Thirty years' experience with gastrinoma. World J Surg 1984;8:427.

766. Malagelada JR, Edis AJ, Adson MA, van Heerden JA, Go VLW. Medical and surgical options in the management of patients with gastrinoma. Gastroenterology 1983;84:1524.

767. Stabile BE, Passaro E. Benign and malignant gastrinoma. Am J Surg 1984;149:144.

768. Mukai K, Greider MH, Grotting JC, Rosai J. Retrospective study of 77 pancreatic endocrine tumors using the immunoperoxidase method. Am J Surg Pathol 1982;6:387.

769. Larsson LI. Classification of pancreatic endocrine tumors. Scand J Gastroenterol 1978;14:15.

770. Heitz PU, Kasper M, Polak JM, Kloppel G. Pancreatic endocrine tumors. Hum Pathol 1982;13:263.

771. Blackburn AM, Bryant MG, Adrian TE, Bloom SR. Pancreatic tumors produce neurotensin. J Clin Endocrinol Metab 1981;52:820.

772. Bloom SR, Adrian TE, Bryant MG, Polak JM. Pancreatic polypeptide: A marker for Zollinger-Ellison syndrome. Lancet 1978;1:1155.

773. Lamers CBH, Diemel JM, Roeffen W. Serum levels of pancreatic polypeptide in Zollinger-Ellison syndrome and hyperparathyroidism from families with multiple endocrine adenamotosis type I. Digestion 1978;18:297.

774. Taylor IL, Rotter J, Walsh JH, Passaro E Jr. Is pancreatic polypeptide a marker for Zollinger-Ellison syndrome? Lancet 1978;1:845.

775. Yamaguchi K, Abe A, Miyakawa S, Ohnami S. Multiple hormone production in endocrine tumors in the pancreas. In: Miyoshi H, ed. Gut hormones. Amsterdam: Elsevier North-Holland Biomedical Press, 1979:343.

776. Adrian TE, Uttenthal LD, Williams SJ, Bloom SR. Secretion of pancreatic polypeptide in patients with pancreatic endocrine tumors. N Engl J Med 1986;315:287.

777. Langstein HN, Norton JA, Chiang HC. V, et al. The utility of circulating levels of human pancreatic polypeptide as a marker of islet cell tumors. Surgery 1990;108:1109.

778. Sheppard BC, Norton JA, Doppman JL, Maton PN, Gardner JD, Jensen RT. Management of islet cell tumors in patients with multiple endocrine neoplasia: A prospective study. Surgery 1989;106:1108.

779. McCarthy DM, Weintraub B. Subunits of human chorionic gonadotropin in the Zollinger-Ellison syndrome. Gastroenterology 1979;76:1198.

780. Stabile BE, Braunstein GD, Passaro E Jr. Serum gastrin and human chorionic gonadotropin in the Zollinger-Ellison syndrome. Arch Surg 1980;115:1090.

781. Bardram L, Agner T, Hagen C. Levels of alpha subunits of gonadotropin can be increased in Zollinger-Ellison syndrome, both in patients with malignant tumors and apparently benign disease. Acta Endocrinol 1988;118:135.

782. Kloppel G, Girard J, Polak JW, Vaitukaitis JL, Kasper M, Heitz PU. Alpha human chorionic gonadotropin and neuron specific enolase as markers for malignancy and neuroendocrine nature of pancreatic endocrine tumors. Cancer Detect Prev 1983;6:161.

783. Norton JA, Jensen RT. Unresolved surgical issues in the management of patients with Zollinger-Ellison syndrome. World J Surg 1991;15:151.

784. Hagn C, Schmid KW, Rischer-Calibrie R, Winkler H. Chromogranin A, B and C in human adrenal medulla and endocrine tissues. Lab Invest 1986;55:405.

785. Lloyd RV, Mervak T, Schmidt K, Warner TGCS, Wilson BS. Immunohistochemical detection of chromogranin and neurospecific enolase in pancreatic endocrine tumors. Am J Surg Pathol 1984;8:607.

786. O'Connor DT, Deftos LJ. Secretion of chromogranin A by peptide-producing endocrine neoplasms. N Engl J Med 1986;314:1145.

787. Sobol RE, Memoli V, Deftos LJ. Hormone-negative, chromogranin A-positive endocrine tumors. N Engl J Med 1989;320:444.

788. Wiedenmann B, Waldherr R, Buhr H, Hille A, Russa P, Huttner WB. Identification of gastroenteropancreatic neuroendocrine cells in normal and neoplastic human tissue with antibodies against synaptophysin, chromogranin A, secretogranin I (chromogranin B), and secretogranin II. Gastroenterology 1988;95:1364.

789. Stabile BE, Howard TJ, Passaro EJ Jr, O'Connor DJ. Source of plasma chromogranin A elevation in gastrinoma. Arch Surg 1990;125:451.

790. Niewenhuijzen-Knuseman AC, Knijnenburg G, Ribiere GB, Bosman FT. Morphology and immunohistochemically-defined endocrine function of pancreatic islet cell tumors. Histopathology 1978;2:389.

791. Regan PT, Malagelada JR. A reappraisal of clinical, roentgenographic, and endoscopic features of the Zollinger-Ellison syndrome. Mayo Clin Proc 1978;53:19.

792. Jensen RT, Gardner JD. Zollinger-Ellison syndrome: Clinical presentation, pathology, diagnosis, and treatment. In: Zakim D, Dannenberg AJ, eds. Peptic ulcer disease and other acid-related disorders. Armonk, NY: Academic Research Associates, 1991;117–211.

793. Richter JF, Pandol SI, Castell DO, McCarthy DM. Gastroesophageal reflux disease in the Zollinger-Ellison syndrome. Ann Intern Med 1981;95:37.

794. Miller LS, Vinayek R, Frucht H, Gardner JD, Jensen RT, Maton PN. Reflux esophagitis in patients with Zollinger-Ellison syndrome. Gastroenterology 1990;98:341.

795. Waxsman I, Gardner JD, Jensen RT, Maton PN. Peptic ulcer perforation as the presentation of Zollinger-Ellison syndrome. Dig Dis Sci 1991;36:19.

796. Wolfe MM, Jensen RT. Zollinger-Ellison syndrome, Current concepts in diagnosis and management. N Engl J Med 1987;317:1200.

797. Wolfe MM, Jain DK, Edgerton JR. Zollinger-Ellison syndrome associated with persistent normal fasting serum gastrin concentrations. Ann Intern Med 1985;103:215.

798. Aoyagi T, Summerskill SHJ. Gastric secretion with ulcerogenic islet cell tumor. Arch Intern Med 1966;117:667.

799. Deveney CW, Deveney KS, Way LW. The Zollinger-Ellison syndrome: 23 years later. Ann Surg 1978;188:384.

800. Deveney CW, Deveney KS, Jaffe BM, Janes RS, Way LW. Use of calcium and secretin in the diagnosis of gastrinoma (Zollinger-Ellison syndrome). Ann Intern Med 1979;87:680.

801. Malagelada JR, Davis CS, O'Fallon WM, Go VLW. Laboratory diagnosis of gastrinoma. Mayo Clin Proc 1982;57:211.

802. Isenberg JI, Walsh JH, Grossman MI. Zollinger-Ellison syndrome. Gastroenterology 1973;65:140.

803. Van Heerden JA, Bernatz PE, Rovelstad RA. The retained antrum-clinical considerations. Mayo Clin Proc 1971;46:25.

804. Korman MG, Scott DG, Hansky J, Wilson H. Hypergastrinemia due to excluded gastric antrum: A proposed method for differentiation from Zollinger-Ellison syndrome. Aust N Z J Med 1972;3:266.

805. Chaudhuri TK, Shirazi SS, Condon RE. Radioisotope scan: A possible aid in differentiating retained gastric antrum from Zollinger-Ellison syndrome in patients with recurrent peptic ulcer. Gastroenterology 1973;65:697.

806. Frucht H, Howard JM, Slaff JE, et al. Secretin and calcium provocative tests in patients with Zollinger-Ellison syndrome: A prospective study. Ann Intern Med 1989;111:713.

807. Isenberg JI, Walsh JH, Passaro E Jr, Moore EW, Grossman MI. Unusual effect of secretin on serum gastrin, serum calcium, and gastric acid secretion in a patient with suspected Zollinger-Ellison syndrome. Gastroenterology 1972;62:626.

808. Cherner JA, Doppman JL, Norton JA, et al. Prospective assessment of selective venous sampling for gastrin to localize gastrinomas. Ann Intern Med 1986;105:841.

809. Lamers CBH, van Tongeren JHM. Comparative study of the use of calcium, secretin, and meal stimulated increase in serum gastrin in the diagnosis of the Zollinger-Ellison syndrome. Gut 1979;18:128.

810. Frucht H, Howard JM, Stark HA, et al. Prospective study of meal provocative gastrin testing in patients with Zollinger-Ellison syndrome. Am J Med 1989;87:528.

811. Ganguli PC, Elder JB, Polak MJ, Pearse AGE. Antral gastrin cell hyperplasia in peptic ulcer disease. Lancet 1974;1:288.

812. Polak JM, Stagg B, Pearse AGE. Two types of Zollinger-Ellison syndrome: Immunofluorescent, cytochemical, and ultrastructural studies of the antral and pancreatic gastric cells in different clinical states. Gut 1972;13:501.

813. Friesen SR, Schimke RN, Pearse AGE. Genetic aspects of Z-E syndrome: Prospective studies in two kindreds—Antral gastrin cell hyperplasia. Ann Surg 1972;176:370.

814. Friesen SR, Tomita T. Pseudo-Zollinger-Ellison syndrome: Hypergastrinemia, hyperchlorohydria without tumor. Ann Surg 1981;194:481.

815. Lamers CBH, Ruland CM, Joosten HJM, Verkooyen HCM, Tongeren JHM, Rehfeld JF. Hypergastrinemia of antral origin in duodenal ulcer. Dig Dis Sci 1978;23:998.

816. Taylor IL, Calam JK, Roth JI, et al. Family studies of hypergastrinemic hyperpepsinogenemic I duodenal ulcer. Ann Intern Med 1981;95:421.

817. Hangen D, Maltz GS, Anderson CM. Marked hypergastrinemia in gastric outlet obstruction. J Clin Gastroenterol 1989;11:442.

818. Fuerle G, Ketterer H, Becker HD, Creutzfeldt W. Circadian serum gastrin concentrations in control persons and in patients with ulcer disease. Scand J Gastroenterol 1972;7:177.

819. Saeed ZA, Doppman JL, Norton J, Maton PN, Gardner JD, Jensen RT. Gastrinoma localization in Zollinger-Ellison syndrome. Intern Med Specialist 1988;9:79.

820. Maton PN, Gardner JD, Jensen RT. Recent advances in the management of gastric hypersecretion in patients with Zollinger-Ellison syndrome. Med Clin North Am 1989;18:847.

821. Fox PS, Hofmann JW, DeCosse JJ, Wilson SD. The influence of total gastrectomy on survival in malignant Zollinger-Ellison tumors. Ann Surg 1974;180:558.

822. Mignon M, Ruszniewski P, Haffar S, Rigaud D, Rene E, Bonfils S. Current approach to the management of the tumoral process in patients with gastrinoma. World J Surg 1986;10:703.

823. Deveney CW, Deveney KE, Stark D, Moss A, Stein S, Way LW. Resection of gastrinomas. Ann Surg 1983;198:546.

824. McCarthy DM. The place of surgery in the Zollinger-Ellison syndrome. N Engl J Med 1980;302:1344.

825. Richardson CT, Peters MN, Feldman M. Treatment of Zollinger-Ellison syndrome with exploratory laparotomy, proximal gastric vagotomy, and H2-receptor antagonists. Gastroenterology 1985;89:357.

826. Norton JA, Sugarbaker PH, Doppman JL, et al. Aggressive resection of metastatic disease in select patients with malignant gastrinoma. Ann Surg 1986;203:352.

827. London JF, Shawker TH, Doppman JL, et al. Prospective assessment of abdominal ultrasound in patients with Zollinger-Ellison syndrome. Radiology 1991;178:763.

828. Wank SA, Doppman HL, Miller DL, et al. Prospective study of the ability of computerized axial tomography to localize gastrinomas in patients with Zollinger-Ellison syndrome. Gastroenterology 1987;92:905.

829. Thompson NW, Vinik AI, Eckhauser FE. Microgastrinomas of the duodenum. Ann Surg 1989;209:396.

830. Maton PN, Miller DL, Doppman HL, et al. Role of selective angiography in the management of Zollinger-Ellison syndrome. Gastroenterology 1987;92:913.

831. Tjon Tham RTO, Falke TAM, et al. CT and MR imaging in advanced Zollinger-Ellison syndrome. Comput Assist Tomogr 1989;13:821.

832. Stark DD, Moss AA, Goldberg HI, et al. Computed tomography and nuclear magnetic resonance imaging of pancreatic islet cell tumors. Surgery 1983;94:1024.

833. Frucht H, Doppman JL, Norton JA, et al. MR imaging of gastrinomas: Comparison with computed tomography, angiography and ultrasound. Radiology 1989;171:713.

834. Legman P, Ruszniewski P, Sibert A, et al. Computed tomograph (CT) and magnetic imaging (MRI) in liver metastases (LM) of digestive endocrinology tumors (DET): A prospective study in 24 patients. Gastroenterology 1989;96:294.

835. Pisegna J, Doppman JL, Metz D, Slimak GG, Gardner JD, Jensen RT. Prospective study of the ability of magnetic resonance (MRI) to detect gastrinomas in patients with Zollinger-Ellison syndrome. Program of American College of Gastroenterology Meeting, 1991.

836. Frucht H, Norton JA, London JF, et al. Detection of duodenal gastrinomas by operative endoscopic transillumination: A prospective study. Gastroenterology 1990;99:1622.

837. Ruszniewski P, Mouyal PA, Combes R, et al. Endoscopic ultrasonography (EUS) is useful for localization of primary gastrinomas. Gastroenterology [Abstract] 1991;100:297.

838. Roche A, Raisonnier A, Gillon-Savouret MC. Pancreatic venous sampling and arteriography in localizing insulinomas and gastrinomas: Procedure and results in 55 cases. Radiology 1982;145:621.

839. Burcharth F, Stage JG, Stadil F, et al. Localization of gastrinoma by transhepatic portal catheterization and gastrin assay. Gastroenterology 1979;77:44.

840. Glowniak JV, Shapiro B, Vinik AI, Glaser B, Thompson NW, Cho KJ. Percutaneous transhepatic venous sampling of gastrin: Value in sporadic and familial islet-cell tumors and G-cell hyperfunction. N Engl J Med 1982;307:293.

841. Miller DL, Doppman JL, Metz D, Maton PN, Jensen RT. Portal venous sampling in Zollinger-Ellison syndrome: Technique, results and complications in 95 procedures. Radiology 1991 (in press).

842. Vinik A, Moattari R, Cho K, Thompson N. Transhepatic portal venous catherization for localization for sporadic and MEN gastrinomas. Surgery 1990;107:246.

843. Doppman JL, Shawker TH, Miller DC. Localization of islet cell tumors. Med Clin North Am 1989;18:793.

844. Norton JA, Shawker TH, Doppman JL, et al. Localization and surgical treatment of occult insulinomas. Ann Surg 1990;212:615.

845. Imamura M, Takashi MP, Isobe Y, Hattori Y, Satomura K, Tobe T. Curative resection of multiple gastrinomas aided by selective arterial secretin injection and intraoperative secretin test. Ann Surg 1989;210:710.

846. Doppman JL, Miller DL, Chang R, et al. Gastrinomas: Localization by means of selective intraarterial injection of secretin. Radiology 1974;174:25.

847. Sigel B, Coelho MCU, Nyhus LM, et al. Detection of pancreatic tumors by ultrasound during surgery. Arch Radiol 1982;117:1058.

848. Charboneau WJ, James EM, van Heerden JA, et al. Intraoperative realtime ultrasonographic localization of pancreatic insulinomas. J Ultrasound Med 1983;2:251.

849. Cromack DT, Norton JA, Sigel et al. The use of high-resolution intraoperative ultrasound to localize gastrinomas: An initial report of a prospective study. World J Surg 1987;11:648.

850. Norton JA, Cromack DT, Shawker TH, et al. Intraoperative ultrasonographic localization of islet cell tumors. Ann Surg 1988;207:160.

851. Comi RJ, Gorden P, Doppman HL, Norton JA. Insulinoma. In: Go VLW, Gardner JD, Brooks FP, et al, eds. The exocrine pancreas: Biology, pathology and diseases. New York: Raven Press, 1986:745–761.

852. Friesen SR. Effect of total gastrectomy on the Zollinger-Ellison tumor: Observation by second-look operations. Surgery 1967;62:609.

853. Friesen SR. Treatment of the Zollinger-Ellison syndrome. Am J Surg 1982;143:331.

854. McArthur KE, Collen MJ, Maton PN. Omeprazole: Effective convenient therapy for Zollinger-Ellison syndrome. Gastroenterology 1985;88:939.

855. Lamers CDHW, Lind T, Moberg S, Jansen JBMJ, Olbe L. Omeprazole in Zollinger-Ellison syndrome: Effects of a single dose and of long term treatment in patients resistant to histamine H2-receptor antagonists. N Engl J Med 1984;310:758.

856. Frucht H, Maton P, Jensen RT. The use of omeprazole in patients with Zollinger-Ellison syndrome. Dig Dis Sci 1991;36:405.

857. Hirschowitz BI, Denen J, Raufman JP, LaMont B, Berman R, Humphries T. A mul-

858. ticenter U.S. study of omeprazole treatment of Zollinger-Ellison syndrome. Gastroenterology [Abstract] 1988;94:188.

858. Delcher JC, Soule JC, Mignon M, et al. Effectiveness of omeprazole in seven patients with Zollinger-Ellison syndrome resistant to histamine H2-receptor antagonists. Dig Dis Sci 1986;31:693.

859. Lloyd-Davis KA, Rutgerssan K, Solvell L. Omeprazole in Zollinger-Ellison syndrome: Four year international study. Gastroenterology 1986;90:1523.

860. Meijer JL, Jansen JB, Lamers CB. Omeprazole in the treatment of Zollinger-Ellison syndrome and histamine H2-antagonist refractory ulcers. Digestion 1989;44:31.

861. Maton PN, McArthur KE, Wank SA, et al. Long-term efficacy and safety of omeprazole in patients with Zollinger-Ellison syndrome. Gastroenterology 1986;90:1537.

862. Vinayek R, Howard JM, Maton PN, et al. Famotidine in the therapy of gastric hypersecretory states. Am J Med 1986;81:49.

863. Collen MJ, Howard JM, McArthur KE, et al. Comparison of ranitidine and cimetidine in the treatment of gastric hypersecretion. Ann Intern Med 1984;100:52.

864. McCarthy DM, Hyman PE. Effect of isopropamide on response to oral cimetidine in patients with Zollinger-Ellison syndrome. Dig Dis Sci 1982;27:353.

865. Miller LS, Doppman JD, Maton PN, Gardner JD, Jensen RT. Zollinger-Ellison syndrome. In: Collen MJ, Benjamin SB, eds. Pharmacology of peptic ulcer disease. Handbook of experimental pharmacology, 1991 (in press).

866. McCarthy DM, Peikin SR, Lopatin RN. Hyperparathyroidism: A reversible cause of cimetidine-resistant gastric hypersecretion. Br Med J 1979;1:765.

867. Gogel HK, Buckman MT, Cadieux D, McCarthy DM. Gastric secretion and hormonal interactions in multiple endocrine neoplasms type I. Arch Intern Med 1985;145:855.

868. Norton JA, Cornelius MJ, Doppman JL, Maton PN, Gardner JD, Jensen RT. Effect of parathyroidectomy in patients with hyperparathyroidism and Zollinger-Ellison syndrome and multiple endocrine neoplasia type 1: A prospective study. Surgery 1987;102:958.

869. Jensen RT. Basis for failure of cimetidine in patients with Zollinger-Ellison syndrome. Dig Dis Sci 1984;29:363.

870. Stadil F, Stage JG. Cimetidine and the Zollinger-Ellison (ZE) syndrome. In: Wastell C, Lance P, eds. Cimetidine. London: Churchill Livingstone, 1978:91–104.

871. Deveney CW, Stein S, Way LW. Cimetidine in the treatment of Zollinger-Ellison syndrome. Am J Surg 1983;146:116.

872. Stabile BE, Ippoliti AF, Walsh JH, Passaro E Jr. Failure of histamine H2-receptor antagonist therapy in Zollinger-Ellison syndrome. Am J Surg 1983;145:17.

873. Jensen RT, Collen MJ, McArthur KE, et al. Comparison of the effectiveness of ranitidine and cimetidine in inhibiting acid secretion in patients with gastric hypersecretory states. Am J Med 1984;77:90.

874. Howard JM, Chremos AN, Collen MJ, et al. Famotidine, a new potent long-acting histamine H2-receptor antagonist: Comparison with cimetidine and ranitidine in the treatment of Zollinger-Ellison syndrome. Gastroenterology 1985;88:1026.

875. Raufman J-P, Collins SM, Pandol SJ, et al. Reliability of symptoms in assessing control of gastrin and secretin in patients with Zollinger-Ellison syndrome. Gastroenterology 1983;84:108.

876. Metz D, Pisegna JR, Fishbeyn VA, Benya RV, Jensen RT. Control of gastric and hypersecretion in the management of Zollinger-Ellison syndrome. World J Surg 1991 (in press).

877. McArthur KE, Raufman JP, Seaman JJ, et al. Cimetidine pharmacokinetics in patients with Zollinger-Ellison syndrome. Gastroenterology 1987;93:69.

878. Ziemniak JA, Madura M, Adamonis AJ, et al. Failure of cimetidine in Zollinger-Ellison syndrome. Dig Dis Sci 1983;28:976.

879. Vinayek R, Amantea MA, Maton PN, Frucht H, Gardner JD, Jensen RT. Pharmacokinetics of oral and intravenous omeprazole in patients with Zollinger-Ellison syndrome. Gastroenterology 1991;101:138.

880. Jensen RT, Collen MJ, Allende HD, et al. Cimetidine induced impotence and breast changes in patients with gastric hypersecretory states. N Engl J Med 1983;308:883.

881. Alumets J, El Munshid HA, Hakanson R, et al. Effect of antrum exclusion on endocrine cells of rat stomach. J Physiol (Lond) 1979;286:145.

882. Maton PN, Lack EE, Collen MJ, et al. The effect of Zollinger-Ellison syndrome and omeprazole therapy on gastric endocrine cells. Gastroenterology 1990;99:943.

883. Lehy T, Mignon M, Cadiot G, et al. Gastric endocrine cell behavior in Zollinger-Ellison patients upon long-term patient antisecretory treatment. Gastroenterology 1989;96:1029.

884. D'Adda T, Corletto V, Pilato FD, et al. Quantitative ultrastructure of endocrine cells of oxyntic mucosa in Zollinger-Ellison syndrome. Gastroenterology 1990;99:17.

885. Maton PN, Frucht H, Vinayek R, Wank SA, Gardner JD, Jensen RT. Medical management of patients with Zollinger-Ellison syndrome. Gastroenterology 1988;94:294.

886. Fraker D, Norton JA, Saeed Z, Maton P, Gardner JD, Jensen RT. A prospective study of pre- and postoperative control of acid secretion in patients with Zollinger-Ellison syndrome. Surgery 1988;104:1054.

887. Saeed ZA, Norton JA, Frank W, et al. Parenteral antisecretory drug therapy in patients with Zollinger-Ellison syndrome. Gastroenterology 1989;96:1393.

888. Vinayek R, Frucht H, London JF, et al. Intravenous omeprazole in patients with Zollinger-Ellison syndrome undergoing surgery. Gastroenterology 1990;99:10.

889. London J, Frucht H, Doppman JL, Maton PN, Gardner JD, Jensen RT. Zollinger-Ellison syndrome in the acute care setting. J Intens Care Med 1989;4:272.

890. Zollinger RM. Gastrinoma: Factors influencing prognosis. Surgery 1985;97:49.

891. Ellison EC, Carey LC, Sparks J, et al. Early surgical treatment of gastrinoma. Am J Med 1987;82:17.

892. Podevin P, Ruszniewski P, Mignon M, et al. Management of multiple endocrine neoplasia type I (MEN I) in Zollinger-Ellison syndrome. Gastroenterology [Abstract] 1990;98:230.

893. Maton PN, Gardner JD, Jensen RT. The incidence and etiology of Cushing's syndrome in patients with Zollinger-Ellison syndrome. N Engl J Med 1986;315:1.

894. Delcore R Jr, Cheung LY, Friesen SR. Characteristics of duodenal wall gastrinomas. Am J Surg 1990;160:621.

895. Norton JA, Doherty GM, Fraker DL. Surgery for endocrine tumors. In: Go VLW, Gardner JD, Brooks FP, Lebenthal E, Diangano EP, Scheele G, eds. Exocrine pancreas. New York: Raven Press, 1991 (in press).

896. Norton JA. Invited commentary. World J Surg 1984;8:572.

897. Moertel CG, Hanley JA, Johnson LA. Streptozotocin alone compared with streptozotocin plus fluorouracil in the treatment of advanced islet-cell carcinoma. N Engl J Med 1980;303:1189.

898. Buchanan KD, O'Hare MMT, Russel CJF, Kennedy TL, Hadden DR. Factors involved in the responsiveness of gastrointestinal apudomas to streptozotocin. Dig Dis Sci 1986;31:511S.

899. Von Schrenck T, Howard JM, Doppman JL, et al. Prospective study of chemotherapy in patients with metastatic gastrinoma. Gastroenterology 1988;94:1326.

900. Ruszniewski PH, Rougier P, Andre-David F, et al. Prospective multicentric study chemotherapy with streptozotocin (STZ) and 5-fluorouracil (5FU) for liver metastases (LM) in Zollinger-Ellison syndrome (ZES). Gastroenterology [Abstract] 1989;96:431.

901. Carrasco CH, Chuang VP, Wallace S. Apudoma metastatic to the liver: Treatment by hepatic artery embolization. Radiology 1983;149:79.

902. Ajani JA, Carrasco CH, Charnsangavej C, et al. Islet cell tumors metastatic to the liver: Effective palliation by sequential hepatic artery embolization. Ann Intern Med 1988;108:340.

903. Maton PN, Gardner JD, Jensen RT. The use of the long acting somatostatin analogue 201-995 in patients with pancreatic endocrine tumors. Dig Dis Sci 1989;34:29.

904. Kvols HM, Buck M, Moertel LG, et al. Treatment of metastatic islet cell carcinoma with a somatostatin analogue (SMS-201-995). Ann. Intern Med 1987;107:162.

905. Maton PN. The use of the long-acting somatostatin analogue, octreotide in patients with islet cell tumors. Gastroenterol Clin North Am 1989;18:897.

906. Reubi JC. Somatostatin analogue inhibits chondrosarcoma and insulinoma tumor growth. Acta Endocrinol 1985;109:108.

907. Shepherd JJ, Senator GB. Regression of liver metastases in patients with gastrin secreting tumor treated with SMS 201-995. Lancet 1986;2:274.

908. Bonfils S, Ruszniewski P, Laucouret H, Castil J, Rene W, Mignon M. Long-term management of Zollinger-Ellison syndrome with SMS 201-995, a long-acting somatostatin analog. Can J Physiol Pharmacol 1986;63:6.

909. Erickson B, Oberg K, Alm G, et al. Treatment of malignant endocrine pancreatic tumors with human leukocyte interferon. Lancet 1986;2:1307.

910. Slimak GG, Pisegna J, Metz DL, Gardner JD, Jensen RT, Maton PN. Use of alpha interferon in patients with metastatic gastrinoma. Gastroenterology [Abstract] 1991;100:299.

911. Whipple AO. The surgical therapy of hyperinsulinism. J Int Chir 1938;3:237.

912. Galbut DL, Markowitz AM. Insulinoma: Diagnosis, surgical management and long-term followup. Am J Surg 1980;139:682.

913. Giercksky KE, Halse J, Mathisen W, et al. Endocrine tumors of the pancreas. Scand J Gastroenterol 1980;15:129.

914. Boden G. Insulinoma and glucagonoma. Semin Oncol 1987;14:253.

915. Fajans SS, Vinik AI. Insulin-producing islet cell tumors. Endocrinol Metab Clin North Am 1989;18:45.

916. Stefanini P, Carboni M, Patrassi N, Basoli A. Beta-islet cell tumor of the pancreas: Results of a study on 1,067 cases. Surgery 1974;75:597.

917. Service FJ, Dale AJ, Elveback LR, Jiang N. Insulinoma: Clinical and diagnostic features of 60 consecutive cases. Mayo Clin Proc 1976;51:417.

918. Glickman MH, Hart MJ, White TT. Insulinoma in Seattle: 39 cases in 30 years. Am J Surg 1980;140:119.

919. Nelson RL, Rizza RA, Service FJ. Documented hypoglycemia for 23 years in a patient with insulinoma. JAMA 1978;240:1891.

920. Boden G. Glucagonomas and insulinomas. Gastroenterol Clin North Am 1989;18:831.

921. Moller DE, Flier JS. Insulin resistance: Mechanisms, syndromes and implications. N Engl J Med 1991;325:938.

922. Grunberger G, Weiner JL, Silverman R, Taylor S, Gorden P. Factitious hypoglycemia due to surreptitious administration of insulin: Diagnosis, treatment and long-term follow-up. Ann Intern Med 1988;108:252.

923. Danforth DN, Gorden P, Brennan MF. Metastatic insulin secreting carcinoma of the pancreas: Clinical course and the role of surgery. Surgery 1984;96:1027.

924. Jensen RT, Norton JA. Pancreatic endocrine tumors. In: Sleisinger MH, Fordtran JS, Scharschmidt BF, Feldman M, eds. Gastrointestinal disease: Pathophysiology, diagnosis, management. Philadelphia: WB Saunders, 1992 (in press).

925. Dunnick NJ, Schaner JL, Doppman JL, et al. Computed tomography in adrenal tumors. AJR 1979;132:43.

926. Vinik AI, Delbridge L, Moattari R, Cho K, Thompson N. Transhepatic portal vein catheterization for localization of insulinomas: A ten-year experience. Surgery 1991;109:1.

927. Doppman JL, Miller DL, Chang R, Gorden P, Norton JA. Insulinomas localization with selective intraarterial injection of calcium. Radiology 1991;178:237.

928. Dunnick NR, Long JA, Krudy A, et al. Localizing insulinomas with combined radiographic methods. AJR 1980;135:747.

929. Doppman JL, Brennan MF, Dunnick NR, Kahn CR, Gorden P. The role of pancreatic venous sampling in the localization of occult insulinoma. Radiology 1981;138:557.

930. Norton JA, Sigel B, Baker AR, et al. Localization of an occult insulinoma by intraoperative ultrasonography. Surgery 1985;97:381.

931. Reubi JC, Lamberts SW, Maurer R. Somatostatin receptors in normal and tumoral tissues. Horm Res 1988;29:65.

932. Norton JA, Doppman JL, Jensen RT. Cancer of the endocrine system. In: DeVita VT, Hellman S, Rosenberg SA, eds. Cancer: Principles and practice of oncology. Philadelphia: JB Lippincott, 1989:1269–1344.

933. Tutt GO Jr, Edis AJ, Servie FJ, van Heerden JA. Plasma glucose monitoring during operation for insulinoma: A critical reappraisal. Surgery 1980;88:351.

934. Kudlow JE, Albisser AM, Angel A, et al. Insulinoma resection facilitated by the artificial endocrine pancreas. Diabetes 1978;27:774.

935. DeMarinis L, Barbarino A. Calcium antagonists and hormone release. I. Effects of verapamil on insulin release in normal subjects and patients with islet-cell tumor. Metabolism 1980;29:599.

936. Murakami K, Taniguchi H, Kobayshi T, Seki M, Olmon M, Baba S. Suppression of insulin release by calcium antagonist in human insulinoma in vivo and in vitro: Its possible role for clinical use. Kobe J Med Sci 1979;25:237.

937. Stehouwer CD, Lems WF, Fischer HR, Hackeng WH. Malignant insulinoma: Is combined treatment with verapamil and the long-acting somatostatin analogue octreotide (SMS 201-995) more effective than single therapy with either drug? Neth J Med 1989;35:86.

938. Blum I, Doron M, Laron Z, et al. Prevention of hypoglycemia attacks by propanolol in a patient suffering from insulinoma. Diabetes 1975;24:535.

939. Hofeldt FD, Dippe SE, Levin SR, Karam JH, Blum MR, Forsham PH. Effects of diphenylhydantoin upon glucose-induced insulin secretion in three patients with insulinoma. Diabetes 1974;23:192.

940. Gorden P, Comi RJ, Maton PN, Go VLW. Somatostatin and somatostatin analogue (SMS 201-995) in treatment of hormone-secreting tumors of the pituitary and gastrointestinal tract and non-neoplastic diseases of the gut. Ann Intern Med 1989;110:35.

941. Dunne MJ, Elton R, Fletcher T, Hofker PH, Shiu J. Somatostatin and gastroenteropancreatic endocrine tumors: Therapeutic characteristics. In: O'Dorisio TM, ed. Somatostatin in the treatment of GEP endocrine tumors. Berlin: Springer-Verlag, 1987:93.

942. Mozell E, Stenzel P, Woltering EA, Rosch J, O'Dorisio TM. Functional endocrine tumors of the pancreas clinical presentation, diagnosis, and treatment. Curr Probl Surg 1990;27:303.

943. Eckhauser FE, Cheung PS, Vinik AI, et al. Nonfunctioning malignant neuroendocrine tumors of the pancreas. Surgery 1986;100:978.

944. Vinik AI, Strodel WE, Eckhauser FE, et al. Somatostatinomas, PPomas, neurotensinomas. Semin Oncol 1987;14:263.

945. O'Dorisio TM, Vinik AI. Pancreatic polypeptide and mixed peptide-producing tumors of the gastrointestinal tract. In: Cohen S, Soloway RD, eds. Hormone-producing tumors of the gastrointestinal tract. London: Churchill Livingstone, 1985:117.

946. Walsh JH. Gastrointestinal hormones. In: Johnson LR, ed. Physiology of the gastrointestinal tract. New York: Raven Press, 1987:1981.

947. Vinik AI, Moattari AR. Treatment of endocrine tumors. Endocrinol Metab Clin North Am 1989;18:483.

948. Kent RB, van Heerden JA, Weiland LH. Nonfunctioning islet cell tumors. Ann Surg 1981;193:185.

949. Shaw JA, Vance RP, Geisinger KR, Marshall RB. Islet cell neoplasms: A fine needle aspiration cytology study with immunocytochemical correlations. Am J Clin Pathol 1990;94:142.

950. Hsiu J-G, D'Amato NA, Sperling MH, et al. Malignant islet-cell tumors of the pancreas diagnosed by fine needle aspiration biopsy: A case report. Acta Cytol 1985;29:556.

951. Lin TH, Tseng HC, Zhu Y, Zhong SX, Chen J, Cui QC. Insulinoma: An immunocytochemical and morphologic analysis of 95 cases. Cancer 1985;56:1420.

952. Sneige N, Ordonez NG, Vaenattukathil S, Samaan NA. Fine needle aspiration cytology in pancreatic endocrine tumors. Diagn Cytopathol 1987;3:35.

953. Schwartz TM. Atropine suppression test for pancreatic polypeptide. Lancet 1978;2:43.

954. Verner JV, Morrison AB. Islet cell tumor and a syndrome of refractory watery diarrhea and hypokalemia. Am J Med 1958;29:529.

955. Matsumoto KK, Peter JB, Schultze RG, et al. Watery diarrhea and hypokalemia associated with pancreatic islet cell adenoma. Gastroenterology 1967;52:695.

956. Verner JV, Morrison AB. Non-B islet tumors and the syndrome of watery diarrhea, hypokalemia and hypochlorhydria. Clin Gastroenterol 1974;3:595.

957. O'Dorisio TM, Mekhjian H, Gaginella TS. Medical therapy of VIPoma. Endocrinol Metab Clin North Am 1989;18:545.

958. Capella C, Polak JM, Butta R, et al. Morphologic patterns and diagnostic criteria of VIP-producing endocrine tumors: A histologic, histochemical, ultrastructural and biochemical study of 32 cases. Cancer 1983;52:1860.

959. Long RG, Bryant MG, Mitchell SJ, Adrian TE, Polak JM, Bloom SR. Clinicopathological study of pancreatic and ganglioneuroblastoma tumors secreting vasoactive intestinal polypeptide (VIPomas). Br Med J 1981;282:1767.

960. Verner JV, Morrison AB. Endocrine pancreatic islet disease with diarrhea: Report of a case due to diffuse hyperplasia of no beta islet tissue with a review of 54 additional cases. Arch Intern Med 1974;1974;133.

961. Bloom SR, Christofides ND, Yiengan T, et al. Peptide histidine isoleucine (PHI) and Verner-Morrison syndrome. Gut 1983;24:473.

962. Krejs GJ. VIPomas syndrome. Am J Med 1987;82:37.

963. Ginsberg AL. The VIP controversy: Stephen R. Bloom vs. Jerry D. Gardner. Dig Dis Sci 1978;23:30.

964. Kane MG, O'Dorisio TM, Krejs GJ. Production of secretory diarrhea by intravenous infusion of vasoactive intestinal peptide. N Engl J Med 1983;309:1482.

965. Laburthe M, Amiranoff B. Peptide receptors in intestinal epithelium. In: Makhlouf GM, ed. The gastrointestinal system: Handbook of physiology. Bethesda: American Physiological Society, 1989:215.

966. Krejs GJ. Comparison of the effect of VIP and PHI on water and ion movement in the canine jejunum in vivo. Gastroenterol Clin Biol 1984;8:868.

967. Mekhjian HS, O'Dorisio TM. VIPoma syndrome. Semin Oncol 1987;14:282.

968. Bloom SR, Long RG, Bryant MG, et al. Clinical, biochemical and pathological studies on 62 VIPomas. Gastroenterology 1980;78:1143.

969. Morris AI, Turnberg LA. Surreptitious laxative abuse. Gastroenterology 1979;77:780.

970. Read NW, Read MG, Krejs GJ, et al. A report of five patients with large volume secretory diarrhea but no evidence of endocrine tumor or laxative abuse. Dig Dis Sci 1982;27:193.

971. Read WN, Krejs G, Read MG, et al. Chronic diarrhea of unknown origin. Gastroenterology 1980;78:264.

972. Maton PN, O'Dorisio TM, Howe BA, et al. Effect of a long-acting somatostatin analogue (SMS 201-995) in a patient with pancreatic cholera. N Engl J Med 1985;312:17.

973. Mallinson CN, Bloom SR, Warin AP, et al. A glucagonoma syndrome. Lancet 1974;2:1.

974. Holst JJ. Glucagon-producing tumors. In: Cohen S, Soloway D, eds. Hormone producing tumors of the gastrointestinal tract. New York: Churchill Livingstone, 1985:57.

975. McGavran M. H, Unger RH, Recant L, et al. A glucagon-secreting alpha-cell carcinoma of the pancreas. N Engl J Med 1966;274:1408.

976. Wilkinson DS. Necrolytic migratory erythema with carcinoma of the pancreas. Trans St. John's Hosp Dermatol Soc 1973;59:244.

977. Guillausseau PJ, Gauillausseau C, Villet R, et al. Les glucagonomas: Aspect cliniques, biologiques, anatomo-pathologiques et therapeutiques (Revue general de 130 cas). Gastroenterol Clin Biol 1982;6:1029.

978. Leichter SB. Clinical and metabolic aspects of glucagonoma. Medicine 1980;59:100.

979. Stacpoole PW. The glucagonoma syndrome: Clinical features, diagnosis, and treatment. Endocr Rev 1981;2:347.

980. Bataille D. The gastrointestinal system. In: Makhlouf GN, ed. Handbook of physiology. Bethesda: American Physiological Society, 1989:455.

981. Abravia C, De Bartolo M, Katzen R, Lawrence AM. Disappearance of glucagonoma rash after surgical resection, but not during dietary normalization of serum amino acids. Am J Clin Nutr 1984;39:351.

982. Yamada T, Chiha T. Somatostatin. In: Makhlouf GN, ed. The gastrointestinal system: Handbook of physiology. Bethesda: American Physiological Society, 1979:431.

983. Ganda PO, Weir GC, Soeldner JS, et al. Somatostatinoma: A somatostatin-containing tumor of the endocrine pancreas. N Engl J Med 1977;296:963.

984. Larsson LI, Hirsch MA, Holst J, et al. Pancreatic somatostatinoma clinical features and physiologic implications. Lancet 1977;1:1666.

985. Krejs GJ, Orci L, Conlon M, et al. Somatostatinoma syndrome (biochemical, morphological, and clinical features). N Engl J Med 1979;301:285.

986. Boden G, Shimoyama R. Somatostatinoma. In: Cohen S, Soloway RD, eds. Hormone-producing tumors of the gastrointestinal tract. New York: Churchill Livingstone, 1985:85.

987. Konomi K, Chijiiwa K, Katsuta T, Yamaguchi K. Pancreatic somatostatinoma: A case report and review of the literature. J Surg Oncol 1990;43:259.

988. Soldati TK, Delnoce G, Garino M, Farin EC, De Paolis P, Balba G. Pancreatic somatostatinoma. Pan Minerva Med 1990;32:141.

989. Rivier J, Spress J, Thorner M, Vale V. Characterization of a growth-hormone releasing factor from a human pancreatic islet cell tumor. Nature 1982;300:276.

990. Thorner MO, Perryman RL, Cronin MJ, et al. Somatotroph hyperplasia. J Clin Invest 1982;70:965.

991. Guillemin R, Brazeau P, Bohlen P, Esch F, Ling N, Wehrenberg W. Growth hormone-releasing factor from a human pancreatic tumor that caused acromegaly. Science 1982;27:774.

992. Berger C, Trouillas J, Bloch B, et al. Multihormonal carcinoid tumors of the pancreas: Secreting growth hormone-releasing factor as a cause of acromegaly. Cancer 1984;54:2097.

993. Sano T, Yamasaki R, Saito H, et al. Growth hormone-releasing hormone (GHRH) secreting pancreatic tumor in a patient with multiple endocrine neoplasia type 1. Surg Pathol 1987;11:810.

994. Moller DE, Moses AC, Jones K, Thorner MO, Vance ML. Octreotide suppresses both growth hormone (GH) and GH-releasing hormone (GHRH) in acromegaly due to ectopic GHRH secretion. J Clin Endocrinol Metab 1989;68:499.

995. Von Werder K, Losa M, Stalla FK, et al. Long-term treatment of a metastasizing GRFoma with a somatostatin analogue (SMS 201-995) in a girl with gigantism. Scand J Gastroenterol 1986;21:238.

996. Christofides ND, Stephanou A, Suzuki H, Yianigou Y, Bloom SR. Distribution of immunoreactive growth hormone-releasing hormone in the human brain and intestine and its production by tumors. J Clin Endocrinol Metab 1984;59:747.

997. Bostwick DG, Quan R, Hoffman AR, Webber RJ, Chang J-R, Bensch KG. Growth-hormone-releasing factor immunoreactivity in human endocrine tumors. Am J Pathol 1984;117;167.

998. Dayal Y, Lin HD, Tallberg K, Reichlin BAS, DeLellis RA, Wolfe JH. Immunocytochemical demonstration of growth hormone-releasing factor in gastrointestinal and pancreatic endocrine tumors. Am J Clin Pathol 1986;85:13.

999. Barkan AL. Acromegaly: Diagnosis and therapy. Endocrinol Metab Clin North Am 1989;18:277.

1000. Barkan AL, Shenker Y, Grekin RJ, et al. Acromegaly from ectopic GHRH secretion by a malignant carcinoid tumor: Successful treatment with long-acting somatostatin analogue SMS Cancer 1986;61:221.

1001. Melmed S, Ziel FH, Braustein GD, et al. Medical management of acromegaly due to ectopic production of GHRH by a carcinoid tumor. J Clin Endocrinol Met 1988;67:395.

1002. Wilson DM, Hoffman AR. Reduction of pituitary size by the somatostatin analogue SMS 201-995 in a patient with an islet cell tumour secreting growth hormone releasing factor. Acta Endocrinol 1986;113:23.

1003. Caplan PH, Koob L, Abellera RM, et al. Cure of acromegaly by operative removal of an islet cell tumor of the pancreas. Am J Med 1978;64:874.

1004. Fuerle GE, Helmstaedter V, Tischbirek K, et al. A multihormonal tumor of the pancreas producing neurotensin. Dig Dis Sci 1981;26:1125.

1005. Gutniak M, Rosenqvist U, Grimelius L. Report on a patient with watery diarrhea syndrome caused by a pancreatic tumour containing neurotensin, enkephalin and calcitonin. Acta Med Scand 1980;208:95.

1006. Bloom SR, Lee YC, Lacroute JM. Two patients with pancreatic apudomas secreting neurotensin and VIP. Gut 1983;24:448.

1007. Wood JR, Wood SM, Lee YC. Neurotensin-secreting carcinoma of the bronchus. Postgrad Med J 1983;59:46.

1008. Shulkes A, Boden R, Cook I, et al. Characterization of a pancreatic tumor containing vasoactive intestinal peptide, neurotensin and pancreatic polypeptide. J Clin Endocrinol Metab 1984;58:41.

1009. Maier W, Schumacher A, Etzrodt H, et al. A neurotensinoma of the head of the pancreas: Demonstration by ultrasound and computed tomography. Eur J Radiol 1982;2:125.

1010. Ferris CF. Neurotensin. In: Makhlouf GN, ed. The gastrointestinal tract: Handbook of physiology. Bethesda: American Physiological Society, 1989:559.

1011. Clark ES, Carney JA. Pancreatic islet cell tumor associated with Cushing's syndrome. Am J Surg Pathol 1984;8:917.

1012. Deftos LJ, McMillan PJ, Sartinano GP, Abuid J, Robinson AG. Simultaneous ectopic production of parathyroid hormone and calcitonin. Metabolism 1976;25:543.

1013. Arps H, Dietel M, Schulz A, Janzarik H, Kloppel G. Pancreatic endocrine carcinoma with ectopic PTH-production and paraneoplastic hypercalcaemia. Virchows Arch [A] 1986;408:497.

1014. Cryer PE, Hill GJ. Pancreatic islet cell carcinoma with hypercalcemia and hypergastrinemia. Cancer 1976;38:2217.

1015. Palmieri GMA, Nordquist RE, Omenn GS. Immunochemical localization of parathyroid hormone in cancer tissue from patients with ectopic hyperparathyroidism. J Clin Invest 1974;53:1726.

1016. Rasbach DA, Hammond JM. Pancreatic islet cell carcinoma with hypercalcemia: Primary hyperparathyroidism or hormonal hypercalcemia of malignancy. Am J Med 1985;78:337.

1017. Bresler L, Boissel P, Conroy T, Grosdidier J. Pancreatic islet cell carcinoma with hypercalcemia: Complete remission 5 years after surgical excision and chemotherapy. Am J Gastroenterol 1991;86:635.

1018. Ajani JA, Levin B, Wallace S. Systemic and regional therapy of advanced islet cell tumors. Gastroenterol Clin North Am 1989;18:923.

1019. Kvols LK, Buck M. Chemotherapy of the metastatic carcinoid and islet cell tumors: A review. Am J Med 1987;82:77.

1020. Herr RR, Jahnke HK, Argoudelis AD. The structure of streptozotocin. J Am Chem Soc 1967;98:4808.

1021. Weiss RB. Streptozotocin: A review of its pharmacology, efficacy, and toxicity. Cancer Treat Rep 1982;66:427.

1022. Rakieten N, Rakieten ML, Nadkani MV. Studies of the diabetogenic action of streptozotocin (NSC-37917). Cancer Chemother Rep 1969;29:91.

1023. Murray-Lyon IM, Eddelsteon ALWF, Williams R, et al. Treatment of multiple hormone producing malignant islet cell tumor with streptozotocin. Lancet 1968;2:895.

1024. Moertel CG, Kvols LK, O'Connell MJ, Rubin J. Treatment of neuroendocrine carcinomas with combined etoposide and cisplatin. Cancer 1991;68:227.

1025. Duncan LA, Marynick SP. Glucagonoma and Dacarbazine. Ann Intern Med 1982;97:930.

1026. Kessinger A, Lemon HM, Foley JF. The glucagonoma syndrome and its management. J Surg Oncol 1977;9:419.

1027. Strauss GM, Weitzman SA, Aoki TT. Dimethyltriazenoimidazole carboxamide therapy of malignant glucagonomas. Ann Intern Med 1979;90:57.

1028. Marynick SP, Fagadau WR, Duncan LA. Malignant glucagonoma syndrome. Response to chemotherapy. Ann Intern Med 1980;93:453.

1029. Prinz RA, Budrinath K, Banerji M, et al. Operations and chemotherapeutic management of malignant glucagon producing tumors. Surgery 1981;90:713.

1030. Awrich AE, Peetz M, Fletcher WS. Dimethyltriazenoimidazole carboxamide therapy of islet cell carcinomas of the pancreas. J Surg Oncol 1981;17:321.

1031. Kurose T, Seino Y, Ishida LT, et al. Successful treatment of metastatic glucagonoma with dacarbazine. Lancet 1984;1:621.

1032. McFadden D, Jaffe BN. Surgical approaches to endocrine-producing tumors of the gastrointestinal tract. In: Cohen S, Soloway RD, eds. Hormone producing tumors of the gastrointestinal tract. New York: Churchill Livingstone, 1985:139.

1033. Valette PJ, Souquet JC. Pnacreatic islet cell tumors metastatic to the liver: Treatment by hepatic artery chemo-embolization. Horm Res 1989;32:77.

1034. Redding TW, Schally AV. Inhibition of growth of pancreatic carcinomas in animal models by analogs of hypothalamic hormones. Proc Natl Acad Sci USA 1984;84:248.

1035. Lamberts SW, Hofland LJ, van Koetsveld PM, et al. Parallel in vivo and in vitro detection of functional somatostatin receptors in human endocrine tumors: Consequences with regard to diagnosis, localization and therapy. J Clin Endocrinol Metab 1990;31:566.

1036. Oberg K, Lindstrom H, Alm G, Lundquist G. Successful treatment of therapy-resistant pancreatic cholera with human leukocyte interferon. Lancet 1985;1:725.

1037. Anderson JV, Bloom SR. Treatment of malignant endocrine tumors with human leukocyte interferon. Lancet 1987;1:97.

1038. Balentine JD. Pathology of oxygen toxicity. New York: Academic Press, 1982.

1039. Wermer P. Endocrine adenomatosis: Peptic ulcer in a large kindred. Am J Med 1963;35:205.

1040. Loeb JN. Polyglandular disorders. In: Wyngaarden JB, Smith LH, eds. Cecil textbook of medicine. Philadelphia: WB Saunders, 1982:1304.

1041. Oberg K, Skogseid B, Eriksson N. Multiple endocrine neoplasia type I. Acta Oncol 1989;28:383.

1042. Radford DM, Ashley SW, Wells SA Jr, Gerhard DS. Loss of heterozygosity of markers on chromosome 11 in tumors with patients with multiple endocrine neoplasia syndrome I. Cancer Res 1991;50:1154.

1043. Larsson C, Skogseid B, Oberg K, et al. Multiple endocrine neoplasia type I gene maps to chromosome 11 and is lost in insulinoma. Nature 1988;332:85.

1044. Bystrom C, Larsson C, Blomberg C, et al. Localization of the MEN-1 gene to a small region within chromosome 11 q 13 by deletion mapping in tumors. Proc Natl Acad Sci USA 1990;87:1968.

1045. Knudson AG. Mutation and cancer: Statistical study of retinoblastoma. Proc Natl Acad Sci USA 1971;68:820.

1046. Bale A. E, Norton JA, Wong EL, et al. Allelic loss on chromosome 11 in hereditary and sporadic tumors related to familial multiple endocrine neoplasia type 1. Cancer Res 1991;51:1154.

1047. Brandi ML, Aurbach GD, Fitzpatrick LA, et al. Parathyroid mitogenic activity in plasma from patients with familial multiple endocrine neoplasia type I. N Engl J Med 1986;314:1287.

1048. Brandi ML. Multiple endocrine neoplasia type I: General features and new insights into etiology. J Endocrinol Invest 1991;14:61.

1049. Zimmering MB, Brandi ML, de Grange DA, et al. Circulating fibroblast growth factor-like substance in familial multiple endocrine neoplasia-type I. J Clin Endocrinol Metab 1990;70:149.

1050. Thakker RV, Bonloux P, Wooding C, et al. Association of parathyroid tumors in multiple endocrine neoplasia type 1 with loss of alleles on chromosome 11. N Engl J Med 1989;321:60.

1051. Bone HG. Diagnosis of multiglandular endocrine neoplasias. Clin Chem 1990;36:711.

1052. Leight GS, Hensley MI. Management of familial hyperparathyroidism. Prog Surg 1987;184:106.

1053. Wells SA Jr, Farndon JR, Dale JK, et al. Long-term evaluation of patients with primary parathyroid hyperplasia managed by total parathyroidectomy and heterotopic auto-transplantation. Ann Surg 1980;192:451.

1054. Prinz RA, Gamvros OI, Seller D, Lynn JA. Subtotal parathyroidectomy for primary chief cell hyperplasia of the multiple endocrine neoplasia type I syndrome. Ann Surg 1981;193:26.

1055. Rizzoli R, Green J, Marx SJ. Primary hyperparathyroidism in familial multiple endocrine neoplasia type I. Long-term follow-up of serum calcium levels after parathyroidectomy. Am J Med 1985;78:467.

1056. Thompson NW, Lloyd RV, Nishiyama RH, et al. MEN-1 pancreas:a histological and immuno-histochemical study. World J Surg 1984;8:561.

1057. Kloppel G, Willemar S, Stamm B, et al. Pancreatic lesions and hormonal profile in pancreatic tumors in multiple endocrine neoplasia type I. Cancer 1986;57:1820.

1058. Thompson NW. Surgical considerations in the MEN-1 syndrome. In: Johnston IDA, Thompson NW, eds. Endocrine surgery. Butterworths, London: 1983:144–163.

1059. Friesen SR, Tomita T, Kimmel JR. Pancreatic polypeptide update: Its role in detection of the tract for multiple endocrine adenopathy syndrome, type I and pancreatic polypeptide-secreting tumors. Surgery 1983;94:1028.

1060. Rasbach DA, van Heerden JA, Telandar RL, et al. Surgical management of hyper-insulinism in the multiple endocrine neoplasia, type I syndrome. Arch Surg 1985;120:584.

1061. Lamers CB, Stadil F, Tongeren JMH. Prevalence of endocrine abnormalities in patients with the Zollinger-Ellison syndrome and their families. Am J Med 1981;64:687.

1062. Eisenberg AA, Wallerstein H. Pheochromocytoma of the suprarenal medulla (paraglioma): A clinicopathological study. Arch Pathol 1932;14:818.

1063. Hazard JB, Hawk WH, Creile G Jr. Medullary (solid) carcinoma of the thyroid-clinicopathologic entity. J Clin Endocrinol Metab 1979;19:704.

1064. Norton JA, Wells SA Jr. Medullary thyroid carcinoma and multiple endocrine neoplasia type-II syndromes. In: Friesen S, ed. Surgical endocrinology. Philadelphia: JB Lippincott, 1988.

1065. Tashjian AH Jr, Howland BG, Melvin KEW, Hill CS Jr. Immunoassay of human calcitonin: Clinical measurement, relation to serum calcium and studies in patients with medullary carcinoma. N Engl J Med 1970;283:890.

1066. Jackson CE, Block MA, Greenawald KA, et al. The two-mutational event theory in medullary thyroid cancer. Am J Hum Genet 1979;31:704.

1067. Wolfe HJ, Melvin KEW, Cervi-Skinner SJ, et al. C-cell hyperplasia preceding medullary thyroid carcinoma. N Engl J Med 1973;189:437.

1068. Sipple JH. The association of pheochromocytoma with carcinoma of the thyroid gland. Am J Med 1961;31:163.

1069. Williams ED. A review of 17 cases of carcinoma of the thyroid and pheochromocytoma. J Clin Pathol 1965;18:288.

1070. Schimke RN, Hartmann WH. Familial amyloid-producing medullary thyroid carcinoma and pheochromocytoma: A distinct genetic entity. Ann Intern Med 1965;63:1027.

1071. Manning PC, Molnar GD, Black BM, Priestly JT, Woolner LB. Pheochromocytoma, hyperparathyroidism and thyroid carcinoma occurring coincidentally. N Engl J Med 1963;268:68.

1072. Williams ED, Pollock DJ. Multiple mucosal neuromata with endocrine tumors: A syndrome alluded to von Recklinghausen's disease. J Path Bacteriol 1989;91:71.

1073. Simpson NE, Kidd KK, Goodfellow PJ, et al. Assignment of multiple endocrine neoplasia type 2a to chromosome 10 by linkage. Nature 1987;328:528.

1074. Sobol H, Narod SA, Nakamura Y, et al. Screening for multiple endocrine neoplasia 2a with DNA polymorphism analysis. N Engl J Med 1989;312:996.

1075. Telenius H, Mathew CGP, Nakamura Y, et al. Application of DNA markers to screening families with multiple endocrine neoplasia 2A. Eur J Surg Oncol 1990;16:134.

1076. Wu JS, Larson NL, Myers S, et al. The genetic defect in multiple endocrine neoplasia type 2A maps next to the centrosome of chromosome 10. Am J Hum Genet 1990;46:624.

1077. Mathew GCP, Easton DF, Nakamura Y, et al. Presymptomatic screening for multiple endocrine neoplasia type 2A with linked DNA markers. Lancet 1991;337:7.

1078. Norum RA, Lafreniere R, O'Neal LW, et al. Linkage of multiple endocrine neoplasia type 2B gene (MEN2B) to chromosome 10 markers linked to MEN2A. Genomics 1990;8:313.

1079. Jackson CE, Norum RH, O'Neal LW, Nikolai TF, DeLaney JP. Linkage between MEN 2B and chromosome 10 markers linked to MEN 2A. Am J Hum Genet [Abstract] 1988;45:154.

1080. Grun R, Eberle F. Ergebn Inner Mediz Kinderheildk 1981;46:151.

1081. Keiser HR, Beaven MA, Doppman J, et al. Sipple's syndrome: Medullary thyroid carcinoma, pheochromocytoma and parathyroid disease. Ann Intern Med 1973;78:561.

1082. Wells SA Jr. Multiple endocrine neoplasia type II: Recent results. Cancer Res 1990;18:71.

1083. Easton DF, Ponder MA, Cummings TA, et al. The clinical and screening-age-at-onset distribution for the MEN-2 syndrome. Am J Hum Genet 1989;44:208.

1084. Wells SA Jr, Baylin SG, Leight GS, et al. The importance of early diagnosis in patients with hereditary medullary thyroid carcinoma. Ann Surg 1982;195:505.

1085. Wells SA Jr, Baylin SB, Gann DW, et al. Medullary thyroid carcinoma: Relationship of method of diagnosis to pathological staging. Ann Surg 1978;188:377.

1086. Melvin KEW, Miller HH, Tashjian AH Jr. Early diagnosis of medullary carcinoma of the thyroid by means of calcitonin assay. N Engl J Med 1971;285:1115.

1087. Wells SA Jr, Baylin SG, Linehan WM, et al. Provocative agents and the diagnosis of medullary carcinoma of the thyroid gland. Ann Surg 1978;188:139.

1088. Valk TW, Frager MW, Gross MD, et al. Spectrum of pheochromocytoma in multiple endocrine neoplasia: A scintigraphic portrayal using ^{131}I-metaiodobenzylguanidine. Ann Intern Med 1981;94:762.

1089. Shapiro B, Fig LM. Management of pheochromocytoma. Endocrinol Metab Clin North Am 1989;18:443.

1090. Wells SA Jr, Baylin SG, Johnsrude IS, et al. Thyroid venous catheterization in the early diagnosis of familial medullary thyroid carcinoma. Ann Surg 1982;196:505.

1091. Hull CJ. Pheochromocytoma: Diagnosis, preoperative preparation and anesthetic management. Br J Aneaesth 1986;58:1453.

1092. Farndon JR, Fagraeus L, Wells SA Jr. Recent developments in the management of phaechromocytoma. In: Johnston IDA, Thompson NW, eds. Endocrine surgery. London: Butterworths, 1983:189–201.

1093. Jackson CE, Talpos GB, Kanbouris A, et al. The clinical course after definitive operation for medullary thyroid carcinoma. Surgery 1983;94:995.

1094. Harsoulis P, Leontsini M, Economou A, et al. Fine needle aspiration biopsy cytology in the diagnosis of thyroid cancer: Comparative study of 213 operated patients. Br J Surg 1986;73:461.

1095. Abu-Nema T, Ayyash K, Tibblin S. Role of aspiration biopsy cytology in the diagnosis of cold solitary nodules. Br J Surg 1987;74:203.

1096. Ramacciotti CE, Pretorius HT, Chu EW, et al. Diagnostic accuracy and use of aspiration biopsy in the management of thyroid nodules. Arch Intern Med 1984;144:11669.

1097. Schroder DM, Chambous A, France CJ. Operative strategy for thyroid cancer: Is total thyroidectomy worth the price? Cancer 1986;58:2320.

1098. Crile G, Pontius KI, Hawk WA. Factors influencing the survival of patients with follicular carcinoma of the thyroid gland. Surg Gynecol Obstet 1985;160:409.

1099. Savino D, Sibley RK, Sumner H. Significance of Hurthle cell in thyroid neoplasms: Reexamination of an old but persistent problem. Lab Invest [Abstract] 1981;44:59.

1100. Caplan RH, Abellera RM, Kisken WA. Hurthle cell tumors of the thyroid gland: A clinicopathologic review and long-term follow-up. JAMA 1984;251:3114.

1101. Gosain AK, Clark OH. Hurthle cell neoplasms. Arch Surg 1984;119:515.

1102. Sokal M, Harmar GI. Chemotherapy for anaplastic carcinoma of the thyroid. Clin Oncol 1978;4:3.

1103. Macfarlane DA. Cancer of the adrenal cortex. Ann R Coll Surg 1958;23:155.

1104. Chun HG, Yagoda A, Kemeny N. Cisplatin for adrenal cortical carcinoma. Cancer Treat Rep 1983;67:513.

1105. Kahler HJ, Heilmeyer L. Klinikund pathophysiologie des karzinoids und karzinoid-syndroms unter besonderer beruck sichtigung der pharmacologie des 5-hydroxyptamins. Ergeb Inn Med Kinderheildk 1961;16:291.

1106. Valimaki M, Harvinen H, Salmela P, Sane T, Sjoblom S-J, Pelkenon R. Is the treatment of metastatic carcinoid tumor with interferon not as successful as suggested? Cancer 1991;67:547.

1107. Bukowski RM, Stephens R, Oishi N, Pedersen R, Chen T. Phase II trials of 5-FU, adriamycin, cyclophosphamide and streptozotocin in metastatic carcinoid. Proc Amer Soc Clin Oncol 1983;2:130.

1108. Hancke S. Localization of hormone-producing gastrointestinal tumors by ultrasonic scanning. Scand J Gastroenterol 1979;53:115.

1109. Wilson SD. The role of surgery in children with Zollinger-Ellison syndrome. Surgery 1982;92:682.

1110. Vogel SB, Wolfe MM, McGuigan JE. Localization and resection of gastrinomas in Zollinger-Ellison syndrome. Ann Surg 1987;205:550.

1111. Delcore R, Hermeck AS, Friesen SR. Selective surgical management of correctable hypergastrinemia. Surgery 1989;106:1094.

1112. Moertel CG, Lavin PT, Hahn RG. Phase II trial of doxorubicin for advanced islet cell carcinoma. Cancer Treat Rep 1982;66:1567.

1113. Bukowski RM, McCracken JD, Balcerzek SP, et al. Phase II study of chlorozotocin in islet cell carcinoma. Cancer Chemother Pharmacol 1983;11:48.

1114. Frame J, Kelsen D, Kemeny N, et al. A Phase II trial of streptozotocin and adriamycin in advanced APUD tumors. Am J Oncol 1988;11:490.

1115. Bonfils S, Ruszniewski P, Haffar S, Laucouret H. Chemotherapy of hepatic metastases (HM) in Zollinger-Ellison syndrome (ZES): Report of a multicenteric analysis. Dig Dis Sci 1986;31:51.

1116. Kvols LK, Buck M, Moertel CG, et al. Treatment of metastatic islet cell tumors with a somatostatin analogue. Ann Intern Med 1987;107:162.

1117. Rothmund M, Angelini L, Brunt M, et al. Treatment of metastatic islet cell tumors with a somatostatin analogue. Ann Intern Med 1990;14:393.

1118. Rayfield EJ, Goldberg IJ, Gregerich EW, et al. Transportal blood sampling for pre-operative localization of insulinoma. Mt Sinai J Med 1983;50:258.

1119. Cho KJ, Vinik AI, Thompson NHD, et al. Localization of the source of hyperinsulinism. AJR 1982;139:237.

Cancer: Principles & Practice of Oncology, Fourth Edition,
edited by Vincent T. DeVita, Jr., Samuel Hellman, Steven A. Rosenberg.
J.B. Lippincott Co., Philadelphia © 1993.

James C. Yang   Eli J. Glatstein

Steven A. Rosenberg   Karen H. Antman

CHAPTER **42**

Sarcomas of Soft Tissues

Soft tissues refer to the extraskeletal connective tissues of the body that connect, support, and surround other discrete anatomic structures. This portion of the body mass lying between the epidermis and parenchymal organs includes the organs of locomotion, such as muscles and tendons, and supportive tissue structures, such as fibrous tissue, fat, and synovial tissue. The soft somatic tissues are ubiquitous and comprise more than 50% of body weight. The more than 400 muscles in the human body comprise about 40% of adult body weight.

Soft tissue sarcomas refer to malignant tumors arising in the soft tissues, and they are grouped together because of similarities in pathologic appearance, clinical presentation, and behavior. A combination of embryologic, functional, and morphologic characterizations define this tumor group.

The Greek word *sarkoma* means a fleshy growth, and virtually all tumors included in the soft tissue sarcomas arise from a common embryonic ancestry, the primitive mesoderm (Table 42–1). Nine to 13 days after fertilization of the ovum, the human embryo undergoes a transition from a phase of increasing cell number to a phase of morphologic organization into the endoderm, ectoderm, and mesoderm, the three primary germ layers of the embryo.[1] Within these layers are established commitments to developmental potentials that far precede morphologic differentiation of the cells.

The primitive mesoderm gives rise to organs such as the kidney, ureter, oviducts, uterus, gonads, and heart and a wide range of hematopoietic, lymphatic, and reticuloendothelial tissues. The primitive mesenchyme, a loose network of cells and intercellular matrix within the mesoderm, is largely responsible for the development of the common connective tissues of the body listed in Table 42–1. Tumors of these connective tissues are referred to as soft tissue sarcomas. Because of similarities in anatomic sites of origin, clinical presentation,

and clinical behavior, tumors arising in Schwann cells, a class of cells surrounding peripheral nerves that arise from the neural tube of the primitive ectoderm, are also included in the category of soft tissue sarcomas.

Malignant tumors are categorized as sarcomas or carcinomas based on whether they arise from connective tissue (*i.e.,* sarcomas) or epithelial tissue (*i.e.,* carcinomas). This differentiation is imprecise, and many sarcomas arise from tissues that fit the morphologic criteria of epithelium. Epithelium is a morphologic, not embryologic, term that is used to designate cellular structures that cover or line surfaces on or in the body and may arise from ectoderm, endoderm, or mesoderm. The endothelium lining the vascular and lymphatic channels and the mesothelium lining the body cavities and visceral organs are two types of epithelium that arise from the mesoderm. These epithelial structures give rise to malignant tumors that resemble and behave like tumors that develop from connective tissue cells. Tumors arising from the endothelium and the mesothelium are included in the category of sarcomas. Sarcomas arise mostly from mesodermal structures and from connective tissue cells. Some sarcomas arise from ectodermal structures, and some arise from epithelium.

This chapter describes the natural history and treatment of the soft tissue sarcomas. All visceral organs contain connective tissue stroma that can undergo malignant transformation. These visceral sarcomas are discussed in the chapters dealing with individual organ systems.

INCIDENCE

Approximately 5800 new cases of soft tissue sarcoma and 3300 deaths from this disease occurred in the United States in 1991.[2]

TABLE 42-1.   Embryonic Derivation of the Soft Tissue and Bony Sarcomas

Fertilized ovum

Blastoderm (day 9–13)

Endoderm   Mesoderm   Ectoderm

GI tract
Lungs, and so on

Skin
Mammary gland, and
so on

Nervous system
Brain
Spinal cord
Adrenal
medulla

Hematopoietic system
Genitourinary system
Heart

Connective tissue and smooth
muscle of viscera

Pleura
Peritoneum
Pericardium
Blood vessels
    wall
    endothelium
Bone
Cartilage
Muscle
Soft connective tissues
    fibrous
    synovial, and so on

Schwann cells

Visceral sarcomas

Soft tissue and bony
sarcomas

The annual age-adjusted incidence was 2 per 100,000 persons. Data from New Zealand suggest that the incidence and mortality from soft tissue sarcomas have been increasing (from 1.3 per 100,000 men in 1955 to 2.2 per 100,000 men in 1977) in that country, although no change in incidence was seen in Denmark during the same period.[3,4] There appears to be no sex or racial pattern for these cancers in the United States.

Soft tissue sarcomas comprise 0.7% of all cancers, although these tumors comprise 6.5% of all cancers in children younger than 15 years of age.[2] Soft tissue sarcomas rank fifth in cancer incidence among children younger than 15, behind leukemia, central nervous system cancers, lymphomas, and sympathetic nervous system cancers. Soft tissue sarcomas rank fifth as a cause of cancer death in this age group behind leukemia, nervous system cancers, renal cancer, and bone cancer.

EPIDEMIOLOGY

Little is known about epidemiologic or etiologic factors of importance in patients with soft tissue sarcomas. There is no proven genetic predisposition to the development of soft tissue sarcomas, although Li and Fraumeni reported four kindreds with pairs of young children (*i.e.*, three sets of siblings and one set of cousins) with soft tissue sarcomas.[5] This incidence exceeded that expected on a chance basis ($p = 0.06$).

This familial cancer syndrome is associated with an increased incidence of soft tissue sarcoma and with breast cancer, osteosarcoma, brain tumors, leukemia, and adrenal carcinoma. Although these kindreds have germline abnormalities of the tumor suppressor gene p53, somatic mutations of p53 are found in only a portion of sporadic, nonfamilial sarcomas.[6,7]

There have been several reports of childhood sarcomas associated with a small increase in incidence of other familial cancers (especially breast cancer) that tended to occur in mothers younger than 30 years of age.[5,8–14] Lymphangiosarcoma of the arm in women after mastectomy and axillary lymph node ablation (Stewart-Treves syndrome) almost certainly does not represent evidence of an etiologic correlation between mammary cancer and sarcoma of soft tissue, but rather is the development of lymphangiosarcoma in lymphedematous arms.[15]

Although Sloane and Hubbel reported an increased incidence of congenital defects in children with soft tissue sarcomas, this association was not seen by Li and Fraumeni.[8,16]

Soft tissue sarcomas are thought to occur with slightly increased frequency in patients with a variety of genetically transmitted diseases, such as the basal cell nevus syndrome, tuberous sclerosis, Werner's syndrome, intestinal polyposis, and Gardner's syndrome.[14,17–21] Patients with multiple neurofibromatosis (von Recklinghausen's disease) have approximately a 15% chance of developing a neurofibrosarcoma.[18]

Although many patients with soft tissue sarcomas present with a recent history of trauma, it is likely that minor trauma merely calls a preexisting lesion to the patient's attention.

Chemical carcinogens, such as 3-methylcholanthrene, and viruses can cause soft tissue sarcomas in experimental animals, but there is no convincing link between these factors and sarcomas in humans. Studies in Sweden in 1979 and 1981 linked environmental exposure to phenoxyacetic acids (a class of herbicides) and chlorophenols (wood preservatives) to a sixfold increase in the risk of developing soft tissue sarcoma.[22,23] These studies were based on small numbers of patients, and a later analysis of more than 350,000 Swedish agricultural and forestry workers potentially exposed to these chemicals failed to confirm this association.[24] A case-control study from New Zealand failed to find an association between exposure to phenoxyherbicides and the incidence of soft tissue sarcomas, and an analysis of data from Denmark also cast doubt on this association.[3,4] Because of the early Swedish reports, there was concern that Vietnam veterans exposed to Agent Orange, a mixture of two commercial phenoxyacetic acid herbicides containing trace amounts of dioxins, might have an increased incidence of soft tissue sarcomas, but two studies failed to show a significant correlation.[25,26]

Sarcomas have a tendency to occur in areas previously exposed to ionizing radiation, although sarcomas in radiation therapy fields are uncommon. In 1977, Adam and Reif could find only 7 cases in the world literature of fibrosarcoma of the chest wall in women undergoing radiation therapy after mastectomy for breast cancer.[27] The latent period of these lesions averaged 15 years after radiation exposure. An additional 7 cases were described by Kuten and colleagues in 1985.[28] Sixteen cases of radiation-induced sarcomas of the chest wall occurred at the M.D. Anderson Cancer Center in Houston between 1944 and 1984, representing 5% of the 331 sarcomas of the chest wall that were seen during that period.[29] Similar findings were reported by O'Neil and colleagues, who reviewed 11 patients with soft tissue fibrosarcomas after irradiation of the chest wall for breast cancer.[30]

Halperin and colleagues reported 5 cases of bone or soft tissue sarcomas occurring more than 5 years after treatment of Hodgkin's disease.[31] Two of these patients had received radiation therapy alone, 2 were treated with a combination of radiation and chemotherapy, and 1 received chemotherapy alone. Four cases of soft tissue sarcoma and 1 case of osteosarcoma occurred, with latent periods of 6 to 11 years. These investigators calculated the risk of developing a sarcoma in 5-year survivors of Hodgkin's disease to be 0.9%.

Osteosarcomas appear to be the most common sarcomas induced by radiation. Arlen and associates summarized 50 cases of postirradiation osteosarcoma, and Martland described osteosarcoma developing after ingestion of radium and mesothorium during the painting of luminous watch dials.[32,33]

Sarcomas are associated with foreign-body implantations in rodents, and sporadic reports of this phenomenon in humans have appeared.[34] Ott tabulated all cases published before 1966.[35] The responsible foreign bodies were mainly metal implants, bullets, shrapnel pieces, and bone transplants, with latent periods of as long as 40 years. The true incidence of foreign-body-induced sarcomas is probably minimal, because no sarcomas were seen among 11,000 women who underwent augmentation mammoplasty with a variety of materials or in 281 patients who underwent prosthetic replacement for facial defects.[36,37]

SITES OF SOFT TISSUE SARCOMAS

Because of the ubiquitous nature of the connective tissues, soft tissue sarcomas can arise anywhere in the body. Visceral sarcomas arise from the connective stroma found in all organs and are rarer than sarcomas originating in somatic sites. Visceral sarcomas are not considered in this chapter. Sites of somatic soft tissue sarcomas from nine reported series are presented in Table 42–2.[38–46] Approximately 60% of sarcomas occur in the extremities. The ratio of lower-extremity to upper-extremity tumors is 3 to 1. About 75% of lower-extremity sarcomas originate at or above the knee. Other sites include the head and neck regions (9%) and the trunk (31%). Within the trunk, approximately 40% of tumors are located in the retroperitoneum, and the remaining tumors are located in the abdominal wall, chest wall, mediastinum, and breast. Treatment approaches for patients with soft tissue sarcomas must consider the site of the origin of the tumor.

PATHOLOGIC CLASSIFICATION

PRINCIPLES OF CLASSIFICATION

Each of the soft tissues can give rise to benign and malignant groups of tumors. The transformation of a benign soft tissue tumor into a malignant sarcoma is rare. Because of the many different soft tissues, a variety of histologically distinct, but often grossly similar, sarcomas have been identified.[47–50] The pathologic classification presented in Table 42–3, based on the putative cell of origin of each tumor, was suggested by

TABLE 42-2. Sites of Soft Tissue Sarcomas

	Sites				
Investigations	*Head and Neck*	*Trunk/ Retroperitoneum*	*Upper Extremity*	*Lower Extremity*	*Total*
Shieber et al, 1961[38]	16	39	20	50	125
Hare et al, 1963[39]	42	34/5	32	48	161
Ferrell et al, 1972[40]	8	19	15	36	78
Sears et al, 1980[41]	12	16	6	26	60
Abbas et al, 1981[42]	24	66/38	42	81	251
Lindberg et al, 1981[43]	26	74	63	137	300
Potter et al, 1985[44]	12	48/36	59	152	307
Torosian et al, 1987[45]	21	92/90	81	208	492
ACS Survey, 1987[46]	406	872/568	594	2110	4550
Total	567	1997	912	2848	6324
(%)	(9)	(32)	(14)	(45)	(100)

TABLE 42-3.   Histologic Classification of Soft Tissue Tumors

I. *Tumors and Tumor-like Lesions of Fibrous Tissue*
  A. Benign
    1. Fibroma
    2. Nodular fasciitis (including intravascular and cranial types)
    3. Proliferative fasciitis
    4. Proliferative myositis
    5. Fibroma of tendon sheath
    6. Elastofibroma
    7. Nuchal fibroma
    8. Nasopharyngeal fibroma
    9. Keloid
  B. Fibrous tumors of infancy and childhood
    1. Fibrous hamartoma of infancy
    2. Myofibromatosis (solitary, multicentric)
    3. Fibromatosis colli
    4. Infantile digital fibromatosis
    5. Infantile fibromatosis (desmoid type)
    6. Giant cell fibroblastoma
    7. Gingival fibromatosis
    8. Calcifying aponeurotic fibroma
    9. Hyalin fibromatosis
  C. Fibromatoses
    1. Superficial fibromatoses
      a. Palmar and plantar fibromatosis
      b. Penile (Peyronie's) fibromatosis
      c. Knuckle pads
    2. Deep fibromatoses
      a. Abdominal fibromatosis
      b. Extra-abdominal fibromatosis
      c. Intra-abdominal fibromatosis
      d. Mesenteric fibromatosis (Gardner's syndrome)
      e. Postradiation fibromatosis
      f. Cicatricial fibromatosis
  D. Malignant
    1. Adult fibrosarcoma
    2. Congenital and infantile fibrosarcoma
    3. Inflammatory fibrosarcoma
    4. Postradiation fibrosarcoma
    5. Cicatricial fibrosarcoma

II. *Fibrohistiocytic Tumors*
  A. Benign
    1. Fibrous histiocytoma
      a. Cutaneous (dermatofibroma)
      b. Deep
    2. Atypical fibroxanthoma
    3. Juvenile xanthogranuloma
    4. Reticulohistiocytoma
    5. Xanthoma
  B. Intermediate
    1. Dermatofibrosarcoma protuberans
    2. Bednar tumor
  C. Malignant
    1. Malignant fibrous histiocytoma
      a. Storiform-pleomorphic
      b. Myxoid (myxofibrosarcoma)
      c. Giant cell (malignant giant cell tumor of soft parts)
      d. Inflammatory (malignant xanthogranuloma, xanthosarcoma)
      e. Angiomatoid

III. *Tumors and Tumor-like Lesions of Adiopose Tissue*
  A. Benign
    1. Lipoma (cutaneous, deep, and multiple)
    2. Angiolipoma
    3. Spindle cell and pleomorphic lipoma
    4. Lipoblastoma and lipoblastomatosis
    5. Angiomyolipoma
    6. Myelolipoma
    7. Intramuscular and intermuscular lipoma
    8. Lipoma of tendon sheath

    9. Lumbosacral lipoma
    10. Interneural and perineural fibrolipoma
    11. Diffuse lipomatosis
    12. Cervical symmetrical lipomatosis (Madelung's disease)
    13. Pelvic lipomatosis
    14. Hibernoma
  B. Malignant
    1. Liposarcoma, predominantly
      a. Well-differentiated
        (1) Lipoma-like
        (2) Sclerosing
        (3) Inflammatory
      b. Myxoid
      c. Round cell (poorly differentiated myxoid)
      d. Pleomorphic
      e. Dedifferentiated

IV. *Tumors of Muscle Tissue*
  A. Smooth muscle
    1. Benign
      a. Leiomyoma (cutaneous and deep)
      b. Angiomyoma (vascular leiomyoma)
      c. Epithelioid leiomyoma (benign leiomyoblastoma)
      d. Intravenous leiomyomatosis
      e. Leiomyomatosis peritonealis disseminata
    2. Malignant
      a. Leiomyosarcoma
      b. Epithelioid leiomyosarcoma (malignant leiomyoblastoma)
  B. Striated muscle
    1. Benign
      a. Adult rhabdomyoma
      b. Genital rhabdomyoma
      c. Fetal rhabdomyoma
    2. Malignant
      a. Rhabdomyosarcoma, predominantly
        (1) Embryonal (including botryoid)
        (2) Alveolar
        (3) Pelomorphic
        (4) Mixed
      b. Ectomesenchymoma (rhabdomyosarcoma with ganglion cell differentiation)

V. *Tumors and Tumor-like Lesions of Blood Vessels*
  A. Benign
    1. Hemangioma
      a. Capillary (including juvenile)
      b. Cavernous
      c. Arteriovenous
      d. Venous
      e. Epithelioid (angiolymphoid hyperplasia, Kimura's disease)
      f. Granulation tissue type (pyogenic granuloma)
    2. Deep hemangioma (intramuscular, synovial, perineural)
    3. Hemangiomatosis
    4. Glomus tumor
    5. Hemangiopericytoma
    6. Papillary endothelial hyperplasia (intravascular vegetant hemangioendothelioma of Masson)
  B. Intermediate
    1. Hemangioendothelioma
      a. Epithelioid
      b. Spindle cell
      c. Malignant endovascular papillary angioendothelioma
  C. Malignant
    1. Hemangiosarcoma
    2. Kaposi's sarcoma
    3. Malignant glomus tumor
    4. Malignant hemangiopericytoma

(continued)

TABLE 42-3. *(Continued)*

VI. *Tumors of Lymph Vessels*
  A. Benign
    1. Lymphangioma
      a. Cavernous
      b. Cystic (cystic hygroma)
    2. Lymphangiomatosis
    3. Lymphangiomyoma and lymphangiomyomatosis
  B. Malignant
    1. Angiosarcoma

VII. *Tumors and Tumor-like Lesions of Synovial Tissue*
  A. Benign
    1. Giant cell tumor of tendon sheath
      a. Localized (nodular tenosynovitis)
      b. Diffuse (florid synovitis)
  B. Malignant
    1. Synovial sarcoma (malignant synovioma), predominantly
      a. Biphasic (fibrous and epithelial)
      b. Monophasic (fibrous or epithelial)
    2. Malignant giant cell tumor of tendon sheath

VIII. *Tumors of Mesothelial Tissue*
  A. Benign
    1. Localized fibrous mesothelioma (subserosal fibroma)
    2. Multicystic peritoneal mesothelioma
    3. Mesothelioma of the genital tract (adenomatoid tumor)
  B. Malignant
    1. Diffuse and localized mesothelioma, predominantly
      a. Epithelial
      b. Fibrous
      c. Biphasic

IX. *Tumors and Tumor-like Lesions of Peripheral Nerves*
  A. Benign
    1. Traumatic neuroma
    2. Morton's neuroma
    3. Neuromuscular hamartoma
    5. Nerve sheath ganglion
    5. Neurilemoma (benign schwannoma)
    6. Neurofibroma, solitary
      a. Localized
      b. Diffuse
      c. Pacinian
      d. Pigmented
    7. Granular cell tumor
    8. Neurofibromatosis (von Recklinghausen's disease)
      a. Localized
      b. Plexiform
      c. Diffuse
    9. Pigmented neuroectodermal tumor of infancy (retinal anlage tumor)
    10. Ectopic meningioma
    11. Nasal glioma
    12. Neurothekeoma
  B. Malignant
    1. Malignant schwannoma, including malignant schwannoma with rhabdomyoblastic differentiation (malignant Triton tumor), glandular malignant schwannoma, and epithelioid malignant schwannoma

    2. Peripheral tumors of primitive neuroectodermal tissues (Neuroepithelioma)
    3. Malignant pigmented neuroectodermal tumor of infancy (retinal anlage tumor)
    4. Malignant granular cell tumor

X. *Tumors of Autonomic Ganglia*
  A. Benign
    1. Ganglioneuroma
    2. Melanocytic schwannoma
  B. Malignant
    1. Neuroblastoma
    2. Ganglioneuroblastoma
    3. Malignant melanocytic schwannoma

XI. *Tumors of Paraganglionic Structures*
  A. Benign
    1. Paraganglioma (solitary, multiple, familial)
  B. Malignant
    1. Malignant paraganglioma

XII. *Tumors and Tumor-like Lesions of Cartilage and Bone-Forming Tissues*
  A. Benign
    1. Panniculitis ossificans
    2. Myositis ossificans
    3. Fibrodysplasia (myositis) ossificans progressiva
    4. Extraskeletal chondroma
    4. Extraskeletal osteoma
  B. Malignant
    1. Extraskeletal chondrosarcoma
      a. Well-differentiated
      b. Myxoid (chordoid sarcoma)
      c. Mesenchymal
    2. Extraskeletal osteosarcoma

XIII. *Tumors and Tumor-like Lesions of Pluripotential Mesenchyme*
  A. Benign
    1. Mesenchymoma
  B. Malignant
    1. Malignant mesenchymoma

XIV. *Tumors and Tumor-like Lesions of Disputed or Uncertain Histogenesis*
  A. Benign
    1. Congenital granular cell tumor
    2. Tumoral calcinosis
    3. Myxoma (cutaneous and intramuscular)
    4. Aggressive angiomyxoma
    5. Amyloid tumor
    6. Parachordoma
  B. Malignant
    1. Alveolar soft part sarcoma
    2. Epithelioid sarcoma
    3. Clear cell sarcoma of tendons and aponeuroses (malignant melanoma of soft parts)
    4. Extraskeletal Ewing's sarcoma

XV. *Unclassified Soft Tissue Tumors and Tumor-like Lesions*

(Enzinger FM, Weiss SW. Soft tissue tumors. 2nd ed. St. Louis: CV Mosby, 1988)

Enzinger and Weiss.[50] Pathologic classifications based on the appearance of the predominant cell in the lesion (*i.e.*, round cell or spindle cell sarcomas) are less useful and should not be employed. Each of the sarcomas tends to reflect the morphologic appearance of the cell of origin, and the tendency of these tumors to dedifferentiate results in a variety of overlapping patterns that can make them difficult to classify.

Competent pathologists often disagree on the cell of origin of an individual tumor.[51,52] The great variation in the reported incidence of various subtypes of soft tissue sarcomas probably reflects differences of opinion among pathologists.

There are tumors arising from the soft tissues that are grossly similar to sarcomas but rarely metastasize. Many of these tumors (*e.g.*, desmoid tumors, dermatofibrosarcoma protuberans) are capable of aggressively invading local tissues in a fashion characteristic of true sarcomas. It is important to differentiate these locally aggressive, nonmetastasizing lesions from those that are truly benign or malignant because of the therapeutic implications. Injury may provoke proliferative lesions in soft tissues. These can mimic soft tissue tumors, and because of their high mitotic rate, they are often difficult to differentiate from malignant lesions. An example is myositis ossificans.

For each histologically distinct malignant sarcoma, the tendency to metastasize depends on the grade of the tumor. Low-grade sarcomas are capable of aggressive, invasive local growth but tend not to disseminate. High-grade tumors are more likely to metastasize. In a survey of 4550 sarcoma patients, Lawrence and colleagues found approximately 33% of the tumors had low-grade classifications, and the others were high-grade lesions.[46] Assigning a pathologic grade to an individual tumor as a means of predicting clinical behavior has not been easy. The general criteria for grading—mitotic rate, nuclear morphology, degree of cellularity, cellular anaplasia or pleomorphism, and the presence of necrosis—are not readily quantifiable. However, sarcomas of the various histologic types can be assigned a numeric grade. The range of grades attributed to the more common types of sarcoma is presented in Figure 42–1.[50]

Costa and colleagues at the National Cancer Institute (NCI) correlated histologic features, such as histologic type, number of mitoses, degrees of necrosis, pleomorphism, cellularity, and matrix of the primary lesion, with the overall prognoses of these patients.[53] Stratified analyses revealed that the degree of necrosis was the single best histopathologic parameter that

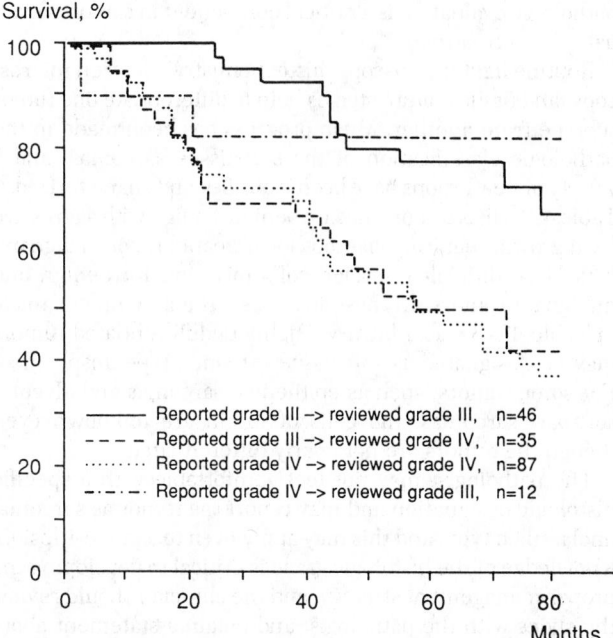

FIGURE 42–2. Comparison of overall survival of patients with high grade sarcomas based on tumor grading by individual referring pathologists and central pathology review by the Scandinavian Sarcoma Group. When compared with the prognosis of patients with agreement on tumor grading (——, grade III; and ··· grade IV), the prognosis of those with disagreement on tumor grade (- - -, III versus IV; - ·-, IV versus III) was best predicted by the central review group. Such review of equivocal cases by pathologists with extensive experience in sarcoma grading can be crucial in estimating prognosis and planning appropriate therapy.

predicted the time to recurrence and the overall survival of patients ($p = 0.025$ and $p = 0.002$, respectively). The investigators proposed a grading system using the degree of necrosis to differentiate aggressive lesions. Grade 2 lesions were high-grade tumors with no or minimal necrosis, and grade 3 lesions were high-grade lesions with moderate or marked necrosis.[53] When using this criterion alone, a significant difference was seen between the prognoses of patients with grades 2 or 3 lesions. This system was independently confirmed by Lack and coworkers, who reviewed 300 extremity sarcomas and found the degree of necrosis to be the most significant determinant in predicting time to recurrence and overall survival.[54] However, there was only a 64% concordance rate in assigning a grade to 87 extremity soft tissue sarcomas that were previously reviewed by Costa and colleagues.[54]

A somewhat more elaborate grading system was proposed by Trojani and associates, using tumor differentiation, mitosis count, and the degree of tumor necrosis to predict the prognoses of patients with high-grade sarcomas.[55] Using this grading system, Coindre and coworkers reported a 75% concordance in grading 25 soft tissue sarcomas between an experienced panel of pathologists and a study group of 15 pathologists who had not been involved in the development of the grading system.[51]

Alvegard and Berg demonstrated that the grading of tumors by pathologists experienced in evaluating sarcomas correlated better with patient prognosis than grading assigned by referring pathologists (Fig. 42–2). This emphasizes that expert

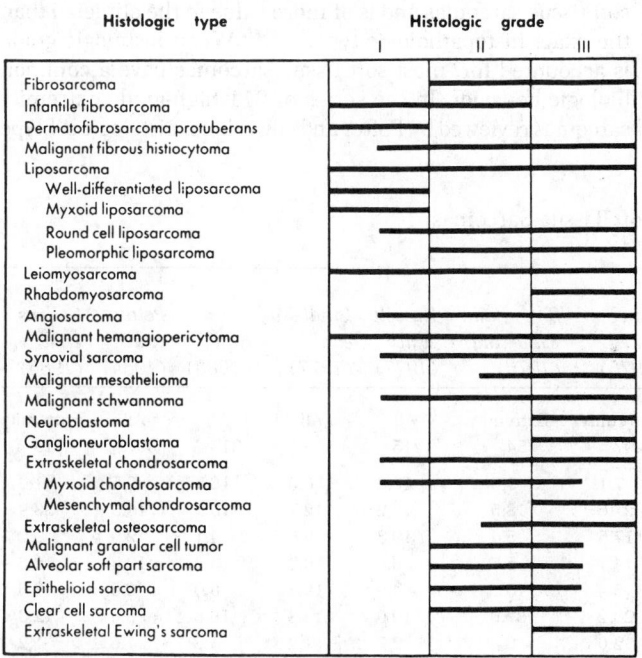

FIGURE 42–1. Soft tissue sarcomas. Estimated range of degree of malignancy based on histologic type and grade. Grade within the overall range depends on specific histologic features such as cellularity, cellular pleomorphism, mitotic activity, amount of stroma, infiltrative or expansive growth, and necrosis. (Enzinger FM, Weiss SW. Soft tissue tumors. 2nd ed. St. Louis: CV Mosby, 1988)

pathologic evaluation is a critical component in sarcoma evaluation and treatment.[56]

Routine light microscopy, histochemistry, electron microscopy, and tissue culture studies help to differentiate one tumor subtype from another. Much progress has been made in the pathologic classification of the soft tissue sarcomas, and a variety of new lesions have been identified and characterized.[50] Table 42–3 lists tumors that are benign, benign with aggressive local growth requiring vigorous local treatment, or malignant. It is often difficult to assign cells of origin for benign and malignant tumors. In these instances, the assignment made in Table 42–3 was arbitrary. Highly undifferentiated tumors may be designated as soft tissue sarcoma, type unspecified. For some tumors, such as epithelioid sarcomas and alveolar soft-part sarcomas, the cells of origin are unknown even though the tumors are not poorly differentiated.

The pathologist may not feel comfortable with a specific histologic designation and may report the tumor as sarcoma, unclassified type, and this may apply even to a grade 1 lesion. Knowledge of the histologic grade is critical to developing the proper management strategy, and the clinician should review the slides with the pathologist and obtain a statement about grade, even if the pathologist does not wish to specify cell type.

HISTOPATHOLOGIC CLASSIFICATION OF MALIGNANT TUMORS

Competent pathologists differ in attaching a histiogenic label to types of soft tissue sarcomas. These disagreements confound attempts to compare reports from different institutions about the incidence of histologic subtypes, frequency of tumors at different anatomic sites, stage of disease at presentation, frequency of local failure with different treatment modalities, and frequency of distant metastasis. This is particularly evident in Table 42–4, which collates the relative frequency of the various histopathologic types in several series.[38-40,44,57-65] The large differences in the incidence of different histopathologic

types almost certainly reflect the differences in diagnostic criteria used by the pathologists. For example, in the series reported by Shieber and Graham and by Ferrell and Frable, there are no lesions that are considered as unclassifiable sarcomas.[38,40] In contrast, Hare and Cerny had 28.5%, Pack and Ariel had 36.4%, and Potter and coworkers had 9.5% unclassifiable sarcomas.[39,44,57] Another example of these disparities is illustrated by the 5.4% incidence of fibrosarcomas in the series by Pack and Ariel, compared with the 37% to 44% incidence of fibrosarcomas in the series reported by Simon and Enneking, Hare and Cerny, and Shieber and Graham.[38,39,57,60]

Changes in histologic classification of lesions, such as the recognition of a separate category of malignant fibrous histiocytomas, generated wide variations in the reported incidence of soft tissue sarcomas. For example, in the five series listed in Table 42–4 published before 1972, no cases of malignant fibrous histiocytomas were reported. Since 1972, this lesion has gained increasing recognition, and the 20.4% incidence reported in the series by Simon and Enneking in 1976 is comparable to the 17.5% incidence reported by Lindberg and associates, 22.8% reported by Potter and coworkers, 15.6% reported by Suit, 14.6% reported by Collin and colleagues, and 25.9% reported by Lawrence and colleagues.[44,47,60,63-65]

Presant and colleagues reviewed 216 consecutive sarcoma patients in the Southeastern Cancer Study Group experience and found concordance in histopathologic diagnoses in only 66% of cases.[52] The diagnoses of the primary member institution and a pathology review panel were compared. Coindre and coworkers reported a 61% concordance among pathologists in assigning histologic type in 25 soft tissue sarcomas.[51] The available evidence indicates that the histopathologic grade is the most important indicator of the biologic behavior of soft tissue sarcomas and is of more value to the clinician than the exact histopathologic type.[50,53-55] When histologic grade is accounted for, most soft tissue sarcomas have a common biologic behavior. In the series of 211 high-grade extremity sarcomas reviewed by Potter and coworkers, histologic subtype

TABLE 42-4. Relative Incidence (%) of Histologic Types of Soft Tissue Sarcomas in Various Studies

Soft Tissue Sarcomas	Shieber and Graham[38] (1962)	Hare and Cerny[39] (1963)	Pack and Ariel[57] (1964)	Martin et al[58] (1965)	Ferrell and Frable[40] (1972)	Shiu et al[59] (1975)	Simon and Enneking[60] (1976)	Russell et al[61] (1977)	Lindberg et al[63] (1977)	Suit[64] (1983)	Potter et al[44] (1984)	Collins et al[65] (1986)
Sites	All	All	All	All	All	Extremity	Extremity	All	All	All	All	Extremity
Total no. of cases	125	200	717	398	117	297	54	1215	166	315	307	315
Unclassified	0	28.5	36.4	14.8	0	7.1	5.6	10.0	6.0	16.5	9.5	1.0
Liposarcoma	16.0	11.5	14.6	26.9	17.0	27.6	18.5	18.2	12.7	15.2	18.3	33.9
Rhabdomyosarcoma	16.0	5.0	13.9	20.6	30.0	17.5	5.6	19.3	9.6	4.1	2.9	9.2
Synoviosarcoma	0.8	2.5	8.4	3.0	2.5	14.1	5.6	6.9	10.2	3.8	19.5	12.6
Neurofibrosarcoma	3.2	0	6.4	0	0	5.4	0	4.9	19.3	6.0	6.8	7.6
Fibrosarcoma	44.0	43.0	5.4	24.1	33.0	20.2	37.0	19.0	13.3	16.8	3.6	12.3
Angiosarcoma	4.8	0	2.6	0.3	0	2.0	0	2.7	1.2	3.2	1.6	1.2
Leiomyosarcoma	6.4	6.5	0	6.3	4.0	2.4	0	6.5	4.2	7.6	11.4	3.8
Mesenchymoma	0	0	0	0	0	0.3	0	0.3	0	0.9	0	0
Malignant fibrous histiocytoma	0	0	0	0	0	1.0	20.4	10.5	17.5	15.6	22.8	14.6
Other	8.8	3.0	12.1	4.0	13.5	2.4	7.4	1.7	6.0	10.2	3.6	3.4

was not a significant determinant of disease-free or overall survival (Fig. 42–3).[66] The difficulties in pathologic classification and its negligible importance in arbitrating therapy compel the treatment of soft tissue sarcomas as a group.

BENIGN TUMORS OF SOFT TISSUE

BENIGN TUMORS OF FIBROUS ORIGIN

There are many variants of fibrous tumors that are nonmalignant and do not metastasize. Most are successfully treated by simple excision and do not recur. Some tumors in this category, such as nodular fasciitis, can be mistaken for true fibrosarcomas. Others, such as extraabdominal desmoid tumors, require special attention because aggressive local therapy is necessary to prevent recurrence.

Fibroma

"Fibroma" has been applied to any benign fibrous growth. Many congenital malformations and reparative tissue growths fall into this category. With increased understanding of the variants of fibrous tissue neoplasms, fewer tumors are called fibromas, and the term is now restricted to benign, encapsulated, fibrous nodules that seldom grow larger than a few centimeters in diameter. A subcutaneous or soft fibroma (*i.e.*, fibroma molle) is a pedunculated subcutaneous growth composed of fibrous tissue and fat covered by epidermis. Fibroma durum is a pedunculated lesion, often arising in the oral mucosa, that may result from malocclusion or malfitting dentures. All of these lesions should be treated by simple excision. They rarely recur.

Elastofibroma

Elastofibroma is a rare lesion that usually occurs under the scapular muscles and frequently attaches to the rib cage.[67–70]

Many are not noticed, and one series found them in 10% of 235 autopsy cases.[68] The lesions are benign and do not recur after simple enucleation.

Palmar and Plantar Fibromatosis

Tumor-like proliferations of the palmar and plantar aponeuroses can give rise to tumor-like nodules.[71–74] Only the palmar fibromatosis (Dupuytren's contracture) is associated with flexion contractures. Heredity affects incidence, and lesions occur six times as often in men as in women. The lesions grow slowly as localized nodular enlargements that can infiltrate the fascia and involve overlying skin and subcutaneous tissue. The lesions are benign, although they have a tendency to recur after simple excision. Consequently, small nodules should be left untouched. If excision is necessary, attempts should be made to widely excise the palmar or plantar fascia.

Juvenile Aponeurotic Fibroma

Juvenile aponeurotic fibroma (*i.e.*, Keasby's tumor) is a form of fibromatosis that affects the palms or soles of children and young adults.[75–77] The lesion can infiltrate and overgrow subcutaneous fat and muscle, but metastases never occur. The lesions invade locally and have a tendency to recur after limited excision. Attempts to achieve negative microscopic margins should be made.

Congenital Generalized Fibromatosis

Generalized fibromatosis, usually present at birth, is characterized by multiple, widely scattered, nodular and infiltrating fibroblastic lesions, diffusely present in the superficial and deep tissues, viscera, and bone.[78–80] The disease is often fatal because of vital organ involvement, but it represents a congenital rather than neoplastic condition.

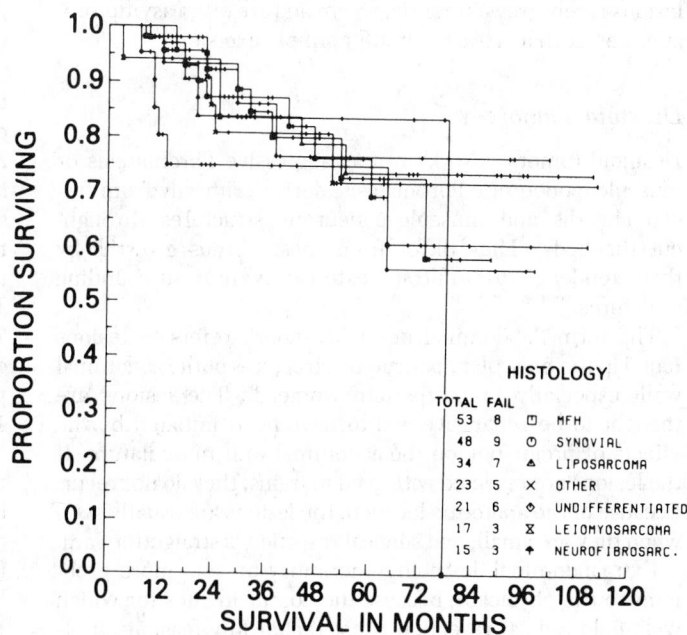

FIGURE 42–3. Actuarial analysis of overall survival for 211 patients with high-grade extremity sarcomas categorized by histologic subtype. There are no significant differences between the groups. (Potter DA, Kinsella T, Glatstein E, et al. High grade soft tissue sarcomas or the extremities. Cancer 1986;58:190–205)

Fibrous Hamartoma of Infancy

Fibrous hamartoma occurs predominantly in boys and presents in the first year of life with a solitary mass in the axilla, upper extremity, head, or neck.[81] These lesions are situated almost exclusively in the dermis or subcutaneous fat and can become large. Local excision is almost always curative, because this lesion does not metastasize.

Fibromatosis Colli

This distinctive form of fibromatosis develops in the sterno-cleidomastoid muscle of newborn or very young children. In many cases, a small lump in the sternocleidomastoid muscle noticed in the newborn disappears spontaneously.[82,83] If the lesion persists for several months after birth, it can grow and produce neck contractures. Lack of treatment can result in large growths, with subsequent spread to the trachea and surrounding organs. These lesions should be excised and often require removal of the entire sternocleidomastoid muscle.

Penile Fibromatosis

Also called Peyronie's disease, penile fibromatosis involves a circumscribed fibrous thickening arising in the connective tissue sheath that separates the corpus cavernosum from the tunic albuginea.[84] It causes pain and curvature of the penis on penile erection. Surgical excision of the fibrous tissue is the preferred treatment.

Nodular Fasciitis

Nodular fasciitis, also called pseudosarcomatous or proliferative fasciitis, should be treated by simple excision. Its morphologic appearance causes it to be confused with fibrosarcoma.[85–88] These lesions generally arise in the subcutaneous fascia or the superficial portions of the deep fascia. The growth of these lesions is frequently rapid. Maximal size is usually achieved within a few weeks, and then growth stops. These lesions rarely grow larger than 5 cm and are often asymptomatic. Fewer than 10% recur after simple excision.

Desmoid Tumors

Desmoid tumors, also known as aggressive fibromatosis or musculoaponeurotic fibromatosis, derive primarily from fascial sheaths and musculoaponeurotic structures throughout the body. They differ from most fibrous growths by their tendency to infiltrate extensively into surrounding structures.[89–105]

The term "abdominal desmoid tumor" refers to lesions found in the muscular aponeurotic structures of the abdominal wall, especially in postpartum women.[92] The lesions are thought to be reparative and to have been initiated by the effects of pregnancy on the abdominal wall musculature. If the lesions are resected with good margins, they do not recur. Because of the anatomic location, the lesions are usually seen when they are small, and surgical resection is straightforward.

Extraabdominal desmoid tumors may present more problems to the physician, because they occur in sites for which wide-field radical resection is not technically feasible; if attempted, irradiation may be associated with appreciable morbidity. These lesions occur around the shoulder girdle, inguinal region, and lower extremities. They are not encapsulated, infiltrate locally, and are destructive but do not metastasize. Histopathologically, these lesions are primarily fibroblastic with elongated, thin, delicate nuclei, which appear virtually normal. Mitotic figures are uncommon, usually less than 1 per 50 high-power fields.

The preferred treatment for extraabdominal desmoid is wide-field resection with negative margins in all dimensions.[106] The local recurrence rate is 50% to 75% of the cases for which margins were close or positive.

In a review of 138 patients at Memorial Sloan-Kettering Cancer Center, Posner found that inadequate surgical resection and presentation with recurrent disease were independent predictive factors for recurrence after surgery. The overall survival rate for these patients was 92% at 5 years, with 11 patients succumbing to tumor-related complications. All 11 patients had lesions in nonextremity sites, leading to obstruction, fistula, sepsis, and malnutrition.[105]

If wide resection is not feasible, radiation therapy may be an effective treatment. James Ewing, in 1928, commented that desmoid tumors slowly responded to irradiation and that this treatment could be considered for lesions not amenable to surgical resection.[93] Successful treatment by irradiation has been reported in an incidental way in describing results of large surgical series.[94]

Benninghoff and Robbins described the treatment of 4 patients with desmoid tumors, 3 of whom were treated after incomplete surgery and 1 for frank recurrent tumor.[95] Radiation doses were modest, but good responses were obtained in 3 of 4 patients. Greenberg and coworkers reported long-term control in 8 of 9 patients with desmoid tumors treated by irradiation alone or in combination with surgery.[96] Wara and associates reported a series of 16 patients with desmoid tumors, 12 of whom were treated for gross tumor (>5 cm).[98] Two died from disease, but the remaining 10 were alive without tumor 2 to 6 years after treatment. Among the 4 patients treated after incomplete surgical resection (no palpable tumor), there was 1 local recurrence at 2 years; the other 3 patients were free of evident disease at 2 to 4 years.

Suit and Russell described the results of treatment of 4 patients with desmoid tumor, 2 of whom had massive local disease and 2 of whom were treated after incomplete surgery.[99] All 4 remained disease free for 5 years. Seventeen patients treated by radiation therapy for desmoid tumors at the Massachusetts General Hospital and followed for more than 12 months were reported by Kiel and Suit.[100] Ten patients were treated by irradiation alone and 7 by irradiation and surgery. There were 3 local failures: 2 of 10 after irradiation and 1 of 7 after irradiation and surgery. However, 2 of the failures developed after doses of only 2200 and 2400 cGy. Among 15 patients who received doses greater than 5000 cGy, there was 1 local failure (follow-up, 12–96 months).

For the patient who has uncertain or minimally positive margins at the first resection, and re-resection is not feasible, the patient should be observed and treatment implemented at the first sign of regrowth. In these circumstances, local failure is not universal; some patients may be able to avoid high-dose radiation treatment. At the Massachusetts General Hospital, 8 patients with uncertain or minimally positive margins after resection were followed, and only one recurred; after re-resection, this patient is free of disease.[100]

There are reports that hormonal or antihormonal medication may achieve long-term remission of desmoid tumors. Kinzbrunner and colleagues described a patient with a 16-kg desmoid tumor of the back that regressed to a 5 × 5 × 2 cm mass in 2 weeks after treatment with tamoxifen (20 mg four times daily).[101] Lanari described a small series of patients with desmoid tumors treated successfully with progesterone.[102] Using another approach, Waddell and Gerner reported that administration of indomethacin and ascorbic acid could cause regression of desmoid tumors.[103] Because of the limited toxicity of these approaches, the use of these agents in the treatment of desmoid tumors deserves further clinical study.

BENIGN TUMORS OF STRIATED MUSCLE

Rhabdomyoma

These are extremely rare benign tumors of skeletal muscle, generally occurring in the tongue, neck muscles, larynx, uvula, nasal cavity, axilla, vulva, and heart.[107,108] These tumors are treated by simple excision.

BENIGN TUMORS OF SMOOTH MUSCLE

Leiomyoma

Leiomyomas rarely occur outside of the uterus and the gastrointestinal tract.[109,110] They can occur in the skin and subcutaneous tissues and probably arise from the smooth muscle of small blood vessels in these tissues. These lesions are treated by simple excision.

Epithelioid Leiomyoma

Epithelioid leiomyoma (*i.e.*, leiomyoblastoma) are most frequently found in the wall of the gastrointestinal tract, especially in the stomach. They are similar to other smooth muscle tumors but may become large and hemorrhagic and exhibit small cystic areas. Simple excision is usually curative.

BENIGN TUMORS OF ADIPOSE TISSUE

Lipomas

Lipomas are among the most common of all benign neoplasms and arise in any location where fat is normally present. These lesions may occur in deep tissue, although they usually arise subcutaneously. They are characteristically multilobulated masses of fatty tissue that vary from small nodules to large masses weighing several kilograms.

Multiple lipomatosis is a condition of diffuse overgrowths that may occur throughout the body. These are not true tumors and are probably a result of fat metabolism disorders.

Spindle cell lipomas are rare benign tumors that occur almost exclusively in the neck and shoulders of males.[111] The major importance of these tumors is their tendency to be confused with liposarcomas.

Angiolipomas are lipomas containing a network of many small capillaries and are usually quite painful.[112] Some angiolipomas are infiltrative and require a wider margin of resection than most lipomas.

The treatment for lipomas is simple enucleation. Recurrence is uncommon after this limited treatment.

Lipoblastomatosis

Lipoblastomatosis, also called adipose hamartomatosis, is found in infants. It consists of lobular soft tissue growths separated by partitions of loose fibrous tissue.[93,113,114] About 10% of these lesions recur after simple local excision, but they have no tendency to metastasize.

Atypical Lipoma

The designation of atypical lipoma is applied to subcutaneous lipomatous neoplasms that display cytologic atypia not seen in most lipomas.[115-118] These lesions occur in the subcutaneous or deep muscular layers. Simple excision cures virtually all subcutaneous lesions, although simple excision of deep muscular lesions often results in local recurrence that may require reexcision. These lesions have no tendency to metastasize and can be controlled by reexcision.

Hibernoma

Hibernomas are unusual lipomas that are thought to arise from vestiges of brown fat, similar to the glandular, brown adipose tissue occurring in certain hibernating animal species.[119] These are benign tumors and should be treated by simple excision.

BENIGN TUMORS OF SYNOVIAL TISSUE

Giant Cell Tumor of Tendon Sheath

Giant cell tumors of tendon sheath, also called localized nodular tenosynovitis, are usually solitary and arise from the tendon sheath, joints or bursae of the hand, palm, or wrist.[120,121] These soft tissue lesions can produce atrophy of the bony cortex or actual erosion into adjacent bone. Simple excision is the treatment of choice. Villonodular synovitis is probably related to giant cell tumor of tendon sheath but almost always occurs in joints and presents with pain and swelling. This benign tumor-like growth erodes the bone and appears to be a primary bone tumor. The synovium of the affected joint is usually diffusely involved, and total synovectomy is the treatment of choice.

Ganglion

Ganglions are multilocular, fibrous-walled cysts, usually occurring on the dorsal aspect of the wrist. These lesions form as a result of synovial tissue that has become pinched off and undergoes degeneration. Simple excision is almost always curative.

BENIGN TUMORS OF NEURAL TISSUE

Neurilemoma

Neurilemomas are benign, encapsulated tumors, also called schwannomas, that almost always occur as solitary lesions.[50,122] The most common site of origin is the eighth cranial nerve (*i.e.*, acoustic neuroma), although cranial peripheral nerves are often affected. This is also the most common benign neoplasm of the spinal canal. These lesions often grow with an easily demonstrable flattened nerve seen along its capsule. These lesions rarely recur if resected locally. Every effort should be made to preserve the nerve involved if this nerve is of clinical significance (*e.g.*, the facial nerve). These lesions arise from Schwann cells, although they are different from neurofibromas.

Neurofibroma

Neurofibromas are thought to arise from Schwann cells, although they differ from neurilemomas in that they tend not to be encapsulated and have a much softer consistency. They may also occur at many different sites. These lesions may be locally infiltrative, although simple excision is almost always curative.

Multiple neurofibromas are a feature of von Recklinghausen's disease, which is an autosomal dominant disorder that affects 1 of 3000 live births.[123-132] In this condition, neurofibromas may occur in virtually all sites of the body and be associated with any peripheral or intraspinal nerves. Plexiform neurofibromas may cause massive enlargement of an extremity. About 10% to 15% of patients with von Recklinghausen's disease develop malignant schwannoma, and these malignant tumors can arise in benign, superficial neurofibromas. Neurofibromas in von Recklinghausen's disease should be removed for cosmetic reasons or if they become painful or undergo rapid enlargement. In a long-term study of 212 patients with neurofibromatosis, 57 developed malignant tumors; 21 patients developed cancers of the central nervous system, 6 developed cancers of the peripheral nervous system, and the remainder developed cancers at other sites.[132]

BENIGN TUMORS OF VASCULAR TISSUE

Hemangioma

Hemangiomas are vascular neoplasms that can occur anywhere in the body.[133-135] About 75% are present at birth, and about 60% occur in the head and neck area. Most hemangiomas of infancy spontaneously regress. Some lesions grow rapidly during the early months of life and may be a source of some concern, although most disappear by about 5 years of age. These lesions may be primarily composed of capillaries or widely dilated veins (*i.e.*, cavernous hemangioma). These lesions do not metastasize, and simple excision is often curative, although it is not necessary except for cosmetic reasons. In some instances, the hemangioma may exhibit rapid growth and abut or compromise vital structures. In these instances, low-dose radiation confined to the hemangioma may be used. Efforts should be made to use techniques that limit the dose to the vascular process itself. Radiation treatment for these lesions is rarely indicated, and even large medical centers probably do not see more than 3 or 4 patients each decade for whom radiation treatment is warranted.

Lymphangioma

Lymphangiomas are similar to hemangiomas, although the vascular spaces do not contain blood cells. These lesions can occur virtually anywhere in the body. Cystic hygromas are lymphangiomas of the neck. The lesions require surgical excision. The extent of the procedure should be dictated by the location and the desire to achieve a reasonable cosmetic result.

Glomus Tumors

The normal glomus is a 1-mm end organ arteriovenous anastomosis.[136-139] This organ enlarges into a painful and tender mass. About 15% occur in the subungual regions, although any location in the skin and soft tissue is possible. Local excision is usually curative, and metastases do not occur. Glomus tumors may be located along the larger vessels. A common syndrome is that of the glomus tumor near the jugular foramen, designated as a glomus jugulare. These lesions are not resectable and are effectively treated by radiation therapy (5000 cGy delivered over about 5 weeks). Lesions regress slowly, but permanent control of the process is regularly achieved.

Infantile Hemangiopericytomas

Although hemangiopericytomas in the adult are more benign in their behavior than most soft tissue sarcomas, these tumors can metastasize and are therefore be considered with malignant lesions.[139,140] However, hemangiopericytomas that occur in infancy appear to be benign lesions without significant metastatic potential. These tumors occur almost exclusively in the skin and may have evidence of infiltrative growth outside the main tumor mass. These lesions generally do not recur after wide local excision.

BENIGN TUMORS OF HISTIOCYTIC TISSUE

The work of Stout and colleagues has significantly improved our understanding and recognition of tumors of presumed histiocytic origin.[49,50] Variants of these tumors have received more than 30 different names in a variety of nomenclature systems. The tumors are composed wholly or in part of cells with the morphologic characteristics of histiocytes and with various fibroblastic components. It is thought that these tumors are of purely histiocytic origin, but histiocytes in these lesions can differentiate toward fibroblastic morphology.

Dermatofibroma

Dermatofibromas, also called sclerosing hemangioma or fibrous xanthoma of skin, are common soft tissue lesions that are usually about 1 cm in diameter and occur in the dermis. Simple excision is always curative.

Fibrous Histiocytoma

Many variants of histiocytoma, also called fibrous xanthoma, exist.[49,50,141] Superficially located histiocytic lesions behave in a benign manner, although deep, benign histiocytomas may invade locally into surrounding tissue. These lesions can occur anywhere in the body. Superficial lesions are always cured by simple excision, but a wider margin of normal tissue should be obtained for deep, benign fibrous histiocytomas. Local recurrence is uncommon.

Atypical Fibrous Histiocytomas

Although superficial fibrous histiocytomas are always totally benign and cured by simple excision, deep fibrous histiocytomas may have a more atypical morphologic appearance and are more ominous in their tendency to recur locally.[142–144] Although superficial lesions may occasionally fit the criteria for atypical histiocytoma (*e.g.*, 3 of 18 atypical fibrous histiocytomas reported by Soule and coworkers), almost all are located deep in soft tissue or muscle.[142] Despite the absence of obvious anaplasia, a rapidly growing, deeply occurring fibrous histiocytoma may achieve a diameter of 6 cm or larger; more than half of these lesions recur after simple excision. These lesions usually do not metastasize, although rare reports of metastases after many local recurrences for lesions with this histology have been reported. Recommended therapy includes wide local excision, with negative microscopic margins in all directions. As a result of inadequate local treatment at first resection, recurrent local extension of these tumors, especially in the retroperitoneal area, can lead to death.

Dermatofibrosarcoma Protuberans

Dermatofibrosarcoma protuberans can occur in any part of the body.[145–150] The exact histogenesis is not known, although a histiocytic origin is likely. These lesions most often begin as indurated nodules in the skin that grow slowly and are often ignored until they are large. They show an extremely aggressive tendency to invade surrounding local tissue; they should be regarded as malignant neoplasms. They do not metastasize, even after multiple recurrences. About 50% recur after simple excision, and a wide excision including a wide margin of surrounding tissue should be achieved in therapy.[150] The first resection is important, because tumor spread at the inadequate first resection may lead to uncontrollable local growth. These benign lesions may ultimately lead to amputation of extremities or even death because of extensive invasion of vital organs.

Many of the comments regarding use of radiation therapy discussed under the treatment of desmoid tumors may apply to these lesions.[96–100] In a review of the NCI experience with locally aggressive but nonmetastasizing soft tissue tumors seen between 1975 and 1982, Glenn and coworkers identified 35 cases that were completely resected. Twenty patients received radiation therapy postoperatively, and one tumor recurred. One recurrence was seen among 15 patients treated by surgery alone. Follow-up in this study ranged from 12 to 97 months, with a median of 36 months.

If surgical treatment of dermatofibrosarcoma protuberans is not feasible or requires a radical procedure, consideration should be given to radiation therapy in combination with conservative surgery or to radiation therapy alone in special circumstances.[151]

BENIGN TUMORS OF MESOTHELIAL TISSUE

Mesothelioma

The cells lining the pleura, peritoneum, and pericardium are mesothelial cells. Although most tumors of mesothelial tissue are malignant, benign tumors can occur, usually in the pleura. These lesions project outwardly from the viscera or parietal pleura into the adjacent cavity but do not infiltrate aggressively into local tissue. They may grow to be quite large, and simple excision is usually curative.

BENIGN TUMORS OF UNCERTAIN TISSUE ORIGIN

Granular Cell Myoblastoma

Granular cell myoblastomas rarely grow larger than 6 cm and can be cured by local excision.[152] If these lesions develop beneath the epidermis or mucous membranes, they can lead to squamous tissue proliferation, possibly mimicking a squamous cell carcinoma.

Mesenchymoma

Mesenchymomas, also referred to as hamartoma or mixed mesodermal tumor, are composed of at least two different mesenchymal elements.[153] Lesions often contain smooth muscle, skeletal muscle, fat, and angiomatous and osseous tissue in various combinations. Although most lesions are malignant, rare benign forms have been described. Benign tumors are generally small, and none of the individual elements contain cells with atypical or anaplastic appearance. Local excision is adequate therapy.

Myxoma

Myxoma is thought to arise from embryonic rests and is composed of spindle cells imbedded in a mucinous intercellular matrix.[154,155] It can occur in any of the soft tissues, bone, or occasionally in the heart and genitourinary tract. When these lesions develop in the soft tissues, they are generally close to a large muscle or aponeurosis. They are cured by local excision. Deep tumors can sometimes infiltrate contiguous structures, but local resection is usually curative.

There are many other less common benign tumors of soft tissue.[50]

DIAGNOSIS

Soft tissue sarcomas most often present as asymptomatic soft tissue masses. Because these lesions arise in compressible tissues and are often far from vital organs, symptoms are few until the lesions are quite large compared with the anatomic part. For example, a sarcoma often presents at 8 to 15 cm in the thigh or buttock, 3 to 4 cm in the wrist, but only 0.5 to 1 cm around the digits. Symptoms generally result from pressure or traction on adjacent nerves or muscles. There are no reliable physical signs to differentiate benign from malignant soft tissue lesions; consequently, all soft tissue lumps that persist or grow should be biopsied. Even soft and pliable subcutaneous lumps thought to be lipomas occasionally prove surprising. Leaving soft tissue lumps in place without biopsy is justified only if they have been present and unchanged for many years before being observed by the physician.

The nature of the biopsy of soft tissue sarcomas is an important aspect of the overall management of these patients. Because the biopsy site must be removed in any definitive resection, care should be taken to place the biopsy incision at a location and orientation that does not compromise subsequent surgical excision.

Adequate and representative tissue must be obtained in any biopsy of a soft tissue mass, and this typically requires an incisional or excisional biopsy. Although in centers with extensive experience with sarcoma, multiple core-needle biopsies can provide adequate pathologic material, aspiration cytology is typically not sufficient.[156] Immunohistochemistry or electron microscopy often is necessary, and these efforts are hampered by insufficient tissue. Inhomogeneity within large tumors can also lead to critical sampling errors, particularly in assigning tumor grade. If uncertainty remains after initial biopsy, do not hesitate to obtain additional tissue. The decision between excisional and incision biopsy is based on tumor size and location.

Soft tissue sarcomas grow in the path of least resistance and push surrounding tissue before them. This surrounding tissue forms a pseudocapsule and always contains invasive prongs of malignant tissue. For this reason, shelling out soft tissue sarcomas is never curative. Excision through the pseudocapsule often spreads tumor into surrounding tissue and can greatly complicate further surgical treatment. Excisional biopsy is an appropriate means of establishing a diagnosis only for soft tissue sarcomas smaller than 3 cm in diameter.

Tumors larger than 3 cm in diameter require an incisional biopsy. This technique allows acquisition of a generous wedge of tissue from the lesion and minimally disrupts the surrounding tissue planes. The incisional biopsy should be performed through a carefully placed small incision that does not compromise subsequent radical excision of the lesion. Impeccable hemostasis is essential, because hematomas resulting from biopsies of soft tissue sarcomas can spread tumor along their paths.

Although most experienced surgeons consider an incisional biopsy preferable to a limited excisional biopsy for the diagnosis of soft tissue sarcomas, a survey of surgical practices in the United States conducted by The American College of Surgeons showed that roughly half of the sarcomas were biopsied by excision.[46] This practice did not change during two intervals surveyed, 1977 to 1978 and 1983 to 1984 (Table 42–5). Only 20% of patients had a diagnosis established by incisional biopsy during these same periods.

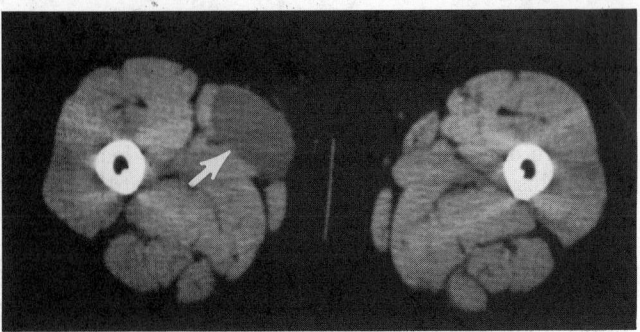

FIGURE 42–4. Computed tomography scan of midthigh region in patient with a myxoid liposarcoma (*white arrow*). Transaxial orientation demonstrates relation to underlying muscle groups.

The importance of the adequate placement of the biopsy incision cannot be overemphasized. Improper placement may preclude proper radical resection of the lesion and may lead to large increases in the radiation fields necessary to encompass all areas of possible spread. Incisions on the extremities should be placed longitudinally to prevent compromise of the muscle group excisions that may subsequently be necessary. At other sites, the incision should be parallel to the long axis of the underlying principal muscle. Biopsies of lesions in the buttocks should be placed as inferiorly as possible to allow subsequent development of skin flaps if hemipelvectomy is necessary.

Planning surgical resection or radiation therapy requires a careful and detailed determination of the pattern of local spread and assessment of the tissues probably involved by microscopic disease. The physical examination determines the approximate size of the lesion, attachment to deep or superficial structures, relation of the tumor to prior biopsy sites, functional status of the part, and presence of prior injury or concurrent medical disease that would confound the execution of the desired surgery or radiation. The radiographic evaluation of the patient with soft tissue sarcoma should include these procedures[157–165]:

1. Xerogram or soft tissue radiograph of the affected part
2. Computed tomography (CT), magnetic resonance imaging (MRI), or ultrasound through the affected region
3. CT or full-chest tomogram
4. Arteriogram in certain instances
5. Radionuclide bone scan

The most important diagnostic procedures in assessing the pattern of involvement of the primary lesion are CT (Fig. 42–4) or MR scans (Fig. 4-5). High-quality CT or MR scans are essential because these techniques permit accurate delineation of the muscle compartment or anatomic structures involved by gross disease.

Chang and colleagues performed a prospective evaluation of preoperative CT and MR scans of patients with extremity sarcomas.[164] Operative findings were correlated with the scans. CT and MRI were found comparable in evaluating the tumor's relation to major neurovascular and skeletal structures. However, MRI demonstrated better visual contrast between tumor and muscle. MRI has the advantage of displaying anatomy in coronal and sagittal views, but CT is restricted to transaxial views. Bland and colleagues reported that MRI was

TABLE 42-5. Biopsy Techniques for Sarcoma Diagnosis

Type of Biopsy	1977–1978		1983–1984	
	No.	*%*	*No.*	*%*
None	319	13.5	380	11.0
Needle	114	4.8	311	9.0
Incisional	466	19.8	753	21.8
Excisional	1210	51.4	1644	47.6
Other	139	5.9	278	8.0
Unknown	107	4.5	91	2.6
Total	2355	100.0	3457	100.0

(Lawrence W Jr, Donegan WL, Natarajan N, et al. Adult soft tissue sarcomas. A pattern of care survey of the American College of Surgeons. Ann Surg 1987;205:349–359)

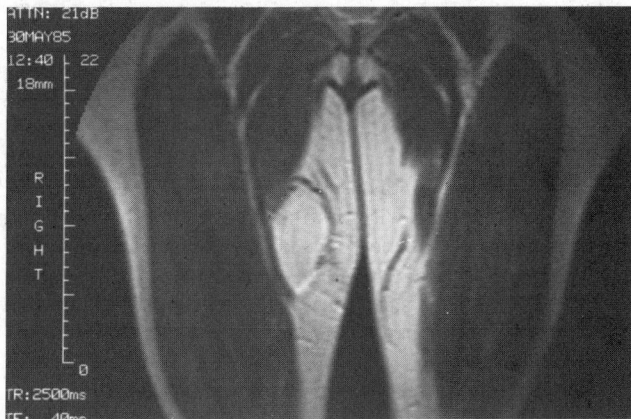

FIGURE 42–5. T1-weighted MRI scan of the same patient shown in Figure 42–3. This scan demonstrates excellent tumor to muscle contrast for this myxoid liposarcoma. The coronal image is helpful in defining the longitudinal extent of the tumor in the thigh.

significantly better than CT in predicting resectability of 53 soft tissue sarcomas in various sites.[165] This was a result of the multiplanar imaging and improved visual contrast afforded by MRI.[165]

Arteriography can also delineate the position and status of major vessels and the local extent of disease, and it is particularly useful for estimating the proximity of tumor to major vessels, for determining the pattern of displacement or deviation of vessels, and for determining the encasement of a vessel by tumor, resulting in abrupt, irregular change in the caliber of the vessel, which is characteristic of neoplastic involvement.[161–163] The late venous phase can show the venous drainage, which should be controlled intraoperatively early in the course of surgery to prevent major embolization of tumor cells. An arteriogram is of minimal benefit in planning the treatment of recurrent tumors or the reoperation of incompletely excised lesions.

Although sarcomas rarely invade bone, assessment of soft tissue reaction in the periosteum and at the margin of soft tissues may be estimated by bone scan.[46,166] A positive scan does not mean that the tumor has invaded bone or periosteum. A positive scan may simply be the consequence of periosteal reaction to the increased blood flow of a nearby tumor. This could serve as a guide to wide resection near the bone or to removing periosteum or a portion of the bone in the area that is positive on scan in the patients treated by surgery alone. Patients with positive bone scans and no radiographic periosteal reactions who are being treated by irradiation and surgery should not have stripping of periosteum unless operative findings reveal fixation of the lesion to the bone.

Sarcomas of soft tissue infrequently metastasizes to regional lymph nodes, and lymphangiography is rarely indicated.[170]

STAGING

The single most important prognostic factor in patients with soft tissue sarcomas is the histologic grade of the primary lesion.[50,53–55,61] Grades are assigned from grade 1 (well-differentiated) to grade 3 (poorly differentiated).

In the staging system for soft tissue sarcomas proposed by the American Joint Committee for Cancer Staging and End Results, the histologic grade is the most important determinant of stage.[61,62] The system is based on four parameters: G or histopathologic grade, T, N, and M. Details of the staging system, which was revised in 1987, are presented in Table 42–6. G1, G2, and G3 lesions are sarcomas that are well-differentiated, moderately differentiated, or poorly differentiated, respectively. T1 lesions are smaller than 5 cm; T2 lesions are equal to or larger than 5 cm. N1 lesions have metastatic disease in regional lymph nodes, and M1 lesions show clinical evidence of distant metastasis. All lesions that are G1 and T1 or T2 and are N0M0 are stage 1. All lesions that are G2 and T1 or T2 and are N0M0 are stage II, and all lesions that are G3 and T1 or T2 and are N0M0 are stage III. All lesions that are N1 become stage IVA, without regard to grade or size. The correlation of this staging system with prognosis

TABLE 42-6. American Joint Committee Staging System for Soft Tissue Sarcomas

T	Primary tumor	
	T1	Tumor less than 5 cm
	T2	Tumor 5 cm or greater
G	Histologic grade of malignancy	
	G1	Low
	G2	Moderate
	G3	High
N	Regional lymph nodes	
	N0	No histologically verified metastases to regional lymph nodes
	N1	Histologically verified regional lymph node metastasis
M	Distant metastasis	
	M0	No distant metastasis
	M1	Distant metastasis

Stage I	
Stage IA G1T1N0M0	Grade 1 tumor less than 5 cm in diameter with no regional lymph node or distant metastases
Stage IB G1T2N0M0	Grade 1 tumor 5 cm or greater in diameter with no regional lymph node or distant metastases
Stage II	
Stage IIA G2T1N0M0	Grade 2 tumor less than 5 cm in diameter with no regional lymph node or distant metastases
Stage IIB G2T2N0M0	Grade 2 tumor 5 cm or greater in diameter with no regional lymph node or distant metastases
Stage III	
Stage IIIA G3T1N0M0	Grade 3 tumor less than 5 cm in diameter with no regional lymph node or distant metastases
Stage IIIB G3T2N0M0	Grade 3 tumor 5 cm or greater in diameter with no regional lymph node or distant metastases
Stage IV	
Stage IVA G1–3T1–2N1M0	Tumor of any grade or size with histologically verified metastasis to regional lymph nodes, but no distant metastases
Stage IVB G1–3T1–2N0–1M1	Clinically diagnosed distant metastases

(Bears OH, Henson DE, Hutter RVP, Kennedy BJ, eds. Manual for staging cancer, American Joint Committee on Cancer. 4th ed. Philadelphia: JB Lippincott, 1992)

TABLE 42-7. Local Control and Disease-free Survival for 220 Patients with Soft Tissue Sarcoma Treated at MGH by Radiation and Surgery According to AJC Stage

| AJC Stage* | No. of Patients | 5-Year Actuarial Results | |
		Local Control	Disease-free Survival
IA	17	1.00	1.00
IB	30	0.93	0.88
IIA	40	0.88	0.83
IIB	66	0.85	0.52
IIIA	33	0.93	0.87
IIIB	69	0.79	0.39
IVA	3	1.00	1.00
Total	258	0.88	0.66

* Excludes patients with distant metastases (stage IVB) and patients with sarcomas arising from thoracic, abdominal, pelvic, and retroperitoneal sites.
(Suit HD, Mankin HJ, Willett G, et al. Limited surgery and external irradiation in soft tissue sarcomas. In: Recent Concepts in Sarcoma Treatment. Proceedings of the International Symposium on Sarcomas. Tarpon Springs, FL, October 8–10, 1987. The Netherlands: Kluwer Academic Publishers, 1988)

in 220 patients with soft tissue sarcomas of all sites, excluding retroperitoneum, treated at the Massachusetts General Hospital is presented in Table 42–7.[62]

The survivals for adults with soft tissue sarcomas by clinical and pathologic stage are shown in Fig. 42–6. For clinical stages I, II, III, and IV, the 5-year estimated survival rates are 79%, 65%, 45%, and 10%, respectively.[46]

An alternate staging system has been proposed by Enneking and colleagues (Table 42–8).[167] In this system, patients are categorized as stage I (low-grade, no metastases), stage II (high-grade, no metastases), or stage III (either grade with regional or distant metastases). Tumors are designated "A" if they are contained within an anatomic compartment and are designated "B" if they extend across fascial planes. The correlation of survival with stage of disease using this scheme in 397 patients with sarcomas of the extremity is shown in Table 42–9.[167] This staging system is practical only for extremity sarcomas.

Factors thought to be of prognostic importance in patients with soft tissue sarcomas are listed in Table 42–10.[44,61,64,16] The site of a soft tissue sarcoma often influences resectability and local control and cure. Lesions in the trunk, especially those in the retroperitoneum, mediastinum, head, and neck, often involve vital structures before they become clinically apparent. They are usually large, and local control by any approach is less likely for these tumors than for tumors on the extremity or torso. In the extremity, the exact site of the lesion has prognostic importance. Proximal lesions are less curable than distal lesions. In the series reported by Simon and Enneking, local recurrences after surgery alone in the buttock, groin, thigh, and areas below the knee were 38%, 14%, 15%, and 0%, respectively (Table 42–11).[60]

Size is an important parameter for freedom from distant metastases and for local control. Among subjects whose treatment controlled the primary lesion, distant control decreased

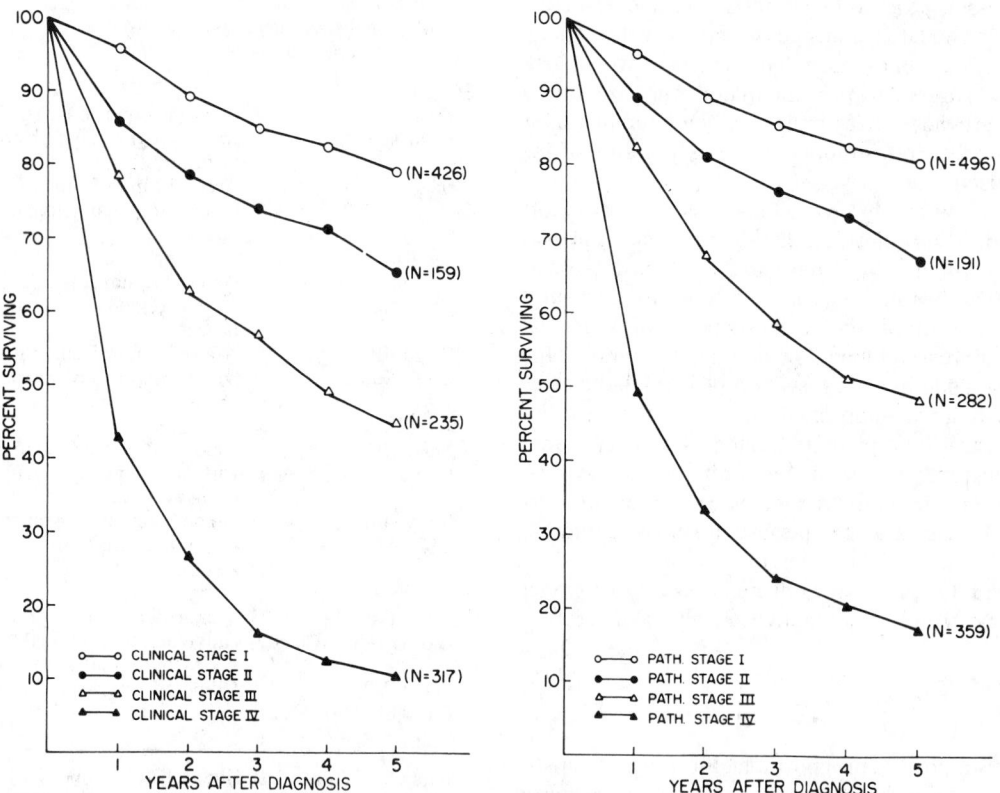

FIGURE 42–6. Overall survival of patients with soft tissue sarcomas according to AJCC clinical and pathologic grading of tumors. There is a strong correlation of survival with each stage of disease.

TABLE 42-8. Enneking System for Staging of Sarcomas of Soft Tissues or Bone

Stage	Characteristic
I	Low grade
IA	Intracompartmental
IB	Extracompartmental
II	High grade
IIA	Intracompartmental
IIB	Extracompartmental
III	Any grade
	N1 or M1

(Enneking WF, Spanier SS, Goodman MA. The surgical staging of musculoskeletal sarcoma. J Bone Joint Surg [Am] 1980;62:1027–1030)

TABLE 42-9. Predicted Survival According to Stages, Based on 397 Extremity Sarcoma Patients

	Probability of Survival	
Stage	2 Years	5 Years
IA	0.99	0.97
IB	0.95	0.89
IIA	0.88	0.73
IIB	0.73	0.45
III	0.37	0.08

(Enneking WF, Spanier SS, Goodman MA. The surgical staging of musculoskeletal sarcoma. J Bone Joint Surg [Am] 1980;62:1027–1030)

rapidly with tumor size (Table 42–12).[44,61,64,169] Size is a major factor in achieving local control by surgery alone for tumors in some anatomic sites (*e.g.,* head, neck, retroperitoneum), and it is a dominant factor in the results of radiation therapy alone. For irradiation combined with surgery, local control did not depend on size for lesions up to 150 mm.

Soft tissue sarcomas rarely spread to regional lymph nodes. In a review of 374 patients referred to the NCI during 24 years, only 3 patients (2.6%) of 113 who had lymph nodes evaluated had evidence of metastases to draining lymph nodes before gross dissemination of disease.[170] In a review of more than 2500 patients in the world literature, Weingrad and Rosenberg analyzed the incidence of lymph node metastases from each of the major histologic types of soft tissue sarcomas (Table 42–13).[170] Approximately 5% of patients with soft tissue sarcomas developed nodal metastases at any point in the course of their disease, although for patients with synovial cell sarcoma and rhabdomyosarcoma the, incidence was higher. Patients with involvement of draining lymph nodes had a substantially poorer prognosis than did those whose lymph nodes were not involved. Mazeron and Suit reported an incidence of regional lymph node involvement of 5.9% for 323 patients with stage M0 soft tissue sarcoma.[171] There was no regional node involvement in patients with grade 1 sarcomas compared with 2% and 12% for grades 2 and 3, respectively. In their series, the 19 patients who had nodal involvement had a 5-year survival rate of 32%.

Rosenberg and coworkers reported an inverse correlation between prognosis and the number of perioperative blood transfusions administered to patients who underwent resections of localized high-grade sarcomas of the extremities.[172] The number of transfusions represented a prognostic variable independent of tumor size. This observation requires confirmation by others.

The histologic cell of origin of soft tissue sarcomas is not of major prognostic importance if lesions of equivalent grade are compared. There appears to be no prognostic importance attached to the age or sex of patients with soft tissue sarcomas, except that fibrosarcomas occurring in children tend to have a better prognosis than those in adult patients, even if allowances are made for grade and size.[173] Liposarcomas may be less aggressive in children.[174]

NATURAL HISTORY OF SOFT TISSUE SARCOMAS

COMMON FEATURES

The poor prognosis of most patients with soft tissue sarcomas is due to the tendency of these lesions to invade aggressively into surrounding tissues and for early hematogenous dissemination, usually to the lungs. Soft tissue sarcomas invade locally along anatomic planes, such as nerve fibers, muscle bundles, fascial planes, and blood vessels. Most patients with soft tissue sarcomas present without obvious clinical metastases. Of 565 soft tissue sarcoma patients admitted to Memorial Sloan-Kettering Cancer Center between 1983 and 1985, 128 (22.7%) had evidence of metastases at presentation.[175] At the Massachusetts General Hospital between 1971 and 1981, 28 (10.3%) of 272 patients who presented with a primary sarcoma were found to have distant metastases.[176] In the American College of Surgeons survey, 1365 (23.5%) of 5812 patients who presented with soft tissue sarcoma had evidence of distant metastases.[46] The lung was the most frequent site of distant metastases, accounting for 33% of the metastatic lesions, followed by bone and liver (Table 42–14).[46]

Because the appropriate diagnosis is often not appreciated or suspected before biopsy, many soft tissue sarcomas are initially treated by shelling out the lesion through the pseudocapsule. In the American College of Surgeons survey, approximately half of sarcomas were biopsied by this procedure or by excision (see Table 42–5). Only 20% of the sarcomas were diagnosed by incisional biopsy. Excisional biopsy is inadequate as sole therapy, and more than 90% of these patients have local recurrences.

In a review of 87 patients with low-grade sarcomas with a median follow-up of 7 years, Marcus found that 14 patients

TABLE 42-10. Prognostic Factors for Patients With Primary Soft Tissue Sarcomas

Histologic grade
Site (proximal vs distal; extremity vs trunk)
Size
Lymph node involvement

TABLE 42-11. Anatomic Site Correlated With Local Recurrence Rate of Soft Tissue Sarcomas of the Extremities

Anatomic Site	No. of Patients	% Total	No. With Recurrence	No. Without Recurrence	% Recurrence
Lower extremity	(53)				
Intrapelvic	2	3	2	0	100
Buttock	8	11	3	5	38
Groin	7	10	1	6	14
Thigh	26	37	4	22	15
Knee	3	4	0	3	0
Below knee	7	10	0	7	0
Upper extremity	(17)				
Shoulder girdle	4	6	2	2	50
Arm	7	10	0	7	0
Below elbow	6	9	1	5	17

(Simon MA, Enneking WF. The management of soft-tissue sarcomas of the extremities. J Bone Joint Surg [Am] 1976;58:317)

had local recurrences, 3 developed distant metastases, and the estimated tumor-related mortality rate at 10 years was 7%.[177] Factors retrospectively associated with poorer disease-free survival were retroperitoneal location, no postoperative radiation therapy, and positive surgical margins. Overall survival was most affected by tumor location, with 50% of the tumor-related deaths occurring in the 8% of patients with retroperitoneal lesions. Even these deaths occurred 7.0 to 9.5 years after diagnosis. Although these results are somewhat better than those from large national surveys, this difference may be due to a low proportion of retroperitoneal tumors and pathologic tumor grading by an institution with extensive sarcoma experience.

The pattern of recurrence in patients with high-grade soft tissue sarcoma is a function of the primary site of the lesion. Potter and associates analyzed 307 patients referred to the NCI between 1975 and 1982 who underwent complete surgical resection of high-grade soft tissue sarcomas, often in combination with chemotherapy and radiation therapy.[44] The pattern of recurrence in the 107 patients is shown in Table 42-15. Patients with retroperitoneal sarcomas had a greater tendency to recur with disseminated disease throughout the abdomen, and patients with truncal sarcomas had a higher local recurrence rate than was seen in patients with primary lesions in the extremities. Among the entire group with recurrences, the lung was the predominant site (52%) of the first isolated recurrence; isolated local recurrence was seen in 20% of patients. In the American College of Surgeons survey, treatment failures in patients without metastases at initial diagnoses and with total gross resections of the soft tissue sarcomas occurred in 452 (37%) of 1209 patients.[46] Isolated locoregional recurrence occurred in 236 (52.2%) of these patients. This high rate may reflect inadequate surgical resection or inadequate adjunctive treatments. At least 25% of the patients had limited local excisions of the primary tumor if no distant disease was documented.

TABLE 42-12. Actuarial Distant Control Rates at 5 Years Among 159 Patients With G2-3 Sarcoma of Soft Tissue With Control of Primary Lesion After Treatment by Radiation and Surgery

Tumor Size (mm)	No. of Patients	Actuarial Distant Control (5 y)
<25	17	0.94
26–49	48	0.77
50–100	55	0.62
101–150	24	0.51
151–200	9	0.42
>200	6	0.17
Total	159	0.65

(Suit HD, Mankin HJ, Wood WC, et al. Treatment of the patient with stage M₀ soft tissue sarcoma. J Clin Oncol 1988;6:854–862)

TABLE 42-13. Incidence of Lymph Node Metastases in Patients With Soft Tissue Sarcomas

Histology	No. of Series	No. of Patients	Incidence of Lymph Node Metastases No.	Incidence of Lymph Node Metastases %
Liposarcoma	7	288	15	5.7
Fibrosarcoma	14	1083	55	5.1
Rhabdomyosarcoma	13	888	108	12.2
Synoviosarcoma	13	535	91	17.0
Unclassifiable	5	125	11	8.8
Neurofibrosarcoma	2	60	0	0

(Weingrad DW, Rosenberg SA. Early lymphatic spread of osteogenic and soft-tissue sarcomas. Surgery 1978;84:231–240)

TABLE 42-14. Clinically Involved Distant Metastatic Sites at Time of Diagnosis of Sarcoma

Metastatic Sites	1977–1978		1983–1984	
	No.	%	No.	%
Bone	126	22.6	191	23.7
Lung	186	33.3	275	34.1
Liver	83	14.9	126	15.7
Brain	19	3.4	22	2.7
Other	144	25.8	193	23.9
Total	558	100.0	807	100.0

(Lawrence W, Donegan WL, Natarajan N, et al. Adult soft tissue sarcomas. A pattern of care survey of The American College of Surgeons. Ann Surg 1987;205:349–359)

The time until local recurrence is fairly constant in most reported series. Cantin and coworkers demonstrated that approximately 80% of all lesions that recur after surgery do so within 2 years.[178] In 54 patients treated surgically by Simon and Enneking, all local recurrences occurred by 30 months after definitive resection.[60] Lindberg and associates also reported that 80% of local recurrences occurred in the first 2 years and 100% by 3 years.[179] Shiu and associates reported 87% of local recurrences within the first 2 years.[59] Gerner and associates reported that 82% of local recurrences were evident by 2 years at Roswell Park Memorial Institute.[180]

Patients undergoing amputation or radical local excision have local recurrence rates of about 20%.[59,60] In older series from Memorial Sloan-Kettering Cancer Center, local recurrences were seen in 59% of patients undergoing conservative excision, compared with 25% for those undergoing radical excision.[178] At the M.D. Anderson Cancer Center, patients undergoing conservative excision had a 77% local recurrence rate, compared with 28% for those undergoing radical excision.[58] These series were not randomized, and these figures are highly influenced by patient selection factors. In general, however, the larger the surgical excisions in all directions from the tumors, the lower are the local recurrence rates.

Spread to draining lymph nodes is an uncommon finding. In a review by Weingrad and Rosenberg of more than 30 series,

5.8% of almost 3000 patients developed lymph node metastases some time during their course (see Table 42–13). These figures reflect the incidence of lymph node metastases at any time during the course of the disease; spread to lymph nodes in the early stages is less frequent. There was a 3.2% incidence of nodal spread in almost 6000 patients analyzed in the American College of Surgeons survey.[46] Mazeron and Suit reported a 5.9% incidence of regional nodal involvement in 323 patients with stage M0 sarcoma.[171] The incidence of lymph node metastases is somewhat higher for epithelioid sarcomas (20–40%), in synovial cell sarcoma (17%), and in rhabdomyosarcoma (12%) than for other histologic types.

Before 1977, when surgery was the primary modality of treatment, the overall 5-year survival rate in most reported series of patients with soft tissue sarcoma was approximately 50% (Table 42–16).[38,39,57–61,168,180–182]

UNIQUE FEATURES OF HISTOLOGIC SUBTYPES

Despite the common biologic behavior of equivalent-grade soft tissue sarcomas, there are some features that are unique to individual histologic types.

Fibrosarcoma

Before 1965, fibrosarcoma was the most common diagnosis of soft tissue sarcoma.[183,184] Since that time, the recognition of a larger variety of subtypes of soft tissue sarcoma has significantly decreased this diagnosis. As stated by Stout and Lattes, "One should try to restrict the term 'fibrosarcoma' to growths that are composed of cells and fibers derived from fibrocytes and exclude all the fibrous growths derived from other types of cells acting as facultative fibroblasts."[49] Although some pathologists differentiate fibroblastic fibrosarcoma from pleomorphic fibrosarcoma largely by the uniformity of the herringbone pattern of the tumor and the number of mitotic figures, this is mainly a reflection of grading.[47] Because of the changing definition of fibrosarcoma, earlier series undoubtedly contain sarcomas that would now be identified as other histologic types.[183–186] Infantile fibrosarcomas are extremely rare. There have been 3 cases of inoperable infantile fibrosarcoma that completely responded to chemotherapy.[187,188]

TABLE 42-15. Frequency of Initial Recurrence Pattern by Site of Primary Sarcoma

Primary Site	Extremity No. (%)	Retroperitoneal No. (%)	Trunk No. (%)	Breast No. (%)	Head and Neck No. (%)	Total No. (%)
Isolated lung	43 (70)	3 (17)	5 (29)	3 (75)	2 (50)	56 (52)
Isolated local	7 (10)	5 (30)	7 (41)	0	2 (50)	21 (20)
Isolated other	11 (15)	1 (6)	2 (12)	1 (25)	0	15 (14)
Multiple	4 (5)	8 (47)	3 (18)	0	0	15 (14)
Total	65 (100)	17 (100)	17 (100)	4 (100)	4 (100)	107 (100)

(Potter DA, Glenn J, Kinsella T, et al. Patterns of recurrence in patients with high-grade soft tissue sarcoma. J Clin Oncol 1985;3:353–366)

TABLE 42-16. Soft Tissue Sarcomas: Results of Surgical Excision Alone

Investigations	No. of Patients	Survival Before 1977 (%)	
		5 Years	10 Years
Task Force, AJC[61]	1215	41	30
Surgery Branch, NCI (before 1975)[181]	66	48	44
Gerner et al[180]	155	50	26
Shieber and Graham[38]	125	27	22
Martin and Ariel[58]	183	40	
Pack and Cerny[57]	717	39	
Hare[39]	200	39	
Shiu et al[59]	297	55	41
Suit et al[168]	100	52	
Simon and Enneking[60]	54	62	
Markhede et al[160]	97	59	

Rhabdomyosarcoma

Rhabdomyosarcoma accounts for about 15% of all sarcomas.[189–194] Because the skeletal muscle accounts for approximately 40% of adult body weight, this tumor, on a per weight basis, is one of the rarest of all tumors. Striated muscle cells are highly differentiated cells that rarely undergo mitosis in the postnatal period, which probably accounts for the low incidence of these malignancies.

The three categories of rhabdomyosarcoma are pleomorphic, alveolar, and embryonal. Many tumors contain several histologic patterns, and the assignment of a specific subtype is often nebulous. Because the alveolar and embryonal types usually occur in childhood, they are often referred to as juvenile-type rhabdomyosarcomas. "Botryoid" indicates the gross appearance of a subset of embryonal rhabdomyosarcomas that have a polypoid or grape-like appearance. Embryonal rhabdomyosarcomas with botryoid features are commonly found in the urogenital tract of infants and children, although these tumors have occurred in the oral and nasal pharynx. Embryonal tumors occasionally are found in adult and elderly patients. Lloyd and associates reported a series of 54 cases of embryonal rhabdomyosarcomas in patients 20 years or older.[194] Embryonal rhabdomyosarcomas are the most common soft tissue sarcomas of children. Discussion of these tumors is presented elsewhere in the text.

Alveolar rhabdomyosarcomas are distinguished by slit-like alveolar spaces in the tumor.

Pleomorphic rhabdomyosarcomas generally present in adulthood, although they can appear in childhood. They are rare adult sarcomas that arise within skeletal muscles. The most common sites of pleomorphic rhabdomyosarcomas are the extremities. These are often highly anaplastic lesions, having small and large cells with one or many bizarre nuclei. Their diagnosis has changed dramatically in recent years. A review by Hajdu of 214 sarcomas originally diagnosed as pleomorphic rhabdomyosarcoma led to a reclassification of 93 of these lesions as other histologic subtypes, mainly malignant fibrous histiocytoma.[47] Differentiation of pleomorphic rhabdomyosarcoma from other pleomorphic sarcomas can be aided by immunohistochemical staining using antibodies specific for constituent proteins of sarcomeric muscle.[195–197]

Leiomyosarcoma

Leiomyosarcomas are malignant neoplasms that arise from smooth muscle. Because these tumors can arise from the walls of small and large blood vessels, they can occur anywhere in the body.[198–201] Leiomyosarcomas also occur in the viscera, arising from smooth muscle (*e.g.*, the uterus) or from vessels in these organs. Leiomyosarcomas commonly arise in the retroperitoneum, where they are highly aggressive neoplasms.

Liposarcoma

Liposarcomas are malignant lesions of adipose tissue.[202–207] The incidence in men exceeds that in women by about 1.5 to 1. Multicentric liposarcomas have been described. In a series of 97 patients with liposarcomas reported by Kindbloom and coworkers, 11 patients had second liposarcomas that developed at sites remote from their first tumors.

Four subtypes of liposarcomas are recognized: well-differentiated, myxoid, lipoblastic (*i.e.*, round cell), and pleomorphic tumors. Some investigators refer to fibroblastic liposarcomas as a fifth subtype. Well-differentiated liposarcomas can exhibit aggressive local invasion and can infrequently metastasize late in their course. Lipoblastic or epithelioid sarcomas are composed of uniform round cells and are highly vascular. These are highly malignant lesions, and like the pleomorphic liposarcomas, they have only a 20% to 30% 5-year survival rate in most reported series.

Synovial Sarcoma

Synovial sarcomas are malignant neoplasms that arise from tendosynovial tissue and occur most commonly in the second through fourth decades.[208–212] The lower extremities are the most common sites of synovial sarcomas. They can occur in any muscle, although not usually close to joints. Although extremities are the most common sites, lesions can occur in the abdominal wall and in other skeletal muscles of the trunk. The two synovial sarcomas generally recognized are the monophasic and biphasic types. Monophasic synovial sarcomas are characterized by sheaths of monotonous spindle cells; the biphasic variety has slit-like spaces or clefts present within the tumor. These clefts are lined by cuboidal or tall columnar epithelial cells and sometimes resemble carcinomas. Calcified areas often appear within the synovial sarcomas and lead to a characteristic x-ray appearance of this type of soft tissue sarcoma. Some investigators consider epithelioid and clear cell sarcomas to be variants of synovial cell sarcoma, although these types are considered separately in this chapter.

Cagle and colleagues reviewed 45 synovial cell sarcoma patients and were able to identify high-risk and low-risk patients based on percent of glandularity and mitotic rates.[213] Low-risk patients, identified as having more than 50% glandular features and less than 15 mitoses per 10 high-power fields, had a 100% survival rate. High-risk patients, with less than 50% glandular features and more than 15 mitoses per 10 high-power fields, had a 37% survival rate.

Neurofibrosarcomas

Neurofibrosarcomas are malignant tumors of neural sheath origin. They have also been referred to as neurogenic sarcomas, malignant schwannomas, and malignant neurilemomas.[131,214] These tumors can occur anywhere in the body.

Neurofibrosarcomas are frequently associated with von Recklinghausen's disease, a chronic, progressive disease inherited as a mendelian-dominant trait and associated with multiple neurofibromas and skin pigment changes, which are characterized as café-au-lait spots.[123–131] About 10% of patients with neurofibromatosis develop sarcomatous changes during their lifetimes, often in preexisting, benign masses.

Angiosarcomas

Hemangiosarcomas and lymphangiosarcomas arise from blood and lymphatic vessels, respectively.[215–221] These are almost uniformly high-grade lesions, but they are uncommon, comprising only 2% of all soft tissue sarcomas. In 1948, Stuart and Treves reported 6 cases of lymphangiosarcoma in lymphedematous arms after radical mastectomy.[15,222–224] In 1972, Woodward and colleagues reported 23 cases of lymphangiosarcoma associated with chronic lymphedema seen at the Mayo Clinic and reviewed the world literature of 163 cases reported up to that time.[222] The cases of postmastectomy lymphangiosarcoma occurred at an average age of 63.9 years and at an average of 10 years and 3 months after mastectomy. Because of the diffuse nature of these tumors, most physicians recommend radical amputation (*i.e.*, shoulder disarticulation, forequarter amputation) for patients who develop lymphangiosarcoma in the upper extremity after mastectomy.[222–224]

Hemangiosarcomas may occur anywhere in the body but often arise in skin and superficial soft tissue, which contrasts sharply with the deep location of most soft tissue sarcomas.[50] Of 366 hemangiosarcomas, 33% arose in the skin and 25% in the soft tissues. Fifty percent of cutaneous hemangiosarcomas are localized in the head and neck region. These are extremely aggressive tumors despite multimodality therapy,

and one series of 72 patients reported by Holden and co-workers had a 12% 5-year survival rate.[225]

Hemangiopericytoma

Malignant hemangiopericytoma is a malignant sarcoma thought to arise from the pericyte cells of smooth muscle origin that lie around small vessels.[139,140,226–228] Benign and malignant hemangiopericytomas exist, and the rarity of these lesions has led to considerable confusion in differentiating benign and malignant variants. Hemangiopericytomas should be treated as other sarcomas. In most series, 5-year survival rates of approximately 50% are recorded.

Kaposi's Sarcoma

In 1872, Kaposi described "multiple idiopathic pigmented sarcomas of the skin" that "arise in the skin, without any known local or systemic cause."[229,230] These tumors are thought to arise from endothelial cells and present as raised pigmented lesions of the skin. Four clinical types of Kaposi's sarcoma have been recognized (Table 42–17).[231] The classic Kaposi's sarcoma occurs in elderly men of Mediterranean or Jewish extraction living in the United States or Europe.[232–235] This is a rare tumor, and in 1965, Reynolds and colleagues reported a series of only 70 patients collected during 38 years.[232] These lesions usually start as a reddish nodule on the lower extremity. The disease is generally indolent and can be palliated with radiation therapy if necessary. Approximately 20% of these patients die as a direct result of Kaposi's sarcoma, usually because of gastrointestinal or pulmonary involvement.[229] Many of these patients developed second malignancies (*e.g.*, lymphomas), and in one series, death from secondary primaries, often lymphoreticular neoplasms, was as great a threat to life as was mortality from the Kaposi's sarcoma itself.[230,236]

In 1950, interest in Kaposi's sarcoma was renewed after a second form of the disease was described by Kaminer and

TABLE 42–17. Comparison of Clinical Manifestations of Kaposi's Sarcoma

Type	Population	Male to Female Ratio	Clinical Characteristics	Course
Classic	Jewish, Italian heritage (age 50–80 y)	15:1	Lower extremity cutaneous lesions	Indolent: 10–15-year survival
African	Young adult (age 25–40 y)	13:1	Lower-extremity nodular cutaneous lesions	Indolent, locally aggressive disease
	Children (age 2–13 y)	3:1	Generalized lymphadenopathy, cutaneous lesions rare	Rapidly progressive: 2–3-year survival
Renal transplant	Iatrogenic immunosuppressed patient	2.3:1	Localized cutaneous or disseminated	Indolent or progressive: fatal in 30%
Epidemic	AIDS patients	20:1	Disseminated mucocutaneous lesion and visceral involvement	Fulminant: <20% 2-year survival

(Adapted from Krigel RL, Friedman-Kien AE. Kaposi's sarcoma in AIDS. In: DeVita VT, Hellman S, Rosenberg, SA, eds. AIDS. Etiology, diagnosis, treatment, and prevention. Philadelphia: JB Lippincott, 1985:185–211)

Murray, who compiled 43 cases of Kaposi's sarcoma in Bantu men in Africa.[237] In some areas of Africa, Kaposi's sarcoma is a common neoplasm, representing between 3% and 9% of all reported malignancies.[235,238] This disease can be more aggressive than the American or European Kaposi's sarcoma. These lesions can respond to chemotherapy with dactinomycin, vincristine, and dacarbazine (DTIC).[230]

Another type of Kaposi's sarcoma is associated with renal transplantation, and the first case was reported in 1969.[239] Since then, a number of renal allograft recipients have been reported to develop Kaposi's sarcoma after the onset of immunosuppressive therapy. The incidence of Kaposi's sarcoma in patients undergoing renal transplantation appears to be 0.4%, which represents between 150 to 200 times the expected incidence of this tumor in the general population. The average time to development of Kaposi's sarcoma after transplantation is about 16 months. The extent of the tumor correlates with the degree of depression of cellular immunity. In some cases the tumors have regressed because of reduction or changes in immunosuppressive therapy.[240–243]

The Kaposi's sarcoma associated with acquired immunodeficiency syndrome (AIDS) has been called epidemic Kaposi's sarcoma. The initial reports of epidemic Kaposi's sarcoma appeared in 1981.[244] The clinical features of these patients are reminiscent of Kaposi's sarcoma of immunosuppressed renal transplant patients, underscoring the opportunistic nature of this tumor. Approximately 48% of homosexual males with AIDS present with or eventually develop Kaposi's sarcoma. Approximately 4% of all heterosexual intravenous drug users with AIDS and about 12% of Haitian AIDS patients develop epidemic Kaposi's sarcoma.[231] None of the hemophiliac patients with AIDS have developed Kaposi's sarcoma. This form of the disease can be extremely virulent, and death from the disease or related complications of immunodeficiency occurs in most patients. Kaposi's sarcoma in AIDS is reviewed in Chapter 59.

Malignant Fibrous Histiocytoma

Malignant fibrous histiocytoma was characterized by O'Brien and Stout as a group of tumors having a common origin from tissue histiocytes.[141,245–250] This diagnosis has achieved great popularity in recent years, and many cases previously diagnosed as pleomorphic rhabdomyosarcoma or undifferentiated fibrosarcoma are now categorized as malignant fibrous histiocytoma. A wide spectrum of fibrous histiocytomas exists, from those that are benign to those that are highly atypical to those that are frankly malignant. In many series, malignant fibrous histiocytoma is the most common diagnosis attached to soft tissue sarcomas.

These tumors are more common in adults, with 40% occurring in the sixth and seventh decades of life and with fewer than 5% occurring in patients younger than 20 years of age.[251–253]

Alveolar Soft Part Sarcoma

Alveolar soft part sarcomas were described by Christopherson in 1952.[254–256] These tumors have a unique histologic appearance, but the cell of origin is unknown. These are true malignant sarcomas with no benign counterpart, although they

tend to have a more protracted course than most other sarcomas. Although most patients ultimately die from the disease, 5-year survival rates of 60% are common. Many patients develop metastatic disease that progresses slowly over the course of 5 to 15 years before death.

The tumor commonly arises in the thigh in adults and in the head and neck region in children.[50] In 143 patients reviewed by the Armed Forces Institute of Pathology, 44% of the tumors arose in the lower extremities, 27% in the head and neck area, 17% in the upper extremities, and 11% in the trunk.[50]

Epithelioid Sarcoma

Epithelioid sarcomas are of unknown origin and occur almost exclusively in the extremities, usually in the hand or foot, associated with aponeurotic structures.[257–262] These tumors differ in their natural history from most other sarcomas in that they have a greater tendency to spread to noncontiguous areas of skin, subcutaneous tissue, fat, and bone. The tumors have a high propensity to spread to draining lymph nodes. Chase and Enzinger reviewed 241 cases of epithelioid sarcoma in which the most common initial sites of metastases were the lymph nodes (48%) and lungs (24%).[262] A more aggressive course was associated with a proximal or axial tumor location, increased tumor size or depth, hemorrhage, mitotic figures, necrosis, or vascular invasion. More favorable behavior was observed if the tumor arose in distal extremities in younger patients or in female patients between the ages of 10 and 49. Long-term survival is similar to or slightly better than for most other soft tissue sarcomas. Recommended therapy for these patients is wide excision, often involving amputation of the extremity and regional lymph node dissection.

TREATMENT

Surgery alone, surgery combined with radiation, surgery combined with radiation and intraarterial chemotherapy, or radiation alone have been used for the treatment of soft tissue sarcomas. There has been an intense and sustained interest in evaluating treatment strategies that preserve limbs of patients with sarcomas of soft tissue of the extremities and reduce the extent of resection for patients who have lesions on the torso or in the head and neck region by combining less than radical surgery with radiation and chemotherapy.

A National Institutes of Health consensus conference in 1984 reviewed a variety of limb-sparing approaches, which included surgery plus adjunctive radiation therapy or chemotherapy, for the treatment of high-grade extremity sarcomas.[263] They concluded that limb-sparing treatment for some of these sarcoma patients was an effective treatment option. The available data indicate that the results of these conservative approaches were equivalent to those obtained by more radical surgical procedures in selected subgroups of patients.

In discussing the rationale for combining these modalities, the results are presented in terms of frequency of local control, survival, and complications. Important technical aspects are delineated for currently employed strategies.

TABLE 42–18. Local Recurrence Rate After Surgery Alone

Investigations	Local Failures/Total No. of Patients (%)		
	Marginal Excision	Wide Excision	Radical Excision
Simon et al[60]	3/6　(50)	7/20　(35)	3/43　(7)
Markehede et al[182] *	16/21　(76)		5/76　(7)
Gerner et al[180]	54/58　(93)	15/25　(60)	3/38　(8)
Shiu et al[59] †			54/297　(18)
Total	73/85　(86)	22/45　(49)	65/454　(14)

* Two patients received preoperative radiation therapy.
† Eighteen patients had adjunctive radiation therapy.

SURGERY

The essential ingredient in any surgical approach designed to maximize local control is to achieve adequate negative surgical margins. Until the late 1940s and the early 1950s, the surgical approach to the patient with sarcoma of a soft tissue was a local excision, which removed the grossly evident tumor mass with little or no margin of adjacent normal tissue. This is a "marginal excision." The local failure rate for this procedure is approximately 86% (range, 50–93%), as indicated in Table 42–18.[59,60,180,182] Improvement to reduce local failure rates emphasized the use of more extensive surgical procedures to obtain wider margins of normal tissue. Wide local excisions, which usually entail only soft tissue resections, are associated with local recurrences of 49% if surgery alone is performed (see Table 42–18). More radical procedures, such as amputation or muscle compartmental excisions, are associated with an even lower local failure rate of 14% (range, 7–18%), as documented in four separate series (see Table 42–18).

Resection of a soft tissue sarcoma requires that the tumor be located so that an acceptably wide margin of normal tissue can be obtained between the edge of the tumor and the adjacent critical, nonresectable structures, such as major nerves, vessels, bone, and important tendons. This guideline does not apply to many anatomic sites, such as the groin, knee, popliteal space, most portions of the leg, the ankle, many sites within the head and neck area, supraclavicular area, some axillary sites, the elbow region, and most of the forearm, wrist, and hand. Because of the inability to obtain a clear margin at those sites and still retain acceptable function, approximately half of patients with extremity sarcomas were subjected to amputation at institutions with a large experience in sarcoma surgery. Table 42–19 shows the proportion of patients with extremity sarcomas treated by radical resection or amputation at the University of Florida in Gainesville or at Memorial Sloan-Kettering Cancer Center in New York City.[59,60]

The combined results of amputation for the treatment of sarcoma of soft tissue from four centers showed that local control was obtained in 40 of 40 patients with lesions of the leg or foot.[59,60,182,264] In these patients, the level of amputation was well above the lesion and, in most instances, above the level of the proximal joint. These results can be taken as the benchmark for local control results for sarcomas of the distal

TABLE 42–19. Local Control of Soft Tissue Sarcomas of the Extremities by Radical Surgery

Series Factors	Simon and Enneking[59]	Shiu et al[60]
Total number of patients	54	297
Radical local resection	25 (46%)	158 (53%)
Amputation	29 (54%)	139 (47%)
Local control		
Radical local resection	88%	72%
Amputation	79%	93%
Overall	83%	82%

extremities. If the level of amputation is closer to the tumor (*e.g.*, thigh lesions), about 10% of patients fail locally. In the University of Florida and Goteborg series, 5% and 89% local failure rates were documented after surgery obtaining adequate and inadequate margins, respectively (Table 42–20).[60,182]

Sites of failure among 464 patients treated by surgery alone at three institutions are shown in Table 40–21.[59,182,265] The total local failure rate was 19%; 35% developed distant metastases. These figures are a fair indication of the best that can be accomplished by surgery alone for soft tissue sarcoma in extremities, although patient selection can influence these results. The proportion of patients amputated in the three centers shown in Table 42–21 were 47%, 16%, and 50%, respectively; which was 41% in the combined study.[59,182,264] An average local control rate of 81% was achieved but only with a high rate of amputation.

The more conservative procedures have been employed in combined-modality treatments to reduce local recurrences but perform limb-sparing surgery. These treatments have been adopted by many institutions with extensive experience in sarcoma surgery. For example, the percentage of limb-sparing procedures being performed at Memorial Sloan-Kettering Cancer Center has increased since 1975, when approximately 50% of all extremity sarcoma patients received amputations. Between 1982 and 1984, 83% of patients had limb-sparing operations, and only 17% had amputations.[266] In recommending a limb-sparing procedure, the physician must inform the patient that the risk of local failure may be higher than for amputation.

Although a local recurrence should be avoided if possible, its true impact is not yet known.[267,268] Any association between local recurrence and distant metastases could be causally re-

TABLE 42–20. Adequacy of Margins of Radical Surgery Related to Local Failure Rate

Investigations	No. Local Failures/ Total Failures (%)	
	Negative Margins	Positive Margins
Simon and Enneking[60]	1/46　(2)	8/8　(100)
Markhede et al[182]	5/76　(7)	16/19　(84)
Total	6/122　(5)	25/27　(89)

TABLE 42–21. Patterns of Failure in Patients With Extremity Sarcomas Treated by Surgery Alone

Investigations	No. of Patients	Follow-up (y)	Amputation (%)	Local Failure ± Distant Metastases (%)	Distant Metastases (%)
Memorial Sloan-Kettering Cancer Center[59] *	297	5–24	139 (47)	54 (18)	88 (30)
University of Goteborg[182] †	97	3–23	17 (16)	20 (21)	46 (27)
University of Florida at Gainesville[265]	70	2–19	35 (50)	14 (20)	27 (39)
Total	464	2–24	191 (41)	88 (19)	161 (35)

* Eighteen patients received adjunctive radiation therapy.
† Series includes four patients with truncal sarcomas; two patients received preoperative radiation therapy.

lated or merely a reflection of more aggressive tumor biology. Resolution of such issues would clarify the risk of conservative surgery in marginal cases.

Technical Aspects of Surgery

Extremity Sarcomas

The categorization of surgical procedures by Enneking is useful in carefully defining the nature of the surgical procedure performed (Table 42–22).[269] There are four types of surgical procedures for soft tissue sarcomas.

Intracapsular excision involves removal of the tumor by directly incising the tumor capsule. This procedure leaves gross tumor behind and is of diagnostic value only.

In *marginal excision*, all gross tumor, including the pseudocapsule, is excised locally. Soft tissue sarcomas tend to grow by radial expansion and compress normal structures around them. This pseudocapsule gives the gross appearance of compartmentalization of the tumor from surrounding structures, but invasion of local tissues occurs through the pseudocapsule. The local recurrence rate after treatment by marginal excision alone is close to 90% (see Table 42–18).

In *wide excision*, the tumor is removed with a margin of normal surrounding tissue in continuity with the tumor. This procedure does not imply removal of entire structures within which the tumor may be found. The local recurrence rate after treatment by wide resection alone is approximately 50%.

In *radical resection*, tumor is removed with all tissue in the anatomic compartment occupied by the tumor. The excision takes place by dissecting along planes that are separated from the tumor and its tissues of origin by at least one uninvolved anatomic plane in all directions. The resected specimen includes the origin and insertion of all muscles and any bones or joints that are contained within the anatomic compartment of resection. This procedure may involve amputation, although nonablative procedures can fulfill the criteria for radical resection (Fig. 42–7). The local recurrence rate after these procedures is approximately 14%.

Amputative Procedures. In the treatment of soft tissue sarcomas of the extremities, a variety of amputative procedures can be employed.

For *amputations of the foot,* amputations of digits, ray amputations, transmetatarsal amputation, and Syme amputations at the level of the ankle joint are accepted procedures for ischemic lesions of the foot, but they infrequently give an adequate margin for soft tissue sarcomas in the foot and should be combined with adjuvant radiation therapy to maximize the changes for obtaining local control.

TABLE 42–22. Surgical Procedures for Soft Tissue Extremity Sarcomas

Margin	How Margin Was Achieved		Plane of Dissection	Microscopic Appearance
	Limb Salvage	Amputation		
Intracapsular	Intracapsular piecemeal excision	Intracapsular amputation	Within lesion	Tumor at margin
Marginal	Marginal en bloc excision	Marginal amputation	Within reactive zone, extracapsular	Reactive tissue ± microsatellites
Wide	Wide en bloc excision	Wide through-bone amputation	Beyond reactive zone through normal tissue within compartment	Normal tissue ± "skips"
Radical	Radical en bloc resection	Radical disarticulation	Normal tissue, extracompartmental	Normal tissue

(Adapted from Enneking, WF. Staging of musculoskeletal neoplasms. In: Current concepts of diagnosis and treatment of bone and soft tissue tumors. Heidelberg: Springer-Verlag, 1984)

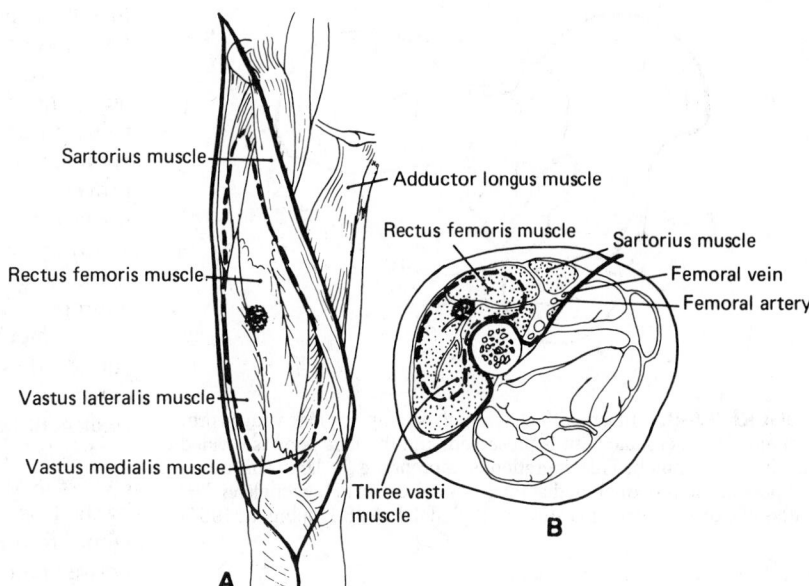

FIGURE 42–7. **(A)** Schematic drawing of the anterior thigh and **(B)** transverse section through the thigh, illustrating the anatomic extent of a radical resection, without amputation, of a soft tissue sarcoma lying within the rectus femoris muscle. (Courtesy of Dr. Martin Malawer)

Below-knee amputation is usually performed about a third the distance between the knee and the ankle and involves division of the tibia and fibula. Muscles to the ankle or foot are transected. This amputation is the treatment of choice for any substantive soft tissue sarcoma of the foot. Because the weight-bearing portions of the foot tolerate radiation therapy poorly, amputation is often the best treatment for these lesions.

Above-knee amputation through the thigh can be performed at any level distal to the lesser trochanter. Major muscle groups of the thigh are transected. This amputation is of little value for tumors occurring above the knee and is often indicated for tumors of the leg.

Hip disarticulation is a form of amputation involving disarticulation of the hip joint with complete removal of the femur. Most muscles attached to the lower extremity are removed entirely. It is often suitable for patients with lesions of the middle and distal thigh.

Hemipelvectomy involves removal of the entire lower extremity and hemipelvis with disarticulation of the sacroiliac joint and pubic symphysis (Fig. 42–8). All major muscles that attach to the lower extremity, except the iliopsoas, are removed. This operation is often applied to the treatment of proximal thigh and buttock lesions. A conventional hemipelvectomy uses a posterior flap of skin and subcutaneous tissue overlying the buttock. For lesions of the buttock, it is possible to construct an anterior flap that includes part of the quadriceps muscles and the femoral vessels. The use of anterior-flap hemipelvectomies has greatly extended the application of this procedure.

Modified hemipelvectomy allows preservation of the iliac wing and improves patient rehabilitation. This procedure is similar to the standard hemipelvectomy, except that the sacroiliac joint is preserved and the iliac bone is excised from an area below the level of the sciatic notch (Fig. 42–9). This operation does involve transection of muscles in the buttock and is not suitable for lesions in this area. Internal hemipelvectomy can be performed with removal of the innominate bone and adjacent muscles but with preservation of the ipsilateral lower extremity.[270]

Extended hemipelvectomy is used if lesions of the iliac wing are too close to the sacroiliac joint to permit its disarticulation. Extension of the standard hemipelvectomy to include excision of the sacral ala at the level of the lateral vertebral bodies adds little in morbidity to this procedure and often adds several centimeters of margin from the tumor.

Amputations of the upper extremities follow the principles enunciated for those of the lower extremities. Below-elbow amputations are often used for the treatment of tumors of the hand and wrist. Above-elbow amputations are used for tumors of the forearm. Disarticulation of the shoulder joint is an operation reserved for distal arm and elbow lesions. Forequarter amputation is applied to the treatment of lesions of the shoulder girdle or the proximal arm. This operation includes removal of the entire upper extremity, including the scapula and clavicle.

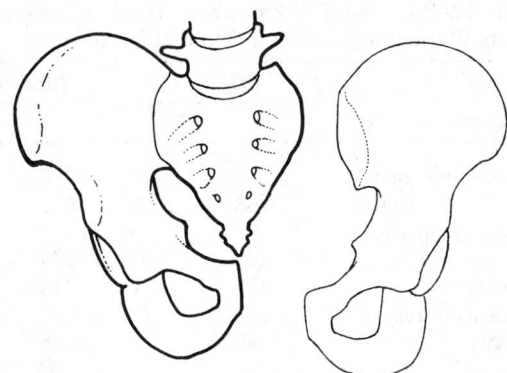

FIGURE 42–8. In a hemipelvectomy, removal of the entire lower extremity including the hemipelvis is performed by disarticulation of the sacroiliac joint and symphysis pubis. This approach may be required for large soft tissue tumors of the buttock and anterior or lateral proximal thigh. (Sugarbaker PH, Nicholson TH. Atlas of extremity sarcoma surgery. Philadelphia: JB Lippincott, 1984)

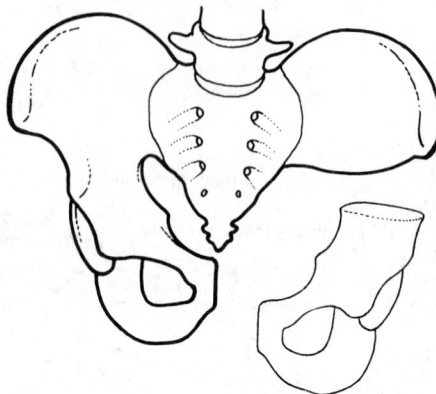

FIGURE 42–9. In a modified hemipelvectomy, the iliac wing is preserved. The sacroiliac joint is preserved, and the iliac bone is divided at the sciatic notch. This operation is appropriate for large soft tissue tumors of the proximal medial thigh. (Sugarbaker PH, Nicholson TH. Atlas of extremity sarcoma surgery. Philadelphia: JB Lippincott, 1984)

Nonamputative Procedures. Nonamputative surgical procedures used in the treatment of patients with soft tissue sarcomas of the extremities should also be known to the surgical oncologist.

Wide excision is one of the most common surgical procedures performed for extremity sarcomas. In the American College of Surgeons survey, approximately half of all sarcomas were treated with this surgical procedure (Table 42–23).[46] As indicated in Table 42–18, this procedure results in a local control rate of 50% if used alone, and wide excision is often employed with adjunctive radiation therapy.

Sound surgical principles must be adhered to (Fig. 42–10). Surgery should include wide excision of all normal tissue in the tumor area, including several centimeters of normal tissue in all directions and excision of all skin and subcutaneous tissue near the tumor. All previous scars, biopsy areas, and areas containing hematoma from previous biopsies should be resected. Surgical excision of the sarcoma should be completed without spilling of tumor, which can severely compromise the ability to deliver effective radiation therapy. A tour-

TABLE 42–23. Surgical Procedures Used in Sarcoma Patients Without Metastases at Time of Diagnosis

	1977–1978		1983–1984	
Procedures	*No.*	*%*	*No.*	*%*
Wide local resection	879	52.4	1412	56.7
Limited local resection	455	27.1	583	23.4
Anatomic compartmental resection	168	10.0	249	14.8
Amputation	108	6.4	138	8.2
More than one type of surgery	69	4.1	108	6.4
Total	1679	100.0	2490	100.0

(Lawrence W, Donegan WL, Natarajan N, et al. Adult soft tissue sarcomas. A pattern of care survey of the American College of Surgeons. Ann Surg 1987;205:349–359)

niquet can be placed on the extremity above the lesion before ligation of the venous outflow, as a first part of the surgical procedure, but there is no convincing evidence that this reduces the distant spread. Because these tumors rarely metastasize to draining nodes, lymph node dissection should be confined to patients with clinically suspicious and biopsy-proven nodal involvement. Current data do not support prophylactic lymph node dissection for sarcoma. For histologies showing a significant incidence of lymphatic metastases (*e.g.,* epithelioid sarcoma), an increased level of suspicion is appropriate.

Placement of metallic clips as a guide to the limits of the surgical dissection is essential in all nonamputative sarcoma resections. The clips identify the entire dissected area in the treatment field for construction of the radiation portals.

Muscle compartmental excision is useful for some anatomic sites (*e.g.,* thigh) containing compartments that are bounded by the fascia and its extensions. Because it is unusual for sarcomas to transgress these fascial boundaries, excision of the entire anatomic compartment containing the tumor is often successful in eradicating all local tumor. These procedures are classified as radical nonamputative excisions (see Table 42–22), and according to the American College of Surgeons survey, they were performed in approximately 10% to 15% of patients (see Table 42–23).[46]

In the thigh, there are three major compartments bounded by the fascia lata and its extensions: the anterior compartment, including the quadriceps muscle (see Fig. 42–8); the medial compartment, including the adductor muscles; the posterior compartment, including the hamstring muscles. The anterior thigh compartment consists of the quadriceps and sartorius muscles and the femoral artery, vein, and nerve. Excision of the anterior compartment leads to significant loss of motion and stability of the knee. In these situations, hamstring transfers can be performed to provide needed muscular movement at the knee. The medial thigh compartment consists of the gracilis, adductor brevis, adductor longus, adductor magnus, and the pectineus muscles. The obturator nerve supplies this compartment. In addition, the profunda femoris artery must be sacrificed when this compartment is resected. The posterior compartment consists of the semimembranosus, semitendinosus, and biceps femoris muscles and the posterior portion of the adductor magnus muscle and the sciatic nerve.

Several atlases of extremity surgery for patients with soft tissue sarcomas detail the performance of these surgical procedures.[160,271]

Truncal Sarcomas

The principles guiding the surgical therapy of extremity lesions apply to truncal sarcomas.[272–277] However, there are unique therapeutic features of these lesions that require special consideration. The anatomic location of most truncal sarcomas precludes surgical excision with margins wide enough to ensure local control, especially for sarcomas in the head and neck region and for mediastinal and retroperitoneal tumors. Surgical excision should be aimed at removing all gross tumor with as much marginal tissue in the expected areas of local spread as is compatible with reasonable morbidity. Radiation therapy should be used in the treatment of virtually all high-grade truncal sarcomas, and the surgeon should outline the margins of resection with metallic clips. For tumors

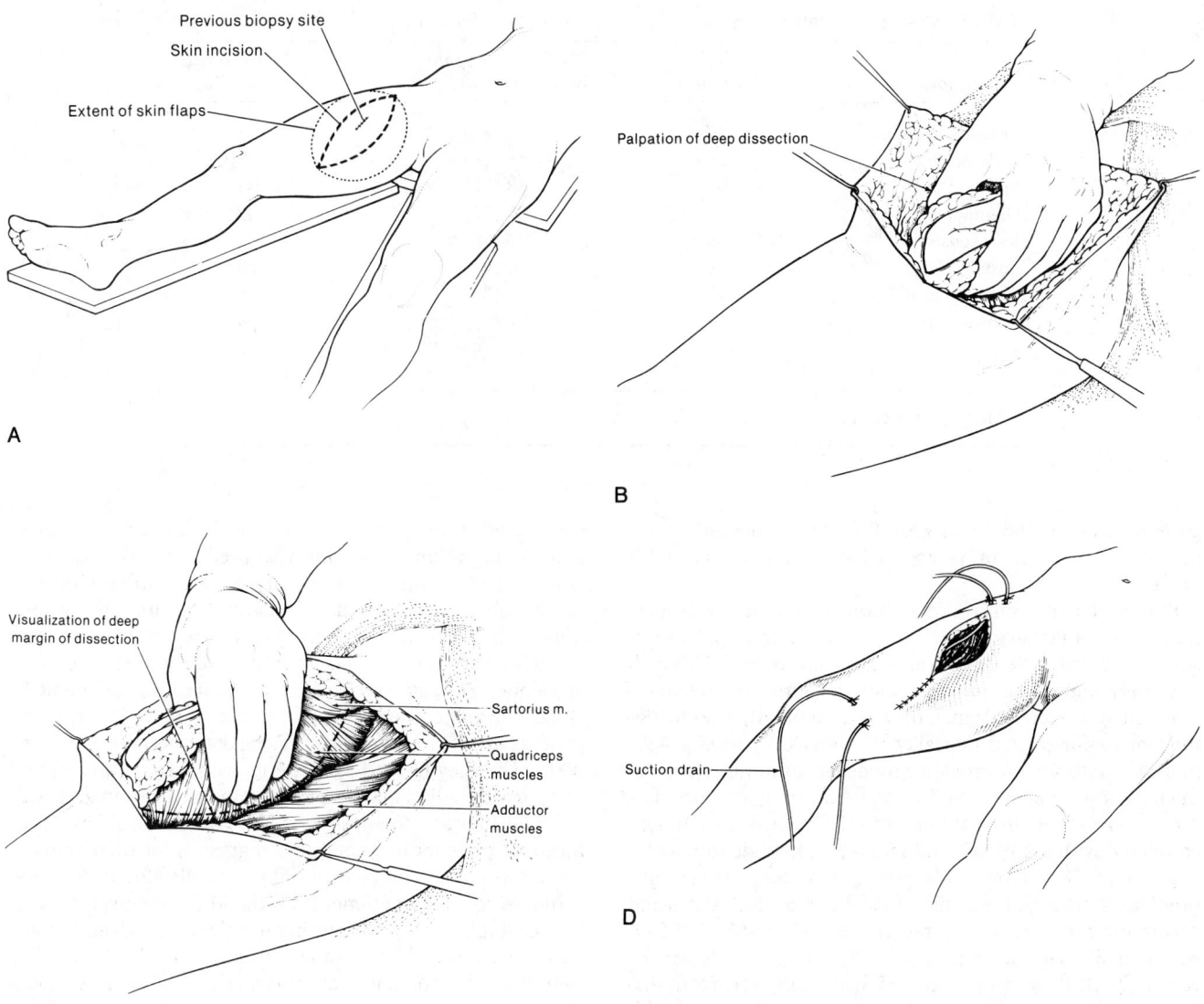

FIGURE 42–10. Wide excision of an anterior thigh sarcoma. **(A)** Elliptical skin incision encompassing previous biopsy incision(s) or drain site(s) is made. Subcutaneous skin flaps are developed to the lateral extent of the muscle margins. **(B)** Palpation of the tumor within the muscle is constantly needed to localize the mass and achieve a margin of at least 2 cm in all directions. Removal of the tumor without visualization of the mass is important. **(C)** Visualization of the deep margin is obtained and the muscle divided. **(D)** The extent of the dissection is marked with clips for subsequent planning of radiation fields. The skin flaps are closed over suction drains to allow apposition of the flaps to the surgical bed.

of the thoracic or abdominal walls, full-thickness excisions, except for skin, are indicated.[275,276,278,279] Replacement of the abdominal wall with synthetic materials does not preclude subsequent radiation therapy.

Sarcomas of the retroperitoneum present a unique surgical challenge.[280–286] These tumors tend not to cause symptoms until they are quite large, with extensive local invasion. Delamater reported a patient with an abdominal liposarcoma that reached 125 kg, and reports of tumors reaching 27 kg are not rare.[287,288] Most retroperitoneal sarcomas weigh several pounds when diagnosed and extensively invade local tissues. The most common diagnoses in the retroperitoneum are liposarcoma and leiomyosarcoma.

Evaluation of patients with retroperitoneal sarcomas should include ultrasound studies, CT, intravenous pyelogram, and

if necessary, gastrointestinal contrast studies. Arteriography can delineate the blood supply of the tumor. Venacavography should be employed if invasion of the vena cava is suspected.

It is rarely possible to achieve negative microscopic margins in the excision of retroperitoneal sarcomas. An attempt should be made to remove all gross tumor, even if this involves resection of a kidney or other intraabdominal structures. In a 20-year retrospective review of 78 patients with retroperitoneal sarcomas treated between 1951 and 1971, Fortner and colleagues reported the necessity of en bloc excision of adjacent organs in 75% of patients.[289] The colon or kidney were the organs most often resected. This was similar to the experience reported by McGrath and coworkers from the Medical College of Virginia, where complete resection of tumors required en bloc excision of adjacent organs in 68% of the

TABLE 42–24.   Treatment Results for Retroperitoneal Sarcomas

Investigations	No. of Patients	No. With Complete Resection (%)	5-Year Overall Survival (%)
Braasch and Mon[280]	37	13 (35)	16
Cody et al[281]	68	45 (66)	25
Storm et al[282]	54	28 (52)	33
Glenn et al[277]	48	37 (77)	43*
Karakousis et al[283]	68	27 (39)	30
Bose[284]	29	6 (21)	20
McGrath et al[285]	47	18 (38)	33
Jaques et al[286]	114	67 (59)	64
Total	465	241 (52)	

* Three-year overall survival rate.

patients; kidney and colon were the organs most often resected.[285] The role of postoperative radiation therapy is unclear.

Reported 5-year survival rates after treatment of retroperitoneal sarcomas vary from 16% to 37% (Table 42–24). Most series included patients with all grades of sarcoma. Although low-grade tumors can have an indolent course, the retroperitoneum is one site in which they can eventually lead to significant tumor-related mortality.[286] Marcus reported a 43% mortality rate for low-grade retroperitoneal tumors, but the median time to death was 7 years.[177] Storm and colleagues reported a 5-year survival rate of 54% for low-grade tumors compared with a 23% survival rate for high-grade tumors.[282] For high-grade and low-grade lesions in this location, a major problem is the high frequency of local recurrence. Abbas and coworkers reported a local recurrence rate of 63%.[290] In a series of 37 patients reported by the NCI, 16 had recurrences.[277] Of these 16 patients, 12 had locally recurrent disease, alone or in conjunction with recurrence in other sites.[277]

The ability to achieve complete resection of all gross disease may improve cure rates. McGrath reported a 70% 5-year survival rate after complete resections, compared with an 8% survival rate for patients undergoing partial excisions or biopsies only.[285] Complete resection of all gross disease was possible in only 49% of the patients in a combined series (see Table 42–24).

The roles of adjuvant radiation therapy and chemotherapy have not been established, and although widely used, there is no evidence that results are better than after surgical resection alone. A prospective randomized trial at the NCI comparing intraoperative radiation therapy with postoperative external-beam irradiation in 35 patients with resectable retroperitoneal soft tissue sarcomas revealed no difference in therapeutic effectiveness.[291] Innovative combined-modality approaches are needed for retroperitoneal sarcomas.

RADIATION THERAPY

Radiation Therapy Alone

Radiation therapy alone in the management of soft tissue sarcomas has been limited to patients who have locally advanced, inoperable, recurrent, or metastatic disease. The radiation doses used have been somewhat low by modern standards, and the intention of therapy was predominantly palliative. Nonetheless, there were reports documenting objective regression and occasional local control of large, inoperable tumors. In 1951, Cade reported that unresectable sarcomas in 6 of 22 patients were locally controlled with radiation therapy alone; they survived from 5 to 26 years after treatment.[292] Windeyer and coworkers reported the results of treating 58 patients with fibrosarcomas.[293] Using doses between 6000 and 8000 cGy, they treated 11 patients with large, unresectable tumors with radiation therapy alone and an additional 11 with radiation therapy for postsurgical recurrences. Fourteen of these 22 patients had complete regression of their tumors, and 27% of the tumors were locally controlled for many years.

In a series of 35 patients from the M.D. Anderson Cancer Center, high-dose radiation therapy alone was given for soft tissue sarcomas.[294] Doses ranged from 7000 to 7500 cGy. The overall local recurrence rate was 66%, and 7 of 10 patients with extremity sarcomas had recurrences. In a series from the Massachusetts General Hospital, 54 patients were treated with primary radiation therapy for soft tissue sarcomas.[295] Of the 26 patients who were treated with doses greater than 6500 cGy, 61% were locally controlled at 4 years. Most lesions smaller than 5 cm were controlled. However, of the 28 patients treated with doses less than 6500 cGy, only 2 patients were alive and free of disease for more than 2 years. An analysis of the experience with radiation therapy alone ($\geq$6500 cGy) reported by Tepper and Suit showed an inverse association between tumor size and ability to obtain local control (Table 42–25).[296] For tumors smaller than 5 cm, 5 to 10 cm, and more than 10 cm, the local control rates with radiation therapy alone were 88%, 53%, and 33%, respectively.

Data demonstrate that the dose required to inactivate a tumor increases with the number of viable tumor cells, and radiation therapy given to microscopic disease is much more effective than treatment of gross disease.[297]

Local control can be achieved by radiation therapy alone, but it usually requires aggressive treatment with very high doses of radiation, which carries significant risks of adverse sequelae. The local control rates achieved with radiation therapy alone appear to be inferior to those obtained with surgery. Radiation therapy should be used as a primary modality only

TABLE 42–25. Relation of Size of Lesion to Local Control Achieved by Radiation Therapy Alone

Size of Lesion	No. of Patients	No. Locally Controlled (%)*
<5 cm	8	7 (88)
5–10 cm	17	9 (53)
>10 cm	10	3 (33)
Total	35	19 (54)

* Tumor dose of ≥6500 rad.
(Tepper JE, Suit HD. Radiation therapy of soft tissue sarcomas. Cancer 1985;55:2273–2277)

for patients who have lesions that are not amenable to standard treatments because of tumor size, anatomic location, medical inoperability, or refusal of a patient to agree to conventional treatment. An exception may be desmoid tumors that cannot be resected; several series have shown that excellent local control was achieved with radiation therapy alone.[298–300]

The contribution of radiation therapy for some sarcomas remains uncertain. Mirabell and colleagues reported 26 patients with positive surgical margins after resection of primary fibromatoses.[301] Without further therapy, only 9 patients had recurrences during a 5-year period. Because the risk of metastasis is negligible for this lesion, close observation is a reasonable policy if patients are reliable and wider resection would result in major functional deficits. Mirabell also reported that 10 patients treated with irradiation for primary control of desmoid tumors achieved local control. Similar data for aggressive fibromatoses were reported by McCollough and associates.[302]

Combining Radiation Therapy and Surgery

The rationale for combining surgery with adjuvant radiation therapy is to employ conservative surgery and moderate-dose radiation therapy to preserve the function of the area involved, especially limbs. Radiation therapy is used to treat microscopic tumor extending into the adjacent tissues beyond the primary tumor mass, achieving the same results as a more radical resection. An advantage of this approach is that the treatment volume for radiation therapy is designed to encompass the surrounding tissues at risk for tumor involvement, such as nerves, vessels, tendons, and bone, which would otherwise

limit the ability to perform an adequate local resection. Theoretically, combined therapy offers a high degree of local control and improved functional and cosmetic results, especially in the extremities. This expectation has been realized in clinical practice in several different series.[43,44,303,304]

In 1951, Cade reported a survival rate of 61% in a series of 80 patients treated with wide excision followed by radiation therapy, compared with 27% (6 of 22) with amputation.[292] He championed the use of radiation therapy in combination with wide local excision. Results of combined-modality treatment from recent literature are shown in Tables 42–26 and 42–27. Although several reports show excellent results from combining limb-sparing surgery with radiation therapy for high-grade sarcomas of the extremities, it is still unclear if radiation therapy should be administered before, during, or after the surgical procedure. It is obvious that combining radiation therapy with conservative surgery has avoided ablative surgical procedures and maintained local control in most patients (85%), and by eliminating the need for generous surgical margins, the functional results are excellent. Additional research is needed to define the contribution of each modality and to relate results to grade, histologic type, tumor size, and anatomic site.

For low-grade sarcomas, local control is the predominant issue, but any potential enhancement of local control by radiation therapy must be weighed against functional deficits and impairment in quality of life caused by radiation therapy. The issues can only be resolved by a randomized prospective study that considers quality of life factors.

PREOPERATIVE RADIATION THERAPY. There are several theoretical advantages of preoperative radiation therapy combined with conservative surgery in the management of soft tissue sarcomas. First, inactivation of tumor cells by radiation therapy may decrease the risks of tumor implantation in the surgical wound and decrease metastatic spread from any tumor cells that enter vascular spaces during surgery. Second, the volume to be treated can be limited to clinically and radiologically evident tumor and the adjacent tissues at risk for microscopic extension, without encompassing all the tissues that are manipulated during the surgical procedure itself. Third, the mass is often smaller at the time of surgery after responding to radiation therapy, which facilitates conservative resection. Fourth, an inoperable sarcoma may be made resectable by regression with radiation therapy.

The major disadvantages of preoperative radiation therapy

TABLE 42–26. Local Control and Survival After Preoperative Radiation Therapy for Extremity Soft Tissue Sarcomas

Investigations	No. of Patients	Follow-up (y)	Local Failure ± Distant Metastases (%)	5-Year Disease-Free Survival (%)
Massachusetts General Hospital[305]	90	1–18	15 (17)	67 (74)
M.D. Anderson[306]	27	≥5	2 (7)	15 (56)
University of Florida[307]	19	1–5	1 (5)	11 (58)
Pooled data	136		18 (13)	93 (68)

TABLE 42–27. Local Recurrence Rate With Conservative Surgery and Postoperative Radiation Therapy

Investigations	No. of Patients	Follow-up (y)	Dose (Gy)	Patients With Local Recurrence (%)	5-Year Disease-Free Survival (%)
University California San Francisco[303]	29	>2	50–75	3 (10)	68
M.D. Anderson[43]	300	2–7	60–75	67 (22)	68
National Cancer Institute[44] *	129	1–8	63	10 (8)	60
Massachusetts General Hospital[304] *	123	1–12	60–68	16 (12)	65
Pooled data	581			96 (17)	

* Extremity sites only.

are the delay in surgical resection (a psychological disadvantage for some patients), a risk of compromising wound healing, and the necessity for the radiation therapist to have planned and executed radiation therapy before surgical resection. Often, an initial excision is carried out by a surgeon who is removing a piece of tissue for diagnosis. In some instances, the diagnosis of a sarcoma comes as a surprise and many of the potential benefits of preoperative radiation therapy cannot be realized because of a suboptimal biopsy procedure. Nonetheless, several series demonstrated that planned preoperative radiation therapy in patients with high-grade sarcomas can yield excellent results (see Table 42–26).[305–307] Radiation-induced shrinkage of an inoperable tumor resulted in some tumors becoming resectable.[294,308,309]

POSTOPERATIVE RADIATION THERAPY. Radiation therapy in combination with surgery is most commonly employed in the postoperative period. For patients for whom postoperative radiation therapy is planned, the amount of surgical resection itself remains a matter of some controversy. Although all gross tumor should be removed, some physicians advocate minimal excision of surrounding normal tissue, and others advocate the widest excision possible that is compatible with reasonable limb function. The crucial issue is that larger surgical excisions remove more normal tissue and require the use of wider radiation fields; wide excisions may ultimately reduce the functional result that can be achieved. For lesions in the groin, popliteal space, ankle, elbow, forearm, wrist, hand, or foot, the margins are necessarily close at some point in the dissection. For lesions that occur in fleshy parts of the body, the margins can be more generous. Expansion of local operations to include vascular reconstruction or bone replacement procedures has been advocated in recent years.[310–314]

The advantages of postoperative radiation therapy include immediate surgery, which can be a psychological advantage for some patients; no radiation-induced delay in wound healing; and an entire specimen available for histopathologic investigation. Moreover, the exact size and pattern of extension of the tumor are interpreted definitively.

The conservative surgical procedure itself has a moderate probability of achieving local control if the surgeon is able to

get around the tumor with a negative margin. Adjuvant radiation therapy can minimize the necessity of wide margins, optimizing function, and maximize the probability of local control. However, in encompassing all tissues manipulated by the surgeon, the postoperative treatment volume is usually larger than that used for preoperative radiation. Moreover, if there is a delay in starting radiation therapy, as for wound healing, there may be a larger number of residual tumor cells. A prolonged delay in wound healing may allow residual microscopic tumor to become palpable.

There are several published series demonstrating the results of surgery with postoperative radiation therapy (see Table 42–27).[43,44,303,304] One of the earliest and largest came from the M.D. Anderson Cancer Center, where more than 300 patients with soft tissue sarcomas were treated.[43] The surgery consisted of conservative excision, usually shelling out, with removal of the gross tumor and a limited amount of normal tissue. Patients received a dose between 6000 and 7000 cGy during 6 to 7 weeks. No attempt was made to include the entire muscle or anatomic compartment in the treatment field. The local recurrence rate for all patients treated with combined conservative surgery and postoperative radiation therapy was 22% and 20% for those with extremity sarcomas. In the patients who had extremity sarcomas, most of the recurrences occurred in the fleshy portions of the extremity, where lesions typically were large and extended for significant distances along fascial planes. The disease-free survival rate at 5 years was 61% for all primary sites. For the extremities, it was 69%; for head and neck sarcomas, it was 63%; but for retroperitoneal disease, the 5-year survival rate was only 33%. Local failure rates ranged from 10% for stage I to 28% for stage III tumors. Distant metastases developed in 5% of patients with stage I, in 29% with stage II, and in 43% with stage III tumors. The investigators reported significant complications in 7% of the patients, including soft tissue necrosis, traumatic fractures of bone within the radiation field, fibrosis with limitation of motion, nerve and vascular injuries, and moderate edema. Nonetheless, of those with extremity tumors undergoing such treatment, 85% of the patients maintained functional limbs.

In a smaller series from the University of California at San

Francisco, 29 patients with extremity sarcomas were treated with surgery and postoperative radiation therapy.[303] Most had grade 3 tumors. The dose usually ranged between 5500 and 7000 cGy. Radiation fields were designed to cover the surgical bed with a generous margin; no effort was made to treat the entire involved muscle group from origin to insertion. The 5-year determinant survival rate was 81%, and the 5-year relapse-free survival rate was 68%. The local control rate was 90%. No patient required amputation due to radiation sequelae. It was demonstrated that radiation can sterilize microscopic disease and reduce the local recurrence rate in patients undergoing simple excision of soft tissue sarcomas. Of the patients undergoing conservative excision and postoperative radiation therapy, 22 had microscopically positive margins of resection, but only 3 of these 22 patients developed local recurrences after postoperative radiation therapy. Of 14 nonirradiated patients treated with conservative surgery alone in whom margins were positive, 11 developed local recurrences.

It is difficult to assess the influences of size, grade, histology, and anatomic site in comparing patients from different series. To overcome some of these potential biases, Rosenberg and colleagues conducted a randomized prospective clinical trial evaluating limb-sparing surgery plus postoperative radiation therapy compared with amputation in patients with high-grade extremity sarcomas at the NCI.[264] The dose of radiation therapy employed for the patients undergoing limb-sparing surgery was usually 6300 cGy. All patients received postoperative adjuvant chemotherapy. Forty-three patients were entered into the trial with an (updated) median follow-up of 11 years. There were 17 patients randomized to amputation and 27 to limb-sparing surgery plus postoperative radiation therapy (1:2 randomization). There were five local recurrences in the group receiving limb-sparing surgery and one (a protocol violator) in the group randomized to radical surgery (Fig. 42–11). Despite this finding, the 10-year overall survival rate for the two groups was approximately equal at 75%.

A randomized, prospective study demonstrated the benefit of radiation therapy for local control of high-grade extremity sarcoma. Yang and colleagues randomized 90 patients to receive surgery and chemotherapy or to receive surgery, chemotherapy, and radiation therapy.[315] With a median follow-up of 5 years, no patient receiving radiation therapy had a local recurrence, but 9 of 46 treated with only surgery and chemotherapy had local recurrences. The low local recurrence rate in patients not receiving radiation therapy may be attributable to their receiving chemotherapy, because several studies have indicated an effect of adjuvant chemotherapy on local recurrence.[316,317] Despite the significant difference in local recurrences, overall survival of the two groups was identical, again raising the question of the impact of local recurrence on survival (Fig. 42–12). A concurrent, prospective quality of life study of these patients indicated that radiation therapy impaired quality of life and limb function, but the magnitude of impairment was small. This confirms that radiation therapy can control local disease in sarcoma patients undergoing limb-sparing surgery, but it suggests that local recurrences may have minimal influence on overall survival. Highly selected patients who have optimal surgery for favorable tumors (and who may receive adjuvant chemotherapy) may be able to safely avoid adjuvant radiation therapy.

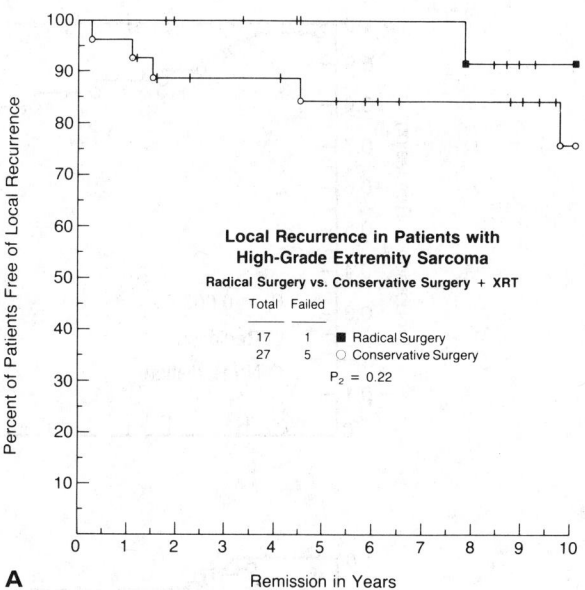

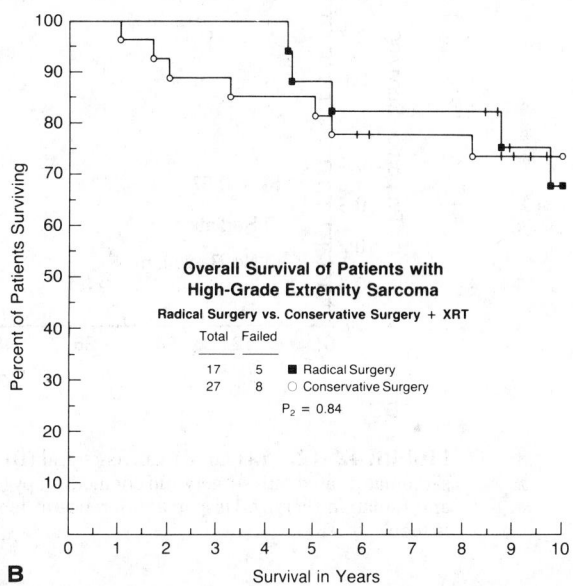

FIGURE 42–11. **(A)** Local recurrence in patients with high-grade extremity sarcoma and a limb-sparing surgical option, who were randomized to receive a limb-sparing resection with radiation therapy rather than amputation (standard therapy at the time). All patients in this trial received postoperative adjuvant chemotherapy. With few patients, there was a small, statistically insignificant difference in local recurrence. **(B)** Updated overall survival of patients in the same study. Long-term survival of patients randomized to limb-sparing surgery versus amputation appears to be similar. This represents the only prospective randomized study of this issue.

Rydholm and associates and the Scandinavian Sarcoma Group have already applied these concepts in a series of 70 patients with high-grade and low-grade sarcomas confined to the subcutaneous space or totally within a deep muscular fascia.[318] These fascial planes had not been violated by previous biopsy; many preoperative diagnoses were made on the grounds of radiographs and fine-needle aspirate. In 56 of the 70 patients, widely negative surgical margins including fascia or wide muscular cuffs were obtained and no adjuvant radia-

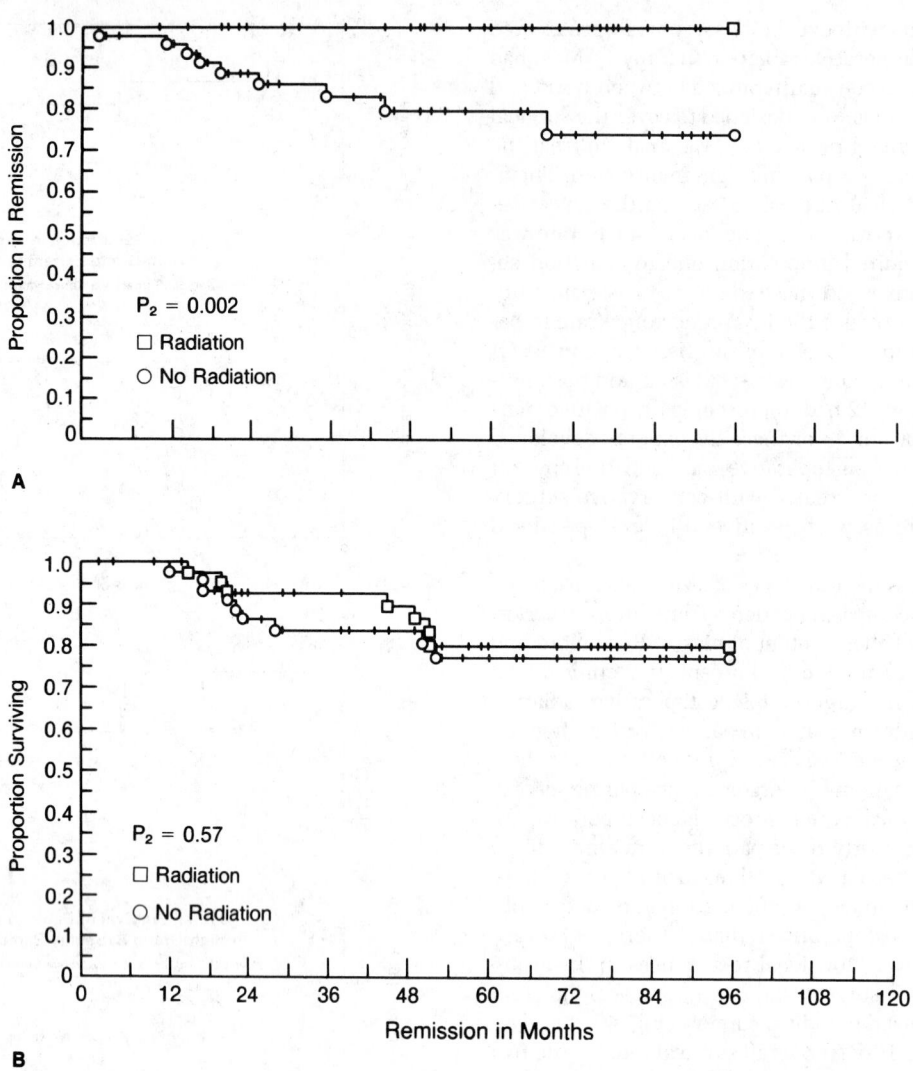

FIGURE 42–12. **(A)** Local recurrence and **(B)** overall survival of patients with high-grade extremity sarcomas treated with surgery and chemotherapy (no radiation therapy) or with surgery, chemotherapy, and radiation therapy. Despite a difference in local recurrence rate, no difference in overall survival is seen.

tion therapy was given. With a median follow-up of 5 years, only 4 (7%) of these patients had local recurrences. Despite the excellent results from this highly experienced group of investigators, the approach remains experimental and controversial and does not represent a recommendation for therapy of patients undergoing limb-sparing procedures.

INTRAOPERATIVE BRACHYTHERAPY. A less commonly employed approach combining surgery and radiation therapy is the use of intraoperative brachytherapy.[319] This approach requires a surgery and radiation therapy team with expertise in this technique. Brennan and colleagues reported a trial

evaluating the efficacy of intraoperative brachytherapy in adult patients with operable soft tissue sarcomas of the extremities or superficial trunk at Memorial Sloan-Kettering Cancer Center.[320] Temporary implants of iridium 192 were employed using after-loading techniques. Usually, this consisted of a single-plane implant. A total of 117 patients were prospectively randomized to receive or not receive intraoperative brachytherapy. With median follow-up of only 16 months, 2 of 52 patients receiving brachytherapy developed local recurrences, compared with 9 of 65 in the group not receiving brachytherapy ($p = 0.06$). No survival differences were seen between the two groups during the short follow-up period. Similar data have been reported by others.[321,322]

The advantages and disadvantages of brachytherapy are somewhat similar to those for preoperative radiation therapy; however, an additional advantage is that the complete treatment is considerably shorter, because the radiation is given during the time of surgery and the immediate week or so thereafter. The treatment necessitates detailed planning and exceptionally close cooperation between the surgeon and the radiation therapist, but the results achieved with brachytherapy in this study are comparable to the best reports of treatment using external-beam radiation therapy.

Technical Aspects of Radiation Therapy

The most commonly employed technique in the treatment of soft tissue sarcomas is the combined use of surgery and postoperative radiation therapy. This approach mandates an adequate resection of all gross disease. A shell-out procedure, which involves the excision of the tumor around its pseudocapsule, is suboptimal. Giuliano and Eilber documented persistent macroscopic tumor in approximately 50% of the patients at the time of reexcision of previous shell-out operative sites.[323] A planned reexcision of the operative sites should always be performed if the initial excision is deemed inadequate.

Radiation portals should be designed to treat muscle groups from origin to insertion to encompass the entire fascial plane, which may be potentially contaminated by tumor cells within postoperative hematomas.[324] Whether this is better than a 5- to 10-cm margin around the tumor bed is unknown. For the occasional tumor involving a subcutaneous primary location without muscle involvement, an 8- to 10-cm margin around the initial tumor volume should be employed. If preoperative radiation therapy is used, an 8- to 10-cm margin around the tumor mass in all dimensions should be obtained.

For primary tumors of the extremities, the only contraindications to limb-sparing surgery and radiation therapy are lesions that are so extensive that negative margins cannot be obtained; gross invasion of a joint; extensive involvement of several compartments of the extremity; or invasion of major neurovascular or bony structures beyond the scope of grafting or reconstruction.

Radiation therapy is often planned postoperatively after wound healing. It is essential to establish the extent of disease as seen by the surgeons who carried out the surgery and the apparent site of origin, possible residual tumor, tumor spillage, or hemorrhage. Ideally, the radiation therapist should directly observe the surgery.

In planning radiation therapy, it is essential to simulate the patient in a treatment position. The extremity is immobilized in a reproducible position at the time of simulation. A cast is usually necessary to immobilize the extremity in the same position each day with respect to the table top (Fig. 42–13). If large fields are needed, the patient should not be turned, because rotation of an extremity around a major joint may occur in more than one plane. If very long fields are required, treat isocentrically with pairs of matching fields, using a shifting match-line technique or the match-line wedge technique.[325] The match-line wedge technique allows shifting the angle of obliquity in such a way that matching may occur in different planes, and this can be an advantage in designing radiation fields that correspond to an anatomic compartment. The match-line wedge technique has some theoretical advantage over shifting the match line 1 cm every 1000 cGy, as is commonly done.

Every attempt is made to define the tumor volume to optimize the radiation portals (Figs. 42–14 and 42–15). Customized, individually shaped blocks are cut out for each patient to optimize the tumor volume, and the process adds secondary collimation beyond what a linear accelerator itself can offer. Generous use of clips placed at the time of surgery to define the extent of resection allow the therapist to see at simulation where the surgeon has been, and in many instances, the clips enable planning of oblique fields, which spare unmanipulated tissues but incorporate tissues that were handled at surgery. It is often surprising to see how far beyond the surgical scar some of the clips may appear. At the time of simulation, the scar is marked with wire to visualize on simulator films how the scar will be treated within the radiation field. If the radiation port strikes the scar perpendicularly, rather than tangentially, tissue-equivalent bolus material should be applied superficially to increase the dose to the scar. This ensures that the skin-sparing effects of high-energy x-rays, applied perpendicularly to the skin, do not work to the patient's disadvantage by underdosing the scar itself.

An attempt is made to spare at least 33% of the circumference of the extremity from the direct radiation field to optimize function and minimize lymphedema. Every effort is made to exclude joints from the radiation field if the surgery permits. If the scar crosses the joint, at least some of the joint is blocked out, unless the joint was entered surgically. Active involvement of the physical therapist with the patient is essential from the beginning to motivate the patient. This is essential to maximize the function of the extremity, muscles, and joints.

Postoperative tumor doses of 6300 cGy at 180 cGy per day are recommended. If there is gross residual disease, an increase in the total dose to approximately 7000 to 7500 cGy can be achieved using shrinking-field techniques to minimize the volume receiving the highest dose. The first volume reduction is made at 4500 cGy, and if a second volume reduction is needed, it can be made at 6300 cGy.

Lesions of the hand and foot are frequently able to be treated with conservative surgery and radiation therapy with excellent functional results.[326] The radiation therapy must be planned carefully, and it frequently necessitates high-energy electrons for at least part of the treatment. Similar principles apply to sarcomas of the head and neck region.

Lesions of the chest or abdominal wall can frequently be treated with high doses of radiation therapy postoperatively using a combination of x-rays and electrons. Doses range from 6000 to 7000 cGy or even higher, depending on the volume and location of the tumor. For retroperitoneal sarcomas, dose limitations usually reflect the tolerance of the small bowel and kidney. Doses in excess of 5500 cGy carry a considerable risk of small bowel injury.

For patients who receive preoperative radiation therapy, a dose of 4500 to 5000 cGy is recommended, at the rate of 180 cGy each day. Additional boosts may be given, intraoperatively or postoperatively, depending on the surgical findings and pathologic margins. The total dose for these patients can reach 7000 cGy.

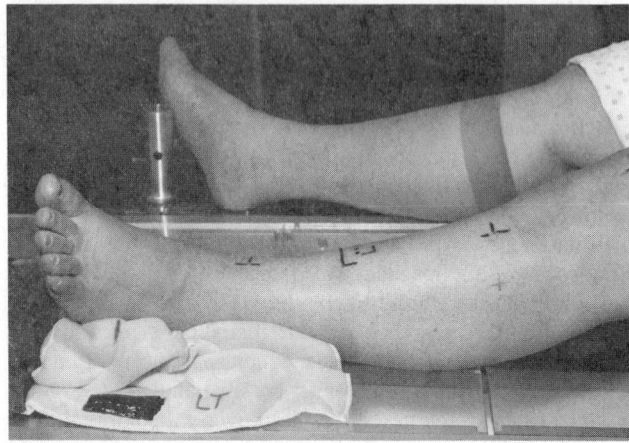

A

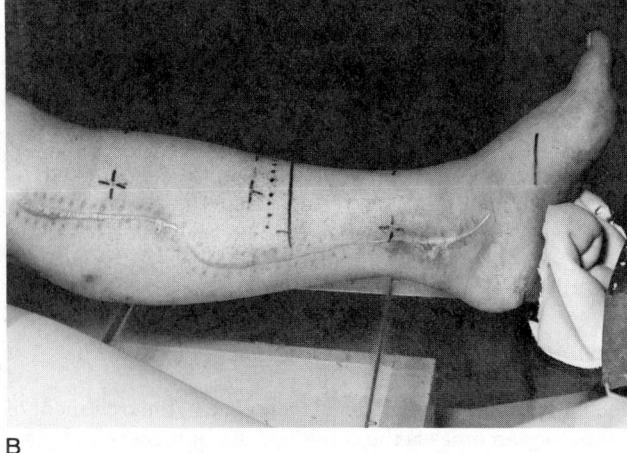

B

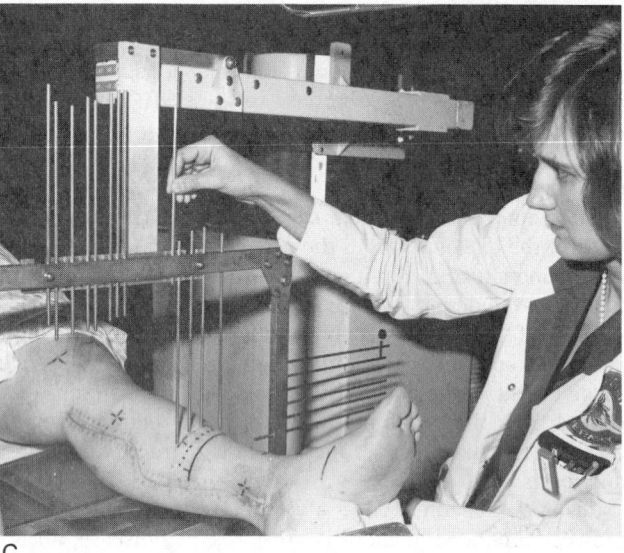

C

FIGURE 42–13. **(A)** Patient with a sarcoma of the left leg. A cast was individually molded to surround her foot and ankle such that the foot will always be in exactly the same position for each day's treatment. This is done at the time of simulation, which is a mock-up procedure during which the positioning and measurements required for treatment are determined, although treatment is not actually carried out. Diagnostic x-ray films are taken that mimic exactly what will be done with the megavoltage x-ray beam. **(B)** Medial view of the left leg. The scar can be seen, and several reference points have been marked on the skin. The cast and its relation to supporting the foot can be seen. **(C)** After positioning, it is important to determine the contour of what is being irradiated. Because the tissues vary in their thickness at any one level and because radiation is continuously attenuating as it transverses tissue, the thickness of the tissue at different levels in the radiation field will result in differing doses. To know what the discrepancies are, contours are taken at various levels. In this view, a mechanical device is being used to outline the contour at various levels in differing directions. After the contours have been determined, dose calculations can be made for the various levels that have been determined.

Intraarterial Chemotherapy, Radiation Therapy, and Surgery

Eilber and associates reported their extensive experience with preoperative intraarterial doxorubicin (Adriamycin) and radiation therapy for sarcomas of the extremity.[327] The rationale for this approach is to deliver regionally an active chemotherapeutic agent that has direct cytotoxic and potentially radiosensitizing effects on the tumor. In their early experience, intraarterial doxorubicin was given at 30 mg/day over 24 hours for 3 consecutive days. On the following day, radiation therapy was started, and 350-cGy fractions were administered daily for 10 days for a total dose of 3500 cGy. At 1 to 2 weeks after completion of irradiation, an en bloc resection of all gross disease was performed.

A total of 77 patients with high-grade extremity sarcomas were treated, and 74 (96%) were able to have limb-salvage surgery. Local tumor recurrence was noticed in only 3 (4%) patients. However, complications occurred in 25 (35%), with 14 (17%) requiring a second operative procedure. These complications consisted mainly of bone fractures and wound slough. Because of this high complication rate, the preoperative radiation therapy regimen was reduced to 1750 cGy in

five fractions. An additional 105 patients were treated with this regimen, and 102 (97%) were able to undergo limb-salvage surgery. Complications were reduced, with reoperation required in 6 (6%) patients. Local recurrences were seen in 9 (8%) patients. With this combined preoperative regimen, more than 96% of the patients with high-grade extremity tumors were able to have nonamputative surgery with acceptable local control.

Denton and colleagues at the University of Alabama reported a local recurrence rate of 3% for 30 patients with soft tissue and bony extremity sarcomas using a similar regimen. The mean follow-up was only 22 months.[328] Results achieved with this approach are comparable to standard multimodality approaches; however, no comparative randomized trials have been performed. Lokich reported the use of preoperative systemic chemotherapy in combination with radiation therapy in 3 patients with bulky soft tissue sarcomas and noticed marked tumor regression in 2 patients.[329]

Other investigators used regional arterial chemotherapy alone or in conjunction with hyperthermic perfusion as a preoperative adjunct or as primary therapy for unresectable tumors.[330–332] The advantages of regional chemotherapy in these approaches have not been definitively demonstrated. Didolkar

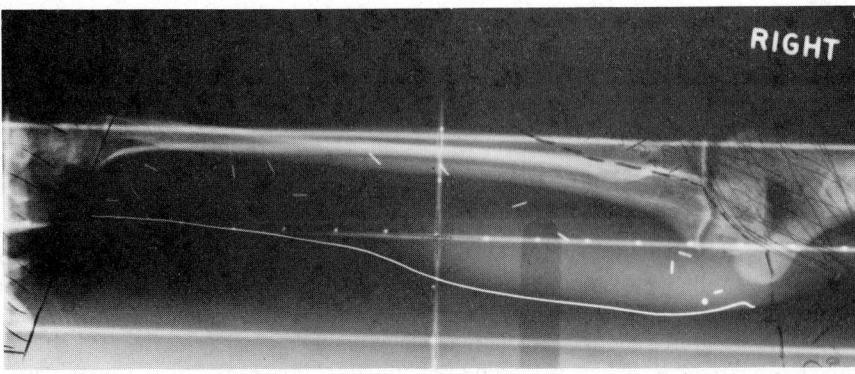

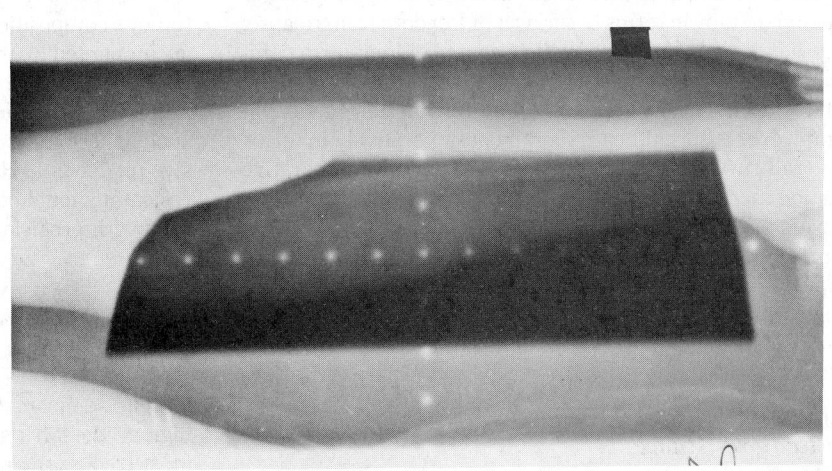

FIGURE 42–14. **(A)** On a different patient, a simulation process is demonstrated. Metallic clips have been placed throughout the course of the surgeon's exploration to show exactly where the surgeon has been. A piece of wire corresponds to the forearm of this particular patient, showing where the scar is in relation to the treatment field. It occurs right at the edge of the tissue being treated. The crossmark represents the center of the radiation field, which is situated in the middle of the soft tissue of the forearm itself. The forearm has been positioned carefully in such a way that the radius and ulna superimpose on the same plane. One edge of the radiation field corresponds to the bony structures themselves, leaving soft tissue above that line which is outside the radiation field. A dotted line represents a customized block that is cut to protect approximately half of the elbow joint, keeping it outside the high-dose radiation volume. **(B)** Port film on the same patient taken with 4 MeV x-rays in the treatment position. This image matches the simulator film seen in **A.**

and colleagues reported that intraarterial doxorubicin achieved similar regional tissue levels as intravenously administered drug in animals.[333] It is difficult to assess the efficacy of preoperative intraarterial chemotherapy from any of these studies.

Fast-Neutron Therapy

At least two reports have emerged on the treatment of locally advanced sarcomas treated with fast-neutron therapy. Salinas and coworkers from the M.D. Anderson Cancer Center reported 20 (69%) of 29 patients with advanced soft tissue sarcomas who achieved local control of their tumors with fast-neutron therapy.[334] Four patients developed complications. Pelton and colleagues from the University of Washington reported that 16 patients with unresectable soft tissue sarcomas were treated with fast neutrons, including 11 who had no evidence of metastatic disease and who were treated with curative intent.[335] These patients received a mixture of neutrons and photons. Local control was achieved in approximately 60%, with no relapses seen after 30 months. Only 4 patients, however, were alive without evidence of disease. A common complication of treatment was severe subcutaneous fibrosis, which in 2 patients necessitated skin grafts. One patient who received abdominal radiation for retroperitoneal sarcomas developed a small bowel obstruction thought to be related to radiation enteritis and fibrosis.

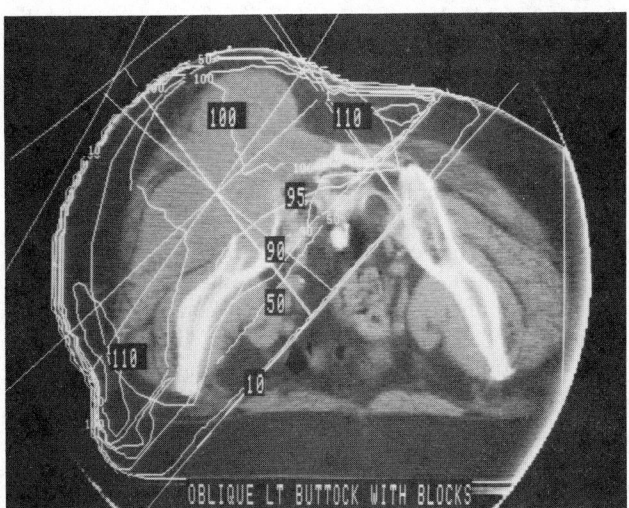

FIGURE 42–15. CT cut for a patient with a large buttock sarcoma. The patient is prone, and the extensive soft tissue mass, which could not be resected, is seen. The patient is being treated with oblique fields designed to treat the entire ilium on the right and as the soft tissue mass. The fields are wedged to account for the contour of the buttock itself, and the fields are slightly offset, so that the 50% isodose lines from each field direction coincide within the pelvis. The numbers represent different isodose curves on this particular slice (one of many sequential cuts), and they relate closely to the soft tissue mass itself. The intention is to take this entire volume to a dose of approximately 7500 cGy. In this case, treatment was carried out twice daily.

Although neutron therapy is still investigational in this country, fast-neutron therapy for patients with inoperable soft tissue sarcomas appears to offer a reasonable chance of local control and potential long-term survival, but its precise role must still be defined.

Intraoperative Radiation Therapy

Intraoperative radiation therapy is used at the time of surgery and permits a high single dose of electron-beam therapy to be delivered directly to the tumor bed, after moving as many incidental structures out of the radiation field as possible. For soft tissue sarcomas, its use has been predominantly for primary tumors in the retroperitoneum; it has not shown any significant benefit over conventional surgery and postoperative radiation therapy in terms of survival or freedom from relapse. Large single doses are potentially a source of long-term complications for ureters and nerves. In a randomized study, the NCI was unable to show the benefit of intraoperative radiation therapy over external-beam therapy postoperatively in terms of overall survival or disease-free survival.[291] Intraoperative radiation therapy was able to reduce the frequency of radiation enteritis in these patients.

Similar data were reported from Massachusetts General Hospital.[336] Because many of these patients developed sarcomatosis of the peritoneum, intraoperative radiation therapy remains investigational.

Radiation Sensitizers, Radiosensitivity, and Radioresistance

For most sarcomas, complete surgical resection is recommended if it can be accomplished without excessive morbidity. If a patient has a sarcoma that is not amenable to resection, it is still possible that radiation therapy alone can control the local disease.

Although radiation therapy may be rejected for treating soft tissue or bony sarcomas because the tumor is thought to be "radioresistant," data demonstrate that this concept is fallacious. Tepper and Suit reported a series of 35 patients who had soft tissue sarcomas that were treated with doses of 6500 cGy or more (see Table 42–25).[296] For lesions smaller than 5 cm, 7 of 8 achieved local control. For lesions between 5 and 10 cm, 9 of 17 achieved local control. For lesions larger than 10 cm, only 3 of 10 achieved local control.

Kinsella and Glatstein from NCI reported a series using a variety of intravenous radiosensitizers in the management of unresectable soft tissue and bony sarcomas.[337] Most tumors were larger than 10 cm; the median size was 14×14 cm. Local control (*i.e.,* freedom from all symptoms and no further growth) was achieved for at least a year in 22 of 29 patients who had extensive disease. Many tumors were radiosensitive but not radioresponsive. Radiosensitive refers to specific parameters (*e.g.,* D_o, D_q, or n) that are obtained from in vitro cell survival curves. Whether the tumor is sensitive or resistant depends on the exact quantitative parameters derived from such studies. Often a tumor is called radioresistant, but the tumor is really radio-unresponsive, because the tumor does not demonstrate any decrease in size (exactly how much is unspecified) seen relatively quickly (also unspecified) after some modest doses of radiation therapy (also unspecified).

The concept of radioresponsiveness of tumors is 40 years old and was useful for differentiating tumors that shrank quickly, such as lymphomas or seminomas, from those that did not. In their review of 29 patients with massive sarcomas treated with hypoxic cell sensitizers or halogenated pyrimidines, the NCI reported patients in whom all the cells were destroyed pathologically, but in whom the mass never regressed. In some instances, the patients survived more than 5 years without any growth of tumor after irradiation.

The role of radiation sensitizers in the management of these tumors is an area of active investigation. The important point is that all the tumor cells can apparently be destroyed, even if the mass does not necessarily regress. A significant component of a sarcomatous mass may be represented by the matrix of stroma of the tumor. Depending on the extent of a tumor's composition, the death of tumor cells is not necessarily accompanied by measurable regression. Some sarcomas can be radiosensitive, but not necessarily radioresponsive. Examples of this phenomenon have been seen in other tumors, such as testicular cancer treated with chemotherapy or massive mediastinal Hodgkin's disease. Radiosensitive and radioresistant should be defined carefully, and the words must be used with precision.

CHEMOTHERAPY

Adjuvant Chemotherapy

Despite adequate local treatment, almost half of patients with high-grade soft tissue sarcomas develop metastatic disease, most frequently in the lungs. This led to intensive efforts to identify adjuvant chemotherapy regimens that can prevent metastatic spread. The studies must be carefully designed to address sarcomas of a specific grade and location and to balance factors such as size and margin status. Due to the scarcity of these tumors, studies of adequate size to detect or exclude a significant benefit of adjuvant chemotherapy are few and somewhat conflicting.

Several nonrandomized trials suggesting an improved outcome with adjuvant chemotherapy used similar agents, including doxorubicin, DTIC, vinca alkaloids, and high-dose methotrexate. Cyclophosphamide was shown to have activity against metastatic sarcoma. The results of combinations of these agents have been reported from prospective, randomized trials of adjuvant therapy for high-grade soft tissue sarcomas of the extremities, head, neck, and trunk. Due to the low risk of metastatic disease in patients with grade 1 lesions, the trials should be confined to lesions of higher grade. Because the prognosis (and possibly the efficacy of adjuvant chemotherapy) for lesions of the extremities differs from that of sarcomas in nonextremity locations, clinical trials should consider these groups separately.

There have been 11 reported prospective, randomized trials of adjuvant chemotherapy for soft-tissue sarcoma.[316,317,338-354] Five combined extremity and nonextremity tumors, but they included data analysis by tumor location.[316,317,342,349,350] Four included only patients with extremity tumors, and two studied only nonextremity tumors.[345,351-355] Data on extremity sarcomas could be obtained from nine trials, and nonextremity tumors were analyzed in seven trials as shown in Table 42–28. Of the results confined to extremity tumors, three studies

TABLE 42–28. Adjuvant Chemotherapy for Sarcoma: Randomized Studies

Investigations*	No. of Patients	Tumor Grades	Chemotherapy Agents†	Median Follow-up (mo)	Disease-free Survival (%)‡		Overall Survival (%)‡	
					No CTX	+CTX	No CTX	+CTX
Extremity								
Alvegard[349] (SSG 1989)	155	2, 3	Dx	40	NR	NR	NR	NR
Antman[350] (DFCI/MGH, ECOG, ISSG 1990)	101	1–3	Dx	54	64	78	67	79
Benjamin[351] (MDA 1987)	46	2, 3	DxVCA	>120	35	(55)§	57	65§
Bramwell[316] (EORTC 1988)	223	1–3	DxVCDt	36	66	77‖	74	81‖
Chang[355] (NCI 1988)	67	2, 3	DxC	85	54	(75)	60	82
Edmunson[342] (Mayo 1984)	48	1–3	DxVCDtA	64	67	86	82	88
Eilber[352] (UCLA 1987)	119	3	Dx	36	58	58‖	75	78‖
Picci[345] (Rizzoli 1988)	77	2, 3	Dx	42	42	(68)¶	68	(88)¶
Ravaud[317] (Bergonie 1990)	36	2, 3	DxVCDt	52	NR	(NR)	NR	(NR)
Nonextremity								
Alvegard[349] (SSG 1989)	26	2, 3	Dx	40	NR	NR	NR	NR
Antman[350] (DFCI/MGH, ECOG, ISSG 1990)	67	1–3	Dx	54	47	53	52	54
Bramwell[316] (EORTC 1988)	125	1–3	DxVCDt	36	50	63‖	71	81‖
Edmunson[342] (Mayo 1984)	13	1–3	DxVCDtA	64	NR	NR	NR	NR
Omura[353] (GOG 1985)	156	NR	Dx	60	45	60	47	60
Ravaud[317] (Bergonie 1990)	23	2, 3	DxVCDt	52	NR	NR	NR	NR
Yang[354] (NCI 1992)	81	2, 3	DxC	59	57	59	65	63

* SSG, Scandinavian Sarcoma Group; DFCI, Dana-Farber Cancer Institute; MGH, Massachusetts General Hospital; ECOG, Eastern Cooperative Oncology Group; ISSG, Intergroup Sarcoma Study Group; MDA, M.D. Anderson Cancer Center; EORTC, European Organization for Research on Treatment of Cancer; NCI, National Cancer Institute; Mayo, Mayo Clinic; UCLA, University of California, Los Angeles; Rizzoli, Istituto Ortopedico Rizzoli, Bologna; Bergonie, Fondation Bergonie, Bordeaux; GOG, Gynecologic Oncology Group. Year of last update is in parnetheses.
† Dx, doxorubicin; V, vincristine; C, cyclophosphamide; A, dactinomycin; Dt, DTIC.
‡ Survival values are estimated 5-year actuarial values (taken from text or published survival curves) unless otherwise noted. Parenthetic values are significantly greater than randomized comparison group, $p \leq 0.05$. All other differences are not significant. CTX, chemotherapy; NR, not reported.
§ Estimated 10-year actuarial survival rates.
‖ Survival rates at last available patient follow-up.
¶ Estimated 4-year actuarial survival rates.

showed a significant survival advantage for doxorubicin-based chemotherapy.[317,345,346] A third study of 67 patients with extremity lesions at the NCI showed a significant overall survival benefit at 5-year follow-up, but due to a few late deaths, the difference was not significant with 9-year median follow-up.[355] The other six studies did not show significant survival differences with the use of adjuvant chemotherapy. Of eight studies with disease-free survival values presented, seven showed superior results with chemotherapy, but only four were statistically significant. Several studies showed a significant impact of chemotherapy on the incidence of local recurrence.[316,317,339,351]

Many of these studies have limited power to detect a difference, and several are open to criticism on methodologic grounds. In two studies, patients received some preoperative chemotherapy before randomization and then were randomized to stop or continue this chemotherapy.[345–347,352] In one trial that showed no effect of chemotherapy, only 75% of randomized patients were eligible, and of those eligible and randomized to chemotherapy, approximately two thirds received 85% or less of the planned chemotherapy dose.[349] Many trials

included patients with low-grade tumors that are unlikely to be chemotherapy responsive.

In some studies, clinically evident doxorubicin cardiotoxicity occurred in as many as 10% of patients (with subclinical or clinical findings in as many as half of patients), and this may have offset any overall survival benefit of adjuvant chemotherapy.[356] In one NCI study, a lower-dose, less toxic doxorubicin regimen was compared with the NCI regimen with demonstrated benefit and was shown to be equally effective.[355,357]

Studies confined to lesions of the head, neck, trunk, and retroperitoneum have uniformly failed to show any statistically significant benefit from a variety of adjuvant regimens, although many are limited by small patient numbers. In the most recent NCI study, the estimated 5-year survival of 88 patients with high-grade tumors randomized to receive or not receive postoperative doxorubicin and cyclophosphamide were 63% and 65%, respectively. Disease-free survival was also similar (59% and 57%).[354]

The use of adjuvant chemotherapy for primary high-grade

adult soft tissue sarcomas remains experimental. Although existing data suggest that there may be an improvement in disease-free survival, this difference is only significant in a few studies and seems confined to sarcomas of the extremities. Many studies continue to include low-grade lesions with high-grade tumors, a practice that can only obfuscate any possible benefit of chemotherapy. Studies showing a survival benefit to adjuvant chemotherapy for node-positive breast cancer and Dukes' stage C colon cancer required many hundreds of randomized patients to attain statistical significance. The existing literature on soft tissue sarcomas can neither prove or exclude a benefit from adjuvant chemotherapy.

TREATMENT OF RECURRENT OR METASTATIC SARCOMAS

Potter and associates reviewed the initial sites of tumor recurrence after primary treatment of soft tissue sarcomas in 307 patients referred to the NCI.[44] These patients underwent complete surgical resection, often in combination with postoperative chemotherapy and radiation therapy. A total of 107 (35%) patients had local recurrences or developed distant metastases; the sites of disease are identified in Table 42–14. The lung was the predominant site of first recurrence in 52% of these patients, followed by isolated local recurrences (20%). The pattern of recurrence depended on the primary site of the sarcoma. Patients with sarcomas of the head and neck, retroperitoneum, and chest or abdominal wall had a higher local recurrence rate than those with extremity sites. In the American College of Surgeons survey, there were 452 (37%) of 1209 treatment failures in patients without metastases at the initial diagnoses who had total gross resections of their soft tissue sarcomas.[46] Among patients with recurrent disease, 236 (52%) had isolated locoregional recurrences, and 83 (18%) had isolated lung recurrences. Approximately 80% of all recurrences became evident within 5 years.

Aggressive surgical management of isolated local recurrences should be attempted. A thorough evaluation for evidence of disseminated disease must be performed before contemplating resection of a local recurrence. In the NCI experience, 20 (96%) of 21 isolated local recurrences were surgically resectable. Figure 42–16 shows the actuarial continuous disease-free and overall survival of patients who were rendered free of disease after resection of a local recurrence. The 3-year survival was 69%. Shiu and associates were able to resect 35 (81%) of 43 isolated locally recurrent extremity sarcomas, with a subsequent 5-year survival rate of 45%.[59] Giuliano and coworkers reported that 35 (92%) of 38 patients surgically rendered free of a local recurrence of an extremity or truncal (excluding retroperitoneal) sarcoma had a 5-year actuarial survival rate of 87%.[358] In the American College of Surgeons survey, the 5-year survival rate after salvage therapy of isolated local failures was 61%.[46]

Metastasectomy for isolated pulmonary recurrences is clearly warranted. Patients who are found to have pulmonary metastases by plain chest x-ray film or chest CT scans should have a thorough evaluation for extrapulmonary tumor, particularly in the primary site, to determine operability. For extremity and truncal sarcoma patients, this can be accomplished by physical examination and CT or MR scans of the

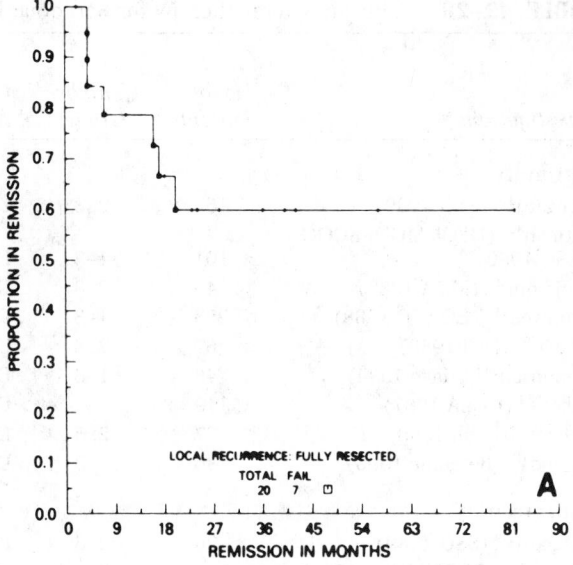

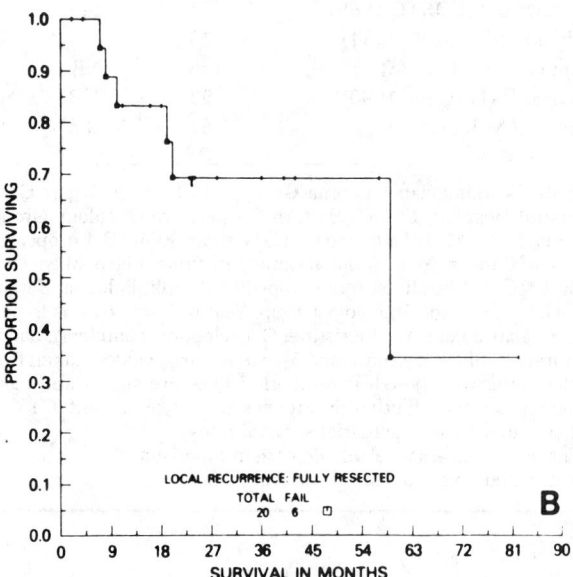

FIGURE 42–16. **(A)** Disease-free survival and **(B)** overall survival in patients with high-grade sarcomas who underwent resection of isolated locally recurrent disease. (Potter DA, Glenn J, Kinsella T, et al. Patterns of recurrence in patients with high-grade soft tissue sarcomas. J Clin Oncol 1985;3:353–366)

primary site. For patients with retroperitoneal sarcomas, an evaluation of the liver should be performed to detect metastases. Patients with extrapulmonary tumors are not candidates for pulmonary resection. In Potter's analysis of NCI patients, 40 (72%) of 56 patients with isolated pulmonary metastases were rendered free of disease after surgery, which resulted in an actuarial 3-year survival rate of 38% (Fig. 42–17).

Pass, Roth, and colleagues reported that the number of metastatic nodules (≤6) seen on preoperative CT scan, the disease-free interval (>1 year), and tumor doubling time (≥20 days) significantly correlated with survival in soft tissue sarcoma patients undergoing their first pulmonary metastasectomy.[359,360] Nevertheless, there were long-term survivors with

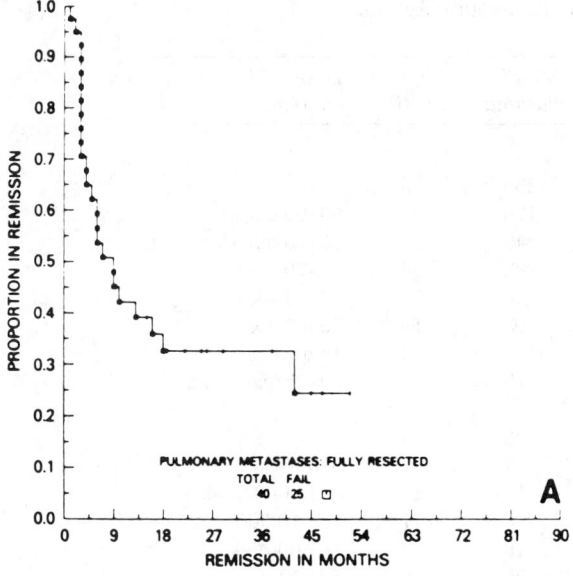

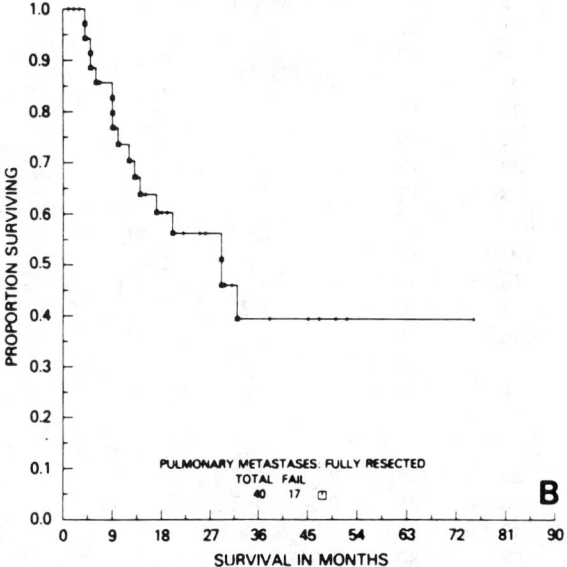

FIGURE 42–17. **(A)** Disease-free survival and **(B)** overall survival in patients with high-grade sarcomas who underwent resection of isolated pulmonary metastases. (Potter DA, Glenn J, Kinsella T, et al. Patterns of recurrence in patients with high-grade soft tissue sarcomas. J Clin Oncol 1985;3:353–366)

poor prognostic parameters, and no single criterion was sufficient to exclude attempted resection. In the American College of Surgeons survey, the 5-year survival rate after pulmonary metastasectomy was 21%.[46] Resection of recurrent pulmonary metastases can result in survival benefit. In the NCI experience, 29 patients had two or more resections for pulmonary metastases, resulting in a 22% 3-year actuarial survival rate after the second thoracotomy.[361] There have been no operative deaths after 254 pulmonary resections for metastases at the NCI since 1978. Because of the minimal morbidity and potential survival benefit of pulmonary metastasectomy, patients treated for primary soft tissue sarcomas should be closely monitored for development of pulmonary

metastases at least every 6 months with lung tomograms or chest CT for 3 years after resection of the primary tumor.[362]

CHEMOTHERAPY FOR DISSEMINATED SOFT TISSUE SARCOMAS

Soft tissue sarcomas constitute a heterogenous class of neoplasms with divergent response rates to available chemotherapy. Regimens including vincristine, dactinomycin, and cyclophosphamide result in response rates of 80% or more in previously untreated embryonal and alveolar rhabdomyosarcoma, and combination chemotherapy is now established in the primary treatment of these lesions. Of the classic adult soft tissue sarcomas, malignant fibrous histiocytoma and synovial sarcomas have the highest response rates to doxorubicin-based combination chemotherapy. The lowest response rates are observed in angiosarcomas, extraskeletal chondrosarcomas, and leiomyosarcomas of gastrointestinal origin. Mesotheliomas and Kaposi's sarcoma differ from the classic soft tissue sarcomas and are not discussed in this section.

Widely divergent response rates for a given drug or combination reflect the mix of histologies included on the trial, dose and schedule of administration, prior therapy, and biases introduced by the small numbers of patients in some studies. Publication bias (*i.e.*, negative studies are rarely reported) probably also plays a role, particularly in nonrandomized studies.

Single-Agent Chemotherapy

Commercially Available Agents

Table 42–29 summarizes the activity of various single agents in soft tissue sarcoma. Single-agent doxorubicin, the most active commercially available single agent, had a response rate of 15% to 35% in various studies.[363–368] A dose-response association has been observed in nonrandomized trials and in combination with other agents in randomized trials, with dose rates of 60 to 70 mg/m^2 every 3 weeks superior to dose rates of 50 mg/m^2 or less every 3 weeks.[364–366,404] Doxorubicin administered by continuous infusion over 4 days in combination regimens has been reported to be less cardiotoxic and equally effective as bolus dosing in some studies.[405–408]

Ifosfamide is a cyclophosphamide analog with one chloroethyl group shifted to the ring nitrogen atom. Preclinical and human phase I and II trials for sarcomas, lymphoma, and small cell lung cancer have shown an apparent lack of cross-resistance with cyclophosphamide.[409–412] Ifosfamide has activity in patients with sarcoma who have failed doxorubicin-containing regimens.[385,391–393,413–415] A European Organization for Research and Treatment of Cancer (EORTC) study showed ifosfamide at 5 g/m^2 to be somewhat superior to cyclophosphamide at 1.5 g/m^2 as single-agent treatment of advanced sarcoma and resulted in less myelotoxicity.[393] The production of acrolein from ifosfamide and the resulting cystitis requires the use of the urothelial protective agent mesna (sodium-2-mecapto-ethane-sulfonate). Mesna has been shown to be superior to N-acetylcystein in preventing hematuria in a randomized trial of sarcoma patients receiving ifosfamide.[416]

DTIC has a single-agent response rate of 18% and is particularly active in leiomyosarcomas. Nausea associated with its administration may be decreased by administration as a continuous infusion.[394]

TABLE 42–29. Commercially Available Chemotherapeutic Agents for Soft Tissue Sarcoma by Class

Investigations	Drug	No. of Patients	% RR*	Dose (mg/m²)
	Anthracyclines			
Total	Doxorubicin	356	26	
Blum[363]		130	34	60–90 q 3 wk
O'Bryan et al[364]		49	31	60–75 q 3 wk
O'Bryan et al[365]		82	28	25–70 q 3 wk
Schoenfeld[366]		66	27	70 q 3 wk
Borden et al[367]		93	19	70 q 3 wk
Borden et al[367]		92	16	15 q wk
Cruz et al[368]		15	13	20–25/day × 3 q wk
	Antimetabolites			
Total	Methotrexate, high-dose	76	13	
Rosen et al[369]		1	1/1	8000/wk
Vaughan et al[370]		14	14	5–12,000/2 wk
Isacoff and Eilber[371]		6	17	1.5–10,000
Karakousis et al[372]		18	5	2–4,000/wk
Von Hoff et al[373]		26	20	>1000
Frei et al[374]		9	0/9	2–10,000/1–4 wk
Total	Methotrexate, standard-dose	81	21	
Andrews[375]		19	10	
Subramanian[376]		41	37	
Buesa[377]		21	0	
Amato[378]	Bleomycin	32	6	
Golbey[379]	Dactinomycin	30	17	
Gold[380]	5-Fluorouracil	8	12	
	Vincas			
Total	Vincristine	103	12	
Selawry[381]		15	40	
Korbitz[382]		7	0	
Total	Etoposide	40	8	
Radice[383]		34	6	
Bleyer[384]		6	16	
	Alkylating agents			
	Ifosfamide†			
Elias[385,386]	High dose	20	35	2.0–4.5 × 4 d
Klein[387]		8	38	2.5–3.5 × 5 d
Czownicki[389]		13	38	1.25–2.5 × 5 d
Niederle[390]		57	30	1.6–3.0 × 5 d
Antman[391]		124	23	2.0–2.5 × 4 d
Wiltshaw[392]	Standard dose	42	38	5.0–8.0 × 1 d
Bramwell[393]		68	18	5.0 × 1 d
Buesa[394]	Dacarbazine (DTIC)	44	18	
Total	Cisplatin	103	12	
Bramwell[395]		17	0	
Karakousis[396]		13	23	
Samson[397]		42	7	
Thigpen[398]		19	5	
Budd[399]		40	15	200 mg/m²
Gershenson[400]		12	42	GYN only
Goldstein[401]	Carboplatin	50	12	
Total	Cyclophosphamide	82	8	
Bergsagel[402]		12	16	
Korst[403]		3	0	
Bramwell[393]		67	8	

* % RR percent response when the denominator includes at least 10 cases.
† In adults by dose per course.

TABLE 42–30. Investigational Chemotherapeutic Agents for Soft Tissue Sarcomas by Class

Drug	References	No. of Patients Evaluable	% Responding
Anthracyclines			
Carminomycin	417	48	27
Azotomycin	418, 419	28	18
AMSA	420–423	9	11
Iclarubicin	424	23	4
Diaziquone (AZQ)	425, 427	108	2
Mitoxantrone	428, 429	115	1
Menogaril	430	21	5
Esorubicin	431	14	7
Epirubicin	432	32	19
Echinomycin	433	34	0
Antimetabolites			
Trimetrexate	434, 435	36	8
Cycloleucine	436–438	118	11
Chlorozotocin	439–445	160	4
Cytembena	446, 447	24	4
PALA/5 fluorouracil	448, 449	23	0
PALA/dipyridamole	450, 451	46	11
Baker's Antifol	452, 453	30	0
Alkylating Agents			
Methyl-CCNU	454, 455	85	6
Hexamethylmelamine	456–458	88	5
Dibromodulcitol	459, 460	34	3
Dianhydrogalacitol	461	28	0
Gallium nitrate	462	31	0
Vinca & Related Compounds			
VM-26	463	33	3
Vindesine	464, 465	3	0
Miscellaneous			
DDMP	466	15	7
Piperazinedione	467–469	22	5
ICRF 159	460	29	5
MGBG	378, 470	54	2
Pyazofurin	470–472	47	0
Maytansine	460, 473	44	0
Bruceantin	460, 473	34	0
Homoharingtonin	474	16	0
Biologicals			
Tumor necrosis factor	475	16	0
Tumor necrosis factor	476	1	0
Interferon-α	477	16	0
Interferon-β	478	20	1
Interleukin-2	479	6	0

Investigational Agents

The studies of single investigational agents in the treatment of advanced sarcoma are shown in Table 42–30. Currently, there are no consistent data to recommend a particular agent without further study.[417–479]

Combination Chemotherapy

Randomized Studies

Most large randomized cooperative group studies have reported response rates of 17% to 30% (Table 42–31). The median survival in these trials is in the range of 12 months, with no significant differences in survival observed. This lack of effect on survival despite differences in response rates probably results from several factors: high response rates (often >50%) are required to impact on survival in patients with advanced disease, many patients not responding to one treatment subsequently receive the other agent or regimen, and the 0.5 to 2 log decrease in tumor cell number represented by many partial or complete responses is often not significant in a patient with an advanced tumor burden of 10^9 to 10^{12} cells. Other endpoints for chemotherapy such as its ability to improve the results of surgery or radiation therapy given preoperatively in patients with bulky disease deserve further study.

The addition of DTIC to doxorubicin has been evaluated in three randomized trials. The Gynecologic Oncology Group (GOG) and the Eastern Cooperative Oncology Group (ECOG) evaluated doxorubicin as a single agent and with DTIC.[367,480–481] The response rate was higher for the combination in both studies, significantly in the ECOG study. In the third Southwest Oncology Group (SWOG) study patients received doxorubicin, cyclophosphamide, and vincristine with DTIC or dactinomycin. The DTIC-containing arm was significantly more active.[482]

SWOG, ECOG, and GOG studies evaluating the addition of cyclophosphamide to an doxorubicin-containing regimen showed no advantage for the addition of cyclophosphamide.[366,483,484] In the ECOG trial, after the dose of doxorubicin was decreased from 70 mg/m² to 50 mg/m² to avoid myelosuppression from cyclophosphamide, the response rate for doxorubicin at 70 mg/m² as a single agent was significantly higher than for the combination with the lower doxorubicin dose.[366]

The EORTC evaluated doxorubicin alone, doxorubicin with ifosfamide, and doxorubicin, cyclophosphamide, DTIC, and vincristine (CYVADIC regimen).[485] There was significantly more myelosuppression and a trend but no significant advantage in response rate or survival for the two combinations. An ECOG study comparing doxorubicin with or without ifosfamide observed a significant difference in response for the ifosfamide arm with a trend for longer survival in the ifosfamide arm.[486]

The SWOG/CALGB study of doxorubicin and DTIC alone compared with the addition of ifosfamide demonstrated response rates of 17% and 32%, respectively.[487] Although the response rate and duration of response were significantly improved for the three-drug arm, myelosuppression (including fatal sepsis) was also significantly worse. Median survival times were 13 and 12 months, respectively.

M.D. Anderson Cancer Center compared CYVADIC at high and intermediate doses, and the EORTC compared full-dose with alternating half-dose therapy.[488] Both studies correlated dose with response.[404]

Two studies randomized patients between different schedules of similar regimens. An adjuvant trial at Memorial Sloan-Kettering Cancer Center corroborated the decreased cardio-

TABLE 42–31. Randomized Chemotherapy Trials for Measurable Soft Tissue Sarcoma

Investigations	Group*	Regiment†	No. of Patients	% CR‡	% RR‡	Comments
Studies Comparing the Addition of DTIC						
Omura et al[480]	GOG	A	80	6	16	Uterine sarcoma only
		AD	66	11	24	
Lerner[481]	ECOG	A	34	3	18	
		AD	32	3	44	Leiomyosarcomas only
Borden et al[367]	ECOG	A q 3 wk	93	6	19	A 15 mg/m²/wk
		A q wk	92	4	16	A 70 mg/2 q 3 wk
		AD	95	6	30	
Benjamin et al[482]	SWOG	ACVD	221	14	52	
		ACVAd	224	12	40	
Studies Evaluating the Addition of Cyclophosphamide						
Schoenfeld et al[366]	ECOG	A	66	6	27	A 70 mg/m²
		ACV	70	4	19	A 50 mg/m²
		CVAd	64	2	11	A none
Baker et al[483]	SWOG	AD	79	14	32	
		ADC	95	13	35	
		ADAd	98	9	24	
Muss et al[484]	GOG	A	50	1	19	
		AC	54	2	20	
Studies Evaluating Vindesine						
Bordon et al[491]	ECOG	A Vindesine	149	4	17	
		A	149	6	18	
Studies Evaluating Dose and Schedule						
Zalupski et al[490]	SWOG	AD	135	7	19	Bolus
		AD	143	10	18	Continuous infusion
Casper et al[489]	MSKCC	A	32			Bolus
		A	39			Continuous infusion
Bodey et al[488]	SWOG	ADCV	27	15	67	A 50 mg/m² C 500 mg/m²
		ADCV	24	33	71	A 80 mg/m² C 800 mg/m²
Pinedo et al[404]	EORTC	ADC	71	20	38	Full dose rate
		AD-CV	74	5	14	Half dose rate
Studies Evaluating Ifosfamide						
Bramwell[393]	EORTC	I	68	2	18	5 g/m²
		C	67	1	8	1.5 g/m²
Antman[487]	ISSG	AD	170	2	17	
		ADI	166	4	32	Myelosuppression more severe
Santoro[485]	EORTC	A	212	4	24	
		AI	202	6	27	Myelosuppression more severe
		ACDV	135	8	28	Nausea vomiting more severe
Blum[486]	ECOG	A	87		20	
		AI	87		35	

* GOG, Gynecologic Oncology Group; ECOG, Eastern Cooperative Oncology Group; SWOG, Southwest Oncology Group; MSKCC, Memorial Sloan Kettering Cancer Center; EORTC, European Organization for Research and Treatment of Cancer; ISSG, Intergroup Sarcoma Study Group.
† A, doxorubicin; Ad, dactinomycin; C, cyclophosphamide; D, DTIC; I, ifosfamide; V, vincristine.
‡ CR, complete response; RR, response rate.

toxicity of continuous-infusion doxorubicin, but patients receiving the continuous infusion had a higher incidence of relapse.[489] A SWOG study compared bolus with continuous-infusion doxorubicin and DTIC. The response rate was identical, but the toxicity (particularly doxorubicin-associated cardiotoxicity and nausea and vomiting from DTIC) was substantially reduced with continuous infusion.[490]

The combination resulting in the highest response rates in soft tissue sarcomas is doxorubicin (60 mg/m^2) and ifosfamide (7.5 g/m^2) with or without DTIC (1 g/m^2). The doses of doxorubicin and DTIC should be given by continuous infusion over 4 days to decrease the risk of cardiotoxicity and the severity of nausea and vomiting. Ifosfamide should be divided and given daily over 3 days and with mesna for bladder protection. Physicians may choose single-agent doxorubicin or doxorubicin and DTIC for palliation for patients who may not tolerate the combination. Ifosfamide is currently the most active salvage agent for patients who have failed a doxorubicin-containing regimen.

Nonrandomized Studies

Nonrandomized, phase II combination chemotherapy trials are described in Table 42–32. Response rates in single-institution phase II trials are superior to similar regimens tested in randomized trials by cooperative groups. This may be due to smaller patient numbers, better patient selection, and higher dose delivery by single institutions. Small single-institution studies with poor results may be less reported. Nevertheless, these trials are helpful in estimating the range of responses for a regimen and in designing randomized trials.

Dose-Intensive Therapy

In laboratory models of sarcomas and other malignancies, the delivery of the highest possible doses of chemotherapy is essential to achieving curative therapy. Theory and experimental and clinical data suggest that sarcoma recurs despite an initial response to chemotherapy because of resistance to the chemotherapy drugs. In the laboratory, resistance to alkylating agents can often be overcome by using a five-fold to ten-fold higher dose.[544] There is ample evidence of a correlation between doxorubicin dose and tumor response from three randomized trials.[366,404,488]

Because the limiting toxicity of higher chemotherapy doses is myelosuppression, several investigators have used hematopoietic growth factors to allow delivery of the full dose on schedule.[517,545,546] Autotransplants have been used to ensure prompt marrow recovery after high doses of chemotherapy. Ewing's sarcoma, rhabdomyosarcoma, and osteosarcoma are optimal tumors for studies of the role of high-dose therapy based on their sensitivity at conventional chemotherapy doses.

Forty-three children with malignant soft tissue sarcomas were treated at the Royal Marsden Hospital in Sutton, England, with a rapid-dose-delivery schedule consisting six courses of vincristine, doxorubicin, and cyclophosphamide followed in 36 patients by high-dose melphalan with autologous bone marrow support. There was one toxic death due to infection and possible cardiomyopathy. Using International Society of Pediatric Oncology (SIOP) staging, there were 11 stage I pa-

tients, 13 stage II patients, 7 stage III patients, and 12 stage IV patients. The actuarial survival rate at 5 years was 57%, and the event-free survival rate was 44% for all stages. For patients with nonmetastatic diseases, the rates were 62% and 53%, respectively. This treatment strategy enables completion of all chemotherapy by 4 months. Radiation and surgery were conservative to minimize late sequelae.[547]

Of 95 patients with sarcoma collected in a review by Pinkerton for the European Bone Marrow Transplant Registry, 64 received high-dose therapy as consolidation after the first complete or partial response. About 20% maintained durable complete responses at more than 40 months. However, 35% of the 40 patients transplanted during complete remission were disease free.[548] At the Dana-Farber Cancer Institute, a high-dose ifosfamide, carboplatin, and etoposide regimen is being studied as consolidation therapy for patients with sarcomas responding to conventional-dose therapy.[385,386]

HORMONE THERAPY

Observing that a higher percentage of premenopausal than postmenopausal patients who developed uterine sarcomas survived for 5 years, some investigators have suggested that estrogen replacement may be efficacious in the treatment of postmenopausal women with sarcomas. Lantta and colleagues documented estradiol and progesterone receptors in two endometrial stromal sarcomas.[549] One of the patients responded to hormone treatment for 2 years. One endometrial stromal sarcoma responded to progesterone, and a second case of endometrial stromal sarcoma responded to medroxyprogesterone after failure of tamoxifen and combination chemotherapy.[550,551] However, of 29 patients with uterine sarcomas treated with 40 mg/day of tamoxifen in a Clinical Oncology Society of Australia study, 0 of 19 patients with leiomyosarcomas, none of 3 with endometrial stromal sarcomas, and 1 of 7 with malignant mixed müllerian tumors had objective responses.[552] Of 60 patients with uterine sarcomas, 48% and 30% were estrogen and progesterone receptor positive, respectively. Only 1 of 28 patients with recurrent disease had a response to hormonal therapy. Receptor status did not affect prognosis.[553]

THERAPY FOR BORDERLINE AND LOW-GRADE SARCOMAS

Desmoids are low-grade fibrosarcomas of the abdominal or chest wall, usually occurring in sites of prior trauma most frequently in women. Optimal treatment remains wide excision and radiation therapy. For recurrent and unresectable disease, tamoxifen has been used with some success.[554–556] Responses have been reported to chemotherapy regimens such as vinblastine (10 mg/week) and methotrexate (50 mg/week).[557] This regimen has produced responses in 2 of 2 patients with disabling fibromatosis and in 2 of 4 patients with neurofibromatosis.[557]

A 12-year-old boy with hemangiomatosis was reported to have normalization of his exercise tolerance, clubbing, pulmonary pressure-volume curve, and of the abnormal vascular pattern on pulmonary angiogram in response to interferon-2α.[558]

(text continues on page 1480)

TABLE 42–32. Nonrandomized Combination Chemotherapy in Untreated Sarcomas

Combination*	Investigations	Institute†	No. of Patients Evaluable	% CR‡
Doxorubicin-based Combinations				
AD	Total		732	9
	Gottlieb[492]	SWOG	100	5
	Baker[483]	SWOG	79	15
	Borden[367]	ECOG	95	6
	Omura[480]	GOG	66	11
	Saiki[493]	SWOG	114	9
	Weh[494]	Hamburg	38	
	Baker[407]	SWOG	278	9
ADC	Total		200	14
	Benjamin[406]	MDAH	46	15
	Blum[495]	DFCI	23	17
	Baker[483]	SWOG	97	11
	Handman[496]	Minneapolis	18	28
	Ikeda[497]	Japan	16	6
ADV	Total		161	7
	Gottlieb[498]	SWOG	107	10
ADVC	Total		399	15
	Yap[499,500]	SWOG	125	17
	Benjamin[482]	MDAH	60	13
	Bui[501]	France	60	7
	Pfeffer[502]	Hadassah	31	13
	Pinedo[404]	EORTC	60	13
	Choi[503]	Hong Kong	12	17
	Bodey[488]	MDAH	51	23
ADVC-AD	Lopez[504]	Rome	40	10
ACV	Schoenfeld[366]	ECOG	70	4
ACVAd	Benjamin[482]	MDAH	224	12
ADAd	Baker[483]	SWOG	98	10
A + methyl-CCNU	Rivkin[505]	SWOG	41	7
A + streptozotocin	Chang[506]	UNCC	14	0
Epirubicin-based Combinations				
ED	Lopez[507]	Rome	52	17
EDI	Casali[508]	Milano	26	8
EP	Jelic[509]	Belgrade	35	20
EI	Elli[510]	Argentina	12	17
Ifosfamide-based Combinations				
IA	Cantwell[511]	Newcastle	16	6
IA	Dombernowshy[512]			
IA	Edmonson[513]	Mayo Clinic	44	2
IA	Loehrer[514]	Indiana	42	7
IA	Mansi[515]	Royal Marsden	54	6
IA	Schutte[516]	EORTC	175	9
IA	Steward[517]	EORTC	51	8
IA	Weh[494]	Hamburg	45	
IA	Wiltshaw[518]	Royal Marsden	60	
IAD	Bramwell[519]	London, Ontario	43	5
IAD	Elias[520]	DFCI	108	10
IC	Elias[386]	DFCI	8	12
IEtoposide	Wellens[521,522]	Duisburg	13	15
IEtoposide, hyperthermia	Issels[523]	Munich	38	16

(continued)

TABLE 42–32. *(Continued)*

Combination*	Investigations	Institute†	No. of Patients Evaluable	% CR‡
Ifosfamide-based Combinations *(continued)*				
IE	Elli[510]	Argentina	12	17
IE	Hoffmann[524]	Leverksen, FRG	55	
IE	Toma[525]	Genoa	38	11
IDE	Casali[508]	Milano	52	10
IP	Biernbaum[526]	Essen	12	17
IP	Budd[527]	SWOG	28	4
IP	Hartlapp[528]			
IP/WLRT	Zamboglou[529]	Dusseldorf	8	75
Cisplatin-based Combinations				
	Total		219	6
AP	Klippenstein[530]	Frankfurt	18	21
APC	Edmonson[531]	Mayo Clinic	20	0
APC	Cormier[532]	Mayo Clinic	20	0
APC	Edmonson[533]	Mayo Clinic	63	0
AP Mitc	Edmonson[533]	Mayo Clinic	63	0
APV	Biernbaum[526]	Essen	16	19
APC/Hmm	Jansen (mixed mesodermal sarcoma)[534]	Rotterdam	6	33
PI	Biernbaum[526]	Essen	12	17
P/D	Piver[535]	RPMI	20	20
Methotrexate Combinations				
	Total		463	5
AM	Presgrave[536]	Austria	36	0
AMV	Kaufman[537]	RPMI	14	7
AMVD	Kaufman[537]	RPMI	5	0
AMVDAd	Shiu[538]	MSKCC	41	0
AMVAd	Shiu[538]	MSKCC	32	0
AM Mustard	Subramanian[376]	Marsen	22	15
AMC	Presant[539]	C. of Hope	105	6
AMC/ADV	Presant[539]	C. of Hope	32	16
AMCDV	Lynch, Shiu[538,540]	MSKCC	36	11
AMCDV	Pfeffer[541]	Jerusalem	24	13
AMC	Lowenbraun[542]		140	3
Dactinomycin-based Combinations				
	Total		298	1
AdVC	Jacobs[543]	UCSF	17	6
AdVC	Schoenfeld[366]	ECOG	64	2
AdVC		Mayo Clinic	61	2
AdL	Cruz[368]	MDAH	25	0
AdLV	Cruz[368]	MDAH	26	0
AdL + cycloleucine	Golbey[379]	RPMI	25	0
AdL = cycloleucine	Golbey[379]	RPMI	40	0
AdM = chlorambucil	Golbey[379]	RPMI	40	0

* A, doxorubicin; Ad, dactinomycin; C, cyclophosphamide; D, DTIC; E, Epirubicin; Hmm, hexamethylmelamine; M, high-dose methotrexate; I, ifosfamide; L, (L-PAM) melphalan; P, cisplatin; V, vincristine; Mitc, mitomycin C; WLRT, whole lung radiation therapy.
† UCSF, University of California, San Francisco; ECOG, Eastern Cooperative Oncology Group; GOG, Gynecologic Oncology Group; SIOP, International Society of Pediatric Oncology; SWOG, Southwest Oncology Group; MDAH, M.D. Anderson Cancer Center; EORTC, European Organization for Research and Treatment of Cancer; MSKCC, Memorial Sloan Kettering Cancer Center; RPMI, Roswell Park Memorial Institute, Rochester, NY.
‡ CR, complete response.

QUALITY OF LIFE ISSUES

Medical decisions should be predicated on an understanding of the influence of treatments on survival. If different treatments result in equivalent survival outcomes, the effects of these treatments on the quality of life may help in choosing the most appropriate treatment for a patient.[559] One example is the treatment of patients with high-grade extremity soft tissue sarcomas in which there is a choice between limb-sparing surgery combined with adjuvant therapy or amputation. In a prospective, randomized NCI study, Rosenberg and colleagues demonstrated that the overall survival rates of these two treatment modalities were equivalent.[264] Although intuition predicts that the limb-sparing approach should result in improved quality of life over amputation and should therefore be offered to a patient, there are few data available to determine the functional capacity and quality of life for patients who have had either treatment.

Sugarbaker and coworkers assessed quality of life for 26 patients undergoing limb-sparing surgery or amputation for soft tissue sarcomas of the extremity.[560] Psychosocial and clinical assessments were used to measure the impact of treatment on psychosocial adjustment, daily activities, economic status, mobility, pain, sexual relationships, and treatment trauma. Analysis of this study revealed no evidence of improved quality of life in patients undergoing limb-sparing surgery plus irradiation compared with amputation.

In a study reported by Weddington and colleagues, the psychological outcome of 33 patients with extremity sarcoma who underwent amputation or limb-sparing surgery were evaluated.[561] A battery of standard psychosocial assessment tests were employed and revealed no psychological advantage of limb-sparing surgery to amputation. These studies appear to indicate that the impact of amputation or limb-sparing surgery are equivalent, an idea that is contrary to intuition. This may be a result of insensitive tools in the assessment of quality of life, which is a difficult concept to measure, or these studies may reflect the ability of an amputee to compensate and adjust to a lost limb. It appears that there is no compelling reason to attempt a limb-sparing approach instead of an amputation for every patient with a high-grade sarcoma, because the impact of these treatments on survival and quality of life are equivalent. If there is concern about obtaining adequate tumor margins with a limb-sparing procedure, amputation should be performed.

Multimodality treatment of soft tissue sarcomas significantly improved patient survival. The optimal combination of surgery, radiation therapy, and chemotherapy has not been defined. Evaluation of the impact of various combined modality treatments on the quality of life of patients becomes an important determinant in optimizing therapy if survival results are not affected.[562]

In an NCI study, the role of adjuvant, postoperative radiation therapy was studied in patients with high-grade extremity sarcomas treated with limb-sparing surgery and adjuvant chemotherapy.[563] A concurrent prospective study of the quality of life evaluated economic status, sexual activity, functional parameters, and indicators of global well-being. There were significantly more local recurrences in patients treated with only surgery and chemotherapy, but the overall survival of the two groups was virtually identical. In this study, quality of life parameters helped to weigh the detriment of those few local recurrences against the detriment of administering high-dose radiation therapy in all cases. Radiation therapy was found to result in a significantly greater degree of pain, edema, and joint stiffness, which tended to abate with time. Because the magnitude of these effects was modest, no difference in activities of daily living was seen. Psychosocial parameters were not consistently influenced by irradiation, and the Functional Living Index (Cancer), a global parameter of quality of life, showed no differences beyond 6 months from surgery. Such studies should not be construed to prescribe one therapy over another, but they define and quantitate the differences between two treatments, allowing some patients to choose a therapy based on personal priorities.

REFERENCES

1. Patten BM. Human Embryology. New York: McGraw-Hill, 1968.
2. Boring CC, Squires TS, Tong T. Cancer statistics, 1991. CA 1991;41:19–39.
3. Smith AH, Pearce NE, Fisher DO, et al. Soft tissue sarcoma and exposure to phenoxyherbicides and chlorophenols in New Zealand. JNCI 1984;73:1111–1117.
4. Lynge E, Storm HH, Jensen OM. The evaluation of trends in soft tissue sarcoma according to diagnostic criteria and consumption of phenoxyherbicides. Cancer 1987;60:1896–1901.
5. Li FP, Fraumeni JF Jr. Soft-tissue sarcomas, breast cancer, and other neoplasms. A familial syndrome? Ann Intern Med 1969;71:747–752.
6. Malkin D, Li FP, Strong LC, et al. Germ line p53 mutations in a familial syndrome of breast cancer, sarcomas and other neoplasms. Science 1990;250:1233–1238.
7. Mulligan LM, Matlashewski GJ, Scrable HJ, et al. Mechanisms of p53 loss in human sarcomas. PNAS 1990;87:5863–5867.
8. Li FP, Fraumeni JF Jr. Rhabdomyosarcoma in children: Epidemiologic study and identification of a familial cancer syndrome. JNCI 1969;43:1365–1373.
9. Li FP, Tucker MA, Fraumeni JF Jr. Childhood cancer in sibs. J Pediatr 1976;88:419–423.
10. Miller RW. Deaths from childhood leukemia and solid tumors among twins and other sibs in the United States, 1960–1967. JNCI 1971;45:203.
11. Chabalko JJ, Creagon ET, Fraumeni JF Jr. Epidemiology of selected sarcomas in children. JNCI 1974;53:675.
12. Remzi D, Kendi S. Rhabdomyosarcoma of the prostate in childhood. Turk J Pediatr 1966;8:143–149.
13. Bottomley RH, Condit PT. Cancer families. Cancer Bull 1968;20:22–24.
14. Fraumeni JF Jr, Vogel CL, Easton JM. Sarcomas and multiple polyposis in a kindred. A genetic variety of hereditary polyposis? Arch Intern Med 1968;121:57–61.
15. Stewart FW, Treves NP. Lymphangiosarcoma in postmastectomy lymphedema: A report of six cases in elephantiasis chirurgica. Cancer 1948;1:64–81.
16. Sloane JA, Hubbel MM. Soft tissue sarcomas in children associated with congenital anomalies. Cancer 1969;23:175–182.
17. Schjweisguth O, Gerard-Marchant R, Lemerle J. Naevomatose baso-cellulaire association a un rhabdomyosarcome congenital. Arch Fr Pediatr 1968;25:1083–1093.
18. Heard G. Malignant disease in von Recklinghausen's neurofibromatosis. Proc R Soc Med 1963;56:502–503.
19. Reed WB, Nickel WR, Campion G. Internal manifestations of tuberous sclerosis. Arch Dermatol 1963;87:715–728.
20. Epstein CJ, Martin GM, Schultz AL, et al. Werner's syndrome. A review of its symptomatology, natural history, pathologic features, genetics and relationship to the natural aging process. Medicine (Baltimore) 1966;45:177–221.
21. Usui M, Ishii S, Yamawaki S, et al. The occurrence of soft tissue sarcomas in three siblings with Werner's syndrome. Cancer 1984;54:2580–2586.
22. Hardell L, Sandstrom A. Case-control study: Soft-tissue sarcomas and exposure to phenoxyacetic acids or chlorophenols. Br J Cancer 1979;39:711–717.
23. Eriksson M, Hardell L, Berg NO, et al. Soft tissue sarcomas and exposure to chemical substances: A case-referent study. Br J Ind Med 1981;38:27–33.
24. Wiklund K, Holm LE. Soft tissue sarcoma risk in Swedish agricultural and forestry workers. JNCI 1986;76:229–234.
25. Greenwald P, Kovasznay B, Collins DN, et al. Sarcomas of soft tissue after Vietnam service. JNCI 1984;73:1107–1109.
26. Kang H, Enzinger F, Breslin P, et al. Soft tissue sarcomas and military service in Vietnam: A case-control study. JNCI 1987;79:693–699.
27. Adam YG, Reif R. Radiation-induced fibrosarcoma following treatment for breast cancer. Surgery 1977;81:421–425.
28. Kuten A, Sapir D, Cohen Y, et al. Postirradiation soft tissue sarcoma occurring in breast cancer patients: Report of seven cases and results of combination chemotherapy. J Surg Oncol 1985;28:168–171.
29. Souba WW, McKenna RJ, Meis J, et al. Radiation-induced sarcomas of the chest wall. Cancer 1986;57:610–615.
30. O'Neil NB, Cocke W, Mason D, et al. Radiation-induced soft tissue fibrosarcoma: Surgical therapy and salvage. Ann Thorac Surg 1982;33:625–628.

31. Halperin EC, Greenberg MS, Suit HD. Sarcoma of bone and soft tissue following treatment of Hodgkin's disease. Cancer 1984;53:232–236.

32. Arlen M, Higinbotham NL, Huvos AG, et al. Radiation-induced sarcoma of bone. Cancer 1971;28:1087–1099.

33. Martland HS, Humphries RE. Osteogenic sarcoma in dial painters using luminous paint. Arch Pathol 1929;7:406–417.

34. Brand KG. Foreign body induced sarcomas. In: Becker FF, ed. Cancer. New York: Plenum Press, 1975:485–511.

35. Ott G. Fremd Körpersarkome. Exp Med Pathol Klin 1970;32:1.

36. De Cholnky T. Augmentation mammaplasty: Survey of complications in 10,941 patients by 265 surgeons. Plast Reconstr Surg 1970;45:573.

37. Rubin LR, Bromberg BE, Walden RH. Long-term human reaction to synthetic plastics. Surg Gynecol Obstet 1971;132:603.

38. Shieber W, Graham P. An experience with sarcomas of the soft tissues in adults. Surgery 1962;52:295.

39. Hare HF, Cerny MF. Soft tissue sarcoma: A review of 200 cases. Cancer 1963;16:1332.

40. Ferrell HW, Frable WJ. Soft part sarcomas revisited. Review and comparison of a second series. Cancer 1972;30:475–480.

41. Sears HF, Hopson R, Inouye W, et al. Analysis of staging and management of patients with sarcoma. Ann Surg 1980;191:488–493.

42. Abbas JS, Holyoke ED, Moore, et al. The surgical treatment and outcome of soft tissue sarcoma. Arch Surg 1981;116:765–769.

43. Lindberg RD, Martin RG, Romsdahl MM, et al. Conservative surgery and postoperative radiotherapy in 300 adults with soft-tissue sarcomas. Cancer 1981;47:2391–2397.

44. Potter DA, Glenn J, Kinsella T, et al. Patterns of recurrence in patients with high-grade soft tissue sarcomas. J Clin Oncol 1985;3:353–366.

45. Torosian MH, Friedrich C, Godbold J, et al. Soft tissue sarcomas: Initial characteristics and prognostic factors in patients with and without metastic disease. Semin Surg Oncol 1988;4:13–19.

46. Lawrence W Jr, Donegan WL, Nachimuth N, et al. Adult soft tissue sarcomas. A pattern of care survey of the American College of Surgeons. Ann Surg 1987;205:349–359.

47. Hajdu SI. Pathology of soft tissue tumors. Philadelphia: Lea & Febiger, 1979.

48. Mirr JM. The soft tissues. In: Coulson WF, ed. Surgical pathology. Philadelphia: JB Lippincott, 1978.

49. Stout AP, Lattes R. Tumors of the soft tissue. In: Atlas of tumor pathology. 2nd series. Washington, DC: Armed Forces Institute of Pathology, 1967.

50. Enzinger FM, Weiss SW. Soft tissue tumors. St. Louis: CV Mosby, 1988.

51. Coindre JM, Trojani M, Contesso G, et al. Reproducibility of a histopathologic grading system for adult soft tissue sarcoma. Cancer 1986;58:306–309.

52. Presant CA, Russell WO, Alexander RW, et al. Soft-tissue and bone sarcoma histopathology peer review: The frequency of disagreement in diagnosis and the need for second pathology opinions. The Southeastern Cancer Study Group experience. J Clin Oncol 1986;4:1658–1661.

53. Costa J, Wesley RA, Glatstein E, et al. The grading of soft tissue sarcomas. Results of a clinicohistopathologic correlation in a series of 163 cases. Cancer 1984;53:530–541.

54. Lack EE, Steinberg SM, White DE, et al. Extremity soft tissue sarcomas: Analysis of prognostic variables in 300 cases and evaluation of tumor necrosis as a factor in stratifying higher-grade sarcomas. J Surg Oncol 1989;41:263–273.

55. Trojani M, Contesso G, Coindre JM, et al. Soft tissue sarcomas of adults. Study of pathological prognostic variables and definition of a histopathological grading system. Int J Cancer 1984;33:37–42.

56. Alvegard TA, Berg NO, et al. Histopathological peer review of high-grade soft tissue sarcoma: The Scandinavian Sarcoma Group experience. J Clin Oncol 1989;7:1845–1951.

57. Pack GI, Ariel IM. Treatment of cancer and allied diseases. In: Tumors of the soft somatic tissues and bone. Vol VIII. New York: Harper & Row, 1964.

58. Martin RG, Butler JJ, Albores-Saavedra J. Soft tissue tumors: Surgical treatment and results. In: Tumors of bone and soft tissue. Chicago: Year Book Medical Publishers, 1965.

59. Shiu MH, Castro EB, Hajdu SI, et al. Surgical treatment of 297 soft tissue sarcomas of the lower extremity. Ann Surg 1975;182:597.

60. Simon MA, Enneking WF. The management of soft tissue sarcomas of the extremities. J Bone Joint Surg [Am] 1976;58:317.

61. Bears OH, Henson DE, Hutter RVP, Kennedy BJ, eds. Manual for staging of cancer, American Joint Committee on Cancer. 4th ed. Philadelphia: JB Lippincott, 1992.

62. Suit HD, Mankin JH, Willett G, et al. Limited surgery and external irradiation in soft tissue sarcomas. In: Recent concepts in sarcoma treatment. Proceedings of the International Symposium on Sarcomas, Tarpon Springs, FL, October 8–10, 1987. The Netherlands: Kluwer Academic Publishers, 1988.

63. Lindberg RD, Martin RG, Romsdahl MM, et al. Conservation surgery and radiation therapy for soft tissue sarcomas. In: Martin RG, Ayala AG, eds. Management of primary bone and soft tissue tumors. Chicago: Year Book Medical Publishers, 1977.

64. Suit HD. Patterns of failure after treatment of sarcoma of soft tissue by radical surgery or by conservative surgery and radiation. Cancer Treat Symp 1983;2:241–246.

65. Collins C, Hadju SI, Godbold J, et al. Localized, operable soft tissue sarcoma of the lower extremity. Arch Surg 1986;121:1425–1433.

66. Potter DA, Kinsella T, Glatstein E, et al. High grade soft tissue sarcomas of the extremities. Cancer 1986;58:190–205.

67. Jarvi OH, Saxen E. Elastofibroma dorsi. Acta Pathol Microbiol Immunol Scand 1961;144:S83–S84.

68. Jarvi OH, Lansimies PH. Subclinical elastofibromas in the scapular region in an autopsy series. Acta Pathol Microbiol Immunol Scand [A] 1975;83:87–108.

69. Jarvi OH, Saxen AE, Hopsu-Havu VK, et al. Elastofibroma: A degenerative pseudotumor. Cancer 1969;23:42–63.

70. Stemmermann GN, Stout AP. Elastofibroma dorsi. Am J Clin Pathol 1962;37:490–506.

71. Conway H. Dupuytren's contracture. Am J Surg 1954;87:10.

72. Luck JV. Dupuytren's contracture. J Bone Joint Surg [Am] 1959;41:635.

73. Skoog T. Dupuytren's contracture: Pathogenesis and surgical treatment. Surg Clin North Am 1967;47:433–444.

74. Allen RA, Woolner LB, Ghormley RK. Soft-tissue tumors of the sole: With special reference to plantar fibromatosis. J Bone Joint Surg [Am] 1955;37:14–26.

75. Allen PM, Enzinger FM. Juvenile aponeurotic fibroma. Cancer 1970;26:857–867.

76. Goldman RL. The cartilage analogue of fibromatosis (aponeurotic fibroma): Further observations based on 7 new cases. Cancer 1970;26:1325–1331.

77. Keasbey LE. Juvenile aponeurotic fibroma (calcifying fibroma). Cancer 1953;6:338–346.

78. Bartlett RC, Otis RD, Haakso AO. Multiple congenital neoplasms of soft tissues. Report of 4 cases in 1 family. Cancer 1961;14:913–920.

79. Beatty EC. Congenital generalized fibromatosis in infancy. Am J Dis Child 1962;103:620.

80. Teng P, Warden MJ, Cohn WL. Congenital generalized fibromatosis (renal and skeletal) with complete spontaneous regression. J Pediatr 1963;62:748–753.

81. Enzinger FM. Fibrous hamartoma of infancy. Cancer 1965;18:241–251.

82. Chandler A. Muscular torticollis. J Bone Joint Surg [Am] 1948;30:566.

83. Brown JB, McDowell F. Wry-neck facial distortion prevented by resection of fibrosed sternomastoid muscle in infancy and childhood. Ann Surg 1950;131:721–733.

84. Smoth BH. Peyronie's disease. Am J Clin Pathol 1966;45:670.

85. Allen PW. Nodular fasciitis. Pathology 1972;4:9–26.

86. Bernstein KE, Lattes R. Nodular (pseudosarcomatous) fasciitis; a nonrecurrent lesion: Clinicopathologic study of 134 cases. Cancer 1982;49:1668–1679.

87. Soule EH. Proliferative (nodular) fasciitis. Arch Pathol 1962;73:437.

88. Hutter RVP, Stewart FW, Foote FW Jr. Fasciitis: A report of 70 cases with follow-up proving the benignity of the lesion. Cancer 1962;15:992–1003.

89. MacKenzie DH. The differential diagnosis of fibroblastic disorders. Oxford: Blackwell Scientific, 1970.

90. Das Gupta TK, Brasfield RD, O'Hara J. Extra-abdominal desmoids. Ann Surg 1969;170:109.

91. Enzinger FM, Shiraki M. Musculoaponeurotic fibromatosis of the shoulder girdle. Cancer 1967;20:113.

92. Brasfield RD, Das Gupta TK. Desmoid tumors of the anterior abdominal wall. Surgery 1969;65:241.

93. Ewing J. Neoplastic disease. Philadelphia: WB Saunders, 1928.

94. Musgrove JE, McDonald JR. Extra-abdominal desmoid tumors: A differential diagnosis and treatment. Arch Pathol 1948;45:513–540.

95. Benninghoff D, Robbins R. The nature and treatment of desmoid tumors. Am J Roentgenol Radium Ther Nucl Med 1964;91:132–137.

96. Greenberg HM, Goebel R, Weichselbaum RR, et al. Radiation therapy in the treatment of aggressive fibromatoses. Int J Radiat Oncol Biol Phys 1981;7:305–310.

97. Kirchmer JT Jr, Woma FJ Jr. Desmoid tumors of the abdominal wall. South Med J 1977;70:1136.

98. Wara WM, Phillips TL, Hill DR, et al. Desmoid tumors—treatment and prognosis. Radiology 1977;124:225–226.

99. Suit HD, Russell WO. Radiation therapy of soft tissue sarcomas. Cancer 1975;36:759–764.

100. Kiel KD, Suit HD. Radiation therapy in the treatment of aggressive fibromatoses (desmoid tumors). Cancer 1984;54:2051–2055.

101. Kinsbrunner B, Ritter S, Domingo J, et al. Remission of rapidly growing desmoid tumors after tamoxifen therapy. Cancer 1983;52:2201–2204.

102. Lanari A. Effect of progesterone on desmoid tumors (aggressive fibromatosis). N Engl J Med 1983;309:1523.

103. Waddell WR, Gerner RE. Indomethacin and ascorbate inhibit desmoid tumors. J Surg Oncol 1980;15:85–90.

104. Khorsand J, Karakousis CP. Desmoid tumors and their management. Am J Surg 1985;149:215–218.

105. Posner MC, Shiu MH, Newsome JL, et al. The desmoid tumor: Not a benign disease. Arch Surg 1989;124:191–196.

106. Kofoed H, Kamby C, Anagnostaki L. Aggressive fibromatosis. Surg Gynecol Obstet 1985;160:124–127.

107. Czernobilsky B, Cornog JL, Enterline HT. Rhabdomyoma: Report of a case with ultrastructural and histochemical studies. Am J Clin Pathol 1968;49:782–789.

108. Morgan JJ, Enterline HT. Benign rhabdomyoma of the pharynx: A case report, review of the literature, and comparison with cardiac rhabdomyoma. Am J Clin Pathol 1964;42:174–181.

109. Lendrum AC. Painful tumors of the skin. Ann R Coll Surg Engl 1947;1:62–67.

110. Stout AP. Solitary cutaneous and subcutaneous leiomyoma. Am J Cancer 1937;29:435–469.

111. Enzinger FM, Harvey DA. Spindle cell lipoma. Cancer 1975;36:1852–1859.

112. Lin JJ, Lin F. Two entities in angiolipoma. A study of 459 cases of lipoma with review of infiltrating angiolipoma. Cancer 1974;34:720–727.

113. Chung EB, Enzinger FM. Benign lipoblastomatosis. An analysis of 35 cases. Cancer 1973;32:482–491.

114. Alba-Greco M, Garcia RL, Vuletin JC. Benign lipoblastomatosis. Ultrastructure and histogenesis. Cancer 1980;45:511.

115. Evans HL, Soule EH, Winkelmann RK. Atypical lipoma, atypical intramuscular lipoma,

and well-differentiated retroperitoneal liposarcoma. A reappraisal of 30 cases formerly classified as well-differentiated liposarcoma. Cancer 1979;43:574–584.

116. Dionne GP, Seemayer TA. Infiltrating lipomas and angiolipomas revisited. Cancer 1974;33:732–738.

117. Enzinger FM. Benign lipomatous tumors simulating a sarcoma. In: Martin RG, Ayala AG, eds. Management of primary bone and soft tissue tumors. Chicago: Year Book Medical Publishers, 1977:11–24.

118. Kindblom LG, Angervall L, Stener B, et al. Intermuscular and intramuscular lipomas and hibernomas: A clinical, roentgenologic, histologic, and prognostic study of 46 cases. Cancer 1974;33:754–762.

119. Mesara BW, Batsakis JC. Hibernoma of the neck. Arch Otolaryngol 1967;85:95.

120. Jones FE, Soule EH, Coventry MB. Fibrous xanthoma of synovium (giant cell tumor of tender sheath, pigmented nodular synovitis). J Bone Joint Surg [Am] 1969;51:76.

121. Gehwheiler JA, Wilson VW. Diffuse biarticular pigmented villonodular synovitis. Radiology 1969;93:137.

122. Slooff JL, Kernohan JW, MacCarty CS. Primary intramedullary tumors of the spinal cord and filum terminale. Philadelphia: WB Saunders, 1964.

123. D'Agostino A. Sarcomas of the peripheral nerves and somatic soft tissues associated with multiple neurofibromatosis. Cancer 1963;16:1015.

124. Buck BE. Congenital neurogenous sarcoma with rhabdomyosarcomatous differentiation. J Pediatr Surg 1977;12:581–582.

125. Hammond JA. Detection of malignant change in neurofibromatosis by gallium-67 scanning. Can Med Assoc J 1978;119:352–353.

126. Herman J. Sarcomatous transformation in multiple neurofibromatosis. Ann Surg 1950;131:206.

127. Hunt K. Neurofibrosarcoma complicating von Recklinghausen's disease. J Ky Med Assoc 1976;74:346–349.

128. Lee C. Malignant degeneration of thoracic neurofibromata. NY State J Med 1972;75: 347–352.

129. Wander JW, Das Gupta TK. Neurofibromatosis. Curr Probl Surg 1977;14:1–81.

130. Riccardi VM. Medical progress. von Recklinghausen neurofibromatosis. N Engl J Med 1981;305:1617–1626.

131. Nambisan RN, Rao U, Moore R, et al. Malignant soft tissue tumors of nerve sheath origin. J Surg Oncol 1984;25:268–272.

132. Sorensen SA, Mulvihill JJ, Nielsen A. Long-term follow-up of von Recklinghausen neurofibromatosis survival and malignant neoplasms. N Engl J Med 1986;314:1010–1015.

133. Allen PW, Enzinger FM. Heamangioma of skeletal muscle: An analoysis of 89 cases. Cancer 1972;29:8–22.

134. Lister WA. The natural history of strawberry nevi. Lancet 1938;1:1429–1434.

135. Modlin JJ. Capillary hemangiomas of the skin. Surgery 1955;38:169–180.

136. Riveros M, Pack GT. The glomus tumors—report of 20 cases. Ann Surg 1951;133: 394.

137. Carroll RE, Berman AT. Glomus tumors of the hand: Review of the literature and report of 28 cases. J Bone Joint Surg [Am] 1972;54:691–703.

138. Shugart RR, Soule EH, Johnson EW. Glomus tumor. Surg Gynecol Obstet 1963;117: 334–340.

139. Stout AP. Tumors featuring pericytes: Glomus tumor and hemangiopericytoma. Lab Invest 1965;5:217–223.

140. Enzinger FM, Smith BH. Hemangiopericytoma. An analysis of 106 cases. Hum Pathol 1976;7:61–82.

141. Soule EH, Enriquez P. Atypical fibrous histiocytoma, malignant fibrous histiocytoma, malignant histiocytoma, and epithelioid sarcoma. A comparative study of 65 tumors. Cancer 1972;30:128.

142. Kempson RL, McGavran MH. Atypical fibroxanthomas of the skin. Cancer 1964;17: 1463–1471.

143. Kauffman SL, Stout AP. Histiocytic tumors (fibrous xanthoma and histiocytoma) in children. Cancer 1961;14:469–482.

144. O'Brien JE, Stout AP. Malignant fibrous xanthomas. Cancer 1964;17:1445–1458.

145. Brenner W, Schaefler K, Habrans C, et al. Dermatofibrosarcoma protuberans metastatic to a regional lymph node. Report of a case and review. Cancer 1975;36:1897–1902.

146. Burkhardt BR, Soule EH, Winkelman RK, et al. Dermatofibrosarcoma protuberans: Study of 56 cases. Am J Surg 1966;111:638–644.

147. Taylor HB, Helwig EB. Dermatofibrosarcoma protuberans: A study of 115 cases. Cancer 1962;15:717–725.

148. McPeak CJ, Druz T, Nicastri AD. Dermatofibrosarcoma protuberans: An analysis of 86 cases—five with metastasis. Ann Surg 1967;166:803.

149. Glenn J, Potter D, Kinsella T, et al. Unpublished results, 1985.

150. Roses DF, Valensi Q, LaTrenta G, et al. Surgical treatment of dermatofibrosarcoma protuberans. Surg Gynecol Obstet 1986;162:449–452.

151. Rinck PA, Habermalz HJ, Loceck H. Effective radiotherapy in one case of dermatofibrosarcoma protuberans. Strahlentherapie 1982;158:681–685.

152. Strong EW, McDivitt RW, Brasfield RD. Granular cell myoblastoma. Cancer 1970;25: 415–422.

153. Le Ber MS, Stout AP. Benign mesenchymomas in children. Cancer 1962;15:598–605.

154. Stout AP. Myxoma, the tumor of primitive mesenchyme. Ann Surg 1948;127:706–719.

155. Enzinger FM. Intramuscular myxoma. Am J Clin Pathol 1965;43:104.

156. Barth RJ, Merino MJ, Solomon D, et al. A prospective study of the value of core needle biopsy and fine needle aspiration in the diagnosis of soft tissue sarcoma. Surgery 1992;112:536–543.

157. Martel W, Abell MR. Radiologic evaluation of soft tissue tumors. A retrospective study. Cancer 1973;32:352–366.

158. Berger PE, Kuhn JP. Computed tomography of tumors of the musculoskeletal system in children. Clinical applications. Radiology 1978;127:171–175.

159. Neifeld JP, Walsh JW, Lawrence W Jr. Computed tomography in the management of soft tissue tumors. Surg Gynecol Obstet 1982;155:535–540.

160. Lawrence W Jr, Neifeld JP, Terz JJ. Manual of soft tissue tumor surgery. New York: Springer-Verlag, 1983.

161. Levin DC, Watson RC, Baltaxe HA. Arteriography in diagnosis and management of acquired peripheral soft-tissue masses. Radiology 1972;103:53–58.

162. Hudson TM, Haas G, Enneking WF, et al. Angiography in the management of musculoskeletal tumors. Surg Gynecol Obstet 1975;141:11–21.

163. De Santos LA, Wallace S, Finklestein JB. Angiography and lymphangiography in peripheral soft tissue sarcomas. In: Martin RG, Ayala AG, eds. Management of primary bone and soft tissue tumors. Chicago: Year Book Medical Publishers, 1977.

164. Chang AE, Matory YL, Dwyer AJ, et al. Magnetic resonance imaging versus computed tomography in the evaluation of soft tissue tumors of the extremities. Ann Surg 1987;205: 340–348.

165. Bland KI, McCoy DM, Kinard RE, et al. Application of magnetic resonance imaging and computerized tomography as an adjunct to the surgical management of soft tissue sarcomas. Ann Surg 1987;205:473–481.

166. Enneking WF. Preoperative staging of sarcomas. Cancer Treat Symp 1985;3:67–70.

167. Enneking WF, Spanier SS, Goodman MA. The surgical staging of musculoskeletal sarcoma. J Bone Joint Surg [Am] 1980;62:1027–1030.

168. Suit HD, Russell WO, Martin RG. Sarcoma of soft tissue: Clinical and histopathologic parameters and response to treatment. Cancer 1975;35:1478–1483.

169. Suit HD, Mankin HJ, Wood WC, et al. Treatment of the patient with stage M_o soft tissue sarcoma. J Clin Oncol 1988;6:854–862.

170. Weingrad DW, Rosenberg SA. Early lymphatic spread of osteogenic and soft-tissue sarcomas. Surgery 1978;84:231–240.

171. Mazeron JJ, Suit HD. Lymph nodes as sites of metastases from sarcomas of soft tissue. Cancer 1987;60:1800–1808.

172. Rosenberg SA, Seipp CA, White DE, et al. Perioperative blood transfusions are associated with increased rates of recurrence and decreased survival in patients with high-grade soft-tissue sarcomas of the extremities. J Clin Oncol 1985;3:698–709.

173. Soule EH, Pritchard DJ. Fibrosarcoma in infants and children: A review of 110 cases. Cancer 1977;40:1711–1721.

174. Shmahler BM, Enzinger FM. Liposarcoma occurring in children. An analysis of 17 cases and review of the literature. Cancer 1983;52:567–574.

175. Brennan MF. Presentation, demographics and prognostic factors of soft tissue sarcoma. In: Shiu MH, Brennan MF, eds. Surgical management of soft tissue sarcoma. Philadelphia: Lea & Febiger, 1989.

176. Suit HD. Patterns of failure after treatment of sarcoma of soft tissue by radical surgery or by conservative surgery and radiation. Cancer Treat Symp 1983;2:241–246.

177. Marcus SG, Merino MJ, Steinberg SM, et al. Long-term outcome of patients with low grade soft tissue sarcomas. Arch Surg 1993 (in press).

178. Cantin J, McNeer GP, Chu FC, et al. The problem of local recurrence after treatment of soft tissue sarcoma. Ann Surg 1968;168:47–53.

179. Lindberg RD, Martin RG, Romsdahl MM. Surgery and postoperative radiotherapy in the treatment of soft tissue sarcomas in adults. Am J Roentgenol Radium Ther Nucl Med 1975;123:123–129.

180. Gerner RE, Moore GE, Pickren JW. Soft tissue sarcomas. Ann Surg 1975;181:803–808.

181. Rosenberg SA, Kent H, Costa J, et al. Prospective randomized evaluation of the role of limb-sparing surgery, radiation therapy, and adjuvant chemoimmunotherapy in the treatment of adult soft-tissue sarcomas. Surgery 1978;84:62–69.

182. Markhede G, Angervall L, Stener B. A multivariate analysis of the prognosis after surgical treatment of malignant soft tissue tumors. Cancer 1982;49:1721–1733.

183. Pritchard DJ, Soule EH, Taylor WF, et al. Fibrosarcoma: Clinicopathologic and statistical study of 199 tumors of soft tissues of extremities and trunk. Cancer 1974;33:888–897.

184. Stout AP. Fibrosarcoma: The malignant tumor of fibroblasts. Cancer 1948;1:30–63.

185. Pritchard DJ, Soule EH, Taylor WF, et al. Fibrosarcoma: Clinicopathological and statistical study of 199 tumors of soft tissues of extremities and trunk. Cancer 1974;33: 880.

186. Castro EB, Hajdu SI, Fortner JG. Surgical therapy of fibrosarcoma of extremities. Arch Surg 1973;107:284.

187. Grier HE, Perez-Atayde AR, Weinstein JH. Chemotherapy for inoperable infantile fibrosarcoma. Cancer 1985;56:1507–1510.

188. Delepine N, Cornille H, Desbois JC, et al. Complete response of congenital fibrosarcoma to chemotherapy. Lancet 1986;1:1453–1454.

189. Soule EH, Geitz M, Henderson EH. Embryonal rhabdomyosarcoma of the limbs and limb girdles. A clinico-pathologic study of 61 cases. Cancer 1969;23:1338–1346.

190. Maurer HM, Moon T, Donaldson M, et al. The intergroup rhabdomyosarcoma study. Cancer 1977;40:2015.

191. Ariel IM, Briceno M. Rhabdomyosarcoma of the extremities and trunk: Analysis of 150 patients treated by surgical resection. J Surg Oncol 1975;7:269–287.

192. Linscheid RL, Soule EH, Henderson ED. Pleomorphic rhabdomyosarcoma of the extremities and limb girdles: A clinico-pathologic study. J Bone Joint Surg [Am] 1965;47: 715–725.

193. Albores-Saavedra J, Martin RG, Smith JL. Rhabdomyosarcoma: A study of 35 cases. Ann Surg 1963;157:186–197.

194. Lloyd RV, Hajdu SI, Knapper WH. Embryonal rhabdomyosarcoma in adults. Cancer 1983;51:557–565.

195. Agamanolis DP, Dasu S, Krill CE. Tumors of skeletal muscle. Hum Pathol 1986;17: 778–795.

196. Osborn M, Hill C, Altmannsberger M, et al. Monoclonal antibodies to titin in conjunction with antibodies to desmin separate rhabdomyosarcomas from other tumor types. Lab Invest 1986;55:101–108.

197. De Jong Ash, Van Kessel-Van Vark M, Alsus-Lutter Che: Hum Pathol 1987;18:298–303.

198. Stout AP, Hill WT. Leiomyosarcoma of the superficial soft tissues. Cancer 11:844–854, 1958.

199. Abwasi OE, Dozois RR, Weiland LH, et al. Leiomyosarcoma of the small and large bowel. Cancer 1978;42:1375.

200. Kevorkian J, Cento DP. Leiomyosarcoma of large arteries and veins. Surgery 1973;73:390.

201. Wile AG, Evans HL, Romsdahl MM. Leiomyosarcoma of soft tissue: A clinicopathologic study. Cancer 1981;48:1022–1032.

202. Enterline HT, Culberson JD, Rochlin DB, et al. Liposarcoma. A clinicopathologic study of 53 cases. Cancer 1960;11:932–950.

203. Spittle MF, Newton KA, Mackenzie DH. Liposarcoma. A review of 60 cases. Br J Cancer 1971;24:696.

204. Kindblom L, Angervall L, Svendsen P. Liposarcoma. A clinicopathologic, radiographic and prognostic study. Acta Pathol Microbiol Immunol Scand 1975;253:1.

205. Ackerman LV. Multiple primary liposarcomas. Am J Pathol 1944;20:789–793.

206. Enzinger FM, Winslow DJ. Liposarcoma. A study of 30 cases. Virchows Arch [A] 1962;335:367–388.

207. Reszel PA, Soule EH, Coventry MB. Liposarcoma of the extremities and limb girdles. A study of 222 cases. J Bone Joint Surg [Am] 1966;48:229.

208. Cadman NL, Soule EH, Kelly PJ. Synovial sarcoma: An analysis of 134 cases. Cancer 1965;18:613–627.

209. Gerner RE, Moore GE. Synovial sarcoma. Ann Surg 1975;181:22–25.

210. Hajdu SI, Shiu MH, Fortner JG. Tendosynovial sarcoma. A clinicopathological study of 136 cases. Cancer 1977;39:1201–1217.

211. Crocker DW, Stout AP. Synovial sarcoma in children. Cancer 1959;12:1123–1133.

212. Mobergen G. Nilsonne U, Friberg S. Synovial sarcoma. Acta Orthop Scand Suppl 1968;11:3.

213. Cagle LA, Mirra JM, Storm FK, et al. Histologic features relating to prognosis in synovial sarcoma. Cancer 1987;59:1810–1814.

214. Storm FK, Eilber FR, Mirra J, et al. Neurofibrosarcoma. Cancer 1980;45:126–129.

215. Girard C, Johnson WC, Graham JH. Cutaneous angiosarcoma. Cancer 1970;26:868–883.

216. Gulesserian HP, Lawton RL. Angiosarcoma of the breast. Cancer 1969;24:1021–1026.

217. Dunegan LJ, Tobon H, Watson CG. Angiosarcoma of the breast: A report of two cases and a review of the literature. Surgery 1976;79:57–59.

218. Woodward AH, Ivins JC, Soule EH. Lymphangiosarcoma arising in chronic lymphedematous extremities. Cancer 1972;30:562–572.

219. Rosai J, Sumner HW, Kostianovsky M, et al. Angiosarcoma of the skin. A clinicopathologic and fine structural study. Hum Pathol 1976;7:83.

220. Maddox JC, Evans L. Angiosarcoma of skin and soft tissue: A study of forty-four cases. Cancer 1981;48:1907–1921.

221. Morales PH, Lindberg RD, Barkley HT. Soft tissue angiosarcomas. Int J Radiat Oncol Biol Phys 1981;7:1655–1659.

222. Woodward AH, Ivins JC, Soule EH. Lymphangiosarcoma arising in chronic lymphadematous extremities. Cancer 1972;30:562–572.

223. Silverberg SG, Kay S, Koss LG. Postmastectomy lymphangiosarcoma: Ultrastructural observations. Cancer 1971;27:100–108.

224. Nemoto T, Stubbe N, Gaeta J, et al. Pathogenesis of lymphangiosarcoma following mastectomy and irradiation. Surg Gynecol Obstet 1969;128:489–494.

225. Holden CA, Spittle MF, Jones EW. Angiosarcoma of the face and scalp, prognosis and treatment. Cancer 1987;59:1046–1057.

226. Mira JG, Chu FCH, Fortner JG. The role of radiotherapy in the management of malignant hemangiopericytoma. Report of eleven new cases and review of the literature. Cancer 1977;39:1254–1259.

227. Stout AP. Hemangiopericytoma (a study of 25 new cases). Cancer 1949;2:1027–1954.

228. O'Brien PH, Brasfield RD. Hemangiopericytoma. Cancer 1965;14:249–252.

229. Hood AF, Farmer ER, Weiss RA. Kaposi's sarcoma. Johns Hopkins Med J 1982;151:222–239.

230. Steis RG, Broder S. The clinical relationship between immunodeficiency diseases and cancer with special emphasis on acquired immunodeficiency syndrome (AIDS) and Kaposi's sarcoma. In: DeVita VT Jr, Hellman S, Rosenberg SA, eds. Important advances in oncology 1985. Philadelphia: JB Lippincott, 1985.

231. Krigel RL, Friedman-Kien AE. Kaposi's sarcoma in AIDS. In: DeVita VT Jr, Hellman S, Rosenberg SA, eds. AIDS: Etiology, diagnosis, treatment and prevention. Philadelphia: JB Lippincott, 1985:185–211.

232. Reynolds WA, Winkelmann RK, Soule EH. Kaposi's sarcoma: A clinicopathologic study with particular reference to its relationship to the reticuloendothelial system. Medicine (Baltimore) 1965;44:419–443.

233. Rothman S. Remarks on sex, age and racial distribution of Kaposi's sarcoma and on possible pathogenetic factors. Acta Union Int Contra Cancrum 1962;18:326–329.

234. Dorffel J. Histogenesis of multiple idiopathic hemorrhagic sarcoma of Kaposi. Arch Dermatol Syph 1932;26:608–634.

235. Oettle AG. Geographical and racial differences in the frequency of Kaposi's sarcoma as evidence of environmental or genetic causes. Acta Unio Int Contra Cancrum 1962;18:330–363.

236. O'Brien PH, Brasfield RD. Kaposi's sarcoma. Cancer 1966;19:1497.

237. Kaminer B, Murray JF. Sarcoma idiopathicum multiplex haemorrhagicum of Kaposi, with special reference to its incidence in the South African Negro, and two case reports. South Afr J Clin Sci 1950;1:1–25.

238. Loethe F. Kaposi's sarcoma in Uganda Africans. Acta Pathol Microbiol Immunol Scand Suppl 1963;161:1–71.

239. Siegel JH, Janic R, Alper JC, et al. Disseminated visceral Kaposi's sarcoma. JAMA 1969;207:1493.

240. Stribling J, Wertzner S, Smith GV. Kaposi's sarcoma in renal allograft recipients. Cancer 1978;42:442.

241. Zisbrod A, Hairnov M, Schanzer H, et al. Kopsi's sarcoma after kidney transplantation. Transplantation 1980;30:383.

242. Penn I. Kaposi's sarcoma in organ transplant recipients. Transplantation 1979;27:8.

243. Myers BD, Kessle E, Levi D, et al. Kaposi's sarcoma in kidney transplant recipients. Arch Intern Med 1974;133:387.

244. Hymes K, Cheung T, Greene JB, et al. Kaposi's sarcoma in homosexual men: A report of eight cases. Lancet 1981;2:598–600.

245. O'Brien JE, Stout AP. Malignant fibrous xanthomas. Cancer 1964;17:1445–1458.

246. Wasserman TH, Stuart ID. Malignant fibrous histiocytoma with widespread metastases. Autopsy study. Cancer 1974;33:141–146.

247. Kearney MM, Soule EH, Ivins JC. Malignant fibrous histiocytoma. A retrospective study of 167 cases. Cancer 1980;45:167–178.

248. Weiss SW, Enzinger FM. Malignant fibrous histiocytoma. An analysis of 200 cases. Cancer 1978;41:2250–2266.

249. Leite C, Goodwin JW, Sinkovics JG, et al. Chemotherapy of malignant fibrous histiocytoma: A Southwest Oncology Group report. Cancer 1977;40:2010–2014.

250. Reagan MT, Clowry LJ, Cox JD, et al. Radiation therapy in the treatment of malignant fibrous histiocytoma. Int J Radiat Oncol Biol Phys 1981;7:311–315.

251. Weiss SW. Malignant fibrous histiocytoma. A reaffirmation. Am J Surg Pathol 1982;6:773–784.

252. Bertoni F, Capanna R, Biagini R, et al. Malignant fibrous histiocytoma. An analysis of 78 cases located and deeply seated in extremities. Cancer 1985;56:356–367.

253. Raney RB, Allen A, O'Neill J, et al. Malignant fibrous histiocytoma of soft tissue in childhood. Cancer 1986;57:2198–2201.

254. Christopherson WM, Foote FW, Stewart FW. Alveolar soft part sarcomas: Structurally characteristic tumors of uncertain histogenesis. Cancer 1952;5:100.

255. Lieberman PH, Foote FW, Stewart FW, et al. Alveolar soft-part sarcoma. JAMA 1966;198:1047–1051.

256. Unni KK, Soule EH. Alveolar soft part sarcoma. An electron microscopic study. Mayo Clin Proc 1975;50:592–598.

257. Bryan RS, Soule EH, Dobyns JH, et al. Primary epithelioid sarcoma of the hand and forearm. A review of thirteen cases. J Bone Joint Surg [Am] 1974;56:458–465.

258. Peimer AC, Smith RJ, Sirota RL, et al. Epithelioid sarcoma of the hand and wrist: Patterns of extension. J Hand Surg [Am] 1977;2:275–282.

259. Prat J, Woodruff JM, Marcove RC. Epithelioid sarcoma. An analysis of 22 cases indicating the prognostic significance of vascular invasion and regional lymph node metastasis. Cancer 1978;41:1472–1487.

260. Enzinger FM. Epithelioid sarcoma. A sarcoma simulating a granuloma or a carcinoma. Cancer 1970;26:1029–1041.

261. Shimm DS, Suit HD. Radiation therapy of epithelioid sarcoma. Cancer 1983;52:1022–1025.

262. Chase DR, Enzinger FM. Epithelioid sarcoma. Am J Surg Pathol 1985;9:241–263.

263. National Institutes of Health Consensus Development Panel on Limb-Sparing Treatment of Adult Soft Tissue Sarcomas and Osteosarcomas. Introduction and conclusions. Cancer Treat Symp 1985;3:1–5.

264. Rosenberg SA, Tepper J, Glatstein E, et al. The treatment of soft tissue sarcomas of the extremities. Prospective randomized evaluations of (1) limb-sparing surgery plus radiation therapy compared with amputation and (2) the role of adjuvant chemotherapy. Ann Surg 1982;196:305–315.

265. Simon MA, Spainer SS, Enneking WF. Management of adult soft-tissue sarcomas of the extremities. Surg Annu 1979;1:363–402.

266. Brennan MF, Shiu MH, Collin C, et al. Extremity soft tissue sarcomas. Cancer Treat Symp 1985;3:71–81.

267. Rooser B, Gustafson P, Rydholm A. Is there no influence of local control on the rate of metastases in high-grade soft tissue sarcoma? Cancer 1990;65:1727–1729.

268. Gustafson P, Rooser B, Rydholm A. Is local recurrence of minor importance for metastases in soft tissue sarcoma? Cancer 1991;67:2083–2086.

269. Enneking WF. Staging of musculoskeletal neoplasms. In: Current concepts of diagnosis and treatment of bone and soft tissue tumors. Heidelberg: Springer-Verlag, 1984.

270. Karakousis CP. Internal hemipelvectomy. Surg Gynecol Obstet 1984;158:279–282.

271. Sugarbaker P. Atlas of extremity surgery. Philadelphia: JB Lippincott, 1985.

272. Greager JA, Das Gupta TK. Adult head and neck soft-tissue sarcomas. Otolaryngol Clin North Am 1986;19:565–572.

273. McKenna WG, Barnes MM, Kinsella TJ, et al. Combined modality treatment of adult soft tissue sarcomas of the head and neck. Int J Radiat Oncol Biol Phys 1987;13:1127–1133.

274. Weber RS, Benjamin RS, Peters LJ, et al. Soft tissue sarcomas of the head and neck in adolescents and adults. Am J Surg 1986;152:386–392.

275. King RM, Pairolero PC, Trastek VF, et al. Primary chest wall tumors: Factors affecting survival. Ann Thorac Surg 1986;41:597–601.

276. Greager JA, Patel MK, Briele HA, et al. Soft tissue sarcomas of the adult thoracic wall. Cancer 1987;59:370–373.

277. Glenn J, Sindelar WF, Kinsella T, et al. Results of multimodality therapy of resectable soft-tissue sarcomas of the retroperitoneum. Surgery 1985;97:316–324.

278. Shiu MH, Flanebaum L, Hajdu SI, et al. Malignant soft tissue tumors of the anterior abdominal wall. Arch Surg 1980;115:152–155.

279. Graeber GM, Snyder RJ, Fleming AW, et al. Initial and long-term results in the management of primary chest wall neoplasms. Ann Thorac Surg 1982;34:664–673.

280. Braasch JW, Mon AB. Primary retroperitoneal tumors. Surg Clin North Am 1967;47: 663.

281. Cody HS, Turnbull AD, Fortner JG, et al. The continuing challenge of retroperitoneal sarcomas. Cancer 1981;47:2147–2152.

282. Storm FK, Sondak VK, Economou JS. Sarcomas of the retroperitoneum. In: Eilber FR, Morton DL, Sondak VK, et al, eds. The soft tissue sarcomas. New York: Grune & Stratton, 1987:239–248.

283. Karakousis CP, Velez AF, Emrich LJ. Management of retroperitoneal sarcomas and patient survival. Am J Surg 1985;150:376–380.

284. Bose B. Primary malignant retroperitoneal tumors: Analysis of 30 cases. Can J Surg 1979;22:215–220.

285. McGrath PC, Neifield JP, Lawrence W, et al. Improved survival following complete excision of retroperitoneal sarcomas. Ann Surg 1984;200:200–204.

286. Jaques DP, Coit DG, Hajdu SI, et al. Management of primary and recurrent soft-tissue sarcoma of the retroperitoneum. Ann Surg 1990;212:51–59.

287. Delamater J. Mammoth tumor. Cleve Med Gazette 1859;1:31.

288. Enzinger FM, Winslow DJ. Liposarcoma. A study of 30 cases. Virchows Arch [A] 1962;335:367–388.

289. Fortner JG, Martin S, Hajdu S, et al. Primary sarcoma of the retroperitoneum. Semin Oncol 1981;8:180–184.

290. Abbas S, Holyoke ED, Moore R, et al. The surgical treatment and outcome of soft-tissue sarcoma. Arch Surg 1981;116:765–769.

291. Kinsella TJ, Sindelar WF, Lack E, et al. Preliminary results of a randomized study of adjuvant radiation therapy in resectable adult retroperitoneal soft tissue sarcomas. J Clin Oncol 1988;6:18–25.

292. Cade SS. Soft tissue tumors: Their natural history and treatment. Proc R Soc Med 1951;19:19–36.

293. Windeyer SB, Dische S, Mansfield CM. The place of radio-therapy in the management of fibrosarcoma of the soft tissues. Clin Radiol 1966;17:32–40.

294. Lindberg RD. Soft tissue sarcoma. In: Fletcher GH, ed. Textbook of radiotherapy. Philadelphia: Lea & Febiger, 1980:922–942.

295. Suit HD. Sarcomas of soft tissue. In: The third annual current approaches to radiation oncology, biology, and physics. San Francisco: University of California, 1983:138–141.

296. Tepper JE, Suite HD. Radiation therapy of soft tissue sarcomas. Cancer 1985;55:2273–2277.

297. Todoroki T, Suit HD. Effect of fractionated irradiation prior to conservation and radical surgery on therapeutic gain in spontaneous fibrosarcoma of the C3H mouse. J Surg Oncol 1986;31:279–286.

298. Leibel SA, Ware WM, Hill DR, et al. Desmoid tumors: Local control and patterns of relapse following radiation therapy. Int J Radiat Oncol Biol Phys 1983;9:1167–1171.

299. Greenberg HM, Goebel R, Weichselbaum RR, et al. Radiation therapy in the treatment of aggressive fibromatoses. Int J Radiat Oncol Biol Phys 1981;7:309–319.

300. Kiel KD, Suit HD. Radiation therapy in the treatment of aggressive fibromatoses (desmoid tumors). Cancer 1984;54:2051–2055.

301. Mirabell R, Suit HD, Mankin HJ, et al. Fibromatoses: From post-surgical surveillance to combined surgery and radiation therapy. Int J Radiat Oncol Biol Phys 1990;18:535–540.

302. McCollough WM, Parons JT, van der Griend R, et al. Radiation therapy for aggressive fibromatoses. J Bone Joint Surg [Am] 1991;73:717–725.

303. Leibel SA, Transbaugh RF, Wara WM, et al. Soft tissue sarcomas of the extremities. Survival patterns of failure with conservative surgery and post-operative irradiation compared to surgery alone. Cancer 1982;50:1076–1083.

304. Suit HD, Mankin HJ, Wood WC, et al. Pre-operative, intra-operative, and post-operative radiation in the treatment of primary soft tissue sarcoma. Cancer 1985;55:2659–2667.

305. Suit HD, Mankin HJ, Schiller AL, et al. Results of treatment of sarcoma of soft tissue by radiation and surgery at Massachusetts General Hospital. Cancer Treat Symp 1985;3:43–47.

306. Lindberg R. Treatment of localized soft tissue sarcomas in adults at M.D. Anderson Hospital and Tumor Institute (1960–1981). Cancer Treat Symp 1985;3:59–65.

307. Enneking WF, McAuliffe JA. Adjunctive preoperative radiation therapy in treatment of soft tissue sarcomas: A preliminary report. Cancer Treat Symp 1985;3:37–42.

308. Atkinson L, Garvan JM, Newton NC. Behavior and management of soft tissue sarcomas. Cancer 1963;16:1552–1562.

309. Suit HD, Proppe KH, Mankin HJ, et al. Pre-operative radiation therapy for sarcoma of soft tissue. Cancer 1981;47:2269–2274.

310. Fortner JG, Kim DK, Shiu MH. Limb-preserving vascular surgery for malignant tumors of the lower extremity. Arch Surg 1977;112:391–394.

311. Imparato AM, Roses DF, Francis KC, et al. Major vascular reconstruction for limb salvage in patients with soft tissue and skeletal sarcomas of the extremity. Surg Gynecol Obstet 1978;147:891–896.

312. Morton DL, Eilber FR, Townsend CM Jr, et al. Limb salvage from a multidisciplinary treatment approach for skeletal and soft tissue sarcomas of the extremity. Ann Surg 1976;184:268–278.

313. Steed DL, Peitzman AB, Webster MW, et al. Limb sparing operations for sarcomas of the extremities involving critical arterial circulation. Surg Gynecol Obstet 1987;164:493–498.

314. Nambisan RN, Karakousis CP. Vascular reconstruction for limb salvage in soft tissue sarcomas. Surgery 1987;101:668–677.

315. Yang JC. Unpublished data, 1992.

316. Bramwell V, Rouesse J, Steward W, et al. European experience of adjuvant chemotherapy for soft tissue sarcoma: Interim report of a randomized trial of CYVADIC versus control. In: Ryan JR, Baker LH, eds. Recent concepts in sarcoma treatment. Dordrecht: Kluwer Academic Publishers, 1988.

317. Ravaud A, Bui NB, Coindre JM, et al. Adjuvant chemotherapy with CYVADIC in high risk soft tissue sarcoma: A randomized prospective trial. In: Salmon SE, ed. Adjuvant therapy of cancer. Vol 6. Philadelphia: WB Saunders, 1990.

318. Rydholm A, Gustafson P, Rooser B, et al. Limb-sparing surgery without radiotherapy based on anatomic location of soft tissue sarcoma. J Clin Oncol 1991;10:1757–1765.

319. Shiu MH, Turnbull AD, Nori D, et al. Control of locally advanced extremity soft tissue sarcomas by function-saving resection and brachytherapy. Cancer 1984;53:1385–1392.

320. Brennan MF, Hilaris B, Shiu MH, et al. Local recurrence in adult soft-tissue sarcoma. Arch Surg 1987;122:1289–1293.

321. Habrand JL, Gerbaulet A, Pejovic MH, et al. Twenty years experience of interstitial iridium brachytherapy in the management of soft tissue sarcomas. Int J Radiat Oncol Biol Phys 1991;20:405–411.

322. Gemer LS, Trowbridge DR, Neff J, et al. Local recurrence of soft tissue sarcoma following brachytherapy. Int J Radiat Oncol Biol Phys 1991;20:587–592.

323. Giuliano AE, Eilber FR. The rationale for planned reoperation after unplanned total excision of soft-tissue sarcomas. J Clin Oncol 1985;3:1344–1348.

324. Tepper JE, Rosenberg SA, Glatstein E. Radiation therapy technique in soft tissue sarcomas of the extremity—policies at the National Cancer Institute. Int J Radiat Oncol Biol Phys 1982;8:263–273.

325. Fraass BA, Tepper JE, Glatstein E, et al. Clinical use of a match-line wedge for adjacent megavoltage radiation field matching. Int J Radiat Oncol Biol Phys 1983;9:209–216.

326. Kinsella TJ, Loefler JS, Fraass BA, et al. Extremity preservation by combined modality therapy in sarcomas of the hand and foot: An analysis of local control, disease-free survival and function result. Int J Radiat Oncol Biol Phys 1983;9:1115–1119.

327. Eilber FR, Guiliano AE, Huth J, et al. Limb salvage for high grade soft tissue sarcomas of the extremity: Experience at The University of California, Los Angeles. Cancer Treat Symp 1985;3:49–57.

328. Denton JW, Dunham WK, Salter M, et al. Preoperative regional chemotherapy and rapid-fraction irradiation for sarcomas of the soft tissue and bone. Surg Gynecol Obstet 1984;158:545–551.

329. Lokich JJ. Preoperative chemotherapy in soft tissue sarcoma. Surg Gynecol Obstet 1979;148:512–516.

330. Stehlin JS, de Ipolyi PD, Giovanella BC, et al. Soft tissue sarcomas of the extremity. Multidisciplinary therapy employing hyperthermic perfusion. Am J Surg 1975;130:643–646.

331. Krementz ET, Carter RD, Sutherland CM, et al. Chemotherapy of sarcomas of the limbs by regional perfusion. Ann Surg 1977;185:555–564.

332. Karakousis CP, Lopez R, Catane R, et al. Intraarterial Adriamycin in the treatment of soft tissue sarcomas. J Surg Oncol 1980;13:21–27.

333. Didolkar MS, Kanter PM, Baffi RR, et al. Comparison of regional versus systemic chemotherapy with Adriamycin. Ann Surg 1978;187:332–336.

334. Salinas R, Hussey DH, Fletcher GH, et al. Experience with fast neutron therapy for locally advanced sarcomas. Int J Radiat Oncol Biol Phys 1980;6:267–272.

335. Pelton JG, Del Rowe JD, Bolen JW, et al. Fast neutron radiotherapy for soft tissue sarcomas: University of Washington experience and review of the world's literature. Am J Clin Oncol 1986;9:397–400.

336. Willet CG, Suit HD, Tepper JE, et al. Intraoperative electron beam radiation therapy for sarcoma of retroperitoneal soft tissue sarcoma. Cancer 1991;68:278–283.

337. Kinsella TJ, Glatstein E. Clinical experience with intravenous radiosensitizers in unresectable sarcomas. Cancer 1987;59:908–915.

338. Rosenberg SA, Tepper J, Glatstein E, et al. Prospective randomized evaluation of adjuvant chemotherapy in adults with soft tissue sarcomas of the extremities. Cancer 1983;52:424–434.

339. Rosenberg SA. Prospective randomized trials demonstrating the efficacy of adjuvant chemotherapy in adult patients with soft tissue sarcomas. Cancer Treat Rep 1984;68:1067–1078.

340. Rosenberg SA, Chang AE, Glatstein E. Adjuvant chemotherapy for treatment of extremity soft tissue sarcomas: Review of National Cancer Institute experience. Cancer Treat Symp 1985;3:83–88.

341. Antman K, Suit H, Amato D, et al. Preliminary results of a randomized trial of adjuvant doxorubicin for sarcomas: Lack of apparent difference between treatment groups. J Clin Oncol 1984;2:601–608.

342. Edmonson JH, Felming TR, Ivins JC, et al. Randomized study of systemic chemotherapy following complete excision of nonosseous sarcomas. J Clin Oncol 1984;2:1390–1396.

343. Baker LH. Adjuvant therapy for soft tissue sarcomas. In: Ryan JR, Baker LO, eds. Recent concepts in sarcoma treatment. Dordrecht: Kluwer Academic Publishers, 1988.

344. Antman K, Amato D, Lerner H, et al. Adjuvant doxorubicin for sarcoma: Data from The Eastern Cooperative Oncology Group and Dana-Farber Cancer Institute/Massachusetts General Hospital studies. Cancer Treat Symp 1985;3:109–115.

345. Picci P, Bacci G, Gherlinzoni F, et al. Results of a randomized trial for the treatment of localized soft tissue tumors of the extremities in adult patients. In: Ryan JR, Baker LO, eds. Recent concepts in sarcoma treatment. Dordrecht: Kluwer Academic Publishers, 1988.

346. Gherlinzoni F, Bacci G, Picci P, et al. A randomized trial for the treatment of high-grade soft-tissue sarcomas of the extremities: Preliminary observations. J Clin Oncol 1986;4:552–558.

347. Eilber FR, Giuliano AE, Huth JF, et al. Adjuvant Adriamycin in high-grade extremity soft-tissue sarcoma—a randomized prospective trial. Proc Am Soc Clin Oncol 1986;5:125.

348. Lerner HJ, Amato DA, Savlov ED, et al. Eastern Cooperative Oncology Group: A comparison of adjuvant doxorubicin and observation for patients with localized soft tissue sarcoma. J Clin Oncol 1987;5:613–617.

349. Alvegard TA, Sigurdsson H, Mouridsen H, et al. Adjuvant chemotherapy with doxorubicin

for high-grade soft tissue sarcoma: A randomized trial of the Scandinavian Sarcoma Group. J Clin Oncol 1989;7:1504–1513.

350. Antman K, Ryan L, Borden E, et al. Pooled result from three randomized adjuvant studies of doxorubicin versus observation in soft tissue sarcoma: 10-year results and review of the literature. In: Salmon SE, eds. Adjuvant therapy of cancer. Vol VI. Philadelphia: WB Saunders, 1990.

351. Benjamin TO, Terjanian TO, Fenoglio CJ, et al. The importance of combination chemotherapy for adjuvant treatment of high-risk patients with soft-tissue sarcomas of the extremities. In: Salmon SE, ed. Adjuvant therapy of cancer. Vol VI. Philadelphia: WB Saunders, 1990.

352. Eilber FR, Giuliano AE, Huth JF, et al. Postoperative adjuvant chemotherapy (Adriamycin) in high-grade extremity soft tissue sarcomas—a randomized prospective trial. In: Salmon SE, ed. Adjuvant therapy of cancer. Vol V. Orlando: Grune & Stratton, 1987.

353. Omura GA, Major FJ, Blessing JA, et al. A randomized clinical trial of adjuvant Adriamycin in uterine sarcomas: A Gynecologic Oncology Group study. J Clin Oncol 1985;3: 1240–1245.

354. Yang JC. Unpublished data.

355. Chang AE, Kinsella T, Glatstein E, et al. Adjuvant chemotherapy for patients with high-grade soft-tissue sarcomas of the extremities. J Clin Oncol 1988;6:1491–1500.

356. Dresdale A, Bonow RO, Wesley R, et al. Prospective evaluation of doxorubicin-induced cardiomyopathy resulting from postsurgical adjuvant treatment of patients with soft tissue sarcomas. Cancer 1983;52:51–60.

357. Ettinghausen SE, Bonow RO, Palmeri ST, et al. Prospective study of cardiomyopathy induced by adjuvant doxorubicin therapy in patients with soft-tissue sarcomas. Arch Surg 1986;121:1445–1451.

358. Giuliano AE, Eilber FR, Morton DL. The management of locally recurrent soft-tissue sarcoma. Ann Surg 1982;196:87–91.

359. Roth JA, Putnam JB, Wesley MN, et al. Differing determinants of prognosis following resection of pulmonary metastases from osteogenic and soft tissue sarcoma patients. Cancer 1985;55:1361–1366.

360. Jablons D, Steinberg SM, Roth J, et al. Metastasectomy for soft tissue sarcoma; Further evidence for efficacy and prognostic factors. J Thorac Cardiovasc Surg 1989;97:695–705.

361. Rizzoni WE, Pass HI, Wesley MN, et al. Resection of recurrent pulmonary metastases in patients with soft-tissue sarcomas. Arch Surg 1986;121:1248–1252.

362. Pass HI, Dwyer A, Makuch R, et al. Detection of pulmonary metastases in patients with osteogenic and soft-tissue sarcomas: The superiority of CT scans compared with conventional linear tomograms using dynamic analysis. J Clin Oncol 1985;3:1261–1265.

363. Blum RH. An overview of studies of Adriamycin (NSC-123127) in the United States. Cancer Chemother Rep 1975;6:247–251.

364. O'Bryan RM, Luce JK, Talley RW, et al. Phase II evaluation of Adriamycin in human neoplasia. Cancer 1973;32:1–8.

365. O'Bryan RM, Baker LH, Gottlieb JE, et al. Dose response evaluation of Adriamycin in human neoplasia. Cancer 1977;39:1940–1948.

366. Schoenfeld D, Rosenbaum C, Horton J, et al. A comparison of Adriamycin versus vincristine and Adriamycin and cyclophosphamide for advanced sarcoma. Cancer 1982;50:2757–2762.

367. Borden EC, Amato D, Enterline HT, et al. Randomized comparison of Adriamycin regimens for treatment of metastatic soft tissue sarcomas. J Clin Oncol 1987;5:840–850.

368. Cruz AB Jr, Thames EA Jr, Aust JB, et al. Combination chemotherapy for soft tissue sarcomas: A phase III study. J Surg Oncol 1979;11:313–323.

369. Rosen G, Caparros B, Nirenberg A, et al. High-dose methotrexate (HDMTX) with citrovorum factor rescue (CFR) in the treatment of radiation-induced sarcomas. Proc Am Assoc Clin Radiol 1981;1983:194.

370. Vaughn C, McKelvey E, Balcerzak S, et al. High-dose methotrexate with leucovorin rescue plus vincristine in advanced sarcoma: A Southwest Oncology Group study. Cancer Treat Rep 1984;68:409–410.

371. Isacoff WH, Eilber F, Tabbarah H, et al. Phase II clinical trial with high-dose methotrexate therapy and citrovorum factor rescue. Cancer Treat Rep 1978;62:1295–1304.

372. Karakousis CP, Rao U, Carlson M. High-dose methotrexate as secondary chemotherapy in metastatic soft-tissue sarcomas. Cancer 1980;46:1345–1348.

373. Von Hoff DD, Rozencweig M, Louie AC, et al. "Single"-agent activity of high-dose methotrexate therapy with citrovorum factor rescue. Cancer Treat Rep 1978;62:233–235.

374. Frie E, Blum R, Pitman S, et al. High-dose methotrexate with leucovorin rescue: Rationale and spectrum of antitumor activity. Am J Med 1979;68:370–375.

375. Andrews N, Wilson W. Phase II study of methotrexate (NSC 740) in solid tumors. Cancer Chemother Rep 1967;51:471–474.

376. Subramanian S, Wiltshaw E. Chemotherapy of sarcoma—a comparison of three regimes. Lancet 1978;1:683–686.

377. Buesa JM, Mouridsen HT, Santoro A. Treatment of advanced soft tissue sarcomas with low-dose methotrexate: A phase II trial by the European Organization for Research on Treatment of Cancer (EORTC) Soft Tissue and Bone Sarcoma Group. Cancer Treat Rep 1984;68:683–694.

378. Amato DA, Borden EC, Shiraki M, et al. Evaluation of bleomycin, chlorozotocin, MGBG, and bruceantin in patients with advanced soft tissue sarcoma, bone sarcoma, or mesothelioma. Invest New Drugs 1985;3:397–401.

379. Golbey R, Li MC, Kaufman RF. Actinomycin in the treatment of soft part sarcomas. [Abstract] James Ewing Society Scientific Program, 1968.

380. Gold G, Hall T, Shnider B, et al. A clinical study of 5-fluorouracil. Cancer 1959;19: 935–939.

381. Selawry OS, Holland JF, Wolman IJ. Effect of vincristine (NSC-67574) on malignant solid tumors in children. Cancer Chemother Rep 1968;52:497–499.

382. Korbitzs BC, Davis HL Jr, Ramirez G, et al. Low doses of vincristine (NSC-67574) for malignant disease. Cancer Chemother Rep 1969;53:249–254.

383. Radice PA, Bunn PA Jr, Ihde DC. Therapeutic trials with VP-16 and VM-26. Cancer Treat Rep 1979;63:1231–1239.

384. Bleyer WA, Chard RL, Krivit W, et al. Epipodophyllotoxin therapy of childhood neoplasia. A comparative phase II analysis of VM26 and VP16-213. Proc Am Assoc Clin Radiol 1978;19:373.

385. Elias AD, Eder JP, Shea T, Begg CB, Frei III E, Antman KH. High dose ifosfamide with mesna uroprotection: A phase I study. J Clin Oncol 1990;8:170–178.

386. Elias AD, Ayash LJ, Eder JP, et al. A phase I study of high-dose ifosfamide and escalating doses of carboplatin with autologous bone marrow support. J Clin Oncol 1991;9:320–327.

387. Klein HO, Wickramanayake PD, Coerper CL, Christian E, Pohl J, Brock N. High-dose ifosfamide and mesna as continuous infusion over five days-a phase I/II trial. Cancer Treat Rev 1983;10(suppl A):167–173.

388. Chawla SP, Rosen G, Lowenbraun S, Morton D, Eilber F. Role of high dose ifosfamide (HDI) in recurrent osteosarcoma. Proc Am Soc Clin Oncol 1990;9:310.

389. Czownicki Z, Utracka-Hutka B. Clinical studies with uromitexan-an antidote against urotoxicity of holoxan. Preliminary results. Nowotwory(Pol) 1981;30:377–383.

390. Niederle N, Scheulen ME, Cremer M, Schutte J, Schmidt CG, Seeber S. Ifosfamide in combination chemotherapy for sarcomas and testicular carcinomas. Cancer Treat Rev 1983;10(suppl A):129–135.

391. Antman KH, Ryan L, Elias A, Sherman D, Grier E. Response to ifosfamide and mesna: 124 previously treated patients with metastatic or unresectable sarcoma. J Clin Oncol 1989;7:126–131.

392. Stuart-Harris R, Harper PG, Kaye SB, Wiltshaw E. High-dose ifosfamide by infusion with mesna in advanced soft tissue sarcoma. Cancer Treat Rev 1983;10(suppl A): 163–164.

393. Bramwell V, Mouridsen HT, Santoro A, et al. Cyclophosphamide vs ifosfamide: Final report of a randomized phase II trial in adult soft tissue sarcoma. Eur J Cancer Clin Oncol 1987;23:311–321.

394. Buesa JM, Mouridsen HT, Oosterom ATV, et al. High-dose DTIC in advanced soft-tissue sarcomas in the adult. A phase II study of the EORTC soft tissue and bone sarcoma group. Ann Oncol 1991;2:307–309.

395. Bramwell VHC, Brugarols A, Mouridsen HT, et al. EORTC. Phase II study of cisplatinum in CYVADIC-resistant soft tissue sarcoma. Eur J Cancer 1979;15:1511–1513.

396. Karakousis CP, Holterman OA, Holyoke E. Cisdichlorodiamineplatinum (II) in metastatic soft tissue sarcomas. Cancer Treat Rep 1979;63:2071–2075.

397. Samson MK, Baker LH, Benjamin RS, Lane M, Plager C. Cisdichlorodiamineplatinum (II) in advanced soft tissue and bony sarcomas. A Southwest Oncology Group study. Cancer Treat Rep 1979;63:2027–2028.

398. Thigpen JT, Blessing JA, Wilbanks GD. Cisplatin as second-line chemotherapy in the treatment of advanced or recurrent leiomyosarcoma of the uterus. Am J Clin Oncol 1986;9:18–20.

399. Budd GT, Metch B, Balcerzak SP, Fletcher WS, Baker LH, Mortimer JE. High-dose cisplatin for metastatic soft tissue sarcoma. Cancer 1990;65:866–869.

400. Gershenon DM, Kavanagh JJ, Copeland LJ, Edwards CL, Stringer CA, Wharton JT. Cisplatin therapy for disseminated mixed mesodermal sarcoma of the uterus. J Clin Oncol 1987;5:618–621.

401. Goldstein D, Cheuvart B, Trump DL, et al. Phase II trial of carboplatin in soft-tissue sarcoma. Am J Clin Oncol 1990;13:420–423.

402. Bergsagel DE, Levin WC. A prelusive clinical trial of cyclophosphamide. Cancer Chemother Rep 1960;8:120–134.

403. Korst DR, Johnson D, Frenkel EP, Challener WL III. Preliminary evaluation of the effect of cyclophosphamide on the course of human neoplasms. Cancer Chemother Rep 1960;7:1–12.

404. Pinedo HM, Branwell VHC, Mouridson MD, et al. CYVADIC in advanced soft tissue sarcoma: A randomized study comparing two schedules. A study of the EORTC Soft Tissue and Bone Sarcoma Group. Cancer 1984;53:1825–1832.

405. Legha S, Benjamin RS, Mackay B, et al. Reduction of doxorubicin cardiotoxicity by prolonged continuous intravenous infusion. Ann Intern Med 1982;96:133–139.

406. Benjamin R, Yap B, Frazier O Jr, et al. Combination chemotherapy for sarcomas with cyclophosphamide and continuous infusion Adriamycin and dacarbazine (CI-CYA-DIC) with surgical intensification. Proc Am Assoc Clin Radiol Am Soc Clin Oncol [Abstract] 1981;22:526.

407. Baker LK, Green S, Ryan J, et al. Combined modality therapy for disseminated soft tissue sarcoma, phase III. Proc Am Soc Clin Oncol 1987;6:138.

408. Brennan MF, Friedrich C, Almadrones L, et al. Prospective randomized trial examining the cardiac toxicity of adjuvant doxorubicin in high grade extremity sarcomas. In: Sydney Salmon, ed. Adjuvant therapy of cancer V. Orlando: Grune & Stratton, 1987: 745–754.

409. Brock N. Pharmacological studies with ifosfamide—a new oxazaphosphorine compound. In: Semonsky M, Hejzler M, Masak S, eds. Advances in antimicrobial and antineoplastic chemotherapy. Proceedings of the Seventh International Congress of Chemotherapy, Prague, 1971. Berlin: Urban & Schwarzenberg, 1972:2:749–756.

410. Cabanillas F, Hagemeister FB, Bodey GP, Freireich EJ. IMVP-16: An effective regimen for patients with lymphoma who have relapsed after initial combination chemotherapy. Blood 1982;60:693–697.

411. Antman KH, Montella D, Rosenbaum C, Schwen M. Phase II trial of ifosfamide with mesna in previously treated metastatic sarcoma. Cancer Treat Rep 1985;69:499–502.

412. Morgan LR, Posey LE, Rainey J, et al. Ifosfamide: A weekly dose fractionated schedule in bronchogenic carcinoma. Cancer Treat Rep 1981;65:693–695.

413. Czownicki Z, Utracka-Hutka B. Contributions to the treatment of malignant tumors with ifosfamide. In: Burkeret H, Voight HC, eds. Proceedings of the International Holoxan Symposium. Dusseldorf: Asta-Werke, 1977:109–111.

414. De Kraker J, Voute PA. Ifosfamide and vincristine in pediatric tumors. A phase II study. Eur Paediatr Haematol Oncol 1984;1:47–50.

415. Magrath I, Sandlund J, Raynor A, Rosenberg S, Arasi V, Miser J. A phase II study of ifosfamide in the treatment of recurrent sarcomas in young people. Cancer Chemother Pharmacol 1986;18(suppl 2):S25–S28.

416. Legha S, Papadopoulos N, Plager C, et al. A comparative evaluation of the uroprotective effect of mercaptoethane sulfonate (mesna) and N-acetylcysteine in sarcoma patients treated with ifosfamide. Proc Am Soc Clin Oncol [Abstract] 1990;9:1205.

417. Perevodchikova NI, Lichinister MR, Gorbunova VA. Phase II clinical study of carminomycin: Its activity against soft tissue sarcomas. Cancer Treat Rep 1977;61:1705–1707.

418. Weiss AJ, Ramirez G, Grage T, Strawitz J, Goldman L, Downing V. Phase II study of azotomycin (NSC-56654). Cancer Chemother Rep 1968;52:611–614.

419. Chang P, Wiernik PHP. Phase II study of azotomycin in sarcomas. Cancer Treat Rep 1979;61:1719.

420. De Jager R, Body JJ, Dupong D, Klastersky J, Kenis Y. Phase I study of oral 4'-(9-acrindylamino-methanseulfonanidide) m-AMSA (C-574). Proc Am Soc Clin Oncol 1979;20:429.

421. Legha SS, Gutterman JU, Hall SW, et al. Phase I clinical investigation of 4'-(9-acridinylamino) methanesulfon-manisiside (NSC 249992), a new acridine derivative. Cancer Res 1978;38:3712–3716.

422. Von Hoff DD, Howser D, Gormley P, et al. Phase I study of methanesulfonamide, N-(4-9-acridinylamino)-3-methoxyphenyl-m-AMSA using a single-dose schedule. Cancer Treat Rep 1978;62:1421–1426.

423. Schneider R, Sklanoff R, Ochoa M. Phase I trial of AMSA (4'-acrindylamino)-methansulfon-manisidide). Proc Am Assoc Cancer Res 1979;20:114.

424. Bertrand M, Multhauf P, Bartolucci A, Ellison D, Gockerman J. Phase II study of aclarubicin in previously untreated patients with advanced soft tissue sarcoma. Cancer Treat Rep 1985;69:725–726.

425. Zidar B, Baker L, Rivkin S, Balcerzak SP, Stephens RL. A phase II study of diaziquone in advanced soft tissue and bony sarcoma. A Southwest Oncology Group Study. Cancer Treat Rep 1985;69:1035–1036.

426. Chan C, Bartolucci A, Brenner D, et al. Phase II trial of diaziquone in anthracycline-resistant adult soft tissue bone sarcoma patients: A Southeastern Cancer Study Group trial. Cancer Teat Rep 1986;70:427–428.

427. Slayton RE, Blessing JA, Clarke-Pearson D. A Phase II trials of Diaziquone (AZQ) in mixed mesodermal sarcomas uterus. A gynecologic oncology group study. Invest New Drugs 1991;9:93–94.

428. Presant C, Gams R, Bartolucci A. Treatment of metastatic sarcomas with mitroxantrone. Cancer Treat Rep 1984;68:813–814.

429. Bull FE, Von Hoff DD, Balcerzak SP, Stephens RL, Panettiere FJ. Phase II trial of mitoxantrone in advanced sarcomas. A Southwest Oncology Group study. Cancer Treat Rep 1985;69:231–233.

430. Buckner JC, Edmonson JH, Ingle JN, Schaid DJ. Evaluation of menogaril in patients with metastatic sarcomas and no prior chemotherapy exposure. Am J Clin Oncol 1989;12:384–386.

431. Giaccone G, Donadio M, Calciati A. Phase II study of esorubicin in the treatment of patients with advanced sarcoma. Oncology 1989;46:285–287.

432. Chevallier B, Montcuquet P, Fachini T, et al. Phase II study of epirubicin in advanced soft tissue sarcoma. Bull Cancer 1990;77:991–995.

433. Taylor SA, Metch B, Balcerzak SP, Hanson KH. Phase II trial of Echinomycin in advanced soft tissue sarcomas. A Southwest Oncology Group study. Invest New Drugs 1990;8:381–383.

434. Quirt I, Eisenhauer E, Knowling M, et al. A phase 2 study of trimetrexate in metastatic soft tissue sarcoma. Proc Am Soc Clin Oncol 1988;7:275.

435. Licht JD, Gonin R, Antman KH. Phase II trial of trimetrexate in patients with advanced soft tissue sarcoma. Cancer Chemother Pharmacol 1991;28:223–225.

436. Johnson R. Preliminary phase I trials with 1-aminocyclopentane carboxylic acid (NSC-1026) (cycloleucine). Cancer Chemother Rep 1963;32:67–71.

437. Aust J, Andrews N, Shcroeder J, Lawton RL. Phase II study of 1-aminocyclopentane-carboxylic acid (NSC 1026) in patients with cancer. Cancer Chemother Rep 1970;54:237–241.

438. Savlov ED, MacIntyre JM, Knight E, Woller J. Comparison of doxorubicin with cyclo-leucine in the treatment of sarcomas. Cancer Treat Rep 1981;65:21–27.

439. Amato DA, Borden EC, Shiraki M, et al. Evaluation of bleomycin, chlorozotocin, MGBG, and bruceantin in patients with advanced soft tissue sarcoma, bone sarcoma, or me-sothelioma. Invest New Drugs 1985;3:397–401.

440. Mouridsen HT, Bramwell VH, Lacave J, et al. Treatment of advanced soft tissue sarcomas with chlorozotocin: A phase II trial of the EORTC soft tissue and bone sarcoma group. Cancer Treat Rep 1981;65:509–511.

441. Kovach JS, Moertel CG, Schutt AF. A phase I study of chlorozotocin (NSC 178248). Cancer 1979;43:2189–2196.

442. Gralla RJ, Tan CTC, Young CW. Phase I trial of chlorozotocin. Cancer Treat Rep 1979;63:17–20.

443. Presant CA, Bartolucci AA. Phase II evaluation of chlorozotocin in metastatic sarcomas. Med Pediatr Oncol 1984;12:25–27.

444. Sordillo PP, Magill GB, Gralla RJ. Chlorozotocin: Phase II evaluation in patients with advanced sarcomas. Cancer Treat Rep 1981;65:513–514.

445. Talley RW, Samson MK, Brownlee RW, Samhouri AM, Fraile RJ, Baker LH. Phase II evaluation of chlorozotocin in advanced human cancers. Eur J Cancer 1981;17:337–343.

446. Baker LH, Samson MK, Izbicki RM. Phase I and II evaluation of cytembena in disseminated epithelial ovarian cancer and sarcomas. Cancer Treat Rep 1976;60:1389–1391.

447. Matejovsky Z. Effects of cytembena in the treatment of malignant musculoskeletal tumors. Neoplasma 1971;18:473–480.

448. Kurzrock R, Yap BS, Plager C, et al. Phase II evaluation of PALA in patients with refractory metastatic sarcomas. Am J Clin Oncol 1984;7:305–307.

449. Presant CA, Ardalan B, Multhauf P. Continuous five-day infusion of PALA and 5-FU. A pilot phase II trial. Med Pediatr Oncol 1983;11:162–163.

450. Baselga J, Magill GB, Curley T, Casper ES. Phase II trial of pala + dipyridamole in patients with metastatic soft tissue sarcoma. Proc Am Assoc Cancer Res [Abstract] 1990;31:1187.

451. Casper ES, Baselga J, Smart TB, Magill GB, Markman M, Ranhosky A. A phase II trial of PALA + dipyridamole in patients with advanced soft-tissue sarcoma. Cancer Chemother Pharmacol 1991;28:51–54.

452. Rodriquez V, Gottlieb J, Burgess MA, et al. Phase I studies with Baker's antifol (NSC 139105). Cancer 1976;38:690–694.

453. Thigpen JT, O'Bryan RM, Benjamin RS, Coltman CA Jr. Phase II trial of Baker's antifol in metastatic sarcoma. Cancer Treat Rep 1977;61:1485–1487.

454. Tranum BP, Haut A, Rivkin SE, et al. A phase II study of methyl-CCNU in the treatment of solid tumors and lymphomas in the Southwest Oncology Group. Cancer 1974;35:1148–1153.

455. Creagan ET, Hahn JH, Ahmann DL, Edmonson JH, Bisel HF, Eagan RT. A comparative clinical trial evaluating the combination of actinomycin D, cyclophosphamide, and vincristine, and a single agent, methyl-CCNU, in advanced sarcomas. Cancer Treat Rep 1976;60:1385–1386.

456. Borden EC, Larson P, Ansfield FJ, et al. Hexamethylmelamine: Treatment of sarcomas and lymphomas. Med Pediatr Oncol 1977;3:401–406.

457. Blum RH, Livingston BB, Carter SK. Hexamethylmelamine: A new drug with activity in solid tumors. Eur J Cancer 1973;9:195–202.

458. Sooriyaarachchi GS, Ramirez G, Roley EL. Hemangiopericytoma of the uterus. J Surg Oncol 1978;10:399–406.

459. Conroy JF, Roda PI, Prasavinichai S. Dibromodulcitin in the treatment of metastic hemangiopericytoma. Am J Clin Oncol 1982;5:453–456.

460. Borden EC, Ash A, Enterline HT, et al. Phase II evaluation of dibromodulcitol, ICRF-159, and maytansine for sarcomas. Am J Clin Oncol 1982;5:417–420.

461. Kimball JC, Cangir A. A phase II trial of dianhydrogalactitol in advanced soft tissue and bony sarcomas, a Southwest Oncology Group Study. Cancer Treat Rep 1979;63:553–554.

462. Saiki J, Stephens R, Fabian C, Kraut E, Fletcher W. Phase II evaluation of gallium nitrate (NSC-15200) in soft tissue and bone sarcomas. Proc Am Assoc Cancer Res 1981;22:525.

463. Bleyer WA, Krivit W, Chard RL, Hammond D. Phase II study of VM-26 in acute leukemia, neuroblastoma, and other refractory childhood malignancies: A report from the Children's Cancer Study Group. Cancer Treat Rep 1979;63:977–981.

464. Currie VE, Wong PP, Krakoff IH, Young CW. Phase I trial of vindesine in patients with advanced cancer. Cancer Treat Rep 1978;62:1333–1336.

465. Rossof AH, Chandra G, Walter J, et al. Phase II trial of vindesine (desacetyl vinblastine amide sulfate) in advanced metastatic cancer. Proc Am Assoc Cancer Res 1979;20:146.

466. Alberto P, De Jager RL, Brugarlas A, Hansen H, Cavalli F, Host H. Phase II study of diamino-dichlorophenyl-methylpyrimidine with folinic acid protection and rescue. Proc Am Assoc Cancer Res 1979;20:323.

467. Benjamin RS, Keating MJ, Valdivieso M, et al. Phase I–II study of piperazinedione in adults with solid tumors and acute leukemia. Cancer Treat Rep 1979;63:939–943.

468. LaGasse L, Thigpen T, Morrison F. Phase II trial of piperazinedione in treatment of advanced endometrial carcinoma, uterine sarcoma, and vulvar carcinoma. Proc Am Soc Clin Oncol 1979;20:388.

469. Thigpen T, Blessing JA, Homesley HD, Hacker N, Curry SL. Phase II trial of piperazinedione in treatment of advanced or recurrent uterine sarcoma, a GOG study. Am J Clin Oncol 1985;8:350–352.

470. Sordillo PP, Magill GB. Phase II evaluation of pyrazofurin in patients with soft-tissue sarcomas. Am J Clin Oncol 1985;8:316–318.

471. Salem PA, Bodey GP, Burgess MA, Murphy WK, Freireich EJ. A phase I study of pyrazofurin. Cancer 1977;40:2806–2809.

472. Gralla RJ, Sordillo PP, Magill GB. Phase II evaluation of pyrazofurin in patients with metastatic sarcoma. Cancer Treat Rep 1978;62:1573.

473. Blum R, Kahlert T. Maytansine: A phase I study of an ansamacrolide with antitumor activity. Cancer Treat Rep 1978;62:435–438.

474. Ajani JA, Dimery I, Chawla SP, et al. Phase II studies of homoharringtonine in patients with advanced malignant melanoma; sarcoma; and head and neck, breast, and colorectal carcinomas. Cancer Treat Rep 1986;70:375–379.

475. Rinehart J, Balcerzak SP, Hersh E. Phase II trial of tumor necrosis factor in human sarcoma: A Southwest Oncology Group study. Proc Am Soc Clin Oncol [Abstract] 1990;9:1229.

476. Robertson PA, Ross HJ, Figlin RA. Tumor necrosis factor induces hemorrhagic necrosis of a sarcoma. Ann Intern Med 1989;111:682–684.

477. Schuff-Werner P, Bartsch H, Schreml W, Nagel GA. Treatment of soft tissue sarcoma with recombinant alpha-interferon. Antiviral Res [Abstract 1] 1984;3:93.

478. Harris JE, Das Gupta T, Vogelzang M, et al. Treatment of soft tissue sarcoma with fibroblast interferon—an American Cancer Society/Illinois Cancer Council study. Cancer Treat Rep 1986;70:293–294.

479. Rosenberg SA, Lotze MT, Muul LM, et al. A progress report on the treatment of 157 patients with advanced cancer using lymphokine-activated killer cells and interleukin-2 or high-dose interleukin-2 alone. N Engl J Med 1987;316:890–897.

480. Omura GA, Major FJ, Blessing JA, et al. A randomized study of Adriamycin with and without dimethyl trazenoimidazole carboxamide in advanced uterine sarcomas. Cancer 1983;52:626–632.

481. Lerner H, Amato D, Stevens C, Borden E, Enterline H. Leiomyosarcoma: The Eastern Cooperative Oncology Group experience with 222 patients. Proc Am Assoc Cancer Res [Abstract C-561] 1983;24:142.

482. Benjamin RS, Gottlieb JA, Baker LH. CYVADIC vs CYVADACT—a randomized trial of cyclophosphamide, vincristine and Adriamycin, plus either dacarbazine or actinomycin D in metastatic sarcomas. Proc Am Assoc Cancer Res 1976;17:256.

483. Baker LH, Frank J, Fine G, et al. Combination chemotherapy using Adriamycin, DTIC, cyclophosphamide, and actinomycin D for advanced soft tissue sarcomas: A randomized comparative trial. J Clin Onc 1987;5:851–861.

484. Muss HB, Bundy B, Di Saia PJ, et al. Treatment of recurrent advanced uterine sarcoma—a randomized trial of doxorubicin vs doxorubicin and cyclophosphamide. Cancer 1985;55:1648–1653.

485. Santoro A, Rouesse J, Steward W, et al. A randomized EORTC study in advanced soft tissue sarcomas (STS): ADM vs. ADM + IFX vs. CYVADIC. Proc Am Soc Clin Oncol [Abstract 1196] 1990;9:309.

486. Blum RH, Edmonson JH. Investigations of ifosfamide (IF) for adult soft tissue sarcomas in ECOG. Eur J Cancer 1991;27:S350.

487. Antman K, Baker L, Balcerzak S, Crowley J, for CALGB and SWOG. A randomized study of doxorubicin and dacarbazine ± ifosfamide and mesna in advanced sarcomas. Proc ECCO 1991.

488. Bodey GP, Rodriquez V, Murphy WK, Burgess A, Benjamin RS. Protected environment-prophylactic antibiotic program for malignant sarcoma: Randomized trial during remission induction chemotherapy. Cancer 1981;47:2422–2429.

489. Casper ES, Gaynor JJ, Hajdu SI, et al. A prospective randomized trial of adjuvant chemotherapy with bolus versus continuous infusion of doxorubicin in patients with high-grade extremity soft tissue sarcoma and an analysis of prognostic factors. Cancer 1991;68:1221–1229.

490. Zalupski M, Metch B, Balcerzak S, et al. Phase III comparison of doxorubicin and dacarbazine given by bolus versus infusion in patients with soft-tissue sarcomas: A Southwest Oncology Group study. JNCI 1991;83:926–932.

491. Borden EC, Amato DA, Edmonson JH, Ritch PS, Shiraki M. Randomized comparison of doxorubicin and vindesine to doxorubicin for patients with metastatic soft-tissue sarcomas. Cancer 1990;66:862–867.

492. Gottlieb JA, Baker LH, Quagliana JM, et al. Chemotherapy of sarcomas with a combination of Adriamycin and dimethyltrazeno-carboxamide. Cancer 1972;30:1632–1638.

493. Saiki J, Baker LH, Rivkin SE, et al. A useful high-dose intermittent schedule of Adriamycin and DTIC in the treatment of advanced sarcomas. Cancer 1986;58:2196–2197.

494. Weh HJ, Zugel M, Wingberg D, et al. Chemotherapy of metastatic soft tissue sarcoma with a combination of Adriamycin and DTIC or Adriamycin and ifosfamide. Onkologie 1990;13:448–452.

495. Blum R, Corson J, Wilson R, et al.: Successful treatment of metastatic sarcomas with cyclophosphamide, Adriamycin and DTIC. Cancer 1980;46:1722–1726.

496. Hamdan H, Savage P, Skubitz K. A pilot study of continuous infusion chemotherapy for soft tissue sarcomas. Proc Am Soc Clin Oncol 1990;9:316.

497. Ikeda K, Ogawa M, Inagaki J, et al. A combination chemotherapy with Adriamycin, cyclophosphamide and DTIC (ACD) for advanced adult soft part sarcoma. Gan To Kagaku Ryoho 1984;11:235–239.

498. Gottlieb JA, Baker LH, O'Brian RM, et al. Adriamycin (NSC 123127) used alone and in combination for soft tissue and bony sarcomas. Cancer Chemother Rep 1975;6:271–282.

499. Yap B, Baker LH, Sinkovics JG, et al. Cyclophosphamide, vincristine, Adriamycin, and DTIC (CYVADIC) combination chemotherapy for the treatment of advanced sarcomas. Cancer Treat Rep 1980;64:93–98.

500. Yap BS, Sinkovics JG, Benjamin RS, et al. Survival and relapse patterns of complete responders in adults with advanced soft tissue sarcomas. Proc Am Soc Clin Oncol [Abstract] 1979;20:352.

501. Bui NB, Chauvergne J, Hocke C, et al. Analysis of a series of sixty soft tissue sarcomas in adults treated with a cyclophosphamide-vincristine-Adriamycin-dacarbazine (CYVADIC) combination. Cancer Chemother Pharmacol 1985;15:82–85.

502. Pfeffer MR, Sulkes A, Biran S. Treatment of advanced soft tissue sarcomas with a modified CYVADIC protocol. Oncology 1984;41:308–313.

503. Choi TK, NG A, Wong J. Doxorubicin, dacarbazine, vincristine, and cyclophosphamide in the treatment of advanced gastrointestinal leiomyosarcoma. Cancer Treat Rep 1985;69:443–444.

504. Lopez M, Di Lauro L, Papaldo P, et al. Alternating combination chemotherapy of advanced soft tissue sarcomas in adults. Am J Clin Oncol 1984;7:539–542.

505. Rivkin SE, Gottlieb JA, Thigpen T, et al. Methyl-CCNU and Adriamycin for patients with metastatic sarcomas. A Southwest Oncology Group study. Cancer 1980;46:446–451.

506. Chang P, Wiernik PH. Combination chemotherapy with Adriamycin and streptozotocin. Clin Pharmacol Ther 1976;20:606–610.

507. Lopez M, Carpano S, DiLauro L, Vici P, Conti EMS. Epirubicin and DTIC for advanced soft tissue sarcomas. Oncology 1991;48:230–233.

508. Casali P, Pastorino U, Zucchinelli, P, et al. Epidoxorubicin plus ifosfamide and decarbazine (EID) in advanced soft tissue sarcomas. Ann Oncology 1992;3(Suppl 2):S125–S126.

509. Jelic S, Vuletic L, Milanovic N, Tomasevic Z, Kovcin V. High-dose epirubicin-cisplatin chemotherapy for advanced soft tissue sarcoma. Tumori 1990;76:467–471.

510. Elli A, Botto G, Mendez A, et al. Ifosfamide plus epidoxorubicin for advanced soft tissue sarcomas. Preliminary report. Proc Am Soc Clin Oncol [Abstract 1227] 1990;9:317.

511. Cantwell BM, Carmichael J, Ghani S, Harris AL. A phase II study of ifosfamide/mesna with doxorubicin for adult soft tissue sarcoma. Cancer Chemother Pharmacol 1988;21:49–52.

512. Dombernowsky P, Mouridsen H, Schutte J, et al. Phase II study of ifosfamide + Adriamycin in advanced soft tissue sarcoma in adults. A preliminary analysis. Cancer Chemother Pharmacol 1986;18(suppl 2):S17.

513. Edmonson JH, Buckner JC, Long HJ, Loprinzi CL, Schaid DJ. Phase II study of ifosfamide-etoposide-mesna in adults with advanced nonosseous sarcomas. JNCI 1989;81:863–866.

514. Loehrer PS, Sledge GJ, Nicaise C, et al. Ifosfamide plus doxorubicin in metastatic adult sarcomas: A multi-institutional phase II trial. J Clin Oncol 1989;7:1655–1659.

515. Mansi JL, Fisher C, Wiltshaw E, MacMillan S, King M, Stuart-Harris R. A phase I–II study of ifosfamide in combination with Adriamycin in the treatment of adult soft tissue sarcoma. Eur J Cancer Clin Oncol 1988;24:1439–1443.

516. Schutte J, Mouridsen HT, Stewart W, et al. Ifosfamide plus doxorubicin in previously untreated patients with advanced soft tissue sarcoma. The EORTC soft tissue and bone sarcoma group. Eur J Cancer 1990;26:558–561.

517. Steward WP, Verweij J, Somers R, et al. Doxorubicin plus ifosfamide with rhGM-CSF in the treatment of advanced adult soft tissue sarcomas—preliminary results of a phase II study from the EORTC soft tissue and bone sarcoma group.

518. Wiltshaw E, Westbury G, Harmer C, McKinna A, Fisher C. Ifosfamide plus mesna with and without Adriamycin in soft tissue sarcoma. Cancer Chemother Pharmacol 1986;18(suppl 2):S10–S12.

519. Bramwell V, Quirt I, Warr D, et al. Combination chemotherapy with doxorubicin, dacarbazine, and ifosfamide in advanced adult soft tissue sarcoma. JNCI 1989;81:1496–1499.

520. Elias A, Ryan L, Sulkes A, Collins J, Aisner J, Antman K. Response to mesna, doxorubicin, ifosfamide, and dacarbazine in 108 patients with metastatic or unresectable sarcoma and no prior chemotherapy. J Clin Oncol 1989;7:1208–1216.

521. Wellens W, Donhuijsen-Ant R, Habets L, et al. Therapie progredienter Sarkome mit Etoposid und Ifosfamide. Aktuel Onkol 1981;4:159–164.

522. Wellens W, Mussgnug G, Havets L, Schafer E, Westerhausen M. The combination ifosfamide/VP 16–213 in therapy of small cell bronchogenic carcinoma and other malignant tumors. In: Burkett H, Nagel G, eds. New experience with the oxazaphosphorines with special reference to the uroprotector uromitexan. Basel: Karger, 1980:81–87.

523. Issels RD, Prenninger SW, Nagele A, et al. Ifosfamide plus etoposide combined with regional hyperthermia in patients with locally advanced sarcomas: A phase II study. J Clin Oncol 1990;8:1818–1829.

524. Hoffmann W, Weidmann B, Migeod F, Konner J, Seeber S. Epirubicin and ifosfamide in patients with refractory breast cancer and other metastatic solid tumours. Cancer Chemother Pharmacol 1990;26(suppl 1):S69–70.

525. Toma S, Palumbo R, Songo G, et al. Doxorubicin (or epidoxorubicin) combined with ifosfamide in the treatment of adult advanced soft tissue sarcomas. Ann Oncol 1992;3(Suppl 2):S119–S123.

526. Bierbaum W, Bremer K, Firusian N, High M, et al. Chemotherapeutische behandlungsmoglichkeiten bei forgeschrittenen sarkomen. Dtsch Med Wochenschr 1981;106:1181–1185.

527. Budd GT, Metch B, Weiss S, et al. SWOG 8641: Ifosfamide and cisplatin in the treatment of metastatic soft tissue sarcoma. Proc Am Soc Clin Oncol [Abstract 1222] 1990;9:316.

528. Hartlapp JH, Munch HJ, Illiger HJ, Wolter H, Jensen JC. Alternatives to CYVADIC combination therapy of soft tissue sarcomas. Cancer Chemother Pharmacol 1986;18(suppl 2):S20–S22.

529. Zamboglou N, Furst G, Pape H, Bannach B, Molls M, Schmitt G. [Results of whole lung irradiation and chemotherapy in comparison with partial lung irradiation in metastasizing, undifferentiated soft tissue sarcomas]. Strahlenther Onkol 1988;164:386–392.

530. Klippenstein TH, Mitrou PS, Kochendorfer KJ, Bergmann L. High-dose Adriamycin (ADM) and cisplatin (DDP) in advanced soft-tissue sarcomas and invasive thymomas: A pilot study. Cancer Chemother Pharmacol 1984;13:78–81.

531. Edmonson JH, Hahn RG, Schutt AJ, Bisel HF, Ingle JN. Cyclophosphamide, doxorubicin, and cisplatin combined in the treatment of advanced sarcomas. Med Pediatr Oncol 1983;11:319–321.

532. Cormier WJ, Hahn RG, Edmonson JH, Eagan RT. Phase II study in advanced sarcoma: Randomized trial of pyrazofurin versus combination cyclophosphamide, doxorubicin and dichlorodiammineplatinum (CAP). Cancer Treat Rep 1980;64:655.

533. Edmonson JH, Long HJ, Richardson RL, et al. Phase II study of a combination of mitomycin, doxorubicin and cisplatin in advanced sarcomas. Cancer Chemother Pharmacol 1985;15:181–182.

534. Jansen RLH, Van der Burg MEL, Verweij J, Stoter G. Cyclophosphamide, hexamethylmelamine, Adriamycin and cisplatin combination chemotherapy in mixed mesodermal sarcoma of the female genital tract. Eur J Cancer Clin Oncol 1987;23:1131–1133.

535. Piver MS, Shashikant BL, Patsner B. Cis-dichlorodiammineplatinum plus dimethyltriazenoimidazole carboxamide as second- and third-line chemotherapy for sarcomas of the female pelvis. Gynecol Oncol 1986;23:371–375.

536. Presgrave P, Woods RL, Tatteresall MH, et al. Combination chemotherapy of adult soft tissue sarcomas with a combination of doxorubicin and methotrexate. Cancer Treat Rep 1987;71:1087–1088.

537. Kaufman JH, Catane R, Douglass HO. Combined Adriamycin, vincristine, and methotrexate in advanced adult soft tissue sarcoma. NY State J Med 1977;77:742–743.

538. Shiu MH, Magill GB, Hopfan S. Recent trends in treatment of soft tissue sarcomas. In: Hajdu SI, ed. Philadelphia: Lea & Febiger, 1979:537–542.

539. Lynch G, Magill GB, Sordillo PP, et al. Combination chemotherapy of advanced sarcomas in adults with cyomad. Cancer 1982;50:1724–1727.

540. Presant CA, Lowenbraun S, Bartolucci AA, et al. Metastatic sarcomas: Chemotherapy with Adriamycin, cyclophosphamide, and methotrexate alternating with actinomycin D, DTIC, and vincristine. Cancer 1981;47:457–465.

541. Pfeffer MR, Sulkes A, Biran S. Cyclophosphamide, Adriamycin, DTIC and vincristine with methotrexate in the treatment of advanced soft tissue sarcomas. Isr J Med Sci 1988;24:599–603.

542. Lowenbraun S, Moffitt JS, Smalley R, et al. Combination chemotherapy with Adriamycin, cyclophosphamide and methotrexate in metastatic sarcomas. Proc Am Soc Clin Oncol 1977;18:289.

543. Jacobs EM. Combination chemotherapy of metastatic testicular germinal cell tumors and soft part sarcomas. Cancer 1970;25:324–332.

544. Frei III E, Antman K, Teicher B, Eder P, Schnipper L. Bone marrow autotransplantation for solid tumors—prospects. J Clin Oncol 1989;7:515–526.

545. Antman KS, Griffin JD, Elias A, et al. Effect of recombinant human granulocyte-macrophage colony-stimulating factor on chemotherapy-induced myelosuppression. N Engl J Med 1988;319:593–598.

546. Steward WP, Verweij J, Somers R, et al. High dose chemotherapy with two schedules of recombinant human granulocyte-macrophage colony-stimulating factor in the treatment of advanced adult soft tissue sarcomas. Proc Am Soc Clin Oncol [Abstract 1240] 1991;10:349.

547. Pinkerton CR, Groot LJ, Barrett A, et al. Rapid VAC high dose melphalan regimen, a novel chemotherapy approach in childhood soft tissue sarcomas. Br J Cancer 1991;64:381–385.

548. Pinkerton CR. Megatherapy for soft tissue sarcomas. EBMT experience. Bone Marrow Transplant 1991;3:120–122.

549. Lantta M, Kahanp K, Karkkainen J, Lehtovirta P, Wahlstrom T, Widholm O. Estradiol and progesterone receptors in two cases of endometrial stromal sarcoma. Gynecol Oncol 1984;18:233–239.

550. Keen CE, Philip G. Progestogen-induced regression in low-grade endometrial stromal sarcoma. Case report and literature review. Br J Obstet Gynaecol 1989;96:1435–1439.

551. O'Brien AA, O'Briain DS, Daly PA. Aggressive endometrial stromal sarcoma responding to medroxyprogesterone following failure of tamoxifen and combination chemotherapy. Br J Obstet Gynaecol 1985;92:862–866.

552. Rome RM, Campbell JJ, Cope TI, et al. Tamoxifen in advanced and recurrent uterine sarcomas: A phase II study. Cancer Treat Rep 1986;70:811–812.

553. Wade K, Quinn MA, Hammond I, Williams K, Cauchi M. Uterine sarcoma: Steroid receptors and response to hormonal therapy. Gynecol Oncol 1990;39:364–367.

554. Posner MC, Shiu MH, Newsome J, Hajdu SI, Gaynor JJ, Brennan MF. The desmoid tumor—not a benign disease. Arch Surg 1989;124:191–196.

555. Mckinnon JG, Neifeld JP, Kay S, Parker GA, Foster WC, W Lawrence Jr. Management of desmoid tumors. Surg Gynecol Obstet 1989;169:104–106.

556. Biron P, Meckenstock R, Bobin JY, et al. Presence of hormone receptors in desmoid tumors. Proc Am Soc Clin Oncol 1990;9:285.

557. Weiss AJ, Lackman RD. Response of various low grade neoplasms of mesothelial origin to chemotherapy. Proc Am Soc Clin Oncol 1990;9:315.

558. White CW, Sondheimer HM, Crouch EC, Wilson H, Fan LL. Treatment of pulmonary hemangiomatosis with recombinant interferon alfa-2a. N Engl J Med 1989;320:1197–1212.

559. Moskowitz AJ, Pauker SG. A decision analytic approach to limb-sparing treatment for adult soft tissue and osteogenic sarcoma. Cancer Treat Symp 1985;3:11–26.

560. Sugarbaker PH, Barofsky I, Rosenberg SA, et al. Quality of life assessment of patients in extremity sarcoma clinical trials. Surgery 1982;91:17–23.

561. Weddington WW, Segraves KB, Simon MA. Psychological outcome of extremity sarcoma survivors undergoing amputation or limb salvage. J Clin Oncol 1985;3:1393–1399.

562. Chang A, Culnane M, Lampert M, et al. Quality of life changes in soft tissue sarcoma patients undergoing multimodality treatment. Proc Am Soc Clin Oncol 1987;6:254.

563. Yang JC. Unpublished data, 1992.

Cancer: Principles & Practice of Oncology, Fourth Edition,
edited by Vincent T. DeVita, Jr., Samuel Hellman, Steven A. Rosenberg.
J.B. Lippincott Co., Philadelphia © 1993.

Karen H. Antman   Frederick P. Li

Harvey I. Pass   Joseph Corson

Thomas DeLaney

CHAPTER **43**

Benign and Malignant Mesothelioma

EPIDEMIOLOGY

The annual incidence of malignant mesothelioma in the United States is approximately 2200 cases or about 12.1 per million white men, and the rate appears to be increasing.[1] Asbestos is the predominant cause of pleural, peritoneal, and probably epididymal mesothelioma in humans. As many as 8 million living persons in the United States have been occupationally exposed to asbestos over the last 50 years during mining and milling of asbestos and diverse manufacturing processes that use the material.[2] Many public and private buildings contain asbestos, including 10% to 15% of U.S. schools that were insulated or sprayed on interior surfaces with asbestos between 1946 and 1972.[3] The public health significance of exposure in these buildings and the cost effectiveness of asbestos removal are controversial.[4]

HISTORY OF ASBESTOS USAGE

The resistance of asbestos to heat and combustion was recognized by ancient civilizations.[5] The Industrial Revolution greatly expanded demand for asbestos as insulating and packing material for machines and power generators. Two world wars further increased the demand for asbestos in ships and other equipment of combat and transport. The availability, durability, and low cost of asbestos additionally expanded its range of uses in industrial and consumer products.[6]

Although Pliny had observed that asbestos mine slaves were less healthy than other slaves, the health hazards of asbestos exposure were generally not recognized until this century.[5] In 1898, pulmonary scarring and eventual death from respiratory failure was observed in asbestos workers from French and English asbestos textile mills.[7] However, the cause of the pulmonary fibrosis remained uncertain, because tuberculosis and other respiratory infections were often epidemic among poor laborers. In 1930, the causal association between asbestos and asbestosis was firmly established by Merewether and Price at the London Chest Hospital.[8] After limits were set on allowable industrial levels of asbestos exposure in England, many thought the asbestos problem had been solved.[5] However, case reports of lung cancer in patients with asbestosis appeared as early as 1935.[9,10] In 1955, Doll reported a case-control study that established the association between asbestos and lung cancer.[11]

MECHANISMS OF CARCINOGENICITY

Two major forms of asbestos exist: curly, pliable, serpentine asbestos (*i.e.*, chrysotile) and rod-like amphiboles (*i.e.*, crocidolite, amosite, anthophyllite, tremolite, actinolyte).[12] Chrysotile, crocidolite, and amosite are mined for their commercial utility; anthophyllite, tremolite, and actinolyte are usually contaminants. Asbestos fibers tend to separate readily and form numerous individual strands, which often are less than 1 μm in diameter. The carcinogenic effects of asbestos appear to result from its physical properties, rather than chemical structure.[13] Long, rod-like fibers of narrow diameter are more likely to induce tumors in laboratory animals.[14] After inhalation, most asbestos is expectorated or swallowed and subsequently excreted in the feces.[6] The remainder can be cleared from the tracheobronchial tree by several mechanisms, including ciliary action in the trachea, ingestion by

1489

macrophages, or penetration through the endothelial lining into interstitial tissues.[6,15,16] Short fibers are cleared more readily than long fibers. Fibers that remain preferentially accumulate in the lower third of the lungs adjacent to the visceral pleura.

Although there appears to be a consensus that serpentine asbestos is less carcinogenic than the rod-like amphiboles, debate continues over whether cases associated with chrysotile asbestos are actually caused by amphibole contamination or are due to chrysotile itself.[17,18]

Asbestos initiates an inflammatory and fibrotic process, mediated in part by cytokines released by activated alveolar macrophages.[19] At a molecular level, protooncogenes such as *PDGFB* (formerly *SIS*), which codes for the platelet-derived growth factor β-chain) are upregulated in alveolar macrophages from fibrotic lungs a factor that enhances mesothelial cell proliferation. Asbestos can transfect DNA into cells.[19] Epidermal growth factor-positive cells have been found in 68% of mesotheliomas examined and correlate with improved survival.[20]

ASBESTOS-ASSOCIATED MESOTHELIOMA

The existence of mesothelioma as a distinct pathologic entity was debated by pathologists before 1960.[21] In the late 1940s, case reports of mesotheliomas in patients with asbestosis began to appear. In 1960, Wagner and colleagues in South Africa reported 33 cases of mesothelioma diagnosed in patients between 31 and 68 years of age in a South African crocidolite mining community.[22] An additional 14 cases appeared in an addendum to the paper. Most of these patients were exposed in childhood through living in the vicinity of asbestos mills and mines; a few had occupational contacts. This study was followed by reports of mesotheliomas in asbestos workers in other parts of the world.

INCIDENCE

The actual annual incidence of mesothelioma is unknown because the neoplasm is difficult to diagnose, even by expert pathologists.[1] Data from death certificates are unreliable for estimating disease frequency despite the usually rapidly fatal outcome of malignant mesothelioma. Cancer deaths are not coded by morphology (*e.g.,* mesothelioma); the cause of mortality is assigned by primary site of the neoplasm (*e.g.,* primary neoplasms of pleural and peritoneum). In a recent study by the Surveillance, Epidemiology and the End Results (SEER) Program of the National Cancer Institute (NCI), only 274 of 1130 white decedents with mesothelioma (approximately 95% diagnosed by microscopy) were recorded as having died of a primary neoplasm of pleura or peritoneum.[23] Most mesothelioma cases were coded as having malignant neoplasm of the lung or unknown site. A reasonable estimate is that 2200 new cases (range, 1000–3000+) of mesothelioma occur annually in the United States.[23–25] Reported rates have increased in the last decade by as much as 50%.[23] Projections suggest that the number of cases will rise moderately into the next century and then decline as a result of recent legislation to reduce asbestos exposure in the workplace and the ambient environment.[25]

In the United States, mesothelioma is approximately three-fold more common in men than in women.[1,23,24] Incidence rises steadily with age, and is approximately ten-fold higher in men between the ages of 60 and 64 years than among those between 30 and 34.

PERSONS AT HIGH RISK

Persons at high risk of developing mesothelioma can be identified by tracing the processing and commercial uses of asbestos. The mineral is mined, milled, and incorporated into a wide range of industrial and commercial products, including insulation, textiles, heat protectors, filters, and construction materials (*e.g.,* spackling, roofing, siding, floor and ceiling tiles).[1,5,6] Workers with high levels of asbestos exposure are miners, millers, producers of asbestos products, and laborers who install plumbing, boilers, and heating equipment in ships, factories, and homes. The risk extends to workers who may not handle asbestos directly but are in proximity to the material, such as carpenters, electricians, and welders in shipyards.

The risk of mesothelioma associated with occupational exposure to asbestos has been examined in case-control studies and cohort studies. In case-control studies, as many as 75% of the cases had asbestos exposure, compared with a small fraction of controls.[1] In cohort studies, the proportion of asbestos workers who died of mesothelioma exceeded 10% in several studies.[26,27] However, mesothelioma risk is difficult to quantitate for several reasons. First, ambient levels of asbestos in most workplaces have not been measured. A "high" level in one study may be called "moderate" or "low" in another. Duration of employment has been used as another surrogate measure of exposure. Second, the time from exposure to the development of mesothelioma is long, usually 3 to 4 decades in most reported studies. Mathematical modeling suggests that risk of mesothelioma increases exponentially by the third to fourth power of time from first exposure, but few cohorts have been followed to the end of life. Third, the composition of the inspired asbestos differed among exposed workers. Evidence suggests that the amphiboles are more carcinogenic, perhaps because of the physical characteristics of these fibers. The long, needle-like fibers appear to lodge more readily in the distal respiratory area, where they persist longer and are transported to the pleura and peritoneum.[14,28]

Despite the obstacles to quantifying risk of mesothelioma, several consistent observations have emerged from studies worldwide. Crocidolite is associated with the high risk of mesothelioma in miners, manufacturers, and workers who install asbestos products.[29] Another amphibole, amosite, appears to carry an intermediate risk. Chrysotile, currently the major form of asbestos in production, shows the weakest association with mesothelioma.[14,30] Occupations with highest risk appear to be insulators, asbestos producers and manufacturers, and the heating and construction tradespeople. The projected lifetime risk among these workers exposed from early adulthood is as high as 20%. Working in proximity to these occupational groups in construction sites confers a relatively lower risk. Some patients with mesothelioma have reported only isolated or brief occupational exposures to asbestos.

Malignant mesothelioma is rarely curable, and screening of asbestos workers for mesothelioma is therefore inappropriate.[31] However, smoking greatly increases the risk of lung cancer (but not mesothelioma) in asbestos workers, and smoking cessation efforts are needed in this high-risk group.[31,32] Clinicians considering the diagnosis of malignant mesothelioma should take a detailed exposure history, emphasizing the period between 20 and 50 years before diagnosis and including possible household contact exposure.[33] Brief exposures may be long forgotten.[34,35]

Exposure in the Home

Mesothelioma in wives and children of asbestos workers has prompted studies that show increased asbestos levels in their homes.[30,36–38] Presumably, asbestos was brought into the home on hair and on clothing to be washed in the family laundry. Asbestos workers were required to shower and change clothing before leaving the work place only after 1972. Asbestos-related neoplasms have been reported in multiple members of some families, but genetic predisposition to the neoplasm remains to be shown.[39,40] The risk of mesothelioma in household contacts of asbestos workers may be as high as 0.4% to 1%, but the rate varies with the level of household contamination and may be overestimated in the reported data.[32]

MESOTHELIOMAS WITHOUT A HISTORY OF ASBESTOS EXPOSURE

No asbestos exposure can be documented in about 30 to 50% of cases of mesothelioma. Quantitation of asbestos fibers in some of these patients has documented background pulmonary fiber levels consistent with the absence of a substantial asbestos exposure.[41]

About 25 published cases of pleural and peritoneal mesothelioma have developed after therapeutic irradiation, and in 2 patients, tumors arose adjacent to deposits of thorium dioxide (thorotrast) still visible on chest radiographs after extravasation during diagnostic procedures years earlier.[42–45] A median of 16 years (range, 7–36 years) elapsed between irradiation and detection of mesothelioma.

A high incidence of mesothelioma (*i.e.*, 22 per 10,000 persons >25 years) observed in the Anatoli region of Turkey has been attributed to zeolite, a silicate ubiquitous in the soil and sometimes sprayed onto homes.[46,47] Erionite is associated with a high incidence of mesothelioma.[48]

MALIGNANT PLEURAL MESOTHELIOMA

PRESENTATION

Malignant pleural mesothelioma most commonly develops in the fifth to seventh decade (median age, 60). A significant proportion of patients with mesothelioma diagnosed between the ages of 20 and 40 report household or neighborhood exposure during childhood.[22,49,50] Children who present with the disease frequently have no apparent asbestos exposure.[51–56]

Men are affected five times as often as women. Dyspnea, nonpleuritic chest wall pain, or both bring patients to medical attention. Examination is remarkable for dullness at one base, and a chest radiograph reveals a large freely movable unilateral pleural effusion. Some patients are asymptomatic, with effusions found incidentally on chest radiographs. Sixty per-

cent have right-sided lesions, and fewer than 5% have bilateral involvement at the time of diagnosis.

A computed tomography (CT) scan or magnetic resonance image (MRI) of the chest to assess the extent of disease is indicated if any treatment is contemplated.[57] Loss of lung volume is evident early on CT scan.[57,58] Scoliosis with contracture of the ipsilateral hemithorax is visible even on a chest radiograph with advanced disease. Despite a history of asbestos contact in 50% to 70% of patients, pleural plaques or interstitial fibrosis are apparent on chest radiographs in approximately 20%, but pleural calcifications are evident on almost half of CT scans and in as many as 87% at autopsy.[57,59]

DIAGNOSIS

Initial misdiagnosis is common. Pathologic opinion appears particularly diverse if litigation is involved. Because a substantial percentage of mesotheliomas develop in patients with no known asbestos exposure and because other malignancies are common in asbestos workers, asbestos exposure should not influence the diagnosis of mesothelioma. Because of the poor prognosis of pleural mesothelioma, a major role of establishing the diagnosis is to exclude the possibility of a more treatable illness. Accurate diagnosis is important in the event of subsequent litigation and for epidemiologic and therapeutic studies.

Diagnostic Surgery

It is sometimes difficult to obtain an accurate histologic confirmation of mesothelioma from pleural fluid cytology or needle biopsy specimens, but the diagnosis of mesothelioma has such a poor prognosis that an unequivocal tissue diagnosis is mandatory. This usually requires surgical intervention with thoracoscopy or thoracotomy, despite the risk of seeding the biopsy site or surgical scar with tumor.[60] For patients who are not candidates for radical surgery, thoracoscopy usually obtains sufficient tissue for histochemical analysis.[61] Later development of chest wall masses from seeding of the biopsy site or surgical scar is an uncommon complication (about 10%) of any diagnostic procedure, but it can usually be avoided by radiotherapy to the scar if appropriate.[60]

If preoperative studies suggest stage I mesothelioma in a good-risk patient with asbestos exposure, most surgeons combine the diagnostic and therapeutic surgical interventions.[62] Generous biopsies can be performed at the inception of the exploration, using frozen sections to differentiate mesothelioma from adenocarcinoma. A sample of uninvaded lung should be obtained for counting asbestos fibers.[34,63]

Bronchoscopy should be performed in all patients with suspected mesothelioma to rule out endobronchial disease, which is rare in mesothelioma.[64] The role of mediastinoscopy in patients with suspected mesothelioma is undefined. Some surgeons think it is unnecessary, because nodes can be removed with the lung. Others think that, because positive nodes indicate stage III disease, surgery is contraindicated. Nevertheless, if radical extrapleural pneumonectomy is contemplated, mediastinoscopy is recommended, because 20% of patients with mesothelioma have mediastinal lymph node involvement.[64]

Cytology, Needle Biopsies, and Sections From Cell Blocks

The results of repeated cytologic examination or biopsy may be negative despite active tumor. If tumor tissue is obtained, light microscopy often provides documentation of malignancy, but it usually does not differentiate adenocarcinoma from mesothelioma. Electron microscopy of needle biopsy or cytocentrifuge specimens from pleural fluid may establish the mesothelial origin of the malignant tumor. Sputum cytology and bronchoscopy may be helpful in documenting an occult bronchogenic adenocarcinoma.

PATHOLOGY

Gross and Microscopic Appearance

Discrete nodules and plaques of firm, grayish tumor coalesce, eventually obliterating the parietal and visceral surfaces. A rind of up to 5 cm thick may encase and constrict the lung with only superficial invasion. The chest wall, pericardium, diaphragm, and interlobar fissures are involved relatively early.[65] At autopsy, tumor invades thoracic lymph nodes in as many as 70% of patients, with occasional extension to cervical nodes.[66] Small hematogenous metastases are documented to liver and lung and less commonly to kidney, adrenal, and bone in 33% to 67% of cases.[66,67] Without careful postmortem examination, hematogenous metastases may be missed.

Extensive sampling of biopsy, pleurectomy, or pneumonectomy specimens is required. A small piece should be fixed in glutaraldehyde for electron microscopy and the remainder promptly fixed in neutral buffered formalin. There are three histologic variants: epithelial, sarcomatoid, and mixed.[65,68] Fifty percent to 60% are epithelial, characterized by tubular, papillary, solid, or vacuolated patterns. The sarcomatoid variant is composed of ovoid or spindle-shaped cells with cellularity and hyperchromatism similar to that of a fibrosarcoma. A biphasic pattern with mixed epithelial and sarcomatoid elements is virtually pathognomonic of malignant mesothelioma, although extensive sampling may be required to demonstrate the minor component.

Differential Diagnosis

Benign inflammatory and reactive processes producing mesothelial hyperplasia or other malignant tumors may mimic mesothelioma but do not invade normal tissues and lack cytologic atypia and hyperchromatism.[66] Adenocarcinomas from primary lung, breast, ovary, stomach, kidney, or prostate cancer frequently metastasize to the pleura and can be extremely difficult to differentiate from epithelial mesothelioma cytologically or histologically. Metastatic adenocarcinoma with extensive pleural involvement may grossly resemble mesothelioma (*i.e.*, pseudomesothelioma).[69] Sarcomatous mesothelioma must be differentiated from fibrosarcoma, malignant fibrous histiocytoma, malignant schwannoma, and hemangiopericytoma. Synovial sarcoma and carcinosarcoma, which may have mixed sarcomatous and epithelial components, usually present as localized masses in the lung.

Autopsy requires skilled performance and experienced interpretation to exclude other occult primary carcinomas. Advanced malignant mesothelioma tends to form peripheral visceral masses, mimicking primary carcinomas.[65] Asbestos counts and postmortem examinations may have legal and epidemiologic value.

HISTOCHEMICAL METHODS. Three methods are in common use to differentiate metastatic adenocarcinomas from epithelial mesotheliomas. The periodic acid-Schiff stain (PAS) used before and after diastase digestion is the single most reliable histochemical method available.[65] Strongly PAS-diastase-positive *neutral* mucopolysaccharides are found in intracellular secretory vacuoles and in intraacinar vacuoles in most adenocarcinomas, but they are rarely found in most mesotheliomas. Their presence is strong but not unequivocal evidence for a diagnosis of adenocarcinoma. Appropriate controls for diastase activity and to differentiate staining of vacuoles from stroma and other structures are essential. Alcian blue at pH 2.5 and colloidal-iron stain *acid* mucopolysaccharides present in mesothelioma and many adenocarcinomas.[66] Disappearance after digestion with hyaluronidase that removes hyaluronic acid in intracellular and secretory vacuoles and intercellular lumens is characteristic of mesothelioma. However, *stromal* hyaluronic acid is a nonspecific finding in many tumors. Under most staining conditions, Mayer's mucicarmine method (*i.e.*, stains neutral and weakly acidic mucopolysaccharides in intracellular and intercellular secretory vacuoles pink or red) is strongly positive in many adenocarcinomas. Mesotheliomas are usually negative but occasionally may stain strongly in some laboratories possibly due to fixation or technical conditions. The method is not completely reliable.

IMMUNOHISTOCHEMISTRY. Immunoperoxidase stains using various antibodies may be effectively applied to paraffin-embedded tumor tissue. Monoclonal antibodies against keratin proteins are strongly reactive in mesothelioma with diffuse cytoplasmic staining and perinuclear accentuation with ring formation.[70] Epithelial and spindle-shaped tumor cells of mixed and sarcomatoid variants are often stained, reflecting the transitional patterns of differentiation observed on electron microscopy.[71] This reactivity is helpful in differentiating mesothelioma from fibrosarcoma, malignant fibrous histiocytoma, and schwannoma, but carcinosarcomas and synovial sarcomas, which have biphasic histology, also express keratin proteins. Adenocarcinomas stain positively, usually with localization to the periphery of the tumor cell. Immunoperoxidase staining for Leu-M1 is usually absent in mesotheliomas but positive in most adenocarcinomas. Staining for carcinoembryonic antigen is usually weak or absent in mesotheliomas and renal, prostate, and some ovarian and endometrial carcinomas, but it is moderate to strong in most other adenocarcinomas.[72,73]

ELECTRON MICROSCOPY. The epithelial variant is composed of polygonal cells with numerous long, slender, branching surface microvilli, desmosomes, abundant tonofilaments, and intracellular lumen formation.[71,74] Primary lung, breast, and upper gastrointestinal tract adenocarcinomas have short stubby surface microvilli, fewer tonofilaments, and microvillus rootlets or lamellar bodies.[75,76] Ovarian and endometrial carcinomas lack intracytoplasmic lumens, but have few tonofilaments and may express features of intestinal metaplasia (*e.g.*, abundant mucin droplets, numerous cilia, dense core granules).[75,76] Elongated nuclei and abundant rough endoplasmic reticulin are found in the sarcomatoid variant. Stromal cells separated by matrix-containing collagen fibers appear spindled or ovoid with sarcomatoid and epithelial features, characteristic of the biphasic nature of mesothelioma.[71,74]

STAGING

Butchart and others have proposed various staging systems that predict survival with statistical significance in some series.[77] The Butchart classification (Table 43–1) suffers from an absence of TNM descriptions and vague statements about lymph node involvement and degrees of chest wall invasion. The International Union Against Cancer (UICC) proposed a TNM staging system that probably is as good an attempt to unify future reporting of mesothelioma as any other system.[78] The weighting system of the individual descriptions as they translate into stage I through IV disease is handled in a similar manner to the new International Staging System used for non-small cell lung cancer, but the impact of nodal disease and long-term survival as a function of organ of invasion or depth of invasion with confined hemothorax disease remains problematic.

Probably the major role of noninvasive procedures is to determine isolated hemithorax disease. A CT or MR scan of the primary tumor to assess the extent of disease is indicated if treatment is contemplated. Characteristic CT findings in almost 100 patients are pleural thickening in 92% (intralobar fissures in 86%), effusions in 74%, and pleural calcifications in 20% to 50%.[44,57,79] A CT scan is helpful in differentiating benign from malignant pleural thickening but does not reliably differentiate primary from metastatic malignancy. Fewer patients have been evaluated by MRI, but the extent of tumor and its invasion of adjacent structures are well documented. Coronal MRI was particularly helpful for evaluating the diaphragm.[80] Although brain, bone, and liver metastases or extension into other serosal surfaces are found in more than half of patients at autopsy, they are sufficiently uncommon at presentation to obviate the need for extensive baseline studies in the absence of symptoms or laboratory abnormalities. However, these studies may identify an occult adenocarcinoma of the lung, a pattern of widespread metastases or a markedly elevated serum or pleural fluid carcinoembryonic antigen (CEA), suggesting a diagnosis other than mesothelioma.[66,81] Although there are no definitive biomarkers for mesothelioma, future studies investigating serial serum levels of tissue polypeptide antigen or thrombomodulin may be of interest.[82,83] Mesotheliomas take up gallium 67.[84]

Pulmonary function tests may document restrictive lung disease resulting from encasement of the lung and assess the potential tolerance for pneumonectomy. Obstructive spirometric changes are unrelated to mesothelioma or asbestosis.[85] Laboratory evaluation is otherwise generally unremarkable except for an elevated platelet count and erythrocyte sedimentation rate.

NATURAL HISTORY

Prognostic variables at presentation significantly associated with a longer survival include age under 55 to 65, 0 to 1 per-

TABLE 43–1. Staging Systems for Malignant Mesothelioma

Butchart Staging Classification

I	Tumor confined within the capsule of the parietal pleura, involving only ipsilateral pleura, lung, pericardium, and diaphragm
II	Tumor invading chest wall or involving mediastinal structures, such as esophagus, heart, opposite pleura
III	Tumor penetrating diaphragm to involve peritoneum; involvement of opposite pleura
	Lymph node involvement outside the chest
IV	Distant blood-borne metastases

UICC Staging Proposal*

I	T1, N0, M0
	T2, N0, M0
II	T1, N1, M0
	T2, N1, M0
III	T3, N0, M0
	T3, N1, M0
	T1, N2, M0
	T2, N2, M0
	T3, N2, M0
IV	Any T, N3, M0
	T4, any N, M0
	Any T, and N, M1
T	(Primary Tumor And Extent)
TX	Primary tumor cannot be assessed
T0	No evidence of primary tumor
T1	Primary tumor limited to ipsilateral parietal or visceral pleura
T2	Tumor invades any of the following: ipsilateral lung, endothoracic fascia, diaphragm, pericardium
T3	Tumor invades any of the following: ipsilateral chest wall muscle, ribs, mediastinal organs or tissues
T4	Tumor extends to any of the following: contralateral pleura or lung by direct extension, peritoneum or intraabdominal organs by direct extension, cervical tissues
N	(Lymph Nodes)
NX	Regional lymph nodes cannot be assessed
N0	No regional lymph nodes metastases
N1	Metastases in ipsilateral bronchopulmonary of hilar lymph nodes
N2	Metastases in ipsilateral mediastinal lymph nodes
N3	Metastases in contralateral mediastinal internal mammary, supraclavicular, or scalene lymph nodes
M	(Metastases)
MX	Presence of distant metastases cannot be assessed
M0	No known distant metastases
M1	Distant metastasis present

* Staging solely on clinical measures is designated cTNM. Staging that can be done on clinical pathologic information is designated as pTNM. Clinical and pathologic groups are identical.

formance status, stage I disease, epithelial histology, lack of chest pain at diagnosis, and a normal platelet count.[86–90]

Shortness of breath and chest pain can be controlled initially by repeated thoracenteses and minor narcotics. Although chest tube drainage and sclerosis are usually unsuccessful, pleural fluid eventually becomes loculated as the tumor obliterates the pleural space.[67] With advanced disease, fatigue and dyspnea increase out of proportion to x-ray findings or pulmonary function values. Because hypoxia results from shunting of desaturated blood through a poorly aerated lung, therapeutic oxygen provides little symptomatic relief.

Mesothelioma tends to be locally invasive. Chest wall masses develop in about 10% of patients over thoracentesis, chest tube drainage, or thoracotomy tracts.[67,91] Direct involvement of esophagus, ribs, vertebrae, nerves, and the superior vena cava cause dysphagia, pain, cord compression, brachial plexopathy, Horner's syndrome, or superior vena cava syndromes, respectively.[92] Fevers and sweats with no documented source of infection are common and often accompanied by significant weight loss, poor performance status, and an early death. Thrombocytosis and other clotting abnormalities occur in 10% to 20% (more frequently in peritoneal mesothelioma).[93,94] Disseminated intravascular coagulation, thrombophlebitis, pulmonary emboli, Coombs-positive hemolytic anemia, and hypercalcemia associated with elevated levels of a parathyroid hormone-like peptide have been reported.[95,96]

The median survival is 4 to 18 months in various series (range, weeks to 16 years). Patients usually die of respiratory failure or pneumonia. Small bowel obstruction from direct extension through the diaphragm develops in about one third, and 10% die of pericardial or myocardial involvement.[50,92]

Localized malignant fibrous tumors of the pleura may resemble sarcomatous mesotheliomas histologically. Of 82 malignant localized tumors, 45% were cured by simple excision.[97] If the nature of the lesion is ambiguous, involvement of the pleura on random biopsy would establish a diagnosis of diffuse, malignant disease.

CYTOGENETICS

Asbestos, a poor mutagen, can be cytotoxic and is associated with chromosomal abnormalities in exposed cells.[39,40,98] Asbestos induces mesothelial proliferation, but in vitro malignant transformation has not been demonstrated.

Ploidy status and the percentage of cells actively synthesizing DNA have been analyzed by flow cytometry in almost 200 malignant mesotheliomas.[99-102] Ploidy and S-phase fraction seem to be consistent in different sections from the same tumor and were not associated with histologic subtype.[100] In the various studies, 60% to 65% were diploid and 27% were near diploid. In contrast, 85% of lung cancers are aneuploid.[99] Significantly shorter survival is associated with a high percentage of S-phase cells but not aneuploidy.[100,101] The number of copies of 7p correlated inversely with survival.[103] Recurring chromosomal changes, including partial deletions of 1p, 3p, 9p and monosomy 4 and 22, suggest a cascade of events involving alterations of genes on more than one chromosome. These regions should be targeted for molecular investigation into the possibility of suppressor genes in mesothelioma.[104-108] Mesotheliomas displayed little genetic instability (heterogeneity) within tumor populations, unlike lung cancers.[105]

HUMORAL FACTORS

Hyaluronic acid has been useful in diagnosis or for following response but is relatively nonspecific.[109] A markedly elevated serum or pleural fluid CEA suggests a diagnosis other than mesothelioma. Hematopoietic growth factors and blood group antigens have been produced by normal and malignant mesothelial cell lines.[110-114]

TREATMENT

Surgery

Although some physicians feel strongly that mesothelioma patients should be referred to institutions with research programs, others advocate supportive care alone after definitive biopsy because reported cures with any treatment remain anecdotal. In 68 patients in Glasgow with mesothelioma managed supportively, the median survival was 30 weeks (*i.e.*, 22 weeks for patients with pain and 44 weeks for patients with dyspnea).[90] A similar median survival of 7 months was recorded by Ruffie and colleagues for 176 patients with mesothelioma treated supportively in Canada.[115] Harvey reported a 6-month median survival for 76 nonsurgically treated patients; 33 had had pleurodesis, chemotherapy, or radiation.[116]

Diffuse malignant mesothelioma is usually associated with chest wall pain and recurrent effusions.[117] Pleurectomy successfully controls recurrent effusions in 88% of patients. Surgery probably has no role in the palliation of the pain associated with chest wall invasion, which is better treated with nonnarcotic analgesics, antiinflammatory agents, or opiates.[117]

Although the staging of mesothelioma has been inconsistent, it is reasonable to consider surgical therapy in patients with stage I disease, defined by Butchart as a tumor confined within the capsule of the parietal pleura, involving only the ipsilateral lung, pericardium, and diaphragm.[77] Stage I disease, however heterogenous, is associated with a longer survival, although this may be solely associated with lead-time bias. Cases in which tumor extends beyond the confines of the parietal pleural capsule, with diffuse invasion of neighboring structures, are probably not amenable to radical surgery.

Preoperative Evaluation

Any patient considered for radical surgical therapy must be able to withstand pneumonectomy and prolonged anesthesia. Cardiac status should be screened by an electrocardiogram, and the patient should be questioned for signs of acquired heart disease that may need further noninvasive investigation. Adequate pulmonary reserve is crucial. The forced expiratory volume (FEV_1) of more than 2 L per second is desirable; if the FEV_1 is less than this, quantitative ventilation-perfusion scanning should be performed to document that residual FEV_1 after pneumonectomy will be greater than 1 L per second. As with primary lung cancer, good-risk patients usually have good nutritional status. Some surgeons think that age over 65 years is a contraindication to surgery.[62]

Surgical Technique

Pleurectomy. Pleurectomy has been strongly advocated by the Memorial Sloan-Kettering Cancer Center (MSKCC) group.[64] Da Valle uses pleurectomy in patients with minimal invasion of the visceral pleura (*i.e.*, free pleural space without tissue invasion) for attempted cure.[62] Extrapleural dissection of the parietal pleura is begun after a generous posterolateral thoracotomy. The pleura is stripped from the apex of the lung to the diaphragm, along with the pericardium, as necessary (Fig. 43–1). Most of the mediastinum and chest wall pleura can be removed, but the diaphragmatic pleura usually cannot be completely resected. Hemostasis is controlled as the procedure is performed, and blood replacement is frequently necessary. Two large intercostal catheters are used to drain blood and to manage peripheral bronchopleural fistulas. Large fistulas are suture ligated to allow maximal expansion of the underlying lung with underwater seal drainage. Operative mortality is low (1–2%), but complications include bronchopleural fistulas, hemorrhage, and subcutaneous emphysema.

Extrapleural Pneumonectomy. Extrapleural pneumonectomy is a more radical procedure, which includes en bloc removal of the parietal pleura, lung, pericardium, and diaphragm (Fig. 43–2 and Table 43–2). The approach can be by posterolateral thoracotomy (in the sixth interspace) or by thoracoabdominal incision (in the sixth or seventh interspace) with subdiaphragmatic blunt dissection of the peritoneum. The latter approach allows easier resection of the diaphragm and avoids the lower thoracotomy counter-incision needed if the posterolateral incision is used. Extrapleural dissection to the hilum, early entry into the pericardium retrosternally to accomplish intrapericardial pneumonectomy, and use of double-lumen anesthesia were described by Da Valle.[62] Diaphragmatic resection is followed by reconstruction using Dacron or Gortex material to prevent abdominal content herniation. Right-sided pericardial resections are usually reconstructed to prevent cardiac herniation. Intercostal tube drainage after pneumonectomy is optional. Operative mortality, earlier reported to be as high as 27% to 31%, is now 5% to 9%. Serious complications have been seen in 25% of the patients, including bronchopleural fistulas and empyema, vocal cord paralysis, chylothorax, arrhythmia, and respiratory insufficiency.[62]

Results of Surgical Treatment

Palliation. There is poor documentation of the results of palliative surgical intervention for mesothelioma. Law controlled 22 of 25 recurrent effusions by pleurectomy and reported objective relief of pain and dyspnea lasting weeks to months.[117,127] In a report by Ruffie, 63 patients had partial decortication and debulking for mesothelioma, which prevented recurrence of pleural effusion in 86% of cases.[115] Brancatisano has verified the efficacy of effusion control in 44 of 45 patients having subtotal parietal pleurectomy.[128]

Survival. Survival figures after pleurectomy or extrapleural pneumonectomy are difficult to interpret due to the different treatment philosophies and ways in which patients are selected for these operations. They should be considered separately. The MSKCC series investigated the use of pleurectomy with selective brachytherapy and postoperative radiation therapy from 1976 to 1988. Forty-one patients received only external-beam irradiation after decortication and pleurectomy, and 54 patients received an implant and external-beam therapy. Median survival for the entire group was 12.6 months, with a 2-year survival rate of 35%. A select group of 27 patients who had pure epithelial histology and who did not require an implant had a median survival of 22.5 months and a 2-year survival rate of 41%.[64] Ruffie reported a median survival of 9.8 months in this group of decorticated patients and Brancatisano's patients survived a median of 16 months.[115,128] Law, in a series of 28 patients, reported a 2-year survival rate of 32% after pleurectomy alone, with a median survival of 20 months.[117,127] The median survival for 23 patients after pleurectomy performed by Da Valle was 11.2 months.[62] Lewis reported an older series of patients with a median survival of 6.7 months after pleurectomy.[129]

Because the degree of tumor debulking varied in the pleurectomy series, the potential impact of radical surgery is

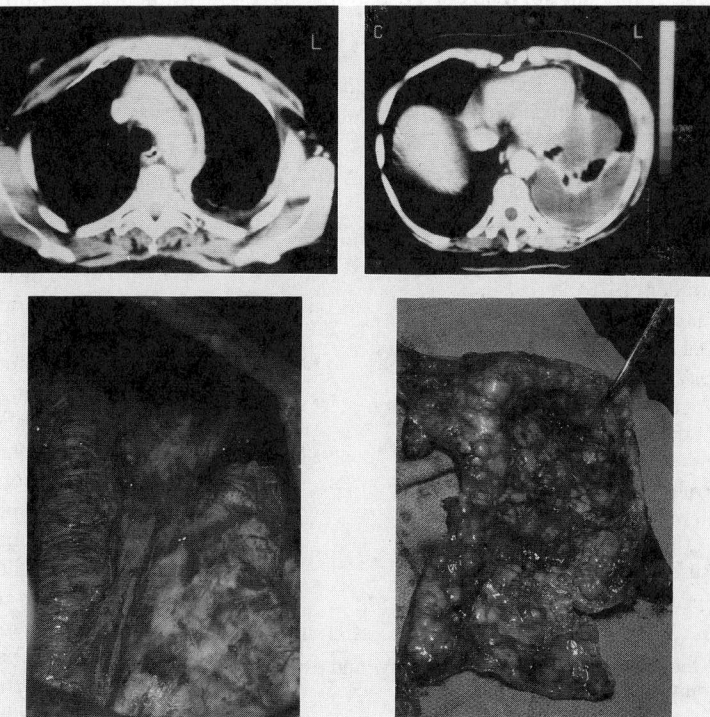

FIGURE 43–1. Pleurectomy for diffuse pleural mesothelioma. Preoperative tomograms demonstrate thickened pleura and fluid; the operative photograph and specimen are depicted below.

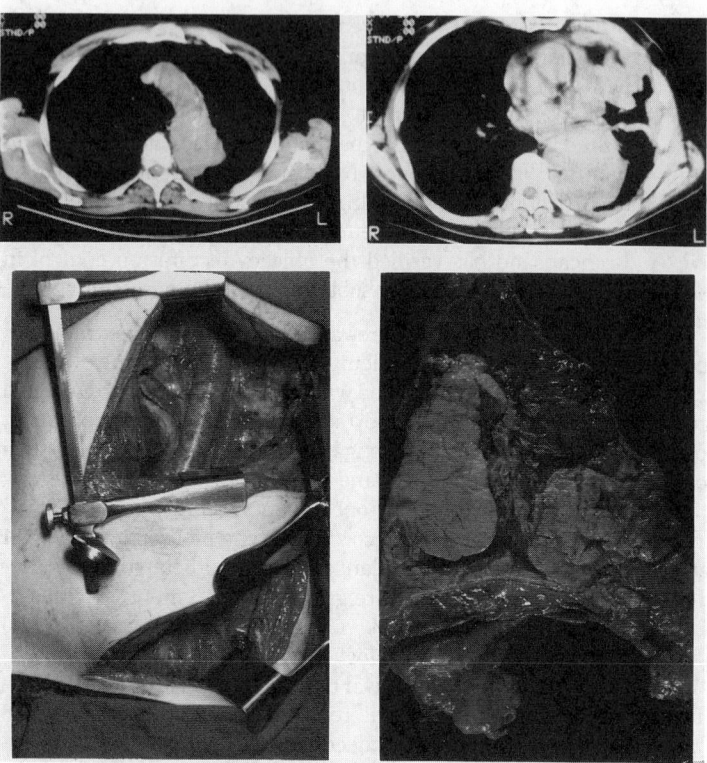

FIGURE 43–2. Left-sided diffuse mesothelioma. Two CT cuts show chest wall, fissure involvement, and aortic arch abutment. The surgical photograph demonstrates the skeletonized aorta, partial pericardectomy, and partial diaphragmatic removal through a counter incision. The surgical specimen is demonstrated in the lower right.

probably more accurately assessed by long-term survival after extrapleural pneumonectomy. Butchart reported a 9% 2-year survival after extrapleural pneumonectomy compared with a 24% 2-year survival and 15% 3-year survival for Da Valle's 33 patients. The Ontario and Quebec group of 23 patients with extrapleural pneumonectomy had a 2-year survival of 17%, and Rusch reported a 2-year survival of 33% with a 10-month median survival for 20 patients having extrapleural

pneumonectomy.[125] This last series is probably one of the most representative of the modern surgical management of mesothelioma; although it is not randomized, it represents a detailed analysis of recurrence patterns after pleurectomy and extrapleural pneumonectomy. The implication from the study was that extrapleural pneumonectomy may alter the natural history of pleural mesothelioma in that relapse occurred predominantly in systemic sites, but lesser operations were characterized predominantly by local and progressive pleural relapses.

Conclusions and Recommendations. To consider any surgical management for patients with pleural mesothelioma, the diagnosis must be certain with immunohistochemical techniques or electron microscopic confirmation. Thoracoscopic techniques will probably be used with greater frequency and earlier to define patients with earlier-stage disease. If repeated semiinvasive attempts do not secure the diagnosis, open biopsy is indicated. In patients with minimal disease or persistent pleural effusion, pleurectomy and decortication usually clinch the definitive diagnosis and palliate the effusion. If the lung and pleura cannot be mobilized easily from the chest wall due to invasion, a generous biopsy specimen should be obtained and the procedure terminated. Extrapleural pneumonectomy, especially with diaphragmatic removal, may be appropriate for selected patients. If the patient has had concomitant diagnosis and pleurectomy, most of the disease is debulked, and baseline computerized tomography after the pleurectomy does not reveal disease that could be scored in response to therapy, it is reasonable to defer further treatment. When local or systemic recurrences can be documented, referral to or participation in a defined treatment protocol should be initiated.

TABLE 43–2. Extrapleural Pneumonectomy for Diffuse Pleural Mesothelioma

Investigations	No. of Patients	Mortality (%)	Median Survival (mo)
Woern (1974)[118]	62	Unspecified	19
Bamler (1976)[119]	17	23	
Butchart (1978)[77]	29	31	4
DeLaria (1985)[120]	11	0	
DaValle (1986)[62]	33		
Vogt-Moykopf (1987)[121]	55	5.5	10.2
Faber (1988)[122]	33	9	13.5
Probst (1989)[123]	111*	6.3	9
Geroulenos (1990)[124]	18	7	20
Rusch (1991)[125]	20	15	10
Sugarbaker (1991)[126]	31	6	21

* Includes patients with pleurectomy and extrapleural pneumonectomy.

Radiation Therapy

PRINCIPLES. The efficacy of irradiation, like that of other treatment modalities, remains uncertain in the definitive treatment of patients with pleural mesothelioma. Its use has not been subjected to randomized clinical trials. Although several series suggest benefit, the variable clinical course of the disease and the frequent use of radiation in conjunction with surgery or chemotherapy make it difficult to assess its contribution to an overall treatment program.

Mesothelioma cells are more sensitive to radiation (*i.e.*, assessed by the surviving fraction after 200 cGy) than non-small cell lung cancer cells, but they are less sensitive than small cell lung cancer cells.[130] The use of irradiation for mesothelioma differs considerably from its use in lung cancer because of the extensive pleural involvement seen in mesothelioma. If irradiation is used for definitive treatment of malignant mesothelioma, treatment of the entire pleura is indicated. This treatment volume is extremely difficult to irradiate to tumoricidal doses without causing significant injury to the normal tissues of adjacent lung, heart, and liver.[131]

Most recent series document occasional regressions of gross disease with modest doses of radiation but do not indicate that survival is significantly altered by irradiation compared with supportive care (Table 43–3). Between 1971 and 1980, 116 patients in good general condition and without evidence of extrathoracic disease were seen at the Brompton and Royal Marsden Hospitals in London.[117,127] Fifty-two patients underwent active treatment, and the other 64 received supportive care, with the choice determined by physician preference. No difference in survival was seen between the two groups, with a 2-year survival rate of about 33% and 4-year survival rates of 0% to 11%. Active treatment consisted of parietal pleurectomy and decortication of the lung for 28 patients, radiation therapy for 12 patients (after surgery in 8), and chemotherapy for the remaining 12 patients (8 of whom had surgery). Radiation consisted of 5000 to 5500 cGy using rotating arc fields designed to treat the pleura and spare underlying lung. One patient showed a dramatic response to radiotherapy with resolution of effusion, pain, and dyspnea. She was well and active 4 years after completion of treatment. Two other patients experienced sustained regression of recurrent pleural effusions after radiotherapy. Although the treatment volume and normal tissue tolerance limit radiation dose, radiation therapy to these large bulky tumors can occasionally produce significant regression and worthwhile palliation.

Another large series from South Africa failed to demonstrate any convincing evidence that currently employed therapies significantly affected the course of the disease. Alberts and colleagues compiled the treatment outcome for 262 patients treated between 1965 and 1985 with chemotherapy, radiotherapy, chemotherapy plus radiotherapy, or decortication plus radiotherapy and chemotherapy.[135] The median survival of 9.6 months was similar for all groups. Only a small group of patients treated with doxorubicin and irradiation with 1000 cGy every 6 weeks for four courses appeared to show prolonged survival, with a median survival of 23 months.

Because of the variable course of the disease, the different radiation treatment techniques used (*e.g.*, anteroposterior-posteroanterior rotational arc, combined photon-electron radiotherapy), and normal tissue constraints on radiation dose, the relation between radiation dose and treatment response is not well established. The series from the Joint Center for Radiation Therapy in Boston included 29 treatment courses for palliation between 1968 and 1980.[91] Relief of pain, dyspnea, and other symptoms was seen in 4 of 6 patients treated with doses of 4000 cGy or more, but only 1 of 23 treatment courses at lower doses achieved successful palliation. Doses of 1500 to 2000 cGy (*i.e.*, the normal tissue tolerance dose of whole lung irradiation) were ineffective in controlling disease in patients with diffuse involvement of the visceral pleura with 1- to 2-mm nodules.

A report from the Peter MacCallum Cancer Institute in Australia described successful palliation in 17 (65%) of 26 evaluable palliative radiation courses.[136] Short-course treatment with 2000 cGy in five fractions appeared to give comparable palliation to that seen with more protracted courses (*i.e.*, 3000–4000 cGy in 10–15 fractions). Fifteen patients were given high-dose radiotherapy with radical therapeutic intent. Twelve completed treatment to 5000 cGy. The median survival of the 12 patients completing treatment was 17 months, with an estimated 2-year survival of 17%.[136] In a series from Thomas Jefferson Medical School in Philadelphia, 2 of 9 patients had local control for 20 and 40 months, respectively,

TABLE 43–3. Radiation Series

Investigations	No. of Patients	Dose (cGy)	Outcome
University of Iowa[132]	3	2000–2500	Symptomatic improvement
Brompton/Royal Marsden[117,127]	12	5000–5500	1 asymptomatic for 4 y
			2 with effusions controlled until demise
Joint Center for Radiation Therapy[91]	6	>4000	4 with significant symptomatic relief
	23	<4000	1 with significant symptomatic relief
Institut Gustave-Roussy[133]	14	3500–5000	4 alive at 1–41 mo
			10 dead at 1–37 (median, 15) mo
Thomas Jefferson Medical School[134]	9	6000	2 with local control at 20 and 40 mo

after 6000 cGy to the entire ipsilateral pleura, mediastinum, and involved areas of lung.[134] Radiation was given in three courses of 2000 cGy over a total of 10 weeks by a split-course technique.

Although information is limited, histologic subtype does not appear to have a major impact on the outcome of irradiated patients. In the early MSKCC series of patients from 1939 to 1972 with disease confined to the hemithorax treated primarily with radiotherapy, 15 patients with the epithelial subtype of mesothelioma had a median survival of 8 months, compared with 9 months in patients with the fibrosarcomatous subtype.[137] Although the volume of disease influences radiotherapeutic outcome in many other sites, its impact on the radiation response of pleural mesothelioma is not well characterized.

The combination of irradiation with debulking surgery can be rationalized if the patient can be rendered with only microscopic residual disease on most pleural surfaces after surgery. Irradiation is more effective at a given dose level for treating microscopic than for gross disease.[138] Higher doses of boost irradiation with brachytherapy or localized external-beam irradiation can be used to sites of residual gross disease. This strategy can maximize local control while minimizing the normal tissue complications from irradiation.

Irradiation has been used to prevent seeding of biopsy tracts and surgical wounds. In one series from Marseilles, irradiation consisting of 2100 cGy in three fractions prevented the development of wound seeding after thoracoscopy or thoracotomy in 24 patients.[139] Before initiation of prophylactic irradiation, wound seeding occurred in 17 (61%) of 33 biopsied patients. None of the patients who had developed growth of nodules in an incision responded to subsequent irradiation.

In considering the use of irradiation in this disease, the potential complications of high-dose irradiation to a large volume should be weighed in the treatment decision. The frequency, type, and severity of radiation complications depend on technique, volume, dose, fractionation, and normal tissue in the field and type and timing of any other treatment, such as chemotherapy. Remarkably, some earlier series reported no acute or chronic complications from the use of radiotherapy alone.[91,133] This may have been a function of limited-volume treatment or short survival. One series reported few complications with radiotherapy after 5000 to 5500 cGy were delivered with an off-axis rotational technique. Among 12 patients, complications included nausea and malaise in 6, transient radiation hepatitis in 1, and mild esophagitis in 1.[117,127] No case of radiation pneumonitis was seen. However, if no attempt has been made to shield lung or if the organ tolerance of other tissues such as the liver has been exceeded, significant complications have occurred. Ball and Cruikshank reported a case of fatal radiation hepatitis in a patient treated for a right pleural mesothelioma and a case of radiation myelitis (after 4000 cGy) in their series of 12 radically irradiated patients.[136] Maasilta reported deterioration in lung function after high-dose irradiation (5500–7100 cGy) given with chemotherapy.[140,141] Forced vital capacity and diffusing capacity showed significant declines at 1.5 to 2 months after radiotherapy and continued to decline over the year after radiation therapy. By radiologic assessment, treatment essentially obliterated lung function on the affected side. Hypoxemia and pathologic physiologic shunting increased in 2 of 6 patients monitored. Lung function

should be evaluated to assess potential tolerance before undertaking hemithorax irradiation. Liver position should be determined and adequate hepatic shielding should be used after 3000 cGy. Maasilta and Hallman reported the association of bronchoalveolar lavage plasmin and surfactant in mesothelioma patients with radiation pulmonary injury.[141,142]

The use of radioactive colloids (*i.e.*, ^{198}Au or ^{32}P in chromic phosphate) instilled into the pleural space has been studied. Pleural effusions have disappeared for as long as 3.5 years.[143] The exact response rate and duration to this approach is unknown. In a series from Hahnemann Medical College, all 6 patients were alive at 12 months or longer after instillation of isotopes.[144] The extent of other treatment and exact length of survival were not reported. Because of the physical characteristics of these isotopes (especially ^{32}P), their effect on bulky disease is limited. ^{32}P is a pure beta (electron) emitter with maximal tissue penetration of 8 mm and the bulk of energy deposited in the first 2 mm. ^{198}Au emits 90% of its energy as beta particles with an energy of 0.96 MeV. These have tissue penetrations of less than 5 mm, although the emitted photons have energies of 0.412 to 1.099 MeV and can penetrate several centimeters. An equally important limitation on the use of radiocolloids is the problem of obtaining optimal distribution of isotope throughout the pleural space. Gordon and colleagues attempted radioisotope instillation in 3 patients, but fluoroscopy or gamma camera measurements indicated that the distribution was suboptimal.[91] Both agents may have limited roles in patients with low-volume disease or in conjunction with surgery in patients with an adequate pleural distribution. The distribution of a radiotracer or contrast material should be tested before the therapeutic administration of these agents.

RADIATION THERAPY TECHNIQUES. Several different radiation therapy techniques have been used to irradiate the pleura to high doses. Because of the diffuse pleural involvement, the target volume is large and includes the pleural surface, diaphragm, and mediastinum. Attempts at radical irradiation must be limited to patients with disease confined to one hemithorax. Field borders must extend above the first rib superiorly; below the diaphragmatic reflection of the pleura inferiorly, which is usually at about the lower border of the twelfth thoracic vertebra; laterally to clear the bony rib cage; and include the full width of the mediastinum. The field size can be increased to include masses extending through the chest wall or diaphragm or to include the whole heart when the pericardium is involved. The demarcation of sites of residual gross disease with surgical clips placed at thoracotomy greatly facilitates planning by allowing accurate, high-dose boost irradiation and lessens the likelihood of normal tissue injury. CT scans can delineate sites of gross disease, but they may miss invasion of tumor into the mediastinum or through the diaphragm and areas of miliary seeding of the pleura.[57,145,146] MRI can delineate mediastinal invasion by mesothelioma and may have an increasing role in radiologic assessment and treatment planning.[80,147]

Radical irradiation has delivered 4000 to 5500 cGy to the entire pleural surface (with the exception of the reflections extending into the fissures in the lung) and the mediastinum. Other structures such as the heart have been included as clinically indicated. This dose has been followed by boost treatment to 5500 to 7100 cGy to focal areas of gross disease through reduced portals. Although some have chosen to irradiate the entire hemithorax with opposed anterior and posterior photon fields to doses of 4000 to 5000 cGy without lung shielding followed by conning down to smaller fields, such techniques can cause irreversible pulmonary injury.[131,136]

Techniques have been developed to spare the lung. One involves the use of an off-axis beam rotational technique to irradiate a maximal area of the pleural space to high dose while shielding underlying lung.[117,127] Several others involve matching photon and electron beams.[134,145,148,149] These involve the use of large, opposed anterior and posterior external-beam portals with central lung blocking. The pleural areas underneath the blocks are treated with electron beams of appropriate energy (10–15 MeV). CT scans are used to define the thickness of the chest wall, delineate patient contour, and plan treatment. Tissue compensators may improve dose distribution. Currently no completely satisfactory technique for high-dose irradiation of the pleura exists. Even careful photon and electron techniques deliver substantial doses to the lung because of the penetrating ability of the electron beams in the lung and contribution from side scattered electrons set in motion during photon irradiation.[149] Advances in sophisticated conformal radiotherapy may improve the available dose distribution.[150]

With fractions of 180 to 200 cGy given five times weekly, reasonable treatment precautions limit the spinal cord dose to 4000 cGy, the esophagus to 4500 to 5000 cGy, the whole lung to 2000 cGy, a functional portion of the liver to 3000 cGy, and 50% of the heart to 4000 cGy. Radiation tolerances may be lowered if irradiation is given in conjunction with chemotherapy, especially doxorubicin, despite separation of the two modalities by weeks or months.

A single report on the use of fast neutrons describes a complete regression of bulk disease without evidence of recurrence 78 months after treatment.[151] In this report, a portion of the disease was treated with cobalt 60 radiation with similar response. Because of the poor depth-dose characteristics of the available neutron beams, only very thin patients could be treated with a pure neutron technique. However, these or other particles may have a role in selected patients in delivering boost treatment to sites of gross disease.

Chemotherapy

SINGLE-AGENT STUDIES. Before the wide availability of CT scans, most mesotheliomas were not strictly measurable. Measurable masses on chest radiographs were frequently obscured by effusions, producing data that are totally unreliable in determining response to therapy. Response rates to standard agents remain difficult to define. Relatively small positive studies are reported promptly, but larger series with lower response rates may never be published. Nevertheless, data from single-agent studies are shown in Table 43–4. Response rates are included in the table if the number of evaluable patients exceeded 10. Doxorubicin appears to have some activity against mesothelioma, although response rates vary considerably. Methotrexate with rescue, 5-azacytidine, and 5-fluorouracil may also have single-agent activity. Cisplatin as a single agent does not appear to be significantly active, with 5 of 49 patients responding in several phase II studies.

COMBINATION CHEMOTHERAPY. Response rates for combination regimens range from 30% to 40% of 10 to 20 patients in single-institution series to 0% to 14% for cooperative group trials of the same combinations (Table 43–5). Response rates for combinations with and without doxorubicin are similar to the 18% response rate of single-agent doxorubicin (see Table 43–4). Doxorubicin and cyclophosphamide with or without dacarbazine yielded response rates of 7% in both arms of a large randomized trial that accrued advanced-disease patients concurrently with a second study for stage I and II mesothelioma.[229] The response rates may be artificially low in this study because good prognosis patients were treated on a competing study. The Cancer and Leukemia Group B randomized patients with measurable mesothelioma to cisplatin and doxorubicin or to cisplatin and mitomycin C. The objective response rates (24%) in patients with measurable disease were similar.[230] Based on the activity of intraperitoneal cisplatin, the Lung Cancer Study Group completed a trial of 47 patients treated with intrapleural cisplatin and cytarabine. Of the 37 patients evaluated, 49% had at least 75% decrease in the size of their effusions.[125]

Surgery With Intraoperative and Postoperative Adjuvant Therapy

Most patients with mesothelioma cannot be rendered free of disease with surgical therapy alone, and local and systemic recurrences lead to ultimate failure. In a MSKCC report of 41 patients who underwent parietal pleurectomy between 1976 and 1982, disease at the completion of surgery remained on the diaphragm (49%), visceral pleura (51%), mediastinum (49%), chest wall (27%), and lung (5%).[245] Seventy-eight percent had residual gross disease after surgery. Radical pleuropneumonectomy can remove more disease in selected patients but may still have residual microscopic or gross tumor after even the most aggressive surgical resection.

In a Dana-Farber Cancer Institute and Brigham and Women's Hospital select series of 44 patients treated from 1980 to 1991, extrapleural pneumonectomy followed by cisplatin, doxorubicin, and cyclophosphamide chemotherapy and external-beam irradiation resulted in a 48% 2-year survival rate.[126] The operative mortality rate was 5%.[126] Those with lymph node involvement or sarcomatous histology had a significantly poorer survival. In a multivariate analysis of their mesothelioma registry, survival was significantly prolonged for patients who underwent pleuropneumonectomy and chemotherapy and radiotherapy.[86]

Rusch at MSKCC has been investigating the combination of pleurectomy and intraoperative intracavitary administration of cisplatin, followed by postoperative systemic therapy with cisplatin and mitomycin C. The results of this study are forthcoming. At the M.D. Anderson Cancer Center, 20 patients initially received cyclophosphamide, doxorubicin, and DTIC. Five whose disease responded partially underwent surgical resection. Follow-up was short at the time of publication.[238]

A completely different approach has been studied in at the NCI. Recognizing the magnitude of the problem of local control, patients undergo debulking of the disease to a minimum of 5 mm by modified extrapleural pneumonectomy or pleurectomy decortication and intraoperative photodynamic therapy. Before surgery, patients receive the photosensitizer di-

TABLE 43–4. Single-Agent Response Rates in Malignant Mesothelioma Studies With More Than 5 Patients

Agent	No. of Patients Evaluable	No. of Patients Responding	Response (%)	References
Anthracyclines				
Doxorubicin	164	29	18	134, 152–162
THP-doxorubicin	15	0		163
Pirarubicin	85	11	14	164–166
Epirubicin	69	8	12	167, 168
Detorubicin	21	9	43	169
Aclacinomycin A	10	1	10	170
Alkylating Agents				
Cyclophosphamide	14	4	28	154, 171–174
Ifosfamide	43	7	16	175, 176
Mechlorethamine	6	2		177–182
Thiotepa	7	1		152, 171, 180, 181, 183
Melphalan	3	2		174, 183
Procarbazine	6	2		184
Mitomycin C	12	2	17	50, 185
Cisplatin	56	8	14	186–192
Cisplatin (weekly)	9	4	44	193
Carboplatin	97	11 (2 CR)	11	194–200
Iproplatin	7	0		198, 199
Vincas				
Vincristine	23	0		201
Etoposide	51	3	6	202–205
Vindesine	37	1	3	206, 207
Antimetabolites				
5-Fluorouracil	28	4	14	154, 156, 208, 209
Methotrexate, high dose	9	4		171
Dideazafolic acid (CB3717)	18	1	6	198, 210
5-Azacytidine	7	0		211, 212
Dihydro-5-azacytadine	55	4 (1 CR)	7	213, 214
Bleomycin	6	1		215, 216
Miscellaneous				
AMSA	19	1	5	217
Cycloleucine	7	2		215
AZQ	20	0	0	218
Biologicals				
BCG (after surgery)	30		Inevaluable	219
RNA (intrapleural)	10	8	80	220
Interferon				
α	13	2	15	221
β	14	0		222
γ (intrapleural)	99	24 (7 CR)	24	223–226
γ (intrapleural)	10	0		225
Interleukin-2 (intrapleural)	24	10	42	225, 227, 228

CR, complete response.

TABLE 43–5. Reported Therapeutic Combinations in Series With More Than 15 Patients

Agents Used	No. of Patients Evaluable	No. of Patients Responding	Response (%)	References
Doxorubicin-containing Combinations				
5-Azacytadine	36	8	27	87, 216, 231
Ifosfamide	27	5	19	232, 233
Cisplatin	54	14	26	230, 234–236
Cisplatin, bleomycin, mitomycin	25	(1 CR) 11	44	237
Cyclophosphamide ± DTIC	81	6	7	229, 238
Cyclophosphamide, DTIC, vincristine	30	8	21	181, 239, 240
Radiotherapy	24	4	16	87, 161
Nondoxorubicin-containing Combinations				
Cisplatin, etoposide	26	3	12	241
Cisplatin, pirarubicin	39	6	15	166, 242
Cisplatin, mitomycin C	32	10	31	230, 243
Rubidizone, decarbazine	23	0	0	244

hematoporphyrin ether. Theoretically, when the sensitizer that is retained by residual tumor tissue is activated by 630-mm light from two argon pump dye lasers, the resulting photochemical reaction results in cytotoxicity. First-generation light dosimetry has been developed for this technique, and total hemothorax illumination uses light-dispersing media. These trials may lead to the use of water-soluble chemoluminescent compounds as a source of photon delivery.

The use of intraoperative brachytherapy to give a boost dose of radiation to residual areas of gross disease after surgical resection has theoretical appeal because of the opportunity to deliver higher doses to residual disease while sparing normal tissue.[64,245] Forty-one patients were treated between 1976 and 1982 with aggressive surgical exploration, permanent ^{125}I implantation if the volume of residual disease was small (4 patients), or temporary ^{192}Ir implantation if disease was more diffuse (11 patients). Nine patients underwent complete resection of all gross disease, and boost was not attempted. Seven patients also had installation of ^{32}P 5 to 7 days postoperatively. All patients received 4500 cGy of external-beam irradiation to the entire hemithorax 4 to 6 weeks postoperatively with a mixed photon-electron technique to minimize the dose to the lung parenchyma. Some patients also received chemotherapy. The median survival for all patients was 21 months (range, 6–32 months), with 2-year survival of 40%. Disease-free survival was only 13% at 2 years. Isolated local failures occurred in 7 (17%), and 22 patients had distant failures. Four patients developed complications of radiotherapy (*e.g.*, pneumonitis, pulmonary fibrosis, pericardial effusion, esophagitis). In principle, intraoperative electron-beam or brachytherapy boosts may improve local control; in practice, little advantage has been demonstrated. The median time to appearance of a local recurrence in this series was 9 months.

A large nonrandomized series from Hamburg has shown some prolongation of life expectancy with multimodal treatment compared with best supportive care.[246] Ninety-three pa-

tients younger than 71 years of age with malignant pleural mesothelioma, a Karnofsky performance status greater than 60, and no other major medical problems underwent aggressive multimodal treatment or best supportive care according to patient preference. Aggressive treatment included surgery (*i.e.*, parietal pleurectomy or extrapleural pneumonectomy) if possible, followed by doxorubicin, vindesine, and cyclophosphamide. Of the 57 patients in the aggressive treatment group who were in partial or complete remission without progression at the completion of the chemotherapy, 16 received 4500 to 6000 cGy using rotating tangential technique to areas of original extension of tumor. The median survival in the treated patients was 13 months, compared with 7 for those receiving best supportive care. The treated patients, however, were younger, had a better performance status at presentation, and were more amenable to surgery.

Combined radiotherapy and chemotherapy may be more effective than radiotherapy or chemotherapy alone. Theoretically, cisplatin or doxorubicin can be used as a radiosensitizer. A small group of South African patients treated with doxorubicin and radiation of 1000 cGy every 6 weeks for four courses survived a median of 23 months.

MALIGNANT PERITONEAL MESOTHELIOMA

PRESENTATION AND DIAGNOSIS

Patients usually present with symptoms and signs of advanced disease, including pain, ascites, weight loss, or an abdominal mass.[247–249] A tumor in the omentum may be palpable as an epigastric mass.

No satisfactory staging system has been proposed for peritoneal mesothelioma, which is usually confined to the abdomen at diagnosis. Chest radiographs reveal pleural plaques in about 50% of patients with peritoneal primaries, compared with 20% in patients with pleural mesothelioma, reflecting the higher level of asbestos exposure in patients with peritoneal disease. Classic findings on CT scan include mesenteric thickening, peritoneal studding, hemorrhage within the tumor mass, and ascites, but patients may have advanced disease with relatively normal CT scans.[250-252] MRI offers the possibility of improved resolution. Given the low incidence of bone, brain, or liver metastasis at presentation, extensive evaluation for metastatic disease is inappropriate without laboratory test abnormalities. Adrenal, intrapulmonary, or bony metastases should raise the possibility of an alternative diagnosis.

Peritoneal fluid from malignant ascites may be a watery transudate or a viscous fluid rich in mucopolysaccharides. No diagnostic significance has been attached to the character of the fluid, although a viscous ascites with high fluid hyaluronidase levels may suggest the diagnosis. Massive ascites may result in confusion of mesothelioma with severe cirrhosis. Cytologic analysis establishes the diagnosis for only 5% to 10% of patients.[249] Definitive diagnosis requires adequate tissue sampling, preferably from peritinoscopy or an open, visually directed biopsy. A generous biopsy specimen is required to perform immunohistochemical stains and electron microscopy. Open biopsy permits inspection of the abdominal cavity for extent of disease with particular attention to the bowel and ovaries to differentiate mesothelioma from more common causes of peritoneal carcinomatosis. Peritoneal mesotheliomas can be confused with adenocarcinomas arising from any abdominal organ, but the pattern of spread and tendency to accumulate in the pelvis readily leads to confusion with adenocarcinoma of the ovary or carcinoma arising from mullerian duct remnants in the peritoneum.

The tumor usually remains confined to the abdomen until late in the course, and even then, it is more likely to spread to one or both pleural cavities than to disseminate hematogenously. Thrombocytosis is common and associated with a poor prognosis. Other common clotting abnormalities include phlebitis, emboli, hemolytic anemia, and disseminated intravascular coagulation. Most patients die without metastases or involvement of the chest.[249] Esophageal achalasia, secondary amyloidosis, and dermatomyositis have been reported.[253-255] The median survival of untreated patients in most series is 4 to 12 months.[95,247,248,256]

PATHOLOGY

Rare, well-differentiated papillary variants found in younger woman and a syndrome of recurrent peritoneal mesothelial cysts have been associated with a prolonged survival despite bulky disease.[257,258] The disease rarely progresses over time to a typical malignant mesothelioma.[259] Treatment should be provided only with clearly documented progression.[259-261]

Multilocular peritoneal inclusion cysts (*i.e.*, cystic mesotheliomas) are associated with prior surgery, endometriosis, or pelvic inflammatory disease.[262] Although predominantly affecting women, men have been affected.[263-267] Local recurrences develop in about half of the patients. Neither lesion size nor proliferation correlate with outcome.[262] Some investigators advocated classifying this lesion as reactive proliferation rather than as malignant.[262]

THERAPY

Surgery

Surgical and autopsy series have shown that peritoneal mesothelioma involves all peritoneal surfaces, often with masses of 5 cm or more.[268,269] Sites of local invasion included the liver, abdominal wall, diaphragm, retroperitoneum, gastrointestinal tract, and bladder. Seeding of laparotomy scars and biopsy tracts has been observed. The tumor is usually confined to the peritoneal cavity at the time of initial diagnosis and remains there for much or all of the subsequent clinical course.[95] Effective local therapy may have a substantial impact on the survival of patients with this disease. Complete surgical resection is rarely feasible and has not been shown to afford survival benefit without additional therapy. Nevertheless, surgical intervention can provide palliation for small bowel obstruction and relief of massive ascites by peritovenous shunting or paracentesis with a Tenckhoff catheter.[270]

Radiation Therapy

Despite its use in the few reported survivors in this disease, the role of radiation therapy remains unclear. Megavoltage external radiotherapy can deliver a homogeneous dose to the entire abdominal cavity and its contents, although critical organ tolerance limits dose in several areas. Several techniques have been described and used predominantly for the therapy of ovarian carcinoma.[271] The first report was the moving-strip technique, which was necessary because of limited field size and dose rate with ^{60}Co units but which was shown to have a higher morbidity than the open-field techniques.[272] The technique reported from the Joint Center for Radiation Therapy (JCRT) uses open fields with a 67% transmission block to attenuate the dose given to the abdomen superior to the L5–S1 interspace.[273] The superior border of the field is placed above the maximal excursion of the diaphragm by 1 to 2 cm as observed by fluoroscopy. The inferior border is placed at the ischial tuberosities. Laterally, the field extends 1 to 2 cm beyond the properitoneal fat stripe. Daily fractions of 120 cGy in the upper abdomen and 180 cGy in the pelvis are given 5 times weekly to opposed anterior and posterior fields, with both fields treated daily. Doses are prescribed to midplane on the central axis. Total doses of 3000 cGy in the upper abdomen and 4500 cGy in the pelvis are given in 5 weeks. Full-thickness kidney blocks are added to anterior and posterior fields after 1800 cGy. When intraperitoneal chemotherapy is used, the transmission block is omitted and a uniform daily dose of 120 cGy is given to a total dose of 3000 cGy. Blocks are also placed over a portion of the heart and the inferior pelvis lateral to the abdominal cavity to protect the femoral heads and soft tissue. Treatment breaks are given when the total leukocyte count drops to 1500 to 2000/μl or the platelet count drops below 75 to 100,000/μl.

Intraperitoneal instillation of radioactive colloidal gold (^{198}Au) was first reported to improve the symptoms of peritoneal mesothelioma in 1955.[274] Nine other patients treated by the administration of colloidal ^{198}Au have been reported.[182] Two of nine were disease free for 3.5 and 5 years, respectively. Four other patients had clinical improvement of symptoms. The concentration of radiocolloid is generally greatest in the pelvis and lateral gutters, but adhesions from prior surgery and tumor can cause adherence of loops of bowel that may result in inhomogenous spread of the radiocolloid.[181,275] Neither [198]Au nor ^{32}P give substantial dose to tumor cells within gross tumor masses. The estimated dose from 20 mCi of ^{32}P is 18,000 cGy at 0.04 mm but only 4300 cGy at 1 mm and 1700 cGy at 2 mm.[276] The distribution of a radiotracer or contrast material should be tested before the therapeutic administration of these agents. The major complication associated with intraperitoneal instillation of radiocolloids is small bowel obstruction, which occurs in 2% to 10% of patients.[277,278] If external-beam irradiation is also given to the pelvis, as many as 33% of patients may develop bowel complications.[273,279]

Chemotherapy

Because the results of intravenous chemotherapy in patients with malignant mesothelioma have been disappointing and because there is a tendency for the disease to remain confined to the peritoneum, interest has focused on the use of intraperitoneal chemotherapy. The primary theoretical obstacle to this form of treatment is the shallow depth of drug penetration into tumor nodules. Advantages include greatly enhanced drug concentrations in the peritoneal cavity and decreased systemic toxicity. Substantial intravenous drug concentrations are obtained from peritoneal absorption of some drugs like cisplatin. The combination of free-surface diffusion and intracapillary drug flow may be more effective than intravenous treatment alone. Intraperitoneal cisplatin and intravenous thiosulfate protection resulted in a 59% complete response rate, but many patients relapsed quickly after treatment, implying incomplete eradication of tumor using cisplatin alone. Mitomycin C, doxorubicin, and epidoxorubicin have been used intraperitoneally.[248,280,281]

Combined-Modality Approaches

Because surgery or radiotherapy alone have resulted in only a few anecdotal long-term mesothelioma survivors, intensive combined-modality approaches are being studied at several institutions. One of four patients treated at Seattle with surgery, radiotherapy, and chemotherapy had no tumor as assessed by follow-up CT scan at the time of publication.[282]

Three sequential series of patients were treated at the Dana-Farber Cancer Institute and JCRT with surgery, radiotherapy, and chemotherapy. One of 3 patients treated with surgery, intravenous cyclophosphamide, doxorubicin, and DTIC (before and after whole-abdominal radiotherapy) remains alive and well 10 years after diagnosis.[248] Patients treated on a phase I trial between 1982 and 1985 were initially evaluated by computerized tomography. The protocol surgeon was unwilling to attempt resection in 7 of 13 patients with bulky tumors. The remaining 6 patients underwent resection of all lesions larger than 1 cm in diameter and placement of a Tenchkoff catheter or a Portacath intraperitoneal access device. Two of the 6 patients had received prior debulking surgery and intravenous chemotherapy. They then received doxorubicin (20–50 mg) total dose and cisplatin (20–100 mg/m^2) separately administered intraperitoneally for a total of 8 to 12 treatments. At the time of second laparotomy for removal of the access device, all 6 patients had at least an objective 50% decrease in the size of the tumor. (None of the seven patients who presented with inoperable tumor had more than a minimal response to intravenous or intraperitoneal chemotherapy.) Chemotherapy was followed by whole-abdominal irradiation in 5 patients. One patient did not receive irradiation because of prior limited-field irradiation for Hodgkin's disease. Currently, 4 of the 6 patients (including 3 of 5 who received irradiation) remain disease-free 8 to 10 years after diagnosis.[248,256] One patient currently requires chronic intravenous hyperalimentation due to malabsorption, but the remaining 3 patients have normal performance status.

A phase II trial began in 1986.[256] Twenty patients have completed therapy. The median survival for the entire treated group is 16.4 months. Intensive multimodality therapy produces a high response rate and may ultimately prolong survival for this otherwise rapidly fatal disease.

MALIGNANT MESOTHELIOMA OF THE TUNICA VAGINALIS TESTIS

There are about 37 cases of malignant mesothelioma of the tunical vaginalis testis reported in the literature.[283,284] Asbestos exposure was documented in about half of the more recently reported cases. Patients usually present with a hydrocele or "hernia." There may be diffuse peritoneal or abdominal lymph node involvement at diagnosis. Mesotheliomas arising in the tunica vaginalis testes appear to have a more indolent disease course.[283,285–287]

MALIGNANT MESOTHELIOMA OF THE PERICARDIUM

There are just over 100 cases of malignant mesothelioma of the pericardium reported in the literature.[288] Asbestos exposure has not been documented in most patients. Children with pericardial mesothelioma have been reported.[289] Patients usually present with a pericardial effusion, congestive heart failure, an anterior mediastinal mass, or tamponade.[288–292] Diffuse pericardial involvement is found at surgery. The diagnosis is often unsuspected before surgery or autopsy.[293–295]

BENIGN MESOTHELIOMA

Benign tumors involving mesothelium arise with some frequency in the pleura and peritoneum, the tunica vaginalis testis, the atrioventricular node of the heart, and rarely in the mediastinum, liver, and adrenal.[296–301] Those of peritoneum, including tunica vaginalis testis and adrenal, are mesothelial derived, but the others are of disputed histogenesis (*e.g.*, atrioventricular node) or appear to arise from submesothelial mesenchymal cells that do not exhibit mesothelial differentiation.

BENIGN FIBROUS TUMORS OF THE PLEURA

Benign fibrous tumors of the pleura are approximately one third as common as diffuse malignant mesotheliomas and are most common in patients between 40 and 70 years of age.[302] Because they appear to arise from subsurface fibrous tissue, rather than from the mesothelial lining, they have also been called submesothelial fibromas, localized fibrous mesothelioma, or solitary fibrous tumor of the pleura.[302-304] Few patients have been exposed to asbestos, approximating the incidence of exposure in the general population. CT scan and MR imaging are useful but non specific. The differential diagnosis between benign and malignant lesions is based on histologic study.[305] Lesions have ranged in diameter from 1 to 36 cm. Associated effusions can be serosanguineous. Hypertrophic pulmonary osteoarthropathy has occurred in about one third of patients, particularly associated with lesions larger than 10 cm. Hypoglycemia has also been associated with large lesions, associated in some cases with tumor production of insulin-like growth factor.[306,307]

Mesotheliomas are often pedunculated, and 80% arise from but usually do not invade the visceral pleura.[97] Benign pleural mesotheliomas usually have a sharp separation between tumor and compressed lung, and resection can be performed without pulmonary resection. Others may require a limited chest wall resection. Although usually cured if completely resected, recurrences have been reported after several decades, and 12% of patients eventually die of extensive local tumor.[59,120,302]

Localized malignant fibrous tumors of the pleura have also been described. Of 82 malignant localized tumors, 45% were cured by simple excision.[97] If the nature of the lesion is ambiguous, involvement of the pleura on random biopsy can establish a diagnosis of diffuse, malignant disease.

BENIGN FIBROUS MESOTHELIOMAS OF THE GENITAL TRACTS

Called benign mesotheliomas in the past, these neoplasms are probably more accurately designated adenomatoid tumors.[308,309] They usually arise in the scrotum and epididymis. Similar tumors histologically also are occasionally described in women. Talc granulomas have been described in proximity to the tumor in one case.[310]

BENIGN MESOTHELIOMA OF THE CARDIAC ATRIOVENTRICULAR NODE

Patients with benign mesotheliomas of the atrioventricular node present most frequently with heart block.[311] Sudden death has been reported despite the implantation of a pacemaker. The diagnosis is often made at autopsy.[312] Patients have ranged newborn to elderly.[313] The histologic origin of the tumor is disputed.[314]

REFERENCES

1. McDonald AD, McDonald JC. Epidemiology of malignant mesothelioma. In: Antman K, Aisner J, eds. Asbestos-related malignancy. Orlando: Grune & Stratton, 1987:31–55.
2. Hogan MD, Hoel DG. Estimated cancer risk associated with occupational asbestos exposure. Risk Analysis 1981;1:67–76.
3. Irving KF, Alexander RG, Bavley H. Asbestos exposures in Massachusetts public schools. Am Ind Hyg Assoc J 1980;41:270.
4. Mossman BT, Bignon J, Corn M, Seaton A, Gee JB. Asbestos: Scientific developments and implications for public policy. Science 1990;247:294–301.
5. Lee DHK, Selikoff IJ. Historical background to the asbestos problem. Environ Res 1979;18:300.
6. Editorial. A physician's guide to asbestos-related diseases. JAMA 1984;252(18):2593–2597.
7. Women Inspectors of Factories. Annual Report for 1898. London: Her Majesty's Stationery Office, 1899.
8. Merewether ERA, Price CV. Report on effects of asbestos dust in the lungs and dust suppression in the asbestos industry. London: Her Majesty's Stationery Office, 1930.
9. Lynch KM, Smith WA. Pulmonary asbestosis. III. Carcinoma of lung in abestosilicosis. Am J Cancer 1935;14:56–64.
10. Gloyne SR. Two cases of squamous carcinoma of the lung occurring in asbestosis. Tubercle 1935;17:5.
11. Doll R. Morality from lung cancer in asbestos workers. Br J Med 1955;12:81.
12. Craighead JE, Mossman BT. The pathogenesis of asbestos-associated disease. N Engl J Med 1982;306:1446.
13. Timbrell V. Physical Factors as etiological mechanisms. In: Biological effects of asbestos. Lyon: International Agency of Research on Cancer, 1973.
14. Stanton MF, Layard M, Tegeris A, EM, May M, Kent E. Carcinogenicity of fibrous glass: Pleural response in relation to fiber dimension. JNCI 1977;58:589–603.
15. Editorial. Asbestos in water. Lancet 1981;2:132.
16. Lee KP, Barras CE, Griffith FD, Waritz RD. Pulmonary response and transmigration of inorganic fibers by inhalation exposure. Am J Pathol 1981;102:314–323.
17. Gibbs AR, Griffiths DM, Pooley FD, Jones JS. Comparison of fibre types and size distributions in lung tissues of paraoccupational and occupational cases of malignant mesothelioma. Br J Ind Med 1990;47:621–626.
18. Rogers AJ, Leigh J, Berry G, Ferguson DA, Mulder HB, Ackad M. Relationship between lung asbestos fiber type and concentration and relative risk of mesothelioma. A case-control study. Cancer 1991;67:1912–1920.
19. Rom WN, Travis WD, Brody AR. Cellular and molecular basis of the asbestos-related diseases. Am Rev Respir Dis 1991;143:408–422.
20. Dazzi H, Hasleton PS, Thatcher N, Wilkes S, Swindell R, Chatterjee AK. Malignant pleural mesothelioma and epidermal growth factor receptor (EGF-R). Relationship of EGF-R with histology and survival using fixed paraffin embedded tissue and the F4, monoclonal antibody. Br J Cancer 1990;61:924–926.
21. Robertson HE. Endothelioma of the pleura. Cancer Res 1924;8:317.
22. Wagner JC, Sleggs EA, Marchand P. Diffuse pleural mesothelioma and asbestos in the North Western Cape Province. Br J Ind Med 1960;17:260.
23. Connelly RR, Spirtas R, Myers MH, Percy CL, Fraumeni JF. Demographic patterns for mesothelioma in the United States. JNCI 1987;78:1053.
24. Enterline PE, Henderson VL. Geographic Patterns for female pleural mesothelioma deaths for 50 states. JNCI 1987;79:1.
25. Walker AM, Loughlin JE, Freidlander ER, Rothman KJ, Dreyer NA. Projections of asbestos-related disease 1980–2009. J Occup Med 1983;25:409–425.
26. Selikoff IJ, Hammonds EC, Seidman H. Mortality experience of insulation workers in the United States and Canada, 1943–76. Ann N Y Acad Sci 1979;330:195–203.
27. Selikoff IJ, Hammond EC, Seidman H. Latency of asbestos disease among insulation workers in the United States and Canada. Cancer 1980;46:2736–2740.
28. Wagner JC, Sleggs EA, Marchand P. The effects of the inhalation of asbestos in rats. Br J Cancer 1974;29:252–269.
29. Wagner JC, Berry G, Polley FD. Mesotheliomas and asbestos type in asbestos textile workers: A study of lung contents. Br Med J 1982;285:603–606.
30. Anderson HA, Lilis R, Daum SM, Fischbein AS, Selikoff IJ. Household-contact asbestos neoplastic risk. Ann N Y Acad Sci 1976;271:311–323.
31. McNeil BJ, Eddy DM. The costs and effects of screening for cancer among asbestos-exposed workers. J Chron Dis 1982;35:351.
32. Selikoff IJ, Churg J, Hammond EC. Asbestos exposure and neoplasia. JAMA 1964;188:142.
33. Carey TS, Hadler NM. The role of the primary physician in disability determination for social security insurance and workers' compensation. Ann Intern Med 1986;104:706–710.
34. Churg A. Fiber counting and analysis in the diagnosis of asbestos-related disease. Hum Pathol 1982;13:381.
35. Thomson JG, Kaschula ROC, MacDonald RR. Asbestos as a modern urban hazard. Afr Med J 1963;37:77.
36. Li FP, Lokich J. Familial mesothelioma after intense asbestos exposure at home. JAMA 1978;240:467.
37. Risberg B, Nickels J, Wagermark J. Familial clustering of malignant mesothelioma. Cancer 1980;45:2422.
38. Vianna NJ, Polan AK. Non-occupational exposure to asbestos and malignant mesothelioma in females. Lancet 1978;1:1061–1063.
39. Lechner D. Effects of asbestos on cultured human lung epithelial and mesothelioma cells. Proc Am Assoc Cancer Res [Abstract 228] 1983;24:58.
40. Mossman BT, Craighead JE. Asbestos-induced epithelial changes in organ cultures of hamster trachea: Inhibition by retinyl methyl ether. Science 1980;207:311.
41. Gibbs AR, Jones JS, Pooley FD, Griffiths DM, Wagner JC. Non-occupational malignant mesotheliomas. IARC Sci Publ 1989;90:219–228.
42. Antman KH, Corson JM, Li FP, et al. Malignant mesothelioma following radiation exposure. J Clin Oncol 1983;1:695–700.
43. Horie A, Hiraoka K, Yamamoto O, et al. An autopsy case of peritoneal malignant mesothelioma in a radiation technologist. Acta Pathol Jpn 1990;40:57–62.
44. Kawashima A, Libshitz HI, Lukeman JM. Radiation-induced malignant pleural mesothelioma. Can Assoc Radiol J 1990;41:384–386.
45. Lerman Y, Learman Y, Schachter P, et al. Radiation associated malignant pleural mesothelioma. Thorax 1991;46:463–464.
46. Artvinli M, Baris YI. Malignant mesothelioma in a small village in the Anatolian region of Turkey: An epidemiologic study. JNCI 1979;63:17.
47. Suzuki Y. Malignant mesothelioma induced by asbestos and zeolite in the mouse peritoneum. Proc Am Assoc Cancer Res 1983;24:240.

48. Gardner MJ, Saracci R. Effects on health of non-occupational exposure to airborne mineral fibres. IARC Sci Publ 1989;90:375–397.

49. Kane MJ, Chahinian AP, Holland JF. Malignant mesothelioma in young adults. Cancer 1990;65:1449–1455.

50. Antman K, Blum R, Greenberger J, et al. Multimodality therapy for mesothelioma based on a study of natural history. Am J Med 1980;68:356–362.

51. Bellocq JP, Chenard NM, Marcellin L, et al. [Malignant peritoneal mesothelioma in a child. Diagnostic difficulties in a locally "non tumoral" form, revealed by cervical lymph node metastasis.] Arch Anat Cytol Pathol 1989;37:240–247.

52. Bento L, Martinez MA, Conde J, Bardaji C, Montes M, Gonzalez A. Mesothelial cysts of the peritoneum in children. Cir Pediatr 1989;2:140–142.

53. Cooper SP, Fraire AE, Buffler PA, Greenberg SD, Langston C. Epidemiologic aspects of childhood mesothelioma. Pathol Immunopathol Res 1989;8:276–286.

54. Geary WA, Mills SE, Frierson HJ, Pope TL. Malignant peritoneal mesothelioma in childhood with long-term survival. Am J Clin Pathol 1991;95:493–498.

55. Lin CM, Lee Y, Ho MY. Malignant mesothelioma in infancy. Arch Pathol Lab Med 1989;113:409–411.

56. Tewari SC, Kurian G, Jayaswal R, Chakravorty S, Chadha SK, Chauhan MS. Malignant mesothelioma in the young (with prosthetic aortic valve an unusual association). J Assoc Physicians India 1989;37:187–189.

57. Grant DC, Seltzer SE, Antman KH, et al. Computer tomography of malignant pleural mesothelioma. J Comput Assist Tomogr 1983;7:626.

58. Mirvis S, Dutcher JP, Haney PJ, et al. CT of malignant pleural mesothelioma. AJR 1983;140:665.

59. Antman KH. Clinical presentation and natural history of benign and malignant mesothelioma. Semin Oncol 1981;8:313–320.

60. Shearn JC, Jackson D. Malignant pleural mesothelioma: Report of 19 cases. J Thorac Cardiovasc Surg 1981;31:53.

61. Menzies R, Charbonneau M. Thoracoscopy for the diagnosis of pleural disease. Ann Intern Med 1991;114:271–276.

62. DaValle MJ, Faber LP, Kittle CF. Extrapleural pneumonectomy for diffuse, malignant mesothelioma. Ann Thorac Surg 1986;42:612.

63. Roggli VL, Greenberg SD, McLarty JL, et al. Asbestos body content of the larynx in asbestos workers: A study of five cases. Arch Otolaryngol 1980;106:533.

64. Martini N, McCormach PM, Baines MS, et al. Pleural mesothelioma. Ann Thorac Surg 1987;43:113.

65. Kannerstein M, Churg C, McCaughery WTE, eds. Asbestos and mesothelioma: A review. New York: Appleton-Century-Crofts, 1978:81.

66. Kannerstein M, Churg J. A critique of the criteria for the diagnosis of diffuse malignant mesothelioma. Mt. Sinai J Med 1977;44:485.

67. Elmes PC, Simpson M. The clinical aspects of mesothelioma. Q J Med 1976;45:427.

68. Winslow DJ, Taylor HB. Malignant peritoneal mesotheliomas. 1960;13:127.

69. Harwood TR, Grecey DR, Yokoo H. Pseudomesotheliomatous carcinoma of the lung. A variant of peripheral lung carcinoma. Am J Clin Pathol 1976;65:159.

70. Corson J, Pinkus G. Cellular localization patterns of keratin proteins in pleural mesothelioma and metastatic adenocarcinomas a diagnostic discriminant. Lab Invest 1991;64:114A.

71. Suzuki Y, Churg C, Kannerstein M. Ultrastructure of human malignant diffuse mesothelioma. Am J Pathol 1976;85:241.

72. Corson JM, Pinkus GSS. Mesothelioma: Profile of keratin proteins and carcinoembryonic antigen; and immunoperoxidase study of 20 cases and comparison with pulmonary adenocarcinomas. Am J Pathol 1982;108:80.

73. Said J, Nash G, Lee M. Immunoperoxidase localization of keratin, proteins, carcinoembryonic antigen, and factor VIII in adenomatoid tumors: Evidence for a mesothelial derivation. Hum Pathol 1982;13:1106.

74. Bolen JW, Thorning D. Mesotheliomas: A light and electron microscopical study concerning the histogenic relationships between the epithelial and the mesenchymal variants. Am J Surg Pathol 1980;4:451.

75. Warhol WJ, Hickey WF, Corson J. Malignant mesothelioma: Ultrastructural distinction from adenocarcinoma. Am J Surg Pathol 1982;6:307.

76. Warhol MJ, Hunter NJ, Corson JM. An ultrastructural comparison of mesotheliomas and adenocarcinomas of the ovary and endometrium. Int J Gynecol Pathol 1982;1:125.

77. Butchart EG, Ashcroft T, Barnsley WC, et al. Pleuropneumonectomy in the management of diffuse malignant mesothelioma of the pleura: Experience with 29 patients. Thorax 1976;31:15.

78. Rusch VS, Ginsberg RJ. New concepts in the staging of mesotheliomas. In: Deslauriers J, Lacquet LK, ed. International trends in general thoracic surgery. Vol. 6. St. Louis: CV Mosby, 1990:336–343.

79. Leung AN, Muller NL, Miller RR. CT in differential diagnosis of diffuse pleural disease. AJR 1990;154:487–492.

80. Lorigan JG, Libshitz HI. MR imaging of malignant pleural mesothelioma. J Comput Assist Tomogr 1989;13:617–620.

81. McDonald AD, Magner D, Eyssen G. Primary malignant mesothelial tumors in Canada, 1960–1968. Cancer 1973;31:869.

82. Pluygers E, Badewyns P, Minette P, Beandoin M, Gourdin P. Biomarker assessments in asbestos-exposed workers as indicators for selective prevention of mesothelioma or bronchogenic carcinoma: Rationale and practical implications. Eur J Canc Prev 1991;1.

83. Collins CL, Ordonez NG, Schaefer R, et al. Thrombomodulin expression in malignant pleural mesothelioma and pulmonary adenocarcinoma. Am J Pathol 1992;141(4):827–833.

84. Nakano T, Maeda J, Iwahashi N, Tamura S, Hada T, Higashino K. Gallium-67 scanning in patients with malignant pleural mesothelioma. Jpn J Med 1990;29:255–260.

85. Weill H. Asbestos-associated diseases. Science, public policy and litigation. Chest 1983;84:601–608.

86. Antman K, Shemin R, Ryan L, et al. Malignant mesothelioma: Prognostic variables in a registry of 180 patients, the Dana-Farber Cancer Institute and Brigham and Women's Hospital experience over two decades 1965–1985. J Clin Oncol 1988;6:147–153.

87. Chahinian AP, Pajak T, Holland J, et al. Diffuse malignant mesothelioma: Prospective evaluation of 69 patients. Ann Intern Med 1982;96:746.

88. Ruffie P, Feld R, Minkin S, et al. Diffuse malignant mesothelioma of the pleura in Ontario and Quebec: A retrospective study of 332 patients. J Clin Oncol 1989;7:1157–1168.

89. Schildge J, Kaiser D, Henss H, Fiebig H, Ortlieb H. [Prognostic factors in diffuse malignant mesothelioma of the pleura.] Pneumologie 1989;43:660–664.

90. Hulks G, Thomas JS, Waclawski E. Malignant pleural mesothelioma in Western Glasgow 1980–86. Thorax 1989;44:496–500.

91. Gordon W, Antman K, Breenberger J, Weichselbaum R, Chaffey J. Radiation therapy in the management of patients with mesothelioma. Int J Radiat Oncol Biol Phys 1982;8:19.

92. Antman KH. Malignant mesothelioma. N Engl J Med 1980;303:200–202.

93. Wojtukiewicz MZ, Zacharski RL, Memoli VA, et al. Absence of components of coagulation and fibrinolysis pathways in situ in mesothelioma. Thromb Res 1989;55:279–284.

94. De Pangher, Manzini V, Brollo A, Bianchi C. Thrombocytosis in malignant pleural mesothelioma. Tumori 1990;76:576–578.

95. Antman K, Pomfret E, Aisner J, McIntyre J, Osteen RT, Greenberger JS. Peritoneal mesothelioma: Natural history and response to chemotherapy. J Clin Oncol 1983;1:386–391.

96. McAuley P, Asa SL, Chiu B, Henderson J, Goltzman D, Drucker DJ. Parathyroid hormone-like peptide in normal and neoplastic mesothelial cells. Cancer 1990;66:1975–1979.

97. England DM, Hochholzer L, McCarthy MJ. Localized benign and malignant fibrous tumors of the pleura. A clinicopathologic review of 223 cases. Am J Surg Pathol 1989;13:640–658.

98. Olofsson K, Mark J. Specificity of asbestos-induced chromosomal aberrations in short-term cultured human mesothelial cells. Cancer Genet Cytogenet 1989;41:33–39.

99. Burmer GC, Rabinovitch PS, Kulander BG, Rusch V, McNutt MA. Flow cytometric analysis of malignant pleural mesotheliomas. Hum Pathol 1989;20:777–783.

100. Dazzi H, Thatcher N, Hasleton PS, Chatterjee AK, Lawson RA. DNA analysis by flow cytometry in malignant pleural mesothelioma: Relationship to histology and survival. J Pathol 1990;162:51–55.

101. Pyrhonen S, Laasonen A, Tammilehto L, et al. Diploid predominance and prognostic significance of S-phase cells in malignant mesothelioma. Eur J Cancer 1991;27:197–200.

102. Tierney G, Wilkinson MJ, Jones JS. The malignancy grading method is not a reliable assessment of malignancy in mesothelioma. J Pathol 1990;160:209–211.

103. Tiainen M, Tammilehto L, Rautonen J, Tuomi T, Mattson K, Knuutila S. Chromosomal abnormalities and their correlations with asbestos exposure and survival in patients with mesothelioma. Br J Cancer 1989;60:618–626.

104. Fletcher JA, Weidner N, Corson JM. Laboratory investigation and genetics in sarcomas. Curr Opin Oncol 1990;2:467–473.

105. Fletcher J, Cibas E, Granados R, et al. Consistent chromosome aberrations and genetic stability in malignant mesotheliomas: Diagnostic relevance. Proc US Can Acad Pathol [Abstract]1991;64:114.

106. Decker HJ, Li FP, Bixenman HA, Sandberg AA. Chromosome 3 and 12p rearranged in a well-differentiated peritoneal mesothelioma. Cancer Genet Cytogenet [Letter] 1990;46:135–137.

107. Flejter WL, Li FP, Antman KH, Testa JR. Recurring loss involving chromosomes 1, 3, and 22 in malignant mesothelioma: Possible sites of tumor suppressor genes. Genes Chromosom Cancer 1989;1:148–154.

108. Hagemeijer A, Versnel MA, Van DE, et al. Cytogenetic analysis of malignant mesothelioma. Cancer Genet Cytogenet 1990;47:1–28.

109. Hillerdal G, Lindqvist U, Engstrom AL. Hyaluronan in pleural effusions and in serum. Cancer 1991;67:2410–2414.

110. Demetri GD, Zenzie BW, Rheinwald JG, Griffin JD. Expression of colony-stimulating factor genes by normal human mesothelial cells and human malignant mesothelioma cells lines in vitro. Blood 1989;74:940–946.

111. Nakamura Y, Ozaki T, Yanagawa H, Yasuoka S, Ogura T. Eosinophil colony-stimulating factor induced by administration of interleukin-2 into the pleural cavity of patients with malignant pleurisy. Am J Respir Cell Mol Biol 1990;3:291–300.

112. Okazaki H, Kano S, Hatake K, et al. [A case of malignant pleural mesothelioma producing colony-stimulating factor (CSF).] Nippon Naika Gakkai Zasshi 1989;78:506–511.

113. Jordon D, Jagirdar J, Kaneko M. Blood group antigens, Lewisx and Lewisy in the diagnostic discrimination of malignant mesothelioma versus adenocarcinoma. Am J Pathol 1989;135:931–937.

114. Kawai T, Suzuki M, Torikata C, Suzuki Y. Expression of blood group-related antigens and Helix pomatia agglutinin in malignant pleural mesothelioma and pulmonary adenocarcinoma. Hum Pathol 1991;22:118–124.

115. Ruffie P, Feld R, Minkin S, et al. Diffuse malignant mesothelioma of the pleura in Ontario and Quebec: A retrospective study of 331 patients. J Clin Oncol 1990;45:40–42.

116. Harvey JC, Fleischman EH, Kagan R, Streeter OE. Malignant pleural mesothelioma: A survival study. J Surg Oncol 1990;45:40–42.

117. Law MR, Hodson ME, Turner-Warurch M. Malignant mesothelioma of the pleura: Clinical aspects and symptomatic treatment. Eur J Respir Dis 1984;65:162.

118. Woern H. Mopeglichkeiten und Ergebnisse der chirurgischen Behandlung des malignen Pleuramesotheliomas. Thoraxchirurgie 1974;22:339–356.

119. Bamler KJ, Maassen W. Malignant pleura mesotheliomas. Thoraxchirurgie 1974;22:386.

120. DeLaria G, Jensik R, Faber LP, Kittle CF. Surgical management of malignant mesothelioma. Ann Thorac Surg 1978;26:375.

121. Voyt-Moykopf I, Etspule W, Bulzebruck H. Das diffuse meligne pleuramesotheliom: Diagnostik, therapie and prognose. Z Herz Thorac Gefabchir 1987;1:67–77.

122. Faber LP. Surgical treatment of asbestos related disease of the chest. Surg Clin North Am 1988;68:525–530.

123. Probst G, Buelzebruck H, Bauer H, Branscheld HG, Vogt-Moykopf I. The role of pleuropneumonectomy in the treatment of diffuse malignant mesothelioma of the pleura. In: Deslauriers J, Lacquet LK, eds. Thoracic surgery: Surgical management of pleural diseases. St. Louis: CV Mosby, 1990:344–350.

124. Geroulanos S, Lampe P, Hafner F, Buchmann P, Largiader F. Malignant pleural mesothelioma: Diagnosis, therapy and prognosis. Schweiz Rundsch Med Prax 1990;79:361–367.

125. Rusch VW, Piantadose S, Holmes EC. The role of extrapleural pneumonectomy in malignant pleural mesothelioma. A Lung Cancer Study Group trial. J Thorac Cardiovsc Surg 1991;102:1–9.

126. Sugarbaker DJ, Lee TH, Coupe G, et al. Extrapelural pneumonectomy, chemotherapy and radiotherapy in the treatment of diffuse malignant pleural mesothelioma. J Thorac Cardiovasc Surg 1991;102:10–15.

127. Law MR, Gregor A, Hodson ME, Bloom HJG, Turner-Warwick M. Malignant mesothelioma of the pleura: A study of 52 untreated patients. Thorax 1984;39:255–259.

128. Brancatisano RR, Joseph MG, McCaughan BC. Pleurectomy for mesothelioma. Med J Aust 1991;154:455–457.

129. Lewis RJ, Sisler GE, Mackenzie JW. Diffuse mixed malignant pleural mesothelioma. Ann Thoracic Surg 1981;3:153–160.

130. Carmichael J, Degraff WG, Gamson J, et al. Radiation sensitivity of human lung cancer cell lines. Eur J Cancer Clin Oncol 1989;25:527–534.

131. Maasilta P. Deterioration in lung function following hemithorax irradiation for pleural mesothelioma. Int J Radiat Oncol Biol Phys 1991;20:433–438.

132. Ehrenhaft JL, Sensenig DM, Lawrence MS. Mesotheliomas of the pleura. J Thorac Cardiovasc Surg 1960;40:393–409.

133. Eschwege F, Schlienger M. La Radiotherapie des mesotheliomes pleuraux malins: A propos de 14 cas irradies a dose elevees. J Radiol Electrol 1973;54:255–259.

134. Dobelbower RR, Strubler KA, Vaisman I. Clinical applications of high energy electron beams: The pancreas, pleura, and spine. In: High energy electrons in radiation therapy. Berlin: Springer-Verlag, 1980:91–97.

135. Alberts AS, Falkson G, Goedhals L, et al. Malignant pleural mesothelioma: A disease unaffected by current therapeutic maneuvers. J Clin Oncol 1988;6:527–535.

136. Ball DL, Cruickshank DG. The treatment of malignant mesothelioma of the pleura: Review of a 5-year experience, with special reference to radiotherapy. Am J Clin Oncol 1990;13:4–9.

137. Wanebo HJ, Martini N, Melamed MR, Hilaris B, Beattie EJ. Pleural mesothelioma. Cancer 1986;38:2481–2488.

138. Todoroki T, Suit HD. Effect of fractionated irradiation prior to conservative and radical surgery on therapeutic gain in a spontaneous fibrosarcoma of the C3H mouse. J Surg Oncol 1986;31:279–286.

139. Boutin C, Irrisson M, Rathelot P, Petite JM. L'extension parietale des mesotheliomas pleuraux malins diffus apres biopsies: Prevention par radiotherapie locale. Presse Med 1983;12:1823.

140. Maasilta P, Kivisaari L, Holsti LR, Tammilehto L, Mattson K. Radiographic chest assessment of lung injury following hemithorax irradiation for pleural mesothelioma. Eur Respir J 1991;4:76–83.

141. Maasilta P, Salonen EM, Vaheri A, Kivisaari L, Holsti LR, Mattson K. Procollagen-III in serum, plasminogen activation and fibronectin in bronchoalveolar lavage fluid during and following irradiation of human lung. Int J Radiat Oncol Biol Phys 1991;20:973–980.

142. Hallman M, Maasilta P, Kivisaari L, Mattson K. Changes in surfactant in bronchoalveolar lavage fluid after hemithorax irradiation in patients with mesothelioma. Am Rev Respir Dis 1990;141:998–1005.

143. Richart R, Sherman CD. Prolonged survival in diffuse pleural mesothelioma treated with Au198. Cancer 1959;12:799–805.

144. Brady LW. Mesothelioma the role for radiation therapy. Semin Oncol 1981;8:329–334.

145. Bricout PB, Engler MJ. Computerized tomography scanning and the planning of high-dose radiotherapy for pleural mesothelioma: A report of five patients. Int J Radiat Oncol Biol Phys 1981;7:821–826.

146. Rusch VW, Godwin JD, Shuman WP. The role of computed tomography scanning in the initial assessment and the follow-up of the malignant pleural mesothelioma. J Thorac Cardiovasc Surg 1988;96:171–177.

147. Shimojo M, Tsuda N, Kamihata H, et al. [Magnetic resonance imaging for cardiovascular masses.] J Cardiol 1989;19:583–592.

148. Kutcher GJ, Kestler C, Greenblatt D, et al. Technique for external beam treatment for mesothelioma. Int J Radiat Oncol Biol Phys 1987;13:1747–1752.

149. Soubra M, Dunscombe PB, Hodson DI, et al. Physical aspects of external beam radiotherapy for the treatment of malignant pleural mesothelioma. Int J Radiat Oncol Biol Phys 1990;18:1521–1527.

150. Takahashi K, Purdy J, Liu YY. Work in progress: Treatment planning system for conformation radiotherapy. Radiology 1983;147:567–573.

151. Blake PR, Catterall M, Emerson PA. Pleural mesothelioma treated by fast neutron therapy. Thorax 1985;40:72–73.

152. Bonadonna G, Beretta G, Tancini G, et al. Adriamycin studies at the Instituto Nazionale Tumori, Milan. Cancer Chemother Rep 1975;6:231–245.

153. Benjamin RS, Wiernik PH, Bachur NR. Adriamycin: A new effective agent in the therapy of disseminated sarcomas. Med Pediatr Oncol 1975;1:63–67.

154. Gerner RE, Moore GE. Chemotherapy of malignant mesothelioma. Oncology 1974;30:152–1555.

155. Gottlieb JA, Baker LH, O'Bryan RM, et al. Adriamycin (NSC 123127) used alone and in combination for soft tissue and bony sarcomas. Cancer Chemother Rep 1975;6:271–282.

156. Harvey VJ, Slevin ML, Ponder BA, et al. Chemotherapy of diffuse malignant mesothelioma: Phase II trials of single-agent 5-fluorouracil and Adriamycin. Cancer 1984;54:961–964.

157. Kucuksu N, Thomas W, Ezdinli E. Chemotherapy of malignant diffuse mesothelioma. Cancer 1976;37:1265–1274.

158. Lerner H, Amato D, Shiraki M, et al. A prospective study of Adriamycin programs in malignant mesothelioma. Proc Am Soc Clin Oncol [Abstract C-901] 1983;2:230.

159. Mischler NE, Chuprevich T, Johnson RO, et al. Malignant mesothelioma presenting in the pleura and peritoneum. J Surg Oncol 1979;11:185–191.

160. O'Bryan RM, Luce JK, Talley RW, et al. Phase II evaluation of adriamycin in human neoplasia. Cancer 1973;32:1–8.

161. Stock RJ, Fu YS, Carter JR. Malignant peritoneal mesothelioma following radiotherapy for seminoma of the testis. Cancer 1979;44:914–919.

162. Van Dyk JJ, VanDer AM. Adriamycin in the treatment of cancer. S Afr Med J 1976;50:61–66.

163. Ruffie P, Salomon C, Herait P, et al. Phase II study of THP-Adriamycin (THP-A) in malignant pleural mesothelioma (MPM). Presented at the First International Mesothelioma Conference. Paris, 1991:40.

164. Kaukel E, Koschel G, Gatzemeyer U, Salewski E. A phase II study of pirarubicin in malignant pleural mesothelioma. Cancer 1990;66:651–654.

165. Sridhar KS, Hussein AM, Feun LG, Zubrod CG. Activity of pirarubicin (4'-0-tetrahydropyranyladriamycin) in malignant mesothelioma. Cancer 1989;63:1084–1091.

166. Koschel G, Calavrezos A, Kaukel E, et al. Phase III randomized comparison of pirarubicin vs. pirarubicin and cisplatin for treatment of pleural mesotheliomas. Proceedings of the Sixth European Congress Against Cancer. 1991;6.

167. Magri MD, Veronesi A, Foladore S, et al. Epirubicin in the treatment of malignant mesothelioma: A phase II cooperative study. The North-Eastern Italian Oncology Group—Mesothelioma Committee. Tumori 1991;77:49–51.

168. Mattson K, Giaccone G, Kirkpatrick A, et al. Epirubicin in malignant mesothelioma: A phase II study of the EORTC lung cancer cooperative group. J Clin Oncol 1992; 10:824–828.

169. Colbert N, Izrael V, Vannetzel JM, et al. A prospective study of detorubicin in malignant mesothelioma. Am Soc Clin Oncol 1985;4:127.

170. Earhart RH, Amato DJ, Chang AY, et al. Phase II trial of 6-diazo-5-oxo-L-norleucine versus aclacinomycin-A in advanced sarcomas and mesotheliomas. Invest New Drugs 1990;8:113–119.

171. Butt WO. Mesothelioma of the pleura. J Can Assoc Radiol 1962;13:40–49.

172. Di Pietro S, Gennari L. Successful cyclophosphamide treatment in a case of diffuse pleural mesothelioma. Tumori 1963;49:69–73.

173. Hichock HT. Mesothelioma of the pleura. Irish J Med Sci 1970;3:453–456.

174. Yap BS, Benjamin RS, Burgess MA, et al. The value of Adriamycin in the treatment of diffuse malignant pleural mesothelioma. Cancer 1978;42:1692–1696.

175. Alberts AS, Falkson G, Zyl LV. Malignant pleural msothelioma: Phase II pilot study of ifosfamide and mesna. JNCI 1988;80:698–700.

176. Zidar BL, Metch B, Balcerzak SP, et al. A phase II evaluation of ifosfamide and mesna in unresectable diffuse malignant mesothelioma: A Southwest Oncology Group study. Cancer 1992;70:2547–2551.

177. Champion P. Two cases of malignant mesothelioma after exposure to asbestos. Am Rev Respir Dis 1971;103:821–826.

178. Cafrey PF, Lucido JL. The clinical and pathologic aspects of pleural mesotheliomas. Surgery 1961;49:690–695.

179. Gray FW, Tom BCK. Diffuse pleural mesothelioma: A survival of one year following nitrogen mustard therapy. J Thorac Cardiovasc Surg 1962;44:73–77.

180. Jara F, Takita H, Rao UN. Malignant mesothelioma: Clinicopathologic observation. N Y State J Med 1977;77:1885–1888.

181. Kaplan WD, Zimmerman RE, Bloomer WD, Knapp RC. Therapeutic intraperitoneal ^{32}P: A clinical assessment of the dynamics of distribution. 1981;138:683–688.

182. Legha SS, Muggia FM. Pleural mesothelioma: Clinical features and therapeutic implications. Ann Intern Med 1977;87:613–621.

183. McGowan L, Bunnag B, Arias LF. Mesothelioma of the abdomen in women; monitoring of therapy by peritoneal fluid study. Gynecol Oncol 1975;3:10–14.

184. Falkson G, DeVilliers PC, Falkson HC. N-isopropyl-L-2-methylhydrazino)-p-toluamide hydrochloride (NSC 77213) for the treatment of cancer patients. Cancer Chemother Rep 1965;46:7–16.

185. Kelsen D, Bajorin D, Mintzer D. Phase II trial of mitomycin C in malignant mesothelioma. Am Soc Clin Oncol [Abstract] 1985;4:146.

186. Dabouis G, Le Mevel B, Corroller J. Treatment of diffuse pleural malignant mesothelioma by cisdichlorodiammine platinum in nine patients. Cancer Chemother Pharmacol 1981;5:209–210.

187. Daboys G, Delajartre MB, Le Mevel BP. Treatment of diffuse pleural malignant mesothelioma by cis-diaminedichloroplatinum: Preliminary results in eleven patients. Med Oncol Soc Nice France 1979;52:98.

188. Glatstein E, Fuks Z, Bagshaw M. Diaphragmatic treatment in ovarian carcinoma: A new radiotherapeutic technique. Int J Radiat Oncol Biol Phys 1977;2:357–362.

189. Hayes DM, Cvitkovic E, Golbey RB, et al. High dose cisplatinum diaminedichloride. Cancer 1977;39:1372–1381.
190. Mintzer D, Kelson D, Frimmer D, et al. Phase II trial of high dose cisplatin in patients with malignant mesothelioma. Proc Am Soc Clin Oncol 1984;3:258.
191. Rossoff AH, Slayton RE, Perlia CP. Preliminary clinical experience with cisdiamine dichloroplatinum (II) (NSC 119875 CACO). Cancer 1972;30:1451–1456.
192. Samson MK, Baker LH, Benjamin RS, et al. Cis-dichlorodiammineplatinnum III in advanced soft tissue and bony sarcomas: A Southwest Oncology Group study. Cancer Treat Rep 1979;63:11–12.
193. Planting A, Goey H, Verweij J. Phase II study of six weekly courses of high dose cisplatin in mesothelioma. Proc Am Assoc Cancer Res [Abstract 1158] 1991;32:194.
194. Raghavan D, Gianoutsos P, Bishop J, et al. Phase II trial of carboplatin in the management of malignant mesothelioma. J Clin Oncol 1990;8:151–154.
195. Vogelzang NJ, Goutsou M, Corson JM, et al. Carboplatin in malignant mesothelioma: A phase II study of the Cancer and Leukemia Group B. Cancer Chemother Pharmacol 1990;27:239–242.
196. Mbidde EK, Harland SJ, Calvert AH, Smith IE. Phase II trial of carboplatin (JM8) in treatment of patients with malignant mesothelioma. Cancer Chemother Pharmacol 1986;18:284–285.
197. Mbidde EK, Smith IE, Harland S. Phase II trial of carboplatin (JM8) in the treatment of patients with mesothelioma (M). Br J Cancer 1986;54:215.
198. Cantwell BMJ, Harris AL, Ghani S. Phase II studies of a novel antifolate CB3717, and the platinum analogues JM8 and JM9, in mesothelioma of pleura and peritoneum. Br J Cancer 1986;54:216.
199. Cantwell BMJ, Franks CR, Harris AL. A phase II study of the platinum analogues JM8 and JM9. Cancer Chemother Pharmacol 1986;18:286–288.
200. Rebattu P, Riou R, Pacheco Y, Clavel M, Perrin-Fayolle M. Phase II study of very high dose cisplatin in the treatment of malignant mesothelioma. Presented at the First International Mesothelioma Conference. Paris, 1991:36.
201. Martensson G, Sorenson S. A phase II study of vincristine in malignant mesothelioma: a negative report. Cancer Chemother Pharmacol 1989;24:133–134.
202. Falkson G, Falkson H. Clinical trial of the oral form 4'-dimethylepipodophyllotoxin-p-D-ethylidene glucoside (NSC 141540) and VP-16-213. Am Assoc Cancer Res 1978;1:160.
203. Nissen NI, Larsen V, Pederson H, et al. Phase I clinical trial of a new antitumor agent, 4'dimethylepipodophyllotoxin-9-(4,6-O-ethylidene-beta-D-glucopyranoside) (NSC 141540). Cancer Chemother Rep 1972;56:769–777.
204. Nissen NI, Dombernowsky P, Hansen HH, et al. Phase I clinical trial of an oral solution of VP16-213. Cancer Treat Rep 1976;60:943–945.
205. Smit EF, Berendsen HH, Postmus PE. Etoposide and mesothelioma. J Clin Oncol [Letter] 1990;8:1281.
206. Boutin C, Irisson M, Guerin J, et al. Phase II trial of vindesin on malignant pleural mesothelioma. Cancer Treat Rep 1987;71:205–206.
207. Kelsen D, Gralla R, Chang E. Vindesine in the treatment of malignant mesothelioma: A phase II study. Cancer Treat Rep 1983;67:821–822.
208. Porter JM, Cheek JM. Pleural mesothelioma: Review of tumor histogenesis and report of 12 cases. J Thorac Cardiovasc Surg 1968;55:882–890.
209. Riddell RJ. Three cases of mesothelioma. Med J Aust 1966;2:554–559.
210. Cantwell MJ, Earnshaw M, Harris AL. Phase II study of a novel antifolate, N-10-propargyl-5,8-dideazafolic acid (CB3717) in malignant mesothelioma. Cancer Treat Rep 1986;70:1335–1336.
211. Vogler WR, Arkun S, Valez-Garcia E. Phase I study of twice weekly-azacytidine. Cancer Chemother Rep 1974;58:895–899.
212. Vogler WR, Miller DS, Keller JW. 5-Azacytidine: A new drug for the treatment of myeloblastic leukemia. Blood 1976;48:331–337.
213. Harmon D, Vogelzang N, Roboz J, et al. Dihydro-5-azacytidine (DHAC) in malignant mesothelioma (Meso) using serum hyaluronic acide (SHA) as a tumor marker: A phase II trial of the CALGB. Proc Am Soc Clin Oncol [Abstract 1248] 1991;10:351.
214. Dhingra HM, Murphy WK, Winn RJ, Raber MN, Hong WK. Phase II trial of 5,6-dihydro-5-azacytidine in pleural malignant mesothelioma. Invest New Drugs 1991;9:69–72.
215. Lerner H, Schoenfeld D, Martin A, Falkson G, Borden E. Malignant mesothelioma: The Eastern Cooperative Oncology Group Experience. Cancer 1983;52:1981–1985.
216. Chahinian AP, Pajak T, Holland J, et al. Evaluation of 63 patients with diffuse malignant mesothelioma. Proc Am Assoc Cancer Res/Am Soc Clin Oncol 1980;21:360.
217. Falkson G, Vorobiof DA, Lerner JH. A phase II study of M-AMSA in patients with malignant mesothelioma with cyclophosphamide, Adriamycin and vincristine. Cancer Chemother Pharmacol 1980;4:135.
218. Eagan R, Frytak S, Richardson R, et al. Phase II trial of diaziquone in malignant mesothelioma. Cancer Treat Rep 1986;70:429.
219. Webster I, Cochrane JWC, Burkhardt KR. Immunotherapy with BCG vaccine in 30 cases of mesothelioma. S Afr Med J 1982;81:277–278.
220. Esposito S. RNA Therapy for pleural mesothelioma. Lancet 1969;2:1203–1204.
221. Christmas TI, Musk AW, Robinson BW. Phase II study of recombinant human alpha interferon therapy in malignant pleural mesothelioma. Proc Am Assoc Cancer Res 1990;31:A1678.
222. Von Hoff DD, Metch B, Lucas JG, Balcerzak SP, Grunberg SM, Rivkin SE. Phase II evaluation of recombinant interferon-beta (IFN-beta ser) in patients with diffuse mesothelioma: A Southwest Oncology Group study. J Interferon Res 1990;10:531–534.
223. Brandely M, Sousell Sante R. A Phase II multicentre study of recombinant interferon (r-IFN-γ) in malignant mesothelioma. Presented at the First International Mesothelioma Conference. [Abstract] Paris, 1991:5.
224. Boutin C, Viallat JR, Astoul P. Treatment of mesothelioma with interferon gamma and interleukin 2. Rev Pneumol Clin 1990;46:211–215.
225. Boutin C. Treatment of malignant mesothelioma using intrapleural gamma interferon. Bull Acad Natl Med [Discussion 427] 1990;174:421–426.
226. Boutin C, Viallat JR, Zandwijk NV, et al. Activity of intrapleural recombinant gamma-interferon in malignant mesothelioma. Cancer 1991;67:2033–2037.
227. Stoter G, Goey SH, Slingerland R, Bolhuis RL, Eggermont AM. Intrapleural interleukin-2 (IL-2) in malignant pleural mesothelioma: A phase I–II study. Proc Am Assoc Cancer Res [Abstract] 1990;31:275.
228. Robinson BWS, Bowman RV, Christmas TI, Manning LS, Musk AW. Clinical experience using immunotherapy (IL-2/LAK cells or interferon alpha 2a) in malignant mesothelioma. Presented at the First International Mesothelioma Conference. Paris, 1991:38.
229. Samson M, Baker L, Wasser L, et al. Randomized comparison of cyclophosphamide, DTIC and adriamycin vs. cyclophosphamide and adriamycin in patients with advanced malignant mesothelioma: A sarcoma intergroup study. Proc Am Soc Clin Oncol 1985;4:128.
230. Chahinian AP, Antman K, Aisner J, et al. Cisplatin with Adriamycin or mitomycin for malignant mesothelioma: A randomized phase II trial. Proc Am Assoc Clin Oncol [Abstract] 1987;6:183.
231. Chahinian AP, Holland JF. Treatment of diffuse malignant mesothelioma: A review. Mt Sinai J Med 1978;45:54–67.
232. Carmichael J, Cantwell BM, Harris AL. A phase II trial of ifosfamide/mesna with doxorubicin for malignant mesothelioma. Eur J Cancer Clin Oncol 1989;25:911–912.
233. Alberts AS, Falkson G, van ZL. Ifosfamide and mesna with doxorubicin have activity in malignant mesothelioma. Eur J Cancer [Letter; comment] 1990;26:1002.
234. Zidar B, Pugh R, Schiffer L, et al. Treatment of six cases of mesothelioma with doxorubicin and cis-platinum. Cancer 1983;52:1788–1791.
235. Ardizzoni A, Rosso R, Salvati F, et al. Activity of doxorubicin and cisplatin combination chemotherapy in patients with diffuse malignant pleural mesothelioma. An Italian Lung Cancer Task Force Phase II study. Cancer 1991;67:2984–2987.
236. Niki Y, Nakayama S, Soga T, et al. [A case of remission induced in diffuse pleural malignant mesothelioma by the treatment with cisplatin and doxorubicin.] Gan To Kagaku Ryoho 1989;16:3635–3638.
237. Breau JL, Boaziz C, Morere JJF, Sadoun D, Israel L. Combination chemotherapy with cisplatinum, Adriamycin, bleomycin and mitomycin C, plus systemic and intrapleural hyaluronidase in 25 consecutive cases of stages II, III pleural mesothelioma. Presented at the First International Mesothelioma Conference. Paris, 1991:5.
238. Dhingra H, Valdivieso M, Tannir N, et al. Combined modality treatment for mesothelioma with Cytoxan, Adriamycin, and DTIC (CYADIC) and adjuvant surgery. Am Soc Clin Oncol [Abstract] 1983;2:205.
239. Spremulli E, Wampler G, Regelson E, et al. Chemotherapy of malignant mesothelioma. Cancer1977;40:2038–2045.
240. Gottlieb JA, Bodney GP, Sinkovics JG, et al. An effective new four-drug combination regimen (CY-VA-DIC) for metastatic sarcomas. Proc Am Assoc Cancer Res/Am Soc Clin Oncol 1974;15:162.
241. Eisenhauer EA, Evans WK, Murray N, Kocha W, Wierzbicki R, Wilson K. A Phase II study of VP-16 and cisplatin in patients with unresectable malignant mesothelioma. An NCI Canada clinical trials group study. Invest New Drugs 1988;6:327–329.
242. Niki Y, Soga T, Nishimura A, et al. [A diffuse, pleural, malignant mesothelioma kept in long remission by chemotherapy combining pirarubicin and cisplatin.] Gan No Rinsho 1990;36:2463–2467.
243. Chahinian AP, Norton L, Szrajer L, et al. Mitomycin C and cisplatin in human malignant mesothelioma xenografts in nude mice: Clinical correlation. Proc Am Assoc Cancer Res [Abstract 597] 1983;24:151.
244. Zidar BL, Benjamin RS, Frank J, et al. Combination chemotherapy for advanced sarcomas of bone and mesothelioma utilizing rubidazone and DTIC: A Southwest Oncology Group Study. Am J Clin Oncol 1983;6:71–74.
245. Hilaris BS, Dattatreyudu NK, Wong E, Kutcher GJ, Martini N. Pleurectomy and intraoperative brachytherapy and postoperative radiation in the management of malignant pleural mesothelioma. Int J Radiat Oncol Biol Phys 1984;10:325–331.
246. Calavrezos A, Koschel G, Husselmann H, et al. Malignant mesothelioma of the pleura. Klin Wochenschr 1988;66:607–635.
247. Moertel C. Peritoneal mesothelioma. Gastroenterology 1972;63:346.
248. Antman K, Osteen R, Klegar K, et al. Early peritoneal mesothelioma: A treatable malignancy. Lancet 1985;2:977–982.
249. van Gelder T, Hoogsteden HC, Versnel MA, de Beer P, Vandenbroucke JP, Planteydt HT. Malignant peritoneal mesothelioma: A series of 19 cases. Digestion 1989;43:222–227.
250. Whitley NO, Brenner DE, Antman KH, Grant K, Aisner J. Computed tomographic evaluation of peritoneal mesotheliomas: An analysis of eight cases. AJR 1982;138:531–535.
251. Cozzi C, Bellomi M, Frigerio LF, et al. Double contrast barium enema combined with non-invasive imaging in peritoneal mesothelioma. Acta Radiol 1989;30:21–24.
252. Fukuda T, Hayashi K, Mori M, et al. [Radiologic manifestations of peritoneal mesothelioma.] Nippon Igaku Hoshasen Gakkai Zasshi 1991;51:643–648.
253. Nensey YM, Ibrahim MA, Zonca MA, Ma CK. Peritoneal mesothelioma: An unusual cause of esophageal achalasia. Am J Gastroenterol 1990;85:1617–1620.
254. Rashchupkina ZP, Karmilov VA, Iudina LI, Burtsev VI. [Malignant mesothelioma of the peritoneum with secondary amyloidosis of the internal organs.] Klin Med (Mosk) 1990;68:99–101.
255. von Hirschhausen R, Clemens M. [Paraneoplastic dermatomyositis in peritoneal mesothelioma.] Med Klin 1990;1:113–115.
256. Weissmann L, Osteen R, Corson J, Herman T, Antman K. Combined modality therapy for intraperitoneal mesothelioma. Proc Am Soc Clin Oncol 1988;7:274:1063.
257. Foyle A, Al-Jabi M, McCaughey WTE. Papillary peritoneal tumors in women. Am J Surg Pathol 1981;5:241.

258. Katsube Y, Mukai K, Silverberg SG. Cystic mesothelioma of the peritoneum: A report of five cases and review of the literature. Cancer 1982;50:1615.

259. Burrig KF, Pfitzer P, Hort W. Well-differentiated papillary mesothelioma of the peritoneum: A borderline mesothelioma. Report of two cases and review of literature. Virchows Arch [A] 1990;417:443–447.

260. Daya D, McCaughey WT. Well-differentiated papillary mesothelioma of the peritoneum. A clinicopathologic study of 22 cases. Cancer 1990;65:292–296.

261. Lammer F, Scherrer C, Hacki WH. [Well-differentiated papillary mesothelioma of the peritoneum. Rare, but prognostically important differential diagnosis.] Schweiz Med Wochenschr 1991;121:954–946.

262. Ross MJ, Welch WR, Scully RE. Multilocular peritoneal inclusion cysts (so-called cystic mesotheliomas). Cancer 1989;64:1336–1346.

263. O'Neil JD, Ros PR, Storm BL, Buck JL, Wilkinson EJ. Cystic mesothelioma of the peritoneum. Radiology 1989;170:333–337.

264. Villaschi S, Autelitano F, Santeusanio G, Balistreri P. Cystic mesothelioma of the peritoneum. A report of three cases. Am J Clin Pathol 1990;94:758–761.

265. Baddoura FK, Varma VA. Cytologic findings in multicystic peritoneal mesothelioma. Acta Cytol 1990;34:524–528.

266. Canty MD, Williams J, Volpe RJ, Yunan E. Benign cystic mesothelioma in a male. Am J Gastroenterol 1990;85:311–315.

267. Kristensen KA, Ostergaard E. Cystic mesothelioma of peritoneum: Occurrence in a man. J Clin Gastroenterol 1990;12:702–704.

268. McCaughey WTE. Criteria for diagnosis of diffuse mesothelial tumors. Ann N Y Acad Sci 1965;132:603.

269. Kannerstein M, Churg J. Peritoneal mesothelioma. Hum Pathol 1977;8:83.

270. Lomas DA, Wallis PJ, Stockley RA. Palliation of malignant ascites with a Tenckhoff catheter. Thorax 1989;44:828.

271. Einhorn N, Hamos KV, et al. Radiation therapy of ovarian carcinoma: Presentation of a six-field technique. Radiother Oncol 1986;7:125–131.

272. Fazekas J, Maier JG. Irradiation of ovarian carcinomas: A prospective comparison of the open-field and moving strip techniques. AJR 1974;120:118–123.

273. Lederman GS, Recht A, Herman T, Osteen R, Corson J, Antman KH. Long-term survival in peritoneal mesothelioma. The role of radiotherapy and combined modality treatment. Cancer 1987;59:1882–1886.

274. Rose RG, Palmer JD, Lougheed MN. Treatment of peritoneal mesothelioma with radioactive colloidal gold. Cancer 1955;8:478–481.

275. Leichner PK, Rosenshein N, Leibel SA, Order SE. Distribution and tissue dose of intraperitoneal administered radioactive chromic phosphate (³²P) in New Zealand white rabbits. Radiology 1980;134:729–734.

276. Cross WG. Table of beta dose distributions. In: Chalk River, Ontario, 1967.

277. Piver SM. Radioactive colloids in the treatment of stage IA ovarian cancer. Obstet Gynecol 1972;40:42–44.

278. Pezner RD, Stevens KR, Tong D, Allen CV. Limited epithelial carcinoma of the ovary treated with curative intent by the intraperitoneal installation of radiocolloids. Cancer 1978;42:2563–2571.

279. Klaassen D, Starreveld A, Shelly W, et al. Levitt M. External beam pelvic radiotherapy plus intraperitoneal radioactive chromic phosphate in early stage ovarian cancer: A toxic combination. Int J Radiat Oncol Biol Phys 1985;11:1801–1804.

280. Hayashi T, Nasu Y, Aramaki K, Johnsen T, Matsuura H. [A case of peritoneal malignant mesothelioma with disappearance of ascites result of intraperitoneal instillation of mitomycin C and oral administration of UFT.] Gan To Kagaku Ryoho 1989;16:2449–2452.

281. Sugarbaker PH, Cunliffe WJ, Graves T, et al. Phase I and pharmacologic studies with early postoperative intraperitoneal epiadriamycin. Fourth International Conference on Advances in Regional Cancer Therapy. Berchtesgaden, Germany, 1989.

282. Taylor RA, Johnson LP. Mesothelioma: Current perspectives. West J Med 1981;134:379–383.

283. Antman K, Cohn S, Green M. Malignant mesothelioma of the tunica vaginalis testis. J Clin Oncol 1984;2:447–451.

284. Carp NZ, Petersen RO, Kusiak JF, Greenberg RE. Malignant mesothelioma of the tunica vaginalis testis. J Urol 1990;144:1475–1478.

285. Kamiya M, Eimoto T. Malignant mesothelioma of the tunica vaginalis. Pathol Res Pract 1990;186:680–684.

286. Rodriguez AJ, Garmendia LJ, Hernandez LI, et al. [Diffuse malignant mesothelioma of the testicular tunica vaginalis. Report of a new case.] Arch Esp Urol 1990;43:897–899.

287. Smith AH, Handley MA, Wood R. Epidemiological evidence indicates asbestos causes laryngeal cancer. J Occup Med 1990;32:499–507.

288. Asoh Y, Nakamura M, Maeda T, et al. [Brain metastasis from primary pericardial mesothelioma. Case report.] Neurol Med Chir (Tokyo) 1990;30:884–887.

289. Eker R, Cantez T, Dogan O, Demiryent M, Celik A, Karabocuoglu M. Pericardial mesothelioma. A pediatric case report. Turk J Pediatr 1989;31:305–309.

290. Taguchi T, Fujiwara Y, Ichiki H, Kohno N, Hiwada K. [A case of malignant pericardial mesothelioma detected by gallium-67 scintigraphy.] Kaku Igaku 1991;28:281–284.

291. Aggarwal P, Wali JP, Agarwal J. Pericardial mesothelioma presenting as a mediastinal mass. Singapore Med J 1991;32:185–186.

292. Pascual MA, Povar J, Munoz J, et al. [Pericardial mesothelioma: Apropos of a case.] Rev Esp Cardiol 1989;42:559–561.

293. Dai RP. [Primary pericardial mesothelioma: A report of four cases.] Chung Hua Fang She Hsueh Tsa Chih 1989;23:90–92.

294. Gurevich MA, Odinokova VA, Smirnov VB, Iankovskaia MO. [Clinico-morphological characteristics of pericardial mesothelioma.] Sov Med 1991;1991:8–11.

295. Torii T, Takasuga H, Mizushima M, Ito J, Kanaya T, Matsushima T. [Primary malignant mesothelioma of the pericardium masquerading as malignant pleural mesothelioma: Report of an autopsy case and review of the reported cases in Japan as to its invasion to neighboring organs.] Kokyu To Junkan 1989;37:1027–1032.

296. De Klerk DP, Nime F. Adenomatoid tumors (mesothelioma) of testicular and paratesticular tissue. Urology 1975;6:635.

297. Fenoglio JJ, Jacobs DW. Ultrastructure of the mesothelioma of the atrioventricular node. 1977;40:721.

298. Scully R, Mark EJ, McNeeley BU. Case record of the Massachusetts General Hospital. N Engl J Med 1982;306:32.

299. Balassiano M, Reichert N, Rosenman Y, Hertcheg E, Lieberman Y, Yellin A. Localized fibrous mesothelioma of the mediastinum devoid of pleural connections. Postgrad Med J 1989;65:788–790.

300. Kottke MK, Hart WR, Broughan T. Localized fibrous tumor (localized fibrous mesothelioma) of the liver. Cancer 1989;64:1096–1102.

301. Simpson PR. Adenomatoid tumor of the adrenal gland. Arch Pathol Lab Med 1990;114:725–727.

302. Briselli M, Mark EJ, Dickersin GR. Solitary fibrous tumors of the pleura: Eight new cases and review of 360 cases in the literature. Cancer 1981;47:2678.

303. Scharifker D, Kaneko M. Localized fibrous "mesothelioma" of pleura (sub-mesothelial fibroma). A clinicopathologic study of 18 cases. Cancer 1979;43:627.

304. Dalton WT, Zolliker AS, McCaughey WTE, et al. Localized primary tumors of the pleura. An analysis of 40 cases. Cancer 1979;44:1465.

305. Majoulet JF, Millant P, Bouillet P, Le BA, Gaillard S. [Radiologic aspect of benign pleural fibrous mesothelioma. Reports of 4 cases.] Ann Radiol (Paris) 1990;33:229–236.

306. Strom EH, Skjorten F, Aarseth LB, Haug E. Solitary fibrous tumor of the pleura. An immunohistochemical, electron microscopic and tissue culture study of a tumor producing insulin-like growth factor I in a patient with hypoglycemia. Pathol Res Pract 1991;187:109–113.

307. Scotte M, Bessou JP, Andro JF, et al. [Hypoglycemic pleural mesothelioma. A case report.] Ann Chir 1990;44:688–691.

308. Davies JH, Notley RG. Adenomatoid tumours of the male genital tract. Review of 5 men presenting with an intrascrotal swelling subsequently diagnosed as an adenomatoid tumor. Eur Urol 1989;16:393–394.

309. Lopez JI, Aranda FI. Absence of estrogen immunoreactivity in adenomatoid tumors of male reproductive system. Pathol Res Pract 1990;186:395–396.

310. Kupryjanczyk J. Adenomatoid tumor of the ovary and uterus in the same patient. Zentralbl Allg Pathol 1989;135:437–444.

311. Corbi P, Jebara V, Fabiani JN, et al. [Benign tumors of the heart (excluding myxoma). Experience with 9 surgically treated cases.] Ann Cardiol Angeiol (Paris) 1990;39:433–436.

312. Subramanian R, Flygenring B. Mesothelioma of the atrioventricular node and congenital complete heart block. Clin Cardiol 1989;12:469–472.

313. Fontaliran F, Guillois B, Colin A, et al. Congenital atrioventricular block and maternal lupus erythematosus. Histologic discovery of tumor of the artrioventricular node. Arch Mal Coeur 1989;82:609–613.

314. Monma N, Satodate R, Tashiro A, Segawa I. Origin of so-called mesothelioma of the atrioventricular node. An immunohistochemical study. Arch Pathol Lab Med 1991;115:1026–1029.

Cancer: Principles & Practice of Oncology, Fourth Edition,
edited by Vincent T. DeVita, Jr., Samuel Hellman, Steven A. Rosenberg.
J.B. Lippincott Co., Philadelphia © 1993.

Martin M. Malawer

Michael P. Link

Sarah S. Donaldson

CHAPTER **44**

Sarcomas of Bone

Malignant tumors arising from the skeletal system are rare, representing only 0.2% of all new cancers. Approximately 2100 new cases in the United States occur annually.[1] Osteosarcoma and Ewing's sarcoma are the two most common bone tumors; they occur mainly during childhood and adolescence.[2-4] Other mesenchymal (spindle cell) neoplasms—fibrosarcoma, chondrosarcoma, and malignant fibrous histiocytoma—that characteristically arise after skeletal maturity are less common.[5-18] These are sometimes associated with underlying benign bony tumors, previous irradiation, or primary bone disease.[5-16]

The surgical, chemotherapeutic, and radiotherapeutic principles developed in the treatment of osteosarcomas form the basis of the management strategy for most of the spindle cell neoplasms. Within the past decade, there has been an explosion of clinical knowledge and experience in the management of bony neoplasms.[18-28] The development of centers with specific interest in these tumors has played an important role in the advancement of biologic understanding, surgical management, and multimodality treatment of these tumors.[24-27] A surgical staging system that permits standardized preoperative evaluation, analysis, and end-result reporting has been developed.[28]

Amputation was once the standard method of treating bony sarcomas, but the past decade has witnessed the development of limb-sparing surgery for most malignant and aggressive benign tumors.[29-39] Advances in orthopedics, bioengineering, radiographic imaging, radiation therapy, and chemotherapy have contributed to safer, more reliable surgical procedures.[40-80] Axial computerized tomography (CT) and magnetic resonance imaging (MRI) permit extremely accurate evaluation of the local anatomy and enhance the possibility of safe resection.[81-88] Limb-sparing surgery is considered safe and routine for a large number of carefully selected patients. An evaluation system to determine a patient's functional status has been developed.[28] This system has enabled evaluation and comparison of the various limb-sparing procedures and types of surgical reconstructions.

Paralleling these advances has been the demonstrated effectiveness of adjuvant chemotherapy in dramatically increasing overall survival, and the bleak 15% to 20% survival rate with surgery alone before the 1970s rose to 55% to 80% with various adjuvant treatment regimens during the 1980s.[49-52,89-91] Multidrug regimens are now considered essential treatment. The timing, mode of delivery, and different combinations of these agents are being investigated at many centers. Preoperative chemotherapy regimens, administered by the intravenous or intraarterial route, and postoperative regimens are being evaluated to determine their effect on the tumor and their impact on the choice of operative procedure and on overall survival.[92-99]

This chapter focuses on malignant spindle cell tumors; Ewing's sarcoma is presented elsewhere. Benign tumors are described briefly, and their significance for the oncologist is explained.[2,3] We emphasize natural history, surgical staging, criteria of patient selection for amputation or limb-sparing surgery, and the technique of limb-sparing procedures. The development, role, timing, and mode of delivery of adjuvant chemotherapy and its relation to stage of disease is discussed. The role of radiation therapy in specific clinical situations is presented.

CLASSIFICATION AND TYPES OF BONE TUMORS

Bone consists of cartilaginous, osteoid, and fibrous tissue and of bone marrow elements. Each tissue can give rise to benign or malignant spindle cell tumors.[2-4] The classification of bone tumors is based on cell type and recognized products of proliferating cells. The classification, described by Lichtenstein in 1954 and modified by Dahlin is presented in Table 44–1.[3,55] Jaffe recommends that each tumor be considered a separate clinical-pathologic entity.[4] Radiographic, histologic, and clinical data are necessary to form an accurate diagnosis and to determine the degree of activity and malignancy of each lesion.

Cartilage tumors are lesions in which cartilage is produced. They are the most common bone tumors. Osteochondroma is the most common benign cartilage tumor; 1% to 2% of solitary osteochondromas become malignant.[56–57] Enchondroma is a benign cartilage tumor that occurs centrally; in an adult, malignant transformation may occur. Chondrosarcoma, the most common malignant cartilage tumor, occurs intramedullarly or peripherally. Ten percent are secondary, arising from an underlying benign lesion.[2] Most chondrosarcomas are low grade, although 10% differentiate into a high-grade spindle cell sarcoma or a rare mesenchymal chondrosarcoma.[2,56]

Osteoid tumors are lesions in which the stroma produces osteoid. The benign forms are osteoid and osteoblastoma. Osteoid osteomas are never malignant. Osteoblastomas rarely metastasize; if they do, it is only after multiple local recurrences.[58] Osteosarcomas are the most common primary malignant tumors of the bone. Histologically, they are composed of malignant spindle cells and osteoblasts that produce osteoid or immature bone. Several variants are now recognized.[59] Parosteal, periosteal, and low-grade intraosseous osteosarcoma are histologically and radiographically distinct from the classic central medullary osteosarcomas and have more favorable prognoses.[60–62]

Fibrous tumors of bone are rare. Desmoplastic fibroma is a locally aggressive, nonmetastasizing tumor, analogous to fibromatosis of soft tissue.[5,6] Fibrosarcoma of bone appears histologically as its soft tissue counterpart. Multiple sections must be obtained to demonstrate the lack of osteoid production. If osteoid is present, the lesion is classified as an osteosarcoma. Malignant fibrous histiocytoma (MFH), the counterpart of soft tissue MFH, has been described in bone.[7–9] It rarely occurs. The pathology of bone and soft tissue MFH is similar, consisting of a storiform pattern with a histiocytic component. Giant cell tumors are of unknown origin; originally called benign, they are now considered to be low-grade sarcomas. They have a high rate of local recurrence and malignant transformation.[63,64]

Tumors presumably arising from bone marrow elements are the round cell sarcomas. The two most common are Ewing's sarcoma and non-Hodgkin's lymphoma, which are discussed in other chapters.

RADIOGRAPHIC EVALUATION AND DIAGNOSIS

Radiographic evaluation, combined with the clinical history and histology, is necessary for accurate diagnosis. Bone scans, angiography, CT scans, and MRI generally are not helpful in determining a diagnosis but are important in delineating the extent of local involvement.

A systematic approach to the radiographic evaluation of skeletal lesions was described by Madewell and colleagues, who studied and correlated several hundred radiographic and pathologic specimens.[65] They considered the radiograph as

TABLE 44–1.   General Classification of Bone Tumors

Histologic Type*	Benign	Malignant
Hematopoietic (41.4%)		Myeloma
		Reticulum cell sarcoma
Chondrogenic (20.9%)	Osteochondroma	Primary chondrosarcoma
	Chondroma	Secondary chondrosarcoma
	Chondroblastoma	Dedifferentiated chondrosarcoma
	Chondromyxoid fibroma	Mesenchymal chondrosarcoma
Osteogenic (19.3%)	Osteoid osteoma	Osteosarcoma
	Benign osteoblastoma	Parosteal osteogenic sarcoma
Unknown origin (9.8%)	Giant cell tumor	Ewing's tumor
		Malignant giant cell tumor
		Adamantinoma
	(Fibrous) histiocytoma	(Fibrous) histiocytoma
Fibrogenic (3.8%)	Fibroma	Fibrosarcoma
	Desmoplastic fibroma	
Notochordal (3.1%)		Chordoma
Vascular (1.6%)	Hemangioma	Hemangioendothelioma
		Hemangiopericytoma
Lipogenic (<0.5%)	Lipoma	
Neurogenic (<0.5%)	Neurilemmoma	

* Distribution based on Mayo Clinic experience.
(Adapted from Dahlin DC. Bone tumors: General aspects and data on 6,221 cases. 3rd ed. Springfield, IL, Charles C. Thomas, 1978; classification based on Lichtenstein: Classification of primary tumors of bone. Cancer 1951;4:335–351)

the gross specimen from which a detailed histologic interpretation could be made and biologic activity accurately diagnosed. According to their system, a bone tumor is evaluated by five radiographic parameters: anatomic site, borders, bone destruction, matrix formation, and periosteal reaction.

Specific anatomic sites of the bone give rise to specific groups of lesions. Johnson explained this by a field theory, which hypothesizes that the most active cells of a certain area of bone give rise to tumors that are characteristic of that area.[66] Figure 44–1 summarizes the anatomic sites of common bone tumors. In general, spindle cell sarcomas are metaphyseal, and round cell sarcomas tend to be diaphyseal.

The border reflects the growth rate and the response of the adjacent normal bone to the tumor. Most tumors have characteristic borders. Benign lesions (*e.g.,* nonossifying fibromas, unicameral bone cysts) have well-defined borders and a narrow transition area that is often associated with a reactive sclerosis. Aggressive or benign tumors (*e.g.,* chondroblastoma, giant cell tumors) tend to have faint borders and wide zones of transition with little sclerosis, reflecting a more rapidly growing lesion. Poorly delineated or absent margins indicate an aggressive or malignant lesion.

Bone destruction is the hallmark of a bone tumor. Bone destruction is described as a geographic, moth-eaten, or permeative pattern.[67] In general, these patterns are found in the tubular bone rather than in the flat bone and represent a combination of cortical and cancellous destruction. These patterns reflect the progressively increasing growth rate of the underlying tumor.

Calcification of the matrix or new bone formation can produce an area of increased density within the lesion. Calcification typically appears as flocculent or stippled rings or clusters. The appearance of the new bone varies from dense

sclerosis that obliterates all evidence of normal trabeculae to small, irregular, circumscribed masses described as "wool" or "clouds." Calcification and ossification may appear in the same lesion. Neither type of matrix formation is diagnostic of malignancy.

Periosteal reaction indicates malignancy but is not pathognomonic of a particular tumor. A combination of periosteal changes is often found. In malignant tumors, periosteal reaction is noncontinuous and thin, with multiple laminations. A parallel or a perpendicular pattern may be present.

The radiographic parameters of benign and malignant tumors are quite different. Benign tumors have round, smooth, well-circumscribed borders. There is no cortical destruction and generally no periosteal reaction. Malignant lesions have irregular, poorly defined margins. There is evidence of bone destruction and a wide area of transition with periosteal reaction. Soft tissue extension is common.

NATURAL HISTORY

Tumors arising in bone have characteristic patterns of behavior and growth that differentiate them from other malignant lesions.[68,88] These patterns form the basis of a staging system and current treatment strategies. These principles and their relation to management, as formulated by Enneking, are described here.[68,88]

BIOLOGY AND GROWTH

A spindle cell sarcomas form a solid lesion that grows centrifugally. The periphery of this lesion is the least mature. Unlike a true capsule that surrounds a benign lesion and is

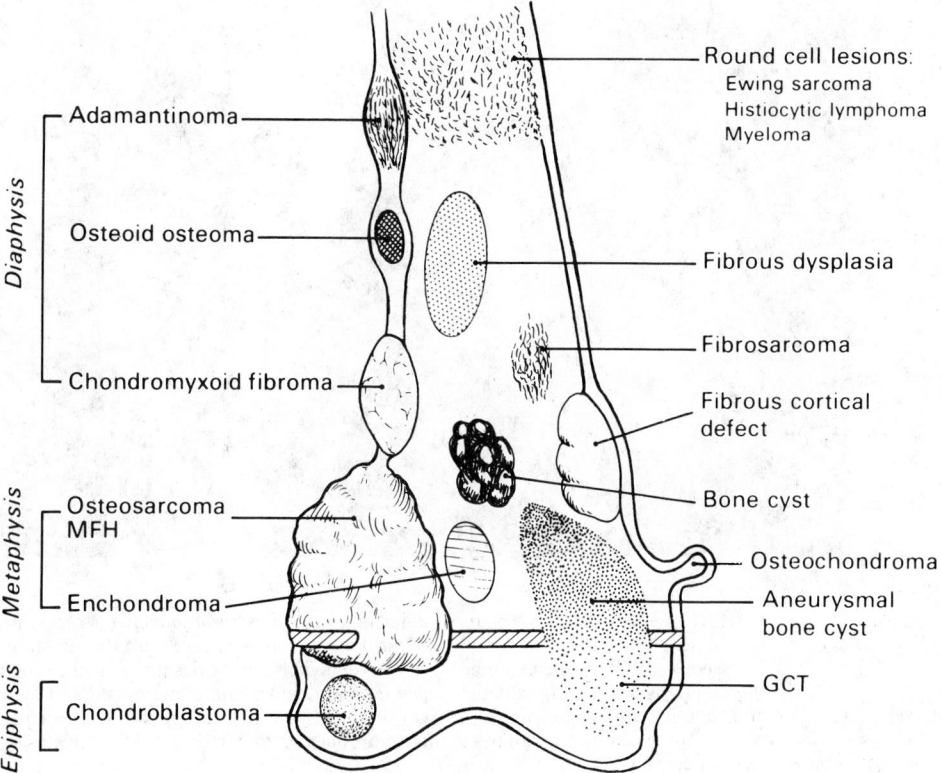

FIGURE 44–1. Common anatomic sites of bone tumors. (Modified from Madewell JE, Ragsdale ED, Sweet DE. Radiographic and pathologic analysis of solitary bone lesions. Radiol Clin North Am 1981;19:715–814)

composed of compressed normal cells, the malignant tumor is generally enclosed by a pseudocapsule and consists of compressed tumor cells and a fibrovascular zone of reactive tissue with a inflammatory component that interdigitates with the normal tissue adjacent to and beyond the lesion. The thickness of the reactive zone varies with the degree of malignancy and histiogenic type. The histologic hallmark of sarcomas is their potential to break through the pseudocapsule to form satellite lesions of tumor cells. This characteristic differentiates a nonmalignant from a malignant mesenchymal tumor.

High-grade sarcomas have a poorly defined reactive zone that may be invaded and destroyed by the tumor (Fig. 44–2). There may be tumor nodules in tissue that appear to be normal and not contiguous with the main tumor. These are called skip metastases. Although low-grade sarcomas regularly demonstrate tumor interdigitation into the reactive zone, they rarely form tumor nodules beyond this area.

The three mechanisms of growth and extension of bone tumors are compression of normal tissue, resorption of bone by reactive osteoclasts, and direct destruction of normal tissue.

Benign tumors grow and expand by the first two mechanisms, and direct tissue destruction is characteristic of malignant bone tumors. Sarcomas respect anatomic borders and remain within one compartment. Local anatomy influences tumor growth by setting the natural barriers to extension. Bone sarcomas usually take the path of least resistance. Most benign bone tumors are unicompartmental; they remain confined and may expand the bone in which they arose. Malignant bone tumors are bicompartmental; they destroy the overlying cortex and go directly into the adjacent soft tissue. The determination of anatomic compartment involvement has become more important with the advent of limb-preservation surgery.

PATTERNS OF SPREAD AND CLASSIFICATION

Based on biologic considerations and natural history, Enneking classified bone tumors into five categories, each of which shares certain clinical characteristics and radiographic patterns and requires similar surgical procedures.[68,118]

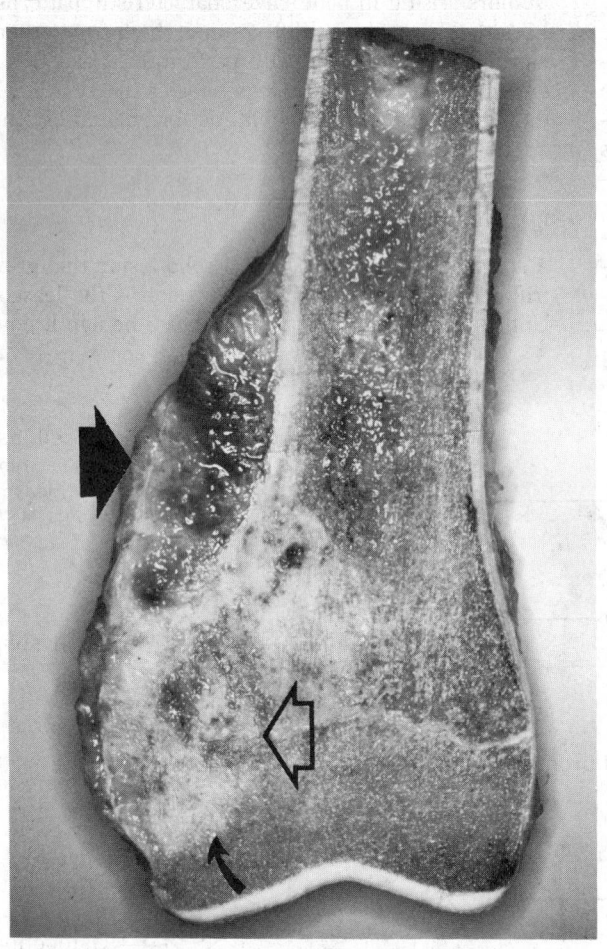
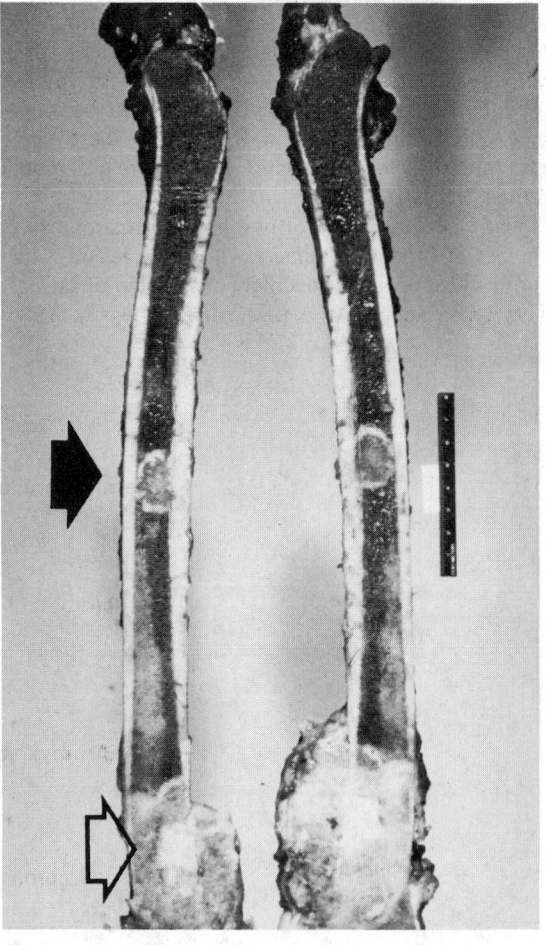

A   B

FIGURE 44–2. Common patterns of local growth of osteosarcoma. Gross specimens of two femoral osteosarcomas. **(A)** Typical osteosarcoma. Most osteosarcomas arise within the metaphysis and have a large extraosseous (soft tissue) component (*solid arrow*). This tumor has arisen within the metaphysis and involves the epiphysis by direct destruction (*open arrow*) through the growth plate and by tracking along the cortex and then back into (*curved solid arrow*) the epiphysis. **(B)** Skip metastasis. A separate tumor (*solid arrow*) nodule not in continuity with the main tumor (*open arrow*) mass is a skip metastasis. This is a poor prognostic sign for survival.

Benign and latent: lesions whose natural history is to grow slowly during normal growth of the person and then stop, with a tendency to heal spontaneously. They never become malignant and, if treated by simple curettage, they heal rapidly. Surgery is not indicated unless they become symptomatic.

Benign and active: lesions whose natural history is one of progressive growth. Simple curettage leaves a reactive rim with some tumor. Curettage has a high recurrence rate. Wide excision through normal bone results in local control in approximately 95% of patients.

Benign and aggressive: lesions that are locally aggressive but do not metastasize. The tumor extends through the capsule into the reactive zone. Local control can be obtained only by removing the lesion with a margin of normal bone beyond the reactive zone.

Low-grade malignant: lesions that have a low potential to metastasize. Histologically there is no true capsule but a pseudocapsule. Tumor nodules exist within the reactive zone but rarely beyond. Local control can be accomplished only by removal of all tumor and reactive tissue with a margin of normal bone. These lesions can be treated successfully by surgery alone.

High-grade malignant: lesions whose natural history is to grow rapidly and to metastasize early. Tumor nodules are often found within and beyond the reactive zone and at some distance in the normal tissue. Surgery is necessary for local control, and systemic therapy is warranted to prevent metastasis.

METASTASES

Bone tumors, unlike carcinomas, disseminate almost exclusively through the blood; bones lack a lymphatic system. There have been rare reports of early lymphatic spread to regional nodes.[18,100] Lymphatic involvement, which has been found in 10% of cases at autopsy, is a poor prognostic sign.[69] McKenna observed that 6 (3%) of 194 patients with osteosarcoma who underwent amputation demonstrated lymph node involvement. None of these patients survived 5 years.[70] Hematogenous spread is manifested by pulmonary involvement in its early stages and secondarily by bony involvement.[70–75] Bone metastasis is occasionally the first sign of dissemination. With the use of adjuvant chemotherapy, the skeletal system has become a more common site of initial relapse.[45,101,102]

SKIP METASTASIS

A skip metastasis is a tumor nodule that is located within the same bone as the main tumor but not in continuity with it. Transarticular skip metastases are located in the joint adjacent to the main tumor.[76] Skip metastases are most often seen with high-grade sarcomas. A skip lesion develops by the embolization of tumor cells within the marrow sinusoids; in effect, they are local micrometastases that have not passed through the circulation (see Fig. 44–2). Transarticular skips are believed to occur through periarticular venous anastomosis. The clinical incidence of skip metastases is less than 1%.[77] These lesions connote a poor prognosis.[76,77]

Wuisman and Enneking reported the natural history of 23 osteosarcomas with skip metastases evaluated at the University of Florida.[102a] Twenty-three patients with documented skip metastases were compared with 224 patients with stage II osteosarcoma without skip metastases. Seventeen skip metastases were in the same bone and six were transarticular. There was no difference in the mean age, sex ratio, or distribution of patients. Only 10 skip metastases were picked up on preoperative staging studies. The remaining 13 were detected only on examination of whole mount macrosections. Skip metastasis has a significant impact on local recurrence (30% versus 10%) and metastatic disease (95% versus 50%). Neither prognosis nor incidence of skip metastasis differed by age for groups older or younger than 21 years. The researchers reported an overall incidence of 6%. They concluded that adjuvant chemotherapy had no effect on patients with skip metastasis.

LOCAL RECURRENCE

Local recurrence of a benign or malignant lesion is due to inadequate removal. The aggressiveness of the tumor determines which surgical procedure is required for local control. Ninety-five percent of all local recurrences, regardless of histology, develop within 24 months of attempted removal.[68,78,79] Local recurrence of a high-grade sarcoma decreases overall survival prospects substantially. Local recurrence in patients who have undergone therapy may be associated with an even poorer prognosis.[74]

JOINT INVOLVEMENT

The articular cartilage is thought to be a natural barrier to direct articular extension by tumor. In a careful study of 45 macrosections of primary bone sarcomas, Simon reported 17 (38%) with articular extension.[80] He described three mechanisms: pericapsular, direct extension along intraarticular structures, and direct extension through the articular cartilage. Pathologic fracture, which opens a direct communication from tumor bone to joint cartilage, is a fourth mechanism (Fig. 44–3).

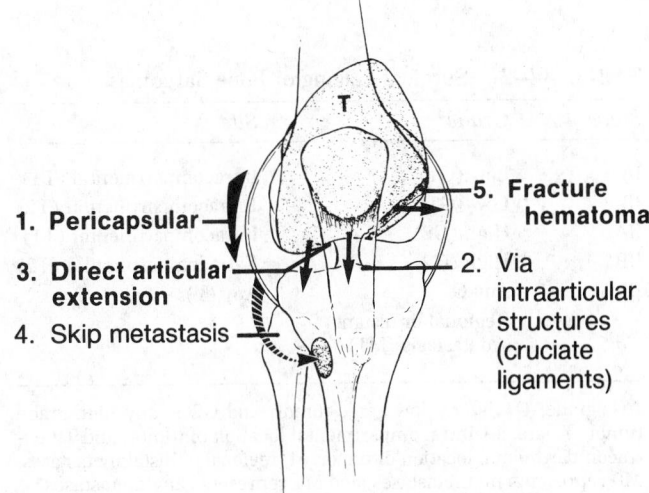

FIGURE 44–3. Mechanisms of articular involvement by high-grade bone sarcomas.

STAGING BONE TUMORS

In 1980, the Musculoskeletal Tumor Society adopted a surgical staging system for bone sarcomas (Table 44–2).[118] The system is based on the fact that mesenchymal sarcomas of bone behave similarly, regardless of histiogenic type. The surgical staging system described by Enneking and colleagues is based on GTM classification: grade (G), location (T), and lymph node involvement and metastases (M) (see Table 44–2).

SURGICAL GRADE

In the staging system, G represents the histologic grade of a lesion and other clinical data. These factors are used to make a surgical determination of low grade (G1) or high grade (G2) (Fig. 44–4).

SURGICAL SITE

T represents the site of the lesion, which may be intracompartmental (T1) or extracompartmental (T2). Compartment is defined as an anatomic structure or space bounded by natural barriers of tumor extension. The significance of T1 lesions is easier to define clinically, surgically, and radiographically than that of T2 lesions, and there is a higher chance of adequate removal of the former by a nonamputative procedure. Low-grade bone sarcomas are usually intracompartmental (T1), and high-grade sarcomas are extracompartmental (T2).

LYMPH NODES AND METASTASES

Lymphatic spread is a sign of wide dissemination (M). Regional lymphatic involvement is equated with distal metastases.

The surgical staging system developed by Enneking and colleagues for surgical planning and assessment of bone sarcomas is summarized:

Stage IA (G1,T1,M0): low-grade intracompartmental lesion, without metastasis
Stage IB (G1,T2,M0): low-grade extracompartmental lesion, without metastasis

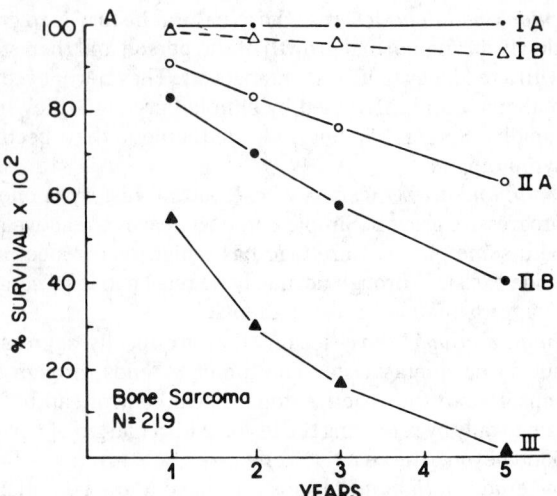

FIGURE 44–4. Survival rates of patients over a 5-year period with bone sarcoma according to stage of disease. (Enneking WF, Spanier SS, Goodman MA. A system for the surgical staging of musculoskeletal sarcoma. Clin Orthop 1980;153:106–120)

Stage IIA (G2,T1,M0): high-grade intracompartmental lesion, without metastasis
Stage IIB (G2,T2,M0): high-grade extracompartmental lesion, without metastasis
Stage IIIA (G1 or G2,T1,M1): intracompartmental lesion, any grade, with metastasis
Stage IIIB (G1 or G2,T2,M1): extracompartmental lesion, any grade, with metastasis

Spanier and coworkers further evaluated and refined stage IIB osteosarcoma and divided them into six categories (E1 to E6) depending on their local growth patterns (Table 44–3)

TABLE 44–3. Definitions of Anatomic Extent for Stage IIB Tumors

Maximal Extent	Definition
E1	Tumor touches but does not elevate or penetrate the periosteum
E2	Tumor elevates but does not penetrate the periosteum
E3	Tumor penetrates into but not through the periosteum
E4	Minimal extraperiosteal extension, not into a defined structure or space, seen as a nodule of tumor of one centimeter or less in fat just outside the periosteum, where muscle does not insert onto bone; the nodule often lies next to a small artery and may represent a small venous embolus that has destroyed the wall of the vein
E5	Tumor invades any one of the following: tendon; ligament; periarticular structures (tumor is covered by synovial tissue); joint (tumor is intraarticular); muscle; bone; or space, such as the popliteal fossa or the axilla
E6	Tumor invades two structures or more

(Spanier SS, Schuster JJ, Vander Griend RA. The effect of local extent of the tumor on prognosis in osteosarcoma. J Bone Joint Surg [Am] 1990;72:643–652)

TABLE 44–2. Surgical Staging of Bone Sarcomas

Stage	Grade*	Site
IA	Low (G1)	Intracompartmental (T1)
IB	Low (G1)	Extracompartmental (T2)
IIA	High (G2)	Intracompartmental (T1)
IIB	High (G2)	Extracompartmental (T2)
III	Any G Regional or distant metastasis (M1)	Any (T)

* G, grade; G1 is any low-grade tumor, and G2 is any high-grade tumor. T, site; T1 intracompartmental location of tumor, and T2 extracompartmental location of tumor. M, regional or distal metastases; M0 represents no metastases, and M1 represents any metastases. (Enneking WF, Spanier SS, Goodman MA. A system for the surgical staging of musculoskeletal sarcoma. Clin Orthop 1980;153:106–120)

and correlated it with prognosis (*i.e.,* disease-free interval) in 51 patients who had osteosarcoma.[102b] E6 was the worse prognostic factor for stage IIB osteosarcoma (*i.e.,* if the tumor invades two or more structures adjacent to the bone, the risk of failure was 5.9 times greater than if the tumor was smaller and more circumscribed). They did not determine any relation to sex, age, or size. They agreed that the most important factor determining prognosis was the initial extent of local disease and that it must be given primary consideration in evaluating and comparing different therapeutic regimens.

PREOPERATIVE EVALUATION

If the plain radiographs suggest an aggressive or malignant tumor, staging studies should be performed before biopsy. All radiographic studies are influenced by surgical manipulation of the lesion, making interpretation more difficult.[39,68] The biopsy site may be in a location that is not optimal for subsequent en bloc removal or radiation therapy.[24,103,104] Bone scintigraphy, MRI, CT, or angiography are required to delineate local tumor extent, vascular displacement, and compartmental localization.[42–46,68,78,82–88]

BONE SCANS

Bone scintigraphy assists in determining polyostotic involvement, metastatic disease, and intraosseous extension of tumor.[42,43,45] Malignant bone tumors, although solitary, may in rare cases present with skeletal metastasis.[46] Skip metastases are rarely detected by bone scans because they are small and localized to the fatty marrow and do not excite cortical response.[76,77]

Appreciation of the intraosseous extension of a bone tumor is important in surgical planning. Watts recommended removal of bone 6 to 7 cm beyond the area of scintigraphic abnormality.[32] This has been accepted as a safe margin for limb-sparing procedures.

COMPUTED TOMOGRAPHY

CT allows accurate determination of intraosseous and extraosseous extension of skeletal neoplasms.[40–44] It accurately depicts the transverse relation of a tumor. By varying window settings, the examiner can study cortical bone, intramedullary space, adjacent muscles, and extraosseous soft tissue extension. CT should include the entire bone and the adjacent joint. Infusion of intravenous contrast material permits identification of the adjacent large vascular structures. CT evaluation must be individualized. To obtain the maximal benefit of image reconstruction, the surgeon should discuss the information desired with the radiologist. Three dimensional reconstruction may be useful.

MAGNETIC RESONANCE IMAGING AND STAGING

MRI has several advantages in the diagnoses of bone sarcomas.[81–88] It has better contrast discrimination than any other modality, and imaging can be performed in any plane (Fig. 44–5). MRI is ideal for imaging the medullary marrow and for the detection of tumor and the extraosseous component.

It has proven especially helpful in several difficult clinical situations, such as detecting small lesions, evaluating a positive bone scan if the corresponding plain radiograph is negative, determining the extent of infiltrative tumors, and detecting skip metastases. MRI has become invaluable in the planning of limb-sparing procedures.[86,88]

ANGIOGRAPHY

The technique of arteriography for bone lesions differs from that used for arterial disease. A minimum of two views (biplane) is necessary to determine the relation of the major vessels to the tumor.[105] Experience with limb-sparing procedures has increased, and it has become essential to determine individual vascular patterns before resection. This is especially crucial for tumors of the proximal tibia, where vascular anomalies are common.[106] Angiography is the most reliable means of determining vascular anatomy and displacement, but MRI and CT better demonstrate extraosseous extension.

CHOOSING A RADIOGRAPHIC METHOD FOR EVALUATION

One or all of the described studies are required in the preoperative evaluation of a bone sarcoma. There are unique benefits to each study. Bloem performed a prospective study comparing results of CT, MRI, scintigraphy, and angiography with 56 resected specimens to determine the appropriate choice of procedures.[106a] MRI was the best single modality to use. It was the most accurate for determining intraosseous extent of tumor, and scintigraphy and CT were often misleading. Angiography was performed only if the primary tumor was in the vicinity of the primary tumor. They also reported CT and MRI were as accurate in evaluation of cortical changes. MRI was superior in detection of muscular involvement in the knee, pelvis, and shoulder compared with CT.

MRI and CT (transverse data), combined with bone scans and angiography, allow the physician to develop a three-dimensional construct of the local tumor area before surgery and formulate a detailed surgical approach.

BIOPSY TECHNIQUE AND TIMING

The biopsy of a suspected bone tumor must be performed with great care and skill.[103,104] This principle cannot be overemphasized. The consequences of a poorly executed biopsy are often the deciding factor in the choice between a limb-salvage procedure or an amputation. Murray and colleagues from M.D. Anderson Cancer Center (MDACC) judged that only 19% of patients referred to that institution for treatment of primary bone sarcomas had properly placed biopsies.[24] All of these patients had open (incisional) biopsies, although 92% of such procedures performed at MDACC over the same period were needle biopsies. Similarly, Mankin compared the results of biopsies performed at the referring institution with those performed at the treatment center.[104] In this study, which involved 329 patients, a major error in diagnosis occurred for 60% of patients from referring hospitals, and 18.2% of the referred patients had to have less than optimal treatment due

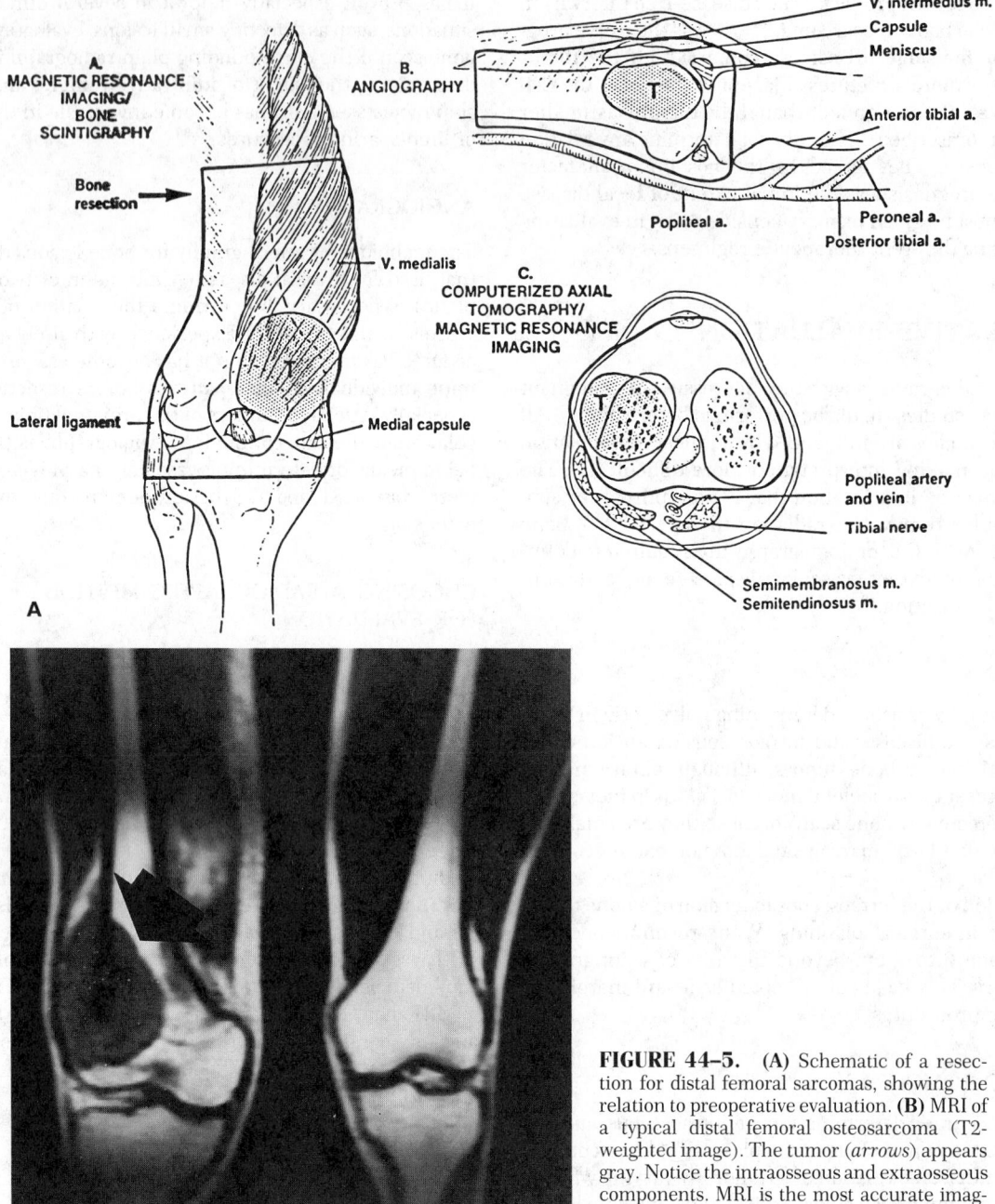

FIGURE 44–5. **(A)** Schematic of a resection for distal femoral sarcomas, showing the relation to preoperative evaluation. **(B)** MRI of a typical distal femoral osteosarcoma (T2-weighted image). The tumor (*arrows*) appears gray. Notice the intraosseous and extraosseous components. MRI is the most accurate imaging modality for determining the intraosseous extent of tumor.

to problems related to the biopsy, and for 8.5% of the total, the prognosis and outcome were adversely affected by the biopsy.

The biopsy should be performed by the surgeon who makes the ultimate decision about the operative procedure. This entails the referral of some patients who are strongly suspected of having primary bony malignancies to a regional cancer center for biopsy.

Trephine or core biopsy is recommended and often obtains an adequate specimen for diagnosis.[107–109] Multiple samples can be obtained from the same puncture site by slightly changing the angle of approach. Radiographs should be obtained to document the position of the trocar. Core biopsy is

preferred if limb-sparing is an option, because it entails less local contamination than open biopsy. Core biopsy is especially helpful in difficult areas, such as the spine, pelvis, and hips. If a core biopsy proves to be inadequate, a small incisional biopsy is performed.

Every precaution should be taken to avoid contamination in performing an open biopsy. A tourniquet is used if feasible. If there is a soft tissue component, there is no need to biopsy the underlying bone. To decrease subsequent hemorrhage, polymethylmethacrylate (PMMA) is used to plug a cortical window; Gelfoam is used for hemostasis in the soft tissue. The overlying pseudocapsule is carefully closed to ensure maximal hemostasis. If it is necessary to biopsy the underlying bone, it is essential to use a small, rounded cortical window. This is especially true for a tumor that requires primary radiation therapy. Large segments do not reossify, often leading to fracture and the need for amputation. Regardless of the technique used, tumor cells contaminate all tissue planes and compartments transversed. All biopsy sites must be removed en bloc if the tumor is resected or irradiated.

Frozen-section analyses are obtained for all biopsy specimens. Many bone tumors can be adequately sectioned with a microtome. The purpose of the initial frozen section is to determine whether enough viable tumor has been obtained to yield satisfactory paraffin sections for interpretation. If not, additional specimens must be obtained. Frozen-section studies may suggest that additional material is necessary for electron microscopy studies or special staining techniques.

Interest has been renewed in frozen-section diagnosis and immediate surgery. Although the idea is attractive, there is no evidence that this procedure increases survival. Its major advantage is to decrease the risk of tumor microextension and contamination in a bloodless field, if a tourniquet has been used.[68,109]

RESTAGING AFTER PREOPERATIVE CHEMOTHERAPY

With the advent of preoperative (*i.e.*, neoadjuvant) chemotherapy for osteosarcoma, a need has developed to serially evaluate the clinical and radiographic response of the tumor before surgery. The staging and preoperative clinical studies previously described are used in evaluating tumor response. These studies are summarized in other reports.[110–114]

CLINICAL EVALUATION

Pain often decreases after the induction of chemotherapy. Alkaline phosphatase levels also decrease. The tumor becomes smaller, especially if significant matrix is not present. Conversely, increase of pain, elevation of alkaline phosphatase, or increasing tumor size are obvious signs of tumor progression.

PLAIN RADIOGRAPHY

There is a good correlation between radiographic response and the amount of necrosis.[112,113] Smith described the radiographic responses seen on serial radiographs: increased ossification of tumor osteoid, marked thickening and new bone formation of the periosteum and tumor border (giving the tumor a more benign appearance), and decrease in soft tissue mass (Fig. 44–6A,B).[113] The healing ossification is usually solid, homogenous, and regular and is easily differentiated from tumor osteoid.[112] There are less significant changes within the intramedullary component, including increased sclerosis and lysis, presumably due to necrosis and hemorrhage.

ANGIOGRAPHY

After chemotherapy, there is a marked decrease in vascularity.[111,112] Chuang evaluated 53 patients and reported that those with a complete angiographic response had more than 90%

necrosis; among those with a partial response, necrosis ranged from 40% to 78%.[112] He concluded that angiographic evaluation was as reliable as pathologic evaluation and that the angiographic features were the best clinical criteria for the evaluation of tumor response.

Carrasco and coworkers from MDACC reported their extensive experience with intraarterial chemotherapy for osteosarcoma (81 patients) and evaluated the angiographic appearance and changes after two and four cycles of preoperative chemotherapy.[112a] They developed a simple radiographic system for angiographic changes. They evaluated the midarterial and parenchymal (capillary) phase:

1. Angiographic response with complete disappearance of tumor vascularity and stain
2. Total disappearance of tumor vascularity with slight persistence of tumor stain (capillary phase)
3. No response and persistence of tumor vascularity and capillary stain

They reported that 40% of the histologic responders (>90% tumor necrosis) and 91% of nonresponders were identified after two cycles. After four cycles, 91% of the responders but only 50% of the nonresponders were identified. The number of courses were not different between the responders and nonresponders. They concluded the disappearance of tumor vascularity after two courses of chemotherapy was highly suggestive of a good histologic response and was unlikely to occur in the histologic nonresponders.

COMPUTED TOMOGRAPHY

The most consistent finding in patients responding to therapy is a decrease in soft tissue mass and the development of a rim-like calcification similar to that seen on plain radiographs (Fig. 44–6C,D).[110] Changes in marrow are not helpful in evaluating response.

BONE SCINTIGRAPHY

Bone scan changes are difficult to evaluate. A decrease in activity generally indicates a favorable response; however, reparative bone formation, signalled by increased activity, may be misleading. Dynamic bone scans (quantitative bone scans), which are based on tumor blood flow and regional plasma clearance by bone and soft tissue, may allow more valid evaluations.[114] Regions that show a greater than 20% decrease in ^{99m}Tc-monodiphosphate plasma clearance are reported to be associated with necrotic tumor.

MAGNETIC RESONANCE IMAGING

MRI is a promising modality for evaluating chemotherapy-induced tumor necrosis. A preliminary report by W.R. Hogeboom and coworkers evaluated 10 patients undergoing preoperative therapy.[112b] They reported variable changes associated with tumor necrosis: decreased tumor size, cystic formation, reactive calcification, and changes in the T2 signal. They emphasized that a marked increase in T2 signal intensity is the result of necrosis, but much more investigation is required to correlate MRI findings with the spectrum of tumor necrosis before it is considered a reliable technique.

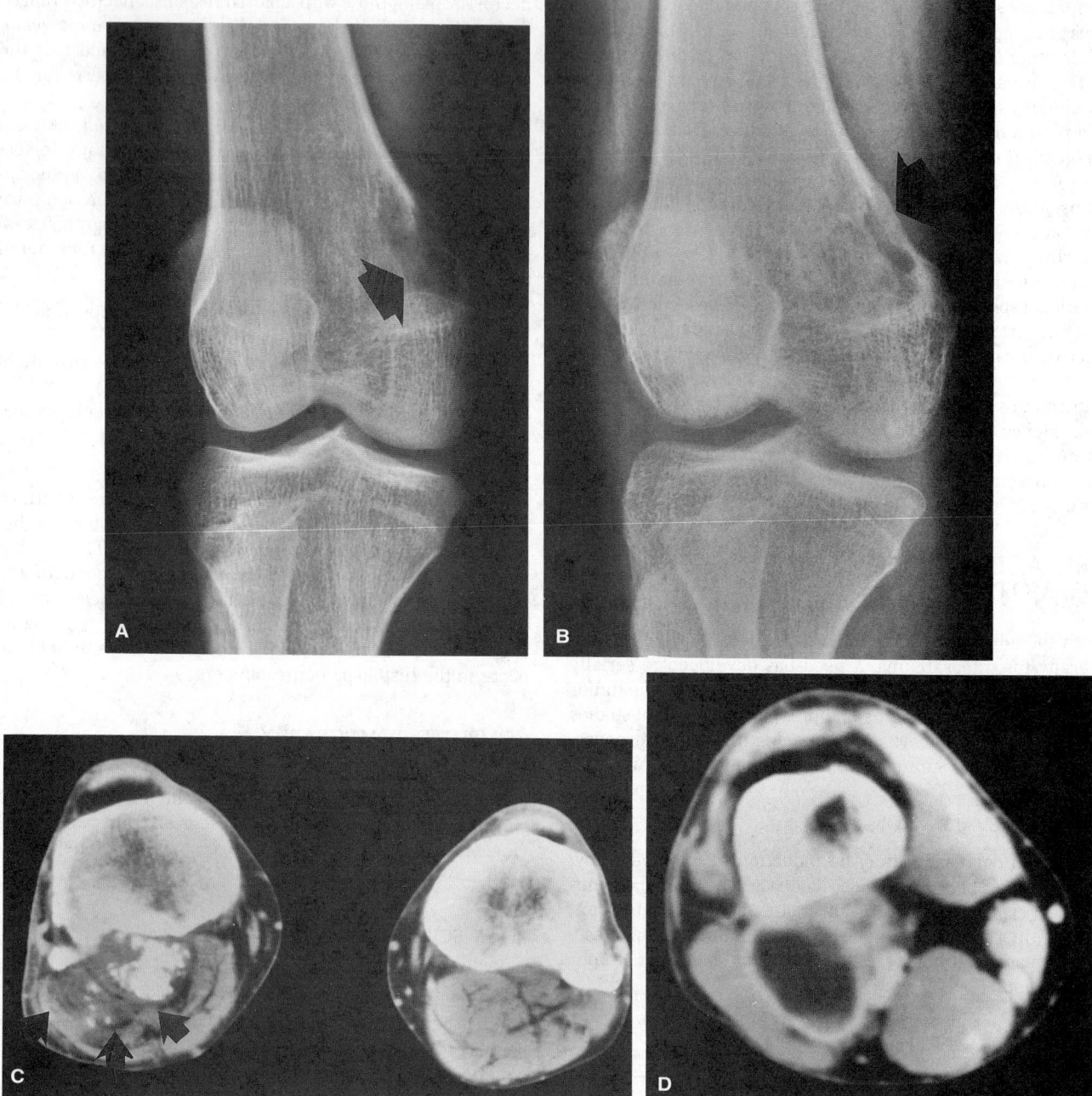

FIGURE 44–6. Response of osteosarcoma to preoperative (neoadjuvant) chemotherapy. **(A)** Plain radiograph of a small distal femoral osteolytic osteosarcoma of the medial femoral condyle. Notice the cortical destruction (*arrow*). **(B)** Plain radiograph after two cycles of intraarterial chemotherapy. Notice the reossification of the medullary space and healing of the cortical defect (*arrow*). These changes are considered typical of tumor necrosis with secondary healing response. This new bone is nontumor reparative bone and not neoplastic. **(C)** CT scan of another patient with a distal femoral osteosarcoma with a large posterior extraosseous component (*arrows*). This patient initially would have required amputation. **(D)** CT scan after two courses of neoadjuvant, intraarterial chemotherapy. There was mark necrosis (*dark center*) with new, nonneoplastic bone rimming associated with some shrinkage of the tumor mass. This patient underwent a limbsparing procedure. Pathologic examination showed 100% tumor necrosis. The rim of reossification is typically seen on CT scans and indicates a good tumor response.

TABLE 44–4. Classification of Surgical Procedures for Bone Tumors

Margin*	Local	Amputation
Intralesional	Curettage or debulking	Debulking amputation
Marginal	Marginal excision	Marginal amputation
Wide	Wide local excision	Wide through bone, amputation
Radical	Radical local resection	Radical disarticulation

* Tumors are classified by the type of margin achieved and whether obtained by a local or ablative procedure.
(Enneking WF, Spanier SS, Goodman MA. A system for the surgical staging of musculoskeletal sarcoma. Clin Orthop 1980;153:106–120)

HISTOLOGY

Serial needle biopsies are unreliable due to the possibility of sampling error.

SURGICAL MANAGEMENT OF SKELETAL TUMORS

Surgical removal, including curettage, resection, and amputation, is the traditional method of managing skeletal neoplasms. Limb-sparing techniques were developed during the early 1970s.[20–22,28–39] Marcove has described cryosurgery for some bony tumors.[115–117] Enneking and colleagues formulated means of classifying of surgical procedures based on the surgical plane of dissection in relation to the tumor (Table 44–4) and the method of accomplishing the removal (Table 44–5). The scheme summarized below permits meaningful comparisons of various operative procedures and gives surgeons a common language.[68,78,118]

1. *Intralesional.* An intralesional procedure passes through the pseudocapsule of the neoplasm directly into the lesion. Macroscopic tumor is left, and the entire operative field is potentially contaminated. Curettage is an intralesional procedure.
2. *Marginal.* A marginal procedure is one in which the entire lesion is removed in a single piece. The plane of dissection passes through the pseudocapsule or reactive zone around the lesion. If performed for a sarcoma, it leaves macroscopic disease.
3. *Wide* (intracompartmental). A wide excision, commonly called en bloc resection, includes the entire tumor, the reactive zone, and a cuff of normal tissue. The entire structure of origin of the tumor is not removed. In patients with high-grade sarcomas, this procedure may leave skip nodules.
4. *Radical* (extracompartmental). The entire tumor and the structure of origin of the lesion are removed. The plane of dissection is beyond the limiting fascial or bony borders.

Any of these procedures may be accomplished by a local (*i.e.*, limb-sparing) procedure or by amputation. Amputation may entail a marginal, wide, or radical excision, depending on the plane in which it passes. An amputation does not necessarily remove all cancer, but it can achieve a specific margin. The local anatomy determines how such a margin is to be obtained. The aim of preoperative staging is to assess local tumor extent and important local anatomy to enable the surgeon to decide how to achieve a desired margin and evaluate the feasibility of surgical procedures. This system allows meaningful comparisons of surgical procedures, end-results reporting, and analysis of combined data. In general, benign bone tumors may be treated adequately by an intralesional procedure (*i.e.*, curettage) or a marginal excision. Malignant tumors require a wide (*i.e.*, intracompartmental) or radical (*i.e.*, extracompartmental) removal, which may be an amputation or an en bloc procedure. Wide excision combined with adjuvant chemotherapy is the treatment of most high-grade bone sarcomas. Radical resections are rarely performed.

LIMB-SPARING SURGERY

Principles and Techniques

Limb salvage surgery is a safe operation for selected patients.[23–36,119–121] This technique may be used for all spindle cell sarcomas, regardless of histogenesis. Between 30% and 80% of patients with osteosarcoma can be treated successfully with this technique.[24,26,28,32,39,118]

The successful management of localized osteosarcomas and other sarcomas requires careful coordination and timing of staging studies, biopsy, surgery, and preoperative and postoperative chemotherapy, and radiation therapy.

TABLE 44–5. Surgical Procedure, Plane or Dissection, and Residual Disease for Musculoskeletal Tumors

Type	Plane of Dissection	Result
Intralesional	Piecemeal debulking or curettage	Leaves macroscopic disease
Marginal	Shell out en bloc through pseudocapsule or reactive zone	May leave either "satellite" or "skip" lesions
Wide	Intracompartmental en bloc with cuff of normal tissue	May leave "skip" lesions
Radical	Extracompartmental en bloc, entire compartment	No residual

(Enneking WF, Spanier SS, Goodman MA. A system for the surgical staging of musculoskeletal sarcoma. Clin Orthop 1980;153:106–120)

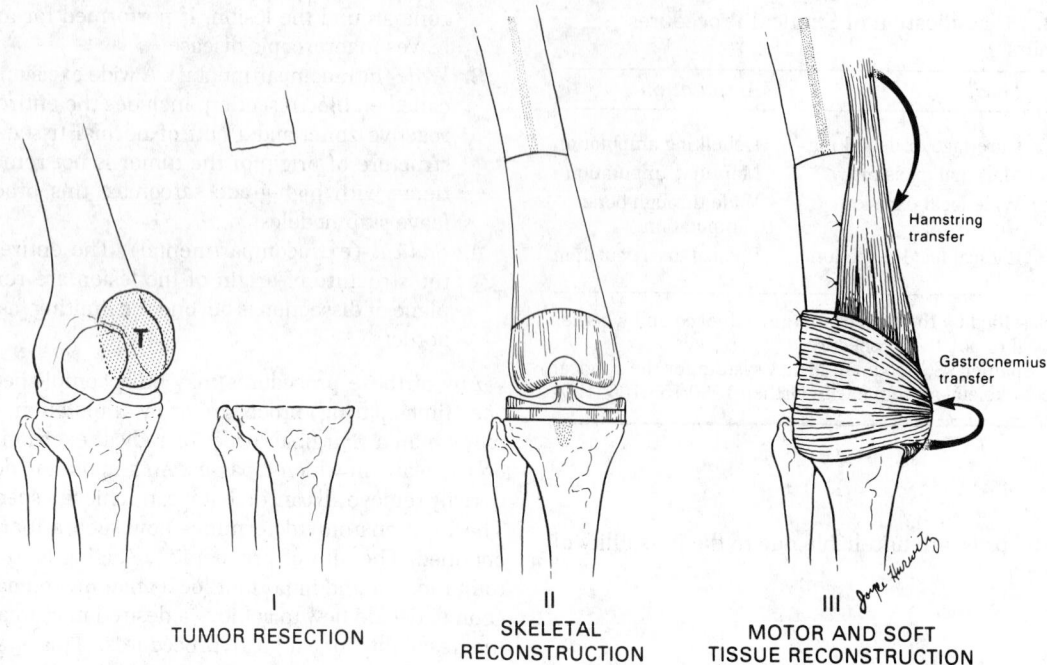

I
TUMOR RESECTION

II
SKELETAL RECONSTRUCTION

III
MOTOR AND SOFT TISSUE RECONSTRUCTION

Hamstring transfer

Gastrocnemius transfer

FIGURE 44–7.   Schematic diagram of the three phases of a limb-sparing procedure.

Successful limb-sparing procedures consist of three surgical phases (Fig. 44–7).[120]

1. *Resection of tumor.* This strictly follows the principles of oncologic surgery. Avoiding local recurrence is the criterion of success and the main determinant of the amount of bone and soft tissue to be removed (Fig. 44–8).
2. *Skeletal reconstruction.* The average skeletal defect after adequate bone tumor resection is 15 to 20 cm. Tech-

niques of reconstruction vary and are independent of the resection, although the degree of resection may favor one technique over the other.

3. *Soft tissue and muscle transfers.* Muscle transfers are performed to cover and close the resection site and to restore motor power. Adequate skin and muscle coverage is mandatory. Distal tissue transfers are not used because of the possibility of contamination.

The surgical guidelines and technique of limb-sparing surgery used by Malawer are summarized[120]:

1. No major neurovascular tumor involvement
2. Wide resection of the affected bone, with a normal muscle cuff in all directions
3. En bloc removal of all previous biopsy sites and all potentially contaminated tissue
4. Resection of bone 3 to 4 cm beyond abnormal uptake, as determined by CT or MRI and bone scan
5. Resection of the adjacent joint and capsule
6. Placement of the tourniquet proximal to the lesion, if possible
7. Adequate motor reconstruction, accomplished by regional muscle transfers
8. Adequate soft tissue coverage

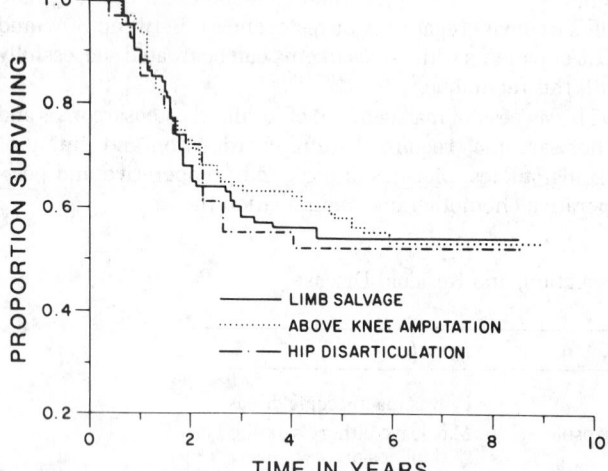

FIGURE 44–8.   Length of survival versus type of operative procedure for 227 patients (pooled data) with high-grade osteosarcoma of the distal femur (Kaplan-Meier analysis). There is no survival difference for patients treated by hip disarticulation, above-knee amputation, or a limb-sparing procedure. (Simon MA, Aschliman MA, Thomas N, et al. Limb-salvage treatment versus amputation for osteosarcoma of the distal end of the femur. J Bone Joint Surg [Am] 1986;68:1331–1337)

Types of Skeletal Reconstruction

Large skeletal defects are reconstructed after tumor resection by several different methods. Osteoarticular defects are most often reconstructed by segmental, custom prostheses that are fixed to the remaining intramedullary bone by PMMA (Fig. 44–9). The newer knee prostheses allow some rotation and flexion and extension, and this mobility decreases the forces on the bone-cement interface and lessens the risk of loosening. There has been interest in combining porous coating to the

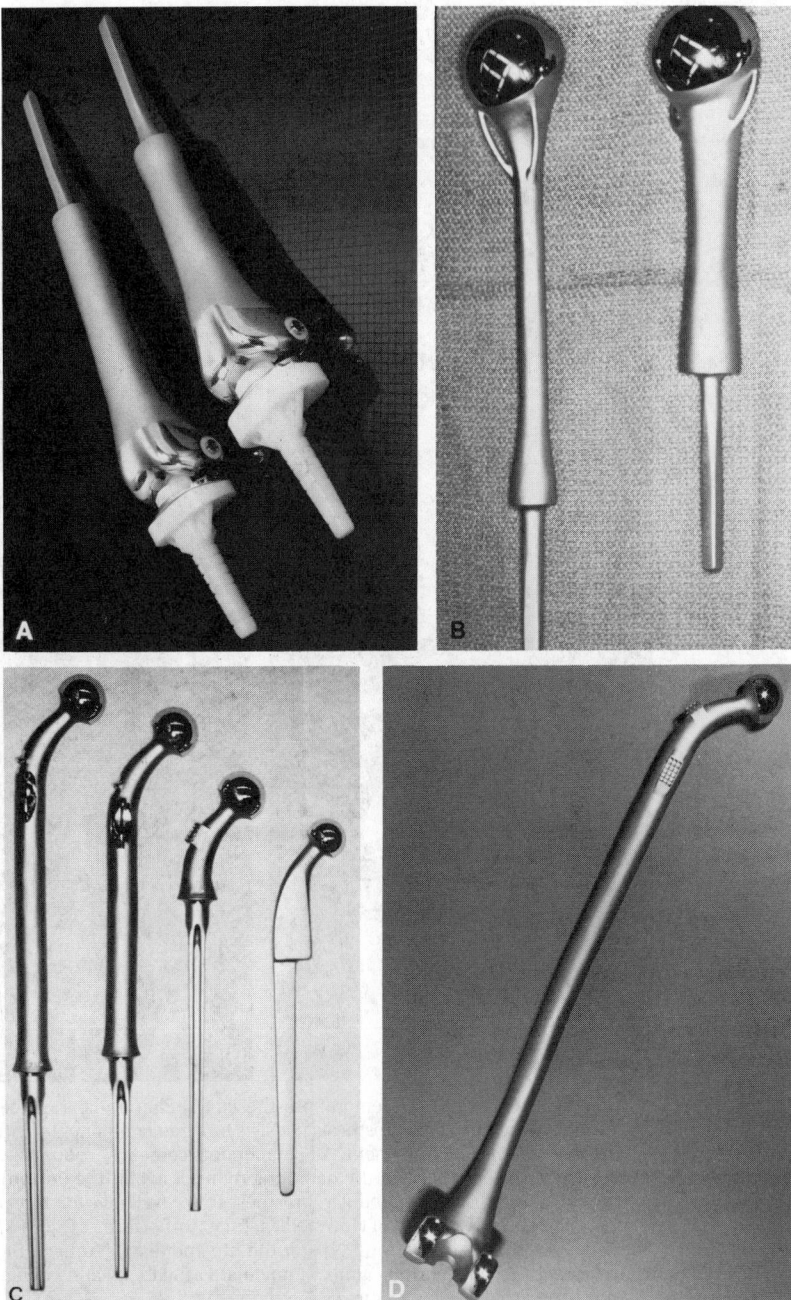

FIGURE 44–9. Prostheses used in selected patients for skeletal reconstruction using limb-sparing procedure. Different lengths are necessary to reconstruct the various resection defects. **(A)** Segmental distal femoral replacements with a total-knee component. **(B)** Segmental proximal humeral replacements. **(C)** Segmental proximal femoral replacements. **(D)** Total femoral replacement.

prosthesis to obtain biologic ingrowth, in the hope of obtaining long-term or permanent fixation.[37,122–124] Titanium, a new alloy with superior metallurgical properties, has been introduced. Most of these devices can be custom made within several weeks. In the hope of eliminating even this delay, modular systems that can be assembled in the operating room are now being evaluated (Fig. 44–10).[37,122] Alternative methods of segmental replacement include large autograft or allograft, used to obtain an arthrodesis, or osteoarticular allografts that may replace the affected joint.[33,122,124,125] Composite allograft (*i.e.,* allograft placed over a prosthesis) has been used. In general, allografts have been used successfully for low-grade sarcomas or giant cell tumors of bone that do not require chemotherapy or radiation therapy.

Contraindications

One contraindication to limb-sparing surgery is major neurovascular involvement. Although vascular grafts may be used, the adjacent nerves are usually at risk, making successful resection less likely. The magnitude of resection in combination with vascular reconstruction is often prohibitive.

Pathologic fractures contraindicate surgery. A fracture through a bone affected by a tumor spreads tumor cells by the hematoma beyond accurately determined limits. The risk of local recurrence increases under such circumstances. If a pathologic fracture heals after neoadjuvant chemotherapy, a limb-salvage procedure may be performed successfully.[125a]

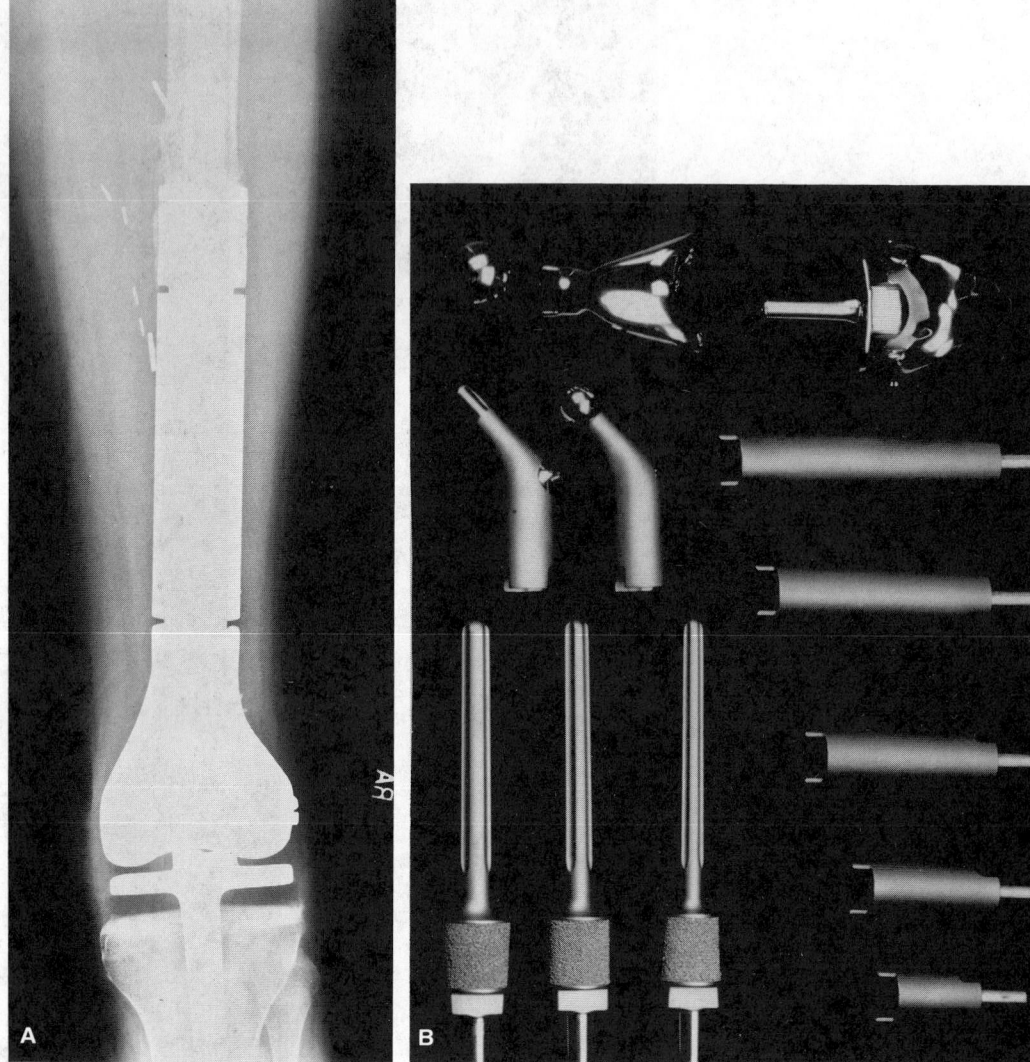

FIGURE 44–10.   Distal femoral prosthesis. **(A)** Plain radiograph of a recently designed modular prosthesis of the distal femur. This prosthesis consists of three components: intramedullary stem, body segment, and a rotating-hinge knee component. All components come in various sizes. This permits immediate construction and use of the prosthesis in the operating room. It avoids the customary 4 to 6 weeks of delay in obtaining a truly custom prosthesis. Modular prostheses are available for the proximal tibia, proximal humerus, and proximal femur. (Courtesy of Howmedica, Inc., Rutherford, NJ). **(B)** Modular Segmental Replacement System (Howmedica, Inc., Rutherford, NJ) for the hip and distal femur. A modular system for large segmental prosthetic replacements permits almost immediate availability and choice of sizes without the need for customization and avoids delays in surgery.

An inappropriate or poorly planned biopsy jeopardizes local tumor control by contaminating normal tissue planes and compartments.

The risk of infection after implantation of a metallic device or allograft in an infected area is prohibitive. Sepsis jeopardizes the effectiveness of adjuvant chemotherapy.

Immature skeletal age contraindicates limb-sparing surgery. The predicted leg-length discrepancy should not be greater than 6 to 8 cm. Expandable prostheses have been used in this situation with success. Upper-extremity reconstruction is independent of skeletal maturity.

There must be enough uninvolved muscle remaining to reconstruct for a functional extremity.

Prognosis

Makley and coworkers reported from the Children's Cancer Study Group in a randomized study of 166 patients the relation of various aspects of surgical management to prognosis for disease-free survival.[125b] They found no advantage to the various aspects of surgical management: interval from first symptom to definitive surgery, interval from biopsy to definitive surgery, surgical sequence, type of surgery, or site of primary tumor.

Evaluation of Limb-Sparing Procedures

A comprehensive and reliable evaluation schema and rating system of limb-sparing procedures have been developed.[126,127]

The system sets forth six primary factors whose specific criteria depend on the unique considerations of six major functional anatomic regions. The primary factors are motion, pain, stability or deformity, strength, emotional acceptance and function, and complications. Extensive analysis using these criteria performed for 1323 patients was presented at the Third International Symposium on limb salvage. The mean follow-up of these patients was 47.8 months. The most common tumors were osteosarcoma, chondrosarcoma, and giant cell tumor; together these account for 70% of all tumors in this group of patients. The functional results are summarized:

1. *Periacetabular pelvic resections.* "Internal hemipelvectomy" had a higher recurrence rate than resection in other anatomic regions. Arthrodesis of the femur to the ilium produced the best results. Prosthetic and allograft reconstruction had an extremely high incidence of complications, especially infection.

2. *Modular versus customized devices.* There were no significant differences in the functional results of modular or customized prostheses. A significant problem with both systems was the lack of soft tissue reattachments.

3. *Resections about the knee.* There were no overall functional differences between arthrodesis, osteoarticular allografts, prosthetic arthroplasty, and rotationplasty. All were better than a prosthetic limb after an above-knee amputation. Each, however, had unique limitations that were not reflected in the overall ratings.

AMPUTATIONS

An amputation provides definitive surgical treatment in patients in whom a limb-sparing resection is not a prudent option. A significant number of patients still require amputation, despite the advent of limb-sparing surgery. Amputations for cancer, compared with those performed for other causes, tend to be at a more proximal anatomic level, to occur in younger people (reflecting the incidence of bone sarcomas), and to be technically more difficult.[128] The resultant psychological and cosmetic losses are more substantial. The amputation experience of the National Cancer Institute (NCI) during the past 30 years has been reviewed; 89% of these procedures were done for sarcomas.[128] Fifty-five percent of the lower-extremity amputations were hip disarticulations or hemipelvectomies. One half of the upper-extremity amputations were interscapulothoracic (*i.e.*, forequarter) resections. Osteosarcoma accounted for one third all amputations. Large lesions around the pelvis or proximal femur usually require amputation, but most sarcomas of the shoulder girdle and knee can now be resected.

CRYOSURGERY

Cryosurgery is the use of liquid nitrogen ($-196°C$) after curettage of a tumor cavity to kill the remaining tumor cells.[115–117,129–132] Necrosis occurs between $-20°C$ and $-40°C$.[128] In general, a double freeze and thaw cycle is required. The aim of this technique is to enhance local tumor control after a careful curettage and avoid resection of the involved bone. Cryosurgery was initially developed by Marcove at Memorial Sloan-Kettering Cancer Center (MSKCC) for the treatment of metastatic bone tumors.[115,117] Marcove ap-

plied this technique to the treatment of aggressive benign tumors, specifically giant cell tumors and to low-grade sarcomas and chordomas.[130–132] The local recurrence rate after cryosurgery for these aggressive benign tumors decreased from 30% to 40% to between 5% and 10%.[115–117] This technique is not used for high-grade sarcomas.

CHEMOTHERAPY FOR BONE SARCOMAS

Before the advent of effective adjuvant chemotherapy, the outlook for patients with osteosarcoma was dismal. Most patients who presented without evidence of metastases and were treated only with surgery ultimately developed metastases and died.[129–133] A review of the literature published in 1972 summarized experience with 1337 patients in 11 studies conducted between 1946 and 1971.[133] Approximately half of the patients developed metastatic disease—usually in the lung—within 6 months after surgery of the primary tumor, and more than 80% developed recurrent disease. Fewer than 20% of the patients survived 5 years. The inescapable conclusion is that 80% of patients presenting without overt metastases had microscopic subclinical metastases at the time of diagnosis. The expectation that fewer than 20% of patients would survive beyond 5 years appeared to be reasonable, and this expectation served as the background for trials of adjuvant chemotherapy conducted in the 1970s and 1980s.

By the late 1970s, the prognosis for patients with osteosarcoma was improving, and this improvement was largely attributed to the beneficial effects of adjuvant chemotherapy. However, investigators from the Mayo Clinic and elsewhere challenged the apparent contribution of adjuvant chemotherapy, reporting that the prognosis of patients treated with or without adjuvant therapy had apparently improved over time.[134–140]

Two randomized, controlled trials were conducted in the mid-1980s by investigators of the Multi-institutional Osteosarcoma Study (MIOS) and investigators from the University of California in Los Angeles (UCLA) to resolve the controversy over the role of adjuvant chemotherapy in osteosarcoma. Both studies included a control group treated only with surgery of the primary tumor and no postsurgical adjuvant chemotherapy. Preliminary and mature results of these studies confirm the favorable impact of adjuvant chemotherapy in the treatment of osteosarcoma.[141–144] Life tables of event-free survival for patients in the control groups of these studies recapitulated the historic experience before 1970.

It is apparent from results of these recent trials that the natural history of osteosarcoma has not changed in the past 20 years; fewer than 20% of patients treated only with surgery of the primary tumor can be expected to survive without relapse. The bleak historic experience that served as the background for many uncontrolled adjuvant trials in the 1970s appears to be equally valid as a control for studies in the 1980s, 1990s, and beyond. Microscopic, subclinical metastatic disease can be presumed to exist in virtually all patients at the time of diagnosis. Although the more favorable results from the Mayo Clinic for patients treated without adjuvant chemotherapy remain unexplained, it is apparent from the MIOS and UCLA studies that the administration of adjuvant chemotherapy has a significant favorable influence on outcome and should be recommended for all patients with osteosarcoma.

ADJUVANT CHEMOTHERAPY

The rationale for adjuvant chemotherapy of osteosarcoma is derived from experimental evidence that microscopic metastatic disease can be eradicated if the treatment is initiated when the total body burden of metastatic tumor is sufficiently low.[145–147]

The strategy of adjuvant chemotherapy after surgical removal of the primary tumor has been applied successfully in the management of other childhood tumors. However, osteosarcoma is a relatively drug-resistant neoplasm, and results of studies of the activity of single agents and drugs in combination against macroscopic osteosarcoma have been disappointing (Table 44–6). Few drugs have produced responses in more than 15% of patients, and most responses are partial. Notable exceptions are the responses observed in trials of doxorubicin (Adriamycin), cisplatin, high-dose methotrexate with leucovorin rescue, and ifosfamide.[148–156] The effectiveness of high-dose methotrexate, however, has not been universally accepted; reported response rates have varied widely, ranging from no response to 80%.[153–155,157,158] The effectiveness of this drug may be dose dependent, because dose escalation has produced responses in patients found previously to be unresponsive to treatment.[159] A steep dose-response re-

TABLE 44–6. Representative Studies and Pooled Data for Single-Agent Chemotherapy Response in Overt, Primary or Metastatic Osteosarcoma

Agent	Responders/ Evaluable Patients	% PR + CR*
Cyclophosphamide	4/28	15
Melphalan	5/32	15
Mitomycin C	3/23	13
Vincristine/vinblastine	0/21	0
Uracil mustard	0/10	0
Hydroxyurea	0/10	0
Procarbazine	0/10	0
DTIC	2/14	14
Doxorubicin	28/109	26
5-Fluorouracil	0/11	0
Cisplatin	8/24	33
Dactinomycin	4/26	15
Methotrexate	0/14	0
High-dose methotrexate plus vincristine and leucovorin		
Every 3 weeks	11/26	42
Every week	9/11	82†
Ifosfamide	6/18	33

* PR, partial response; CR, complete response. CR is less than 10% of total response rate in all major trials.
† May include some patients who concurrently received surgery or coned down irradiation to metastases.
(Adapted with permission from Bode U, Levine AS. The biology and management of osteosarcoma. In: Levine AS, ed. Cancer in the young. New York: Masson Publishing USA, 1982;575–602)

lation may also pertain to doxorubicin.[148,160] The combination of bleomycin, cyclophosphamide, and dactinomycin (BCD regimen) is used, although its effectiveness has been disputed.[161]

Logic dictates that the application of agents inactive against macroscopic osteosarcoma should not influence the natural history of this disease. Experimental evidence, however, suggests that eradication of microscopic metastases is possible, even with drugs that are marginally effective or ineffective against gross macroscopic tumors.[145–147,162] The hopeless prognosis for patients with osteosarcoma encouraged the enthusiastic application of the available agents, singly or in combination, as adjuvant therapy for patients with nonmetastatic osteosarcoma. Results of some of the important adjuvant chemotherapy trials of the 1970s and early 1980s are summarized in Table 44–7.

Concerns have been raised that adjuvant chemotherapy for osteosarcoma may delay but not prevent relapse. However, the results of many of the adjuvant studies reported in Table 44–7, some with follow-up beyond 10 years, suggest that life tables of event-free survival have stable plateaus beyond 4 years and that relapses after 3 years are infrequent. Most patients surviving 3 years without evidence of recurrence are probably cured.

Examination of the results of chemotherapy trials reveals a trend in the direction of improved outcome for patients treated on more intensive chemotherapy regimens. Considering that so few drugs have demonstrable activity against macroscopic osteosarcoma, the results reported in adjuvant trials are remarkable. Approximately 60% to 65% of patients with osteosarcoma treated with modern intensive adjuvant chemotherapy regimens survive without recurrence. The development of adjuvant regimens has been largely empiric, and newer, more intensive regimens have resulted in additional improvements in outcome. Further improvements in results of treatment will probably result from the development of new active agents. The activity of ifosfamide has been demonstrated, and this drug is now incorporated into newer regimens under study with promising preliminary results.[181]

PRESURGICAL CHEMOTHERAPY

Presurgical chemotherapy has been used with increasing frequency during the past decade in the management of osteosarcoma. This strategy evolved concurrently with limb-sparing procedures. Initial attempts at limb salvage at the MSKCC in 1973 involved the fabrication of customized endoprostheses for selected patients undergoing en bloc resection. While the prosthesis was being made (requiring as long as 3 months), chemotherapy was administered to prevent tumor progression.[178] Retrospectively, patients treated with presurgical chemotherapy fared better than did patients treated during the same period with immediate surgery and postoperative adjuvant therapy.[179]

On histologic evaluation, the response in the primary tumor to preoperative chemotherapy was found to be a powerful prognostic factor; unfavorable responders were likely to develop distant metastases despite continued use of chemotherapy with the same agents after surgery.[182] The prognostic significance of tumor response to preoperative chemotherapy has been confirmed in studies conducted by the German So-

TABLE 44–7. Results of Representative Trials of Adjuvant Therapy for Osteosarcoma

Investigations*	Adjuvant Regimen*	No. of Patients	Relapse Free (%)
DFCI[163,164]	HDMTX, VCR (study I)	12	42
NCI[165]	HDMTX, VCR ± BCG†	39	38
CALGB[160,166,167]	ADRIA	88	39
CALGB[168]	ADRIA ± HDMTX†	62	50
DFCI[164]	ADRIA + VCR ± HDMTX (study II)	22	59
DFCI[164,169]	ADRIA + VCR + HDMTX (weekly) (study III)	46	60
CCSG[170]	ADRIA + VCR + (HDMTX vs IDMTX)*	166	38
SWOG[171–173]	COMPADRI I (CTX, VCR, ADRIA, PAM)	43	49
SWOG[172,173]	COMPADRI II (CTX, VCR, ADRIA, PAM, HDMTX)	53	35
SWOG[172,173]	COMPADRI III (CTX, VCR, ADRIA, PAM, HDMTX)	84	38
St. Jude[174]	ADRIA + HDMTX + CTX (OSTEO 72)	26	50
St. Jude[174]	ADRIA + HDMTX + CTX (OSTEO 77)	50	56
Roswell Park[175,176]	ADRIA + CDDP	22	61
Mayo Clinic[140]	HDMTX + VCR vs no adjuvant therapy‡	38	40 (chemotherapy)
			44 (no chemotherapy)
MIOS[141,142]	BCD + HDMTX + ADRIA + CDDP vs no adjuvant therapy§	36 randomized	63 (chemotherapy)
		165 nonrandomized	12 (no chemotherapy)
UCLA[144]	BCD + HDMTX + VCR + ADRIA (+intraarterial ADRIA + XRT) vs no adjuvant therapy§	59	55 (chemotherapy)
			20 (no chemotherapy)
EORTC[139,177]	Whole-lung irradiation vs no adjuvant treatment‖	86	43 (with treatment)
			28 (no treatment)
Mayo Clinic[138]	Whole-lung irradiation (+dactinomycin) vs no adjuvant treatment*	53	40
MSKCC[178–180]	HDMTX + VCR + ADRIA + CTX (T4 + T5 pooled)	52 (<21 years)	48

* HDMTX, high-dose methotrexate (5 g/m² or more) + leucovorin rescue; VCR, vincristine; BCG, bacillus Calmette-Guérin; ADRIA, doxorubicin (Adriamycin); IDMTX, intermediate-dose methotrexate (750 mg/m²) + leucovorin rescue; CTX, cyclophosphamide; PAM, phenylalanine mustard; CDDP, cisplatin; BCD, bleomycin, cyclophosphamide, dactinomycin combination; DFCI, Dana-Farber Cancer Institute; NCI, National Cancer Institute; CALGB, Cancer and Acute Leukemia Group B; CCSG, Children's Cancer Study Group; SWOG, Southwest Oncology Group; MIOS, Multiinstitutional Osteosarcoma Study; UCLA, University of California, Los Angeles; EORTC, European Organization for Research on Treatment of Cancer; MSKCC, Memorial Sloan-Kettering Cancer Center.
† Randomized study; no significant difference in relapse-free survival for patients on each treatment arm of study.
‡ Randomized study; no significant difference in relapse-free survival for patients receiving and not receiving adjuvant HDMTX.
§ Randomized study; difference in results of treatments highly significant ($p < 0.01$).
‖ Randomized study; difference in results of treatments significant at 6% level.

---

ciety for Pediatric Oncology (GPO),[183–185] and in studies from the Instituto Rizzoli,[186] the Children's Cancer Study Group,[187] and the MDACC.[180] Patients at high risk for recurrent disease can be identified early in treatment based on the poor response of the primary tumor to presurgical chemotherapy.

Although the initial impetus for presurgical chemotherapy was limb salvage, several theoretical advantages of presurgical chemotherapy apply to all patients with osteosarcoma (Table 44–8).[179] Because chemotherapy is administered soon after biopsy and diagnosis, treatment of the micrometastases known to be present in most patients can be instituted early. This offers a substantial advantage over the traditional adjuvant approach, in which the administration of systemic chemotherapy is delayed by a month or more for surgery and wound healing. Earlier administration of systemic treatment may reduce the emergence of drug-resistant cells in the micrometastases.[189–190] For the surgeon, presurgical chemotherapy has some advantages, because it allows time for fabrication of a prosthesis and may effect a reduction of bulky tumors, increasing the feasibility of limb-salvage surgery in selected patients.

ASSESSMENT OF TUMOR RESPONSE

Assessment of the response of primary tumors has been based on clinical and radiographic data, but the histologic appearance of the resected tumor specimen after presurgical chemotherapy has emerged as the standard for measuring response.[180,182,187,191] Several systems for grading the effect of preoperative chemotherapy have been proposed, all of which are based on the degree of cellularity and necrosis in the resected specimen. The grading system designed at MSKCC by Huvos has been used widely (Table 44–9).[180,182] Grade III and IV responses, indicating extensive to complete response in the primary tumor, are favorable. Grade I and II responses, indicating minimal destruction of the tumor, are unfavorable

TABLE 44-8. Considerations for Presurgical and Postsurgical Chemotherapy Regimens

Timing of Chemotherapy	Advantages	Disadvantages
Preoperative chemotherapy	Early institution of systemic therapy against micrometastases	High tumor burden (not optimal for first-order kinetics)
	Reduced chance of spontaneous emergence of drug-resistant clones in micrometastases	Increased probability of the selection of drug-resistant cells in primary tumor, which may metastasize
	Reduction in tumor size, increasing the change of limb salvage	Delay in definitive control of bulk disease; increased chance for systemic dissemination
	Provides time for fabrication of customized endoprosthesis	
	Less chance of viable tumor being spread at the time of surgery	Psychological trauma of retaining tumor
	Individual response to chemotherapy allows selection of different risk groups	Risk of local tumor progression with loss of a limb-sparing option
Postsurgical chemotherapy	Radical removal of bulk tumor decreases tumor burden and increases growth rate of residual disease, making S-phase-specific agents more active and optimizing conditions for first-order kinetics	Delay of systemic therapy for micrometastases
		No preoperative in vivo assay of cytotoxic response
	Decreased probability of selecting a drug-resistant clone in the primary tumor	Possible spread of viable tumor by surgical manipulation

(Fig. 44-11). In studies using the Huvos Grading System, patients with a favorable response (grade III or IV) fare extremely well, but those with an unfavorable histologic response to preoperative chemotherapy (grade I or II) are likely to develop distant metastases. An update of data from MSKCC trials suggest that modification of the Huvos system is in order. It is apparent that only grade IV response predicts an excellent outcome; patients with grade II and III responses fare equally, with an intermediate prognosis; and patients demonstrating only minimal response to chemotherapy have the worst outcome.[193] The Huvos grading system has served as a model for other systems for grading tumor response.

The grading system formerly used by the GPO identifies six categories of response.[191] In the COSS-80 study, favorable response was defined as greater than 50% tumor destruction after presurgical chemotherapy, but in GPO studies, 90% destruction is required. The grading system favored by investigators at the MDACC divides response into three categories: no effect or doubtful effect with less than 40% tumor destruction; partial effect with 40% to 60% tumor destruction; and definite effect, in which more than 60% of the tumor is destroyed and fibrovascular regeneration is present.[192] Grading systems are necessarily imprecise and subject to sampling errors. However, with scrupulous attention to adequate sectioning from many sites of the surgical specimen, the degree of response can be reliably and reproducibly assessed.

TABLE 44-9. Histologic Grading of the Effect of Preoperative Chemotherapy on Primary Osteosarcoma

Grade	Effect
I	Little or no effect identified
II	Area of acellular tumor osteoid, necrotic, or fibrotic material attributable to the effect of chemotherapy, with other areas of histologically viable tumor
III	Predominant areas of acellular tumor osteoid, necrotic, or fibrotic material attributable to the effect of chemotherapy with only scattered foci of histologically viable tumor cells identified
IV	No histologic evidence of viable tumor identified within the entire specimen

(Reproduced with permission from Rosen G, et al. Primary osteogenic sarcoma: Eight-year experience with adjuvant chemotherapy. J Cancer Res Clin Oncol [Suppl] 1983;106:55–67)

TAILORING OF CHEMOTHERAPY

One of the most compelling rationales for presurgical chemotherapy is its use as an in vivo drug trial to determine the drug sensitivity of an individual tumor and to customize postoperative chemotherapy. Results of studies from the MSKCC and elsewhere suggest that patients whose tumors are re-

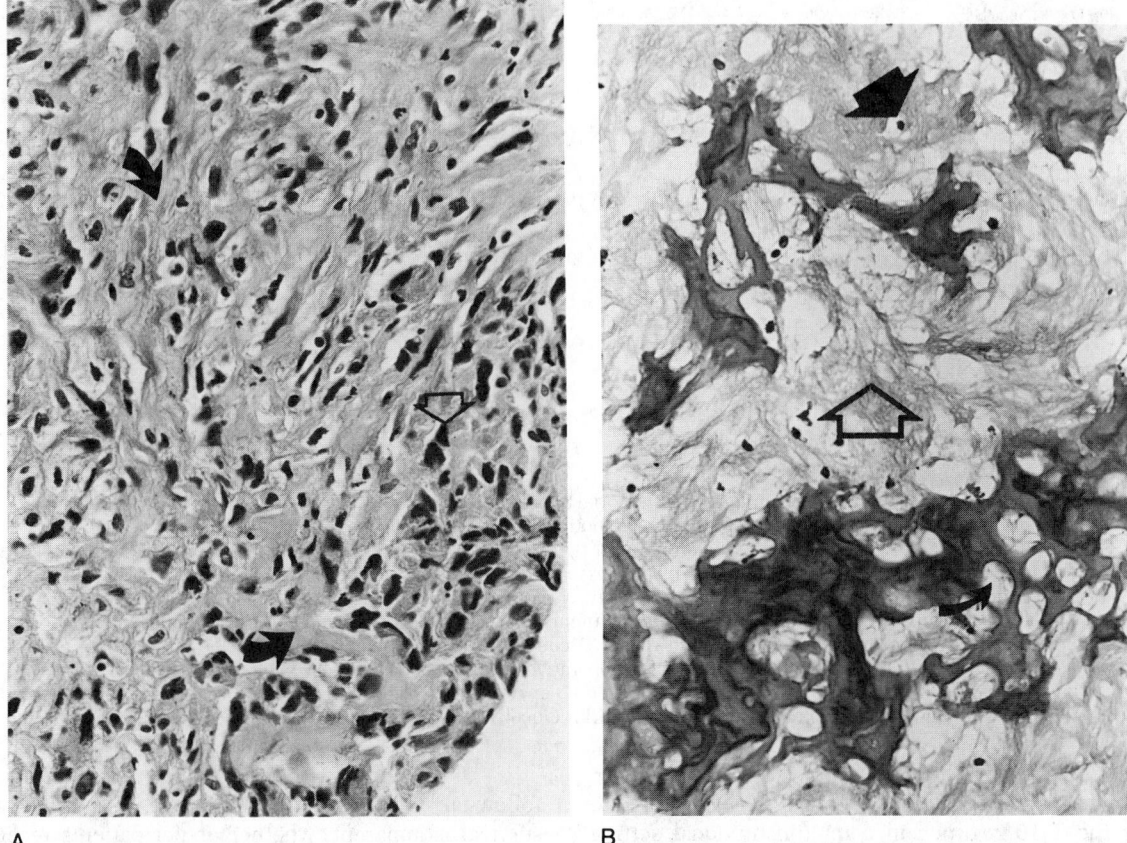

A   B

FIGURE 44–11. Two histologic effects of preoperative chemotherapy. **(A)** The section demonstrates a typical high-grade osteosarcoma (hematoxylin & eosin stain; original magnification ×200). Notice the typical osteoid (*solid curved arrows*) being made by malignant stroma cells (*open arrow*). **(B)** Photomicrograph demonstrating complete tumor cell necrosis. There are no viable cells remaining in this section; the lacunae are empty, and only the extracellular matrix (osteoid and tumor bone) remains. Osteosarcomas may not shrink much despite complete necrosis due to the persistence of their extracellular matrix.

sponsive to presurgical therapy are destined to do well when the same therapy is continued postoperatively. Patients whose tumors are unresponsive to the presurgical regimen have a much less favorable outlook and may benefit from a change in chemotherapeutic agents.

This strategy was pioneered at MSKCC in the T-10 protocol (Fig. 44–12A).[180,194] Patients were treated preoperatively with high-dose methotrexate, the BCD combination, and doxorubicin. Those with favorable (grades III and IV) histologic responses continued to receive the same agents postoperatively (T-10B regimen). Patients demonstrating unfavorable (grades I and II) histologic responses were treated on regimen T-10A, consisting of doxorubicin and cisplatin with the BCD combination (without high-dose methotrexate) postoperatively (Fig. 44–12B). Although only 39% of patients achieved a favorable histologic response to presurgical chemotherapy (51% if only patients younger than 21 were analyzed), virtually all of the favorable responders were projected to survive free of recurrence.[180,194] The patients whose primary tumors demonstrated an unfavorable histologic response were switched to the cisplatin-containing regimen, and almost 85% were initially projected to remain relapse free at 3 years. Overall, in preliminary reports, 90% of patients treated on the T-10 regimen with tailored therapy were projected to remain disease free at 3 years. Moreover, a significant difference in outcome could no longer be detected between favorable and unfavorable responders to presurgical chemotherapy, supporting the contention that poor responders were "salvaged" by the administration of alternative chemotherapy postoperatively. Because of these favorable preliminary results, the T-10 protocol served as a model for many of the osteosarcoma treatment studies launched in the 1980s, virtually all of which featured the use of presurgical chemotherapy and tailoring of treatment based on responsiveness of the primary tumor.

NEOADJUVANT CHEMOTHERAPY

Results reported from representative trials using presurgical chemotherapy are summarized in Table 44–10. Responses in the primary tumor have been variable with favorable responses observed in 30% to 85% of patients. The overall results are excellent, but comparable to adjuvant studies that used regimens of equal intensity without any preoperative chemotherapy (see Table 44–7). The importance of tailoring therapy (*i.e.,* postoperative chemotherapy is individualized based on response of the primary tumor) in this strategy remains to be defined.

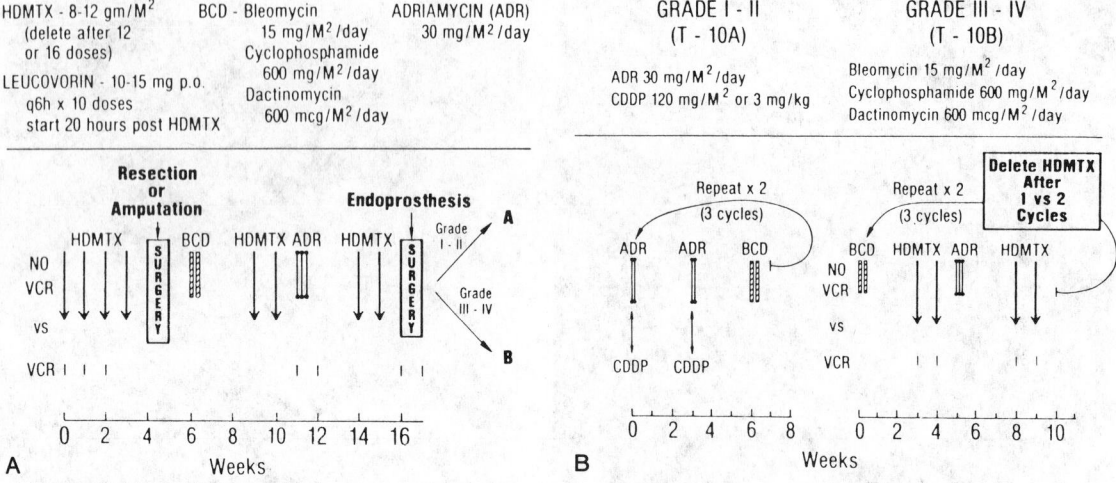

FIGURE 44–12. The T-10 regimen from Memorial Sloan-Kettering Cancer Center. **(A)** All patients receive the initial 16-week regimen. The presurgical chemotherapy regimen features four weekly courses of high-dose methotrexate and leucovorin rescue followed by resection of amputation. Patients undergoing endoprosthetic replacement receive 16 weeks of presurgical chemotherapy. **(B)** Postoperative chemotherapy is determined by the histologic grade of response of the primary tumor to presurgical chemotherapy. Patients achieving an unfavorable response in the primary tumor (grades I and II) receive T-10A regimen postoperatively, featuring doxorubicin, cisplatin, and the BCD combination. Patients achieving a favorable response (grades III and IV) receive the T-10B regimen postoperatively and continue to receive high-dose methotrexate with doxorubicin and the BCD combination. (Rosen G, et al. Primary osteogenic sarcoma: Eight-year experience with adjuvant chemotherapy. J Cancer Res Clin Oncol 1983;106[Suppl]:55–67)

The Children's Cancer Study Group (CCSG) attempted to duplicate the T-10 regimen in a multiinstitutional setting (CCSG 782).[187] Results were not as favorable as those initially reported from MSKCC; only 30% of the patients demonstrated favorable responses in the primary tumor. These patients fared extremely well, with 90% projected to remain disease free at 2 years. The remaining poor-responding patients did not benefit from a change in therapy postoperatively. Overall, 61% of patients in the CCSG study were projected to remain free of recurrent disease at 2 years—a disappointing result compared with the initial results reported from MSKCC.

The COSS-82 trial of the GPO also tested the strategy of tailoring treatment.[185] As in the CCSG trial, results suggest that patients demonstrating poor response of the primary tumor are destined to do poorly and that treatment of poor responders with salvage regimens (as in the T-10 protocol) is inadequate to improve their prognosis. Investigators of the GPO concluded that active agents should not be withheld from the initial therapy of newly diagnosed patients.

At the Instituto Rizzoli overall results have improved over time concurrent with the adoption of the strategy of presurgical chemotherapy.[186,197] However, the Rizzoli investigators conclude that the improvement in prognosis more likely reflects improved effectiveness of the agents used rather than the use of presurgical chemotherapy, because a group of patients treated concurrently at the same institution without the benefits of presurgical chemotherapy fared just as patients treated with presurgical chemotherapy.[197] As in the CCSG and COSS-82 trials, favorable responders in the Rizzoli trial had a better overall outcome; however, change in the postoperative chemotherapy for poor responders did not alter their unfavorable prognosis.

An update of results of the MSKCC studies indicates that the promising preliminary results have eroded with additional follow-up.[193] Moreover, no difference in overall disease-free survival is apparent, whether or not patients received presurgical chemotherapy as part of their management. Although histologic response to preoperative chemotherapy strongly predicted subsequent disease-free survival and overall survival, with longer follow-up, the MSKCC investigators were unable to demonstrate an improvement in disease-free survival for poor responders who received a modification of their postoperative chemotherapy compared with a similar group of patients treated without such tailoring of treatment.[193]

Whether the administration of presurgical chemotherapy (with or without tailoring of treatment based on tumor response) results in an improvement in outcome for patients with chemotherapy remains to be demonstrated conclusively. A study designed to test this question is currently being conducted by the Pediatric Oncology Group.

Although responsiveness of the primary tumor to presurgical chemotherapy is a powerful predictor of outcome, the likelihood that an individual patient will respond favorably cannot be predicted at the time of diagnosis. Because it is apparent that most poor responders relapse and that modifications of postsurgical chemotherapy fail to influence this unfavorable outcome, strategies are needed to predict favorably and poorly responding patients before the initiation of therapy so that more aggressive approaches can be used for poor-prognosis patients earlier in treatment. Analysis of tumor DNA content or expression of a multidrug resistance gene (*MDR*) in primary tumors before therapy may prove to be useful for this purpose.[198]

INTRAARTERIAL CHEMOTHERAPY

Presurgical chemotherapy may be administered directly into the arterial supply of the tumor to maximize drug delivery to

TABLE 44–10. Results of Representative Trials Incorporating Presurgical Chemotherapy for Osteosarcoma

Investigations*	Regimen*	No. of Patients	Relapse Free (%)
MSKCC[179,180,193]	HDMTX + VCR + ADRIA + BCD (T-7)	54 (under 21 years)	74
MSKCC[179,180,194]	HDMTX + VCR + ADRIA + BCD ± CDDP (depending on response) (T-10)	79 (under 21 years)	76
GPO[183,184]	ADRIA + HDMTX + (BCD or CDDP) ± interferon (COSS 80)†	116	68
Mount Sinai[195]	HDMTX + ADRIA + CDDP	25	77
CCSG[187]	HDMTX + VCR + ADRIA + BCD ± CDDP (depending on response) (CCSG-782)	192	61
GPO[185]	HDMTX + ADRIA + CDDP + IFOS (COSS-82)	125	58
EOIS[196]	ADRIA + CDDP ± HDMTX‡	231	63 (−HDMTX) 48 (+HDMTX)
Rizzoli[186]	IA CDDP + (HDMTX vs IDMTX) + ADRIA ± BCD (depending on response)§	127	51% (overall) (58%) (HDMTX) (42%) (IDMTX)
M.D. Anderson[188]	(IA CDDP vs HDMTX) + ADRIA (postoperative therapy determined based on response to preoperative therapy) (TIOS I)	43	60
M.D. Anderson	IA CDDP + ADRIA ± CTX (depending on response) (TIOS III)	24	

* HDMTX, high-dose methotrexate (12 g/m^2 or more) + leucovorin rescue; IDMTX, intermediate-dose methotrexate (750 mg/m^2) + leucovorin rescue; VCR, vincristine; ADRIA, doxorubicin (Adriamycin); BCD, bleomycin, cyclophosphamide, dactinomycin combination; CDDP, cisplatin; IA, intraarterial administration; CTX, cyclophosphamide.
MSKCC, Memorial Sloan-Kettering Cancer Center; GPO, German Society for Pediatric Oncology; CCSG, Children's Cancer Study Group; EOIS, First European Osteosarcoma Intergroup Study; Rizzoli, Instituto Ortopedico Rizzoli; M.D. Anderson, M.D. Anderson Cancer Center.
† Randomized study; no significant difference in relapse-free survival for patients on each treatment arm of study.
‡ Randomized study; favors treatment without HDMTX. (Some patients treated only adjuvantly).
§ Randomized study; difference in results of treatments significant at 7% level.

the tumor vasculature.[186,192,199,200] Doxorubicin and cisplatin have been delivered by prolonged intraarterial infusion to the extremities. Pharmacokinetic studies have shown that intraarterial chemotherapy produces high local drug concentrations.[199] Dramatic responses in the primary tumors have been observed in these patients, facilitating limb-salvage surgery. Significant skin and muscle necrosis, however, can occur as an inadvertent complication of intraarterial infusion.[201] The technique has appropriately been limited to centers with excellent angiographic support facilities.

The rationale for the use of intraarterial therapy is not self-evident for several reasons. Even in the prechemotherapy era, control of the primary tumor in patients with extremity primaries was rarely a problem; it was micrometastatic disease in the lung that ultimately killed the patient. Improvements in the outcome of patients with osteosarcoma have resulted directly from improvements of systemic chemotherapy for micrometastatic disease rather than from better local control measures, although the rate of limb salvage has increased dramatically.

Strategies that improve drug delivery to the primary tumor at the expense of drug delivery to micrometastatic disease are counterintuitive. Most intraarterial regimens use single-agent chemotherapy for the first 2 to 3 months of treatment, but improvements in outcome for patients with osteosarcoma have resulted from the application of multiagent chemotherapy.

There is little evidence to suggest that responses observed from intraarterial administration are superior to those seen with systemic intravenous administration of the same agents. In the COSS-86 study of the GPO, responses observed in primary tumors of patients receiving intraarterial chemotherapy were not superior to responses seen in patients given the same agents intravenously.[202] Nor is it certain that the administration of intraarterial chemotherapy translates into superior overall outcome for patients as determined by improvement in relapse-free survival. An update of studies from the MDACC, where intraarterial chemotherapy was pioneered, indicates that the overall disease-free survival for pediatric patients treated with intraarterial cisplatin, definitive surgery, and postoperative adjuvant chemotherapy is projected to be 60%—a disappointing result from a single-institution trial compared with results achieved in other multiinstitutional trials with or without presurgical or intraarterial chemotherapy (see Tables 44–7 and 44–10).[188]

INFLUENCE OF REGIONAL CHEMOTHERAPY ON THE CHOICE OF SURGICAL PROCEDURE

A relatively new concept in the management of extremity sarcomas is the use of regional chemotherapy employing the intraarterial route (Fig. 44-13).[172,189,190,201,206] To improve the

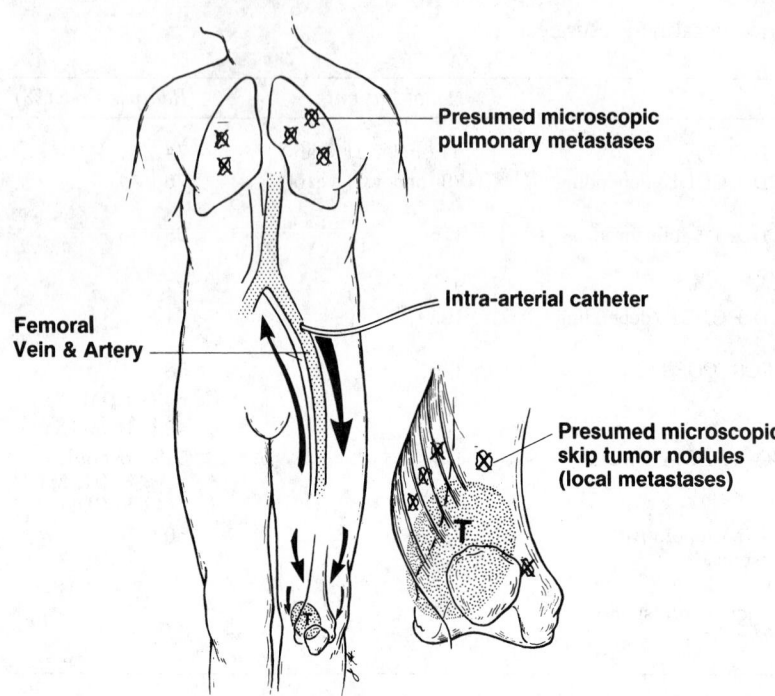

Presumed microscopic pulmonary metastases

Intra-arterial catheter

Femoral Vein & Artery

Presumed microscopic skip tumor nodules (local metastases)

FIGURE 44–13. Postulated mechanism of the regional effect of neoadjuvant chemotherapy. The chemotherapeutic agent is delivered to the tumor at a presumed high dose and then becomes systemic to treat the probable micrometastases in the lungs. (Malawer MM, Buch R, Reaman G, et al. Impact of two cycles of preoperative chemotherapy with intraarterial cisplatin and intravenous doxorubicin on the choice of surgical procedure for high-grade bone sarcomas of the extremities. Clin Orthop Rel Res 1991;270:214–222)

results of preoperative intravenous chemotherapy, further downstage the tumor, and increase the limb-sparing procedure rate, some surgeons and oncologists began using intraarterial chemotherapy preoperatively. Presumably, this allows a higher cytotoxic concentration of chemotherapy to be directed to the primary tumor. Doxorubicin and cisplatin are the two most common drugs evaluated using this technique. A large experience has been reported from UCLA, MDACC, Chil-

dren's Hospital in Washington, and the Rizzoli Institute in Italy.[138,143,155,172,187,189–191,201–206]

Malawer and colleagues reported an 82% conversion rate for patients with extremity osteosarcomas that would have required amputation (14 of 17 patients) before treatment and subsequently obtained a good clinical response to intraarterial chemotherapy, resulting in a limb-sparing procedure being performed (Fig. 44–14).[206a] Only 1 patient deemed initially resectable progressed during the preoperative (intraarterial) phase of treatment. It is the subjective impression of many surgeons that intraarterial chemotherapy results in a higher limb-sparing rate for extremity sarcomas, although no difference in overall survival has been demonstrated. We think that only rarely should a patient be treated by primary amputation without determining the patient's response to preoperative (intraarterial or intravenous) chemotherapy.

AMPUTATION V. LIMB-SPARING SURGERY

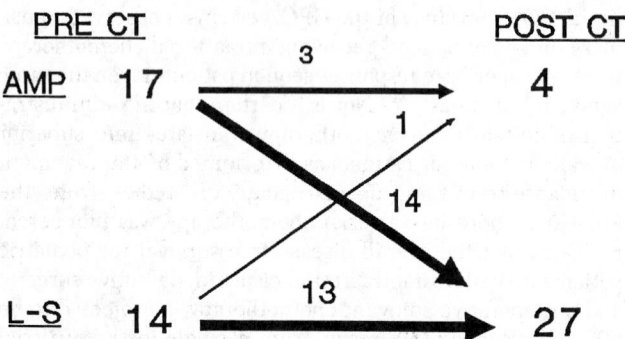

PRE CT — POST CT

AMP 17 → 4
3
1
14
13
L-S 14 → 27

FIGURE 44–14. The impact of neoadjuvant chemotherapy on the choice of surgical procedure: surgical decisions made before receiving chemotherapy (PRE CT) compared with actual surgical procedure performed after induction with intraarterial chemotherapy (POST CT). Initially 17 (55%) of 31 patients would have required an amputation, compared with only 4 (13%) of 31 amputations actually performed (limb salvage rate of 87%). Notice that 14 (82%) of 17 patients were converted from an amputative decision to a limb-sparing procedure. (Malawer MM, Buch R, Reaman G, et al. Impact of two cycles of preoperative chemotherapy with intraarterial cisplatin and intravenous doxorubicin on the choice of surgical procedure for high-grade bone sarcomas of the extremities. Clin Orthop Rel Res 1991;270:214–222)

RADIATION THERAPY FOR BONE TUMORS

In keeping with the multidisciplinary, multimodality approach to the treatment of bone tumors, all patients should be evaluated by a radiation oncologist and by an orthopedic and medical (or pediatric) oncologist before decisions concerning therapy are made. Close communication between members of the care team is crucial. Tumors of the axial skeleton and facial bones are treated by a combination of limited surgery and radiation therapy. Ewing's sarcoma and peripheral primitive neuroectodermal tumors of bone may be managed by definitive radiation treatment, complete surgical excision, or combined surgical and radiation therapy approaches and are discussed elsewhere in this text. In general, radiation therapy is not used in the primary treatment of osteosarcoma. Patients who refuse definitive surgery, require palliation, or have tumors in axial locations may require radiation therapy.

TREATMENT PLANNING

Optimal radiation therapy of bone tumors requires careful planning (Table 44–11). Planning begins with tumor localization and accurate definition of the clinical and radiographic extent of tumor and of all tissue at risk for microscopic involvement. Precise, three-dimensional definition is required. This evaluation is identical to that done for surgical evaluation (see Preoperative Evaluation). These composite studies are used to establish the maximal tumor dimensions.

With the clinical physicist, decisions are made about the optimal choice of irradiation beam (*e.g.,* photon, electron), technique (*e.g.,* external-beam, brachytherapy, intraoperative therapy), beam modifiers (*e.g.,* compensators, wedge filters), and immobilization system. All patients should undergo simulation and be treated with megavoltage therapy units. There is no role for orthovoltage (low kV x-rays) in the management of primary tumors of bone.

Patient immobilization is essential to optimal radiation therapy. The patient should be placed in a comfortable position on the treatment table. The precise patient set-up should be planned using three points for reproducibility.[207] Immobilization devices such as casts, shells, vacuum pillows, and sandbags are frequently necessary.[208] Molding techniques that require a cast of the anatomic site to be treated are generally preferred if treatment fields are complex and the irradiation course is lengthy.

DOSE AND VOLUME CONSIDERATIONS

Large treatment volumes that include the entire clinical and radiographic extent of tumor plus a generous margin for microscopic or subclinical extension of disease are needed. For tumors that tend to spread along the medullary canal (*e.g.,* lymphoma, Ewing's sarcoma), the standard radiation field has included the entire bone, with a boost of radiation to the area of bulky disease. Current protocols suggest that irradiation to an involved field only may be sufficient for children with small round cell bone tumors who have responded to induction chemotherapy. If large fields are needed, it is desirable to use an extended source-to-skin distance to enable the entire radiation field to fit into one portal. If extended distances are not possible and two radiation fields must be abutted, this should be done through areas of microscopic rather than gross disease. Matchlines should be routinely moved every 1000 cGy.

TABLE 44–11. Guidelines for Optimal Radiation Therapy in the Treatment of Bone Sarcomas

---

Tumor localization
Simulation
Patient immobilization
Megavoltage irradiation
High radiation dose
Large treatment fields, with use of shrinking and cone-downed fields
Beam-shaping devices
Beam modifiers—compensators, wedges
Multiple fields treated each day

The irradiated field should encompass at least the same volume of tissue that would be resected plus an allowance of approximately 2 cm for patient movement and dose fall-off at the margin of the field. Extremity fields should be planned with a strip of tissue purposely out of the beam to allow lymphatic and venous return and to decrease morbidity. This nonirradiated strip should overlie the lymphatic drainage, which is located medially in the lower and upper extremities.

Because high doses are often necessary in the treatment of malignant bone tumors, a shrinking field technique is advised. This allows treatment to a large volume of subclinical disease with a moderate radiation dose, while the area of gross tumor is treated to a higher, sterilizing dose.

Additional principles involve the use of multiple beam-shaping devices so that shaped fields can be designed to conform to the individual tumor volume and patient anatomy. Multiple fields should be used to optimize the radiation dosage, and all fields must be treated every day. Beam modifiers, including compensating filters and wedge filters, should be employed to account for individual variations in patient thickness. The use of multiple small radiation fractions per day (*i.e.,* hyperfractionation) may allow the administration of higher tumor doses while simultaneously protecting sensitive nearby normal structures, such as the spinal cord, from the late effects of radiation therapy.

If chemotherapy and radiation therapy are being used, it is important to avoid the concomitant administration of drugs, such as doxorubicin and dactinomycin, that may act as radiosensitizers in normal tissues.

COMPLICATIONS OF IRRADIATION

The complications of irradiation are directly related to treatment dose and volume. Reactions occurring during the early stages of treatment are usually reversible and not of major significance. These include erythema, dry desquamation of the skin, and epilation. More serious late reactions may include fibrosis, contracture, atrophy, impaired growth, secondary fracture, and radiation-induced sarcoma. If pelvic treatment is required, it is important to consider ovarian transposition in young women whenever possible, techniques to move the small bowel out of the pelvis, and avoidance of treating the entire bladder if cyclophosphamide or ifosfamide are also being used. Fibrosis and contracture can be minimized and possibly avoided by embarking on an active physical therapy program during radiation therapy; the program should be continued after irradiation. Whenever possible, the radiologists should avoid treating across a joint space and avoid treating an open epiphysis. The risk of secondary fracture increases if there has been extensive destruction of bone such that remodeling and repair do not reconstitute the affected part. For tumors of weight-bearing bones, partial weight bearing and protective bracing are important until reossification occurs.

IRRADIATION FOR BENIGN BONE TUMORS

Some benign bone tumors are difficult to differentiate from their malignant counterparts. They have a significant rate of local recurrence and may undergo malignant transformation. The oncologist may be called to aid in establishing the correct diagnosis of a benign bone tumor or to treat local recurrence.

In general, benign tumors are managed surgically and are not considered for irradiation. However, specific indications for considering irradiation may include one or multiple recurrences and inability to completely resect.

There are several guidelines to consider in contemplating a course of irradiation for benign disease. Determine the consequences of no treatment and the natural history of the benign disease. Determine the risk-benefit ratio of radiation treatment and other therapies. Consider radiation treatment if surgical approaches have not succeeded in alleviating the condition and if the risk of other therapies is greater than the risk of radiation therapy. Determine the potential long-term risk of radiation treatment; the quality of radiation, dose, volume, time, underlying organs at risk, and any underlying disease. Obtain informed consent.[209]

Several benign tumors that deserve special consideration are discussed in the following sections.

Solitary and Multiple Osteochondromas

Osteochondromas are the most common benign bone tumor. These tumors are characteristically sessile or pedunculated, arising from the cortex of a long tubular bone adjacent to the epiphyseal plate. Osteochondromas are usually solitary, except in patients with multiple hereditary exostosis. Plain radiographs are usually diagnostic, and no additional tests are required. Sessile osteochondromas are difficult to diagnose, especially if they occur in unusual sites such as the distal posterior femur, where they must be differentiated from a parosteal osteosarcoma. Bone scintigraphy and CT scans are helpful in differentiating these two entities.

Osteochondromas "grow" with the person until skeletal maturity is reached. Growth of an osteochondroma during adolescence therefore does not signify malignancy. Pain is not a sign of malignancy in childhood or adolescence, although in adulthood, it is a significant warning sign. Pain in a child may be due to a local bursitis, mechanical irritation of adjacent muscles, or pathologic fracture.

Between 1% and 2% of solitary osteochondromas undergo malignant transformation; patients with multiple hereditary exostosis are at higher risk.[2,4,56,57] Malignant tumors arising from a benign osteochondroma are usually low-grade chondrosarcomas. Proximal osteochondromas are more likely to undergo malignant transformation than distal lesions. Surgical removal is recommended only for symptomatic osteochondromas and for those arising along the axial skeleton and pelvic or shoulder girdle.

Enchondromas

Enchondromas are composed of mature hyaline cartilage that arises within a bone (Fig. 44–15). They may be solitary or multiple (*i.e.*, Ollier's disease) and have been reported in most bones.[3,4] Their biologic potential is often overestimated or underestimated. Pathologic interpretation of cartilage tumors is more difficult than for other bone tumors; it is particularly difficult to differentiate a benign enchondroma from a grade I chondrosarcoma.[10,11,210] Malignant transformations do occur, but the rate is difficult to determine.[211] Lesions of the pelvis, femur, and ribs are generally at higher risk for malignant transformation than lesions at more distal sites.

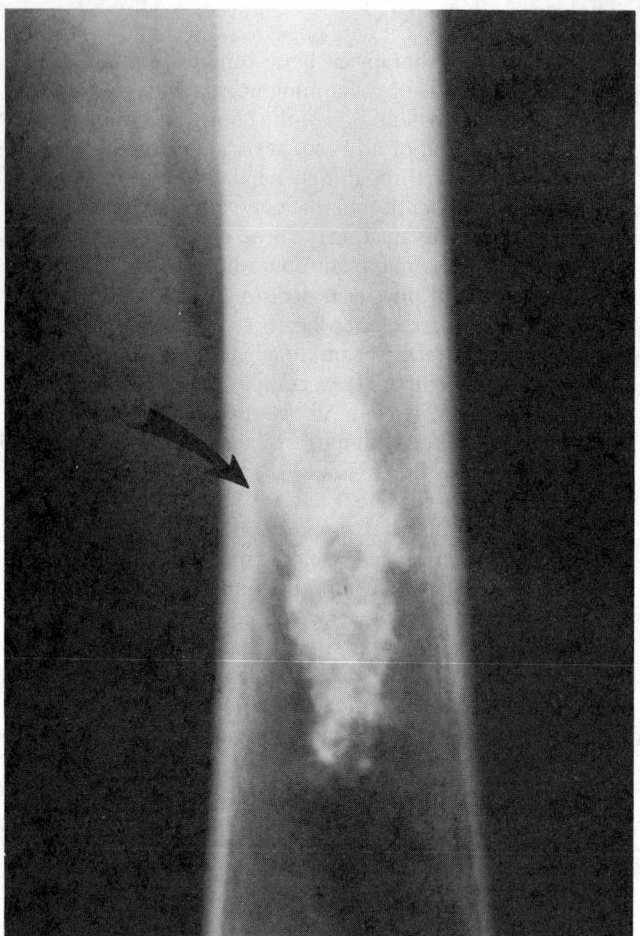

FIGURE 44–15. Enchondroma. Typical enchondroma occurring in the diaphysis of the femur. There is minimal cortical response to the tumor without evidence of bony destruction. Endosteal scalloping (*arrow*) indicates an active lesion. The differentiation from a low-grade intramedullary chondrosarcoma is based on clinical symptoms, histology, and radiographic changes.

Pain is a sign of local aggressiveness and possible malignancy. Enchondromas of the hands and feet are benign, regardless of pathology, but cartilage tumors of the pelvic or shoulder girdle are often malignant, even though the histology appears benign.[3] Plain radiographs may be helpful in this differentiation. Radiographic scalloping is a sign of local aggressiveness. Bone scintigraphy is not helpful in differentiating a low-grade chondrosarcoma from an "active" enchondroma. Patient age is an important indicator of possible malignancy; enchondromas rarely undergo malignant transformation before skeletal maturity. Painful, benign-appearing proximal enchondromas in adults are often malignant, despite their histology. The correlation of symptoms, plain radiographic findings, and histology is crucial.

Chondroblastoma, Osteoblastoma, and Osteoid Osteoma

Chondroblastoma and osteoblastoma are characterized by immature but benign chondroid and osteoid production, respectively. Both may undergo malignant transformation in rare cases.[58,211] Osteoid osteomas are small (<1 cm), painful, bone-forming tumors that are always benign (Fig. 44–16). The oncologist must be aware of these entities and be able to differentiate them from their malignant counterparts, chondrosarcoma and osteosarcoma. Chondroblastomas appear radiographically in the epiphysis of a child; conversely, primary chondrosarcomas are rarely epiphyseal and occur in adults. Although osteoblastomas may be found in any bone, the spine and skull account for 50% of all reported cases. Osteoblastomas must be differentiated from osteosarcomas and osteoid osteoma.

Chondroblastomas and osteoblastomas are considered aggressive, benign lesions with a high recurrence rate after simple curettage.[2-4,211] Local control can be obtained by primary resection; however, routine resection cannot be recommended for tumors adjacent to a joint. Marcove reports a 5% to 10% local recurrence rate if curettage is combined with cryosurgery.[211] This method has avoided the need for resection and extensive reconstruction in selected patients. Osteoid osteomas are treated by simple excision. Because surgical removal is the treatment of choice for these benign bone lesions, the role of radiation therapy is limited. For nonresectable tumors, radiation therapy has been associated with long-term control, but most radiation oncologists do not believe irradiation plays a role in the management of these conditions.[209]

Aneurysmal Bone Cyst

Aneurysmal bone cysts (ABCs) are benign tumors of childhood, occurring typically before skeletal maturity.[2-4] They never become malignant. ABCs often involve the metaphyseal regions of the long bones or the vertebrae. Radiographically, ABCs are eccentric, lytic, and expansile, characterized by cortical destruction and periosteal elevation (see Fig. 44–16). ABCs can grow rapidly and appear extremely aggressive. Differentiation from a primary malignancy may be difficult. Differential diagnosis includes giant cell tumor and telangiectatic osteosarcoma. ABCs may contain some osteoid, but careful examination reveals this to be reactive and not neoplastic. Approximately one third of ABCs arise in conjunction with another (underlying) bony neoplasm.[211,214] The classic treatment is simple curettage and bone graft, which has a recurrence rate of 20% to 35%.[4] Wide curettage may decrease the recurrence rate to approximately 10%. Marcove recommends curettage and cryosurgery as the primary treatment. Radiation therapy is recommended in surgically inaccessible sites.[3,214,215] Megavoltage doses of 2500 to 3000 cGy in 18 to 24 days have been associated with a decrease in local recurrence from 32% to 8% and are generally recommended.[180,181,209,214,215]

Desmoplastic Fibroma

Desmoplastic fibroma is an extremely rare bone tumor; only 50 cases have been reported.[211] It is characterized by abundant collagen formation and a fibrous stroma without evidence of mitosis or pleomorphism. It presents radiographically as an osteolytic lesion with well-defined margins. The basic differential diagnosis is primary fibrosarcoma of bone. Treatment is en bloc resection; curettage has a significant rate of local recurrence.

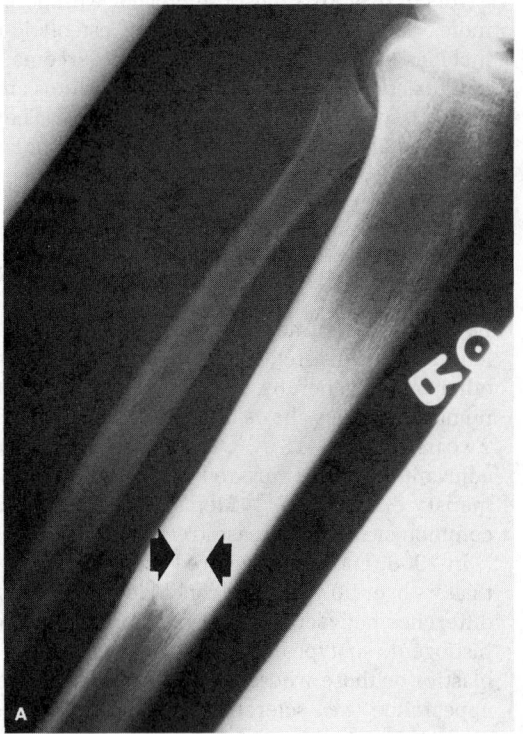 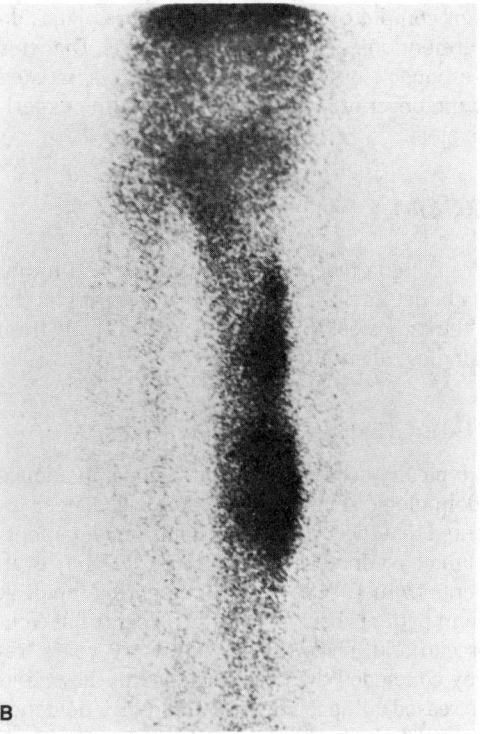

FIGURE 44–16. Osteoid osteoma. **(A)** Osteoid osteomas are characteristically a small lesion, represented radiographically as a small radiolucent nidus between 1 and 10 mm in diameter (*arrow*) surrounded by a large amount of reactive, nonneoplastic sclerotic bone. Tomograms are often necessary to demonstrate the nidus. **(B)** Bone scans will always demonstrate marked uptake that corresponds with the nidus and the reactive bone. The main radiologic differential is a sclerosing osteosarcoma.

Histiocytosis X

Langerhans' cell histiocytosis is a more descriptive and currently accepted term to describe the disease commonly referred to as histiocytosis X. The solitary or multifocal osseous lesions (Greenberger stage IA and IB) were formerly referred to as eosinophilic granuloma.[217] Histiocytosis X can be difficult to diagnose and may mimic radiographically a primary bone malignancy.

Almost any bone can be involved. Radiographically, it appears as a lytic, destructive defect, with poorly defined margins. Periosteal elevation occurs in half of all cases. This combination of characteristics strongly resembles that of Ewing's sarcoma or osteomyelitis. If arising in a flat bone, specifically the pelvis, there may be a large soft tissue component. Solitary lesions are treated by curettage.

The indications for radiation therapy include lesions of the mandible, gingiva and maxilla, where loose or painful teeth cause symptoms or reluctance to eat; lesions of weight-bearing bone at risk of fracture (*e.g.*, lytic lesion of femoral head, where curettage is not appropriate); local recurrence after surgery; local lesions showing no clinical or radiographic signs of healing after curettage or excision; expansile lesions producing symptoms or compromise of critical structures (*e.g.*, spinal cord compression or pressure on the ocular globe or optic nerve); lesions producing cosmetic deformity (*e.g.*, facial, orbital, or skull bones); painful lesions despite chemotherapy; and diabetes insipidus. Low radiation doses in the range of 600 to 1000 cGy are generally recommended and produce complete responses in approximately 90% of sites irradiated.[215-222] Local recurrences have been reported after 450 cGy, but they are rare after 600 cGy.[217] Vertebral lesions causing partial or complete collapse (*e.g.*, vertebra plana) do not require treatment unless they are symptomatic. Diabetes insipidus may respond to local irradiation if therapy is initiated promptly after the onset of symptoms, although this experience is not universal.[218,219]

OSTEOSARCOMA

Osteosarcoma is a high-grade, malignant spindle cell tumor arising within a bone. Its differentiating characteristic is the production of "tumor" osteoid or immature bone directly from a malignant spindle cell stroma.[2,3,59,220]

CLINICAL CHARACTERISTICS

Osteosarcoma typically occurs during childhood and adolescence. An epidemiologic study from the Swedish Cancer Institute documented that the mean and median ages of patients with osteosarcoma have increased since 1971.[220a] They evaluated 227 patients from 1971 to 1984 and reported the peak incidence to be in patients between 10 to 19 years of age but observed the mean and median to be 29 and 20 years, respectively. They concluded the true incidence in the age of patients had increased, although the overall annual incidence of 2.1 cases per million had not changed. When osteosarcoma occurs in patients older than 40 years, it is usually associated with a preexistent condition, such as Paget's disease, irradiated bones, multiple hereditary exostosis, or polyostotic fibrous dysplasia.[2,220-224] Bones of the knee joint and the proximal humerus are the most common sites, accounting for 50% and 25%, respectively, of all osteosarcomas.[211] Approximately 80% to 90% of osteosarcoma occur in the long tubular bones.[2,4,56,221,226-228] The axial skeleton is rarely affected. Less than 1% are found in the hands and feet.[2]

With the exception of serum alkaline phosphatase levels, which are elevated in 45% to 50% of patients, laboratory findings are usually not helpful.[226] Elevated alkaline phosphatase is not diagnostic, because it is also associated with other skeletal diseases. Pain is the most common complaint. Physical examination demonstrates a firm, soft tissue mass fixed to the underlying bone with slight tenderness. There is no effusion in the adjacent joint, and motion is normal. Incidence of pathologic fracture is less than 1%. Systemic symptoms are rare.

RADIOGRAPHIC CHARACTERISTICS

Typical radiographic findings are increased intramedullary radiodensity due to tumor bone or calcified cartilage, an area of radiolucency due to nonossified tumor, a pattern of permeative destruction with poorly defined borders, cortical destruction, periosteal elevation, and extraosseous extension with soft tissue ossification.[226-228] This combination of characteristics is not seen in other lesions. Wilner classified 600 radiographs of osteosarcoma seen at MSKCC into three broad categories: sclerotic osteosarcoma (32%), osteolytic (22%), and mixed (46%) (Fig. 44–17).[228] Although there was no statistically significant difference among overall survival rates among these types, the patterns are important to recognize. The sclerotic and mixed type offer few diagnostic problems. Errors of diagnosis most often occur with pure osteolytic tumors. The differential diagnosis of osteolytic osteosarcoma includes giant cell tumor, ABC, fibrosarcoma, and MFH.[229] In a series of 305 osteosarcomas, De Santos and Edeiken reported that 42 (13.5%) were purely lytic. They usually presented as ill-defined lesions with moderate or large soft tissue components. Nine of the lesions had benign radiographic features.

CLINICAL AND PROGNOSTIC CONSIDERATIONS

Before the era of adjuvant chemotherapy, treatment of osteosarcoma consisted of amputation. Metastasis to lungs and other bones generally occurred within 24 months. A large number of series shows an overall survival of 5% to 20% at 2 years (Fig. 44–18).[71-74] This pattern has been altered by adjuvant chemotherapy and aggressive thoracotomy for pulmonary disease.[45,101,230] Metastases may now appear at less common sites, and disease-free intervals are longer.[230]

In 1968, Lockshin reviewed the experience of 100 investigators over 50 years and concluded there was no significant difference between survival rates of patients with the three histiogenic subtypes (*i.e.*, osteoblastic, chondroblastic, fibroblastic) or those whose lesions had a different radiographic appearance (*i.e.*, sclerotic, osteolytic, or mixed).[231] Size of tumor, patient age, and degree of malignancy did not correlate with survival.[231] The most significant variable was anatomic site. Patients with pelvic and axial lesions had a lower survival rate than those with tumors of the extremities, probably due to surgical inaccessibility and incomplete removal. Patients

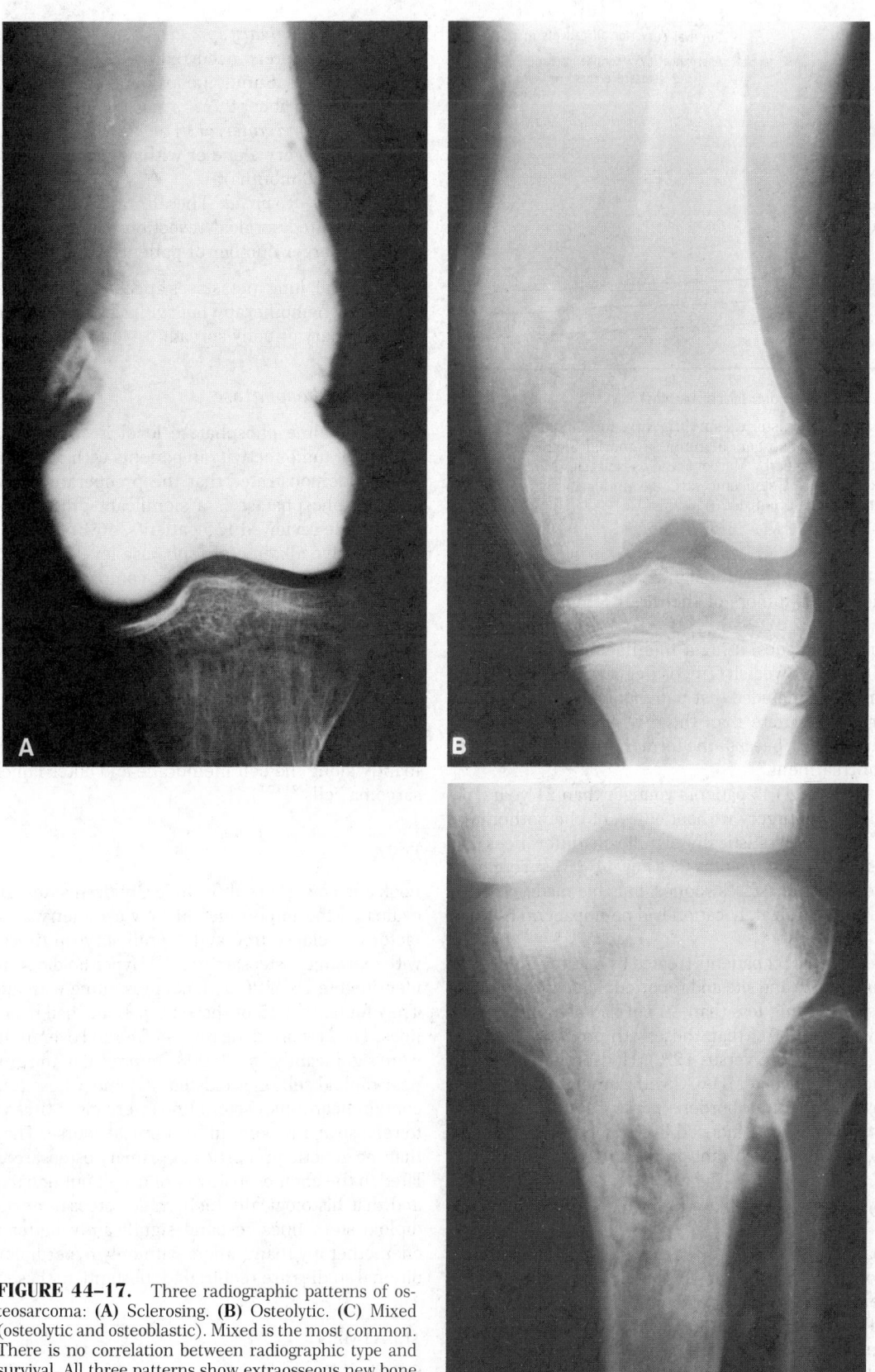

FIGURE 44–17. Three radiographic patterns of osteosarcoma: **(A)** Sclerosing. **(B)** Osteolytic. **(C)** Mixed (osteolytic and osteoblastic). Mixed is the most common. There is no correlation between radiographic type and survival. All three patterns show extraosseous new bone formation. This is pathogenomic of a bone-forming neoplasm.

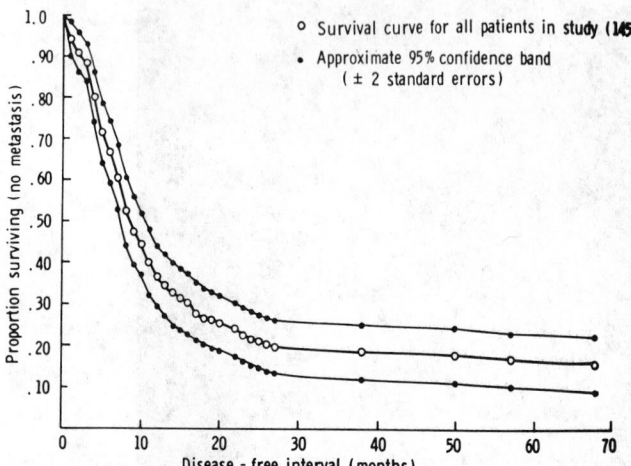

FIGURE 44–18.   The historical survival curve for 145 patients with osteosarcoma treated by surgery alone at Memorial-Sloan Kettering Cancer Center, as reported by Marcove and associates. (Marcove RC, Mick V, Hajek JV, et al. Osteogenic sarcoma under the age of 21. J Bone Joint Surg [Am] 1966;48:1–26)

with tumors of the tibia had a significantly higher survival rate than those with tumors of the distal femur (35% versus 16%).

Larsson and colleagues, using a multifactorial analysis of all patients from the Swedish Cancer Registry between 1958 to 1968, similarly concluded that patients with tibial lesions had a better survival rate than those with femoral lesions (38.1% versus 15.1%), because the former were less advanced at the time of treatment.[232]

Marcove, reviewing 145 patients younger than 21 years of age who underwent surgery without adjuvant chemotherapy at MSKCC, found no statistically significant differences in race, sex, or duration of symptoms (see Fig. 44–18).[71] Younger patients developed metastases sooner, but this made no difference in overall survival. Location had no impact on 5-year survival.

Brostrom evaluated 52 patients treated by surgery alone.[233] He studied tumor size and site and reported that patients with distal lesions measuring less than 10 cm had a significantly higher survival ($p < 0.01$) than those with proximal lesions greater than 10 cm (43% versus 12%). Hudson, after evaluating 98 patients treated at MDACC with three different protocols, reported that tumor burden ($p = 0.04$) and the percentage of tumor necrosis induced by induction therapy ($p = 0.01$) were the most important prognostic factors.[233a]

Changing Pattern of Metastasis

The classic pattern and time frame of metastatic dissemination of osteosarcoma has been somewhat modified by the use of adjuvant chemotherapy and thoracotomy. Bacci and coworkers evaluated the pattern of metastatic spread of osteosarcoma in 193 patients at the Rizzoli Orthopaedic Institute.[234] Thirty patients treated with surgery alone were compared with 163 patients treated with adjuvant chemotherapy:

1. *Site of initial relapse.* No difference was found in sites of first relapse; approximately 90% of cases in both groups occurred in the lungs.

2. *Extrapulmonary spread.* After chemotherapy, extrapulmonary spread occurred in 10% of patients, usually in bony sites. Simultaneous bone and lung metastases occurred in about 2%.
3. *Disease-free interval.* The time to metastases differed with surgery alone or with adjuvant chemotherapy (13 versus 8 months).
4. *Pattern of spread.* The alteration of metastatic spread permitted surgical resection of pulmonary metastases in a larger number of patients (51% versus 29%).

In general, lung metastases appear later and are fewer after adjuvant chemotherapy but with variable difference on extrapulmonary or bony spread.

Alkaline Phosphatase

Serum alkaline phosphatase level is an important biologic marker of tumor activity in patients with osteosarcoma.[235,236] Francis demonstrated that the preoperative serum level of alkaline phosphatase is a significant prognosticator of survival.[226] He reviewed 155 patients, 46% of whom had normal preoperative alkaline phosphatase levels. Of the 2-year survivors, 85% had normal levels, compared with 12% of those dying of disease. Of the 10-year survivors, 93% had normal alkaline phosphatase levels. Scranton and coworkers found similar findings; 16 (42%) of 38 patients had elevated alkaline phosphatase levels before definitive surgery; 12 (54%) of 22 patients with normal levels survived, but only 3 (18.7%) of 16 of those with elevated levels survived.[237] Electromicroscopy has demonstrated that alkaline phosphatase is found predominantly along the cell membrane and outer lamella of osteosarcoma cells.[235,236]

DNA

Look and coworkers at St. Jude Children's Research Hospital evaluated the importance of flow cytometry as a prognostic factor on relapse-free and overall survival times in patients with extremity osteosarcoma.[238] Hyperdiploid stem lines were identified in 25 of 26 patients presenting without metastasis. They found that 15 of these 26 patients had near-diploid cell lines. They reported the relapse-free and overall survival times were significantly ($p < 0.003$) improved in the group in which near-diploid cell lines existed. Patients whose tumors did not contain near-diploid stem lines were eight times more likely to relapse at any point in the clinical course. They concluded that the genetic properties of primary osteosarcoma were related to the chemosensitivity of occult pulmonary metastases and that histologically high-grade osteosarcomas with near-diploid stem lines respond significantly better to adjuvant chemotherapy than tumors with only hyperdiploid lines. Additional studies are required to substantiate these findings.[238a]

TREATMENT

Surgical Resection of Localized Extremity Osteosarcoma

The traditional procedure for localized osteosarcoma has been amputation one joint above the tumor-containing bone or, occasionally, transmedullary amputation.[2,3,71–73] Within the past decade, parallel developments in radiology, orthopedics, and oncology have made nonamputative procedures an option for 50% to 80% of patients.[20-33] A significant impetus for these developments was the introduction of effective chemotherapeutic agents in the early 1970s.[47-52]

Springfield and coworkers from the University of Florida compared limb-sparing surgery with amputation in 53 patients with stage IIB osteosarcoma.[239] For ethical reasons, the patients were not randomized. There was no difference in survival between amputation and resection or between radical or wide surgical margins. There were three local recurrences. They recommended a wide surgical resection for adequate local control. They recommended amputation if the major neurovascular bundle was involved. They concluded that local recurrence was due to an extremely aggressive tumor or to skip metastases. The unique features of evaluation, management, and resection of tumors are described in the following sections.

SHOULDER GIRDLE. A surgical classification of shoulder girdle resections is shown schematically in Fig. 44–19.[241,242] This classification is useful for all limb-sparing procedures of the shoulder girdle. It is recommended that osteosarcomas arising from the proximal humerus be treated by a type VB

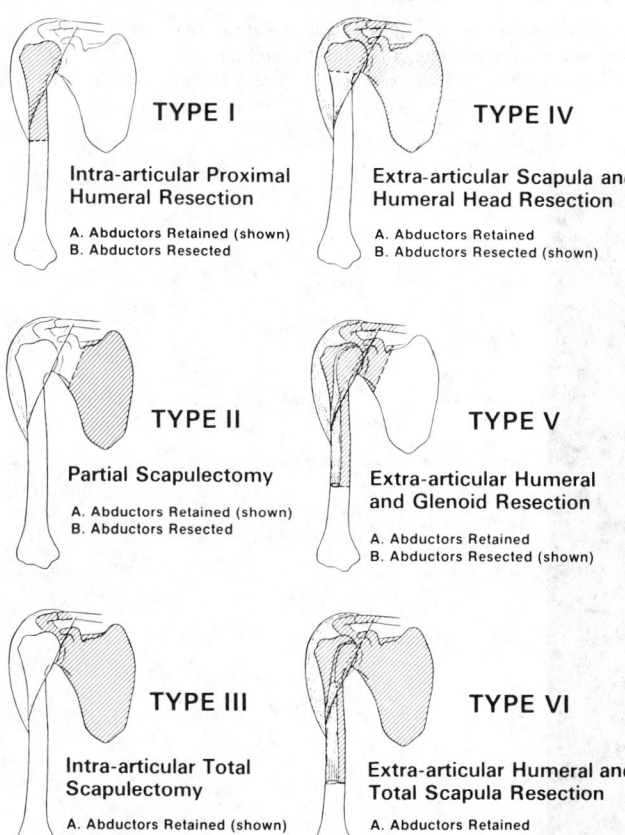

TYPE I

Intra-articular Proximal Humeral Resection

A. Abductors Retained (shown)
B. Abductors Resected

TYPE II

Partial Scapulectomy

A. Abductors Retained (shown)
B. Abductors Resected

TYPE III

Intra-articular Total Scapulectomy

A. Abductors Retained (shown)
B. Abductors Resected

TYPE IV

Extra-articular Scapula and Humeral Head Resection

A. Abductors Retained
B. Abductors Resected (shown)

TYPE V

Extra-articular Humeral and Glenoid Resection

A. Abductors Retained
B. Abductors Resected (shown)

TYPE VI

Extra-articular Humeral and Total Scapula Resection

A. Abductors Retained
B. Abductors Resected (shown)

FIGURE 44–19. Schematic of proposed surgical classification of shoulder girdle resections. In general, types I–III are for benign or low-grade tumors, and types IV–VI are for high-grade tumors. A and B denote the status of the abductor mechanism: A, intact; B, partially or completely excised. Types I–III and types IV–VI are intraarticular and extraarticular resections, respectively.

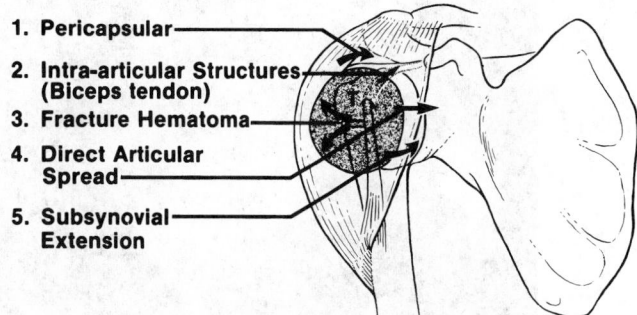

1. **Pericapsular**
2. **Intra-articular Structures** (Biceps tendon)
3. **Fracture Hematoma**
4. **Direct Articular Spread**
5. **Subsynovial Extension**

FIGURE 44–20. Mechanisms of local tumor spread for sarcomas of the shoulder. (Malawer MM, Buch R, Reaman G, et al. Impact of two cycles of preoperative chemotherapy with intraarterial cisplatin and intravenous doxorubicin on the choice of surgical procedure for high-grade bone sarcomas of the extremities. Clin Orthop Rel Res 1991;270:214–222)

resection (see Fig. 44–19). Figure 44–20 illustrates the types of local spread for a sarcoma involving the shoulder joint.

PROXIMAL HUMERUS. Adequate resection of the proximal humerus requires removal of 15 to 20 cm of the humerus and shoulder joint with the deltoid, rotator cuff, and portions of the biceps and triceps muscles (Figs. 44–21 and 44–22).[240] The procedure involves suspension of the arm, motor reconstruction, and provision of adequate soft tissue coverage (Fig. 44–23).

Proximal humeral lesions should not be biopsied through the deltopectoral interval, because this contaminates the subscapularis and pectoralis muscles and the area adjacent to the axillary sheath. Biopsy under fluoroscopy through the anterior third of the deltoid by a trocar is preferred. Angiography is the most useful preoperative study. If the neurovascular bundle is clear of tumor, resection is feasible. All other structures can be removed. The major contraindications to local resection are tumor involvement of the lymph nodes or chest wall, pathologic fracture, or massive soft tissue contamination.

Resectability is determined by early exploration of the neurovascular structures by division of the pectoralis major. This approach does not jeopardize formation of an anterior flap in patients who require forequarter amputation. Preservation of the musculocutaneous nerve is important. The short biceps muscle, responsible for elbow flexion, is the most important muscle left after resection. Extraarticular resection of the glenohumeral joint by medial scapulosteotomy is safer than intraarticular resection.

A custom prosthesis is used for reconstruction. Soft tissue reconstruction and suspension are essential to avoid postoperative pain, instability, and fatigability (see Fig. 44–23). Suspension by Dacron tape and muscle transfers are effective. Hand and wrist functions are normal after resection. Shoulder motion is minimal but stable, and scapulothoracic motion provides some internal and external rotation. Cosmesis is acceptable and can be enhanced with use of a shoulder pad.

DISTAL FEMUR. Adequate en bloc resection includes 15 to 20 cm of the distal femur and proximal tibia and portions of the adjacent quadriceps (Fig. 44–24).[120] Biplane angiography is crucial to determine popliteal vessel involvement.

(text continues on page 1542)

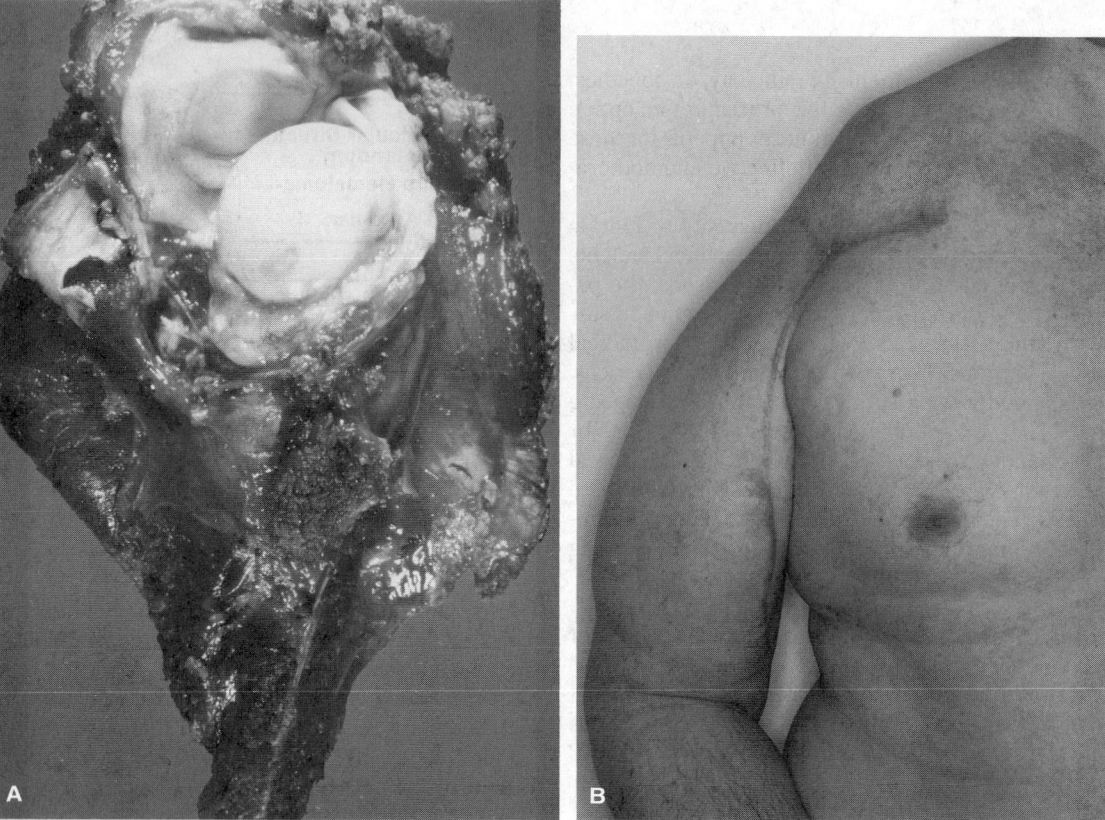

FIGURE 44–21. Osteosarcoma of the proximal humerus treated by a type V shoulder-girdle resection. **(A)** Gross specimen demonstrates the glenohumeral joint. This resection was extraarticular due to the high risk of tumor involvement of the joint. **(B)** Clinical appearance 2 years after surgery. The patient has a stable shoulder with normal elbow and hand function.

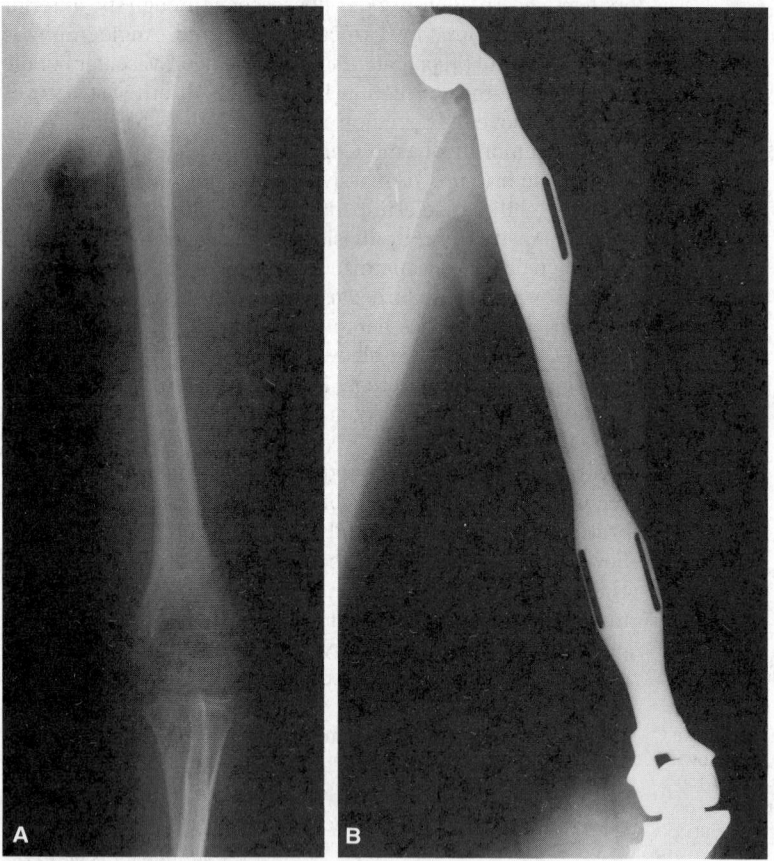

FIGURE 44–22. Osteosarcoma involving the entire humeral shaft, determined by bone scan and MRI. **(A)** Plain radiograph before chemotherapy. **(B)** This patient was treated by a custom total humeral resection and reconstruction by a custom total humeral prosthesis, including a hinge-elbow joint, showing the advancements made in design and manufacture of a custom prosthesis.

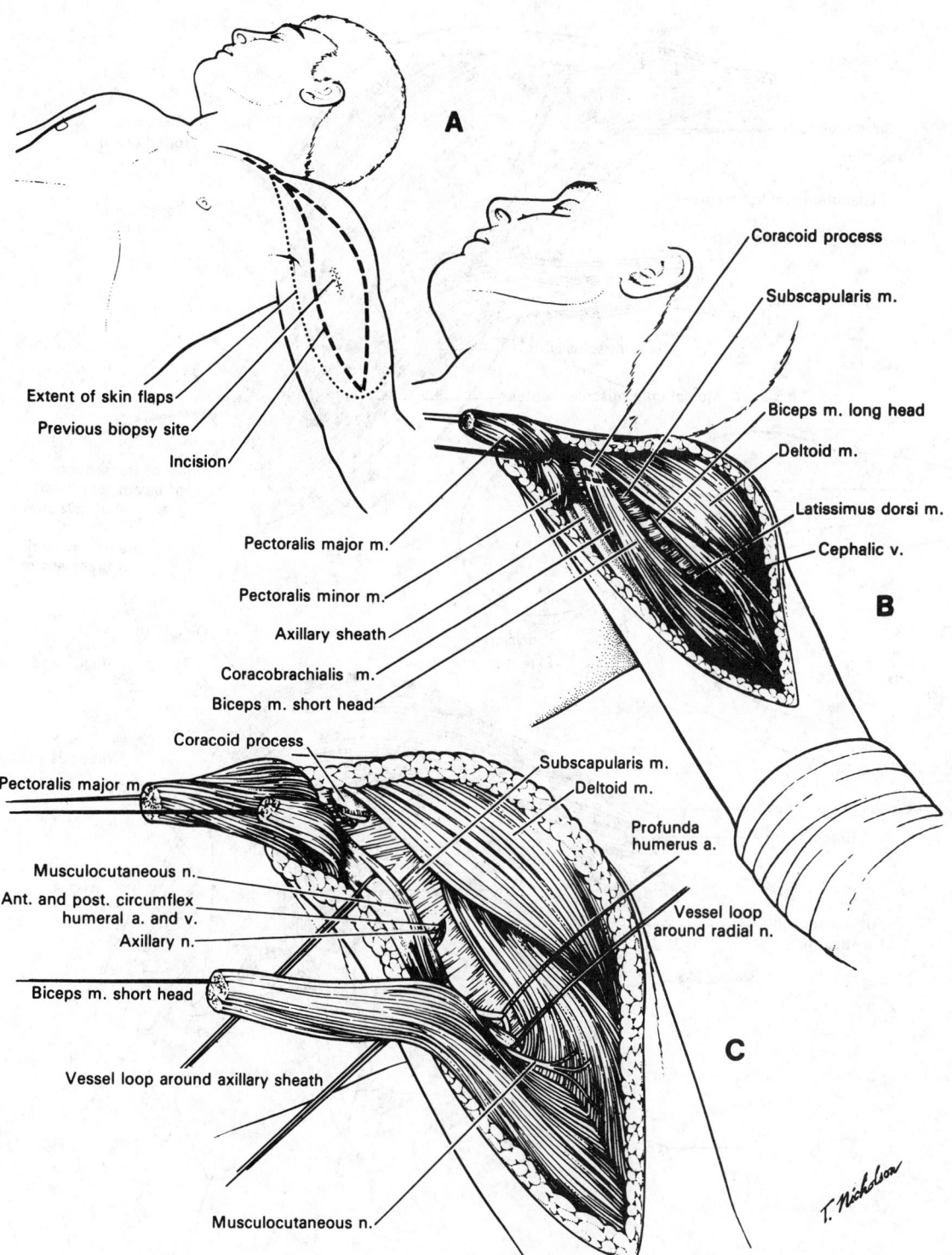

A

Extent of skin flaps
Previous biopsy site
Incision

Coracoid process
Subscapularis m.

Biceps m. long head
Deltoid m.
Latissimus dorsi m.
Cephalic v.

B

Pectoralis major m.
Pectoralis minor m.
Axillary sheath
Coracobrachialis m.
Biceps m. short head
Coracoid process
Pectoralis major m.

Subscapularis m.
Deltoid m.
Profunda humerus a.

Musculocutaneous n.
Ant. and post. circumflex humeral a. and v.
Axillary n.
Biceps m. short head

Vessel loop around radial n.

Vessel loop around axillary sheath

C

Musculocutaneous n.

T. Nicholson

FIGURE 44–23.   Technique of shoulder girdle resection for high-grade sarcomas of the proximal humerus.

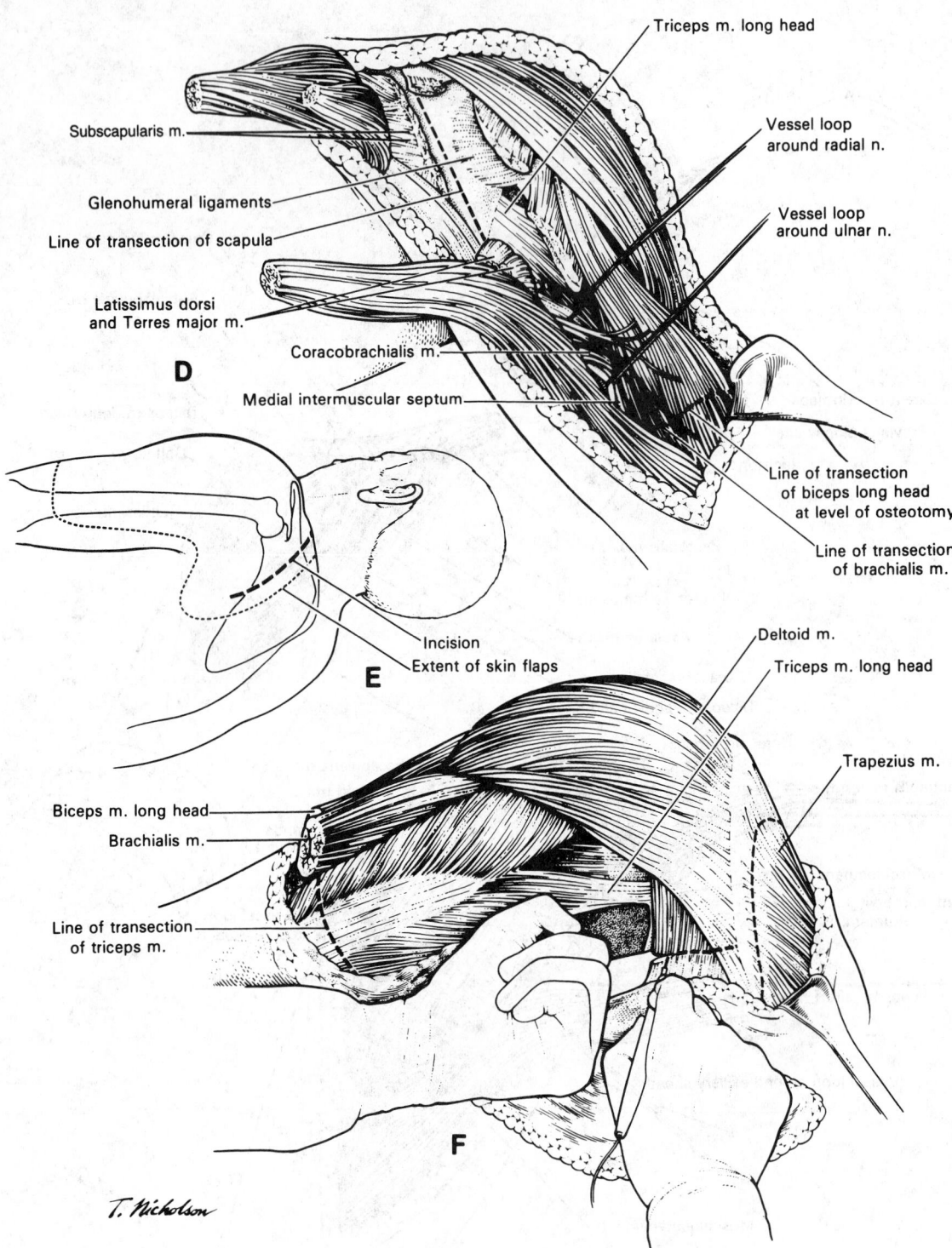

Triceps m. long head

Subscapularis m.

Vessel loop
around radial n.

Glenohumeral ligaments

Vessel loop
around ulnar n.

Line of transection of scapula

Latissimus dorsi
and Terres major m.

Coracobrachialis m.

Medial intermuscular septum

Line of transection
of biceps long head
at level of osteotomy

Line of transection
of brachialis m.

D

Incision
Extent of skin flaps

E

Deltoid m.

Triceps m. long head

Trapezius m.

Biceps m. long head

Brachialis m.

Line of transection
of triceps m.

F

T. Nicholson

FIGURE 44–23. *(Continued)*

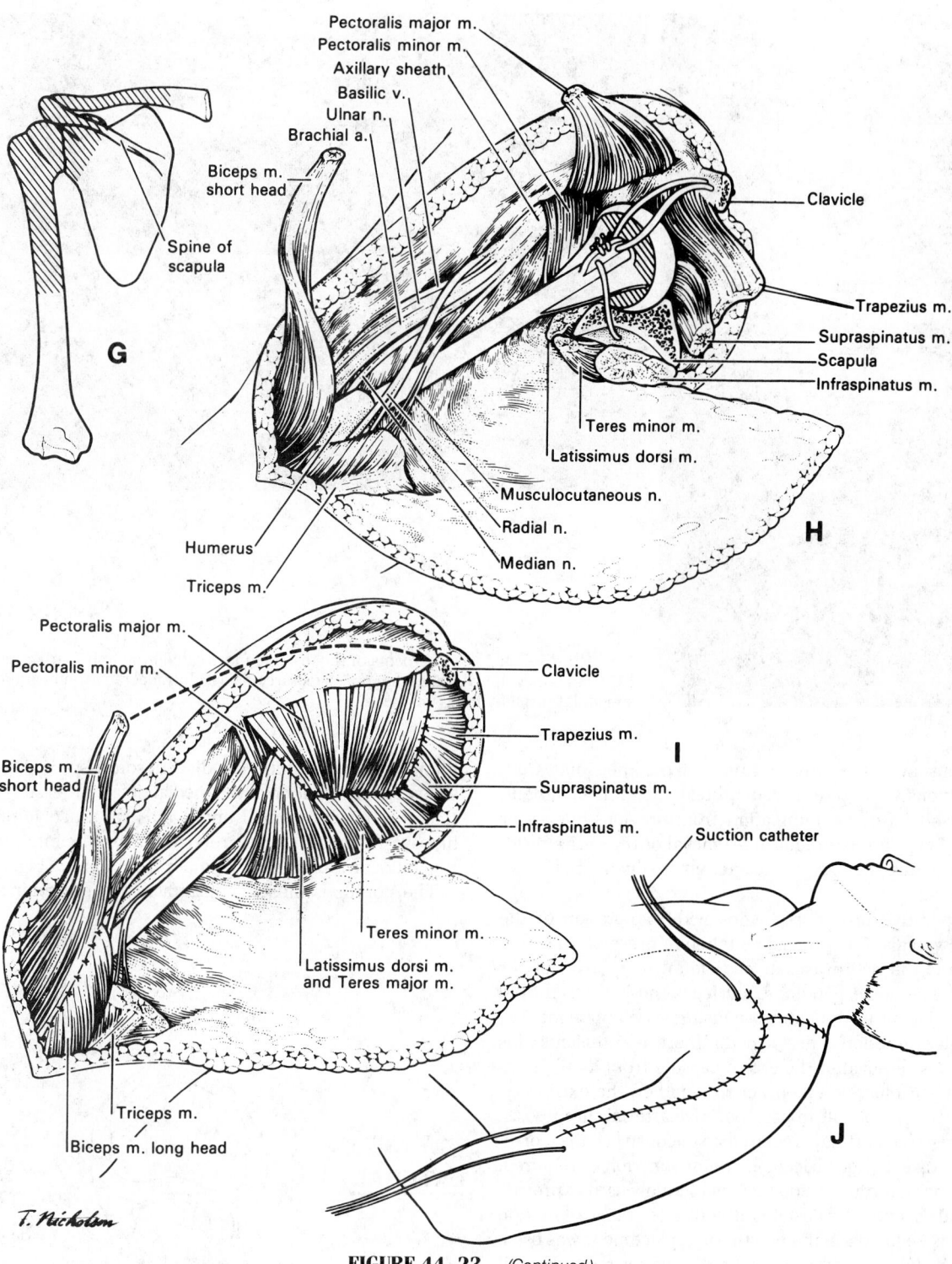

Pectoralis major m.
Pectoralis minor m.
Axillary sheath
Basilic v.
Ulnar n.
Brachial a.
Biceps m. short head
Spine of scapula
Clavicle
Trapezius m.
Supraspinatus m.
Scapula
Infraspinatus m.
Teres minor m.
Latissimus dorsi m.
Musculocutaneous n.
Radial n.
Median n.
Humerus
Triceps m.

G

H

Pectoralis major m.
Pectoralis minor m.
Clavicle
Trapezius m.
Biceps m. short head
Supraspinatus m.
Infraspinatus m.
Teres minor m.
Latissimus dorsi m. and Teres major m.
Triceps m.
Biceps m. long head

I

Suction catheter

J

T. Nicholson

FIGURE 44–23. *(Continued)*

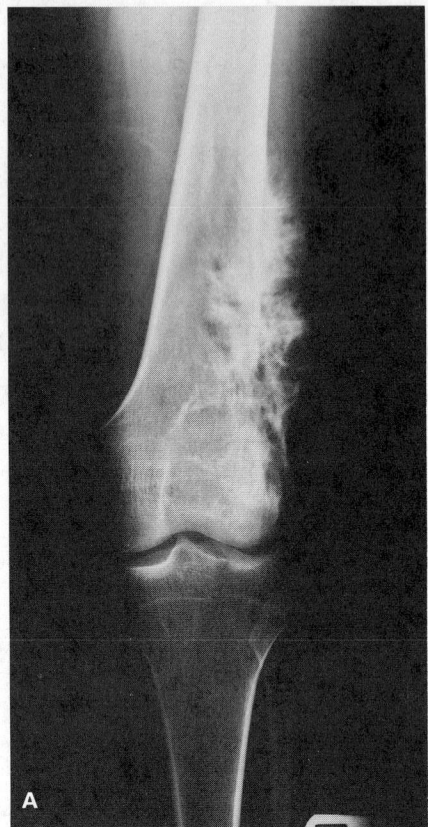
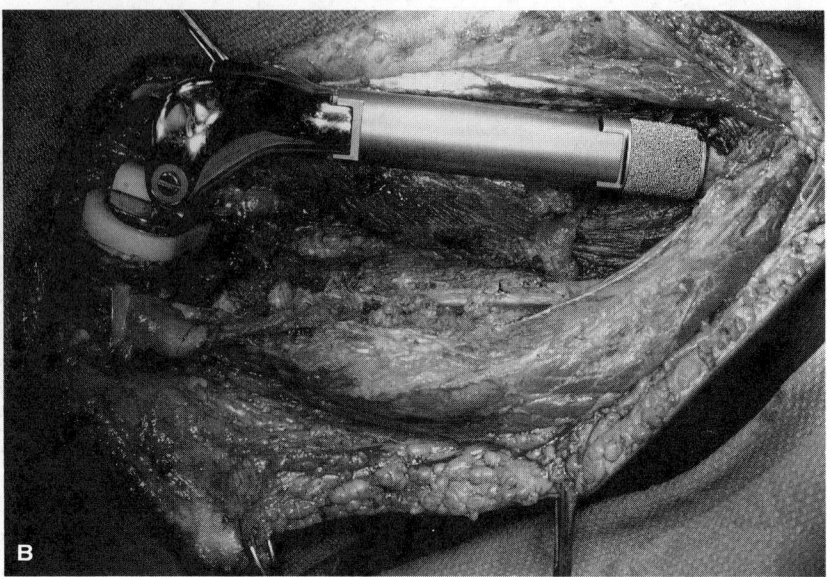

FIGURE 44–24. Osteosarcoma of the distal femur treated by a limb-sparing resection. **(A)** Plain radiograph of a distal femoral osteosarcoma. **(B)** Intraoperative photograph shows a modular distal femoral prosthesis.

Biopsy must avoid the sartorial canal and the knee joint. Contraindications to resection are popliteal vessel involvement, massive soft tissue contamination from previous biopsy, or fracture. Large tumors requiring removal of the entire quadriceps or hamstrings can be adequately reconstructed by an arthrodesis.

The operative procedure begins with exploration of the popliteal vessels. Care should be taken to preserve the sural vessels and the neurovascular pedicle to the gastrocnemius muscles. The corresponding quadriceps muscle is removed en bloc adjacent to the extraosseous tumor component. Extraarticular resection is performed if there are effusions; this necessitates removal of the entire capsule from its tibial insertion. Care must be taken not to lengthen the extremity, because this may result in postoperative arterial thrombosis. Hamstring transfers are required to reconstruct the corresponding resected quadriceps if motor function is required. A gastrocnemius transposition flap is routinely used to provide additional coverage.[243] Postoperatively, knee range of motion exercise is begun early if a prosthetic replacement was used. If an arthrodesis is performed, a long-leg cast is required until incorporation of the grafts. Hip and ankle motion are usually normal. A cane and brace are routinely recommended for 12 months.

PROXIMAL TIBIA. Limb-sparing procedures often are not feasible for tumors of the proximal tibia.[244] It is more difficult to obtain an adequate margin of resection and a good functional result with lesions of the proximal tibia, which tend to have a higher incidence of local complications than do distal femoral tumors. These problems are directly related to the ana-

tomic constraints: minimal adjacent soft tissue and the normal subcutaneous location of the medial tibial border. It is essential that the biopsy is small and avoids the knee joint. A core biopsy of medial flare is preferred to avoid contamination of the anterior musculature and peroneal nerve (Fig. 44–25).

The popliteus muscle adjacent to the posterior aspect of

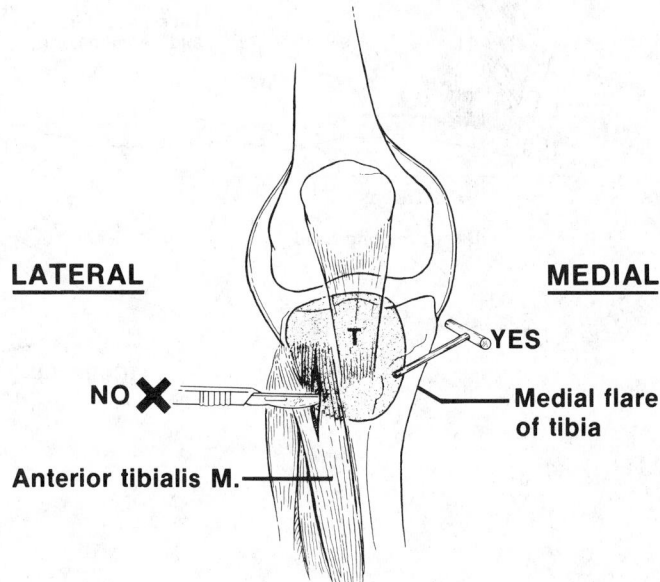

FIGURE 44–25. Biopsy technique for proximal tibial sarcomas. The biopsy should always be performed medially to avoid contamination of the anterior tibial muscles.

the tibia prevents direct tumor involvement of the neurovascular bundle.[244,245] Lateral angiography is essential to demonstrate this interval. A large posterior tumor component makes resection unadvisable. The anteroposterior projection is useful to delineate anomalous vascular patterns. Adequate resection of the proximal tibia requires ligation of the anterior tibial artery and, in most cases, the peroneal artery. The remaining posterior tibial artery leaves a viable extremity in a young person.[244] An anomalously absent posterior tibial artery, which occurs in 5% of patients, is a contraindication for resection.[246] Tumor extension often involves the tibiofibular capsule.[244] Extraarticular resection of the proximal tibiofibular joint en bloc with the tibia is required to obtain a safe margin. The average resection length is 15 to 18 cm.

Reconstruction is by prosthetic replacement, arthrodesis, or allograft (Fig. 44–26). The medial gastrocnemius is routinely transferred to provide soft tissue coverage of the reconstructed area.[243] Dacron tape is used to reattach the patella to the transferred gastrocnemius and prosthesis. Postoperative management is similar to that used for distal femoral resections.[244]

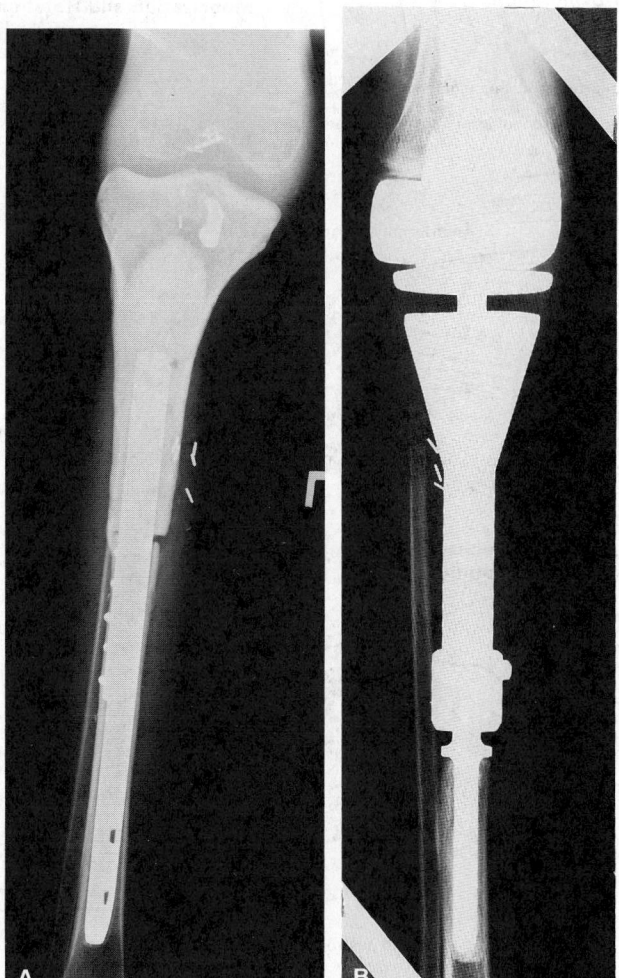

FIGURE 44–26. Two methods of reconstruction after resection of the proximal tibia. **(A)** Allograft replacement. **(B)** Expandable custom prosthesis used for the skeletal immature patient.

PROXIMAL FIBULA. Tumors of the proximal fibula require the same evaluation as proximal tibial lesions.[246] Unique considerations are early soft tissue extension, proximity to the lateral tibial condyle, necessity of ligation of the anterior and peroneal arteries, sacrifice of the peroneal nerve, and tumor infiltration of the tibiofibular joint capsule. Large tumors are often unresectable. Biplane angiography is necessary to determine anomalous vascular patterns and vascular displacement. Bone scintigraphy with multiple rotation views of the proximal tibia or MRI is essential to determine bony involvement of the adjacent tibial plateau. Contraindications to resection are direct tibial involvement, an anomalously absent posterior tibial artery, and intraarticular knee joint extension. Due to the multiple musculotendinous attachment of the proximal fibula, muscle infiltration generally occurs along muscle planes beyond visible borders.

Adequate resection includes the fibula, the tibiofibular joint, the anterior and lateral muscle compartments, and a portion of the lateral gastrocnemius, soleus, and intermuscular septum (Fig. 44–27). Wide excision of all adjacent muscle groups is mandatory (Fig. 44–28). No reconstruction of the bony defect is required. The lateral collateral ligament is reattached to the lateral joint capsule. A lateral gastrocnemius transposition flap is used to close the resultant defect.[243] After surgery, the only functional deficit is a drop foot, treated by an orthosis. Knee function is normal.[246]

Osteosarcoma of the Pelvis and Proximal Femur

Osteosarcomas of the pelvis and proximal femur (Fig. 44–29) are less common than those occurring at other anatomic areas, accounting for 10% and 5%, respectively, of all osteosarcomas.[211] Tumors arising from these structures are often large, involve important structures, and are difficult to resect. Hemipelvectomy is often required for pelvic tumors, and modified hemipelvectomy is used for tumors of the proximal femur.[128] The limb-sparing options, if feasible, are all functionally superior to amputation at this level.[126,127] A poorly planned biopsy often contaminates the extrapelvic structures, making a hemipelvectomy the only safe option. The technique of pelvic biopsy is shown in Fig. 44–30. Detailed anatomic and surgical considerations are discussed in the section on chondrosarcomas, which more commonly arise in these sites.

Limb-Sparing Surgery or Amputation

Limb-sparing surgery is now considered the preferred treatment for a significant number of patients with osteosarcomas and other high-grade bone sarcomas.[23,107,119,122,128] Amputations are reserved principally for patients in whom the primary tumor is deemed unresectable.[128] Extensive data have been obtained within the past 5 years about the crucial factors in the decision to perform a limb-sparing procedure or an amputation.[107–109,126,127] The major considerations and goals to be met in choosing a limb-salvage procedure are summarized[23]:

1. *Local recurrence.* The chance of local recurrence should not be higher than that associated with amputation.
2. *Survival.* Overall survival should not be jeopardized due to treatment delay or an ineffective (adjuvant) treatment program.

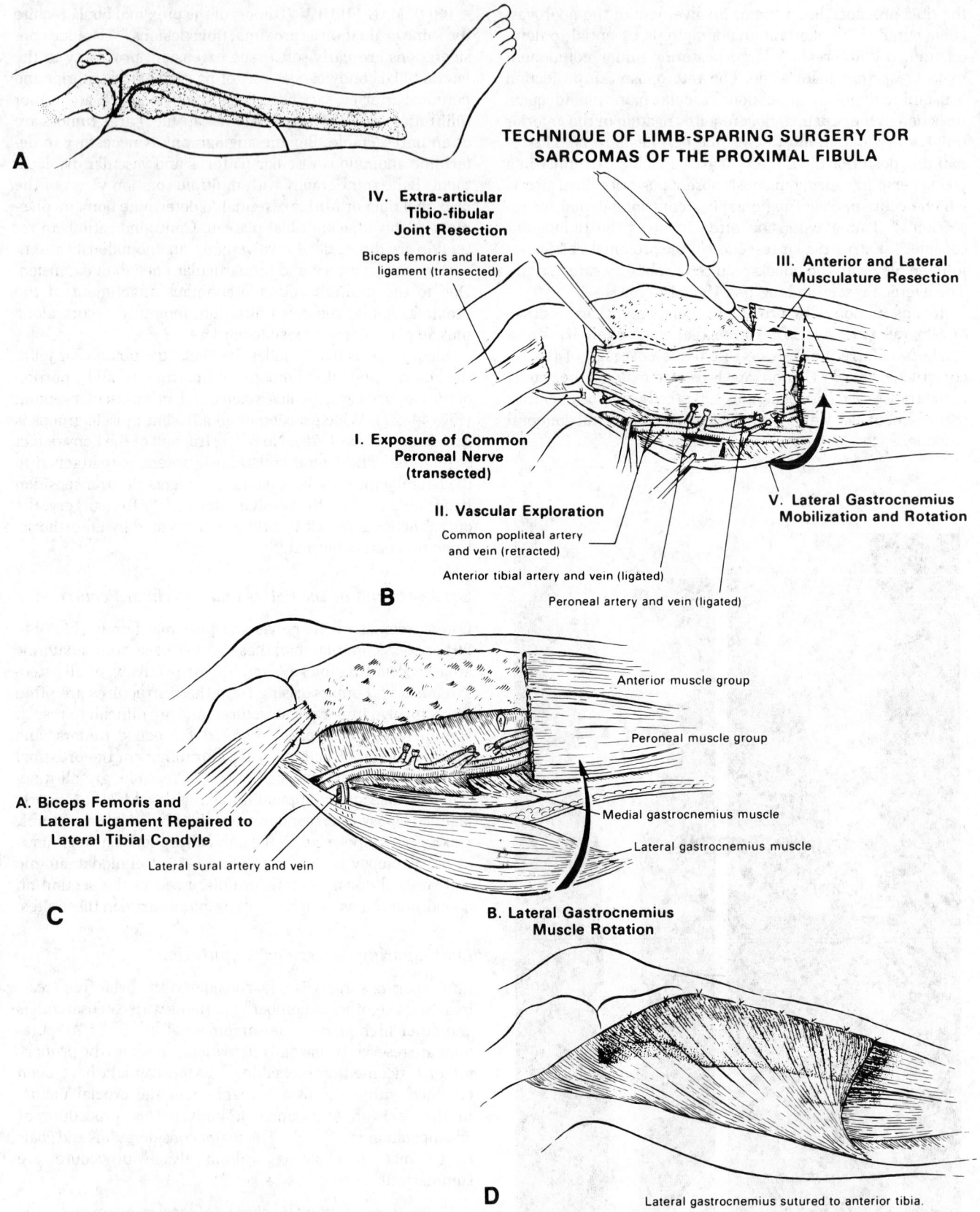

TECHNIQUE OF LIMB-SPARING SURGERY FOR SARCOMAS OF THE PROXIMAL FIBULA

IV. Extra-articular Tibio-fibular Joint Resection

Biceps femoris and lateral ligament (transected)

III. Anterior and Lateral Musculature Resection

I. Exposure of Common Peroneal Nerve (transected)

II. Vascular Exploration

Common popliteal artery and vein (retracted)

Anterior tibial artery and vein (ligated)

Peroneal artery and vein (ligated)

V. Lateral Gastrocnemius Mobilization and Rotation

B

Anterior muscle group

Peroneal muscle group

Medial gastrocnemius muscle

Lateral gastrocnemius muscle

A. Biceps Femoris and Lateral Ligament Repaired to Lateral Tibial Condyle

Lateral sural artery and vein

C

B. Lateral Gastrocnemius Muscle Rotation

Lateral gastrocnemius sutured to anterior tibia.

D

FIGURE 44–27. Technique of limb-sparing surgery for sarcomas of the proximal fibula. **(A)** Utilitarian incision. **(B)** Steps of resection of tumor. **(C)** Resection defect. Notice that both the anterior tibial and peroneal arteries have been ligated and the anterior and lateral muscle compartments removed. The defect is closed routinely by a lateral gastrocnemius muscle transfer. **(D)** Bony reconstruction is not necessary. (Malawer MM. Surgical management of aggressive and malignant tumors of the proximal fibula. Clin Orthop 1984;186:172–181)

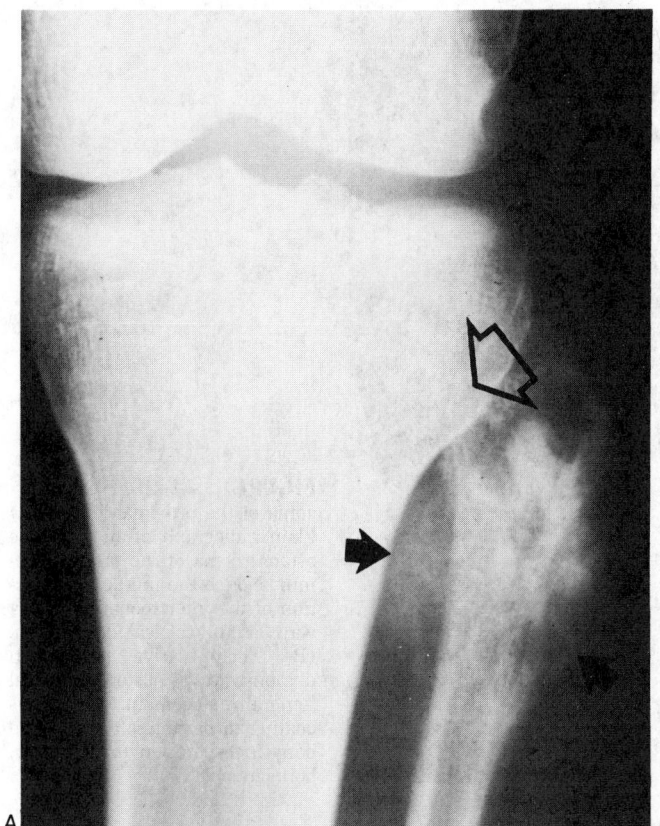
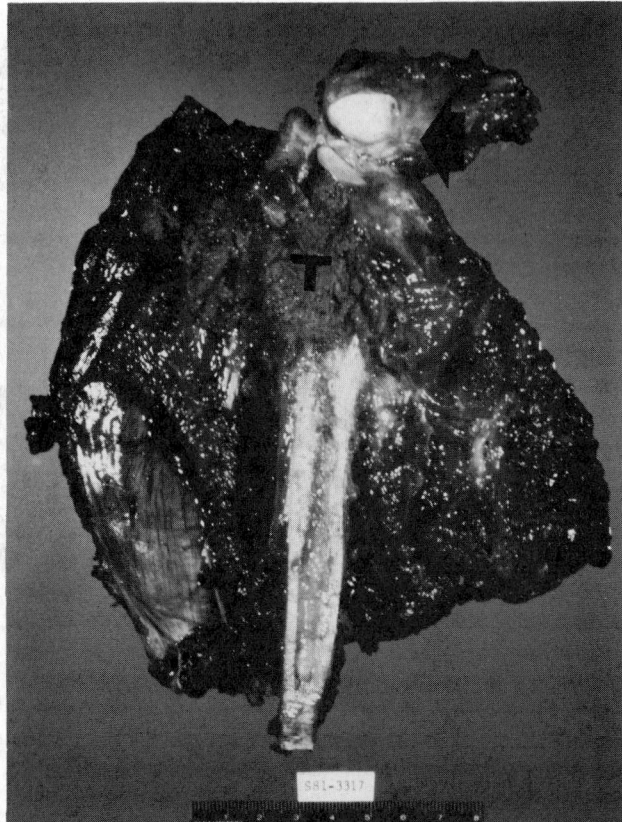

FIGURE 44–28. **(A)** Osteosarcoma of the proximal fibula. Plain radiograph of the knee demonstrates an osteosarcoma of the proximal fibula. Notice the large soft tissue component (*solid arrows*) and the intimate relation to the proximal tibiofibular joint. Tumors arising from the proximal fibula can often be treated by a limb-sparing procedure. **(B)** Gross specimen of a fibula resection for an osteosarcoma. An extraarticular resection was performed. The tibiofibular joint (*solid arrow*) was opened and demonstrated pericapsular tumor extension. This is a common finding and emphasizes the need for routine extraarticular resection for sarcomas of the proximal fibula. T, tumor. (Malawer MM. Surgical management of aggressive and malignant tumors of the proximal fibula. Clin Orthop 1984;186:172–181)

3. *Function.* The means of reconstruction should be functional, with minimal long-term morbidity and need for additional surgery. The psychological impact and duration of rehabilitation must be considered.

Many studies have demonstrated that the risk (<5%) of local recurrence in patients who have undergone limb-sparing surgery is the same or less than the risk in those treated by amputation.[23,26–28,126] However, these are carefully selected patients, and the procedures have been performed in institutions whose staff is familiar with the techniques. The reported continuous disease-free survival rates are the same or better than those in large series of patients undergoing amputation alone.[26,27,30,33,36,38,52,53] If the criteria for patient selection are met, despite the variations among institutions, limb-salvage is a safe procedure. Eilber and colleagues from UCLA reported 78% (64 of 83) consecutive patients with malignant skeletal tumors who were treated by a limb-sparing resection, with no difference in overall survival compared with those treated by amputation.[26] The overall local recurrence rate was 2.7%. Eckardt and associates, from the same institution, subsequently reported their experience specifically with stage IIB osteosarcoma for the period 1972 to 1984.

Seventy-eight (67%) of 116 patients were treated by a limb-sparing resection, with a local recurrence rate of 3.8%.[23]

The functional advantages of limb-sparing surgery merit careful consideration. Preservation of the upper humerus after resection of a proximal humeral sarcoma, for example, leaves a normal hand and elbow that are far superior to any prosthesis. Except for lack of shoulder motion, function is essentially normal. The advantage of such a procedure over forequarter amputation is obvious. Similarly, the functional advantages of preservation of the lower extremity after proximal femoral resection or pelvic resection are far superior to a hemipelvectomy. Initially, there was concern regarding the functional outcome of limb-sparing procedures about the knee, but Enneking reported that resections followed by reconstruction at this site by several different modalities all had a higher functional rating than an amputation in a multiinstitutional study using a standard evaluation scheme.[122]

Effect of Chemotherapy on Surgical Decisions

The initial impetus to limb-sparing surgery in the mid-1970s was the introduction of doxorubicin and methotrexate. Surgeons decided that adjuvant therapy might allow something

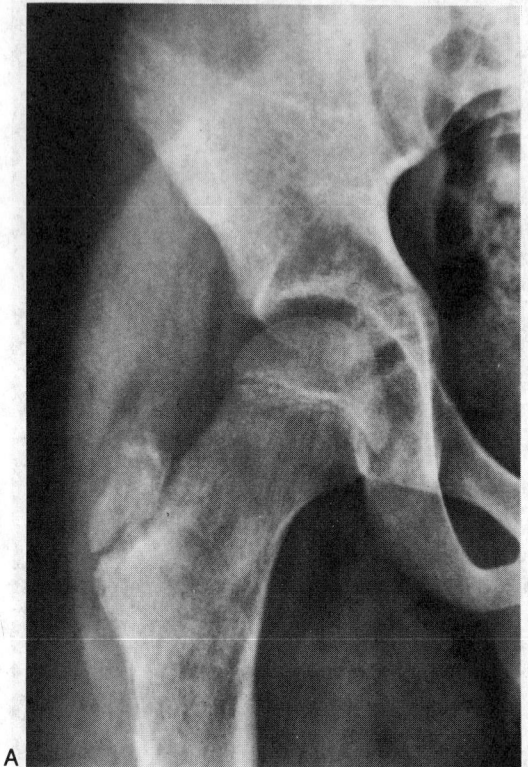
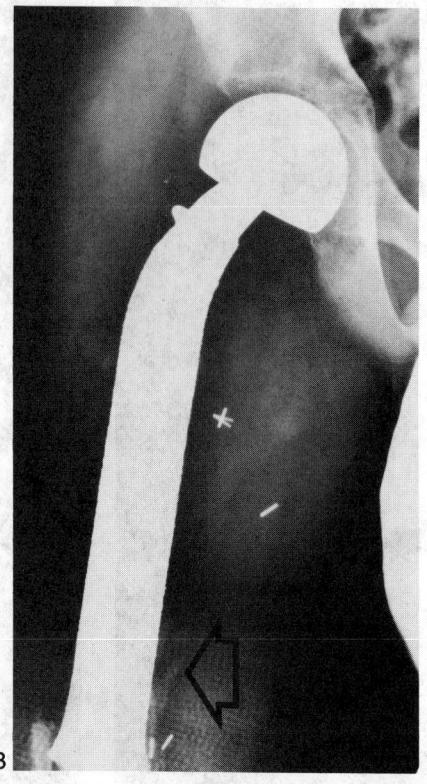

FIGURE 44–29. Osteosarcoma of the proximal femur. **(A)** Plain radiograph of an osteolytic osteosarcoma of the proximal femur. Notice the mottled destruction of the intertrochanteric area with lateral cortical destruction. **(B)** Postoperative radiograph demonstrates a custom proximal femoral replacement with porous coating to permit soft tissue and bony incorporation (*open arrow*, bone graft).

less than radical surgery. Most surgeons now think that adjuvant chemotherapy permits limb-sparing surgery to be performed more safely, with a lower local recurrence rate. Can a narrower surgical margin be a safe one with adjuvant chemotherapy? Although many surgeons believe this is possible, some evidence suggests that adjuvant chemotherapy has a beneficial effect, and other data suggest that it does not.[26,74]

Eilber and colleagues reported an encouragingly low 2.6% (5 of 183 patients) local recurrence rate for high-grade bone and soft tissue tumors and concluded that it was due to multimodal therapy (*i.e.*, preoperative irradiation and intraarterial and postoperative chemotherapy) that destroys microscopic disease at the periphery of the primary tumor.[26] The exact modality responsible for the favorable outcome was undetermined, but these researchers doubted that it was related to more accurate surgery. Conversely, Picci and associates evaluated by detailed mapping 50 osteosarcoma (Fig. 44–31)

specimens from patients who had followed two different intravenous preoperative regimens. They reported a high incidence (63%) of viable tumor within the extraosseous soft tissue.[248] They concluded that a wide surgical margin is required because viable tumor is often at the periphery.

Because all preoperative chemotherapeutic agents entail the risk of increased local morbidity, skin breakdown, infection, and possible tumor progression and the possibility of losing a nonamputative option, additional studies are needed to determine the relation of preoperative chemotherapy to the choice of surgical margin.

Clinical Presentations of Osteosarcoma and Treatment Considerations

LOCALIZED EXTREMITY DISEASE. Management requires the expertise of a multidisciplinary team familiar with

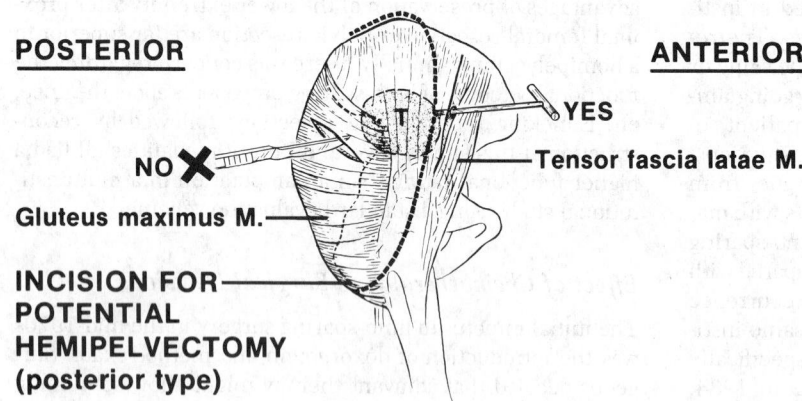

FIGURE 44–30. Biopsy technique for buttock and iliac tumors. The potential posterior hemipelvectomy flap (*dotted line*) should never be violated. A small biopsy from the lateral aspect is recommended.

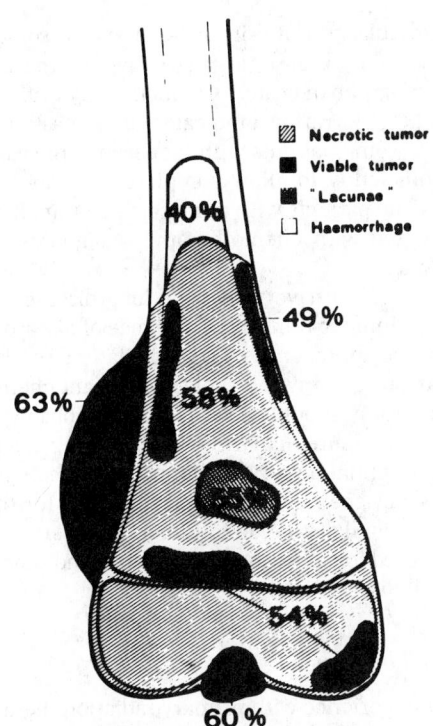

☒ Necrotic tumor
■ Viable tumor
■ "Lacunae"
▢ Haemorrhage

40%

49%

63% 58%

54%

60%

FIGURE 44–31. The percentage of viable tumor in each preferential site found in patients with viable tumor after preoperative treatment for osteosarcoma as for 50 patients. (Picci P, Bacci G, Companacci M, et al. Histological evaluation of necrosis in osteosarcoma induced by chemotherapy, regional mapping of viable and nonviable tumor. Cancer 1985;56:1515–1521)

the various management options. Patients with a suspected diagnosis of osteosarcoma (based on radiographic findings) should be referred to centers with treatment programs before biopsy.

The patient with a primary tumor of the extremity without evidence of metastases requires surgery to control the primary tumor and chemotherapy to control micrometastatic disease. The choice between amputation and limb-sparing resection must be made by an experienced orthopedic oncologist. Most distal femoral, proximal tibial, and proximal humerus osteosarcomas can be treated by limb-sparing resection. Routine amputations are no longer performed, and all patients should be evaluated for limb-sparing options. Intensive, multiagent chemotherapeutic regimens have provided the best results to date (see Tables 44–7 and 44–10). Patients who are judged unsuitable for limb-sparing options may become suitable candidates for limb-sparing operations after neoadjuvant chemotherapy. The management of these patients mandates close cooperation between chemotherapist and surgeon. Malawer recommends all patients be treated with neoadjuvant chemotherapy before making a surgical decision.

PELVIC TUMORS AND VERTEBRAL BODY TUMORS. In some pelvic and most vertebral primary tumors, complete resection is often not possible. Most pelvic osteosarcomas can be treated by hemipelvectomy; more centrally located pelvic tumors, especially those involving the sacrum, are unresectable. Only a few pelvic osteosarcomas can be treated by limb-sparing resection (internal hemipelvectomy). Contraindica-

tions to resection are unusually large extraosseous extensions with sacral plexus or major vascular involvement. Rarely, vertebral and sacral resections have been attempted.[203–205] In general, these tumors cannot be resected with negative margins and are best treated by radiation therapy and chemotherapy. Some success has been achieved with systemic or intraarterial chemotherapy, which is administered to convert apparently inoperable tumors into lesions that can be ablated surgically.[206,247a] In 1991, Tienghi and coworkers reported their results of 26 patients with pelvic osteosarcoma treated with infusional and postoperative intravenous chemotherapy. Only 1 patient remained disease free.[248a] This emphasizes the difficulty of treatment for pelvic osteosarcoma.

Patients with primary tumors of the axial skeleton have had poor outcomes because local control was rarely achieved. The prognosis for these patients may improve with a more aggressive surgical approach and more effective chemotherapy. Patients whose tumors can be completely resected should be approached with curative intent; radiation therapy provides significant palliation in patients with unresectable primary tumors.

Sundaresan and coworkers from MSKCC reviewed their experience of 35 years with vertebral osteosarcomas and reported their results of 24 patients.[248b] All lesions were stage IIB. They concluded that surgical resection should be part of the treatment strategy and not simple decompression and irradiation. Otherwise, local recurrence and dissemination is almost certain to occur. They observed the initial presentation was usually pain associated with neurologic deficit. The plain radiograph usually showed a mixed osteoblastic and osteolytic involvement of the anterior vertebral structures. CT and MRI is required and almost always demonstrates an extraosseous component. The researchers strongly recommended a two-stage surgical procedure after the diagnosis was established. The first stage should be a partial anterior spondylectomy followed by combination chemotherapy while monitoring the patient's tumor response. If the tumor remains under control, the remainder of the tumor should be resected by a posterior approach (*i.e.*, total spondylectomy) with additional stabilization by instrumentation, bone graft, or cementation. External-beam irradiation is given postoperatively.

METASTATIC PULMONARY DISEASE AT DIAGNOSIS. Metastatic disease detected at initial diagnosis does not preclude a curative treatment strategy, although the presence of extrathoracic metastases makes it extremely unlikely. In general, the surgical principles outlined for the treatment of relapsing patients apply equally to the patient presenting with macroscopic metastases. Newly diagnosed patients have not been exposed to chemotherapy and are likely to have drug-resistant tumors, and several options are therefore available for them.

For the patient presenting with resectable disease (*i.e.*, usually fewer than 15 pulmonary nodules and a primary tumor of the extremity), the traditional approach has been resection of all evidence of macroscopic disease by median sternotomy and limb amputation or resection, followed by intensive adjuvant chemotherapy. The tumor burden is reduced to a minimum before the application of adjuvant therapy. Some investigators favor treatment with chemotherapy, followed weeks or months later by definitive surgery for residual macroscopic disease in primary and metastatic sites.[249,250] Arguments advanced to justify this approach are similar to those used to support the strategy of preoperative chemotherapy in general, and the theoretical advantages and disadvantages of this strategy as discussed for patients with nonmetastatic osteosarcoma apply here as well. The risk for the patient with metastases is that growth of tumor nodules in the face of chemotherapy may render small, operable metastases unresectable and prevent cure. Primary treatment with chemotherapy may be appropriate, however, in patients with inoperable metastases, which may respond sufficiently to allow complete resection. Patients with widespread unresectable metastases are also best treated first with chemotherapy, with definitive surgery reserved for those achieving a satisfactory response. Because these patients usually require surgery for the primary tumor as a palliative procedure, early surgery may be recommended despite unresectable pulmonary disease.

RECURRENT DISEASE AFTER CURATIVE ATTEMPT. Historically, patients developing recurrent disease had a poor prognosis and were treated palliatively; most patients died within 1 year of the development of metastatic disease. Because more than 85% of metastases occur in the lung, surgical resection of tumor nodules can be readily accomplished. With the advent of thoracic CT scanning, metastatic nodules can be detected when quite small and more easily resectable, although the surgeon usually discovers more lesions at thoracotomy than anticipated from the CT scan.[251] In many patients, the lungs are likely to be the only site of metastases, especially in cases in which recurrences appear more than 1 year after diagnosis and in which the metastatic lesion is solitary. These recurrent tumors are likely to behave more indolently and may not further metastasize. These patients have been cured by thoracotomy alone.

Complete surgical resection of all overt metastatic disease is a prerequisite for long-term salvage after relapse.[252–255] Patients not treated by thoracotomy have little hope for cure, because complete responses of macroscopic metastases to chemotherapy are rare.[253,254] The completeness of surgical resection is an important determinant of outcome, because patients left with measurable or microscopic disease at the resection margins are unlikely to be cured.[253]

CHEMOTHERAPY AND METASTATIC DISEASE. Many investigators have recommended adjuvant chemotherapy after thoracotomy for the management of metastatic osteosarcoma to destroy residual microscopic tumor deposits after surgical treatment of overt metastases.[249,256–258] For patients who develop recurrent disease within 1 year of initial surgery, the possibility of microscopic metastatic disease is quite high, and additional chemotherapy is indicated. Long-term survival has been reported for some patients with recurrent osteosarcoma who were treated only with surgery without further chemotherapy.[253–255] These survivors were more likely to be patients suffering late relapses with solitary pulmonary nodules.

If overt metastatic disease is discovered, a thorough search for all metastatic lesions is essential. The discovery of unresectable extrathoracic metastases or unresectable pulmonary disease is a contraindication to aggressive thoracotomy, and the patient should be treated palliatively. Radiation therapy may be particularly useful in this context. In some patients with unresectable disease, an aggressive approach with curative intent may be indicated. Chemotherapy, with or without radiation therapy, rarely eradicates all metastatic disease; nonetheless, some patients with inoperative metastases may respond sufficiently to allow complete resection of disease later, and some patients with unresectable pulmonary metastases are cured with chemotherapy or high-dose radiation therapy alone.

Patients found to have resectable lung disease should undergo thoracotomy to remove all evidence of disease. Bilateral disease may be approached by staged bilateral thoracotomies or a median sternotomy. The role of adjuvant chemotherapy after thoracotomy should be studied; it is probably indicated for patients with more than three lesions appearing 6 months to 1 year after initial surgery and for patients whose metastatic disease has not been completely resected or for those with evidence of pleural disruption by tumor. Repeat thoracotomies may be required for subsequent recurrence and should be performed if all disease can be resected.

Radiation Therapy

Significant experience with primary radiation therapy for osteosarcomas was obtained in the 1950s and early 1960s. Primary radiation therapy with delayed amputation gained acceptance in 1955, when Cade advocated initial therapy with irradiation and delayed amputation for patients in whom there was no evidence of metastasis 4 to 6 months after radiation therapy.[259] This approach was designed to circumvent amputation in most patients who were destined to suffer an early relapse. Radiation doses were 7000 to 8000 cGy in 7 to 9 weeks at 1000 cGy each week. There were a few patients in Cade's series who were not subjected to delayed amputation who were controlled with irradiation alone, and amputation was eventually performed. The 5-year survival rate was 21.8%. Other investigators followed a similar regimen, using various radiation doses and schedules (Table 44–12). Subsequent surgical specimens of many of the patients managed in this fashion were found to have no histologic evidence of their tumor.[260–265] The ability of high radiation doses to sterilize some tumors was associated with significant necrosis of normal tissue.

Results of preoperative irradiation were subsequently evaluated. Overall success with preoperative irradiation followed by ablative surgery was suboptimal; most patients relapsed shortly after treatment. This led Jenkin and colleagues at Princess Margaret Hospital to recommend limiting irradiation to patients who had unresectable tumors or those being treated for palliation only.[266–267] Beck and coworkers observed no survival advantage for preoperative irradiation followed by surgery over surgery alone; only 43% of their patients obtained any palliative benefit from radiation therapy.[268] Disappointingly, no benefit has been observed from irradiation delivered under conditions of local tissue hypoxia, split-course radiation therapy, or with hydrogen peroxide or cytotoxic drug therapy.[269–271]

Radiation therapy has been successful in several clinical situations: facial lesions, palliation, and as a postoperative adjuvant.

TABLE 44–12. Series of Primary Radiation Followed by Delayed Surgery for Osteosarcoma

No. of Patients	Dose	Machine	Survival (%)	References
133	7000–8000 cGy/7–9 wk, 1000 cGy/wk	2 MV	21.8	243
10	10,000 cGy, 180 cGy/fraction	^{60}Co	60	245
92	6000–8000 cGy in 230-cGy fractions	or 2 MV	21.8	244a
16	1600–10,500 cGy in 200-cGy fractions	Orthovoltage and 2 MV	75 (1–16 y) Follow-up	244b
54	Variable	Variable	27.5	244c
23	1800–12,000 cGy/2–29 wk	Orthovoltage and 2 MV	26	244d
27	5000–6000 cGy in 25–30-cGy fractions		0	247
27	5000–6000 cGy/5–6 wk repeated × 1 7000–8000 cGy/8–9 wk	Orthovoltage or 1–4 Mv	23	249

OSTEOSARCOMA OF THE MAXILLA OR MANDIBLE. Osteosarcoma arising from facial bones, specifically the maxilla or mandible, have a different biology and natural history from those located elsewhere in the body. There is a lower risk of dissemination. Tumors arising in these sites have a high rate of local recurrence if treated by surgery alone. Clark and associates reported 66 patients with maxillary or mandibular primary tumors; 43 died, most with primary local recurrences.[272] Chambers and Mahoney suggested preoperative radiation therapy for such patients.[273] They reported a 73% survival rate at 5 years among 33 patients treated with high-dose radiation therapy (*i.e.*, interstitial technique or external-beam) followed immediately by wide surgical excision (*i.e.*, hemimandibulectomy and resection of surrounding soft tissues). Long-term survival after surgery alone ranged between 35% to 45%.[274] Surgical excisions associated with a high local recurrence rate are explained by difficulties in achieving adequate surgical margins. The increased survival after combined-modality treatment supports the fact that high radiation doses can eradicate microscopic disease. De Fries and colleagues and Abbiyik reported similar improved survival rates using a combination of preoperative irradiation, resection, and chemotherapy.[275,276] Conversely, Livolsi reported 5 patients irradiated in the postoperative period for osteosarcoma of the maxilla, all of whom died.[277] The long delay between the completion of surgery and the start of postoperative radiation therapy may have contributed to the poor results.

PALLIATION. Radiation therapy is extremely beneficial for patients requiring palliation of metastatic bony sarcomas, tumors at axial sites (which are unresectable), and advanced, inoperable lesions of the pelvis or extremities. A novel approach using high-dose-per-fraction irradiation and intraarterial 5'-bromodeoxyuridine (BUDR) as a radiosensitizer was undertaken by the Stanford Group.[278] Pulsed 48-hour BUDR infusions were performed before each 600-cGy radiation fraction, with a total radiation dose to the primary site of 4200 to 4800 cGy in 5 weeks in seven or eight fractions. Infusions of methotrexate-leucovorin were administered simulta-

neously. Local control was achieved in 7 (78%) of the 9 patients treated.[279] However, local tissue toxicity was excessive and included subcutaneous fibrosis, nonhealing traumatic fractures, peroneal neuropathy, and atrophy. Because the patients were treated with an unusual fractionation scheme using large fractions and intravenous chemotherapy, the specific role of BUDR in local control with its excessive toxicity was not established.

Kinsella used intravenous radiosensitizers of BUDR, iododeoxyuridine (IUDR), or misonidazole with high-dose radiation therapy, with various fractionation schemes and usually with chemotherapy, in patients with large, unresectable primary or metastatic sarcomas.[280] Twenty-one (75%) of 29 patients achieved local control, defined as freedom from symptoms and absence of growth. These studies demonstrated the efficacy of radiation therapy in obtaining long-term local control and palliation. The results lend support to additional clinical investigations using radiation sensitizers with high-dose radiation therapy.

ADJUVANT PULMONARY IRRADIATION. Variable results have been achieved from the use of adjuvant pulmonary irradiation in patients with primary osteosarcoma.[281,283-287] Breur and associates performed a randomized trial comparing amputation plus adjuvant whole-lung irradiation with amputation alone in 86 patients.[240,264-266] The midplane pulmonary lung dose was 1750 cGy in 10 fractions in 12 days, which, with lung correction, equalled slightly less than 2000 cGy. They found a significant benefit in the 3-year disease-free survival in the group that received adjuvant radiation therapy among patients younger than 17 years of age. Forty-eight percent of these patients survived without disease, compared with 28% in the group receiving surgery alone. This study is now being extended to the European Organization for Research on the Treatment of Cancer (EORTC) in a trial comparing amputation and lung irradiation with surgery and adjuvant chemotherapy and with all three treatments.[283-287] Their study, EORTC-SIOP 03 trial 20781, revealed a 4-year disease-free survival rate of 24% and overall survival rate of 43%, with no difference between the treatment arms.[286] For patients who subsequently developed lung metastases, successful pulmonary surgery could be done more frequently among patients who had elective lung irradiation of 2000 cGy than the other group. In this study, elective lung irradiation had an equal effect and provided the same survival as those receiving adjuvant chemotherapy (*i.e.*, methotrexate, vincristine, doxorubicin, cyclophosphamide).[286]

The French Bone Tumor Study Group gave the combination of intensive chemotherapy (*i.e.*, mitomycin C, vincristine, methotrexate, doxorubicin, dacarbazine, cyclophosphamide) and prophylactic lung irradiation of 2000 cGy after primary local treatment of surgery or radiation therapy to patients with osteosarcoma of the extremities.[287] They reported a 5-year survival rate of 66% and disease-free survival rate of 58%, but there was impairment of pulmonary function, which had not been seen when lung irradiation was given without simultaneous chemotherapy. Conversely, Rab and colleagues used a lower midplane radiation dose of 1500 cGy with concomitant dactinomycin in a randomized study and failed to show a survival benefit over amputation alone.[288] No toxicity was seen. Similarly, Jenkin found no benefit from 1500 cGy in 14 days of pulmonary irradiation with simultaneous dactinomycin.[289] Caceres and associates found no advantage over adjuvant doxorubicin alone.[290] Today, lung irradiation is rarely performed in the United States.

VARIANTS OF CLASSIC OSTEOSARCOMA

Dahlin has identified 11 variants of the classic osteosarcoma.[59] These accounted for 268 (28%) of 1021 cases reviewed at the Mayo Clinic. Osteosarcoma arising in the jaw bones, the most common variant, is characterized by well-differentiated cells with a low metastatic potential.[59] Excluding tumors arising secondary to Paget's disease, irradiation, or dedifferentiation of a chondrosarcoma, parosteal and periosteal osteosarcomas are the most common variants of classic osteosarcoma arising in the extremities, unlike classic osteosarcoma, which arises within a bone (intramedullary), both arise on the surface of the bone (juxtacortical).

Parosteal Osteosarcoma

Parosteal osteosarcoma is a distinct variant of conventional osteosarcoma, accounting for 4% of all osteosarcoma.[60] It arises from the cortex of a bone and generally occurs in an older persons. It has a better prognosis than classical osteosarcoma.

CLINICAL CHARACTERISTICS. There is a slight predominance of parosteal osteosarcoma in women. The distal posterior femur is involved in 72% of all cases; the proximal humerus and proximal tibia are the next most frequent sites. Parosteal osteosarcoma metastasizes slowly and has an overall survival rate of 75% to 85%.[60,291] Unni and colleagues found that all patients who died of tumor lived more than 5 years. The natural history of parosteal osteosarcoma is progressive enlargement and late metastasis. Parosteal osteosarcoma presents as a mass and occasionally is associated with pain. In contrast with conventional osteosarcoma, duration of symptoms varies from months to years. Unni reported that 50 of 79 patients had complaints of greater than 1 year, and one third of this group had pain for more than 5 years.[291] Tumor size, location, and duration of symptoms did not correlate with survival.[60]

RADIOGRAPHIC FINDINGS. Radiographs characteristically show a large, dense, lobulated mass broadly attached to the underlying bone without involvement of the medullary canal (Fig. 44–32). If old enough, the tumor may encircle the entire bone. The periphery of the lesion is characteristically less mature than the base. Ahuja emphasized that intramedullary extension is difficult to determine from plain radiographs.[60] Unni emphasized that high-grade foci did not usually alter the radiographic appearance of these tumors.[291]

PATHOLOGY AND GRADING. Parosteal osteosarcoma is characterized by well-formed lamellar or woven bone with a mature spindle cell stroma with few signs of malignancy. The cellularity of the spindle cell components varies; generally, it is not anaplastic and there are few mitoses.[2–4,59,60] The dif-

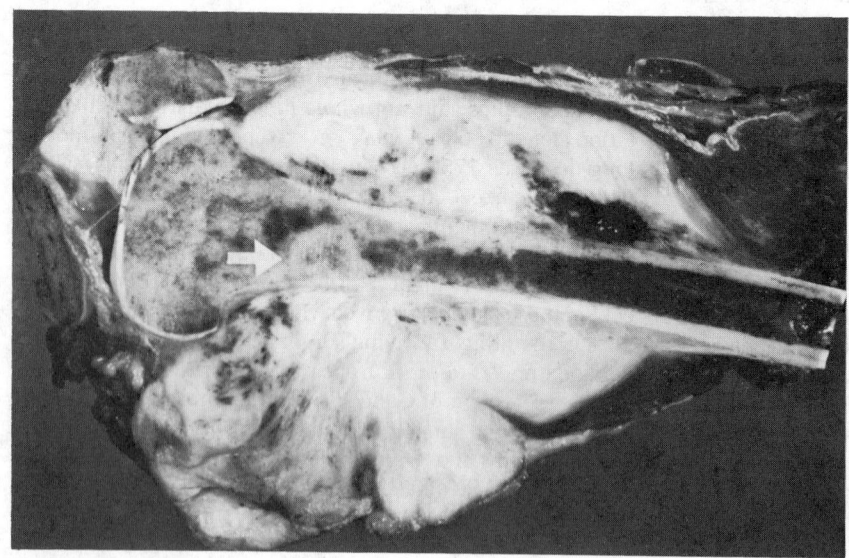

FIGURE 44–32. Parosteal osteosarcoma with intramedullary extension (*arrow*). Large parosteal osteosarcoma of the distal femur treated by an above-knee amputation. The patient refused treatment for 4 years before amputation. Intramedullary extension is a sign of advanced disease.

ferential diagnoses are osteochondroma, myositis ossificans, and conventional osteosarcoma. Cortical tumors of the posterior femur should always be suspected of malignancy; this is a rare location for a benign osteosarcoma. Unlike sarcoma, myositis ossificans is rarely attached to the underlying bone. The periphery is more mature, radiographically and histologically.

Ahuja reviewed all the parosteal osteosarcoma at MSKCC from 1934 to 1975 and described three grades: grade I (low grade), grade II (intermediate), and grade III (high grade).[60] He emphasized the importance of evaluating the fibroblastic, cartilaginous, and osseous components independently. Of the tumors of 24 patients, 8 were grade I, 10 were grade II, and 6 were grade III. Unni from the Mayo Clinic reviewed 79 patients and reported 18 (23%) were grade II and 7 (9%) had high-grade foci.[291] Neither Unni nor Ahuja could differentiate the three grades on plain radiographs. The survival rate of patients with grade III tumors is similar to that of patients with conventional osteosarcoma.

Intramedullary involvement does not necessarily imply a worse prognosis, although this may be the case in patients with high-grade lesions.[60] Eleven (46%) of 24 patients reviewed by Ahuja had medullary involvement; all patients with medullary involvement who had local resections had local recurrences.

TREATMENT. Wide excision of the tumor is the treatment of choice. This may be accomplished by an amputation or a limb-sparing procedure. There has been no experience reported of preoperative chemotherapy or radiation therapy. Parosteal osteosarcomas are often amenable to limb preservation due to their distal location, low grade, and lack of local invasiveness. If the adjacent neurovascular bundle is free of tumor, resection is feasible. Vascular displacement is not a contraindication for resection. The major surgical decision usually is whether to remove the entire end of the bone and the adjacent joint or to preserve the joint. Small lesions can be resected with joint preservation. If the medullary canal is involved, the joint usually cannot be preserved. A second factor mitigating against joint preservation is extensive cortical involvement. Techniques of resection and reconstruction are similar to those described for conventional osteosarcoma. The major difference is that only a small amount of soft tissue usually needs to be resected; consequently, a good functional result is obtained. Grade III parosteal lesions warrant systemic therapy due to the risk of metastasis.

Periosteal Osteosarcoma

Periosteal osteosarcoma is a rare cortical variant of osteosarcoma that arises superficially on the cortex, usually on the tibial shaft.[61] Radiographically, it is a small, radiolucent lesion with some evidence of bone spiculation. The cortex is characteristically intact with a scooped-out appearance and a Codman's triangle (Fig. 44–33). Histologically, periosteal osteosarcomas are relatively high-grade chondroblastic osteosarcomas composed of malignant cartilage with areas of anaplastic spindle cells and osteoid production. Unni and col-

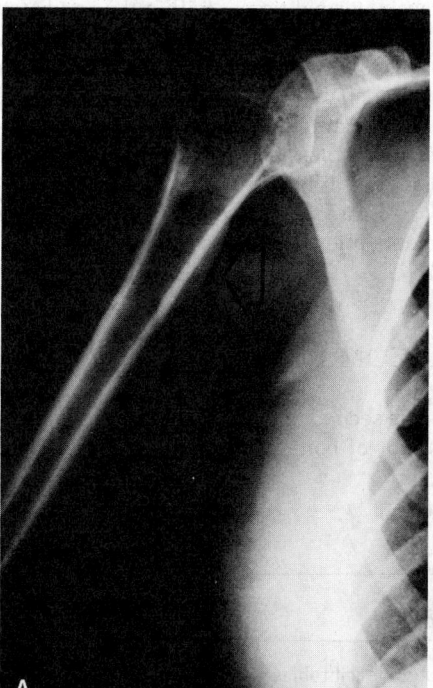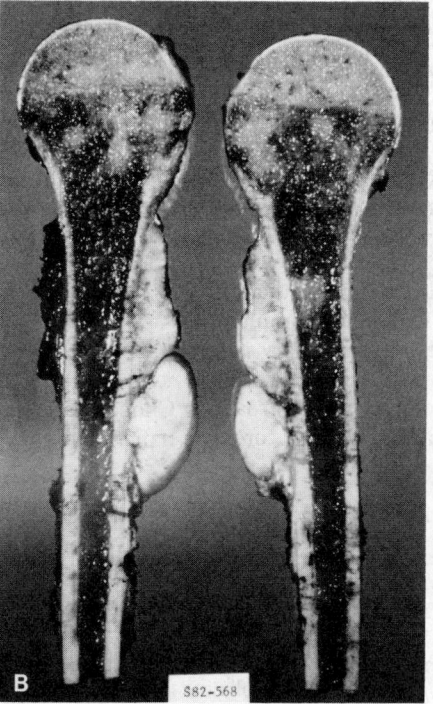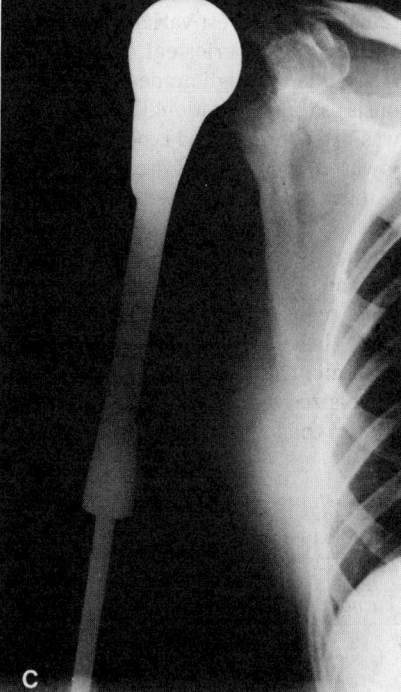

FIGURE 44–33. Periosteal osteosarcoma. **(A)** Typical radiograph of a periosteal osteosarcoma of the humerus. Notice the cortical location with a scooped-out defect of the lateral aspect of the shaft and the diaphyseal location. **(B)** Longitudinal section of the gross specimen after a limb-sparing resection. The tumor seems to arise on the outer cortex without any evidence of cortical involvement. **(C)** Postoperative radiograph. A custom prosthesis was used to reconstruct the defect. (Dunham WK, et al. Periosteal osteosarcoma. Cancer 1985;55:165–171)

leagues, in a report of 23 cases, found periosteal osteosarcomas to be one third as frequent as the parosteal variant.[61] The largest tumor measured 2.5 × 3.5 cm. Four of the 23 patients died of metastatic disease. Treatment is similar to that of other high-grade lesions. En bloc resection should be performed if feasible; otherwise, amputation is indicated. Table 44–13 compares the significant characteristics of periosteal tumors with those of conventional osteosarcoma.

Paget's Sarcoma

Approximately 1% of patients with Paget's disease develop a primary bone sarcoma.[223,224] Greditzer reported 41 sarcomas among 4415 patients with Paget's disease followed at the Mayo Clinic; 35 were osteosarcomas, and 6 were fibrosarcomas.[224] The average patient age was 64, and the most common sites were the pelvis, femur, and humerus. One half were osteolytic; the remainder had a mixed pattern. Cortical destruction and a soft tissue component were the most common signs found; periosteal elevation was rare. Most patients with this condition present with pain; a patient with known Paget's disease who complains of increasing pain, especially if it is well localized, should be evaluated radiographically. The diagnosis is usually made by plain radiography and confirmed by biopsy. Traditionally, fewer than 8% of patients survive, and most deaths occur within 2 years.[225] Treatment is similar to that recommended for adolescent patients with osteosarcoma without metastatic disease.

High-Grade Surface Osteosarcoma

High-grade surface osteosarcomas (*i.e.*, peripheral, conventional) is the rarest variant of surface osteosarcomas.[292] The parosteal and periosteal osteosarcomas have a better prognosis, and the high-grade surface variant has the same prognosis as the conventional, intramedullary lesion. This variant was previously called type III parosteal osteosarcoma. Schajowicz and coworkers studied the different surface osteosarcomas.[292] They reported that only 7 (9%) of 80 surface osteosarcomas were considered to be high-grade variants. The median age of patients was 13.5 years (younger than for other surface lesions), and most tumors were located in the diaphyseal region of the bone. The femur was the most common site. These tumors may show extensive intramedullary involvement. Radiographically, it appears as a small or moderate-sized lesion with slight to heavy calcification. The broad base of the lesion abuts the cortex. The radiographic features often are misleading and may suggest the periosteal variant. The preoperative diagnosis may be difficult. However, the young age, diaphyseal location, and highly malignant histologic features indicate the correct diagnosis. Wide excision with limb-preservation has been reported. Adjuvant chemotherapy is warranted due to its high rate of metastases.

Small Cell Osteosarcoma

Small cell osteosarcoma is a rare variant of osteosarcoma that resembles Ewing's sarcoma and is often classified as an "atypical" Ewing's sarcoma.[293,294] Characteristically, there are areas of osteoid and some chondroid formation. Differentiation from Ewing's sarcoma or the typical osteosarcoma is important, because its response to treatment is poorly defined. Sim and colleagues recommend surgery, but at the Pediatric Branch of the NCI, these tumors, like other pediatric round cell tumors, are treated by a combination of radiation therapy and chemotherapy.[293,294]

Radiation-Induced Osteosarcoma

Osteosarcomas that arise in a previously irradiated field and that meet the general criteria of a radiation-induced sarcoma (*i.e.*, latent for 5–20 years, documented secondary sarcoma, and occurring in a documented irradiated field) are rare. Amendola and coworkers from the University of Michigan reviewed 22,306 patients treated with irradiation between 1934 to 1983 and reported 23 patients with radiation-associated sarcomas.[295] The incidence was 0.1%. The median latent period was 13 years (range, 3–34 years). All sarcomas originated in previously normal tissues within the irradiated field. There were 5 bone sarcomas and 18 soft tissue sarcomas. The radiation dose ranged from 2500 to 7200 cGy. Their data suggested that intensive chemotherapy may have shortened the latency period. The treatment of radiation-induced osteosarcoma is wide resection if possible combined with adjuvant chemotherapy. The unique difficulty to the surgeon is the difficulty a previously irradiated field presents when choosing the best local treatment option. Increased local complications may be anticipated.

CHONDROSARCOMA

Chondrosarcoma is the second most common primary malignant spindle cell tumor of bone.[2] Chondrosarcomas form a

TABLE 44–13. Radiographic and Clinical Differential of Classic, Parosteal, and Periosteal Osteosarcoma

Type of Tumor	Common Anatomic Site	Location	Radiographic Appearance	Histology	Metastases
Classic	Distal femur, proximal tibia	Intramedullary	Destructive, osteoblastic/osteolytic	High grade (fibroblastic, chondroblastic and osteoblastic)	Early
Parosteal	Posterior distal femur	Cortical	Dense, homogenous new bone	"Mature" bone and fibroblastic stroma, low grade	Late
Periosteal	Proximal tibia and humerus	Cortical	"Scooped-out" lesion with calcification	Chondroblastic high grade	Intermediate

heterogenous group of tumors whose basic neoplastic tissue is cartilaginous without evidence of direct osteoid formation. Occasionally, bone formation occurs from differentiation of cartilage. If there is evidence of direct osteoid or bone production, the lesion is classified as an osteosarcoma. There are five types of chondrosarcoma: central, peripheral, mesenchymal, differentiated, and clear cell.[2–4,10] The classic chondrosarcomas are central (arising within a bone) or peripheral (arising from the surface of a bone). The other three are variants and have distinct histologic and clinical characteristics.

Central and peripheral chondrosarcomas can arise as primary tumors or secondary to underlying neoplasm (Fig. 44–34). Seventy-six percent of primary chondrosarcomas arise centrally.[2,10–12,212] Secondary chondrosarcomas most often arise from benign cartilage tumors. The multiple forms of benign osteochondromas or enchondromas have a higher rate of malignant transformation than the corresponding solitary lesions.[11,12,57,210]

CENTRAL AND PERIPHERAL CHONDROSARCOMAS

Clinical Characteristics

Half of all chondrosarcomas occur in patients older than 40.[2,211] Only 3.8% occur in patients younger than 20.[2] The most common sites are the pelvis (31%), femur (21%), and shoulder girdle (13%).[11,12,210–211] Chondrosarcomas are the most common malignant tumors of the sternum and scapula. The clinical presentation varies. Peripheral chondrosarcomas may become quite large without causing pain, and local symptoms develop only because of mechanical irritation. Pelvic chondrosarcomas are often large and present with referred pain to the back or thigh, sciatica secondary to sacral plexus irritation, urinary symptoms from bladder neck involvement, or unilateral edema due to iliac vein obstruction, or as a painless abdominal mass. Conversely, central chondrosarcomas

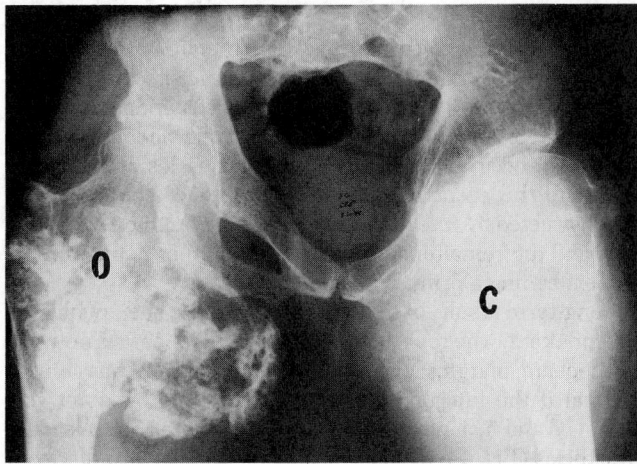

FIGURE 44–34. Radiograph of a patient with multiple hereditary osteochondromas. Notice the large sessile, lobulated osteochondroma (O) on the patient's right and a secondary (peripheral) chondrosarcoma (C) on the left. Secondary osteochondromas characteristically arise from benign underlying osteochondromas. Radiographically, they have poorly defined borders associated with a large soft tissue component with calcifications. This patient underwent a left modified hemipelvectomy.

present with dull pain. A mass is rare. Pain, which indicates active growth, is an ominous sign of a central cartilage lesion. This cannot be overemphasized. An adult with a plain radiograph suggestive of a "benign" cartilage tumor but associated with pain probably has a chondrosarcoma.

Histology and Grading

Chondrosarcomas are graded I, II, and III. Most chondrosarcomas are grade I or II.[1,10–12,210–212] The metastatic rate of moderate grade lesions is 15% to 40%; for high-grade lesions, it is 75%.[1,10–12,85,210] Grade III lesions have the same metastatic potential as osteosarcomas.[11,212]

Because cartilage tumors are difficult to grade histologically, some investigators have attempted to apply cytologic, histochemical and biochemical analysis to evaluate these lesions.[10,210,211,296,297] Sanerkin described a combination of cytologic and histologic criteria.[210] He emphasized that cytologic analysis evaluates nuclear abnormalities better than conventional histologic sections, and histologic evaluation of the bone-tumor interface is the best predictor of local aggressiveness. Krocberg performed a retrospective study of DNA content of 45 chondrosarcomas as an indicator of malignancy by evaluating diploid (normal DNA content) and hyperploid (abnormal increase in DNA) and correlating this to 10-year survival.[298] Regardless of tumor grade, size, and location, patients with diploid content had better prognoses than those with hyperploid DNA. A preliminary report on assessing the malignancy of cartilage tumor by flow cytometry to determine the percentage of diploid, tetraploid, and aneuploid cells indicates that it may be a promising method of grading chondrosarcomas.[299]

Radiographic Diagnosis and Evaluation

Central chondrosarcomas have two distinct radiologic patterns.[300] One is a small, well-defined lytic lesion with a narrow zone of transition and surrounding sclerosis with faint calcification. This is the most common malignant bone tumor that may appear radiographically benign. The second type has no sclerotic border and is difficult to localize. The key sign of malignancy is endosteal scalloping. It is difficult to diagnose on plain radiographs and may go undetected for a long period. In contrast, peripheral chondrosarcoma is recognized easily as a large, calcified mass protruding from a bone (see Fig. 44–34). Its differential diagnosis includes large benign osteochondroma, parosteal osteosarcoma, and juxtacortical myositis ossificans. Correlation of clinical, radiographic, and histologic data is essential for accurate diagnosis and evaluation of the aggressiveness of cartilage tumor. Proximal or axial location, skeletal maturity, and pain point toward malignancy, even though the cartilage may appear "benign."

Prognosis

Metastatic potential tends to correlate with the histologic grade of the lesion.[10–12,212] Marcove reported long-term follow-up of 113 chondrosarcomas of the proximal femur and pelvis.[212] The survival rates in patients with grade I, II, and III lesions were 47%, 38%, and 15%, respectively; the overall survival rate was 52%. There was no significant difference between grades I and II; however, the mortality rate for grade III was significantly higher ($p < 0.02$) than for the other two. Eleven of 59 deaths occurred after 5 years. He emphasized that the meaningful survival interval should be considered 10 or 15 years. There was no relation between prognosis and grade, age, sex, or location. There was no statistical difference between primary and secondary chondrosarcomas. Adequacy of surgical removal was the main determinant of recurrence. In general, chondrosarcomas occurring during childhood have a worse prognosis than those occurring in adulthood.[301]

In a review of 125 chondrosarcomas at the Instituto Ortopedico Rizzoli, Gitellis reported that adequacy of treatment was the main determinant of local recurrence, length of survival, and length of disease-free interval.[13] Patients adequately treated had a 6% local recurrence rate, but the recurrence rate among those inadequately treated was 69%. The 10-year survival rates were 78% (adequately treated) and 61% (inadequately treated). There was no relation between local recurrence and grade.

Peripheral chondrosarcomas have a lower grade than central lesions. Gitellis and associates reported that 43% of peripheral lesions were grade I, compared with 13% of central lesions.[13] Ten-year survival rates among those with peripheral lesions were 77%, compared with 32% among those with central lesions. Secondary chondrosarcomas arising from osteochondromas also have a low malignant potential; 85% are grade I. Garrison reported only 3% of 75 patients with secondary chondrosarcoma from an osteochondroma developed metastases, although 12% died of local recurrence.[57]

Treatment

Treatment of chondrosarcoma is surgical removal.[10,12,212,278,279,301,302] There have been no reports of effective adjuvant chemotherapy. Resection guidelines for high-grade chondrosarcomas are similar to those for osteosarcoma. The shoulder and pelvic girdle are the most common sites for chondrosarcoma. These sites, combined with the fact that chondrosarcomas tend to be low grade, make them amenable to limb-sparing procedures. Lesions of the ribs and sternum are treated by wide excision. Cryosurgery, a technique using liquid nitrogen after thorough curettage of the lesion, has been used for central, low-grade chondrosarcomas.[116,117] There have been a few reports of effective radiation therapy for axial chondrosarcomas, and most encouraging reports used fractionated proton radiation therapy for the low-grade chondrosarcomas arising at the base of the skull.[303] The Massachusetts General Hospital group report a 5-year local control rate of 82%, and a 10-year local control rate of 58% among 28 patients with low-grade base of skull chondrosarcomas treated to approximately 69 CGE (cobalt GY equivalent) using the proton beam.[303] High-grade chondrosarcomas warrant consideration of adjuvant chemotherapy.

Limb-Sparing Procedures for Specific Anatomic Sites

The four most common sites of chondrosarcomas are the pelvis, proximal femur, shoulder girdle, and diaphyseal portions of long bones.

Pelvis. The pelvis consists of three areas: ilium, periacetabulum, and pubic rami (Fig. 44–35). Each site may be re-

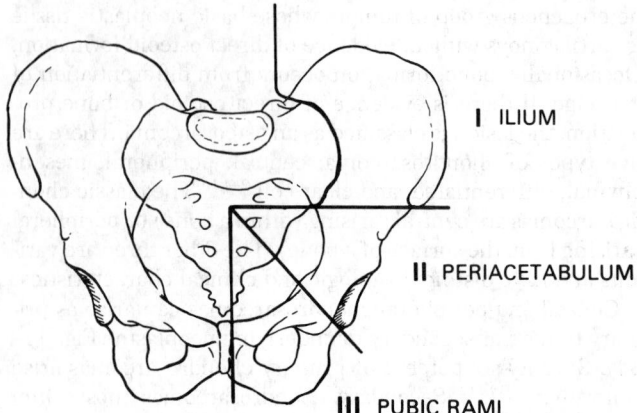

FIGURE 44–35.   Segmental resection for pelvic tumors.

sected independent of the others.[29,279] Resections are classified type I (iliac wing), type II (acetabulum), and type III (pubic rami, pelvic floor). Bone scan most accurately determines specific bony involvement, and CT and MRI can delineate the extraosseous component (Fig. 44–36). Contraindications to resection are vascular (*e.g.*, iliac artery and vein), peritoneal, and sacroiliac joint or sarcoplexus involvement.

The retroperitoneal space is explored first to determine resectability. Type I resection is performed by a supraacetabular osteotomy and disarticulation of the sacroiliac joint. Type II resection may require removal of the femoral head; intraarticular involvement of the hip joint by tumor is evaluated by arthrotomy before finalizing the surgical plan. Types II and III resections require mobilization of the iliac vessels and femoral nerve. Care must be taken to protect these structures. The type III procedure requires mobilization of the bladder and urethra before resection. Bilateral pelvic floor resection may be used for chondrosarcomas arising from the midline of the symphysis pubis, in which case urethral resection and reconstruction may be required. Partial cystectomy may be necessary.

Despite the magnitude of resection, pelvic reconstruction is less complex than that at other anatomic sites. Type I and III resections do not require bony reconstruction. In type I, the abductor musculature is closed to the abdominal wall muscles, and in type III, the perineal muscles are approximated to the adductor muscles. The periacetabular area is reconstructed by intentionally creating a nonunion of the femur and the remaining portion of the ilium or pubic rami or by performing a primary arthrodesis.

Long-term results of these procedures have been published by Enneking, who reported that local recurrence was only 4% if adequate margins were obtained.[29] Function was almost normal if the hip joint was preserved. If the hip joint was removed and fusion was obtained, results were good. A saddle prosthesis (Fig. 44–37) permits reconstruction after periacetabular resections with minimal morbidity.[304]

Proximal Femur. Chondrosarcoma of the proximal femur can often be treated successfully by resection and prosthetic replacement. A lateral trephine biopsy is recommended. Care must be taken to avoid intraarticular contamination. A posterior approach should be avoided because of potential con-

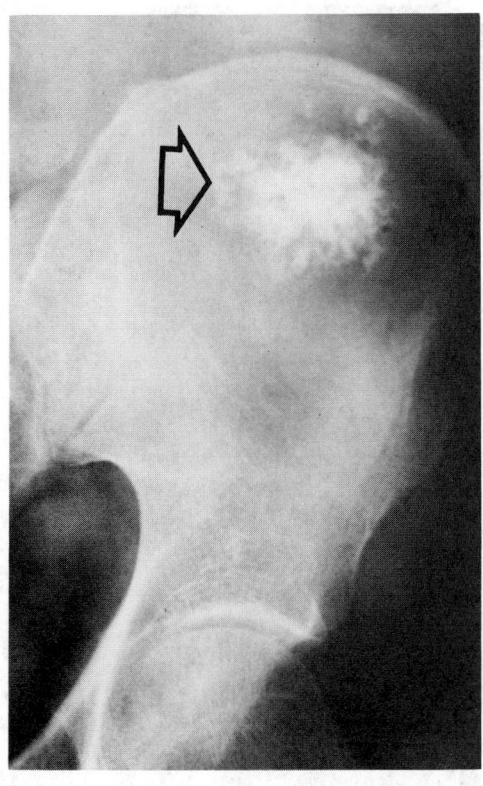

A

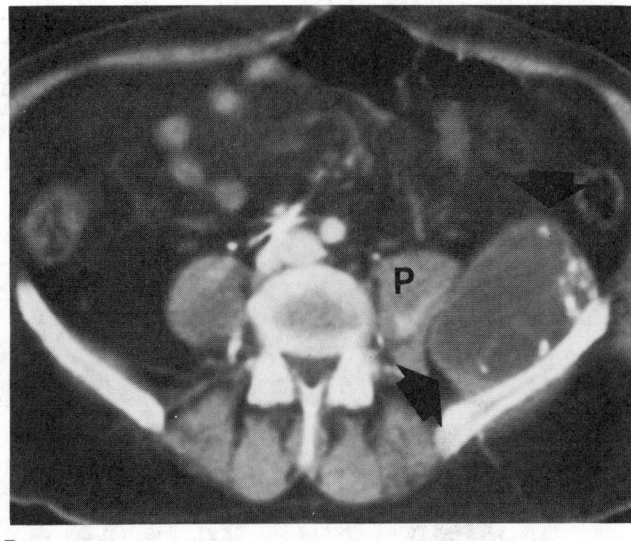

B

FIGURE 44–36. Chondrosarcoma of the pelvis. (**A** Plain radiograph demonstrates a small area of calcification within the ilium, suggesting a small intraosseous chondrosarcoma. (**B**) CT scan of the same area that surprisingly demonstrated a large chondrosarcoma (*solid arrows*) arising from the ilium, displacing the psoas muscle medially. The small area of calcification (*small solid arrow*) correlated with the plain radiograph (**A**).

tamination of the posterior flap in the event a hemipelvectomy is required.

Shoulder. The technique of resection of chondrosarcomas of the proximal humerus is similar to that described for osteosarcomas. In low-grade, intracompartmental (stage IA) tumors, preservation of the deltoid, rotator cuff musculature, and glenoid is possible, and there are several alternatives for reconstruction. Endoprosthesis, fibula autografts, and allografts have high rates of success.[34–39,125–127]

Segmental Resection for the Tibia, Femur, Humerus. Central diaphyseal chondrosarcomas can be adequately treated by segmental resection without sacrificing the adjacent joint. Because the ends of the bones are not involved, function is excellent. Reconstruction is performed by allografts or autografts combined with internal fixation.

Cryosurgery

Marcove pioneered the technique of cryosurgery for bone tumors. This method involves thorough curettage and cryotherapy of the cavity with liquid nitrogen.[115–117] With increasing experience, he expanded the indications to low-grade intramedullary cartilage tumors and to some high-grade lesions. Employing these indications, he has treated 30 chondrosarcomas with only one local recurrence. The major advantages of cryosurgery are preservation of bone stock and the avoidance of resection.

Radiation Therapy

Unresectable or inoperable chondrosarcomas arising within the axial skeleton and pelvic or shoulder girdle can be controlled and, in some cases, cured by radiation therapy. For

chondrosarcomas of the facial bones and skull, a combination of radiation therapy and surgery have been successful.

Although chondrosarcomas have been considered radioresistant, data show that some are radiocurable.[309] Among 38 patients undergoing radical irradiation, with or without concurrent chemotherapy, at the Princess Margaret Hospital, 5- and 10-year actuarial survival rates of 41% and 36%, respectively, were achieved. Median survival was 46 months.[309] The best results, a 48% 5-year actuarial survival rate, were obtained in the group with favorable (well and moderately differentiated) histology. Conversely, for those with unfavorable (mesenchymal and poorly differentiated) histology the 5-year survival rate was only 22%. Radical radiation therapy was defined as a minimum of 4000 cGy in 4 or more weeks of megavoltage therapy. Of the 38 patients treated, 17 developed local recurrence. The investigators recommend 5000 cGy in 4 weeks with treatment to the whole bone if possible and, if not, at least a 5-cm margin of normal bone. They found tumor regression continued slowly for 2 to 3 years after therapy.

McNaney and colleagues from MDACC reported 20 patients with chondrosarcoma treated with photons or neutrons, with or without chemotherapy.[310] The doses of radiation administered ranged from 4000 to 7000 cGy. Thirteen (65%) of 20 patients were surviving at a median of 30 months after treatment. Among the 11 patients treated with radiation therapy alone, 6 (54%) survived. Six patients, all of whom had received photon therapy alone, developed local failures. There were no local failures among the 4 patients treated with a mixed beam of photons and neutrons.

After radical irradiation, clinical regression of tumor is slow and may take months to complete. Radiographically, the affected bone never returns to normal. The combination of ex-

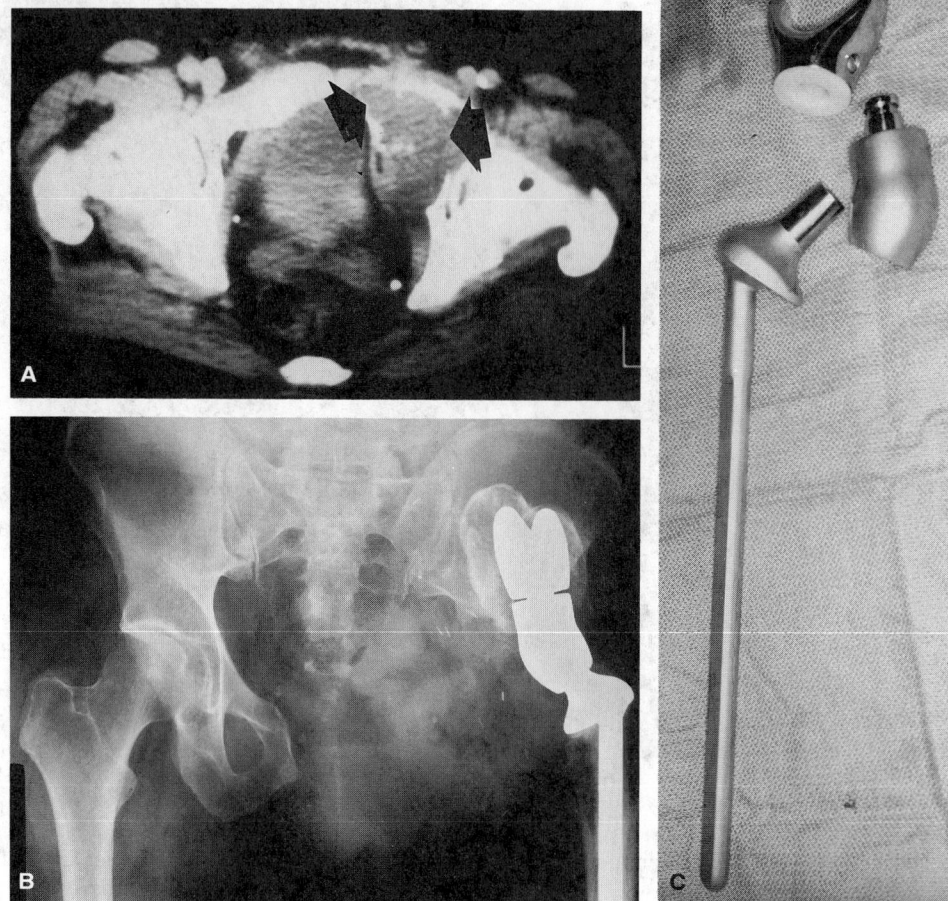

FIGURE 44–37. Limb-sparing resection for a large periacetabular chondrosarcoma involving the pelvic floor. **(A)** CT scan shows acetabular destruction by a large tumor mass (*arrows*) with involvement of the pubic rami. **(B)** The patient was treated by an internal hemipelvectomy (type II and III resection). **(C)** A custom-made saddle prosthesis was used for the reconstruction. This is a new type of pelvic prosthesis that has made pelvic reconstruction more reliable with less morbidity than other techniques.

tremely slow regression of tumor with a persistent radiologic defect makes follow-up and assessment of response difficult. Unfortunately, there are no rebiopsy data to document long-term sterilization of these tumors. Radiation therapy for chondrosarcoma can provide palliation. In such cases, high doses (approximately 5000 cGy in 4 to 5 weeks or its equivalent) are necessary; low doses for symptomatic relief are ineffective.[311]

Ryall and associates used irradiation and the radiosensitizer Razoxane (ICRF-159) in 8 patients with 12 chondrosarcomas. Seven tumors in 5 patients achieved complete or partial remission after 4500 to 6000 cGy. Two of the responders were disease free 2.5 years after treatment.[312]

Data on the relation between dose and tumor control probability are lacking; however, it seems apparent that prolonged local control requires a high radiation dose. Treatment planning requires documentation by CT of the extent of soft tissue disease.

There is some experience using radioactive ^{35}S for treatment of metastatic chondrosarcoma.[2,287] ^{35}S is selectively taken up by chondrocytes and bone marrow, causing tumor necrosis. Because of reports of associated ^{35}S-induced bone marrow suppression and severe aplastic anemia, this technique is not recommended.[2,313]

Treatment of the Maxilla, Mandible, and Skull

The treatment of chondrosarcomas of the maxilla, mandible, and skull entails irradiation and surgery, a combination that has a better potential for improving local control than surgery alone. Local recurrence rates as high as 85% have been reported for head and trunk lesions.[311,314] Among 18 patients with tumors of the head and neck, the MSKCC group reported local recurrence in 11 (61%).[315] The high local recurrence rate reflects the anatomic constraints on the surgical procedure. Austin-Seymour and associates reported an improved actuarial 5-year disease-free survival rate of 76% and local control rate of 82% for 28 patients receiving focused proton beam radiation therapy for low-grade chondrosarcomas of the base of the skull.[303]

VARIANTS OF CHONDROSARCOMA

Clear Cell Chondrosarcoma

Clear cell chondrosarcoma, the rarest form of chondrosarcoma, is a slow growing, locally recurrent tumor resembling a chondroblastoma but with some malignant potential.[305] It usually occurs in adults. The most difficult clinical problem is early recognition. It is often confused with chondroblastoma.

Metastases occur only after multiple local recurrences. Primary treatment is wide excision. Systemic therapy is not required.

Mesenchymal Chondrosarcoma

Mesenchymal chondrosarcoma is a rare, aggressive variant of chondrosarcoma characterized by a biphasic histologic pattern (*i.e.*, small, compact cells intermixed with islands of cartilaginous matrix).[306–308] These tumors have a predilection for flat bones; long, tubular bones are rarely affected.[211] They tend to occur in the younger age group and have a high rate metastatic potential. Harwood reported 8 of 17 patients died within 1 year of diagnosis.[306] The 10-year survival rate is 28%.[306] This entity responds favorably to radiation therapy. It is hypothesized that the round cell component, similar to other round cell sarcomas, is relatively radiosensitive. Treatment is surgical removal combined with adjuvant chemotherapy. Radiation therapy is recommended if the tumor cannot be completely removed.[306]

Approximately 10% of chondrosarcomas may dedifferentiate into a fibrosarcoma or osteosarcoma.[2,10,11,56] This occurs in older persons and is highly fatal. Surgical treatment is similar to that described for other high-grade sarcomas. Adjuvant therapy is warranted.

GIANT CELL TUMOR OF BONE

Giant cell tumor (GCT) of bone is an aggressive, locally recurrent tumor with a low metastatic potential.[14–16,63–64,211,313] It consists of spindle-shaped and ovoid cells uniformly interspersed with multinucleated giant cells. GCT refers to the de novo, malignant GCT, not the tumor that arises from the transformation of a giant cell tumor previously thought to be benign. These two lesions are separate clinical entities.

CLINICAL CHARACTERISTICS

GCTs occur slightly more often in female than male patients. Pain, mass, local tenderness, and decreased motion in the adjacent joint are the most common clinical symptoms. Eighty percent of GCTs in the long bones occur after skeletal maturity, and 75% of these develop around the knee joints.[2,3,63] Effusion or pathologic fracture, uncommon with other sarcomas, are common with GCT. The tumors occasionally occur in the vertebrae (2–5%) or the sacrum (10%).[2–4]

GRADING AND PATHOLOGIC CHARACTERISTICS

Jaffe attempted to grade GCTs: grade I (completely benign), grade II (borderline), and grade III (frankly sarcomatous).[4] Grades I and II do not correlate well with biologic behavior. There is also a poor correlation between the histologic pattern and the tendency for recurrence or malignant transformation.[14,15,63,211] Nineteen percent to 25% of giant cell tumors have some osteoid production.[211] If osteoid formation is found, care must be exercised in differentiating a GCT from an osteosarcoma. Conversely, an osteosarcoma with giant cells may be misinterpreted as a benign GCT. There is no correlation between osteoid formation and increased risk of recurrence or metastasis. Necrosis or hemorrhage is often found. Neither is related to malignant potential or local recurrence rate.[63]

NATURAL HISTORY

Although GCTs are rarely malignant de novo (2–8%), they may undergo transformation and demonstrate malignant potential histologically and clinically after multiple local recurrences.[14–16,177,288] Between 8.6% and 22% of known GCTs become malignant after local recurrence.[14–16,211,314] This rate decreases to less than 10% if patients who have undergone radiation therapy are excluded from the series. Hutter found that 40% of malignant GCTs were malignant at the first recurrence.[15] The remainder had become malignant by the second or third recurrence; each recurrence increases the risk of malignant transformation of typical GCT, especially if the transformation occurs after radiation therapy. Local recurrence of a GCT is determined by the adequacy of surgical removal rather than histologic grade.

RADIOGRAPHIC AND CLINICAL EVALUATION

Giant cell tumors are eccentric lytic lesions without matrix production. They have poorly defined borders with a wide area of transition. They are juxtaepiphyseal with a metaphyseal component. Although the cortex is expanded and appears destroyed at surgery, it is usually found to be attenuated but intact. Periosteal elevation is rare; soft tissue extension is common.

TREATMENT

Treatment of GCT of bone is surgical removal. Resection is curative for 90% of these tumors.[14,15,308] Curettage, with or without bone grafts, has a recurrence rate of 40% to 75%.[14–16,63,316] Johnson and Dahlin reported a recurrence rate of 29% within 1 year of curettage and of 54.1% within 5 years.[16] Although en bloc excision offers a reliable cure, routine resection is not recommended.[316] Primary resection of a joint has a significant morbidity. It is recommended for GCT of the proximal radius and fibula, distal ulna, tubular bones of hand and foot, coccyx, sacrum, and pelvic bones. Under certain situations, it is reasonable to perform a curettage. Goldenberg recommends that small tumors with an intact cortex and symptoms of less than 2 to 3 months' duration be treated by curettage.[63] If the lesion heals, resection is avoided. Curettage does not rule out a later curative resection.

The current technique of curettage is more extensive than previously performed. Curettage is accomplished through a large cortical window, equal to the length of the bony defect, using mechanical curettage and a mechanical burr. This extensive technique has been called "curettage/resection" and has significantly decreased the rate of local recurrence to approximately 15% to 25%. Bone graft and PMMA are used to reconstruct the surgical defect.

Amputation is reserved for massive recurrence, malignant transformation, or infection. Due to the biologic propensity for malignant transformation, irradiation is reserved for specific lesions, usually lesions of the spine, which cause bone destruction in a confined area and can lead to spinal cord compression and severe deformity.[107a] Treatment of GCT of the vertebrae and sacrum must be individualized. A combination of surgical excision and cryosurgery or radiation therapy is required to eradicate the tumor and prevent neurologic impairment.[106–107a]

Cryosurgery

Cryosurgery has been used more successfully for GCTs than for any other type of bone tumor.[115-117,317] Marcove developed the technique of cryosurgery because of the high recurrence rates after curettage and the significant risk of sarcomatous degeneration in tumors treated by irradiation. He found cryosurgery effective in eradicating the tumor while preserving joint motion and avoiding resection or amputation. He reported a 17-year experience of 100 GCTs treated by thorough curettage and cryosurgery.[117] He found a recurrence rate of 16% in the first 50 cases and 2% in the following 50 cases. The major complications of cryosurgery are necrosis of the adjacent bones, which may develop a late pathologic fracture, and delayed union. Rate of secondary pathologic fracture has been decreased by a combination of PMMA augmentation, bone graft, internal fixation of the cavity, and postoperative use of a long-leg brace with a quadrilateral socket.[317,318] Persson from Sweden reported curettage with PMMA augmentation of the bony defect with bony necrosis due to the heat of polymerization. This technique may provide better local control than curettage alone.[319]

Radiation Therapy

The indications for irradiation include inoperable and incompletely resected lesions and locally recurring lesions despite definitive surgery. These situations are most likely to occur in the spine.[320] Doses of 4500 to 5500 cGy in 5 to 6 weeks using megavoltage equipment are recommended.[181,215,295,321,322]

There has been a long and justified apprehension that some patients may develop a malignant and fatal neoplasm after irradiation.[324,325] This concern was supported by Dahlin from the Mayo Clinic, who reported that malignant degeneration ultimately appeared in 37 patients treated with irradiation alone or in combination with a surgical procedure.[323] The average time for malignant change was approximately 9 years. McGrath presented data from the Bristol Tumor Registry that substantiate this concern.[324] Neither of these studies break down the radiation dose to bone in patients who did or did not develop malignancies. It is known that some of these patients were treated with orthovoltage radiation, and multiple courses were given.

The Princess Margaret Hospital group reported that local tumor has been controlled in 13 of 14 patients with giant cell tumor treated with one course of megavoltage radiation. The disease of 12 patients was controlled for longer than 5 years.[321] The researchers observed no instance of malignant transformation. Larsson and colleagues reported 3 patients with giant cell tumor of the spine and sacrum treated by moderate doses of radiation therapy; all have done well.[320]

MALIGNANT FIBROUS HISTIOCYTOMA

CLINICAL CHARACTERISTICS

Malignant fibrous histiocytoma (MFH) is a high-grade bone tumor histologically similar to its soft tissue counterpart.[7-9] It is a disease of adulthood. The most common sites are the metaphyseal ends of long bones, especially around the knee. Alkaline phosphatase values are normal. Pathologic fracture is common. Huvos emphasized that a lytic metaphyseal lesion with a pathologic fracture in an adult with a normal serum alkaline phosphatase level suggests a primary MFH rather than an osteosarcoma or fibrosarcoma.[9] MFH disseminates rapidly. Spanier reported that 9 of 11 patients died of the tumor. The average disease-free survival was 6 months.[7] She reported one third of patients (3 of 9) with pulmonary metastasis had lymph node dissemination. She hypothesized that lymphatic spread was due to the histiocytic component of the tumor.

RADIOGRAPHIC CHARACTERISTICS

MFH is an osteolytic lesion associated with marked cortical disruption, minimal cortical or periosteal reaction, and no evidence of matrix formation.[9] The extent of the tumor routinely exceeds plain radiographic signs. McCarthy and associates reporting on 35 patients with MFH, found that four tumors were multicentric and four were associated with bone infarcts.[8]

TREATMENT

There have been few reports about the efficacy of chemotherapy for MFH of bone.[213,326,327] Bacci and colleagues reported 12 patients treated by surgery and chemotherapy, compared with 18 patients treated with surgery alone over the same time at the Instituto Ortopedico Rizzoli.[326] The disease-free survival rates were 59% (7 of 12) and 5% (1 of 18), respectively. Heeten reported 3 patients with MFH treated by preoperative chemotherapy; a grade IV response (100% necrosis) was obtained in all 3.[327]

Earl and coworkers from the Royal National Orthopedic Hospital evaluated the chemosensitivity of MFH of bone.[328] Eighteen patients were treated with preoperative and postoperative chemotherapy consisting of methotrexate, ifosfamide, and doxorubicin. Four patients had 100% tumor necrosis; 2 patients had more than 90%, and the remainder had between 50% and 70% tumor necrosis. Of 13 patients presenting with localized disease (median, 24 months), only 1 patient had died at the time of the report. They concluded that MFH of bone was a chemosensitive lesion and suggested long-term studies to determine if there is a survival advantage to adjuvant chemotherapy.

Due to the extremely poor prognosis of MFH, chemotherapy is thought to be justified. Although there are only limited data, there are striking similarities to the results seen with osteosarcoma. The primary approach to treatment of MFH of bone is radical surgical resection combined with adjuvant chemotherapy.

FIBROSARCOMA OF BONE

CLINICAL CHARACTERISTICS

Fibrosarcoma of bone is a rare entity characterized by interlacing bundles of collagen fibers (*i.e.*, herringbone pattern) without any evidence of tumor bone or osteoid formation.[5] Fibrosarcoma occurs in middle age. The long bones are most affected. Fifteen percent of tumors are found in the bones of the head and neck.[211] Fibrosarcomas occasionally arise in conjunction with an underlying disease, such as fibrous dysplasia, Paget's disease, bone infarcts, osteomyelitis, and post-irradiation bone and giant cell tumor.[5] Fibrosarcoma may be central or cortical (*i.e.*, periosteal). The histologic grade is a good prognosticator of metastatic potential. Huvos reported overall survival rates of 27% and 52% for central and peripheral lesions, respectively.[5] Late metastases do occur, and 10- and 15-year survival rates vary. Periosteal tumors usually have a better prognosis than central lesions.

RADIOGRAPHIC DIAGNOSIS AND TREATMENT

Fibrosarcoma is a radiolucent lesion that shows minimal periosteal and cortical reaction. The radiographic appearance closely correlates with the histologic grade of the tumor.[5] Low-grade tumors are well defined, but high-grade lesions demonstrate indistinct margins and bone destruction similar to osteolytic osteosarcoma. Plain radiographs often underestimate the extent of the lesion. Pathologic fracture is common (30%) because of the lack of matrix formation. Differential diagnosis includes GCT, aneurysmal bone cyst, MFH, and osteolytic osteosarcoma.[5,6]

Fibrosarcoma of bone is primarily managed surgically. Irradiation is recommended for inoperable tumors and for patients with postsurgical residual disease and for palliation.

CHORDOMA

CLINICAL PRESENTATION AND DIAGNOSIS

Chordoma is a rare neoplasm arising from notochordal remnants in the midline of the neural axis and involving the adjacent bone. The ends of the spine are the most common sites. The sacrococcus and the base of the skull (35%) near the sphenooccipital area are most commonly involved, accounting for 50% and 35%, respectively, of all chordomas.[211] Histologically, the physaliferous cell is pathognomonic. Large areas of syncytial strands of cells lying in a mass of mucus

are typically present. Myxoid chondrosarcoma and metastatic carcinoma must be differentiated. This tumor is highly fatal due to the high rate of local recurrence and local complications.[329–332] Death is most commonly due to local disease.[329] Gray and colleagues reviewed 222 cases from the literature and observed that only 2 patients were disease free at 10 years.[332] Average survival was 5.7 years. Mindell emphasized the main malignant potential of chordomas resides in their critical locations adjacent to important structures, their locally aggressive nature, and their extremely high rate of recurrence.[329] Chordomas at the base of the skull are often described as chondroid chordomas. Patients with these lesions at this site tend to survive longer than those with sacrococcygeal tumors.

The most common complaint of patients with sacrococcygeal tumors is dull pain; constipation is an occasional symptom. Bladder and sensory loss are late complaints. Clinical suspicion is the key to early diagnosis. Rectal examination characteristically reveals a large presacral mass. Sphenooccipital tumors present with signs of cranial nerve or pituitary dysfunction. CT and MRI are essential for accurate evaluation (Fig. 44–38). Myelography is used to determine intraspinal extension. A transrectal biopsy should not be performed because of potential contamination. A small midline posterior incision or trocar biopsy is recommended.

TREATMENT

Surgery

The first surgical procedure has the best chance of cure.[331,332] Inadequate surgery results in local recurrence, with little chance of subsequent surgical removal. Sacrococcygeal tumors are best removed by a combined abdominosacral approach, as described by Localio and colleagues.[302,303] They emphasized wide excision of the sacrum one level higher than the lesion. A lateral position is used. The rectum can be mobilized and the iliac vessels controlled anteriorly. The rectum may be removed with the sacrum if necessary. Guterberg and

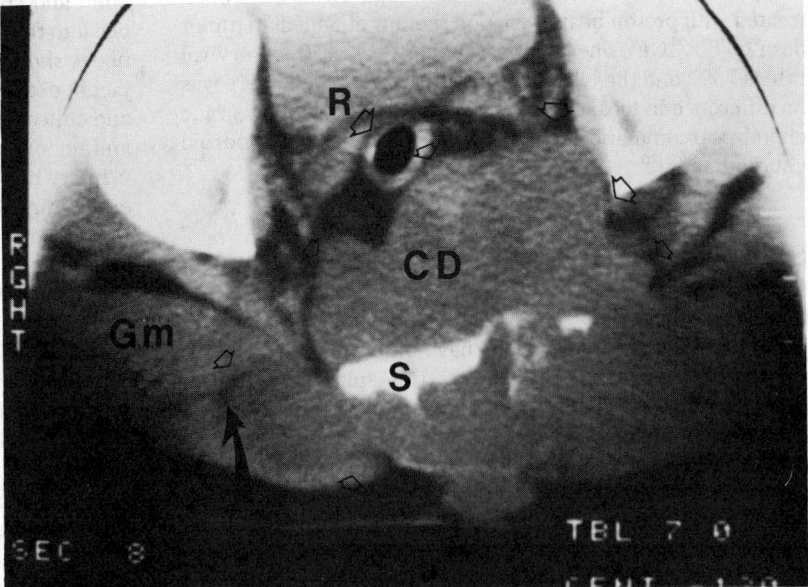

FIGURE 44–38. Computed tomography of a chordoma arising within the sacrum (s). There is destruction of the body of the sacrum with a huge soft tissue component (outlined by *small arrows*). The tumor (CD) extends to the rectum (R) and is infiltrating the gluteus maximus (Gm) muscle (*black arrow*). These are typical findings of a sacrococcygeal chordoma, which explains the difference in obtaining local control. Differential diagnosis includes metastatic carcinoma and giant cell tumor of the sacrum.

associates reported that if only half of the first sacral vertebra remains bilaterally, the pelvic girdle is still stable enough to allow immediate mobilization.[333] Recently De Vries reported 2 long-term survivors (7 and 10 years) after cryosurgery of sacral chordomas.[334]

Radiation Therapy

Because local recurrence is common with chordomas, radiation therapy is an integral treatment modality, particularly for tumors of the base of skull and sphenooccipital region. Results of conventional radiation therapy have been disappointing. Heffelfinger and colleagues reported 36 patients with nonchondroid varieties of chordomas of the base of skull, none of whom were rendered free of disease by surgery, irradiation, or a combination thereof.[335] However, the chondroid variant is more sensitive; of 19 patients with chondroid chordomas, 7 were alive, and 6 were disease free. Other investigators reported 5 patients with cervical chordomas, only one who was alive and disease free 5 years after irradiation and surgery.[336]

Amendola and associates reported 21 patients with a 5-year survival rate of 50% but a disappointing 10-year survival rate of only 20%. This is not surprising, because chordomas are relatively slow growing.[337] Long-term survival free of tumor regrowth over 10 years is relatively rare.[338] Amendola emphasized the importance of using CT in planning the radiation field, high radiation doses (*i.e.*, 5500–7000 cGy with megavoltage equipment), and use of irradiation immediately after surgery to prolong local control, rather than reserving it until recurrence. The Massachusetts General Hospital (MGH) experience of 48 patients is similar to that reported by others; 50% of the patients survived 5 years or more.[339] Radiation doses varied from 4500 to 8040 cGy, but even with high doses, there was a 45% incidence of local recurrence.

Investigators at MGH and the University of California now advocate using precision heavy-charged-particle irradiation, particularly for chordoma of the basisphenoid region and cervical spine. The MGH experience now includes 68 patients, 40 with chordomas and 28 with low-grade chondrosarcomas of the basisphenoid region and cervical spine who have been treated with proton-beam radiation therapy at a median tumor dose of 69 CGE. The actuarial 5-year disease free survival rate is 76%, and the local control rate is 82%.[340,341] There was no difference in local control between patients with low-grade chondrosarcoma and those with chondroid or nonchondroid chordoma.[303,340]

SMALL ROUND CELL SARCOMAS OF BONE

Round cell sarcomas of bone behave differently and require different therapeutic management from spindle cell sarcomas.[342,343] These tumors consist of poorly differentiated small cells without matrix production. They present radiographically as osteolytic lesions. These lesions are best treated with irradiation and chemotherapy; surgery is reserved for special situations. Non-Hodgkin's lymphoma and Ewing's sarcoma are the two most common small cell sarcomas. The differential diagnosis of all round cell sarcomas includes metastatic neu-

roblastoma, metastatic undifferentiated carcinoma, histiocytosis, small cell osteosarcoma, osteomyelitis, and multiple myeloma.

LYMPHOMAS OF BONE

CLINICAL PRESENTATION AND DIAGNOSIS

Diffuse large cell lymphoma of bone (previously called reticulum cell sarcoma of bone) accounts for only 5% of the primary bone tumors. Lymphoma presenting in bone is usually a sign of disseminated (stage IV) disease; occasionally, it may be a true solitary lesion defined as "involvement of single extralymphatic organ or site (stage IE)."[342,343] Reimer at the NCI reported that only 1 of 12 patients presenting with bone lymphomas had a true solitary lesion.[342] Sweet and colleagues from the University of Chicago reported that 50% of so-called solitary lesions were associated with disease elsewhere.[343] Sweet presented a useful algorithm for the evaluation and treatment of bone lymphomas. He emphasized that all patients with a presumed solitary lymphoma of bone should undergo a thorough evaluation for other involvement.[343]

Treatment is based on extent of disease. Stage IE lesions have traditionally been treated with radiation therapy, with a reported 90% cure rate.[342] The role of surgery is limited to obtaining adequate tissue for diagnosis and treatment of pathologic fracture. The technique of biopsy is important to avoid secondary fracture through potentially irradiated bone. Biopsy for a suspected round cell tumor should always include a frozen section and additional material for electron microscopy, tissue culture, and immunophenotyping. Patients presenting with pathologic fractures require fixation. To prevent late fractures, all patients treated with radiation therapy should be protected with a brace until reossification occurs.

RADIATION THERAPY

Local control of the primary tumor with retention of good function of the affected part is commonly achieved after radiation therapy. Radiation therapy is administered to the entire bone and soft tissue extent with a dose of 4000 cGy and a boost to the original tumor area to 5000 cGy. Regional lymph nodes should be included in the radiation port if they are adjacent to the area treated or if clinically involved. Mendenhall and colleagues from the University of Florida, achieved local and regional control in all irradiated sites of 21 patients with primary bone lymphoma.[344] Two patients relapsed in apparently uninvolved regional lymph node sites that had not been included in the primary treatment portal.

Patients with lymphoma of the bone should be considered as having systemic disease and accordingly require chemotherapy. Investigators from Dana-Farber Cancer Center reported 11 children who had been treated with irradiation and chemotherapy consisting of APO (doxorubicin, prednisone, cyclophosphamide), with an 8-year actuarial lymphoma-free survival of 100% and a disease-free survival rate of 79%, for an overall actuarial survival rate of 90%.[345] There were no relapses. This is consistent with experience from the Bone Tumor Center, Bologna, Italy, where 23 (88%) of 26 patients survived disease free after irradiation and chemotherapy with doxorubicin, vincristine, and cyclophosphamide, with no local relapses at 7.5 years (median) of follow-up.[346] In the Dana-Farber experience, 2 patients developed second bone tumors, 5 and 7.5 years after beginning therapy. Because of the success from intensive combination chemotherapy, investigators have begun to question the need for primary radiation therapy among children responding to multiagent chemotherapy.[347,348] Current pediatric protocols using multiagent chemotherapy for non-Hodgkin's lymphoma do not routinely use radiation therapy for those with primary lymphoma of the bone.

REFERENCES

1. Silverberg E, Lubera, J. Cancer statistics, 1987. CA 1987;37:2–20.
2. Dahlin DC. Bone tumors: General aspects and data on 6,221 cases. 3rd ed. Springfield: Charles C Thomas, 1978.
3. Lichtenstein L. Bone tumors. 5th ed. St. Louis: CV Mosby, 1977.
4. Jaffe HL. Tumors and tumorous conditions of the bone and joints. Philadelphia, Lea & Febiger, 1958.
5. Huvos AG, Higinbotham NL. Primary fibrosarcoma of bone. A clinicopathologic study of 130 patients. Cancer 1975;35:837–847.
6. Wilner D. Fibrosarcoma. In: Wilner D, ed. Radiology of bone tumors and allied disorders, I. Philadelphia: WB Saunders, 1982:2291–2324.
7. Spanier SS, Enneking WF, Enriquez P. Primary malignant fibrous histiocytoma of bone. Cancer 1975;36:2084–2098.
8. McCarthy EF, Matsuno T, Dorfman HD. Malignant fibrous histiocytoma of bone: A study of 35 cases. Hum Pathol 1979;10:57–70.
9. Huvos AG. Primary malignant fibrous histiocytoma of bone. Clinicopathologic study of 18 patients. N Y State J Med 1976;76:552–559.
10. Shives TS, Wold LE, Dahlin DC, Beabout JW. Chondrosarcoma and its variants. In: Sim FH, ed. Diagnosis and treatment of bone tumors: A team approach. Thorofare, NJ: Slack, 1983:211–217.
11. Marcove RC. Chondrosarcoma: Diagnosis and treatment. Orthop Clin North Am 1977;8:811–819.
12. Pritchard DJ, Lunke RJ, Taylor WF, et al. Chondrosarcoma: A clinicopathologic statistical analysis. Cancer 1980;45:149–157.
13. Gitellis S, Bertoni F, Chieti PP, Campanacci M. Chondrosarcoma of bone. J Bone Joint Surg [Am] 1981;1248–1256.
14. Dahlin DC, Cupps RE, Johnson EW Jr. Giant cell tumor: A study of 195 cases. Cancer 1970;25:1061–1070.
15. Hutter VP, Worcester JN Jr, Francis KC, et al. Benign and malignant giant cell tumor of bone. A clinicopathological analysis of the natural history of the disease. Cancer 1962;15:653–690.
16. Johnson EW Jr, Dahlin DC. Treatment of giant cell tumor of bone. J Bone Joint Surg [Am] 1959;41:895–904.
17. Nascimento AG, Huvos AC, Marcove RC. Primary malignant giant cell tumor of bone: A study of eight cases and review of the literature. Cancer 1979;44:1393–1402.
18. Weingard DN, Rosenberg SA. Early lymphatic spread of osteogenic and soft-tissue sarcomas. Surgery 1978;84:231–240.
19. Enneking WF, Spanier SS, Goodman MA. A system for the surgical staging of musculoskeletal sarcoma. Clin Orthop 1980;153:106–120.
20. Marcove RC, Rosen G. En bloc resection for osteogenic sarcoma. Cancer 1980;45:3040–3044.
21. Malawer MM. Distal femoral osteogenic sarcoma, principles of soft tissue resection and reconstruction in conjunction with prosthetic replacement (adjuvant surgery). In: Chao EYS, ed. Design and application of tumor prosthesis for bone and joint reconstruction. New York: Thieme-Stratton, 1983:297–309.
22. Morton DL, Eilber FR, Townsend CM Jr, et al. Limb salvage from a multidisciplinary treatment approach for skeletal and soft tissue sarcomas of the extremity. Ann Surg 1976;184:268–278.
23. Enneking WF, Dunham WK. Resection and reconstruction for primary neoplasms involving the innominate bone. J Bone Joint Surg 1978;60:731–746.
24. Marcove RC, Lewis MM, Rosen G, et al. Total femur and total knee replacement: A preliminary report. Clin Orthop 1977;126:147–152.
25. Eilber FR, Morton DL, Eckardt J, et al. Limb-salvage for skeletal and soft tissue sarcomas: Multidisciplinary preoperative therapy. Cancer 1984;53:2579–2584.
26. Eilber FR, Eckhardt J, Morton DL. Advances in the treatment of sarcomas of the extremity: Current status of limb salvage. Cancer 1984;54:2695–2701.
26a. Weisenburg TH, Eilber FR, Grant TT, et al. Multidisciplinary "limb salvage" treatment of soft tissue and skeletal sarcomas. Int J Radiat Oncol Biol Phys 1981;7:1495.
27. Simon MA, Aschliman MA, Thomas N, et al. Limb-salvage treatment versus amputation for osteosarcoma of the distal end of the femur. J Bone Joint Surg [Am] 1986;68:1331–1337.
28. Enneking WF. Modification of the system for functional evaluation of surgical management of musculoskeletal tumors. In: Enneking WF, ed. Limb-sparing surgery for musculoskeletal tumors. New York: Churchill Livingstone, 1987:626–639.
29. Enneking WF, Dunham WK. Resection and reconstruction for primary neoplasms involving the innominate bone. J Bone Joint Surg [Am] 1978;60:731–746.
30. Marcove RC, Lewis MM, Rosen G, et al. Total femur and total knee replacement. A preliminary report. Clin Orthop 1977;126:147–152.
31. Mankin HJ, Fogelson FS, Thrasher AZ, et al. Massive resection and allograft transplantation in the treatment of malignant bone tumors. N Engl J Med 1976;294:1247–1255.
32. Watts HG. Introduction to resection of musculoskeletal sarcomas. Clin Orthop 1980;153:31–38.
33. Enneking WF, Shirley PD. Resection-arthrodesis for malignant and potentially malignant lesions about the knee using an intramedullary rod and local bone graft. J Bone Joint Surg [Am] 1977;59:223–235.
34. Janeck CJ, Nelson CL. Enbloc resection of shoulder girdle: Technique and indications. Report of a case. J Bone Joint Surg [Am] 1972;54:1754–1758.
35. Francis KC, Worcester JN Jr. Radical resection for tumors of the shoulder with preservation of a functional extremity. J Bone Joint Surg [Am] 1962;44:1423–1429.
36. Marcove RC, Lewis MM, Huvos AG. En bloc upper humeral-interscapular resection, the Tikhoff-Linberg procedure. Clin Orthop 1977;124:219–228.
37. Chaos EYS, Ivins JC. Design and application of tumor prosthesis for bone and joint reconstruction—The design and application. New York: Thieme-Stratton, 1983.
38. Malawer MM, Sugarbaker PH, Lambert M, et al. Limb-salvage surgery for tumors of the proximal humerus and shoulder girdle. The Tikhoff-Linberg procedure and its modifications. Surgery 1955;97:518–528.
39. Sim FH, Bowman WE, Chao EYS. Limb salvage surgery and reconstructive techniques. In: Sim FH, ed. Diagnosis and treatment of bone tumors: A team approach. Thorofare, NJ: Slack, 1983:75–105.
40. De Santos LA, Bernardino ME, Murry JA. Computed tomography in the evaluation of osteosarcoma: Experience with 25 cases. AJR 1979;132:535–540.
41. Destouet JM, Gilula LA, Murphy W. Computed tomography of long bone osteosarcoma. Radiology 1979;131:439–445.
42. Mckillop JH, Etcubanas E, Goris ML. The indications for and limitations of bone scintigraphy in osteogenic sarcoma: A review of 55 patients. Cancer 1981;48:1133–1138.
43. Levine E. Computed tomography of musculoskeletal tumors. Crit Rev Diagn Imaging 1981;16:279–309.
44. Rosenthal DI. Computed tomography in bone and soft tissue neoplasms: Application and pathologic correlation. Crit Rev Diagn Imaging 1982;18:243–278.
45. Goldstein H, McNeil BJ, Zufall E, et al. Changing indications for bone scintigraphy in patients with osteosarcoma. Radiology 1980;135:177–180.
46. Bacci G, Picci P, Calderoni P, et al. Full-lung tomograms and bone scanning in the initial work-up of patients with osteogenic sarcoma. A review of 126 cases. Eur J Cancer Clin Oncol 1982;18:967–971.
47. Jaffe N, Link MP, Cohen D, et al. High-dose methotrexate in osteogenic sarcoma. NCI Monogr 1981;56:201–206.
48. Cortes EP, Holland JF, Wang JJ, et al. Amputation and Adriamycin in primary osteosarcoma. N Engl J Med 1974;291:998–1000.
49. Rosen G, Marcove RC, Caparros B, et al. Primary osteogenic sarcoma. The rationale for preoperative chemotherapy and delayed survey. Cancer 1979;43:2163–2177.
50. Rosen G, Caparros B, Huvos AC, et al. Preoperative chemotherapy for osteogenic sarcoma: Selection of postoperative adjuvant chemotherapy based upon the response of the primary tumor to preoperative chemotherapy. Cancer 1982;49:1221–1230.
51. Muggia F, Catani R, Lee YJ, et al. Factors responsible for therapeutic success in osteosarcoma. In: Jones S, Salmon S, eds. Adjuvant therapy for cancer. 2nd ed. New York: Grune & Stratton, 1979.
52. Cortes EP, Holland JP. Adjuvant chemotherapy for primary osteogenic sarcoma. Surg Clin North Am 1981;61:1391–1404.
53. Rosen G, Murphy ML, Huvos AG, et al. Chemotherapy, en bloc resection and prosthetic replacement in the treatment of osteogenic sarcoma. Cancer 1976;37:1–11.
54. Goorin AM, Frei E II, Abelson HT. Adjuvant chemotherapy for osteosarcoma: A decade of experience. Surg Clin North Am 1981;61:1379–1389.
55. Lichtenstein L. Classification of primary tumors of bone. Cancer 1951;4:335–341.
56. Spjut HJ, Dorfman HD, Fechner DE, Ackerman LV. Tumors of bone and cartilage. In: Atlas of tumor pathology, fasc. 5, 2nd series. Washington, DC: Armed Forces Institute of Pathology, 1971.
57. Garrison RC, Unni KK, Mcleod RA, et al. Chondrosarcoma arising in osteochondroma. Cancer 1982;49:1890–1897.
58. Merryweather R, Middlemiss JH, Sanerkin NG. Malignant transformation of osteoblastoma. J Bone Joint Surg [Br] 1980;62:381–384.
59. Dahlin DC, Unni KK. Osteosarcoma of bone and its important recognizable varieties.
60. Ahuja SC, Villacin AB, Smith J, et al. Juxtacortical (parosteal) osteogenic sarcoma. J Bone Joint Surg [Am] 1977;59:632–647.
61. Unni KK, Dahlin DC, Beabout SW. Periosteal osteogenic sarcoma. Cancer 1976;37:2476–2485.
62. Unni KK, Dahlin DC, McLeod RA, Pritchard DJ. Interosseous well-differential osteosarcoma. Cancer 1977;40:1337–1347.
63. Goldenberg RR, Campbell CJ, Bonfiglio M. Giant cell tumor of bone. An analysis of two hundred and eighteen cases. J Bone Joint Surg [Am] 1970;52:619–664.
64. Johnson EW, Dahlin DC. Treatment of giant cell tumor of bone: An evaluation of 24 cases treated at the Johns Hopkins hospital between 1925–1955. Orthopedics 1969;62:187–191.
65. Madewell JE, Ragsdale BD, Sweet DE. Radiographic and pathologic analysis of solitary bone lesions. Radiol Clin North Am 1981;19:715–814.
66. Johnson LC. A general theory of bone tumors. Bull N Y Acad Med 1953;19:164–171.
67. Lodwick GS. The bone and joints. In: Enneking WF, ed. Atlas of tumor radiology. Chicago: Year Book Medical Publishers, 1971.
68. Enneking WF. Musculoskeletal tumor surgery, vol. I. New York: Churchill Livingstone, 1983:1–60.

69. Jeffree GM, Price CHG, Sissins HA. The metastatic spread of osteosarcoma. Br J Cancer 1975;32:87–107.

70. McKenna RJ, Schwinn CP, Soong KY, Higinbotham NL. Sarcomata of the osteogenic series (osteosarcoma, fibrosarcoma, chondrosarcoma, parosteal osteosarcoma and sarcomata arising in abnormal bone: An analysis of 552 cases. J Bone Joint Surg [Am] 1966;48:1–26.

71. Marcove RC, Mike V, Hajack JV, et al. Ostegenic sarcoma under the age of twenty-one. J Bone Joint Surg [Am] 1970;52:411–423.

72. Sweetnam R. Surgical management of primary osteosarcoma. Clin Orthop 1975;111: 57–64.

73. Campanacci M, Bacci G, Bertoni F, Picci P, Minutillo A, Franceschi C. The treatment of osteosarcoma of the extremities: Twenty years' experience at the Instituto Ortopedico Rizzoli. Cancer 1981;48:1569–1581.

74. Campanacci M, Bacci G, Bertoni F, et al. The treatment of osteosarcoma of the extremity: Twenty years' experience at the Instituto Orthopedico Rizzoli. Cancer 1981;48:1569–1581.

75. Brostrom L-A. On the natural history of osteosarcoma. Aspects of diagnosis, prognosis and endocrinology. Acta Orthop Scand Suppl 1980;183:1–38.

76. Enneking WF, Kagan A. Intramarrow spread of osteosarcoma. In: Management of primary bone and soft tissue tumors. Chicago: Yearbook Medical Publishers, 1976: 171–177.

77. Malawer MM, Dunham WF. Skip metastases in osteosarcoma: Recent experience. J Surg Oncol 1983;22:236–245.

78. Enneking WF, Spanier SS, Malawer MM. The effect of the anatomic setting on the results of surgical procedure for soft parts sarcoma of the thigh. Cancer 1981;47: 1005–1022.

79. Simon MA, Spanier SS, Enneking WF. The management of soft tissue tumors of the extremities. J Bone Joint Surg [Am] 1976;60:317.

80. Simon MA. Intra-articular extension of adult primary bone sarcomas: Implications for limb-sparing surgical procedures. In: Chao, EYS, Ivins JS, eds. Tumor prosthesis for bone and joint reconstruction. The design and application. New York: Thieme-Stratton, 1983.

81. Bohndorf, K, Reiaer M, Lochner B, et al. Magnetic resonance imaging of primary tumours and tumour-like lesions of the skeleton. Skeletal Radiol 1986;15:511–517.

82. Cohen MD, Weetman RM, Provisor AJ, et al. Efficacy of magnetic resonance imaging in 139 children with tumors. Arch Surg 1986;121:522–529.

83. Turner DA. Nuclear magnetic resonance in oncology. Semin Nucl Med 1985;15: 210–223.

84. Zimmer WD, Berquist TH, McLeod RA, et al. Bone tumors: Magnetic resonance imaging versus computed tomography. Radiology 1985;155:709–718.

85. Powers JA. Magnetic resonance imaging in marrow diseases. Clin Orthop 1985;206: 79–85.

86. Sundaram M, McGuire MH, Herbold DR. Magnetic resonance imaging of osteosarcoma. Skeletal Radiol 1987;16:23–29.

87. Easton EJ, Powers JA. Musculoskeletal magnetic resonance imaging. Thorofare, NJ: Slack, 1986.

88. Pettersson H, Springfield DS, Enneking WF. Radiologic management of musculo-skeletal tumors. New York: Springer-Verlag, 1986.

89. Link MP. Adjuvant therapy in the treatment of osteosarcoma. In: DeVita VT, Hellman S, Rosenberg SA, eds. Important advances in oncology. Philadelphia: JB Lippincott, 1986:193–207.

90. Link MP, Goorin AM, Miser AW, et al. The effect of adjuvant chemotherapy on relapse-free survival in patients with osteosarcoma of the extremity. N Engl J Med 1986;314:1600–1606.

91. Eilber F, Giliano A, Eckardt J, et al. Adjuvant chemotherapy for osteosarcoma: A randomized prospective trial. J Clin Oncol 1987;5:21–26.

92. Edmonson J, Creagan E, Gilchrist G. Phase II study of high dose methotrexate in patients with unresectable metastatic osteosarcoma. Cancer Treat Rep 1981;65:5438–5439.

93. Rosen G, Nirenberg A. Chemotherapy for osteogenic sarcoma: An investigative method, not a recipe. Cancer Treat Rep 1982;66:1687–1697.

94. Dahlin DC. The problems in assessment of new treatment regimens of osteosarcoma. Clin Orthop 1980;153:81–85.

95. Goorin A, Perez-Atayde A, Gebhardt A, et al. Weekly high-dose methotrexate and doxorubicin for osteosarcoma: The Dana Farber Cancer Institute/The Children's Hospital—study III. J Clin Oncol 1987;5:1178–1184.

96. Ettinger LJ, Douglas HO, Mindell ER, et al. Adjuvant adriamycin and cisplatin in newly diagnosed, non-metastatic osteosarcoma of the extremity. J Clin Oncol 1986;4: 353–362.

97. Rosen G, Marcove RC, Huvos AG, Caparros BI, Lane JM, Nirenberg A, Cacavio A, Groshen S. Primary osteogenic sarcoma: 8-Year experience with adjuvant chemotherapy. J Cancer Res Clin Oncol 1983;106:55–67.

98. Winkler K, Beron G, Kotz R, et al. Neoadjuvant chemotherapy for osteogenic sarcoma: Results of a Cooperative German/Austrian study. J Clin Oncol 1984;2:617–624.

99. Winkler K, Beron G, Delling G, et al. Neoadjuvant chemotherapy of osteosarcoma: Results of a randomized cooperative trial (COSS-82) with salvage chemotherapy based on histological tumor response. J Clin Oncol 1988;6:329–337.

100. Tobias JD, Pratt CB, Parham DM, et al. The significance of calcified regional lymph nodes at the time of diagnosis of osteosarcoma. Orthopedics 1985;8:49–52.

101. Giuliano AE, Feig S, Eilber F. Changing metastatic patterns of osteosarcoma. Cancer 1984;54:2160–2164.

102. Jaffee N, Smith E, Abelson H, Frei E. Osteogenic sarcoma. Alterations in the pattern of pulmonary metastases with adjuvant chemotherapy. J Clin Oncol 1983;1:251–254.

102a. Wuisman P, Enneking WF. Prognosis of patients who have osteosarcoma with skip metstasis. J Bone Joint Surg [Am] 1990;72:60–68.

102b. Spanier SS, Schuster JJ, Vander Griend RA. The effect of local extent of the tumor on prognosis in osteosarcoma. J Bone Joint Surg [Am] 1990;72:643–652.

103. Enneking WF. The issue of the biopsy. [Editorial] J Bone Joint Surg [Am] 1982;64: 1119–1120.

104. Mankin HJ, Lange TA, Spanier S. The hazards of biopsy in patients with malignant primary bone and soft-tissue tumors. J Bone Joint Surg [Am] 1982;64:1121–1127.

105. Hudson TM, Hass G, Enneking WF, Hawkins EF. Angiography in the management of musculoskeletal tumors. Surg Gynecol Obstet 1975;141:11–21.

106. Malawer MM, McHale KA. Limb-sparing surgery for high grade malignant tumors of the proximal tibia: Surgical technique and a new method of extensor mechanism reconstruction. Presented at the 4th International Symposium on Limb-salvage Surgery in Musculoskeletal Oncology, Kyoto, Japan, 1987.

106a. Bloem JL, Taminiau AHM, Eulderink F, Hermans J, Pauwels EKJ. Radiologic staging of primary bone sarcoma: MR imaging, scintigraphy, angiograhpy and CT correlated with pathologic examination. Radiology 1988;169:805–810.

107. Moore TM, Meyers MH, Patzakis MJ, et al. Closed biopsy of musculoskeletal lesions. J Bone Joint Surg [Am] 1979;61:375–380.

107a. Savino R. Gherlinzoni F, Morandi M, et al. Surgical treatment of giant-cell tumor of the spine. J Bone Joint Surg [Am] 1983;65:1283–1289.

108. Schajowicz F, Derqui JC. Puncture biopsy in lesions of the locomotor system. Review and results in 4050 cases, including 941 vertebral punctures. Cancer 1968;21:5331–5487.

109. Springfield DS, Goodman MA. Biopsy of musculoskeletal lesions. Orthopedics 1980;3: 868–870.

110. Mail JT, Cohen MD, Mirkin LD, Provisor AJ. Response of osteosarcoma to preoperative intravenous high-dose methotrexate chemotherapy: CT evaluation. AJR 1985;144: 89–93.

111. Jaffe N, Knapp J, Chuang VP, Wallace S, et al. Osteosarcoma: Intraarterial treatment of the primary tumor with *cis*-diammine-dichlorplatinum II (CDP): Angiographic, pathologic, and pharmacologic studies. Cancer 1983;51:402–407.

112. Chuang VP, Benjamin R, Jaffe N, et al. Radiographic and angiographic changes in osteosarcoma after intra-arterial chemotherapy. AJR 1982;139:1065–1069.

112a. Carrasco CH, Charnsangavel C, Raymond AK, et al. Osteosarcoma: Angiographic assessment of response to preoperative chemotherapy. Radiology 1989;170:839–842.

112b. Hogeboom WR, Hoekstra HJ, Mooyaart EL, Oosterhuis JE, Postma A, Veth RPH, Koops HS. Magnetic resonance imaging (MRI) in evaluating in vivo response to neoadjuvant chemotherapy for osteosarcomas of the extremities. Eur J Surg Oncol 1989;15:424, 430.

113. Smith J, Heelan RT, Huvos AG, et al. Radiographic changes in primary osteogenic sarcoma following intensive chemotherapy. Radiology 1982;143:355–360.

114. Sommer H-J, Knop J, Heise U, Winkler K, Delling G. Histomorphometric changes of osteosarcoma after chemotherapy, Correlation with ^{99}Tc methylene diphosphonate functional imaging.

115. Marcove RC, Lyden JP, Huvos AC, Bullough PB. Giant cell tumor treated by cryo-surgery. Report of 25 cases. J Bone Joint Surg [Am] 1973;55:1633–1644.

116. Marcove RC, Stovell P, Huvos AC, Bullough P. The use of cryosurgery in the treatment of low and medium grade chondrosarcoma: A preliminary report. Clin Orthop 1977;122:147–156.

117. Marcove RC. A 17-year review of cryosurgery in the treatment of bone tumors. Clin Orthop 163:231–233.

118. Enneking WF, Spanier SS, Goodman MA. A system for the surgical staging of mus-culoskeletal sarcoma. Clin Orthop 1980;153:106–120.

119. Marcove RC, Rosen G. En bloc resection for osteogenic sarcoma. Cancer 1980;45: 3040–3044.

120. Malawer MM. Distal femoral osteogenic sarcoma, principles of soft tissue resection and reconstruction in conjunction with prosthetic replacement (adjuvant surgery). In, Chao EYS, ed. Design and application of tumor prosthesis for bone and joint reconstruction. New York: Thieme—Stratton, 1983:297–309.

121. Morton DL, Eilber FR, Townsend CM Jr, Grant TT, et al. Limb salvage from a mul-tidisciplinary treatment approach for skeletal and soft tissue sarcomas of the extremity. Ann Surg 1976;184:268–278.

122. Enneking WF. Concluding material. In: Enneking WF, ed. Limb-sparing surgery for musculoskeletal tumors. New York: Churchill Liningstone, 1987:624–639.

123. Malawer MM, Meller I. Porous-coated segmental prosthesis for large tumor defects—a prosthesis based upon immediate fixation (PMA) and extracortical bone fixation: Analysis of 20 consecutive patients. Annual meeting of the Musculoskeletal Tumor Society, Toronto, 1987.

124. Heck DA, Chao EY, Sim FH, et al. Titanium fibermetal segmental replacement prostheses and radiographic analysis and review of current status. Clin Orthop 1987;204:266–285.

125. Mankin HJ, Fogelson FS, Thrasher AZ, et al. Massive resection and allograft trans-plantation in the treatment of malignant bone tumors. N Engl J Med 1976;294:1247–1255.

125a. Malawer MM. Unpublished data.

125b. Makley JT, Krailo M, Ertel IJ, et al. The relationship of various aspects of surgical management to outcome in childhood nonmetastatic osteosarcoma: A report from the Children's Cancer Study Group. J Pediatr Surg 1988;23:146–151.

126. Enneking WF. A system for the functional evaluation of the surgical management of musculoskeletal tumors. In Enneking WF, ed. Limb-sparing surgery for musculoskeletal tumors. New York: Churchhill Livingstone, 1987.

127. Miller G. Opening remarks. In Enneking WF, ed. Limb-sparing surgery for musculoskeletal tumors. New York: Churchill Livingstone, 1987.

128. Malawer MM, Baker A. Amputations for tumor. In: Evarts CM, ed. Surgery of the musculoskeletal system. 2nd ed. New York: Churchill Livingstone, 1989.

129. Marcove RC, Mike V, Hajek JV, Levin AG, Hutter RVP. Osteogenic sarcoma under the age of twenty-one. A review of one hundred and forty-five operative cases. J Bone Joint Surg [Am] 1970;52:411–423.

130. Mike V, Marcove RC. Osteogenic sarcoma under the age of 21: Experience at Memorial Sloan-Kettering Cancer Center. In: Terry WD, Windhorts D, eds. Immunotherapy of cancer: Present status of trials in man. New York: Raven Press, 1978.

131. Gehan EA, Sutow WW, Uribe-Botero G, Romsdahl M, Smith TL. Osteosarcoma: The M.D. Anderson experience, 1950–1974. In: Terry WD, Windhorst D, eds. Immunotherapy of cancer: Present status of trials in man. New York: Raven Press 1978.

132. Uribe-Botero G, Russell W, Sutow W, Martin R. Primary osteosarcoma of bone: A clinicopathologic investigation of 243 cases, with necropsy studies in 54. Am J Clin Pathol 1977;67:427–435.

133. Friedman MA, Carter SK. The therapy of osteogenic sarcoma: Current status and thoughts for the future. J Surg Oncol 1972;4:482–610.

134. Taylor WF, Ivins JC, Dahlin DC, Edmonson JH, Pritchard DJ. Trends and variability in survival from osteosarcoma. Mayo Clin Proc 1978;53:695–700.

135. Taylor WF, Ivins JC, Dahlin DC, Pritchard DJ. Osteogenic sarcoma experience at the Mayo Clinic, 1963–1974. In: Terry WD, Windhorts D, eds. Immunotherapy of cancer: Present status of trials in man. New York: Raven Press, 1978.

136. Taylor WF, Ivins J, Pritchard D, Dahlin DC, Gilchrist GS, Edmonson JH. Trends and variability in survival among patients with osteosarcoma: A 7-year update. Mayo Clin Proc 1985;60:91–104.

137. Strander H, Adamson U, Aparisi T, et al. Adjuvant interferon treatment of human osteosarcoma. Recent Results Cancer Res 1979;68:40–44.

138. Rab GT, Ivins JC, Childs DS, Cupps RE, Pritchard DJ. Elective whole lung irradiation in the treatment of osteogenic sarcoma. Cancer 1976;38:939–942.

139. Breur K, Cohen P, Schweisguth O, Hart A. Irradiation of the lungs as an adjuvant therapy in the treatment of osteosarcoma of the limbs: An EORTC randomized study. Eur J Cancer 1978;14:461–471.

140. Edmonson JH, Green SJ, Ivins JC, et al. A controlled pilot study of high-dose methotrexate as post surgical adjuvant treatment for primary osteosarcoma. J Clin Oncol 1984;2:152–156.

141. Link MP, Goordin AM, Miser AW, et al. The effect of adjuvant chemotherapy on relapse-free survival in patients with osteosarcoma of the extremity. N Engl J Med 1986;314:1600–1606.

142. Link MP, Shuster JJ, Goorin AM, et al. Adjuvant chemotherapy in the treatment of osteosarcoma: Results of the Multi-institutional Osteosarcoma Study. In: Ryan J, Baker LO, eds. Recent concepts in sarcoma treatment. Proceedings of the International Symposium on Sarcomas, Tarpon Springs, Florida, October 8–10, 1987. Dorecht, The Netherlands: Kluwer Academic Publishers, 1988:283–290.

143. Link MP, Goorin AM, Horowitz M, Meyer WH, Belasco J, Baker A, Ayala A, Shuster J. Adjuvant chemotherapy of high grade osteosarcoma of the extremity: Updated results of the Multi-institutional Osteosarcoma Study. Clin Orthop 1991;Sept(270):8–14.

144. Eilber F, Giuliano A, Eckardt J, Patterson K, Moseley S, Goodnight J. Adjuvant chemotherapy for osteosarcoma: A randomized prospective trial. J Clin Oncol 1987;5:21–26.

145. Laster WR Jr, Mayo JG, Simpson-Herren L, Griswold DP Jr, Lloyd HH, Schabel FM Jr, Skipper HE. Success and failure in the treatment of solid tumors. II. Kinetic parameters and "cell cure" of moderately advanced carcinoma 755. Cancer Chemother Rep 1969;53:169–188.

146. Schabel FM. Rationale for adjuvant chemotherapy. Cancer 1977;39:2875–2882.

147. Schabel FM Jr. The use of tumor growth kinetics in planning "curative" chemotherapy of advanced solid tumors. Cancer Res 1969;29:2384–2389.

148. Cortes EP, Holland JF, Wang JJ, Sinks LF. Doxorubicin in disseminated osteosarcoma. JAMA 1972;221:1132–1138.

149. Nitschke R, Starling KA, Vats T, Bryan H. Cis-diamminedichloroplatinum (NSC-119875) in childhood malignancies: A Southwest Oncology Group study. Med Pediatr Oncol 1978;4:127–132.

150. Ochs JJ, Freeman AL, Douglass HO, Higby DS, Mindell ER, Sinks LF. Cis-dichlorodiammineplatinum (II) in advanced osteogenic sarcoma. Cancer Treat Rep 1978;62:239–245.

151. Baum ES, Gaynon P, Greenberg L, Krivitt W, Hammond D. Phase II study of cis-dichlorodiammineplatinum (II) in childhood osteosarcoma: Children's Cancer Study Group report. Cancer Treat Rep 1979;63:1621–1627.

152. Gasparini M, Rouesse J, van Oosterom A, et al. Phase II study of cisplatin in advanced osteogenic sarcoma. Cancer Treat Rep 1985;69:211–213.

153. Jaffe N, Farber S, Traggis D, et al. Favorable response of metastatic osteogenic sarcoma to pulse high-dose methotrexate with citrovorum rescue and radiation therapy. Cancer 1973;31:1367–1373.

154. Pratt C, Howarth C, Ransom J, et al. High dose methotrexate used alone and in combination for measurable primary and metastatic osteosarcoma. Cancer Treat Rep 1980;64:11–20.

155. Jaffe N, Frei E, Traggis D, Watts H. Weekly high-dose methotrexate-citrovorum factor in osteogenic sarcoma. Pre-surgical treatment of primary tumor and overt pulmonary metastases. Cancer 1977;39:45–50.

156. Marti C, Kroner T, Remagen W, Berchtold W, Cserhati M, Varini M. High-dose ifosfamide in advanced osteosarcoma. Cancer Treat Rep 1985;69:115–117.

157. Edmonson J, Creagan E, Gilchrist G. Phase II study of high dose methotrexate in patients with unresectable metastatic osteosarcoma. Cancer Treat Rep 1981;65:538–539.

158. Grem J, King S, Wittes R, Leyland-Jones B. The role of methotrexate in osteosarcoma. JNCI 1988;80:626–655.

159. Rosen G, Nirenberg A. Chemotherapy for osteogenic sarcoma: An investigative method, not a recipe. Cancer Treat Rep 1982;66:1687–1697.

160. Cortes EP, Holland JF, Wang JJ, Sinks LF, Blom J, Senn H, Bank A, Glidewell O. Amputation and Adriamycin in primary osteosarcoma. N Engl J Med 1974;291:998–1000.

161. Mosende C, Gutierrez M, Caparros B, Rosen G. Combination chemotherapy with bleomycin, cyclophosphamide and dactinomycin for the treatment of osteogenic sarcoma. Cancer 1977;40:2779–2786.

162. Frei E, Jaffe N, Skipper HE, Gero MG. Adjuvant chemotherapy of osteogenic sarcoma: Progress and perspectives. In: Salmon SE, Jones SE, eds. Adjuvant therapy of cancer. Amsterdam: Elsevier/North Holland Biomedical Press, 1977:49–64.

163. Jaffe N, Frei E, Traggis D, Bishop Y. Adjuvant methotrexate and citrovorum-factor treatment of osteogenic sarcoma. N Engl J Med 1974;291:994–997.

164. Goorin A, Delorey M, Gelber RD, Price K, Vawter G, Jaffe N, Watts H, Link M, Frei E, Abelson HT. The Dana-Farber Cancer Institute/The Children's Hospital adjuvant chemotherapy trials for osteosarcoma: Three sequential studies. Cancer Treat Rep 1986;3:155–159.

165. Rosenberg SA, Chabner BA, Young RC, et al. Treatment of osteogenic sarcoma. I. Effect of adjuvant high-dose methotrexate after amputation. Cancer Treat Rep 1979;63:739–751.

166. Cortes EP, Holland JF, Glidewell O. Amputation and Adriamycin in primary osteosarcoma: A 5-year report. Cancer Treat Rep 1978;62:271–277.

167. Cortes EP, Holland JF, Glidewell O. Adjuvant therapy of operable primary osteosarcoma—Cancer and Leukemia Group B experience. Recent Results Cancer Res 1979;68:16–24.

168. Cortes E, Necheles TF, Holland JF, Carey RW, Blom J, Brunner K, Falkson G, Weinberg V. Adjuvant chemotherapy for primary osteosarcoma: A Cancer and Leukemia Group B experience. In: Salmon S, Jones S. eds. Adjuvant therapy of cancer, III. New York: Grune & Stratton, 1981:201–210.

169. Goorin A, Perez-Atayde A, Gebhardt M, et al. Weekly high dose methotrexate and doxorubicin for osteosarcoma: The Dana Farber Cancer Institute/The Children's Hospital—study III. J Clin Oncol 1987;5:1178–1184.

170. Krailo M, Ertel I, Makley J, et al. A randomized study comparing high-dose methotrexate with moderate-dose methotrexate as components of adjuvant chemotherapy in childhood nonmetastatic osteosarcoma: A report from the Children's Cancer Study Group. Med Pediatr Oncol 1987;15:69–77.

171. Sutow WW, Sullivan MP, Fernbach DJ, Cangir A, George SL. Adjuvant chemotherapy in primary treatment of osteogenic sarcoma. A Southwest Oncology Group study. Cancer 1975;36:1598–1602.

172. Sutow WW, Gehan EA, Dyment PG, Vietti T, Miale T. Multidrug adjuvant chemotherapy for osteosarcoma: Interim report of Southwest Oncology Group studies. Cancer Treat Rep 1978;62:265–269.

173. Herson J, Sutow WW, Elder K, Vietti TJ, Falletta JM, Crist WM, Vats TS, Miale T. Adjuvant chemotherapy in nonmetastatic osteosarcoma: A Southwest Oncology Group study. Med Pediatr Oncol 1980;8:343–352.

174. Pratt CB, Champion JE, Fleming ID, Rao B, Kumar PM, Evans WE, Green AA, George S. Adjuvant chemotherapy for osteosarcoma of the extremity. Long-term results of two consecutive prospective protocol studies. Cancer 1990;65:439–445.

175. Ettinger LJ, Douglass HO, Higby DJ, Mindell ER, Nime F, Ghoorah J, Freeman AI. Adjuvant Adriamycin and cis-diamminedichloroplatinum (cis-platinum) in primary osteosarcoma. Cancer 1981;47:248–254.

176. Ettinger LJ, Douglass HO, Mindell ER, Sinks L, Tebbi CK, Risseeuw D, Freeman AI. Adjuvant Adriamycin and cisplatin in newly diagnosed, non-metastatic osteosarcoma of the extremity. J Clin Oncol 1986;4:353–362.

177. van der Schueren E, Breur K. Role of lung irradiation in the adjuvant treatment of osteosarcoma. Recent Results Cancer Res 1982;80:98–102.

178. Rosen G, Murphy ML, Huvos AG, Gutierrez M, Marcove RC. Chemotherapy, en bloc resection, and prosthetic bone replacement in the treatment of osteogenic sarcoma. Cancer 1976;37:1–11.

179. Rosen G, Marcove RC, Caparros B, Nirenberg A, Kosloff C, Huvos AG. Primary osteogenic sarcoma. The rationale for preoperative chemotherapy and delayed surgery. Cancer 1979;43:2163–2177.

180. Rosen G, Marcove RC, Huvos AG, Caparros BI, Lane JM, Nirenberg A, Ccavio A, Groshen S. Primary osteogenic sarcoma: Eight-year experience with adjuvant chemotherapy. J Cancer Res Clin Oncol 1983;106:55–67.

181. Miser J, Arndt C, Smithson W, et al. Treatment of high grade osteosarcoma (OGS) with ifosamide (Ifos), mesna, Adriamycin (ADR), and high dose methotrexate (HDMTX). Proc Am Soc Clin Oncol 1991;10:310.

182. Huvos A, Rosen G, Marcove RC. Primary osteogenic sarcoma. Pathologic aspects in 20 patients after treatment with chemotherapy, en bloc resection and prosthetic bone replacement. Arch Pathol Lab Med 1977;101:14–18.

183. Winkler K, Beron G, Kotz R, et al. Neoadjuvant chemotherapy for osteogenic sarcoma: Results of a cooperative German/Austrian study. J Clin Oncol 1984;2:617–624.

184. Winkler K, Beron G, Kotz R, et al. Adjuvant chemotherapy in osteosarcoma—effects of cisplatinum, BCD, and fibroblast interferon in sequential combination with HD-MTX and Adriamycin. Preliminary results of the COSS 80 study. J Cancer Res Clin Oncol 1983;106:1–7.

185. Winkler K, Beron G, Delling G, et al. Neoadjuvant chemotherapy of osteosarcoma: Results of a randomized cooperative trial (COSS-82) with salvage chemotherapy based on histological tumor response. J Clin Oncol 1988;6:329–337.

186. Bacci G, Picci P, Ruggieri P, et al. Primary chemotherapy and delayed surgery (neoadjuvant chemotherapy) for osteosarcoma of the extremities. The Instituto Rizzoli experience in 127 patients treated preoperatively with intravenous methotrexate (high versus moderate doses) and intraarterial cisplatin. Cancer 1990;65:2539–2553.

187. Provisor A, Nachman J, Krailo M, Ettinger L, Hammond D. Treatment of non-metastatic osteogenic sarcoma of the extremities with pre- and post-operative chemotherapy. Proc Am Soc Clin Oncol 1987;6:217.

188. Hudson M, Jaffe MR, Jaffe N, et al. Pediatric osteosarcoma: Therapeutic strategies, results and prognostic factors derived from a 10-year experience. J Clin Oncol 1990;8:1988–1997.

189. Goldie JH, Coldman AJ. A mathematical model for relating the drug sensitivity of tumors to their spontaneous mutation rate. Cancer Treat Rep 1979;63:1727–1733.

190. DeVita VT. The relationship between tumor mass and resistance to chemotherapy. Cancer 1983;51:1209–1220.

191. Salzer-Kuntschik M, Delling G, Beron G, Sigmund R. Morphological grades of regression in osteosarcoma after polychemotherapy. Study COSS 80. J Cancer Res Clin Oncol 1983;106:21–24.

192. Jaffe N, Prudich J, Knapp J, et al. Treatment of primary osteosarcoma with intra-arterial and intravenous high-dose methotrexate. J Clin Oncol 1983;1:428–431.

193. Meyers PA, Heller G, Healey J, et al. Chemotherapy for non-metastatic osteogenic sarcoma: The Memorial-Sloan-Kettering experience. J Clin Oncol 1992;10:5–15.

194. Rosen G, Caparros B, Huvos AG, et al. Preoperative chemotherapy for osteogenic sarcoma: Selection of postoperative adjuvant chemotherapy based on the response of the primary tumor to preoperative chemotherapy. Cancer 1982;49:1221–1230.

195. Weiner M, Harris M, Lewis M, Jones R, Sherry H, Feuer EJ, Johnson J, Lahman E. Neoadjuvant high-dose methotrexate, cisplatin, and doxorubicin for the management of patients with nonmetastatic osteosarcoma. Cancer Treat Rep 1986;70:1431–1432.

196. Bramwell V, Burgers M, Sneath R, Jelliffe A, van Oosterom A, Voute T, Freedman L, van Glabbeke M. Preliminary report of the First European Osteosarcoma Intergroup study. Proc Am Soc Clin Oncol 1988;7:273.

197. Avella M, Bacci G, McDonald DJ. Adjuvant chemotherapy with six drugs (Adriamycin, methotrexate, cisplatinum, bleomycin, cyclophosphamide, and dactinomycin) for non-metastatic high grade osteosarcoma of the extremities. Results of 32 patients and comparison to 127 patients concomitantly treated with the same drugs in a neoadjuvant form. Chemioterapia 1988;7:133–137.

198. Look AT, Douglass EC, Meyer WH. Clinical importance of near-diploid tumor stem lines in patients with osteosarcoma of an extremity. N Engl J Med 1988;318:1567–1572.

199. Jaffe N, Knapp J, Chuang VP, et al. Osteosarcoma: Intra-arterial treatment of the primary tumor with *cis*-diammine-dichloroplatinum II (CDP): Angiographic, pathologic and pharmacologic studies. Cancer 1983;51:402–407.

200. Jaffe N, Robertson R, Ayala A, et al. Comparison of intra-arterial *cis*-diamminedichloroplatinum II with high dose methotrexate and citrovorum factor rescue in the treatment of primary osteosarcoma. J Clin Oncol 1985;3:1101–1104.

201. Eilber FR, Eckardt J, Morton DL. Advances in the treatment of sarcomas of the extremity. Current status of limb salvage. Cancer 1984;54:2695–2701.

202. Winkler K, Bielack S, Delling G, et al. Effect of intraarterial versus intravenous cisplatin in addition to systemic doxorubicin, high-dose methotrexate, and ifosfamide on histologic tumor response in osteosarcoma (study COSS-86). Cancer 1990;66:1703–1710.

203. Martin NS, Williamson J. The role of surgery in the treatment of malignant tumors of the spine. J Bone Joint Surg [Br] 1970;52:227–237.

204. Sterner B. Total spondylectomy in chondrosarcoma arising in the seventh thoracic vertebra. J Bone Joint Surg [Br] 1971;53:288–295.

205. Sterner BL, Johnson OE. Complete removal of three vertebra for giant cell tumor. J Bone Joint Surg [Br] 1971;53:278–287.

206. Maobiglet GM, Benjamin R, Patt YZ, et al. Intra-arterial *cis*-platinum for patients with inoperable skeletal tumors. Cancer 1981;48:1–4.

206a. Malawer MM, Buch R, Reaman G, et al. Impact of two cycles of preoperative chemotherapy with intraarterial cisplatin and intravenous doxorubicin on the choice of surgical procedure for high-grade bone sarcomas of the extremities. Clin Orthop Rel Res 1991;270:214–222.

207. Martinez A, Donaldson SS, Bagshaw MA. Special set-up and treatment techniques for the radiotherapy of pediatric malignancies. Int J Radiat Oncol Biol Phys 1977;2:1007–1016.

208. Watkins DMB. Radiation therapy mold technology. Toronto: Pergamon Press, 1981.

209. Order SE, Donaldson SS. Radiation therapy of benign disease. Berlin: Springer-Verlag, 1990.

210. Sanerkin NG. The diagnosis and grading of chondrosarcoma of bone. A combined cytologic and histologic approach. Cancer 1980;45:582–594.

211. Huvos AG. Bone tumors. Diagnosis, treatment and prognosis. Philadelphia: WB Saunders, 1979.

212. Marcove RC, Mike V, Hutter RVP, et al. Chondrosarcoma of the pelvis and upper end of femur. J Bone Joint Surg [Am] 1972;54:561–572.

213. Bacci G, Springfield D, Picci P, et al. Adjuvant chemotherapy for malignant fibrous histiocytoma in the femur and tibia. J Bone Joint Surg [Am] 1985;67:620–625.

214. Nobler MP, Higginbotham NL, Phillips RF. The cure of aneurysmal bone cyst: Irradiation superior to surgery in an analysis of 33 cases. Radiology 1968;90:1185–1192.

215. Cassady JR. Radiation therapy in less common primary bone tumors. In: Jaffe N, ed. Solid tumors in childhood. Littleton, MA: PSG Publishing, 1979:205–214.

216. Anonsen CK, Donaldson SS. Langerhans' cell histiocytosis of the head and neck. Laryngoscope 1987;97:537–542, 1987

217. Greenberger JS, Crocker AC, Vawter G, et al. Results of treatment of 127 patients with systemic histiocytosis (Letterer-Siwe syndrome, Schuller-Christian syndrome and multifocal eosinophilic granuloma). Medicine (Baltimore) 1981;60:311–338.

218. Greenberger JS, Cassady JR, Jaffe N, et al. Radiation therapy in patients with histiocytosis: Management of diabetes insipidus and bone lesions. Int J Radiat Oncol Biol Phys 1979;5:1749–1755.

219. Gramatovici R, D'Angio GJ. Radiation therapy in soft-tissue lesions in histiocytosis X (Langerhans' cell histiocytosis). Med Pediatr Oncol 1988;16:259–262.

220. Dahlin DC, Conventry MB. Osteosarcoma, a study of 600 cases. J Bone Joint Surg [Am] 1967;49:101–110.

220a. Stark A, Kricbergs S, Nilsonne U, Silversward C. The age of osteosarcoma patients is increasing. An epidemiological study of osteosarcoma in Sweden 1971 to 1984. J Bone Joint Surg [B] 1990;72:89–93.

221. Richter MP, D'Angio GJ. The role of radiation therapy in the management of children with histiocytosis X. Am J Pediatr Hematol Oncol 1981;3:161–163.

222. Selch MT, Parker RG. Radiation therapy in the management of Langerhans cell histiocytosis. Med Pediatr Oncol 1990;8:151–154.

223. Wick MR, Siegal GP, Unni KK, et al. Sarcomas of bone complicating osteitis deformas (Paget's disease), 50 years' experience. Am J Surg Pathol 1981;5:47–59.

224. Greditzer HG, McLeod RA, Unni KK, et al. Bone sarcomas in Paget's Disease. Radiology 1983;146:337–333.

225. Huvos AG, Wooard HQ, Cahan WG, et al. Postradiation osteogenic sarcoma of bone and soft tissues, a clinicopathologic study of 66 patients. Cancer 1982;55:1244–1255.

226. Francis KC, Kohn H, Malawer MM. Osteogenic sarcoma. J Bone Joint Surg [Am] 1976;55:754.

227. Enneking WF. Musculoskeletal tumor society, VII. New York: Churchill Livingstone, 1983:1021–1125.

228. Wilner D. Osteogenic sarcoma (osteosarcoma). In: Wilner D, ed. Radiology of bone tumors and allied disorders. Philadelphia: WB Saunders, 1982:1897–2095.

229. De Santos LA, Edeiken B. Purely lytic osteosarcoma. Skeletal Radiol 1982;9:1–7.

230. Jaffe N, Smith E, Abelson HT, et al. Osteogenic sarcoma: Alterations in the pattern of pulmonary metastases with adjuvant chemotherapy. J Clin Oncol 1983;1:251–254.

231. Lockshin MD, Higgins TT. Prognosis in osteogenic sarcoma. Clin Orthop 1968;58:85–101.

232. Larsson SE, Lorentzon R, Wedron H, Boquist L. The prognosis in osteosarcoma. Int Orthop 1981;5:305–310.

233. Brostrom L, Strander H, Nisonne U. Survival in osteosarcoma in relation to tumor size and location. Clin Orthop 1982;167:250–254.

233a. Hudson M, Jaffe MR, Jaffe N, et al. Pediatric osteosarcoma: Therapeutic strategies, results, and prognostic factors derived from a 10-year experience. J Clin Oncol 1990;8:1988–1997.

234. Bacci G, Avella M, Picci P, Briccoli A, Dallari D, Campanacci M. Metastatic patterns in osteosarcoma. Tumori 1988;74:421–427.

235. Levine AM, Rosenberg SA. Alkaline phosphatase levels in osteosarcoma tissue are related to prognosis. Cancer 1979;44:2291–2293.

236. Levine AM, Trich T, Rosenberg SA. Osteosarcoma cells in tissue culture: II. Characterization and location of alkaline phosphatase activity. Clin Orthop 1975;3:33–41.

237. Scranton PE Jr, DeCicco FA, Totten RS, Yunis EJ. Prognostic factors in osteosarcoma. A review of 20 years experience at the University of Pittsburgh Health Center Hospitals. Cancer 1975;36:2179–2191.

238. Look AT, Douglass EC, Meyer WH. Clinical importance of near-diploid tumor stem lines in patients with osteosarcoma of an extremity. N Engl J Med 1988;318:1567–1572.

238a. Bauer HCF, Kricbergs A, Silversward C. Prognostication including DNA analysis in osteosarcoma. Acta Orthop Scand 1989;60:353–360.

239. Springfield DS, Schmidt R, Grahm-Pole J, Marcus RB Jr, Spanier SS, Enneking WF. Surgical treatment for osteosarcoma. J Bone Joint Surg [Am] 1988;70:1124–1130.

240. Malawer MM, Sugarbaker, PH, et al. The Tikhoff-Linberg procedure and its modifications, In: Sugarbaker PH, ed. Atlas of sarcoma surgery. Philadelphia: JP Lippincott, 1984.

241. Malawer MM, Meller I, Dunham WK. A new surgical classification system for shoulder-girdle resections, analysis of 38 patients. Clin Orthop Rel Res 1991;267:33–43.

242. Malawer MM, Meller I, Dunham WK. Proposed surgical classification of shoulder girdle resections for bone and soft tissue tumors: Description of a new system and analysis of 38 patients. American Society of Shoulder and Elbow Surgery, New Orleans, 1987.

243. Malawer MM, Price WM. Gastrocnemius transposition flaps in conjunction with limb-sparing surgery for primary sarcomas around the knee. Plast Reconstr Surg 1984;73:741–750.

244. Malawer MM, McHale KA. Limb-sparing surgery for high grade tumors of the proximal tibia and a new method of extensor mechanism reconstruction. 4th International Symposium on Limb-salvage in Musculoskeletal Oncology. Kyoto, Japan, 1987.

245. Hudson TM, Springfield DS, Schiebler M. Popliteus muscle as a barrier to tumor spread: Computer tomography and angiography. J Comput Assist Tomogr 1984;8:498–501.

246. Malawer MM. Surgical management of aggressive and malignant tumors of the proximal fibula. Clin Orthop 1984;186:172–181.

247. Rosen G. Preoperative chemotherapy in osteogenic sarcoma. In: Enneking WF, ed. Limb-sparing surgery for musculoskeletal tumors. New York: Churchill Livingstone, 1987:260–267.

247a. Sundaresan N, Rosen G, Fortner JG, et al. Preoperative chemotherapy and surgical resection in the management of posterior paraspinal tumors. J Neurosurg 1983;58:446–450.

248. Picci P, Bacci G, Companacci M, et al. Histological evaluation of necrosis in osteosarcoma induced by chemotherapy, regional mapping of viable and nonviable tumor. Cancer 1985;56:1515–1521.

248a. Tienghi A, Fiorentini G, Monti T, Graziani G, Bardella D, Margangolo M. Neo-adjuvant locoregional chemotherapy (NALC) in pelvic osteosarcoma (PO). Ann Oncol 1990;1:97.

248b. Sundaresan N, Rosen G, Huvos AG, Krol G. Combined treatment of osteosarcoma of the spine. Neurosurgery 1988;23:714–719.

249. Rosen G, Huvos AG, Mosende C, Beattie EJ, Exelby PR, Capparos B, Marcove RC. Chemotherapy and thoracotomy for metastatic osteogenic sarcoma. A model for adjuvant chemotherapy and the rationale for timing of thoracic surgery. Cancer 1978;41:841–849.

250. Pratt C, Champion J, Senzer N, et al. Treatment of unresectable or metastatic osteosarcoma with cisplatin or cisplatin-doxorubicin. Cancer 1985;56:1930–1933.

251. Cregan E, Frytak S, Pairolero P, Hahn RG, Muhm JR. Surgically proven pulmonary metastases not demonstrated by computed chest tomography. Cancer Treat Rep 1978;62:1404–1405.

252. Telander R, Pairolero P, Pritchard D, Sim F, Gilchrist G. Resection of pulmonary metastatic osteogenic sarcoma in children. Surgery 1978;84:335–341.

253. Putnam JB, Roth J, Wesley M, Johnston M, Rosenberg SA. Survival following aggressive resection of pulmonary metastases from osteogenic sarcoma: Analysis of prognostic factors. Ann Thorac Surg 1983;36:516–523.

254. Goorin A, Delorey M, Lack E, et al. Prognostic significance of complete surgical resection of pulmonary metastases in patients with osteogenic sarcoma: Analysis of 32 patients. J Clin Oncol 1984;2:425–431.

255. Meyer WH, Schell MJ, Kumar APM, Rao BN, Green AA, Champion J, Pratt CB. Thoracotomy for pulmonary metastatic osteosarcoma. An analysis of prognostic indicators of survival. Cancer 1987;59:374–379.

256. Weichselbaum R, Cassady J, Jaffe N, Filler R. Preliminary results of aggressive multimodality therapy for metastatic osteosarcoma. Cancer 1977;40:78–83.

257. Beattie E, Martini N, Rosen G. The management of pulmonary metastases in children with osteogenic sarcoma with surgical resection combined with chemotherapy. Cancer 1975;35:618–621.

258. Pappo A, Meyer W, Marina N, Mahmoud H, Pratt C. Chemotherapy for recurrent osteosarcoma (OS): Is it worth it? In, Proc Am Soc Clin Oncol 1992;11:368.

259. Cade S. Osteogenic sarcoma: A study based on 133 patients. J R Coll Surg Edinb 1955;1:79–111.

260. Lee ES, MacKenzie DH. Osteosacoma: A study of the value of preoperative megavoltage radiotherapy. Br J Surg 1964;51:252–274.

261. Farrell C, Reventos A. Experience in treating osteosarcoma at the Hospital of the University of Pennsylvania. Radiology 1964;83:1080–1083.

262. Sweetnan R, Knowelden J, Seedon H. Bone sarcoma: Treatment by irradiation, amputation, or a combination of the two. Br Med J 1971;2:363–367.

263. Phillips TL, Sheline GE. Radiation therapy of malignant bone tumors. Radiology 1969;92:1537–1545.

264. Allen CV, Stevens KR. Preoperative irradiation for osteogenic sarcoma. Cancer 1973;31:1365–1366.

265. Gaitan-Yanguas M. A study of the response of osteogenic sarcoma and adjacent normal tissues to radiation. Int J Radiat Oncol Biol Phys 1981;7:593–595.

266. Jenkin RD. Radiation treatment of Ewing's sarcoma and osteogenic sarcoma. Can J Surg 1977;20:530–536.

267. Jenkin RDT, Allt WEC, Fitzpatrick PJ. Osteosarcoma. An assessment of management with particular reference to primary irradiation and selective delayed amputation. Cancer 1972;30:393–400.

268. Beck JC, Wara WM, Bovill EG, et al. The role of radiation therapy in the treatment of osteosarcoma. Radiology 1976;120:163–165.

269. Suit HD. Radiation therapy given under conditions of local tissue hypoxia for bone and soft tissue sarcoma. In: M.D. Anderson Hospital: Tumors of bone and soft tissue. Chicago: Year Book Medical Publishers, 1965:143–163.

270. Scanlon PW. Split-dose radiotherapy for radioresistant bone and soft tissue sarcoma: Ten years' experience. AJR 1972;114:544–552.

271. Lee ES. Treatment of bone sarcoma. Proc R Soc Med 1971;64:1179–1180.

272. Clark JL, Unni KK, Dahlin DC, et al. Osteosarcoma of the jaw. Cancer 1983;51:2311–2316.

273. Chambers RG, Mahoney WD. Osteogenic sarcoma of the mandible: Current management. Am Surg 1970;36:463–471.

274. Suit HD. Role of therapeutic radiology in cancer of bone. Cancer 1975;35:930–935.

275. De Fries HO, Perlin E, Leibel SA. Treatment of osteogenic sarcoma of the mandible. Arch Otolaryngol 1970;105:358–359.

276. Akbiyik N, Alexander LL. Osteosarcoma of the maxilla treated with radiation therapy and surgery. J Natl Med Assoc 1981;73:355–356.

277. Livolsi VA. Osteogenic sarcoma of the maxilla. Arch Otolaryngol 1977;103:485–488.

278. Goffinet DR, Kaplan HS, Donaldson SS, et al. Combined radiosensitizer infusion and irradiation of osteogenic sarcoma. Radiology 1975;117:211–214.

279. Martinez A, Goffinet DR, Donaldson SS, et al. Intra-arterial infusion of radiosensitizer (BUdR) combined with hypofractionated irradiation and chemotherapy for primary treatment of osteogenic sarcoma. Int J Radiat Oncol Biol Phys 1985;2:123–128.

280. Kinsella TJ, Glatstein E. Clinical experience with intravenous radiosensitizers in unresectable sarcomas. Cancer 1987;59:908–915.

281. Weichselbaum RR, Cassady JR. Radiation therapy in osteosarcoma. In: Jaffe N, ed. Solid tumors in childhood, 1979:183–190.

282. Newton KA, Barrett A. Prophylactic lung irradiation in the treatment of osteogenic sarcoma. Clin Radiol 1978;29:493–496.

283. Breur K, Cohen P, Schweisguth O, et al. Irradiation of the lungs as an adjuvant therapy

284. Breur K, Schweisguth O, Cohen P, et al. Prophylactic irradiation of the lungs to prevent development of pulmonary metastases in patients with osteosarcoma of the limbs. NCI Monogr 1981;56:233–236.

285. Breur K, van der Schueren E. Adjuvant therapy in the management of osteosarcoma: Need for critical reassessment. Recent Results Cancer Res 1978;68:5–15.

286. Burgers JMV, van Glabbeke M, Busson A, et al. Osteosarcoma of the limbs. Report of the EORTC-SIOP 03 trial 20681 investigating the value of adjuvant treatment with chemotherapy and/or prophylactic lung irradiation. Cancer 1988;61:1024–1031.

287. French Bone Tumor Study Group. Age and dose of chemotherapy as major prognostic factors in a trial of adjuvant therapy of osteosarcoma combining two alternating drug combinations and early prophylactic lung irradiation. Cancer 1988;61:1304–1311.

288. Rab GT, Luins JC, Child DS, et al. Elective whole lung irradiation in the treatment of osteogenic sarcoma. Cancer 1976;38:949–952.

289. Jenkin RDT. The Treatment of osteosarcoma with radiation: Current indications. In: Management of primary bone and soft tissue tumors. Chicago: Year Book Medical Publishers, 1976:151–162.

290. Caceres E, Zaharia M, Moran M, et al. Adjuvant whole lung radiation with or without Adriamycin treatment in osteogenic sarcoma. Cancer Treat Rep 1978;62:297–299.

291. Unni KK, Dahlin DC, Beaubout SW, Ivins JC. Parosteal osteogenic sarcoma. Cancer 1976;37:2466–2475.

292. Schajowicz F, McGuire MH, Araujo S, Muscolo DL, Gitelis S. Osteosarcoma arising on the surfaces of long bones. J Bone Joint Surg [Am] 1988;70:555–564.

293. Martin SE, Dwyer A, Kissane JM, et al. Small-cell osteosarcoma. Cancer 1982;50:990–996.

294. Sim FH, Unni Ku, Beaubout JW, et al. Osteosarcoma with small cells simulating Ewing's tumor. J Bone Joint Surg [Am] 1979;61:207–215.

295. Amendola BE, Amendola MA, McClatchey KD, Miller CH Jr. Radiation-associated sarcoma: A review of 23 patients with postradiation sarcoma over a 50-year period. Am J Clin Oncol 1989;12:411–415.

296. Mankin HJ, Cantley KD, Lipielo L, et al. The biology of human chondrosarcoma. I. Description of the cases, grading, and biochemical analyses. J Bone Joint Surg [Am] 1980;62:160–176.

297. Mankin HJ, Cantley KD, Schiller AL, et al. The biology of human chondrosarcoma. II. Variations in chemical composite among types and subtypes of benign and malignant cartilage tumors. J Bone Joint Surg [Am] 1980;62:176–188.

298. Krocberg A, Zelterberg A, Soderberg G. A comparative study of cellular DNA content and clinicopathologic features. Cancer 1982;50:577–583.

299. Alho A, Connor JF, Mankin HJ, Schiller AL, Campbell C. Assessment of malignancy of cartilage tumors using flow cytometry. A preliminary report. J Bone Joint Surg [Am] 1983;65:779–785.

300. Edeiken J. Bone tumors and tumor-like conditions. In: Edeiken J, ed. Roentgen diagnosis of diseases of bone. 3rd ed. Baltimore: Williams & Wilkins, 1981:30–414.

301. Aprin H, Riserborough EJ, Hall JE. Chondrosarcoma in children and adolescents. Clin Orthop 1982;166:226–232.

302. Steel HH. Partial or complete resection of the hemipelvis: An alternative to hindquarter amputation for periacetabular chondrosarcoma of the pelvis. J Bone Joint Surg [Am] 1978;60:719–730.

303. Austin-Seymour M, Munzenrider J, Goitein M, et al. Fractionated proton radiation therapy of chordoma and low-grade chondrosarcoma of the base of the skull. J Neurosurg 1989;70:13–17.

304. Aboulafia AJ, Faulks C, Li W, Buch R, Matthews J, Malawer MM. Reconstruction using the saddle prosthesis following excision of malignant periacetabular tumors. In: Brown, KLB, ed. Complications of limb salvage, prevention, management and outcome. Montreal: ISLOS, 1991.

305. Unni KK, Dahlin DC, Beaubout JW, Sim FH. Chondrosarcoma: Clear-cell variant. A report of 16 cases. J Bone Joint Surg [Am] 1976;57:676–683.

306. Harwood AR, Krajbich JI, Fornasier VL. Mesenchymal chondrosarcoma: A report of 17 cases. Clin Orthop 1981;158:144–148.

307. Huvos AG, Rosen G, Dabska M, Marcove RC. Mesenchymal chondrosarcoma: A clinicopathologic analysis of 35 patients with emphasis on treatment. Cancer 1983;51:1230–1237.

308. Mankin HJ, Doppelt SH, Sullivan TR, Tomford WW. Osteoarticular and intercalary allograft transplantation in the management of malignant tumors of bone. Cancer 1982;50:613–630.

309. Krochak R, Harwood AR, Cummings BJ, et al. Results of radical radiation for chondrosarcoma of bone. Radiother Oncol 1983;1:109–115.

310. McNaney D, Lindberg RD, Ayala AG, et al. Fifteen year radiotherapy experience with chondrosarcoma of bone. Int J Radiat Oncol Biol Phys 1982;8:187–190.

311. Harwood AR, Krajbich JI, Fornasier VL. Radiotherapy of chondrosarcoma of bone. Cancer 1980;45:2769–2777.

312. Ryall RDH, Bates T, Newton KA, et al. Combination of radiotherapy and RA 20X and (ICRF 159) for chondrosarcoma. 1979;44:891–895.

313. Marcove RC. The surgery of tumors of bone and cartilage. 2nd ed. New York: Grune & Stratton, 1984.

314. Nascimento AG, Huvos AC, Marcove RC. Primary malignant giant cell tumor of bone study of eight cases and review of the literature. Cancer 1979;44:1393–1402.

315. Arlen M, Tollefsen HR, Huvos AS, et al. Chondrosarcoma of the head and neck. Am J Surg 1970;120:456–460.

316. Campanacci M, Giunti A, Olmi R. Giant-cell tumors of bone: A study of 209 cases with long-term follow-up in 130. Ital J Orthop Traumatol 1977;1:249–277.

317. Marcove RC, Weiss L, Vaghaiwall M, Pearson R. Cryosurgery in the treatment of

giant cell tumor of bone: A report of 52 consecutive cases. Clin Orthop 1978;134: 275–289.

318. Malawer MM, Dunham WK, Zaleski T, Zielinski CJ. The management of aggressive and low grade malignant bone tumors by cryosurgery: analysis of 40 consecutive cases. In: Enneking WF, ed. Limb-sparing surgery for musculoskeletal tumors. New York: Churchill Livingstone, 1987:498–510.

319. Persson BM, Wouters HW. Curettage and acrylic cementation in surgery of giant cell tumor of bone. J Bone Joint Surg [Am] 1976;120:125–133.

320. Larsson SE, Lorenzton R, Boquist L. Giant cell tumors of the spine and sacrum causing neurological problems. Clin Orthop 1975;111:201–211.

321. Bell RS, Harwood AR, Goodman SB, et al. Supervoltage radiotherapy in the treatment of difficult giant cell tumors of bone. Clin Orthop 1983;174:208–216.

322. Harwood AR, Fornasier VL, Rider WD. Supervoltage irradiation in the management of giant-cell tumor of bone. Radiology 1977;125:223.

323. Dahlin DC, Cupps RE, Johnson EW. Giant cell tumor: A study of 195 cases. Cancer 1970;25:1061–1070.

324. McGrath PH. Giant cell tumor of the bone: An analysis of fifty-two cases. J Bone Joint Surg [Br] 1972;54:216–229.

325. Tountas AA, Fornasier VL, Harwood AR, et al. Post-irradiation sarcoma of bone. Cancer 1979;43:182–187.

326. Bacci G, Springfield D, Picci P, et al. Adjuvant chemotherapy for malignant fibrous histiocytoma in the femur and tibia. J Bone Joint Surg [Am] 1985;67:620–625.

327. Heeten GJ, Koops HS, Kamps WA, et al. Treatment of malignant fibrous histiocytoma of bone, a plea for primary chemotherapy. Cancer 1985;56:37–40.

328. Earl HM, Morittu MD, Pringle J, Kemp H, Souhami. Sensitivity of malignant fibrous histiocytoma of bone (MFHB). Ann Oncol (in press).

329. Mindell ER. Current concept review. Chordoma. J Bone Joint Surg [Am] 1981;63: 501–505.

330. Localio AS, Eng K, Ranson JHC. Abdominosacral approach for retrorectal tumors. Am Surg 1980;179:555–560.

331. Localio AS, Francis KC, Rossano PC. Abdominosacral resection of sacrococcygeal chordoma. Ann Surg 1967;166:394–400.

332. Gray SW, Singhabhandhu B, Smith RA, Skandalakis JE. Sacrococcygeal chordoma: Report on a case and review of the literature. Surgery 1975;78:573.

333. Guterberg B, Romanus B, Sterner BL. Pelvic strength after major amputation of the sacrum. An experimental study. Acta Orthop Scand 1976;47:635–642.

334. DeVries J, Oldhoff J, Hadders, HN. Cryosurgery treatment of sacrococcyceal chordoma: Report of four cases. Cancer 1986;58:2348–2354.

335. Heffelfinger MJ, Dahlin DC, MacCarthy CS, et al. Chordomas and cartilaginous tumors of the skull base. Cancer 1973;32:410–420.

336. Sundaresian N, Galicich JH, Chu FCH, et al. Spinal chordoma. J Neurosurg 1979;50: 312–319.

337. Amendola BE, Amendola MA, Oliver E, et al. Chordoma: Role of radiation therapy. Radiology 1986;158:839–843.

338. Cummings BJ, Hodson ID, Bush RS. Chordoma: The results of megavoltage radiation therapy. Int J Radiat Oncol Biol Phys 1983;9:633–642.

339. Rich TA, Schiller A, Suit HD, et al. Clinical and pathologic review of 48 cases of chordoma. Cancer 1985;56:182–187.

340. Austin-Seymour M, Munzenrider J, Goitein M, et al. Proton radiation therapy of chordoma and low grade chondrosarcoma of the base of the skull and cervical spine. Int J Radiat Oncol Biol Phys 1986;12(suppl 1):98.

341. Raffel C, Wright DC, Gutin PH, et al. Cranial chordomas: Clinical presentation and results of operative and radiation therapy in twenty-six patients. Neurosurgery 1985;17: 703–710.

342. Reimer RR, Chabner BAC, Young RC, et al. Lymphoma presenting in bone. Results of histopathology, staging and therapy. Ann Intern Med 1977;87:50–55.

343. Sweet DL, Moss DP, Simon MA, et al. Histiocytic lymphoma (reticulum-cell sarcoma) of bone. Current strategy for orthopedic surgeons. J Bone Joint Surg [Am] 1981;63: 79–84.

344. Mendenhall NP, Jones JJ, Kramer BS, et al. The management of primary lymphoma of bone. Radiother Oncol 1987;9:137.

345. Loeffler JS, Tarbell NJ, Kozakewich H, et al. Primary lymphoma of bone in children: Analysis of treatment results with Adriamycin, prednisone, Oncovin (APO), and local radiation therapy. J Clin Oncol 1986;4:496–501.

346. Bacci G, Jaffe N, Emiliani E, et al. Therapy for primary non-Hodgkin's lymphoma of bone and a comparison of results with Ewing's sarcoma. Ten years' experience at the Instituto Orthopedico Rizzoli. Cancer 1986;57:1468–1472.

347. Coppes MJ, Patte C, Couanet D, et al. Childhood malignant lymphoma of bone. Med Pediatr Oncol 1991;19:22–27.

348. Furman WL, Fitch S, Hustu HO, et al. Primary lymphoma of bone in children. J Clin Oncol 1989;7:1275–1280.

Cancer: Principles & Practice of Oncology, Fourth Edition,
edited by Vincent T. DeVita, Jr., Samuel Hellman, Steven A. Rosenberg.
J.B. Lippincott Co., Philadelphia © 1993.

Bijan Safai

CHAPTER **45**

Cancers of the Skin

The skin is the largest organ of the body and consists of three layers: epidermis, dermis, and subcutis (*i.e.*, hypodermis). It is a specialized structure with a wide range of functions that include protection from the environment, synthesis of vitamin D, production of a large number of cytokines, antigen presentation, thermoregulation, and sensation of touch and temperature. Several different cell and tissue types, originating from all three embryonic layers, participate in the formation of the three layers of the skin and its associated appendages. These cell and tissue elements can transform to produce a large number of benign and malignant growths (Tables 45–1 and 45–2). This chapter summarizes the nonmelanoma skin cancers and precancerous conditions.

EPIDEMIOLOGY

Nonmelanoma skin cancers are the most common cancers in the U.S. white population. More than 600,000 new cases are diagnosed annually, according to the data from the American Cancer Society.[1] The mortality rate for the nonmelanoma skin cancers is approximately 2100 per year.[1] Because most skin cancers are diagnosed and treated in private office settings or outpatient clinics, the available statistics are thought to grossly underestimate the actual number of nonmelanoma skin cancer cases.

Basal cell carcinoma is the most frequently diagnosed skin cancer in whites, accounting for approximately 75% to 80% of all reported cases.[2] Squamous cell carcinoma is the second most common skin cancer and is estimated to represent 20% to 25% of all reported skin cancer cases.[2]

Persons with fair skin who sunburn easily are more sus-

ceptible to developing basal cell carcinoma on the sun-exposed areas of their skin. Basal cell carcinoma occurs less often in darkly pigmented persons, in whom squamous cell carcinoma is the most common skin cancer. Basal cell carcinoma is seen more frequently in men than in women, and it mostly occurs later in life. However, recent observations indicate an increased incidence of basal cell carcinoma in younger age groups.

Other skin cancers, such as soft tissue sarcomas involving the dermis and subcutis and the adnexal carcinomas, are much less frequent and, although they are encountered in clinical practice, are not as common as basal cell carcinoma or squamous cell carcinoma.

ETIOLOGY AND PATHOGENESIS OF SKIN CANCERS

The two major factors influencing the development of skin cancers are exposure to ultraviolet radiation and type of skin (Table 45–3). Chemical carcinogens have been extensively studied, especially in laboratory animals, as etiologic factors for cutaneous malignancies. Ionizing radiation and primary chronic irritation play major roles in skin cancers. Attention has recently been focused on viruses that may cause skin cancers, specifically human papillomavirus causing skin and mucous membrane carcinomas. Host genetic makeup and host immunity also play roles in the development of skin cancers.

EXPOSURE TO ULTRAVIOLET LIGHT AND SKIN TYPE

Ample evidence supports the combined influence of ultraviolet (UV) light and skin type on the incidence of skin cancer. There is a higher incidence of skin cancer in albinos than in normally pigmented persons living in Africa. The incidence of skin cancer is higher in Australia than in Scandinavian

We acknowledge the significant contribution of Keon Menzies.

1567

TABLE 45–1.   Tumors Arising From Epidermal Cells

Keratinocytic Tumors

Benign
- Seborrheic keratosis
- Epidermal nevi
- Clear cell acanthoma
- Kyrle's disease
- Epidermal cyst
- Trichilemmal cyst
- Birt-Hogg-Dube syndrome
- Becker's nevus
- Warty dyskeratoma

Premalignant
- Actinic (solar) keratosis
- Large cell acanthoma
- Chondrodermatitis nodularis helicis
- Cutaneous horn
- Radiation dermatitis
- Bowen's disease
- Erythroplasia of Queyrat
- Bowenoid papulosis
- Epidermodysplasia verruciformis
- Leukoplakia
- Organoid (sebaceous) epidermal nevi
- Porokeratosis
- Fibroepithelioma of Pinkus
- Keratoacanthoma

Malignant
- Basal cell carcinoma
- Squamous cell carcinoma

Tumor of Merkel's Cells

Merkel's cell carcinoma

Tumors of Langerhans Cells

Histiocytosis X
Letterer-Siwe disease
Hand-Schüller-Christian disease
Eosinophilic granuloma

Tumors of Melanocytic Origin

Benign
- Melanocytic nevi

Premalignant
- Dysplastic nevi
- Congenital nevi

Malignant
- Malignant melanoma

Tumors of Epidermal Appendages

Tumors of hair follicles
Benign
- Inverted follicular keratosis
- Trichodiscoma
- Tumors of the follicular infundibulum
- Trichilemmoma
- Trichofolliculoma
- Trichoepithelioma
- Pilomatricoma

Tumors of hair follicles (Continued)
Malignant
- Trichilemmocarcinoma
- Pilomatrix carcinoma

Tumors of sebaceous glands
Benign
- Fox-Fordyce anomaly
- Organoid (sebaceous) nevi
- Sebaceous gland hyperplasia
- Sebaceous adenoma
- Sebaceous epithelioma

Malignant
- Sebaceous carcinoma

Tumors of apocrine glands
Benign
- Supernumerary nipple
- Apocrine hidrocystoma
- Syringocystadenoma papilliferum
- Hidradenoma papilliferum

Premalignant
- Extramammary Paget's disease

Malignant
- Apocrine adenocarcinoma

Tumors of eccrine glands
Benign
- Poroma
- Syringoma
- Chondroid syringoma
- Hidrocystoma
- Spiradenoma
- Hidradenoma
- Cylindroma

Primary malignant
- Syringoid eccrine carcinoma
- Mucinous eccrine carcinoma
- Clear cell carcinoma
- Microcystic eccrine carcinoma
- Adenoid cystic carcinoma
- Aggressive digital papillary adenocarcinoma
- Eccrine adenocarcinoma

Secondary malignant
- Porocarcinoma
- Malignant syringoacanthoma
- Malignant chondroid syringoma
- Spiradenocarcinoma
- Hidradenocarcinoma
- Cylindrocarcinoma

TABLE 45–2. Tumors Arising in the Dermis and Subcutis

Fibrous or Connective Tissue Tumors
Benign
  Dermatofibroma
  Keloid (Hypertrophic scars)
  Angiofibroma
Malignant
  Dermatofibrosarcoma protuberans
  Atypical fibroxanthoma
  Malignant fibrous histiocytoma
  Epithelioid sarcoma

Neural Sheath Tumors
Neurofibroma
Neurofibromatosis
Malignant neurofibroma
Schwannoma (Neurilemmoma)
Malignant schwannoma
Granular cell tumor
Malignant granular cell tumor

Vascular Tumors
Benign
  Angiokeratomas
  Pyogenic granuloma
  Lymphangioma
  Glomus tumors

Malignant
  Angiosarcoma
  Endovascular papillary angioendothelioma
  Spindle cell hemangioendothelioma
  Epithelioid vascular tumor
  Malignant angioendothelioma
  Kaposi's Sarcoma

Tumors Arising From Smooth Muscle
Benign
  Leiomyomas
Malignant
  Leiomyosarcomas

Tumors of Adipose Tissue Involving The Skin
Benign
  Lipoma
Malignant
  Liposarcoma
  Lipoblastoma

countries, where the population has similar skin, but UV light exposure is different. Squamous cell carcinoma usually occurs in the sun-exposed areas of head and neck. Persons with outdoor occupations, such as sailors and farmers, have a higher incidence of skin cancers than those with indoor occupations. Epidemiologic studies worldwide suggest that UV radiation is the most important etiologic agent for skin cancers.[3,4] The incidence of nonmelanoma skin cancers directly correlates with the proximity to the equator. A quantitative association has been observed between the lifetime sun exposure and the risk of developing nonmelanoma skin cancers. In outdoor workers, the most common sites for skin cancers are on the head, neck, and dorsum of the hands, which are the sites of maximal chronic sun exposure. Chronic UV exposure has changed from occupational to a more recreational pattern, and younger and younger persons are being diagnosed with skin cancers.

TABLE 45–3. Skin Type Assessment

Skin Type	Sunburn and Tanning History
I	Always burns, never tans
II	Always burns, minimal tan
III	Burns often, tans gradually (light brown)
IV	Burns minimally, tans well (moderate brown)
V	Burns rarely, tans profusely (dark brown)
VI	Never burns, deeply pigmented (black)

There is considerable environmental concern about the depletion of the ozone layer by certain chemicals. The ozone layer acts as a strong barrier in absorbing a major portion of UV radiation and preventing it from reaching the earth.[5] The chemicals responsible for the depletion of the ozone layer include chlorofluorocarbons, which are found in aerosol sprays and refrigerators. It is thought that the depletion of ozone over the next few years will rapidly increase the incidence of skin cancers.

Persons with light complexions have a higher chance of developing skin cancers than those with darker skin, who are protected from solar damage by the melanin pigment in the skin. Cutaneous malignancies are rare in dark-skinned persons, but African albinos have a high incidence of skin cancers on sun-exposed areas.

UV light may influence the development and progression of skin cancers by affecting the host immune system. The classic work of Kripke and colleagues showed that UV-induced cancers in mice are highly antigenic and that most are rejected by the host's immune system after transplantation into a normal, genetically identical animal.[6,7] However, the primary host in whom the tumor was induced by UV light becomes tolerant to the tumor and allows its rapid growth. Kripke's work indicates the development of suppressor factors and cells that suppress the host's immune system and prevent rejection of UV-induced skin cancer. These observations have not yet been confirmed in humans, but it is likely that UV light affects Langerhans cells in human skin, which may alter the host immune system, allowing the development and progression of skin cancer.

CHEMICAL CARCINOGENESIS

Most information about cutaneous carcinogenesis has been obtained from studies using laboratory animals, especially mice. After topical application of a carcinogen at regular intervals, the animals develop multiple squamous papillomas, most of which regress spontaneously. Some of the lesions develop the cytologic criteria of malignant cells, and these tumors may become locally invasive.

Three stages of progression have been identified for chemical carcinogenesis: initiation, promotion, and carcinogenesis. During the initiation phase, the DNA configuration of the cells undergoes some basic changes.[8] The process of initiation may remain unchanged for the life of the tissue, or it may progress to malignancy. The epidermal cells in psoriasis share many features with initiated cells. The initiated cells are usually terminally differentiated but may lose their pattern of differentiation and retain their ability to multiply. For the promoter to be effective and cause malignancies, the cell must have been initiated previously. Most promoters usually cause inflammation and hyperplasia, and their effects are reversible. Promoters can induce tumors only after initiation.[9] Some initiators and promoters are listed in Table 45-4.

Tar, which contains polycyclic aromatic hydrocarbons, is an initiator, and it has been used for treating psoriasis.[10] Nitrogen mustard is an accepted treatment for cutaneous T-cell lymphoma. Phorbol esters, which are found in croton oil, are known promoters. Anthralin, used in the treatment of psoriasis, and benzoyl peroxide, used in the treatment of acne, are also known promoters. Long-term use of these agents in humans has not been associated with an increased incidence of malignancy.[10,11] No chemical carcinogen has been identified that gives rise to basal cell carcinoma or malignant melanoma in animals, but experiments with cutaneous chemical carcinogenesis in laboratory animals cannot be directly applied to humans.

The well-documented cases of scrotal carcinoma in chimney sweepers offer the classic description of chemical carcinogenesis in man.[12] Arsenic is recognized as a chemical carcinogen. Increased incidence of cancers are reported in localities where there is a high level of arsenic in the drinking water.[13] Medical exposure to arsenic in the form of Fowler's solution, Donovan's solution, and Asiatic pills in the treatment of asthma and syphilis predisposes to the development of arsenical keratosis, skin cancer, and possibly lung cancer.

IONIZING RADIATION

Exposure to ionizing radiation can induce cutaneous malignancies in humans, usually basal cell carcinoma, squamous

TABLE 45-4. Initiators and Promoters Used in Dermatologic Therapy

Initiators	Promoters
Ultraviolet light	Ultraviolet light
Tar (polycyclic aromatic hydrocarbons)	Phenol
Nitrogen mustard	Anthralin
Psoralen	Phorbol esters
	Benzoyl peroxide

cell carcinoma, and spindle cell carcinoma.[14] Radiation-induced cancers of the skin have been reported in patients receiving ionizing radiation as therapy. In the past, acne, facial hair, and tinea capitis were treated with x-ray therapy. Patients receiving these types of therapy later developed severe radiodermatitis in the form of skin atrophy, telangiectasia, hypopigmentation, or hyperpigmentation. Some of these patients developed large, invasive, deforming skin cancers. These inappropriate uses of x-ray therapy have been discontinued, but accidental exposure to x-rays and exposure for medical reasons continues to cause radiation dermatitis. Occupational exposure and the resultant radiodermatitis and skin cancers, such as squamous cell carcinoma on the fingers of dentists, is no longer seen. The use of fractionated doses of radiation has reduced the long-term side effects of radiation therapy.

CHRONIC IRRITATION OR INFLAMMATION

Skin cancers can develop in areas of chronic inflammation or irritation. Examples of such tumors include cancers developing in the area of chronic osteomyelitis sinus, lupus erythematosus, decubitus ulcers, scars of burns, and sinus formation.[15-21] Chewing tobacco or betel nuts can cause squamous cell carcinoma of the oral cavity and lip.

VIRAL ONCOGENESIS

Many malignant neoplasms are caused by viruses in animals. In humans, such associations have rarely been documented. Human papillomavirus (HPV) has been identified in lesions of verrucous carcinoma, bowenoid papulosis, and in situ epidermoid carcinoma.[22-24] Many papillomavirus subtypes have been identified, and HPV types 5, 8, 14, 16, 17, and 33 are associated with various epidermal carcinomas and carcinoma of the cervix.[25,26] It is possible that other inducing factors are needed to produce the malignant tumor from some of these papillomaviruses. These papillomaviruses appear potentially oncogenic in humans.[27] There are other viruses, such as human T-cell lymphotrophic virus-I in leukemia-lymphoma and Epstein-Barr virus in Burkitt's lymphoma and nasopharyngeal carcinoma, that may be associated with some of the human malignancies, but conclusive information is not available.

IMMUNOLOGIC FACTORS

The concept of immune surveillance suggests that many potentially fatal tumor cells are continuously being detected and destroyed by the immune system before they can form large enough tumors to permit clinical detection. Antibody-mediated and cell-mediated cytotoxic antitumor responses have been detected in animal tumors, but in humans, the detection of immunologic reactivity against malignant tumors and the value of destruction of tumor cells by immune cells are not well documented. The findings of tumor immunology are applicable to several areas of cutaneous oncology.

The work of Kripke and coworkers indicates that a suppressor T cell and suppressor factor are produced in mice, in response to the effect of UV radiation on the immune system.[6,7] Immunoregulation and carcinogenesis have been extensively investigated in murine systems, but the interaction between UV light and the human immune system is not well delineated.

Patients with primary or secondary immunodeficiencies are prone to develop de novo cutaneous malignant neoplasms.[28] Those receiving immunosuppressive therapy (*e.g.,* renal transplant recipients) also develop cutaneous malignant tumors.[29–32] Patients with lymphoreticular malignancies have a higher incidence of nonmelanoma skin cancers, and these skin cancers behave more aggressively in the immunocompromised host.[32–35] It appears that there is some association between the host's immune status and the development of skin cancer, but this relation is not well understood.

GENETIC FACTORS

Several genetically inherited syndromes increase susceptibility for the development of skin cancers. These genodermatoses include xeroderma pigmentosum, nevoid basal cell carcinoma, familial dysplastic nevus syndrome, Bazex's syndrome, and multiple self-healing epithelioma of Ferguson-Smith. Some other genodermatoses, such as Torre's syndrome, Cowden's syndrome, Gardner's syndrome, Peutz-Jeghers syndrome, dyskeratosis congenita, and Carney's syndrome, manifest with some nonmalignant skin lesions and are usually associated with internal malignancies.

CLASSIFICATION OF SKIN TUMORS

To describe the various tumors of the skin in an orderly fashion, the cellular origin and the location in the three layers are followed. Tables 45–1 and 45–2 summarize the tumor of the skin based on their cell of origin, biologic behavior, and location in the three layers of the skin.

BENIGN TUMORS ARISING FROM EPIDERMAL KERATINOCYTES

Benign tumors are commonly diagnosed. They rarely give rise to malignant tumors, but they may be confused with some of the malignant lesions. It is important for clinicians to be able to recognize and differentiate them from malignant skin tumors.

SEBORRHEIC KERATOSIS

Seborrheic keratosis or basal cell papilloma is a common benign lesion produced by the overgrowth of epidermal keratinocytes. It occurs most often on the trunk, face, and neck of middle-aged and elderly persons. Lesions may be found on the extremities but not on the palms and soles. Essential diagnostic features include multiple domed or flat-topped, round or ovoid, verrucous papules that are brown to black. These slightly raised, sharply demarcated lesions appear to be stuck on the surface of the skin. Histologic features are characteristic and consist of acanthosis, hyperkeratosis, and papillomatosis with keratin horn and pseudocysts. The lesion consists mostly of squamous and basaloid epidermal cells. Histologic types include acanthotic, hyperkeratotic, reticulated (adenoidal), clonal and irritated (inflamed) lesions. Other types

include melanoacanthoma, dermatosis papulosis nigra, stucco keratosis, and seborrheic keratoses of the Leser-Trélat sign. Leser-Trélat sign is characterized by a sudden appearance of innumerable new lesions of seborrheic keratosis, which may be a sign of an internal malignancy.[36] Rare transformations of seborrheic keratosis to basal cell carcinoma and squamous cell carcinoma have been reported.[37]

Differential diagnosis consists of intraepidermal epithelioma, verruca vulgaris, dermal nevus, pigmented basal cell carcinoma, well-differentiated squamous cell carcinoma, and malignant melanoma. If histologic confirmation is necessary for differential diagnosis, shave excision is the method of choice. Because of its relatively superficial location, seborrheic keratoses may be removed by curettage and light electrodesiccation or by cryosurgery with liquid nitrogen or carbon dioxide ice.

EPIDERMAL NEVI

Epidermal nevi are benign, congenital, hyperplastic lesions with a smooth or hyperkeratotic surface. They typically appear at birth or in early childhood. Epidermal nevi are uncommon. Lesions may be solitary or multiple, or they may form a plaque covering a large area of skin, usually in an asymmetric or linear distribution. The lesions vary in color from skin color to deeply pigmented brown to black. Clinical variants include nevus verrucosus, linear epidermal nevus, systematized epidermal nevus, ichthyosis hystrix, inflammatory linear epidermal nevus, and epidermal nevus syndrome.[38] Epidermal nevus syndrome or large verrucous epidermal nevus may present with widespread involvement but predominantly on one side of the body. It frequently coexists with central nervous system and skeletal abnormalities.[39] Epidermal nevi remain benign and require treatment only if cosmetically indicated. There have been rare cases of transformation to carcinomas.[40]

CLEAR CELL ACANTHOMA

Clear cell acanthoma appears as a solitary, pink to red, scaly nodule on the lower leg.[41] The lesion is slow growing, sharply delineated, and 1 to 2 cm in diameter. Lesions appear stuck on, like seborrheic keratosis, and vascular, like granuloma pyogenicum. The growth is usually asymptomatic, but the thin, crusty cover may ooze some moisture. Multiple lesions are uncommon.[42] Histologically, the lesion consists of a proliferating population of slightly enlarged keratinocytes with abundant, clear cytoplasm, rich in glycogen. The nuclei appear normal. The lesion is usually excised for histologic diagnosis.

KYRLE'S DISEASE

Kyrle's disease (*i.e.,* hyperkeratosis follicularis et parafollicularis in cutem penetrans) appears as multiple hyperkeratotic lesions with inflammation and crusting.[43] The lesions are seen mostly on the lower extremities but appear on upper limbs, trunk, soles, and rarely on other areas of the body. It is thought that the condition is produced by the hyperkeratotic lesions penetrating from the epidermis into the dermis, forming a keratotic plug that stimulates inflammatory and foreign-body giant cell reactions. The histologic picture includes hyperkeratosis, mainly around hair follicles, lichenoid reactions, and lymphocytic infiltration.[44]

Kyrle's disease and perforating folliculitis are clinically and histologically hard to differentiate. Uremic follicular hyperkeratosis is used to describe lesions that have features of Kyrle's disease and perforating folliculitis.[45] Unlike the rarity of Kyrle's disease, this new entity is fairly common and occurs mostly in patients with diabetes and renal failure.[46] These lesions must be differentiated from actinic keratosis and squamous cell carcinoma, and they require biopsy and histologic confirmation. No effective treatment is available, but cryotherapy may be of some value.

CYSTS

Cysts are relatively common lesions occurring in young and middle-aged persons, and they are usually of great concern to patients. Two of the more common forms are epidermal cyst and trichilemmal (*i.e.*, pilar) cyst.

Epidermal cysts are single or multiple lesions, mostly found on the face, neck, chest, and back. They arise spontaneously or may form as a result of trauma. A cyst normally enlarges to about 1 to 5 cm, but remains as a firm, asymptomatic mass unless it becomes infected. Histologically, epidermal cysts are intradermal or subcutaneous cavities lined with normal surface epidermis and filled with fluid and epithelial debris. Development of basal cell carcinoma, squamous cell carcinoma, and Bowen's disease from epidermal cysts have been reported.[47–49] Effective treatment requires complete removal of the cyst and its sac.

Trichilemmal cysts are clinically indistinguishable from epidermal cysts. Trichilemmal cysts may be single or multiple lesions, frequently seen on the scalp but rarely on the face and neck. Histologically, the pilar cyst is lined by epithelium resembling hair follicle epithelium. The absence of the granular layer differentiates it from the epidermal cyst, which consists of all the layers of the epidermis.[50,51] Trichilemmal cysts may have a more hyperplastic presentation, and they are referred to as proliferating trichilemmal cysts.[52,53] Malignant degeneration with metastasis of proliferating trichilemmal cysts has been reported.[54] Treatment is surgical excision of the entire cyst.

BIRT-HOGG-DUBE SYNDROME

Birt-Hogg-Dube syndrome is inherited as an autosomal dominant trait and consists of the triad of trichodiscoma, fibrofolliculoma, and acrocordan.[55–57] The patient has multiple, asymptomatic, flesh-colored papules on the face, mainly around the nose. Histologically, the lesions may show proliferation of the superficial hair follicle (*i.e.*, trichodiscoma) or proliferation of the dermal part of the hair follicle (*i.e.*, fibrofolliculomas) or features of fibrous skin tags (*i.e.*, acrochordon). Lesions are removed only if cosmetically indicated.

BECKER'S NEVUS

Becker's pigmented hairy epidermal nevus (*i.e.*, Becker's melanosis) is a relatively common condition presenting with a patch of hyperpigmented, coalescing macules on the shoulders and upper extremities, mostly in young men.[58] Hyper-

trichosis is frequently associated with the tan or brown patches. This condition is usually preceded by a sunburn of the involved area. Histologically, the skin appears normal except for an increased number of melanocytes, especially in the dermis, and the increased melanin in the basal layer of the epidermis.[59] The hair follicles appear normal, but the diameter of the hair may be thicker than normal. There is no need for treatment except if cosmetically indicated.

WARTY DYSKERATOMA

Warty dyskeratoma presents in middle-aged patients as a solitary lesion on the scalp, face, or neck, but it may occur in unexposed skin and the oral mucosa.[60,61] It occurs as a slightly elevated, circumscribed papule or nodule with a raised border and keratotic umbilicated or pore-like center. The lesion typically grows to about 1 to 10 mm in diameter. Common complaints are itching, burning sensation, recurrent drainage, and bleeding due to trauma. Histologically, the lesion appears as a large, cup-shaped invagination with a keratotic and parakeratotic plug. The upper portion of the invagination shows numerous acantholytic and dyskeratotic cells. One or more pilosebaceous structures are commonly associated with warty dyskeratoma, but they are not etiologic, because lesions may also occur on the oral mucosa. In older patients, these lesions are frequently associated with premalignant and malignant lesions, such as solar keratosis, squamous cell carcinoma, basal cell carcinoma, and adnexal carcinomas. Differential diagnosis includes Darier's disease, sebaceous cyst, solar keratosis, basal cell carcinoma, verrucae, nevocellular nevus, and folliculitis. Surgical excision is the most commonly recommended treatment approach.

PREMALIGNANT TUMORS OF THE EPIDERMIS

Because of the absence of good epidemiologic data, it is difficult to determine with certainty whether a lesion is a true precancerous lesion and gives rise to a malignant condition or if the association is a coincidental finding. An example of this is keratoacanthoma, which is usually a benign, self-healing lesion, but it may predispose the patient to squamous cell carcinoma.

ACTINIC OR SOLAR KERATOSIS

Actinic or solar keratoses are common asymptotic lesions seen mostly on sun-exposed areas of light-skinned persons. The lesions are commonly multiple and appear on sun-damaged skin as skin-colored to yellow-brown, firm, raised papules with scaly, rough, keratotic surfaces and erythematous bases. Unlike seborrheic keratosis, actinic keratosis appears to arise from within the epidermis, rather than being "stuck on" the skin. Common sites for actinic keratosis are the face, dorsum of the hands, the upper chest, upper back, and lower lip. The lesions are typically a few millimeters to 1 cm in diameter. In Australia, 40% of persons over age 40 have one or more actinic keratoses.[62] Histologic features include epidermal dysplasia sparing the skin appendages, hyperkeratosis and inflammation with lymphocytic infiltration, and evidence of actinic elastosis and telangiectasia in the dermis. Abnormal keratinocytes appear less basophilic than normal keratinocytes and vary in size and shape.

Approximately 20% to 25% of actinic keratoses eventually transform into carcinoma in situ and finally into invasive squamous cell carcinoma years after their initial appearance (Fig. 45–1).[63,64] If induration, erythema, or erosion are observed, possible progression to squamous cell carcinoma should be suspected. If malignant transformation is suspected, shave excision of the lesion and histologic examination are recommended. Lesions may transform into squamous cell carcinoma more rapidly in patients who are immunosuppressed or have genetic defects of DNA repair enzymes (*e.g.,* xeroderma pigmentosum). The report from Australia indicates a much lower number, approximately 1%, developing into basal cell carcinoma.[62]

Differential diagnosis includes seborrheic keratoses, lichenoid keratoses, warts, pigmented basal cell carcinomas, lentigo maligna, malignant melanomas, and early squamous cell carcinomas. Existing lesions are treated by curettage and electrodesiccation or liquid nitrogen cryotherapy. Multiple and widespread lesions may be treated with application of a cream or solution containing 5-fluorouracil (5-FU) for approximately 3 weeks, but this treatment may produce considerable discomfort.[65] Dermatoabrasion may be an alternative. Some reports indicate spontaneous regression of lesions.[66] Protection against excessive sun exposure by the use of protective clothing and sunscreens helps to prevent actinic keratosis.

CHEMICAL AND OTHER KERATOSES

Other keratoses that may be considered as premalignant cutaneous dysplasia are arsenical keratosis (Fig. 45–2) induced by exposure to arsenic, tar keratoses induced by exposure to tars and other polycyclic aromatic hydrocarbons, thermal keratoses induced after prolonged (≤20 years) exposure to infrared radiation that causes chronic cutaneous thermal damage, chronic radiation keratoses induced by exposure to x-rays, and chronic cicatrix keratoses or scar keratoses that may degenerate to scar carcinoma with metastatic potential.

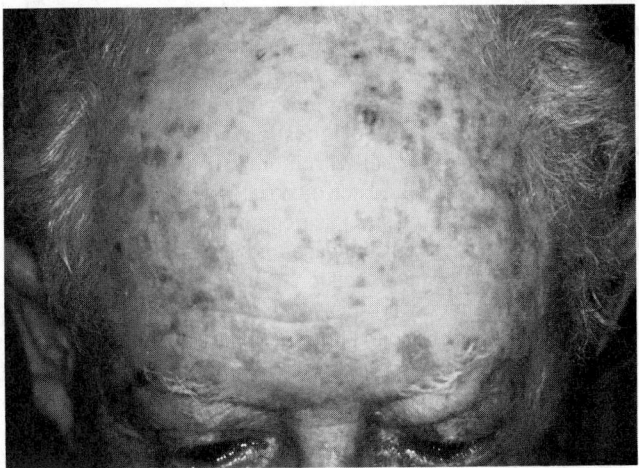

FIGURE 45–1. Severely sun-damaged skin, solar keratosis, basal cell carcinoma, and squamous cell carcinoma on sun-exposed skin of a white man.

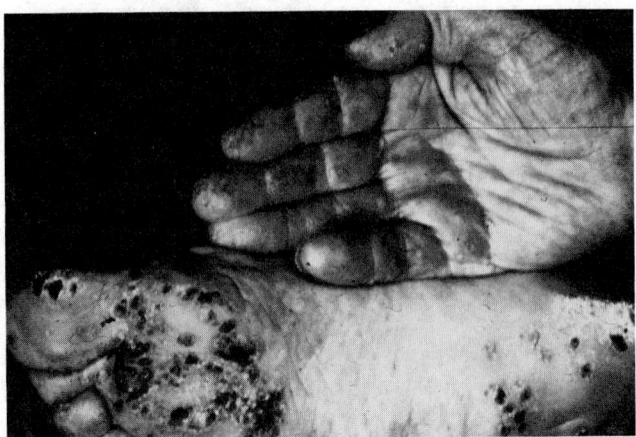

FIGURE 45–2. Arsenic keratosis on the palm and sole.

LARGE CELL ACANTHOMA

Large cell acanthoma occurs mostly on sun-exposed skin as a sharply demarcated, slightly hyperkeratotic, scaly, pigmented lesion, usually less than 1 cm in diameter.[67] Most lesions are solitary, but some multiple lesions are seen.[68] It is clinically similar to actinic keratosis, but this rare lesion is easily differentiated histologically from actinic keratosis by the presence of large keratinocytes with proportionally large nuclei scattered in a disordered arrangement of epidermal cells.[69] Another differential diagnosis is Bowen's disease. The management of large cell acanthoma is similar to actinic keratosis.

CHONDRODERMATITIS NODULARIS HELICIS

Chondrodermatitis nodularis helicis is most commonly seen in elderly men and appears as tender, painful, inflamed, scaly, erythematous papules or nodules on the apex of the ear.[70–72] Lesions are occasionally ulcerated and crusted. Advanced cases show significant cartilage destruction and distortion of the pinna. A few of these patients develop squamous cell carcinoma if left untreated. Histologic features include actinic damage in the epidermis and dermis, but the essential feature for diagnosis is inflammation and damage of underlying cartilage by a lymphocytic infiltration. Management includes use of a topical or intralesional corticosteroid and, if not effective, surgical excision.

CUTANEOUS HORN

Cutaneous horn appears as a protuberant, raised, hard, hyperkeratotic nodule with an erythematous base commonly occurring on the sun-exposed areas of white-skinned persons (Fig. 45–3). It usually develops due to the underlying dysplasia or frank neoplasm, and it is therefore considered a marker of skin cancer. The histopathology of the underlying lesion includes actinic keratosis, seborrheic keratosis, filiform verruca, trichilemmoma, basal cell carcinoma, or squamous cell carcinoma.[73–75] A histopathologic study indicates that 39% of underlying lesions were premalignant and malignant epidermal lesions, and 61% were benign lesions.[75] The lesion with a portion of the base should be removed for histologic ex-

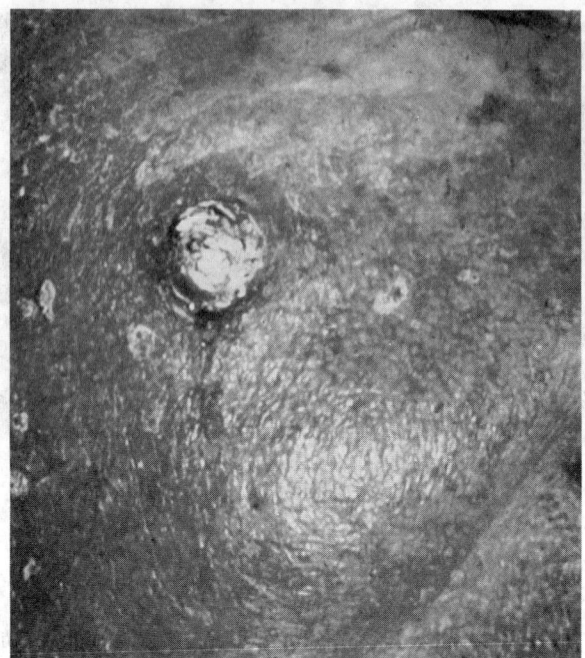

FIGURE 45–3. Cutaneous horn on severely sun-damaged facial skin.

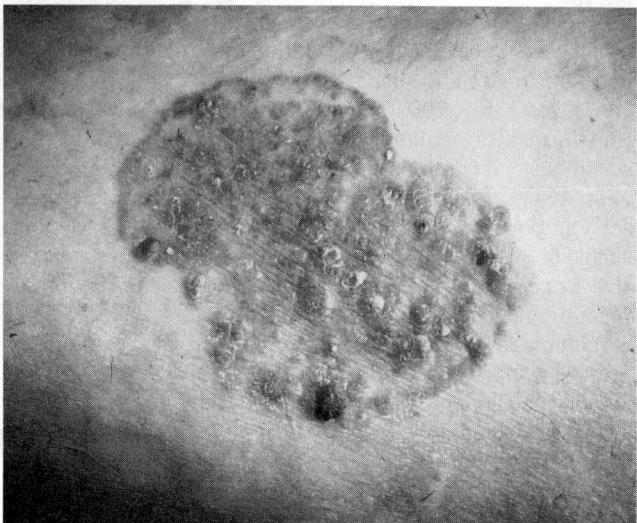

FIGURE 45–4. Bowen's disease on the trunk.

amination. Final treatment is usually determined by the pathology of the underlying tissue.

RADIATION DERMATITIS

Radiation dermatitis is the term used to describe skin damage due to x-irradiation, whether exposure occurs as a result of occupational hazard or therapeutic treatments.[76] Involved skin is dry, scaly, erythematous, thin, and discolored. Areas of telangiectasia, hyperpigmentation and hypopigmentation, and hyperkeratosis and ulceration are common. Histologically, the damaged area shows atrophy and loss of polarity of epidermal keratinocytes, changes in elastic and collagen bundles of the dermis, and destruction of hair follicles, sebaceous glands, and sweat glands. There is a potential for developing actinic keratosis, basal cell carcinoma, and squamous cell carcinoma on this kind of skin.[77,78] Management includes removal of any overlying skin lesion and continuous skin care. Soft tissue sarcomas may develop in the irradiated tissue.[79,80]

BOWEN'S DISEASE

Bowen's disease or intraepidermal carcinoma in situ is an intraepidermal squamous cell carcinoma that may involve any area of the skin but tends to favor sun-exposed areas of the face, neck, and extremities (Fig. 45–4). In one third of the patients, the lesions may be multiple. Bowen's disease is papulosquamous and appears as a slowly enlarging, sharply defined, round to irregular plaque with a rough, scaly, hyperkeratotic, erythematous surface. Other surface characteristics include pigmentation, fissures, erosion, and ulceration. Similar to in situ epidermoid carcinoma, Bowen's lesions may progress to invasive squamous cell carcinoma. This transformation to squamous cell carcinoma is reported in 3% to 5% of the cases, with most cases remaining as carcinoma in situ.[81,82]

The cause of Bowen's disease is unknown, but UV radiation, HPV-induced epidermodysplasia verruciformis, and history of ingestion of inorganic arsenic (*e.g.*, water or medication) are considered etiologic factors.[23,83,84] Bowen's disease has been seen on nonexposed areas of the skin in younger persons without a history of arsenic ingestion and without HPV infections.

Histologic features of Bowen's disease include gross dysplasia of the upper layers of epidermal cells with the basal cell layer relatively normal, individual cell keratinization, and giant keratinocytes with atypical mitoses. It has been suggested that patients with Bowen's disease are more likely to develop other cancers, including basal cell carcinoma, adnexal carcinoma, melanoma, or cancers of the lung, gastrointestinal tract, genitourinary tract, and the reticuloendothelial system, but the role of Bowen's disease as a marker of internal malignancies is unclear. A report from the Armed Forces Institute of Pathology indicates that as many as 80% of the cases of Bowen's disease have other cutaneous and noncutaneous malignancies.[85] Another report suggests that as many as 29% of the patients have internal malignancies.[86]

Many of the published reports contain major deficiencies, such as lack of sufficient control groups.[87] In view of the existing controversies, it is recommended that patients with Bowen's disease have a complete clinical examination combined with the necessary diagnostic workup. Differential diagnosis includes basal cell carcinoma, psoriasis, extramammary Paget's disease, and actinic keratosis. Excisional biopsy of the most indurated area is recommended for histologic confirmation of Bowen's disease and detection of squamous cell carcinoma. Surgical excision of the entire lesion provides the highest cure rate. Cryotherapy or curettage and desiccation have been recommended, but there is a higher chance of recurrence.

ERYTHROPLASIA OF QUEYRAT

Erythroplasia of Queyrat is a clinicopathologic variant of Bowen's disease, occurring almost exclusively on the glans penis of uncircumcised, middle-aged and older men (Fig. 45–

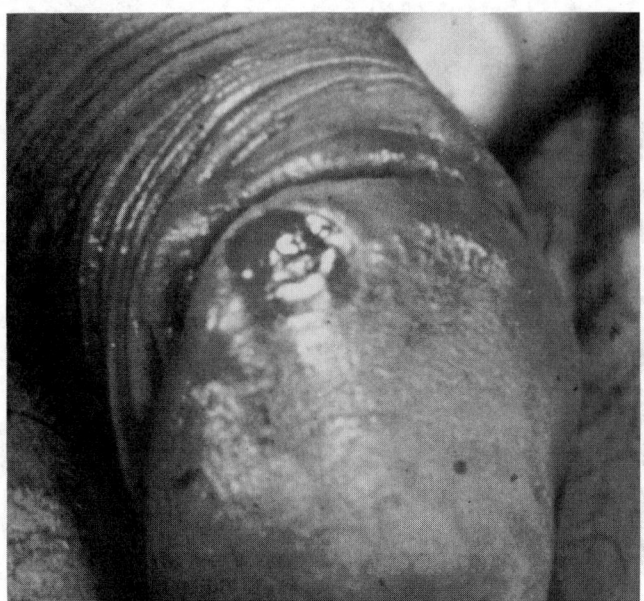

FIGURE 45–5. Erythroplasia of Queyrat occurring as in situ epidermoid carcinoma on the penis.

5). It may occur on the penile shaft, scrotum, and the vulva, but it is questionable whether these presentations are Bowen's disease of the anogenital region. The lesion appears as an asymptomatic, sharply demarcated, bright red, shiny plaque with a smooth, velvety surface.[88,89] The histologic features are identical to Bowen's disease, especially of the anogenital region. However, the rate of transformation into invasive squamous cell carcinoma is much higher for Bowen's disease, and the resultant squamous cell carcinoma tends to be more aggressive.[88,90] Cryotherapy and curettage and electrodesiccation have been used. It is advisable to use surgical excision of the tumor with microscopic control of the margin (Mohs' micrographic surgery) and to circumcise the penis.

BOWENOID PAPULOSIS

Bowenoid papulosis is a multicentric anogenital dysplasia that presents as verrucous or lichenoid pink to reddish-brown papules, erythematous macules, or leukoplakia-like lesions in young men and women.[23,91–94] Lesions of the oral mucosa have been reported.[95] Although pruritus and inflammation with tenderness and pain are occasionally reported, most patients with bowenoid papulosis have no symptoms. The lesions typically present as inconspicuous, noncondylomatous papules with mostly smooth and only slightly papillomatous surfaces. The lesions are 0.2 to 3.3 cm in diameter, with small papules coalescing into large pigmented plaques.[94,96] Bowenoid papulosis is a cutaneous manifestation of the sexually transmitted HPV. It is mostly linked with HPV type 16, but types 18, 34, and 39 have also been linked to its pathogenesis. This condition normally follows a benign but persistent course over many years. Occasional spontaneous regression, particularly in pregnant women, and progression to anogenital carcinoma has been reported.[91,97–101] These lesions are frequently confused with genital warts.

The histology is similar to Bowen's disease. Bowenoid papulosis does not show the full-thickness epidermal involvement and disorderly keratinocyte maturation characteristic of Bowen's disease and in situ squamous cell carcinoma. It has dysplastic keratinocytes scattered throughout the epidermis in a background of orderly keratinocyte maturation. These atypical keratinocytes have crowded nuclei that appear large, hyperchromatic, and pleomorphic, and are often in metaphase. The epidermis exhibits papillated hyperplasia with focally prominent, hypergranular areas. There are atypical mitotic figures, individual cell necrosis, dyskeratosis, and multinucleated keratinocytes scattered in the epidermis. If podophyllin has been used topically for the treatment of these lesions, histologic sections may exhibit a pattern of pseudoepitheliomatous hyperplasia with bizarre keratinocytic forms, because podophyllin causes metaphase arrest.

The clinical features usually differentiate bowenoid papulosis from Bowen's disease. Bowenoid papulosis usually presents in young, sexually active men and women between 20 and 40 years of age, and the lesions appear as multiple, small papules.[23,91–94,96] Bowen's disease occurs in patients older than 50 years of age and is usually a single plaque.[81,82] The lesions respond well to local destructive therapy, such as electrodesiccation, laser surgery, cryosurgery, and ablation.[102] Topical treatment with 5-FU and intramuscular or intralesional interferons have also been used in the treatment of bowenoid papulosis.[103] Recurrences after treatment are common, due to the life-long nature of HPV infections. Patients with this condition, especially women, and their sexual partners are at high risk for anogenital carcinomas and should have frequent evaluations.

EPIDERMODYSPLASIA VERRUCIFORMIS

Epidermodysplasia verruciformis is a rare, chronic, and often hereditary disease characterized by widespread eruption of flat, wart-like lesions and reddish-brown plaques with slightly scaly surfaces and irregular borders.[104–106] The wart-like lesions are mainly distributed on the hands, feet, and face, sometimes in a linear arrangement, and the pigmented plaques preferentially involve the trunk, neck, and proximal parts of the extremities. These premalignant lesions have many characteristics of actinic keratoses. Malignant transformation to squamous cell carcinoma in predominantly sun-exposed areas occurs in 30% of patients. Most patients show defects in cell-mediated immunity characterized by anergy to dinitrochlorobenzene and common skin antigens, depressed lymphocyte blastogenic reactivity to mitogens, abnormal T-lymphocyte populations, and decreased number of T lymphocytes.[83,107–109] However, the humoral immune system is left intact.[110]

The cause is attributed to rare types of human papillomavirus (HPV), mostly type 5, 8, 12, and 14. HPV appears to take advantage of the immunologic state to induce epidermodysplasia verruciformis.[107–112] The occurrence of HPV infections and epidermodysplasia verruciformis in immunosuppressed renal allograft recipients, in an immunosuppressed patient with systemic lupus erythematous, and in a patient with Hodgkin's disease provides support for this hypothesis.[111–114] Another line of evidence comes from the family members of patients with epidermodysplasia verruciformis, in whom the wart-like lesions started to appear but eventually regressed.[106] However, there are patients with epidermodys-

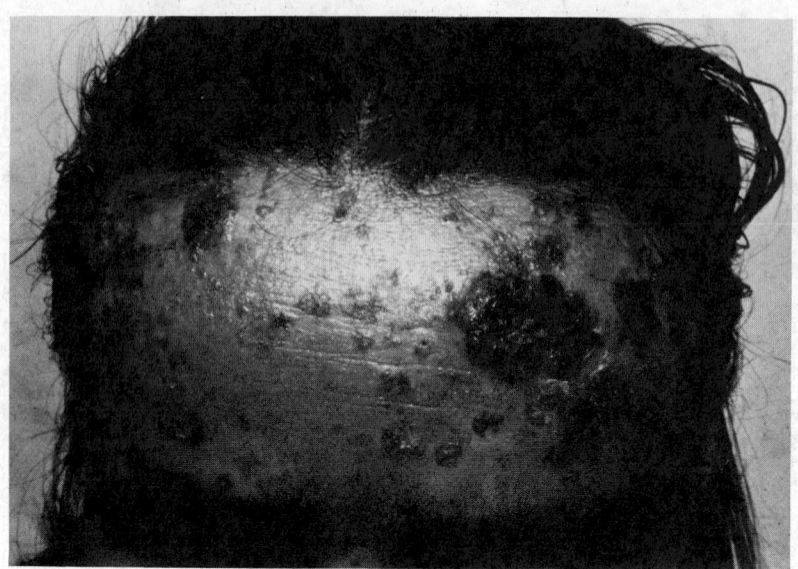

FIGURE 45–6. Multiple lesions of in situ superficial squamous cell carcinoma on the face of a woman with epidermodysplasia verruciformis.

plasia verruciformis without immune dysfunction.[115,116] Some investigators believe that the impaired cellular immunity could be a result of the HPV infection. The etiologic factors associated with the development of epidermodysplasia verruciformis are HPV infection, impaired cellular immunity, and the genetic makeup of the host. It is important for HPV-infected, immunosuppressed patients to have regular dermatologic examinations.

Epidermodysplasia verruciformis is an extremely protracted disease that usually begins in infancy or early childhood (5–11 years) with various types of warts and plaques. Later, it may progress to form verrucous plaques and nodules or transform to in situ squamous cell carcinoma. The rate of appearance of new lesions varies considerably, with some lesions disappearing in some areas as more appear in other areas. Malignant tumors typically develop in the third or fourth decade of life in approximately one third of the patients. These patients are not inconvenienced by these transformations, which are neither painful nor itchy. Malignant lesions are numerous and continue to progress as noninvasive in situ carcinoma without metastasis (Fig. 45–6). They are locally destructive if not treated. There is no effective therapy for epidermodysplasia verruciformis, but aromatic retinoids, such as etretinate and etretin, may have some beneficial effects.[83] Interferons produce only partial responses during therapy, with lesions returning in the same locations after therapy is discontinued.[116] Surgical removal, electrosurgical approaches, and cryotherapy are used.

LEUKOPLAKIA

Leukoplakia appears as white patches on the mucous membranes of the oral mucosa and vulva.[117] Leukoplakia is a clinical description. About 20% of the patients have histologies that consist of epithelial dysplasia and hyperkeratosis of the mucosa. Approximately 15% of the dysplastic cases develop carcinoma in situ, and 3% to 6% develop invasive squamous cell carcinoma within the involved area.[117,118] Differential diagnosis includes lichen planus, candidiasis, hairy leukoplakia, white sponge nevus, pachyonychia congenita, and dyskeratosis congenita.

ORGANOID OR SEBACEOUS NEVI

Organoid or sebaceous nevi are skin lesions composed of abnormal numbers of pilosebaceous structures and apocrine glands. These congenital lesions appear as raised, yellowish papules that grow gradually to develop a papillomatous surface.[119,120] They usually occur on the scalp and are present at birth. Basal cell carcinoma has been reported in as many as 10% of patients, and squamous cell carcinoma occurs rarely.[121] Syringocystadenoma papilliferum derived from the apocrine gland and basal cell carcinomas may be associated with organoid nevus (Fig. 45–7). Histologically, the lesion consists

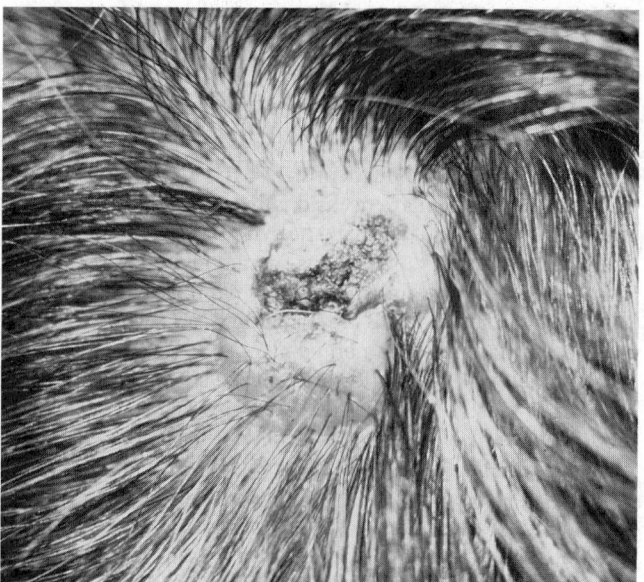

FIGURE 45–7. Basal cell carcinoma at a previous site of a sebaceous nevus.

of large numbers of skin appendages, including sebaceous, eccrine, and apocrine glands, hair follicles, and smooth muscle. Because of these structures, the term organoid nevus appears more appropriate. In syringocystadenoma papilliferum, cystic lesions of the epidermis are lined by a double layer of columnar epithelium showing decapitation secretion, suggesting apocrine gland origin.[119] After histologic confirmation of the diagnosis, the lesion is usually removed by surgical excision.

POROKERATOSIS

Porokeratosis describes a variety of epidermal disorders that share a dyskeratotic histologic pattern.[122] Except for the punctate type, porokeratosis is characterized by a distinct peripheral, raised, hyperkeratotic ridge that corresponds histologically to a parakeratotic column, called the coronoid lamella, which is a keratin-filled invagination of the epidermis. The central portion is typically flattened or of normal thickness but rarely acanthotic. The disseminated superficial actinic type is the most common and is reported in some instances to be inherited as an autosomal dominant trait.[123] The skin lesions are small, multiple, circular patches with slightly raised borders, usually on sun-exposed areas.[124] This type has been reported in renal transplant recipients and after chemotherapy for other malignancies, suggesting that immunosuppression may be involved in the development of porokeratosis.[125–127] The plaque type was originally described by Mibelli and typically begins in childhood. The lesions have atrophic centers and raised rims, and they tend to expand peripherally. This clinical picture and the lack of sweating in the center is characteristic of this condition.[125,128]

The linear nevoid variant may be widely distributed or may be localized to a segment of the body.[129] Clinically, the lesions resemble those of linear verrucous epidermal nevus. The disseminated palmoplantar variety typically presents on the palms and soles of adolescents and young adults and later may involve other areas of the body.[130] This type lacks the history of sun exposure. The punctate type is confined to the palms and soles and presents as numerous, moderately tender, 1- to 2-mm keratotic plugs.[131] Various types of malignancies, including squamous cell carcinoma, basal cell carcinoma, and Bowen's disease, have been reported to develop within porokeratotic lesions.[128,132–134] Differential diagnosis includes verruca vulgaris and solar keratosis, which may also have the coronoid lamella structure. The punctate type may be impossible to differentiate from plantar and palmar warts. Specimens for histologic diagnosis must include the peripheral raised ridge. Porokeratosis of Mibelli (plaque type) and disseminated superficial actinic porokeratosis should be treated with surgical excisions and close observation because of the possibility of progression to malignancy. The other types may be controlled with cryotherapy.

FIBROEPITHELIOMA OF PINKUS

Fibroepithelioma of Pinkus is usually seen on the back and appears as flesh-colored skin tags. Characteristic histologic features consist of a network of anastomosing epithelial strands connected to the overlying epidermis and admixed with a fibrous stroma. The network may be a few layers thick.

Acanthosis of the epidermis and horn cysts make the lesion resemble seborrheic keratosis. Basal cell carcinomas are reported to develop in a small percentage of these fibroepithelial tumors.[78,135] Management is by surgical excision for histologic diagnosis.

KERATOACANTHOMA

Keratoacanthoma is a rapidly growing hyperkeratotic papule that presents on sun-exposed skin of middle-aged and elderly persons.[136] Clinically and histologically, this lesion resembles squamous cell carcinoma and is sometimes associated with actinic keratosis. They usually spontaneously regress or involute in about 6 months, but some may show atypical features and behave more aggressively. It is difficult to differentiate between keratoacanthoma and squamous cell carcinoma.[137–140] Keratoacanthoma behaves more aggressively in immunosuppressed hosts.

The lesion initially appears as a rapidly growing, reddish papule and reaches full size in 1 to 3 months. Most lesions remain between 1 to 2 cm, are firm, and have a raised rolled border and a central keratin plug (Fig. 45–8). At the end of the growth phase, the lesion becomes quiescent for a while, and then slowly undergoes spontaneous regression, leaving an ugly scar. Keratoacanthoma usually appears as an isolated lesion, although multiple eruptive and multiple self-healing lesions have been reported.[141,142] The most common sites for lesions are sun-exposed skin of the face, head and neck, and the dorsum of the hands in persons older than 40 years of age.

Histologically, keratoacanthoma is diagnosed by a central keratin plug with a surrounding proliferation of squamous epithelium extending down into the dermis. Histologic confirmation is only possible if the biopsy of the lesion includes the lateral border and the central crater. A wedge resection of the lesion from one side to the other, deep into the subcutaneous

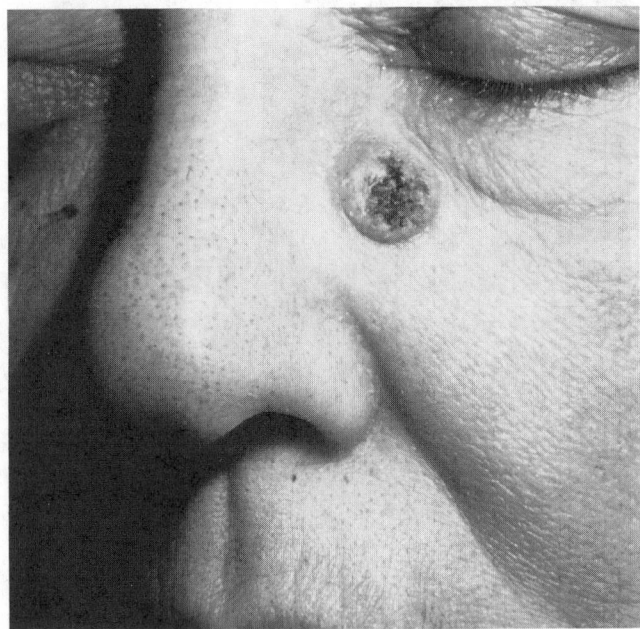

FIGURE 45–8. Keratoacanthoma. Notice the central crater.

fat, should be forwarded for histologic examination. This biopsy procedure may result in regression of the lesion. If the lesion persists longer or if more acceptable cosmetic results are required, it is best to surgically excise the lesion. Shave excision down to the deep dermis is effective for the treatment of keratoacanthoma. In cases of aggressive keratoacanthoma or if squamous cell carcinoma cannot be ruled out, complete surgical excision with appropriate margins is recommended.

MALIGNANT EPIDERMAL TUMORS

BASAL CELL CARCINOMA

Basal cell carcinoma is the most common cancer among whites, accounting for most of the 600,000 new cases of non-melanoma skin cancer in the United States each year.[1] Basal cell carcinoma rarely metastasizes and is easily treated and cured.[143] It appears on sun-exposed areas in fair-skinned persons who have had long-standing sun exposure. It is usually seen in elderly persons and those suffering from xeroderma pigmentosum, Bazex's syndrome, basal cell nevus syndrome, and linear basal cell nevi.[78,121,144–147] Its incidence increases with age, but because of easy access to the sunbelt areas and outdoor recreational activities and because it has become fashionable to be suntanned, basal cell carcinoma is now seen more often in younger persons. It is no longer surprising to see basal cell carcinoma in patients in their third or fourth decade of life.

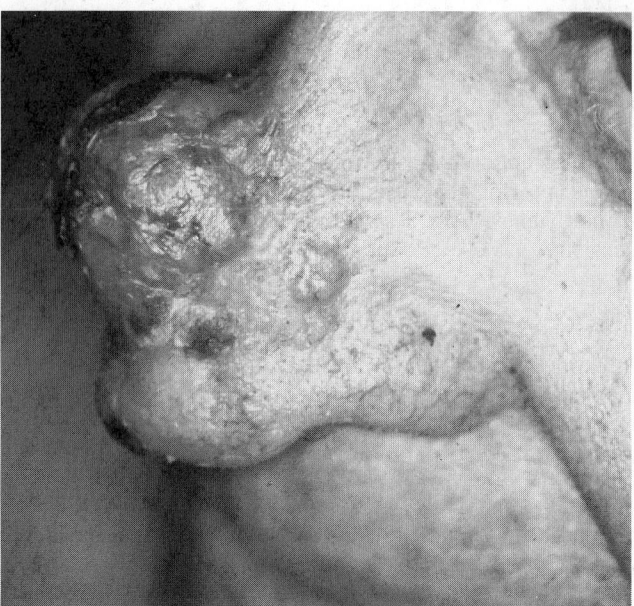

FIGURE 45–10. Large, tumorous basal cell carcinoma on the nose. Notice the concomitant sun-damaged skin.

Most basal cell carcinomas occur on sun-exposed areas such as the face (Figs. 45–9 and 45–10), especially the nose, the nasolabial fold, and the inner canthus areas. Solitary basal cell carcinomas are seen in the geographic areas with temperate climate. Multiple tumors and tumors on areas other than the face are seen usually in tropical and equatorial regions. Basal cell carcinoma occurs more commonly in men than in women, with the incidence increasing with age and with the latitude.[62,148]

Clinical Presentation

Basal cell carcinoma appears as a slowly growing, shiny, skin-colored to pink, translucent, raised papule. Telangiectasia is seen on the surface of the lesion. As the lesion enlarges, it may ulcerate and develop a rolled border and crusted center. The lesion may then regress to a smaller and less visible size.

Several clinicopathologic variants of basal cell carcinoma have been described.[78,149–152] They are nodular, multiple superficial, cystic, adenoid, pigmented, and morphea types. Pigmented basal cell carcinoma may be confused with malignant melanoma. Some basal cell carcinomas may have a hyperkeratotic surface and scaly appearance and may be confused with actinic keratosis, sebaceous keratosis, squamous cell carcinoma, and Bowen's disease. The morphea-type basal cell carcinoma has a scar-like sclerotic appearance and lacks telangiectasia and translucency, and the usual distinct border is not seen. The lesion is larger and more indurated in palpation than on inspection. Another form of basal cell carcinoma is the so-called basosquamous cell carcinoma.[153] This lesion has biologic behavior and pathologic features intermediate between basal cell and squamous cell carcinomas.

Most basal cell carcinomas are diagnosed when the tumors are a few millimeters to 1 to 2 cm in diameter (Figs. 45–11 and 45–12). However, much larger, ulcerated tumors may be

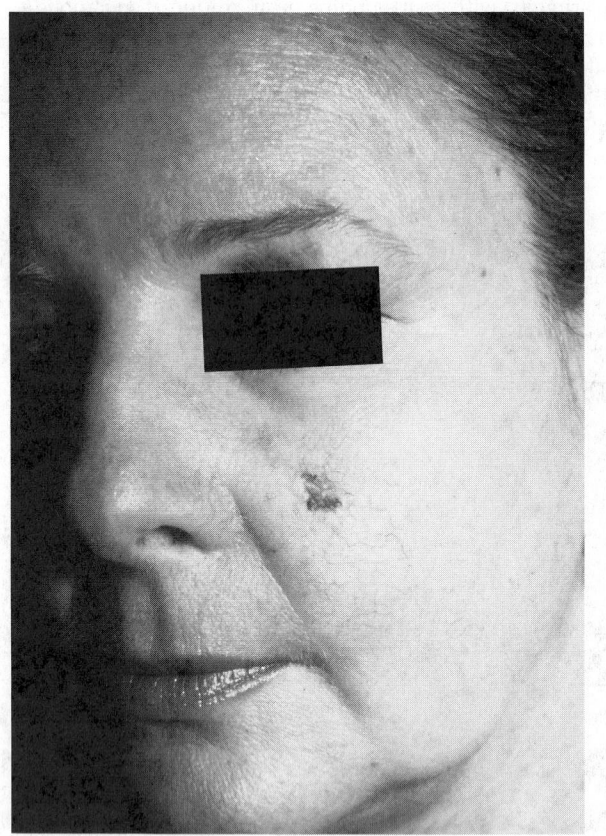

FIGURE 45–9. Basal cell carcinoma on the face of a white woman.

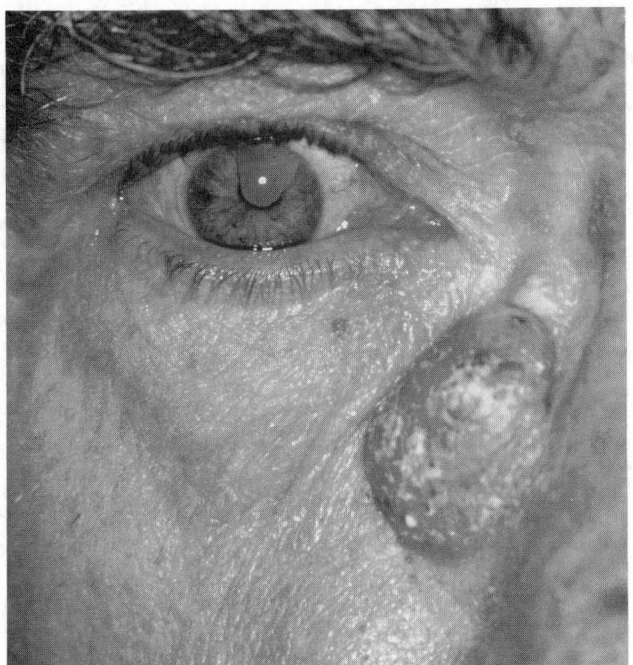

FIGURE 45–11. Nodular basal cell carcinoma.

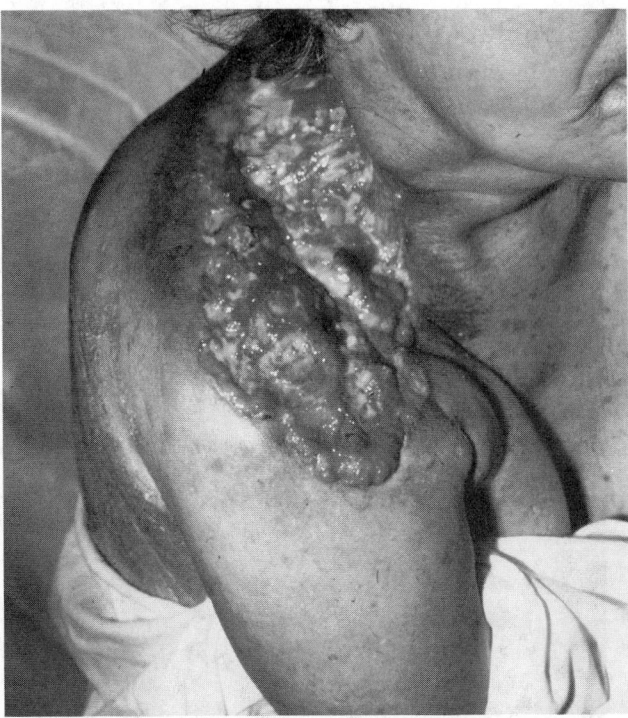

FIGURE 45–13. Large, invasive, ulcerative basal cell carcinoma.

seen (Fig. 45–13). Basal cell carcinoma does not usually metastasize, but it can invade underlying tissues and organs slowly and cause destruction of skin, cartilage, soft tissue, and bone.[154,155] Rarely, if basal cell carcinoma reaches the bone or blood circulation, it may metastasize.[143] The world literature indicates fewer than 300 cases of metastatic basal cell carcinoma. After it reaches metastatic levels, it behaves as aggressively as other types of cancers and can spread to vital organs such as lymph nodes and lung.

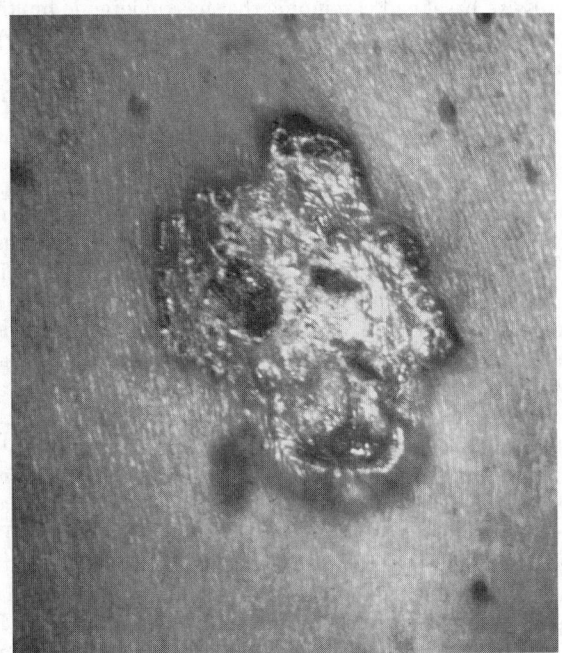

FIGURE 45–12. Ulcerated basal cell carcinoma.

Pathogenesis

Most reports indicate the importance of fair complexion, blue eyes, and fair hair in the development of basal cell carcinoma. This is especially true if the people have fair complexions and live in a sunny region, such as Scandinavians who live in Australia.[62,148,156,157] The role of genetic susceptibility to the development of basal cell carcinoma has been suggested and is well documented in cases of xeroderma pigmentosum (Fig. 45–14) and basal cell nevus syndrome.[78,144,146,147] The proven role of genetic markers is that of inheritance of the fair complexion. Although few recent reports indicate a possible role for the major histocompatibility complex, there are no confirmed data proving the role of HLA antigens (*e.g.*, DR-5) in the development of basal cell carcinoma.[158]

The association of chronic UV light exposure and development of basal cell carcinoma is well accepted.[62,148,156,157] It is the cumulative effect of UV light over many years that causes the development of basal cell carcinoma. After the necessary level of sun exposure (threshold) is reached, the exposed person continues to develop basal cell carcinomas; the process appears to be irreversible. The chance of developing basal cell carcinoma directly relates to the number of previous basal cell carcinomas.[159] For example, a person who has had 10 basal cell carcinomas has the chance to develop one new tumor each year thereafter. Other conditions that may predispose to the development of basal cell carcinoma include other primary malignancies, especially lymphoreticular types, immunodeficiency states, and trauma, such as traumatic injuries or small pox vaccination.[78,158,160–162] Although basal cell carcinomas are most commonly seen on the sun-exposed areas of the skin, many basal cell carcinomas are seen in less exposed areas, such as the nasolabial fold and the inner canthus,

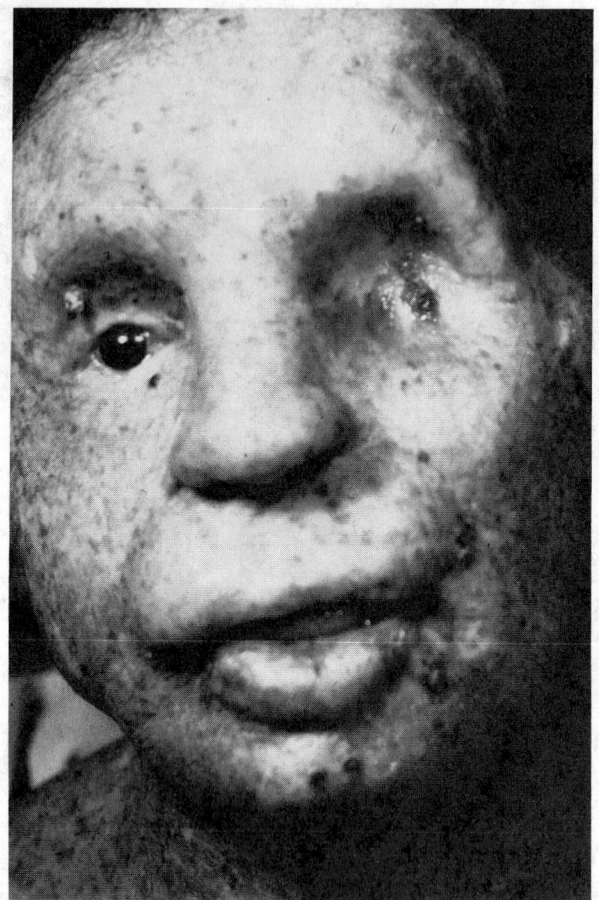

FIGURE 45–14. Severe solar damage, basal cell carcinoma, and squamous cell carcinoma developed in a man with xeroderma pigmentosum who lost one of his eyes.

suggesting that other factors (*e.g.*, embryologic closure lines) may contribute to the development of the tumor.

Basal cell carcinomas are reported only on hair-bearing skin, but in cases of basal cell nevus syndrome and linear basal cell nevi, basal cell carcinomas may be seen on the soles and palms.[146] These observations suggest that the tumors may originate from epithelial cells of hair follicles. Ionizing radiation, whether received from the environment or as part of therapeutic modalities, can promote the development of basal cell carcinoma. X-irradiated skin shows evidence of chronic dermatitis several years later and may give rise to basal cell or squamous cell carcinomas.[76–78,163,164] In the 1950s and 1960s, x-irradiation was used for the treatment of acne and hypertrichosis. Many patients who received therapeutic x-rays developed radiation dermatitis and multiple skin cancers of the face 20 to 30 years later.

Histopathology

In all forms of basal cell carcinomas, the histologic features include masses of compactly arranged basaloid cells resembling cells in the basal layer of epidermis extending down from the epidermis into the dermis (Fig. 45–15).[152,165,166] There is usually a variable dermal stroma reaction. In the sclerosing type of basal cell carcinoma, the cells are more fusiform and are admixed with a more pronounced stromal

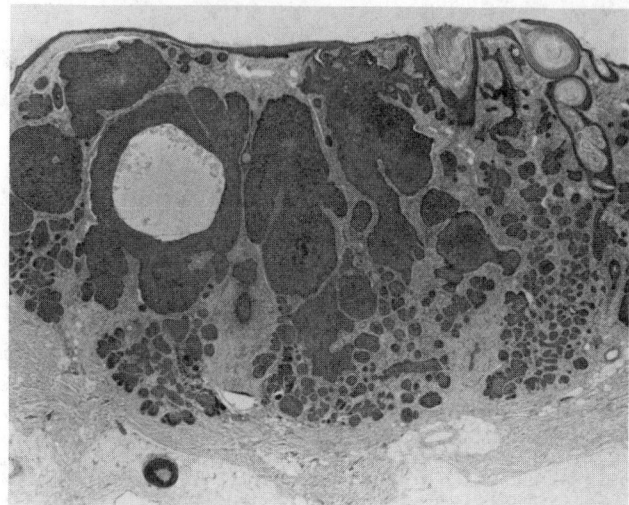

FIGURE 45–15. Histologic section of basal cell carcinoma.

reaction. In most cases, especially in the nodular, cystic, and adenoid types, there is a clear peripheral palisading of the dark epithelial cells that is characteristic of basal cell carcinoma. The differential diagnosis includes trichoepithelioma, which may also show some palisading of the cells.[167] Pigmented basal cell carcinoma is due to aggregation of melanin within the tumor. Basosquamous cell carcinoma consists of a fibrous stroma admixed with a downward proliferation of epithelial cells that lack palisading and have some of the features of squamous cell carcinoma and more frequent mitosis.[149,153]

Metastasizing Basal Cell Carcinoma

Basal cell carcinoma usually spreads by direct extensions from the primary tumor site and has little tendency to metastasize.[143,168] Fewer than 300 cases have been reported in the world literature. Metastatic disease usually arises from a more aggressive basal cell carcinoma that has undergone multiple recurrences after treatment. The tumor invades and destroys the underlying tissues, and when metastases reach vital organs, they behave aggressively.[154,155]

Management of Basal Cell Carcinoma

Several methods are available for the treatment of basal cell carcinoma (Table 45–5).[167,169,170] The choice is usually based on the location, type of lesion, and experience of the physician. Smaller lesions can be treated with surgical excision or curettage and desiccation.[171,172] Radiation therapy, although used less frequently, is the most appropriate treatment for basal cell carcinoma of the eyelid, nose, and lips. Cryosurgery and topical use of 5-FU have also been suggested, but the cure rate is not as high as with other techniques. Tumors with poorly defined margins and recurrent basal cell carcinomas are best treated by microscopically controlled excisional surgery that is known as Mohs' micrographic surgery.[173–175] This technique allows the removed tissue to be mapped in relation to the underlying site. Additional tissue removal is carried out at sites where tumor cells are present microscopically. The treatment is considered complete when there is no tumor found in removed tissue. Cure rates of 90% to 95% are

TABLE 45–5. Management of Nonmelanoma Skin Cancer

Type of Cancer	Therapy
Basal Cell Carcinomas	
Superficial	Topical chemotherapy, cryotherapy, curettage and electrodesiccation, excision, laser vaporization, irradiation, Mohs' micrographic surgery (for multicentric or >2–3 cm)
Nodular-ulcerative	Cryotherapy, curettage and electrodesiccation, excision, irradiation, Mohs' micrographic surgery (high-risk anatomic site, aggressive clinical or histologic pattern, or >2–3 cm)
Morphea	Excision, Mohs' micrographic surgery
Basosquamous	Excision, Mohs' micrographic surgery
Recurrent	Irradiation, Mohs' micrographic surgery
Squamous Cell Carcinoma	
In situ epidermoid cancer	Cryotherapy, laser vaporization, curettage and electrodesiccation, excision, irradiation, Mohs' micrographic surgery
Invasive cancer	Excision, irradiation, Mohs' micrographic surgery
Verrucous carcinoma	Excision, Mohs' micrographic surgery
Adnexal Cancer	
Eccrine, apocrine, and sebaceous carcinomas	Excision, Mohs' micrographic surgery
Extramammary Paget's disease	
Merkel's cell tumor	

achieved with most methods of treating primary basal cell carcinoma. Mohs' surgery has a cure rate of 96% to 99%.[173–175]

Recurrent lesions are larger than 1 to 2 cm, are located over embryologic cleavage planes, or are the sclerosing type. Some lesions are more aggressive and have multiple recurrences, and Mohs' surgery is the treatment of choice. The superficial spreading type of basal cell carcinoma usually recurs, no matter what method of treatment is chosen, because there are small nests of basaloid cells away from the visible margin of the tumor.

Intralesional injection of interferon has been used for treating basal cell carcinoma.[176] The available data are not convincing, and this approach is still experimental. Systemic retinoids have also been used in the treatment of multiple skin cancers and basal cell carcinomas, but the results are not promising. Avoidance of excessive and long periods of sun exposure are effective in the prevention of this cancer.

SQUAMOUS CELL CARCINOMA

Squamous cell carcinoma is a malignant skin cancer arising from epidermal keratinocytes with the potential for metas-

tasis. Squamous cell carcinomas are usually seen in fair-skinned persons who have had excessive sun exposure and developed actinic keratosis (see Fig. 45–1).[62,78,148,156,157] It is more common in men than women. The incidence is estimated to be 20% to 25% of that of basal cell carcinoma. The true incidence of basal cell and squamous cell carcinomas is not available because many practitioners remove and treat these forms of skin cancer without reporting them to the appropriate cancer registry. Any figure is likely to be an underestimation. In Australia, where data are perhaps more accurate, the incidence of squamous cell carcinoma is 166 per 100,000 people, 652 per 100,000 for basal cell carcinoma, and 19 per 100,000 for melanoma.[62,148] In blacks and whites who are treated with PUVA, the incidence of basal cell and squamous cell carcinoma is approximately the same.[177,178]

Pathogenesis

As in basal cell carcinoma, it is the cumulative amount of lifetime UV exposure that influences the development of squamous cell carcinoma.[179–181] Albinos are at especially high risk for developing squamous cell carcinoma early in life if they are exposed to excessive amounts of UV light, indicating the protective value of pigmentation.[182] Occupational and nonoccupational exposure to sunlight are significant risk factors. It is reported that there is an increased incidence of squamous cell carcinoma in persons who have been treated with PUVA.[183] PUVA treatment has been available in the United States for the past 17 years and consists of the systemic intake of psoralen, which is a photosensitizing drug, and exposure to long-wave UV radiation (UVA of 320–360 nm).[177,178] In Europe, however, the use of this photochemotherapy has not been associated with increased squamous cell carcinoma.[184]

The incidence of squamous cell carcinoma is increased among patients who are on immunosuppressive therapy for organ transplantation.[111,185] In these patients, the ratio of basal cell carcinoma to squamous cell carcinoma is reversed, suggesting that the immune system may influence the control of early squamous cell carcinoma. Chronic ulceration, chronic sinus disease, chronic inflammation, and scar tissues increase the chance of developing squamous cell carcinoma. Exposure to ionizing radiation can result in the development of squamous cell carcinoma several years later.

Certain topical agents used for the treatment of chronic skin conditions are carcinogenic and perhaps cause squamous cell carcinoma. Tar causes skin cancer in laboratory animals, but there is no evidence for tar causing skin cancer in humans.[11] Squamous cell carcinoma was considered an occupational hazard among cotton spinners due to contact with the cotton oil. Industrial exposure to chemicals (*e.g.*, cutting oils) is now recognized as a risk factor for squamous cell carcinoma. The historic reports of scrotal malignancies in chimney sweeps was assumed to be due to contact with carcinogenic soot.[12] Arsenic was also recognized to be a carcinogen producing skin cancer and cancers of other organs. In the presteroid era, arsenic was used in the treatment of many diseases.[84,186]

Human papillomavirus has been found in some squamous cell carcinomas.[97,98,185,187–189] HPV types 16 and 18 were found in cancers of the cervix.[91] HPV infections are normally found in patients who are not immunosuppressed.

Clinical Presentation

Squamous cell carcinoma usually appears on the areas of the skin that are damaged by sun exposure. The most common sites of squamous cell carcinoma are the face, neck, back, forearm, and dorsum of the hand of an elderly, white patient with sun-damaged skin (Figs. 45–1 and 45–16 through 45–19). The primary lesion manifests as a red, indurated papule that appears de novo or on an actinic keratosis and expands rapidly, producing a large nodule that eventually ulcerates and metastasizes to a local draining lymph node. Bowen's disease, cutaneous horn (Fig. 45–20), chondrodermatitis nodularis helicis, chronic ulcers, scar tissues, and radiodermatitis may be precursor sites of squamous cell carcinomas (Figs. 45–21 and 45–22) and basal cell carcinomas.[62–64,77,78] The patient may have several primary lesions developing at the same time or in a rapid succession. Tumors arising from sun-damaged skin have relatively lower rates of metastasis, but tumors arising on the mucocutaneous surface or those arising from skin with previous tissue changes (*e.g.*, scars of burns, sites of trauma) tend to be more aggressive, invade locally, and metastasize rapidly.

Squamous cell carcinoma of mucocutaneous sites usually occurs in patients with a history of heavy smoking and heavy alcohol intake.[190] These lesions may arise from an area of leukoplakia or an indurated or ulcerated plaque and metastasize rapidly. Chewing tobacco and betel nuts can influence the development of oral squamous cell carcinoma. Verrucous carcinoma may occur in the oral cavity or sole of the foot and may present as a persistent, firm or vegetating plaque on these areas.

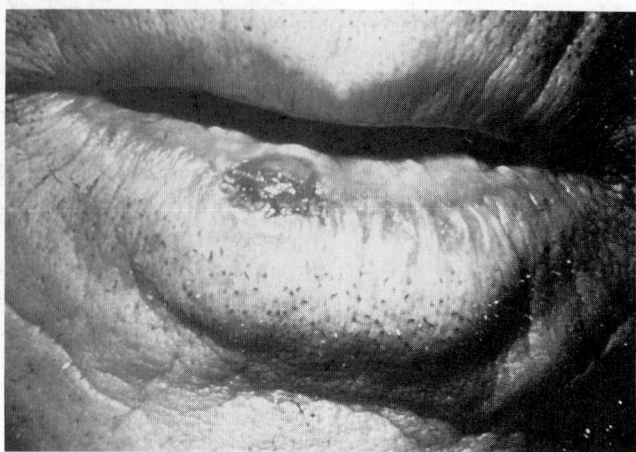

FIGURE 45–17.   Squamous cell carcinoma on the lower lip.

Giant condylomata of Buschke-Lowenstein usually presents as warty lesions on male genitalia. This condition is associated with HPV.[191] Squamous cell carcinoma may develop in a preexisting condition of Buschke-Lowenstein condylomata. Epithelioma cuniculatum usually presents as a small ulcer with peripheral hyperkeratosis on the soles of the feet.[192] This lesion is difficult to eradicate.

Squamous cell carcinoma arising in patients receiving photochemotherapy appears similar to those seen in normal persons and occurs on normal-appearing skin as small crusted nodules.[183] In immunosuppressed patients, it is important to perform skin biopsies on suspected lesions of basal cell carcinoma, squamous cell carcinoma, or actinic keratosis.

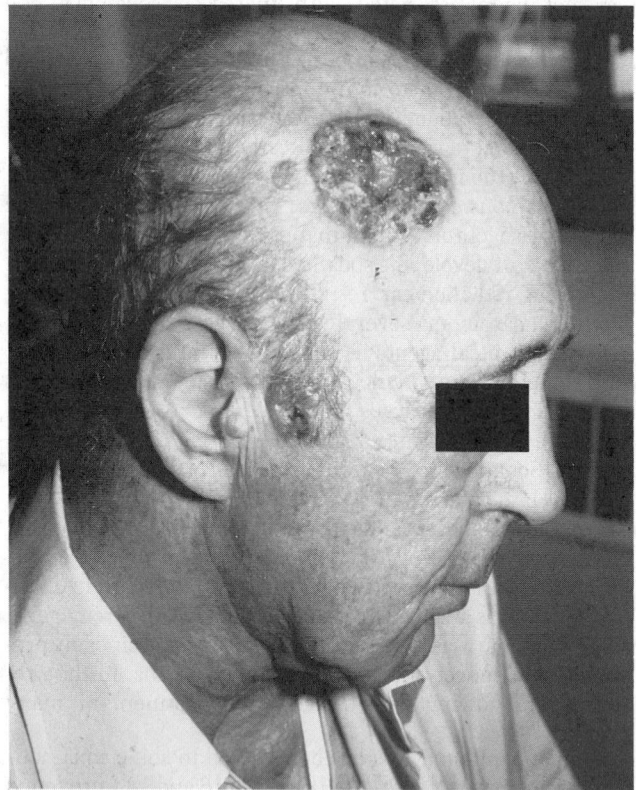

FIGURE 45–16.   Large, ulcerated squamous cell carcinoma on the face and scalp.

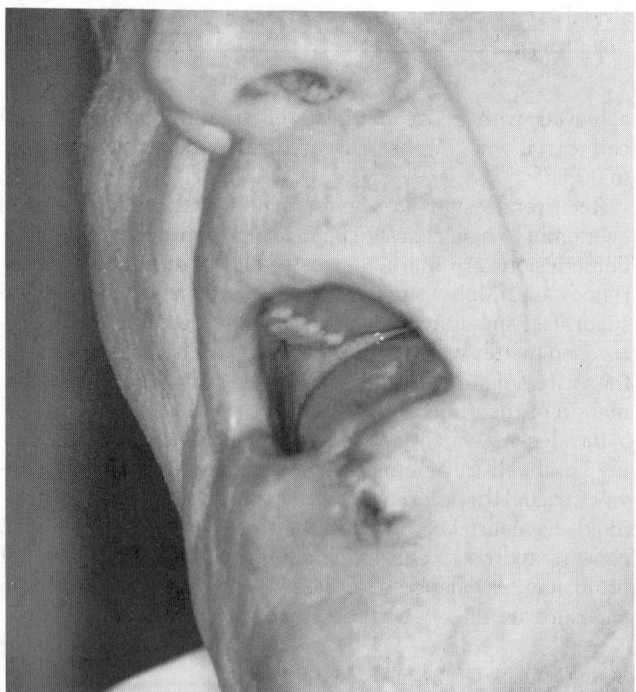

FIGURE 45–18.   Large, invasive squamous cell carcinoma on the lower lip.

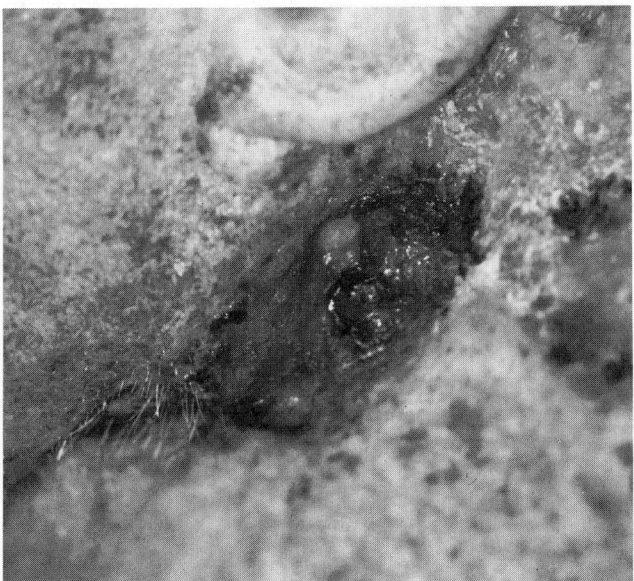

FIGURE 45–19. Large, ulcerated, invasive squamous cell carcinoma on the neck and face.

Classification and Prognosis

The characteristic features of squamous cell carcinoma include proliferation of atypical squamous cells invading the underlying dermis producing an irregular, disorganized architecture. Individually keratinized cells and horn cysts are present. In verrucous carcinoma, giant condyloma of Buschke-Lowenstein, and epithelioma cuniculatum, there is hyperplasia

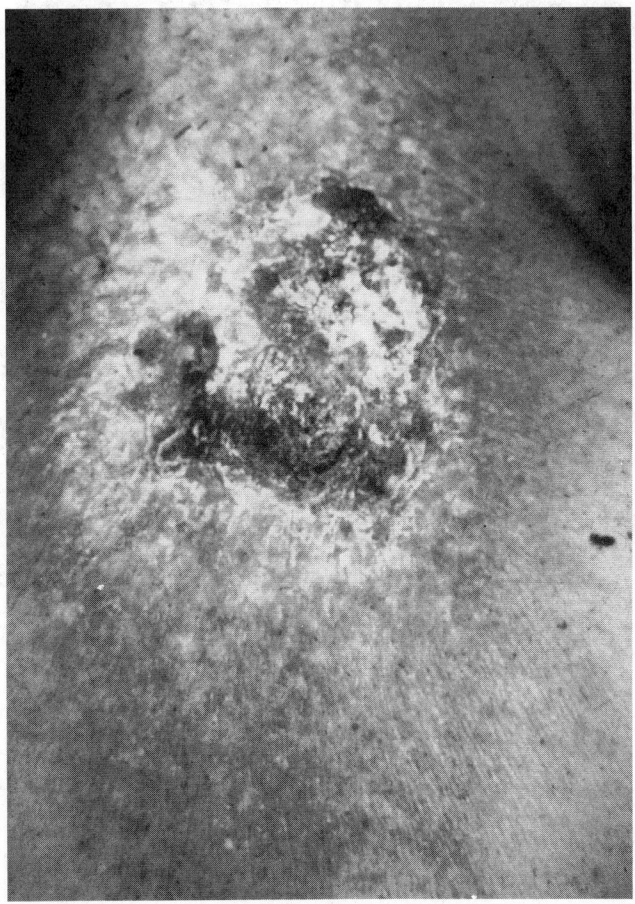

FIGURE 45–21. Squamous cell carcinoma at the site of radiation dermatitis.

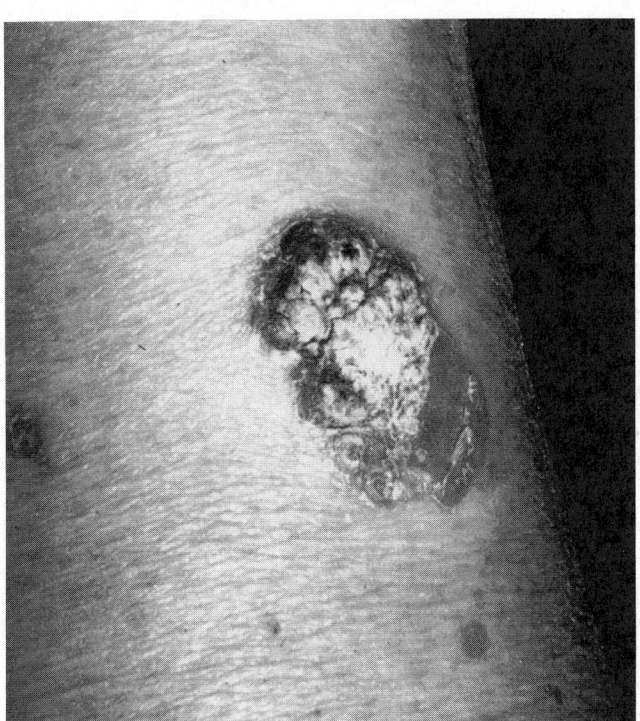

FIGURE 45–20. Squamous cell carcinoma manifesting with a cutaneous horn.

of the mucous membrane epidermis but no evidence of invasion into the dermis.[190–192] Mitotic figures are infrequent.

Attempts have been made to classify squamous cell carcinoma based on the percentage of the undifferentiated cells and to relate this to the prognosis. There are four grades (1–4) of squamous cell carcinoma.[193] Grade 1 has fewer than 25% undifferentiated cells, and grade 4 has more than 75%. The higher the number of undifferentiated cells, the worse is the prognosis. Differential diagnosis of squamous cell carcinoma includes keratoacanthoma, spindle cell melanoma, and soft tissue sarcoma with spindle cells. Antikeratin antibodies can be used to identify and confirm the keratinocyte origin of a given tumor.[194] This is even possible in formalin-fixed, paraffin-embedded specimens. Antibodies against S-100 proteins or NKIC3 indicate a possible melanoma.

Management

Most practitioners use similar treatment modalities for basal cell carcinoma and squamous cell carcinoma (see Table 45–5).[195] Squamous cell carcinoma requires a more aggressive approach, such as wider excision. Tumors on the mucous membranes must be excised with good margins; Mohs' micrographic surgery may be used.[173,196] Close follow-up for recurrences and metastatic spread is highly recommended. In most cases, surgery is preferred to radiation therapy.

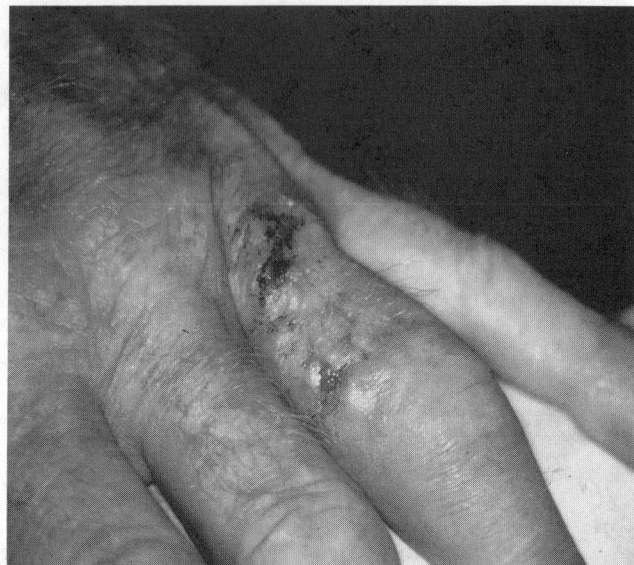

FIGURE 45–22. Squamous cell carcinoma on the finger secondary to radiation exposure.

CANCER-ASSOCIATED GENODERMATOSES

Several inherited dermatoses are associated with the development of cutaneous malignancies. These include xeroderma pigmentosum, nevoid basal cell carcinoma, familial dysplastic nevus syndrome, and multiple self-healing epithelioma of Ferguson-Smith.

XERODERMA PIGMENTOSUM

Xeroderma pigmentosum is a rare disease that occurs in approximately 1 in 250,000 persons in the general population. It is inherited as an autosomal recessive trait and is characterized by severe sun sensitivity, photophobia, cutaneous pigmentary changes, advanced solar damage, multiple skin cancers (*e.g.*, basal cell carcinoma, squamous cell carcinomas, malignant melanoma), and ocular or neurologic changes.[147]

The defect in these patients includes the inability of mast cell strains to excise UV-induced pyrimidine dimers, which results in unrepaired UV-damaged DNA and the development of skin cancers. The remaining repair capability is expressed as unscheduled DNA synthesis and is confirmed by complementary methods of DNA-incising capacity and post-UVL-exposed colony-forming ability. There are nine complementation groups that vary greatly in the degree of defect of unscheduled DNA repair.

The severity of the disease correlates closely with the residual repair capacity. Avoidance of the sun and use of total sunblocks as early in life as possible should be initiated. With the use of sunscreens and other protection mechanisms, these patients live much longer, and they usually die of neurologic involvement and infection rather than UV-induced cancer. Neurologic involvement and progressive mental dysfunction are seen in more than 50% of those who live longer.

Diagnosis of xeroderma pigmentosum is confirmed by a DNA repair study of a fibroblast culture. The best treatment is protection from UV exposure. Actinic keratosis and various skin cancers should be treated appropriately. The use of topical 5-FU or cryotherapy for multiple lesions is helpful. Radiation therapy is not recommended, although the fibroblasts are not sensitive to x-ray damage. Oral retinoid therapy has been used, but the value of this approach requires proof.

BASAL CELL NEVUS SYNDROME

Basal cell nevus syndrome is inherited as an autosomal dominant gene with complete penetrance and variable expression.[146] It is a relatively common genodermatosis, but almost 67% of the patients have no family history, suggesting a high rate of spontaneous mutation. Clinical features are seen in skin, bone, optic tissue, and in the central nervous system. Skin lesions consist of basal cell carcinoma that have atypical features resembling skin tags or pink or flesh-colored, small papules and palmar and plantar pits. Bone cysts are seen in the mandible, and abnormalities of the ribs occur. The ophthalmic evidence includes coloboma or cataracts. Other manifestations include intracranial calcification, ocular hypertelorism, enlarged occipitofrontal head circumference, and increased risk of medulloblastoma and meningioma.

It is thought that the expression of the autosomal dominant gene requires solar radiation. Skin lesions usually develop in large numbers between puberty and age 35. They may become nodular or ulcerative and aggressive. After basal cell carcinoma appears, various modes of therapy should be used to remove the tumors completely. Radiation therapy is not recommended.

FAMILIAL DYSPLASTIC NEVUS SYNDROME

Familial dysplastic nevus syndrome is described elsewhere in this book. The syndrome has an autosomal dominant pattern and consists of large numbers of nevi in the family members of patients with malignant melanoma.

MULTIPLE SELF-HEALING EPITHELIOMA OF FERGUSON-SMITH

Multiple self-healing epithelioma of Ferguson-Smith is an autosomal dominant condition in which affected patients develop crops of raised nodules, most of which regress spontaneously and leave depressed scars. Two large families have been carefully studied. Sporadic cases are also seen. Lesions are seen in early adult life on sun-exposed areas. The histologic features are indistinguishable from squamous cell carcinoma, but the clinical history resembles keratoacanthoma.

TORRE'S SYNDROME

Torre's syndrome includes cutaneous lesions of sebaceous adenoma, sebaceous carcinoma, and basal cell carcinoma in association with carcinoma of the gastrointestinal tract, especially the colon. Multiple keratoacanthomas may also exist. Full colonoscopy and careful long-term follow-up is recommended.

COWDEN'S SYNDROME

Cowden's syndrome presents as multiple hair follicle tumors, mainly tricholemmomas. Oral papillomas are associated with breast carcinoma. The syndrome is thought to be inherited as an autosomal dominant condition. Thyroid carcinoma, ocular and neurologic abnormalities, gastrointestinal problems, and skeletal abnormalities are reported.

GARDNER'S SYNDROME

Gardner's syndrome is an autosomal dominant condition manifesting with cutaneous cysts, bony abnormalities, and colonic polyps that may progress to carcinoma. Adrenal, thyroid, and ovarian carcinomas and carcinoids are also associated with Gardner's syndrome.

CARNEY'S SYNDROME

Carney's syndrome consists of myxomas, endocrine dysfunction, pigmentary abnormalities and breast and endocrine cancers. The exact mode of this rare syndrome is not as yet well established.

TUMORS ARISING FROM EPIDERMAL MERKEL'S CELL

MERKEL'S CELL CARCINOMA

Merkel's cell carcinoma, formerly called trabecular carcinoma, is an uncommon, highly malignant, primary cutaneous neuroendocrine carcinoma arising from Merkel's cells located in the basal layer of the epidermis and in the hair follicles.[197,198] Merkel's cells are associated with sensory neurites in the dermal papillae, forming mechanoreceptor in the skin. The neoplastic Merkel's cells are characteristically small, round to polygonal, undifferentiated tumor cells with scanty cytoplasm. These tumor cells exhibit different histologic patterns.[199] The most common pattern is the solid type, which is composed of irregular groups of tumor cells interconnected by strands of connective tissue. The trabecular type is characterized by well-defined cords of cells that form invading columns or cords between collagen bundles. The diffuse type exhibits poor cohesion and a lymphoma-like diffuse type of growth.

This lesion occurs mostly in white, elderly persons, with an equal incidence in men and women. It is usually localized to the sun-exposed areas of the head and neck but does occur on the extremities, trunk, and genitalia in a random distribution. The clinical presentation is a rapidly growing, painless, firm, nontender, shiny, bluish-red, intracutaneous nodule 0.5 to 5 cm in diameter. The tumor arises in the dermis and extends into the subcutis. The epidermis is infrequently involved, and the overlying skin is intact and rarely ulcerated. There is a high incidence of distant metastases, regional lymph node involvement, and locoregional recurrences, resulting in poor prognosis even after treatment.[199–202] The prognosis of Merkel's cell carcinoma shows a sex differentiation, with 3-year survival rates of 35.6% for men and 67.6% for women.[201] The three reported instances of spontaneous regression occurred in women.[203,204] The recommended treatment is wide surgical excision of the tumor and prophylactic regional node dissec-tion. Postoperative radiation therapy to the local site and regional lymph nodes is helpful.[205,206] Chemotherapy is considered effective in some reports.[207]

TUMORS ARISING FROM EPIDERMAL LANGERHANS CELLS

HISTIOCYTOSIS X

Langerhans cells are bone marrow-derived dendritic cells that reside in the upper layer of the epidermis. Proliferation of Langerhans cells results in development of a clinically heterogenous group of diseases commonly called histiocytosis X. Three distinct variants have been described: Letterer-Siwe disease, Hand-Schüller-Christian disease, and eosinophilic granuloma.

Letterer-Siwe Disease

Letterer-Siwe disease is seen in children younger than 2 years of age and manifests with fever, lymphadenopathy, hepatosplenomegaly, pulmonary involvement, cutaneous eruption, and thrombocytopenia. Skin eruptions are in the form of seborrheic dermatitis or purpuric red-brown papules.

Hand-Schüller-Christian Disease

Hand-Schüller-Christian disease occurs in children between the ages of 2 and 6 years with the triad of exophthalmos, diabetes insipidus, and bony involvement of the skull. This is a more chronic progressive form of histiocytosis X than Letterer-Siwe disease, which is acute, fulminant, rapidly progressive, and usually fatal.

Eosinophilic Granuloma

Eosinophilic granuloma is commonly seen in children and young adults with solitary bone lesions or involvement of other organs.

Overlap of these three diseases makes classification difficult. Staging according to the extent of disease and the type of organ(s) involved is reported to have prognostic value. More detailed descriptions of these conditions can be found in other chapters of this book.

TUMORS ARISING FROM SKIN APPENDAGES

Skin appendages or adnexa include eccrine and apocrine sweat glands, hair follicles, sebaceous glands, and nail beds. Many adnexal tumors have been described, but these tumors are rare and often are difficult to diagnose clinically because of lack of distinguishable features.[208,209] Histologically, most of these tumors present a diagnostic dilemma to the pathologist. To identify the origin of these tumors, histochemical staining, ultrastructural studies, antikeratin antibodies, antibodies to epithelial membrane antigen (EMA), and carcinoembryonic antigen (CEA) have been used. The antigen tests are positive in sweat glands and negative in hair follicles. Most of the skin appendage tumors are slow growing and benign. Those considered malignant are mostly locally invasive. There are rare cases of metastasizing and highly malignant tumors. Morphologic criteria may not correlate with biologic behavior of the tumors.

TUMORS OF HAIR FOLLICLES

Many tumors may arise from various segments of the hair follicle (see Table 45–1 and Fig. 45–23).[210] These tumors proliferate but do not metastasize. Some of the more frequent types are summarized here.

INVERTED FOLLICULAR KERATOSIS

Inverted follicular keratosis usually appears as a firm, gray, flat plaque on the face that is indistinguishable from seborrheic keratosis and may sometimes be similar to verruca vulgaris.[211] It is suspected to be a virally induced lesion, but no HPV has been found in this tumor. Histologically, it is thought to be a proliferation of the keratinocytes of the follicular infundibulum or the intraepidermal part of the hair follicle. Under low-power light microscopy, a papillomatous mass of keratinocytes is seen. Squamous eddies and keratin cyst within a hair follicle sometimes gives a true pattern of inverted follicular keratosis.

TRICHODISCOMA

Trichodiscoma usually appears as multiple, skin-colored papules on the face. It is sometimes seen in family members.[55–57,212] It is thought that the lesion arises from the dermal component of the hair disk, giving a regular dome-shaped fibrovascular histology in the papillary dermis with a hair follicle at the margin.

TUMORS OF THE FOLLICULAR INFUNDIBULUM

Tumors of the follicular infundibulum appear as smooth, raised, skin-colored papules on the face. They are thought to arise from the infundibulum of the hair follicle, which is the area above the entry point of the sebaceous duct into the hair canal.[213] Histologically, the tumor is composed of pale epithelial cells rich in glycogen.

TRICHILEMMOMA

Trichilemmoma (*i.e.*, trichilemmocarcinoma) appears as single or multiple small nodules on the face and is usually asymptomatic. Hair may be seen in these lesions. The lesions resemble common warts. In women with multiple lesions of this type, Cowden's syndrome must be considered. Tumors originate from the outer part of the hair root sheath. Histologically, tumors contain large, lobulated, palisading epithelial cells with pale cytoplasm high in glycogen content.[73] These tumors are CEA and EMA negative and can be differentiated from tumors of eccrine origin that may have similar histology but are CEA and EMA positive. Malignant trichilemmoma (*i.e.*, trichilemmocarcinoma) has been reported with local lymph node metastasis.[214,215]

TRICHOFOLLICULOMA

Trichofolliculoma presents as multiple, skin-colored papules with tufts of hair emerging from some of the lesions. The lesions may coalesce to form plaques several centimeters in diameter. The histology consists of poorly formed hair follicles that are easily diagnosable from other hair follicles in these tumors.[216] A variant called sebaceous trichofolliculoma is composed of lobules of sebaceous epithelium with acini and duct formations.[217]

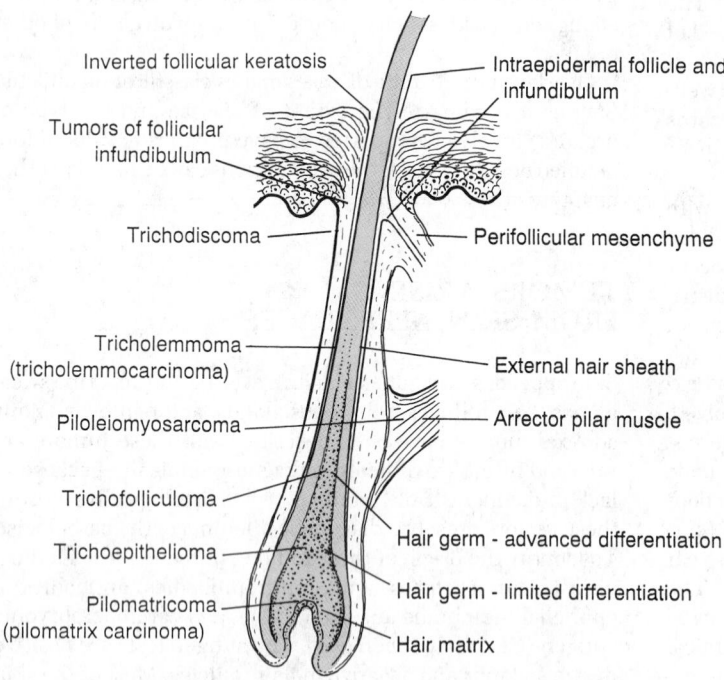

FIGURE 45–23. Schematic diagram of tumors arising from the hair follicle.

TRICHOEPITHELIOMA

Trichoepithelioma may be single or multiple and appears as nondescript skin-colored papules on the face, especially the nasolabial fold, eyelids, and central face. The tumors are inherited as an autosomal dominant trait. The tumor arises from the hair shaft deep in the sebaceous gland attachment. Histologically, this tumor has some of the features of morphea-type basal cell carcinoma and should be differentiated from it.[218]

PILOMATRICOMA

Pilomatricoma (*i.e.*, calcifying epithelioma of Malherbe) arises from the hair matrix.[219] The tumor may be single or multiple and appears mostly during the first decades of life and are occasionally familial. The tumor manifests as a solid, hard nodule a few centimeters in diameter. The histologic picture is fairly specific; darkly stained basaloid cells are seen in some areas, and in other areas, the cells have changed and developed configurations of shadow or ghost cells. Around these ghost cells, calcification usually usually makes the nodule firm. A fibrous stroma is seen around both cell types and calcification. Giant cells are frequent. Malignant transformation to pilomatrix carcinoma is rare.[219-221] Malignant tumors may invade locally but do not metastasize.

TUMORS OF SEBACEOUS GLANDS

Tumors of sebaceous glands are rare and mostly benign, but they may progress to malignancy.

FOX-FORDYCE ANOMALY

Fox-Fordyce anomaly is a condition in which sebaceous glands are found on mucosal surfaces, mostly in the oral mucosa.[222] Sebaceous glands are usually present on skin and not on mucous membranes. These mucosal sebaceous glands appear as yellowish papules. Histologically, they consist of collections of sebaceous glands.

ORGANOID OR SEBACEOUS NEVI

Organoid or sebaceous nevi are skin lesions composed of abnormal numbers of skin appendages with a high tendency of basal cell carcinoma developing secondarily to this lesion (see Fig. 45-7).[119-121] The term organoid nevus is more accurate because skin appendages other than sebaceous gland, such as eccrine gland and smooth muscle, may be present. However, because of its appearance and the presence of sebaceous glands in this tumor, it may still be referred to as sebaceous epidermoid nevus.

SEBACEOUS GLAND HYPERPLASIA

Sebaceous gland hyperplasia is a common skin lesion of the face of most elderly persons. The lesion appears as multiple, raised, yellowish papules with depressed centers and some telangiectasia.[223] Differential diagnosis includes basal cell carcinoma. Histopathologic features include collections of layers of sebaceous gland shadows.

SEBACEOUS ADENOMAS AND EPITHELIOMAS

Sebaceous adenomas and epitheliomas are two conditions that present as yellow or white raised papules on the face. Collections of sebaceous gland cells with foamy cytoplasm are seen in the sebaceous gland adenoma.[224] In sebaceous gland epithelioma, the histopathology consists of masses of compact sebaceous cells, some of which are the small, dark, basaloid type.[225] Differential diagnosis includes hair follicle tumors and basal cell carcinoma. The possibility of Muir-Torre syndrome should be considered.

SEBACEOUS CARCINOMA

Sebaceous carcinoma occurs most frequently on the upper eyelids of women in their sixties, but it may also be seen on the scalp and face.[225,226] On the eyelid, it may appear as a chronic conjunctivitis or chalazion.[227-229] On the face, it may have the appearance of a yellowish, raised papule or plaque that is translucent with a greasy surface.[230,231] Pathologic features include lobules of cells with foamy cytoplasm and basaloid cells with large numbers of mitotic figures. The tumors may extend to subcutaneous tissue and may perforate through the fascia and muscles and then rapidly metastasize. The histologic differential diagnosis includes squamous cell carcinoma, Paget's disease, and malignant melanoma. Special stains for fat, anticytokeratins, and EMA are helpful in the histologic diagnosis. Radiation therapy and chemotherapy have been used, but surgical excision with microscopic control of the margin is the best approach.[232-234]

TUMORS OF APOCRINE GLANDS

SUPERNUMERARY NIPPLE

Supernumerary nipple appears as a firm nodule on the area near the nipple. It is similar to an intraepidermal nevus or skin tag. Pathologic features consist of ectopic breast tissue, dilated mammary glands, hair follicles, and isolated smooth muscles.[235]

APOCRINE HIDROCYSTOMA

Apocrine hidrocystoma or cystadenoma appears as translucent bluish papules occurring most commonly on the face.[236] Differential diagnosis is pigmented basal cell carcinoma or nevus. Pathologic features include cystic structures lined with a row of tall columnar cells and a layer of myoepithelial cells in the periphery.

SYRINGOCYSTADENOMA PAPILLIFERUM

Syringocystadenoma papilliferum or papillary syringoadenoma presents as highly verrucous lesions appearing mostly on the scalp and face. The lesion may develop on an organoid nevus.[119] More than 50% are reported at birth and 25% at puberty. Histopathology consists of invaginated cystic structures lined with two layers of columnar epithelial cells and a plasma cell-rich stroma. Rare cases of transformation into adenocarcinoma with regional lymph node metastases have been reported.[237]

HIDRADENOMA PAPILLIFERUM

Hidradenoma papilliferum is found exclusively in women on the vulvar area and appears as a palpable lesion on the labia majora. It may also be found in the perineal and perianal regions. Histopathology is similar to syringocystadenoma papilliferum, except that there is no plasma cell infiltration. One case of malignant transformation has been reported. It developed into a fatal, metastasizing squamous cell carcinoma.[238]

PAGET'S DISEASE

Paget's disease of the skin is identified as atypical cells present within the epidermis. It may clinically and pathologically be confused with Bowen's disease.[239] Paget's disease may occur frequently on the areola and nipple (*i.e.,* mammary Paget's disease) or less commonly on the vulva, scrotum, or perineal and perianal areas (*i.e.,* extramammary Paget's disease). Characteristic histologic features of Paget's disease are large epithelioid (Paget's) cells with dark hyperchromatic nuclei, cytologic atypia, and frequent mitotic figures within the epidermis.

After confirmation of the diagnosis by skin biopsy for histologic examination, the extramammary Paget's disease is usually treated with wide excision of the involved area. In cases of Paget's disease of the breast, surgical approach of the skin and underlying carcinoma is recommended.

Extramammary Paget's disease is a rare form of adenocarcinoma observed mostly in the skin of the anogenital and axillary regions, and less frequently in the esophagus, oral mucosa, tongue, bronchial epithelium, urethra, buttocks, thighs, chest, external auditory canal, and eyelid. The lesions appear as a solitary, well-defined patch with an eczematous surface. Differential diagnosis includes psoriasis and eczematous dermatosis. It shares histologic resemblances to mammary Paget's disease, showing characteristic large anaplastic Paget's cells with round or ovoid nucleus and clear cytoplasm, occurring singly or in small groups within the epidermis.[240] Although mammary Paget's disease is an epidermal manifestation of an underlying mammary duct adenocarcinoma, extramammary Paget's disease arises from an underlying adenocarcinoma or from intraepithelial precursors, and it occurs in areas with a high density of apocrine or eccrine glands. There is controversy about whether Paget's cells originate from the ductal carcinoma or from the epidermis. Extramammary and mammary Paget's disease are presumed to be variants of epithelial carcinoma, possessing the potential to develop from or to be the cause of an underlying adenocarcinoma.

Treatment of extramammary Paget's disease depends on the area of involvement, but it is usually by wide local excision or Mohs' micrographic surgery with or without subsequent radiation therapy.[241] Depending on the area involved, a split skin graft may be necessary.

APOCRINE ADENOCARCINOMAS

Apocrine adenocarcinoma is a rare tumor that usually occurs in the areas with apocrine glands, such as the axillae and the anogenital region. It has developed in other sites, such as the auditory meatus, where ceruminal glands are found. Apocrine gland carcinoma may locally invade or metastasize to regional lymph nodes. The histopathology is that of adenocarcinoma with various degrees of differentiation. Even in poorly differentiated tumors, recognition of an apocrine structure is usually possible in some sections. The tumor shows high activity for apocrine enzymes such as acid phosphatase, β-glucuronidase, and indoxyl acetate esterase, but there is no activity of eccrine enzymes such as phosphorylase and succinic dehydrogenase.

TUMORS OF ECCRINE GLANDS

Eccrine sweat glands can be the source of many benign or malignant tumors (Fig. 45–24). Secondary eccrine gland carcinomas arise directly from eccrine glands through a malignant transformation. These malignant tumors are rare and usually develop from a preexisting eccrine appendage tumor of lesser maturity.[209] There is at least one recognizable tumor for each morphologic region. The diagram simplifies the locations where various tumors originate (see Fig. 45–24 and Table 45–1).

BENIGN TUMORS

Poroma

Poromas are benign neoplasms arising from the outer cells of the intraepidermal duct and the uppermost region of the straight intradermal duct. Variants of poromas or poroid neoplasms include hidroacanthoma simplex, eccrine poroma, dermal duct tumor, and poroid hidradenoma.[242–250] Hidro-

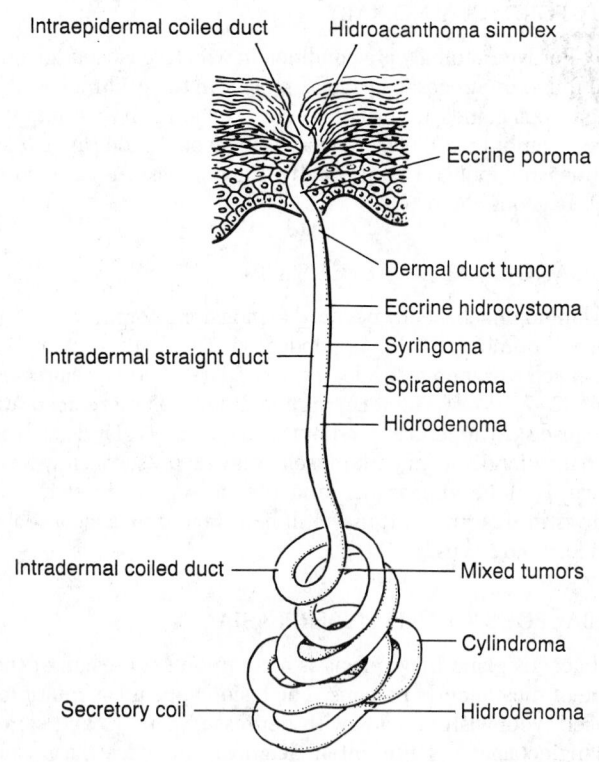

Intraepidermal coiled duct

Hidroacanthoma simplex

Eccrine poroma

Dermal duct tumor

Eccrine hidrocystoma

Syringoma

Spiradenoma

Hidrodenoma

Intradermal straight duct

Intradermal coiled duct

Mixed tumors

Cylindroma

Secretory coil

Hidrodenoma

FIGURE 45–24. Schematic diagram of tumors arising from the eccrine gland.

acanthoma simplex and eccrine poroma are confined within the epidermis. Dermal duct tumor is detached from the epidermis and occurs as an intradermal nodule.[248] Poroid hidradenoma has features of poroma and hidradenoma. This variant is a wholly intradermal neoplasm with solid and cystic components of a typical hidradenoma, but on closer examination, the same cells as those in hidroacanthoma simplex, eccrine poroma, and dermal duct tumor are observed. The four poroid neoplasms have similar architectural aspects and identical cytologic features, and a sharp demarcation among types of poromas is not always possible.

The poroid cells are slightly smaller than keratinocytes and have plump, oval to round nuclei, inconspicuous nucleoli, and scant cytoplasm. There is little variation in size and shape of cells seen within poromas. Poromas also contain cuticular cells, which are larger than poroid cells, having slightly larger nuclei with more pronounced chromatin. They are situated around the lumen of eccrine ducts. One of these two cell types tends to predominate in poromas, giving these neoplasms a monomorphous appearance.

Hidroacanthoma simplex appears as a small plaque on the face and is benign.[242] Malignant hidroacanthoma simplex has been reported, but it is controversial if these are truly malignant because hidroacanthoma simplex has some histologic features of carcinoma in situ.[196,243,251] Eccrine poroma appears as raised, pink to red nodules most often on the soles of the feet. Malignant transformation of this tumor to porocarcinoma is rarely reported.[246,249–251] Porocarcinomas are mostly located on the lower extremities and may metastasize. In the malignant form, mitotic figures, duct formation, and atypical cells in the vascular slit-like spaces are seen. The malignant form should be differentiated from Paget's disease, squamous cell carcinoma, and other carcinomas. Management is surgical excision. The behavior of malignant poromas is relatively unpredictable, and microscopically checked surgical excision is advised for this malignant neoplasm.

Syringoma

Syringomas or eccrine mixed tumors are benign tumors of the luminal cells of the intradermal portion of the eccrine duct. The disease presents as multiple, smooth, firm, dome-shaped, slightly yellow or skin-colored papules that are 1 to 5 mm in diameter. Lesions are usually found on the lower eyelids and upper parts of the cheeks. They occur with much less frequency on the neck, chest, axillae, pubic area, scalp, and periumbilical region. Histologically, the tumor consists of well-circumscribed nodules in the upper dermis containing small solid nests, cords, and tubules of neoplastic epithelial cells randomly distributed throughout a prominent stroma of markedly thickened, closely packed bundles of collagen.[252] Epithelial cells have dark-staining nuclei with scanty cytoplasm or with abundant pale-staining cytoplasm. A variant called clear cell syringoma consists mostly of solid aggregates of the epithelial cell with abundant cytoplasm.[253]

Syringomas are usually diagnosed in middle-aged or older persons. This tumor often make its first appearance at puberty or in adolescence. Women are affected twice as often as men. Japanese women have an unusually high incidence that is sixfold greater than white or black women.[254] Patients with Down's syndrome also have a high incidence, with females affected more often than male patients.[255]

Another form of syringomas, an eruptive type, presents as numerous widespread crops of syringomas and is found most often in pubescent girls, almost exclusively on the anterior aspects of the neck, trunk, axillae, and inner aspects of extremities.[255,256] The crops of syringomas appear episodically and erupt over 2 to 3 years, after which the neoplasms persist without further growth. During this growth period, papules may be so numerous that they become confluent to form plaques. These lesions have identical histology to those of conventional syringoma.

The differential diagnosis is desmoplastic trichoepithelioma. In rare cases, syringomas may transform to syringomatous carcinoma.[257–261]

Chondroid Syringoma

Chondroid syringoma presents as well-encapsulated, spherical or lobulated, dermal or subcutaneous nodules on the head and neck areas, and the lesions may reach large sizes.[262,263] Twice as many men as women are affected. The lesions are also called mixed tumors because they have epithelial components that may differentiate into eccrine, apocrine, and follicular structures. Pathologic features include a mixed collection of cells in an ill-defined peripheral border. Some lesions contain more tubular structures, and others are more solid. The tubular structures are embedded in a dense fibrous stroma. The tubular structures are lined by eccrine secretory cells. Rarely, areas suggestive of apocrine glands are seen. Malignant chondroid syringomas have been reported rarely.[264–270] The tumor occurs on the extremities and may arise from a preexisting benign mixed tumor or may be malignant from the onset. It can recur locally and metastasize.

Eccrine Hidrocystoma

Eccrine hidrocystoma appears mostly on the face as solitary or multiple small translucent nodules with some bluish to dark brown-black pigmentation.[271] Histologic examination reveals a single cyst lined by two layers of cuboidal rather than columnar (as in apocrine) cells and does not show evidence of decapitation secretion. The lesions are usually located within the papillary dermis.

Eccrine Spiradenoma

Eccrine spiradenoma presents as deeply seated nodules on any part of the skin but most frequently on the face, scalp, neck, trunk, and arms, and it often causes spontaneous pain.[272–274] This lesion occurs with equal distribution among men and women. Tumors may be solitary, or multiple nodules may be grouped together and confined to a circumscribed region where they may become confluent or remain discrete. The epidermis overlying these dermal or subcutaneous nodules may show no change in color or may be pink or bluish, but it is rarely ulcerated.

Malignant forms (*e.g.,* spiradenocarcinoma) are rare.[275–278] This carcinoma occurs within a preexisting spiradenoma or may appear as a satellite nodule. The rapidly expanding nodule may cause inflammation and ulceration of the lesion. One patient died of widespread metastasis and local recurrence.[277] Spiradenomas arises from intradermal straight duct of eccrine glands. The histology consists of cords of epithelial cells in an edematous stroma. The cords contain two cell types: small basaloid cells with dark-staining nuclei lying at the periphery of slit-like tubular lumens and larger cells with pale nuclei lying within the cords. The cords and stroma form encapsulated lobules with the dermis and with no interconnection to the epidermis. The cells show high levels of phosphorylase activity, indicating their eccrine origin. In malignant tumors, some areas with typical spiradenoma structures are replaced with broad, confluent sheets of cells without intervening cords and tubular structures. These solid areas have many mitotic figures and show patterns similar to squamous metaplasia, spindle cell sarcoma, and poorly differentiated adenocarcinoma.[275-277] Large cyst formations are also found in malignant areas of spiradenoma.

The differential diagnosis includes cylindroma, lymphangioma, and other vascular neoplasms. Management consists of surgical excision.

Eccrine Hidradenoma

Eccrine hidradenoma manifests clinically as reddish-blue nodules on any area of skin but mostly on the face. This tumor arises from the secretory coil of the eccrine duct as a well-circumscribed tumor within the dermis and with no epidermal connection. It may show differentiation that is reminiscent of the lower portion of the intradermal straight duct.

Histopathologic examination reveals two main cell types: small cuboidal cells with basophilic cytoplasm and round nucleus (*i.e.*, duct lining cells) and larger cells with clear cytoplasm and small, dark nuclei (*i.e.*, secretory coil cells). The proportions of these cell types vary among lesions. These cells form a well-defined tumor mass with occasional cystic or duct-like formations. The clear cells in hidradenoma are similar to the cells seen in tricholemmoma or clear cell carcinoma of the kidney. However, the presence of tubular lumens and cystic spaces is characteristic of hidradenomas and may be used for differential diagnosis. The clear cells are derived form the secretory coil that is active in secretion and resorption. These clear cells are more prone to malignant transformations.[279-286] Clear cell hidradenocarcinomas are discussed later. Hidradenomas mostly contain cells of eccrine origin, but cells with apocrine secretory features may be seen in some areas. Surgical excision is the treatment of choice.

Cylindroma

Cylindroma (*i.e.*, turban tumor) is postulated to have eccrine, apocrine, and pilar differentiation, but new information indicates that it is a benign neoplasm arising from the intradermal coiled duct of eccrine glands.[287,288] This lesion may be solitary, but most often it presents as multiple, firm, smooth, dome-shaped, movable, pink to red papules or nodules that are 3 to 30 mm in diameter. Ulceration is uncommon and is usually a consequence of trauma. Women are affected four times more frequently than men. About 10% of all cylindromas are hereditary in an autosomal dominant fashion with variable penetrance; carriers of the trait may not necessarily manifest the disease.

Lesions usually appear in early adult life, but the onset may be as early as childhood or adolescence. Papules, nodules, and tumors occur mainly on the scalp, but they may be found on the face and upper part of the trunk. If tumors are widespread in the skin, the clinical picture, at first glance, may resemble neurofibromatosis. The neoplasm grows slowly but persistently, with new tumors continuously appearing and becoming confluent in some areas. If nodules of cylindromas cover the entire scalp and are heaped up, they resemble a turban.

The nonhereditary expression of cylindroma (90% of patients) usually appears as a solitary lesion arising on a hair-bearing area. If cylindromas occur on extremities, the patients also tend to have lesions on the scalp.

Histologically, cylindromas are composed of islands of epithelial cells surrounded by prominent thick rims of hyalinized basement membrane material. Globules of the same material are found within islands of neoplastic cells. Nodules are well circumscribed but not encapsulated, are situated in the dermis and subcutis, and lack foci of necrosis. Aggregations of epithelial cells vary considerably in size and shape, but cells are close to one another in a pattern resembling a jigsaw puzzle. These aggregates are composed of a centrally located population of neoplastic epithelial cells with large nuclei and abundant cytoplasm surrounded by a peripheral population of cells with smaller nuclei and scanty cytoplasm. Tubules may be found in some of these islands of epithelial cells. The lumen of these tubules are lined by cells with cuticular features like those of normal eccrine or apocrine ducts. Scalp tumors may extend to the fascia and the periosteum. The epidermis is not involved, but it is usually thinned due to the pressure of the underlying tumor. Cylindromas may contain zones that are almost indistinguishable from spiradenomas, giving further evidence for its eccrine origin.[288]

Cylindromas have rarely progressed to cylindrocarcinoma.[289-291] Most of the cases have developed from long-standing tumors of cylindroma. Histologically, the tumors are similar to cylindromas but are marked by large numbers of mitotic figures and atypical mitoses. Cylindrocarcinomas are aggressive, with metastases to lymph nodes, bone, and visceral organs.

PRIMARY ECCRINE GLAND CARCINOMAS

Primary eccrine gland carcinomas may arise from preexisting, less mature eccrine gland tumors or may develop de novo from eccrine glands within the skin. Primary eccrine gland carcinomas include syringoid eccrine carcinoma, mucinous eccrine carcinoma, clear cell carcinoma, microcystic eccrine carcinoma, adenoid cystic carcinoma, aggressive digital papillary adenocarcinoma, and eccrine adenocarcinoma.

The clinical features of these tumors are nonspecific, and the final diagnosis is always based on histology. The tumors usually are located on the head, neck, or extremities and manifest as slow-growing nodules or infiltrated plaques.[292] These are rare tumors, with only about 200 cases reported in the world literature. Several different subtypes have been described (see Fig. 45–24 and Table 45–1).

Syringoid Eccrine Carcinoma

Syringoid eccrine carcinoma appears as a solitary, firm, plaque-like, verrucous tumor on the head or face of elderly persons. The lesion may secrete fluid and resemble syringocystadenoma papilliferum. Scalp lesions may cause alopecia. The common benign lesions of syringoma are multiple papules distributed on the lower eyelids, and the benign lesions of eruptive syringoma are located on the neck, chest, umbilicus, or genitalia. Syringoma may be associated with Down's syndrome, Marfan's syndrome, or Ehlers-Danlos syndrome. Histology consists of tubulocystic proliferations with epithelial cord, the so-called tadpole picture, which is also seen in benign syringoma and hence the name syringoid eccrine carcinoma. Slight cellular atypia, nuclear hyperchromatism, deep invasion, and numerous crowded tubulocystic structures signify that the tumor is not benign syringoma. Syringoid eccrine carcinomas may be locally destructive or metastasize widely.[257-261]

Mucinous Eccrine Carcinoma

Mucinous eccrine carcinoma appears as a solitary, slow-growing, painless nodule, most frequently on the eyelids, but it may appear on the head, neck, or elsewhere on the body.[293-299] Local recurrences are reported, but metastasis is rare. Small cystic structures and tubular cords formed by basaloid cells are common. These structures resemble eccrine ducts. The cells show features of low-grade malignant tumors. There is a mucinous degeneration of the stroma that stains with Alcian blue.

Clear Cell Carcinoma

Clear cell carcinoma (*i.e.*, malignant clear cell hidradenoma, clear cell hidradenocarcinoma, or malignant clear cell acrospiroma) is a solitary tumor of the face, head, hand, or foot.[282-285] Widespread metastases are common.[282,286] These tumors may appear de novo as malignant tumors or develop as a malignant transformation of benign clear cell hidradenoma (*i.e.*, acrospiroma). The histology is similar to the benign condition except for cellular atypia and invasive borders. Clear cells, produced by large amounts of glycogen, are admixed with large oval or spindle-shaped cells. Large cystic spaces, lined with these clear cells, may be found in some tumors.

Microcystic Eccrine Carcinoma

Microcystic eccrine carcinoma manifests as an indurated, ill-defined, slow-growing, solitary nodule or plaque on the upper lip and cheek of middle-aged women.[300-304] The surface may appear smooth or crusted. Local recurrence is common, but metastasis is rare. Histologic examination reveals small cystic spaces, eccrine duct-like structures, and keratinous cysts in a fibrous stroma. The best sign of malignancy in these tumors is the deep infiltration with perivascular, perineural, and muscular invasions. The lesions may look like morphea-type basal cell carcinoma. Lesions are CEA positive, indicating the sweat gland origin. Differential diagnosis includes syringoma, desmoplastic trichoepithelioma, and papillary eccrine adenoma.

Adenoid Cystic Carcinoma

Adenoid cystic carcinoma is an extremely rare, indolent tumor that preferentially occurs on the scalp but may occur elsewhere.[305-308] Alopecia may be associated with this condition. It presents as crusted verrucous plaques or deep-seated nodules. Metastasis was reported in only 1 patient.[309] The histologic features of this tumor are similar with those of adenoid cystic carcinoma of the salivary gland.[310] The microscopic picture shows dermal nodules with no epidermal contact. As the name implies, there are many cystic spaces with areas of solid tissue. Small basaloid cells with scanty cytoplasm are the prominent cell type, but numerous fibroblasts and lymphocytic infiltrates can be found. These are in a fibrous stroma. The tumor shows an infiltrative growth pattern extending into the dermis or the subcutis. The adenoid cystic variant of basal cell carcinoma may present a diagnostic problem for this adnexal carcinoma.[310]

Aggressive Digital Papillary Adenocarcinoma

Aggressive digital papillary adenocarcinoma is a rare eccrine tumor with an acral location. These tumors present most often in older persons as a solitary, asymptomatic, slowly enlarging mass, most frequently on a digit or adjacent tissue.[311,312] The lesion is freely movable. Some patients may experience pain or tenderness, and the surface of the lesion may be ulcerated and bleeding. Deep infiltration of the underlying soft tissue results in a high local recurrence rate with a possibility of metastases to lymph nodes, bone, and visceral organs. Locally aggressive tumors are hard to differentiate from those that may metastasize. The histologic picture shows poor glandular differentiation, presence of necrosis, prominent cellular atypia, and invasion of the underlying tissue and bone. Lesions show a tubuloalveolar pattern with cystic spaces and atypical cells forming glandular structures. The epidermis is usually intact, except if ulceration and bleeding occur. Cells stain positive for CEA and S-100, showing their eccrine origin.

Differential diagnosis includes giant tumor of the tendon sheath, inclusion cyst, glomus tumor, metastatic tumor, pyogenic granuloma, and cavernous hemangioma. Treatment is wide excision or amputation of the digit. Chemotherapy is ineffective. After metastasis occurs, the prognosis is poor.

Eccrine Adenocarcinoma

Eccrine adenocarcinomas manifest as enlarging ulcerated nodules with no distinct clinical features.[261,313-319] Histologic examination reveals solid masses with various glandular differentiations resembling normal eccrine glands and ducts in a well-differentiated tumor. The poorly differentiated form of eccrine adenocarcinoma is highly malignant and may metastasize rapidly. Differentiation from metastatic adenocarcinoma may be impossible, but after visceral carcinomas are ruled out, the diagnosis of eccrine adenocarcinoma should be considered.

SECONDARY ECCRINE CARCINOMAS

Some of the benign eccrine gland tumors may transform and become malignant. Rapid enlargement, change in color, pain, or ulceration are usually signs of malignant transformation. In some instances, a benign-appearing lesion is removed but histologically is proven to consist of a small area of malignant degeneration.

Several secondary eccrine carcinomas arising from benign eccrine tumors are described (see Fig. 45–24 and Table 45–1). These include spiradenocarcinoma, cylindrocarcinoma, porocarcinoma, malignant chondroid syringoma, malignant syringoacanthoma, and hidradenocarcinoma. These malignant degenerations are discussed in the sections describing their benign counterparts. The bulk of tumor cells in all these tumors (*e.g.*, poromas, spiradenomas, cylindromas) are CEA negative, but in the malignant phenotype in which the tumor has undergone ductal differentiation, the cells are CEA positive.

TUMORS ARISING FROM THE DERMIS

Various cellular elements existing within the dermis may give rise to a variety of benign and malignant tumors. Because of their localization, these lesions clinically appear as subcutaneous nodules with a normal overlying epidermis. Accurate diagnosis is only possible after surgical excision and histologic evaluation. The most common of these lesions are summarized in Table 45–2. Detailed descriptions of these conditions can be found in other chapters in this book.

LYMPHORETICULAR TUMORS AND RELATED CONDITIONS

Skin is an immunologic organ and as such participates in the traffic and housing of immune cells. It is not surprising to see that malignant transformation of some of these cells may take place within the skin. The group of diseases classified under the cutaneous T-cell lymphomas appears to have special tropism for the epidermal tissues (*i.e.*, epidermotropism), and they originate and remain within the skin for a long period. The nonepidermotropic cutaneous T-cell lymphomas and the cutaneous B-cell lymphomas are other lymphoreticular malignancies involving skin. Other forms of lymphomas and leukemias may spread to skin and produce skin infiltrates.

TUMORS METASTATIC TO SKIN

Skin metastasis is rare, discovered in 0.2% to 9% of autopsies of cancer patients. The incidence of skin metastasis is associated with the type of primary cancer and with the sex of the patient. The site of metastasis to skin varies, and an increased frequency of metastasis to certain sites of skin is reported for some cancers.[244,320,321] Skin metastasis usually occurs if the disease is widespread with metastasis to multiple sites. Skin metastasis is usually a poor prognostic sign, but sometimes it is seen before the primary malignancy is recognized.

The frequency of skin metastasis in women is 69% for breast cancer, 9% for large intestine cancer, 5% for melanoma, 4% for lung cancer, 4% for ovarian cancer, 2% for sarcoma, 2% for uterine cervical cancer, 2% for pancreatic cancer, 1% for squamous cell carcinoma of oral cavity, and 1% for bladder cancer. In men, the frequency of cutaneous metastasis is 24% for lung, 19% for large intestine, 13% for melanoma, 12% for squamous cell carcinoma of oral cavity, 6% for kidney cancer, 6% for stomach cancer, 3% for esophageal cancer, 3% for sarcoma, 2% for pancreatic cancer, 2% for urinary bladder cancer, 2% for salivary gland tumors, 2% for breast cancer, and 1% each for prostate, thyroid, liver, and squamous cell carcinoma of skin.

Some skin metastases have certain morphologic and clinical features that differentiate them from other lesions. Neuroblastoma may appear as multiple, firm, nontender, mobile, bluish, subcutaneous nodules, described by the term "blueberry muffin." In breast cancer, the metastasis may present as inflammatory carcinoma, or it may appear in several other forms. Hypernephroma may clinically resemble Kaposi's sarcoma pyogenic granuloma. The primary sources of skin metastasis in women younger than 40 are, in descending order, breast cancer, melanoma, colon cancer, and ovarian cancer; in women older than 40, they are breast, colon cancer, lung cancer, ovarian cancer, and melanoma; for men younger than 40, the primary sources are melanoma, colon cancer, and lung cancer; for men older than 40, the sources are lung cancer, colon cancer, oral squamous cell carcinoma, and melanoma.

PRINCIPLES OF DIAGNOSIS AND TREATMENT

In many skin tumors, the clinical diagnosis is obvious and most dermatologists feel reasonably confident about the clinical impression. However, surveys of prehistologic diagnoses of basal cell carcinoma and malignant melanoma indicate that even among trained dermatologists there can be a wide margin of error in clinical diagnosis.

There are instances for which a definitive clinical diagnosis cannot be easily entertained, and a series of differential diagnoses are usually considered. The problem is much greater for skin appendage tumors and tumors arising from soft tissues of the skin. It is essential to develop a systematic approach in the diagnosis and management of skin tumors and use all the available resources to reduce the margin of error and select the appropriate treatment.

As part of the evaluation of patients with a malignant skin tumor the following input should be obtained: duration of the lesion, associated symptoms (*e.g.*, pain, itching), and recent changes; occupational and recreational history and history of prior sun exposure; type of skin and ethnic background; medical history including radiation exposure, history of arsenic ingestion, chronic ulcer, burn scars, osteomyelitis, and the presence of other coexisting diseases (*e.g.*, carcinomas, organ transplantation, immunodeficiency); and family history of skin and other cancers.

A complete skin examination, including examination of the scalp, ears, palms, soles, interdigital areas, and mucous membranes, should be undertaken. The extent of sun damage to skin should be assessed, evaluating the level of solar elastosis, scaling, erythema, telangiectasia, and solar lentigines. The size, location, shape, color, and other morphologic characteristics of the tumor should be recorded and marked on an anatomic chart. Regional and distant lymph nodes should be assessed. Clinical photographs are valuable in the field of skin cancers. Photographs should be taken whenever possible with a centimeter scale and date adjacent to the lesion before any procedure. This should become part of the routine procedures in all dermatology clinics. Biopsy specimens are processed for routine histologic studies. Special stains, antibodies for cell markers using immunoperoxidase, and ultrastructural studies are used for confirming certain diagnoses.

Other tests, such as blood screening for anemia, lymphoreticular disorders, anergy panel, immunosuppression, coagulation disorders, and markers of malignancies, may be necessary in some cases. Chest radiography, lymphangiography, computed tomography, liver and spleen scans, and magnetic resonance imaging should only be performed if indicated. After completion of these evaluations, a final diagnosis can be entertained and treatment can be planned.

BIOPSY AND TREATMENT PLANNING

Biopsy of a skin tumor allows microscopic examination of the tissue specimen and usually results in an accurate histologic diagnosis. The histologic diagnosis permits the physician to choose the appropriate therapy.

Biopsy

Four different biopsy techniques are used for skin lesions suspected for malignant tumors. Shave biopsy uses a scalpel to slice a superficial portion of the tumor. Punch biopsy uses a cylindrical instrument with an internal diameter of 2 to 8 mm to remove a deeper portion of the tumor down to the level of dermis or subcutaneous tissue. In incisional biopsy, a portion of the tumor is removed with a scalpel. In excisional biopsy, the entire lesion with a small border of normal skin is excised with a scalpel.

The selected technique should yield the primary specimen for an accurate diagnosis. For example, superficial specimens using a skin biopsy is adequate for the diagnosis of noduloulcerative, cystic, or superficial basal cell carcinoma. However, the diagnosis of squamous cell carcinoma may be missed in a superficial shave biopsy, because squamous cell carcinoma extends into the papillary dermis. A punch biopsy, incisional biopsy, or excisional biopsy are more appropriate in such cases. For pigmented skin lesions for which the differential diagnoses includes pigmented basal cell carcinoma and malignant melanoma, incisional or excisional biopsies are recommended. Punch biopsy should not be performed on possible melanomas, because tumor cells can be driven deeper into the dermis. In the case of morphea basal cell carcinoma, it is best to perform a punch or incisional biopsy. Shave biopsy does not provide sufficient tissue for differentiation of this entity from benign processes such as scar lesions or trichoepithelioma.

Keratoacanthomas are considered to be benign neoplasms, but the histologic picture of keratoacanthomas can be confused with squamous cell carcinoma. The diagnosis of keratoacanthoma can only be differentiated from squamous cell carcinoma based on the gross architectural pattern. Therefore biopsy of any lesion suspected for keratoacanthoma must include both opposite edges plus the central portion of the lesion. A wedge-shaped incision of the lesion from the center of the lesion to both opposite edges provides a sufficient specimen. For adnexal tumor or subcutaneous tumors, incisional or excisional biopsies are recommended. Biopsies are usually performed in an outpatient setting with the use of local anesthetic such as 1% or 2% lidocaine. These are usually uncomplicated procedures with little morbidity.

Treatment Planning

There are several acceptable choices for the treatment of cutaneous malignancies. These include curettage and electrodesiccation, excision, Mohs' micrographic surgery, cryotherapy, radiation therapy, topical chemotherapy, and laser vaporization. After the histologic diagnosis has been confirmed, several factors must be considered to determine the appropriate therapeutic approach. The size of the lesion, the anatomic location, the clinical nature, histologic characteristics, general health and age of the patient, and whether the lesion is primary, recurrent, or metastatic should be considered.

The size of the tumor is important in deciding the treatment plan and assessing the final outcome. In the case of basal cell carcinoma, the larger the tumor, the greater is the chance of recurrence. This is even true when Mohs' micrographic surgery is used.[173,322] Lesions larger than 2 to 3 cm have a much lower rate of cure than those smaller than 1 cm.

The location of the tumor also plays an important role in the final outcome of the treatment. Skin areas located along the embryonal fusion planes have the potential for deep invasion and higher rates of recurrences. These areas include the midface under the eyes, periauricular and postauricular areas, the paranasal, nasolabial, and inner canthal areas. For these high-risk areas, select the type of treatment that gives the highest cure rate and least chance of recurrence, such as Mohs' micrographic surgery. The anatomic function of the area and the final cosmetic appearance of the wound are also important in selecting the method of treatment.

The longer the tumor has been present, the greater is the chance for deeper invasion. The duration of the tumor correlates with the biologic behavior of the tumor. Tumors with well-defined borders and slow growth pattern have less chance of recurrence than tumors with ill-defined borders and multicentric, aggressive natures.

Tumors with histologic patterns of basosquamous or morphea types have a higher rate of recurrence and should be treated with modalities with higher cure rates. Another factor that should be considered in selecting a treatment modality is the pattern of spread of the tumor. The inadequacy of the standard histopathologic methods should be kept in mind when interpreting the reports about the margins of the tumor. Routine histopathologic methods allow pathologists to evaluate selected portions of the surgical specimen, and they are therefore offering an incomplete analysis of all the surgical margins.

The general health of the patient must be carefully considered. For patients with coagulopathy, a less invasive procedure should be selected and, if necessary, the problem should be temporarily corrected before surgery (*e.g.*, infusion of platelets before surgery in cases of thrombocytopenia). In elderly, debilitated patients, procedures requiring one or two office visits are preferred to those needing 10 to 15 visits. In patients with immunodeficiency states, the chance of infection is increased and the tumor may be more aggressive.

If tissue preservation is important (*e.g.*, eyelids, vermilion border of the lip, the tip of the nose), less destructive methods are usually recommended. These include radiation therapy or Mohs' micrographic surgery.

CURETTAGE AND ELECTRODESICCATION

Curettage and electrodesiccation are commonly used to treat basal cell carcinoma, superficial squamous cell carcinoma, and precancerous and benign lesions. Treatment is based on the difference in the consistency between the tumor and the normal surrounding tissues.

Curettage is performed with the use of a curet, which is a pencil-like instrument with a round or oval tip, sharpened on one side. Using the curet, the tumor is debulked down to the normal tissue, which is indicated by the sound and texture. Normal skin is firm and has a gritty sound on curettage. Electrodesiccation is used to destroy any residual tumor cells and produce hemostasis. A biopsy is recommended before the use of curettage and electrodesiccation. If possible, a shave biopsy is preferred, because it is easier to perform curettage after shave biopsy than after a punch or incisional biopsy. This technique is frequently used for the treatment of basal cell carcinoma, superficial squamous cell carcinoma, selected cases of Bowen's disease, keratoacanthomas, and hypertrophic actinic keratoses.

The cure rate with this approach is 77% to 97%. Immediately after the procedure, 12% to 30% of patients have nests of basal cell carcinoma in the treated areas. The inflammatory reaction after the procedure or possibly an immunologic reaction may be responsible for the destruction of these tumors after curettage and electrodesiccation. The cure rate for this technique also depends on patient selection. It is important to avoid high-risk patients who have more aggressive histology, larger tumors, longer duration of disease, or tumors located in high-risk anatomic areas. Morphea-like basal cell carcinomas are not suitable for treatment with this technique. Lesions larger than 1 cm, especially on the face, have an increased tendency to recur.[323] Tumors that are present longer have a tendency to become more infiltrative and break down into smaller more invasive cords with a more fibrotic stromal reaction. This type of histology is more resistant to curettage and electrodesiccation and causes more recurrences. It is also likely that older tumors may invade deeply across a broad front until they reach a tissue barrier of skin. In these cases, tumors extend deceptively beyond the reach of the curet.

Curettage and electrodesiccation is best used in superficial and nodular basal cell carcinoma of low recurrence areas. It is not effective for morphea basal cell carcinoma, recurrent basal cell carcinoma, or squamous cell carcinoma. This technique should not be used in certain areas because of cosmetic considerations, such as wound contracture around eyes and mouth. In the hands of skilled experienced practitioners, the cure rate can be as high as 95% to 97%.[324–327] A high recurrence rate is reported if less experienced dermatology residents performed the procedure.

In the current technique, the curet is used to define the size, shape, and extent of the tumor and then excise the area with a 2- to 3-mm margin.[328] Electrodesiccation is used to destroy tiny pockets of tumor cells and an extra rim of tissue at the base and periphery of the defect produced by curettage and to produce hemostasis. A high-frequency (500,000–1,000,000 Hz), highly damped alternating current of high voltage (>2000 V) and low amperage (100–1000 mA) is used for electrodesiccation. The electrical resistance of the skin generates sufficient heat to produce tissue injury at the point of contact. The heat causes dehydration of the cells and instantaneous cell death. Because of the low amperage, there is sharp delineation between normal and destroyed tissue. Increasing the current (amperage) causes more heat, deeper penetration, and excessive tissue destruction and scarring. Hemostasis results from thrombosis of affected vessels.

CRYOTHERAPY

The first report of cryotherapy in the treatment of malignant tumors of the skin appeared in 1963 by Cooper.[329] Although Cooper is recognized as the father of cryosurgery, the use of this technique began after the turn of the century.[330]

Cryotherapy takes advantage of the cryonecrosis that is achieved by cellular and microvascular response to subzero temperatures. Using liquid nitrogen (−195.5°C), freezing temperatures are achieved in viable tissues, transforming water into ice. Some changes in cells in subzero temperatures include the formation of extracellular and intracellular ice, abnormal concentration and crystallization of electrolytes, and denaturation of lipoprotein complexes that are lethal to the cells.[331] The more severe effect of cryotherapy is thought to be on the microvasculature of the skin and the tumor tissues. With proper selection of the tumor size and location, it is possible to achieve a high cure rate, excellent would healing, and cosmetically acceptable results (Fig. 45–25).

This technique is especially useful for patients with pacemakers, those with adverse reactions to local anesthetic, and those who are poor surgical risks. It can be used for the treatment of lesions smaller than 2 cm that are located on the eyelid, nose, ear, chest, back, or tip of the nose. It is recommended for the treatment of recurrent tumors and tumors with definable margins. A 3- to 5-mm tumor-free margin is used to increase the cure rate. The involved region is anesthetized with local anesthetic, and the freezing time is decided based on the size of the tumor. Open spray takes a longer period than spray through a plastic cone. The freeze-thaw time is usually 1:2 for direct spray or 1:4 for spray through plastic cone. The temperature of the tissue is controlled by a thermocoupler inserted under the tumor. A temperature of −50°C is thought to be sufficient for cryotherapy. A double freeze-thaw cycle is recommended for safe and accurate treatment.

Cryotherapy is not an option for the treatment of morphea-type basal cell carcinoma. It cannot be used in patients with abnormal cold intolerance (*e.g.*, cryoglobulinemia, Raynaud's disease) or on tumors located in certain anatomic areas such as free margin of eyelid, vermilion border of the lip, ala nasi, anterior and posterior ear, or scalp and for tumors larger than 3 cm. Tumors located on the nasolabial fold or inner canthi require wider margins of freezing to increase the cure rate. The morbidity of cryotherapy is moderate and includes edema, oozing, erosions, hemorrhaging, and secondary infections. The cosmetic result is good except for hypopigmentation or hyperpigmentation. The latter condition usually fades within a few months after therapy.

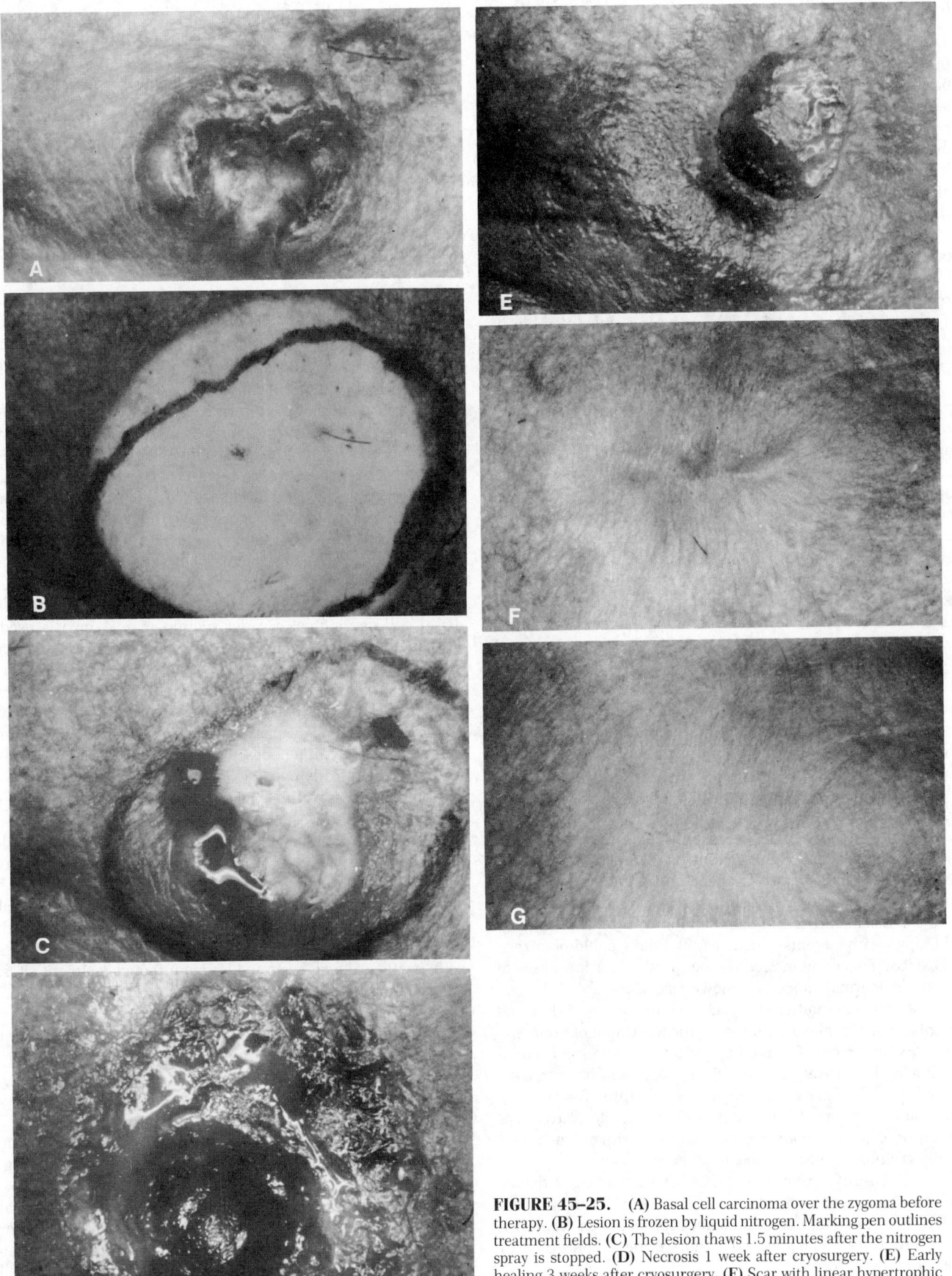

FIGURE 45–25. (A) Basal cell carcinoma over the zygoma before therapy. (B) Lesion is frozen by liquid nitrogen. Marking pen outlines treatment fields. (C) The lesion thaws 1.5 minutes after the nitrogen spray is stopped. (D) Necrosis 1 week after cryosurgery. (E) Early healing 3 weeks after cryosurgery. (F) Scar with linear hypertrophic element 3 months after cryosurgery. (G) One year after cryosurgery, there is a hypopigmented scar with no hypertrophy.

CHEMOTHERAPY

Topical chemotherapy has been used for the treatment of precancerous (*e.g.*, actinic keratoses) and cancerous (*e.g.*, basal cell carcinoma) lesions of the skin.[332–334] Many chemicals have been tried, including salicylic acid, pyrogallic acid, podophyllin, thiotepa, BCNU, 5-FU, and retinoids. With the exception of 5-FU, which has been effective, these agents have been unsatisfactory. BCNU is effective in the treatment of cutaneous T-cell lymphoma, and retinoids are still in clinical trials.

5-FU blocks the action of the enzyme thymidylate synthetase, which catalyzes the methylation of 2-dioxyuridylic acid to thymidylic acid. 5-FU prevents DNA synthesis and cellular reproduction by inhibition of the production of thymidylic acid. The inhibition of nucleic acid synthesis is most notable in rapidly proliferating neoplastic cells, compared with normal cells with a normal rate of metabolism.

5-FU is used topically as a cream or lotion once or twice per day for several weeks and produces a severe inflammatory response in the precancerous and malignant areas. 5-FU is available in concentrates of 1%, 2%, and 5% and can be used to achieve desired levels of inflammation. The lotion is best applied by a soft brush and the cream with fingertip. Topical steroid cream can be used to alleviate the inflammation without lessening the efficacy of 5-FU. It is not necessary to induce extreme discomfort in patients' skin to obtain results. Mild to moderate erythema is sufficient. If no erythema occurs with the 1% 5-FU cream, the concentration should be increased to 2% or 5%. Facial areas, the dorsum of the hand, and lower extremities are often treated with 5-FU. Concomitant use of topical 13-all-*trans*-retinoic acid (*i.e.*, tretinoin cream) enhances the effect of topical 5-FU.[335] Sun exposure may induce more severe reactions and photosensitivity. After the completion of the treatment with 5-FU, a careful examination of the skin is recommended to identify and biopsy any persistent or newly developed lesions.

Complications of treatment with 5-FU includes allergic reaction to the vehicle, erythema, and pigmentary changes. 5-FU is quite effective in the treatment of actinic keratoses and superficial basal cell carcinoma. It has been shown to be ineffective in other forms of cancer, including other types of basal cell carcinoma.

5-FU has been tried in combination with topical immune therapy with agents such as 2,4-dinitrochlorobenzene (DNCB). This combination has been used in a few cases of in situ epidermal cancer and Bowen's disease.[336]

Systemic chemotherapy, such as the use of 5-FU and cisplatin, has not been effective in the treatment of nonmelanoma skin cancer. Chemotherapy for squamous cell carcinoma and adnexal tumors of the skin has been unsuccessful.[337,338] This approach may be helpful for treating metastatic tumors. Isotretinoin, a vitamin A derivative, has been used in the treatment of advanced primary squamous cell carcinoma, but not enough data are available.[339]

Topical use of tretinoin cream has been effective in reducing sun damage to the skin.[340] Use of this agent for over a year results in thickened epidermis and new collagen formation in the dermis.[341] This work has not yet been confirmed by other investigators.

Many believe that 5-FU is not a good modality for the treatment of basal cell carcinoma because it may result in a tumor-free surface while the tumor underneath continues to grow. Other investigators have reported the use of 5-FU in the treatment of in situ epidermal carcinoma, but this approach is not accepted by other clinicians.[342–344]

Nitrogen mustard is an accepted modality in the treatment of cutaneous T-cell lymphomas.[345] Topical application of BCNU has been used occasionally in the treatment of cutaneous T-cell lymphoma.[346] Methotrexate was used to treat basal cell carcinoma alone or in combination with demecolcine and thiocolchicine but was not effective.[335,347,348] Dactinomycin, cytosine arabinoside, and spiramycin were ineffective in treating basal cell carcinoma.[347,348]

SURGICAL EXCISION

Surgical excision is an effective treatment approach for all forms of skin tumors in most anatomic locations (Fig. 45–26). Surgical excision is performed in an elliptical shape along the Langer's cleavage lines, and in most instances, primary closure of the wound is possible and results in good cosmetic healing. The procedure is usually performed under local anesthesia with the use of scalpel and curved scissors. Surgical margins of excision vary according to the type of tumor; a 3- to 5-mm margin is acceptable for basal cell carcinomas that do not metastasize, but a margin of several centimeters is considered sufficient for Merkel cell carcinoma and squamous cell carcinoma. For recurrent basal cell carcinoma or morphea basal cell carcinoma, a wider margin (*e.g.*, 1 cm) is used. Although specific guidelines about the margin of resection for tumors such as squamous cell carcinoma, Merkel's cell carcinoma, or eccrine carcinoma have not been developed, it is accepted that wider margins should be taken with tumors that are larger or extend deeper into the skin and underlying tissue. Local draining lymph nodes are examined and removed only if they are clinically palpable.

Split-thickness or full-thickness skin grafts are sometimes necessary for the closure of wounds if the tumor is large and primary closure is not possible or if primary closure may result in undesirable cosmetic appearance (*e.g.*, excision of tumors from the lip, nose, or eyelid).

Split-thickness grafts are usually obtained with a mechanical dermatome and are used to cover large surgical defects with minimal vascularity, such as periosteum.[349] Split-thickness skin grafts are well accepted by noninfected recipient sites. However, the color of split-thickness graft is not matched, and it creates a donor site that heals slowly by secondary intention. Full-thickness grafts are used when a good color match is important, and the donor sites require primary closure.

Split- and full-thickness grafts are immobilized after surgery to prevent movement and bleeding. It usually takes 5 to 7 days to accept the graft and 2 to 3 months for the tissue to mature and become cosmetically acceptable skin (Fig. 45–27).

A skin flap is another choice for the closure of surgical excision site. Skin flaps are attached on one side to the donor area and carry their own blood supplies. While attached to the base by a pedicle, the separated skin is advanced or rotated to cover the surgical defect. Rotation flaps are simple and are

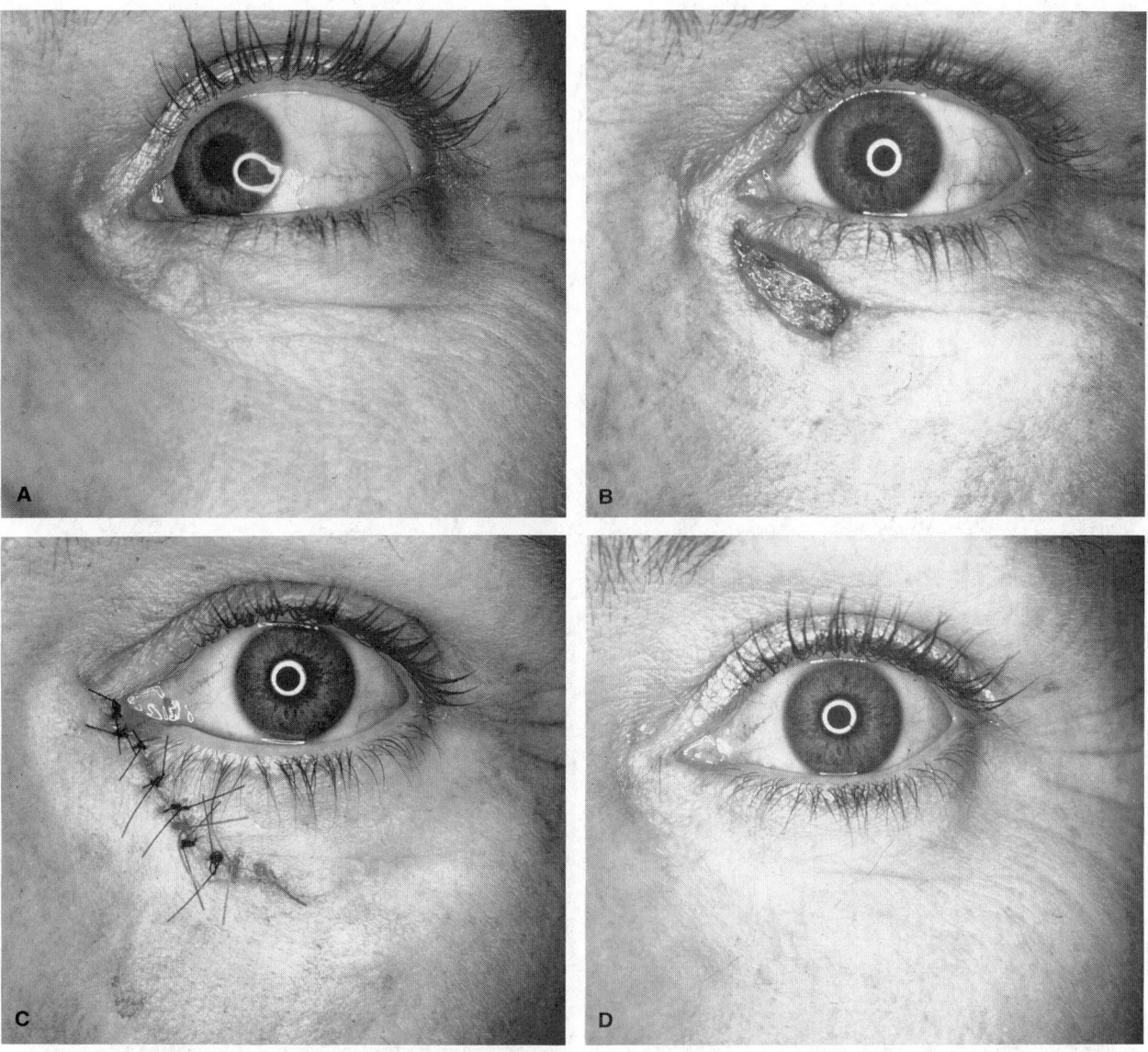

FIGURE 45–26. **(A)** Primary basal cell carcinoma in an infraorbital site close to the inner canthus. **(B)** Surgical excision of the tumor. **(C)** Primary closure. **(D)** Same patient 9 months after surgery.

commonly used to cover surgical defects. They can be designed to fit the desired anatomic site.

With advancement of microvascular surgery, the tissue transfer from one part of the body to another can be achieved by anastomosing the donor artery and vein to the recipient artery and vein. The technique of surgical excision allows microscopic evaluation of the entire tumor and its margins. The technique can be performed with minimal discomfort and complications and with good cosmetic results. It can be performed on the trunk, extremities, cheeks, forehead, chin, and scalp. For important anatomic sites, such as lesions located on the alar rim of the nose, lip, or eyelids, special care should be taken to prevent distortion if the tissue and poor cosmetic results.

The decision to preform surgical excision should be made only after consideration of all other therapeutic modalities available.

RADIATION THERAPY

Indications and Applications

Most skin cancers are radiosensitive, and this method of treatment is one of the most effective therapies for selected skin tumors. This approach is usually recommended for patients who are poor surgical risks or are elderly debilitated or when the tumor is large. The advantages of radiation therapy include acceptability by most patients, because there is no pain involved, no hospitalization required, and patients can continue to function normally in their own environment during the course of therapy. Radiation therapy does not cause keloid formation, contracture, or ectropion. Radiation therapy allows the uninvolved tissue to be preserved and produces a much lesser degree of defect. Among the disadvantages of this method are multiple patient visits and loss of hair follicles and sweat glands at the site of therapy. The decision about

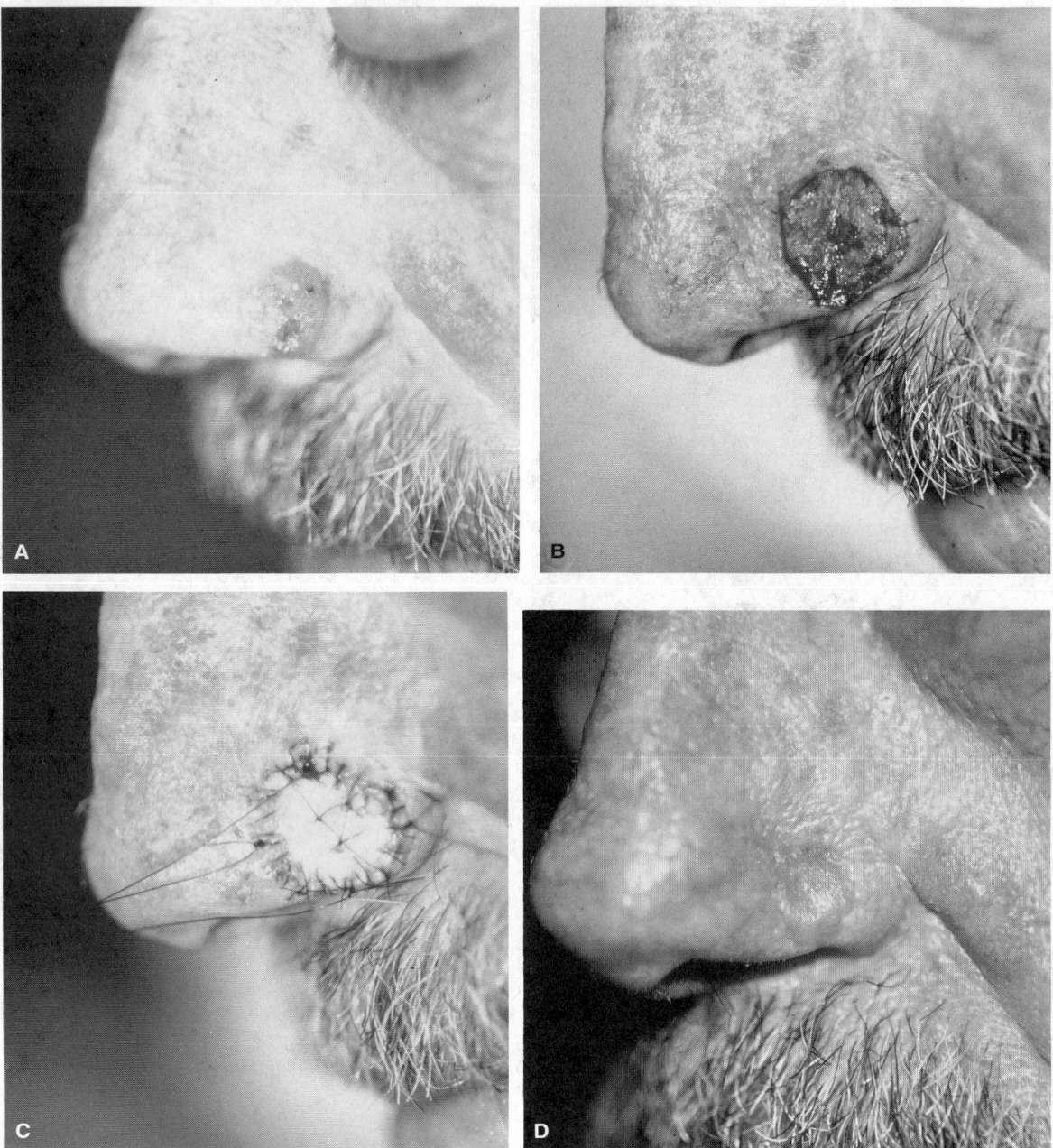

FIGURE 45–27.   **(A)** Basal cell carcinoma of the ala nasi. **(B)** The site after surgery. **(C)** Full-thickness graft. **(D)** The same patient 6 months after surgery.

whether to use radiation therapy or other modalities is based on the size and anatomic location of tumor, histology of the neoplasm, age of the patient, recurrence rates, and the anticipated cosmetic results.

Radiation therapy is usually the best choice of treatment for skin cancers located on the nose, eye, lip, eyelid, and inner and outer canthi (Figs. 45–28 through 45–31). Skin tumors along the embryonal fusion planes can also be treated and cured with this modality. Radiation therapy is usually recommended for primary basal cell carcinoma and squamous cell carcinoma, but it can be used for recurrent lesions as well (Fig. 45–32). It is not appropriate to treat recurrent skin cancers with radiation therapy if the tumor was initially treated

with this approach. Morphea basal cell carcinoma is ill defined in depth and borders and not suitable for radiation treatment, but it is radiosensitive.

The cure rate for radiation therapy is 96.4% for basal cell carcinoma and 91.9% for squamous cell carcinoma, if therapy is performed by an experienced specialist.[350] Similar results were reported by another group.[351] The selection of appropriate treatment modality for a given tumor and the experience of the physician administrating the treatment are important in the final outcome.

The cosmetic results of radiation therapy is good and acceptable to the patients. However, as time passes, chronic radiation dermatitis may take place in the form of atrophy,

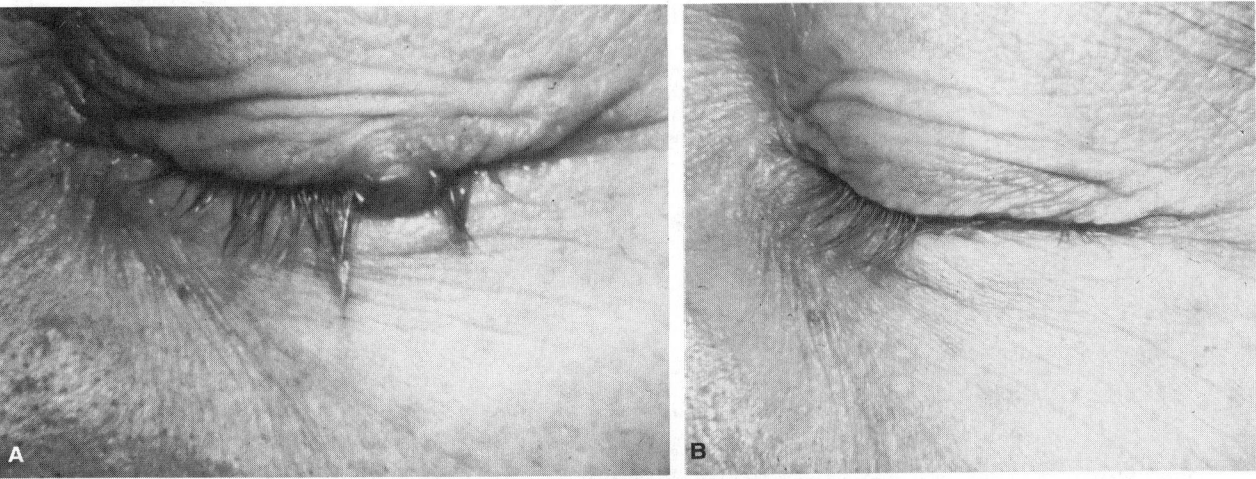

FIGURE 45–28. **(A)** Basal cell carcinoma on the margin of the upper eyelid. **(B)** Same patient 1 year after treatment with x-ray therapy.

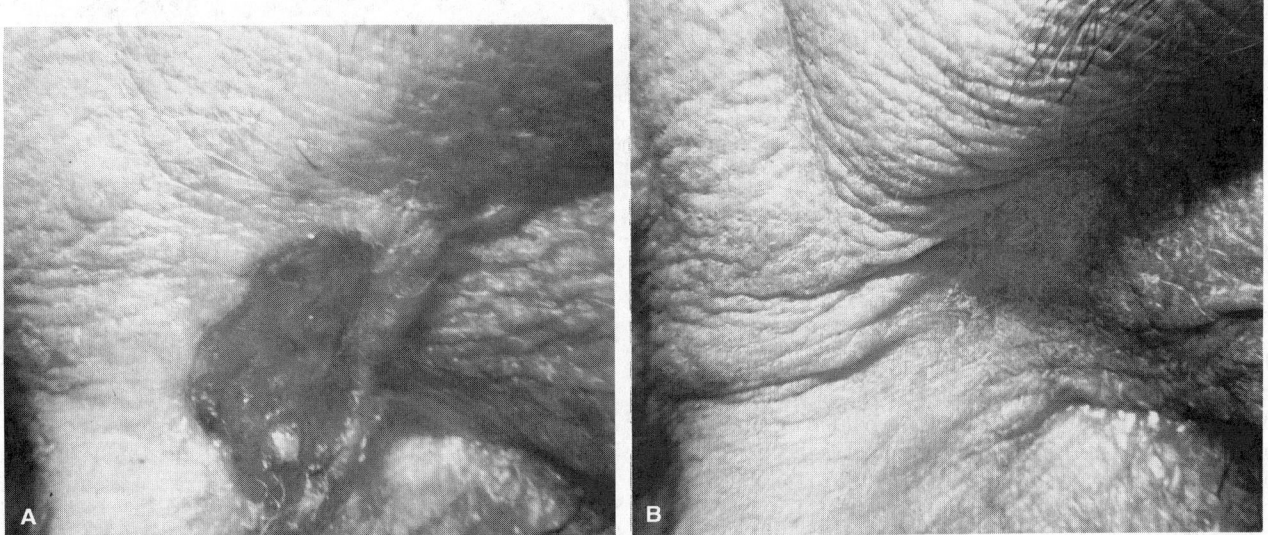

FIGURE 45–29. **(A)** Basal cell carcinoma of the left inner canthus. **(B)** After using 10 x-ray treatments of 400 cGy each for a total dose of 4000 cGy and an HVL of 0.5 mm of aluminum.

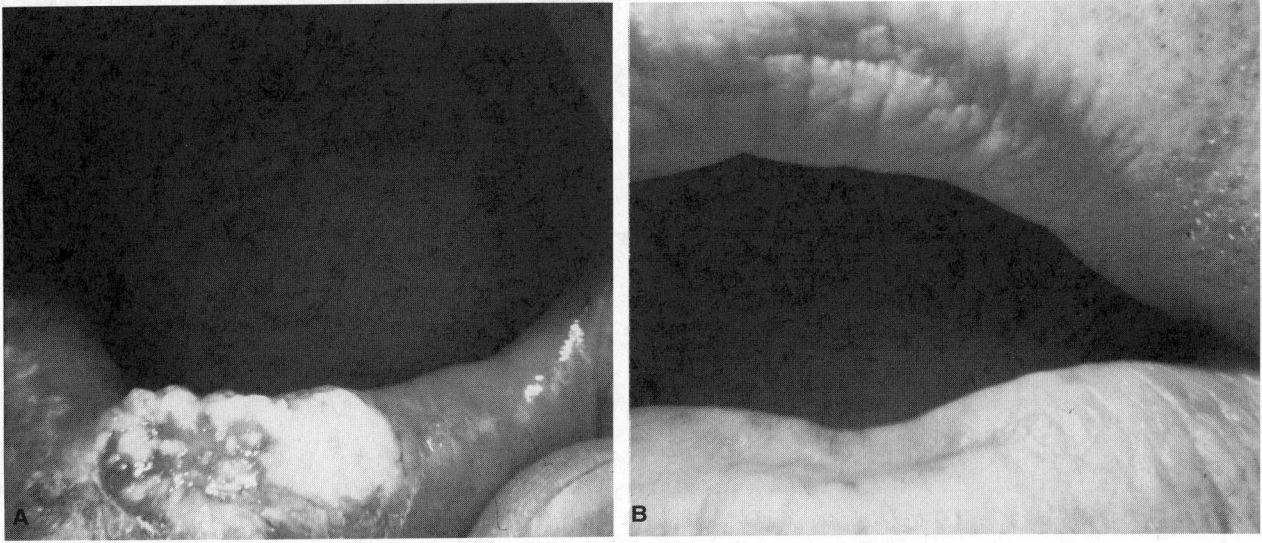

FIGURE 45–30. **(A)** Squamous cell carcinoma on the lower lip of a smoker. **(B)** The same patient after using 10 radiation treatments of 450 cGy each for a total dose of 4500 cGy and an HVL of 1 mm of aluminum.

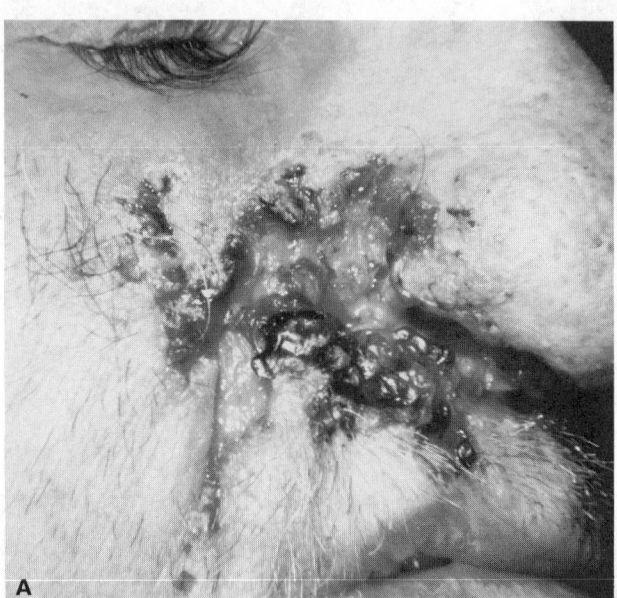 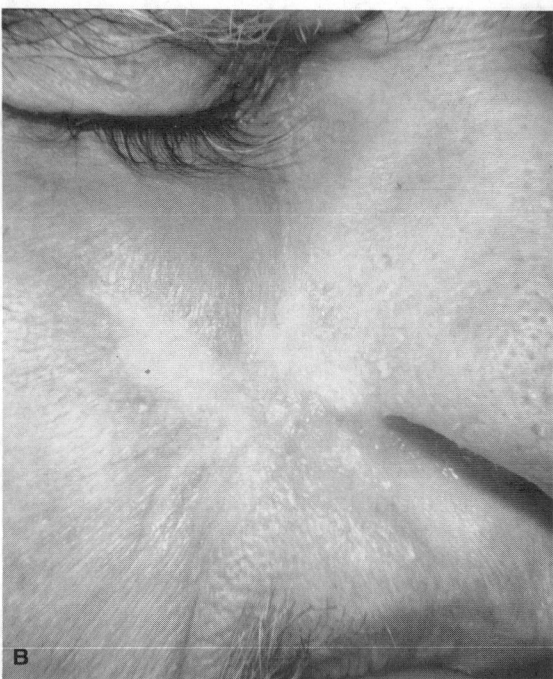

FIGURE 45–31. **(A)** Recurrent basal cell carcinoma of right nosolabial fold. **(B)** The same patient after using 10 treatments of 360 cGy each for a total of 3600 cGy and an HVL of 2 mm of aluminum.

telangiectasia, hyperpigmentation, or hypopigmentation, and radiation-induced precancerous lesions may appear. Radiation therapy is therefore recommended for selected cases, and only for patients 50 years of age or older.

A biopsy should always be performed for histologic diagnosis before initiation of radiation therapy. History of prior treatment, specifically the use of x-ray therapy, should be obtained for skin cancers or for other skin conditions such as acne, removal of hair, tinea capitis. The tumor is evaluated, and a lead shield with a portal exposure to fit the tumor and at least

a 0.5 cm of normal tissue is produced. Wider margins are necessary for recurrent lesions and for lesions located at the embryonal fusion plane. The clinical margin for the tumor should be well defined, even if multiple biopsies are necessary. The tumor is exposed to x-rays through the port in the lead shield by touching the lead glass cone of the x-ray machine to the lead shield, reducing the scattered radiation. Specially sensitive areas, such as thyroid glands, gonads, and eyes, are covered with lead shields before each treatment. Protection from the exit dose of radiation is also recommended. An in-

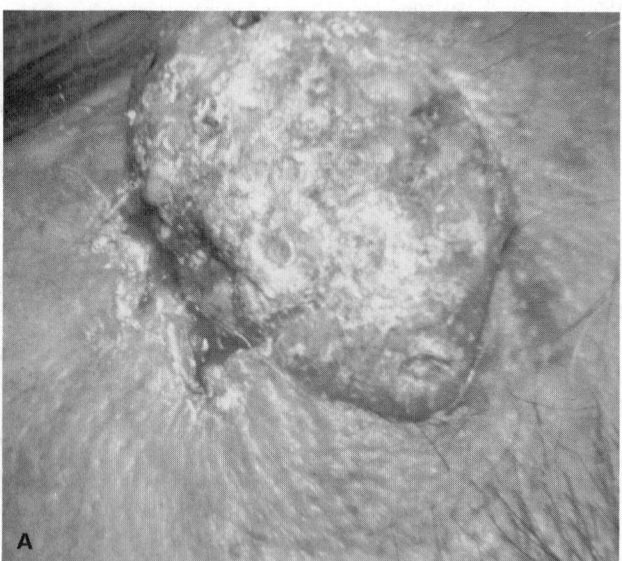 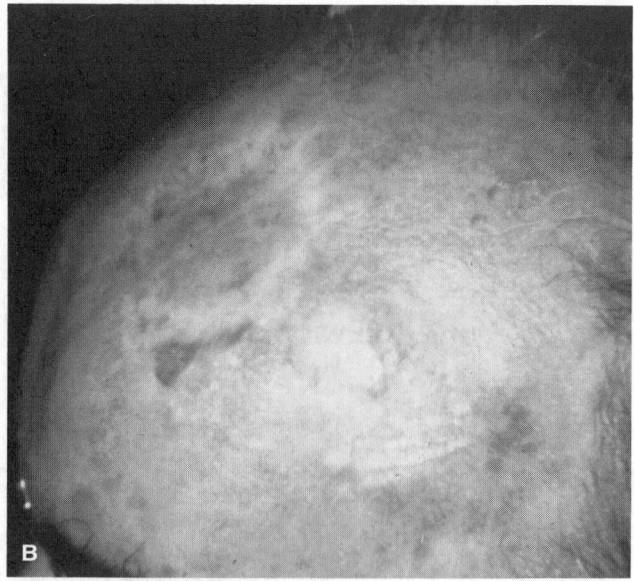

FIGURE 45–32. **(A)** The 5-cm fungating tumor is a recurrent basal cell carcinoma at the site of an old surgical graft. **(B)** The same patient after using 10 treatments of 400 cGy each for a total dose of 4000 cGy and an HVL of 2 mm of aluminum. The surgical graft scar is adjacent to the lesion.

ternal nasal shield, gum shield, and eye shield are used when treating these organs.

Immediate side effects include erythema and exudative reaction at treatment sites, loss of eyelashes when treating eyelids, and mucositis when treating the nose. The treatment is repeated until the appropriate amount of radiation is administered to the skin tumor.

Radiation Technology

The goal of radiation is to selectively destroy the tumor tissue and spare the normal surrounding area. Modern radiologic technology has made it possible to select the quality, dose, and fractionation of the radiation so that only the neoplastic tissue is destroyed.

The quality of radiation is determined by the amount of kilovoltage and by the type of filter used. The half-value layer (HVL) is the thickness of a given filter material that reduces the intensity of a beam of photons to 50% of the original exposure. The thickness of tissue or tissue depth measured in millimeters that absorbs 50% of the surface dose is called half-value depth ($D_{\frac{1}{2}}$). In the treatment of each skin cancer, the amount of kilovoltage and the thickness and type of the filter is selected so that the $D_{\frac{1}{2}}$ is equal to the thickness of the tumor, and the tissue underlying the tumor is minimized. Softer radiation reaching normal tissue causes a less chronic radiation reaction.

$D_{\frac{1}{2}}$ is determined by kilovoltage, the HVL, the distance between the anode (target) of the x-ray tube and the target-to-skin distance, and by the size of the field. Based on the available calculation, the intensity or dose rate of radiation at a given point is inversely proportional to the square of its distance from the target. The dose to the base of the lesion is equal to one half of the surface dose. If the depth (thickness) of the tumor is known, the appropriate quality of radiation can be selected from precalibrated table available for each x-ray machine. An x-ray machine producing superficial x-rays with a $D_{\frac{1}{2}}$ of 7 to 10 mm is sufficient for most skin tumors. Most basal cell carcinomas and squamous cell carcinomas infiltrate to the depth of 2 to 5 mm.[352] A total dose of 2000 to 3000 cGy for the depth of the tumor is recommended for the treatment of most skin cancers that correspond to 4000 to 6000 cGy on the surface. To prevent radiation sequela of short or long term, the entire dose of x-rays is fractionated into smaller doses and is administered over 3 to 4 weeks. For example, to achieve a good cosmetic result and high cure rate, a 4000-cGy dose could be divided into 10 fractions of 400 cGy each. Fractionation of the dose can be achieved in many different ways, but all approaches give a high cure rate and low recurrence rate. For smaller lesions (*e.g.*, eyelids), the physician can use the so-called contact x-ray, which could be produced by 50 to 60 kV, an HVL of 2 to 4 mm of aluminum, and a short distance from target to skin (1.5–3 cm).[353] This approach allows most x-rays to be absorbed by the tumor and a rapid drop down of radiation to normal tissue.

Another x-ray machine that is now commonly used is a soft x-ray unit with beryllium windows. These machines range from 10 to 100 kV and have lower inherent filtration that allows higher dose rates. Modern units have predetermined and fixed kV-filter combinations and special mechanisms to prevent errors of delivery.

Another effective approach is the use of electron-beam irradiation in the treatment of superficial skin tumors. The depth of penetration of electrons depends on the amount of the voltage used to produce them (2–15 MeV).[354,355] Because of limited depth of penetration electron-beam irradiation does not affect deep tissues and produces excellent cosmetic results. Electrons are more precise than x-rays, give better cosmetic results, and are useful in treating certain skin cancers like large carcinomas located on the scalp or lesions overlying cartilage or in elderly persons, for whom there is a risk of bone and cartilage necrosis if low-energy photons are used.[354] However, the electron beam is not widely available, is more costly, and requires a lengthy recalibration for each patient.

Radium molds and implants have been used in the past for the treatment of skin cancers, but because of the hazards, they are no longer in use.

CHEMOSURGERY AND MOHS' MICROGRAPHIC SURGERY

The combination of surgical and microscopic approaches to eradicate skin tumors was initially formulated by Frederick Mohs. When he was a medical student, he observed that injection of 20% zinc chloride into tissues resulted in fixation and preservation of histologic structure when later viewed under a microscope. This observation led him to develop the technique of chemosurgery for the treatment of skin cancers.[173–175,356] Zinc chloride paste is used to fix the tumor in situ. The tumor is then serially removed, and a careful map of the area and the specimen are developed and color coded. The excised tumor is divided into several segments, and horizontal sections are prepared by the frozen-tissue technique and evaluated for the presence of tumors by light microscopy. The lateral and deep margins of resected tumors are examined, and the areas with tumor involvement are marked on the color-coded maps of the removed tissue. These steps are repeated for the areas identified as involved with tumor until all the margins are free of the tumor, and the entire neoplastic mass is removed (Figs. 45–33 and 45–34). The fixed-tissue technique, which is effective but time consuming, has been eliminated and replaced by the frozen-section technique of cryosectioning. This technique has recently been renamed as Mohs' micrographic surgery.[173–175]

Mohs' micrographic surgery is indicated for tumors of skin that are difficult to treat using other methods. The technique's greatest success has been in the treatment of difficult basal cell carcinomas and squamous cell carcinomas (Fig. 45–35). This technique has been used to treat other cancers that have a high recurrence rate using conventional surgery and other therapeutic modalities (Fig. 45–36). In these cases, it is sensible to combine the step-wise surgical removal with precise microscopic control of removed tumor tissue to achieve a more complete removal and higher cure rate.

Mohs' micrographic surgery is currently used to treat some of the more difficult skin cancers, including basal cell carcinoma, squamous cell carcinoma, erythroplasia of Queyrat, bowenoid papulosis, Bowen's disease, verrucous carcinoma, keratoacanthoma, microcytic adnexal carcinoma, sebaceous carcinoma, extramammary Paget's disease, malignant melanoma, Merkel's cell carcinoma, dermatofibrosarcoma protuberans, atypical fibroxanthoma, leiomyosarcoma, and an-

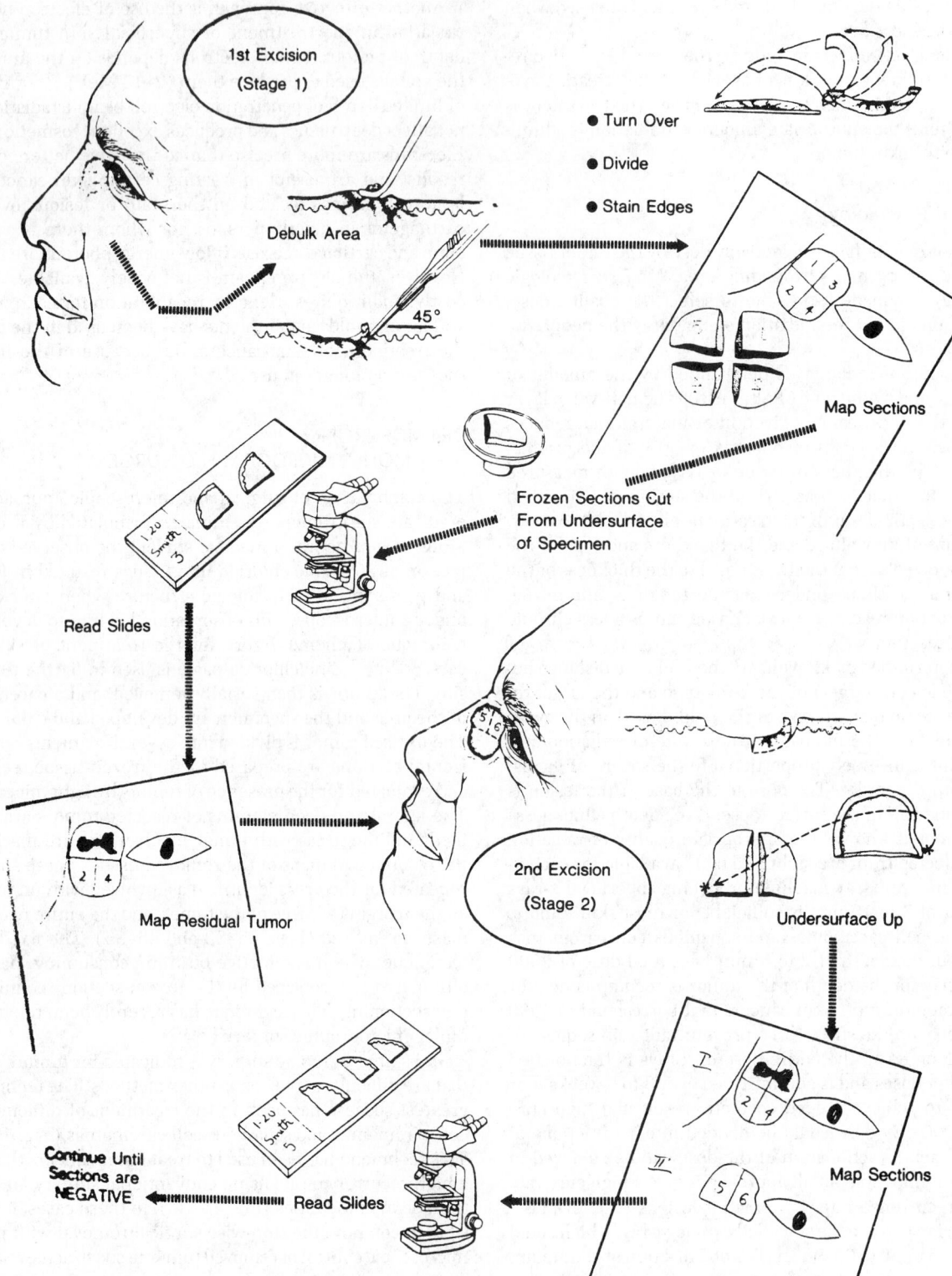

FIGURE 45–33. Schematic representation of the technique of Mohs' surgery.

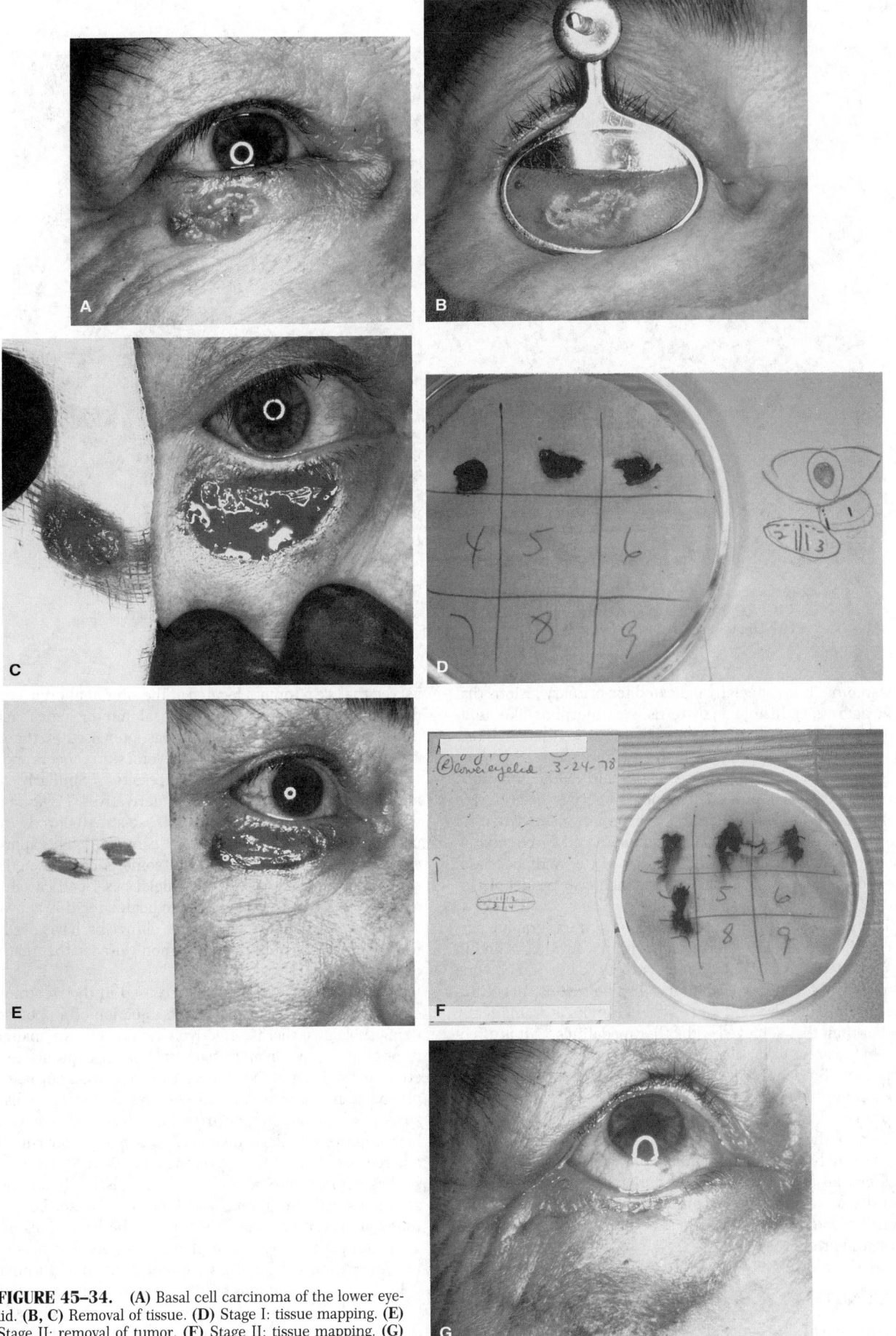

FIGURE 45–34. **(A)** Basal cell carcinoma of the lower eyelid. **(B, C)** Removal of tissue. **(D)** Stage I: tissue mapping. **(E)** Stage II: removal of tumor. **(F)** Stage II: tissue mapping. **(G)** Seven months after surgery.

1603

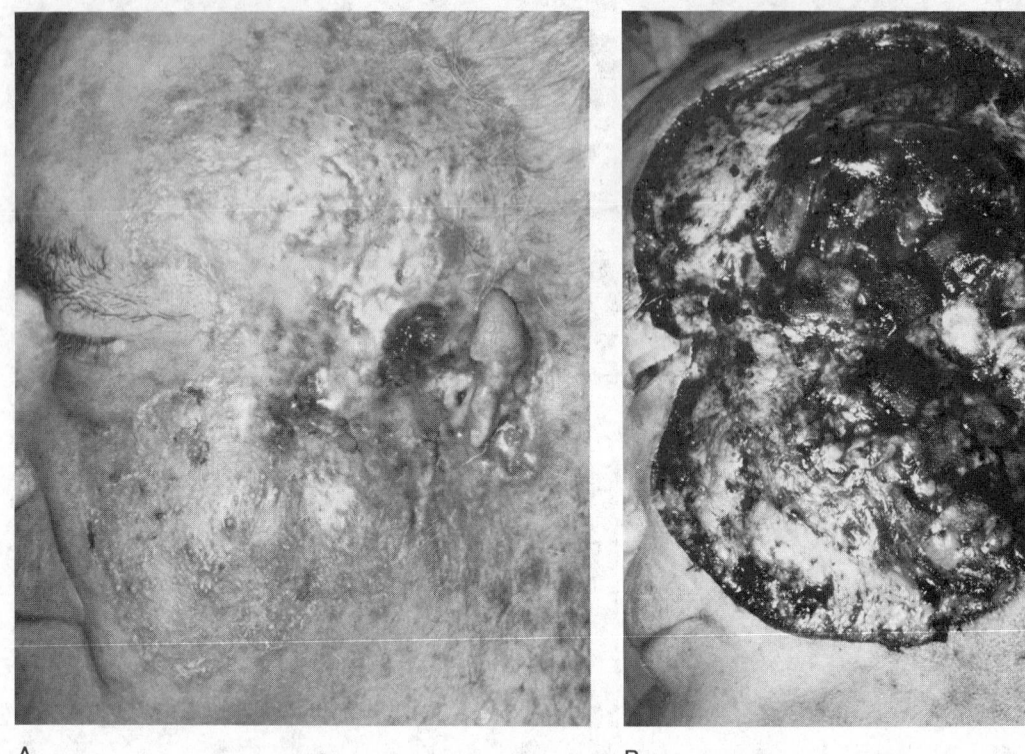

A   B

FIGURE 45–35.   (A) Extensive infiltrating, destructive morpheaform basal cell carcinoma of the left cheek.
(B) The tumor extends far beyond the clinical margins defined by Mohs' micrographic surgery.

giosarcoma. It is especially indicated for primary lesions that have aggressive histologic patterns (*e.g.,* morphea-like, infiltrative) or primary lesions located on the areas that are likely to have subclinical spread or high recurrence rate.

Normal tissue preservation is essential for functional and cosmetic reasons. Mohs' micrographic surgery is the preferred technique if tissue-sparing surgery is important, as when removing basal cell carcinoma or squamous cell carcinoma located on the embryonal fusion planes of the midface, nasal area, or periauricular areas that are high risk for deeply invasive tumors.

There are several advantages for Mohs' micrographic surgery. The procedure is performed within a few hours and in an outpatient setting, and the defect produced by the technique can heal by secondary intention or can be reconstructed immediately. The cure rate for recurrent tumors is dramatically higher than that achieved with other modalities.[357] It is effective in the areas of high recurrence, in cosmetically important areas, and for deeply invasive tumors, because the horizontal sectioning and examination of the entire lateral and deep margins ensures complete removal of the tumor.

Because the defect of removing a large invasive tumor could be extremely large and potentially devastating to the patient, it is crucial to discuss the procedure, the expected defects, and the possibilities for reconstruction. Photographs of previously treated cases and the end results are helpful in demonstrating the procedure.

IMMUNOTHERAPY AND EXPERIMENTAL MODALITIES

Destruction of skin cancer by the local cell-mediated reaction was initially described by Klein.[358] He and his associates ob-

served that skin tumors located at the sites of allergic contact dermatitis were destroyed by the local immunologic reaction, and DNCB, a sensitizing agent, was later used by the same investigators in the treatment of several skin cancers and precancerous lesions with acceptable results.[358] Similarly, recall antigens, such as purified protein derivatives, *Candida,* pertussis, *Trichophyton,* and streptokinase-streptodornase, were used in the treatment of some skin cancers.[359] This approach was effective in the treatment of some uncomplicated skin cancers. Actinic keratosis, superficial basal cell carcinoma, and Bowen's disease are good candidates for this approach. Although other investigators and clinicians have used this technique, it has not become commonly used in the treatment of skin cancers.

Photodynamic therapy has been used in the treatment of skin cancers.[360] It is based on the injection of a photosensitizing substance that is selectively retained by the malignant tumor but not by normal tissue.[361,362] After exposure to penetrating visible light, the photosensitizing substance undergoes photodynamic activation and destroys the tumor cells and spares the surrounding normal skin. Most studies have used hematoporphyrin derivative (*i.e.,* dihematoporphyrin ether) and red laser light with a wavelength of 600 to 700 nm. These studies demonstrated effectiveness in basal cell carcinoma, squamous cell carcinoma, and Bowen's disease. Long-term follow-up is not yet available. One of the limitations of this approach is the generalized photosensitivity that may occur in some patients receiving systemic injection of porphyrin.

Intralesional injections of interferon (interferon α-2a) into basal cell carcinoma may provide a short-term remission of the tumor.[176] Long-term results are not yet known. Although there has been limited morbidity, the repeated injections

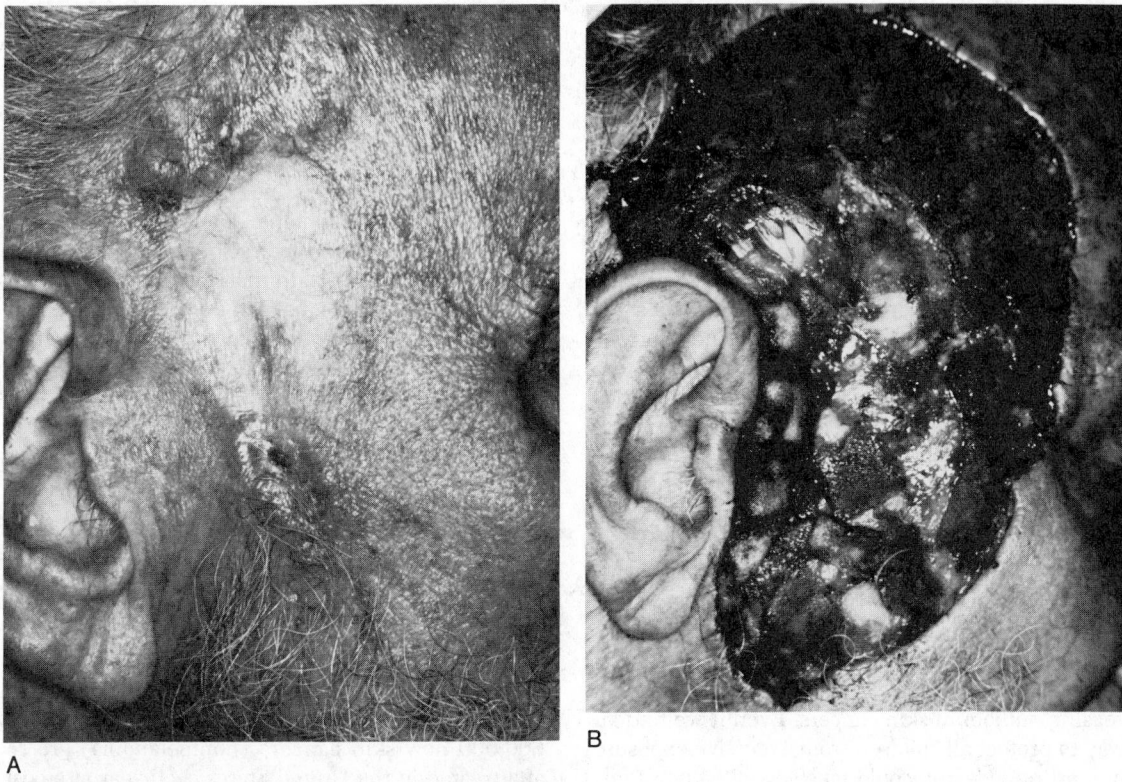

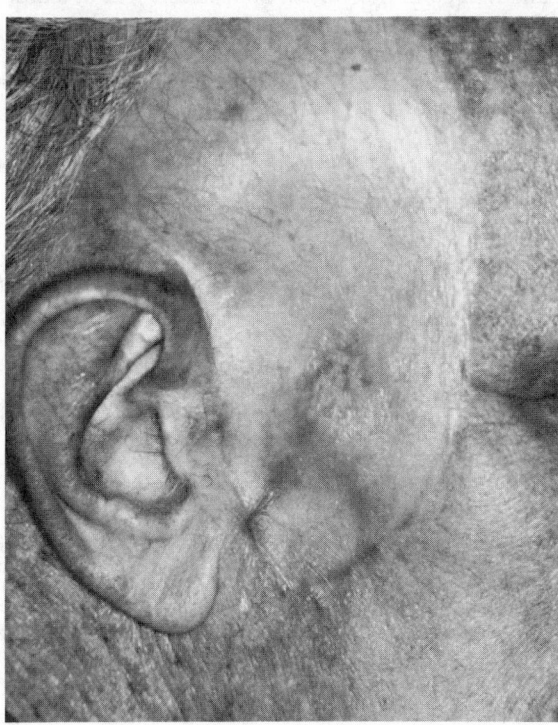

FIGURE 45–36. **(A)** Recurrent basal cell carcinoma of the right cheek after three previous treatments with electrodesiccation and curettage. **(B)** Considerable extension of the wound after six stages of Mohs' micrographic surgery. **(C)** Four months postoperatively. The defect was covered by a full-thickness skin graft after surgery.

needed to eradicate the tumor could be a limiting factor and increase the cost of the therapy. Newer developments in this field may allow the use of biologic factors to become a standard therapy for skin cancers in the future.

TRENDS IN DIAGNOSIS AND TREATMENT

Basal cell carcinoma and squamous cell carcinoma are the most common cancers in the white population. Although the mortality rate from these cancers is low, they exert a heavy burden on the health care system in developed countries. All indicators point to a continued increase in the incidence of skin cancers and their heavy burden on the health care system because of the availability of outdoor recreational activities and sunbathing all year round and because of the cultural norms of our society.

Severe sun exposure and UV damage to the skin continues for years. The problem is compounded by the rapid and continuous depletion of the ozone layer due to the release of ozone-damaging chemicals in the industrialized world. Although the government has placed a ban on production and release of these chemicals, the depletion of ozone will continue for many years. Another important factor is the continuous increase in the aging population, which is accompanied by an increasing number of skin cancers. Even if we find an effective way to protect all children from excessive exposure to UV light starting today, it would take several generations to eliminate those who have been severely damaged. Most likely, in most of these cases the initiation and promotion has occurred in the sun exposed persons and it will continue to cause skin cancers in a significant proportion of the aging population.

Currently, the most logical and effective approach is to identify the risk population for skin cancer, provide early diagnosis guidelines, and educate the public about preventing additional sun exposure. Early diagnosis of skin cancers can only be achieved with public educational programs indicating the importance of early diagnosis and treatment. In the past 6 years, public education and awareness has been increased by free skin cancer screening offered to the public every May or June in the United States. Considerable experience has been gained about the optimal means of public education, and awareness has increased greatly, but a significant workload is generated due to the large numbers of normal persons who have to be seen and reassured.

Excessive sun damage can be prevented with commercially available sunscreens. Sunscreens have protected against further development of UV-induced papillomas in hairless mice, and it is possible that the same is true for humans, but some questions remain unanswered about sunscreen use for humans.[363] Increased pigmentation in persons with white skin could be an alternative approach. Several laboratories are experimenting with a melanocyte-stimulating hormone analog, which produces greater melanization of the skin after topical or systemic application.[364]

Another possible approach is the reversal of actinic damage before the development of skin cancers. It is thought that UV-induced photoaging is a precursor of actinic keratosis, which is a precursor of nonmelanoma skin cancers. By reversing photoaging, it may be possible to prevent development of nonmelanoma skin cancers. Even delay in progression to the malignant stage could be valuable. It is reported that after 1 year of using UV protection measures, approximately 25% of actinic keratoses are reversed.[66] Daily topical use of retinoic acid (0.1%) has reversed the aging process of facial skin over a period of 4 to 5 months.[365]

Work is in progress to develop more effective modes of therapy for skin cancers, including the development of newer types of lasers for the management of precancerous and cancerous skin lesions and the use of newer biologic agents, such as interferon. It is certain that over the next few years other biologic agents will be used in the treatment of skin cancers. Further development is needed of photodynamic therapy, specifically the use of hematoporphyrin derivative and UV light. The use of gene therapy is in the preclinical stages and may soon become available for clinical trails. Culturing of basal cell carcinoma opens a new avenue for the study of the biochemistry and molecular biology of the disease.[366] Drugs can be tested on these cell lines before going into clinical trials.

FINANCIAL CONSIDERATIONS OF TREATMENT

The cost of management and care of precancerous and malignant cutaneous diseases caused by UV light accounts for a significant portion of the health care budget. More than 600,000 new skin cancers (nonmelanoma) are recognized and treated in the United States each year at a cost of more than 1 billion dollars. Because the aging population is increasing in size, because of uncertainties about the biologic effect of depletion of the ozone, and because of the continued cultural and habitual exposure to sunlight, we will continue to be faced with increasing numbers of skin cancers and associated expenses.

The prudent approach is to develop new measures to prevent further depletion of the ozone, increase public and medical practitioners' awareness about skin cancers and the importance of early diagnosis, and continue investigations into prevention, control, and care of more advanced disease.

REFERENCES

1. Boring CC, Squires TS, Tong T. Cancer Statistics, 1992. CA 1992;42:19–38.
2. Yiannias JA, Goldberg LH, Carter-Campbell S, et al. The ratio of basal cell carcinoma to squamous cell carcinoma in Houston, Texas. J Dermatol Surg Oncol 1988;14:886–889.
3. MacKie RM, Elwood JM, Hawk JLM. Links between exposure to ultraviolet radiation and skin cancer. J R Coll Physicians Lond 1987;21:91–96.
4. Council on Scientific Affairs. Harmful effects of ultraviolet radiation. JAMA 1989;262:380–384.
5. National Institutes of Health. Summary of the consensus development conference on sunlight, ultraviolet radiation, and the skin. J Am Acad Dermatol 1991;24:608–612.
6. Kripke ML, Sass ER, eds. Anitgenicity of murine skin tumors induced by UV light. JNCI 1974;53:1333–1336.
7. Kripke ML. Immunology and photocarcinogenesis. J Am Acad Dermatol 1986;14:149–155.
8. Brookes P, Lawley PD. Evidence for binding of polynuclear aromatic hydrocarbons to the nucleic acids of mouse skin: Relation between carcinogenic hydrocarbons and their binding to DNA. Nature 1964;202:781–784.
9. Marks F, Furstenberger G. Experimental evidence that skin carcinogenesis is a multistep phenomenon. Br J Dermatol 1986;115:1.
10. Jones SK, MacKie RM, Hole DJ, et al. Further evidence for the safety of tar in psoriasis. Br J Dermatol 1985;113:97–101.
11. Yuspa SH. Chemical carcinogenesis related to the skin. Prog Dermatol 1981;15:1.
12. Potter M. Percivall Pott's contribution to cancer research. NCI Monogr 1963;10:1.
13. Yeh S. Relative incidence of skin cancer in Chinese in Taiwan with special reference to arsenical cancer. NCI Monogr 1963;10:81.
14. Traenkle HL. X-ray induced cancer in man. NCI Monogr 1963;10:423–440.

15. Bowers RF, Young JM. Carcinoma arising in scars, osteomyelitis and fistulae. Arch Surg 1960;80:564.

16. Cruickshank AH, McConnell EM, Miller DG. Malignant degeneration in burn scars, chronic ulcers and sinuses. J Clin Pathol 1963;16:573.

17. Giblin T, Pickrell K, Pitts W, et al. Malignant degeneration in burn scars: Marjolin's ulcer. Ann Surg 1965;162:291.

18. Sedlin ED, Fleming JL. Epidermoid carcinoma arising in chronic osteomyelitic foci. J Bone Joint Surg [Am] 1963;45:827.

19. Hejna WF. Squamous cell carcinoma developing in the chronic draining sinuses of osteomyelitis. Cancer 1965;18:128.

20. Mustoe T, Upton J, Marcellino V, et al. Carcinoma in chronic pressure sores: A fulminant disease process. Plast Reconstr Surg 1986;77:116.

21. Rattner H, Bluefarb SM, Johnson HJ. Squamous cell epithelioma superimposed on a patch of chronic discoid lupus erythematosus. Arch Dermatol 1956;73:601.

22. Lutzner MA. The human papillomaviruses. Arch Dermatol 1983;119:631.

23. Ikengerg H, Gissmann L, Gross G, et al. Human papillomavirus type 16-related DNA in genital Bowen's disease and in bowenoid papulosis. Int J Cancer 1983;32:563–565.

24. Oblek S, Jablonska S, Orth G. HPV-associated intraepithelial neoplasia of external genitalia. Clin Dermatol 1985;3:104.

25. Meanswell CA, Cox MF, Blackledge G, et al. HPV 16 DNA in normal and malignant cervical epithelium: Implications for the aetiology and behavior of cervical neoplasia. Lancet 1987;1:703–707.

26. . Human papillomaviruses and cervical cancer: A fresh look at the evidence. Lancet 1987;1:725–726.

27. Ostrow RS, Bender M, Niimura M, et al. Human papillomavirus DNA in cutaneous primary and metastasized squamous cell carcinomas from patients with epidermodysplasia verruciformis. Proc Natl Acad Sci USA 1982;79:1634.

28. Walder BK, Robertson MR, Jeremy D. Skin cancer and immunosuppression. Lancet 1971;2:1282.

29. Hoxtell EO, Mandel JS, Murray SS, et al. Incidence of skin carcinoma after renal transplantation. Arch Dermatol 1977;113:436.

30. Koranda FC, Dehmel EM, Kahn G, et al. Cutaneous complications in immunosuppressed renal homograft recipients. JAMA 1974;229:419.

31. Penn I, Halgrimson CG, Starzl TE. De novo malignant tumors in organ transplant recipients. Transplant Proc 1971;3:773.

32. Westburg SP, Stone OJ. Multiple cutaneous squamous cell carcinomas during immunosuppressive therapy. Arch Dermatol 1973;107:893.

33. Berg JW. The incidence of multiple primary cancers: 1. Development of further cancers in patients with lymphoma, leukemias and myeloma. JNCI 1967;38:741.

34. Turner JE, Callen JP. Aggressive behavior of squamous cell carcinoma in a patient with preceding lymphocytic lymphoma. J Am Acad Dermatol 1981;4:446.

35. Weimar VM, Ceilley RI, Goeken JA. Aggressive behavior of basal and squamous cell cancers in patients with chronic lymphocytic lymphoma or chronic lymphocytic leukemia. J Dermatol Surg Oncol 1979;5:609.

36. Gitlin MC, Pirozzi DJ. The sign of Leser-Trelat. Arch Dermatol 1975;111:792–793.

37. Gallimore AP. Malignant transformation of a clonal seborrhoeic keratosis. Br J Dermatol 1991;124:287–290.

38. Su WPD. Histopathologic varieties of epidermal nevus. Am J Dermatopathol 1982;4:161–170.

39. Solomon LM, Fretzin DF, Dewald RL. The epidermal nevus syndrome. Arch Dermatol 1977;113:767–769.

40. Levin A, Amazon K, Rywlin AM. A squamous cell carcinoma that developed in an epidermal nevus: Report of a case and review of the literature. Am J Dermatopathol 1984;6:51–55.

41. Degos R, Civatte J. Clear cell acanthoma. Experience of 8 years. Br J Dermatol 1970;83:248–254.

42. Trau H, Fisher BK, Schewach-Millet M. Multiple clear cell acanthoma. Arch Dermatol 1980;116:433–434.

43. Carter VH, Constantine VS. Kryle's disease: I. Clinical findings in five cases and review of the literature. Arch Dermatol 1968;97:624–632.

44. Constantine VS, Carter VH. Kryle's disease: II. Histopathologic findings in five cases and review of the literature. Arch Dermatol 1968;97:633–639.

45. Gracia-Bravo B, Rodriguez-Pichardo A, Camacho F. Uraemic follicular hyperkeratosis. Clin Exp Dermatol 1985;10:448–454.

46. Hood AF, Hardegen GL, Zarate AR, et al. Kyrle's disease in patients with chronic renal failure. Arch Dermatol 1982;118:85–88.

47. Delacretaz J. Keratotic basal cell carcinoma arising from an epidermoid cyst. J Dermatol Surg Oncol 1977;3:310–311.

48. McDonald LW. Carcinomatous change in cysts of skin. Arch Dermatol 1963;87:208–211.

49. Shelly WB, Wood MG. Occult Bowen's disease in keratinous cysts. Br J Dermatol 1981;105:105–108.

50. Cotton DWK, Kirkham N, Young BJJ. Immunoperoxidase antikeratin staining of epidermal and pilar cysts. Br J Dermatol 1984;111:63–68.

51. McGavran MN, Binnington B. Keratinous cysts of the skin: Identification and differentiation of pilar cysts from epidermal cysts. Arch Dermatol 1966;94:499–508.

52. Baptista AP, Silva LGE, Born MC. Proliferating trichilemmal cyst. J Cutan Pathol 1983;10:178–187.

53. Brownstein MN, Arluk DK. Proliferating trichilemmal cyst: A simulant of squamous cell carcinoma. Cancer 1981;48:1207–1214.

54. Saida T, Oohara K, Hori Y, et al. Development of a malignant proliferating trichilemmal cyst in a patient with multiple trichilemmal cysts. Dermatologica 1983;166:203–208.

55. Birt AR, Hogg GR, Dube WJ. Herediatry multiple fibrofolliculomas with trichodiscomas and acrochordons. Arch Dermatol 1977;113:1674–1677.

56. Fujita WH, Barr RJ, Headley JL. Multiple fibrofolliculmas with trichodiscomas and acrochordons. Arch Dermatol 1981;117:32–35.

57. Ubogy-Rainey Z, James WD, Lupton GP, et al. Fibrofolliculomas, trichodiscomas, and acrochordons the Birt-Hogg-Dube syndrome. J Am Acad Dermatol 1987;16:452–457.

58. Copeman PWM, Wilson JE. Pigmented hairy epidermal nevus (Becker). Arch Dermatol 1965;92:249–251.

59. Tate PR, Hadge SJ, Owen LG. A quantitative study of melanocytes in Becker's nevus. J Cutan Pathol 1980;7:404–409.

60. Tanay A, Mehregan AH. Warty dyskeratoma. Dermatologica 1969;138:155–164.

61. Harriest TJ, Murphy GF, Mihm MC Jr. Oral warty dyskeratoma. Arch Dermatol 1980;116:929–931.

62. Marks R. Non-melanoma skin cancer and solar keratoses in Australia. Eur J Epidemiol 1985;1:319–322.

63. Montgomery H. Precancerous dermatosis and epithelioma in situ. Arch Dermatol Syphilol 1939;39:387.

64. Brownstein MH, Rabinowitz AD. The precursors of cutaneous squamous cell carcinoma. Int J Dermatol 1979;18:1–16.

65. Bercovitch L. Topical chemotherapy of actinic keratoses of the upper extremity with tretinoin and 5-fluorouracil: A double-blind controlled study. Br J Dermatol 1987;116:549–552.

66. Marks R, Foley P, Goodman G, et al. Spontaneous remission of solar keratoses. The case for conservative management. Br J Dermatol 1986;115:649–655.

67. Rahbari H, Pinkus H. Large cell acanthoma: One of the actinic keratoses. Arch Dermatol 1978;114:49–52.

68. Rabinowitz AD. Multiple large cell acanthoma. J Am Acad Dermatol 1983;8:840–845.

69. Sanchez Yus E, De Diego V, Urrutia S. Large cell acanthoma. Am J Dermatopathol 1988;10:197–208.

70. Santa Cruz DJ. Chondrodermatitis nodularis helicis: A transepidermal perforating disorder. J Cutan Pathol 1980;7:70–76.

71. Goette DK. Chondrodermatitis nodularis chronica helicis: A perforating necrotic granuloma. J Am Acad Dermatol 1980;2:148–154.

72. Bard JW. Chondrodermatitis nodularis chronica helicis. Dermatologica 1981;163:376.

73. Brownstein MH, Shapiro EE. Trichilemmal horn: Cutaneous horn overlying trichilemmoma. Clin Exp Dermatol 1979;4:59–63.

74. Sandbank M. Basal cell carcinoma at the base of cutaneous horn (cornu cutaneum). Arch Dermatol 1971;104:97–98.

75. Yu RCH, Pryce DW, Macfarlane AW, et al. A histopathological study of 643 cutaneous horns. Br J Dermatol 1991;124:449–452.

76. Goldschmidt H, Sherwin WK. Reactions to ionizing radiation. J Am Acad Dermatol 1980;3:551–579.

77. Lazar P, Cullen SI. Basal cell epithelioma and chronic radiodermatitis. Arch Dermatol 1963;88:172–175.

78. McGibbon DH. Malignant epidermal tumors. J Cutan Pathol 1985;12:224–238.

79. Seo IS, Warner TFCS, Warren JS, et al. Cutaneous postirradiation sarcoma. Ultrastructural evidence of pluripotential mesenchymal cell derivation. Cancer 1985;56:761–767.

80. Souba WW, McKenna RJ Jr, Meis J, et al. Radiation-induced sarcomas of th chest wall. Cancer 1986;57:610–615.

81. Kao GF. Carcinoma arising in Bowen's disease. Arch Dermatol 1986;122:1124–1126.

82. Ackerman AB. Bowenoid papulosis. J Am Acad Dermatol 1981;4:608.

83. Lutzner MA, Blanchet-Bradon C, Orth G. Clinical observations, virologic studies, and treatment trials in patients with epidermodysplasia verruciformis, a disease induced by specific human papillomaviruses. J Invest Dermatol 1984;83:18–25S.

84. Bettley FR, O'Shea JA. The absorption of arsenic and its relation to carcinoma. Br J Dermatol 1975;92:563–568.

85. Graham JH, Helwig EB. Bowen's disease and its relationship to systemic cancer. Arch Dermatol 1959;80:133–159.

86. Callen JP, Headington J. Bowen's amd non-Bowen's squamous intraepidermal neoplasia of the skin. Arch Dermatol 1980;116:422–426.

87. Arbesman H, Ransohoff DF. Is Bowen's disease a predictor for the development of internal malignancy? JAMA 1987;257:516–518.

88. Graham JH, Helwig EB. Erythroplasia of Queyrat. Cancer 1973;32:1396–1414.

89. Goette DK. Erythroplasia of Queyrat. Arch Dermatol 1974;110:271–273.

90. Mikail GR. Cancers, precancers, and pseudocancers on the male genetalia. J Dermatol Surg Oncology 1980;6:1027–1035.

91. Obalek SJ, Jablonska S, Beaudenon MB, et al. Bowenoid papulosis of the male and female genitalia: Risk of cervical neoplasia. J Am Acad Dermatol 1986;14:433–444.

92. Wade TR, Kopf AW, Ackermann AB. Bowenoid papulosis of the penis. Cancer 1978;42:1890–1903.

93. Wade TR, Kopf AW, Ackermann AB. Bowenoid papulosis of the genitalia. Arch Dermatol 1979;115:306–308.

94. Schwartz RA, Janniger CK. Bowenoid papulosis. J Am Acad Dermatol 1991;24:261–264.

95. Karatochvil FJ, Cioffi GA, Auclair PL, et al. Virus-associated dysplasia (bowenoid papulosis?) of the oral cavity. Oral Surg Oral Med Oral Pathol 1989;68:312–316.

96. Patterson JW, Kao GF, Graham JH, et al. Bowenoid papulosis: A clinicopathologic study with ultrastructural observations. Cancer 1986;57:823–836.

97. Rudlinger R, Buchmann P. HPV 16-positive bowenoid papulosis and squamous cell carcinoma of the anus in an HIV-positive man. Dis Colon Rectum 1989;32:1042–1045.

98. Bonnekoh B, Mahrle G, Steigleder GK. Transition of bowenoid papulosis (HPV-16) into cutaneous squamous cell carcinoma in two patients. Z Hautkr 1987;62:773–784.

99. Skinner MS, Sternberg WH, Ichinose H, et al. Spontaneous regression of bowenoid atypia of the vulva. Obstet Gynecol 1973;42:40–46.

100. Friedrich EG. Reversible vulvar atypia: A case report. Obstet Gynecol 1972;39:173–181.

101. Berger BW, Hori Y. Multicentric Bowen's disease of the genitalia: Spontaneous regression of lesions. Arch Dermatol 1978;114:1698–1699.

102. Landthaler M, Haina D, Brunner R, et al. Laser therapy of bowenoid papulosis and Bowen's disease. J Dermatol Surg Oncol 1986;12:1253–1257.

103. Gross G, Roussaki A, Papendick U. Efficacy of interferons on bowenoid papulosis and other precancerous lesions. J Invest Dermatol 1990;95:152S–157S.

104. Lutzner M. Epidermodysplasia verruciformis: An autosomal recessive disease characterized by viral warts and skin cancer. Bull Cancer 1978;65:169–182.

105. Androphy E, Dvoretzky I, Lowry D. X-linked inheritance of epidermodysplasia verruciformis. Arch Dermatol 1981;121:864–868.

106. Jablonska S, Orth G, Jarzabek-Chorzelska M. Twenty-one years of follow-up studies of familial epidermodysplasia verruciformis. Dermatologica 1979;158:309.

107. Glinski W, Obalek S, Jablonska S, et al. T cell defect in patients with epidermodysplasia verruciformis due to human papilloma virus type 3 and 5. Dermatologica 1981;162:141–147.

108. Majewski S, Skopinska-Rozewska E, Jablonska S, et al. Partial defect of cell mediated immunity in patients with epidermodysplasia verruciformis. J Am Acad Dermatol 1986;15:996.

109. Majewski S, Malejczyk J, Jablonska S, et al. Natural cell-mediated cytotoxicity against various target cells in patients with epidermodysplasia verruciformis. J Am Acad Dermatol 1990;22:423–427.

110. Obalek S, Glinski W, Hagtek M, et al. Comparative studies on cell-mediated immunity in patients with different warts. Dermatologica 1980;161:73–83.

111. Pfister H, Iftner TH, Fuchs PG. Papillomaviruses from epidermodysplasia verruciformis patients and renal allograft recients. Papillomaviruses: Molecular and clinical aspects. UCLA Symp Mol Cell Biol 1985;32:85–100.

112. Rudlinger R, Smith JW, Bunney MH, et al. Human papillomavirus infections in a group of renal transplant recipients. Br J Dermatol 1986;115:681–692.

113. Tanigaki T, Kanda R, Sato K. Epidermodysplasia verruciformis (L-L, 1922) in a patient with systemic lupus erythematous. Arch Dermatol Res 1986;278:247–248.

114. Gross G, Ellinger K, Roussaki A, et al. Epidermodysplasia verruciformis in a patient with Hodgkin's disease: Characterization of a new papillomavirus type and interferon treatment. J Invest Dermatol 1988;91:957–962.

115. Claudy A, Touraine J, Mitanne D. Epidermodysplasia verruciformis induced by a new human papillomavirus (HPV-8): Report of a case without immune dysfunction. Effects of treatment with an aromatic retinoid. Arch Dermatol Res 1982;27:213–219.

116. Androphy E, Dvoretzky I, Maluish A, et al. Response of warts in epidermodysplasia verruciformis to treatment with systemic and intralesional alpha interferon. J Am Acad Dermatol 1984;11:197–202.

117. Waldron CA, Shafer WG. Leukoplakia revisited. A clinicopathologic study of 3256 oral leukoplakias. Cancer 1975;36:1386–1392.

118. Silverman S Jr, Gorsky M, Lozada F. Oral leukoplakia and malignant transformation. A follow-up study of 257 patients. Cancer 1984;53:563–568.

119. Wilson JE. Naevus sebaceous. Br J Dermatol 1970;82:99–117.

120. Morioka S. The natural history of nevus sebaceous. J Cutan Pathol 1985;12:200–213.

121. Domingo J, Helwig EB. Malignant neoplasms associated with the nevus sebaceous of Jadassohn. J Am Acad Dermatol 1979;1:545–556.

122. Chernosky ME. Porokeratosis. Arch Dermatol 1986;122:869–870.

123. Chernosky ME, Anderson DE. Disseminated superficial actinic porokeratosis. Genetic aspects. Arch Dermatol 1969;99:408–412.

124. Schwarz T, Seiser A, Gschnait F, Disseminated superficial "actinic" porokeratosis. J Am Acad Dermatol 1984;11:724–730.

125. MacMillian AL, Roberts SOB. Porokeratosis of Mibelli after renal transplantation. Br J Dermatol 1974;90:45–54.

126. Lederman JS, Sober AJ, Lederman GS. Immunosuppression: A cause of porokeratosis? J Am Acad Dermatol 1985;13:75–79.

127. Neumann RA, Knobler RM, Metze, et al. Disseminated superficial porokeratosis and immunosuppression. Br J Dermatol 1988;119:375–380.

128. Brodkin RH, Ricket RR, Fuller FW, et al. Malignant disseminated porokeratosis (DSAP). Arch Dermatol 1987;123:1521–1526.

129. Rahbari H, Cordero AA, Mehregan AH. Linear porokeratosis. Arch Dermatol 1974;109:526–528.

130. Shaw JC, White CR Jr. Porokeratosis plantaris, plamaris et disseminata. J Am Acad Dermatol 1984;11:454–460.

131. Himmelstein R, Lynnfield YL. Punctate porokeratosis. Arch Dermatol 1984;120:263–264.

132. Coskey RJ, Mehregan A. Bowen disease associated with porokeratosis of Mibelli. Arch Dermatol 1975;111:1480–1481.

133. Lozinski AZ, Fisher BK, Walter JB, et al. Metastatic squamous cell carcinoma in linear porokeratosis of Mibelli. J Am Acad Dermatol 1987;16:448–451.

134. Shrum JR, Cooper PH, Greer KE, et al. Squamous cell carcinoma in disseminated superficial actinic porokeratosis. J Am Acad Dermatol 1982;6:58–62.

135. Pinkus H. Premalignant fibroepithelial tumors of the skin. Arch Dermatol 1953;67:598–615.

136. Rook A, Whimster I. Keratoacanthoma. A 30-year retrospect. Br J Dermatol 1979;100:41–47.

137. Walinsky S, Silvers DV, et al. Spontaneous regression of a giant keratoacanthoma. Cancer 1978;41:12–16.

138. Golddenhersh MA, Olsen TG. Invasive squamous cell carcinoma initially diagnosed as giant keratoacanthoma. J Am Acad Dermatol 1984;10:372–378.

139. Chalet MD, Connors RC, Ackerman AB. Squamous cell carcinoma vs. keratoacanthoma: Criteria for histologic differentiation. J Dermatol Surg 1975;1:16–17.

140. Kern WH, McCray MK. The histopathologic differentiation of keratoacanthoma and squamous cell carcinoma of the skin. J Cutan Pathol 1980;7:318–325.

141. Sullivan JJ, Donoghue MF, Kynaston B, et al. Multiple keratoacanthomas. Aust J Dermatol 1980;21:16–24.

142. Winkelmann RK, Brown J. Generalized eruptive keratoacanthoma. Arch Dermatol 1968;97:615–623.

143. Domarus HV, Stevens PJ. Metastatic basal cell carcinoma: Report of five cases and review of 170 cases in the literature. J Am Acad Dermatol 1984;10:1043–1060.

144. Rahbari H, Mehregan AH. Basal cell epithelioma (carcinoma) in childern and adolescents. Cancer 1982;49:350–353.

145. Plosila M, Kiistala R, Niemi KM. The Bazex syndrome: Follicular atrophoderma with multiple basal cell carcinomas, hypotrichosis, and hypohidrosis. Clin Exp Dermatol 1981;6:31–37.

146. Gorlin RJ. Nevoid basal cell carcinoma syndrome. J Med 1992;66:98–113.

147. Khatri ML, Shafi M, Mashina A. Xeroderma pigmentosum. J Am Acad Dermatol 1992;26:75–78.

148. Giles G, Marks R, Foley P. The incidence of non-melanocytic skin cancer in Australia. Br Med J 1988;296:13–17.

149. Kuflik EG. Clinical variants of basal cell carcinoma. Cutis 1981;28:403–408.

150. Miller SJ. Biology of basal cell carcinoma (part I). J Am Acad Dermatol 1991;24:1–13.

151. Miller SJ. Biology of basal cell carcinoma (part II). J Am Acad Dermatol 1991;24:161–175.

152. Sexton M, Jones DB, Maloney ME. Histologic pattern analysis of basal cell carcinoma. J Am Acad Dermatol 1990;23:1118–1126.

153. Borel DM. Cutaneous basosquamous carcinoma. Review of the literature and report of 35 cases. Arch Pathol 1973;95:293–297.

154. Gormley DE, Hirsch P. Aggresive basal cell carcinoma of the scalp. Arch Dermatol 1978;114:782–783.

155. Jacobs GH, Rippey JJ, Altini M. Prediction of aggressive behavior in basal cell carcinoma. Cancer 1982;49:533–537.

156. Urbach F. Geographic distribution of skin cancer. J Surg Oncol 1971;3:219.

157. Hall AF. Relationship of sunlight, complexion and heredity to skin carcinogenesis. Arch Dermatol Syphilol 1950;61:589.

158. Myskowski PL, Pollack MS,, Schorr E, et al. Human leukocyte antigen associations in basal cell carcinoma. J Am Acad Dermatol 1985;12:997–1000.

159. Robinson JK. Risk of developing another basal cell carcinoma: A 5-year prospective study. Cancer 1987;60:118.

160. Abram H, Barsky S. Pigmented basal cell epithelioma arising in the scar of an onchocerciasis nodule. Int J Dermatol 1984;23:658–660.

161. Rich JD, Shesol BF, Horne DW. Basal cell carcinoma arising in a smallpox vaccination site. J Clin Pathol 1980;33:134–135.

162. Korula R, Hughes CF. Squamous cell carcinoma arising in a sternotomy scar. Ann Thorac Surg 1991;51:667–669.

163. Schwartz RA, Burgess GH, Milgrom H. Breast carcinoma and basal cell epitheliomaa after x-ray therapy for hirsutism. Cancer 1979;44:1601–1605.

164. Anderson NP, Anderson HE. Development of basal cell epitheliomas as a consequence of radiodermatitis. Arch Dermatol Syphilol 1951;63:586–596.

165. Sexton M, Jones DB, Maloney ME. Histologic pattern analysis of basal cell carcinoma. Study of a series of 1039 consecutive neoplasms. J Am Acad Dermatol 1990;23:1118–1126.

166. Pollack SW, Goslen JB, Sheretz, et al. The biology of basal cell carcinoma. A review. J Am Acad Dermatol 1982;7:569–577.

167. Brooke JD, Fitzpatrick JE, Golitz LE. Papillary mesenchymal bodies: A histologic finding useful in differentiating trichoepitheliomas from basal cell carcinomas. J Am Acad Dermatol 1989;21:523–528.

168. Lo JS, Snow SN, Reizner GT, et al. Metastatic basal cell carcinoma: Report of twelve cases with a review of the literature. J Am Acad Dermatol 1991;24:715–719.

169. Drake LA, Ceilley RI, Cornelison RL, et al. Guidelines of care for basal cell carcinoma. J Am Acad Dermatol 1992;26:117–120.

170. McGrouther DAM. Treatment of basal cell carcinoma. A plastic surgeon's view. Br J Dermatol 1987;117:399.

171. Spiller WF, Spiller RF. Treatment of basal cell carcinoma by curettage and electrodesiccation. J Am Acad Dermatol 1984;11:808.

172. Cott RE, Wood MG, Johnson BL. Use of curettage and shave excision in office practice. J Am Acad Dermatol 1987;16:1243–1251.

173. Swanson N. Mohs' surgery. Arch Dermatol 1983;119:761–773.

174. Hruza GJ. Mohs' micrographic surgery. Otolaryngol Clin North Am 1990;23:845–864.

175. Mikhail GR. Mohs' micrographic surgery. Philadelphia: WB Saunders, 1991.

176. Greenway HT, Cornell RC, Tanner DJ, et al. Treatment of basal cell carcinoma with intralesional interferon. J Am Acad Dermatol 1986;15:437–443.

177. Lindelof B, Sigurgeirsson B, Tegner E, et al. PUVA and cancer: A large-scale epidemiological study. Lancet 1991;338:91–93.

178. Chaung TY, Heinrich LA, Schultz MD, et al. PUVA and skin cancer. J Am Acad Dermatol 1992;26:173–177.

179. Aubry F, McGibbon B. Risk factors of squamous cell carcinoma of the skin: A case-control study in the Montreal region. Cancer 1985;55:907–911.

180. Kwa RE, Campana K, Moy RL. Biology of cutaneous squamous cell carcinoma. J Am Acad Dermatol 1992;26:1–26.

181. Johnson TM, Rowe DE, Nelson BR, et al. Squamous cell carcinoma of the skin (excluding lip and oral mucosa). J Am Acad Dermatol 1992;26:467–484.

182. Luande J, Henschke CI, Mohammed N. The Tanzanian human albino skin: Natural history. Cancer 1985;55:1823.

183. Stern RS, Laird N, Melski J, et al. Cutaneous squamous cell carcinoma in patients treated with PUVA. N Engl J Med 1984;310:1156–1161.

184. Henseler T, Christophers E, Honigsmann H, et al. Skin tumors in the European PUVA study. J Am Acad Dermatol 1987;16:108–116.

185. Benton EC, Bunney MH, Barr BB, et al. Skin cancers and their relationship to human papilloma virus infection in a group of renal allograft recipients. Br J Dermatol [Abstract] 1988;118:270.

186. Arhelger SW, Kremem AJ. Arsenical epitheliomas of medicinal origin. Surgery 1951;30:977.

187. Eliezri YD, Silverstein SJ, Nuovo GJ. Occurrence of human papillomavirus type 16 DNA in cutaneous squamous and basal cell neoplasms. J Am Acad Dermatol 1990;23:836–842.

188. Obalek S, Favre M, Jablonska S, et al. Human papillomavirus type 2-associated basal cell carcinoma in two immunosuppressed patients. Arch Dermatol 1988;124:930–934.

189. Eliezri YD, Silverstein SJ, Nuovo GJ. Occurrence of human papillomavirus type 16 DNA in cutaneous squamous and basal cell neoplasms. J Am Acad Dermatol 1990;23:836–842.

190. Headington JT. Verrucous carcinoma. Cutis 1978;21:207–211.

191. Okagaki T, Clark BA, Zachow KR, et al. Presence of human papillomavirus in verrucous carcinoma (Ackerman) of the vagina. Immunocytochemical, ultrastructural and DNA hybridization studies. Arch Pathol Lab Med 1984;108:567–570.

192. Kao G, Graham JH, Helwig EB. Carcinoma cuniculatum. Cancer 1982;49:2395–2403.

193. Broders S. Practical points in the microsurgic grading of carcinoma. N Y State J Med 1932;32:667–680.

194. Kahn H, Baumal R, From L. Role of immunohistochemistry in the diagnosis of undifferentiated tumors involving the skin. J Am Acad Dermatol 1986;14:1063.

195. Robbinson JK. What are adequate treatment and follow-up care for nonmelanoma cutaneous cancer? Arch Dermatol 1987;123:331–332.

196. Mohs FE, Sahl W. Chemosurgery for verrucous carcinoma. J Dermatol Surg Oncol 1979;5:302.

197. Toker C. Trabecular carcinoma of the skin. Arch Dermatol 1972;105:107–110.

198. Bayrou O, Avril MF, Charpentier P, et al. Primary neuroendocrine carcinoma of the skin. J Am Acad Dermatol 1991;24:198–207.

199. Pilloti S, Rilke F, Bartoli C, et al. Clinicopathologic correlations of cutaneous neuroendocrine Merkel cell carcinoma. J Clin Oncol 1988;6:1863–1873.

200. Goepfert H, Rammler D, Silva E, et al. Merkel cell carcinoma (endocrine carcinoma of the skin) of the head and neck. Arch Otolaryngol Head Neck Surg 1984;110:707–712.

201. Meland NB, Jackson IT. Merkel cell tumor diagnosis, prognosis, and management. Plast Reconstr Surg 1986;77:632–638.

202. Hitchcock CL, Bland KI, Laney RG,III, et al. Neuroendocrine (Merkel cell) carcinoma of the skin: Its natural history, diagnosis, and treatment. Ann Surg 1988;207:201–207.

203. Kayashima K, Ono T, Johno M, et al. Spontaneous regression in Merkel cell (neuroendocrine) carcinoma of the skin. Arch Dermatol 1991;127:550–553.

204. O'Rourke MGE, Bell JR. Merkel cell tumor with spontaneous regression. J Dermatol Surg Oncol 1986;12:994–997.

205. Cotlar AM, Gate JO, Gibbs FA. Merkel cell carcinoma: Combined surgery and radiation therapy. Am Surg 1986;52:159–164.

206. Shaw JHF, Rumball E. Merkel cell tumor: Clinical behavior and treatment. Br J Surg 1991;78:138–142.

207. Crown J, Lipzstein R, Cohen S, et al. Chemotherapy of metastatic Merkel cell cancer. Cancer Invest 1991;9:129–132.

208. Cotton D. Troublesome tumors: I. Adnexal tumors of the skin. J Clin Pathol 1991;44:543–548.

209. Hashimoto K, Mehregan AH, Kumakiri M. Tumors of skin apendages. Boston: Butterworths, 1987.

210. Headington JT. Tumors of the hair follicle. Am J Pathol 1976;85:480–505.

211. Spielogel RL, Austin C, Ackerman AB. Inverted follicular keratosis is not a specific keratosis but a verruca vulgaris (or seborrheic keratosis) with squamous eddies. Am J Dermatol 1983;5:427–442.

212. Starink TM, Kisch LS, Meijer CJ. Familial multiple trichodiscomas. Arch Dermatol 1985;121:888–891.

213. Mehregan AH. Tumor of follicular infundibulum. Dermatologica 1971;142:177–183.

214. Arico M, LaRocca E, Noto G, et al. Proliferating trichilemmal tumor with lymph node metastases. Br J Dermatol 1989;121:793–797.

215. Ten Seldam REJ. Tricholemmocarcinoma. Aust J Dermatol 1977;18:62–67.

216. Gray FHR, Helwig EB. Trichofolliculoma. Arch Dermatol 1962;86:619–625.

217. Pelwig G. Sebaceous trichofolliculoma. J Cutan Pathol 1980;7:395–403.

218. Takei Y, Fukushiro S, Ackerman AB. Criteria for histologic differentiation of desmoplastic trichoepithelioma (sclerosing epithelial hamartoma) from morphea-like basal cell carcinoma. Am J Dermatopathol 1985;7:207–221.

219. Wick MR, Coffin CM. Sweat gland and pilar carcinomas. In: Wick MR, ed. Pathology of unusual malignant cutaneous tumors. New York: Marcel Dekker, 1985.

220. Manivel C, Wick MR, Muka K. Pilomatrix carcinoma: An immunohistochemical comparison with benign pilomatrixoma and other benign cutaneous lesions of pilar origin. J Cutan Pathol 1986;13:22–29.

221. Tateyama H, Eimoto T, Tada T, et al. Malignant pilomatricoma. Cancer 1992;69:127–132.

222. Chambers SO. The structure of Fordyce's disease as demonstrated by wax reconstruction. Arch Dermatol Syphilol 1928;18:666–672.

223. Banse-Kupin L, Morales A, Barlow M. Torre's syndrome: Report of two cases and review of the literature. J Am Acad Dermatol 1984;10:803–817.

224. Troy JL, Ackerman AB. Sebaceoma: A distinctive benign neoplasm of adnexal epithelium differentiating toward sebaceous cells. Am J Dermatopathol 1984;6:7–13.

225. Wolfe JT, Wick MR, Campbell RJ. Sebaceous carcinoma of the oculocutaneous adnexa and extraocular skin In: Wick MR, ed. Pathology of unusual malignant cutaneous tumors. New York: Marcel Dekker, 1985:77–106.

226. Wick MR, Goellner JR, Wolfe JT, et al. Adnexal carcinomas of the skin. II. Extraocular sebaceous carcinomas. Cancer 1985;56:1163–1172.

227. Dixon RS, Mikhail GR, Slater HC. Sebaceous carcinoma of the eyelid. J Am Acad Dermatol 1980;3:241–243.

228. Rao NA, Hidayat AA, McLean IW, et al. Sebaceous carcinomas of the ocular adnexa: A clinicopathologic study of 104 cases, with five-year follow-up data. Hum Pathol 1982;13:113–122.

229. Wolfe JT, Yeatts RP, Wick MR, et al. Sebaceous carcinoma of the eyelid. Am J Surg Pathol 1984;8:597–606.

230. King DT, Hirose FM, Gurevitch AW. Sebaceous carcinoma of the skin with visceral metastases. Arch Dermatol 1979;115:862.

231. Pricolo VE, Rodil JV, Vezeridis MP. Extraorbital sebaceous carcinoma. Arch Surg 1985;120:853–855.

232. Pardo FS, Wang CC, Albert D, et al. Sebaceous carcinoma of the ocular adnexa: Radiotherapeutic management. Int J Radiat Oncol Biol Phys 1989;17:643–647.

233. Whittington R, Browning ME, Farrell GR, et al. Radiation therapy and chemotherapy in malignant sweat gland tumors. J Am Acad Dermatol 1986;15:1093–1097.

234. Tan KC, Cheah ST. Surgical treatment of sebaceous carcinoma of eyelids with clinicopathological correlation. Br J Plast Surg 1991;44:117–121.

235. Mehregan AH. Supernumerary nipple. A histologic study. J Cutan Pathol 1981;8:96–104.

236. Hassan MO, Khan MA, Kruse TV. Apocrine cystadenoma. Arch Dermatol 1979;115:194–200.

237. Numata M, Hosoe S, Itoh N, et al. Syringadenocarcinoma papilliferum. J Cutan Pathol 1985;12:3–7.

238. Shenoy YMV. Malignant perianal papillary hidradenoma. Arch Dermatol 1961;83:965–967.

239. Guldhammer B, Norgaard T. The differential diagnosis of intraepidermal malignant lesions using immunohistochemistry. Am J Dermatopathol 1986;8:295–301.

240. Ordóñez NG, Awalt H, MacKay B. Mammary and extramammary Paget's disease: An immunohistochemical and ultrastructural study. Cancer 1987;59:1173–1183.

241. Coldiron BM, Goldsmith BA, Robinson JK. Surgical treatment of extramammary Paget's disease: A report of six cases and a reexamination of Mohs' micrographic surgery compared with conventional surgical excision. Cancer 1991;67:933–938.

242. Rahbari H. Hidroacanthoma simplex: A review of 15 cases. Br J Dermatol 1983;109:219–225.

243. Ishikawa K. Malignant hidroacanthoma simplex. Arch Dermatol 1971;114:529–532.

244. Strayer DS, Santa Cruz DJ. Carcinoma in situ of the skin: A review of histopathology. J Cutan Pathol 1981;7:244–259.

245. Bottles K, Sagebiel RW, McNutt NS, et al. Malignant eccrine poroma: Case report and review of the literature. Cancer 1984;53:1579–1585.

246. Shaw M, McKee PH, Lowe D, et al. Malignant eccrine poroma. A study of 27 cases. Br J Dermatol 1982;107:675–680.

247. Gschnait F, Horn F, Lindlbauer R, et al. Malignant eccrine poroma. J Cutan Pathol 1980;7:349–353.

248. Hu CH, Marques AS, Winkelmann RK. Dermal duct tumor: A histochemical and electron microscopic study. Arch Dermatol 1978;114:1659–1664.

249. Mishima Y, Marioka S. Oncogenic differentiation of the intraepidermal eccrine sweat duct: Eccrine poroma, poroepithelioma, and porocarcinoma. Dermatologica 1969;138:238.

250. Pinkus H, Mehregan A. Epidermotropic eccrine carcinoma. Arch Dermatol 1963;88:597.

251. Bardach H. Hidroacanthoma simplex with in situ porocarcinoma. J Cutan Pathol 1978;5:236.

252. Hashimoto K, Gross B, Lever W. Syringoma: Histochemical and electron microspic studies. J Invest Dermatol 1966;46:150.

253. Feibelman CE, Maize JC. Clear cell syringoma. A study by conventional and electron microscopy. Am J Dermatopathol 1984;6:139–150.

254. Butterworth T, Strean LP, Beerman H, et al. Syringoma and mongolism. Arch Dermatol 1964;91:483–487.

255. Urban C, Cannon J, Cole R. Eruptive syringomas in Down's syndrome. Arch Dermatol 1981;117:374.

256. Hashimoto K, DiBella RJ, Borsuk GM, et al. Eruptive hidradenoma and syringoma: Histological, histochemical, and electron microspic studies. Arch Dermatol 1967;96:511–519.

257. Cooper PH, Mills SE, Leonard DD. Sclerosing sweat duct (syringomatous) carcinoma. Am J Surg Pathol 1985;9:422–433.

258. Weber P, Gretzula J, Garland L, et al. Syringoid eccrine carcinoma. J Dermatol Surg Oncol 1987;13:1.

259. Moy RL, Rivkin JE, Lee H, et al. Syringoid eccrine carcinoma. J Am Acad Dermatol 1991;24:864–867.

260. Lipper S, Peiper SC. Sweat gland carcinoma with syringomatous features: A light microscopic and ultrastructural study. Cancer 1979;44:157–163.

261. Mehregan AH, Hashimoto K, Rahbari H. Eccrine adenocarcinoma. A clinico-pathologic study of 35 cases. Arch Dermatol 1983;119:104–114.

262. Headington J. Mixed tumors of skin: Eccrine and apocrine types. Arch Dermatol 1961;84:989.

263. Hirch P, Helwig EG. Chondroid syringoma. Mixed tumor of the skin salivary gland type. Arch Dermatol 1961;84:835–847.

264. Botha JBC, Kahn LB. Aggressive chondroid syringoma. Report of a case in an unusual location and with local recurrence. Arch Dermatol 1978;114:954–955.

265. Harrist TJ, Aretz TH, Mihm MC Jr, et al. Cutaneous malignant mixed tumor. Arch Dermatol 1981;117:719–724.

266. Hilton JMN, Blackwell JB. Metastasizing chondroid syringoma. J Pathol 1973;109:167–170.

267. Webb JN, Stott WG. Malignant chondroid syringoma of the thigh. Report of a case with electron microscopy of the tumour. J Pahtol 1975;116:43–46.

268. Redono C, Rocamora A, Villoria F, et al. Malignant mixed tumor of the skin. Malignant chondroid syringoma. Cancer 1982;49:1690–1696.

269. Matz LR, McCully DJ, Stokes BAR. Metastasizing chondroid syringoma: Case report. Pathology 1969;1:77.

270. Ishimura E, Iwamoto H, Kobashi Y, et al. Malignant chondroid syringoma. Report of a case with widespread metastasis and review of the pertinenet literature. Cancer 1983;52:1966–1973.

271. Cordero AA, Montes LF. Eccrine hidrocystoma. J Cutan Pathol 1976;3:292–293.

272. Mambo NC. Eccrine spiradenoma: Clinical and pathologic study of 49 tumors. J Cutan Pathol 1983;10:312–320.

273. Tsur H, Lipskier E, Fisher BK. Multiple linear spiradenomas. Plast Reconstruct Surg 1981;68:100–102.

274. Schmoeckel C, Burg G. Congenital spiradenoma. Am J Dermatopathol 1992;10:541–545.

275. Evans HL, Daniel Su WP, Smith L, et al. Carcinoma arising in eccrine spiradenoma. Cancer 1979;43:1881–1884.

276. Cooper PH, Frierson HF Jr, Morrison G. Malignant transformation of eccrine spiradenoma. Arch Dermatol 1985;121:1445.

277. Dabska M. Malignant transformation of eccrine spiradenoma. Pol Med J 1972;11:388.

278. Yaremchuck MJ, Elias LS, Graham RR, et al. Sweat gland carcinoma of the hand: Two cases od malignant eccrine spiradenoma. J Hand Surg 1984;9A:910–914.

279. Keasbey LE, Hadley GC. Clear cell hidradenoma. Three cases with widespread metastases. Cancer 1954;7:934–952.

280. Kersting DW. Clear cell hidradenoma and hidradenocarcinoma. Arch Dermatol 1963;87:323–333.

281. Hernandez-Perez E, Cruz FA. Clear cell hidradenocarcinoma. Dermatologica 1976;153:249–252.

282. Headington JT, Neiderhuber JE, Beals TF. Malignant clear cell acrospiroma. Cancer 1978;41:641.

283. Hernandez-Perez E, Cruz FA. Clear cell hidroadenocarcinoma: Report of an unsual case. Dermatologic 1976;153:249.

284. Czarnecki DB, Aarons I, Dowling JP, et al. Malignant clear cell hidradenoma: A case report. Acta Dermatovenereol 1982;62:173–176.

285. MacKenzie DH. A clear-cell hidradenocarcinoma with metastases. Cancer 1957;10:1021–1023.

286. Keasbey LE, Hadley GG. Clear-cell hidradenoma. Report of three cases with widespread metastases. Cancer 1954;7:934–952.

287. Cotton DNK, Braye SG. Dermal cylindromas originate from the eccrine sweat gland. Br J Dermatol 1984;111:53–61.

288. Goette DK, McConnell MA, Fowler VR. Cylindroma and eccrine spiradenoma coexistent in the same lesion. Arch Dermatol 1982;118:273–274.

289. Urbanski SJ, From L, Abramowicz A, et al. Metamorphosis of dermal cylindroma: Possible relation to malignant transformation. J Am Acad Dermatol 1985;12:188–195.

290. Lyons JB, Rouillard LM. Malignant degeneration of turban tumour of scalp. Trans St John's Hosp Dermatol Soc 1961;46:74–77.

291. Bondeson L. Malignant dermal eccrine cylindroma. Acta Derm Venereol (Stockh) 1979;59:92–94.

292. Glatt HJ, Proia AD, Tsoy EA, et al. Malignant syringoma of the eyelid. Ophthalmology 1984;91:987–990.

293. Headington JT. Primary mucinous carcinoma of skin. Cancer 1977;39:1055.

294. Santa Cruz D, et al. Primary mucinous carcinoma of the skin. Br J Dermatol 1978;98:645.

295. Wright J, Font R. Mucinous sweat gland adenocarcinoma of eyelid. Cancer 1979;44:1757.

296. Gardner T, O'Grady R. Mucinous adenocarcinoma of the eyelid: A case report. Arch Ophthalmol 1984;102:912.

297. Yeung K, Stinson J. Mucinous (adenocystic) carcinoma of sweat glands with widespread metastases. Cancer 1977;39:2556.

298. Mendoza S, Helwig E. Mucinous (adenocystic) carcinoma of the skin. Arch Dermatol 1971;103:68.

299. Baandrup U, Sogaard H. Mucinous (adenocystic) carcinoma of the skin. Dermatologica 1982;164:338.

300. Cooper PH, Dahl M. Sclerosing carcinomas of sweat ducts (microstic adnexal carcinoma). Arch Dermatol 1986;122:261–264.

301. Glodstein DJ, Barr RJ, Santa Cruz DJ. Microcystic adnexal carcinoma. A distinct clinicopathologic entity. Cancer 1982;50:566–572.

302. Lupton GP, McMarlin SL. Microscystic adnexal carcinoma. Report of a case with 30-year follow-up. Arch Dermatol 1986;122:286–289.

303. Nickoloff BJ, Fleischmann HE, Carmel J, et al. Microcystic adnexal carcinoma. Immunohistologic observations suggesting dual (pilar and eccrine) differentiation. Arch Dermatol 1986;122:290–294.

304. Fleischmann HE, Rath RJ, Wood C, et al. Microscystic adnexal carcinoma treated by microscopically controlled excision. J Dermatol Surg Oncol 1984;10:873–875.

305. Salzman MJ, Eades E. Primary cutaneous adenoid cystic carcinoma: A case report and reviiw of the Cancers. Plast Reconstr Surg 1991;88:140–144.

306. Cooper PH, Adelson G, Holthaus W. Primary cutaneous adenoid cystic carcinoma. Arch Dermatol 1984;120:774–777.

307. Seab JA, Graham JH. Primary cutaneous adenoid cystic carcinoma. J Am Acad Dermatol 1987;17:113–118.

308. Perzin K, Gullane P, Conley J. Adenoid cystic carcinoma involving the external auditory canal: A clinicopahtologic study of 16 cases. Cancer 1982;50:2873.

309. Sanderson KV, Batten JC. Adenoid cystic carcinoma of the scalp with pulmonary metastasis. Proc R Soc Med 1975;68:649–650.

310. Wick MR, Swanson PE. Primary adenoid cystic carcinoma of the skin. A clinical, histological, and immunocytochemical comparison with adenoid cystic carcinoma of salivary glands and adenoid basal cell carcinoma. Am J Surg Pathol 1986;8:2–13.

311. Kao GF, Helwig EB, Graham JH. Aggressive digital papillary adenoma and adenocarcinoma. A clinicopathological study of 57 patients, with histochemical, immunopathological, and ultrastructural observations. J Cutan Pathol 1987;14:129.

312. Ceballos PI, Penneys NS, Acosta R. Aggressive digital papillary adenocarcinoma. J Am Acad Dermatol 1990;23:331–334.

313. Teloh H, Balkin R, Grier J. Metastasizing sweat-gland carcinoma: Report of a case. Arch Dermatol 1957;76:80.

314. Grant R. Sweat gland carcinoma with metastases. JAMA 1960;173:490.

315. Miller W. Sweat gland carcinoma. Am J Clin Pathol 1967;47:767.

316. Dave V. Eccrine sweat gland carcinoma with metastases. Br J Dermatol 1972;86:95.

317. Chow C, Campbell P, Burry A. Sweat gland carcinoma in children. Cancer 1984;53:1222.

318. Wick M, et al. Adnexal carcinomas of the skin. I. Eccrine carcinoma. Cancer 1985;56:1147.

319. Cruz DJS. Sweat gland carcinomas: A comprehensive review. Semin Diagn Pathol 1987;4:38–74.

320. Brownstein MH, Helwig EB. Pattern of cutaneous metastases. Arch Dermatol 1972;105:862–868.

321. Reingold IM. Cutaneous metastases from internal carcinoma. Cancer 1966;19:162–168.

322. Mohs FE. Chemosurgery, microscopically controlled surgery for skin cancer. Springfield: Charles C Thomas, 1978.

323. Dubin N, Kopf AW. Multivariate risk score for recurrence of cutaneous basal cell carcinoma. Arch Dermatol 1983;119:373.

324. Chernosky ME. Squamous cell and basal cell carcinoma: Preliminary study of 3816 primary skin cancers. South Med J 1978;71:802.

325. Freeman RG, Knox JM, Heaton CL. The treatment of skin cancer: A statistical study of 1341 skin tumors comparing results obtained with irradiation, surgery, and curettage followed by electrodesiccation. Cancer 1964;17:535.

326. Spiller WF, Spiller RF. Treatment of basal cell epithelioma by curettage and electrodesiccation. J Am Acad Dermatol 1984;11:808.

327. Knox J, Lyles TW, Shapiro EM, et al. Curettage and electrodesiccation in the treatment of skin cancer. Arch Dermatol 1960;82:197.

328. Johnson TM, Tromovitch TA, Swanson NA. Combined curettage and excision: A treatment method for primary basal cell carcinoma. J Am Acad Dermatol 1991;24:613–617.

329. Cooper IS. Cryogenic surgery: New method of destruction or extirpation of benign and malignant tumors. N Engl J Med 1963;268:743.

330. Whitehouse HH. Liquid air in dermatology: Its indications and limitations. JAMA 1907;49:371.

331. Zacarian SA. Cryosurgery for skin cancer and cutaneous disorders. St. Louis: CV Mosby, 1985.

332. Belisario JC. Topical cytotoxic therapy for cutaneous cancer and precancer. Arch Dermatol 1965;92:293.

333. Street ML, White JW, Gibson LE. Multiple keratoacanthomas treated with oral retinoids. J Am Acad Dermatol 1990;23:862–866.

334. Dillaha CJ, Jansen GT, Honeycutt WM, et al. Selective cytotoxic effects of topical 5-fluorouracil. Arch Dermatol 1983;119:774.

335. Peck GL. Topical tretinoin in actinic keratosis and basal cell carcinoma. J Am Acad Dermatol 1986;15:829–835.

336. Raat JH, Krown SE, Pinske CM, et al. Treatment of Bowen's disease with topical dinitrochlorobenzene and 5-fluorouracil. Cancer 1976;37:1633.

337. Coker DD, Elias EG, Virvathana T, et al. Chemotherapy for metastatic basal cell carcinoma. Arch Dermatol 1983;119:44.

338. Woods RL, Stewart JF. Metastic basal cell carcinoma: Report of a case responding to chemotherapy. Cancer 1983;52:1583.

339. Lippman S, Meyskens F. Treatment of advanced squamous cell carcinoma of the skin with isotretinoin. Ann Intern Med 1987;107:499.

340. Weiss JS, Ellis CN, Headington JT, et al. Topical tretinoin improves photoaged skin: A double-blind vehicle-controlled study. JAMA 1988;259:527–532.

341. Kligman AM, Grove GL, Hirose R, et al. Topical tretinoin for photoaged skin. J Am Acad Dermatol 1986;15:836–859.

342. Dillaha CJ, Jansen GT, Honeycutt WM, et al. Selective cytotoxic effect of topical 5-fluorouracil. Arch Dermatol 1963;88:247.

343. Fulton JE, Carter DM, Hurley HJ. Treatment of Bowen's disease with topical 5-fluorouracil under occlusion. Arch Dermatol 1968;97:178.

344. Jansen GT, Honeycutt WM, Dillaha CJ. Bowenoid condition of the skin: Treatment with topical 5-fluorouracil. South Med J 1967;60:185.

345. Waldrof DS. Mycosis fungoides—response with topical nitrogen mustard. Arch Dermatol 1968;97:608.

346. Zackheim H, Epstein EH Jr, McNutt NS, et al. Topical carmustine (BCNU) for mycosis fungoides and related disorders: Ten-year experience. J Am Acad Dermatol 1983;9:363.

347. Klein E, Stoll H, Milgrom H, et al. Tumors of the skin. IV. Double blind study of effects of local administration of anti-tumor agents in basal cell carcinoma. J Invest Dermatol 1965;44:351–353.

348. Klein E, Stoll H, Milgrom H, et al. Tumors of the skin V. Local administration of anti-tumor agents to multiple superficial basal cell carcinoma. J Invest Dermatol 1965;45:489–495.

349. Stegman S, Tromovitch T, Glogau R. Grafts. In: Stegman S, ed. Basics of dermatologic surgery. Chicago: Year Book Medical Publishers, 1982.

350. Knox JM, Freeman RG, Duncan WC, et al. Treatment of skin Cancer. South Med J 1967;60:241.

351. Kopf AW. Computer analysis of 3531 basal cell carcinomas of the skin. J Dermatol 1979;6:267.

352. Atkinson HR. Skin carcinoma depth and dose homogeneity in dermatological x-ray therapy. Aust J Dearmatol 1962;6:208.

353. Domonkos AN. Treatment of eyelid carcinoma. Arch Dermatol 1965;91:364.

354. Grosch E, Lambert HE. The treatment of difficult cutaneous basal and squamous cell carcinomata with electrons. Br J Radiol 1979;52:472.

355. Viravathana T, Prempree T, Sewchand W, et al. Technique and dosimetry in the management of extensive basal cell carcinomas od the head and neck region by irradiation with electron beams. J Dermatol Surg Oncol 1980;6:290.

356. Mohs FE. Chemosurgery for skin cancer: Fixed and fresh tissue technique. Arch Dermatol 1976;11:211.

357. Menn H, Robins P, Kopf A, et al. The recurrent basal cell epithelioma. Arch Dermatol 1971;103:628.

358. Klein E, Holterman OA, Helm F, et al. Immunologic approaches to the management of primary and secondary tumors involving the skin and soft tissues: Reviews of a ten-year program. Transplant Proc 1975;7:297.

359. Holterman OA, Papermaster BW, Walker MJ, et al. Regression of cutaneous neoplasms following delayed-type hypersensitivity challenge reactions to microbial antigens or lymphokines. J Med 1975;6:157.

360. Pennington DG, Waner M, Knox A. Photodynamic therapy for multiple skin cancers. Plast Reconstr Surg 1988;82:1067–1071.

361. Dougherty TJ, Weishaupt KR, Boyle DG. Photoradiation therapy of human tumors. In: Regan JD, Parrish JA, eds. The science of photomedicine. New York: Plenum Press, 1982:625.

362. Dougherty TJ. Photodynamic therapy (PDT) of malignant tumors. Crit Rev Oncol Hematol 1984;2:83.

363. Klingman LH, Akin FJ, Kligman AM. Sunscreens prevent ultraviolet photocarcinogenesis. J Am Acad Dermatol 1980;3:30–35.

364. Kolata G. Futuristic treatments for the hair and skin. N Y Times Med Sci 1987;15:24.

365. Weiss JS, Ellis CN, Headington JT, et al. Topical tretinoin improved photoaged skin. JAMA 1988;259:527–531.

366. Brusk MM, Santschi CH, Bell T, et al. Culture of basal cell carcinoma. J Invest Dermatol 1992;98:45–49.

Cancer: Principles & Practice of Oncology, Fourth Edition,
edited by Vincent T. DeVita, Jr., Samuel Hellman, Steven A. Rosenberg.
J.B. Lippincott Co., Philadelphia © 1993.

Charles M. Balch
Alan N. Houghton
Lester J. Peters

CHAPTER **46**

Cutaneous Melanoma

Cutaneous melanoma is becoming a more common disease. In 1991, an estimated 32,000 persons developed melanoma, and almost 6500 died. The incidence of melanoma has increased during the past decade at a rate faster than that for any other cancer except lung cancer in women. The reasons for this increase are unclear, but factors may include increased recreational exposure to sunlight, an increased amount of ultraviolet irradiation from the midrange sunbeam spectrum (UVB) that reaches the earth's surface, and earlier detection of melanoma. This disease is largely confined to whites, in whom the age-adjusted incidence rate in the United States is about 12 per 100,000 persons and is threefold higher (30 per 100,000) in some geographic areas.[1-3] In 1935, only 1 in 1500 persons developed melanoma. The incidence dropped dramatically to 1 in 250 in 1980 and to 1 in 135 in 1987. Assuming present trends, the incidence will be 1 in 90 persons by the year 2000 (Fig. 46-1).[4]

Fortunately, most new patients are diagnosed early in the disease's clinical course, when it can be cured with simple surgical treatment. More than 90% of melanomas can be recognized as malignant by experienced observers; therefore, it behooves each physician to know the clinical characteristics of melanoma so that biopsies can be performed on suspicious moles or skin lesions as early as possible. Histologic verification and microstaging are essential before embarking on treatment. The options for therapy range from very conservative surgical treatment for early lesions to more radical approaches for biologically aggressive melanomas. Judgment, experience, and knowledge of the prognostic factors are essential for choosing the most appropriate treatment for individual patients.

CLINICAL CHARACTERISTICS

HIGH-RISK POPULATIONS

The typical melanoma patient has a fair complexion and a tendency to sunburn rather than tan, even after a brief exposure to sunlight.[5,6] The importance of these features was delineated in a case-control study in which 287 women with melanoma were compared with 574 age-matched controls.[5] Red hair was associated with a tripling of relative risk, blond hair with a 60% risk increase, and fair skin with a doubling of risk. There was a more than threefold increase in risk for those patients with more than 20 nevi.

A patient with a melanoma has a higher risk for developing a second primary melanoma than an individual in the general population has for developing a melanoma.[7] This risk varies from 3% to 5% in different series,[8-10] a risk 900-fold that of the general population.[11] A patient who has multiple dysplastic nevi or has a familial form of melanoma has an even greater risk for developing multiple primary melanomas.[8,12,13]

Familial melanomas are uncommon but have been well documented, and individuals in such families constitute an identifiable high-risk group.[9,13-18] Between 4% and 10% of patients describe a history of melanoma among their first-degree relatives.[14] Clark and colleagues described an autosomal dominant hereditary occurrence of melanoma,[19] originally termed the B-K mole syndrome and now referred to as the dysplastic nevus syndrome, familial type.[20] Patients with this syndrome typically have between 10 and 100 pigmented lesions located predominantly on the trunk, buttocks, or lower extremities. Genetic factors may play an important role

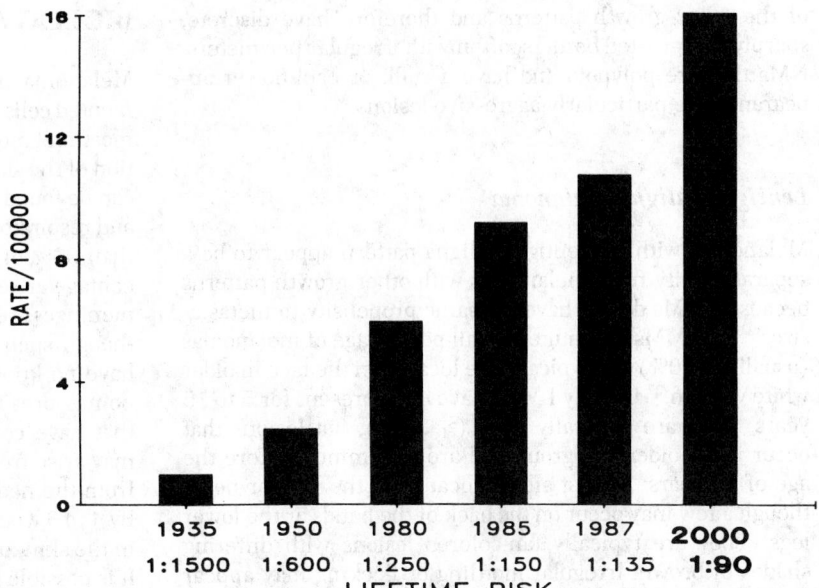

FIGURE 46–1. Past, current, and projected lifetime risk of a person in the United States developing malignant melanoma. (Rigel DS, Kopf AW, Friedman RJ. The rate of malignant melanoma in the US: Are we making an impact? J Am Acad Dermatol 1987;17:1050)

in the predisposition to melanoma, perhaps by genes controlling some aspect of immune response to melanoma antigens.[14,21,22] Melanoma-prone patients appear to have increased frequencies of certain blood, complement, and HLA phenotypes.[14,21,23-26]

SIGNS AND SYMPTOMS

Melanomas can be located anywhere on the body, but they occur most commonly on the lower extremities in women and on the back in men. Some of the clinical characteristics of melanoma are illustrated in Color Figure 46–2.[27-30] Typical features of cutaneous melanoma include variegation, an irregular raised surface, an irregular perimeter with indentations, and ulceration of the surface epithelium. Although melanomas may have a variety of clinical appearances, the common denominator is their changing nature. Any pigmented lesion that undergoes a change in size, configuration, or color should be considered a melanoma, and an excisional biopsy should be performed.

GROWTH PATTERNS

A convenient way to categorize melanomas is by their growth patterns.[27,31,32] These growth patterns represent distinct pathologic entities and have unique clinical features that can be recognized by the experienced clinician. The different categories of melanoma are all distinct from benign lesions, and each category portends a different prognosis. Histologic confirmation is essential before making any definitive treatment plans. The four major growth patterns are superficial spreading melanoma (SSM), nodular melanoma (NM), lentigo maligna melanoma (LMM), and acral lentiginous melanoma (ALM).

Superficial Spreading Melanoma

About 70% of melanomas are SSMs.[27,31-33] The lesions generally arise in a preexisting nevus. A history of slowly evolving change of the precursor lesion for more than 1 to 5 years is not uncommon, with more rapid growth developing months before diagnosis. SSMs can occur at any age after puberty. A typical SSM first appears as a deeply pigmented area in a brown junctional nevus. The lesion may take on a lacy appearance. Often, patches of regression are recognizable by an amelanotic area. Early in its evolution, an SSM is generally a flat lesion. It may develop an irregular surface, usually asymmetrically, depending on the vertical growth phase that develops as it enlarges. As the lesion grows, the surface may become glossy. Characteristically, there is notching or indentation of the perimeter, especially as the SSM enlarges.

Nodular Melanoma

The nodular growth pattern is the second most common growth pattern in most series (15–30% of patients).[27,31-33] NMs are more aggressive tumors and usually develop more rapidly than SSMs. They can occur at any age (but usually in middle age) and are most common on the trunk or head and neck. Men tend to have more NMs than women, whereas the opposite is true for SSMs. NMs are usually 1 to 2 cm in diameter but can be much larger. They begin more commonly in uninvolved skin than in preexisting nevi.

NMs are generally darker than SSMs, more uniform in coloration, and more raised or dome-shaped. The typical NM is a blue-black lesion that often resembles a blood blister or hemangioma. It may have other shadings of red, gray, or purple. About 5% of NMs lack pigment altogether (*i.e.*, are amelanotic) and have a fleshy appearance. NMs are often symmetrical but sometimes appear as irregularly shaped plaques. They lack the radial (horizontal) growth phase that is typical of the other growth patterns and therefore have discrete, sharply demarcated borders, often with irregular perimeters. NMs that are polypoid and have a stalk or cauliflower appearance are particularly aggressive lesions.[34]

Lentigo Maligna Melanoma

Melanomas with the lentigo maligna pattern appear to be a separate entity from melanomas with other growth patterns because LMMs do not have the same propensity to metastasize.[32,35,36] LMMs constitute a small percentage of melanomas (usually 4–10%) and typically are located on the face in older white women.[37] Usually LMMs have been present for 5 to 15 years. They are generally large (> 3 cm), flat lesions that occur in an older age group and are uncommon before the age of 50 years. Almost all are located on the face or neck, though a few may occur on the back of the hands or the lower legs. They are typically tan-colored lesions with differing shades of brown. Irregular mottling or flecking may appear as the lesions enlarge, with areas of dark brown or black in some parts and areas of regression in others. LMMs can have convoluted borders with prominent notching and indentation, which generally represent areas of regression. The diagnosis of LMM requires the presence of sun-related changes in both the epidermis and dermis.[32,36,37]

Acral Lentiginous Melanoma

Melanomas with the acral lentiginous growth pattern characteristically occur on the palms or soles or beneath the nail beds.[28,38–42] Not all plantar or volar melanomas are ALMs; a minority are SSMs or NMs.[43–46] ALMs occur in only 2% to 8% of white patients with melanoma[47] but in a substantially higher proportion (35–60%) of dark-skinned patients, including black, Asian, and Hispanic patients.[41,48–51]

Most ALMs are located on the sole of the foot.[40] They are generally large, with an average diameter of about 3 cm.[39] ALMs generally occur in older people, with the average patient's age in the 60s. Their evolution is short, ranging from a few months to several years, with an average of 2.5 years. Initially, these lesions appear as tan or brown flat stains on the palm or sole and often resemble LMMs. The haphazard array of color is characteristic. A minority of such lesions take on a flesh-colored appearance that can be misdiagnosed as granuloma. Ulceration is not uncommon, and fungating masses can result from neglected lesions. As with LMMs, these lesions often have irregular, convoluted borders. ALMs are much more aggressive than LMMs and are more likely to metastasize.

ALMs include subungual melanoma, an infrequently seen presentation of cutaneous melanoma.[43–45,52,53] It develops in only 2% to 3% of white patients but in a higher proportion of dark-skinned patients. It occurs equally in men and women and is most often diagnosed in older patients (median age of 55 to 65 years). More than three fourths of subungual melanomas involve either the great toe or the thumb. The most common sign of an early subungual melanoma is a brown to black discoloration under the nail bed.

BIOLOGY OF MELANOMA

Melanoma arises from melanocytes, which are dendritic pigmented cells found usually within epithelial surfaces. In adults, most melanocytes are located at the epidermal-dermal junction of the skin and in the choroid of the eye, but melanocytes can be found in the meninges, along mucosa of the alimentary and respiratory tracts, and even in lymph node capsules. More than 90% of melanomas arise in the skin, and a small percentage arise in the eye. Primary melanoma can occur in the meninges, respiratory tract, gallbladder, and other sites, although such incidences are rare. About 4% of melanomas have no known primary site. Although most of these melanomas presumably come from primary lesions in the skin that have completely regressed, some primary melanomas may arise from undiagnosed internal sites. Melanocytes arise from the neural crest early in the development of the fetus. By 4 to 6 weeks, they have migrated to their final destinations in the skin, uveal tract, meninges, and ectodermal mucosa.[54] It is possible that the ability of melanoma cells to metastasize rapidly and widely is determined by traits that facilitate the migration of melanocyte precursors through tissues before reaching epithelial tissues.

The melanocyte is a specialized cell type that synthesizes the pigment melanin using the enzyme tyrosinase in organelles called melanosomes. The presence of melanosomes, as detected by electron microscopy, or of pigment in an undifferentiated tumor can assist in the diagnosis of melanoma. Gene products other than tyrosinase regulate pigmentation. The techniques of molecular genetics have been used to identify the gene encoding tyrosinase and other genes specifically expressed in melanocytes.[55] Some of these gene products are potential targets for immunotherapies and chemically mediated cytotoxic therapies.[56–59] For example, some intermediates in the melanin synthetic pathway can be cytotoxic. This phenomenon has led to research into new strategies for treatment with compounds that can augment the production of toxic metabolites in the melanin pathway.[57–59]

Antigenic markers have been used to investigate the differentiation of melanocytes and the pathogenesis of melanoma.[60,61] Markers of melanocytic cells are useful to confirm the histologic diagnosis when the clinical pattern does not fit a diagnosis of melanoma or when melanoma is suspected in an undifferentiated tumor. Two widely used markers are S-100 protein and HMB-45, both of which can be detected by antibodies in paraffin-embedded tissues.[62] S-100 is expressed by almost all melanomas, but is expressed by sarcomas, nerve sheath tumors, and a subset of carcinomas. HMB-45 is more specific for melanocytic cell but is not always positive in metastatic melanomas. HMB-45 and S-100 are most effective when applied as part of a panel of markers, including cytokeratins, leukocyte common antigen, and other specialized markers.

Melanoma has emerged as an excellent paradigm to study events of malignant transformation and tumor progression. Clark and colleagues have proposed a model of tumor progression for melanoma.[63] The model defines lesions that represent putative steps in progression from normal melanocyte to melanoma. Lesions range from benign to most malignant in the following progression:

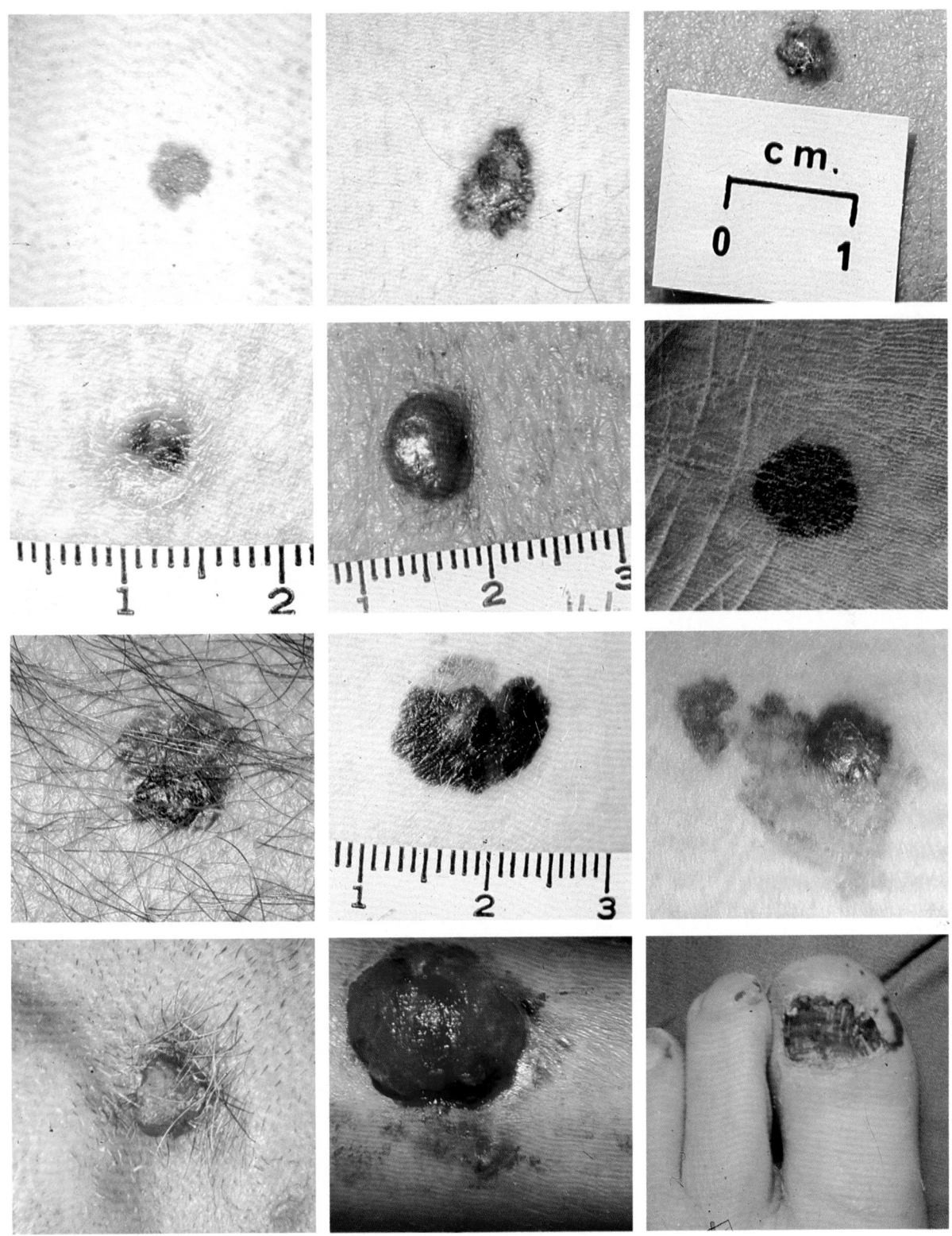

COLOR FIGURE 46–2. The clinical spectrum of cutaneous melanoma. The features include any combination of variegation, irregular surface, irregular perimeter, and ulceration.

common acquired nevus → dysplastic nevus

→ primary melanoma (superficial or radial growth phase)

→ primary melanoma (deep or vertical growth phase)

→ metastatic melanoma.

The common acquired and dysplastic nevi are benign proliferative lesions, and each subsequent step displays properties of increasing malignant potential. For instance, cells in deep primary melanoma lesions (vertical growth phase) have the ability to invade into underlying tissue, and a subpopulation of these cells presumably has competence for metastasis. This model has formed a framework for identifying high-risk premalignant lesions and for characterizing specific molecules involved in the pathogenesis of melanoma.

Studies of melanoma cell growth, adhesion, and differentiation may lead to novel pharmacologic or biologic approaches for therapy. Normal melanocytes require exogenous growth factors for proliferation. Each of these growth factors bind to cell-surface receptors with tyrosine kinase activities, including basic fibroblast growth factor (bFGF), insulin or insulin-like growth factors, hepatocyte growth factor, and kit ligand.[64–66] Melanoma cells can grow in the absence of any exogenous growth supplements, suggesting that they produce their own growth factors. One of the best characterized melanoma growth factors is bFGF. Melanoma cells, but not melanocytes, produce their own bFGF, and bFGF production appears to be an early event in melanoma progression. Antisense oligodeoxynucleotides or antibodies against bFGF have been used to inhibit bFGF production by melanoma cells, leading to inhibition of melanoma cell growth.[67,68] Autocrine production of bFGF alone does not appear to be sufficient to cause malignant transformation of melanocytes.[69] Melanoma cells express a variety of cell-surface adhesion molecules that could play a role in cell invasion and metastasis. Several of these cell-surface markers might be useful in predicting prognosis (*e.g.,* propensity for distant metastases), including the intercellular adhesion molecule-1, the ganglioside GD2, and the β3 integrin subunit.[70,71]

GENETIC ALTERATIONS IN MELANOMA

Specific genetic alterations have been implicated in the pathogenesis of melanoma. At least four distinct genes located on chromosomes 1, 6, 7, and 9 may play a role in melanoma. Genes located on different chromosomes also may contribute to melanoma progression. These findings suggest that melanoma is the result of a complex series of genetic events. Clues to the location or identity of genes involved in melanoma have come from genetic investigations of familial melanoma and from cytogenetic studies of pigmented lesions and melanomas.

Familial melanoma is a syndrome accounting for 4% to 10% of melanoma cases in the United States. Studies of heritable forms of melanoma, performed in families that have frank dysplastic nevus syndromes, have suggested that melanoma in this setting can be inherited in a highly penetrant, autosomal dominant mode.[72,73] DNA markers have been used to map a melanoma susceptibility gene to chromosome 1p in six kindreds.[74] A familial melanoma gene on chromosome 1p remains unconfirmed. Two other studies of different family groups have failed to detect a melanoma gene on chromosome

1p.[75,76] One difficulty has been the inability to define reproducible criteria for the diagnosis of the dysplastic nevus syndrome. These preliminary findings suggest that familial melanoma may be a heterogenous set of syndromes influenced by different genes.

Cytogenetic studies have shown that chromosomes in metastatic melanoma cells are highly aneuploid, whereas normal melanocytes are diploid. The occurrence of nonrandom chromosome alterations suggests that there are genes at these chromosomal locations that are necessary for malignant transformation and melanoma progression. The chromosomes most frequently involved in melanoma are 1, 6, and 7.[77–83] A review of the literature by Fountain and colleagues reported that chromosomes 1, 6, and 7 were rearranged in, respectively, 83%, 66%, and 61% of melanomas.[84] Chromosome 9 is the next most common chromosome to show rearrangements and is altered in almost half of all melanomas.[83] Alteration in chromosome 9 may be an early event in the pathogenesis of melanoma because alterations are found in some nevi, including dysplastic nevi.[85–87] Chromosomes 2, 3, 10, and 11 are involved in about one third of melanomas. In addition to nonrandom chromosomal abnormalities in melanomas, genetic analysis has shown widespread loss of genes throughout chromosomes in cultured melanomas.[88] About one fourth of genetic loci examined have shown a loss of genes. There is evidence that melanoma arises from a single transformed cell and is therefore clonally derived.[89] Genetic alterations appear to start early within the primary lesion, or even in precursor lesions, but widespread genetic alterations continue during metastasis.[89]

Sites of specific chromosomal alterations in cancer have provided clues to the location of tumor suppressor genes.[90] The most prevalent tumor suppressor locus identified in human cancer so far, p53, appears to be mutated only very infrequently in melanomas.[91] Evidence for a tumor suppressor locus on chromosome 6 has come from in vitro experiments that have introduced a normal copy of chromosome 6 into melanoma cell lines by microcell hybridization.[92] Expression of the normal chromosome 6 suppressed the malignant phenotype, reversing cell morphology, anchorage-independent growth in soft agar, and tumorigenicity in mice.

Selective chromosomal alterations may predict clinical course and prognosis. This approach has proved useful in the management of hematopoietic malignancies but has not been applied readily to solid tumors. Preliminary investigations have suggested that abnormalities in chromosomes 7 and 11 correlate with survival of patients with stage IV metastatic melanoma.[93] Although these results need to be confirmed, they suggest that cytogenetic analyses of melanoma could be useful in predicting clinical course.

EPIDEMIOLOGY

Exposure to sunlight (*i.e.,* UVB irradiation) is considered the major cause of cutaneous melanoma.[94] That the association is causal is supported by the demographic pattern of occurrence in humans, by the observation that DNA is sensitive to damage by solar radiation,[95] by sporadic induction of melanomas in animals through dual exposure to chemical carcinogens and UVB light,[96,97] and by evidence that the immune system may be depressed by UVB rays.[98]

In humans, the following patterns of melanoma occurrence suggest that sunlight is a cause of melanoma:

1. There is an inverse relation between incidence of melanoma and degree of skin pigmentation.
2. Incidence rates are higher in persons residing closer to the equator.[99,100]
3. The incidence of certain types of melanomas increases in anatomic sites exposed to sunlight.[101]
4. Migration studies suggest that risk is increased by moving to an area of more intense sun exposure.[102]
5. The risk for melanoma increases with increasing recreational exposure to the sun.

Inability to tan, higher frequency of sunburns, and younger age at first sunburn also have been associated with a predisposition to melanoma.[5] Finally, LMMs occur almost exclusively in sun-exposed parts of the body and in elderly persons, suggesting cumulative sunlight exposure as a contributing etiologic factor.

Several observations are not consistent with UVB irradiation as a sole cause of melanoma.[103] First, the incidence of melanoma does not increase consistently across geographic areas with increasing sunlight, although the relation may be skewed by the variable mix of people with different ethnic backgrounds and skin color. Second, melanoma affects white-collar, educated, urban workers more often than outdoor or blue-collar workers. Third, most melanomas occur in relatively young persons who have not had years of constant exposure to sunlight. Finally, some melanomas occur in relatively unexposed anatomic sites such as the palms, soles, bathing trunk areas, and mucous membranes. These observations are inconsistent with assigning cumulative sunlight exposure as the only etiologic factor, although it is possible that brief, intense exposure may contribute to or initiate carcinogenic events.

For SSMs and NMs, the pattern of risk suggests that susceptibility to sunburn determines the risk to the same or greater degree than the actual incidence of sunburn events does. Cumulative sunlight exposure has not been a consistent finding in many epidemiologic studies. No major environmental factors other than UVB irradiation have been identified as contributing substantially to the increasing incidence of cutaneous melanoma. The inheritable combination of light skin color and freckling suggests that genetically determined host susceptibility may play a more important role in the etiology of cutaneous melanoma than previously appreciated. The above characteristics are consistent with the two-step model of UVB-ray carcinogenesis, in which the initiation and promotion events result in melanoma in a genetically susceptible subpopulation of individuals.

The incidence of and mortality from cutaneous melanoma are rising steadily among white populations throughout the world.[48,94,104] In most studies, the incidence is doubling every 6 to 10 years. It is estimated that the incidence of melanoma among white persons in the United States will be 1 in 90 persons by the year 2000 (see Fig. 46–1).[5] In Queensland, Australia, the incidence has increased from 15 per 100,000 persons (the highest incidence in the world) in the 1963 to 1968 period to 28.4 per 100,000 in the 1979 to 1980 period.[105,106] In Sweden, the incidence has increased from 2.5 per 100,000 in 1958 to 11.6 per 100,000 in 1980.[107] Compare this high incidence in a fair-skinned population to the incidence of only 0.8 melanomas per 100,000 persons in China.[48,108,109]

CHANGES IN THE NATURAL HISTORY OF MELANOMA

The incidence of melanoma has been increasing rapidly, especially during the past two decades. A detailed analysis involving 7040 stage I melanoma patients treated over 30 years demonstrated major changes in the clinical and the pathologic features of the disease.[110] Over this period, there was a steady increase in the proportion of patients initially diagnosed as having localized disease (73% before 1960 compared with 81% by 1990). Melanomas have become thinner, less invasive, less ulcerative, and more curable. Most melanomas seen at many institutions measure less than 1 mm in thickness,[110,111] and more melanomas exhibit a radial growth phase with a superficial spreading growth pattern. The median thickness of melanomas decreased from about 3.0 mm before 1960 to less than 1.0 mm since 1985 (Fig. 46–3).[110] There was a significant increase during this period of extremity melanomas and a corresponding decrease of head and neck melanomas.[110] No significant change in site distribution was observed for trunk melanomas. The changes that have occurred probably

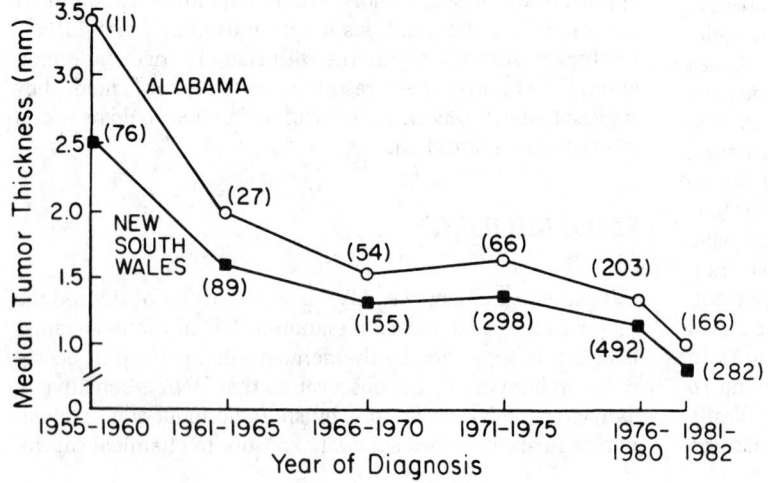

FIGURE 46–3. Changes in the median tumor thickness of melanomas treated from 1955 to 1982. The number of patients is shown in parentheses. (Balch CM, Shaw HM, Soong S-j, et al. Changing trends in the clinical and pathologic features of melanoma. In: Balch CM, Milton GW, eds. Cutaneous melanoma: Clinical management and treatment results worldwide. Philadelphia: JB Lippincott, 1985:313)

STAGING SYSTEMS

MICROSTAGING

Microstaging is an integral part of the staging and clinical management of melanoma. Two methods have been used. The Breslow microstaging method measures the thickness of the lesion using an ocular micrometer. The total vertical height (not just the depth) of the melanoma is measured, from the granular layer to the area of deepest penetration.[112] If the lesion is ulcerated, measurements should be made from the surface of the ulcer to the deepest part of the lesion. The Clark microstaging method categorizes levels of invasion that reflect increasing depth of penetration into the dermal layers of the subcutaneous fat (*i.e.*, levels II, III, IV, or V).[27]

Although the tumor thickness and the level of invasion can predict the risk for metastases, data from several institutions have demonstrated that tumor thickness is a more accurate and reproducible prognostic parameter than interpreting the level of invasion. Significant regression of the tumor invalidates the prognostic value of these microstaging methods.

ORIGINAL THREE-STAGE SYSTEM

The original and most widely used system involves three stages: stage I for localized melanoma, stage II for regional metastases, and stage III for distant metastases.[113,114] It is simple and easy to recall but, unfortunately, does not include important disease criteria (*e.g.*, tumor thickness) that allow for more accurate staging. A major limitation of this system is that 85% or more of melanoma patients diagnosed now have clinically localized disease (stage I). This disproportionate number of patients in one stage defeats the purpose of a classification system designed to categorize metastatic risk.

NEW STAGING SYSTEM ADOPTED BY THE AMERICAN JOINT COMMITTEE ON CANCER

The American Joint Committee on Cancer (AJCC) has worked for more than 10 years to develop uniform staging systems for all cancer types. In its extensive retrospective studies of melanoma, many factors influencing treatment results were identified. Based on these factors, a four-stage system was adopted (Table 46–1).[115,116] This system divides patients with clinically localized melanomas into two groups according to microstaging criteria, with the result that the metastatic risk categories are more evenly grouped among four stages (Fig. 46–4). It is a useful and practical classification for clinicians treating melanoma.

PROGNOSTIC FEATURES OF MELANOMA

Many factors are known to predict the risk for metastatic disease in melanoma. A prognostic factors analysis of melanoma is therefore essential to identify the dominant variables that can be used for evaluating results of clinical research trials involving adjunctive systemic therapy and for making

TABLE 46–1. New Staging System for Melanoma Adopted by the American Joint Committee on Cancer

Stage	Criteria
IA	Localized melanoma ≤0.75 mm or level II* (T1N0M0)
IB	Localized melanoma 0.76–1.5 mm or level III* (T2N0M0)
IIA	Localized melanoma 1.5–4 mm or level IV* (T3N0M0)
IIB	Localized melanoma >4 mm or level V* (T4N0M0)
III	Limited nodal metastases involving only one regional lymph node basin, or fewer than 5 in-transit metastases without nodal metastases (any T, N1M0)
IV	Advanced regional metastases (any T, N2M0) or any patient with distant metastases (any T, any N, M1 or M2)

* When the thickness and level of invasion criteria do not coincide with a T classification, thickness should take precedence. (Adapted from American Joint Committee on Cancer, Manual for Staging of Cancer, 4th ed. Beahrs OH, Henson DE, Hutter RVP, and Kennedy BJ, eds. Philadelphia: JB Lippincott, 1992:145)

surgical decisions. In evaluating treatments, it is important to account for those prognostic variables that can categorize patients accurately into different risk groups for metastatic disease. Otherwise, differences (or lack of differences) between treatment regimens may not be due to the treatments themselves but may reflect imbalances of prognostic factors.

This section reviews a prognostic factors analysis involving more than 8500 patients with cutaneous melanoma treated at the University of Alabama in Birmingham (UAB) and the University of Sydney Melanoma Unit (SMU) over 25 years (1955–1980).[117] The median follow-up of all patients was 8 years.

CLINICALLY LOCALIZED MELANOMA
(AJCC STAGES I AND II)

Characteristics of 6515 patients with localized melanoma were analyzed by single and multifactorial statistical analysis to determine which clinical and pathologic features of melanoma would predict the risk for metastases.[117]

Anatomic Location of Primary Lesion

Melanomas were divided evenly among the four major anatomic locations; 52% were on the upper and lower extremities, and 47% occurred on the trunk or head and neck. Patients with melanomas on the extremities had a better survival rate than those with melanomas of the trunk or head and neck (*p* < 0.00001), and those with melanomas on the upper extremities had a slightly better survival rate than those with melanomas on the lower extremities (*p* = 0.08). Analysis of anatomic subsites revealed some further differences in prognosis. Among those with melanomas in the head and neck region, patients with melanomas located on the scalp had worse prognoses than those with lesions on the face or neck. These differences remained even after accounting for sex and tumor thickness.[35,117] There was no sex difference in prognosis for patients with lesions on these head and neck subsites. There was no survival difference between patients with back lesions

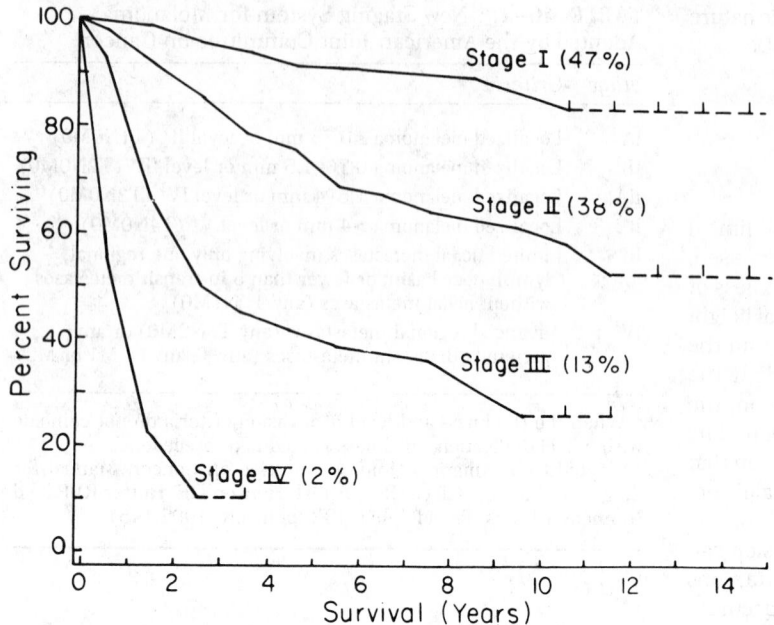

FIGURE 46–4. Fifteen-year survival results for more than 4000 melanoma patients treated at the University of Alabama in Birmingham and the University of Sydney. Patients are subgrouped according to the new four-stage system adopted by the American Joint Committee on Cancer. The distribution of patients is shown in parentheses. Patients with clinically localized melanomas (stage I by the original three-stage system) have now been divided into two stages according to tumor thickness and level of invasion (the newly designated stages I and II). (Ketcham AS, Balch CM. Classification and staging systems. In: Balch CM, Milton GW, eds. Cutaneous melanoma: Clinical management and treatment results worldwide. Philadelphia: JB Lippincott, 1985:55)

and those with chest lesions, even when subgrouped by sex. Female patients with melanomas on the back had a better survival rate than did male patients with back melanomas (p = 0.016). Patients with melanomas located on the hands and feet had significantly worse prognoses than those with lesions on the arms or legs.[117–119] Women with extremity melanomas had better prognoses than men did ($p < 0.00001$). Part of this sex difference in prognosis could be accounted for by the higher proportion of men with ulcerated melanomas (29% versus 19%).

Gender

Numerous studies of melanoma patients have shown that women have a better survival rate than men.[48,117–125] In the UAB-SMU analysis, women had a statistically significant survival advantage over men ($p < 0.00001$). A primary reason for better survival rates in women was that their melanomas

occurred more commonly on the extremities (a more favorable prognostic site) and were less frequently ulcerated.

Tumor Thickness

The total vertical height of a melanoma is the single most important prognostic factor in stages I and II melanoma.[120,126–128] It is a quantitative parameter that can define subsets of patients with different survival rates ($p < 0.00001$). Numerous groups of thickness subsets have been analyzed for their prognostic value (*e.g.*, < 1 mm, 1 to 4 mm, > 4 mm), and only one subset was found to be more discriminating than those originally advocated by Breslow.[128] As demonstrated by actuarial survival curves, a more significant survival difference was found using the 4 mm rather than the 3 mm criterion.[117,120] There are apparently no natural breakpoints.[129] Instead, statistically defined subgroups vary from one data set to another depending on the number of patients, the duration

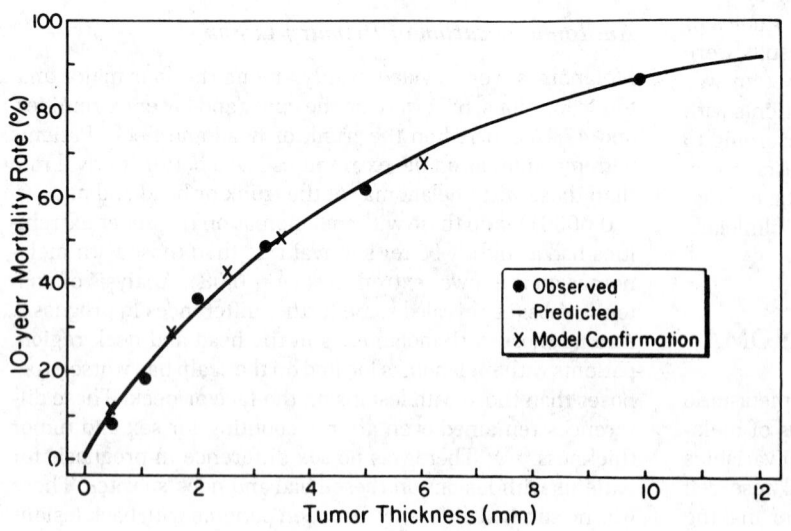

FIGURE 46–5. Observed and predicted 10-year mortality based on a mathematic model derived from tumor thickness.[117] The mathematic model is 9(T) = 1 − 0.966.e − 0.2016T and is described in more detail by Soong.[130] The solid line represents the 10-year mortality predicted by the model; the closed circles represent the actual observed mortality for 2627 patients. The accuracy of the model was confirmed by applying it to 747 AJCC stage I and II melanoma patients from the WHO Melanoma Group (data that were not used in the derivation of the model). Mortality for these patients is indicated by the Xs. The linear nature of the curve demonstrates that there are no natural breakpoints; rather, there is a continuous correlation of survival with tumor thickness. (Balch CM, Soong S-j, Shaw HM, et al. An analysis of prognostic factors in 4000 patients with cutaneous melanoma. In: Balch CM, Milton GW, eds. Cutaneous melanoma: Clinical management and treatment results worldwide. Philadelphia: JB Lippincott, 1985:321)

of follow-up, and the distribution of other factors (*e.g.,* ulceration, anatomic site of primary lesion, sex). The large number of patients in the UAB-SMU series has permitted the derivation of a simple nonlinear mathematic model that describes the relation between tumor thickness and 10-year mortality as a continuous event (Fig. 46–5).[130]

Level of Invasion

There is an inverse correlation between increasing level of melanoma invasion and survival. The level of invasion is a significant prognostic factor by single-factor analysis ($p < 0.00001$) and differentiates patients at various risks for metastases.

Comparison of Level of Invasion With Thickness as a Prognostic Indicator

A direct comparison of the level of invasion and tumor thickness microstaging methods was made by subdividing each level of invasion into thickness categories. Within levels III, IV, and V, gradations of thickness influenced survival (Fig. 46–6). Converse relations were not observed when analyzing sets of melanoma thickness subdivided by levels of invasion. For example, the 5-year survival rates for patients with level III, IV, or V lesions that measured 1.5 to 4.0 mm were not significantly different. These observations demonstrate that the measurement of tumor thickness is a more accurate prognostic factor than level of invasion.[48,118,119,120–123,126,127,131–135]

Ulceration

Ulcerated melanomas appear to be more aggressive lesions biologically because they invade through the epidermis rather than pushing it upward. The presence of ulceration in microscopic sections of melanoma was a significant adverse determinant of survival ($p < 0.00001$) in the UAB-SMU study.[117] Patients with stages I and II melanoma with ulceration had a 10-year survival rate of 50%, whereas those without ulceration had a 79% 10-year survival rate ($p < 0.0001$). Men had a higher proportion of ulcerated lesions than women (26% versus 20%). There was a positive correlation between ulceration and thickness ($p < 0.0001$). The median tumor thickness for patients with ulcerated lesions was 2.6 mm, whereas those without ulcerated lesions had a median tumor thickness of 0.8 mm. Lesions more than 1.5 mm thick were associated with a 46% incidence of ulceration.

Growth Pattern

Patients with SSM and LMM lesions had the best survival rate, whereas those with NM lesions had the worst. The most statistically significant difference among these groups was between SSM and NM ($p < 0.0001$). When patients with SSM and NM were matched for lesion thickness and their 10-year survival rates calculated, no difference was found between growth patterns as prognostic factors (Fig. 46–7). Patients with SSMs appear to have better prognoses than those with NMs only because the former are thinner lesions. Those with LMMs constituted only a small number of patients (4%).

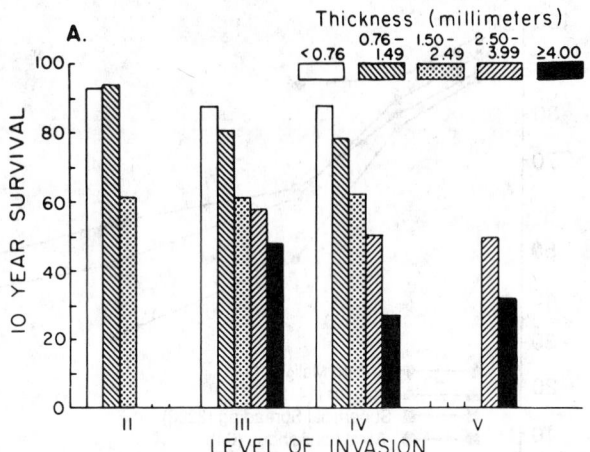

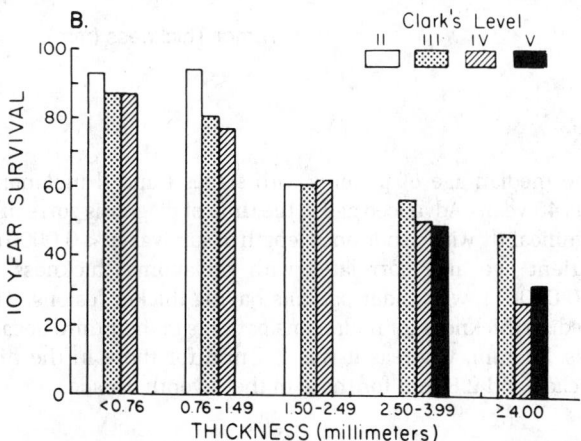

FIGURE 46–6. Comparison of two microstaging methods: tumor thickness versus level of invasion. **(A)** Ten-year survival rates for AJCC stages I and II melanoma patients according to levels of invasion and subgrouped by tumor thickness. There were statistically significant differences in survival rates for patients with lesions of various thicknesses within levels III, IV, and V. **(B)** Ten-year survival rates for AJCC stages I and II melanoma patients according to tumor thickness subgrouped by levels of invasion. There were no statistically significant differences in survival rates for patients with lesions of various levels of invasion within each thickness subgroup. (Balch CM, Soong S-j, Shaw HM, et al. An analysis of prognostic factors in 4000 patients with cutaneous melanoma. In: Balch CM, Milton GW, eds. Cutaneous melanoma: Clinical management and treatment results worldwide. Philadelphia: JB Lippincott, 1985:332)

These lesions were all located on the face or neck and were generally thinner lesions. When matched thickness for thickness, patients with LMM lesions had better prognoses than the other growth pattern groups.[35,36] Even patients with LMM lesions 3 mm thick or greater had an 80% 10-year survival rate. It should be emphasized that other characteristics of LMM lesions (*e.g.,* face and neck locations, chronic skin damage, older patients) may contribute to the distinctiveness of this growth pattern as much as its histologic appearance. ALMs constituted only 2% of all cases. When matched by lesion thickness, patients with ALM lesions had worse prognoses than those of any growth pattern (see Fig. 46–7).

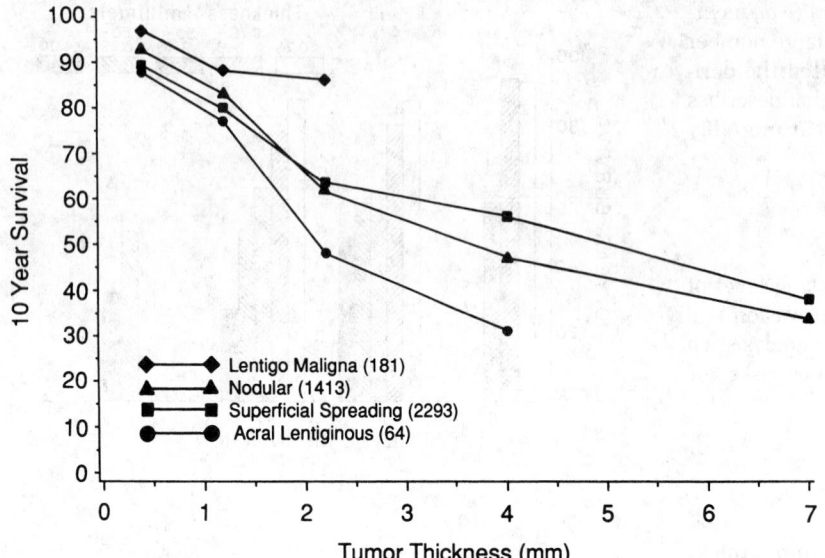

FIGURE 46–7.   Ten-year survival rates for stages I and II melanoma patients according to growth pattern and tumor thickness. Among patients with melanomas of equivalent tumor thickness, those with nodular and superficial spreading melanomas had similar survival rates, those with lentigo maligna melanomas had a much more favorable prognosis, and those with acral lentiginous melanomas had the worst prognosis. The number of patients is shown in parentheses. (Balch CM, Soong S-j, Shaw HM, et al. An analysis of prognostic factors in 4000 patients with cutaneous melanoma. In: Balch CM, Houghton AN, Milton GW, Sober AJ, Soong S-j, eds. Cutaneous melanoma. 2nd ed. Philadelphia: JB Lippincott, 1992:165)

Age

The median age of patients with stages I and II melanoma was 45 years. Advanced age at the time of diagnosis correlated significantly with a shortened length of survival ($p < 0.00001$). Patient age also correlated with melanoma thickness ($p < 0.00001$), with older patients having thicker lesions. The median thickness for melanoma patients in their third decade was 1.1 mm, whereas it was 1.5 mm for those in the fifth decade and 2.8 mm for those in the seventh decade.

Multifactorial Analysis

The above clinical and pathologic parameters were simultaneously compared for their prognostic strength using multifactorial analysis. The influence of these factors on survival was examined using a cohort of 4568 patients with AJCC stages I and II melanoma for whom information was available for all prognostic factors being analyzed. The dominant factors predicting survival were thickness of the melanoma, melanoma ulceration (presence or absence), and anatomic location (upper extremity, lower extremity, trunk, or head and neck). Four other variables correlated to a lesser extent with survival in certain subgroups of patients: (1) the type of initial surgical management (primary excision alone versus excision plus elective lymph node dissection), (2) pathologic stage (I, II, or III), (3) level of invasion, and (4) sex.

Most other major studies using multifactorial analysis have established tumor thickness to be the most important prognostic factor in their series of patients with stages I and II melanoma.[48,118,119,121,123,131–137] Similarly, ulceration was found to be another strong predictor of survival in seven other patient series.[119,122,123,132,133,135,136,138] Three of these series confirmed that anatomic location of the primary lesion was another major predictor of survival.[118,119,132]

Other factors analyzed by multifactorial analysis that emerged as important variables overall or within selected subgroups in other series included sex[121,122,137] and age of the patient[132] and such tumor features as lymphocytic infiltra-

tion,[122,131] tumor diameter,[122,123,134] cell type,[122,135] microscopic satellites,[138] mitotic activity,[118,123,131–137]and level of invasion.[132] The timing of the biopsy before first definitive treatment was found to have a significant influence on survival in one series.[122] Flow cytometry analyses of DNA content (aneuploidy versus diploidy) correlated with survival in several recent studies.[138a]

METASTATIC MELANOMA IN REGIONAL LYMPH NODES
(AJCC STAGE III)

Twelve prognostic factors of melanoma were examined in a series of 1698 patients with nodal metastases who were treated at UAB and SMU during the past 30 years.[117]

Sex

Most patients with AJCC stage III melanomas were men (69%), whereas they constituted a minority of stages I and II patients (48%). There were no differences in survival rates among male and female stage III melanoma patients, even when the data were cross-analyzed by other categories.

Anatomic Location of Primary Lesion

Primary melanomas accompanied by nodal metastases occurred in anatomic locations distributed throughout the body, with 55% arising in axial locations (trunk or head and neck). Patients with melanomas on the trunk constituted the largest group (35% of the entire series). There was no statistically significant difference in survival rates for patients with stage III melanoma when subgrouped by anatomic sites. Those with melanomas of the extremities had the best survival rates.

Age

The median age of the entire stage III patient population was 46 years. Older stage III melanoma patients tended to have a worse prognosis than younger patients. For example, only 20% of patients were alive after 5 years if they were older than 50 years at the time of the initial diagnosis, compared with 38% of patients who developed melanoma when they were 50 years old or younger. This difference was statistically significant ($p = 0.0001$). Significant differences appeared when the data were subgrouped further by gender. Men 50 years or younger had a much higher survival rate than older men ($p = 0.0006$), whereas the difference between younger and older women was not as great ($p = 0.02$).

Number of Metastatic Nodes

There was a direct correlation between number of metastatic nodes and survival. Patients with one metastatic node had a better survival rate than patients with two metastatic nodes or more.[139] Data from patients with different numbers of nodal metastases were analyzed for survival differences. The greatest differences in this series were between patients with one metastatic node, patients with two to four nodes, and patients with five or more nodes (Fig. 46–8). Thirty-seven percent of patients had one metastatic node, 38% had two to four, and 25% had five or more. Their 10-year survival rates were 40%, 18%, and 9%, respectively ($p < 0.001$). Ten-year survival rates demonstrated that only patients with one positive node had a reasonable prospect of cure (40% were alive at 10 years), whereas only about 15% of patients with two or more metastatic nodes were alive at 10 years.

Ulceration

Ulceration was the most important predictor of the risk for subsequent nodal metastases in patients with AJCC stages I and II melanoma, and it continued to be an important predictive factor once nodal metastases had occurred.[139,140] The 3-year survival for patients with stage III ulcerative melanomas was only 29%, compared with 61% for nonulcerative melanomas ($p = 0.0002$). For each category of nodal metastasis, the presence of ulceration in the primary lesion implied a worse prognosis than if the melanoma had an intact overlying epithelium. Patients with one positive node and no ulceration of the primary melanoma had the most favorable prognoses of any stage III patient group, having a 50% 10-year survival rate.

Tumor Thickness

The median thickness for stage III melanomas was 3.4 mm, compared with 1.2 mm for stages I and II lesions ($p < 0.001$). Forty percent of patients with stage III disease had thick melanomas (> 4 mm thick). A significant relation was identified between thickness and ulceration. Patients with nonulcerative melanomas of 4 mm or less had a more favorable 5-year survival rate compared with patients whose lesions were greater than 4 mm thick (37% versus 24%, respectively); patients with ulcerated melanomas greater than 4 mm had only an 18% 10-year survival rate.

Multifactorial Analysis

Each of the above prognostic factors was examined for its predictive value for metastatic risk and survival in stage III melanoma patients.[117,139] By single-factor analysis, the most significant prognostic variables were (1) the number of metastatic nodes, (2) the presence or absence of ulceration of the primary melanoma, (3) tumor thickness of the primary melanoma (< or > 4 mm), and (4) the patient's age. The multifactorial analysis showed that the number of metastatic nodes ($p = 0.0001$), the anatomic site of the primary melanoma ($p < 0.0151$), and tumor ulceration ($p = 0.0661$) were the dominant prognostic variables. Tumor thickness and patient age strongly correlated with prognosis in the combined UAB and SMU data ($p = 0.0001$), but the SMU data did not include the number of metastatic nodes as a variable in the multifactorial analysis.

The number of metastatic nodes was first shown to be of prognostic significance in a multifactorial analysis by Cohen and associates.[141] Later, Day and associates[142] and Callery and associates[143] demonstrated that tumor thickness and the number of metastatic nodes were dominant and independent

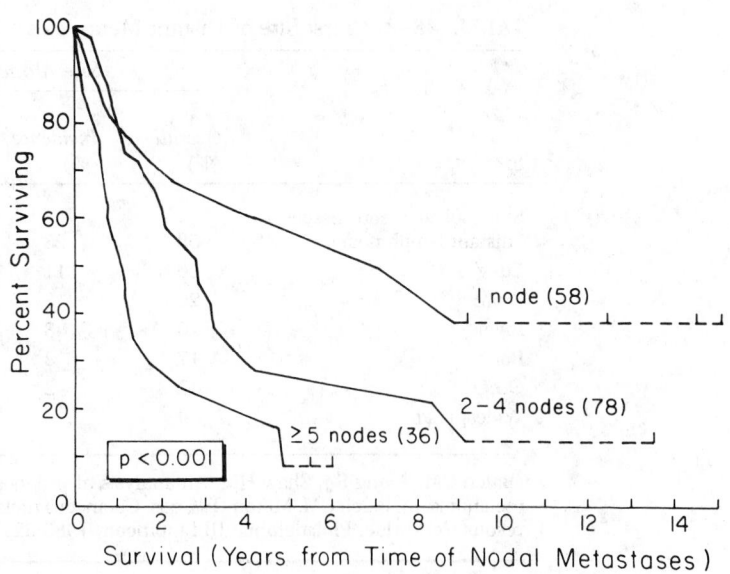

FIGURE 46–8. Survival for all stage III (AJCC) melanoma patients according to the number of metastatic nodes. (Balch CM, et al. A multifactorial analysis of melanoma patients with lymph node metastases [stage II]. Ann Surg 1981;193:377)

variables in stage III patients. Cascinelli and colleagues identified the extent of nodal metastases (*i.e.*, confined to or invading through the lymph node capsule) and the number of metastatic nodes as the most significant factors in a multifactorial analysis of 530 stage III patients.[121,144]

METASTATIC MELANOMA AT DISTANT SITES
(AJCC STAGE IV)

The data for 200 patients with distant metastases treated at UAB were analyzed for predictive factors affecting survival rates.[145]

Site of Distant Metastases

The locations of distant metastases were an important prognostic factor when examined by single-factor analysis (p = 0.0001). The skin, subcutaneous tissues, and distant lymph nodes were the most common first sites of relapse, which occurred in 59% of patients. In 23% of patients, nonvisceral metastases at these sites were the sole manifestation of disease (14% for skin, 5% for subcutaneous sites, and 4% for distant lymph nodes). The median survival duration for the entire patient group was 7 months, with 25% alive at 1 year. There was no difference in survival among patients with metastases at any combination of these three sites. The next most common site of first relapse was the lungs (36% of patients). Patients with isolated lung metastases had the longest median survival duration (11 months) of patients with metastases at site. The brain, liver, and bone were the next most common sites of first relapse. The median duration of survival for these patients was very poor, ranging from 2 to 6 months, with a 1-year survival rate of only 8% to 10%.

The presence of visceral metastases had an overriding influence on survival, because those patients with combined visceral and nonvisceral metastases had the same poor prognoses as those with visceral metastases alone.

Number of Metastatic Sites

Patients with a single distant metastasis had longer survivals than patients with metastases at two or more sites (see Fig. 46–8). Number of metastatic sites was the most significant factor predicting survival in patients with distant metastases by single-factor analysis (p < 0.00005). The median survival was 7 months for patients with one metastatic site, 4 months for those with two sites, and 2 months for those with three or more metastatic sites.

Similarly, the 1-year survival rate was 36% for patients with one metastatic site and 13% for patients with two sites, with no 1-year survival for patients with three or more sites. Within the single-site group, patients with metastases in the lung, skin, subcutaneous tissue, or distant lymph nodes had a better survival rate than patients with metastases at any other single site (Table 46–2).

Sex

Once melanoma progressed to distant metastases, there was no correlation between the sex of the patient and the clinical courses (p = 0.98). Survival curves for male and female AJCC stage IV melanoma patients were superimposable.

Remission Duration

The length of remission was not a statistically significant factor, by single-factor analysis, in predicting the clinical course of disease when the survival rates were calculated from the onset of distant metastases (p = 0.25).

Multifactorial Analysis

Each of the prognostic factors was examined for its predictive value for metastatic risk and survival rate.[145] Only the number of metastatic sites and the location of the sites (visceral, nonvisceral, or both) correlated with survival rates in a single-factor analysis. When all factors were analyzed in a Cox regression analysis, the dominant factors for stage IV mela-

TABLE 46–2. First Site of Distant Metastases

Site	Site Alone			Plus Other Sites	
	Overall (%)	Incidence (%)	Median Survival (mo)	Incidence (%)	Median Survival (mo)
Skin, subcutaneous tissues, distant lymph nodes	59	23	7.2	36	5.0
Lung	36	11	11.4	25	4.0
Brain	20	8	5.0	12	1.4
Liver	20	3	2.4	17	2.0
Bone	17	3	6.0	14	4.0
Other	12	2	2.2	10	2.0
Widespread	4		2.4		2.4

(Balch CM, Soong S-j, Shaw HM. An analysis of prognostic factors in 400 patients with cutaneous melanoma. In: Balch CM, Milton GW, eds. Cutaneous melanoma: Clinical management and treatment results worldwide. Philadelphia: JB Lippincott, 1985:321)

noma patients were as follows: (1) the number of metastatic sites (one, two, or three or more; $p = 0.00001$), (2) the remission duration (< 12 months versus > 12 months; $p = 0.019$), and (3) the site of metastases (visceral versus non-visceral; $p = 0.019$). These results were the same even after accounting for palliative chemotherapy. There were no histologic criteria of the primary melanomas that predicted the patients' clinical courses once they developed distant metastases.

Another multifactorial analysis of stage IV patients was performed by Presant and colleagues.[146] They found significant determinants of survival to include high performance (activity) status, no liver involvement, female sex, and bone involvement only.

MANAGEMENT OF THE PRIMARY MELANOMA

INDICATIONS AND TECHNIQUES OF BIOPSY

Biopsies for melanomas can be either excisional or incisional.[147] Whichever technique is used, full-thickness biopsy into the subcutaneous tissue must be performed to permit microstaging of the lesion (for thickness and level of invasion). Shave or curette biopsies should never be used for lesions suspected of being melanomas.

Excisional Biopsies

An excisional biopsy is indicated for a suspicious lesion that is not large (*i.e.*, < 1.5 cm in diameter) and is located in an area in which the amount of skin excised is not crucial (*e.g.*, on the trunk). The lesion should be excised with an elliptical incision including a narrow margin (2 mm) of normal-appearing skin. Taking slightly larger margins (*e.g.*, 1 cm) of

skin may be insufficient for a malignant lesion and excessive for a benign one.

The direction of the biopsy incision is important, because a biopsy that is not oriented properly may necessitate a skin graft when an elliptical incision and primary closure might have been possible. The biopsy incision should be oriented so that it can be reexcised with optimal skin margins and minimal skin loss if the lesion proves to be malignant. The excisional biopsy technique is illustrated in Figure 46–9.

Incisional Biopsies

Incisional biopsies should be performed when the amount of skin removed is crucial (*e.g.*, face, hands, feet). They may be indicated for large lesions, for which an excisional biopsy would be a formidable procedure. An incisional biopsy can be made with a scalpel, but usually a 6-mm punch biopsy is preferred to take a full-thickness core of skin and subcutaneous tissues from the most raised or irregular area of the lesion.

The biopsy specimen should not be taken at the periphery of the lesion unless there are areas of raised nodularity at this location. No decrease in survival rates or increase in local recurrence rates has been observed in our experience with the incisional approach[147] and in the experience of others.[148,149] Moreover, an incisional biopsy is a simple, expedient office procedure and provides representative tissue if taken properly. Such an approach is more cost-effective than inpatient biopsies, especially those taken under general anesthesia.

SURGICAL MARGINS OF EXCISION

Local control of a primary melanoma requires wide excision of the tumor or biopsy site with a margin of normal-appearing skin. Until recently, the routine surgical approach was to excise all primary melanomas with a 3- to 5-cm margin and

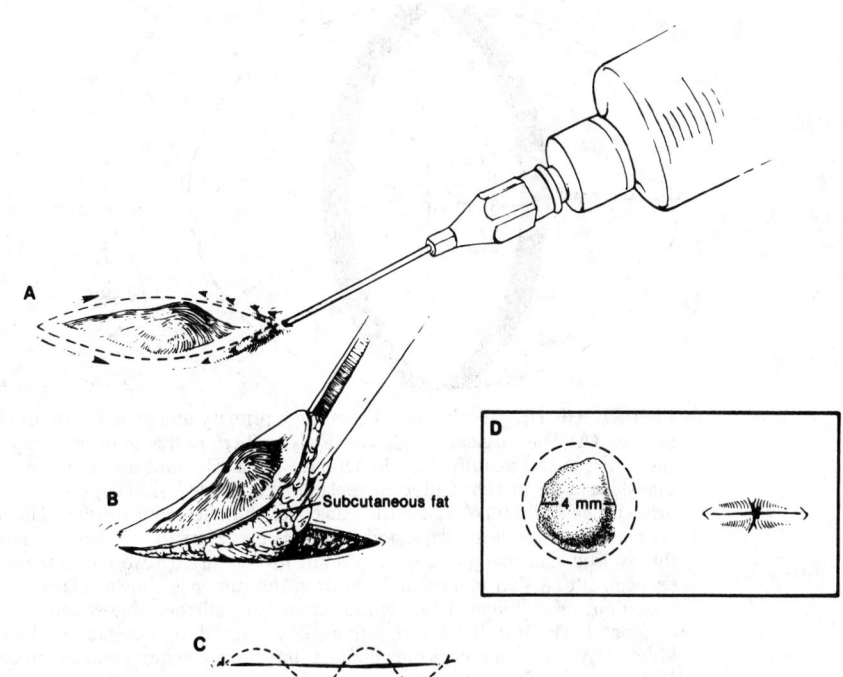

FIGURE 46–9. Technique of excisional biopsy for melanoma. **(A)** The suspicious lesion is first injected with local anesthetic around but not into the lesion itself. **(B)** The entire lesion is excised with a narrow rim (1 to 2 mm) of normal-appearing skin around it, including the underlying subcutaneous fat. Care is taken to avoid crushing the specimen with forceps. **(C)** The incision is closed after hemostasis is completed. This can be performed with a subcuticular closure using synthetic absorbable sutures or with simple interrupted nylon sutures. **(D)** An alternative approach for small lesions. An excision with a 6-mm punch is an inexpensive and expedient office procedure. The lesion is completely excised with the punch biopsy instrument, and the skin edges are closed with a single 4-0 nylon suture. (Urist MM, Balch CM, Milton GW. Surgical management of the primary melanoma. In: Balch CM, Milton GW, eds. Cutaneous melanoma: Clinical management and treatment results worldwide. Philadelphia: JB Lippincott, 1985:74)

apply a split-thickness skin graft to the defect. It has become increasingly clear that the risk for local recurrence correlates more with the tumor thickness than with the margins of surgical excision.[127,150–153] Therefore, it seems more rational to excise melanomas using surgical margins that vary according to tumor thickness and ulceration, because these factors correlate best with the risk for local recurrence.

The earliest lesion is a melanoma in situ.[154] This is a noninvasive tumor that does not metastasize but is capable of recurring locally.[155] Although the natural history of these noninvasive lesions is not completely understood, there is a risk for local recurrence as an in situ or invasive melanoma if they are not reexcised after biopsy.[155,156] It is recommended that the biopsy site of an in situ melanoma be excised, usually with a 0.5- to 1-cm margin of skin.

For thin melanomas (< 1.00 mm in thickness), there has been only minimum risk for local recurrence in all reported patient series,[127,147,148,150,152,156–158] despite wide variations in margins of excision. In other words, survival is not influenced by the size of the resection margins. This does not mean that reexcision is unnecessary, but that the minimal standards for a safe margin have not been established in any scientific study. A wide excision consisting of at least a 1-cm margin of skin is recommended by many melanoma surgeons.[127,147,152,156,157,159–161] This can be performed as a generous elliptical excision and a primary skin closure (Fig. 46–10). In a recent study of 936 patients with melanomas less than 1 mm thick, there was no local recurrence, despite the fact that 61% of patients had conservative margins (< 2 cm) of excision.[147] For intermediate and thick melanomas (> 1.0 mm thick), a margin of 2 to 3 cm is usually employed. The risk for local recurrence may exceed 10% to 20% for those melanomas more than 4 mm thick.[127,152,158,161] Because LMMs have a low risk for recurrence and generally occur on the

face, they can be safely excised with a 1-cm margin of excision.

Results of the first randomized study involving surgical margins for melanomas less than 2 mm thick have been reported recently by the World Health Organization (WHO) Melanoma Group.[162] In a study of 612 evaluable patients who were randomly assigned to either a 1-cm or 3-cm surgical margin of excision, there were no local recurrences in the group with melanomas less than 1 mm thick. There were three local recurrences in the group of patients with melanomas 1.0 to 2.0 mm thick, and all 3 patients had received narrow excisions.[162a] These results demonstrate conclusively that a narrow excision for thin melanomas (< 1.0 mm) is safe, but no conclusion could be reached about the safety of excising melanomas more than 1.0 mm in thickness. A randomized prospective study conducted by the Intergroup Melanoma Committee has evaluated 2- to 4-cm radial margins of excision for intermediate thickness melanomas (1.0–4.0 mm). The trial has been closed to patient accrual, and the preliminary results indicate that a 2 cm excision margin is safe.

Special Sites

FINGERS AND TOES. A melanoma located on the skin of a digit or beneath the fingernail must be removed by a digital amputation. When such a biopsy-confirmed lesion is located on the finger (especially the thumb), it is important to save as much of the digit as possible to maximize function. The amount that can be saved depends on the extensiveness of the lesion (*i.e.*, amount of nail bed or paronychial involvement) and the location of its proximal border. In general, amputations of digits are performed proximal to the distal joint of the thumb and at the middle interphalangeal joint of

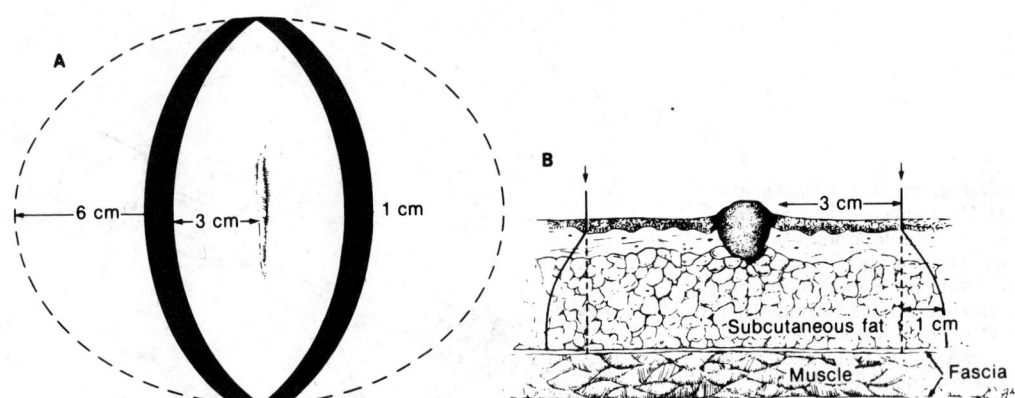

FIGURE 46–10.   Technique of excising a primary melanoma with an elliptical excision and primary skin closure. **(A)** The surgical margin consists of a 3-cm radius of normal-appearing skin surrounding the biopsy site or the lateral margin of the intact melanoma. The long axis of the incision should be three to four times the width of the incision. After the melanoma is excised, skin flaps are raised in a plane above the deep fascia for a sufficient distance to close the skin edges without undue tension. The most extensive area of mobilization is near the center of the flaps, and it often is necessary to mobilize the skin flaps for a distance twice that of the excised skin margin. A suction drain in the surgical wound may be needed. **(B)** Cross-section of the excision site. A skin margin of 3 cm from the tumor is shown. Flaps of gradually increasing thickness are raised for an additional 1 to 2 cm to remove any surrounding subdermal lymphatics. Excising the fascia is optional. (Urist MM, Balch CM, Milton GW. Surgical management of the primary melanoma. In: Balch CM, Milton GW, eds. Cutaneous melanoma: Clinical management and treatment results worldwide. Philadelphia: JB Lippincott, 1985:78)

the fingers, as long as the lesions are small and confined to the nail bed. For a melanoma located on a toe, an amputation of the entire digit at the metatarsal-phalangeal joint is indicated; this generally does not cause any significant morbidity.

SOLE OF THE FOOT. A melanoma on the plantar surface often involves a sizable defect in a weight-bearing area. If possible, a portion of the heel or ball of the plantar surface should be retained to bear the greatest burden of pressure. If possible, the deep fascia over the extensor tendons should be preserved as a base for the skin coverage.

EAR. For a small suspicious lesion of the helix, the preferred initial procedure for diagnosis is excisional biopsy followed by a wedge reexcision if the diagnosis of melanoma is confirmed. A partial amputation may be necessary for larger lesions. A total amputation of the ear should be restricted to patients with widespread local disease or those with recurrence after partial amputation.

FACE. Facial lesions usually cannot be excised with more than a 1-cm margin because of adjacent vital structures. In these cases, the surgeon should use his best judgment based on the width and thickness of the melanoma and its exact location on the face. The expected local recurrence rate after surgery is 4%. Radiation therapy has been used with some success for LMMs located on the face.[163]

ROLE OF RADIATION THERAPY

Superficial contact radiation therapy has been used in Europe for more than 60 years in the treatment of cutaneous melanoma. This technique results in very high incident doses of radiation, often in excess of 10,000 cGy, with very rapid fall-off (about 50% at 1 mm), and is therefore suitable only for superficial lesions. Conventional radiation therapy has little role in the initial treatment of primary melanoma, except perhaps for the LMM variety. Harwood reported in 1983 on a series of 28 patients with LMM treated definitively with conventionally fractionated radiation therapy at Princess Margaret Hospital from 1958 to 1982.[163] Only 2 patients had recurrences, although some lesions took up to 24 months to regress completely after radiation.

LOCAL RECURRENCES AND THEIR MANAGEMENT

A local recurrence is defined as any tumor that occurs within 5 cm of the scar of a previously excised melanoma. This definition is important in analyzing the risk factors involved and the influence of the surgical margins of excision of the primary melanoma. Local recurrences should be considered as retained extensions of the primary tumor. They are distinct from satellites and in-transit metastases that are intralymphatic in origin and occur between the primary tumor site and the regional lymph nodes.

Risk Factors in Local Recurrences

In general, patients with the highest risk for local recurrence have melanomas that have metastasized or melanomas with poor prognostic features. One analysis of local recurrence

demonstrated that AJCC stages I and II patients with the highest risk had melanomas with any of the following features: thickness of 4 mm or more (13% of patients), ulceration (11.5%), or location on the foot, hand, scalp, or face (5–12%).[147]

The overall risk for local recurrence is very low and is about 3.2% in collected series involving 3520 patients.[147] Local recurrences usually develop within 5 years after the primary melanoma excision but sometimes occur as late as 10 years afterward.[153,164]

Management of Local Recurrences

Comparative studies of treatment alternatives have not been performed for local recurrences. There are three options: (1) surgical excision, (2) isolated limb perfusion with regional chemotherapy and hyperthermia, or (3) radiation therapy. A single local recurrence, especially in a patient with a previously excised melanoma having favorable prognostic features, can probably be excised with a generous surgical margin and no further treatment. On the other hand, a patient who has multiple recurrences (either simultaneous or sequential) or poor prognostic features of the primary melanoma (*e.g.,* tumors > 4 mm thick, especially with ulceration) might be considered for isolated limb perfusion, because the risks of additional recurrences and in-transit metastases are substantially increased.[165] In patients for whom surgical excision is not feasible, or whose lesions have recurred on multiple occasions, radiation therapy with or without adjuvant hyperthermia should be considered. Our recommendation for treatment of local recurrences is the same as that for metastatic dermal or subcutaneous metastases.

Local recurrences imply a poor prognosis and are usually the first sign that metastases will develop, because most patients with local recurrences subsequently develop metastatic disease.[147,158,166] In a study of 95 patients with local recurrences, the median survival was 3 years, with a 10-year survival rate of only 20%.[147]

REGIONAL METASTATIC MELANOMA

DIAGNOSIS AND CLINICAL EVALUATION

Regional metastases are the most common indication of metastatic melanoma. The physician managing melanoma must be vigilant in making the diagnosis and instituting prompt treatment because some patients can be cured. Moreover, effective palliation can be provided even to those who are not curable. Any adenopathy suspected of harboring metastatic disease should be investigated. If the index of suspicion for metastatic disease is low, the node may be monitored by frequent examination until a diagnosis can be made. In some instances, either fine-needle aspiration or open biopsy is warranted if the examination is equivocal or close follow-up is not possible.

Surgical excision of metastatic nodes is the only effective treatment for cure or local disease control. Some surgeons prefer to excise only clinically demonstrable metastatic nodes. This type of excision has been termed a therapeutic or delayed lymph node dissection. Other surgeons choose to excise the nodes even when they appear normal because of the risk for occult or microscopic metastases. This excision has been termed an elective lymph node dissection (ELND) (called an immediate or prophylactic lymph node dissection). Surgical treatment for established nodal metastases is best described by discussing each of the major lymph node basins where metastatic melanoma can occur. Later sections describe the management of in-transit metastases and the rationale for ELND for micrometastases in the lymph nodes.

ILIOINGUINAL NODAL METASTASES

Rationale

The surgical technique for ilioinguinal lymph node dissection has been described and illustrated.[167–170] There are two contiguous node-bearing basins in the ilioinguinal area that might contain metastatic melanoma. The first is composed of the femoral nodes located within the femoral triangle. The second nodal basin is composed of the iliac and obturator lymph nodes.

In patients with demonstrable nodal metastases, a combined dissection of the iliac and femoral lymph nodes is recommended because at least 25% of patients with femoral nodal metastases have iliac nodal involvement as well.[171,172] There is some controversy concerning the benefit of iliac lymph node dissection. Some surgeons have stated that patients with melanoma of the lower extremities cannot be cured if their nodal metastases extend above the inguinal ligament and that a combined ilioinguinal lymph node dissection is associated with a higher risk for leg edema and wound complications compared with excision of the inguinal nodes alone.[173] Other surgeons have demonstrated that some patients with iliac nodal metastases can be cured or experience prolonged survival (with a 9% to 30% 5-year survival rate) with ilioinguinal lymph node dissection, particularly those patients with microscopic metastases in the inguinal nodes.[171,172,174,175] Excision of the obturator lymph nodes is important, because they can be metastatically involved.[170,176]

Complications and Their Management

In an analysis of 58 patients who underwent inguinal groin dissections, the short-term complications were infrequent and of short duration.[177] Leg edema was a frequent long-term complication (in 26% of patients) but was largely confined to the thigh, and only 8% of patients had edema of the lower leg. Seroma occurred in 23% of patients despite the use of suction catheters, but treatment with simple incision and drainage is generally straightforward. Pain (5% of patients) and functional deficit (3%) were uncommon. Only 1 patient (2%) had persistent severe edema. A wound complication extended hospitalization by an average of 2.1 days. Increasing age was the only risk factor for the development of more wound complications. Residual edema can be a debilitating result of inguinal node dissection.

Three series using preventive measures such as perioperative antibiotics, elastic stockings, leg elevation exercises, and diuretics have shown a decreased incidence of leg edema after groin dissection.[169,177,178] Vigorous prophylactic measures are important because it is difficult to reverse the progression of

edema. The patients in one series who followed this prophylactic regimen had a strikingly lower incidence of leg edema than those who did not (7% versus 46%; $p < 0.004$).[178]

AXILLARY NODAL METASTASES

Rationale

The most important feature of axillary node dissection is the completeness of the dissection, including the level III lymph nodes medial to the pectoralis minor muscle. A partial axillary node dissection is simply not in the patient's best interest; moreover, there is little additional morbidity or operative time involved in a complete axillary node dissection. The surgical technique for axillary node dissection has been described and illustrated by others.[167,179–181]

Complications and Their Management

The complication rate for axillary node dissection is low. The most frequent complication is wound seroma.[177,179,180] In a series of 98 radical axillary node dissections in melanoma patients treated at UAB,[177] wound-related complications included infections (7% of patients), seroma (27%), nerve dysfunction or pain (22%), and hemorrhage (1%). Wound-related complications extended the average hospitalization by less than 1 day. Long-term complications included arm edema (1% of patients), pain at the operative site (6%), and functional deficit (9%). Analysis of risk factors showed that increasing age was significantly associated with wound complications, whereas being female or obese only approximated statistical significance as predictive factors.

CERVICAL NODAL METASTASES

Rationale

Metastases to lymph nodes from primary melanomas in the head and neck area through the lymphatics are fairly predictable.[167] Melanomas occurring anterior to the pinna of the ear generally metastasize to the parotid, submandibular, submental, upper jugular, and posterior triangle (spinal accessory and transverse cervical) lymph nodes. Lesions occurring inferior to the lateral fissure of the lip will spread to cervical lymph nodes rather than to parotid nodes. Melanomas occurring on the scalp posterior to the pinna of the ear usually spread to occipital, postauricular, posterior triangle, or jugular chain nodes.

Radical neck dissection is recommended when nodal metastases are clinically evident. The surgical technique for this operation has been published previously.[167,182–185]

Modified Neck Dissection

Although there has never been a comparative study of modified versus radical neck dissection for melanoma, many surgeons have adopted the modified approach because of favorable results in patients with squamous cell carcinoma.[185,186] Modified neck dissection is generally reserved for patients undergoing elective neck dissection, but patients with limited metastatic disease are considered, except when it occurs in the posterior triangle near the spinal accessory nerve. Several variations of a basic technique have been described.[186-191] In comparison with the radical neck dissection discussed above, the only differences in the modified neck dissection are the sparing of the spinal accessory nerve and the sternomastoid muscle.

There are two advantages to modified neck dissection. First, there is better shoulder function and no shoulder drop. Second, the cosmetic result is better. Studies evaluating the functional results of modified neck dissection have shown a good cosmetic result; however, 30% of patients do not retain full spinal accessory nerve function.[192]

Complications and Their Management

A review of complications after radical neck dissection for melanoma revealed that short-term complications (seroma, pain, and skin slough) were common (10–19% of patients). Long-term problems such as neck pain and functional deficit occurred in only 6% to 7% of patients.[177]

A chylous leak can occur even when great care is used to detect leaks before closing the neck wound. Once the leakage rate is less than 50 ml daily, it usually stops within 7 to 10 days.

PAROTID LYMPH NODE DISSECTION

Rationale

Parotid lymph node metastases may be extraglandular or intraglandular. The most common extraglandular nodal metastases are in the preauricular nodes and the nodes located about the tail of parotid. Metastatic intraglandular nodes are generally found within the substance of the parotid gland and are usually located superficial to the seventh cranial nerve.

Melanomas arising on the scalp or face, anterior to the pinna of the ear, and superior to the commissure of the lip are at risk to metastasize to parotid lymph nodes.[193] This parotid chain of nodes is contiguous to the cervical nodes; for this reason, it is generally advisable to combine neck dissection with parotid lymph node dissection if there are metastases to the parotid nodes. The exception to this rule might be a tumor arising immediately over the parotid gland and requiring wide local excision, thereby necessitating parotid dissection to avoid injury to the seventh cranial nerve. Details of the surgical technique have been published.[167,194,195]

Complications and Their Management

Complications after parotidectomy are uncommon when the principles outlined above are followed. The incidence of facial nerve injury is proportional to the extent of dissection and the type and amount of tumor.[196-198] For elective dissection of parotid tumors in general, temporary paralysis of the facial nerve is reported in 10% to 20% of patients and permanent paralysis in 1% to 3%. When recognized during surgery, facial nerve injury should be repaired by primary anastomosis or nerve grafting from the contralateral greater auricular nerve. Seromas and salivary fistulas are uncommon and usually are self-limited. Gustatory sweating (Frey's syndrome) occurs more often than is generally reported but presents problems in only about 5% of patients.[197]

MANAGEMENT OF IN-TRANSIT METASTASES

DIAGNOSIS

In-transit metastases are located between the primary melanoma and the first major regional nodal basin. They probably originate from melanoma cells trapped in lymphatics. Although they may occur in deeper lymphatics, in-transit metastases usually are observed as subcutaneous or intracutaneous metastases (*i.e.*, satellitosis).

The number and location of in-transit metastases and the presence or absence of regional nodal metastases have implications for survival. Those patients with few in-transit metastases have better prognoses than those with multiple lesions. In the Tulane Medical Center series, patients with four or fewer lesions had better outcomes than those with five or more lesions.[199] Regional nodal metastases occur in about two thirds of patients with in-transit metastases and, if present, are associated with a lower survival rate.[200,201]

The reported incidence of in-transit metastases varies. This variation is due in part to the different definitions of in-transit metastases, the referral patterns of the reporting institution, and the proportion of patients with high-risk melanomas. The centers that practice isolated limb perfusion report a substantially higher incidence of in-transit metastases than those that do not. The actual incidence is probably 2% in most surgical practices. The reported incidence of 10% to 20% in some series reported in the 1960s and early 1970s[173,174,202,203] probably results from the fact that most melanomas diagnosed at that time were thicker, more likely to be ulcerated, and associated with a higher risk for nodal metastases than are the melanomas diagnosed in the 1980s.

TREATMENT OPTIONS

The treatment for in-transit metastases is not standardized. The treatment chosen depends primarily on the number and location of lesions in the integument, the presence of metastases elsewhere, the risk of the treatment, and whether previous metastases have been treated successfully. Aggressive local treatment is more effective than available systemic treatment.

Surgery

Surgery may be considered for one or a few lesions. Even with multiple lesions, excision of larger metastases (*i.e.*, those lesions greater than 2 cm) may prevent or relieve symptoms. A regional lymph node dissection usually is performed in patients with in-transit metastases, if it was not done previously, because there is a substantial risk of nodal metastases. Amputation of an extremity is rarely indicated, and then only when other treatments have failed and the patient is symptomatic with pain, bleeding, or odor.

Isolated Limb Perfusion

Isolated limb perfusion is probably the treatment of choice for most patients with in-transit metastases involving an extremity. Sometimes dramatic results can occur in terms of local disease control and prolongation of life.[165] One prospective controlled clinical trial provides evidence that prophylactic perfusion increases survival rates.[204]

Regional Chemotherapy Infusion

Intraarterial infusion of dacarbazine (DTIC) or cisplatin can reduce tumor burden in some patients.[205-207] It may be considered for lesions of the extremities if isolated limb perfusion has previously failed or is unavailable. Partial response rates of 40% to 50% have been reported, but the response durations were short.

Radiation Therapy

In-transit metastases too extensive for surgical excision often can be controlled effectively by radiation therapy. Wide fields and the use of an electron beam of 6 to 9 MeV with an appropriate bolus to eliminate skin sparing are recommended. Postoperative irradiation is indicated after excision of in-transit metastases that recurred after previous excision. Our recommendation for treatment for local recurrences is the same as that for dermal or subcutaneous metastases.

Intralesional Immunotherapy

Some of the first successful treatments using nonspecific immunotherapy were for in-transit metastases. Immunotherapy has been administered as intralesional injections of a variety of agents, including bacillus Calmette-Guérin (BCG), vaccinia virus, and DNCB.[208-210]

Systemic Chemotherapy

In most instances, systemic DTIC chemotherapy (alone or in combination with other agents) offers little chance of success for controlling in-transit metastases. Nevertheless, tumor growth can be temporarily arrested in a few patients but usually for only a few months. Systemic chemotherapy may be considered for multiple lesions, especially if the lesions are symptomatic and if other treatment alternatives cannot be used or have failed.

ELECTIVE LYMPH NODE DISSECTION

RATIONALE

The issue of ELND is probably one of the most important controversies in the management of patients with melanoma. Two randomized prospective studies of extremity melanomas did not demonstrate any survival advantage for ELND, whereas three nonrandomized studies involving melanomas from all anatomic sites showed a statistically significant improvement in survival for a subgroup of intermediate thickness melanomas.[211] Although surgeons are in unanimous agreement that all melanoma patients do not need ELND, there is still a continuing debate that centers around two issues. First, is it possible to identify accurately a subgroup of melanoma patients at high risk for microscopic regional nodal metastases? Second, if such a high-risk group can be identified, what is the optimal timing of dissection (immediate versus

delayed)? Prospective randomized studies are in progress to resolve this issue. In the meantime, it is justified to consider ELND in selected intermediate thickness melanoma patients in whom the benefit is sufficiently high and the morbidity sufficiently low to justify in an individual patient.

Theoretically, elective lymphadenectomy has the major advantage of treating a nodal metastasis at a relatively early stage in its natural history, when the tumor burden is generally less than several million cells. The disadvantage is that some patients may be subjected to surgery when they do not have nodal metastases. Conversely, the advantage of delayed lymphadenectomy is that only patients with demonstrable metastases undergo major operations. The great disadvantage, however, is that treatment is delayed until the metastases are clinically palpable, a time when the tumor burden is much greater (*i.e.*, many billions of metastatic cells). As a consequence, the chances for cure are diminished. By the time regional nodal metastases can be detected clinically, 70% to 85% of patients have distant micrometastases of which they will eventually die.[139]

SELECTION OF PATIENTS

Lymphadenectomy

Before defining risk factors for occult metastatic disease in melanoma patients with clinically normal lymph nodes, it is important to categorize patients biologically into three groups: (1) those patients with melanoma localized to the primary lesion site, (2) those with local disease plus possible regional nodal micrometastases, and (3) those with local disease plus distant micrometastases irrespective of whether they have nodal micrometastases. The intuitive surgical strategies are wide excision of the primary lesion site as the sole procedure for patients in the first group and removal of regional nodes containing microscopic or occult metastases for patients in the second group. Regardless of the surgical treatment at the primary and regional sites, the survival of patients in the third category is dictated by the presence of micrometastases at distant sites.

Tumor thickness provides a quantitative estimate of the risk for occult metastatic melanoma at regional and distant sites (Fig. 46–11). Melanoma thickness is the most important but not the sole guide for selecting patients who might benefit from ELND.[127] The major advantage of using tumor thickness for these surgical decisions is that it can provide a quantitative estimate of the risk for occult metastatic melanoma in regional and distant sites.[112,117,120,126-128] Thin melanomas (< 0.76 mm) are associated with localized disease and a 95% or greater cure rate. ELND would provide no therapeutic benefit in such patients. Patients with intermediate thickness melanomas (0.76 mm to 4 mm) have an increased risk (up to 60%) of harboring occult regional metastases, but have a relatively low risk (< 20%) of distant metastases (see Fig. 46–11). Patients with these lesions might therefore benefit from ELND.[112,126,127,211-216] Patients with thick melanomas (> 4 mm) are at high risk for regional nodal micrometastases (> 60%) and for occult distant disease (> 70%) at the time of initial presentation.[112,120,127,140,211,214] These patients do poorly as a group, because the distant metastases in most instances negate the benefit of surgically excising the regional

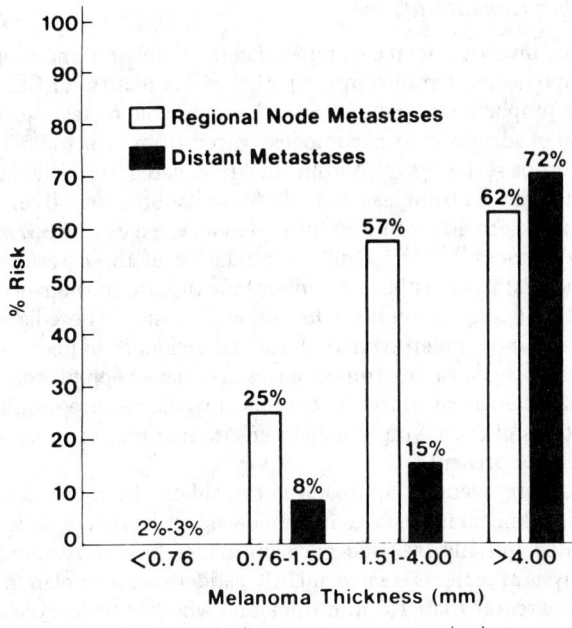

FIGURE 46–11. Estimated biologic risk that microscopic metastases become clinically evident in regional nodes (within 3 years) and at distant sites (within 5 years) for melanomas subgrouped by thickness categories. (Balch CM. Surgical management of regional lymph nodes in cutaneous melanoma. J Am Acad Dermatol 1980;3:511)

lymph nodes. The treatment goal of removing these nodes is palliative, and the operation might be deferred until nodal metastases become clinically evident. Some surgeons prefer to perform ELND as expectant palliation in patients with thick melanomas to avoid the probability (about 30%) of a second operation for lymph node metastases.[214] ELND might be justified as a staging procedure to document the pathologic status of the lymph nodes in patients with thick melanomas before entry into clinical trials involving systemic adjuvant chemotherapy or immunotherapy.

The anatomic site of the melanoma is an important criterion in predicting the risk for regional nodal micrometastases. Patients with melanomas on the extremities have more favorable prognoses, whereas those with melanoma on the trunk or head and neck area have a higher risk for microscopic metastatic disease, even with equivalent tumor thicknesses. Extremity melanomas in women have the lowest biologic potential for metastasis compared with lesions of equivalent thickness on the extremities of men, and patients with melanomas located on the trunk or head and neck area fare worse regardless of sex.[124,125,211,217] Finally, ulcerative melanomas have a higher risk for micrometastases than their nonulcerated counterparts, even when matched for other prognostic parameters such as tumor thickness.[126,213,218,219]

The growth pattern is important to consider in this decision-making process. Patients with LMMs have a low biologic risk for metastases, so ELND is not recommended.[217,220] The decision to perform ELND is made selectively based on the estimated risk for nodal metastases in regional lymph nodes and at distant sites.

ELND for extremity melanomas in women usually is not recommended unless the tumor thickness is at least 1.5 mm

or more.[211] Conversely, ELND is recommended more liberally for patients at higher risk, such as men with extremity melanomas and men or women with melanomas located on the trunk or head and neck area. A recommendation for ELND might be considered in these latter patients whose tumor thickness is as low as 1.0 mm. In patients with melanomas more than 4 mm thick, the risk for distant microscopic metastases is so high that it negates any potentially curative benefit of a regional operation.

Tumor thickness should not be the sole criterion for making surgical treatment decisions. Other factors, such as the presence or absence of tumor ulceration, the patient's sex and age, the anatomic location of the melanoma, and the operative risk should all be considered when making the decision to perform ELND on any individual patient.

Identifying the Regional Lymph Nodes At Risk

Because melanomas located on the trunk and on the head and neck area have unpredictable lymphatic drainage, it is difficult to decide which nodal basin is at risk for metastatic disease. In many patients, this problem has been surmounted by performing a radionuclide cutaneous scan that can locate accurately the nodes that are the primary drainage site for a melanoma located anywhere on the trunk.[221-224] All of the regional nodes should be removed, or a policy of monitoring multiple nodal sites at risk should be followed. An ELND of two nodal basins (*e.g.*, bilateral axillary dissection) for trunk melanomas may be warranted in select cases, but removing more than two nodal basins or performing a bilateral cervical dissection as an ELND is never indicated. A bilateral inguinal dissection is usually not performed electively because of its attendant side effects, especially edema of the extremities and genitalia.

Results of Treatment

Results of a prospective but nonrandomized trial of ELND involving 1319 surgically treated patients at the SMU have demonstrated an improved survival rate for those with intermediate thickness melanomas ranging from 0.76 to 4.0 mm (Fig. 46–12).[126,211,212,215] For patients with extremity melanomas, the benefit was greater in men than women.[211,217] A similar analysis of 676 patients treated at UAB during the past 25 years also demonstrated a benefit of ELND for patients who have intermediate thickness melanomas ranging from 1.5 to 4.0 mm (see Fig. 46–12).[35,112,126,140,211,217] Men with melanomas in the 0.76 to 1.5 mm range had the same trend toward an improved survival rate, but this was not statistically significant, largely because the sample size was smaller (Table 46–3). A retrospective data analysis from the Duke Medical Center and the Memorial Sloan-Kettering Cancer Center demonstrated an improved survival rate for patients with intermediate thickness melanomas who undergo ELND,[213,216] although a similar analysis from the University of Pennsylvania did not.[220]

Patients with melanomas located on axial sites (*i.e.*, trunk and head and neck) have a higher risk for metastases than those patients with extremity melanomas.[211,212] There have been no randomized prospective trials of the benefits of ELND for axial melanomas. It is incorrect in our view to extrapolate the data from extremity melanomas and apply it to the treat-

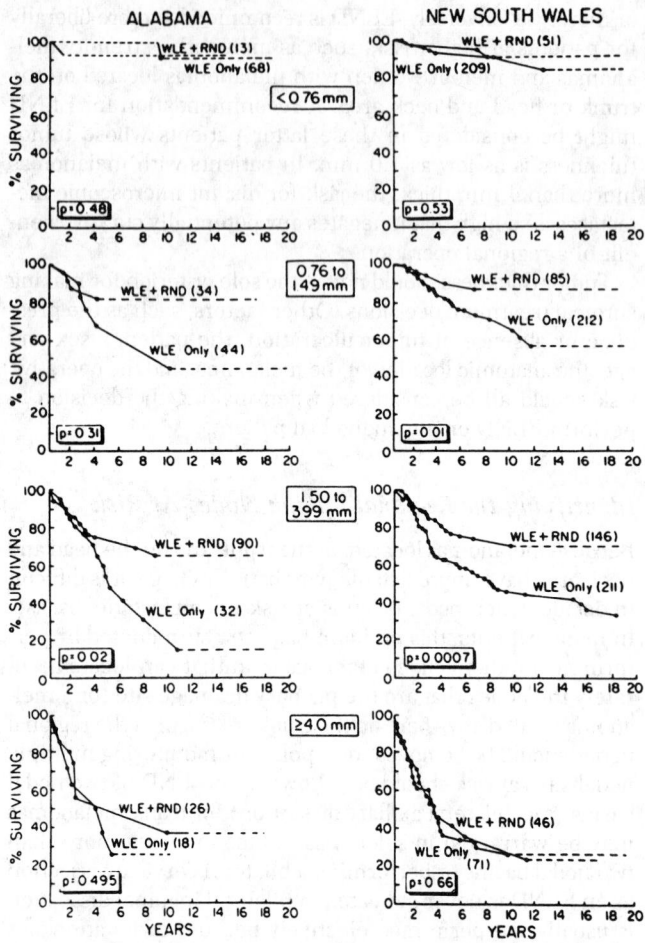

FIGURE 46–12. Actuarial survival curves calculated over 20 years for clinical AJCC stages I and II melanoma patients at the University of Alabama in Birmingham and the University of Sydney. Patients are subgrouped by tumor thickness and initial surgical management (wide local excision [WLE] + elective lymph node dissection [ELND]). The number of patients in each group is shown in parentheses. The p values were calculated for differences between each pair of survival curves. The benefit of ELND was greatest in patients with tumors 1.50 to 3.99 mm thick. For 0.76- to 1.49-mm melanomas, the differences were significant only for the Australian patients. The survival curves did not begin to diverge significantly until 5 to 8 years postoperatively. Patients with thin melanomas (< 0.76 mm) and thick melanomas (> 4.00 mm) did not benefit from an ELND. (Balch CM, Cascinelli N, Milton GW, et al. Elective lymph node dissection: Pros and cons. In: Balch CM, Milton GW, eds. Cutaneous melanoma: Clinical management and treatment results worldwide. Philadelphia: JB Lippincott, 1985:135)

ment of patients with axial melanomas. The results from the UAB and SMU data demonstrate an improved survival rate for patients with axial melanomas of intermediate thickness (0.76 to 4 mm) who underwent ELND. The risk for regional nodal metastases is greater and the benefit of ELND is even more apparent in this patient group than in those with extremity melanomas (see Table 46–3).[35,211,212,217] Hansen and McCarten, in a retrospective analysis of 50 patients with head and neck melanomas, also demonstrated an apparent improved survival rate with ELND for melanomas exceeding 1.5 mm in thickness.[225]

Other Considerations

Some investigators have argued that the number of metastatic lymph nodes identified by the pathologist is small after ELND. The proportion of patients with demonstrable metastatic disease in surgically excised nodes ranged from 10% to 25% in different series.[226–228] Within thickness categories, this incidence ranged from less than 5% for melanomas less than 1.5 mm thick to 40% or more for melanomas exceeding 3.0 mm in thickness.[127,214,216] One interpretation of these results is that most patients have no metastatic disease in their nodes and are being overtreated with surgical excision. These figures significantly underestimate the actual incidence of nodal metastases, because micrometastases may have been present in unsampled areas of the specimens. It would require multiple sections of each lymph node to ensure that micrometastases were not present.

A more accurate approach is to analyze the incidence of regional nodal metastases in a follow-up evaluation of patients treated initially by wide excision alone. In a retrospective analysis of patients treated at UAB, patients whose melanomas were greater than 1.5 mm thick and who had wide excision of their melanomas as their only initial surgical management had a 57% risk that nodal micrometastases would become clinically detectable within 3 years of diagnosis (see Fig. 46–11).[127] This percentage is more than double the incidence of occult nodal metastases found by examining randomly sectioned lymph nodes after ELND and is substantiated in part by the studies of Lane and colleagues[229] and Das Gupta,[230] who examined serial sections of nodes removed electively and found occult metastases in 42%.

Results of Randomized Clinical Trials Involving ELND

Two prospective trials to evaluate ELND in the treatment of stage I and stage II melanoma have been performed: an international cooperative study conducted by the WHO Melanoma Group[231–233] and a study by surgeons at the Mayo Clinic.[234] These studies demonstrated that all patients did not benefit from ELND. The question remains, however, whether any subgroup of patients might benefit. Both studies included melanomas of all thicknesses and did not specifically address the potential benefit of ELND in the subgroup of intermediate thickness melanomas described above.

The WHO Melanoma Group study involved 553 patients with stages I and II primary melanoma in the distal two thirds of the limbs. Of these patients, 286 (52%) were randomized to receive wide excision of the primary melanoma as initial treatment and node dissection only if regional node metastases became clinically detectable; 267 (48%) received wide excision plus ELND. The two groups were matched according to the major prognostic criteria. No differences in survival were noted between the two groups. Because subgroups of patients may have benefited from ELND, survival was evaluated according to prognostic criteria: sex, invasion levels III and IV, tumor thickness, and ulceration. No significant survival differences were reported in any of these subgroups. A separate analysis of the data demonstrated a 22% increase in 10-year survival in a small subgroup with intermediate-risk lesions.[211]

TABLE 46–3. Ten-Year Survival Rates of Clinical Stage I Melanoma Patients Treated at the Sydney Melanoma Unit, Australia, and the University of Alabama, Birmingham

Tumor Thickness (mm)	Extremity Melanomas			Trunk and Head and Neck Melanomas		
	WLE Only	WLE and ELND	p Value	WLE Only	WLE and ELND	p Value
<0.76	94% ± 5% (n = 142)	100% ± 0% (n = 26)	0.230	86% ± 6% (n = 135)	83% ± 8% (n = 38)	0.343
0.76–1.49	74% ± 8% (n = 125)	92% ± 4% (n = 66)	0.042	56% ± 10% (n = 131)	80% ± 7% (n = 51)	0.049
1.50–3.99	54% ± 7% (n = 114)	80% ± 6% (n = 107)	0.005	33% ± 6% (n = 129)	64% ± 7% (n = 129)	0.0008
≥4.0	30% ± 10% (n = 33)	44% ± 13% (n = 34)	0.400	22% ± 9% (n = 56)	26% ± 13% (n = 38)	0.806

ELND, elective (prophylactic) lymph node dissection; WLE, wide local excision.
(Balch CM, Cascinelli N, Milton GW, Sims FH. Elective lymph node dissection: Pros and cons. In: Balch CM, ed. Cutaneous melanoma. 2nd ed. Philadelphia: JB Lippincott, 1992:345)

Surgeons at the Mayo Clinic conducted a clinical study from 1972 to 1976 in which 171 stage I melanoma patients were randomized into one of three treatment groups. Sixty-two patients had their nodes left intact, 55 patients had ELND that was delayed 30 to 60 days after the primary melanoma excision, and 54 patients had elective lymphadenectomy concomitantly with the primary melanoma excision.[234] Patients with lesions of the head and neck and midline trunk were excluded. Compared with the two groups of patients who underwent ELND, patients who did not have ELND were older, more often men, and had worse prognostic features (*i.e.*, deeper invasion, thicker lesions, and more nodular lesions). The subgroup that received immediate ELND had more sites involving the trunk than did the other subgroups. None of these differences was statistically significant, although the subgroup with intact nodes was biased toward an unfavorable prognosis. Six characteristics were analyzed: initial surgical treatment, age, sex, anatomic site, tumor thickness, and growth pattern. The only factors that were significantly related to survival were tumor thickness ($p < 0.0001$) and growth pattern ($p = 0.02$).

When overall survival and disease-free survival of the three surgical treatment groups were compared, there were no significant differences.[234] The 5-year survival rate was 85% when the nodes were left intact, 85% when the nodes were removed immediately, and 91% when delayed ELND was performed. Survival and disease-free survival were significantly related to the thickness of the lesion.

The Mayo Clinic and the WHO Melanoma Group studies indicated no benefit from routine ELND for patients with stages I and II melanoma involving the extremities. There are legitimate differences in interpreting the results of the two trials.[211,217] These differences can be resolved only by continuing to perform randomized clinical trials using stratification criteria, extending these studies to all anatomic sites but confining the patient eligibility to intermediate thickness melanomas. Multiinstitutional surgical trials are being conducted in North America and Europe to assess the optimal timing of lymphadenectomy (immediate versus delayed if necessary) in a randomized prospective manner for intermediate thickness melanomas.

THE ROLE OF ADJUVANT RADIATION THERAPY

The role of radiation therapy as a surgical adjuvant after therapeutic node dissection or as an alternative to ELND in the regional treatment of patients with intermediate to thick melanomas has not been defined clearly. The rationale for its consideration in this context is that ELND, although effectively reducing regional recurrence rates, carries varying degrees of morbidity and does not offer any survival advantage in patients with thick primary tumors.[211,215] On the other hand, therapeutic dissection of pathologically involved nodes is associated with a local recurrence rate of up to 50% in patients with head and neck melanomas.[185,235]

Because of the management problems associated with uncontrolled locoregional disease and the extent of elective dissections required for scalp and facial primary sites, a study was initiated at the M.D. Anderson Cancer Center in 1983 to evaluate the role of radiation therapy in the treatment of clinically uninvolved lymph drainage areas. The study evaluated the use of radiation therapy in patients at high risk for nodal metastases and as an adjunct to surgery in patients undergoing therapeutic nodal dissections.

The preliminary results of this trial indicate an apparent advantage in terms of locoregional recurrence for adjuvant radiation therapy and were published by Ang and colleagues in 1990.[236] The following is an update of the study. Through August 1991, 153 patients were entered and divided into three groups. Group I consisted of 67 patients with primary lesions more than 1.5 mm in thickness (median 3.0 mm) or at Clark's level III or greater who had no clinically palpable lymphadenopathy. After wide local excision, these patients received radiation therapy to the tumor bed and draining lymphatics of 3000 cGy Dmax delivered in 5 fractions over 2.5 weeks with electron beams of appropriate energy. This group of patients had an overall 5-year rate of locoregional control of 87%, and 5-year survival of 63%. All patients with level III lesions less than 1.5 mm thick survived 5 years, and 82% of those whose primary lesion was 1.6 to 4 mm in thickness were 5-year survivors with adjuvant radiation therapy (Fig. 46–13). These results are similar to those obtained with elective nodal dissections for intermediate thickness melanomas (see Fig. 46–13).

Group II consisted of 29 patients with previously untreated disease who presented with clinically positive lymphadenopathy. These patients mostly received postoperative radiation therapy (3000 cGy Dmax delivered in 5 fractions over 2.5 weeks); the remainder received preoperative treatment (200 cGy Dmax delivered in 4 fractions over 2 weeks). These patients achieved a 5-year locoregional control rate of 96% and a 5-year survival of 44%. Survival was inversely proportional to the number of pathologically involved lymph nodes.

Group III consisted of 57 patients who presented with recurrent regional or local disease, but without evidence of distant metastases. These patients were treated in the same manner as group II patients. Their 5-year locoregional control rate was 88%, and the survival rate was 39%.

These results demonstrate that adjuvant radiation therapy, either alone in clinically node-negative patients or as a surgical adjuvant in pathologically node-positive patients, can achieve locoregional control in excess of 85%. This is substantially better than rates previously reported with surgery alone in comparable patients. The radiation therapy schedule used was not associated with any significant morbidity. In total, 3 of the 153 patients treated have sustained mild to moderate sequelae. There have been no severe complications. Although these data are impressive, proof of a therapeutic benefit from adjuvant radiation therapy can be obtained only from a prospective randomized trial. Such a trial, based on our pilot study, is under development by the Radiation Therapy and Oncology Group (RTOG).

METASTATIC MELANOMA AT DISTANT SITES

SITES AND PATTERNS OF METASTASES

Melanoma can metastasize to almost every major organ and tissue. Average survival is very short when metastases are detected in multiple visceral sites. Autopsy series have revealed that the lung is involved in 70% to 87% of cases, liver in 54% to 77%, bowel in 26% to 58%, brain in 36% to 54%, heart in 40% to 45%, adrenals in 36% to 54%, kidney in 35% to 48%, and bone in 23% to 49% (Table 46–4).[236,237] Most patients die with disseminated disease involving multiple organ sites; the actual cause of death is often respiratory failure or brain complications.[238,239] In clinical series, metastases to the lung, liver, brain, and bone occur in 11% to 36% of patients, well below the frequencies detected in autopsy series.[145,238–246] Metastases to the heart, adrenals, pancreas, and kidney have been detected only infrequently in clinical series (< 1% of cases), although abdominal visceral metastases are identified at higher frequencies with the use of computed tomography (CT) scans and magnetic resonance imaging (MRI). These studies suggest that clinical evaluation of patients often underestimates the extent of metastatic disease and actual tumor burden.

The site of first distant metastasis is an important prognostic variable (see Table 46–4). After treatment for primary or regional disease, the most frequent distant sites for first recurrence are the skin, subcutaneous tissues, and distant lymph nodes (up to 59% of patients; see Table 46–4).[117,247] This pattern of recurrence confirms the importance of a careful physical examination in monitoring patients with AJCC stage I, II, or III melanoma who are free of disease. The median survival of patients with skin, subcutaneous tissue, and distant

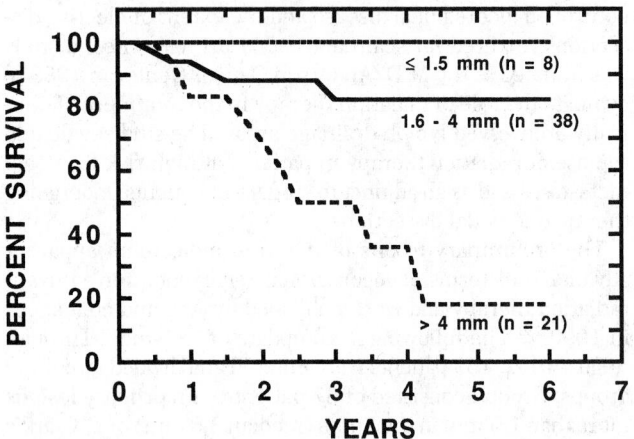

FIGURE 46–13. Survival of patients at The University of Texas M.D. Anderson Cancer Center receiving elective irradiation of the draining lymphatics of primary cutaneous melanomas of the head and neck, as a function of tumor thickness. All patients had primary lesions invading to Clark's level III or greater.

TABLE 46–4. Common Distant Sites of Metastatic Melanoma

Site	Clinical Series* (%)	Autopsy Series* (%)
Skin, subcutaneous, lymph nodes	42–59	50–75
Lungs	18–36	70–87
Liver	14–20	54–77
Brain	12–20	36–54
Bone	11–17	23–49
GI tract	1–7	26–58
Heart	<1	40–45
Pancreas	<1	38–53
Adrenals	<1	36–54
Kidneys	<1	35–48
Thyroid	<1	25–39

* From references 145, 238, 240, 241, 242, 243, 244, 245, 246, and 250.
(Adapted from Balch CM, Milton GW. Diagnosis of metastatic melanoma at distant sites. In: Balch CM, Milton GW, eds. Cutaneous melanoma: Clinical management and treatment results worldwide. Philadelphia: JB Lippincott, 1985:221)

lymph node metastases is 7 months, but there is wide variability of survival in this group of patients. The second most frequent site for first relapse is the lung (up to 36% of patients); patients with lung involvement have a median survival of 11 months. The liver, brain, and bone comprise the next most frequent sites of recurrence (median survival for these patients ranges from only 2 to 6 months). In general, patients with visceral metastases (with or without skin, subcutaneous tissue, or lymph node involvement) do very poorly. In the UAB series, more than 80% of patients with visceral metastases were dead within 1 year and almost all died within 2 years.[117] Patients with lung metastases as their only visceral metastatic site generally fared better (median survival 11.4 months) than patients with tumors at other visceral sites. In the series from UAB, median survival of patients with a single distant metastatic site was 7 months, with two sites 4 months, and with three sites 2 months.[117,145] Disease-free intervals of 1 year[145] and 2 years[248] have been associated with longer survival.

DIAGNOSTIC EVALUATION OF METASTATIC DISEASE

The evaluation for metastatic disease in patients who are clinically free of tumors should include a careful physical examination, chest x-ray films, and liver function tests. Serum lactate dehydrogenase (LDH) is a useful marker for widespread metastases, especially for the detection of liver disease.[243,249,250] Blood in the stool and abdominal and gastrointestinal symptoms should be investigated as possible indications of metastases. Particular attention should be paid to signs or symptoms of central nervous system involvement. In all patients with systemic melanoma metastases, there should be a high index of suspicion for associated brain, spinal cord, or meningeal metastases. Extensive radiographic evaluation of patients with AJCC stage I, II, or III melanomas who are free of disease rarely reveals metastases. Chest tomography, upper gastrointestinal series, barium enema, abdominal ultrasound, intravenous pyelogram, brain CT scan, and radionuclide scans of brain, bone, and liver rarely reveal metastases in the absence of symptoms, signs, or abnormal standard test results (*e.g.*, chest x-ray films, hemogram, liver function tests including LDH).[244,251-260] The rate of false-positive tests makes extensive evaluations costly. Likewise, conventional scanning with ^{67}Ga is not a sufficiently sensitive or specific screening test, although it can detect metastatic melanoma.[261-265]

Although metastases can remain stable for months, even without treatment, progression of existing tumors or appearance of new tumors can occur rapidly, sometimes accompanied by precipitous clinical deterioration. Patients need to be evaluated at frequent intervals by medical personnel who are familiar with the patient's diagnosis and conditions. Despite the poor prognoses and the availability of prognostic indicators for patients with systemic metastases, it is often difficult to predict the course of an individual patient's disease. Periods of stability without evident tumor growth can be interrupted by a medical emergency (*e.g.*, seizure due to intracranial hemorrhage from a brain metastasis or acute gastrointestinal bleeding from a small bowel lesion).

TREATMENT MODALITIES

Patients with systemic metastases (AJCC stage IV) have poor prognoses. The mean survival is about 6 months,[117,145,248] and cure is not a realistic aim. Treatment of this group of patients should include careful evaluation for the potential role of surgery, radiation therapy, and systemic therapy.[266] General guidelines for choosing treatment modalities are presented in Table 46–5. Selection of treatment options should take into account the general medical condition of the patient, the potential for prevention or relief of symptoms, and improve-

TABLE 46–5. Treatment Options for Systemic Metastatic Melanoma

Treatment Option	Site of Metastases	Comments
Surgery	Superficial lesions Brain Symptomatic visceral Occasional lung	Best for solitary lesions, especially symptomatic; low-risk patients
Radiation therapy	Superficial lesions Brain Bone	Treatment of symptomatic lesions
Chemotherapy	Systemic metastases	Skin, subcutaneous tissue, lymph node, and lung lesions most responsive
Limb perfusion	Local recurrences	Restricted to extremity lesions; requires major surgery
Hyperthermia	Liver lesions Large superficial lesions	Experimental treatment
Intralesional therapy	Skin lesions	Experimental treatment; can be locally effective for dermal metastases
Systemic immunotherapy	Systemic metastases	Experimental treatment

(Adapted from Houghton AN, Balch CM. Treatment for advanced melanoma. In: Balch CM, ed. Cutaneous melanoma. 2nd ed. Philadelphia: JB Lippincott, 1992:468)

ment in the quality of life. The median age of patients with melanoma, about 45 years, is young compared with the age of most adult cancer patients. Careful consideration must be given to the impact of prognosis and treatment for these patients, who are frequently primary providers for their families and have full-time occupations.

NO TREATMENT

The option of no treatment is important, especially in asymptomatic patients, those who are terminally ill, or those at advanced ages. There are two groups of patients for whom no treatment is a major consideration. The first group consists of asymptomatic patients with tumors in favorable sites, such as the lung or bone (but not brain). The physician may elect to observe these lesions if they are growing slowly and are not causing symptoms. Quality of life is maintained in this instance, and treatment can be deferred until the lesions begin to progress, either by size or multiplicity, or until the patients develop symptoms. The second group consists of patients who are terminally ill or very old and for whom the benefit-to-risk ratio is small. The decision to forego treatment can be difficult; it is often best made by the patients themselves with the assistance of close relatives or medical or nursing advisors. A patient should not be denied treatment when there is a reasonable expectation that the treatment will be successful and the risk or toxicity is low.

SURGERY

Surgery is an effective palliative treatment for isolated metastases, especially because melanoma often metastasizes sequentially and effective chemotherapy is not available. Surgical excision of metastatic melanoma probably gives the patient the best, quickest, and longest lasting palliation. On some occasions, the palliative effect can last for 5 to 10 years.[242,267-269] The favorable experience with surgical resection of distant metastases in selected patients treated at four institutions is shown in Table 46–6.

The limitation of surgery is that it is a local form of treatment, and the patient will eventually die from metastatic disease elsewhere. Careful patient selection is important. Observation for several weeks may provide relevant information about the rate of tumor growth and the presence of other multiple metastases, which could emerge during the observation period. Surgery should be confined to situations involving accessible lesions that are limited in size and number and in which the operation can be safely performed. Some examples of accessible lesions include isolated visceral metastases (especially brain) and occasional lung metastases. Most amenable to this approach are gastrointestinal metastases that cause obstructions, and superficially located lesions in the skin, subcutaneous tissues, or distant lymph nodes. Liver metastases are associated with such a short survival (*i.e.*, 2–4 months) that surgical excision generally is not indicated.

The choice of surgical excision as a means of palliation depends on the site of the disease and the duration of anticipated survival. If the patient's life is likely to be measured in weeks, the surgical ablation of a large growth is not justified, whereas longer anticipated survival makes excision of gross disease worth considering. Each case has to be considered on its own merits.

RADIATION THERAPY

Over the past two decades, a large number of retrospective clinical studies on the role of radiation therapy for metastatic and recurrent melanoma have been published and are reviewed by Peters and colleagues.[270] These studies involved a variety of metastatic sites (*e.g.*, cutaneous, lymph nodes, brain, bone, lung, and other viscera), and no general conclusions can be drawn from them. In the treatment of cutaneous and lymph node metastases, most investigators observed improved response rates with higher fractional doses.[271-280] The interpretation of the role of fraction is complicated by the variability in total dose administered and by the heterogeneity of the clinical material. Bentzen and colleagues[281] recently undertook an analysis of the role of fraction size correcting for total dose and tumor volume, using the data base of Overgaard and colleagues[279] and more recently accrued cases. They found that the probability of local control increased with size of dose per fraction, at least up to 900 cGy (Fig. 46–14). However, the use of high fractional doses limits the total dose that can be administered without causing injury to many late-reacting normal tissues.[282] The optimal size of dose per fraction represents a trade-off between the probability of sterilizing the melanoma versus the probability of causing normal tissue damage. Using subcutaneous fibrosis as the normal tissue end-

TABLE 46–6.   Median Survival of Melanoma Patients After Complete Surgical Resection of Distant Metastases

	Survival in Months (No. of Patients)			
Site	*M.D. Anderson Cancer Center*[242]	*Memorial Hospital*[268]	*Univ. of Alabama Hospitals*[269]	*Roswell Park Institute*[267]
Skin, subcutaneous	23 (64)	25 (12)	17 (13)	31 (25)
Lung	16 (26)	19 (17)	9 (17)	9 (13)
Brain	15 (16)	7.5 (5)	8 (17)	5 (4)
GI (excluding liver)	18 (9)	15 (12)	8 (5)	8 (3)
Overall 2-year survival	15%	21%	16%	31%

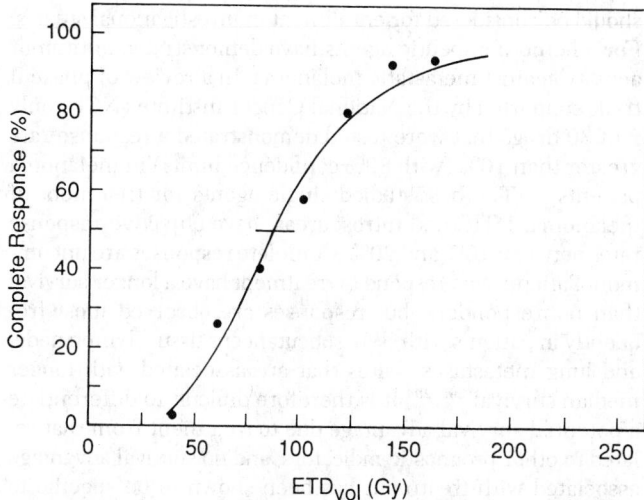

FIGURE 46–14. Dose-response relation showing the probability of achieving complete response as a function of volume-corrected extrapolated total dose (ETD_{vol}). The horizontal bar indicates the 95% confidence limits of the 50% complete response probability. (Overgaard J, et al. Some factors of importance in the radiation treatment of malignant melanoma. Radiother Oncol 1986;5:187)

point, Bentzen and colleagues calculated the therapeutic ratio as a function of dose per fraction.[281] The therapeutic ratio increased rapidly between 200 and 500 cGy and gradually thereafter. However, the lower confidence limit for the therapeutic ratio showed a peak in the range of 500 to 600 cGy which would, therefore, define the safest dose per fraction to be used when damage to connective tissue is dose limiting. Although this analysis supports the use of larger than conventional fractional doses, at least for the treatment of subcutaneous and lymph nodal metastases, a recent RTOG study failed to demonstrate any significant advantage of a treatment regimen consisting of 4 fractions of 800 cGy compared with one consisting of 20 fractions of 250 cGy.[283] A total of 137 patients were entered into this study, which included all metastatic sites other than the abdomen or brain. Most metastases were in soft tissues, skin, or lymph nodes. Tumors were stratified according to whether they were greater or less than 5 cm in largest diameter, but otherwise size was not recorded or corrected in the analysis. Total response rates were 59.7% with the 4 × 800 cGy regimen, and 57.8% with the 20 × 250 cGy regimen.

In summary, the question of optimal fraction in the treatment of melanoma remains controversial. It is certain that no single fraction size is optimal for all patients because of variability of the radiobiologic characteristics of individual tumors. Although most retrospective studies and the elegant analysis of Bentzen and colleagues[281] support the use of larger than standard dose fractions, no advantage was observed in the randomized RTOG trial.[283] We believe that the appropriate recommendation for dose fractionation should be based on considerations of normal tissue tolerance. The treatment should be convenient for the patient, at least as effective as standard treatment, and used at sites where hypofractionated treatment is well tolerated. The hypofractionated regimen is not recommended when the dose-limiting normal tissue is the central nervous system or the abdominal viscera because of the poor tolerance of these organs to large-dose fractions.

EXPERIMENTAL THERAPIES

Because the results achieved in melanoma by standard radiation therapy are less than optimal regardless of fractionation schedule, a variety of experimental therapies have been proposed and tested.

Hyperthermia

A good review of the value of hyperthermia as an adjuvant to radiation therapy in the management of malignant melanoma was published in 1987 by Overgaard and Overgaard.[284] These authors reported that in patients with subcutaneous or lymph node metastases, the response to radiation therapy was significantly improved by the addition of hyperthermia to a temperature of 43°C for 30 minutes. When the two treatments were given immediately sequentially ("simultaneously"), no improvement in therapeutic ratio was observed, because normal tissue reactions were exacerbated to the same extent as tumor response was improved. When hyperthermia was delayed until 3 to 4 hours after administration of each of three radiation therapy doses of 800 cGy, a significant improvement in therapeutic ratio was observed. Many other researchers have reported increased response rates with adjuvant hyperthermia in the treatment of malignant melanoma, and their work is reviewed by Meyer and colleagues.[285] With the exception of a study by Overgaard and Overgaard,[284] few attempts have been made to measure the therapeutic ratio, and improvement in this parameter has not been demonstrated in a randomized trial.

Clinical hyperthermia is limited by the technical difficulty associated with heating large or deep-seated tumors. Nonetheless, for accessible superficial lesions, it seems reasonable to use adjuvant hyperthermia when it is available.

High Linear Energy Transfer Irradiation

On radiobiologic grounds, fast neutron radiation therapy would be expected to achieve results equal to, or possibly better than, high dose per fraction x-ray or gamma-ray radiation therapy. The largest series of patients reported for whom such therapy has been employed is from the Hammersmith Hospital in London. In a series of 68 patients with 87 recurrent or metastatic lesions, Blake and colleagues reported a 71% complete response rate that was durable for the remainder of the patients' lives in 91% of cases.[286] A high complication rate of 22% was observed; however, most of these complications occurred in treatments of lower limb, groin, and axilla. Further studies of the value of fast neutron radiation therapy using somewhat lower biologically effective doses than those employed at Hammersmith are under way in the United States. No data from these studies are available.

Radiosensitizers

Both hypoxic and aerobic cell sensitizers are being studied as radiation therapy adjuvants for metastatic melanoma. Dische reported complete and sustained remission in 5 of 7 cases of recurrent cutaneous or lymph node disease treated with high-dose radiation therapy (5200–5600 cGy in 20 fractions) in conjunction with the hypoxic cell sensitizer Ro-03-8799 (pimonidazole).[287] Because a significant proportion of hypoxic cells has been demonstrated in autochthonous metastases of human melanoma,[288] further studies using sensitizers specific to hypoxic cells are indicated.

Another class of sensitizers is being tested by the RTOG in the treatment of brain metastases. In this study, the halogenated pyrimidine iododeoxyuridine is the sensitizer. The drug is incorporated into the DNA of cells during the S phase of the cell cycle and is therefore preferentially incorporated into brain metastases relative to the surrounding normal brain. No data on the results of this trial are available.

Photodynamic Therapy

The principle of photodynamic therapy is based on the cytotoxic effects of visible light on cells that have taken up dyes extracted from hematoporphyrin. Several such dyes are selectively retained in neoplastic tissue, affording a therapeutic advantage when these tissues can be illuminated with visible light. Photodynamic therapy is of particular interest in the treatment of dermal metastases from malignant melanoma. It is too early to assess the value of this approach in relation to other therapies. For a recent review of photodynamic therapy, see DeLaney and Glatstein.[289]

Thermal Neutron Capture Therapy

When the isotope boron 10 is irradiated with thermal neutrons, it undergoes nuclear disintegration and releases an α particle with a range of 10 to 14 μm, allowing highly selective irradiation of cells that concentrate the isotope. Mishima and associates recently reported on the first human treatment with neutron capture therapy using the melanoma-seeking drug ^{10}B1-para-boronophenylalanine HCl (^{10}B1-BPA HCl).[290] The patient had a metastatic lesion in the left occipital region. A ^{10}B tumor concentration of 24 μg/g was achieved in the tumor, and the lesion was then irradiated with thermal neutrons from a nuclear reactor. Complete regression of the lesion occurred and had been maintained for 10 months at the time the report was published. The ability to target ^{10}B selectively to melanoma by incorporating the isotope into a precursor of melanin synthesis makes this approach an attractive one for future development.

Radiolabeled Antibodies

The use of radiolabeled antibodies specific to melanoma antigens is an appealing concept, especially for adjuvant systematic therapy for a disease in which cytotoxic chemotherapy is of limited efficacy. Major problems relating to antibody specificity, stability, radionuclide specific activity, antigenic heterogeneity, and modulation of expression must be resolved before the full potential of this approach is realized. This strategy is discussed in more detail in the section on monoclonal antibodies.

Chemotherapy

Systemic therapy for melanoma, both as adjuvant therapy and for treatment of disseminated (stage IV) disease, remains unsatisfactory. Patients with high-risk or metastatic disease should be considered for enrollment in investigational studies. Few chemotherapeutic agents have demonstrated antitumor activity against metastatic melanoma. In a review of phase II trials supported by the National Cancer Institute (NCI), only 2 of 30 drugs that were tested demonstrated a response rate greater than 10% (with 80% confidence limits) in melanoma patients.[291] The best-studied single agents for treatment of melanoma, DTIC and nitrosoureas, have objective response rates between 10% and 20%. Complete responses are uncommon. Patients who respond to treatment have a longer survival than nonresponders, but responses are observed most frequently in patients with skin, subcutaneous tissue, lymph node, and lung metastases—sites that are associated with longer median survival.[292–294] It is therefore difficult to differentiate a potential survival advantage due to treatment from that related to other prognostic indicators, and no survival advantage associated with treatment has been shown to be specific to treatment and independent from other prognostic factors.

The evaluation of experimental systemic treatments for melanoma should take into account the following two prognostic factors for metastatic disease: (1) sites of tumor (skin, subcutaneous tissues, lymph nodes, and lung versus non-lung visceral sites), and (2) number of organs or tissues involved with disease (one, two, three or more). Occasionally, individual skin or subcutaneous lesions that are small (< 1 cm in diameter) can wax and wane without treatment. It is therefore important to choose sizable indicator lesions that can be confidently measured. Spontaneous regression that would fit the criterion for objective response to treatment (*i.e.*, greater than 50% decrease in the product of the greatest perpendicular diameters of measurable lesions, lasting at least 1 month) occurs infrequently when measurable indicator lesions are used.

SINGLE-AGENT CHEMOTHERAPY. DTIC remains the most active single agent for the treatment of systemic melanoma. The response rate is about 20% (Table 46–7), and patients with skin, subcutaneous tissue, and lymph node involvement respond most frequently.[292–316] Lung metastases are also responsive to DTIC, but liver, bone, and brain metastases respond infrequently. The median duration of response is 5 to 6 months. Complete responses were observed in about 5% of 580 patients entered into phase III trials, and most of these complete responses occurred in subcutaneous and lymph node metastases.[308] A minority (31%) of patients who achieved complete response survived and remained disease-free at 6 years. Overall, about 2% of patients treated with DTIC sustain long-term complete responses.

DTIC is typically well tolerated. The major side effects of DTIC used to be nausea and vomiting, but effective antiemetic regimens can control this toxicity in a high proportion of patients.[317,318] Ondansetron or a combination of lorazepam, dexamethasone, and metoclopramide appear to be effective antiemetic regimens. Other side effects of DTIC include local pain at the injection site, neutropenia, and thrombocytopenia, which are usually mild and occur between days 10 and 21, and flu-like symptoms and diarrhea. Photosensitivity reactions occur infrequently. Dose-related and life-threatening liver failure due to hepatic necrosis and venoocclusive disease has been seen in rare cases. DTIC may be given as a 1-day, 5-day, or 10-day regimen. Recommended doses are as follows: (1)

TABLE 46–7. Active Chemotherapy for Metastatic Melanoma

Agent	No. of Evaluable Patients	Response		References
		No. of CR + PR (%)	95% CI (%)	
Dacarbazine (DTIC)	1936	382 (20)	18–22	291–316
Carmustine (BCNU)	122	22 (18)	11–25	319–321
Lomustine (CCNU)	270	35 (13)	9–17	322–324, 326
Tauromustine (TCNU)	42	7 (17)	6–31	331
Fotemustine	153	37 (24)	17–31	329, 330
Cisplatin	188	43 (23)	17–29	332–339
Carboplatin	43	7 (16)	5–27	340
Vincristine	52	6 (12)	3–20	341–347
Vinblastine	62	8 (13)	5–21	348–357
Vindesine	273	39 (14)	10–18	358–369
Taxol	65	12 (18)	9–28	370–372
Dibromodulcitol	205	28 (14)	9–18	373–381
Detorubicin	42	8 (19)	7–31	382
Piritrexim	31	7 (23)	8–37	383

CR, complete response; PR, partial response; CI, 95% confidence interval for response rates.

850–1000 mg/m² given intravenously for 1 day every 3 to 4 weeks; (2) 250 mg/m²/day given intravenously for 5 days every 3 weeks; or (3) 2 to 4.5 mg/kg/day given intravenously for 10 days repeated every 4 weeks. There is no evidence that response rates or duration are affected by schedule or daily dose. With the advent of effective antiemetic regimens, the 1-day schedule repeated every 3 to 4 weeks is acceptable and often is least intrusive to the patient. It is generally well tolerated and should be administered in an appropriate outpatient setting. Dose can be escalated as tolerated, depending on neutropenia and thrombocytopenia, because hematologic toxicity is not usually cumulative. Blood counts should be followed carefully during treatment.

The nitrosoureas are a second group of agents with defined activity against melanoma (see Table 46–7). Response rates are generally between 10% and 20%. Hematologic toxicity of the nitrosoureas can be more severe than with DTIC and is cumulative. Carmustine (BCNU), lomustine (CCNU), semustine (methyl-CCNU), and fotemustine are the best studied of this class.[319–331] Sites of responses are similar to those responding to DTIC (*e.g.*, skin, subcutaneous tissues, lymph nodes, lungs). Because the central nervous system is a common site for metastasis, it was hoped that the lipid-soluble nitrosoureas would induce frequent responses at brain sites. This generally has not been the case, with the possible exception of fotemustine. Fotemustine was synthesized to facilitate penetration into cells and through the blood–brain barrier by addition of an amino acid analogue 1-amino-ethyl-phosphonic acid chain onto a chlorethyl-nitrosourea to take advantage of cellular amino acid transport systems. Although response rates of fotemustine are similar to those observed with other nitrosoureas and with DTIC, fotemustine was reported to induce 9 partial responses in 36 patients with brain metastases, an observation that needs to be confirmed.[330] Recently, a new nitrosourea, tauromustine (TCNU), has demonstrated activity in melanoma.[331]

Activity against melanoma has been detected with several other classes of agents (see Table 46–7). Cisplatin and the related compound carboplatin have measurable, although generally limited, activity against melanoma.[332–340] The vinca alkaloids vindesine, vincristine, and vinblastine have marginal activity against metastatic melanoma, with response rates in the range of 12% to 14%.[341–369] Both these classes have been used widely in combination therapies for melanoma. Taxol, a plant product derived from the Western yew tree (*Taxus brevifolia*), promotes microtubule assembly. Because of limited supply, clinical trials with taxol have been restricted, but preliminary findings in melanoma are encouraging and need to be extended.[370–372] Dibromodulcitol (mitolactol), a lipid-soluble agent with alkylating properties, has been shown to have activity in melanoma.[373–381] It has been suggested that a daily dose schedule is more effective than an intermittent dose schedule. Two other agents, the semisynthetic anthracycline detorubicin and the dihydrofolate reductase inhibitor piritrexim, have been reported to have activity in single phase II trials, but these studies need to be confirmed.[382,383]

HIGH-DOSE CHEMOTHERAPY WITH OR WITHOUT AUTOLOGOUS BONE MARROW TRANSPLANTATION. Increasing dose is one strategy to overcome resistance to therapy. Because single agents have only limited activity in melanoma, dose could be a factor in establishing more respectable complete response rates in melanoma, particularly with alkylating agents. Most studies exploring high-dose chemotherapy have been phase I–II trials using autologous bone marrow rescue. Several drugs have been evaluated, including alkylating agents (*e.g.*, melphalan, thiotepa), DTIC, and nitrosoureas.[384–400]

High-dose chemotherapy trials with autologous bone marrow rescue have generally involved small numbers of patients (Table 46–8). Responses have been observed in 38% of patients treated with high-dose BCNU.[389] High-dose melphalan

TABLE 46–8. Results of High-Dose Chemotherapy Trials With Autologous Bone Marrow Transplantation

Agent	No. of Patients	Response (%)	CR (%)	Median Response Duration (mo)	References
Melphalan	48	58	19	3–6	390–392
Thiotepa	51	57	8	3	393
BCNU	29	38	13	6	389
DTIC + melphalan or ifosfamide	37	49	14	4	400
BCNU combinations*	38	50	8	2–4	385, 394–396, 399

CR, complete response.
* BCNU plus varying combinations of melphalan, cisplatin, and cyclophosphamide.

or thiotepa has induced responses in 50% to 60% of patients.[390-393] High-dose BCNU has been added to varying combinations of melphalan, thiotepa, cyclophosphamide, or cisplatin, with a 50% overall response rate.[385,394-396,398,399] High doses of DTIC plus melphalan or ifosfamide have produced responses in 49% of patients.[400] Although these results are encouraging, they cannot be considered a meaningful advance. Toxicity of these regimens is substantial, and they are associated with fatalities (in up to a third of cases at very high doses). Although advances in hematopoietic growth factors suggest that this approach can be extended, life-threatening toxic reactions can occur at extramedullary sites (e.g., liver, lung). The least encouraging aspect of these trials has been the low rate of long-term responses. In trials with adequate follow-up, median durations of response have been short, in

the range of 3 to 6 months, and meaningful remissions in non-lung visceral lesions have been infrequent.

There has been considerable interest in the past few years in the dose-response relation of cisplatin in the treatment of melanoma. The aggregate of studies has not found a dose-response relation after systemic treatment with doses of up to 200 mg/m² (Table 46–9). In general, response rates with high doses of cisplatin, either alone or in combination, are not discernibly improved over standard doses.[320-339] However, a regimen of cisplatin (60 to 150 mg/m²) in combination with WR 2721 (ethiofos), a thiol derivative that protects normal host tissues, has been reported to give an objective response rate of 45% (23 of 51 patients, including patients with metastatic sites in the liver).[335,401,402] Median duration of response was only 3 months. A recent update showed a 55%

TABLE 46–9. Cisplatin-based Chemotherapy in Melanoma

Regimen	No. of Evaluable Patients	No. of Responses (%)	Complete Response (%)	References
Single-Agent Therapy				
Cisplatin (all doses)	18	43 (23)	3	332–339
<100 mg/m²	10	1 (10)	0	333
100–149 mg/m²	125	28 (22)	2	320, 334, 335
≥150 mg/m²	53	14 (26)	6	335–339
Combination Chemotherapy				
Cisplatin (all doses)	1279	363 (28)	7	321, 406–409, 442–447, 449, 451, 453–469, 470–473, 476, 478, 479, 482, 484
<100 mg/m²	764	199 (26)	5	321, 406, 407–409, 442, 447, 452, 456–462, 464, 465, 467–469, 470, 472, 473, 478, 479, 482
100–149 mg/m²	389	126 (32)	10	443–446, 451, 453, 455, 457, 430–457
≥150 mg/m²	126	38 (30)	10	449, 451, 454, 475, 476, 484

(Adapted from Steffens TA, Bajoin DF, Chapman PB, et al. A phase II trial of high-dose cisplatin and dacarbazine: Lack of efficacy of high-dose cisplatin-based therapy for metastatic melanoma. Cancer 1991;68:1230)

response rate (5 complete and 15 partial responses) in 36 patients treated with 150 mg/m² cisplatin plus WR 2721; the median duration of response was 6 months.[402] This regimen is given as a rapid 30-minute infusion every 3 to 4 weeks, and it has been suggested that the schedule of treatment might be important, because most high-dose regimens of cisplatin with lower response rates have used divided dose schedules.[402] The cisplatin/WR 2721 regimen is being tested in an Eastern Cooperative Oncology Group randomized trial.

Regional administration of cisplatin has allowed very high doses to be administered. Regional perfusion of high-dose cisplatin, 100 to 200 mg/m², with hyperthermia (38–40.5°C) in limbs with in-transit disease produced responses in 67% of 15 patients (95% confidence interval, 43–91%).[403] Complete responses were observed in 6 patients (40%), but only 3 responses were durable (> 2 years). Toxicity was severe at doses of more than 150 mg/m². In this study, very high plasma levels in the isolated limb were achieved, with doses (areas under the curve) generally 10-fold higher than similar doses given systemically. Despite treatment with extraordinary doses, durable responses were achieved in a minority of patients with favorable sites of disease. Intrahepatic arterial chemoembolization using cisplatin combined with polyvinyl sponges has been reported to produce responses in 46% of 30 patients with liver metastases from ocular melanoma.[404,405] Liver metastases from ocular melanoma rarely respond to systemic therapy with cisplatin-based combination regimens or to intrahepatic infusion of cisplatin alone, suggesting that tissue injury or necrosis produced by embolization might overcome cisplatin resistance.

COMBINATION THERAPY FOR SYSTEMIC METASTATIC MELANOMA. The role of combination chemotherapy in treatment of advanced melanoma is not entirely clear. This is because the history of combination chemotherapy for melanoma is not orderly. There have been many single and unconfirmed reports of initial high response rates, followed by confirmatory trials or randomized studies that find response rates that are similar to DTIC. For example, despite an initial encouraging report of high response rates for a combination of cisplatin, vinblastine, and bleomycin (PVB), confirmatory trials and randomized studies comparing PVB with DTIC showed no advantage for the combination.[406–409] Because toxicity of DTIC is minimal when treatment is accompanied by effective antiemetic therapy, it is important to demonstrate meaningful therapeutic gains of potentially more toxic and expensive combination regimens.

Combination chemotherapy trials for melanoma can be categorized into two types. The first approach has been to develop combinations of agents that have demonstrated single-agent activity. Despite an impression that combination regimens containing cisplatin are generally superior to DTIC alone, this has not been formally established (see Table 46–9). The overall response rates in combination regimens containing either low-dose or high-dose cisplatin are not detectably greater than DTIC. Clinical trials of DTIC in combination with nitrosoureas, vinca alkaloids, interferon-α, or cisplatin have response rates of 13% to 32%, in the range of rates with these single agents used alone.[410–436] The lack of clearly additive or synergistic antitumor effects of combinations has been disappointing.[410–442] This is perhaps due to the marginal activity of most of these drugs and suggests that resistance mechanisms of melanoma cells crosses these different classes of drugs.

Three groups of combination regimens in Table 46–10 are worth noting. First, combinations of DTIC, a vinca alkaloid, and cisplatin have had an overall response rate of 32% in reported trials.[420–436] Without direct comparison with DTIC, it is not possible to affirm that these combination regimens are definitely better than DTIC, and they certainly involve more toxicity. One regimen of this sort is the CVD combination developed at the M.D. Anderson Cancer Center: cisplatin 20 mg/m² intravenously on days 1 to 5, vinblastine 1.6 mg/m² intravenously on days 1 to 5, and DTIC 800 mg/m² on day 1.[436] A combination regimen, often called the Dartmouth regimen, comprised of DTIC, BCNU, cisplatin and ta-

TABLE 46–10. Results of Combination Regimens Containing DTIC

Regimen	No. of Evaluable Patients	% Response Rate (95% CI)	Complete Response (%)	References
DTIC Plus:				
Nitrosourea	302	21 (16–25)	7	294, 297, 410–416
Vinca alkaloid	223	18 (13–23)	4	311, 315, 325, 410, 417–420
Interferon-α	387	27 (23–31)	9	421–430
Nitrosourea + vinca alkaloid	1114	23 (20–25)	6	307, 308, 311, 431–440
Cisplatin + vinca alkaloid	255	32 (26–38)	7	441–447
Cisplatin + tamoxifen	23	13 (0–27)	9	476
Nitrosourea + cisplatin + tamoxifen	141	46 (38–54)	11	402, 477–480

95% CI, 95% confidence interval for response rates.

moxifen, has a reported response rate of 46% (95% confidence interval, 38–54%) in 141 evaluable patients in sequential phase II studies.[439-441] The reported complete response rate was 11% (95% confidence interval, 6–17%).[402] Again, no direct comparison with DTIC has been made. Toxicity is generally greater than observed with DTIC and includes occasional severe neutropenia and thrombocytopenia, which can be related to cumulative dose (especially for BCNU). This regimen was initially published by Del Prete and colleagues, with follow-up studies from McClay and colleagues.[439-441] The doses of drugs are as follows: cisplatin 25 mg/m^2 and DTIC 220 mg/m^2 administered intravenously daily for 3 days every 4 weeks, BCNU 150 mg/m^2 intravenously once every 8 weeks, and tamoxifen 10 mg orally twice a day throughout therapy.[440] Because tamoxifen has no demonstrated activity against melanoma and might contribute to toxicity (in particular deep vein thrombosis and pulmonary embolism), it was eliminated from the combination in a follow-up study.[441-443] Responses were observed in only 10% (2 of 20) of patients.[367]

In a subsequent study by the same group, adding tamoxifen increased the response rate back to 53%.[402] This intriguing observation suggested that tamoxifen might be critical for the activity of the combination. In clonogenic assays, the combination of tamoxifen with cisplatin, but not BCNU, has been reported to be synergistic.[442] A pilot study of escalated doses of tamoxifen (160 mg daily) with DTIC, BCNU, and cisplatin produced a possible increase in hematologic toxicity, and 7 responses (including 4 complete responses) were observed in 15 patients.[402] The basis for the possible increased activity of this regimen is a mystery. If this regimen has an improved response rate, BCNU and tamoxifen may be crucial. This is suggested by a phase II trial of cisplatin, DTIC, and tamoxifen (without BCNU) in which there were responses in only 3 of 23 patients (13% response rate; 95% confidence interval, 0–27%), a result consistent with response rates observed with cisplatin plus DTIC or DTIC alone.[437-438] Results of a randomized study comparing the Dartmouth regimen with DTIC are needed to assess further the efficacy of the Dartmouth regimen. A third combination regimen uses DTIC plus interferon-α (see below for a discussion of interferon-α therapy). The mean overall response rate in these trials is 27%.[410-419] Results of randomized trials are conflicting. A small randomized trial showed a significantly higher response rate in patients treated with DTIC plus interferon-α compared with DTIC alone.[419] However, a preliminary report from a larger randomized trial showed no response rate advantage for combinations of DTIC plus interferon-α versus DTIC, but did demonstrate a significant prolongation of response duration for the combination.[418]

A second approach has been to combine defined active agents (*e.g.*, DTIC, nitrosoureas) with agents having little or no known activity against melanoma.[444,445] It is not surprising that these trials have usually shown discouraging results, particularly noticeable in confirmatory studies after preliminary reports of high response rates. Response rates with these combination regimens are not distinctly better than single-agent DTIC or the same combination of active drugs used without the inactive agent (*e.g.*, regimens containing DTIC, nitrosourea, vinca alkaloid, and bleomycin compared with the same drugs without bleomycin). For example, a regimen of CCNU, procarbazine (minimal single-agent activity), and vincristine was originally reported to have a response rate of 48% in 44 patients, with 25% of patients achieving complete responses. However, a confirmatory trial by the NCI of Canada observed only a 12% response rate (2% complete responses) with the same regimen in 65 patients.[444,445]

Biologic Therapy

There is evidence that the immune system can influence the pathogenesis of melanoma. Several biologic agents have been tested in patients with metastatic melanoma and have demonstrated antitumor activity (Table 46–11). The rapid evo-

TABLE 46–11. Clinical Trials With Recombinant Interferon-α

Interferon Type	Dose (mU/m^2)	Weekly Schedule	No. of Evaluable Patients	No. of PR + CR (%)	CR	References
α2a	12–50	tiw	96	22 (23)	4	494
α2a	18–36	qd	17	4 (24)	0	495
α2a	15–50	—	18	2 (11)	2	496
α2a	10	biw	12	1 (8)	0	497
α2a	18–36	tiw	62	5 (8)	0	498
α2b	10–50	qd $\times$ 5	23	4 (17)	2	499
α2b	10	tiw	45	10 (22)	4	501
α2b	20	qd $\times$ 5	12	0 (0)	0	502
α2b	—	—	24	7 (29)	2	503
α2b	30	qd $\times$ 5	27	1 (4)	0	504
α2b	20	qd $\times$ 5	26	3 (12)	2	505
α2c	$\leq$30	qd	10	2 (20)	1	506
α2c	5–30	qd	8	1 (12)	1	507
Total			380	60 (16)	18	

PR, partial response; CR, complete response.

lution of recombinant DNA technology to produce cytokines such as interferons and interleukins and of hybridoma methodology to develop monoclonal antibodies has allowed purified reagents to be produced in large quantities for clinical trials. The availability of these agents and the development of assays to measure them are allowing better studies about their pharmacology, mechanisms of action, and effects on various components of the immune system. Among this class of agents, the type I interferons (specifically recombinant interferon-α) and interleukin-2 (IL-2) have been studied most extensively. Other treatments under intensive investigation are monoclonal antibodies and active immunotherapy by vaccination.

INTERFERON-α. Interferon-α is an active agent in the treatment of metastatic melanoma.[446] Initial clinical investigations of interferon-α in patients with cancer used a purified preparation obtained from virus-stimulated buffy coat leukocytes.[447] The purification of small quantities of interferon-α required huge amounts of blood products and resulted in a final product that was less than 2% pure. Production was made more complicated by the fact that the interferon-α family consists of at least 20 proteins with a high degree of identity (> 80%) in amino acid sequences. The isolation of genes coding for leukocyte interferon-α allowed clinical studies of the pure (> 95%) recombinant materials to begin in 1983.

Although responses were observed infrequently in trials using purified natural interferon-α, trials using recombinant human interferon-α have confirmed that these agents have antitumor activity against melanoma (see Table 46–11).[448-463] Toxicity is manifested mainly by flu-like symptoms, myalgia, headache, chills, fever, and anorexia, with an accompanying drop in performance status during treatment with higher doses. Neutropenia can occur, and increases in serum transaminase levels occasionally require cessation of therapy. Continued treatment generally is associated with a decrease in side effects. Objective response rates average about 15% (see Table 46–11). Trials using daily or 3 times weekly schedules generally show more activity than trials using interrupted or intermittent schedules. As with other treatments, most responses have been partial and short-lived and occur mainly in skin, subcutaneous tissue, lymph node, and lung sites. Complete responses have been observed in about 5% of treated patients. Occasional durable complete responses have been observed.[446,450] An optimal dose of interferon-α has not been established, although there is a trend in favor of higher doses, suggested by a higher proportion of complete responses and a tendency toward longer durations of response.[448,449] Another notable feature of treatment with interferon-α is delay in response after starting treatment, a pattern different from most other therapies.[446] For example, a remarkable patient reported by Kirkwood and colleagues initially progressed after starting interferon-α but then achieved a complete response at 12 months.[446] Interferon-α is being evaluated in combination with cytotoxic agents, with other immunologic agents such as IL-2 and monoclonal antibodies, and in adjuvant trials.

Interferon-β binds to the same cell surface receptor as interferon-α. Side effects of interferon-β are similar to interferon-α, but it is unclear whether there might be a difference in clinical efficacy.[464] Interferon-γ, also called immune interferon, binds to distinct receptors and has several biologic properties that are distinct from interferon-α. Little activity against melanoma has been observed in preliminary clinical studies of interferon-γ.[465-468]

INTERLEUKIN-2 AND ADOPTIVE IMMUNOTHERAPY. A large body of evidence has demonstrated that rejection of established tumors can be mediated by cellular immune responses. Observations in experimental animal models, using both immunogenic and poorly immunogenic tumors, showed that high doses of IL-2 could induce tumor regressions of established micrometastases in liver and lung.[469-474] When lymphocytes are activated by IL-2, they acquire enhanced lytic activity for tumor cells and are called lymphokine-activated killer (LAK) cells.[470] The addition of LAK cells to treatment with high doses of IL-2 has produced higher therapeutic efficacy in animal models than either treatment alone.[471-474]

These experimental studies in animal models led Rosenberg and colleagues to design phase I trials to evaluate IL-2 and activated lymphocytes individually and then in combination.[475] Clinical trials of high-dose bolus injections of IL-2, with or without the addition of LAK cells, have demonstrated reproducible responses in patients with metastatic melanoma, with response rates of 10% to 25% using several doses and schedules of administration.[475-494] Table 46–12 lists results of studies using IL-2 alone or combined with adoptive cellular therapy with LAK cells. Activity of IL-2 was first described by Rosenberg and colleagues at the NCI Surgery Branch in Maryland using bolus injection of IL-2 and subsequently was confirmed by other groups. Partial responses are typically of short duration, but durable complete responses have been observed in a small proportion of patients. The toxic effects of high-dose IL-2 can be severe and are dependent on dose and schedule. They include oliguria, pulmonary insufficiency, central nervous system changes, arrhythmias, hypotension, and, infrequently, myocardial infarction.[495-498] Toxicities generally clear rapidly with the exception of neurologic effects, which can reverse more slowly. Treatment-associated mortality has been observed in 1% to 2% of patients, usually related to myocardial infarction and central catheter sepsis.

Continuous intravenous infusion of IL-2 is biologically more active than bolus IL-2, as measured by the height of rebound lymphocytosis after treatment and the activity of circulating lymphocytes during treatment. However, response rates of IL-2 administered by continuous infusion generally have been inferior to clinical results with bolus IL-2 administration, and bolus IL-2 is the preferred schedule of administration. Response rates are similar with and without LAK cells, suggesting that any effect of LAK cells is marginal. Data from the NCI Surgery Branch show a possible advantage for durable responses in patients treated with LAK, but this observation remains to be confirmed.[478] A report from Mitchell and colleagues has suggested that the addition of low-dose cyclophosphamide to low-dose infusion IL-2 can result in a response rate greater than 20%.[493,494]

T lymphocytes may play a crucial role in tumor regression produced by treatment with IL-2. This has been demonstrated in animal models.[499,500] Cytotoxic T lymphocytes that specifically kill or proliferate in response to autologous melanoma cells can be isolated from patients with advanced melanoma.[434,512] Regressing tumors biopsied after IL-2 therapy show infiltration of T lymphocytes.[513] Animal models have

TABLE 46–12.   Clinical Trials With Interleukin-2

Schedule	No. of Evaluable Patients	No. of Responses (%)	No. of Complete Responses (%)	95% Confidence Interval (%)	References
Bolus I.V.					
IL-2 alone	175	31 (18)	4 (2)	12–23	522, 525, 526, 532, 534, 536
IL-2/LAK	164	24 (15)	8 (5)	9–20	519–522, 525–527, 534, 536
IL-2/TIL*	20	11 (55)	1 (5)	33–77	559, 560
Continuous I.V.					
IL-2 alone	85	8 (9)	0 (0)	3–16	523, 531, 533, 535
IL-2/LAK	147	18 (12)	2 (1)	7–17	523, 528–530, 533
IL-2/TIL*	21	5 (24)	1 (5)	6–42	561
IL-2/CTX	38	9 (27)	2 (5)	11–38	537, 538
Bolus/Continuous I.V.					
IL-2/LAK	50	7 (14)	1 (2)	4–24	524

* IL-2/TIL was administered with cyclophosphamide.
LAK, lymphokine-activated killer cells; TIL, tumor-infiltrating lymphocytes; CTX, cyclophosphamide.

shown substantial antitumor activity of adoptive immunotherapy using lymphocytes isolated from tumor sites (tumor-infiltrating lymphocytes, or TILs).[514] Animals primed with either cyclophosphamide or total body irradiation were injected with IL-2-expanded TIL and treated with IL-2.[514] Much lower doses of IL-2 were needed to attain the equivalent antitumor effects seen in animals treated with high-dose IL-2 plus LAK cells. Based on these preclinical studies, clinical evaluation of adoptive immunotherapy with TIL and IL-2 were initiated.[515,516] A trial from the NCI Surgery Branch observed 11 responses in 20 patients (55%) treated with bolus IL-2 and TIL in conjunction with cyclophosphamide.[515,516] A trial using continuous infusion IL-2 and TIL plus cyclophosphamide observed a 24% response rate in 21 patients, consistent with the lower response rate of continuous infusion IL-2.[517]

MONOCLONAL ANTIBODIES. The diagnosis and treatment of melanoma with monoclonal antibodies has been treated in detail elsewhere.[518,519] Two strategies are being pursued for monoclonal antibody (MoAb) treatment of melanoma: treatment with MoAb alone to activate the host immune system, and treatment with MoAb conjugated to cytotoxic agents, either radioisotope or plant toxins (*e.g.*, ricin A chain).

Clinical trials have been performed with unconjugated MoAbs and MoAbs conjugated to radionuclides or toxins. Phase I studies of mouse MoAb alone have shown that MoAb can reach tumor sites after systemic administration.[520–525] Responses have been observed after treatment with several MoAbs against the gangliosides GD2 and GD3.[520,521,525–531] However, responses have not been observed after treatment with unconjugated MoAb against two glycoprotein antigens (p97 and the high molecular weight proteoglycan antigen).[521,523,524,532] Responses have been reported after treat-

ment with MoAb conjugated to radionuclide or the A chain of the plant toxin ricin.[533–536]

The most intensively studied MoAbs have been anti-GD3 MoAbs, particularly MoAb R24.[520,525–528] Several other MoAbs against GD3 have been investigated, including MoAbs MG-21 and ME36.1.[529,530] These anti-GD3 MoAbs are notable because they are efficient at mediating activation of human complement and triggering killing of melanoma cells in the presence of human peripheral blood mononuclear cells (antibody-dependent cellular cytotoxicity). MoAb R24 can induce inflammatory responses specifically within tumor sites after intravenous administration.[520,525,527] Toxicity generally has been mild to moderate after treatment with low doses. The maximum tolerated doses have not been defined for most unconjugated MoAbs. However, the maximum tolerated dose of MoAb R24 resulted in malignant hypertension, associated with markedly excessive serum levels of catecholamines, at cumulative doses of more than 1200 mg/m^2 administered over 5 to 7 days.[537] This side effect is probably caused by weak reactivity of MoAb with the adrenal medulla, an organ that has a developmental origin that is similar to melanocytes. No other severe end-organ symptom has been observed, for example, to be related to reactivity of R24 with melanocytes in the skin or eye.

Trials of MoAb have been limited until recently by difficulties in production of MoAb for clinical use. However, several phase I trials have been performed. Responses have been observed with anti-GD3 MoAb in phase I trials at 5 different institutions (Table 46–13).[520,526–530,538] Most trials have been performed using systemic administration, but in one trial, isolated limb perfusion with R24 was performed.[528] Most responses have been observed at lower doses (≤ 30 mg/m^2 daily). Durable responses in soft tissue or visceral lesions have been observed in a small number of patients, in some cases

TABLE 46–13. Phase I Trials of Unconjugated Monoclonal Antibodies Against GD2 and GD3 Ganglioside Antigens

MoAb	Antigen	Route	No. of Evaluable Patients	Response	References
R24	GD3	I.V.	21	4 PR	564, 569
R24	GD3	I.V.	5	2 PR	570
R24	GD3	I.V.	6	1 CR	595
				1 PR	
R24 (high-dose)	GD3	I.V.	7	NR	590
R24	GD3	ILP	12	1 PR	572
MG21	GD3	I.V.	8	1 CR	573
Me36.1	GD2/GD3	I.V.	13	1 CR	574
3F8	GD2	I.V.	9	2 PR	566
L72	GD2	IL	8	4 PR	575

CR, complete response; IL, intralesional; ILP, isolated limb perfusion; I.V., intravenous; MoAb, monoclonal antibody; NR, no response; PR, partial response.

lasting more than 2 years.[530,530a] MoAb 3F8 against the related ganglioside GD2 has shown antitumor activity against melanoma in phase I trials.[521] Anti-GD2 MoAbs but not anti-GD3 MoAbs can produce neurologic symptoms, particularly severe pain.[521] This toxicity is observed even at low doses and may be related to reactivity of anti-GD2 MoAb with peripheral nerve fibers. This side effect may limit the application of some anti-GD2 MoAbs in melanoma.

A pilot trial of MoAb fragments against the glycoprotein p97 antigen and conjugated to the radionuclide iodine 131 has been reported.[533] Up to 500 mCi of radioisotope was administered, and the primary dose-limiting toxic effects (thrombocytopenia and neutropenia) were due to marrow irradiation. Ricin, a natural product of beans from the plant *Ricinus communis*, is a potent inhibitor of protein synthesis. Ricin is composed of two chains, designated A and B, that are disulfide linked. The A chain is able to inhibit protein synthesis. The ricin A chain has been conjugated to MoAbs, and phase I trials have demonstrated generally mild toxicity (*e.g.,* flu-like symptoms, hepatic enzyme elevations).[534–536] A phase II study in 46 patients with melanoma has been completed; 1 complete response and 3 partial responses were observed.[536]

Because most antimelanoma MoAbs are of mouse origin, they have generally induced a human immunoglobulin (Ig) G response to the mouse immunoglobulin.[520,521,523,524,537–539] This immune resistance to mouse MoAb can effectively prevent the MoAb from reaching tumor sites. Two methods are being explored to bypass the human antimouse immunoglobulin response. First, genes coding for mouse MoAbs can be genetically manipulated to construct humanized MoAbs composed of mouse antigen-binding regions ligated to human immunoglobulin sequences.[540,541] These engineered humanized MoAbs should be reaching clinical trials shortly. A second approach is to derive human MoAbs from melanoma antigens. Human MoAbs to the gangliosides GD2 and GD3 have been isolated, and a pilot trial of intralesional injection of a human IgM anti-GD2 MoAb showed partial and complete regression of injected skin lesions.[531]

ACTIVE IMMUNIZATION: TUMOR VACCINES. Tumor vaccines have a long history, but the search for effective methods to induce active immunity against tumors has been difficult. Repeated attempts have been made to inhibit the outgrowth of tumors and to influence the natural history of melanoma by immunization with tumor cells or extracts of tumor cells. More recently, purified antigens, recombinant vaccines, genetically modified melanoma cells, and antiidiotype antibodies have entered into clinical trials. Evidence is mounting that vaccination can induce immune responses to melanoma. Trials have been initiated to evaluate potential efficacy of vaccines as adjuvant therapy in high-risk patients. Table 46–14 lists the strategies that are being taken to construct melanoma vaccines. At this point, there is no consensus on which approaches are most promising. Most clinical studies have been performed in patients after resection of regional

TABLE 46–14. Strategies for Immunization

I. Whole Melanoma Cells
  A. Autologous cells
  B. Allogeneic cells
  C. Neuraminidase-treated cells
  D. Haptenized cells
II. Melanoma Cell Lysates
  A. Viral oncolysates
    1. Vaccinia virus
    2. Newcastle disease virus
    3. Vesicular stomatitis virus
  B. Shed melanoma cell supernatant
III. Purified Antigens
  A. Gangliosides
IV. Recombinant Vaccines
  A. v-P97ny
V. Gene Therapy
  A. Expression of tumor necrosis factor and interleukin-2 in melanoma cells
VI. Antiidiotype Monoclonal Antibodies
  A. Anti-HMW-MAA
  B. Anti-GD3 ganglioside

lymph node metastases or high-risk primary lesions and in patients with advanced metastatic disease. Responses have been observed in a few patients with advanced disease, but these appear to be infrequent. Patients who develop evidence of immune responses have improved disease-free survival and overall survival.[541-549] This does not mean that vaccines improve the clinical course (*e.g.*, patients who a priori have a better prognosis may be more likely to develop an immune response to vaccination) but is consistent with the hypothesis that an immune response induced by vaccination can prevent cancer recurrence.

Problems exist in the construction of tumor vaccines, including weak immunogenicity of tumor antigens, heterogeneity of antigen expression in tumors, and the ability of tumors to escape an immune response.[60,61,70] Most melanoma antigens on tumor cells are not tumor-specific (*i.e.*, present only on cancer cells) but are shared with certain normal cells.[60,70]

Early specific vaccination trials in melanoma (as opposed to nonspecific vaccination with BCG) used immunization with unmodified, irradiated allogeneic or autologous melanoma cells, either alone or in combination with BCG and other nonspecific immunomodulators. In these trials, it has been difficult to show that vaccination had any benefit or elicited any specific immune responses.[550-553] One exception has been immune responses to gangliosides, the major acidic glycolipid of melanoma cells, in some patients immunized with selected allogeneic melanoma cells.[543,544]

Efforts have been made to improve immunogenicity of allogeneic tumor cells by using the enzyme neuraminidase to remove sialic acid residues from the cell surface.[554,555] Strategies have been developed to augment the immune response to tumor antigens by infecting tumor cells with nonpathogenic viruses. Viral proteins presented on the cell membrane of tumors have been shown to augment the immunogenicity of tumor antigens.[546,547,549] Several centers have investigated the immunogenicity of lysates derived from tumor cells infected with Newcastle disease virus, vaccinia virus, and vesicular stomatitis virus. Prospective randomized clinical trials are under way to evaluate the potential efficacy of viral oncolysates in an adjuvant setting. Another approach to increasing immune response has been to alter tumor cells by binding haptens to autologous tumor cells.[556] Genetic alteration of melanoma cells, called gene therapy, is being investigated to augment the immune response against weakly immunogenic melanoma antigens. Cells have been altered to secrete the immunologically active molecules tumor necrosis factor and IL-2, and clinical studies of vaccination with genetically modified cells have been initiated.[557,558]

An effort is under way to immunize patients with purified or partially purified preparations of potentially immunogenic molecules from melanoma cells. The rationale for this approach comes from the identification of antigens on melanoma cells that can be recognized by antibodies in sera or lymphocytes from patients with melanoma. Gangliosides have been shown to induce antibody responses after immunization.[543,544] Of particular interest, the ganglioside GM2 can induce IgM antibody responses in up to 90% of immunized patients, and prospective randomized studies have been started to evaluate GM2 and other ganglioside vaccines. Another strategy has been to use supernatants containing a mixture of shed melanoma antigens for immunization.[544]

Other molecules that are recognized by the humoral immune response of melanoma patients, the antigens, have been isolated, and genes encoding these antigens have been cloned.[56,559] These genes are being used to construct recombinant DNA vaccines. A vaccine has been constructed by expressing the p97 melanoma antigen in vaccinia virus vector, and clinical trials have been initiated.[559] In preclinical studies, the p97 glycoprotein antigen was immunogenic in primates immunized with the recombinant vaccine. The identification of melanoma antigens recognized by T lymphocytes opens avenues for the construction of vaccines to elicit specific cellular immune responses.[560]

A final approach has been to mimic melanoma antigens using antiidiotype MoAb. Certain antiidiotype monoclonal antibodies can function as "images" of tumor antigens to elicit immune responses. Antiidiotype monoclonal antibodies have been shown to mimic the high molecular weight proteoglycan melanoma antigen and the ganglioside GD3.[561-564] Clinical trials have been initiated with antiidiotype vaccines in patients with stages III and IV melanomas.

There are several agents that might be used to augment nonspecifically the immunogenicity of vaccines. First, immune adjuvants can augment the level, duration, and quality of the immune response elicited by specific antigens. The standard adjuvant, alum, has not been shown to be very effective. BCG is an effective adjuvant for vaccines with GM2 ganglioside.[544] Detoxified endotoxin, liposomes, saponin, muramyl peptides, and other substances are being actively investigated as adjuvants. A clinical trial using allogeneic melanoma cell lysates and an adjuvant containing detoxified endotoxin (DETOX) observed 4 responses in 25 patients with metastatic melanoma.[565]

A second issue has been the phenomenon of suppressor lymphocytes. Studies in mice bearing transplantable tumors have demonstrated that a population of T lymphocytes can actively suppress specific immune responses, and suppression mediated by these T lymphocytes can be abrogated by low doses of cyclophosphamide.[566] Studies in humans suggest that low-dose cyclophosphamide can enhance humoral and cell-mediated response to tumor antigens, and some vaccine trials have incorporated pretreatment with cyclophosphamide.[566-569] Responses have been observed occasionally in patients treated with autologous melanoma cell vaccine plus low-dose cyclophosphamide.[565,570]

INTRALESIONAL THERAPY. A high proportion of skin lesions have been shown to regress after injection with nonspecific immunomodulatory agents such as BCG. The first study of this kind was done by Morton in 1971, and subsequent investigations confirmed that injection of BCG into superficial cutaneous lesions leads to responses at the injected sites (in about two thirds of lesions) and occasionally at uninjected sites (in 21% of lesions in proximity to injected lesions).[571-575] Other agents, including purified protein derivative, methanol extracted residue, and dinitrochlorobenzene, have produced similar results.[576-579] Intralesional therapy is most likely to induce regressions of small dermal lesions; the response of subcutaneous or large tumors is substantially lower.

Combinations of Biologic Agents and Chemotherapy

Exploration of combinations of biologic agents and chemotherapy for treatment of melanoma is an active area of investigation. Combinations of chemotherapy and immunologic agents have a long history. Early clinical trials of chemotherapy combined with nonspecific immunomodulators such as BCG, *Corynebacterium parvum*, or levamisole did not demonstrate any beneficial effects. Recent in vitro and preclinical studies in animals have suggested that combinations of recombinant cytokines or monoclonal antibodies (*e.g.,* IL-2 and interferon-α, monoclonal antibody and IL-2, tumor necrosis factor and interferon-γ) are additive or synergistic. Clinical trials of cytokines with and without chemotherapy have been initiated.[580–583]

Phase I–II studies have evaluated combinations of IL-2, interferon, and chemotherapy, including cisplatin, DTIC, and cyclophosphamide.[493,494,515,516,584–592] The combination of DTIC and interferon-α is discussed in the section on combination chemotherapy. Preliminary results of a series of small studies using combinations of IL-2, interferon-α, and cisplatin either alone or in combination chemotherapy regimens have reported overall response rates of 40% in 169 patients (95% confidence interval, 32–47%).[588–592] These preliminary results need to be extended in larger prospective trials. Combinations of IL-2 and interferon (interferon-α or interferon-β) have been examined in preliminary trials.[593–603] There is a suggestion that response rates to the combination may be higher than with either cytokine alone, particularly at higher dose levels, but toxicity may be additive.

Biologic agents that induce inflammation are beginning to be explored. Inflammatory monoclonal antibodies are being used in combination with IL-2, interferon-α, macrophage colony-stimulating factor, or tumor necrosis factor-α.[604] The proinflammatory cytokines tumor necrosis factor-α and interferon-γ have synergistic effects in vitro and have been studied clinically in combination in a phase I trial.[605] A preliminary report of the combination of tumor necrosis factor-α, interferon-γ, and melphalan administered as a regional limb perfusion was reported to induce complete response in 89% of patients with in-transit metastases, although substantial toxicity was observed.[606]

Endocrine Therapy

There appears to be little role for single-agent endocrine therapy in the treatment of melanoma. Clinical reports of responses to tamoxifen are mainly anecdotal, and extensive trials have demonstrated minimal or no activity for tamoxifen, the antiandrogen cyproterone acetate, or medroxyprogesterone acetate.[606] Tamoxifen has been proposed to have synergistic effects with a combination of DTIC, BCNU, and cisplatin.[441,443]

Status of Adjuvant Therapy

Advances in melanoma treatment over the past decade have evolved primarily from more detailed knowledge about prognostic factors of primary and metastatic lesions. Within the larger group of melanoma patients who undergo potentially curative treatment by surgical resection, subgroups can be identified who are at high risk for recurrence and for development of systemic metastases. Patients with thick primary melanomas (> 4.0 mm thick), in-transit lesions, and regional lymph node involvement are at particular risk. Once distant metastases develop, most patients die of their diseases. The investigation of adjuvant systemic treatment that can prevent melanoma recurrence remains a critical area of investigation. The rationale and general principles for adjuvant treatment of cancer are based on the premise that treatment, whether chemotherapy or immunotherapy, is more effective when the tumor cell population is small. Randomized trials using DTIC, nitrosoureas, a variety of combination chemotherapy regimens, BCG, *Corynebacterium parvum*, transfer factor, and combinations of immunotherapy and chemotherapy have not demonstrated any advantage for treatment.

Adjuvant treatment for melanoma should be considered within clinical research protocols. It is recommended that the option of experimental adjuvant treatment be considered for patients with AJCC stage II or III melanoma who are free of disease but are at high risk for recurrence. Investigations of adjuvant treatment include the following:

1. *Interferon.* No randomized trial has observed significant advantage for treatment with interferons. The Eastern Cooperative Oncology Group has a trial of adjuvant therapy with high-dose interferon-α2b compared with observation in stage II–III high-risk patients. Preliminary results suggest a survival advantage for the treated group, but the data have not reached maturity to support statistical significance.[607] Severe hepatic and neurologic toxicity were observed frequently in the 110 patients in the treatment arm. Two ongoing randomized intergroup trials are comparing high-dose and low-dose interferon-α with observation: a WHO randomized trial in AJCC stage III patients and a North Central Oncology Treatment Group trial in high-risk patients. A recent randomized trial of interferon-γ by the Southwest Oncology Group was closed because of possible adverse effects in the interferon-γ treatment arm.[608]

2. *Active immunization.* Various approaches to melanoma vaccination have been reviewed above. None of the randomized trials has demonstrated a survival or disease-free survival advantage in vaccinated patients. Small randomized studies of adjuvant vaccination with neuraminidase-treated allogeneic melanoma cells with BCG or with the ganglioside GM2 plus BCG have not demonstrated any benefit.[543,544,553] Survival advantage has been demonstrated in patients who develop specific immune responses to vaccination, but this observation does not establish that vaccination is causally related to improved survival.[543–549] There are several randomized trials ongoing to evaluate vaccination in an adjuvant setting, including studies using viral oncolysates and allogeneic melanoma cell lysates plus DETOX. Trials evaluating novel melanoma vaccine constructs are also under way (see Table 46–14).

3. *Levamisole.* Several randomized trials have been conducted with levamisole as an adjuvant agent. Three trials have shown no significant advantage of adjuvant therapy with levamisole over placebo.[609–615] A randomized trial of combination chemotherapy by the Southwest Oncol-

ogy Group demonstrated no advantage when levamisole was included with chemotherapy.[613] A recent randomized trial from the NCI of Canada Clinical Trials Group demonstrated a significant improvement in survival in groups treated with levamisole or levamisole plus BCG compared with an untreated control arm, providing the only evidence of adjuvant activity of levamisole.[610]

4. *Chemotherapy.* This option includes treatment with combination chemotherapy regimens that have activity against advanced metastatic melanoma. High-dose chemotherapy with autologous bone transplant has been evaluated in adjuvant trials. Agents with the best established activity against advanced melanoma, DTIC, and nitrosoureas, either alone or in combinations, have not shown any statistical advantage in survival or disease-free survival in adjuvant trials.

5. *Regional perfusion* of chemotherapy with or without hyperthermia has not shown any reduction in mortality in clinical studies to date when used as adjuvant therapy in patients at high-risk for locoregional recurrence.

6. *Other modalities.* A recent retrospective analysis of randomized trials from several centers suggested a survival advantage in patients with resected locoregional metastatic melanoma who were treated with *Corynebacterium parvum* compared with patients treated with BCG.[616] A small randomized study of megestrol acetate versus observation suggested a survival advantage for treated patients that approached significance (p = 0.06).[617]

MANAGEMENT OF SPECIFIC SITES OF METASTASES

Skin, Subcutaneous Tissues, and Distant Lymph Nodes

The most common sites of distant metastases are the skin and subcutaneous tissues.[145,242,243] Lesions are generally 0.5 to 2.0 cm in diameter and are readily detectable by physical examination. Occasionally, it may be clinically difficult to differentiate a cutaneous metastasis from a second primary melanoma. Distant metastases can occur in any lymph node chain and generally are asymptomatic. Superficial nodal metastases are easily diagnosed by physical examination. They usually can be detected on chest x-ray films, with CT scans or tomograms used as confirmatory tests, whereas abdominal metastatic nodes generally are detected by CT scans or ultrasonography.[255,618-621]

If distant nodal metastases are isolated (one or a few), surgical excision is the treatment of choice, providing a safe, quick, and effective treatment (see Table 46-6). They usually should be excised before they become bulky and symptomatic and require even more extensive surgery. These lesions should be excised with a rim of normal-appearing tissue (usually 0.5–1.0 cm) to minimize the risk of recurrence. Sequential metastases can be excised surgically unless they are multiple or appear in rapid succession. For multiple or recurrent lesions, radiation therapy may be considered as a second option.[270-281,283] For most dermal, subcutaneous, and lymph node metastases, we recommend treatment with 6 fractions of 600 cGy given twice weekly. The overall reported probability of a complete or partial response to radiation therapy in these sites is about 65%. This response rate is rather meaningless when tumor size is not considered. For lesions of 1 cm or less, response to radiation is almost universal, and about two-thirds of the tumors undergo complete and durable regression.[281] Conversely, a complete response was obtained in only about 20% of lesions greater than 5 cm in diameter in the RTOG study.[283] The use of radiation therapy should, therefore, be considered before metastatic deposits reach massive proportions.

Palliative radiation therapy is occasionally indicated for symptomatic nodal metastases in the mediastinum or retroperitoneum. When treating these sites, we recommend using a conventional fractionation regimen because of the poor tolerance of the thoracic spinal cord and abdominal viscera to large dose fractions. Systemic therapy, either experimental or standard, may be considered for widespread multiple lesions or symptomatic deep lymph nodes not accessible to radiation therapy. About 40% of patients with metastases localized in skin, subcutaneous tissues, or lymph nodes without visceral involvement survive more than 1 year, and 5% to 10% of these patients are alive at 5 years.

Lung, Pleura, and Mediastinum

The second most common initial sites of metastasis are the lungs and pleura (see Table 46-2). These lesions are evaluated by chest x-ray films preoperatively and during follow-up, whereas suspicious intrathoracic metastases are evaluated further by tomograms, CT scans, or bronchoscopy.

For screening purposes, standard chest x-ray films are sufficiently sensitive and cost-effective to be used for all melanoma patients. The yield of the more expensive pulmonary tomograms or CT scans is too low and the cost too high to justify when the chest x-ray films are normal.[244,619,622] Evaluation of suspicious metastases begins when one or more lesions are seen on chest x-ray films, the usual presentation of pulmonary metastases from melanoma.[145,243,623-625] Most patients have multiple pulmonary nodules; only 22% have solitary nodules.[626] Hilar and mediastinal adenopathy frequently accompany pulmonary metastases.[627]

Whole-lung tomograms or CT scans of the chest are of value in evaluating suspicious chest lesions or in determining whether the metastatic disease seen on chest x-ray films is also present elsewhere in the chest.[619,628-631] Bronchoscopy with biopsy may be considered in a few patients when the diagnosis of pulmonary lesions is in doubt. For solitary pulmonary metastases in asymptomatic patients, surgical excision may be indicated if no new lesions appear during an observation period of 3 to 4 weeks and if the tumor has a slow growth rate.[632] Whole-lung tomograms or CT scans are essential, for often a patient with a solitary lesion appearing on chest x-ray films actually has other pulmonary or intrathoracic lesions as well.[626,630,633] The operation is safe (< 1% mortality), but careful patient selection is important because only a minority of patients benefit. Surgical lesion of solitary pulmonary metastases is justified in selected patients, because truly long-term survival can be achieved.[242,267-269,633-638] The median postoperative survival ranges from 16 to 24 months, with 5-year survival rates of 12% to 21% in some large series. Not all institutions, however, have had such favorable results (see Table 46-6).[639,640]

Another justification for excising solitary pulmonary lesions is to confirm that they do not represent a second primary malignancy or a benign process. This situation can occur in up to one third of patients whose workups culminate in thoracotomies.[633,635] Patients who are not considered for surgery, such as those with multiple, slow-growing tumors, might be followed with no treatment at all while the tumors are asymptomatic. If the pulmonary metastases grow rapidly, especially if multiple visceral sites are involved or if the patient is symptomatic, an initial course of chemotherapy might be given. The response rate of DTIC chemotherapy is particularly poor for pulmonary metastases, and there is no evidence that the drug prolongs life.[250,641]

Brain and Spinal Cord

The brain is the initial site of metastases in 12% to 20% of melanoma patients and is usually associated with widespread visceral disease (Fig. 46–15).[145,240,246,250,642-646] At autopsy, cerebral metastases are present in 36% to 54% of patients.[230-240,241,250] The hemispheres generally are involved equally, with the cerebrum, usually the frontal lobe, involved most frequently, followed by the cerebellum, base of the brain, and spinal cord. Hydrocephalus is associated with about 33% of posterior fossa lesions. Cerebral metastases are solitary in only about 25% of patients.[246,645-648] An unusual feature of cerebral metastases is their propensity for hemorrhage, which occurs much more frequently than with other histologic types of metastases. Hemorrhage occurs in 33% to 50% of patients with melanoma metastases involving the brain.[645,649-651]

Headaches, alterations of mental status, and focal neurologic deficits are the most common symptoms of brain metastases.[245,646,648,649,652,653] Seizures are more common in patients with melanoma metastases in the brain than in patients with other types of brain tumors but occur in only about 25% of the melanoma patients with brain involvement.[649,652-654] It is common for these melanoma patients to present with subarachnoid or intracerebral hemorrhages.[645,649,650,655-660]

Routine brain scans are not useful for detecting occult metastases in asymptomatic patients in any disease stage. This was demonstrated in five separate series involving 504 patients with local or regional disease; not a single true-positive brain scan was obtained.[245,252,254,661,662] In patients with stage IV melanomas, cerebral metastases were detected by brain scan in 11% to 16% of patients studied, but all patients with positive scans had antecedent symptoms.[245,258,645,663]

The radiologic diagnosis of symptomatic melanoma metastases of the central nervous system has been reviewed in several published series.[510,650] The best single test for the diagnosis of intracerebral metastases is either an MRI or CT scan with contrast enhancement.[645,650,653,664-666] Compared with CT scans, MRI appears to have a better ability to distinguish hemorrhage from tumor. Leptomeningeal metastases can occur, usually in association with other distant metastases.[667,668]

Corticosteroids are the mainstay of initial treatment for brain metastases, the most effective being dexamethasone (up to 100 mg/day). This can reduce the edema around the tumor and relieve symptoms in most patients, at least temporarily.[669-671] Eighty-six percent of patients with multiple brain lesions treated with radiation therapy remained steroid dependent, whereas only 33% of patients with solitary lesions treated with surgery with or without radiation have remained steroid dependent.[654] Lack of improvement or exacerbation of symptoms during a trial of steroids can be due to intratumor hemorrhage with intracerebral hematoma.

Radiation therapy is the treatment of choice for multiple tumors. Chemotherapy generally is not effective for brain metastasis from melanoma.[250,643,652,670] Surgical excision is preferred for solitary and surgically accessible lesions. A craniotomy is a relatively safe procedure (with operative mortality of less than 5%) that alleviates symptoms in most patients and prevents further neurologic damage in patients with demonstrable metastases. It should be considered for some patients with symptomatic brain metastases, even when there is limited disease at other sites, because their estimated life span can exceed 2 to 3 months and their neurologic status usually improves. Whole-brain irradiation is generally given postoperatively.[242,269,643,644]

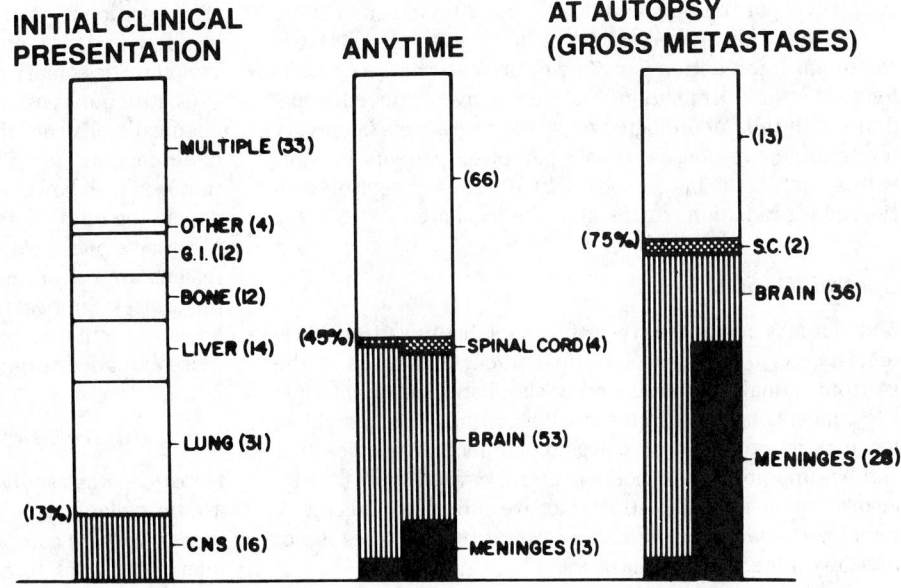

FIGURE 46–15. Incidence of central nervous system metastases in patients with advanced melanoma. The graph represents 122 patients and 53 autopsies. Central nervous system metastases sites were the first sites of relapse in 13% of patients. They occurred later in the clinical course in 45% of patients with metastases at other sites, and were present in 75% of patients at autopsy. The overlapping proportions indicate patients with more than one site of metastases. (Amer MH, Sarraf MA, Baker LH, et al. Malignant melanoma and central nervous system metastases: Incidence, diagnosis, treatment and survival. Cancer 1978;42:660)

Survival in different series averages about 7 months for surgically treated patients (see Table 46–6) and ranges from 2 to 20 months.[242,258,267–269,642–644,646–649,672–675] Satisfactory improvement in neurologic condition occurs in most patients. Survival results are influenced by remission duration, neurologic status at time of surgery, and presence of metastases at other sites.[676] Although long-term survival is uncommon, a few patients will live 3 to 5 years or more after surgery.[246,647,674,677–679]

Radiation therapy should be considered if the lesions are multiple or located in an area that would preclude a safe operation. Brain metastases present a challenging radiotherapeutic management problem. Although about 60% to 70% of patients receiving whole-brain radiation therapy experience measurable improvement in their performance status, benefit is usually of short duration and essentially all patients die with active intracranial disease. No modification of fractionation schedule[275,680,681] has been shown to be consistently superior to the reference standard of 3000 cGy in 10 fractions over 2 weeks for melanoma that is metastatic to the brain. There is a subset of good-prognosis patients treated with a high-dose accelerated fractionation regimen who may have derived a survival benefit.[682] We currently recommend 3000 cGy in 10 fractions to the whole brain as best standard treatment for patients with multiple metastases.

When surgical removal of brain metastases is possible, this should be performed and followed by whole-brain irradiation. A recent study from the M.D. Anderson Cancer Center demonstrated that combined treatment provided significantly improved survival over surgery alone.[683] If surgical margins are inadequate, a coned-down boost to the resection site to deliver a dose of 4500 cGy is justified. Patients with solitary brain metastases that are unresectable are candidates for treatment by stereotaxic radiosurgery, in which a large single ablative dose is given to a small volume encompassing the gross disease.[684]

Surgical decompression of obstructing spinal cord lesions is indicated in selected patients, although there is evidence that radiation therapy might be an effective alternative in some patients.[653,685] To maximize spinal cord tolerance in patients with a significant life expectation, we recommend treatment with conventional fractionation to a total dose of 4500 cGy at 250 cGy per fraction or 5000 cGy at 200 cGy per fraction.

High doses of corticosteroids should be given as well. Early treatment intervention is essential, because the best results for surgery and irradiation treatments have occurred in patients with mild neurologic symptoms; there have been very few treatment responses in totally paraplegic patients. Patients with symptomatic but nonobstructive disease might be considered for radiation treatment of the local area.[277]

Gastrointestinal Tract

Melanoma is one of the types of tumors that most frequently metastasize to the gastrointestinal tract. Metastases to the gastrointestinal tract usually occur simultaneously in multiple sites, most commonly in the small intestines. The individual lesions are exophytic or polypoid submucosal nodules that can be umbilicated or undergo central cavitation.[695–699] Metastases in the gastrointestinal tract are difficult to detect with radiologic studies, so the routine use of these studies is not indicated for screening purposes.

Early involvement of the gastrointestinal tract usually causes vague and subtle symptoms. The most common clinical manifestations are due to the following: chronic bleeding with anemia, anorexia, and weight loss; obstruction of the small bowel with abdominal pain, nausea, and vomiting; or acute bleeding with hematemesis or melena.[244,250,688,691–697]

Intussusception is a frequent cause of obstructive symptoms and other abdominal complaints, and numerous cases have been reported in the literature.[688,695,696,698] Intussusception usually follows a chronic or subacute course, characterized by an insidious onset. The triad of abdominal cramps, nausea without vomiting, and abdominal distention was the most consistent symptom in one series.[698]

The diagnosis of gastrointestinal metastases is usually made by barium contrast radiographs or by endoscopy. Several reviews have been written about the radiologic detection of metastatic melanoma involving the gastrointestinal tract.[688–690,699] All patients undergoing an upper gastrointestinal series for abdominal complaints should have a small bowel follow-through examination, because metastases are most likely to be present in this area. If the small bowel series is normal but there is a strong clinical suspicion of metastases, then a small bowel enteroclysis can be performed.

One of the most common symptoms of gastrointestinal metastases is chronic bleeding. In anemic patients, this can be treated with repeated blood transfusions. Systemic therapy can be considered for patients with multiple gastrointestinal lesions, and surgical excision is the treatment of choice for solitary metastases, if the patient's condition permits and there are no other visceral metastases.

Surgery is recommended for most patients with the acute complications of obstruction, massive bleeding, or perforation. These complications cannot be treated by other modalities, and the only alternative is to allow the patient to die. The final decision depends on the patient's overall condition, but symptoms can be successfully alleviated in most cases, and survival after surgical excision of the metastases averages 4 to 8 months.[240,242,244,267–269,691–696,698] In patients with multiple gastrointestinal metastases, only lesions causing immediate symptoms should be removed unless those remaining are relatively few and can be safely excised. Survival of 2 to 5 years after excision of gastrointestinal metastases has been reported in a few patients, most of whom had palliative excision for symptomatic solitary or intestinal metastases.[240,242,267–269,691–696]

Obstruction is usually due to large polypoid lesions that mechanically obstruct the bowel or act as leading points for intussusception.[693,696,698] These submucosal lesions generally are removed with bowel resections or, occasionally, enterotomies, depending on the sites and numbers of lesions.

Massive or repeated episodes of bleeding requiring transfusions are uncommon and are likely to result from gastric metastases. Surgical treatment generally consists of segmental bowel resection or partial gastrectomy, although sometimes more extended surgery is required.[242,246,267–269,691–693,695]

Liver, Biliary Tract, and Spleen

Hepatic metastases occur in 10% to 20% of patients with metastatic melanoma in different clinical series but are present in most cases at autopsy.[145,240,246,250,700] It is unusual for isolated liver metastases to occur in patients with cutaneous melanoma. Patients with liver metastases generally have widespread melanoma. The prognoses of these patients are poor (*i.e.*, median survival of 2 to 4 months), and treatment options are few.

Screening tests for liver metastases should consist only of a history, physical examination, and measurement of serum liver chemistries. These are sufficiently accurate and the most cost-effective of all available tests. There are now numerous studies that document the futility of using liver scintiscans, ultrasound studies, or CT scans to screen for occult liver metastases in melanoma patients.[244,245,252,254,661,662,701] They are neither warranted nor cost-effective as screening tests in patients with localized or regional melanoma.

The patterns of abnormal liver chemistries that suggest liver metastases are elevated LDH or alkaline phosphatase levels in the presence of normal or only slightly elevated serum glutamic-oxaloacetic transaminase or bilirubin levels.[243,250,663,702] An elevated LDH level is a clinically useful and specific indicator for metastatic melanoma.[703] When liver metastases are suspected, the confirmatory radiologic tests to be considered include ultrasound, CT scan, radionuclide liver scan, or hepatic arteriogram.[518] Most comparative studies have found that abdominal CT scans are somewhat more accurate and reliable than ultrasound and radionuclide liver scans for evaluation of liver masses.[255,704-706]

Metastatic melanoma involving the gallbladder or bile ducts is present in 4% to 20% of patients at autopsy.[246,250,251] Patients with symptoms of gallbladder metastases should be considered for cholecystectomy if metastasis is confined to the gallbladder and if they are medically fit and have life expectancies exceeding several months.[688,707-710] Short-term relief of symptoms is usually successful, but all reported patients have died within a year.[708-710]

Melanoma is one of the few tumors that metastasizes to the spleen.[240,244,246] It may rarely cause splenomegaly but is more often diagnosed as an incidental finding on a liver-spleen scan or abdominal CT scan or at laparotomy. Most patients with splenic metastases (up to 88%) have concomitant liver or pancreatic metastases.

Bone

Bone metastases occur infrequently (11% to 17%) in most clinical series but are more commonly observed in autopsy series (see Table 46–4).[240,246,711,712] Skeletal metastases generally occur in patients with widespread metastatic disease but occasionally represent the first evidence of recurrence.[711,712] The life span of these patients is short, but effective palliative treatment can be achieved in many cases, so it is worthwhile to pursue the diagnosis. In the asymptomatic melanoma patient, particularly with AJCC stage I or II disease, the yield of occult bone metastases on bone scan is too low to justify it as a screening procedure.[245,252,661-663,713]

Bone metastases from melanoma are medullary in location and destructive in nature. They generally appear osteolytic on x-ray films and provoke little if any bone formation. Patterns of bone metastases have been described previously.[711,712,714] Axial metastases account for up to 80% of bone lesions and are most common in the spine.[246,711,712] When they involve the vertebral body, there are often compression fractures that may lead to neurologic symptoms such as radicular back pain, paresthesia or paresis of the legs, or urinary retention. Only about 10% of lytic lesions occur in weight-bearing bones, which could result in pathologic fractures.[246,712]

Skeletal radionuclide scintigraphy has established itself over radiographic skeletal surveys as the initial test for evaluating suspected bone metastases. Scan abnormalities are nonspecific and must be correlated with radiographic studies and patient histories (for fractures, trauma, arthritis) to differentiate between benign and malignant causes.

The life span of melanoma patients with bone metastases is 4 to 6 months on the average and even shorter when other sites are involved.[145,711,712] The treatment chosen depends on the degree of symptoms, the location and magnitude of bone lesions, and the expected life span. Symptomatic metastases generally involve non-weight-bearing bones, particularly the spine or ribs. In these cases, radiation therapy to the lesions usually gives relief for up to 6 months; however, the fields should generally be restricted to the area of symptomatic involvement. A high-dose, short-course schedule minimizes patient travel time and hospitalization.[277,824] The available chemotherapy generally is not effective for palliation of skeletal metastases.[531]

Irradiation is effective in palliating the pain of bone metastases in most patients. A fractionation schedule of 3000 cGy in 10 fractions is usually recommended, although it has not been established as optimal in any comparative study. More abbreviated schedules, such as 2000 cGy in 5 fractions, are effective but are not recommended for spinal or pelvic bone metastases requiring large fields because of their acute gastrointestinal toxicity. Pathologic fractures in long bones should be stabilized before radiation therapy is given. In weight-bearing long bones judged radiographically to be at risk for pathologic fracture, prophylactic internal fixation is advisable. Radiation therapy should begin immediately after surgery in these patients to minimize the period of hospitalization. In this clinical situation, we recommended a radiation dose of 3600 cGy in 6 fractions. The higher biologic dose for pathologic fractures is recommended because bone healing requires more regression of metastatic tumor than does simple pain relief.

Kidneys and Urinary Tract

Although metastatic melanoma frequently appears in the kidneys and urinary tract at autopsy, metastases in these sites rarely cause clinically recognizable symptoms, and usually these symptoms are terminal manifestations of the disease. Solitary or symptomatic metastases that are amenable to treatment do occur occasionally.

Renal metastases generally occur as multiple, small (3 to 10 mm) cortical nodules that are usually asymptomatic but can cause hematuria or melanuria. Some may be large enough to cause obstructive lesions with hydronephrosis or bleeding.[717] Although patients with bladder metastases commonly have multiple subepithelial pedunculated or sessile lesions, solitary lesions can occur.[718-722]

Kidney and urinary tract metastases generally are asymptomatic until the terminal stages of disease, and death usually occurs within 1 to 4 months after the clinical diagnosis is made. Metastatic melanoma can occasionally mimic primary renal or bladder carcinomas, both endoscopically and radiographically.[729] The most common symptom prompting a urinary tract investigation is gross or microscopic hematuria.[240,246] In most patients, the diagnosis of metastases can be made by intravenous pyelogram, cystogram, cystoscopy, or imaging scans (CT or sonar). Occasionally, cytologic examination of the urine reveals melanoma cells.[723]

Bladder metastases can be treated by transurethral resection or partial cystectomy, depending on their number, sizes, and locations.[718] Symptoms usually can be relieved, but survival after treatment averages only 3 to 6 months. Patients rarely survive longer than 1 year.

Kidney and ureteral metastases causing bleeding or obstruction can be treated by ureteronephrectomy in selected patients or by a ureteral stent if the patient is not a candidate for surgery.[717,724] In most cases, survival averages only 4 months. Prostate and urethral metastases can cause hematuria, dysuria, or hesitancy.[725] Symptomatic prostate metastases rarely occur but can be treated by transurethral resection or open prostatectomy.[717,725]

METASTATIC MELANOMA FROM UNKNOWN PRIMARY SITE

A small proportion of melanoma patients present with metastatic diseased lymph nodes or distant sites but no detectable primary site. Patients presenting with occult primary melanoma comprise between 1% and 12% of patients with metastatic disease.[139,726–732] About two thirds of these patients present with tumors in lymph nodes (most frequently in the axilla) and one third with distant metastases (most frequently in the skin, subcutaneous tissues, lungs, and brain). All patients with occult primary melanoma should be examined carefully for potential sequestered primary lesions, especially in the eye and scalp. In this group of patients, it is important to get a careful history of previous treatment for nevi. About 10% to 20% of patients describe previous nevi within the lymphatic drainage areas of metastatic lymph nodes. About one third of patients have had treatment for pigmented lesions, often by nondiagnostic procedures such as curettage or diathermy.[236,733] Any biopsy specimens from previously excised pigmented lesions that are available should be reevaluated by an experienced pathologist, because occasionally these turn out to be well-differentiated primary melanomas on review. Two thirds of patients give no history of suspicious pigmented lesions.

The survival rate of patients with unknown primary lesions is no different from that of patients with metastatic cutaneous melanoma when matched for prognostic factors. When appropriate, surgical management should be considered first. Lymphadenectomy for nodal disease can be associated with long-term survival similar to the results seen in patients with cutaneous metastases to lymph nodes; survival is generally better if only one node is involved than if multiple nodes contain tumors. Two-year survival rates of 30% to 40% can be observed in patients with skin and subcutaneous metastases from cutaneous and unknown primary sites.[236,729] A small proportion of melanoma patients present with metastatic disease either in lymph nodes or at distant sites, and no primary site can be detected. Patients presenting with occult primary melanoma comprise between 1% and 12% of patients with distant metastatic disease.[139,726–732]

REFERENCES

1. McLeod GR, David NC, Little JH, et al. Melanoma in Queensland, Australia: Experience in the Queensland Melanoma Project. In: Balch CM, Milton GW, eds. Cutaneous melanoma: Clinical management and treatment results worldwide. Philadelphia: JB Lippincott, 1985:379.
2. Roush GC, Schymurs M, Holford TR. Risk for cutaneous melanoma in recent Connecticut birth cohorts. Am J Publ Health 1985;75:679.
3. Redman JC, Mora DB. Malignant melanomas of the skin diagnosed and treated in Albuquerque, New Mexico in 1980. J Dermatol Surg Oncol 1982;8:41.
4. Rigel DS, Kopf AW, Friedman RJ. The rate of malignant melanoma in the US: Are we making an impact? J Am Acad Dermatol 1987;17:1050.
5. Armstrong BK, English DR. Epidemiologic studies. In: Balch CM, Houghton AN, Milton GW, Sober AJ, Soong S-j, eds. Cutaneous melanoma. 2nd ed. Philadelphia: JB Lippincott, 1992:12–22.
6. Gellin GA, Kopf AW, Garfinkel L. Malignant melanoma: A controlled study of possibly associated factors. Arch Dermatol 1969;99:43.
7. Scheibner A, Milton GW, McCarthy WH, et al. Multiple primary melanoma: A review of 90 cases. Aust J Dermatol 1982;23:1.
8. Bellet RE, Vaisman I, Mastrangelo MJ, et al. Multiple primary malignancies in patients with cutaneous melanoma. Cancer 1977;40:1974.
9. Lynch HT, Frichot BC III, Lynch J, et al. Family studies of malignant melanoma and associated cancer. Surg Gynecol Obstet 1975;141:517.
10. Moseley HS, Giuliano AE, Storm FK, et al. Multiple primary melanoma. Cancer 1979;43:939.
11. Veronesi U, Cascinelli N, Bufalino R. Evaluation of the risk of multiple primaries in malignant cutaneous melanoma. Tumori 1976;62:127.
12. Elder DE, Goldman LI, Goldman SC, et al. Dysplastic nevus syndrome: A phenotypic association of sporadic cutaneous melanoma. Cancer 1980;46:1787.
13. Wallace DC, Exton LA, McLeod GRC. Genetic factor in malignant melanoma. Cancer 1971;27:1262.
14. Acton RT, Balch CM, Budowle B, et al. Immunogenetics of melanoma. In: Reisfeld RA, Ferrone S, eds. Melanoma antigens and antibodies. New York: Plenum, 1982:1.
15. Greene MH, Reimer RR, Clark WH Jr, et al. Precursor lesions in familial melanoma. Semin Oncol 1978;5:85.
16. Lynch HT, Frichot BC III, Lynch JF. Familial atypical multiple mole-melanoma syndrome. J Med Genet 1978;15:352.
17. Reimer RR, Clark WH Jr, Greene MH, et al. Precursor lesions in familial melanoma: A new genetic preneoplastic syndrome. JAMA 1978;239:744.
18. Wallace DC, Beardmore GL, Exton LA. Familial malignant melanoma. Ann Surg 1973;177:15.
19. Clark WH Jr, Reimer RR, Greene M, et al. Origin of familial malignant melanomas from heritable melanocytic lesions: The B-K mole syndrome. Arch Dermatol 1978;114:732.
20. Elder DE, Green MH, Guerry D, et al. The dysplastic nevus syndrome: Our definition. Am J Dermatopathol 1982;4:455.
21. Acton RT, Balch CM, Barger BO, et al. The occurrence of melanoma and its relationship with host, lifestyle and environmental factors. In: Costanzi JJ, ed. Malignant melanoma 1. The Hague: Martinus Nijhoff, 1983:151.
22. Clark DA, Necheles T, Nathanson L, et al. Apparent HL-A5 deficiency in malignant melanoma. Transplantation 1973;15:326.
23. Barger BO, Action RT, Soong S-j, et al. Increase of HLA-DR4 in melanoma patients from Alabama. Cancer Res 1982;42:4276.
24. Budowle B, Barger BO, Balch CM, et al. Associations of properdin factor B with melanoma. Cancer Genet Cytogenet 1982;5:247.
25. Pandey JP, Johnson AH, Funderberg HH, et al. HLA antigens and immunoglobulin allotypes in patients with malignant melanoma. Hum Immunol 1981;2:185.
26. Walter G, Brachtel R, Hilling M. On the incidence of blood group O and Gm phenotypes in patients with malignant melanoma. Hum Genet 1979;49:71.
27. Clark WH Jr, Ainsworth AM, Bernardino EA, et al. The developmental biology of primary human malignant melanomas. Semin Oncol 1975;2:83.
28. Fitzpatrick TB, Milton GW, Balch CM, Shaw HM, McCarthy WH, Sober AJ. Clinical characteristics. In: Balch CM, Houghton AN, Milton GW, Sober AJ, Soong S-j, eds. Cutaneous melanoma. 2nd ed. Philadelphia: JB Lippincott, 1992:223–233.
29. Mihm MC Jr, Fitzpatrick TB, Lane-Brown MM, et al. Early detection of primary cutaneous malignant melanoma: A color atlas. N Engl J Med 1973;289:989.
30. Sober AJ, Fitzpatrick TB, Mihm MC Jr, et al. Early recognition of cutaneous melanoma. JAMA 1979;242:2795.
31. Clark WH Jr, From L, Bernardino EA, et al. The histogenesis and biologic behavior of primary human malignant melanomas of the skin. Cancer Res 1969;29:705.
32. McGovern VJ, Murad TM. Pathology of melanoma: An overview. In: Cutaneous melanoma: Clinical management and treatment results worldwide. Philadelphia: JB Lippincott, 1985:29.
33. Mihm MC Jr, Clark WH Jr, Fromm L. The clinical diagnosis, classification and histogenetic concepts of the early stages of cutaneous malignant melanomas. N Engl J Med 1971;284:1078.
34. Manci EA, Balch CM, Murad TM, et al. Polypoid melanoma, a virulent variant of the nodular growth pattern. Am J Clin Pathol 1981;75:810.
35. Urist MM, Balch CM, Soong S-j, et al. Head and neck melanoma in 536 clinical stage I patients: A prognostic factors analysis and results of surgical treatment. Ann Surg 1984;200:769.
36. McGovern VJ, Shaw HM, Milton GW, et al. Is malignant melanoma arising in a Hutchinson's melanotic freckle a separate entity? Histopathology 1980;4:235.

37. Clark WH Jr, Mihm MC Jr. Lentigo maligna and lentigo-maligna melanoma. Am J Pathol 1969;55:39.

38. Arrington JH III, Reed RJ, Ichinose H. Plantar lentiginous melanoma: A distinctive variant of human cutaneous malignant melanoma. Am J Surg Pathol 1977;1:131.

39. Coleman WP III, Loria PR, Reed RJ, et al. Acral lentiginous melanoma. Arch Dermatol 1980;116:773.

40. Krementz ET, Reed RJ, Coleman WP, et al. Acral lentiginous melanoma: A clinicopathologic entity. Ann Surg 1982;195:632.

41. Seiji M, Takahashi M. Acral melanoma in Japan. Hum Pathol 1982;13:607.

42. Sondergaard K, Olsen G. Malignant melanoma of the foot: A clinicopathological study of 125 primary cutaneous malignant melanomas. Acta Pathol Microbiol Immunol Scand [Abstract] 1980;88:275.

43. Feibleman CE, Stoll H, Maize JC. Melanomas of the palm, sole and nailbed: A clinicopathologic study. Cancer 1980;46:2492.

44. Paladugu RR, Winberg CD, Yonemoto RH. Acral lentiginous melanoma: A clinicopathologic study of 36 patients. Cancer 1983;52:161.

45. Patterson RH, Helwig EB. Subungual malignant melanoma: A clinical-pathologic study. Cancer 1980;46:2074.

46. Hughes LE, Horgan I, Taylor BA, et al. Malignant melanoma of the hand and foot: Diagnosis and management. Br J Surg 1985;72:813.

47. Lopansri S, Mihm MC Jr. Clinical and pathological correlation of malignant melanoma. J Cutan Pathol 1979;6:180.

48. Balch CM, Cascinelli N, Drzewiecki KT, et al. A comparison of prognostic factors worldwide. In: Balch CM, Houghton AN, Milton GW, Sober A, Soong S-j, eds. Cutaneous melanoma. 2nd ed. Philadelphia: JB Lippincott, 1992;188.

49. Balch CM, Urist MM, Maddox WA, et al. Melanoma in the Southern United States: Experience at the University of Alabama in Birmingham. In: Balch CM, Milton GW, eds. Cutaneous melanoma: Clinical management and treatment results worldwide. Philadelphia: JB Lippincott, 1985.

50. Reintgen DS, McCarty KM Jr, Cox E, et al. Malignant melanoma in black American and white American populations: A comparative review. JAMA 1982;248:1856.

51. McCarthy WH, Shaw HM, Milton GW, et al. Melanoma in New South Wales, Australia: Experience at the Sydney Melanoma Unit. In: Balch CM, Milton GW, eds. Cutaneous melanoma: Clinical management and treatment results worldwide. Philadelphia: JB Lippincott, 1985:371.

52. Pack GT, Oropeza R. Subungual melanoma. Surg Gynecol Obstet 1967;124:571.

53. Papachristou DN, Fortner JG. Melanoma arising under the nail. J Surg Oncol 1982;21:219.

54. Le Douarin N. Migration and differentiation of neural crest cells. Curr Top Dev Biol 1980;61:31.

55. Hearing VT. Enzymatic control of pigmentation in mammals. FASEB J 1991;5:2902.

56. Vijayasaradhi S, Bouchard B, Houghton AN. The melanoma antigen gp75 is the human homologue of the mouse *brown* locus product. J Exp Med 1990;171:1375.

57. Wick MM, Byers L, Frei E III. L-Dopa: Selective toxicity for melanoma cells in vitro. Science 1977;197:468.

58. Pawelek JM, Lerner AB. 5,6-dihydroxyindole is a melanin precursor showing potent cytotoxicity. Nature 1978;276:627.

59. Morrison ME, Yagi MJ, Cohen G. In vitro studies of 2,4-dihydroxyphenylalanine, a prodrug targeted against malignant melanoma cells. Proc Natl Acad Sci USA 1985;82:2960.

60. Houghton AN, Eisinger M, Albino AP, et al. Surface antigens of melanocytes and melanomas: Markers of melanoma differentiation and melanoma subsets. J Exp Med 1982;156:1755.

61. Houghton AN, Real FX, Davis LJ, et al. Phenotypic heterogeneity of melanoma: Relation to the differentiation program of melanoma cells. J Exp Med 1987;164:812.

62. Barnhill RL, Mihm MC Jr. Histopathology of malignant melanoma and its precursor lesions. In: Balch CM, Houghton AN, Milton GW, Sober AJ, Soong S-j, eds. Cutaneous melanoma. 2nd ed. Philadelphia: JB Lippincott, 1992:234.

63. Clark WH Jr, Elder ED, Guerry D IV et al. The precursor lesions of superficial spreading and nodular melanoma. Hum Pathol 1984;15:1147.

64. Rodeck U, Melber K, Kath R, et al. Constitutive expression of multiple growth factor genes by melanoma cells but not normal melanocytes. J Invest Dermatol 1991;97:20.

65. Halaban R. Growth factors and tyrosine protein kinases in normal and malignant melanocytes. Cancer Metastasis Rev 1991;10:129.

66. Herlyn M, Houghton AN. Biology of melanocytes and melanoma. In: Balch CM, Houghton AN, Milton GW, Sober AJ, Soong S-j, eds. Cutaneous melanoma. 2nd ed. Philadelphia: JB Lippincott, 1992:234.

67. Becker B, Meier CB, Herlyn M. Proliferation of human malignant melanomas is inhibited by antisense oligodeoxynucleotides targeted against basic fibroblast growth factor. EMBO J 1989;8:3685.

68. Halaban R, Kwon BS, Ghosh S, et al. bFGF as an autocrine growth factor for human melanomas. Oncogene Res 1988;3:177.

69. Dotto GP, Moellmann G, Ghosh S, et al. Transformation of murine melanocytes by basic fibroblast growth factor cDNA and oncogenes and selective suppression of the transformed phenotype in a reconstituted cutaneous environment. J Cell Biol 1989;109:3115.

70. Houghton AN, Herlyn M, Ferrone S. Melanoma antigens. In: Balch CM, Houghton AN, Milton GW, Sober AJ, Soong S-j, eds. Cutaneous melanoma. 2nd ed. Philadelphia: JB Lippincott, 1992:234.

71. Albeda SM, Mette SP, Elder DE, et al. Integrin distribution in malignant melanoma: Association with the β3 subunit with tumor progression. CA

72. Lynch HT, Frichot BC III, Lynch JF. Familial atypical multiple mole melanoma syndrome. J Med Genet 1978;15:352.

73. Greene MH, Goldin LR, Clark WH Jr, et al. Familial cutaneous malignant melanoma: Autosomal dominant trait possibly linked to the Rh locus. Proc Natl Acad Sci USA 1983;80:6071.

74. Bale SJ, Dracopoli NC, Tucker MA, et al. Mapping the gene for hereditary cutaneous malignant melanoma-dysplastic nevus to chromosome 1p. N Engl J Med 1989;320:1376.

75. van Haeringen A, Bergman W, Nelen MR, et al. Exclusion of the dysplastic nevus syndrome locus from the short arm of chromosome 1 by linkage studies in Dutch families. Genomics 1989;5:61.

76. Cannon-Albright LA, Goldgar DE, Wright EC, et al. Evidence against the reported linkage of the cutaneous melanoma-dysplastic nevus syndrome locus to chromosome 1p36. Am J Hum Genet 1990;46:912.

77. Becher R, Gibas Z, Karakousis C, et al. Nonrandom chromosome changes in malignant melanoma. Cancer Res 1983;43:5010.

78. Trent JM, Rosenfeld SB, Meyskens FL. Chromosome 6q involvement in human malignant melanoma. Cancer Genet Cytogenet 1983;9:177.

79. Pathak S, Drwinga HL, Hsu TC. Involvement of chromosome 6 in rearrangements in human malignant melanoma cell lines. Cytogenet Cell Genet 1983;36:573.

80. Balaban G, Herlyn M, Guerry D, et al. Cytogenetics of human malignant melanoma and premalignant lesions. Cancer Genet Cytogenet 1984;11:429.

81. Balaban GB, Herlyn M, Clark WH Jr, et al. Karyotypic evolution in human malignant melanoma. Cancer Genet Cytogenet 1986;19:113.

82. Limon J, Dal Cin P, Sait SNJ, et al. Chromosome changes in metastatic human melanoma. Cancer Genet Cytogenet 1988;30:201.

83. Pedersen MI, Bennett JW, Wang N. Nonrandom chromosome structural aberrations and oncogene loci in human malignant melanoma. Cancer Genet Cytogenet 1986;20:11.

84. Fountain JW, Bale SJ, Housman DE, Dracopoli NC. Genetics of melanoma. Cancer Surv 1990;9:645.

85. Richmond A, Fine R, Murray D, et al. Growth factor and cytogenetic abnormalities in cultured nevi and malignant melanomas. J Invest Dermatol 1986;86:295.

86. Cowan JM, Halaban R, Francke U. Cytogenetic analysis of melanocytes from premalignant nevi and melanomas. JNCI 1988;80:1159.

87. Parmiter AH, Balaban G, Clark WH Jr, et al. Possible involvement of the chromosome region 10q24–26 in early stages of melanocyte neoplasia. Cancer Genet Cytogenet 1988;30:313.

88. Dracopoli NC, Houghton AN, Old LJ. Loss of polymorphic restriction fragments in malignant melanoma: Implications for tumor heterogeneity. Proc Natl Acad Sci USA 1985;82:1470.

89. Dracopoli NC, Alhadeff B, Houghton AN. Loss of heterozygosity at autosomal and X-linked loci during tumor progression in a patient with melanoma. Cancer Res 1987;47:3995.

90. Cavenee WK, Dryja TP, Phillips RA, et al. Expression of recessive alleles by chromosomal mechanisms in retinoblastoma. Nature 1983;305:779.

91. Volkenandt M, Schlegel U, Nanus DM, Albino AP. Mutational analysis of the human p53 gene in malignant melanoma. Pig Cell Res 1991;4:35.

92. Trent JM, Stanbridge EJ, McBride HL, et al. Tumorigenicity in human melanoma cell lines controlled by introduction of human chromosome 6. Science 1990;247:568.

93. Trent JM, Meyskens FL, Salmon SE, et al. Relation of cytogenetic abnormalities and clinical outcome in metastatic melanoma. N Engl J Med 1990;22:1508.

94. Lee JAH. The causation of melanoma. In: Balch CM, Milton GW, eds. Cutaneous melanoma: Clinical management and treatment results worldwide. Philadelphia: JB Lippincott, 1985:303.

95. Lee JAH. Melanoma and exposure to sunlight. Epidemiol Rev 1982;4:110.

96. Berkelhammer J, Oxenhandler RW. Evaluation of premalignant and malignant lesions during the induction of mouse melanomas. Cancer Res 1987;47:1251.

97. Pawlowski A, Haberman HF, Menon IA. Junctional and compound pigmented nevi induced by 9,10-dimethyl-1,benzanthracene in skin of albino guinea pigs. Cancer Res 1976;36:2813.

98. Kripke ML, Fisher MS. Immunologic parameters of ultraviolet carcinogenesis. JNCI 1976;57:211.

99. Crombie IK. Variation of melanoma incidence with latitude in North America and Europe. Br J Cancer 1979;40:774.

100. Lee JAH. Melanoma in cancer epidemiology and prevention. In: Schottenfeld D, Fraumeni JF Jr, eds. Cancer, epidemiology and prevention. Philadelphia: WB Saunders, 1982:984.

101. Elwood JM, Gallagher RP. Site distribution of malignant melanoma. Can Med Assoc J 1983;128:1400.

102. Katz L, Ben-Tuvla S, Steinitz R. Malignant melanoma of the skin in Israel: Effect of migration. In: Magnus K, ed. Trends in cancer incidence. Washington, DC: Hemisphere, 1982:419.

103. Newell GR. Is ultraviolet irradiation the sole cause of melanoma? Melanoma Lett 1987;5:4.

104. Jensen OM, Bolander AM. Trends in malignant melanoma of the skin. World Health Stat Q 1980;33:2.

105. Greene A. Incidence and reporting of cutaneous melanoma in Queensland. Aust J Dermatol 1982;23:105.

106. McLeod GR, Davis NC, Little JH, et al. Melanoma in Queensland, Australia: Experience in the Queensland Melanoma Project. Personal communication, 1990.

107. Eldh J, Boeryd B, Suurkula M, et al. Melanoma in Sweden: Experience at the University of Goteborg. In: Balch CM, Milton GW, eds. Cutaneous melanoma: Clinical management and treatment results worldwide. Philadelphia: JB Lippincott, 1985:469.

108. Crombie IK. Radical differences in melanoma incidence. Br J Cancer 1979;40:185.

109. Lam K-H, Wong J. Melanoma in Hong Kong. Experience at the Queen Mary Hospital. In: Balch CM, Milton GW, eds. Cutaneous melanoma: Clinical management and treatment results worldwide. Philadelphia, JB Lippincott, 1985:495.

110. Balch CM, Soong S-j, Shaw HM, et al. Changing trends in the clinical pathological features of melanoma. In: Balch CM, Houghton AN, Milton GW, Sober A, Soong S-j, eds. Cutaneous melanoma. 2nd ed. Philadelphia: JB Lippincott, 1992:40.

111. Balch CM, Soong S-j, Milton GW, et al. A comparison of prognostic factors and surgical results in 1,786 patients with localized (stage I) melanoma treated in Alabama, USA, and New South Wales, Australia. Ann Surg 1982;196:677.

112. Breslow A. Thickness, cross-sectional areas and depth of invasion in the prognosis of cutaneous melanoma. Ann Surg 1970;172:902.

113. Goldsmith HS. Melanoma: An overview. CA 1979;29:194.

114. McNeer G, Das Gupta TK. Prognosis in malignant melanoma. Surgery 1964;56:512.

115. Beahrs OH, Myers MH. Manual for staging of cancer: American Joint Committee on Cancer. Philadelphia: JB Lippincott, 1983:117.

116. Ketcham AS. Classification and staging. In: Balch CM, Houghton AN, Milton GW, Sober A, Soong S-j, eds. Cutaneous melanoma, 2nd ed. Philadelphia: JB Lippincott, 1992:213.

117. Balch CM, Soong S-j, Shaw HM, Urist MM, McCarthy WH. An analysis of prognostic factors in 8500 patients with cutaneous melanoma. In: Balch CM, Houghton AN, Milton GW, Sober A, Soong S-j, eds. Cutaneous melanoma. 2nd ed. Philadelphia: JB Lippincott, 1992:165.

118. Day CL Jr, Sober AJ, Kopf AW. A prognostic model for clinical stage I melanoma of the lower extremity: Location on foot as independent risk factor for recurrent disease. Surgery 1981;89:599.

119. Day CL Jr, Sober AJ, Kopf AW. A prognostic model for clinical stage I melanoma of the upper extremity: The importance of anatomic subsites in predicting recurrent disease. Ann Surg 1981;193:436.

120. Balch CM, Murad TM, Soong S-j, et al. A multifactorial analysis of melanoma: Prognostic histopathological features comparing Clark's and Breslow's staging methods. Ann Surg 1978;188:732.

121. Cascinelli N, Morabito A, Bufalino R, et al. Prognosis of stage I melanoma of the skin. Int J Cancer 1980;26:733.

122. Drzewiecki KT, Andersen PK. Survival with malignant melanoma: A regression analysis of prognostic factors. Cancer 1982;49:2414.

123. Schmoeckel C, Bockelbrink A, Bockelbrink H, et al. Low-and high-risk malignant melanoma. I. Evaluation of clinical and histological prognosticators in 585 cases. Eur J Cancer Clin Oncol 1983;19:227.

124. Shaw HM, McGovern VJ, Milton GW, et al. Histologic features of tumors and the female superiority in survival from malignant melanoma. Cancer 1980;45:1604.

125. Shaw HM, McGovern VJ, Milton GW, et al. Malignant melanoma: Influence of site of lesion and age of patient in the female superiority in survival. Cancer 1980;46:2731.

126. Balch CM, Soong S-j, Milton GW, et al. A comparison of prognostic factors and surgical results in 1,786 patients with localized (stage I) melanoma treated in Alabama, USA, and New South Wales, Australia. Ann Surg 1982;196:677.

127. Balch CM, Murad TM, Soong S-j, et al. Tumor thickness as a guide to surgical management of clinical stage I melanoma patients. Cancer 1979;43:883.

128. Breslow A. Thickness, cross-sectional areas and depth of invasion in the prognosis of cutaneous melanoma. Ann Surg 1970;172:902.

129. Day CL Jr, Lew RA, Mihm MC Jr, et al. The natural break points for primary-tumor thickness in clinical stage I melanoma. N Engl J Med 1981;305:1155.

130. Soong S-j. A computerized mathematical model and scoring system for predicting outcome in patients with localized melanoma. In: Balch CM, Houghton AN, Milton GW, Sober A, Soong S-j, 1992:200.

131. Day CL Jr, Sober AJ, Kopf AW, et al. A prognostic model for clinical stage I melanoma of the trunk: Location near the midline is not an independent risk factor for recurrent disease. Am J Surg 1981;142:247.

132. Eldh J, Boeryd B, Peterson LE. Prognostic factors in cutaneous malignant melanoma in stage I: A clinical, morphological and multivariate analysis. Scand J Plast Reconstr Surg 1978;12:243.

133. Prade M, Bognel C, Charpentier P, et al. Malignant melanoma of the skin: Prognostic factors derived from a multifactorial analysis of 239 cases. Am J Dermatopathol 1982;4:411.

134. Schmoeckel C, Bockelbrink A, Bockelbrink H, et al. Low- and high-risk malignant melanoma. II. Multivariate analyses for a prognostic classification. Eur J Cancer Clin Oncol 1983;19:237.

135. Van der Esch EP, Cascinelli N, Preda F, et al. Stage I melanoma of the skin: Evaluation of prognosis according to histologic characteristics. Cancer 1981;48:1668.

136. Cox EB. Prognostic factors in malignant melanoma. In: Seigler HF, ed. Clinical management of melanoma. The Hague: Martinus Nijhoff, 1982:279.

137. Hacene K, Le Doussal V, Brunet M, et al. Prognostic index for clinical stage I cutaneous malignant melanoma. Cancer Res 1983;43:2991.

138. Day CL Jr, Sober AJ, Kopf AW, et al. A prognostic model for clinical stage I melanoma of the upper extremity: The importance of anatomic subsites in predicting recurrent disease. Ann Surg 1981;193:436.

138a. Kheir SA, Bines SD, Vonroenn JH, Soong-S-j, Urist MM, Coon JS. Prognostic significance of DNA aneuploidy in stage I cutaneous melanoma. Ann Surg 1988;207:455.

139. Balch CM, Soong S-j, Murad TM, et al. A multifactorial analysis of melanoma. III. Prognostic factors in melanoma patients with lymph node metastases (stage II). Ann Surg 1981;193:377.

140. Balch CM, Soong S-j, Murad TM, et al. A multifactorial analysis of melanoma. II.

141. Cohen MH, Ketcham AS, Feix EL, et al. Prognostic factors in patients undergoing lymphadenectomy for malignant melanoma. Ann Surg 1977;186:635.

142. Day CL Jr, Sober AJ, Lew RA, et al. Malignant melanoma patients with positive nodes and relatively good prognoses: Microstaging retains prognostic significance in clinical stage I melanoma patients with metastases to regional nodes. Cancer 1981;47:955.

143. Callery C, Cochran AJ, Roe DJ. Factors prognostic for survival in patients with malignant melanoma spread to the regional lymph nodes. Ann Surg 1982;196:69.

144. Cascinelli N, Nava M, Vaglini M, et al. Melanoma in Italy. Experience at the National Cancer Institute of Milan. In: Balch CM, Milton GW, eds. Cutaneous melanoma: Clinical management and treatment results worldwide. Philadelphia: JB Lippincott, 1985:447.

145. Balch CM, Soong S-j, Murad TM, et al. A multifactorial analysis of melanoma. IV. Prognostic factors in 200 melanoma patients with distant metastases (stage III). J Clin Oncol 1983;1:126.

146. Presant CA, Bartolucci AA (for the Southeastern Cancer Study Group). Prognostic factors in metastatic malignant melanoma: The Southeastern Cancer Study Group experience. Cancer 1982;49:2192.

147. Singletary SE, Balch CM, Urist MM, McCarthy WH, Cascinelli N. Surgical treatment of primary melanoma. In: Balch CM, Houghton A, Milton GW, Sober A, Soong S-j, eds. Cutaneous melanoma. 2nd ed. Philadelphia: JB Lippincott, 1992:269.

148. Bagley FH, Cady B, Lee A, et al. Changes in clinical presentation and management of malignant melanoma. Cancer 1981;47:2126.

149. Jones WM, Williams WJ, Roberts MM, et al. Malignant melanoma of the skin: Prognostic value of clinical features and the role of treatment in 111 cases. Br J Cancer 1968;22:437.

150. Cascinelli N, van der Esch EP, Breslow A, et al. Stage I melanoma of the skin: The problem of resection margins. Eur J Cancer 1980;16:1079.

151. Day CL Jr, Mihm MC Jr, Sober AJ, et al. Narrower margins for clinical stage I malignant melanoma. N Engl J Med 1982;306:479.

152. Elder DE, Guerry D IV, Heiberger RM, et al. Optimal resection margin for cutaneous malignant melanoma. Plast Reconstr Surg 1983;71:66.

153. Milton GW, Shaw HM, Farago GA, et al. Tumour thickness and the site and time of first recurrence in cutaneous malignant melanoma (stage I). Br J Surg 1980;67:543.

154. Ackerman AB. Malignant melanoma in situ. The fat, curable stage of malignant melanoma. Pathology 1985;17:298.

155. Jones RE Jr, Cash ME, Ackerman AB. Malignant melanomas mistaken histologically for junctional nevi. In: Ackerman AB, ed. Pathology of malignant melanoma. New York: Masson, 1981:93.

156. Kelly JW, Sagebiel RW, Calderon W, et al. The frequency of local recurrence and microsatellites as a guide to re-excision margins for cutaneous malignant melanoma. Ann Surg 1984;6:759.

157. Breslow A, Macht SD. Optimal size of resection margin for thin cutaneous melanoma. Surg Gynecol Obstet 1977;145:691.

158. Roses DF, Harris MN, Rigel D, et al. Local and in-transit metastases following definitive excision for primary cutaneous malignant melanoma. Ann Surg 1983;198:65.

159. Schmoeckel C, Bockelbrink A, Bockelbrink H, et al. Low- and high-risk malignant melanoma: Prognostic significance of the resection margin. Eur J Cancer Clin Oncol 1983;19:237.

160. Cosimi AB, Sober AJ, Mihm MC. Conservative surgical management of superficially invasive cutaneous melanoma. Cancer 1984;53:1256.

161. Milton GW, Shaw HM, McCarthy WH. Resection margins of melanoma. Aust NZ J Surg 1985;55:225.

162. Veronesi U, Cascinelli N, Adamus J, et al. Primary cutaneous melanoma 2 mm less in thickness. Results of a randomized study comparing wide with narrow surgical excision: A preliminary report. N Engl J Med 1988;318:1159–1162.

162a. Veronesi U, Cascinelli N. Narrow excision (1-cm margin): A safe procedure for thin cutaneous melanoma. Arch Surg 1991;126:438–441.

163. Harwood AR. Conventional fractionated radiotherapy for 51 patients with lentigo maligna and lentigo maligna melanoma. Int J Radiat Oncol Biol Phys 1983;9:1019.

164. Briele HA, Beattie CW, Ronan SG, et al. Late recurrence of cutaneous melanoma. Arch Surg 1983;118:800.

165. Krementz ET, Ryan RF, Muchmore JH, Carter RD, Sutherland CM, Reed RJ. Hyperthermic regional perfusion for melanoma of the limbs. In: Balch CM, Houghton AN, Milton GW, Sober A, Soong S-j. Cutaneous melanoma, 2nd ed. Philadelphia: JB Lippincott, 1992:403.

166. Elias EG, Didolkar MS, Goel IP, et al. A clinicopathologic study of prognostic factors in cutaneous malignant melanoma. Surg Gynecol Obstet 1977;144:327.

167. Karakousis CP. Groin dissection. In: Balch CM, Houghton AN, A, Soong S-j, eds. Cutaneous melanoma. 2nd ed. Philadelphia: JB Lippincott, 1992:392.

168. Das Gupta TK. Radical groin dissection. Surg Gynecol Obstet 1969;129:1275.

169. Holmes EC, Moseley HS, Morton DL, et al. A rational approach to the surgical management of melanoma. Ann Surg 1977;186:481.

170. Karakousis CP. Ilioinguinal lymph node dissection. Am J Surg 1981;141:299.

171. Dasmahapatra KS, Karakousis CP. Therapeutic groin dissection in malignant melanoma. Surg Gynecol Obstet 1983;156:21.

172. Finck SJ, Giuliano AE, Mann BD, et al. Results of ilioinguinal dissection for stage II melanoma. Ann Surg 1982;196:180.

173. McCarthy JG, Haagensen CD, Herter FP. The role of groin dissection in the management of melanoma of the lower extremity. Ann Surg 1974;179:156.

174. Fortner JG, Booher RJ, Pack GT. Results of groin dissection for malignant melanoma in 220 patients. Surgery 1964;55:485.

175. Karakousis CP, Lawrence JE, Rao UR. Groin dissection in malignant melanoma. Am J Surg 1986;152:491.

176. Harris MN, Gumport SL, Berman IR, et al. Ilioinguinal lymph node dissection for melanoma. Surg Gynecol Obstet 1973;136:33.

177. Urist MM, Maddox WA, Kennedy JE, et al. Patient risk factors and surgical morbidity after regional lymphadenectomy in 204 melanoma patients. Cancer 1983;51:2152.

178. Karakousis CP, Heiser MA, Moore RH. Lymphedema after groin dissection. Am J Surg 1983;145:205.

179. Chretien PB, Ketcham AS, Hoye RC, et al. Axillary dissection with preservation of the pectoralis major muscle. Ann Surg 1971;173:554.

180. Harris MN, Gumport SL, Maiwandi H. Axillary lymph node dissection for melanoma. Surg Gynecol Obstet 1972;135:936.

181. Ames FC, Balch CM, McCarthy W. Axillary lymph node dissection. In: Balch CM, Houghton AN, Milton GW, Sober A, Soong S-j. Cutaneous melanoma. 2nd ed. Philadelphia: JB Lippincott, 1992:384.

182. Bakamjian VY, Miller SH, Poole AG. A technique for radical dissection of the neck. Surg Gynecol Obstet 1977;144:419.

183. Beahrs OH. Surgical anatomy and technique of radical neck dissection. Surg Clin North Am 1977;57:663.

184. Martin HE, Del Balle B, Ehrlich H, et al. Neck dissection. Cancer 1951;4:441.

185. Byers RM. Cervical and parotid node dissections. In: Balch CM, Houghton AN, Milton GW, Sober A, Soong S-j, eds. Cutaneous melanoma. 2nd ed. Philadelphia: JB Lippincott, 1992:376.

186. Turkula LD, Woods JE. Limited or selective nodal dissection for malignant melanoma of the head and neck. Am J Surg 1984;148:446.

187. Becker GD, Parell GJ. Technique of preserving the spinal accessory nerve during radical neck dissection. Laryngoscope 1979;89:827.

188. Bocca E, Pagnataro O. A conservative technique in radical neck dissection. Ann Otol Rhinol Laryngol 1967;76:975.

189. Calearo CV, Teatini G. Functional neck dissection: Anatomical grounds, surgical technique, clinical observations. Ann Otol Rhinol Laryngol 1983;92:215.

190. Jesse RH, Ballantyne AJ, Larson D. Radical or modified neck dissection: A therapeutic dilemma. Am J Surg 1978;136:516.

191. Lingeman RE, Helmus C, Stephens R, et al. Neck dissection: Radical or conservative. Ann Otol Rhinol Laryngol 1977;86:737.

192. Schuller DE, Reiches NA, Hamaker RC, et al. Analysis of disability resulting from treatment including radical neck dissection or modified neck dissection. Head Neck Surg 1983;6:551.

193. Storm FK, Eilber FR, Sparks FC, et al. A prospective study of parotid metastases from head and neck cancer. Am J Surg 1977;134:115.

194. Beahrs OH, Adson MA. The surgical anatomy and techniques of parotidectomy. Am J Surg 1958;95:885l.

195. Woods JE. Parotidectomy: Points of technique for brief and safe operation. Am J Surg 1983;145:678.

196. Dunn EJ, Kent T, Hines J, et al. Parotid neoplasms: A report of 250 cases and review of the literature. Ann Surg 1976;184:500.

197. Powell ME, Clairmont AA. Complications of parotidectomy. South Med J 1983;76:1109.

198. Woods JE. The facial nerve in parotid malignancy. Am J Surg 1983;146:493.

199. Sutherland CM, Mather FJ, Krementz ET. Factors influencing survival among patients with regional melanoma treated by regional perfusion. Surg Gynecol Obstet 1987;164:111.

200. Stehlin JS Jr, Smith JL Jr, Jing B, et al. Melanomas of the extremities complicated by in-transit metastases. Surg Gynecol Obstet 1966;122:3.

201. Treidman L, McNeer G. Prognosis with local metastasis and recurrence in malignant melanoma. Ann NY Acad Sci 1963;100:123.

202. Moore GE, Gerner RE. Malignant melanoma. Surg Gynecol Obstet 1971;132:427.

203. Stehlin JS Jr, Clark RL. Melanoma of the extremities: Experiences with conventional treatment and perfusion in 339 cases. Am J Surg 1965;110:366.

204. Ghussen F, Nagel K, Groth W, et al. A prospective randomized study of regional extremity perfusion in patients with malignant melanoma. Ann Surg 1984;200:764.

205. Calvo DB III, Patt YZ, Wallace S, et al. Phase I–II trial of percutaneous intra-arterial cis-diamminedichloroplatinum (II) for regionally confined malignancy. Cancer 1980;45:1278.

206. Einhorn LH, McBride CM, Luce JK, et al. Intra-arterial infusion therapy with 5-(3,3-dimethyl-1-triazeno) imidazole-4-carboxamide (NSC-45388) for malignant melanoma. Cancer 1973;32:749.

207. Savlov ED, Hall TC, Oberfield RA. Intra-arterial therapy of melanoma with dimethyl triazeno imidazole carboxamide (NSC-45388). Cancer 1971;28:1161.

208. Karakousis CP, Choe KJ, Holyoke ED. Biologic behavior and treatment of intransit metastasis of melanoma. Surg Gynecol Obstet 1980;150:29.

209. Morton DL, Eilber FR, Holmes EC, et al. BCG immunotherapy of malignant melanoma: Summary of a seven-year experience. Ann Surg 1974;180:634.

210. Shingleton WW, Seigler HF, Stocks LH, et al. Management of recurrent melanoma of the extremity. Cancer 1975;35:574.

211. Balch CM, Milton GW, Cascinelli N, Milton GW, Sim FH. Elective node dissection: Pros and cons. In: Balch CM, Houghton AN, Milton GW, Sober A, Soong S-j, eds. Cutaneous melanoma. 2nd ed. Philadelphia: JB Lippincott, 1992:345.

212. Milton GW, Shaw HM, McCarthy WH, et al. Prophylactic lymph node dissection in clinical stage I cutaneous malignant melanoma: Results of surgical treatment in 1319 patients. Br J Surg 1982;69:108.

213. Reintgen DS, Cox EB, McCarty KM Jr, et al. Efficacy of elective lymph node dissection in patients with intermediate thickness primary melanoma. Ann Surg 1983;198:379.

214. Schneebaum S, Briele HA, Walker MJ, et al. Cutaneous thick melanoma: Prognosis and treatment. Arch Surg 1987;122:707–711.

215. McCarthy WH, Shaw HM, Milton GW. Efficacy of elective lymph node dissection in 2,347 patients with clinical stage I malignant melanoma. Surg Gynecol Obstet 1985;161:575.

216. Wanebo HJ, Woodruff J, Fortner JG. Malignant melanoma of the extremities: A clinicopathologic study using levels of invasion (microstage). Cancer 1975;35:666.

217. Balch CM. The role of elective lymph node dissection in melanoma: Rationale, results and controversies. J Clin Oncol 1988;6:163, 392.

218. Balch CM, Wilkerson JA, Murad TM, et al. The prognostic significance of ulceration of cutaneous melanoma. Cancer 1980;45:3012.

219. McGovern VJ, Shaw HM, Milton GW, et al. Ulceration and prognosis in cutaneous malignant melanoma. Histopathology 1982;6:399.

220. Elder DE, DuPont G, VanHorn M, et al. The role of lymph node dissection for clinical stage I malignant melanoma of intermediate thickness (1.51–3.99 mm). Cancer 1985;56:413–418.

221. Fee HJ, Robinson DS, Sample WF, et al. The determination of lymph shed by colloid fold scanning in patients with malignant melanoma: Preliminary study. Surgery 1978;84:626.

222. Sullivan DC, Croker BP, Harris CC, et al. Lymphoscintigraphy in malignant melanoma: Tc-antimony sulfur colloid. AJR 1981;137:847.

223. Meyer CM, Lecklitner ML, Logic JR, et al. Technetium-99m sulfur colloid cutaneous lymphoscintigraphy in the management of truncal melanoma. Radiology 1979;131:205.

224. Lamki LM, Logic JR. Defining lymphatic draining patterns with cutaneous lymphoscintigraphy. In: Balch CM, Houghton AN, Milton GW, Sober AJ, Soong S-j, eds. Cutaneous melanoma. 2nd ed. Philadelphia: JB Lippincott, 1992:367.

225. Hansen MG, McCarten AB. Tumor thickness and lymphocytic infiltration in malignant melanoma of the head and neck. Am J Surg 1974;128:557.

226. Goldsmith HS, Shah JP, Kim DH. Prognostic significance of lymph node dissection in the treatment of malignant melanoma. Cancer 1970;26:606.

227. Gumport SL, Harris MN. Results of regional lymph node dissection for melanoma. Ann Surg 1974;179:105.

228. Sugarbaker EV, McBride CM. Melanoma of the trunk: The results of surgical excision and anatomic guidelines for predicting nodal metastasis. Surgery 1976;80:22.

229. Lane N, Lattes R, Malm J. Clinicopathological correlations in a series of 117 malignant melanomas of the skin of adults. Cancer 1958;11:1025.

230. Das Gupta TK. Results of treatment of 269 patients with primary cutaneous melanoma: A five-year prospective study. Ann Surg 1977;186:201.

231. Veronesi U, Adamus J, Bandiera DC, et al. Inefficacy of immediate node dissection in stage I melanoma of the limbs. N Engl J Med 1977;297:627.

232. Veronesi U, Adamus J, Bandiera DC, et al. Stage I melanoma of the limbs: Immediate versus delayed node dissection. Tumori 1980;66:373.

233. Veronesi U, Adams J, Bandiera DC, et al. Delayed regional lymph node dissection in stage I melanoma of the skin of the lower extremities. Cancer 1982;49:2420.

234. Sim FH, Taylor WF, Pritchard DJ, et al. Lymphadenectomy in the management of stage I malignant melanoma: A prospective randomized study. Mayo Clin Proc 1986;61:697.

235. Bowsher WG, Taylor BA, Hughes LE. Morbidity, mortality and local recurrence following regional node dissection for melanoma. Br J Surg 1986;73:906.

236. Ang KK, Byers RM, Peters LJ, Maor MH, Wendt CD, Morrison WH, Goepfert H. Regional radiotherapy as adjuvant treatment for head and neck malignancy melanoma. Arch Otolaryngol Head Neck Surg 1990;116:169–172.

237. Lee YT. Malignant melanoma: Patterns of metastasis. Can J Physician 1980;30:137.

238. Budman DR, Camacho E, Wittes RE. The current causes of death in patients with malignant melanoma. Eur J Cancer 1978;14:327.

239. Patel JK, Didolkar MS, Pickren JW, et al. Metastatic pattern of malignant melanoma: A study of 216 autopsy cases. Am J Surg 1978;135:807.

240. Amer MH, Al-Sarraf M, Vaitkevicius VK. Clinical presentation, natural history and prognostic factors in advanced melanoma. Surg Gynecol Obstet 1979;149:687.

241. De la Monte SM, Moore GW, Hutchins GM. Patterned distribution of metastases from malignant melanoma in humans. Cancer Res 1983;43:3427.

242. Feun LG, Gutterman J, Burgess MA, et al. The natural history of resectable metastatic melanoma (stage IVA melanoma). Cancer 1982;50:1656.

243. Finck SJ, Giuliano AE, Morton DL. LDH and melanoma. Cancer 1983;51:840.

244. Meyer JE, Stolbach L. Pretreatment radiographic evaluation of patients with malignant melanoma. Cancer 1978;42:125.

245. Roth JA, Eilber FR, Bennett LR, et al. Radionuclide photoscanning: Usefulness in preoperative evaluation of melanoma patients. Arch Surg 1975;110:1211.

246. Das Gupta T, Brasfield R. Metastatic melanoma: A clinicopathological study. Cancer 1964;17:1323.

247. Sacre R, Lejeune FJ. Patterns of metastases distribution in 173 stage I and II melanoma patients. Anticancer Res 1982;2:47.

248. Nambisan RN, Alexiou G, Reese PA, et al. Early metastatic patterns and survival in malignant melanoma. J Surg Oncol 1987;34:248.

249. Garg R, McPherson TA, Lentle B, et al. Usefulness of an elevated serum lactate dehydrogenase value as a marker for hepatic metastases in malignant melanoma. Can Med Assoc J 1979;120:1114.

250. Einhorn LH, Burgess MA, Vallejos C, et al. Prognostic correlations and response to treatment in advanced metastatic malignant melanoma. Cancer Res 1974;34:1995.

251. Muss HB, Richards F II, Barnes PL, et al. Radionuclide scanning in patients with advanced malignant melanoma. Clin Nucl Med 1979;4:516.

252. Aranha GV, Simmons RL, Gunnarsson A, et al. The value of preoperative screening procedures in stage I and II malignant melanoma. J Surg Oncol 1979;11:1.

253. Thomas JH, Panoussopoulous D, Liesmann GE, et al. Scintiscans in the evaluation of patients with malignant melanoma. Surg Gynecol Obstet 1979;149:574.

254. Evans RA, Bland KI, McMurtrey MJ, et al. Radionuclide scans not indicated for stage I melanoma. Surg Gynecol Obstet 1980;150:532.

255. Doiron MJ, Bernardino ME. A comparison of non-invasive imaging modalities in the melanoma patient. Cancer 1981;47:2581.

256. Au FC, Maier WP, Malmud LS, et al. Preoperative nuclear scans in patients with melanoma. Cancer 1984;53:2095.

257. Iscoe N, Kersey P, Gapski J, et al. Predictive value of staging investigations in patients with clinical stage I malignant melanoma. Plast Reconstr Surg 1987;80:233.

258. Lewi HJ, Roberts MM, Donaldson AA, et al. The use of cerebral computer assisted tomography as a staging investigation of patients with carcinoma of the breast and malignant melanoma. Surg Gynecol Obstet 1980;151:385.

259. Ardizzoni A, Grimaldi A, Repetto L, et al. Stage I–II melanoma: The value of metastatic workup. Oncology 1987;44:87.

260. Zartman GM, Thomas MR, Robinson WA. Metastatic disease in patients with newly diagnosed malignant melanoma. J Surg Oncol 1987;35:163.

261. Milder MS, Frankel RS, Bulkley BG, et al. Gallium-67 scintigraphy in malignant melanoma. Cancer 1973;32:1350.

262. Romolo JL, Fischer SG. Gallium-67 scanning compared with physical examination in the preoperative staging of melanoma. Cancer 1979;44:468.

263. Berkerman C, Hoffer PB, Bitran JD. The role of gallium-67 in the evaluation of cancer. Semin Nucl Med 1984;14:296.

264. Rossleigh MA, McCarthy WH, Milton GW, et al. The role of gallium-67 studies in the management of malignant melanoma. Med J Aust 1984;140:401.

265. Kirkwood JM, Meyers JE, Vlock DR, et al. Tomographic gallium-67 citrate scanning: Useful new surveillance for metastatic melanoma. Ann Surg 1983;198:102.

266. Houghton AN, Legha S, Bajorin DF. Treatment for advanced melanoma. In: Balch CM, Houghton AN, Milton GW, Sober A, Soong S-j, eds. Cutaneous melanoma. 2nd ed. Philadelphia: JB Lippincott, 1992:468.

267. Hena MA, Emrich LJ, Nambisan RN, et al. Effect of surgical treatment of stage IV melanoma. Am J Surg 1987;153:270.

268. Overett TK, Shiu MH. Surgical treatment of distant metastatic melanoma: Indications and results. Cancer 1985;56:1222.

269. Wornom IL, Smith JW, Soong S-j, et al. Surgery as palliative treatment for distant metastases of melanoma. Ann Surg 1986;204:181.

270. Peters LJ, Byers RM, Ang KK. Radiotherapy for melanoma. In: Balch CM, Houghton AN, Milton GW, Sober AJ, Soong S-j, eds. Cutaneous melanoma. 2nd ed. Philadelphia: JB Lippincott, 1992:509–521.

271. Habermalz HJ, Fischer JJ. Radiation therapy of malignant melanoma: Experience with high individual treatment doses. Cancer 1976;38:2258.

272. Hornsey S. The relationship between total dose, number of fractions and fraction size in the response of malignant melanoma in patients. Br J Radiol 1978;51:905.

273. Katz HR. The results of different fractionation schemes in the palliative irradiation of metastatic melanoma. Int J Radiat Oncol Biol Phys 1981;7:907.

274. Lobo PA, Liebner EJ, Chao JJ, et al. Radiotherapy in the management of malignant melanoma. Int J Radiat Oncol Biol Phys 1981;7:21.

275. Strauss A, Dritschilo A, Nathanson L, et al. Radiation therapy of malignant melanomas. An evaluation of clinically used fractionation schemes. Cancer 1981;47:1262.

276. Trott KR, von Lieven H, Kummermehr J, et al. The radiosensitivity of malignant melanomas. II. Clinical studies. Int J Radiat Oncol Biol Phys 1981;7:15.

277. Adam JS, Habeshaw T, Kirk J. Response rate of malignant melanoma to large fraction irradiation. Br J Radiol 1982;55:605.

278. Doss LL, Memula N. The radioresponsiveness of melanoma. Int J Radiat Oncol Biol Phys 1982;8:1131.

279. Overgaard J, von der Masse H, Overgaard MA. A randomized study comparing two high-dose per fraction radiation schedules in recurrent or metastatic melanoma. Int J Radiat Oncol Biol Phys 1985;11:1837.

280. Overgaard J, Overgaard M, Hansen V, et al. Some factors of importance in the radiation treatment of malignant melanoma. Radiother Oncol 1986;5:183.

281. Bentzen SM, Overgaard J, Thames HD, Overgaard M, Hansen PV, van der Masse H. Clinical radiobiology of malignant melanoma. Radiother Oncol 1989;16:169.

282. Thames HD, Withers HR, Peters LJ, Fletcher GH. Changes in early and late radiation responses with altered dose fractionation: Implications for dose-survival relationships. Int J Radiat Oncol Biol Phys 1982;8:219.

283. Sause WT, Cooper JS, Rush S, Ago CT Cosmatos D, Coughlin CT, et al. RTOG 83-05: A randomized trial evaluating fraction size in external beam radiation therapy in treatment of melanoma. Int J Radiat Oncol Biol Phys 1991;20:429.

284. Overgaard J, Overgaard M. Hyperthermia as an adjuvant to radiotherapy in the treatment of malignant melanoma. Int J Hyperthermia 1987;3:483.

285. Meyer JL, Kapp DS, Fessemdem P. Hahn GH. Hyperthermic oncology: Current biology, physics and clinical results. Pharmacol Ther 1989;42:251.

286. Blake PR, Catterall M, Errington RF. Treatment of malignant melanoma by fast neutrons. Br J Surg 1985;75:517.

287. Dische S. Radiotherapy using the hypoxic cell sensitizer Ro 03-8799 in malignant melanoma. Radiother Oncol 1987;10:11.

288. Chapman JD, Urtasun RC, Frank AJ, Raleigh JA, Meeker BE, McKinnon SA. The measurement oxygenation status of individual tumors. In: Paliwal BR, Fowler JF, Herbert DE, Kinsella TJ, Orton CG, eds. Prediction of response in radiation therapy: The physical and biological basis. New York: American Institute of Physics, 1989:49.

289. DeLaney TF, Glatstein E. Photodynamic therapy of cancer. Compr Ther 1988;14:43.

290. Mishima Y, Ichilhashi M, Hatta S, Honda Ch, Yamamura K, Nakagawa T, et al. First human clinical trial of melanoma neutron capture: Diagnosis and therapy. Strahlenther Onkol 1989;165:251.

291. Marsoni S, Hoth D, Simon R. Clinical drug development. An analysis of phase II trials, 1970–1985. Cancer Treat Rep 1987;71:71.

292. Comis RL. DTIC (NSC-45388) in malignant melanoma: A perspective. Cancer Treat Rep 1976;64:1123.

293. Luce JK. Chemotherapy of malignant melanoma. Cancer 1972;30:1604.

294. Costanza ME, Nathanson L, Schoenfeld D, et al. Results with methyl-CCNU and DTIC in metastatic melanoma. Cancer 1977;40:1010.

295. Wagner DE, Ramirez G, Weiss AJ. Combination phase I–II study of imidazole carboxamide (NSC-45388). Oncology 1971;26:310.

296. Nathanson L, Wolter K, Horton J. Characteristics of prognosis and response to an imidazole carboxamide in malignant melanoma. Clin Pharmacol Ther 1971;12:955.

297. Costanza ME, Nathanson L, Lenhard R, et al. Therapy of malignant melanoma with an imidazole carboxamide and bischloroethyl nitrosourea. Cancer 1972;30:1457.

298. Moon JH, Gailanai S, Cooper MR, et al. Comparison of the combination of 1,3-bis (2-chloroethyl)-1-nitrosourea (BCNU) and vincristine with two dose schedules of 5-(3,3-dimethyl-1-triazeno) imiadazole 4-carboxamide (DTIC) in the treatment of disseminated malignant melanoma. Cancer 1975;35:368.

299. Van der Merwe AM, Falkson G, Van Eden EB. Metastatic malignant melanoma. Imidazole carboxamide in its treatment. Med Proc 1971;17:399.

300. Luce JK, Thurman WG, Isaacs BL, Talley RW. Clinical trials with the antitumor agent 5-(3,3-dimethyl-1-triazeno) imidazole-4-carboxamide (NSC-45388). Cancer Chemother Rep 1970;54:119–124.

301. Gerner RE, Moore GE. Study of 5-(3,3-dimethyl-1-triazeno) imidazole-4-carboxamide (NSC-45388) in patients with disseminated melanoma. Cancer Chemother Rep 1973;57:83.

302. Gottlieb JA, Serpick AA. Clinical evaluation of 5-(3,3-dimethyl-1-triazeno) imidazole 4-carboxamide in malignant melanoma and other neoplasms: Comparison of twice weekly and daily administration schedules. Oncology 1971;25:255.

303. Burke PJ, McCarthy NWH, Milton GW. Imidazole carboxamide therapy in advanced malignant melanoma. Cancer 1971;27:744.

304. Cowan DH, Bersagel DE. Intermittent treatment of metastatic malignant melanoma with high-dose 5-(3,3-dimethyl-1-triazeno)-imidazole-4-carboxamide (NSC-45388). Cancer Chemother Rep 1971;55:175.

305. Vogel CL, Comis RL, Ziegler JL, Kiryabwire JW. Study of 5-(3,3-dimethyl-1-triazeno) imidazole-4-carboxamide (NSC-45388) given intravenously in the treatment of malignant melanoma in Uganda. Cancer Chemother Rep 1973;55:143.

306. Costanza J. DTIC (NSC-45388) studies in the Southwest Oncology Group. Cancer Treat Rep 1976;60:189.

307. Pritchard KI, Quirt IC, Cowan DH et al. DTIC therapy in metastatic malignant melanoma: A simplified dose schedule. Cancer Treat Rep 1980;64:1123.

308. Hill GJ II, Krementz ET, Hill HZ. Dimethyl triazeno imidazole carboxamide and combination therapy for melanoma. IV. Late results after complete response to chemotherapy. Cancer 1984;53:1299.

309. Einhorn LH, Burgess MA, Vallejos C, et al. Prognostic correlations and response to treatment in advanced metastatic melanoma. Cancer Res 1974;34:1995.

310. Thatcher N, Anderson H, James R, et al. DTIC by 24 hour infusion for metastatic melanoma. Proceedings of the First International Conference on Skin Melanoma (Venice), 1985;1:156.

311. Carter RD, Krementz ET, Hill GJ II, et al. DTIC (NSC-45388) and combination therapy for melanoma. I. Studies with DTIC, BCNU, CCNU, vincristine, and hydroxyurea. Cancer Treat Rep 1976;60:601.

312. Bellet RE, Mastrangelo MJ, Laucius JF, et al. Randomized prospective trial of DTIC (NSC-45388) alone versus BCNU (NSC-409962) in the treatment of metastatic malignant melanoma. Cancer Treat Rep 1976;60:595.

313. Carter SK, Friedman MA. 5-(3,3-dimethyl-1-triazeno) imidazole-4-carboxamide (DTIC, DIC, NSC-45388): A new tumor agent with activity against malignant melanoma. Eur J Cancer 1972;8:85.

314. Salem PA, Sinno B, Hajj A, et al. High dose intermittent therapy with 5-(3,3-dimethyl-1-triazeno) imidazole-4-carboxamide (DTIC) in melanoma and other solid tumors. Proc Am Assoc Cancer Res 1976;17:116.

315. Ahmann DL, Hahn RG, Bisel HF, et al. Clinical evaluation of 5-(3,3-dimethyl-1-triazeno) imidazole-4-carboxamide (NSC-45388), melphalan (NSC-8806) and hydroxyurea (NSC-32065) in the treatment of disseminated malignant melanoma. Cancer Chemother Rep 1972;56:369.

316. Carbone PP, Costello W. Eastern Cooperative Oncology Group studies with DTIC (NSC-45388). Cancer Treat Rep 1976;60:193–198.

317. Tyson LB, Clark RA, Gralla RJ, et al. High-dose metoclopramide: Control of dacarbazine-induced emesis in a preliminary trial. Cancer Treat Rep 1982;66:2108.

318. Clark RA, Tyson LB, Gralla RJ, et al. Antiemetic therapy: Management of chemotherapy-induced nausea and vomiting. Semin Oncol Nurs 1989;5:53.

319. Ramirez G, Wilson W, Grage T, et al. Phase II evaluation of 1,3-bis(2-chloroethyl-nitrosourea) (BCNU; NSC-409962) in patients with solid tumors. Cancer Chemother Rep 1972;56:787.

320. DeVita VT, Carbone PP, Owens AH Jr, et al. Clinical trials with 1,3,-bis(2-chloroethyl)-1-nitrosourea, NSC-409962. Cancer Res 1965;25:1875.

321. Ahmann DL. Nitrosoureas in the management of disseminated malignant melanoma. Cancer Treat Rep 1976;60:747.

322. Beretta G, Pancera G, Locatelli C, et al. Lomustine (CCNU) and epirubicin as alternative treatments to dacarbazine (DIC) for advanced malignant melanoma. Proceedings of the First International Conference on Skin Melanoma (Venice), 1985;1:148.

323. Ahmann DL, Hahn RG, Bisel HF. A comparative study of 1-(2-chloroethyl)-3-cyclohexyl-1-nitrosourea (NSC-79037) and imidazole carboxamide (NSC-45388) with

vincristine (NSC-67574) in the palliation of disseminated malignant melanoma. Cancer Res 1972;32:2432.

324. Hoogstraten B, Gottlieb JA, Caoili E, et al. CCNU (1-(2,chloroethyl)-3-cyclohexyl-1-nitrosourea, NSC-79037) in the treatment of cancer. Cancer 1973;32:38.

325. Ahmann DL, Hahn RG, Bisel HF. Evaluation of 1-(2-chloroethyl-3-4-methyl-cyclo-hexyl)-1-nitrosourea (methyl-CCNU, NSC-95441) versus combined imidazole carboxamide (NSC-45388) and vincristine (NSC-67574) in palliation of disseminated melanoma. Cancer 1974;33:615.

326. Wasserman TH, Slavik M, Carter SK. Review of CCNU in clinical cancer therapy. Cancer Treat Rev 1974;1:131.

327. Young RC, Canellos GP, Chabner BA, et al. Treatment of malignant melanoma with methyl-CCNU. Cancer Pharmacol Ther 1974;15:617.

328. Wasserman TH, Slavik M, Carter SK. Methyl-CCNU in clinical cancer therapy. Cancer Treat Rev 1974;1:251.

329. Jacquillat C, Khayat D, Banzet P, et al. Final report of the French multicenter Phase II study of the nitrosourea fotemustine in 153 evaluable patients with disseminated malignant melanoma including patients with cerebral metastases. Cancer 1990;66:1873.

330. Khayat D, Lokiec F, Bizzari J-P, et al. Phase I clinical study of the new amino acid-linked nitrosourea S10036 administered on a weekly schedule. Cancer Res 1987;47:6782.

331. Nolte H, Lindgaard-Nedsen E, Bloomquist E, et al. Phase II evaluation of tauromustine in disseminated malignant melanoma. Proc Am Soc Clin Oncol 1988;7:249.

332. Al-Sarraf M, Fletcher W, Oishi N, et al. Cisplatin hydration with and without mannitol diuresis in refractory disseminated malignant melanoma: A Southwest Oncology Group study. Cancer Treat Rep 1982;66:31.

333. Goodnight JE Jr, Moseley HS, Eilber FR, et al. Cis-dichlorodiammineplatinum (II) alone and combined with DTIC for treatment of disseminated malignant melanoma. Cancer Treat Rep 1979;63:2005.

334. Schilcher RB, Wessels M, Niederle N, Seeber S, Schmidt CG. Phase II evaluation of fractionated low and single high dose cisplatin in various tumors. J Cancer Res Clin Oncol 1984;107:57.

335. Glover D, Glick J, Weiler C, Fox K, Grabelsky S, Guerry D. High dose cis-platinum (DDP) and WR-2721 in metastatic melanoma. Proc Am Soc Clin Oncol 1987;7:247.

336. Song SY, Chary KK, Higby DJ, Henderson ES, Klein E. Cisdiamminedichloride platinum (II) in the treatment of metastatic malignant melanoma. Clin Res 1977;25:411.

337. Chary KK, Higby DJ, Henderson ES, Swinerton KD. Phase I study of high-dose cis-dichlorodiammineplatinum (II) with forced diuresis. Cancer Treat Rep 1977;61:367.

338. Mortimer JE, Chestnut T, Higano CS, Goodman G. High dose cisplatin in metastatic melanoma: Comparison of two schedules. Proc Am Soc Clin Oncol 1988;7:254.

339. Kim S, McClay E, Kirmani S, et al. Biweekly intravenous (IV) cisplatin with sodium thiosulfate. Proc Am Soc Clin Oncol 1990;9:88.

340. Evans L, Casper ES, Rosenbluth R. Phase II trial of carboplatin in advanced malignant melanoma. Cancer Treat Rep 1987;71:171.

341. Rumke PH. The use of chemotherapy in the management of patients with malignant melanoma. Dev Oncol 1984;25:190.

342. Costa G, Hreshchyshyn MM, Holland JF. Initial clinical studies with vincristine. Cancer Chemother Rep 1962;24:39.

343. Holland JF, Scharlay C, Gailanai S, et al. Vincristine treatment of advanced cancer: A cooperative study of 392 cases. Cancer Res 1264;33:1258.

344. Gubisch NJ, Norena D, Perlia CP, et al. Experience with vincristine in solid tumors. Cancer Chemother Rep 1963;32:19.

345. Shaw RK, Brunner JA. Clinical evaluation of vincristine (NSC-67574). Cancer Chemother Rep 1964;42:45.

346. Reitmeier RJ, Moertel CG, Blackburn CM, et al. Vincristine (NSC-67574) therapy of adult patients with solid tumors. Cancer Chemother Rep 1964;34:21.

347. Smart CR, Ottoman RE, Rochlin DB, et al. Clinical experience with vincristine (NSC-67574) in tumors of the central nervous system and other malignant diseases. Cancer Chemother Rep 1968;52:733.

348. Frei E, Franzino A, Shnider BI, et al. Clinical studies of vinblastine. Cancer Chemother Rep 1961;12:125.

349. Armstrong JG, Dyke RW, Fouts PJ, et al. Hodgkin's disease, carcinoma of the breast and other tumors treated with vinblastine sulfate. Cancer Chemother Rep 1962;18:49.

350. Acute Leukemia Group B, Eastern Cooperative Group. Neoplastic diseases: Treatment with vinblastine. Arch Intern Med 1965;111:846.

351. Bond WH, Rohn RJ, Bates LH, et al. Treatment of neoplastic diseases with an improved oral preparation of vinblastine sulfate. Cancer 1966;19:213.

352. Hodes ME, Rohn RJ, Bond WH, Yardley JM, Corpening WS. Vincaleukoblastine. IV. A summary of two and one half years' experience in the use of vinblastine. Cancer Chemother Rep 1962;16:401.

353. Hill JM II, Loeb E. Treatment of leukemia, lymphoma, and other malignant neoplasms with vinblastine. Cancer Chemother Rep 1961;15:41.

354. Falkson G, Van Dyk JJ, Verwoerd HF. The chemotherapy of malignant melanoma. S Afr Med J 1968;42:89.

355. Wright TL, Hurley J, Korst DR, et al. Vinblastine in neoplastic disease. Cancer Res 1963;23:169.

356. Smart CR, Rochlin DB, Nahum AM, et al. Clinical experience with vinblastine sulfate (NSC-49842) in squamous cell carcinoma and other malignancies. Cancer Chemother Rep 1964;34:31.

357. Bleehan NM, Jellifee AM. Vinblastine sulfate in the treatment of malignant disease. Br J Cancer 1965;19:268.

358. Currie VE, Wong PP, Krakoff IH, et al. Phase I trial of vindesine in patients with advanced cancer. Cancer Treat Rep 1978;62:1333.

359. Camacho FJ, Young CW, Wittes RE. Phase II trial of vindesine in patients with malignant melanoma. Cancer Treat Rep 1980;64:179.

360. Retsas S, Peat I, Ashford R, et al. Updated results of vindesine as a single agent in the therapy of advanced malignant melanoma. Cancer Treat Rev 1980;7(Suppl):87.

361. Carmichael J, Atkinson RJ, Calman KC, Mackie RM, Naysmith AM, Smyth JF. A muticentre phase II trial of vindesine in malignant melanoma. Eur J Cancer Clin Oncol 1982;18:1293.

362. DiBella NJ, Berris R, Garfield D, Fink K, Speer J, Sakamoto A. Vindesine in advanced breast cancer, lymphoma and melanoma. Invest New Drugs 1984;2:323.

363. Quagliana JM, Stephens RL, Baker LH, Costanzi JJ. Vindesine in patients with metastatic malignant melanoma. J Clin Oncol 1984;2:316.

364. Smith IE, Hedley DW, Powles TJ, et al. Vindesine: A phase II study in the treatment of breast carcinoma, malignant melanoma and other solid tumors. Cancer Treat Rep 1978;62:1427.

365. Nelimark RA, Peterson BA, Vosika GJ, et al. Vindesine for metastatic malignant melanoma. Eur J Cancer Clin Oncol 1983;18:1293.

366. Rumke P, Everall JD, Mulder JH, et al. EORTC phase II trial of vindesine in advanced melanoma. Eur J Cancer Clin Oncol 1983;19:1173.

367. Arseneau JC, Mellette SJ, Kuperminc M, et al. Phase II study of vindesine in metastatic malignant melanoma. Cancer Treat Rep 1981;65:355.

368. Wagstaff J, Anderson HA, Shiu W, et al. Phase II study of vindesine infusion in visceral metastatic malignant melanoma. Cancer Treat Rep 1983;67:839.

369. Mayol XF, Beltran J, Rubio-Bazan R, et al. Multicenter phase II trial with 5-day continuous infusion of vindesine in metastatic malignant melanoma. Cancer Treat Rep 1983;68:1199.

370. Wiernik PH, Schwartz EL, Einzig A, et al. Phase I trial of taxol given as a 24-hour infusion every 2 days: Responses observed in metastatic melanoma. J Clin Oncol 1987;5:1232.

371. Einzig A, Trump DL, Sasloff J, et al. Phase II pilot study of taxol in patients with malignant melanoma. Proc Am Soc Clin Oncol 1988;7:249.

372. Legha SS, Ring S, Papadopoulos N, et al. A phase II trial of taxol in metastatic melanoma. Cancer 1990;65:2478.

373. Andrews NC, Weiss AJ, Ansfield FJ, et al. Phase I study of dibromodulcitol (NSC-104800). Cancer Chemother Rep 1971;55:61.

374. Phillips RW, Brook J. Clinical experience with dibromodulcitol (NSC-104800) in solid tumors. Cancer Chemother Rep 1971;55:567.

375. Andrews NC, Weiss AJ, Wilson W, et al. Phase II study of dibromodulcitol (NSC-104800). Cancer Chemother Rep 1974;58:653.

376. Bellet RE, Catalano RB, Mastrangelo MJ, et al. Positive phase II trial of dibromodulcitol in patients with metastatic melanoma refractory to DTIC and nitrosoureas. Cancer Treat Rep 1978;69:2095.

377. Simmonds MA, Lipton A, Harvey HA, et al. Phase II study of mitolactol in metastatic malignant melanoma. Cancer Treat Rep 198;69:65.

378. Amato DA, Bruckner H, Guerry D IV, et al. Phase II evaluation of dibromodulcitol and actinomycin D, hydroxyurea and cyclophosphamide in previously untreated patients with malignant melanoma. Invest New Drugs 1987;5:293.

379. Medina W, Kirkwood JM. Phase II trial of mitolactol in patients with metastatic melanoma. Cancer Treat Rep 1985;69:723.

380. Murray N, Silver H, Shah A, et al. Phase II study of mitolactol in advanced malignant melanoma. Cancer Treat Rep 1985;69:723.

381. Malden LT, Coates AS, Milton GW, et al. Mitolactol chemotherapy for malignant melanoma. Cancer Treat Rep 1984;68:1045.

382. Friustaci S, Gafprini G, Galligioni E, et al. Phase II trial of Esorubicin in patients with advanced melanoma. Cancer Treat Rep 1987;71:325.

383. Feun LG, Gonzalez R, Savaraj N, et al. Phase II study of piritrexim in metastatic melanoma using intermittent, low dose administration. J Clin Oncol 1986;4:179.

384. Phillips GL, Fay JW, Herzig GP, et al. Intensive 1,3-bis(2-chloroethyl)-1-nitrosourea (BCNU) with autologous bone marrow transplantation therapy of refractory cancer: A preliminary report. Exp Hematol 1979;7:372.

385. Thomas MR, Robinson WA, Glode LM, et al. Treatment of advanced malignant melanoma with high-dose chemotherapy and autologous bone marrow transplantation: Preliminary results—phase I study. Am J Clin Oncol 1982;5:611.

386. Lazarus HM, Herzig RH, Graham-Pole J, et al. Intensive melphalan chemotherapy and cryopreserved autologous bone marrow transplantation for the treatment of refractory cancer. J Clin Oncol 1983;1:359.

387. Spitzer G, Dicke K, Zander AR, et al. High-dose chemotherapy with autologous bone marrow transplantation. Cancer 1984;54:216.

388. Tchekmedyian NS, Tait N, van Echo D, et al. High-dose chemotherapy without autologous bone marrow transplantation in melanoma. J Clin Oncol 1991;9:1811.

389. Phillips GL, Fay JW, Herzig GP, et al. Intensive 1,3-bis(2-chloroethyl)-1-nitrosourea (BCNU), NSC-409962 and cryopreserved autologous marrow transplantation for refractory cancer: A phase I–II study. Cancer 1983;52:1792.

390. Lazarus HM, Herzig RH, Wolff SN, et al. Treatment of metastatic malignant melanoma with intensive melphalan and autologous bone marrow transplantation. Cancer Treat Rep 1985;69:473.

391. McElwain TJ, Hedley DW, Burton G, et al. Marrow autotransplantation accelerates hematological recovery in patients with malignant melanoma treated with high-dose melphalan. Br J Cancer 1979;40:72.

392. McElwain TJ, Hedley DW, Gordon MY, et al. High dose melphalan and non-cryopreserved autologous bone marrow treatment of malignant melanoma and neuroblastoma. Exp Hematol 1979;7(Suppl):360.

393. Wolff SN, Herzig RH, Fay JW, et al. High dose thiotepa with autologous bone marrow

transplantation for metastatic melanoma: Results of phase I–II studies of the North American Bone Marrow Transplantation Group. J Clin Oncol 1989;7:245.

394. Antman K, Eder JP, Elias A, et al. High dose combination alkylating agent preparative regimen with autologous bone marrow support: The Dana-Farber Cancer Institute/ Beth Israel Hospital experience. Cancer Treat Rep 1987;71:119.

395. Ciobanu N, Dutcher J, Gucalp R, et al. High dose chemotherapy with autologous bone marrow transplantation for malignant melanoma after failure of interleukin-2 and lymphokine activated killer cells. Proc Am Soc Clin Oncol 1989;8:281.

396. Slease RB, Benear JB, Selby GB, et al. High dose combination alkylating agent therapy with autologous bone marrow rescue for refractory solid tumors. J Clin Oncol 1988;6:1314.

397. Eder JP, Antman K, Elias A, et al. Cyclophosphamide and thiotepa with autologous bone marrow transplantation in patients with solid tumors. JNCI 1990;80:1221.

398. Shea TC, Antman KH, Eder JP, et al. Malignant melanoma: Treatment with high-dose combination alkylating chemotherapy and autologous bone marrow support. Arch Dermatol 1988;124:878.

399. Moormeier JA, Williams SF, Kaminer LS, et al. High-dose tri-alkylator chemotherapy with autologous stem cell rescue in patients with refractory malignancies. JNCI 1990;82:29.

400. Thatcher N, Lind M, Morgenstern G, et al. High dose double alkylating agent chemotherapy with DTIC, melphalan or ifosphamide and marrow rescue for metastatic malignant melanoma. Cancer 1989;63:1296.

401. Glover D, Glick JH, Weiler C, et al. WR 2721 and high-dose cis-platin: An active combination in the treatment of metastatic melanoma. J Clin Oncol 1987;5:574.

402. Mastrangelo MJ, Berd D, Bellet RE. Aggressive chemotherapy for melanoma. PPO Updates 1991;5:1.

403. Coit DG, Bajorin DF, Menedez-Botet C, et al. A phase I study of hyperthermic isolation limb perfusion using cisplatin for metastatic melanoma. Proc Am Soc Clin Oncol 1991;10:294.

404. Mavligit G, Carrasco C, Papadopoulos N, et al. Regression of ocular melanoma metastatic to the liver after chemoembolization with cis-platinum and polyvinyl sponge. Proc Am Soc Clin Oncol 1987;6:830.

405. Mavligit GM, Charnsangavej C, Carrasco CH, et al. Regression of ocular melanoma metastatic to the liver after hepatic arterial chemoembolization with cisplatin and polyvinyl sponge. J Am Med Assoc 1988;260:974.

406. Nathanson L, Kaufman SD, Carey RW. Vinblastine infusion, bleomycin, and cis-dichlorodiammine-platinum chemotherapy in metastatic melanoma. Cancer 1981;48:1290.

407. Nathanson L, Wittenberg BK. Pilot study of vinblastine and bleomycin combinations in the treatment of metastatic melanoma. Cancer Treat Rep 1980;64:133.

408. National Cancer Institute of Canada Melanoma Group. Vinblastine, bleomycin, and cis-platinum for the treatment of metastatic malignant melanoma. J Clin Oncol 1984;2:131.

409. Luikart SD, Kennealey GT, Kirkwood JM. Randomized phase III trial of vinblastine, bleomycin, and cis-dichlorodiammine-platinum versus dacarbazine in malignant melanoma. J Clin Oncol 1984;2:164.

410. Kirkwood JM, Ernstoff MS, Guiliano A, et al. Interferon-α2a and dacarbazine in melanoma. JNCI 1990;82:1062.

411. McLeod GRC, Thomson DB, Hersey P. Recombinant interferon alpha-2b in advanced melanoma: A phase I–II study in combination with DTIC. Int J Cancer 1987;1(Suppl):31.

412. Breier S, Pensel R, Roffe C, et al. High dose DTIC with recombinant interferon-α2b for the treatment of metastatic malignant melanoma. Proc Am Soc Clin Oncol 1990;9:821.

413. Vorobiof DA, Falkson G, Voges CW. DTIC versus DTIC and recombinant interferon-α2b in treatment of patients with advanced malignant melanoma. Proc Am Soc Clin Oncol 1989;8:284.

414. Bajetta E, Negretta E, Giannotti B, et al. Phase II study of interferon-α2a and dacarbazine in metastatic melanoma. Proc Am Soc Clin Oncol 1989;8:286.

415. Mickiewicz E, Estevez R, Rao F, et al. Interferon-α2b for the treatment of metastatic melanoma. Proc Am Soc Clin Oncol 1990;9:281.

416. Kerr R, Pippen P, Mennel R, et al. Treatment of metastatic malignant melanoma with a combination of interferon-α2a and dacarbazine. Proc Am Soc Clin Oncol 1989;8:288.

417. Mulder NH, Schraffordt S, Koops H, et al. Dacarbazine and α-interferon for disseminated metastatic melanoma. Proc Am Soc Clin Oncol 1990;9:279.

418. Sertoli MR. DTIC with or without recombinant interferon α-2A at different dosages in the treatment of stage IV melanoma patients: Preliminary results of a randomized clinical trial. Proc Advances Biol Clin Management Melanoma 1991;34:138.

419. Falkson CI, Falkson G, Falkson HC. Improved results with the addition of interferon α-2b to dacarbazine in the treatment of 6 patients with malignant melanoma. J Clin Oncol 1991;9:1403.

420. Hill II JG, Metter GE, Krementz ET, et al. DTIC and combination therapy for melanoma. II. Escalating schedules of DTIC with BCNU, CCNU, and vincristine. Cancer Treat Rep 1979;63:1989.

421. McKelvey EM, Luce JK, Talley RW, et al. Combination chemotherapy with bis-chloroethyl nitrosourea (BCNU), vincristine and dimethyl triazeno imidazole carboxamide (DTIC) in disseminated malignant melanoma. Cancer 1977;39:1.

422. Berretta G, Bajetta E, Bonadonna G, et al. Polichemioterapia con 5 (3,3-dimetiltriazeno)-imidazole-4-carboxamide (DTIC; NSC-45388), 1,3-bis (2-chloretil)-1-nitrosourea (BCNU; NSC-409962) e vincristina (NSC-67574) nel melanoma in fase metastatizzata. Tumori 1973;59:239.

423. Berretta G, Bonadonna G, Cascinelli N, et al. Comparative evaluation of three com-

bination regimens for advanced malignant melanoma: Results of an international cooperative study. Cancer Treat Rep 1976;60:33.

424. Cohen SM, Greenspan EM, Ratner LH, et al. Combination chemotherapy of malignant melanoma with imidazole carboxamide, BCNU, and vincristine. Cancer 1977;39:41.

425. Luce JK, Torin LB, Price H. Combination dimethyltriazeno imidazole carboxamide (NSC-45388), vincristine (NSC-67574; VCR) and 1,3-bis (2-chloroethyl)-1-nitrosourea (NSC-409962; BCNU) chemotherapy of disseminated malignant melanoma. Proc Am Assoc Cancer Res 1970;11:50.

426. Einhorn LH, Furnas B. Combination chemotherapy for disseminated malignant melanoma with DTIC, vincristine and methyl-CCNU. Cancer Treat Rep 1977;61:881.

427. Carmo-Pereira J, Costa FO, Pimentel P. Combination cytotoxic chemotherapy for metastatic cutaneous malignant melanoma with DTIC, BCNU and vincristine. Cancer Treat Rep 1976;60:1381.

428. Kleeberg UR, Schreml W. Polychemotherapie des metastasierenden melanomas. Vincristin, carmustin, dacarbazin. Deutsch Med Wochenschr 1976;101:890.

429. Berretta G, Bonadonna G, Bajetta E, et al. Combination chemotherapy (NSC-45388) in advanced malignant melanoma, soft tissue sarcomas and Hodgkin's disease. Cancer Treat Rep 1976;60:1381.

430. Gunderson S. Dacarbazine, vindesine and cisplatin combination chemotherapy in advanced malignant melanoma. Cancer Treat Rep 1987;71:997.

431. Carey RW, Anderson JR, Green M, et al. Treatment of metastatic malignant melanoma with vinblastine, dacarbazine and cisplatin: a report from the Cancer and Leukemia Group B. Cancer Treat Rep 1986;70:329.

432. Verschraegen CF, Kleeberg UR, Mulder J, et al. Combination of cisplatin, vindesine and dacarbazine in advanced malignant melanoma: A phase II study of the EORTC Malignant Melanoma Cooperative Group. Cancer 1988;62:1061.

433. Ringborg U, Jungnelius J, Hansson J, Strander H. DTIC-vindesine-cisplatin in disseminated malignant melanoma: A phase II study. Proc Am Soc Clin Oncol 1987;6:212.

434. Wussow P, Hartman F, Block B, Schmoll HJ, Deicher H, Peter HH. Treatment of advanced malignant melanoma with dacarbazine, vindesine and dacarbazine (DVP). Proceedings of the Fourth European Conference on Clinical Oncology and Cancer Nursing (Paris), 1987:238.

435. Gundersen S. Dacarbazine, vindesine and cisplatin combination chemotherapy in advanced malignant melanoma: A phase II study. Cancer Treat Rep 1987;71:997.

436. Legha SS, Ring S, Papadopoulos N, Plager C, Chawla S, Benjamin R. A prospective evaluation of a triple-drug regimen containing cisplatin, vinblastine and DTIC (CVD) for metastatic melanoma. Cancer 1989;64:2024.

437. Steffens TA, Bajorin DF, Chapman PB, et al. A phase II trial of high-dose cisplatin and dacarbazine: Lack of efficacy of high-dose cisplatin-based therapy for metastatic melanoma. Cancer 1991;68:1230.

438. Buzaid AC, Murren JR, Durivage HJ. High-dose cisplatin with dacarbazine and tamoxifen in the treatment of metastatic melanoma. Cancer 1991;68:1238.

439. Del Prete SA, Maurer LH, O'Donnell J. Combination chemotherapy with cisplatin, carmustine, dacarbazine, and tamoxifen in metastatic melanoma. Cancer Treat Rep 1984;68:1403.

440. McClay EF, Mastrangelo MJ, Bellet RE. Combination chemotherapy and hormonal therapy in the treatment of malignant melanoma. Cancer Treat Rep 1987;71:465.

441. McClay EF, Mastrangelo MJ, Sprandio JD, et al. The importance of tamoxifen to a cisplatin-containing regimen in the treatment of metastatic melanoma. Cancer 1989;63:1292.

442. McClay EF, Albright K, Jones J, et al. Modulation of cisplatin resistance by tamoxifen in human malignant melanoma. Proc Advances in the Biology and Clinical Management of Melanoma 1991;43:101.

443. McClay EF, Sprandio JD, Mastrangelo MJ, et al. Importance of tamoxifen to a combination chemotherapy regimen for melanoma. Proc Am Soc Clin Oncol 1988;7:251.

444. Carmo-Pereira J, Kosta SO, Henriques E. Combination cytotoxic chemotherapy with procarbazine, vincristine and lomustine in disseminated malignant melanoma: Eight years follow-up. Cancer Treat Rep 1984;68:1211.

445. Shelley W, Quirt I, Bodurtha A, et al. Lomustine, vincristine and procarbazine in the treatment of metastatic melanoma. Cancer Treat Rep 1985;69:941.

446. Kirkwood JM, Ernstoff M. Potential application of the interferons in oncology: Lesions drawn from studies of human melanoma. Semin Oncol 1986;13:48.

447. Krown SE, Burk MW, Kirkwood JM, et al. Human leukocyte (α) interferon in metastatic malignant melanoma: The American Cancer Society phase II trial. Cancer Treat Rep 1984;68:723.

448. Creagan ET, Ahmann DL, Green SJ, et al. Phase II study of recombinant leukocyte A interferon (rIFN-αA) in disseminated malignant melanoma. Cancer 1984;54:2844.

449. Creagan ET, Ahmann DL, Green SJ, et al. Phase II study of low-dose recombinant leukocyte A interferon in disseminated malignant melanoma. J Clin Oncol 1985;2:1002.

450. Creagan ET, Ahman DL, Frytak S, et al. Recombinant leukocyte A interferon (rIFN-α2A) in the treatment of disseminated malignant melanoma: Analysis of complete and long-term responding patients. Cancer 1986;58:2576.

451. Jacquillat C, Mural J, Chelq C, et al. Treatment of metastatic malignant melanoma with Roferon A. Proceedings of the Third European Conference on Clinical Oncology and Cancer Nursing (Stockholm), 1985;3:183.

452. Hersey P, Hasic E, MacDonald M, et al. Effects of recombinant leukocyte interferon (rIFN-αA) on tumor growth and immune responses in patients with metastatic melanoma. Br J Cancer 1985;51:815.

453. Thompson DB, McLeod GR. Pilot efficacy study of recombinant leukocyte A interferon (Ro 22-8181; IFN-rA) in patients with metastatic melanoma. Proceedings of the

Third European Conference on Clinical Oncology and Cancer Nursing (Stockholm), 1984;3:47.

454. Legha SS, Papadopoulos NEJ, Plager C, et al. Clinical evaluation of recombinant interferon-α2A (Roferon-A) in metastatic melanoma using two different schedules. J Clin Oncol 1987;5:1240.

455. Kirkwood JM, Ernstoff MS, Davis CA, et al. Comparison of intramuscular and intravenous recombinant interferon in melanoma and other cancers. Ann Intern Med 1985;103:32.

456. Robinson WA, Kirkwood J, Harvey H et al. Effective use of recombinant α2a-interferon in metastatic malignant melanoma. Proc Am Soc Clin Oncol 1984;3:60.

457. Robinson WA, Mughal TI, Thomas MR, et al. Treatment of metastatic melanoma with recombinant interferon α2. Immunobiology 1986;172:275.

458. Coates A, Rallings M, Hersey P, et al. Phase II study of recombinant α-2 interferon in advanced malignant melanoma. J Interferon Res 1986;6:1.

459. Dorval T, Palangie T, Jouve M, et al. Treatment of metastatic malignant melanoma with recombinant interferon alpha-2b. Invest New Drugs 1987;5:561.

460. Hawkins MJ, McCune CS, Speyer JL, et al. Recombinant α-2 interferon (SCH 30500) in patients with metastatic malignant melanoma: An ECOG pilot study. Proc Am Soc Clin Oncol 1984;3:51.

461. Miller RL, Steis RG, Clark JW, et al. Randomized trial of recombinant α-2B-interferon with or without indomethacin in patients with metastatic malignant melanoma. Cancer Res 1989;49:1871.

462. Kokaschka EM, Micksche M, Babits R, et al. Phase I study with high dose recombinant α-2 interferon in chemotherapy-resistant malignant melanoma patients. Antiviral Res 1984;3:105.

463. Kuzmits R, Kokoschka EM, Micksche M, et al. Phase II results with recombinant interferons: Renal cell carcinoma and malignant melanoma. Oncology 1985;42:26.

464. Hawkins MJ, Horning S, Konrad MW, et al. Phase I evaluation of a synthetic mutant of β-interferon. Cancer Res 1985;45:5914.

465. Creagan ET, Ahmann DL, Long HJ, et al. Phase II study of recombinant interferon-gamma in patients with disseminated malignant melanoma. Cancer Treat Rep 1987;71:843.

466. Ernstoff MS, Trautman T, Davis CA, et al. A randomized phase I/II study of cutaneous versus intermittent intravenous interferon gamma in patients with metastatic malignant melanoma. J Clin Oncol 1987;5:1804.

467. Gutterman JU, Rosenblum MG, Rios A, et al. Pharmacokinetic study of partially pure gamma-interferon in cancer patients. Cancer Res 1984;44:4164.

468. Kurzrock R, Quesada JR, Talpaz M, et al. Phase I study of multiple doses intramuscularly administered recombinant gamma interferon. J Clin Oncol 1986;4:1101.

469. Truitt RL, Gale RP, Bortin MM. Cellular immunotherapy of cancer. Prog Clin Biol Res 1987;244:1.

470. Grimm EA, Mazumder A, Zhang HZ, et al. Lymphokine-activated killer phenomenon: Lysis of natural killer resistant fresh solid tumor cells by interleukin-2-activated autologous human peripheral blood lymphocytes. J Exp Med 1982;155:1823.

471. Mule JJ, Shu S, Schwarz SL. Successful adoptive immunotherapy of established pulmonary metastases with LAK cells and recombinant interleukin 2. Science 1984;255:1487.

472. Rosenberg SA, Mule JJ, Spiess PJ, et al. Regression of established pulmonary metastases and subcutaneous tumor mediated by the systemic administration of high-dose recombinant interleukin 2. J Exp Med 1985;161:1169.

473. Mule JJ, Shu S, Rosenberg SA. The antitumor efficacy of lymphokine-activated killer cells and recombinant interleukin 2 in vivo. J Immunol 1985;135:646.

474. Lafreniere R, Rosenberg SA. Successful immunotherapy of experimental hepatic metastases with lymphokine-activated killer cells and recombinant interleukin 2. Cancer Res 1985;45:3755.

475. Rosenberg SA, Lotze MT, Muul LM. Special report: Observations on the systemic administration of autologous lymphokine-activated killer cells and recombinant interleukin-2 to patients with metastatic cancer. N Engl J Med 1985;313:1485.

476. Dutcher JP, Creekmore S, Weiss GR, et al. Phase II study of high dose interleukin-2 and lymphokine activated killer cells in patients with melanoma. Proc Am Soc Clin Oncol 1987;6:970.

477. Rosenberg SA, Lotze MT, Muul LM, et al. A progress report on the treatment of 157 patients with advanced cancer using lymphokine-activated killer cells and interleukin-2 or high-dose interleukin-2 alone. N Engl J Med 1987;316:889.

478. Rosenberg SA, Lotze MT, Yang JC, Aebersold PM, et al. Experience with the use of high-dose interleukin-2 in the treatment of 652 cancer patients. Ann Surg 1989;210:474.

479. West WH, Tauer KW, Yanelli JR, et al. Constant infusion recombinant interleukin 2 adoptive immunotherapy of advanced cancer. N Engl J Med 1987;316:898.

480. Bar MH, Sznol M, Atkins MB, et al. Metastatic melanoma treated with combined bolus and continuous infusion interleukin-2 and lymphokine-activated killer cells. J Clin Oncol 1990;7:1138.

481. Dutcher JP, Creekmore S, Weiss GR, et al. A phase II study of interleukin-2 and lymphokine-activated killer cells in patients with metastatic melanoma. J Clin Oncol 1989;7:477.

482. Parkinson DR, Abrams JS, Wiernik PH, et al. Interleukin-2 therapy in patients with metastatic malignant melanoma. J Clin Oncol 1990;8:1650.

483. Mittelman A, Gafney L, Penichet K, et al. A phase I dose escalation study of recombinant interleukin-2 and lymphokine-activated killer cells in patients with advanced cancer. Proc Am Soc Clin Oncol 1987;6:237.

484. Dutcher JP, Gaynor ER, Boldt DH, et al. A Phase II study of high-dose continuous infusion interleukin-2 with lymphokine-activated killer cells in patients with metastatic melanoma. J Clin Oncol 1991;9:641.

485. Dillman RO, Barth N, Oldham RK, et al. Continuous interleukin-2 and lymphokine-activated killer cells in advanced cancer. Proc Am Soc Clin Oncol 1989;8:188.

486. Dillman RO, Oldham RK, Tauer KW, et al. Continuous interleukin-2 and lymphokine-activated killer cells for advanced cancer: A National Biotherapy Study Group Trial. J Clin Oncol 1991;9:1233.

487. Perez EA, Scudder SA, Meyers F, et al. Weekly 24 hour continuous infusion interleukin-2 for metastatic melanoma and renal carcinoma. Proc Am Soc Clin Oncol 1989;8:190.

488. Whitehead RP, Kopecky KJ, Samson MK, et al. A phase II study of IV bolus recombinant interleukin-2 in metastatic malignant melanoma: A Southwest Oncology Group Study. Proc Am Soc Clin Oncol 1989;8:284.

489. Richards JM, Bajorin DF, Vogelzang NJ, et al. Treatment of metastatic melanoma with continuous intravenous IL-2 ± LAK cells: A randomized trial. Proc Am Soc Clin Oncol 1990;9:279.

490. McCabe MS, Stablein D, Hawkins MJ. The modified group C experience: Phase III randomized trials of IL-2 vs IL-2/LAK in advanced renal cell carcinoma and advanced melanoma. Proc Am Soc Clin Oncol 1991;10:213.

491. Dorval T, Mathiot C, Fridman WH. A phase II trial of recombinant interleukin-2 in patients with metastatic melanoma. Proc Am Soc Clin Oncol 1991;10:297.

492. Blair S, Flaherty L, Valdivieso M, et al. Comparison of high dose interleukin-2 with combined chemotherapy/low dose IL-2 in metastatic malignant melanoma. Proc Am Soc Clin Oncol 1991;10:294.

493. Mitchell MS, Kempf RA, Harel W, et al. Effectiveness and tolerability of low-dose cyclophosphamide and low-dose intravenous interleukin-2 in disseminated melanoma. J Clin Oncol 1988;6:409.

494. Mitchell MS, Kempf RA, Harel W, et al. Low-dose cyclophosphamide and low-dose interleukin-2 for malignant melanoma. Bull NY Acad Med 1989;65:128.

495. Lotze MT, Matory YL, Raynor AA, et al. Clinical effects and toxicity of interleukin-2 in patients with cancer. Cancer 1986;58:2764.

496. Ognibene FP, Rosenberg SA, Lotze MT, et al. Interleukin-2 administration causes reversible hemodynamic changes and left ventricular dysfunction similar to those seen in septic shock. Chest 1988;94:750.

497. Webb DE, Austin HA, Belldegrun A, et al. Metabolic and renal effects of interleukin-2 immunotherapy for metastatic cancer. Clin Nephrology 1988;30:141.

498. Szybalski W. X-ray sensitization by halopyrimidines. Cancer Chemother Rep 1974;58:539–557.

499. Hatanaka H, ed. Neutron capture therapy, Proceedings of the Second International Symposium on Neutron Capture Therapy, Teikyo University, Tokyo, October 1985. Niigata, Japan: Nishimura, 1986.

500. Greenberg PD, Kern DE, Cheever MA. Therapy of disseminated murine leukemia with cyclophosphamide and immune Lyt 1 + 2-T cells: Tumor eradication does not require participation of cytotoxic T cells. J Exp Med 1985;161:4303.

501. Anichini A, Fossati G, Parmiani G. Clonal analysis of cytotoxic T lymphocyte response to autologous human metastatic melanoma. Int J Cancer 1985;35:683.

502. De Vries JE, Spits H. Cloned cytolytic T lymphocyte (CTL) lines reactive with autologous melanoma cells. I. In vitro generation, isolation, and analysis of phenotype and specificity. J Immunol 1984;132:510.

503. Herin M, Lemoine C, Weynant P, et al. Production of stable cytolytic T lymphocyte (CTL) against autologous human melanoma. Int J Cancer 1987;39:390.

504. Hersey P, MacDonald M, Schibeci S, et al. Clonal analysis of cytotoxic T lymphocytes (CTL) against autologous melanoma: Classification based on phenotype, specificity, and inhibition of monoclonal antibodies to T cell structures. Cancer Immunol Immunother 1986;22:15.

505. Fossati G, Anichini A, Parmiani G. Melanoma cell lysis by human CTL clones: Differential involvement of T3, T8 and HLA antigens. Int J Cancer 1987;39:689.

506. Anichini A, Fossati G, Parmiani G. Heterogeneity of clones from a human metastatic melanoma detected by autologous cytotoxic T lymphocyte clones. J Exp Med 1986;163:215.

507. Itoh K, Tilden AB, Balch CM. Interleukin 2 activation of cytotoxic T lymphocytes infiltrating into human metastatic melanoma. Cancer Res 1986;46:3011.

508. Itoh K, Platsoucas CD, Balch CM. Autologous tumor-specific cytotoxic T lymphocytes in the infiltrate of human metastatic melanoma. J Exp Med 1988;168:1419.

509. Muul LM, Spiess PJ, Director EP, et al. Identification of specific cytolytic immune responses against autologous tumors in humans bearing malignant melanoma. J Immunol 1987;138:989.

510. Mukherji B, MacAlister TJ. Clonal analysis of cytotoxic T cell response against human melanoma. J Exp Med 1983;158:240.

511. Knuth A, Danowski B, Oettgen HF, et al. T cell mediated cytotoxicity against autologous malignant melanoma: Analysis with interleukin 2 dependent T cell cultures. Proc Natl Acad Sci USA 1984;81:3511.

512. Topalian SL, Solomon D, Rosenberg SA. Tumor-specific cytolysis by lymphocytes infiltrating human melanoma. J Immunol 1989;142:3714.

513. Cohen PJ, Lotze MT, Roberts JR, et al. The immunopathology of sequential tumor biopsies in patients treated with interleukin-2. Correlation of response with T-cell infiltration and HLA-DR expression. Am J Pathol 1987;129:208.

514. Rosenberg SA, Spiess PJ, Lafreniere R. A new approach to adoptive immunotherapy of cancer with tumor-infiltrating lymphocytes. Science 1986;233:1318.

515. Topalian S, Solomon D, Avis FP, et al. Immunotherapy of patients with advanced cancer using tumor infiltrating lymphocytes in recombinant interleukin-2: A pilot study. J Clin Oncol 1988;6:838.

516. Rosenberg SA, Packard BS, Aebersold PM, et al. Use of tumor-infiltrating lymphocytes and interleukin-2 in the immunotherapy of patients with metastatic melanoma: A preliminary report. N Engl J Med 1988;319:1676.

517. Dillman RO, Oldham RK, Barth NM, et al. Continuous interleukin-2 and tumor-infiltrating lymphocytes as treatment of advanced melanoma: A National Biotherapy Study Group Trial. Cancer 1991;68:1.

518. Houghton AN, Chapman PB, Bajorin DF. Antibodies in cancer therapy: Clinical application. 22.3 Melanoma. In: Devita VT Jr, Hellman S, Rosenberg SA. Biologic therapy of cancer. Philadelphia: JB Lippincott, 1991:533.

519. Houghton AN, Scheinberg DA. Monoclonal antibodies: Potential applications to the treatment of cancer. Semin Oncol 1986;13:165.

520. Houghton AN, Mintzer D, Cordon-Cardo C, et al. Mouse monoclonal IgG3 antibody detecting GD3 ganglioside: A phase I trial in patients with malignant melanoma. Proc Natl Acad Sci USA 1985;82:1242.

521. Goodman GE, Beaumier P, Hellstrom I, et al. Pilot trial of murine monoclonal antibodies in patients with advanced melanoma. J Clin Oncol 1985;3:340.

522. Cheung N-K, Lazarus H, Miraldi FD, et al. Ganglioside GD2 specific monoclonal antibody 3F8: A phase I study in patients with neuroblastoma and malignant melanoma. J Clin Oncol 1987;5:1430.

523. Oldham RK, Foon KA, Morgan AC, et al. Monoclonal antibody therapy of malignant melanoma: In vivo localization in cutaneous metastasis after intravenous administration. J Clin Oncol 1984;2:1235.

524. Schroff RW, Woodhouse CS, Foon KA, et al. Intratumor localization of monoclonal antibody in patients with melanoma treated with antibody to a 250,000 dalton melanoma-associated antigen. JNCI 1985;74:299.

525. Vadhan-Raj S, Cordon-Cardo C, Carswell E, et al. Phase I trial of a mouse monoclonal antibody against GD3 ganglioside in patients with melanoma: Induction of an inflammatory response at tumor sites. J Clin Oncol 1988;6:1636.

526. Dippold WG, Berhard H, Dienes HP, et al. Treatment of patients with melanoma by monoclonal ganglioside antibodies. Eur J Cancer Clin Oncol 1988;21:S65.

527. Dippold WG, Knuth A, Meyer zum Buchenfelde KH. Inflammatory tumor response to monoclonal antibody infusion. Eur J Cancer Clin Oncol 1985;21:97.

528. Coit D, Houghton AN, Cordon-Cardo C, et al. Isolation limb perfusion with monoclonal antibody R24 in patients with malignant melanoma. Proc Am Soc Clin Oncol 1988;7:962.

529. Goodman GE, Hellstrom I, Hummel D, et al. Phase I trial of monoclonal antibody MG-21 directed against a melanoma-associated GD3 ganglioside antigen. Proc Am Soc Clin Oncol 1987;6:823.

530. Lichtin A, Iliopoulos D, Guerry D, et al. Therapy of melanoma with an anti-melanoma ganglioside monoclonal antibody: A possible mechanism of a complete response. Proc Am Soc Clin Oncol 1988;7:247.

530a. Houghton, AN. Personal communication.

531. Irie RF, Morton DL. Regression of cutaneous metastatic melanoma by intralesional injection with human monoclonal antibody to ganglioside GD2. Proc Natl Acad Sci USA 1986;83:8694.

532. Schroff RW, Morgan AC Jr, Woodhouse CS, et al. Monoclonal antibody therapy in malignant melanoma: Factors effecting in vivo localization. J Biol Response Mod 1987;6:457.

533. Larson SM, Carrasquillo JA, Krohn KA, et al. Localization of 131-I labeled p97-specific Fab fragments in human melanoma as a basis for radiotherapy. J Clin Invest 1983;72:2101.

534. Vitteta ES, Fulton RJ, May RD, et al. Redesigning nature's poisons to create antitumor reagents. Science 1987;238:1098.

535. Spitler LE, Del Rio M, Khentigan A, et al. Therapy of patients with malignant melanoma using a monoclonal antimelanoma antibody-ricin A chain immunotoxin. Cancer Res 1987;47:1717.

536. Spitler LE. Clinical trials of immunotoxin. Second International Congress on Monoclonal Antibody 1987;1:26.

537. Bajorin DB, Chapman PB, Wong G, et al. A phase I trial of high-dose R24 mouse monoclonal antibody in patients with metastatic melanoma. Proc Am Assoc Cancer Res 1991;32:265.

538. Raymond J, Kirkwood J, Vlock D, et al. A phase IB trial of murine monoclonal antibody R24 (anti-GD3) in metastatic melanoma. Proc Am Soc Clin Oncol 1991;10:298.

539. Schroff RW, Foon KA, Beatty SM, et al. Human anti-mouse immunoglobulin response in patients receiving monoclonal antibody therapy. Cancer Res 1985;45:879.

540. Morrison SL, Oi V. Transfer and expression of immunoglobulin genes. Ann Rev Immunol 1984;2:239.

541. Reichmann L, Clark MR, Waldmann H, et al. Reshaping antibodies for therapy. Nature 1988;332:323.

542. Yamaguchi H, Furukawa K, Fortunato S, et al. Cell surface antigens of human melanoma recognized by human monoclonal antibodies. Proc Natl Acad Sci USA 1987;84:2416.

543. Morton DL, Nizze RJ, Gupta RK, et al. Active specific immunotherapy of malignant melanoma. In: Kim JP, Jim BS, Park J-G, eds. Current status of cancer control and immunobiology. Seoul, Korea, 1987:152.

544. Livingston PO, Natoli EJ, Calves MJ, et al. Vaccines containing purified GM2 ganglioside elicit GM2 antibodies in melanoma patients. Proc Natl Acad Sci USA 1987;84:2911.

545. Bystryn J-C, Oratz R, Harris MN, et al. Immunogenicity of a polyvalent melanoma antigen vaccine in humans. Cancer 1988;61:1065.

546. Hersey P, Edwards A, Coates A, et al. Evidence that treatment with vaccinia melanoma cell lysates (VMCL) may improve survival of patients with stage II melanoma. Cancer Immunol Immunother 1987;25:257.

547. Hersey P, Edwards A, Coates A, et al. Evidence that treatment with vaccinia melanoma cell lysates (VMCL) may improve survival of patients with stage II melanoma. Cancer Immunol Immunother 1987;25:257.

548. Jones PC, Sze LL, Liu PY, et al. Prolonged survival for melanoma patients with elevated IgM antibody to oncofetal antigen. JNCI 1981;66:249.

549. Wallack MK, Bash JA, Leftheriotis E, et al. The positive relationship of clinical and serologic responses to vaccinia melanoma oncolysate. Arch Surg 1987;122:1460.

550. Livingston PO, Oettgen HF, Old LJ. Specific active immunotherapy in cancer treatment. In: Mihich E, ed. Immunological approaches to cancer therapeutics. New York: John Wiley & Sons, 1982:363.

551. Livingston PO, Takeyama H, Pollack MS, et al. Serological responses of melanoma patients to vaccines derived from allogeneic cultured melanoma cells. Int J Cancer 1983;31:567.

552. Livingston PO, Kaelin K, Pinsky CM, et al. The serologic response of patients with stage II melanoma to allogeneic melanoma cell vaccines. Cancer 1985;56:2194.

553. Fisher RI, Terry WD, Hodes RJ, et al. Adjuvant immunotherapy or chemotherapy for malignant melanoma. Surg Clin North Am 1981;61:1267.

554. Seigler HF, Cox E, Mutzner F, et al. Specific active immunotherapy for melanoma. Ann Surg 1979;190:366.

555. Cox EB, Vollmer RT, Seigler HF. Melanoma in the Southeastern United States: Experience at the Duke Medical Center. In: Balch CM, Milton GW, eds. Cutaneous melanoma: Clinical management and treatment results worldwide. Philadelphia: JB Lippincott, 1985:407.

556. Berd D, Murphy G, McGuire HC Jr, Mastrangelo MJ. Immunization with haptenized, autologous tumor cells induces inflammation of human melanoma metastases. Cancer Res 1991;51:2731.

557. Gansbacher B, Gee C, Houghton AN, et al. Retroviral lymphokine gene transfer induced secretion of interleukin-2 or interferon-gamma by human melanoma cells. Proc Am Assoc Cancer Res 1991;32:255.

558. Rosenberg SA. Immunotherapy and gene therapy of cancer. Gottlieb Award lecture. Proc Adv Biol Clin Management Melanoma 1991;43:61.

559. Estin CD, Stevenson US, Plowman GD, et al. Recombinant vaccinia virus vaccine against the human melanoma antigen p97 for use in immunotherapy. Proc Natl Acad Sci USA 1987;85:1052.

560. Van der Bruggen P, Traversari C, Chomez P, et al. A gene encoding an antigen recognized by cytolytic T lymphocytes on a human melanoma. Science 1991;254:1643.

561. Kageshita T, Chen ZJ, Kim J-W, et al. Murine anti-idiotypic monoclonal antibodies to syngeneic antihuman high molecular weight-melanoma associated antigen monoclonal antibodies: Development, characterization and clinical application. Pigment Cell Res 1988;1(Suppl):185.

562. Kusama M, Kageshita T, Tsujisaki M, et al. Syngeneic antiidiotypic antisera to murine antihuman high molecular weight melanoma-associated antigen monoclonal antibodies. Cancer Res 1987;47:4312.

563. Mittelman A, Chen ZJ, Kageshita T, et al. Active specific immunotherapy in patients with melanoma: A clinical trial with mouse antiidiotypic monoclonal antibodies elicited with syngeneic anti-high-molecular weight-melanoma-associated antigen monoclonal antibodies. J Clin Invest 1990;86:2136.

564. Chapman PB, Houghton AN. Induction of IgG antibodies against GD3 ganglioside in rabbits by an anti-idiotypic monoclonal antibody. J Clin Invest 1991;88:186.

565. Mitchell MS, Harel W, Kempf RA, et al. Active-specific immunotherapy for melanoma. J Clin Oncol 1990;8:856.

566. North RJ. Cyclophosphamide-facilitated adoptive immunotherapy of an established tumor depends on elimination of tumor-induced suppressor T-cells. J Exp Med 1982;35:1063.

567. Livingston PO, Hoffman MK, Enker WE. Inhibition of suppressor cell activity in melanoma patients by cyclophosphamide. Proc Am Soc Clin Oncol 1984;3:58.

568. Berd D, Mastrangelo MJ, Engstrom PF, et al. Augmentation of the human immune response by cyclophosphamide. Cancer Res 1982;42:4862.

569. Berd D, Danna V, Maguire HC, et al. Induction of cell mediated immunity to autologous melanoma cells and regression of metastases after treatment with a melanoma cell vaccine preceded by cyclophosphamide. Cancer Res 1986;46:2572.

570. Berd D, Maguire HC Jr, McCue P, Mastrangelo MJ. Treatment of metastatic melanoma with an autologous tumor-cell vaccine: Clinical and immunologic results in 64 patients. J Clin Oncol 1990;8:1858.

571. Morton DL. Immunological studies with human neoplasms. J Reticuloendothel Soc 1971;10:137.

572. Mastrangelo MJ, Bellet RE, Berd D. Immunology and immunotherapy of human cutaneous malignant melanoma. In: Clark WH Jr, Goldman LI, Mastrangelo MJ, eds. Human malignant melanoma. New York: Grune & Stratton, 1979:355.

573. Pinsky CM, Hirshaut Y, Oettgen HF. Treatment of malignant melanoma by intratumoral injection of BCG. NCI Monogr 1973;39:255.

574. Mastrangelo MJ, Sulit HL, Prehn LM. Intralesional BCG in the treatment of metastatic malignant melanoma. Cancer 1976;37:684.

575. Klein E, Holterman OA. Immunotherapeutic approaches to the management of neoplasms. NCI Monogr 1972;35:379.

576. Klein E, Holterman OA, Helm F et al. Immunologic approaches to the management of primary and secondary tumors involving the skin and soft tissues. Review of a ten year program. Transplant Proc 1975;7:297.

577. Tisman G, Wu SJG, Safire GE. Intralesional PPD in malignant melanoma. Lancet 1975;1:161.

578. Krown SE, Hilal E, Pinsky CM. Intralesional injection of the methanol extraction residue of Bacillus Calmette-Guerin (MER) into cutaneous metastases of malignant melanoma. Cancer 1978;42:2648.

579. Cohen MH, Feliz E, Jessup J, et al. Treatment of metastatic melanoma by intralesional injection of BCG, organic chemicals and *C. parvum*. In: Crispen RG, ed. Neoplasm immunity mechanisms. Philadelphia: Franklin Institute Press, 1975:121.

580. Cameron RB, McIntosh JK, Rosenburg SA. Synergistic antitumor effects of combination immunotherapy with recombinant interleukin-2 and recombinant hybrid interferon-α in the treatment of established murine hepatic metastases. Cancer Res 1988;48:5810.

581. Rosenberg SA, Schwarz S, Spiess P. Combination immunotherapy of cancer: Synergistic antitumor interactions of interleukin-2, interferon-α and tumor-infiltrating lymphocytes. JNCI 1988;80:1392.

582. Rosenberg SA, Lotze MT, Yang JC, et al. Combination therapy with interleukin-2 and interferon-α for the treatment of patients with advanced cancer. J Clin Oncol 1989;7:1863.

583. Eisenthal A, Cameron RC, Uppenkamp I, et al. Effect of combined therapy with lymphokine activated killer cells, interleukin-2 and specific monoclonal antibody on established B16 melanoma lung metastases. Cancer Res 1988;48:7140.

584. Shiloni E, Pouillart P, Janssens A, et al. Sequential dacarbazine chemotherapy followed by recombinant interleukin-2 in metastatic melanoma: A pilot multicentre phase I–II study. Eur J Cancer Clin Oncol 1989;25(Suppl 3):45.

585. Papadopoulos NEJ, Howard J, Murray JL, et al. Phase I–II DTIC and interleukin 2 (IL2) trial for metastatic malignant melanoma. Proc Am Soc Clin Oncol 1989;8:290.

586. Shiloni E, Pouillart P, Janssens A, et al. Sequential dacarbazine chemotherapy followed by recombinant interleukin-2 in metastatic melanoma: A pilot multicentre phase I–II study. Eur J Cancer Clin Oncol 1989;25:45.

587. Stoter G, Aamdal S, Rodenhuis S, et al. Sequential administration of recombinant human interleukin-2 and dacarbazine in metastatic melanoma: A multicentric phase II study. J Clin Oncol 1991;9:1687.

588. Richards JM, Ramming K, Bitran JD, et al. Combination of chemotherapy and biologic therapy for the treatment of melanoma. Clin Res [Abstract] 1990;38:844.

589. Sznol M, Clark J, Smith J, et al. A phase II study of IL-2/LAK in combination with chemotherapy and interferon-alfa in patients with metastatic melanoma and renal cell carcinoma. Proc Am Soc Clin Oncol [Abstract] 1990;9:759.

590. Sznol M, Clark J, Smith J, et al. A pilot evaluation of interleukin-2 (IL-2) and lymphokine-activated killer (LAK) cells in combination with chemotherapy and α-interferon. Proc Am Soc Clin Oncol [Abstract] 1989;8:742.

591. Demshak PA, Mier JW, Robert NJ, et al. Interleukin-2 and high-dose cisplatin in patients with metastatic melanoma: A pilot study. J Clin Oncol 1991;1821.

592. Khayat D. Cisplatin, IL-2 and interferon. Proc Adv Biol Clin Management Melanoma, Houston, 1991:29.

593. Pichert G, Jost LM, Fierz W, et al. Clinical and immune modulatory effects of alternative weekly interleukin-2 and interferon alfa-2a in patients with advanced renal cell carcinoma and melanoma. Br J Cancer 1991;63:287.

594. Rosenberg SA, Lotze MT, Yang JC, et al. Combination therapy with interleukin-2 and α-interferon for the treatment of patients with advanced cancer. J Clin Oncol 1989;7:1863.

595. Bergmann L, Weidmann E, Mitrou PS, et al. Interleukin-2 in combination with interferon-α in disseminated malignant melanoma and advanced renal cell carcinoma: A phase II study. Onkologie 1990;13:137.

596. Sznol M, Mier JW, Sparano J, et al. A phase I study of high-dose interleukin-2 in combination with interferon-α2b. J Biol Response Modifiers 1990;9:529.

597. Mittelman A, Huberman B, Fallon S, et al. Phase I study of recombinant interleukin-2 (IL-2) and recombinant human interferon α (IFN-Roche) in patients (pts) with melanoma, renal cell carcinoma (Ca), colorectal CA and malignant B-cell disease. Proc Am Soc Clin Oncol 1989;8:179.

598. Budd GT, Osgood B, Barna B, et al. Phase I clinical trial of interleukin 2 and α-interferon: Toxicity and immunologic effects. Cancer Res 1989;49:6432.

599. Lee KH, Talpaz M, Rothberg JM, et al. Concomitant administration of recombinant human interleukin-2 and recombinant interferon α-2A in cancer patients: A phase I study. J Clin Oncol 1989;7:1726.

600. Mittelman A, Huberman M, Puccio C, et al. A phase I study of recombinant human interleukin-2 and α-interferon-2a in patients with renal cell cancer, colorectal cancer, and malignant melanoma. Cancer 1990;66:664.

601. West W, Schwartzberg L, Blumenchein G, et al. Continuous infusion interleukin-2 (IL-2) plus SC interferon α-2B (IFN) in advanced malignancy. Proc Am Soc Clin Oncol [Abstract] 1990;9:738.

602. Huberman M, Mittelman A, Fallon B, et al. Preliminary observations from a phase I study of recombinant human interleukin-2 (IL2) and roferon-a (recombinant human α-IFN) in patients with malignant b-cell disease, renal and colorectal cancer, and melanoma. Proc Am Soc Clin Oncol [Abstract] 1988;7:653.

603. Krigel R, Poiesz B, Comis R, et al. A phase I study of recombinant interleukin-2 (RIL-2) plus recombinant beta ser 17 interferon (IFN-beta ser). Proc Am Soc Clin Oncol 1986;5:225.

604. Bajorin DF, Chapman PB, Wong G, et al. Phase I evaluation of a combination of monoclonal antibody R24 and interleukin 2 in patients with metastatic melanoma. Cancer Res 1990;50:7490.

605. Urba WJ, Kopp WC, Clark JW, et al. The in vivo immunomodulatory effects of recombinant interferon gamma plus recombinant tumor necrosis factor-α. J Clin Oncol 1991;9:1831.

606. Lienard D, Ewalenko P, Delmotte J-J, Renard N, LeJeune FJ. High dose recombinant tumor necrosis factor α in combination with interferon gamma and melphalan in isolation perfusion of the limbs for melanoma and sarcoma. J Clin Oncol 1992;10:52.

607. Kirkwood JM. Rationale for use of interferon in the therapy of high risk melanoma. Eur J Cancer 1992 (in press).

608. Meyskens FL, Kopecky K, Samson M, et al. Recombinant human interferon-γ: Adverse effects in high-risk stage I and II cutaneous malignant melanoma. JNCI 1990;82:1071.

609. Spitler LE, Sagebiel R. A randomized trial of levamisole versus placebo as adjuvant therapy in malignant melanoma. N Engl J Med 1980;303:1143.

610. Quirt IC, Shelley WE, Pater JL, et al. Improved survival in patients with poor-prognosis malignant melanoma treated with adjuvant levamisole: A phase III study by the National Cancer Institute of Canada Clinical Trials Group. J Clin Oncol 1991;9:729.

611. Gonzalez RL, Spitler LE, Sagebiel RW, et al. Effect of levamisole as a surgical adjuvant therapy for malignant melanoma. Cancer Treat Rep 1978;62:1703.

612. Loutfi A, Shakr A, Jerry M, et al. Double-blind randomized prospective trial of levamisole/placebo in stage I cutaneous malignant melanoma. Clin Invest Med 1987;10:325.

613. Costanzi JJ, Fletcher WS, Balcerzak SP, et al. Combination chemotherapy plus levamisole in the treatment of disseminated malignant melanoma: A Southwest Oncology Group study. Cancer 1984;53:833.

614. Stevenson HC, Green I, Hamilton JM, et al. Levamisole: Known effects on the immune system, clinical results, and future application to the treatment of cancer. J Clin Oncol 1991;9:2052.

615. Parkinson DR. Levamisole as adjuvant therapy for melanoma: Quo vadis? J Clin Oncol 1991;9:716.

616. Lipton A, Harvey HA, Balch CM, et al. Corynebacterium parvum versus Bacille Calmette-Guerin adjuvant immunotherapy of stage III malignant melanoma. J Clin Oncol 1991;9:1151.

617. Creagan ET, Ingle JN, Schutt AJ, et al. A prospective randomized control trial of megestrol acetate among high risk patients with resected malignant melanoma. Am J Clin Oncol 1989;12:152.

618. Bernardino ME, Goldstein HM. Gray scale ultrasonography in the evaluation of metastatic melanoma. Cancer 1978;42:2529.

619. Heaston DK, Putman CE. Radiographic manifestations of thoracic malignant melanoma. In: Seigler HF, ed. Clinical management of melanoma. The Hague: Martinus Nijhoff, 1982:62.

620. Braman SS, Whitcomb ME. Endobronchial metastasis. Arch Intern Med 1975;135:543.

621. Feldman L, Kricun ME. Malignant melanoma presenting as a mediastinal mass. JAMA 1979;241:396.

622. Curtis A McB, Ravin CE, Deering TF, et al. The efficacy of full-lung tomography in the detection of early metastatic disease from melanoma. Diagn Radiol 1982;144:27.

623. Chen JTT, Dahmash NS, Ravin CE, et al. Metastatic melanoma to the thorax: Report of 130 patients. AJR 1981;137:293.

624. Gromet MA, Ominsky SH, Epstein WL, et al. The thorax as the initial site for systemic relapse in malignant melanoma: A prospective survey of 324 patients. Cancer 1979;44:776.

625. Simeone JF, Putman CE, Greenspan RH. Detection of metastatic malignant melanoma by chest roentgenography. Cancer 1977;39:1993.

626. Webb WR, Gamsu G. Thoracic metastasis in malignant melanoma: A radiographic survey of 65 patients. Chest 1977;71:176.

627. Webb WR. Hilar and mediastinal lymph node metastases in malignant melanoma. AJR 1979;133:805.

628. Chang AE, Schaner EG, Conkle DM, et al. Evaluation of computed tomography in the detection of pulmonary metastases: A prospective study. Cancer 1979;43:913.

629. Mintzer RA, Malave SR, Neiman HL, et al. Computed vs. conventional tomography in evaluation of primary and secondary pulmonary neoplasms. Radiology 1979;132:653.

630. Neifeld JP, Michaelis LL, Doppman JL. Suspected pulmonary metastases: Correlation of chest x-ray, whole lung tomograms, and operative findings. Cancer 1977;39:383.

631. Schaner EG, Chang AE, Doppman JL, et al. Comparison of computed and conventional whole lung tomography in detecting pulmonary nodules: A prospective radiologic-pathologic study. AJR 1978;131:51.

632. Morton DL, Joseph WL, Ketcham AS, et al. Surgical resection and adjunctive immunotherapy for selected patients with multiple pulmonary metastases. Ann Surg 1973;178:360.

633. Cahan WG. Excision of melanoma metastases to lung: Problems in diagnosis and management. Ann Surg 1973;178:703.

634. Cline RE, Young WG Jr. Long term results following surgical treatment of metastatic pulmonary tumors. Am Surg 1970;36:61.

635. McCormack, Martini N. The changing role of surgery for pulmonary metastases. Ann Thorac Surg 1979;28:139.

636. Thayer JO Jr, Overholt RH. Metastatic melanoma to the lung: Long-term results of surgical excision. Am J Surg 1985;149:558.

637. Vidne BA, Richter S, Levy MJ. Surgical treatment of solitary pulmonary metastasis. Cancer 1976;38:2561.

638. Morrow CE, Vassilopoulos PP, Grage TB. Surgical resection for metastatic neoplasms of the lung: Experience at the University of Minnesota Hospitals. Cancer 1980;45:2981.

639. Mathisen DJ, Flye MW, Peabody J. The role of thoracotomy in the management of pulmonary metastases from malignant melanoma. Ann Thorac Surg 1979;27:295.

640. Wilkins EW Jr, Head JM, Burke JF. Pulmonary resection for metastatic neoplasms in the lung: Experience at the Massachusetts General Hospital. Am J Surg 1978;135:480.

641. Presant CA, Bartolucci AA, Smalley RV, et al. Cyclophosphamide plus (3,3-dimethyl-l-triazeno)-imidazole-4-carboxamide (DTIC) with or without Corynebacterium parvum in metastatic malignant melanoma. Cancer 1979;44:899.

642. Vieth RG, Odom GL. Intracranial metastases and their neurosurgical treatment. J Neurosurg 1965;23:375.

643. Amer MH, Al-Sarraf M, Baker LH, et al. Malignant melanoma and central nervous

system metastases: Incidence, diagnosis, treatment and survival. Cancer 1978;42: 660.

644. Fell DA, Leavens ME, McBride CM. Surgical versus nonsurgical management of metastatic melanoma of the brain. Neurosurgery 1980;7:238.

645. Ginaldi S, Wallace S, Shalen P, et al. Cranial computed tomography of malignant melanoma. AJR 1981;136:145.

646. Pennington DG, Milton GW. Cerebral metastasis from melanoma. Aust NZ J Surg 1975;45:405.

647. Bullard DE, Cox EB, Seigler HF. Central nervous system metastases in malignant melanoma. Neurosurgery 1981;8:26.

648. Posner JB, Chernik NL. Intracranial metastases from systemic cancer. Adv Neurol 1978;19:579.

649. Bremer AM, West CR, Didolkar MS. An evaluation of the surgical management of melanoma of the brain. J Surg Oncol 1978;10:211.

650. Enzmann DR, Kramer R, Norman D, et al. Malignant melanoma metastatic to the central nervous system. Radiology 1978;127:177.

651. Gildersleeve N Jr, Koo AH, McDonald CJ. Metastatic tumor presenting as intracerebral hemorrhage: Report of 6 cases examined by computed tomography. Radiology 1977;124:109.

652. Carella RJ, Gelber R, Hendrickson F, et al. Value of radiation therapy in the management of patients with cerebral metastases from malignant melanoma: Radiation Therapy Oncology Group brain metastases study I and II. Cancer 1980;45:679.

653. Posner JB. Management of central nervous system metastases. Semin Oncol 1977;4: 81.

654. Byrne TN, Cascino TL, Posner JB. Brain metastases from melanoma. J Neurooncol 1983;1:313.

655. Hayward RD. Malignant melanoma and the central nervous system: A guide for classification based on the clinical findings. J Neurol Neurosurg Psychiatry 1976;39:526.

656. Hayward RD. Secondary malignant melanoma of the brain. Clin Oncol 1976;2:227.

657. McCann WP, Weir BKA, Elvidge AR. Long-term survival after removal of metastatic malignant melanoma of the brain: Report of two cases. J Neurosurg 1968;28:483.

658. McNeel DP, Leavens ME. Long-term survival with recurrent metastatic intracranial melanoma: Case report. J Neurosurg 1968;29:91.

659. Scott M. Spontaneous intracerebral hematoma caused by cerebral neoplasms: Report of eight verified cases. J Neurosurg 1975;42:338.

660. Wolpert SM, Zimmer A, Schechter MM, et al. The neuroradiology of melanomas of the central nervous system. AJR 1967;101:178.

661. Felix EL, Sindelar WF, Bagley DH, et al. The use of bone and brain scans as screening procedures in patients with malignant lesions. Surg Gynecol Obstet 1975;141:867.

662. Thomas JH, Panoussopoulous D, Liesmann GE, et al. Scintiscans in the evaluation of patients with malignant melanomas. Surg Gynecol Obstet 1979;149:574.

663. Muss HB, Richards F II, Barnes PL, et al. Radionuclide scanning in patients with advanced malignant melanoma. Clin Nucl Med 1979;4:516.

664. Bardfeld PA, Passalaqua AM, Braunstein P, et al. A comparison of radionuclide scanning and computed tomography in metastatic lesions of the brain. J Comput Assist Tomogr 1977;1:315.

665. Holtas S, Cronqvist S. Cranial computed tomography of patients with malignant melanoma. Neuroradiology 1981;22:123.

666. Solis OJ, Davis KR, Adair LB, et al. Intracerebral metastatic melanoma: CT evaluation. Comput Tomogr 1977;1:135.

667. Wasserstrom WR, Glass JP, Posner JP. Diagnosis and treatment of leptomeningeal metastases from solid tumors: Experience with 90 patients. Cancer 1982;49:759.

668. Fleisher M, Wasserstrom WR, Schold SC, et al. Lactic dehydrogenase isoenzymes in the cerebrospinal fluid of patients with systemic cancer. Cancer 1981;47:2654.

669. Fletcher JW, George EA, Henry RE, et al. Brain scans, dexamethasone therapy, and brain tumors. JAMA 1975;232:1261.

670. Gottlieb JA, Frei E III, Luce JK. An evaluation of the management of patients with cerebral metastases from malignant melanoma. Cancer 1972;29:701.

671. Ruderman NB, Hall TC. Use of glucocorticoids in the palliative treatment of metastatic brain tumors. Cancer 1965;18:298.

672. Atkinson L. Melanoma of the central nervous system. Aust NZ J Surg 1978;48:14.

673. Cooper JS, Carella R. Radiotherapy of intracerebral metastatic malignant melanoma. Radiology 1980;134:735.

674. Hafstrom L, Jonsson P-E, Stromblad L-G. Intra-cranial metastases of malignant melanoma treated by surgery. Cancer 1980;46:2088.

675. Winston KR, Walsh JW, Fischer EG. Results of operative treatment of intracranial metastatic tumors. Cancer 1980;45:2639.

676. Galicich JH, Sundearesan N, Arbit E, et al. Surgical treatment of single brain metastasis: Factors associated with survival. Cancer 1980;45:381.

677. Bauman ML, Price TR. Intracranial metastatic malignant melanoma: Long-term survival following subtotal resection. South Med J 1972;65:344.

678. Mandybur TI. Intracranial hemorrhage caused by metastatic tumors. Neurology 1977;27:650.

679. Reyes V, Horrax G. Metastatic melanoma of the brain: Report of a case with unusually long survival period following surgical removal. Ann Surg 1950;131:237.

680. Ziegler JC, Cooper JS. Brain metastases from malignant melanoma: Conventional vs. high-dose-per-fraction radiotherapy. Int J Radiat Oncol Biol Phys 1986;12:1839.

681. Vlock DR, Kirkwood JM, Leutzinger C, et al. High dose fraction radiation therapy for intracranial metastases of malignant melanoma. Cancer 1982;49:2289.

682. Choi KN, Withers R, Rotman M. Metastatic melanoma in brain: Rapid treatment or large dose fractions. Cancer 1985;56:10.

683. Skibber JM, Soong S-j, Austin L, Balch CM, Urist MM, Peters LJ, Sawaya R. Cranial irradiation after surgical excision of brain metastases in melanoma patients. 1992 (in press).

684. Loeffler JS, Alexander ED, Kooy HM, Wen PY, Fine HA, Black PM. Radiosurgery for brain metastases. PPO Updates 1991;5(2):1–12.

685. Young RF, Post EM, King GA. Treatment of spinal epidural metastases: Randomized prospective comparison of laminectomy and radiotherapy. J Neurosurg 1980;53:741.

686. Booth JB. Malignant melanoma of the stomach: Report of a case presenting as an acute perforation and review of the literature. Br J Surg 1965;52:262.

687. Das Gupta TK, Brasfield RD. Metastatic melanoma of the gastrointestinal tract. Arch Surg 1964;88:969.

688. Goldstein HM, Beydoun MT, Dood GD. Radiologic spectrum of melanoma metastatic to the gastrointestinal tract. AJR 1977;129:605.

689. Oddson TA, Rice RP, Seigler HF, et al. The spectrum of small bowel melanoma. Gastrointest Radiol 1978;3:419.

690. Thompson WH. Radiographic manifestations of metastatic melanoma to the gastrointestinal tract, hepatobiliary system, pancreas, spleen and mesentery. In: Seigler HF, ed. Clinical management of melanoma. The Hague: Martinus Nijhoff, 1982:133.

691. Fraser-Moodie A, Hughes RG, Jones SM, et al. Malignant melanoma metastases to the alimentary tract. Gut 1976;17:206.

692. Giler S, Kott I, Urca I. Malignant melanoma metastatic to the gastrointestinal tract. World J Surg 1979;3:375.

693. Goodman PL, Karakousis CP. Symptomatic gastrointestinal metastases from malignant melanoma. Cancer 1981;48:1058.

694. Harris MN. Massive gastrointestinal hemorrhage due to metastatic malignant melanoma of small intestine. Arch Surg 1964;88:1049.

695. Klausner JM, Skornick Y, Lelcuk S, et al. Acute complications of metastatic melanoma to the gastrointestinal tract. Br J Surg 1982;69:195.

696. Macbeth WAAG, Gwynne JF, Jamieson MG. Metastatic melanoma in the small bowel. Aust NZ J Surg 1969;38:309.

697. Shah SM, Smart DF, Texter EC Jr, et al. Metastatic melanoma of the stomach: The endoscopic and roentgenographic findings and review of the literature. South Med J 1977;70:379.

698. Karakousis C, Holyoke ED, Douglass HO Jr. Intussusception as a complication of malignant neoplasm. Arch Surg 1974;109:515.

699. Beckly DE. Alimentary tract metastases from malignant melanoma. Clin Radiol 1974;25:385.

700. Felix EL, Bagley DH, Sindelar WF, et al. The value of the liver scan in preoperative screening of patients with malignancies. Cancer 1976;38:1137.

701. Seigler HF, Fetter BF. Current management of melanoma. Ann Surg 1977;186:1.

702. Garg R, McPherson TA, Lentle B, et al. Usefulness of an elevated serum lactate dehydrogenase value as a marker of hepatic metastasis in malignant melanoma. Can Med Assoc J 1979;120:1114.

703. Bernardino ME, Thomas JL, Barnes PA, et al. Diagnostic approaches to liver and spleen metastases. Radiol Clin North Am 1982;20:469.

704. MacCarty RL, Stephens DH, Hattery RR, et al. Hepatic imaging by computed tomography: A comparison with ^{99m}Tc-sulfur colloid, ultrasonography, and angiography. Radiol Clin North Am 1979;17:137.

705. Smith TJ, Kemeny MM, Sugarbaker PH, et al. A prospective study of hepatic imaging in the detection of metastatic disease. Ann Surg 1982;195:486.

706. Snow JH Jr, Goldstein HM, Wallace S. Comparison of scintigraphy, sonography, and computed tomography in the evaluation of hepatic neoplasms. AJR 1979;132:915.

707. Balthazar EJ, Javors B. Malignant melanoma of the gallbladder. Am J Gastroenterol 1975;64:332.

708. Bowdler DA, Leach RD. Metastatic intrabiliary melanoma. Clin Oncol 1982;8:251.

709. McFadden PM, Krementz ET, McKinnon WMP, et al. Metastatic melanoma of the gallbladder. Cancer 1979;44:1802.

710. Shimkin PM, Soloway MS, Jaffe E. Metastatic melanoma of the gallbladder. AJR 1972;116:393.

711. Fon GT, Wong WS, Gold RH, et al. Skeletal metastases of melanoma: Radiographic, scintigraphic, and clinical review. AJR 1981;137:103.

712. Stewart WR, Gelberman RH, Harrelson JM, et al. Skeletal metastases of melanoma. J Bone Joint Surg [Abstract] 1978;60:645.

713. Devereux D, Johnston G, Blei L, et al. The role of bone scans in assessing malignant melanoma in patients with stage III disease. Surg Gynecol Obstet 1980;151:45.

714. Steiner GM, MacDonald JS. Metastases to bone from malignant melanoma. Clin Radiol 1972;23:52.

715. Tong D, Gillick L, Hendrickson FR. The palliation of symptomatic osseous metastases: Final results of the study by the Radiation Therapy Oncology Group. Cancer 1982;50: 893.

716. Harrelson JM. Orthopaedic considerations in the treatment of malignant melanoma. In: Seigler HF, ed. Clinical management of melanoma. The Hague: Martinus Nijhoff, 1982:435.

717. McKenzie DJ, Bell R. Melanoma with solitary metastasis to ureter. J Urol 1968;99: 399.

718. Das Gupta T, Grabstald H. Melanoma of the genitourinary tract. J Urol 1965;93:607.

719. deKernion JB, Golub SH, Gupta RK, et al. Successful trans-urethral intralesional BCG therapy of a bladder melanoma. Cancer 1975;36:1662.

720. Goldstein HM, Kaminsky S, Wallace S, et al. Urographic manifestations of metastatic melanoma. Radiology 1974;121:801.

721. Sheehan EE, Greenberg SD, Scott R Jr. Metastatic neoplasms of the bladder. J Urol 1963;90:281.

722. Weston PAM, Smith BJ. Metastatic melanoma in the bladder and urethra. Br J Surg 1964;51:78.

723. Woodard BH, Ideker RE, Johnston WW. Cytologic detection of malignant melanoma in urine. Acta Cytol 1978;22:350.

724. Nakazono M, Iwata S, Kuribayashi N. Disseminated metastatic ureteral melanoma: A case report. J Urol 1975;114:624.

725. Lowsley OS. Melanoma of the urinary tract and prostate gland. South Med J 1951;44: 487.

726. Baab GH, McBride CM. Malignant melanoma: The patient with an unknown site of primary origin. Arch Surg 1975;110:896.

727. Chang P, Knapper WH. Metastatic melanoma of unknown primary. Cancer 1982;49: 1106.

728. Das Gupta T, Bowden L, Berg JW. Malignant melanoma of unknown primary origin. Surg Gynecol Obstet 1963;117:341.

729. Giuliano AE, Moseley HS, Morton DL. Clinical aspects of unknown primary melanoma. Ann Surg 1980;191:98.

730. Milton GW, Shaw HM, McCarthy WH. Occult primary malignant melanoma: Factors influencing survival. Br J Surg 1977;64:805.

731. Reintgen DS, McCarty KS, Woodard B, et al. Metastatic malignant melanoma with an unknown primary site. Surg Gynecol Obstet 1983;156:335.

732. Mundth ED, Guralnick EA, Raker JW. Malignant melanoma: A clinical study of 427 cases. Ann Surg 1965;162:15–28.

733. Elder DE. Metastatic melanoma. Pigment Cell 1987;8:182.

Cancer: Principles & Practice of Oncology, Fourth Edition,
edited by Vincent T. DeVita, Jr., Samuel Hellman, Steven A. Rosenberg.
J.B. Lippincott Co., Philadelphia © 1993.

Jose A. Sahel

John D. Earle

Daniel M. Albert

CHAPTER **47**

Intraocular Melanomas

Melanomas are the commonest primary intraocular malignancy in the white population. They arise from uveal melanocytes, mature melanin-producing and melanin-containing cells, residing in the uveal stroma. These cells originate from the neural crest and possess long, dendrite-like processes. Melanomas may also arise in the conjunctiva. Proliferations of cells other than uveal melanocytes can arise in the eye; the epithelia of the iris, ciliary body, and retina can undergo reactive or neoplastic proliferations, forming adenomas or adenocarcinomas.[1-5] This chapter deals exclusively with uveal melanomas, with particular emphasis on the current therapeutic issues and controversies.

EPIDEMIOLOGY

The annual age-adjusted incidence of noncutaneous melanomas as reported in the Surveillance, Epidemiology, and End Results (SEER) Program during the period of 1973 to 1977 was 0.7 per 100,000 population in the United States.[6] Similar data were reported from epidemiologic studies conducted in New England (0.65 per 100,000 residents from 1984 to 1985),[7] the Swedish West Coast (0.72 per 100,000 from 1956 to 1975),[8] and Iceland (0.7 per 100,000 in men and 0.5 per 100,000 in women from 1955 to 1979).[9]

In the Third National Cancer Survey, conducted from 1969 to 1971, the annual age-adjusted incidence of intraocular melanomas in the United States was estimated at 0.6 per 100,000.[10] The precise anatomic origin of ocular melanomas was unspecified in about 25% of cases. Seventy-three percent of the tumors arose within the globe (mainly from the choroid), and 2% developed from the conjunctiva. Melanoma accounted for 70% of all primary eye malignancies, followed in frequency by the childhood tumor retinoblastoma (13%). In persons older than 20 years of age, melanoma was the reported diagnosis for 80% of all primary ocular cancers.[10] Data from the Missouri Department of Health,[11] China,[12] the SEER Program,[6] New England,[7] Iceland,[9] Finland,[13] and the Ocular Melanoma Task Force[14] are similar to those reported by the Third National Cancer Survey.[10] (Few studies have provided reliable, long-term survival rates. The Finnish study showed that the 5-, 10-, and 15-year survival rates were 65%, 52%, and 46%, respectively.[13]) The annual age-adjusted incidence of ocular melanomas is about one eighth that of skin melanoma in the United States.[13] The recently observed increase in the incidence of cutaneous melanomas has not been observed for uveal melanomas.[15-19] Although the incidence increases steadily by decade, with a peak in the seventh decade, uveal melanoma cases can occur before the age of 20 years, as illustrated by 101 of the 6359 cases on file at the Registry of Ophthalmic Pathology at the Armed Forces Institute of Pathology (AFIP), 40 of 3706 consecutive patients seen at Wills Eye Hospital, and several other reports.[7,12,20-27] Most studies show a median age at diagnosis of about 55 years, with rates decreasing after the age of 70 years.[13,23,28,29]

White persons have an eightfold greater risk for ocular melanoma than black persons (compared with a sixfold greater risk for skin melanomas)[10,14,30-32] and a threefold greater risk than certain Asian populations.[5,15] Although Scotto and associates found that the overall risk for ocular melanomas did not vary by sex,[5] Jensen,[23] Gislason and colleagues,[9] and others[7,16,33] noted a predominance of men. Ocular and skin melanoma show similar age patterns, with more women affected at younger ages and more men affected later in life.[5] The Third National Cancer Survey indicated a left-sided excess of 18% for ocular melanomas in men and a right-sided excess in women.[10]

ETIOLOGY AND HISTOGENESIS

As for most human cancers, the specific causes of ocular melanomas are unknown. However, epidemiologic, electron microscopic, and experimental data allow the characterization of risk factors, predisposing conditions, and hypothetical genetic or oncogenic causes.

PREDISPOSING CONDITIONS

Ocular melanocytosis and oculodermal melanocytosis (nevus of Ota) predipose to the development of uveal melanomas. In 4.6% of reported cases of nevus of Ota, malignant transformation was recorded,[36–38] and except for a single anecdotal case,[35] the melanoma occurred in the affected eye. Rare cases of uveal melanomas have been reported in patients with neurofibromatosis.[38,39]

Evidence that nevi are the origin of most choroidal melanomas has been provided by Yanoff and Zimmerman and others.[3,40,41] Yet a nevus-like configuration associated with choroidal melanoma may in some instances be explained by other mechanisms, such as flattening of normal uveal melanocytes or tumor cells; a secondary proliferative effect of the malignancy; or common oncogenic stimuli.[3,42,43] The last two mechanisms have been postulated in a few cases of bilateral, diffuse melanocytic tumors of the uvea in patients with systemic carcinoma.[3,44,45] In some instances, a familial increased occurrence of uveal melanoma has been recorded.[28,46–48]

Data on the occurrence of uveal melanocytic tumors in patients with the dysplastic nevus syndrome are controversial but generally support periodic ophthalmoscopic examination of these patients.[49–53] The association between uveal melanomas and other cancers is controversial. Turner and coworkers showed that the overall prevalence of nonbasal cell cancers in uveal melanoma patients was twice the expected number based on an age- and sex-matched population.[54] A link between cutaneous and uveal melanoma was suspected based on their association in three cases of primary uveal and cutaneous melanomas among 333 patients. A family history of cutaneous or uveal melanoma was present in 14 and 2 patients, respectively.[54] Lischko and associates conducted a case-control study among 197 New England cases with 385 matched control subjects and 337 cases (from the United States) with 800 control subjects.[55] They concluded that the association of prior malignancies with uveal melanomas is weak. In a similar study of 407 uveal melanoma patients from the Western United States compared with 870 control subjects, Holly and colleagues found no excess of prior cancers.[56] Cytogenetic studies of uveal melanoma tissues from 19 patients suggest that recessive alleles at some chromosome 2 loci may be important in the oncogenesis of these tumors.[57]

ONCOGENIC STIMULI

Certain electron microscopic and biomolecular studies of ocular melanomas suggest a possible etiologic role of viruses.[58] Viruses such as the feline sarcoma virus have been used successfully in the induction of ocular melanoma in animals.[58–61] In a study of a single population of chemical workers, a statistically significant and higher than expected incidence of ocular melanomas was found.[62] Nicotine has been incriminated in the unusual incidence of uveal melanomas in men.[63] Various chemicals, including nickel bisulfamide, platinum, methylcholanthrene, ethionine, N-2-fluorenylacetamide, radium, and N-methyl-N-nitrosourea, have been reported to induce ocular melanocytic tumors in animals.[59–70] A possible connection between levodopa therapy in Parkinson's disease and malignant melanoma has been mentioned.[71]

The role of hormonal factors and pregnancy has been suggested in some publications. Hartge and coworkers reported a case-controlled study comparing 238 women with uveal melanoma with 223 matched control women.[72] They showed that women with a past medical history of pregnancy or hormonal substitutive treatment with estrogens had an increased risk (relative risk of 1.4),[72] whereas a past medical history of oophorectomy had a decreased influence on relative risk (0.6), and oral contraceptives had none.[72] The role of pregnancy in the growth of uveal melanoma has been documented by Seddon and associates[73] and Shields and colleagues.[74] Whether the growth observed clinically is secondary to cellular growth or other factors, such as fluid retention and vascular engorgement, is unclear.

A case-controlled study lends support to the etiologic role of sunlight exposure.[75] A study of host factors (Northern European ancestry, light skin color, ten or more cutaneous nevi), ultraviolet radiation, and the risk for uveal melanoma indicated that personal attributes are strong independent risk factors.[76] Holly and associates proved that light skin color and easily sunburned skin increased the risk for uveal melanoma twofold, whereas ultraviolet exposure increased this risk fourfold and sevenfold, if intensive.[77] These data, which contradict previous studies,[10,78] confirm the high association between light iris color and the presence of iris melanocytic lesions.[79]

HISTOPATHOLOGY, PROGNOSTIC PARAMETERS, AND NATURAL HISTORY

CHOROIDAL AND CILIARY BODY MELANOMAS: CYTOLOGIC AND HISTOLOGIC CLASSIFICATION

The accurate histologic diagnosis of uveal melanoma is, in most instances, easily made by the experienced histopathologist. Rarely, differentiation from metastatic carcinoma may be facilitated by immunohistochemical labeling of S100 protein. This technique is not helpful in differentiating other neural crest-derived tumors, such as schwannomas, neurofibromas, and leiomyomas.[3] The S100 immunophenotypes of uveal melanoma differ considerably from cutaneous melanoma.[80] HMB-45 immunostaining may be a useful adjunct in the differentiation between uveal melanomas and nevi.[81] Otherwise, immunocytochemistry has not provided reliable characterization of uveal melanoma using cutaneous melanoma antibodies or antihuman leukocyte antigen antibodies or allowed preparation of reliable monoclonal antibodies.[82–85]

In 1931, Callender recognized major cell types in the spectrum of cells composing uveal melanomas, and this finding provided a cytologic classification clearly correlated with prognosis after enucleation.[86] The different cell types are shown in Table 47-1 and discussed in the following sections.[3,86,87]

TABLE 47–1. Histopathologic Classification of Choroidal and Ciliary Body Melanocytic Tumors

Iris

Pretreatment Clinical Classification (cTNM)

Primary Tumor (T)

TX   Minimum requirements to assess the primary tumor cannot be met
T0   No evidence of primary tumor
T2   Tumor involving not more than one quadrant, with extension into the anterior chamber angle
T3   Tumor involving more than one quadrant, with extension into the anterior chamber angle
T4   Tumor with extraocular extension

Regional Lymph Nodes (N)

NX   Minimum requirements to assess the regional lymph nodes cannot be met
N0   No evidence of regional lymph node involvement
N1   Evidence of involvement of the regional lymph nodes

Distant Metastases (M)

MX   Minimum requirements to assess the presence of distant metastases cannot be met
M0   No evidence of distant metastases
M1   Evidence of distant metastases

Ciliary Body

Pretreatment Clinical Classification (cTNM)

Primary Tumor (T)

TX   Minimum requirements to assess the primary tumor cannot be met
T0   No evidence of primary tumor
T1   Tumor limited to the ciliary body
T2   Tumor with extension into the anterior chamber and/or iris
T3   Tumor with extension into the choroid
T4   Tumor with extraocular extension

Regional Lymph Nodes (N)

NX   Minimum requirements to assess the regional lymph nodes cannot be met
N0   No evidence of regional lymph node involvement
N1   Evidence of involvement of the regional lymph nodes

Distant Metastases (M)

MX   Minimum requirements to assess the presence of distant metastases cannot be met
M0   No evidence of distant metastases
M1   Evidence of distant metastases

Choroid

Pretreatment Clinical Classification (cTNM)

Primary Tumor (T)

TX   Minimum requirements to assess the primary tumor cannot be met
T0   No evidence of primary tumor
T1   Tumor not more than 10 mm in its greatest dimension, and/or with an elevation of not more than 3 mm
T1A   Tumor not more than 7 mm in its greatest dimension and with an elevation of not more than 2 mm
T1B   Tumor more than 7 mm but not more than 10 mm in its greatest dimension and with an elevation of more than 2 mm but not more than 3 mm
T2   Tumor more than 10 mm but not more than 15 mm in its greatest dimension and with an elevation of more than 3 mm but not more than 5 mm
T3   Tumor more than 15 mm in its greatest dimension or with an elevation of 5 mm or more
T4   Tumor with extraocular extension
    Note: When dimension and elevation show a difference in classification, the highest category should be used for classification.

Regional Lymph Nodes (N)

NX   Minimum requirements to assess the regional lymph nodes cannot be met
N0   No evidence of regional lymph node involvement
N1   Evidence of involvement of regional lymph nodes

Distant Metastases (M)

MX   Minimum requirements to assess the presence of distant metastases cannot be met
M0   No evidence of distant metastases
M1   Evidence of distant metastases

Spindle A cells are uniform, cohesive cells with small, slender, spindle-shaped nuclei often showing longitudinal folds in the nuclear membrane. The nucleoli are not distinct, and mitotic figures are rare. The cell borders are difficult to identify.

Spindle B cells are plumper, cohesive spindle cells with larger ovoid nuclei containing a coarse chromatin network and a conspicuous nucleolus. Mitotic figures are seen more frequently. The cell borders are difficult to discern. Spindle A and B cells may be arranged in rows or palisades, constituting the fascicular pattern, which is now regarded as having no prognostic significance.[3,88] A careful reappraisal of 90 pure spindle A melanomas by McLean and colleagues found that 15 had features of benignity, whereas the other 75 had larger, hyperchromatic nuclei with frequent mitotic activity associated with histologic features of malignancy (*e.g.,* invasiveness) and greater size.[89] In the revised AFIP classification of uveal melanomas, the spindle A and B subtypes are no longer separated.[89]

Epithelioid cells were described by Callender as larger, more pleomorphic, poorly cohesive, polygonal cells with abundant eosinophilic cytoplasm.[86] The nuclei are round and contain large single or multiple nucleoli. Mitotic figures are abundant. A subtype consisting of small cells with less cytoplasm and a smaller nucleus is now included in this category, because it has other typical features of epithelioid cells, such as large eosinophilic nucleoli and lack of cohesiveness.[90] According to Callender's cytologic characterization, uveal melanomas are divided into the following three categories:

1. Spindle cell melanomas, type A, B, or both, accounting for 30% of intraocular tumors
2. Mixed cell melanomas containing spindle and epithelioid cells
3. Epithelioid cell melanomas accounting for 5% of intraocular tumors

The major cell types described by Callender are part of a continuous spectrum, and the pathologist's identification of a particular cell type involves subjective judgment.[91,92] In the Collaborative Ocular Melanoma Study (COMS), it was found useful to include an "intermediate" category of cells that share characteristics of spindle B and epithelioid cells.[93]

This issue was also addressed by Gamel and McLean, who described a more objective method of assessing uveal melanomas histopathologically.[94] This method, which uses computerized cytomorphology, mainly entails evaluating the inverse of the standard deviation of the nucleolar area and, more recently, measurement of the mean of the ten largest nucleoli. This measure appears to be the best objective determination of a tumor's malignant potential ($p > 0.001$).[95-98] Studies by Gamel and associates and others have corroborated the well-documented prognostic value of Callender's classification, especially as to the pejorative significance of high epithelioid cell content.[30,86,88,90,95-102]

Several attempts to evaluate the growth and malignant potential of uveal melanomas have been made recently using DNA cell cycle studies, for example, bromodeoxyuridine uptake or Ki-67 antibody as a marker of cycling cells[102,103] and DNA or RNA content by flow cytometry.[103,106] The value of these methods and the usefulness of silver-stained nucleolar-organizer regions must still be prospectively compared with cytomorphometric determinations and conventional cytology by an experienced pathologist.[103-108]

Paul and coworkers reviewed 2652 cases accessioned at the AFIP by 1959 and found that 95% of patients with spindle A tumors, 85% of those with spindle B tumors, 60% of those with mixed cell tumors, and 83% of those with epithelioid tumors were alive 5 years after enucleation.[30] At 16 years after enucleation, the survival rates were 85%, 80%, 46%, and 34%, respectively.[62] McLean and colleagues, in a review of 3432 cases from the AFIP, found that the overall mortality from metastasis 15 years after enucleation was 46%.[102] The mortality of patients with mixed cell melanomas was three times that of patients with pure spindle cell lesions.

In Jensen's series of 302 reported cases from Denmark that had been observed for 25 years, 150 (50%) of the patients died from metastatic melanoma.[23,109,110] Fewer than 1% of patients with spindle A tumors died from metastatic disease; 83% with mixed cell tumors were dead; and in 71% of patients with epithelioid tumors, the cause of death was metastatic melanoma.

After the studies of Rosenberg and coworkers on the prognostic and therapeutic value of tumor-infiltrating lymphocytes, a reappraisal of the well-known lymphocytic infiltration of some uveal melanomas has been undertaken.[111-115] Analysis of tumor-infiltrating lymphocytes detected in five tumors (among 27 melanomas studied) has shown the predominance of cytotoxic T cells and the predominant expression of T-cell receptor V α7.[111,112]

The role of infiltrating lymphocytes in the regression of animals with tumors is a current avenue of investigation.[100-102]

NATURAL HISTORY

Growth Rate

Little is known about the natural history of uveal melanomas; until recently, all patients underwent enucleation immediately after the diagnosis.[3,116,117] Data on the growth pattern of small melanomas from series of patients observed by Gass and others have contributed to the knowledge of the rate of intraocular tumor growth before treatment.[110,118-121]

These findings and other selected reports[122,123] suggest a Gompertzian (expotential) growth curve, as postulated by Manschot and associates.[124] The doubling time of uveal tumors may vary from 2 months or less[119-125] to several years.[117-119] In rapidly growing tumors, a high mitotic activity and the presence of epithelioid cells have been documented.[119,123,125] Rarely, spontaneous regression of a choroidal melanoma has been reported.[126]

Intraocular Spread

Small melanomas usually grow from a discoid to a hemispheric shape. They progressively obliterate the choriocapillaris and displace Bruch's membrane and the retina inward. When Bruch's membrane is disrupted, the tumor grows in the subretinal space in a mushroom configuration.[3,127-136] The retinal pigment epithelium overlying the tumors undergoes early changes, including drusen formation and orange pigment (lipofuscin) accumulation.[3,127-133] The neurosensory retina is detached frequently and, in some instances, infiltrated by tumor cells, which can seed into the vitreous.[132]

Anterior choroidal and ciliary body tumors are more likely to affect the lens and to seed the posterior chamber. The zonule, lens, iris, anterior chamber, and angle may be involved. Secondary glaucoma may result from obstruction of the outflow pathways by tumor cells, cell debris, and phagocytic cells swollen with ingested cell debris (melanomalytic glaucoma).[133,134] The tumor may infiltrate through the scleral spur into the trabecular network.

Although the sclera is stated to be an effective barrier against extraocular extension, scleral infiltration by tumor cells along ciliary vessels and nerves and along the vortex veins is frequent (32.3% of large melanomas in a series reported by Shammas and Blodi).[135] Approximately 5% of melanomas grow diffusely in the plane of the uvea or circumferentially along the root of the iris. They induce a slight thickening of the uvea (approximately 3–5 mm) and are often unsuspected or are diagnosed late in the course of the tumor, when secondary glaucoma or extraocular spread occur. Such extraocular extension may occur adjacent to or through the optic nerve or can occur anteriorly about the limbus.[136]

Extraocular Extension

Although extrascleral extension may be observed with small tumors,[137,138] it is more likely to occur when the tumor has reached a larger size. In a study by Shammas and Blodi, extrascleral extension was observed in 18% of tumors exceeding 10 mm in diameter.[138] The overall incidence of transcleral extension was determined to about 13% among 1842 malignant melanomas studied by Starr and Zimmerman.[139] Others series have compiled similar data.[140,141] Starr and Zimmerman noted a tenfold increase in the incidence of postoperative recurrence if the tumor extended to the surgical margin. The depth of the scleral extension may have a prognostic significance.[142] Other paths of extraocular spread include the optic nerve[143,144] and the lumen of the vortex veins.[145]

Because of the absence of lymphatics in the eye, lymphatic spread has not been demonstrated; this is in contrast to cutaneous melanomas.[146] Hematogenous dissemination to the liver is a frequent form of metastatic spread.[3,15,147,148] The respective roles of nonspecific trapping and of cell-surface antigens in the invasiveness and dissemination of uveal melanomas remain poorly explored fields of investigation.[149-154]

Some clones of melanoma cells with a preferential propensity for liver metastasis mediated by cell-surface properties have been characterized.[155,156] Patients with preexisting liver damage are more likely to be affected.[157,158] Metastases to other sites (lungs, heart, gastrointestinal tract, lymph nodes, pancreas, skin, central nervous system, bones, spleen, adrenal glands, kidneys, ovaries, and thyroid gland) generally occur in association with liver metastases.[133] In a recent survey of metastases from proton beam-treated melanomas, liver involvement was documented in almost all patients[159]; the overall 1-year survival was 13%.[159]

In a series of studies, Zimmerman and McLean found that most deaths from metastatic disease occurred in the first 5 years after enucleation, with a peak mortality in the second and third years (about 8% per year), and compared these data with the natural course of untreated melanomas.[3,90,116,160] In a conclusion that remains controversial, they incriminated enucleation as a risk factor and suggested two principal mechanisms: (1) dissemination of tumor cells during traumatic operations, as demonstrated experimentally by Fraunfelder and colleagues,[161] and (2) decreased host resistance to disseminated tumor cells. This latter mechanism has been called by Niederkorn and coworkers the "loss of intraocular induced concomitant immunity" mediated by cytotoxic T lymphocytes.[115,162,163] Zimmerman's and McLean's assumptions have been challenged by several investigators. Seigel and associates concluded that the statistical data can be interpreted differently and that there was no evidence to suggest that the existing pattern of treatment be altered.[164] Manschot and Van Peperzeel,[124] Kersten and Blodi,[165] and Davidorf[166] pointed out that most melanomas are diagnosed only when they have reached a relatively large size and concomitantly have given rise to metastases, and only then are they enucleated. The clinical consequences of these controversies have been employment of less traumatic techniques for enucleation and new impetus to the search for alternative treatments.[129,167]

PROGNOSTIC ASSESSMENT OF CHOROIDAL AND CILIARY BODY MELANOMAS

In most studies, the second most important prognostic parameter after the number of epithelioid cells is the largest tumor diameter.[3,90,100,101,135,169] This is followed, according to Seddon and colleagues, by the location of the anterior margin of the tumor, the invasion of the line of transsection, and the degree of pigmentation.[100,101,135] In a study of 253 choroidal and ciliary body melanomas for which a follow-up of 5 years or more was available, Shammas and Blodi identified the following eight factors that significantly influenced prognosis:

Age of the patient at enucleation
Location of the tumor
Location of the anterior border of the tumor
Largest tumor diameter in contact with the sclera
Height of the tumor
Integrity of Bruch's membrane
Cell type
Scleral infiltration by tumor cells

Using a multivariate analysis, McLean and coworkers reached similar conclusions for small melanomas.[102] Parameters that significantly influenced prognosis were cell type,

largest dimension, scleral extension, and mitotic activity. A single factor analysis identified three additional factors of significance: degree of scleral invasion, optic nerve invasion, and pigmentation. In most of the studies, increased pigmentation has been associated with increased mortality.[15,30,102,110,135] In a multivariant analysis, however, these three parameters appear statistically related to cell type and tumor size,[55,100,101,168,169] but a close interval by interval analysis of the prognostic value of size and cell type shows a decline over time after tumor excision.[170]

In summary, all studies show that the prognosis of a patient with a choroidal or ciliary body melanoma treated by enucleation is *adversely affected* if the following occur:

The tumor contains epithelioid cells.
The tumor involves the ciliary body.
The largest tumor dimension exceeds 10 mm.
The tumor extends to the sclera.
Numerous mitotic figures are present.

Many of these prognostic parameters are lacking in patients treated conservatively (*i.e.*, by methods other than enucleation). Because of reports with a brief follow-up period, bias in patient selection and sample size, and use of different survival analysis models, the comparison of survival rates with either conservative approaches or enucleation remains a subject of intense controversy.[167,169–172] The survival rates in large series after 5 years do not differ significantly: the reported tumor-related mortality 5 years after radiation therapy ranges from 11% to 25%,[169–181] whereas preliminary assumptions based on a log normal model may indicate a poorer life prognosis after 10 years for patients treated conservatively.[172] COMS, a prospective, multicenter study, should provide answers to this crucial and controversial issue.[173]

Several studies have established a correlation between rapid tumor regression after radiation therapy and poor prognosis for life.[175–178] Rapid regression of tumor height after irradiation appears to be a risk factor for metastasis.[175] That can possibly be correlated with a less differentiated cell type found in rapidly regressing tumors. However, this hypothesis is difficult to support because (1) cytologic study of such melanomas would depend on needle biopsy, which is rarely performed before radiation therapy; (2) in those rare cases, cytologic aspiration does not provide a reliable characterization of the cell type; and (3) histologic study of enucleated eyes after irradiation may not reflect accurately the cytologic features of the tumor before irradiation, particularly in mixed cell tumors.

DISTINGUISHING FEATURES OF IRIS MELANOMAS

Malignant melanoma of the iris is rare compared with melanomas of the rest of the uvea; the estimated ratios range from 1 in 6 to 1 in 30.[15,182–187] The average age at diagnosis of iris melanocytic tumors, including nevi, is 40 to 50 years.[109,110,127–130,185–187] Many patients (17–33%) give a long history of a noticeable pigmented iris lesion before clinical diagnosis. This observation is widely interpreted as suggesting that such tumors arose from preexisting nevi.[184,185,188–192] Zimmerman and others believe that the difference in size between tumors of the iris and other uveal tumors is the most critical feature affecting tumor behavior.[161,193,196] Iris melanomas are comparatively small lesions, generally much smaller than the posterior uveal tract tumors that come to clinical attention.[166,193-196] Iris melanomas grow more slowly than posterior uveal melanomas. Kersten and colleagues,[194] applying the scheme proposed by Apple and Blodi for choroidal melanomas,[197] suggested that the slow growth rate is related to the small size of iris melanomas. This slow growth and the high proportion of spindle A cells probably account for the low number of recurrences, metastasis, or death from disease several years or decades after the onset of symptoms.[194,198] The literature has continued to stress the relatively benign behavior and good prognosis of iris melanomas compared with melanomas of the choroid and ciliary body. Those melanomas in the ciliary body and choroid are associated with a mortality tenfold higher than the mortality from iris melanomas.[90] Green, reviewing 783 cases from the literature, noted 18 (2.29%) reported deaths from metastatic disease.[4] In two recent clinicopathologic studies, 138 and 107 patients, respectively, with a previous diagnosis of iris melanomas had no tumor-related deaths.[182,188] These series emphasize that many lesions previously called melanomas are actually nevi. Jakobiec and Silbert reclassified 138 lesions with an initial histopathologic diagnosis of melanoma into a nine-part classification, including three malignant categories; on reexamination using their criteria, only 13% of lesions were judged malignant.[182] In a similar series of 107 such tumors,[188] a ten-part classification derived from Jakobiec and Silbert was applied. Only 10% of the lesions were considered melanomas. The argyrophilic-stained nucleolar organizer region-associated count may provide an accurate prediction of the malignant nature and potential or iris melanocytic lesions.[199,199a] However, the low malignant potential of iris melanocytic tumors is accepted by most authors.[192-194,198,200,201] Moreover, the prognostic assessment of iris melanoma should consider that local spread of some melanocytic tumors, even with "benign" cytology, may lead to sight-threatening complications, such as refractory secondary glaucoma, and that incomplete or inappropriate surgery may increase both local and systemic malignant potential.[182,191,192,198,202,203]

DIAGNOSIS OF UVEAL MELANOMAS

CHOROIDAL AND CILIARY BODY MELANOMAS

The diagnosis of choroidal and ciliary body melanomas has reached a high degree of accuracy at eye centers where experienced clinicians and modern ancillary testing facilities are available.[204-210] This point is well illustrated by a comparison of the misdiagnosis rates among the eyes on file at the AFIP: 19% (of 529 eyes) until 1962, 20% (of 208 eyes) between 1963 and 1970, and 6.4% (of 744 eyes) between 1970 and 1980.[204-207] During the 11-year period of the last study, the rate of misdiagnosis declined from 12.5% to 1.4%.[207] Between 1954 and 1977, the misdiagnosis rate was 2.6% (of 244 eyes) at the Mayo Clinic.[208] In this series, in addition, six clinically unsuspected melanomas were found.[208] This high rate of correct clinical diagnosis is particularly impressive, because only outpatient procedures (including clinical ex-

amination, ultrasound, and fluorescein angiography) were used. No biopsies were performed, as is done for many other tumors. A review of 395 eyes enucleated during a 50-year period, based on the pathology files of Ohio State University, revealed a misdiagnosis rate of 10.9% from 1931 to 1959, which decreased to 1.7% from 1960 to 1981. Nine percent of choroidal melanomas were unsuspected preoperatively, and all of these were in eyes with opaque media.[209] In a series of 400 consecutive patients referred to the oncology unit of the Wills Eye Hospital with an incorrect diagnosis of melanoma (*i.e.*, patients proved to have pseudomelanomas), the correct diagnosis was reached through clinical evaluation in 397 cases (99%).[210] In that series, the most commonly encountered conditions mimicking a melanoma included suspicious choroidal nevi (26.5%), peripheral disciform degeneration (11%), congenital hypertrophy of the retinal pigment epithelium (9.5%), and choroidal hemangioma (8%). Most metastatic carcinomas had been diagnosed correctly by the referring ophthalmologists.[210] A high rate of accuracy was recently reported in the multicenter COMS.[211]

The cornerstone of diagnosis of posterior uveal melanoma remains clinical examination, particularly indirect ophthalmoscopy through a dilated pupil. Fundus contact lens examination and the use of a three-mirror lens can be extremely helpful.[127-130] Scleral transillumination as advocated by Reese is also a useful aid.[128] Pigmented conjunctival lesions, such as conjunctival melanoma, staphylomas, scleral ectasia, hematoma, cellular blue nevi, and ocular melanocytosis, may mimic extraocular extension of uveal melanomas.[212] Visual field studies are of little help in diagnosis or in distinguishing melanomas from choroidal nevi.[42,91,129,213,216] Although clinical examination by an experienced observer remains the most important test in establishing the presence of an ocular melanoma, ancillary diagnostic testing can be extremely valuable.[46,127-130,215]

Fluorescein angiography and monochromic photography have proved useful in differentiating subretinal or choroidal hemorrhage and hemangioma from melanoma. Although no angiographic pattern is pathognomonic for choroidal melanomas, features of value include early mottling, fluorescence, orange pigment over the margin of the tumor, progressive fluorescence of the lesion with late staining, and multiple pinpoint leaks that increase in size. Breaks in Bruch's membrane and retinal invasion can be detected from abnormalities such as a "double circulation" pattern.[44,127-130,215-218]

The combined use of A- and B-mode ultrasound techniques is valuable in confirming the clinical diagnosis of choroidal melanoma, especially in the presence of opaque media.[129,130,173,205,210,219-228] The B-mode ultrasound characteristics useful in differentiating melanomas from metastases or hemangiomas are acoustic hollowness, choroidal excavation, and orbital shadowing. Small tumors elevated less than 2 to 3 mm cannot be evaluated accurately. In large tumors, ultrasound provides valuable size data for serial measurements.[220,226] However, a difference between ultrasonographic and histopathologic measurements of tumor thickness was demonstrated, probably resulting from tumor shrinkage after laboratory preparation.[220] Extrascleral extension can be detected by contact B-mode ultrasound.[221] Ultrasound is an important follow-up tool after conservative treatment of uveal melanoma.[229] Recent reports on the usefulness of color-coded

Doppler imaging are promising in characterization and follow-up studies.[230–232]

The usefulness of radioactive phosphorus (phosphorus 32) in determining malignancy is more controversial. It probably has limited indications for use in routine cases in which adequate support for a diagnosis of ocular melanoma has been obtained with less complicated procedures.[129,130,233–236]

Radiologic examination, including computed tomography (CT), is useful in evaluating the presence and size of extraocular extension of tumor.[237–239]

Images of uveal melanoma were included in early reports of magnetic resonance imaging (MRI) studies.[240] This imaging modality has become more useful with the increase in its availability, the use of thin-section imaging, the development of surface coils, and the employment of contrast material (gadolinium).[240–246] Typically, pigmented melanomas are hyperintense on T1-weighted images with enhancement by gadolinium.[205,243–246] Therefore, this method is promising in the detection, the characterization, and the delimitation of difficult cases. Phosphorus 31 magnetic resonance spectroscopy may be helpful in this respect soon.[247,248] Nevertheless, ultrasonography is currently the main imaging modality employed in intraocular melanomas.

Immunologic testing does not yet offer reliable results.[249–255] Using the indirect immunoperoxidase method, Felberg and coworkers found that 78% of patients with uveal malignancy had tumor-associated antibodies (TAA), whereas 24% of control subjects tested positive for TAA.[249] Unfortunately, TAA assays could not be used to separate primary from secondary uveal tumors. Studies of monoclonal antibodies, as discussed earlier, are not yet convincing.[252,254] Radioimmunoscintigraphy using technetium 99m (^{99m}Tc)-labeled monoclonal antibodies are too preliminary to be considered as reliable diagnostic tools.[253,255] However, surveillance of melanoma-associated antigens and carcinoembryonic antigens may be useful for monitoring recurrence or metastatic disease.[251,256,257]

In a review of 51 consecutive patients who had undergone enucleation for a choroidal melanoma and 50 patients with simulating lesions, Char and colleagues found that the ophthalmoscopic examination was the most accurate diagnostic modality, allowing correct diagnosis of choroidal melanomas in all patients with clear media.[258] Subretinal fluid, orange pigmentation, and collar button configuration occurred more often with melanomas than with other lesions. In 63% of melanoma patients, fluorescein angiography was diagnostic, and in 82%, A- and B-mode ultrasonography was diagnostic.[258]

In some dubious cases, fine-needle aspiration biopsy has been proposed.[129,130,259] However, the interpretation of aspirates may be difficult, even in the hands of an experienced pathologist, and subsequent tumor cell seeding in the needle track has been reported.[260,261] Nevertheless, in selected cases, this technique has proved useful to differentiate benign from malignant lesions.[129,130,259,262] The lack of histologic data before conservative treatment of most uveal melanomas imposes a major limitation on an understanding of tumor response to irradiation and the accurate adaptation of conservative approaches and on the estimate of prognosis for such examinations.

Despite ancillary examinations, the differential diagnosis of small tumors may be difficult. Careful follow-up study of such patients at short intervals with photography, fluorescein angiography, and ultrasound is advocated to demonstrate tumor growth.[42,66,129,130,204,263]

Patients with suspected intraocular melanoma should undergo a physical examination and metastatic workup. Clinical laboratory studies should include routine blood studies, chest radiography, and liver enzyme measurements. CT should be performed if other tests suggest liver involvement.[127–130,147,148,157,173,205,264–266] Liver ultrasonography and liver-spleen scans may be useful.

IRIS MELANOMAS

Iris tumors are visible not only to the ophthalmologist but also to the patient, family, and friends.[127–130,193] Patients frequently are aware of a spot on the iris that has been present for many years but has only recently shown growth. The ophthalmologist can examine the lesion carefully with a slit-lamp biomicroscope and gonioscopy, and with the aid of serial iris fluorescein photography, can determine the size and vasculature of the tumor.[130,267] Iris tumors are usually small, discrete lesions replacing the normal architecture of the iris stroma, but they may be extensive (*e.g.*, diffuse or ring), infiltrative, or even multiple, such as the hypopigmented, multifocal nodules composing the picture of tapioca melanomas.[3,127–130,182] Only a few clinical findings—increased vascularity, involvement of the ciliary body, secondary glaucoma, and documented tumor growth—are helpful in distinguishing benign from malignant iris melanocytic tumors.[182,185,187,195,196,269–271] The differential diagnosis includes entities characterized by diffuse increased pigmentation, including melanosis, siderosis bulbi, heterochromia iridis, foreign bodies encapsulated by fibrous tissue, iris cysts, essential iris atrophy, peripheral anterior synechia, tumors of the retinal pigment epithelium, leiomyomas, granulomas—as seen in tuberculosis, herpes, or sarcoidosis—metastatic neoplasms, syphilitic gummas, and nevoxanthoendothelioma.[152,195,196,269–272]

TREATMENT OF UVEAL MELANOMAS

PRETREATMENT CLINICAL STAGING

It is useful to discuss the treatment of choroidal and ciliary body melanomas in terms of the following tumor sizes: (1) small 2 to 2.5 mm elevated <16 mm base; (2) medium ≥2.5 to ≤10.0 mm elevated ≤16 mm base; (3) large >10 mm elevated >16 mm base *or* at least 2 mm elevated *and* >16 mm base.[3,127–139,205] This division by size is referred to in the remainder of this chapter.

Comparisons of results from various series would benefit from more uniform staging of uveal tumors. The American Joint Committee on Cancer has developed a staging classification of uveal melanomas based on the tumor, node, metastasis (TNM) system (see Table 47-1).[3,273] However, this classification is not widely used for various reasons, including the rarity of detectable metastases at the time of diagnosis, particularly lymphatic lesions. Moreover, in contrast to the Reese-Ellsworth classification of retinoblastomas,[128] this classification is of marginal help in predicting the visual outcome of conservative approaches, because of such factors as the distance to the optic nerve and macula. Moreover, as mentioned earlier, the lack of histopathologic data in most patients managed conservatively has given emphasis to evaluation of the tumors based solely on patterns of tumor growth before and tumor regression after radiation therapy. Therefore, the comparison of data from most retrospective and often incomplete studies would increase the current confusion and controversies.

TREATMENT OF CHOROIDAL AND CILIARY BODY MELANOMAS

In the late nineteenth century, enucleation became the standard and almost universally accepted treatment for all choroidal or ciliary body melanomas.[276] Early enucleation continues to have its ardent advocates[124,180,275]; however, in recent years enucleation has been reassessed as a conventional means of treating malignant melanomas of the choroid and ciliary body. This reassessment has.resulted from (1) the development of newer and more precise diagnostic tests for recognizing malignant melanomas and the serial documentation of their size; (2) more information about clinical and pathologic features that determine survival; (3) additional observations about the natural course of untreated ciliary body and choroidal melanomas; (4) therapeutic developments other than enucleation to treat these tumors without destroying the eye; and (5) disagreements regarding the value and risks of enucleation.[3,61,90,100,101,116,118,126,160-167,173,174,180,197,205]

Currently, most authors agree that the goals for treating a uveal melanoma should be to destroy or inactivate the neoplasm, to maintain useful vision in the involved eye, to use a treatment with few side effects, and, most important, to provide the patient with the best prognosis for life among the treatment alternatives that are available.[127-130,173,174,205] Beyond these basic statements, many controversies will continue until results from prospective, randomized treatment trials are collected.[129,167,173,205] Therefore, the treatment ultimately selected is determined currently by the specific findings in the individual patient with regard to tumor size, location, and growth rate, the preferences of the ophthalmologist, and the desires of the patient.

SMALL MELANOMAS

The choices open to the physician treating a small choroidal or ciliary body melanoma include observation; some method of local treatment, including radiation therapy, photoradiation, cryotherapy, ultrasonic hyperthermia, local resection; and enucleation.

Observation

An accumulating body of evidence indicates that the risks to these patients in observing these tumors are low (Table 47-2).[91,117-119,126,129,130,214,215,277-280] Serial examination every 3 months without intervention seems appropriate if the tumor is asymptomatic or appears dormant; if the diagnosis is equivocal; if no growth is seen on serial ophthalmoscopic, photographic, and ultrasound examinations; in elderly, seriously ill patients; or for a tumor in the patient's only useful eye when the tumor is growing slowly.[129,176,210,215,277-281]

If the tumor shows progression, particularly rapid growth or an increase in size beyond 10 mm in diameter and 3 mm in elevation, or if the lesions results in significant impairment of vision, treatment is indicated.

Photocoagulation

In this method, the xenon arc, the argon laser, photoradiation with red light after photosensitization with hematoporphyrin derivatives, or dye laser after phthalocyanine photosensitization can be used.[129,130,281-296] Some success with photocoagulation has been documented histologically in small series.[128,130,288] The following criteria for selecting patients with melanoma for photocoagulation treatment were suggested by Meyer-Schwickerath[281] and Vogel[282] and adapted by Shields and others[29,205,294]:

1. The diagnosis of melanoma and evidence of growth should be documented thoroughly.

TABLE 47–2. Observation Versus Enucleation of Small Tumors of the Choroid and Ciliary Body

Aspect Evaluated	Char et al[118]	Gass[263]*	Shields[222]	Davidorf et al[280]	McLean et al[90]	Shammas et al[135]	Barr et al[278]	Thomas et al[279]	Seddon et al[100]
No. of eyes	20	100	150	38	37	129	16	27	267
Management	Observation: enucleation if growth	Observation: enucleation or further follow-up if growth	Observation: enucleation if growth	Enucleation	Enucleation	Enucleation	Enucleation	Enucleation	Enucleation
Follow-up	1–19 y before enucleation; average 4.5 y after enucleation	>8 y	2–5 y	>5 y	6 y	5 y	6 y	10 y	8 y
Evidence of growth	45%	36%	10–15%						
Deaths from metastases	—	3%	—	5% 5 y 19% 10 y	25%	8% 5 y 10% 10 y	11%	10%	12% 5 y 18% 10 y

* Gass assumed that tumors exhibiting no growth over 5 years were actually nevi.

2. The tumor should not be greater than 5 diopters in elevation and 6 disk diameters at its greatest diameter.
3. The tumor must be surrounded completely without damaging the fovea or the optic disk.
4. The patient must have clear ocular media and a sufficient mydriasis to enable photocoagulation to be performed.
5. The tumor surface should not have large overlying retinal vessels.

Photocoagulation requires several outpatient treatment sessions and is carried out after mydriasis and (for xenon photocoagulation) induction of retrobulbar anesthesia. A double confluent row of heavy coagulation is repeated three times at monthly intervals to encircle the tumor and to obliterate the choroidal vasculature supplying the gray discoloration and a surrounding atrophic choroidal scar.

Long-term complications of photocoagulation include retinal vascular obstruction, visual field defect, macular pucker, cystoid macular edema, choroid neovascularization, vitreous hemorrhage, and retinal detachment.[129,205,282,294] Recurrences may appear, usually within 2 years of treatment. In a 20-year follow-up of 54 patients with uveal melanomas, Vogel reported that 63% were alive, although only 46% were considered cured by photocoagulation.[282] Twenty percent of patients subsequently underwent enucleation. Of the 20 patients (37%) who died, 8 did so as a result of metastatic disease, 3 died from other causes, and 9 died from undetermined causes.[282] Shields reported that among 35 patients treated between 1976 and 1979, 25 retained useful vision, 5 had poor vision, and 5 subsequently underwent enucleation.[129] There were no tumor-related deaths. Comparison of xenon arc and argon laser photocoagulation in 38 consecutive patients with a minimal follow-up of 58 months showed that recurrences were less frequent and appeared later after xenon photocoagulation irradiation.[286] Photocoagulation seems best suited for small posterior melanomas located within 3 mm of the optic disk or fovea. In such lesions (photocoagulation-induced) retinopathy may cause visual loss.[129,130,205] The patient's desire to avoid radiation therapy or enucleation may be the deciding factor for using this modality. Photocoagulation is also helpful in the treatment of secondary serious macular detachments.[297] Reports on hematoporphyrin and phthalocyanine phototherapy are too preliminary.[261–264,267,272,273]

Radiation

For lesions meeting the clinical criteria for choroidal melanomas that are no larger than about 10 mm in height or 16 mm in diameter, brachytherapy is an acceptable therapeutic option. Before 1930, Moore used radon 222 seed to treat choroidal melanomas.[298] In the 1960s, Stallard popularized cobalt ^{60}Co as a brachytherapy source.[299] Although dosimetry was still relatively crude, the use of standardized plaques became common because of the long half-life of [60]Co. Results in a large series of patients managed in similar fashion became available, demonstrating the equivalence with enucleation within the limits of balancing the prognostic factors in these retrospective analyses. Markoe and associates used the Cox proportional hazards model to compare results in 100 patients treated with ^{60}Co plaques with results in enucleated patients.[300] Survival was better for the plaque-treated patients, although

the findings were not statistically significant. Vision deteriorated in a roughly linear fashion: approximately 40% had better vision than 20/200 visual acuity at 5 years.[300]

In 1976, Sealy and coworkers first reported using iodine ^{125}I for choroidal melanomas.[301] In 1979, Packer and Rotman suggested ^{125}I as the isotope of choice for brachytherapy of choroidal melanomas, based on the ease of shielding the adjacent structures and the safety of medical personnel.[302] Of 58 patients, 8 failed locally, and 45 remained alive without disease. Thirty-eight percent had deterioration of vision of two or more lines on the Snellen chart.[303] Garretson and colleagues reported results in 26 patients treated with ^{125}I plaques who were followed for a minimum of 2 years (mean, 45 months).[304] One patient died at 21 months. Visual acuity remained within two Snellen lines of preoperative levels in 54%. Of the 12 patients who lost more than two lines of acuity, 8 developed retinal changes, and 3 developed cataracts. Enucleation accounted for the loss of vision in the last patient. Enucleation was necessary in a single patient because of tumor growth.

Lommatzsch has published results comparable with those achieved with ^{125}I or ^{60}Co plaque using β-particles from ruthenium 106 and rhubidium 106.[305] He notes a 10-year survival of 67% in 309 cases.[306]

The COMS, involving some 42 clinical centers and 6 central units carefully monitoring quality, is conducting two randomized clinical trials. The first trial compares enucleation with ^{125}I brachytherapy for melanomas 2.5 to 10 mm in height and as much as 16 mm in diameter. Eligible patients randomized to irradiation receive treatment with ^{125}I sources in a gold-backed plaque shielding the posterior tissues. A dose of 100 Gy is delivered at 50 to 125 cGy/hour at the apex of the tumor (for tumors 5–10-mm high and to 5 mm for tumors 2.5–5-mm high). The second trial tests the value of preoperative external-beam irradiation (2000 cGy in five fractions) versus enucleation alone for patients with large tumors.[173]

More than 1000 patients were entered into these controlled trials through 1991. Heavy-charged particle beams are being investigated, using cyclotron-produced protons at Massachusetts General Hospital and synchrocyclotron-generated helium ions at the Lawrence Laboratory at Berkeley. These beams were selected because of their sharp penumbra and the Bragg peak, describing the greater deposition of energy at a depth. Both facilities use careful patient evaluation before treatment and sophisticated immobilization procedures that allow precise positioning of ports guided by radiographic confirmation of the tumors, the bases of which are marked by tantalum rings sutured to the sclera around the margin demonstrated by transillumination and indirect ophthalmoscopy. For treatment, generally 4000 to 10,000 cGy (^{60}Co equivalent dose corrected for relative biologic effect [RBE] with a factor of 1.1) is delivered in five fractions over 8 to 10 days at Harvard. At Berkeley, 7000 or 8000 cGy (^{60}Co equivalent dose corrected for RBE 1.3) is delivered over five fractions.

With a relatively short follow-up period, Saunders and coworkers have reported that irradiation failed locally in 5 of 75 patients, and 18% had neovascular glaucoma.[307] Twenty patients received a 70-Gy equivalent dose. Because of the high local failure rate, the dose was increased to 80-Gy equivalent for the remaining 55 patients. The mean follow-up at the time of the reporting was only 18 months. Local recurrence was detected in 4 of 20 patients treated with 70-Gy equivalent, and 1 of the 55 patients treated to 80-Gy equivalent has recurred (mean follow-up in the latter group was 14 months). Of the 42 patients followed for more than 1 year, 10 had vision worse than 20/200.[307]

Between 1975 and 1981, 128 patients were treated at the Massachusetts General Hospital cyclotron. The results are reported with a median follow-up of 5.4 years. Vision seemed to be declining linearly, with 69% of patients having at least 20/200 visual acuity at 5 years. Eight eyes were enucleated because of complications (6%), and metastases developed in 20.5% of patients.[308] Poorer outcome was seen for thicker tumors and tumors located nearer the optic disk and fovea.[309]

Other Local Nonsurgical Techniques

Preliminary reports on the experimental use of microwave, ferromagnetic, or ultrasonically induced hyperthermia described tumor regression in most patients.[310-317] This technique has been used in association with radiation in some instances, with good results in tumor control with lower doses of irradiation.[312-317]

Lincoff and coworkers obtained discouraging results with cryotherapy of ocular melanomas in 4 patients.[318] There are anecdotal reports of successful treatments for small peripheral melanomas.[129,277,319,320] Documented evidence for the efficacy of these alternative approaches is scant.

Local Resection

Peyman and coworkers developed a technique of local sclerochorioretinal resection for choroidal melanomas.[321-325] After a series of photocoagulation treatments around the tumor to create a firm chorioretinal adhesion or an area of bare sclera, the tumor is surgically removed, along with the adjacent sclera and retina. The defect is replaced by a scleral graft. Peyman and coworkers suggested that surgical candidates should have the following:

1. No evidence of metastatic disease
2. The ability to tolerate general anesthesia
3. A tumor base no larger than 12 mm and tumor location at least three disk diameters from the optic disk
4. Exudative retinal detachment no larger than one third of the fundus
5. Clear media

After local resection, one third of the eyes needed enucleation because of complications, including vitreous hemorrhage and retinal detachment.[11-35] Shields and associates advocate the use of partial lamellar sclerouvectomy in selected cases.[326] Most authors report that patients treated by local resection are also amenable to radiation therapy and that early visual loss is far more frequent after surgical resection.[129,130,205,327] The risk of leaving viable tumor cells in the eye after resection is a matter of concern. For these reasons, this technique has not been adopted widely.

Iridocyclectomy has proved useful in the treatment of ciliary body melanomas in several series.[129,130,328,329] In the series of Forrest and associates of 107 iridocyclectomies for ciliary body melanoma, 6% of the patients had subsequent enucleation; most problems related to surgical management or to the tumor area occurred within 4 years of surgery.[328] Foulds and Damato,

who promoted this method, have employed the approach for many years with good results.[329,330] In contrast to resection of choroidal melanomas, iridocyclectomy is widely accepted for the treatment of ciliary body melanomas.[329,330]

Enucleation

In the case of patients with a healthy second eye, enucleation is advised if the tumor shows evidence of rapid progression and invasion of the optic nerve or extraocular extension is suspected.[119,130,205] Other complications, including loss of central vision, failure of previous conservative treatment, and the patient's desires, may make enucleation the treatment of choice.

TREATMENT OF LARGE MELANOMAS OF THE CHOROID AND CILIARY BODY

Most clinicians agree that it would be inadvisable to treat cases of large melanoma by methods other than enucleation.[125,130,331] Possible exceptions include patients with the tumor occurring in their only seeing eye, occasional patients in whom vision can be salvaged by irradiation, and patients who refuse enucleation.[337] Abramson and Ellsworth recommend local irradiation in these latter difficult cases.[331,332]

Some authors recommend external irradiation before enucleation,[333-338] but convincing evidence for the usefulness of this therapy is still lacking.[338-340] This method is being evaluated currently in the COMS.[173,341]

Zimmerman and associates have suggested that when enucleation is carried out, the "no-touch" technique of Fraunfelder should be considered.[3,342] This method was designed to minimize the possibility of seeding of tumor cells into the blood vessels during enucleation. The authors claim that this technique avoids intraocular pressure elevations higher than 15 mm before complete freezing occurs around the tumor. Subsequently, cryotherapy prevents the flow of fluid and blood to or from the tumor before the manipulation necessary for enucleation. Although most surgeons do not use the no-touch technique, it is increasingly recognized that enucleation should be carried out by a surgeon skilled and experienced in the procedure and that surgery should be done with a minimum of unnecessary manipulation.[127-130,205,343]

TREATMENT OF MEDIUM-SIZED MELANOMAS OF THE CHOROID AND CILIARY BODY

Treatment of medium-sized tumors is the subject of current controversy. Although general agreement exists that observation of small melanomas carries little risk and that large melanomas should be enucleated, there is less consensus regarding medium-sized melanomas. Good results with radiation therapy using various modalities have been reported.[119,130,176,343-350] This method is unequivocally advocated in patients in whom the tumor occurs in their only seeing eye, in patients whose eyes retain useful vision, and in patients who refuse enucleation. However, in most instances, both treatment options remain possible, and personal choice is often the deciding factor. For these reasons, a nationwide, prospective, randomized comparison of radiation versus enucleation has been undertaken under the auspices of the National

Eye Institute "in order to demonstrate that either radiation or enucleation offers a better chance for survival, or that there is no difference in survival."[173,341] In this multicenter study, tumors 2.5 to 10 mm in height and no more than 16-mm basal diameter are randomized. Immunotherapy and chemotherapy have not been established as significantly useful modalities for primary or adjuvant treatment of medium-sized melanomas of the choroid or ciliary body.[351–354] However, in view of the likelihood of subclinical metastases being present at the time of diagnosis, a systemic treatment should be tested when an effective agent becomes available.

TREATMENT OF TUMORS WITH EXTRASCLERAL EXTENSION

Patients with extrascleral extension of an intraocular tumor have a poor prognosis.[139] Affeldt and coworkers reported that two thirds of 60 patients followed up after enucleation for uveal melanoma with extrascleral extension eventually died from metastatic disease.[355] Attempts should be made to detect extraocular extension preoperatively with ultrasound, CT, and MRI. At the time of surgery, the episcleral surface should be inspected carefully. These visual and imaging findings should be confirmed subsequently by frozen-section study.[3] Excision of adjacent Tenon's capsule and orbital tissue is then performed. The indications for primary or secondary exenteration remain controversial, because no clear evidence exists for an increase in life expectancy after exenteration compared with enucleation. Of 15 patients who underwent exenteration in the series reported by Starr and Zimmerman, only 1 survived longer than 13 months.[139] Affeldt and colleagues concluded that exenteration within 2 months after enucleation is beneficial.[355] In 1977, Shammas and Blodi initially reported good results of exenteration, particularly if the operation was performed promptly after recognition of residual tumor in the orbit.[138] However, a subsequent study of long-term results at the same institution showed little improvement in survival.[356] The usefulness of exenteration remains disputed.[356–359] Hykin and coworkers advocate postenucleation orbital radiation therapy in patients with extrascleral extension.[360]

METASTATIC DISEASE

Metastatic disease is observed in about 2% of patients at the time of diagnosis.[14,147,148,361] Fournier and coworkers[362] and Gronemeyer and coworkers[363] have suggested that local resection of solitary hepatic metastases in patients with uveal melanoma may be an effective palliative treatment and possibly lead to longer survival. Other authors have reported prolonged periods of remission after hepatic artery embolization.[366] Experimental studies using immunologic approaches are in progress,[365] but these tentative treatments are still anecdotal. Currently, metastatic melanoma is incurable and usually is treated palliatively with chemotherapy and radiation therapy (see Chap. 46).[205,366–369]

TREATMENT OF IRIS MELANOMA

In the past 30 years, gradual recognition of the better prognosis of iris melanoma has led to a conservative approach.

Every effort is made to avoid enucleation in most cases.[128–130,182,189,190] Different options are possible, according to the clinical situation.

OBSERVATION

If the following factors are present, surgical intervention is not necessary:

1. There is no clinical evidence that the lesion is progressing.
2. There is a lack of pronounced neovascularization.
3. The lesion is not producing any visual disturbances.
4. No significant complications, such as hemorrhage into the anterior chamber, trabecular involvement, secondary glaucoma, and an obvious extension outside the eye, are evident.
5. The lesion arises in the only seeing eye.
6. The lesion is situated near the pupil.

CONSERVATION EXCISION

The anecdotal nature of reports on photocoagulation of iris melanomas does not allow definitive conclusions to be drawn.[370,371] Surgery should be considered if there is evidence of rapid tumor growth, the tumor interferes with vision, and the tumor induces noncontrollable secondary glaucoma.[129,130,271,372]

In 1958, Reese pointed out that iris melanoma, with or without ciliary body involvement, seldom metastasizes or spreads by seeding.[128] Iris melanomas are capable of local extension and infiltration. Subsequently, interest developed in the use of iridectomy, iridocyclectomy, and corneoscleroiridocyclectomy, with grafting, as alternatives to enucleation.[128–130] Although some authors advocate diagnostic needle biopsy of the iris lesion,[182,203,372] this procedure is usually not performed because of the risk of tumor dissemination.

The object of excisional iridectomy is to remove the tumor entirely without allowing tumor cells to disseminate in the eye or in the incision. The procedure is similar to that described by Reese, in which a limbal incision is made that is large enough to allow removal of the lesion by basal iridectomy under direct observation.[128] Iridectomy of peripheral tumors should be performed before the lesion extends to the trabecular meshwork. Some authors emphasize the local and systemic risks of delaying the removal of a growing tumor.[271,373] If the trabecular meshwork is involved in the quadrant of the tumor, inducing secondary glaucoma, iridotrabeculectomy is indicated. When the iris tumor extends to the ciliary body, iridocyclectomy must be considered, as was advocated by Raubitschek[376] and Verhoeff[375] many years ago and introduced into clinical practice through the efforts of Muller and associates[376] and Stallard.[377,378] A basic technique for resecting the iris tumor together with involved ciliary body has been reported by Jones.[379] Many patients requiring more extensive surgery than iridectomy for iris tumor removal also require an operation more extensive than iridocyclectomy. Examples are patients in whom the tumor not only invades the ciliary body but also fills the chamber angle and is adjacent to the tissue in the angle or to the cornea itself. In such cases, the surgeon should consider corneoscleroiridocyclectomy with or without a corneoscleral graft.[129,130,329] Surgical complications include intraocular hemorrhage, hypotony, subluxation of the lens, cataract, late detachment of the retina, corneal edema, macular edema, and vitreous loss. If the excision is incomplete, tumor may recur. Therefore, the finding of spindle B cells should lead to frequent and extremely thorough follow-up examinations. If similar numbers of epithelioid cells are disclosed histopathologically, their lack of cohesiveness argues toward enucleation in view of a high risk for recurrence and exteriorization.[182]

ENUCLEATION

Enucleation for an iris melanoma is not exceptional but must be considered in individual cases if the following conditions exist:

1. The melanoma is clearly growing and involves more than half the iris and anterior chamber angle.
2. The tumor, growing in a blind eye, is too bulky to be removed by excision.
3. There is a secondary glaucoma refractory to medical treatment, particularly after vision is lost.
4. Histopathologic features point toward a high risk for recurrence or exteriorization, or both.
5. Extraocular extension is present.
6. The tumor has recurred after previous iridectomy or iridocyclectomy and is judged unsuitable for further treatment.

In the case of extraocular spread or metastatic disease, or both, the treatment is the same as for advanced choroidal or ciliary body melanomas.

REFERENCES

1. Rawles ME. Origin of pigment cells from neural crest in mouse embryos. Physiol Zool 1947;20:248–266.
2. Zimmerman LE. Melanocytes, melanocytic nevi, and melanocytomas. Invest Ophthalmol Vis Sci 1965;4:11–41.
3. Zimmerman LE. Malignant melanoma of the uveal tract. In: Spencer WH, ed. Ophthalmic pathology. Vol 3. Philadelphia: WB Saunders, 1986:2072–2139.
4. Green WR. The uvea. In: Spencer WH, ed. Ophthalmic pathology. Vol 3. Philadelphia: WB Saunders, 1986:1352–2072.
5. Scotto, J, Fraumeni JF, Lee JAH. Melanomas of the eye and other noncutaneous sites. JNCI 1976;56:489–491.
6. Young JL, Percy CL, Asire AJ, et al. Cancer incidence and mortality in the United States, 1973–1977. Cancer Inst Monogr 1981;57:1–187.
7. Egan KM, Seddon JM, Gradoudas ES, et al. Uveal melanoma in New England: Profile of cases diagnosed in 1984 to 1985. Invest Ophthalmol Vis Sci 1987;28(Suppl):144.
8. Abrahamson M. Malignant melanoma of the choroid and the ciliary body, 1956–1975. Acta Ophthalmol (Copenh) 1982;61:600–610.
9. Gislason I, Magnussen G, Tulinius H. Malignant melanoma of the uvea in Iceland, 1955–1979. Acta Ophthalmol (Copenh) 1985;63:385–394.
10. Cutler SJ, Young JL, eds. Third National Cancer Survey: Incidence data. NCI Monogr 1975;41:1–454.
11. Chang JC. Personal communication. St. Louis, Missouri Department of Social Services, Division of Health, October 4, 1983.
12. Kuo PK, Puliafito CA, Wang KM, et al. Uveal melanoma in China. Int Ophthalmol Clin 1982;22:57–71.
13. Teikari JM, Rairio I. Incidence of choroidal melanoma in Finland in the years 1973–1980. Acta Opthlamol (Copenh) 1985;63:661–665.
14. Graham BJ, Duane TD. Meetings, conferences, symposia: Report of the Ocular Melanoma Task Force. Am J Ophthalmol 1981;90:728–733.
15. Haukulin T, Teppo L, Saxen F. Cancer of the eye: A review of trends and differentials. World Health Stat Q 1978;31:143–158.
16. Jensen QA, Prause JU. Malignant melanomas of the human uvea in Denmark: Incidence and a 25-year follow-up of cases diagnosed between 1943 and 1952, In: Lommatzsch PK, Blodi FC, eds. Intraocular tumors. Berlin: Springer-Verlag, 1983:85–92.
17. Strickland D, Lee JHA. Melanomas of the eye: Stability of rates. Am J Epidemiol 1981;113:700–702.
18. Swerdlow AJ. Epidemiology of eye cancer in adults in England and Wales, 1962–1977. Am J Epidemiol 1983;118:294–300.
19. Houghton, A, Flannery J, Viola MV. Malignant melanoma in Connecticut and Denmark. Int J Cancer 1980;25:95–104.
20. Rosenbaum PS, Boniuk M, Font RL. Diffuse uveal melanoma in a 5-year-old child. Am J Ophthalmol 1988;106:601–6060.
21. Barr CC, McLean IW, Zimmerman LE. Uveal melanoma in children and adolescents. Arch Ophthalmol 1981;95:2133–2134.
22. Shields CL, Shields JA, Milite J, et al. Uveal melanoma in teenagers and children. Ophthalmology 1991;98:1662–1666.
23. Jensen OA. Malignant melanoma of the uvea in Denmark, 1943–1952: A clinical, histopathological and prognostic study. Acta Ophthalmol 1963;75(Suppl):1–200.
24. Apt L. Uveal melanomas in children and adolescents. Int Ophthalmol Clin 1962;2:403–410.
25. Fledelius H, Land A. Malignant melanoma of the choroid in an 11-month-old infant. Acta Ophthalmol 1975;53:1 160–166.
26. Jones ST. Choroidal malignant melanoma in a child. Br J Ophthalmol 1967;51:489–491.
27. Verdauger J. Prepubertal and pubertal melanomas in ophthalmology. Am J Ophthalmol 1965;60:1002–1011.
28. Raivo I. Uveal melanoma in Finland: An epidemiological, clinical, histological and prognostic study. Acta Ophthalmol 1977;133(Suppl):3–64.
29. Egan KM, Seddon JM, Glynn RJ, et al. Epidemiologic aspects of uveal melanoma. Surv Ophthalmol 1988;32:239–251.
30. Paul EV, Parnell BL, Fraker M. Prognosis of malignant melanomas of the choroid and ciliary body. Int Ophthalmol Clin 1968;5:387–402.
31. Malik MOA, El Sheikh EH. Tumors of the ey and adnexa in the Sudan. Cancer 1979;44:293–303.
32. Miller B, Abraham C, Cole CG, et al. Ocular malignant melanoma in South African blacks. Br J Ophthalmol 1981;65:720–722.
33. Swerlow AJ. Epidemiology of melanoma of the ey in the Oxford region, 1952–78. Br J Cancer 1983;47:311–313.
34. Albert DM, Scheie HG. Nevus of Ota with malignant melanoma of the choroid. Arch Ophthalmol 1963;69:774–777.
35. Body FC. Ocular melanocytes and melanoma. Am J Ophthalmol 1975;80:389.
36. Dutton JJ, Anderson RL, Schelper RL, et al. Orbital malignant melanoma and oculodermal melanocytes: Report of two cases and review of the literature. Ophthalmology 1984;91:946–507.
37. Gonder JR, Shields JA, Albert DM, et al. Uveal malignant melanoma associated with ocular and oculodermal melanocytosis. Ophthalmology 1982;89:953–960.
38. Yanoff M, Zimmerman LE. Histogenesis of malignant melanomas of the uvea: III. The relationship of congenital ocular melanocytosis and neurofibromatosis to uveal melanomas. Arch Ophthalmol 1967;77:331–336.
39. Gartner S. Malignant melanoma of the choroid in von Recklinghausen's disease. Am J Ophthalmol 1940;23:73–78.
40. Yanoff M, Zimmerman LE. Histogenesis of malignant melanomas of the uvea: II. Relationship of uveal nevi to the malignant melanomas. Cancer 1967;20:497–507.
41. Volker HE, Naumann GO. Multicentric primary malignant melanomas of the choroid: Two separate malignant melanomas of the choroid and two uveal nevi in one eye. Br J Ophthalmol 1978;62:408–413.
42. Sahel JA, Albert DM. Choroidal nevi. In: Ryan SJ, ed: Retina. Vol 1. St Louis: CV Mosby, 1989:625–637.
43. Albert DM, Lahav M, Packer S, et al. Histogenesis of malignant melanomas of the uvea: Occurrence of nevus-like structures in experimental choroidal tumors. Arch Ophthalmol 1974;92:318–323.
44. Gass JDM. Stereoscopic atlas of macular diseases. St Louis: CV Mosby, 1987:182–195.
45. Margo CE, Paven PR, Gendelman D, et al. Bilateral melanocyte uveal tumors associated with systemic non-ocular malignancy: Malignant melanomas or benign paraneoplastic syndrome. Retina 1987;7:137–141.
46. Walker JP, Weiter JJ, Albert, DM, et al. Uveal malignant melanoma in three generations of the same family. Am J Ophthalmol 1979;88:723–726.
47. Lynch H, Anderson D, Krush A. Heredity and intraocular malignant melanoma: Study of two families and review of 45 cases. Cancer 1968;21:119–125.
48. Reese AB. Tumors of the eye. 3rd ed. Hagerstown, MD: Harper & Row, 1976:177–178.
49. Reese AB. Association of uveal nevi with skin nevi. Arch Ophthalmol 1952;48:271–275.
50. Albert DM, Chang MA, Lamping KA, et al. The dysplastic nevus syndrome: A pedigree with primary malignant melanomas of the choroid and skin. Ophthalmology 1985;92:1728–1734.
51. Albert DM, Searl SS, Forget B, et al. Uveal findings in patients with cutaneous melanoma. Am J Ophthalmol 1987;95:474–479.
52. Rodriquez-Sains RS. Ocular findings in patients with dysplastic nevus syndrome. Ophthalmology 1986;93:661–665.
53. Taylor MR, Guerry D IV, Dondl EE, et al. Lack of association between intraocular melanoma and cutaneous dysplastic nevi. Am J Ophthalmol 1984;98:478–482.
54. Turner BJ, Statkowski RM, Ausberger JJ, et al. Other cancers in uveal melanoma patients and their families. Am J Ophthalmol 1989;107:601–608.
55. Lischko AM, Seddon JM, Gragoudas ES, et al. Evaluation of prior primary malignancy as a determinant of uveal melanoma: A case-control study. Ophthalmology 1989;96:1716–1721.
56. Holly EA, Ashton DA, Ahn DK, et al. No excess prior cancer in patients with uveal melanoma. Ophthalmology 1991;98:608–611.

57. Mukai S, Dryja TP. Loss of alleles at polymorphic loci on chromosome 2 in uveal melanoma. Cancer Genet Cytogenet 1986;22:45–53.

58. Albert DM. The association of viruses with uveal melanoma. Trans Am Ophthalmol Soc 1980;77:367–421.

59. Albert DM, Shadduck JA, Lin HS, et al. Animal models for the study of uveal melanomas. Int Ophthalmol Clin 1980;20:143–160.

60. Albert DM. Need for animal models of human diseases of the eye. Am J Pathol 1980;101:177–185.

61. Albert DM. Ocular melanoma: A challenge to visual science. Invest Ophthalmol Vis Sci 1982;23:550–580.

62. Albert DM, Puliafito CA, Fulton AB, et al. Increased incidence of choroidal malignant melanoma occurring in a single population of chemical workers. Am J Ophthalmol 1980;89:323–337.

63. Keeny AH, Waddell WJ, Perraut TC. Carcinogenesis and nicotine in malignant melanoma of the choroid. Trans Am Ophthalmol Soc 1987;80:131–142.

64. Albert DM, Gonder JR, Papale J, et al. Induction of ocular neoplasms in Fischer rats by introcular injection of nickle subsulfide. Invest Ophthalmol Vis Sci 1982;22:768–782.

65. Evgenyeva TP. Pigmented tumors in rats induced by introduction of platinum and cellophane films into the chamber of the eye. Buill Eksp Biol Med (Moscow) 1972;74:76–77.

66. Patz A, Wulff LB, Rogers SW. Experimental production of ocular tumors. Am J Ophthalmol 1959;48:98–111.

67. Benson WR. Intraocular tumor after ethionine and N-2-fluorenyl-acetamide. Arch Pathol 1962;73:404–406.

68. Taylor GH, Dougherty TF, Mays CW, et al. Radium-induced eye melanomas in dogs. Radiat Res 1972;51:361–373.

69. Albert DM, Puliafito CA, Haluska FG, et al. Induction of ocular neoplasms in Wistar rats by N-methyl-N-nitrosourea. Exp Eye Res 1986;42:83–86.

70. Folberg R, Baron J, Reeves RD, et al. Animal model of conjunctival primary acquired melanomas. Ophthalmology 1989;96:1006–1013.

71. Van Rens GH, DeJohn P, Demols E, et al. Uveal malignant melanoma and levodopa therapy in Parkinson's disease. Ophthalmology 1982;89:1464–1466.

72. Hartge P, Tucker MA, Shields JA, et al. Case-control study of female hormones and eye melanoma. Cancer Res 1989;49:4622–2625.

73. Seddon JM, MacLaughlin DT, Albert DM, et al. Uveal melanomas presenting during pregnancy and the investigation of estrogen receptors in melanomas. Br J Ophthalmol 1982;66:695–704.

74. Shields CL, Shields JA, Eagle RC Jr, et al. Uveal melanoma and pregnancy. Ophthalmology 1991;98:1667–1673.

75. Tucker MA, Shields JA, Hartge P, et al. Sunlight exposure as risk factor for malignant melanoma. N Engl J Med 1985;313:789–792.

76. Seddon JM, Gragoudas ES, Glynn RJ, et al. Host factors, UV radiation, and risk of uveal melanoma: A case control study. Arch Ophthalmol 1990;108:1274–1280.

77. Holly EA, Aston DA, Char DH, et al. Uveal melanoma in relation to ultraviolet light exposure and host factors. Cancer Res 1990;50:5773–5777.

78. Edwood JM, Lee JA, Walter SD, et al. Relationship of melanoma and other skin cancer mortality to latitude and ultraviolet radiation in the United States and Canada. Int J Epidemiol 1972;3:325–332.

79. Kliman GH, Augsburger JJ, Shields JA. Association between iris color and iris melanocytic lesions. Am J Ophthalmol 1985;100:547–548.

80. Kan-Mitchell J, Rao N, Albert DM, et al. S-100 immunopheotypes of uveal melanomas. Invest Ophthalmol Vis Sci 1990;31:1492–1496.

81. Beckenkamp G, Schafer HJ, Von Domarus D. Immunocytochemical parameters in ocular malignant melanomas. Eur J Cancer Clin Oncol 1988;24:542–645.

82. Van Der Pol JP, Jager MJ, DeWolff-Rouendaal D, et al. Heterogeneous expression of melanoma-associated antigens in uveal melanomas.

83. Bomanji J, Garner A, Prasad J, et al. Characterization of ocular melanoma with cutaneous melanoma antibodies. Br J Ophthalmol 1987;71:647–650.

84. Natali PG, Bigotti A, Necotra MR, et al. Analysis of the antigenic profile of uveal melanoma lesions with anti-cutaneous melanoma-associated antigen and anti-HLA monoclonal antibodies. Cancer Res 1989;49:1269–1274.

85. Damato BE, Campbell AM, McGuire BJ, et al. Monoclonal antibodies to uveal melanoma. Eye 1987;1:686–690.

86. Callender GR. Malignant melanotic tumors of the eye: A study of histologic types in 111 cases. Trans Am Acad Ophthalmol Otolaryngol 1931;36:131–142.

87. Zimmerman LE, Sobin LH. International histological classification of tumors: Histological typing of tumors of the eye and its adnexa. No. 24. Geneva: World Health Organization, 1980.

88. McLean IW, Foster WD, Zimmerman LE, et al. Modification of Callender's classification of uveal melanoma at the Armed Forces Institute of Pathology. Am J Ophthalmol 1983;96:502–509.

89. McLean IW, Zimmerman LE, Evans RM. Reappraisal of Callender's spindle A type of malignant melanoma of the choroid and ciliary body. Am J Ophthalmol 1978;86:557–564.

90. McLean IW, Foster MD, Zimmerman LE. Uveal melanoma: Location, size, cell type and enucleation as risk factors in metastasis. Hum Pathol 1981;13:123–132.

91. Gass JDM. Problems in the differential diagnosis of choroidal nevi and malignant melanomas. Am J Ophthalmol 1977;83:299–323.

92. Gamel JW, McLean IW. Quantitative analysis of the Callender classification of uveal melanoma cells. Arch Ophthalmol 1977;95:686–691.

93. Collaborative Ocular Melanoma Study manual of procedures. National Technical Information Service. NTIS PB90-115536. Springfield, VA, 1989.

94. Gamel JW, McLean IW. Modern developmenst in histopathologic assessment of uveal melanomas. Ophthalmology 1984;91:679–684.

95. Gamel JW, McLean IW, Greckey RA, et al. Objective assessment of the malignant potential of intraocular melanomas with standard microslides stained with hematoxylin-eosin. Hum Pathol 1985;16:689–692.

96. Donoso LA, Augsburger JJ, Shields JA, et al. Metastatic uveal melanoma: Correlation between survival time and cytomorphology of primary tumors. Arch Ophthalmol 1986;104:76–82.

97. Wilder HC, Callender GR. Malignant melanoma of the choroid: Further studies on prognosis by histologic type and fiber content. Am J Ophthalmol 1939;22:851–855.

98. Seddon JM, Polivogianis L, Hsieh CC, et al. Death from uveal melanoma: Number of epithelioid cells and inverse SD of nucleolar areas as prognostic factors. Arch Ophthalmol 1987;105:801–806.

99. McCurdy JB, Gamel JW, McLean IW. A simple, efficient, and reproducible method for determining the malignant potential of uveal melanoma. Invest Ophthalmol Vis Sci 1991;32(ARVO Suppl):1197.

100. Seddon JM, Albert DM, Lavin PT, et al. A prognostic factor study of disease-free interval and survival following enucleation for uveal melanoma. Arch Ophthalmol 1983;101:1894–1899.

101. Lavin PT, Albert DM, Seddon JM, et al. A deficit survival analysis to assess the history of uveal melanoma. J Clin Dis 1984;37:481–487.

102. McLean IW, Foster WD, Zimmerman LE. Prognostic factors in small malignant melanomas of the choroid and ciliary body. Arch Ophthalmol 1977;95:48–58.

103. Bardenstein DS, Char DH, Kaleta-Michaels S, et al. Ki-67 and bromodeoxyuridine labelling of human choroidal melanoma cells. Curr Eye Res 1991;10:479–484.

104. Char DH. DNA cell cycle studies in uveal melanoma. Trans Am Ophthalmol Soc 1989;86:561–580.

105. Rennie IG, Ress RC, Parsons MA, et al. Estimation of DNA content in uveal melanomas by flow cytometry. Eye 1989;3:611–617.

106. Chen TC, Char DH, Waldman F, et al. Flow cytometry measurement of nuclear RNA content in uveal melanoma. Ophthalmic Res 1990;22:187–193.

107. McLean IW, Gamel JW. Prediction of metastasis of uveal melanoma: Comparison of spectrophotometric determination of DNA. Invest Ophthalmol Vis Sci 1988;29:507–511.

108. Marcus DM, Minkovitz JB, Wardwell SD, et al. The value of nucleolar organizer regions in uveal melanoma. Am J Ophthalmol 1990;110:527–534.

109. Jensen OA. Malignant melanomas of the human uvea: Recent follow-up of cases in Denmark, 1943–1952. Acta Ophthalmol 1970;46:1113–1128.

110. Jensen OA. Malignant melanomas of the human uvea: 25-year follow-up of cases in Denmark, 1943–1952. Acta Ophthalmol 1982;60:161–182.

111. Durie FH, Campbell AM, Lee WR, et al. Analysis of lymphocytic infiltration in uveal melanoma. Invest Ophthalmol Vis Sci 1990;31:2106–2110.

112. Nitta R, Oksenberg JR, Rao NA, et al. Predominant expression of T cell receptor V alpha 7 in tumor infiltrating lymphocytes of uveal melanoma. Science 1990;248:671–674.

113. Knisely T, Niederkorn JY. Immunologic evaluation of spontaneous regression of an intraocular murine melanoma. Invest Ophthalmol Vis Sci 1990;31:247–257.

114. Richardson JT, Burns RP, Misfeldt ML. Association of uveal melanocyte destruction in melanoma-bearing swine with large granular lymphocyte cells. Invest Ophthalmol Vis Sci 1989;30:2455–2460.

115. Niederkorn JY, Benson JL. Differential expression of tumor-specific cytotoxic T lymphocyte activity and delayed type hypersensitivity in the anterior chamber of the eye. Invest Ophthalmol Vis Sci 1991;32(ARVO Suppl):937.

116. Curtin VT, Cavender JC. Natural course of selected malignant melanomas of the choroid and ciliary body. Mod Prob Ophthalmol 1974;12:523–527.

117. McLean IW, Foster MD, Zimmerman LE, et al. Inferred natural history of uveal melanoma. Invest Ophthalmol Vis Sci 1980;19:760–770.

118. Char DH, Heilborn DL, Juster RR, et al. Choroidal melanoma growth patterns. Br J Ophthalmol 1983;67:575–578.

119. Gass JDM. Comparison of uveal melanoma growth rates with mitotic index mortality. Arch Ophthalmol 1985;103:924–931.

120. Char DH, Hogan MJ. Management of small elevated pigmented choroidal lesions. Br J Ophthalmol 1977;61:54–58.

121. Curtin VT. Choroidal and ciliary body malignant melanomas. Mod Prob Ophthalmol 1979;20:115–120.

122. Friberg TR, Finchberg E, McQuaig S. Extremely rapid growth of a primary choroidal melanoma. Arch Ophthalmol 1983;11:1376–1377.

123. Sahel JA, Pesavento R, Frederick AR Jr, et al. Uveal melanoma arising de novo over a 16-month period. Arch Ophthalmol 1988;106:381–385.

124. Manschot WA, van Peperzeel HA. Choroidal melanoma: Enucleation or observation? A new approach. Arch Ophthalmol 1980;98:71–77.

125. Augsburger JJ, Gonder JR, Amsel J, et al. Growth rates and doubling time of posterior uveal melanomas. Ophthalmology 1984;91:1709–1715.

126. Lambert JR, Char DH, Howes E Jr, et al. Spontaneous regression of a choroidal melanoma. Arch Ophthalmol 1986;104:732–734.

127. Brini A, Dhermy P, Sahel J. Oncology of the eye and adnexa: Atlas of clinical pathology. In: Monographs in Ophthalmology Series. Vol. 13. Dordrecht: Kluwer, 1990:143.

128. Reese AB. Tumors of the eye. 3rd ed. Hagerstown, MD: Harper & Row, 1976:174–262.

129. Shields JA. Diagnosis and management of intraocular tumors. St Louis: CV Mosby, 1983:75–254.

130. Char DH. Clinical ocular oncology. New York: Churhill Livingstone, 1989:91–166.

131. Font RL, Zimmerman LE, Armaly MF. The nature of the orange pigment over a

choroidal melanoma: Histochemical and electron microscopic observation. Arch Ophthalmol 1974;91:359–365.

132. Dunn WJ, Lambert HM, Kincaid MC, et al. Choroidal melanoma with early vitreous seeding. Retina 1988;8:155–192.

133. Yanoff M. Glaucoma mechanism in ocular malignant melanomas. Am J Ophthalmol 1970;70:898–904.

134. El Baba F, Hagler WS, De la Cruz A, et al. Choroidal melanoma with pigment dispersion into the vitreous and melanomalytic glaucoma. Ophthalmology 1988;956:370–376.

135. Shammas HF, Blodi FC. Prognostic factors in choroidal and ciliary body melanomas. Arch Ophthalmol 1977;95:63–69.

136. Font RL, Spaulding AG, Zimmerman LE. Diffuse malignant melanoma of the uveal tract: A clinicopathologic report of 56 cases. Trans Am Acad Ophthalmol Otolaryngol 1968;72:877–894.

137. Duffin RM, Straatsma BR, Foos RY, et al. Small malignant melanoma of the choroid with extraocular extension. Arch Ophthalmol 1981;99:1027–1020.

138. Shammas HF, Blodi FC. Orbital extension of choroidal and ciliary body melanomas. Arch Ophthalmol 1977;93:2002–2005.

139. Starr HJ, Zimmerman LE. Extrascleral extension and orbital recurrence of a malignant melanoma of the choroid and ciliary body. Int Ophthalmol Cent V 1962;2:369–385.

140. Affeldt JC, Minckler DS, Azen SP, et al. Prognosis in uveal melanoma with extrascleral extension. Arch Ophthalmol 1980;98:1975–1979.

141. Pach JM, Robertson DM, Taney BS, et al. Prognostic factors in choroidal and ciliary body melanomas with extrascleral extension. Am J Ophthalmol 1988;101:325–331.

142. Packard RBS. Pattern of mortality in choroidal malignant melanoma. Br J Ophthalmol 1980;64:565–573.

143. Shammas HF, Blodi FC. Peripapillary choroidal melanomas: Extension along the optic nerve and its sheaths. Arch Ophthalmol 1978;96:440–444.

144. Chess J, Albert DM, Bellows AR, et al. Uveal melanoma: Case report of extension through the optic nerve to the surgical margin in the orbital apex. Br J Ophthalmol 1984;68:272–275.

145. Ruiz RS. Early treatment in malignant melanomas of the choroid. In: Brockhurst RJ, Boruchoff SA, Hutchinson BT, et al, eds. Controversy in ophthalmology. Philadelphia: WB Saunders, 1977:604–610.

146. Lock-Anderson J, Partoft S, Jensen MG. Patterns of the first lymph node metastases in patients with cutaneous malignant melanoma of axial localization. Cancer [Abstract] 1988;62:9.

147. Pack JM, Robertson DM. Matastases from untreated uveal melanomas. Arch Ophthalmol 1986;104:1624–1625.

148. Wagoner MD, Albert DM. The incidence of metastases from untreated ciliary body and choroidal melanoma. Arch Ophthalmol 1982;100:939–940.

149. Fornabio DM, Alterman AL, Stackpole CW. Matastatic dissemination of B16 melanoma: Evidence that metastases can result from non-specific trapping of disseminated cells. Invasion Metastasis 1988;8:1–16.

150. Albelda SM, Mette SP, Elder DE, et al. Integrin distribution in malignant melanoma: Association of the B3 subunit with tumor progression. Cancer Res 1990;50:6757–6764.

151. Kath R, Jambrosio J, Holland L, et al. Development of invasive and growth factor independent cell variants from primary melanoma. Cancer Res 1991;51:4853–4858.

152. Hart IR, Brich M. Cell adhesion receptors in melanoma progression and metastasis: The biology of melanoma. In: The 35th Annual Clinical Conference and 24th Annual Special Pathology Program: Advances in the biology and clinical management of melanoma. Houston, November 20–23, 1991:8.

153. Raz A. Tumor cell migration and the metastatic cascade: The biology of melanoma. In: The 35th Annual Clinical Conference and 24th Annual Special Pathology Program: Advances in the biology and clinical management of melanoma. Houston, November 20–23, 1991:9–10.

154. Price JE, Zhang RD. Melanoma brain metastasis. The biology of melanoma. In: The 35th Annual Clinical Conference and 24th Annual Special Pathology Program: Advances in the biology and clinical management of melanoma. Houston, November 20–23, 1991:10, 11.

155. Fidler IJ, Nicholson CJ. Organ selectiveity for implantation survival and growth of B16 melanoma. JNCI 1976;57:1199–1201.

156. Donoso LA, Nagy RM, McFall RC, et al. Metastatic choroidal melanoma: Hepatic binding protein reactivity toward a liver metastasizing clone. Arch Ophthalmol 1983;101:787–790.

157. Zimmerman LE. Gamma-glutamyl transpeptidase in the prognosis of patients with uveal melanomas. Am J Ophthalmol 1983;96:409–411.

158. Pascal SG, Saulenas AM, Fourner GA, et al. An investigation into the association between liver damage and metastatic uveal melanoma. Am J Ophthalmol 1985;100:448–453.

159. Gragoudas ES, Egan KM, Seddon JM, et al. Survival of patients with metastases from uveal melanoma. Ophthalmology 1991;98:383–390.

160. Zimmerman LE. Does enucleation of the eye containing a malignant melanoma prevent or accelerate the dissemination of tumor cells? Br J Ophthalmol 1978;62:420–425.

161. Fraunfelder FT, Boozman FW, Wilson RS, et al. No-touch technique for intraocular malignant melanomas. Arch Ophthalmol 1977;95:1616–1620.

162. Niederkorn JY, Streihlen JW. Intracamerally induced concommitant immunity: Mice harboring progressively growing intraocular tumors are immune to spontaneous metastases and secondary tumor challenge. J Immunol 1983;131:2587–2594.

163. Niederkorn JY. Enucleation-induced metastasis of intraocular melanoma in mice. Ophthalmology 1984;91:692–700.

164. Seigel D, Myers M, Ferris F III, et al. Survival rates after enucleation of eyes with malignant melanoma. Am J Ophthalmol 1979;87:761–765.

165. Kersten RC, Blodi FC. Prognosis of choroidal melanomas. Ophthal Forum 1983;1:21–27.

166. Davidorf FH. The melanoma controversy: A comparison of choroidal, cutaneous, and iris melanomas. Surv Ophthalmol 1981;25:373–377.

167. Albert DM. Towards resolving the ocular melanoma controversy. Arch Ophthalmol 1979;97:431–432.

168. Kidd MN, Cyness RW, Patterson CC, et al. Prognostic factors in malignant melanomas of the choroid: A retrospective survey of cases occurring in Northern Ireland between 1965 and 1980. Trans Ophthalmol Soc UK 1986;105:114–121.

169. Seddon JM, Egan KM, Gragoudas ES. Choroidal melanoma: Prognosis. In: Ryan SJ, ed. Retina. Vol 1. St Louis: CV Mosby, 1989:363–373.

170. Gamel JW, McLean IW, Greenberg RA. Interval by interval Cox model analysis of 3480 cases of intraocular melanoma shows a decline in the prognostic value of size and cell type over time after tumor excision. Cancer 1988;61:574–579.

171. Seddon JM, Gragnodas ES, Egan KM, et al. Relative survival rates after alternative therapy for uveal melanoma. Ophthalmology 1990;97:769–777.

172. Augsburger JJ, Gamel JW. Log normal distribution of uveal melanoma deaths following cobalt 60 plaque. Invest Ophthalmol Vis Sci 1991;32(ARVO Suppl):980.

173. COMS Group: Collaborative ocular melanoma study manual of procedures. National Technical Information Service, Springfield, VA, 1989. NTIS Accession No. PB90-115536.

174. Shields JA. Introduction to the management of posterior uveal melanomas. In: Ryan SJ, Ogden TE, Schchat AP, eds. Retina. Vol 1. St Louis: CV Mosby, 1989:683–686.

175. Augsburger JJ, Gamel JW, Shields JA, et al. Post-irradiation regression of choroidal melanomas as risk factor for death from metastatic disease. Ophthalmology 1987;94:1173–1177.

176. Abramson DH, Servodidio CA, McCormick B, et al. Changes in height of choroidal melanomas after plaque therapy. Br J Ophthalmol 1990;74:359–362.

177. Guthoff R, Hasse J, Von Domarus D, et al. Regression behavior of choroidal melanoma after radiotherapy: A new prognosis parameter. Klin Monatsbl Augenheilkd 1990;196:6–10.

178. Glynn RJ, Seddon JM, Gragoudas ES, et al. Evaluation of tumor regression and other prognostic factors for early and late metastasis after proton irradiation of uveal melanoma. Ophthalmology 1989;96:1566–1573.

179. Grange JD, Thacoor S, Bienvelez B, et al. Comparative study of the speed of tumor regression in 127 uveal melanomas treated with ^{106}Ru/^{106}Ru: Correlations between cytologic analysis, histopathology of enucleated eyes and tumor regression on one hand, vital prognosis on the other hand. Ophthalmologie 1990;4:221–224.

180. Manschot WA, Van Strik R. Choroidal melanoma: Analysis of published therapeutic results. Forschr Ophthalmol 1987;84:183–186.

181. Adams KS, Abramson DH, Ellsworth RM, et al. Cobalt plaques versus enucleation for uveal melanoma: Comparison of survival rates. Br J Ophthalmol 1988;72:494–497.

182. Jakobiec FA, Silbert G. Are most iris "melanomas" really nevi. Arch Ophthalmol 1981;99:2117–2132.

183. Holland G. Zur Klinik und Pathologie der Pigmenttumoren der Iris. Klin Monatsbl Augenheilkd 1967;150:359–370.

184. Rones B, Zimmerman LE. The prognosis of primary tumors of the iris treated by iridectomy. Arch Ophthalmol 1964;60:193–205.

185. Ashton D. Primary tumors of the iris. Br J Opththalmol 1964;48:65–68.

186. Heath P. Tumors of the iris: Classification and clinical follow-up. Trans Am Ophthalmol Soc 1964;62:51.

187. Duke JR, Dunn SN. Primary tumors of the iris. Arch Ophthalmol 1958;59:204.

188. Colt CA, Sahel JA, Seddon JM. unpublished data.

189. Reese AB. Tumors of the eye. 3rd ed. Hagerstown, MD: Harper & Row, 1976:229–262.

190. Cleasby GW. Malignant melanom of the iris. Arch Ophthalmol 1958;60:403–417.

191. Arentsen JJ, Green WR. Melanoma of the iris: Report of 72 cases treated surgically. Ophthalmic Surg 1975;6:23–32.

192. Green WR. The uveal tract. In: Spencer WH, ed. Ophthalmic pathology. Vol 3. Philadelphia: WB Saunders, 1986:1300–1342.

193. Zimmerman LE. Histologic considerations in the management of tumors of the iris and ciliary body. Ann Inst Barraquer 1972;10:27–56.

194. Kersten RC, Tse D, Andersen DR. Iris melanoma: Nevus or malignancy? Surv Ophthalmology 1985;29:423–433.

195. Shields JA. Melanocytic tumors of the iris. In: Shields JA, ed. Diagnosis and management of intraocular tumors. St Louis, CV Mosby, 1983:

196. Char DH. Anterior uveal tumors. In: Char DH, ed. Clinical ocular oncology. New York: Churchill Livingstone, 1989:

197. Apple D, Blodi FC. Pathologic observations and clinical approach to uveal melanomas. In: Nicholson D, ed. Ocular pathology update. New York: Masson Publishing, 1980:213–226.

198. Sunba MN, Rahj AHS, Morgan G. Tumors of the anterior uveal tract: I. Metastasizing malignant melanoma of the iris. Arch Ophthalmol 1980;98:82–85.

199. Deuble K, McCartney A. Nucleolar organizer regions in iris melanocytic tumors: An accurate predictor? Eye 1990;4:743–750.

199a. Marcus DM, Mawn LA, Egan KM, Albert DM. Nucleolar organizer regions in iris nevi and melanoma. Am J Ophthalmol 1992;114:202–207.

200. Geisse LJ, Robertson DM. Iris melanomas. Am J Ophthalmol 1985;99:638.

201. McGalliard JN, Johnston PB. A study of iris melanoma in Northern Ireland. Br J Opthalmol 1989;73:591.

202. Planten JT. An unnecessary mistake. Ophthalmologica 1970;160:369.

203. Grossniklaus HE, Brown RH, Stulting RD, et al. Iris melanoma seeding through a trabeculectomy site. Arch Ophthalmol 1990;1287:

204. Ferry AP. Lesions mistaken for malignant melanoma of the posterior uvea: A clinicopathologic analysis of 100 cases with ophthalmoscopically visible lesions. Arch Ophthalmol 1964;72:463–469.

205. Shields JA, Zimmerman LE. Lesions simulating malignant melanoma of the posterior uvea. Arch Ophthalmol 1973;89:466–471.

206. Zimmerman LE. Problems in the diagnosis of malignant melanomas of the choroid and ciliary body. Am J Ophthalmol 1973;75:917–929.

207. Chang M, Zimmerman LE, McLean IW. The persisting pseudomelanoma problem. Arch Ophthalmol 1984;102:726–727.

208. Robertson DM, Campbell RJ. Errors in the diagnosis of malignant melanoma of the choroid. Am J Opthalmol 1979;87:269–275.

209. Daviddorf FH, Letson AD, Weiss ET, et al. Incidence of misdiagnosed and unsuspected choroidal melanomas. Arch Ophthalmol 1983;101:410–412.

210. Shields JA, Augsberger JJ, Brown GC. The differential diagnosis of posterior uveal melanoma. Ophthalmology 1980;87:518–522.

211. Collaborative Melanoma Study Group. Accuracy of diagnosis of choroidal melanoma in the Collaborative Ocular Melanoma Study: COMS Report No. 1. Arch Ophthalmol 1990;108:1268–1273.

212. Donoso LA, Shields JA, Nagy RM. Epibulbar lesions simulating extraocular extension of uveal melanoma. Am J Ophthalmol 1982;14:1120–1123.

213. Flindall RJ, France SM. Visual field studies of benign choroidal melanoma. Arch Ophthalmol 1969;81:41–44.

214. Augsburger JJ, Schroeder RP, Territo C, et al. Clinical parameters predictive of enlargement of melanocytic choroidal lesions. Br J Ophthalmol 1989;73:911–917.

215. Shields JA, Shields CL, Donoso LA. Management of posterior melanoma. Surv Ophthalmol 1991;36:161–195.

216. Augsburger JJ, Golden MI, Shields JA. Fluorescein angiography of choroidal malignant melanomas with retinal invasion. Retina 1986;4:232–241.

217. Cantrill HL, Cameron JD, Ramsay, et al. Retinal vascular changes in malignant melanoma of the choroid. Am J Ophthalmol 1984;97:411–418.

218. Leff SR, Augsburger JJ, Shields JA. Focal fluorescence of choroidal melanoma. Br J Ophthalmol 1986;70:104–106.

219. Coleman DJ, Abramson DH, Jack RL, et al. Ultrasonic diagnosis of tumors of the choroid. Am J Ophthalmol 1974;91:344–364.

220. Nicholson DH, Frazier-Byrne S, Chin MT, et al. Echographic and histologic tumor height measurements in uveal melanoma. Am J Ophthalmol 1985;100:456–457.

221. Martin JA, Robertson DM. Extrascleral extension of choroidal melanoma diagnosed by ultrasound. Ophthalmology 1983;90:1334–1339.

222. Shields JA. Current approaches to the diagnosis and management of choroidal melanomas. Surv Ophthalmol 1977;21:443–463.

223. Shields JA, McDonald PR, Leonard BC, et al. The diagnosis of uveal malignant melanoma in eyes with opaque media. Am J Ophthalmol 1977;83:95–105.

224. Dixon PA, Abrams GW, Caya JG. Acoustic analysis of the cytologic structure of malignant melanomas with standardized echography. In: Ossoinig KC, ed. Ophthalmic echography. Proceedings of the 10th SIDUO Congress, St. Petersburg Beach, Florida, November 7–10, 1984. Martinus Nijhoff, Dr W Junk Publi, Dordrecht Doc Opthalmol Proc Series, 1987;48:347–356.

225. Ossoinig KC, Reshef DS, Harrie RP, Hasenfratz GC. Acoustic tissue differentiation with standardized echography in reference to melanomas and pseudomelanomas. In: Ossoinig KC, ed. Ophthalmic echography. Proceedings of the 10th SIDUO Congress, St Petersburg Beach, Florida, November 7–10, 1984. Martinus Nijhoss, Dr Junk Publ, Dordrecht Doc Opthalmol Proc Series, 1987;48:363–364.

226. Char DH, Kroll S, Stone RD, Harrie R, Kerman B. Ultrasonographic measurement of uveal melanoma thickness: interobserver variability. Br J Ophthalmol 1990;74:183–185.

227. Coleman DJ, Silverman RH, Rondeau MJ, Lizzi FL, McLean IW, Jakobiec FA. Correlations of acoustic tissue typing of malignant melanoma and histopathologic features as a predictor of death. Am J Ophthalmol 1990;110:380–388.

228. Gosbell AD, Barry WR, Favilla I, Burgess F. Volume measurement of intraocular tumors by cross-sectional ultrasonographic scans. Aust/NZ J Ophthalmol 1991;19:327–333.

229. Abramson DH, Servodidio CA, McCormick B, Fass D, Zang E. Changes in height of choroidal melanomas after plaque therapy. Br J Ophthalmol 1990;74:359–362.

230. Lieb WE, Cohen SM, Marton DA, et al. Color Doppler imaging of the eye and orbit: Technique and normal vascular anatomy. Arch Ophthalmol 1991;109:527–531.

231. Lieb WE, Shields JA, Cohen SM, et al. Color Doppler imaging in the management of intraocular tumors. Ophthalmology 1990;97:1660–1664.

232. Guthoff RF, Berger RW, Winkler P, Helmke K, Chumbley LC. Doppler ultrasonography of malignant melanomas of the uvea. Arch Ophthalmol 1991;109:537–541.

233. Wollensak J, Heinrich M. In vivo and in vitro measurement of P32 untake inthe ocular tissue in cases of malignant melanoma. Graefes Arch Clin Exp Ophthalmol 1981;217:35–44.

234. McLean IW, Shields JA. Prognostic value of ^{33}P uptake in posterior uveal melanomas. Ophthalmology 1980;87:543–548.

235. Boniuk M, Ruiz RS. Viewpoints: The ^{33}P test in the diagnosis of ocular melanoma. Surv Ophthalmol 1980;24:671–678.

236. Goldberg B, Kara GB, Previtte LR. The use of radioactive phosphorus (^{32}P) in the diagnosis of ocular tumors. Am J Ophthalmol 1980;90:817–828.

237. Mafee MF, Peyman GA, McKusick MA. Malignant uveal melanoma and similar lesions studied by computed tomography. Radiology 1985;156:403–408.

238. Peyster RG, Augsburger JJ, Shields JA, et al. Choroidal melanoma: Comparison of CT, fundoscopy and ultrasound. Radiology 1985;136:675–680.

239. Augsburger JJ, Peyster RG, Markoe AM, et al. Computed tomography of posterior uveal melanomas. Arch Ophthalmol 1987;105:1512–1516.

240. Sobel DF, Kelly W, Kjos BO, et al. MR imaging of orbital and ocular disease. AJNR 1983;6:259–264.

241. Mafee MF, Peyman GA, Grisdano JF, et al. Malignant melanoma and stimulating lesions: MR imaging evaluation. Radiology 1986;160:773–780.

242. De Keiser RJ, Vielvoye GJ, de Wolff-Rouendahl D. Nuclear magnetic resonance imaging of intraocular tumors. Am J Ophthalmol 1986;102:438–441.

243. Chambers RB, Davidorf FH, McAdoo JF, Chakeres DW. Magnetic resonance imaging of uveal melanomas. Arch Ophthalmol 1987;105:917–921.

244. Bond JB, Haik BG, Mihara F, Gupta KL. Magnetic resonance imaging of choroidal melanoma with and without gadolinium contrast enhancement. Ophthalmology 1981;98:459–466.

245. Raymond WR, Char DH, Norman D, Protzko EE. Magnetic resonance imaging evaluation of uveal tumors. Am J Ophthalmol 1991;5:633–641.

246. Peyster RG, Augsburger JJ, Shields JA, Hershey BL, Eagle R Jr, Haskin ME. Intraocular tumors: Evaluation with MR imaging. Radiology 1988;168:773–779.

247. Kurhanewicz J, Winguth SD, Char DH, et al. ^{31}P magnetic resonance spectroscopy of animal uveal melanoma. Invest Ophthalmol Vis Sci 1990;31:1745–1753.

248. De Potter P, Von Weymarn C, Zografos L. In vivo phosphorus 31 magnetic resonance spectroscopy of human uveal melanomas and other intraocular tumors. Am J Ophthalmol 1991;111:276–288.

249. Felberg NT, Donoso LA, Federman JL. Tumor-associated antibodies in the serum of patients with ocular melanoma. Ophthalmology 1980;87:529–533.

250. Felberg NT, Pro-Landazuri JM, Shields JA, et al. Tumor-associated antibodies in the serum of patients with ocular melanoma. Arch Ophthalmol 1979;97:256–259.

251. Donoso LA, Felberg NT, Edelberg K, et al. Metastatic uveal melanoma: An ocular melanoma-associated entigen in the serum of patients with metastatic disease. J Immunol 1986;7:273–283.

252. Ringens PJ, Van Haperen R, Vennegoor C, et al. Monoclonal antibodies in detection of choroidal melanoma. Graefe Arch Clin Exp Ophthalmol 1989;227:287–290.

253. Schaling DF, Van Kroonenburgh MJPG, Borsje RA, et al. Radioimmuno-scintigraphy with melanoma-associated monoclonal antibody fragments in choroidal melanoma. Graefe Arch Clin Exp Ophthalmol 1989;227, 3:291–294.

254. Whitmore WG, Witkin SS, Ellsworth RM. Circulating melanoma-associated antigens in ocular melanoma. Am Ophthalmol 1988;20:212–217.

255. Schaling DF, Van Der Pol JP, Jager MJ, Van Kroonenburgh MJPG, Oosterhuis JA, Ruiter DJ. Radioimmunoscintigraphy and immunohistochemistry with melanoma-associated monoclonal antibodies in choroidal melanoma: A comparison of the clinical and immunohistochemical results. Br J Ophthalmol 1990;74:538–541.

256. Meyer E, Navon D, Zonis S. The role of carcinoembryonic antigen in surveillance of patients with choroidal malignant melanoma: A prospective study. Ann Ophthalmol 1987;19:24–25.

257. Meyer F, Navon D, Zonis S. The role of carcinoembryonic antigen in surveillance of patients with choroidal malignant melanoma: A prospective study. Ann Ophthalmol 1987;19:24–25.

258. Char DH, Stone RD, Irvine AR, et al. Diagnosis modalities in choroidal melanoma. Am J Ophthalmol 1980;89:223–230.

259. Augsburger JJ, Shields JA, Folberg R, et al. Fine needle aspiration biopsy in the diagnosis of intraocular cancer: Cytologic-histologic correlations. Ophthalmology 1985;92:39–49.

260. Karcioglu ZA, Gordon RA, Karcioglu GC. Tumor seeding in ocular fine needle aspiration biopsy. Ophthalmology 1985;92:1763–1767.

261. Glasgow BJ, Brown HH, Zargoza AM, Foos RY. Quantitation of tumor seeding from fine needle aspiration of ocular melanomas. Am J Ophthalmol 1988;105:538–546.

262. Char DH, Miller TH, Crawford JB. Cytopathologic diagnosis of benign lesions simulating choroidal melanomas. Am J Ophthalmol 1991;112:70–75.

263. Gass JDM. Observation of suspected choroidal and ciliary body melanomas for evidence of growth prior to enucleation. Ophthalmology 1980;87:523–528.

264. Felberg NT, Shields JA, Maguire J, et al. Gamma-glutamyl transpeptidase in the prognosis of patients with uveal malignant melanoma. Am J Ophthalmol 1983;95:467–473.

265. Donoso LA, Nagy RG, Brochman RJ, et al. Metastatic uveal melanoma: Hepatic cell-surface enzymes, isoenzymes, and serum sialic acid levels in early metastatic disease. Arch Ophthalmol 1983;101:791–794.

266. Donoso LA, Bend D, Augsberger JF. Metastatic uveal melanoma: Pretherapy serum liver enzyme and liver scan abnormalities. Arch Ophthalmol 1985;103:796–798.

267. Jakobiec FA, Depot MJ, Henkind P, et al. Fluorescein angiographic patterns of iris melanocytic tumors. Arch Ophthalmol 1982;100:1288–1299.

268. Ferry AP. Lesions mistaken for malignancy of the iris. Arch Ophthalmol 1985;74:9–18.

270. Shields JA, Sanborn GE, Augsburger JJ. The differential diagnosis of malignant melanoma of the iris: A clinical study of 300 patients. Ophthalmology 1983;90:716–720.

271. Territo C, Shields CL, Shields JA, Augsburger JJ, Schroeder RP. Natural course of melanocytic tumors of the iris. Ophthalmology 1988;95:1251.

272. Gupta K, Hoepher JA, Streeten BW. Pseudomelanoma of the iris in herpes simplex keratitis. Ophthalmology 1986;93:1524–1527.

273. Beras OH, Myers MH. Manual for staging of cancer. 2nd ed. Philadelphia: JB Lippincott, 1983:197–208.

274. Fuchs E. Das sarcom des uvealtractus. Wein: Wilhelm, Braumueller, 1882.

275. Kersten RC. Management of choroidal malignant melanoma at Iowa. Ophthalmologica 1984;189:24–35.

276. Char DH. Therapeutic options in uveal melanomas. Am J Ophthalmol 1984;98:796–799.

277. Char DH. Management of choroidal melanoma and retinoblastoma. In: Kanski JJ, Morse PM, eds. Disorders of the vitreous, retina, and choroid. Butterworth international medical review in ophthalmology. London: Butterworth, 1983:122–146.

278. Barr CC, Sipperley JO, Nicholson DH. Small melanomas of the choiroid. Arch Ophthalmol 1978;96:1580–1582.

279. Thomas JV, Green WR, Waumenee AE. Small choroidal melanomas: A long-term follow-up study. Arch Ophthalmol 1979;97:861–864.

280. Davidorf FH, Lang JR. The natural history of malignant melanoma of the choroid and ciliary body: Small versus large tumors. Trans Am Acad Ophthalmol Otolaryngol 1975;79:310–320.

281. Meyer-Schwickerath G. The preservation of vision by treatment of intraocular tumors with light coagulation. Arch Ophthalmol 1961;66:458–466.

282. Vogel MH. The application of photocoagulation in the treatment of the choroid. Ophthalmic Forum 1983;1:46–47.

283. Foulds WS, Danato BF. Low-energy long-exposure laser therapy in the management of choroidal melanoma. Graefes Arch Clin Exp Ophthalmol 1986;224:26–31.

284. Lin LH, Ni C. Hematoporphyrin phototherapy for experimental intraocular malignant melanoma. Arch Ophthalmol 1983;101:301–303.

285. Gomer CJ, Doinon DR, White L, et al. Hematoporphyrin derivative photoradiation-induced damage to normal and tumor tissue of the pigmented rabbit eye. Curr Eye Res 1984;3:229–237.

286. Tse DT, Dutton JJ, Weingeist TA, et al. Hematoporphyrin photoradiation therapy for intraocular and orbital malignant melanoma. Arch Ophthalmol 1984;102:833–838.

287. Bruce RA Jr. Evaluation of hematoporphyrin photoradiation therapy to treat choroidal melanomas. Lasers Surg Med 1984;4:59–64.

288. Vogel MH. Histopathologic observations of photocoagulated malignant melanomas of the choroid. Am J Ophthalmol 1972;74:466–474.

289. Jaffe GJ, Mieler WF, Burke JM, Williams GA. Photoablation of ocular melanoma with a high-powered argon endolaser. Arch Ophthalmol 1989;107:113–118.

290. Phillips AMR, Browne BH, Allan D, Szczesny PJ, Lee WR, Foulds WS. Haematoprophyrin photosensibilization treatment of experimental choroidal melanoma: Annual Congress of the Ophthalmology Society, United Kingdom, April 1987. Eye 1987;1:680–685.

291. Bruce RA, McCaugnan JS. Lasers in uveal melanoma. Ophthalmol Clin North Am 1989;2:597–604.

292. Shukla M, Gerke E, Bornfeld N, Meyer-Schwickerath G. Tumor regression after photocoagulation of malignant melanomas of the choroid: An ultrasonographic study. Ophthalmologica 1987;194:119–125.

293. Jalkh AE, Trempe CL, Nasrallah FP. Treatment of small choroidal melanomas with photocoagulation. Ophthalmic Surg 1988;19:738–742.

294. Shields JA, Glazer LC, Mieler WF, Shields CL, Gottlieb MS. Comparison of xenon ard and argon laser photocoagulation in the treatment of choroidal melanomas. Am J Ophthalmol 1990;109:647–655.

295. Bauman WC, Mones JM, Tritten JJ, et al. Transpupillary phthalocyanine photodynamic therapy of experimental posterior malignant melanoma. Invest Ophthalmol Vis Sci 1991;32(suppl):713.

296. Ozler SA, Nelson JS, De Queiroz JL, et al. Photodynamic therapy of experimental choroidal melanoma model using chloroaluminum sulfonated phtalocyanine. Invest Ophthalmol Vis Sci 1991;32:1196.

297. Folk JC, Weingeist TA, Coonan P, Blodi CF, Folberg R, Kimura AE. The treatment of serous macular detachment secondary to choroidal melanomas and nevi. Ophthalmology 1989;96:547–551.

298. Moore RF. Choroidal sarcoma treated by the intraocular insertion of radon seeds. Br J Ophthalmol 1930;14:14–152.

299. Stallard HB. Radiotherapy for malignant melanoma of the choroid. Br J Ophthalmol 1966;50:147–155.

300. Markoe AM, Brady LW, Shields JA, et al. Malignant melanoma of the eye: Treatment of posterior uveal lesions by Co-60 plaque radiotherapy versus enucleation. Radiology 1985;156:801–803.

301. Sealy R, Le Roux PLM, Rapley F, et al. The treatment of ophthalmic tumors with low energy sources. Br J Urol 1976;49:551–554.

302. Packer S, Rotman M. Radiotherapy of choroidal melanoma with iodine-125. Ophthalmology 1980;87:582–590.

303. Bosworth JL, Packer S, Rotman M, Ho T, Finger PT. Choroidal melanoma I-125 plaque therapy. Radiology 1988;169:249–251.

304. Garretson BR, Robertson DM, Earle JD. Choroidal melanoma treatment with iodine-125 brachytherapy. Arch Ophthalmol 1987;105:1394–1397.

305. Loammatsch PK. B-irradiation of choroidal melanoma within 106R/106Rh applicators: 16 years' experience. Arch Ophthalmol 1983;101:713–717.

306. Lommatzsch PK. Results after beta-irradiation (106 Ru/106Rh) of choroidal melanomas: 20 years' experience. Am J Clin Oncol 1987;10:146–151.

307. Saunder WH, Char DH, Quivey JM. Precision high-dose radiotherapy: Helium ion treatment of uveal melanoma. Int J Radiat Oncol Biol Phys 1985;11:227–233.

308. Gragoudas ES, Seddon JW, Eagan KM, et al. Long-term results of proton beam radiated uveal melanomas. Ophthalmology 1987;94:395–453.

309. Seddon JM, Gragoudas ES, Polivogianis L, et al. Visual outcome after proton beam irradiation of uveal melanoma. J Ophthalmol 1986;93:666–674.

310. Finger PT, Packer S, Svitra PP, et al. Hyperthermic treatment of intraocular tumors. Arch Ophthalmol 1986;102:1477, 1481.

311. Burgess JE, Char DH, Svitra PP, et al. Effects of hyperthemia on experimental choroidal melanoma. Br J Ophthalmol 1985;69:854–860.

312. Finger PT, Packer S, Sviltra PP, et al. Thermoradiotherapy for intraocular tumors. Arch Ophthalmol 1985;103:1574–1578.

313. Riedel KG, Svitra PP, Seddon JM, et al. Proton beam irradiation and hyperthermia: Effects on experimental choroidal melanoma. Arch Ophthalmol 1985;103:1862–1869.

314. Coleman DJ, Lizzi FL, Burgess SE, et al. Ultrasonic hyperthermia and radiation in the management of intraocular malignant melanoma. Am J Ophthalmol 1986;101:635–642.

315. Finger PT, Packer S, Paglione RW, Gatz JF, Ho TK, Bosworth JL. Thermoradiotherapy of choroidal melanoma: Clinical experience. Ophthalmology 1989;96:1384–1388.

316. Mieler WF, Jaffe GJ, Steevens RA. Ferromagnetic hyperthermia and iodine 125 brachytherapy in the treatment of choroidal melanoma in a rabbit model. Arch Ophthalmol 1989;107:1524–1528.

317. Swift PS, Stauffer PR, Fries PD, et al. Microwave hypertehrmia for choroidal melanoma in rabbits. Invest Ophthalmol Vis Sci 1990;31:1754–1760.

318. Lincoff H, McLean T, Long R. The cryosurgical treatment of intraocular tumors. Am J Ophthalmol 1977;63:389–390.

319. Abramson DH, Lisman RD. Cryopexy of a choroidal melanoma. Ann Ophthalmol 1979;11:1418–1421.

320. Hidayat AA, LaPiana FG, Kramer KK, et al. The effect of rapid freezing on uveal melanomas. Am J Ophthalmol 1987;103:66–80.

321. Peyman GA, Ericson ES, Axelrod AJ, et al. Full-thickness eyewall resection in primates: An experimental approach to the treatment of choroidal melanoma. Arch Ophthalmol 1973;89:410–412.

322. Peyman GA, Apple DJ. Local excision of a choroidal malignant melanoma: Full-thickness eyewall resection. Arch Ophthalmol 1974;92:216–218.

323. Peyman GA. Eyewall resection. Ophthalmic Forum 1983;4:38–41.

324. Peyman GA, Juarez CL, Diamond FG, et al. Ten-year experience with eyewall resection for uveal malignant melanomas. Ophthalmology 1984;91:1720–1723.

325. Peyman GA, Gremillon CM. Eyewall resection in the management of uveal neoplasms. Jpn J Ophthalmol 1989;33:458–471.

326. Shields JA, Shields CL, Shah P, Sivalingram V. Partial lamellar sclerouvectomy for ciliary body and choroidal tumors. Ophthalmology 1991;98:971–983.

327. Augsbuerger DJ, Lowry JC, Eisenman R. Matched group study of surgical resection versus cobalt-60 plaque radiotherapy for primary choroidal or ciliary body melanoma. Ophthalmic Surg 1990;21:682–688.

328. Forrest AW, Keyser RB, Spencer WH. Iridocyclectomy for melanomas of the ciliary body: A follow-up study of pathology and surgical mortality. Trans Am Acad Opthalmol 1978;85:1237–1249.

329. Damato B, Foulds Ws. Ciliary body tumors and their management. Trans Ophthalmol Soc UK 1986;103:256–264.

330. Foulds WS, Damato BE. Surgical resection of choroidal melanomas. In: Ryan SJ, ed. Retina. Vol 1. St Louis: CV Mosby, 1989:713–720.

331. Blodi FC. Ophthalmology. JAMA 1980;243:2202–2203.

332. Abramson DH, Ellsworth RM. Treatment of choroidal melanomas. Bull NY Acad Med 1978;54:849–854.

333. Char DH, Phillips TL. Pre-enucleation irradiation of uveal melanoma. Br J Ophthalmol 1986;69:177–179.

334. Augsburger JJ, Eagle RC, Chiu M., Shields JA. The effect of pre-enucleation radiotherapy on mitotic activity of choroidal and ciliary body melanomas. Ophthalmology 1987;94:1627–1630.

335. Jager MJ, Van Der Pol JP, De Wolff-Rouendaal D, De Jong PTVM, Ruiter DJ. Decreased expression of HLA class II antigens on human uveal melanoma cells after in vivo x-ray irradiation. Am J Ophthalmol 1988;105, 1:78–86.

336. Rousseau AP, Deschenes J, Pelletier G, Tremblay M, Larochelle-Belland M. Effect of pre-enucleation radiotherapy on the viability of human choroidal melanoma cells. Can J Ophthalmol 1989;24:10–14.

337. Mooy CM, De Jong PTVM, Van Der Kwast TH, Mulder PGH, Jager MJ, Ruiter DJ. Ki-67 immunostaining in uveal melanoma: The effect of pre-enucleation radiotherapy. Ophthalmology 1990;97:1275–1280.

338. Krissig I, Rohrbach M, Lincoff H. Irradiation of choroidal melanomas before enucleation? Retina 1989;9:101–104.

339. Char DH, Phillips TL, Andejeski Y, Crawford JB, Kroll S. Failure of prenucleation radiation to decrease uveal melanoma mortality. Am J Ophthalmol 1988;106:21–26.

340. Kenneally CZ, Farber MG, Smith ME, Deviveni R. In vitro melanoma cell growth after preenucleation radiation therapy. Arch Ophthalmol 1988;106:223–224.

341. Straatsma BR, Fine SL, Earle JD, Hawkins BS, Diener-West M, McLaughlin JA. The collaborative ocular melanoma study research group: Enucleation versus plaque irradiation for choroidal melanoma. Ophthalmology 1988;95:1000–1004.

342. Wilson RS. Ocular melanoma. Surgical experience with "no touch" enucleation. South Med J 1983;76:202–204.

343. Davidorf FH, McAdoo JF. Enucleation for choroidal melanoma. In: Ryan SJ, ed. Retina. Vol 1. St Louis: CV Mosby, 1989:687–691.

344. Augsburger JJ, Gamel JW, Lauritzen K, Brady LW. Cobalt-60, plaque radiotherapy vs enucleation for posterior uveal melanoma. Am J Ophthalmol 1990;109:585–592.

345. Egan KM, Gragoudas ES, Seddon JM, et al. The risk of enucleation after proton beam irradiation of uveal melanoma. Ophthalmology 1989;96:1377–1383.

346. Char DH, Castro JR, Kroll SM, Irvine AR, Quivey JM, Stone RD. Five-year follow-up of hemium ion therapy for uveal melanoma. Arch Ophthalmol 1990;108:209–214.

347. Gragoudas ES, Seddon JM, Egan K, et al. Ophthalmology 1987;94:349–353.

348. Zografos L, Gaillaud C, Perret C, et al. Conservative treatment of uveal melanomas at Lausanne University Eye Clinic. 80 Jahreskongr Scheiz Ophthalmol Ges, Engelberg, September 9–12, 1987. Klin Monatsbl Augenheildk 1988;192:572–578.

349. Grange JD, Gerard JP, Ragab M, et al. Place of beta-ray brachytherapy in the conservative treatment of choroidal and ciliary body melanomas. Ophthalmologie 1989;3:175–179.

350. Lommatzch PK, Kirsch IH. 106RU/106RH plaque radiotherapy for malignant melanomas of the choroid. Doc Ophthalmol 1988;68:225–238.
351. Smith GM. Ocular melanoma and immunotherapy. Ophthalmologica (Basel) 1979;178:111–113.
352. The TH, De Gast GC, Huiges HA, et al. Immunologic aspects of melanoma. Ophthalmologica (Basel) 1977;175:25–27.
353. Stark WJ, Rosenthal AR, Mullins GM, et al. Simultaneous bilateral uveal melanomas responding to BCNU therapy. Trans Am Acad Ophthalmol Otolaryngol 1971;75:70–83.
354. Liu HS, Refojo MF, Albert DM. Experimental combined systemic and local chemotherapy for intraocular malignancy. Arch Ophthalmol 1980;98:905–908.
355. Affeldt JC, Minckler DS, Azen SP, et al. Prognosis of malignant melanoma of the choroid and ciliary body. Int Ophthalmol Clin 1962;5:389–402.
356. Kersten RC, Tse D, Anderson RL, et al. Role of orbital exenteration in malignant melanoma with extrascleral extension. Ophthalmology 1985;92:436–443.
357. Rini FJ, Jakobiec FA, Hornblass A, Beckerman BL, Anderson RL. The treatment of advanced choroidal melanoma with massive orbital extension. Am J Ophthalmol 1987;104:634–640.
358. Shields CL, Shields JA, Yarian DL, Augsberger JJ. Intracranial extension of choroidal melanoma via the optic nerve. Br J Ophthalmol 1987;71:172–176.
359. Shields JA, Shields CL. Massive orbital extension of posterior uveal melanoma. J Ophthalmol Plast Reconstr Surg 1991;7:238–251.
360. Hykin PG, McCartney ACE, Plowman PN, Hungerford JL. Postenucleation orbital radiotherapy for the treatment of malignant melanoma of the choroid with extrascleral extension. Br J Ophthalmol 1990;74:36–39.
361. Gragoudas ES, Seddon JM, Egan KM, et al. Metastasis from uveal melanoma after proton beam irradiation. Ophthalmology 1988;95:992–999.
362. Fournier GA, Albert DM, Arrigg CA, et al. Resection of solitary metastasis: Approach to palliative treatment of hepatic involvement with choroidal melanoma. Arch Ophthalmol 1984;102:80–82.
363. Gronemeyer U, Enger Mann R, Thiede A. Erfolgreiche Entfernung siner Lebersmetastase 15 Jahre nach Enukleation wegen Aderhaut melanom. Fortschr Ophthalmol 1984;81:363–364.
364. Carrasco CH, Wallace S, Charnsangavny C, et al. Treatment of hepatic metastases in ocular melanoma: Embolization of the hepatic artery with polyvinyl spone and asplatin. JAMA 1986;255:3152–3151.
365. Harning R, Szalay J. A treatment for metastasis of murine ocular melanoma. Invest Ophthalmol Vis Sci 1988;29:1505–1510.
366. Schiller JH, Storer B, Bittner G, Willson JK, Borden EC. Phase II trial of a combination of interferon-beta and interferon-gamma in patients with advanced malignant melanoma. J Interferon Res 1988;8:581–589.
367. Creagan ET. Interferon trials in the management of malignant melanoma and other neoplasms: An overview. In: Nathanson L, ed. Basic and clinical aspects of malignant melanoma. 1987:167–194.
368. McCutcheon IE, Baranco RA, Katz DA, Saris SC. Adoptive immunotherapy of intracerebral metastases in mice. J Neurosurg 1990;72:102–109.
369. The 35th Annual Clinical Conference and 24th Annual Special Pathology Program. Advances in the biology and clinical management of melanoma. Symposium 3. Treatment for distant metastases. November 20–23, 1991.
370. Wilson RS, Fraunfelder FT, Hanna C. Recurrent tapioca melanoma of the iris and ciliary body treated with argon laser. Am J Ophthalmol 1976;82:213–217.
371. Cleasby GW, van Wertenbrugge JA. Treatment of iris melanoma by photocoagulation: A case report. Ophthalmic Surg 1987;18:42–44.
372. Char DH, Crawford JB, Gonzales J, Miller T. Iris melanoma with increased intraocular pressure: Differentiation of focal solitary tumors from diffuse or multiple tumors. Arch Ophthalmol 1989;107:548.
373. Hungerford J. Prognosis in ocular melanoma. Br J Ophthalmol [Editorial] 1989;73:689.
374. Raubitschek E. Uber Iristumoren. Klin Monatsbl Augenheikd 1914;52:683–694.
375. Verhoeff FH. Sarcoma of the iris. Trans Am Ophthalmol Soc 1933;31:270–271.
376. Muller HK, Sollner F, Lund OE. Erfahrunger bei der operativen von Tumeren der Iris wurzel und des Ciliarkorpers. Berl Dtsch Ophthalmol Ges Heidelberg 1961;63:194–199.
377. Stallard HB. Partial cyclectomy. Br Ophthalmol 1961;45:797–802.
378. Stallard HB. Partial iridocyclectomy and sclerectomy. Br J Ophthalmol 1966;50:656–659.
379. Jones IS. Iridocyclectomy and corneoscleroiridocyclectomy. In: Reese AB, ed. Tumors of the eye. 3rd ed. Hagerstown, MD: Harper & Row, 1976:238–239.

Cancer: Principles & Practice of Oncology, Fourth Edition,
edited by Vincent T. DeVita, Jr., Samuel Hellman, Steven A. Rosenberg.
J.B. Lippincott Co., Philadelphia © 1993.

Victor A. Levin

Philip H. Gutin

Steven Leibel

CHAPTER **48**

Neoplasms of the Central Nervous System

INCIDENCE AND CLASSIFICATION

Extrapolating available Surveillance, Epidemiology, and End Results (SEER) registry data for 1978 to 1984, the combined incidence of all recorded primary intracranial and spinal axis tumors is between 2 and 19 in 100,000 per year, depending on age.[1] There is an early peak (3.1 in 100,000) between 0 and 4 years, a trough (1.8 in 100,000) between 15 and 24 years, and then a steady rise in incidence that reaches a plateau (17.9–18.7 in 100,000) between 65 and 79 years of age.

The diversity in primary intracranial and spinal axis tumors partly results from the diversity of phenotypically distinct cells capable of transformation into tumors. Table 48–1 shows the hypothetical 15 cell types that can give rise to these tumors. The relative frequency of the seven commonest families of intracranial tumors is given in Table 48–2, and the distribution of spinal tumors is shown in Table 48–3.[2] The commonest tumors are those that are derived from glial precursors (astrocytes, ependymocytes, and oligodendrocytes). The existence of histologically mixed astrocytoma-oligodendroglioma and the less common astrocytoma-ependymoma implies that astrocytomas, oligodendrogliomas, and ependymomas may arise from common stem or progenitor cells. The facts that these tumors arise in different locales within the cranium and the spinal axis and that various types predominate at different ages suggest that differing molecular and genetic mechanisms may underly tumorigenesis at different times in the life span.

Central nervous system (CNS) tumors are the most prevalent solid neoplasms of childhood, the second leading cancer-related cause of death in children younger than 15 years of age, and the third leading cancer-related cause of death in

adolescents and adults between the ages of 15 and 34 years. However, most intracranial tumors occur in people older than 45 years. Table 48–4 lists the frequency of intracranial tumors by tumor type and age at first presentation. Glioblastoma rarely occurs in people younger than 15 years but dramatically increases after the age of 45. The incidence of most glial tumors, other than glioblastoma multiforme, actually decreases with increasing age. There is some concern that the incidence of anaplastic astrocytoma and glioblastoma multiforme is increasing in the elderly population,[3] although incorrect ascertainment preceding the widespread availability of computed tomography (CT) scans in the late 1970s may account for some of the presumed increase in incidence.[4,5]

A similar age-related increase in prevalence occurs with differentiated or "benign" meningiomas that increase from 0.2% of all primary intracranial tumors in patients younger than 24 years of age to 39% of tumors in patients older than 65 years.[6] Table 48–4 shows a different pattern for malignant meningiomas, which increase from 0.2% in children to 2.4% in adults older than 60 years of age.

The overall incidence of primary spinal cord tumors is approximately 15% of that of brain tumors. For gliomas, the age-adjusted incidence is 0.11% to 0.14%; for meningiomas, 0.08% to 0.28%, depending on sex (females higher than males); and for nerve sheath tumors, 0.07% to 0.13%.[7] As shown in Table 48–3, the frequency of specific spinal cord tumors is strikingly different from that of the brain tumors. Gliomas constitute approximately 23% of spinal tumors, and most are ependymomas with a predilection for the cauda equina. Schwannomas and meningiomas account for approximately 60% of spinal tumors, with schwannomas being

1679

TABLE 48–1. Classification of Primary Intracranial Tumors by Cell of Origin

Normal Cell	Tumor
Astrocyte	Astrocytomas, glioblastoma multiforme
Ependymocyte	Ependymoma, ependymoblastoma
Oligodendrocyte	Oligodendroglioma
Arachnoidal fibroblasts	Meningioma
Nerve cell or neuroblast	Ganglioneuroma, neuroblastoma, retinoblastoma
External granular cell or neuroblast	Medulloblastoma
Schwann cell	Schwannoma (neurinoma)
Melanocyte	Melanotic carcinoma
Choroid epithelial cell	Choroid plexus papilloma or carcinoma
Pituitary	Adenoma
Endothelial or "stromal" cell	Hemangioblastoma
Primitive germ cells	Germinoma, pinealoma, teratomas, cholesteatoma
Pineal parenchymal cell	Pineocytoma
Notochordal remnant	Chordoma

slightly more frequent; both types occur most often in adult life. Other less common spinal tumors are the lipomas, dermoids, and hemangioblastomas.

TUMORIGENESIS

Several cytogenetic studies have demonstrated an increased copy number of chromosomes 7 and 22 and nonrandom losses associated with chromosomes 9p, 10, and 17p in human gliomas.[8,9] The amplification of genetic material suggests the presence of a protooncogene, whereas the loss of genomic loci implies a possible tumor-suppressor gene. With respect to the increasing malignancy of gliomas, it has been shown that chromosomal loss of chromosome 17p is an early event seen in all grades of astrocytoma malignancy[10] and that the *p53* gene, which is one of the tumor-suppressor genes that

TABLE 48–2. Frequency of Primary Intracranial Brain Tumors

Type	Frequency (%)
Gliobastoma multiforme	30
Astrocytoma	20
Other gliomas (ependymoma, oligodendroglioma, medulloblastoma)	7
Meningioma	18
Nerve sheath (*e.g.*, neurinoma)	9
Pituitary	5
Other (unspecified)	11

(Modified from the Office of Biometry and Epidemiology [Tables 3–1C, 3–5, and 3–6A], 1977)

TABLE 48–3. Distribution of Primary Spinal Tumors

Histology	Sloff et al[2]	Preston-Martin[7]
Neurilemmoma	29.0	22.0
Meningioma	25.5	42.0
Ependymoma	12.8	15.1
Sarcoma	11.9	
Astrocytoma	6.5	11.2
Other gliomas		1.9
Vascular tumors	6.2	
Chordomas	4.0	
Epidermoids	1.4	
Other	2.7*	5.6

* Lipoma and subarachnoid seeding from primary intracranial tumor.

maps to p13 of chromosome 17, is mutated frequently.[11] The loss of chromosome 9p appears to represent an intermediate event that occurs in most higher-grade astrocytomas,[12] whereas the loss of a portion of chromosome 10 is a late event seen primarily in glioblastoma multiforme tumors.[13] Some evidence suggests that losses on chromosome 19 may be involved in oligodendrogliomas.[14] Ependymomas are associated with a duplication of the long arm of chromosome 12 and losses on chromosome 22.[15]

For meningiomas, multiple deletions of chromosome 22 and constitutional heterozygosity have been observed in a high percentage of cases.[16–18] The neurofibromatosis type II (*NF2*) gene is located on chromosome 22. Recent evidence suggests that the *NF2* gene is centromeric to break points in meningiomas, suggesting the suspected meningioma tumor-suppressor and *NF2* genes are separate entities.[18] Interestingly, for females, alterations on chromosome 22 are much larger than any alterations seen for males with meningiomas.[18,19]

For CNS tumors of children, the commonest genomic alteration identified by karyotypic and molecular analyses is the short arm of chromosome 17 (17p).[20–22] Medulloblastomas have shown extra copies of chromosome 11 and marker chromosomes 8q+, 17p+, and 20q+,[23] and unbalanced translocations resulting in a partial 1q trisomy and 6q monosomy.[24] Nonrandom alterations were observed also in chromosomes 1, 6, 10, 11, 13, and 22. Additionally, amplification of c-*MYC* and epidermal growth factor receptor (EGF-R) has been observed to be associated with medulloblastomas and pediatric gliomas, respectively.[25,26] Although a limited number of specimens were examined in each of the studies, the results indicate that losses in genomic material or the amplification of protooncogenes occur in pediatric brain tumors, similar to those observed for adult tumors. These results strongly implicate the loss of function of tumor-suppressor genes and the possible consequences of germ line mutations.

In addition to chromosomal abnormalities, cytokine and receptor aberrations are seen in gliomas. For instance, transforming growth factor-α (TGF-α)-producing cells are seen throughout all grades of astrocytoma, but amplified EGF-R and TGF-α are seen more often in higher-grade astrocytomas.[27] The amplification of chromosome 22 may also be associated with increased expression of platelet-derived growth factor-β (PDGF-β). PDGF-α maps to chromosome 7, which

TABLE 48–4. Frequency of Intracranial Tumors as a Function of Age Range

Histology	Age Ranges (y)						
	0–9	10–19	20–29	30–39	40–49	50–59	60–74
Astrocytoma	60	59	76	81	86	87	91
"Low-grade"	9.8	7.1	7.1	4.9	2.5	1.5	1.8
"Astrocytoma"	28.0	31.7	40.4	41.9	38.2	31.1	28.8
Anaplastic	18.5	10.9	11.0	12.8	9.6	8.3	11.0
Mixed	2.5	2.7	2.8	3.4	2.2	2.1	0.7
Glioblastoma	1.3	7.4	14.4	18.2	32.9	44.2	51.0
Medulloblastoma	21.0	10.0	5.5	2.3	1.0	0.1	0.0
Ependymoma*	8.7	2.7	4.3	1.8	0.8	1.3	0.5
Oligodendroglioma	1.1	4.0	5.0	6.4	6.2	3.6	1.6
Embryonal/teratoid†	1.0	1.3	0.3	0.3	0.0	0.0	0.0
Meningioma‡	0.2	0.4	1.2	1.7	1.2	2.0	2.4

* Includes differentiated and anaplastic ependymoma.
† Includes germinoma, mixed embryonal pinealomas, and malignant teratomas.
‡ Underestimate, because SEER does not include many "benign" tumors in its registry; these are probably malignant meningiomas.
(Data based on unpublished SEER program search, 1978–1984)

is also amplified. Increased expression of basic FGF is seen in gliomas and may be important as an autocrine and angiogenic factor in high-grade gliomas. Pediatric glioblastomas and medulloblastomas have been shown to have amplification of EGF-R in similar proportions to that observed in adult tumors.[26] These results suggest that the activation of cytokines and their receptors, by any of several mechanisms, may play an important role in primary tumor initiation or progression, or both.

GENETIC FACTORS

For most brain tumors, a genetic predisposition is lacking. Some exceptions are NF1 and NF2, tuberous sclerosis, Li-Fraumeni syndrome, familial polyposis (Turcot's syndrome), and Osler-Weber-Rendu syndrome; the last two are rare. Li-Fraumeni syndrome is an autosomal dominant disorder characterized by the appearance of diverse tumors (malignant glioma, breast cancer, soft tissue sarcoma, osteosarcoma, leukemia, and adrenocortical carcinoma) that often occur at a young age. Noncancerous skin fibroblasts and lymphocytes derived from people with Li-Fraumeni syndrome have germ line p53 mutations.[28,29] Careful study of familial clusters of specific CNS tumors and CNS tumors with other neoplasms is stimulating careful molecular genetic analysis that leads to the elucidation of the critical cascades that underlie CNS malignancies.

NF1 is relatively common, with an incidence of 1 in 3500. Patients with NF1 develop cutaneous lesions (café-au-lait spots), subcutaneous neurofibroma, anterior optic nerve gliomas, and other brain tumors. NF1 is associated with a gene on chromosome 17q (*NF1* gene).[30,31]

NF2 is inherited as an autosomal dominant disorder with incomplete penetrance. It has an incidence of 1 in 50,000. Acoustic schwannomas, especially bilateral acoustic schwannomas; bony and mesenchymal abnormalities; and a spectrum of gliomas from well-differentiated astrocytoma to glioblas-

toma multiforme have been observed in NF2 families. Cytogenetic and linkage studies have implicated the *NF2* gene on chromosome 22q.[19] However, a specific transcribed gene responsible for the genesis of NF2 has not been identified.

Another phakomatosis associated with brain tumors is tuberous sclerosis, a hereditary disease with cutaneous, neurologic, cardiac, and kidney abnormalities. Tuberous sclerosis is normally obvious in children. It is characterized by acneiform skin lesions, angiofibromas, periungual fibromas, epilepsy, periventricular hamartomas composed of abnormal glia, and in some patients, mental retardation. Gliomas may be associated with tuberous sclerosis; the commonest type is an uncommon ganglioglioma. Potential genetic loci on 9q and 11q have been suggested.[32]

With greater sophistication in genetic investigations, specific abnormalities of the genome likely will be found for each specific brain tumor histology. As more is learned about oncogene function and the specific association of chromosomal alterations to structural proteins and enzymes, it is likely that the genetics of tumor development and the entire panoply of tumor growth control will be understood.

CHEMICAL INDUCTION AND EPIDEMIOLOGY

The epidemiology of primary CNS tumors has provided hints but few definitive observations with respect to environmental or occupational causes. Although brain tumors can be experimentally induced in a high proportion of rodents by the use of certain chemicals, the association of chemical exposure and brain tumors is limited to a few occupations. A higher than expected increase in the incidence of brain tumors has been observed as a result of purported exposure to pesticides, herbicides, and fertilizers,[33] various petrochemical industries,[34] and health professions.[35] Whether these statistical observations are credible is difficult to determine. Aside from a known association between vinylchloride and gliomas, there are no common chemical or environmental threads among these observations.[34]

VIRAL INFECTION AND CNS NEOPLASIA

Viruses have been implicated directly in the development of gliomas only in rats, dogs, and monkeys. In all cases, direct CNS injection of the virus is required. In rats, the avian sarcoma virus produces glial tumors[36]; in dogs, Rous sarcoma virus leads to gliosarcomas[37]; in owl monkeys, a human polyoma virus (JC virus) produces glial neoplasms[38]; and in hamsters, JC virus produces medulloblastomas.[39] Although a direct association between virus exposure and CNS tumors has not been established in humans, patients with primary CNS lymphoma have been observed to have a high incidence of infection with Epstein-Barr virus (EBV) and evidence of EBV in their tumor tissue.[40] Common viral exposure could explain the occasional glioma cluster observed in schools and communities. However, it is extremely difficult to pinpoint mutations due to a virus to validate this hypothesis.

TRAUMA AND CNS NEOPLASIA

CNS neoplasia, like most cancers, appears to be unassociated with prior trauma. It has been suggested that the incidence of meningiomas is higher in patients with a prior history of head trauma, but this hypothesis was not supported by a prospective study.[41] Trauma could be a progression event; however, this theory would be difficult to prove.

CNS NEOPLASIA AFTER RADIATION, CHEMOTHERAPY, AND IMMUNOSUPPRESSION

The incidence of CNS tumors after treatment for a prior malignancy is small. The literature contains several examples of astrocytomas occurring 3 to 7 years after craniospinal axis irradiation and chemotherapy for acute lymphocytic leukemia (ALL) and craniopharyngioma[42,43]; unfortunately, none of the reports contain sufficient information to determine risk assessment. In non-Hodgkin's lymphoma, 2% of 44 second malignancies were an astrocytoma.[44] As in the cases discussed previously, no measure of risk assessment is possible, although such infrequent reporting would suggest that these are uncommon or rare events. Meningiomas have been reported in association with scalp irradiation for tinea capitis, the risk for meningiomas being as high as 21% in one study.[45,46]

For unknown reasons, transplant recipients and patients with acquired immunodeficiency syndrome (AIDS) have substantially increased risks for primary CNS lymphoma but not gliomas.

ANATOMIC AND CLINICAL CONSIDERATIONS

The clinical presentation of the various tumors is best appreciated by considering the relation of signs and symptoms to anatomy.[47]

INTRACRANIAL TUMORS

Intracranial tumors produce symptoms primarily by two mechanisms: mass effect (and increased intracranial pressure), due entirely to the tumor or to the tumor and surrounding edema, or infiltration and destruction of normal tissue.

General Signs and Symptoms

Typical infiltrative intracerebral tumors, such as the various grades of astrocytoma and oligodendroglioma and some of the more primitive neuroectodermal tumors, can produce headache, gastrointestinal upset such as nausea and vomiting, personality changes, and slowing of psychomotor function. These may be the only clinical indications of tumor.

Because headache is a common presenting symptom in patients with intracranial tumor, clinical patterns and their localizing value must be appreciated. Brain parenchyma does not have pain-sensitive structures, and tumor pain (headache) has been attributed to local swelling and distortion of pain-sensitive nerve endings associated with blood vessels, primarily in the meninges. Tumors grow at different rates and, therefore, achieve variable size before signs and symptoms occur. But once a tumor has achieved a critical volume causing compression and displacement of brain, the onset and demise of headache seem to correlate with changes in intracranial pressure.

Headaches can vary in severity and quality; they often occur in the early morning hours or on first awakening. Patients sometimes complain of an uncomfortable feeling in the head rather than headache. Although there is not an exact relation between the location of tumor headache and the location of the tumor, some rules are worth remembering. More often than not, frontal and temporal tumors produce headache in frontal, retroorbital, or temporal regions, whereas infratentorial tumors tend to produce occipital and retroauricular headache. Occasionally, however, retroorbital headaches are observed with infratentorial tumors.

Gastrointestinal symptoms are common. Patients complain of loss of appetite, queasiness, nausea, and, occasionally, vomiting. Vomiting appears more commonly in children and in patients harboring infratentorial rather than supratentorial tumors. Although textbooks discuss projectile vomiting as an infrequent generalized symptom of brain tumors, in these authors' experience, it is common in children but rare in adults. From reports in the literature and discussions with experienced neurosurgeons, it seems as though there is a lower incidence of vomiting currently compared with past years; this may reflect the fact that patients are diagnosed earlier than in previous years and receive glucocorticoids that can modify dramatically many of the generalized signs and symptoms of brain tumors.

Sometimes the only presenting symptoms are changes in personality, mood, mental capacity, and concentration. Occasionally, merely a slowing of psychomotor activity is the antecedent symptom of intracranial tumor. Patients with brain tumors tend to sleep longer at night and nap during the day. These changes in function and activity often are apparent to the family and the examiner but not to the patient; in other instances, only the patient recognizes the changes in mental function. None of these symptoms are unique to brain tumors;

they could easily be confused with depression, neurasthenia, or other psychological problems.

Focal Cerebral Syndromes

Although fewer than 10% of patients presenting with seizures have a brain tumor as the cause of the seizure, seizures are a presenting symptom in approximately 20% of patients with supratentorial brain tumors. With rapidly growing infiltrative malignant gliomas, they are likely to take the form of focal motor or sensory seizures, although generalized seizures are also common. In patients with slowly growing astrocytomas, oligodendrogliomas, or meningiomas, generalized seizures may antedate the clinical diagnosis by months to years. The value of the focal seizure as a means of tumor localization is high, sufficiently so that tumor should be considered causative until proved otherwise.

The distribution of infiltrative parenchymal tumors in the brain is directly related to the mass of the lobe or region. Frontal tumors occur more commonly than parietal tumors, which, in turn, occur more often than temporal lobe tumors, and so forth. Anatomic or regional involvement by tumors, although not completely stereotypic as it is with CNS vascular disease, nonetheless has certain features that distinguish them and help the clinician localize the tumor or, at least, to consider the diagnosis.

The frontal lobe syndrome varies markedly from patient to patient. It can range from personality change to headache and mild slowing of contralateral hand movements and to contralateral spastic hemiplegia, marked elevation in mood, or loss of initiative and dysphasia (if it is the dominant lobe). Assuming the normal pattern of left hemisphere dominance, unilateral tumors affecting the right frontal lobe can cause left hemiplegia, slight elevation in mood, difficulty in adapting to new situations, loss of initiative, and even occasional primitive grasp and sucking reflexes. Left frontal lobe tumors can cause right hemiplegia and nonfluent dysphasia with or without some apraxia of lip, tongue, or hand movements.

Bifrontal disease, a condition usually associated with infiltrative gliomas and primary CNS lymphomas, can cause varying degrees of bilateral hemiplegia, spastic bulbar palsy, severe impairment of intellect, lability of mood, dementia, and prominent primitive grasp, suck, and snout reflexes.

Temporal lobe syndromes, like frontal lobe syndromes, can range from symptoms that are detectable only on careful testing of perception and spatial judgment to severe impairment of recent memory. Homonymous quadrantanopsia, auditory hallucinations, and even aggressive behavior can occur as a result of tumors of either temporal lobe. Involvement of the nondominant temporal lobe can also result in minor perceptual problems and spatial disorientation. Dominant temporal lobe involvement can lead to dysnomia, impaired perception of verbal commands, and even a full-blown, fluent Wernicke-like aphasia. Bilateral disease, involving both temporal lobes, is rare in comparison with the bilaterality of frontal lobe tumors that readily cross through the corpus callosum. This is fortunate, because bitemporal tumor involvement is devastating. It produces impairment of memory, especially recent memory, and can lead to dementia.

Parietal lobe syndromes affect sensory and perceptual functions more than motor modalities, although mild hemi-paresis is sometimes seen with extensive parietal lobe tumors. Tumors impinging on either parietal lobe can produce a decrease in the perception of cortical sensory stimuli that may vary from mild sensory extinction, observable only by testing, to a more severe sensory loss with deep tumors that leads to hemianesthesia or other hemisensory abnormalities. Homonymous hemianopsia or visual inattention also may occur. In addition, involvement of the nondominant parietal lobe can lead to perceptual abnormalities and, in severe cases, to anosognosia and apraxia for self-dressing. Unilateral dominant parietal lobe tumors lead to alexia, dysgraphia, and certain types of apraxia.

Occipital lobe tumors can produce contralateral homonymous hemianopsia or visual aberrations that take the form of imperception of color, object size, or object location. Bilateral occipital disease can produce cortical blindness.

The classic disconnection syndromes associated with corpus callosum lesions are seen rarely in patients with brain tumors. Even though infiltrative gliomas often cross the corpus callosum in the region of the genu or the splenium, the involvement of additional structures complicates neurologic interpretation, obscuring classic disconnection syndromes. With respect to partial lesions, interruption of association fibers in the anterior part of the corpus callosum usually causes a failure of the left hand to carry out spoken commands. Lesions in the splenium of the corpus callosum interrupt visual fibers connecting the right occipital lobe and left angular gyrus, resulting in an inability of patients to read or name colors.

Symptoms related to thalamic tumors vary as a function of tumor size and whether the tumor produces secondary blockage of cerebrospinal fluid (CSF) flow and hydrocephalus. Occasionally, tumors in the thalamus and, less commonly, in the basal ganglia, can reach 3 to 4 cm in diameter before the patient has symptoms severe enough to seek medical attention. Patients typically present with headaches resulting from hydrocephalus and increased intracranial pressure secondary to trapping of the lateral horn of one of the ventricles. In addition or independently, patients can present with a mild sensory abnormality on the contralateral side, which is detected only by testing of sensory extinction or, rarely, severe neuropathic pain syndrome. Patients may complain of intermittent paresthesias on the contralateral side; because they are episodic and seizure-like, anticonvulsant drugs are used sometimes and actually may be beneficial. With more involvement of the basal ganglia, contralateral intention tremor and hemiballistic-like movement disorders can be observed. Thalamic tumors usually do not present in a manner typical of thalamic strokes, unless bleeding into the tumor has occurred.

Focal Infratentorial Syndromes

The brain stem, composed of the medulla oblongata and the pons, has both nuclear groups and traversing axons. Tumors invading or compressing the brain stem can produce dire consequences; even a small increase in size, for example, 1 to 2 mm, may lead to death or devastating signs and symptoms. Tumors can be primarily intrinsic or intrinsic with exophytic components in the fourth ventricle, peripontine cisterns, or in both locations. Cranial nerve involvement, therefore, can be at the nuclear level or of the cranial nerve as it leaves the brain stem.

The commonest tumor of the brain stem is an astrocytoma (glioma), the initial clinical manifestations of which are palsies involving cranial nerves VI and VII on one side in 90% of patients. These usually are followed by involvement of long tracts resulting in hemiplegia, unilateral limb ataxia, ataxia of gait, paraplegia, hemisensory syndromes, gaze disorders, and, occasionally, hiccups. Less commonly, long-tract signs precede the cranial nerve abnormalities; this is more likely with confined intrinsic brain stem lesions.

The midbrain, juxtaposed between the pons and the cerebral hemispheres, encompasses the tectum, the cerebral peduncles, and the cerebral aqueduct. If the midbrain is involved, obstructive hydrocephalus can occur, producing vomiting, drowsiness, and cerebellar signs. Patients with medullary tumors have a more rapidly progressive course and are more likely to have deficits in cranial nerves VI (usually late), VII, IX, and X, and dysarthria, personality change, and head tilt. Unlike the expansive posterior fossa tumors, headache, vomiting, and papilledema occur late.

Fourth ventricular tumors, because of their location, tend to produce obstructive hydrocephalus early in their development. This produces profound headache and vomiting and associated disturbances of gait and balance. With rapidly progressing lesions, cerebellar herniation may develop.

Tumors of the cerebellum have valuable localizing signs and symptoms. In slowly growing tumors, the initial symptoms may be headache and nausea, which are caused by increased intracranial pressure, and mild imbalance in gait or ataxia of a limb. In more rapidly growing cerebellar tumors, there may be prominent morning headache, vomiting, a stumbling gait with frequent falling, nystagmus and dizziness, and visual symptoms caused by papilledema. Abnormal posturing of the head is seen often in children but not in adults. In children, the head is tilted back and away from the side of the tumor. Posturing of the head is curious in that it indicates unilateral

cerebellum-foramen magnum herniation. Bilateral sixth cranial nerve palsies are uncommon. Midline lesions in and around the cerebellar vermis lead to truncal and gait ataxia, whereas lesions in a cerebellar hemisphere lead to unilateral appendicular ataxia, most readily observed in upper extremity movements.

Tumors of the base of the skull, although not particularly common, nevertheless are important because many are curable by surgery. Table 48–5[48] summarizes the salient clinical features of seven of the more common clinical syndromes.

A classic base-of-skull tumor presentation is that associated with acoustic neurilemmomas (schwannoma), the most frequent cause of the cerebellopontine angle syndrome. Almost all such patients have involvement of the auditory or vestibular portions of cranial nerve VIII; more than 50% have facial weakness, disturbance of taste, and sensory loss of the face; approximately 40% have ataxia of gait; and fewer than 25% have unilateral appendicular ataxia. Deafness and vestibular dysfunction due to damage to the auditory and vestibular nerve branches are characteristic of these tumors. Finally, these tumors can attain an extremely large size before they are discovered.

Another group of tumors that present with distinct signs and symptoms is that which occurs in or near the sella turcica. Table 48–6 summarizes the location, tumors, and some of the salient features of sellar and parasellar tumors.[49]

Many patients present with defects of the visual field, less commonly with blindness and optic atrophy. The visual field abnormality is usually a partial or complete bitemporal hemianopsia associated with intrasellar tumors such as pituitary adenomas. With lesions that expand from below the optic chiasm, the upper temporal quadrants are affected first. Patients can also present with scotomata in either eye. With long-standing, slowly progressive disease, unilateral or bilateral optic atrophy can be observed. Expansion of tumor may

TABLE 48–5. Differential Diagnosis of Tumors at the Base of the Skull

Site of Lesion	Associated Tumors	Clinical Findings
Anterior parts	Carcinomas invasive from frontal and ethmoid sinuses; meningiomas	Unilateral anosmia, frontal lobe syndrome, seizures
Superior orbital	Meningiomas, carcinoma of nasopharynx	Lesions of cranial nerves III, IV, V, VI with ophthalmoplegia, pain, and hypesthesia in VI distribution
Cavernous sinus	Chondromas, meningiomas, sellar and parasellar tumors	Cranial nerves III, IV, VI, and sometimes V involvement with ophthalmoplegia
Apex of the petrous temporal bone	Cholesteatoma, chondroma, meningioma, neurinoma, sarcoma	Cranial nerves V and VI involvement with sensory and motor findings and diplopia
Sphenoid and petrous bones	Meningioma, chondroma, nasopharyngeal carcinoma, metastasis	Lesions of cranial nerves III, IV, VI resulting in ophthalmoplegia; fifth may be associated with trigeminal neuralgia syndrome
Jugular foramen	Glomus jugular tumors, neurinomas, chondromas, cholesteatoma, meningioma, nasopharyngeal carcinoma	Cranial nerves IX, X, XI producing difficulty with swallowing and speaking and weakness of neck muscles
Cerebellopontine angle	Neurinoma, meningioma, cholesteatoma, metastasis of cerebellar tumors	Cranial nerve VII lesions: loss of hearing, vertigo, and nystagmus; cerebellar: ataxia; cranial nerves V, VII, occasionally IX and XII; brain stem symptoms and signs of increased intracranial pressure

(Adapted from Bingas B. Tumours of the base of the skull. In: Vinken PJ, Bruyn GW, eds. Handbook of clinical neurology: Tumours of the brain and skull. Vol 17. Amsterdam: North Holland, 1974:136)

TABLE 48–6. Clinical Syndromes Associated With Tumors of Sellar Region

| Tumor | Disorders | | Incidence and Degree | Syndromes |
	Anterior Pituitary Gland	Hypothalamus		
In the Sella				
Adenoma				
Active	+			Cushing's disease, acromegaly, gigantism
Inactive	+	+/−		Forbes-Albright syndrome, hypopituitarism
Chondroma	+			
Metastasis	+			
Craniopharyngioma			Regular Clinical	
Intrasellar	+			
Intrasellar and suprasellar	+	+		
Close to Sella				
Suprasellar craniopharyngioma		+	Regular Clinical	Adiposogenital dystrophy (Frohlich)
Suprasellar meningioma		+/−		
Suprasellar epidermoid				
Optic pathway glioma		+/−	Rare	Russell's syndrome
Hypothalamic glioma		+	Frequent	Precocious puberty
Hypothalamic hamartoma		+	Clinical	
Pineal tumors		+	Frequent Clinical	
Tumors with aqueductal obstruction and hydrocephalus		+		Cushingoid
Remote From Sella				
Cerebral hemispheres	+/−	+/−	Rare	
Meningioma glioma			Latent	

(Fahlbusch R, Marguth F. Endocrine disorders associated with intracranial tumors. In: Vinken PJ, Bruyn GW, eds. Handbook of clinical neurology: Tumours of the brain and skull. Part I, Vol 16. Amsterdam: North Holland, 1974:345)

involve the hypothalamus and compression of the third ventricle, leading to obstructive hydrocephalus and signs of increased intracranial pressure, such as headache and nausea and vomiting.

Some of the pituitary tumors produce secondary signs and symptoms, because they elaborate hormones that create various syndromes of endocrine hyperactivity (Table 48–7). A few pituitary tumors produce no detectable hormones or produce hormones in quantities that assume no clinical significance. Currently, it is uncommon for patients with endocrine-active tumors to present with large tumors; it is more common for patients with endocrine-inactive tumors to seek medical attention because of optic chiasmal compression-hypopituitarism as a consequence of a large mass. Compression leads to detectable hyposecretion of specific cells, with production of growth hormone being the most sensitive, followed closely by gonadotropins. Cells producing thyroid-stimulating hormone and corticotropin are much more resistant, and their function is impaired only at a later stage of growth.

Table 48–8 summarizes the differential diagnosis of tumors by location in children and adults.[50]

Acute and Life-Threatening Syndromes Caused by Intracranial Tumors

Because the brain and the spinal cord are surrounded by a rigid skull and dural membranes, expanding lesions within or abutting the brain or spinal cord can cause displacement of vital structures. This can lead, in the brain, to respiratory arrest and death and, in the spinal cord, to paraplegia or quadriplegia.

TABLE 48–7. Clinical Syndromes Produced by Endocrine-Activity Pituitary Adenomas

Hormone Produced	Clinical Syndrome
Prolactin	Amenorrhea and galactorrhea, impotence
Growth hormone	Gigantism and acromegaly
Corticotropin	Cushing's disease, Nelson's syndrome (after adrenalectomy)
Thyroid-stimulating hormone (rare)	Hyperthyroidism

TABLE 48–8. Differential Diagnosis of Tumors by Location and Age at Onset of Symptoms

Location	Child	Adult
Supratentorial	Astrocytoma	Metastatic
	Glioblastoma	Glioblastoma
	Oligodendroglioma	Astrocytoma
	Sarcoma	Meningioma
	Neuroblastoma	Oligodendroglioma
	Mixed glioma	Mixed glioma
Infratentorial	Astrocytoma	Metastatic
	Medulloblastoma	Astrocytoma
	Ependymoma	Glioblastoma
	Brain stem glioma	Ependymoma
		Brain stem glioma
Sellar and parasellar	Craniopharyngioma	Pituitary
	Optic glioma	Meningioma
	Epidermoid	
Base of the skull		Neurinoma
		Meningioma
		Chordoma
		Carcinoma
		Dermoid, epidermoid

To understand the sequence of events leading to temporal lobe-tentorial (uncal) herniation and cerebellar-foramen magnum herniation, a visual image of intracranial anatomy is needed. The tentorium cerebelli forms a rigid tissue partition between the cerebral hemispheres above and the cerebellum and brain stem below. Through this opening passes the midbrain centrally and cranial nerve III anterolaterally.

Immediately lateral to cranial nerve III lies the medial portion of the temporal lobe called the *uncus*. An expanding mass lesion situated above the tentorium may displace the uncus medially and inferiorly beneath the tentorium. Table 48–9 summarizes the neurologic findings and pathologic causes for the events that constitute the temporal lobe-tentorial herniation syndrome.[51]

A rapid increase in the volume of the supratentorial compartment leading to herniation can be caused by many different factors. A rapidly growing glioblastoma can present in this manner, although it is more usual for it to occur as a terminal or near-terminal event after ineffective therapy for the tumor. It can also occur when there is a dramatic increase in the amount of edema associated with metastasis to the brain or with hyponatremia and hypoosmolar syndromes. The injudicious use of parenteral hypoosmolar 5% dextrose in water often is sufficient to produce an abrupt increase in brain edema and temporal lobe herniation. These authors also have seen temporal lobe herniation follow a group of shortly spaced seizures. Presumably, the seizures, which are associated with hypoventilation, produce local hypoxia around the tumor with a resultant increase in brain edema.

Mass lesions in the infratentorial compartment can displace brain tissue upward through the tentorium, but more commonly force brain tissue downward through the foramen magnum. In this situation, the cerebellar tonsils move caudally through the foramen magnum, and in doing so, wedge against the medulla, causing the findings summarized in Table 48–10.

Cerebellar-foramen magnum herniation frequently results from, or is contributed to by, obstructive hydrocephalus. In such instances, emergency removal of fluid from the more cephalad ventricular system may relieve symptoms and be life saving. Surgical intervention is indicated only if the reason

TABLE 48–9. Temporal Lobe-Tentorial (Uncal) Herniation

Neurologic Findings	Pathologic Causes
Pupillary dilation and ptosis	Compression of ipsilateral oculomotor nerve between herniating tissue and petroclinoid ligament
Ipsilateral hemiplegia	Compression of contralateral cerebral peduncle against tentorium (Kernohan's notch)
Contralateral hemiplegia	Compression of ipsilateral cerebral peduncle; when associated with compression of contralateral peduncle, bilateral corticospinal tract signs
Homonymous hemianopia	Compression of posterior cerebral artery against the tentorium can lead to occipital ischemia or infarction and contralateral homonymous hemianopia; occasionally bilateral field cuts
Midbrain syndrome: Cheyne-Stokes respirations, stupor and coma, bipyramidal signs, decerebrate rigidity, dilated fixed pupils, gaze paresis, altered oculocephalic reflexes	Crushing of midbrain between herniating temporal lobe and leaf of tentorium associated with vascular occlusion and perivascular hemorrhages
Coma, rising blood pressure, and bradycardia	These late signs occur from rising intracranial pressure and hydrocephalus as the aqueduct is compressed and the subarachnoid space becomes compromised

(Adapted from Adams RD, Victor M. Principles of neurology. New York: McGraw-Hill, 1977:586)

TABLE 48–10. Cerebellar-Foramen Magnum Herniation

Neurologic Findings	Pathologic Causes
Head tilt, stiff neck, posturing of neck, or paresthesias over the neck	Downward displacement of inferior hemispheres through the foramen magnum; may be unilateral or bilateral
Tonic extensor spasms of limbs and body (cerebellar "fits") and later coma	Compressive effects of cerebellum or hydrocephalus on the upper brain stem
Respiratory arrest	Medullary compression

(Adapted from Adams RD, Victor M. Principles of neurology. New York: McGraw-Hill, 1977:586)

for the herniation is treatable. In the instance of cerebellar-foramen magnum herniation aggravated by acute obstructive hydrocephalus, ventriculoperitoneal shunting is often necessary. Care must be taken, however, because too rapid a change in the CSF dynamics can lead to a rapid and damaging movement of the brain, which can lead to occlusion of posterior cerebral arteries and brain stem injury.

These two herniation syndromes will lead to death, unless there is prompt intervention. The immediate intravenous administration of hyperosmotic agents, such as mannitol or urea, and large doses of synthetic glucocorticoids, such as dexamethasone or methylprednisolone, should be given promptly to reduce intracranial pressure and to avert impending death.

Hemorrhage into a tumor is not as common as might be expected, although the incidence of intratumor hemorrhage may increase because of iatrogenic thrombocytopenia associated with the current use of chemotherapy in the treatment of brain tumors. Primary tumors that most commonly bleed de novo are glioblastoma and oligodendrogliomas; of the metastatic tumors, those from the lung, melanoma, hypernephroma, and choriocarcinoma are most likely to be associated with intratumoral hemorrhage. Signs and symptoms of intratumoral hemorrhage may be temporized by the use of osmotic agents and glucocorticoids, but if extensive and life threat-

ening, operation and decompression are indicated. Under no circumstances should a lumbar puncture be performed in any of the acute herniation syndromes. In fact, lumbar puncture should never be done indiscriminately. The indications for lumbar puncture are discussed in another section of this chapter.

SPINAL AXIS

To understand the clinical presentation of tumors of the spinal axis, the local anatomy (Fig. 48–1) and how tumors might present with respect to anatomy must be appreciated. The cranial dura is firmly adherent to the skull (with the exception of dural duplications of the falx and tentorium), and no extradural space normally exists between dura and skull. An entirely different anatomic relation in the spinal canal accounts for a well-defined extradural space containing epidural fat and blood vessels. By way of the intervertebral foramina, this extradural space communicates with adjacent extraspinal compartments, for example, the mediastinum and the retroperitoneal space. With rare exceptions, extradural tumors are metastatic, reaching the extradural space through intervertebral foramina.

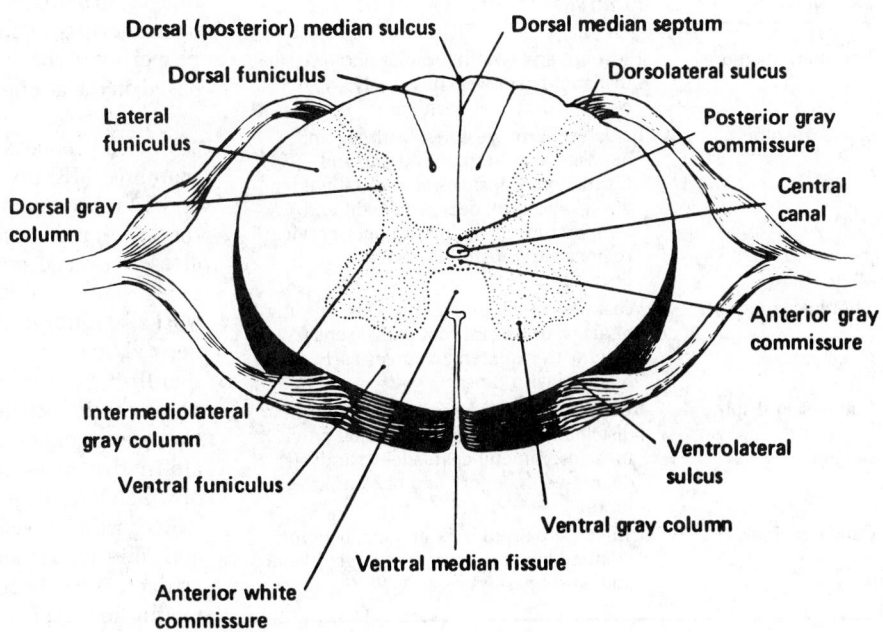

FIGURE 48–1. Cross-section of thoracic spinal cord shows relation of spinal nerves to intraspinal tracts.

Tumors arising inside of the dural tube (intradural tumors) may originate within the spinal cord (intramedullary), or they may take origin outside the spinal cord (extramedullary). The two common extramedullary intradural tumors, neurilemmoma (schwannoma) and meningioma, are attached, respectively, to sensory nerve roots and to dura and involve the spinal cord by compression.

Neurology of Spinal Cord Tumors

A spinal tumor produces two effects: local (focal) and distal (remote). Local effects indicate the tumor's location along the spinal axis, and distal effects reflect involvement of motor and sensory long tracts within the spinal cord. Table 48–11 summarizes the clinical findings useful in localizing a spinal cord tumor.

Distal effects are common to all spinal tumors sooner or later, and symptoms and signs are confined to structures innervated below the spinal cord level of involvement. Although neurologic manifestations commonly begin unilaterally, a full-blown Brown-Séquard's syndrome of cord hemisection can occur but is rare. More characteristic are motor changes: weakness and spasticity, if the tumor lies above the conus medullarus, or weakness and flaccidity, if at or below the conus. Typically, sensory impairment begins distally in the feet. Impairment of bladder function occurs later in tumors above the conus, but may be an early manifestation of tumors in or below the conus. The upper level of impaired long-tract function usually is several segments below the actual site of tumor involvement.

Local manifestations may reflect involvement of bone, with pain constituting the cardinal symptom of metastatic tumors. Involvement of spinal roots produces pain, sensory impairment, and weakness with atrophy in the appropriate radicular

TABLE 48–11.   Clinical Manifestations of Spinal Cord Tumors

Location	Findings
Foramen magnum	Eleventh and twelfth cranial nerve palsies; ipsilateral arm weakness early; cerebellar ataxia; neck pain
Cervical spine	Ipsilateral arm weakness with leg and opposite arm in time; wasting and fibrillation of ipsilateral neck, shoulder girdle, and arm; decreased pain and temperature sensation in upper cervical regions early; pain in cervical distribution
Thoracic spine	Weakness of abdominal muscles; sparing of arms; unilateral root pains; sensory level with ipsilateral changes early and bilateral with time
Lumbosacral spine	Root pain in groin region and sciatic distribution; weakened proximal pelvic muscles; impotence; bladder paralysis; decreased knee jerk and brisk ankle jerks
Cauda equina	Unilateral pain in back and leg, becoming bilateral when the tumor is large; bladder and bowel paralysis

distribution. Less often, involvement of spinal gray matter produced by extensive pressure from extramedullary tumors or direct damage by intramedullary tumors causes segmental sensory and motor changes.

Historically, tumors at or near the foramen magnum have been diagnosed incorrectly more often than have spinal tumors at any other site, because foramen magnum tumors can mimic such diverse conditions as multiple sclerosis, amyotrophic lateral sclerosis, and cervical disk disease. The frequency of delayed diagnoses of these tumors justifies the dictum that myelography or magnetic resonance imaging (MRI) is indicated as a diagnostic measure in any neurologic disease that can be accounted for by a lesion at or below the foramen magnum.

Occasionally, a cervical intramedullary tumor will mimic syringomyelia, with dissociated sensory loss, weakness, and wasting in the arms and hands and variable long-tract involvement. In most instances, the clinical presentation of a spinal tumor does not indicate if it is extradural or intradural.

The rate at which symptoms develop can be helpful in distinguishing extradural from intradural tumor, with a history of days to a few weeks characterizing metastatic extradural tumors, and a longer course, often many months, reflecting the slower growth of intradural tumors. A history of previously diagnosed cancer or other system involvement also is helpful.

NEURODIAGNOSTIC TESTS

NEUROIMAGING

The diagnosis of intracranial tumor requires radiographic confirmation. Fortunately, the great strides in radiology have yielded technologic advances best adapted for the brain and the spinal cord. Nuclear imaging, arteriography, and pneumoencephalography have been supplanted by the much more sensitive and descriptive techniques of MRI and CT. Both techniques are applicable to demonstrate intracranial and spinal lesions. Both CT and MRI produce cross-sectional digital images. In both, the depicted anatomy and pathology are based on numeric computerized representations of certain physical properties of the tissue.[52] The CT image is composed of pixels based on the attenuation of x-rays that are, in turn, dependent on the electron density of the tissue being studied. The MRI scan also produces an image based on pixels, but unlike CT scanning, MRI pixel intensity is based on proton density, T1 and T2 relaxation times, and flow (blood flow). The MRI scan, therefore, represents a complex interrelation of four parameters. Data acquisition also can be manipulated by the operator to a greater degree than can be done with CT scans. CT and MRI also differ in that MR data can be acquired in any plane desired, including oblique planes, in a primary fashion such that there is no compromise of spatial or contrast detail. CT scans can be acquired only in the axial or half-axial planes. Computer-generated reformations are required to generate alternative views, such as orthogonal and off-axis images, all of which have degradation of both spatial and contrast detail.

Because MRI scanning can generate images in any plane and offers high resolution and contrast without associated bone artifact, it has been shown to be superior to CT scan in detecting and localizing brain tumors and evaluating edema, hydrocephalus, or hemorrhage.[53] Unfortunately, MRI is not superior to CT in specificity.

Availability of modern imaging equipment varies with the economies of various communities. If MRI is unavailable, a CT scan after administration of iodinated contrast material is the imaging method of choice.

Intraaxial CNS tumors normally produce edema that is partially correlated with the rapidity of tumor growth. An exception is the benign cerebral meningioma, a slow-growing tumor that can produce profound edema. The so-called vasogenic edema associated with brain tumors is fluid that has leaked through an incompetent blood–brain barrier and is seen on the CT scan as relatively low attenuation compared with nor-

mal brain. On MRI, edema appears as an area of low-signal intensity on T1-weighted images and high-signal intensity on T2-weighted images.

Mass lesions in the brain can obstruct the ventricular system, resulting in hydrocephalus. MRI is perhaps slightly superior to CT in evaluating hydrocephalus and its causes, because more planes of view are available to the radiologist. Dilation of one or both of the lateral ventricles and not the rest of the ventricular system suggests obstruction at the foramen of Monro as is seen with colloid cysts or gliomas in this region. Dilation of a temporal horn of the ventricular system suggests a tumor in the ventricular atrium "trapping" the temporal horn. Dilation of only the lateral and third ven-

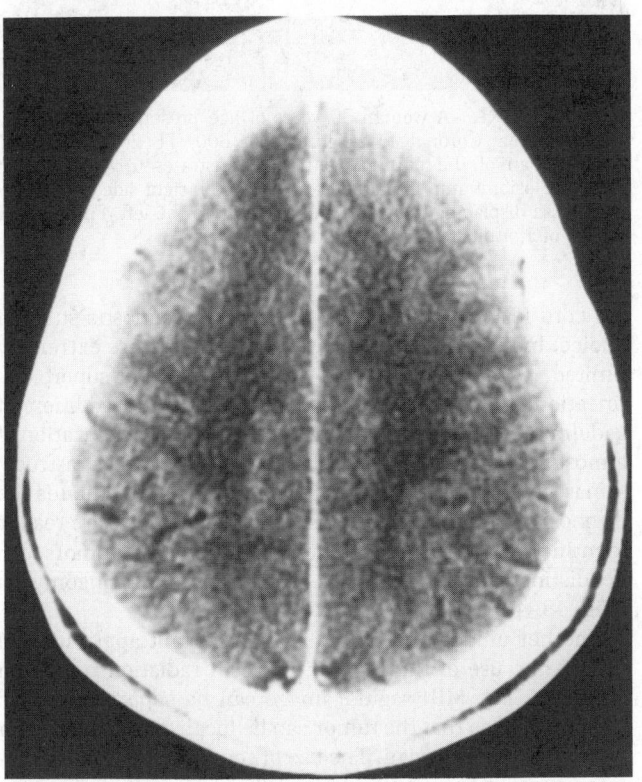

A

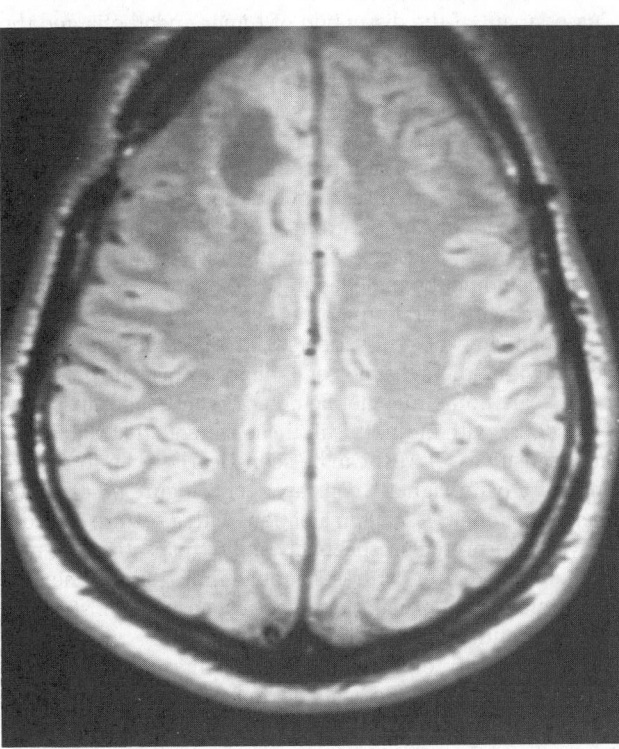

B

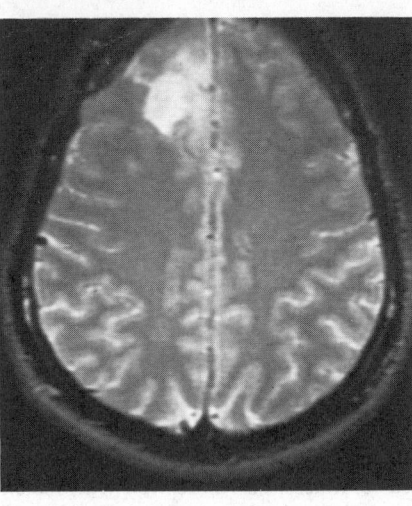

C

FIGURE 48–2. A young man presented with a single focal seizure that generalized into a major motor seizure. **(A)** A postcontrast axial CT demonstrates a poorly defined area of low density involving the most anterior portion of the corona radiata extending anteriorly to the gray matter on the right. No contrast enhancement, sulcal effacement, or mass effect is present. **(B)** After this CT scan, a T2-weighted (TR 2000, TE 20) axial MRI scan was performed that shows an area of decreased signal intensity at the gray-white junction at the most anterior medial aspect of the right frontal lobe. **(C)** On the second echo (TR 2000, TE 60), the lesion exhibits high signal intensity. On biopsy, the tumor was found to be a well-differentiated astrocytoma.

tricles points to a lesion of the aqueduct; when all the ventricles are dilated, communicating hydrocephalus caused by tumor seeding to the meninges or by the reaction to previous therapy should be considered.

Brain tumors occasionally bleed, and this bleeding can be insignificant or can cause dramatic clinical consequences. Metastatic brain tumors that tend to bleed are melanoma, renal cell carcinoma, choriocarcinoma, and thyroid carcinoma. Of the primary CNS tumors, glioblastoma and oligodendrogliomas are more commonly associated with hemorrhage than are other primary tumors. Acute hemorrhage appears as high attenuation on CT, but subacute hemorrhage may be harder to detect by CT. On MRI, acute hemorrhage is of low-signal intensity on T1 and T2; the subacute hemorrhage poorly seen on CT produces a bright signal on both T1- and T2-weighted MRI scans.

Assessment of the disruption of tumor endothelia and the passage of contrast material compared with the intact blood–brain barrier is an important step in radiologic evaluation. The use of contrast agents in CT and MRI scanning provides, in some patients, improved tumor visualization[54] and, in all patients, an improved ability to discern tumors from other pathologic entities, to discern one tumor type from another, and even to discern higher from lower grade malignancies.[55] There are few situations when administration of contrast agents should not be included in the radiologic evaluation of the patient with a brain tumor.

Approximately 50% of patients with low-grade gliomas may present with tumors that do not exhibit contrast enhancement on CT scan. Some may not be detected on CT because they are isodense with brain. It is in these patients that the differential sensitivity of MRI can be seen clearly, even in the absence of a paramagnetic contrast agent. Figure 48–2 shows an example of a CT scan on a patient with a seizure disorder that was interpreted prospectively and retrospectively as normal before and after contrast agent administration. The MRI scan is clearly abnormal. Stereotactic biopsy demonstrated a well-differentiated astrocytoma.

The possibility of obtaining high-quality coronal images without artifact associated with beam hardening through bone makes MRI particularly attractive for evaluating the base of the skull and the posterior fossa. Figure 48–3 is an example of a high-quality MRI scan on a patient with pituitary adenoma. Although this lesion would be identified readily on CT, the relation to the optic chiasm and infundibulum would certainly not be identified as clearly.

In the posterior fossa, the lack of artifact and the availability of sagittal and coronal planes make MRI uniquely suited for detecting and characterizing neoplasms. Both intraaxial and extraaxial masses are distinguished easily, and their relation to the ventricular cisternal systems is assessed easily.

In the evaluation of intracranial tumors, cerebral angiography is used much less frequently than in the past. Angiography may be used to confirm an impression on MRI or CT that the lesion in question is a vascular malformation or an aneurysm rather than a neoplasm. In certain situations, for example, with large meningiomas, angiography may be useful before surgery to determine the blood supply so that it can be embolized during the angiographic procedure or obliterated during the surgical procedure, or both.

In the evaluation of intramedullary and extramedullary spi-

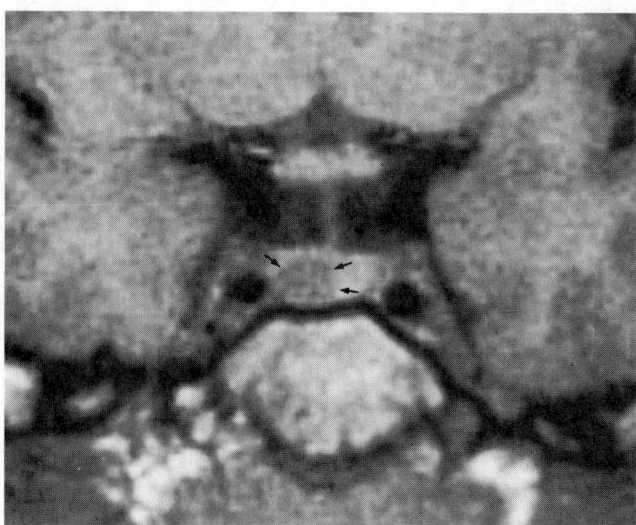

FIGURE 48–3. A woman 30 years of age presented with hyperprolactinemia. Coronal T1-weighted (TR 600, TE 20) 3-mm-thick section scan of the pituitary gland demonstrates (*arrows*) a low-intensity lesion 9 mm in diameter involving the right side of the pituitary fossa displacing the gland and the stalk to the left. Findings are typical of a pituitary microadenoma.

nal cord lesions, high-quality MRI is the diagnostic study of choice. Indications for myelography currently are extremely limited, because multiplanar MRI can provide superb delineation of the spinal cord contour, and the addition of gadolinium-DTPA provides enhancement and visualization of almost all intrinsic tumors (such as ependymomas, astrocytomas, meningiomas, and schwannomas) and facilitates the diagnosis of leptomeningeal disease.[56] Tumor cysts are readily identified on MRI, and currently spinal cord tumors can be distinguished much more reliably from syringomyelia (Fig. 48–4).

Another unique and particularly important application of MRI is the use of the sagittal image in radiation treatment planning. The MRI sagittal image can be superimposed on the port film so that the tumor can be localized accurately for appropriate port design. The use of the MRI scan is now routine in treatment planning of any base-of-skull or posterior fossa lesion.

TANGENT SCREEN, PERIMETRY, AUDIOMETRY, AND ELECTROENCEPHALOGRAPHY

Testing for abnormalities of the visual system is part of the neurologic examination. However, the results of confrontation visual field testing need quantitation to provide greater accuracy and to follow the effects of treatment. Formal visual field testing is done using tangent screens, and scotomas and field defects are diagnosed with perimetry. Figure 48–5 schematically represents the common visual field abnormalities and their anatomic localization.

Quantitation of deafness is performed by formal audiometric testing. This can be helpful in the diagnosis of acoustic neurinomas. The electrical equivalent of auditory signals can be observed by recording over the brain stem. These signals, called *auditory evoked responses*, correlate well with lesions in the brain stem and can be used to follow patients with brain

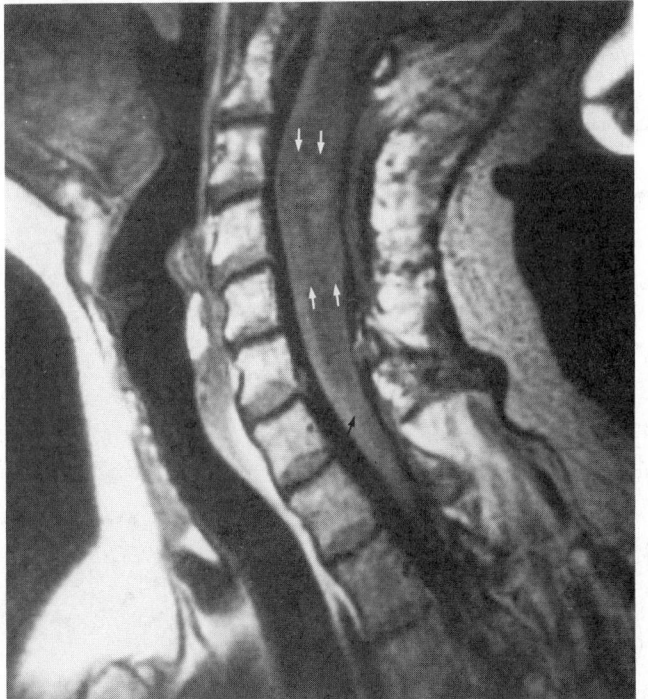

A

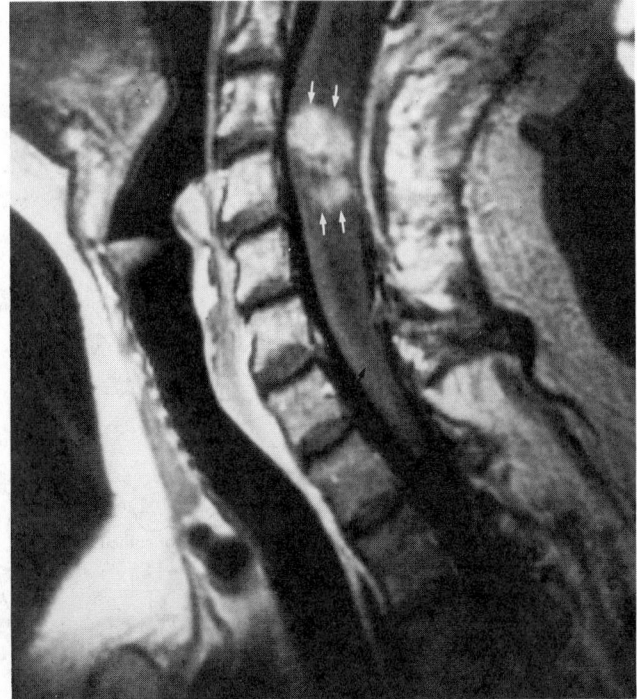

B

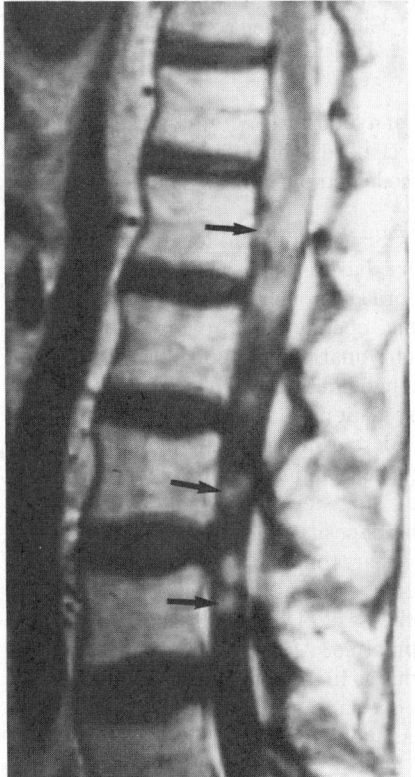

C

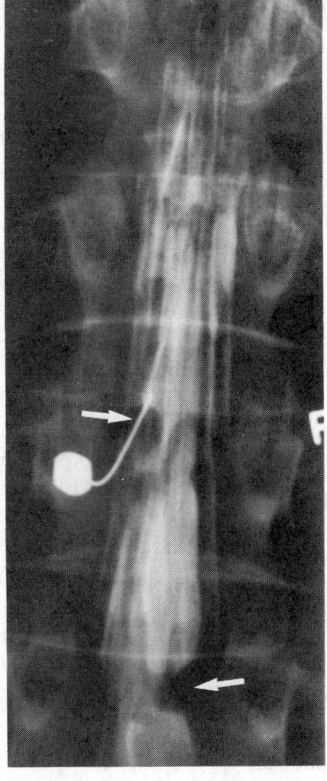

D

FIGURE 48–4. A 39-year-old man with a known cerebral glioblastoma multiforme developed spinal cord symptoms. **(A)** A T1-weighted (TR 600, TE 20) sagittal scan of the thoracolumbar spine shows mild heterogeneity of signal near the conus, but is otherwise normal. **(B)** A T2-weighted (TR 2000, SE 35,70) sagittal scan provides no additional information. **(C)** A T1-weighted (TR 600, SE 20) image after Gd-DTPA administration clearly shows high signal-enhancing tumor (*black arrows* show some of lesions) immediately caudad to the conus resulting in a high-grade partial block and multiple additional drop metastases. **(D)** A water-soluble contrast myelogram demonstrates the drop metastases (*white arrows* show some of lesions) and incompletely delineates the mass adjacent to the conus. (Courtesy of Gordon Sze, Department of Radiology, Yale University School of Medicine, New Haven, Connecticut)

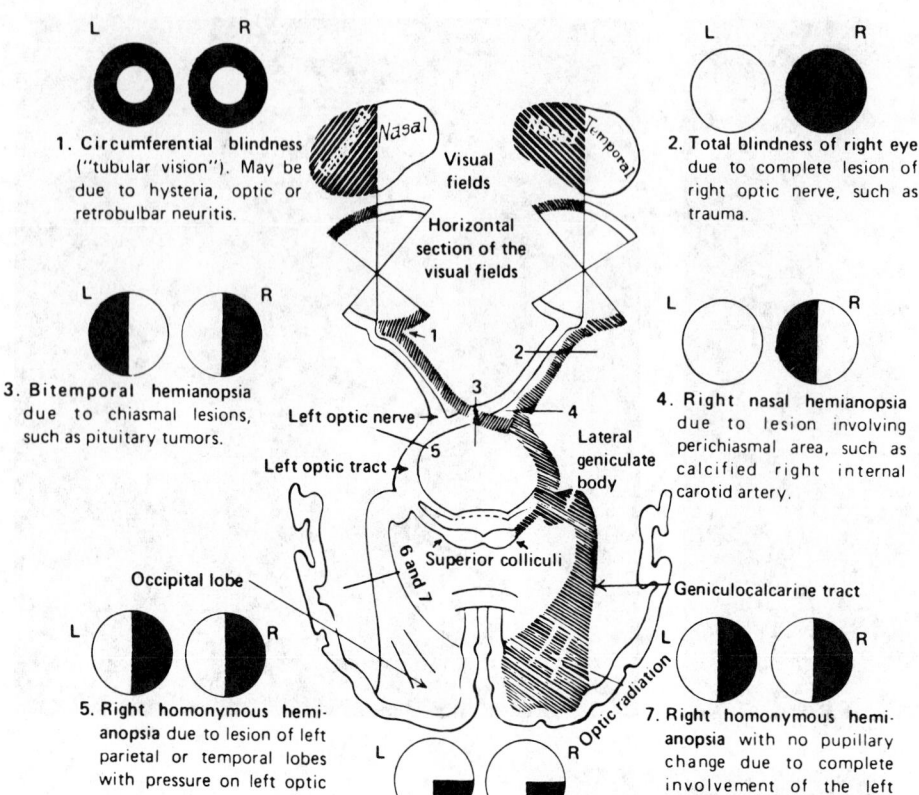

FIGURE 48–5. Schematic representation of the visual pathways and the effects lesions can have on the visual fields. (Chusid JG. Correlative neuroanatomy and functional neurology. Los Altos, CA: Lange, 1973)

stem tumors. Similar evoked potentials measured over the visual cortex after visual stimuli are less valuable in the evaluation or follow-up study of patients with brain tumors, but can help distinguish multiple sclerosis from tumor.

The electroencephalogram once had a place in the diagnosis and follow-up study of intracranial neoplasms. Its major value is in the diagnosis of seizure disorders and in following the rare patient whose neurologic deterioration may be related to subclinical seizures rather than tumor growth.

TUMOR AND CEREBROSPINAL FLUID MARKERS

For patients with intracranial and spinal tumors, examination of peripheral blood and CSF has been found to be helpful for diagnosis and for therapy monitoring. Pituitary tumors often produce endocrinologic abnormalities measurable by sensitive radioimmunoassays. Polycythemia associated with a tumor of the posterior fossa (cerebellum) may be useful as presumptive evidence for the diagnosis of hemangioblastoma. Some parasellar and pineal region embryonal tumors secrete unique hormones and proteins; β-human chorionic gonadotrophic hormone (β-HCG) and α-fetoprotein (AFP) are examples of hormones associated with trophoblastic tissue and yolk sac, respectively.[57,58] Finally, measurement of polyamines such as putrescine in the CSF is helpful in following patients with tumors located near the ventricle or spinal subarachnoid space; however, it is not widely used.[59]

INDICATIONS FOR AND INTERPRETATION OF CEREBROSPINAL FLUID EXAMINATION

Lumbar puncture in a patient with headache, papilledema, and a presumed diagnosis of tumor is risky, because it in-

creases the possibility of a fatal cerebellum-foramen magnum or temporal lobe-tentorial herniation. Lumbar puncture should follow rather than precede neuroimaging studies, such as MRI and CT scanning.

The examination of CSF is useful in following patients with intracranial tumors that have a propensity to seed the subarachnoid space and spread through the CSF pathways. Typically, medulloblastoma, ependymoma, choroid plexus carcinoma, and some embryonal pineal and suprasellar region tumors have a high enough likelihood of spread to justify CSF examinations. In these patients, it is important to obtain a lumbar puncture for CSF to examine for malignant cells (cytology), protein, and glucose and specific markers such as β-HCG and AFP. These tests determine if malignant cells are in the CSF and if tumor deposits have reached sufficient size to begin to block CSF subarachnoid pathways. A high protein concentration with normal glucose levels and normal cytology is seen in tumors of the base of the skull, such as acoustic neurinoma, and in spinal cord tumors. The appearance of xanthochromic CSF, due to high protein content, with an absence of erythrocytes is characteristic of spinal cord tumors obstructing the subarachnoid space and producing stasis of the CSF in the caudal lumbar sac.

Evaluation of Patients With Intracranial Tumors During Therapy

Critical to the evaluation of the efficacy of any therapy for brain tumors is the reliability of the measurement of tumor growth (deterioration) or tumor regression (response). Before MRI, sequential neurologic examinations, CT scans, and radionuclide scans were used to evaluate for response and regrowth.[60] Later, with improvement in CT scanners and to reduce the cost of therapy evaluations, contrast-enhanced CT scanning became the major method to evaluate patients for response and regrowth. Contrast-enhanced MRI scans are replacing CT scans in many instances. However, the extreme sensitivity of the MRI to changes in brain water content and small enhancing lesions can be confusing in the evaluation of tumor regrowth and progression. The use of magnetic resonance spectroscopy and diffusion-perfusion algorithms may improve the ability to assess tumor regrowth in the postirradiation period.

To interpret the results of therapy correctly and to improve patient care, understanding factors other than cell division is important; these are discussed in the following sections.

FACTORS THAT MAY PRODUCE CLINICAL DETERIORATION

The commonest causes of neurologic deterioration in brain tumor patients undergoing radiation therapy or chemotherapy, or both, are growth of the tumor or increased peritumoral edema. Both cause increased pressure in the cranial cavity that is transmitted primarily to the adjacent brain; in turn, hydrostatic pressure on the brain can lead to impairment of cerebral blood flow. The clinical result can be progressive impairment of functioning brain with resultant neurologic deficits. These manifestations may include signs and symptoms of increased intracranial pressure and temporal lobe or cerebellar herniation (see Tables 48–5 and 48–6).

Neurologic deterioration, without neuroimaging evidence of tumor growth, can occur for any of the following reasons:

1. Obstructive hydrocephalus can occur secondary to tumor in the ventricular system at the aqueduct of Sylvius, fourth ventricle, or foramen of Monro or communicating hydrocephalus due to infiltrative tumor (carcinomatosis, CNS leukemia, and arachnoiditis).
2. Hemorrhage into a tumor may occur.
3. Fluid imbalance, particularly hyponatremia caused by excessive administration of parenteral dextrose in water solutions, may develop.
4. Hypertension can accentuate intratumoral and peritumoral edema.
5. Reactive peritumoral edema (or demyelination) may develop early in the course of radiation therapy.
6. An "early-delayed" syndrome, observed in about 20% to 25% of patients completing a course of cranial irradiation, can be distinguished from tumor regrowth only by waiting and finding that the patient's condition improves without further treatment.[61] This encephalopathy responds to corticosteroids and resolves within several weeks without specific sequelae. This syndrome is not unique to patients with brain tumors, and is observed in leukemic children after prophylactic cranial irradiation.
7. Radiation necrosis can occur within 6 months to 10 years or longer after radiation therapy and can produce neurologic impairment that may be indistinguishable from tumor recurrence.
8. Seizures may suggest that the tumor is growing and may result in an increase in the neurologic deficit apart from any direct effect of the tumor. Recovery from any increase in weakness and mental dullness may take several hours to a week in postictal patients who are already brain injured. Even subclinical seizures can cause deterioration, persisting for hours to days, which resolves with control of the seizures. The electroencephalogram is usually diagnostic in these patients, and the treatment is better control of seizures. Patients receiving long-term chemotherapy often require higher doses of anticonvulsants or widely fluctuating dosages caused by drug-induced hepatic changes.
9. Infection and fever often exacerbate neurologic signs and symptoms, regardless of the site of infection. The more common causes of infection include pneumonia secondary to aspiration or atelectasis and urinary tract infections; meningitis and cerebral abscess are less common.
10. Metabolic disorders, anemia, fatigue, and emotional depression can cause clinical deterioration, including increase in focal deficit on testing, that is difficult to distinguish from tumor progression. Such conditions generally produce no alteration of neuroimages.

In these authors' experience, at least 10% of patients who eventually respond to therapy become significantly worse at the end of a first course of chemotherapy, and transient deterioration is observed occasionally even during the second year of continuous chemotherapy. Paradoxically, this clinical worsening early in therapy may result from an increase in tumor bulk resulting from "effective" therapy. Several factors contribute: cell mass may increase when doomed cells form giant cells or undergo one or more successful cell divisions before dying; the CNS also has an inefficient mechanism for disposing of dead cells produced by chemotherapy or irradiation; and edema, probably caused by irritative products of cell lysis, may be present within the tumor mass and in adjacent brain.

GLUCOCORTICOID USAGE

Administration of glucocorticoids is usually begun before surgery for brain tumor. If an adequate surgical decompression is achieved, the steroid dose can be tapered off rapidly and discontinued within the first week or two after the operation. Some patients require steroid maintenance because a large volume of tumor remains, because tumor occupies the brain stem or spinal cord, or because of steroid dependence resulting from long-term prior usage.

Patients who no longer require corticosteroids after surgery may need them during or after radiation therapy. Reactive edema may occur during irradiation, and there may be a transient period of drowsiness and increased deficit for 6 to 16 weeks after treatment. In both instances, signs and symptoms usually resolve within a few weeks; observation of the subsequent clinical course is often the only way to differentiate these reactions from tumor progression.

The lowest dosage of glucocorticoid that maintains patients at their maximum level of comfort and function should be sought. Ordinarily, this is determined by decreasing the dosage until symptoms increase or become apparent, then increasing the dosage until they subside. If deterioration is secondary to tumor growth or treatment-induced effects, glucocorticoids may have to be increased to keep the patient comfortable. For example, 3 mg/day of dexamethasone may have the desired effect for a patient with stabilized disease; however, a deteriorating patient may require dexamethasone doses of 64 mg/day or more.

The efficacy of chemotherapy and radiation therapy can be affected by glucocorticoid dosage. A decrease in steroid requirement suggests improvement, assuming that the previous dosage was actually required. An increase in dosage suggests deterioration. Because increased glucocorticoid dosage may improve neurologic status and reduce the image size on an MRI and CT scan, an attempt should be made to document tumor recurrence before increasing glucocorticoid dosage.

SURGERY

GENERAL CONSIDERATIONS

No other modality can reduce tumor bulk as quickly as surgery, and advances in imaging, pharmacologic agents for brain edema, neuroanesthesia, and surgical magnification, illumination, and instrumentation have made operative approaches to tumors in even the most remote corners of the CNS possible and reasonably safe. The goal of brain tumor surgery is to resect and cure the tumor completely. If surgical cure is not possible, such as in most gliomas, tumor bulk reduction and consequent decompression of the brain is the next goal and, when possible, should be the first therapeutic modality for the tumor.

An extremely important byproduct of cytoreductive surgery is the acquisition of adequate tissue for histopathologic examination. Only rarely should brain tumors be treated with irradiation or chemotherapy without a definitive tissue diagnosis. In patients with tumors that are believed to be inaccessible by open craniotomy or in patients for whom open craniotomy is deemed unhelpful, a needle biopsy should be performed with guidance from CT, MRI, or ultrasound. CT-guided stereotaxy is the easiest method for obtaining tissue with a needle.

SURGICAL PLANNING

The intrinsic characteristics of a tumor's appearance and its relative position in the brain as shown on a technically adequate MRI scan can most often narrow the diagnostic possibilities to one or two choices, and a view of the tumor in several planes simplifies surgical planning.

Cerebral angiography is important in surgical planning for tumors that may encircle critical cerebral blood vessels, such as basal meningiomas, or for tumors that can be extremely vascular, such as hemangioblastomas, meningiomas, and glomus tumors. Angiography done in temporal proximity (24–96 hours) to the planned surgical procedure can be combined with embolization of the tumor's blood supply, in many instances making the surgical procedure technically easier.

The final selection of a surgical approach is made after adequate imaging, after developing a differential diagnosis, and after assessing the patient's general condition. In the era of modern neuroanesthesia, it is rare that a craniotomy must not be done because of poor general medical status. The design of an appropriate scalp incision and bone flap is the final preoperative decision.

PREOPERATIVE AND ANESTHETIC MANAGEMENT

Patients undergoing surgery for supratentorial tumors should be placed on anticonvulsants, and corticosteroids commonly (dexamethasone) should be administered for a few days preoperatively, when possible, to reduce cerebral edema and thereby facilitate cerebral retraction for perfect exposure. Blood levels of anticonvulsants should be monitored to ensure that the therapeutic range has been achieved. Anticonvulsants should also be continued for at least 1 year. Corticosteroids should be continued into the postoperative period and then tapered, when possible. The anesthetic agents are selected for their lack of effect on intracranial pressure. In general, the head is held rigidly with pin fixation to minimize movement as the surgeon is looking through the operating microscope, where the slighest movement is dramatically amplified. As the procedure is about to commence, mannitol (1 g/kg body weight) is administered and hyperventilation to a Pco_2 of 25 to 30 mm Hg is accomplished for definitive reduction of the intracranial pressure in preparation for brain retraction. These authors routinely administer bromodeoxyuridine intravenously during the induction of anesthesia to obtain a labeling index of the tumor on the fixed tissue postoperatively.[62]

CRANIOTOMY FOR SUPRATENTORIAL TUMORS

The bony opening is designed so that it is generous enough to facilitate surgery. The bone flap is centered over the tumor or positioned to provide access to the route of approach. In all instances, the scalp flap is designed to accommodate the bone flap fully, and the vascular supply to the scalp is given careful consideration in the design.

After the scalp incision is made and the scalp flap reflected, burr holes are drilled and connected with a hand or power saw. The bone flap can be turned back, attached to the temporal muscle (osteoplastic flap) or its blood supply, or removed completely (free flap). The dura is opened only after the brain has been softened completely by mannitol diuresis and intraoperative hyperventilation. Sometimes a few minutes' wait is necessary to secure maximum decompression, and this brief pause can be critical to the success of the subsequent surgical approach.

The dura is reflected back, and the approach to the tumor is made. The surgeon can be confused by a field of normal-appearing cortex when seeking to expose a small subcortical lesion. In this situation, intraoperative ultrasonography is invaluable in delineating the position of a small tumor, and a cortical incision can be made directly over the lesion, thereby minimizing cortical injury. Tumor removal is usually done with grasping instruments, sponges, and suction, but removal of firm, adherent, or calcified tumor tissue can be difficult and is simplified by use of the Cavitron ultrasonic aspirator (CUSA), which ultrasonically disrupts the tumor at its tip and sucks it away. Tumor in locations where access is limited (for example, the third ventricle) and space to use graspers and other equipment is not available sometimes can be dealt with best by use of the CO_2 laser, which can vaporize tumor tissue with a "hands off" technique. Tumor removal with a laser is slow, however, and is reserved for special circumstances.

In the rare situations when brain swelling is worrisome at the time of closure, a catheter is left in the subdural space to measure the intracranial pressure. All patients are monitored in the intensive care unit for at least 1 night after surgery, and a CT scan is done within 48 hours to evaluate the success of the tumor resection. Serum electrolyte levels and osmolality are measured often in the postoperative period to ensure that the patient is relatively dehydrated through the first several days and to detect the possible onset of inappropriate secretion of antidiuretic hormone or diabetes insipidus.

CRANIOTOMY FOR POSTERIOR FOSSA TUMORS

The occiput and, commonly, the dorsal aspects of C1 and C2 are exposed. A generous craniotomy is done unilaterally or bilaterally to accommodate an approach through the vermis or through, over, or around the cerebellar hemisphere. A laminectomy of C1 and sometimes C2 is done in certain midline approaches to improve tumor exposure or extend the decompression. The CO_2 laser occasionally is more valuable than the CUSA in posterior fossa tumor resections because of the tight working space.

STEREOTACTIC TUMORS BIOPSY

For intrinsic tumors of the deep midline, for example, pontine or corpus callosum gliomas, for deep tumors of the dominant hemisphere, or for diffuse nonfocal tumors, surgical resection is not practical. In these situations, needle biopsy for diagnosis is essential. There is no longer any reason to perform a full craniotomy for the purpose of biopsy only. Tissue can be obtained through a needle directed by hand through a burr hole under CT scan guidance or a needle directed by many devices that incorporate ultrasound images. However, in these authors' opinion, nothing is as simple or accurate as CT- or MRI-directed stereotactic biopsy.

A number of image-guided stereotactic systems are available.[63,64] Figure 48–6 shows the general sequence of events using the Brown-Roberts-Wells guidance technique. Typically, the patient undergoes a CT scan with a rigid array of bars affixed tightly to the skull to minimize movement. In adults, local anesthesia usually is used; children usually require general anesthesia. The CT scan image demonstrates the lesion in which the biopsy will be performed and also the localizing rods, thereby relating the target to a volume encompassed by the rods. By digitizing the position of the target and the position of the rods, this relation is formalized, and the coordinates for a trajectory to the target are created in a way specific to the individual stereotactic system used.

The target is approached through a burr hole or a (smaller) twist drill hole. The biopsy instrument is guided to the target by use of an adjustable stereotactic arc that is placed on the head in fixed relation to the former position of the localizing rods used for the CT scan. A fragment of tissue is aspirated or grasped for removal, and a frozen section confirms the acquisition of diagnostic material and most often also suggests a working diagnosis. Experienced surgeons obtain diagnostic tissue in more than 95% of patients, and these patients stay only 1 night in the hospital.[64] The principal risk of the surgery, hemorrhage at the biopsy site, occurs in few patients.[64] Occasionally, cerebral edema is exacerbated by the procedure.

RADIATION THERAPY

GENERAL CONSIDERATIONS

Most primary CNS neoplasms are unifocal and, therefore, they are potentially curable with effective local forms of therapy. However, most of these lesions infiltrate for a considerable distance into surrounding normal CNS tissue, and their borders are poorly demarcated, even by CT scan or MRI. Therefore, it is often necessary to irradiate a substantial amount of normal tissue within the target volume to relatively high doses, and the tolerance of these tissues to irradiation becomes a limiting factor. As local treatments become more aggressive, as in the case of malignant gliomas, the incidence of radiation injury will probably increase.

TOLERANCE OF THE BRAIN

Adverse reactions associated with cranial irradiation differ in their pathogenesis and can be classified according to their time of presentation into (1) acute reactions that occur during or shortly after radiation therapy; (2) early-delayed reactions that appear within a few weeks to 2 or 3 months after irradiation; and (3) late-delayed injuries that develop several months to years after treatment.[65]

Acute reactions are thought to be caused by radiation-induced edema and to include symptoms of increased intracranial pressure if the whole brain is treated or if there is an intensification of preexisting neurologic symptoms or signs when the treatment is confined to the location of the lesion. Symptoms are generally mild and self-limited and, if necessary, can be treated effectively with corticosteroids. A dose of 60 Gy in conventional daily dose fractions of 1.8 to 2 Gy, five times per week, can be given to all or part of the brain without significant acute morbidity. Hyperfractionated irradiation schedules of 0.9 to 1.2 Gy, two or three times daily, to doses as high as 81.6 Gy, and accelerated fractionation programs of 1.6 to 2 Gy given two or three times daily to approximately 60 to 70 Gy delivered to a portion of the brain are also acutely tolerable. Individual dose fractions as much as 6 Gy to the whole brain are well tolerated, provided that the total administered dose is reduced coincident with the increase in fraction size. Severe complications, however, have been observed with higher dose fractions.[66]

The early-delayed reaction, characterized by somnolence or an exacerbation of preexisting signs and symptoms, is thought to result from temporary demyelination caused by the effects of radiation on oligodendroglial cells[61] or radiation-induced changes in capillary permeability.[67] In addition, early vascular abnormalities and tumor necrosis may induce clinical and radiographic changes that are indistinguishable from tumor progression.[68] Although signs and symptoms are usually mild, corticosteroid therapy and intensive medical support may be required. The appearance of new findings during this early posttreatment interval does not always indicate that the tumor has recurred or that a change in therapy is needed.

Late-delayed radiation injuries constitute the most serious aftereffects of therapeutic irradiation on the brain and vary in their appearance and severity from asymptomatic white matter changes to potentially fatal necrosis. The late-delayed reaction presents as a focal or as a diffuse white matter injury

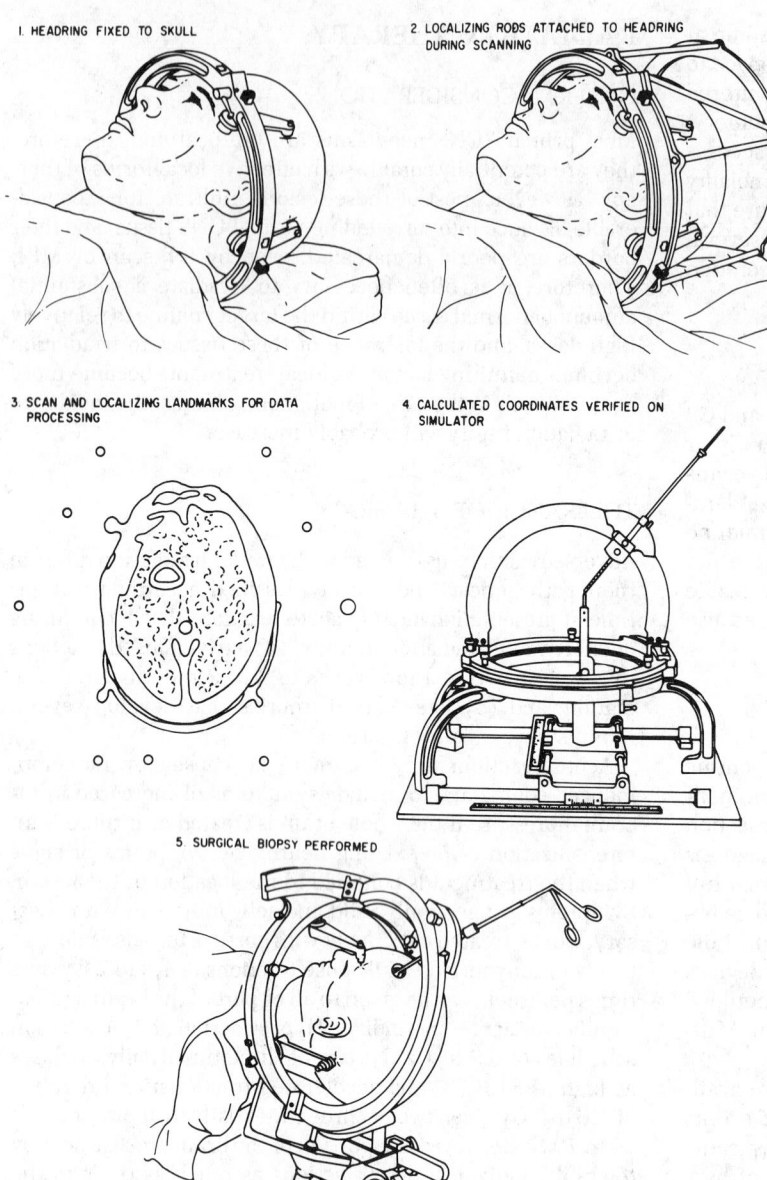

1. HEADRING FIXED TO SKULL

2. LOCALIZING RODS ATTACHED TO HEADRING DURING SCANNING

3. SCAN AND LOCALIZING LANDMARKS FOR DATA PROCESSING

4. CALCULATED COORDINATES VERIFIED ON SIMULATOR

5. SURGICAL BIOPSY PERFORMED

FIGURE 48–6. Steps and typical equipment used for CT-guided stereotactic biopsy. The equipment depicted is part of the Brown-Roberts-Wells guidance technique. (Weiss MH. Clinical neurosurgery. In: Proceedings of the Congress of Neurological Surgeons. Baltimore: Williams & Wilkins, 1983)

that may occur together in the same patient. The clinical presentation depends on the site and volume of the brain exposed. Patients with focal radiation necrosis present with localizing neurologic signs, often accompanied by symptoms of increased intracranial pressure. Focal hypodensity or a contrast-enhancing mass with surrounding vasogenic edema may be seen on CT scan. MR images show a contrast-enhancing mass with focal hyperintensity on T2-weighted images. Diffuse white matter injury typically occurs after large-volume or whole-brain irradiation. Clinical features include seizure disorders and varying degrees of neuropsychological impairment. Diffuse white matter hypodensity is seen on CT scan, often accompanied by a focal enhancing mass, whereas T2-weighted MR images show diffuse periventricular white matter hyperintensity.[69] Late radiation injury has been attributed to vascular injury or to a direct effect on glial cells, and multiple mechanisms are probably involved.[65] Rarely, therapeutic irradiation causes an intracranial vessel occlusive vasculopathy[70,71] or secondary neoplasia.[71]

The tolerance of the brain depends on the size of the dose per fraction and the total dose administered. The probability of injury increases with larger daily doses and doses in excess of 60 Gy delivered in 30 fractions over approximately 6 weeks. Sheline and associates suggested that the threshold doses for brain injury are approximately 35 Gy for 10 fractions, 60 Gy for 35 fractions, and 76 Gy for 60 fractions.[72] They further demonstrated that the isoeffective dose (termed *neuret*) formula should have an exponent of $N = -0.41$ and an exponent of $T = -0.03$ (where N is the number of fractions and T is the total time in days), but they warned that this formula may not be applicable to extremely small or large numbers of fractions or to extremely short or long overall treatment times.

Approximately 4% to 9% of patients treated for brain tumors develop clinically detectable focal radiation necrosis, and this form of injury may be found in as many as 15% to 22% of patients at autopsy. A review by Marks and colleagues of 139 patients who received irradiation for primary brain tumors with at least 45 Gy in daily dose fractions of 1.8 to 2 Gy disclosed 7 patients with brain necrosis.[73] A recalculation of their data, assuming a daily dose of 1.8 Gy given five times per week, demonstrated that the incidence of necrosis was directly related to dose. Of 51 patients who received total doses of 57.6 Gy or less, there were no cases of necrosis. Two of 60 patients (3%) who received between 57.6 and 64.8 Gy developed necrosis, and 5 of 28 patients (18%) who received 64.8 to 75.6 Gy developed necrosis.[74]

Several additional factors may affect the radiation tolerance of the brain. Children younger than 2 to 3 years of age are thought to be more susceptible to injury than are adults because of incomplete development of the CNS.[72] Vasculopathy associated with endocrine disorders,[75] CNS infection,[76] and cerebral edema[77] also appear to potentiate the effects of radiation.

The risk of injury may be amplified by some chemotherapeutic agents.[78] The most dramatic illustration of the toxicity of combined modality therapy was observed in children with acute lymphoblastic leukemia treated with prophylactic brain irradiation and methotrexate administered intravenously and intrathecally. Two delayed syndromes, necrotizing leukoencephalopathy and mineralizing microangiopathy, have been recognized in children who received 24 Gy in 1.5 to 2 Gy daily increments, which without chemotherapy are well below tolerance levels. Although necrotizing leukoencephalopathy has not been reported with a dose of 24 Gy in the absence of chemotherapy and occurs in fewer than 1% to 2% of patients receiving intrathecal and high-dose intravenous methotrexate, the incidence with all three therapies combined is as high as 45%.[79] It is currently recognized that methotrexate is most toxic when given during or after radiation therapy, and attention to this detail has reduced the frequency of this complication significantly.

Because radiation-induced changes are often indistinguishable from tumor recurrence on CT and MRI, the clinical diagnosis of radiation necrosis may be difficult to confirm. Thallium 201 single-photon emission computed tomography (SPECT)[80] and F-18 fluorodeoxyglucose positron emission tomography (PET)[81] studies may help separate patients with radiation necrosis from those with recurrent tumor. However, a biopsy may be required to confirm the diagnosis, especially when the injury occurs at or near the tumor site.

Corticosteroids may improve or stabilize the neurologic symptoms associated with the effects of radiation injury. Surgical resection is often beneficial to patients with favorably situated, focal radiation-induced lesions who deteriorate neurologically and become dependent on corticosteroids.[81]

Decreased levels of intellectual function have been observed after cranial irradiation in children and adults with acute lymphoblastic leukemia, small cell lung carcinoma, and primary brain tumors. IQ decrements and perceptual and learning disabilities seen after CNS prophylaxis in children with acute lymphoblastic leukemia have long been attributed to cranial irradiation. However, a recent study comparing the long-term cognitive outcome of children treated with 18 or 24 Gy and intrathecal methotrexate or intrathecal and intravenous methotrexate without cranial irradiation failed to demonstrate an overall decline in verbal, performance, or full-scale IQ in any of the three groups, although 22% to 30% of children in each group showed at least a 15-point decline in IQ during the study period. The authors proposed that ecologic factors

or continuation-phase chemotherapy rather than radiation therapy might account for the IQ changes.[82]

Neuropsychological deterioration has been recognized in long-term surviving patients with small cell lung carcinoma who receive prophylactic cranial irradiation. These patients are treated with a variety of chemotherapeutic agents that may enhance the effects of radiation on the CNS. The risk and severity of impairment appear to be related to radiation dose and fraction size and to the type, sequence, and dose intensity of the chemotherapeutic agents used.[83]

Children irradiated for brain tumors have IQ decrements and behavioral disturbances. Most require formal psychological intervention and special education programs. Young age at treatment, supratentorial tumor sites, the use of whole-brain irradiation, poorly controlled seizure disorders, the presence of sensorimotor deficits, and the addition of chemotherapy have a negative influence on IQ.[84] The risk and severity of neuropsychological dysfunction are also affected by psychological stress, reduced school attendance, and the adequacy of rehabilitative efforts.[85]

Cranial irradiation also leads to intellectual impairment in adults. Unlike in children, however, only a limited amount of quantitative information is available, especially for patients treated with radiation therapy alone. Impairment is most pronounced in those patients who have had chemotherapy and whole-brain irradiation.[85] Decrements in tests of new learning ability, recent memory, abstraction, and problem solving have been observed,[86] and early return to work after treatment may lead to improvement or recovery of neuropsychological function.[87]

Radiation therapy may cause hypothalamic-pituitary dysfunction, and the incidence and degree of hormone suppression appear to be dose related, with a threshold of approximately 25 to 30 Gy.[88] Growth hormone deficiency is the most frequent endocrine dysfunction observed after radiation therapy. Children who undergo irradiation to the hypothalamic-pituitary axis should be evaluated for pituitary function before, and periodically after, irradiation. Early detection of a deficiency permits appropriate hormonal replacement therapy before irreversible damage has occurred.

TOLERANCE OF THE SPINAL CORD

Radiation myelopathy may present as a transient early-delayed or as a more ominous late-delayed reaction. Transient radiation myelopathy is clinically manifested by momentary, electrical shock-like paresthesias or numbness radiating from the neck to the extremities, precipitated by neck flexion (Lhermitte's sign). The syndrome develops after an average latent period of 3 to 4 months and gradually resolves over the ensuing 3 to 6 months without the need for specific therapy. These findings have been attributed to transient demyelination caused by radiation-induced inhibition of myelin-producing oligodendroglial cells in the irradiated cord segment.[89] An alternative hypothesis suggests that radiation induces a transient disruption of the blood–spinal cord barrier, resulting in vasogenic edema, which in turn leads to demyelination.[67]

Radiation myelopathy is one of the most feared complications in clinical radiotherapy. In addition to its obvious neurologic sequelae, about 50% of patients die from secondary complications.[90] The latent period between the completion of radiation therapy and the onset of symptoms is bimodal in distribution, with the first peak occurring at 12 to 14 months and the second occurring at 24 to 28 months. A dual mechanism of injury has been suggested to explain the bimodal distribution of presentation. The earlier peak is associated with demyelination and white matter necrosis due to a direct effect on oligodendroglial cells, whereas the later peak results from intramedullary microvascular injury. The signs and symptoms that accompany radiation myelopathy are irreversible. They may be partial in some patients, whereas in others there is progressive functional loss that becomes complete over several months. Less commonly, radiation myelopathy is manifested by the acute onset of paraplegia or quadriplegia that evolves over several hours or a few days, resulting from infarction of the cord. Myelopathy may also be heralded by lower motor neuron dysfunction due to selective injury to anterior horn cells.[91]

The diagnosis of radiation myelopathy requires a history of radiation therapy in doses sufficient to result in injury. The portion of the cord irradiated must be slightly above the dermatome level of expression of the lesion, and the latent period from the completion of treatment to the onset of injury must be consistent with that observed in radiation myelopathy. There are no confirmatory laboratory tests or imaging studies that distinguish radiation myelopathy from other spinal cord lesions, and the diagnosis is often one of exclusion.

The medical and legal consequences of radiation myelopathy are such that treatment with radiation therapy is often compromised to keep the spinal cord dose within a "safe" level.[92] A dose of 50 Gy in 25 fractions over 5 weeks usually is considered to be safe, the risk of myelopathy being less than 0.5%.[92] The dose of 40 to 45 Gy commonly given to the spinal cord in head and neck irradiation appears to be well below the steep portion of the dose-response curve.[92] It is estimated that with conventionally fractionated irradiation (1.8–2 Gy per fraction, five fractions per week), the incidence of myelopathy is 5% for doses in the range of 57 to 61 Gy and 50% for doses of 68 to 73 Gy.[93] At doses higher than the tolerance threshold, the risk of injury increases with the length of cord irradiated.[94] There is no convincing evidence that the cervical and thoracic cord differ in their radiosensitivity. The belief that the cervical cord is more tolerant than the thoracic cord probably arose from differences in biologic dose resulting from the practice of treating with one field per day, which was common through the mid-1970s.[93]

Various isoeffect formulas have been proposed for the spinal cord. Wara and coworkers derived an Ellis-type formula with an exponent of N = −0.377 and an exponent of T = −0.058.[95] Van der Kogel and Berendsen concluded that the isoeffect formula should have an N exponent of −0.4 and that for treatment times as long as 6 weeks, the time factor was essentially negligible.[96] These formulas suggest that in addition to the total dose given, radiation myelopathy is related to the size of the individual daily dose and predict that spinal cord tolerance will continue to increase with decreasing fraction size. However, data indicate that reducing the fraction size to lower than 2 Gy does not alter the dose response significantly,[97] and that extrapolating from a conventionally fractionated cord dose to an equivalent hyperfractionated cord dose using any isoeffect formula should be approached with caution.[93]

TUMOR TARGET VOLUME AND TREATMENT TECHNIQUES

The appropriate volume to encompass within the radiation treatment portal varies according to the specific histopathologic tumor type and, with certain histologies, is a topic of considerable controversy. Because their tendency to infiltrate beyond the lesional borders visualized by neuroimaging studies is limited, certain tumors, such as benign meningiomas, pituitary adenomas, craniopharyngiomas, and acoustic neurilemmomas, may be treated with narrow margins of surrounding normal tissue. In contrast, the astrocytic gliomas require larger margins for uncertainty because of their tendency to infiltrate beyond the identifiable tumor periphery. Improved imaging techniques and a better understanding of recurrence patterns have fostered the use of limited radiation portals rather than whole-brain irradiation for malignant gliomas. Comparisons of CT and MRI studies with clinical and pathologic findings have shown that (1) malignant gliomas are localized, and microscopic invasion of the perilesional brain is limited at the time of initial diagnosis[98]; (2) only 1.1% of patients present with multiple lesions[99]; (3) after initial treatment, most of these lesions, when they recur, do so at their original location[100]; and (4) isolated tumor cell infiltration may extend to the periphery of T2-weighted MRI abnormalities.[101] Clinical studies have failed to demonstrate that irradiating the whole brain is superior to treating more limited fields,[74] and patients surviving for extended periods after whole-brain irradiation, especially in combination with chemotherapy, may suffer considerable treatment-related morbidity.[85] Until the primary tumor can be controlled with greater frequency, and the patterns of failure in such patients suggest that local fields are unjustified, there is little rationale for treating the whole brain.

The radiation-beam energy and field arrangements are selected after consideration of the location of the tumor within the brain and the geometry of the target volume. The *tumor volume* is defined as a three-dimensional reconstruction of the tumor contour based on operative findings and data from CT and MRI studies. The *target volume* consists of the volume of tissue that must be irradiated to encompass the tumor volume with a margin of surrounding tissue considered to be at risk for microscopic tumor spread and to account for patient movement and daily set-up uncertainties. Depending on tumor size and location, treatment portals may be coaxially opposed or designed in a more complex fashion, using multiple or rotational fields with wedge filters. Three-dimensional conformal radiation therapy is a new method of treatment planning and delivery designed to enhance the conformation of the dose to the target volume, while maximally restricting the dose delivered to the normal tissue outside the treatment volume. In the future, this approach may improve the outcome of patients with brain tumors by allowing higher than traditional radiation doses to be administered safely. Megavoltage equipment with energies ranging from cobalt 60 to 15 MeV photons is used to administer radiation therapy. Treatment is generally given in daily fractions of 1.72 to 2 Gy/day five times per week. The total doses referred to in this chapter assume that this "conventional" fractionation scheme is used unless otherwise specified.

Certain neoplasms, such as medulloblastomas and primitive

neuroectodermal tumors, require treatment to the entire craniospinal axis. Patients are treated prone in an immobilization cast to ensure daily positional reproducibility. The intracranial contents, including the upper one or two segments of the cervical cord, are treated through opposed lateral fields. The spine is treated through one or two posterior fields, depending on the size of the patient. The collimator for the lateral cranial fields is angled to match the divergence of the upper border of the adjacent spinal field, and the treatment couch is angulated so that the inferior border of the cranial field is perpendicular to the superior edge of the spinal field. Individualized focused blocks protect the normal extracranial head and neck tissues from the primary radiation beam. The cranial and posterior spine fields may be abutted, but a gap of 0.5 to 1 cm is often left between the fields. When two posterior spinal fields are used, as is usually the case, a gap is calculated so that the 50% isodose lines meet at the level of the spinal cord. All junction lines are moved 0.5 to 1 cm daily or at least every 10 Gy to avoid overdosing or underdosing segments of the cord. This is accomplished by expanding the lateral cranial fields and moving the posterior spine fields caudally without changing their dimensions. A fixed block is placed at the inferior margin of the caudal spinal field to keep the lower margin of the irradiated volume at the same location. Several modifications of this approach are used in clinical practice.

CHEMOTHERAPY

GENERAL PHARMACOLOGIC CONSIDERATIONS

The use of anticancer agents in the treatment of intracranial and spinal tumors is established for many primary tumors. For parenchymal CNS tumors, however, controversy surrounds the concept of limited antitumor efficacy for agents with restricted blood–brain barrier permeability.[102] Supporting the concept is the fact that many infiltrative primary CNS tumors (*e.g.*, gliomas) have cellular regions within the brain with apparently intact normal-appearing brain capillaries. In addition, the actual extent of capillary breakdown accounting for the leakage responsible for positive-contrast CT and radionuclide brain scans is small.[103] Although drug delivery to portions of any primary tumor would be expected to occur to the same extent as with non-CNS tumors, delivery (by diffusion) to infiltrative regions distant from leaky tumor capillaries would be expected to be compromised. Diffusion, being a slow process, cannot achieve significant drug concentrations, unless plasma drug levels are sustainable for prolonged periods, and the diffusing drug is relatively stable in the tumor tissue as it diffuses.

A secondary supporting argument is that most agents with antitumor activity against CNS tumors readily cross the blood–brain barrier.[104] For example, all of the nonsugar-containing chloroethylnitrosoureas (CENUs) such as BCNU, CCNU, PCNU, and ACNU have shown efficacy as single agents, whereas sugar-containing CENUs are less effective.[47] Procarbazine, another commonly used agent, also crosses the blood–brain barrier and is active.[105] Agents such as bleomycin, doxorubicin, cisplatin, vincristine (VCR), and mithramycin have shown no activity or have activity limited to primitive childhood and embryonal tumors.

Whether ease of blood–brain barrier passage constitutes an absolute or relative advantage is somewhat academic, given the paucity of chemotypes with demonstrable antitumor activity. Even a small pharmacokinetic disadvantage takes on disproportionate importance when the selective cytotoxicity of a drug is small. This may well be the case with many of the drugs used, because they share narrow therapeutic indices because of dose-limiting systemic toxicity.

Finally, with respect to drugs for CNS tumors, many of the available anticancer drugs can be toxic to the CNS if given at extremely high doses or when given in a manner to circumvent the blood–brain barrier.[106] The blood–brain barrier exists to protect the brain from many potentially toxic compounds. If the blood–brain barrier did not exist, CNS toxicity rather than myelotoxicity or gastrointestinal toxicity would be dose limiting for most drugs.

Pharmacokinetic considerations for intracranial nonparenchymal tumors and extramedullary spinal tumors are less dependent on the ability to cross the blood–brain barrier readily, because many of these tumors gain blood supply from meningeal blood vessels that are significantly more permeable than those of the brain.

REGIONAL DRUG DELIVERY CONSIDERATIONS

Under most circumstances regional drug delivery produces greater drug exposure than does systemic intravenous or oral administration. With respect to intracranial and spinal tumors, the regional delivery takes the form of intra-CSF therapy, intraarterial infusion, and intratumoral therapy.

Therapy by the CSF route (usually by ventricular reservoir) is a form of regional drug delivery that is used to treat meningeal neoplasia resulting from primary or secondary tumor invasion of the subarachnoid space and, less commonly, one of the ventricular cavities. It is often, but not always, associated with malignant cells floating in the CSF.

The advantages of intra-CSF therapy are high local drug levels; low systemic toxicity; and the ability to increase the frequency of treatments. However, delivery of drugs through the CSF can be dangerous and is associated with a high morbidity rate. The drugs commonly used are methotrexate, cytarabine, and thiotepa. All three drugs have been reported to produce CNS damage ranging from fever and chills to leukoencephalopathy and myelitis. Efficacy is limited when gross lesions exist (≥5 mm diameter) or when CSF pathways are blocked and CSF flows are diverted.

Of concern in the use of CSF therapy is that slow clearance of drug can lead to increased neurotoxicity. Normally, these authors find, after injection into a ventricular reservoir and pumping the reservoir five times, the CSF distribution and flow of radionuclide-labeled albumin in the ventricle is well distributed and the half-time from ventricle to cisterna magnum is approximately 60 minutes. In many instances, obvious hydrocephalus is not apparent by neuroimaging, but a physiologic slowing of CSF flow (and presumably CSF absorption) is present. This slowing of CSF flow can lead to poor distribution in the subarachnoid CSF for drugs with high capillary clearance, such as cytarabine, and a greater likelihood of serious CNS toxicity for a drug such as methotrexate.

Another form of regional therapy is the intraarterial administration of anticancer drugs through carotid or vertebral arteries. The advantage of this approach is an increased uptake during the first passage of drug through tumor capillaries. Increased efficacy would be expected for patients whose tumors reside within the perfusion territory of the infused artery. Contrary to what may be thought, systemic toxicity will not be reduced unless the total administered dose is reduced, because the actual amount of drug taken up into the tumor is a small fraction of the injected dose. On the other hand, focal brain and retinal morbidity are increased, as was demonstrated by the clinical trials with BCNU[107] and cisplatin.[108] Controversial results of clinical trials do not commend this form of treatment, except under controlled experimental conditions.

Intratumoral therapy is regional therapy that is applicable for cystic tumors with a narrow rim of surrounding tumor. Pharmacokinetic considerations implicate problems with maintenance of tumor cavity drug levels; diffusion distances from the cavity to the outer margin of tumor; nonspecific biodegradation and binding of drug or drug products; and the need for repeat treatments. Modern clinical trials evaluating this form of regional therapy have not been published.

CEREBRAL ASTROCYTOMAS

PATHOLOGY CLASSIFICATION

This section deals primarily with classification of astrocytomas of varying degrees of aggressiveness, ranging from juvenile pilocytic astrocytoma to glioblastoma multiforme. The slower growing or less aggressive lesions are often referred to as *low grade* or *benign,* and the more rapidly progressive neoplasms are referred to as *high grade* or *malignant.* With the exception of juvenile pilocytic astrocytomas, subependymomas, and the limited number of astrocytomas that can be completely resected, even "benign" astrocytomas are highly lethal. For low-grade astrocytomas, Bloom reported 10-year survival rates of 6% to 10%.[109] Laws and associates had 10- and 20-year survival rates of about 21% and 16% for subtotally resected low-grade cerebral astrocytomas[110]; expected survival for a comparable group of age- and sex-matched normal subjects would have been approximately 95% at 10 years. Liebel and associates had 10-year survival rates of 35% and 11%, depending on whether radiation therapy was used.[111]

Many classification systems for astrocytomas have been advanced that have advocated the presumed cell of origin or the degree of malignancy, or both. The most widely used grading system has been that of Kernohan and Sayre, in which the astrocytomas are graded from I to IV, with grade IV being the most malignant.[112] Although the grades I and II of Kernohan and Sayre have significantly longer median survival times than grades III and IV, the system is not prognostically useful for separating grades I and II from grades III and IV.[110,113] Some of the randomized trials reported during the last decade for malignant gliomas have failed to find a difference in survival for grade III compared with grade IV. In the Radiation Therapy Oncology Group (RTOG) and Eastern Cooperative Oncology Group (ECOG) prospective randomized trial of 626 patients, the median survival time for grade III astrocytoma was 10 months compared with 9 months for grade IV.[114] On the other hand, when these same patients were histologically grouped as astrocytoma with anaplastic foci versus glioblastoma multiforme, there were marked differences in both median survival time and 18-month survival rates; these were 28 months

and 62%, respectively, for anaplastic astrocytoma versus 8 months and 15% for glioblastoma multiforme. Similar differences between anaplastic astrocytoma (or malignant astrocytoma) and glioblastoma multiforme have been reported in older retrospective studies from the University of California at San Francisco (UCSF),[115] Stanford,[116] and Jefferson[117] medical centers.

For most purposes, a three-tier system is satisfactory.[118] Daumas-Duport and colleagues proposed a grading system that assigned a point system to nuclear atypia, mitoses, endothelial proliferation, and necrosis.[119,120] Grade I tumors had none of these features, grade II had one feature, grade III had two features, and grade IV had three or more features. In their initial evaluation, this grouping led to distinct and separate median survival curves. A subsequent review of 251 cases at the Massachusetts General Hospital found no statistical difference in survival between grades II and III.[121] Necrosis was found to be a significant predictor of short survival, in agreement with previous studies.[122]

RATIONALE FOR SURGERY

Data from animal experiments suggest, and a large clinical experience with tumors at many sites would confirm, that maximal surgical resection improves the results of subsequent radiation therapy and chemotherapy. This principle would seem to transfer to the treatment of astrocytomas. Gross total surgical resection was among the dominant factors favoring longer survival in a large series of patients with grade I or II astrocytomas treated at the Mayo Clinic.[123] The second Brain Tumor Study Group trial of radiation therapy and chemotherapy regimens showed a correlation between the extent of surgical resection and subsequent survival in patients with the more malignant astrocytomas.[124] Salcman's review of older literature reporting on the results of treatment of more than 600 patients with such malignant gliomas who received only surgical treatment confirms this correlation.[125] Andreou and coworkers approached this problem from a different perspective, looking at the impact of the amount of tumor present on the postoperative CT scan and "useful survival" (Karnofsky performance score [KPS] > 30) and demonstrating a significant inverse correlation.[126] This same inverse condition of postoperative enhancing tumor volume with survival was confirmed in a much larger group of patients studied by the Brain Tumor Cooperative Group (BTCG),[127] whereas Winger and associates showed that the extent of resection was a significant independent variable for survival in 285 consecutive patients treated for malignant gliomas.[128]

A number of factors might be responsible for the improved clinical outcome when astrocytomas are aggressively resected. An assiduous resection can remove 90% of a typical astrocytoma, thereby decompressing the brain and substantially reducing the tumor cell burden. A large tumor mass left in the brain can serve as a nidus for cerebral edema after radiation therapy because of the indolent removal of dead cells from the brain.[129,130] In addition, aggressive surgical resection reduces (1) the number of separate cell populations in these heterogenous tumors, thereby eliminating some already radioresistant and chemoresistant populations; (2) the probability of further mutation toward resistance by lowering the overall number of tumor cells; and (3) the number of cells in regions remote from blood vessels, regions where chemotherapeutic agents cannot penetrate and where hypoxia can (theoretically) confer radioresistance.[131]

SURGICAL PRINCIPLES FOR CEREBRAL ASTROCYTOMAS

The goal of every craniotomy for a cerebral astrocytoma is gross total resection, and adequate exposure should be accomplished for this purpose, although sometimes aggressive resection proves impossible at the time of the operation. Tumors are approached through an incision in the crest of an overlying gyrus, the selection of which is aided by intraoperative ultrasound images. Self-retaining retractors are placed to retract gently both sides of the cortical incision (generally about 3 cm in length), and then the operating microscope is brought in for the approach through the subcortical white matter to the tumor. The tumor is resected with suction, two-point coagulation forceps, grasping instruments, the CO_2 laser, or the CUSA, the resection proceeding from the inside out, so that surrounding normal white matter is disturbed minimally. The glistening peritumoral white matter is seen easily through the microscope as each of the tumor's margins are reached, and it is at this interface that the resection is stopped. Hemostasis is sometimes difficult but must be perfect. Hemispheric tumor cysts can be drained and, when possible, fenestrated into an adjacent ventricle to prevent reaccumulation. Tumors not amenable to resection because of their location or their diffuseness should be biopsied stereotactically. Again, there is no indication for a craniotomy when the purpose is merely to biopsy (and not resect) a tumor.

The introduction of cortical mapping procedures into brain tumor surgery has made feasible the extensive resection of tumors in functionally critical areas. By use of intraoperative cortical stimulation, motor- and speech-associated cortex can be mapped, and safe routes to deep-lying tumors and safe resection limits determined.[132] A principal disadvantage of surgery that incorporates mapping of speech is that the patient cannot be given general anesthesia, and the surgeon must, therefore, anticipate unexpected patient movement and inferior brain relaxation during the operation.

REOPERATION FOR CEREBRAL ASTROCYTOMAS

Evidence is accumulating that reoperation for resection of cerebral astrocytomas at the time of their recurrence can be efficacious.[125,133,134] The rationale cited earlier for the aggressive initial resection of cerebral astrocytomas seems to fit equally well the prospect for re-resection at recurrence. This is only true, however, if there is some treatment modality (*e.g.*, chemotherapy and brachytherapy) that the patient can receive after the reoperation, and most often there is.

Salcman proposes from experience with reoperation of all patients who were to receive further therapy for recurrence of malignant glioma that relatively nonselective approach might be rational, given that reoperation is safe and of potential benefit despite the patient's age, performance status, tumor grade, or interval between initial surgery and recurrence.[125] Salcman emphasizes that reoperation is technically more demanding than the initial surgery, because tissues are

compromised by previous therapy and, consequently, the postoperative infection rate is high.

Young and coworkers argue for more rigid selection criteria when choosing candidates for reoperation on recurrent malignant gliomas.[133] They found that patients with a KPS higher than 60 and an interval between the initial surgery and recurrence of at least 6 months had the longest survival times after reoperation. Harsh and associates looked at the effect of reoperation on the subsequent high-quality survival (KPS of at least 70) of patients with recurrent malignant gliomas.[134] Age and preoperative KPS have effects on the duration of high-quality survival in this study, with relative youth and high performance scores being advantageous. Because their data suggest that reoperation can significantly enhance the effects of chemotherapy on recurrent brain tumors, Harsh and associates would not suggest confining reoperation to young patients in excellent condition, but would suggest instead simply using these factors as guidelines in the broader therapeutic picture.

RADIATION THERAPY

The differentiated or low-grade astrocytomas constitute a heterogenous group of tumors, and the variability in their behavior has led to uncertainties regarding their therapy and prognosis. Approximately 10% to 35% of astrocytomas are amenable to total surgical resection.[135] The local control rate for completely resected cystic cerebellar astrocytomas approaches 100%, and postoperative irradiation is not recommended.[111,113] Similarly, the 5- and 10-year survival rates for patients with juvenile pilocytic astrocytomas are almost 100% after complete or "radical subtotal" resection.[135,136] In contrast, patients with supratentorial nonpilocytic "ordinary" astrocytomas or mixed oligoastrocytomas who undergo total or radical subtotal resection do not do as well. In a series of 23 such patients, 14 of whom received postoperative irradiation, the 5- and 10-year survival rates were 52% and 21%, respectively.[135]

The 5- and 10-year survival rates for patients with low-grade cerebral astrocytomas treated by subtotal resection alone range from 0% to 25%.[137] For incompletely resected and irradiated juvenile pilocytic astrocytomas, Wallner and coworkers reported 10- and 20-year progression-free survival rates of 74% and 41%, respectively.[136] Unfortunately, the authors had no data relative to incompletely resected and nonirradiated lesions. Shaw and associates found that patients with supratentorial pilocytic astrocytomas who underwent subtotal resection or biopsy and irradiation survived longer than nonirradiated patients.[135] However, the number of patients treated with surgery alone was small, and, therefore, the efficacy of radiotherapy for this tumor is uncertain.

Retrospective reviews suggest that postoperative irradiation is valuable for other types of astrocytomas that are incompletely resected. Leibel and colleagues found that the 5- and 10-year recurrence-free survival rates with incomplete resection alone were 19% and 11%, respectively, whereas, with the addition of postoperative irradiation to doses of 50 to 55 Gy, the survival rates increased to 46% and 35%.[111] For adults, the 5-year survival rate was 10% after surgery alone and 32% with combined therapy. Fazekas reported a 5-year survival of 41% with postoperative irradiation compared with 13% with surgery alone, even though the nonirradiated patients represented a prognostically more favorable subgroup.[113] Shaw and coworkers found that survival was directly related to dose.[135] Patients receiving at least 53 Gy had a significantly longer survival than those receiving less than 53 Gy or surgery alone ($p = 0.04$).

Therapeutic recommendations currently are based on the results of retrospective studies. Postoperative irradiation is not indicated for pilocytic astrocytomas when a complete or near-complete resection has been performed. After subtotal resection, either immediate irradiation or close follow-up may be recommended, deferring treatment until there is disease progression. Postoperative irradiation appears to be beneficial for patients with incompletely removed, unfavorable astrocytomas. Radiation therapy has also been recommended for completely resected, unfavorable lesions.[135] A dose of 55 Gy is administered using conventional fractionation. Limited radiation fields are used that encompass the lesion defined by CT scan with a 2- to 3-cm margin of normal tissue and the T2-weighted MRI abnormality with a 1- to 2-cm margin, whichever volume is larger. A combined North Central Cancer Treatment Group, RTOG, and ECOG study is addressing the question of whether there is a relation between dose and tumor control in adult patients with supratentorial astrocytomas. Patients are randomized to receive 50.4 Gy in 28 fractions or 64.8 Gy in 36 fractions. An adequate dose in children younger than 5 years of age is likely to lead to unacceptable neurologic sequelae, and radiation therapy is delayed until there is evidence of disease progression. When radiation therapy is necessary, the dose is reduced to 50 Gy.

Although it is generally agreed that patients with neurologic impairment, tumor progression, or malignant transformation should undergo radiation therapy, it is common for some practitioners to defer treatment in asymptomatic patients or in those with seizures who are medically controlled. Proponents of this approach argue that with CT and MRI, the disease is diagnosed early in its natural history and that it is not certain whether there is an advantage of early irradiation over delayed irradiation or whether radiation therapy even alters the prognosis.[138] The effect of this policy on patient outcome is not known, but it is being prospectively tested in adults by the BTCG and the Southwest Oncology Group and in children by the Children's Cancer Study Group (CCSG) and the Pediatric Oncology Group (POG).

Retrospective studies indicate that the prognosis of patients with anaplastic astrocytomas is superior to that of patients with glioblastoma multiforme and that the addition of radiation therapy confers a significant survival improvement over surgery alone.[115,116] The BTCG conducted the first clinical trial in which patients with malignant gliomas were randomized to receive postoperative irradiation or supportive care only.[139] Ninety percent of the 222 evaluable patients had glioblastoma multiforme. The median survival time for patients receiving supportive care alone was 14 weeks, whereas those treated with radiation therapy had a median survival time of 36 weeks ($p = 0.001$). The 1-year survival rates were 24% with radiation therapy and 3% for the nonirradiated patients. Similar findings were reported by the Scandinavian Glioblastoma Study Group. In that study, nearly 30% of the irradiated patients maintained a full or partial working capacity, although none of the untreated patients maintained this level of performance.[140] Combining data from a series of BTCG trials, Walker and

colleagues demonstrated a stepwise prolongation of survival with increasing dose.[141] The median survival times for patients in the 50-, 55-, and 60-Gy subgroups were 28, 36, and 42 weeks, respectively (difference in survival between the 50- and 60-Gy groups was significant, $p = 0.004$). A combined RTOG and ECOG study failed to demonstrate a further survival improvement when 60 Gy was compared with 70 Gy.[142] These data led to the practice of treating patients with anaplastic astrocytomas and glioblastoma multiforme with a dose of 60 Gy in single daily fractions of 1.72 to 2 Gy, five times per week.

The amount of tissue to include within the treatment volume is the subject of considerable discussion. The BTCG and RTOG malignant glioma trials use partial brain fields defined by the extent of tumor on neuroimaging studies. In the BTCG protocols, the target volume is defined as a 3-cm margin of tissue surrounding the perimeter of the CT- and MRI-defined contrast-enhancing lesion. The RTOG protocols use a shrinking field approach. Initially, the treatment volume includes the contrast-enhancing lesion and surrounding edema on the preoperative CT-MRI study with a 2-cm margin. Subsequently (after 46 Gy of a 60-Gy course), the target volume is reduced to include the enhancing lesion only (without edema) with a 2.5-cm margin.

The response of malignant gliomas to standard radiation therapy techniques is limited by their striking inherent radioresistance and the radiosensitivity of the surrounding normal brain tissue. In addition to pursuing more effective chemotherapy programs (see chemotherapy section), several new approaches, including the use of chemical radiation sensitizers, heavy particle irradiation, altered fractionation schemes, and interstitial brachytherapy, have been examined. Hypoxic cell radiation sensitizers, such as misonidazole[143] and high-linear-energy transfer radiations, have been used to overcome the effects of hypoxia. These approaches have not yet improved survival over that produced by conventional irradiation. Proton irradiation is being used selectively to boost malignant gliomas to higher than conventional doses.

The halogenated pyrimidine analogs are radiosensitizers that are selectively incorporated into rapidly dividing cells undergoing DNA synthesis.[144] When integrated into DNA in the place of thymidine before radiation, cells become more than three times more sensitive to radiation, depending on concentration, exposure time, and percentage of thymidine replaced by the analog. Two halogenated pyrimidines, bromodeoxyuridine (BUDR) and iododeoxyuridine (IUDR), are undergoing clinical testing currently.

In a phase I–II study conducted by the Northern California Oncology Group (NCOG), 310 patients with malignant gliomas received BUDR in weekly 96-hour infusions of 0.8 mg/m^2/day during a 6-week course of irradiation. This was followed by 1 year of PCV chemotherapy consisting of lomustine (CCNU), 110 mg/m^2 orally on day 1; procarbazine, 60 mg/m^2 orally on days 8 to 21; and vincristine, 1.4 mg/m^2 intravenously on days 8 and 29. The median survival times for patients with anaplastic astrocytoma and glioblastoma multiforme were 252 and 64 weeks, respectively.[145,146] Compared with historical controls, the survival of patients with anaplastic astrocytoma using this regimen was particularly encouraging. This and other studies[147,148] suggest that halogenated pyrimidine radiosensitization in malignant gliomas is measurable, and methods to improve the degree of radio-sensitization are under investigation.[149] A randomized study comparing BUDR-, IUDR-, and hydroxyurea-sensitized radiation therapy (all arms followed by PCV) in patients with anaplastic astrocytoma is being conducted at UCSF.

Hyperfractionated irradiation is the use of two or more treatments per day with fraction sizes smaller than conventional dose fractions to deliver a higher dose in the same overall treatment time as conventionally fractionated therapy. With hyperfractionation, tumor control probabilities should improve without increasing the risk of late complications. Further, with a 4- to 8-hour interval between doses, there is greater probability that rapidly proliferating tumor cells will be irradiated during more radiosensitive phases of the cell cycle and become "self-sensitized" by redistribution. Target cells for late sequelae proliferate slowly, and, therefore, for these tissues little redistribution or self-sensitization occurs.[150]

In a dose-escalation study reported by Urtasun and associates,[151] patients received 61.4, 71.2, and 80 Gy in fractions of 0.9 to 1.1 Gy three times daily. The median survival times for the three dose subgroups were 45.8, 37.2, and 60.5 weeks, respectively. The survival difference between the two highest dose levels was significant ($p = 0.003$). In an RTOG randomized phase II dose-escalation study, patients were given 64.8, 72, 76.8, or 81.6 Gy in 1.2-Gy twice-daily fractions. Patients receiving 72 Gy had the longest median survival, and no further improvement in outcome was observed at the higher dose levels.[152] Based on these data, the RTOG is conducting a randomized trial comparing hyperfractionated irradiation (72 Gy) with conventionally fractionated radiation therapy (60 Gy; BCNU is given in both arms).

Another fractionation option, accelerated fractionation, attempts to reduce the overall treatment time by giving conventional-sized dose fractions two or three times daily. This treatment schedule may improve the therapeutic ratio by reducing the opportunity for tumor cell repopulation during treatment, thereby increasing the probability of tumor control for a given dose level.[150] Several trials using accelerated regimens have been conducted, but none has shown a survival benefit over conventional irradiation.[153,154] These studies indicate that although rapid regeneration does not appear to explain the radioresistance of malignant gliomas, the overall treatment time can be shortened. This outcome may be especially appropriate in patients with relatively short survival expectancies.[153] Further, altered fractionation schedules provide an opportunity to integrate chemosensitizers and hypoxic cell sensitizers in a novel fashion.

Most gliomas are localized to a single area of the brain,[99,100] and they should be controllable if sufficiently high radiation doses can be delivered without damaging the surrounding normal brain tissue. One approach to augmenting the radiation dose is with interstitial brachytherapy. Iodine 125 and iridium 192 sources are most commonly used in clinical practice, and stereotactic techniques have been devised for the placement of afterloading catheters that are removed after the prescribed dose has been accrued. Well-circumscribed, peripheral, solitary supratentorial lesions measuring as large as 5 cm are best suited for implantation. Further, candidates must have good neurologic function and a KPS of at least 70. Based on these criteria, about one third of patients with newly diagnosed malignant gliomas are candidates for this procedure.[155]

Several studies have demonstrated survival improvements in patients with glioblastoma multiforme when external irradiation is combined with brachytherapy. Gutin and coworkers reported the results of an NCOG trial that evaluated brachytherapy as an adjunct to external irradiation and chemotherapy in patients with newly diagnosed supratentorial malignant gliomas.[156] Patients received involved field external irradiation to 60 Gy with concomitant hydroxyurea (300 mg/m^2 orally every other day) followed by an implant to deliver an additional minimum tumor dose of 50 to 60 Gy. Patients were then given PCV chemotherapy every 6 to 8 weeks for 1 year. Although the median survival time of patients with glioblastoma multiforme (88 weeks) compared favorably with that of historical controls, there was no apparent gain observed in performing implantation at diagnosis in patients with nonglioblastoma multiforme (median survival time, 157 weeks). Loeffler and associates reported the outcome of 35 patients with glioblastoma multiforme who underwent partial brain external irradiation (59.4 Gy in 33 fractions) followed by an additional 50 Gy given by interstitial implantation.[157] Survival rates at 1 and 2 years were 87% and 57%, respectively, for patients receiving brachytherapy compared with 40% and 12.5%, respectively, for a control group matched by radiographic and patient characteristics ($p < 0.001$). The BTCG is conducting a randomized study comparing interstitial implantation (60 Gy at 10 Gy per day) preceding external irradiation (60.2 Gy at 1.72 Gy per fraction) and BCNU with external irradiation and BCNU alone. Brachytherapy has also been shown to improve the survival and quality of life of patients with recurrent malignant gliomas who meet the criteria of implantation.[158]

To amplify the effects of interstitial implantation, brachytherapy is being combined with a variety of dose-modifying agents, including interstitial hyperthermia, halogenated pyrimidine analogs, hypoxic cell radiosensitizers, and cisplatin chemotherapy. A randomized trial testing the addition of interstitial microwave hyperthermia to the brachytherapy boost after external irradiation in newly diagnosed patients with glioblastoma multiforme is being conducted at UCSF.[156] However, as local control has improved with brachytherapy, peripheral and distant CNS relapses are becoming more common.[159] This observation suggests that efforts designed only to enhance the effects of brachytherapy may not lead to a significant additional survival gain.

CHEMOTHERAPY

It is unfortunate that only a few patients with astrocytoma receive chemotherapy; most patients are never offered the option. Nonetheless, astrocytomas have been the most extensively treated of primary intracranial tumors.

Controlled (randomized) clinical trials have demonstrated the efficacy of a number of drugs when combined with irradiation as adjuvant therapy. Table 48–12 summarizes the results of controlled (randomized) clinical trials of adjuvant chemotherapy.[114,160–170] Efficacy has been shown for BCNU, CCNU, PCNU, procarbazine, streptozotocin, and the combination of CCNU, procarbazine, and PCV.

The era of controlled clinical trials for malignant astrocytomas began with the inception of the Brain Tumor Study Group in 1967. The European Organization for Research on

TABLE 48–12. Survival Time for Studies That Combined Irradiation and Chemotherapy for Patients With Anaplastic Astrocytoma or Glioblastoma Multiforme With Karnofsky Performance Scores of 60 or Higher

Treatment	Percentage of Glioma Multiforme	Survival Percentile in Weeks	
		50%	25%
BCNU[114,160–162]	45–89	43–55	75–78
CCNU[163–166]	41–100	43–55	
MeCCNU[160]	82	42	73
STZ[168]	79	43	78
PCB[161]	89	47	83
CDDP[167]	77	53	
CCNU-PCB[164]	63	50	
BCNU-PCB[169]	79	50	
HU-BCNU-PCB-VM-26[169]	78	50	
MeCCNU-DTIC[114]	68	42	
"8-in-1-day"[170]	74	47	73

BCNU, carmustine; CCNU, lomustine; MeCCNU, methyl CCNU; STZ, streptozotocin; DTIC, dacarbazine; VM-26, teniposide; CDDP, *cis*-diaminedichloroplatinum; PCB, procarbazine; HU, hydroxyurea.

Treatment of Cancer then established a comparable group. In addition, other national and regional cooperative groups have conducted controlled chemotherapy trials. Tables 48–12 to 48–14 summarize selected data from some of these groups. Differences in reports are sometimes confusing, for instance, some groups report survival or time to tumor progression (TTP) from initiation of therapy, whereas others use the original surgery date for untreated patients. Some groups define histologic groups and separate glioblastoma multiforme from anaplastic astrocytoma, and others combine the two groups under the heading of malignant glioma.

In addition to histology, other factors influence the likelihood and duration of response. Major known factors are age, performance status, and extent of surgical resection at onset of therapy. For instance, younger patients are more likely to respond and for a longer period; better performance status

patients do best; and patients who have more extensive surgical resection do better than those who do not have surgery or who have biopsy only.[125,199]

With consideration for these covariants, it is still clear that adjuvant chemotherapy after surgery and radiation therapy for glioblastoma and anaplastic astrocytomas increases both TTP and survival, more so for the patients with anaplastic gliomas than for glioblastoma. There is less precise information with respect to response because of differing criteria used by the various groups. However, most investigators agree on the definition of deterioration or tumor progression: TTP and survival are more universal measures for controlled clinical trials. TTP is a more pure measure of efficacy, because at time of initial progression, many patients receive other forms of therapy. Survival, however, is a better measure of the social usefulness of the life attained by the therapy.

Chemotherapy appears to benefit mostly the lower 50th percentile of patients, and especially those below the 25th percentile. This is reasonable, because in vitro tumor drug sensitivity assays suggest that approximately 60% of patients are resistant to a given agent.[200,201]

Nitrosourea-based drug combinations appear superior to monotherapy, although even this conclusion is based on only one controlled study by the NCOG. In that study, postradiation therapy BCNU was compared with the PCV combination.[171] The greatest benefit for chemotherapy, based on TTP and survival, was in PCV-treated anaplastic astrocytomas. For glioblastoma multiforme patients, TTP and survival at the 50th percentile were for PCV at 37 and 53 weeks and for BCNU at 34 and 57 weeks, respectively; for the 25th percentile, they were for PCV at 72 and 94 weeks and for BCNU at 43 and 71 weeks, respectively. This was more significant ($p = 0.009$) for anaplastic tumors. TTP and survival at the 50th percentile were for PCV at 126 and 157 weeks and for BCNU at 63 and 82 weeks, respectively; for the 25th percentile, they were for PCV at 6.1 years and were not attained (>7.7 years) and for BCNU at 2.7 years and 4.1 years, respectively. At the dose schedule used, substituting BUDR for hydroxyurea during radiation therapy appears to offer no advantage.[182,183a] For glioblastoma, no survival advantage is seen; for anaplastic gliomas, the mean survival is higher (4.6 versus 3 years), but because only 50% of patients have died, it is too soon to be certain of the statistical trend.

TABLE 48–13. Survival for Adequately Treated Glioblastoma Multiforme Patients With Karnofsky Performance Scores of 60 or Higher Treated on NCOG Protocols

Treatment	Percentile in Weeks*	
	50%	25%
RT + HU-BCNU[171]	57 (34)	71 (43)†
RT + HU-PCV[171]	53 (37)	94 (72)
FU-CCNU-RT + HU + MISO-PCB-VCR-BCNU-FU[172]	50 (41)	NA (59)†
RT + BUDR-PCV[173]	62 (43)	88 (69)

NCOG, Northern California Oncology Group; BCNU, carmustine; HU, hydroxyurea; PCV, lomustine (CCNU), procarbazine (PCB), vincristine (VCR); FU, fluorouracil; RT, radiation therapy; MISO, misonidazole; BUDR, bromodeoxyuridine; NA, not available.
* Time to tumor progression in parentheses.
† Not significant.

TABLE 48–14. Survival for Adequately Treated Anaplastic Gliomas Other Than Glioblastoma Multiforme in Patients With Karnofsky Performance Scores of 60 or Higher Treated on NCOG Protocols

Treatment	Percentile in Weeks*	
	50%	25%
RT + HU-BCNU[171]	82 (63)	214 (142)†
RT + HU-PCV[171]	157 (126)	NA (317)
RT + BUDR-PCV[171a]	252 (148)	NA (NA)‡

NCOG, Northern California Oncology Group; BCNU, carmustine; HU, hydroxyurea; PCV, lomustine (CCNU), procarbazine (PCB), vincristine (VCR); RT, radiation therapy; BUDR, bromodeoxyuridine; NA, not available.
* Time to tumor progression in parentheses.
† p = 0.009.
‡ Not significant.

More approaches need to be considered to improve the results cited in Tables 48–12 to 48–14. As a rule, new protocols for controlled trials usually come from phase II studies of chemotherapy efficacy against recurrent or progressive astrocytomas. Table 48–15 summarizes many of the published studies and several studies completed recently but not published. In many ways, Table 48–15 is disappointing. As was the case with adjuvant therapy of previously untreated astrocytomas, the nitrosoureas, alone and in combination, are the most active for recurrent and progressive tumors. It is disappointing that drugs designed specifically for gliomas, such as diaziquone (AZQ) and spiromustine, are only mediocre agents in the clinic.[180–182,184] Table 48–15 shows that even though the number of patients benefiting from chemotherapy is high in some studies, nevertheless, among the response and stable tumor patients, the duration of benefit has shown only modest gains during the last decade. This failure of chemotherapy is probably a function of de novo and emergent resistance of tumor cell subclones.

The use of the combination of polyamine inhibitors for anaplastic astrocytomas is encouraging. Alpha-difloromethylornithine–methyl-bisguanylhydrazone (DFMO-MGBG),[194] DFMO,[183a] and DFMO-BCNU[193] have been used with good results. For DFMO-MGBG patients with recurrent or progressive disease who had been heavily pretreated with nitrosoureas, approximately 50% responded or stabilized on the combination for a median time to progression (MTP) of 52 weeks (the MTP for the stable group alone was 50 weeks). Since that study, additional patients have been treated; as of September 1, 1987, 21 of 29 patients with anaplastic astrocytomas have stabilized or responded, with a median duration of 49 weeks. As a single agent, DFMO appears to have similar activity to the DFMO-MGBG combination. In both instances, the MTP for recurrent anaplastic gliomas achieving response and stable disease was almost 1 year. The difference in response rates (72% versus 46%) may reflect too lenient entry requirements for the DFMO patients and a subsequent high number of patients who went off therapy before the first evaluation at 8 weeks.[194a]

DFMO-BCNU, a combination found active in cultured cells and against rodent tumors, was found active against recurrent

TABLE 48–15. Chemotherapy of Recurrent and Progressive Supratentorial Astrocytomas

Treatment	Percentage of Response and Stable Tumor (MTP, wk)*		
	GM	AA	GM + AA†
Single Agents			
BCNU[104,174]	29 (22)	64 (22)	
CCNU[175,176]			42 (23)
PCNU[177]	33 (8)	69 (28)	
PCB[105,178]	27 (30)	28 (49)	50 (26)
BIC[179]	20 (na)	23 (22)	
AZQ, 24 h[180]	50 (18)	47 (16)	
AZQ, bolus[181,182]			24 (24)
Melphalan (oral)[183]	0 (NA)	7 (NA)	
Melphalan (IV)[183a]	0 (NA)	0 (NA)	
Spiromustine[184]			27 (5)
Cisplatin[185a,186]		73 (8)	83 (12)
Carboplatin[185a,186]	43 (14)	54 (16)	
DFMO[183a]		21 (NA)	44 (48)
Betaseron[187]	51 (18)	50 (16)	
Combinations			
BCNU-VCR[188]			41 (17)
BCNU-PCB[60]		46 (17)	56 (23)
CCNU-PCB-VCR[189,190]	45 (15)	65 (27)	
BCNU-FU[191]		89 (32)	
BCNU-FU-HU-MP[192]		55 (23)	71 (46)
BCNU-FU, PCB, CCNU-PCB[183a]		95 (41)	
DFMO-BCNU[193]	30 (8)	57 (76)	
DFMO-MGBG[194]		72 (49)	
TG-PCB-DBD-CCNU-FU-HU[195]	61 (40)	92 (65)	
PCB-FU-HU-MP[183a]	33 (16)	50 (20)	
AZQ-BCNU[196,197]	0–28 (9)	80 (37)	
AZQ-PCB[196]	31 (25)	53 (42)	
Cytoxan-VCR[198]	60 (15)	78 (35)	
Carboplatin-FU-PCB[199a]	32 (20)	57 (36)	

GM, glioblastoma multifome; AA, anaplastic astrocytoma; BCNU, carmustine; CCNU, lomustine; PCB, procarbazine; TG, 6-thioguanine; DBD, dibromodulcitol; MTP, median time to progression; AZQ, diaziquone; DFMO, alpha-difloromethylornithine; VCR, vincristine; FU, fluorouracil; HU, hydroxyurea; MP, mercaptopurine; MGBG, methyl-bisguanylhydrazone; NA, not available.
* Time to tumor progression in parentheses.
† GM and AA were not analyzed separately, because histologies were not separated or too few patients were found in each group to separate activity by histology.

gliomas with a median survival of 92 weeks.[193] These studies open new therapeutic opportunities, because these polyamine inhibitors can interact with other agents to improve their efficacy.

Another encouraging finding may be a recently completed study[195] conducted in an attempt to overcome tumor resistance to CCNU. In that study, 6-thioguanine, dibromodulcitol, and procarbazine were given before CCNU to enhance tumor cell kill by interfering with DNA repair. The results were dramatic for the anaplastic gliomas, when 95% of patients who had failed radiation therapy responded or stabilized for an MTP of 15 months, and 25% did not fail until 33 months; 61% of glioblastoma patients with response or stable disease had an MTP of 9.3 months.[195] Of those who failed earlier nitrosourea therapies, 38% of anaplastic glioma patients and 58% of glioblastoma patients benefited, with MTPs of 10.6 and 5.1 months, respectively.

Intravenous cisplatin and carboplatin have shown only modest activity with respect to TTP, although response and stable rates appear high.[185,186] This may reflect poor tumor and adjacent brain penetration of these drugs and their inability to kill tumor cells at a distance from the main tumor mass. Betaseron, an interferon-β, attained 50% response and stable rates in a cooperative study; however, the duration of benefit is low, with MTPs of 16 to 18 weeks.[187]

Autologous bone marrow transplantation (ABMT) has had few practitioners, generally because of a low rate of observed complete responses to any form of chemotherapy. Single-agent BCNU was used years ago with no definable gains over conventional-dose nitrosourea therapy.[202] Other researchers have used thiotepa[203] and etoposide.[204,205] Although neither thiotepa nor etoposide alone has shown remarkable activity against gliomas, various combinations of the three agents are being evaluated.[206,207] It is currently unclear whether ABMT has a place in the management of cerebral gliomas.

BRAIN STEM GLIOMAS

CLINICAL AND PATHOLOGIC CONSIDERATIONS

Tumor involvement of the brain stem is due, in order of decreasing frequency, to astrocytoma, glioblastoma, and ependymoma. These tumors can be primarily central, diffuse, and infiltrative or focally infiltrative with or without an exophytic; the latter carry a better prognosis. Cranial nerve involvement can be at the nuclear level or of the cranial nerve as it leaves the brain stem. The initial manifestations of a brain stem glioma are unilateral palsies of cranial nerves VI and VII in approximately 90% of patients. Cranial nerve involvement is usually followed by long tract signs, such as hemiplegia, unilateral limb ataxia, ataxia of gait, paraplegia, hemisensory syndromes, gaze disorders, and, occasionally, hiccups. Less commonly, long tract signs precede the cranial nerve abnormalities; this is more likely with confined central intrinsic lesions.

If the tumor is a well-differentiated or an anaplastic astrocytoma, it is likely to involve the midbrain and produce hydrocephalus, vomiting, drowsiness, and cerebellar signs; if the tumor is a glioblastoma, it more often involves the medulla. Children with glioblastoma characteristically have a rapidly progressive course and are likely to have deficits in cranial nerves VI, VII, IX, and X and dysarthria, personality change, and head tilt. Unlike expansive posterior fossa tumors, headache, vomiting, and papilledema occur late.

As a group, the prognosis is poor, with 5-year survival rates varying between 0% and 38% and a median survival of less than 1 year in most series.[208–210] Certain patients do better than others. For instance, patients with type II tumors do better than those with infiltrative type I tumors. Moderately anaplastic exophytic tumors do better than higher-grade anaplastic tumors.

SURGERY

Modern imaging of the CNS with MRI scanning has improved the capability for definitive diagnosis of brain stem tumors. Lesions previously difficult to distinguish from brain stem glioma, for example, clivus tumors, foramen magnum meningiomas, multiple sclerosis, occult arteriovenous malformations, and brain stem abscesses, usually can now be excluded. Still, biopsy of brain stem gliomas for confirmation of the diagnosis and for definite tumor grading should be performed when possible. Biopsy of brain stem gliomas accessible through the floor of the fourth ventricle or presenting on the lateral surface of the pons can be accomplished safely, and associated symptomatic cysts can be drained. Attempt at complete resection of these tumors is contraindicated. Stereotactic needle biopsy of brain stem gliomas using CT and MRI guidance seems to have a low complication rate, so this method is being used increasingly, with the consequence that fewer patients are being treated without a tissue diagnosis.[211]

RADIATION THERAPY

Radiation therapy, the primary treatment for brain stem tumors, improves survival and can stabilize or reverse neurologic dysfunction in 75% to 90% of patients.[212,213] Traditionally, brain stem gliomas have been treated with up to doses of 50 to 60 Gy (1.8 Gy/fraction/day) through parallel opposed portals with the tumor dose calculated at the midline on the central axis of the beam. Sagittal MRI offers improved target definition and allows the radiation portals to be tailored to the contour of the lesion. The irradiated volume includes a margin of normal tissue of approximately 2 cm around the tumor. According to a multiinstitutional survey by Freeman and Suissa,[209] the 1-, 2-, and 5-year survival rates of children treated with conventional radiation therapy techniques were 50%, 29%, and 23%, respectively.[214,215]

Because of the relatively poor results obtained with conventional radiation dose-fractionation schedules and the observation that these tumors recur locally, hyperfractionated irradiation, designed to deliver higher tumor doses, is being evaluated.[216] Consistent, although modest, improvements in outcome have been observed when patients treated with hyperfractionation regimens of up to doses of 70.2 to 72 Gy (1–1.17 Gy twice daily) have been compared with historical control patients treated with conventional or low-dose hyperfractionated irradiation.[217–219] In a trial reported by Edwards and coworkers, 53 patients (19 adults and 34 children) with brain stem gliomas were treated with hyperfractionated irradiation to 72 Gy using 1 Gy twice daily, 5 days per week, with an interfraction interval of 4 to 8 hours.[219] The median survival time was 74 weeks (adults, 92 weeks, and children, 64 weeks). No increase in acute or delayed radiation-induced neurotoxicity was observed with this fractionation schedule, and the dose was subsequently escalated to 78 Gy. Although the outcome of children treated with this protocol is better than that observed in studies using conventional radiation therapy alone or with chemotherapy, it cannot be determined currently whether this is due to the fractionation schedule used, patient selection, or improvements in tumor localization and treatment planning using MRI.[219] Although these questions can be addressed only in a randomized trial, the data provide further evidence that higher doses can be safely administered to brain tumors using hyperfractionation regimens.

CHEMOTHERAPY

As with cerebral astrocytomas, chemotherapy is primarily nitrosourea based.[221] The use of chemotherapy, adjuvant to irradiation, has been infrequent. The CCSG randomly compared radiation therapy with radiation therapy followed by CCNU, PCV, and prednisone.[222] The mean survival was 11 months, and there was no difference between the two groups. In another trial, 5-fluorouracil and CCNU before radiation therapy and hydroxyurea and misonidazole during radiation therapy were evaluated[223]; in that study, TTP (32 weeks) and survival (44 weeks) were not better than the initial CCSG study.

For recurrent or progressive brain stem gliomas, few therapies have been evaluated.[221] Some benefit has been demonstrated, but the extent of benefit was not well established. In a recent study, 5-fluorouracil, CCNU, hydroxyurea, and 6-mercaptopurine were used to treat children and adults with recurrent or progressive brain stem gliomas.[224] Sixty-nine percent of 13 patients had response or stabilization, with a relapse-free survival of 25 weeks; the overall survival was 27 weeks. This finding is somewhat worse than would be expected for supratentorial gliomas. These authors conducted a phase II study of recurrent malignant gliomas with a combination of BCNU and DFMO. In that study, 3 of 5 patients benefited, with the 3 continuing at 1 to 3 years.[193] Although not curative, some of these chemotherapeutic leads should be exploited.

CEREBELLAR ASTROCYTOMAS

CLINICAL AND PATHOLOGIC CONSIDERATIONS

Astrocytomas arising in the cerebellum are considered separately, because their prognosis is consistently better than astrocytomas arising in the cerebrum or brain stem. These tumors, which occur most often during the first two decades of life, arise in the vermis or more laterally in a cerebellar hemisphere. Cerebellar astrocytomas usually are well circumscribed; they can be cystic, solid, or an admixture of polycystic and solid.

Histologically, most astrocytomas are low grade and lack features commonly associated with anaplasia; many are pilocytic in appearance and, histologically, some are juvenile pilocytic astrocytomas. In a series on 451 children reported from the Hospital for Sick Children of Toronto, cerebellar astrocytomas accounted for 25% of all posterior fossa tumors; 99 of 111 (89%) of the cerebellar astrocytomas were low grade, with nearly all vermian in origin.[225]

Because most of these tumors arise in the vermis, the clinical presentation is similar to medulloblastoma, with truncal ataxia, headache, nausea and vomiting, and in the young, split cranial sutures and head enlargement from raised intracranial pressure.

SURGERY

Cystic cerebellar astrocytomas are exposed through a posterior fossa craniectomy. The cyst is located with a cannula and then exposed by an incision through the cerebellar folia. Self-retaining retractors are placed into the cyst and then, with the aid of the operating microscope, the cyst is examined and the vascular, firm mural module identified, dissected, and removed. The nonneoplastic cyst wall is not excised.

Solid cerebellar astrocytomas are separated carefully from surrounding cerebellar white matter, again using the improved visualization offered by the operating microscope. The texture and appearance of the tumor are usually distinct and the separation from white matter usually is not difficult, so the only barrier to complete resection becomes deep penetration of the tumor into the dentate nucleus, cerebellar peduncles, or brain stem.

RADIATION THERAPY

See the discussion in the section on cerebral astrocytomas; the same principles apply. Completely resected cerebellar astrocytomas do not require radiation therapy. The remainder receive total doses of 50 to 60 Gy, depending on the histologic features and the age of the patient.

CHEMOTHERAPY

Because surgery alone or surgery and irradiation is often curative, chemotherapy has been limited to cases of recurrence or if the tumor is histologically highly anaplastic. For these tumors, the authors' approach has been to use nitrosourea-based therapies.

Chemotherapy adjuvant to surgery and radiation has not been commonly advocated for these tumors. The authors' experience is anecdotal (Table 48–16), but appears consistent with chemotherapy results for cerebral gliomas.[226] All patients received a nitrosourea; however, the chemotherapy combinations varied depending on which program was being used at the time for supratentorial gliomas. For patients at recurrence, chemotherapy provided palliation, with relapse-free survivals in 50% of patients at 18 months and 25% of patients surviving longer than 32 months.[226] As with the adjuvant chemotherapy patients, all were treated on a protocol being used at the time for cerebral gliomas. Among these patients, 5 of 18 (28%) developed metastases to the leptomeninges (3 of 5) or intracranial extracerebral parenchymal sites (2 of 5). All leptomeningeal disseminations occurred in conjunction with locoregional recurrences. In many patients, therefore, combined systemic and intraventricular therapy may be needed for tumor control.

OPTIC, CHIASMAL, AND HYPOTHALAMIC GLIOMAS

CLINICAL AND PATHOLOGIC CONSIDERATIONS

Nearly all gliomas of the optic nerve and chiasm are discovered in patients before the age of 20 years, and most before the age of 10 years.[227] In some patients there is a family kindred of neurofibromatosis. Lewis and colleagues prospectively evaluated 217 patients with neurofibromatosis and found that gliomas along the anterior visual pathway occurred in 15% and were occasionally bilateral.[228] Sixty-seven percent of these tumors were not suspected clinically or obvious on ophthalmologic examination.

TABLE 48–16. Chemotherapy for Recurrent
Cerebellar Astrocytomas[226]

Age (y)	Diagnosis	Treatment(s)	Survival in Months
Adjuvant Chemotherapy			
25	GM	RT-BUDR-PCV	+45
8	GM	RT-8422	+22
15	GM	RT-8422	+19
13	AA	RT-PCV	22
13	AA	RT-CYCLE	+52
Chemotherapy at Progression			
19	GM	8522, ACNU, PCB	+20
29	AA	BCNU, PCV, 8422	18
38	AA	BFHM	10
25	AA	CYCLE, AraC, TEPA	32
11	AA	BCNU, CYCLE	+112
33	AA	BCNU	6
4	MG	CCNU	+152
31	MG	CYCLE	10
38	LG	PCV	5
42	JPA	CYCLE, HME	30

GM, glioblastoma multiforme; AA, anaplastic astrocytoma; MG, meningioma; LG, low grade; JPA, juvenile pilocytic astrocytoma; RT, radiation therapy; PCV, lomustine (CCNU) + procarbazine (PCB) + vincristine; CYCLE, carmustine (BCNU), 5-fluorouracil, CCNU, PCB; BTRC 8422 is 6-thioguanine, PCB, dibromodulcitol, CCNU, vincristine; BTRC 8522 is 6-thioguanine, PCB, dibromodulcitol, CCNU, 5-fluorouracil, hydroxyurea; HME, elliptinium; BUDR, bromodeoxyuridine; ACNU, intraventricular nimustine; AraC, intraventricular cytarabine; TEPA, intraventricular thiotepa; BFHM is BCNU, 5-fluorouracil, hydroxyurea, 6-mercaptopurine.

With respect to tumor location, Housepian and associates reported that 25% involved one optic nerve, 73% the chiasm, and 3% the optic tracts.[229] In another series, 25% involved the chiasm alone, 33% the chiasm and hypothalamus, and 42% the chiasm and optic nerves or tracts.[230] Clinically, these tumors produce loss of visual acuity (70%), strabismus and nystagmus (33%), visual field impairment (bitemporal hemianopsia, 8%), developmental delay, macrocephaly, ataxia, hemiparesis, proptosis, and precocious puberty. Funduscopic evaluation demonstrates a range of findings from normal optic disks through venous engorgement to disk pallor due to atrophy. Tumors involving the chiasm often grow to involve the hypothalamus, causing a diencephalic syndrome that is characterized by emaciation (especially in children between 3 months and 2 years of age), motor overactivity, and euphoria.

Pathologically, these tumors range from primarily piloid and stellate astrocytes (commonest), with or without oligodendroglia, through the gamut of malignant astrocytomas to glioblastoma multiforme (rare). Typically, optic gliomas appear as fusiform expansions of any part of the nerve; they tend to bridge through the optic foramen and expand as dumbbell-shaped tumors within the skull. The nerve can be infiltrated by tumor originating in the chiasm, the walls of the third ventricle, or the hypothalamus. The tumors found in patients with neurofibromatosis often affect a single optic nerve and are grossly normal in appearance, although infiltrated by tumor and surrounded by a fibrous stroma.

Diagnosis is best made by MRI scan and should use images in the sagittal plane. The CT scan is satisfactory for diagnosis but is not as sensitive or descriptive as the MRI scan. The MRI also shows hypothalamic involvement more clearly.

SURGERY

Unilateral tumors of the optic nerve (as opposed to the chiasm) should be resected, particularly when there is profound visual loss or when proptosis is disfiguring.[231] A transcranial approach to the orbit is preferred, permitting complete resection of the tumor-infiltrated nerve from the chiasm to the globe and sparing the globe for an optimum cosmetic effect.[231] The involved nerve is inspected through a unilateral craniotomy, and the nerve is sectioned at the chiasm. The orbit is then unroofed, and the optic nerve's attachment to the globe is exposed and divided, allowing the tumor to be removed.

Biopsy of smaller tumors of the optic nerve, chiasm, or the nerve and chiasm must sometimes be accomplished when radiographic studies cannot exclude meningioma or other diagnoses definitively. Subtotal resection of larger tumors of these structures is occasionally necessary for decompression, but resection of the chiasm with resultant blindness is never indicated.

RADIATION THERAPY

Treatment of optic nerve and chiasmal gliomas is controversial, because some patients with incomplete surgical resections have been followed for 10 to 20 years without progression.[227] The literature suggests, however, that untreated optic gliomas, especially those involving the chiasm or extending into the hypothalamus or optic tracts, progress locally or are fatal in 75% of patients. Tenny and coworkers found that only 21% of patients who were followed after biopsy or exploration survived compared with 64% of those who received radiation therapy.[232] In general, optic nerve gliomas have a better prognosis than those involving the chiasm, and tumors confined to the anterior chiasm have a better outcome than those that involve adjacent structures (posterior chiasmal tumors).[233–236]

Routine postoperative irradiation is not indicated for most gliomas confined to the optic nerve. In contrast, radiation therapy can prevent tumor progression, improve disease-free survival, and stabilize or improve vision in patients with chiasmal lesions. Wong and colleagues reported that 6 of 27 (22%) chiasmal gliomas that did not receive radiation therapy progressed locally, whereas 9 of 20 (45%) failed that received radiation therapy.[234] Three of these recurrences occurred in the adults with extremely aggressive, nonresponsive tumors. Further, 87% of the irradiated patients who received a dose of 50 to 55 Gy were controlled compared with 55% of those who received 46 Gy or less. Radiation therapy significantly improved the relapse-free survival but not the overall survival. In another series collected from the literature, local control was achieved in 154 of 189 (81%) irradiated anterior chiasmal tumors, whereas 92 of 142 (65%) posterior tumors were controlled. Vision improved in 61 of 210 (29%) evaluable patients and remained stable in 118 of 210 (56%) patients.[233]

Although some clinicians advocate deferring irradiation in asymptomatic patients until there are signs of disease progression, others recommend that radiation therapy be given early in the course of the disease to minimize the risk of visual deterioration.[234,237] The radiation portals are tailored to the tumor volume and designed to avoid irradiation of the lens of the eye. A three-field or bicoronal arc technique may be used to treat smaller lesions. A dosage of 50 to 55 Gy in daily 1.8-Gy fractions is recommended.

For hypothalamic tumors, radiation therapy produced radiographic improvement in 11 of 24 (46%) with an MTP of 70 months.[239] Those patients who did not receive radiation therapy initially had an MTP of 30 months.

CHEMOTHERAPY

There are few published chemotherapy trials in this group of patients. Chemotherapy has been used successfully to delay the initiation of radiation therapy in young children.[238] Packer and associates treated 24 children (median age 1.6 years) with a combination of dactinomycin and VCR.[230] Six of the cases involved the chiasm, 8 involved the chiasm and hypothalamus, and 10 involved the chiasm and visual pathways. At a median follow-up period of 4.3 years, 38% of patients had progressed.[230]

Petronio and coworkers reported on 19 infants or children with chiasmatic and hypothalamic gliomas treated with chemotherapy after surgical or radiologic diagnosis.[240] Of the 12 tumors in which a biopsy was obtained, there were 7 juvenile pilocytic astrocytomas, 2 astrocytomas, 2 anaplastic astrocytomas, and 1 subependymal giant cell astrocytoma. The children were between 3 months and 15 years of age when treated. The chemotherapy included one of three regimens: 1 with dactinomycin and VCR; 1 with the combination of BCNU, 5-fluorouracil, hydroxyurea, and 6-mercaptopurine; and 15 with the combination of 6-thioguanine, procarbazine, dibromodulcitol, CCNU, and VCR (BTRC 8422 protocol). Fifteen of 18 initially treated with chemotherapy responded or stabilized; the median follow-up period exceeded 1.5 years (range, 1.4 months to 5.8 years). The four patients who progressed responded to radiation therapy.

Rodriguez and colleagues reported a series of 33 hypothalamic gliomas,[239] some of whom were included in the Petronio series.[240] Chemotherapy at presentation or recurrence was beneficial in 10 of 16 (62%) patients.

OLIGODENDROGLIOMAS

CLINICAL AND PATHOLOGIC CONSIDERATIONS

Oligodendrogliomas have a relatively flat "peak" incidence between 25 and 49 years. Although they are commonest (80%) in the cerebral hemispheres, approximately 15% occur in the third or lateral ventricles or protrude into a ventricle from the thalamus.[241] Grossly, these tumors are often well demarcated, and in 20% they are cystic. They have a 10% likelihood of spreading through the CSF pathways. Like astrocytomas, they vary in malignancy. Attempts have been made to grade oligodendrogliomas on an A through D scale[241]; however, grades A through C vary little, and B and C are virtually identical with respect to survival such that these subdivisions seem

unnecessary; a designation of *differentiated* or *highly anaplastic* may be sufficient. These tumors often have both astrocytic or ependymal elements seen at biopsy; such tumors are called *mixed gliomas*.

Clinically, these tumors present in the typical fashion of hemispheral astrocytomas. However, two features distinguish them from astrocytomas: the antecedent history, averaging 7 to 8 years, tends to be longer, and seizures are more common, occurring in 70% to 90% of patients by the time of diagnosis. Provisional diagnosis may be made by CT or MRI neuroimaging, but histologic confirmation is necessary and almost always possible. Approximately 50% of oligodendrogliomas have scattered calcification, usually related to intrinsic blood vessels, which are evident by CT scan.

At recurrence or autopsy, approximately 60% of oligodendroglioma and most mixed oligoastrocytoma patients demonstrate histologically an anaplastic astrocytoma or glioblastoma multiforme. This may belie a common origin of both types of tumors to the O2A progenitor cell.

SURGERY

The surgical resection of hemispheric oligodendrogliomas follows the same principles as discussed earlier for cerebral astrocytomas, with gross total removal being the goal when this is consistent with good neurologic outcome. The margins of oligodendrogliomas can appear to be more distinct than those of astrocytomas, but generally they are infiltrative, and surgical cure remains unlikely. Oligodendrogliomas often recur in the previous operative site. Under these circumstances, reoperation may be advisable, particularly when followed by chemotherapy.

RADIATION THERAPY

The role of postoperative irradiation in patients with differentiated oligodendrogliomas is controversial and contradictory. The lack of randomized trials precludes the statement of firm recommendations. Some authors recommend immediate postoperative irradiation for patients with incompletely resected lesions,[242,243] some advise that only patients with anaplastic tumors or mixed oligoastrocytomas receive radiation therapy,[244] and others advocate that radiation therapy be deferred until there is evidence of tumor progression or recurrence.[245] Data from three recent retrospective series suggest that the median survival time is increased from 23 to 60 months to 38 to 132 months by the addition of postoperative irradiation.[242,243,246,247]

Wallner and associates reviewed the outcome of 42 patients and observed 5- and 10-year survival rates of 61% and 33%, respectively; relapse-free survival rates were only 33% and 25%.[242] The 10-year survival rate for patients with pure oligodendrogliomas who received at least 45 Gy was 56% compared with 18% for nonirradiated patients ($p = 0.092$). The survival rates for patients with irradiated mixed oligoastrocytomas were virtually identical to those for the irradiated pure tumors. Wallner and coworkers concluded that adjunctive radiation therapy increased the time to tumor recurrence and the number of long-term survivors.[242] Lindegaard and colleagues found that radiation therapy prolonged the median survival time but did not influence the overall cure rate when given after subtotal resection, whereas it did not appear to be indicated after total resection.[243] On the other hand, Bullard and associates could find no evidence that postoperative radiation therapy was beneficial.[246]

Based on the poor long-term prognosis associated with these tumors and data that suggest that radiation therapy may be beneficial, these authors continue to recommend postoperative irradiation after incomplete resection. It is reasonable, however, to defer treatment in asymptomatic children until there are signs of tumor progression. Radiation therapy is given using fields that encompass the tumor volume with a 2- to 3-cm margin. A dose of 55 to 60 Gy is used in adults, and the dose is reduced to 50 Gy in children.

CHEMOTHERAPY

As with radiation trials, prospective clinical chemotherapy trials of oligodendroglioma patients have not been published. There are, however, individual patients reported within trials for malignant astrocytomas. In those reports, chemotherapy was limited to the treatment of recurrent, well-differentiated, and moderately anaplastic oligodendrogliomas and the primary treatment of the highly anaplastic oligodendrogliomas with surgery, radiation therapy, and chemotherapy.

Because many of these isolated patients came from the authors' own published reports, they reviewed their experience during the last decade. Table 48–17 summarizes TTP and survival results of treatment of oligodendrogliomas and mixed tumors that had been treated at recurrence. In their series, the median time to first recurrence for the oligodendrogliomas was 2.4 years; those treated with chemotherapy (primarily nitrosourea based) at recurrence had a median survival of an additional 1.4 years. These results are similar to those for well-differentiated (moderately anaplastic) astrocytomas. For the mixed tumors, the median time to first recurrence was 1.8 years, and the median time from recurrence to death was an additional 1.6 years for those treated with chemotherapy

TABLE 48–17. Patients With Oligodendroglioma and Oligoastrocytoma Tumors Treated for Recurrence With Chemotherapy* at UCSF between 1977 and 1987

Tumors	Percentiles	
	50%	25%
Oligodendroglioma (median age 37)		
Time to first tumor recurrence (n = 21)	2.4 y	3.8 y
Time from recurrence to death (n = 12)	1.4 y	2.8 y
Mixed Oligoastrocytoma (median age 35)		
Time to first tumor recurrence (n = 53)	1.8 y	4.9 y
TIme from recurrence to death (n = 20)	1.6 y	>2.0 y†

* Chemotherapy included nitrosourea-based therapies, the combination of PCV, procarbazine, DFMO-MGBG, and thiotepa. In addition, 20–25% had a reoperation after recurrence before starting chemotherapy.
† The 25% has not been reached, because 10 in 20 have not failed yet.

at recurrence. Cairncross and MacDonald have advocated the combination of CCNU, procarbazine, and VCR.[248] They believe that oligodendrogliomas are more sensitive to chemotherapy than are anaplastic astrocytomas, although survival differences are measurable in months, not years, between the two groups. Based on these results, they have initiated prospective trials.

EPENDYMOMA

CLINICAL AND PATHOLOGIC CONSIDERATIONS

Ependymomal tumors arise from cells of ependymal lineage and, therefore, have a propensity for occurring in the obliterated central canal of the spinal cord, the filum terminale, and white matter adjacent to a ventricular surface (usually a highly angulated surface).[50] Sixty percent of intracranial ependymomas are infratentorial, and 40% are supratentorial.[249] Of infratentorial sites, the fourth ventricle is the commonest site. Extension into the subarachnoid space occurs in 50% of these cases, and encasement of the medulla and upper cervical cord can occur. Of supratentorial ependymomas, 50% are primarily intraventricular, and the remainder are parenchymal, arising from ependymal rests. Most of the intraventricular tumors arise in the lateral ventricles, and fewer (25%) occur in the third ventricle .

Ependymomas can be classified in various ways. Ependymomas are either differentiated (ependymoma or myxopapillary ependymoma) and, therefore, low grade or, less commonly, they are anaplastic and higher grade and more likely to disseminate through the CSF pathways.

Clinical presentations are dependent on the location of tumor. Intraventricular tumors often cause increased intracranial pressure and hydrocephalus. As a result, headache, nausea and vomiting, papilledema, ataxia, and vertigo are found in most patients at presentation. Focal neurologic signs and symptoms are more often seen with extraventricular supratentorial ependymomas.

Either MRI or CT scanning is sufficient to make the anatomic diagnosis before surgery. The presence of calcium in a fourth ventricular tumor is highly suggestive but not diagnostic of an ependymoma. Surgical exploration and biopsy are essential for the selection of appropriate treatment. For anaplastic ependymomas, staging myelography and examination of the CSF for cytologic evidence of malignancy are essential.

The inclusion of ependymoblastomas, which are known for their propensity to disseminate throughout the CNS, tends to overestimate the risk of seeding.[252,253] In a literature review, Vanuytsel and Brada found that the overall incidence of spinal seeding was 6.9%.[254] It was 1.6% for supratentorial tumors and 9.7% for infratentorial lesions, 8.4% for high-grade tumors, and 4.5% for low-grade lesions. No patient with high-grade supratentorial lesions developed spinal seeding, whereas 15.7% of those with high-grade infratentorial tumors developed spinal dissemination. For low-grade tumors, 2.7% of patients with supratentorial lesions developed seeding compared with 5.5% for those with infratentorial lesions. The incidence of spinal seeding was related directly to local tumor control, regardless of tumor grade. The incidence of spinal dissemination was 3.3% in locally controlled patients and 9.5% in those with uncontrolled primary lesions ($p < 0.05$).

SURGERY

Approximately half of hemispheric ependymomas arise from the wall of the lateral ventricle, and half appear to be intraparenchymal, arising perhaps from remote fetal ependymal cell rests.[250] Hemispheric ependymomas tend to be cystic and, even when not, are often well circumscribed from surrounding brain, allowing gross total resection. A wide craniotomy permits a transcortical exposure of the tumor through a cortical incision placed to avoid injury to vital brain tissue. The tumor is removed using the operating microscope, and every effort is made to minimize bleeding into the ventricular cavity. At the end of the resection, the ventricular system is gently irrigated free of blood and blood clots to prevent mechanical obstruction to CSF flow, to prevent the blockage of the CSF absorptive bed (arachnoid granulations), and to reduce the irritation of bloody CSF to the brain.

Ependymomas arising from the floor of the fourth ventricle are approached through a wide bilateral suboccipital craniectomy and laminectomy of C1. The tumor is exposed by retracting the cerebellar tonsils laterally and splitting the inferior aspect of the vermis, although often a tongue of tumor is visible over the dorsal aspect of the medulla and upper cervical spinal cord before the tonsils are retracted. The dorsal convexity of the tumor comes into view as the cerebellar vermis is divided, and its attachment to the floor of the fourth ventricle can then be exposed progressively and evaluated. Firm attachment precludes a gross total resection, as does infiltration of the tumor into the cranial nerves of the cerebellopontine angle through the foramen of Luschka. Tumor is removed to the extent possible using illumination and magnification afforded by the operating microscope.

There would appear to be a relation between residual ependymoma left by the surgeon and a poorer outcome after radiation therapy.[251] In ependymomas, as in most of the gliomas, a maximal surgical resection should be carried out when possible.

RADIATION THERAPY

It is well established that postoperative irradiation improves the survival of patients with intracranial ependymomas, and 5-year survival rates with doses of 45 Gy or more range from 40% to 87%.[74] Tumor grade has been considered to be the most important determinant of tumor behavior and prognosis. The 5-year survival for patients with low-grade tumors ranges from 60% to 80%, whereas for anaplastic ependymomas, it is only 10% to 47%.[74] Most series fail to distinguish patients with malignant ependymomas from those with ependymoblastomas that are classified as primitive neuroectodermal tumors and have an especially poor prognosis. Analyses suggested that when these lesions are excluded, tumor grade has less prognostic value.[252]

The risk of seeding, however, was independent of whether prophylactic spinal irradiation was given.[254] For high-grade lesions, spinal dissemination occurred in 9.4% of patients receiving craniospinal irradiation and in 6.7% of those treated with local radiation therapy only. Similarly, for low-grade tumors, spinal seeding occurred in 9.3% after craniospinal irradiation, whereas 2.2% developed seeding without prophylactic treatment.

The recommended treatment volumes for supratentorial low-grade ependymomas vary from generous local fields to the whole brain, whereas for low-grade infratentorial tumors they include local fields, the whole brain with cervical spine extension, and craniospinal axis irradiation. Wallner and coworkers reviewed the outcome of low-grade ependymomas treated with local irradiation after surgery; only 1 in 16 patients, who was eventually found to have a local recurrence, developed spinal dissemination.[255] The 5- and 10-year survival rates for those who received more than 45 Gy (approximately 50 Gy in most instances) were 67% and 57%, respectively. Recurrence at the primary tumor site was the most frequent pattern of failure. Based on this series and data from others and the greater precision in determining tumor extent currently available through high-quality diagnostic imaging, low-grade supratentorial ependymomas are treated using a generous target volume with a dose of at least 54 Gy. Spinal CT and MRI studies, myelography, and CSF evaluation are not obtained routinely in these patients. Patients with low-grade infratentorial lesions are treated similarly. The remainder of the craniospinal axis is treated only if pretreatment CSF cytology studies reveal malignant cells or if radiographic studies show evidence of tumor spread.

Most authors agree that in the case of anaplastic ependymomas, the entire craniospinal axis should be treated, although some recommend whole-brain irradiation with an additional boost for high-grade supratentorial lesions located away from the CSF pathways.[253] A dose of 54 Gy is given to the primary tumor site and 35 to 40 Gy to the remainder of the axis. If spread within the brain is demonstrated, the entire brain receives 54 Gy. Spinal imaging studies are routinely performed, and any area of gross involvement is boosted to 50 Gy. Despite the apparent superiority of craniospinal irradiation in some series,[256] the findings that local recurrence is the primary pattern of failure,[253,255,257,258] that subarachnoid failure is rare in the absence of local failure,[256,257] and that spinal metastases may not be prevented by prophylactic treatment[253,254] have led some investigators to question the routine use of craniospinal irradiation in anaplastic lesions. Future clinical trials probably will focus on more aggressive local therapy to improve primary tumor control in both low- and high-grade ependymomas and will address the necessity of spinal prophylaxis in high-grade lesions.

CHEMOTHERAPY

Because the need for chemotherapy for these tumors has been limited and, before the MRI era, they were hard to assess, most chemotherapeutic trials are anecdotal. For primary treatment of anaplastic ependymomas, these authors have been using craniospinal axis irradiation with oral hydroxyurea followed by six courses of polydrug chemotherapy (BTRC 8422) with 6-thioguanine, procarbazine, dibromodulcitol, CCNU, and VCR. Since 1984, they have treated 17 consecutive children and adults with this regimen. As of October 1991, they have had 9 failures, an MTP of 3.4 years, and a 5-year disease-free survival of 42%.

Table 48–18 summarizes some published and unpublished series of chemotherapy for recurrent differentiated or anaplastic ependymomas. The authors have, for many years, treated recurrent ependymomas with BCNU or dibromodulcitol as monotherapy.[259] Results were better than those achieved for anaplastic astrocytomas. Subsequent to those trials, they used the drug combination of 6-thioguanine, procarbazine, dibromodulcitol, CCNU, and VCR (BTRC 8422A); they achieved an 82% response and stable rate for an MTP of 21.3 months.

Goldwein and colleagues retrospectively analyzed 16 recurrent ependymoma patients treated with a variety of agents alone and in combination (VCR, cisplatin, CCNU, procarbazine, VP-16, and ifosfamide).[260] Approximately 20% of patient trials led to a partial response or stable disease (more common 7 to 1), for an approximate median of 6 to 10 months.

Gaynon and associates of the CCSG used carboplatin every 4 weeks and found a response and stable disease rate of 28% (4 in 14) with a duration of 6+, 17+, 12, and 15 months.[261] Those who did not receive prior cisplatin were more likely to respond to carboplatin. Bertolone and coworkers evaluated cisplatin and found 6 of 8 (75%) benefiting, with an MTP of 3.8 months.[185] Ettinger and colleagues, also of the CCSG, used AZQ on a 5-day every 3-week schedule in 12 children with recurrent or metastatic disease. One 35+ month response was reported.[262]

MENINGIOMAS

CLINICAL AND PATHOLOGIC CONSIDERATIONS

Meningiomas arise from arachnoidal cells in the meninges, especially in areas of the arachnoid villi. In some series, meningiomas constitute 39% of primary CNS tumors.[46] The most frequent locations of these tumors are along the sagittal sinus

TABLE 48–19. Sites of Predilections of Meningiomas Within the Intracranial Regions

Site	Number
Parasagittal	65
Convexity	54
Sphenoidal ridge	53
Olfactory groove	29
Suprasellar	28
Posterior fossa	23
Spinal	18
Periocular	12
Temporal fossa	8
Falx	7
Choroidal	6
Gasserian	5
Multiple	2
Combined with neurinomas	2
Intraorbital	1

(Cushing H, Eisenhardt L. Meningiomas. Vol 1. Their classification, regional behavior, life history and surgical end results. Springfield: Charles C. Thomas, 1938:73)

and over the cerebral convexity. Table 48–19 summarizes the frequency of these tumors according to location.[263] Meningiomas are extraaxial, intracranial (and sometimes spinal) tumors that produce symptoms and signs through compression of adjacent brain tissue and cranial nerves. They often also produce hyperostosis. Table 48–20 summarizes the symptoms and signs associated with these tumors.

Histologically, most meningiomas are differentiated, with low proliferative capacity and limited invasiveness. Less commonly, meningiomas are more anaplastic with a higher

TABLE 48–18. Chemotherapy for Recurrent Ependymoma and Anaplastic Ependymomas

Treatment*	Percentile of TTP (mo) 50%	25%
BCNU (11/14)[183a]	13	24
DBD (9/12)[259]	16	20
AZQ (5/12)[262]	10	16
Carboplatin (4/14)[261]	14	NA
Cisplatin (6/8)[220]	3.8	4.3
VCR-CDDP-CCNU-PCB-VP-16-IFSO combinations (8/37)[260] †	9	10
6-TG-PCB-DBD-CCNU-VCR (9/11)[258a]	21.6	NA

TTP, time to tumor progression; BCNU, carmustine; NA, not available or attained; AZQ, diaziquone; VCR, vincristine; CDDP, cisplatin; CCNU, lomustine; PCB, procarbazine; VP-16, etoposide; 6-TG, 6-thioguanine; DBD, dibromodulcitol.
* (Responder + Stable)/All patients.
† 16 patients were treated on 37 different trials.

TABLE 48–20. Neurologic Findings Associated With Meningiomas as a Function of Their Location

Site	Presentation
Sphenoidal ridge	Nonpulsating, painless unilateral exophthalmos; unilateral visual loss; ophthalmoplegia; ICP
Cerebral convexity	Altered mentation; ICP; seizures
Intraventricular	Hydrocephalus; headache; mental changes; visual field abnormalities
Olfactory groove	Central scotoma; ipsilateral optic atrophy; contralateral papilledema; ipsilateral loss of smell; altered mentation; focal motor abnormalities
Tuberculum sellae	Loss of vision; bitemporal hemianopia; papilledema or optic atrophy
Other basilar sites	See Table 48–5
Cerebellar convexity	ICP; cerebellar findings
Cerebellopontine angle	Cerebellar findings; hearing loss
Foramen magnum	No findings; spastic paresis and sensory findings in upper extremities

ICP, increased intracranial pressure.

proliferative capacity and are invasive. Even though the difference in the 30-minute bromodeoxyuridine labeling index in situ for the differentiated meningiomas may be less than 1% versus 3% to 4% for anaplastic meningiomas,[264] biologically, the anaplastic meningiomas behave considerably differently than the more differentiated meningiomas.

SURGERY

The perception that meningiomas are surgically resectable gives these tumors an undeserved reputation of benignity. Although meningiomas usually are well circumscribed and do not invade adjacent brain, they can occur virtually anywhere in the CNS, and access is sometimes only by deep retraction. In addition, these tumors may be extremely vascular and can surround important structures such as cranial nerves and major arteries at the skull base. Such characteristics can preclude a smooth operation, and a total removal is commonly not possible. Simpson reported on a large series of surgically resected meningiomas and documented that even when there was a perceived total resection, the recurrence rate was 9%.[265] A more modern series from Massachusetts General Hospital shows that a "total resection" is followed by 7% recurrence rate at 5 years, 20% at 10 years, and 32% at 15 years.[266]

Nevertheless, in dramatic contrast to the more common cerebral gliomas, certain meningiomas are surgically resectable, and the neurosurgeon is usually more favorably disposed toward tackling a meningioma than operating on another glioma. The neurosurgeon's zeal must be tempered with an understanding of the risks of removing a particular meningioma in a particular location and an understanding of the impact of this meningioma on the well-being of the particular patient, because these tumors are often exceedingly slow-growing and the patients are often elderly. The presence of a meningioma is not an absolute indication for surgery; when surgery is undertaken in an elderly patient, partial removal is sometimes adequate.

Preoperative Planning

The preoperative preparation of the patient, the surgical planning, and the intraoperative anesthetic management are as described in the earlier surgery section. However, the planning of surgery for meningiomas must be extremely assiduous, because a detailed knowledge of surgical anatomy is necessary in these tumors. A preoperative angiogram to assess overall tumor vascularity and to identify arterial feeders is often important. In many instances, the angiography procedure is combined with embolization of the tumor's blood supply. The angiogram is done within 24 to 96 hours of the operative procedure, so that alternative vascular routes to the tumor do not have time to develop.

Surgical Principles

Those feeding arteries that could not be occluded by embolization are addressed first at the operation, if they are accessible. These arteries are meningeal and cerebral in origin. The tumor is retracted from surrounding normal brain progressively as the tumor bulk is reduced by the use of the CUSA

or, for extremely vascular tumors, the cutting loop of the electrocoagulation unit or the CO_2 laser. Meningiomas at individual sites pose special surgical problems.

At the cerebral convexity, a large bone flap is made around the tumor, a dural incision circumscribes the tumor, and the dura attached to the tumor is used to retract the tumor from the brain as microdissection frees the adhesions between the tumor and surrounding brain.

Parasagittal meningiomas abut the midline; difficulties in removal are related to critical draining veins, to involvement of the sagittal sinus with tumor, and to the often massive overlying bony erosion or hyperostosis or both. A patent sagittal sinus cannot be transected for a complete tumor removal except in its anterior one third, so a careful study of the preoperative arteriogram looking for the patency of the sinus and for the position of the draining veins in the region is critical. Some clinicians advocate opening the sagittal sinus for removal of tumor that has grown through its wall, and others advocate resecting and grafting the involved sagittal sinus wall. In the authors' opinion, these dangerous maneuvers are not usually indicated, because recurrence-free survivals after subtotal resection of these lesions are extended,[266] and because the tumor may grow to occlude the sinus completely, thereby making complete resection possible later with a lesser risk to life.

Falx meningiomas do not involve the sagittal sinus but occupy the falx below the sinus, often becoming bilateral. Major complications of resection of falx meningiomas relate to interruption of draining veins and consequent cerebral edema and venous infarction.

Olfactory groove meningiomas grow extremely large before their neurologic sequelae lead to their discovery. Surgery is carried out through a large bifrontal bone flap based low on the forehead. The broad sessile base of the tumor is attacked first with its blood supply, then the tumor's bulk is reduced by internal coring and dissection, with attention to protection of the optic nerves, carotid artery, and anterior cerebral arteries on the tumor's posterior aspect.

Tuberculum sellae meningiomas are smaller at presentation because of their proximity to the optic apparatus. Attention to the safety of the optic apparatus and the anterior cerebral and carotid arteries is equally critical.

Sphenoid ridge meningiomas vary in approach, depending on whether they occupy the outer, middle, or inner third of the sphenoid bone. Outer third tumors can be a problem purely of tumor mass, purely of massive temporal hypertosis from en plaque tumor invading bone, or a combination of both. When it is present, the tumor mass insinuates itself in the sylvian tissue, and its removal through a frontotemporal craniotomy is complicated by the tumor's adherence (on its medial aspect) to sylvian veins. Surgical cure is not possible. Middle third tumors grow into both the frontal and temporal fossae in a globular fashion. The approach is through a frontotemporal craniotomy, with the base of the tumor approached first to eliminate the blood supply. Surgical cure is likely. Inner third tumors arise from the anterior clinoid process and compress the optic nerve and encase the carotid and middle cerebral arteries. In addition, medial sphenoidal meningiomas can grow diffusely into the cavernous sinus and optic canal. Only in those situations where the tumor presents early because of optic nerve compression is total removal even feasible. Most commonly, a complete resection is not possible, and the surgeon stops when the risk of the surgery exceeds potential benefits.

Tentorial meningiomas arise from the broad surface or free edge of the tentorium and are approached under the temporal lobe or under the occipital lobe, depending on their placement. In all instances, the principle of removal is incision of the tentorium around the tumor and gradual bulk reduction and separation of the tumor from surrounding brain. Venous sinuses and critical draining veins, particularly the vein of Labbé, must be protected.

Cerebellopontine angle or lateral posterior fossa meningiomas arise from the petrous bone and are exposed through a posterior fossa craniectomy by retracting the cerebellum medially. Involvement of cranial nerves VII and VIII can occur, and ventrally situated tumors may be marked by extreme adherence to the brain stem; no attempt at complete removal is justifiable in this situation.

Clival meningiomas have been approached under the temporal lobe, through the posterior fossa and temporal bone, and even transorally. Because these tumors involve cranial nerves and important arterial perforators to the brain stem, a conservative approach, internal decompression of the tumors, seems prudent sometimes. If possible, however, total removal should be attempted in the young patient at the first operation, because adhesions will preclude surgical cure at a subsequent reoperation.

RADIATION THERAPY

The need for adjunctive radiation therapy is determined by the extent of surgical resection and the histopathologic features of the tumor (benign versus malignant). The risk of recurrence for completely resected meningiomas is small, and postoperative irradiation is not usually recommended. In contrast, the risk of relapse after subtotal resection ranges from 33% to 60% at 5 years to more than 90% at 15 years.[247,266] Several reports suggest that postoperative irradiation prolongs the interval to recurrence, prevents tumor regrowth in some patients, and improves the survival of patients with incompletely resected meningiomas. Barbaro and associates compared the outcome of 54 patients who were treated with subtotal resection and radiation therapy with a group of 30 patients who underwent subtotal resection alone.[267] Sixty percent of the nonirradiated patients developed recurrence, whereas 32% of the irradiated patients recurred. The median time to recurrence was 10.4 years for the irradiated patients compared with 5.5 years for the nonirradiated group ($p < 0.05$). Taylor and coworkers found that 69% of their patients relapsed after subtotal excision alone, whereas only 15% of those treated with subtotal excision and postoperative irradiation recurred ($p = 0.01$).[268] The 10-year survival rate was 81% for patients treated with combined therapy compared with 49% for nonirradiated patients. The actuarial 5-, 10-, and 15-year relapse-free survival rates for patients undergoing subtotal resection and irradiation reported by Graholm and colleagues were 78%, 67%, and 56%, respectively.[269] These results compare favorably with the relapse-free survival rates of 63%, 45%, and 9% reported by Mirimanoff and associates for incompletely resected, nonirradiated patients.[266]

It is controversial whether patients should be treated with radiation therapy after their initial subtotal resection or when signs of disease progression appear. Some clinicians have found that patients with benign meningiomas do equally well with either approach[270]; others suggest that initial postoperative irradiation is preferable, because recurrence has an adverse influence on outcome, and many patients who recur after initial subtotal excision alone may not be salvaged by subsequent treatment.[268] Postoperative irradiation often is deferred in elderly patients and in those in poor medical condition until there is evidence of symptomatic progression.[268] When a surgical resection is not feasible, radiation therapy may relieve symptoms and substantially decrease the rate of tumor progression.[269]

Malignant meningiomas behave in a more aggressive manner than their benign counterparts. Chan and Thompson found that the mean survival of 6 patients treated with surgery alone was only 7.2 months, compared with 5.1 years for 12 patients treated with surgery and postoperative irradiation.[271] Six of the 9 patients with malignant histology reported by Graholm and coworkers died within 5 years.[269] The recurrence rate among 53 patients with malignant meningiomas collected from six series in the literature was 49%. The recurrence rates were 33% for patients treated with complete resection alone, 12% for those undergoing complete resection and radiation therapy, 55% for patients treated by subtotal resection and irradiation, and 100% for those treated by subtotal resection alone.[257] These data suggest that all patients with malignant meningiomas should be offered postoperative irradiation, regardless of the extent of resection.

The tumor volume for radiation therapy, defined by CT scan or MRI and modified by the neurosurgeon's description of the site of residual disease, is treated with a margin of 1.5 to 2 cm. Extensive base-of-skull tumors and malignant meningiomas require more generous margins. A dose of 55 Gy in daily fractions of 1.8 to 2 Gy is recommended for benign meningiomas, whereas the dose is increased to 60 Gy for malignant lesions.

CHEMOTHERAPY

There is currently no place for chemotherapy for newly diagnosed and nonirradiated meningiomas, because chemotherapy is not required except in the most intransigent recurrences. For patients who present with histologically malignant meningiomas or recurrent, surgically inaccessible, more-differentiated meningiomas, the situation is only slightly different. Because of the potentially lethal consequences of these two situations, the authors have been treating with aggressive surgery, focal irradiation, and cytotoxic chemotherapy.

The authors have evaluated the combinations of cyclophosphamide, doxorubicin, and VCR (9 patients); DTIC and doxorubicin (5 patients); and high-dose ifosfamide with mesna (2 patients). Little objective activity was noted for the first, 1 in 5 responses in the second, and 1 in 2 in the third. Grunberg and colleagues reported on the use of mifepristone, an antiprogesterone, in 14 patients with recurrent meningiomas; 5 in 14 showed objective response after 6 to 12 months of daily oral therapy.[272] A randomized trial for incompletely resected meningiomas is being advanced to better determine the relative merits of mifepristone chemotherapy.

PRIMARY CNS LYMPHOMA

CLINICAL AND PATHOLOGIC CONSIDERATIONS

Primary non-AIDS CNS lymphomas are often B-cell lymphomas of the histiocytic (large cell or large cell immunoblastic) type. In some patients, EBV has been found in biopsy material.[40] In the past, most patients with primary CNS lymphoma had no predisposing immunosuppressive disorder. However, primary CNS non-Hodgkin's lymphoma has been seen with inherited immunosuppression (ataxia-telangiectasia, Wiskott-Aldrich syndrome, and severe combined immunodeficiency disease [SCID]), acquired immunosuppression (systemic lupus erythematosus, tuberculosis, and vasculitis), drugs that are immunosuppressants (transplant patients), and EBV.[40,273–275] Unfortunately, these tumors are taking on greater importance because of their association with immunodeficiency states.

Before the AIDS era, CNS lymphomas represented only 1% of all lymphomas. In transplant recipients, CNS lymphomas accounted for 50% of lymphomas. As a result of the AIDS epidemic, primary CNS lymphoma has become more prevalent and, by some estimates, it will become the commonest primary CNS tumor during the 1990s.[276]

Clinically, these tumors are more prevalent among men. Before AIDS, they had their peak incidence in the fourth to sixth decades. Because of AIDS-associated CNS lymphomas, the age for the peak incidence is decreasing, with these tumors becoming more common in the third and fourth decades. The average time from onset of disease to diagnosis is approximately 1 to 2 months. In a recent literature review, Murray and associates found that 52% of cases were supratentorial, 34% were multiple, 12% were cerebellar, 2% were in the brain stem, and fewer than 0.5% were spinal.[277]

Because the level of clinical concern determines how quickly diagnosis is made and how long symptoms are allowed to progress, patterns of presentation vary from series to series. The following categories of symptoms have been observed: (1) those due to increased intracranial pressure, such as headache, nausea, and vomiting; (2) those associated with deficits in higher cortical function, including personality change, psychiatric manifestations, and dementia; (3) focal neurologic deficits; and (4) seizures. Most prevalent are symptoms and signs of confusion, lethargy, and memory loss followed by focal findings of hemiparesis or dysphasia.

The contrast-enhanced CT and MRI appearance of these lesions is sometimes distinctive. Multiple lesions and homogenous enhancement of signal in the paraventricular regions, basal ganglia, thalamus, or corpus callosum suggest CNS lymphoma. Sometimes, the extent of disease appears disproportionate to the neurologic deficit. Many tumors have minimal, if any, mass effect. The differential diagnosis of AIDS-associated CNS lymphoma must include the many opportunistic fungal and parasitic infections also common to AIDS, especially toxoplasmosis. However, as with gliomas, the diagnosis is made by biopsy.

CSF examination is sometimes helpful to identify specific cytoplasmic immunoglobulins. Although specific CSF abnormalities are seen in fewer than 30% of patients with primary CNS lymphomas, pleocytosis, increased protein, hypogalycorrhachia, positive cytology, and specific monoclonal antibody staining of surface markers may be helpful.

SURGERY

Because a tissue diagnosis is essential and surgery is not curative for patients with multiple lesions or with small and poorly accessible lesions in, for example, the thalamus, corpus callosum, or deep dominant hemisphere, these patients may receive only a CT-stereotactic biopsy. Large single hemispheric lesions should be surgically reduced, as should the largest of multiple lesions, when intracranial pressure cannot be controlled otherwise. CSF shunting procedures are sometimes necessary when there is diffuse meningeal tumor invasion and consequent communicating hydrocephalus.

RADIATION THERAPY

Primary CNS lymphomas are clinically aggressive tumors, and although they are limited to one "extranodal site," their behavior is comparable with that of disseminated high-grade systemic lymphomas.[278] Survival times from the onset of symptoms vary from 1 to 3.3 months with supportive care alone and 0.9 to 4.6 months after surgical resection (without adjuvant therapy).[279,280] Although radiation therapy generally results in prompt clinical and radiographic improvement, the duration of response is surprisingly short, and local recurrence usually ensues. The median survival time after treatment with radiation therapy ranges from 10 to 18 months,[281] and the 5-year disease-free survival rate is only 3%.[74] Because of the multifocal nature of CNS lymphomas, their predilection for leptomeningeal infiltration, and their tendency to be more widespread than indicated by imaging studies, the entire intracranial contents are included within the treatment fields. Several retrospective reviews suggest that there is a direct relation between radiation dose and outcome. Pollack and co-workers found that patients treated with doses of 40 to 50 Gy to the whole brain survived longer than those who received lower doses.[282] Further, Murray and colleagues observed that patients who received 50 Gy or more to the primary tumor site had a better outcome than those given less than 50 Gy.[283]

To examine the efficacy of high-dose radiation therapy, the RTOG conducted a prospective study in which patients were given 40 Gy to the whole brain followed by an additional 20 Gy to the primary lesion. The median survival time of the 41 evaluable patients was 11.6 months; the 1- and 2-year survival rates were 48% and 28%, respectively. Age and KPS were the most important predictors of outcome. Patients who were older than 60 years of age or had a KPS of less than 60 had an especially poor prognosis (median survival time 5.6–7.6 months) compared with younger and more functionally intact patients (median survival time 21–23 months).[284] These results suggest that even 60 Gy is inadequate and provide convincing evidence that more aggressive therapeutic regimens are needed.

Usually, it is recommended that patients with solitary lesions receive 40 to 50 Gy to the whole brain, supplemented by an additional 10 to 15 Gy to the primary tumor site using conventional fractionation schedules. Because of the risk of ocular involvement and the efficacy of orbital irradiation in affected patients,[285] inclusion of the posterior orbits within the whole-brain irradiation field has been recommended.[282] Although craniospinal axis irradiation may be of value in patients with primary leptomeningeal lymphoma, its efficacy in other patients is unproved.[74] In most situations, spinal irradiation has been replaced by intrathecal chemotherapy. The prognosis of AIDS patients with CNS lymphomas is much poorer than in non-AIDS-related CNS lymphoma. The median survival time may be as brief as 2 months, and patients often die from other causes.[276,286] For these patients, a dose of 40 Gy in 3 weeks to the whole brain provides satisfactory palliation.

CHEMOTHERAPY

Chemotherapy is of proved efficacy in the treatment of systemic lymphoma. A variety of agents and approaches have been used to treat primary CNS lymphoma with variable results. In some patients, glucocorticoids cause the temporary disappearance of contrast-enhancing lesions on CT. This effect may result from the direct cytolytic effect of glucocorticoids or from stabilization of the blood–brain barrier. This usually is a short-lived response. Unfortunately, chemotherapy trials have been sporadic and often have involved few patients.

Early studies used chemotherapy at the time of recurrence or progression. More recently, chemotherapy was given adjuvant to radiation therapy. Regimens used include nitrosoureas; procarbazine; mustard compounds; high-dose methotrexate; high-dose cytosine arabinoside; cytoxan, doxorubicin, VCR, and prednisone (CHOP); VCR, cytoxan, procarbazine or 6-mercaptopurine (VENP or VEMP); dexamethasone, high-dose cytosine arabinoside, and cisplatin (DHAP)[287]; PCV[288]; and osmotic blood–brain barrier opening with cytoxan, methotrexate, procarbazine, and dexamethasone.[289] Reports indicate that all regimens are capable of producing remission, although the resilence of remission in terms of duration is variable.

McLaughlin and associates reported on 10 patients treated with DHAP.[287] They found 2 in 4 had a complete response at initial treatment and 4 in 6 treated at relapse also achieved complete response. Chamberlain and Levin reported 10 patients treated with radiation therapy and concomitant hydroxyurea followed by PCV. Median and 25% survival times were 30 and 50 months.[288]

Neuwelt and colleagues reported on the use of osmotic blood–brain barrier disruption using intraarterial mannitol in association with intraarterial methotrexate (1–5 g) with leucovorin rescue and intravenous cyclophosphamide (30 mg/kg).[289] During the next 14 days, the patients received oral procarbazine (100 mg/day) and dexamethasone (24 mg/day). Of 13 patients treated at recurrence, the median survival was 17 months. For the 17 patients treated at initial presentation, the median survival was 55 months (radiation was used for tumor progression or recurrence).

Some of the best results have been obtained by DeAngelis and associates, using high-dose intravenous methotrexate and intraventricular methotrexate before radiation therapy.[281] Patients received preradiation therapy methotrexate (1 g/m^2) and intraventricular methotrexate; whole-brain and tumor-boosted radiation therapy; and postradiation therapy, two courses of cytarabine (3 g/m^2 for 2 days). Of 32 patients studied, the median survival was 42 months compared with 21 months for those receiving radiation therapy only.[290]

Given the scarcity of non-AIDS primary CNS lymphomas, it is clear that randomized cooperative trials are necessary to consolidate these observations and provide a more rational basis for future treatments.

PRIMITIVE NEUROEPITHELIAL TUMORS

CLINICAL AND PATHOLOGIC CONSIDERATIONS

The treatment of primitive neuroepithelial tumors is controversial and complex. Much of the controversy is based on the failure to understand that there are multiple entities included within this pathologic diagnosis. Controversy surrounds the classification of these tumors.[291] Primitive cells that remain undifferentiated or exhibit varying degrees of neuronal or glial differentiation, or both, are the hallmark of these tumors. Conceptually, these tumors can be viewed as developmentally aberrant brain cells. Therefore, primitive neuroepithelial tumors can be divided into the following classification schema: medulloepithelioma, neuroblastoma, spongioblastoma, ependymoblastoma, pineoblastoma, and medulloblastoma. With the exception of medulloblastoma, primitive neuroepithelial tumors are rare.

It has been proposed that all neoplasms showing primitive poorly differentiated neuroepithelial cells be called *primitive neuroectodermal tumors*, regardless of location or cell type. Because of the infrequency of these tumors and the controversy surrounding an all-inclusive classification schema currently, it is best to refer to each histiotype separately.

Clinically, however, these tumors share some common and disquieting features. Primarily, they are proliferative and malignant tumors that tend to spread throughout the neuraxis like medulloblastoma. As a result, a complete evaluation of the CNS, including contrast-enhanced CT scans of the entire brain, CSF cytology, and metrizamide myelography, must be performed before the initiation of treatment.

SURGERY

The initial therapy for primitive neuroectodermal tumors is surgical bulk reduction whenever feasible. Surgical principles are the same as those for astrocytoma described earlier.

RADIATION THERAPY

Because of their propensity to spread throughout the subarachnoid space, primitive neuroectodermal tumors are treated with craniospinal axis irradiation. The doses are similar to those given for medulloblastoma. The primary tumor should receive 54 Gy at 1.8 Gy/day, with the remainder of the axis receiving 30 to 40 Gy, depending on the age of the patient. These tumors appear to be less radiocurable than medulloblastomas. In a series of 14 patients reported by Gaffney and coworkers, the 5-year survival rate was 25%.[292] Two of the three long-term survivors received craniospinal irradiation, and all had chemotherapy. None of the patients with more than 90% primitive elements in their pathology specimen survived 5 years.

Within this category is a distinct pathologic and clinical entity that differs from other primitive neuroectodermal tumors, namely the primary cerebral neuroblastoma. Berger and colleagues found that 7 of the 11 patients treated with local irradiation to a dose of 50 Gy were alive with no evidence of tumor progression.[293] Of the 6 patients with cystic tumors, none had recurrent disease, whereas 4 of the 5 patients with solid tumors recurred. Based on this analysis, it is recommended that patients with primary cerebral neuroblastomas receive craniospinal axis irradiation only if there is evidence of tumor spread beyond the site of origin. If the tumor is localized, focal irradiation is the treatment of choice.

CHEMOTHERAPY

Because primitive neuroectodermal tumors are an uncommon type of tumor, there are no controlled chemotherapy trials. Reports of isolated cases and small series indicate that drugs active against medulloblastoma have activity in primitive neuroectodermal tumors (see medulloblastoma chemotherapy section that follows).

MEDULLOBLASTOMA

CLINICAL AND PATHOLOGIC CONSIDERATIONS

Medulloblastoma appears more similar to the primitive neuroectodermal tumors of childhood than to the gliomas. Although the cell of origin of these tumors is controversial, it is probable that medulloblastoma takes its origin from germinative neuroepithelial cells in the roof of the fourth ventricle.[50] Consistent with its embryonal nature is the fact that the peak incidence occurs in the first decade of life (see Table 48–4); 50% to 60% of medulloblastomas occur in the first decade, with a peak between 5 and 9 years. A second but lesser peak occurs between 20 and 30 years.

The typical location for childhood medulloblastoma is in the cerebellum, mostly in the midline and posterior vermis (Fig. 48–7); many encroach on the cisterna magna and the fourth ventricle. In adolescents and adults, there is an increasing tendency for tumors to be laterally placed in the cerebellar hemispheres. Regardless of where in the cerebel-

lum they occur, the tendency for metastatic spread (within craniospinal intradural axis) of medulloblastoma is relatively high. At presentation, as many as 30% of patients have positive cytology or myelographic evidence of spinal metastasis.[294,295] Extra-CNS metastasis is less common and occurs in fewer than 5% of patients; most metastases are to long bones.[294]

Based on bromodeoxyuridine 30-minute labeling indices, medulloblastoma would be considered a highly proliferative tumor because its labeling index is approximately 14%, as opposed to gliomas, which range between less than 1% to 10%.[264]

The overall disease-free 5-year survival for medulloblastoma is approximately 50%.[222,294,296–299] However, the extent of disease at initial diagnosis defines risk. When risk factors are considered, survival is altered dramatically. Poor risk is defined as less than a 75% resection (probably >1 cc residual); invasion of the brain stem; metastasis to the spinal cord, cerebrum, and leptomeninges or seeding of the cerebellum; positive CSF cytology 2 weeks after surgery; and age younger than 4 years.[222,296,297] Of the poor-risk factors, two need explanation. Resection of less than 75% is an imprecise measure of remaining tumor—CT and MRI measurement of residual tumor volume would be better. However, in most patients, if the surgeon can remove more than 75% of tumor, the resection is usually a gross total resection. Poor risk associated with age 4 years and younger may relate more to the restricted irradiation to the developing CNS and its negative impact on tumor control. Most radiation therapists will not treat with full doses of craniospinal irradiation at 4 years.

The disease-free survival of poor-risk patients with craniospinal irradiation with or without chemotherapy is approximately 25% to 30%.[298] Good-risk patients, on the other hand, have 5-year disease-free survivals of 66% to 70%.[299,300]

At relapse, the major site of first recurrence is the posterior

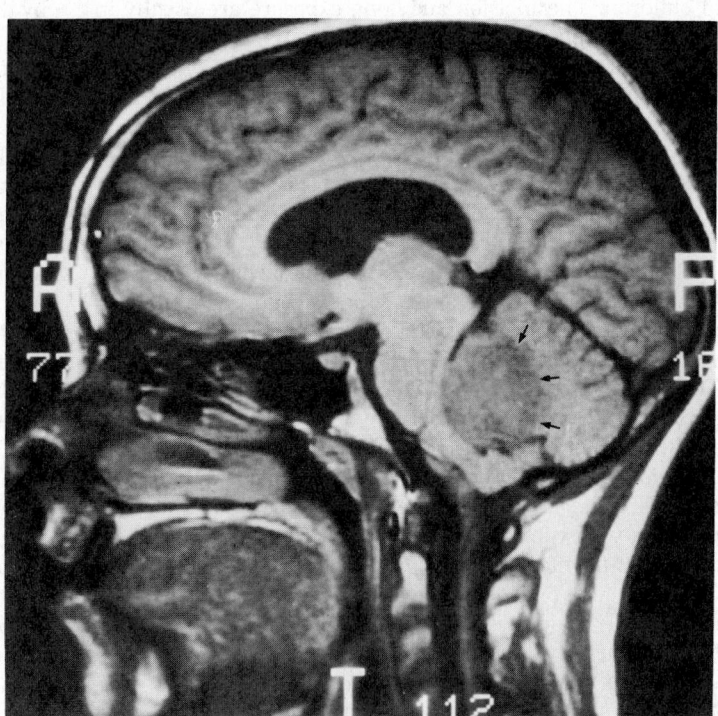

FIGURE 48–7. This young girl presented with headache and gait ataxia. A T1-weighted sagittal MRI scan (TR 600, TE 20) demonstrated a large, low-intensity mass involving the inferior aspect of the cerebellum in the midline and extending to and filling the fourth ventricle. There is arcuate stretching and displacement of the medulla and secondary hydrocephalus. The well-circumscribed nature and location of the tumor is fairly characteristic for medulloblastoma.

fossa in more than 50% of patients, the frontal lobe in nearly 20%, bone in 10% to 15%, and other cerebral and suprasellar regions in 10% to 15%.[294,300]

The incidence of systemic metastasis varies between 10% and 30%,[297,298] although the 10% incidence is most similar to the authors' experience. Most extra-CNS metastases are to long bones and ribs, with lymph nodes being a distant second site. In the series by Park and associates[297] and by Lowery and colleagues,[298] the median time to the development of extra-CNS metastasis was 10 to 12 months; in the authors' more recent study, it was 18 months.[301] In the Park study, 17% of ventriculoperitoneal-shunted patients developed systemic metastases, whereas only 4% in unshunted patients did so. In Lowery's series, 30% of patients developed systemic metastases, and none had been shunted previously. These authors' experience is that, except in patients with rampant disease, they did not find an association between ventriculoatrial or ventriculoperitoneal shunting, with or without an in-line filter, and systemic metastases. Bone metastases can occur as the only evidence of recurrence in nonshunted patients years after their initial presentation with CNS disease.

SURGERY

Although hydrocephalus associated with medulloblastoma obstructing the fourth ventricle can be relieved with a preresection CSF shunt, it is more usual to defer shunting and control increased intracranial pressure with corticosteroids. In as many as 60% of patients, aggressive resection of the tumor relieves hydrocephalus. An occipital burr hole is commonly placed at surgery, before the posterior fossa exposure is done, to allow cannulation of the ventricles for drainage of CSF to lower the increased intracranial pressure so that the dura can be opened safely.

Surgery for medulloblastoma is carried out in the prone or the sitting position. The prone position is preferred, especially in children. The incision and bony exposure are usually in the midline, but a paramedian incision and unilateral bony removal are done when the tumor is limited to one hemisphere, particularly in adults. The more commonly used midline craniectomy extends down through the foramen magnum, and a laminectomy of C1 (and rarely, C2) is performed to decompress herniated cerebellar tonsils or to remove a caudally extending tongue of tumor over the dorsum of the spinal cord.

After the dura is opened, the cerebellar tonsils are retracted laterally, and it is in the foramen of Magendie that the purplish-gray tumor usually is first seen. The floor of the fourth ventricle is separated from the tumor by a cottonoid pledget. The pledget is advanced to protect the floor of the fourth ventricle as the tumor is resected.

The thinned cerebellar vermis is progressively incised in the midline until the dorsum of the tumor is exposed. The tumor is usually soft and moderately vascular and is readily removed with suction irrigation, the CUSA, or laser, using the operating microscope for magnification and illumination. Clinical studies of cooperative groups show that an aggressive (gross total) removal is associated with an improved prognosis for the patient.[297] Dissection is continued laterally to remove tumor from the cerebellar hemispheres and ventrally to remove tumor from the fourth ventricle. When the obstructive hydrocephalus has been relieved, the CSF can be seen flowing from the aqueduct of Sylvius superiorly. It is rare for medulloblastoma to invade the floor of the fourth ventricle; when it does, careful use of the laser can be attempted to remove it. Closure is carried out in multiple layers, with particular attention to a tight dural closure to decrease the risk for pseudomeningocele (bulging wound) formation and the risk for aseptic meningitis and consequent communicating hydrocephalus from spilled blood products. Postoperative CSF shunting for hydrocephalus remains necessary in about 30% to 40% of patients.

RADIATION THERAPY

Medulloblastomas commonly infiltrate the subarachnoid space and have a striking propensity to spread throughout the CSF. As many as 25% to 30% of patients have clinically unsuspected cytologic and radiographic evidence of CNS dissemination at the time of diagnosis,[302,303] and for this reason, radiation therapy is directed to the entire craniospinal axis. Doses of 54 to 55 Gy to the primary tumor site and 35 to 36 Gy to the remainder of the craniospinal axis are generally recommended.[304] These doses usually are reduced by about 10 Gy for children younger than 2 or 3 years of age. Five-year survival rates in recent series range from 50% to 65% or higher.[74] The prognosis is affected by local tumor extent, completeness of surgical resection, presence of CSF dissemination, and age at diagnosis.[299] Although medulloblastoma is considered to be one of the most radiosensitive tumors of the CNS, local recurrence remains the primary cause of failure.[74]

Although modern radiation therapy techniques have greatly improved the prognosis for patients with medulloblastoma, the maximum benefit that can be achieved with conventional radiation therapy has probably been reached. Adjunctive chemotherapy programs are being pursued actively to further improve the outcome. Randomized trials have been conducted by the International Society of Pediatric Oncology (SIOP)[299] and the CCSG.[300] Each study compared radiation therapy plus chemotherapy with radiation therapy alone. The SIOP study used a regimen of weekly VCR during radiation therapy followed by eight courses of VCR and CCNU, cycled every 6 weeks. Patients in the CCSG study received similar chemotherapy plus prednisone. Neither trial demonstrated an overall improvement in outcome with the addition of chemotherapy. The 5-year disease-free survival rates in the CCSG and SIOP studies were 59% and 55%, respectively, for radiation therapy plus chemotherapy, and 50% and 43%, respectively, for radiation therapy alone. Chemotherapy did, however, appear to benefit certain patients with more advanced stages of disease, including those having only partial or subtotal tumor excision, those with brain stem involvement, and those with advanced T (T3 and T4) and M (M1–M3) stages. Based on these findings, patients with medulloblastoma have been separated into "low-stage" or "good-risk" and "high-stage" or "poor-risk" subgroups, and different study questions are being examined in each group.

Clinical studies in good-risk patients have been directed at decreasing treatment-related morbidity, including neuropsychological dysfunction, impaired growth of the spine, and hypothalamic-pituitary dysfunction, by reducing the dose of prophylactic irradiation to areas remote from the primary tumor site. A pilot study from the Children's Memorial Hospital and Northwestern University in Chicago found that there were no isolated spinal relapses in children given 24 Gy to the craniospinal axis.[305] However, a randomized trial conducted by CCSG and POG, which compared 23.4 Gy with the standard 36 Gy craniospinal prophylactic dose in good-risk children, was closed prematurely when an interim analysis demonstrated an excessive number of overall treatment failures and isolated neuraxis recurrences in the low-dose arm.[306]

The combination of low-dose craniospinal axis irradiation and chemotherapy also is being examined. It is expected that future studies will examine the use of more aggressive chemotherapy and seek to improve local control using approaches such as hyperfractionated irradiation. Efforts to decrease the morbidity of craniospinal axis irradiation should continue, provided that disease control is not compromised.

CHEMOTHERAPY

Medulloblastomas are responsive to a variety of antineoplastic agents, including VCR, nitrosoureas, procarbazine, dibromodulcitol, cyclophosphamide, methotrexate, platinum compounds, and various drug combinations. Table 48–21 summarizes some of the single agents and their observed response rates for CNS medulloblastoma when treated at recurrence or for progressive disease. For extra-CNS disease, these same agents have activity, although drugs such as cyclophosphamide, methotrexate, doxorubicin, and VCR may be more active than the nitrosoureas and procarbazine.

Table 48–22 summarizes some of the drug combinations that have been used for recurrent or progressive CNS medulloblastoma. It is not possible to compare the durability of these responses, because some reports pool the primitive neuroectodermal tumor patients with medulloblastoma, whereas others do not provide individual lengths of response,

TABLE 48–21. Efficacy of Single-Agent Chemotherapy for Recurrent and Progressive CNS Medulloblastoma

Treatment	Response*
Doxorubicin[308]	0/6 (0%)
PCNU[313]	0/4 (0%)
Etoposide (VP-16)[329]	0/4 (0%)
AZQ[182,208]	6/21 (28%)
BCNU[188,309]	2/6 (33%)
Carboplatin[261,317]	12/34 (35%)
Methotrexate (I.V.)[319–321]	5/13 (38%)
Cisplatin[314–316]	11/27 (40%)
Melphalan I.V.[330]	6/12 (50%)
Dibromodulcitol[259]	15/29 (51%)
Vincristine[322–327]	11/15 (73%)
Procarbazine[105]	3/4 (75%)
CCNU[174,175,310–312]	12/15 (80%)
Cyclophosphamide[318]	7/7 (100%)
Teniposide (VM-26)[328]	1/1 (100%)

VM-26, teniposide; AZQ, diaziquone; BCNU, carmustine; I.V., intravenous; CCNU, lomustine; VP-16, etoposide.
* Complete response plus partial response plus stable disease.

TABLE 48–22. Efficacy of Combination Chemotherapy for Recurrent and Progressive CNS Medulloblastoma

Treatment	Response
VCR-Pred-PCB(OPP)[335]	3/12 (25%)
VCR-CYT[336]	4/8 (50%)
6-TG-PCB-DBD-CCNU-VCR[258a]	6/10 (60%)
CCNU-PCB-VCR(PCV)[331]	10/16 (62%)
VM-26-CCNU-Pred[333]	2/3 (67%)
"8-in-1-day"[339]	6/9 (67%)
MOPP[334]	14/19 (73%)
VCR-MTX-BCNU[332]	8/8 (100%)
VCR-BCNU-Dex-MTX(I.V.)[337]	8/8 (100%)
CCNU-VCR-CPDD[338]	6/6 (100%)

VCR, vincristine; Pred, prednisone; PCB, procarbazine; MOPP, mustagen + Oncovin + Procarbazine + prednisone; CYT, cytoxan; 6-TG, 6-thioguanine; DBD, dibromodulcitol; CCNU, lomustine; VM-26, teniposide; MOPP, mechlorethamine, VCR, PCB, Pred; MTX, methotrexate; BCNU, carmustine; Dex, dexamethasone; CPDD, cisplatin.

an MTP, or Kaplan-Meier curves. This is unfortunate, because those studies suggest an MTP range of 10 to 19 months among the better single agent and combination chemotherapy programs.[338] It is clear, however, that better treatments are needed for recurrent and progressive disease. Whether well-founded or not, current emphasis appears to be with drug combinations such as cyclophosphamide, teniposide, and cisplatin or CCNU, VCR, and cisplatin. Whether these approaches provide long-standing benefit or short-term gain awaits more careful adjuvant studies. Problems with drug delivery of these agents to the CNS may compromise long-term benefits and ultimate cure.

As adjuvant therapy to surgery and irradiation, chemotherapy has shown inconsistent but sometimes dramatic benefit. Part of the problem resides with an agreement for the definition of good and poor risk and the tendency of some investigators to pool data from medulloblastoma with other primitive neuroectodermal tumors. Another constraint is that patients who receive craniospinal irradiation do not tolerate high-dose aggressive chemotherapy protocols well because of reduced bone marrow reserves. In an attempt to improve the tolerance to cytotoxic agents, these authors and others conducted trials to evaluate reduced craniospinal radiation therapy doses.

The authors conducted a nonrandomized trial of preradiation procarbazine and hydroxyurea during reduced craniospinal irradiation.[296] In that study they found that, after 2 weeks of oral procarbazine and irradiation with hydroxyurea, reducing the craniospinal radiation dose to 25 Gy to the spinal axis and 25 to 35 Gy to the whole brain was not detrimental with respect to disease-free survival or recurrence patterns in good- and poor-risk patients. When this group was compared with historical controls treated with conventional doses, Halberg and associates[307] found no increase in tumor recurrence in the brain or spinal axis. The 5-year disease-free survival rates for good- and poor-risk patients were 77% and 39%, respectively. In both groups, 70% of recurrences were in the posterior fossa only.

In a nonrandomized study, Packer and coworkers evaluated 108 children treated between 1975 and 1989 for medulloblastoma and other primitive neuroectodermal tumors.[340] Before 1982, children received surgery and radiation therapy, but after 1982 they also had chemotherapy with CCNU, VCR, and cisplatin. There was no difference in disease-free survival rates for children with standard risk factors; however, there was a significant difference in the 5-year survival rate for poor-risk patients treated before 1982 (35%) compared with those treated later (87%) ($p < 0.001$).

A randomized postoperative trial with postirradiation nitrogen mustard, PCV, procarbazine, and prednisone (MOPP) versus radiation therapy alone for newly diagnosed medulloblastoma found that patients treated with irradiation plus MOPP had a statistically significant increase in overall survival rate at 5 years compared with patients treated with radiation therapy alone (74% versus 56%; $p = 0.06$).[341]

The authors recently presented preliminary results of a study that opened in 1984.[342] In that study, they gave combination chemotherapy with 6-thioguanine, procarbazine, dibromodulcitol, CCNU, and VCR before and for as many as 8 cycles every 6 weeks after radiation therapy in children and adults with high-risk (more than 25% residual tumor, brain stem invasion, positive CSF cytology, positive myelogram) medulloblastoma. Radiation therapy consisted of 54 Gy to the posterior fossa and 24 Gy to the craniospinal axis. Of the 30 patients evaluable (25 children and 5 adults), there were 17 failures, a 5-year disease-free survival of 30%, and an MTP of 4.3 years. Seven pineoblastomas were also treated, with four failures to date, an MTP of 1.6 years, and 38% 5-year disease-free survival.

Hyperfractionated radiation therapy regimens, although potentially less damaging to the CNS, may lead to more bone marrow damage and less tolerance to systemic chemotherapy.

One approach that is being evaluated consists of aggressive preradiation therapy chemotherapy. The advantage of this approach is that it unequivocally defines response; the disadvantage is that some drugs may fail to achieve adequate levels in patients with poor risk due to CSF spread of tumor cells.

Kretschmar and colleagues treated 21 newly diagnosed children with poor-risk medulloblastoma on a 9-week-postoperative, preradiation therapy chemotherapy regimen of PCV and cisplatin.[343] The children older than 2 years of age then received radiation therapy. Of 13 children with measurable disease after surgery, 5 showed a definite response (1 complete response, 4 partial responses, and 5 minor responses) on CT scan. They also evaluated mustagen, Oncovin Procarbazine, and prednisone (MOP) in 6 infants until the age of 2 years, at which time they were referred for irradiation. Four of the 6 infants were disease free at 19, 32, 35, and 57 months from diagnosis.

"Eight-in-1-day" therapy has also been evaluated before radiation therapy.[339] Of 21 eligible medulloblastoma patients who received at least two courses of chemotherapy, 12 (57%) responded (including 3 complete responses and 3 partial responses). The MTP for the combined medulloblastoma-primitive neuroectodermal tumor group was 2 years.

In another study, Kovnar and associates treated 11 newly diagnosed children with measurable residual disease and characteristics indicative of poor prognosis with preradiation

therapy cisplatin and etoposide.[344] There were 2 of 11 complete responses, 8 partial responses, and 1 stable disease determined radiographically in the series.

For extracranial metastases, the best results appear with aggressive combination chemotherapy. In this situation, issues of CNS drug delivery are not important, and many drugs are active. Initially, these authors evaluated the combination of cyclophosphamide, doxorubicin, and VCR; 7 patients treated responded for a median duration of 17 months, and 2 continue at 34 and 62 months without evidence of disease.[300] Other combinations with good activity are cyclophosphamide and VCR[345]; VCR, dactinomycin, and cyclophosphamide[346]; cisplatin, cyclophosphamide, and VP-16; and DTIC and doxorubicin.[183a]

PINEAL REGION TUMORS

CLINICAL AND PATHOLOGIC CONSIDERATIONS

The pineal gland is located in the posterior portion of the third ventricle. Tumors in this region are rare, accounting for fewer than 1% of intracranial tumors, although in children they constitute 3% to 8% of intracranial tumors.[347] The peak incidence of germ cell tumors is the second decade, and few present after the third decade.[348] Table 48–23 summarizes the types of tumors found in the pineal region.[349] In all series, germinomas are the commonest histology, accounting for 33% to 50% of pineal tumors (the higher frequencies are seen in Japan). Gliomas are second commonest, accounting for about 25% of pineal tumors; astrocytomas are the commonest of the glial neoplasms arising at this site.

Neurologic signs and symptoms are caused by obstructive hydrocephalus and involvement of ocular pathways. Major symptoms are headache, nausea and vomiting, lethargy, and diplopia. Signs are primarily ocular but can include ataxia and hemiparesis. The major ocular manifestation is paralysis of conjugate upward gaze (Parinaud's syndrome), although pupillary and convergence abnormalities are seen, as are skew deviation and papilledema.

Determination of tumor histology and extent of disease is

TABLE 48–23. Classification of Pineal Region Tumors

I. Tumors of germ cell origin
  A. Germinoma (atypical teratoma, dysgerminoma, seminoma)
  B. Embryonal carcinoma
    1. Extraembryonic structures
      a. Endodermal sinus tumors (yolk sac tumor)
      b. Choriocarcinoma
    2. Embryonic endoderm, mesoderm, ectoderm
      a. Immature teratoma
      b. Mature teratoma
II. Tumors of pineal parenchymal cells
  A. Pineoblastoma
  B. Pineocytoma
III. Tumors of glial and other cell origin
IV. Nonneoplastic cysts and masses

(Adapted from Herrick MK. Pathology of pineal tumors. In: Neuwelt EA, ed. Diagnosis and treatment of pineal region tumors. Baltimore: Williams & Wilkins, 1984:31)

critical for optimal management of pineal region tumors. Figure 48–8 is a schema the authors use to evaluate and stage patients with pineal region tumors.

The prognosis for these tumors varies depending on the histology and size of tumor and the extent of disease at presentation. Typically, patients with mature teratomas do well with surgery alone; germinomas do best with radiation, although preradiation therapy chemotherapy may increase the cure rate and reduce the total radiation dose; gliomas respond to therapy in a manner discussed in earlier sections; and the remaining tumors respond variably to chemotherapy and radiation therapy, leading to survivals ranging from months to years before recurrence.

SURGERY

Because pineal tumors are near the center of the brain, they are among the most difficult brain tumors to remove, and it is this factor that creates some controversy in their management. Some authors promulgate decompressing the nearly invariable obstructive hydrocephalus with a shunt and then irradiating the tumor without a tissue diagnosis. However, because of an increasingly favorable experience with microsurgical approaches to the pineal region, the current recommendation is to obtain a tissue diagnosis and, when possible, to carry out a gross total resection of the tumor.[350] Resection is particularly important for pineal masses that may be relatively radioresistant or that do not require radiation therapy, such as teratomas, arachnoid cysts, and meningiomas.

Many surgical approaches to the pineal region have been described: (1) through the dilated lateral ventricle; (2) through the posterior corpus callosum; (3) under the occipital lobe; and (4) through the posterior fossa over the cerebellum.[351] The most commonly used microsurgical approaches are currently the infratentorial supracerebellar approach described first by Horsley, later by Krause, and recently resurrected and modernized by Stein, and the supratentorial approach under the occipital lobe described by Poppen and popularized re-

cently by Clark.[351] Both have been associated with low morbidity and mortality in experienced hands.

The place of CT-guided (stereotactic) biopsy in the diagnosis of pineal region tumors is unclear. Although such biopsies have been described as relatively safe, there is a risk that tissue sampling of these heterogenous tumors may not depict accurately the correct histologic nature of the tumor.[352] Without an accurate histologic diagnosis, treatment planning may be erroneous or inadequate. In its favor is the advantage of rapid tissue diagnosis and shortened hospital stay.

RADIATION THERAPY

With certain exceptions, such as benign teratomas, radiation therapy has an established role in the treatment of pineal and suprasellar tumors of pineal parenchymal or germ cell origin. Because of their location and infiltrative nature, complete surgical extirpation often is not possible. In the past, high mortality and morbidity rates associated with biopsy or attempted resection, especially with older surgical techniques, often led to the use of radiation therapy without histologic confirmation. In such instances, response to low-dose radiation therapy, measurement of AFP and β-HCG, and CSF cytology were used to provide diagnostic information. There has been a tendency to increase the use of biopsy and attempted resection. Although surgery theoretically might be expected to increase the incidence of CSF seeding, there is no proof that this will occur. A review of older literature suggests that the incidence of spinal seeding increased from 3% for tumors in which biopsy was not obtained to 23% when biopsy was obtained from the tumors.[74] However, Linstadt and associates found no instances of failure in the spinal axis in 13 patients with biopsy-proved germinomas, only one of whom received prophylactic spinal irradiation.[353]

Five-year survival rates with radiation therapy range from 44% to 78% and vary with histology and extent of disease, age, radiation volume, and dose to the primary site.[74] Accord-

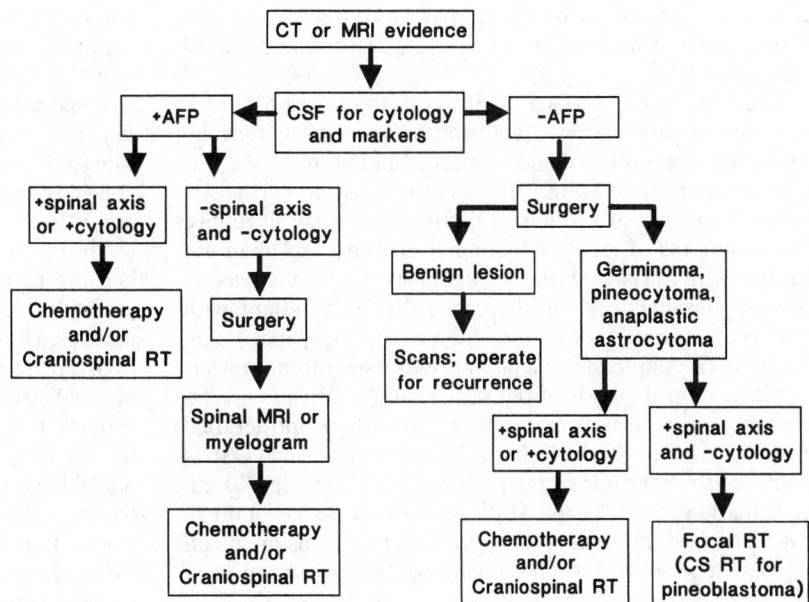

FIGURE 48–8. Treatment and evaluation schema for pineal region tumors. (Modified from Edwards MSB, Hudgins RJ, Wilson CB, et al. Pineal region tumors in children. J Neurosurg 1988;68:689)

ing to a multiinstitutional survey by Wara and coworkers, the survival of patients with pineal parenchymal cell tumors or malignant teratomas was 21% (3 of 14) compared with 72% (26 of 36) for those with germinomas.[354] This survey and the report of Jenkin and colleagues[355] indicated that patients younger than 25 to 30 years of age have survival rates of 65% to 80% compared with 35% to 40% for older patients. This finding may reflect the increased incidence of true germinomas in younger patients.

Germinomas are infiltrative tumors that tend to spread along the ventricular walls or throughout the leptomeninges. The incidence of CSF seeding ranges from 7% to 12%. Because of these features, the use of fields encompassing the entire ventricular system, the whole brain, and even the entire craniospinal axis has been recommended. In a literature review, Salazar and colleagues found a recurrence-free survival rate of 76% for patients with whole-brain irradiation compared with 61% for irradiation to the ventricular system and 51% for smaller volumes.[356] Further analysis of those data showed a 90% survival rate for patients treated with whole-brain irradiation and a tumor dose of least 50 Gy. If smaller fields were used or the dose to the primary tumor site was less than 50 Gy, the survival was 33%. With less than whole-brain irradiation, recurrences at the margin of the irradiated volume were reported in the older literature. However, the frequency of such recurrences should be reduced with the availability of CT and MRI for treatment planning. Linstadt and associates concluded that the risk for spinal metastases from germinomas was too small to justify routine prophylactic spinal irradiation, but recommended its use when there is tumor spill at surgery or in those patients with malignant CSF cytology or known subependymal or leptomeningeal metastases.[353]

At some institutions, if the histologic diagnosis is unknown and CSF cytology and myelography are negative, radiation therapy is administered at a dose of about 25 Gy at 1.8 Gy/fraction to the primary tumor site with a generous margin that includes at least the third ventricle. The CT or MRI scan is then repeated. If substantial regression has occurred, it is assumed that the lesion is a germinoma, and the whole brain is given an additional dose of approximately 25 Gy. If there is little or no response by CT or MRI, an additional 30 Gy is given to the primary field or a surgical resection is carried out, if possible.

The paradigm described by Edwards and Levin for management of pineal region tumors differs somewhat from the approach just discussed and is outlined in Figure 48–8.[350] If hydrocephalus is present, patients are placed on corticosteroids. A shunt is placed only if corticosteroids fail to relieve the symptoms of raised intracranial pressure. An open operation with the goal to resect the tumor is preferred to a CT-guided stereotactic biopsy. Occasionally, in a patient with widely disseminated disease, a stereotactic biopsy may be indicated. The approach (supratentorial versus infratentorial) is planned on the basis of the MRI scan. At the time of craniotomy, an external ventricular drain with an intracranial pressure monitor is placed in the lateral ventricle and CSF is removed to lower intracranial pressure and measure CSF tumor markers (β-HCG and AFP). A tumor biopsy is obtained, and, based on the findings at operation and the histologic diagnosis, a decision is reached regarding the aggressiveness of tumor resection.

Additional therapy is planned based on the histology, CSF markers, staging CT and MRI, and myelogram; localized germinomas (two-cell pattern) are treated with 25 Gy to the ventricular system and an additional 25 Gy to the tumor with a 1.5- to 2-cm margin. If the germinoma is disseminated, systemic chemotherapy or craniospinal irradiation is administered. Nongerminomatous malignant germ cell tumors, whether localized or disseminated, are treated with systemic chemotherapy (for six courses), followed by restaging studies. After restaging, localized tumors receive focal radiation therapy, and disseminated tumors receive craniospinal irradiation (54 Gy to the primary tumor, 45 Gy to the ventricular system, 35 Gy to the spinal cord, and 45 Gy to any localized spinal cord lesions).

Biopsy-verified tumors with little or no tendency to metastasize to the spinal cord, such as teratomas, embryonal cell carcinomas, pineocytomas, and low-grade gliomas, are treated by resection or with local radiation fields only. Craniospinal axis irradiation is reserved for tumors that have a strong tendency toward cord involvement (such as pineoblastoma), for those with positive CSF cytology, or for those with radiographic evidence of spinal cord involvement.

CHEMOTHERAPY

Chemotherapy for glial neoplasms is similar to that covered in earlier sections. The chemotherapy for germ cell tumors is in flux but is encouraging. For germinomas, complete responses before radiation therapy or at recurrence have been observed with cisplatin and bleomycin[357]; cyclophosphamide alone[358,359] or the combination of cyclophosphamide, vinblastine, and bleomycin[358]; the combination of cisplatin and etoposide[360]; and dactinomycin, methotrexate, vinblastine, and cisplatin.[348,350]

For nongerminoma malignant germ cell tumors (*e.g.*, embryonal, endodermal sinus, and mixed tumors), the benefits of chemotherapy are far less impressive, with partial rather than complete responses and recurrence within months to years being the norm. Chemotherapies with activity include combinations of cyclophosphamide, vinblastine, and bleomycin[358]; cisplatin, VCR, and bleomycin[361]; cisplatin and etoposide[362]; and cisplatin, bleomycin, and teniposide.[362a] Occasional patients with recurrent germ cell tumors who have failed the combination of cisplatin, bleomycin, and vinblastine therapies have responded to the authors' BTRC 8422 protocol (6-thioguanine, procarbazine, dibromodulcitol, CCNU, and VCR).

The results with chemotherapy have appeared paradoxical, because patients with systemic seminoma treated with cisplatin, bleomycin, and vinblastine have developed brain metastases while receiving chemotherapy.

Given the rarity of CNS germ cell tumors and the similarity of small trials reported in the literature, it is obvious that cooperative group trials are necessary to determine which of the existing chemotherapy combinations are most active. Second-generation studies could then address modifications based on a reasonable data base rather than the few anecdotal studies in the literature. Much study needs to be done to elucidate the best drug combinations and use of chemotherapy in these patients.

PITUITARY ADENOMAS

CLINICAL AND PATHOLOGIC CONSIDERATIONS

Pituitary gland tumors tend to produce neuroendocrine or neurologic symptoms and signs. Anatomically, tumors arising from the pituitary gland can compress the pituitary, grow out of the sella to compress and invade the optic chiasm, and, if growth is unabated, extend into the temporal lobe, third ventricle, and the posterior fossa. The chief finding in most patients is visual loss initially characterized by a bitemporal hemianopia. Headache occurs in about 20%. Less frequent are ocular palsies due to compression or invasion of the cavernous sinus.

Neuroendocrine abnormalities can be associated with tumor compression of the pituitary gland or hypersecretion of hormones, or both. Table 48–7 summarizes some of the more common syndromes and their endocrine abnormalities. Sexual impotence in men and amenorrhea and galactorrhea in women are commonly associated with hyperprolactinemia. Growth hormone hypersecretion is associated with acromegaly or gigantism, depending on the age of the patient. Corticotropin hypersecretion results in Cushing's disease. Elements of hypothyroidism, adrenal insufficiency, and growth hormone deficiency may follow compression of the pituitary gland by growth of an adenoma.

The diagnosis of a pituitary tumor is based on sensitive radioimmunoassays, CT scans, and, most recently, MRI. Figure 48–3 shows an MRI scan of a pituitary adenoma before surgery.

Pituitary adenomas are classified as endocrine inactive or endocrine active. Most secrete one or, occasionally, two hormones. The reported incidence of the various types of pituitary adenomas depends on the institution's referral patterns. Of 800 patients operated on at UCSF between 1970 and 1981, 630 of 800 (79%) were endocrine active; of these, 331 of 630 (52%) were prolactin secreting, 27% growth hormone secreting, 20% corticotropin secreting, and only 0.3% were thyroid-stimulating hormone secreting.[363] Undifferentiated cell adenomas are considered to be nononcocytic (null) or oncocytic (oncocytoma) tumors.

Of prognostic importance are the functional status of the tumor and how large or invasive it is. Table 48–7 is the grade and staging system used at UCSF.[363]

SURGERY

The goal of surgery for the larger (usually, but not always, endocrine inactive) pituitary tumors is to decompress the visual pathways and reduce tumor bulk, whereas the goal for hypersecreting adenomas is normalization of the hypersecretion with preservation of remaining normal pituitary function. For larger nonsecreting pituitary adenomas, surgical cure is not possible or necessary, because radiation therapy adjuvant to surgery is usually curative. In contrast, the hypersecreting adenoma should be resected in its entirety, whenever possible, because the effects of hypersecretion can be devastating, and response to radiation therapy is slow and less predictable.

The operative approach of choice for most pituitary tumors is transsphenoidal, because it is safer and better tolerated than the alternative transcranial (frontal craniotomy) approach.[364] The transsphenoidal approach is possible for tumors occu-

pying the sella turcica and even in those with fairly large medial suprasellar extension as long as the tumor is soft (the usual case) and can drop into the sella with progressive resection. Tough, woody suprasellar tumors and those with extension laterally into the middle fossa or anteriorly beneath the frontal lobes must be resected by craniotomy.

RADIATION THERAPY

Microadenomas of the pituitary, usually diagnosed because of endocrine hypersecretion, may be totally resected. There is no indication for radiation therapy, unless there is persistent hormone elevation. Macroadenomas, particularly the endocrine inactive lesions, may invade into adjacent structures, such as the cavernous sinus, the optic chiasm, or the third ventricle. Subtotal resection and postoperative irradiation can relieve mass effect, shrink the remaining tumor, prevent regrowth, and lower hormone levels. Further, radiation therapy alone or in conjunction with medical treatment is an effective alternative to primary treatment for patients who are medically inoperable or who refuse surgery.

Radiation therapy controls tumor growth in more than 90% of patients with nonfunctioning, prolactin-secreting, and growth hormone-secreting adenomas. Sheline and Tyrrell demonstrated that patients with large, nonfunctioning adenomas or prolactin-secreting adenomas associated with visual field deficits had a 60% recurrence rate (using visual field changes as an endpoint) within 5 years after incomplete resection alone.[365] The recurrence rate was reduced to about 4% by the addition of radiation therapy, whereas 7% treated with radiation therapy alone recurred. Approximately two thirds of patients who presented with modest visual field defects, involving not more than one quadrant, who were treated by surgery or radiation therapy alone had return of normal vision in the involved eyes. With larger visual field defects, restoration of vision was better in patients who received preradiation therapy surgical decompression than in those treated by radiation therapy alone. In patients with acromegaly and visual field defects, normal vision was achieved by irradiation alone in about two thirds of patients.

Radiation therapy is less effective in controlling endocrine hypersecretion than in controlling the growth of pituitary adenomas. Radiation therapy decreases serum growth hormone concentrations to normal levels (usually defined as <10 ng/ml in the radiation therapy and surgery literature) in 80% to 85% of acromegalic patients. However, several years may be required for the levels to normalize.[364] The probability of normalization is related to the pretreatment growth hormone level. Radiation therapy is most effective in tumors with relatively small preradiation therapy growth hormone elevations (30–50 ng/ml), whereas the response is less predictable with higher growth hormone levels.[75] Radiation therapy controls hypercortisolism in 50% to 75% of adults and 80% of children with Cushing's disease. Response occurs within 6 to 9 months of treatment.[366,367]

Data on control of prolactin secretion by conventional radiation therapy are more difficult to interpret. Irradiation decreases prolactin levels by 75% to 90% on the average, and the response occurs over several years. However, normal levels are only attained in about 30% of patients when radiation therapy is used as primary treatment or after incomplete surgical resection.[368-370] Bromocriptine may be administered to reduce temporarily the prolactin level in patients with incompletely resected macroadenomas who are receiving radiation therapy. The drug is then periodically withdrawn to determine whether the prolactin level has returned to normal. Medical treatment with dopamine agonists alone does not appear to represent adequate therapy for prolactin-secreting adenomas. Bromocriptine does not produce a permanent reduction in tumor size and prolactin concentration after the course of therapy is completed and, unlike radiation therapy, does not reduce the risk of tumor expansion during pregnancy. Further, it commits the patient to a lifetime of medicinal use and its potential side effects.[371]

Pituitary adenomas may be treated using several different techniques. One approach is to use bilateral coronal arcs with moving wedge filters. The usual treatment plan includes two 110° arcs with 30° wedge filters. The field size is chosen to include the target volume in the 95% isodose line. The neck is placed in the flexed position so that the plane of rotation is behind the eyes. During simulation, markers are placed on the eyelids. Three tattoo marks are placed on the skin and used for alignment with laser beams to ensure daily positional reproducibility. For large tumors, a three-field technique with lateral opposed wedged portals and a superior or vertex field may be used. The total dose is carried to 45 Gy in 25 fractions of 1.8 Gy, calculated at the 95% isodose line. This combination of fraction size and total dose provides long-term tumor control in more than 90% of cases, and, therefore, a larger dose is not indicated.[372] Further, radiation-induced injury to optic apparatus or adjacent brain with this dose-fractionation scheme is rare, whereas larger fractions or greater total doses lead to a higher incidence of injury. The optic chiasm appears especially sensitive to radiation injury in patients with acromegaly. Bloom and Kramer reported five instances of visual complication in 40 acromegalic patients.[75] The complications were largely in patients receiving daily increments of 2 Gy and total doses of 50 Gy. Hypopituitarism, however, may develop as a late complication years after completion of radiation therapy.[364] Hypopituitarism is more likely to occur in patients who have had surgery and postoperative radiation therapy than in those who have been treated by radiation therapy or surgery alone.[373] Because hypopituitarism is largely correctable by hormone replacement therapy, patients treated for pituitary adenomas should be observed by an endocrinologist for the remainder of their lives.

CRANIOPHARYNGIOMAS

CLINICAL AND PATHOLOGIC CONSIDERATIONS

Craniopharyngiomas occur primarily in children. These tumors arise from cell rests that are remnants of Rathke's pouch at the juncture of the infundibular stalk and the pituitary gland. Most of these tumors become symptomatic only after they have attained a diameter of about 3 cm. They are usually cystic at the time of presentation. They may compress the optic chiasm or pituitary gland and extend up into the third ventricle. The cyst is high in proteinaceous material and calcium and is seen easily by CT scan or MRI.

Clinically, craniopharyngiomas produce increased intracranial pressure and hypopituitary-hypothalamic-chiasmal

dysfunction. Symptoms vary and, in children, may include obesity, delayed development, decreased vision and optic atrophy, field defects, and papilledema.

SURGERY

Craniopharyngiomas usually are approached by a microsurgical procedure done through a right frontal craniotomy. Large craniopharyngioma cysts that enter and enlarge the sella turcica can be drained and resected through a transsphenoidal procedure.

The goal of most surgeons in the surgery of craniopharyngioma is total removal, but some do a more conservative operation and depend on the excellent results with radiation therapy discussed later. Aggressive removal nearly guarantees some injury to the pituitary gland and stalk, with subsequent temporary or permanent diabetes insipidus and elements of hypopituitarism. Patients injured in this manner must take replacement hormones and use inhaled desmopressin acetate spray for the control of diabetes insipidus for life. However, patients whose vision was affected by the craniopharyngioma can expect improvement after surgery. The mortality of craniopharyngioma resection should be extremely low.

In Europe, a few centers are treating craniopharyngioma cysts with stereotactic puncture and the instillation of colloidal therapeutic radioisotopes, particularly yttrium 90.[374] Such treatments are being tried in this country also with colloidal phosphorus 32. Intracystic therapy may be a good treatment for craniopharyngioma cysts recurring after conventional external-beam irradiation.

RADIATION THERAPY

Although debate exists regarding the extent to which total excision should be attempted, numerous reports demonstrate that local tumor control and survival after subtotal removal, consisting of extensive resection or of limited biopsy and cyst aspiration and irradiation, is comparable with that achieved by radical excision.[375-378] The local control rates after complete resection, subtotal resection alone, and incomplete resection and postoperative irradiation are 70%, 26%, and 75%, respectively.[379] Ten-year survival rates range from 24% to 100% for complete resection, 31% to 52% for subtotal resection, and 62% to 84% for incomplete resection and irradiation.[375-377,380,381] Patients undergoing conservative treatment including biopsy and cyst drainage and irradiation appear to enjoy a better quality of life and demonstrate less psychosocial impairment than those initially treated with more extensive resections.[377] Further, conservative therapy is associated with less hypothalamic-pituitary dysfunction[382] and a lower incidence of persistent diabetes insipidus[390] than when a total or near-total excision is attempted. More extensive resections using a subfrontal approach may be associated with frontal lobe and visual perceptual dysfunction.[383]

The radiation therapy target volume is based largely on CT scanning using relatively small margins around demonstrated tumor. The technique varies according to size and location of residual tumor, but most patients are treated by bicoronal arcs with moving wedge filters, similar to the method used for pituitary adenomas. The total dose is 55 Gy, given in daily

1.8-Gy increments. In children younger than 3 years of age, it is recommended that, if possible, irradiation be delayed until the child is older.

CEREBELLOPONTINE ANGLE NEURILEMMOMAS

CLINICAL AND PATHOLOGIC CONSIDERATIONS

The major tumors occurring in this region are the acoustic nerve tumors and meningiomas. Meningiomas have been discussed previously; therefore, the discussion that follows is limited to acoustic neurilemmomas (schwannoma and neurofibroma). These tumors originate on cranial nerve VIII, almost always on the vestibular division, at the point where the nerve acquires its reticulin and Schwann cell investment. Within the skull, this transition zone occurs in the internal auditory foramen and causes local erosion of the internal auditory meatus. Slow growth characterizes these tumors; therefore, they can grow to substantial size before clinical symptoms lead to diagnosis. They often occupy the posterior fossa at the angle between the cerebellum and the pons. By compression, they can affect cranial nerves VII, V, and, less often, IX and X alone or in various combinations. When large enough, they can compress the medulla and obstruct the CSF, leading to hydrocephalus.

Acoustic neurilemmomas are commonest in the fifth decade and can be associated with familial neurofibromatosis. In the latter instance they occur earlier, in late childhood and adolescence, and may be bilateral.

In a series from the Massachusetts General Hospital, auditory and vestibular branch involvement was found to occur in 98% of patients, facial weakness with disturbances of taste in 56%, sensory loss over the face in 56%, gait abnormality in 41%, and appendicular ataxia in 20%.[51]

Diagnosis by skull x-ray examination is suggestive, but definitive diagnosis is most effectively made with MRI or CT scan done in conjunction with the CSF administration of metrizamide contrast.

SURGERY

The aim of surgery for acoustic neurilemmomas is complete resection, with the surgical approach chosen after consideration of the patient's age and residual hearing and the size and location of the tumor.[384] When useful hearing is present, the suboccipital approach is taken because of the possibility of hearing preservation postoperatively, particularly in smaller tumors. In patients with poor hearing, the translabyrinthine approach, which produces deafness in the operated-on ear, is used for its lower overall morbidity. Occasionally, tumors that reside purely within lateral portions of the internal acoustic canal are approached through the middle cranial fossa.[384]

The translabyrinthine route requires only a small incision behind the ear through which the petrous bone is gradually removed with a high-speed drill until the facial nerve is identified and exposed to the point where it can be separated from the tumor and protected. The dura of the posterior fossa is seen easily and can be opened to gain access to the intradural component of the tumor.

The transoccipital approach requires a unilateral posterior fossa craniectomy, after which the dura is opened and the cerebellum is retracted medially to expose the cerebellopontine angle. The lower cranial nerves are protected while tumor is removed, and the porus acusticus is unroofed in an effort to identify the facial nerve, and in smaller tumors, the acoustic nerve as well. Once the facial nerve is identified, the remainder of the tumor is removed in a usually lengthy and involved operation that fully exploits the surgeon's microsurgical skill.

Complete removal of acoustic neurilemmomas through the posterior fossa can be predicted in almost every instance, and life-threatening complications are rare except in patients with extremely large tumors. As mentioned earlier, preservation of the acoustic nerve is rare in even small tumors, but the facial nerve is in continuity at the end of most acoustic tumor resections. Therefore, any postoperative paresis or paralysis tends to be temporary. When the facial nerve is divided during surgery, it is sutured together when possible, or a nerve graft is placed between the stumps. Facial paralysis with no evidence of recovery within a few months is treated by surgical reinnervation, wherein another cranial nerve, usually a branch of the accessory nerve, is joined to the facial nerve peripherally. Bilateral acoustic tumors are seen with NF2 and present difficult problems in surgical decision making.[385] In general, a conservative approach is taken, treating the largest tumor when symptoms absolutely require it. Bilateral aggressive tumor resections lead to complete deafness and confer the possibility of bilateral facial nerve paralysis, a cosmetic and functional problem.

RADIATION THERAPY

There have been few reports on the role of radiation therapy for treatment of acoustic neurilemmomas. A review by Wallner and colleagues disclosed 62 patients who were thought to have had a total resection and did not receive irradiation.[386] The recurrence rate in this group was only 3% (2 of 62). The 15-year actuarial survival and relapse-free survival rates were 98% and 94%, respectively. Thirty patients underwent subtotal resection, defined as removal of less than 90% of the tumor. Six of the 13 (46%) patients with subtotally resected lesions recurred, whereas only 1 of 17 (6%) of those treated with subtotal resection and postoperative irradiation to a dose higher than 45 Gy relapsed. The 15-year relapse-free survival rate for patients treated with subtotal resection and radiation therapy (>45 Gy) was 94% compared with 41% for nonirradiated patients ($p = 0.01$); the corresponding 15-year survival rates were 100% and 67%, respectively ($p = 0.016$). There were no recurrences among 3 patients in whom biopsy was obtained at the time of surgery that was followed by irradiation. On the other hand, 4 of 7 patients who were irradiated for disease progression after having had resection alone subsequently developed a second recurrence. Based on these data, it was concluded that postoperative irradiation should be given after subtotal resection to reduce the risk of local tumor progression. The target volume includes a narrow margin around the residual tumor. Treatment is given using a homolateral pair of angled beams with wedge filters in daily increments of 1.8 to 2 Gy to a total of 50 to 55 Gy. Stereotactic radiosurgery has been used as an alternative to surgery in selected patients with small acoustic neurilemmomas.[387]

GLOMUS JUGULARE TUMORS

CLINICAL AND PATHOLOGIC CONSIDERATIONS

Glomus jugulare tumors arise from glomus tissue in the adventitia of the jugular bulb (glomus jugulare) or along Jacobson's nerve in the temporal bone, sometimes multifocally. The tumor invades temporal bone diffusely, but growth is characteristically slow. Sometimes they are endocrine active, with a carcinoid or pheochromocytoma-like syndrome.[388]

Because glomus jugulare tumors occur in the jugular foramen, they commonly cause lower cranial nerve palsies and early symptoms of hoarseness and difficulty swallowing. Later, facial weakness, hearing loss, and atrophy of the tongue become prominent. Pulsating tinnitus also may be a presenting symptom, and a pulsating mass can sometimes be seen behind the eardrum.

A presumptive radiologic diagnosis of glomus tumor can be made by CT or MRI scanning, with jugular neurilemmoma being the main differential diagnosis. Because glomus tumors incite a tremendous blood supply, particularly by way of the ascending pharyngeal artery, cerebral angiography provides the definitive diagnosis. Because preoperative tumor embolization is essential to surgical removal of glomus tumors, the diagnostic angiogram should be performed just before surgery when possible.

Histopathologically, numerous vascular channels are distinctive. The background is composed of clear cells clumped in a fibrous matrix. A small percentage of glomus tumors are malignant.

SURGERY

The treatment of glomus jugulare tumors is controversial, with advocates for radiation,[389] surgery, and the combination.[390] Most clinicians would agree that a resection should be attempted and that in most instances gross surgical resection, if not a cure, is a realistic goal.

Surgery on glomus tumors is most often performed by a neurosurgeon and a head and neck surgeon together after preoperative embolization. The base of the skull in the region of the jugular foramen is first exposed, and neurovascular structures are identified and mobilized through a high transverse cervical incision. When the incision is extended behind the pinna and a mastoidectomy is completed, the facial nerve can be protected, and the entire tumor bulb, the jugular bulb, and the internal jugular vein can be seen passing through the base of the skull. Finally, after a suboccipital craniectomy, the sigmoid sinus above and the jugular vein below can be ligated, and the segment between them excised with the attached tumor. Complications of this procedure include CSF leak and cranial nerve (particularly facial) palsy.

RADIATION THERAPY

Even though glomus tumors are histologically benign, radiation therapy is effective and has been recommended for symptomatic lesions that cannot be totally resected or as primary treatment.[389,391–393] These tumors regress slowly after irradiation, and the success of radiation therapy is measured by the amelioration of symptoms and the absence of disease progression. The dose required for control is relatively modest.

Kim and associates reported a series of 40 patients with such lesions and added a literature survey.[394] The control rate with subtotal resection and postoperative irradiation was 85%. When radiation therapy only was used for inoperable or recurrent tumors, control was achieved in 88%. Their composite data, including cases from the literature, showed a 25% recurrence rate for doses lower than 40 Gy, whereas only 1.4% recurred with doses of 40 Gy or higher.

Based on these data, a dose of 45 Gy in 5 weeks is recommended. Although a dose of 50 Gy has been advocated for more advanced tumors, there is no evidence that such lesions require higher doses.[393] Treatment is usually delivered through a homolateral pair of angled, wedged portals, depending on the precise location of the lesion.

CHORDOMAS

CLINICAL AND PATHOLOGIC CONSIDERATIONS

Chordomas occur along the pathway of the primitive notochord, which extends, in human embryos, from the tip of the dorsum sellae to the coccyx. Chordomas are extradural, multilobulated tumors, varying in consistency from extremely soft to woody and cartilaginous. They are pseudoencapsulated and may invade through the basal dura.

The typical chordoma is composed of cord-like rows of distended, vacuolated (physaliferous) cells. A variant, the chondroid chordoma, has distinctly chondroid elements and may be less aggressive.[395] None of the histopathologic characteristics of tumor aggressiveness (cellularity, pleomorphism, and mitoses) seems to be predictive in chordoma.

The diagnosis of clivus chordomas cannot be made without radiologic tests and often is delayed because symptoms are nonspecific and vague. At onset there is usually headache and intermittent diplopia. These vague symptoms often are not reported, allowing the tumor to grow to an enormous size before the diagnosis is made. Gradually, headache (upper clivus tumors) and neck pain (lower clivus tumors) worsen. Superiorly placed tumors proceed to cause diplopia and facial numbness as the cavernous sinus and Meckel's cave are invaded. Lower clivus tumors compress the lower cranial nerves and later the brain stem.

The differential diagnosis of cranial chordoma includes basal meningioma, neurilemmoma (schwannoma), nasopharyngeal carcinoma, pituitary adenoma, and craniopharyngioma. MRI scanning usually results in a working diagnosis of chordoma, but surgical biopsy (and resection) is mandatory.

SURGERY

Surgery for cranial chordomas is obligatory to obtain diagnostic tissue, to enhance the effectiveness of subsequent radiation therapy, and to improve the patient's clinical condition. With an aggressive surgical resection, a favorable effect on the severe headaches and neurologic deficits associated with chordomas can be anticipated.

Intracranial chordomas occur at the base of the skull, a region relatively remote from surgical access. Consequently, a variety of innovative approaches have been developed by neurosurgeons and head and neck surgeons, and these procedures are commonly done with both types of specialist in attendance.

For midline lesions of the upper clivus that extend into the sella or sphenoid sinus, or both, a transseptal, transsphenoidal approach (as for pituitary tumors) is best. Large, compressive, transdural extensions of these upper clivus tumors into the interpeduncular cistern must be removed through a transcranial, subtemporal, intradural approach. For the more lateralized upper clival tumor and some lateralized midclival tumors, an approach through a sphenoethmoidectomy (to which may be added a maxillectomy) is useful. For midline tumors of the midclivus and lower clivus, a transoral resection is commonly used. A combination of exposures sometimes is necessary for extremely large tumors.

A potentially serious complication of the transsphenoidal, transsphenoethmoid, and transoral approaches is CSF leakage and consequent meningitis. Therefore, every attempt must be made to keep the dura intact during these procedures. Because dural invasion by cranial chordomas may occur 50% of the time, inadvertent entry of the dura during tumor resection is sometimes unavoidable. Careful intraoperative patching of the leak with fat and muscle grafts followed by postoperative spinal CSF drainage is essential.

Cranial chordomas often recur after surgery and radiation therapy. In this situation, reoperation directed toward symptomatic improvement is the only treatment option. Reoperations are complicated by surgical scarring and tissue compromise from irradiation.

RADIATION THERAPY

Chordomas and low-grade chondrosarcomas of the base of skull, clivus, and axial skeleton are not amenable to complete surgical resection. With conventional megavoltage irradiation (median dose of 50 Gy), the local control rate for these lesions is only 27%.[396] Although higher doses appear to improve the local control rate, the proximity of dose-limiting critical structures, such as the optic nerves, the chiasm, other cranial nerves, the brain stem, the temporal lobes, and the spinal cord, limit the dose that can be delivered safely to these lesions.[397] Charged-particle beams such as protons and helium ions, which feature sharp lateral beam edges and a finite range in tissue, may be used to deliver higher doses than are possible with conventional photon irradiation while keeping the dose to neighboring critical structures at a safe level. The depth of penetration can be tailored to the clinical situation by varying the energy of the beam or by interposing bolus material in the beam path. Charged-particle beams can be made to stop in front of a critical structure, such as the spinal cord, and in combination with other lateral or oblique beams, a target volume may be "wrapped" around a critical structure. Precise tumor and normal tissue identification and beam delivery techniques, highly reproducible patient positioning, and accurate compensation for tissue inhomogeneities in the beam path are required.

Available data suggest that the higher doses that are achievable with charged-particle irradiation result in higher local control rates than have been observed with conventional radiation therapy techniques. Austin-Seymore and coworkers reported the outcome of 68 patients with chordomas or low-grade chondrosarcomas of the clivus treated postoperatively at the Harvard Cyclotron Laboratory at Massachusetts General Hospital with a 160-MeV proton beam.[396] The median dose was 69 cobalt Gy equivalent (CGE; the dose in proton Gy multiplied by 1.1, the relative biologic effectiveness [RBE] for protons compared with cobalt 60), with a range of 56.9 to 75.6 CGE. Local control was achieved in 90% of patients (61 of 68), with follow up ranging from 17 to 152 months (median of 34 months). The 5-year actuarial local control and disease-free survival rates were 82% and 76%, respectively. Treatment was complicated by unilateral or bilateral blindness in 3 patients, and 9 patients developed pituitary insufficiency requiring hormone replacement. A study comparing 66.6 CGE with 72 CGE is in progress.

Berson and colleagues reviewed the results of 45 patients with chordomas and chondrosarcomas of the base of skull and cervical spine treated at the University of California Lawrence Berkeley Laboratory with helium ion or neon beams.[398] Total doses ranged from 59.4 to 80 Gy equivalent (GyE; the physical dose multiplied by the RBE; 1.2–1.3 for helium and 2–3.3 for neon). After initial subtotal resection, 23 patients were treated with charged particles alone, and 13 were treated with photons and particles combined. Nine patients were treated for recurrent disease. The 5-year actuarial local control and survival rates were 59% and 62%, respectively. The 2-year actuarial local control rate for patients treated at initial diagnosis was 78% compared with 33% for those with recurrent tumors ($p < 0.01$). The 2-year local control rate for tumor volumes of less than 20 ml was 80%, whereas it was 33% for larger lesions ($p < 0.05$). Complications included unilateral or bilateral blindness in 5 patients, and 4 patients developed brain stem injury.

HEMANGIOBLASTOMAS AND HEMANGIOMAS

CLINICAL AND PATHOLOGIC CONSIDERATIONS

Hemangioblastoma accounts for approximately 2% of intracranial tumors, arising most often in the cerebellar hemispheres and vermis. Usually solitary, these tumors can be multiple and may also occur in the brain stem, spinal cord, and supratentorial compartment. Cerebellar hemangioblastoma can be sporadic or occur as a familial disorder as part of the von Hippel-Lindau complex that is transmitted as an autosomal dominant disorder with varying degrees of penetrance. Other entities associated with familial hemangioblastoma are hypernephroma, polycystic kidneys, pancreatic cysts, pheochromocytoma, and erythrocytosis.

Cerebellar hemangioblastomas usually are recognized in the third decade causing symptoms of increased intracranial pressure and symptoms and signs of cerebellar dysfunction. Gait disturbance and imbalance are particularly common. Clinical progression is slow, because these tumors enlarge extremely slowly.

The hemangioblastoma probably arises during embryonic life from primitive endothelial cells around the fourth ventricle. The tumor is composed of numerous capillary and sinusoidal channels lined with endothelial cells. Interspersed are nests of lipid-laden pseudoxanthoma cells. The tumor is usually cystic and contains proteinaceous, xanthochromic fluid. The cyst contains a red (vascular) firm mural nodule, the apparent source of the fluid. The cyst wall is a glial non-neoplastic reaction to the secreted fluid. Occasional hemangioblastomas (brain stem and spinal cord, particularly) are without cysts.

SURGERY

In most instances, the diagnosis can be made by CT scan or MRI. Angiography, to confirm the diagnosis, is usually done before surgery. Cerebellar hemangioblastoma tumors are readily approached and excised, with the cyst drained and the entire solid portion carefully dissected and removed. Solid hemangioblastomas of the brain stem are exceedingly vascular, and their removal is associated with high mortality; even biopsy can be associated with precipitous bleeding and significant morbidity. Such tumors are sometimes irradiated with or without a confirmatory biopsy.

RADIATION THERAPY

Radiation therapy is recommended for patients with unresectable, incompletely excised, and recurrent hemangioblastomas and for those patients who are medically inoperable. Sung and coworkers reported their experience of 23 patients treated with radiation therapy for cerebellar hemangioblastoma.[399] About half of their patients received doses of 36 Gy or lower, and the remainder (12 of 23) received 40 to 55 Gy in 4 to 6.5 weeks. The 5-, 10-, and 15-year survival rates for the lower dose group were 54.5%, 27.3%, and 8.1%, respectively, whereas the survival rates for the higher dose group were 90.5%, 56.5%, and 56.5%, respectively. These findings are similar to those reported by Smalley and associates.[400] In their series, 19 patients had gross residual disease after initial surgery or recurrent tumors, whereas 6 had only microscopic disease. The overall 5-, 10-, and 15-year survival rates were 85%, 58%, and 58%, respectively, and the recurrence-free survival rates were 76%, 52%, and 42%, respectively. Eight of the 19 patients with gross disease were locally controlled. In-field disease control rates were significantly higher in patients who received at least 50 Gy ($p = 0.06$) or a time-dose-fractionation (TDF) of more than 75 Gy (equivalent to 46–48.6 Gy at 1.8–2 Gy per fraction, 5 days per week [$p = 0.004$]) than in those who received lower doses. Five of the 6 patients treated for microscopic disease were controlled. Based on these data, doses of at least 50 to 55 Gy in 5.5 to 6 weeks appear to be warranted.

CHOROID PLEXUS PAPILLOMA AND CARCINOMA

CLINICAL AND PATHOLOGIC CONSIDERATIONS

Choroid plexus papilloma and carcinoma are rare tumors that occur most often in children younger than 12 years of age, although they can occur at any age. Nearly half of these tumors are found in patients younger than 20 years of age. The tumor is an irregularly lobulated reddish mass, which on histopathologic examination is apparently normal choroid plexus. Rarely, these tumors show malignant features and are then classified as choroid plexus carcinoma.

In children, choroid plexus papillomas most often occur in the lateral ventricles. In adults, the fourth ventricular papilloma is commonest. Third ventricle tumors are exceedingly rare. Because papillomas tend to grow slowly within ventricles, they expand to fill the ventricle and block CSF flow. In addition, papillomas are thought to secrete CSF. Choroid plexus papillomas (and carcinomas) can produce hydrocephalus secondary to obstruction of the CSF; by CSF overproduction by the tumor; or by damage to the CSF resorptive bed from recurrent hemorrhages. As a result, increased intracranial pressure without focal findings is the commonest presentation; fourth ventricular tumors can also be associated with focal findings of ataxia and nystagmus.

Although choroid plexus papillomas and carcinomas extensively seed throughout the ventricular and subarachnoid spaces, seeding from papillomas is usually subclinical, whereas that from carcinomas is frequent and dramatically symptomatic. These tumors are seen easily by CT scan and MRI. In patients with anaplastic changes, the authors advocate staging by myelography and examination of the CSF.

Therapy for anaplastic tumors should be approached in a manner similar to medulloblastoma and malignant ependymomas. Because of the aggressive nature of the more anaplastic tumors, therapy must be equally aggressive, requiring radiation therapy and, in some instances, intraventricular chemotherapy.

SURGERY

The treatment of choroid plexus papillomas is total surgical excision. Choroid plexus tumors of the lateral ventricle are approached through a high parietal cortical incision and transcortical approach to the ventricular trigone. The predilection of these tumors for the left side makes this worrisome. Hydrocephalus is the rule and simplifies the exposure when retraction into the ventricle is established. Tumor arteries and veins are identified by use of the operating microscope and then coagulated, after which smaller tumors are removed intact and larger tumors are removed piecemeal. In half of the patients, hydrocephalus is relieved by tumor resection, but persistent hydrocephalus requires shunting.

Choroid plexus papillomas of the third ventricle are exceedingly rare but can be approached through various surgical exposures of the third ventricle. The problems of removal of fourth ventricular choroid plexus tumors are similar to those associated with suboccipital removal of medulloblastomas or ependymomas, as discussed earlier.

RADIATION THERAPY

Choroid plexus papillomas usually are considered to be radioresistant, but information regarding the use and response to irradiation is anecdotal. Naguib and coworkers reported a case of an inoperable choroid plexus papilloma with extensive involvement of the mastoid bone.[401] This patient received 49.5 Gy in 32 treatments during a 33-day period. Serial CT scans showed that 16 months after completion of the radiation therapy, the mass was markedly reduced in size. Such anecdotes suggest that radiation therapy to the primary tumor site may be offered for inoperable choroid plexus papillomas and carcinomas.[402,403] With choroid plexus carcinoma, consideration must be given to treating the entire craniospinal axis, although data to support this approach are lacking. With a negative myelogram and negative CSF cytology, an alternative approach is to treat primary tumor with radiation therapy in conjunction with intrathecal and systemic chemotherapy.

CHEMOTHERAPY

Usually, chemotherapy is not used for choroid plexus papillomas. For the more anaplastic tumors, however, the authors have increasingly used chemotherapy adjuvant to surgery and irradiation to prevent the inevitable recurrence and CSF dissemination common to the choroid plexus carcinomas. As with many of the less common tumors discussed, there are no chemotherapeutic guidelines and few reports to guide the therapist.

Initially, the authors used chemotherapy only for recurrent disease. They have used combinations of cyclophosphamide, doxorubicin, and VCR and nitrosourea-based combinations. They have seen transient responses and disease control with both. They have also used intraventricular chemotherapy with low-dose methotrexate (2–3 mg/day for 5 days) or cytosine arabinoside (30 mg/day for 3 days), or both, to stave subarachnoid spread. As a result of this experience, the authors currently advocate the use of adjuvant chemotherapy with a nitrosourea-based combination after irradiation and the use of concomitant intraventricular chemotherapy. During irradiation, they have used intraventricular cytosine arabinoside and methotrexate after irradiation. Further study and additional approaches should be considered.

SPINAL AXIS TUMORS

CLINICAL AND PATHOLOGIC CONSIDERATIONS

Some of the clinical features of spinal axis tumor localization and diagnosis have been discussed previously. Most primary spinal axis tumors produce symptoms and signs as a result of spinal cord and nerve root compression rather than because of parenchymal invasion.

The reported frequency of primary spinal cord tumors is between 10% and 19% of all primary CNS tumors.[404] Although most spinal axis tumors are extradural, most *primary* spinal axis tumors are intradural. Of intradural tumors, the intradural extramedullary neurilemmomas and meningiomas are the commonest (see Table 48–3). Neurilemmomas and meningiomas are normally intradural, but occasionally they may present as extradural tumors. Other intradural extramedullary tumors are vascular tumors, chordomas, and epidermoids.

Intramedullary tumors have the same cellular origins as the other CNS tumors discussed previously. In terms of frequency, ependymomas occur in about 40% of patients with intramedullary tumors; next most common are the astrocytomas of low- and mid-anaplasia. These are followed in frequency by less common histologies such as oligodendroglioma, ganglioglioma, medulloblastoma, and various hemangiomas and hemangioblastomas.

Table 48–24 classifies spinal axis tumors by location. Although different tumor types exhibit a predilection for certain spinal regions, taken altogether, spinal tumors are distributed

TABLE 48–24. Classification of Spinal Tumors by Their Location in Relation to the Spinal Cord and Dura Mater

Location	Usual Tumor Types
Extradural	Metastatic (carcinoma, lymphoma, melanoma, sarcoma), chordoma
Intradural	
Extramedullary	Schwannoma,* meningioma
Intramedullary	Astrocytoma, ependymoma†

* May extend along nerve root into extradural and extraspinal spaces.
† Ependymomas originating from the filum terminale and involving the cauda equina, not intramedullary in the strictest sense, are included here by custom.

almost evenly along the spinal axis. Approximately 50% of spinal tumors involve the thoracic spinal canal, 30% involve the lumbosacral spine, and the remainder involve the cervical spine, including the foramen magnum. Some tumors, such as the neurilemmomas, occur with greatest frequency in the thoracic region, although they can be found throughout the spine and often extend through an intervertebral foramen to acquire a dumbbell configuration.

Meningiomas are dural based and arise preferentially at the foramen magnum and in the thoracic spine. Astrocytomas are distributed throughout the spinal cord, and most ependymomas involve the conus medullaris and the cauda equina. Spinal chordomas are characteristically sacral.

Clinically, patients with spinal axis tumors present as a sensorimotor spinal tract syndrome; a painful radicular-spinal cord syndrome; or a central syringomyelic syndrome. In the *sensorimotor presentation,* symptoms and signs are in response to compression of the spinal cord. The onset is gradual over weeks to months, initial presentation is asymmetric, and motor weakness predominates. The level of impairment determines the muscle groups involved. Because of external compression, dorsal column involvement occurs with paresthesia and abnormalities of pain and temperature on the side contralateral to the motor weakness.

Radicular spinal cord syndromes occur because of external compression and infiltration of spinal cord roots. The main symptom is sharp, knife-like pain in the distribution of a sensory nerve root. The intense pain is often of short duration, with pain that is more aching in nature persisting for longer periods. The pain typically is exacerbated by coughing and sneezing or other maneuvers that increase intracranial pressure. Local paresthesia and impairment of sensations of pain and touch are common, as are weakness and muscle wasting. These findings commonly antedate cord compression by months.

Spinal tumors, particularly intramedullary tumors, can produce *syringomyelic dysfunction* by destruction and cavitation within the central gray matter of the cord. This produces lower motor neuron destruction and attendant segmental muscle weakness, wasting, and loss of reflexes. There is also a dissociated sensory loss of pain and temperature sensation with preservation of touch. With extension of the lesion, however, touch, vibration, and position sense are affected.

Finally, many patients with spinal axis tumors or supratentorial tumors that show a tendency toward drop metastases tend to lead to leptomeningeal neoplasia. Choucair and colleagues found that 1.2% of glioblastomas and 1.5% of anaplastic gliomas had metastatic spread of their supratentorial tumors to the spinal cord at some time during the course of their disease.[99]

SURGERY

General Considerations

The use of the operating microscope is as essential for spinal cord tumor surgery as it is for brain tumor surgery. In addition, other surgical adjuncts, such as intraoperative ultrasound, the CO_2 laser, and the CUSA, are equally valuable for the resection of spinal cord tumors. The ultrasound is particularly useful for examining the spinal cord through an intact or open dura to assess the level of maximum tumor involvement or to differentiate tumor cysts from solid tumor masses.

Surgical Planning

MRI scanning is invaluable for the diagnosis, localization, and characterization of spinal tumors (see Fig. 48–4). In all but vascular tumors (*e.g.*, hemangioblastoma), where angiography is needed, or tumors that cause extensive bony destruction (*e.g.*, metastasis), where CT scanning might be helpful, a technically excellent MRI scan is most often sufficient for preoperative planning for spinal tumors. Determination of the spinal level of the tumor and its exact relation to the spinal cord is important in localization. Corticosteroids are given before, during, and after spinal cord tumor surgery to help control spinal cord edema.

Removal of Intradural Extramedullary Tumors

Meningiomas and neurilemmomas (schwannomas) occur in the intradural extramedullary spinal compartment. Most of these tumors can be completely resected (cured), because through a laminectomy exposure they can be easily separated and rotated away from the spinal cord, which is already displaced, but not invaded, by tumor.

Neurilemmomas arise from spinal rootlets (most often dorsal rootlets), and their removal includes sections of those rootlets involved. Neurilemmomas can grow along the nerve root in a dumbbell fashion through a neural foramen; and although some of these extraspinal tumor extensions can be removed by extending the initial laminectomy exposure laterally, some must be resected at a separate operation through a thoracotomy, a costotransversectomy, or a retroperitoneal approach.

Meningiomas in most patients can be removed through a posterior (laminectomy) approach, because they are commonly lateral or anterolateral, and even the more anteriorly placed tumors cause enough lateral displacement of the spinal cord to allow access for resection without traction on the spinal cord. The uncommon tumor directly anterior to the spinal cord must sometimes be approached anteriorly, arterolaterally, or posterolaterally. Anteriorly situated meningiomas at the foramen magnum are sometimes unresectable because of their encasement of the vertebral artery.

Removal of Intramedullary Tumors

The commonest intramedullary tumors are ependymoma and astrocytoma. Hemangioblastoma is another (infrequent) tumor occurring in the spinal intramedullary compartment. Surgery is the principal treatment for all these tumors, with the exception of anaplastic astrocytomas.

Intramedullary tumors are approached through a laminectomy exposure, and after the dura is opened, a longitudinal myelotomy is made over the widened region of spinal cord and the incision deepened several millimeters to the tumor surface. Dissection planes around the tumor are sought microsurgically and, in the case of ependymomas, usually found and extended gradually around the tumor's surface, because removal of the central tumor bulk (by CO_2 laser or CUSA) causes the tumor to collapse. Usually, such tumors are completely removed. Tumors with indefinite dissection planes (usually low-grade astrocytomas) cannot be removed completely, but bulk reduction can cause long-term palliation. If frozen section shows a tumor to be malignant, surgery is aborted, and radiation therapy is the treatment.

Hemangioblastomas are extremely vascular tumors, so the tumor margins are addressed first where feeding arteries are coagulated, and the tumor is dissected and removed en bloc. The dorsal location of most of these tumors and the commonly associated cyst simplifies the removal to some extent.

RADIATION THERAPY

Radiation therapy is recommended for incompletely resected neoplasms of the spinal axis. As a rule, doses of 50 to 55 Gy are used so that the risk of radiation injury to the cord is less than that from the neoplasm itself. However, for lesions involving only the cauda equina and in situations in which irreversible and complete transverse myelopathy already has occurred, higher doses are permissible. The tumor usually is treated with a margin of 2 to 3 cm. Extension of the portals to include the thecal sac has been suggested for ependymomas that are removed piecemeal.[405] Ependymomas of the cord have a longer natural history than astrocytomas. Although most astrocytomas that recur do so within 3 years of treatment, recurrence of ependymomas may be delayed for as long as 12 years.[406]

Adjunctive radiation therapy is not necessary when ependymomas are removed completely in an en bloc fashion. However, 75% of patients (3 of 4) reported by Wen and associates recurred locally or with spread to the thecal sac after complete resection alone when the tumor was excised piecemeal.[405] All 7 nonirradiated patients with incompletely excised lesions reported by Barone and Elvidge[407] and Schuman and coworkers[408] recurred. In contrast, postoperative radiation therapy appears to improve tumor control and disease-free survival in patients with incompletely resected ependymomas. Sloof and colleagues[409] found their irradiated patients survived nearly twice as long as those who were not irradiated. Five- and 10-year survival rates in irradiated patients with localized ependymomas range from 60% to 100% and 86% to 93%, respectively, whereas 10-year relapse-free survival rates vary from 43% to 58%. Local control rates range from 60% to 100% in most reported series.[406] Myxopapillary ependymomas that arise exclusively in the conus medullaris have a better prognosis than the cellular ependymomas that arise in the cord.[405]

The 5- and 10-year survival rates for irradiated patients with low-grade astrocytomas of the spinal cord vary from 60% to 90% and 40% to 90%, respectively; the 5- and 10-year relapse-free survival rates are 66% and 53%, respectively.[406] Approximately 50% to 65% of astrocytomas are controlled locally. Patients with malignant gliomas have a much poorer prognosis; none of the patients with anaplastic astrocytoma or glioblastoma multiforme survived longer than 8 months.

CHEMOTHERAPY

There have been no reports of controlled clinical trials of chemotherapy for primary spinal axis tumors. Drugs active against intracranial astrocytomas, oligodendrogliomas, ependymomas, medulloblastoma, and germ cell tumors may logically be assumed to be equally efficacious against these same histologies in the spinal cord. Along with reports of chemotherapy activity against intracranial tumors, anecdotal patients have been included.

The authors' experience suggests that palliation is possible for astrocytomas using nitrosourea-based chemotherapy regimens. No therapy is clearly superior. For drop metastases from ependymomas, they have used BCNU and dibromodulcitol as single agents and various combinations with some benefit.[138,183a] For drop metastases from medulloblastoma, various drugs have been found to be beneficial. Specifically, cyclophosphamide, carboplatin, methotrexate, procarbazine, teniposide, and VCR have been used alone or in various combinations. These drugs would be expected to produce palliation for weeks to many months.

Although leptomeningeal spread is a common complication of primary spinal axis tumors, the use of intraventricular and intrathecal chemotherapy is limited to the treatment of microscopic deposits. Biodistribution in the subarachnoid CSF can be limited in the face of intradural extramedullary tumors. In addition, deposits of 5 mm in diameter or larger are not likely to benefit because of limitations in diffusion coupled with transcapillary loss of drug in the tumor.[410]

REFERENCES

1. SEER search performed for this chapter between 1978–1984.
2. Sloof JL, Kernohan JW, MacCary CS. Primary intramedullary tumors of the spinal cord and filum terminale. Philadelphia: WB Saunders, 1964.
3. Davis DL, Hoel D, Percy C, et al. Is brain cancer mortality increasing in industrial countries? Ann NY Acad Sci 1990;609:791.
4. Boyle P, Maisonneuve P, Saracci R, Muir CS. Is the increased incidence of primary malignant brain tumors in the elderly real? JNCI [Editorial] 1990;82:1594.
5. Greig NH, Ries LG, Yancik R, Rapoport SI. Increasing annual incidence of primary malignant brain tumors in the elderly. JNCI 1990;82:1621.
6. Percy AK, Elveback LR, Okazaki H, et al. Neoplasms of the central nervous system: Epidemiologic considerations. Neurology 1972;22:40.
7. Preston-Martin S. Descriptive epidemiology of primary tumors of the spinal cord and spinal meninges in Los Angeles County, 1972–1985. Neuroepidemiology 1990;9:106.
8. Bigner SH, Mark J, Burger PC, et al. Specific chromosomal abnormalities in malignant human gliomas. Cancer Res 1988;48:405.
9. Jenkins RB, Kimmel DW, Moertel CA, et al. A cytogenetic study of 53 human gliomas. Cancer Genet Cytogenet 1989;39:253.
10. James CD, Carlbom E, Nordenskjold M, et al. Mitotic recombination of chromosome 17 in astrocytomas. Proc Natl Acad Sci USA 1989;86:2858.
11. Cavenee WK, Scrable HJ, James CD. Molecular genetics of human cancer predisposition and progression. Mutat Res 1991;247:199.
12. Bigner SH, Mark J, Burger PC, et al. Specific chromosomal abnormalities in malignant human gliomas. Cancer Res 1988;48:405.
13. James CD, Carlbom E, Dumanski JP, et al. Clonal genomic alterations in glioma malignancy stages. Cancer Res 1988;48:5546.
14. Ransom DT, Ritland SR, Jenkins RB, et al. Loss of heterozygosity studies in human gliomas. Cancer Res 1991;32:302.
15. Neville BG, Berry AC, Stoddart Y. A case of malignant spinal cord ependymoma in association with a duplication of part of the long arm of chromosome 12. J Med Genet 1985;22:154.
16. Collins VP. The molecular genetics of meningiomas. Brain Pathol 1990;1:19.
17. Dumanski JP, Carlbom E, Collins VP, Nordenskjold M. Deletion mapping of a locus on human chromosome 22 involved in the oncogenesis of meningiomas. Proc Natl Acad Sci USA 1987;84:9275.
18. Dumanski JP, Rouleau GA, Nordenskjold M, Collins VP. Molecular genetic analysis of chromosome 22 in 81 cases of meningioma. Cancer Res 1990;50:5863.
19. Menon AG, Ponder BAJ, Seizinger BR. The neurofibromatosis genes: Molecular cloning to cellular function. Cancer Cells 1991;3:147.
20. Griffin CA, Hawkins AL, Packer RJ, et al. Chromosome abnormalities in pediatric brain tumors. Cancer Res 1988;48:175.
21. Raffel C, Gilles FE, Weinberg KI. Reduction to homozygosity and gene amplification in central nervous system primitive neuroectodermal tumors of childhood. Cancer Res 1990;50:587.
22. James CD, He J, Carlbom E, et al. Loss of genetic information in central nervous system tumors common to children and young adults. Genes Chromosom Cancer 1990;2:94.
23. Friedman HS, Schold C Jr. Rational approaches to the chemotherapy of medulloblastoma. Neurol Clin North Am 1985;3:843.
24. Stratton MR, Darling J, Cooper CS, Reeves BR. A case of cerebellar medulloblastoma with a single chromosome abnormality. Cancer Genet Cytogenet 1991;53:101.
25. Bigner SH, Friedman HS, Vogelstein B, et al. Amplification of c-*myc* gene in human medulloblastoma cell lines and xenografts. Cancer Res 1990;50:2347.
26. Wasson JC, Saylors RL, Zeltzer P, et al. Oncogene amplification in pediatric brain tumors. Cancer Res 1990;50:2987.
27. Yung WK, Zhang X, Steck PA, Hung MC. Differential amplification of the TGF-alpha gene in human gliomas. Cancer Commun 1990;2:201.
28. Malkin D, Li FP, Strong LC, et al. Germ line p53 mutations in a familial syndrome of breast cancer, sarcomas, and other neoplasms. Science 1990;250:1233.
29. Srivastava S, Zou ZQ, Pirollo K, et al. Germ-line transmission of a mutated p53 gene in a cancer-prone family with Li-Fraumeni syndrome. Nature 1990;348:747.
30. Wallace MR, Marchuk DA, Anderson LB, et al. Type I neurofibromatosis gene: Identification of a large transcript disrupted in three NF1 patients. Science 1990;249:181.
31. Cawthon RM, Weiss R, Xu G, et al. A major segment of the neurofibromatosis type 1 gene: cDNA sequence, genomic structure, and point mutations. Cell 1990;62:193.
32. Sampson JR, Yates JR, Pirrit LA, et al. Evidence for genetic heterogeneity in tuberous sclerosis. J Med Genet 1989;26:511.
33. Musicco M, Filippini G, Bordo BM, et al. Gliomas and (occupational) exposure to carcinogens: Case-control study. Am J Epidemiol 1982;116:782.
34. Moss AR. Occupational exposure and brain tumors. J Toxicol Environ Health 1985;16:703.
35. McLaughlin JK, Malker HS, Blot WJ, et al. Occupational risks for intracranial gliomas in Sweden. JNCI 1987;78:253.
36. Copeland DD, Bigner DD. Glial-mesenchymal tropism of in vivo avian sarcoma virus neuro-oncogenis in rats. Acta Neuropathol (Berl) 1978;41:23.
37. Wodinski I, Kensler CJ, Rall DP. The induction and transplantation of brain tumors in neonate beagles. Proc Am Assoc Cancer Res [Abstract] 1969;99.
38. Major EO, Vacante DA, Traub RG, et al. Owl monkey astrocytoma cells in culture spontaneously produce infectious JC virus which demonstrates altered biological properties. J Virol 1987;61:1435.
39. Matsuda M, Yasui K, Nagashima K, Mori W. Origin of the medulloblastoma experimentally induced by human polyomavirus JC. JNCI 1987;79:585.
40. Hochberg RH, Miller G, Schooley RT, et al. Central nervous system lymphoma related to Epstein-Barr virus. N Engl J Med 1983;309:745.
41. Annegers JF, Laws ER Jr, Kurland LT, et al. Head trauma and subsequent brain tumors. Neurosurgery 1979;4:203.
42. Malone M, Lumley H, Erdohazi M. Astrocytoma as a second malignancy in patients with acute lymphoblastic leukemia. Cancer 1986;57:979.
43. Sogg RL, Donaldson SS, Yorke CH. Malignant astrocytoma following radiotherapy of a craniopharyngioma. J Neurosurg 1978;48:622.
44. Poster DS, Bruno S. The occurrence of second primary neoplasms in patients with non-Hodgkin's lymphomas. IRCS Med Sci Cancer 1980;8:554.
45. Rubinstein AB, Shalit MN, Cohen M, et al. Radiation-induced cerebral meningioma: A recognizable entity. J Neurosurg 1984;61:966.
46. Spallone A, Gagliardi FM, Vagnozzi R. Intracranial meningiomas related to external cranial irradiation. Surg Neurol 1979;12:153.
47. Levin VA, Wilson CB. Clinical characteristics of cancer in the brain and spinal cord. In: Crook ST, Prestayko A, eds. Cancer and chemotherapy: Introduction to neoplasia and antineoplastic chemotherapy. Vol 2. New York: Academic Press, 1981:167.
48. Bingas B. Tumours of the base of the skull. In: Vinken PJ, Bruyn GW, eds. Handbook of clinical neurology; Tumors of the brain and skull. Vol 17. Amsterdam: North Holland, 1974:136.
49. Fahlbusch R, Marguth F. Endocrine disorders associated with intracranial tumors. In: Vinken PJ, Bruyn GW, eds. Handbook of clinical neurology: Tumors of the brain and skull. Vol 16. Amsterdam: North Holland, 1974:345.
50. Russell DJ, Rubinstein LJ. Pathology of tumors of the nervous system. 4th ed. Baltimore: Williams & Wilkins, 1977.

51. Adams RD, Victor M. Principles of neurology. New York: McGraw-Hill, 1977:586.
52. Brant-Zawadzki M, Norman D, eds. Magnetic resonance imaging of the central nervous system. New York: Raven Press, 1987.
53. Brant-Zawadski M, Badami JP, Mills CM, et al. Primary intracranial tumor imaging: A comparison of magnetic resonance and CT. Radiology 1984;150:435.
54. Berry I, Brant-Zawadski M, Osaki L, et al. Gd-DPTA in clinical MR of the brain: II. Extraxial lesions and normal structures. Am J Roentgenol 1986;147:1223.
55. Butler AR, Horii SC, Kricheff I, et al. Computed tomography in astrocytomas: A statistical analysis of the parameters of malignancy and the positive contrast enhanced CT scan. Radiology 1978;129:433.
56. Dillon WP, Norman D, Newton TH, et al. Intradural spinal cord lesions: Gd-DTPA enhanced MR imaging. Radiology 1989;170:229.
57. Edwards MSB, Davis RL, Laurent JP. Tumor markers and cytologic features of cerebrospinal fluid. Cancer 1985;56:1773.
58. Inoue HK, Naganuma H, Ono N. Pathobiology of intracranial germ-cell tumors: Immunochemical, immunohistochemical, and electron microscopic investigations. J Neurooncol 1987;5:105.
59. Marton LJ, Edwards MS, Levin VA, et al. CSF polyamines: A new and important means of monitoring medulloblastoma. Cancer 1981;47:757.
60. Levin VA, Crafts D, Wilson CB, et al. BCNU and procarbazine treatment for malignant brain tumors. Cancer Treat Rep 1976;60:243.
61. Hoffman WF, Levin VA, Wilson CB. Evaluation of malignant glioma patients during the postirradiation period. J Neurosurg 1979;50:624.
62. Hoshino T, Nagashima T, Murovic J, et al. In situ cell lanetics studies on human neuroectodermal tumors with bromodeoxyuridine labeling. J Neurosurg 1986;64:453.
63. Heilbrun MP. Computed tomography-guided stereotactic systems. Clin Neurosurg 1984;31:564.
64. Apuzzo MLJ, Chandrasoma PT, Cohen D, et al. Computed imaging stereotaxy: Experience and perspective related to 500 procedures applied to brain masses. Neurosurgery 1987;20:930.
65. Leibel SA, Sheline GE. Tolerance of the brain and spinal cord to conventional irradiation. In: Gutin PH, Leibel SA, Sheline GE, eds. Radiation injury to the nervous system. New York: Raven Press, 1991:239.
66. Young DF, Posner JB, Chu F, et al. Rapid-course radiation therapy of cerebral metastases: Results and complications. Cancer 1974;34:1069.
67. Delattre JY, Rosenblum MK, Thaler HT, et al. A model of radiation myelopathy in the rat: Pathology, regional capillary permiability changes and treatment with dexamethasone. Brain 1988;111:1319.
68. Graeb DA, Steinbok P, Robertson WD. Transient early computed tomographic changes mimicking tumor progression after brain tumor irradiation. Radiology 1982;144:813.
69. Valk PE, Dillon WP. Radiation injury of the brain. AJNR 1991;12:45.
70. Brant-Zawadzki MB, Anderson M, De Armond SJ, et al. Radiation-induced large intracranial vessel occlusive vasculopathy. AJR 1980;134:51.
71. Bernstein M, Laperriere N. Radiation-induced tumors of the nervous system. In: Gutin PH, Leibel SA, Sheline GE, eds. Radiation injury to the nervous system. New York: Raven Press, 1991:455.
72. Sheline GE, Wara WM, Smith V. Therapeutic irradiation and brain injury. Int J Radiat Oncol Biol Phys 1980;6:1215.
73. Marks JE, Baglan RJ, Prassad SC, et al. Cerebral radio-necrosis: Incidence and risk in relation to dose, time, fractionation and volume. Int J Radiat Oncol Biol Phys 1981;7:243.
74. Leibel SA, Sheline GE. Radiation therapy for neoplasms of the brain. J Neurosurg 1987;66:1.
75. Bloom B, Kramer S. Conventional radiation therapy in the management of acromegaly. In: Black PM, Zervas NT, Ridgeway ED, eds. Secretory tumors of the pituitary gland. Vol 1. New York: Raven Press, 1984:179.
76. Rottenberg DA, Chernik MD, Deck MDF, et al. Cerebral necrosis following radiotherapy of extracranial neoplasms. Ann Neurol 1977;1:339.
77. Burger PC, Mahaley MS Jr, Dudka L, et al. The morphologic effects of radiation administered therapeutically for intracranial gliomas: A postmortem study of 25 cases. Cancer 1979;44:1256.
78. DeAngelis LM, Shapiro WR. Drug/radiation interactions and central nervous system injury. In: Gutin PH, Leibel SA, Sheline GE, eds. Radiation injury to the nervous system. New York: Raven Press, 1991:361.
79. Bleyer WA, Griffin TW. White matter necrosis, mineralizing microangiopathy, and intellectual abilities in survivors of childhood leukemia. In: Gilbert HA, Kagan AR, eds. Radiation damage to the nervous system. New York: Raven Press, 1980:155.
80. Kim KT, Black KL, Marciano D, et al. Thallium-201 SPECT imaging of brain tumors: Methods and results. J Nucl Med 1990;31:965.
81. Gutin PH. Treatment of radiation necrosis of the brain. In: Gutin PH, Leibel SA, Sheline GE, eds. Radiation injury to the nervous system. New York: Raven Press, 1991:271.
82. Mulhern RK, Fairclough D, Ochs J. A prospective comparison of neuropsychologic performance of children surviving leukemia who received 18-Gy, 24-Gy, or no cranial irradiation. J Clin Oncol 1991;9:1348.
83. Johnson BE, Becker B, Goff WB, et al. Neurologic, neuropsychologic, and computed cranial tomographic scan abnormalities in 2- to 10-year survivors of small-cell lung cancer. J Clin Oncol 1985;12:1657.
84. Mulhern RK, Ochs J, Kun LE. Changes in intellect associated with cranial radiation therapy. In: Gutin PH, Leibel SA, Sheline GE, eds. Radiation injury to the nervous system. New York: Raven Press, 1991:325.
85. Eiser C. Intellectual abilities among survivors of childhood leukemia as a function of CNS irradiation. Arch Dis Child 1978;53:391.
86. Hochberg FH, Slotnick B. Neuropsychologic impairment in astrocytoma survivors. Neurology 1980;30:172.
87. Maire J Ph, Coudin B, Guerin, J, et al. Neuropsychologic impairment in adults with brain tumors. Am J Clin Oncol 1987;10:156.
88. Shalet SM, Beardwell CG, Pearson D, et al. The effect of varying doses of cerebral irradiation on GH production in childhood. Clin Endocrinol 1976;5:287.
89. Jones A. A transient radiation myelopathy (with reference to Lhermitte's sign of electrical paresthesia). Br J Radiol 1964;37:727.
90. Schultheiss TE, Stephens LC, Peters LJ. Survival in radiation myelopathy. Int J Radiat Oncol Biol Phys 1986;12:1765.
91. Reagen TJ, Thomas JE, Colby MY Jr. Chronic radiation myelopathy: Its clinical aspects and differential diagnosis. JAMA 1968;203:128.
92. Marcus RB Jr, Million RR. The incidence of myelitis after irradiation of the cervical spinal cord. Int J Radiat Oncol Biol Phys 1990;19:3.
93. Schultheiss TE. Spinal cord radiation "tolerance": Doctrine versus data. Int J Radiat Oncol Biol Phys 1990;19:219.
94. Abbatucci JS, Delozier T, Quint R, et al. Radiation myelopathy of the cervical spinal cord: Time, dose and volume factors. Int J Radiat Oncol Biol Phys 1978;4:239.
95. Wara WM, Phillips TL, Sheline GE, et al. Radiation tolerance of the spinal cord. Cancer 1975;35:1558.
96. Van der Kogel AJ, Barendsen GW. Late effects of spinal cord irradiation with 300 kV x-rays and 15 MeV neutrons. Br J Radiol 1974;47:393.
97. Ang KK, Van der Kogel AJ, van der Scheuren E. Lack of evidence for increased tolerance of rat spinal cord with decreasing fraction doses below 2 Gy. Int J Radiat Oncol Biol Phys 1985;11:105.
98. Burger PC, Dubois PJ, Schold SC Jr, et al. Computerized tomographic and pathologic studies in untreated, quiescent, and recurrent glioblastoma multiforme. J Neurosurg 1983;58:159.
99. Choucair AK, Levin VA, Gutin PH, et al. Development of multiple lesions during radiation therapy and chemotherapy in patients with gliomas. J Neurosurg 1986;65:654.
100. Hochberg FH, Pruitt A. Assumptions in the radiotherapy of glioblastoma. Neurology 1980;30:907.
101. Kelly PJ, Dauman-Duport C, Kispert DB, et al. Imaging-based stereotaxic serial biopsies in untreated intracranial glial neoplasms. J Neurosurg 1987;66:865.
102. Levin VA. Pharmacokinetics and CNS chemotherapy. In: Hellmann K, Carter SK, eds. Fundamentals of cancer chemotherapy. New York: McGraw-Hill, 1986:28.
103. Levin VA, Patlak CS, Landahl HD. Heuristic modeling of drug delivery to malignant brain tumors. J Pharmacokinet Biopharm 1980;8:257.
104. Levin VA. Chemotherapy of primary brain tumors. Neurol Clin North Am 1985;3:855.
105. Kumar ARV, Renaudin J, Wilson CB, et al. Procarbazine hydrochloride in the treatment of brain tumors. J Neurosurg 1974;40:365.
106. Weiss HD, Walker MD, Wiernik PH. Neurotoxicity of commonly used antineoplastic agents. N Engl J Med 1974;291:75.
107. Feun LG, Wallace S, Yung WK, et al. Phase I trial of intracarotid BCNU and cisplatin in patients with malignant intracerebral tumors. Cancer Drug Deliv 1984;1:239.
108. Stewart DJ, Grahovac Z, Benoit B, et al. Intracarotid chemotherapy with a combination of 1,3-*bis*-(2-chloroethyl)-1-nitrosourea (BCNU), *cis*-diaminedichloroplatinum (cisplatin), and 4'-O-demethyl-1-O-(4,6-O-2-thenylidene-beta-D-glucopyranosyl) epipodophyllotoxin (VM-26) in the treatment of primary and metastatic brain tumors. Neurosurgery 1984;15:828.
109. Bloom HJG. Intracranial tumors: Response and resistance to therapeutic endeavors, 1970–1980. Int J Radiat Oncol Biol Phys 1982;8:1083.
110. Laws ER Jr, Taylor WF, Clifton MB, et al. Neurosurgical management of low-grade astrocytoma of the cerebral hemispheres. J Neurosurg 1984;61:665.
111. Leibel SA, Sheline GE, Wara WM, et al. The role of radiation therapy in the treatment of astrocytomas. Cancer 1975;35:1551.
112. Kernohan JW, Sayre GP. Tumors of the central nervous system. In: Atlas of tumor pathology. Section 10, Fascicle 35. Washington, DC: Armed Forces Institute of Pathology, 1952.
113. Fazekas JT. Treatment of grade I and II brain astrocytomas: The role of radiotherapy. Int J Radiat Oncol Biol Phys 1977;2:661.
114. Chang CH, Horton J, Schoenfeld D, et al. Comparison of postoperative radiotherapy and combined postoperative radiotherapy and chemotherapy in the multidisciplinary management of malignant gliomas. Cancer 1983;52:997.
115. Sheline GE. Radiation therapy of primary tumors. Semin Oncol 1975;2:29.
116. Marsa GW, Goffinet DR, Rubinstein LJ, et al. Megavoltage irradiation in the treatment of gliomas of the brain and spinal cord. Cancer 1975;36:1681.
117. Kramer S. Radiation therapy in the management of malignant gliomas. In: Cancer of the central nervous system. Proceedings of the Seventh National Cancer Conference. Philadelphia: JB Lippincott, 1983:823.
118. Fulling KH, Nelson JS. Cerebral astrocytic neoplasms in the adult: Contribution of histologic examination to the assessment of prognosis. Semin Diagn Pathol 1984;1:152.
119. Daumas-Duport C, Scheithauer BW, Kelly PJ. A histologic and cytologic method for the spatial definition of gliomas. Mayo Clin Proc 1987;62:435.
120. Daumas-Duport C, Scheithauer B, O'Fallon J, Kelly P. Grading of astrocytomas, a simple and reproducible method. Cancer 1988;62:2152.
121. Kim TS, Halliday AL, Hedley-Whyte ET, Convery K. Correlates of survival and the Daumas-Duport grading system for astrocytomas. J Neurosurg 1991;74:27.
122. Nelson JS, Tsukada Y, Schoenfeld D, Fulling K, Lamarche J, Peress N. Necrosis as a prognostic criterion in malignant supratentorial, astrocytic gliomas. Cancer 1983;52:550.

123. Laws ER, Taylor WF, Clifton MB, et al. Neurosurgical management of low-grade astrocytoma of the cerebral hemispheres. J Neurosurg 1984;61:665.

124. Waller MD, Alexander E Jr, Hunt WE, et al. Evaluation of BCNU and/or radiotherapy in the treatment of anaplastic gliomas: A cooperative clinical trial. J Neurosurg 1978;49:333.

125. Salcman M. Malignant glioma management. Neurosurg Clin North Am 1990;1:49.

126. Andreou J, George AE, Wise A, et al. CT prognostic criteria of survival after malignant glioma surgery. Am J Neuroradiol 1983;4:488.

127. Wood JR, Green SB, Shapiro WR. The prognostic importance of tumor size in malignant gliomas: A computed tomographic scan study by the Brain Tumor Cooperative Group. J Clin Oncol 1988;6:338.

128. Winger MJ, MacDonald DR, Cairncross JG. Supratentorial anaplastic gliomas in adults. J Neurosurg 1989;71:487.

129. Kumar ARV, Hoshino T, Wheeler KT, et al. Comparative rates of dead tumor cell removal from brain, muscle, subcutaneous tissue, and peritoneal cavity. JNCI 1974;52:1751.

130. Gutin PH, Leibel SA, Wara WM, et al. Recurrent malignant gliomas: Improved survival following interstitial brachytherapy with high-activity iodine-125 sources. J Neurosurg 1987;67:864.

131. DeVita VT Jr. The relationship between tumor mass and resistance to chemotherapy: Implication for surgical adjuvant treatment of cancer. Cancer 1983;51:1209.

132. Berger MS, Kincaid J, Ojemann GA, et al. Brain mapping techniques to maximize resection, safety, and seizure control in children with brain tumors. Neurosurgery 1989;25:786.

133. Young B, Oldfield EH, Markesbery WR, et al. Reoperation for glioblastoma. J Neurosurg 1981;55:917.

134. Harsh GR IV, Levin VA, Gutin PH, Seager M, Silver P, Wilson CB. Reoperation for recurrent glioblastoma and anaplastic astrocytoma. Neurosurgery 1987;21:615.

135. Shaw EG, Daumas-Duport C, Scheithauer BW, et al. Radiation therapy in the management of low-grade supratentorial astrocytomas. J Neurosurg 1989;70:853.

136. Wallner KE, Gonzales MF, Sheline GE, et al. Treatment results of juvenile pilocytic astrocytoma. Neurosurgery 1988;69:171.

137. Shaw EG, Scheithauer BW, Gilbertson DT. Postoperative radiotherapy of supratentorial low-grade gliomas. Int J Radiat Oncol Biol Phys 1989;16:663.

138. Cairncross JG, Laperriere NJ. Low-grade glioma: To treat or not to treat? Arch Neurol 1989;46:1238.

139. Walker MD, Alexander E, Hunt WE, et al. Evaluation of BCNU and/or radiotherapy in the treatment of anaplastic gliomas. J Neurosurg 1978;49:333.

140. Kristiansen K, Hagen S, Kollevold T, et al. Combined modality therapy of operated astrocytomas grade III and IV—confirmation of the value of postoperative irradiation and lack of potentiation of bleomycin on survival time: A prospective multicenter trial of the Scandinavian Glioblastoma Study Group. Cancer 1981;47:649.

141. Walker MD, Strike TA, Sheline GE. An analysis of dose-effect relationship in the radiotherapy of malignant gliomas. Int J Radiat Oncol Biol Phys 1979;5:1725.

142. Nelson DF, Diener-West M, Horton J, et al. Combined modality approach to treatment of malignant gliomas: Reevaluation of RTOG 7401/ECOG 1374 with long-term follow-up. NCI Monogr 1988;6:279.

143. Bleehen NM. Studies of high grade cerebral gliomas. Int J Radiat Oncol Biol Phys 1990;18:811.

144. Djordjevic B, Szybalski W. Genetics of human cell lines: III. Incorporation of 5-bromo- and 5-iododeoxyuridine into the deoxyribonucleic acid of human cells and its effect on radiation sensitivity. J Exp Med 1960;112:509.

145. Levin VA, Wara WM, Gutin PH, et al. Initial analysis of NCOG 6G82-1: Bromodeoxyuridine (BUdR) during irradiation followed by CCNU, procarbazine, and vincristine (PCV) chemotherapy for malignant gliomas. Proc Am Soc Clin Oncol [Abstract] 1990;9:91.

146. Phillips TL, Levin VA, Ahn DK. Evaluation of bromodeoxyuridine in glioblastoma multiforme: A Northern California Oncology Group phase II study. Int J Radiat Oncol Biol Phys 1991;21:709.

147. Kinsella TJ, Collins J, Rowland J, et al. Pharmacology and phase I/II study of continuous intravenous infusions of iododeoxyuridine and hyperfractionated radiotherapy in patients with glioblastoma multiforme. J Clin Oncol 1988;6:871.

148. Hegarty TJ, Thornton AF, Diaz RF, et al. Intra-arterial bromodeoxyuridine radiosensitization of malignant gliomas. Int J Radiat Oncol Biol Phys 1990;19:421.

149. Rodriquez R, Kinsella TJ. Halogenated pyrimidines as radiosensitizers for high grade glioma revisited. Int J Radiat Oncol Biol Phys 1991;21:859.

150. Withers HR. Biologic basis for altered fractionation schemes. Cancer 1985;55:2086.

151. Urtasun RC, Fulton D, Huyser-Wierenga D, et al. Dose intensity in radiotherapy: "Is more better" for patient with malignant glioma? Proc Am Soc Clin Oncol [Abstract] 1989;8:84.

152. Nelson DF, Curran WJ, Nelson JS, et al. Hyperfractionation in malignant glioma report on a dose searching phase I/II protocol of the Radiation Therapy Oncology Group (RTOG). Proc Am Soc Clin Oncol [Abstract] 1990;9:90.

153. Simpson WJ, Platts ME. Fractionation study in the treatment of glioblastoma multiforme. Int J Radiat Oncol Biol Phys 1976;1:639.

154. Keim H, Potthoff PC, Schmidt K, et al. Survival and quality of life after continuous accelerated radiotherapy of glioblastomas. Radiother Oncol 1987;9:21.

155. Florell RC, MacDonald DR, Irish WD, et al. Selection bias, survival, and brachytherapy for glioma. J Neurosurg 1991;76:179.

156. Gutin PH, Prados MD, Phillips TL, et al. External irradiation followed by an interstitial high activity iodine-125 implant "boost"'" in the initial treatment of malignant gliomas: NCOG Study 6G-82-2. Int J Radiat Oncol Biol Phys 1991;21:601.

157. Loeffler JS, Alexander E, Wen P, et al. Results of stereotactic brachytherapy used in the initial management of patient with glioblastoma. JNCI 1990;82:1918.

158. Leibel SA, Gutin PH, Wara WM, et al. Survival and quality of life after interstitial implantation of removable high-activity iodine-125 sources for the treatment of patients with recurrent malignant gliomas. Int J Radiat Oncol Biol Phys 1989;17:1129.

159. Loeffler JS, Alexander E, Hochberg FH, et al. Clinical patterns of failure following stereotactic interstitial irradiation for malignant gliomas. Int J Radiat Oncol Biol Phys 1990;19:1455.

160. Walker MD, Green SB, Byar DP, et al. Randomized comparison of radiotherapy and nitrosoureas for the treatment of malignant glioma after surgery. N Engl J Med 1980;303:1323.

161. Green SB, Byar DP, Walker MD, et al. Comparison of carmustine, procarbazine, and high-dose methylprednisolone as additions to surgery and radiotherapy for the treatment of malignant glioma. Cancer Treat Rep 1983;67:1.

162. Nelson DF, Schoenfeld D, Weinstein AS, et al. A randomized comparison of misonidazole sensitized radiotherapy plus BCNU and radiotherapy plus BCNU for treatment of malignant glioma after surgery: Preliminary results of an RTOG study. Int J Radiat Oncol Biol Phys 1983;9:1143.

163. Paoletti P, Cuna GRD, Knerich R, et al. Multidisciplinary treatment for central nervous system tumors with nitrosourea compounds. ACTA Neurochir 1978;41:287.

164. Eyre HJ, Quagliana JM, Eltringham JR, et al. Randomized comparisons of radiotherapy and CCNU versus radiotherapy, CCNU plus procarbazine for the treatment of malignant gliomas following surgery. J Neurooncol 1983;1:171.

165. Adinolfi D, Buoncristiani P, Casotto A, et al. Multidisciplinary treatment for brain tumors. J Neurosurg Sci 1978;22:111.

166. EORTC Brain Tumor Group. Effect of CCNU on survival rate of objective remission and duration of free interval in patients with malignant brain glioma—final evaluation. Eur J Cancer 1978;14:851.

167. Feun LG, Steward DJ, Maor M, et al. A pilot study of *cis*-diaminedichloroplatinum and radiation therapy in patients with high-grade astrocytomas. J Neurooncol 1983;1:109.

168. Deutsch M, Green SB, Strike TA, et al. Results of a randomized trial comparing BCNU plus radiotherapy, streptozotocin plus radiotherapy, BCNU plus hyperfractionated radiotherapy, and BCNU following misonidazole plus radiotherapy in the postoperative treatment of malignant glioma. Int J Radiat Oncol Biol Phys 1989;16:1389.

169. Shapiro WR, Green SB, Burger PC, et al. Randomized trial of three chemotherapy regimens and two radiotherapy regimens and two radiotherapy regimens in postoperative treatment of malignant glioma: Brain Tumor Cooperative Group Trial 8001. J Neurosurg 1989;71:1.

170. Rozental JM, Robins HI, Finlay J, Healy B, et al. "Eight-in-one-day" chemotherapy administered before and after radiotherapy to adult patients with malignant gliomas. Cancer 1989;63:2475.

171. Levin VA, Silver P, Hannigan J, Wara WM, Gutin PH, Davis RL, Wilson CB. Superiority of post-radiotherapy adjuvant chemotherapy with CCNU, procarbazine, and vincristine (PCV) over BCNU for anaplastic gliomas: NCOG 6G61 Final Report. Int J Radiat Oncol Phys Biol 1990;18:321.

171a. Levin VA. Unpublished observations, 1992.

172. Levin VA, Wara WM, Davis RL, et al. NCOG protocol 6G91: Seven drug chemotherapy and irradiaion for patients with glioblastoma multiforme. Cancer Treat Rep 1986;70:739.

173. Phillips TL, Levin VA, Ahn DK, et al. Evaluation of bromodeoxyuridine in glioblastoma multiforme—a Northern California Cancer Center phase II study. Int J Radiat Oncol Biol Phys 1991;21:709.

174. Wilson CB, Gutin PH, Boldrey EB, et al. Single-agent chemotherapy of brain tumors. Arch Neurol 1976;33:739.

175. Fewer D, Wilson CB, Boldrey EB, et al. Phase II study of 1-(2-chloroethyl)-3-cyclohexyl-1-nitrosourea (CCNU) in the treatment of brain tumors. Cancer Chemother Rep 1972;56:421.

176. Rosenblum ML, Reynolds AF, Smith KA, et al. Chloroethyl-cyclohexyl-nitrosourea (CCNU) in the treatment of malignant brain tumors. J Neurosurg 1973;39:306.

177. Levin VA, Resser K, McGrath L, et al. PCNU treatment for recurrent malignant gliomas. Cancer Treat Rep 1984;68:969.

178. Rodriguez LA, Prados M, Silver P, Levin VA. Re-evaluation of procarbazine for the treatment of recurrent malignant CNS tumors. Cancer 1989;64:2420.

179. Levin VA, Crafts D, Wilson CB, et al. Imidazole carboxamides. Relationship of lipophilicity to activity against intracerebral murine glioma 26 and preliminary phase II clinical trial of 5-(3,3-bis chloroethyl)-1-triazeno)-imidazole-4-carboxamide (NSC-82196) in primary and secondary brain tumors. Cancer Chemother Rep 1975;59:107.

180. Chamberlain MC, Prados MD, Silver P, Levin VA. A phase I/II study of 24 hour intravenous AZQ in recurrent primary brain tumors. J Neurooncol 1988;6:319.

181. Decker DA, Al-Sarraf M, Kresge C, et al. Phase II study of aziridinylbenzoquinone (AZQ NSC-182986) in the treatment of malignant gliomas recurrent after radiation: Preliminary report. J Neurooncol 1985;3:19.

182. Schold SC, Friedman HS, Bjornsson TD, et al. Treatment of patients with recurrent primary brain tumors with AZQ. Neurology 1984;34:615.

183. Chamberlain MC, Prados MD, Silver P, et al. A phase II trial of oral melphalan in recurrent primary brain tumors. Am J Clin Oncol 1988;11:52.

183a. VA Levin, et al. Unpublished observations, 1987 and 1991.

184. Prados MD, Rodriguez L, Seager M, et al. Phase II study of spirohydantoin mustard for the treatment of recurrent malignant gliomas. Cancer Treat Rep 1987;71:1105.

185. Bertolone SJ, Baum ES, Krivit W, Hammond GD. A phase II study of cisplatin therapy in recurrent childhood brain tumors. J Neurooncol 1989;7:5.

185a. Spence AM, et al. Unpublished observations, 1991.

186. Yung WKA, Mechtler L, Gleason MJ. Intravenous carboplatin for recurrent malignant gliomas: A phase II study. J Clin Oncol 1991;9:860.

187. Yung WKA, Prados MD, Levin VA, et al. Intravenous recombinant interferon-beta, betaseron, in patients with recurrent malignant gliomas: A phase I/II study. J Clin Oncol 1991;9:1945.

188. Fewer D, Wilson CB, Boldrey EB, et al. Chemotherapy of brain tumors: Clinical experience with carmustine amd vincristine. JAMA 1972;222:549.

189. Gutin PH, Wilson CB, Kumar ARV, et al. Phase II study of procarbazine, CCNU, vincristine combination chemotherapy in the treatment of malignant brain tumors. Cancer 1975;35:1398.

190. Levin VA, Edwards MS, Wright DC, et al. Modified procarbazine, CCNU, and vincristine (PCV 3) combination chemotherapy in the treatment of malignant brain tumors. Cancer Treat Rep 1980;64:237.

191. Levin VA, Hoffman WF, Pischer TL, et al. BCNU–5-fluorouracil combination in the treatment of recurrent malignant brain tumors. Cancer Treat Rep 1978;62:2071.

192. Levin VA, Phuphanich S, Liu H-C, et al. Phase II study of combined BCNU, 5-fluorouracil, hydroxyurea, and 6-mercaptopurine (BFHM) for the treatment of malignant gliomas. Cancer Treat Rep 1986;70:1271.

193. Prados M, Rodriguez L, Chamberlain M, Silver P, Levin VA. Treatment of recurrent gliomas with 1,3-*bis*(2-chloroethyl)-1-nitrosourea and α-difluoromethylornithine. Neurosurgery 1989;24:806.

194. Levin VA, Chamberlain MC, Prados MD, et al. Phase I-II study of eflornithine and mitoguazone combined in the treatment of recurrent primary brain tumors. Cancer Treat Rep 1987;71:459.

194a. Levin VA, Prados MD, Yung WK, Gleason MJ, Ictech S, Malec M. Treatment of recurrent gliomas with eflornithine. JNCI 1992;84:1432.

195. Levin VA, Prados MD, Davis RL, et al. Treatment of recurrent gliomas with a polydrug protocol designed to combat nitrosourea resistance. J Clin Oncol 1992;10:766.

196. Schold SC Jr, Mahaley MS Jr, Vick NA, et al. Phase II diaziquone-based chemotherapy trials in patients with anaplastic supratentorial astrocytic neoplasms. J Clin Oncol 1987;5:464.

197. Yung WKA, Harris MI, Bruner JM, Feun LG. Intravenous BCNU and AZQ in patients with recurrent malignant gliomas. J Neurooncol 1989;7:237.

198. Longee DC, Friedman HS, Albright RE, et al. Treatment of patients with recurrent gliomas with cyclophosphamide and vincristine. J Neurosurg 1990;72:583.

199. Byar DP, Green SB, Strike TA. Prognostic factors for malignant glioma. In: Walker MD, ed. Oncology of the nervous system. Boston: Martinus Nijhoff, 1983:379.

199a. Yung WKA, et al. Unpublished observations, 1991.

200. Rosenblum ML, Gerosa MA, Wilson CB, et al. Stem cell studies of human brain tumors. J Neurosurg 1983;58:170.

201. Thomas DGT, Darling JL, Paul EA, et al. Assay of anti-cancer drugs in tissue culture: Relationship of relapse free interval (RFI) and in vitro chemosensitivity in patients with malignant cerebral glioma. Br J Cancer 1985;51:525.

202. Goodwin W, Crowley J. A retrospective comparison of high-dose BCNU with autologous marrow rescue plus radiotherapy vs IV BCNU plus radiation therapy in high grade gliomas: A Southwest Oncology Group review. Proc Annu Meet Am Soc Clin Oncol [Abstract] 1989;8:A352.

203. Ahmed T, Feldman E, Helson L, et al. Phase I-II trial of high-dose thiotepa (HDT) with autologous bone marrow transplantation (ABMT) and localized radiotherapy (RT) for patients (pts) with astrocytoma grade III-IV. Proc Annu Meet Am Assoc Cancer Res [Abstract] 1990;31:A1023.

204. Long J, Leff R, Daly M, et al. Phase II trial of high-dose etoposide (E) and autologous bone marrow transplantation for treatment of progressive glioma. Proc Annu Meet Am Soc Clin Oncol [Abstract] 1989;8:A360.

205. Glannone L, Wolff SN. Phase II treatment of central nervous system gliomas with high-dose etoposide and autologous bone marrow transplantation. Cancer Treat Rep 1987;71:759.

206. Finlay JL, August C, Packer R, et al. High-dose multi-agent chemotherapy followed by bone marrow "rescue" for malignant astrocytomas of childhood and adolescence. J Neurooncol 1990;9:239.

207. Finlay JL. High-dose chemotherapy with bone marrow rescue in children and young adults with malignant brain tumors. Proc Annu Meet Am Assoc Cancer Res [Abstract] 1991;32:A1078.

208. Allen JC, Bloom J, Ertel I, et al. Brain tumors in children: Current cooperative and institutional chemotherapy trials in newly diagnosed and recurrent disease. Sem Oncol 1986;13:110.

209. Freeman CR, Suissa S. Brain stem tumors in children: Results of a survey of 62 patients treated with radiation. Int J Radiat Oncol Biol Phys 1986;12:1823.

210. Eifel PJ, Cassady JR, Belli JA. Radiation therapy of tumors of the brainstem and midbrain in children: Experience of the Joint Center For Radiation Therapy and Children's Hospital Medical Center (1971–1981). Int J Radiat Oncol Biol Phys 1987;13:847.

211. Coffey RJ, Lunsford LD. Stereotactic surgery for mass lesions of the midbrain and pons. Neurosurgery 1985;17:12.

212. Eifel PJ, Cassady JR, Belli JA. Radiation therapy of tumors of the brainstem and midbrain in children: Experience of the Joint Center for Radiation Therapy and Children's Hospital Medical Center. Int J Radiat Oncol Biol Phys 1987;13:847.

213. Kim TH, Chin HW, Pollan S, et al. Radiotherapy of primary brain stem tumors. Int J Radiat Oncol Biol Phys 1980;6:51.

214. Albright AL, Guthkelch AN, Packer RJ, et al. Prognostic factors in pediatric brain-stem gliomas. J Neurosurg 1986;65:751.

215. Stroink AR, Hoffman HJ, Hendrick EB, et al. Diagnosis and management of pediatric gliomas. J Neurosurg 1986;65:745.

216. Halperin EC. Pediatric brain stem tumors: Patterns of treatment failure and their implications for radiotherapy. Int J Radiat Oncol Biol Phys 1985;11:1293.

217. Packer RJ, Allen JC, Goldwein JL, et al. Hyperfractionated radiotherapy for children with brainstem gliomas: A pilot study using 7,200 cGy. Ann Neurol 1990;27:167.

218. Freeman CR, Krischer J, Sanford RA, et al. Hyperfractionated radiation therapy for brain stem tumors: Results of treatment at the 7020 cGy dose level of Pediatric Oncology Group Study No. 8495. Cancer 1991;68:474.

219. Edwards MSB, Wara WM, Urtasun RC, et al. Hyperfractionated radiation therapy for brain-stem glioma: A phase I-II trial. J Neurosurg 1989;70:691.

220. Bertolone SJ, Baum ES, Krivit W, Hammond GD. A phase II study of cisplatin therapy in recurrent childhood brain tumors. J Neurooncol 1989;7:5.

221. Fulton DS, Levin VA, Wara WM, et al. Chemotherapy of pediatric brain stem tumors. J Neurosurg 1981;54:721.

222. Jenkin D. Posterior fossa tumors in childhood: Radiation treatment. Clin Neurosurg 1983;30:203.

223. Levin VA, Edwards MS, Wara WM, et al. 5-fluorouracil and CCNU followed by hydroxyurea, misonidazole and irradiation for brain stem gliomas: A pilot study of the Brain Tumor Research Center and the Children's Cancer Group. Neurosurgery 1984;14:679.

224. Rodriguez LA, Prados M, Fulton D, Edwards MSB, Silver P, Levin V. Treatment of recurrent brain stem gliomas and other CNS tumors with 5-fluorouracil, CCNU, hydroxyurea and 6-mercaptopurine. Neurosurgery 1988;22:691.

225. Humphreys RP. Posterior cranial fossa brain tumors in children. In: Youmans JR, ed. Youmans' neurological surgery. Philadelphia: WB Saunders, 1982:2747.

226. Chamberlain MC, Silver P, Levin VA. Poorly differentiated gliomas of the cerebellum—a study of 18 patients. Cancer 1990;65:337.

227. Walsh FB, Hoyt WF. Clinical neuro-opthalmology. Baltimore: Williams & Wilkins, 1969:2076.

228. Lewis RA, Gerson LP, Axelson KA, Riccardi VM, Whitford RP. von Recklinghausen neurofibromatosis: II. Incidence of optic gliomata. Ophthalmology 1984;91:929.

229. Housepian EM, Trokel SL, Jakobiec FO, et al. Tumors of the orbit. In Youmans JR, ed. Youmans' neurological surgery. Philadelphia: WB Saunders, 1982:3024.

230. Packer RJ, Sutton LN, Bilaniuk LT, et al. Treatment of chiasmatic/hypothalamic gliomas of childhood with chemotherapy: An update. Ann Neurol 1988;23:79.

231. Housepian EM. Surgical treatment of unilateral optic nerve gliomas. J Neurosurg 1969;31:604.

232. Tenny RT, Laws ER, Young BR, Rush JA. The neurosurgical management of optic gliomas: Results in 104 patients. J Neurosurg 1982;57:452.

233. Bataini JP, Delanian S, Ponvert D. Chiasmal gliomas: Results of irradiation management and review of literature. Int J Radiat Oncol Biol Phys 1991;21:615.

234. Wong JYC, Uhl V, Wara WM, Sheline GE. Optic gliomas: A re-analysis of the University of California, San Francisco experience. Cancer 1987;60:1847.

235. Danoff BF, Kramer S, Thompson N. The radiotherapeutic management of optic nerve gliomas in children. Int J Radiat Oncol Biol Phys 1980;6:45.

236. Flickinger JC, Torres C, Deutsch M. Management of low-grade gliomas of the optic nerve and chiasm. Cancer 1988;61:635.

237. Horowich A, Bloom HJG. Optic gliomas: Radiation therapy and prognosis. Int J Rad Oncl Biol Phys 1985;11:1067.

238. Rosenstock JG, Packer RJ, Bilaniuk L. Chiasmatic optic glioma treated with chemotherapy. J Neurosurg 1985;63:862.

239. Rodriguez LA, Edwards MSB, Levin VA. Management of hypothalamic gliomas in children: An analysis of 33 cases. Neurosurgery 1990;26:242.

240. Petronio J, Edwards MSB, Prados M, et al. Management of chiasmal and hypothalamic gliomas of infancy and childhood with chemotherapy. J Neurosurg 1990;74:701.

241. Ludwig CL, Smith MT, Godfrey AD, et al. A clinicopathologic study of 323 patients with oligodendrogliomas. Ann Neurol 1986;19:15.

242. Wallner KE, Gonzales M, Sheline GE. Treatment of oligodendrogliomas with or without postoperative irradiation. J Neurosurg 1988;68:684.

243. Lindegaard K-F, Mork SJ, Eide GE, et al. Statistical analysis of clinicopathological features, radiotherapy, and survival in 170 cases of oligodendroglioma. J Neurosurg 1987;67:224.

244. Halperin EC, Kun LE, Constine LS, Tarbell NJ. Pediatric radiation oncology. New York: Raven Press, 1989:58.

245. Reedy DP, Bay JW, Hahn JF. Role of radiation therapy in the treatment of cerebral oligodendroglioma: An analysis of 57 cases and a literature review. Neurosurgery 1983;13:499.

246. Bullard DE, Rawlings CE, Phillips B, et al. Oligodendroglioma: An analysis of the value of radiation therapy. Cancer 1987;60:2179.

247. Karlsson UL, Leibel SA, Wallner K, et al. Brain tumors. In: Perez CA, Brady LW, eds. Principles and practice of radiation oncology. 2nd ed. Philadelphia: JB Lippincott 1992:515.

248. Cairncross JG, MacDonald DR. Chemotherapy for oligodendroglioma: Progress report. Arch Neurol 1991;48:225.

249. Kernohan JW, Sayre GP. Tumors of the central nervous system. In: Atlas of tumor pathology. Section 10, Fascicle 35. Washington, DC: Armed Forces Institute of Pathology, 1952.

250. Svien HJ, Mabon RF, Kernohan JW, et al. Ependymoma of the brain: Pathologic aspects. Neurology 1953;3:1.

251. Healey EA, Barnes PD, Kupsky WJ, et al. The prognostic significance of post-operative residual tumor in ependymoma. Neurosurgery 1991;28:666.

252. Ross GW, Rubinstein LJ. Lack of histopathological correlation of malignant ependymomas with postoperative survival. J Neurosurg 1989;70:31.

253. Goldwein JW, Corn BW, Finlay JL, et al. Is craniospinal irradiation required to cure

children with malignant (anaplastic) intracranial ependymomas? Cancer 1991;67: 2766.

254. Vanuytsel L, Brada M. The role of prophylactic spinal irradiation in localized intracranial ependymoma. Int J Radiat Oncol Biol Phys 1991;21:825.

255. Wallner KE, Wara WM, Sheline GE, et al. Intracranial ependymomas: Results of treatment with partial or whole brain irradiation without spinal irradiation. Int J Radiat Oncol Biol Phys 1986;12:1937.

256. Salazar OM, Castro-Vita H, Van Houtte P, et al. Improved survival in cases of intracranial ependymoma after radiation therapy: Late report and recommendations. J Neurosurg 1983;59:652.

257. Marks JE, Adler SJ. A comparative study of ependymomas by site of origin. Int J Radiat Oncol Biol Phys 1982;8:3.

258. Shaw EG, Evans RG, Scheithauer BW, et al. Postoperative radiotherapy of intracranial ependymoma in pediatric and adult patients. Int J Radiat Oncol Biol Phys 1987;13: 1457.

258a. Prados M, Levin VA, Edwards MSB. Unpublished observations, 1991.

259. Levin VA, Edwards MSB, Gutin PH, et al. Phase II evaluation of dibromodulcitol in the treatment of recurrent medulloblastoma, ependymoma, and malignant astrocytoma. J Neurosurg 1984;61:1063.

260. Goldwein JW, Leahy JM, Packer RJ, et al. Intracranial ependymomas in children. Int J Radiat Oncol Biol Phys 1990;99:1497.

261. Gaynon PS, Ettinger LJ, Baum ES, et al. Carboplatin in childhood brain tumors: A Children's Cancer Study Group phase II trial. Cancer 1990;66:2465.

262. Ettinger LJ, Ru N, Krailo M, et al. A phase II study of diaziquone in children with recurrent or progressive primary brain tumors: A report from the Children's Cancer Study Group. J Neurooncol 1990;9:69.

263. Cushing H, Eisenhardt L. Meningiomas: Their classification, regional behavior, life history, and surgical end results. Springfield: Charles C Thomas, 1938:73.

264. Hoshino T, Nagashima T, Murovic J, et al. Cell kinetic studies of in situ human brain tumors with bromodeoxyuridine. Cytometry 1985;6:627.

265. Simpson D. The recurrence of intracranial meningiomas after surgical treatment. J Neurol Neurosurg Psychiatry 1957;20:22.

266. Mirimanoff RO, Dosoretz DE, Linggood RM, et al. Meningioma. Analysis of recurrence and progression following neurosurgical resection. J Neurosurg 1985;62:18.

267. Barbaro NM, Gutin PH, Wilson CB, et al. Radiation therapy in the treatment of partially resected meningiomas. Neurosurgery 1987;20:525.

268. Taylor BW, Marcus RB Jr, Friedman WA, et al. The meningioma controversy: Postoperative radiation therapy. Int J Radiat Oncol Biol Phys 1988;15:244.

269. Graholm J, Bloom HJG, Crow JH. The role of radiotherapy in the management of intracranial meningiomas: The Royal Marsden Hospital experience with 186 patients. Int J Radiat Oncol Biol Phys 1990;18:755.

270. Solan MJ, Kramer S. The role of radiation therapy in the management of intracranial meningiomas. Int J Radiat Oncol Biol Phys 1985;11:675.

271. Chan RC, Thompson GB. Morbidity, mortality, and quality of life following surgery for intracranial meningiomas. J Neurosurg 1984;60:52.

272. Grunberg SM, Weiss MH, Spitz IM, et al. Treatment of unresectable meningiomas with the antiprogesterone agent mifepristone. J Neurosurg 1991;74:861.

273. Schneck SA, Penn I. De novo brain tumors in renal transplant recipients. Lancet 1971;1:983.

274. Pitchenik AE, Fischl MA, Walls KW. Evaluation of cerebral-mass lesions in acquired immunodeficiency syndrome. N Engl J Med 1983;308:1099.

275. Payan MJ, Gambarelli D, Routy JP, et al. Primary lymphoma of the brain associated with AIDS. Acta Neuropathol 1984;64:78.

276. Rosenblum ML, Levy RM, Ziegler JL. Primary central nervous system lymphomas in patients with AIDS. Ann Neurol 1988;23(suppl):S13.

277. Murray K, Kun L, Cox J. Primary malignant lymphoma of the central nervous system. J Neurosurg 1986;65:600.

278. DeAngelis LM, Yahalom J, Rosenblum M, Posner JB. Primary CNS lymphoma: Managing patients with spontaneous and AIDS-related disease. Oncology 1987;1:52.

279. Jellinger K, Radaskiewicz TH, Slowik F. Primary malignant lymphomas of the central nervous system in man. Acta Neuropathol (Berlin) 1975;95:102.

280. Henry JM, Heffner RR Jr, Dillard SH, et al. Primary malignant lymphomas of the central nervous system. Cancer 1974;34:1293.

281. DeAngelis LM, Yahalom J, Heinemann MH, et al. Primary central nervous system lymphoma: Combined treatment with chemotherapy and radiotherapy. Neurology 1990;40:80.

282. Pollack IF, Lunsford ID, Flickinger JC, Dameshek HL. Prognostic factors in the diagnosis and treatment of primary central nervous system lymphoma. Cancer 1989;63: 939.

283. Murray K, Kun L, Cox J. Primary malignant lymphoma of the central nervous system: Results of treatment of 11 cases and review of the literature. J Neurosurg 1986;65: 600.

284. Nelson DF, Martz KL, Bonner H, et al. Definitive radiation therapy in the treatment of primary non-Hodgkin's lymphoma of the central nervous system, non-AIDS related. Report of RTOG study 8315. Int J Radiat Oncol Biol Phys 1992;23:9.

285. Margolis L, Fraser R, Lichter A, Char DH. The role of radiation therapy in the management of ocular reticulum cell sarcoma. Cancer 1980;45:688.

286. Goldstein JD, Dickson DW, Moser FG, et al. Primary central nervous system lymphoma in acquired immunodeficiency syndrome. Cancer 1991;67:2756.

287. McLaughlin P, Velasquez WS, Redman JR, et al. Chemotherapy with dexamethasone, high-dose cytarabine, and cisplatin for parenchymal brain lymphoma. JNCI 1988;80: 1408.

288. Chamberlain MC, Levin VA. Adjuvant chemotherapy for primary lymphoma of the central nervous system. Arch Neurol 1990;47:1113.

289. Neuwelt EA, Goldman D, Dahlborg SA, et al. Primary central nervous system lymphoma treated with osmotic blood-brain barrier disruption and combination chemotherapy: Prolonged survival and preservation of cognitive function. Proc Annu Meet Am Soc Clin Oncol [Abstract] 1990;9:A1047.

290. DeAngelis LM, Yahalom J. Combined modality treatment of primary central nervous system lymphoma (PCNSL). Proc Annu Meet Am Soc Clin Oncol [Abstract] 1991;10: A368.

291. McComb RD, Burger PC. Pathologic analysis of primary brain tumors. Neurol Clin North Am 1985;3:711.

292. Gaffney CC, Sloane JP, Bradley NJ, Bloom HJG. Primitive neuroectodermal tumours of the cerebrum: Pathology and treatment. J Neurooncol 1985;3:23.

293. Berger MS, Edwards MD, Wara WM, et al. Primary cerebral neuroblastoma: Long-term follow-up review and therapeutic guidelines. J Neurosurg 1983;59:418.

294. Bloom HJG. Medulloblastoma in children: Increasing survival rates and further prospects. Int J Radiat Oncol Biol Phys 1982;8:2023.

295. Deutsch M. The impact of myelography on the treatment results for medulloblastoma. Int J Radiat Oncol Biol Phys 1984;10:999.

296. Levin VA, Rodriguez LA, Edwards MSB, et al. Treatment of medulloblastoma with procarbazine hydroxyurea, and reduced radiation doses to whole brain and spine. J Neurosurg 1988;68:383.

297. Park TS, Hoffman HJ, Hendrick EB, et al. Medulloblastoma: Clinical presentation and management—experience at the Hospital For Sick Children, Toronto, 1950–1980. J Neurosurg 1983;58:543.

298. Lowery GS, Kimball JC, Patterson RB, et al. Extraneural metastases from cerebellar medulloblastoma. Am J Pediatr Hematol Oncol 1982;4:259.

299. Tait DM, Thornton-Jones H, Bloom HJG, et al. Adjuvant chemotherapy for medulloblastoma: The first multi-centre control trial of the International Society of Pediatric Oncology (SIOP I). Eur J Cancer 1990;26:464.

300. Evans AE, Jenkin RD, Sposto R, et al. The treatment of medulloblastoma: Results of a prospective randomized trial of radiation therapy with and without CCNU, vincristine, and prednisone. J Neurosurg 1990;72:572.

301. Chamberlain MC, Silver P, Edwards MSB, Levin VA. Treatment of extraneural metastatic medulloblastoma with a combination of cyclophosphamide, adriamycin, and vincristine (CAV). Neurosurgery 1988;23:476.

302. Deutsch M. The impact of myelography on the treatment results of medulloblastoma. Int J Radiat Oncol Biol Phys 1984;10:999.

303. Allen JC, Epstein F. Medulloblastoma and other primary CNS malignant neuroectodermal tumors: The effect of age and extent of disease on prognosis. J Neurosurg 1982;57:446.

304. Kun LE, Constine LS. Medulloblastoma-caution regarding new treatment approaches Int J Radiat Oncol Biol Phys 1991;20:897.

305. Brand WN, Schneider PH, Tokars RP. Long-term results of a pilot study of low-dose cranial-spinal irradiation for cerebellar medulloblastoma. Int J Radiat Oncol Biol Phys 1987;13:1641.

306. Deutsch M, Thomas P, Boyett J, et al. Low-stage medulloblastoma: A Children's Cancer Study Group (CCSG) and Pediatric Oncology Group (POG) randomized study of standard vs reduced neuraxis irradiation. Proc Am Soc Clin Oncol [Abstract] 1991;10: 124.

307. Halberg FE, Wara WM, Fippin LF, et al. Low-dose craniospinal radiation therapy for medulloblastoma. Int J Radiat Oncol Biol Phys 1991;20:651.

308. Benjamin RS, Wiernik PH, Bachur NR. Adriamycin chemotherapy: Efficacy, saftey, and pharmacologic basis of an intermittent single high-dose schedule. Cancer 1974;33: 19.

309. Shapiro WR. Chemotherapy of primary malignant brain tumors. Cancer Child 1975;35: 965.

310. Ward HWC. Central nervous system tumors of childhood treated with CCNU, vincristine and radiation. Med Pediatr Oncol 1978;4:315.

311. Garrett MJ, Hughs HJ, Ryall RDH. CCNU in brain tumors. Clin Radiol 1974;25:183.

312. Ward HWC. CCNU in the treatment of recurrent medulloblastoma. Br Med J 1974;1: 642.

313. Hancock C, Allen J, Tan CTC. Phase II trial of PCNU in children with recurrent brain tumors and Hodgkin's disease. Cancer Treat Rep 1984;68:441.

314. Walker RW, Allen JC. Treatment of recurrent primary intracranial childhood tumors with *cis*-diamine-dichloroplatinum. Ann Neurology 1983;14:371.

315. Bertolone SJ, Baum E, Krivit W, et al. Phase II trial of cisplatinum diamino-dichloride (CPDD) in recurrent childhood brain tumors: A CCSG trial. Proc Am Assoc Cancer Res 1983;2:72.

316. Sexauer CL, Kahn A, Burger PC, et al. *Cis*-platinum in recurrent pediatric brain tumors: A POG phase II study. Cancer 1985;56:1497.

317. Allen JC, Walker R, Luks E, et al. Carboplatin and recurrent childhood brain tumors. J Clin Oncol 1987;5:459.

318. Allen JC, Helson L. High-dose cyclophosphamide chemotherapy for recurrent CNS tumors in children. J Neurosurg 1981;55:749.

319. Rosen G, Ghavimi F, Nirenberg A, et al. High-dose methotrexate with citrovorum factor rescue for the treatment of central nervous system tumors in children. Cancer Treat Rep 1977;61:681.

320. Djerassi I, Kim JS, Shulman K. High-dose methotrexate-citrovorum factor rescue in the management of brain tumors. Cancer Treat Rep 1977;61:691.

321. Mooney C, Souhami R, Pritchard J. Recurrent medulloblastoma: Lack of response to high-dose methotrexate. Cancer Chemother Pharmacol 1983;10:135.

322. Haddy TB, Ferbach DJ, Watkins WL, et al. Vincristine in uncommon malignant disease in children. Cancer Chemother Rep 1964;41:41.

323. Lassman LP, Pearce GW, Gang J. Effect of vincristine sulfate on the intracranial gliomata of childhood. Br J Surg 1966;53:774.

324. Lampkin BC, Maurer AM, McBride BH. Response of medulloblastoma to vincristine sulfate: A case report. Pediatrics 1967;39:761.

325. Smart CR, Ottoman RE, Rochlin DB, et al. Clinical experience with vincristine in tumors of the central nervous system and other malignant diseases. Cancer Chemother Rep 1968;52:733.

326. Afra D. Vincristine therapy in malignant glioma recurrencies. Neurochirurgia 1973;16:189.

327. Rosenstock JG, Evans AE, Schut L: Response to vincristine of recurrent brain tumors in children. J Neurosurg 1976;45:135.

328. Skylansky BD, Mann-Kaplan RS, Reynolds BF, et al. 4'-demethyl-epipodophyllotoxin-D-thenylidene-glucoside (PTG) in the treatment of malignant intracranial neoplasms. Cancer 1974;33:460.

329. Bleyer WA, Krivit W, Chard RL. Phase II study of VM26 in leukemia, neuroblastoma, and other refractory childhood malignancies: A report from the Children's Cancer Study Group. Cancer Treat Rep 1979;63:977.

330. Friedman HS, Schold SC Jr, Mahaley MS Jr, et al. Phase II treatment of medulloblastoma and pineoblastoma with melphalan: Clinical therapy based on experimental models of human medulloblastoma. J Clin Oncol 1989;7:904.

331. Crafts DC, Levin VA, Edwards MS, et al. Chemotherapy of recurrent medulloblastoma with combined procarbazine, CCNU, vincristine. J Neurosurg 1978;49:589.

332. Thomas P, Duffner PK, Cohen ME, et al. Multimodality therapy for medulloblastoma. Cancer 1980;45:666.

333. Seiler RW. Combination chemotherapy with VM26 and CCNU in primary malignant brain tumors of children. Helv Paediatr Acta 1980;35:51.

334. van Eys J, Baram TZ, Cangir A, et al. Salvage chemotherapy for recurrent primary brain tumors in children. J Pediatr 1988;113:601.

335. Cangir A, Ragab AH, Steubner P, et al. Combination chemotherapy with vincristine, procarbazine, prednisone with or without nitrogen mustard (MOOP vs OPP) in children with recurrent brain tumors. Med Pediatr Oncol 1984;12:1.

336. Freidman HS, Mahaley MS, Schold SC Jr, et al. The efficacy of vincristine and cyclophosphamide in the therapy of recurrent medulloblastoma. Neurosurgery 1986;18:335.

337. Thomas PR, Duffner PK, Cohen ME, et al. Multimodality therapy for medulloblastoma. Cancer 1980;45:666.

338. Lefkowitz IB, Packer RJ, Siegel KR, et al. Results of treatment of children with recurrent medulloblastoma/primitive neuroectodermal tumors with lomustine, cisplatin, and vincristine. Cancer 1990;65:412.

339. Pendergrass TW, Milstein JM, Geyer JR, et al. Eight drugs in 1 day chemotherapy for brain tumors: Experience in 107 children and rationale for preirradiation chemotherapy. J Clin Oncol 1987;5:1221.

340. Packer RJ, Sutton LN, Goldwein JW, et al. Improved survival with the use of adjuvant chemotherapy in the treatment of medulloblastoma. J Neurosurg 1991;74:433.

341. Krischer JP, Ragab AH, Kun L, et al. Nitrogen mustard, vincristine, procarbazine, and prednisone as adjuvant chemotherapy in the treatment of medulloblastoma: A Pediatric Oncology Group Study. J Neurosurg 1991;74:905.

342. Prados M, Levin VA, Edwards MS, Wara W. Combined chemotherapy/radiotherapy for pediatric brain tumors: The UCSF experience [Abstract No. A48]. International Symposium on Pediatric Neuro-Oncology. June 1—3, 1989, Seattle, WA, 1989.

343. Kretschmar CS, Tarbell NJ, Kupsky W, et al. Pre-irradiation chemotherapy for infants and children with medulloblastoma: A preliminary report. J Neurosurg 1989;71:820.

344. Kovnar EH, Kellie SJ, Horowitz ME, et al. Preirradiation cisplatin and etoposide in the treatment of high-risk medulloblastoma and other malignant embryonal tumors of the central nervous system: A phase II study. J Clin Oncol 1990;8:330.

345. Christ WM, Ragab AH, Vietti TJ, et al. Chemotherapy of childhood medulloblastoma. Am J Dis Child 1976;13:639.

346. Nathanson L, Kovacs SG. Chemotherapeutic response in metastatic medulloblastoma: Report of two cases and a review of the literature. Med Pediatr Oncol 1978;4:105.

347. Hoffman HJ. Pineal region tumors. Prog Exp Tumor Res 1987;30:281.

348. Matsutani M, Takakura K, Sano K. Primary intracranial germ cell tumors: Pathology and treatment. Prog Exp Tumor Res 1987;30:307.

349. Herrick MK. Pathology of pineal tumors. In: Neuwelt EA, ed. Diagnosis and treatment of pineal region tumors. Baltimore: Williams & Wilkins, 1984:31.

350. Edwards MSB, Levin VA. Chemotherapy of third ventricle tumors. In: Appuzzo M, ed. Third ventricular tumors. Baltimore: Williams & Wilkins, 1987:838.

351. Schmidek HH, Waters A. Pineal masses: Clinical features and management. In: Wilkins RH, Rengachary SS, eds. Neurosurgery. New York: McGraw-Hill, 1985:688.

352. Pecker J, Scarabin J-M, Vallee B, et al. Treatment in tumours of the pineal region: Value of stereotaxic biopsy. Surg Neurol 1979;12:341.

353. Linstadt D, Wara WM, Edwards MSB, et al. Radiotherapy of primary intracranial germinomas: The case against routine craniospinal irradiation. Int J Radiat Oncol Biol Phys 1988;17:291.

354. Wara WM, Jenkin RDT, Evans A, et al. Tumors of the pineal and suprasellar region: Children's Cancer Study Group results, 1960-1975—a report from the Children's Cancer Study Group. Cancer 1979;43:698.

355. Jenkin RDT, Simpson WJK, Keen CW, et al. Pineal and suprasellar germinomas: Results of radiation treatment. J Neurosurg 1978;48:99.

356. Salazar OM, Castro-Vita H, Bakos RS, et al. Radiation therapy for tumors of the pineal region. Int J Radiat Oncol Biol Phys 1979;5:491.

357. Matsukado Y, Abe H, Tanaka R, et al. Cisplatin, vinblastine and bleomycin (PVB) combination chemotherapy in the treatment of intracranial malignant germ cell tumors—a preliminary report of a phase II study—The Japanese Intracranial Germ Cell Tumor Study Group. Gan No Rinsho 1986;32:1387.

358. Allen JC, Kim JH, Packer RJ. Neoadjuvant chemotherapy for newly diagnosed germ-cell tumors of the central nervous system. J Neurosurg 1987;67:65.

359. Jereb B, Zupancic N, Petric J. Intracranial germinoma: Report of seven cases. Pediatr Hematol Oncol 1990;7:183.

360. Mizuno M, Yoshida J, Noda S. Combined chemotherapy of CDDP and etoposide in intracranial germinomas. Gan To Kagaku Ryoho 1989;16:3457.

361. Miyamachi K, Aida T, Abe H. Five cases of primary intracranial germ cell tumor treated by combination chemotherapy with cisplatin. No Shinkei Geka 1988;16:1053.

362. Kobayashi T, Yoshida J, Sugita K, et al. Combination chemotherapy with cisplatin and etoposide for intracranial germ cell tumors [Abstract No. A5]. International Symposium on Pediatric Neuro-Oncology. June 1–3, 1989, Seattle, WA, 1989.

362a. Edwards MSB, Ablin A. Unpublished observations, 1987.

363. Wilson CB. Surgical management of endocrine-active pituitary adenomas. In: Walker MD, ed. Oncology of the nervous system. Boston: Martinus-Nijhoff, 1983:117.

364. Eastman RC, Gorden P, Roth J. Conventional supervoltage irradiation is an effective treatment for acromegaly. J Clin Endocrinol Metab 1979;48:931.

365. Sheline GE, Tyrrell JB. Pituitary tumors. In: Perez CA, Brady LW, eds. Principles and practice of radiation oncology. Philadelphia: JB Lippincott, 1987:1108.

366. Orth DN, Liddle GW. Results of treatment in 108 patients with Cushing's syndrome. N Engl J Med 1971;285:243.

367. Jennings AS, Liddle GW, Orth DN. Results of treating childhood Cushing's disease with pituitary irradiation. N Engl J Med 1977;297:957.

368. Grossman A, Besser GM. Prolactinomas. Br Med J 1985;290:182.

369. Kleinberg DL, Noel GL, Frantz AG. Galactorrhea: A study of 235 cases including 48 with pituitary tumors. N Engl J Med 1977;296:589.

370. Sheline GE, Grossman A, Jones AE, Besser GM. Radiation therapy of prolactinomas. In: Black PM, Zervas NT, Ridgway ED, Martin JB, eds. Secretory tumors of the pituitary gland. New York: Raven Press, 1984:1–35.

371. Halberg FE, Sheline GE. Radiotherapy of pituitary tumors. Endocrinol Metab Clin North Am 1987;16:667.

372. McCollough WM, Marcus RB Jr, Rhoton AL Jr, et al. Long-term follow-up of radiotherapy for pituitary adenoma: The absence of late recurrence after ≥ 4500 cGy. Int J Radiat Oncol Biol Phys 1991;21:607.

373. Feek CM, McLelland J, Seth J, et al. How effective is external pituitary irradiation for growth hormone secreting pituitary tumors? Clin Endocrinol 1984;20:401.

374. Coffey, RJ, Lunsford LD. The role of stereotactic techniques in the management of craniopharyngiomas. In: Rosanblum ML, ed. The role of surgery in brain tumor management. Philadelphia: WB Saunders, 1991:161.

375. Richmond IL, Wara WM, Wilson CB. Role of radiation therapy in the management of craniopharyngiomas in children. Neurosurgery 1980;6:513.

376. Sung DI, Chang CH, Harisiadis L, et al. Treatment results of craniopharyngiomas. Cancer 1981;47:847.

377. Fischer EG, Welch K, Belli JA, et al. Treatment of craniopharyngiomas in children, 1972–1981. J Neurosurg 1985;62:496.

378. Weiss M, Sutton L, Marcial V, et al. The role of radiation therapy in the management of childhood craniopharyngioma. Int J Radiat Oncol Biol Phys 1989;17:1313.

379. Wen B-C, Hussey DH, Staples J, et al. A comparison of the roles of surgery and radiation therapy in the management of craniopharyngiomas. Int J Radiat Oncol Biol Phys 1989;16:17.

380. Danoff BF, Cowchock FS, Kramer S. Childhood craniopharyngioma: Survival, local control, endocrine and neurologic function following radiotherapy. Int J Radiat Oncol Biol Phys 1983;9:171.

381. Carmel PW, Antunes J, Chang CH. Craniopharyngiomas in children. Neurosurgery 1982;11:382.

382. Thomsett MJ, Conte FA, Kaplan SL, Grumbach MM. Endocrine and neurologic outcome in childhood craniopharyngioma: Review of effect of treatment in 42 patients. J Pediatr 1980;97:728.

383. Cavazzuti V, Fischer EC, Welch K, et al. Neurological and psychophysiological sequelae following different treatments of craniopharyngiomas in children. J Neurosurg 1983;59:409.

384. Jackler RK, Pitts LH. Acoustic neuroma. In: Rosenblum ML, ed. The role of surgery in brain tumor management. Neurosurg Clin North Am 1990;1:199.

385. Martuza RL, Ojemann RG. Bilateral acoustic neuromas: Clinical aspects, pathogenesis, and treatment. Neurosurgery 1982;10:1.

386. Wallner KE, Sheline GE, Pitts LH, et al. Efficacy of irradiation for incompletely excised acoustic neurilemomas. J Neurosurg 1987;67:858.

387. Flickinger JC, Lunsford LD, Coffey RJ, et al. Radiosurgery of acoustic neurinomas. Cancer 1991;67:345.

388. Farriro JB III, Hyams VL, Benke RH, et al. Carcinoid apudoma arising in glomus jugulare tumors. Laryngoscope 1980;90:110.

389. Simko TG, Griffin TW, Gerdes AJ, et al. The role of radiation therapy in the treatment of glomus jugulare tumors. Cancer 1978;42:104.

390. Gardner G, Cocke EW Jr, Robertson JT, et al. Glomus jugulare tumors: Combined treatment. I. J Laryngol Otol 1981;95:437.

391. Cummings BJ, Beale FA, Garrett PG, et al. The treatment of glomus tumors of the temporal bone by megavoltage radiation. Cancer 1984;53:2635.

392. Springate SC, Weichselbaum RR. Radiation or surgery for chemodectoma of the temporal bone: A review of local control and complications. Head Neck 1990;12:303.

393. Million RR, Cassisi NJ. Chemodectomas (glomus body tumors). In: Million RR, Cassisi NJ, eds. Management of head and neck cancer. Philadelphia: JB Lippincott, 1984:567.

394. Kim JA, Elkon D, Lim ML, et al. Optimum dose of radiotherapy for chemodectomas of the middle ear. Int J Radiat Oncol Biol Phys 1980;6:815.

395. Heffelfinger MJ, Dahlin DC, MacCarty CS, et al. Chordomas and cartilaginous tumors at the skull base. Cancer 1973;32:410.

396. Austin-Seymore M, Munzenrider J, Goitein M, et al. Fractionated proton radiation therapy of chordoma and low-grade chondrosarcoma of the base of the skull. J Neurosurg 1989;70:13.

397. Phillips T, Newman H. Chordomas. In: Deeley T, ed. Modern radiotherapy and oncology: Central nervous system tumors. Boston: Butterworths, 1974:184.

398. Berson AM, Castro JR, Petti P, et al. Charged particle irradiation of chordoma and chondrosarcoma of the base of skull and cervical spine: The Lawrence Berkeley Laboratory Experience. Int J Radiat Oncol Biol Phys 1988;15:559.

399. Sung DI, Chang CH, Harisiadis L. Cerebellar hemangioblastomas. Cancer 1982;49:553.

400. Smalley SR, Schomberg PJ, Earle JD, et al. Radiotherapeutic considerations in the treatment of hemangioblastomas of the central nervous system. Int J Radiat Oncol Biol Phys 1990;18:1165.

401. Naguib MG, Chou SH, Mastri A. Radiation therapy of a choroid plexus papilloma of the cerebellopontine angle with bone involvement. J Neurosurg 1981;54:245.

402. Ausman JI, Schrontz C, Chason J, et al. Aggressive choroid plexus papilloma. Surg Neurol 1984;22:472.

403. Carpenter DB, Michelsen WJ, Hays AP. Carcinoma of the choroid plexus: Case report. J Neurosurg 1982;56:722.

404. Connolly ES. Spinal cord tumors in adults. In: Youmans JR, ed. Youmans' neurological surgery. Philadelphia: WB Saunders, 1982:3196.

405. Wen B-C, Hussey DH, Hitchon PW, et al. The role of radiation therapy in the management of ependymomas of the spinal cord. Int J Radiat Oncol Biol Phys 1991;20:781.

406. Linstadt DE, Wara WM, Leibel SA, et al. Postoperative radiotherapy of primary spinal cord tumors. Int J Radiat Oncol Biol Phys 1989;16:1397.

407. Barone B, Elvidge A. Ependymomas: A clinical survey. J Neurosurg 1970;33:428.

408. Schuman R, Alvord E, Leech R. The biology of childhood ependymomas. Arch Neurol 1975;32:731.

409. Sloof J, Kernohan J, MacCarty C. Primary intramedullary tumors of the spinal cord and filum terminale. Philadelphia: WB Saunders, 1964.

410. Forman AD, Levin VA. Intraventricular therapy. In: Perry MC, ed. The chemotherapy source book. Baltimore: Williams & Wilkins, 1991:213.

Cancer: Principles & Practice of Oncology, Fourth Edition,
edited by Vincent T. DeVita, Jr., Samuel Hellman, Steven A. Rosenberg.
J.B. Lippincott Co., Philadelphia © 1993.

Philip A. Pizzo   David G. Poplack
Marc E. Horowitz   Daniel M. Hays
Larry E. Kun

CHAPTER **49**

Solid Tumors of Childhood

Despite their rarity, childhood cancers have enlightened the epidemiology, genetics, etiology, and treatment of pediatric and adult malignancies. There are, however, striking and important differences in the types of malignancies that occur in children or adults.

EPIDEMIOLOGY OF CHILDHOOD CANCER

Approximately 6500 to 7200 new cases of childhood cancer are diagnosed each year in the United States. Cancer is second only to accidents as the leading cause of death in children younger than 15 years of age. Table 49–1 lists the incidences of the most common childhood cancers. Leukemias and lymphomas comprise almost 48% of pediatric cancers, followed by tumors of the central nervous system (20%), the sympathetic nervous system, soft tissues, kidney, bone, liver, eye, and germ cells. These malignancies often have a high growth fraction and a propensity for rapid growth. Carcinomas are rare during childhood. Pediatric tumors are characterized by unique age peaks, and some have sex, genetic, race, and geographic predilections.

Age is important in pediatric cancer in at least three ways. First, as shown in Table 49–2, the predominant type of childhood cancer varies according to the age of the child. The incidence of several cancers peaks soon after birth (*e.g.*, neuroblastoma, retinoblastoma), suggesting the role of prenatal events, but the incidence of other tumors (*e.g.*, lymphomas, bone tumors) increases with age, suggesting that postnatal events are important. Second, histologically identical malignancies can behave differently at different ages. For example, neuroblastoma, the most common tumor of infancy, has an excellent prognosis if it occurs in infants younger than 1 year of age, but it has a dismal prognosis in older children. Whether

these differences reflect biologic properties of the host or the tumor is an unresolved but important issue. Third, the age of the child at diagnosis may predict the tumor's malignant potential. For example, sacrococcygeal tumors rarely have malignant elements if they are diagnosed at birth. However, if diagnosis is delayed until after the child is 2 months old or older (because the mass is intrapelvic and not directly visible), 50% to 70% of these tumors are malignant.

Sex influences the incidence and outcome of certain pediatric cancers. Most pediatric neoplasms have a male predominance (see Table 49–1), although for some tumors, such as Ewing's sarcoma and rhabdomyosarcoma, this does not become apparent until after the age of 13 years. Teratomas are an exception, because almost 75% occur in girls, but their potential for malignancy is higher in boys.

Race influences the distribution and outcome of several pediatric cancers. The cancer rate for black children is approximately 20% less than that for white children. For example, Ewing's sarcoma rarely occurs in American and African blacks. Testicular cancer is unusual in black children, and the early age peak observed in white children with acute lymphocytic leukemia (ALL) is not observed in blacks. However, the prognosis for black children who do develop ALL appears to be worse than for white children, probably because of the predominance of T-cell leukemia in black patients.

During recent years, the geographic diversity of cancer has become better appreciated. For example, although Burkitt's lymphoma accounts for almost half of the childhood cancers in Uganda, it is rare outside of the "Burkitt's belt." Conversely, neuroblastoma appears to be exceedingly rare in the Burkitt's belt. Retinoblastoma accounts for only 1% of the childhood cancers in the United States but is far more common in India. Hepatic tumors, which are rare in the United States, are considerably more frequent in the Far East. The distribution of

TABLE 49–1.   Incidence of Childhood Cancers

Malignancy	Rate (per million/y)	Ratio Sex (M:F)	Ratio Race (W:B)	Peak Age (y)
Leukemias				
Acute lymphocytic	24.7	1.3	2.4	2–5
Acute nonlymphocytic	5.0	1.2	1.0	<2
Lymphomas				
Non-Hodgkin's	9.3	2.9		6–16
Hodgkin's	7.5	3.0	1.6	>10
Central Nervous System Tumors				
Gliomas	13.4	>1.0	1.1	Constant
Medulloblastoma	4.9	1.6	0.8	5–10
Ependymoma	2.1	>1.0	2.6	<5
Solid Tumors				
Neuroblastoma	8.0	1.4	1.6	<3
Wilm's tumor	6.9	0.9	0.9	<5
Retinoblastoma	3.0	<1.0	0.8	<3
Rhabdomyosarcoma	3.7	>1.2	0.9	Bimodal: 2–6 and 14–18
Ewing's sarcoma	2.1	>1.0	>1.0	10–18
Osteosarcoma	3.1	>1.0	1.2	10–18
Primary hepatic	1.6	>1.3		Bimodal: <2 and >14
Germ cell teratoma	0.4	0.3	0.8	Bimodal: <2 and >14

Hodgkin's disease by subtype also appears to vary geographically, with the more aggressive varieties predominating in developing countries. Some of these differences reflect racial and genetic factors, whereas others are due to variations in the environment and various oncogenic cofactors, like Epstein-Barr virus (EBV), hepatitis B virus, and human T-cell lymphotropic virus (HTLV).

The most famous geographic cluster of childhood cancer was the putative concentration of childhood leukemia in a single parish in Niles, Illinois, in 1963. Several clusters have been described over the years to suggest an association of the malignancy with environmental factors (*e.g.*, viruses, chemical pollution). Most have not held up to detailed investigation, but the recent cluster of leukemia in Woburn, Massachusetts, implicating chemical water pollution is noteworthy and suggests the need for continuing vigilance and research.

Ecogenetics is the study of the interaction between environmental and genetic factors in carcinogenesis, particularly of genetic variations in response to environmental agents. Table 49–3 details environmental agents that interact with genetic traits or defects to produce a malignant phenotype. Environmental factors include chemicals, radiation, and viruses. The genetic predisposition may be created by a sporadic mutation or familial transmission.

GENETICS AND BIOLOGY

The importance of genes and inheritance is exemplified in many childhood cancers. In some families, several members are affected by the same tumor or by various types of cancers.

Certain human tumors are clearly inheritable. For example, approximately 40% of retinoblastomas appear to be inherited as an autosomal dominant trait with high penetrance. Wilms' tumor and neuroblastoma may also be bilateral and inheritable. Despite this dominant pattern of transmission, it is gene loss that leads to malignancy. The genetic information in the "retinoblastoma locus" on chromosome 13q14 acts to suppress the development of retinoblastoma, and if both alleles are lost (*i.e.*, a recessive mutant), the normal suppression of this tumor is lost and retinoblastoma occurs. In familial retinoblastoma, a loss of both retinoblastoma alleles is transmitted, leading to the expression of disease. In patients who have one copy of the allele, which can effectively suppress the development of retinoblastoma, the mutation, loss, or inactivation of this allele produces retinoblastoma.

Similar modes of genetic oncogenesis appear to occur in patients with Wilms' tumor, osteosarcoma, hepatoblastoma, and rhabdomyosarcoma (Table 49–4). The Li-Fraumeni syndrome, in which there is an increased incidence of breast cancer and other malignancies in the mothers of some children with rhabdomyosarcoma or osteosarcoma, is associated with the loss of genetic material or mutation on chromosome 17 (p53 region).

Some genetic disorders are associated with an increased incidence of cancer. For example, children with trisomy 21 (Down's syndrome) have a 10-fold increase in the incidence of acute lymphocytic leukemia; those with Klinefelter's syndrome (*i.e.*, XXY) have a greater than 60-fold increase in their incidence of breast cancer. Patients with chromosome fragility and defective DNA repair (*e.g.*, xeroderma pigmentosa, Bloom's syndrome, Fanconi's anemia) have an increased risk of cancer.

TABLE 49–2. Predominant Pediatric Cancers by Age and Site

Tumors	Newborn (<1 y)	Infancy (1–3 y)	Children (3–11 y)	Adolescents and Young Adults (12–21 y)
Leukemias	Congenital leukemia AML AMMoL CML, juvenile	ALL AML CML, juvenile	ALL AML	AML ALL
Lymphomas	Very rare	Lymphoblastic	Lymphoblastic Undifferentiated	Lymphoblastic Undifferentiated (Burkitt's, Hodgkin's)
Solid Tumors				
Central nervous system	Medulloblastoma Ependymoma Astrocytoma Choroid plexus papilloma	Medulloblastoma Ependymoma Astrocytoma Choroid plexus papilloma	Cerebellar astrocytoma Medulloblastoma Astrocytoma Ependymoma Craniopharyngioma	Cerebellar astrocytoma Astrocytoma Craniopharyngioma Medulloblastoma
Head and neck	Retinoblastoma Rhabdomyosarcoma Neuroblastoma Multiple endocrine neoplasia	Retinoblastoma Rhabdomyosarcoma Neuroblastoma	Rhabdomyosarcoma Lymphoma	Lymphoma Rhabdomyosarcoma
Thoracic	Neuroblastoma Teratoma	Neuroblastoma Teratoma	Lymphoma Neuroblastoma Rhabdomyosarcoma	Lymphoma Ewing's Rhabdomyosarcoma
Abdominal	Neuroblastoma Mesoblastic nephroma Hepatoblastoma Wilms' (>6 mos)	Neuroblastoma Wilms' Hepatoblastoma Leukemia	Neuroblastoma Wilms' Lymphoma Hepatoma	Lymphoma Hepatocellular carcinoma Rhabdomyosarcoma
Gonadal	Yolk sac tumor of testis (endodermal sinus tumor) Teratoma Sarcoma Botryoides Neuroblastoma	Rhabdomyosarcoma Yolk sac tumor of testis Clear cell sarcoma kidney	Rhabdomyosarcoma	Rhabdomyosarcoma Dysgerminoma Teratocarcinoma, teratoma Embryonal carcinoma of testis Embryonal cell and endodermal sinus tumors of ovary
Extremity	Fibrosarcoma	Fibrosarcoma Rhabdomyosarcoma	Rhabdomyosarcoma Ewing's	Osteosarcoma Rhabdomyosarcoma Ewing's sarcoma

ALL, acute lymphoblastic leukemia; AML, acute myelogenous leukemia; AMMoL, acute myelomono-cytic leukemia; CML, chronic myelogenous leukemia.

Many translocations specific for malignancies have been identified. Some translocations are associated with oncogenes (*MYC* and the 8:14 translocation of Burkitt's lymphoma), and some oncogenes are uniquely associated with certain tumors (*MYCN* [previously N-*myc*] in neuroblastoma). The genome of every normal cell contains at least 30 protooncogenes. Although the gene product of every oncogene is not known, it is apparent that some of their products play a role in the regulation of cell growth. The activation or mutation of oncogenes or their translocation next to sites important in growth regulation contribute to malignancy (Table 49–5). Although many of the examples in which alteration of growth factors and differentiation contribute to the expression of neoplasia have been in pediatric tumors, the genetic mechanism being elucidated has relevance for adult tumors (Table 49–6).

Certain pediatric tumors are frequently associated with congenital disorders, malformations, or syndromes (Table 49–7). Patients with these disorders should be followed with the awareness that they may be at risk for developing a cancer. Because congenital findings may be associated with an inheritable malignancy, such as retinoblastoma and multiple endocrine neoplasia syndromes, genetic counseling of the patient and family is important.

Genetic disorders that alter the immune system (*e.g.*, ataxia-telangiectasia, Wiskott-Aldrich syndrome) are associated with an increased risk of cancer. The increased occurrence of lymphoma in adult patients and leiomyomas and leiomyosarcomas in children with acquired immunodeficiency syndrome (AIDS) emphasizes the integral association between immunoregulation and cancer.

TABLE 49–3. Ecogenetics of Tumors of the Young

Environmental Agent	Genetic Trait	Tumor or Outcome
Ionizing radiation	Ataxia-telangiectasia with lymphoma	Radiation toxicity
	Retinoblastoma	Sarcoma
	Nevoid basal cell carcinoma syndrome	Basal cell carcinoma
Ultraviolet radiation	Xeroderma pigmentosum	Skin cancer, melanoma
	Cutaneous albinism	Skin cancer
	Hereditary dysplastic nevus syndrome	Melanoma
Stilbestrol	X0 Turner's syndrome	Adenosquamous endometrial carcinoma
Androgen	Fanconi's pancytopenia	Hepatoma
Iron	Hemochromatosis	Hepatocellular carcinoma
Tyrosine	Tyrosinemia	Hepatocellular carcinoma
Monosaccharides	Glycogen storage disease type I	Hepatic adenoma
Epstein-Barr virus?	Purtilo X-linked lymphoproliferative syndrome	Burkitt's and other lymphomas
Papillomavirus type 5	Epidermodysplasia verruciformis	Skin cancer

(Mulvihill JJ. Clinical genetics of pediatric cancer. In: Pizzo PA, Poplack DG, eds. Principles and practice of pediatric oncology. Philadelphia: JB Lippincott, 1993)

In addition to genetically mediated or transmitted factors, prenatal exposure to certain drugs or substances have been associated with a heightened risk for developing cancer. For example, the fetal alcohol or hydantoin syndromes have been associated with neuroblastoma, and prenatal exposure to diethylstilbestrol increases the risk for adolescent girls to develop a clear cell adenocarcinoma of the vagina.

Some pediatric tumors have the interesting biologic property of undergoing spontaneous regression. This is most common in neuroblastoma, but it has also been observed in retinoblastoma, histiocytosis, sacrococcygeal teratoma, and hepatoblastoma. Study of the genetic controls that affect this differentiation process are central to developing new treatment modalities for these neoplasms. For example, *MYCN*

amplification correlates with the stage of neuroblastoma, and lowering *MYCN* expression in vitro with *cis*-retinoic acid causes differentiation of these cells into more mature neural cells. This suggests that future therapeutic strategies should focus on the differentiation of tumor cells rather than their destruction.

UNUSUAL CLINICAL MANIFESTATIONS

Although most children with cancer come to medical attention because of growing masses, the signs and symptoms of cancer can sometimes be subtle, nonspecific, or confusing and can result in delays in diagnosis and treatment (see Table 49–7).

TABLE 49–4. Pediatric Malignancies With Recognized or Likely Recessive Genetic Alterations

Tumor	Chromosomal Alterations
Neuroblastoma	1p36
Embryonal tumors of Beckwith-Wiedemann syndrome	11p
Retinoblastoma	13q14
Osteosarcoma	13q14
Astrocytoma	17q12
Acoustic neuroma and meningioma	22
Meningioma	22

(Israel, MA. Cancer cell biology. In: Pizzo PA, Poplack DG, eds. Principles and practice of pediatric oncology. 2nd ed. Philadelphia: JB Lippincott, 1993)

TABLE 49–5. Cancer-Associated Genes Implicated in Selected Pediatric Malignancies

Malignancy	Genes
Leukemia	p53, *ABL, FMS, KRAS, MYB, MYC, NRAS, SRC*
Lymphoma	*BCL, MYB, MYC, RAS*
Glioma	p53, *ERBB2, FES, MYB, MYC, NEU, NRAS, RAF, ROS, SIS*
Wilms' tumor	*WT1, MYB, MYCN*
Neuroblastoma	*MYB, MYC, MYCN, NRAS, SRC*
Retinoblastoma	*RB, MYCN, SRC*
Germ cell tumors	*HST, MYC, MYCN*
Rhabdomyosarcoma	p53, *FOS, KRAS, MYB, MYC, NRAS, REL, SRC*
Osteogenic sarcoma	*RB, MET, SIS, SRC*
Ewing's sarcoma	*DBL, ETS, MYC, RAF, SRC*
Peripheral neuroectodermal tumors	*ETS, MYC, RAF, SRC*

TABLE 49–6.   Childhood Cancers Associated With Congenital Syndromes or Malformations

Syndrome or Anomaly	Tumor
Aniridia	Wilms' tumor
Hemihypertrophy	Wilms' tumor, hepatoblastoma, adrenocortical carcinoma
Genitourinary abnormalities (including testicle maldescent)	Wilms' tumor, Ewing's sarcoma, nephroblastoma, testicular carcinoma
Beckwith-Wiedemann syndrome	Wilms' tumor, neuroblastoma, adrenocortical carcinoma
Dysplastic nevus syndrome	Melanoma
Nevoid basal cell carcinoma syndrome	Basal cell carcinoma, medulloblastoma, rhabdomyosarcoma
Poland's syndrome	Leukemia
Trisomy 21 (Down's syndrome)	Leukemia, retinoblastoma
Blooms' syndrome	Leukemia, gastrointestinal carcinoma
Severe combined immune deficiency disease	EBV-associated B-lymphocyte lymphoma/leukemia
Wiscott-Aldridge syndrome	EBV-associated B-lymphocyte lymphoma
Ataxia-telangiectasia	EBV-associated B-lymphocyte lymphoma, gastric carcinoma
Retinoblastoma	Wilms' tumor, osteosarcoma, Ewing's sarcoma
Fanconi's anemia	Leukemia, squamous cell carcinoma
Multiple endocrine neoplasia syndromes (MEN-I, -II, -III)	Andenomas of islet cells, pituitary, parathyroid, and adrenal glands
	Submucosal neuromas of the tongue, lips, eyelids
	Pheochromocytomas, medullary carcinoma of the thyroid
	Malignant schwannoma, nonappendiceal carcinoid
Neurofibromatosis (von Recklinghausen's syndrome)	Rhabdomyosarcoma, fibrosarcoma, pheochromocytomas, optic glioma, meningioma

Several pediatric tumors are biologically active and produce a variety of oncofetal proteins and other substances that may have diagnostic or prognostic value. These indicators, listed in Table 49–8, are measured in serum or in urine. Only rarely do these substances directly affect the patient.

Some pediatric cancers may present with bilateral involvement (*e.g.*, Wilms' tumor, retinoblastoma), making thorough examination important before any surgical procedures are performed. Some nonmalignant processes can also be confused with a cancer (*e.g.*, histoplasmosis with lymphoma, osteomyelitis with bone tumors), and some cancers can mimic other malignancies (*e.g.*, neuroblastoma mimics ALL in the bone marrow or peripheral blood).

PROGNOSTIC FACTORS

Most pediatric cancers can be divided into good and poor prognostic categories. Although the stage, site, and extent of

disease have provided the traditional means for classifying patients, additional refinements have been achieved using tumor histology, immunologic typing, and molecular analysis. The identification of risk groups permits therapy to be tailored so that patients likely to do well can receive less intensive and less toxic regimens, and more intensive therapies can be restricted to patients with a poorer prognosis. However, prognostic factors are dynamic and, in some cases, artificial, because improvements in therapy may modify or even nullify previously important risk factors.

Histologic variants of specific pediatric neoplasms have been recognized and correlated with prognosis. For example, Wilms' tumors can now be divided into favorable and unfavorable histologic variants, which correlate with prognosis; 57% of patients with unfavorable histology die of their tumors, compared with 7% of patients with favorable histology. Similar prognostic correlations can be achieved with immunologic classification; children with the common acute leukemia antigen, CALLA, on their lymphoblasts fare better than those lacking this antigen. Molecular analysis has determined the gene rearrangements in children with null cell leukemias, further clarifying the cell lineage and guiding treatment. Pathologic diagnosis and molecular analysis have become particularly important in defining the small, round cell tumors of childhood (*i.e.*, neuroblastoma, rhabdomyosarcoma, Ewing's sarcoma, lymphoma, peripheral neuroectodermal tumors), clarifying important prognostic features and directing new therapeutic approaches. For example, recognition that peripheral neuroepithelial tumors share a t(11;22) abnormality and an oncogene profile with Ewing's sarcoma, rather than with the histologically similar neuroblastoma, has helped to define appropriate treatment regimens.

MANAGEMENT OF PEDIATRIC TUMORS

The successful management of pediatric cancer requires a carefully orchestrated team of a pediatric oncologist; a surgeon; a radiotherapist; diagnostic specialists in radiology, nuclear medicine, pathology, and clinical laboratory data; pediatric, medical, and surgical subspecialty consultants; nurses; pharmacists; and the supportive care services of specialists in physical, respiratory, recreation, and occupational therapy. Because the child with cancer is under enormous physical and emotional stress, appropriate psychosocial resources for the patient and family are important for optimal therapy.

Therapy for certain pediatric tumors has become more specialized, raising the question of whether all children with cancer should be treated at pediatric cancer centers. The complexity of most treatment protocols and the support services necessary to deliver and monitor them has consistently demonstrated a significant survival advantage for children treated in a specialty center over those treated in a community hospital. An alternative is a shared management plan in which the daily primary care is coordinated by community physicians who work under the guidance of a specialty treatment center.

Although the major modalities of therapy—surgery, radiation, and chemotherapy—are the same for pediatric and adult neoplasms, several features distinguish their application in children.

TABLE 49–7. Nonspecific Clinical Findings Associated With or as the Sole Manifestation of a Childhood Cancer

Clinical Findings	Tumor
Eye or orbit	
Strabismus	Retinoblastoma
Leukokoria ("cat's eye")	Retinoblastoma
Heterochromia—anisocoria and Horner's syndrome	Neuroblastoma
Opsoclonus—myoclonus ("dancing eyes") or acute cerebellar encephalopathy	Neuroblastoma
Proptosis	Neuroblastoma, lymphoma, retinoblastoma, rhabdomyosarcoma
Chronic sinusitis or otitis media	Rhabdomyosarcoma, nasopharyngeal carcinoma
Chronic diarrhea (Verner-Morrison syndrome)	Neuroblastoma, MEN-II
Skin	
"Blueberry muffin" nodules	Neuroblastoma
Seborrheic dermatitis	Histiocytosis
Nodular "blueberry" lips	MEN-II
Hypertension	Neuroblastoma, carcinoid, APUD tumors, pheochromocytoma, Wilms'
Virilization	Hepatoblastoma, arrhenoblastoma, adrenal rest tumors, gonadoblastoma
Feminization	Chorioepithelioma, teratoma, hepatoblastoma, adrenal tumor, nongestational choriocarcinoma, embryonal cell carcinoma, granulosa thecal cell tumors

SURGERY

Two principles guide management. First, with rare exception, no child should be considered to have disease that is so far advanced that cure can be ruled out. Second, although there should be no hesitation to perform a radical procedure for cure, every attempt should be made to minimize disability and deformity. With the use of preoperative or neoadjuvant chemotherapy or radiation therapy, tumors resectable with difficulty or loss of function (*i.e.,* hepatoma, rhabdomyosarcoma) have been converted into more readily resectable lesions. Limb-sparing procedures provide important alternatives for children with extremity lesions and have become increasingly important with improvements in survival.

Attention should be given to the general principles of pediatric and cancer surgery. Care must be used to avoid excessive blood loss because the common tumors of childhood are large and vascular, originating in vascular organs (*e.g.,* hepatoma) or surrounding major blood vessels, such as the vena cava and aorta (*e.g.,* neuroblastoma, Wilms' tumor). Surgical technique must be meticulous, and presurgical planning must anticipate a vascular catastrophe. Blood replacement must be readily accomplished. If rapid transfusion is necessary, the blood should be warmed to 37°C and its pH

TABLE 49–8. Biological Markers for Pediatric Tumors

Tumors	AFP	hCG	Ferritin	Catecholamines	NSE	LDH	Alkaline Phosphatase	Polyamine	Cystathionine	CEA
Germ cell tumor	+	+				+				+
Liver tumor	+	+	+						+	+
Neuroblastoma			+	+	+	+			+	+
Ewing's sarcoma						+				
Osteosarcoma						+	+			
Medulloblastoma					+			+		
Lymphoma						+				

AFP, α_1-fetoprotein; hCG, human chorionic gonadotropin; NSE, neuron-specific enolase; LDH, lactate dehydrogenase; CEA, carcinoembryonic antigen; +, reported to be elevated in some or all patients with active disease.

buffered to 7.4 to avoid the potential for a cardiac arrest that can occur when large volumes of cold, relatively acid, bank blood (10°C, pH 7.0) are administered to the small child. The surgeon and anesthesiologist must be aware that what is considered insignificant blood loss in an adult may be life-threatening in a small child whose circulating blood volume is small. For example, the loss of 400 ml of blood in a 1-year-old child represents half of the child's blood volume.

Another important difference between children and adults is the greater heat loss that occurs when a child is anesthetized, primarily because of the proportionally large body surface area of children. Hypothermia, cardiac irritability, metabolic acidosis, and clotting abnormalities can result from excessive heat loss. To avoid this, the operating room and the child should be kept warm and monitored carefully.

RADIATION THERAPY

As with adults, the primary goal of radiation therapy in children is to deliver an effective tumoricidal dose while sparing as much normal tissue as possible. This goal is more difficult to achieve in young children because of potential growth retardation and second malignancies.

To deliver technically acceptable irradiation, careful treatment planning and simulation are essential, as is immobilization and sedation, particularly for the young or uncooperative child. Ketamine anesthesia is particularly useful in young children, especially for those who require multiple treatments.

Although children often tolerate the acute radiation reactions better than adults, late changes in skeletal and soft tissue development are important and unique consequences. Treatment planning should attempt to create symmetry wherever possible, particularly in visible areas, such as the head and neck, and in the spine. Inadequate attention to symmetric irradiation of growing bone results in abnormal development that may not become apparent until the child enters the pubertal growth phase (*e.g.*, vertebral asymmetry resulting in scoliosis). Soft tissues, teeth, and visual structures may fail to develop normally after irradiation. Decreased muscle mass can lead to imbalance and relative asymmetry. Blood vessels and other structures with the radiation field, such as the thyroid and pituitary glands, may develop imperfectly. Brain tissue is particularly susceptible to late effects, especially if radiation is combined with neurotoxic drugs like methotrexate. Similarly, radiation therapy may exacerbate chemotherapy-induced toxicities, such as doxorubicin-induced cardiomyopathy or cyclophosphamide-related hemorrhagic cystitis. The most sobering consideration is that therapeutic irradiation increases the risk of second tumors.

CHEMOTHERAPY

One of the most important differences between pediatric and adult neoplasms is their general chemosensitivity and the possibility that a cure can be attained with combination chemotherapy. Analyses confirm continued improvements during the last decade in the numbers of children with cancer who are being cured. The drugs used in children are usually the same as those used in adults. Combination chemotherapy is the rule, and for the most part, higher dosages of chemotherapeutic agents are employed in children (except new-borns), because their tolerance of the acute side effects of chemotherapy is greater than that of adults. Many chemotherapeutic regimens in children consist of more intensive and frequent drug administrations, with less dose modifications for myelosuppression or infection, than in adults. However, appropriate dose adjustment and modification is necessary on a regular basis to account for the normal growth of children. Brain growth relative to body surface area is completed by the age of 3 years, and dosages of intrathecal drugs should have an upper limit based on age rather than body surface area.

Many chemotherapy regimens for children are given over prolonged periods, frequently from 1 to 3 years. Efforts are being directed at defining good-risk patients for whom shorter durations of therapy may suffice. Nonetheless, for many children extended courses of treatment are necessary. In attempting to adjust schedules so that school attendance and daily activities can be normal, many treatment protocols use oral drugs for patients who are receiving maintenance therapy. However, absorption of oral chemotherapy may result in decreased bioavailability of the chemotherapeutic agent, which can contribute to treatment failure, and children, particularly adolescents, may not take medications, necessitating careful monitoring of pediatric cancer patients.

Because long-term survival is achievable for children and because growing organs may be more susceptible to long-term damage, careful consideration must be given to the chemotherapeutic agents used in children. The magnitude of long-term complications from regimens administered a decade ago are only now being appreciated. The pediatric oncologist should anticipate the future impact of current strategies.

SUPPORTIVE CARE

The treatment program for the child with cancer cannot focus only on tumor reduction and the physical side effects of therapy. Every attempt must be made to ensure that the child survives as a functional member of the family and society, and a comprehensive support matrix must offer the child every opportunity to grow and mature as normally as possible. This requires a coordinated school program with educational monitoring and psychological counseling; psychosocial support for the patient, siblings, and family; and occupational recreational, and physical therapy.

WILMS' TUMOR

EPIDEMIOLOGY AND GENETICS

The annual incidence of Wilms' tumor is 7 per million children younger than 16 years of age, a statistic that varies little from one part of the world to another. One child in 10,000 develops Wilms' tumor. In 1991, approximately 460 new cases of Wilms' tumor occurred in the United States, accounting for 5% to 6% of childhood cancers. The tumor occurs equally in boys and girls worldwide, but a slight preponderance of girls was seen in the National Wilms' Tumor Study (NWTS). The median age at diagnosis in the NWTS experience was 39 months for patients with unilateral tumors and 26 months for those with bilateral tumor.

Congenital anomalies associated with Wilms' tumor include aniridia, hemihypertrophy, malformation of the genitalia (*e.g.,* cryptorchidism, hypospadias, pseudohermaphroditism, gonadal dysgenesis), the Beckwith-Wiedemann, Drash, and Perlman malformation syndromes, and neurofibromatosis.

Case reports and the records of the NWTS-1 document the occurrence of familial Wilms' tumor in about 1% of patients. The mode of inheritance is thought to be autosomal dominant with variable penetrance. According to the two-hit mutation model, the pathogenesis of Wilms' tumor lies in the loss of a functioning gene by mutations at homologous loci. Cytogenetic characterization of somatic and tumor cells from patients with Wilms' tumor has identified the location of this gene at band p13 of chromosome 11. Although the somatic cells of most patients are karyotypically normal, those with aniridia often have a deletion at 11p13 or half-normal levels of catalase, an enzyme mapped to that region of chromosome 11. This constitutional chromosomal abnormality, the first hit, may involve enough of the chromosome to be cytogenetically detectable, as is the case with associated aniridia, or may involve only a point mutation at the Wilms' tumor locus. A candidate recessive gene at 11p13 has been cloned and, unlike the genes in retinoblastoma, appears to be inactivated in only a subset of Wilms' tumors, especially those whose histopathology is reminiscent of intralobar nephroblastomatosis. It seems likely, based in detailed family studies, that more than a single gene is involved in the molecular pathogenesis of Wilms' tumor.

PATHOLOGY

Wilms' tumor usually presents as a large mass, the surface of which is smoother than the more irregular and nodular neuroblastoma. The tumor mass is often surrounded by a fibrous pseudocapsule composed of compressed, atrophic renal tissues and may contain cystic areas and necrosis and hemorrhage. Calcification is uncommon. The tumors are most often unicentric, but in the NWTS experience, 7% are multifocal in one kidney, and 5.4% involved both kidneys at the time of presentation or subsequently. Rarely, the tumor is extrarenal, occurring in the retroperitoneum, pelvis, or inguinal region. Local extension of tumor through the capsule and into the perinephric fat is common. Tumor invades the renal vein in 10% of patients, and tumor thrombus may extend to the right atrium. Spread to the lymph nodes of the renal hilum or the perinephric lymph nodes occurs in approximately 20% of patients and is prognostically unfavorable.

As a consequence of its derivation from the metanephric blastema, the histologic spectrum of Wilms' tumor is broad. The typical histologic pattern is triphasic, which includes blastemal, epithelial, and stromal cells, with undifferentiated spindle cells surrounding epithelial cell tubules of various sizes and shapes, sometimes forming abortive glomeruli. Biphasic patterns composed of stromal and blastemal cells and monophasic tumors consisting of one cell type are also encountered. A monophasic epithelial Wilms' tumor with papillary or tubular differentiation may be difficult to differentiate from an undifferentiated renal cell carcinoma. Because Wilms' tumor rarely poses a problem in recognition, ultrastructural and immunohistochemical studies, often essential for other childhood tumors, have little utility. Ultrastructurally, the tumor is characterized by numerous desmosomes, cilia, and distinctive flocculent densities surrounding the tumor cells.

There is a subgroup of patients with Wilms' tumor who have *anaplastic tumors.* Anaplasia is categorized as the presence of hyperdiploid mitotic figures, a threefold or greater nuclear enlargement or hyperchromasia of enlarged nuclei. Two sarcomatous variants, clear cell sarcoma and rhabdoid tumor, also confer poor prognoses. Anaplasia is recognized by hyperdiploid miotic features, threefold or greater nuclear enlargement, and hyperchromasia of enlarged nuclei. Even a single focus of anaplasia correlates with an adverse prognosis. These histologic markers of hyperploidy have been supported by flow cytoflurometric studies of DNA content in Wilms' tumors. Anaplasia occurs in approximately 5% of the tumors, is rare (2%) in children younger than 2 years, and increasingly frequent in older children, until the incidence reaches 13% in those older than 5 years. Relapses were seen in 27 (55%) of 49 NWTS-1 and NWTS-2 stage I, II, and III children with anaplastic tumors, and relapses occurred in 101 (14%) of 720 patients with nonanaplastic or "favorable histology" tumors. Stage I patients with anaplastic tumors do as well as those with histologically favorable tumors.

Clear cell sarcoma of the kidney, a distinct entity, occurs in the same age group as Wilms' tumor, but it has a poorer prognosis, with relapse common even in the stage I patients. The tumor consists of nests of polygonal to stellate cells with small nuclei, inconspicuous nucleoli, and pale vesicular cytoplasm, which form cords separated by a fine vascular network. This variant of Wilms' tumor has been associated with a high rate of skeletal metastasis and was originally called the "bone-metastasizing renal tumor of childhood."

Rhabdoid tumor of the kidney is a monomorphous tumor with cells containing prominent acidophilic cytoplasm, similar to rhabdomyoblasts, but it does not contain ultrastructural features of muscle and immunohistochemical markers. This tumor is not associated with rhabdomyosarcoma. The cell of origin is unknown, and it may occur outside the kidney. The median age at diagnosis of the cases seen in the NWTS was 13 months (range, 2 months to 5 years). Simultaneous primitive neuroectodermal tumors of the brain have developed in children with this variant. The outlook for children with rhabdoid tumor of the kidney is poor. Fewer than 20% of the patients survive, and aggressive chemotherapy has not altered this.

Nephroblastomatosis, a small cluster of blastemal cells, tubules, or stromal cells that is usually situated at the periphery of the renal lobe is thought to be the precursor lesion of Wilms' tumor. Its presence in a kidney biopsy specimen demands close follow-up to detect possible evolution of bilateral Wilms' tumor.

Congenital mesoblastic nephroma is a tumor of the newborn or young infant. It is composed of bundles of spindle cells with an interdigitating margin that extends into the renal parenchyma. Although these tumors are usually curable by surgery alone, there are subtypes that contain more cystic components and have a higher mitotic index, indicating a metastatic potential. The tumor has been diagnosed in utero by ultrasound and may be associated with polyhydramnios. This tumor is curable by a standard surgical approach that results in a histologically proven complete resection. Rarely, the tumor may infiltrate the perirenal structures, including the liver. Care must be taken in the resection of tumor infringing on the capsule of the liver, because hemostasis may be difficult to achieve and uncontrollable bleeding may result.

CLINICAL PRESENTATION AND NATURAL HISTORY

Wilms' tumor most frequently presents as an asymptomatic flank or abdominal mass, usually detected on a routine physical examination or discovered by parents when bathing the child. The differential diagnosis includes hydronephrosis, neuroblastoma, and other tumors that present with an abdominal component or organomegaly, such as leukemia, lymphoma, and hepatoma. Wilms' tumor is rare after the age of 7 years. A characteristic presentation of rapid abdominal enlargement, anemia, hypertension, and occasionally, fever with egg-shell calcification visible on plain x-ray films has been attributed to sudden subcapsular hemorrhage. Of 164 patients, 68% presented with abdominal mass, 29% with abdominal pain, 26% with hematuria, 18% with fever, and 14% with anorexia. Elevated blood pressure affects approximately 25% of patients and is caused by elevated renin.

On physical examination, the abdominal mass of Wilms' tumor is smoother in outline and usually more confined to one side of the abdomen than the irregular and nodular mass of neuroblastoma (Table 49–9). However, Wilms' tumor may be bilateral or may grow large enough that it can be felt on both sides of the abdomen. Tumor involvement can be extensive, with infiltration through the renal capsule or invasion into the renal vein (8–40%) through the vena cava to the heart.

Metastatic disease is evident at diagnosis in approximately 15% of patients with Wilms' tumor. The most common sites of hematogenous metastasis are the lung (85%) and liver (15%). Brain metastasis is a rare form of recurrence. With the exception of those with clear cell sarcoma, bone metastasis is uncommon. The regional lymph nodes are involved in 15% to 25% of patients. Positive nodes are associated with unfavorable histology (*i.e.*, anaplasia) and a relatively poor prognosis. For patients with node-positive Wilms' tumor of a favorable histologic pattern, the mortality rate is 17%, compared with a 97% survival rate for patients with negative nodes.

EVALUATION

The child with an abdominal mass should be examined thoroughly to arrive at the most likely preoperative diagnosis, assess the local and distant extent of the tumor, and prepare the patient for surgery.

Physical evaluation for evidence of concomitant congenital anomalies should be sought (see Table 49–9). Distended ab-

TABLE 49–9. Characteristic Features of Wilms' Tumor and Neuroblastoma

Characteristic Features	*Wilms' Tumor*	*Neuroblastoma*
Age at presentation	3.6 y (rare before 6 mo)	<2 y (most common tumor of infancy)
Associated congenital anomalies	Aniridia, hemihypertrophy, genitourinary abnormalities	Rare: Beckwith-Wiedemann syndrome, nisidioblastosis, von Recklinghausen's syndrome
Clinical presentation	Smooth, bulging flank mass; may enlarge rapidly; usually confined to one side	Firm and irregular flank mass frequently crossing the midline of abdomen, often fixed
Radiologic findings	Intrarenal mass with calyceal distortion and displacement but little change in axis of the kidney	Outward and downward displacement of kidney, "dropping lily," with microcalcifications

A

Wilms' Tumor (Left Kidney)

B

Neuroblastoma Paraspinal
Microcalcification Tumor

Tumor markers	None	Vanillylmandelic acid, homovanillic acid, catechols, ferritin, neuron-specific enolase
Metastases	Lungs, lymph nodes, liver, brain, bone (rare)	Liver, bone, bone marrow, lymph nodes

dominal veins may indicate occlusion of the inferior vena cava by tumor thrombus. Routine laboratory studies should also include tests for urine catecholamines. The most sensitive tests are not necessarily the best because the successful treatment of Wilms' tumor is founded on the chest x-ray films and intravenous pyelograms (IVP). Abdominal ultrasound can provide an accurate assessment of the mass and detect tumor thrombi in renal veins. Ultrasound can delineate tumor extension to the inferior vena cava or right atrium. Abdominal computed tomography (CT) provides the most precise means to assess the tumor. Magnetic resonance imaging (MRI) is useful for diagnosing and staging Wilms' tumor and may replace other techniques because it is noninvasive and does not employ ionizing radiation.

The metastatic workup should include four-view chest x-ray films. The use of lung CT is controversial and not advocated by the NWTS for low-risk children. Should a patient with low-stage disease whose only site of metastasis is a lung nodule, visible on CT scan but not chest x-ray films, be upstaged and treated more aggressively? There are no data to support such an approach, and most stage I and II patients assessed by chest x-ray films alone are cured. Moreover, focal atelectasis or granulomas are indistinguishable from metastatic tumor. Treatment for stage IV patients with lung disease includes irradiation of the entire thorax; whether patients with lung metastases demonstrated only by CT scan require this therapy is unknown. A decision analysis concluded that there was no advantage in routine chest CT scans and the NWTS

Committee does not recommend this for low-risk children. Postoperatively, patients with a histologic diagnosis of clear cell sarcoma should be staged with bone scan and CT of the brain. This is unnecessary for other variants of Wilms' tumor. The diagnosis of rhabdoid tumor of the kidney warrants brain CT because of its association with brain metastases and primary brain tumors.

STAGING AND PROGNOSTIC FACTORS

A clinicopathologic grouping that determined the extent of tumor at diagnosis and surgery was used in NWTS-1 and NWTS-2. Analysis of these clinical trials resulted in the staging system shown in Table 49–10. Unfavorable histologic types, distant metastasis, and lymph node involvement continue to affect prognosis adversely. Conversely, analysis of NWTS-3 indicated that children younger than 2 years of age who had stage I tumors smaller than 250 g with favorable histology had the best outcome.

TREATMENT

The advances in treating Wilms' tumor reflect integration of improved methods of surgery, radiation therapy, and chemotherapy. Optimal treatment of the patient requires that the pediatric, radiation, and surgical oncologists begin to coordinate their efforts during the initial diagnostic and staging workup.

TABLE 49–10. Staging Systems for Wilms' Tumor

Clinical Grouping (NWTS-1 and NWTS-2)*	*Clinical Staging (NWTS-3)*
I. Tumor limited to the kidney and completely resected. The surface of the renal capsule is intact. The tumor was not ruptured before or during removal. There is no residual tumor apparent beyond the margins of resection.	I. Tumor limited to the kidney and completely resected. The surface of the renal capsule is intact. The tumor was not ruptured before or during removal. There is no residual tumor apparent beyond the margins of excision.
II. Tumor extends beyond the kidney but is completely resected. There is local extension of the tumor: penetration beyond the pseudocapsule into the perirenal soft tissues or periaortic lymph node involvement. The renal vessel outside the kidney substance is infiltrated or contains tumor thrombus. There is no residual tumor apparent beyond the margins of resection.	II. Tumor extends beyond the kidney but is completely excised. There is regional extension of the tumor: penetration through the outer surface of the renal capsule into the perirenal soft tissues. Vessels outside the kidney substance are infiltrated or contain tumor thrombus. The tumor may have been biopsied or there has been local spillage of tumor confined to the flank. There is no residual tumor apparent at or beyond the margins of excision.
III. Residual nonhematogenous tumor confined to the abdomen. Any of the following may occur: A. The tumor has ruptured before or during surgery, or a biopsy has been performed. B. Implants are found on peritoneal surfaces. C. Lymph nodes are involved beyond the abdominal periaortic chains. D. The tumor is completely resectable because of local infiltration into vital structures.	III. Residual nonhematogenous tumor confined to the abdomen. Any of the following may occur: A. Lymph nodes on biopsy are found to be involved in the hilus, the periaortic chains, or beyond. B. There has been diffuse peritoneal contamination by the tumor such as by spillage of tumor beyond the flank before or during surgery, or by tumor growth that has penetrated through the peritoneal surface. C. Implants are found on the peritoneal surfaces. D. The tumor extends beyond the surgical margins either microscopically or grossly. E. The tumor is not completely resectable because of local infiltration into vital structures.
IV. Hematogenous metastases. Deposits beyond group III in lung, liver, bone, and brain. V. Bilateral renal involvement either initially or subsequently.	IV. Hematogenous metastases. Deposits beyond stage III in lung, liver, bone, and brain. V. Bilateral renal involvement at diagnosis. An attempt should be made to stage each side according to the above criteria on the basis of extent of disease before biopsy.

* The clinical group (stage) is defined by the surgeon in the operating room and is confirmed by the pathologist. In NWTS, patients are categorized by stage and histology (favorable or unfavorable).

Surgery

The goal of surgery is to remove the primary tumor, even if there are distant metastases. Two questions require consideration preoperatively. Is the mass too large for safe resection without tumor rupture? Is there any evidence for bilateral involvement?

Approximately 5% to 15% of patients have tumors that are too large for safe primary surgical resection. These tumors cross the midline, appear to be fixed to adjacent structures, or are not visualized on IVP. In the past, radiation therapy was used to achieve preoperative tumor shrinkage, and although it was effective, it frequently delayed surgery. Preoperative chemotherapy (1.0 mg/m^2 of vincristine for infants and 1.5 mg/m^2 for children, administered every 5–7 days) can substantially shrink the tumor mass in 80% of patients within 2 to 3 weeks, making subsequent surgery safe and effective.

If preoperative chemotherapy or radiation therapy is being considered, a definitive diagnosis should first be established by a needle biopsy or an open biopsy through a small retroperitoneal incision. Biopsy by one of these methods minimizes the possibility of tumor contaminating the entire abdominal cavity and eliminates the possibility of a false diagnosis and unnecessary therapy.

The possibility of bilateral Wilms' tumors (5% of cases) should be determined preoperatively. The prognosis for patients with bilateral disease is good (approximately an 87% survival rate), even if the tumors are not entirely resectable. Surgery should remove all tumor only if adequate renal parenchyma can be left on one or both sides. Treatment for bilateral Wilms' tumor should be individualized, and many different approaches have been successful. For example, in patients with a large tumor on one side and a small tumor on the other, nephrectomy is indicated for the larger lesion and partial nephrectomy for the smaller one. In patients with two large primary tumors, biopsy followed by chemotherapy and second-look surgery and, if possible, resection of the residual tumors should be considered. Bilateral nephrectomy and renal transplant has not been especially successful, and this approach is indicated only if all other measures have failed.

In patients deemed surgically resectable, good exposure should be obtained with a generous transabdominal incision that, if necessary, should extend into the thorax. The renal vein should be ligated before beginning extensive dissection, although this does not appear to affect prognosis. Avoid rupture of the tumor during surgery because operative spill, which occurs in 16% of cases, appears to increase the risk of abdominal recurrence. This liability may be overcome if the peritoneal surfaces are irradiated after the spill. Perhaps the greatest hazard in the resection of Wilms' tumor is hemorrhage due to injury to the vena cava. The vena cava should be isolated above and below the tumor so that damage to it can be quickly controlled. Tumors that invade the liver capsule usually are totally resectable, because they rarely penetrate deeply into the liver parenchyma.

After the tumor is removed with a long segment of ureter, the hilar and local paraaortic lymph nodes should be biopsied, and any enlarged or suspicious nodes should be removed. Although lymph node biopsy is important in staging, retroperitoneal lymph node dissection is not of proven value and has potential morbidity.

Tumor extending into the vena cava can usually be removed with venotomy and traction. If the tumor segment in the inferior vena cava is completely obstructed, it is best left in situ. If the tumor embolus extends into the heart, a median sternotomy and midline abdominal incision provides exposure of the right atrium and the intrapericardial portion of the inferior vena cava. Extracorporeal circulation is necessary in these cases. Intracardiac extension of Wilms' tumor of favorable histology does not impact adversely on survival. If resection is not possible, shrinkage with chemotherapy or radiation therapy should be pursued and patients managed as if stage III.

For large or hemorrhagic tumors, surgical resection may be accomplished more effectively after embolization of the renal artery with Gelfoam particles, which reduce renal vascularity and shrink tumor bulk. This procedure should be considered if the patient presents with gross hematuria but has a resectable primary tumor.

During surgery, the contralateral kidney should be carefully examined after it has been mobilized and its capsule has been opened. If, after resection of the primary tumor, an easily removable contralateral lesion is found, it should be excised if sufficient renal tissue can be left behind to maintain renal function. If this cannot be safely guaranteed, the contralateral nodule should be biopsied.

The liver and the remainder of the abdomen should be inspected for metastases, and the tumor bed or areas of extension or residual disease should be outlined with metallic clips. Although tumor resection is important, a small volume of residual tumor does not appear to adversely affect prognosis. Heroic efforts to remove the last vestiges of tumor are not indicated.

Surgical extirpation of pulmonary nodules is beneficial if the resection can be accomplished without compromising pulmonary function. Similarly, surgical resection has been successful in eradicating liver and brain metastases.

Radiation Therapy

The role of radiation therapy has become more sharply defined in recent years. Improved chemotherapy has eliminated postoperative irradiation for early-stage disease. Radiation therapy is used conservatively because of the toxic effects of large irradiation fields in very young children. There is a potential for growth disturbances, and hepatic, pulmonary, or cardiac damage can result from irradiation used in conjunction with chemotherapy. Because of the anticipated long survival of patients with Wilms' tumor, there is appropriate concern about the risk of developing second malignancies.

Radiation therapy has been effective in virtually eliminating abdominal failure because of microscopic or gross residual disease. In conjunction with chemotherapy, irradiation has achieved a high proportion of disease control in cases with pulmonary metastases. Preoperative radiation therapy had proven the value of diminishing large tumors before resection, diminishing operative spill and improving disease-free survival. The efficacy and reduced toxicity of preoperative chemotherapy has supplanted preoperative radiation.

The use of postoperative radiation therapy is dictated by operative stage and histology. The NWTS-1 and NWTS-2 trials showed that postoperative radiation therapy is not necessary for stage I patients, regardless of age, who have favorable histologic patterns, if they are treated with adjuvant vincristine and dactinomycin. Results from NWTS-3 demonstrated that stage II patients with favorable histology did not benefit from radiation therapy. Neither stage I or II patients with favorable histology require postoperative radiation therapy.

Patients with favorable stage III tumors (and some include stage II patients with intraoperative spillage), based on NWTS-3 findings, should receive limited (*e.g.*, 1080 cGy) postoperative radiation with the addition of doxorubicin (Adriamycin) to the vincristine plus dactinomycin regimen.

Postoperative radiation therapy is recommended for all patients with unfavorable histologic patterns, regardless of stage, and for patients with stage IV tumors. Abdominal treatment in stage IV presentations should be defined by the extent of abdominal disease. Radiation treatment of pulmonary metastases is independent of "abdominal stage."

Radiation therapy ports should be tailored to the extent of disease found at surgery. Whole-abdominal irradiation is used only in patients with abdominal spill (Fig. 49–1). Residual disease or documented lymph node involvement requires tumor bed irradiation, usually as hemiabdominal therapy, to encompass the initial tumor and paraaortic volume. It is important to include the full width of the vertebrae, to encompass the retroperitoneal nodes, and to avoid asymmetric closure of the vertebral epiphyses.

Radiation to extrarenal and extraabdominal sites has been integrated into treatment planning for patients with stage IV Wilms' tumor. Patients with pulmonary metastases should receive doxorubicin with 1200 cGy of whole-lung irradiation, with only the growth centers of the humeri blocked. If this treatment follows abdominal or renal fossa irradiation, care must be taken to avoid normal tissues, such as the remaining kidney or liver. Patients with hepatic, brain, or bone involvement are treated with irradiation.

Chemotherapy

Wilms' tumor was found to be responsive to dactinomycin in the 1960s. Other active agents include vincristine, doxorubicin, cyclophosphamide, and cisplatin, which have response rates of 63%, 60%, 27%, and 16%, respectively. Successive studies by single institutions, collaborative groups, and the NWTS have identified the following principles of treatment:

1. *Stage I with favorable histology or anaplastic and stage II with favorable histology:* Chemotherapy with dacti-

nomycin and vincristine is superior to either alone. Radiation therapy is not needed.
2. *Stage III with favorable histology and stage IV with favorable histology:* Chemotherapy with dactinomycin, vincristine, and doxorubicin and postoperative irradiation.
3. *Stage II, III, and IV anaplastic tumors:* Chemotherapy with dactinomycin, vincristine, doxorubicin, and possibly cyclophosphamide (pending results from NWTS IV) and postoperative irradiation.
4. *Stage I through IV clear cell sarcoma:* Chemotherapy with doxorubicin, vincristine, and dactinomycin and irradiation.
5. *Stage V (bilateral) Wilms' tumor:* The goal is to preserve enough functioning renal parenchyma, usually by removing the kidney with the major involvement and only a portion of the less affected kidney. Bilateral nephrectomy and kidney transplantation is a last resort. Postoperative radiation therapy should be considered for both renal fossae, although lack of residual disease may make this unnecessary. The adjuvant schedules and radiation treatment should be dictated by the histology and extent of residual disease.

The results of NWTS-3 are summarized in Table 49–11. Because relapse after 2 years from diagnosis is rare, most disease-free children at this point are cured. NWTS-4, now underway, will determine if there is an advantage to single-dose or divided-dose dactinomycin and doxorubicin. It will also evaluate a 6-month treatment for patients with stage II, III, or IV tumors. The International Society of Pediatric Oncology (SIOP) focused on the preoperative treatment of Wilms' tumor with radiation therapy or with chemotherapy. Results have been excellent. The group found that residual tumor at the time of surgery is a negative prognostic indicator.

The acute and long-term toxic effects of therapy have influenced treatment. Seventeen toxic deaths in NWTS-2 resulted primarily from leukopenia (7) and liver failure (41). Because 4 of 47 infants (<1 year old) died of leukopenia, chemotherapy doses have been decreased by 50% for this age group. Long-term side effects of the disease and its treatment include cardiomyopathy caused by the interaction between doxorubicin and radiation, skeletal growth disturbances after irradiation, and radiation-induced nephritis in the remaining kidney.

Most children in the United States with Wilms' tumor are treated on the NWTS. Although almost 90% of Wilms' tumor patients are curable and tolerate therapy well, the child with this disease deserves to be managed by a team experienced in pediatric cancer.

NEUROBLASTOMA

Neuroblastoma represents frustration and hope to those who treat cancer in children. Cure is elusive for most children (>1 year old) with this disease who present with disseminated tumor. Despite improved chemotherapeutic regimens that can effect complete responses, recurrence is common in older patients. However, because the molecular genetics of this tumor are better understood than most other human cancers, there is an implicit promise of more effective and less toxic treatments.

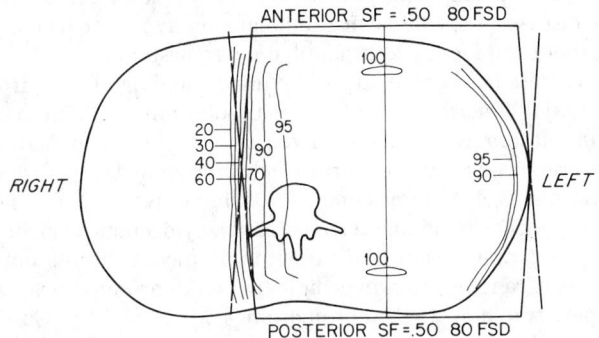

FIGURE 49–1. Dosimetry for hemiabdominal irradiation. Notice inclusion of the paraaortic lymph nodes and full width of the vertebral body within the 90% volume. Dosimetry depicts dose configuration for a field identical but contralateral to that shown.

TABLE 49–11. Results in Randomized NWTS-3 Patients

Stage/ Histology	Regimen	No. of Patients	4-Year Survival Relapse-Free (%)	4-Year Survival Overall (%)
I/FH	AMD + VCR (10 wk)	306	89.0 }	95.6 }
I/FH	AMD + VCR (6 mo)	301	91.8 } $p = 0.19$	97.4 } $p = 0.15$
II/FH	AMD + VCR (+RT)	70	90.0 }	91.1 }
II/FH	AMD + VCR (−RT)	67	87.4 }	94.9 }
II/FH	AMD + VCR + ADR (+RT)	71	86.9 } $p = 0.89$	89.6 } $p = 0.73$
II/FH	AMD + VCR-ADR (−RT)	70	87.9 }	93.6 }
III/FH	AMD + VCR (1000 cGy)	71	71.4 }	85.2 }
III/FH	AMD + VCR (2000 cGy)	70	76.8 }	85.1 }
III/FH	AMD + VCR-ADR (1000 cGy)	68	82.0 } $p = 0.22$	90.9 } $p = 0.90$
III/FH	AMD + VCR-ADR (2000 cGy)	66	85.9 }	86.7 }
IV/FH	AMD + VCR + ADR	64	71.9 }	78.4 }
IV/FH	AMD + VCR + ADR + CPM	56	77.9 } $p = 0.43$	86.6 } $p = 0.29$
I–III/UH	AMD + VCR + ADR	69	67.1 }	68.3 }
I–III/UH	AMD + VCR + ADR + CPM	61	62.4 } $p = 0.86$	68.4 } $p = 0.88$
IV/UH	AMD + VCR + ADR	12	58.3 }	58.3 }
IV/UH	AMD + VCR + ADR + CPM	17	52.9 } $p = 0.70$	52.9 } $p = 0.69$

FH, favorable histology; UH, unfavorable histology; AMD, dactinomycin; VCR, vincristine; ADR, doxorubicin; CPM, cyclophosphamide; p values indicate results of test for the two or four regimens in brackets.
(Green DM, et al. Wilms' tumor [nephroblastoma, renal embryoma]. In: Pizzo PA, Poplack DG, eds. Principles and practice of pediatric oncology. 2nd ed. Philadelphia: JB Lippincott, 1993)

EPIDEMIOLOGY AND GENETICS

Neuroblastoma is the fourth most common pediatric malignancy, with an annual incidence of 10 cases per million children. In the United States, it comprises 8% to 10% of cancers diagnosed in children under 15 years of age or approximately 525 new cases annually. The incidence is significantly less in African than in American black children, raising the possibility that environmental factors are important and may be responsible for the increased incidence of neuroblastoma between 1943 and 1980. Alcohol, hair-coloring products, and certain medicines used during pregnancy may be prenatal risk factors for neuroblastoma, but none have been confirmed.

The median age at diagnosis of neuroblastoma is approximately 2 years. Half of all malignancies diagnosed in the first month of life and a third during the first year are neuroblastoma. The mortality of neuroblastoma occurring in the first year of life is far lower than that in the older child, suggesting the unique biology of this tumor. Microscopic nodules of primitive neuroblasts, usually larger than 3 mm and occasionally invading blood vessels, referred to as "neuroblastoma in situ," have been observed at autopsy in infants dying before 3 months old of other causes at 40 to 200 times the expected incidence. Autopsy examination of the adrenal glands of 92 18-week to 20-week fetuses demonstrated "neuroblastoma in situ" in all. It is clear that a normal phase in the embryogenesis of the adrenal gland, which is histologically similar to neuroblastoma, may persist into the first year of life. It is not understood how this relates to the observed spontaneous regression of neuroblastoma, especially stage IVS, or to the high rate of cure of the less than 1-year-old infant with a tumor indistinguishable from the usually fatal lesion seen in older children.

Molecular geneticists are studying neuroblastoma as a paradigm for elucidating the biology of differentiation and its relation to oncogenesis. The two-hit hypothesis, which postulates that malignancy is a function of prezygotic and postzygotic mutations, may be relevant to neuroblastomas. Neuroblastoma has been associated with the genetic diseases neurofibromatosis, Beckwith-Wiedemann syndrome (i.e., omphalocele, macroglossia, visceromegaly, neonatal hypoglycemia), nisidiroblastosis, and trisomy 18 and with teratogenic syndromes caused by in utero exposure to alcohol and hydantoins. These associations are rare, indicating that they may be coincidental. Although familial neuroblastoma, characterized by multiple primaries, very young age at presentation (i.e., 9 months versus 22 months for neuroblastoma in the general population), and autosomal dominant inheritance, is uncommon, its existence establishes that a germline mutation may promote tumorigenesis. Siblings and offspring of nonfamilial neuroblastoma patients are at low risk for developing the disease. A specific constitutional karyotypic abnormality has not been identified in familial neuroblastoma.

Progress has been made in the understanding of the chromosomal abnormalities of the neuroblastoma cell. Human neuroblastomas are characterized cytogenetically by partial monosomy for the short arm of chromosome 1 (1p−) and abnormality of chromosome 17. Double-minutes (DM) and homogeneously staining regions (HSR), cytogenetic evidence of gene amplification, and variability in modal chromosome number, ranging from hypodiploidy (<46 chromosomes) to hypertetraploidy (>92 chromosomes), are evident. Chromosome 1 abnormalities, specifically deletions at 1p22, are a common feature of a diverse group of pediatric solid tumors. The amplified genes identified within neuroblastoma cells as HSR and DM are designated as *MYCN* (previously designated

N-*myc* and homologous to v-*myc*). This gene is normally present in a single copy on chromosome 2. The number of copies of the *MYCN* oncogene is related to the clinical aggressiveness of the tumor and is a prognostic indicator independent of stage and age, the number of copies does correlate with the stage of the tumor and progression-free survival at 18 months from diagnosis. Amplification of *MYCN* has been detected in 30% of untreated neuroblastomas. Amplification can be detected in 5% to 10% of patients with low stages of disease or IVS and 30% to 40% of those with more advanced stages. The *MYCN* copy number is an intrinsic biologic property of each patient's tumor, remaining consistent within the tumor, in tumors at different sites, and over time, uninfluenced by treatment. The product of *MYCN* gene is yet to be identified, but it is probably related to the growth of the neuroblastoma cell.

Other oncogenes implicated in pathogenesis include *RAS*, identified initially in human neuroblastoma cell line SK-N-SH, and *SRC*, which expresses the enzyme tyrosyl kinase. Expression of *HRAS* (previously Ha-*ras*) appears to correlate with lower stage of disease and more differentiated tumors.

The DNA index of neuroblastoma cells, analyzed by flow cytometry, has been shown by investigators at St. Jude Children's Research Hospital to correlate with outcome. Tumors that are hyperdiploid are more likely to have lower stages of disease and be more chemotherapy responsive than those with a diploid DNA index.

The status of the immune system in patients with neuroblastoma has been studied. Although mild lymphopenia and leukopenia have been demonstrated at diagnosis, no general humoral or cellular immune defects have been detected. Natural killer cell activity is depressed in neuroblastoma patients. Clinical trials using the methanol-extracted residue of bacillus Calmette-Guérin (BCG), with BCG-treated and neuraminidase-treated tumor cells, to provoke an antitumor immune response in patients have not demonstrated the benefit for this immunotherapy.

Monoclonal antibodies have been raised to antigens on the surface of human neuroblastoma cells to develop reagents that have immunodiagnostic and immunotherapeutic utility. The cell-surface glycosphingolipid diganglioside GD_2 is an abundant antigen on neuroblastoma cells. Monoclonal antibodies to GD_2 recognize neuroblastoma cells relatively specifically without cross-reacting with normal marrow or lymphoid cells. With this monoclonal antibody, Cheung and coworkers were able to detect as few as 0.01% neuroblastoma cells in the marrow. They were able to identify neuroblastoma cells in the bone marrow in 74% of 35 neuroblastoma patients, and conventional histologic techniques and clonogenic assays detected 27% and 55%, respectively. Shedding of GD_2 into the plasma of patients with neuroblastoma may be useful for monitoring responses to therapy. ^{131}I-tagged monoclonal antibodies to GD_2 can ablate human neuroblastoma xenograft tumors in nude mice. Monoclonal antibodies to other neuroblastoma antigens include 5A7 to a cytoplasmic antigen and CE7, KP-NAC8, 5G3, 6–19, and UJ13A to cell-surface antigens. ^{131}I-coupled monoclonal antibodies have been administered as treatment for neuroblastoma. Responses were seen in patients with disseminated disease, but those with large tumor masses were resistant to this therapy. Substantial bone marrow toxicity was incurred, and issues of delivery and dosimetry must be addressed before the potential of this approach can be realized. Monoclonal antibodies may be useful in purging tumor cells from bone marrow for use in autologous bone marrow transplant regimens.

Neuroblastoma has a biologic characteristic unique among human cancers, the capacity to spontaneously differentiate and regress. Residual microscopic tumor left in the bed of a resected, localized neuroblastoma rarely results in recurrence of the disease. Disseminated neuroblastoma has spontaneously regressed in a subset of very young children with disease metastatic to the liver, skin, or bone marrow, but not involving bone, a condition designated as stage IVS neuroblastoma by D'Angio, Evans, and Koop. Histologic evidence of neuroblastoma having differentiated into mature ganglion cells is found in tumors removed from patients during second-look surgical procedures after induction chemotherapy and in older children with isolated mediastinal or abdominal masses, detected incidentally and found to be pure ganglioneuroma. Potential markers for determining disease may be nerve growth factor and the neurosecretory proteins chromogranin and neuropeptide Y.

This phenomenon stimulated laboratory investigation into the mechanisms of differentiation of neuroblastoma cells. In cultured neuroblastoma cells, agents such as prostaglandin E_1, 3',5'-cyclic nucleotide phosphodiesterase inhibitors, thyroid hormone, and Bu_2cAMP that increase the intracellular cAMP levels, decrease the mitotic rate and increase the degree of differentiation. Differentiating agents, including cyclophosphamide, vincristine, the phosphodiesterase inhibitor papaverine, and the thymidylate synthetase inhibitor trifluromethyl-2-deoxyuridine, used in the treatment of neuroblastoma have resulted in good antitumor responses, but the role of the differentiating agents could not be ascertained because the patients received simultaneous high-dose chemotherapy.

Retinoic acid differentiates neuroblastoma cells in vitro. It probably interacts through a cytoplasmic protein that binds retinoic acid or by the glycosylation of cell surface constituents. Clinical studies with this agent are being initiated as a component of multimodal therapy.

PATHOLOGY AND BIOLOGIC MARKERS

Neuroblastoma is thought to be derived from the embryonic neural crest. The presumptive stem cell of the neural crest, the sympathogon, differentiates into sympathoblasts, the cells of origin of neuroblastoma, and into its more mature forms, ganglioneuroblastoma and ganglioneuroma, and the chromaffin or nonchromaffin paraganglionic cells, the progenitors of pheochromocytomas and paragangliomas. As a "small, round, blue cell" tumor, neuroblastoma consists of dense nests of cells separated by fibrovascular bundles. Hemorrhage, necrosis, and calcification are frequent. Other microscopic features include Homer-Wright neural rosettes with a central fibrillar core and a fibrillary intercellular matrix that can be shown ultrastructurally to be neural cell processes. In the more-differentiated tumor, ganglion cells are present. They are large cells with prominent nucleoli and generous cytoplasm that are scattered throughout a fibrillar matrix. Ganglioneuroblastoma contains areas of neuroblastoma and ganglion cells; ganglioneuroma has ganglion cells, Schwann cells, and nerve bundles. It is important for the pathologist to take multiple sections of a ganglioneuroma to exclude neuroblastoma.

TABLE 49–12. Immunohistochemistry in the Differential Diagnosis of Neuroblastoma

	Small Blue Round Cell Neoplasms				
Stains	*Neuroblastoma*	*Lymphoma*	*Ewing's Sarcoma*	*Rhabdomyosarcoma*	*Primitive Neuroectodermal Tumors*
Neurofilament	+	–	±	–	–
Synaptophysin	+	–	–	–	–
Neuron-specific enolase	+	–	–*	–*	+
β_2-microglobulin	–	–	–	–	+
LCA (T-200 protein)	–	+	–	–	–
Vimentin	–	±	+	+	+
Myoglobin	–	–	–	+	–
Myosin	–	–	–	+	–
Actin	–	–	–	+	–
Desmin	–	–	–	+	–

* Extraosseous Ewing's sarcoma variants of Ewing's sarcoma and rhabdomyosarcoma stain for neuron-specific enolase.
(Brodeur RM, Castleberry RP. Neuroblastoma. In: Pizzo PA, Poplack DG, eds. Principles and practice of pediatric oncology. 2nd ed. Philadelphia: JB Lippincott, 1993)

The characteristic electron microscopic finding of neuroblastoma is the dense core granule (*i.e.*, catecholamine or neurosecretory granule), which is a 50- to 200-mm membrane-bound unit found in the periphery of the cytoplasm. The ultramicroscopic appearance of the neural rosettes is that of peripherally clustered tumor nuclei surrounding a mass of neuritic processes or neuropil.

Neuroblastoma can be difficult to differentiate from other small, round cell tumors of childhood, including Ewing's sarcoma, lymphoma, rhabdomyosarcoma, and other peripheral neurally derived neoplasms, such as the peripheral neuroepithelioma or Askin's tumor. Table 49–12 lists some of the features that help to differentiate these tumors. Neuroblastoma exhibits formaldehyde-induced fluorescence as the catecholamine metabolites from isoquinolone compounds when exposed to formaldehyde, and glyoxylic acid provides a rapid and sensitive assay. Identification of specific cellular constituents, such as enzymes (*i.e.*, neuron-specific enolase) or surface antigens, by sensitive immunoperoxidase techniques, in which paraffin-embedded, formaldehyde-fixed tissues may be used with specific antisera, have become an integral part of the pathologist's workup of the small, round, blue cell tumor.

An often useful adjunct to tissue examination in the diagnosis of neuroblastoma is detection of tumor markers in the blood or urine. The most commonly used is the urinary excretion of tumor-produced catecholamines. Urinary vanillylmandelic acid (VMA) and homovanillic acid (HVA) are elevated in at least 65% of neuroblastoma patients. If both metabolites are sought, more than 90% of patients are identified. Pretreatment measurements correlate with prognosis. Higher levels of catecholamine metabolites are found in patients with more extensive disease. For stage IV patients, a ratio of VMA to HVA of more than 1.5 is associated with a better prognosis. Patients whose neuroblastomas arise from the dorsal root ganglions are nonsecretors of catecholamines. The most reliable method for detection of catecholamine metabolites is a 24-hour urine test. The LaBrosse spot test, which screens for VMA in the urine, is associated with a relatively high false-negative rate because it requires a high concentra-

tion of VMA in the samples. Dietary restrictions are not necessary for a reliable 24-hour urine catecholamine quantitation, but catecholamine medications should be avoided. In Japan, mass screening of infants 6 to 7 months old using VMA spot tests has been successful in the early detection of neuroblastoma, and studies are underway in North America and Europe.

Neuron-specific enolase is elevated in most neuroblastoma patients. Higher levels in those with more advanced disease are prognostic of a poorer outcome. Serum ferritin elevation correlates with a poorer prognosis. Cystathionine is elevated in the urine of at least 50% of neuroblastoma patients. As with the other biomarkers, lower levels were associated with a better prognosis.

CLINICAL PRESENTATION AND DIAGNOSIS

Neuroblastoma can occur anywhere along the sympathetic nervous system. The most common site of primary tumor is within the abdomen, in an adrenal gland (40%) or in a paraspinal ganglion (25%); thoracic (15%) and pelvic (5%) primaries account for the rest. Thoracic primaries are more common in children younger than 1 year old (Table 49–13). Metastatic disease is identified in half the infants and two thirds of the older children at diagnosis. (Table 49–14). The most common sites of metastases are lymph nodes, bone

TABLE 49–13. Primary Site of Neuroblastoma According to Age

Primary Site of Tumor	*Percentage of Patients by Age at Diagnosis*	
	≤12 Mo	*>13 Mo*
Head and neck	5	2–3
Thoracic	20	10–15
Abdominal	55	70–75
Pelvic	5	5
Other (or unknown)	15	2–13

TABLE 49–14. Extent of Disease at Diagnosis According to Age

Stage at Diagnosis	No. of Patients by Age at Diagnosis		
	≤1 Year	>1 Year	Total
Localized	93 (39)*	83 (19)	176 (26)
Regional	43 (18)	54 (13)	97 (15)
Disseminated	61 (25)	290 (68)	351 (52)
IVS	44 (18)	0 (0)	44 (7)
Total	241	427	668

* Numbers in parentheses are percentages.
(Courtesy of JJ Shuster, PhD, Pediatric Oncology Group Statistical Office. From Brodeur GM, Castleberry RP. Neuroblastoma. In: Pizzo PA, Poplack DG, eds. Principles and practice of pediatric oncology. 2nd ed. Philadelphia: JB Lippincott, 1993)

marrow, bone, liver, and subcutaneous tissue. Lung metastases are rare.

The signs and symptoms at presentation depend on the primary and metastatic sites. The most common presentation, that of a large abdominal or flank mass that is firm, irregular, and crosses the midline, must be differentiated from Wilms' tumor. Thoracic neuroblastoma presents as a posterior mediastinal mass and is usually found coincidentally when a chest radiograph is obtained for other reasons, although it occasionally causes respiratory symptoms or signs of thoracic spinal cord compression from local extension (Fig. 49–2). Neuroblastoma arising from the cervicothoracic ganglion is often confused with benign lymphadenopathy, but the presence of Horner's syndrome or heterochromia irides from sympathetic dysfunction suggests the true diagnosis. Pelvic neuroblastoma arising from the organ of Zuckerkandl may present as a palpable mass alone or with symptoms related to bladder or vascular compression.

Several unusual presentations of neuroblastoma are noteworthy. First, the firm, subcutaneous, blue-tinged nodules, reminiscent of the blueberry muffin sign associated with congenital rubella, are most often encountered in the neonate with neuroblastoma. Second is the opsoclonus-polymyoclonus syndrome of acute cerebellar and truncal ataxia and dancing eyes, which is associated with persistent neurologic sequelae but limited tumor; it indicates a favorable prognosis. A third unusual symptom is that of intractable, watery diarrhea and hypokalemia (*i.e.,* Kerner-Morrison syndrome) caused by va-

soactive intestinal peptide produced by ganglioneuroblastoma and measured in the plasma of these patients. Olfactory neuroblastoma (*i.e.,* esthesioneuroblastoma) arises in the nasal cavity and presents with obstruction. It is most commonly seen in adults and is most probably a peripheral neuroepithelioma.

Neuroblastoma has an unusual predisposition to periorbital metastasis, which presents with proptosis and ecchymosis. This is secondary to sphenoid bone involvement or invasion of the retrobulbar tissues. Intracranial metastasis other than direct extension from bony lesions of the skull are rare. The so-called cerebral neuroblastoma is a supratentorial tumor of primitive neuroectoderm that is more closely related to a family of primary central nervous system (CNS) tumors.

Bone marrow involvement with neuroblastoma is common and may be difficult to differentiate from acute leukemia or other solid tumors, like rhabdomyosarcoma, metastatic to marrow. Neuroblastoma cells are more likely to be periodic acid-Schiff (PAS)-negative and form rosettes, but the clinical tests and tissue histopathology usually confirm the diagnosis.

In some neuroblastoma patients, no primary tumor site can be found. This is most common in the unique syndrome (stage IVS) that occurs in infants younger than 1 year old. It is characterized by small or undetectable tumors, usually of the adrenal, with skin, hepatic, or bone marrow (but not bone) metastases that may undergo spontaneous regression. Hepatic enlargement may be significant, causing symptoms that necessitate therapeutic intervention.

A bone marrow aspirate and a biopsy may provide tumor for diagnostic pathologic studies and adjunctive laboratory analysis such as flow cytometry for establishing the DNA index, which may be clinically useful. The international staging system calls for two aspirates and biopsies, one from each iliac crest, to enhance diagnostic sensitivity.

Evidence is accumulating that there are three genetic subsets of neuroblastoma based on chromosomal abnormalities and *MYCN*. One consists of younger patients (<1 year) who have a hyperdiploid or near-triploid karyotype with few chromosomal abnormalities and a good prognosis. A second group is older and has a near-diploid karyotype without consistent chromosomal abnormalities and more advanced, albeit slowly progressing, disease. The third group of patients, with rapidly advancing tumor that is almost always fatal (<5% survival) are older and have advanced tumor stages with near-diploid or tetraploid karyotype with deletions or LoH of 1p36, amplified *MYCN* or both.

Although other small, round, blue cell tumors metastatic to

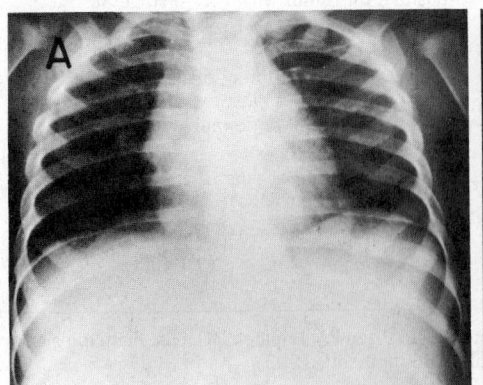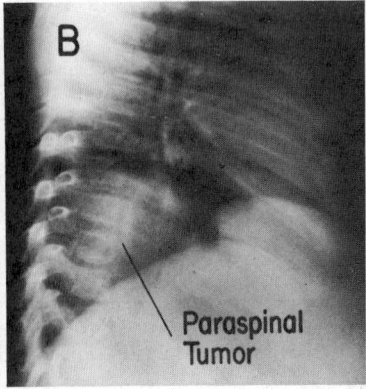

Paraspinal Tumor

FIGURE 49–2. Chest roentgenograph in (A) frontal and (B) lateral projections, demonstrating paravertebral pleural displacement. Size of the thoracic component can be appreciated on the lateral projection.

the bone marrow may have similar histologic features, a diagnosis of neuroblastoma may be confirmed if abnormal urine catecholamine excretion is found in conjunction with the marrow findings, and this often obviates a major surgical procedure. A careful search of many slides must be undertaken before the marrow can be declared uninvolved. Examination of slides of the buffy coat made from 1 to 2 ml of heparinized marrow may increase the yield.

CT is the best imaging modality for neuroblastoma and should be performed for every patient to determine the location and extent of the primary and metastatic lesions. CT detects abdominal neuroblastoma with an extremely high sensitivity, and calcifications are seen in approximately 85% of patients. The IVP is less sensitive than a CT scan in the evaluation of an abdominal mass and should not be done routinely. Bilateral adrenal calcifications detected in an otherwise asymptomatic child with an abnormal birth history are probably due to neonatal adrenal hemorrhage. Experience with MRI of neuroblastoma visualizes the tumor in many planes, demonstrates the vascular anatomy, and improves the definition of the intraspinal extension, aiding the determination of resectability.

Nuclear medicine scans of use in evaluating neuroblastoma include the technetium 99m methylene diphosphonate bone scan, which is more sensitive than the conventional skeletal survey. Bone scanning agents are frequently taken up by ex-

traosseous tumor, further aiding in the metastatic workup. ^{131}I-meta-iodobenzylguanidine (MIBG), which has been used in the diagnosis and treatment of pheochromocytoma because of its preferential uptake by cells with adrenergic secretory vesicles, allows the imaging of most neuroblastomas and should be performed if available.

The laboratory evaluation of neuroblastoma should include a complete blood count and coagulation studies. Coagulopathy is not uncommon in patients with disseminated disease and may be caused by intravascular coagulation. Hypocoagulability and hypercoagulability have been reported.

STAGING

There have been several staging systems for neuroblastoma (Table 49–15). Because of the prognostic influence of regional lymph node involvement and the importance of the initial surgical procedure in determining further treatment, the Pediatric Oncology Group (POG) adopted a modification of the staging system advocated by Hayes and coworkers at St. Jude Children's Research Hospital based on the surgical-pathologic staging of patients with clinically localized disease, a concept originally advocated by Pinkel in 1958. It is important that investigators working in this field be able to compare results of treatment protocols, and an international working group has been established to develop a common system. The In-

TABLE 49–15. Comparison of Staging Systems for Neuroblastoma

CCSG System[116]	POG System[6]	International (INSS)[124]
Stage I. Tumor confined to the organ or structure of origin.	Stage A. Complete gross resection of the primary tumor, with or without microscopic residual disease. Intracavitary lymph nodes not adhered to the primary tumor must be histologically free of tumor. Nodes adhered to the surface of or within the primary may be positive.	Stage 1. Localized tumor confined to the area of origin; complete gross excision, with or without microscopic residual disease; identifiable ipsilateral and contralateral lymph nodes negative microscopically.
Stage II. Tumor extending in continuity beyond the organ or structure of origin, but not crossing the midline. Regional lymph nodes on the ipsilateral side may be involved.	Stage B. Grossly unresected primary tumor. Nodes and nodules the same as in stage A.	Stage 2A. Unilateral tumor with incomplete gross excision; identifiable ipsilateral and contralateral lymph nodes negative microscopically. Stage 2B. Unilateral tumor with complete or incomplete gross excision; with positive ipsilateral regional lymph nodes; identifiable contralateral lymph nodes negative microscopically.
Stage III. Tumor extending in continuity beyond the midline. Regional lymph nodes may be involved bilaterally.	Stage C. Complete or incomplete resection of primary. Intracavitary nodes not adhered to primary must be histologically positive for tumor. Liver as in stage A.	Stage 3. Tumor infiltrating across the midline with or without regional lymph node involvement or unilateral tumor with contralateral regional lymph node involvement or midline tumor with bilateral lymph node involvement.
Stage IV. Remote disease involving the skeleton, bone marrow, soft tissue and distant lymph node groups (see stage IVS)	Stage D. Dissemination of disease beyond intracavitary nodes (*i.e.*, extracavitary nodes, liver, skin, bone marrow, bone).	Stage 4. Dissemination of tumor to distant lymph nodes, bone, bone marrow, liver, or other organs (except as defined in stage 4S).
Stage IVS. As defined in stage I or II, except for the presence of remote disease confined to the liver, skin, or marrow (without bone metastases).	Stage DS. Infants <1 year of age with stage IVS disease (see CCSG).	Stage 4S. Localized primary tumor as defined for stage 1 or 2 with dissemination limited to liver, skin, or bone marrow.

(Brodeur GM, Castleberry RP. Neuroblastoma. In: Pizzo PA, Poplack DG, eds. Principles and practice of pediatric oncology. 2nd ed. Philadelphia: JB Lippincott, 1993)

ternational Staging System is based on clinical, radiographic, and surgical assessment. Table 49–15 describes this system.

THERAPY

Successful treatment of the child with neuroblastoma requires a carefully considered multidisciplinary approach. The initial diagnostic workup establishes whether the disease is disseminated or localized. In the patient with localized disease, the operation is key to defining the local extent of tumor and to completely resecting the tumor. Radiation therapy plays a role in the treatment of the patient with localized disease and the palliative management of the patient with disseminated disease unresponsive to chemotherapy. Chemotherapy is central in the management of those with unresectable local tumor or metastatic disease.

Surgery

The surgical approach depends on tumor site, disease stage, and age of the patient. Among those with cervical, mediastinal, and to a lesser extent, pelvic tumors, complete excision is usually feasible and should be aggressively pursued. The same approach is occasionally possible for a primary abdominal tumor, particularly if it is small or laterally placed. Most localized abdominal neuroblastomas extend centrally and surround the major branches of the aorta, making the tumors unresectable by conventional surgical procedures. Every large series contains some long-surviving patients in whom these tumors were literally "carved" away from the central vessels, but there are more patients for whom this did not result in cure. In general, abdominal tumors are biopsied, and a second or third attempt is made to remove them after intensive chemotherapy or radiation therapy. If complete gross resection can be carried out during a second or third procedure, the patient will probably survive. These procedures may be instrumental in creating a favorable-prognosis group.

Among patients with metastatic disease, an early aggressive attempt to resect the primary tumor does not increase survival. In patients in whom metastatic disease can be controlled, successful secondary excisions of the primary tumors produce relatively extensive survival times.

In patients with functional neuroblastomas, early excision of the major tumor mass is essential to ameliorate symptoms. Surgery for patients with stage IVS disease should be conservative. After all disseminated disease is eliminated by chemotherapy or spontaneously, the remaining primary tumor mass is usually excised, although this has never been demonstrated to be necessary. Surgical procedures have been devised to relieve intraabdominal pressure in patients with stage IVS disease by employing plastic sheets to create an artificial ventral "hernia."

Radiation Therapy

In general, dosages of radiation for neuroblastoma range from 1500 to 3000 cGy, depending on the child's age, tumor location, and volume. Radiation therapy appears to have a clearly defined role for children with regional lymph node metastases (INSS stages 2B and 3). It has been used successfully in neonates with Evans stage IVS who developed respiratory distress secondary to hepatomegaly or for children with cord compression due to dumbbell lesions. However, fractionated radiation has not improved survival for children with metastatic disease, although local therapy can provide pain relief for children with advanced disease.

Chemotherapy

Neuroblastoma is usually chemoresponsive and sometimes curable. The complete and partial response rates vary for the most common single agents: cyclophosphamide (59%), cisplatin (46%), epipodophyllotoxins (30%), vincristine (24%), dacarbazine (14%), melphalan (24%), and ifosfamide (20%). Combination schedules are employed and, with surgery and radiation therapy, they can be combined to delineate multimodal risk-based therapy (Fig. 49–3).

Treatment of Low-Risk Patients

Infants and children with localized and resected tumors (INSS stage 1), partially resected tumors (INSS stage IIA), with regional disease (INSS 2B or 3), or INSS 4S disease are in this category of low risk.

Children with INSS stage 1 have a survival exceeding 90% with surgery alone. Neither radiation or chemotherapy are administered initially to these patients. However, postoperative chemotherapy (*i.e.*, sequential cyclophosphamide and doxorubicin) is indicated for children with INSS stage 2A, 2B, and 3 tumors and is associated with survival rates of 85%, 87%, and 89%, respectively.

Treatment of Intermediate-Risk Patients

Children with metastatic disease to regional lymph nodes only (INSS stage 2B or 3) or infants with INSS stage 4 disease are the intermediate-risk category. Children with stage 2B and 3 disease are treated with chemotherapy (*e.g.*, cyclophosphamide and doxorubicin, high-dose cisplatin and tenoposide with cyclophosphamide and doxorubicin and with radiation therapy. Similarly, infants with INSS stage 4 require intensive combination chemotherapy and radiation and may achieve survival rates ranging between 60% to 75%.

Treatment of High-Risk Patients

Most children with neuroblastoma fall into the high-risk category. They include children older than 2 years of age with disseminated (INSS stage 4) disease. Survival for this group of patients remains around 15% despite several therapeutic approaches. These children now receive intensive chemotherapy in conjunction with autologous bone marrow transplantation, and although this approach appears to improve early survival, relapses continue to occur. Most of these children are initially responsive to chemotherapy and achieve an initial remission. This suggests that drug-resistant tumor cells are present from the outset or that mutations evolve rapidly with treatment. Schedules that modulate multidrug resistance together with dose intensity may offer some hope.

New strategies are needed for children with advanced neuroblastoma, and the use of biologic agents is being studied. Included are the hematopoietic cytokines (*e.g.*, granulocyte or granulocyte-macrophage colony-stimulating factors) that can permit more timely delivery or higher doses of chemotherapy, the use of adoptive immunotherapy with tumor-

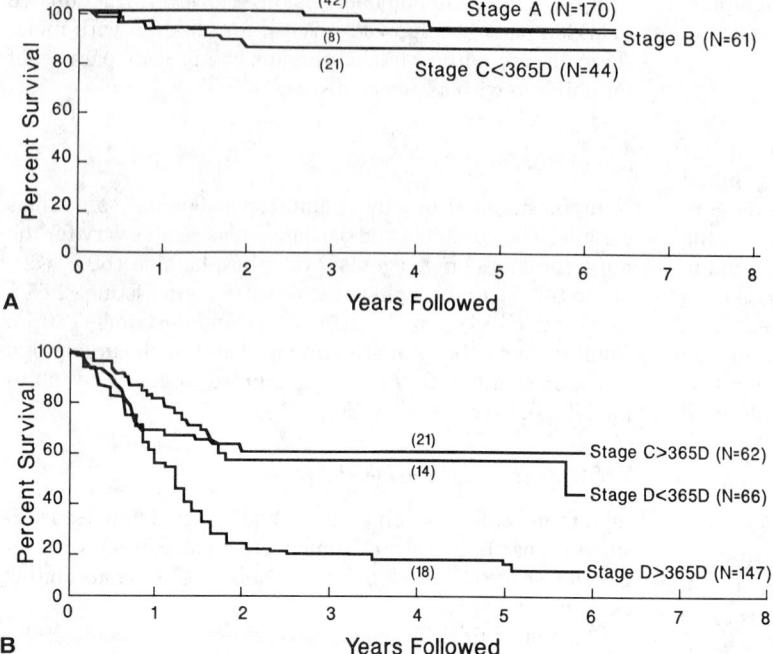

FIGURE 49–3. Survival in 550 consecutive patients with neuroblastoma treated from 1981 to 1989 on POG protocols. Based on POG stage and age (≤1 or >1 year), three prognostic groups emerged: **(A)** low risk and **(B)** intermediate and high risk.

infiltrating lymphocyte, differentiating agents, and monoclonal antibodies.

RETINOBLASTOMA

Retinoblastoma, the most common primary tumor of the eye in children, has many distinguishing features. Arising from the nuclear layer of the retina, tumors may be multifocal, bilateral, congenital, inherited, or acquired. Patients may have unique chromosomal abnormalities, and tumors can undergo spontaneous regression. Patients with the inherited form of retinoblastoma appear to be at increased risk for second, nonocular malignancies.

The estimated annual incidence of retinoblastoma is 1 in 15,000 to 34,000 live births. According to the Third National Cancer Survey and the Surveillance, Epidemiology, and End Results (SEER) group, there are approximately 11 new cases of retinoblastoma per million children younger than 5 years of age. There are approximately 200 new cases each year in the United States, 90% of which are diagnosed in children (see Table 49–1). The disease is bilateral in 40 to 60 cases. Although retinoblastoma accounts for only 1% of pediatric tumors, it serves as an important model for understanding the genetics of oncogenesis.

EPIDEMIOLOGY AND GENETICS

The mean age of presentation for retinoblastoma is 17 months, with 80% diagnosed before the age of 4 years. Although the tumor has been described in adults, it is rare in children older than 5 years. Retinoblastoma occurs in hereditary, nonhereditary, and chromosomal deletion forms. The retinoblastoma gene may be transmitted from parent to child or acquired as a new mutation. No family history of retinoblastoma is found in 90% of patients.

The hereditary form of retinoblastoma accounts for ap-

proximately 40% of cases, and it is inherited as a highly penetrant, autosomal dominant trait. A two-mutation hypothesis explains the genetics of inherited retinoblastoma. The first mutation occurs in the germinal cells, and the second occurs in the somatic cells. In the sporadic form of the disease, both mutations occur in the somatic cells. It is presumed that the timing of the mutational event in embryonic development determines whether the entire retinal anlage or only that of one eye is affected. Most patients with the hereditary form of retinoblastoma have bilateral disease, although unilateral disease occurs in almost 25% of these patients. Overall, approximately 30% of patients with retinoblastoma have bilateral disease, and 70% have unilateral involvement. Eleven patients with bilateral retinoblastoma subsequently developed pineoblastoma, suggesting that genetic susceptibility to transformation can be conferred to ectopic neuroblastic photoreceptors in the pineal gland (*i.e.*, trilateral retinoblastoma).

Most patients with retinoblastoma lack appreciable chromosomal abnormalities in most autosomal cells. A deletion on the long arm of chromosome 13 within band 13q14 has been observed in a few patients with retinoblastoma, some of whom have a syndrome that includes mental retardation, microcephaly, skeletal abnormalities, and dysmorphic features. Using recombinant DNA probes, which are homologous to unique loci on human chromosome 13, a specific retinoblastoma locus (*RB1*) has been defined, confirming that chromosome loss or loss and reduplication can lead to the expression of a recessive mutation. Dryja and coworkers examined tumor tissue obtained from 8 patients with retinoblastoma, none of whom had a family history of this disease. Four of the eight tumors demonstrated chromosome 13 homozygosity, which had no correlation with the degree of tumor differentiation or whether the tumors were multifocal or unifocal.

The tight linkage of the retinoblastoma (*RB1*) gene locus to the genetic locus of esterase D, assigned to 13q14, has demonstrated that the two independent genetic events consist of the loss or inactivation of wild-type alleles. The *RB* gene is 200,000 base pairs and encodes a 928 amino acid product that is a nuclear phosphoprotein with DNA-binding activity. Within the 13q14 band locus of the retinoblastoma gene, the loss of one *RB* allele is insufficient for tumorigenesis, but the loss of both alleles by nondisjunction or point mutation is associated with tumor production.

The genetic susceptibility for oncogenesis in patients with the inheritable form of retinoblastoma is further underscored by the fact that these patients have an increased risk for developing second malignancies that are unrelated to radiation or chemotherapy exposure. The predominant second cancers include osteosarcoma, fibrosarcoma, Ewing's sarcoma, and Wilms' tumor. Patients with bilateral retinoblastoma have a 15% to 20% chance of developing a second, nonocular neoplasm 1 to 40 years after their treatment for retinoblastoma. Fibroblasts from patients with the genetic form of retinoblastoma have increased radiation sensitivity and defective DNA repair. Fibroblasts from siblings of patients with retinoblastoma also have this radiation sensitivity pattern. The complementary sequences to the retinoblastoma gene have been cloned and demonstrate deletion at the 13q14 *RB* locus in some patients with osteosarcoma, offering an explanation for the close association of these two malignancies.

The incidence of second malignancies increases over time. For irradiated patients, the incidence of second tumor was 20% at 10 years, 50% at 20 years, and approximately 90% at 30 years. For nonirradiated patients, the incidence of second malignancies was 10% at 10 years, 30% at 20 years, and 68% at 32 years. Based on a series of 882 patients, the cumulative index of second malignancies was 2% at 12 years and 4.2% at 18 years after diagnosis. This incidence was doubled in patients with the genetic form of retinoblastoma.

Genetic counseling is important for patients with the genetic form of retinoblastoma. Assuming that the mutation is a germinal event, the risk for bearing an affected child may be as high as 50%. This is straightforward if there is a family history of the disease but more difficult for sporadic cases, because these may be heritable or nonheritable. Bilateral cases, even without a family history, are always the hereditary type, and the offspring of affected patients have a 50% risk of having retinoblastoma. Of the unilateral cases, 10% to 12% have the hereditary form, and the first child of a survivor has a 5.6% chance of having the disease (Fig. 49–4)

Parents of an affected child should always have a funduscopic examination. If a child with retinoblastoma is born to physically sound parents, the risk of a second child having retinoblastoma is 1% if the first child had unilateral retinoblastoma and 6% if the child had bilateral disease. The use of restriction fragment length polymorphism may facilitate diagnosis and permit prenatal and postnatal prediction of susceptibility to the heritable form of retinoblastoma.

Nonprogressive retinal lesions (*i.e.*, retinomas) have been described in patients presumed to carry the retinoblastoma gene. These retinomas consist of translucent, gray, elevated masses that extend from the retina into the vitreous cavity and are frequently associated with calcified foci and pigment-epithelium hyperplasia. In a recent survey of 34 patients with retinomas and 5 with phthisis bulbi, which is associated with retinoblastoma, 67% had a family history of retinoblastoma, and 23 (68%) of their offspring developed retinoblastomas. Although retinoma may represent a mutation of a more mature retinoblast, making it nonmalignant, its detection should

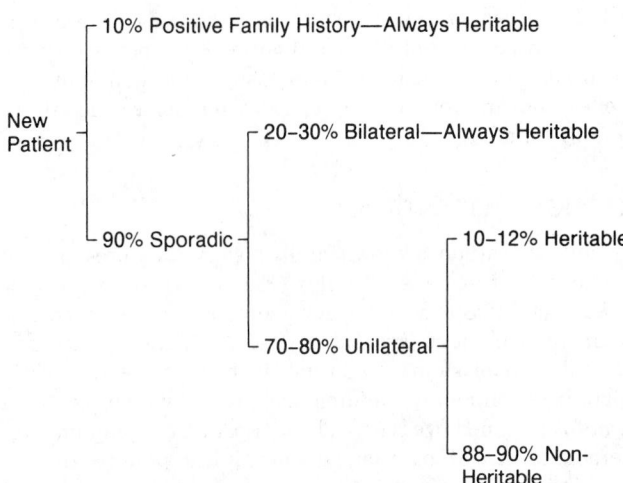

FIGURE 49–4.   Flow diagram of statistical probabilities for a newly diagnosed patient with retinoblastoma. (Donaldson SS, Egbert PR. Retinoblastoma. In: Pizzo PA, Poplack DG, eds. Principles and practice of pediatric oncology. 2nd ed. Philadelphia: JB Lippincott, 1993)

prompt genetic counseling and follow-up of the affected person.

PATHOLOGIC AND ANATOMIC CONSIDERATIONS

Retinoblastoma, putatively arising from the outer layer of the retina, consists of small, round cells with scanty cytoplasm and chromatin-rich nuclei. Histologic examination shows similarity with neuroblastoma and medulloblastoma, including aggregation around blood vessels, necrosis, calcification, and Flexner-Winter stained rosettes. Tumors are often multifocal, averaging four to five lesions in as many as 84% of the patients. This multifocality and the predilection of retinoblastoma to invade the optic nerve influences treatment planning.

Endophytic and exophytic local extension of retinoblastoma are recognized. Endophytic growth is characterized by extension into the vitreous cavity, and exophytic growth invades the subretinal space, with consequent retinal detachment. With endophytic extension, tumor fragments can break away from the main tumor mass to form vitreous seeds, which is a poor prognostic finding.

Most patients with retinoblastoma have disease restricted to the eye and orbit. Local tumor growth usually involves the choroid or the sclera if subretinal seeds cross Brach's membrane. The highly vascular choroid is involved in more than 25% of patients and, although this serves as a potential site for dissemination, it is not as serious as scleral involvement. Scleral involvement usually occurs by direct extension from the choroid or by spread along emissary veins.

Glaucoma can result from tumor growth in a retinal detachment that pushes the iris forward to occlude the trabecular network. It can also result if a neovascular membrane grows on the iris and over the trabecular network, blocking the egress of aqueous fluid. Iris neovascularization may be exacerbated by radiation therapy.

Of particular concern is extension of retinoblastoma cells through the lamina cribrosa and into or along the optic nerve. If the tumor extends just 10 to 22 mm along the optic nerve, invasion into the meninges is usually a consequence, a particularly poor prognostic feature.

Slightly more than half of the deaths with retinoblastoma

are due to distant tumor metastases, although 47% of deaths are a consequence of direct intracranial extension. As with neuroblastoma, hematogenous metastases most often involve bones, bone marrow, and lymph nodes; pulmonary metastases are uncommon.

CLINICAL PRESENTATION

In children without a known family history, 75% present with leukocoria or "cat's eye" reflex (Fig. 49–5), strabismus, or poor vision due to vascular involvement, vitreous seeds, or retinal detachment (see Table 49–7). In patients with unilateral retinoblastoma, strabismus is the most frequent early sign. Less commonly, children may present with proptosis, a painful inflamed eye, cervical adenopathy, or symptoms referable to sites of metastatic disease. It is imperative that infants and children with these symptoms undergo a careful ophthalmologic evaluation. Young children do not complain of loss of vision, and intraocular tumors are not painful unless there is also glaucoma or inflammation. Any child with a known family history of retinoblastoma or retinomas should be examined at birth and at regular intervals thereafter. Of 158 infants with retinoblastoma diagnosed during the first 6 months of life (mean age, 3.6 years), 60% had leukocoria, and 68% had bilateral disease. Many of these patients had advanced disease despite their early evaluation.

In young children suspected of having retinoblastoma, examination of the retina may need to be performed under general anesthesia. This is particularly important if tumor involvement includes the ora serrata or if the tumor cannot be visualized because of retinal detachment or vitreous hemor-

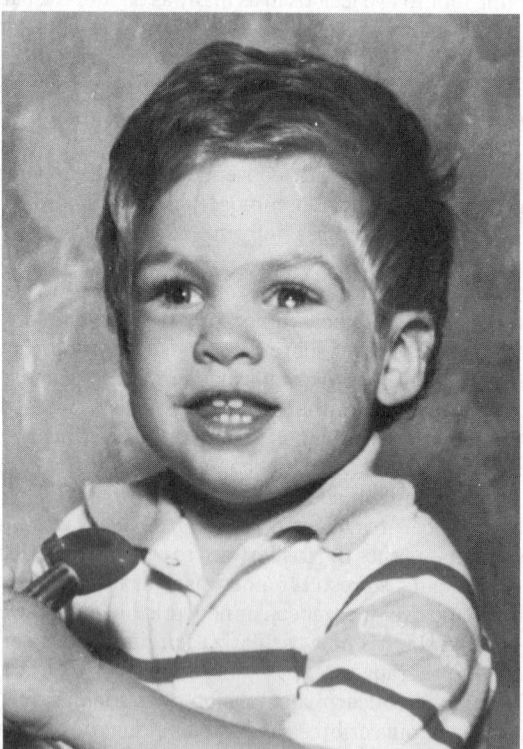

FIGURE 49–5.   Child exhibiting leukokoria in the left eye, the most common presenting sign of retinoblastoma. (Donaldson SS, Egbert PR. Retinoblastoma. In: Pizzo PA, Poplack DG, eds. Principles and practice of pediatric oncology. 2nd ed. Philadelphia: JB Lippincott, 1993)

rhage obscuring the tumor mass. The differential diagnosis includes visceral larva migrants (*i.e.*, *Toxocara* granuloma), Coats' disease, retrolental fibroplasia, and persistent hyperplastic primary vitreous. Findings of calcification, which occurs in 50% to 75% of patients, or vitreous seedings are compatible with retinoblastoma. Orbital CT scan can detect calcification in more than 80% of patients, and in children younger than 3 years of age in whom the diagnosis is suspected, CT-detected calcification is virtually diagnostic. Two dimensional B-scan ultrasonography is of particular value in demonstrating mass lesions in the posterior segment of the fundus, because retinoblastoma has a high internal acoustic reactivity due to the pressure of calcium and the interface between necrotic and viable areas.

EVALUATION

Examination of the child with retinoblastoma should determine the extent of local disease and metastatic disease. Careful examination of both retinas by direct and indirect ophthalmoscopy is essential, and the extent of orbital disease and intracranial extension should be assessed by CT scan. Two-dimensional B-scan ultrasonography can help in determining whether there is a mass in the posterior segment. Because of intraocular calcifications, CT of the orbit is more sensitive than plain films of the skull. MRI can determine the extent of orbital and CNS involvement. Patients should have a lumbar puncture for cytocentrifuge CSF examination, a bone marrow aspirate, and a biopsy. Patients with extensive orbital involvement should have bone scans. Lactic acid dehydrogenase may be elevated in the aqueous humor of patients with retinoblastoma.

Because of the predominance of intraocular disease and because of improved survival, treatment planning and staging has been focused on the management of local disease and on preserving the eye and vision. The most widely used staging system for retinoblastoma assesses the likelihood of local tumor control and preservation of vision but does not predict survival. As outlined in Table 49–16, this grouping system divides patients according to the likelihood of preserving vision after radiation therapy based on tumor size, the number and location of lesions, and vitreous seeding. In this system, tumor size is expressed by comparison with the optic disk (1.5 mm diameter). Each eye should be evaluated separately to assess the most effective therapy and to determine if there is any potential for preserving or restoring useful vision. Although this system is useful in guiding management of intraocular disease, it does not predict survival for patients with advanced (group V) disease at presentation.

A histologically based staging system, which considers intraocular and extraocular tumor extension and which correlates with patient survival, has been adopted by St. Jude Children's Research Hospital (Table 49–17). This staging system permits the integration of multimodal treatment planning for patients with advanced local disease, but it is based on results of enucleation.

TREATMENT

Treatment Planning

Treatment planning must consider unilateral or bilateral involvement; the size, number, and location of local tumors;

TABLE 49-16. Reese-Ellsworth Clinical Grouping System for Retinoblastoma

Group I: Very Favorable
1. Solitary tumor, less than 4 disk diameters* in size, at or beyond equator.
2. Multiple tumors, none over 4 disk diameters in size, all at or behind equator.

Group II: Favorable
1. Solitary tumor, 4 to 10 disk diameters in size, at or behind equator.
2. Multiple tumors, 4 to 10 disk diameters in size, at or behind equator.

Group III: Doubtful
1. Any lesion anterior to equator.
2. Solitary tumors larger than 10 disk diameters behind equator.

Group IV: Unfavorable
1. Multiple tumors, some larger than 10 disk diameters.
2. Any lesion extending anteriorly to ora serrata.

Group V: Very Unfavorable
1. Massive tumors involving over half the retina.
2. Vitreous seeding.

* 1 disk diameter = 1.6 mm.
(Reese AB, Ellsworth RM. The evaluation and current concepts of retinoblastoma therapy. Trans Am Acad Ophthalmol Otolaryngol 1963;67:164–172)

TABLE 49-17. St. Jude Children's Research Hospital Staging System

I. Tumor (unifocal or multifocal) confined to retina
  A. Occupying 1 quadrant or less
  B. Occupying 2 quadrants or less
  C. Occupying more than 50% of retinal surface
II. Tumor (unifocal or multifocal) confined to globe
  A. With vitreous seeding
  B. Extending to optic nerve head
  C. Extending to choroid
  D. Extending to choroid and optic nerve head
  E. Extending to emissaries
III. Extraocular extension of tumor (regional)
  A. Extending beyond cut end of optic nerve (including subarachnoid extension)
  B. Extending through sclera into orbital contents
  C. Extending to choroid and beyond cut end of optic nerve (including subarachnoid extension)
  D. Extending through sclera into orbital contents and beyond cut end of optic nerve (including subarachnoid extension)
IV. Distant metastases
  A. Extending through optic nerve to brain
  B. Blood-borne metastases to soft tissue and bone
  C. Bone marrow metastases

(Pratt CB. Management of malignant solid tumors in children. Pediatr Clin North Am 1972;19:1141–1155)

tumor extension into the choroid, sclera, or optic nerve; and evidence of extraocular disease. The goal of therapy for patients with localized disease (Ellsworth-Reese stages I and II or St. Jude stages I, IIA, and IIB) is local control with surgery or radiation therapy. Unfortunately, most children with unilateral involvement present with far advanced disease and with little potential for preserving vision. Patients with advanced local disease may require postoperative treatment to the orbit or contiguous extension sites of the CNS. The management of patients with bilateral disease depends on the extent and group of disease in each eye. It is no longer appropriate to enucleate the most severe eye in patients with bilateral involvement. With modern radiation therapy, vision may be spared.

Surgery

ADVANCED UNILATERAL DISEASE. Most children with sporadic unilateral retinoblastoma have advanced intraocular disease at the time of presentation, often with little or no vision in the affected eye. Although the potential for visual preservation exists with irradiation, at least 50% of patients with advanced local disease subsequently require enucleation, because of irradiation-induced complications or inadequate local tumor control. Enucleation is the treatment of choice for children with advanced unilateral disease, especially if there is involvement of the optic nerve head or if the child has glaucoma. If enucleation is performed, at least 10 mm of the optic nerve should be resected to remove any disease that may have extended along the nerve. If microscopic exami-

nation detects evidence of tumor along the nerve tract, local irradiation should be administered. An artificial eye can be fitted in 6 weeks. In children younger than 3 years of age, the orbit ceases to grow normally after enucleation and, as the face grows, the orbit becomes more sunken.

LIMITED DISEASE. Patients with limited unilateral or bilateral tumors (<4 disk diameters) may be candidates for photocoagulation or cryotherapy instead of enucleation combined with radiation. Photocoagulation by the technique of Meyer-Schwicherath obliterates small tumors and destroys their blood supply. This procedure requires direct visualization of the tumor and is best restricted to posterior tumor masses. The tumor mass must be easily differentiated from the optic nerve head or macula, must not involve the choroid, and must not have a large nutrient vessel. The technique is used in cases with residual or recurrent disease after irradiation. Although successful, photocoagulation can be complicated by retinal detachment and hemorrhage.

Cryotherapy has been occasionally successfully used for primary treatment; it is more often employed for excision of residual or recurrent disease after irradiation. It is applied by a probe placed directly on the conjunctiva or sclera through a small incision in the conjunctiva. The position of the probe is guided by ophthalmoscopy, and the tumor can be observed to whiten as it freezes. Of 138 retinoblastomas treated in one study, the overall success with cryotherapy was 70%, with a 93% survival rate. Cryotherapy was useful as a primary modality in small (<4 disk diameters or <3 mm in diameter and 2 mm thick) tumors (20 of 21 cured) and for radiation failures (58 of 66). Successful cryotherapy is limited by the size, location, and elevation of the tumor. It is ineffective in the treatment of vitreous seeds. Peripheral lesions may not be effectively treated by cryotherapy.

BILATERAL DISEASE. The treatment plan for patients with bilateral disease depends on the extent of tumor involvement in each eye. If one eye has lost vision or has clearly established optic nerve head involvement, it should be enucleated, and the less involved eye should be irradiated. If vision is present and imaging studies show no obvious optic nerve involvement, both eyes may be treated by irradiation. For group I, II, and III patients with bilateral retinoblastoma treated with irradiation, tumors were controlled in 73% to 80% of the cases. If both eyes are severely affected at the time of presentation, it is preferable to administer a trial of bilateral irradiation, because the possibility for some preservation or restoration of vision exists.

Although the 5-year survival rates for patients presenting with group IV or V disease is 88%, the chance for satisfactory tumor control and preservation of vision is low (29%). Recent experience with improved radiation therapy techniques and liberal use of phototherapy or cryotherapy have resulted in disease control in almost 80%, including group IV cases. With group V disease, primary irradiation control has been reportedly anecdotally.

Radiation Therapy

The purpose of radiation therapy in retinoblastoma is the control of local disease while preserving vision. However, the advantages of this approach must be weighed against its potential short-term and long-term complications. Because most patients have multiple tumors in one or both eyes, radiation fields must include the entire anatomic extent of the retina, the anterior border of which is the ora serrata. This is important because tumor cells from the posterior retina may be channeled into the region of the ora serrata and result in local failure if not included in the radiation field.

Radiation treatment planning requires the joint efforts of the radiation therapist, ophthalmologist, and anesthesiologist. Several techniques for external-beam irradiation have been employed. Concerns about including the lacrimal gland and direct conjunctival effects limit general use of anterior fields to cases with advanced disease (including vitreous seeding). Modern techniques permit accurate lateral field arrangements, which assure adequate coverage of the retina, diminish direct irradiation of the optic lens, and limit the degree of late xerophthalmia (Fig. 49–6). Young children should be anesthetized, usually requiring ketamine to ensure immobilization and relatively fixed ocular positioning. Excellent results have been reported by using a technically precise lateral photon field or by magnetic fixation of the eye using a low-vacuum contact lens that is attached to a small iron pin. Alternatively, a Comberg lens that has a radiopaque marker on the anterior surface of the cornea can be used for the setup.

No firm radiation dose-response relation has been proved for retinoblastoma. Most clinical series report doses between 4500 to 5400 cGy delivered over 4 to 6 weeks.

The regression patterns after radiation therapy include a "cottage cheese" appearance due to calcium deposition or shrinkage and a homogenous, gray, nonvascular mass with an annulus of atrophic pigment around the bone. Determination of tumor sterilization requires experience and serial ophthalmologic examinations.

Localized radiation, using radioactive plaques or particle radiation, although useful in patients with recurrent tumors, is comparable to cryotherapy or phototherapy. Local modifications, such as addressing less than the full retinal surface, should be used for primary control only in the unusual unilateral, limited-size, unifocal tumors. Patients who have residual orbital or optic nerve tumor after surgery should receive wide-field (*i.e.*, orbit and optic nerve) irradiation after enucleation. In general, a dosage of 4500 to 5400 cGy is delivered in 1800 to 200-cGy fractions over 5 to 6 weeks. At higher doses, optic atrophy may occur. Full cranial or craniospinal irradiation is indicated for patients with brain or dural extension.

Chemotherapy

Although chemotherapy was first used in patients with retinoblastoma in 1953, its role remains undefined. Because effective local control and survival is achieved in 90% of patients with surgery and radiation, chemotherapy is best restricted to patients with locally extensive (*e.g.*, choroidal or optic nerve), regional, or distant disease. Unfortunately, responses have been unsatisfactory. Patients with CNS extension and meningeal disease may benefit from intrathecal or intraventricular methotrexate. The agents that have been most extensively used in retinoblastoma include triethanolamine (TEM), vincristine, nitrogen mustard, cyclophosphamide, doxorubicin, and methotrexate. TEM has most often been administered by an intracarotid route, usually before the start of irradiation, although without proven efficacy. Ifosfamide has produced short-term, partial responses, and combinations of cyclophosphamide and dactinomycin, cyclophosphamide and doxorubicin, and cisplatin and VM-26 have been associated with mixed or partial responses. Preirradiation chemotherapy has been used for children with extensive intraocular tumors.

PRIMARY HEPATIC TUMORS

Primary malignancies of the liver, although infrequent in childhood, pose a considerable therapeutic and diagnostic challenge. One to two hepatic tumors per million children occur annually in the United States, with hepatoblastoma predominating in children younger than 5 years of age and hepatocellular carcinoma (HCC) in older children. As with Wilms' tumor, hepatoma most often presents as an asymptomatic abdominal mass that is found in a routine physical examination or discovered coincidentally by parents. Fewer than 25% of patients experience symptoms of abdominal pain, weight loss, or malaise, but when these symptoms occur, they are usually associated with advanced disease. The primary objective is to differentiate a hepatic malignancy from benign hepatic tumors, nonneoplastic hepatomegaly, and other causes of abdominal enlargement, particularly Wilms' tumor and neuroblastoma.

From a survey of 656 hepatic tumors in children, 423 (64%) were malignant, 54% were hepatoblastomas, 35% were hepatocellular sarcomas, and 11% were sarcomas (Table 49–18). Hemangiomas and hamartomas account for approximately 75% of the benign liver tumors, and almost 90% of these lesions occur in infants younger than 6 months. Benign vascular tumors can reach considerable size in infancy and

A OPPOSED PAIR, NORMALIZED TO d1/2 OF OPEN AREA

CENTERED AT ORA SERRATA

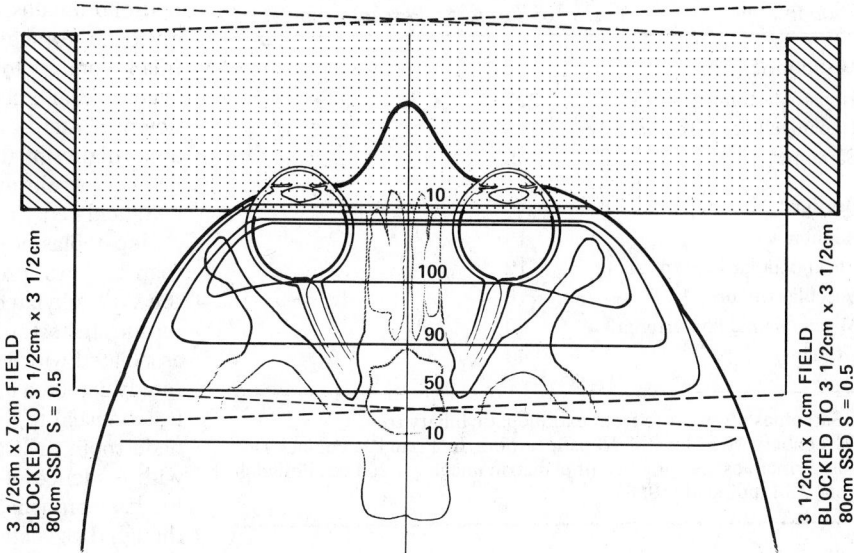

B SINGLE FIELD NORMALIZED TO d3 OF OPEN AREA

CENTERED AT ORA SERRATA

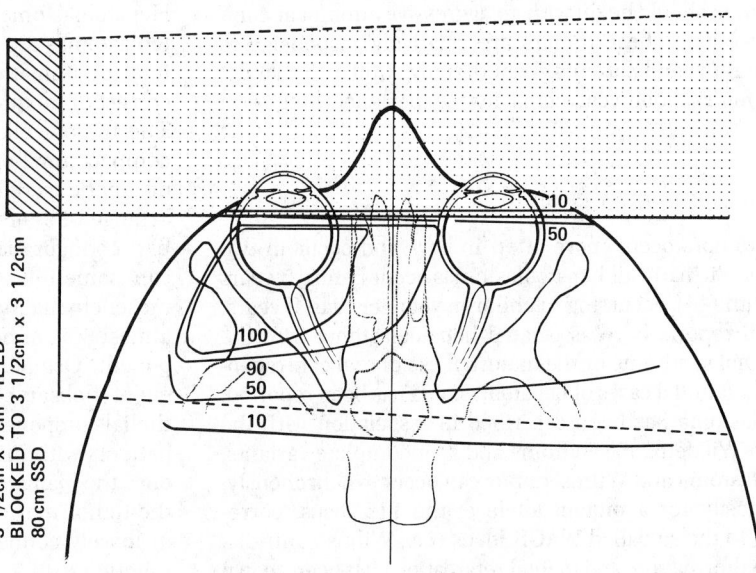

FIGURE 49–6. Isodose curves from a 4-MV linear accelerator for a 3.5 × 7 cm field blocked to an effective field of 3.5 × 3.5 cm, with the anterior border of the treatment field located at the ora serrata. Using the beam-splitting technique, the lens and pituitary receive less than 10% of the given dose. **(A)** For bilateral treatment, using equally weighted opposed lateral fields, the dose is calculated at the midplane with the retina lying within the 90% isodose curve. **(B)** For unilateral treatment, the dose is calculated to a depth of 3 cm. The retina lies within the 90% isodose curve, and the opposite eye receives 50% to 70% of the given dose.

may have an alarming clinical presentation, including high-output congestive heart failure due to arteriovenous shunting, hemorrhage, and bleeding with evidence of platelet consumption (the Kasabach-Merritt syndrome), and shock may occur after the rupture of a vascular tumor mass. Cavernous hemangioma, characterized by vascular spaces lined by a single layer of flat endothelial cells, often with evidence of old and new thrombus formation, and hemangioendotheliomas, composed of many small vascular channels lined by one or more layers of endothelial cells, are the two most important benign lesions that should be differentiated from malignant hepatic tumors. Although hemangioendotheliomas can be found at multiple sites within the liver, the metastatic potential

of these tumors is exceedingly low. Benign hemangiomas can be treated with steroids and, if they fail to respond, low doses of radiation are generally successful in causing shrinkage; surgical resection is rarely necessary.

Hepatic sarcoma is a rare malignancy that constitutes approximately 10% of the primary hepatic tumors of childhood. The most common presenting symptom is abdominal pain. Evaluation should include a thorough determination of the extent of abdominal disease to guide resection and a search for metastases, especially in lung and bone. Tumors are classified as undifferentiated (*i.e.,* embryonal) sarcomas if there is no evidence of specific differentiation and the malignant elements are mesenchymal, having a myxoid background and

TABLE 49–18. Frequency of Benign and Malignant Hepatic Tumors in Children: Selected North American Series

Tumor Type	No. of Tumors	Percentage of Total
Malignant		
Hepatoblastoma	227	34.6
Hepatocellular carcinoma	148	22.5
Sarcoma*	45	6.8
Benign		
Adenoma	13	2
Focal nodular hyperplasia	12	2
Vascular tumors	118	18
Mesenchymal hamartoma	53	8
Other	40	6

* Sarcomas often arose from extrahepatic biliary tree.
(Greenberg M, Filler RM. Hepatic tumors. In: Pizzo PA, Poplack DG, eds. Principles and practice of pediatric oncology. 2nd ed. Philadelphia: JB Lippincott, 1993)

stellate cells. If there is evidence of differentiation, a more specific diagnosis may be assigned, such as rhabdomyosarcoma if striated muscle cells are present.

Treatment should begin with an aggressive attempt at complete resection. These tumors are relatively responsive to chemotherapy, and patients given therapy similar to that developed for rhabdomyosarcoma may experience long-term survival.

EPIDEMIOLOGY AND GENETICS

Hepatic tumors occur more often in boys and occur in two age peaks. Virtually all hepatoblastomas occur before 5 years of age, with 65% occurring in children younger than 2 years. Anecdotal reports have associated hepatoblastoma with the fetal alcohol syndrome or the maternal use of oral contraceptives. Four familial cases of hepatoblastoma has been reported. Hepatoblastoma has been described in association with the Beckwith-Wiedemann syndrome and its incomplete variants. Hepatoblastoma and Wilms' tumor can occur synchronously. Homozygosity for a mutant allele at the 11p locus, corresponding to the so-called WAGR locus (*i.e.,* Wilms', aniridia, genital malformation, and mental retardation) has been shown in biopsy tissue and in explants from 2 patients with hepatoblastoma.

HCC rarely occurs in infants and has its peak childhood incidence during adolescence. HCC is associated with preexisting cirrhosis and chronic hepatitis caused by the hepatitis B virus (HBV), an association that is particularly prominent in countries where there is a high prevalence of HBV infection, such as Japan. HBV sequences are integrated into the DNA of the HCC cells. Perinatal transmission of HBV has been associated with the onset of HCC 6 to 7 years later, suggesting that the latency period may be shorter in children than in adults. Epidemiologic studies suggest that control of HBV transmission and infection (*i.e.,* by vaccination) may eventually decrease the incidence of HCC in adults and children.

A variety of syndromes and congenital malformations have been associated with primary hepatic tumors, including hemihypertrophy, osteopetrosis, DeToni-Fanconi syndrome, neurofibromatosis, ataxia-telangiectasia, lipid storage disease, glycogen storage disease, hereditary tyrosinemia, biliary atremia secondary to extrahepatic biliary atresia, and the homozygous ZZ and heterozygous phenotypes of α_1-antitrypsin deficiency states. Recent studies have demonstrated an abnormality of the p53 gene at the DNA, RNA, or protein level. The relevance of this pathogenesis of HCC remains to be elucidated.

Hepatoblastoma has presented with virilization in fewer than 25 boys. Prolonged use of anabolic steroids, especially the C17 alkylated forms (*e.g.,* oxymetholone, methyltestosterone, testosterone enanthate, methandienone) have been associated with HCC. Although α-fetoprotein (AFP) is commonly detected in the serum of patients with hepatoblastoma, it is unusual to find evidence of elevated levels of choriogonadotropin (hCG). However, hCG can be detected in children with evidence of virilization, and immunoperoxidase staining has confirmed that hepatoma cells produce the hCG, although these cells may not be the same ones producing AFP. Estrogen and progesterone receptors have been found in hepatoblastoma.

PATHOLOGY

Hepatoblastoma and HCC are epithelial neoplasms. Hepatoblastomas are generally divided into tumors that consist of fetal or immature hepatic epithelial cells and tumors that consist of mixtures of epithelial and mesenchymal elements. The tumor cells have a high nuclear to cytoplasmic ratio, compact amphophilic or basophilic cytoplasm, and evidence of miotic activity. Most commonly, the tumor cells are arranged in cords two to three cells thick and have a sheet-like configuration. Acinar or pseudoglandular components can sometimes be defined, although a mixed epithelial-mesenchymal variant of hepatoblastoma, accounting for almost 30% of hepatoblastomas, can have a spindle cell component. Osteoid and extramedullary hematopoiesis are frequently observed in these mixed tumors. Although the epithelial component appears to be a prognostic determinant for patients with mixed hepatoblastomas, embryonal cells influence the malignant potential of these tumors. Less commonly, the tumor may appear more anaplastic, consisting of sheets of loosely connected cells with scant cytoplasm and a high mitotic rate.

HCC in children may be histologically identical to that seen in adults, although an important variant has been recently defined. This rare tumor, called fibrolamellar carcinoma, occurs primarily in younger patients (mean age, 25; range, 5–35 years) and is characterized by deeply eosinophilic neoplastic hepatocytes, many of which contain intracellular hyaline globules and distinct pale bodies surrounded by fibrous bands, often with a lamellar configuration. Fibrolamellar carcinoma presents as a single tumor nodule and has a much more favorable prognosis (median survival, 32 months) than other forms of HCC. Nonetheless, it is important to differentiate fibrolamellar carcinomas from benign hepatic adenomas, because survival depends on surgical resection.

HCC has a distinctive ultrastructural appearance characterized by large, round, centrally placed nuclei, prominent nucleoli, abundant large mitochondria, and microvilli on the plasma membrane.

By the time of presentation, tumor masses are usually quite large, regardless of histologic type, and frequently involve the right lobe of the liver. Spread to other parts of the liver usually occurs by direct extension, but it may take place through intrahepatic vascular or lymphatic channels. Extrahepatic tumor spread usually occurs by way of the regional lymph nodes in the porta hepatis, and the lungs are the primary sites of metastatic disease.

CLINICAL PRESENTATION

A palpable abdominal mass in the right upper quadrant is the predominant finding in more than 90% of patients with primary hepatic tumors. Usually, there are no other physical signs or symptoms. Severe osteopenia with back pain and pathologic features of weight-bearing bones can occur. Iso sexual precocity, although uncommon, can be seen in approximately 3% of the hepatoblastomas that secret β-hCG.

Abdominal pain is more frequent in patients with HCC, and the mean duration of symptoms before presentation is only 1 to 2 months. Hemoperitoneum with an acute abdominal crisis may be the primary presentation.

In patients with localized hepatic tumors, most routine laboratory tests are normal. Anemia or thrombocytopenia are important findings because they may indicate that the mass is a benign vascular tumor with associated bleeding or platelet consumption. Thrombocytosis can be seen in hepatoblastoma and HCC. Polycythemia, with hemoglobin levels higher than 16 g/100 ml may occur in patients with HCC due to the extrarenal production of erythropoietin. In patients with hepatic tumors, the SGOT and alkaline phosphatase levels may be slightly elevated, but the serum bilirubin is elevated in only 5% of patients with hepatoblastoma, compared with almost 25% of those with HCC.

An α-globulin, AFP is produced normally by embryonic hepatocytes and is present in the serum for the first few days after birth. Elevated AFP has been described in 40% of children with HCC and in 67% of children with hepatoblastomas. The protein is not specific for hepatic tumors and can be elevated in the serum of children with embryonal testicular carcinoma and teratomas. Cystanthininuria has been described in children with primary hepatic neoplasms, but it can be found in patients with neuroblastoma. Serum ferritin levels are elevated in 97% patients with HCC, but they are also elevated in 87% patients with uncomplicated cirrhosis. Although not useful diagnostically, serum ferritin levels have been observed to fall with tumor response and to rise with tumor progression. Rarely, the serum hCG levels may be elevated in patient with virilization and hepatomas. The level of unsaturated vitamin B_{12}-binding protein is elevated in the fibrolamellar variant of HCC and increases with disease progression.

Because the primary goal of the initial evaluation is to define the extent of disease and to differentiate a primary hepatic tumor from the other abdominal masses that may occur in children, a chest x-ray film, abdominal radiograph, and IVP should be obtained. Ultrasound radionuclide liver scan, CT, and to a lesser extent, arteriography are important in delin-

eating the contour and extent of the tumor. Hepatoblastoma and HCC have diffused hyperechoic patterns, unlike benign lesions, which are usually less echogenic. CT scanning is important in defining the extent of tumor and potential operability. Characteristically, tumor masses have lower attenuation than surrounding tissue, although tumors may be isodense. CT scanning is of particular value in assessing the left lobe of the liver, a site hard to define by arteriography. MRI appears to be able to image parenchymal structure and vascular structures, making it the most accurate imaging study and a replacement for angiography.

TREATMENT PLANNING

The staging system, based on surgical resectability, correlates with outcome (Table 49-19 and Fig. 49-7). This approach is verified by the fact that cure of primary hepatic neoplasms requires complete resection. From a surgical viewpoint, the liver can be divided into lobes and segments according to its vascular supply. The right lobe of the liver contains about 70% of the total liver mass, and each segment of the left lobe represents an additional 15%. Because of the liver's remarkable ability to regenerate, it is possible to remove as much as 85% of the total liver at one time and still expect complete regeneration of liver cell mass within 3 weeks in infants and within 3 months in children after surgery. Tumors contained in one lobe of the liver and those arising in the right lobe that do not extend beyond the medial segment of the left lobe are amenable to surgical resection. Improvements in anesthesia and surgical techniques and in vigilant management before, during, and after surgery have minimized the hazards of hepatic resection.

Surgery

BIOPSY. Although excision is preferred, some tumors may be unresectable, because many liver segments are involved or because the hepatic arterial and venous inflow and outflow tracts are involved with tumors. In such cases, preoperative chemotherapy, with or without radiation, may render the tumor resectable. Before beginning such therapy, histologic di-

TABLE 49-19. Clinical Grouping of Malignant Hepatic Tumor

Designation	Criteria
Group I	Complete resection of tumor by wedge resection lobectomy or by extended lobectomy as initial treatment
Group IIA	Tumors rendered completely resectable by initial irradiation or chemotherapy
Group IIB	Residual disease confined to one lobe
Group III	Disease involving both lobes of the liver
Group IIIB	Regional node involvement
Group IV	Distant metastases, irrespective of the extent of liver involvement

(Greenberg M, Filler R. Hepatic tumors. In: Pizzo PA, Poplack DG, eds. Principles and practice of pediatric oncology. 2nd ed. Philadelphia: JB Lippincott, 1993)

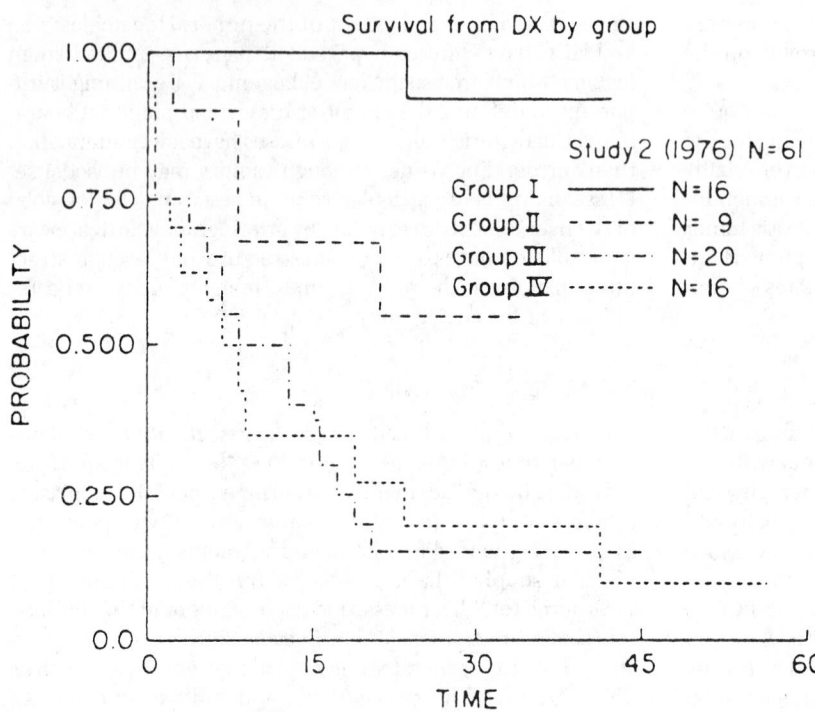

Survival from DX by group

Study 2 (1976) N=61

Group I ———— N=16
Group II - - - - - N= 9
Group III - · - · - N=20
Group IV ········· N= 16

FIGURE 49–7. Life table analysis of survival in a mixed population of children with hepatoblastoma and hepatocellular carcinoma. Survival probability is correlated with clinical grouping 0 to 60 months after diagnosis and treatment. (Greenberg M, Filler RM. Hepatic tumors. In: Pizzo PA, Poplack DG, eds. Principles and practice of pediatric oncology. 2nd ed. Philadelphia: JB Lippincott, 1993)

agnosis is essential. Although an open liver biopsy has been employed, a needle biopsy is satisfactory and avoids the need for general anesthesia, although hemorrhage may occur. Some recommend preoperative chemotherapy in patients with an elevated AFP who have CT scans and anteriograms suggesting hepatoma.

OPERATIVE TECHNIQUE. The recommended procedure for hepatic resection in children is similar to that used in adults. A thoracoabdominal approach is preferred because it offers excellent exposure and precludes the development of negative intrathoracic pressure, which may cause the aspiration of air into an open venous system. This approach provides excellent visualization of the entire supradiaphragmatic inferior vena cava, into which an internal venous shunt can be placed so that liver blood flow can be isolated in the event of catastrophic hemorrhage.

After the porta hepatis is dissected, the vessels and ducts to the lobe to be excised are ligated and divided. The liver is mobilized by dividing the diaphragmatic attachments, and the diaphragm may be divided radially to the vena cava. Tapes are passed around the vena cava above and below the liver to ensure control of excessive bleeding. Before the hepatic veins are isolated, the liver capsule is incised along a lobar or segmental division, and the liver substance is divided bluntly. Bridging vessels and bile ducts are ligated as they are encountered. Because of the short extrahepatic length of the hepatic veins in children, they should be approached by dissection through the liver substance rather than at their exit from the liver. With this technique, inadvertent venous injury, which can result in difficult to control bleeding, can be minimized. Large vessels and ducts are individually ligated on the raw surface of the remnant lobe. Sump and Penrose drains are placed in the liver bed, and the incision is closed.

If the gallbladder remains, it should be drained with a cholecystostomy.

Profound hypothermia with circulatory arrest has been used as an adjunct to surgery in a difficult hepatectomy. Before division of the liver, cardiopulmonary bypass is instituted and hypothermia is induced. With the child's body temperature at 20°C, the circulation can be stopped for as long as 60 minutes, and resection and repair of vascular structures can be performed in a bloodless operative field. Alternatively, a normothermic, isolated hepatic circulatory arrest in which the lower thoracic aorta, porta hepatis, and the vena cava above or below the liver are clamped to effectively stop liver circulation has been used as an adjunct to hepatic resection. Hemodilution is another procedure that produces an essentially bloodless exposure and permits the return of the patient's own erythrocytes after surgery. These techniques should be considered for children with large tumors or with tumors adjacent to the hepatic veins.

INTRAOPERATIVE MANAGEMENT. The most frequent and serious intraoperative problem is hemorrhage. Even without uncontrolled bleeding, the loss of one blood volume (up to 800 ml in a 10-kg child) is not unusual. Accurate measurement of blood lost in surgical sponges and by suction and measurement of intraarterial blood pressure, central venous pressure, and urine output is necessary to estimate replacement volumes. Because hypothermia tends to cause cardiac irritability, metabolic acidosis, and abnormal blood clotting mechanisms, blood administered during surgery should be warmed to 37°C. Unless the procedure is performed with induced hypothermia, the child's normal body temperature should be maintained by providing a warm operating room temperature and by the use of a warming blanket. Adjusting the pH 7.0 of bank blood to pH 7.4 decreases the incidence of cardiac arrest, which can be triggered by the rapid infusion of large volumes of cold, relatively acidic blood.

PREOPERATIVE CHEMOTHERAPY OR RADIATION THERAPY. Preoperative chemotherapy or radiation therapy (1200–2000 cGy) has been used to reduce the size of the primary tumors before resection. The use of continuous-infusion doxorubicin and cisplatin has shrunk tumors in 35% to 95% of patients. Ten of these patients had initially unresectable tumors, but after chemotherapy, the tumors were completely resectable. Although the experience with HCC is more limited, preoperative chemotherapy with doxorubicin and cisplatin is recommended before resection in all patients.

POSTOPERATIVE MANAGEMENT. Despite advances in surgical techniques, surgical morbidity and mortality rates are still high. Between 11% and 25% of the patients die during or after hepatic resections. Blood loss was the most common intraoperative and postoperative complication. A single blood-stained dressing may represent significant blood loss in an infant, but too vigorous volume replacement may result in pulmonary edema. Other postoperative complications include subphrenic abscess, wound infection, biliary fistula, and small bowel obstruction.

Hepatic resection may result in a variety of metabolic derangements, particularly hypoglycemia and coagulopathies. These problems can usually be avoided by the continuous intravenous infusion of 10% dextrose postoperatively, with daily infusion of albumen for the first postoperative week and the administration of vitamin K.

Radiation Therapy

The role of preoperative and postoperative radiation therapy is less defined than that for surgery and chemotherapy. When employed, doses range between 1200 and 2000 cCy. Although used for preoperative therapy in patients failing to respond to chemotherapy, radiation therapy may be better used for the treatment of microscopic residual disease after resection.

Adjuvant Chemotherapy

Approximately 50% of children with hepatoblastomas or HCC appear to be cured after complete tumor resection. In general, children with hepatoblastoma do better than those with HCC. The use of preoperative chemotherapy in patients with inoperative tumors should further improve these results. Metastatic disease is an important cause of death in patients with residual tumor. The Children's Cancer Study Group (CCSG) and POG evaluated combination chemotherapy consisting of pulses of vincristine, cyclophosphamide, and doxorubicin, alternating every 3 weeks with vincristine, cyclophosphamide, and 5-fluorouracil (5-FU) for 1 year. Of 16 patients who received adjuvant therapy after complete surgical resection, only 1 patient developed distant metastases, compared with 7 of 11 historic controls who did not receive adjuvant chemotherapy. Among the regimens recommended are cisplatin (20 mg/m²/day) by continuous infusion for 5 days with doxorubicin (25 mg/m²/day) for 3 days. Treatments are given every 3 to 4 weeks for six cycles, beginning 3 to 4 weeks after surgery, permitting regeneration of hepatic tissue.

GERM CELL TUMORS

The germ cell tumors of infants and children reflect the transformation of primordial cells that have failed to migrate to their predestined location. The totipotent germ cells normally arise from the yolk sac of the 4-week-old human embryo and migrate along the gonadal ridge to the gonadal anlage before their final descent into the pelvis. During embryogenesis, some of these germ cells fail to complete this migration and come to rest along the dorsal midline of the embryo. The primordial germ cells give rise to an undifferentiated cell line and a primitive, committed germ cell line. The undifferentiated germ cell undergoes differentiation into embryonic (*i.e.,* somatic cells) or the extraembryonic cells of yolk sac, chorion, and allantoin cells. Malignant transformation of these cells gives rise to tumors that reflect their embryonic features. Tumors of the embryonic germ cells are the teratomas and consist of each of the embryonic cell layers of ectoderm, mesoderm, and endoderm. However, tumors of extraembryonic cells have trophoblastic features, as in choriocarcinoma, or characteristics of the yolk sac endoderm and extraembryonic mesoderm, as in embryonal adenocarcinoma of the infantile testis (Fig. 49–8).

EPIDEMIOLOGY AND GENETICS

Germ cell tumors comprise approximately 3% of childhood neoplasms and have a bimodal age distribution. Almost 67% arise in extragonadal sites. Extragonadal teratomas and yolk sac tumors of the testis occur in infants and young children. Ovarian teratomas and dysgerminomas have their peak incidence during adolescence.

Karyotypic analysis has demonstrated several nonrandom structural changes, most commonly is chromosomes 1 and 12 but also in chromosomes 5, 7, 9, 17, 21, and 22. An isochromosome 12p[i(12p)] has been identified in various histologic subtypes of germ cell tumors. Familial inheritance of testicular and other germ cell tumors have been described. The malignant potential of histologically benign-appearing teratomas may be suggested by the DNA index, aneuploidy, and presence of the *MYC* oncogene.

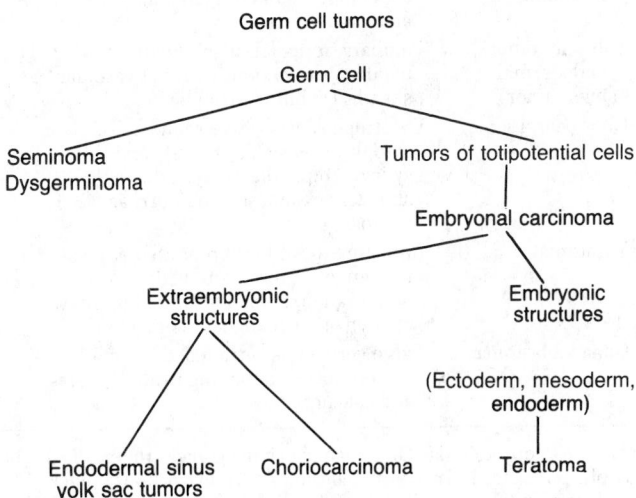

FIGURE 49–8. Histogenesis of germ cell tumors.

ANATOMIC AND PATHOLOGIC CONSIDERATIONS

The classification and comparative pathology of germ cell tumors are shown in Tables 49–20 and 49–21.

Teratomas

Teratomas are composed of tissues that are derived from three germinal layers, the endoderm, mesoderm, and ectoderm. They may be solid or cystic and are classified histologically as mature, immature, and malignant. Mature teratomas consist of well-differentiated tissues (*e.g.*, brain, skin, gastrointestinal, bone) and are benign. Immature teratomas contain embryonic tissue, usually neuroglia or neural tube-like structures, in addition to mature tumors. Teratomas with malignant potential may contain elements of germinoma, choriocarcinoma, endodermal sinus tumor, or embryonal carcinoma. There may be a mixture of mature, embryonic and unequivocally malignant elements, making examination of multiple histologic sections mandatory.

Teratomas in infants and young children are primarily extragonadal. Of 245 patients with 254 teratomas admitted to the Boston Children's Hospital Medical Center from 1928 to 1982, 49% were detected in the newborn period. Sacrococcygeal teratomas were most common (40%), followed by ovary (37%), head and neck (6%), retroperitoneum (5%), mediastinum (4%), CNS (4%), testes (3%), and liver or trunk (1%) teratomas.

Fifty percent to 75% of sacrococcygeal teratomas are diagnosed at birth, and almost 75% occur in girls. Although every teratoma has the potential to become malignant, 48% are benign, 23% have immature but nonmalignant components, and 29% are malignant. Most tumors are diagnosed within the first 2 months after birth (90% at birth) and are almost invariably benign.

Sacrococcygeal tumors can be external or internal (*i.e.*, presacral), 44% of them have an external component and an intrapelvic or intraabdominal extension. In 10% of patients, they can be entirely presacral. Tumors that are entirely or predominantly external have a lower malignant potential than presacral tumors, 8% of which are malignant, or intrapelvic or intraabdominal tumors, approximately 20% of which are malignant.

Sacrococcygeal teratomas vary in size from small localized lesions to massive tumors. Rarely, the tumor is so large in utero that a cesarean section is necessary for delivery, and death of the child due to uncontrolled hemorrhage has been reported during vaginal delivery if the tumor ruptures.

Germinoma

Germinomas are uniform in appearance, consisting of large, round cells with vesicular nuclei and clear or finely granular eosinophilic-staining cytoplasm separated by vascular fibrous septal-containing lymphocytes and focal granulomas.

The most common sites in children are the ovary, anterior mediastinum, and pineal gland, and the tumor is the predominant histologic type found in dysgenic gonads and undescended testes. Germinomas account for 10% of ovarian tumors in children and 15% of all germ cell tumors.

Embryonal Carcinoma and Endodermal Sinus Tumor

Endodermal sinus tumor (*i.e.*, yolk sac tumor) is the most common malignant germ cell tumor found in children. It is

TABLE 49–20. Comparative Characteristics of Germ Cell Tumors by Pathologic Types

Tumor Type	Characteristic Histology	Frequency	Most Common Locations	AFP	HCG	PLAP
Germinoma	Large round cells, vesicular nuclei, clear eosinophilic cytoplasm; monotonous pattern	+	Ovary, anterior mediastinum, pineal, undescended testes	−	−	+
Embryonal carcinoma	Poorly differentiated, epithelial appearance; solid or glandular, anaplasia, necrosis	++	Testes, young adult	+	±	±
Yolk sac tumor (endodermal sinus tumor)	Papillary, reticular or solid pattern; papillary projections with perivascular sheaths (Schiller-Duval bodies)	+++	Testes, infant: sacrococcygeal, ovary	+	−	−
Choriocarcinoma	Cytotrophoblasts (large round cells, clear cytoplasm, vesicular nuclei) and syncytiotrophoblasts (syncytia with abundant cytoplasm); hemorrhage, necrosis	+	Mediastinal, ovary, pineal	−	+	−
Teratoma	Immature to well-differentiated tissues foreign to anatomic site with lack of organization; benign or immature may contain other malignant components	++++	Sacrococcygeal midline structures	−	−	−
Gonadoblastoma	Large germ cells surrounded by smaller Sertoli's cells containing hyaline bodies and calcium	+	Dysgenic gonads	−	−	−

AFP, α-fetoprotein; HCG, human chorionic gonadotropin; PLAP, placental alkaline phosphatase.
(Ablin A, Isaacs H Jr. Germ cell tumors. In: Pizzo PA, Poplack DG, eds. Principles and practice of pediatric oncology. 2nd ed. Philadelphia: JB Lippincott, 1993)

TABLE 49–21. Comparative Clinical Presentations of Germ Cell Tumors

Tumor	Age	Relative Frequency (%)	Symptoms	Findings	Pathology
Extragonadal					
Sacrococcygeal	Infants	41	Constipation, neurologic abnormalities of bladder or lower extremities	Presacral mass with or without extension to buttocks or pelvis and abdomen	65% benign 5% immature 30% malignant
Mediastinal		6	Cough, wheeze, dyspnea	Anterior mediastinal mass	Benign or malignant
Abdominal	<2 y	5	Secondary to pressure pain, GU obstruction, constipation	Often retroperitoneal; also stomach, omentum, liver	Benign or malignant
Intracranial	Children	6	Headache, paralysis of upward gaze, incoordination	Pineal or supracellular tumors; AFP or hCG in CSF	Any type germ cell tumor
Head and neck	Infants	4	Pressure-related; respiratory or swallowing difficulty	Large mass on physical examination	Usually benign
Vagina	<3 y	1	Blood-tinged vaginal discharge	Polypoid mass from vagina	Usually malignant
Gonadal					
Ovarian	10–14 y	29	Abdominal pain, nausea, vomiting, constipation, GU symptoms	Abdominal pelvic mass; calcifications in 50%; often + AFP or hCG	Any type germ cell tumor
Testicular	Infants, postpubertal	7	Painless swelling of testis or painful torsion	Testicular mass; metastases to lung in infants	Any type germ cell tumor; 82% malignant, 18% benign. Infants mostly yolk sac tumors

GU, genitourinary; AFP, α-fetoprotein; hCG, human chorionic gonadotropin.
(Ablin A, Isaacs H Jr. Germ cell tumors. In: Pizzo PA, Poplack DG, eds. Principles and practice of pediatric oncology. 2nd ed. Philadelphia: JB Lippincott, 1993)

characterized by a labyrinthine glandular pattern consisting of flat epithelial cells and rounded papillary processes with a central capillary (*i.e.*, Schiller-Duval body). The tumor represents a proliferation of yolk sac endoderm and extraembryonic mesenchyme. It was first recognized as a distinct entity by Teilum, because of its similarity to the endodermal sinus found in rat placenta. Although most yolk sac tumors present as infant testicular tumors, yolk cell tumors occurring as pure or component portions of mixed germ cell tumors are rather common in the ovaries of young girls and in several extragonadal sites, including the sacrococcygeal area, pelvis, mediastinum, liver, retroperitoneum, vagina, and CNS.

Choriocarcinoma, Gonadoblastoma, and Polyembryoma

Choriocarcinoma is an uncommon, highly malignant tumor consisting of gestational forms arising from placenta and nongestational forms arising from extraplacental tissues in a nongravid woman. In an infant, choriocarcinoma may present as a congenital tumor arising from a maternal placental primary tumor and transmitted to the fetal bloodstream; it presents as a mediastinal or ovarian tumor in young children or as a placental tumor in the pregnant adolescent. Choriocarcinomas consist of cytotrophoblasts, which are large round cells with clear cytoplasms and variable vesicular nuclei, and syncytiotrophoblasts, which are larger cells with vacuolated cytoplasm and irregular nuclei that form syncytia.

Gonadoblastoma is a rare germ cell tumor that occurs almost exclusively during the first 20 years of life in patients with dysgenic gonads, usually in association with a Y chromosome. Almost 33% of these tumors are associated with germinomas. Gonadoblastomas consist of large germ cells surrounded by smaller round, darkly staining Sertoli's cells, forming microfollicles consisting of hylanine bodies and calcium deposits.

Polyembryoma is a rare tumor that consists of embryoid bodies comparable to presomatic embryos. They stain positive for AFP and hCG, suggesting embryonic and extraembryonic differentiation.

TREATMENT

Clinical Evaluation and Treatment Planning

Depending on the anatomic site, histologic type, and stage, surgery is combined with radiation or chemotherapy in the management of children with germ cell tumors. The surgical considerations are tailored to each tumor.

Radiation Therapy

Radiation therapy, even in limited doses, can be highly curative for several germ cell tumors. However, in the more common yolk sac tumors and embryonal carcinomas or the malignant teratomas of extragonadal origin, the role of radiation therapy is less certain. Few patients with malignant sacrococcygeal teratomas have been long-term survivors. Similar data support the use of regional radiation therapy for other extragonadal tumors poorly controlled with surgery or chemotherapy.

Doses of radiation for germinomas may be limited to 2500 cGy for patients with microscopic disease or to 3500 cGy for large tumors. With endodermal sinus tumors, effective local control has only been achieved at doses of 4000 to 4500 cGy or higher.

Chemotherapy

Methotrexate was the first chemotherapeutic agent to demonstrate efficacy against germ cell tumors, producing a 47% complete response rate in gestational choriocarcinoma. Several agents have been evaluated, singly and in combination, with remarkable results in some germ cell tumors. Among the agents that have been used are vincristine, dactinomycin, cyclophosphamide, vinblastine, bleomycin, cisplatin, doxorubicin, ifosfamide, and VP-16. The most commonly employed combinations are vincristine, dactinomycin, and cyclophosphamide (VAC), vinblastine, dactinomycin, and bleomycin (VAB), or cisplatin, vinblastine, and bleomycin (PVB). For testicular tumors in adults, PVB combinations have been the standard, with complete response rates of 70% and overall response rates of 100%. Combinations of PVB plus doxorubicin have also been employed. For ovarian germ cell tumors in adults, PVB combinations have proven superior to VAC regimens for patients with endodermal sinus tumor and those with stage III or IV disease of any cell type.

Similar regimens have been employed for germ cell tumors occurring in children. Adjuvant VAC chemotherapy has been most extensively used, particularly for children with ovarian tumors and endodermal sinus tumors. Other combinations have demonstrated efficacy, particularly those with cisplatin, bleomycin, and doxorubicin in addition to vincristine, dactinomycin, and cyclophosphamide.

Vinblastine, bleomycin, cisplatin, dactinomycin, cyclophosphamide, and doxorubicin were evaluated in treating 79 children with poor-risk germ cell tumors; 39% had evidence of metastatic disease at diagnosis. Approximately 69% of these patients had complete responses and 27% attained partial responses. After 4 years, 45% of the patients are free of disease.

Epipodophyllotoxin and ifosfamide have been evaluated as salvage agents for adults and children with germ cell tumors, particularly in conjunction with high-dose cisplatin. More intensive regimens using high doses of melphalan, VP-16, and cyclophosphamide have been administered in conjunction with autologous bone marrow reconstitution. Regimens using ifosfamide and VP-16 in conjunction with cisplatin, bleomycin, cyclophosphamide, dactinomycin, doxorubicin, and vinblastine are being explored.

Specific Management Strategies

SACROCOCCYGEAL TUMORS. For infants with external masses in the sacrococcygeal area, the differential diagnosis includes meningomyelocele, chordoma, duplication of the rectum, neurogenic tumors, lipoma, vestigial tail, and hemangioma. In infants without external masses, asymmetric intergluteal folds warrant a careful rectal examination to search for a presacral lesion. The incidence of malignancy if the diagnosis is established before the infant is 2 months of age is 10% for boys and 7% for girls. If diagnosis is delayed until the infant is older than 2 months, 67% of boys and 47% of girls develop malignant tumors. A careful rectal examination is essential in the evaluation of these infants. With more advanced presacral or intrapelvic involvement, particularly if the diagnosis is delayed, infants may develop bowel or bladder dystonia as a consequence of the tumor mass. Albeit rarely, invasion of the lumbosacral plexus or spinal cord may result in lower extremity weakness and pain. Approximately 20% of infants with advanced local involvement have pulmonary metastases at the time of diagnosis.

Radiographic examination of the pelvis may demonstrate calcification in the tumor mass or the destruction of the sacrum. Barium enema, a CT scan, and an IVP should be performed to evaluate the intrapelvic extent of tumor. A chest x-ray film should always be obtained to assess the presence of metastatic disease.

The serum AFP level is elevated in malignant sacrococcygeal tumors. Of 61 infants with teratoma, the AFP level was normal in 96% with mature lesions but was elevated in 97% of those with malignant elements. It is important to monitor AFP levels, even in patients whose sacrococcygeal tumor was initially benign, because late recurrences may develop. Serum ferritin may be elevated in patients with germ cell tumors and, although not tumor specific, may serve as another biologic marker.

The operative approach depends on whether the tumor is primarily extrapelvic or there is intrapelvic or intraabdominal extension. For lesions that are predominantly external, a one-stage posterior sacral approach, in which the coccyx and possibly the lower sacrum are removed, is the treatment of choice. For lesions that extend into the pelvis, a two-stage procedure is usually necessary. An anterior approach through the abdomen is taken so that the superior extent of the tumor can be defined and removed. For the second stage, the child is positioned face downward, and a V-shaped incision is made over the upper buttocks. The lower sacrum is divided, and with the coccyx attached to the specimen, the previously mobilized intrapelvic mass is delivered. The lower part of the mass is separated from the rectum, and the skin is incised posteriorly behind the mass so that the tumor can be removed intact. The major surgical complication is massive bleeding. In most children, anal and urinary sphincter functions are not impaired.

The success of therapy correlates most closely with the histologic type and the surgical resectability of the primary tumor. With few exceptions, patients with benign, resectable tumors survive with surgery alone. If local, benign recurrence takes place, reexcision can be curative. In contrast, fewer than 10% of children whose tumors have malignant components or who have surgically unresectable tumors survive.

MEDIASTINAL GERM CELL TUMORS. Mediastinal tumors are usually located in the anterior superior mediastinum, but they rarely can be located posteriorly. Occurrence in the mediastinum is related to the fact that the urogenital ridge in the embryo extends past C6 to L4. These tumors are often asymptomatic but may result in tracheobronchial compression hemoptysis or hormone production.

In boys, most lesions are endodermal sinus tumors, but pure and malignant-element teratomas have been described. Chest CT scanning is the imaging procedure of choice, and the differential diagnosis must include thymomas, thymic cysts, lymphomas, lymphangiomas, lipomas, bronchial and enteric cysts, and neurogenic tumors.

Most mediastinal germ cell tumors can be approached by a unilateral thoracotomy or a median sternotomy. Complete excision is necessary except for immature teratomas with neuroglial elements in young children; in older children, this can be highly malignant.

ABDOMINAL GERM CELL TUMORS. The primary sites of abdominal germ cell tumors are in the retroperitoneum, but they can involve the stomach, omentum, and liver. Patients may present with vague abdominal complaints or bleeding, and abdominal germ cell tumors must be differentiated from Wilms' tumor, neuroblastoma, lymphoma, or rhabdomyosarcoma.

HEAD AND NECK TUMORS. The oral cavity is the site of almost 6% of germ cell neoplasms. They are usually found at birth, and most are benign. Intracranial germ cell tumors account for 0.5% to 2% of brain tumors in children. They arise in the pineal area and can involve the suprasellar and infrasellar regions.

TESTICULAR TUMORS. Approximately 7% of germ cell tumors and 1% of all childhood cancers arise in the testes. About 77% of testicular tumors originate from germ cells; 25% of these are benign. The most common malignant germ cell tumors of the testes have been described as infantile adenocarcinoma of the testes, embryonal carcinoma, orchioblastoma, adenocarcinoma with clear cells, and embryonal adenocarcinoma. Unifying terms for these malignancies are endodermal sinus tumor or yolk sac tumor. Choriocarcinomas and seminomas are unusual in children; the youngest patient described being 8 years old. Although testicular tumors account for less than 1% of childhood tumors, they are much less common in American and African blacks and in Asians. An increased incidence of congenital anomalies, particularly of the genitourinary tract, is associated with patients with testicular germ cell tumors.

Most infants and young boys with cancer of the testes present with a painless mass that usually has been growing slowly for months. Almost all of these children, particularly those with endodermal sinus tumors, are younger than 2 years of age. Testicular tumors rarely occur in adolescents.

Almost 25% of infants with a malignant tumor have a hydrocele, making transillumination potentially misleading. Physical examination usually reveals a hard, painless testicular mass, 2 cm in diameter or larger, not involving the scrotal wall or spermatic cord. The possibility of distant spread, particularly to lymph nodes in the inguinal and supraclavicular regions and retroperitoneum, should be carefully assessed. The scrotum should be carefully examined for evidence of direct extension to the scrotal skin and to determine if the mass is in the testis or in a paratesticular site.

Although endodermal sinus tumors tend to remain confined to the testes for a relatively long period, early diagnosis is critical. The relative rarity of these tumors and a lack of awareness that testicular cancer can occur in infants makes delays in diagnosis of as long as 3 months common.

After a testicular mass is suspected, a biopsy should be done as soon as possible. An inguinal incision should be made, and the spermatic cord should be exposed and occluded at the internal abdominal ring with a noncrushing vascular clamp before manipulation of the testis. If a gross diagnosis of neoplasm can be made when the testis is delivered into the wound, radical orchiectomy is performed by ligating and dividing the spermatic cord at the internal ring and removing the mass with the entire cord. If the testicular mass is obviously benign (*e.g.*, hydrocele), appropriate treatment is provided and the testis is returned to the scrotum. If the diagnosis is uncertain, the testis is walled off with sponges and an incisional biopsy is performed. Frozen-section diagnosis is used to determine additional treatment. It is unnecessary to excise a portion of the scrotum unless the tumor has been previously biopsied in situ or if the extragonadal tissues are grossly involved. If retroperitoneal lymph node dissection is contemplated, placement of a nonabsorbable suture on the ligated spermatic cord aids in defining the distal end of the inguinal dissection during lymphadenectomy.

The physician must determine whether the tumor is restricted to the scrotum and, if not, whether the retroperitoneal lymph nodes or distant sites are involved. This dictates retroperitoneal node dissection, radiation, or chemotherapy. The major sites of metastases for testicular germ cell cancers are the lungs, liver, lymph nodes, and CNS.

A variety of staging systems are used, and in evaluating reports from different centers, the distinction between clinical staging and pathologic staging should be recognized, although they are usually the same for boys with this neoplasm.

Virtually all patients with embryonal adenocarcinoma of the testis and 90% of patients with nonseminomatous testicular tumors have elevated serum levels of hCG and AFP. Measurement of AFP and hCG before and after surgery, and then at least monthly, can assess tumor burden or recurrence.

Ultrasonography can help in defining testicular and adnexal masses. CT scans of the chest and abdomen and a bone scan are part of the metastatic workup, and MRI of the pelvis produces optimal visualizations of pelvic structures.

Retroperitoneal node dissection has been recommended for accurate pathologic staging of testicular tumors. For example, of adults with stage I embryonal carcinoma, 53% actually had stage II disease after retroperitoneal lymphadenectomy. However, for endodermal sinus tumor, the results of node dissection have been quite different. Positive nodes were found in only 4 of 53 node dissections in clinical stage I patients. Therefore, node dissection for staging purposes is useful only for those children in whom retroperitoneal node involvement is suspected by ultrasound, MRI, or CT scan or for patients without lung metastases in whom AFP of hCG remains elevated.

After radical orchiectomy and clinical staging are completed, further therapy, possibly including retroperitoneal node dissection, chemotherapy, and irradiation, is considered. Approximately 80% of children have stage I disease, and 20% have stage II or stage III disease.

The value of node dissection in the treatment of endodermal sinus tumor is not clear cut. Current data suggest that radical orchiectomy alone is comparable to orchiectomy plus retroperitoneal node dissection for children younger than 36 months of age with stage I embryonal carcinoma or endodermal sinus tumor. However, other data describe a cure rate (84%) after orchiectomy plus node dissection that is almost twice the cure rate after orchiectomy alone (48%). These discrepancies may be due to inclusion of older patients in the early studies, histologic differences in the study populations, and the fact that less radical orchiectomies are performed than in the past. On the basis of current data, retroperitoneal lymphadenectomy is not recommended for patients with stage I disease, particularly if serum markers are positive before surgery and fall at the expected rate after inguinal orchiectomy.

If retroperitoneal lymph nodes are the site of metastatic disease (stage II), lymphadenectomy appears to increase survival. Considerable controversy surrounds the value of bilateral or unilateral lymphadenectomy. The cross-communications between the lymphatic channels of the testes support the need for bilateral retroperitoneal node dissection, but few patients have had negative ipsilateral nodes and positive contralateral nodes. Survival figures for patients with germ cell neoplasms receiving unilateral or bilateral adenectomies were comparable. Unilateral dissection is recommended if no gross tumor is discovered. When ipsilateral nodes are grossly positive, bilateral adenectomy is advised, or a modified (superior aspect only) node dissection on the contralateral side can be performed, minimizing the possibility of retrograde ejaculation, a disturbing complication of bilateral adenectomy if both second lumbar sympathetic ganglia are excised. Although some reports raise doubts about the safety of this procedure in small children, experience indicates that retroperitoneal node dissection is well tolerated. A simple midline, paramedian, or transverse abdominal incision generally gives adequate exposure in children.

Approach to the Child With an Undescended Testicle. Although the incidence of an undescended testis is 0.23%, the risk for developing testicular cancer in these cases is 20 to 40 times that in a normal testis. Almost 20% of the tumors that occur in cryptorchid patients do so in the descended testis. This suggests that there may be a genetic predisposition to develop testicular cancer in patients with an undescended testis or that a basic defect in gonadogenesis accounts for failure of the testis to descend and for subsequent oncogenesis.

Tumors of all germ cell types can arise in cryptorchid testis and can occur in adulthood (median age, 38 years). However, seminomas appear to be more common in the undescended testis than in the scrotal testis.

There is debate about orchiopexy in the child with an undescended testis. Although it is clear that orchiopexy does not prevent the development of testicular cancer, especially because it can arise in the contralateral descended testis, it does make the testis more accessible for palpation and monitoring. Because these patients have a higher risk of developing cancer, periodic evaluation is important. If the diagnosis of a cryptorchid testis is not made until after puberty, when dysgenesis and atrophy are probable, orchiectomy is recommended.

OVARIAN TUMORS. Gynecologic malignancies are extremely rare in children and adolescents and differ in their clinical presentation and histology from those occurring in adults. Ovarian tumors are the most common, but only account for 1% of cancers in girls younger than 17 years of age; nonovarian malignant tumors are even less common. The peak incidence is between 10 and 14 years of age. Unlike the pattern in adults, approximately 90% of pediatric gynecologic tumors are immature, and only 10% are differentiated carcinomas.

The ovary descends from the abdomen into the bony pelvis during puberty, and in younger children and in most adolescents, an ovarian tumor presents as an abdominal mass. The longer infundibular pedicle in the child facilitates torsion of an enlarged ovary, resulting in abdominal pain. In the adolescent, abdominal pain can be due to endometriosis, a diagnosis that is frequently overlooked. Symptoms can include constipation or genitourinary complaints. Rarely, tumors may produce hCG and can mimic signs of pregnancy. Nonneoplastic cysts comprise 25% to 35% of the ovarian masses, of which half are follicular and half are simple, parovarian, or luteal. In an infant, an adnexal mass is likely to be a nonneoplastic cyst. Mesonephric duct cysts (*e.g.,* Gartner's duct cysts) and paramesonephric duct cysts can present as abdominal or pelvic masses. If associated with symptoms or if the cystic mass is larger than 4 cm, laparoscopy or laparotomy is indicated.

The remaining 65% to 75% of ovarian tumors are true neoplasms, of which 33% are malignant. Germ cell tumors account for 60% to 89% of the ovarian tumors in children and adolescents (compared with 20% in adults) and are more likely to be malignant in younger children and infants. With increasing age, tumors of the sex cord stroma (*e.g.,* granulosa-theca cell tumor, Sertoli-Leydig cell tumors) and tumors of common epithelial origin increase in frequency; in adolescents 15 to 17 years old, almost 33% of ovarian neoplasms are epithelial tumors. Most benign tumors occur in prepubertal patients, and most malignant tumors occur after 13 years of age.

A calcified ovarian mass is found in almost half of the patients, particularly those with benign teratomas. These can be demonstrated with pelvic ultrasound, and abdominal and chest CT scans should be performed to rule out evidence of metastatic disease. Levels of hCG can be elevated with embryonal carcinoma and choriocarcinoma, and AFP increases in patients with endodermal sinus tumor.

The staging for ovarian tumors in children is modified from the International Federation of Gynecology and Obstetrics:

Stage I   Disease is limited to one or both ovaries, with the capsule intact and peritoneal fluid negative for malignant cell.

Stage II   Disease includes or is beyond the ovarian capsule with local pelvic extension. Retroperitoneal nodes and peritoneal fluid are negative for malignant cells.

Stage III Positive retroperitoneal nodes or malignant cells are in the peritoneal fluid or abdominal extension.

Stage IV   Extraabdominal dissemination exists.

In children, the ovaries are in the abdomen, and if there are malignant ascites, they are classified as stage III disease.

Approaches to management are based on the patient's tumor type and extent.

Mature Cystic (Dermoid) or Solid Teratoma. These benign neoplasms account for approximately 40% of ovarian tumors and are the most common tumors in older adolescents. These tumors are frequently unilateral in children, but in adults, almost 25% are bilateral. Approximately 40% to 50% of mature teratomas are calcified, and diagnosis is usually suggested by a plain abdominal radiograph and ultrasonography. Malignant degeneration is rare in children. Therapy consists of oophorocystectomy with the preservation of as much ovarian tissue as possible. Oophorectomy is indicated only if there is torsion, rupture, or if the mass is so large that normal ovarian tissue cannot be reconstructed.

Immature Teratomas. Immature teratomas account for 7.4% of childhood ovarian neoplasms and most commonly occur around the age of 11 years. The tumors are composed of variable amounts of incompletely differentiated germ cell elements, most commonly of neural origin. Immature teratomas may not be clinically or grossly differentiated from benign cysts or solid teratomas, and scrupulous histologic examination is important. Teratomas containing immature elements can become malignant, and survival is closely correlated with stage. Approximately 50% of patients with immature teratomas have measurable levels of AFP. These tumors tend to be radioresistant, and treatment has included surgery (*i.e.,* salpingo-oophorectomy for unilateral lesions) and chemotherapy.

Dysgerminomas. Dysgerminomas comprise 16% of germ cell tumors. They are rare before the age of 10 and occur most frequently in prepubertal and young adolescent girls; almost 50% of these tumors occur before the age of 20. These tumors are usually surrounded by a dense capsule and may be bilateral in 5% to 10% of patients. Dysgerminomas are endocrinologically inactive; hormonal symptoms signal an undetected teratocarcinoma with chorioepitheliomatous elements. Dysgerminomas are generally considered low-grade malignancies, although spread may occur if the tumor extends through the capsule and involves lymph nodes or blood vessels.

Treatment planning should take into account that dysgerminomas are highly radiosensitive tumors. If the tumor is well encapsulated, a salpingo-oophorectomy is recommended and has been associated with a 96% survival. More advanced disease may require hysterectomy and bilateral oophorectomy. Wide-field, low-dose irradiation or chemotherapy (VAC or PVB) are indicated if the tumor has penetrated through the ovarian capsule. Better results may be attained with bleomycin, etoposide, and cisplatin (BEP). Disease has recurred 5 to 34 years after treatment.

Embryonal Cell Carcinoma. This carcinoma accounts for 6% of ovarian neoplasms, is highly malignant, and occurs primarily in girls 13 to 14 years of age. Almost 60% of these tumors are associated with endocrinologic manifestations, including precocious puberty, abnormal vaginal bleeding, and hirsutism. Both hCG and AFP are detectable in patients with this tumor. Because the survival for patients whose tumor has been completely resected, usually with salpingo-oophorectomy, is only 50%, adjuvant chemotherapy (VAC) is indicated.

Endodermal Sinus or Yolk Sac Tumors. Like embryonal cell carcinomas, yolk sac tumors are highly malignant germ cell tumors, primarily occurring in older adolescents. Elevated AFP is detectable in virtually all cases. The fact that fewer than 20% of patients with localized and completely resected tumors are curable with surgery alone is testimony to the malignant potential of these tumors. All patients, even those with completely resectable tumors, should receive adjuvant chemotherapy. Mixed germ cell tumors are infrequent and are treated according to the most malignant element present.

Mesenchymal Sex Cord Stromal Tumors. Stromal tumors account for approximately 13% of ovarian tumors in children. The granulosa-theca cell tumor is the most common type and most often presents with precocious pseudopuberty and an abdominal mass, particularly in premenarcheal girls. Postmenarcheal girls may present with menstrual abnormalities or with virilization. Unlike the typical thecal tumor in adults, the histologic picture in children consists of a diffuse or solid pattern with larger cells and prominent luteinization of cellular components; Call-Exner bodies and "coffee bean" nuclei are inconspicuous. This tumor follows a benign course in children and is usually effectively treated with a unilateral salpingo-oophorectomy. Sertoli cell tumor (*i.e.,* androblastoma) is extremely rare and is benign and effectively treated with a salpingo-oophorectomy.

Epithelial ovarian neoplasms are rarely found in premenarcheal girls, and even if they occur in adolescents, their malignant potential is less than in adults. Because of their rarity, specific therapeutic guidelines distinct from those used in adults are not defined.

CERVICAL AND VAGINAL TUMORS. Vaginal or cervical neoplasms are rare in children. In infants and young children, vaginal tumors are more likely to be rhabdomyosarcoma (botryoides variant) than carcinomas. However, with increasing age, evidence of cervical intraepithelial neoplasias has been observed with frequencies of up to 31 of 1000 female adolescents. The current recommendation is for sexually active adolescents to have PAP smears annually.

In the early 1970s, an increased frequency of clear cell adenocarcinoma was observed in young women whose mothers had received diethylstilbestrol (DES) in an attempt to prevent fetal wastage. Although the survival rate for women with clear cell adenocarcinomas is 80% to 90%, this is closely correlated with the extent and stage of disease at diagnosis, and in utero exposure to DES should be recognized as a significant risk factor. It is important to recognize that the incidence of vaginal adenosis and adenocarcinoma depends on the age of the fetus at the time of in utero exposure to DES and the dose and duration of DES treatment. As many as 20% to 90% of exposed girls can have vaginal adenosis, defined as mucinous columnar cells or metaplastic squamous cells, with or without mucinous droplets in the vaginal scrapings. Current recommendations call for all exposed girls to have pelvic examinations by an experienced gynecologist by the age of 14 or after menarche. This should include careful examination, cytologic samplings of the cervix and vagina, iodine staining of the vagina, and colposcopy and biopsy of suspicious lesions. Follow-up examinations should be performed annually. The treatment of clear cell sarcoma requires radical surgery, including vaginectomy, hysterectomy, and lymphatic resection.

RHABDOMYOSARCOMA

Rhabdomyosarcoma, arising from mesenchymal cells that initiate striated muscle differentiation, accounts for approximately 5% to 8% of all solid tumors in children. It is the most common soft tissue sarcoma in children younger than 15 years, with an annual incidence of 4.5 per million white children and 1.3 per million black children. Survival for children with rhabdomyosarcoma, like that for children with Wilms' tumor, has greatly improved since the incorporation of chemotherapy into treatment programs. With current multidisciplinary regimens, approximately two thirds of the patients are surviving 3 years from diagnosis.

Rhabdomyosarcoma can occur in infants, children, or adolescents, and because its presentations are varied, it should not be considered as a single entity. The extent of the tumor at diagnosis, its histology, and the primary site are each important factors for treatment planning and prognosis. During the last decade, many hundreds of patients have been entered into multi-institutional trials organized by the Intergroup Rhabdomyosarcoma Study (IRS), and much of our present understanding of the natural history, pathology, and treatment of rhabdomyosarcoma is derived from these studies.

EPIDEMIOLOGY AND GENETICS

Rhabdomyosarcoma appears to have two age peaks of occurrence, the first in children between 2 and 6 years of age and the second during adolescence, between 14 and 18 years. The early peak is primarily due to the occurrence of tumors in the head and neck region and the genitourinary tract. The late peak is predominately accounted for by primary tumors of the male genitourinary tract; tumors of the head and neck region, trunk, and extremity are common in this group. Orbital tumors occur at any age.

As with other pediatric malignancies, rhabdomyosarcoma has been associated with several congenital disorders, including neurofibromatosis, Gorlin's basal cell nevus syndrome, and the fetal alcohol syndrome. A few families have been described with an increased frequency of breast and other cancers in the relatives of children with rhabdomyosarcoma. This Li-Fraumeni syndrome has recently been associated with a germ line mutation in the p53 tumor suppressor gene located on chromosome 17. Other familial associations have been reported, including an excess incidence of rhabdomyosarcoma in the siblings of children with brain tumors and adrenal cortical carcinoma.

There has been work on the characterization of the molecular and cytogenetic lesions of rhabdomyosarcoma. Translocation t(2;13) (q37;q14) is a common finding in alveolar rhabdomyosarcoma, and a loss of heterogeneity on the short arm of chromosome 11 has been described. Work with human rhabdomyosarcoma cell lines led to the identification of intracellular peptides that modulate cell growth, the transforming growth factors and the insulin-like growth factor-2. The DNA content of rhabdomyosarcoma tumor cells is associated with histology; the prognosis associated with hyperdiploidy (usually found in embryonal tumors) is the best, that associated with near-tetraploid tumors (often alveolar) is intermediate, and the prognosis of diploid tumors is the worst.

Human rhabdomyosarcoma xenograft lines were grown in the flanks of immunosuppressed mice to investigate the mechanisms of resistance of rhabdomyosarcoma to cytotoxic chemotherapy. Vincristine resistance may be related to the production of an altered tubule subunit. The level of activity of a DNA repair enzyme correlates with the sensitivity of the rhabdomyosarcoma xenograft lines to the nitrosourea, methyl-CCNU. Human xenograft tumors have been invaluable for the rational development of new approaches to the treatment of rhabdomyosarcoma. The identification of melphalan as an active agent in the xenograft model has had its activity confirmed in phase II clinical studies.

PATHOLOGY

The head and neck are sites for approximately 38% of rhabdomyosarcomas, and the orbit is the most common single location. The next most common sites are the genitourinary tract (21%), extremities (18%), trunk (7%), and retroperitoneum (7%). The sites of primary involvement are related to the age of the child. Histologic subtype of rhabdomyosarcomas vary according to age and site.

Since the description in 1946 of rhabdomyosarcoma as a tumor of skeletal muscle, significant advances have been made in the histopathologic classification of this tumor and in correlating subtypes with clinical behavior and prognosis. Three major subtypes of rhabdomyosarcoma exist: embryonal, alveolar, and pleomorphic. The embryonal histologic subtype accounts for approximately 50% to 60% of childhood rhabdomyosarcoma and is characterized by variable numbers of large acidophilic myoblast cells and a large number of primitive round cells and spindle-shaped cells showing little myoblastic differentiation. The tumor stroma is usually loose and edematous. Compared with fetal tissue, the embryonal variant most closely resembles the developing muscle of a 1- to 7-week-old fetus. Although cross-striations can facilitate the diagnosis, they often are not visible by light microscopy. Sarcoma botryoides, although grossly differentiated by polypoid, edematous, and myxoid appearance, is histologically similar to embryonal rhabdomyosarcoma. The characteristic feature of the botryoides variant is the cambium layer of Nicholoson, a multilayered band of spindle cells with relatively little cytoplasm that lies parallel to and just below the mucosal surface of the tumor.

Alveolar rhabdomyosarcoma, the second most common subtype, is distinguished by a unique tissue pattern reminiscent of pulmonary alveoli. Tumor cells and giant multinucleated cells line septa and protrude into an open alveolar space. The alveolar subtype typically occurs in older children and young adults, is much more likely to occur in the extremities or perineal sites, is more likely to spread to the lymph nodes, and has a worse prognosis than the more common embryonal rhabdomyosarcoma.

Pleomorphic rhabdomyosarcoma is rarely seen in children and occurs primarily in adults 30 to 50 years old. It is a more differentiated tumor composed of haphazardly and compactly arranged spindle cells and multinucleated giant cells.

A pathologic classification was developed by the IRS. This classification divides tumors into favorable and unfavorable histologies by cytologic features rather than the tissue pattern. There are two unfavorable histologic categories. The first, called anaplastic, is similar to that described for Wilms' tumor and is characterized by the presence of enlarged, bizarre mitotic figures and diffuse nuclear hyperchromatism with pleomorphism. It can be found focally or diffusely throughout the tumor. The second, called monomorphous, is characterized by round cells of uniform size with constant cytologic features. Tumors that contain neither anaplastic nor monomorphic features are histologically favorable. Of 405 cases evaluated from the first IRS trial, 330 (81.5%) were categorized as favorable, and 75 (18.5%) were categorized as unfavorable. This histologic grading was used to evaluate the prognosis of 261 patients with localized rhabdomyosarcoma on the second IRS trial, and 89% of the 211 patients with favorable histologic subtypes survived, compared with 72% of those with unfavorable cytologic features. If the cytologic and tissue patterns are evaluated by light microscopy, a group of patients with a less favorable prognosis can be defined. Of 171 patients with completely resected rhabdomyosarcoma, 40 (23%) had unfavorable cytologic features or the alveolar subtype. The recurrence rate for these patients was 43%, compared with 15% for patients whose tumors did not have these unfavorable features. Analyses may permit the selection of patients who are at increased risk for tumor recurrence and who may profit from additional or more intensive therapy. However, the IRS criteria have not yet been fully validated.

An independent study at the National Cancer Institute (NCI) and St. Jude Children's Research Hospital evaluated the IRS cytologic criteria in conjunction with the classic histologic classification (*i.e.*, embryonal or alveolar) and other criteria (*e.g.*, solid variant of alveolar rhabdomyosarcoma) and demonstrated that the monomorphous or solid variant of alveolar rhabdomyosarcoma is associated with an aggressive clinical course, as is alveolar rhabdomyosarcoma of any cytologic type. Although various percentages of alveolar histologic features have been used by pathologists to diagnose "alveolar" rhabdomyosarcoma, it now is apparent that any amount confers a poor prognosis. Therefore, the "0% standard" is being used in IRS-III to diagnose alveolar rhabdomyosarcoma for the assignment of treatment. The current classification that is being used in IRS studies is presented in Table 49–22.

CLINICAL PRESENTATION

Rhabdomyosarcoma may occur at any body site containing striated muscle or its mesenchymal anlage. In infants, a frequent presentation is a grape-like, clustered polypoid vaginal mass, the botryoides variant of embryonal rhabdomyosarcoma. In young patients, the most common presentation is a mass in the head and neck region or genitourinary tract. In adolescence, rhabdomyosarcoma often presents as a painless extremity or truncal mass or as a nontender scrotal swelling

TABLE 49–22. IRS Staging Systems for Rhabdomyosarcoma

		Proposed Staging System for IRS-IV					
Clinical Grouping System		*Stage*	*Sites**	*Tumor Size*	*Lymph Nodes*	*Metastases*	*5-Year Progression-Free Survival (%)*
Group I	Localized disease, completely resected Regional nodes not involved A. Confined to muscle or organ of origin B. Contiguous involvement-infiltration outside the muscle or organ of origin, as through fascial planes	I	GU Non-BP, HN Non-PM, Orbits	a, b†	N0, N1	M0	73
Group II	Regional disease A. Grossly resected tumor with microscopic residual disease. No evidence of gross residual tumor. No clinical or microscopic evidence of regional node involvement B. Regional disease, completely resected (regional nodes involved completely resected with no microscopic residual) C. Regional disease with involved nodes, grossly resected, but with evidence of microscopic residual	II	All other	a	N0	M0	65
Group III	Incomplete resection or biopsy with gross residual disease	III	All other	b a, b	N0 N1	M0 M0	44
Group IV	Metastatic disease present at onset	IV	Any site	a, b	N0, N1	M1	20

* GU Non-BP, genitourinary, not bladder-prostate; HN Non-PM, head and neck non-parameningeal; N0, regional nodes not involved by tumor, N1, regional nodes involved by tumor; M0, no distant metastases, M1, distant metastases.
† a, ≤5 cm; b, >5 cm.
‡ Except clinical group I paratestis, clinical group I and II orbital.

that may be separate from the testis. Intraabdominal lymph node metastases, which occur in as many as 26% of patients with paratesticular rhabdomyosarcoma, may sometimes present as an abdominal mass. The only sites not recognized by the IRS as probable primary tumors are brain, bone, and lung.

Rhabdomyosarcoma may present as a tumor mass or it may be discovered coincidentally during the evaluation of more nonspecific clinical symptoms. For example, a retroperitoneal rhabdomyosarcoma may present as an abdominal mass, with or without ascites, or it may present as an acute abdomen mimicking acute appendicitis. Rhabdomyosarcoma of the biliary tract, which is usually the botryoides type, most frequently presents with asymptomatic, direct hyperbilirubinemia due to biliary obstruction, but it may present with symptoms of acute cholecystitis or "relapsing hepatitis."

Rhabdomyosarcoma is the most common malignancy involving the bladder, prostate, or vagina in children. The clinical presentation may be as an asymptomatic abdominal or perineal mass, with tumor encroachment or obstruction. Symptoms include increased frequency of urination, urinary retention, or hematuria.

Rhabdomyosarcoma is the most common nonocular orbital tumors in children, usually presenting with proptosis, but rarely with evidence of direct extension into the CNS, perhaps because of its early diagnosis or containment by the bony orbit. Tumors of the middle ear may present as a polypoid or botryoid mass associated with ear pain and chronic otitis media, as a hemorrhagic discharge from the ear canal, or with evidence of a cranial nerve palsy. Contiguous extension into the CNS by primary parameningeal rhabdomyosarcoma may result in cranial nerve palsies, increased intracranial pressure, and meningeal symptoms. Tumors of the nasopharynx can be subtle in their presentation, including airway obstruction, sinusitis, epistaxis, local pain, and dysphagia. The rich lymphatics of the nasopharynx contribute to contiguous and distant spread. The CNS is the most common site of invasion by nasopharyngeal rhabdomyosarcoma.

Rhabdomyosarcoma spreads by direct extension to contiguous structures, such as parameningeal extension to the CNS, or by lymphatic and hematogenous metastasis. The margins of the primary tumor are often indistinct because of its pseudocapsule and are difficult to define on physical examination and at surgery. The incidence of lymph node metastases varies according to primary site in most series. There appears to be a particularly high incidence of lymph node involvement associated with primary lesions of the genitourinary tract (20%), paratesticular region (26%), extremity, and perineum (10–17%), but the incidence of lymph node metastasis from other sites appears to be lower (*e.g.*, 4% in the orbit).

The most common sites of hematogenous spread are lungs, bone, bone marrow, and liver. Because this occurs at initial diagnosis in 10% to 20% of patients, pretreatment examination should include a careful evaluation of the extent of the primary tumor and a detailed investigation of potential metastatic sites. In addition to special radiographic studies of the primary site, patients should have a bone scan, chest CT scan, bilateral bone marrow biopsies, and aspirates. Patients with head and neck primaries should have a head CT scan and spinal fluid examination. An MR scan is useful for defining the extent of the primary lesion and its resectability.

STAGING

The staging system for rhabdomyosarcoma used most commonly is the IRS clinical-pathologic grouping system, which is based on the extent of the extirpative surgery, except in cases of distant dissemination (see Table 47–22). Although this has been a useful approach to directing treatment, it obviates analysis of the local characteristics of the tumor, such as size and invasiveness, and incorporates results of therapy (*e.g.*, extent of operative resection) in outcome analysis. The IRS Committee analyzed IRS-II patients retrospectively restaged using a presurgical system. They confirmed the validity of staging by the degree of involvement of contiguous organs or structures, tumor size larger than 5 cm, and the presence of metastatic disease. IRS-IV is evaluating a prospective TNM staging system.

TREATMENT

Treatment Planning

The therapeutic plan for patients with rhabdomyosarcoma is determined by the primary site of involvement, histologic classification, and the clinical group or stage. Certain primary sites, such as the orbit, parameningeal sites, vagina, and prostate, are usually best managed by an initial biopsy followed by primary irradiation and adjuvant chemotherapy. The management of limited trunk, extremity, and paratesticular lesions usually includes the removal of all gross disease followed by adjuvant chemotherapy with irradiation as needed.

Among patients with bladder or prostate lesions, the overall bladder salvage rate on the same IRS regimens has been approximately 35%, and the mortality rate has been 20% to 30%, which is higher than the mortality associated with standard primary surgical approaches. Primary uterine tumors usually affect older patients and apparently not very responsive to chemotherapy. Primary chemotherapy has achieved its goal in eliminating anterior pelvic exenteration for patients with vaginal tumors.

Because the prognosis and approach to management vary according to the primary tumor sites, the general principles of management are considered first and then applied to specific sites of disease.

Surgery

The efficacy of radiation therapy and chemotherapy has had a major impact on the surgical procedures now recommended for rhabdomyosarcoma. Before the development of these modalities, radical operations were the only means to achieve tumor control, and even with extensive and often disabling surgery, local recurrence rates were high and cure rates were low. Some limited surgical procedures are now adequate, and the timing and extent of these procedures are important for retaining high rates of survival and improving functional results.

The exact role of surgery varies with the location, size, and extent of the tumor at presentation. Surgical extirpation is indicated if removal of the primary tumor imposes no major functional disability or if excision of the primary tumor permits the elimination of postoperative irradiation by completely excising the tumor or permits a reduction in the dose without increasing functional deficit by eliminating all but microscopic disease. This approach is especially appropriate in the treatment of rhabdomyosarcoma of the extremity, for which group I and II tumors without lymph node metastases have a much better prognosis than group III tumors. However, patients with large, invasive extremity tumors without evidence of metastatic disease do poorly even after amputation.

If only partial tumor removal is possible, particularly if removal would result in significant long-term disability, initial surgery should be limited to biopsy, preferably with sampling of regional lymph nodes. This is especially true in the treatment of orbital tumors, for which biopsy followed by irradiation and chemotherapy has resulted in excellent long-term survival. Sampling of clinically uninvolved regional nodes is recommended for tumors of the genitourinary tract, paratesticular region, extremities, and perineum. Node groups with apparent involvement are biopsied regardless of the primary site, except for patients with stage IV disease.

Preoperative chemotherapy or radiation therapy to reduce the size of the tumor, followed by removal of the residual tumor at a second operation, is currently under evaluation in the treatment of genitourinary rhabdomyosarcomas. The goals of this approach are the preservation of bladder function and achievement of long-term survival.

Radiation Therapy

Reports in the 1960s established the efficacy of high-dose, wide-field irradiation to achieve local control of rhabdomyosarcomas in children. With megavoltage equipment, orbital rhabdomyosarcoma could be controlled in 90% of patients with appropriate doses and volumes of radiation therapy.

Local control was achieved in 96% of the 27 patients treated with conservative, function-preserving surgery plus combination chemotherapy and high-dose, large-volume radiation therapy, with doses of 5500 to 6500 cGy to the primary tumor site. This approach has been confirmed in many studies.

The IRS analyzed the role of radiation therapy in the local tumor control of 524 children with rhabdomyosarcoma and showed that radiation therapy was not required for patients whose primary tumor was totally excised and who had no microscopic residual disease (group I).

For more advanced disease, radiation therapy is important for local and regional disease control. Overall local tumor control in patients with local residual disease (stages II and III) is well documented in 75% to 90% of those treated with adequate irradiation and chemotherapy.

Both principles of treatment include wide volumes, using prechemotherapy or preoperative tumor extent to determine irradiation fields. Wide margins are important; 60% local of regional failure in parameningeal tumors are due primarily to inadequate irradiation volumes. Inclusion of regional lymph nodes with documented involvement is important; irradiation of clinically uninvolved nodes is controversial.

A local control rate of more than 95% can be achieved for microscopic disease (stage II) with 4000 cGy. For patients with "gross" or "bulky" disease (stage III), doses in excess of 4500 to 5500 cGy are required. Daily fractions of 150 to 180 cGy are effective and well tolerated.

In selected patients, brachytherapy may be of value. Particularly for pelvic tumors, the use of intracavitary irradiation may facilitate disease control with less damage to surrounding normal tissues. IRS-IV is evaluating hyperfractioned radiation therapy to learn whether it can improve local control of bulky lesions without increasing morbidity.

Chemotherapy

Before the routine use of systemic chemotherapy, the long-term survival for children with rhabdomyosarcoma was poor, and cure was largely restricted to a few favorable anatomic sites, such as the orbit. The utility of adjuvant chemotherapy in patients who had been rendered disease-free with surgery or radiation therapy has been convincingly demonstrated. The survival rate for patients receiving vincristine plus dactinomycin was 82%, compared with 47% for patients not receiving chemotherapy.

Many chemotherapeutic agents have single-agent activity in rhabdomyosarcoma (Table 47–23), although the most commonly used regimens include combinations of vincristine, dactinomycin, and cyclophosphamide. Refinements of the chemotherapy regimens for rhabdomyosarcoma have been generated by the IRS studies. Data accrued from the first of these cooperative trials (IRS-I) supported the following conclusions:

1. Adjuvant chemotherapy with vincristine, dactinomycin, and oral cyclophosphamide (VAC) eliminates the need for postoperative radiation therapy in patients whose tumors were totally excised and who had no evidence of residual microscopic disease (group I).
2. A two-drug regimen (vincristine plus dactinomycin) was as effective as three drugs (VAC) for patients with grossly resected but microscopic residual disease (group II) treated with irradiation.
3. Doxorubicin did not improve the outcome when added to pulse VAC (vincristine, dactinomycin, and intravenous cyclophosphamide) for patients with gross residual

TABLE 49–23. Response of Rhabdomyosarcoma to Single Agents

Drug	No. of Evaluable Patients	CR	PR	% CR + PR/ Total
Dactinomycin	14		6	43
Cyclophosphamide	26	2	11	42
Vincristine	42	3	10	31
Doxorubicin	40	2	11	33
Cisplatin	19	1	3	21
VP-16 (etoposide)	5		1	20
DTIC	9		2	22
Methotrexate	6	1	2	50
Melphalan (newly diagnosed)	13		10	77
Melphalan (recurrent)	13		2	8
Ifosfamide	8		2	25

CR, complete response (100% disappearance); PR, partial response (50–99% disappearance).

(group III) or disseminated (group IV) disease. However, doxorubicin was given at a relatively low dose intensity.

The relapse-free survival rates at 3 years were 82% to 84% for group I, 63% to 72% for group II, 54% to 61% for group III, and 17% to 23% for group IV patients (Table 49–24). Several conclusions were drawn from the data generated in IRS-II:

1. The chemotherapy regimen for group I patients could be simplified, because a two-drug regimen (vincristine plus dactinomycin) appeared as effective (83% 2-year relapse-free survival) as the three-drug VAC regimen (87% 2-year relapse-free survival).
2. A moderately more intensive regimen of vincristine and dactinomycin was as good as or better (81% 2-year relapse-free survival) than a pulse VAC regimen of vincristine, dactinomycin, and intravenous cyclophosphamide (70% 2-year relapse-free survival) for group II patients, all of whom had postoperative irradiation.
3. Treatment of groups III and IV patients remains a problem. In this trial, the addition of doxorubicin to the VAC regimen did not result in a major improvement in survival. The preliminary results for group IV patients showed the 3-year survival in IRS-II to be 32%, compared with 17% to 23% in IRS-I.

IRS-III, which investigated the contribution of cisplatin and etoposide to the therapeutic regimen, is complete and is being analyzed. IRS-IV is comparing VAC with vincristine, dactinomycin, and ifosfamide (VAI) and vincristine, ifosfamide, and etoposide (VIE) in patients with stage II and III disease. Stage IV patients are treated with new pairs of drugs in an upfront phase II "window." The pairs include ifosfamide and doxorubicin, ifosfamide and etoposide, and vincristine and melphalan.

For patients with advanced disease, new approaches to treatment are being explored. The most prominent are new drugs, such as cisplatin, VP-16, and DTIC, added to the current chemotherapy regimen of vincristine, dactinomycin, cyclophosphamide, and doxorubicin, and the intensification of chemotherapy, particularly doxorubicin and cyclophosphamide, with or without total-body irradiation and autologous bone marrow rescue. General conclusions from the St. Jude Children's Research Hospital study of preirradiation chemotherapy in the treatment of rhabdomyosarcoma are that the approach does not jeopardize overall survival and does allow the assessment of chemotherapy response independently. Those patients with chemotherapy-resistant tumors were unlikely to be locally controlled with irradiation. This identifies subsets of patients who may be approached with experimental techniques, such as hyperfractionation or brachytherapy.

Analysis of many studies suggests that many of the patients who are disease-free at 2 years will remain in remission. However, if relapse occurs, the long-term survival rate is poor (2%), emphasizing the need to maximize primary treatment regimens and to develop better salvage protocols.

Management of Specific Tumors

HEAD AND NECK PRIMARY TUMORS. Embryonal tumors (78%) predominate in the head and neck region, including the botryoid variant in the pharynx, larynx, maxillary sinus, and middle ear. Alveolar tumors are found in 9.5% of cases; extraosseous Ewing's sarcoma is found in 2.5%; and 10% are undifferentiated.

Before the routine use of chemotherapy and adequate irradiation, the long-term survival of patients with head and neck primaries was poor (9–15%), with metastases occurring by the hematogenous and lymphatic routes. After combined modality therapy, the 3-year disease-free survival for patients with rhabdomyosarcoma of the head and neck region (groups I–III) rose to 66%.

Despite these improvements, the potential long-term complications of therapy are of concern because the mean age of children with head or neck rhabdomyosarcoma is less than 10 years. The use of high-dose local radiation therapy and prophylactic whole-brain irradiation can cause major complications for these children, and the facial, dental, mucosal, and endocrine complications of high-dose radiation therapy, especially if administered with chemotherapy, are well known.

EYE AND ORBIT TUMORS. The orbit is the most common site for rhabdomyosarcomas of the head and neck region, accounting for approximately 25% of these tumors. Since the institution of multimodality therapy for orbital rhabdomyosarcomas, 91% of patients are disease-free at 3 years. Orbital tumors are usually confined to the orbit and surrounding structures and rarely metastasize to distant sites, local nodes, or the CNS if properly irradiated. Although most orbital tumors are only biopsied and are classified as group III tumors, orbital exenteration is unnecessary because of the efficacy of radiation therapy and chemotherapy, except for local recurrence after conventional therapy.

TABLE 49–24. Actuarial Survival at Three Years: Results of The Intergroup Rhabdomyosarcoma Studies I and II

Prognostic Factors	IRS-I	IRS-II
Clinical Group		
I	79	88
II	68	77
III	42	68
IV	18	32
Histologic Type		
Embryonal		69
Alveolar		56
Other		66
Primary Site		
Orbit	91	93
Genitourinary (GU)	74	
GU (mainly group III)		64
Cranial parameningeal	53	71
Other head or neck	59	69
Trunk	53	57
Extremity	53	56
Retroperitoneum-pelvis	39	46
Total	686	956

Whether radiation should be administered before or in conjunction with systemic chemotherapy is controversial. The IRS protocols used simultaneous therapy. The total radiation dose is comparable to that prescribed for other sites, and the minimal volume usually includes the entire bony limits of the orbit. For treatment of limited disease, this field usually extends from the supraorbital ridge superiorly, to the infraoptic foramen interiorly, and across the midline to the inner canthus of the opposite eye. To avoid chronic keratoconjunctivitis, radiation therapy should be delivered with the eyelids open. Because the preauricular and upper cervical nodes appear to be negative in most cases, their inclusion in the irradiated field is unnecessary.

Adjuvant chemotherapy is necessary for all patients with orbital rhabdomyosarcoma. Treatment with radiation alone results in hematogenous metastases in approximately 33% of the patients. The most common therapy uses vincristine plus dactinomycin.

Ninety percent of the children whose orbits have been irradiated for rhabdomyosarcoma developed evidence of a cataract 1 to 4 years after completion of therapy. Enophthalmos, stenosis of the lacrimal duct, keratoconjunctivitis, photophobia, or conjunctivitis were seen in 20% of these patients. Secondary surgery was necessary in approximately 33% of these patients to improve functional results after radiation therapy; enucleation was required in 8% of patients.

PARAMENINGEAL RHABDOMYOSARCOMA. The parameningeal sites include the middle ear, auditory canal, mastoid, nasal cavity, paranasal sinuses, pharynx, pterygopalatine fossa, and the infratemporal fossa. Patients with parameningeal tumors who were enrolled in the IRS-I protocol had a significantly lower 3-year relapse-free survival rate (46%) than those with other head and neck primaries. The reason for treatment failure in 35% of these patients was tumor invasion into the CNS. None of the patients who developed this pattern of relapse survived. Detailed analysis of these patients suggested that these local treatment failures were probably a reflection of inadequate radiation dose (*i.e.*, 13 of 19 patients received <5000 cGy) and volume (*e.g.*, 11 of 19 patients had less than adequate volume). After using adequate treatment fields and doses of more than 5000 cGy, parameningeal tumor extension occurred in less than 5% of the patients. Rhabdomyosarcoma arising in a parameningeal site has a propensity for contiguous extension into the CNS, but radiation ports that include potential extension sites control the tumor in many patients. Current treatment planning includes higher radiation doses and more carefully planned radiation ports based on extensive imaging studies before chemotherapy. These modifications have produced a significant reduction in local failures and CNS extension in patients with primary parameningeal rhabdomyosarcoma. Intrathecal chemotherapy for patients with parameningeal disease is probably unnecessary if the radiation ports are adequate, and it has been eliminated from IRS-IV.

OTHER HEAD AND NECK TUMORS. Rhabdomyosarcoma can arise in the scalp, neck, parotid, oropharynx, larynx, or cheek. Surgical resection with margins that are sufficient to eliminate the need for radiation therapy are rarely possible without unacceptable functional or cosmetic consequences.

Primary radiation and chemotherapy form the cornerstone of management for these patients. Of 36 patients with primaries in these areas (groups I–III), 27 (75%) have remained disease-free for 3 or more years after therapy. Four of 5 failures received no irradiation or less than 1500 cGy. Only 2 of 37 patients with nonorbital, nonparameningeal primaries of the head (excluding the neck) on IRS-I relapsed.

PRIMARY TUMORS OF THE TRUNK. The trunk is the primary site in 7% to 9% of patients. The prognosis for this group, influenced by the type, extent, and location of the tumor at diagnosis, is not as favorable as that for patients with head and neck primaries. Of 30 patients, 14 tumors occurred on the chest wall, 10 were paraspinal, and 6 were on the abdominal wall; 15 of the 30 patients remained disease free at 5+ years. The prognosis appeared to be best for patients with paraspinal tumors (7 of 10 surviving disease free) and poorest for those with chest wall tumors (5 of 15 survived disease free). Only 3 of 12 patients with alveolar tumors have remained disease free, in contrast to 12 of 18 patients with nonalveolar tumors. Of 18 patients with retroperitoneal tumors treated with multimodality therapy, 14 had a greater than 50% tumor response; however, only 4 remained alive and free of active tumor.

Patients with localized tumors of the trunk (groups I and II) fare better (9 of 14 surviving disease free) than those with extensive local or disseminated tumor at diagnosis (6 of 16 disease-free survivors). Because of the poorer prognosis for patients with gross residual disease, complete surgical removal of the tumor is recommended and should be possible in many of these patients without unacceptable consequences. Such procedures are frequently recognized as incomplete, because microscopic residual disease is found in the detailed examination of the specimen. If the tumor is completely excised with adequate margins and there is no microscopic disease, postoperative irradiation is unnecessary. Use of electron-beam irradiation and interstitial techniques and the judicious use of photon irradiation to minimize normal tissue damage are particularly important. Because the major reason for failure in this group is distant dissemination, adjuvant chemotherapy is essential.

PRIMARY TUMORS OF THE EXTREMITY. Approximately 16% of rhabdomyosarcomas occur in the extremities. In contrast to tumors of the head and neck region, rhabdomyosarcoma of the extremity is more common in adolescents, is associated with a high incidence of relapse, and has a low survival rate. Early studies suggested that upper-extremity and distal lesions had a better prognosis than lower-extremity and proximal lesions, an observation that is supported in the IRS-I study, in which 44% of patients with lower-extremity lesions relapsed, compared with 30% of those with upper-extremity disease.

Rhabdomyosarcoma of the extremity is distinct in two important ways: the high incidence of alveolar cells (44% versus 16% for all other sites) and the high incidence of lymph node metastasis (17% versus none for orbit lesions and 3% for head and neck primaries). The importance of histologic types is reflected in the higher relapse rate (65%) for patients with stage I or II disease whose extremity tumors were alveolar, compared with 33% for patients with nonalveolar tumors, although their initial response rates were similar.

Although wide surgical resection should be performed if it can be accomplished without causing a major functional defect, amputation, especially of the upper extremity, is rarely required. Delayed amputation may be necessary if significant uncorrectable growth discrepancy occurs in the lower extremity after cure of the lesion. Because of the high incidence of regional lymphatic spread, a lymph node biopsy is recommended. The radiation guidelines are similar to those for other sites, although care must be taken to avoid circumferential irradiation with its attendant risk of long-term vascular and lymphatic complications.

The major problem in the treatment of patients with alveolar rhabdomyosarcoma continues to be the failure to control systemic disease. Current regimens for patients with extremity lesions use more intensive chemotherapy schedules.

PRIMARY TUMORS OF THE GENITOURINARY SYSTEM. The genitourinary tract is the primary site of approximately 20% of rhabdomyosarcomas. The principal genitourinary sites are the prostate, bladder, vagina, and paratesticular tissues. The overall survival was 70% to 75% for patients with genitourinary primaries. The overall survival of patients with genitourinary tumors is related to stage; relapse rate is 19% for patients with localized, grossly resected bladder and prostate tumors, compared with 39% for patients with group III or IV disease at diagnosis. The most common histologic type is embryonal; the botryoid variant occurs frequently in these sites. Lymph node metastases are common but site specific. For example, 26% of patients with paratesticular primaries have paraaortic node involvement, compared with a lower incidence for vaginal primaries. The role of retroperitoneal node dissection is an area of controversy, particularly in view of its long-term complications. It is generally recommended that regional nodes be sampled, especially in patients with paratesticular primaries, and if they are positive, patients should receive radiation therapy to that region.

Although the survival of patients with tumors at these sites has improved markedly with the addition of combination chemotherapy to pelvic surgery and radiation therapy, the long-term sequelae of these therapies in young children are significant. The use of primary chemotherapy (*i.e.*, pharmacologic debulking) followed by limited surgery and irradiation has been evaluated for treatment of the primary tumors of the genitourinary tract. This sequencing has eliminated anterior pelvic exenteration for many children with vaginal tumors. Among patients with localized bladder or prostate lesions, the overall bladder salvage rate on the IRS regimens has been approximately 35%; the mortality rates of 20% to 30% with attempted bladder salvage seems higher than that associated with standard primary exenteration approaches. Primary uterine tumors are a distinct group (older age) and apparently not very responsive.

Radiation therapy seeks to include the pelvic disease with maximal sparing of the femoral heads, acetabulum, and bowel. Coordination of radiation with cyclophosphamide is important to minimize short-term and long-term bladder complications. Mesna administered with cyclophosphamide is usually successful in preventing hemorrhagic cystitis even if the bladder is irradiated. Rotational and multiple-field techniques should

be used. Brachytherapy may be possible in selected cases. Dose and volume considerations are comparable to other sites. If paraaortic node biopsies and lymphangiogram are negative, irradiation of these regional nodes may be omitted. If positive, the lymph nodes should be included in the radiation fields.

EWING'S SARCOMA AND PERIPHERAL PRIMITIVE NEUROECTODERMAL TUMOR

In 1921, James Ewing described a vascular, hemorrhagic bone tumor composed of small, round cells without associated osteoid formation that usually occurred in the midshaft of the long bones or in the flat bones of the trunk. Although Ewing's sarcoma, the second most common primary bone tumor of childhood, was originally thought to arise from the endothelial cell, recent evidence suggests that it is derived from primitive neural tissue. Molecular and cytogenetic studies of this tumor produced important clues regarding the molecular pathogenesis of this disease. Multimodality therapy has increased the proportion of long-term disease-free survivors from less than 15% to more than 50% during the past 20 to 30 years.

EPIDEMIOLOGY AND BIOLOGY

Ewing's sarcoma occurs most frequently in the second decade of life and is rare before 5 or after 30 years of age (Fig. 49–9). The incidence in males is equal to that in females until age 13 years, when, as with osteosarcoma, males predominate. As with osteosarcoma, epidemiologic studies demonstrate that

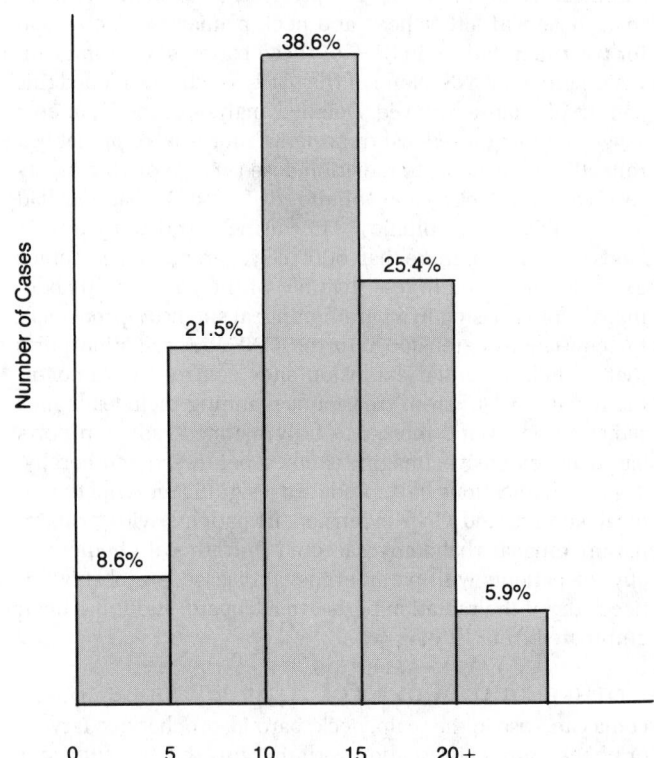

FIGURE 49–9. Age distribution of 303 patients with Ewing's bone sarcoma in the Intergroup Ewing's Sarcoma Study.

taller persons are more likely to develop Ewing's sarcoma, suggesting that its development is in some way linked to growth.

The annual incidence of Ewing's sarcoma in the United States is 1.7 cases per million white children younger than 15 years of age. A striking epidemiologic finding is the exceedingly low incidence of Ewing's sarcoma in African and American blacks and Chinese. Ewing's sarcoma has not been associated with congenital syndromes, but an association with skeletal anomalies (*i.e.,* enchondroma, aneurysmal bone cyst) and genitourinary anomalies (*i.e.,* hypospadias, duplication of the renal collecting system) has been reported. Ewing's sarcoma has been associated with retinoblastoma.

A chromosomal translocation, t(11:22), is a characteristic abnormality of Ewing's sarcoma. In a series of 13 karyotyped tumors, 9 demonstrated this translocation and two others contained a deletion on chromosome 22. The translocation is indistinguishable from that reported in peripheral neuroepithelioma by Whang-Peng and colleagues, suggesting that these entities have a common histogenesis. This is further supported by the demonstration of neuroectoderm-associated antigens on Ewing's cell lines in culture and identical patterns of protooncogene expression as seen in peripheral neuroepithelioma. Because of this realization tumors that once would have been diagnosed as Ewing's sarcoma are now often designated as peripheral neuroepithelioma or synonymously peripheral primitive neuroectodermal tumors (PPNET) based on any hint of neural differentiation at light or electron microscopic levels. For this reason, Ewing's sarcoma and PPNET are discussed together in this section. Table 49–25 compares the biologic features of Ewing's sarcoma and PPNET with neuroblastoma.

PATHOLOGY

Ewing's sarcoma is an undifferentiated round cell tumor possessing no unique morphologic markers. It is diagnosed only after the exclusion of the other small, round, blue cell tumors of childhood, which include primary sarcoma of bone (including small cell osteosarcoma and mesenchymal and myxoid chondrosarcoma), primitive sarcoma of bone, rhabdomyosarcoma, lymphoma, neuroblastoma, and peripheral neuroepithelioma. Refinements in electron microscopic, immunocytochemical, cytogenetic, and molecular genetic techniques have increased the sensitivity with which these tumors can be identified, consequently shrinking the numbers of cases left in the Ewing's "waste basket."

Biopsy should ensure that adequate tissue is obtained for these special studies. Tissue for electron microscopy is best fixed in glutaraldehyde and in alcohol for immunocytochemistry. The core-needle biopsy may compromise an accurate diagnosis, but a fine-needle aspirate is not acceptable as the sole biopsy sample.

By light microscopy, Ewing's sarcoma is a diffuse mass of homogenous tumor cells. There is often a biphasic population, with larger, clear cells and smaller, darker cells. Marked vascularity and widespread coagulative necrosis are typical features. The tumor infiltrates bone with surprisingly little destruction. Tumor margins are usually infiltrative or "pushing." A filigree pattern in which finger-like processes of compact, basophilic cells intertwine correlates with poorer survival.

The cells of Ewing's sarcoma are approximately the size of histiocytes, two to three times the size of a small lymphocyte, and have a centrally placed ellipsoid or spherical nucleus with a delicate nuclear membrane. The nuclear chromatin is usu-

TABLE 49–25. Comparison of Peripheral Neuroectodermal Tumors With Neuroblastoma and Ewing's Sarcoma

Variable	Neuroblastoma	PNET	Ewing's Sarcoma
Clinical Presentation			
Age	<4	Adolescence	Adolescence
Site	Abdominal	Thoracic, extremity, pelvis	Thoracic, extremity, pelvis
Biologic Markers			
Cytologic features of neural differentiation	+	±	−
EM features of neural differentiation	+	±	−
Neurotransmitters	Adrenergic	Cholinergic	Cholinergic
Surface HLA expression	−	+	+
Cytogenetic Characteristics			
Chromosomal translocation	−	t(11;22)(q24;q11–12)	t(11;22)(q24;q11–12)
Gene amplification	+	−	−
Oncogene Expression			
MYCN	+	−	−
MYC	−	+	+

(Israel MA, Miser JS, Triche TJ, et al. Neuroepithelial tumors. In: Pizzo PA, Poplack DG, eds. Principles and practice of pediatric oncology. Philadelphia: JB Lippincott, 1989:629)

ally faintly stippled, and the nucleoli are inconspicuous. The cytoplasm of Ewing's sarcoma is devoid of organelles, but cytoplasmic glycogen is usually demonstrable by electron microscopy or the PAS stain with light microscopy. A large cell variant consisting of larger, more pleomorphic cells with conspicuous nucleoli demonstrates the same clinical behavior as typical Ewing's sarcoma. An unusual pattern of intramyofiber skeletal muscle invasion by tumor cells seen in a few patients is a negative prognostic factor.

Like neuroblastoma and Ewing's sarcoma, PPNET are highly cellular and consist of a monotonous pattern of primitive-appearing round cells, most of which lack any evidence of neural differentiation. Electron microscopy may reveal evidence of dense core granules, neurites, neurotubules, and neurofilaments in prominent Golgi's apparatus. Immunocytochemical staining is often positive for neuron-specific enolase.

Ewing's sarcoma is a diagnosis of exclusion that is made with decreasing frequency by pathologists who, using electron microscopy and immunocytochemistry, diligently search for clues to a tumor's histogenesis. This can be a source of frustration for the oncologist who must determine treatment for patients with tumors that have limited "history," such as primitive sarcomas of bone and peripheral neuroepithelioma. A rational approach is to treat the Ewing's family of tumors in a uniform manner until there are data to indicate that specific subsets have biologic and clinical differences that warrant a unique approach.

NATURAL HISTORY AND EVALUATION

Although Ewing's sarcoma most commonly presents in the femur and bones of the pelvis, it can affect any bone. Unlike osteosarcoma, it often originates in the axial skeleton. Table 49–26 lists the distribution and frequency of primary sites of

TABLE 49–26. Distribution of Primary Sites in Ewing's Sarcoma

Primary Site	Frequency (%)	
Pelvis/sacrum	20.5	
Pelvis		17.2
Sacrum		3.3
Proximal extremity	31.4	
Humerus		10.6
Femur		20.8
Distal extremity	27.1	
Tibia		10.6
Fibula		12.2
Radius + ulna		2.0
Hands + feet		2.3
Other	14.1	
Rib		6.9
Vertebrae		4.9
Skull/face		2.8
Scapula		4.0
Clavicle		1.7
Other		0.7

patients enrolled in the first Intergroup Ewing's Sarcoma Study.

Most patients with Ewing's sarcoma seek medical attention because of pain and swelling of the affected bone or region. Systemic symptoms, such as fatigue, weight loss, and intermittent fever, may be present, especially in patients with metastatic disease. The duration of symptoms before presentation may be measured in weeks or months and is often prolonged in patients who have primary sites in the axial skeleton. When intratumor hemorrhage and necrosis occur, the tumor can become fluctuant, erythematous, and warm, mimicking infection. Frequently the entire medullary cavity of the affected bone is involved with the tumor (Table 49–27).

Extension through the bony cortex and into the soft tissues often results in a large soft tissue mass that, particularly with axial lesions, may be larger than the intraosseous component (Fig. 49–10).

Less common presentations of Ewing's sarcoma include primary rib tumor associated with a pleural effusion and respiratory symptoms, mandibular lesions presenting with chin and lip parasthenias, primary vertebral tumor with symptoms of nerve root or spinal cord compression, and sacral primary with neurogenic bladder.

The chest wall is the most common site for PPNET. The trunk, abdomen, and pelvis are other primary sites. PPNET usually present as sometimes painful masses, and when invading the chest wall, they are often associated with a malignant pleural effusion. If the tumor involves the paraspinal region, extension into the spinal cord must be considered. PPNET arising in the extremities or pelvis are similar to Ewing's sarcoma, with bony involvement of a soft tissue mass and pain.

The incidence of metastatic disease at the time of presentation in patients with Ewing's sarcoma or PPNET ranges from 14% to 50%, depending on the thoroughness of the metastatic workup and the referral base of the reporting institutions. Metastasis is predominantly hematogenous, although lymph node involvement may occur. The lung is the most common site of metastatic disease at presentation and the most frequent site of initial relapse. CNS involvement is detected in fewer than 1% of patients and is the site of first relapse in fewer than 5% of patients. More commonly, the CNS is involved as a result of direct intracranial or intraspinal extension of bony metastatic disease.

The importance of the initial diagnostic biopsy in a patient with a suspected Ewing's sarcoma should be emphasized. The soft tissue component of the tumor is often viable and yields a better specimen than the frequently necrotic intramedullary component of the tumor. Electron microscopy and immunocytochemistry must be employed for an accurate diagnosis. The surgical or pediatric oncologist should tell the pathologist the suspected diagnosis before surgery. Improper placement of the initial biopsy may obviate subsequent limb-sparing surgery.

The diagnostic evaluation should include a CT scan of the primary tumor and lungs. The use of MRI complements the CT scan in defining the primary tumor. Experience with this technology suggests that it may be overly sensitive, exaggerating the size of the lesion, resulting in overly generous radiation ports. Until experience with MRI accumulates, it should not replace the CT. A radionuclide bone scan is essen-

TABLE 49–27. Typical Radiographic Characteristics of Bone Tumors

Feature	Osteosarcoma	Ewing's Sarcoma
Location in bone	Metaphyseal	Diaphyseal
Involvement of long bones	Yes	Yes
Involvement of flat bones	Rare	Yes
Diffuse medullary cavity involvement	Rare	Common ("moth-eaten" or permeative involvement)
New bone formation	Yes	No—only as secondary phenomenon
Periosteal reaction	Yes ("Codman's triangle") or spiculation	Yes ("onionskin" appearance)
	Not prominent but may be present	Yes

tial to find bony metastases. The bone marrow should be assessed with a bone aspirate and biopsy. In the event of a pelvic lesion, bone marrow distant from the primary site must be sampled to determine if there has been dissemination. Although there is no specific serum marker for Ewing's sarcoma, lactate dehydrogenase is frequently elevated in those with more advanced disease, which has negative prognostic implications.

There is no uniformly accepted staging system for Ewing's sarcoma. A system based on a TNM concept is more appropriate for this disease than a system based on the extent of disease after a surgical procedure, because the approach to the local control of this tumor is rarely surgical. Experience suggests that the size of the lesion has prognostic importance. In several studies, the prognosis of those with lesions less than 5 to 10 cm in the maximal diameter was better than for those with larger tumors. Node involvement (N) is rare. The

presence of metastatic disease (M) dramatically reduces the likelihood of survival.

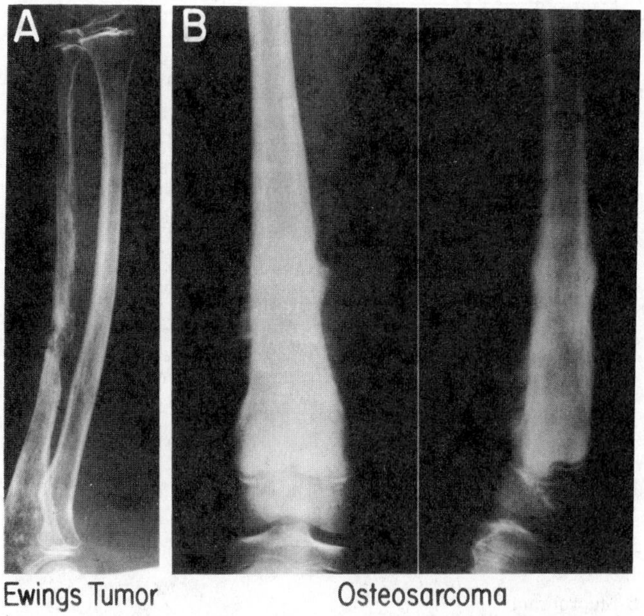

The most favorable prognostic factors are a distal primary tumor, normal serum lactate dehydrogenase, and absence of metastatic disease at presentation. Pelvic and sacral sites for primary tumors and metastatic disease are the least favorable factors. A partial or complete response to initial chemotherapy is a strong predictor of long-term disease control.

TREATMENT

Every patient with Ewing's sarcoma or PPNET should be treated with curative intent. Even patients with widely metastatic disease can, if not cured, have excellent responses to therapy, which may translate into years of disease control. Successful treatment requires close coordination among the surgeon, chemotherapist, and radiotherapist to ensure the most effective approach to controlling the primary lesion and the inevitable dissemination of the tumor.

Surgery

With surgical therapy alone, the long-term survival rates of patients in most early series were less than 10%, with failure usually caused by distant metastatic disease. The success of adjuvant chemotherapy in preventing distant failure in patients with Ewing's sarcoma and the effectiveness of radiation therapy in controlling the primary site of disease have resulted in abandoning surgery as the sole primary modality of therapy. Before improved irradiation equipment, patients whose initial treatment included surgery lived longer than patients who did not have surgery. A retrospective analysis revealed that 57 of the 334 patients had partial or complete resection of the tumor, and patients whose tumors had been resected lived longer than those who did not have surgery. Although these data must be cautiously evaluated for their potential selection bias, they do suggest that the role of surgery in the primary management of Ewing's sarcoma deserves evaluation. Balanced against this is the excellent local control attained with megavoltage irradiation and the low frequency of therapy-induced functional deficits if careful treatment planning was used. There are, however, no controlled data that compare the advantages and disadvantages of surgery and irradiation for the primary treatment of Ewing's sarcoma.

The indications for primary surgical resection of Ewing's

Ewings Tumor   Osteosarcoma

FIGURE 49–10. Radiographs of typical osteosarcoma and Ewing's tumor. **(A)** Ewing's tumor of the ulna. Notice the diaphyseal involvement with no tumor-related new bone and extensive permeative appearance. **(B)** Classic osteosarcoma of the femur in frontal and lateral projections. Typical metaphyseal location, new bone formation, lack of permeation, Codman's triangle, and spiculation are evident.

sarcoma used at some institutions include a lesion in an expendable bone, such as the rib, clavicle, fibula, or individual bones of the feet. Surgery usually follows initial chemotherapy, which can be expected to significantly debulk the lesion. Amputation may be indicated if there is an unmanageable pathologic fracture, but many of fractures heal during initial chemotherapy, allowing subsequent irradiation. If the tumor arises at or below the knee in a young child (<6 years) and a major uncorrectable functional deformity is expected from radiation therapy, amputation or limb-sparing surgery with an expandable prosthesis should be considered.

The two goals of therapy, local and distant tumor control and preservation of function, guide the management of an individual lesion. If a major functional loss, such as sacrifice of the peroneal nerve in resection of a fibular lesion, is likely to result from surgery, irradiation is usually preferred.

Radiation Therapy

James Ewing initially described the tumor's susceptibility to radium. It has since been recognized that this tumor is highly responsive to radiation therapy. Before the availability of chemotherapy, local control of Ewing's sarcoma was attained in 44% to 86% of patients with radiation doses greater than 4000 to 5000 cGy, even though long-term survival was low (16–25%).

With the addition of effective chemotherapy and local irradiation, local recurrence of Ewing's sarcoma is approximately 10% for distal extremity lesions and 20% to 40% for patients with proximal extremity or pelvis primaries. Coordinated therapy has increased the control of microscopic systemic disease and markedly increased survival. In a report of 193 patients treated on the first Intergroup Ewing's Sarcoma Study, the overall local control rate was 90%, and the survival had increased to 56% at 3+ years. These results have been corroborated in other studies.

Local control with primary irradiation and chemotherapy appears to depend on tumor size. Failure occurred in 2 of 20 patients with lesions less than 8 cm in diameter, compared with 9 of 30 patients with larger primary tumors. Disease-free survival rates differed even more: 72% of patients with lesions smaller than 8 cm at 5 years and 22% of patients with larger lesions. Local failures with pelvic primary tumors were only 8% for lesions less than 5 cm, compared with 17% for larger lesions. There are significant differences in local control and survival with lesions with volumes greater or smaller than 100 ml.

Radiation therapy is the primary mode of therapy for most local lesions. In conjunction with chemotherapy, doses of more than 5000 to 5500 cGy achieve tumor control in 80% to 85% of patients. Overall survival and local control have been improved by adding chemotherapy to irradiation.

To maintain function, a meticulous radiation technique is required. Necessary technical aspects include megavoltage apparatus, immobilization techniques for daily reproduction, and the use of beam-modifying devices, including compensators, wedge filters, and individually constructed blocks. Appropriate treatment of an extremity lesion includes the preservation of an unirradiated strip of skin and soft tissue to prevent late lymphedema and contractures. With the use of moderate-dose radiation therapy and systemic chemotherapy,

the functional results achieved in 29 patients who survived 2 years showed that only 18% of the patients had a severe functional deficit if doses of 5000 cGy were combined with chemotherapy.

Second cancers occur in the radiation field in 3% to 18% of patients. The incidence appears to be related to total radiation dose, to radiation energy (orthovoltage), and to the use of chemotherapy.

Integrated Radiation Therapy and Chemotherapy

Current treatment protocols for Ewing's sarcoma often begin with three to five cycles of chemotherapy before irradiation. This allows for the assessment of the response to chemotherapy. Early institution of radiation therapy should be considered in a patient with progressive spinal cord compression or airway obstruction caused by the tumor. Doxorubicin and dactinomycin, commonly used chemotherapeutic agents in Ewing's sarcoma, interact with radiation, potentially exacerbating local toxicity and necessitating treatment interruptions, with negative consequences for local control. These problems may be decreased by delaying irradiation for a few days after the drugs are given and carefully planning radiation treatment.

Chemotherapy

Before the use of adjuvant chemotherapy, long-term survival of patients with Ewing's sarcoma was rare. In the largest prechemotherapy series, only 36 (9.6%) of 374 patients treated with surgery or radiation therapy survived for 5 years. As with Wilms' tumor and rhabdomyosarcoma, single-agent chemotherapy trials were initiated in the 1960s with highly encouraging results. As shown in Table 49–28, many agents appear to be active against Ewing's sarcoma, with cyclophosphamide and doxorubicin consistently the most active. Few new agents have been developed for this or other pediatric cancers, possibly because drugs are tested against tumors resistant to multiple drugs and radiation.

In 1973, a multiinstitutional randomized trial, the first Intergroup Ewing's Sarcoma Study (IESS-I), was initiated. Patients without evidence of metastatic disease were treated on one of three treatment regimens. Local tumor control was

TABLE 49–28. Phase II Studies in Ewing's Sarcoma

Agent	Response (No. Responding/Total)	Response Rate (%)
Cyclophosphamide	19/37	51
Doxorubicin	24/58	41
Ifosfamide	10/31	32
Vincristine	3/10	30
Dactinomycin	3/9	33
BCNU	6/18	33
5-Fluorouracil	5/16	31
Etoposide	3/10	30
Cisplatin	2/27	7
Melphalan (high dose)	9/11	82
Ifosfamide/etoposide	16/17	94

planned with radiation therapy to the entire involved bone in doses ranging from 4500 to 4400 cGy, depending on the patient's age, followed by a boost of 1000 cGy to gross radiographically demonstrable tumor. Daily dose fractionation was 200 cGy, delivered 5 days each week. In addition to local therapy, patients were randomly assigned to receive adjuvant VAC with doxorubicin (regimen 1); VAC without doxorubicin (regimen 2); or VAC plus bilateral pulmonary irradiation, which consisted of midplane dose of 1500 to 1800 cGy (regimen 3). The duration of chemotherapy was 1.5 to 2 years. The survival of patients on this study are listed in Table 49–29. Important results included the following:

1. The survival rate after 3 years was 56% for the entire group.
2. The addition of doxorubicin to VAC significantly improved the disease-free survival at 2 years (72% versus 36%).
3. The addition of pulmonary irradiation to VAC decreased pulmonary recurrence if compared with VAC alone, but it was less effective than the combination of VAC plus doxorubicin.
4. The local control and disease-free survival was related to treatment and to primary site. Pelvic, humeral, and femur lesions had the poorest outcome; rib lesions were intermediate; and the best results were seen in patients with primary lesions below the knee and in the skull or spine.
5. A filigree histologic pattern was associated with a poorer prognosis.

Of 44 patients with metastatic disease or advanced regional disease treated with VAC plus doxorubicin and irradiation to primary and metastatic sites, 31 (70%) responded completely. Of these, 18 (41%) remained disease free at a median of 34 months.

The second Intergroup Ewing's Sarcoma Study (IESS II) evaluated the role of a more intensive regimen, which relied heavily on the two most active agents, cyclophosphamide and doxorubicin.

The current combined POG and CCSG protocol is a randomized study to determine whether ifosfamide and etoposide can improve outcome for patients with Ewing's sarcoma or PPNET of bone. Future studies will probably incorporate the

hematopoietic growth factors to learn whether increased dose intensity can improve outcome.

Single-institution studies have played a major role in the development of therapy for Ewing's sarcoma. These studies furthered the concepts of dose intensity and preirradiation chemotherapy. In one study, 79% of patients with localized disease treated with aggressive chemotherapy and local irradiation or surgery were free of disease at a median of 41 months from beginning therapy.

NCI investigators tested a strategy that maximized the use of cyclophosphamide and doxorubicin to achieve complete remission followed by irradiation to the primary and metastatic sites of disease, which was followed by total-body irradiation. Improved outcome was correlated to a higher dose intensity of doxorubicin delivered in that study and autologous bone marrow reconstitution to prevent systemic recurrence. Although most patients achieved a complete response, this has not been maintained in the patients presenting with metastatic disease. A study in progress is testing the efficacy of the intensive vincristine, doxorubicin, and cyclophosphamide regimen in combination with the noncross-resistant pair, ifosfamide and etoposide, and irradiation to the primary site.

Hayes and coinvestigators at the St. Jude Children's Research Hospital, using a cytokinetically based, sequential, moderate-dose cyclophosphamide and doxorubicin regimen based on their experience with neuroblastoma, report complete responses in patients with metastatic disease and a disease-free survival rate comparable to that achieved with more intense regimens. This approach was tested by the POG in a larger group of patients with disappointing results.

Although several groups have been successful in achieving complete responses, the actuarial disease-free survival curves have continued to drop years after diagnosis. The disheartening experience of diagnosing a relapse in a Ewing's sarcoma patient as much as 10 to 15 years after the initial treatment is all too familiar to those who treat this disease. This phenomenon is not commonly seen with the other childhood sarcomas. It is possible that the molecular abnormality that gives rise to this tumor is predisposed by a somatic defect that favors oncogenesis and that the late recurrence is, in fact, a new tumor.

LESS COMMON SARCOMAS

Approximately 25% to 45% of all soft tissue sarcomas in children have a histologic pattern other than rhabdomyosarcoma, comprising almost 3% of all tumors in children. Although these types of sarcomas are more commonly seen in adults, the prognosis may be better for children. The difference in prognosis is most pronounced for infants and younger children whose tumors often have a benign behavior and excellent prognosis with surgery alone. Soft tissue sarcomas that occur in adolescents often have a behavior similar to those in adults.

The most common sites for soft tissue sarcomas are the extremities and trunk, especially the retroperitoneum. The usual approach to the treatment of these tumors in adults is wide surgical excision. Radiation therapy is usually added postoperatively. Although debated, the role of adjuvant chemotherapy appears to be useful for adult patients with resectable, high-grade soft tissue sarcomas of the extremities.

TABLE 49–29. Correlation of Local Control and Disease-Free Survival With Site of Primary Disease

Site	No. of Patients	Local Control (%)	Disease-Free Survival (%)
Pelvis	37	31 (84)	14 (38)
Humerus	24	19 (79)	12 (50)
Femur	43	40 (93)	22 (51)
Tibia	22	20 (91)	15 (68)
Fibula	25	24 (96)	17 (68)
Ribs	10	9 (90)	6 (60)
Skull and spine	12	12 (100)	12 (100)
Others	20	18 (90)	14 (70)

The utility of adjuvant chemotherapy in children is being studied by POG because similar histologic patterns may have a different biologic behavior in children.

Most of the information about the treatment of children with nonrhabdomyosarcomatous soft tissue sarcomas comes from retrospective analyses of the experiences of a single institutions. Although valuable, careful prospective multiinstitutional studies are needed to determine the roles of radiation therapy and chemotherapy in the treatment of these diseases. The POG is addressing these issues in a prospective multiinstitutional trial. The ability to surgically extirpate the tumor is the most important prognostic factor. In a retrospective review of 62 cases of childhood soft tissue sarcomas other than rhabdomyosarcoma treated at St. Jude, 84% survived with no evidence of disease if the tumor could be completely removed, but only 1 of 26 patients survived if gross tumor remained after resection.

FIBROSARCOMA

Although rare, fibrosarcoma is one of the most common nonrhabdomyosarcomatous soft tissue sarcomas in children and adolescents. It occurs most frequently in the extremity, often in the distal segments. The incidence of fibrosarcoma has two age peaks, one in infants and children younger than 5 years of age, and the second in patients 10 to 15 years of age. It appears that fibrosarcoma in infants has a more benign course.

Fibrosarcoma is a spindle cell tumor with a characteristic herringbone pattern or regularly interweaving fascicles of parallel arrays of tumor cells. Important features are evidence of mitoses, nuclear pleomorphism, and increased basophilia of individual, sometimes anaplastic, tumor cells. Cells are densely packed, but reticulin stain reveals a regular pattern of stromal collagen fibers not easily appreciated by light microscopy. The differential diagnosis includes fibromatosis (which can be exceedingly aggressive locally, but which does not metastasize), nodular fasciitis, myositis ossificans, and inflammatory pseudotumor among the nonmalignant conditions and neurofibrosarcoma and poorly differentiated embryonal rhabdomyosarcoma among malignant tumors.

Of 52 cases of congenital fibrosarcoma, 37 occurred on an extremity and 15 on the trunk. Of the patients with extremity tumors, 92% were free of metastatic disease, and 95% were alive, despite a 27% local recurrence rate. Congenital fibrosarcomas of the trunk appear to be more aggressive, with 20% of patients developing metastases, and 26% dying of their disease. The standard therapy for fibrosarcoma is surgical extirpation by wide local excision, usually without additional therapy. The use of irradiation and chemotherapy in the local management of congenital fibrosarcoma is restricted to situations in which surgical removal is not possible.

There is no evidence that adjuvant chemotherapy is indicated in the treatment of congenital fibrosarcoma and nonmetastatic fibrosarcoma of young children. Several recent reports document that at least some of these tumors are sensitive to chemotherapy, and for patients who have unresectable metastatic or primary disease, chemotherapy may be useful. Several combinations of chemotherapy have been used: vincristine, doxorubicin, and cyclophosphamide; vincristine, dactinomycin, and cyclophosphamide; ifosfamide and eto-

poside have resulted in complete regressions of metastatic fibrosarcoma.

NEUROFIBROSARCOMA

Neurofibrosarcomas, malignant tumors of nerve sheath origin, account for approximately 5% to 10% of all nonrhabdomyosarcomatous soft tissue sarcomas in children. Neurofibrosarcoma occurs in association with a dominantly inherited syndrome, neurofibromatosis (*i.e.*, von Recklinghausen's disease) in about 50% of patients. Approximately 5% to 16% of patients with von Recklinghausen's disease develop neurofibrosarcoma.

Although superficially similar in appearance to fibrosarcoma, neurofibrosarcoma is a more aggressive tumor. The cells are usually more variable in size and shape, a herringbone pattern is absent, and typical features of adult neurofibrosarcomas often can be found in some areas of the tumor (*e.g.*, myxoid stroma, palisading of nuclei, and occasionally well-defined organoid arrays of nuclei). These features, common in benign schwannomas, are far less conspicuous in the malignant counterpart, but can be diagnostic if present. Diagnosis is best established by electron microscopy. The most common primary sites of neurofibrosarcoma appear to be the extremities (42%), retroperitoneum (25%), and trunk (21%).

As with fibrosarcoma, surgery plays a key role in the management of children with neurofibrosarcoma. Postoperative irradiation may be indicated if surgery does not attain negative margins. The role of chemotherapy in the treatment of patients with neurofibrosarcoma is unclear. Experience with extremity tumors in a few adults at the NCI suggests that a regimen of doxorubicin and cyclophosphamide may be effective in the adjuvant treatment of localized, grossly removed neurofibrosarcoma. Although chemotherapy can produce tumor regressions in patients with gross local and metastatic disease, no regimen appears to enhance disease-free survival in patients with advanced disease. The combination of ifosfamide and etoposide, a regimen highly active in the treatment of recurrent small, round cell tumors of neural origin, has produced partial tumor regressions in 2 of the 4 patients with recurrent neurofibrosarcoma who were evaluated.

MALIGNANT FIBROUS HISTIOCYTOMA

Although malignant fibrous histiocytoma (MFH) was the most common histologic diagnosis in the NCI series of adults with extremity sarcomas, accounting for 53 (25%) of 211 patients, it is much less common in children. At St. Jude, only 5 (8%) of the 62 cases of nonrhabdomyosarcomatous soft tissue sarcoma were diagnosed as MFH. The typical microscopic appearance of MFH resembles fibrosarcoma, but it is differentiated by marked cellular pleomorphism, multiple cell types (especially lipid-laden tumor cells), and a more malignant appearance. A storiform pattern of tumor cells, described as radiating fascicles of tumor cells at right angles from one another, is virtually diagnostic of this tumor.

Because of the rarity of this tumor in childhood, the approach to treatment of this malignancy is based on the adult experience. The accepted initial management is wide local excision of the tumor. Limb-sparing operations with radiation to the tumor bed have been as successful as amputations for tumors in the extremities. The role of adjuvant chemotherapy is not yet established in children with MFH. Of 7 patients with MFH, 2 had their tumor completely removed and were then treated with adjuvant chemotherapy; both were alive 1.4 and 9 years later. Comparable survivals without adjuvant chemotherapy have also been described.

Vincristine, dactinomycin, and cyclophosphamide, with or without doxorubicin, has produced objective tumor regressions in patients with advanced disease. Four of the 5 patients with group III or IV disease had complete or partial tumor regressions, and 2 remained disease free at 4.6 and 5.4 years. Responses to ifosfamide plus etoposide have been reported.

SYNOVIAL SARCOMA

Synovial sarcoma accounted for 29% of the nonrhabdomyosarcomatous soft tissue sarcomas at St. Jude Children's Research Hospital. The most common anatomic location is the lower extremity, often in the thigh and the knee; the next most common site is the upper extremity. Approximately 15% to 20% occur on the head, neck, or trunk.

Synovial cell sarcomas can have two components, a spindle cell fibrous stroma virtually indistinguishable from fibrosarcoma and a distinct glandular component with absolute epithelial differentiation.

Significant prognostic features are small tumor size (<5-cm diameter); a primary site in the hand, foot, or knee; a younger age; and a predominant epithelioid pattern. The disease-free survival rate for adult patients with localized tumors of the extremities is approximately 70%. Eight of the 18 patients treated at St. Jude were long-term survivors.

Because this tumor is relatively rare in children, the optimal treatment guidelines have not yet been established. Wide local excision is the treatment of choice to control the primary tumor. Radiation therapy may improve control with microscopically inadequate margins; treatment planning should seek to ensure normal function and normal growth by maximal sparing of bone and normal soft tissue. The effectiveness of irradiation in the control of bulky disease has not been established.

The benefit of adjuvant chemotherapy in the treatment of synovial sarcoma in children and young adults is not clear, but adjuvant cyclophosphamide and doxorubicin administered postoperatively to adult patients was beneficial. Tumor regressions in patients with advanced disease have been documented with several chemotherapy regimens. Although these treatment plans have usually included cyclophosphamide and doxorubicin, a regimen of vincristine, dactinomycin, and cyclophosphamide has been advocated. Objective tumor regressions have been seen with the combination regimen of ifosfamide and etoposide.

HEMANGIOPERICYTOMA

Hemangiopericytoma, a tumor that presumably arises from the pericyte cells that surround vascular channels, accounts for approximately 3% of all soft tissue sarcomas in children. It can be benign or malignant. The most common primary sites are the extremities, especially the lower extremities; the retroperitoneum is the second most common site of disease,

followed by the head and neck region and the trunk. The most common sites of secondary disease are the lungs and bone.

The behavior of this tumor in older children is similar to that of hemangiopericytoma in adult patients. The overall 5-year survival rate for adults varies from 30% to 70%. The therapeutic approach is wide local excision. Adjuvant chemotherapy has been of value in adults with this disease. As with other soft tissue sarcomas, radiation therapy is used if complete surgical removal of the tumor cannot be accomplished.

Responses to chemotherapy have been reported with the use of vincristine, cyclophosphamide, doxorubicin, dactinomycin, methotrexate, mitoxantrone, and other alkylating agents. Although there is no randomized study confirming the role of adjuvant chemotherapy is this disease, the high incidence of metastatic disease and relative chemoresponsiveness of the tumor had led many investigators to treat these patients with chemotherapy after extirpation of the primary tumor.

Hemangiopericytoma may rarely occur in infants, and although similar in histologic appearance to the adult form, infantile hemangiopericytoma usually follows a more benign course. These tumors usually arise in the subcutis; however, occasionally they may have extensive local infiltration or metastasize. The treatment of choice for infantile hemangiopericytoma is surgery alone if the tumor is localized; however, complete regression of metastatic disease in patients with this entity has been seen with chemotherapy.

ALVEOLAR SOFT PART SARCOMA

Alveolar soft part sarcoma (ASPS) is a rare sarcoma that usually occurs in patients between the ages of 15 and 35 years. Although 6 of the 62 patients in the St. Jude series had ASPS, the actual incidence in children and adolescents is probably lower. The tumor usually occurs in the skeletal muscle of the extremities in adults, but the head and neck region is a common site in children.

The most distinctive feature of ASPS is the presence of PAS-positive, diastase-resistant inclusions in the cytoplasm, which show a regular crystalline structure. That some inclusions closely resemble neurosecretory granules provokes suspicion that the tumor may be neuroepithelial, but immunocytochemistry is inconclusive in this regard.

Alveolar soft part sarcoma usually presents as a slow-growing, painless mass. The clinical course of patients with ASPS is indolent but usually progressive. The most common sites of metastatic disease are lung, brain, bone, and lymph nodes.

The initial therapeutic approach is complete local excision alone, with radiation and chemotherapy reserved for the treatment of recurrent disease. Many patients eventually relapse and subsequently die of disease. This ominous fact strongly suggests that new approaches to the prevention of relapses are needed in the treatment of this disorder.

LEIOMYOSARCOMA

Leiomyosarcoma is rare in childhood, accounting for less than 2% of soft tissue sarcomas in children. The most common primary sites of disease are the retroperitoneum vascular tissue, peripheral soft tissue, and the gastrointestinal tract.

The tumor cells are elongate, with cigar-shaped nuclei and brightly eosinophilic cytoplasm (due to the content of myofilaments), and they are closely packed in parallel arrays. The appearance is superficially similar to fibrosarcoma, but the eosinophilic nuclei, resembling smooth muscle in normal tissues, and usual monotonous regularity of tumor cells are distinct.

The most common approach to the treatment is local excision. The role of chemotherapy and radiation therapy in children is undefined. If complete extirpation of the tumor can be achieved, the prognosis is usually good for tumors arising outside of the gastrointestinal tract; however, tumors arising in this site generally have a poor prognosis. Leiomyosarcomas of the colorectal region in children, although extremely rare, appear to have a relatively good prognosis if the tumor can be successfully excised.

LIPOSARCOMA

Although primarily a disease of adults, with a peak age of incidence between 40 and 60 years, liposarcomas may occur in children, most often in the early part of the second decade of life. The tumor rarely affects infants and young children, in whom its behavior is usually benign. The two most common primary sites are the extremities and the retroperitoneum. The tumor may be well-differentiated, myxoid, round cell, or pleomorphic (in increasing degree of malignancy and decreasing survival). Most tumor cells are fibroblastic; only rare cells show conspicuous lipoblastic differentiation. The distinction from MFH can be difficult, but the presence of a myxoid stroma, conspicuous small blood vessels, and scant mitotic activity are all typical of liposarcoma.

The treatment of choice for localized liposarcoma is wide local excision. Local recurrences may ultimately result in the death of the patient because of extension of the tumor into vital structures. The role of adjuvant chemotherapy in the treatment of liposarcomas of childhood is undefined. Radiation appears to be effective in the control of microscopic disease in adults.

HISTIOCYTOSES

The histiocytoses are an uncommon group of clinically diverse syndromes that share a histopathology characterized by granuloma formation with the infiltration and proliferation of histocytes. The classic clinical triad of the histiocytosis X syndromes includes a solitary lytic lesion of bone (*i.e.*, eosinophilic granuloma); a chronic disorder characterized by exophthalmos, diabetes insipidus, and skeletal lesions (*i.e.*, Hand-Schüller-Christian syndrome); and an acute fulminant disseminated disorder of young children manifested by skin lesions, hepatosplenomegaly, lymphadenopathy, mastoiditis, osteolytic lesions, pneumonitis, anemia, thrombocytopenia, and fever (*i.e.*, Letterer-Siwe disease). The clinical and biologic diversity has made it difficult to characterize and classify histiocytosis as a neoplastic or nonneoplastic disorder and has contributed to the controversy about its appropriate management.

BIOLOGIC CONSIDERATIONS

The infiltration and accumulation of cells in the monocyte or macrophage series into a target tissue can be a primary or secondary event, and not all diseases associated with histiocytic infiltration are classified as histiocytoses.

Histiocytes arise from the uncommitted bone marrow stem cell and differentiate along the granulocyte-macrophage axis. One of the primary functions of normal histiocytes is phagocytoses of aged erythrocytes, microbes, or tumor cells, and erythrophagocytosis is a common finding in many of the histiocytoses of childhood. The characteristic findings of histiocytoses may be the result of diverse pathogenic mechanisms. For example, in "histiocytosis-X," now known as Langerhans' cell histiocytosis, the proliferation and accumulation of histiocytes is the result of immunologic stimulation of the Langerhans' cell. It does not appear that these histiocytes are truly malignant, and improvement has been noticed with the administration of thymic extracts. In the cases of infection-associated hemophagocytic syndrome, the macrophage appears to be reacting to a foreign antigen, and this histiocytosis reverses when the infection and its antigenic stimulation abates. Other histiocytoses may represent a genetic abnormality (*e.g.*, familial erythrophagocytic lymphohistiocytosis) or a clonal neoplastic proliferation (*e.g.*, malignant histiocytosis).

PATHOLOGY

To clarify this diverse group of histiocytoses, the Histiocytosis Society has developed a classification system based on pathologic examination that divides the histiocytoses into three classes.

In class I histiocytoses, the central cell has the histopathologic feature of the Langerhans' cell and this designation replaces those syndromes previously referred to as histiocytosis X (*i.e.*, eosinophilic granuloma, Hand-Schüller-Christian syndrome, and Letterer-Siwe disease). The lesions associated with Langerhans' cell histiocytosis are granulomatous and are highlighted by the presence of Langerhans' cells with Birbeck's granules, which can be seen by electron microscopy.

Class II histiocytoses include all the other nonmalignant histiocytoses in which the mononuclear phagocyte is not a Langerhans' cell. These are reactive histiocytoses that are usually associated with a mixed lymphohistiocytic infiltrate, generally in the sinusoids, cortex, and paracortex, but without effacement of nodal architecture. The infiltrating histiocytes appear normal, and they have low nuclear to cytoplasmic ratios, mature nuclear chromatin, inconspicuous nucleoli, and abundant cytoplasm. The two disorders categorized in class II histiocytoses, the infection-associated hemophagocytic syndrome (IAHS) and familial erythrophagocytic lymphohistiocytosis (FEL), are denoted by erythrophagocytosis and the secondary accumulation of histocytes.

Class III histiocytosis is a true neoplasm, of which malignant histiocytosis is the best known disease. Lymph nodes in class III histiocytosis are characterized by nodal effacement and infiltration with cells containing reticular chromatic patterns, prominent nucleoli, and basophilic cytoplasm. Erythrophagocytosis may be observed in class III histiocytosis, but it is not a prominent as in class II.

CLINICAL PRESENTATION, DIAGNOSIS, AND TREATMENT

Class I Histiocytoses

As seen in Table 49–30, the Langerhans' cell histiocytosis has a variable presentation and clinical course and can undergo regression and exacerbation within the same patient. In acute disseminated histiocytosis, the skin is involved in 70% to 100% of patients and is characterized by a scaling, eczematoid rash over the trunk, neck, groin, and scalp. Scalp lesions are not infrequently misdiagnosed as a seborrheic dermatitis. There is often a petechial component, and in rare cases, skin lesions can antedate more widespread disease. A syndrome referred to as regressing atypical histiocytosis has been described and is characterized by noduloulcerative skin lesions composed of atypical histiocytes, monocytes, and multinucleated giant cells with erythrophagocytosis. However, these patients have cutaneous disease only, and the skin lesions are indolent and characterized by spontaneous regressions and recurrences. Recognition of this disorder is important to avoid unnecessary treatment.

Lytic bone lesions serve as the clinical hallmark of Langerhans' histiocytoses and occur with a frequency comparable to skin disease, most commonly involving the flat bones and vertebrae, frequently with pain and functional impairment.

In approximately 33% of patients, there is evidence of bilateral osteomastoiditis with bilateral suppurative discharge. Skeletal survey is a more reliable diagnostic and follow-up tool in these patients than radionuclide bone scans.

Histiocytic infiltration into the reticuloendothelial system results in generalized lymphadenopathy. Enlargement of the liver and spleen, particularly if associated with functional abnormalities, carries an ominous prognosis. Although hepatosplenomegaly is infrequent in initial presentation, it develops in almost half of patients with disseminated histiocytosis, sometimes with jaundice and occasionally with the onset of cirrhosis. Similarly, pulmonary findings are infrequent at initial diagnosis, but some pulmonary manifestations, particularly a diffuse interstitial infiltrate, develop during the disease course in almost 67% of patients. Buccal and gingival infiltration occurs in about 40% of patients and is manifested as loose or floating teeth. More ominous are hematologic abnormalities, including anemia and thrombocytopenia.

Of patients with generalized disease, 25% to 50% develop diabetes insipidus during their disease course. Nonetheless, the classic Hand-Schüller-Christian syndrome, which includes diabetes insipidus, exophthalmos, and geographic skull lesions, is found in fewer than 10% of patients with disseminated histiocytosis. The presence of diabetes insipidus is rarely associated with radiographic abnormalities of the sella turcica.

TABLE 49–30. Clinical, Prognostic, and Therapeutic Aspects of the Major Childhood Histiocytoses

Variable	LCH or Class I	IAHS or Class II	FEL or Class II	MH or Class III
Clinical presentation	Wide spectrum, from mild discomfort related to lesions (lytic bone lesions, chronic otitis, diabetes insipidus) to generalized symptoms including fever and weight loss	Pancytopenia, hepatosplenomegaly, fever coagulopathy	Irritability, fever, wasting sometimes with a coagulopathy and hepatosplenomegaly	Variable, from systemic disease (*e.g.*, acute leukemia) to a localized mass lesion
Diagnostic findings	Birbeck's granules in lesional cells	Morphologically normal macrophages, documented infection, and negative family history	Morphologically normal macrophages and negative search for infection, sometimes positive family history	Malignant macrophages
Prognosis	Variable, but a self-resolving disease process in most cases	Excellent, providing underlying infection is controlled and immunosuppression can be reversed	Extremely poor; uniformly rapidly fatal	Up to 75% survival at 40 months reported with appropriate therapy for patients with MH or THL; prognosis is poor for patients with acute monocytic leukemia
Recommended treatment	None to mild radiation or chemotherapy (vinblastine or etoposide and steroids) for certain lesions	Avoidance of immunosuppressive therapy; etoposide is being explored experimentally	Experimental (etoposide); bone marrow transplantation	Doxorubicin in a combination chemotherapy regimen for MH or THL; appropriate therapy for acute monocytic leukemia

LCH, Langerhans' cell hystiocytosis; IAHS, infection-associated hemophagocytic syndrome; FEL, familial erythrophagocytic lymph histiocytosis; MH, malignant histiocytosis; THL, true histiocytic lymphoma.
(Ladisch S, Jaffe ES. The histiocytoses. In: Pizzo PA, Poplack DG, eds: Principles and practice of pediatric oncology. 2nd ed. Philadelphia: JB Lippincott, 1993)

Increasingly recognized are the delayed neurologic manifestations that include hyperreflexia, ataxia, vertigo, nystagmus, and dysarthria.

Diagnosis requires biopsy and electron microscopy to determine the presence of Birbeck's granules and to eliminate other disorders that may cause lytic bone lesions, especially metastatic neuroblastoma.

Two prognostic features stand out. First, mortality is higher for children younger than 2 years of age at the time of diagnosis. Second, organ dysfunction, especially if multiple organ systems are involved, decreases survival. Particularly ominous is hepatic involvement at the time of initial diagnosis. These factors influence approaches to therapy.

The treatment of patients with monostotic bone lesions is the most straightforward and includes surgical biopsy or curettage. Low-dose megavoltage irradiation (500–1000 cGy) is recommended only for lesions that are surgically inaccessible, including vertebral bodies or sites adjacent to major growth plates.

The treatment of patients with generalized involvement is more controversial. Which patients should be treated? If treatment is undertaken, should it be with chemotherapy or immunotherapy? What should be the intensity and duration of therapy? These questions are complicated by the clinical diversity of Langerhans' cell histiocytosis and the chance that the disease may undergo a spontaneous regression. While treating the underlying process, care should be taken to avoid iatrogenic morbidity. Symptomatic or palliative therapy should not be overlooked, because disabling problems, such as diabetes insipidus, progressive destruction of a weight-bearing bone, extensive and progressive mandibular involvement, mastoid disease, and proptosis, can often be resolved with a short course of local irradiation.

Current systemic treatment options include chemotherapy, immunotherapy, and low-dose, total-body irradiation. A variety of drugs (*e.g.*, chlorambucil, vinblastine, etoposide, methotrexate, with or without prednisone) yield complete and partial response rates of 40% to 60%. The overall response rates to combination chemotherapy do not appear to be clearly superior to single-drug schedules in most series, although one study suggested that combination therapy was preferable for children younger than 2 years of age who had extensive disease. Conversely, combination regimens are likely to be associated with more toxicity. Some investigators recommend withholding chemotherapy from patients who have multifocal disease limited to the skeleton or skin. Recent data suggest that early intervention may offset the onset of delayed, particularly neurologic, complications. Patients with more extensive disease, particularly those with evidence of hepatic dysfunction, require chemotherapy with agents such as vinblastine (for infants <1 year of age) or vinblastine or etoposide plus prednisone and 6-mercaptopurine for older children. Children who fail to respond to chemotherapy may benefit from low-dose cyclosporine alone or in combination with chemotherapy, perhaps because of its ability to affect a reduction in cytokine production.

Class II Histiocytoses

FEL is an autosomal-recessive disorder characterized by fever, irritability, leptomeningeal involvement, hepatosplenomegaly, and abnormal liver dysfunction, with bone marrow findings of histiocytic and lymphocytic infiltration and with prominent erythrophagocytosis. FEL occurs primarily in young infants, and families with several affected members have been described. Unlike histiocytosis X, FEL is differentiated by a variety of immunologic abnormalities, including depressed antibody levels, anergy, and defective lymphocyte proliferation. In one family, plasma-mediated inhibition of cellular immunity was described, which correlated with the plasma triglyceride level, raising the question of whether the immune abnormalities were primary or secondary phenomena. Clinical and immunologic improvement was observed with plasma-exchange transfusion in a patient with FEL. An increase of acidic glycosphingolipids and a decrease of α-galactosidase activity suggest that FEL may be associated with unique quantitative and qualitative abnormalities of the hepatic gangliosides.

FEL is a rapidly progressive disorder and is frequently complicated by thrombocytopenia and a disseminated intravascular coagulopathy. Progressive neurologic deterioration and brain atrophy with perivascular infiltration of the brain and meninges by lymphocytes and histiocytes can occur. An X-linked histiocytosis has been described in which there is nodal infiltration by macrophages and plasma cells with hypergammaglobulinemia.

Because of its rapidly fulminant course and lymphohistiocytic infiltration suggesting a malignant neoplasm, cytotoxic therapy has been employed for FEL. Although transient improvements have been observed with combination regimens similar to those used for acute leukemia, remissions are rarely sustained, and the patients die. Two approaches have been explored as alternatives to chemotherapy: plasma exchange and bone marrow transplantation. Plasma exchange is based on the presence of circulating immunosuppressive activity in patients with FEL. After exchange transfusion, a reduction in plasma-inhibiting activity and some reversal of the depressed cellular immunity was observed, but these responses were not sustained. Bone marrow transplantation is based on the hypothesis that FEL represents an uncontrolled proliferation of lymphocytes and histiocytes. Bone marrow transplantation has been successful for a few patients, but additional experience is necessary.

IAHS is considered a class II histiocytosis. The clinical appearance of IAHS is similar to FEL, and the diagnosis rests on presence of an infection and a negative family history for this disease. Like FEL, there is striking erythrophagocytosis in the bone marrow of children with IAHS, and with the absence of Birbeck's granules on electron microscopy, this differentiates IAHS from Langerhans' cell histiocytosis.

The keys to the successful therapy of children with IAHS are the discovery of the infectious agent and the avoidance of immunosuppressive therapy. Although cytotoxic therapy is generally contraindicated for IAHS, etoposide may be beneficial in halting disease progression. However, caution is appropriate because of the secondary leukemias observed in patients treated with etoposide.

Class III Histiocytosis

Acute monocytic leukemia and malignant histiocytosis fall into the category of class III histiocytosis. Malignant histiocytosis is a nonfamilial, rapidly fatal disorder characterized by fever, generalized tender lymphadenopathy, hepatosplenomegaly, subcutaneous inflammatory infiltration, pancytopenia, and a Coombs-positive hemolytic anemia. A characteristic finding is erythrophagocytosis in the bone marrow, liver, and spleen, along with histiocytic infiltration of the subcapsular and medullary regions of lymph nodes. Immunochemical analysis has demonstrated that malignant histiocytosis cells stain positively for the S-100 protein (a CNS-specific protein), that many contain evidence of κ or λ chains, and that many are lysosome negative, suggesting that they are derived from T-zone histiocytes rather than from the monocyte-macrophage axis. Cytogenetic analysis of malignant histiocytes from the bone marrow of an infant with malignant histiocytosis revealed a translocation [t(8:16)(p11′3)], which disappeared after clinical remission.

For patients with malignant histiocytosis and FEL, intervention is clearly necessary. However, a continuing issue is whether this should be with prednisone alone or with regimens including vincristine and cyclophosphamide. Prolonged responses have been observed in some patients with malignant histiocytosis treated with combination chemotherapy, including vincristine, prednisone, cyclophosphamide, doxorubicin, vinblastine, bleomycin, methyl-CCNU, etoposide, and cytosine arabinoside, although the overall mortality rate of these patients remains quite high (68%).

Additional insights into the immunology and classification of the histiocytoses are necessary, and continued exploration of immune replacement or its mediation are important objectives.

CARCINOMAS AND OTHER LESS COMMON TUMORS OF CHILDHOOD

Many of the tumors that are common in adults occur only rarely in children. Principles for evaluation and management are generally similar to those for adults. Some insights about the pediatric aspects of those tumors are offered here.

HEAD AND NECK TUMORS

Nasopharyngeal Carcinoma

Nasopharyngeal carcinoma is a rare neoplasm in North America. It is more common in black than white teenagers. In children, rhabdomyosarcoma and non-Hodgkin's lymphomas are much more common nasopharyngeal tumors. Nasopharyngeal carcinoma appears to be closely associated with EBV infection. Management includes irradiation (6000–7000 cGy) and chemotherapy (*e.g.*, 5-FU, methotrexate, bleomycin, cisplatin). In patients with localized involvement, a disease-free survival rate of 78% has been reported.

Oropharyngeal Tumors

Squamous cell carcinoma of the tongue and oral cavity are extremely rare in children, but the incidence is increasing because of the use of smokeless tobacco products. It has been estimated that as many as 8% to 30% of male high-school and college students regularly use smokeless tobacco, often be-

ginning at 12 years of age. The use of these products should be discouraged by physicians caring for teenagers and young adults.

Ameloblastoma

Ameloblastoma or adamtanoma is a rare tumor that arises in the mandible, maxilla, or rarely, long bones. The primary therapeutic modalities are surgery and irradiation. The role of chemotherapy is not established.

Laryngeal Tumors

The most common childhood tumor involving the larynx is rhabdomyosarcoma, and squamous cell tumors of the larynx occur only rarely. Juvenile papillomatosis is a benign overgrowth of epithelial cells, primarily affecting the larynx and responsive to surgery or, in recurrent cases, radiation therapy or interferon.

TUMORS OF THE LUNG AND THORAX

Lung Cancer

Although rare, more that 100 cases of primary lung cancers in children have been reported, including bronchogenic carcinoma, usually of the undifferentiated or adenocarcinomatous type, occurring primarily in adolescents. Bronchial adenomas have been described, the primary treatment for which is surgical resection.

Pulmonary blastoma, a rare subpleural neoplasm has been described in children. It can metastasize and may respond to combination chemotherapy.

Thymoma

To be considered a tumor of the thymus gland, neoplastic epithelial cells must be demonstrable, because many malignant and nonmalignant processes are associated with thymomas. Included are Hodgkin's and non-Hodgkin's lymphomas, germ cell tumors, carcinoids, thymolipomas, myasthenia gravis, autoimmune diseases (*e.g.*, polymyositis, systemic lupus erythematosus, rheumatoid arthritis), and endocrine disorders (*e.g.*, hyperparathyroidism, Addison's syndromes, panhypopituitarism).

Thymomas are usually slowly growing tumors found in the anterior mediastinum. Diagnosis may be heralded by nonspecific symptoms, including cough, dyspnea, and in advanced cases, evidence of a superior vena cava syndrome. Thymomas are locally invasive, and metastases can occur in lymph nodes, bone, liver, kidney, or brain.

Thymomas are generally radiosensitive and treatment includes 3500 to 4500 cGy given over 3 to 6 weeks. Thymomas have responded to doxorubicin, cisplatin, and alkylating agents. Most authorities reserve chemotherapy for patients not responding to local therapy. Survival rates appear to be 65% to 83% for patients with locally confined tumors and 30% to 54% for invasive tumor.

Breast Cancer

Most breast tumors in pediatric patients are benign, the most common being the fibroadenomas that occur in adolescents.

Although these tumors can become quite large (*e.g.*, cystosarcoma phyllodes), they are usually benign.

Although uncommon, carcinomas of the breast have been described in boys and girls. They do not appear to be different from adult tumors, and the recommendations for therapy are the same.

ENDOCRINE TUMORS

Endocrine tumors comprise 4% to 5% of childhood neoplasms, most which are benign or low-grade malignancies. Most of these tumors do not secrete hormones, with 40% to 45% arising from gonadal origins, 30% from the thyroid, and 20% from the pituitary gland. Less commonly, tumors involve the parathyroids, adrenal gland, and the gastroenteropancreatic unit. Although most of these tumors are sporadic and of embryonic origin, a smaller percentage may be familial (*e.g.*, medullary carcinomas of the thyroid, pheochromocytoma), among which are the genetically transmitted syndromes of multiple endocrine neoplasia (MEN).

Most thyroid cancers in children are papillary or follicular, usually presenting as an asymptomatic solitary nodule or cervical adenopathy. Although a trial of thyroid suppression is recommended by some, the 14% to 40% incidence of carcinoma in children with thyroid nodules should prompt surgical resection. The 10-year survival is better for younger patients with thyroid carcinoma (83%) than for adults (60%).

Adrenal carcinomas are rare in childhood (<0.5% of pediatric tumors) and occur primarily in children younger than 8 years old. These tumors are endocrinologically active, causing Cushing's syndrome, virilization, or feminization; aldosterenomas are rare in children.

One of the primary objectives is to differentiate carcinoma from a benign adenoma. Carcinomas are usually larger and more inhomogenous by CT and ultrasound at the time of diagnosis. Tumors weighing less than 100 g have an excellent prognosis, but those weighing more than 500 g have a poor prognosis. Surgery is the treatment of choice, and awareness that tumors may be bilateral in as many as 10% of patients is important. For patients with extensive local or metastatic disease in kidney, lymph nodes, liver, lung, mesentery, brain, or bone, chemotherapy with 5-FU, dactinomycin, cyclophosphamide, and op′DDD should be administered. Inhibitors of steroid synthesis (*e.g.*, aminoglutethimide, metapyrone, ketoconazole) or glucocorticoid antagonists (*e.g.*, RU486) may be useful. If hypoaldosteronism or hypocortisolism develops, after treatment with mitolane, fludrocortisone or hydrocortisone replacement may be necessary. Studies are in progress using suramin, an antiparasitic agent that, as a side-effect, can cause the necrosis of the adrenal cortex. Preliminary results are encouraging.

MEN syndromes are exceedingly rare in pediatrics but have been described in families. MEN type I consists of tumors of the pituitary, parathyroid, and pancreas (in particular, the Zollinger-Ellison syndrome); MEN type II consists of medullary carcinoma of the thyroid and pheochromocytoma (MEN-IIa) and a familial syndrome that includes mucosal neuromas and a Marfan-like body habitus (MEN-IIb) (Table 49–31).

RENAL CELL CARCINOMA

Renal cell carcinoma (*e.g.*, clear cell carcinoma, renal cell adenocarcinoma, hypernephroma) is the most common primary kidney tumor in adults, but it is rare in children, occurring with an annual incidence of 4 per million. Renal cell carcinoma has been seen in patients with the von Hippel-Lindau syndrome, tuberous sclerosis, and a constitutional

TABLE 49–31. Comparison of Clusters of Involved Tumors in MEN Syndromes

Site of Origin	MEN-I	MEN-IIa	MEN-IIb*
Pituitary gland	Prolactinoma Somatotropinoma Corticotropinoma		
Thyroid gland		C-cell hyperplasia Medullary carcinoma	Medullary carcinoma
Parathyroid glands	Parathyroid hyperplasia, adenoma	Parathyroid hyperplasia, adenoma	
Adrenal cortex	Adrenal adenoma, hyperplasia		
Adrenal medulla		Pheochromocytoma	Pheochromocytoma
Gastroenteropancreatic unit	Gastrinoma Insulinoma VIPoma Glucagonoma		
Other	PPoma Lipomas Carcinoids		Mucosal neuromas, ganglioneuromas

* Characterized also by marfanoid habitus.
(Chrousos GP. Endocrine tumors. In: Pizzo PA, Poplack DG, eds. Principles and practice of pediatric oncology. 2nd ed. Philadelphia: JB Lippincott, 1993)

chromosome translocation. There is a high frequency of abnormalities, t(3:8)(p14″4), of chromosome 3.

The four patterns of pathology are papillary, solid, cystic, and sarcomatous, although these have little prognostic impact. The cellular morphology includes clear cell, granular cell, and sarcomatoid types.

Unlike Wilms' tumor, in which the presenting mass is often asymptomatic, renal cell carcinoma usually presents with abdominal or flank pain and hematuria. The average age of patients with renal cell carcinoma is 11 years, but it has been described in children as young as 14 months.

The most important prognostic factor is stage. Children with stage I disease had a 100% survival rate; stage II had a 66% survival rate; stage III had 43% survival rate; and stage IV had a 12% survival rate. This is related to the therapeutic approaches. Radical nephrectomy with resection of the kidney, adrenal gland, surrounding perinephric fat, Gerota's fascia, and regional lymph nodes is the treatment for localized renal cell carcinoma. The role of radiation therapy is unclear for children, although some physicians have advocated 4000 to 4500 cGy postoperatively for children with stage II disease. Chemotherapy has not been particularly successful, but interferon and the use of interleukin-2 (IL-2) with lymphokine-activated killer (LAK) cells have been successful in adults; data for children are lacking.

GASTROINTESTINAL TRACT CARCINOMAS

Carcinomas of the stomach, colon, gallbladder, and pancreas have been described in children, although their incidence is strikingly low. These tumors are usually not suspected in children. Because the tumors are so rare in children, the treatments are similar to those used in adults.

CANCERS OF THE SKIN

Melanoma is the most common skin cancer in children, followed by basal cell and squamous cell carcinomas. Ionizing irradiation is an important risk factor and contributes to the regional distribution of these cancers.

The familial occurrence of melanoma in patients with the dysplastic nevus syndrome is recognized. These nevi are usually located on the trunk but can occur in the scalp or extremities. Approximately 10% of patients with these lesions develop melanomas.

The clinical appearance of melanomas and their local and metastatic spread is similar in children to that of adults. Biopsy is necessary for diagnosis, but whether it is incisional or excisional depends on the location and size of the lesion. If the lesion is a melanoma, a wide excision is necessary. Curettage or cryotherapy can be used for basal cell or squamous cell carcinomas. As in adults, chemotherapy has been used for patients with melanoma who have evidence of regional lymph node involvement. The use of IL-2 and LAK cells in adults with melanoma suggests therapeutic utility for children or adolescents with evidence of extensive disease.

Pediatricians should recommend decreased sun exposure, the use of sunscreens for children and teenagers, and the removal of congenital nevi.

REFERENCE

Pizzo PA, Poplack DG, eds. Principles and practice of pediatric oncology. 2nd ed. Philadelphia: JB Lippincott, 1993.

Cancer: Principles & Practice of Oncology, Fourth Edition,
edited by Vincent T. DeVita, Jr., Samuel Hellman, Steven A. Rosenberg.
J.B. Lippincott Co., Philadelphia © 1993.

David G. Poplack   Ian T. Magrath
Larry E. Kun   Philip A. Pizzo

CHAPTER **50**

Leukemias and Lymphomas of Childhood

There have been major advances in the treatment of children with leukemia and lymphoma during the past 30 years. The record of therapeutic achievements in these diseases constitutes one of the true success stories of modern clinical oncology. Perhaps the most dramatic example is the improvement in the outlook for children with acute lymphoblastic leukemia (ALL), a disorder that was uniformly fatal only 40 years ago. More than half of the children with this disease now are alive and free of disease more than 5 years after initial diagnosis, and most of these patients are considered cured. Forty years ago the major concern was developing better methods of inducing complete remission; today the focus has shifted to issues facing long-term survivors. The situation is somewhat different for children with acute myelogenous leukemia (AML). Although the outlook for these patients has improved, curative therapy for most of these children remains elusive. In contrast, progress in treating the childhood non-Hodgkin's lymphomas (NHL) has been particularly striking. Before the 1970s, fewer than 30% of children obtained long-term, disease-free survival. Currently, 60% to 80% of children with NHL are considered curable.[1]

Improvement in therapy for these disorders has resulted from innovative application of the principles of combination chemotherapy and the combined-modality approach. Intensive biologic, immunologic, and cytogenetic characterization has contributed significantly to our understanding of these disorders. For example, information about the differentiation status of malignant lymphoid cells, derived in part from technical advances such as immunophenotyping with monoclonal antibodies and determination of immunoglobulin and T-cell receptor gene rearrangements, has provided a more rational

means of classifying these disorders. Similarly, application of the type of molecular biologic methods that led to the demonstration of oncogene expression in Burkitt's lymphoma cells is likely to help elucidate the cause of lymphoid and nonlymphoid malignancies.

EPIDEMIOLOGY AND ETIOLOGY

Acute leukemia is the most common malignancy in children. Each year in the United States, approximately 2000 cases are diagnosed. ALL accounts for three fourths of these cases; AML makes up most of the remaining cases. Chronic myelogenous leukemia (CML) is rare and comprises fewer than 5% of childhood leukemias.[2]

ALL has a peak incidence in children between 2 and 6 years of age. The increased peak incidence of ALL in whites in the United States is not observed in blacks. This difference is largely responsible for the observation that acute leukemia is almost twice as common in white than in nonwhite children.

In AML, there is no peak age of incidence in childhood. The two forms of CML in childhood tend to occur at somewhat different ages. The median age of onset for the juvenile form is approximately 2 years of age, whereas the Philadelphia chromosome-positive (Ph-positive) type more commonly appears in older children.[3] AML and CML occur with similar frequencies in whites and nonwhites.

ALL occurs more commonly in boys; this pattern is particularly striking in pubertal children. In contrast, among children younger than 5 years of age, AML occurs more commonly in girls, and between 5 to 15 years, the incidence in each sex is equal; thereafter, males are affected more frequently.

1792

There has been considerable interest in reports of "leukemic clusters," which are a greater than expected number of leukemia cases within a given geographic area or period. Most studies have been unable to confirm this phenomenon.

A variety of possible causative factors for leukemia have been examined, including environmental and genetic factors, viruses, and immunodeficiency states. Irradiation and exposure to toxic chemicals are the most studied environmental factors. The increased incidence of leukemia observed in survivors of atomic bomb explosions in Hiroshima and Nagasaki in 1945 is well known. Persons closest to the hypocenters of these explosions had the highest incidence of leukemia. The type of leukemia that developed corresponded to the age at exposure; ALL was more common in children. There is an increased risk to children exposed to diagnostic radiation, particularly in the first trimester. A higher incidence of leukemia was found in several early studies in which irradiation was used to treat thymic enlargement in neonates, tinea capitis infection, or ankylosing spondylitis.

The use of alkylating agents to treat childhood malignancy has been associated with the development of leukemia in adulthood (*e.g.*, Hodgkin's disease). Therapy-induced leukemia is more common in those persons who also have received concomitant radiation therapy. Chronic exposure to toxic chemicals (*e.g.*, benzene) has been associated with the development of leukemia, usually AML.

There is considerable controversy about the potential risks associated with exposure to ionizing radiation from routine nuclear power plant emissions. Although an association between exposure to electromagnetic fields and the development of childhood ALL has been reported, it has not been confirmed.

There is evidence for the role of genetic factors in leukemogenesis. The incidence of leukemia is increased in children with certain constitutional chromosomal abnormalities. Children with trisomy 21 (*i.e.*, Down's syndrome) have approximately 15 times greater risk of developing leukemia than persons in the general population. ALL is most commonly observed, although AML may occur, particularly in neonatal cases. The *ETS2* oncogene, which has been implicated in leukemogenesis may be found on chromosome 21. The development of leukemia in children with Down's syndrome is believed to reflect the presence of an unstable genome that is more susceptible to other leukemogenic factors. The observation that fibroblasts from Down's syndrome children are transformed more readily in vitro by SV40 virus supports this thesis. The same observation has been made in fibroblasts of children with Fanconi's syndrome, a rare, recessively transmitted disorder characterized by a variety of congenital abnormalities that is frequently associated with the development of AML. Patients with Bloom's syndrome, another recessively transmitted chromosomal fragility disorder, characterized by short stature and photosensitive telangiectatic erythema, also have a higher incidence of leukemia, usually AML. The development of leukemia in these patients may be a consequence of genetic recombination of somatic cell chromosomes.

Patients with ataxia-telangiectasia, an immunodeficiency disease in which abnormalities of chromosomes 14 and 7 have been observed, are at an increased risk of lymphoid malignancy, including ALL. The loci of three rearranging T-cell receptor genes, α (chromosome 14), β, and γ (chromosome 7), are at chromosomal positions susceptible to breakage and rearrangement in patients with ataxia-telangiectasia. The extent to which immune deficiency contributes to the genetic predisposition of patients to develop malignancy is unknown.

The risk of leukemia is increased in children with Klinefelter's syndrome and the trisomy G syndrome. Leukemia also has been associated with a variety of less-well-characterized chromosomal abnormalities. The increased risk of leukemia in children born to relatively older women may be related to the existence of subtle karyotypic abnormalities present in aging mothers. An increased risk of leukemia has been observed in several genetically determined congenital syndromes that are not associated with known karyotypic abnormalities, including the Rubinstein-Taybi syndrome, Schwachman's syndrome, Poland's syndrome, and neurofibromatosis.

The development of leukemia in more than one family member has been documented. The risk of leukemia is two to four times greater among siblings of leukemic children than in the general population. Those at highest risk for the development of leukemia are identical twins of children with the disease. Their risk may be as high as 25%, but it diminishes with age, and after the age of 7 years, the risk of leukemia for the unaffected twin returns to that of the general population. Although these observations strongly imply a genetic basis for the increased risk of leukemia, other factors, such as common exposure to a leukemogenic prenatal or postnatal event, cannot be excluded.

Recent attention has been focused on the p53 oncogene, a recessive tumor-suppressor gene.[4-7] Somatic p53 mutations have been reported in ALL but with a low frequency. Studies of familial ALL have identified nonhereditary p53 mutations in a few cases. It does not appear, however, that a mutant p53 gene is the cause of increased susceptibility to leukemia in most familial cases.

There has been intense interest in the possible role of viruses in the development of human leukemia. Certain retroviruses can cause leukemia in avian, murine, bovine, feline, and nonhuman primate species.[8] HTLV-I and HTLV-II, the human T-cell leukemia and lymphoma viruses, appear to play a role in the development of adult T-cell leukemia and hairy cell leukemia. No definite link has been confirmed between HTLV-I infection and children with ALL. The role of DNA viruses, particularly the Epstein-Barr virus (EBV), in lymphoid malignancy has been studied.

Infection with human immunodeficiency virus has been associated with a variety of malignancies, including lymphoma, angiogenic sarcoma, and leiomyosarcoma. Cases of B-lineage ALL have been reported.[9]

An association between immunodeficiency and the development of leukemia has been established. Children with the Wiskott-Aldrich syndrome, congenital hypogammaglobulinemia, or severe combined immunodeficiency disease have an increased incidence of lymphoid malignancy, including leukemia. Presumably, impaired immune surveillance permits the development of malignancy. The increased risk of leukemia in ataxia-telangiectasia patients probably is related to impaired immunity and genetic factors. Chronic use of immunosuppressive agents has been associated with the development of leukemia. The role that immune dysfunction plays in the development of leukemia in patients without a recognized immunodeficiency syndrome is unknown. Abnormalities in the immune system of newly diagnosed patients with ALL have been observed, but whether they precede or are a consequence of the leukemia is unclear.

ACUTE LYMPHOBLASTIC LEUKEMIA

CLINICAL PRESENTATION AND DIAGNOSIS

The presenting signs and symptoms of the child with ALL (Table 50–1) reflect the degree to which the bone marrow has been infiltrated with leukemic lymphoblasts and the extent of extramedullary spread. The most common symptoms and physical findings result from anemia, thrombocytopenia, and neutropenia and include pallor and fatigue, anorexia, petechiae, purpura, bleeding, and infection. Localized or generalized lymphadenopathy, hepatomegaly, and splenomegaly are the consequence of extramedullary leukemic spread. Overt symptoms of CNS leukemia are relatively rare at the time of initial diagnosis. Leukemic infiltration of the periosteum and bone frequently occurs, and bone pain, often manifesting as a limp or refusal to walk, is common in young children. The duration of symptoms in children presenting with ALL varies from days to months.

Because children most frequently present with relatively nonspecific symptoms, ALL clinically may mimic several childhood conditions, including infectious mononucleosis, id-

iopathic thrombocytopenic purpura, pertussis and parapertussis, chronic viral infections (*e.g.,* cytomegalovirus, acute infectious lymphocytosis) and rheumatoid arthritis. ALL may be confused with aplastic anemia. Rarely, it may present as the hypereosinophilic syndrome. ALL must be differentiated from other pediatric malignancies that may involve bone marrow, including non-Hodgkin's lymphoma, rhabdomyosarcoma, retinoblastoma, and neuroblastoma.

Replacement of normal bone marrow elements by leukemic cells produces an abnormal hemogram in most newly diagnosed patients (see Table 50–1). Anemia and thrombocytopenia occur in more than two thirds of patients. The peripheral leukocyte count may be normal or low, but approximately one third of patients have an initial leukocyte count of more than 20,000/mm³. An increased leukocyte count at diagnosis connotes a poor prognosis. Leukemic cells may be seen in the peripheral blood, but morphologic assessment of these cells is often misleading. Careful examination of a bone marrow aspirate is mandatory to make a diagnosis. On rare occasions, a bone marrow biopsy may be necessary. Although the presence of greater than 5% lymphoblasts indicates leukemia, most laboratories require a minimum of 25% leukemic blast cells in the bone marrow aspirate to confirm the diagnosis.[3] A definitive diagnosis requires careful morphologic examination of marrow aspirate smears stained with Romanovsky stain and detailed cytochemistry studies using myeloperoxidase or Sudan black, periodic acid-Schiff (PAS), and nonspecific esterase stains. Immunophenotyping, biochemical analysis (*e.g.,* TdT determination), and cytogenetic analyses should also be performed (Tables 50–2 and 50–3).

In addition to a detailed history, physical examination, and hematologic evaluation, newly diagnosed leukemia patients require other laboratory studies, including uric acid and electrolyte level determinations, kidney and liver function studies,

TABLE 50–1. Symptoms, Physical Findings, and Laboratory Features in Children with ALL

Clinical or Laboratory Feature	Patients (%)
Symptoms and Physical Findings	
Fever	61
Bleeding (*e.g.,* petechiae or purpura)	48
Bone pain	23
Lymphadenopathy	50
Splenomegaly	62
Hepatosplenomegaly	68
Laboratory Features	
Leukocyte count (/mm³)	
<10,000	53
10,000–49,000	30
>50,000	17
Hemoglobin (g/dl)	
<7.0	43
7.0–11.0	45
>11.0	12
Platelet count (/mm³)	
<20,000	28
20,000 to 99,000	47
>100,000	25
Lymphoblast morphology	
L1	84
L2	15
L3	1

(Miller DR. Acute lymphoblastic leukemia. Pediatr Clin North Am 1980;27:269–291)

TABLE 50–2. Morphologic, Cytochemical, and Biochemical Characteristics Helpful in Differentiating ALL From AML

Characteristic	ALL	AML
Nuclear-cytoplasmic ratio	High	Low
Nuclear chromatin	Clumped	Spongy
Nucleoli	0–2	2–5
Granules	−	+
Auer rods	−	+/−
Cytoplasm	Blue	Blue-gray
Cytochemical reaction		
Peroxidase	−	+
Sudan Black B	−	+
Periodic acid-Schiff	+/−	−
Naphthyl ASD chloracetate esterase	−	+/−
α-Napthyl acetate esterase	−	+/−
α-Napthyl butyrate esterase	−	−
Terminal deoxynucleotidyl transferase (TdT)	+*	−

* TdT is usually negative in typical FAB L3 ALL.
(Poplack DG. Clinical manifestations of acute lymphoblastic leukemia. In: Hoffmann R, ed. Hematology, basic principles and practice. New York: Churchill Livingstone, 1990:776–784)

TABLE 50–3. Monoclonal Antibodies Commonly Used to Immunophenotype Leukemia

CD	Antibody	Predominant Reactivity
T Cell		
CD1	T6	Thymocytes
CD2	T11	Pan-T
CD3	T3	Pan-T
CD4	T4/Leu-3	T helper/inducer
CD5	T101/Leu-1	Pan-T, B-cell CLL
CD7	Leu-9	Pan-T
CD8	T8/Leu-2	T cytotoxic/suppressor
CDw29	4B4	T4+/4B4+ (helper//inducer)
		T4+/2H4+ (suppressor/inducer)
B Cell		
CD19	B4	Pan-B
CD20	B1	Pan-B
CD21	B2	C3dR
CD24	BA1	Pan-B
	PCA-1	Plasma cells
Myeloid		
CD11c	Leu-M5	Monocytes, hairy cell
CD13	My7	Pan-myeloid
CD14	Leu-M3/MY4/MO2	Monocytes
CD15	Leu-M1	Monocytes, granulocytes
CD33	My9	Pan-myeloid
Miscellaneous		
CD9	BA2	Hematopoietic Progenitor/leukemic blasts
CD10	CALLA/J5	ALL/Burkitt's/follicular lymphoma
CD34	My10/HPCA-1	Hematopoietic progenitor cells/HTLV-infected cells
CD41a	Plt-1	Platelets/megakaryocytes
CD45	T-200/LCA	Pan-leukocyte
	T9	Transferrin receptor/proliferating cells

(CD classification number, corresponding antibodies and their predominant reactivity are listed with permission of Jane Trepel, PhD, Medicine Branch, National Cancer Institute. Other data from Poplack DG. Clinical manifestations of acute lymphoblastic leukemia. In: Hoffmann R, ed. Hematology, basic principles and practice. New York: Churchill Livingstone, 1990:776–784)

and appropriate radiologic studies. Hyperuricemia, a consequence of increased purine metabolism in leukemia cells, often exists at diagnosis or is provoked by initiation of treatment. Adequate hydration, alkalinization, and treatment with the xanthine oxidase inhibitor allopurinol are required to prevent uric acid nephropathy. Leukemic cell lysis frequently produces elevated serum lactate dehydrogenase (LDH) levels. Liver function tests may be abnormal at diagnosis, presumably the result of leukemic infiltration of the liver. A variety of metabolic abnormalities may be seen on initial presentation, including hyperkalemia, hypomagnesemia, and hypocalcemia or hypercalcemia. Low serum levels of immunoglobulins have been reported in as many as 30% of newly diagnosed patients

with ALL. Whether this represents a preexisting condition or is a consequence of the disease is not clear. Leukemic cells are capable of suppressing immunoglobulin synthesis in vitro, suggesting that in some patients this mechanism may play a role.

Chest x-ray films may reveal the presence of a mediastinal mass, particularly in high-risk patients. Leukemic infiltrates of the periosteum and bone may produce changes in the radiologic appearance of the long bones. Bone lesions may be observed radiographically even if there is no pain, and rarely, the bone lesions of ALL mimic osteomyelitis.

EXTRAMEDULLARY LEUKEMIA

Extramedullary leukemic spread may be clinically overt or detectable only by invasive diagnostic procedures. Extramedullary disease is important because it may cause local morbidity and because an extramedullary relapse frequently heralds bone marrow relapse, presumably as a result of spread to the bone marrow from the involved site. Current treatment strategies aim to prevent extramedullary relapse and to treat it aggressively if it occurs.

The two most important sites of extramedullary spread are the central nervous system (CNS) and the testes. Ovarian leukemia, perhaps because of inaccessibility to detailed physical examination, is rarely detected. Extramedullary disease can also occur in the liver, spleen, kidneys, gastrointestinal tract, and lung.

Central Nervous System Leukemia

The significance of CNS leukemia became apparent in the late 1950s and 1960s, when the CNS became the most frequent site of initial relapse because of better systemic treatment and longer survival. The incidence of CNS disease was as high as 75% to 80%. CNS disease was difficult to eradicate, and almost invariably, was rapidly followed by bone marrow relapse. The recognition of this latter phenomenon led to the development of effective CNS preventive therapy that improved the prognosis of children with this disease.

CNS leukemia is thought to develop by hematogenous seeding of circulating leukemic cells or by direct spread of leukemic cells from involved cranial bone marrow. CNS leukemia initially involves the meninges; deeper invasion of the brain parenchyma occurs in more advanced disease. Overt CNS leukemia occurs in fewer than 5% of children at diagnosis and rarely is symptomatic.[10] Symptomatic patients manifest a variety of signs and symptoms of increased intracranial pressure, including headaches, nausea, vomiting, lethargy, irritability, nuchal rigidity, and papilledema. Cranial nerve palsies may occur (most commonly of the sixth or seventh cranial nerves), often as an isolated event. More unusual presentations include the hypothalamic-obesity syndrome, diabetes insipidus, ataxia due to cerebellar involvement, and symptoms related to subdural or epidural leukemic infiltration. Any unexplained neurologic sign or symptom in a patient with ALL requires evaluation to exclude CNS leukemia.

The diagnosis of CNS disease is made by cytologic examination of cerebrospinal fluid (CSF) obtained by lumbar puncture. CSF should be examined after cytocentrifugation, a technique that concentrates the leukemic cells and increases diagnostic sensitivity tenfold. Relying solely on the demonstration of a pleocytosis in CSF is insufficient and potentially misleading. In symptomatic patients, CSF pressure is usually elevated, and hypoglycorrhachia and increased CSF protein levels are common. The heightened awareness of the possibility of CNS relapse has made surveillance lumbar punctures routine. As a result, CNS leukemia is more commonly diagnosed in the asymptomatic patient, in whom CSF pressure and chemistries may be normal and CSF leukemic cell counts relatively low. Although skull x-ray films, the computed tomography (CT) brain scan, head magnetic resonance imaging (MRI), and the electroencephalogram may occasionally be abnormal for the patient with overt CNS leukemia, none of these tests is reliable for diagnosis.

Testicular Leukemia

The incidence of testicular leukemia increased in the 1970s with improved survival of ALL patients. The testes constitute an important site of relapse, and although clinically demonstrable testicular disease is rarely evident at the initial diagnosis, occult testicular involvement has been reported in as many as 25% of newly diagnosed boys. Overt testicular recurrence, presenting as painless testicular enlargement, may occur in as many as 15% of boys undergoing chemotherapy. In one earlier study, testicular infiltration was reported in approximately 40% of boys who had successfully completed a 2.5-year to 3-year course of treatment.[11,12] Although the overall incidence of testicular disease appears to be significantly lower on current therapeutic protocols, biopsy-proven, occult testicular leukemia has been found in as many as 15% of asymptomatic boys on completion of chemotherapy, an observation consistent with relatively high incidence of late, overt relapses in these patients.

Testicular disease is more likely to occur in boys with a high initial leukocyte count ($>20,000/mm^3$), prominent lymphadenopathy and splenomegaly, T-cell disease, or significant thrombocytopenia ($>30,000/mm^3$).[13] The diagnosis of clinically suspected testicular leukemia is made by wedge biopsy. Testicular recurrence frequently is followed by systemic relapse, particularly if the testicular relapse has occurred during or immediately after maintenance chemotherapy. Isolated testicular relapse occurring 6 months or longer after cessation of therapy is associated with a relatively good prognosis if treated appropriately.

MORPHOLOGIC CLASSIFICATION

The considerable variation in the morphologic appearance of ALL cells led to numerous attempts to subclassify the disease. The system proposed by the French-American-British (FAB) cooperative working group, which divides lymphoblasts into three categories, has been most useful.[14] L1 lymphoblasts are smaller, with little cytoplasm and inconspicuous nucleoli or none at all. L2 lymphoblasts are larger, with abundant cytoplasm and prominent nucleoli. Leukemic cells of the L3 type are cytomorphologically identical to Burkitt's lymphoma cells. Approximately 85% of childhood ALL cases have L1 lymphoblasts, 14% are L2, and 1% are L3. The L2 lymphoblast is the most common type in adults. Concordance among observers using this system is high, and the FAB classification has prog-

nostic value.[14,15] L1 lymphoblasts are associated with a higher remission induction rate and prolonged remission and survival. L2 cells convey a poor prognosis independently of other prognostic variables. Patients with the L3 variety have the least favorable prognosis. With the possible exception of L3 cells, which ordinarily possess surface immunoglobulin and other B-cell markers, there is no apparent correlation between FAB classification and immunologic cell-surface markers.[14]

DIAGNOSIS AND CLASSIFICATION

Immunophenotypes

Immunologic techniques have permitted the identification of distinct immunologic subtypes of ALL and have confirmed that ALL is a heterogenous disease in which leukemic transformation and clonal expansion may occur at different stages in lymphoid differentiation. Initially, using standard immunologic methods for surface membrane characterization, three forms of ALL were identified. Between 1% and 2% had lymphoblasts with B-cell characteristics, and most patients were found to have lymphoblasts that lacked definable T-cell or B-cell markers. Further classification using heterologous antisera and monoclonal antibodies detected a common leukemia-associated antigen (CALLA) on the leukemic cells of approximately 80% of the children with "non-T, non-B-cell" leukemia and designated these as having "common ALL" to differentiate them from the antigen-negative, non-T, non-B-cell group with "null cell" ALL.

Clinical differences were apparent among the immunologic subtypes of ALL. Children with common ALL had a relatively good prognosis, faring better than those with null cell ALL. T-cell ALL was found to have distinctive clinical features, frequently occurring in older boys presenting with a high initial leukocyte count and a mediastinal mass. T-cell ALL is associated with a poor prognosis, but it is unclear whether any immunologic subtype is a significant independent prognostic variable.

More sophisticated immunologic methods have revealed that most non-T, non-B lymphoblasts are actually early B cells. These cells are capable of differentiating in vitro into cells with B-cell markers, may possess intracytoplasmic immunoglobulin, and demonstrate immunoglobulin gene rearrangement indicative of precursor cells committed to the B-cell lineage.[16] Approximately 20% to 30% of B-cell precursor ALL cases have lymphoblasts that are cytoplasmic μ ($C\mu$) heavy chain positive. These pre-B-cell ALL cases represent a relatively mature stage of development and are differentiated from $C\mu$-negative early pre-B-cell cases of ALL.[17] Pre-B-cell ALL has a worse prognosis than the early pre-B-cell type.[17]

Using recombinant DNA technology for analysis of immunoglobulin gene rearrangement in precursor-B-cell ALL and monoclonal antibodies for immunophenotyping different B-cell antigens, investigators have defined distinct stages of differentiation for pre-B-cell ALL.[17] Monoclonal antibodies also have been used to define different subsets of normal thymocytes that correspond to different stages of intrathymic differentiation.[18] Typing with these antibodies has demonstrated that T-cell leukemias may be derived from these different stages of differentiation.

Molecular biologic analysis of the genes encoding the T-cell receptor have provided a useful marker of T-cell differentiation in an analogous fashion to immunoglobulin gene rearrangement in pre-B-cell ALL.[19] Although most ALL cells can be readily classified as B-cell or T-cell lineage, some leukemic cells coexpress cell surface marker antigens or molecular markers, suggesting that traditional views of lineage classification may be overly restrictive.[19,20] For example, immunoglobulin gene rearrangement may occur in cases of T-cell ALL, and conversely, T-cell receptor gene rearrangement occurs in some cases of B-lineage ALL (Fig. 50–1).

There are also numerous reports of ALL cases in which the leukemic cells express characteristics of more than one he-

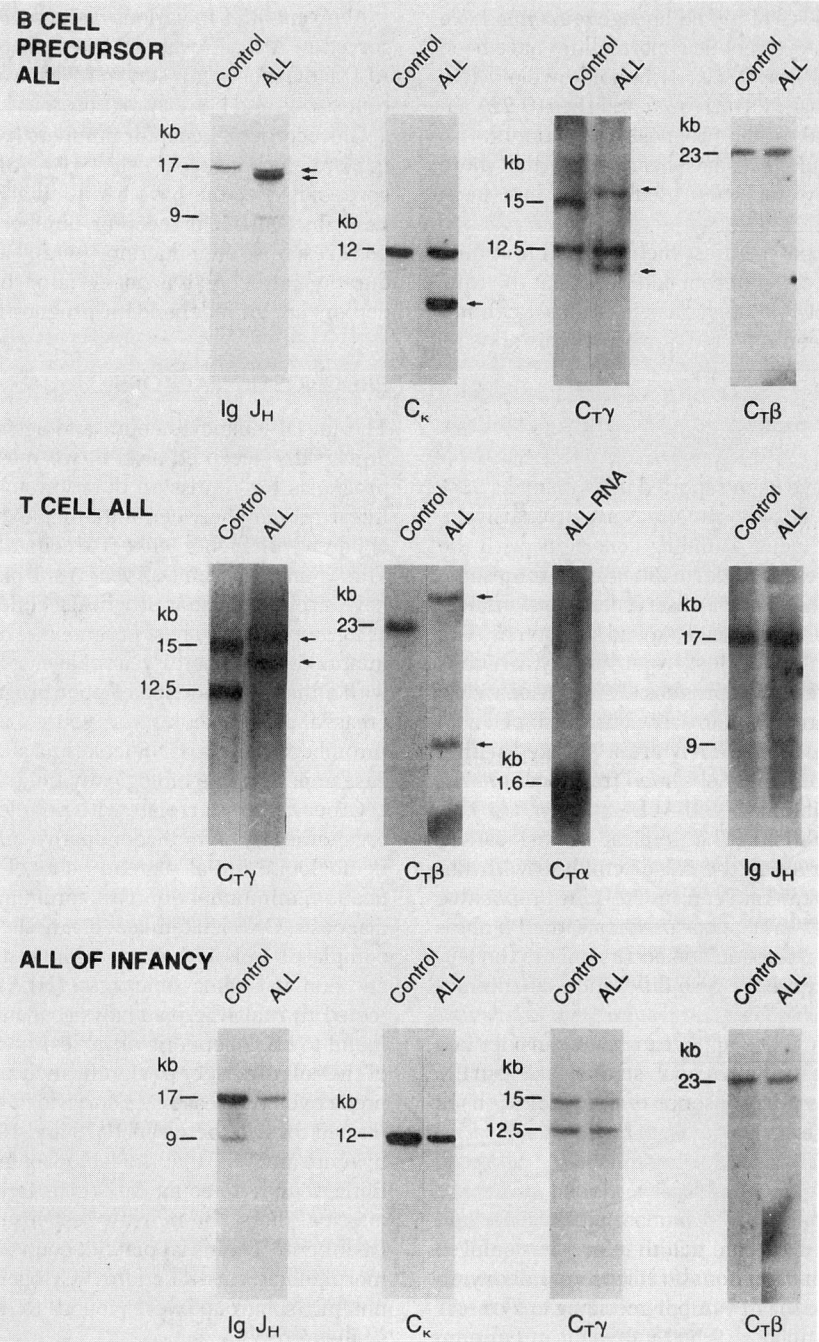

FIGURE 50–1. Examples of patterns of immunoglobulin and T-cell receptor gene rearrangement in acute lymphoblastic leukemia of childhood shown by Southern and Northern analysis. (Reproduced with permission from Carolyn Felix, MD). **(A)** B-cell precursor ALL. This case demonstrates rearrangement of both alleles of the immunoglobulin heavy chain gene, one allele of the κ light chain gene, and both alleles of the T-cell receptor γ gene. The T-cell receptor β gene remains in germline configuration. **(B)** T-cell ALL. This case illustrates rearrangement of both alleles of the T-cell receptor; γ and β line configuration of the immunoglobulin heavy chain gene is shown. **(C)** ALL of infancy (B-cell precursor). This case demonstrates the germline configuration both of immunoglobulin heavy and light chain genes and of the γ and β T-cell receptor genes. Rearrangements are indicated by arrows and germline bands by dash marks.

matopoietic lineage.[21-23] The incidence of cases that express myeloid and lymphoid markers has been reported to be as high as 25%.[24] It is not clear whether they represent leukemias that have developed from normal multilineage potential precursors or represent cases occurring from aberrant or inappropriate gene activation and thus have not been derived from a corresponding normal stage of hematopoietic development. Guidelines for the diagnosis of mixed lineage leukemia have been proposed.[25] Certain cytogenetic abnormalities have been associated with mixed lineage (*i.e.*, lymphoid-myeloid leukemias), including the t(4;11)(q21;q23) and the t(9;22) abnormalities. In most studies, the prognosis for patients with acute mixed-lineage leukemias has been poor, and more intensive chemotherapy for these leukemias has been advocated.[23]

At relapse, most patients manifest their original immunophenotypes. Expression of a different cell lineage at the time of relapse is a rare event. Although changes in blast cell immunophenotype have been reported at relapse, this appears to be the exception.

Cytogenetics

Abnormal karyotypes have been reported in as many as 90% of children with ALL.[26] The abnormalities are ordinarily restricted to the leukemia cells, a finding consistent with the clonal nature of the disease. Abnormalities in chromosome number and structure have been observed. Approximately 67% of patients have diploid or pseudodiploid karyotypes. The remaining 33% of patients manifest hyperdiploidy, which is associated with a relatively good prognosis.[27] Translocations, the most common structural abnormality observed, occur in approximately 40% of patients. They are associated with a poor prognosis. More commonly observed translocations include the t(8;14) (specific for B-cell ALL), t(9;22), t(4;11), and t(1;19) abnormalities. The typical translocation, t(9;22)(q34;q11), observed in the 5% of children with Ph-positive ALL, is similar to that seen in CML. In Ph-positive ALL, however, a disorder with a poor prognosis, the Ph chromosome is not found in remission and occurs only in the leukemic lymphoid line. There are also differences at the molecular level.[27]

Chromosomal abnormalities appear to have considerable prognostic importance. Chromosomal studies are usually normal during remission; the presence of aneuploid cells is thought to herald relapse.

Biochemistry

Study of several enzymes indicate that they may be useful in the diagnosis and classification of ALL. Terminal deoxynucleotidyl transferase (TdT), a DNA polymerizing enzyme, is not found in normal lymphocytes but is present in lymphoblasts of T-cell and non-T, non-B-cell types. TdT expression is variable in B-cell ALL. TdT determination may help to differentiate ALL from AML, in which it is rarely present. TdT activity, however, has no prognostic significance in ALL.

Several purine pathway enzymes, whose activity is abnormal in certain childhood immunodeficiency states, have specific patterns of expression that correlate with immunologic subtypes of ALL.[28] For example, T-cell lymphoblasts have ele-

vated adenosine deaminase (ADA), but lower 5'-nucleotidase and purine nucleoside phosphorylase activity than non-T, non-B lymphoblasts.[28] These findings raised the possibility that selective therapy, aimed at taking advantage of these enzyme abnormalities, might be of value. Deoxycoformycin, an ADA inhibitor, has undergone clinical trials and has been used for in vitro marrow purging.

Abnormalities in various lysozomal enzymes have been observed in ALL. Elevated LDH activity has been observed in ALL at diagnosis; low serum LDH levels correlate with longer remissions and better prognoses.

Glucocorticoid receptor numbers have been correlated with in vitro glucocorticoid sensitivity. A lower number of glucocorticoid receptors have been found on T-cell lymphoblasts. Low glucocorticoid receptor numbers are associated with a poor response to induction therapy and a shorter remission duration, although it is not certain whether glucocorticoid receptors are an independent prognostic factor.

PROGNOSTIC FACTORS

The initial leukocyte count and age at diagnosis of ALL are universally accepted as the two most reliable indicators of prognosis for remission duration and survival.[29] There is a linear relation between initial leukocyte count and outcome; children with higher leukocyte counts have a poorer prognosis. Very young children (<2 years) and older patients (>10 years) have a relatively poor prognosis; children in the intermediate age group have the best prognosis. The worse prognosis is for infants younger than 1 year of age.[30,31] These children present with a higher incidence of poor prognostic features (*e.g.*, increased initial leukocyte count, massive organomegaly, thrombocytopenia, CNS leukemia at diagnosis) and their disease appears to be biologically unique.[30]

Other factors correlate with prognosis, including sex, race, organomegaly, lymphadenopathy, mediastinal mass, initial hemoglobin, initial platelet count, FAB morphologic classification, immunophenotype, serum immunoglobulin levels at diagnosis, CNS leukemia at diagnosis, the rapidity of attaining complete remission, chromosomal status, serum LDH level, and human leukocyte antigen (HLA) type.[27,29,32] When subjected to multivariate analysis, many of these features are found to be dependent variables.[27,29,32] A retrospective study of the relative order of significance and association of factors predictive for disease-free survival in a group of 1419 children treated for ALL between 1978 and 1982 revealed, after multivariate analysis, that the factors of greatest importance were initial leukocyte count, sex (girls fare better than boys), mediastinal mass, the marrow response on day 14 of induction treatment, age, initial platelet count, hepatomegaly, and FAB morphologic classification.[29] Cytogenetics and immunophenotypic subgroup were found to be important in other studies.[17,27]

The prognostic importance of some factors may vary somewhat from study to study, which may be caused by differences in treatment and in the patient populations.

Most current protocols use prognostic criteria (*e.g.*, initial leukocyte count, age at diagnosis) to stratify patients at diagnosis into different risk groups. Staging of this type permits selective application of treatment to different risk groups. High-risk patients are treated with more aggressive chemotherapy regimens, but low-risk patients receive less-intensive therapy, designed to be equally effective but avoid the toxicities and complications of aggressive therapy.

No single system of ALL staging has been universally accepted. An example is shown in Figure 50–2 that illustrates the event-free survival curves for patients treated on a Children's Cancer Study Group (CCSG) series of protocols that stratified patients into five risk groups: good, average, poor (primarily on the basis of initial leukocyte count, age at diagnosis, and FAB classification), infants, and patients presenting with lymphomatous features, a group at high risk of treatment failure, particularly CNS relapse.[29]

TREATMENT

As our understanding of ALL has increased, evaluation and treatment of children with this disease has become more complex. An appropriate patient workup requires sophisticated techniques (*e.g.*, immunophenotyping, cytogenetic analysis, molecular genotyping, biochemical assays) and stratification of patients into risk groups for appropriate therapy. Recognition of the biologic heterogeneity of ALL makes it inappropriate to define a standard ALL treatment regimen. Combination chemotherapy remains the primary therapeutic modality. Current treatment is divided into four phases: remission induction, CNS preventive therapy, consolidation, and maintenance.

Remission Induction

The first goal of ALL treatment is induction of complete remission, defined as the lack of any evidence of leukemia on physical examination and hematologic evaluation. The bone marrow must be normocellular, with fewer than 5% lymphoblasts, and peripheral blood counts should be within the range of normal values. There must be no detectable CNS or other extramedullary disease. It has been estimated that patients with clinically overt ALL have approximately 10^{12} leukemic

cells, and patients in remission have fewer than 10^{10} blast cells. In these terms, remission induction requires a reduction in the number of leukemic cells by at least 99%. Although prednisone and vincristine traditionally have been the most widely used two-drug combination, capable of inducing remission in approximately 80% to 90% of patients, it is now clear that this combination is inadequate. The addition of a third agent, L-asparaginase or daunorubicin, raises the induction rate to 90% to 100% and significantly prolongs remission. The addition of a fourth induction agent, usually the anthracycline daunorubicin, together with intensive consolidation therapy, improves remission duration, even in patients with poor-risk factors.[33] Most induction regimens last approximately 4 weeks. There is evidence that the rapidity of cytoreduction correlates with remission duration (Fig. 50–3).

Central Nervous System Prophylaxis

The concept of CNS preventive therapy is based on the assumption that undetectable CNS leukemia is present in most patients at the time of diagnosis, residing in that "sanctuary site" protected by the blood-brain barrier from cytotoxic concentrations of most systemically administered antileukemic agents. Studies in the 1960s aimed at prevention of CNS leukemia demonstrated that administration of 2400 cGy of cranial irradiation and intrathecal methotrexate after remission induction reduced the incidence of overt CNS leukemia from more than 60% to 10% or less.

Although this approach was universally adopted in the 1970s, the adverse effects of CNS irradiation on neurologic and intellectual functions prompted a reappraisal of this strategy. There is now a large body of data documenting long-term side effects, including CT-detected brain abnormalities, impaired intellectual and psychomotor function, and neuroendocrine dysfunction, in a proportion of patients treated with 2400 cGy of cranial irradiation and intrathecal chemotherapy. This has stimulated a search for safer methods of CNS prophylaxis. Several approaches have been studied, in-

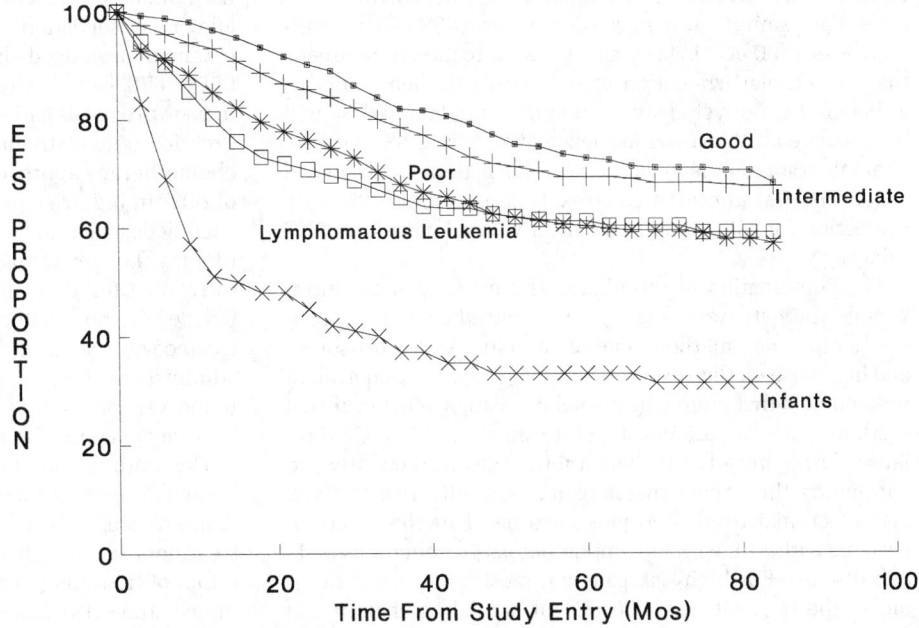

FIGURE 50–2. Event-free survival of 3507 children with ALL stratified according to prognostic groups and treated by the Children's Cancer Study Group. (Reproduced with permission of WA Bleyer, MD, and H Sather, PhD)

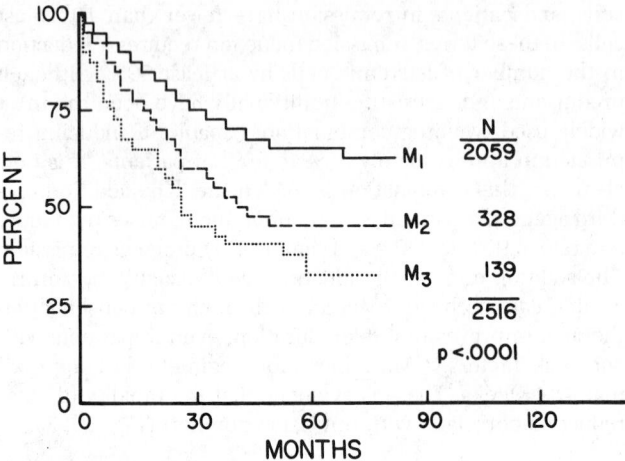

FIGURE 50–3. Disease-free survival from completion of induction treatment according to day 14 bone marrow status in 2516 children with ALL. Day 14 bone marrow status was a highly significant independent predictor of disease-free survival. (Miller D, Coccia P, Bleyer W, et al. Early response to induction therapy as a predictor of disease-free survival and late recurrence of childhood acute lymphoblastic leukemia: A report from the Childrens Cancer Study Group. J Clin Oncol 1989;7:1807–1815)

cluding using lower doses of cranial irradiation (1800 cGy) with intrathecal methotrexate; periodic intrathecal methotrexate during maintenance with intensive systemic chemotherapy; triple intrathecal chemotherapy with methotrexate, cytosine arabinoside, and hydrocortisone; intermediate-dose methotrexate alone or with concomitant intrathecal methotrexate; or high-dose systemic methotrexate alone.

The risk of developing CNS leukemia depends on certain predictive factors at presentation. Characteristics associated with an increased risk of CNS leukemia include a high initial leukocyte count, T-cell disease, thrombocytopenia, profound lymphadenopathy or hepatosplenomegaly, and patients who are very young or black.[10,30] The recognition of different risk groups led to the concept of tailoring CNS preventive therapy, using equally effective, less-intensive CNS treatment if possible. For example, it is now evident that 1800 cGy is as effective as 2400 cGy in providing CNS protection in regimens that use cranial irradiation plus intrathecal chemotherapy, although it is not yet clear if reduction in radiation dose will be associated with a lower incidence of adverse CNS sequelae. Cranial irradiation is not necessary for patients with a good prognosis; intrathecal methotrexate alone offers adequate protection for this group of children with a low risk of CNS relapse.[34]

The combination of intrathecal and moderate-dose intravenous methotrexate, maintenance intrathecal triple chemotherapy (*i.e.*, methotrexate, cytarabine, hydrocortisone), and high-dose methotrexate alone appear to provide equivalent protection to that offered by cranial irradiation and intrathecal methotrexate for patients at an intermediate risk of CNS relapse. Triple intrathecal chemotherapy given frequently and continuing throughout maintenance is as effective as 2400 cGy of cranial irradiation plus intrathecal methotrexate in patients with ALL without lymphomatous presentations or T-cell disease. For high-risk patients, most published data indicate the necessity of 1800 cGy of cranial irradiation and

intrathecal methotrexate to prevent CNS relapse.[10] A study employing very-high-dose methotrexate infusions, high-dose cytarabine, and sequential intrathecal chemotherapy with methotrexate and cytarabine demonstrated effective CNS preventive therapy for high-risk patients without using cranial irradiation. Although this study requires confirmation, the results raise the possibility that the need for cranial irradiation in high-risk patients may be obviated by the use of aggressive chemotherapy.[35]

Consolidation and Maintenance Therapy

After remission induction, additional treatment is necessary. Without maintenance treatment, most patients relapse within 1 to 2 months. Methotrexate and 6-mercaptopurine are the two drugs most frequently administered during maintenance. Usually, 6-mercaptopurine is given on a daily basis; methotrexate is given intermittently (*e.g.*, once or twice weekly). The value of adding agents to standard 6-mercaptopurine and methotrexate maintenance therapy has been controversial, and the data have been somewhat contradictory. The addition of intermittent pulses of vincristine and prednisone appears to prolong remission, although the value of this approach after intensive induction therapy is unclear. The intensive, weekly use of L-asparaginase may add to the effectiveness of maintenance treatment. Other approaches include repeated pulses of an intensive combination of agents periodically during maintenance and sequential intensive multiagent therapy.[36]

The choice of an appropriate maintenance regimen may also differ for different risk groups. Although 6-mercaptopurine and methotrexate may be adequate for certain good-risk patients, more intensive maintenance therapy appears to be optimal in treating poor-risk patients.

To improve cytoreduction early in maintenance, many regimens now include a period of intensified therapy shortly after remission induction with drugs that minimize the development of cross-resistance. Intensive remission "consolidation" therapy of this type has improved treatment success even in patients with poor prognoses.[36–39] A West German study that used intensive induction and consolidation and "reinduction" and "reconsolidation" phases of therapy early in maintenance obtained prolonged disease-free survival in approximately 65% to 70% of children, with significantly improved results in poor-prognosis patients.[37] Similarly, a study employing early "reinforcement" therapy followed by a rotational combination chemotherapy approach produced an event-free survival rate of 69% in high-risk patients.[38]

Drug dosage is an important consideration in maintenance therapy. Longer remissions occurred in patients randomized to receive full-dose maintenance therapy with 6-mercaptopurine, methotrexate, and cyclophosphamide than in those treated with the same agents administered at half dose. Orally administered 6-mercaptopurine and methotrexate have profound variations in bioavailability, suggesting that this may be a mechanism of treatment failure for some patients.

The optimal duration of maintenance treatment is not known. Most centers treat patients for 2.5 to 3 years. A randomized study demonstrated that 5 years of maintenance treatment has no advantage over 3 years.[40] The optimal duration of treatment appears to be different for girls and boys; in one study, 1.5 years of therapy was sufficient for girls but inadequate for boys. It is likely that the intensity of therapy has bearing on the optimal duration of treatment. Because much of the information on which the current policy of 2.5 to 3 years of maintenance therapy is based was derived from less-intensive therapeutic regimens than many currently in use, additional study of this important question is needed.

The outlook for patients who successfully complete a full 2.5-year to 3-year course of treatment is good. Approximately 80% of these patients can expect to remain disease free. The greatest number of relapses occur in the first year after discontinuing chemotherapy. After 4 years "off" treatment, relapse is unusual.

Treatment of Relapse

BONE MARROW RELAPSE. Bone marrow relapse is the most frequent form of treatment failure in patients with ALL. Reinduction of remission is possible in most patients who suffer an initial marrow relapse, but most patients experience subsequent relapse and eventually die of the disease. Nevertheless, many patients can achieve prolonged second remissions, justifying an aggressive treatment approach to the child in relapse. Multidrug induction regimens are the most effective. The best results have been obtained with a four-drug combination, which includes vincristine, prednisone, L-asparaginase, and daunorubicin and produces remission in 90% of patients.

Other factors influence the remission induction rate for relapsed patients. Children whose relapses occur more than 6 months after completion of chemotherapy regimens have a better chance of achieving and maintaining prolonged second remission than do children who relapse while receiving maintenance therapy. Second remissions are more readily induced in patients who receive suboptimal induction or maintenance therapy as initial treatment for their disease or who had longer first remissions.

A second course of CNS preventive therapy is necessary for patients in second remission. Without additional CNS prophylaxis in these patients, almost 50% suffer CNS relapses. In previously irradiated patients, intrathecal chemotherapy is an effective form of second CNS prophylaxis.

Unfortunately, second or subsequent remissions, particularly in children relapsing on treatment, are usually short. However, it has been reported that prolonged second remissions (>2 years) can be obtained with aggressive chemotherapy in 10% to 30% of patients who relapse on therapy and in approximately one third of patients who relapse after elective cessation of therapy.[41-43]

Bone marrow transplantation is another approach used to treat relapse patients (Fig. 50-4). An early report from the Seattle transplant group on the long-term follow-up of a group of patients with ALL who received allogeneic bone marrow transplantation indicated that, with a minimum follow-up of more than 5 years, 27% of the patients transplanted in second or subsequent remissions and 15% of patients transplanted during relapse were alive and free of disease.[44] A report from Seattle confirmed other studies that have reported long-term disease-free survival for 40% or more of patients transplanted during second remission.[45-47] Allogeneic bone marrow transplantation is feasible for the approximately one third of relapsed patients who have an HLA-identical sibling. Bone mar-

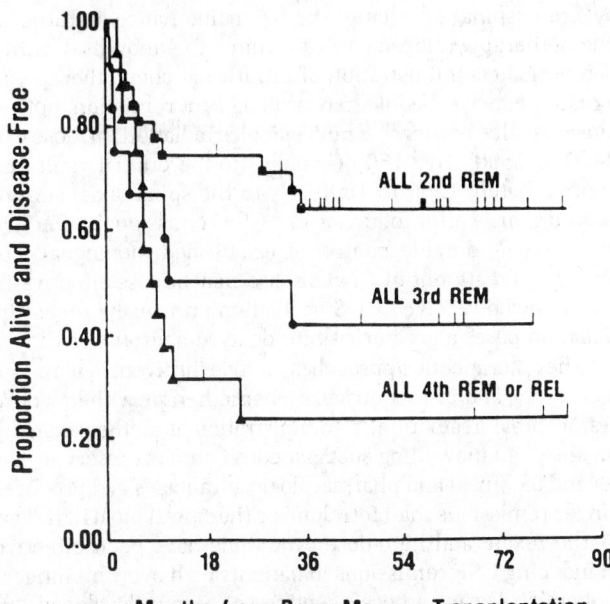

FIGURE 50-4. Disease-free survival of children receiving transplants for ALL. Patients were stratified according to their disease status at the time of transplantation. (Brochstein JA, Kernan NA, Groshen S, et al. Allogeneic bone marrow transplantation after hyperfractionated total-body irradiation and cyclophosphamide in children with acute leukemia. N Engl J Med 1987;317:1618–1624)

row transplantation is considered the treatment of choice for patients in second bone marrow remission whose initial relapse occurred while undergoing chemotherapy or within 3 months of its completion.[41,48] An analysis performed by the International Bone Marrow Transplant Registry indicates that patients with late relapses (>36 months after attainment of first remission or after completion of maintenance therapy) should probably receive chemotherapy, with bone marrow transplantation reserved for subsequent relapses.[48-50]

Methods of crossing the histocompatibility barrier are being studied in several centers and, if successful, ultimately may increase the applicability of bone marrow transplantation. Autologous transplantation with remission marrow treated in vitro with leukemia-specific monoclonal antibodies is being investigated. Relapse-free survival can be achieved in approximately 20% to 30% of relapsed patients using this approach.[51,52] Other approaches being studied for patients without a histocompatible sibling donor include the use of partially matched, related donors or unrelated matched donors identified through comprehensive bone marrow typing banks. The effectiveness of these marrow transplant approaches and their eventual role for therapy of ALL requires additional study.

CENTRAL NERVOUS SYSTEM RELAPSE. Although CNS preventive therapy has dramatically reduced its incidence, CNS relapse remains a significant cause of treatment failure in ALL. CNS relapse may occur as an isolated relapse, concomitant with bone marrow relapse or with recurrence in another extramedullary site (*e.g.*, testes). Intrathecal methotrexate, alone or together with cytosine arabinoside and hydrocortisone, produces CNS remission (*i.e.*, clearance of CSF lymphoblasts) in more than 90% of patients. Unless followed by craniospinal irradiation or by maintenance intrathecal chemotherapy, relapse ensues within 3 to 4 months. Continued periodic administration of intrathecal chemotherapy on a maintenance schedule may prolong CSF remission, but relapse usually occurs.[10] Craniospinal irradiation, at doses of 2400 to 2500 cGy (150 cGy daily) to the cranial vault and approximately 1200 to 1800 cGy to the spinal axis, administered shortly after induction of a CSF remission, is effective in achieving durable control of established meningeal leukemia.[10] Treatment of CNS disease may be less effective in patients who received CNS irradiation previously; repeat irradiation poses a greater risk for delayed neurotoxicity.[53]

Other therapeutic approaches include intraventricular chemotherapy and intraventricular chemotherapy with low-dose craniospinal irradiation.[10] Administration of methotrexate by means of an indwelling subcutaneous Ommaya reservoir has several technical and pharmacologic advantages and produces longer remissions than intralumbar therapy alone. High-dose methotrexate and high-dose cytarabine have been effective in inducing CSF remissions in patients with overt meningeal leukemia. New intrathecal agents are also being developed.[54,55] Because isolated CNS relapse often heralds a bone marrow relapse, intensification of systemic therapy at the time of isolated CNS relapse is considered essential.

TESTICULAR RELAPSE. Testicular relapse requires treatment with radiation therapy. Unilateral disease frequently has been followed by relapse in the contralateral testis, particularly in patients with early testicular relapse during therapy.[6] Bilateral testicular radiation therapy is indicated for all patients. A dosage of 2400 cGy is considered adequate, although rare cases of local recurrence have been reported. In the past, testicular recurrence frequently was followed by systemic relapse and was associated with a poor prognosis. The practice of intensifying systemic therapy or reinducing patients at the time of isolated testicular relapse has produced a dramatic improvement, and prolonged disease-free survival is now possible.[56,57]

Supportive Care

The provision of optimal supportive care is a vital element in the treatment of the child with ALL. Appropriate use of blood component therapy; an aggressive approach to detection, prevention, and management of infectious complications; maintenance of the metabolic and nutritional needs of the patient; and comprehensive, continuous psychosocial support for patient and family are mandatory.

Late Effects of Treatment

The increased survival of children with ALL has focused attention on the late effects of antileukemia therapy. Recognition of adverse sequelae is particularly important now that it is possible to define good-risk patients for whom less intensive but equally effective therapy may be designed.

The effects of CNS preventive therapy on neurologic and intellectual function have been of particular concern. The awareness of adverse sequelae has stimulated a search for equally effective alternative approaches to CNS preventive therapy. Children treated for overt CNS disease are at a higher risk for neurologic and neuropsychologic sequelae of treatment.[53] Careful monitoring of patients at risk for possible adverse CNS sequelae, with periodic neurologic examination, CT or MRI brain scans, and psychometric testing is advocated.[53]

The reproductive capacity of children exposed to prolonged antileukemic therapy has been evaluated, and most boys and girls treated with conventional chemotherapy (not including cyclophosphamide) appear to maintain gonadal function and undergo normal pubertal progression. However, boys who have received testicular irradiation have a high rate of testicular endocrine failure and may require androgen replacement therapy. As survival times increase, more patients face the prospect of parenthood. Although scarce, the available evidence suggests no increase in birth defects in the offspring of mothers or fathers previously treated for ALL.

Damage to other systems (*e.g.,* elevated liver enzymes) may occur during therapy, but long-term toxic effects after treatment are unusual. Although treatment with anthracyclines carries the possibility of cardiac toxicity, most protocols use limited cumulative doses of this agent. Some patients, however, who receive anthracyclines for ALL treatment may be at a significant risk for late-onset congestive heart failure. A study from the Dana-Farber Cancer Institute indicated that over half of a group of long-term ALL survivors had evidence of abnormal left ventricular function.[58] These results and those of other studies increased concern about late anthracycline cardiotoxicity and emphasized the need for careful cardiac monitoring and follow-up of children at risk.[59]

Second malignancies have been reported in ALL, but the incidence has been exceedingly low. There are, however, an increasing number of brain tumors (mostly secondary malignant gliomas) diagnosed in children after cranial irradiation.[60] Reports from St. Jude Children's Research Hospital indicated an unexpectedly high number of cases of secondary acute myelogenous leukemia in patients treated with intensive chemotherapy that included exposure to epipodophyllotoxins.[60a] These leukemias have been characterized by the presence of an 11q23 chromosomal abnormality. These reports and those of secondary leukemias occurring in other cancer patients treated with epipodophyllotoxins led to questions about the role of these compounds in the treatment of newly diagnosed patients with ALL.[61-63]

For many children with ALL, most therapy can be administered on an outpatient basis. Despite its length, treatment is usually compatible with a reasonably normal lifestyle. Most patients do not experience significant late sequelae and tolerate treatment well.

Treatment Obstacles

Despite the dramatic improvement in therapy, many treatment obstacles must be overcome before a cure becomes a reality for all patients.

Continued efforts must be made to define more precisely those clinical and biologic features of greatest prognostic value, permitting improved delineation of patient subgroups requiring more or less intensive therapy. The most important problem is the need for improved treatment of patients in the poor-risk category. Although efforts to intensify therapy for these patients appear promising, greater understanding of the disease that affects them is needed. The group of patients failing current therapy is known to be biologically heterogenous, manifesting differences in clinical presentation and in the cytogenetic, immunologic, and molecular features of their disease. The application of molecular biologic methods to the study of drug resistance may ultimately provide valuable information about the mechanisms of treatment failure. Studies of the role of expression of the multidrug resistance gene, *MDR1*, in patients with ALL who have experienced treatment failure are in progress.[64]

The causes of treatment failure must be identified. More than one third of children with ALL relapse, most during maintenance therapy. Recent studies, suggesting that variation and limitations in drug bioavailability may be partially responsible for treatment failure during maintenance, require confirmation.

Molecular biologic techniques are being applied to detect minimal residual disease. In the past, most methods lacked sufficient sensitivity, but studies using polymerase chain reaction technology demonstrate an enhanced ability to detect residual leukemic cells and suggest that this approach may be useful in identifying patients at risk for relapse.[65-68]

Because attention also must focus on the development of more effective treatment for the relapsed patient, the role of bone marrow transplantation in the treatment of ALL is likely to increase. Recent successes in the use of partially mismatched donors offers the possibility of totally crossing the HLA barrier. The role of autologous marrow transplantation may expand as newer methods of in vitro purging (*e.g.*, radiolabeled monoclonal antibodies or biologics) become available.

An exciting potential application for biologics in ALL treatment is in the area of molecularly cloned hematopoietic growth factors. Preclinical and early clinical studies with granulocyte-macrophage colony-stimulating factor (GM-CSF) and granulocyte colony-stimulating factor (G-CSF) confirm the potential of these agents to shorten the duration and severity of chemotherapy-induced myelosuppression. These agents may allow intensified chemotherapy for patients with ALL at high risk of treatment failure.

ACUTE MYELOGENOUS LEUKEMIA

AML represents approximately 20% of all cases of acute leukemia in children. Considerable progress has been made in the treatment of childhood AML in the past decade. The prognosis for children with this disease, although appreciably greater than that for adults, is significantly worse than for children with ALL. AML shares many features with the adult form of the disease (see Chap. 54). With some minor differences, the biology of AML is similar in children and adults, with the possible exception of neonatal leukemia.

Approximately 50% to 70% of children are classified as having AML, and 20% to 40% have acute myelomonocytic leukemia.[69] The FAB system of morphologic classification in equally applicable to childhood AML. There is some evidence that patients in the FAB M5a (acute monoblastic leukemia) and M5b (acute monocytic leukemia) subcategories have a less favorable prognosis.[70] The responses to treatment of the other FAB subtypes are similar.

Mixed-lineage leukemia has been reported in cases presenting as childhood AML. In one series, approximately 15% of cases of AML expressed lymphoid antigens. Most of these cases were FAB M1 or M2 and expressed the T-cell antigen CD7 and CD2.[71] The clinical significance of mixed lineage is not clear.[20] Acute megakaryocytic leukemia (M7), recently added to the FAB classification system, occurs more commonly in children with Down's syndrome. M7 is frequently associated with myelofibrosis.

Definable cytogenetic abnormalities are present in more than two thirds of AML cases. There are some cytogenetic differences between childhood and adult AML. The −5, 5q−, and −7 abnormalities often seen in adults are rare in children. The 11q23 translocation occurs frequently in infants and often is associated with biphenotypic leukemia. This translocation is also found in cases of secondary AML arising as a consequence of epipodophyllotoxin therapy. A t(1;22) has been associated with acute megakaryocytic leukemia in infants.

Chromosomal patterns appear to have prognostic implications. Trisomy 8, t(8;21), inv(16), and t(9;11) are associated with a high rate of complete remission; abnormalities of chromosome 7 (*e.g.*, monosomy 7) are associated with a low rate of remission induction. The t(9;11) and the t(15;17) (found in M3 disease) are associated with prolonged remission duration.

Information about the influence on prognosis of other factors such as age, sex, and leukocyte count has been somewhat conflicting. Very young age (<1 year) and high leukocyte count (>20,000/mm^3) are unfavorable prognostic factors for attaining complete remission.[69,72] Cases of M1 subtype that lack Auer rods have a low remission induction rate.[73] Remission rates are also low in cases of treatment-related secondary AML or AML that develop after a myelodysplastic syndrome. Age at diagnosis, initial leukocyte count, and FAB classification affect remission duration.[69] Children older than 2 years of age have a better prognosis than younger children, with those between 3 and 10 years of age having the best prognosis. The poor prognosis for children younger than 2 years may be related to the observation that the M4 and M5 FAB categories occur more often in these children (Table 50–4).[70]

Because AML and ALL have similar clinical presentations but quite different therapies and prognoses, it is important for the clinician to differentiate them. In addition to use of special stains (*e.g.*, myeloperoxidase, Sudan black, PAS, specific esterase), determination of TdT activity (usually lacking in AML) and immunophenotyping with myeloid-specific monoclonal antibodies are important.[74] After the diagnosis of AML is established, the FAB subtype should be determined, because this classification system has prognostic value and because certain FAB subcategories present unique clinical problems. For example, patients with the M3 (promyelocytic leukemia) subtype frequently develop a disseminated intravascular coagulation-like syndrome. Cytogenetic analysis of the initial bone marrow specimen should also be performed.

As in adults, the most effective regimens for remission induction include cytosine arabinoside plus an anthracycline (usually daunorubicin) in a two-drug combination or with additional drugs such as 6-thioguanine, prednisone, vincristine, or 5-azacytidine. To induce a complete remission, it is usually necessary to produce profound marrow aplasia. An exception may be patients with M3 (acute promyelocytic leukemia) who

TABLE 50–4. Frequencies of FAB Subtypes in Childhood Acute Nonlymphocytic Leukemia

		Incidence (%)	
FAB Type	Common Name	Age <2 Years	Age >2 Years
M1	Acute myeloblastic leukemia without maturation	15–20	25
M2	Acute myeloblastic leukemia with maturation		25–30
M3	Acute promyelocytic leukemia (hypergranular variant)		5
M3V	Acute promyelocytic leukemia (microgranular variant)		
M4	Acute myelomonocytic leukemia	30	25
M4Eo	Acute myelomonocytic leukemia with eosinophilia		
M5	Acute monocytic leukemia	50–55	15
M6	Erythroleukemia		≤5
M7	Acute megakaryocytic leukemia		≤5

(Adapted from Grier H, Weinstein H. Acute myelogenous leukemia. In: Pizzo PA, Poplack DG, eds. Principles and practice of pediatric oncology. 2nd ed. Philadelphia: JB Lippincott, 1993)

have a high remission induction rate if treated with all-*trans*-retinoic acid. With induction chemotherapy, the potential for morbidity and mortality from infection may be great, necessitating aggressive supportive care measures. Induction morbidity may be higher with doxorubicin (Adriamycin) than with daunomycin. In most centers, complete remission can be induced in approximately from 75% to 85% of children.

CNS leukemia appears to be more common at diagnosis in AML than in ALL, occurring in 5% to 20% of patients.[75] CNS disease appears to be more common in patients with very high initial leukocyte counts and with the monocytic and myelomonocytic subtypes.[75] Several studies have indicated benefit of CNS preventive therapy.[70,76] Most centers rely on intrathecal chemotherapy with methotrexate or with cytosine arabinoside. Cranial irradiation is not used in most frontline AML protocols.

As in ALL, maintenance chemotherapy has been employed in childhood AML to prolong the duration of the initial remission. Although a variety of strategies have been used, most regimens produced median remissions of less than 2 years. Studies using intensive treatment have demonstrated improvement, with approximately 40% of children achieving prolonged event-free survival.[70,76–79] It is not clear that, after intensive induction and consolidation therapy, maintenance therapy provides additional therapeutic benefit.[80]

Many centers perform bone marrow transplantation for patients who achieve an initial remission and have a histocompatible sibling donor (see Chap. 66). This approach is promising. The CCSG compared bone marrow transplantation with conventional AML maintenance chemotherapy in a nationwide study. The results demonstrated a statistically significant better disease-free survival rate at 3 years for transplantation (49%) than for chemotherapy (36%).[80a] Because some intensive chemotherapy programs have achieved results similar to those obtained for transplantation, there is controversy about the optimal postremission strategy. Most centers suggest marrow transplantation for patients who have an appropriately matched HLA-compatible allogeneic sibling donor.

Studies evaluating the role of autologous marrow transplantation for patients with AML suggest that this strategy may have a role in first or subsequent remission. Purging has been accomplished with chemotherapeutic agents (*e.g.*, 4-hydroperoxycyclophosphamide) or monoclonal antibodies. Autologous marrow transplantation provides a potential transplant option for patients who lack a histocompatible donor. This strategy has produced significant long-term survival of patients transplanted during second remission.[81–84] Whether autologous bone marrow transplantation offers an advantage over chemotherapy alone in children with AML in first remission is currently being assessed in a randomized study of the Pediatric Oncology Group (POG).

Recent studies have demonstrated high complete remission induction rates in patients with acute promyelocytic leukemia (M3) treated with all-*trans*-retinoic acid.[85–87] The therapeutic benefit associated with all-*trans*-retinoic acid therapy has stimulated investigation into the possible therapeutic role of other differentiation agents in the treatment of AML. In vitro studies indicate differentiation of M1 and M2 subtypes with a combination of all-*trans*-retinoic acid and other differentiating agents (*e.g.*, low-dose cytarabine, G-CSF). Clinical trials of these combinations are beginning.

NEONATAL LEUKEMIA

Neonatal leukemia occurs in the first month of life. It is a rare disorder, and most cases are AML. Neonatal or so-called congenital leukemia may be associated with Down's syndrome or other chromosomal abnormalities. Congenital leukemia frequently presents with infiltration of the skin, usually nodular, which may be ecchymotic as a result of concomitant thrombocytopenia. Leukemic infiltration of the lungs, liver, and spleen are common. The initial leukocyte count is frequently greater than 100,000/mm³. The prognosis for neonatal leukemia has been poor. Although complete remissions have been obtained, they are usually short, and long-term survivors have not been reported. There is, however, little experience treating these children with the type of intensive combination chemotherapy regimens used to treat older children with AML.

Patients with neonatal leukemia and Down's syndrome pose a unique problem. A number of these children have had disease that resolved spontaneously over weeks or months. Some researchers have suggested that this disorder represents a defect in the regulation of granulopoiesis and should be considered a myeloproliferative syndrome. However, some patients with this transient disorder have experienced recurrences that proved fatal. The relation between these processes is unclear.

CHRONIC MYELOGENOUS LEUKEMIA

CML is relatively rare in childhood, accounting for 1% to 5% of childhood leukemias.[2] The two major forms are the adult form, which typically is seen in adolescents, and the juvenile form, which occurs mainly in infants. Adult CML is discussed in depth in Chapter 55. The juvenile form of the disease occurs less frequently and differs biologically and clinically from adult CML (Table 50–5).

Juvenile CML is a disease of infancy, rarely occurring after 5 years of age. Typically, it presents with symptoms of fatigue, pallor, and recurrent infection. An eczematoid facial rash, prominent and frequently suppurative lymphadenopathy, thrombocytopenia, and hemorrhagic manifestations at diagnosis also differentiate juvenile CML from the adult form. The Philadelphia chromosome, a hallmark of adult CML, is lacking in juvenile CML. The leukocyte count is usually less than 100,000/mm³. These features, the presence of thrombocytopenia, and a relatively low myeloid to erythroid ratio, which reflects the hyperplasia of both lines in the bone marrow, are useful in differentiating juvenile from adult CML.[2]

In juvenile CML, in vitro bone marrow culture yields a predominance of monocytic colonies, suggesting that it is a form of myelomonocytic leukemia. Juvenile CML is also associated with several erythroid abnormalities, including a persistently high fetal hemoglobin level and other findings similar to those seen in fetal erythrocytes, suggesting that there is disordered regulation of erythropoiesis. Immunologic abnormalities have been noticed. Unlike adult CML, which has its characteristic chronic phase, the juvenile form of the disease follows a course of progressive deterioration that does not have a terminal blastic phase. In its later stages, profound erythroid hyperplasia is seen.

Treatment for juvenile CML is totally unsatisfactory; most patients survive less than 1 year after diagnosis. Chemotherapeutic intervention has not altered the natural history of this disease. Bone marrow transplantation has been attempted successfully and is appropriate to consider.

NON-HODGKIN'S LYMPHOMA

The childhood non-Hodgkin's lymphomas differ in many respects from their adult counterparts.[88] For example, pediatric lymphomas are virtually always diffuse rather than nodular,

TABLE 50–5. Features of the Adult and Juvenile Forms of Chronic Myelogenous Leukemia

Feature	Adult Form	Juvenile Form
Age at onset (median)	14.2 years	22.5 months
Sex (M:F)	6:1	2.1
Philadelphia chromosome	Present	Absent
Physical findings		
Facial rash	Absent	Present
Lymphadenopathy	Occasional	Frequent, with tendency to suppuration
Splenectomy	Marked	Mild to moderate
Hemorrhagic manifestations	Absent	Frequent
Hematologic findings		
Initial leukocyte count	Usually >100,000/mm³	Usually <100,000/mm³
Thrombocytopenia at diagnosis	Uncommon	Frequent
Monocytosis	Absent	Usually present
Fetal hemoglobin levels	Normal	30–70%
Erythrocyte I antigen	Normal	Reduced
Erythrocyte enzymes	?	Increased fetal enzyme systems Decreased carbonic anhydrase
Ineffective erythropoiesis	Absent	Present
Marrow M:E ratio	10:1–50:1	2:1–5:1
Leukocyte alkaline phosphatase	Decreased	Decreased or lower limit of normal
Serum vitamin B₁₂ level	Increased	Increased
Colony-forming characterizations	Predominantly granulocytic	Almost exclusively monocytic
Urine and serum muramidase	Slightly elevated	Markedly elevated
Immunologic abnormalities	None	Increased immunoglobulin levels High incidence of antinuclear and anti-IgG antibodies
Response to busulfan	Good	Poor
Median survival	2.5–3 years	<9 months
Terminal phase	Blast crisis	Erythroid hyperplasia; intense normoblastemia

(Adapted from Altman AJ. Chronic leukemias of childhood. Pediatr Clin North Am 1988;35[4]:765–787)

and they are more often extranodal than nodal. Immunophenotypic studies indicate that B-cell lymphomas account for about 80% of adult NHL, but in childhood, approximately 40% of NHLs are of T-cell origin. Most childhood NHLs arise from lymphoid precursors, and almost all are included in the National Cancer Institute's (NCI) category of "high grade" lymphomas. Only a small fraction (predominantly in older children) fall into the intermediate-grade category, and essentially none are considered low grade. In contrast, high-grade lymphomas are relatively uncommon in adults, who usually have low-grade lymphomas. Childhood lymphomas are rapidly fatal if untreated, but expeditiously instituted chemotherapy results in cure of a high proportion of patients.

Childhood NHL, like adult NHL, has the propensity for early, widespread, noncontiguous dissemination. Leukemic presentation and the development of primary CNS relapse are common, and this has given rise to diagnostic confusion because in the presence of bone marrow involvement the clinical syndromes of "leukemia" and "lymphoma" are not sharply separable. Lymphoblastic lymphomas are indistinguishable cytomorphologically from acute lymphoblastic leukemias. Better definition of individual pathologic entities on the basis of their cytogenetic and molecular characteristics is likely to improve this situation. For example, it has already become clear through detailed pathobiologic characterization that the so-called B-cell ALL is the same entity as small, noncleaved cell lymphoma and should be treated as such. The separation of lymphoblastic lymphoma from ALL is more difficult. An arbitrary and widely used clinical definition is that 25% of bone marrow cells must be blasts for a diagnosis of ALL. Such a definition appears to be of little biologic or prognostic significance.

EPIDEMIOLOGY

NHL is approximately 1.5 times as common as Hodgkin's disease in children younger than 15 years; Hodgkin's disease has a higher incidence in children and young adults older than 16 years. The average annual incidence in the United States of NHL is approximately 9 cases per 1 million white children younger than 15 years old and approximately 5 per 1 million black children. There is a male preponderance, with a male to female ratio of 2.5:1 to 3:1. The peak incidence occurs between the ages of 7 to 11 years. Involvement before the age of 3 is uncommon.

Although the precise cause of NHL is unknown, it is clear that the disease results from genetic changes, the likelihood of which is influenced by environmental factors. Several inherited and acquired conditions predispose to the development of NHL. The association between inherited immunodeficiency disease and NHL is well documented; NHL accounts for more than half of all malignancies that occur in children with inherited immunodeficiency syndromes, including ataxiatelangiectasis, Wiscott-Aldrich syndrome, common variable immunodeficiency disease, severe combined immunodeficiency disease (SCID), and the X-linked lymphoproliferative syndrome.[89] In some of these immunodeficiency states, chromosomal abnormalities or the genetic instability associated with the chromosomal abnormality contribute to the increased risk of lymphoid malignancy. For example, translocations involving the long arm of chromosome 14 at band q32 are fre-

quently encountered in ataxia-telangiectasia. Translocations that involve the immunoglobulin heavy chain locus are common in neoplasms of B-cell origin, and it seems probable that the greater activity of the enzyme system that mediates immunoglobulin gene rearrangement in ataxia-telangiectasia accounts for the increased likelihood of developing an NHL-associated chromosomal translocation. In the X-linked recessive syndrome described by Purtilo, fatal infectious mononucleosis, NHL (including immunoblastic and small, noncleaved cell lymphoma), hypogammaglobulinemia, and aplastic anemia may occur. Epstein-Barr virus EBV appears to be relevant to the pathogenesis of many of the lymphomas that develop in the inherited immunodeficiency states, because EBV genomes are frequently found in the tumor cells.

Acquired immunodeficiency is associated with the development of lymphoma. Patients undergoing chronic immunosuppressive therapy after organ allografting have an increased risk of lymphoproliferative syndromes that are almost invariably EBV associated. Patients with human immunodeficiency virus (HIV) infection have a markedly increased risk of lymphomas, some of which have the typical histologic pattern and chromosomal abnormalities of Burkitt's lymphoma. Whatever the cause of the immunosuppression, lymphomas confined to the CNS are much more common than in immunocompetent persons. In patients with HIV infection, CNS lymphomas appear to be invariably associated with EBV. This is not the case for systemic HIV-associated lymphomas, approximately 40% of which are EBV associated.

EBV and malaria have been implicated in the development of Burkitt's lymphoma in African children, and evidence suggests that the form of the disease that is endemic in equatorial Africa (with an average annual incidence of between 5 and 15 per 100,000 children younger than 15 years) represents a separate molecular subtype.[90] A retrovirus, HTLV-I, has been implicated in the pathogenesis of one form of adult T-cell leukemia-lymphoma that is prevalent in Japan, the Caribbean, and parts of the southern United States. However, retroviruses have not been linked to the pathogenesis of childhood lymphomas.

Chronic treatment with hydantoin drugs, including phenytoin (Dilantin), has been associated with development of pseudolymphomas and true malignant lymphomas, including Hodgkin's disease and NHL. NHL has developed as a second malignancy in patients treated with chemotherapy, particularly if in addition to radiation therapy, for Hodgkin's disease. Recently, epidemiologic evidence from Kansas and Nebraska has been collected that suggests that high exposure to certain herbicides is linked to lymphomagenesis. Plants containing phorbol esters have been implicated in the pathogenesis of Burkitt's lymphoma in equatorial Africa.

PATHOLOGIC AND IMMUNOLOGIC CLASSIFICATION

The histologic classification of pediatric NHL is much less complicated than the classification of adult NHL, because there are only three major categories. Unfortunately, these three categories have different names in different classification schemes.[88] In the NCI working formulation, the categories are small, noncleaved cell lymphoma, lymphoblastic lymphoma, and large cell lymphoma (Table 50–6). The corresponding categories in the older Rappaport scheme are un-

TABLE 50–6. Distribution of Histopathologic Types of Diffuse Lymphomas in Childhood

Histologic Classification	Approximate Frequency (%)
Lymphoblastic (convoluted and nonconvoluted)	30–40
Small non-cleaved (Burkitt's and non-Burkitt's, pleomorphic)	40–50
Large cell	15

(Magrath IT. Malignant non-Hodgkin's lymphomas. In: Pizzo PA, Poplack DG, eds. Principles and practice of pediatric oncology. Philadelphia: JB Lippincott, 1993)

differentiated lymphoma, lymphoblastic lymphoma, and histiocytic (also referred to as large cell) lymphoma. Each of these categories can be further divided on the basis of histology, immunophenotype, or both.

An indication that these histologic categories are biologically meaningful is provided by the observation that they correspond to different, although overlapping clinical syndromes. Lymphoblastic lymphomas characteristically present with supradiaphragmatic disease, particularly anterior superior mediastinal (thymic) involvement. Small, noncleaved cell lymphomas usually present with intraabdominal disease. Lymphoblastic and small noncleaved cell lymphomas are approximately equal in frequency and account for some 85% of childhood NHL. Large cell lymphomas do not have a characteristic clinical syndrome and may occur at a variety of nodal and extranodal sites, including Waldeyer's ring, lymph nodes, abdomen, chest, skin, and bone.

Immunologic classification is extremely important in childhood NHL. Lymphoblastic lymphomas are predominantly neoplasms of the precursors of functional T cells and, much less commonly, of B-cell precursors. Regardless of phenotype, lymphoblastic lymphomas almost always contain TdT. Studies using monoclonal antibodies capable of delineating the various stages of intrathymic differentiation indicate that the malignant T cells in lymphoblastic lymphoma generally bear the immunophenotypic stamp of intermediate or late thymocytes. In contrast, T-cell ALL lymphoblasts often display the characteristics of early thymocytes. A small subset of lymphoblastic lymphomas—those that present as isolated bone or lymph node involvement—have the immunophenotype of common acute lymphoblastic leukemia, a pre-B-cell phenotype. All small, noncleaved cell lymphomas, including Burkitt's and non-Burkitt's subtypes, are of B-cell origin and express various B-cell markers, including CD19, CD20, and surface immunoglobulin, predominantly IgM (associated with kappa or lambda light chains). They also express HLA-DR antigens and usually express the CALLA antigen, but they do not contain TdT. Many large cell tumors also express B-cell characteristics, but the recently described anaplastic large cell lymphomas, most of which bear T-cell surface antigens, are characterized by the uniformly high level of expression of the CD30 (Ki-1) antigen.

Pathogenesis

As is the case for all malignant tumors, NHL probably arises as a consequence of the accumulation of genetic abnormalities in a cell. The small chance that a genetic lesion able to contribute to lymphomagenesis will arise coupled to the need for multiple genetic abnormalities usually results in monoclonality of the tumor cells (although clonal evolution subsequently occurs). It is probable that dysfunction of oncogenes and antioncogenes are required, and such functional abnormalities are produced by a restricted set of changes in the genome that may include chromosomal translocation, point mutation, deletion, or amplification. Particularly characteristic of the lymphoid neoplasms is involvement of the antigen receptor genes in the molecular abnormalities.[88] An increasing number of chromosomal translocations in lymphoid malignancy have been shown to involve deregulation of "master" genes involved in the regulation of other genes (*i.e.*, transcription factors). In addition to changes in cellular genes, the expression of adventitious genes provided by viruses may contribute to the ultimate functional changes that give rise to neoplasia.

Lymphoblastic Lymphoma

The genetic changes in lymphoblastic malignancies are quite heterogenous but often result in the deregulation of master genes.[89a] Translocations sometimes produce the juxtaposition of such genes to the T-cell antigen receptor genes on chromosomes 7 (β) and 14 (α,δ), such as t(7;9), t(7;10), t(7;11), t(10;14), and t(11;14). A master gene known as *TAL1* or *SCL* is deregulated by chromosomal translocation (and juxtaposition to the T-α receptor on chromosome 14) or interstitial deletion within chromosome 1, on which *TAL1/SCL* gene is situated. These deletions have been described in some 20% of T-cell leukemias, suggesting that mechanisms other than chromosomal translocation may be more frequently employed in T-cell malignancies. Genetic abnormalities have not been described in the pre-B-cell variety of lymphoblastic lymphoma but may be similar to those reported in pre-B leukemia, such as t(1;19). There has been no clear separation of the genetic changes associated with lymphoblastic leukemias and lymphoblastic lymphomas.

Small, Noncleaved Cell Lymphoma

Small, noncleaved cell lymphoma is divided into two subtypes: Burkitt's lymphoma and non-Burkitt's lymphoma. It is not clear that this histologic distinction is meaningful in children, because most small, noncleaved cell lymphomas in this age group are Burkitt's lymphomas.[88,90] In adults, the non-Burkitt's subtype is differentiated from Burkitt's lymphoma at a molecular level. In older patients, small, noncleaved cell lymphomas may bear a quite different chromosomal abnormality, the 14;18 translocation associated with the follicular lymphomas and about 25% of large cell lymphomas. All small, noncleaved cell lymphomas are derived from B-cell lineage.

Burkitt's cells manifest a characteristic cytogenetic abnormality in which genetic material is exchanged between the q24 band of the long arm of chromosome 8, at the location of the c-*MYC* gene, and the q32 band of chromosome 14, t(8;14), the site of the immunoglobulin heavy chain genes.[90] Rarely, "variant" translocations can be demonstrated, t(8;22) or t(2;8), which involve the same band on chromosome 8 and one of the light chain immunoglobulin genes on the partner chromosome (κ on 2p12, and λ on 22q12). As a consequence of these translocations, the expression of *MYC*, a master gene involved in cell proliferation, is deregulated. In effect, *MYC* is expressed as if it were an immunoglobulin gene. Cells bearing a deregulated *MYC* gene are probably unable to enter a resting phase, and in the presence of additional genetic events, become fully malignant neoplastic clones.

Burkitt's lymphoma was originally described in equatorial Africa, and the disease there differs in several respects from the North American form of the disease and from the disease in most other parts of the world (Table 50–7). Apart from the much higher incidence rate in Africa (hence the term "endemic"), the typical presentation of African Burkitt's lymphoma, a large tumor of the maxilla or mandible, with or without orbital involvement, is rarely seen in the "sporadic" form of the disease seen in the United States. Moreover, bone marrow involvement is much more common in the American form of the disease than the African. The endemic and sporadic forms of the disease also differ biologically. EBV DNA and the EBV nuclear antigen are usually in the tumor cells in African children but are much less frequently encountered in North American patients. Although the cytogenetic findings are similar in endemic and sporadic tumors, there is a difference in the location of the breakpoint on chromosome 8. In endemic tumors, the breakpoint occurs a variable distance upstream of the gene, but in sporadic tumors, it is usually within the gene or its flanking sequences. Although genetic factors cannot be completely excluded, it seems probable that Burkitt's lymphoma is composed of a mixture of molecular subtypes and that the incidence of each type depends on the environment.

Large Cell Lymphomas

It appears that at least some large cell lymphomas have a similar pathogenesis (*i.e.*, contain the same genetic abnormalities) as the small, noncleaved cell lymphomas. However, little is known of the pathogenesis of the remaining large cell lymphomas. The anaplastic or Ki-1 subtype appears to arise from perifollicular activated lymphocytes of T-cell or B-cell lineages and frequently bears a nonrandom translocation involving chromosome band 5q35. The partner chromosome varies (*i.e.*, usually 2, but sometimes 3 or 1), and other translocations, such as t(2;13), have been described.

CLINICAL PRESENTATION

Childhood NHL can arise in almost any organ or tissue but involves peripheral lymph nodes in approximately 15% of patients.[88] Although systemic symptoms including fever, night sweats, and weight loss may be observed, these are relatively uncommon features, except in anaplastic large cell lymphomas. Symptoms usually reflect the presence of a tumor mass, except in the small number of patients with a leukemic presentation of a small, noncleaved cell lymphoma. The most frequent site of involvement at presentation is the abdomen, and most intraabdominal NHLs are small, noncleaved cell lymphomas. Pain, a palpable mass, or generalized abdominal swelling are the most common reasons for seeking medical assistance, and occult or overt bleeding from the gastrointestinal tract, with consequent anemia, is often observed. Intussusception is a frequent presentation in the younger child and is usually caused by a small intestinal tumor that often proves to be totally resectable. Involvement of the terminal ileum or ascending cecum occurs in approximately 40% of patients with small, noncleaved cell lymphomas.[88]

The chest is the next most frequently involved site, and approximately 70% of patients with lymphoblastic lymphoma have a mediastinal mass. However, large cell lymphomas, but rarely small, noncleaved cell lymphomas, may also present with a mediastinal mass.[38] Mediastinal enlargement usually presents with dyspnea, particularly if there is an associated pleural effusion, dysphagia, or superior vena cava obstruction.

Childhood NHL may present with involvement of a variety of other sites, including peripheral lymphadenopathy (frequently cervical or supraclavicular in lymphoblastic lymphoma), tonsils, nasopharynx, or other portions of Waldeyer's ring (with or without involvement of cervical lymph nodes), bone marrow, bones, skin, gonads, breast, face, or CNS. These

TABLE 50–7. Differences Between Endemic and Sporadic Burkitt's Lymphoma

Endemic	*Sporadic*
Common (100 per 1 million children)	Rare (1–2 per 1 million children)
Distribution relates to climate and geography	Distribution apparently unrelated to climate and geography
Nearly always associated with EBV (95%)	Uncommonly associated with EBV (15%)
t(8:14) common	t(8:14) common
No IgM secretion	Secretion of IgM
Chromosome 8 breakpoints upstream of c-*MYC*	Chromosome 8 breakpoints within c-*MYC*
Jaw tumors common, marrow involvement rare	Jaw tumors rare, marrow involvement common
Multiple relapses not incompatible with eventual prolonged disease-free survival	Survival uncommon after relapse

EBV, Epstein-Barr virus; CTX, cyclophosphamide; COM, cyclophosphamide, vincristsine, methotrexate.
(Magrath IT. Malignant non-Hodgkin's lymphomas. In: Pizzo PA, Poplack DG, eds. Principles and practice of pediatric oncology. Philadelphia: JB Lippincott, 1993)

tumors grow rapidly, and clinical symptoms have rarely existed for more than 6 to 8 weeks before presentation.

PRETREATMENT EVALUATION AND STAGING

The diagnosis of NHL can only be definitively established by biopsy and, wherever possible, immunophenotyping and cytogenetics. Because of the extremely rapid growth rate of the NHLs that occur in children, particularly of the small, noncleaved cell lymphomas, a rapid and expeditious assessment of disease extent is essential. In addition to a detailed history and physical examination, a complete blood count with careful examination of the peripheral smear for circulating blasts should be performed. Blood chemistries, including electrolytes, BUN, creatinine, liver function tests, and serum calcium and uric acid, should be performed routinely. In patients with the largest tumor burdens, marked abnormalities in renal function and uric acid levels may be detected. Measurement of serum LDH is a useful correlate of tumor burden. The level of soluble interleukin-2 receptor in serum appears to be a reliable prognostic factor, particularly for B-cell lymphomas.

Posterior and lateral chest x-ray films should be obtained to assess mediastinal, hilar, pericardial, or pleural involvement. The trachea and bronchi should be evaluated for patency and displacement. CT scan of the mediastinum is much more valuable in documenting the extent of chest disease than chest x-ray films, and CT scans of the abdomen are usually performed, although in very young children, ultrasound examination may be more valuable in view of the lack of retroperitoneal fat. Sometimes these studies provide complementary information. A particularly valuable whole-body screening study for the small, noncleaved cell lymphomas is the ^{67}Ga scan. Bilateral bone marrow biopsies and aspirates are advocated to maximize detection of marrow involvement. Lumbar puncture should be performed and a cytocentrifuged CSF specimen examined for malignant cells, but because intrathecal therapy is normally given to all patients, CSF examination can be performed at the same time intrathecal therapy is first administered. Mandatory and optional staging procedures for the child with NHL are shown in Table 50–8.

Because treatment consists of chemotherapy, there is no role for a staging laparotomy. However, laparotomy may be necessary for biopsy of an abdominal mass at the time of presentation, and in patients with regionally limited disease, the most common site is the terminal ileum and cecum. Complete resection of the offending tumor mass may be feasible and the safest surgical procedure. Patients who have the mass completely resected, even those with positive mesenteric nodes, have an excellent prognosis.

The Ann Arbor staging system is of limited value in childhood NHL; most pediatric lymphomas are extranodal, and unlike Hodgkin's disease, NHL in children is not orderly or predictable in its pattern of spread or relapse, and prognosis is not readily determined by the number of sites affected. The most widely used staging system in pediatric NHL is that used at St. Jude Children's Research Hospital (Table 50–9). This and similar systems differ from the Ann Arbor scheme in that they do not differentiate between primary nodal and extranodal presentations, and they recognize the poor prognosis (in American NHL) of bone marrow involvement and CNS disease. A quite widely used staging scheme, originally designed

TABLE 50–8. Staging Procedures for Non-Hodgkin's Lymphoma

Mandatory

Complete blood count, platelet count, differential
Chest x-ray films (posteroanterior and lateral)
Bone marrow aspirates and biopsy
Lumbar puncture with cytocentrifuge examination
 of cerebrospinal fluid
Liver function tests
Serum electrolytes, BUN, creatinine, and uric acid levels
Chest and abdominal CT scan

Optional (depending on clinical circumstances)

Bone scan and skeletal survey
Intravenous urogram
Barium studies on the gastrointestinal tract
Myelography
MRI
Lymphangiography*
Ultrasonography

---

* Rarely indicated.

---

for African Burkitt's lymphoma, includes a separate stage, AR, that includes patients with more than 90% resection of intraabdominal disease.

Some institutions no longer use a recognized staging system. For example, the CCSG classifies children with NHL on the basis of whether they have localized or nonlocalized disease. In this definition, patients with localized disease have tumor limited to a single extranodal site, with or without positive regional nodes, or to lymph nodes in one or two adjacent lymphatic regions. All other tumors, including mediastinal disease, are classified as nonlocalized disease. Localized disease in this system corresponds to stage I and stage II disease in the St. Jude system and includes children with a particularly favorable prognoses. This system, although less elaborate, effectively separates patients with limited disease from those with extensive tumor involvement. As treatment results continue to improve, the utility of these staging systems as predictors of prognosis will diminish. Currently, they remain essential for meaningful comparison of results obtained in clinical trials and will continue to be necessary as long as treatment is predicated on the extent of disease.

TREATMENT

At the time of presentation, it is essential to recognize conditions requiring emergency treatment, such as airway or vascular obstruction, paraplegia, compression of optic nerves, cardiac tamponade, gastrointestinal perforation or bleeding, and uricosemia. Patients with extensive intraabdominal disease may have multiple causes of renal failure, including uricosemia and renal outflow tract obstruction. Before the initiation of chemotherapy in all patients with high tumor burdens, it is essential to initiate allopurinol and to establish good diuresis. If this is not possible, hemodialysis may be necessary to rectify biochemical abnormalities and to avoid severe

TABLE 50–9. Clinical Staging Systems for Childhood Lymphomas

Stage	Memorial Sloan-Kettering (Wollner)	St. Jude Children's Research Hospital (Murphy)	Stage	National Cancer Institute (Ziegler, Magrath)
I	One single site	A single tumor (extranodal) or single anatomic area (nodal) with the exclusion of mediastinum or abdomen	A	Single solitary extraabdominal site
II	Two or more sites on the same side of the diaphragm	A single tumor (extranodal) with regional node involvement Two or more nodal areas on the same side of the diaphragm Two single (extranodal) tumors with or without regional node involvement on the same side of the diaphragm A primary GI tract tumor, usually in the ileocecal area, with or without involvement of associated mesenteric nodes only	B	Multiple extraabdominal sites
III	Disseminated disease without marrow or CNS involvement	Two single tumors (extranodal) on opposite sides of the diaphragm Two or more nodal areas above and below the diaphragm All the primary intrathoracic tumors (mediastinal, pleural, thymic) All extensive primary intraabdominal disease All paraspinal or epidural tumors regardless of other tumor site(s)	C	Intraabdominal tumor
IV	Any of the above with bone marrow and/or CNS involvement	Any of the above with initial CNS or bone marrow involvement	D	Intraabdominal tumor with involvement of ≥ extraabdominal site
			AR	Intraabdominal tumor with >90% of tumor surgically resected

and possibly fatal worsening after rapid tumor lysis. The syndrome of rapid tumor lysis is characterized by azotemia, hyperphosphatemia, and hypocalcemia as a result of the liberation of tumor breakdown products into the bloodstream.[88] In uricosemia, alkaline diuresis is normally recommended, but after near normalization of serum uric acid levels, alkalinization should be stopped, because phosphates, which are released by lysed tumor cells and may produce renal tubular obstruction, are less soluble in alkaline urine.

Because one of the potentially most devastating consequences of rapid tumor lysis is hyperkalemia, potassium is not normally administered to patients undergoing chemotherapy. Hyperkalemia is essentially unknown in the presence of a good diuresis. Establishment and maintenance of a high urine flow is the key to the successful management of patients with massive tumor burdens and the potential for tumor lysis. Normally, 4 to 5 L/m^2 per day can be safely administered to these patients if careful monitoring is performed. This is best conducted in a critical care unit.

Chemotherapy

Before the 1970s, the overall survival of children with NHL was poor; few patients survived 5 years after diagnosis, and most survivors had limited disease. Although the use of surgery or radiation therapy was modestly effective in patients with limited disease (*e.g.*, a single extraabdominal, extrathoracic tumor site or totally resected abdominal tumor), as many as

two thirds of patients experienced relapse. The pattern of relapse, with frequent recurrences at sites distant from the radiation field, including bone marrow, suggested that failure occurred because of widespread occult disease. The addition of combination chemotherapy to treat patients with limited disease raised the overall survival figures for this group to approximately 90%, making radiation therapy superfluous because it adds potential toxicity without apparent therapeutic advantage.[91] Radiation and surgery also have no role in treating patients with advanced disease. Systemic combination chemotherapy is indicated for all patients with childhood NHL. Using the most effective modern regimens, 85% to 95% of patients achieve complete remissions, and 90% of patients with limited disease and 60% to 80% of patients with extensive disease are cured. Relapse does not occur with any significant frequency beyond 2 years, and in patients with small, noncleaved cell lymphomas, relapse is rare beyond 10 months.

For purposes of treatment, childhood NHL is usually divided into lymphoblastic and nonlymphoblastic lymphomas, which includes small, noncleaved cell and large cell lymphomas. Lymphoblastic lymphomas are most often treated with regimens similar to that initially designed for the treatment of high-risk ALL. The most frequently used are modifications of the LSA$_2$-L$_2$ protocol designed at the Memorial Sloan-Kettering Cancer Center. This approach stems from a randomized trial performed by the CCSG. In this study, the LSA$_2$-L$_2$ protocol was compared with the COMP regimen, which includes cyclophosphamide, vincristine, methotrexate, and prednisone, and was modified from regimens developed for patients with Burkitt's lymphoma. Most patients in both treatment groups also received radiation therapy to sites of bulky disease. For nonlocalized lymphoblastic leukemia, 76% of patients treated with LSA_2-L_2 were disease free at 2 years, compared with 26% of patients treated with COMP. For nonlocalized nonlymphoblastic lymphoma, 57% of patients treated with COMP achieved 2-year disease-free survival, compared with 28% of children who received LSA_2-L_2 therapy. For patients with localized disease, histologic subtype did not appear to have prognostic significance. In this group, the less toxic four-drug COMP regimen was as effective as the more intensive ten-drug LSA_2-L_2 treatment (89% versus 84%). Similar results to those obtained with LSA_2-L_2 have been reported for another leukemia-type protocol, the APO regimen (Table 50-10), but patients with Burkitt's lymphoma fared badly with this regimen.

These results were originally interpreted as indicating that patients with lymphoblastic lymphoma and nonlymphoblastic lymphoma should be treated differently, but it has become clear that lymphoblastic lymphomas may be treated with lymphoma-type regimens, although patients with small, noncleaved cell lymphoma should not be treated with a leukemia-type regimen. Anthracyclines appear to be an important component of successful treatment protocols for lymphoblastic lymphomas. Regimens based on repeated alkylating agent therapy that also contain anthracyclines appear to be as successful as LSA_2-L_2. For example, an NCI regimen containing cyclophosphamide, vincristine, prednisone, and doxorubicin alternating with prolonged methotrexate infusions has been shown to be effective for lymphoblastic and nonlymphoblastic lymphomas, producing a disease-free survival at 3 years of approximately 60%, and the POG ACOP+ regimen has been shown to produce similar results to LSA_2-L_2. The results of one small series of lymphoblastic lymphoma patients treated with an ALL-like approach that omitted anthracyclines was reported. This protocol, which included cytarabine and VM-26 and was not as complicated as LSA_2-L_2, had a predicted disease-free survival rate at 4 years of 73%.[90a]

CNS prophylaxis is incorporated into all protocols, but there is no evidence that cranial irradiation is necessary, and most pediatric oncologists now use only intrathecal therapy. The optimal duration of therapy for lymphoblastic lymphoma remains unknown.

Treatment regimens for the nonlymphoblastic lymphomas, most of which are B-cell tumors, usually incorporate cyclophosphamide, vincristine, and intermediate-dose or high-dose methotrexate. Patients with limited disease are usually treated with a combination of cyclophosphamide, vincristine, prednisone, and methotrexate (COMP) or doxorubicin (*e.g.,* CHOP). In patients with extensive disease, other drugs (*e.g.,* VM-26, ifosfamide, cytarabine, BCNU) are usually employed. The most successful regimens, such as those of the French Society of Pediatric Oncology, the Berlin-Frankfurt-Münster group (BFM), and the recent NCI and Dana-Farber protocols (Fig. 50–5), include more than four drugs. The last three protocols have treatment durations of approximately 12 weeks, but produce disease-free survival rates in excess of 70% for patients with extensive disease. It seems that excellent results can be obtained with intensive, short-duration regimens containing a backbone of cyclophosphamide, high-dose methotrexate, vincristine, and high-dose cytarabine. Doxorubicin, ifosfamide, and the epipodophyllotoxins are also included in most of these regimens. A modified version of the French protocol used in a small group of patients with CNS disease at presentation proved to be highly successful. Until this report, little progress in improving survival rates had been made in treating this subgroup.

Patients with anaplastic large cell lymphomas have been treated successfully (*i.e.,* anticipated long-term survival rate of approximately 70%) with the BFM and LSA_2-L_2 protocols. There appears to be little point in treating these patients with the much longer LSA_2-L_2 regimen if intensive, short-duration therapies are equally successful.

CENTRAL NERVOUS SYSTEM PREVENTIVE THERAPY

In the past, the CNS was an initial site of relapse in almost one third of children with NHL. Some form of CNS preventive therapy is warranted for most patients. CNS spread is less common in patients with limited disease (stage I or II), and it has been suggested that CNS preventive therapy can be avoided in some patients with limited disease without producing a significant increase in subsequent CNS relapse. Included in this group are patients with totally resected abdominal disease and non-Burkitt's, nonmediastinal, limited nodal disease that is not close to the meninges. However, this policy has not been subjected to clinical trial, and for this reason, most centers treat all patients with CNS preventive therapy.

Intrathecal therapy with or without cranial irradiation has been used. Although the relative efficacy of each form of CNS preventive therapy has not been carefully studied in a randomized fashion, it is now clear that intrathecal chemotherapy alone is highly effective and cranial irradiation is unnecessary. The CCSG compared LSA_2-L_2 with COMP. The use of intrathecal chemotherapy alone was associated with an incidence of isolated CNS disease of only 6%. In the NCI study described earlier, the inclusion of intrathecal chemotherapy with methotrexate and cytosine arabinoside reduced the incidence of primary CNS relapse from approximately 20% to 2%.

Radiation Therapy

Although radiation therapy plays an important role in the treatment of adult non-Hodgkin's lymphomas, its role in pediatric NHL is limited. Specific emergency situations, including acute respiratory distress, superior vena cava syndrome, spinal cord compression, orbital proptosis, and cranial nerve palsy, may be effectively treated with radiation therapy. However, because irradiation may contribute to the development of toxicity (*e.g.,* esophagitis, cardiac failure after irradiation of a mediastinal mass), its role should be limited only to emergencies for which chemotherapy alone is not effective. In the small, noncleaved cell lymphomas, the effectiveness of chemotherapy has significantly limited the need for radiation therapy. One of the few exceptions may be the treatment of intraparenchymal brain disease. Although it has been traditional to include irradiation in the treatment of patients with localized disease, a randomized study, largely confined to patients with nonlymphoblastic lymphoma, demonstrated that irradiation added toxicity without therapeutic benefit.[91] At 4

TABLE 50–10. Chemotherapy Regimens Used for Childhood Non-Hodgkin's Lymphoma

LSA_2-L_2 (Modified)	COMP	NCI 77-04

LSA_2-L_2 (Modified)

Induction

Cyclophosphamide, 1.2 g/m² I.V., day 1

Vincristine, 2.0 mg/m² I.V. (maximum dose, 2.0 mg), days 3, 10, 17, and 24

Methotrexate, 6.25 mg/m² I.V., days 5, 31, and 34

Daunomycin, 60 mg/m² I.V., days 12 and 13

Prednisone, 60 mg/m² PO (maximum dose, 60 mg), days 3–30

Consolidation

Cytosine arabinoside, 100 mg/m² I.V. daily for 5 days (Mon–Fri) for 2 wk

Thioguanine, 50 mg/m² PO 8–12 h after each cytosine arabinoside injection

Asparaginase, 6000 IU/m² IM daily for 14 days after completion of cytosine arabinoside and thioguanine

Methotrexate, 6.25 mg/m² IT twice, 3 days apart, beginning 2 to 3 days after last dose of asparaginase

Carmustine, 60 mg/m² I.V. single dose given 2 to 3 days after completion of methotrexate

Maintenance

1. Thioguanine, 300 mg/m² PO, days 1–4
2. Hydroxyurea, 2.4 g/m² PO, days 1–4
   Daunomycin, 45 mg/m² I.V., day 5
3. Methotrexate, 10 mg/m² I.V., days 1–4
   Carmustine, 60 mg/m² I.V., day 5
4. Cytosine arabinoside, 150 mg/m² I.V., days 1–4
   Vincristine, 2.0 mg/m² I.V. (maximum dose, 2.0 mg), day 5
5. Methotrexate, 6.25 mg/m² IT, 2 doses given 3 days apart

Repeat maintenance cycles 1–5

COMP

Induction

Cyclophosphamide, 1.2 g/m² I.V., day 1

Vincristine 2.0 mg/m² I.V. (maximum dose, 2.0 mg), days 3, 10, 17, and 24

Methotrexate, 6.25 mg/m² IT, days 5, 31, 34

Methotrexate, 300 mg/m² I.V. (60% of dose as I.V. push, 40% as 4-h infusion) on day 12

Prednisone, 60 mg/m² PO (maximum dose, 60 mg), days 3–30

Maintenance

Cyclophosphamide, 1.0 g/m² I.V., day 1

Vincristine, 1.5 mg/m² I.V. (maximum dose, 2 mg), days 1 and 4

Methotrexate, 6.25 mg/m² IT, day 1 (excluded from first maintenance cycle)

Methotrexate, 300 mg/m² I.V. (60% of dose as I.V. push, 40% as 4-h infusion), day 15

Prednisone, 60 mg/m² PO (maximum dose, 60 mg), days 1–5 (excluded from first maintenance cycle)

Repeat maintenance cycle every 28 days

NCI 77-04

CYCLE 1

Systemic Therapy

Cyclophosphamide, 1.2 g/m² I.V., day 1

Methotrexate (begins on day 10), 300 mg/m² I.V. (over first hour), then 60 mg/m² I.V. hourly for next 41 h, followed by calcium leucovorin 48 mg/m² I.V., then 12 mg/m² I.V. every 6 h until plasma methotrexate levels $<5 \times 10^{-8}$ M.

Intrathecal Therapy

Cytosine arabinoside, 30 mg/m² IT, days 1, 2, 3, and 7

Methotrexate, 12.5 mg/m² IT (maximum dose, 12.5 mg), day 10, 6–8 hours after commencement of systemic methotrexate infusion

CYCLES 2 TO 6

Systemic Therapy (Begins When Granulocyte Count ≥ 1500/mm³)

Cyclophosphamide, 1.2 g/m² I.V., day 1

Adriamycin, 40 mg/m² I.V., day 1

Vincristine, 1.4 mg/m² I.V., day 1 (maximum dose 2.0 mg)

Prednisone, 40 mg/m² I.V. or PO, days 1–5

Methotrexate and calcium leucovorin day 10, as in cycle 1

Intrathecal Therapy

CYCLES 2 AND 3

Cytosine arabinoside, 30 mg/m² IT, days 1 and 2

Methotrexate, 12.5 mg/m² IT (maximum dose 12.5 mg), day 3 and on day 10 6–8 h after commencement of systemic methotrexate infusion

CYCLES 4, 5, AND 6

Cytosine arabinoside, 45 mg/m² IT, day 1

Methotrexate 12.5 mg/m² IT (maximum dose 12.5 mg), day 10

Patients with Burkitt's lymphoma/undifferentiated lymphoma, stages A, B, AR, stop therapy after 6 cycles. All other patients are treated for a total of 15 cycles.

CYCLES 7 TO 15

Cyclophosphamide, 1.2 mg/m² I.V., day 1

Adriamycin, 40 mg/m² I.V., day 1

Vincristine, 1.4 mg/m² I.V. (maximum dose 2.0 mg), day 1

Prednisone, 40 mg/m² I.V. or PO, days 1–5

Methotrexate and calcium leucovorin on day 14 as in cycle 1

Cycles are repeated on day 28 or when granulocyte count is ≥1500/mm³ and platelet count ≥75,000/mm³

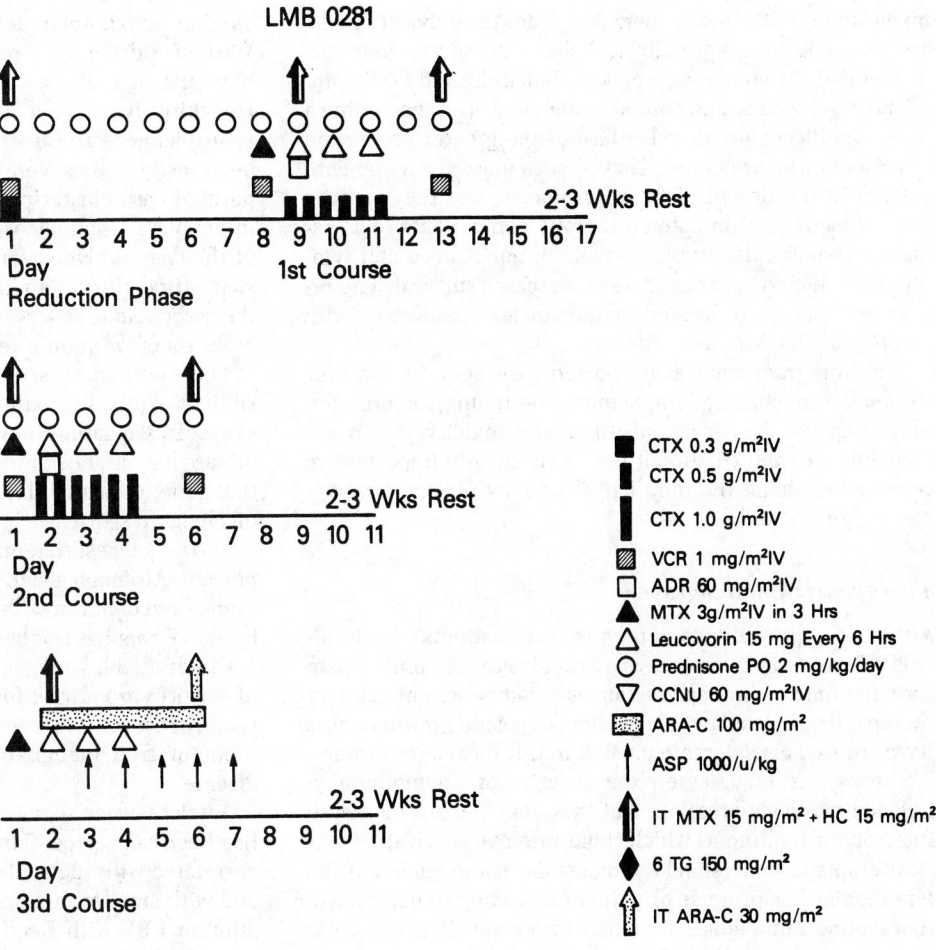

LMB 0281

■	CTX 0.3 g/m²IV
▮	CTX 0.5 g/m²IV
▎	CTX 1.0 g/m²IV
▨	VCR 1 mg/m²IV
□	ADR 60 mg/m²IV
▲	MTX 3g/m²IV in 3 Hrs
△	Leucovorin 15 mg Every 6 Hrs
○	Prednisone PO 2 mg/kg/day
▽	CCNU 60 mg/m²IV
▨	ARA-C 100 mg/m²
↑	ASP 1000/u/kg
⇑	IT MTX 15 mg/m² + HC 15 mg/m²
◆	6 TG 150 mg/m²
⇑	IT ARA-C 30 mg/m²

FIGURE 50–5. The LBM-02 protocol of the SFOP for B cell lymphoblastic lymphomas stages I and II (large nasopharyngeal primaries in stage II are included). Cyclophosphamide is given at the doses shown daily in two fractions. Maintenance courses are given monthly. During maintenance ara-C is given as two SC fractions; otherwise it is given as a continuous intravenous infusion. (Schema prepared from information in Patte C, Philip T, Rodary C, et al. Improved survival rate in children with stage III and IV B cell non-Hodgkin's lymphoma and leukemia using multi-agent chemotherapy: Results of a study of 114 children from the French Pediatric Oncology Society. J Clin Oncol 1986;4:1219–1226)

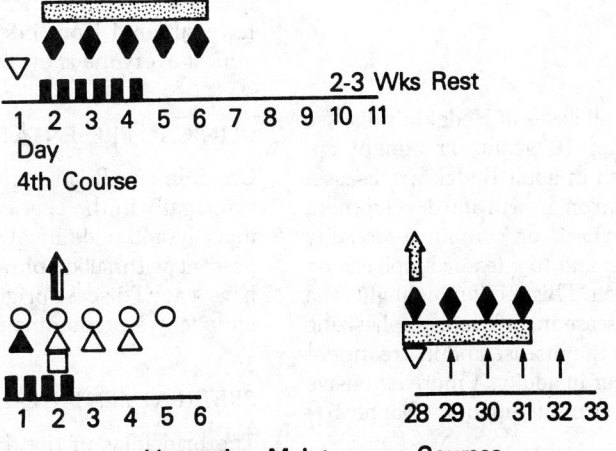

Alternating Maintenance Courses

years, 88% of the patients in this study are projected to be disease-free survivors; no significant difference has been found in the rate of locoregional failure. Previous studies suggesting benefit using local radiation therapy in more advanced childhood NHL used less effective systemic chemotherapy.[91a] Although no randomized trial has been conducted recently using patients with advanced disease, the excellent results obtained in several treatment protocols using chemotherapy alone has

led to the exclusion of radiation therapy in most current studies.

Complications of Therapy

Treatment of children with NHL may be associated with acute and chronic complications. The acute risks of multiagent systemic chemotherapy include infection as a complication of myelosuppression and hemorrhage from thrombocytopenia, and the toxic effects of individual chemotherapy include cardiomyopathy, hemorrhagic cystitis, hepatitis, and CNS complications. Sterility and second malignancies are becoming a more significant problem because of the greater proportion of patients who are cured. These issues must always be considered in the design of future protocols, and they provide good reasons to eliminate all therapy components (*e.g.,* radiation therapy, doxorubicin in small, noncleaved cell lymphomas) that do not contribute to increased survival. The report of increased second malignancies associated with epipodophyllotoxins is worrisome.

One important trend is to shorten treatment duration for the nonlymphoblastic lymphomas. Shortening the duration of therapy has the advantage of reducing toxicity, patient inconvenience, and treatment cost. It is equally important to consider reducing the duration of therapy for the lymphoblastic lymphomas.

Therapeutic Challenges

Although improvements in the results of patients with localized or extensive disease have markedly reduced enthusiasm for bone marrow transplantation as a component of primary therapy, the molecularly cloned hematopoietic growth factors have aroused considerable interest in this form of treatment. These agents may lessen the severity of chemotherapy-induced myelosuppression, and they may permit increased intensity of treatment, which could improve survival.

Attempts to understand the molecular pathogenesis of the lymphomas has promise of ultimately leading to quite novel therapeutic approaches in which tumor-specific molecular targets are identified. Unfortunately, it is likely to be many years before such approaches enter the clinic.

HODGKIN'S DISEASE

Approximately 10% to 15% of all cases of Hodgkin's disease occur in patients younger than 16 years. Treatment approaches differ from those used in adult Hodgkin's disease. The adverse effects of irradiation on growth and development in children have led to an emphasis on combined-modality therapy with limited irradiation and to a lesser emphasis on stage-specific therapy in children. This section highlights the salient features of Hodgkin's disease in children, emphasizing those aspects that differentiate the disease and its treatment in children from those that occur in adults. A more extensive discussion of Hodgkin's disease can be found in Chapter 51.

EPIDEMIOLOGY

The incidence of Hodgkin's disease increases throughout the pediatric age range. Most pediatric cases occur in children 11 years of age or older. Hodgkin's disease is rarely seen in children younger than 4.[92] Among prepubertal children, there is a striking predominance of boys. In early adolescence, the number of girls with Hodgkin's disease increases significantly.

The cause of Hodgkin's disease remains obscure. Although an increased incidence of Hodgkin's disease has been noticed in children with inherited immunodeficiency syndromes, in-

cluding ataxia-telangiectasia, Chediak-Higashi syndrome, Wiskott-Aldrich syndrome, and congenital agammaglobulinemia, it is not as common in these conditions as non-Hodgkin's lymphoma.

Suspicion of an infectious cause for Hodgkin's disease has been fostered by several reported associations, including reports of case clustering, a higher incidence in patients with infectious mononucleosis, and the bimodal incidence curve of the disease. However, there is no conclusive evidence of space-time clusters in children, and it remains possible that the associations observed result from the interplay of factors other than common infections.

There is an increased incidence of Hodgkin's disease among siblings of affected patients, especially if they are of the same sex. An association between certain HLA antigens and the disease has also been reported. These two observations suggest that genetic factors play a role. A difference in the age peaks of Hodgkin's disease in industrialized and underdeveloped countries suggest that environmental factors may also be important. Although a significant association between tonsillectomies and children with Hodgkin's disease has been reported by some, this has not been confirmed.

Children and young adults receiving phenytoin for control of seizures are at risk for a lymphoma-like syndrome, which usually reverses with cessation of the drug, and the development of true malignant lymphomas, including Hodgkin's disease.

A link between socioeconomic status and Hodgkin's disease has been suggested. The incidence of Hodgkin's disease is correlated with higher family income and educational status and with smaller family size. There appears to be an association of EBV with Reed-Sternberg cells. EBV is most often associated with mixed cellular Hodgkin's disease, but its exact role in pathogenesis is unknown. The association does raise questions about the increased incidence among persons who have suffered from infectious mononucleosis, even though almost everyone is eventually infected with this virus.

CLINICAL PRESENTATION

Children usually present with disease above the diaphragm, principally in the cervical or mediastinal nodes; isolated axillary lymph node involvement is infrequent.[92] Patients who present with subdiaphragmatic involvement often prove to have stage I disease originating in inguinal lymph nodes with lymphocyte-predominant histology.

PRETREATMENT EVALUATION

The principles of the diagnostic workup for the child with Hodgkin's disease are similar to those for adults (see Chap. 51). Lymphangiography is a feasible procedure in most children, and its diagnostic accuracy in the pediatric population has been substantiated; there is a greater than 90% correlation between lymphangiographic and histopathologic results. Because the dye persists in lymph nodes, lymphangiography is also a valuable means of assessing the results of therapy. Lymphangiography may reveal disease in lymph nodes that are not enlarged, and for this reason, the yield of lymphangiography is approximately 15% above that of CT alone. In the young child, lymphangiography is understandably a more difficult procedure, but this is offset by the lesser need of lymphangiography for the detection of pathologic nodes not detectable by CT, because few patients are currently treated by irradiation alone, particularly young children.

Indications for staging laparotomy are controversial, and arguments for and against its use are considered in Chapter 51. At Stanford University, where staging laparotomy was introduced, this procedure is no longer systematically performed in children. Laparotomy can provide more information about the extent of disease. In reviews of staging laparotomies with splenectomy in pediatric populations, resultant changes in the clinical stage affected approximately 15% to 50% of patients.[93] Approximately 20% of all clinical stage I patients have occult infradiaphragmatic disease at laparotomy, and in stage II cases that are clinically supradiaphragmatic, the incidence of histologically positive disease is 30%. In lymphocyte-predominant disease limited to the neck, the yield of laparotomy is sufficiently low to obviate its use.

Although information provided by a staging laparotomy and splenectomy may be unobtainable by other means, there has been considerable concern about the morbidity of the procedure in the pediatric population. The major risk is overwhelming postsplenectomy sepsis, which in the past occurred in as many as 10% of children with Hodgkin's disease. The use of polyvalent pneumococcal vaccine or prophylactic antibiotic therapy has markedly reduced the incidence of postsplenectomy infection in children at risk, but current treatment trends and the demonstration that similarly good results can be obtained without splenectomy weigh against its use.[92]

Because laparotomy is primarily a means of identifying otherwise occult disease in the abdomen, its value is primarily as a means of guiding local or regional therapy.[94] When combined-modality therapy is to be used, it is highly questionable whether the patient should be subjected to laparotomy and splenectomy. The use of chemotherapy and extended-field, low-dose irradiation in all children with Hodgkin's disease without the use of staging laparotomy has resulted in 85% survival, and the relapse-free survival rate for clinical stages I, II, and III approaches 90%.[95] It is possible that chemotherapy alone may provide results close to those achieved with combined-modality therapy (see section on therapy).

Staging is largely used these days as a guide to the treatment approach. With the possible exception of stage IV disease, it has lost its importance as a prognostic indicator, as has histologic subtype. Few prognostic factors have retained importance in the modern era of highly effective therapy for Hodgkin's disease, although age appears to be significant. Children have a better outcome than adults, although the reasons for this may be multiple and not necessarily a consequence of the biology of the disease.

THERAPY

Because the results of the treatment of Hodgkin's disease in children have been excellent, a major consideration in current treatment approaches is to limit morbidity. Available data indicate that the use of combined-modality therapy for patients in all stages of disease, except perhaps those with stage I or certain presentations of stage IV disease, results in high survival rates and a low risk of relapse.[95,96] Gratifying results, for example, were obtained for 57 children of all stages treated at the Sick Children's Hospital, Toronto (*i.e.*, 10-year survival rate of 85%, relapse-free survival rate of 80%), in whom no staging laparotomy was performed and three cycles of MOPP were given before and three after low-dose extended-field irradiation.[97]

The universal application of this approach, however, may inappropriately expose patients to added complications from both modalities.[98] Complications of irradiation in childhood include impairment of growth and development of bones, muscles, and soft tissues; thyroid dysfunction; and an increase in the risk of second malignancies, particularly solid tumors.[92] Irradiation is responsible for a 10% to 20% increase in the late appearance of heart disease (*e.g.*, valvular, coronary). Late complications of chemotherapy include infertility and second malignancies. MOPP chemotherapy results in a high incidence of sterility in postpubertal men, although it is likely that prepubertal boys will have a lower incidence of infertility. Ovarian function may also be compromised, although younger prepubertal and pubertal girls appear to be less susceptible to these effects than older, postpubertal women.

The risk of AML after MOPP treatment alone during the first 10 years after therapy is approximately 8%, and it may be exacerbated by previous or concurrent extensive irradiation. However, in the Stanford experience with combined-modality therapy (with less use of MOPP), the risk of secondary leukemia is 3% at 10 years. Beyond 10 years, the risk of developing secondary leukemia is negligible, although the risk of other tumors, including NHL and breast cancer, which appears beyond 15 years after therapy, appears to persist indefinitely, and the overall risk of a second neoplasm may be as high as 30% at 20 years with current regimens. Chemotherapy regimens other than MOPP, such as ABVD (doxorubicin, bleomycin, vincristine, DTIC), may achieve similar disease control with less risk of secondary tumors. However, the use of ABVD carries the potential risk of severe pulmonary damage from bleomycin and anthracycline-induced cardiac failure. The latter complication is not only an acute side effect. Recent reports have indicated that cardiac failure can occur many years after the cessation of treatment, and in patients treated with mediastinal irradiation, this could prove to be an important late complication. The combined use of MOPP and ABVD may be more effective than either alone, although there are fewer data about the long-term side effects of combined regimens.

In view of the potential risks associated with chemotherapy and radiation therapy, consideration should be given to whether there are subgroups of patients for whom one or other modality may be more appropriate or even whether chemotherapy alone may produce similar results to combined-modality therapy. The possibility of developing more effective chemotherapy regimens that are associated with a lower incidence of late effects has always been a goal of medical oncologists with a special interest in Hodgkin's disease. The vinblastine, bleomycin, and methotrexate regimen used at Stanford as adjuvant (after irradiation) therapy in patients with limited disease, for example, has not been associated with infertility. A variety of approaches designed to reduce the complications of therapy have been recommended. For example, reduction in radiation volume by using high-dose involved-field techniques rather than extended-field irradiation may be sufficient for patients with favorable stage I presentations, and although relapse rates will be higher, those who relapse are likely to be salvaged by chemotherapy. A group of 28 children with stage I or II disease treated at St Bartholomew's hospital for whom clinical staging was followed by limited-volume irradiation (involved field or mantle) achieved a survival rate (96% at 10 years) at least equal to 48 patients treated at Stanford University (86% at 10 years) using pathologic staging followed primarily by extended-field irradiation. Freedom from relapse at 10 years was 90% in the Stanford series and 83% in the London series.[99] Alternatively, intermediate-dose, involved-field radiation therapy combined with chemotherapy employing MOPP, ABVD, or MOPP plus ABVD, can also reduce the radiation volume, but this approach, at least if MOPP is used as the chemotherapy regimen, is associated with a significant risk of secondary leukemia.

The use of chemotherapy alone has been studied, and as with any approach using chemotherapy, the constitution of the drug regimen was important.[42,43,45] The details of each of these strategies and the controversies surrounding them are discussed in detail in Chapter 51. No single approach is accepted by all oncologists as optimal, and the achievement of an appropriate balance between maximizing disease-free survival and minimizing treatment complications for the child with Hodgkin's disease must take into consideration the stage of disease and the age of the patient.

Most pediatric patients with Hodgkin's disease are beyond puberty. For this group, growth changes are of relatively less concern and an approach based on extended-field irradiation for patients with pathologic stage I or IIA disease, with chemotherapy reserved for children who relapse after initial irradiation, is more acceptable to those who feel strongly that irradiation should be an important component of treatment.[92] For stage I disease, local irradiation may be adequate, because it can produce a disease-free survival rate of approximately 85%, and most relapsing patients can be salvaged with chemotherapy. Older children with stage III disease have traditionally been treated with combined-modality therapy, but many consider that all stage III patients should receive chemotherapy alone.[92,96] In older patients with extensive mediastinal disease, B symptoms, or disease beyond stage IIIA, there is general agreement on the use of primary chemotherapy, although many prefer to add involved-field irradiation.[92,95,96]

Defining optimal treatment for the younger child has been more difficult. Such children with pathologic stage I lymphocyte-predominant disease limited to the neck, particularly the upper neck, have an excellent disease-free survival rate after involved-field or limited extended-field ("minimantle") treatment. Treatment of this favorable-prognosis group reduces the likelihood of significant cardiac, pulmonary, and structural effects from irradiation, and by eliminating chemotherapy, it prevents the adverse sequelae associated with combined-modality treatment.

In patients with stage II disease managed with local fields only, relapse rates of more than 30% are common, even with surgical staging. Although relapsing patients still appear to respond well to chemotherapy, the excellent overall survival must be balanced against the eventual, rather high proportion of patients who receive combined-modality therapy. In young children with extensive disease, most centers favor primary chemotherapy with involved-field or extended-field irradiation

using limited radiation doses (1500–2500 cGy) to diminish the pronounced growth changes associated with large-volume, full-dose radiation therapy. This approach produces an excellent outcome with significant reduction in the risk of major deficits in growth and development.[95,96] In addition to the previously described Toronto study,[97] a series of children were treated at Stanford with 1500 to 2500 cGy of total nodal irradiation followed by six cycles of MOPP, which produced a relapse-free survival rate of 93%.[98]

In a disease in which irradiation has historically been of such importance, it is only with reluctance that this modality is abandoned. However, as doses of radiation are lowered without loss of efficacy in combined-modality approaches, the possibility that chemotherapy alone can achieve the same good results without the late complications of combined-modality therapy becomes more acceptable. Longo and coworkers reported the results of a randomized trial in adults, in which MOPP combination chemotherapy (54 evaluable patients) was compared with radiation therapy (51 patients) in patients with stages IB, IIA, IIB, or IIIA Hodgkin's disease. MOPP alone was significantly superior in patients with stages IIIA, massive mediastinal disease, patients with no B symptoms, patients with an erythrocyte sedimentation rate above 20 mm, patients with more than four sites of disease, or patients younger than 40. The overall projected 10-year disease-free survival rates were 60% for patients randomized to receive radiation therapy and 86% for patients randomized to receive MOPP chemotherapy ($p_2 = 0.009$), and the projected 10-year overall survival rates were 76% and 92%, respectively ($p_2 = 0.051$).[100]

Encouraging results with chemotherapy alone have been obtained in children. For example, an Australian group reported 92% failure-free survival (median follow-up, 45 months) for 53 children staged clinically and treated with chemotherapy alone with MOPP or ChlVPP (chlorambucil, prednisone, vinblastine, procarbazine).[101] Eighteen of 19 patients with massive mediastinal disease achieved remissions and none relapsed, and there were only four adverse events among 38 children with stage I or II disease. These data need to be complemented by long term follow-up, because knowledge of the actual survival and incidence of late effects is necessary for drawing final conclusions with respect to these divergent approaches to treatment. However, the potential avoidance of the complications associated with laparotomy and splenectomy, the obviation of radiation-induced dysmorphia, and the lower risk of second malignancies than for combined-modality therapy makes the further exploration of chemotherapy-alone approaches attractive.

In adults, some series have suggested that ABVD is more affective than MOPP alone and as effective as ABVD and MOPP combined. Whether ABVD, the MOPP plus ABVD hybrid regimen used in Vancouver, or another regimen will prove to provide optimal efficacy with the least likelihood of sterility and secondary malignancies remains to be seen, and it is one of the major issues to be resolved in the treatment of Hodgkin's disease. Few studies using ABVD for children have been conducted, but the CCSG reported a pilot study of children with stage III or IV disease treated with 12 cycles of ABVD followed by low-dose irradiation (2100 cGy). Early results are gratifying: event-free survival was 87% at 3 years, although 9% of patients developed significant pulmonary toxicity (*i.e.*, 2 of 6 patients died). It is too early to determine the incidence of second malignancies, late cardiac toxicity, or infertility. The duration of treatment in this study may be longer than is necessary, and this is likely to be an important factor in late effects. Regimens including fewer cycles must be studied. Variations in the chemotherapy regimen are not the only approach to the reduction of late effects. Alternative approaches to the prevention of infertility, such as the use of gonadotropin releasing hormone analogs in pubertal and post pubertal children, may be employed in the future, but it is difficult to envision early intervention for the prevention of secondary malignancies.

Although many issues remain to be resolved in the treatment of childhood Hodgkin's disease, the fact that there is so much focus on the late complications of therapy is a tribute to the success that has been achieved in the treatment of this disease. Overall 5- and 10-year survival rates have progressively improved, and most centers are achieving rates of approximately 90% in series including all stages of disease. It is difficult to justify staging laparotomy, and it is becoming increasingly clear that chemotherapy should be the primary modality of treatment in all stages except perhaps stage I. It will be important to establish whether even low-dose local or regional irradiation adds any therapeutic advantage to chemotherapy alone.

REFERENCES

1. Anderson JR, Wilson JF, Jenkin DJ, et al. Childhood non-Hodgkin's lymphoma: The results of a randomized therapeutic trial comparing a 4-drug regimen (COMP) with a 10-drug regimen LSA$_2$-L$_2$. N Engl J Med 1983;308:559–565.
2. Smith KL, Johnson W. Classification of chronic myelocytic leukemia in children. Cancer 1974;34:670–679.
3. Altman AJ. Chronic leukemias of childhood. Pediatr Clin North Am 1988;35(4):765–787.
4. Malkin D, Li F, Strong L, et al. Germline p53 mutations in a familial syndrome of breast cancer, sarcomas, and other neoplasms. Science 1990;250:1233.
5. Felix C, Nau M, Takahaski T, et al. Identification of p53 gene abnormalities in acute lymphoblastic leukemia of childhood: Nonhereditary p53 mutation in the Li-Fraumeni syndrome. J Clin Invest 1992;89(2):640–647.
6. Felix CA, D'Amico D, Mitsudomi T, et al. Absence of hereditary p53 mutations in ten familial leukemia pedigrees. J Clin Invest 1992;90:653–658.
7. Till M, Rapson N, Smith P. Family studies in acute leukemia in childhood: A possible association with autoimmune disease. Br J Cancer 1979;49:62–71.
8. Kirsch I. Molecular biology of the leukemias. Pediatr Clin North Am 1988;35:693–722.
9. Rossi G, Gerla R, Cadeo G, et al. Acute lymphoblastic leukaemia of B cell origin in an anti-HIV positive intravenous drug abuser. Br J Haematol 1988;68:140–141.
10. Bleyer WA, Poplack DG. Prophylaxis and treatment of leukemia in the central nervous system and other sanctuaries. Semin Oncol 1985;12:131–1148.
11. Russo A, Schiliro G. The enigma of testicular leukemia: A critical review. Med Pediatr Oncol 1986;14:300–306.
12. Bowman WP, Aur RJA, Hustu HO, et al. Isolated testicular relapse in acute lymphocytic leukemia of childhood: Categories and influence on survival. J Clin Oncol 1984;2:924–929.
13. Miller LP, Miller DR. Acute lymphoblastic leukemia in children: current status, controversies, and future perspective. Crit Rev Oncol Hematol 1986;1:129–197.
14. Bennett JM, Catovsky D, Daniel MT, et al. French-American-British (FAB) Cooperative Group: The morphological classification of acute leukemias-concordance among observers and clinical correlation. Br J Haematol 1981;47:553–561.
15. Miller DR, Krailo M, Bleyer WA, et al. Prognostic implications of blast cell morphology in childhood acute lymphoblastic leukemia: A report from the Children's Cancer Study Group. Cancer Treat Rep 1985;69:1211–21.
16. Korsmeyer SJ, Arnold A, Bakshi A, et al. Immunoglobulin gene rearrangement and cell surface antigen expression in acute lymphocytic leukemia of T-cell and B-cell precursor origins. J Clin Invest 1983;71:301–313.
17. Crist WM, Grosse CE, Pullen J, et al. Immunologic markers in childhood acute lymphocytic leukemia. Semin Oncol 1985;2:105–121.
18. Foon KA, Todd RF III. Immunologic classification of leukemia and lymphoma. Blood 1986;68:1–31.
19. Felix CA, Wright JJ, Poplack DG, et al. T cell receptor α-, β-, and γ-Genes in T-cell and pre-B cell acute lymphoblastic leukemia. J Clin Invest 1987;80:545–556.
20. Mirro J, Zipf TF, Pui C, et al. Acute mixed lineage leukemia: Clinicopathologic correlations and prognostic significance. Blood 1985;65:1115–1123.
21. Williams M, Innes DJ, Borowitz M, et al. Immunoglobulin and T cell receptor gene rearrangements in human lymphoma and leukemia. Blood 1987;69:79.
22. Stass S, Mirro JJ. Lineage heterogeneity in acute leukaemia: Acute mixed-lineage leukaemia and lineage switch. Clin Haematol 1986;15:811.
23. Altman A. Clinical features and biological implications of acute mixed lineage (hybrid) leukemias. Am J Pediatr Hematol Oncol 1990;12:123–133.
24. Wiersma S, Ortega J, Sobel E, et al. Clinical importance of myeloid-antigen expression in acute lymphoblastic leukemia of childhood. N Engl J Med 1991;324:800–808.
25. Hurwitz C, Loken M, Graham M, et al. Asynchronous antigen expression in B lineage acute lymphoblastic leukemia. Blood 1988;72:299–307.
26. Williams DL, Raimondi S, Rivera G, et al. Presence of clonal chromosome abnormalities in virtually all cases of acute lymphoblastic leukemia. N Engl J Med 1985;10:640–641.
27. Look AT. The emerging genetics of acute lymphoblastic leukemia: Clinical and biologic implications. Semin Oncol 1985;12:92–104.
28. Poplack DG, Blatt J, Reaman G. Purine pathway enzyme abnormalities in acute lymphoblastic leukemia. Cancer Res 1981;41:4821–4823.
29. Hammond GD, Sather H, Bleyer WA, et al. Stratification by prognostic factors in the design and analysis of clinical trials for acute lymphoblastic leukemia. Haematology and Blood transfusion. In: Buchner T, Schellong G, Hiddemann W, Urbanitz D, Ritter J, eds. Acute leukemias. Berlin: Springer-Verlag, 1987:161–166.
30. Reaman G, Zeltzer P, Bleyer WA, et al. Acute lymphoblastic leukemia in infants less than one year of age: A cumulative experience of the Children's Cancer Study Group. J Clin Oncol 1985;3:1513–1521.
31. Crist W, Pullin J, Boyett J, et al.: Clinical and biologic features predict a poor prognosis in acute lymphoid leukemias in infants: A Pediatric Oncology Group study. Blood 1986;67:135–140.
32. Sather HN. Statistical evaluation of prognostic factors in ALL and treatment results. Med Pediatr Oncol 1986;14:158–165.
33. Steinherz PG, Gaynon P, Miller DR, et al. Improved disease-free survival of children with acute lymphoblastic leukemia at high risk for early relapse with the New York regimen—a new intensive therapy protocol: A report from the Children's Cancer Study Group. J Clin Oncol 1986;4:744–752.
34. Bleyer WA, Coccia PF, Sather HN, et al. Reduction in central nervous system leukemia with a pharmacokinetically derived intrathecal methotrexate dosage regimen. J Clin Oncol 1983;1:317–325.
35. Poplack D, Reaman G, Bleyer W, et al. Successful prevention of central nervous system (CNS) leukemia without cranial radiation in children with high risk acute lymphoblastic leukemia (ALL): A preliminary report. Proc Am Soc Clin Oncol 1989;8:828.
36. Riehm H, Gadner H, Henze G, et al. Acute lymphoblastic leukemia: Treatment results in three BFM studies (1970–1981). In: Murphy SB, Gilbert JR, eds. Leukemia research: Advances in cell biology and treatment. New York: Elsevier Biomedical, 1983:251–263.
37. Henze G, Langermann HJ, Fengler R, et al. Acute lymphoblastic therapy study BFM 70/81 in children and adolescents: Intensified reinduction therapy for patients with different risk for relapse. Klin Pediatr 1982;194:195–203.
38. Rivera G, Raimondi S, Hancock M, et al. Improved outcome in childhood acute lymphoblastic leukaemia with reinforced early treatment and rotational combination chemotherapy. Lancet 1991;337:61–66.
39. Tubergen D, Gilchrist G, Coccia P, et al. The role of intensified chemotherapy in intermediate risk acute lymphoblastic leukemia (ALL) of childhood. CCG-105. Proc Am Soc Clin Oncol 1990;9:835.
40. Nesbit ME, Sather HN, Robison LL, et al. Randomized study of 3 years versus 5 years of chemotherapy in childhood acute lymphoblastic leukemia. J Clin Oncol 1983;1:308–316.
41. Butturine A, Rivera GK, Bortin MM, et al. Which treatment for childhood acute lymphoblastic leukaemia in second remission? Lancet 1987;1:429–432.
42. Henze G, Fengler R, Hartmann R, et al. Chemotherapy for bone marrow relapse of childhood acute lymphoblastic leukemia. Cancer Chemother Pharmacol 1989;24:S16–19.
43. Henze G, Fengler R, Hartman R, et al. BFM group treatment results in relapsed childhood acute lymphoblastic leukemia. In: Buchner S, Hiddemann W, Ritter J, eds. Haematology and blood transfusion, acute leukemias II. Berlin: Springer-Verlag 1990:619–626.
44. Thomas ED, Sanders JE, Flowinoy N, et al. Marrow transplantation for patients with acute lymphoblastic leukemia: A long-term follow-up. Blood 1983;62:1139–1141.
45. Sanders JE, Thomas ED, Buckner CD, et al. Marrow transplantation for children with acute lymphoblastic leukemia in second remission. Blood 1987;70:324–326.
46. Sanders J, Thomas E, Buckner C, et al. Marrow transplantation for children with acute lymphoblastic leukemia in second remission. Blood 1987;70:324–326.
47. Barrett A, Horowitz M, Gale R, et al. Marrow transplantation for acute lymphoblastic leukemia: Factors affecting relapse and survival. Blood 1989;74:862–871.
48. Gale R, Butturini A. Bone marrow transplantation in acute lymphoblastic leukemia. In: Champlin R, ed. Bone marrow transplantation. Boston: Kluwer Academic Publishers, 1990:223–233.
49. Champlin R, Gale R. Acute lymphoblastic leukemia: Recent advances in biology and therapy. Blood 1989;73:2051–2066.
50. Rivera G, Santana V, Mahmoud H, et al. Acute lymphoblastic leukemia of childhood: The problem of relapses. Bone Marrow Transplant 1989;4:80–85.
51. Kersey J, Weisdorf D, Nesbit M, et al. Comparison of autologous and allogeneic bone marrow transplantation for treatment of high-risk refractory acute lymphoblastic leukemia. N Engl J Med 1987;317:461–467.

52. Sallan S, Niemeyer C, Billett A, et al. Autologous bone marrow transplantation for acute lymphoblastic leukemia. J Clin Oncol 1989;7:1594–11601.
53. Poplack DG, Brouwers, P. Adverse sequelae of central nervous system therapy. Clin Oncol 1985;4:263–285.
54. Berg SL, Balis FM, Zimm S, et al. Phase I/II trial and pharmacokinetics of intrathecal diaziquone in refractory meningeal malignancies. J Clin Oncol 1992;10:143–148.
55. Adamson PC, Balis FM, Arndt CA, et al. Intrathecal 6-mercaptopurine: Preclinical pharmacology, phase I/II trial, and pharmacokinetic study. Cancer Res 1991;51:6079–6083.
56. Smith S, Wofford M, Shuster J, et al. Treatment of testicular leukemia in children with acute lymphoblastic leukemia (ALL): A Pediatric Oncology Group study. Proc Am Soc Clin Oncol 1990;9:841.
57. Uderzo C, Zurlo M, Adamoli L, et al. Treatment of isolated testicular relapse in childhood acute lymphoblastic leukemia: An Italian multicenter study. J Clin Oncol 1990;8:672–677.
58. Lipshultz S, Colan S, Gelber R, et al. Late cardiac effects of doxorubicin therapy for acute lymphoblastic leukemia in childhood. N Engl J Med 1991;324:808–815.
59. Yeung S, Yoong C, Spink J, et al. Functional myocardial impairment in children treated with anthracyclines for cancer. Lancet 1991;337:816–818.
60. Shapiro S, Mealey JJ. Late anaplastic gliomas in children previously treated for acute lymphoblastic leukemia. Pediatr Neurosci 1989;15:176–180.
60a. Pui C-H, Behm F, Raimondi S, et al. Secondary acute myeloid leukemia in children treated for acute lymphoblastic leukemia. N Engl J Med 1989;321:136–142.
61. Pui C-H, Behm F, Raimondi S, et al. Secondary acute myeloid leukemia in children treated for acute lymphoid leukemia. N Engl J Med 1989;321:136–142.
62. Kreissman S, Gelber F, Sallan S, et al. Secondary acute myeloid leukemia (AML) in children treated for acute lymphoblastic leukemia (ALL). Proc Am Soc Clin Oncol 1990;9:846.
63. Ratain M, Kaminer L, Bitran J, et al. Acute nonlymphocytic leukemia following etoposide and cisplatin combination chemotherapy for advanced non-small cell carcinoma of the lung. Blood 1987;70:1412–1417.
64. Rothenberg M, Mickley L, Cole D, et al. Expression of the mdr-1/P-170 gene in patients with acute lymphoblastic leukemia. Blood 1989;74:1388–1395.
65. Yamada M, Wasserman R, Lange B, et al. Minimal residual disease in childhood B-lineage lymphoblastic leukemia. Persistence of leukemic cells during the first 18 months of treatment. N Engl J Med 1990;323:448–455.
66. Yokota S, Hansen-Hagge T, Ludwig W-D, et al. Use of polymerase chain reactions to monitor minimal residual disease in acute lymphoblastic leukemia patients. Blood 1991;77:331–339.
67. Neale G, Menaarguez J, Kitchingman G, et al. Detection of minimal residual disease in T-cell acute lymphoblastic leukemia using polymerase chain reaction predicts impending relapse. Blood 1991;78:739–747.
68. Wright JJ, Poplack DG, Bakhshi A, Reaman G, Cole D, Jensen JP, Korsmeyer SJ. Gene rearrangements as markers of clonal variation and minimal residual disease in acute lymphoblastic leukemia. J Clin Oncol 1987;5:735–741.
69. Lampkin BC, Woods W, Strauss R, et al. Current status of the biology and treatment of acute non-lymphocytic leukemia in children (Report from the ANLL Strategy Group of Children's Cancer Study Group). Blood 1983;61:215–228.
70. Weinstein HJ, Mayer RJ, Rosenthal DS, et al. Chemotherapy for acute myelogenous leukemia in children and adults: VAPA update. Blood 1983;62:315–319.
71. Pui CH, Raimondi S, Head D, et al. Characterization of childhood acute leukemia with multiple myeloid and lymphoid markers at diagnosis and relapse. Blood 1991;78:1327.
72. Creutzig U, Ritter J, Riehm H, et al. Improved treatment results in childhood acute myelogenous leukemia: A report of the German cooperative study AML-BFM-78. Blood 1985;65:298.
73. Creutzig U, Ritter J, Schellong G. Identification of two risk groups in childhood acute myelogenous leukemia after therapy intensification in study AML-BFM-83 as compared with study AML—AML-BFM-78. Blood 1991;75:1932.
74. Griffin JD, Mayer RJ, Weinstin HJ, et al. Surface marker analysis of acute myeloblastic leukemia: Identification of differentiation-associated phenotypes. Blood 1983;62:557–563.
75. Pui CH, Dahl GV, Kalwinsky DK, et al. Central nervous system leukemia in children with acute nonlymphoblastic leukemia. Blood 1985;66:1062–1067.
76. Grier HE, Gelber RD, Camitta BM, et al. Prognostic factors in childhood acute myelogenous leukemia. J Clin Oncol 1987;5:1026.
77. Grier HE, Gelber RD, Camitta BM, et al. Prognostic factors in childhood acute myelogenous leukemia. J Clin Oncol 1987;5:1026.
78. Woods WG, Ruyman FB, Lampkin B, et al. The role of timing of high-dose cytosine arabinoside intensification and of maintenance therapy in the treatment of children with acute nonlymphocytic leukemia. Cancer 1990;66:1106.
79. Ravindranath U, Steuber CP, Krischer J, et al. High dose cytarabine for intensification of early therapy of childhood acute myeloid leukemia: A Pediatric Oncology Group study. J Clin Oncol 1991;9:572.
80. Champlin R, Gale RP. Acute myelogenous leukemia: Recent advances in therapy. Prolonged survival in acute myelogenous leukemia without maintenance chemotherapy. Blood 1987;69:1551.
80a. Nesbit M, Buckley L, Lampkin B, et al. Comparison of allogeneic bone marrow transplantation (BMT) with maintenance chemotherapy in previously untreated childhood acute non-lymphocytic leukemia (ANLL). Proc Am Soc Clin Oncol [Abstract] 1987;6:163.
81. Reiffers J, Gaspard MH, Maraninchi D, et al. Comparison of allogeneic or autologous bone marrow transplantation and chemotherapy in patients with acute myeloid leukemia in first remission: A prospective controlled trial. Br J Haematol 1989;71:57.
82. Lowenberg B, Verdonck JL, Dekker AW, et al. Autologous bone marrow transplantation in acute myeloid leukemia in first remission: Results of a Dutch prospective study. J Clin Oncol 1990;8:287.
83. Lenarsky C, Weinberg K, Peterson J, et al. Autologous bone marrow transplantation with 4-hydroperoxycyclophosphamide purged marrows for children with acute-nonlymphoblastic leukemia in second remission. Bone Marrow Transplant 1990;6:425.
84. Ball ED, Mills LE, Cornwell GG III, et al. Autologous bone marrow transplantation for acute myeloid leukemia using monoclonal antibody-purged bone marrow. Blood 1990;75:1199.
85. Huang ME, Ye UC, et al. Use of all-*trans* retinoic acid in the treatment of acute promyelocytic leukemia. Blood 1988;72:567.
86. Castaigne S, Chomienne C, et al. All-*trans* retinoic acid as a differentiation therapy for acute promyelocytic leukemia. I. Clinical results. Blood 1990;76:1704.
87. Smith MA, Adamson PC, Balis FM, et al. Phase I and pharmacokinetic evaluation of all-*trans* retinoic acid in pediatric patients. J Clin Oncol 1992;10(11):1666–1673.
88. Magrath I, Malignant non-Hodgkin's lymphomas in children. In: Pizzo PA, Poplack DG, eds. Principles and practice of pediatric oncology. Philadelphia: JB Lippincott, 1992.
89. Seibel N, Cossman J, Magrath I. Lymphoproliferative disorders. In: Pizzo PA, Poplack DG, eds. Principles and practice of pediatric oncology. Philadelphia: JB Lippincott, 1992.
89a. Rabbitts, TH. Translocations, master genes, and differences between the origins of acute and chronic luekemias. Cell 1991;67:641–646.
90. Magrath IT. The Pathogenesis of Burkitt's Lymphoma. Adv Cancer Res 1990;55:133–270.
90a. Dahl GV, Rivera, G, Pui CH, et al. A novel treatment of childhood lymphoblastic non-Hodgkin's lymphoma: Early and intermittent use of teniposide plus cytarabine. Blood 1985;66:1110.
91. Link MP, Donaldson SS, Berard CW, et al. Results of treatment of childhood localized non-Hodgkin's lymphoma with combination chemotherapy with or without radiotherapy. N Engl J Med 1990;322, 1169–1174.
91a. Mott MG, Chessells JM, Willoughby ML, et al. Adjuvant low dose radiation in childhood T cell leukaemia/lymphoma (report from the United Kingdom children's cancer study group—UKCCSG). Br J Cancer 1984;50:457.
92. Mauch PM, Weinstein H, Botnick L, et al. An evaluation of long-term survival and treatment complications in children with Hodgkin's disease. Cancer 1983;51:925–932.
93. Donaldson SS, Kaplan HS. A survey of pediatric Hodgkin's disease at Stanford University: Results of therapy and quality of survival. In: Rosenberg SA, Kaplan HS, eds. Malignant lymphomas: Etiology, immunology, pathology, treatment. New York: Academic Press, 1982.
94. Russell KJ, Donaldson SS, Cox RS, Kaplan HS. Childhood Hodgkin's disease: Patterns of relapse. J Clin Oncol 1984;2:80–87.
95. Jenkin D, Doyle D. Paediatric Hodgkin's disease—late results and toxicity. Int J Radiat Oncol Biol Phys 1987;13:92.
96. Lange B, Littman P. Management of Hodgkin's disease in children and adolescents. Cancer 1983;51:1371–1377.
97. Jenkin D, Doyle J, Berry M, et al. Hodgkin's disease in children: Treatment with MOPP and low dose, extended field irradiation without laparotomy. Late results and toxicity. Med Pediatr Oncol 1990;18:265–272.
98. Donaldson SS, Kaplan HS. Complications of treatment of Hodgkin's disease in children. Cancer Treat Rep 1981;66:977–989.
99. Donaldson SS, Whitaker SJ, Plowman PN, et al. Stage I–II pediatric Hodgkin's disease: Long-term follow-up demonstrates equivalent survival rates following different management schemes. J Clin Oncol 1990;8:1128–1137.
100. Longo DK, Glatstein E, Diffey PL, et al. Radiation therapy versus combination chemotherapy in the treatment of early-stage Hodgkin's disease: Seven-year results of a prospective randomized trial. J Clin Oncol 1991;9:906–917.
101. Ekert H, Waters KL, Smith P, et al. Treatment with MOPP or ChlVPP chemotherapy only for all stages of childhood Hodgkin's disease. J Clin Oncol 1988;6:1845–1850.

Cancer: Principles & Practice of Oncology, Fourth Edition, edited by Vincent T. DeVita, Jr., Samuel Hellman, Steven A. Rosenberg. J.B. Lippincott Co., Philadelphia © 1993.

Vincent T. DeVita, Jr

Samuel Hellman

Elaine S. Jaffe

CHAPTER **51**

Hodgkin's Disease

HISTORY

Thomas Hodgkin's historic paper, "On Some Morbid Appearances of the Absorbent Glands and Spleen," was read before the Medical and Chirurgical Society on January 10 and 24, 1832.[1,2] Hodgkin described six cases of his own and a case described by Thomas Carswell in 1828. A watercolor of the morbid anatomy of this case was on display during Hodgkin's presentations. Like many later discoverers of new diseases, Hodgkin was certain that others must have noticed the disorder; he commented to fellow anatomists that such cases "can scarcely have failed to have fallen under their observation in the course of cadaveric inspection," and such observations had been made.

Hodgkin recognized that he was dealing with a primary disease of the lymphatic glands and not a secondary response to inflammation. His certainty about this was remarkable in its day, especially because he was aware that two of his patients had other illnesses (i.e., tuberculosis, syphilis) that might have accounted for the pathology. Also remarkable is the fact that Hodgkin described the entity based on the natural history of the disease without the aid of a microscope. Subsequent analysis of material from Hodgkin's patients (preserved in the Gordon Museum at Guy's Hospital Medical School, London) confirmed that 4 of 7 patients had Hodgkin's disease; Carswell's case could not be confirmed without tissue, and in the remaining two cases, syphilis and lymphosarcoma were thought to be the causes of the adenopathy.[1]

Hodgkin's contribution would have fallen into oblivion if not for the unselfish behavior of Sir Samuel Wilks. In the course of his description of primary and secondary amyloidosis, also a first, he reported a variant associated with "a peculiar enlargement of lymphatic glands frequently associated with diseases of the spleen." He first thought his observation

was original, but by the time he completed writing his paper, he became aware of Hodgkin's work through mention of it in another paper by Bright and diligently tracked it down, noting, "It is only to be lamented that Dr. Hodgkin did not affix a distinct name to this disease, for by so doing, I should not have experienced so long an ignorance (which I believe I share with many others) of a remarkable class of cases."[3] Wilks' paper in 1865 was entitled, "Enlargement of the Lymphatic Glands and Spleen (or, Hodgkin's Disease)," thereby immortalizing Thomas Hodgkin.[4] Nuland questions whether Sir Samuel's seemingly unselfish act was as generous as it appears. He suggests that Sir Richard Bright called to his attention Dr. Hodgkin's priority and pressured his acknowledgment.[5]

Hodgkin's description was the first of a distinct malignancy of the lymphatic system, preceding the description of leukemia by Craigie,[6] Bennett,[7] and Virchow[8] by 61 years and reticulum cell sarcoma by Roulet[9] by 98 years. These important descriptions were largely microscopic delineations of causes of adenopathy other than Hodgkin's disease. Another feat similar to that of Dr. Thomas Hodgkin was not to follow for 126 years, until Burkitt described the lymphoma that bears his name, based on its unique clinical presentation in patients in central Africa.[10]

The history of the discovery of the pathognomonic giant cells of Hodgkin's disease was reviewed by Kaplan.[1] Wilks had the benefit of a microscope and had histologically examined some cases, but observed only that "the microscope showed masses of cells and fibres as of new tissue."[4] Greenfield contributed the first low-power drawings of the appearance of those cells in 1878.[11] Goldmann, using Ehrlich's staining procedures, recognized the acidophilic nature of the nucleolus of the cells in 1892.[12] Sternberg also described the cells in 1898.[13] However, it was Reed who most clearly illus-

1819

trated the appearance of the multinuclear giant cells with excellent drawings from her 8 patients cases in 1902, and the cells have since been known as Reed-Sternberg cells.[14] The malignant nature of the disease was generally agreed on after the clonal origin of the malignant cell was confirmed by cytogenetic analysis of cell lines by Seif and Spriggs in 1967.[15]

ETIOLOGY AND EPIDEMIOLOGY

In the United States, Hodgkin's disease is diagnosed in 7 of every 100,000 people annually. There is a bimodal incidence pattern for Hodgkin's disease in economically advantaged countries.[16,17] In economically underdeveloped countries, the overall incidence of Hodgkin's disease is lower than in developed countries, but incidence before the age of 15 is higher, with only a modest increase throughout adolescence and young adulthood. Associated with this disparity is a difference in the distribution of histologic subgroups, with nodular sclerosing Hodgkin's disease underrepresented in less developed countries. In Japan, the first peak of Hodgkin's disease usually seen in developed countries is absent. The pattern of Hodgkin's disease varies as the level of development changes within a specific region. Examination of longitudinal data from the Connecticut cancer registry revealed the evolution from an "intermediate" to a typical "developed" pattern between the years 1935 and 1980.[18] There is an increased risk of Hodgkin's disease with increasing educational level of the patient. The relative risk varied from 0.7 to 1.8, depending on the educational level.[18]

The potential infectious nature of Hodgkin's disease has been a topic of discussion since its earliest description. *Mycobacterium tuberculosis* was first suspected to be the etiologic organism because of the high incidence of tuberculosis in patients with this disease.[19-22] Since that time, considerable epidemiologic evidence in support of an infectious cause, particularly a virus, has been found. In several studies that addressed the possibility of an increased risk of Hodgkin's disease associated with infectious mononucleosis, a disease caused by the Epstein-Barr virus (EBV), there was a modest threefold excess in the incidence of Hodgkin's disease among patients with a prior history of mononucleosis over that in controls.[23-27] Serologic and molecular biologic data also provide support for an etiologic role of EBV in Hodgkin's disease. There have been several reports of Hodgkin's disease developing in association with serologically documented primary EBV infection. In serologic studies, the proportion of Hodgkin's patients who have IgG antibody to EBV viral capsid antigens (indicative of prior infection) is similar to controls, but data from the Boston-Worcester case control study show that in young adults with a history of infectious mononucleosis there is a significantly higher geometric mean titer of antibodies against the capsid antigen than controls.[18] The results could reflect reactivation of the virus after development of Hodgkin's disease, but a follow-up study suggested otherwise. Using the resources of five serum banks with 240,000 specimens, 43 patients were identified from whom blood had been drawn and stored an average of 50 months before diagnoses, with results similar to the previous findings. These results imply that, at least for a subset of patients with Hodgkin's disease, endogenous immune stimulation plays a role.

For a short period, there was concern that Hodgkin's disease might be contagious because of reports of clustering of the disease, but that concern has been effectively dispelled.[18] The clustering was first reported by Vianna and associates among high school students exposed to the disease.[28,29] Population-based studies, using cancer registries in Connecticut and California, convincingly made the argument that the reported clusters occurred by chance alone, and a study that repeated the methodology of Vianna and coworkers in a different location also failed to confirm their findings.[31,32] An alternative hypothesis suggested an association between the incidence of Hodgkin's disease and childhood factors that decrease exposure to infectious agents at an early age. Studies showed that the risk of Hodgkin's disease was higher under certain circumstances. Risk-reducing factors that decreased or delayed early exposure to infections included fewer siblings, single-family houses, early birth order, and fewer playmates. The incidence of clinical mononucleosis is also associated with these factors, because the disease becomes clinically relevant only after early childhood. It appears that the infection has different consequences depending on the patient's age at infection and that infection by EBV may parallel that of another agent, with EBV as a cofactor.[33]

Other, unexplained factors are associated with an increased risk of acquiring Hodgkin's disease, including increased risk among woodworkers, elevated rates after tonsillectomy and appendectomy, the familial association of Hodgkin's disease, and its linkage with certain HLA antigens.[34-41]

PATHOLOGY CLASSIFICATION

Hodgkin's disease is unique among cancers because the tumor palpated by the physician largely contains normal lymphocytes, plasma cells, and fibrous stroma of the lymph node, with only a scattering of the characteristic malignant cells of Hodgkin's disease, the Reed-Sternberg cells and their mononuclear variants. The diagnosis of Hodgkin's disease should rarely be made in the absence of Reed-Sternberg cells, although the presence of such a cell by itself is not pathognomonic of the disease. Cells simulating Reed-Sternberg cells have been found in reactive lymphoid hyperplasias, such as infectious mononucleosis, non-Hodgkin's lymphomas, and nonlymphoid malignancies, including carcinomas and sarcomas.[42-45] The historic evolution of the diagnosis and classification of Hodgkin's disease is shown in Table 51–1.

Since the detailed descriptions by Sternberg and Reed, Hodgkin's disease has been recognized as a form of lymphoreticular malignancy with distinctive clinical and pathologic features.[13,14] Histologically, there is a polymorphous admixture of cytologically abnormal cells (*i.e.*, Reed-Sternberg cells and their mononuclear variants) and a variety of apparently normal reactive elements. The Reed-Sternberg cell is large, with two or more mirror-image nuclei, each containing a single, prominent nucleolus (Fig. 51–1).

In the first clinically useful subclassification of Hodgkin's disease developed by Jackson and Parker, cases were divided into three groups: paragranuloma, granuloma, and sarcoma.[50] This classification identified the 10% of patients with the most favorable and least favorable prognoses (*i.e.*, paragranuloma and sarcoma, respectively), but approximately 80% remained

TABLE 51–1. Landmarks in the Description of Hodgkin's Disease

Investigations	Year	Observation
Hodgkin[2]	1832	"On some morbid appearances of the absorbent glands and spleen"
Wilks[4]	1865	"Cases of the enlargement of the lymph glands and spleen (or Hodgkin's disease)"
Langhans[46]	1872	First description of histologic features of Hodgkin's disease, including a description of giant cells and intense fibrous bands
Greenfield[11]	1878	
Pell[47]	1887	Described cyclic fever in Hodgkin's disease
Sternberg, Reed[13,14]	1898, 1902	First definitive description of Hodgkin's disease and clear illustrations of the cells bearing their names
Parker, Jackson, Fitzhugh[48]	1932	Described the absence of response to tuberculin in the presence of tuberculosis in Hodgkin's disease
Jackson, Parker[44]	1937	First histopathologic classification of Hodgkin's disease
Lukes[49]	1963	Described the current histopathologic classification of Hodgkin's disease

TABLE 51–2. Histologic Classifications of Hodgkin's Disease

Jackson, Parker[44] (1944)	Lukes, Butler, Hicks[45] (1966)
Paragranuloma (10%)*	Lymphocytic predominant (15%)
	Nodular sclerosis (70%)
Granuloma (80%)	Mixed cellularity (10%)
	Lymphocyte depleted (5%)
	Diffuse fibrosis type
	Reticular type
Sarcoma (10%)	

* The figures in parentheses indicate the percentage of patients in various subcategories in the National Cancer Institute population.

in the category of granuloma. A major advance occurred in 1966, when Lukes, Hicks, and Butler proposed a new histologic classification that appeared to correlate well with clinical stage and aggressiveness of disease.[45] This scheme was later simplified into the Rye classification, which is now widely employed by pathologists and clinicians. These two classifications are compared in Table 51–2. In the Rye classification, Hodgkin's disease is divided into four categories: lymphocyte predominant, mixed cellularity, lymphocyte depleted, and nodular sclerosis. Although the initial basis of this classification

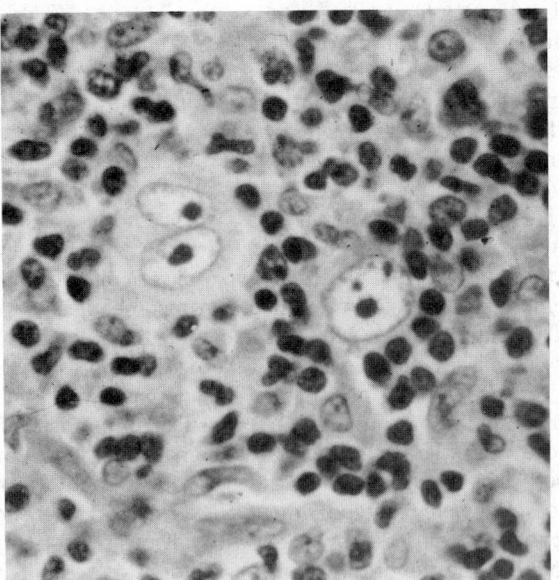

FIGURE 51–1. Characteristic Reed-Sternberg cell and mononuclear variant of Hodgkin's disease (hematoxylin & eosin stain; original magnification × 400).

was to divide cases according to the relative proportion of neoplastic mononuclear cells and Reed-Sternberg cells according to reactive elements, especially lymphocytes, in recent years, certain of the forms, such as lymphocyte-predominant Hodgkin's disease, have been shown to have distinctive morphologic, phenotypic, and clinical features. Nodular sclerosing Hodgkin's disease has long been regarded as unique. Its clinical and morphologic features were first hinted at by Greenfield in 1878 but not clearly described until 85 years later by Lukes and colleagues in 1963.[11,49]

The original Lukes and Butler scheme subdivided lymphocyte-predominant Hodgkin's disease (LPHD) into nodular and diffuse subtypes. This distinction was obliterated by the Rye modification but appears to be important in the light of new information that consistently links the nodular subtype to the B-cell arm of the immune system. In LPHD, the lymph node architecture is usually effaced, although a remnant of normal lymph node may remain. The cellular proliferation is composed of benign-appearing lymphocytes with or without benign histiocytes. The growth pattern may be diffuse but is more frequently nodular, and the nodules are considerably larger than those of follicular lymphomas. It is often necessary to examine multiple sections to identify diagnostic Reed-Sternberg cells, and some authorities question whether such cells are necessary for diagnosis in this form.[50] However, L and H variant cells are frequent and are the most characteristic cellular element in the nodular form of LPHD. These cells often have multilobated nuclei and have been called "popcorn" cells because of their resemblance to a popped kernel of corn. Fibrosis is usually not seen. This subtype is more common in male than in female patients and often occurs in the younger age groups (<35 years of age). Most patients have clinically localized disease and are asymptomatic, and the prognosis is usually favorable.

Progressive transformation of germinal centers is linked and often associated with LPHD of the nodular subtype. The nodal architecture is altered by large nodules that contain dispersed follicular center cells in clusters and ill-defined islands; Reed-Sternberg cells and L and H variants are absent. Progressive transformation of germinal centers can be seen with LPHD, precede it, or follow it in other sites.[51–53] The association of this lesion with nodular LPHD has supported the concept that the latter may be closely linked with the B-cell system. The diagnosis of progressive transformation of germinal centers should alert the clinician to the possible development of LPHD. The L and H cells express a B-cell phenotype. In paraffin sections, they are CD20 (Leu-26) positive and CD15 (Leu-M1) negative.[53–56] This phenotype is encountered in most cases of diffuse LPHD, indicating that most cases of the diffuse type represent progression from the nodular variant.[57]

Diffuse large cell lymphomas of B-cell type have been associated with the nodular variant of LPHD.[58] Both processes may occur in the same anatomic site, so-called composite lymphoma, or the large cell lymphomas may occur after the diagnosis of Hodgkin's disease.[59,60] Many of these patients seem to have a better prognosis than those with de novo large cell lymphoma, suggesting it may be a unique variant.[58] The B-cell phenotype lends further support to the B-cell origin of nodular LPHD. Although these lymphomas have been shown to be clonal, clonality has not been proven for the L and H cells of nodular LPHD, phenotypically or genotypically.

In lymphocyte-depleted Hodgkin's disease (LDHD), Reed-Sternberg cells and "pleomorphic" variant cells are plentiful in proportion to normal lymphocytes. The original Lukes and Butler scheme included two subtypes of LDHD: diffuse fibrosis and reticular. The reticular subtype contained sheets of pleomorphic neoplastic cells, making differentiation from a high-grade non-Hodgkin's lymphoma difficult.[61] The currently lower incidence of LDHD than previously reported suggests that some cases previously diagnosed as LDHD may have represented large cell immunoblastic lymphomas.[62] LDHD had been considered as a distinct clinicopathologic entity occurring in older patients with minimal peripheral adenopathy and widespread abdominal disease.[63] However, this syndrome is now in question because misclassification of high-grade diffuse lymphomas such as Hodgkin's disease was common in older series. This same difficulty may be responsible for the association of a significantly worse prognosis with the lymphocyte-depleted type found in these same studies.[62] Using stringent criteria, LDHD accounts for only 5% of all patients in current series.

Most cases of LDHD are the diffuse fibrosis subtype. In this subtype, diffuse fibroblastic proliferation may be prominent, and the process may even have a sarcomatous appearance. Normal lymphocytes are sparse, but neutrophils may be conspicuous, and foci of necrosis are common. Reed-Sternberg cells and variants are present but may be difficult to detect due to the marked fibroblastic reaction. LDHD is the most common category associated with the acquired immunodeficiency syndrome (AIDS). These patients usually have widespread disease with involvement of liver and bone marrow.[64–66] The absence of an effective lymphocytic response may contribute to aggressive clinical and pathologic behavior.

The nodular sclerosis category is distinctive morphologically and clinically. There are two histologic features that differentiate this form of Hodgkin's disease from all others. The first is a variant of the Reed-Sternberg cell, the so-called lacunar cell.[67,68] In formalin-fixed tissue, the abundant pale cytoplasm often retracts and gives the appearance of a cell in space. The second feature, seen in most cases, is a thickened capsule with a proliferation of orderly collagenous bands that divide the lymphoid tissue into circumscribed nodules (Fig. 51–2). In some cases, the sclerosis is absent or minimal, but

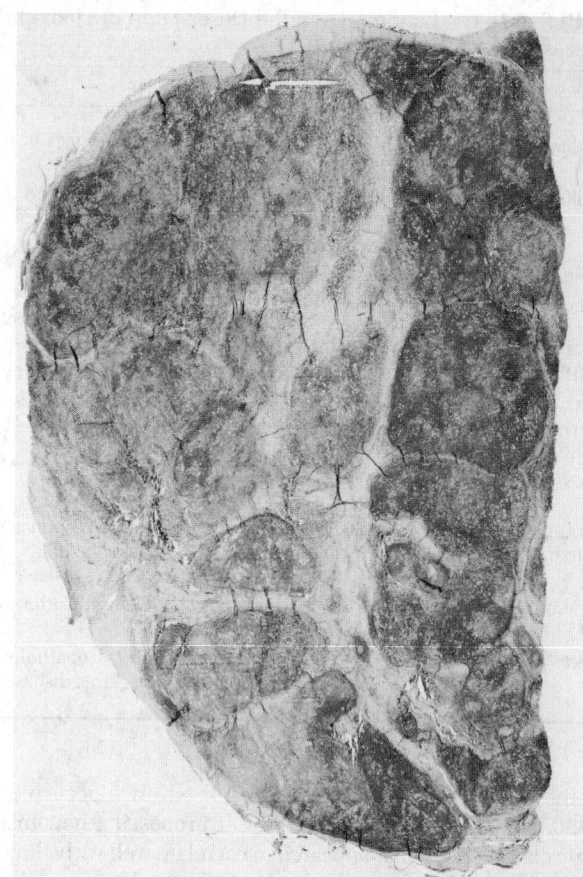

FIGURE 51–2. Lymph node involved by nodular sclerosing Hodgkin's disease. Cellular nodules are surrounded by dense fibrous bands (hematoxylin & eosin stain; original magnification × 8).

the presence of numerous lacunar cells, often in focal nodular aggregates, led some investigators to refer to this as the "cellular phase of nodular sclerosis." Strum and Rappaport observed progression from the cellular phase to classic nodular sclerosis with fibrous bands in sequential biopsies.[69] Nodular sclerosis is the only form of Hodgkin's disease that is more common in female than male patients. It most frequently occurs in adolescents and young adults and is unusual in patients older than 50 years of age. The process has a striking propensity to involve lower cervical, supraclavicular, and mediastinal lymph nodes.

This category can be subclassified according to the frequency of the malignant cells relative to normal lymphocytes. In the lymphocyte-depleted subtype, malignant cells are extremely numerous. Marked necrosis accompanied by acute inflammatory cells is seen in the center of cellular nodules. The neoplastic "histiocytes" palisading this necrosis may, to the unwary, mimic necrotizing granulomas. Fibrous bands may be inconspicuous, although capsular fibrosis is evident. Because of the frequent sheets of malignant cells, this subtype also has been referred to as the syncytial variant. The lymphocyte-depleted subtype, although not clearly an independent prognostic indicator, correlates with advanced stage at presentation and the presence of B symptoms.[62,70,71] Bulky mediastinal disease often is associated with this subtype.[72] MacLennan and coworkers proposed a subclassification scheme for nodular sclerosing Hodgkin's disease, which they believe has clinical and prognostic significance.[73] The type II of Bennett overlaps with the lymphocyte-depleted forms and the syncytial variant.

Mixed-cellularity Hodgkin's disease is characterized by an inflammatory background rich in lymphocytes, plasma cells, eosinophils, and histiocytes.[74,75] The Reed-Sternberg cells and their mononuclear counterparts are of the classic variety with prominent inclusion-like nucleoli, representing 5 to 15 cells per high-power field. Because of the inflammatory background, the differential diagnosis often includes peripheral T-cell lymphoma, and immune markers may be necessary to resolve this point. A relatively high percentage of patients have stage III or IV disease. To some extent, mixed-cellularity Hodgkin's disease has been used to include all cases of Hodgkin's disease that do not readily fall into another category.[45] This wastebasket approach should be avoided, and such cases should be considered "unclassifiable" or "not further subclassified."

Needle-core biopsies of the liver and bone marrow are frequently obtained for staging Hodgkin's disease. To diagnose involvement, the examiner should see atypical mononuclear cells or Reed-Sternberg cells in the appropriate inflammatory environment. In a patient with an established primary diagnosis, Reed-Sternberg cells are not required. However, a polymorphous cellular infiltrate in the absence of atypical cells with prominent nucleoli is a nonspecific finding and should not be considered evidence of disease. In the bone marrow, the atypical cells are frequently distributed in a markedly fibrotic background. The marrow may be replaced by diffuse fibrosis, and atypical cells may be difficult to observe.[76] Bone marrow aspirates are usually not useful in the diagnosis of Hodgkin's disease in the bone marrow. Bone marrow involvement in LPHD is rare and is usually not associated with fibrosis.

Most subtypes of Hodgkin's disease preferentially involve the T-cell-dependent zones of the lymphoid system.[71] In partially involved lymph nodes, the paracortex and the periarteriolar lymphoid sheath and marginal zone of the splenic white pulp are preferentially involved. The thymus gland is frequently involved by nodular sclerosing Hodgkin's disease and may undergo cystic degeneration secondary to involvement.[77] A thymic cyst should be carefully examined microscopically for evidence of occult Hodgkin's disease. Hodgkin's disease tends to involve axial or central lymph node groups. Mesenteric lymph nodes, Waldeyer's ring, and epitrochlear lymph nodes are rarely involved.

A nonnecrotizing epithelioid granulomatous reaction frequently accompanies Hodgkin's disease.[68–78] It may be found in involved lymph nodes and may be extensive enough to obscure the presence of Hodgkin's disease. Sarcoid-like granulomas can be seen throughout the lymphoreticular system in the spleen, liver, and bone marrow. This granulomatous response by itself does not indicate evidence of occult involvement. Patients with granulomas have, stage for stage, better prognoses than patients without this reaction.[75] The granulomas may represent a positive response to the disease.

CELLULAR ORIGIN OF HODGKIN'S DISEASE

The precise cellular origin of Hodgkin's disease is not firmly established, but theories have included derivation from a B lymphocyte or a macrophage-reticulum cell line.[79–82] Origin from a cell of the immune system is strengthened by the observation that Hodgkin's disease is characterized by a functional deficit in T-cell-mediated immune responses early in the course of the disease and before therapy, which persists in cured patients.[83–85] The lymphocytes within Hodgkin's lesions are usually identifiable as predominantly CD4-positive T cells.[86] In the past, a B-cell origin had been proposed based on the presence of surface or cytoplasmic immunoglobulins.[87] However, evidence of monoclonality and synthesis of immunoglobulin associated with Reed-Sternberg cells is lacking. The immunoglobulin is probably passively absorbed by means of IgG Fc receptors on the neoplastic cells and later internalized into the cytoplasm. Internalization of cytophilic antibody occurs in vitro, and similar binding in vivo may produce immunoglobulin on the surface of and within the neoplastic cells.[81]

A hypothesis that received some support was that the Reed-Sternberg cells might be related to the "histiocytic" system, in particular to an antigen-presenting cell rather than a phagocytic cell.[88] Although Reed-Sternberg cells have Ia antigens and Fc receptors, they have never been observed to be phagocytic, and they lack the lysosomal enzymes characteristic of phagocytic cells. The cytochemical profile of Reed-Sternberg cells does resemble that of interdigitating reticulum cells, which is also involved in antigen presentation to T cells. Interdigitating reticulum cells are usually identified in the lymph node paracortex, where Hodgkin's disease is observed to begin in pathologic sections. An interesting feature is the tendency of Reed-Sternberg cells to be rosetted by normal lymphocytes, particularly T cells.[89] This simulates a phenomenon normally demonstrated by T cells and histiocytes.

A useful diagnostic feature, which does not necessarily shed light on the cell of origin of Hodgkin's disease, is the presence of the CD15 antigen in Reed-Sternberg cells and their mononuclear counterparts. Anti-CD15 antibodies, such as Leu-M1, also react with normal granulocytes.[90] Leu-M1 detects a sugar sequence containing lacto-*N*-fucopentose. This reagent works in paraffin-embedded sections and has considerable clinical utility. It is positive in most cases, with the exception of the lymphocyte-predominant variant, which is usually negative.

Established Hodgkin's disease-derived cell lines share many of the phenotypic characteristics of freshly isolated Reed-Sternberg cells.[91] A monoclonal antibody, Ki-1 (CD30), prepared against the cell lines also reacts with Hodgkin's cells in frozen sections of involved nodes.[92] It was hoped that this antibody might shed light on the origin of Reed-Sternberg cells, but subsequent studies showed that it detects an activation antigen without lineage specificity.[93] The CD30 antigen is also expressed on some activated T cells, B cells, EBV-transformed cell lines, and the cells of large cell anaplastic lymphomas, sometimes referred to as Ki-1-positive lymphomas.[94–96]

Although Reed-Sternberg cells do not express lineage-specific markers, they do express antigens characteristic of activated T or B lymphocytes. The cells express interleukin-2 (IL-2) receptors, transferrin receptors, HLA-DR antigens, and Ki-1, all features of activated lymphocytes.[97] The application of molecular probes added support for a lymphoid origin. Clonal rearrangements of antigen receptor genes, most commonly the immunoglobulin genes, have been shown in several instances, especially in cases containing numerous malignant cells or enriched for malignant cells.[98-101] One patient with lymphoid papulosis, a benign cutaneous eruption that can progress to lymphoma, had a t(8:9) translocation in the lymphocytes in the skin lesion and in the cells of a T-cell lymphoma that developed later.[102] This was associated with tumor-specific rearrangement of the α-chain of the T-cell receptor. This patient developed Hodgkin's disease, and the same T-cell receptor rearrangement and translocation were identified in the Reed-Sternberg cells, suggesting a clonal origin from a T-cell line for all these disorders.

One study identified the *BCL2* oncogene in about a third of tested specimens of Hodgkin's tissue using the polymerase chain reaction technique, which suggested a B-cell origin.[103] Another more definitive study showed that although cytogenetic abnormalities are common in Reed-Sternberg cells, the t(14:18) translocation, so common to B-cell lymphomas, is unusual, and *BCL* expression is likely related to bystander normal lymphocytes that carry the 14:18 translocation, which can also be detected in reactive lymphoid tissue.[103a] Another study using antibodies specific for the protein of the *p53* suppressor oncogene found expression common in all types of Hodgkin's disease and neoplastic CD30-positive lymphomas, but not in LPHD, again providing confusing information about the cellular lineage of the Reed-Sternberg cell.[104]

A hypothesis that may explain these diverse bits of evidence of a multilineage origin of the Reed-Sternberg cell is that the malignant cell represents an in vivo hybridoma that occurs in response to the stimulus of an unidentified viral infection that promotes fusion of the interdigitating reticular cell and B, T, or both lymphocytes.[105,106] This hypothesis proposes that the multiple and varied expression of the genome of the Reed-Sternberg cell and its mononuclear variant could represent components of lymphoid cells incorporated into the malignant cell, including the EBV genome, and the described translocations. Using molecular hybridization techniques, the EBV genome was identified in as many as a third of the tissue samples of Hodgkin's and was localized by in situ hybridization to the malignant cells.[107-110] Evidence was provided for clonality of the viral genome in these cases, suggesting that it was incorporated before or at a early stage in the neoplastic transformation. However, these observations are not inconsistent with the incorporation of the EBV genome and that of an infected lymphocyte into an in vivo hybridoma.

In contrast to the other subtypes of Hodgkin's disease, there is a general consensus that the nodular subtype of LPHD is derived from the B-cell system rather than the T-cell system. Affected lymph nodes contain large numbers of polyclonal B lymphocytes, and this subtype of Hodgkin's disease often coexists or is preceded by progressive transformation of germinal centers.[53] The atypical Reed-Sternberg variant cells in this subtype express CD20 and contain the J chain, further supporting a B-cell derivation.[54,111-113] It appears that the cell of origin of Hodgkin's disease may vary in different histologic subtypes, with B and T lymphocytes and interdigitating reticular cells becoming malignant or fusing under different circumstances, suggesting that Hodgkin's disease may represent a generic lymph node reaction to an insult to the immune system.

IMMUNOLOGIC ABNORMALITIES

Hodgkin's disease is associated with a complex deficiency in cellular immunity.[79,81,85,114-116] The panoply of alterations includes impairment of delayed cutaneous hypersensitivity, enhanced immunoglobulin production, high levels of circulating immune complexes, production of antilymphocyte and anti-Ia antibodies, decreased natural killer cell cytotoxicity, enhanced sensitivity to suppressor monocytes and suppressor T cells, and a variety of other disorders of serum factors, including high levels of circulating IL-2 receptors.[85,117,118] In vitro, peripheral blood lymphocytes show spontaneous DNA and IgG synthesis and depressed proliferative response to T-cell mitogen stimulation with impairment of lymphokine production. The data suggest immunosuppression secondary to chronic overstimulation by cytokines, a hypothesis that fits the inflammatory histologic picture, but it is difficult to explain the persistence of these abnormalities in cured patients.

Increasing numbers of long-term survivors provided the opportunity to restudy anergy and in vitro lymphocyte responsiveness in patients who have been successfully treated. Studies at the National Cancer Institute (NCI) in a population of uniformly staged and treated patients showed that anergy did not influence prognosis within a given stage; after successful treatment, anergy to recall antigens was reversible, although response to neonantigens remained suppressed.[83,84,119-121] Fisher and coworkers have shown that, although the total number of circulating lymphocytes in patients who have been in remission for anywhere from 1.3 to 12.8 years (mean, 6.5 years) was not different from normals, the percentage of E-rosetting cells and the response to concanavalin-A and phytohemagglutinin were significantly depressed compared with normal controls.[123] Patients with normal numbers of T cells had depressed in vitro responses to antigens and were abnormally sensitive to the suppressor effects of concanavalin-A-activated lymphocytes and suppressor monocytes compared with normal controls. This defect persisted for long disease-free periods.[122,123] That this defect seems to be related to the disease itself is reinforced by the fact that patients with other types of lymphomas treated with a similar chemotherapy regimen did not have evidence of this defect.[122,124]

Lymphopenia is common in advanced stages of Hodgkin's disease and is also induced by treatment, particularly by radiation therapy. Its most profound effect is in depressing the CD4:CD8 ratio. Radiation therapy-induced lymphopenia returns to normal within 12 to 111 months after cessation of treatment.[124] Because the CD8-positive population appears relatively unaffected by radiation therapy and the CD4-positive lymphocyte population regenerates slowly after treatment is discontinued, the profound deficiency in helper T cells induced by radiation therapy may explain some clinical consequences of immunodeficiency, with an excess of herpes zoster infections during the first and second years after cessation of radiation therapy.[124-127]

Unlike the defects in delayed hypersensitivity, most studies of humoral response have shown that the antibody response of B cells and that B-cell numbers are normal in all but patients with the most advanced Hodgkin's disease. B-cell function is affected by treatment. Although splenectomy alone does not alter B-cell function, the combination of splenectomy and chemotherapy or combined splenectomy, chemotherapy, and radiation therapy does diminish B-cell function, as measured by antibody response to several bacterial antigens.[128,129]

In a study of 51 patients who were vaccinated with the 14-valent pneumococcus vaccine, combined with *Hemophilus influenzae* type B and meningococcus type C, responses were compared with normal control samples and with control patients rendered asplenic for reasons other than the staging of Hodgkin's disease.[130,131] The geometric mean of natural antibodies to these bacterial polysaccharides was not significantly different among the three groups. Persistence of antibody levels in Hodgkin's disease patients was also similar to that of healthy controls, asplenic controls, and patients treated with radiation therapy only. Patients who received chemotherapy or chemotherapy plus radiation therapy had more significant and rapid declines in antibody levels, to 10% to 20% of peak levels, and declines in the levels of natural antibodies. Timing of splenectomy was not important to the development of antibody response, but the timing of initiation of treatment was significant. Patients receiving chemotherapy or combined-modality therapy less than 10 days after vaccination had significantly lower antibody responses. The investigators concluded that the antibody response in patients with untreated Hodgkin's disease was normal and unaffected by the stage or the procedures used for staging the disease. Vaccination of all patients 10 to 14 days before the initiation of chemotherapy is therefore appropriate.[130,131] Because there is no response to booster vaccinations within the first year, boosters are not recommended, although no data are available to evaluate the effect of booster vaccination later. Neither immunization nor antibiotic prophylaxis can be guaranteed to prevent the development of sepsis due to encapsulated microorganisms in patients with Hodgkin's disease whose staging included splenectomy and who have been heavily treated with chemotherapy or radiation therapy. Vaccinated patients and antibiotic-treated patients should remain alert to the risk.

The data indicate that the functional defect in the immune system in Hodgkin's disease appears simultaneously with the appearance of the disease itself. The defect is aggravated by treatment, particularly radiation therapy, and persists in a variable, time-dependent manner, with some recovery occurring after treatment is discontinued. With the exception of rare cases of autoimmune hemolytic anemia and autoimmune thrombocytopenia, a mildly increased incidence of herpes zoster, and the rare occurrence of overwhelming sepsis related to splenectomy and therapy, the immune system of patients with Hodgkin's disease appears to function quite well, given the large number of immune defects that have been described. Opportunistic infections are relatively rare, and second malignancies appear to be more a function of the use of a combined chemotherapy and radiation therapy regimen than the underlying immune defect itself. Placed in the context of the defect found in patients with AIDS, these immunologic abnormalities are more important in the development of the disease itself than as a complicating factor.

CLINICAL IMMUNOLOGIC DISORDERS IN HODGKIN'S DISEASE

Compared with lymphocytic lymphomas, monoclonal protein spikes are less common in Hodgkin's disease.[132] In a study of 71 patients with Hodgkin's disease, unexplained positive Coombs' test results were observed for 7 male patients; all had extensive disease (stages III and IV), and 6 had constitutional symptoms.[133] The Coombs' test results were positive at initial diagnosis for 3 patients and at the time of relapse for 4. Only 3 patients in this group had overt hemolysis. The antibody was characterized in 3 patients, all of whom fulfilled the criteria for IgG with anti-I[t] specificity. This antibody may be unique for Coombs-positive hemolytic anemia associated with Hodgkin's disease.[134]

Idiopathic thrombocytopenic purpura (ITP) is uncommonly associated with Hodgkin's disease.[135-137] ITP occurs usually at the time of the diagnosis or later. ITP associated with Hodgkin's disease appears to be more severe and resistant to treatment than ITP alone or associated with other illnesses. Only 6 of 23 patients, for example, responded to steroids, although 6 of 10 patients who underwent splenectomy specifically for ITP appeared to have a good and durable response.[128,129] ITP occurred after splenectomy had been performed for staging purposes in 11 patients. This finding indicates that the antibody responsible for thrombocytopenia can be produced in sites other than the spleen. Most patients develop ITP while in remission after successful radiation therapy or chemotherapy, and the occurrence of ITP does not necessarily indicate relapse. Because most reported cases occurred after splenectomy, the combination of corticosteroids and immunosuppressive drugs is required for treatment, and most patients respond well to this treatment.

Autoimmune neutropenia is rarely associated with Hodgkin's disease. The three reported cases occurred in the absence of active disease after splenectomy, suggesting that the spleen plays no role in this disorder and that splenectomy should not be considered as a form of treatment.[138]

NATURAL HISTORY AND DISEASE EVOLUTION

Hodgkin's disease was first reported to spread by contiguity by the Swiss radiotherapist Gilbert.[139-141] His work was expanded by Peters, Kaplan, and others, who tested the value of prophylactic radiation therapy to lymph nodes adjacent to those involved with disease.[142-145] With the advent of bipedal lymphography in the early 1960s and routine use of staging laparotomy, a better understanding of the evolution of this disease has been reached.[144-150] Although Hodgkin's disease is still thought to be unifocal in origin with spread to contiguous lymph nodes, at some point in the natural history of the disease, the malignant cells become more aggressive, may invade blood vessels, and spread to other organs in a manner similar to visceral malignancies.[145] The champion of this hypothesis was the late Henry Kaplan who was strongly influenced by data of Peters that showed Hodgkin's could be cured by regional radiation therapy, including radiation therapy to contiguous uninvolved nodes. This hypothesis fails, however, to account for some obvious exceptions to the notion of contiguous spread, such as the tendency of the disease to skip the mediastinum but involve the left supraclavicular and periaortic nodes in the abdomen; the involvement of the spleen early in the disease, without other organ involvement, despite the fact that the spleen has no afferent lymphatics; and the involvement of two disconnected sites, such as both axillae.

Sir David Smithers offered another plausible hypothesis.[151] He proposed that Hodgkin's disease, although unifocal in origin, spread quite early through vascular and lymphatic channels like other malignancies, but that its unique pattern of distribution could be explained by the malignant cells involving preferential sites, such as lymph nodes and spleen and only later involving other organs as the disease became more aggressive. Smithers' hypothesis provides an explanation for all of the exceptions to the theory of relentless contiguous spread. To account for the curability of early Hodgkin's disease by regional radiation therapy, Smithers' suggests that radiation therapy works by killing the malignant cell and disrupting its preferential sites of involvement.

Patients with nodular sclerosing Hodgkin's disease tend to have upper thoracic disease that remains localized for longer periods in lymph nodes and adjacent structures. LPHD often presents as solitary peripheral lymph node involvement; extensive workup on such patients may not reveal other sites of disease. However, patients who present with apparently localized LDHD usually do have other, often subdiaphragmatic sites of involvement.

Subdividing lymphocyte-predominant disease into nodular and diffuse forms has resulted in the recognition of quite different clinical behaviors. The diffuse form acts like other Hodgkin's disease types, with relapse infrequent; when it occurs, it occurs early in the posttreatment period. The nodular form is commonly associated with relapses, independent of initial stage, and relapse occurs even after long relapse-free periods.[152]

Histologic evolution of Hodgkin's disease appears to occur concomitantly with progression of disease. For example, as the disease advances there is progressive loss of lymphocytes and an increase in the number of malignant cells and fibrosis. One type of the disease probably begins as LPHD and evolves into mixed cellularity and eventually to LDHD. The reticular form of this LDHD appears to be diminishing due to its correct classification as a diffuse lymphocytic or immunoblastic lymphoma. The nodular sclerosing form of the disease probably begins as a cellular phase that proceeds to the classic picture, showing subdivision of the nodes by fibrous bonds, and then to diffuse fibrosis and necrosis. Histologic characteristics and stage are often correlated. Lymphocyte-predominant and nodular sclerosing disease are more commonly diagnosed in stages I and II, but mixed-cellularity and lymphocyte-depleted disease are more commonly seen in the advanced stages.

DIAGNOSIS AND STAGING

Hodgkin's disease usually arises in lymph nodes. The initial diagnosis of Hodgkin's disease can only be made with a biopsy. Occasionally, multiple biopsies are necessary for proper diagnosis, because reactive hyperplasia of lymph nodes adjacent to those involved by tumor may lead to enlargement and encourage biopsy of a node that is easily accessible but uninvolved.[153] Needle aspiration of lymph nodes is inadequate for initial diagnosis, because it is not usually possible to subclassify the disease among the lymphomas with the limited amounts of biopsy material provided.

Staging is used to differentiate patients who can benefit from extended-field radiation therapy from those who require systemic treatment. Staging systems are anatomic descriptions that describe sites of tumor involvement in relation to the diaphragm. The first useful staging for Hodgkin's disease was developed by Peters and colleagues.[141,154] In 1965, a new staging system was developed at a meeting in Rye, New York, a system that added the designation stage IV to the Peters classification for patients with disseminated disease outside the lymph node system.[155] This was modified at the Ann Arbor Staging Conference in 1970.[156] The Ann Arbor version modified the previous classification in two major ways. First, based on data indicating that localized extensions did not alter prognosis if adequately irradiated, patients whose disease spread contiguously from lymph nodes to adjacent organs were not considered to have diffuse dissemination but were classified only by the extent of lymph node involvement (stages I–III) followed by the subscript *E*, which denoted direct extension.[157] Second, involvement of the spleen is indicated by the subscript *S*. In all systems, patients are classified further as *A* or *B* on the basis of the absence or presence of constitutional symptoms, such as fever higher than 38°C for 3 consecutive days, night sweats, or unexplained loss of more than 10% of body weight in the prior 6 months. At the Ann Arbor meeting, it was decided that pruritus, previously considered an important systemic symptom, did not by itself have prognostic impact and was not sufficient to include a patient in the B category.

In 1989, a new classification was proposed, known as the Cotswald system (Table 51–3).[158] It was developed because of the increasing use of new diagnostic techniques such, as computed tomography (CT) scanning and magnetic resonance

TABLE 51–3. The Cotswald Staging Classification for Hodgkin's Disease

Stage I	Involvement of a single lymph node region or a lymphoid structure (*e.g.*, spleen, thymus, Waldeyer's ring)
Stage II	Involvement of two or more lymph node regions on the same side of the diaphragm (*i.e.*, the mediastinum is a single site, hilar lymph nodes are lateralized). The number of anatomic sites should be indicated by a subscript (*e.g.*, II$_2$)
Stage III	Involvement of lymph node regions or structures on both sides of the diaphragm: III$_1$: With or without splenic hilar, celiac, or portal nodes III$_2$: With paraaortic, iliac, mesenteric nodes
Stage IV	Involvement of extranodal site(s) beyond that designated E:
A:	No symptoms
B:	Fever, drenching sweats, weight loss
X:	Bulky disease: >⅓ the width of the mediastinum >10 cm maximal dimension of nodal mass
E:	Involvement of a single extranodal site, contiguous or proximal to a known nodal site
CS:	Clinical stage
PS:	Pathologic stage

(Lister TA, Crowther D, Sutcliffe SB, et al. Report of a committee convened to discuss the evaluation and staging of patients with Hodgkin's disease: Cotswald meeting. J Clin Oncol 1989;7:1630–1636; J Clin Oncol [Erratum] 1990;8:1602)

imaging (MRI), and because of the greater appreciation of the influence of tumor bulk as a separate prognostic indicator within any given stage. It recognizes mediastinal adenopathy of greater than one third of the widest internal diameter of the chest or any tumor mass greater than 10 cm in diameter by the designation X. With the new schema, patients with residual abnormalities after treatment, which cannot be confirmed as benign or malignant, are designated as CRu (u for unconfirmed).

Table 51–4 outlines the recommended staging procedures.[159] Staging starts with a detailed history and physical examination. The history must be careful to determine the presence or absence of systemic symptoms. Physical examination should determine the extent of lymph node involvement. Basic laboratory tests include evaluation of renal and hepatic function, complete blood count, erythrocyte sedimentation rate, and serum lactate dehydrogenase and alkaline phosphatase levels. Roentgenographic studies include the chest radiograph and thoracic CT scan to evaluate mediastinal lymphadenopathy and any extension of such adenopathy into the surrounding viscera. If the chest x-ray film is normal, a CT scan is usually unnecessary. Abdominal involvement is evaluated using the lower-extremity lymphogram and abdominal CT.

With the advent of CT, the routine use of the bipedal lymphogram has been questioned, but it is still the superior staging tool because its sensitivity and specificity are superior to CT scans and because it can determine abnormal architecture of nodes and enlargement.[160–163] Although more labor intensive, the lymphogram has other important features. It can be used as a guide to ensure the removal of involved nodes during laparotomy and confirm their removal afterward, and it can identify abnormal nodes when they are not enlarged. It also is an inexpensive way of monitoring response to treatment. The CT scan is easier to administer and more valuable in the assessment of hepatic portal, mesenteric, and celiac lymph nodes.

Bone marrow biopsy, not aspiration, is required, because

TABLE 51–4. Required Evaluation Procedures in Staging Hodgkin's Disease

1. Adequate surgical biopsy, reviewed by an experienced hematologist
2. A detailed history recording duration and the presence or absence of fever, unexplained sweating and its severity, unexplained pruritus, and unexplained weight loss
3. A careful and detailed physical examination; special attention to all node-bearing areas, including Waldeyer's ring and determination of size of liver and spleen
4. Necessary laboratory procedures
   a. Complete blood count, including an erythrocytic sedimentation rate
   b. Serum alkaline phosphatase level
   c. Evaluation of renal function
   d. Evaluation of liver function
5. Radiologic studies
   a. Chest radiograph (posteroanterior and lateral)
   b. Chest and abdominal computed tomography scan
   c. Bilateral lower-extremity lymphogram
   d. Views of skeletal system to include thoracic and lumbar vertebrae, the pelvis, proximal extremities, and any areas of bone tenderness

Hodgkin's of the marrow is often spotty and associated with fibrosis. Bone marrow biopsy is particularly important in symptomatic patients and in those with bone lesions, bone pain, hypercalcemia, or an elevated level of serum alkaline phosphatase.[164–168]

Isotopic scanning of the liver, spleen, and bone may be helpful in defining sites of additional disease. Gallium scanning may be useful, especially the higher-dose (7–10 mCi) imaging on a triple-peak Anger camera. Single-photon emission CT (SPECT) has resulted in the occasional finding of unexpected disease but is more useful in determining suspected recurrence in previously treated patients.[169] Data suggest that lymphomatous involvement of lymph nodes may have a different MRI pattern than fibrosis. This finding, like gallium scanning, may be important in evaluating patients for residual disease or recurrence after treatment.

STAGING LAPAROTOMY

Staging laparotomy is less important than it was 10 years ago.[159,170] It was originally developed by the Stanford group to provide information about the patterns of involvement in subdiaphragmatic Hodgkin's disease.[149] Its justification is that if it alters stage, which it often does, it will alter therapy. The latter should not often be the case, however, because the major determinant of the decision to proceed to laparotomy is whether radiation therapy alone will be used for treatment. Because more stages of Hodgkin's disease are being treated with chemotherapy alone or in combination with radiation therapy, laparotomy need not be done in these patients.[171]

If laparotomy is done, it must be carried out by physicians skilled in the technique, who perform it in a consistent fashion and in conjunction with the treating physician.[172,173] It should include a detailed inspection of the abdomen. The removed spleen should be sectioned in 0.3-cm slices. If disease is identified in the spleen, the total number of nodules should be enumerated. The weight of the spleen should be determined. Examination of the liver should include a wedge biopsy of the right lobe, three needle biopsies of the right and left lobes, and a biopsy of any grossly abnormal hepatic lesions. After inspection and palpation of the nodal groups, a biopsy should be taken of the right and left paraaortic and iliac nodes, regardless of their character on palpation and even if they appear normal on lymphography. Suspicious nodes identified on lymphography should be removed. Lymph nodes should be removed from the splenic hilar, porta, hepatic, mesenteric, and iliac regions. At one time, oophoropexy, the placement of the ovaries out of their normal position to shield them from pelvic irradiation, was recommended routinely for young female patients. This no longer is an indication for laparotomy or necessary for treatment, because the use of pelvic irradiation has been almost eliminated. Iliac bone marrow biopsy should be performed at the time of operation. The early studies employing routine staging laparotomy observed that alterations in clinical stage were made as frequently as 35% of the time as a result of the findings obtained at surgical staging.[174–177] After physical examination and chest x-ray films, approximately 90% of patients are categorized as having early-stage disease (stage I or II). After lymphography, one third of these patients are shown to have more advanced disease. Another one third of patients with clinically diagnosed early-stage disease are placed in higher stages after laparotomy. In the average institution, after all staging procedures are completed, 60% of patients are considered to have stages III or IV disease, and 40% have stages I or II.[159]

Staging laparotomy is a major surgical procedure with established morbidity and mortality.[179–181] Institutions with the most extensive experience report mortality statistics as low as 0.1%, but much higher rates have been reported.[181,182] Morbidity may include wound infection, subphrenic abscess, pulmonary embolus, stress ulcer, gastrointestinal bleeding, pulmonary infection, and wound dehiscence. Staging laparotomy and splenectomy in children require special consideration. Although the complication rate is similar to that observed in adults, there is an increased incidence of severe, sudden, overwhelming infection in children after staging laparotomy and splenectomy.[178–180,183–186] The risk of this complication increases as age decreases below 10 years. It seems prudent to be selective in the use of such procedures in young patients.[187,188]

No evidence suggests that splenectomy improves the ability to administer chemotherapy or radiation therapy, increases the response rate, or alters the survival rate.[189–192] Several studies reported a disconcerting increase in secondary leukemias in patients who have undergone splenectomy compared with similarly treated patients who have not had surgical staging.[193,194] There is no good explanation for this finding, but the consistency of the data between studies suggests it is a real risk. Laparotomy does, however, treat the involved spleen. The reduction of the irradiated field required may permit the physician to avoid irradiating a significant portion of the stomach, intestine, left kidney, and left lower lobe of the lung. Posttreatment laparotomy as a guide to further management has had mixed results and should not be considered a routine procedure.[195,196]

PATTERNS OF CLINICAL PRESENTATION

The clinical presentation of Hodgkin's disease varies in different geographic locations and clinical settings. Reviews of patients seen at the Harvard Joint Center for Radiotherapy in Boston (JCRT) may serve as an example (Table 51–5).[197,198] In this group, 57% of patients were male, 24% had systemic symptoms, 85% were younger than 40 years of age, and 60% had lymphocyte-predominant histology. The predominant sites of lymph node involvement were the mediastinum (59%), left neck (58%), and right neck (55%). One of these sites of involvement existed in 92% of the patients seen. Some sites were positively correlated with each other while others were not (Figs. 51–3 and 51–4), suggesting possible clinical evolution of the disease.[198] Epitrochlear, popliteal, and mesenteric nodes are uncommonly involved. The spleen is involved in approximately 25% of patients.

Liver involvement without splenic involvement is rare in Hodgkin's disease. The risk of liver involvement increases as the size of the involved spleen increases. Liver involvement is also unusual in patients who have normal-sized spleens, even if the spleens are involved in Hodgkin's disease.[141] Bone marrow involvement with Hodgkin's disease is associated with extensive tumor and usually with systemic symptoms.[199,200] Leukopenia, anemia, or thrombocytopenia are rarely seen, although an elevated alkaline phosphatase level may give some

TABLE 51–5. Upstaging of Stage I and II Patients by Clinical Parameters

Subgroup	No. of Patients	PS III-IV (%)	p Value (Logistic Regression)
Sex			
M	296	85 (29%)	0.003
F	256	46 (18%)	
Symptomatic stage			
A	444	94 (21%)	0.027
B	108	37 (34%)	
Sites			
1	171	28 (17%)	0.003
≥2	381	103 (27%)	
Age			
≤39	481	110 (23%)	0.081
≤40	71	21 (30%)	
Histology			
LP/NS	403	91 (23%)	Not significant
MC/LD	149	40 (27%)	

PS, pathologic stage; LP, lymphocyte predominant; NS, nodular sclerosing; MC, mixed cellularity; LD, lymphocyte depleted.
(Mauch P, Larson D, Osteen R, et al. Prognostic factors for positive surgical staging in patients with Hodgkin's disease. J Clin Oncol 1990;8:257–265)

hint of bone marrow involvement. The bones themselves may be involved, especially in patients with advanced disease. Rarely, there is invasion of the bone from adjacent lymphadenopathy. The bone lesions are usually osteolytic but may be osteoblastic. Radioisotopic bone scans may reveal focal areas of increased uptake although conventional radiographs

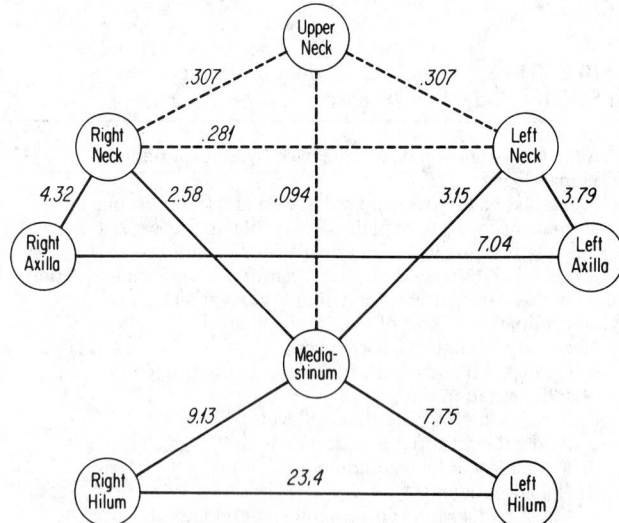

FIGURE 51–3. Patterns of presentation of Hodgkin's disease. Solid lines indicate positive associations, and dotted lines indicate negative associations. Odds ratios are written next to the lines for statistically significant associations ($p \leq 0.01$). (Mauch P, Kalish LA, Kadin M, et al. Patterns of presentation of Hodgkin's disease: Implications for etiology and pathogenesis. Cancer 1992 [in press])

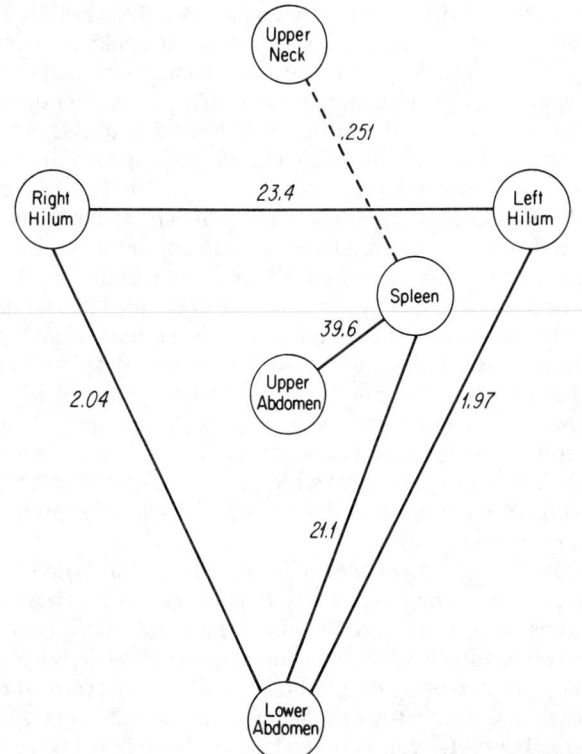

FIGURE 51–4. Patterns of presentation of Hodgkin's disease. Solid lines indicate positive associations, and dotted lines indicate negative associations. Odds ratios are written next to the lines for statistically significant associations ($p \leq 0.01$). (Mauch P, Kalish LA, Kadin M, et al. Patterns of presentation of Hodgkin's disease: Implications for etiology and pathogenesis. Cancer 1992 [in press])

are normal.[201] Such findings are not always evidence of involvement and should be confirmed histologically if possible. Involvement of the bone should not be equated with involvement of the marrow unless there is other evidence of widely disseminated disease. Musshoff and Boutis demonstrated long-term disease-free survival in patients with isolated bone lesions if treated appropriately with radiation therapy.[202]

Involvement of the skin, subcutaneous tissue, and breast can occur with Hodgkin's disease.[203] The disease rarely involves the central nervous system, although invasion of the epidural space can occur by extension through the intervertebral foramina from paraaortic lymph nodes, with neurologic symptoms and pain as the predominant clinical features.[204–206] Unlike other malignant lymphomas, Hodgkin's disease rarely arises in the gastrointestinal tract. Compression of the ureters from lymphadenopathy may occur. Unusual urologic complications of Hodgkin's disease are lipoid nephrosis and amyloid nephrosis, which may occur although no other clinical manifestations of persistence or recurrence are detected.[207,208] They have been reported to regress after effective antitumor treatment. Pleural effusions with low specific gravity and low protein content are usually simple transudates. Neither these nor exudative pleural effusions are indicative of pleural invasion of Hodgkin's disease. Such a diagnosis requires histologic confirmation by pleural biopsy or open thoracotomy. These effusions are often the consequence of hilar or pulmonary involvement. Pericardial in-

volvement may occur as a result of direct invasion from mediastinal lymphadenopathy.

TREATMENT

RADIATION THERAPY

The extreme radiation responsiveness of the lymphomas was noticed shortly after the discovery of x-rays. In 1902, Pusey reported a series of patients with Hodgkin's disease treated with irradiation. In the early part of the century, therapy was limited by the equipment available.[209] The machines had poor depth-dose characteristics and caused extensive skin reactions, limiting their usefulness. Despite this drawback, there was abundant interest in irradiating this tumor. Teschendorf,[210] Voorhoeve,[211] and Kruchen[212] described therapy for these patients. It was Gilbert who laid the foundation for the principles of modern radiation therapy, despite the availability of only orthovoltage radiation therapy.[139,140] Gilbert recognized the importance of treating all involved disease with the maximal dose possible if cure was the goal. He suggested treating adjacent sites, to the extent possible, because of the frequency of adjacent recurrences. These are the principles of radiation therapy today. Gilbert's technique was followed in Toronto and reported by Peters in 1950.[141] She reported patients who were alive as long as 20 years after treatment, indicating that patients could be cured with irradiation, because there were no recurrences in patients who were disease-free 10 years after treatment.[142] The concept of irradiation of adjacent nodal groups with lower doses of radiation was used by Peters.

In 1963, Easson and Russell published an article entitled, "The Cure of Hodgkin's Disease."[213] This work reported the long-term results of local treatment of Hodgkin's disease and localized non-Hodgkin's lymphomas. The paper emphasized that Hodgkin's disease could be cured. Other investigators in the early 1950s and 1960s reported the results of localized irradiation, but it was Kaplan and his group at Stanford who systematically studied the role of radiation therapy in the treatment of Hodgkin's disease and devised new techniques using supervoltage techniques to treat the disease.[214–219] These pioneering studies form the basis of much of what we know today about the curability of Hodgkin's disease.

The information in Figure 51–5 comes from a compilation of studies demonstrating a dose-response association.[220] Although low doses of radiation cause tumors to disappear, high doses are required to ablate them permanently. Hodgkin's disease, like other tumors, has a dose-response curve. This was an important concept, because the prevailing attitude at the time was that, because the disease was responsive to radiation but still incurable, low doses should be given to make local nodal masses regress while "saving" the radiation tolerance for the required subsequent therapies after the disease reappeared. This philosophy of treatment confirmed the self-fulfilling prophecy of the incurability of Hodgkin's disease. However, as seen in the figure, after high doses were given, local recurrence was uncommon.

The Stanford group provided evidence, suspected by Gilbert and Peters, of the orderliness and continuity of the initial presentation of Hodgkin's disease and of its subsequent extension.[217,219] The adaptation of modern supervoltage tech-

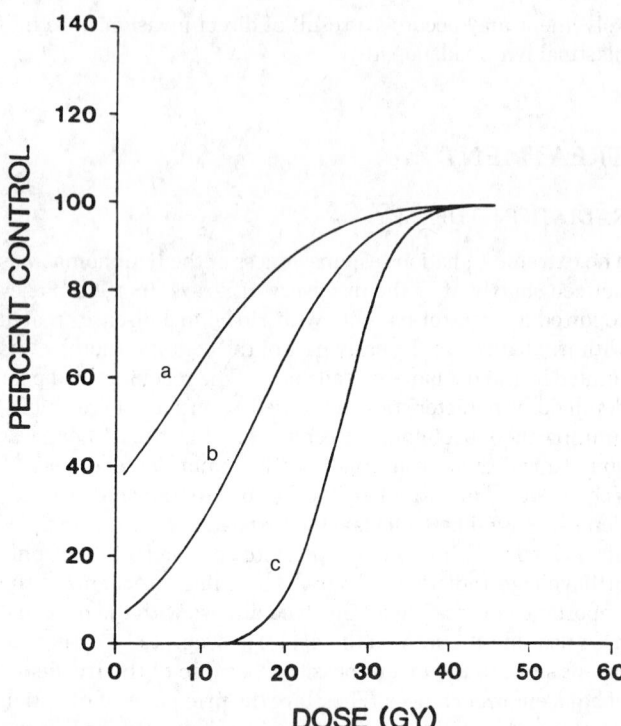

FIGURE 51–5. Dose-response curves (kV and MV data) for subclinical (curve a), <6-cm (curve b) and 6-cm (curve c) nodes. Higher doses are required for equal probabilities of control as disease burden increases. (Vijayakumar S, Myrianthopoulos LC. An updated dose-response analysis in Hodgkin's disease. Radiother Oncol 1992;24:1–13)

niques for the treatment of Hodgkin's disease for the first time allowed high doses of radiation to be given in extensive volumes, and careful beam direction and shielding allowed the treatment to be tolerated by normal tissues.

It is recommended that local tumor masses receive "boost therapy" to a minimal dose of 4000 to 4400 cGy, but apparently uninvolved areas treated for subclinical disease appear to be controlled adequately with doses of 3000 to 3500 cGy. Other data suggest that 3000 cGy may be sufficient.[221] The dose-time relation for Hodgkin's disease is less well known. Because of normal tissue tolerance, patient acceptance, and tumor control, tumor doses of between 150 and 220 cGy per day given five times each week appear to be appropriate. If a significant interruption in treatment occurs, it appears that larger doses should be given.[222] Supervoltage methods must be used to deliver the wide-field radiation required. This method has the advantages of spared skin, increased depth dose, and sharp beam edges with reduced lateral scatter.

A basic tool for the treatment of patients with Hodgkin's disease is the modern linear accelerator, which provides x-ray beams in the 4- to 8-MeV range. Although cobalt units can be used, conventionally available cobalt units have significant limitations. When used at distances of less than 80 cm, they tend to have poor depth-dose characteristics. They often have far less well defined beam edges, because of the large source and short treatment distances. This latter factor causes significantly greater irradiation of adjacent and apparently shielded tissues.

Hodgkin's disease treatment may be divided into three volumes to be irradiated: the mantle, the paraaortic area, and

the pelvis.[223] The mantle technique, well described by the Stanford group, is an attempt to treat in continuity the lymph nodes of the neck, axilla, and mediastinum—including the occipital and preauricular lymph nodes—in one contiguous treatment volume. To do this, a wide field is placed on the patient and individually made blocks are fashioned to shield the normal tissues that are not to be treated. For this technique to be done accurately, a supervoltage linear accelerator is required and a treatment-planning simulator or localizer must be available. This must allow the duplication of therapy fields using diagnostic-quality radiation so that detailed radiographs can be made for the fabrication of the blocks. Such a simulator film is shown in Figure 51–6 with the appropriate block outlines. The check films are made on the supervoltage machine. However, because of the radiation energy, this film, although useful for check purposes, is much less satisfactory than the simulator films. The blocks can be made to conform to the divergent x-ray beam so that the edge of the field can be as sharp as possible.

The mantle treatment irradiates a large volume of normal tissues, and care must be taken to limit the unnecessary normal tissue irradiation while ensuring adequate irradiation of the tumor volume. This procedure requires careful evaluation and planning, using diagnostic x-ray films, CT scans, simulation, and dosimetric calculations and measurements. The normal tissue tolerances of the lung and heart have been evaluated in the course of treatment of Hodgkin's disease.[224–226] Whole-lung irradiation, to a maximal dose of 1650 cGy in 150-cGy fractions, is used frequently if the ipsilateral hilum is involved with tumor. The whole heart should not be treated unless evidence of pericardial involvement exists. Under normal circumstances, a significant portion of the cardiac silhouette can be shielded. It is important that the match-line between the mantle and the paraaortic area does not allow overlap of a portion of the spinal cord. If this overlap occurs, the dose that is received can cause significant neurologic

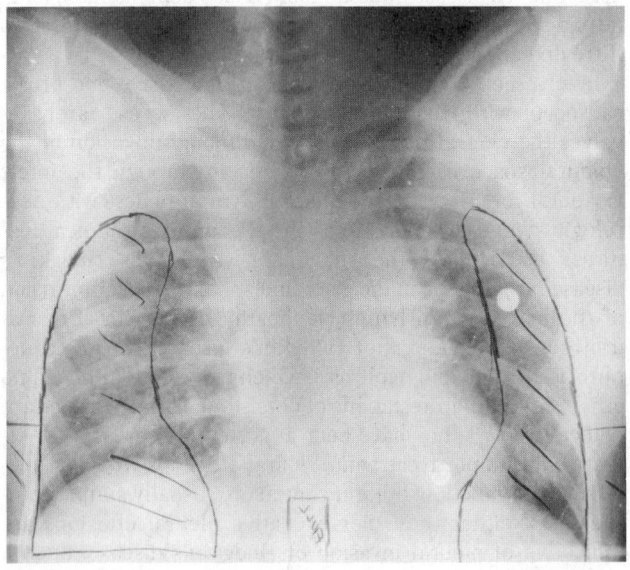

FIGURE 51–6. Simulated film for radiation treatment fields in a patient with mediastinal Hodgkin's disease. Dark lines indicate shielding blocks.

damage. The geometry involved in proper field arrangement for the match-line can be more complicated than is immediately apparent. Techniques to match these fields properly have been described.[227] Farah reported excellent results using a combined mantle and paraaortic field, avoiding any question of overlap at the match-line.[228] The dose per fraction is reduced to 160 cGy, resulting in a shorter treatment course. Treatments of the paraaortic nodes and pelvis are frequently done together as described by the Stanford group.[229,230] It is the experience of others that this treatment is better tolerated if divided into a paraaortic field and a separate pelvic field. In either circumstance, the paraaortic field must be wide enough to include the paraaortic lymph nodes as demonstrated on the lymphogram.

Most modern radiotherapeutic techniques have been influenced by the results of laparotomy. Laparotomy is only of value if the results may alter therapy. It allows removal of the spleen and the placement of radiopaque clips on the splenic pedicle, so that the radiation therapy field may be tailored accurately to this volume. The normal right side of the paraaortic field, as shown in Figure 51–7, does not treat the porta hepatitis; if it is to be treated, the field must be extended laterally. The same considerations for field overlap apply between the paraaortic and pelvic fields; however, these fields are less critical, because this overlap area is below the level of the spinal cord. Considerations for the pelvic field include the treatment of the lymph nodes with as little radiation as possible to important sacral and pelvic bone marrow. The need for pelvic treatment has been markedly reduced, because stages I and II supradiaphragmatic Hodgkin's disease can be treated without pelvic irradiation, and for stage III disease, total nodal irradiation has a limited role. If the pelvic field is to be treated, the amount of marrow irradiated may be greatly reduced by careful blocking and by the use of linear accelerators rather than cobalt units. Adequate covering of the inguinal and femoral lymph nodes must be ensured, and the testes should be shielded. For women, a central block can be placed and the ovaries moved to the midline by tacking them in front or in back of the uterus, a technique first described by Trueblood and colleagues.[231]

Although individual preference in technique may have a role, most important are the general principles of careful beam definition, detailed patient positioning, use of simulators, individually constructed shielding techniques, and verification of dose, usually using thermoluminescent dosimetry. Small technical considerations, such as the position of the arm, can greatly influence the amount of normal tissue treated and must be considered carefully. Maximal cure with minimal complications can occur only if all the technical aspects of radiation therapy are considered carefully. This fact has been substantiated in a review of the pattern of radiation treatment that related recurrence to technical inadequacies. The facility at which treatment was given significantly affected recurrence rate. Even among university medical centers, technical differences had a significant effect on relapse-free survival. The rates of in-field or marginal recurrence varied from 0% to 11% at different centers among patients with identical-stage disease, and the relapse rate varied from 10% to 39%. These differences did not relate to variations in staging procedures. The portal films of a random sample of patients treated for curative intent were reviewed, and in more than one third of the cases, the treatment portal films did not adequately cover the disease, and more than half of these patients had relapses. For patients with adequate portals, relapse rate was only 14% over a 4-year period.[226,232]

Results of Radiation Therapy

With the results of radiation therapy reported by Peters and associates[142,143] and Easson and Russell,[213] the question of whether uninvolved areas should be irradiated became an important one. In 1966, Peters carefully analyzed her data in an attempt to answer this question.[144] Review of these data makes it difficult to prove that irradiation of the uninvolved lymph nodes in stage I or IIA disease affects the outcome. The Stanford group conducted a randomized, prospective clinical trial (L1) that compared local irradiation with extended-field irradiation for treating stages I and II disease.[141] This study showed no significant difference between involved-field and extended-field irradiation with respect to survival or freedom from relapse. A similar national collaborative study also failed to show significant differences.[233] These studies preceded the use of staging laparotomy and also failed to consider the paraaortic area as a contiguous site for supraclavicular node disease.

A new trial was introduced at Stanford (H1) in which the alternatives for stages I and IIA disease were involved-field irradiation and total nodal irradiation (TNI).[235] This study was

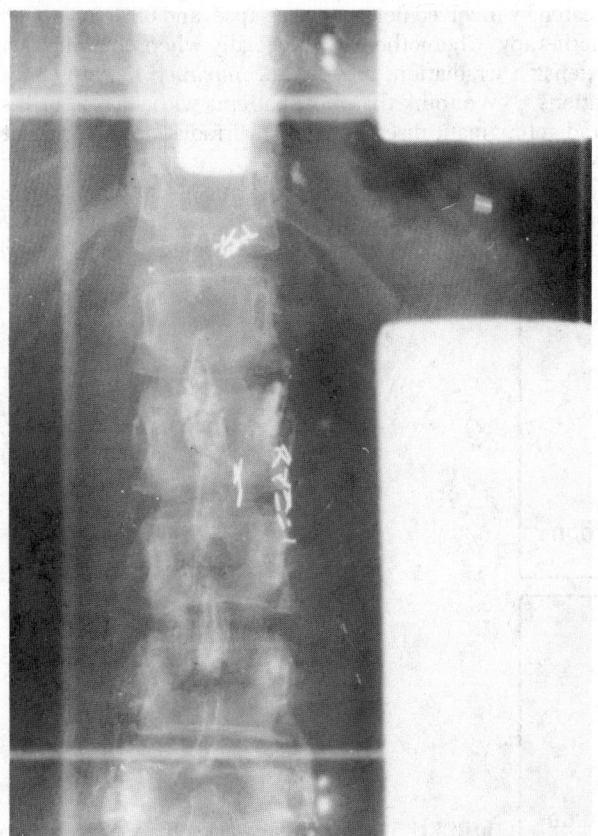

FIGURE 51–7.   Normal paraaortic field used in treating a patient with Hodgkin's disease below the diaphragm. The porta hepatic nodes were not involved.

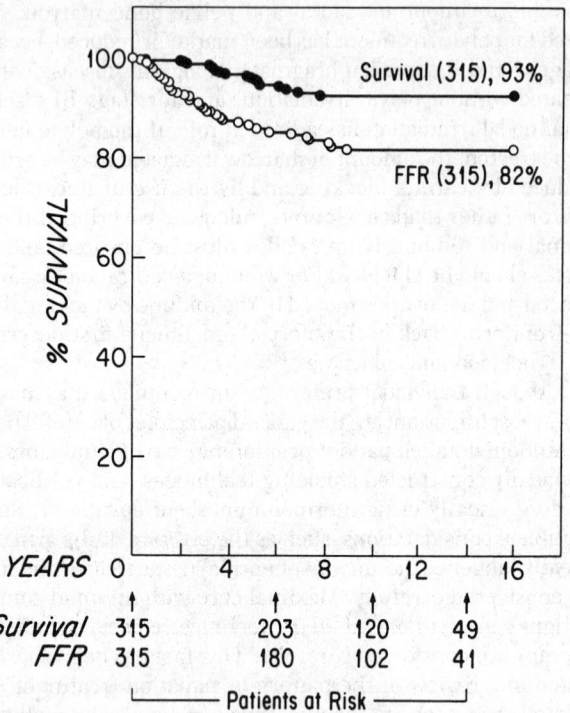

FIGURE 51–8. Survival and freedom from first relapse (FFR) rates for pathologic stage IA and IIA patients treated with mantle and para-aortic–splenic pedicle irradiation. Median follow-up time was 9 years. (Mauch P, Tarbell N, Weinstein, et al. Stage IA and IIA supradiaphragmatic Hodgkin's disease: Prognostic factors in surgically staged patients treated with mantle and para-aortic irradiation. J Clin Oncol 1988;6:1576–1583)

started 1 year before the introduction of laparotomy at Stanford; therefore, most of the patients in this study had staging laparotomies. Results of this study showed a highly significant difference in relapse-free survival in favor of TNI, although overall survival was not affected.[141]

TNI is far more extensive than the intended irradiation of subclinical contiguous disease in stages I and IIA patients. For supradiaphragmatic disease, pelvic irradiation can probably be eliminated. This deletion would greatly reduce the amount of bone marrow irradiated and limit the dose to the gonads. Such a technique for supradiaphragmatic stages I and IIA patients has been recommended at the JCRT.[164,197] The results of such treatment are shown in Figure 51–8. Relapse-free and overall survival rates for stages IA and IIA patients are 82% and 93%, respectively. Review of the 315 patients treated in this manner with a median follow-up of 9 years reveals a 3% rate of pelvic nodal recurrences. This result indicates that the pelvis can be spared irradiation, and the patient still derives the value of extended-field irradiation. This method permits adequate chemotherapy dosage and a decreased likelihood for tumor induction or fatal infection.[234] These studies were done in laparotomy-staged patients in whom the spleen had been removed.

As long-term follow-up increases, it appears that freedom from relapse depends on initial therapy but that survival of patients with early-stage Hodgkin's disease does not, because salvage chemotherapy is so good that overall survival is unaffected. Figure 51–9 describes the results of patients treated at Stanford with involved fields compared with those treated by extended-field irradiation. Chemotherapy with a regimen of nitrogen mustard, vincristine, procarbazine, and prednisone (MOPP) for these radiation therapy failures is quite successful (Table 51–6).[236–238]

The goal of treatment is to cure the most patients with the least therapy to avoid complications. Only 32% of patients treated by involved fields avoid relapse, and 68% require chemotherapy. Chemotherapy, especially when combined with extensive irradiation, may be accompanied by late complications.[239] We think that most patients with stages I or II supradiaphragmatic disease treated by irradiation should receive extended-field irradiation.

Data from the M.D. Anderson Cancer Center,[240] the European Organization for the Research and Treatment of Cancer (EORTC),[241] St. Bartholomew's Hospital,[242] and Memorial

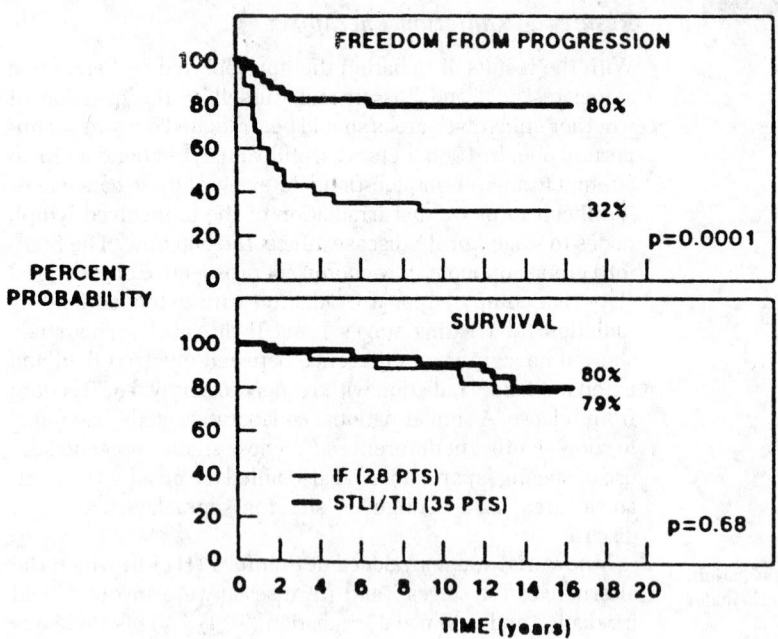

FIGURE 51–9. Involved-field (IF) versus extended-field irradiation. (Rosenberg SA, Kaplan HS. The evolution and summary results of the Stanford randomized clinical trials of the management of Hodgkin's disease: 1962–1984. Int J Radiat Oncol Biol Phys 1985;11:5–22)

TABLE 51–6. MOPP for Hodgkin's Disease Relapse After Initial Radiation Therapy

Investigations	Initial Stage	No. of Patients	5-Year Relapse-Free Survival (%)	5-Year Survival (%)
Timothy et al[236]	IA–IIIA	33	85	92
Portlock[237]	IA–IIIA	46	50	58
Mauch et al[238]	IA–IIIA	28	70	70

Hospital pediatric studies[243] have indicated that relapse-free survival was similar in laparotomy-staged patients treated with a mantle field only, compared with those treated more extensively. In these studies, the patients were usually selected for having no or only minimal mediastinal involvement. The EORTC included only patients younger than 40 years of age with nodular sclerosis or lymphocyte-predominant histology, an erythrocyte sedimentation rate of less than 70, and only one or two sites of involvement. These data must be used with caution for patients with more extensive disease.

Although treatment of the paraaortic field is not associated with significant long-term toxic effects, it does cause acute symptoms. It increases the amount of bone marrow irradiated, and in the pediatric patient, it significantly damages growth in the axial spine. It is desirable to avoid the use of the para-aortic field, which may be possible for clinically staged IA patients with lymphocyte-predominant histology and high neck involvement.[244] Its use in patients with more extensive disease results in a greater number of relapses. Although overall survival may be the same, more patients are exposed to chemotherapy. The appropriate treatment of Hodgkin's disease by stage is discussed later in this chapter.

A separate subgroup of patients with stage I or II disease has a higher likelihood for relapse. These patients have large mediastinal masses.[245] Review of such patients at the JCRT revealed that, of 315 stage IA and IIA patients treated with mantle or paraaortic fields, 35 had mediastinal masses greater than one third of the total chest diameter (Table 51–7). Patients relapsed within the initial treatment volume and in adjacent, untreated lymph nodes, and extranodal relapse occurred primarily in the lung. These patients are more likely to experience recurrence, even at involved sites separate from the mediastinum.

TABLE 51–7. Influence of Mediastinal Hodgkin's Disease Treated With Mantle and Paraaortic Irradiation After Relapse

Extent of Disease	No. of Patients	14-Year Relapse Free Survival (%)
No mediastinal disease	142	87
Mediastinal disease		
≤1/3	138	85
>1/3	35	53

(Mauch P, Gorshein D, Cunningham J, et al. Influence of mediastinal adenopathy on site and frequency of relapse in patients with Hodgkin's disease. Cancer Treat Rep 1982;66:809–817)

Investigators disagree about the best treatment for patients with large mediastinal masses. Significant numbers of patients with large mediastinal masses who fail to respond to irradiation only may be salvaged with chemotherapy, and their ultimate results are similar to patients treated by combined modalities initially. However, treatment with initial irradiation often requires extensive irradiation of the heart and lung to include the large mediastinal mass, which can be the source of significant morbidity. Despite this drawback, with the careful use of thoracic CT scanning, patients may be selected for radiation therapy only.[246] It appears that the treatment of patients with large mediastinal masses needs to be individualized to maximize cure while avoiding unnecessary complications of irradiation or combined-modality treatment.

The prognostic importance of large mediastinal masses has been reported repeatedly.[247–250] Most patients with stage I or IIA disease have no or little mediastinal involvement. For this group, the relapse-free survival rate is 86%, and the overall survival rate is 93%, using a technique that spares the pelvis from irradiation.[251] There appears to be a subgroup of patients with disease limited only to the mediastinum. These patients rarely (2 of 22) have large masses and enjoy excellent prognoses, with an 85% relapse-free rate and 100% overall actuarial survival rate at 8 years.[250–253]

Extensive mediastinal involvement causes several additional problems for patients. They appear to be anesthesia risks, with difficulty occurring during extubation, and the risk-benefit ratio of laparotomy increases.[254] Although this risk can be greatly reduced by irradiating the mass before exploratory laparotomy, the treatment involves a significant amount of heart and lung. This provides another reason for treating these patients with primary chemotherapy, restricting radiation to a limited role as a boost technique at the end of the chemotherapy. Review of three sequential staging and treatment programs—pathologic staging and radiation therapy, pathologic staging and combined-modality treatment, and clinical staging and combined-modality treatment—showed the group receiving only radiation therapy to have the poorest freedom from relapse. They are successfully salvaged with chemotherapy, resulting in similar overall survival rates (Fig. 51–10).[253]

Although the data for subdiaphragmatic-presentation stages I and IIA disease are far more limited, the results of extended-field treatment appear equally satisfactory.[255] In the JCRT experience, there were 15 such patients, with two recurrences. The question of the importance of histology is not certain. It is thought that mixed-cellularity and lymphocyte-depleted disease are more likely present with higher-stage disease when carefully evaluated.

The first curative attempt at treatment of stage III disease

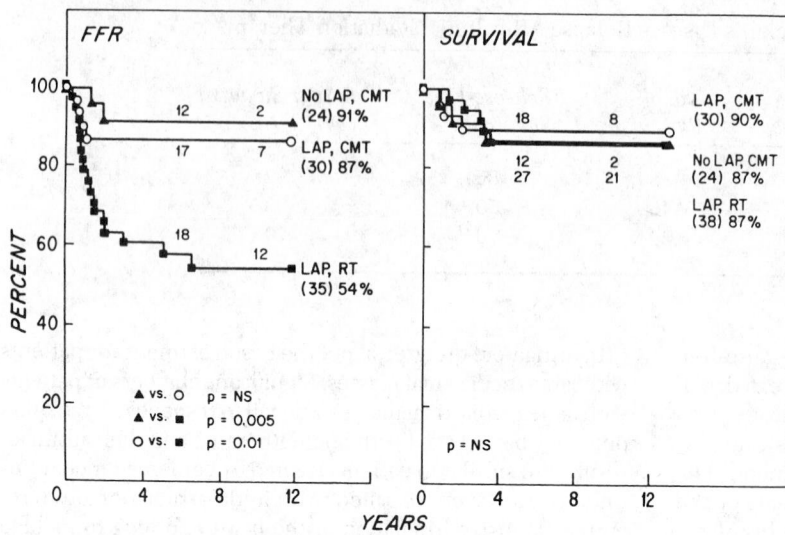

FIGURE 51–10. Actuarial freedom from first relapse (FFR) and survival rates of clinical stage IA and IIB Hodgkin's disease patients undergoing staging laparotomy and radiation therapy, staging laparotomy and combined radiation therapy and chemotherapy (CMT), or CMT without staging laparotomy. (Leopold KA, Canellos GP, Rosenthal D, et al. Stage IA–IIIB Hodgkin's disease: Staging and treatment with large mediastinal adenopathy. J Clin Oncol 1989;7:1059–1065)

was presented in the Stanford (L2) protocol. This protocol compared the conventional low-dose irradiation (*i.e.*, palliative therapy for a disease that was considered to be incurable) with radical irradiation to all lymph node-bearing areas (TNI), including the spleen. Relapses occurred earlier and more frequently in the palliatively treated groups, but their ultimate survival was not statistically significantly lower, presumably because of the success of salvage drug therapy. The success of TNI was the first demonstration that some stage III patients could be cured with irradiation only.[214] Figure 51–11 reveals the actuarial survival and relapse-free survival rates for laparotomy-staged IIIA patients from the JCRT. Despite the increased accuracy of staging, more than 50% of the patients so treated experience relapse.[256] Although many of these patients can be salvaged by subsequent combination chemo-

therapy, initial treatment with combined-modality therapy is associated with an overall improvement in survival.

Attempts to subdivide these patients into stages IIIA1 and IIIA2 demonstrate the important prognostic significance of this substaging. But even stage IIIA1 patients have a significant likelihood of failure if treated with irradiation only (Fig. 51–12). Perhaps the only group associated with an excellent relapse-free survival rate are the stage IIIA2 patients with fewer than five splenic nodules, because in the JCRT experience, patients treated with radiation only had a 70% rate of freedom from first relapse and an overall survival rate of 100%. Total lymphoid irradiation in the hands of the Stanford group has been associated with a better relapse-free survival rate for stage III patients. These data are better than those from Yale or the JCRT.[257] Possible reasons for this difference include a

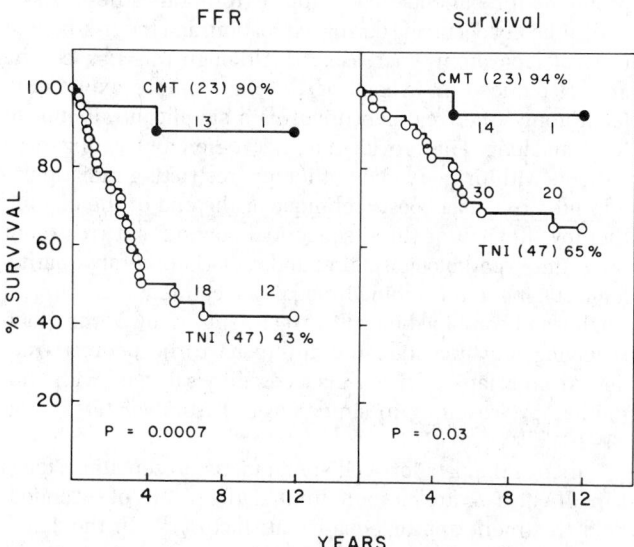

FIGURE 51–11. Actuarial relapse-free survival and survival rates for laparotomy-determined stage IIIA patients treated with combined-modality therapy (CMT) or total nodal irradiation (TNI). (Mauch P, Gorshein D, Cunningham J, et al. Influence of mediastinal adenopathy on site and frequency of relapse in patients with Hodgkin's disease. Cancer Treat Rep 1982;66:809–817)

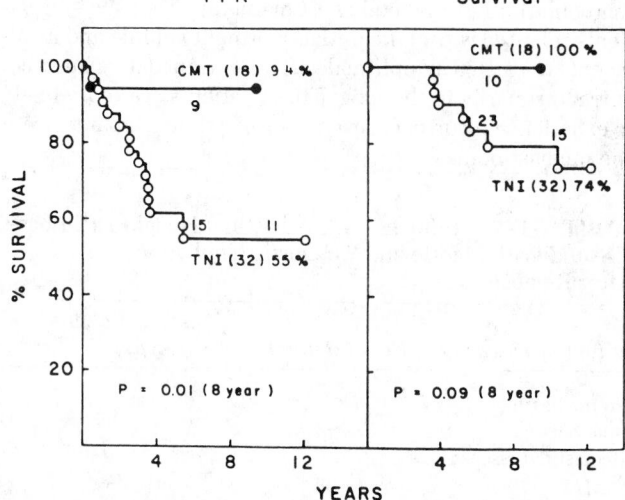

FIGURE 51–12. Freedom from relapse (FFR) and actuarial survival rates after total nodal irradiation (TNI) or combined-modality therapy (CMT) for pathologic stage IIIA1 Hodgkin's disease. (Mauch P, Gorshein D, Cunningham J, et al. Influence of mediastinal adenopathy on site and frequency of relapse in patients with Hodgkin's disease. Cancer Treat Rep 1982;66:809–817)

larger proportion of nodular sclerosis patients seen at Stanford and the routine irradiation of the liver employed there for treating patients with splenic involvement.

Treatment of stages IIB and IIIB Hodgkin's disease with irradiation alone can result in some cases of long-term, relapse-free survival (*i.e.*, approximately 30% in the Stanford L1 and L2 protocols using TNI). Although there is general agreement that radiation therapy alone is unsatisfactory treatment for stage IIIB disease, some data suggest that, in surgical stage IIB disease, irradiation alone may have the same results as combined-modality treatment.[141,256,258] A recent report combines the Stanford and JCRT results for these patients. In this series, 103 patients were treated with radiation therapy only; at 7 years, the rate of freedom from relapse was 74%, and the overall survival rate was 87%. Although the rate of freedom from relapse with combined-modality treatment was better (84%), the overall survival was the same.[259]

Complications of Radiation Treatment

Complications of treatment are related to the technique used, dose administered, and irradiated volume. Most of the complications associated with irradiation are seen in the mantle field.[260] Although no immediate changes are usually apparent on the chest radiograph or in clinical function, a paramediastinal pulmonary density that outlines the irradiated field may be seen on the x-ray film with time. These signs are usually without symptoms, although the patients occasionally may develop dry cough or dyspnea on exertion.

A more important potential complication is acute radiation pneumonitis. This side effect depends on the volume of the lung irradiated and the total dose given. Some changes in pulmonary function after irradiation can be seen if looked for carefully, but symptomatic radiation pneumonitis is much less common if the pulmonary volume irradiated is restricted. If whole-lung irradiation is required, the dose should be restricted to less than 1650 cGy. For example, of 315 patients with stage IA or IIA disease treated with mantle (and paraaortic) irradiation at the JCRT, only 16 (5.1%) developed symptomatic radiation pneumonitis.[251] Symptoms associated with this condition include shortness of breath, cough, and occasional fever. If a large volume of lung has been irradiated to high doses, these changes may become progressive and sometimes fatal.

Several techniques have been used to reduce pulmonary complications. Radiation therapy has been given to large pulmonary masses and interrupted at approximately 1500 cGy to allow time for the mass to shrink; the radiation was continued using smaller fields after a 2- or 3-week hiatus. Similarly, whole-lung irradiation has been given to patients with hilar lymph node involvement, using transmission blocks that allow only a portion of the dose to reach the lungs or fields that include the whole lungs but only to tolerable doses.[141] These techniques have allowed pulmonary irradiation without complications, although long-term follow-up reveals some persistent effects.[261]

Cardiac complications of radiation therapy in Hodgkin's disease were first reported by the Stanford group.[225] When the whole heart is irradiated to doses of greater than 3000 cGy, as many as 50% of the patients develop pericardial complications.[224] By limiting the volume of pericardium irradiated,[259] keeping the radiation fraction less than 250 cGy, and limiting the total dose, such complications have become uncommon, with only 9 cases of pericarditis in 315 patients treated in the JCRT series.[251] It is important to avoid treating the whole pericardium, but if whole-pericardium irradiation is required, the dose must be limited. Technique is also important. If patients are treated primarily through anterior portals, a much larger dose is received by the anterior-placed heart. These techniques have resulted in significant cardiac complications and should be avoided.[262] New methods of cardiac evaluation have revealed abnormal ventricular ejection fractions in some patients long after mediastinal irradiation.[263,264] The symptom complex seen is largely that of pericarditis and, in some patients, continued pericardial fluid causing tamponade or eventual pericardial fibrosis. These conditions can be treated surgically.

Evidence suggests that early coronary artery disease may be a consequence of mediastinal irradiation.[265] One large epidemiologic study shows no significant increase in cardiac-related deaths in Hodgkin's disease patients.[266] However, long-term follow-up data from Stanford revealed disturbing results.[267] Review of the records of 2232 patients treated between 1961 and 1990 revealed 88 deaths, 54 from acute myocardial infarction and 34 from other cardiac complications. The relative risk of death from heart disease is 3.1 compared with age and sex matched controls. The risk was reduced, but still significant, in those who had received less than 3000 cGy to the mediastinum. The relative risk increased with periods of observation, with risk of acute myocardial infarction highest with irradiation of patients younger than 20 years of age ($p<0.01$). A significant decrease in long-term survival occurred as a result of cardiac toxicity.

The most common neurologic complication seen with irradiation is Lhermitte's sign. This transient complication of radiation therapy consists of numbness, tingling, or "electric" sensations, which are produced or exacerbated by head flexion. Carmel and Kaplan reported an incidence of 15% among their patients treated with mantle fields.[224] These symptoms are transitory and are not associated with permanent sequelae. The pathogenesis is unknown. Spinal cord transection can occur when a portion of the spinal cord is included in the mantle and paraaortic fields. If overlap is avoided, this complication does not occur at the doses of 3600 to 4000 cGy used. Radiation fibrosis in the brachial plexus rarely occurs. This complication usually arises if high doses of radiation are given to large neck and axillary tumor masses. Progressive motor and sensory loss have been recorded in patients who have received large doses. Rare malignant tumors of nerve sheaths have been reported long after radiation therapy.[268] These tumors usually are associated with irradiation and chemotherapy.

The thyroid gland is irradiated with the mantle, resulting in about 30% of patients developing an elevated thyroid-stimulating hormone level without T_3 or T_4 reduction.[269] With prompt supplemental thyroid treatment, clinical hypothyroidism has occurred in less than 5% of these patients.[251] Rarely, hyperthyroidism and exophthalmos are seen. Thyroid neoplasms rarely are seen with therapeutic doses of radiation.[270]

Complications related to paraaortic fields are uncommon, and if the doses and fields are as described, gastrointestinal complications are rare. In 315 patients receiving paraaortic field irradiation, there were 8 with complications (*i.e.*, small bowel obstructions) at the JCRT.[251] This 2.5% incidence is similar to that seen with laparotomy without radiation therapy. Pelvic treatment alone may cause persistent thrombocytopenia or leukopenia. This complication is rare with current techniques that use well-collimated linear accelerators and judicious blocks. Infectious complications of treatment occur if TNI and splenectomy are used.

CHEMOTHERAPY

Hodgkin's disease is curable by combination chemotherapy. Single-drug therapy plays a small role in the treatment of newly diagnosed patients, because experienced oncologists usually can select a combination drug program from the options displayed in the tables in this chapter that fit the condition of the patient; the use of drugs in combination is required to effect substantial remission rates and to ensure durable remissions.[271–315] Although remissions are attainable with single agents, they rarely last.

Nitrogen mustard was first used as treatment for lymphomas in 1943 by Goodman and associates.[316] The results, published after World War II, were exciting; they showed marked dissolution of lymph nodes in patients with Hodgkin's disease, but recurrence proved to be the rule. The period between 1942 and 1963 saw the introduction of several new drugs—other alkylating agents, corticosteroids, the antifols, the vinca alkaloids, and a drug almost entirely specific for Hodgkin's disease, procarbazine.[316–323] All were used in the first attempts to cure advanced Hodgkin's disease by combination chemotherapy.

The early studies with single agents did not provide any evidence of the capacity of chemotherapy to cure Hodgkin's disease. Figure 51–13 compares the only available series of untreated patients (all stages included) with the results using alkylating agents alone and with a modern series using all the drugs applied in combination programs given in sequence.[324–326] The shapes of the curves are similar. Median survival was approximately 1 year, and fewer than 5% of patients were alive at 5 years.

The first intensive, four-drug combination program for Hodgkin's disease used vincristine, methotrexate, cyclophosphamide, and prednisone (MOMP) given for 2.5 months.[327] The goal of this pilot protocol was to test the safety of such an approach. Only 14 patients were studied. The data showed the approach was safe and associated with a high complete remission rate (80%). The administration of a two-drug combination, vinblastine and chlorambucil, produced a complete remission rate of approximately 40%. However, this was not a significant improvement over the response achieved with vinblastine alone, and no information on the durability of these remissions—the hallmark of the capacity to cure—was given.[327,328]

In 1964, as experience with procarbazine accrued, the MOMP program was modified in several ways. The duration of treatment was lengthened to 6 months, and procarbazine was substituted for methotrexate.[327] This program was named MOPP.[70,327–333] Each of the agents in the MOPP regimen was selected based on its antitumor activity as a single agent, and the drugs were given in full doses and according to their op-

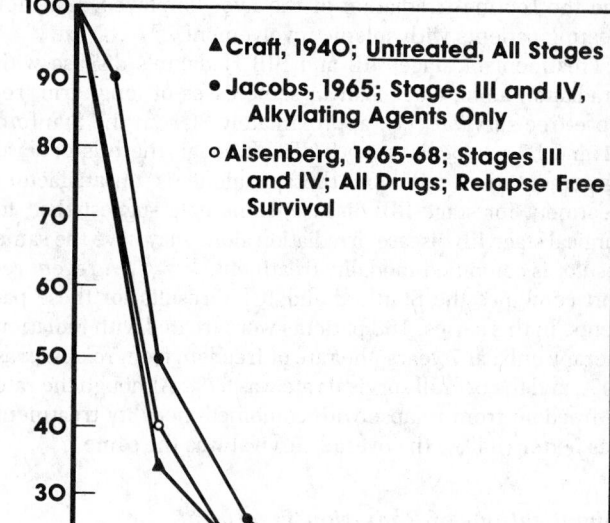

FIGURE 51–13. Two survival curves of patients with advanced Hodgkin's disease treated with single-agent chemotherapy compared with a group left untreated. (DeVita VT. Consequences of the chemotherapy of Hodgkin's disease. Cancer 1981;47:1–13)

timal schedule, with the exception that rest intervals were spaced between cycles and timed, according to available cell kinetics data, to allow marrow recovery between cycles of treatment.[334] Drugs were selected to minimize overlapping toxicity to any single organ. Vincristine was selected over its analog vinblastine, even though vinblastine was the favored drug, because vincristine has less marrow toxicity (although vincristine produced more neurotoxicity). The four drugs were given over a 2-week period. A complete cycle of MOPP took 29 days and consisted of a 2-week treatment period and a 2-week recovery period. A minimum of six cycles was given until the patients achieved a complete remission or tumor grew despite treatment.

Three features of MOPP were unique at the time. The goal of the program was to cure rather than to palliate, as had been the practice in the preceding 2 decades; the cyclic use of combination chemotherapy for 6 months exceeded the duration of any prior treatment of adult tumors; and it was the first regimen to make use of the sliding scale to adjust drug doses for marrow suppression. The sliding scale was designed to permit the administration of each cycle on time, with maximal allowable doses of each agent, and to preserve the dose rate and the integrity of the drug combination.[328] Provisions for delaying subsequent cycles were made only if toxicity was severe enough to require omission of drugs from that cycle. The sliding scale had an interesting effect on dosing in the MOPP regimen and later in other studies of combination chemotherapy. Usually, after two cycles at full or near-full doses,

TABLE 51–8. Twenty-Year MOPP Follow-Up Study by the National Cancer Institute

Number of evaluable patients	188
Number of complete responders	157 (84%)
Number of induction failures	31 (16%)
Number of relapses	56 (34%)
Number continuously free of disease	101 (54%)
Number dead	98 (52%)
Of Hodgkin's disease	68
Free of disease	30
Number alive	90 (48%)
With Hodgkin's disease	2
Free of disease	88

patients had significant myelosuppression, and doses in the third cycle had to be reduced according to the sliding scale to administer the third cycle on schedule and preserve the integrity of the combination (*i.e.*, give some of all four drugs). The impact of reducing doses in the third cycle was to allow the use of full or near-full doses in the fourth or later cycles. The net effect was preservation of dose rate by maintaining tight intervals between cycles.

At NCI, then and now, the dose of vincristine was given on the basis of body surface area and only modified for severe neurotoxicity. The lamentable current practice of capping the dose at a total of 2 mg has no scientific or medical justification and results in a top dose suitable only for persons smaller than $1.43m^2$. These types of dose reduction have a deleterious impact on outcome. The standard practice was to administer a minimum of six cycles of treatment or enough cycles to attain a complete remission plus two additional cycles. The average duration of administration for six cycles in the NCI program was 5.8 months, and the omission of any drugs from the program was rare.

The MOPP regimen was considered high-dose, long-duration chemotherapy in 1964. However, subsequent calculations of its dose intensity, using the methods of Hryniuk and Bush[335] and DeVita and colleagues[336] show that it had a dose intensity of 70% of a hypothetical version of MOPP that would use the same four drugs in their full doses continuously, without rest intervals, over 6 months.[336] This type of inadvertent reduction in dose intensity is true of all cyclically administered drug combinations. The early results of the use of MOPP have been confirmed by others, and the durable remissions have been maintained in the NCI study over the past 20 years.[337] Table 51–8 shows the results of the original series after more than 20 years of follow-up. Eighty-four percent of patients attained complete remissions. Of those patients, 64% remain continuously disease-free (Fig. 51–14), and of all treated patients, 54% remain free of disease after a 20-year follow-up. Forty-eight percent of the total population is alive. The relapse-free survival curve illustrates that most negative events took place in the first 4 years of follow-up, after which the curve flattened and relapses were uncommon. The latest relapse in the MOPP study occurred 11 years after treatment was discontinued.

Only 5 (2.5%) patients died of treatment-related toxic effects. Despite the neurotoxicity associated with full doses of vincristine (*i.e.*, 1.4 mg/m² with no dose capping), no patients were permanently paralyzed using a sliding-scale adjustment based on the actual appearance of neurotoxic side effects.

The major factors negatively affecting complete response rate in the original study were B symptoms, male sex, advanced-stage disease, and lower than projected rate of vincristine administration for the first six cycles. The most important variables affecting complete remission duration were B symptoms, age, rapidity with which complete response was achieved (patients requiring five cycles or less had significantly longer remissions), number of external sites of disease, and liver or pleural involvement. The impact of being symptom free is dramatic in the NCI study. All asymptomatic patients with stages IIIA (10 patients) and IVA (13 patients)

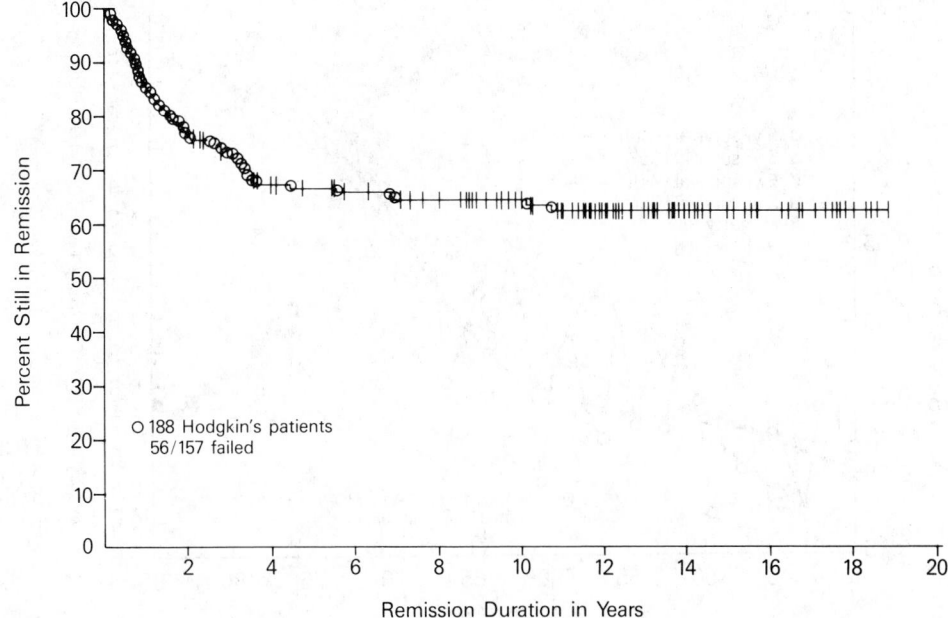

FIGURE 51–14. Remission durations of 188 patients with Hodgkin's disease.

O 188 Hodgkin's patients
56/157 failed

Percent Still in Remission

Remission Duration in Years

attained complete remissions, and only 2 experienced relapses in more than 20 years of follow-up.

In the 1960s, it was fashionable to give additional continuous "maintenance" chemotherapy after a maximal response was attained to maintain this response, especially because there was little expectation of cure. An NCI study in which patients who achieved complete remission were randomized to additional treatment with MOPP, no further treatment, or treatment with the nitrosourea (BCNU) showed maintenance treatment to be ineffective. Since then, nine studies of maintenance treatment in patients who attained a remission with MOPP showed that it adds nothing to long-term relapse-free survival and survival, and maintenance chemotherapy is not recommended if patients have achieved a complete remission, received a minimum of six cycles of treatment, or two additional cycles of treatment have been given after complete remission was documented.[321–340] As a consequence of the development of a standard treatment for advanced Hodgkin's disease, national mortality decreased approximately 63% during the succeeding decade, and survival rates have increased dramatically. The introduction of MOPP chemotherapy into practice and its effect on national survival and mortality data are illustrated in Figure 51–15.[338]

In the 25 years since the inception and confirmation of the efficacy of the MOPP program, clinical trials of treating advanced Hodgkin's disease have taken three major directions: the development of modifications of MOPP, aimed at retaining efficacy while reducing toxicity; the development of new combinations constructed of drugs with different mechanisms of action and presumed to be noncross-resistant to the drugs in the MOPP program; and the use of these noncross-resistant drug combinations in alternating cycles with MOPP or MOPP modifications to avoid early treatment failures and circumvent the development of drug resistance.[337,341]

The first series of studies that followed the NCI report showed MOPP to be superior to a single agent (*i.e.*, nitrogen mustard) used continuously for 6 months in a controlled trial and superior to a new five-drug combination and to the same five drugs used in a strict sequence, even though the complete remission rates with the latter two regimens was similar to that with MOPP.[271,273] This provided important early evidence that complete remission rates alone did not necessarily reflect the true quality of a remission; duration of remission, after all therapy is discontinued, is the most important indicator of the quality of the induction program. Investigators from Stanford University replicated the results of MOPP, using it as reported from the NCI.[339] However, they thought the toxicity of vincristine at doses used at NCI was too severe, and they recommended the now widely adopted practice of limiting the dose of vincristine to no more than 2 mg/dose regardless of body weight or surface area. Omitting prednisone from MOPP reduced the effectiveness, as was shown in one controlled trial comparing MOPP with MOP.[274] Although one uncontrolled study from Stanford did not confirm this observation, the population of patients at Stanford was composed largely of patients who had relapsed after radiation therapy and is not comparable to most other studies.[340]

In a decade of studies designed to reduce the side effects of MOPP by substituting or adding additional drugs, three four-drug combinations emerged: MVPP, ChlVPP, and BCVPP (Table 51–9) with effects equivalent to MOPP but with different and sometimes fewer side effects, making them useful as alternative treatments.[286,287,292–296] ChlVPP (chlorambucil, vinblastine, procarbazine, prednisone) is an attractive variant of the MOPP program. It substitutes chlorambucil for nitrogen mustard and vinblastine for vincristine. It produces somewhat less nausea and vomiting and much less neurotoxicity, although the degree of myelosuppression is similar. The complete remission rate and fraction of patients who survive continuously free of disease appear equivalent to MOPP. The LOPP variant substitutes chlorambucil for nitrogen mustard. In a controlled trial comparing LOPP with MOPP, the programs were found to be equivalent, but the results with both arms were inferior to those reported elsewhere, a difference

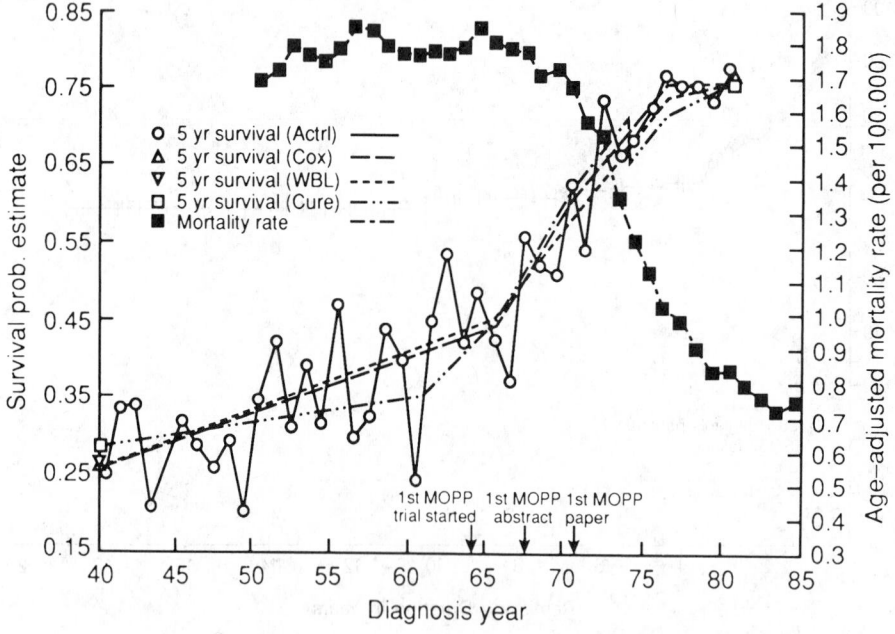

FIGURE 51–15. Hodgkin's disease. The 5-year modeled and actuarial survival rates by the diagnosis year and the U.S. mortality rate by the diagnosis year. (Fuer EJ, Kessler LG, Baker SG, et al. The impact of breakthrough clinical trials on survival in population based tumor registries. J Clin Epidemiol 1991;44:141–153)

TABLE 51–9. Combination Chemotherapy Programs Effective in the Treatment of Advanced-Stage Hodgkin's Disease

Drugs	*Recommended Dose (mg/m²)*	*Route*	*Days**
MOPP regimen			
Nitrogen mustard	6	I.V.	1, 8
Vincristine	1.4	I.V.	1, 8
Procarbazine	100	PO	1–14
Prednisone†	40	PO	1–14
MVPP regimen			
Nitrogen mustard	6	I.V.	1, 8
Vinblastine	6	I.V.	1, 8
Procarbazine	100	PO	1–14
Prednisone	40	PO	1–14
LOPP regimen			
Chlorambucil	6	PO	1–14
Vincristine	1.4	I.V.	1, 8
Procarbazine	100	PO	1–14
Prednisone	40	PO	1–14
ChlVPP regimen			
Chlorambucil	6	PO	1–14
Vinblastine	6	I.V.	1, 8
Procarbazine	100	PO	1–14
Prednisone	40	PO	1–14
ABVD regimen			
Doxorubicin	25	I.V.	1, 15
Bleomycin	10	I.V.	1, 15
Vinblastine	6	I.V.	1, 15
Dacarbazine	375	I.V.	1, 15
MOPP/ABVD regimen			
Alternating months of MOPP and ABVD			
MOPP/ABV hybrid regimen			
Nitrogen mustard	6	I.V.	1
Vincristine	1.4	I.V.	1
Procarbazine	100	PO	1–7
Prednisone	40	PO	1–14
Doxorubicin	35	I.V.	8
Bleomycin	10	I.V.	8
Vinblastine	6	I.V.	8

* Each cycle lasts 28 days.
† In the original report, prednisone was given only on cycles 1 and 4; it is now given with every cycle.
(Longo D. The use of chemotherapy in the treatment of Hodgkin's disease. Semin Oncol 1990;17: 716–735)

apparently related to inadequate dosing.[282] The results with MVPP, which substitutes vinblastine for vincristine, appear equivalent to those with MOPP but with less neurotoxicity and more myelotoxicity. Interpretation of long-term results of MVPP are complicated by the use of two- and four-drug maintenance treatment in all responders. ChlVPP and MVPP are reasonable alternatives to MOPP, especially for older patients who are less able to tolerate the neurologic side effects of vincristine or for patients with intractable nausea and vomiting related to nitrogen mustard.

The BCVPP regimen substitutes vinblastine and cyclophosphamide for vincristine and nitrogen mustard and adds the nitrosourea BCNU. The Eastern Cooperative Oncology Group (ECOG) conducted a randomized comparison of BCVPP and MOPP in a population of patients with advanced disease, of whom 35% were asymptomatic.[277] Unfortunately, MOPP was used in reduced doses and at wider intervals, with a capping of the vincristine dose at 2 mg. The complete response rates for the two regimens were identical, but the duration of complete remission with BCVPP was significantly longer than with the reduced-dose version of MOPP in previously untreated patients. Life-threatening hematologic toxicity was slightly more severe with BCVPP, probably because of the addition of BCNU, but BCVPP treatment produced less gastrointestinal and neurologic toxicity. Follow-up of this population indicates a higher incidence of acute leukemia in the BCVPP arm than the MOPP arm, which is probably due to the addition of the nitrosourea. The addition of BCNU with greater acute toxicity and long-term side effects makes this combination too toxic for routine use.

In other commonly tested MOPP variants, known by the acronym CVPP, various doses of parenteral cyclophosphamide and vinblastine were combined with various doses of oral procarbazine and prednisone in a variety of schedules. The overall complete remission rate in collected studies is approximately 70% (range, 62–74%), and the actuarial 4-year relapse-free survival rates range from 50% to 60%.[302,341,342] These results do not represent an improvement over MOPP, MVPP, or ChlVPP, because toxicities are similar to that of MOPP, with the exception of peripheral neuropathy and extravasation sequelae. The Cancer and Leukemia Group B (CALGB) studied four-drug regimens in which CCNU was substituted for nitrogen mustard in the CVPP regimen. These studies produced a 68% (average) complete response rate and four-year relapse-free survival rates of 50% to 70%.[341,343,344]

The Southwest Oncology Group (SWOG) conducted a study comparing MOPP with MOPP plus bleomycin.[345,351] In the first SWOG study, the complete response rate with MOPP was 70% and 87% for MOPP plus bleomycin. MOPP plus bleomycin was therefore thought to be the superior treatment, and this program was selected as the control for the next study, which compared it with a new version of MOPP referred to as MOPP-BAP, in which half of the dose of nitrogen mustard was replaced with half of the dose of doxorubicin (Adriamycin).[276] The complete response rate with MOPP plus bleomycin in the second study was not comparable to that of the first SWOG study, decreasing to 67%; it also was inferior to the complete response rate for MOPP-BAP (77%). Based on these results, MOPP-BAP was said to be superior; however, superiority once again came at the expense of a sharp decline in each study in the complete response rate for the control arm (the "best therapy" of the prior study). The complete response rate of MOPP-BAP was not significantly better than that of the MOPP-alone arm in the original SWOG study. Although these trends could be accounted for if the later studies began to include more patients with poorer prognostic factors, the data indicate the opposite. Alterations in doses and schedules seem the more likely explanation, with physicians reducing drug doses as they learn to anticipate the toxicity. The addition of drugs to MOPP, ChlVPP, or MVPP has not made them more useful than the original programs used in adequate doses. Adding drugs adds significant risks and precludes the use of these drugs later if initial treatment fails.

The first new regimen of importance was the ABVD regimen (doxorubicin, bleomycin, vinblastine, dacarbazine) developed by Bonadonna and others.[346–348] In the first comparison of ABVD with MOPP as initial therapy for advanced disease, a 71.5% complete remission rate was obtained with the former, which was not significantly different from the 63% remission rate obtained with the latter. No significant differences in the disease-free or overall survival rates were seen, but ABVD was found to be effective in MOPP failures. ABVD and ABVD variants were subsequently used with MOPP in alternating cycles to improve outcome. Table 51–10 enumerates studies comparing alternating cycles of the two noncross-resistant combinations with MOPP and ABVD.[290,306,307,312–315]

These trials were developed to test the utility of the Goldie-Coldman hypothesis (see Chapter 16). Hodgkin's disease served as a useful model because it is one of the few cancers for which more than one effective drug treatment was available for testing. Interpretations of the data in Table 51–10 should be approached at two levels, the first to evaluate the biologic significance of the Goldie-Coldman hypothesis. Failure to validate the hypothesis should have important implications in the design of future clinical trials in Hodgkin's disease. The second level is a more practical one and relates to the selection of appropriate treatment for patients with advanced Hodgkin's disease to maximize the chances for cure at the time of initial treatment. The data show only a marginal advantage, at best, for eight-drug over four-drug programs, and the studies suffer from design problems.

Bonadonna and associates randomized 88 stage IV patients to alternating monthly cycles of MOPP and ABVD or to MOPP alone.[278–281] The patients received 12 monthly cycles of MOPP—twice the usual duration of treatment—or six cycles of MOPP alternating monthly with six cycles of ABVD. Complete remissions were obtained in 74.4% of the patients with MOPP alone and 88.9% of the patients treated with MOPP and ABVD; the difference was not significant. Greater differences in complete response rate in favor of MOPP and ABVD were noted in patients over age 40 who had no prior radiation therapy, those with lymphocyte-depleted histology or B symptoms, more than three nodal sites involved, or those with bulky tumor. None of these differences were significant. Disease-free and overall survival significantly favored MOPP plus ABVD. The 8-year freedom from progression rates were 35.9% and 64.6% for the MOPP and MOPP plus ABVD groups, respectively. Of the total of 72 complete responders, 45.1% in the MOPP group and 72.6% in the MOPP plus ABVD group were continuously disease free at 8 years. The total survival of the complete responders was significantly different, in favor of MOPP plus ABVD only if death from Hodgkin's disease was considered. If all deaths were considered, the differences were not significant (*i.e.*, 61.9% for MOPP; 76.2% for MOPP plus ABVD) after 8 years of observation.

The toxicity of MOPP plus ABVD was less acceptable to patients than that of MOPP alone. Only 7% of MOPP patients refused to complete treatment, compared with 22% of MOPP plus ABVD patients. The doses in the MOPP arm were, however, markedly reduced, and the results with MOPP in this study were inferior to those at NCI and in prior MOPP studies from the Milan group. The major problem appears to have been the duration of the MOPP program. Patients were unable to tolerate continuous exposure to the MOPP drugs, particularly vincristine, for 12 months, and as a consequence, the dose intensity of MOPP was markedly reduced.

A similar study testing the utility of alternating cycles of two noncross-resistant drug combinations was conducted at the NCI.[315] MOPP was compared, in a randomized trial, with MOPP and CABS (CCNU, doxorubicin, bleomycin, streptozotocin), a program shown to be noncross-resistant to MOPP. In this study, cycles of CABS were alternated with MOPP, but in both arms of the study, the projected number of cycles for remission induction was 6 instead of 12, as in the Milan trial. At total of 127 patients were randomized, 64 to MOPP and 63 to MOPP and CABS, of whom 59 and 56, respectively, were evaluable. The complete response rate was equivalent

TABLE 51–10. Controlled Trials of Alternating, Cyclic Combination Treatment of Advanced Hodgkin's Disease

Investigations	Regimen	Complete Response (%)	Relapse-Free Survival (%)	Failure-Free Survival (%)	Overall Survival (%)
NCI, Milan[281]	MOPP	74	50	45	64
	vs				
	MOPP/ABVD	89	73*	65*	84
NCI, Bethesda[315]	MOPP	91	65	68	80
	vs				
	MOPP/CABS	92	72	54	72
ECOG[290]	BCVPP	73	56	47	68
	vs				
	BCVPP + RRx	67	61	49	63
	vs				
	MOPP/ABVD	80	61	61	75
CALGB[352]	MOPP	62	48	47	66
	vs				
	ABVD	82	64	57	74
	vs				
	MOPP/ABVD	83*	64	66	76
Intergroup[353]	MOPP → ABVD	73	72	65	82
	vs				
	MOPP/ABV	82*	79*	77*	89*
Canadian[307]	MOPP/ABV	85	75		84
	vs				
	MOPP/ABVD	82	70		84

* $p < 0.05$.

and excellent for both programs, 92% for MOPP and 88% for MOPP and CABS. After more than 5 years of follow-up, the relapse free and overall survival results of both programs were equal and equivalent to or slightly better than the original MOPP study. Dose intensity of the MOPP program in this study exceeded that of the original NCI MOPP study because dose escalation was allowed.

The CALGB recently reported the early results of a comparison of MOPP with ABVD and with MOPP plus ABVD in a group of patients with previously untreated advanced Hodgkin's disease (stages IIIA–IVB).[306] MOPP plus ABVD patients received 6 cycles of each regimen for a total of 12 cycles but, unlike the Milan trial, both four-drug programs were given over 8 rather than 12 months. An extraordinary rate of dose reduction in the MOPP arm was allowed. In addition to capping the vincristine dose, doses of vincristine were reduced by 30% by the third cycle, and the doses of nitrogen mustard and procarbazine were reduced by 56% and 61%, respectively, by the third cycle. Calculations of dose intensity have not been reported, and the impact of prolonging the intervals between cycles was not assessed. The results are mixed and do not support the use of eight drugs over adequate doses of a four-drug program. For example, the complete response rate for MOPP plus ABVD was 82%, compared with 69% for the reduced version of MOPP. However, the complete response rate for ABVD (81%) was identical to that with MOPP plus ABVD. Failure-free survival of 36 months was significantly better with MOPP plus ABVD (64%) than with MOPP (48%), but it

was identical to that obtained with ABVD alone (64%). No significant difference in disease-free or overall survival among the regimens has emerged after a follow-up of only 5 years. The data suggest an early failure-free survival advantage for MOPP plus ABVD compared with the reduced version of MOPP but no advantage of MOPP plus ABVD over ABVD given at standard doses.

The ECOG compared MOPP plus ABVD, as used by the Milan group, with their BCVPP regimen, alone or with low-dose radiation therapy added to initially involved sites in patients with advanced Hodgkin's disease.[290] In an interim evaluation of 294 patients, complete response rates among the therapeutic options were found to be similar (68–76%), and no differences in disease-free survival of complete responders (66%) was observed. Because there was no advantage to adding radiation therapy to sites involved by tumor, the two BCVPP arms were combined, and significant advantages were then observed for MOPP plus ABVD in the rates of complete responses, progression free survival, and overall survival. These data do not support the idea that alternating cycles of noncross-resistant combinations provided better results than with adequately used four-drug combination. The data also strongly support the view that investigator bias in regard to anticipated toxicity can radically alter dosing practices and outcome. They suggest that future clinical trials should explore dose modification in initial treatment programs to improve cure rate.

The other two trials shown in Table 51–10 compare different versions of alternating regimens with one another without a four-drug control. The most interesting program studied is that of Connors and Klimo, which featured a MOPP plus ABVD variant in which dacarbazine is omitted, the dose of doxorubicin increased, and all drugs other than prednisone are given within 8 days (MOPP plus ABV hybrid).[307,311,312,314] Partial responders received radiation therapy to nodal areas with residual disease. Complete responses were attained in the original study in 96% of 74 evaluable patients, and the actuarial relapse-free survival rate for complete responders, after more than 5 years off treatment, was 90%. However, the complete response rate includes the 15% of the patients who had radiation therapy to residual disease, and almost 40% of the patients in this study population were in the favorable, asymptomatic group. Longer-term results are more in line with those reported with other drug combination programs. Compared with MOPP plus ABVD in a randomized trial in Canada, the two programs have proven to be equivalent although MOPP plus ABV is somewhat less difficult for patients to tolerate. The Milan group is also testing alternating half cycles of MOPP plus ABVD compared with their original MOPP plus ABVD program; early results show identical response rates and equal durability of responses. The last study in Table 51–10 compares MOPP plus ABVD to the same two programs in sequence with six to eight cycles of MOPP followed by three cycles of ABVD.[307] MOPP plus ABVD was superior to the sequence. This result is not surprising, because the ultimate outcome depends on the initial complete remission rate, which is lower with reduced-dose versions of MOPP. Salvage data from the CALGB trial comparing MOPP plus ABVD with MOPP or with ABVD have some bearing on the interpretation of this study. In the CALGB study, patients who failed ABVD were induced into durable complete remissions twice as often with MOPP as those who failed MOPP and were subsequently treated with ABVD. This suggests that in the Intergroup study the reverse sequence, ABVD followed by MOPP, might be superior to MOPP followed by ABVD.

Two uncontrolled studies routinely added radiation therapy after chemotherapy to sites known to be involved with tumor. Wagener and associates studied 50 advanced-stage patients in a nonrandomized trial in which MOPP was alternated with CAVmP (cyclophosphamide, doxorubicin, VM-26, prednisone).[310] Three cycles of each regimen were given on an alternating schedule, after which consolidation radiation therapy was given to initially involved sites. The complete response after chemotherapy was only 68%; 87% were in complete remission after radiation therapy. The actuarial 3-year survival rate of the total group of complete responders was 94%, and the rate of relapse-free survival was 73%. The investigators concluded that the treatment was no more effective than MOPP in achieving complete remission but that it may be superior in terms of survival. No direct comparison has been made with MOPP. Prosnitz and colleagues periodically update results from a study of a regimen for advanced Hodgkin's disease using combination chemotherapy followed by low-dose irradiation to the initial sites of disease.[308] However, the results of the only controlled trial comparing this approach with radiation therapy alone (see Table 51–10) do not support the use of radiation therapy in adequately dosed patients.[272]

Impact of Dose Intensity on Outcome

Dosing practices in clinical studies have been inconsistent and ignored, despite the fact that retrospective studies of dose intensity consistently show an impact on outcome. Although drugs are added and substituted at will and schedules manipulated frequently, the total dose and dose rate themselves are virtually never examined prospectively as independent variables, nor is actual data on dose intensity given at the time of publication.[337] A retrospective report by Carde and colleagues from Stanford University found that lower doses in the MOPP program correlated with poorer outcome.[349] The dose and dose rate of nitrogen mustard, vincristine, and procarbazine in MOPP, as used at Stanford, were important variables in the ability to attain complete remission and in survival. A regression analysis showed that the mean of the total dose and the dose rate of three cytotoxic agents combined had a significant impact on complete remission rate, particularly in patients with B symptoms, strongly supporting the contention that dose and preservation of the integrity of the combination are important. Patients who received less than 65% of the projected total dose of nitrogen mustard had significantly poorer survival than those who received more than 65% of the projected dose. Another report from Stanford indicated that MOPP failures often achieved good palliation with the use of a single alkylating agent as salvage treatment, which also suggested that significant underdosing with alkylating agents was occurring during their initial treatment with MOPP.[355] These data are bolstered by other reports showing a positive correlation between dose intensity of nitrogen mustard, complete remission rates, and survival free of disease.[356–359]

To compare results across studies in Hodgkin's disease, the NCI group followed the practice of Hryniuk and Bush, converting doses to mg/m²/week, to obtain an average dose intensity over the 6-month standard MOPP treatment duration.[335] Calculating dose intensity has several advantages over the prevalent practice of comparing percentages of projected dose delivered. Although the percent of projected dose delivered may be high and similar across studies, the projected dose within each study may vary, rendering the comparison useless. A good example is vincristine, for which the percent projected dose delivered is high in most trials, but dose intensity is low because of the routine capping at 2 mg/dose.

Examples of the impact of ad hoc alterations in the MOPP program on dose intensity are shown in Table 51–11.[291] Ver-

TABLE 51–11. Alterations in Relative Dose Intensity of the MOPP Regimen

MOPP Versions	Cycle Intervals (wk)			
	4	5	6	8
I MOPP, standard	1	0.80	0.67	0.50
II VCR total, 2 mg PCZ scaled up; 14 days	0.92	0.74	0.61	0.46
III VCR total, 2 mg PCZ scaled up; 10 days	0.82	0.66	0.55	0.41

VCR, vincristine; PCZ, procarbazine.

TABLE 51–12. MOPP Regimens for Hodgkin's Disease: Dose Intensity and Outcome

Investigations	Relative Dose Intensity vs NCI MOPP	Actual Relative Dose Intensity	Complete Remission (%)	% Patients Free of Disease (%)
NCI/DeVita	1.0	0.85	84	55 (15)
Stanford/Carde	0.95	0.64*	72	30 (5)†
BNLI/Goldman	0.82		52	30 (5)
SEG/Huguley	0.82	0.64	46	16 (2)
CALGB/Nissen	0.81		74	37 (5)
ECOG/Bakemeier	0.77	0.60	73	37 (5)
Milan/Bonadonna	0.76	0.53–0.66	74	36 (8)
SWOG/Frei	0.70		78	31 (5)

* Actual relative dose intensity from a prior study.
† Estimate made from patients with marrow stage IV.

sion I is used at NCI. It has the highest intended dose intensity of any reported program and is used here as the reference standard. Giving version I with an extra week between cycles results in a 20% reduction in the average dose intensity per cycle. Version II, used in most clinical studies, limits the dose of vincristine to a total of 2 mg; procarbazine is scaled up in dose slowly, a practice used in the clinic to reduce nausea and vomiting. If given with the usual 1-week delay between cycles, version II results in a 25% decrease in average dose intensity. MOPP, in practice and in most clinical trials cited, is more often given at 5-week intervals, with a resulting decrease in dose intensity of up to 34%, a reduction in the range that causes a loss of over half of the cure rate in most animal studies. In some human studies, additional significant changes are made, such as omission of a drug entirely, usually vincristine or procarbazine, from the combination, as was done in the Milan study.

Table 51–12 shows data on intended and actual dose intensity of MOPP. It was possible to estimate actual dose intensity in only five of the eight studies shown. There is no consistent effect of intended or actual dose intensity on the complete response rate, a phenomenon seen in animal studies of drug-curable tumors as well.[291] This is an important source of error, because physicians often judge the effectiveness of a new therapy in curable human tumors by its response rate; however, the relation between dose intensity and the fraction of patients who remain free of disease, which is the best indicator of the quality of remission, is more revealing. Reductions in the actual dose intensity of 29% and 38% in the ECOG and Milan studies, respectively, may result in 33% and 35% decreases in overall disease-free survival. Regression analysis yields a correlation coefficient of 0.88 ($p<0.02$) (Fig. 51–16). The difference in outcome between MOPP and the next three programs shown in Figure 51–16 is significant at the $p<0.001$ level.

In the Milan trial comparing MOPP with MOPP plus ABVD, the complete remission and overall survival rates are not significantly different between the two programs, but the relapse-free survival was superior for MOPP plus ABVD.[281] The results with MOPP were poor. Fifty percent of patients in the MOPP arm of the Milan study experienced relapses in the first 24

months, compared with only 34% of patients at NCI over a 14-year follow-up period. In the Milan study, 35% of patients experienced a 50% reduction of the dose of vincristine, and for 9% of patients, the integrity of the combination was entirely disrupted because vincristine was permanently discontinued. The CALGB trial, comparing MOPP with ABVD and with MOPP plus ABVD, suffers from similar dose reductions in the MOPP but not the ABVD arm.

A major reason for treatment failure in Hodgkin's disease may be *underdosing* rather than resistance in the more traditional sense. To test this hypothesis in a clinical trial, all variables but dose must be controlled. The NCI has developed a protocol to test a dose intensified version of MOPP known as Dose Intense MOPP (DIMOPP) in newly diagnosed patients with stage III or IVB disease.[350] The dose intensity of the alkylating agent is increased by two thirds and that of vincristine and procarbazine by one third. The program is given with the support of colony-stimulating factors. This study and others reporting the use of colony-stimulating factors to support standard or increased dosing present opportunities for physicians to finally address the issue of dosing.[351,354]

Chemotherapy for Advanced Hodgkin's Disease

If adjusted for dosing differences, there appear to be no significant differences in long-term outcome when a program from among the following is well administered: MOPP, MVPP, ChlVPP, BCVPP, ABVD, MOPP plus ABVD, and MOPP plus ABV (see Table 51–9). One of these programs should be used as the initial treatment for previously untreated patients with advanced Hodgkin's disease, without the addition of radiation therapy, except in patients with massive mediastinal involvement. The failure to detect a major difference favoring the eight-drug program makes it essential to develop clinical trials examining other variables to improve primary treatment. The choice of a four- or eight-drug program also affects which drugs are available for salvage. If equivalent cure rates can be attained with full doses of a four-drug program, patients who fail can be treated with the alternative program drugs to reduce the body burden of tumor to prepare them for high-dose chemotherapy with marrow or stem cell support.

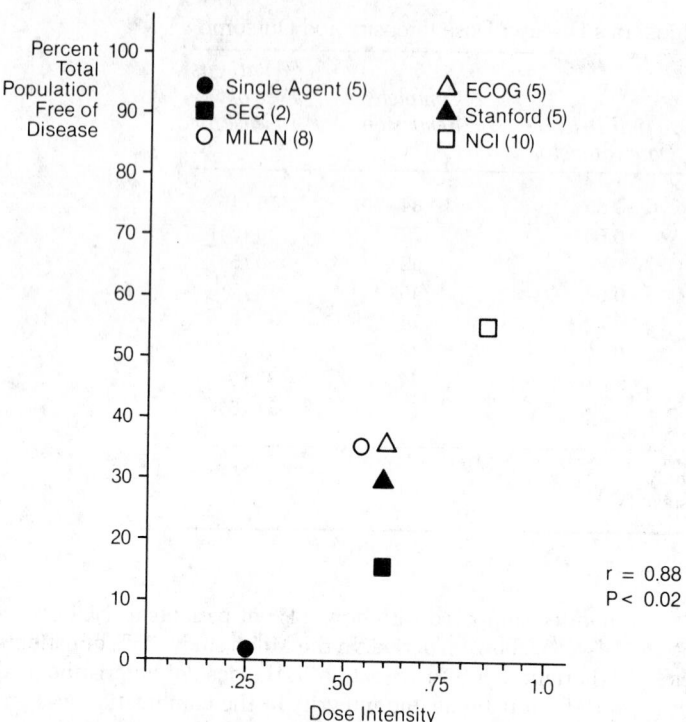

Percent Total Population Free of Disease

● Single Agent (5)   △ ECOG (5)
■ SEG (2)   ▲ Stanford (5)
○ MILAN (8)   □ NCI (10)

r = 0.88
P < 0.02

Dose Intensity

FIGURE 51–16. Relative dose intensity compared with disease-free survival rates of patients with Hodgkin's disease in MOPP programs.

The choice of program should be based largely on toxicity. The acute toxicities of MOPP and ABVD are roughly equivalent but different. The unwarranted fear most physicians have of vincristine-induced neuropathy and the slightly greater nausea and vomiting associated with MOPP often lead to greater dose reductions than with ABVD, with loss of therapeutic effect. A physician is advised to select a program that he or she can faithfully administer in full doses. The most useful MOPP substitute is the ChlVPP regimen, which, if given on the basis of body surface area, appears to preserve dose intensity because it produces fewer acute side effects and to produce equivalent long-term results to MOPP.

The worldwide experience with ChlVPP is minimal. The long-term leukemogenic effect of substituting chlorambucil for nitrogen mustard, while retaining procarbazine, is not yet clear but not likely to be less than with MOPP. MOPP and ChlVPP are reported to be more leukemogenic than ABVD. The limiting and irreversible cardiopulmonary toxicity associated with the use of doxorubicin and bleomycin in ABVD is significant, especially in a young population, and may be an especially serious concern if ABVD is coupled with radiation therapy to the mediastinum. Of the alternating programs, MOPP and ABV is the least emetogenic, because dacarbazine has been omitted, and it is given over a shorter period than MOPP plus ABVD (8 versus 12 months). Because it appears equivalent to MOPP plus ABVD, it may be the program of choice if alternating cyclic chemotherapy is chosen.[307]

Salvage Chemotherapy for Advanced Hodgkin's Disease

One of the most difficult problems faced by oncologists is the proper approach to managing patients with Hodgkin's disease who experience relapse after their primary treatment. It was first observed in 1979 that the length of the prior remission had a marked effect on the ability of patients to respond to subsequent treatment and sustain the response.[360] Patients whose initial remission was longer than 1 year had a greater chance of achieving a second complete remission than newly diagnosed patients of the same stage (95% versus 80%), and their remissions appeared durable. Only about 20% of those who relapsed in less than 1 year attained a second complete remission, and they had a higher risk of relapse. These were important observations for several reasons. They defined subsets of patients with different prognoses who required different approaches to salvage therapy, and they provided information useful in the evaluation of new salvage programs. They also indicated for the first time that drug resistance was probably not the cause of recurrence in patients who had long initial remissions, because they often responded to a second round of the same treatment. The data suggest that undertreatment, particularly underdosing during remission induction, may have led to recurrence, and they provide further support for the notion that dose intensity plays an important role in the outcome of drug-treated patients.[361]

This idea has been significantly bolstered by the results of autologous bone marrow (ABMT) support programs.[362-366] We updated our experience with the long-term follow-up of patients who relapsed from one of several MOPP-based chemotherapy programs at the NCI and were retreated with MOPP.[367] Patients with long initial remissions had a relapse-free survival rate of 45% beyond 10 years, but the development of second cancers and other treatment-related complications reduced the overall survival by almost one half. The disease-free survival rate beyond 11 years from relapse of patients with long initial remissions was only 24%; for those with short initial remissions, it was 11% (Fig. 51–17). The difference was statistically significant. Although long-term survival compatible with cure is possible in patients who relapse after at least 1 year in remission, only about one quarter of the group

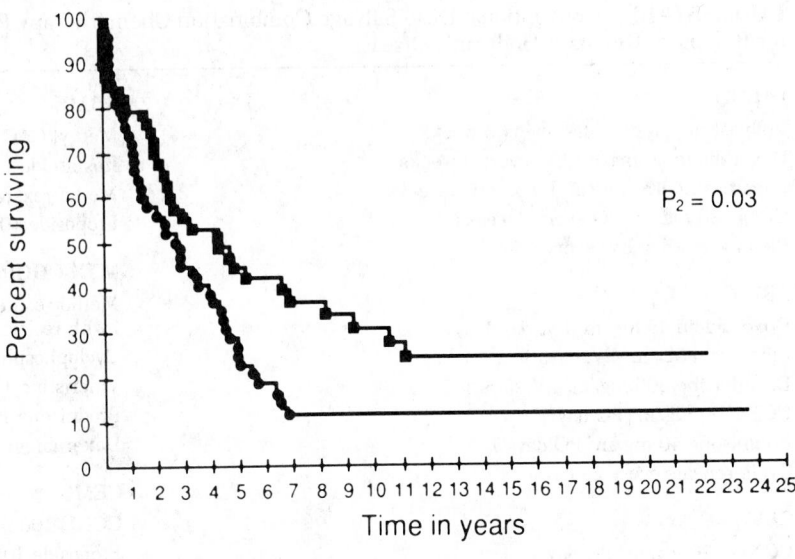

FIGURE 51–17. Kaplan-Meier plot of overall survival from the date of first relapse of patients whose initial remission was shorter than 1 year (●) compared with those whose initial remission was longer than 1 year (■). Survival for patients with short initial remissions is projected to be 11% at 22 years, which is significantly poorer ($p_2 = 0.027$) than the 24% observed for patients with longer initial remissions. (Longo DL, Duffey PL, Young RC, et al. Conventional-dose salvage combination chemotherapy in patients relapsing with Hodgkin's disease after combination chemotherapy: The low probability for cure. J Clin Oncol 1992;10:210–218)

achieve it. The recently published follow-up results from Milan on long-term outcome after ABVD salvage conform to these data.[369] The addition of ABMT or peripheral blood stem cells to support intensification of chemotherapy as salvage treatment has changed the options available for relapsed patients.[362–366] Despite the fact that the patients in ABMT studies were generally resistant to multiple standard drug combinations, the complete remission rates in the various published programs approximates 50%, and a quarter to a half of successfully treated patients remain free of disease, although the follow-up period is still short, with a median of about 3 years.

For the most part, these patients are treated with preparative regimens that contain classes of drugs to which they already have been exposed. The only major new variable is dose intensity—the drugs are given at three to ten times their conventional doses. A major variable that affects outcome is the ability of conventional dose programs to sufficiently reduce tumor volume before transplantation; "responsive failures" make up most of the long-term survivors in transplant programs. Patients who fail a second treatment with a standard program or fail high-dose chemotherapy in the setting of bone marrow support or support with autologous peripheral blood stem cells are candidates for "third-line" programs. Treatment under these circumstances is rarely curative and should be given in the setting of a formal clinical trial, because it provides a way to identify new drug activity that can be used to improve the treatment of newly diagnosed patients.

Patients who fail treatment and are candidates for salvage chemotherapy can be divided into four groups, and their treatment selected accordingly: those initially treated with radiation therapy who recur with systemic disease, patients with advanced disease who fail to attain a complete remission, those who attain a complete remission but whose remission lasts less than 1 year, and patients who relapse after a remission of more than 1 year. Patients who fail radiation therapy should be treated with standard combination chemotherapy as previously outlined. Their response to treatment with chemotherapy is as good as, and in some cases better than, equiv-

alently staged, newly diagnosed patients.[61] Patients who fail to attain a complete remission after treatment with one of the standard programs have the poorest prognosis. Although they sometimes respond to a noncross-resistant standard program (Table 51–13), the remissions are usually brief. This reduction in tumor volume should be exploited, if possible, to prepare them for a program that employs intensive chemotherapy with autologous stem cell or bone marrow support. For patients whose complete remission lasted longer than 1 year, retreatment with the same or a noncross-resistant standard drug combination represents an option that results in satisfactory long-term results compatible with cure in about a quarter of cases.

Because dosing is the most important issue in administering the second set of induction chemotherapy, the choice of which regimen to use should be guided more by the physician's knowledge of the capacity of the particular patient to tolerate the primary treatment. If the patient was treated with MOPP, for example, and marrow suppression was so severe that full doses were not possible, a second six cycles of MOPP is not likely to be any easier to administer, and the selection of ABVD would be a better choice, although marrow sensitivity to drugs is often a generic problem and it would be prudent to augment the treatment with the use of colony stimulating factors. If a patient experienced severe neurotoxicity from the initial treatment with MOPP, MVPP or ChlVPP could be used for retreatment instead of MOPP or ABVD, because vinblastine is substituted for vincristine in these regimens and the general results are roughly equivalent. If nausea and vomiting were the obstacles to administering full doses, as they are occasionally, ChlVPP could be the superior choice for retreatment.

Because the use of high-dose chemotherapy with marrow or stem cell support may reduce the cumulative exposure of the removed bone marrow to drugs and consequently decrease long-term side effects, it is not unreasonable to consider these intensive treatment programs as salvage therapy even for patients who relapse after long remissions, although there are no data on such an approach. It seems wiser to offer patients

TABLE 51–13. Conventional Dose Salvage Combination Chemotherapy Programs for Relapsed, Resistant Hodgkin's Disease

VABCD

Vinblastine 6 mg/m² I.V. every 3 weeks
Doxorubicin 40 mg/m² I.V. every 3 weeks
Dacarbazine 800 mg/m² I.V. every 3 weeks
CCNU 80 mg/m² PO every 6 weeks
Bleomycin 15 U I.V. every 1 week

ABDIC

Doxorubicin 45 mg/m² I.V. day 1
Bleomycin 5U/m² I.V. days 1–5
Dacarbazine 200 mg/m² I.V. days 1–5
CCNU 50 mg/m² PO day 1
Prednisone 40 mg/m² PO days 1–5
Cycle repeats every 28 days

CBVD

CCNU 120 mg/m² PO day 1
Bleomycin 15 U I.V. days 1–22
Vinblastine 6 mg/m² I.V. days 1–22
Dexamethasone 3 mg/m² PO days 1–21
Cycle repeats every 6 weeks

PCVP

Vinblastine 3 mg/m² I.V. every 2 weeks
Procarbazine 70 mg/m² PO every other day
Cyclophosphamide 70 mg/m² PO every other day
Prednisone 8 mg/m² PO every other day
Therapy lasts 1 year

CEP

CCNU 80 mg/m² PO day 1
Etoposide 100 mg/m² PO days 1–5
Prednimustine 60 mg/m² PO days 1–5

EVA

Etoposide 200 mg/m² PO days 1–5
Vincristine 2 mg I.V. day 1
Doxorubicin 50 mg/m² I.V. day 1

MOPLACE

Cyclophosphamide 750 mg/m² I.V. day 1
Etoposide 80 mg/m² I.V. days 1–3
Prednisone 60 mg/m² PO days 1–14
Methotrexate 120 mg/m² I.V. days 15, 22 with rescue
Cytarabine 300 mg/m² I.V. days 15, 22
Vincristine 2 mg I.V. days 15, 22 every 4 weeks

MIME

Methyl GAG 500 mg/m² I.V. days 1–14
Ifosfamide 1 mg/m² I.V. days 1–5
Methotrexate 30 mg/m² I.V. day 3
Etoposide 100 mg/m² I.V. days 1–3, every 3 weeks

MTX-CHOP

Methotrexate 30 mg/m² I.V. every 6 hours for 4 days, days 1, 8 with rescue
Cyclophosphamide 750 mg/m² I.V. day 15
Vincristine 1 mg/m² I.V. days 15, 22
Prednisone 100 mg/m² PO days 22–26
Doxorubicin 50 mg/m² I.V. day 15 every 4 weeks

CEM

CCNU 100 mg/m² PO day 1
Etoposide 100 mg/m² PO days 1–3, 21–23
Methotrexate 30 mg/m² PO days 1–8, 21, 28 every 6 weeks

CEVD

CCNU 80 mg/m² PO day 1
Etoposide 120 mg/m² PO days 1–5, 22–26
Vindesine 3 mg/m² I.V. days 1, 22
Dexamethasone 3 mg/m² PO days 1–8, then
  1.5 mg/m² PO days 9–26 every 6 weeks

CAVP

CCNU 90 mg/m² PO day 1
Melphalan 7.5 mg/m² PO days 1–5
Etoposide 100 mg/m² PO days 6–10
Prednisone 40 mg/m² PO days 1–10 every 6 weeks

EVAP

Etoposide 120 mg/m² I.V. days 1, 8, 15
Vinblastine 4 mg/m² I.V. days 1, 8, 15
Cytarabine 30 mg/m² I.V. days 1, 8, 15
Cisplatin 40 mg/m² I.V. days 1, 8, 15 every 4 weeks

(Longo D. The use of chemotherapy in the treatment of Hodgkin's disease. Semin Oncol 1990;17: 716–735)

whose prior remission was shorter than 1 year the opportunity to use their temporary responsiveness to chemotherapy as a way of reducing tumor volume before intensive therapy and marrow or stem cell support.

These data and others indicate the importance of adequate dosing in the successful treatment of advanced Hodgkin's disease. With the advent of colony-stimulating factors to maintain or increase doses of drugs, it may be possible to reduce the primary failure rate in newly diagnosed patients, which also should have the added benefit of reducing the risk of long-term complications.[370–373] Some new studies have incorporated this approach in their design.[361]

For third-line therapy, the selection of a particular salvage treatment program for a patient no longer responsive to standard regimens is complicated by the heterogeneity of the available data. The literature is summarized in Table 51-

13.[347,348,368,374,376,377,382-388] The problem of small patient numbers in all studies is compounded by the extensive mixture of important disease variables and prior response duration. However, the same general theme runs through these data. The best results are attained in patients who experience relapse asymptomatically, who have recurrent nodal disease, and who had attained a prior complete remission of long duration.

The CEP (lomustine, etoposide, prednimustine) salvage program, developed by the Milan group, is the most interesting among those in Table 51–13. It works as well or better than any other regimen, and all the drugs are administered by the oral route.[379-381] CEP has been used effectively with MOPP or ABVD in alternating cycles in patients who fail to respond to ABVD or MOPP, respectively. ABDIC and VABCD contain doxorubicin, bleomycin, dacarbazine, CCNU, and prednisone and resemble ABVD except for the inclusion of a nitrosourea.[375,386] They are most useful in patients not responding to MOPP but may not be superior to ABVD alone; no data are available for comparison. The patient population in the VABCD study was more uniform and the results easier to interpret. Fifteen patients, for example, had stage IV disease, 11 with systemic symptoms. Eight complete remissions occurred in this group and 5 patients remained disease free at the time of the report.

B-CAVE has three of the ABVD drugs plus the nitrosourea, CCNU, but not dacarbazine.[378] Forty-four percent of patients who did not respond to the MOPP regimen had complete remissions, and a quarter of these patients had not progressed at 4 years, although not all were disease free.

No other program has emerged as a major improvement over these regimens. For those who fail to respond to MOPP, the choices are ABVD, ABVD-like combinations, or CEP. For patients who do not respond to ABVD, CEP appears to be the treatment of choice, although the PCVP program (procarbazine, cyclophosphamide, vinblastine, prednisone), which resembles the MOPP program, may be a useful alternative crossover regimen after ABVD failure.[382] Physicians are urged to use these programs in their recommended doses and schedules.

TREATMENT OF STAGE IIIA DISEASE

Several studies support the use of combination chemotherapy alone for treatment of stage IIIA patients who do not have bulky mediastinal disease. A 94% 10-year disease-free survival rate was reported for patients with asymptomatic disease in the original NCI study. Lister[298] and Crowther[299] reported essentially identical results for patients with stage IIIA disease (96% and 91%, respectively) using MVPP. Results in the Lister study were significantly better than the 60% 10-year disease-free survival rate obtained with TNI alone, and the results of the chemotherapy-alone arm were identical to that obtained with combined-modality therapy in the Crowther study. It appears that combination chemotherapy alone is optimal for patients with stage IIIA disease. However, for asymptomatic patients with bulky mediastinal masses or other sites massively involved by tumor, combined-modality treatment is superior to either modality alone.

In the Cotswald system, stage IIIA is divided into IIIA1 and IIIA2 by the extent of disease. IIIA1 is a laparotomy designation of cases, many which would have been clinical stage IIA. In this subgroup, results with radiation therapy alone appear equivalent to chemotherapy.

CHEMOTHERAPY ALONE AND COMBINED-MODALITY TREATMENT IN EARLY-STAGE DISEASE

One principle that has emerged from preclinical animal studies is that curability is inversely related to tumor burden. After there was sufficient evidence that drugs could cure advanced disease, it was logical to explore the use of chemotherapy in early-stage Hodgkin's disease. Adding chemotherapy to radiation therapy in early-stage Hodgkin's disease patients improves disease control, but overall survival is not significantly higher than with radiation therapy alone in patients treated with combined modality therapy, because of the ability to salvage radiation failures with drugs.[389-392] Usually, disease-free survival is about 10% better for patients receiving combined-modality therapy, but about 10% to 20% of these patients die of secondary acute leukemia and solid tumors related to the combined use of chemotherapy with radiation therapy.[393-395]

A prospective randomized study from Stanford suggests that combination chemotherapy may permit the reduction in radiation fields. Horming and colleagues found that patients receiving involved-field radiation therapy plus six cycles of VBM (vinblastine, bleomycin, methotrexate) chemotherapy had a somewhat better freedom from progression and comparable survival than those treated with total or subtotal nodal irradiation.[396] Most of the 67 patients in this small study had stage IA or IIA disease. It is not clear whether VBM, which has not been tested in advanced-stage disease or without radiation therapy, would be effective adjuvant therapy in the subgroup of stage IIB patients felt by the Stanford group to require combined-modality treatment. The virtue of the VBM regimen is its limited toxicity. It spares fertility and is thought to be less carcinogenic than other available standard options.

The first reported experience with combination chemotherapy in early-stage Hodgkin's disease was from the NCI project in Uganda, East Africa, where there were limited diagnostic and radiation therapy facilities.[397] Forty-eight Ugandan children with early clinical stages of Hodgkin's disease were treated with MOPP combination chemotherapy; 42 (88%) achieved a complete response, and 75% of the children were alive and free of disease at 8 years.

Henry Ekert and his colleagues in Australia and New Zealand demonstrated the efficacy of an approach based on the use of combination chemotherapy in clinically staged children.[398] They treated 38 children with stage I or II Hodgkin's disease with MOPP or ChlVPP. Thirty-seven (97%) of these children obtained a complete response to therapy; 1 patient relapsed and was induced into a durable second remission by salvage therapy. The overall survival rate was 94%, and the disease-free survival rate was 97%.

Two prospective randomized studies examined whether combination chemotherapy alone is superior to combined modality therapy in patients with early-stage Hodgkin's disease. Investigators at the University of Maryland Cancer Center randomized 36 patients with stage IB to IIIA disease to receive extended-field radiation therapy followed by MOPP combination chemotherapy or to receive MOPP alone.[399] With a median follow-up of over 6 years, no significant differences occurred between the combined-modality group (75% of patients alive and free of disease) and the group treated with MOPP alone (80% of patients alive and free of disease). However, overall toxicity of the two regimens was different. Viral and fungal infections occurred more frequently in the combined-modality group. Four of the 17 patients treated with combined-modality therapy had toxicities related to the use of radiation therapy; constrictive pericarditis produced limited exercise capacity in 2 patients, and 2 patients developed hypothyroidism. There were three second neoplasms: two squamous cell lung cancers (one on each arm of the study) and one acute leukemia in a patient who had received irradiation and chemotherapy. The study was too small to lead to any conclusions; it provides no evidence that combined-modality therapy is more efficacious than combination chemotherapy alone, and it appears to be associated with more late toxicities.

Pavlovsky and his colleagues performed a prospective, randomized study of clinical stage I and II patients with Hodgkin's disease, comparing CVPP (cyclophosphamide, vincristine, procarbazine, prednisone) chemotherapy alone to CVPP chemotherapy with involved-field radiation therapy administered between the third and fourth cycles of chemotherapy.[400] Although patients were said to be clinically staged, this examination did not include lymphography in one third of the patients. About one third of the patients probably had more advanced stage disease. Another caveat in interpreting this study is related to the fact that the cyclophosphamide and vinblastine were arbitrarily given only once per cycle (intravenously on day 1) in this highly treatable group of patients. This is half as frequent as the usual administration of these agents. Chemotherapy was administered in markedly attenuated doses. Nevertheless, in the patients without poor prognostic factors, those randomized to receive CVPP alone had an 88% complete response rate, 77% 7-year disease-free survival rate, and 92% overall survival rate at 7 years. No significant differences existed between dose-attenuated CVPP alone and dose-attenuated CVPP plus involved-field radiation therapy. The treatment outcome in patients with bulky mediastinal disease favored the use of combined-modality therapy.

These studies provide no evidence that combined-modality therapy is superior to combination chemotherapy alone in the treatment of early-stage Hodgkin's disease.

Two prospective randomized studies compared the efficacy of radiation therapy alone with combination chemotherapy alone in early-stage Hodgkin's disease. Cimino and colleagues randomized 89 patients with pathologic staged IA or IIA disease to receive subtotal nodal radiation therapy or six cycles of MOPP chemotherapy.[401] Complete responses were obtained in all patients treated with radiation therapy and in 40 (91%) of 44 patients treated with MOPP. The disease-free survival and overall survival rates of patients treated with radiation therapy were 74% and 94%, respectively. For patients treated with MOPP, disease-free and overall survival rates were 73% and 87%, respectively. There were no significant differences between the two arms. Relapse on both arms was more common in patients with massive mediastinal disease.

In a follow-up report, it was observed that patients relapsing from chemotherapy-induced complete remission were less responsive to salvage therapy and that their survival from the time of relapse was 15%, compared with 85% for the group

relapsing from radiation therapy. This difference was statistically significant, but because the number of patients relapsing is small, the overall results of the study are not altered. As would be expected, infertility was a problem for more patients treated with MOPP chemotherapy. All the men were azoospermic, and half the women developed amenorrhea after MOPP therapy, compared with 0% and 10%, respectively, after irradiation.

The NCI began a prospective, randomized trial comparing subtotal nodal radiation with MOPP in early-stage Hodgkin's disease in 1978.[402,403] The study population included 136 patients with stage IA, IB, IIA, IIB, or IIIA1 Hodgkin's disease. Patients had exploratory laparotomy to complete their staging in most cases (92%). Patients with peripheral stage IA disease (usually defined as stage I disease located above the clavicles) were not randomized and were treated with radiation therapy, because their survival with this approach is 95% or better in most series, and one of these patients failed treatment. Patients with stage IA (central), IB, IIA, IIB, or IIIA1 disease were randomized to receive subtotal nodal radiation therapy (*i.e.*, mantle and paraaortic fields) or MOPP combination chemotherapy precisely as it was administered to patients with advanced-stage disease, with no dose reduction.

In the randomized portion of the NCI study, 49 (96%) of the 51 patients who received radiation therapy achieved complete remissions, but 17 (35%) of the complete responders relapsed, 7 within the treatment portals, 5 outside a treatment portal, and 5 within and outside a treatment portal. Ten (20%) patients randomized to receive radiation therapy died, 7 of Hodgkin's disease and 3 free of Hodgkin's disease. Fifty-two (96%) of the 54 evaluable patients who were randomized to receive MOPP chemotherapy achieved a complete response. A significantly smaller fraction (7 patients, 13%) relapsed, all in previously involved sites of disease. Four (7%) patients died, 3 of Hodgkin's disease and 1 free of disease. Figure 51–18 shows the disease-free survival of the complete responders on the randomized portion of the study. The 10-year disease-free survival rate for MOPP-treated patients was 86%; for radiation therapy-treated patients, it was 60%. The difference between these curves is statistically significant in favor of MOPP treatment ($p_2=0.009$). Figure 51–19 shows the overall survival for all randomized patients. The 10-year overall survival rate for MOPP-treated patients is 92%; for radiation therapy-treated patients, it is 76%. The difference between the curves is on the borderline for statistical significance in favor of MOPP treatment ($p_2=0.051$).

In our study, 8 (47%) of 17 patients relapsing after radiation therapy are alive and free of disease after salvage therapy. Three (43%) of the 7 patients relapsing from a MOPP-induced complete response are alive and free of disease after salvage therapy. Although the number of patients relapsing in our study, as in the Cimino study, is small, we do not see evidence that relapsed patients are more refractory to salvage therapy if their primary treatment was combination chemotherapy. Analysis of prognostic factors in the NCI study demonstrated that the advantage of MOPP over radiation therapy was highly significant in two groups of patients: those with massive mediastinal involvement and those with stage IIIA disease. All 11 such patients treated with MOPP are alive and free of disease in their first remission. On the other hand, 6 of 8 patients with massive mediastinal or stage IIIA disease who

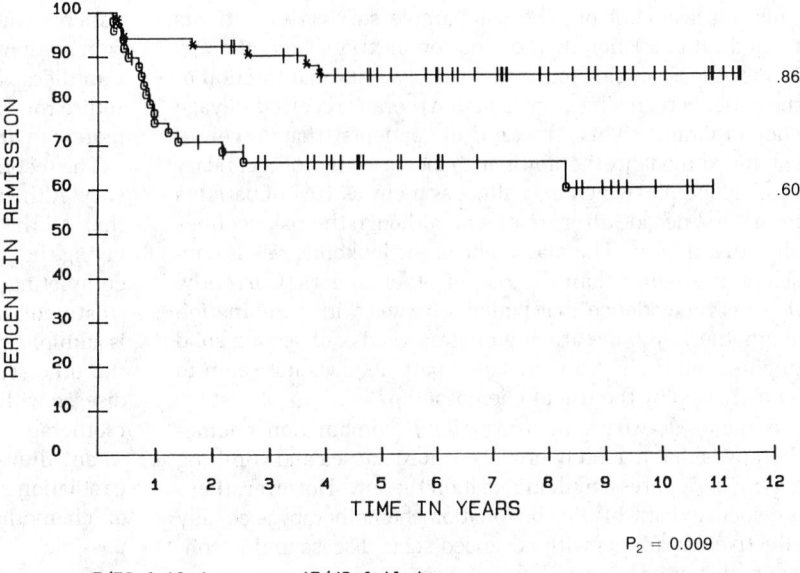

FIGURE 51–18. Kaplan-Meier plot of disease-free survival of patients randomized to receive MOPP (∗) or radiation therapy (○) who achieved complete response on the NCI early stage Hodgkin's disease study. The disease-free survival rate was significantly higher among patients treated with MOPP chemotherapy. (Longo DL, DeVita VT. The use of combination chemotherapy in the treatment of early stage Hodgkin's disease. In: DeVita VT, Hellman S, Rosenberg SA, ed. Important advances in oncology. Philadelphia: JB Lippincott, 1992:155–166)

were randomized to receive radiation therapy relapsed, and 5 died (p_2=0.0004 for disease-free survival; p_2=0.0015 for overall survival—both in favor of MOPP). When these two subsets of patients are excluded from both arms of the randomized study, the differences between MOPP and irradiation in disease-free and overall survival rates are no longer significant. In the subsets of patients treated with radiation therapy today, MOPP combination chemotherapy and radiation therapy are equally effective.

These data are sufficiently good to allow the use of combination chemotherapy for patients with early-stage disease, but this population is highly curable by radiation therapy, the delivery of which is better standardized in the United States than chemotherapy. Reducing drug doses arbitrarily in this population reduces the cure rate, and if there is any risk of this occurring, radiation therapy is the better choice for the patient. Theoretically, these data substantiate the inverse rule,

because the complete response rate increased from ±80%, achievable in advanced-stage patients, to 96% in early-stage patients with reduced body burden of tumor. There is a commensurate decrease in the relapse rate, from between 35% and 45% to 13%.

The major reason to fear radiation therapy is the development of second solid tumors, although the recently reported risk of premature death from coronary artery disease adds another dimension of concern.[267] By 15 years after treatment, 13% of patients have developed a second solid tumor, and it appears that the risk continues to increase with time.[194] Irradiated patients appear to be at significantly increased risk for lung cancer, melanoma, breast cancer, thyroid cancer, sarcomas, and gastric cancer. Although patients treated with radiation therapy alone have a low risk of developing secondary acute leukemia, about one third of radiation-treated patients relapse and require combination chemotherapy for op-

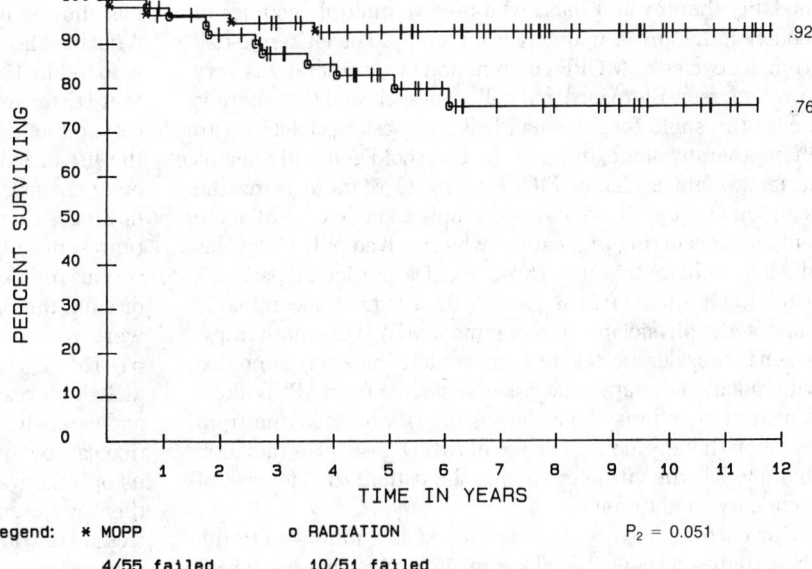

FIGURE 51–19. Kaplan-Meier plot of overall survival of patients randomized to receive MOPP (∗) or radiation therapy (○) on the NCI early stage Hodgkin's disease study. MOPP-treated patients had a survival advantage of borderline statistical significance. (Longo DL, DeVita VT. The use of combination chemotherapy in the treatment of early stage Hodgkin's disease. In: DeVita VT, Hellman S, Rosenberg SA, ed. Important advances in oncology. Philadelphia: JB Lippincott, 1992:155–166)

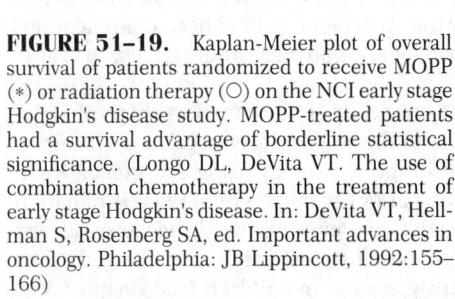

timal disease control. The comparable survival of patients treated with radiation therapy and combination chemotherapy is due at least in part to the fact that a substantial fraction of the patients relapsing after radiation therapy received salvage chemotherapy. This fraction of patients that received combined-modality therapy is at an increased risk of secondary acute leukemia, which may affect as many as 10% of patients in the first decade after treatment, although the risk declines after that time.[394] The magnitude of the leukemic risk is considerably smaller than the risk of other tumors. Currently, there is no evidence that patients treated with combination chemotherapy alone are at an increased risk of second solid tumors, and the risk in irradiated patients does not seem to be increased by the use of chemotherapy.

A major drawback to using MOPP combination chemotherapy is that it acutely produces more nausea and vomiting and myelosuppression than radiation therapy. However, there is evidence that ChlVPP combination chemotherapy is equally effective in patients with advanced-stage disease and is considerably better tolerated. By inference and according to the experience reported by Ekert in children with clinical early-stage disease, ChlVPP should be effective in adults with clinical early-stage disease who have an extraordinary fear of nausea and vomiting.

The major chronic toxic effect of concern with MOPP chemotherapy is infertility, which affects 80% of men and most women older than 26 years of age. Interviews with patients who entered the NCI randomized study suggested that this toxicity may be relevant only for a fraction of patients. Among the 21 men evaluated who were treated with MOPP chemotherapy, only 4 wanted children. Among 30 women treated with MOPP, 10 desired to have children, and 6 were successful. Nevertheless, for patients in whom fertility status is an overriding concern, ABVD chemotherapy appears considerably less toxic to the male and female gonads and should be as effective as MOPP chemotherapy in early-stage disease. Primary fertility-sparing chemotherapy is a valid option for this patient subset.

The concern about secondary acute leukemia in patients treated with MOPP alone is overstated. The major risk of acute leukemia is in patients who are treated with combined-modality therapy and those who receive multiple courses of induction therapy or maintenance therapy. The leukemic risk from six cycles of MOPP combination chemotherapy is very low. Pedersen-Bjergaard and colleagues showed that there is a dose threshold for the small leukemic risk associated with chemotherapy alone and that the threshold generally begins at about eight cycles of MOPP.[402] In 28 years of using the regimen at the NCI, we have seen only a single case of acute leukemia occurring in a patient who received only six cycles of MOPP chemotherapy. However, if a particular patient's fear of acute leukemia is greater than fear of second solid tumors, the physician can recommend ABVD chemotherapy, which is considerably less leukemogenic, even when combined with radiation therapy. The risk of leukemia from ABVD alone is near zero and may be as low as the risk of leukemia from radiation therapy alone. The use of ABVD, instead of radiation therapy, has the virtue of sparing the patient the late risk of secondary solid tumors.

Our current study design, developed as a follow-up to the prior studies, uses ABVD alone for induction therapy for all patients with early-stage disease, and after complete remission, patients are randomized to receive involved-field radiation therapy or to receive no further treatment to assess the future role of radiation therapy in patients who respond completely to drugs.[350]

The techniques of combining irradiation and chemotherapy vary. Although some studies administer all the radiation and then all the chemotherapy, others divide the chemotherapy, giving the radiation after two or three drug cycles, and then completing the chemotherapy. An important principle of treatment is to be sure that at least one treatment modality is administered with appropriate time-dose considerations and the other serves as an adjuvant. For patients with stage II disease with a large mediastinal mass, the full course of chemotherapy should be administered and the irradiation reserved as an adjuvant to the initial site of bulky disease. Extensive irradiation given before chemotherapy may limit the amount of chemotherapy given. This pitfall should be avoided if possible.

HODGKIN'S DISEASE IN HIV-POSITIVE PATIENTS

Although some controversy exists concerning whether Hodgkin's disease is part of the spectrum of AIDS, most epidemiologic studies indicate no evidence to suggest the incidence is higher than might be expected in this young population.[405–410] However, HIV-positive patients with Hodgkin's disease usually present with advanced stage, advanced histology, B symptoms, and unusual patterns of tumor involvement. In contrast to HIV-negative patients, Hodgkin's disease tissues from HIV-positive patients are depleted of helper T lymphocytes and infiltrated with suppressor T cells. Response to chemotherapy has been poor because of poor tolerance to the marrow suppressive effect of drugs and the mucosal toxicity of radiation therapy.[411–413] Outcome is most influenced by whether the HIV-positive patient has clinical manifestations of AIDS at the time of diagnosis.

COMPLICATIONS OF THERAPY

The availability of large populations of long-term survivors has allowed investigators to describe numerous side effects. A detailed list of reported complications in long-term survivors is found in Table 51–14 and reviewed in detail elsewhere.[396] More extensive discussions of the complications of treatment can be found in Chapter 63. Despite the extensive nature of the list of side effects, the lives of long-term survivors are quite normal, because many side effects represent minor annoyances that are easily corrected, occur in few patients, or represent only the potential for future problems. The most serious problem is the risk of developing secondary leukemia or solid tumors in the treatment field. These complications were reviewed previously and are summarized in Table 51–15.

Risk increases dramatically if combination chemotherapy and extensive radiation therapy are used together. This practice can be avoided in most cases by using each modality in its optimal way. The patient is done a disservice if radiation therapy doses or fields are compromised, because salvage treatment with chemotherapy is effective, or if chemotherapy is given concomitantly, except in children (see Chapter 50).

TABLE 51–14. Long-Term Complications in Patients Cured of Hodgkin's Disease

Complication	Etiology and Risk Factors	Management and Prevention
Immunologic dysfunction	Underlying disease, therapy	Appropriate vaccinations
Herpes zoster-varicella	Underlying disease, therapy	Systemic antiviral therapy, zoster immune globulin
Pneumococcal sepsis	Splenectomy, functional asplenia after radiation therapy (RT)	Pretherapy pneumonococcal vaccine, selected antibiotic prophylaxis, avoid unneccessary staging splenectomy
Nonlymphocytic leukemia	Therapy, older than 40 y	Avoid combined-modality therapy for HD. Supportive care, low-dose chemotherapy, aggressive therapy ± bone marrow transplant
Myelodysplastic syndromes	Therapy, older than 40 y	Same as above
Non-Hodgkin's lymphoma	Therapy	Aggressive combination chemotherapy
Solid tumors	Direct or indirect RT exposure	Conventional management
Thymic hyperplasia	Underlying disease, therapy	Resection
Hypothyroidism	Direct or indirect RT exposure	Hormone replacement, thyroid suppression during therapy (?)
Thyroid cancer	Direct or indirect RT exposure, chronic thyroid stimulation	Thyroid suppression
Male infertility	Therapy, underlying disease	Attempt sperm storage, testicular shielding during RT, suppression of spermatogenesis during CT (?), alternative chemotherapy regimens
Male impotence	Therapy, underlying disease	Counseling, trial of testosterone
Female infertility	Therapy	Oophoropexy, ovarian suppression during therapy (?), cyclic estrogen replacement
Female dyspareunia	Therapy, underlying disease	Counseling, cyclic estrogen replacement
Pericarditis, acute	Mediastinal RT, recall with chemotherapy (CT) after RT	Appropriate RT shielding and technique, avoid doxorubicin after RT, antiinflammatory medication, pericardiocentesis
Pericarditis, chronic	Mediastinal RT	Appropriate RT shielding and technique, pericardiectomy
Cardiomyopathy	Mediastinal RT, doxorubicin, recall with CT after RT	Appropriate RT shielding and technique, avoid doxorubicin after RT, monitor for early signs of toxicity, limit cumulative doxorubicin dose, supportive medical management
Pneumonitis, acute	Direct or indirect RT, bleomycin, nitrosoureas, recall with CT after RT	Appropriate RT shielding and technique, monitor for early signs of toxicity, avoid known toxic drugs, avoid excessive pO_2
Pneumonitis, chronic	Same as above	Supportive management
Avascular necrosis	Steroid therapy, underlying disease (?)	Antiinflammatory medications, joint surgery
Growth retardation	Pediatric RT	Minimize RT, use symmetric RT fields
Dental caries	Salivary change after RT	Maintain good oral hygiene, daily fluoride treatments

Using chemotherapy in full doses minimizes the number of drugs and programs that patients need to be exposed to as well. The problem of fertility and treatment is discussed in Chapter 63.

NEW DRUGS AND BIOLOGICS

The testing of new agents for Hodgkin's disease presents a challenging problem.[414] Because treatment of newly diagnosed patients has been so successful and some patients are curable with second-line therapy or with high doses of chemotherapy with ABMT support, the patient who fails to respond to all available treatment is a poor subject for new agent testing. Bone marrow reserve is usually minimal, and the advanced nature of the disease makes long-term observation difficult. This is a problem faced by oncologists for all tumors that respond well to chemotherapy, such as childhood leukemia and testicular cancer. Patients with advanced Hodgkin's disease should be referred to institutes conducting trials on new drug or biologic therapies.[415–423]

Treatment with biologics should be considered as an alter-native to chemotherapy because the side effects of the two modalities are often different. The experience with biologics in Hodgkin's disease is not extensive. Some useful responses and one complete remission have been reported with the use of isotopic immunoglobulins directed against ferritin.[424] Improvement in labeling with isotopes other than iodine 131 may improve the effectiveness of this approach. The use of IL-2 plus lymphokine-activated killer cells in Hodgkin's disease is in its early stages. Some investigators have begun to combine less toxic analogs of active drugs with standard agents in standard combinations to test retention of efficacy with reduced overall toxicity as a way of introducing new agents. Given the heterogeneity of previously treated patients, few useful data have emerged from this approach.

RECOMMENDATIONS FOR TREATMENT OF HODGKIN'S DISEASE BY STAGE

Although the use of laparotomy should be considered as part of the treatment plan, it is unnecessary for patients who receive chemotherapy, regardless of the results of abdominal

TABLE 51–15. Risk Factors for Secondary Acute Myelocytic Leukemia After Therapy for Hodgkin's Disease

Therapy Category	Relative Risk	% Cumulative Risk at 10 Years
Radiation therapy (RT) alone	Very low	0
Induction chemotherapy alone		
MOPP	Low	2–3
BCNU regimens	Intermediate	3–6
ABVD	Low	?
Combined-modality therapy		
Limited field RT plus MOPP	Low	2–3
Extensive RT plus MOPP	High	4–8
Salvage therapy	High	5–15
Age greater than 40 y	Very high	25–40
Maintenance therapy		
All therapy	High	5–10
Prolonged alkylating agents	Very high	10–30

exploration. It appears that certain early-stage presentations have such a low incidence of abdominal disease that laparotomy is not needed, and these patients may receive radiation therapy alone without surgical staging. Clinical stage I male patients with lymphocyte-predominant or nodular sclerosing histology or with high neck disease and all supradiaphragmatic female stage I patients may receive radiation therapy to the mantle only, without laparotomy, unless there is bulky mediastinal disease. For most of the remainder of the stage I and II patients, laparotomy is required if irradiation alone is contemplated.

Patients with pathologic stage I or IIA Hodgkin's disease with supradiaphragmatic disease and without large mediastinal masses should be treated with mantle irradiation. For most patients, paraaortic fields should be included. Exceptions to this rule may be patients without evidence of any mediastinal disease and nodular sclerosis or lymphocyte-predominant histology. Continued use of the paraaortic field in these patients is uncertain and must be left to individual judgment.

Clinical stage I or IIA patients with massive mediastinal masses should be spared laparotomy and splenectomy and treated with combination chemotherapy initially and then with irradiation to the mediastinum. Laparotomy is not indicated because it does not significantly alter therapy and does have an added anesthesia risk. Full-dose chemotherapy should be given with the radiation volume restricted. The total dose of radiation under these circumstances may be reduced to 3500 to 4000 cGy.

Presentations as subdiaphragmatic disease is almost invariably diagnosed by laparotomy. This disease should be treated with paraaortic and pelvic irradiation for pelvic or inguinal presentation. Patients who present with disease in the periaortic nodes produce a complicated problem, because appropriate treatment would be TNI. Because of complications associated with this technique, especially if chemotherapy must be given for failure, the physician should consider seriously whether they should be treated with primary chemotherapy.

Patients with stage IIB disease should be treated with sub-total nodal radiation. Combined-modality therapy probably should not be used in unless they patients have bulky mediastinal disease or their B symptoms do not abate with the mantle radiation therapy field. Patients with clinical stage IIB disease who have not been evaluated by laparotomy should be treated primarily with chemotherapy.

Radiation therapy alone is not indicated in most stage III patients. The possible exception is stage IIIA patients having only upper abdominal and minimal (<5 tumor nodules) splenic involvement (stage IIIA1); irradiation is administered after laparotomy and splenectomy. For the remainder of stage IIIA patients, chemotherapy alone is the treatment of choice. Irradiation should not be added in these groups: it should be used only in patients with massive mediastinal involvement.

Radiation therapy should be limited in children. The data indicate that the paraaortic fields can be omitted in pathologic stage I or IIA pediatric Hodgkin's disease patients.[244] A treatment volume reduction, even further than the mantle, is desirable, because the radiation produces significant retardation of bone growth. This drawback must be balanced against the risks of recurrence, especially in the very young. The irradiated volume must be limited, and care should be taken to attempt symmetric irradiation to limit the deformities produced by unilateral asymmetric bone growth. For young children, we recommend chemotherapy, with avoidance of irradiation as much as possible. For the young adolescent with supradiaphragmatic presentation after pathologic staging, mantle fields offer the best treatment success with the fewest complications.

Although the data on the successful treatment of early-stage disease with chemotherapy allows substitution of combination chemotherapy for radiation therapy, chemotherapy for stage I and II patients should be used selectively, usually in patients who have limited access to sophisticated radiation therapy equipment and techniques and in some growing children.

REFERENCES

1. Kaplan HS. Hodgkin's disease. 2nd ed. Cambridge: Harvard University Press, 1980.
2. Hodgkin T. On some morbid appearances of the absorbent glands and spleen. Med Chir Trans 1832;17:68–114.
3. Bright R. Observations on abdominal tumours and intumescence. Guy's Hosp Rep 1838;3:401–460.
4. Wilks S. Cases of enlargement of lymphatic glands and spleen (or Hodgkin's disease), with remarks. Guy's Hosp Rep 1865;11:56–67.
5. Nuland SB. The lymphatic contiguity of Hodgkin's disease: A historical study. Bull N Y Acad Med 1981;57:776–789.
6. Craigie D. Case of disease of the spleen, in which death took place in consequence in the presence of purulent matter in the blood. Edinburgh Med Surg J 1845;64:400–413.
7. Bennett JH. Case of hypertrophy of the spleen and liver in which death took place from suppuration of the blood. Edinburgh Med Surg J 1845;64:413–423.
8. Virchow R. Weisses Blut, neue Notizen aus den Geb der Naturund Heikunde. (Froriep's neue Notizen) 1845;36:151–156.
9. Roulet F. Dasprinare Retothelsarkom der Lymphkonten. Virchows Arch [A] 1930;277:15–47.
10. Burkitt D. A sarcoma involving the jaws in African children. Br J Surg 1958;46:218–223.
11. Greenfield WS. Specimens illustrative of the pathology of lymphadenoma and leucocythemia. Trans Pathol Soc London 1878;29:272–304.
12. Goldmann EE. Beitrug zu der Lehre von dem malignen Lymphom. Zentralbl Allg Pathol 1892;3:665–690.
13. Sternberg C. Uber eine Eigenartige unter dem Bilde der Pseudoleukamie verlaufende Tuberculose des lymphatichon Apparates. Z Heilk 1898;19:21–90.
14. Reed DM. On the pathological changes in Hodgkin's disease, with especial reference to its relation to tuberculosis. Johns Hopkins Hosp Rev 1902;10:133–196.
15. Seif GSF, Spriggs AI. Chromosome changes in Hodgkin's disease. JNCI 1967;39:557–470.

16. MacMahon B. Epidemiological evidence of the nature of Hodgkin's disease. Cancer 1957;10:1045–1054.

17. Correa P, O'Conor GT, Berard CW, et al. International comparability and reproducibility in histologic subclassification of Hodgkin's disease. JNCI 1973;50:1429–1435.

18. Mueller NE. Hodgkin's disease. In: Schnottenfeld D, Fraumeni J, eds. Cancer epidemiology and prevention. 2nd ed. New York: Oxford University Press, 1992.

19. Steiner PE. Hodgkin's disease: Search for infective agent and attempts at experimental reproduction. Arch Pathol 1934;17:749–763.

20. L'Esperance ES. Experimental inoculation of chickens with Hodgkin's nodes. J Immunol 1929;16:37–60,.

21. Van Rooyan CE. Etiology of Hodgkin's disease with special reference to *B. tuberculosis avis*. Br Med J 1933;1:50–51.

22. Van Rooyan CE. Recent experimental work on the etiology of Hodgkin's disease. Br Med J 1934;2:519–524.

23. Miller RW, Beebe GW. Infectious mononucleosis and the empirical risk of cancer. JNCI 1973;50:315–321.

24. Connolly RR, Chistene BW. A cohort study of cancer following infectious mononucleosis. Cancer Res 1974;34:1172–1178.

25. Rosdahl N, Larsen SO, Clemmensen J. Hodgkin's disease in patients with previous mononucleosis, 30 years' experience. Br Med J 1974;2:253–256.

26. Munoz N, Davidson RJ, Witthoff B, et al. Infectious mononucleosis and Hodgkin's disease. Int J Cancer 1978;22:10–13.

27. Nonoyama M, Kawai Y, Huang CH, et al. Epstein-Barr virus DNA in Hodgkin's disease, American Burkitt's lymphoma and other human tumors. Cancer Res 1974;34:1228–1231.

28. Vianna NJ, Greenwald P, Davies JNP. Extended epidemic of Hodgkin's disease in high school students. Lancet 1971;1:1209–1210.

29. Vianna JH, Polan AK. Epidemiological evidence for transmission of Hodgkin's disease. N Engl J Med 1973;289:499–502.

30. Smith PG, Pike MC, Kinlam LJ, et al. Contacts between young patients with Hodgkin's disease: A case control study. Lancet 1977;2:59–62.

31. Zack MM, Heath CW Jr, Andrews MD, et al. High school contact among persons with leukemia and lymphoma. JNCI 1977;59:1343–1349.

32. Gutterman S, Cole P, Levitan TR. Evidence against transmission of Hodgkin's disease in high schools. N Engl J Med 1979;300:1000–1011.

33. Gutensohn N, Cole P. Childhood social environment and Hodgkin's disease. N Engl J Med 1981;304:135–140.

34. Milham S Jr, Hesser J. Hodgkin's disease in woodworkers. Lancet 1967;2:136–137.

35. Vianna NJ, Greenwald P, Davies JNP. Tonsillectomy and Hodgkin's disease: The lymphoid tissue barrier. Lancet 1971;1:431–432.

36. Bierman HR. Human appendix and neoplasia. Cancer 1968;21:109–118.

37. Hyams L, Wynder EL. Appendectomy and cancer risk: An epidemiological evaluation. J Chronic Dis 1968;21:319–415.

38. Graff KS, Simon RM, Yankee RA, et al. HLA antigens in Hodgkin's disease: Histopathologic and clinical correlations. JNCI 1974;52:1087–1090.

39. Chakaavarti A, Hallaran SL, Bale SJ et al. Etiological heterogeneity in Hodgkin's disease: HLA linked and unlinked determinants of susceptibility independent of histological concordance. Genet Epidemiol 1986;3:407–415.

40. Gutterman S, Barton JW III, Eby NL. Increased sex concordance of sibling pairs with Becket's disease, Hodgkin's disease, multiple sclerosis, and sarcadosis. Am J Epidemiol 1987;126:365–369.

41. Robertson SJ, Lowman JT, Gutterman S et al. Familial Hodgkin's disease: A clinical and laboratory investigation. Cancer 1987;59:1314–1319.

42. Lukes RJ, Tindle BH, Parker JW. Reed-Sternberg-like cells in infectious mononucleosis. Lancet 1969;2:1000–1004.

43. Strum SB, Dark JK, Rappaport H. Observations of cells resembling Sternberg-Reed cells in conditions other than Hodgkin's disease. Cancer 1970;26:176–190.

44. Jackson H Jr, Parker F Jr: Hodgkin's disease. II. Pathology. N Engl J Med 1944;231:35–44.

45. Lukes RJ, Butler JJ, Hicks ED. Natural history of Hodgkin's disease as related to its pathologic picture. Cancer 1966;19:317–344.

46. Langhans T. Das Maligne Lymphosarkom (Pseuddukamie). Virchows Arch [A] 1872;54:509–537.

47. Pell PK. Zur Symptomatologie der sogenannten Pseudoleukemie II. Pseudoleukemie oder chronisches Ruckfallsfieber? Klin Wochenschr 1887;24:644–646.

48. Parker F Jr, Jackson H Jr, Fitzhugh G, et al. Studies of diseases of the lymphoid and myeloid tissues: IV. Skin reactions to human and avian tuberculin. J Immunol 1932;22:277–282.

49. Lukes RJ. Relationship of histologic features to clinical stages in Hodgkin's disease. AJR 1963;90:944–955.

50. Wright MD. Lymphocyte predominance Hodgkin's disease. N Engl J Med 1988;319:246 [Letter to the Editor re Regula DP Jr, Hoppe RT, Weiss LM. Nodular and diffuse types of lymphocyte predominance Hodgkin's disease. N Engl J Med 1988;318:214–219].

51. Poppema S, Kaiserling E, Lennert K. Hodgkin's disease with lymphocyte predominance, nodular type (nodular paragranuloma) and progressively transformed germinal centers—a cytohistological study. Histopathology 1979;3:295.

52. Poppema S, Kaiserling E, Lennert K. Nodular paragranuloma and progressively transformed germinal centers. Ultrastructural and immunohistologic findings. Virchows Arch [B] 1979;31:211–225.

53. Burns BF, Colby TV, Dorfman RF. Differential diagnostic features of nodular L&H Hodgkin's disease, including progressive transformation of germinal centers. Am J Surg Pathol 1984;8:253–261.

54. Pinkus GS, Said JW. Hodgkin's disease, lymphocyte predominance type, nodular—a distinct entity? Unique staining profile for L&H variants of Reed-Sternberg cells defined by monoclonal antibodies to leukocyte common antigen, granulocyte-specific antigen, and B-cell-specific antigen. Am J Pathol 1985;118:1–6.

55. Coles FB, Cartun RW, Pastuszak WT. Hodgkin's disease, lymphocyte-predominant type: Immunoreactivity with B-cell antibodies. Mod Pathol 1988;1:274–278.

56. Pinkus GS, Said JW. Hodgkin's disease, lymphocyte predominance type, nodular—further evidence for a B cell derivation. Am J Pathol 1985;133:211–217.

57. Hansmann M-L, Stein H, Dallenbach F, Fellbaum C. Diffuse lymphocyte-predominant Hodgkin's disease (diffuse paragranuloma). A variant of the B-cell-derived nodular type. Am J Pathol 1991;138:29–36.

58. Sundeen JT, Cossman J, Klein M. Lymphocyte predominant Hodgkin's disease nodular subtype with coexistent "large cell lymphoma": Histological progression or composite malignancy? Am J Surg Pathol 1988;12:599–606.

59. Miettinen M, Franssila KO, Saxén E. Hodgkin's disease, lymphocytic predominance nodular. Increased risk for subsequent non-Hodgkin's lymphomas. Cancer 1983;51:2293–2300.

60. Chittal SM, Alard C, Rossi J-F, et al. Further phenotypic evidence that nodular, lymphocyte-predominant Hodgkin's disease is a large B-cell lymphoma in evolution. Am J Surg Pathol 1990;14:1024–1035.

61. Miller TP, Byrne GE, Jones SE. Mistaken clinical and pathologic diagnoses of Hodgkin's disease: A Southwest Oncology Group study. Cancer Treat Rep 1982;66:645–651.

62. Kant JA, Hubbard SM, Longo DL, et al. The pathologic and clinical heterogeneity of lymphocyte depleted Hodgkin's disease. J Clin Oncol 1986;4:284–294.

63. Neiman RS, Rosen PJ, Lukes RJ. Lymphocyte-depletion Hodgkin's disease. A clinicopathological entity. N Engl J Med 1973;288:751–755.

64. Schoeppel SL, Hoppe RT, Dorfman RF, et al. Hodgkin's disease in homosexual men with generalized lymphadenopathy. Ann Intern Med 1985;102:68–70.

65. Ioachim HL, Cooper MC, Hellman GC. Lymphomas in men at high risk for acquired immune deficiency syndrome (AIDS). Cancer 1985;56:2831–2842.

66. Jaffe ES, Clark J, Steis R, et al. Lymph node pathology of HTLV and HTLV-associated neoplasms. Cancer Res 1985;45:4662S–4664S.

67. Anagnostou D, Parker JW, Taylor CR, et al. Lacunar cells of nodular sclerosing Hodgkin's disease. An ultrastructural and immunohistologic study. Cancer 1977;39:1032–1043.

68. Kadin ME, Glatstein E, Dorfman RF. Clinicopathologic study of 117 untreated patients subject to laparotomy for the staging of Hodgkin's disease. Cancer 1971;27:1277–1294.

69. Strum SB, Rappaport H. Interrelations of the histologic types of Hodgkin's disease. Arch Pathol 1971;91:127–134.

70. DeVita VT Jr, Simon RM, Hubbard SM, et al. Curability of advanced Hodgkin's disease with chemotherapy: Long-term follow-up of MOPP treated patients at NCI. Ann Intern Med 1980;92:587–595.

71. Mann RB, Jaffe, ES, Berard CW. Malignant lymphomas—a conceptual understanding of morphologic diversity. A review. Am J Pathol 1979;94:105–191.

72. Mauch P, Gorshein D, Cunningham J, et al. Influence of mediastinal adenopathy on site and frequency of relapse in patients with Hodgkin's disease. Cancer Treat Rep 1982;66:809–817.

73. MacLennan KA, Bennett MH, Tu A, et al. Relationship of histopathologic features to survival and relapse in nodular sclerosing Hodgkin's disease. A study of 1659 patients. Cancer 1989;64:1686–1693.

74. Lukes RJ. Criteria for involvement of lymph node, bone marrow, spleen, and liver in Hodgkin's disease. Cancer Res 1971;31:1755–1764.

75. Colby TV, Hoppe RT, Warnke RA. Hodgkin's disease: A clinicopathologic study of 659 cases. Cancer 1981;49:1848–1858.

76. Grogan TM. Hodgkin's disease. In: Jaffe ES, ed. Surgical pathology of lymph nodes and related organs. Philadelphia: WB Saunders, 1985:86–134.

77. Rosai J, Levine GD. Tumors of the thymus. In: Atlas of tumor pathology. 2nd series, fasc. 13. Washington, DC: Armed Forces Institute of Pathology, 1975.

78. Kadin ME, Donaldson SS, Dorfman RF. Isolated granulomas in Hodgkin's disease. N Engl J Med 1970;283:859–861.

79. Order SE, Hellman S. Pathogenesis of Hodgkin's disease. Lancet 1972;1:571–573.

80. DeVita VT. Lymphocyte reactivity in Hodgkin's disease: A lymphocyte civil war. N Engl J Med 1973;289:801–802.

81. Kadin ME, Stites DP, Levy R, et al. Exogenous immunoglobulin and the macrophage origin of Reed-Sternberg cells in Hodgkin's disease. N Engl J Med 1978;299:1208–1214.

82. Kaplan HS, Gartner S. "Sternberg-Reed" giant cells of Hodgkin's disease: Cultivation in vitro, heterotransplantation, and characterization as neoplastic macrophages. Int J Cancer 1977;19:511–525.

83. Corder MP, Young RC, DeVita VT. Delayed hypersensitivity in patients with cancer. N Engl J Med 1971;285:522–524.

84. Corder MP, Young RC, Brown RS, et al. Phytohemagglutinin induced lymphocyte transformation: The relationship to prognosis of Hodgkin's disease. Blood 1972;39:595–602.

85. Slivarck DJ, Ellis TM, Nawrocki, et al. The impact of Hodgkin's disease on the immune system. Semin Oncol 1990;17:673–682.

86. Poppema S, Bhan AK, Reinherz EL, et al. In situ immunologic characterization of cellular constituents in lymph nodes and spleens involved by Hodgkin's disease. Blood 1982;59:226–232.

87. Garvin AJ, Spicer SS, Parmley RT, et al. Immunohistochemical demonstration of IgG in Reed-Sternberg and other cells in Hodgkin's disease. J Exp Med 1974;139:1077–1083.

88. Kadin ME. Possible origin of the Reed-Sternberg cell from an interdigitating reticulum cell. Cancer Treat Rep 1982;66:601–608.

89. Braylan RC, Jaffe ES, Berard CW. Surface characteristics of Hodgkin's lymphoma cells. Lancet 1974;2:1328–1329.

90. Hsu S, Jaffe ES. Leu M1 and peanut agglutinin stain the neoplastic cells of Hodgkin's disease. Am J Clin Pathol 1984;82:29–32.

91. Diehl V, Kirschner HH, Burrighter H, et al. Characteristics of Hodgkin's disease-derived cell lines. Cancer Treat Rep 1982;66:615–632.

92. Stein H, Gerdes J, Schwab U, et al. Identification of Hodgkin's and Sternberg-Reed cells as a unique cell type derived from a newly detected small-cell population. Int J Cancer 1982;30:445–459.

93. Andreesen R, Osterholz J, Lohr GW, et al. A Hodgkin cell-specific antigen is expressed on a subset of auto- and alloactivated T (helper) lymphoblasts. Blood 1984;63:1299–1302.

94. Hecht TT, Longo DL, Cossman J, et al. Production and characterization of a monoclonal antibody that finds Reed-Sternberg cells. J Immunol 1984;134:4231.

95. Stein H, Mason DY, Gerdes J, et al. The expression of the Hodgkin's disease associated antigen Ki-1 in reactive and neoplastic lymphoid tissue: Evidence that Reed-Sternberg cells and histiocytic malignancies are derived from activated lymphoid cells. Blood 1985;66:848–858.

96. Dichl Von Kalle C, Fonatsch, et al. The cell of origin in Hodgkin's disease. Semin Oncol 1990;17:660–672.

97. Hsu S, Yang K, Jaffe ES. Phenotypic expression of Hodgkin's and Reed-Sternberg cells in Hodgkin's disease. Am J Pathol 1985;118:209–217.

98. Weiss L, Strickler JG, Hu E, et al. Immunoglobulin gene rearrangements in Hodgkin's disease. Hum Pathol 1986;17:1009–1014.

99. Sundeen JT, Lipford E, Uppencamp M, et al. Rearranged antigen receptor genes in Hodgkin's disease. Blood 1987;70:96–103.

100. Greisser H, Feller A, Lennert K. Rearrangement of the B chain of the T-cell receptor and immunoglobulin genes in lymphoproliferative disorders. J Clin Invest 1986;78:1179–1184.

101. Brinker MG, Poppema S, Buys C, et al. Clonal immunoglobulin gene rearrangements in tissues involved by Hodgkin's disease. Blood 1987;70:186–189.

102. Davis TH, Morton CC, Miller-Cassman R, et al. Hodgkin's disease, lymphomatoid papulosis, and cutaneous T-cell lymphoma derived from a common T-cell clone. N Engl J Med 1992;326:1115–1122.

103. Stetler-Stevenson M, Crush-Stanton S, Cossman J. Involvement of the *bcl-2* gene in Hodgkin's disease. JNCI 1990;82:855–858.

103a. Poppema S, Kaleta J, Hepperle B. Chromosomal abnormalities in patients with Hodgkin's disease: Evidence for frequent involvement of the 14q chromosomal region but infrequent bcl-2 gene rearrangement in Reed-Sternberg cells. JNCI 1992;84:1789–1793.

104. Doglioni C, Pelosio P, Mombello A, et al. Immunohistochemical evidence of abnormal expression of the antioncogene-encoded p53 phosphoprotein in Hodgkin's disease and CD30⁺ anaplastic lymphomas. Hematol Pathol 1991;5:67–73.

105. Sinkovics JG. Hodgkin's disease revisited: Reed-Sternberg cells as natural hybridomas. Crit Rev Immunol 1991;11:33–63.

106. Drexler HG, Gignac SM, Hoffbrand AV, Minowada J. Formation of multinucleated cells in a Hodgkin's disease-derived cell line. Int J Cancer 1989;43:1083–1090.

107. Mueller N, Evans A, Harris NL, et al. Hodgkin's disease and Epstein-Barr virus. Altered antibody pattern before diagnosis. N Engl J Med 1989;320:689–695.

108. Anagnostopoulos I, Herbst H, Niedobitek G, et al. Demonstration of monoclonal EBV genomes in Hodgkin's disease and KI-1-positive anaplastic large cell lymphoma by combined Southern blot and in situ hybridization. Blood 1989;74:810–816.

109. Weiss LM, Movahed LA, Warnke RA, et al. Detection of Epstein-Barr viral genomes in Reed-Sternberg cells of Hodgkin's disease. N Engl J Med 1989;320:502–506.

110. Pallesen G, Hamilton-Dutoit SJ, Rowe M, et al. Expression of Epstein-Barr virus latent gene products in tumour cells of Hodgkin's disease. Lancet 1991;337(8737):320–322.

111. Wu T-C, Mann RB, Charache P, et al. Detection of EBV gene expression in Reed-Sternberg cells of Hodgkin's disease. Int J Cancer 1990;46:801–804.

112. Stein H, Hansmann L, Lennert K, et al. Reed-Sternberg and Hodgkin cells in lymphocyte-predominant Hodgkin's disease of nodular subtype contain J chain. Am J Clin Pathol 1986;86:292–297.

113. Timens W, Visser L, Poppema S. Nodular lymphocyte predominance type of Hodgkin's disease is a germinal center lymphoma. Lab Invest 1986;54:457–461.

114. Levy RA, Kaplan HS. Impaired lymphocyte function in untreated Hodgkin's disease. N Engl J Med 1974;290:181–186.

115. Kaplan HS, Smithers DW. Auto-immunity and homologous disease in mice in relation to the malignant lymphomas. Lancet 1959;2:1–4.

116. Schwartz RS, Beldotti L. Malignant lymphomas following allogenic disease: Transition from an immunological to a neoplastic disorder. Science 1965;149:1511–1514.

117. Romagraaic S, Ferrini PW, Ricci M. The immune defect in Hodgkin's disease. Semin Hematol 1985;22:41–45.

118. Pizzolo G, Chilosi M, Vinouz F, et al. Soluble interleukin-2 receptors in the serum of patients with Hodgkin's disease. Br J Cancer 1987;55:427–428.

119. Bjorkholm M, Holm H, Mellstedt H. Immunologic profile in patients with cured Hodgkin's disease. Scand J Haematol 1977;18:361–368.

120. Young RC, Corder MP, Haynes HA, et al. Delayed hypersensitivity in Hodgkin's disease. A study of 103 patients. Am J Med 1972;52:63–71.

121. King GW, Yanes B, Hurtubise PE, et al. Immune function of successfully treated lymphoma patients. J Clin Invest 1976;57:1451–1460.

122. Van Haelen CP, Fisher RR. Increased sensitivity of T-cells to regulation by normal suppressor cells persist in long-term survivors with Hodgkin's disease. Am J Med 1982;72:385–390.

123. Fisher RI, DeVita VT, Bostick F, et al. Persistent immunologic abnormalities in long-term survivors of advanced Hodgkin's disease. Ann Intern Med 1980;92:595–599.

124. Fisher RI. Implications of persistent T-cell abnormalities for the etiology of Hodgkin's disease. Cancer Treat Rep 1982;66:681–687.

125. Fuks Z, Strober S, Bobrove AM, et al. Long-term effects of radiation on T and B lymphocytes in peripheral blood of patients with Hodgkin's disease. J Clin Invest 1976;58:803–814.

126. Van Rijswijk RE, Sybesma JP, Kater L. A prospective study of the changes in the immune status following radiotherapy for Hodgkin's disease. Cancer 1984;53:62–69.

127. Van Rijswijk RE, Sybesma JP, Kater L. A prospective study of the changes in the immune status before, during and after multiple agent chemotherapy for Hodgkin's disease. Cancer 1983;53:637–644.

128. Weitzman SA, Aisenberg AC, Siber GR, Smith DH. Impaired humoral immunity in treated Hodgkin's disease. N Engl J Med 1977;297:245–248.

129. Minor DR, Schiffman G, McIntosh LS. Response of patients with Hodgkin's disease to pneumococcal vaccine. Ann Intern Med 1979;90:887–892.

130. Hays DM, Ternberg JL, Chen TT, et al. Complications related to 234 staging laparotomies performed in the intergroup Hodgkin's disease in childhood study. Surgery 1984;96:471–478.

131. Donaldson SS, Vosti KL, Berberich FR, et al. Response to pneumococcal vaccine among children with Hodgkin's disease. Rev Infect Dis 1981;3:S133–S143.

132. Ko HS, Pruzanski W. M components associated with lymphoma: A review of 62 cases. Am J Med Sci 1976;272:175–183.

133. Levine AM, Thorton P, Forman SJ, et al. Positive Coombs' test in Hodgkin's disease. Significance and implications. Blood 1980;55:607–611.

134. Booth PB, Jenkins WJ, Marsh WL. Anti-It: A new antibody of the I blood group system occuring in certain Melanesian sera. Br J Haematol 1966;12:341–344.

135. Waddell CC, Cimo PL. Idiopathic thrombocytopenia purpura occurring in Hodgkin's disease after splenectomy. A report of two cases and review of the literature. Am J Haematol 1979;7:381–387.

136. Jones SE. Autoimmune disorders and malignant lymphoma. Cancer 1973;31:1092–1098.

137. Berkman AW, Woog JJ, Kickler TS, et al. Serial determinations of anti-platelet antibodies in a patient with Hodgkin's disease and autoimmune thrombocytopenia. Cancer 1983;51:2057–2060.

138. Heyman MR, Walsh TJ. Autoimmune neutropenia in Hodgkin's disease. Cancer 1987;59:1903–1905.

139. Gilbert R. La roentgentherapie de la granulomatose maligne. J Radiol Electrol 1925;9:509–513.

140. Gilbert R. Radiotherapy in Hodgkin's disease (malignant granulomatosis): Anatomic and clinical foundations: Governing principles: Results. AJR 1939;41:198–241.

141. Kaplan HS. Hodgkin's disease. 2nd ed. Cambridge: Harvard University Press, 1980.

142. Peters MV. A study of survival in Hodgkin's disease treated radiologically. AJR 1950;63:299–311.

143. Peters MV, Middlemiss KCH. A study of Hodgkin's disease treated by irradiation. AJR 1958;79:114–121.

144. Peters MV. Prophylactic treatment of adjacent areas in Hodgkin's disease. Cancer Res 1966;26:1232–1243.

145. Kaplan HS. The radical radiotherapy of regionally localized Hodgkin's disease. Radiology 1962;78:553–561.

146. Kinmouth JB, Taylor GW, Harper RK. Lymphography: A technique for its clinical use in the lower limbs. Br Med J 1955;1.930–942.

147. Lee BJ, Nelson JH, Schwarz G. Evaluation of lymphangiography, inferior venacavography and intravenous pyelography in the clinical staging and management of Hodgkin's disease and lymphosarcoma. N Engl J Med 1964;271:327–337.

148. Glatstein E, Guernsey JM, Rosenberg SA, et al. The value of laparotomy and splenectomy in the staging of Hodgkin's disease. Cancer 1969;24:709–718.

149. Glatstein E, Trueblood HW, Enright LP, et al. Surgical staging of abdominal involvement in unselected patients with Hodgkin's disease. Radiology 1970;97:425.

150. Kaplan HS. On the natural history, treatment and prognosis of Hodgkin's disease. Harvey Lectures, 1968–1969. New York: Academic Press, 1970:215–259.

151. Smithers D. Hodgkin's disease. Edinburgh: Churchill-Livingstone, 1973.

152. Regula DP, Hoppe RT, Weiss LM. Nodular and diffuse types of lymphocyte predominant Hodgkin's disease. N Engl J Med 1988;318:214–219.

153. Slaughter DP, Economou SG, Southwick HW. The surgical management of Hodgkin's disease. Ann Surg 1958;148:705–710.

154. Peters MV, Hasselbach R, Brown TC. The natural history of the lymphomas related to the clinical classification. In: Zarafonetis CJD, ed. Proceedings of the International Conference on Leukemia-Lymphoma. Philadelphia: Lea & Febiger, 1968:357–370.

155. Lukes RJ, Craver LF, Hall TC, et al. Report of the nomenclature committee. Cancer Res 1966;26:311.

156. Carbone PP, Kaplan HS, Musshoff K, et al. Report of the committee on Hodgkin's disease staging. Cancer Res 1971;31:1860–1861.

157. Musshoff K, Ronemann H, Bourlis L, et al. Die extranodulare Lymphogranulomatose. Diagnose, Therapie und Prognose bei zwei unterschiedlichen Formen de Organ Befalls. Ein Beitrag zur Stadienein teilung des morbus Hodgkin. Fortschr Geb Roentgenstr Nuklearmed Erganzungsband 1968;109:776–786.

158. Lister TA, Crowther D, Sutcliffe SB, et al. Report of a committee convened to discuss the evaluation and staging of patients with Hodgkin's disease: Cotswald meeting. J Clin Oncol 1989;7:1630–1636; J Clin Oncol [Erratum] 1990;8:1602.

159. Urba W, Longo DL. Hodgkin's disease: Medical progress. N Engl J Med 1992;326:678–687.

160. Mansfield CM, Fabian G, Jener S, et al. Comparison of lymphography and computer

tomography scanning in evaluating abdominal disease in stages III and IV Hodgkin's disease. Cancer 1990;66:2295–2299.

161. Castellino R, Hoppe RT, Black N. Computed tomography, lymphography and staging laparotomy; correlations in initial staging of Hodgkin's disease. AJR 1984;143:37–41.

162. Hoppe RD, Diehl LF, Lysar M, et al. Hodgkin's disease: Clinical utility of CT in initial staging and treatment. Radiology 1988;169:17–22.

163. Castellino RA. Imaging techniques for staging abdominal Hodgkin's disease. Cancer Treat Rep 1982;66:697–700.

164. Redman HC, Glatstein E, Castellino RA, et al. Computed tomography as an adjunct in the staging of Hodgkin's disease and non-Hodgkin's lymphomas. Radiology 1977;124:381–385.

165. Breeman RS, Castellino RA, Harell GS, et al. CT-pathologic correlations in Hodgkin's disease and non-Hodgkin's lymphoma. Radiology 1978;126:159–166.

166. Jones SE, Tobias DA, Waldman RS. Complete tomographic scanning in patients with lymphoma. Cancer 1978;41:480–486.

167. Aisenberg AC. The staging of Hodgkin's disease. J Exp Clin Cancer Res 1983;2:209–212.

168. Mellor JA, Simmons AV, Barnard DL, et al. A retrospective evaluation of mediastinal tomograms, isotope liver scans and isotope bone scans in the staging and management of patients with lymphoma. Cancer 1983;52:2227–2229.

169. Tumeh SS, Rosenthal DS, Kaplan WD, et al. Lymphoma: Evaluation with Ga-67 SPECT. Radiology 1987;164:111–114.

170. Delaney TF, Glatstein E. The role of the staging laparotomy in the management of Hodgkin's disease. In: DeVita VT Jr, Hellman S, Rosenberg SA, eds. Cancer: Principles and practice of oncology, vol. 1. Philadelphia: JB Lippincott, 1987:1–44.

171. John RE. Is staging laparotomy routinely indicated in Hodgkin's disease? Ann Intern Med 1971;75:459.

172. Kinsella TJ, Glatstein E. Staging laparotomy and splenectomy for Hodgkin's disease: Current status. Cancer Invest 1983;1:87–91.

173. Lacher MJ. Routine staging laparotomy for patients with Hodgkin's disease is no longer necessary. Cancer Invest 1983;1:93–99.

174. Piro AJ, Hellman S. Laparotomy alters treatment in Hodgkin's disease. NCI Monogr 1973;36:307–311.

175. Kaplan HS, Dorfman RF, Nelson TS, et al. Staging laparotomy and splenectomy in Hodgkin's disease: Analysis of indications and patterns of involvement in 285 consecutive, unselected patients. NCI Monogr 1973;36:291–301.

176. Desser RK, Golomb HM, Ultmann JE, et al. Prognostic classification of Hodgkin's disease in pathologic stage III, based on anatomic considerations. Blood 1977;49:883–893.

177. Stein RS, Golomb HM, Diggs CH, et al. Anatomic substages of stage III-A Hodgkin's disease. Ann Intern Med 1980;92:159–165.

178. Rosner F, Zarrabi MH. Late infections following splenectomy in Hodgkin's disease. Cancer Invest 1983;1:57–65.

179. Coker DD, Morris DM, Coleman JJ, et al. Infection among 210 patients with surgically staged Hodgkin's disease. Am J Med 1983;75:97–109.

180. Notter DT, Grossman PL, Rosenberg SA, et al. Infections in patients with Hodgkin's disease: A clinical study of 300 consecutive adult patients. Rev Infect Dis 1980;2:761–800.

181. Desser RL, Ultmann JE. Risk of severe infection in patients with Hodgkin's disease or lymphoma after diagnostic laparotomy and splenectomy. Ann Intern Med 1972;77:143–147.

182. Meeker WR, Richardson JD, West W, et al. Critical evaluation of laparotomy and splenectomy in Hodgkin's disease. Arch Surg 1972;105:222.

183. Jenkin RRT, Berry MP. Hodgkin's disease in children. Semin Oncol 1980;7:202–211.

184. Chilcote RR, Baehner RH, Hammond D. Septicemia and meningitis in children splenectomized for Hodgkin's disease. N Engl J Med 1976;295:798–800.

185. Slaven R, Nelson TS. Complications of staging laparotomy for Hodgkin's disease. NCI Monogr 1973;36:457.

186. Donaldson SS, Kaplan HS. Complications of treatment of Hodgkin's disease in children. Cancer Treat Rep 1982;66:977–989.

187. Mauch PM, Weinstein H, Botnick L, et al. An evaluation of long-term survival and treatment complications in children in Hodgkin's disease. Cancer 1983;51:925–932.

188. Lange B, Littman P. Management of Hodgkin's disease in children and adolescents. Cancer 1983;51:1371–1377.

189. Salzman JR, Kaplan HS. Effect of splenectomy on hematologic tolerance during total lymphoid radiotherapy of patients with Hodgkin's disease. Cancer 1971;27:471–478.

190. Panattiere RJ, Coltman CA. Splenectomy effects on chemotherapy in Hodgkin's disease. Arch Intern Med 1973;131:363–366.

191. Panattiere RJ, Coltman CA, Delaney FC. Splenectomy, chemotherapy and survival in Hodgkin's disease. Arch Intern Med 1977;137:341–343.

192. Ihde DC, DeVita VT, Canellos GP, et al. Effect of splenectomy on tolerance to combination chemotherapy in patients with lymphoma. Blood 1976;47:211–222.

193. Kaldor JM, Day NE, Clarke A, et al. Leukemia following Hodgkin's disease. N Engl J Med 1990;322:7–13.

194. Tucker MA, Coleman CN, Cox RS, et al. Risk of second cancers after treatment for Hodgkin's disease. N Engl J Med 1988;318:76–81.

195. Sutcliffe SB, Wrigley PFM, Timothy AR, et al. Posttreatment laparotomy as a guide to management in patients with Hodgkin's disease. Cancer Treat Rep 1982;6:759–765.

196. Kostraba NC, Peterson BA, Kennedy BJ, et al. Laparotomy in the reevaluation of patients with advanced Hodgkin's disease. Cancer Treat Rep 1981;65:685–687.

197. Mauch P, Tarbell N, Weinstein, et al. Stage IA and IIA supradiaphragmatic Hodgkin's

198. Myers CE, Chabner BA, DeVita VT, et al. Bone marrow involvement in Hodgkin's disease: Pathology and response to MOPP chemotherapy. Blood 1974;44:197–204.

199. Mauch P, Kalish LA, Kadin M, et al. Patterns of presentation of Hodgkin's disease: Implications for etiology and pathogenesis. Cancer (in press).

200. Rosenberg SA. Hodgkin's disease of the bone marrow. Cancer Res 1971;31:1733–1736.

201. Ferrant A, Rodhain J, Michaux L, et al. Detection of skeletal involvement in Hodgkin's disease: A comparison of radiography bone scanning and bone marrow biopsy in 38 patients. Cancer 1975;35:1346–1353.

202. Musshoff K, Boutis L. Therapy results in Hodgkin's disease. Cancer 1968;21:1100–1113.

203. Rubins J. Cutaneous Hodgkin's disease: Indolent causes and control with chemotherapy. Cancer 1978;42:1219–1221.

204. Sapozink MD, Kaplan HS. Intracranial Hodgkin's disease. Report of 12 cases and review of the literature. Cancer 1982;52:1301–1307.

205. Valtysson G, Fisher-Beckfield P, Carbone PP. Cerebellar degeneration with Hodgkin's disease. Cancer 1979;29:246–249.

206. Young RC, Howser DM, Anderson T, et al. Central nervous system complications of non-Hodgkin's lymphoma. The potential role for prophylactic therapy. Am J Med 1979;66:246–249.

207. Moorthy AV, Zimmerman SW, Burkholder PM. Nephrotic syndrome in Hodgkin's disease. Evidence for pathogenesis alternative to immune complex deposition. Am J Med 1976;61:471–477.

208. Yum MN, Edwards JL, Kleit S. Glomerular lesions in Hodgkin's disease. Arch Pathol 1975;99:645–649.

209. Pusey WA. Cases of sarcoma and of Hodgkin's disease treated by exposures to x-rays: A preliminary report. JAMA 1902;38:166–170.

210. Teschendorf W. Veber Bestrahlung der ganzen menschluchen Korpers bel Blutkrankheiten. Strahlenther Onkol 1927;26:720–729.

211. Voorhoeve N. La lymphogranulomatose maligne. Acta Radiol 1925;4:567–589.

212. Kruchen C. Beltrag zur Rontgentheraple der Lymphogranulomatose mit besonder Berucksichtigung der neuren klinischen Ergelnisse. Strahlenther Onkol 1929;31:623–670.

213. Easson EC, Russell MH. The cure of Hodgkin's disease. Br Med J 1963;1:1704.

214. Kaplan HS. Long-term results of palliative and radical radiotherapy of Hodgkin's disease. Cancer Res 1966;26:1250–1252.

215. Kaplan HS. Role of intensive radiotherapy in the management of Hodgkin's disease. Cancer 1966;19:356–367.

216. Kaplan HS. Clinical evaluation and radiotherapeutic management of Hodgkin's disease and the malignant lymphomas. N Engl J Med 1968;278:892–899.

217. Kaplan HS. On the natural history, treatment and prognosis of Hodgkin's disease. Harvey Lectures 1968–1969. New York: Academic Press, 1970:215–259.

218. Kaplan HS. Evidence for a tumoricidal dose level in the radiotherapy of Hodgkin's disease. Cancer Res 1966;26:1221–1224.

219. Rosenberg SA, Kaplan HS. Evidence for an orderly progression in the spread of Hodgkin's disease. Cancer Res 1966;26:1225–1231.

220. Vijayakumar S, Myrianthopoulos LC. An updated dose-response analysis in Hodgkin's disease. Radiother Oncol 1992;24:1–13.

221. Hanks GE, Kinzie JJ, Herring DR, et al. Patterns of care outcome studies in Hodgkin's disease: Results of the national practice and implications for management. Cancer Treat Rep 1982;66:805–808.

222. Landberg T, Liden K, Forslo H. Split-course radiation therapy of mediastinal Hodgkin's disease. TSD and CRE concepts. Acta Radiol 1973;12:33–39.

223. Page V, Gardner A, Karsmark CJ. Physical and dosimetric aspects of the radiotherapy of the malignant lymphomas. I. The mantle technique. Radiology 1970;96:609–618.

224. Carmel RJ, Kaplan HS. Mantle irradiation in Hodgkin's disease. An analysis of technique, tumor irradiation and complications. Cancer 1976;37:2812–2825.

225. Kaplan HS, Stewart HR. Complications of intensive megavoltage radiotherapy for Hodgkin's disease. NCI Monogr 1973;36:439–444.

226. Stewart HR, Cohn KE, Fajardo LF, et al. Radiation-induced heart disease: A study of twenty-five patients. Radiology 1967;89:302–310.

227. Lutz WP, Larsen RD. Technique for match mantle and para-aortic fields. Int J Radiat Oncol Biol Phys 1983;9:1753–1756.

228. Farah R, Ultmann J, Griem M, et al. Extended mantle radiation therapy for pathologic stage I and II Hodgkin's disease. J Clin Oncol 1988;6:1047–1052.

229. Page V, Gardner A, Karsmark CJ. Physical and dosimetric aspects of the radiotherapy of malignant lymphoma. II. The inverted Y technique. Radiology 1970;96:619–626.

230. Lutz WR, Larsen RD. Technique to match mantle and para-aortic fields. Int J Radiat Oncol Biol Phys 1979;5(suppl 2):159.

231. Trueblood HW, Enright LP, Roy GR, et al. Preservation of ovarian function in pelvic irradiation for Hodgkin's disease. Arch Surg 1970;100:236–237.

232. Kinzle JJ, Hanks GE, Maclean CJ, et al. Patterns of care study: Hodgkin's disease relapse rates and adequacy of portals. Cancer 1983;52:2223–2226.

233. Collaborative Group Study. Survival and complications of radiotherapy following involved and extended field therapy of Hodgkin's disease. Stage I and II-A collaborative study. Cancer 1976;38:288–305.

234. Mauch PM, Canellos GP, Rosenthal DS, et al. Reduction of fatal complications from combined modality therapy in Hodgkin's disease. J Clin Oncol 1985;3:501–505.

235. Rosenberg SA, Kaplan HS. The evolution and summary results of the Stanford randomized clinical trials of the management of Hodgkin's disease: 1962–1984. Int J Radiat Oncol Biol Phys 1985;11:5–22.

disease: Prognostic factors in surgically staged patients treated with mantle and para-aortic irradiation. J Clin Oncol 1988;6:1576–1583.

236. Timothy AR, et al. Hodgkin's disease: Combination chemotherapy for relapse following radical radiotherapy. Int J Radiat Oncol Biol Phys 1979;5:165–169.

237. Portlock CS. Impact of salvage treatment on initial relapses in patients with Hodgkin's disease stages I–III. Blood 1978;51:825–833.

238. Mauch P, Ryback M, Rosenthal D, et al. The influence of initial pathologic stage on the survival of patients who relapse from Hodgkin's disease. Blood 1980;56:892–897.

239. Mauch PM, Canellos GP, Rosenthal DS, et al. Reduction of fatal complications from combined modality therapy in Hodgkin's disease. J Clin Oncol 1985;3:501–505.

240. Hagemeister FB, Fuller LM, Sullivan JA, et al. Treatment of patients with stages I and II non-mediastinal Hodgkin's disease. Cancer 1982;50:2307–2313.

241. Carde P, Burgers JM, Henry-Amar M, et al. Clinical stages I and II Hodgkin's disease: A specifically tailored therapy according to prognostic factors. J Clin Oncol 1988;6: 239–252.

242. Ganesan TS, Wrigley PFM, Murray PA, et al. Radiotherapy for stage I Hodgkin's disease: 20 years' experience at St. Bartholomew's Hospital. Br J Cancer 1990;62: 314–318.

243. Mandell LR, Tan C, Groshen S, et al. Can para-aortic radiation be omitted in pathologically staged IA and IIA pediatric Hodgkin's disease? (in press)

244. Mauch P, Larson D, Osteen R, et al. Prognostic factors for positive surgical staging in patients with Hodgkin's disease. J Clin Oncol 1990;8:257–265.

245. Mauch P, Goodman R, Hellman S. The significance of mediastinal involvement in early stage Hodgkin's disease. Cancer 1978;42:1039–1045.

246. Hoppe RT. The management of stage II Hodgkin's disease with a large mediastinal mass: A prospective program emphasizing irradiation. Int J Radiat Oncol Biol Phys 1985;11:349–355.

247. Thar TL, Million RR, Hausner RJ, et al. Hodgkin's disease stage I and II. Relationship of recurrence to size of disease, radiation dose and number of sites involved. Cancer 1979;43:1101–1105.

248. Hoppe RT, Coleman CN, Kaplan HS, et al. Hodgkin's disease, pathologic stage I and II, the prognostic importance of initial sites of disease and extent of mediastinal involvement. Proc Am Soc Clin Oncol 1980;21:471.

249. Velentjas E, Barrett A, McElwain TJ, et al. Mediastinal involvement in early-stage Hodgkin's disease. Eur J Cancer 1980;16:1065–1068.

250. Mauch P, Gorshein D, Cunningham J, et al. Influence of mediastinal adenopathy on site and frequency of relapse in patients with Hodgkin's disease. Cancer Treat Rep 1982;66:809–817.

251. Leslie NT, Mauch P, Hellman S. Stage IA to IIB supradiaphragmatic Hodgkin's disease: Long-term survival and relapse frequency. Cancer 1985;55:2072–2078.

252. Mauch PM, et al. Stage IA–IIA supradiaphragmatic Hodgkin's disease: Prognostic factors in surgically staged patients treated with mantle and para-aortic irradiation. (in press)

253. Leopold KA, Canellos GP, Rosenthal D, et al. Stage IA–IIIB Hodgkin's disease: Staging and treatment with large mediastinal adenopathy. J Clin Oncol 1989;7:1059–1065.

254. Piro AJ, Weiss DR, Hellman S. Mediastinal Hodgkin's disease: A possible danger for intubation anesthesia. Int J Radiat Oncol Biol Phys 1976;1:415–419.

255. Krikorian JG, Portlock CS, Mauch PM. Hodgkin's disease presenting below the diaphragm: A review. J Clin Oncol 1986;4:1551–1562.

256. Mauch P, Goffman T, Rosenthal DS, et al. Stage III Hodgkin's disease: Improved survival with combined modality therapy as compared with radiation therapy alone. J Clin Oncol 1985;3:1166–1173.

257. Rosenberg SA, Kaplan HS, Gladstein EJ, et al. Combined modality therapy of Hodgkin's disease. A report of the Stanford trials. Cancer 1978;42:991–1000.

258. Goodman R, Mauch P, Piro A, et al. Stages IIB and IIB Hodgkin's disease: Results of combined modality treatment. Cancer 1977;40:8489.

259. Crnkovich MJ, Leopold K, Hoppe RT, et al. Stage I to IIB Hodgkin's disease: The combined experience at Stanford University and the Joint Center for Radiation Therapy. J Clin Oncol 1987;5:1041–1049.

260. Hellman S, Mauch P, Goodman RL, et al. The place of radiation therapy in the treatment of Hodgkin's disease. Cancer 1978;42:971–978.

261. Zucali R, Pagnoni AN, Zanini M, et al. Radiological and spirometric evaluation of mediastinal and pulmonary late effects after radiotherapy and chemotherapy for Hodgkin's disease. J Eur Radiother 1981;2:169.

262. Appelfield MM, Slawson RG, Spicer KM, et al. Long-term cardiovascular evaluation of patients with Hodgkin's disease treated by thoracic mantle radiation therapy. Cancer Treat Rep 1982;66:1003–1013.

263. Mauch P, Hellman S, Belli JA. Cardiac effects of mediastinal irradiation. N Engl J Med 1983;309:378.

264. Burns RJ, Bar-Schlomo BZ, Druck MN, et al. Detection of radionuclide cardiomyopathy by gated radionuclide angiography. Am J Med 1983;74:297–303.

265. Annest LS, Anderson RP, Li W, et al. Coronary artery disease following mediastinal radiation therapy. J Thorac Cardiovasc Surg 1983;85:257–263.

266. Bowin JF, Hutchinson GB. Coronary heart disease after irradiation for Hodgkin's disease. Cancer 1982;49:2470–2475.

267. Hancock SL, Hoppe RT. Heart disease mortality after treatment of Hodgkin's disease. Proc Am Soc Clin Oncol 1952;1155:337.

268. Foley KM, Woodruff J, Ellis F, et al. Radiation induced malignant and typical schwannomas. Ann Neurol 1979;7:311–318.

269. Kinsella TJ, Fraass BE, Glatstein E. Late effects of radiation therapy in the treatment of Hodgkin's disease. Cancer Treat Rep 1982;66:991–1001.

270. McDougall IR, Coleman CN, Burke JS, et al. Thyroid carcinoma after high-dose external radiotherapy for Hodgkin's disease. Cancer 1980;45:2056–2060.

271. Stutzman L, Glidewell O. Multiple chemotherapeutic agents for Hodgkin's disease. JAMA 1973;225:1202–1211.

272. Luce JK, Frei E, Gehan EA, et al. Chemotherapy of Hodgkin's disease. Arch Intern Med 1973;131:391–395.

273. Huguley CM, Durant JR, Moores RR, et al. A comparison of nitrogen mustard, vincristine, procarbazine and prednisone (MOPP) vs nitrogen mustard in advanced Hodgkin's disease. Cancer 1975;36:1227–1240.

274. British National Lymphoma Investigation: Value of prednisone in combination chemotherapy of stage IV Hodgkin's disease. Br Med J 1975;3:413–414.

275. Goldman JM. Combination chemotherapy for stage IV Hodgkin's disease (report #14). Clin Radiol 1981;32:531–535.

276. Jones SE, Haut A, Weick JK, et al. Comparison of Adriamycin-containing chemotherapy (MOP-BAP) with MOPP-bleomycin in the management of advanced Hodgkin's disease. Cancer 1983;51:339–347.

277. Bakemeier RF, Anderson JR, Costello W, et al. BCVPP chemotherapy for advanced Hodgkin's disease: Evidence for greater duration of complete remission, greater survival and less toxicity than with a MOPP regimen. Ann Intern Med 1984;101:447–456.

278. Straus DJ, Myers J, Lee BJ, et al. Treatment of advanced Hodgkin's disease with chemotherapy and irradiation. Am J Med 1984;76:270–278.

279. Haybittle JL, Eastering MJ, Hudson BV, et al. Review of British National Lymphoma Investigation studies of Hodgkin's disease: Development of a prognostic index. Lancet 1985;1:967–972.

280. Santoro A, Bonadonna G, Bonfante V, et al. Alternating drug combinations in the treatment of advanced Hodgkin's disease. N Engl J Med 1982;306:770–775.

281. Bonadonna G, Valagussa P, Santoro A. Alternating non-cross-resistant combination chemotherapy with ABVD or MOPP in stage IV Hodgkin's disease: A report of eight year results. Ann Intern Med 1986;104:739–746.

282. Hancock BW, Hudson GV, Hudson BV, et al. British National Lymphoma investigation randomized study of MOPP against LOPP in advanced Hodgkin's disease—long-term results. Br J Cancer 1991;63:578–582.

283. Somers R, Henry-Amar M, Carde P, et al. MOPP vs alternating MOPP/ABVD in advanced Hodgkin's disease (HD). Proc Am Soc Clin Oncol 1988;7:236.

284. Canellos GP, Propert K, Cooper R, et al. MOPP vs ABVD vs MOPP alternating with ABVD in advanced Hodgkin's disease: A prospective CALGB trial. Proc Am Soc Clin Oncol 1988;7:230.

285. Brusamolino E, Lazzarino M, Canevari A, et al. Alternating non-cross-resistant chemotherapy (MOPP-ABVD) in advanced Hodgkin's disease. Proc Am Soc Clin Oncol 1988;7:239.

286. Nicholson WM, Beard MEJ, Crowther D, et al. Combination chemotherapy in generalized Hodgkin's disease. Br Med J 1970;3:7–10.

287. Sutcliffe SB, Wrigley PFM, Peto J, et al. MVPP chemotherapy regimen for advanced Hodgkin's disease. Br Med J 1978;1:679–683.

288. Wagstaff J, Steward W, Jones M, et al. Factors affecting remission and survival in patients with advanced Hodgkin's disease treated with MVPP. Hematol Oncol 1986;4: 135–147.

289. Morgenfeld M, Somoza N, Magnasco J, et al. Combined chemotherapy cyclophosphamide, vinblastine, procarbazine and prednisone (CVPP) versus CVPP plus CCNU (CCVPP) in Hodgkin's disease. Cancer 1979;43:1579–1586.

290. Glick J, Tsiatis A, Chen M, et al. Improved survival with MOPP-ABVD compared to BCVPP ± radiotherapy for advanced Hodgkin's disease: 6-year ECOG results. Blood 1990;76(Suppl 1):351a.

291. DeVita VT, Hubbard SM, Longo DL. Treatment of Hodgkin's disease. JNCI Monogr 1990;10:19–28.

292. Durant JR, Gams RA, Velez-Garcia E, et al. BCNU, velban, cyclophosphamide, procarbazine, and prednisone (BVCPP) in advanced Hodgkin's disease. Cancer 1978;42: 2101–2110.

293. Gams RA, Durant JR, Bartolucci AA. Chemotherapy for advanced Hodgkin's disease: Conclusions from the Southeastern Cancer Study Group. Cancer Treat Rep 1982;66: 899–905.

294. McElwain TJ, Toy J, Smith E, et al. A combination of chlorambucil, vinblastine, procarbazine and prednisolone for treatment of Hodgkin's disease. Br J Cancer 1977;36: 276–280.

295. Selby P, Patel P, Milan S, et al. ChlVPP combination chemotherapy for Hodgkin's disease: Long-term results. Br J Cancer 1990;62:279–285.

296. Vose J, Armitage J, Weisenburger D, et al. ChlVPP—an effective and well-tolerated alternative to MOPP therapy for Hodgkin's disease. Am J Clin Oncol 1988;11:423–426.

297. Longo D. The use of chemotherapy in the treatment of Hodgkin's disease. Semin Oncol 1990;17:716–735.

298. Lister TA, Dorreen MS, Faux M, et al. The treatment of stage IIIA Hodgkin's disease. J Clin Oncol 1983;1:745–749.

299. Crowther D, Wagstaff J, Deakin D, et al. A randomized study comparing chemotherapy alone with chemotherapy followed by radiotherapy in patients with pathologically staged IIIA Hodgkin's disease. J Clin Oncol 1984;2:892–897.

300. Gams RA, Omura GA, Velez-Garcia E, et al. Alternating sequential combination chemotherapy in the management of advanced Hodgkin's disease. A Southeastern Cancer Study Group trial. Cancer 1986;58:1963–1968.

301. Cooper MR, Pajak TF, Nissen N, et al. A new effective four-drug combination of CCNU (1-3-cyclohexyl-1-nitrosourea) (NSC-79038), vinblastine, prednisone, and procarbazine for the treatment of advanced Hodgkin's disease. Cancer 1980;46:654–662.

302. Cooper MR, Pajak TF, Gottlieb AJ, et al. The effects of prior radiation therapy and age on the frequency and duration of complete remission among various four-drug treatment for advanced Hodgkin's disease. J Clin Oncol 1984;2:748–755.

303. Propert KJ, Cooper MR, Spurr C, et al. Combination chemotherapy with vinca alkaloids and alkylating agents for stage III and IV Hodgkin's disease (HD): Ten years of follow-up (CALGB 7251). Proc Am Soc Clin Oncol 1986;5:192.

304. Vinciguerra V, Propert KJ, Coleman M, et al. Alternating cycles of combination chemotherapy for patients with recurrent Hodgkin's disease following radiotherapy a prospectively randomized study by the Cancer and Leukemia Group B. J Clin Oncol 1986;4:838–846.

305. Druker BJ, Canellos GP. Chlorambucil, vinblastine, procarbazine and prednisone (ChlVPP): An effective but less toxic regimen than MOPP for advanced stage Hodgkin's disease (HD). Proc Am Assoc Cancer Res 1986;27:198.

306. Canellos GP, Anderson JR, Propert KJ, et al. Chemotherapy of advanced Hodgkin's disease with MOPP, ABVD, or MOPP alternating with ABVD. N Engl J Med 1992;327: 1478–1484.

307. Connors JM, Klimo P, Adams G, et al. MOPP/ABV hybrid versus alternating MOPP/ABVD for advanced Hodgkin's disease. Proc Am Soc Clin Oncol 1992;11:317.

308. Prosnitz LR, Farber LR, Scott J, et al. Combined modality therapy for advanced Hodgkin's disease: 15-year follow-up data. J Clin Oncol 1988;6:603–612.

309. Wagener DJT, Marion J, Burgers V, et al. Sequential non-cross-resistant chemotherapy regimens (MOPP and CAVmP in Hodgkin's disease stage IIIB and IV. Cancer. 1983;52: 1558–1562.

310. Klimo P, Connors JM. MOPP/ABV hybrid program: Combination chemotherapy based on early introduction of seven effective drugs for advanced Hodgkin's disease. J Clin Oncol 1985;3:1174–1182.

311. Connors JM, Klimo P. MOPP/ABV hybrid chemotherapy for advanced Hodgkin's disease. Semin Hematol 1987;24:35–40.

312. Viviani S, Bonadonna G, Santoro A, et al. Alternating versus hybrid MOPP-ABVD in Hodgkin's disease. The Milan experience. Ann Oncol 1991;2:55–62.

313. Longo DL, Russo A, Duffey PL, et al. Treatment of advanced-stage massive mediastinal Hodgkin's disease: The case for combined modality treatment. J Clin Oncol 1991;9: 227–235.

314. O'Reilly SE, Hoskins P, Klimo P, Connors JM. MACOP-B and VACOP-B in diffuse large cell lymphomas and MOPP/ABV in Hodgkin's disease. Ann Oncol 1991;2(suppl 1):17–23.

315. Longo DL, Duffey PL, DeVita VT, et al. Treatment of advanced-stage Hodgkin's disease: Alternating noncrossresistant MOPP/CABS is not superior to MOPP. J Clin Oncol 1991;9:1409–1420.

316. Goodman LS, Wintrobe MM, Dameshek W, et al. Nitrogen mustard therapy. Use of methyl bis (B-chloreothyl) amine hydrochloride and tris (B-chloroethyl) amine hydrochloride for Hodgkin's disease lymphosarcoma, leukemia, and certain allied and miscellaneous disorders. JAMA 1946;132:126–132.

317. Alpert LP, Petersen SK. The use of nitrogen mustard in the treatment of lymphomata. Bull U S Army Med Dept 1947;7:187–194.

318. Dameshek W, Weisfuse L, Stein T. Nitrogen mustard therapy in Hodgkin's disease. Analysis of 50 consecutive cases. Blood 1949;4:338–379.

319. Bollag W, Grunberg E. Tumor inhibitory effects of a new class of cytotoxic agents: Methyl hydrazine derivatives. Experientia 1963;19:751.

320. Mathe G, Schweisguth O, Schneider M, et al. Methylhydrazine in the treatment of Hodgkin's disease. Lancet 1963;2:1077.

321. Martz G, D'Alessandri A, Keel HJ, et al. Preliminary clinical results with a new antitumor agents RO 4-6467 (NSC 77213). Cancer Chemother Rep 1963;33:5–14.

322. Falkson G, de Villieb PC, Falkson HC. N-Isopropyl-(2-methyl-hydrazine)-p-toluamide (MIH). Proc Soc Exp Biol Med 1965;120:561–565.

323. DeVita VT, Serpick A, Carbone PP. Preliminary clinical studies with ibenzmethyzin. Clin Pharmacol Ther 1966;7:542–546.

324. Craft CB. Results with roentgen ray therapy in Hodgkin's disease. Bull Staff Meet Univ Miami Hosp 1940;11:391–409.

325. Jacobs EM, Peters FC, Luce JK, et al. Mechlorethamine HCL and cyclophosphamide in the treatment of Hodgkin's disease. Cancer Chemother Rep 1963;27:27–32.

326. Aisenberg AC, Qazi R. Improved survival in Hodgkin's disease. Cancer 1976;37:2323–2329.

327. DeVita VT, Serpick A. Combination chemotherapy in the treatment of advanced Hodgkin's disease. Proc Am Assoc Cancer Res 1967;8:13.

328. DeVita VT, Serpick AA, Carbone PP. Combination chemotherapy in the treatment of advanced Hodgkin's disease. Ann Intern Med 1970;73:891–895.

329. Lowenbraun S, DeVita VT, Serpick AA. Combination chemotherapy with nitrogen mustard, vincristine, procarbazine, and prednisone in previously treated patients with Hodgkin's disease. Blood 1970;36:704–717.

330. DeVita VT. Consequences of the chemotherapy of Hodgkin's disease. Cancer 1981;47: 1–13.

331. Frei E III, Luce JK, Gamble JF, et al. Combination chemotherapy in advanced Hodgkin's disease: Induction and maintenance of remission. Ann Intern Med 1973;79:376–382.

332. Canellos GP, Young RC, DeVita VT, et al. Combination chemotherapy of advanced Hodgkin's disease in relapse following extensive radiotherapy. Clin Pharmcol Ther 1972;13:750–754.

333. Cadman E, Bloom AF, Prosnitz A, et al. The effective use of combined modality therapy for the treatment of patients with Hodgkin's disease who relapsed following radiotherapy. Am J Clin Oncol 1983;6:313–318.

334. DeVita VT. Cell kinetics and the chemotherapy of cancer. Cancer Chemother Rep 1971;3:23–33.

335. Hryniuk W, Bush H. The importance of dose intensity in chemotherapy of metastatic breast cancer. J Clin Oncol 1984;2:1281–1288.

336. DeVita VT, Hubbard SM, Longo DL. The chemotherapy of lymphomas: Looking back, moving forward—the Richard and Hinda Rosenthal Foundation Award Lecture. Cancer Res 1987;47:5810–5824.

337. Longo DL, Young RC, Wesley M, et al. Twenty years of MOPP chemotherapy for Hodgkin's disease. J Clin Oncol 1986;4:1295–1306.

338. Fuer EJ, Kessler LG, Baker SG, et al. The impact of breakthrough clinical trials on survival in population based tumor registries. J Clin Epidemiol 1991;44:141–153.

339. Moore ME, Jones SE, Bull JM, et al. MOPP chemotherapy for advanced Hodgkin's disease: Prognostic factors in 81 patients. Cancer 1973;32:52–60.

340. Jacobs C, Portlock CS, Rosenberg SA. Prednisone in MOPP chemotherapy for Hodgkin's disease. Br Med J 1976;2:1469.

341. Morgenfeld M, Somoza N, Magnasco J, et al. Combined chemotherapy cyclophosphamide, vinblastine, procarbazine and prednisone (CVPP) vs CVPP plus CCNU (CCVPP) in Hodgkin's disease. Cancer 1979;43:1579.

342. Diggs Ch, Wiernik PH, Levi JA, et al. Cyclophosphamide, vinblastine, procarbazine and prednisone with CCNU and vinblastine maintenance for advanced Hodgkin's disease. Cancer 1977;39:1949.

343. Gibbs GE, Peterson BA, Kennedy BJ, et al. Long-term survival of patients with Hodgkin's disease. Arch Intern Med 1981;141:897.

344. Nissen IN, Pajak FT, Glidewell O, et al. A comparative study of a BCNU containing 4-drug program versus MOPP versus 3-drug combinations in advanced Hodgkin's disease. Cancer 1979;43:31–40.

345. Coltman CA Jr, Jones SE, Grozea PN, et al. Bleomycin in combination with MOPP in the management of advanced Hodgkin's disease: A Southwest Oncology Group experience. In: Sikic BI, Rosenscweig M, Carter SK, eds. Bleomycin chemotherapy. Orlando, FL: Academic Press, 1985:137–153.

346. Santoro A, Bonadonna G. Prolonged disease-free survival in MOPP-resistant Hodgkin's disease after treatment with Adriamycin, bleomycin, vinblastine and dacarbazine (ABVD). Cancer Chemother Pharmacol 1979;2:101–105.

347. Santoro A, Bonfante V, Bonadonna G. Salvage chemotherapy with ABVD in MOPP-resistant Hodgkin's disease. Ann Intern Med 1982;96:139–143.

348. Papa G, Mandelli F, Anselmo AP, et al. Treatment of MOPP-resistant Hodgkin's disease with Adriamycin, bleomycin, vinblastine and dacarbazine (ABVD). Eur J Cancer 1982;9:803–806.

349. Carde P, MacKintosh R, Rosenberg SA. A dose and time response analysis of the treatment of Hodgkin's disease with MOPP therapy. J Clin Oncol 1983;1:146–153.

350. DeVita VT. The influence of information on drug resistance on protocol design. Ann Oncol 1991;2:53–106.

351. Devereau S, Linch DC, Gribben JG, et al. GM-CSF accelerates neutrophil recovery after autologous bone marrow transplantation for Hodgkin's disease. Bone Marrow Transplant 1989;4:49–54.

352. Anderson J, Canellos GP. MOPP vs. ABVD vs. MOPP alternating with ABVD in advanced Hodgkin's disease. [Abstract] Presented at the International Conference on Malignant Lymphoma, Lugano, 1990.

353. Glick J, Tsiatis A, Schilsky R, et al. A randomized phase III trial of MOPP/ABVD hybrid vs. sequential MOPP-ABVD in advanced Hodgkin's disease: Preliminary results of the Intergroup Trial. Proc Ann Meet Am Soc Clin Oncol [Abstract] 1991;10:A941.

354. Gulati S, Bennett CL. Granulocyte macrophage colony-stimulating factors as adjunct therapy in relapsed Hodgkin's disease. Ann Intern Med 1992;116:177–82.

355. Mead GM, Harker WG, Kushlan P, et al. Single-agent palliative chemotherapy for end-stage Hodgkin's disease. Cancer 1982;50:829–835.

356. Ruud ENVR, Clemens H, Dekker AW, et al. Dose intensity of MOPP chemotherapy and survival in Hodgkin's disease. J Clin Oncol 7:1776–1782, 989.

357. Gobbi PG, Cavalli C, Rossi A, et al. The role of dose and rate of administration of MOPP drugs in 97 retrospective Hodgkin's patients. Haematologica 1987;72:523–528.

358. Rosso R, Venturini M, Mariani GL. The importance of dose intensity in cancer chemotherapy. Forum. Trends Exp Clin Med 1991;1:264–275.

359. Lagarde P, Bonichon H, Eghbali I, et al. Influence of dose intensity and density on therapeutic and toxic effects in Hodgkin's disease. Br J Cancer 1989;59:645–649.

360. Fisher RI, DeVita VT, Hubbard SM, et al. Prolonged disease-free survival in Hodgkin's disease with MOPP reinduction after first relapse. Ann Intern Med 1979;90:761–763.

361. DeVita VT, Hubbard SM, Longo DL. The chemotherapy of lymphomas: Looking back and moving forward. The Richard and Hinda Rosenthal Foundation Award Lecture. Cancer Res 1987;47:5810–5824.

362. Kessinger A, Bierman PJ, Vose JM, Armitage JO. High-dose cyclophosphamide, carmustine, and etoposide, followed by autologous peripheral stem cell transplantation for patients with relapsed Hodgkin's disease. Blood 1991;77:2322–2325.

363. Vose JM, Bierman PJ, Armitage JO. Hodgkin's disease: The role of bone marrow transplantation. Semin Oncol 1990;17:749–757.

364. Phillips GL, Reece DE, Barnett MJ, et al. Allogeneic marrow transplantation for refractory Hodgkin's disease. J Clin Oncol 1989;7:1039–1045.

365. Desch CE, Lasala MR, Smith TJ, Hillner BE. The optimal timing of autologous bone marrow transplantation in Hodgkin's disease patients after a chemotherapy relapse. J Clin Oncol 1992;10:200–209.

366. Armitage JO, Bierman PJ, Vose JM, et al. Autologous bone marrow transplantation for patients with relapsed Hodgkin's disease. Am J Med 1991;91:605–611.

367. Longo DL, Duffey PL, Young RC, et al. Conventional-dose salvage combination chemotherapy in patients relapsing with Hodgkin's disease after combination chemotherapy: The low probability for cure. J Clin Oncol 1992;10:210–218.

368. Vinciguerra V, Coleman M, Jarowski CI, et al. A new combination chemotherapy for resistant Hodgkin's disease. JAMA 1977;237:33–35.

369. Viviani S, Santoro A, Negretti E, et al. Salvage chemotherapy in Hodgkin's disease. Results in patients relapsing more than twelve months after first complete remission. Ann Oncol 1990;1:123–127.

370. Goldman JM, Dawson AA. Combination chemotherapy for advanced resistant Hodgkin's disease. Lancet 1975;2:1224–1227.

371. Longo DL, Duffey PL, Young RC, et al. Conventional-dose salvage combination che-

motherapy in patients relapsing with Hodgkin's disease after combination chemotherapy: The low probability for cure. J Clin Oncol 1992;10:210–218.

372. Devereau S, Linch DC, Gribben JG, et al. GM-CSF accelerates neutrophil recovery after autologous bone marrow transplantation for Hodgkin's disease. Bone Marrow Transplant 1989;4:49–54.

373. Taylor KM, Jagannath S, Spitzer G, et al. Recombinant human granulocyte colony-stimulating factor hasten granulocyte recovery after high-dose chemotherapy and autologous bone marrow transplantation in Hodgkin's disease. J Clin Oncol 1989;7:1791–1799.

374. Weiss J, von Roemling H, Peters HJ, et al. Chemotherapie bei Vorbehandeltem morbus Hodgkin mit Lomustin, Bleomycin, Vinblastin und Dexamethason. Dtsch Med Wochenschr 1983;108:1428–1432.

375. Tannir N, Hagemeister F, Valasquez W, et al. Long-term follow-up with ABDIC salvage chemotherapy of MOPP-resistant Hodgkin's disease. J Clin Oncol 1983;1:432–439.

376. Einhorn LH, Williams SD, Stevens EE, et al. Treatment of MOPP-refractory Hodgkin's disease with vinblastine, doxorubicin, bleomycin, CCNU, and dacarbazine. Cancer 1983;51:1348–1352.

377. Piga A, Ambrosetti A, Todeschini G, et al. Doxorubicin, bleomycin, vinblastine and dacarbazine (ABVD) salvage of mechlorethamine, vincristine, prednisone, and procarbazine (MOPP)-resistant advanced Hodgkin's disease. Cancer Treat Rep 1984;58:947–951.

378. Harker GW, Kushlan P, Rosenberg SA. Combination chemotherapy for advanced Hodgkin's disease after failure of MOPP, ABVD and B-CAV-e. Ann Intern Med 1984;10:440–446.

379. Bonadonna G, Viviani S, Valagussa P, et al. Third-line salvage chemotherapy in Hodgkin's disease. Semin Oncol 1985;12:23–25.

380. Santoro A, Viviani SS, Valagussa P, et al. CCNU, etoposide and prednimustine (CEP) in refractory Hodgkin's disease. Semin Oncol 1986;13:23–26.

381. Cervantes F, Reverter JC, Montserrat E, et al. Treatment of advanced resistant Hodgkin's disease with lomustine, etoposide, and prednimustine. Cancer Treat Rep 1986;70:665–667.

382. Mandelli F, Cimino G, Mauro FR, et al. Prognosis and management of patients affected by multi-pretreated Hodgkin's disease. Haematology 1986;71:205–208.

383. Richards MA, Waxman JH, Ganesan TS, et al. EVA treatment for recurrent or unresponsive Hodgkin's disease. Cancer Chemother Pharmacol 1986;18:51–53.

384. Garbes ID, Gomez GA, Tan T, et al. Salvage chemotherapy for advanced Hodgkin's disease. Med Pediatr Oncol 1987;15:45–48.

385. Hagemeister FBN, Tannir N, McLaughlin P, et al. MIME chemotherapy (Methyl-GAG, ifosfamide, methotrexate, etoposide) as treatment for recurrent Hodgkin's disease. J Clin Oncol 1987;5:556–561.

386. Tseng A, Jacobs C, Coleman CN, et al. Third-line chemotherapy for resistant Hodgkin's disease with lomustine, etoposide, and methotrexate. Cancer Treat Rep 1987;71:475–478.

387. Schulman P, Propert K, Cooper MR, et al. Phase II study of MOPLACE in previously treated Hodgkin's disease. Proc Soc Clin Oncol 1987;6:A742.

388. Levi JA, Wiernik PH, Diggs CH. Combination chemotherapy of advanced previously treated Hodgkin's disease with streptozotocin, CCNU, Adriamycin and bleomycin. Med Pediatr Oncol 1977;3:33–40.

389. Hoppe RT, Coleman CN, Cox RS et al. The management of stage I–II Hodgkin's disease with irradiation alone or combined modality therapy: The Standford experience. Blood 1982;59:455–465.

390. Hagemeister FB, Fuller LM, Velasques WS, et al. Stage I and II Hodgkin's disease: Involved-field radiotherapy versus extended-field radiotherapy versus involved-field radiotherapy followed by six cycles of MOPP. Cancer Treat Rep 1982;66:789–798.

391. Nissen NI, Nordentoft AM. Radiotherapy versus combined modality treatment of stage I and II Hodgkin's disease. Cancer Treat Rep 1982;66:799–803.

392. Anderson H, Deakin DP, Wagstaff J, et al. A randomized study of adjuvant chemotherapy after mantle radiotherapy in supradiaphragmatic Hodgkin's disease PS IIA–IIB: A report from the Manchester Lymphoma Group. Br J Cancer 1985;49:695–702.

393. Coleman DN, Williams CJ, Flint A, et al. Hematologic neoplasia in patients treated for Hodgkin's disease. N Engl J Med 1977;297:1249–1252.

394. Blayney DW, Longo DL, Young RC, et al. Decreasing risk of leukemia with prolonged follow-up after chemotherapy and radiotherapy for Hodgkin's disease. N Engl J Med 1987;316:710–714.

395. Tucker MA, Coleman CN, Cox RS, et al. Risk of second cancers after treatment for Hodgkin's disease. N Engl J Med 1988;318:75–81.

396. Horning SJ, Hoppe RT, Hancock SL, Rosenberg SA. Vinblastine, bleomycin, and methotrexate: An effective adjuvant in favorable Hodgkin's disease. J Clin Oncol 1988;6:1822–1831.

397. Olweny CLM, Katongole-Mbidde E, Kiive C, et al. Childhood Hodgkin's disease in Uganda: A 10-year experience. Cancer 1978;42:787–792.

398. Ekert H, Waters KD, Smith PJ, et al. Treatment with MOPP or ChlVPP chemotherapy only for all stages of childhood Hodgkin's disease. J Clin Oncol 1988;6:1845–1850.

399. O'Dwyer PJ, Wiernik PH, Steward MB, Slawson RG. Treatment of early stage Hodgkin's disease: A randomized trial of radiotherapy plus chemotherapy versus chemotherapy alone. In: Cavalli F, Bonadonna G, Rozencweig M, eds. Malignant lymphomas and Hodgkin's disease: Experimental and therapeutic advances. Boston: Martinus Nijhoff, 1985:329–336.

400. Pavlovsky S, Maschio M, Santarelli MT, et al. Randomized trial of chemotherapy versus chemotherapy plus radiotherapy for stage I–II Hodgkin's disease. JNCI 1988;80:1466–1473.

401. Cimino G, Biti GP, Anselmo AP, et al. MOPP chemotherapy versus extended field radiotherapy in the management of pathological stages I–IIA Hodgkin's disease. J Clin Oncol 1989;7:732–737.

402. Longo DL, Glatstein E, Duffey PL, et al. Radiation therapy versus combination chemotherapy in the treatment of early stage Hodgkin's disease: Seven-year results of a prospective randomized trial. J Clin Oncol 1991;9:897–901.

403. Pedersen-Bjergaard J, Specht I, Larsen SO, et al. Risk of therapy-related leukaemia and preleukaemia after Hodgkin's disease. Relation to age, cumulative dose of alkylating agents, and time from chemotherapy. Lancet 1987;2:83–88.

404. Longo DL, DeVita VT. The use of combination chemotherapy in the treatment of early stage Hodgkin's disease. In: DeVita VT, Hellman S, Rosenberg SA, ed. Important advances in oncology. Philadelphia: JB Lippincott, 1992:155–166.

405. Biggar RJ. Cancer in acquired immunodeficiency syndrome: An epidemiologic assessment. Semin Oncol 1990;17:251–260.

406. Freter CD. Acquired immunodeficiency syndrome-associated lymphoma. NCI Monogr 1990;10:45–54.

407. Zielgler H, Beckstead JA, Volberding PA, et al. Non-Hodgkin's lymphoma in 90 homosexual men. Relation to generalized lymphadenopathy and acquired immunodeficiency syndrome. N Engl J Med 1984;311:565–570.

408. Remick SC, Diamond C, Migliozzi JA, et al. Primary central nervous system lymphoma in patients with and without the acquired immune deficiency syndrome: A retrospective analysis and review of literature. Medicine (Baltimore) 1990;69:345–360.

409. Serrano M, Bellas C, Campo E, et al. Hodgkin's disease in patients with antibodies to human immunodeficiency virus. Cancer 1990;65:2248–2254.

410. Prior E, Goldberg AF, Conjalka MS, et al. Hodgkin's disease in homosexual men. An AIDS-related phenomenon? Am J Med 1986;81:1085.

411. Gill PS, Levine AM, Kiarlo M, et al. AIDS-related malignant lymphomas: Results of prospective drug trials. J Clin Oncol 1987;5:1322.

412. Unger PD, Strauchen JA. Hodgkin's disease in AIDS complex patients. Cancer 1986;58:821.

413. Bookman MA, Longo DL. Complications in patients treated for Hodgkin's disease. Cancer Treat Rev 1986;13:77–111.

414. Louie AC, Cavalli F, Rozensweig M. New agents for Hodgkin's and non-Hodgkin's lymphoma in malignant lymphomas and Hodgkin's disease: Experimental and therapeutic advances. In: Cavalli F, Bonadonna G, Rozensweig M, eds. Malignant lymphomas in Hodgkin's disease: Experimental and therapeutic advances. Boston: Martinus Nijhoff, 1985:493–511.

415. Warrell RP, Coonley CJ, Straus DJ, et al. Treatment of patients with advanced malignant lymphoma using gallium nitrate administered as a seven-day continuous infusion. Cancer 1983;51:1982–1987.

416. Knight WAT, Fabian C, Costanzi J, et al. Methylglyoxal-bis-guanylhydrazone (methyl GAG, MGBG) in lymphoma and Hodgkin's disease. Invest New Drugs 1983;1:235–237.

417. Espana P, Kaplan R, Robichaud K, et al. Phase II study of spiroglimanium (spiro G) in lymphoma patients. Proc Am Soc Clin Oncol 1982;1:166.

418. Weick JK, Jones SE, Ryan DH. Phase II study of amacrine (m-AMSA) in advanced lymphomas: A Southwest Oncology Group study. Cancer Treat Rep 1983;67:489–492.

419. Case ED, Hayes DM. Phase II study of arizidinybenzoquinone in refractory lymphoma. Cancer Treat Rep 1983;67:993–996.

420. Coltman CA, McDaniel TM, Balcerzak SP, et al. Mitoxantone hydrochloride (NSC-310739) in lymphoma. A Southwest Oncology Group study. Invest New Drug 1983;1:65–70.

421. Warrell RP, Kempen SJ. Clinical evaluation of a new anthracyline antibiotic aclacinomycin-A in patients with advanced malignant lymphoma. Am J Clin Oncol 1983;6:81–84.

422. Coonley CJ, Warrell RP, Straus DJ, et al. Clinical evaluation of 4-demethoxydaunorubicin in patients with advanced malignant lymphoma. Cancer Treat Rep 1983;67:949–950.

423. Rosenweig M, Crespeigne N, Kenis Y. Phase I trial with 4-deoxydoxorubin (esonibicen). Invest New Drug 1983;1:309–313.

424. Vriesendorp HM, Herpst JM, Germack MA, et al. Phase I–II studies of yttrium-labeled antiferritin treatment for end-stage Hodgkin's disease, including Radiation Therapy Oncology Group 87-01. J Clin Oncol 1991;9:918–928.

Cancer: Principles & Practice of Oncology, Fourth Edition,
edited by Vincent T. DeVita, Jr., Samuel Hellman, Steven A. Rosenberg.
J.B. Lippincott Co., Philadelphia © 1993.

Dan L. Longo   Peter Mauch

Vincent T. DeVita, Jr   Walter J. Urba

Elaine S. Jaffe

CHAPTER **52**

Lymphocytic Lymphomas

EPIDEMIOLOGY

Malignant lymphomas are the seventh most common causes of death from cancer in the United States.[1] In 1992, approximately 41,000 new cases were diagnosed, and there were approximately 19,400 deaths from the disease. Because of the young average age (42 years) of the lymphoma population, the total in person-years of life lost each year ranks the lymphomas fourth in terms of economic impact among cancers in the United States. There are two major subgroups of lymphoma: Hodgkin's disease and the non-Hodgkin's lymphomas. The term non-Hodgkin's lymphomas does not adequately describe the larger of these two subsets, and because approximately 98% of these lymphomas are of lymphocyte origin, we call them lymphocytic lymphomas. This designation is also not perfect; it is inaccurate in a small fraction of cases and redundant in the rest. As we use the term, lymphocytic lymphomas are those lymphomas that are not Hodgkin's disease.

The incidence of lymphocytic lymphomas is increasing each year; the 50% increase in incidence between 1973 and 1988 reported by the American Cancer Society was one of the largest increases reported for any cancer.[2,3] A large portion of this increase has been attributed to the lymphocytic lymphomas developing in association with the acquired immunodeficiency syndrome (AIDS). The Centers for Disease Control indicate that 3% of all adult patients with AIDS develop lymphoma.[4] In support of this hypothesis is the reported increase in lymphocytic lymphomas among men between the ages of 20 and 54 in San Francisco, which parallels an increase in Kaposi's sarcoma. None of the other geographic areas included in the Surveillance, Epidemiology and End Results (SEER)

Program had such large increases in incidence of lymphocytic lymphoma for men in this age group. The rates for 20- to 54-year-old men in San Francisco County are five times higher than those in SEER areas excluding this region. The inescapable conclusion is that the incidence of AIDS-related lymphomas is increasing. However, the large increase in younger men does not account for the 57% increase in the overall incidence of lymphocytic lymphomas. Increases have been seen for other age groups; the group older than 65 years of age has had a 55% increase in incidence. Although the age-adjusted incidence of lymphomas has increased most for high-grade lymphomas (0.4 to 1.7 per 100,000), as would be expected for AIDS-related lymphomas, the incidence of low- and intermediate-grade lymphomas has also increased.

In the United States, there is a steady increase in the incidence of lymphocytic lymphomas from childhood through 80 years of age. They are more common in males than females (16.6 versus 11.2 per 100,000).[3,5–7] The incidence is higher in whites than blacks (13.7 versus 8.6 per 100,000). Unlike Hodgkin's disease, for which new treatment regimens have been rapidly implemented in the oncologic community and rapid decreases in mortality (50% reduction since 1973) have been observed, there has been a slight increase in mortality rates for the lymphocytic lymphomas. This increase, which occurred despite marked improvements in therapy, remains unexplained.

The lymphocytic lymphomas are found worldwide. Their overall incidence, and the incidence of the various histologic subtypes varies in different parts of the world. Burkitt's lymphoma occurs more frequently in tropical Africa; immunoproliferative small intestine disease in the Middle East; and adult T-cell leukemia-lymphoma in southwest Japan and the Caribbean basin.[8]

ETIOLOGY

A hereditary influence on the incidence of lymphomas is suggested by their higher incidence in patients with inherited immunologic deficiency diseases and by a small increase in the incidence in families of patients with immunologic disorders.[9] One study found a significant increase in the incidence of lymphomas in patients with collagen vascular diseases compared with the general population and adjusted for age.[10] This increased incidence approached 10% in patients with long-standing Sjögren's syndrome who tend to develop diffuse aggressive lymphomas or immunoblastic lymphomas.[11-13] An association between the class I major histocompatibility complex (MHC) antigen HLA-B12 and lymphoma has been reported.[14,15] Klinefelter's syndrome and the Chediak-Higashi syndrome have been associated with an increased risk of lymphoreticular malignancy.[16,17] Several other diseases predispose to the development of lymphomas (Table 52–1). Lymphoma-like syndromes have been found in patients who take phenytoin; in most cases, the disease regresses after the patient stops taking phenytoin, but a small fraction develop malignant lymphomas of several different varieties, including Hodgkin's disease.[18]

Environmental exposures, viruses, chromosomal aberrations, and congenital or acquired immunosuppression have been associated with the development of lymphocytic lymphomas. Despite these associations, the actual cause of most lymphocytic lymphomas remains unknown.

ENVIRONMENTAL EXPOSURE

The increased incidence of lymphoma among Midwestern farmers born after 1900 and dying before age 65 has raised the possibility that relatively recent changes in agricultural techniques and practices, such as the increased use of pesticides and fertilizers after World War II, may play a role in the cause of lymphoid neoplasia.[19] This is supported by case-control studies indicating that occupational exposure to phenoxyherbicides is associated with a twofold to fivefold increase in the risk of developing a lymphocytic lymphoma.[20,21] A dose-response association between lymphoma risk and acres

TABLE 52–1.   Disease Associated With Lymphoma Predisposition

Klinefelter's syndrome
Chediak-Higashi syndrome
Ataxia-telangiectasia syndrome
Wiscott-Aldrich syndrome
Swiss-type agammaglobulinemia
Common variable immunodeficiency disease
Acquired hypogammaglobulinemia
Iatrogenic immunosuppression (*e.g.*, treatment with anti-CD3 or cyclosporine)
Sjögren's syndrome
Rheumatoid arthritis and systemic lupus erythematosus
Acquired immunodeficiency syndrome
Phenytoin therapy
X-linked lymphoproliferative syndrome

sprayed with herbicides has been reported.[22] The carcinogens are presumed to be 2,3-dichlorophenoxyacetic acid (2,4-D) or 2,4,5-trichlorophenoxyacetic acid (2,4,5-T) and their congeners.[23] A case-control study showed that the risk for non-Hodgkin's lymphoma was increased by 50% among Vietnam veterans.[24] Although Agent Orange, a 1:1 mixture of 2,4-D and 2,4,5-T, was originally implicated, the fact that the greatest risk of lymphoma was found among Navy veterans, most of whom were stationed on ocean-going vessels with little opportunity for exposure to Agent Orange, rather than land-based troops in areas exposed to the defoliant, argues against Agent Orange being the causative agent. A 4.2-fold increased risk for developing lymphoma was reported for employees in the U.S. flour industry.[25] The risk was particularly high among persons working in maintenance and elevator departments of mills. Although environmental exposures are associated with lymphoma, the nature of the risky exposure is poorly defined.

It appears that ionizing radiation can cause malignant lymphoma in humans, but the mechanism of neoplastic transformation and the conditions under which it occurs have not been clearly delineated. An increased prevalence of lymphocytic lymphoma was demonstrated in survivors of the atomic bomb in Hiroshima who were exposed to 100 cGy or more.[26,27] An increased incidence of lymphoma has been demonstrated in patients irradiated for ankylosing spondylitis.[28] In both groups, the ratio of observed to expected cases of lymphoma was 2:1. Patients with Hodgkin's disease treated with radiation therapy and chemotherapy have an increased risk of developing secondary large cell lymphomas, often involving the gastrointestinal tract.

IMMUNOSUPPRESSION

Except for the higher incidence of Hodgkin's disease in siblings and the influence of phenytoin on the development of lymphomas, it is difficult to separate the influence of inheritance from immunosuppression, which is probably of etiologic importance even without an inherited background. For example, lymphomas occur with an increased frequency in many congenital and acquired immunodeficiency diseases.

Patients who are chronically immunosuppressed by drugs, particularly those who have received organ transplants, have a higher incidence of cancer, particularly aggressive lymphoproliferative disorders.[29,30] These lesions may range from benign polyclonal B-cell hyperplasias related to Epstein-Barr virus (EBV) infection to frankly malignant monoclonal B-cell lymphomas. Non-B-cell tumors do occur, but comprise 15% or fewer of all tumors. Posttransplantation lymphomas differ from those developing in the general population; extranodal involvement is found in 69% rather than 24% to 48%, respectively, and central nervous system (CNS) involvement is also more common (28% versus 1%). The immunosuppressive regimen influences the incidence of secondary lymphomas; 11% of second cancers are lymphomas after azathioprine- or cyclophosphamide-based therapy, compared with 26% since cyclosporine-based regimens came into use.[31] The secondary lymphomas occur earlier using cyclosporine-based regimens, with a median of 15 months compared with 48 months for the other regimens. The use of anti-CD3 (OKT3) monoclonal antibodies led to an increase in the incidence of lymphomas to 64% of all secondary tumors and to a decrease in the time to disease occurrence (mean, 7 months).[31,32] The higher the dose of OKT3, the higher was the risk of lymphoma.

It is unlikely that the development of lymphoma is agent specific; the risk for developing a lymphoma probably relates more to the extent of immunosuppression. The clinical outcome for these patients varies, but most fare poorly. Anecdotal instances of complete remissions after removal of immunosuppression or treatment with acyclovir have been reported. Most patients require aggressive therapy for eradication of their disease.[33,34] There may be responses to biologic agents when the tumors are in the polyclonal or oligoclonal phase of their natural history. The antibodies, anti-CD21 and anti-CD24, successfully controlled the B-cell lymphoproliferative syndrome in all 16 patients with oligoclonal proliferation after marrow or organ transplantation, and 11 remained free of disease for a median of 3 years after treatment.[35] Interferon-α (IFN-α) plus intravenous immunoglobulin was active in 5 of these patients.[36]

The increased incidence of lymphoma in patients with graft-versus-host disease, in recipients of mismatched T-cell-depleted bone marrow, in patients with iatrogenic immunosuppression, and in patients with AIDS and autoimmune diseases argues strongly for immune dysregulation in the genesis of lymphoma. Chronic antigenic stimulation has been implicated in the development of lymphomas in certain animals, but there are no convincing data in humans. Some patients with nontropical sprue develop primary T-cell lymphomas in the gastrointestinal tract, perhaps related to the gluten stimulation. The immunoglobulin gene rearrangements in about 25% of patients with chronic lymphocytic leukemia (and by inference, diffuse small lymphocytic lymphomas) result in the production of immunoglobulins that share κ chain idiotypes, the structures unique to the antigen recognition site.[37] These tumors rearrange variable region κ genes nonstochastically. This may represent evidence that tumors in different people result from the transformation of a B cell that recognizes a common or similar antigen.

VIRAL CAUSES

There is convincing evidence that viruses cause certain types of lymphomas in rodents, birds, cats, and cows.[38–41] Marek's disease, a lymphoma of chickens, is caused by a herpes-like DNA virus and can now be prevented by a vaccine.[42] A horizontally transmitted C-type retrovirus is a highly infectious cause of bovine lymphosarcoma.[43] Inbreeding appears to play an important role in the viral initiation of these animal cancers.

In humans, there is a strong association between EBV and Burkitt's lymphoma; molecular biologic techniques have established that 98% of endemic cases of Burkitt's lymphoma contain the EBV genome, but only 15% to 20% of nonendemic Burkitt's lymphomas contain the virus.[44] The lymphomas occurring in patients after organ transplantation or with congenital immune deficiencies are usually associated with EBV.[45] Most patients infected with EBV harbor the virus in latent form in B lymphocytes, which are infected by their cell surface receptor for the C3d component of complement (*i.e.*, CD21). The polyclonal B-cell infection is normally controlled by T lymphocytes that eliminate the infected B cells.[46] The viral

nuclear proteins (*e.g.*, EBNA-2, EBNA-3s) and membrane proteins (*e.g.*, LMP-1) that induce proliferation of B cells also display epitopes on the cell surface that can be recognized by T cells. When T-cell deficiency exists, EBV-infected B cells can proliferate, and usually one clone escapes regulation and becomes autonomously proliferating. Males with X-linked lymphoproliferative syndrome fail to recognize EBV, which results in fatal infectious mononucleosis, acquired hypogammaglobulinemia or agammaglobulinemia, virus-associated hemophagocytic syndrome, or malignant lymphocytic lymphoma.[47] EBV has been found in patients with Hodgkin's disease and lymphomatoid granulomatosis, but its etiologic role in these diseases is speculative.

Approximately 50% of the lymphomas occurring in human immunodeficiency virus (HIV)-infected persons harbor the EBV genome.[48] The EBV sequences in a benign lymph node from an HIV-infected patient without AIDS is associated with an increased incidence of concurrent lymphoma at another site and is a marker for the increased risk of developing lymphoma.[49]

Lymphomagenesis seems to require immunodeficiency and cellular proliferation followed by cytogenetic and molecular events. Infection with EBV is postulated to occur early and leads to polyclonal expansion; after a second event, a single clone emerges from the nonmalignant cells.[50] Studies performed during the development of lymphoproliferative disorders support the notion that originally there is a polyclonal population of cells. The immunoglobulin (Ig) genes are present in germline configuration, and there is variability of fragment size in the EBV genome. After a second event, there is evolution into a monoclonal population with a single rearranged Ig gene and a single-size EBV episome.[51] During the polyclonal phase of proliferation, EBV DNA is present in an episomal and linear configuration; the latter form indicates active viral replication. It is at this polyclonal stage that acyclovir treatment and anti-B-cell antibodies have induced remission in lymphoproliferative disorders; these treatments are ineffective after monoclonal proliferations occur and the EBV genome is present only as an episome. The second event required to establish malignancy is thought to be related to protooncogene activation through cytogenetic events, often involving c-*MYC*. These observations support a role for EBV in the development of certain lymphomas in humans, but studies have not proven causality.

The most convincing evidence for a viral cause of human malignant lymphoma is in adult T-cell leukemia-lymphoma (ATL). In 1987, Poiesz and colleagues identified a unique C-type RNA tumor virus in certain patients with mature T-cell malignancies.[52] This retrovirus was called human T-cell leukemia-lymphoma virus (HTLV-I). HTLV-I is a unique, exogenously acquired retrovirus that is not closely related to any known animal retroviruses in terms of antigenicity, amino acid sequence, or nucleic acid sequence homology. Although HTLV-I was first isolated from the neoplastic cells of patients thought to have an aggressive variant of mycosis fungoides, it subsequently was recognized that the disease in these patients was identical to ATL as described in Japan.[53]

Other members of this family of human retroviruses have been described. HTLV-II was identified in a patient with atypical T-cell hairy cell leukemia, but it has been isolated from only a few patients, and it is not clearly associated with a distinct clinicopathologic disease entity.[54] HTLV-III (renamed HIV-1) is a member of a distinct family of viruses and has been shown to be the causative agent of AIDS.[55,56] HTLV-V is the putative etiologic virus for certain cutaneous T-cell lymphomas (CTCL).[57] Data on its epidemiology are not available.

The precise mechanism by which HTLV-I infection leads to malignant transformation in vivo is unknown. HTLV-I does not contain an oncogene, nor do the malignancies arising in various patients have common integration sites. HTLV-I, however, can immortalize lymphoid cells in culture and induce malignancy in an infected human host. A proposed model for HTLV-I-mediated transformation starts with infection of the cell through an unidentified cell surface receptor, followed by viral replication. Viral replication is associated with production of *trans*-activating factors (tax) that lead to expression of a variety of cytokines and receptors including interleukin-1 (IL-1), IL-2, and IL-2 receptor. Data suggest that tax induces *REL* expression, a transcription factor that participates in cell activation. Autocrine stimulation would lead to the polyclonal expansion of infected cells and increase the likelihood of an unidentified secondary event that leads to malignant transformation, monoclonal expansion, and the clinical syndrome of ATL.

Because many patients in endemic areas are infected with HTLV-I, but few develop ATL, there appear to be host factors that affect transformation of lymphocytes by HTLV-I, and strong evidence supporting such host-related genetic factors is emerging. HTLV-I has been isolated from the neurons of patients suffering from tropical spastic paraparesis, a disease epidemiologically similar to ATL.[58] A preliminary study in Japan of patients infected with HTLV-I appears to demonstrate that patients developing ATL have a high prevalence of certain HLA antigens (A26, DQw3), and those developing myelopathy express a distinct HLA haplotype (*e.g.*, A11 or A26, Bw52 or Bw54, Cw1, DQw3).[59] Such strong linkage disequilibrium suggests that the MHC is involved in the pathogenesis of HTLV-I-related disease.

CYTOGENETICS AND MOLECULAR BIOLOGY

Cytogenetic analysis of metaphase chromosomes from lymphocytic lymphomas indicates that more than 90% have chromosomal abnormalities.[60,61] For many, the chromosomal abnormality correlates with histologic subtype, immunophenotype, and with the clinical features of the lymphocytic lymphomas (Table 52–2). The most common abnormalities are sets of reciprocal translocations.[62] Two reciprocal translocations are each involved in more than 10% of all lymphocytic lymphomas; t(8;14)(q24;q32) or one of its variants, t(8;22)(q24;q11) and t(2;8)(p11;q24), are observed in more than 90% of Burkitt's lymphomas, and the t(14;18)(q32;q21) translocation has been detected in 80% to 85% of the follicular lymphomas. These reciprocal translocations result in DNA segments moving from a distant chromosome into the DNA sequences comprising the immunoglobulin genes. This translocation deregulates the expression of the translocated nonimmunoglobulin gene. This nonimmunoglobulin gene is often an oncogene, and overproduction of its protein product leads to disordered cellular growth.

A variety of cytogenetic abnormalities that involve the T-cell receptor β or γ genes on chromosome 7 or the T-cell receptor α or δ genes on chromosome 14 have been reported.[63] The t(11;14)(q13;q32) and t(3;22)(q27;q11) translocations occur in 2% to 10% of lymphocytic lymphomas. The t(11;14) translocation and its molecular counterpart, *BCL1* rearrangement, has been found in 50% of diffuse intermediately differentiated lymphomas, and the t(3;22) translocation is usually found in patients with diffuse large cell lymphomas. Several other reciprocal translocations have been described in fewer than 2% of lymphocytic lymphomas (see Table 52–2). Perhaps the most well known is the t(2;5)(p23;q35), identified in the CD30 or Ki-1 positive anaplastic large cell lymphoma.[64]

There are several other cytogenetic abnormalities that have been called "recurring other aberrations" or ROA by Offit that are also listed in Table 52–2.[65] These include abnormalities of chromosomes 6q, 1p, 1q, and 17 and trisomies of 7, 3 and 12. None of these abnormalities appears to be specific for one histologic subtype.

Efforts have been made to relate cytogenetic defects to natural history.[65] Because patients usually received heterogenous treatments and were not balanced for other known prognostic factors, it is difficult to ascertain a distinct contribution of cytogenetics to outcome. However, it appears that chromosome 1 defects or the presence of more than four chromosomal abnormalities is associated with shorter survival among patients with diffuse large cell lymphoma. The appearance of additional genetic aberrations during the natural history of a low-grade lymphoma signifies a worsening prognosis. The acquisition of increasing numbers of clones bearing trisomy 7, trisomy 3, and del(13q32) or trisomy 18 in t(14,18)-bearing lymphomas is associated with evolution to a more aggressive histology.[66] Further refinement of cytogenetic techniques and more detailed study will provide more clinically useful information, but currently, the status of the chromosomes within a patient's tumor has little influence on our treatment selection.

ONCOGENES

The major impact of cytogenetics has been in increasing our understanding of the molecular events associated with lymphomagenesis. For example, the t(8;14), t(11;14), and t(14;18) translocations bring certain DNA segments into proximity with the immunoglobulin genes. These DNA segments appear to contain protooncogenes or growth-regulating genes that under certain conditions can lead to the disordered growth of the affected cell. In most cases, the translocated gene comes under the influence of the immunoglobulin enhancer element, resulting in amplified expression of the translocated gene's product. Almost all patients with endemic or nonendemic Burkitt's lymphoma have a reciprocal translocation between chromosome 8 and chromosome 14, 2, or 22. The t(8;14) translocation moves the *MYC* oncogene into the immunoglobulin heavy chain locus, and the t(8;22) or t(2;8) brings *MYC* into juxtaposition with one of the light chain loci, λ or κ, respectively.[67] This results in the constitutive expression of *MYC*, which codes for a DNA-binding protein that is thought to be important in the regulation of cell proliferation.

TABLE 52–2. Cytogenetic-immunophenotypic Correlations in Lymphocytic Lymphoma

Phenotype	Rearrangement	Involved Genes or Sequences*		Phenotype	Rearrangement
B(sIg +)	t(8;14)(q24;q32)	MYC	IgH	Ki-1+ anaplastic large cell lymphoma	t(2;5)(p23;q32)
	t(2;8)(p11–12;q24)	Ig κ	MYC		
	t(8;22)(q24;q11)	MYC	Ig λ		
	t(14;18)(q32;q21)	BCL2	IgH		
	t(11;14)(q13;q32)	BCL1	IgH		
	t(1;14)(q21–25;q32)			Variable or unspecified	del(1)(p32–36)
	t(3;14)(p21;q32)				del(1)(p13)
	t(8;14)(q22;q32)				dup(1q)
	t(1;14)(q42;q32)				i(1q)
	t(3;22)(q27–28;q11)				t(1;17)(pllorq11;pllorq11)
	t(10;14)(p11;q32)				del(1)(q21), del(1)(q32), del(1)(q42)
	t(11;14)(q21;q32)				t(2;18)(p11;q21)
	t(11;14)(q23;q32)				del(2)(q32)
					del(3)(p21)
	t(11;14)(p13;q11)†	TCL2	TCRδ		del(4)(p13–14)
	t(11;14)(p15;q11)†	TAL1	TCRδ		del(5)(p13)
	t(8;14)(q24;q11)	MYC	TCRα		i(6p)
	inv(14)(q11q32)	TCRα	IgH		del(6)(q14–27)
	inv(14)(q11q32)	TCRα	TCL1		del(7)(p13–14)
	t(10;14)(q24;q11)	TCL3	TCRδ		i(7q)
	t(1;14)(p32;q11)	TCL5	TCRδ		del(7)(q32)
	t(7;19)(p34–36;p13)†	TCRβ	LYL1		del(9)(p13)
	t(7;9)(q34–36;q34)†	TCRβ			del(10)(q23–24)
	t(7;9)(q34–36;q32)†	TCRβ	TCL4		dup(11)(q13 → q23), dup(11)(q13 → q25)
	t(7;7)(p15;q11)	TCRγ			del(11)(q23)
	t(14;14)(q11;q32)				del(12)(p11–12)
	t(7;14)(q34–36;q11)				del(12)(q22)
	t(7;14)(p15;q11)				dup(12)(q13 → q22)
	t(7;11)(q34–36;p13)†				del(13)(q22)
	del(6)(p21p23)				del(14)(q22q24)
					i(17q)
					i(18q)
					del(22)(q11–12)

* MYC, cellular protooncogene, homolog of the transforming sequence of the avian myelocytomatosis virus DNA-binding protein; IgH, immunoglobulin heavy chain gene; Ig κ, immunoglobulin kappa light chain gene; Ig λ, immunoglobulin lambda light gene; BCL2, B-cell leukemia-lymphoma gene-2 24-kD protein thought to prevent cell death; BCL1, DNA sequences isolated from the translocation breakpoint protein related to the cyclin family of cell cycle control genes; TCL2, DNA sequences isolated from the translocation breakpoint (T-cell leukemia-lymphoma gene-2); TCRδ, T-cell receptor delta chain gene; TCRα, T-cell receptor alpha chain gene; TCL6, T-cell leukemia-lymphoma gene-6; TAL1, DNA sequences isolated from the translocation breakpoint; TCL1, DNA sequences isolated from the translocation breakpoint (T-cell leukemia-lymphoma gene-1); TCL3, DNA sequences isolated from the translocation breakpoint (T-cell leukemia-lymphoma gene-3); TCL5, DNA sequences isolated from the translocation breakpoint (T-cell leukemia-lymphoma gene-5); LYL1, lymphoid leukemia gene-1; TCRβ, T-cell receptor beta chain gene; TCL4, DNA sequences isolated from the translocation breakpoint (T-cell leukemia-lymphoma gene-4); TCRγ, T-cell receptor gamma chain gene.
† These rearrangements have been identified only in T-cell acute lymphoblastic leukemia.
(Modified from LeBeau MM. Seminars in Oncology 1990;17:20–29)

The t(14;18) translocation brings the B-cell leukemia-lymphoma-2 gene (BCL2) from chromosome 18 into the immunoglobulin heavy chain joining region on chromosome 14.[68] When this segment of DNA is transcribed, both gene sequences are found on the same mRNA, a so-called hybrid transcript. The coding regions of the BCL2 gene are left intact so that the BCL2/IG hybrid heavy chain transcript produced continues to encode a normal BCL2 protein. Expression of this hybrid mRNA can be increased by as much as a log over that of normal B cells.[69] Only the BCL2-encoded portion of the hybrid mRNA is translated, and this leads to production of excessive levels of BCL2 protein. BCL2-encoded mRNA levels are normally high during pre-B-cell development, but with maturation, there is down regulation of expression.[70] The

BCL2 protein is an integral inner mitochondrial membrane protein that can block apoptosis, or programmed cell death, of certain B-cell lymphoma cell lines.[71]

When the *BCL2/IG* fusion gene is introduced into the germline of mice (*i.e.*, transgenic mice), there is a polyclonal expansion of resting but responsive IgM-positive, IgD-positive B cells that display prolonged cell survival but no increase in cell cycling.[72] An indolent lymphoid follicular hyperplasia is seen in these mice, which may progress to a malignant diffuse large cell lymphoma.[73] There is a long latency in progression from polyclonal to monoclonal disease and histologic conversion, which suggests secondary genetic changes in addition to the inserted transgene.

Half the high-grade lymphomas contained rearranged *MYC* genes. It was also demonstrated that retroviral insertion of *BCL2*-encoded complementary DNA into human B-cell lines that constitutively overexpress *MYC* and promotes proliferation and tumorigenicity.[74] Taken together, these findings suggest that BCL2 protein provides a survival advantage to B cells and may contribute to neoplasia by permitting a clone to persist until other oncogenes, such as *MYC*, are activated, resulting in cell transformation.

The t(14;18) translocation is found in 85% of follicular lymphomas and in as many as 35% of diffuse large cell lymphomas.[68] Serial examination of tumor specimens during histologic progression from a follicular low-grade lymphoma to an intermediate-grade diffuse lymphoma shows an identical breakpoint in the *BCL2* translocation, indicating that most of the *BCL2*-positive large cell lymphomas probably arose from a *BCL2*-positive follicular small cleaved cell lymphoma.[75] Although the presence of a *BCL2* translocation does not affect the prognosis of a low-grade tumor, its presence in a more aggressive lymphoma may have negative prognostic significance.[76,77] However, the presence of t(14;18) in patients with aggressive lymphoma in relapse has been associated with more prolonged survival, and some of these patients follow a clinical course more similar to indolent lymphomas, with response to therapy followed by relapse occurring over multiple courses of salvage therapy. Techniques that detect the presence of the t(14;18) translocation have found some utility as sensitive indicators of minimal residual disease in the bone marrow or peripheral blood and as a measure of the efficacy of in vitro purging of bone marrow before autologous transplant.[78,79] The use of the t(14;18) translocation or BCL2 protein as a marker of residual disease depends on the assumption that the DNA rearrangement is not found in normal tissue. Early studies failed to detect BCL2 protein in nodes that contained only normal tissue or reactive follicular hyperplasia, but studies using polymerase chain reaction have shown *BCL2* rearrangements in 54% of lymph nodes and tonsils with follicular hyperplasia.[80,81] No *BCL2* rearrangements were detected in reactive lymph nodes without follicular hyperplasia or in bone marrow cells. The implications of these findings are discussed further in the section on treatment of advanced-stage indolent lymphomas.

The t(11;14) translocation involves *BCL1* on chromosome 11 and the immunoglobulin heavy chain gene on 14.[77] Rearrangement deregulates a nearby oncogene called *PRAD1* (parathyroid adenomatosis).[82] *PRAD1*, which is found on 11q13, was identified as a chromosomal breakpoint region rearranged with the parathyroid hormone gene in a subset of

parathyroid adenomas. *PRAD1* codes for a cyclin protein. Cyclin genes are involved in regulation of cell cycle progression. *BCL1* and *PRAD1* are no more than 130 kb apart. *PRAD1*-encoded mRNA was abundantly expressed in 7 of 7 cases of diffuse intermediately differentiated or centrocytic lymphomas. The linkage of a cell cycle-regulated gene to the expression of immunoglobulin in a B cell may lead to uncontrolled growth.

MICROSCOPIC AND FUNCTIONAL ANATOMY OF NORMAL LYMPHOID TISSUES

The principal cellular component of lymphoid tissue is the lymphocyte.[83] Lymphoid cells are widely distributed throughout the body, singly and in centers of aggregation.[84] The primary lymphoid organs in which these cells are generated include the bone marrow and thymus. The secondary lymphoid organs populated by differentiated lymphoid cells include lymph nodes, spleen, Waldeyer's ring (the oropharyngeal lymphoid tissues), and lymphoid aggregates in the lamina propria and submucosa of the respiratory and gastrointestinal tracts. In the gastrointestinal tract, they are referred to as Peyer's patches. Lymphoid elements associated with epithelium in the respiratory and gastrointestinal tracts are sometimes referred to as the mucosa-associated lymphoid tissues (MALT) and gut-associated lymphoid tissues.[85] Lymphoid cells also populate bone marrow, as cohabitants of the numerous hematopoietic elements. In addition to these major sites, lymphoid cells are distributed as normally inconspicuous interstitial elements in essentially all tissues except the CNS.

Other cells of the lymphoreticular system include reticular supporting cells, dendritic and interdigitating reticulum cells, and cells of the monocyte-macrophage series. The reticular cells provide the basic three-dimensional matrix of lymph nodes by virtue of their long cytoplasmic processes joined by tight junctions or desmosomes. Within this matrix, the functional cells of the lymphoid and monocyte-macrophage series migrate, proliferate, and serve as the primary arm of the host immunologic defense apparatus. The lymphoreticular system is the anatomic basis of cellular and humoral immunity.

Normally, the lymphoid and monocytic cells of the lymphoreticular system originate in the bone marrow and from there migrate by way of the blood and lymphatic vessels to populate other lymphoreticular tissues.[83] T cells are processed through the thymus gland, and B cells are processed through the mammalian equivalent of the avian bursa of Fabricius, probably the fetal liver. Although T cells and B cells comprise the two major components of the lymphocyte series, there are minor populations of other lymphocytes, such as natural killer (NK) cells, that may develop independently. Evidence suggests that thymocytes and NK cells share a common progenitor. Monocytes also originate in the bone marrow and, like lymphocytes, circulate and eventually populate extramedullary tissues as cells of the monocyte-histiocytic series.[86] These three populations of lymphoreticular cells (*i.e.*, T cells, B cells, monocyte-macrophages) serve different functions and are to some degree compartmentalized anatomically (Fig. 52–1). The malignant lymphomas frequently mirror these normal anatomic distributions in their spread throughout the lym-

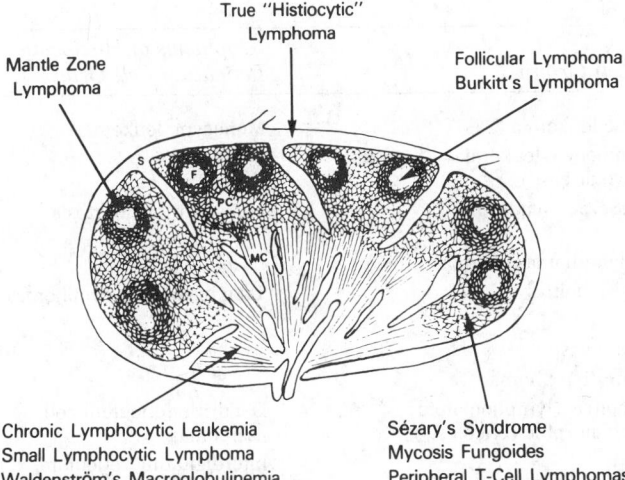

True "Histiocytic"
Lymphoma

Mantle Zone
Lymphoma

Follicular Lymphoma
Burkitt's Lymphoma

Chronic Lymphocytic Leukemia
Small Lymphocytic Lymphoma
Waldenström's Macroglobulinemia

Sézary's Syndrome
Mycosis Fungoides
Peripheral T-Cell Lymphomas

FIGURE 52–1. Schematic diagram of a normal lymph node, illustrating anatomic and functional compartments of the immune system. Malignant lymphomas can be related to these compartments. S, sinuses; F, follicles; PC, paracortex; MC, medullary cords. (Modified from Mann RB, Jaffe ES, Berard CW, et al. Malignant lymphomas: A conceptual understanding of morphologic diversity. Am J Pathol 1979;94:1–3)

phoreticular system.[87] The pattern of spread by the lymphomas is not random, but mimics patterns of normal lymphocyte circulation and distribution.

Functionally, T cells are the basis of the cell-mediated immune system.[88] Cytotoxic T cells directly lyse specific target cells, such as tumor cells or virally infected cells. Other subpopulations of T cells have regulatory functions and act as helpers or suppressors for B cells, macrophages, and other T cells. T lymphocytes recognize antigen when it is associated with the membrane-bound products of the MHC. Some T cells (CD4-positive cells) predominantly recognize antigen in association with class II MHC antigens, and other T cells (CD8-positive cells) recognize antigen in association with class I MHC antigens.

B cells form the basis of the humoral immune system.[89] They express membrane-bound immunoglobulin and, as differentiated B cells or plasma cells, secrete immunoglobulin. The ability to phagocytize particulate material is the hallmark of macrophages and monocytes.[90] These cells play a major role in the processing of antigens and their presentation to lymphocytes. Dendritic reticulum cells and interdigitating reticulum cells are thought to be related to monocyte-macrophages. Although these cells are involved in antigen presentation, they do not serve a phagocytic function.[91,92] The dendritic reticulum cells are localized in lymphoid follicles, and interdigitating reticulum cells are the antigen-presenting cells of the T-cell system and are found in the paracortex. Langerhans cells, most conspicuous in the skin but also found in other sites such as lymph nodes, are closely related to interdigitating reticulum cells and present antigen to T lymphocytes.[93]

IDENTIFICATION OF LYMPHOID CELLS

Normal and neoplastic cells of the immune system can be differentiated by characteristic surface markers. The neo-plastic cells frequently retain the phenotypic markers of their normal counterparts. These features can be used to aid in the characterization and subclassification of lymphoid malignancies (Table 52–3). Surface markers are antigens that may be present initially or can be acquired during differentiation. Many of these markers have been functionally characterized and are now recognized as specific membrane receptors or other structures of functional significance, but other antigens are without recognized specific functions.

In 1975, Kohler and Milstein developed a technique for producing an unlimited supply of an antibody of predefined specificity.[94] The resulting monoclonal antibody is one of extraordinary specificity directed against a single antigenic determinant. This technology has produced an ever-increasing battery of reagents that can identify the antigenic determinants of lymphoreticular cells.

These monoclonal antibodies have replaced a complex variety of assays that were previously used to detect lymphocyte surface markers or receptors.[95] A somewhat bewildering aspect of this technology is the enormous number of monoclonal antibodies published and available through commercial and private sources. In many cases, monoclonal antibodies bear different names but immunoprecipitate identical antigens and are of identical specificity. For example, OKT3 and anti-Leu-4 recognize the same antigen, CD3. An international nomenclature has been developed that follows the pattern used for the naming of HLA-related antigens, and the use of such commonly agreed-on terminology is invaluable in comparing reagents and results. Monoclonal antibodies of comparable specificity belong to the same group or "cluster of differentiation" and bear the same "CD" name (Table 52–4).

Monoclonal antibodies can be used in immunofluorescence or immunohistochemical assays to identify normal and neoplastic lymphoid cells. As currently performed, the cell preparation is incubated with an antibody to the molecule of interest, the unbound antibody is washed off, and the bound antibody is detected by fluorescence or a linked enzymatic reaction that gives a colored product. The advantage of immunohistochemical or immunocytochemical techniques (*i.e.*, those on which tissue sections or cytologic preparations from cell suspensions, respectively, are used) is that the in situ organization, cell morphology, and immunologic phenotype can be seen. This is useful because neoplasms rarely are pure populations of neoplastic cells; a variety of normal cell types are usually present. In trying to decide whether a lymphoma is of B- or T-cell origin, a positive result with an antibody to CD3 suggests T-cell origin only if the tumor cells are positive; many B-cell lymphomas contain large numbers of infiltrating T cells. Although not a substitute for hematoxylin-eosin stain morphologic examination, the use of immunohistochemistry is a valuable adjunct to accurate diagnosis.[96]

Complementary information can be gained using flow cytometry to quantitate the expression of surface antigens on cells.[97] Labeling of cells is conceptually the same as in immunohistochemistry, except that the second antibody is conjugated to a fluorescent molecule, such as fluorescein, phycoerythrin, or rhodamine, instead of an enzyme. Cells in suspension are passed single file through a glass chamber through which laser light of an appropriate wavelength is passed. The amount of fluorescence on a given cell, which is sensed quantitatively, is directly proportional to the number

TABLE 52–3.   Cellular Origin of Malignant Lymphomas

Neoplasms of B-Cell Origin	Neoplasms of T-Cell Origin	Neoplasms of Histiocytic Reticulum Cell Origin
Chronic lymphocytic leukemia (98%)	Chronic lymphocytic leukemia (2%)	Monocytic leukemia
	Large granular lymphocyte leukemia‡ (T gamma lymphoproliferative disease)	
Small lymphocytic (well-differentiated) lymphoma	Mycosis fungoides/Sézary syndrome	Malignant histiocytosis
Lymphocytic lymphoma, intermediate or small cleaved cell types (mantle zone lymphoma)	Diffuse aggressive lymphomas of adults (15%)	
	Peripheral T-cell lymphomas	True histiocytic lymphomas
	Mixed cell type	
	Large cell, immunoblastic	
Follicular lymphomas	Adult T-cell leukemia/lymphoma	
Diffuse aggressive lymphomas of adults (85%)	Angiocentric lymphomas (lymphomatoid granulomatosis polymorphic reticulosis)	Dendritic reticulum cell sarcomas
Mixed cell type		
Large cell type*		Interdigitating reticulum cell sarcomas
Large cell immunoblastic		
Small noncleaved cell*		
Burkitt's (small noncleaved cell) lymphoma		
Acute lymphocytic leukemias (75%)†	Acute lymphocytic leukemias (25%)†	
Lymphoblastic lymphomas (10%)†	Lymphoblastic lymphomas (85%)†	

* Majority of cases, 95%.
† These malignancies are of stem cell origin; they have an immature phenotype, but are committed to B- or T-cell differentiation, respectively.
‡ Bears certain T-cell markers, but is probably of NK cell origin.

of antibody molecules bound and therefore proportional to the amount of surface antigen expressed. Measurement of cell size is made at the same time. Current flow cytometers allow the quantitation of two (or three) antigens on a single cell through the concurrent use of two antibodies tagged with molecules that fluoresce at different wavelengths. The flow cytometer provides enumerations of cell size, number, and fluorescent intensity that can be plotted together in various ways. A flow cytometer is used to look at a statistically significant, reproducible sample of tens of thousands of cells in seconds. This allows characterization of a given preparation with numerous antibodies. The optical system is unbiased and sensitive (*i.e.*, it can detect a few thousand molecules on the cell surface with a high-affinity antibody), and the output can be stored in computers as raw data, allowing sophisticated manipulation and analysis.

Most antibodies currently available work only in suspension or in frozen preparations, because the processing for paraffin sections can alter the antigenic determinants significantly. However, some antigens are preserved in paraffin, and the major cell types (*i.e.*, T cells, B cells, mononuclear phagocytes) can be recognized in paraffin sections.[98,99]

T cells have been especially well characterized with monoclonal antibodies; they can be used to identify the cell's stage of differentiation and its functional capabilities (Fig. 52–2).[100] T cells can be divided into two major subsets, the helper/inducer and suppressor/cytotoxic cells.[101,102] Helper T cells are required for the terminal differentiation of a B cell into a plasma cell and provide help for immunoglobulin secretion. Suppressor cells can inhibit antibody production. Helper cells also promote the differentiation of cytotoxic T cells. In normal peripheral blood, the CD4:CD8 ratio is approximately 2:1,

and in normal lymph nodes, it is approximately 3.5 or 4:1. Most malignancies of T-cell origin preferentially express a CD4- or a CD8-positive phenotype. However, these antigens are not clonal markers and should not be interpreted as such. For unknown reasons, most mature T-cell malignancies have a CD4-positive phenotype.[103,104]

Monoclonal antibodies can also be used to delineate developmental stages of T-cell differentiation.[105,106] Early T cells lack CD4 and CD8 antigens and later coexpress them. Immature T cells express transferrin receptors identified by CD71.[107] This marker has no lineage specificity, because most proliferating cells have such receptors. Two of the earliest markers with some lineage specificity include the E-rosette receptor (CD2) and CD7. Both of these markers can be expressed before rearrangement of the T-cell antigen receptor.[108] This feature raises a question about marker specificity, and some researchers have reported expression of CD2 and CD7 in acute myelogenous leukemia blasts.[109] The CD1 (T6) antigen is found on cortical thymocytes, but is absent on mature T cells.[105] This antigen is expressed on Langerhans cells of the skin.[93] The CD5 antigen found on all normal T cells is also expressed on a subpopulation of normal B cells.[110] It is useful in the characterization of B-cell malignancies, because it is expressed in some tumors (*e.g.*, B-cell CLL) but not others.[111]

The hallmark of a B lymphocyte is the expression of surface immunoglobulin, which consists of one or more heavy chains and only one type of light chain per lymphocyte. Reactive B-cell proliferations are polyclonal, with a ratio of kappa:lambda expression of approximately 2:1. B-cell lymphomas are monoclonal and express only a single light chain type. When all the cells express a given light chain, the correlation with

TABLE 52–4. Selected CD Markers Expressed on Lymphoid and Hematopoietic Cells

CD Designation	Common Names	Molecular Weight	Primary Reactivity
CD1	Leu-6, T6	43–49	Cortical thymocytes, Langerhans cells
CD2	Leu-5, T11	50	SRBC receptor on T cells; cytoadhesion molecule binding to LFA-3
CD3	Leu-4, T3	20–25	T cells; constant element of T-cell receptor complex
CD4	Leu-3a, T4	59	Helper subset of T cells; cytoadhesion structure binding to MHC class II molecules
CD5	Leu-1, T1, T101	67	T cells and minor subset of B cells (B-CLL)
CD7	Leu-9, 3A1	40	T cells; expressed on prethymic T-cell precursor in bone marrow
CD8	Leu-2a, T8	33	Suppressor subset of T cells; cytoadhesion structure binding to MHC class I molecules
CD10	CALLA, J5	100	Membrane-associated neutral endopeptidase; the common acute lymphoblastic leukemia antigen
CD11a	LFA-1	180/95	Leukocytes, cell adhesion molecule
CD11b	Mo1	155/95	Monocytes, granulocytes, NK cells; C3bi receptor
CD11c	Leu-M5, S-HCL3, KiM1	150/95	α chain of the α/β glycoprotein complex; leukocyte cytoadhesion molecule expressed on monocytes, hairy cell leukemia
CD14	MY4	55	Macrophages
CD15	Leu-M1, My1		X-hapten; expressed in mature granulocytes, Reed-Sternberg cells
CD16	FcRIII	50–65	NK, granulocytes, macrophages Fc receptor for immunoglobulin G
CD18			β-chain to CD11a, b, c
CD19	B4, Leu-12	95	B cells, expressed at time of Ig heavy chain gene rearrangement; member of Ig supergene family
CD20	B1, Leu-16, L26	35–37	B cells, expressed at time of Ig light chain gene rearrangement; L-26 epitope is preserved in paraffin sections
CD21	B2	140	B cells; C3d receptor (CR2); serves as Epstein-Barr virus receptor
CD22	Leu-14, SHCL-1	135	Mature B cells; member of Ig supergene family
CD23	FcεRII	45–50	Fc receptor for immunoglobulin E
CD25	Tac, IL-2R	55	α-chain of IL-2 receptor complex; low affinity IL-2 receptor; activated T cells
CD30	Ki-1, BerH2 Hefi-1	105	Activated T cells, B cells; found in Reed-Sternberg cells and cells of large cell anaplastic lymphoma; related to the TRK oncogene and nerve growth factor receptor
CD38	T10, Leu-17	45	Plasma cells, activated T cells
CD45	LCA, T29/33	180–220	Common leukocyte antigen; various isoforms are preferentially expressed on different subsets (*e.g.*, CD45R0 [UCHL-1] expressed on memory T cells); functions as a tyrosine phosphatase
CD52	CAMPATH-1	21–28	Lymphocytes and other white cells
CD54	ICAM-1		Cell adhesion molecule
CD56	Leu-19	220/135	NK cells; N-CAM, neural cell adhesion molecule
CD68	KP1, KiM7	110	Macrophages; antigens preserved in paraffin sections
CD71	T9	95	Transferrin receptor; highly expressed on rapidly growing cells
CD74		41/35/33	Invariant chain associated with Ia molecules

malignancy is excellent. However, when using sensitive techniques, such as immunoglobulin gene rearrangement studies, the clinician must be cautious in equating monoclonality with malignancy. Under some conditions, particularly with immunodeficiency, a monoclonal population may be detected and may undergo spontaneous regression.[112]

Fewer monoclonal antibodies have been developed against B cells and B-cell subsets (Fig. 52–3).[113] Monoclonal antibodies with broad reactivity against normal B cells include CD20 (B1), CD19 (B4), and CD22 (Leu-14). These antigens are usually absent at the plasma cell stage. However, they are expressed in immature B cells before the acquisition of immunoglobulin on the cell membrane.[114,115] The so-called common acute lymphoblastic leukemia antigen (CALLA, CD10) was initially described on tumor cells from approxi-

mately 70% of patients with acute lymphoblastic leukemias.[116] Immunoglobulin gene rearrangement studies demonstrated that these cells were committed to B-cell differentiation, despite their lack of surface of cytoplasmic immunoglobulin.[117] CD10 is also expressed on Burkitt's lymphoma cells and most follicular lymphomas.[111,118] Although normal peripheral blood B cells do not stain with J5 (antibody to CD10), follicular center cells are positive when sensitive techniques are used.[119] CD10 is neither tumor specific nor lineage specific. It is present on neoplastic cells from 10% to 20% of cases of T-cell lymphoblastic lymphoma and leukemia.[106,118] It also occurs at a low-density on normal peripheral blood polymorphonuclear leukocytes.[120]

Most monoclonal antibodies react with monocytes, and macrophages also react with cells of the granulocytic series.

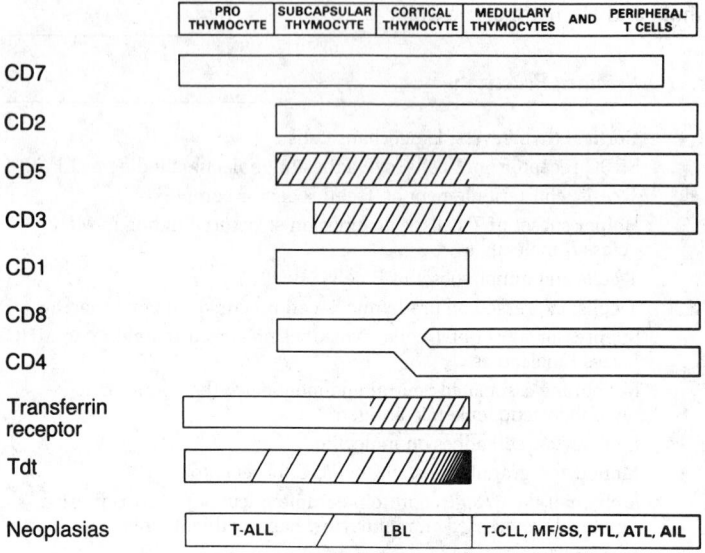

FIGURE 52–2. Monoclonal antibodies can be used to identify different developmental and functional T-cell subpopulations. Monoclonal antibodies are identified according to CD groups established by international nomenclature panel. Neoplasias of T-cell origin can be related to sequential stages of T-cell differentiation. (Modified from Cossman J, Chused T, Fisher R, et al. Diversity of immunologic phenotypes of lymphoblastic lymphoma. Cancer Res 1983;43:4486)

Included in this category are the monoclonal antibodies to CD11 and CD15.[121-123] Antibodies with greater specificity for the monocyte-macrophage fraction include the CD14 group, but these stain many B cells as well.[124] Antibodies to CD68 (KP1) react with macrophages in paraffin and frozen sections.[125]

Several monoclonal antibodies can detect the so-called common leukocyte antigen (CD45).[126,127] This antigen is expressed on all normal lymphoreticular cells. Although these antibodies are not useful in classifying lymphoreticular malignancies, they are useful in differentiating malignant lymphomas from nonlymphoid neoplasms such as carcinomas and sarcomas. All of these antibodies react with an antigen of approximately 200,000 daltons. However, they vary in their ability to stain paraffin-embedded or cryostat sections.

Terminal deoxynucleotidyl transferase (TdT) is a DNA polymerase that catalyses the addition of deoxyribonucleotide triphosphate to the 3′-hydroxy end of single-stranded poly- or oligodeoxyribonucleotide primers.[128] This enzyme is present in immature lymphoid cells of T-cell and B-cell origin. The enzyme is found in low levels in normal bone marrow. Mature peripheral blood B and T lymphocytes and phytohemagglutinin-stimulated lymphocytes do not contain detectable TdT. This enzyme has been identified in the cells of almost all patients with ALL and lymphoblastic lymphoma and in the cells of some patients with chronic myelogenous leukemia in lymphoid blast crisis.[129] TdT determinations may be performed on fresh or frozen tissues in cell suspension and can be identified biochemically or with antisera reactive with TdT antigenically.[130]

The demonstration of various hydrolytic enzymes by cytochemical and histochemical techniques has been useful in

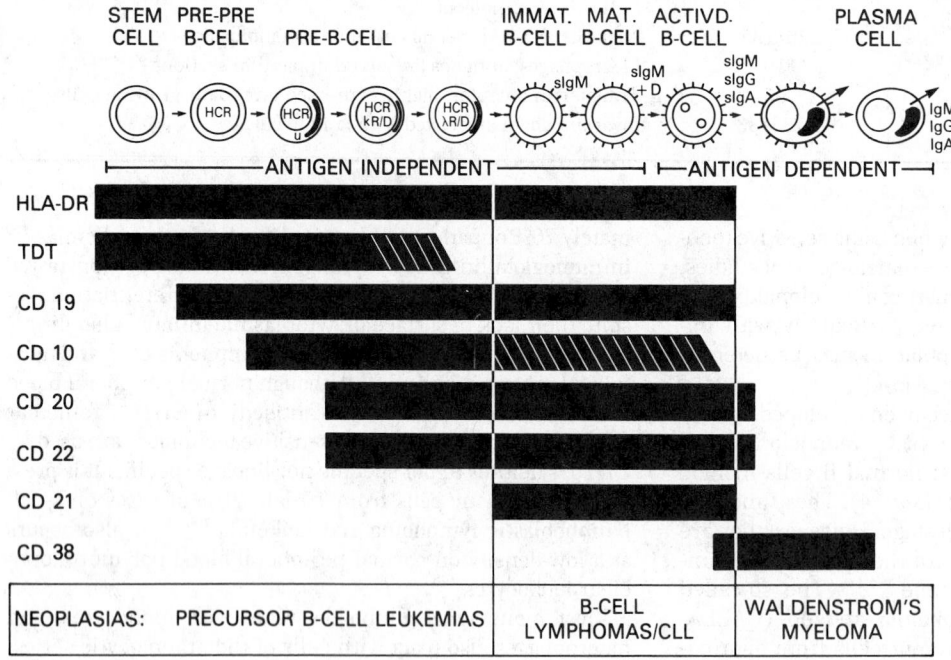

FIGURE 52–3. Diagram demonstrating the molecular genetic and immunophenotypic correlates of normal B-cell differentiation. Monoclonal antibodies are identified according to CD groups established by international nomenclature panel. Steps of heavy and light chain immunoglobulin gene rearrangement are shown. B-cell malignancies are associated with the sequential stages of B-cell differentiation. HCR, heavy chain rearrangement; kappa R/D, kappa light chain rearrangement or deletion; lambda R/D, lambda light chain rearrangement or deletion; μ, mu heavy chain synthesis.

identifying certain cells of the lymphoreticular system.[131] The most helpful assays are those for nonspecific esterase (NSE), acid phosphatase (AP), and tartrate-resistant phosphatase (TRAP). Diffuse activity for NSE and AP is characteristic of monocytes-macrophages; antigen-presenting cells have a more punctate and localized reaction pattern. Normal T lymphocytes display punctate reactivity for NSE (at an acid pH) and AP. However, some reactivity may be seen in normal and neoplastic B lymphocytes. These cytochemical markers are not reliable for the determination of immunologic phenotype of lymphoid cells. TRAP is a characteristic feature of the cells of hairy cell leukemia.[132]

GENE REARRANGEMENT

The technology of molecular biology has provided new methods for detecting lineage, clonality, and minimal residual disease in malignant lymphomas. B cells undergo specific rearrangements of their immunoglobulin genes and T cells their T-cell receptor genes as they are committed to a particular lineage.[133–136] The genes of cells that have not initiated this process are in a germline configuration. As a consequence, the detection of a rearrangement can be used as a tool to determine lineage.[137,138] For example, the cellular origin of hairy cell leukemia was long a subject of speculation, because it had features suggestive of monocytes and B cells. The demonstration of immunoglobulin light chain gene rearrangements resolved the issue.[138] Lymphomas generally can be assigned to T- or B-cell groups by Southern analysis with probes for the T-cell receptor and immunoglobulin subunits. However, certain pitfalls have emerged. Although the finding of rearranged light chain genes appears to be diagnostic of B lineage, heavy chain genes are occasionally rearranged in T or myeloid neoplasms.[139,140] Similarly, the presence of rearranged T-cell receptor genes is not entirely specific for T-cell lineage. Rearranged β chain genes have been seen in otherwise clear cut B-cell lymphomas, and the T-γ gene is problematic as a clonal marker, because its limited number of variable regions gives rise to distinct bands on Southern analysis even in polyclonal populations.[141,142] Nevertheless, only hematopoietic cells rearrange these genes, and therefore, this kind of analysis can be helpful in differentiating between poorly differentiated carcinoma and lymphoma.

The DNA sequences involved in these rearrangements are detected by the Southern blot technique. Intact cellular DNA is isolated and cut into many small fragments by restriction enzymes that are highly specific for certain nucleotide sequences. The restriction fragments can be size separated with agarose gel electrophoresis, and a fragment containing a particular sequence can be detected by using a radioactively labeled, cloned DNA probe that is complementary to the sequence of interest. Because of the innumerable possible rearrangements in a population of normal polyclonal lymphocytes, no single rearrangement pattern would predominate, and a probe would label a smear of fragments of all sizes. However, the nature of the Southern method is such that if more than 1% to 5% of the cells are of monoclonal origin, a single restriction fragment is labeled above the background. In this way, a change in a restriction fragment size from the germline can be used as a marker for a clone of cells derived from a particular lymphocyte.[112] Because each clone

has a unique rearrangement pattern, Southern blot analysis is particularly useful in examining sequential specimens. After establishing the rearrangement pattern of the primary lesion, it is possible to determine whether subsequent biopsies contain a clonal population of lymphoid cells and whether the clone is identical to the original one.

Another important potential clinical use is in staging and in the detection of even small numbers of lymphoma cells. For example, clonal populations of T lymphocytes can be detected in lymph nodes from patients with mycosis fungoides that had been called negative for involvement by standard surgical pathology techniques.[143] However, demonstration of a clonal population of lymphocytes is not always proof of malignancy. Lymphomatoid papulosis is a chronic, often self-remitting illness that is limited to the skin, usually without clinical progression to malignancy, despite containing clonally rearranged T cells.[144]

Clonal populations must be viewed with caution, particularly in the setting of immunodeficiency. Patients with the Wiskott-Aldrich syndrome may develop transient serum monoclonal spikes, and in one study, a clonal proliferation of B cells was identified by gene rearrangement in a lymph node from 1 patient.[112] However, this patient never developed a malignant lymphoproliferative disorder. EBV can immortalize B cells in vitro and in vivo, and in the setting of immunodeficiency, these clones may be expanded and identifiable by Southern blot analysis.[145] However, if immunocompetence can be restored, the clones may regress, as has been demonstrated in renal transplant recipients.[33] A second mutational event is probably required for the true malignant transformation of such expanded B-cell clones.

The physician must be careful to use the information these techniques provide only with the benefit of relevant clinical information. The finding of a faint T-β gene rearrangement in a pleural effusion from a patient with a known T-cell lymphoma, in which the rearranging band matches the size of that in the previous biopsy, can be interpreted as diagnostic of lymphoma in the pleural fluid. The same finding in a patient with AIDS is of unknown significance. As these techniques become more widely available, clinical correlation studies will need to be done. For example, it is unknown whether the demonstration of occult disease in lymph nodes of mycosis fungoides patients has any effect on prognosis or whether it is simply a reflection of the ability of the neoplastic cells to circulate throughout the lymphoid system.

Molecular biology techniques have been made dramatically more sensitive for detecting few residual tumor cells, particularly those expressing chromosomal translocations for which there are probes available (e.g., t[14;18] in follicular lymphoma). The polymerase chain reaction (PCR) technique uses in vitro enzymatic synthesis to amplify specific DNA sequences.[146] The reaction is based on the annealing and extension of two oligonucleotide primers that flank the target region in double-stranded DNA. The technique provides extraordinary sensitivity because 20 cycles of the reaction amplify a specific sequence up to 1 million times, enabling the detection of 1 in 10^5 cells bearing that sequence.[147] Cells from 85% or more of cases of follicular lymphoma contain specific sequences as a consequence of the t(14;18)(q32;q21) that transposes the *BCL2* gene from its normal position on chromosome 18 to join it to the gene for the immunoglobulin heavy chain of the joining region (*IGHJ*) on chromosome 14.[148,149] Using primers that recognize sequences specific to the breakpoint, DNA from cells bearing that translocation are amplified but not DNA from unrearranged *BCL2* or *IGHJ* genes in normal cells.

This technique is currently employed to monitor the completeness of purging of tumor cells from bone marrow in extracorporeal depletion experiments, and if applied carefully to bone marrow and lymph node aspirates, it could alter the criterion for determining complete remission in lymphoma.

NORMAL AND MALIGNANT T-CELL AND B-CELL DEVELOPMENT

With a combination of cell surface phenotyping, enzyme histochemistry, and Southern and Northern molecular biology techniques, it is possible to roughly map the stages of differentiation of lymphoid cells and relate the stages to the phenotypes of particular lymphocytic lymphomas (see Figs. 52–2 and 52–3).[150]

T cells arise from a pluripotent stem cell by way of a lymphoid stem cell and undergo maturation in the thymus. The earliest committed T cells express surface receptors for transferrin receptor (CD71) and CD38 and contain terminal transferase. These cells are located in the thymic cortex and comprise about 5% of all thymocytes. With further maturation, these cells lose CD71, acquire CD1, and concurrently express CD38, CD4, and CD8 antigens. The cells contain no terminal transferase, but the message for rearranged β chains of the T-cell antigen receptor and CD3, the nonpolymorphic 7-chain receptor-associated molecule, is detectable in the cytoplasm, but protein is not yet expressed on the cell surface. A fraction of these cells express low-affinity IL-2 receptors. The CD4- and CD8-positive cells (also called double-positive thymocytes) comprise 80% to 85% of thymocytes in the cortex. In the medulla, which makes up about 10% of the thymocyte population, the phenotype of the thymocytes is indistinguishable from peripheral mature T cells. These cells lose CD1, express CD3 and antigen receptors (mainly α chain–β chain heterodimers), and lose CD8 to become class II MHC-restricted helper T cells or CD4 to become class I MHC-restricted suppressor T cells. Throughout their maturation in the thymus, T cells express CD2 and CD7.

Malignancies arising in early or subcapsular cortical thymocytes are usually T-cell ALL. Lymphoblastic lymphomas may have the phenotype of early or common cortical thymocytes. All the other T-cell lymphomas arise from cells with mature or postthymic phenotype. Most tumors arising from mature cells bear CD4 and include ATL, mycosis fungoides, Sézary's syndrome, angiocentric immunoproliferative lesions, most so-called peripheral T-cell lymphomas (*i.e.*, diffuse large cell, immunoblastic and mixed lymphomas by Working Formulation terminology), and about half of the cases of T-cell CLL. A few peripheral T-cell lymphomas, about half of the cases of T-cell CLL, and some cases of T-γ lymphoproliferative disease (*i.e.*, large granular lymphocytic leukemia, T-cell CLL) express CD8. T-γ lymphoproliferative disease is heterogenous, including some CD3-positive and some CD3-negative cases. Its rarity interferes with completely thorough subclassification. However, even those that express CD3 have more similarity to a subset of NK cells than T cells in that

they may also express OKM1, CD15, CD38, Fc receptors, asialo-GM1, CD57, and CD56. Those expressing CD3 are usually associated with neutropenia, rheumatoid arthritis, and autoantibody formation, and the CD3-negative tumors are less frequently associated with neutropenia and autoimmune phenomena.[151]

Somewhat less is known about B-cell development and the role of the host in shaping it. Fewer B-cell-specific antibodies are available, and most of what is known about B-cell maturation relates to the steps of immunoglobulin gene rearrangement and expression of surface immunoglobulin. The earliest B cell expresses class II MHC (HLA-DR), CD10, and CD19 on the surface, terminal transferase intracellularly, and has rearranged its heavy chain genes. Subsequently, the cell expresses CD20 and nonsequentially produces cytoplasmic μ heavy chains, rearranges κ light chain genes, rearranges λ light chain genes, and loses terminal transferase. This represents the pre-B-cell stage of development. The cell becomes recognizable as an immature B cell after it loses CD10 expression and expresses surface IgM. The cell then expresses surface CD21 (C3d receptor) and has surface IgD and IgM on the membrane. All subsequent steps in B-cell development are driven by exposure to antigen. After contacting antigen, the immunoglobulin genes undergo a class switch and express the isotype they ultimately secrete. Then they lose CD21, CD20, and surface immunoglobulin, and acquire PC-1 and PCA-1, which are plasma cell markers, and they secrete immunoglobulin. This is the life history of follicular center B cells, the cells most commonly giving rise to lymphocytic lymphomas (see Fig. 52–3).

There is another subpopulation of B cells whose relation to follicular center B cells is unclear. Many of the events in the maturation of follicular center B cells after exposure to antigen are assisted by factors produced by helper T cells. Immunoglobulin class switch is T-cell mediated. However, mantle zone B cells appear to be more independent of the influence of T cells; they express CD5, a pan T-cell marker and do not appear capable of switching to immunoglobulin isotypes other than IgM after exposure to antigen.

Most cases of ALL originate from pre-B cells. Burkitt's lymphoma and leukemia arise from the surface IgM-positive immature B cell. Most follicular and diffuse B-cell lymphomas arise from mature or activated B cells. Waldenström's macroglobulinemia and multiple myeloma originate from cells near terminal differentiation. CLL cells express CD5, as do cells of diffuse intermediately differentiated lymphocytic lymphoma, which are also CD10 positive. This may mean that these tumors derive from mantle zone rather than follicular center B cells.

Although it is possible to phenotype malignancies of lymphocytes, the correlation of the phenotype with histology is not complete. Diffuse large cell lymphomas seem to be the most heterogenous, including tumors of B-cell, T-cell, and histiocyte origin. The clinical course of disease is not accurately predicted by the stage of developmental arrest of a particular tumor. For example, ATL is a tumor of mature, postthymic T cells, but it is every bit as aggressive clinically as a lymphoblastic lymphoma, which is derived from a more immature cell. Although phenotyping can be useful in certain ways, it does not provide information that is more valuable to the clinician than the interpretation of hematoxylin and eosin stained tissue examined under a light microscope by an experienced hematopathologist.

PATHOLOGY OF LYMPHOCYTIC LYMPHOMAS

The classification of neoplastic lymphoid disorders has undergone significant evolution over the past 150 years (Table 52–5).[152-164] The Rappaport classification (Table 52–6) has been the most popular classification for clinicians in the United States.[162,165] Rappaport first divided lymphomas by pattern, whether nodular or diffuse, and then by cytologic subtypes. Tumors were termed poorly or well-differentiated lymphocytic based on the degree to which the neoplastic cells resembled normal lymphocytes. Lymphomas composed of large cells with abundant cytoplasm were termed "histiocytic" and were thought to be derived from histiocytes or phagocytic cells. The term "undifferentiated" was used for lymphomas of intermediate cell size that failed to demonstrate evidence of "lymphoid" or "histiocytic" origin.

Although the Rappaport classification was quite popular among clinicians, it became the subject of considerable controversy, for it was proposed at a time when relatively little was known about the normal immune system. As scientists discovered the functional and ontogenetic heterogeneity of the normal immune system, researchers questioned the sci-

TABLE 52–5. Landmarks in the Description of the Lymphocytic Lymphomas

Investigations	Observation
Craigie, 1845[152]	Described the first cases of leukemia
Bennett, 1845[153]	
Virchow, 1845[154]	Differentiated lymphosarcoma from leukemia and included cases described by Hodgkin in the lymphosarcoma group
Billroth, 1871[155]	Coined phrase "malignant lymphomas"
Dreschfeld, 1892[156]	Developed histologic criteria for diagnosing lymphosarcoma
Kundradt, 1893[157]	
Brill et al, 1925[158]	Described giant follicular lymphoma and considered it a benign disease ("Brill-Symmers disease")
Symmers, 1927[159]	
Roulet, 1930[160]	Developed histologic criteria for diagnosing reticulum cell sarcoma and considered it a malignancy of the supporting cells of the lymph node
Gall, Mallory, 1942[161]	Developed criteria for differentiating benign hyperplasia from malignant follicular lymphoma
Rappaport et al, 1956[162]	Described different cell types within follicular lymphomas and named them "nodular lymphomas"
Burkitt, 1958[163]	Described lymphoma of the jaw in Africa, which bears his name
Uchiyama et al, 1977[164]	Described adult T-cell leukemia-lymphoma
Poiesz et al, 1980[52]	Identified HTLV-I as first human retrovirus and the causative agent of adult T-cell leukemia-lymphoma

entific validity of the Rappaport approach. The concepts of well differentiated and poorly differentiated were inaccurate as applied in the Rappaport scheme, as was the use of the term "histiocytic" for a tumor of transformed lymphoid cells.

New classifications attempted to address the scientific inaccuracies of the Rappaport scheme and to relate these tumors more closely to the normal immune system (see Table 52–6).[165-171] For example, the classification of Lukes and Collins proposed that immunologic subtypes could be recognized by morphologic features alone.[168] Although certain features, such as follicle formation by the neoplastic cells, were found to be reliable indicators of follicular B-lymphocyte origin, cytologic features were shown to be unreliable for predicting T- or B-cell phenotype in the diffuse lymphomas.[172,173]

The use of six different pathologic classifications for lymphocytic lymphomas throughout the world makes the international analysis and comparison of clinical trials extremely difficult. A new scheme, called the Working Formulation, is based on an international study comparing the six major systems (Tables 52–6 and 52–7).[174] The basic approach is similar to that of the Rappaport scheme in that lymphomas are classified on the basis of follicular or diffuse pattern and cytologic composition. Although immunologic terminology is not used, correlations with established immunologic phenotypes can be drawn. It has been proposed that this formulation not be viewed as an alternative classification, but rather as a common language that can be used by all clinical investigators to translate from one classification scheme to another. This system is employed throughout this chapter, and we attempt to relate these tumors to the normal immune system if this information is available. The popularity of the Rappaport classification was due to its reproducibility, the fact that it is easily learned, and to the information provided to clinicians, allowing them to relate histology to some reasonable assessment of the likely clinical course. The Working Formulation provides the same clinical information by grouping lymphomas into low-, intermediate-, or high-grade neoplasms based on their untreated or minimally treated natural history (see Table 52–6). Although this has proven to be a useful scheme, we feel that minor modifications are needed to include disease entities that were left out of the original formulation and to improve grouping of the histologic subtypes according to their natural history and the strategies used for their treatment (Table 52–8).

A diagnosis of lymphocytic lymphoma in the Working Formulation is based on morphologic features only, but it has predictive value for survival.[175,176] Low-grade lymphomas are usually characterized by an indolent clinical course and relatively long survival with or without aggressive therapy. Malignant cells are usually found at sites where the normal counterparts of these lymphocytic lymphoma cells are located.[177] For example, follicular lymphomas are derived from follicular B lymphocytes, demonstrate a striking capacity to home to B-cell-dependent portions of the lymphoid system, and have a nondestructive growth pattern.[87] The cells readily circulate or disseminate, and patients with this type of lymphocytic lymphoma usually have stage III or IV disease. However, privileged sites such as testis or CNS are rarely involved by these tumors. Cytologic atypia or anaplasia is not typical of low-grade lymphocytic lymphoma. Follicular lymphomas may respond to normal immunoregulation, unlike the high-grade

TABLE 52–6.   Comparison of Commonly Used Classifications for the Lymphocytic Lymphomas

Modified Rappaport Classification (1966)[166,167]		Lukes and Collins Classification (1974)[168]		Kiel Classification (1974)[169,170]	
Nodular		Undefined cell type		Low-grade malignancy	
Lymphocytic, well differentiated	A*	T-cell type, small lymphocytic	A	Lymphocytic, chronic lymphocytic-leukemia	A
Lymphocytic, poorly differentiated	B	T-cell type, Sézary-mycosis fungoides (cerebriform)		Lymphocytic, other	A
Mixed, lymphocytic and histiocytic	C	T-cell type, convoluted lymphocytic	I	Lymphoplasmacytoid	A
Histiocytic	D	T-cell type, immunoblastic sarcoma (T cell)	H	Centrocytic	E
Diffuse		B-cell type, small lymphocytic	A	Centroblastic-centrocytic, follicular without sclerosis	B, C, D
Lymphocytic, well differentiated with plasmacytoid features	A	B-cell type, plasmacytoid lymphocytic	A	Centroblastic-centrocytic, follicular with sclerosis	
Lymphocytic, well differentiated with plasmacytoid features	A	Follicular center cell, small cleaved	B–E	Centroblastic-centrocytic, follicular and diffuse, without sclerosis	
Lymphocytic, poorly differentiated	E	Follicular center cell, large cleaved	D–G	Centroblastic-centrocytic, follicular and diffuse, with sclerosis	
Lymphoblastic, convoluted	I	Follicular center cell, small noncleaved	J	Centroblastic-centrocytic, diffuse	F
Lymphoblastic, nonconvoluted	I	Follicular center cell, large noncleaved	D–G	Low-grade malignant lymphoma, unclassified	
Mixed, lymphocytic and histiocytic	F	Immunoblastic sarcoma (B cell)		High-grade malignancy	
Histiocytic without sclerosis	G	Subtypes of follicular center cell lymphomas	H	Centroblastic	G
Histiocytic with sclerosis	G	1. Follicular		Lymphoblastic, Burkitt's type	J
Burkitt's tumor	J	2. Follicular and diffuse		Lymphoblastic, convoluted cell type	I
Undifferentiated	J	3. Diffuse		Lymphoblastic, other (unclassified) immunoblastic	H
		4. Sclerotic with follicles		High-grade malignant lymphoma, unclassified	
Malignant lymphoma, unclassified		5. Sclerotic without follicles		Malignant lymphoma, unclassified (unable to specify "high grade" or "low grade")	
Composite lymphoma		Histiocytic		Composite lymphoma	
		Malignant lymphoma, unclassified			

* Letters indicate equivalent or related category in the Working Formulation as shown in Table 52–7.

lymphomas, which are consistently autonomous. Patients with follicular lymphoma may have a history of lymph nodes that wax and wane in size, often for many years before diagnosis.[178] Host immunity has been invoked to explain this phenomenon, and in some cases, the clinical regression has been preceded by bacterial or viral infection. In contrast, the intermediate- and high-grade lymphomas usually have an aggressive and unrelenting natural history unless treated vigorously.[179] Extranodal sites and privileged sites are more frequently involved, and B symptoms are more common.

A further complication in the classification of lymphocytic lymphoma is that a significant fraction of patients with lymphocytic lymphoma have divergent histologies in the same or different biopsy sites, as many as 33% in some series.[180,181] Commonly, there is a follicular pattern in one site and diffuse pattern in another; in such cases, survival is intermediate between the two.[181] Histologic progression from a low-grade lymphoma to one of higher grade during the clinical course is also common in B-cell lymphomas. At the National Cancer Institute (NCI), 37% of patients with a follicular pattern of lymphocytic lymphoma had progression to a diffuse pattern when rebiopsied (>3 months) after initial staging.[182] With

modern therapy, eradication of the diffuse aggressive component with only the residual low-grade follicular component remaining is now seen. The term "composite lymphoma" has been used to describe various cases with more than one histologic type; a strict definition of composite lymphoma is a lymphoma consisting of the two distinctly different and well-delineated varieties of lymphoma occurring in a single anatomic site or mass.[183] Most composite lymphomas do not represent two distinct tumors but are different manifestations of the same clonal proliferation. True composite lymphomas, such as the coexistence of Hodgkin's disease and lymphocytic lymphoma in a single site, are identified rarely.

LOW-GRADE LYMPHOMAS

Malignant Small Cell Lymphocytic Lymphoma

Diffuse small lymphocytic lymphoma (*i.e.*, diffuse well-differentiated lymphoma) composed of well-differentiated small lymphocytes is the solid tumor counterpart of CLL.[184] If patients with the usual peripheral blood manifestations of CLL are excluded, these neoplasms constitute approximately 5% of all lymphocytic lymphomas. The patients, even when

TABLE 52–7. Working Formulation of Lymphocytic Lymphoma for Clinical Use: Recommendations of an Expert International Panel and Comparisons to the Rappaport Scheme

Working Formulation	Rappaport Terminology
Low Grade	
A. Malignant lymphoma, small lymphocytic	Diffuse well-differentiated lymphocyte
Consistent with chronic lymphocytic leukemia	
B. Malignant lymphoma, follicular, predominantly small cleaved cell	Nodular poorly differentiated lymphocytic
Diffuse areas	
Sclerosis	
C. Malignant lymphoma, follicular mixed, small cleaved and large cell	Nodular mixed lymphocytic histiocytic
Diffuse areas	
Sclerosis	
Intermediate Grade	
D. Malignant lymphoma, follicular	Nodular histiocytic
Predominantly large cell	
Diffuse areas	
Sclerosis	
E. Malignant lymphoma, diffuse small cleaved cell	Diffuse poorly differentiated lymphocytic
F. Malignant lymphoma, diffuse mixed, small and large cell sclerosis	Diffuse mixed lymphocytic-histiocytic
Epitheliod cell component	
G. Malignant lymphoma, diffuse	Diffuse histiocytic
Large cell	
Cleaved cell	
Noncleaved cell	
Sclerosis	
High Grade	
H. Malignant lymphoma large cell, immunoblastic	Diffuse histiocytic
Plasmacytoid	
Clear cell	
Polymorphous	
Epithelioid cell component	
I. Malignant lymphoma lymphoblastic	Diffuse lymphoblastic
Convoluted cell	
Nonconvoluted cell	
J. Malignant lymphoma small noncleaved cell	Diffuse undifferentiated
Burkitt's	
Follicular areas	

aleukemic or subleukemic, often have focal involvement of the bone marrow, liver, and other visceral sites at presentation and usually generalized asymptomatic lymphadenopathy.[185] With time, the natural history of this disease seems to be progression to CLL. In most patients, the malignant cells are monoclonal B lymphocytes and, as in CLL, the neoplastic cells express the p65 membrane protein CD5.[111,186] In one study of small lymphocytic lymphoma and CLL, the lymphoma cells usually expressed LFA-1 (CD11a), a cell adhesion molecule that could affect the propensity of recirculating tumor cells to take up residence in a lymph node.[187] CLL cells usually

failed to express these homotypic adhesion molecules. The neoplastic cells of small lymphocytic lymphoma and CLL, like normal medullary cord B lymphocytes, may exhibit some functional differentiation toward plasma cells and can be readily induced to secrete monoclonal immunoglobulin after exposure to the phorbol ester 12-O-tetradecanoylphorbol-13-acetate.[188] The monoclonal protein synthesized and expressed on the cell surface is usually IgM, and the κ light chain is found more often than λ.

The disorder known as Waldenström's macroglobulinemia can be most readily viewed as a form of small lymphocytic

TABLE 52–8. National Cancer Institute Clinical Schema for Lymphocytic Lymphomas Based on Natural History of Untreated or Palliatively Treated Patients

Low Grade or Indolent (median survival measured in years)
Small lymphocytic
Follicular, small cleaved cell
Follicular, mixed
Diffuse, small cleaved cells*
Diffuse, intermediately differentiated (or mantle zone)†
Cutaneous T cell†

Intermediate Grade or Aggressive (median survival measured in months)
Follicular, large cell
Diffuse mixed
Diffuse large cell
Diffuse immunoblastic‡

High Grade (median survival measured in weeks)
Diffuse small noncleaved cell (Burkitt's)
Diffuse small noncleaved cell (non-Burkitt's)
Lymphoblastic
Adult T-cell leukemia-lymphoma†

---

* Working Formulation intermediate-grade tumor with an indolent natural history.
† Omitted from the Working Formulation.
‡ Working Formulation high-grade tumor with an aggressive natural history.

---

neoplasia with immunoglobulin secretion as its sine qua non (see Chap. 54). The cells spontaneously secrete immunoglobulin, resulting in a monoclonal IgM serum spike. These cases represent approximately 15% of all small lymphocytic lymphomas. Morphologically, the cells usually demonstrate plasmacytoid features, often exhibiting a spectrum even within a single patient. Unlike CLL and small lymphocytic lymphomas without plasmacytoid differentiation, the cells are CD5 negative. Clinically, the disease presents a spectrum from CLL-like features to a form characterized predominantly by lymphadenopathy and hepatosplenomegaly. Heavy-chain diseases corresponding to the three most plentiful classes of immunoglobulins are also discussed in the chapter on plasma cell neoplasms.

Small lymphocytic lymphomas may contain moderate numbers of larger cells or prolymphocytes, which may accumulate in growth centers, sometimes imparting a pseudofollicular appearance at low power.[189] If the mitotic rate is less than 30 mitoses per 20 high-powered fields, the prognosis is not adversely affected.[189] However, emergence of a monomorphic proliferation of the larger lymphoid cells indicates progression to a diffuse large cell lymphoma, the so-called Richter's syndrome.[190] This transformation occurs in approximately 1% of patients, but a larger proportion of patients undergo a gradual acceleration in the clinical course of their disease over time. Immunologic studies have shown that these large cells bear the same surface determinants as the small lymphoid cells of the original disease.[191]

Mucosal-Associated Lymphoid Tissue Lymphomas

It has been proposed that extranodal small lymphocytic malignancies represent a distinct clinicopathologic entity related to MALT.[192,193] MALT lymphomas are distinctive morphologically, phenotypically, and clinically. Formerly, they were often diagnosed as pseudolymphomas because they contain normal germinal centers and have a somewhat polymorphous cytologic composition.[194] However, phenotypic analysis has shown that the small lymphocytic component is monoclonal. Unlike most small lymphocytic lymphomas, the MALT lymphomas are consistently CD5 negative.[195]

Recognition of the MALT lymphoma concept may be important because a distinctive clinical behavior has been associated with these tumors. Unlike other small lymphocytic malignancies, they seem to have a low risk of dissemination to lymph nodes, bone marrow, or peripheral blood, but they have a high risk of relapse in diverse extranodal sites. The most common sites of involvement include lung, stomach, salivary glands, and lacrimal glands, but almost every extranodal site is at risk.[195] The clinical course is usually indolent, characterized by multiple recurrences over years, but with limited mortality.

Monocytoid B-cell lymphomas appear closely related to MALT lymphomas. Although this process was first described in lymph nodes, it carries a high risk of extranodal disease.[196] These low-grade lymphomas are similar phenotypically, morphologically, and clinically. A close association with Sjögren's syndrome has been demonstrated.[196]

Follicular Lymphomas

Follicular (*i.e.*, nodular) lymphomas are those in which the neoplastic cells form circumscribed aggregates that morphologically resemble germinal centers (Fig. 52–4).[197] The nodular pattern may exist throughout the tumor, or it may be manifested only in a portion of the lymphoma that elsewhere is composed of diffuse cellular proliferation.[180,198] Follicular lymphoma can be differentiated from reactive follicular hyperplasia by the total effacement of lymph node architecture by nodular proliferation. The nodules vary little in size and shape and are crowded together with little intervening normal lymphoid parenchyma. They also lack well-defined lymphoid cuffs. In areas of the nodules, the neoplastic cells may be confined to the nodules with normal-appearing cells in the internodular tissue or present between the nodules. In the former situation, the neoplasms may be mistaken for benign follicular hyperplasia unless careful scrutiny is given to the cells composing the nodules. Although normal germinal centers are composed of cytologically heterogenous populations representing the entire spectrum of proliferating B cells, neoplastic nodules appear more homogenous and "clonal." Other useful differential features include polarization and the presence of a "starry sky" pattern in reactive germinal centers but not in follicular lymphomas. Nodular lymphomas are neoplasms of follicular B cells.[172,199]

The cells of follicular lymphomas can be predominantly small cleaved cells (poorly differentiated lymphocytic), large noncleaved, or large cleaved cells (histiocytic), or a mixture of cell types, such as mixed small cleaved and large cell (mixed

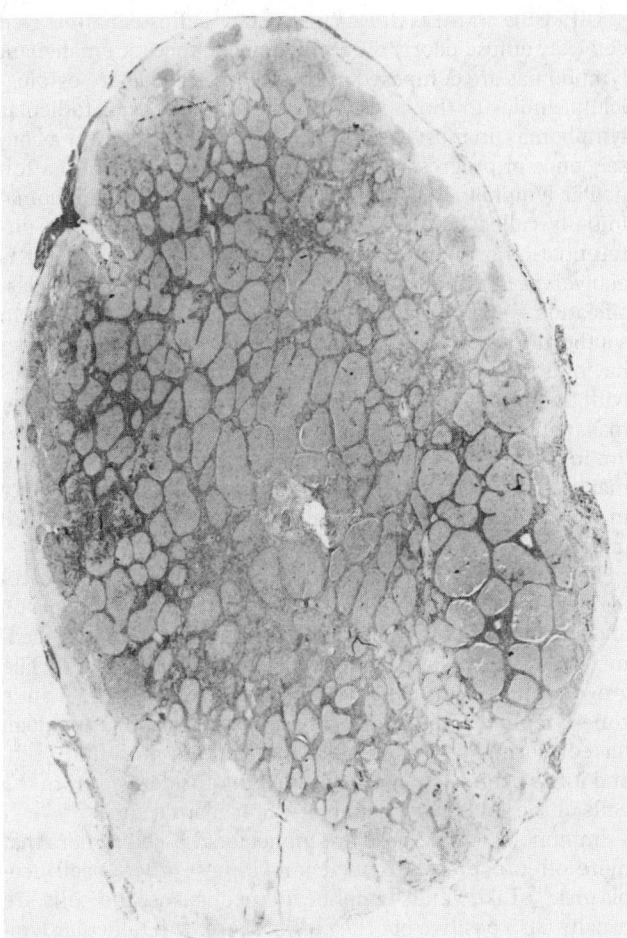

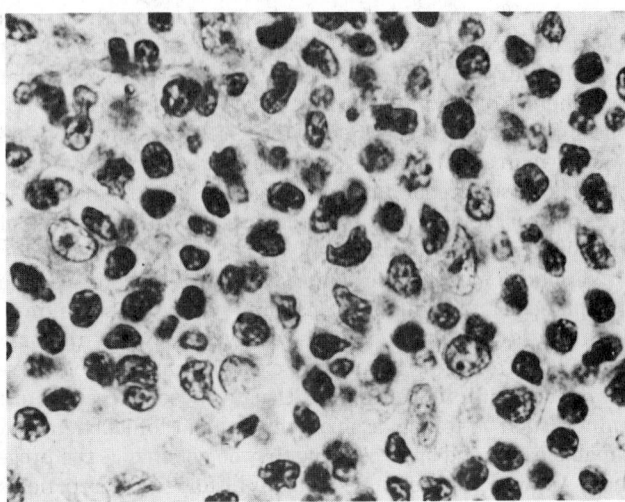

FIGURE 52–5. Follicular lymphoma: predominantly small cleaved cell type. Atypical lymphocytes are indented and angular (hematoxylin & eosin stain; original magnification × 1000).

FIGURE 52–4. Effacement of architecture by monotonous nodularity in follicular lymphoma (hematoxylin & eosin stain; original magnification × 10). Compare this with the predominately cortical location of follicles in a normal lymph node shown in Figure 52–1.

lymphocytic-histiocytic). The larger cells appear to be the replicative component of the process, and the smaller lymphoid cells are more indolent and perhaps more motile.

FOLLICULAR, PREDOMINANTLY SMALL CLEAVED CELL LYMPHOMA. Follicular, predominantly small cleaved cell lymphoma (*i.e.*, nodular poorly differentiated lymphocytic lymphoma) is the most common type of follicular lymphoma, accounting for approximately 60% of cases. The neoplastic cells usually are small, cleaved, indented lymphocytes with few large cells (Fig. 52–5). Mitotic figures are rare. Monoclonal populations of lymphocytes identical to those found in involved lymph nodes are present in the peripheral blood of many patients with follicular lymphomas who do not otherwise have morphologic evidence of leukemia.[200] When leukemia does appear, the lymphoid cells in the peripheral blood exhibit notches in the nucleus ("buttock cells"). The process has been referred to as lymphosarcoma cell leukemia.[201] However, this term should be avoided because it has been used with biologically and clinically diverse malignant lymphomas that happen to have a leukemic phase.

FOLLICULAR, MIXED SMALL CLEAVED AND LARGE CELL LYMPHOMA. In follicular, mixed small cleaved and large cell (nodular mixed) malignant lymphoma, representing approximately 30% of cases, the large nucleolated cells are more abundant, numbering more than five per high-powered field and, in some cases, appearing to be admixed in almost equal numbers with smaller lymphoid cells.[202] As with most follicular lymphomas, patients usually have easily detectable disseminated disease at presentation, but it is not uncommon to find only the smaller cleaved lymphoid cells in sites distant from the nodes of origin, such as liver or bone marrow. In bone marrow, the characteristic paratrabecular location of the lymphoid infiltrates is useful in differentiating involvement by follicular lymphoma from normal lymphoid nodules that are usually within the marrow space and perivascular in location. This observation underscores the belief that the smaller cells are the migratory component of the normal and malignant lymphoid system and that the large cells are the replicative forms.

FOLLICULAR, PREDOMINANTLY LARGE CELL LYMPHOMA. Follicular, predominantly large cell (nodular histiocytic) malignant lymphoma is the least common form of follicular lymphoma and accounts for only 10% of cases.[203] The motile small lymphoid cells, seen in appreciable numbers in the other nodular lymphomas, are few in these tumors, and the patients often appear to have localized tumors. Despite their earlier clinical stage at diagnosis, they had the least favorable prognosis of all follicular lymphomas, because the localized appearance was deceptive and frequent recurrences and progression to diffuse large cell tumors occurred.

VARIATIONS IN PATTERN AND CYTOLOGY OF FOLLICULAR LYMPHOMAS. In many cases of follicular lymphoma, the nodular growth pattern is seen in only part of the lesion. In such cases, the clinical consequences of the diffuse component vary depending on the cytologic composition of the tumor.[204] In lymphomas composed predominantly of small cleaved cells, the presence of even a major diffuse component does not adversely affect prognosis.[198] However, in follicular lymphomas of the mixed small cleaved and large cell type, if the diffuse phase exceeds 50% of the lesion, the tumor appears to behave in a more aggressive manner. In follicular lymphomas composed predominantly of large cells, even if the diffuse component is only focal, the prognosis approximates that of the diffuse aggressive lymphomas.[203]

Variations in histologic composition can be seen in a single lymph node and in different anatomic sites at the same time. As many as one third of patients with lymphocytic lymphoma who undergo staging laparotomy exhibit some histologic discordance in different sites.[205,206] Usually these differences are minor, such as follicular small cleaved and follicular mixed small cleaved and large cell, and they do not change the prognosis. However, in some cases major histologic discrepancies can be seen, such as follicular mixed small cleaved and large cell and diffuse large cell. In such cases, treatment should be based on the most aggressive histologic subtype encountered.

The natural history of follicular lymphomas results in progression in time from a follicular to a diffuse growth pattern, and a cytologic shift from small, relatively slowly proliferating cells to large, more rapidly proliferating cells. The clinical implications of these histologic transformations are discussed in the following sections.

BIOLOGY OF FOLLICULAR LYMPHOMAS. Follicular lymphomas are monoclonal B-cell lymphomas that express only a single light chain, usually κ, with one or more heavy-chain determinants, most commonly IgM, usually without IgD.[199,207] IgG is the predominant heavy-chain class in fewer than half the cases. The cells are intimately associated with dendritic reticulum cells, the presence of which correlates with a follicular growth pattern.[208] The cells express the B-cell antigens CD19, CD20, and CD22. They also usually express CALLA or CD10. In contrast with the small lymphocytic malignancies, they are consistently CD5 negative.[111]

Suspensions prepared from follicular lymphomas may contain 50% or more T lymphocytes, and these cells are within and between the neoplastic nodules.[209] The T cells are phenotypically normal with a normal lymph node CD4:CD8 ratio, and there is no evidence that they are part of the neoplastic proliferation. However, they are not functionally inert and retain a capacity to modulate immunoglobulin synthesis by the neoplastic B lymphocytes.[210] The presence of numerous T cells in these lesions correlates with the likelihood of responding to antiidiotypic antibody therapy.[211]

Immunologic studies have revealed that most patients with follicular lymphomas exhibit "clonal excess" and excess of cells in the peripheral expressing one light chain in the blood derived from the neoplastic clone.[200] This observation may provide a useful parameter to determine response to treatment or for early detection of recurrence. It also implies that, because of the propensity of the malignant cells to circulate, truly localized disease in follicular lymphomas is extremely rare. PCR analysis of peripheral blood showed that circulating cells with the t(14;18) translocation of follicular lymphoma are present in patients who have been in continuous remission for more than 10 years.[78]

DIFFUSE, SMALL CLEAVED CELL. Diffuse small cleaved cell (*i.e.*, diffuse poorly differentiated lymphocytic) malignant lymphomas are composed of lymphoid cells that are cytologically similar to the small cleaved lymphocytes of follicular lymphomas. In most cases, this neoplasm is not simply a consequence of progression to a diffuse growth pattern in a follicular lymphoma. Most cases represent a B-cell lymphoma, initially called lymphocytic lymphoma of intermediate differentiation or mantle zone lymphoma.[212-214] This tumor is equivalent to diffuse centrocytic lymphoma in the Kiel classification.[215] This lesion seems somewhat more common in southern Europe than in the United States. The clinical behavior is heterogenous, and clinical aggressiveness correlates with the mitotic rate.[213,216] Like the other low-grade lymphomas, patients usually present with disseminated disease and are in the middle-aged or older-aged groups. A male predominance is usually seen. Although there is some heterogeneity in the clinical behavior, sustained complete remissions are uncommon.[216,217]

The term "intermediate" indicates that the tumors cytologically appear intermediate between the small lymphocytic and small cleaved lymphomas. In some cases, there is an admixture of small round and small cleaved lymphocytes. The growth pattern is diffuse or vaguely nodular. The term "mantle zone lymphoma" stems from the observation that residual, naked, normal-appearing germinal centers are often seen, and it has been postulated that the tumor is derived from the cells of the follicular lymphoid cuff or mantle zone.[218]

Immunologically, these are monoclonal B-cell tumors that more often express λ than κ, unlike most other B-cell neoplasms.[216] Like small lymphocytic neoplasms, the cells are usually CD5 positive but they often share with follicular lymphoma the expression of CD10.[111] Correlating with the vaguely nodular growth pattern, a residual meshwork of dendritic reticulum cells may be seen.[208] Because not all mantle zone lymphomas have a mantle zone pattern of growth, the term "mantle cell lymphomas" was recently proposed as an alternative.[219] Cytogenetic and molecular studies finding a high frequency of t(11;14) have lent support to the concept that mantle cell lymphomas are a distinct clinicopathologic entity.

Mycosis Fungoides and Sézary Syndrome

Mycosis Fungoides and Sézary syndrome are referred to collectively as the CTCL. This spectrum of rare T-cell disorders is discussed more fully in Chapter 53.

INTERMEDIATE-GRADE LYMPHOMAS

For clinical purposes, these lymphomas can be thought of as a single group because they share a common clinical presentation and natural history and require similar treatment strategies. They include diffuse mixed cell, diffuse large cell, and immunoblastic lymphomas. They are most common in adults but occur in all age groups and present in nodal (65%) and extranodal (35%) sites. These tumors tend to disseminate rapidly and, unlike the low-grade lymphomas, involve privileged sites such as the CNS and testis. They also have a destructive growth pattern, and regardless of the immunologic phenotype, they uncommonly involve T-cell-dependent or B-cell-dependent zones.[171] Their prognosis is distinctly unfavorable unless modern intensive chemotherapeutic regimens can induce a sustained complete remission. If a complete remission is attained and maintained beyond 2 years, the likelihood of being cured is high.

Immunologically, these lymphomas are heterogenous and are composed of morphologically transformed B (85%) and T (15%) lymphocytes. In fewer than 5% of the patients true histiocytic markers can be demonstrated. Originally, using only limited studies, a large proportion of these tumors appeared to be "null," lacking markers of T or B lymphocytes. However, using a large battery of techniques, including Southern hybridization for immunoglobulin gene rearrangement and T-cell receptor gene rearrangement, the cellular origin can be identified in more than 95% of cases.[220]

Morphologic and immunologic studies have attempted to develop clinically useful subclassifications of these intermediate-grade lymphomas. Most morphologic studies have shown that diffuse lymphomas composed of follicular center cells (*i.e.*, mixed small cleaved and large cell, large cleaved, and large noncleaved) have a somewhat better prognosis than other diffuse aggressive lymphoma.[174] However, these differences have not always achieved statistical significance and should not be interpreted to imply that less than intensive chemotherapy is required for these aggressive lymphomas.[221] Reproducibility of these fine morphologic distinctions among different observers or by the same observer is another problem in developing useful subclassification schemes. Immunologic studies have been useful in illustrating the heterogeneity of this group of tumors. One of the problems of antibody phenotyping is the detection of heterogeneity that simply does not appear to have clinical correlation. T-cell intermediate-grade lymphomas may have a poorer prognosis than their B-cell counterparts, but other evidence suggests that immunologic phenotype has not yet proved useful in delineating clinical and prognostic subtypes.[222,223]

Diffuse, Mixed Small and Large Cell Lymphomas

In approximately 75% of patients, the neoplastic cells of diffuse mixed ("histiocytic") malignant lymphomas are cytologically identical to those of follicular mixed lymphomas, and it is likely that the tumors are diffuse outgrowths of formerly follicular proliferations. B-cell markers, similar to those found on the cells of follicular lymphomas, may be demonstrable on the cells of these diffuse tumors, and the term "histiocytic" is a misnomer for the large nucleolated transformed B cell. Adequate biopsy sampling may even reveal focal residual nodularity. Many of these tumors are composed of large monoclonal B cells and admixed phenotypically normal T cells.[224] The term T-cell-rich B-cell lymphoma has been popularized for this lesion.[225] These lesions frequently contain the *BCL2* translocation.[226] The T-cell component is believed to represent a host response comparable to that seen in many follicular lymphomas. In extranodal sites, particularly in the retroperitoneum and mesentery, these follicular center cell lymphomas may be associated with extensive sclerosis. These patients have an age distribution similar to those with nodular lymphomas, and the disease is often of advanced clinical stage at the time of diagnosis, with occult disease in the liver, bone marrow, and extranodal sites. The natural history of these diffuse lymphomas is more aggressive than their follicular counterparts, but potential for cure exists with appropriate therapy.

In some diffuse lymphomas of mixed cell type (approximately 25%), the cells do not resemble those of nodular lymphomas but appear instead to be a pleomorphic mixture of large and small atypical lymphoid cells. The small cells are atypical but distinctively lymphoid, and the larger cells have prominent central nuclei and abundant cytoplasm. An inflammatory background composed of epithelioid histiocytes, plasma cells, and eosinophils may be present. Binucleated forms of large atypical cells may simulate Reed-Sternberg cells, and these cases may be misdiagnosed as Hodgkin's disease, if the fact that the small lymphoid cells also have a neoplastic appearance, in contrast to Hodgkin's disease, is not recognized. In most cases, the malignant cells bear markers of mature or "peripheral" T lymphocytes.[227,228] Cases in which the epithelioid component is conspicuous have been called "lymphoepithelioid cell lymphomas" or "Lennert's lymphoma" because Lennert first described these tumors and postulated that they might be related to Hodgkin's disease.[229-231] With time, the epithelioid cell component, which is nonneoplastic, is lost, and the tumor may progress to one predominantly composed of the large nucleolated cells, so-called large cell immunoblastic lymphoma. Unlike Hodgkin's disease, these peripheral T-cell lymphomas occur in middle-aged or elderly patients and often present with disseminated disease.[101,232] Clinically, they should be approached as other diffuse aggressive lymphocytic lymphomas.

Diffuse, Large Cell Lymphoma

Diffuse, large cell (*i.e.*, diffuse histiocytic) malignant lymphoma represents one of the two subtypes in the Working Formulation derived from diffuse "histiocytic" lymphoma of Rappaport. These lymphomas are composed of large lymphoid cells with nuclear diameters greater than those of admixed "starry sky" histiocytes. The cells may have cytologic features of large noncleaved or large cleaved follicular center cells. In the noncleaved variant (Fig. 52–6), the nuclei are vesicular with reticulated chromatin and two to three distinct nucleoli, often apposed to the nuclear membrane. The cytoplasm is abundant and slightly amphophilic. The cells of the large cleaved variant have finely dispersed nuclear chromatin, inconspicuous and basophilic nucleoli, and sparse eosinophilic cytoplasm. Sclerosis is frequent in the large cleaved cell variant. Mitoses are usually readily identified in both subtypes. As expected from the follicular center cell characteristics, most cases are of B-cell origin.[220] In some cases, a lymphoma with a follicular pattern can be identified in another anatomic site, and biopsies obtained for staging may indicate other evidence of an underlying follicular lymphoma, such as paratrabecular small cleaved or mixed lymphoid infiltrates in the bone marrow. Cases with this morphology may carry the t(14;18) translocation, further supporting a relation to follicular lymphoma.[233]

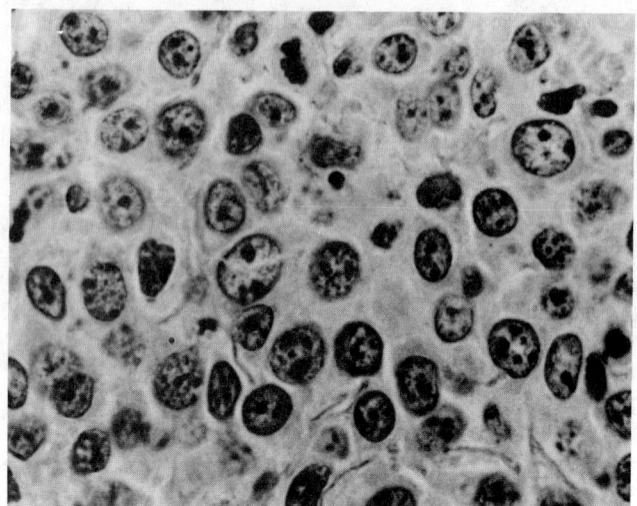

FIGURE 52–6. Malignant lymphoma: diffuse, large cell type. Cells resemble large noncleaved follicular center cells and have multiple, prominent, often membrane-bound nucleoli (hematoxylin and eosin; original magnification × 1000).

Diffuse, Large Cell, Immunoblastic Lymphoma

The category of diffuse, large cell, immunoblastic (diffuse histiocytic) lymphoma is composed of all diffuse histiocytic lymphomas in the Rappaport scheme that do not have the cytologic features of large follicular center cells. Various subtypes are described in the Working Formulation.[174] These are all high-grade (intermediate-grade according to their behavior in most combination chemotherapy clinical trials) neoplasms and commonly exhibit a high mitotic rate.

The *plasmacytoid* subtype is composed of large pleomorphic cells with abundant, deeply amphophilic and pyroninophilic cytoplasm, eccentric nuclei, and prominent central nucleoli. The *clear cell* subtype is composed of cells with abundant, optically clear cytoplasm and distinct nuclear membranes. The *polymorphous* category was proposed to include lymphomas composed of a pleomorphic population of large lymphoid cells, reflecting the morphologic diversity of T-cell lymphomas described in Japan and elsewhere. The term "epithelioid" is used to refer to those large cell lymphomas with a high content of epithelioid histiocytes and represents part of the spectrum of Lennert's lymphomas or lymphoepithelioid cell lymphomas. Similar tumors with a more mixed lymphoid composition are also included in the diffuse, mixed-cell category.

The correlation between morphologic appearance and immunologic subtype is less predictable in these neoplasms. Although plasmacytoid features could indicate a B-cell phenotype, T-cell lymphomas with plasmacytoid features have been described.[173,234] Similarly, the features of the clear cell, polymorphous, and epithelioid subtypes of immunoblastic lymphomas have been most often associated with lymphomas of T-cell origin but can also be encountered in B-cell neoplasms. Moreover, no clinical significance could be demonstrated for these subtypes of large cell immunoblastic lymphoma. The use of these additional descriptive terms is optional.

A variant of immunoblastic lymphoma, large cell anaplastic lymphoma, is characterized by the propensity of the malignant cells to invade lymphoid sinuses.[235] Because of the sinusoidal location of the tumor cells, misdiagnosis as malignant histiocytosis or metastatic carcinoma is common. In most cases studied, the malignant cells express some T-cell antigens, although the cells have a markedly aberrant phenotype. T-cell gene rearrangement has also been shown in some instances. A consistent feature is the expression of the Hodgkin's disease-associated antigen CD30 detected by Ki-1 and Hefi-1 (see Chap. 51).[235,236] This antigen, although present on the malignant cells of Hodgkin's disease, is also found in activated T and B lymphocytes. CD30 bears homology to the nerve growth factor receptor and the related protooncogene *TRK*.[237] This tumor can present in all age groups; but appears relatively common in children and young adults.[235] A high incidence of cutaneous disease has been reported. It is associated with the t(2;5)(p23;q35) translocation.[238] It may follow a more indolent course than other immunoblastic lymphoma types, especially if the disease involves only the skin.

HIGH-GRADE LYMPHOMAS

Diffuse Lymphoblastic Lymphoma

Diffuse lymphoblastic lymphoma is a form of lymphocytic lymphoma common in adolescents and young adults, and it demonstrates a marked male preponderance.[239–241] The neoplastic cells appear blastic with finely distributed nuclear chromatin, small nucleoli, scant cytoplasm, and numerous mitotic figures. The nuclei in some cases are round to oval, but a variable percentage have nuclei with marked lobulations and convolutions. Many of these patients have mediastinal masses, and a relation to the thymus gland was suggested on clinical grounds long before the discovery of T- and B-cell systems.[242] Progression to ALL is a frequent phenomenon in these patients. The enzyme TdT is a ubiquitous feature of all lymphoblastic malignancies and has been demonstrable in virtually all cases studied.[130] The cells from 85% of cases have T-cell surface markers and share many characteristics with the cells from the 20% to 30% of ALL cases of the T-cell type.[106] However, most lymphoblastic lymphoma patients have a slightly more differentiated phenotype than seen in T-cell ALL (see Fig. 52–2). Even in patients who present with soft tissue involvement, a careful workup often reveals occult marrow involvement. There is also a high risk of infiltration of the leptomeninges, with neoplastic cells demonstrable in the cerebrospinal fluid, particularly as a first site of relapse. And as in T-cell ALL, the CNS should be treated prophylactically. Although the disease may appear circumscribed at the time of diagnosis, progression to systemic disease is such a common feature that these patients are now treated with regimens similar to those used for T-cell ALL. This approach has significantly improved the prognosis for this high-grade tumor.

In as many as 10% of patients, the neoplastic cells demonstrate a phenotype similar to that of common ALL or pre-B-cell ALL and are immature lymphoid cells committed to the B-cell lineage.[106] Morphologically, these are indistinguishable from the more frequent T-cell lymphoblastic lymphomas. Clinical differences, however, have been observed in that patients with B-cell tumors usually do not present with mediastinal disease, and isolated lytic bone lesions and skin lesions have been reported.[106,242]

Diffuse Small Noncleaved Cell Lymphoma

Small noncleaved cell (*i.e.*, diffuse, undifferentiated) lymphomas are high-grade malignancies with a high growth fraction and include Burkitt's and non-Burkitt's subtypes. Cytologically, these tumors are composed of cells that resemble small noncleaved follicular center cells. Burkitt's lymphoma is composed of uniform cells of moderate size (15–25 μm) with round to oval nuclei, coarsely reticulated chromatin, and two to five prominent basophilic nucleoli.[243] Each cell possesses a distinct rim of amphophilic and intensely pyroninophilic cytoplasm with the methyl green pyronin stain. Mitoses are numerous, and a starry sky pattern is characteristic but not pathognomonic, because it can be encountered in any rapidly proliferating lymphoma. The growth pattern is usually diffuse, but selective involvement of germinal centers can be seen, further supporting a relation to the B-cell system.[244]

All cases of Burkitt's lymphoma exhibit B-cell markers. The cells usually express a μ heavy chain with a single light-chain type and CD10.[116] The presence of C3d receptors (CD21) varies and correlates with the presence or absence of the EBV genome.[245] Endemic Burkitt's lymphomas, which are usually EBV positive, express C3d receptors, and 85% of nonendemic cases are EBV and C3d receptor negative. The chromosomal abnormalities of Burkitt's lymphoma were previously discussed. The morphologic features of endemic and nonendemic Burkitt's lymphoma are identical. The endemic cases present at a lower median age (7 years) than nonendemic cases (11 years) and more often present in the face and jaw bones. An intraabdominal mass involving the ileocecal region or ovaries is the most common clinical presentation for nonendemic cases. Other extranodal sites frequently involved include kidney, testis, thyroid, and distal long bones. The staging scheme used for Burkitt's lymphoma differs from that used for the other lymphocytic lymphomas. It relates general prognosis to overall tumor burden and bone marrow involvement. As a high-grade lymphoma with a high growth fraction, Burkitt's lymphoma is potentially curable with appropriate combination chemotherapy.[246]

Small noncleaved cell lymphomas of the non-Burkitt's type show a greater degree of nuclear pleomorphism than that considered acceptable to diagnose Burkitt's lymphoma, but they are also high-grade lymphoid neoplasms.[247,248] The mean nuclear diameter is similar to that of Burkitt's lymphoma, 15 to 35 μm, but with greater variation within the tumor cell population; occasional giant cell forms and bizarre cells may be present. The cytologic characteristics are similar to those of Burkitt's, but with greater variation in nuclear shape, chromatin condensation, and nucleolar prominence and number. There is usually a single distinct eosinophilic nucleolus. Small noncleaved cell non-Burkitt's lymphomas present most often in adults (median age, 34 years), and the site of presentation is usually nodal with peripheral lymphadenopathy not uncommon. However, small noncleaved cell lymphomas with nuclear pleomorphism also occur in children, and in this age group, they are virtually indistinguishable clinically and biologically from classic Burkitt's lymphoma.

Neoplastic cells from approximately 95% of cases express B-cell surface markers. Translocations involving the *MYC* oncogene are rare, unlike Burkitt's lymphoma.[249] Both variants of small noncleaved cell lymphomas are the most frequent form of lymphoma seen in association with HIV infection. It has been postulated that the pathogenesis of high-grade B-cell lymphomas in the setting of HIV infection is similar to that of classic Burkitt's lymphoma in Africa.[250] In both settings, polyclonal B-cell proliferation occurs in the absence of effective T-cell regulation, possibly leading to the emergence of a malignant clone.

A mature T-cell phenotype is identified in rare cases of small noncleaved non-Burkitt's lymphoma. This immunologic heterogeneity in concert with some clinicopathologic diversity suggests that, in contrast to Burkitt's lymphoma, this morphologic subtype is not a homogenous clinicopathologic entity.

Adult T-Cell Leukemia-Lymphoma

ATL is a characteristic clinicopathologic entity associated with HTLV-I.[53] The pathologic spectrum of the associated lymphomas is broad and includes several diffuse subtypes in the Rappaport classification and the Working Formulation.[251] The most characteristic morphologic feature is the presence of highly pleomorphic and polylobated cells in the peripheral blood. Polylobated and multinucleated cells can also be seen in the lymph nodes, and by this criterion, many cases have been classified as large cell immunoblastic in the Working Formulation. Approximately 65% of patients present with peripheral blood involvement, and a leukemic phase develops in almost 100% at some time during the clinical course. Other common clinical features include generalized lymphadenopathy, hepatosplenomegaly, cutaneous involvement, hypercalcemia, and lytic bone lesions. Biopsies of lytic lesions do not necessarily show involvement by tumor, and marked osteoclastic activity is seen in lytic lesions and in routine bone marrow biopsies. These observations support the concept that a lymphokine secreted by neoplastic cells, osteoclast activity factor or an osteoclast activating factor-like substance, is responsible for these manifestations. This factor is probably IL-1. The skin lesions are papulonodular with or without ulceration. In two thirds of patients with cutaneous involvement, epidermal infiltration resembling Pautrier's microabscesses is observed. However, most cases can readily be differentiated from mycosis fungoides or Sézary's syndrome on clinical and epidemiologic grounds.

ATL is a postthymic T-cell neoplasm that usually expresses a helper cell surface phenotype. However, in vitro the cells actually function as suppressor cells and suppress immunoglobulin synthesis by B cells.[252] They are strongly positive for acid phosphatase, and the activity is not always entirely inhibited by tartrate.[251] TRAP activity is not pathognomonic of hairy cell leukemia.

MISCELLANEOUS RARE LYMPHOPROLIFERATIVE DISEASES

Angioimmunoblastic Lymphadenopathy

In 1975, a new clinicopathologic entity called angioimmunoblastic lymphadenopathy (AILD) was described.[253,254] It was initially construed as a hyperimmune disorder, but questions have been raised about its potentially neoplastic nature. The mean age of patients is approximately 68 years. The disease has an acute onset with generalized lymphadenopathy. Hepatosplenomegaly and constitutional symptoms occur in most cases. Rashes, a positive Coombs' test, and polyclonal hypergammaglobulinemia are commonly found.

Essential pathologic features include complete architectural effacement; proliferation of arborizing small blood vessels; polymorphous cellular proliferation of lymphocytes, immunoblasts, plasma cells, with or without histiocytes and eosinophils; and absence of germinal centers or a few residual "burned out" or hyalinized germinal centers. Other frequent, but not essential, histologic features are an overall hypocellular appearance with amorphous acidophilic interstitial material. Usually all lymph nodes are involved, and it is important to make the diagnosis only in the appropriate clinical context. Although the disease is progressive and often fatal (median survival, 15 months), the cells are not morphologically malignant. However, as many as 50% of patients are found to have overt lymphomas during the clinical course or at autopsy.[255] The lymphomas are classified as large cell immunoblastic in the Working Formulation.

Cytotoxic treatment has not proved effective in controlling the disease or in preventing progression to lymphoma. Infectious complications often supervene, leading to a high morbidity and mortality after therapy. Corticosteroid therapy, with or without cyclophosphamide, does provide temporary control in some cases.

The polyclonal hypergammaglobulinemia and plasmacytosis found in AILD suggested that it might be a hyperimmune disorder of the B-cell system. However, the immunoblastic cells in AILD and the malignant lymphomas that supervene are Ig negative, and Japanese investigators have described a variant of peripheral T-cell lymphoma that bears a marked resemblance to this lesion.[256] It has been suggested that AILD is a peripheral T-cell lymphoma derived from helper T cells. Cytogenetic investigations that have shown clonal abnormalities in several patients supported a malignant nature for this disease, even early in its course.[257] Clonal rearrangements of the T-cell receptor β chain gene have provided additional evidence for T-cell origin in some cases and further suggest a neoplastic nature.[258,259] However, immunoglobulin gene rearrangements have been found, and sequential analysis has shown spontaneous regression of T-cell and B-cell clones. Others have argued that AILD may be an immunoregulatory disorder.[259] The B-cell clones may be secondary to the expansion of EBV-immortalized B cells as a consequence of the associated immunodeficiency in this disease.[260]

Angiocentric Immunoproliferative Lesions

Although lymphomatoid granulomatosis (LYG), polymorphic reticulosis (PMR), and midline malignant reticulosis (MMR) were initially described as discrete entities in different anatomic sites, they represent the same histologic process. MMR and PMR are associated with the clinical entity lethal midline granuloma and involve the nose, paranasal sinuses, nasopharynx, and palate.[261,262] LYG was first described in the lung, but it also involves the nasopharyngeal sites listed in many patients.[263] Other frequent sites of involvement include skin, kidneys, central and peripheral nervous systems, and gastrointestinal tract. The lesion common to all is an angiocentric and angiodestructive atypical lymphoreticular infiltrate. The vascular involvement often leads to necrosis, which may be extensive. Atypical lymphoid cells are admixed with plasma cells, eosinophils, and histiocytes. Because of these common histologic features, it has been proposed that these lesions represent the same nosologic entity, and the term "angiocentric immunoproliferative lesions" (AIL) has been proposed.[103,264]

LYG was initially described as a benign disorder with a limited risk of progressing to a malignant lymphoma. Similarly, MMR and PMR were believed to be locally invasive and destructive lesions with a low risk of peripheral dissemination. In some series, as many as 50% of patients progress to lymphomas of the large cell immunoblastic type.[265] Moreover, the median survival of LYG patients in one series was only 14 months, and survival was found to be inversely proportional to the number of large, atypical lymphoreticular cells.[266] These observations have prompted the suggestion that these disorders, at least in some cases, may be neoplastic at onset. In the cases studied, the lymphoid cells have had a mature T-cell phenotype, and these processes may represent variants of peripheral T-cell lymphoma.[103,264,267]

Most cases present in adult life (median age, 50 years) and the male to female ratio is 2:1. Presenting complaints are usually related to the involved organs: cough, shortness of breath, and nasal discharge. Systemic symptoms, including fever, weight loss, and malaise, are also common. Approximately 75% of patients with localized upper airway disease respond to radiation therapy without local recurrence or peripheral dissemination. Cyclophosphamide and prednisone have been used in LYG, with as many as 50% sustained complete remissions.[265] Patients who have recurrences or undergo histologic progression require more aggressive multiagent systemic chemotherapy, but survival rates for these patients, who have usually received prior therapy, have been low.

A grading scheme was proposed for AIL.[264] Grade I lesions have a polymorphic cellular composition and no cellular atypia. Grade II lesions demonstrate some cytologic atypia. Grade III lesions represent clear-cut angiocentric lymphoma. Most patients with grade I disease achieved control of their disease with cyclophosphamide and prednisone, unlike patients with grade II disease, most of whom progressed to overt lymphoma within 2 years and died from refractory disease. Patients with grade III disease treated aggressively at onset had a high complete remission rate and prolonged disease-free survival.[264]

EBV is strongly associated with this disease.[268–271] Moreover, by Southern blot analysis the EBV appears to be clonal. Surprisingly, studies to evaluate the clonality of the T-cell antigen receptor genes have not shown clonal arrangements.[270,271] This observation may suggest that the process is not truly of T-cell origin or that the T-cell component is reactive and not neoplastic. In some cases, the cells have exhibited NK cell markers.[272]

True Histiocytic Lymphoma and Malignant Histiocytosis

Malignancies of mononuclear phagocytes include acute monocytic leukemia, malignant histiocytosis, and true histiocytic sarcoma. These three malignancies represent a spectrum in terms of their degree of dissemination and can be conceptually related to different stages of maturation and differentiation in the mononuclear phagocytic series.[273] Acute monocytic leukemia is related to a bone marrow-derived monoblast. This malignancy arises in the bone marrow compartment with secondary involvement of the peripheral blood and usually results in a markedly elevated white blood cell count. Unlike acute myeloid leukemia, there is a somewhat higher incidence of involvement of nonhematopoietic sites, with frequent involvement of skin and gingiva. Hepatosplenomegaly (25%) and lymphadenopathy (50%) are relatively common.[274]

Malignant histiocytosis represents a malignancy of mononuclear phagocytes that are intermediate in differentiation between monocytes and monoblasts and fixed tissue histiocytes. In many instances, the syndromes of acute monocytic leukemia and malignant histiocytosis may merge, and the distinction may be arbitrary and somewhat semantic. Malignant histiocytosis is a systemic malignancy that involves the entire reticuloendothelial system. Within the lymphoreticular system there is preferential involvement of sites normally populated by histiocytes, such as lymph node sinuses, splenic red pulp, and hepatic sinusoids. Bone marrow involvement is common, and although abnormal cells can be seen in the peripheral blood, if peripheral blood involvement is extensive, a diagnosis of acute monocytic leukemia should be considered. Other frequent sites of involvement include skin and bone.

The end point of the spectrum is histiocytic sarcoma or true histiocytic lymphoma, which represents a malignancy of the mononuclear phagocytic series at the stage of the fixed tissue histiocyte. The lesions in histiocytic sarcoma represent localized, relatively discrete tumefactions.[275] In addition to the reticuloendothelial system, common sites of involvement include skin and bone.[276]

Histiocytic sarcomas initially confined to the skin may pursue an indolent clinical course, with spontaneous regression of lesions in some cases.[276] The entity initially described as regressing atypical histiocytosis may represent histiocytic sarcoma with this characteristic presentation.[277] Alternatively, the clinical and pathologic features of these cutaneous lesions are remarkably similar to lymphomatoid papulosis, a chronic self-remitting T-cell lesion of the skin. Poppema had suggested a histiocytic derivation for lymphomatoid papulosis, and because of the high content of lysosomal enzymes in activated T cells, it is not surprising that the distinction between a histiocytic and T-cell origin has been a difficult one.[278] The current molecular and phenotypic evidence supporting a T-cell derivation for lymphomatoid papulosis is strong, and the natures of "regressing atypical histiocytosis" and isolated histiocytic sarcomas of the skin need to be reassessed in light of this new information.[144]

In the absence of special studies, morphologic evidence of phagocytosis by the neoplastic cells, most commonly erythrophagocytosis, has been proposed as a criterion for determining derivation from mononuclear phagocytes. However, phagocytosis is not reliably seen in most mononuclear phagocytic malignancies. Moreover, it is not a specific finding and has been described in lymphoid, plasmacytic, and even epithelial tumors.[267] Even if phagocytosis is observed, it is virtually always clinically insignificant. The clinical syndrome of histiocytic medullary reticulosis, characterized by hepatosplenomegaly, pancytopenia, and jaundice, has been proposed as a manifestation of malignant histiocytosis.[165,279] However, most observers now believe that it is usually a manifestation

of a hemophagocytic syndrome, usually seen in association with immunodeficiency or another hematopoietic malignancy.[280,281] This syndrome appears pathogenetically related to excessive production of lymphokines capable of stimulating mononuclear phagocytes.[282]

Because of the misinterpretation of hemophagocytic syndromes in the past as "malignant histiocytosis," many reports of malignant histiocytosis actually represent hemophagocytic syndromes. This appears to be true for many cases of malignant histiocytosis reported in association with ALL. AIL, including LYG, PMR, and MMR, is often associated with a hemophagocytic syndrome as a terminal event that has been misdiagnosed as malignant histiocytosis.[281] These lesions are now recognized as a variant of peripheral T-cell lymphoma. Because of the underlying T-cell malignancy, there may be an associated immunodeficiency and subsequent development of a hemophagocytic syndrome. Alternatively, the hemophagocytic syndrome could be due to lymphokine production by neoplastic cells. Familial erythrophagocytic lymphohistiocytosis is another disorder in which the terminal phase of the disease appears to be a hemophagocytic syndrome. The underlying condition appears to be a poorly characterized immunodeficiency.

True histiocytic lymphomas preferentially involve lymph nodes sinuses. However, this feature is not specific and can be seen in certain T-cell immunoblastic lymphomas. Many instances of so-called malignant histiocytosis appear to represent this variant of Ki-1-positive or large cell anaplastic lymphoma.[236]

Enzyme cytochemistry and histochemistry remain a reliable adjunct to morphology in the diagnosis of malignancies of the mononuclear phagocytic system. The cells have diffuse activity for nonspecific esterase, which is usually at least partially fluoride sensitive. Preferable methods for detection of esterase activity include the α-naphthyl butyrate esterase reaction because activity is not observed in myeloid cells. Myeloid cells also react minimally or not at all with α-naphthyl acetate esterase. The use of the naphthyl ASD acetate requires the use of fluoride to differentiate myeloid and mononuclear phagocytic cells. Activity for acid phosphatase and β-glucuronidase is usually present as well. In all cases, the activity should be relatively diffuse throughout the cytoplasm and not punctate. Punctate reactivity localized to the Golgi region is more characteristic of lymphoid rather than mononuclear phagocytic cells. Caution should be exercised in the use of enzyme cytochemistry because these enzymes are not specific for mononuclear phagocytes and can be seen in certain carcinomas and sarcomas.

Proliferative lesions of antigen-presenting cells are relatively rare. The principal proliferative lesion of the dendritic cell system is histiocytosis X. Most authorities do not consider histiocytosis X to be a malignancy, but rather consider it to be a proliferative lesion, possibly secondary to immunodeficiency.[283,285] The cells of histiocytosis X have the characteristics of Langerhans cells, including CD1 expression and Birbeck granules. Unlike normal Langerhans cells, the cells also express antigens associated with phagocytic histiocytes such as MY4 (CD14) and Leu-M5 (CD11c).

Although the cells of histiocytosis X may sometimes appear cytologically atypical, even with abnormal mitotic figures, histologic features are said not to be an important prognostic indicator in this disease. Prognosis is best correlated with age at presentation and extent of organ system involvement.[284,285] Patients under 2 years of age tend to have a poor prognosis, but those older than 6 years have an excellent prognosis. Clinical staging schemes useful in prognosis correlate with the extent of organ system involvement. The greater the number of organ systems involved, the poorer the prognosis.

Some rare tumors have a proposed derivation from dendritic reticulum cells or interdigitating reticulum cells.[286-288] These lesions are based in lymph nodes and are often associated with an inflammatory background, necrosis, or both. They tend to present as local disease, and although they may be characterized by local recurrence, systemic spread has not been a feature. Because of the rarity of these lesions, it is difficult to make definitive statements about their clinical course.

Castleman's Disease

The eponym of Castleman's disease has been applied to three histologically and clinically distinct lesions. Although these disorders share some morphologic similarities, it is likely that they differ in their pathogenesis and require different therapeutic approaches.[289]

Castleman's disease was initially described as a localized mass lesion to be differentiated from malignant lymphoma or thymoma.[290] The localized form consists of two histologic subtypes: the hyaline vascular variant and the plasma cell type.[291] The hyaline vascular form is by far the most common, representing approximately 90% of cases. Patients are usually asymptomatic, and the process is often detected as an incidental finding or from symptoms secondary to compression by the mass. It occurs primarily in adults with an equal incidence in men and women. Surgical excision is the treatment of choice, and radiotherapy has not been effective. The most common sites of presentation include the mediastinum (52%), abdomen (26%), neck, axilla, or other nodal locations.[289]

The hyaline vascular form of Castleman's disease is composed of altered germinal centers that contain prominent vascular tufts composed of hyperplastic arterioles and sometimes of capillaries. The follicles lack the normal cellular components of the germinal center and are atrophic or regressed in appearance. The follicles are surrounded by a cuff of small lymphocytes that demonstrate an onion skin configuration. The interfollicular region is expanded as well, with numerous postcapillary venules. Plasma cells are relatively sparse.

The plasma cell variant is much less common. Histologically, it resembles a florid follicular hyperplasia with sheets of plasma cells in the interfollicular region. The prominent vascular changes of the hyaline-vascular form are not observed. There are clinical differences as well. Patients are much more likely to be symptomatic from their disease. The clinical presentation includes fever, fatigue, weight loss, with a hemolytic anemia in 90%. Laboratory abnormalities include increased erythrocyte sedimentation rate and polyclonal hypergammaglobulinemia in approximately 80%. These clinical and laboratory abnormalities appear to be mediated in large part by IL-6, which is produced in the germinal centers of the hyperplastic lymph nodes in large quantities.[292] Surgical excision is still the treatment of choice.

Multicentric or generalized Castleman's disease differs from both of the localized forms.[289] Histologically, it often shows some of the vascular lesions characteristic of the hyaline vascular form, but it also contains a marked plasmacytosis, as in the plasma cell variant. In a few cases, a monoclonal population of plasma cells may be identified by immunohistochemical studies.[289] An association with the POEMS syndrome (*i.e.*, *p*olyneuropathy, *o*rganomegaly, *e*ndocrinopathy, *M* protein, *s*kin changes) has been postulated. Additional evidence differentiating the generalized disease from the localized forms is provided by gene rearrangement studies, which have a high incidence of clonal rearrangements (predominantly of the *IG* genes) in the generalized disease, but not in the localized forms.[293] Clinically, the disease occurs in older age groups. Patients present with severe systemic symptoms, generalized lymphadenopathy, and often hepatosplenomegaly.[294,295] There is a 50% mortality, with a median survival of 27 months. Causes of death include sepsis, malignant lymphoma, and other malignancies. Kaposi's sarcoma has also been reported, and it is likely that some cases of the generalized form of Castleman's disease represent the persistent generalized lymphadenopathy syndrome associated with HIV infection. The generalized form of Castleman's disease is not a histologic entity, and the diagnosis should only be made in the appropriate clinical context. Other causes of the lymphadenopathy should be excluded.

DIFFERENTIAL DIAGNOSIS

SUPERFICIAL LYMPH NODE PRESENTATIONS

Eighty percent or more of adult patients with lymphomas present to their physicians with superficial adenopathy. It may have been detected by the patient or found as a result of a physical examination for another reason. Most patients are asymptomatic, although 20% of patients with the lymphocytic lymphomas and as many as 40% of patients with Hodgkin's disease may have some combination of fever higher than 101.5°F, night sweats, or unexplained weight loss of more than 10% of total body weight in the last 6 months, the so-called B symptoms.[296,297] Patients with low-grade lymphomas often give a history of waxing and waning adenopathy over periods extending from months to years before diagnosis, with an average duration of 5 months.

Lymph node enlargement is usually painless, rubbery, discrete, and located in the neck region. Isolated axillary or inguinal lymph node presentations occur but are less common. It is not possible to make accurate distinctions between the various lymphomas by the size, shape, or feel of the lymph nodes. The diagnosis depends on excision of the entire enlarged node and histologic examination by an experienced pathologist. Node aspiration or needle biopsy are inappropriate diagnostic tests. The distribution of peripheral adenopathy can yield diagnostic information (Table 52–9). Involvement of Waldeyer's ring occurs in fewer than 1% of patients with Hodgkin's disease but is identified in 15% to 33% of patients with the lymphocytic lymphomas and often is associated with lymphomas of the gastrointestinal tract.[296-298] Epitrochlear node involvement is unusual in Hodgkin's disease but relatively common in patients with follicular lymphomas. The duration of signs and B symptoms, if present, and a family

TABLE 52–9. Comparison of Lymphocytic Lymphomas and Hodgkin's Disease

Characteristics	Lymphocytic Lymphoma	Hodgkin's Disease
Presentation	Often extranodal	Usually nodal
Pattern of spread	Hematogenous; noncontiguous nodal spread	Contiguous nodal spread
Extent of disease	Rarely localized nodal disease	Commonly localized nodes
Marrow involvement	Common	Uncommon
Liver involvement	Common	Uncommon
Spleen involvement	Uncommon	Common
Mediastinum	Uncommon (except in lymphoblastic)	Common
Mesenteric disease	Common	Uncommon
Waldeyer's ring	Occasionally	Almost never
Epitrochlear nodes	Occasionally	Almost never
Gastrointestinal involvement	Common	Almost never
Central nervous system involvement	Occasionally	Almost never
Abdominal masses	Common	Uncommon
Skin involvement	Occasionally	Almost never

history of similar or related illnesses such as mononucleosis and immunologic disorders should be documented. During the physical examination, the status of lymph nodes in all peripheral sites, including the spleen, should be determined and recorded for each site separately.

The differential diagnosis of adenopathy depends on the age of the patient; the size, shape, and feel of the lymph nodes; and the location of the adenopathy (Fig. 52–7). Palpable lymph nodes can be a normal finding on careful examination, particularly in the neck region. Soft, flat, elliptical nodes of 0.5 to 1.0 cm are commonly palpable in the submandibular and submental regions and are found by careful examination in as many as 50% of normal people in the superficial jugular or posterior cervical chain.[299] In young patients, superficial adenopathy in the head and neck region is most often related to acute infectious illnesses of the mouth or pharynx. Mononucleosis is a common cause of cervical adenopathy, and although it is often associated with pharyngitis, adenopathy can occur without pharyngeal symptoms. Toxoplasmosis can mimic mononucleosis as well; these disorders can be easily diagnosed by standard methods if suspected. Adenopathy resulting from infection usually causes firm, sometimes tender spherical enlargement of nodes that can be easily confused with lymphomas if they are nontender. A spherical lymph node larger than 1 cm in diameter, thought to be due to an infectious process, and that does not diminish in size over a 4-week period of observation after resolution of the acute pro-

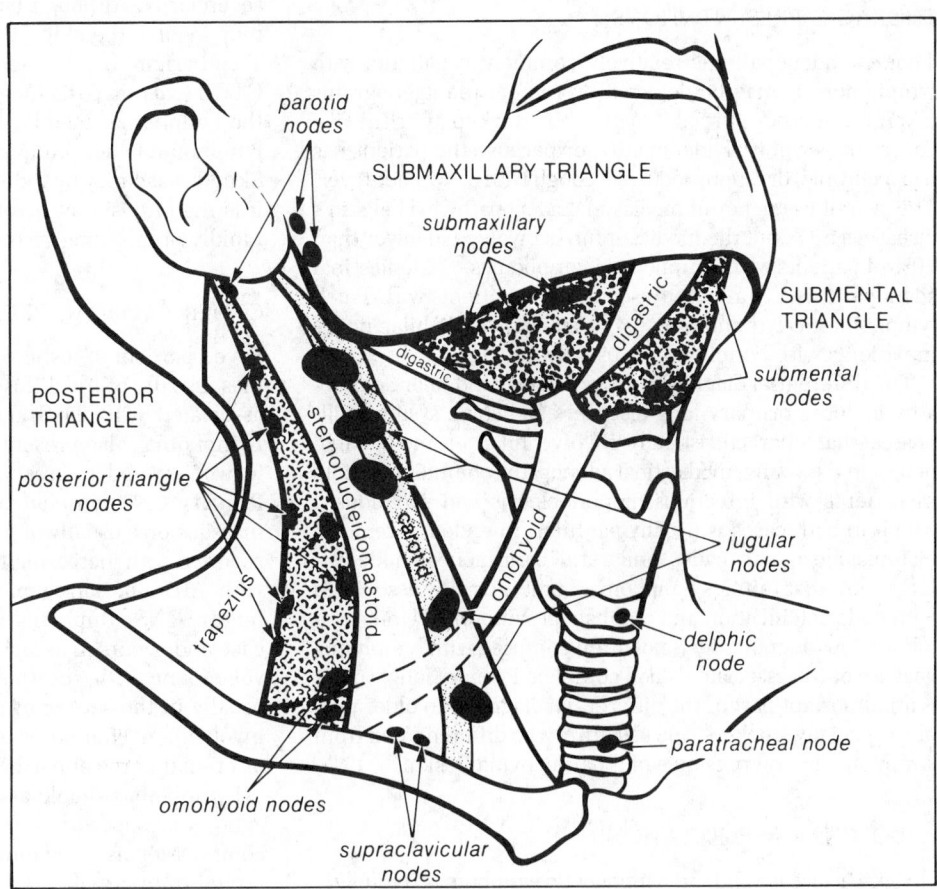

FIGURE 52–7. Anatomic subdivisions of the neck, depicting lymph node areas. (Adapted from Sade HH. Palpable cervical lymph nodes. JAMA 1958;168:496)

cess should be biopsied. Discrete, hard lymph nodes, particularly if fixed or matted, are more worrisome and should be biopsied promptly for diagnosis, particularly in older people. Hard lymph nodes in the submandibular or submental region in older people are more likely related to tumors of the floor of the mouth or larynx. Nasopharyngeal cancers often drain to, and present as, enlarged posterior cervical lymph nodes. Thyroid carcinoma can mimic lymphoma, although the lymph nodes involved with thyroid cancer generally are firmer and are often found in the submental and superficial jugular region, an area less commonly involved in isolation by lymphomas.

Because supraclavicular lymph nodes drain regions of the lung and retroperitoneal space, they can enlarge secondary to lymphomas or other tumors or infectious processes originating in these areas. Isolated axillary lymph node enlargement can be related to local phenomena in the hands or arms, such as infections, trauma (*e.g.,* cat scratch), or insect bites. The clinical presentation affects the likelihood of a specific diagnosis. For example, a young man with an enlarged axillary lymph node is most likely to have a lymphoma or a malignant melanoma, but in a woman, the same two tumors or breast cancer are the most likely diagnoses. Isolated inguinal adenopathy is often difficult to separate from the normal 0.5- to 1.0-cm elliptical lymph nodes found in the region of the inguinal ligament, which are influenced by disorders that occur on the legs and feet. Concomitant enlargement of nodes in the femoral triangle or adenopathy along the external iliac chain should make inguinal adenopathy more suspicious and decrease the threshold for biopsy.

THORACIC PRESENTATIONS

Thoracic adenopathy is relatively common in patients with lymphomas. It may be detected by routine roentgenograms taken for another purpose, such as the workup after the discovery of peripheral adenopathy, or because the patient has had a chronic, dry, nonproductive cough with or without fever. The overall frequency of mediastinal adenopathy in Hodgkin's disease is 50%, but the mediastinum is involved in fewer than 20% of patients with lymphocytic lymphomas.[300] Mediastinal adenopathy is a common presentation in patients with T-cell lymphoblastic lymphomas.[301,302] Involvement of hilar nodes in patients with lymphomas is usually unilateral.

The differential diagnosis of mediastinal and hilar adenopathy includes primary lung disorders and some systemic illnesses that characteristically involve hilar or mediastinal nodes. In the young, mediastinal adenopathy commonly occurs in patients with infectious mononucleosis and sarcoidosis, which in both cases is usually panhilar. In endemic regions, histoplasmosis can cause unilateral paratracheal node enlargement that mimics lymphoma, but it is usually associated with node calcification and esophageal symptoms. Unilateral tuberculous adenopathy is not often confused with lymphoma because of the associated Ghon complex. Primary lung cancer is an important part of the differential diagnosis in older people, especially smokers, and usually can be differentiated from lymphoma by the presence of a parenchymal lesion.

ABDOMINAL PRESENTATIONS

Hodgkin's disease and the lymphocytic lymphomas frequently involve retroperitoneal lymph nodes or the primary lymphatic tissue of the gut and its mesenteric drainage sites. Patients who present with abdominal lymphoma usually have a painless mass discovered on physical examination or pain associated with a palpable mass. Some patients present only with splenomegaly and most often have one of the lymphomas, commonly hairy cell leukemia.[303] Rarely, previously untreated patients may present with perforation of a viscus or hemorrhage from the upper or lower gastrointestinal tract. Previously unsuspected abdominal lymphomas are found more often after the staging workup is completed in patients who have superficial lymph node presentations. Patients whose abdominal disease alone prompts their visit to their physicians most often have one of the lymphomas. It is distinctly unusual to be able to palpate significant abdominal adenopathy in patients with Hodgkin's disease because mesenteric lymph node involvement is uncommon. This is not the case for lymphocytic lymphomas. The so-called Mediterranean lymphoma often presents with disease in the abdomen. Pathologically, these tumors resemble diffuse plasma cell tumors and often are associated with aberrant production of immunoglobulin heavy chains and malabsorption.[304] Abdominal presentations of lymphocytic lymphoma may mimic any type of intraabdominal disease. About two thirds of the lymphocytic lymphomas that involve the gastrointestinal tract originate in the stomach, 25% from the small intestine, and the remainder from the colon and rectum.[305]

CUTANEOUS PRESENTATIONS

Lymphocytic lymphomas may involve the skin primarily or secondarily. Although lymphomas of B-cell or T-cell origin may involve the skin, it is more common for them to be of T-cell origin. Involvement of skin by lymphomas other than CTCL (*e.g.,* mycosis fungoides or Sézary's syndrome) makes the lymphoma stage IV, but the prognosis of the underlying lymphoma is not dramatically affected by cutaneous spread. Skin disease may be indolent regardless of histologic grade if it is the only site of involvement or may be a component of rapidly progressing systemic disease.

OTHER CLINICAL PRESENTATIONS

Seven percent of testicular masses in older men are lymphomas, usually of the diffuse aggressive variety. They often are associated with CNS and Waldeyer's ring involvement.[306] Lymphomas also present as solitary thyroid nodules, usually in women and in association with Hashimoto's thyroiditis. Primary CNS lymphomas presenting as single or multiple mass lesions, usually of intermediate or high grade, are being reported with increasing frequency, particularly in association with AIDS or iatrogenic immunosuppression. More commonly, CNS lymphoma is composed of leptomeningeal disease and occurs in association with bone or bone marrow involvement with intermediate- or high-grade lymphomas, usually in the setting of rapidly progressive disease.[307] CNS involvement commonly presents with symptoms of headache or cranial nerve abnormalities.

Lymphomas should also be included in the differential diagnosis of superior vena cava syndrome, acute spinal cord compression, isolated tumor nodules of the skin, bone tumors, orbital tumors, salivary gland enlargement, sinus problems, and unexplained cytopenias. Some of these manifestations occur with considerable frequency in patients with widespread advancing tumor but are uncommon as initial presentations of the disease.

NATURAL HISTORY AND STAGING OF THE LYMPHOCYTIC LYMPHOMAS

NATURAL HISTORY

With the advent of modern treatment, patients with lymphoma are rarely left untreated, and the natural history is interrupted, often successfully, by treatment. However, there are studies in which patients were followed without treatment or after palliative treatment.[308] What is immediately apparent from these studies is that the natural history of the lymphocytic lymphomas is quite different from that of Hodgkin's disease, but there is a problem in comparing Hodgkin's disease with the lymphocytic lymphomas. Although the behavior of Hodgkin's disease is less affected by the histologic subtype, the lymphocytic lymphomas are a collection of several different diseases with various presentations and natural histories, categorized as low-, intermediate-, and high-grade neoplasms in the Working Formulation. However, certain generalizations are probably appropriate. In contrast to patients with Hodgkin's disease, those with lymphocytic lymphomas most frequently present with advanced disease, commonly with liver or bone marrow involvement. Unlike Hodgkin's disease, in which 50% to 60% of patients have localized disease, only 10% to 15% of lymphocytic lymphoma patients appear to have stage I or II disease.[309–311] Other differences from Hodgkin's disease are also seen. Fewer patients have systemic symptoms, and localized extralymphatic involvement is more common and often occurs as an isolated site of involvement (stage IE) or with adjacent nodes (stage IIE). There is no difference in prognosis for patients with stage I or II localized nodal lymphocytic lymphomas compared with those with extranodal involvement.[312,313]

The clinical features of both diseases are compared in Table 52–9. Lymphocytic lymphomas are probably unifocal in origin, but they remain localized so briefly that widespread disease is the rule at the time of diagnosis rather than the exception. This is particularly true of the low-grade lymphomas. Now that it is accepted that most of the common types of the adult lymphomas originate from a monoclonal population of B cells and the anatomic compartmentalization of these cells in lymph nodes is understood more clearly, certain generalizations can be made about the histologic type of disease to the clinical course of patients with lymphomas.

The most common histologic subgroups are the follicular lymphomas. Patients in this group make up almost half of all cases in most series. The propensity for follicular lymphomas to be associated with widespread disease coincides with the normal tendency of the small untransformed follicular center B cell to migrate in the circulation. These cells have a very small growth fraction, and despite wide dissemination, the follicular small cleaved cell variety of lymphoma is usually clinically indolent. An undetermined fraction of the patients can be left untreated, and approximately 25% evidence waxing and waning adenopathy for months to years before unsightly or painful lymph node enlargement or compression of a vital organ requires treatment.[314] In a few low-grade lymphomas,

spontaneous regression can occur and last for many years.[178] Involvement of the bone marrow and liver does not impart the same adverse prognosis as involvement of these organs by Hodgkin's disease or higher-grade lymphocytic lymphomas.

Although intermediate-grade or aggressive lymphomas are most often of B-cell origin, they have a vastly different natural history than nodular lymphomas.[315] In keeping with the lack of motility of transformed follicular B cells, the diffuse large cell lymphomas more often appear to be clinically localized, although the recurrence rate after local treatment indicates otherwise. Unlike patients with follicular small cleaved cell lymphoma, after tumor is identified in organs such as the bone marrow, liver, and bone, patients with diffuse large cell lymphomas have aggressive, rapidly fatal illnesses unless treated successfully.

There is evidence for a link between follicular small cleaved cell lymphomas and the diffuse large cell lymphomas of B-cell origin. The NCI analyzed a series of 515 patients with lymphocytic lymphomas for their frequency of histologic evolution.[182,315] Among patients with follicular lymphoma who had a repeat biopsy more than 3 months after the initial diagnostic biopsy, histologic progression was found in 41%. At Stanford, the actuarial risk of histologic conversion is about 50% at 8 years.[316] An autopsy study of patients at the NCI who initially were diagnosed as having follicular lymphomas revealed that fewer than 10% had evidence of exclusively follicular disease at autopsy. Survival after conversion is short unless complete remission is achieved with chemotherapy. These data indicate that a substantial number of patients have follicular lymphomas that evolve to a diffuse variety as part of the natural history of their disease.

A likely evolution of the lymphoma can be constructed as follows. The follicle-associated cells of B-cell lymphomas (see Fig. 52–1), which initially retain the characteristic of forming follicles, are close to normal tissue in their growth characteristics and migrate easily while minimally differentiated. This accounts for the ease of detectability of these cells in other organs and in the peripheral blood and for the indolent natural history. Their growth rate and invasive potential, for unknown reasons, remain low, and in time, those that are not clonogenic probably die. In time, the malignant clonogenic B cells take on the morphologic characteristics of transformed lymphocytes and presumably acquire additional genetic alterations related to the more rapid proliferation. This transformation may occur slowly over several years or so rapidly that the evolution antedates diagnosis. These transformed cells are less motile, which accounts for the difficulty in detecting them outside the site of origin with normal staging procedures, but they are more invasive, have a higher growth fraction, and are rapidly fatal if growth is unchecked. It also seems likely that the follicular small cleaved cell lymphoma subtype evolves to follicular mixed and follicular large cell lymphomas as the percentage of large cells increases until effacement of the lymph node occurs, and a pathologic picture of diffuse large cell lymphoma is observed. As with the evolution of the histologic effacement of a lymph node in Hodgkin's disease, the reasons for the varying rate of transformation from nodule-forming indolent lymphocytes to large transformed cells are unknown. However, increased cytogenetic abnormalities have been observed with histologic progression.[66,317] Lymphomas of diffuse small lymphocytic cells disseminate widely at an early stage but have an indolent course, in keeping with their benign histologic appearance. They evolve to large cell B neoplasms with much less frequency and usually kill patients by causing bone marrow failure, with hypogammaglobulinemia leading to fatal infections.

STAGING

Classification Systems

The standard staging system for the lymphocytic lymphomas is the same as that proposed for Hodgkin's disease at the Ann Arbor Conference in 1971 (Table 52–10).[318] This system reflects the number of sites of involvement and their relation to the diaphragm, the existence of B symptoms, and the presence of extranodal disease. Patients can be assigned a clinical stage and a pathologic stage. The clinical stage is based on initial tissue biopsy studies, physical examination, bone marrow biopsy, and radiographic evaluation. The pathologic stage includes information obtained by means of invasive procedures such as additional extranodal tissue biopsies, laparoscopy-directed biopsies or, rarely, staging laparotomy, and splenectomy. Some of these factors are relevant to the low-grade lymphomas, but their major relevance is in the intermediate-grade lymphomas. These clinical prognostic factors are much more important in determining treatment outcome than Ann Arbor stage.

Although the Ann Arbor staging scheme is extremely useful in defining patient composition for clinical trials, it is not as prognostically important for the lymphocytic lymphomas as it is for Hodgkin's disease. For the low-grade lymphomas, it is important to identify patients with stage I or II disease, because radiation therapy may be curative. Careful staging is required to identify the 10% to 15% of patients with limited-stage disease. Formerly, it was thought to be unimportant to differentiate stage III from stage IV disease in the remaining 85%, but recent treatment advances may make this a relevant distinction.

The Ann Arbor staging classification is inadequate for the diffuse intermediate- and high-grade lymphomas. Localized disease is rare (<20% of all patients) for these lymphomas. To say that a patient has a stage II diffuse large cell lymphoma conveys little useful prognostic information. The patient may have small cervical and axillary lymph nodes and an excellent

probability of successful treatment outcome or may have a bulky abdominal disease refractory to treatment. The actual stage of a patient without localized disease (*i.e.,* stage II intermediate or high grade; stage III or IV of any histologic subtype) is probably less important than the presence or absence of several other clinical prognostic factors.[319–327] These factors include performance status, systemic symptoms, tumor burden (*i.e.,* an abdominal mass more than 10 cm in diameter or three or more extranodal sites of disease), bone marrow involvement, and serum LDH and β_2-microglobulin levels. Some series have suggested that age over 55 years is a poor prognostic factor, and others include the speed of response to therapy as a prognostic factor, but these are not universally used in patients with aggressive histology lymphoma.[321,328]

A modification of the Ann Arbor Classification was proposed at the Cotswolds Meeting.[329] One reason for modifying the original scheme was to recognize the prognostic significance of tumor burden. The changes do not make the classification any more relevant to the lymphocytic lymphomas, but the goal of incorporating well-described prognostic factors in the staging classification also makes sense for the lymphocytic lymphomas. For intermediate-grade lymphomas, a three-stage system seems most appropriate. Stage I is the same as Ann Arbor stage I; stage II is the involvement of two of more lymph node regions or localized extralymphatic organ or site (IIE) with none of the poor prognostic factors (*e.g.,* poor performance status, B symptoms, mass more than 10 cm, three or more extranodal sites, marrow involvement, LDH >500); and stage III is stage II with one or more of the poor prognostic factors (Table 52–11).

The lymphocytic lymphomas are a diverse group of lymphoid neoplasms with varied natural histories and patterns of clinical presentation, and it is not possible to recommend a uniform approach to disease staging that can be applied to all patients. Staging issues depend on the individual patient, the histologic subtype of lymphoma, and its likely distribution (Table 52–12). Recommendations for staging procedures modified from those made at the Ann Arbor symposium are shown in Tables 52–13 and 52–14.[330,331]

Clinical Staging

The date the lymph node enlargement was first observed and the rate of subsequent tumor growth should be documented. This information may influence the choice of therapy and, in patients with low-grade lymphomas, influence the decision to institute treatment at all. The history should determine the

TABLE 52–10. Ann Arbor Staging Classification for Hodgkin's Disease

Stage	Characteristics
I	Involvement of a single lymph node region (I) or a single extralymphatic organ or site (IE)
II	Involvement of two or more lymph node regions on the same side of the diaphragm (II) or localized involvement of an extralymphatic organ or site (IIE)
III	Involvement of lymph node regions on both sides of the diaphragm (III) or localized involvement of an extralymphatic organ or site (IIIE) or spleen (IIIS) or both (IIISE)
IV	Diffuse or disseminated involvement of one or more extralymphatic organs with or without associated lymph node involvement. The organ(s) involved should be identified by a symbol: A, asymptomatic; B, fever, sweats, weight loss > 10% of body weight.

TABLE 52–11. National Cancer Institute Modified Staging for Intermediate- and High-Grade Lymphomas

Stage	Characteristics
I	Localized nodal or extranodal disease (Ann Arbor stage I or IE)
II	Two or more nodal sites of disease or a localized extranodal site plus draining nodes with none of the following: performance status ≤ 70, B symptoms, any mass > 10 cm in diameter (particularly gastrointestinal), serum lactate dehydrogenase > 500, three or more extranodal sites of disease
III	Stage II plus any poor prognostic features

TABLE 52–12. Histologic and Pathologic Stages of Lymphocytic Lymphomas

Grade	Stage I (%)	Stage II (%)	Stage III and IV (%)	Common Extranodal Sites*
High grade				
Small noncleaved cell	13	21	66	Gastrointesinal tract, lung/pleura, marrow (14%)
Lymphoblastic	7	20	75	Liver, spleen, lung/pleura, skin, marrow (50%)
Large cell, immunoblastic	23	29	48	Liver, spleen, Waldeyer's ring or GI tract, marrow (12%)
Intermediate grade				
Large cell, diffuse	16	30	54	Liver, spleen, Waldeyer's ring or GI tract, lung/pleura, marrow (10%)
Mixed cell, diffuse	19	26	55	Liver, spleen, Waldeyer's ring or GI tract, bone marrow (14%)
Small cleaved cell, diffuse	9	19	72	Liver, spleen, Waldeyer's ring or GI tract, skin, marrow (32%)
Large cell, follicular	15	12	73	Liver, spleen, Waldeyer's ring or GI tract, marrow (34%)
Low grade				
Mixed cell, follicular	15	12	74	Liver, spleen, marrow (30%)
Small cleaved cell, follicular	8	10	82	Liver, spleen, marrow (51%)
Small lymphocytic	3	8	89	Liver, spleen, marrow (71%)

*Percentages indicate incidence of each stage at presentation.

presence or absence of systemic B symptoms and the presence of symptoms that suggest extralymphatic involvement (*e.g.,* bone pain, gastrointestinal complaints). Particular attention should be given to recording the site and size of all abnormal lymph nodes, including the epitrochlear, femoral, and popliteal sites that are not usually involved in Hodgkin's disease. The presence or absence of hepatosplenomegaly needs to be determined, because unlike Hodgkin's disease, enlargement of these organs in patients with lymphocytic lymphoma correlates with tumor involvement. Preauricular nodal enlargement is often associated with disease in the Waldeyer's ring area, making indirect laryngoscopy an absolute requirement

of the staging workup in these patients. Waldeyer's ring involvement is often associated with involvement of the intestine, and gastrointestinal contrast studies are indicated if the patient appears to have localized disease. Primary lesions in extranodal sites such as bone or skin are frequently associated with involvement of regional nodes. Many patients with skin lesions that occur as primary or secondary lesions have multiple cutaneous lesions that may be remote from one another. A careful inspection of the skin and a biopsy of suspicious lesions are necessary, especially in patients with diffuse lymphomas.

The correlation between peripheral blood counts and bone

TABLE 52–13. Required Evaluation Procedures for Staging Lymphocytic Lymphomas

1. Adequate surgical biopsy, reviewed by an experienced hematopathologist
2. Detailed history recording duration and the presence or absence of fever, unexplained sweating and its severity, unexplained pruritus, and unexplained weight loss
3. Detailed physical examination; special attention to all node-bearing areas, including Waldeyer's ring (indirect laryngoscopy is the procedure of choice) and determination of size of liver and spleen
4. Necessary laboratory procedures
   a. Complete blood count, including an erythrocytic sedimentation rate
   b. Serum alkaline phosphatase
   c. Evaluation of renal function
   d. Evaluation of liver function
   e. Serum lactate dehydrogenase and β_2-microglobulin levels
5. Radiologic studies include
   a. Chest roentgenogram (posteroanterior and lateral)
   b. Bilateral lower extremity lymphogram
   c. Abdominal-pelvic computed tomography scan
6. Bilateral bone marrow needle biopsies (not just aspirates; biopsy should be performed before aspirate, if both are done together)

TABLE 52–14. Procedures Required Under Certain Circumstances for Staging Lymphocytic Lymphomas

1. Computed tomography (CT) scans of the thorax if any abnormality is found or suspected on the routine chest roentgenogram
2. Abdominal ultrasonogram, inferior cavography, intravenous pyelogram or upper and lower gastrointestinal contrast studies to supplement lymphographic findings or investigate sites of unexplained symptoms
3. Plain bone radiographs of symptomatic or tender areas
4. Head or spinal CT for neurologic signs or symptoms
5. Exploratory laparotomy and splenectomy, if management decision depends on identification of abdominal involvement (decision to proceed with laparotomy requires knowledge of treatment plan used at the institution of record)
6. Magnetic resonance imaging to detect bone marrow involvement
7. Gallium whole-body scans
8. Skeletal scintigrams
9. Useful ancillary procedures not required for staging
   a. Hepatic and spleen scintigrams
   b. Serum chemistries including serum calcium and uric acid for overall management of patient
   c. Assessment of the patient's delayed hypersensitivity response to recall antigens

marrow involvement with lymphoma is poor. Abnormal blood counts are found in only 37% of patients with bone marrow infiltration by lymphoma and approximately one half of patients with abnormal blood counts have uninvolved bone marrows. Examination of the peripheral smear in patients with lymphoma may yield evidence of malignant cells in approximately 10% of patients; these patients usually have low-grade, small lymphocytic or follicular center cell lymphomas. However, small numbers of occult circulating monoclonal B cells can be identified by immunologic analysis of the ratio of expression of κ or λ light chains on peripheral blood lymphocytes by flow cytometry; significant deviations from the normal 2:1 κ:λ ratio suggest the presence of an abnormal cell (*i.e.,* clonal excess).[332] Southern hybridization looking for rearranged immunoglobulin genes or PCR analysis may also detect lymphoma cells.[333] Southern analysis has been reported to detect as few as 1 in 100 malignant cells, an improvement of approximately 10-fold over methods using clonal excess.[333] Despite this theoretical advantage, no diagnostic gain was identified when comparing the two methods for detection of occult lymphoma in the peripheral blood.[334]

Lymphoma cells can be detected in the peripheral blood of many patients in whom morphologic analysis of a peripheral blood smear is negative. The incidence of peripheral blood involvement at diagnosis is influenced by histologic subtype and stage. Horning and coworkers documented gene rearrangements in 34% of patients with low-grade lymphomas (80% in the small lymphocytic subtype) and 8% in patients with intermediate-grade lymphoma at diagnosis.[333] Occult lymphoma was identified in 12% of patients with stage I or II disease and in 35% of patients with stage IV disease (45% if the bone marrow was involved). The incidence of occult lymphoma reached almost 50% in patients with recurrent disease. PCR analysis is even more sensitive, capable of detecting 1 in 10^5 to 10^6 cells.[148]

Although more sensitive techniques can detect occult disease more frequently, there are insufficient data to enable us to base therapeutic decisions on the presence of malignant cells in the peripheral blood. Although 10% to 15% of patients with stage I or II disease have circulating lymphoma cells, it is not clear that local radiotherapy should be withheld solely on that basis. Nor does the presence of these cells necessarily portend clinical relapse. Among 63 patients with low-grade lymphoma in clinical remission, only 6 had rearrangements in one study. Nineteen patients relapsed, but only 1 relapsed patient had a gene rearrangement in the peripheral blood before relapse. The other patients with circulating abnormalities had been followed a median of 2 years without relapsing.

Serum chemistries are important because the creatinine may indicate renal insufficiency, suggesting obstruction from retroperitoneal tumor; the uric acid and lactate dehydrogenase (LDH) can be indirect indicators of tumor burden and can be of prognostic value and enable the physician to assess the need for hydration before treatment. Tumor lysis syndrome is an avoidable complication of treatment that is most commonly observed in the treatment of high-grade lymphomas or aggressive lymphomas that are growing rapidly. Liver enzymes, bilirubin, and alkaline phosphatase elevations can occasionally be a sign of liver or bone involvement. Serum β_2-microglobulin may be a good predictor of complete response and time to treatment failure in patients with low-grade lymphomas.[325]

Chest roentgenograms yield positive information in about one fourth of patients. The most frequent abnormality is hilar or mediastinal adenopathy (18% of patients), followed by pleural effusions (8%) and parenchymal involvement (4%). Parenchymal lesions and pleural effusions usually require pathologic verification. A chylous or transudative effusion that lacks malignant cells does not change the pathologic stage of the patient. As in Hodgkin's disease, pulmonary parenchymal lesions are usually associated with concurrent hilar or bulky mediastinal lymph node involvement. If only one hemithorax is involved, the parenchymal lesions can be considered an extension from the lymph nodes and do not necessarily change the patient's stage, except for the E designation.

The use of chest computed tomography (CT) scans is not well defined. In patients with stage III and IV disease, routine CT scans are not performed because systemic treatment is already indicated. If the chest x-ray film is definitely abnormal, CT can confirm this and often identify additional sites of involvement. These sites are usually in the chest and rarely change the stage of disease. If radiation therapy is contemplated, CT of the chest is indicated for optimal design of the treatment portals. CT is also useful for monitoring the response to treatment of mediastinal, pericardial, and hilar disease, which may be difficult to follow on routine chest x-ray films. In a patient with a normal radiograph, a CT scan is not required for routine staging purposes.[335]

As in Hodgkin's disease, an accurate noninvasive evaluation of the abdomen remains a problem. Bipedal lymphangiography had been the standard procedure for this task. In experienced hands, lymphangiography has an overall accuracy of 90% for the evaluation of the paraaortic and iliac lymph node regions.[336,337] However, because of the differing natural histories, it is not as reliable in patients with lymphocytic lymphomas as it is in patients with Hodgkin's disease. A negative lymphangiogram in 147 patients with Hodgkin's disease was associated with only one false-negative study for paraaortic or iliac lymph nodes. Bone marrow and liver involvement were found in only 1% and 3% respectively, and no cases of mesenteric adenopathy were found. There was involvement of the spleen or splenic hilar nodes in 24% and 19% of patients, respectively. In lymphocytic lymphomas, there is a much higher incidence of involvement of upper abdominal nodes (particularly mesenteric nodes), even if the lymphangiogram is negative. In the follicular subtypes, approximately 50% of patients have disease in the upper abdomen even in the presence of a negative lymphangiogram. For diffuse intermediate-grade lymphomas, a negative lymphangiogram is a more reliable indicator of the absence of subdiaphragmatic disease, because 10% or fewer of these patients have abdominal disease.

Even though it provides a better architectural assessment of the paraaortic and pelvic nodes than the CT scan, the lymphangiogram is complemented by the CT scan's ability to visualize other abdominal structures.[337,338] Because it provides such an accurate assessment of lymphomatous involvement of the abdominal and pelvic lymph nodes and is so useful in routine follow-up, the lymphangiogram remains a valuable study. The lymphangiogram is an accurate predictor of the likelihood of finding intraabdominal lymphoma in extranodal sites or in splenic, portal, or mesenteric sites. As many as 80% of patients with positive lymphangiograms have disease in the liver or lymph nodes outside the paraaortic region at laparotomy, and 18% to 50% of patients with negative lymphangiograms have similar findings.

The standard test for diagnosing mesenteric, porta hepatic, and splenic hilar nodal involvement is the abdominopelvic CT scan.[339] This test is particularly useful for patients with follicular lymphomas in whom mesenteric nodal involvement is common. The abdominopelvic CT scan can also identify retrocrural nodal involvement, and it is more accurate than the lymphangiogram in determining the size of nodal disease. Involvement of the kidney, bone, and bulky splenic and liver disease, frequently present in patients with aggressive large cell lymphomas, can also be seen on CT scanning but not on bipedal lymphangiography.[338,340,341] CT scanning appears to document disease below the diaphragm in approximately 10% of patients with a negative lymphangiogram.[331] Lymphangiography has a similar incidence of abnormal findings in patients with negative abdominopelvic CT scans.[341] The two studies appear to be complementary in defining the extent of abdominal disease. A reasonable course of action is to perform the CT scan initially and perform a lymphangiogram if this study is entirely negative. However, a lymphangiogram should be performed on most patients. The dye is retained for many months and is useful in following response to therapy with just a flat plate of the abdomen.

The role of magnetic resonance imaging (MRI) in the identification of lymphomatous involvement of abdominal nodes, kidney, liver, and spleen still must be determined. It does appear to be valuable for the detection of bone marrow involvement in patients with lymphoma. When marrow involvement is suspected, even when random marrow biopsies have been negative, the MRI can be used to identify focal areas of involvement which can then be confirmed by biopsy.[342,343]

Gallium 67 (^{67}Ga) scanning is not performed routinely in all patients at most centers. It is of limited use for diagnostic purposes because of its low sensitivity, 18% in one study.[344] In this study, only 1 of 122 patients had their disease upstaged. Although the reliability of ^{67}Ga imaging has been improved by increasing the dose to between 8 and 11 mCi, using spot imaging, double or triple peak angle cameras, single photon emission computed tomography (SPECT), and delayed view of the abdomen, its utility for the diagnosis or staging of lymphocytic lymphomas has not been extensively assessed.[345] ^{67}Ga is more frequently taken up by tumors of intermediate or high grade.[345–347] The sensitivity of ^{67}Ga imaging is affected by tumor location. Lesions within or near the spleen and liver frequently are missed because of the normal uptake by the liver. The normal uptake exhibited by the cecum and sigmoid colon can mask involved sites particularly the iliac region. ^{67}Ga scanning is well suited for the evaluation of the mediastinum and most useful in the evaluation of patients with residual radiographic abnormalities, particularly in the mediastinum or abdomen.[345,347] Because ^{67}Ga is taken up in cells by the transferrin receptor, a potential surrogate measure of cellular proliferation, the conversion of a group of nodes from low to high ^{67}Ga intensity may herald progression to more aggressive histology. ^{67}Ga scanning may be a useful radiographic marker to measure response to chemotherapy and to

identify early relapse.[347–349] We do not recommend ^{67}Ga scanning routinely in the initial staging workup or during treatment. Baseline ^{67}Ga scanning should be considered in the initial workup of patients with intermediate-grade lymphomas and bulky disease, for whom evaluation of response might be anticipated to be complicated by a residual mass after chemotherapy. Patients whose tumor mass remains ^{67}Ga positive after combination chemotherapy have an extremely poor prognosis with additional conventional treatment, and they should be considered for high-dose chemotherapy and rescue with autologous bone marrow transplantation (ABMT).[348]

Bone lesions are found in 5% to 15% of all patients at presentation and are more common in patients with diffuse large cell lymphomas. Bone scans have a sensitivity and specificity greater than 95% and have replaced routine roentgenographic studies in detecting occult bone lesions.[350] Routine bone scanning for all patients is not recommended, because it is rare that a change in stage or treatment is required based on its results alone. However, if there is bone pain, a bone scan is recommended. A positive bone scan should be confirmed by plain films and the area biopsied if needed for determination of treatment.

Approximately 50% of patients with lymphocytic lymphoma have bone marrow or hepatic involvement on presentation.[351] The incidence of bone marrow metastasis is highest in patients with the small cell lymphocytic lymphomas, follicular or diffuse (40–100%, depending on the type) and lowest in those with diffuse large cell lymphoma (5–15%). Each subtype of disease tends to have an identifiable pattern of bone marrow involvement.[351] The follicular lymphomas are characterized by a paratrabecular location of involvement, but T-cell lymphomas infiltrate the marrow space. Bone marrow involvement in patients with diffuse, aggressive lymphomas is usually widespread and may be associated with focal or diffuse myelofibrosis. Although bone marrow involvement is less frequent in diffuse large cell lymphoma, its detection is important because of its strong correlation with subsequent spread of disease to the CNS. As many as 35% of patients with large cell lymphomas and positive bone marrow biopsies develop CNS spread.[352] Some of these patients have solitary relapses in the CNS, but most have widespread advanced disease. Cytologic examination of the spinal fluid should be performed in all patients with diffuse types of lymphoma with bone marrow involvement, because therapy of the CNS is indicated if positive.[353]

As with Hodgkin's disease, aspiration of the bone marrow is inadequate for staging purposes. Marrow aspirates are insensitive and detect disease in less than 30% of all biopsy-positive marrows. In view of the clinical importance of bone marrow evaluation and the focal nature of metastases, more than one biopsy should be obtained for evaluation. For patients having two biopsies, as many as 30% have positive findings in a single biopsy.[309] Assuming an even chance of obtaining the positive biopsy on the first attempt, a second biopsy should increase the number of positives by up to 15%. Overall, bilateral bone marrow biopsies can be expected to advance the stage in approximately 25% of patients to stage IV, because some of those with marrow disease were previously classified as stage IV on the basis of other extranodal sites. The shift to stage IV predominantly occurs in patients with stage III disease and in those with follicular and small cell lymphocytic lymphomas.

Lymphomatous involvement of the bone marrow can be detected by morphologic assessment alone if there is 5% or greater infiltration by malignant cells. Newer techniques, such as flow cytometric analysis, clonal excess, and Southern blot analysis, have improved the detection level to 1%.[334] The PCR technique for the t(14;18) translocation is capable of reproducibly detecting one tumor cell with a *BCL2* rearrangement in 10^5 to 10^6 normal cells.[148] Studies of limited numbers of patients have shown that morphologically normal peripheral blood and bone marrow may show infiltration with lymphoma when assessed by PCR.[148,149,354]

The utility of PCR for staging the bone marrow has been examined in 152 patients with advanced-stage lymphocytic lymphomas referred to a tertiary care center for bone marrow transplantation.[79] In this skewed population, PCR appeared to add little to morphologic analysis when both tests were performed before therapy. Among 88 patients with low-grade lymphoma, nine marrows that were positive by morphologic assessment were negative by PCR. All nine marrows and lymph node samples obtained from the same patients lacked PCR-amplifiable breakpoints. Therefore, PCR cannot be used alone because 15% of low-grade lymphomas lack the t(14;18) translocation and understaging would result. However, PCR did detect disease in some patients whose marrows were read as negative for lymphoma. Therefore, PCR would upstage 10% of patients from stage III to stage IV disease.

Unless upstaging affects therapy, there is little reason to go to the added expense of PCR analysis. What effect PCR will have on the staging of patients with stage I and II disease is unknown. Between 10% and 15% of these patients contain cells in their peripheral blood with immunoglobulin gene rearrangements detected by Southern analysis, and it is likely that a higher incidence would be found if PCR was used to test the peripheral blood or bone marrow of these patients.[333] Whether detection of the malignant cells in the peripheral blood or bone marrow by PCR should change our approach to these patients requires further study.

One study indicated that PCR analysis can detect *BCL2* rearrangements in hyperplastic lymph tissues from nontumor-bearing persons.[81] The meaning of this is unclear, but if "nonmalignant" cells undergo rearrangement of *BCL2*, the PCR amplification of *BCL2* sequences would have little value as a diagnostic or staging tool. However, it does not appear that *BCL2* rearrangements in "nonmalignant" cells explain the findings discussed previously. Normal bone marrow and bone marrow from more than 200 specimens from patients with non-*BCL2*-containing tumors, were always negative for *BCL2*, and in each case for which bone marrow and lymph node samples were available, PCR detected the same breakpoint in both.

These data suggest that PCR may be a valuable tool in detecting minimal residual disease after chemotherapy. When multiple marrow aspirates and biopsies obtained at the bone marrow harvest are examined for minimal residual disease by morphology and PCR, patients with overt or minimal histologic involvement were all positive by PCR. Patients with no involvement morphologically were also all positive by PCR. However, involvement of the bone marrow by lymphoma can be patchy. Although all bone marrows were positive by PCR,

unless overt involvement was present, not all marrow samples obtained from the same patient at different sites were positive. Only 50% to 60% of the individual samples were positive. Bone marrow biopsies and aspirates were equally effective in permitting PCR analysis. This sampling problem must be addressed before this technique can be used widely. A positive finding from a good lab may well be an important finding, but there is a real question about how many negative findings are needed to be confident of the absence of disease.

Hepatic involvement with lymphocytic lymphoma has been identified in 11% to 42% of patients.[302,355–359] The frequency of identification of liver involvement increases as the size (*i.e.*, from percutaneous biopsies to peritoneoscopy-directed biopsies to staging laparotomies) and number of biopsy specimens increases. Regardless of the biopsy technique, patients with diffuse large cell lymphoma have a much lower incidence of liver metastases than patients with lymphoma in the other major histologic categories of disease. The need for liver biopsy should be determined by the likelihood that the findings will affect treatment. Most patients upstaged after peritoneoscopy-directed liver biopsies were from stage III to stage IV. Because liver involvement is rarely seen in a patient with a negative lymphangiogram, it does not seem sensible to biopsy the liver under these circumstances. Because of the use of effective combination chemotherapy for most stages of aggressive large cell lymphomas and because of the lack of consistent evidence that other subtypes of intermediate- and low-grade lymphomas are adversely affected by minimal initial treatment, the use of percutaneous liver biopsies should be limited to special circumstances.

Staging laparotomy and splenectomy were routinely performed in patients with lymphocytic lymphoma in several centers in the late 1960s and early 1970s. They provided considerable information on the patterns and distribution of disease and uniform staging for early clinical trials. However, staging laparotomy is no longer performed routinely in patients with lymphocytic lymphomas. The current treatment strategies have reduced the number of clinical situations in which a staging laparotomy is required.[302,309,355–359]

For intermediate-grade lymphomas, which often involve the gastrointestinal tract, laparotomies may be performed for diagnostic purposes, and if feasible, complete resection with appropriate staging can be performed. Primary gastric lymphomas are not resected if the extent of tumor requires a total gastrectomy because the morbidity of the procedure is high. However, masses involving other gastrointestinal sites may have improved outcome after resection. Laparotomy upstages a small but significant percentage of patients with low-grade lymphomas. Most upgrades are from stage III to stage IV disease because of occult disease in the liver. Because an advance from stage III to stage IV has minimal impact on therapy, invasive procedures to document hepatic disease are not routinely warranted for patients with stage III disease. Even in patients with stage I or II disease, laparotomy is not performed. Patients with lymphocytic lymphomas tend to be older than those with Hodgkin's disease, and they experience more operative complications. Patients with early-stage low-grade disease are treated with radiation therapy with the full understanding that one third or more have occult disease in the abdomen. Although surgical mortality is approximately 0.5%, significant morbidity, primarily pneumonia, pulmonary embolism, pancreatitis, subdiaphragmatic abscesses, or gastrointestinal bleeding, has been reported in 11% to 40% of patients in three larger series.[302]

The primary factor that accounts for the limited need for laparotomy in lymphocytic lymphoma is the high yield of less morbid procedures and the recognition that precise definition of involvement probably has limited importance in treatment planning for most patients. Laparotomy has been used as a diagnostic tool in patients with residual abdominal masses after treatment. One study showed that CT scans, lymphograms, and gallium scans overpredict for residual disease, and more patients are actually in complete remission than appears to be the case after routine restaging.[360] An NCI study of reexploration of residual abdominal masses that had been stable for at least two cycles of chemotherapy demonstrated that the procedure was not necessary because the abdomens of 21 of the 22 patients did not contain residual lymphoma.[361]

IMMUNOLOGIC ABNORMALITIES IN PATIENTS WITH LYMPHOMA

Clinically apparent immunologic abnormalities, especially of T cells, may precede the development of malignant lymphomas, but for most lymphoma patients the usual measures of immunity are normal. Because the early studies of delayed hypersensitivity in lymphoma patients did not reveal distinct abnormalities in patients with lymphocytic lymphomas, there have been fewer studies in these patients and data are surprisingly scarce. Interpretation of results of available studies needs to be qualified as well because investigators have not allowed for differences among the various histologic subtypes and stages of lymphocytic lymphoma.

The most common immunologic abnormality found in patients with lymphoma is a monoclonal immunoglobulin peak in the serum. A clinically significant monoclonal gammopathy occurs in 6% to 8% of patients with diffuse lymphomas but in 1% or fewer of the patients with follicular lymphomas.[362] These incidence figures reflect the origin of the diffuse lymphomas from the immunoglobulin-producing cells of the medullary cords (see Fig. 52–1). This region is thought to be the site of origin of the cells of Waldenström's macroglobulinemia, chronic lymphocytic leukemia, and the diffuse small lymphocytic lymphomas. With increasingly sophisticated detection methods, it appears that most patients with B-cell lymphoma have microgram or milligram quantities of monoclonal immunoglobulin (M-component) in the serum that is identical in isotype and idiotype to that borne by the malignant cells.[363] However, most patients with an M-component in their serum do not have a lymphoma. Among 1246 patients identified in a screening process to have serum M-components, only 67 (0.05%) had lymphomas.[364] Thirty-three had an elevated level of IgM, 20 had elevated IgG levels, 5 had elevated IgA levels, and 1 had a Bence Jones protein spike. Most patients had diffuse lymphomas. Nine patients had Hodgkin's disease. An associated decrease in the normal serum globulin levels was found in one third of the patients. Seven patients had cryoglobulinemia, and 6 patients had cold agglutinins. The malignant B cells of lymphoma patients do not serve any normal or abnormal immunologic functions, and the paraprotein is not present in sufficient quantity to affect antibody

responses to neoantigens. Rare lymphomas may produce factors with biologic activity. For example, there have been reports of patients with lymphoma and leukopenia whose tumor cells produced an inhibitor of myelopoiesis.[365]

Other immune disorders found in patients with lymphoma include Coombs'-positive autoimmune hemolytic anemia (AIHA) in 1% to 2% of patients and idiopathic thrombocytopenia purpura in fewer than 1.0%.[366] AIHA was associated with splenomegaly, systemic symptoms, and 8 of 9 patients with diffuse lymphomas had widely disseminated disease. No patient in this series died of the autoimmune disorder, which could usually be controlled with the drugs used to treat the underlying lymphoma.

Although patients with systemic symptoms or malnutrition may have generalized immunosuppression, there is no consensus that a particular abnormality can be related to the lymphoma.[367] Jones and colleagues demonstrated pretreatment abnormalities in 38 patients with diffuse large cell lymphoma.[368] These abnormalities, which included low IgA levels, poor skin test reactivity, and low lymphocyte counts, were more common in patients who had advanced-stage disease or B symptoms. Patients with follicular lymphoma had only skin test abnormalities, and the defects were more selective (*e.g.,* only 2 of 6 antigens failed to elicit a response). Similar findings were reported by Advani and associates.[369] Because skin tests are an in vivo measure of CD4-positive helper T-cell function, it appears that lymphoma is associated with some compromise of helper T cells. Other investigators have demonstrated mildly defective in vitro function of helper T cells from patients with lymphoma, but increases of in vitro function of peripheral blood T cells from lymphoma patients have also been reported.[370-372] All of this work is highly phenomenologic. Variations in outcome between assay systems do not allow definitive conclusions, but for most patients with lymphoma, immune defects do not seem to be an important cause of the disease. Nevertheless, rare patients do manifest significant immune abnormalities that appear to be a consequence of the disease rather than a cause of it. Certain T-cell malignancies, most notably some patients with CTCL, continue to provide immune functions such as helper activity or suppressor activity.[373,374] Patients with HTLV-I-related ATL have functional helper T-cell deficits that are comparable to those seen in HIV infection and are associated with a significant risk of opportunistic infections from a variety of pathogens, including *Pneumocystis carinii.*[375]

TREATMENT OF LYMPHOCYTIC LYMPHOMAS

The treatment approach to a particular patient with a lymphocytic lymphoma is determined by the tumor histology, the stage of disease, and the physiologic status of the patient.

The influence of tumor histology on the natural history of the lymphocytic lymphomas was described earlier. Years of clinical trials have established that the histologic diagnosis is perhaps the best single predictor of the outcome of the disease. The Working Formulation divides the lymphocytic lymphomas into histologic grades: low, intermediate, and high. The classification employed at the NCI also divides the lymphocytic lymphomas into three groups, but it has additions and minor alterations to the Working Formulation (see Table 52–8). The changes in the Working Formulation include addition of diffuse intermediately differentiated (or mantle zone) lymphoma, diffuse small cleaved cell lymphomas, and CTCL to the low-grade group; adult T-cell leukemia lymphoma to the high-grade group, and switching the immunoblastic lymphomas from the high-grade to the intermediate-grade group. We think that when treatment selection is considered, this classification is the most useful. The intermediate-grade lymphomas (including immunoblastic subtypes) tend to do well with standard combination chemotherapy, but the high-grade aggressive lymphomas require specialized leukemia-like therapy, including CNS prophylaxis, to achieve the best results. The primary determinant of the treatment approach to an individual patient is the natural history of the particular histologic subtype of lymphocytic lymphoma.

The second major determinant is the extent of disease. The staging issues vary with the natural history (*i.e.*, histologic subtype) of the lymphoma. For the indolent lymphomas, it is important to identify the 10% to 15% of patients with stage I or II disease, because radiation therapy may be curative. It is currently controversial as to whether it is also important to differentiate between stage III and stage IV disease in the remaining 85%; some studies suggest that this is an important distinction.[376–379]

Localized disease (stage I) is diagnosed in fewer than 20% of presenting patients with intermediate-grade lymphomas, but it is important to document because it affects therapy. The actual stage of a patient without localized disease (*i.e.,* II, III, IV) is probably less important than several other prognostic factors that are discussed later. For the high-grade lymphomas, most patients have disseminated disease at diagnosis, and there is no evidence that clinical staging makes an impact on the treatment approach, which in all cases, includes high-dose combination chemotherapy.

The final determinant of the treatment approach to an individual patient is their physiologic status. There is no question that the treatments for lymphoma are toxic, but the toxicities are usually dose-related and predictable. The age range for patients with lymphoma is quite large, and many patients are older than 65 years at the time of diagnosis. Lymphomas that occur in older patients are disproportionately those that may be curable with aggressive combination chemotherapy programs. Advanced age is not a contraindication to using an effective combination chemotherapy program. Clinical experience suggests that older patients may experience somewhat more myelotoxicity than younger patients when drug doses are administered on the basis of body surface area. Older patients are more sensitive to the marrow-suppressive effects of radiation therapy. However, myelotoxicity from chemotherapeutic agents is related to dose, and there is usually a particular dose of drugs that can be safely administered to a patient whose marrow is extremely sensitive. It has been our practice to administer the first cycle of drugs to older patients in full doses or rarely at 80% to 90% of the full dose and to modify subsequent cycles based on the nadir counts, similar to what is done in younger patients.

There is some evidence that the speed of response is an important factor in long-term disease-free survival, and the poorer treatment outcome that has been seen in some series of older patients may be related more to the delivery of in-

adequate doses of drugs in the first few cycles of treatment than to any feature of the tumor in an older patient.[328] Patients with aggressive lymphomas who do not achieve complete remissions have a short and unpleasant life because of the lymphoma. Patients with potentially curable disease should not be treated gently out of fear of toxic effects, which in most patients are completely reversible. The alternative to effective therapy—gentle palliation—has a uniformly fatal outcome and offers the patient treatment- and disease-related toxicity with no prospect for prolonged survival. Treatment priorities must be adjusted to the seriousness of the disease. With the most recent treatment programs, treatment-related death is far less common than treatment-induced long-term complete remission. A different philosophy would be appropriate in the same patient if the diagnosis was a low-grade lymphoma.

The existence of serious underlying medical problems may complicate the choice of therapy for patients with lymphoma. Patients with severe chronic obstructive pulmonary disease, renal failure, cardiomyopathy, or severe hepatic dysfunction should probably not receive bleomycin, high-dose methotrexate, or doxorubicin, respectively.

Another increasingly common clinical dilemma is the treatment of an intermediate- or high-grade lymphoma in the setting of an underlying immunodeficiency. Lymphomas are the most common malignancy seen in immunodeficient patients. Intensive treatment may be associated with complete responses, but the probability of long-term survival often depends more on the natural history of the underlying immune defect than on the lymphoma.

If an underlying medical problem alters the choice of therapy, it is probably best to choose an alternate regimen that does not contain the threatening drug rather than to modify a program on an ad hoc basis by omitting the dangerous drug. No one knows the contribution to the overall success of a program that is related to the effects of an individual agent in that program or whether the modified regimen would have the potential to induce long-term disease-free survival. Without such information, it would seem prudent to use an alternative regimen with a known (although perhaps lower) success rate than to create a new program with no record of success.

TREATMENT OF LOW-GRADE LYMPHOCYTIC LYMPHOMAS

The tumors that comprise the low-grade lymphomas are listed in Table 52–8. Experience in treating patients with diffuse small lymphocytic lymphoma, diffuse small cleaved cell lymphoma, and diffuse intermediately differentiated lymphoma is not extensive, and most of the information about these entities is hidden in larger studies including the more common subtypes such as follicular small cleaved cell and follicular mixed lymphomas. However, there is no evidence that the rarer forms of low-grade lymphomas (except CTCL) require an approach distinct from that used to treat the more common varieties.

There is no area of lymphoma treatment that is more controversial than the treatment of patients with low-grade lymphomas. The central question is whether any treatment can induce long-term disease-free survival and alter the natural history of this indolent neoplasm in patients with advanced-stage disease. However, there is no significant controversy about treating patients with early-stage disease; radiation therapy is potentially curative in this setting. The major decision in early-stage patients relates to the extent of irradiation required and whether the addition of combination chemotherapy improves survival. Although some authors maintain that there are no curative treatments for patients with advanced-stage lymphoma, there are studies indicating that intensive treatment may be curative for certain subsets (particularly stage III) of patients with advanced-stage disease.[376–380] If a lymph node biopsy reveals a low-grade lymphoma, the initial response should not be one of therapeutic nihilism resulting in no or conservative treatment, but it should be considered a call to perform complete staging because the patient is potentially curable if stage I or II disease is found.

Early-Stage Low-Grade Indolent Lymphoma

Clinical trials with early-stage low-grade lymphomas (Ann Arbor stages I, II) are composed mainly of patients with follicular small cleaved cell and follicular mixed lymphomas, because the other low-grade histologic varieties are rare and are rarely localized at presentation. Several studies have demonstrated the efficacy of radiation therapy in the treatment of clinically staged patients with localized disease.[381–385] In an extensively staged group of patients from Stanford (41% had staging laparotomies), actuarial survival of patients with clinical stage I or II follicular lymphoma at 5, 10, and 15 years was 84%, 68%, and 42%, respectively (Fig. 52–8).[381] Freedom from relapse at 5 and 10 years was 62% and 54%, respectively. Eighty percent of patients who were 40 years old or younger appeared to be cured with involved-field, extended-field, or total nodal radiation (TNI) therapy. There were no recurrences in this subgroup of patients after 4 years. There was no plateau on the freedom from relapse curve for patients older than 40 years, and the survival for this subgroup of patients was significantly less than for the younger patients.

In the Princess Margaret experience with more than 200 stage I and II follicular lymphomas, the overall survival rate at 10 years was 60% with a relapse-free survival rate of approximately 55% for patients receiving adequate radiotherapy.[383] Prognostic factors in this study included age, stage, histology, tumor bulk, and presence of B symptoms. In the NCI series, overall survival and disease-free survival rates at 10 years were 69% and 48%, respectively.[384] Patients with stage I disease appeared to have a plateau on the disease-free survival curve, with no relapses after 7 years, but there appeared to be a continua of relapses past 18 years for stage II patients. Similar to the Stanford University study, the disease-free and overall survival rates of patients younger than 45 years appeared significantly greater than for patients older than 45. Despite the apparent incurability of most patients who present with advanced disease, these studies indicate that a significant proportion of patients with early-stage disease may be cured, particularly if they are young (≤45 years) and have small-volume stage I disease.

There is some controversy regarding the appropriate radiotherapy field size for the treatment of the early-stage low-grade lymphomas. Because patients with these lymphomas who are treated with less than TNI often relapse in nodal sites distant from the field edge, some physicians have suggested

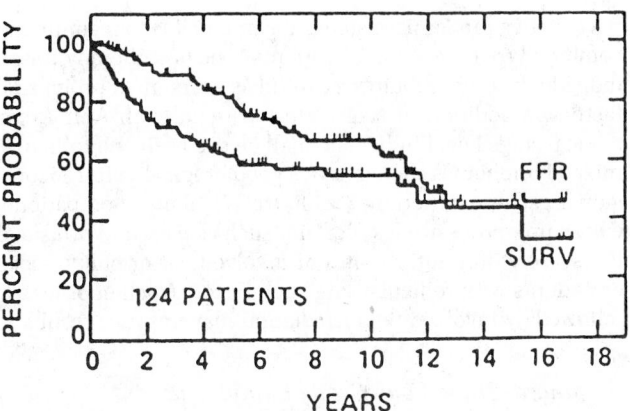

FIGURE 52–8. Survival and freedom from progression curves for extensively staged patients with stage I or II follicular lymphoma managed with radiation therapy at Stanford University.

the use of TNI or total-lymphoid irradiation (TLI) for these patients.[386,387] Support for this approach can be found in the Stanford study, which found that freedom from relapse was higher in patients treated with TLI than for those treated with involved-field or extended-field irradiation. However, if only patients who underwent laparotomy are considered, there is no difference in survival or freedom from relapse for patients receiving involved-field irradiation or TLI.[381] The more extensive the staging evaluation, the less extensive the radiation therapy needs to be. It is not recommended that patients undergo staging laparotomy simply to receive less radiation therapy. The data supporting more extensive irradiation are based on small numbers of patients, and current practice is to employ extended-field radiotherapy in these patients. This should provide adequate therapy while minimizing the potential adverse consequences of extensive irradiation on subsequent treatment that is eventually required for many patients who relapse.

A role for combination chemotherapy alone or in combination with radiotherapy in patients with early-stage low-grade lymphoma has not been established. Three randomized studies failed to demonstrate that the use of chemotherapy plus radiation therapy is superior to radiation therapy alone.[387–389] However, it is difficult to draw conclusions from these studies because each trial only included 4 to 26 patients with low-grade histologies, and the power to detect any significant difference between treatment groups was low. Investigators at M.D. Anderson Cancer Center have investigated a combined-modality approach in sequential nonrandomized trials.[390,391] Patients with clinically staged stage I or II low-grade lymphoma received sequential chemotherapy with cyclophosphamide, vincristine, prednisone, and bleomycin (COP-Bleo regimen), or if adverse prognostic features (*e.g.*, high LDH, extranodal sites, bulky nodes) were present, they received the same regimen plus doxorubicin (CHOP-Bleo). Among 44 patients, the 5-year overall survival and failure-free survival rates were 89% and 74%, respectively.[391] These results are superior to those of historic controls receiving involved-field radiotherapy alone.[390] The results from a nonrandomized series of stage I and II patients treated at St. Bartholomew's Hospital with radiotherapy alone or in combination with CVP indicate identical overall survivals but a markedly superior freedom from relapse among the group that received adjuvant chemotherapy.[385]

Without a randomized study, it is impossible to recommend combined treatment for all patients. The best therapy for an individual patient requires a careful assessment of prognostic factors in addition to stage. Most patients with Ann Arbor clinical stage I or II follicular small cleaved cell and follicular mixed lymphomas should have a good prognosis after locoregional radiation therapy (>3000 cGy) alone. For patients whose prognoses are less certain, such as patients with stage II disease with multiple sites of involvement or bulky nodes or patients with follicular large cell histology, chemotherapy followed by involved-field irradiation may improve results.

Advanced-Stage Low-Grade Lymphoma

The optimal treatment strategy for patients with advanced-stage low-grade lymphoma (Ann Arbor stages III, IV) is controversial.[380,392] Treatment generally follows one of two divergent approaches—an aggressive approach that may include extensive radiation therapy, combination chemotherapy, or both, and a conservative approach that consists of no initial treatment followed by palliative single-agent chemotherapy or involved-field radiotherapy when treatment is needed. This dichotomy exists because more than 20 years of painstaking clinical investigation have failed to prove that immediate aggressive therapy improves patient survival compared with conservative therapy.[380] This is despite repeated demonstrations that the advanced-stage low-grade lymphomas are responsive to single and multiple-agent chemotherapy, radiation therapy, and combined-modality treatment approaches.[380] Unfortunately, the responses last only a median of 2 years; in many studies, 10% or fewer patients with low-grade lymphomas remain in remission for 5 years.[393] This is an unusual advanced malignancy, because even without durable complete remissions, median survival is more than 9 years in many series.[394–396] However, the paradox of the low-grade lymphomas is that all patients ultimately die of their disease and usually do so earlier than patients with aggressive lymphomas.[392]

Figure 52–9 illustrates the survival of 147 previously untreated patients enrolled at St. Bartholomew's Hospital in various protocols, ranging from no initial therapy to conservative treatment with single alkylating agents.[396] Only 53 of 147 patients remain alive; 94 patients have died, and only 18 patients died of causes unrelated to lymphoma. This pattern has been seen so often that it is the expected outcome for patients with advanced-stage low-grade lymphomas. One can immediately see positive aspects for the elderly patient (>65 years), but for the younger patient, this curve implies almost certain death from lymphoma. A variety of strategies have been used in an attempt to alter this inexorable natural history.

DIVERSE APPROACHES. The experience with single-agent or combination chemotherapy or TLI or whole-body irradiation (TBI) alone at several selected institutions is summarized in Table 52–15. Complete responses have been observed with all treatment modalities, but continual relapse at a rate of approximately 10% to 15% per year is found regardless of therapy. Combination chemotherapy induces complete remissions more rapidly than single-agent chemotherapy, but if single-agent chemotherapy is given for adequate periods (≥1 year), there is no difference in complete response rate, disease-free survival, or overall survival compared with combination regimens such as CVP. The use of newer combination regimens appears to increase the complete response rate, but they have not been compared directly with single-agent therapy. Neither TLI nor TBI resulted in durable complete remissions when used alone. For the most part, relapses after chemotherapy occur in previously involved sites and relapses after radiation therapy are in previously unirradiated areas.[412] It is logical to combine both modalities. Randomized trials comparing chlorambucil or CVP to CVP plus TLI and combination chemotherapy (CVP) with the same regimen with TBI failed to show significant improvements in relapse-free or overall survival after the addition of radiotherapy (see Table 52–15).[398,408,413,414] When the Stanford group examined actuarial survival and disease-free survival of 114 patients with stage IV low-grade lymphoma randomized to four treatment protocols (*i.e.*, single alkylating agent, TBI plus boost, combination chemotherapy, and combined-modality [TLI and CVP]), there were no significant differences in complete remission rates or actuarial freedom from progression (Fig. 52–10).[380] The disease-free survival was only 25% at 8 years, but 76% of patients survived 8 years, and 55% survived 10 years. The median survival of all patients was between 10 and 11 years (Fig. 52–11).

The failure to detect treatment-related improvements in disease-free and overall survival and the observations that many patients not eligible for these trials or relapsing after a remission obtained from a previous therapy exhibited stable disease or even underwent spontaneous regression led Rosenberg and his colleagues to follow selected asymptomatic patients with advanced-stage disease without treatment.[314,394] Eighty-three patients were carefully selected based on features felt to be consistent with a good prognosis or because they were felt to be too old or had medical problems precluding more aggressive therapy.[394] Patients were excluded if they had bulky peripheral adenopathy, massive retroperitoneal adenopathy with ureteral deviation or obstruction, B symptoms, or splenomegaly causing symptoms or cytopenia. On comparison of these eligibility criteria with patients on their treatment protocols, 56% of the patients referred to Stanford were

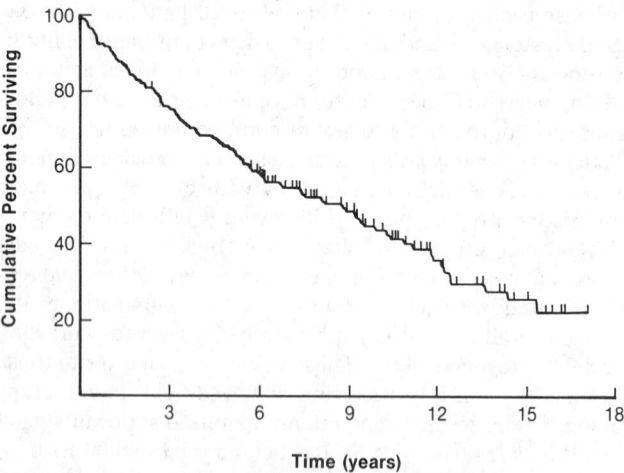

FIGURE 52–9. Overall survival rates for 147 previously untreated patients with stage III or IV indolent lymphoma managed with various treatments at St. Bartholomew's Hospital.

TABLE 52–15. Treatment of Advanced-Stage Low-Grade Lymphomas

Treatment	No. of Patients	Complete Response (%)	Remission Duration (median, months)	Actuarial Survival (median, months)	References
Single alkylating agent	13	46	25+	30	397
	20	65	50	60+	398, 399
	31	13	12	48+	400
	33	33	40	60+	401
Combination chemotherapy					
CVP	49	67	16	83	402
CVP	23	83	50	60+	398
COPP	27	56	84	90	403
BVCP	53	53	26	90	403
CHOP	92	68	?	?	404
CHOP-Bleo	96	77	30	96	405
BACOP	9	89	?	?	406
M-BACOD	10	60	?	?	407
Total-body irradiation (TBI)	33	85	26	26+	408
	31	84	24	48+	409
	28	85	30	48+	410
	17	71	12	48+	399
Combined modality					
CVP vs	23	78	36	—	
CVP + TLI	20	65	48	96+	398
CVP vs	16	67	15+	24+	
CVP + TBI	16	64	15+	24+	408
ProMACE-MOPP + TLI	51	71	45+	60+	411

candidates for no initial therapy. Treatment was withheld until the rate of growth or total bulk of disease was deemed excessive or the patient developed systemic symptoms, anemia, thrombocytopenia, or involvement of new extranodal sites.

Fifty-one of 83 patients eventually required treatment, with a median time to therapy of 33 months. The most common

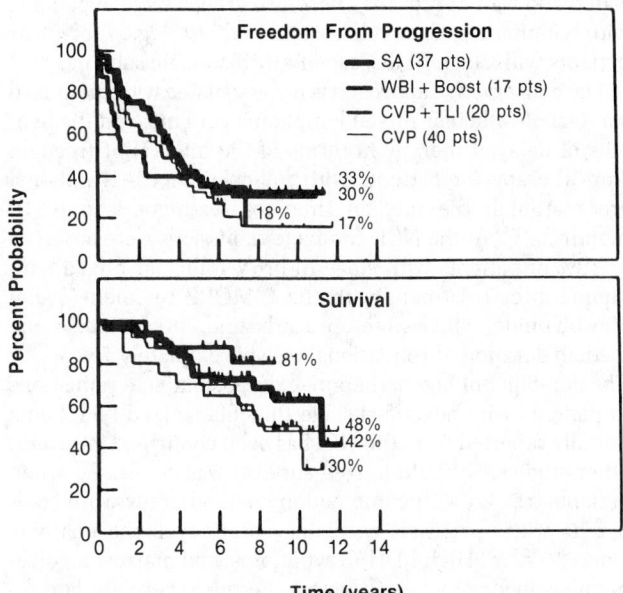

FIGURE 52–10. Freedom from progression (*top panel*) and survival (*bottom panel*) curves of patients with advanced-stage indolent lymphoma treated with different strategies at Stanford University.

reason for initiating therapy was slowly progressive lymphadenopathy, and treatment usually consisted of single alkylating agents. The length of time a patient could be followed without treatment depended on the histologic subtype; patients with follicular mixed lymphoma required treatment significantly earlier (16.5 months) than patients with follicular small cleaved (48 months) or small lymphocytic subtypes (72 months). The five-year survival rate for patients with follicular mixed disease (66%) was shorter than patients with follicular small cleaved (92%) and small lymphocytic subtypes (92%). Overall survival for patients was 82% at 5 years and 73% at 10 years. The median survival of 11 years compares favorably to the results achieved with a variety of different treatments (see Table 52–15). A comparison of similar patients on treatment protocols performed concurrently at Stanford failed to detect an effect of treatment on survival.

An interesting feature of the low-grade lymphocytic lymphomas is their propensity over time to progress to a more aggressive lymphoma. Although some cases may represent outgrowth of a higher-grade tumor that was initially present but undetected at diagnosis (*i.e.*, divergent histologies), most cases represent true transformation from a low-grade subtype. The histology usually changes to a diffuse pattern or a large cell type.[182,316] The transformation rate varies from study to study, but histologic transformation is found in approximately 30% of patients who are rebiopsied and in as many as 90% of patients with lymphoma at postmortem who were initially diagnosed with a low-grade lymphoma.[415] Treatment had been implicated as the cause of histologic progression, but the Stanford study clearly documents that histologic transformation occurs in untreated patients at the same frequency as

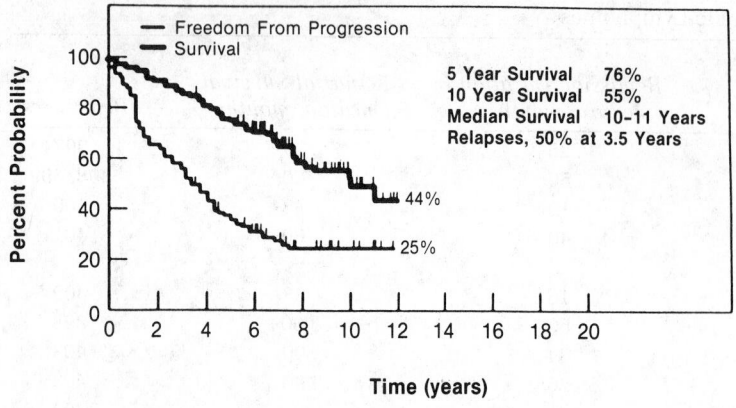

FIGURE 52–11. Data for the patients from Figure 52–10 who received different treatments were merged to obtain freedom from progression and survival curves for all the treatment groups.

in treated patients. The median time to transformation is approximately 57 months. No features have been identified that allow the clinician to predict which patient will undergo transformation. After transformation has occurred, treatment with regimens active against intermediate-grade lymphomas is needed. Complete responses can be achieved, but they appear to be less durable than complete remissions obtained after treatment of de novo large cell lymphomas. Patients who have received previous chemotherapy for their low-grade lymphoma fare particularly poorly.[182,416]

Another interesting feature of the low-grade lymphomas is the occurrence of spontaneous regressions.[178,394] Spontaneous regressions, even complete regressions, were observed in 30% of patients with follicular small cleaved lymphoma followed without initial therapy.[394] The median duration of the spontaneous remissions was more than 13 months, and some patients maintained their remissions for more than 6 years. Regressions in peripheral nodes and intraabdominal sites were observed. Other investigators, including those at the NCI, have seen occasional spontaneous regression of low-grade lymphomas, but not with the frequency reported in this study.

There appear to be several advantages to no initial therapy or the "watch and wait" approach. Foremost is that asymptomatic patients avoid the side effects of therapy, including myelosuppression and the possibility of second tumors. A few patients experience spontaneous regressions and do not require therapy, and a significant number of patients transform to a higher-grade lymphoma, some of whom may be curable with combination chemotherapy.

Several findings color the catholicity of the Stanford experience. In many centers, patients with low-grade lymphomas do not fare as well without therapy as the selected group of Stanford patients. For example, patients with advanced-stage disease at the Memorial Sloan-Kettering Cancer Center[417] had a median survival of only 4 years with conservative treatment, and O'Brien and colleagues[418] reported a median survival of 5 years in initially untreated patients. Although their median time to treatment of 33 months was similar to the Stanford trial, only 11% of patients in the study have not required therapy at 5 years. No spontaneous regressions were observed in this trial. Despite the shorter median survival, there was no survival disadvantage for untreated patients compared with their counterparts receiving treatment with single-agent or combination chemotherapy or with irradiation.

There are certain disadvantages associated with the con-

servative approach.[392,419] Many patients are adversely affected by the constant and visible enlargement of lymph nodes, which serves as an ever-present reminder of their illness and the uncertainties associated with no therapy. When therapy is finally given, it is often in the form of chronic administration of daily oral alkylating agents with or without radiation therapy, treatment that seriously depletes the nonrenewable marrow stem cell pool and can lead to subsequent intolerance to combination chemotherapy or to secondary acute leukemia or myelodysplastic syndromes.[420–425] This conservative therapy may be associated with even greater iatrogenic problems than aggressive cyclic combination chemotherapy. A subset of patients with low-grade lymphomas can be successfully watched, but even in the Stanford study, this represented only 50% to 60% of the patient population. Therefore, 40% to 50% of patients require immediate therapy because of symptoms or bulky disease.

Data suggest that at least two groups of patients with low-grade lymphoma that would otherwise appear eligible for no initial therapy actually may experience long-term disease-free survival after appropriate therapy, and on that basis, they should be considered for immediate therapy rather than a watch and wait approach. These two groups include patients with lymphomas of the follicular mixed histologic subtype or patients with stage III disease of any histologic subtype.

The conservative approach is not associated with prolonged survival of follicular mixed lymphoma patients, and the benefits of delayed therapy in terms of the interval of freedom from therapy for patients with follicular mixed lymphoma are marginal; the median time to treatment is only 16 months.[380,394] At the NCI, complete remissions were observed in 72% of patients with stage III or IV follicular mixed lymphoma after treatment with the C-MOPP regimen (cyclophosphamide, vincristine, procarbazine, prednisone): the median duration of remissions was approximately 7 years.[426] The durability of chemotherapy-induced complete remissions in patients with advanced-stage follicular mixed lymphoma initially reported from the NCI has been confirmed in several other studies.[405,426] Prolonged survival was confirmed when patients treated with combination chemotherapy were compared with patients receiving oral cyclophosphamide alone.[400,427–429] High LDH, B symptoms, and marrow involvement are poor prognostic factors. Because there are late relapses (6–8 years) in these patients, it is difficult to predict confidently the potential for cure. However, even if cure is not achieved in most of these patients, the long initial complete remissions deserve attention because they minimize the number of treatments that patients need and potentially decrease the risk for development of a second hematologic malignancy.

The application of the more sophisticated measures of complete remission (*i.e.,* measurement of clonal excess in peripheral blood cells) confirms that remissions in follicular mixed lymphoma are durable and complete.[430,431] The circulating abnormal clone that is readily detectable in almost 70% of patients with advanced-stage follicular lymphoma disappears with the achievement of clinical complete remission in patients with follicular mixed lymphoma. In follicular small cleaved cell lymphoma, clinical complete remission is often not accompanied by clearing the malignant clone, and it now appears that this may be the harbinger of relapse.[431] The same data are not available using PCR amplification of the *BCL2* translocation.

There has been little experience with the more recently developed lymphoma treatment programs in advanced-stage follicular mixed lymphoma, but extrapolating from the effects of C-MOPP in diffuse large cell lymphoma and the general correlation between the presence of a large cell component and curability with combination chemotherapy, it seems likely that the second- and third-generation combination chemotherapy programs would be excellent therapy for patients with advanced-stage follicular mixed lymphoma. We currently recommend that patients with advanced-stage follicular mixed lymphoma receive initial therapy at diagnosis with a regimen found to be effective for intermediate-grade lymphoma.

The cell cycle kinetics of the individual histologic subtypes is rather distinct.[432] Follicular small cleaved cell lymphomas have the lowest growth fraction and the lowest percentage of cells expressing the transferrin receptor, a rough immunologic correlate of growth fraction. Follicular mixed lymphomas may have a higher growth fraction and more transferrin receptor-positive cells than follicular small cleaved cell lymphomas, and the follicular and diffuse large cell lymphomas have the highest growth fraction of tumors of follicular center cell origin. As the fraction of large cells in the follicular lymphoma rises, the growth fraction of the tumor increases, the clinical pace of disease becomes more rapid, and the tumor becomes more susceptible to eradication by combination chemotherapy.

The behavior of the follicular lymphomas is analogous to bone marrow, another stem cell compartment with two stem cells. In this analogy, the tumor has two stem cell populations, the small cleaved lymphocytic stem cell that is not in cycle, but is renewable and sensitive to inhibition but not eradication by combination chemotherapy, and a second stem cell that becomes more prominent as the fraction of large cells increases and is nonrenewable, in cell cycle, and sensitive to combination chemotherapy.[420] The explanation for the more indolent growth and the more remote curability of the follicular small cleaved cell lymphomas relates to cell kinetics and the resistance of the stem cell. The analogy to bone marrow seems appropriate. Although most chemotherapeutic agents at conventionally tolerable doses can produce transient cytopenias, the marrow stem cell population usually fully recovers and repopulates the marrow to the normal level. Similarly, the stem cell for follicular small cleaved cell lymphoma usually responds to chemotherapy but continues to regrow

and repopulate. A large fraction of follicular mixed lymphoma patients are curable with combination chemotherapy, which correlates with the larger fraction of large cells and the kinetic advantage to treating a nonrenewable stem cell population. This model is speculative but has the advantage of accurately describing the clinical spectrum and response to treatment of the follicular lymphomas. If the stem cell compartment of follicular small cleaved cell lymphomas is analogous to that of the bone marrow, it is possible that treatment capable of ablating bone marrow may also ablate follicular lymphoma. This model provides conceptual support for treating follicular small cleaved cell lymphoma with a high-dose therapy, perhaps with TBI and ABMT.

Patients with stage III disease may also experience long-term disease-free survival. The Stanford experience with TLI (TBI in some) in patients with stage III disease (approximately 50% had staging laparotomies) is instructive.[376,377] The 10-year relapse-free survival rate for stage III patients treated with radiation therapy at Stanford was 40%, with an apparent plateau on the disease-free and overall survival curves (Fig. 52–12). For those with limited stage III disease (*i.e.,* no B symptoms, less than five sites of involvement, maximum size of disease <10 cm), the 15-year freedom from relapse rate was 88%.[377] Most patients relapsed in previously unirradiated lymph node groups, suggesting that the addition of epitrochlear, mesenteric, and Waldeyer's ring fields might have further improved the outcome. Similar excellent results were reported by Cox and colleagues for a study in which the dis-

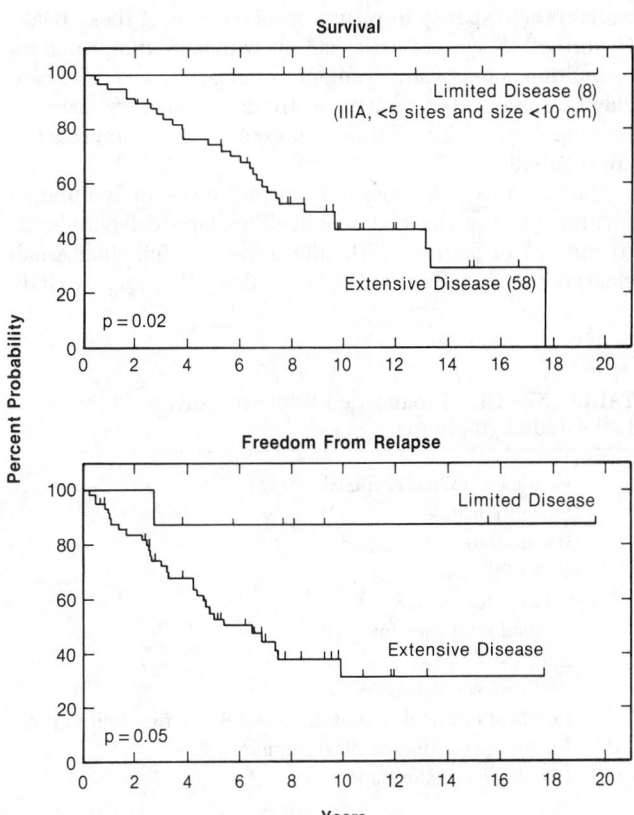

FIGURE 52–12. Disease-free and overall survival curves for patients with stage III indolent lymphoma treated with radiation therapy at Stanford University.

ease-free survival rate was 61% and the actuarial survival rate was 78% at 5 years.[378]

Investigators at M.D. Anderson Cancer Center reported durable remissions in patients with stage III follicular lymphoma using a sequential chemotherapy-radiotherapy sandwich program with CHOP-Bleo and involved-field radiotherapy of 3000 cGy to the abdomen and pelvis and 4000 cGy to peripheral nodes and mediastinum if it is involved.[379,433] This approach resulted in an 81% complete remission rate, a 5-year survival rate of 75%, and 5-year disease-free survival rate of 52% for all patients. Stage III patients without large cell histology, in whom there was no bulky abdominal disease and who had normal LDH levels, did particularly well.

These data strongly suggest that patients with asymptomatic stage III disease, with nonbulky disease involving limited sites should be considered for immediate therapy and are not appropriate candidates for "watch and wait," which merely allows them to progress from a potentially curable to an incurable tumor burden. Extensive radiotherapy with or without chemotherapy is a reasonable option.

Several attempts have been made to discover other useful prognostic factors for patients with low-grade lymphomas.[325–327,403,434–436] The factors that have been most often identified as predictors of complete remission rate or overall survival are listed in Table 52–16. The data are difficult to interpret because the different studies include patients with a variety of stages of disease that are staged according to the institution's own standards (*i.e.*, no liver biopsies or bone marrow examinations in some), and that are untreated, minimally treated, or aggressively treated. These differences may explain the disparity in results observed among these trials. Nevertheless, symptomatic patients with large tumor masses or multiple sites of involvement are clearly a group of candidates suitable for immediate therapy. However, current treatment cures few of these patients, and new approaches are required.

Application of the more recent advances in lymphoma treatment (*e.g.*, active regimens in diffuse large cell lymphoma treatment) to patients with advanced-stage follicular small cleaved cell lymphoma has been slow. However, CHOP,

TABLE 52–16. Prognostic Factors for Advanced-Stage Low-Grade Lymphoma

Histology (follicular mixed)
Stage III disease
B symptoms
Bulk of disease
   Large tumor mass
   Number of sites involved
Age
Performance Status
Levels of lactate dehydrogenase and B_2-microglobulin
Extent of bone marrow involvement
Histologic transformation
Sex
Aggressive chemotherapy
Anemia

CHOP-Bleo, BACOP (bleomycin, doxorubicin, cyclophosphamide, vincristine, prednisone), and M-BACOD (methotrexate, bleomycin, doxorubicin, cyclophosphamide, vincristine, dexamethasone) have been used in patients with advanced-stage follicular small cleaved cell lymphoma (see Table 52–15). Few patients have been treated, and long-term follow-up is often incomplete. Complete response rates appear higher, and they are attained more quickly than if single agent or more conservative regimens were used. There may be a modest improvement in disease-free survival, but there is still a pattern of continual relapse with no evidence of a plateau.

One exception is the Eastern Cooperative Oncology Group trial that demonstrated that COPP (cyclophosphamide, vincristine, procarbazine, prednisone) induced complete remissions in 56% of patients with advanced follicular small cleaved cell lymphoma, and 57% of the complete remissions lasted more than 5 years.[403] The results of treatment in advanced-stage follicular small cleaved cell lymphoma may be improved by using more active combination chemotherapy programs. None of these putative improvements in complete remission rates or duration have translated into survival advantages for treated patients. Because the median survival of even palliated patients is more than 8 years, such a stringent criterion for efficacy takes many years to meet. Nevertheless, survival without disease off all treatment is also an important goal, and the availability of a treatment approach that can achieve durable complete remissions in most patients would probably change the clinical approach to these patients even before the demonstration of a survival advantage.

In an effort to examine the alternative approaches to low-grade lymphoma treatment prospectively, the NCI initiated a prospective randomized study comparing conservative treatment (no initial therapy) with aggressive combined-modality therapy with ProMACE/MOPP flexitherapy followed by low-dose (2400 cGy) TLI.[411] The patients randomized to receive initial treatment test the hypothesis that the reason for the inability of drug combination programs to produce a significant fraction of long-term disease-free survivors is due to the failure in dose escalation. The group receiving no initial therapy is closely followed to determine the overall survival; the fraction of patients with low-grade follicular lymphomas that can be followed without drug treatment; the number of patients that evolve to follicular mixed, follicular, or diffuse large cell lymphoma over time; and the success of delayed aggressive treatment in achieving long-term disease-free survival. Clinically aggressive tumor masses are biopsied at intervals to determine the histology. If therapy is required and the histology remains low-grade, small-field palliative radiation therapy is used as long as possible. If chemotherapy is required for control of systemic symptoms or for histologic evolution, patients are crossed over to the same treatment as those initially randomized to ProMACE/MOPP flexitherapy.

More than 100 patients have been entered on this study since 1978.[411] Eighty-four percent of all patients presenting with low-grade histologic subtypes were eligible for randomization to aggressive or conservative therapy. The other 16% had serious enough symptoms at presentation that local treatment was not thought to be appropriate. Among the patients randomized to aggressive combination chemotherapy, 74% achieved complete remissions, and 67% of those achieving complete remission remain in their initial remission with a median follow-up of more than 6 years. This is in contrast to a median remission duration in previous treatment programs of about 2 years (see Table 52–15). With median follow-up more than twice as long as the average remission duration from previous treatments, only 33% of the complete responders have relapsed.

Fifty-three percent of the patients randomized to conservative treatment were crossed over to aggressive therapy a median of 23 months after randomization. Among the 47% of patients who have not required systemic treatment, 39% required local irradiation to control symptomatic local disease. The 53% of patients who have crossed over to receive aggressive therapy did so a median of 23 months after randomization. About 40% of those crossing over did so because of progressive systemic symptoms, 33% because of histologic conversion to diffuse large cell or other aggressive lymphoma, and 27% because they had exhausted the limits of local irradiation for symptom control. The complete remission rate after crossover was only 40%, significantly less than the complete remission rate seen in patients who received therapy at diagnosis. Only 4 of the complete responders have relapsed, but there is not enough information to predict whether the responses will be as durable with delayed treatment as with immediate treatment. There is no significant difference in overall survival between the two groups, but there is considerable difference between the two approaches in terms of patients alive and free of disease. Nevertheless, it appears that improvements in therapy can result in prolonged disease-free survival in some patients with follicular and low-grade lymphomas.

The conclusion that emerges from this study is that aggressive therapy at diagnosis may be curative. It appears that delaying therapy until symptoms demand systemic intervention substantially reduces the chances for a successful treatment outcome. More data on the negative impact of delaying treatment were generated by a retrospective analysis of patients treated at the University of Chicago.[437] Initial aggressive therapy achieved a complete remission rate of 71%, but aggressive therapy delivered after initial conservative management achieved a complete remission rate of only 25%. It appears that delaying aggressive therapy results in some patients becoming less responsive to therapy. It may be that the decision about a palliative or curative approach must be made at diagnosis. Failing to decide between these options initially is to decide, because palliation is all that can be done if the decision is delayed.

Although PCR analysis has not been performed on patients after ProMACE/MOPP flexitherapy, there is a strong possibility that malignant cells persist at completion of therapy, even in complete responders. After CHOP chemotherapy, all patients harbor *BCL2*-positive cells in their marrow even when by morphologic assessment they appear to be in complete remission.[79] These residual lymphoma cells may be resistant to standard-dose chemotherapy and responsible for the constant relapse rates seen in patients with advanced low-grade lymphoma. This has led some researchers to employ high-dose chemotherapy with ABMT, an approach that is effective salvage therapy for many patients with intermediate-or high-grade lymphomas.[438]

There have been two major obstacles to ABMT for patients with low-grade lymphomas. First is the observation that a very long natural history can be expected even without therapy, making the excessive treatment-related toxicities associated with transplantation unacceptable. However, the long survival may be reassuring to many older patients with low-grade lymphoma, but to our younger patients, little solace can be derived from the survival curve in Figure 52–9. Moreover, improvements in transplant techniques and supportive therapy have made ABMT a safe procedure.[439] The foreshortened life expectancy with conservative management and the low (4%) mortality from high-dose therapy programs has been used to justify high-dose experimental therapy for younger patients. The second obstacle has been the high incidence of bone marrow involvement with indolent lymphoma. It is possible to exclude patients with involved marrows, as some studies did, but this limits the approach to a rather small fraction of patients with advanced-stage lymphocytic lymphoma.

Trials have used bone marrow that has been "purged" of malignant cells by multiple cycles of ex vivo treatment with specific antibody and complement.[440–442] High-dose chemotherapy with ABMT has been tested by several groups in patients with low-grade lymphomas.[442,443] Schouten and colleagues treated 10 patients after histologic transformation of their low-grade lymphoma.[443] These patients were heavily pretreated and tolerated the ABMT rather poorly; only 1 of the 10 patients remains alive and in a complete remission. Much better results were observed in 8 patients whose tumors had retained their original low-grade histology after relapse from their initial response. All 8 patients achieved complete remissions; 6 patients remained in their initial complete remissions from 1 to 5 years, and all 8 were alive at the time of the report. All bone marrows were free of tumor at the time of harvest and no in vitro purging was attempted.

Investigators at the Dana-Farber Cancer Institute treated 69 patients with low-grade lymphomas in sensitive relapse or incomplete first remission with cyclophosphamide 60 mg/kg on two successive days followed by 1200 cGy of TBI and reinfusion of bone marrow that had been purged of malignant cells with the anti-CD20 (B1) monoclonal antibody alone or as part of a cocktail with anti-B5 and anti-CD10 (CALLA), all with complement.[441] Patients were in complete remission or had achieved a minimal disease state (all involved lymph nodes ≤2 cm and bone marrow involvement <20%) before marrow harvest. There were 51 patients with low-grade lymphomas at the time of ABMT and 18 patients whose tumors had undergone histologic transformation. More than 85% of the patients were 50 years of age or younger. After a short follow-up, there was no significant difference in 2-year disease-free survival between patients with low-grade or transformed lymphomas, with 53% and 88% of patients disease-free, respectively. There were 23 relapses, most in previously involved sites, suggesting that resistant lymphoma, not reinfusion of malignant cells with the marrow, was responsible for the relapse. The only significant prognostic factor for disease-free survival was the state of disease at the time of transplant; patients in complete remission did significantly better than partial responders. Rohatiner and colleagues used identical induction and purging regimens in 38 patients who were in their second or subsequent remissions.[442] There were two treatment-related deaths. Median follow-up is only 22 months, but 26 patients remain in remission. Despite bone marrow involvement in almost one half of all patients, ABMT with purged marrow can be performed safely and most patients remain disease free for at least 2 years.

Interesting results regarding purging were reported by Gribben and his colleagues.[79] Among more than 200 patients who had undergone ABMT with in vitro purged marrow, there were 114 whose tumors contained the t(14;18) translocation and who had marrow samples from before and after purging available for PCR analysis. All marrow samples were PCR positive for tumor before purging. No lymphoma cells could be detected after purging in 57 patients. The disease-free survival in these 57 PCR-negative patients was significantly superior to the 57 patients whose marrows could not be cleared of lymphoma cells by purging (Fig. 52–13). The risk of relapse in patients with residual detectable lymphoma cells was 10 times higher than that for patients receiving lymphoma-free marrows. Patients with the least bone marrow involvement and patients who were in complete remission at the time of transplant did well, but the most important prognostic factor was the ability to purge the marrow completely of malignant cells. Follow up is still relatively short, but relapse rates of 7% for recipients of PCR-negative compared with 46% for PCR-positive marrows are impressive.

These data imply that successful purging is an important aspect of therapy. The fact that most patients, even after ABMT, relapse in previously involved sites would seem to argue against the transferred marrow as the source of relapse, but it is possible that it is the microenvironment that is important to relapse and that the most conducive microenvironment is in previously involved sites. These data suggest that a reasonable endpoint for experimental therapy designed to cure this disease is attainment of a completely PCR-negative state in the bone marrow. Others may argue with this approach, because it is clear that the presence of PCR-positive cells in the peripheral blood does not preclude a healthy, long-term survival.[78] PCR-positive cells have been found in the peripheral blood of patients who have been in continuous complete remissions for more than 10 years. Appearance of PCR-positive cells did not predict for progression of disease. The value of their presence as a predictor of relapse has to be verified in prospective trials, but until further information is obtained, we think a reasonable goal of curative therapy in young patients with low-grade lymphoma is the induction of a PCR-negative state.

BIOLOGIC THERAPY. Biologic therapy has been extensively tested in patients with low-grade lymphomas.[444,445] Nonspecific immune stimulants such as bacillus Calmette-Guérin and levamisole have failed to have reproducible effects on complete remission rates or remission duration.[444] The interferons have activity against the lymphocytic lymphomas.[446,447] Interferon has little antitumor activity in intermediate- or high-grade lymphomas, but response rates of approximately 46% (11% complete remissions) are seen in patients with low-grade lymphomas.[446,447] The median time to achieve remission is approximately 3 months; most remissions are partial and last for a median of 8 months. Three preparations of IFN-α (*i.e.*, natural or lymphoblastoid; recombinant IFN-α2a and IFN-α2b) have been used at doses ranging from 1 million units daily to 50×10^6 U/m² 3 times weekly. The highest response rates have been reported at the highest doses, but the higher the IFN dose, the more severe is the toxicity, and few patients can tolerate 50×10^6 U/m² for any significant period.

Combined treatment with IFN-α and chemotherapy has not improved complete remission rates.[448–450] Hawkins and colleagues administered COPA (cyclophosphamide, vincristine, prednisone, doxorubicin) with IFN-α and described excessive myelosuppression at IFN doses of 12×10^6 U/m² or larger.[448] Chlorambucil and IFN-α can be given safely for prolonged periods, but randomized trails have shown that overall response rates with the combination are not superior to chlorambucil alone.[450,451] When patients achieving complete remissions after chlorambucil alone or with IFNα are randomized to maintenance therapy with IFNα or no additional therapy, lower relapse rates were observed in IFN-treated patients.[450,451] It is too early to determine whether there is an effect on overall survival, but the early data are promising.

Several phase II studies of IL-2 with or without lymphokine-activated killer (LAK) cells have been performed in heavily pretreated patients with refractory lymphoma, and responses have been seen in about 27% of treated patients with low-grade lymphoma.[452–455] IL-2 exhibits little activity in patients with intermediate- or high-grade lymphomas or Hodgkin's disease. Responses have been observed in patients receiving IL-2 at high and low doses, by bolus and continuous intravenous infusion, and with or without LAK cells. The responses are usually partial and have a median duration less than 1 year, although long-lasting remissions have been observed. As is the case with IFN-α, the single agent response rate of IL-2 is lower than that expected with chemotherapy in the same patients, but the probability that these biologic agents work by mechanisms entirely different from chemotherapeutic agents makes them attractive for potential combination with other forms of therapy and as therapeutic options to be used much earlier in the course of disease when the host's immune system is minimally compromised.

Monoclonal antibodies have been used with some success

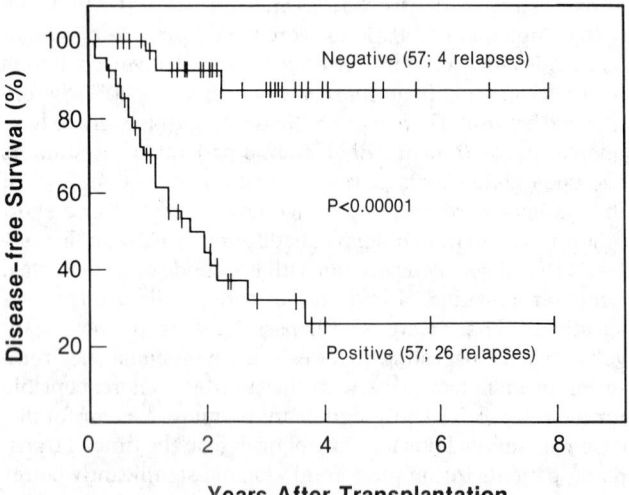

FIGURE 52–13. Disease-free survival rates for patients with indolent lymphoma whose marrow could be purged of polymerase chain reaction-amplified t(14;18)-bearing cells compared with those of patients with indolent lymphoma whose marrow could not be completely purged. This study was conducted at the Dana-Farber Cancer Institute.

in patients with lymphocytic lymphomas. There are four major classes of mechanisms by which monoclonal antibodies may kill tumor cells: by activating host immune system tumor cell lysis mechanisms (*e.g.*, complement, antibody-dependent cellular cytotoxicity); by triggering or interfering with the function of a physiologically important receptor; by targeting biologically active moieties to tumor cells (*e.g.*, toxins, isotopes, drugs, cytokines); and by eliciting an antitumor response indirectly by inducing autoantibodies or by activating cellular responses to the tumor antigen (*i.e.*, antibody functioning as a biologic response modifier).

Since 1980, patients with B-cell lymphoma have been treated with murine or rat monoclonal antibodies directed against the idiotype of the surface immunoglobulin, CD20 (1F5), a panlymphoid cell antigen (CAMPATH-1), and the Epstein-Barr virus receptor (OKB-7).[456-460] With the exception of a single patient (the *first* patient) treated with antiidiotypic antibody, whose response was complete and lasted 50 months with no further therapy, few patients treated with antibody alone experience tumor regressions that meet criteria for partial responses, and such responses are generally short-lived. There are many reasons for this lack of efficacy. There have been essentially no studies of antibodies in lymphoma patients that have taken a particular antibody and developed it in a fashion analogous to the development of other directly acting antitumor agents. In most cases, maximal tolerated doses have not been determined, and optimal pharmacokinetic parameters are unknown. In some cases (particularly in solid tumors), expression of the target antigen is heterogenous in the tumor cell population. Antibodies cannot activate killing mechanisms or exert direct effects on cells to which they cannot bind. Often the target antigen is shed, downmodulated, or altered during the course of antibody therapy. Circulating antigen makes it extremely difficult for the antibody to find the tumor-bound target. Any change in the tumor that makes it more difficult for the antibody to bind to it compromises the efficacy of the therapy. Murine and rat antibodies commonly elicit a host antibody response, usually within 2 weeks of the first exposure to the therapeutic antibody. This represents yet another distracting influence to systemically administered antibody. Murine and rat antibodies activate human effector mechanisms variably, but often poorly.

Antiidiotype therapy is an elegant approach to tumor-specific therapy. Most other tumor-associated target antigens are not tumor specific. However, there have been technical and logistic problems in the implementation of this clever idea. First, each patient's tumor is derived from a single clone. This implies that each tumor requires the generation of a special reagent specific for a particular patient. The labor involved in generating a unique hybridoma for each patient is onerous. Second, the capacity to change the structure of their immunoglobulin molecule appears to be an essential adaptive feature of human B cells. Alteration in the idiotype of a particular tumor occurs even in the absence of therapy, and it appears that most tumors that have lost responsiveness to antiidiotype therapy have developed an idiotype-negative tumor that nevertheless expresses a clonally related immunoglobulin molecule, which has somatically mutated its antigen combining site.[461,462] This genetic flexibility allows us to make antibodies to antigens that have not been invented yet, which is wonderful for our defense system. However, it

means that a single-pronged attack on an idiotypic determinant is unlikely to have a lasting impact on the growth of a B-cell tumor. Strategies to circumvent these two problems include the development of panels of antiidiotypic antibodies that are common to many tumors so that treatment does not have to be individualized, and treatment with multiple antiidiotypic antibodies together or in series minimize the problem of idiotype negative variants.[463]

The problem of antigenic heterogeneity could be overcome by the use of "cocktails" composed of several antibodies. This approach has not yet been tried in humans. Another strategy to overcome heterogeneity is the use of radiolabeled antibody. ^{131}I-labeled antibodies are capable of eradicating a subpopulation of tumor cells lacking the target antigen when they are interspersed with tumor cells bearing the target antigen in mice with lymphoma.[464] Data suggest that the dose rate of radiation delivered to tissue by antibodies may result in antitumor effects better than with the delivery of a maximal tolerated dose of external-beam irradiation.[465]

There have been several studies using radiolabeled antibodies to treat lymphoma in humans. Press and colleagues administered ^{131}I-labeled anti-CD37 (MB-1) antibody to several patients with relapsed lymphoma.[466] With initial tracer doses of antibody, they found that in 5 patients with splenomegaly and high tumor burdens the antibody did not distribute to tumor in a way that would result in the tumor receiving more radioactivity than normal organs. However, 4 other patients showed good tumor localization of the tracer. These 4 patients received 232 to 608 mCi of labeled antibody that was thought to deliver 850 to 4260 cGy of radiation to sites of tumor. Because of the difficulties with dosimetry, these values must be considered estimates. All 4 patients achieved complete remissions, and 2 patients remain in remission at 8+ and 11+ months. However, myelosuppression occurred 3 to 5 weeks after treatment in all cases and required ABMT in two cases. Two patients became hypothyroid. The improved antitumor effects of radiolabeled antibodies have come at the cost of toxicity, but the toxic effects may be anticipated and effectively managed in most cases. There is no evidence to suggest that a maximal tolerated dose of radiation delivered by antibody is superior to a maximal tolerated dose of radiation delivered by external-beam in patients with lymphoma.

De Nardo and colleagues treated 20 B-cell lymphoma patients with ^{131}I-labeled Lym-1 antibody.[467,468] They reported that 65% of the patients obtained responses; three were complete. The response rate was dose related. Patients were more likely to respond after receiving 100 mCi or greater doses of [131]I. Rosen and colleagues treated 5 patients with CTCL with ^{131}I-labeled T101.[469] Patients had subjective improvement in pruritus and objective responses lasting 3 weeks to 3 months. At the highest doses (144–150 mCi), myelosuppression was dose limiting. It appears that the cytoreductive power of antibodies has been augmented by conjugating them to radioisotopes.

One of the most potent ways of augmenting the efficacy of monoclonal antibody therapy is to conjugate the antibody to a toxin or chemotherapeutic agent. The preclinical data on the use of immunotoxins are enormous, but there are many fewer relevant clinical studies. Stone and colleagues treated 23 B-cell lymphoma patients with an anti-CD22 antibody conjugated to ricin A chain. The maximal tolerated dose for bolus therapy was 75 mg/m^2.[470] Only 1 patient had an antitoxin response, and no patient had a response to the antibody. Perhaps all the B cells that make such antibodies express CD22 and are eliminated by the immunotoxin, an idea that needs more extensive study. About half the patients achieved short-term partial responses. Nadler and colleagues used an anti-CD19 antibody (anti-B4) conjugated to an intact ricin molecule whose B chain binding site is blocked in 19 lymphoma patients.[471] One of the problems with the A chain ricin toxin has been its relatively inefficient internalization, which is facilitated greatly by the B chain. They administered the immunotoxin by 7-day continuous infusion and have not reached the maximal tolerated dose at 70 μg/kg/day. There have been one complete and four partial responses at the suboptimal doses used. About half the patients developed an antibody response to the immunotoxin.

NEW ACTIVE AGENTS IN INDOLENT LYMPHOMA. New active agents include the purine analogs 2-deoxycoformycin, fludarabine, and 2'-chlorodeoxyadenosine, and there are new methods of administering older drugs, such as oral etoposide and idarubicin (Table 52–17). The three purine analogs are structurally similar compounds that share important features but have distinct mechanisms of action.[472] They are inactive against most common solid tumors and are effective against the same indolent lymphoproliferative disorders, hairy cell leukemia, chronic lymphocytic leukemia, and low-grade lymphocytic lymphomas. Deoxycoformycin is a potent irreversible inhibitor of adenosine deaminase, and when administered at low doses (4–5 mg/m^2 given every other week), it has almost a 50% response rate in patients with low-grade lymphomas.[472,473] One third of the responses were complete. Fludarabine is an analog of the antiviral agent vidarabine, which is resistant to deamination. It appears to function analogously to ara-C. Phase II studies of fludarabine at 18 to 25 mg/m^2 for 5 days have shown overall response rates of 50% in previously treated patients; complete remissions are seen in approximately 20% of patients.[474,475] 2'-Chlorodeoxyadenosine is a synthetic purine analog that is resistant to degradation by adenosine deaminase. It can kill dividing and nondividing cells, a property that makes it particularly suited for neoplasms with a low growth fraction, such as the indolent lymphomas. Kay and colleagues administered 2'-chlorodeoxyadenosine by continuous infusion at a dose of 0.1 mg/kg/day for 7 days.[476] This dose and schedule induced a 95% complete remission rate in patients with hairy cell leukemia. An overall response rate of 43% was achieved in 40 patients with low-grade lymphomas refractory to or re-

lapsed from previous chemotherapy. Complete responses were seen in 20% of patients.

All three analogs appear to have similar activity in patients with low-grade lymphomas. Although complete responses are observed and some of them have been long-lasting, they are usually temporary, and none of these agents appears to be curative for previously treated patients. Treatment earlier in the natural history of the disease is under investigation, as are combinations with alkylators, anthracyclines, and biologicals. All three drugs are potentially valuable as palliative therapy for relapsing patients.

Etoposide is an effective drug against lymphocytic lymphomas and is a component of many current front-line regimens for the treatment of large cell lymphoma. Hainsworth and his colleagues showed that oral etoposide given at 50 mg/m^2 daily for 21 days results in a 67% partial remission rate, with a median time to progression of 8 months, in patients with low-grade tumors.[477] Responses were seen in patients with disease resistant to regimens containing etoposide given by intravenous infusion. Similar results were described using oral 4-demethoxydaunorubicin (idarubicin).[478,479] These newer drugs and methods are potentially useful for the palliation of patients who have become resistant to other treatments, and they are currently being evaluated as components of front-line therapy.

MANAGEMENT STRATEGY. No initial therapy is an acceptable management approach to patients with advanced-stage follicular small cleaved cell lymphoma, but there is mounting evidence that aggressive treatment at diagnosis may permit a large fraction of patients to enjoy prolonged disease-free survival. Patients younger than 50 years for whom a median survival of 10 years or less represents a significant foreshortening of life expectancy; patients without intercurrent illness; patients with B symptoms, abnormal liver function tests, effusions, or other suggestions of more aggressive disease; and patients initially treated conservatively who undergo histologic conversion to a more aggressive lymphoma should probably receive treatment with one of the newer combination chemotherapy programs with or without TNI for those who achieve complete remission (unnecessary in patients with converted histology).

The decision about whether to treat aggressively should not be indefinitely delayed after diagnosis. Postponing the decision until symptoms demand treatment appears to substantially reduce the efficacy of the treatment program. Those who believe that they must manage patients conservatively should consider the use of cyclical combination chemotherapy such as CVP to control the disease, because the use of chronic oral alkylating agents such as chlorambucil, although it is well tolerated, is associated with irreversible damage to the marrow stem cells, the possible development of a myelodysplasia or secondary leukemia, and a reduction in the capacity to deliver curative therapy if histologic progression should occur. CVP is not associated with chronic marrow damage.

Patients with follicular mixed lymphoma fare worse with a conservative approach and appear to be curable with the chemotherapy programs that have been used in patients with aggressive lymphoma.

Patients with diffuse indolent histologic subtypes may be best managed symptomatically because there are not yet con-

TABLE 52–17. Newer Treatments for Lymphoma

New Single Aspects	Complete Response (%)	Partial Response (%)	References
Deoxycoformycin	20	40	472, 473
Fludarabine	22, 20	26, 32	474, 475
2'-Chlorodeoxyadenosine	20	22	476
Oral etoposide	0	67	477
Oral idarubicin	0, 22	26, 36	478, 479

vincing data that therapy leads to cure. The efficacy of fludarabine in CLL makes it an attractive agent for testing in small lymphocytic and mantle zone lymphoma.

TREATMENT OF AGGRESSIVE LYMPHOMAS

The aggressive lymphomas include diffuse large cell (all varieties, including immunoblastic), diffuse mixed, and follicular large cell lymphomas. They constitute about 60% of all lymphocytic lymphomas. Most are of B-cell origin, but about 20%, including some diffuse mixed, diffuse large cell, and immunoblastic lymphomas, are of T-cell origin and are sometimes called peripheral T-cell lymphomas. The designation "peripheral" refers to the cell-surface phenotype mimicking mature postthymic or peripheral T cells (*i.e.*, CD4 or CD8 positive but not both) and differentiates the cells from cortical thymocytes or thymic T cells, which are positive for both CD4 and CD8. However, the term peripheral T-cell lymphoma is of little use in that it does not describe a discrete clinicopathologic entity.[480,481]

The Ann Arbor staging classification is used to stage patients with lymphocytic lymphoma. However, unlike Hodgkin's disease, which has a pattern of spread well suited to an anatomic site lymph node-based staging schema, lymphocytic lymphomas have a propensity to originate in extranodal sites or to spread hematogenously early in their course. Although the Ann Arbor staging classification defines prognosis quite poorly in patients with aggressive lymphoma, there has been no unanimity on what features should be used to identify prognostic groups. There are data suggesting that features of the tumor itself, clinical factors, and treatment-related variables contribute significantly to patient survival.

Several features of the tumor itself may influence treatment outcome, including cell-surface phenotype, growth fraction, and cytogenetic abnormalities. In several series, patients with T-cell tumors fare more poorly than patients with B-cell tumors.[482,483] In one series, the poorer prognosis for patients with T-cell tumors was found only in patients with stage IV disease, but there were only 8 patients with T-cell tumors of stage IV extent, too few cases from which to extrapolate broadly.[222] Other groups have not found significant differences between patients with B-cell or T-cell aggressive lymphomas.[220,223] As suggested by Stein and colleagues, it may be that apparent differences based on T-cell or B-cell phenotype are related to differences in the treatment regimen.[484] At the NCI, we have not found significant differences in outcome based on T- or B-cell phenotype in patients treated with the ProMACE-based regimens. Miller and colleagues suggested that large cell lymphomas that do not express HLA-DR antigens have a poorer prognosis than those that do.[485] However, the Eastern Cooperative Oncology Group has not found such a correlation.[486] There is no consensus that immunologic phenotype should be used to determine prognosis of aggressive lymphoma patients.

The assessment of proliferation index by staining of tissue with Ki-67, by counting mitoses, or by flow cytometric assessment of S-phase fraction seems to be able to separate good-prognosis (*i.e.*, low proliferation index) from poor-prognosis (*i.e.*, high proliferation index) patients.[487–490] There is evidence that the study of cell adhesion molecules on the surface of the tumor may reveal its propensity to spread.[490–492]

Tumors expressing high amounts of CD44, the lymphocyte homing receptor, appear to be more likely to spread than those expressing low or no CD44. Such data have not been generated on homogenously staged and treated patients. However, there are sufficient data on the role of Ki-67 staining that it would seem necessary to include this feature of the tumor in any new staging system that is developed.

Another feature of the tumor that appears to have prognostic importance is cytogenetic abnormalities.[493] One convincing study demonstrated that patients with follicular lymphoma that progressed to a diffuse aggressive histology developed an extra chromosome 7, an additional chromosome 17, or an isochromosome 17.[66] These patients appear to have a poorer prognosis than patients without these genetic abnormalities. Cabanillas and colleagues observed a similar poor prognosis for patients with diffuse large cell lymphoma presenting with chromosome 7 or 17 abnormalities, at least some of whom may have had a clinically silent period of follicular lymphoma.[494] Schouten and colleagues at the University of Nebraska confirmed and extended those observations.[495,496] Patients with chromosome 6 abnormalities had a higher incidence of immunoblastic histology and were more likely to have B symptoms. Shorter survival was seen among patients whose tumors had abnormalities in chromosome 17 and 5 or had extra chromosomes 6 and 18. In multivariate analysis, these cytogenetic correlations were stronger than the usual clinical prognostic factors. It appears that any new staging system may also need to consider cytogenetic features of the tumor cells, if such data can be generated in a clinically appropriate time frame.

Clinical prognostic factors for aggressive histology lymphoma have been surrogate measures of the physiologic reserve of the patient (*e.g.*, performance status, age) or tumor bulk (*e.g.*, large masses, multiple extranodal sites, high LDH, B symptoms). In patients with good physiologic reserve and low tumor burden, the response to therapy is excellent. If physiologic reserve is poor and tumor burden is large, response and survival are lower. Several research groups analyzed their treatment results and derived prognostic factor models that separate patients into distinct groups.[320,322–324,497–500] Although the criteria defining poor prognosis differ somewhat in their specifics across the models generated by separate groups, they tend to produce similar groupings when the various models are applied to a single large population of patients distinct from those from whom the criteria were initially derived.[322,500]

A major difficulty has been to obtain a reliable measure of tumor burden. Swan and colleagues from M.D. Anderson Cancer Center suggested that serum β_2-microglobulin might be a reliable serum marker for tumor burden.[501] In their 86 patients in whom LDH and β_2-microglobulin were measured, these factors seemed to be independent prognostic factors. All 27 patients with LDH levels of 250 U/L or less and β_2-microglobulin levels of 3 mg/L or less were alive in first remission; 75% of the group with both markers elevated were dead. Other candidate soluble markers associated with tumor burden have been suggested, such as serum soluble IL-2 receptors, urinary neopterin levels, serum CA 125, but the data in support of β_2-microglobulin are currently stronger.[502–504] A major international collaborative project is underway to pool data on patients with aggressive lymphoma and devise a new clinical staging system.[505]

A third category of prognostic factors includes treatment-related variables, such as the delivered dose intensity of therapy. Treatment-related variables are more difficult to assess because their independence from pretreatment characteristics is not entirely clear.

Treatment of Localized Aggressive Lymphomas

The treatment of choice for localized aggressive histology lymphoma is primary combination chemotherapy with or without involved-field radiation therapy. CHOP or modified ProMACE-MOPP regimens have obtained the best results.[506–509] Cabanillas and colleagues reported that stage I patients treated with CHOP had a 100% 5-year disease-free survival rate, and stage II patients had an 80% 5-year survival rate.[506] Connors and colleagues used three cycles of CHOP followed by involved-field radiation therapy in 78 patients with stage I or stage II (without poor prognostic factors) disease.[508] The complete response rate was 99%, and the long-term survival rate was 85%.

The role of adjuvant radiation therapy is unclear. Jones and colleagues reported an amalgamation of the Arizona and Vancouver experiences.[510] All the Vancouver patients received radiation therapy to the involved field after completing CHOP chemotherapy (usually three cycles). At Arizona, radiation therapy was used in certain patients whose tumor masses were not responding promptly to chemotherapy or who required significant dose modifications of their chemotherapy. Patients who were not treated with radiation therapy usually received eight cycles of CHOP. When patients who received radiation therapy were compared with those who did not, there were no significant differences in relapse rate or survival. The relapse rate among those who received radiation therapy was 14% (15 of 107); for those who did not receive radiation therapy, 24% (8 of 33) relapsed. The 10% difference in relapse rate is worrisome, although not statistically significant.

At the NCI, we administered four cycles of chemotherapy with ProMACE-MOPP with the myelotoxic drugs reduced about 25% from the standard ProMACE-MOPP regimen used in patients with advanced-stage disease; after completing the chemotherapy, patients then received 4000 cGy to the involved field in 20 fractions over 4 weeks.[509] Forty-seven of 49 patients with stage I or IE aggressive histology lymphoma achieved complete remissions, and all 47 complete responders have remained in complete remission, with a median follow-up of about 4 years. The only deaths are the 2 patients who failed to achieve an initial complete response and a 68-year-old woman who died free of disease during her second operation for coronary artery disease after having been in complete remission over 3 years. With a long-term survival rate of 94% with minimal toxicity, we concluded that the combined-modality regimen was effective and well tolerated and have little enthusiasm about asking whether the results would be as good without radiation therapy.

Results using radiation therapy alone are clearly inferior to chemotherapy or combined-modality results in localized aggressive lymphoma when patients are clinically staged. In the classic series of Stanford, the 5-year survival rate for patients with stage I or IE disease was 65%, and for patients with stage II or IIE disease, the rate was 25%.[511] Those results were not due to technical deficiencies that have been improved over the last 20 years. Reddy and colleagues reported a 10-year relapse-free survival rate of 66% for stage I diffuse aggressive lymphoma patients treated with radiation therapy alone.[512] Hagberg and colleagues reported a 60% 10-year disease-free survival rate for clinically staged patients.[513] However, when patients are staged pathologically by performing an exploratory laparotomy, radiation therapy results are improved. Vokes and colleagues[514] from the University of Chicago reported a 70% 10-year survival rate for laparotomy-staged stage I patients, and Hallahan and colleagues[515] reported a 91% 10-year disease-free survival rate among stage I patients pathologically staged. The Stanford group found that the use of larger radiation fields resulted in some improvement in outcome in clinically staged patients.[516] However, even better results were obtained by combined-modality therapy.[517] The five-year survival rate of stage I patients was 81%, but with a subset of 21 patients who received chemotherapy sandwiching radiation therapy, there were no relapses and no deaths.

The morbidity associated with an exploratory laparotomy does not seem to be justified in patients with clinical early-stage disease. The results with radiation therapy alone in pathologically staged patients are not superior to the results of combination chemotherapy in clinically staged patients. When patients relapse from a radiotherapy-induced complete response, they do so in sites not previously involved with lymphoma or in extranodal sites, suggesting that more extensive radiation therapy would not have been of value. There is evidence that patients who relapse after radiation therapy-induced complete response are refractory to salvage combination chemotherapy; relapse is usually fatal.[515,518] The problem with the use of radiation therapy alone is that aggressive-histology lymphoma appears to disseminate hematogenously early in the natural history of the disease. Aggressive lymphoma is best viewed as a systemic disease requiring systemic therapy. Primary combination chemotherapy is of proven efficacy. The role of adjuvant involved-field radiation therapy is not universally agreed on, but its use appears to permit the delivery of fewer cycles of chemotherapy to obtain excellent results. It appears that primary chemotherapy followed by radiation therapy is generally associated with a better outcome than the opposite sequence.

Each year, there are dozens of reports of one or more cases of localized aggressive histology lymphoma involving a particular organ or extranodal site. We think that all patients can be approached with a standard staging evaluation, and if they are found to have localized disease, they can be managed with primary chemotherapy and involved-field radiation therapy. It is helpful to know certain disease predilections; for example, Waldeyer's ring involvement may be accompanied by gastrointestinal tract involvement, and sinus involvement can lead to CNS disease. A systematic approach to staging should reveal any occult sites of disseminated disease that would necessitate more aggressive therapy. The job of the oncologist is to protect the patient with an unusual site of lymphoma from being managed idiosyncratically by a well-meaning subspecialist whose expertise is not lymphoma management.

A particularly common site of localized aggressive lymphoma is the gastrointestinal tract. For patients with palpable abdominal masses, there are at least 15 studies in the literature demonstrating superior survival when patients have surgical resection of the primary lesion followed by systemic chemotherapy (see examples in the reference list[519-522]). However, this conclusion may be based on an unintentional bias related to the clinical decision to operate, which was not standardized. None of the studies involving surgical debulking have been prospective randomized trials. Nevertheless, the data supporting surgical debulking in aggressive lymphoma appears to be at least as good as data supporting surgical debulking in Burkitt's lymphoma. Use of radiation therapy alone after surgery, use of surgery alone, or failure to remove as much of the disease as possible appears to be associated with suboptimal cure rates.[523-526]

Fifteen percent to 20% of primary gastrointestinal lymphomas involve the colon; about 60% involve the stomach; and about 15% involve the small bowel. Small intestinal involvement with lymphoma can be due to distinct clinical entities. In Western countries, segmental involvement of the small bowel can be surgically debulked and treated similar to the more common gastric and colonic lesions. However, in the Middle East, there are two forms of small intestinal lymphoma, immunoproliferative small intestinal disease (IPSID) with or without secretion of immunoglobulin α heavy chains. Both entities commonly involve the mesenteric nodes. The nonsecreting IPSID has a predilection for extension into the gastric mucosa. In α-heavy-chain disease, the lymphoma commonly involves the entire length of the small bowel making surgical resection impractical.[527] Both forms of IPSID respond well to state-of-the-art chemotherapy.[528] The surgical debulking of gastric lymphomas is controversial. Although removal of the tumor may improve response to therapy, the morbidity and mortality associated with total gastrectomy are too great, and results with effective chemotherapy programs suggest that gastric sparing is associated with an excellent prognosis.[529] However, if the disease can be totally removed with a subtotal gastrectomy, such a procedure may be indicated.

Ann Arbor stage II patients are heterogenous. Some with bulky disease or other poor prognostic factors behave more like advanced-stage patients, and others with less tumor bulk respond to treatments that are successful in localized disease. We recommend that patients with localized aggressive lymphoma not undergo laparotomy to stage the extent of disease. Although the best treatment program has not been defined conclusively by prospective randomized trial, we suggest that clinically staged patients with fewer than three sites of disease and no bulky masses receive CHOP or modified ProMACE-MOPP combination chemotherapy for four to six cycles followed by involved-field radiation therapy. Patients with three or more sites of disease, any bulky mass (>10 cm), or other poor-prognostic factors should be managed similarly to patients with advanced-stage disease.

Treatment of Advanced-Stage Aggressive Lymphomas

We define advanced-stage aggressive lymphoma as all Ann Arbor stage III or IV patients plus patients with stage II disease with one or more of the poor prognostic factors, such as three or more sites of disease, bulky disease, B symptoms, poor performance status, or high serum LDH levels. The treatment of choice for advanced-stage aggressive lymphoma is combination chemotherapy. Treatment has improved since the mid-1970s. Before the introduction of combination chemotherapy, 5-year survival was essentially zero. The first significant improvement in treatment outcome came with the use of MOPP and C-MOPP, which induced complete responses in about 45% of patients, and most patients who achieved complete remission remained disease free for as long as 24 years.[179] After a median follow-up of 15 years, 37% of patients remain free of disease. The durability of the complete remissions stood in contrast to the brief remissions seen in patients with indolent lymphoma. It is the experience among physicians who treat lymphoma patients that those with aggressive lymphoma are frequently cured of disease. A patient diagnosed with an aggressive lymphoma has a greater likelihood of living 10 years than a patient diagnosed with an indolent lymphoma. Research on the development of curative programs for indolent lymphoma has proceeded much more slowly, partially because of the widespread use of a palliative approach to its treatment.

On the other hand, treatment programs for aggressive lymphoma have progressed to the point that more than 60% of patients with advanced-stage disease are being cured (Tables 52–18 and 52–19). Treatment programs have become more aggressive but only a little more toxic and have produced substantial increases in the fraction of patients achieving complete response. Unlike indolent lymphoma patients who may live several years with active disease, survival with aggressive lymphoma is short. The only chance for prolonged survival in patients with aggressive lymphoma is to obtain a durable complete response.

During the 17 years since the initial success of C-MOPP was reported, the development of new chemotherapy programs has burgeoned. The treatment outcome with these regimens has generally fallen into three groups. The first group of regimens includes C-MOPP, BACOP (in two different dose schedules), COMLA, and CHOP.[179,406,530-534] They produce complete response rates of 45% to 55% and long-term survival rates of 30% to 35%. The second group of regimens includes M-BACOD, m-BACOD, COP-BLAM, CAP-BOP, ACOMLA, ProMACE/MOPP flexitherapy, and ProMACE-MOPP.[534-541] They produce complete response rates of 70% to 75% and long-term survival rates of 45% to 50%. The third group of regimens includes COP-BLAM III, Mega-COMLA, MACOP-B, ProMACE-CytaBOM, F-MACHOP, VACOP-B, and LNH-84.[538,541-547] They produce complete response rates over 80% and long-term survival rates of 60% to 65%.

A fourth group may have begun. Gulati and his colleagues at Memorial Sloan-Kettering Cancer Center have conducted a pilot study with poor-prognosis patients using high-dose therapy with cyclophosphamide plus TBI followed by ABMT.[548] All the patients achieved complete responses, and 79% are long-term disease-free survivors. A common thread through the development of improved treatment approaches is the augmentation of the dose intensity of the treatment program (Table 52–20).

Despite the accumulated experience suggesting that the likelihood of a favorable treatment outcome has improved over the last 17 years, there has been some resistance to this idea. Critics have pointed out the absence (until recently) of controlled trials showing that one regimen is superior to another. Others observed that some of the regimens have been reported by referral centers whose patient population may not reflect the same proportion of poor-prognosis patients seen

TABLE 52–18. The Most Active Chemotherapy Programs for Intermediate-Grade Lymphoma

COP-BLAM	Day 1	Day 10	Day 14	Days 15–21
Cyclophosphamide 400 mg/m² I.V.	X			No therapy
Doxorubicin 40 mg/m² I.V.	X			
Vincristine 1 mg/m² I.V.	X			
Procarbazine 100 mg/m² PO	X-------------X			
Prednisone 40 mg/m²	X-------------X			
Bleomycin 15 mg I.V.			X	

COP-BLAM III		Day 1		Day 2	Day 3	Day 4	Day 5

Cycle A

		Day 1		Day 2	Day 3	Day 4	Day 5
Vincristine 1 mg/m²/day I.V. infusion		X---------------------X					
Bleomycin 7.5 mg/m² I.V. bolus, then 7.5 mg/m²/day I.V. infusion		X---X					
Cyclophosphamide 350 mg/m² I.V.		X					
Doxorubicin 35 mg/m² I.V.		X					
Prednisone 40 mg/m² PO		X		X	X	X	X
Procarbazine 100 mg/m² PO		X		X	X	X	X

Cycle B

Like Cycle A without bleomycin and without day 2 of vincristine infusion

Week	1	3	7	10	13	16	19	22	25	28	31	34
Cycle	A	B	A	B	A	B	A	B	A	B	A	B

CAP-BOP	Day 1	Day 7	Day 15	Day 21
Cyclophosphamide 650 mg/m² I.V.	X			
Doxorubicin 50 mg/m² I.V.	X			
Procarbazine 100 mg/m² PO	X-------------X			
Vincristine 1.4 mg/m²			X	
Bleomycin 10 U/m² SC			X	
Prednisone 100 mg PO			X-------------X	
Cycles repeated every 3–4 weeks				

ProMACE-CytaBOM	Day 1	Day 8	Day 14	Day 15–21
Cyclophosphamide 650 mg/m² I.V.	X			No therapy
Doxorubicin 25 mg/m² I.V.	X			
Etoposide 120 mg/m² I.V.	X			
Cytarabine 300 mg/m² I.V.		X		
Bleomycin 5 mg/m² I.V.		X		
Vincristine 1.4 mg/m² I.V.		X		
Methotrexate 120 mg/m² I.V.		X with leucovorin rescue		
Prednisone 60 mg/m² PO	X---------------------------X			
Cotrimoxazole 2 PO bid throughout 6 cycles of therapy				

MACOP-B	Week	1	2	3	4	5	6	7	8	9	10	11	12
Cyclophosphamide 350		X		X		X		X		X		X	
Doxorubicin 50 mg/m² I.V.		X		X		X		X		X		X	
Vincristine 1.4 mg/m² I.V.			X		X		X		X		X		X
Methotrexate 400 mg/m² I.V.*			X			X				X			
Bleomycin 10 mg/m² I.V.					X				X				X
Prednisone 75 mg/m² PO od		X---taper											
Cotrimoxazole 2 PO bid		X---X											

(continued)

TABLE 52–18. *(Continued)*

VACOP-B	Week	1	2	3	4	5	6	7	8	9	10	11	12
Etoposide 50 mg/m² I.V. day 1				X				X				X	
100 mg/m² PO days 2, 3				X				X				X	
Doxorubicin 50 mg/m² I.V.		X		X		X		X		X		X	
Cyclophosphamide 350 mg/m² I.V.		X				X				X			
Vincristine 1.2 mg/m² I.V.*			X		X		X		X		X		X
Bleomycin 10 U/m² I.V.			X		X		X		X		X		X
Prednisone 45 mg/m² PO daily × 1 wk, then qod × 11 wk													
Cotrimoxazole double strength PO bid × 14 wk													
Ketoconazole 200 mg PO daily × 1 wk, then qod × 11 wk													
Cimetidine 600 mg PO bid × 1 wk, then qod × 11 wk													

LNH-84	Day 1	Day 2	Day 3	Day 4	Day 5
Induction					
Adriamycin 75 mg/m²	X				
Cyclophosphamide 1200 mg/m²	X				
Vindesine 2 mg/m²	X				X
Bleomycin 10 mg	X				X
Prednisone 60 mg/m²	X	X	X	X	X
Methotrexate 12 mg IT			X		

	Week	8	9	10	11	12	13	14	15	16	17	18	19	20	21
Consolidation															
Methotrexate 3 g/m²		X		X											
Ifosfamide 1.5 g/m²						X		X							
Etoposide 300 mg/m²						X		X							
L-asparaginase 50,000 U/m²									X	X					
Cytarabine 100 mg/m² × 4 d													X		X

F-MACHOP	Hours	0	12	36	42	48	60	66
Vincristine 0.5 mg/m²		X	X					
Cyclophosphamide 800 mg/m²				X				
5-Fluorouracil 15 mg/kg				X	X			
Cytosine arabinoside 1000 mg/m²					X	X		
Adriamycin 60 mg/m²						X		
Methotrexate 500 mg/m²							X	X
Prednisone 60 mg/m²	from day 1 to day 14							
Folinic acid 20 mg/m² I.V. q 12 h × 4 starting on hour 84								

* With leucovorin rescue.

in a population of patients not referred to secondary and tertiary care centers. It has been disconcerting that the originally reported results may not be replicated by others. For example, the MACOP-B regimen in the hands of its originators induced a complete response rate of 84% and an 8-year overall actuarial survival rate of 62%.[545] In other series, results varied widely with MACOP-B. Schneider and colleagues obtained a complete response in only 20 (53%) of 38 HIV-negative patients with diffuse large cell lymphoma, and the survival rate at short follow-up was 50%.[549] Similarly, SWOG investigators using MACOP-B reported complete responses in 54 (50%) of 109 patients with aggressive lymphoma, and a 51% survival rate at 3 years.[550] Vitolo and colleagues reported a 71% complete response rate (127 of 180) in patients with diffuse large cell lymphoma, and the overall survival rate was 60% at 3 years.[551]

Although lower response rates are often expected in group studies, one of the poorest results with MACOP-B was reported from a single-institution study, and an excellent result confirming the original report came from a multicenter study.

TABLE 52–19. Prospect for Long-term Survival With Recent Treatment Programs for Diffuse Aggressive Lymphoma

Regimen*	Complete Responses (CR)		Relapse Rate (RR)		Potential for Long-Term Survival (CR) × (1-RR)
ProMACE/MOPP flexitherapy	60/75	(80%)	21/60	(35%)	52%
m-BACOD	59/86	(70%)	15/59	(25%)	52%
COP-BLAM	24/33	(73%)	4/24	(17%)	61%
CAP-BOP	37/51	(73%)	11/37	(30%)	51%
COP-BLAM III	43/51	(84%)	4/43	(9%)	76%
MACOP-B	104/125	(84%)	23/104	(21%)	66%
ProMACE/CytaBOM	80/95	(84%)	20/80	(25%)	63%
F-MACHOP	88/113	(78%)	17/88	(19%)	63%
LNH-84	553/737	(75%)	139/553	(25%)	56%

* These studies were conducted and reported at different times. The relapse rates cannot be considered to have reached the maximal level, because the denominators probably still include some patients who remain at risk of relapse. The calculated potential for long-term disease-free survival for these treatment programs probably overestimates the actual potential for cure in some studies, particularly those with the shortest patient follow-up. The dose and schedule of drugs in the regimens is given in Table 52–18.

One of the most active regimens, LNH-84, was originally described by results obtained in a multicenter study. The observed variability in outcome in different series using the same treatment regimen defies simple answers.

One important issue in the interpretation of clinical results is the degree to which the technology of delivering the regimen has been mastered. This issue has been effectively addressed in the radiation therapy community, in which the lack of standardization of technical issues was found to have a dramatic effect on the treatment outcome. The issue has not been addressed in a meaningful way for the delivery of chemotherapeutic agents, but systematic and periodic adjustments to published regimens are frequently made. Sometimes body surface area is rounded down (*i.e.*, calculated at 1.84, rounded to 1.8). A calculated dose of 11.5 mg of a drug may be delivered at 10 mg if the drug is packaged in 10-mg vials. Delays in

TABLE 52–20. Nine-Drug Relative Dose Intensities of 15 Primary Programs for Diffuse Aggressive Lymphomas

Regimen*	Duration of Treatment (mo)	Percentage of Long-Term Survival	9 Drugs	Drug Exposure During First 2 Weeks
MACOP-B	3	62	0.51	5/6
ProMACE-CytaBOM	4.5	69	0.48	8/8
ProMACE-MOPP	6	54	0.44	6/7
ProMACE/MOPP flexitherapy	8	48	0.43	5/7
M-BACOD	7	48	0.42	5/6
COP BLAM III	9	65	0.40	6/6
BACOP	6	35	0.39	3/5
COP BLAM I	6	55	0.39	6/6
MOPP	6	35	0.36	4/4
COMLA	9	<33	0.28	2/4
CHOP	6	<30	0.26	4/4
LNH-84	4	67	0.70	5/5
F-MACHOP	5	68	0.64	7/7
VACOP-B	3	60	0.43	5/6
High-dose chemotherapy plus total-body irradiation	—	79	ablation	—

*The dose and schedule of drugs in the regimens is given in Table 52–18.

treatment not mandated by resolving toxicities are frequently made. All of these seemingly minor adjustments can accumulate to produce a serious compromise in dose intensity.

A major problem in the reporting of clinical trial results is that the actual dose intensity with which a regimen is delivered is not routinely given. A paper attempting to confirm a result may claim that the regimen was given as originally reported, but no objective data are presented to confirm the assertion. SWOG reported their results in a series of 78 patients treated with ProMACE-CytaBOM.[552] Ninety-seven patients were initially entered on the study from 43 institutions, but 19 patients (20%) were found in retrospect to be ineligible. The complete response rate in the eligible patients was 65%, 21% lower than that obtained at the NCI, a difference that was found to be statistically significant.[553] The SWOG researchers stated that 84% of the ProMACE-CytaBOM cycles were given "precisely as described and consistent with explicit rules for dose modification." However, SWOG capped vincristine at 2 mg rather than delivering the protocol dose of 1.4 mg/m^2. In contrast to the claim, none of the cycles were given as originally reported. It is not clear whether there were other significant modifications. In an effort to make objective comparisons, the SWOG investigators reported actual dose intensity of the therapy but used a method that did not account for delays in treatment and has been said to overestimate the delivered dose intensity.[554] This makes comparisons between the SWOG and NCI cohorts difficult. The use of the SWOG method for both cohorts found that SWOG patients received at least 12% less dose intense therapy. It is not known whether this magnitude of difference is biologically significant. Analysis of response rates by prognostic subset should control for the often claimed differences in prognostic factor composition between referral and cooperative group patient populations. Statistically significant differences between the complete response rates in the two cohorts were still seen after taking distinct prognostic factors into account. Perhaps there are quantifiable differences in drug delivery that may account for the differences in outcome. In the SWOG group, the average number of patients treated at any center was fewer than 3. There may be important aspects of delivering a regimen that are gained with experience. These factors should be examined before a failure to confirm high response rates is used to justify the use of an older treatment regimen for patients with a curable tumor.

Those who believe that the therapy for advanced-stage aggressive histology lymphoma has not improved obtained support for their view from the results of SWOG's randomized comparison of CHOP, m-BACOD, MACOP-B, and ProMACE-CytaBOM reported at the 1992 meeting of the American Society of Clinical Oncology.[555] The study shows no difference among the regimens. This conclusion is based on CHOP results at least 15% better than any previously published (overall survival of 45% rather than 30%), and results with the other regimens 15% to 20% poorer than previously reported. The expected 30% difference was not seen. Those who wish to place their faith in the results of this study must do so in preference to an increasing body of data showing that dose intensity is an important determinant of treatment outcome in this disease. In every tumor type in which chemotherapy is curative, there is evidence for a dose-response association with the outcome.

Meyer and colleagues reviewed the evidence from previously published randomized studies to assess the role of dose intensity in treatment outcome.[556] None of the studies directly addressed the role of dose intensity, but a metaanalysis of 14 trials involving over 2300 patients revealed that patients receiving the regimen with a higher projected dose intensity in a comparative trial were about one third more likely to achieve complete remission than those on the lower dose intensity regimen.

We previously analyzed the influence of projected dose intensity on the likelihood of survival among published regimens.[557] It is difficult to compare the dose intensity of regimens composed of different agents. However, for a hypothetical nine-drug regimen with optimal doses of all the agents, each regimen can be assigned a relative dose intensity in proportion the hypothetical standard. As shown in Figure 52–14, there is a significant linear relation between projected relative dose intensity and long-term survival. This method of examining results is interesting but limited. Some studies have begun reporting actual dose intensity data, which may provide a better idea of the role of dose intensity in outcome.

Kwak and colleagues reviewed the outcome of 115 patients treated at Stanford with CHOP, M-BACOD, or MACOP-B and found that an actual relative dose intensity of doxorubicin delivered in the first 12 weeks of therapy greater than 75% of the projected dose was the single most important predictor of survival.[558] Other clinical prognostic factors included performance status, high LDH levels, and extranodal sites of disease. However, this is the first study to demonstrate the prognostic significance of delivered dose intensity in aggressive lymphoma. It is tempting to suggest that administration of a higher dose intensity of doxorubicin would improve the outcome of patients who received lower-dose-intensity doxorubicin, but the data do not permit that extrapolation. It is presumed that doxorubicin was dose modified on the basis of encountered toxicity. There may be other biologic features of the lymphoma or the patient that affected the ability to deliver full doses of therapy. Higher doses of doxorubicin may not have improved the response. Nevertheless, the results certainly support the notion that dose intensity is an important determinant of treatment outcome, even though this treatment-related variable is not a prognostic factor in the usual sense of the term. Classic prognostic factors are features of the patient or the tumor determined before therapy.

Epelbaum and colleagues reviewed the contribution of dose intensity to the treatment outcome of 95 patients treated with CHOP.[559] They found that age over 60 years, advanced stage, male sex, and receiving less than the median dose intensity of any of the four drugs were significantly associated with a poorer survival. Using multivariate analysis, the average relative dose intensity below the median was the strongest prognostic factor predicting poor survival, followed by age over 60 years. Dose intensity appears to contribute to CHOP treatment outcome.

Banavali and colleagues attempted to improve on CHOP by altering the schedule of administration.[560] They administered cyclophosphamide (600 mg/m^2 given intravenously weekly for eight doses), doxorubicin (50 mg/m^2 given intravenously, weeks 1 and 5), vincristine (1.4 mg/m^2 given intravenously weekly for eight doses), and prednisone (40 mg/m^2 given orally daily for 4 weeks, then tapered). This was followed by

Percent Alive
Disease Free

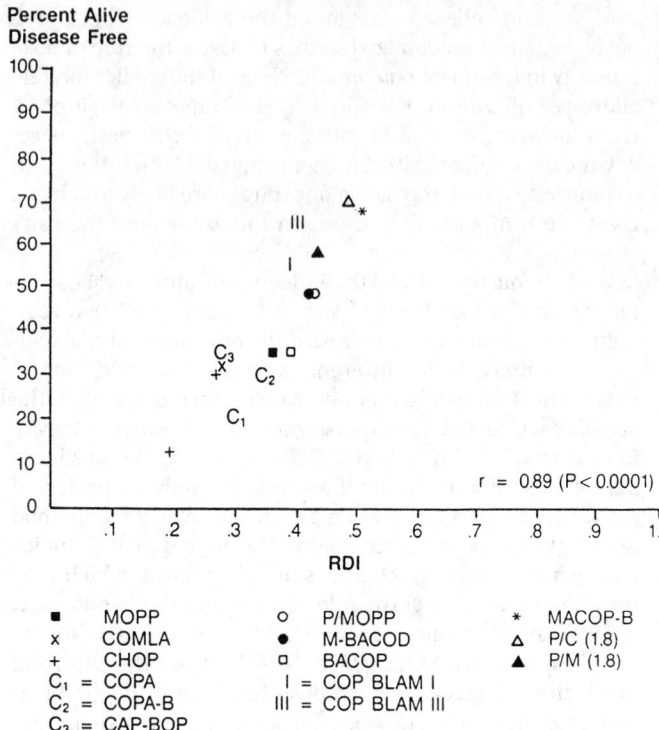

FIGURE 52–14. Relation between normalized nine-drug relative dose intensity (RDI) and disease-free survival of patients with diffuse large cell lymphomas. The 14 most extensively studied treatment programs for diffuse large cell lymphomas use nine drugs in some combination. Each regimen was evaluated for its relative dose intensity based on delivery of full doses of all nine drugs, although none of the programs achieved this ideal; they used four to eight drugs. The regimen that had the highest relative dose intensity was MACOP-B. Its dose intensity was arbitrarily rated as 1, and the other regimens were normalized to MACOP-B, giving a normalized nine-drug relative dose intensity. The long-term survival of each regimen was plotted against the normalized nine-drug relative dose intensity. A statistically significant correlation was found between dose intensity and disease-free survival.

CHOP therapy for 4 weeks every 2 months for 12 to 18 months. The dose intensity of cyclophosphamide, vincristine, and prednisone in the first 8 weeks were significantly augmented over standard CHOP. The complete response rate in 108 patients was 78%, with a 5-year survival rate of 53%. These results compare favorably to the 50% complete response rate and 30% long-term survival rate previously reported for CHOP. Similar increments in response rates and survival were found with Mega-COMLA compared with COMLA.[543] The dose intensity of the cyclophosphamide was doubled by shortening the cycle to 6 weeks from 12. In a small number of patients, the complete response rate was 80%, and 25% of the complete responders relapsed within a median follow-up of 26 months. Conclusions are difficult because of the sporadic use of radiation therapy and CHOP consolidation therapy. However, the results appeared to be an improvement over conventional COMLA.

Improving the dose intensity of CHOP-bleo did not appear to improve the treatment outcome in a series of patients treated at the M.D. Anderson Cancer Center.[561] Nonconcurrent series of patients were treated with conventional doses or maximal tolerated doses (with laminar flow room support) of CHOP-bleo. The conventional-dose regimen was given at about 80% of the dose intensity of the high-dose regimen. Yet the complete response rates (75% for conventional dose; 81% for high dose) and overall survival (53% for conventional dose; 48% for high dose) were not significantly different. There were more good-prognosis patients on the conventional-dose regimen, but it appears that the 20% difference in dose intensity did not translate into an improved outcome. It seems clear that lowering the dose intensity of a regimen can adversely alter its efficacy. The administration of half-dose CHOP to patients, as was routinely done for patients over age

65, resulted in long-term survival in only 12% of patients, compared with 41% in those given full-dose CHOP. Of course, it is also possible that this poorer result was related to differences in the older patient population.

No prospective randomized study with dose intensity as the only variable has been conducted. However, two prospective randomized trials comparing two regimens with substantial overlap in active agents show significant advantages to the regimen with the higher dose intensity. At the NCI, we compared ProMACE-MOPP to ProMACE-CytaBOM in 193 patients with advanced-stage aggressive lymphoma.[541] The complete response rate was significantly higher for ProMACE-CytaBOM (86%) than ProMACE-MOPP (74%), and the projected 8-year survival rate was significantly higher for ProMACE-CytaBOM (69%) than ProMACE-MOPP (53%) (Fig. 52–15). The two regimens share six drugs; five of the six are delivered with greater dose intensity in ProMACE-CytaBOM, and the sixth, methotrexate, has been demonstrated by the Dana-Farber group to make no significant impact on outcome when its dose intensity is reduced (M-BACOD and m-BACOD are similar in efficacy but differ in methotrexate dose intensity).[563] It is possible that the cytarabine and bleomycin in ProMACE-CytaBOM are more active than the mechlorethamine and procarbazine in ProMACE-MOPP, but it seems more likely that the advantage to ProMACE-CytaBOM is related to dose intensity. This is the first randomized study in aggressive lymphoma to demonstrate the superiority of one doxorubicin-containing regimen over another.

Comparison of ProMACE-MOPP to the early NCI study of ProMACE/MOPP flexitherapy allows some evaluation of the Goldie-Coldman hypothesis.[540,562] The Goldie-Coldman hypothesis predicted that earlier exposure of the tumor to non-cross-resistant agents would result in a lower probability of

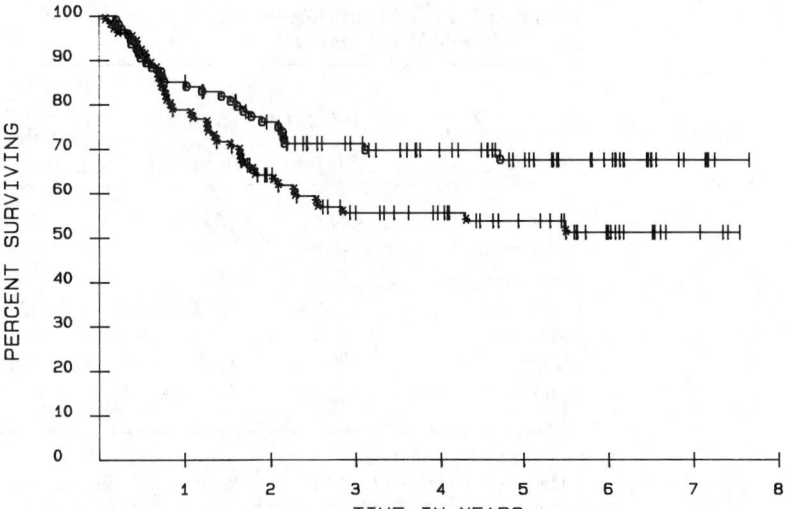

FIGURE 52–15. Survival for patients with advanced-stage lymphoma treated with ProMACE-MOPP (*), for which 44 of 99 failed, or ProMACE-CytaBOM (O), for which 28 of 94 failed, is plotted from the first treatment date to the death date. Four patients died of intercurrent conditions unrelated to lymphoma or its treatment and are censored. All deaths related to lymphoma or lymphoma treatment are plotted. Mantel-Haenszel test for a difference between treatments showed that $p_2 = 0.046$.

developing drug resistance. If this were true, ProMACE-MOPP, which brings the MOPP drugs into the first cycle, should be more effective than ProMACE/MOPP flexitherapy, in which exposure to the MOPP drugs is delayed for 2 or 3 months. However, the results of the two regimens were almost identical: complete response rates were 75% and 74%, and long-term survival rates were 50% and 53% for ProMACE/MOPP flexitherapy and ProMACE-MOPP, respectively. These results represent an excellent internal standard for the consistency of the NCI treatment effects, but they appear to cast some doubt on the ability to improve treatment on the basis of the Goldie-Coldman predictions.

The European Organization for Research and Treatment of Cancer conducted a prospective randomized trial comparing their CHOP-related regimen, CHVmP (in which teniposide replaces vincristine) to the same regimen with vincristine and bleomycin added (CHVmP+VB).[563] CHVmP+VB was significantly better than CHVmP in complete response rate and survival. The complete response rate to CHVmP+VB was 80%, and the 5-year survival rate was 53%. These values were significantly better than the 50% complete response rate and 29% survival rate seen on the CHVmP arm. The improved outcome is clearly related to adding two active agents without compromising the doses of the other four drugs and with no significant additional toxicity. The durability of the complete remissions was comparable with the two regimens, suggesting that the major benefit was obtained because more patients achieved a complete response.

Pilot studies of newer regimens suggest that survival of patients with aggressive lymphoma is improving, and a feature of all the newer regimens is increased dose intensity. COP-BLAM III achieves high-dose intensity partially through the use of infusional drug delivery. MACOP-B involves the weekly delivery of agents. ProMACE-CytaBOM delivers eight active drugs 2 weeks out of 3. F-MACHOP consists of seven drugs administered sequentially within the first 3 days of a treatment cycle. All of these regimens achieve complete responses in 80% or more of patients, and long-term survival rates of 60% or more.

Another treatment experience that favors a role for dose intensity is that of Gulati and colleagues who used myeloab-

lative doses of therapy to treat a group of poor-prognosis patients at Memorial Sloan-Kettering Cancer Center.[548] CHOP therapy and other less aggressive conventional-dose regimens had obtained a 20% survival rate for patients with high LDH levels, large abdominal masses, and B symptoms. However, when treated with high-dose cyclophosphamide plus TBI and ABMT, survival was 79%. This study and those plotted in Figure 52–14 support the conclusion that there is a linear relation between dose intensity and treatment outcome. The data imply that further augmentation of dose intensity may lead to improvements in treatment outcome. However, it may also be true that the dose intensity–survival curve is about to change slopes or plateau and that additional increases in dose intensity would not improve survival.

Although these data seem to support the importance of dose intensity in the treatment of aggressive lymphoma, proof requires a prospective randomized trial in which the only variable is the delivered dose intensity. The availability of colony-stimulating factors may permit dose escalation of the myelotoxic agents, but most of the agents active in lymphoma produce thrombocytopenia and neutropenia. The approved colony-stimulating factors are not effective at preventing or promoting the recovery from thrombocytopenia.

There are other ways of augmenting dose intensity than increasing the doses of the myelotoxic agents. The major variables in dose intensity are amount of drug delivered and time between drug administrations. It is possible to increase dose intensity by increasing individual doses or by administering the drugs closer together. Weekly therapy or continuous infusion therapy are two approaches to augmenting dose intensity that do not require intensive marrow support with factors or transplantation. At the NCI, we have shortened the ProMACE-CytaBOM treatment cycle to 2 weeks by lowering the dose of the myelotoxic agents but have increased their dose intensity by moving their delivery closer together. Table 52–21 compares the delivered dose intensity of the short-cycle ProMACE-CytaBOM with standard ProMACE-CytaBOM. Each agent was delivered with significantly higher dose intensity in the 2-week cycle regimen. Of the first 45 patients, 41 (92%) achieved a complete response, and 7 (17%) of the complete responders relapsed, with a median follow-

TABLE 52–21. Mean Dose Intensity of Short Course Versus Standard ProMACE-CytaBOM

Drugs*	Short ProMACE-CytaBOM		Increased Actual Dose Intensity† Compared With Standard P-C	ProMACE-CytaBOM	
	Delivered	(Projected)		Delivered	(Projected)
Cyclophosphamide	220.4	(237.5)	27%	173.7	(217)
Doxorubicin	9.5	(10)	44%	6.6	(8.3)
Etoposide	47.6	(50)	46%	32.7	(40)
Vincristine	.64	(.70)	60%	0.40	(.46)
Methotrexate	53.1	(60)	52%	34.9	(40)
Ara-C	136	(150)	65%	82.6	(100)
Bleomycin	2.3	(2.5)	64%	1.4	(1.7)

P-C, ProMACE-CytaBOM.
* The dose and schedule of the drugs is given in Table 52–18.
† Mean dose intensity is measured in units of mg/m²/week.

up of 18 months. Although it is still early in the course of this pilot study, it is clear that dose intensity has been increased, myelotoxicity is actually somewhat reduced, and high response rates have been maintained. A randomized study comparing the two methods of delivering ProMACE-CytaBOM would probably represent a true test of the dose intensity question.

Toxicities of Therapy for Aggressive Lymphomas

All of the effective treatment programs for the aggressive lymphomas produce myelosuppression. In general, the degree of myelosuppression is a function of the manner in which the drugs are given. The recommended doses are normalized to body surface area, but these starting guidelines may be adjusted up or down based on the response of the individual patient. We recommend 10% upward adjustment of doses if the patient does not develop a leukocyte nadir below 2000/mm³ or a platelet nadir below 100,000/mm³. More commonly, it is necessary to reduce the doses of myelotoxic agents because of granulocyte nadirs below 500/mm³ or platelet count nadirs below 20,000/mm³ or prolonged duration of nadir. The regimens are published with a sliding scale for modification of each agent based on nadir depth or duration. Patients with cytopenias based on bone marrow involvement should not undergo dose reduction but should receive full dose therapy with appropriate hospitalization and expectant management of febrile neutropenia and thrombocytopenia.

If a patient does not experience myelosuppression during treatment for aggressive lymphoma, the patient is not receiving enough therapy. Infectious complications from myelosuppression occurring in the MACOP-B, VACOP-B, and ProMACE-CytaBOM regimens appear to be significantly reduced by including cotrimoxazole prophylaxis. The treatment-related mortality rate from MACOP-B and VACOP-B was 3%. The treatment-related mortality rate for ProMACE-CytaBOM was 6% because of deaths early in the study from *Pneumocystis carinii* pneumonia.[564] After institution of cotrimoxazole prophylaxis, there were no toxic deaths in the last 59 patients. Another useful effect of the antibiotic treatment was a significant reduction in episodes of febrile neutropenia.[541] Many

patients with a history of sulfa allergy are able to tolerate the cotrimoxazole, perhaps because of the concomitant administration of prednisone. However, for patients who cannot take sulfa, monthly aerosolized pentamidine has been used anecdotally with success in preventing interstitial pneumonitis, but it does not reduce episodes of febrile neutropenia. No patient should receive ProMACE-CytaBOM without some form of *Pneumocystis* prophylaxis.

Other toxic effects depend on the regimen. MACOP-B and m-BACOD induce mucositis in 40% or more of patients. This side effect can be reduced in frequency and severity with the use of prophylactic ketoconazole, careful oral hygiene, removal of dentures, particularly if they are ill fitting, and the use of acyclovir in patients with perioral herpes simplex infection. VACOP-B, F-MACHOP, and ProMACE-CytaBOM are associated with much lower rates of mucositis. Skin rashes may occur in 2% to 10% of patients, usually related to bleomycin or procarbazine. Bleomycin, particularly when used with methotrexate, may contribute to mucositis, but the most serious toxic effect is the induction of pulmonary infiltrates in as many as 20% of patients on the m-BACOD program; other regimens are associated with a frequency of 5% or less. Vincristine may be associated with paresthesias or gait disturbances, all of which are reversible. The most serious toxic effect of vincristine other than skin infiltration with local necrosis is obstipation. Stool softeners and laxatives may prevent or ameliorate vincristine-induced bowel problems.

Doxorubicin is contraindicated in patients with congestive heart failure, but the dose and schedule employed in most of the regimens is rarely associated with the induction of heart failure in the absence of a preexisting cardiomyopathy. Mitoxantrone can effectively replace doxorubicin in some lymphoma treatment programs without loss of efficacy, and mitoxantrone is much less cardiotoxic (conversion factor: 1 mg mitoxantrone = 5 mg doxorubicin).[565]

Prednisone administered intermittently may uncover latent diabetes or make glucose control in known diabetics somewhat more difficult. Continuous prednisone for more than a month, as used in MACOP-B and VACOP-B, can be associated with peptic ulcer disease. Prophylaxis with H₂-blockers may be prudent. The doses of cyclophosphamide used in most lymphoma regimens only rarely induce hemorrhagic cystitis. Substitution of an alternative alkylating agent such as chlorambucil may be done in this setting.

Treatment of the Older Patient With Aggressive Lymphoma

The age range for patients with aggressive lymphoma is quite large, and many patients are older than 65 at diagnosis. Advanced age is not a contraindication to using an effective combination chemotherapy program. Age is generally a surrogate measure for physiologic reserve. A 50-year-old patient with diabetes, hypertension, and a myocardial infarction within the last year may do considerably more poorly than an 80-year-old patient who mowed his own grass until last month. Prognostic factor analysis may demonstrate that age makes a significant impact on outcome, but this piece of data may have diverse contributions. For example, some studies have given older patients 50% of the projected dose of a regimen to avoid toxicity. In other studies, deaths from intercurrent illness have not been identified specifically and may look like treatment-related deaths or treatment failures. Vose and colleagues analyzed 112 patients older than 60 years at diagnosis and found that their complete response, disease-free survival, and overall survival rates were not different from those of younger patients if deaths unrelated to lymphoma or its treatment were excluded.[566] SWOG data demonstrate that anticipatory dose reductions compromise treatment efficacy.[567] Although there are no prospective studies on this topic, clinical experience suggests that older patients may experience somewhat more myelotoxicity than younger patients when drug doses are administered on the basis of body surface area. Although the myelotoxicity from the drugs is dose related, it should be possible to find a dose of the drugs that can be safely administered.

Some investigators have attempted to develop special treatment programs for older patients.[568,569] Most of these therapies are lower in drug dose intensity than standard regimens, and they are associated with poorer results. We recommend that older patients receive standard chemotherapy regimens. If there are legitimate concerns about toxicity because of an existing comorbid condition, a 10% to 20% dose reduction may be used initially. However, further treatment should be based on toxicities actually experienced by the patient rather than making anticipatory dose reductions. Many older patients are willing to cope with acute toxicity for the prospect of prolonged disease-free survival.

TREATMENT OF HIGHLY AGGRESSIVE LYMPHOMAS

The highly aggressive lymphomas are the diffuse small noncleaved cell lymphomas, which include Burkitt's and non-Burkitt's subsets, lymphoblastic lymphoma, and HTLV-I-related adult T-cell lymphoma. These are rare tumors in adults. The diffuse small noncleaved cell lymphomas and lymphoblastic lymphomas are more common in children than in adults, and the most successful approaches to their treatment in adults are those that have been proven effective in children. HTLV-I-related ATL is moderately common in regions where the virus is endemic. It has been estimated that the cumulative lifetime risk of developing ATL among HTLV-I-infected persons in Saga, Japan, is about 4.5% for men and 2.6% for women.[570] Because the highly aggressive lymphomas are frequently disseminated at diagnosis, the application of a rigid staging schema is not useful.

The diffuse small noncleaved cell lymphomas (non-Burkitt's) have often been lumped together with diffuse large cell lymphomas in series reporting treatment results. These lymphomas account for fewer than 10% of the cases of diffuse lymphomas. In the older literature, they were called diffuse undifferentiated lymphomas. The small number of homogenously treated patients prohibits making definitive conclusions about their response to treatment. In the last 14 years, the NCI has obtained a complete response rate of 84% for patients with this histology treated with ProMACE-based chemotherapy regimens; 14% of the complete responders have relapsed, and the long-term survival rate is 67%.

Much depends on the reproducibility of the histologic diagnosis. Burkitt's and non-Burkitt's varieties are often difficult to differentiate. The major difference involves the degree of homogeneity of the nuclear size; Burkitt's tumors are highly homogenous, and non-Burkitt's are more heterogenous. Both tumor types have a high growth fraction and may show rapid clinical progression. A review of the molecular genetics of these two entities lent credence to the notion that they can be reliably separated. Seventeen of 18 Burkitt's tumors were found to have *MYC* rearrangements; none of 11 non-Burkitt's tumors had *MYC* rearrangements.[571] These genetic results and the excellent clinical results obtained with second- and third-generation aggressive lymphoma treatment regimens may mean that the subtle histologic differences in these entities are biologically and clinically significant.

McMaster and colleagues devised a high-intensity, brief-duration combination chemotherapy program for diffuse small noncleaved cell lymphomas that includes cyclophosphamide, doxorubicin, etoposide, vincristine, bleomycin, methotrexate, and prednisone.[572] In 20 adult patients (16 were stage IV), the complete response rate was 85%, and with a median follow-up of 29 months, 65% of patients remain disease free. On the basis of current information, this program or one of the more recent regimens used in aggressive histology lymphoma appear to be excellent choices for the therapy of this rare lymphoma subtype.

Several treatment programs have been effective for patients with Burkitt's lymphoma. Straus and colleagues treated 28 adult patients with an intensive chemotherapy program also used in patients with lymphoblastic leukemia.[573] Fifty-nine percent of the HIV-negative patients with Burkitt's lymphoma were long-term disease-free survivors. The CHOMP regimen of Magrath has a similar level of efficacy; almost 60% of patients can be cured.[574] Patients in whom bulky disease could be surgically removed have an even better outcome (81% 3-year survival).

Schwenn and colleagues performed a pilot study with high-intensity short-duration therapy for children with advanced-stage Burkitt's lymphoma.[575] The regimen included cyclophosphamide, high-dose methotrexate, high-dose cytarabine, and vincristine; the complete response rate for the first 20 patients was 95%, and the survival rate at a median follow-up of 3 years is 75%. This regimen is promising because of the high response rate and because of the short duration of the therapy. Most of the other effective regimens in Burkitt's lymphoma have treated patients for 1 to 2 years.

Lymphoblastic lymphoma is overwhelmingly a tumor of thymocyte origin. It is difficult to differentiate from acute lymphoblastic leukemia on morphologic grounds. Many workers use the degree of bone marrow involvement as the criterion to separate lymphoblastic lymphoma from lymphoblastic leukemia; leukemia is present if neoplastic cells account for 25% or more of the marrow cells. Lymphoblastic lymphoma has a high propensity to involve the mediastinum (presumably related to thymus origin or tropism), the bone marrow, and the CNS and has a high male preponderance.[576] Lymphoma treatment regimens may induce responses, but the responses are generally short.[577]

Many of the regimens that are active in Burkitt's lymphoma are also active in lymphoblastic lymphoma, including CHOMP. The APO regimen and the LSA$_2$-L$_2$ regimen are the most widely used and result in long-term survival of as many as 75% of patients.[578,579] Application of these regimens to adults has been slow, and the results have not been uniform. Complete response rates are high, but it appears that adults require early CNS prophylaxis to minimize the risk of CNS relapse.[580] However, when the dose of systemic therapy is modified to accommodate early CNS prophylaxis, systemic relapse is more common. The high relapse rate seen in adults with lymphoblastic lymphoma has prompted some workers to perform high-dose therapy with autologous or allogeneic bone marrow transplantation in patients in first remission. Among 36 adult patients treated with an LSA$_2$-L$_2$-type protocol, 18 patients in first remission underwent high-dose cyclophosphamide therapy plus TBI and autologous marrow reinfusion.[581] Fourteen of the 18 patients are alive and continue in remission a median of 46 months off therapy. These promising results suggest that the optimal treatment approach in the adult would be to use CHOMP, APO, or LSA$_2$-L$_2$ to obtain a complete response and then administer high-dose cyclophosphamide plus TBI followed by ABMT.

HTLV-I-related ATL is a rare disease that is highly responsive to chemotherapy. However, aggressive therapy is poorly tolerated because of the underlying immunodeficiency in ATL patients. Aggressive treatment generally leads to a treatment-related death from opportunistic infection. The clinical events in HTLV-I-related ATL are not very different from those seen in patients with HIV-associated lymphoma. Long-term disease-free survival has not been reported for ATL patients. The clinical syndrome has different prognostic factors based on whether a leukemia picture or a lymphoma picture predominate: leukocyte count and percentage of neoplastic cells in the circulation are prognostic factors for leukemic patients; serum calcium level is prognostic for lymphoma patients.[582] Waldmann pioneered the clinical use of antibodies directed against the IL-2 receptor with some transient responses.[583] Yttrium 90-labeled antibodies have shown more significant antitumor effects in a few patients. There is evidence that IL-1 may be an autocrine stimulating factor for ATL.[584] If this is true, there may be clinical efficacy with the use of the naturally occurring IL-1 antagonists. It seems unlikely that a chemotherapy-based approach can be successful unless it becomes possible to reverse the underlying immunodeficiency. Biologic approaches to treatment may hold more promise for success.

CENTRAL NERVOUS SYSTEM LYMPHOMA

Lymphomas may involve the CNS in two ways: primary CNS lymphoma, which causes mass lesions and usually is not associated with systemic lymphoma, and secondary lymphoma, which most often involves the meninges without mass lesions and usually occurs in the setting of relapsed or growing systemic lymphoma, usually involving bone or bone marrow, testes, or sinuses. Primary CNS lymphoma is increasing in frequency. It complicates the course of immunodeficiency diseases, including AIDS, which are increasing in frequency, but also there is an increase in the incidence of primary CNS lymphoma in immunocompetent persons.[585] Secondary CNS lymphoma is decreasing in frequency, largely due to the incorporation of high-dose methotrexate in the treatment programs and the use of CNS prophylaxis in patients with known risk factors for secondary CNS involvement.

Primary CNS lymphoma accounts for about 2% of brain tumors and 2% of all lymphomas. Most CNS lymphomas are of B-cell origin and are diffuse aggressive lymphomas histologically. In immunosuppressed patients, EBV is frequently detected and implicated in the cause. It appears on CT scan as a lesion of increased density in at least two thirds of patients and uniformly enhances with contrast, usually homogenously.[586] The lymphoma often occurs in the frontal lobes or involves deep central brain structures and may produce multiple lesions, leading to confusion with metastatic carcinoma.

The most common symptoms of CNS lymphoma are headache, visual disturbances (*e.g.*, blurred or double vision), mental changes (*e.g.*, memory loss, dementia, personality changes), nausea, vomiting, and seizures. The major neurologic findings are hemiparesis, papilledema, visual field defects, and cranial nerve palsies. The cerebrospinal fluid usually has a high protein level but no malignant cells.

CNS lymphoma is responsive to radiation therapy, but intracranial relapses are common, and the median survival is 12 to 18 months, not much greater than the survival of other primary brain neoplasms.[587] After surgical removal of as much tumor as possible, patients are usually treated with whole-brain irradiation to about 4000 cGy, with a boost to the primary lesion of about 1500 cGy. Some have advocated irradiating the spinal axis, but with a clinical failure rate in the spinal cord of only 4%, this practice seems unwarranted. About 90% of primary CNS lymphoma relapses are in the CNS; fewer than 10% of patients have relapses outside the CNS. Improved survival has been reported with the use of chemotherapy in addition to radiation therapy, including VEPA (cyclophosphamide, doxorubicin, vincristine, prednisone), high-dose methotrexate, and DHAP (dexamethasone, high-dose cytarabine, cisplatin).[588–590] Efforts to osmotically open the blood-brain barrier have been claimed to improve outcome.[591] Chamberlain and Levin administered irradiation with hydroxyurea as a radiation sensitizer and then gave adjuvant chemotherapy with procarbazine, CCNU, and vincristine.[592] The median survival of their 10 patients was 30 months, which seems significantly longer than that seen with radiation therapy alone. However, most of the reported treatment experiences are elaborate anecdotes without appropriate controls, and although there is appropriate optimism about the use of drugs, it is not yet clear whether systemic chemotherapy with or without radiation therapy is superior to radiation therapy alone. Nevertheless, efforts to improve the results with radiation therapy are needed.

Secondary CNS lymphoma usually occurs in patients with diffuse lymphoma. If a patient with indolent lymphoma develops CNS signs and symptoms, it usually represents histologic progression to aggressive lymphoma. The usual treatment approach is to administer methotrexate, cytarabine, or thiotepa alone or in combination into the spinal canal by repeated spinal taps (which requires concurrent cranial irradiation to treat the meninges over the convexities) or by way of an indwelling Ommaya reservoir.[593] The CNS disease is usually treated at the same time that therapy is administered for peripheral disease. Meningeal lymphoma can usually be eradicated, but survival is limited due to uncontrolled systemic disease. CNS symptoms can be produced by expanding nodal or extranodal masses that cause cord compression. This complication occurs in about 2% of lymphoma cases and is best managed by local radiation treatment together with systemic treatment, if the symptoms have an acute onset, but combination chemotherapy alone may be used if the symptoms developed gradually and have not progressed to complete cord block. The decision about whether to use radiation therapy is usually aided by obtaining a MR scan to better define the anatomy of the spinal cord involvement.

Orbital lymphomas are rare and can be a site of spread to or from the CNS. Local control may be achieved with radiation therapy, but CNS relapse is common. Orbital lymphomas should be treated with combined-modality therapy.

HIV-ASSOCIATED LYMPHOCYTIC LYMPHOMAS

Within 5 years of the original description of AIDS, it was found that HIV infection was associated with an increased incidence of malignant lymphoma.[594] Lymphocytic lymphomas occur approximately 60 times more frequently in AIDS patients than in the general population.[595] Approximately 3% of all cases of AIDS reported to the Centers for Disease Control had an associated lymphocytic lymphoma. Nineteen percent were primary lymphomas of the brain. Lymphomas occurred in all risk groups, but most occurred in homosexuals. This is probably due to the high prevalence of homosexuals in the U.S. AIDS population, but the incidence of lymphoma is also highest in hemophiliacs and homosexuals and lowest in intravenous drug abusers and persons who acquired HIV by heterosexual contact.[595] The incidence of lymphoma in AIDS patients appears to be increasing. Pluda and coworkers estimate that the probability of AIDS patients on antiretroviral therapy developing a lymphoma by 36 months is 29%.[596,597] The rising incidence is probably related to the prolonged immunosuppression that accompanies the increased survival, which is a consequence of the improvements in treating HIV-associated infectious complications and HIV itself. However, the possibility of a direct etiologic role for antiretroviral therapy in lymphomagenesis cannot be excluded. These data predict that almost 4000 excess cases of lymphocytic lymphoma occurred in 1992 because of HIV infection. This represents almost 10% of all cases of lymphocytic lymphomas.

Lymphomas occur in patients across the entire spectrum of HIV infection.[594,598-604] They are seen in patients with AIDS, AIDS-related complex, progressive generalized lymphadenopathy and in asymptomatic HIV-positive patients. In the early descriptions of lymphoma in AIDS patients, most had already experienced an AIDS-defining illness, such as an opportunistic infection or Kaposi's sarcoma at the time the lymphoma was identified, but some reports described a greater occurrence in HIV-positive asymptomatic patients.[594,600,605,606] Currently, the initial AIDS-defining illness is lymphoma in 3% of all HIV-infected patients.

The spectrum of lymphomas observed in HIV-infected patients is different from that seen in the nonimmunosuppressed population but similar to what is observed in patients with congenital immunodeficiencies or those receiving immunosuppressive therapy after organ transplantation. The most common histologic subtypes are diffuse small noncleaved cell, immunoblastic, and large cell lymphomas.[598-604] Most tumors are high grade according to the Working Formulation and are of B-cell origin; only rare T-cell tumors have been identified. Low-grade lymphomas have been described, but they do not necessarily occur at a higher frequency than in the normal population. The lymphomas occurring in the less symptomatic population (*i.e.*, higher CD4 cell count) are most often of the diffuse small noncleaved cell type, and those occurring in patients with AIDS (*i.e.*, lowest CD4 cell count) tend to be extranodal presentations of immunoblastic and large cell histologic subtypes.[604-607]

Although the exact pathogenesis of AIDS-related lymphomas is unknown, many interrelated factors appear to be involved. As in other lymphomas, EBV and the *MYC* oncogene have been implicated.[608] However, EBV is found in fewer than 50% of HIV-related lymphomas, and *MYC* gene rearrangements are found in a minority of tumors.[48] Shiramizu and colleagues performed a molecular analysis of 40 HIV-positive lymphomas to determine clonality, EBV infection, and the status of the *MYC* oncogene.[608] All were B-cell tumors whose cells were not infected with HIV. Six different tumor types were identified. They observed polyclonal lymphomas that were EBV positive or EBV negative; they observed monoclonal EBV-positive and EBV-negative tumors that had unrearranged, germline *MYC;* and they identified monoclonal EBV-positive and EBV-negative tumors that had undergone characteristic rearrangements of the *MYC* oncogene. There appear to be multiple mechanisms of lymphomagenesis in AIDS patients.

The clinical characteristics of patients with HIV-associated lymphoma differ markedly from those seen in the healthy population.[598-605] The median age at diagnosis is 38 years, compared with 56 years for HIV-negative patients. Patients present with advanced symptomatic disease with frequent involvement of extranodal sites. Between 64% and 83% of patients have stage III or IV disease, and 65% to 91% have involvement of extranodal sites. The most frequently involved extranodal sites include the CNS in 26% (*i.e.*, parenchymal, leptomeningeal), bone marrow in 22%, gastrointestinal tract in 17%, and liver in 12%.[603,606] Involvement with lymphoma has been identified in some unusual sites: lung, oral cavity, Waldeyer's ring, rectum, salivary glands, heart, bone, kidney, adrenal, and orbit.[7,15]

As many as 30% of patients present with stage IE disease, and most of these patients have primary lymphoma of the brain. These patients tend to be the sickest; they have the lowest CD4 cell counts; they have usually already had one or more opportunistic infections; and a significant number of them are not diagnosed with lymphoma until postmortem examination. The delay in diagnosis is probably related to the combination of an insufficient suspicion of the possibility and the difficult differential diagnosis. Most patients with primary CNS lymphoma have symptoms.[603] Focal findings such as hemiparesis or aphasia occur in 35%, seizures in 15%, and cranial nerves palsies in 10%. However, more subtle symptoms, such as confusion, lethargy, or memory loss, may be the only abnormality. It is important to remain alert to the possibility of primary CNS lymphoma in HIV-infected patients.

Radiologic studies are not diagnostic, and lymphoma can easily be confused with toxoplasmosis, a common opportunistic pathogen in AIDS patients. Both can present as space-occupying, contrast-enhancing lesions that may be associated with edema. Lymphomas are more often solitary and usually bigger than the lesions of toxoplasmosis, but this is not absolute. The diagnosis of lymphoma may be strongly suspected by scans, but a definitive diagnosis can only be obtained by brain biopsy. Current practice is to empirically treat equivocal lesions as if they were toxoplasmosis for 1 week, after which a repeat CT scan is performed and followed by a brain biopsy if improvement is not observed.[603]

The treatment of primary CNS lymphoma in an immuno-competent person is unsatisfactory. The use of radiotherapy can be associated with complete remissions, but long-term survival of these patients is rare. AIDS patients with CNS lymphoma are usually extremely ill at diagnosis with poor performance status, and 50% or more die of opportunistic infections.

AIDS patients with disseminated lymphoma have been treated with standard combination chemotherapy regimens that have proven to be effective in nonimmunosuppressed patients with intermediate-grade lymphomas.[598–604,609,610] This approach has been unsuccessful with few long-term disease-free survivors. Many regimens have been used, and complete remission rates of approximately 50% and median survival of 5 to 7 months have been produced. Treatment is poorly tolerated in most of these patients, many of whom have bone marrow involvement and most of whom have poor bone marrow reserve. Multiple dose reductions were given, and limited numbers of cycles could be given. Opportunistic infections occurred in more than half the patients during treatment without *Pneumocystis carinii* pneumonia (PCP) prophylaxis, and although the incidence of PCP can be reduced by as much as 50% if prophylaxis is employed, it cannot be eliminated. Relapse from complete remission is common (33–50%), and in the early studies, relapse in the CNS was not uncommon. Attempts to use more aggressive chemotherapy appear to have actually reduced overall survival in at least two trials. Granulocyte-macrophage colony-stimulating factor (GM-CSF) administered after chemotherapy reduces the granulocyte nadir, reduces the number of days that granulocytes are below 500/mm³, and reduces the frequency of hospitalization for fever and granulocytopenia.[609]

A study employed low-dose M-BACOD with CNS prophylaxis followed by antiretroviral therapy for 42 patients.[610] A complete remission rate of 46% was observed, with a median overall survival of only 5.6 months. There were 4 relapses in the 16 complete remissions but none in the CNS. Opportunistic infections occurred in 21% of patients despite PCP prophylaxis, and deaths on study were split equally between lymphoma and infection.

Treatment of HIV-related lymphoma is difficult, because the patient has two fatal conditions. Current standard regimens are probably as effective against AIDS-related lymphomas as they would be against the same lymphomas in non-immunosuppressed patients if they could be given with the same intensity, but they cannot. By decreasing the intensity, the regimen is made more tolerable, but it becomes less effective (*e.g.*, complete remission rates ≤50%). Colony-stimulating factors may improve this somewhat. Alternatively, infusional regimens that may have lower toxicity because of lower peak plasma concentrations of drugs may maintain antitumor efficacy at acceptable toxicity. CNS prophylaxis is an essential component of treatment. Prophylaxis against opportunistic infection, if possible, should improve the outcome. The optimal use of antiretrovirals is unknown and principally untested. What they can add, beyond more toxicity, during lymphoma-directed chemotherapy is unknown.

If patients are optimally treated and they survive without a fatal infection, a few patients survive for more than 1 year without lymphoma. Patients with CD4 numbers higher than 200/mm³, good performance status, and with lymphoma as their initial AIDS-defining condition have the greatest likelihood of surviving tumor free. However, these patients eventually die of some other complication of AIDS. Biologic approaches that may exert antitumor effects without worsening the immunosuppression have not been extensively tested. In light of the antitumor effects that accompany reversal of immunosuppression in some transplant patients, the best approach to managing AIDS-associated lymphoma may be to focus efforts on immune restoration so that existing active chemotherapy regimens may be administered more safely.

SALVAGE TREATMENT OF LYMPHOMAS

Patients with indolent lymphoma who relapse from complete remission with an indolent lymphoma histology usually receive symptomatic treatment. If indolent lymphoma patients relapse with an aggressive lymphoma, an attempt at curative therapy with an aggressive lymphoma treatment program appears warranted. However, some of these patients may have acquired genetic abnormalities that adversely affect the probability of cure.

The advent of high-dose therapy with or without radiation therapy followed by ABMT, peripheral blood stem cell, or allogeneic bone marrow transplantation has changed the prognosis of patients with relapsed aggressive histology lymphoma from uniformly fatal to potentially curable.[611] Clinical experience with high-dose therapy is rapidly growing. However, it remains somewhat difficult to estimate the fraction of all patients who may benefit from this approach because of variability in patient selection criteria. Nevertheless, several consistent findings have been made. First, patients have a higher likelihood of cure if they enter the high-dose phase of therapy with no or minimal residual disease. Second, high-dose cyclophosphamide plus TBI is a well-tolerated and effective marrow ablative regimen in lymphoma, and it appears that certain other agents, such as etoposide, carboplatin, and cytarabine, may be added to it without significant increase in toxicity. It is not yet clear that such manipulations of the preparative regimen have a favorable impact on treatment outcome. Third, allogeneic transplantation may have a higher rate of treatment-related fatality; but a graft-versus-lymphoma effect may make second remission more durable. Fourth, patients with disease progression in the days before high-dose therapy are unlikely to benefit from the therapy and are significantly more likely to have fatal complications.

Only a subset of relapsed patients are selected for such rigorous, life-threatening treatment. Age over 55 years disqualifies about half of all relapsed patients. It appears that the probability of success is related mainly to two features: response to initial therapy and response to conventional-dose salvage therapy before the transplantation. Gribben and colleagues found that 60% of responding patients had complete responses to high-dose therapy, and none experienced treatment-related death.[612] Resistant relapsers had an approximately 10% complete response rate, and 31% of them died of treatment-related complications. Approximately 30% to 60% of complete responders relapse. Because of the selection process for choosing suitable candidates, about 20% of relapsed patients with aggressive lymphoma can be salvaged with high-dose therapy. Such data strongly support augmentation of dose intensity to yield better results in the primary treatment of aggressive lymphoma.

Several approaches are being taken to improve the results. Efforts are being made to induce a complete response with conventional-dose regimens before taking the patient to high-dose therapy. DHAP produced responses in 58% of patients, and complete responses in 15%.[613] CEPP(B) (cyclophosphamide, etoposide, procarbazine, and prednisone or bleomycin) produced complete responses in 31%.[614] MIME (methyl GAG, ifosfamide, methotrexate, etoposide) produced complete responses in 33%, and a variety of other regimens have been tested with roughly comparable response rates.[615] It remains unclear whether the combination of conventional-dose and high-dose therapy is superior to high-dose therapy alone. In light of the patient selection that takes place before entry onto high-dose protocols, it is not clear whether high-dose therapy is as much of a treatment advance as it may appear.

To address this important question, the PARMA cooperative group has undertaken a prospective randomized trial in which patients with aggressive lymphoma who relapsed after a prior complete response are enrolled at the time of their first or second relapse. Patients older than 60 years and those with CNS or bone marrow relapses are excluded. All patients receive two cycles of DHAP. Responding patients are then randomly allocated to receive four additional cycles of DHAP or high-dose BEAC (carmustine, etoposide, cytarabine, cyclophosphamide) and ABMT.[616] Preliminary data on the first 128 patients have shown no significant differences in the 1-year survival or toxic death rates. This important study should shed light on the contribution of high-dose therapy to the salvage treatment of aggressive lymphoma.

A second modification in salvage therapy that is being evaluated is in the myeloablative regimen. The PARMA group are using BEAC; Moormeier et al[617] tested three alkylating agents together (cyclophosphamide, thiotepa, carmustine) without irradiation; and Glenn and associates[618] are studying BECH (carmustine, etoposide, cyclophosphamide, hydroxyurea). It is too early to say whether these and the other reported preparative regimens have improved efficacy; no controlled trials have been performed.

A third strategy for improvement involves evaluation of bone marrow purging techniques using chemotherapeutic agents or antibody cocktails plus complement, toxins, isotopes, or attached magnetic beads. Patients who relapse after ABMT usually do so in previously involved sites of disease. There is not much evidence that any tumor cells contaminating the donor bone marrow influence sites of relapse. There is no evidence that bone marrow purging techniques make an impact on survival in relapsed patients with aggressive histology lymphoma. Evidence supporting a role for purging in patients with indolent lymphoma was previously discussed.

Although high-dose therapy may be life threatening, Freedman and colleagues reported a toxic death rate of only 4% among 100 patients with relapsed lymphoma sensitive to conventional-dose salvage therapy who were subsequently treated with high-dose cyclophosphamide plus TBI.[439] This toxic death rate for patients with sensitive relapse is comparable to that seen with conventional-dose combination chemotherapy used in primary treatment.

Perhaps the most serious risk from high-dose therapy is the problem of marrow graft failure. Marrow purged with drugs in vitro may be slow to engraft. The number of salvage chemotherapy cycles delivered before marrow harvest may contribute to slow engraftment.[619] Different approaches to promoting engraftment are being explored. For example, the use of peripheral blood stem cells with or without a source of marrow may reduce the number of days of granulocytopenia and thrombocytopenia.[620] Pretreatment with GM-CSF increases the number of circulating stem cells, making stem cell harvest by cytapheresis more efficient.[621] These procedures make bone marrow purging techniques of less relevance because peripheral blood stem cells are not as commonly contaminated by tumor cells. Administration of GM-CSF after transplantation also modestly accelerates engraftment and can permit the use of high doses of single-agent and combination chemotherapy without hematopoietic support. The capacity of IL-1 to promote platelet recovery after high doses of carboplatin therapy may lead to cocktails of colony-stimulating factors that affect all lineages.[622-625]

Another strategy under evaluation for the treatment of relapsed patients with aggressive lymphoma is the reversal of drug resistance mediated by the p170 glycoprotein. Salmon and associates found expression of the p170 glycoprotein efflux pump in three of six samples from relapsed lymphoma patients.[626] They administered high-dose verapamil to 18 patients with refractory lymphoma in addition to CVAD combination chemotherapy (cyclophosphamide bolus on day 1, infusional doxorubicin and vincristine for 4 days, and oral dexamethasone).[627] There were five complete and eight partial responses; median response duration was about 6 months. Unfortunately, the investigators never established that the patients were resistant to CVAD, and it is therefore unclear whether verapamil added anything to this combination.

At the NCI, an infusional combination chemotherapy program called EPOCH (infusional etoposide, doxorubicin, and vincristine, bolus cyclophosphamide, oral prednisone) is being evaluated in relapsed patients.[628] When patients stop responding to the regimen, another cycle of the therapy is given together with r-verapamil, a stereoisomer that reverses drug resistance but has little effect on the heart. This study should assist in evaluating the degree to which p170 is involved in drug resistance in lymphoma.

TREATMENT OF RARE PROLIFERATIVE DISORDERS OF THE LYMPHATIC SYSTEM

Angioimmunoblastic lymphadenopathy is a rare disease with histologic features that resemble Hodgkin's disease without the Reed-Sternberg cells. In some series, life expectancy is less than 1 year.[629] The disease is idiopathic, and it is associated with diffuse adenopathy, polyclonal serum immunoglobulin elevations, and often a history of allergic or autoimmune disease.[630] Transient responses have been obtained after plasmapheresis, but more typically the disease evolves into an aggressive lymphoma. The cells can express elevated levels of *NRAS*-encoded mRNA, the significance of which is unknown.[631] The disease may respond to prednisone or to combination chemotherapy. It bears features suggestive of excess cytokine production or responsiveness (*e.g.*, polyclonal gammopathy). Inhibiting cytokine action with cyclosporin A may be therapeutic, but there is insufficient clinical experience to recommend its routine use.

Castleman's disease (*i.e.*, angiofollicular lymph node hyperplasia) is most often an asymptomatic condition diagnosed incidentally in young men on chest x-ray film as enlarged mediastinal nodes. Sometimes the adenopathy is accompanied by systemic symptoms of fever and weight loss. There is a systemic form of the illness associated with malaise, fever, adenopathy, hepatosplenomegaly, rashes, hypergammaglobulinemia, and occasionally CNS symptoms.[294] Many of the manifestations of the disease may be related to the overproduction of IL-6. The median survival was only 30 months. A case report of a successfully treated case suggests that aggressive therapy may be lifesaving.[632]

Angiocentric immunoproliferative lesions (AIL) are a collection of entities classified as peripheral T-cell disorders and include lymphomatoid granulomatosis, midline granuloma, lymphomatoid papulosis, and polymorphic reticulosis.[633] The disease is characterized by extranodal sites of involvement such as the skin, lungs, kidneys, sinuses, and other organs. The lesions are composed of T cells, and they are divided into three histologic grades ranging from benign to frankly malignant. Treatment of grade 1 lesions with cyclophosphamide and prednisone resulted in a 45% long-term survival; the survival rate for patients with grade 2 lesions was 33%. Most of the deaths in grade 1 and 2 patients were from treatment-refractory lymphoma. Grade 3 lesions, which were considered frank lymphoma and treated like aggressive histology lymphomas, had an 87% long-term survival. It appears that even the low-grade AIL could benefit from aggressive therapy with a lymphoma regimen, because they evolve to lymphoma with a high frequency, and their previous treatment appears to result in the emergence of drug-resistant neoplasms. Such a clinical trial is under way.

Acknowledgments

This research was partially sponsored by the National Cancer Institute, Department of Health and Human Services, under contract N01-C0-74102 with Program Resources, Inc./DynCorp. The contents of this publication do not necessarily reflect the views or policies of the Department of Health and Human Services, nor does mention of trade names, commercial products, or organizations imply endorsement by the U.S. Government.

REFERENCES

1. Cancer facts and figures 1992. New York: American Cancer Society, 1992:4.
2. Devesa SS, Silverman DT, Young JL Jr, et al. Cancer incidence and mortality trends among whites in the United States, 1947–84. JNCI 1987;79:701–770.
3. Ries LAG, Hankey BF, Miller BA, et al. Cancer statistics review, 1973–1988. NIH Pub. No. 91-2789. Bethesda: National Cancer Institute, 1991.
4. Opportunistic non-Hodgkin's lymphomas among severely immunocompromised HIV-infected patients surviving for prolonged periods on antiretroviral therapy—United States. MMWR 1991;40:591–600.
5. Cantor KP, Fraumeni JF. Distribution of non-Hodgkin's lymphoma in the United States between 1950 and 1975. Cancer Res 1980;40:2645–2652.
6. Third National Cancer Survey, 1969 Incidence. Preliminary report. Bethesda: Department of Health, Education and Welfare, 1971:71.
7. Higginson J, Muir CS. Epidemiology. In: Holland JF, Frei E, eds. Cancer medicine. Philadelphia: Lea & Febiger, 1973:241.
8. Shih L-Y, Liang D-C. Non-Hodgkin's lymphomas in Asia. Hematol Oncol Clin North Am 1991;5:983–1001.
9. Vianna NJ, Davies JNP, Polan AK, et al. Familial Hodgkin's disease: An environmental and genetic disorder. Lancet 1974;ii:854–857.
10. Miller DG. The association of immune disease and malignant lymphoma. Ann Intern Med 1967;66:507–521.
11. Zulman J, Jaffe R, Talal N. Evidence that the malignant lymphoma of Sjogren's syndrome is a monoclonal B-cell neoplasm. N Engl J Med 1978;299:1215–1220.
12. Talal N, Sokoloff L, Barth W. Extra salivary lymphoid abnormalities in Sjögren's syndrome (reticulum cell sarcoma, "pseudolymphoma," macroglobulinemia). Am J Med 1967;43:50–65.
13. Kassan SS, Thomas TL, Moutsopoulos HM, et al. Increased risk of lymphoma in Sicca syndrome. Ann Intern Med 1978;89:888–892.
14. Kissmeyer-Nielsen F, Bjorn-Jensen K, Femara RB, et al. HLA phenotypes in Hodgkin's disease: Preliminary report. Transplant Proc 1971;3:1287.
15. Dick FR, Fortuny I, Theologides A, et al. HL-A and lymphoid tumors. Cancer Res 1972;32:2608–2611.
16. MacSween RNM. Reticulum cell sarcoma and rheumatoid arthritis in a patient with XY/XXY/XXX/Y Klinefelter's syndrome and normal intelligence. Lancet 1965;1:460–461.
17. Tan C, Etcubanas E, Lieberman P, et al. Chediak-Higashi syndrome in a child with Hodgkin's disease. Am J Dis Child 1971;121:135–139.
18. Hyman GA, Sommers SC. The development of Hodgkins's disease and other lymphomes during anticonvulsant therapy. Blood J Haematol 1966;28:416–437.
19. Weisenburger DD. Lymphoid malignancies in Nebraska: A hypothesis. Nebr Med J 1985;70:300–305.
20. Hardell L, Eriksonn M, Lenner P, Lundgren E. Malignant lymphoma and exposure to chemicals, especially organic solvents, chlorophenols, and phenoxyacids: A case-control study. Br J Cancer 1981;43:169–176.
21. Hoar SD, Blair A, Holmes FF, et al. Agricultural herbicide use and risk of lymphoma and soft tissue sarcoma. JAMA 1986;256:1141–1147.
22. Wigle DT, Semercin RM, Wilkins K, et al. Mortality study of Canadian male farm operators: Non-Hodgkin's lymphoma and agricultural practices in Saskatchewan. 1990;JNCI 82:575–582.
23. Veneus P, Faggiario F, Tedeschi M, Ciccone G. Incidence rates of lymphomas and soft-tissue sarcomas and environmental measurements of phenoxyherbicides. JNCI 1991;83:362–363.
24. The Selected Cancers Cooperative Study Group. The association of selected cancers with service in the U.S. Military in Vietnam. I. Non-Hodgkin's lymphoma. Arch Intern Med 1990;150:2473–2483.
25. Alavanja MD, Blair A, Masters MN. Cancer mortality in the U.S. flour industry. JNCI 1990;82:840–848.
26. Anderson RE, Nishiyama H, Yohei I, et al. Pathogenesis of radiation related leukemia and lymphoma. Speculations based primarily on experience of Hiroshima and Nagasaki. Lancet 1972;1:1060–1062.
27. Miller RW. Delayed radiation effects in atomic bomb survivors. Science 1969;166:569–574.
28. Court-Brown WM, Doll R. Leukemia and aplastic anemia in patients irradiated for ankylosing spondylitis. Medical Research Council Special Report Series, No. 295. London: Her Majesty's Stationery Office, 1957.
29. Penn I. The incidence of malignancies in transplant recipients. Transplant Proc 1975;7:323–326.
30. Matas AJ, Hertel BF, Rosai J, et al. Post-transplant malignant lymphoma. Distinctive morphologic features related to its pathogenesis. Am J Med 1976;61:716–720.
31. Penn I. Cancers complicating organ transplantation. New Engl J Med 1990;323:1767–1769.
32. Swinnen LJ, Costanzo-Nordin MR, Fisher SG, et al. Increased incidence of lymphoproliferative disorder after immunosuppression with the monoclonal antibody OKT3 in cardiac-transplant receipts. New Engl J Med 1990;323:1723–1728.

33. Starzl TE, Nalesnik MA, Porter KA, et al. Reversibility of lymphomas and lymphoproliferative lesions developing under cyclosporine-steroid therapy. Lancet 1984;1: 583–587.

34. Hanto DW, Frizzera G, Gajl-Peczalska KJ, et al. Epstein-Barr virus-induced B-cell lymphoma after renal transplantation: Acyclovir therapy and transition from polyclonal to monoclonal B-cell proliferation. N Engl J Med 1982;306:913–918.

35. Fischer A, Blanche S, LeBidois J, et al. Anti-B-cell monoclonal antibodies in the treatment of severe B-cell lymphoproliferative syndrome following bone marrow and organ transplantation. N Engl J Med 1991;324:1451–1456.

36. Shapiro RS, Chauvenet A, McGuire W, et al. Treatment of B-cell lymphoproliferative disorders with interferon alpha and intravenous gamma globulin. N Engl J Med 1988;318:1334.

37. Kipps TJ, Fong S, Tomhave E, et al. High-frequency expression of a conserved kappa light-chain variable-region gene in chronic lymphocytic leukemia. Proc Natl Acad Sci USA 1987;84:2916–2920.

38. Kaplan HS. Etiology of lymphomas and leukemia: Role of C-type RNA viruses. Leukemia Res 1978;2:253–271.

39. Dmochowski L. Viral studies in human leukemia and lymphoma. In: Zarafonetis CJD, ed. Proceedings of the international conference on leukemia-lymphoma. Philadelphia: Lea & Febiger, 1968:97.

40. Kawakami TG, Theilan GH, Dungworth DL, et al. "C" type viral particles in plasma of cats with feline leukemia. Science 1967;158:1049–1050.

41. Kawakami TG, Hull SD, Buckley DH, et al. C-type virus associated with Gibbon lymphosarcoma. Nature New Biol 1972;235:170–171.

42. Rapp F. Viruses an etiologic factor in cancer. Semin Oncol 1976;3:49–63.

43. Van der Maaten MJ, Miller JM, Booth AD. Replicating type-C virus particles in monolayer cell cultures from cattle with lymphosarcoma. JNCI 1974;52:491–497.

44. Purtilo DT, Stevenson M. Lymphotropic viruses as etiologic agents of lymphoma. Hematol Oncol Clin North Am 1991;5:901–923.

45. List AF, Greco FA, Vogler LB. Lymphoproliferative diseases in immunocompromised hosts: The role of Epstein-Barr virus. J Clin Oncol 1987;5:1673–1689.

46. Tosato G, Blaese RM. Epstein-Barr virus infection and immunoregulation in man. Adv Immunol 1985;37:99–149.

47. Harrington DS, Weisenburger DD, Purtilo DT. Malignant lymphoma in the X-linked lymphoproliferative syndrome. Cancer 1987;59:1419–1429.

48. Boyle MJ, Sewell WA, Scully TB, et al. Subtypes of Epstein-Barr virus in human immunodeficiency virus-associated non-Hodgkin lymphoma. Blood 1991;78:3004–3011.

49. Shibata D, Weiss LM, Nathwani BN, et al. Epstein-Barr virus in benign lymph node biopsies from individuals infected with the human immunodeficiency virus is associated with concurrent or subsequent development of non-Hodgkin's lymphoma. Blood 1991;77:1527–1533.

50. Klein G. Lymphoma development in mice and humans: Diversity of initiation is followed by convergent cytogenetic evolution. Proc Natl Acad Sci USA 1979;76:2442–2446.

51. Patton DF, Wilkowski CW, Hanson CA, et al. Epstein-Barr virus-determined clonality in post transplant lymphoproliferative disease. Transplantation 1990;49:1080–1084.

52. Poiesz BJ, Ruscetti FW, Gazdar AF, et al. Detection and isolation of type C retrovirus particles from fresh and cultured lymphocytes of a patient with cutaneous T-cell lymphoma. Proc Natl Acad Sci USA 1980;77:7415–7419.

53. Blayney DW, Jaffe ES, Blattner WA, et al. The human T-cell leukemia/lymphoma virus associated with American adult T-cell leukemia/lymphoma. Blood 1983;62:401–405.

54. Kalyanaraman VS, Sarngadharan MG, Robert-Guroff M, et al. A new subtype of human T-cell leukemia virus (HTLV-II) associated with a T-cell variant of hairy cell leukemia. Science 1982;218:571–573.

55. Kanki PJ, Barin F, M'Boup S, et al. New human T-lymphotropic retroviruses related to simian T-lymphotropic virus type III (STLV-III-HGM). Science 1986;232:238–243.

56. Clavel F, Guetard D, Brun-Vezinet F, et al. Isolation of a new human retrovirus from West African patients with AIDS. Science 1986;233:343–346.

57. Manzari V, Gismondi A, Barillari G, et al. HTLV-V. A new human retrovirus in Tac-negative human T-cell lymphoma/leukemia. Science 1987;238:1581–1583.

58. Jacobson S, Raine CS, Mingioli ES, et al. Isolation of an HTLV-I-like retrovirus from patients with tropical spastic paraparesis. Nature 1988;331:540–543.

59. Sonoda S. Relationship of HTLV-I-related adult T-cell leukemia and HTLV-I associated myelopathy to distinct HLA haplotypes. Jikken Igaku 1987;5:769–771.

60. Fifth International Workshop on Chromosomes in Leukemia-lymphoma. Correlation of chromosome abnormalities with histologic and immunologic characteristics in non-Hodgkin's lymphoma and adult T cell leukemia-lymphoma. Blood 1987;70:1554–1564.

61. LeBeau MM. Chromosomal abnormalities in Non-Hodgkin's lymphomas. Semin Oncol 1990;17:20–29.

62. Offit K, Chaganti RSK. Chromosomal abberrations in non-Hodgkin's lymphoma. Biologic and clinical correlations. Hematol Oncol Clin North Am 1991;5:853–869.

63. Schouten HC, Sanger WG, Weisenburger DD, et al. For the Nebraska Lymphoma Study Group: Chromosomal abnormalities in patients with non-cutaneous T-cell non-Hodgkin's lymphoma. Eur J Cancer 1990;26:618–622.

64. Rimokh R, Magaud J-P, Berger F, et al. A translocation involving a specific breakpoint (q35) on chromosome 5 is characteristic of anaplastic large cell lymphoma (Ki-lymphoma). Br J Haematol 1989;71:31–36.

65. Offit K, Wong G, Filippa DA, et al. Cytogenetic analysis of 434 consecutively ascertained specimens of non-Hodgkin's lymphoma: Clinical correlations. Blood 1991;77:1508–1515.

66. Armitage JO, Sanger WG, Weisenberger DD, et al. Correlation of secondary cytogenetic abnormalities with histologic appearance in non-Hodgkin's lymphomas bearing t(14;18)(q32;121). JNCI 1988;80:576–580.

67. Taub R, Kirsch I, Morton C, et al. Translocation of the c-*myc* gene into the immunoglobulin heavy chain locus in human Burkitt's lymphoma and murine plasmacytoma cells. Proc Natl Acad Sci USA 1982;79:7837–7841.

68. Tsujimoto Y, Yunis JJ, Onaroto-Showe L, et al. Molecular cloning of the chromosomal breakpoints of B-cell leukemias with the t(11;14) chromosomal translocation. Science 1984;224:1403–1406.

69. Cleary ML, Smith SD, Sklar J. Cloning and structural analysis of cDNAs for *bcl-2* and a hybrid *bcl-2*/immunoglobulin transcript resulting from the t(14;18) translocation. Cell 1986;47:19–28.

70. Graniger WB, Seto M, Boutain B, et al. Expression of *bcl-2* and *bcl-2*-Ig fusion transcripts in normal and neoplastic cells. J Clin Invest 1987;80:1512–1515.

71. Hockenberry D, Nunez G, Milliman C, et al. *Bcl-2* is an inner mitochondrial membrane protein that blocks programmed cell death. Nature 1990;348:334–336.

72. McDonnell TJ, Deane N, Platt EM, et al. *Bcl-2*-immunoglobulin transgenic mice demonstrate extended B cell survival and follicular lymphoproliferation. Cell 1989;57:79–88.

73. McDonnell TJ, Korsmeyer SJ. Progression from lymphoid hyperplasia to high grade malignant lymphoma in mice transgenic for the t(14;18). Nature 1991;349:254–256.

74. Nunez G, Seto M, Seremetis S, et al. Growth- and tumor-promoting effects of deregulated *bcl-2* in human B-lymphoblastoid cells. Proc Natl Acad Sci USA 1989;86:4589–4593.

75. Zelenetz AD, Chen TT, Levy R. Histologic transformation of follicular lymphoma to diffuse lymphoma represents tumor progression by a single malignant B cell. J Exp Med 1991;173:197–207.

76. Hardy R, Horning SJ. Molecular biologic studies in the clinical evaluation of non-Hodgkin's lymphoma. Hematol Oncol Clin North Am 1991;5:891–900.

77. Yunis JJ, Mayer MG, Arnescu MA, et al. *Bcl-2* and other genomic alterations in the prognosis of large-cell lymphoma. N Engl J Med 1989;320:1047–1054.

78. Price CGA, Meerabux J, Murtaugh S, et al. The significance of circulating cells carrying t(14;18) in long remission from follicular lymphoma. J Clin Oncol 1991;9:1527–1532.

79. Gribben JG, Freedman AS, Neuberg D, et al. Immunologic purging of marrow assessed by PCR before autologous bone marrow transplantation for B-cell lymphoma. N Engl J Med 1991;325:1525–1533.

80. Ngan B-Y, Chen-Levy Z, Weiss LM, et al. Expression in non-Hodgkin's lymphoma of the *bcl-2* protein associated with t(14;18) chromosomal translocation. N Engl J Med 1988;318:1638–1644.

81. Limpens J, de Jong D, van Krieken JHJM, et al. *bcl-2*/J$_H$ rearrangements in benign lymphoid tissues with follicular hyperplasia. Oncogene 1991;6:2271–2276.

82. Rosenberg CL, Wong E, Petty EM, et al. *PRAD1*, a candidate *bcl-1* oncogene: Mapping and expression in centrogenic lymphoma. Proc Natl Acad Sci USA 1991;88:9638–9642.

83. Greaves MF, Owen JJT, Raff MC. T and B lymphocytes: Origins, properties, and roles in immune responses. New York: American Elsevier, 1974.

84. Weiss L. The cells and tissues of the immune system. Structure, functions, interactions. Englewood Cliffs, NJ: Prentice-Hall, 1972.

85. Bienenstock J, Befus D. Gut- and bronchus-associated lymphoid tissue. Am J Anat 1984;170:437–445.

86. Golde D, Cline MJ. A review and reevaluation of the histiocytic disorders. Am J Med 1973;55:49–60.

87. Mann RB, Jaffe ES, Berard CW. Malignant lymphomas a conceptual understanding of morphologic diversity. A review. Am J Pathol 1979;94:105–191.

88. Royer HD, Reinherz EL. T lymphocytes: Ontogeny, function, and relevance to clinical disorders. N Engl J Med 1987;317:1136–1142.

89. Cooper MD. Current Concepts. B lymphocytes: Normal development and function. N Engl J Med 1987;317:1452––1456.

90. Van Furth R, Raeburn JA, van Zwet TL. Characteristics of human mononuclear phagocytes. Blood 1979;54:485–500.

91. Steinman RM, Nussenzweig MC. Dendritic cells: Features and functions. Immunol Rev 1980;53:127–147.

92. Tew JG, Thorbecke GJ, Steinman RM. Dendritic cells in the immune response: Characteristics and recommended nomenclature. J Reticuloendothel Soc 1982;31:371–380.

93. Wood GS, Turner RR, Shiruba RA, et al. Human dendritic cells and macrophages: In situ immunophenotypic definition of subsets that exhibit specific morphologic and microenvironmental characteristics. Am J Pathol 1985;119:73–82.

94. Kohler G, Milstein C. Continuous cultures of fused cells secreting antibody of predefined specificity. Nature 1975;256:495–497.

95. Ajuti F, Cerottini JC, Coombs RRA, et al. Identification, enumeration and isolation of bone marrow derived and thymus derived T lymphocytes from human peripheral blood. Special technical report. Scand J Immunol 1974;3:521–532.

96. Jaffe ES, Cossman J. Immunodiagnosis of lymphoid and mononuclear phagocytic neoplasms. In: Rose NR, Friedman H, Fahey JL, eds. Manual of clinical laboratory immunology. 3rd ed. Washington, DC: American Society of Microbiology, 1986:779.

97. Lovett EJ, Schnitzer B, Keren DF, et al. Application of flow cytometry to diagnostic pathology. Lab Invest 1984;540:115–140.

98. Norton AJ, Isaacson PG. Lymphoma phenotyping in formalin-fixed paraffin wax-embedded tissues. Range of antibodies and staining patterns. Histopathology 1989;14: 437–446.

99. Norton AJ, Isaacson PG. Lymphoma phenotyping in formalin-fixed paraffin wax-embedded tissues. Profiles of reactivity in the various tumor types. Histopathology 1989;14:557–579.

100. Reinherz EL, Haynes BF, Nadler LM, et al. Leukocyte typing II. Human T lymphocytes, vol 1. New York: Springer-Verlag, 1987.

101. Broder S, Waldmann TA. The Sezary syndrome. A malignant proliferation of helper T cells. J Clin Invest 1976;58:1297–1306.

102. Broder S, Waldmann TA. The suppressor cell network in cancer. N Engl J Med 1978;299: 1281–1284.
103. Jaffe ES. Pathologic and clinical spectrum of post-thymic T-cell malignancies. Cancer Invest 1984;2:413–426.
104. Weiss LM, Crabtree GS, Rouse RV, et al. Morphologic and immunologic characterization of 50 peripheral T cell lymphomas. Am J Pathol 1985;118:316–324.
105. Reinherz EL, Kung PC, Goldstein G, et al. Discrete stages of human intrathymic differentiation: Analysis of normal thymocytes and leukemic lymphoblasts of T-cell lineage. Proc Natl Acad Sci USA 1980;77:1588–1592.
106. Cossman J, Chused T, Fisher R, et al. Diversity of immunologic phenotypes of lymphoblastic lymphoma. Cancer Res 1983;43:4486–4490.
107. Goding JW, Burns GF. Monoclonal antibody OKT-9 recognizes the receptor for transferin on human acute lymphocytic leukemic cells. J Immunol 1982;127:1256–1258.
108. Pittaluga S, Uppenkamp M, Cossman J. Development of T3/T cell receptor gene expression in human pre-T neoplasms. Blood 1985;69:1062–1067.
109. Greaves MF, Chan LC, Furley AJW, et al. Lineage promiscuity in hematopoietic differentiation and leukemia. Blood 1986;67:1–11.
110. Caligaris-Cappio F, Gobbi M, Bofill M, et al. Infrequent normal B lymphocytes express features of B-chronic lymphocytic leukemia. J Exp Med 1982;155:623–628.
111. Cossman J, Neckers LM, Hsu SM, et al. Low grade lymphomas: Expression of developmentally regulated B-cell antigens. Am J Pathol 1984;114:117–124.
112. Arnold A, Cossman J, Bakhski A, et al. Immunoglobulin gene rearrangements as unique clonal markers in human lymphoid neoplasms. N Engl J Med 1983;309:1593–1599.
113. Reinherz EL, Haynes BF, Nadler LM, et al. Leukocyte typing II. Human B lymphocytes, vol 2. New York: Springer-Verlag, 1987.
114. Nadler LM, Korsmeyer SJ, Anderson KC, et al. B cell origin of non-T cell acute lymphoblastic leukemia. J Clin Invest 1984;74:332–340.
115. Loken MR, Shah VO, Dattilio KL, et al. Flow cytometric analysis of human bone marrow: II. Normal B lymphocyte development. Blood 1987;70:1316–1324.
116. Greaves MF, Brown G, Rapson NT, et al. Antisera to acute lymphoblastic leukemia cells. Clin Immunol Immunopathol 1975;4:67–84.
117. Korsmeyer SJ, Arnold A, Beach A, et al. Immunoglobulin gene rearrangement and cell surface antigen expression in acute lymphocytic leukemias of T-cell and B-cell precursor origins. J Clin Invest 1983;71:301–313.
118. Ritz J, Nadler LM, Bhan AK, et al. Expression of common acute lymphoblastic leukemia antigen (CALLA) by lymphomas of B cell and T cell lineage. Blood 1981;58:648–652.
119. Hsu SM, Jaffe ES. Phenotypic expression of B lymphocytes. Identification with monoclonal antibodies in normal lymphoid tissues. Am J Pathol 1984;114:387–395.
120. Cossman J, Neckers LM, Leonard WJ, et al. Polymorphonuclear neutrophils express the common acute lymphoblastic leukemia antigen. J Exp Med 1983;157:1064–1069.
121. Breard J, Reinherz EL, Kung PC, et al. A monoclonal antibody reactive with peripheral blood monocytes. J Immunol 1980;124:1943–1948.
122. Todd RF, Nadler LM, Schlossman SF. Antigens on human monocytes by monoclonal antibodies. J Immunol 1981;126:1435–1442.
123. Hanjan SN, Kearney JF, Cooper MD. A monoclonal (MMA) that identifies a differentiation antigen on human myelomonocytic cells. Clin Immunol Immunopathol 1982;23:172–188.
124. Reinherz EL, Haynes BF, Nadler LM, et al. Leukocyte typing II. Human myeloid and hematopoietic cells, vol 3. New York: Springer-Verlag, 1988.
125. Pulford KA, Rigney EM, Micklen KJ, et al. KP1: A new monoclonal antibody that detects a monocyte/macrophage associated antigen in routinely processed tissue sections. J Clin Pathol 1989;42:414–421.
126. Battifora H, Trowbridge IS. A monoclonal antibody useful for the differential diagnosis between malignant lymphoma and nonhematopoietic neoplasms. Cancer 1983;51: 816–821.
127. Warnke RA, Gatter KC, Phil D, et al. Diagnosis of human lymphoma with monoclonal antileukocyte antibodies. N Engl J Med 1983;309:1275–1281.
128. Bollum FJ. Terminal deoxynucleotidyl transferase as a hematopoietic cell marker. A review. Blood 1979;54:1203–1215.
129. Kung PC, Long JC, McCaffrey RP, et al. Terminal deoxynucleotidyl transferase in the diagnosis of leukemia and malignant lymphoma. Am J Med 1978;64:788–794.
130. Braziel RM, Keneklis T, Donlon JA, et al. Terminal deoxynucleotidyl transferase in non-Hodgkin's lymphoma. Am J Clin Pathol 1983;80:655–659.
131. Braziel RM, Hsu SM, Jaffe ES. Lymph nodes, spleen, and thymus. In: Spicer SS, ed. Histochemistry in pathologic diagnosis. New York: Dekker, 1986:203.
132. Yam LT, Li CY, Lam KW. Tartrate-resistant acid phosphatase isoenzyme in the reticulum cells of leukemic reticuloendotheliosis. N Engl J Med 1971;284:357–360.
133. Tonegawa S. Somatic generation of antibody diversity. Nature 1983;301:575–581.
134. Yanagi Y, Yoshihai Y, Leggett K, et al. A human T cell-specific cDNA clone encodes a protein having extensive homology to immunoglobulin chains. Nature 1984;308: 145–149.
135. Hedrick SM, Cohen DI, Nielsen EA, et al. Isolation of cDNA clones encoding T-cell specific membrane-associated proteins. Nature 1984;308:149–153.
136. Hood L, Kronenberg M, Hunkapiller T. T cell antigen receptors and the immunoglobulin supergene family. Cell 1985;40:225–229.
137. Flug F, Pier-Giuseppe P, Bonetti F, et al. T-cell receptor gene rearrangements as markers of lineage and clonality in T-cell neoplasms. Proc Natl Acad Sci USA 1985;82: 3460–3464.
138. Korsmeyer SJ, Greene WC, Cossman J, et al. Rearrangement and expression of immunoglobulin genes and expression of Tac antigen in hairy cell leukemia. Proc Natl Acad Sci USA 1983;80:4522–4526.
139. Cheng GY, Minden M, Toyonaga B, et al. T cell receptor and immunoglobulin gene rearrangements in acute myeloblastic leukemia. J Exp Med 1986;163:414–424.
140. Ha K, Minden M, Hozumi N, et al. Immunoglobulin chain gene rearrangement in a patient with T cell acute lymphoblastic leukemia. J Clin Invest 1984;73:1232–1236.
141. Pelicci PG, Knowles DM, Dalla-Favera R. Lymphoid tumors displaying rearrangements of both immunoglobulin and T cell receptor genes. J Exp Med 1985;162:1015–1024.
142. Uppenkamp M, Pittaluga S, Lipford EH, et al. Limited diversity and selection of rearranged gamma genes in polyclonal T cells. J Immunol 1987;138:1618–1620.
143. Weiss LM, Hu E, Wood GS, et al. Clonal rearrangements of T cell receptor genes in mycosis fungoides and dermatopathic lymphadenopathy. N Engl J Med 1985;313: 539–544.
144. Weiss LM, Wood GS, Trela M, et al. Clonal T cell populations in lymphomatoid papulosis: Evidence of a lymphoproliferative origin for a clinically benign disease. N Engl J Med 1986;315:475–479.
145. Shearer WT, Ritz J, Finegold MK, et al. Epstein-Barr virus associated B cell proliferations of diverse clonal origins after bone marrow transplantation in a 12-year-old boy with severe combined immunodeficiency. N Engl J Med 1985;312:1151–1159.
146. Templeton NS. The polymerase chain reaction: History, methods and applications. Diagn Mol Pathol 1992;1:58–72.
147. Stetler-Stevenson MA, Crush-Stanton S, Cossman J. Involvement of *bcl-2* gene in Hodgkin's disease. JNCI 1990;82:855–858.
148. Stetler-Stevenson MA, Raffeld M, Cohen P, et al. Detection of occult follicular lymphoma by specific DNA amplification. Blood 1988;72:1822–1825.
149. Lee M-S, Chang K-S, Cabanillas F, et al. Detection of minimal residual cells carrying t(14;18) by DNA sequence amplification. Science 1987;237:175–178.
150. Urba WJ, Longo DL. Cytologic, immunologic, and clinical diversity in non-Hodgkin's lymphoma: Therapeutic implications. Semin Oncol 1985;12:250–267.
151. Chan WC, Link S, Mawle A, et al. Heterogeneity of large granular lymphocyte proliferations: Delineation of two major subtypes. Blood 1986;68:1142–1153.
152. Craigie D. Case of disease of the spleen, in which death took place in consequence in the presence of purulent matter in the blood. Edinb Med Surg J 1845;64:400–412.
153. Bennett JH. Case of hypertrophy of the spleen and liver in which death took place from suppuration of the blood. Edinb Med Surg J 1845;64:413–423.
154. Virchow R. Weisses Blut, neue Notizen aus den Geb der naturund Heikunde. Froriep's Neue Notizen 1845;36:151.
155. Billroth T. Multiple lymphome. Erfolgreiche Behandlung mit Arsenik. Wien Med Wochenschr 1871;21:1066–1068.
156. Dreschfeld J. Clinical lecture on acute Hodgkin's Disease. Br Med J 1892;1:893–896.
157. Kundrat H. Uber. Lympho-sarcomatosis. Wien Klin Wochenschr 1893;6:211–213.
158. Brill NE, Baehr G, Rosenthal N, et al. Generalized giant lymphfollicle hyperplasia of lymph nodes and spleen, a hitherto undescribed type. JAMA 1925;84:668–671.
159. Symmers D. Follicular lymphadenopathy with splenomegaly. A newly recognized disease of lymphatic system. Arch Pathol Lab Med 1927;3:816–820.
160. Roulet F. Das primäre Retothelsarkom der Lymphkonten. Virchows Arch [A] 1930;277: 15–47.
161. Gall EA, Mallory TB. Malignant lymphoma. A clinical pathologic survey of 618 cases. Am J Pathol 1942;18:381–429.
162. Rappaport H, Winter WJ, Hicks EB. Follicular lymphoma. A re-evaluation of its position in the scheme of malignant lymphomas, based on a survey of 253 cases. Cancer 1956;9: 792–821.
163. Burkitt D. A sarcoma involving the jaws in African children. Br J Surg 1958;46:218–223.
164. Uchiyama T, Yodoi J, Sagawa K, et al. Adult T-cell leukemia: Clinical and hematologic features of 16 cases. Blood 1977;50:481–492.
165. Rappaport H. Tumors of the hematopoietic system. In: Atlas of tumor pathology, sect III, fasc 8. Washington, DC: Armed Forces Institute of Pathology, 1966.
166. Dorfman RF. Classification of non-Hodgkin's lymphomas. Lancet 1974;1:1295–1296.
167. Bennett MH, Farrer-Brown G, Henry K, et al. Classification of non-Hodgkin's lymphomas. Lancet 1974;2:405–406.
168. Lukes RJ, Collins RD. Immunologic characterization of human malignant lymphomas. Cancer 1974;34:1488–1503.
169. Lennert K, Mohri N, Stein H, et al. Malignant lymphomas other than Hodgkin's disease. Berlin: Springer-Verlag, 1978.
170. Lennert K, Mohri N, Stein H, et al. The histopathology of malignant lymphoma. Br J Haematol 1975;31(suppl 1):193–203.
171. Mathe G, Rappaport H, O'Conor GT, et al. Histological and cytological typing of neoplastic diseases of hematopoietic and lymphoid tissues. In: WHO international histological classification of tumors, no. 14. Geneva: World Health Organization, 1976.
172. Jaffe ES, Shevach EM, Frank MM, et al. Nodular lymphoma: Evidence for origin from follicular B lymphocytes. N Engl J Med 1974;290:813–819.
173. Jaffe ES, Strauchen JA, Berard CW. Predictability of immunologic phenotype by morphologic criteria in diffuse aggressive non-Hodgkin's lymphomas. Am J Clin Pathol 1982;77:46–49.
174. National Cancer Institute sponsored study of classifications of non-Hodgkin's Lymphomas. Summary and description of a working formulation for clinical usage. Cancer 1982;49:2112–2135.
175. Rosenberg SA. Current concepts in cancer. Non-Hodgkin's lymphoma: Selection of treatment on the base of histologic type. N Engl J Med 1979;301:924–928.
176. Jaffe ES. Relationship of classification to biologic behavior of non-Hodgkin's lymphoma. Semin Oncol 1986;13:3–9.
177. Jaffe ES. Follicular lymphomas: Possibility that they are benign tumors of the lymphoid system. JNCI 1983;70:401–403.
178. Krikorian JG, Portlock CS, Cooney DP, et al. Spontaneous regression of non-Hodgkin's lymphomas. A report of nine cases. Cancer Res 1980;46:2093–2099.
179. DeVita VT Jr, Canellos GP, Chabner BA, et al. Advanced diffuse histiocytic lymphoma, a potentially curable disease. Lancet 1975;1:248–250.

180. Warnke RA, Kim H, Fuks Z, et al. The coexistence of nodular and diffuse patterns in nodular non-hodgkin's lymphomas: Significance and clinicopathologic correlation. Cancer 1977;40:1229–1233.

181. Fisher RI, Jones RB, DeVita VT Jr, et al. Natural history of malignant lymphomas with divergent histologies at staging evaluation. Cancer 1981;47:2022–2025.

182. Hubbard SM, Chabner BA, DeVita VT Jr, et al. Histologic progression in non-Hodgkin's lymphoma. Blood 1982;59:258–264.

183. Kim H, Hendrickson MR, Dorfman RF. Composite lymphoma. Cancer 1977;40:959–976.

184. Dick FR, Maca RD. The lymph node in chronic lymphocytic leukemia. Cancer 1978;41:283–292.

185. Pangalis GA, Nathwani BN, Rappaport H. Malignant lymphoma, well differentiated lymphocytic. Its relationship with chronic lymphocytic leukemia and macroglobulinemia of Waldenström. Cancer 1977;39:999–1010.

186. Royston I, Majda JA, Baird SM, et al. Human T-cell antigens defined by monoclonal antibodies: The 65,000-dalton antigen of T-cells (T65) is also found on chronic lymphocytic leukemia cells bearing surface immunoglobulin. J Immunol 1980;125:725–731.

187. Inghirami G, Wieczorek R, Zhee B-Y, et al. Differential expression of LFA-1 molecules in non-Hodgkin's lymphoma and lymphoid leukemia. Blood 1988;72:1431–1434.

188. Cossman J, Necker LM, Braziel RM, et al. In vitro enhancement of immunoglobulin gene expression in chronic lymphocytic leukemia. J Clin Invest 1984;73:587–592.

189. Evans HL, Butler JJ, Youness EL. Malignant lymphoma, small lymphocytic type. A clinicopathologic study of 84 cases with suggested criteria for intermediate lymphocytic lymphoma. Cancer 1978;41:1440–1455.

190. Richter MN. Generalized reticular cell sarcoma of lymph nodes associated with lymphatic leukemia. Am J Pathol 1928;4:285–292.

191. Trump DL, Mann RB, Phelps R, et al. Richter's syndrome: Diffuse histiocytic lymphoma in patients with chronic lymphocytic lymphoma. A report of 5 cases and review of the literature. Am J Med 1980;68:539–548.

192. Isaacson PG, Spencer J. Malignant lymphoma of mucosa-associated lymphoid tissue. Histopathology 1987;11:445–462.

193. Isaacson PG, Spencer J. Malignant lymphoma of mucosa associated lymphoid tissue (MALT). In: Jones DB, Wright DH, eds. Lymphoproliferative diseases. Immunology in medicine series. Norwell: Kluwer-Academic, 1990;15:123–143.

194. Harris NL. Extranodal lymphoid infiltrates and mucosa-associated lymphoid tissue (MALT). Am J Surg Pathol 1991;15:879–884.

195. Sundeen JT, Longo DL, Jaffe ES. CD5 expression in B-cell small lymphocytic malignancies: Correlations with clinical presentation and sites of disease. Am J Surg Pathol 1992;16:130–137.

196. Sheibani K, Burke JS, Swartz WG, et al. Monocytoid B-cell lymphoma. Clinicopathologic study of 21 cases of a unique type of low-grade lymphoma. Cancer 1988;62:1531–1538.

197. Nathwani BN, Winberg CD, Diamond LW, et al. Morphologic criteria for the differentiation of follicular lymphoma from florid reactive follicular hyperplasia. A study of 80 cases. Cancer 1981;48:1794–1806.

198. Garvin AJ, Simon R, Young RC, et al. The Rappaport classification on non-Hodgkin's lymphomas: A closer look using other proposed classifications. Semin Oncol 1980;7:234–243.

199. Leech JH, Glick AD, Waldron JA, et al. Malignant lymphomas of follicular center cell origin in man. I. Immunologic studies. JNCI 1975;54:11–21.

200. Ault KA. Detection of small numbers of monoclonal B lymphocytes in the blood of patients with lymphoma. N Engl J Med 1979;300:1401–1405.

201. Come SE, Jaffe ES, Anderson JC, et al. Leukemic progression of non-Hodgkin's lymphoma: Clinicopathologic features and therapeutic implications. Am J Med 1980;69:667–674.

202. Nathwani BN, Metter GE, Miller TP, et al. What should be the morphologic criteria for the subdivision of follicular lymphomas? Blood 1986;68:837–845.

203. Osborne CK, Norton L, Young RC, et al. Nodular histiocytic lymphoma: An aggressive nodular lymphoma with potential for prolonged disease-free survival. Blood 1980;56:198–203.

204. Hoppe RT. Histologic variation in non-Hodgkin's lymphomas: Commentary. Cancer Treat Rep 1981;65:935–939.

205. Kim H, Dorfman RF. Morphological studies of 84 untreated patients subject to laparotomy for the staging of non-Hodgkin's lymphomas. Cancer 1974;33:657–674.

206. Lotz MJ, Chabner B, DeVita VT, et al. Pathological staging of 100 consecutive untreated patients with non-Hodgkin's lymphomas. Extramedullary sites of disease. Cancer 1976;37:266–270.

207. Levy R, Warnke R, Dorfman RF, et al. The monoclonality of human B-cell lymphomas. J Exp Med 1977;145:1014–1028.

208. Harris NL, Nadler LM, Bhan AK. Immunohistologic characterization of two malignant lymphomas of germinal center type (centroblastic/centrocytic and centrocytic) with monoclonal antibodies: Follicular and diffuse lymphomas of small-cleaved-cell type are related but distinct entities. Am J Pathol 1984;117:262–272.

209. Jaffe ES, Braylan RC, Nanba K, et al. Functional markers: A new perspective on malignant lymphomas. Cancer Treat Rep 1977;61:953–962.

210. Braziel RM, Sussman E, Neckers LM, et al. Induction of immunoglobulin secretion in follicular non-Hodgkin's lymphomas: Role of immunoregulatory T cells. Blood 1985;66:128–134.

211. Lowder JN, Meeker TC, Campbell M, et al. Studies on B lymphoid tumors treated with monoclonal anti-idiotype antibodies: Correlations with clinical responses. Blood 1987;69:199–210.

212. Berard CW, Dorfman RF. Histopathology of malignant lymphomas. In: Roschberg SA, ed. Clinics in hematology, vol 3. Philadelphia: WB Saunders, 1974:39.

213. Weisenburger DD, Nathwani BN, Diamond LW, et al. Malignant lymphoma, intermediate lymphocytic type: A clinical-pathologic study of 42 cases. Cancer 1981;48:1415–1425.

214. Weisenburger DD, Kim H, Rappaport H. Mantle-zone lymphoma: A follicular variant of intermediate lymphocytic lymphoma. Cancer 1982;49:1429–1438.

215. Swerdlow SH, Habeshaw JA, Murray LJ, et al. Centrocytic lymphoma: A distinct clinicopathologic and immunologic entity. Am J Pathol 1983;113:181–197.

216. Bookman MA, Lardelli P, Jaffe ES, Duffey PL, et al. Lymphocytic lymphoma of intermediate differentiation: Morphologic, immunophenotypic, and prognostic factors. JNCI 1990;82:742–748.

217. Jaffe ES, Bookman MA, Longo DL. Lymphocytic lymphoma of intermediate differentiation-mantle zone lymphoma: A distinct subtype of B-cell lymphoma. Hum Pathol 1987;18:877–880.

218. Nanba K, Jaffe ES, Braylan RC, et al. Alkaline phosphatase-positive malignant lymphomas. Am J Clin Pathol 1977;68:535–542.

219. Raffeld M, Jaffe ES. *Bcl-1*, t (11;14) and mantle cell derived lymphomas. Blood 1991;78:259–263.

220. Cossman J, Jaffe ES, Fisher RI. Immunologic phenotypes of diffuse, aggressive, non-Hodgkin's lymphomas. Correlation with clinical features. Cancer 1984;54:1310–1317.

221. Fisher RI, Hubbard SM, DeVita VT Jr, et al. Factors determining our ability to cure aggressive forms of diffuse lymphomas. Blood 1981;58:45–51.

222. Armitage JO, Vose JM, Linder J, et al. Clinical significance of immunophenotype in diffuse aggressive non-Hodgkin's lymphoma. J Clin Oncol 1989;7:1783–1790.

223. Kwak LK, Wilson M, Weiss LM, et al. Similar outcome of treatment of B-cell and T-cell diffuse large-cell lymphomas: The Stanford experience. J Clin Oncol 1991;9:1426–1431.

224. Jaffe ES, Longo DL, Cossman J, et al. Diffuse B cell lymphomas with T cell predominance in patients with follicular lymphoma or "pseudo T cell lymphoma." Lab Invest 1984;50:27A–28A.

225. Ramsay AD, Smith WJ, Isaacson PG. T-cell rich B-cell lymphoma. Am J Surg Pathol 1988;12:433–443.

226. Medeiros LJ, Lardelli P, Stetler-Stevenson M, et al. Genotypic analysis of diffuse, mixed cell lymphomas: Comparison with morphologic and immunophenotypic findings. Am J Clin Pathol 1991;95:547–555.

227. Jaffe ES, Shevach EM, Sussman EH, et al. Membrane receptor sites for the identification of lymphoreticular cells in benign and malignant conditions. Br J Cancer 1975;31:107–120.

228. Waldron JA, Leech JH, Glick AD, et al. Malignant lymphoma of peripheral T lymphocyte origin. Cancer 1977;40:1604–1617.

229. Lennert K, Mestdagh J. Lymphogranulomatoses mit constant hohem Epitheloidzellgehalt. Virchows Arch [A] 1968;344:1.

230. Burke JS, Butler JJ. Malignant lymphoma with a high content of epithelioid histiocytes (Lennert's lymphoma). Am J Clin Pathol 1976;66:1–9.

231. Kim H, Jacobs C, Warnke RA, et al. Malignant lymphoma with a high content of epithelioid histiocytes. A distinct clinicopathologic entity and a form of so-called "Lennert's lymphoma." Cancer 1978;41:620–635.

232. Levine AM, Taylor CR, Schneider DR, et al. Immunoblastic sarcoma of T-cell versus B-cell origin: I. Clinical features. Blood 1981;58:52–61.

233. Lipford E, Wright JJ, Urba W, et al. Refinement of lymphoma cytogenetics by the chromosome 18q21 major breakpoint region. Blood 1987;70:1816–1823.

234. Muller-Hermelink HK, Steinmann G, Stein H, et al. Malignant lymphoma of plasmacytoid T-cells. Morphologic and immunologic studies characterizing a special type of T-cell. Am J Surg Pathol 1983;7:849–862.

235. Kadin ME, Sako D, Berliner N, et al. Childhood Ki-1 lymphoma presenting with skin lesions and peripheral lymphadenopathy. Blood 1986;68:1042–1049.

236. Stein H, Mason DY, Gerdes J, et al. The expression of Hodgkin's disease associated antigen Ki-1 in reactive and neoplastic lymphoid tissue: Evidence that the Reed-Sternberg cells and histiocytic malignancies are derived from activated lymphoid cells. Blood 1985;66:848–858.

237. Durkop H, Latza U, Hummel M, et al. Molecular cloning and expression of a new member of the nerve growth factor receptor family that is characteristic for Hodgkin's disease. Cell 1992;68:421–428.

238. Mitchell AB, Wilbur AF, Richard AL, et al. Morphology in Ki-1 (CD30)-positive non-Hodgkin's lymphoma is correlated with clinical features and the presence of a unique chromosomal abnormality, t(2;5) (p23;q35). Am J Surg Pathol 1990;14:305–316.

239. Barcos MP, Lukes RJ. Malignant lymphoma of convoluted lymphocytes: A new entity of possible T cell type. In: Sinks LF, Godden JO (eds): Conflicts in childhood cancer: An evaluation of current management: Proceedings. New York: Alan R Liss, 1975:147.

240. Nathwani BN, Kim H, Rappaport H. Malignant lymphoma, lymphoblastic. Cancer 1976;38:964–983.

241. Smith JL, Barker CR, Clein GP, et al. Characterization of malignant mediastinal lymphoid neoplasm (Sternberg sarcoma) as thymic in origin. Lancet 1973;1:74–77.

242. Sander CA, Medeiros LJ, Abruzzo LV, et al. Lymphoblastic lymphoma presenting in cutaneous sites: A clinicopathologic analysis of six cases. J Am Acad Dermatol 1991;25:1023.

243. Banks PM, Arseneau JC, Gralnick HR, et al. American Burkitt's lymphoma: A clinicopathologic study of 30 cases: II. Pathologic correlations. Am J Med 1975;58:322–329.

244. Mann RB, Jaffe ES, Braylan RC, et al. Nonendemic Burkitt's lymphoma: A B-cell tumor related to germinal centers. N Engl J Med 1976;295:685–691.

245. Magrath IT, Freeman CB, Pizzo P, et al. Characterization of lymphoma-derived cell lines: Comparison of cell lines positive and negative for Epstein-Barr virus nuclear antigen: II. Surface markers. JNCI 1980;64:477–483.

246. Ziegler JL. Treatment results of 54 American patients with Burkitt's lymphomas are similar to the African experience. N Engl J Med 1977;297:75–80.

247. Grogan TM, Warnke RA, Kaplan HS. A comparative study of Burkitt's and non-Burkitt's "undifferentiated" malignant lymphomas: Immunologic, cytochemical, ultrastructural, cytologic, histopathologic, clinical and cell culture features. Cancer 1982;49:1817–1828.

248. Miliauskas JR, Berard CW, Young RC, et al. Undifferentiated non-Hodgkin's lymphomas (Burkitt's and non-Burkitt's types). The relevance of making this histologic distinction. Cancer 1982;50:2115–2121.

249. Yano T, Van Krieken JHJM, Magrath IT, et al. Histogenetic correlations between subcategories of small non-cleaved cell lymphomas. Blood 1992;79:1282–1290.

250. Croce CM, Tsujimoto Y, Erikson I, et al. Biology of disease: Chromosome translocations and B cell neoplasia. Lab Invest 1984;51:258–267.

251. Jaffe ES, Blattner WA, Blayney DW, et al. The pathologic spectrum of HTLV-associated leukemia/lymphoma in the United States. Am J Surg Pathol 1984;8:263–275.

252. Broder S, Bunn PA Jr, Jaffe ES, et al. T-cell lymphoproliferative syndrome associated with human T-cell leukemia/lymphoma virus. Ann Intern Med 1984;100:543–557.

253. Lukes RJ, Tindle BH. Immunoblastic lymphadenopathy. A hyper-immune entity resembling Hodgkin's disease. N Engl J Med 1975;292:1–8.

254. Frizzera G, Moran EM, Rappaport H. Angioblastic lymphadenopathy: Diagnosis and clinical course. Am J Med 1975;59:803–818.

255. Nathwani BN, Rappaport H, Moran EM, et al. Malignant lymphomas arising in angioimmunoblastic lymphadenopathy. Cancer 1978;41:578–606.

256. Watanabe S, Shimosato Y, Shimoyama M. Adult T-cell lymphoma with hypergammaglobulinemia. Cancer 1980;41:2472–2483.

257. Kaneko Y, Larson RA, Variakojis D, et al. Nonrandom chromosome abnormalities in angioimmunoblastic lymphadenopathy. Blood 1982;60:877–887.

258. Weiss LM, Strickler JG, Dorfman RF, et al. Clonal T cell populations in angioimmunoblastic lymphadenopathy and angioimmunoblastic lymphadenopathy-like lymphoma. Am J Pathol 1986;122:392–397.

259. Lipford EH, Smith HR, Pittaluga S, et al. Clonality of angioimmunoblastic lymphadenopathy and implications for its evolution to malignant lymphoma. J Clin Invest 1987;79:637–642.

260. Weiss LM, Jaffe ES, Liu XF, et al. Detection and localization of Epstein-Barr viral genomes in angioimmunoblastic lymphadenopathy and angioimmunoblastic lymphadenopathy-like lymphoma. Blood 1992;79:1789–1795.

261. Kassel SH, Echevarria RA, Guzzo FP. Midline malignant reticulosis (so-called lethal midline granuloma). Cancer 1969;23:920–935.

262. De Remee RA, Weiland LH, McDonald TJ. Polymorphic reticulosis, lymphomatoid granulomatosis: Two diseases or one? Mayo Clin Proc 1978;53:634–640.

263. Liebow AA, Carrington CB, Friedman RJ. Lymphomatoid granulomatosis. Hum Pathol 1972;3:457–558.

264. Jaffe ES, Lipford EH Jr, Margolick JB, et al. Lymphomatoid granulomatosis and angiocentric lymphoma. A spectrum of post-thymic T cell proliferations. Semin Respir Med 1989;10:167–172.

265. Fauci AS, Haynes BF, Costa J, et al. Lymphomatoid granulomatosis, prospective clinical and therapeutic experience over ten years. N Engl J Med 1982;306:68–74.

266. Katzenstein A, Carrington CB, Liebow AA. Lymphomatoid granulomatosis: A clinical-pathologic study of 152 cases. Cancer 1979;43:360–373.

267. Nichols PW, Koss M, Levine AM, et al. Lymphomatoid granulomatosis: A T-cell disorder. Am J Med 1982;72:467–471.

268. Harabuchi Y, Yamanaka N, Kataura A, et al. Epstein-Barr virus in nasal T-cell lymphomas in patients with lethal midline granuloma. Lancet 1990;335:128–130.

269. Katzenstein AL, Peiper SC. Detection of Epstein-Barr virus genomes in lymphomatoid granulomatosis: Analysis of 29 cases by the polymerase chain reaction technique. Mod Pathol 1990;3:435–441.

270. Ho FCS, Srivastava G, Loke SL, et al. Presence of Epstein-Barr virus DNA in nasal lymphomas of B and T cell type. Hematol Oncol 1990;8:271–281.

271. Medeiros LJ, Peiper SC, Elwood L, et al. Angiocentric immunoproliferative lesions: A molecular analysis of eight cases. Hum Pathol 1991;22:1150–1157.

272. Chan JKC, Ng CS, Path MRC, et al. Most nasal/nasopharyngeal lymphomas are peripheral T-cell neoplasms. Am J Surg Pathol 1987;11:418–429.

273. Jaffe ES. Malignant histiocytosis and true histiocytic lymphomas. In: Jaffe ES, ed. Surgical pathology of lymph nodes and related organs. Philadelphia: WB Saunders, 1985:381.

274. Sultan C, Imbert M, Richard MF, et al. Pure acute monocytic leukemia. A study of 12 cases. Am J Clin Pathol 1977;68:752–757.

275. Van der Valk P, Meijer CJLM, Willemze R, et al. Histiocytic sarcoma (true histiocytic lymphoma): A clinicopathologic study of 20 cases. Histopathology 1984;8:105–123.

276. Willemze R, Rinter DJ, Wilem A, et al. Reticulum cell sarcomas (large cell lymphomas) presenting in the skin. High frequency of true histiocytic lymphoma. Cancer 1982;50:1367–1379.

277. Flynn KJ, Dehner LP, Gajl-Peczalska KJ, et al. Regressing atypical histiocytosis: A cutaneous proliferation of atypical neoplastic histiocytes with unexpectedly indolent biologic behavior. Cancer 1982;49:959–970.

278. Poppema S, Van Voorst Vader PC, Rozenboom-Uiterwijk T, et al. Lymphomatoid papulosis. Case report providing evidence for a monocyte-macrophage origin of the atypical cells. Cancer 1983;52:1178–1182.

279. Scott RB, Robb-Smith AHT. Histiocytic medullary reticulosis. Lancet 1939;2:194–198.

280. Risdall RJ, McKenna RW, Nesbit ME, et al. Virus-associated hemophagocytic syndrome—A benign histiocytic proliferation distinct from malignant histiocytosis. Cancer 1979;44:993–1002.

281. Jaffe ES, Costa J, Fauci AS, et al. Malignant lymphoma and erythrophagocytosis simulating malignant histiocytosis. Am J Med 1983;75:741–749.

282. Simrell CR, Margolick JB, Crabtree GR, et al. Lymphokine-induced phagocytosis in angiocentric immunoproliferative lesions (AIL) and malignant lymphoma arising in AIL. Blood 1985;65:1469–1476.

283. Favara BE, McCarthy RC, Mierau GW. Histiocytosis X. In: Finefold M, ed. Pathology of neoplasia in children and adolescents. Philadelphia: WB Saunders, 1986:126.

284. Nezelof C, Frileux-Herbert F, Cronies-Sachet J. Disseminated histiocytosis X, analysis of prognostic factors based on a retrospective study of 50 cases. Cancer 1979;44:1824–1838.

285. Lahey ME. Prognostic factors in histiocytosis X. Am J Pediatr Hematol Oncol 1981;3:57–60.

286. Monda L, Warnke R, Rosai J. A primary lymph node malignancy with features suggestive of dendritic reticulum cell differentiation. A report of 4 cases. Am J Pathol 1986;122:562–572.

287. Feltkamp CA, van Heerde P, Feltkamp-Vroom TM, et al. A malignant tumor arising from interdigitating cells; light microscopical, ultrastructural, immuno- and enzyme histochemical characteristics. Virchows Arch [A] 1981;393:183.

288. Chan W, Zaatari G. Lymph node interdigitating reticulum cell sarcoma. Am J Clin Pathol 1986;85:739–744.

289. Frizzera G. Castleman's disease and related disorders. Semin Diagn Pathol 1988;5:346–364.

290. Castleman B, Iverson L, Menendez V. Localized mediastinal lymph node hyperplasia resembling thymoma. Cancer 1956;9:822–830.

291. Keller AR, Hochholzer L, Castleman B. Hyaline-vascular and plasma-cell types of giant lymph node hyperplasia of the mediastinum and other locations. Cancer 1972;29:670–683.

292. Yashizaki K, Matsuda T, Nishimoto N, et al. Pathogenic significance of interleukin-6 (IL-6/BSF-2) in Castleman's disease. Blood 1989;74:1360–1367.

293. Hanson CA, Frizzera G, Patton DF, et al. Clonal rearrangement for immunoglobulin and T-cell receptor genes in systemic Castleman's disease. Association with Epstein-Barr Virus. Am J Pathol 1988;131:84–91.

294. Frizzera G, Peterson BA, Bayrd ED, et al. A systemic lymphoproliferative disorder with morphologic features of Castleman's disease: Clinical findings and clinicopathologic correlations in 15 patients. J Clin Oncol 1985;3:1202–1216.

295. Weisenburger DD, Nathwani BN, Winberg CD, et al. Multicentric angiofollicular lymph node hyperplasia: A clinicopathologic study of 16 cases. Hum Pathol 1985;16:162–172.

296. Kaplan HS. Hodgkin's disease. 2nd ed. Cambridge, MA: Harvard University Press, 1980:689.

297. Rosenberg SA, Diamond HD, Jaslowitz B, et al. Lymphosarcoma: A review of 1269 cases. Medicine (Baltimore) 1961;40:31–84.

298. Banfi A, Bonadonna G, Riece SB, et al. Malignant lymphomas of Waldeyer's ring: Natural history and survival after radiotherapy. Br Med J 1972;2:140.

299. Sage HH. Palpable cervical lymph nodes. JAMA 1958;168:496–498.

300. Filly R, Blank N, Castellino RA. Radiographic distribution of intrathoracic disease in previously untreated patients with Hodgkin's disease and non-Hodgkin's lymphoma. Radiology 1976;120:277–281.

301. Simone JV, Verzosa MS, Rudy JA. Initial features and prognosis in 363 children with acute lymphoblastic leukemia. Cancer 1975;36:2099–2108.

302. Bitran JD, Golomb HM, Ultmann JE, et al. Non-Hodgkin's lymphoma, poorly differentiated lymphocytic and mixed cell types: Results of sequential staging procedures, response to therapy, and survival of 100 patients. Cancer 1978;42:88–95.

303. Golomb H. "Hairy" cell leukemia: An unusual lymphoproliferative disease. Cancer 1978;42:946–956.

304. Rappaport H, Ramot B, Hulu N, et al. The pathology of so-called Mediterranean abdominal lymphoma with malabsorption. Cancer 1972;29:1502–1511.

305. Dragosics B, Bauer P, Radaszkiweicz T. Primary gastrointestinal lymphomas. A retrospective clinicopathologic study of 150 cases. Cancer 1985;55:1060–1073.

306. Buskirk SJ, Evans RG, Banks PM, et al. Primary lymphoma of the testis. Int J Radiat Oncol Biol Phys 1982;8:1699–1703.

307. Young RC, Howser DM, Anderson T, et al. Central nervous system complications of non-Hodgkin's lymphoma. The potential role for prophylactic therapy. Am J Med 1979;66:435–443.

308. Jones SE, Fuks Z, Bull M, et al. Non-Hodgkin's lymphomas: IV. Clinicopathologic correlation in 405 cases. Cancer 1973;31:806–823.

309. Chabner BA, Johnson RE, Young RC, et al. Sequential non-surgical and surgical staging of non-Hodgkin's lymphoma. Ann Intern Med 1976;85:149–154.

310. Anderson T, Chabner BA, Young RC, et al. Malignant lymphoma: I. The histology and staging of 473 patients at the National Cancer Institute. Cancer 1982;50:2699–2709.

311. DeVita VT, Canellos GP. Treatment of the lymphomas. Semin Hematol 1972;9:193–209.

312. Reddy S, Saxena VS, Pellettiere EV, et al. Early nodal and extra nodal non-Hodgkin's lymphomas. Cancer 1977;40:98–104.

313. Paryani S, Hoppe RT, Burke JS, et al. Extralymphatic involvement in diffuse non-Hodgkin's lymphomas. J Clin Oncol 1983;1:682–688.

314. Portlock CS, Rosenberg SA. No initial therapy for stage III and IV non-Hodgkin's lymphomas of favorable histologic types. Ann Intern Med 1979;90:10–13.

315. DeVita VT. Human models of human disease: Breast cancer and the lymphomas. Int J Radiat Oncol Biol Phys 1979;5:1855–1867.

316. Acker B, Hoppe RT, Colby TV, et al. Histologic conversion in the non-Hodgkin's lymphomas. J Clin Oncol 1983;1:11–16.

317. Rowley JD. Consistent chromosome abnormalities in human leukemia and lymphoma. Cancer Invest 1983;3:267–280.

318. Carbone PP, Kaplan HS, Musshoff K, et al. Report of the committee on Hodgkin's disease staging. Cancer Res 1971;31:1860–1861.

319. Ciampi A, Bush RS, Gospodarowicz M. An approach to classifying prognostic factors related to survival experience for non-Hodgkin's lymphoma patients: Based on a series of 982 patients: 1967–1975. Cancer 1981;47:621–627.

320. Jagannath S, Velasquez WS, Tucker SL, et al. Tumor burden assessment and its implication for a prognostic model in advanced diffuse large-cell lymphoma. J Clin Oncol 1986;2:859–865.

321. Vose JM, Armitage JO, Weisenberger DD, et al. The importance of age in survival of patients treated with chemotherapy for aggressive non-Hodgkin's lymphomas. J Clin Oncol 1988;6:1838–1844.

322. Coiffier B, Gisselbrecht C, Vose JM, et al. Prognostic factors in aggressive malignant lymphomas: Description and validation of a prognostic index that could identify patients requiring a more intensive therapy. J Clin Oncol 1991;9:211–219.

323. Hoskins PJ, Ng V, Spinelli JJ, et al. Prognostic variables in patients with diffuse large-cell lymphoma treated with MACOP-B. J Clin Oncol 1991;9:220–226.

324. Shipp MA, Harrington DP, Klatt MM, et al. Identification of major prognostic subgroups of patients with large cell lymphoma treated with m-BACOD or M-BACOD. Ann Intern Med 1986;104:757–765.

325. Litan P, Swan F, Cabanillas F, et al. Prognostic value of serum β_2-microgloulin in low-grade lymphoma. Ann Intern Med 1991;114:855–860.

326. Gallagher CJ, Gregory WM, Jones AE, et al. Follicular lymphoma: Prognostic factors for response and survival. J Clin Oncol 1986;4:1470–1480.

327. Soubeyran P, Eghbali H, Bonichon F, et al. Low-grade follicular lymphoma: Analysis of prognosis in a series of 281 patients. Eur J Cancer 1991;27:1606–1613.

328. Armitage JO, Weisenburger DD, Hutchins M, et al. Chemotherapy for diffuse large cell lymphoma: Rapidly responding patients have more durable remissions. J Clin Oncol 1986;4:160–164.

329. Lister TA, Crowther D, Sutcliffe SB, et al. Report of a committee convened to discuss the evaluation and staging of patients with Hodgkin's disease: Cotswold meeting. J Clin Oncol 1989;7:1630–1636.

330. Young RC, Anderson T, DeVita VT. The treatment of Hodgkin's disease: Emphasizing programs at the Clinical Center, National Institutes of Health. Curr Probl Cancer 1977;1:1–29.

331. Moormeier JA, Williams SF, Golomb HM. The staging of non-Hodgkin's lymphomas. Semin Oncol 1990;17:43–50.

332. Smith BR, Weinberg DS, Robert NJ, et al. Circulating monoclonal B lymphocytes in non-Hodgkin's lymphoma. N Engl J Med 1984;311:1476–1481.

333. Horning SJ, Galili N, Cleary M, et al. Detection of non-Hodgkin's lymphoma in the peripheral blood by analysis of antigen receptor gene rearrangements: Results of a prospective study. Blood 1990;75:1139–1145.

334. Berliner N, Ault K, Martin P, et al. Detection of clonal excess in lymphoproliferative disease by kappa/lambda analysis: Correlation with immunoglobulin gene DNA rearrangements. Blood 1986;67:80–85.

335. Khoury MB, Godwin JD, Halvorsen R, et al. Role of chest CT in non-Hodgkin's lymphoma. Radiology 1986;158:659.

336. Marglin S, Castellino RA. Lymphographic accuracy in 632 consecutive, previously untreated cases of Hodgkin's disease and non-Hodgkin's lymphoma. Radiology 1981;140:351–353.

337. Castellino RA, Dunnick NR, Goffinet DR, et al. Predictive value of lymphography for sites of supradiaphragmatic disease encountered at staging laporotomy in newly diagnosed Hodgkin's disease and non-Hodgkin's lymphoma. J Clin Oncol 1983;1:532–536.

338. Castellino RA, Marglin SI. Imaging of abdominal and pelvic lymph nodes: Lymphography or computed tomography. Invest Radiol 1982;17:433–443.

339. Lee JK, Stanley RJ, Sagel SS, et al. Accuracy of computed tomography in detecting intraabdominal and pelvic adenopathy in lymphoma. AJR 1978;131:311–315.

340. Neumann CH, Finberg H, Rosenthal DS. The role of computerized body tomography of the abdomen in the management of lymphoma patients. Postgrad Radiol 1982;2/3:225–239.

341. Benson WJ, Ding JC, Cooper IA. Abdominal CT and lymphography in the initial staging of non-Hodgkin's lymphomas. Aust N Z J Med 1987;17:253–254.

342. Shields AF, Porter BA, Churchley S, et al. The detection of bone marrow involvement by lymphoma using magnetic resonance imaging. J Clin Oncol 1987;5:225–230.

343. Hoane BR, Shields AF, Porter BA, et al. Detection of lymphomatous bone marrow involvement with magnetic resonance imaging. Blood 1991;78:728–738.

344. Longo DL, Schilsky RL, Blei L, et al. Gallium-67 scanning has limited usefulness in staging patients with non-Hodgkin's lymphoma. Am J Med 1980;68:695–700.

345. Anderson KC, Leonard RC, Canellos GP, et al. High dose gallium imaging in lymphoma. Am J Med 1981;75:327–331.

346. Moran EJ, Ultmann JE, Ferguson DJ. Staging laparotomy on non-Hodgkin's lymphoma. Br J Cancer 1975;31:228–236.

347. Israel O, Front DM, Lam M, et al. Gallium 67 imaging in monitoring response to treatment. Cancer 1988;61:2439–2443.

348. Kaplan WD, Jochelson MS, Herman TS, et al. Gallium-67 imaging: A predictor of residual tumor viability and clinical outcome in patients with diffuse large-cell lymphoma. J Clin Oncol 1990;8:1966–1970.

349. Weeks JC, Yeop BY, Canellos GP, Shipp MA. Value of follow-up procedures in patients with large-cell lymphoma who achieve a complete remission. J Clin Oncol 1991;9:1196–1203.

350. Anderson KC, Kaplan WD, Leonard RCF, et al. Role of ^{99m}Tc methylene diphosphonate bone imaging in the management of lymphoma. Cancer Treat Rep 1985;69:1347–1351.

351. Chabner BA, Fisher RI, Young RC, et al. Staging of non-Hodgkin's lymphoma. Semin Oncol 1980;7:285–291.

352. Levitt LJ, Dawson DM, Rosenthal DS, et al. CNS involvement in the non-Hodgkin's lymphomas. Cancer 1980;45:545–552.

353. Bunn PA Jr, Schein PS, Banks PM, et al. Central nervous system complications in patients with diffuse histiocytic and undifferentiated lymphoma: Leukemia revisited. Blood 1976;47:3–10.

354. Crescenzi M, Seto M, Herzig GP, et al. Thermostable DNA polymerase chain amplification of t(14;18) chromosome breakpoints and detection of minimal residual disease. Proc Natl Acad Sci USA 1988;85:4869–4873.

355. Veronesi U, Musumeci R, Pizzetti F, et al. The value of staging laparotomy in non-Hodgkin's lymphomas (with emphasis on the histiocytic type). Cancer 1974;33:446–459.

356. Castellani R, Bonadonna G, Spinelli P, et al. Sequential pathologic staging of untreated non-Hodgkin's lymphomas by laparoscopy and laparotomy combined with marrow biopsy. Cancer 1977;40:2322–2328.

357. Goffinet DR, Warnke R, Dunnick NR, et al. Clinical and surgical (laparotomy) evaluation of patients with non-Hodgkin's lymphomas. Cancer Treat Rep 1977;61:981–992.

358. Chabner BA, Johnson RE, DeVita VT, et al. Sequential staging in non-Hodgkin's lymphoma. Cancer Treat Rep 1977;61:993–997.

359. Heifetz LJ, Fuller LM, Rogers RW, et al. Laparotomy findings in lymphangiogram staged I and II non-Hodgkin's lymphomas. Cancer 1980;45:2778–2786.

360. Fuks JA, Aisner J, Wiernik PH. Restaging laparotomy in the management of non-Hodgkin's lymphomas. Med Pediatr Oncol 1982;10:429–438.

361. Surbone A, Longo DL, DeVita VT Jr, et al. Residual abdominal masses in aggressive non-Hodgkin's lymphoma after combination chemotherapy: Significance and management. J Clin Oncol 1988;6:1832–1837.

362. Moore DF, Migliore PH, Shullenberg CC, et al. Monoclonal macroglobulinemia in malignant lymphoma. Ann Intern Med 1970;72:43–47.

363. Levy RL, Miller RA. Biological and clinical implications of lymphocyte hybridomas: Tumor therapy with monoclonal antibodies. Ann Rev Med 1983;34:107–116.

364. Ko HS, Pruzanski W. M components associated with lymphoma: A review of 62 cases. Am J Med Sci 1976;272:175–183.

365. Balentine L, Skikne BS, Park CH, et al. Malignant lymphocytic lymphoma: Demonstration of a serum inhibitor of myelopoiesis and response to combination chemotherapy. Cancer 1983;52:35–38.

366. Jones SE. Autoimmune disorders and malignant lymphoma. Cancer 1973;31:1092–1098.

367. Anderson TC, Jones SE, Soehnlen BJ, et al. Immunocompetence and malignant lymphoma: Immunologic status before therapy. Cancer 1981;48:2702–2709.

368. Jones SE, Griffith K, Dombrowski P, et al. Immunodeficiency in patients with non-Hodgkin's lymphomas. Blood 1977;49:335–344.

369. Advani SH, Dinshaw KA, Nair CN, et al. Immune dysfunction in non-Hodgkin's lymphomas. Cancer 1980;45:2843–2848.

370. Silver BA, Bostick-Bruton FW, Neckers L, et al. Deficient helper cell function as a cause of diminished pokeweed mitogen blastogenic responses in patients with non-Hodgkin's lymphomas. Cancer 1984;54:2936–2942.

371. Gajl-Peczalska KJ, Chartrand SL, Bloomfield CD. Abnormal immunoregulation in patients with non-Hodgkin's malignant lymphomas. Clin Immunol Immunopathol 1982;23:366–378.

372. Whisler RL, Balerzak SP, Murray JL. Heterogeneous mechanisms of impaired lymphocyte responses in non-Hodgkin's lymphomas. Blood 1981;57:1081–1087.

373. Broder S, Edelson RL, Lutzner MA, et al. Sezary syndrome: A malignant proliferation of helper T cells. J Clin Invest 1976;58:1297–1306.

374. Broder S, Uchiyama T, Muul L, et al. Activation of leukemic prosuppressor cells to become suppressor effector cells. Influence of cooperating normal T cells. N Engl J Med 1981;302:1382–1387.

375. Longo DL, Broder S. Human T-cell leukemia/lymphoma virus (HTLV) associated adult T-cell leukemia. Med Grand Rounds 1984;3:239.

376. Glatstein E, Fuks Z, Goffinet DR, et al. Non-Hodgkin's lymphoma of stage III extent. Is total lymphoid irradiation appropriate treatment? Cancer 1976;37:2806–2812.

377. Paryani SB, Hoppe RT, Cox RS, et al. The role of radiation therapy in the management of stage III follicular lymphomas. J Clin Oncol 1984;2:841–848.

378. Cox JD, Komaki R, Kun LE, et al. Stage III nodular lymphoreticular tumors (non-Hodgkin's lymphomas): Results of central lymphatic irradiation. Cancer 1981;47:2247–2252.

379. Flippen T, McLaughlin P, Conrad FG, et al. Stage III nodular lymphomas. Preliminary results of a combined chemotherapy/radiotherapy program. Cancer 1983;51:987–993.

380. Rosenberg SA. The low-grade non-Hodgkin's lymphomas: Challenges and opportunities. J Clin Oncol 1985;3:299–310.

381. Paryani SB, Hoppe RT, Cox RS, et al. Analysis of non-Hodgkin's lymphomas with nodular and favorable histologies, stages I and II. Cancer 1983;52:2300–2307.

382. Gomez GA, Barcos M, Krishnamsetty RM, et al. Treatment of early-stages I and II-nodular, poorly differentiated lymphocytic lymphoma. Am J Clin Oncol 1986;9:40–44.

383. Gospodarowicz MK, Bush RS, Brown TC. Prognostic factors in nodular lymphomas: A multivariate analysis based on the Princess Margaret Experience. Int J Radiat Oncol Biol Phys 1984;10:489–497.

384. Lawrence TS, Urba WJ, Steinberg SM, et al. Restrospective analysis of stage I and II indolent lymphomas at the National Cancer Institute. Int J Radiat Oncol Biol Phys 1988;14:417–424.

385. Richards MA, Gregory WM, Hall PA, et al. Management of localized non-Hodgkin's lymphoma: The experience at St. Bartholomew's Hospital 1972–1985. Hematol Oncol 1989;7:1–18.

386. Fuks Z, Glatstein E, Kaplan HS. Patterns of presentation and relapse in the non-Hodgkin's lymphomata. Br J Cancer 1975;31:286–297.

387. Monfardini S, Banfi A, Bonadonna G, et al. Improved five-year survival after combined radiotherapy-chemotherapy for stage I–II non-Hodgkin's lymphoma. Int J Radiat Oncol Biol Phys 1980;6:125–134.

388. Landberg TG, Hakansson LG, Moller TR, et al. CVP remission maintenance in stage I or II non-Hodgkin's lymphomas: Preliminary results of a randomized study. Cancer 1979;44:831–838.

389. Toonkel LM, Fuller LM, Gamble JF, et al. Laparotomy staged I and II non-Hodgkin's lymphomas: Preliminary results of radiotherapy and adjunctive chemotherapy. Cancer 1980;45:249–260.

390. McLaughlin P, Fuller LM, Velasquez WS, et al. Stage I–II follicular lymphoma. Treatment results for 76 patients. Cancer 1986;58:1596–1602.

391. McLaughlin P, Fuller L, Redman J, et al. Stage I–II low-grade lymphomas: A prospective trial of combination chemotherapy and radiotherapy. Ann Oncol 1991;2(suppl 2):137–140.

392. Longo DL, Young RC, DeVita VT Jr. What is so good about the good prognosis lymphomas? In: Williams CJ, Whitehouse JMA, eds. Recent advances in medical oncology. Edinburgh: Churchill Livingstone, 1982:223.

393. Matis LA, Young RC, Longo DL. Nodular lymphomas: Current concepts. Crit Rev Oncol Hematol 1986;5:171–197.

394. Horning SJ, Rosenberg SA. The natural history of initially untreated low-grade non-Hodgkin's lymphomas. N Engl J Med 1984;311:1471–1475.

395. Anderson T, DeVita VT Jr, Simon RM, et al. Malignant lymphoma II. Prognostic factors and response to treatment of 473 patients at the National Cancer Institute. Cancer 1982;50:2708–2721.

396. Lister TA. The management of follicular lymphoma. Ann Oncol 1991;2(suppl 2):131–136.

397. Kennedy BJ, Bloomfield CD, Kiang DT, et al. Combinations versus successive single agent chemotherapy in lymphocytic lymphoma. Cancer 1978;41:23–28.

398. Portlock CS, Rosenberg SA, Glatstein E, et al. Treatment of advanced non-Hodgkin's lymphomas with favorable histologies. Preliminary results of a prospective trial. Blood 1976;47:747–756.

399. Hoppe RT, Kushlan P, Kaplan HS, et al. The treatment of advanced stage favorable non-Hodgkin's lymphoma: A preliminary report of a randomized trial comparing single agent chemotherapy, combination chemotherapy, and whole body radiation. Blood 1981;58:592–598.

400. Lister TA, Cullen MH, Beard MEJ, et al. Comparison of combined and single-agent chemotherapy in non-Hodgkin's lymphoma of favorable histological type. Br Med J 1978;6112:533–537.

401. Portlock CS, Fischer DS, Cadman E, et al. High-dose pulse chlorambucil in advanced, low-grade non-hodgkin's lymphoma. Cancer Treat Rep 1987;71:1029–1031.

402. Anderson T, Bender RA, Fisher RI, et al. Combination chemotherapy in non-Hodgkin's lymphomas: Results of long-term follow-up. Cancer Treat Rep 1977;61:1057–1066.

403. Ezdinli EZ, Anderson JR, Melvin F, et al. Moderate versus aggressive chemotherapy of nodular lymphocytic poorly differentiated lymphoma. J Clin Oncol 1985;3:769–775.

404. Jones SE, Grozea PN, Metz EN, et al. Superiority of adriamycin-containing combination chemotherapy in the treatment of diffuse lymphoma. A Southwest Oncology Group study. Cancer 1979;43:417–425.

405. Romaguera JE, McLaughlin P, North L, et al. Multivariate analysis of prognostic factors in stage IV follicular low-grade lymphoma: A risk model. J Clin Oncol 1991;9:762–769.

406. Skarin AT, Rosenthal DS, Malloney WC, et al. Combination chemotherapy of advanced non-Hodgkin's lymphoma with bleomycin, Adriamycin, cyclophosphamide, vincristine and prednisone (BACOP). Blood 1977;49:759–770.

407. Licht JD, Bosserman LD, Anderson JW, et al. Treatment of low-grade and intermediate-grade lymphoma with intensive combination chemotherapy results in long-term disease-free survival. Cancer 1990;66:632–639.

408. Young RC, Johnson RE, Canellos GP, et al. Advanced lymphocytic lymphoma. Randomized comparisons of chemotherapy and radiotherapy alone or in combination. Cancer Treat Rep 1977;61:1153–1159.

409. Choi NC, Timothy AR, Kaufman SA, et al. Low dose fractionated whole body irradiation in the treatment of advanced non-Hodgkin's lymphoma. Cancer 1979;43:1636–1642.

410. Thar TL, Million RR, Noyes WD. Total body irradiation in non-Hodgkin's lymphoma. Int J Radiat Biol 1979;5:171–176.

411. Young RC, Longo DL, Glatstein E, et al. The treatment of indolent lymphomas: Watchful waiting v. aggressive combined modality treatment. Semin Hematol 1988;25(suppl 2):11–16.

412. Schein PS, Chabner BA, Canellos GP, et al. Non-Hodgkin's lymphoma: Patterns of relapse from complete remission after combination chemotherapy. Cancer 1975;35:354–357.

413. Portlock CS. Management of the indolent non-Hodgkin's lymphomas. Semin Oncol 1980;7:292–301.

414. Brereton HD, Young RC, Longo DL, et al. A comparison between combination chemotherapy and total body radiation plus combination chemotherapy in non-Hodgkin's lymphoma. Cancer 1979;43:2227–2231.

415. Garvin AJ, Simon RM, Osborne CK, et al. An autopsy study of histologic progression in non-Hodgkin's lymphoma: 192 cases from the National Cancer Institute. Cancer 1983;52:393–398.

416. Armitage JO, Dick FR, Corder MP. Diffuse histiocytic lymphoma after histologic conversion: A poor prognostic variant. Cancer Treat Rep 1981;65:413–418.

417. Straus DJ, Gaynor JJ, Lieberman PH, et al. Non-Hodgkin's lymphomas: Characteristics of long-term survivors following conservative treatment. Am J Med 1987;82:247–256.

418. O'Brien MER, Easterbrook P, Powell J, et al. The natural history of low grade non-Hodgkin's lymphoma and the impact of a no initial treatment policy on survival. Q J Med 1991;292:651–660.

419. Chabner BA. Nodular non-Hodgkin's lymphoma: The case for watchful waiting. Ann Intern Med 1979;90:115–117.

420. Botnick LE, Hannon EC, Hellman S. Limited proliferation of stem cells surviving alkylating agents. Nature 1976;262:68–70.

421. Hellman S, Reincke V, Botnick LE, et al. Functional organization of the hematopoietic stem cell compartment: Implications for cancer and its therapy. J Clin Oncol 1983;1:227–284.

422. Dumont J, Thiery JP, Mazabrand A, et al. Acute myeloid leukemia following non-Hodgkin's lymphoma: Danger of prolonged use of chlorambucil as maintenance therapy. Nouv Rev Fr Hematol 1980;22:391–404.

423. Cameron S. Chlorambucil and leukemia. N Engl J Med 1977;296:1065.

424. Casciata DA, Scott DA. Acute leukemia following prolonged cytotoxic agent therapy. Medicine (Baltimore) 1979;58:32–47.

425. Lerner HJ. Acute myelogenous leukemia in patients receiving chlorambucil as long term adjuvant chemotherapy for stage II breast cancer. Cancer Treat Rep 1978;62:1136–1138.

426. Longo DL, Young RC, Hubbard SM, et al. Prolonged initial remission in patients with nodular mixed lymphoma. Ann Intern Med 1984;100:651–656.

427. Ezdinli EZ, Costello WG, Icli F, et al. Nodular mixed lymphocytic-histiocytic lymphoma (NM): Response and survival: Eastern Cooperative Oncology Group. Cancer 1980;45:261–267.

428. Merchant N, McLaughlin P, Fuller L, et al. Follicular (nodular) mixed lymphoma: A review of 65 cases. Proc Am Soc Clin Oncol 1984;3:249.

429. Peterson BA, Anderson JR, Frizzera G, et al. Combination chemotherapy prolongs survival in follicular mixed lymphoma (FML). Proc Am Soc Clin Oncol 1990;9:259.

430. Sobel RE, Dillman RO, Collins H, et al. Applications and limitations of peripheral blood lymphocyte immunoglobulin light chain analysis in the evaluation of non-Hodgkin's lymphoma. Cancer 1985;56:2005–2010.

431. Lindemalm C, Mellstedt H, Biberfeld P, et al. Clonal blood B-cell excess in relation to prognosis in untreated non-leukemic patients with non-Hodgkin's lymphoma. In: Cavalli F, Bonadonna G, Rozencweig M, eds. Malignant lymphomas and Hodgkin's disease: Experimental and therapeutic advances. Boston: Martinus-Nijhoff, 1985:225.

432. Hansen H, Koziner B, Clarkson B. Marker and kinetic studies in the non-Hodgkin's lymphomas. Am J Med 1981;71:107–123.

433. McLaughlin P, Fuller LM, Velasquez WS, et al. Stage III follicular lymphoma: Durable remissions with a combined chemotherapy-radiotherapy regimen. J Clin Oncol 1987;5:867–874.

434. Leonard RCF, Hayward RL, Prescott RJ, et al. The identification of discrete prognostic groups in low grade non-Hodgkin's lymphoma. Ann Oncol 1991;2:655–662.

435. Bastion Y, Berger F, Bryon P-A, et al. Follicular lymphomas: Assessment of prognostic factors in 127 patients followed for 10 years. Ann Oncol 1991;2(suppl 2):123–129.

436. Cabanillas F, Smith T, Bodey GP, et al. Nodular malignant lymphomas. Factors affecting complete response rate and survival. Cancer 1979;44:1983–1989.

437. Samuels B, Ultmann J, Pearson M, et al. Favorable non-Hodgkin's lymphoma: A fifteen year experience. Proc Am Soc Clin Oncol 1987;6:206.

438. Philip T, Armitage JO, Spitzer G, et al. High dose therapy and autologous bone marrow transplantation after failure of conventional chemotherapy in adults with intermediate grade or high grade non-Hodgkin's lymphoma. N Engl J Med 1987;316:1493–1498.

439. Freedman AS, Takvorian T, Anderson KC, et al. Autologous bone marrow transplantation in B-cell non-Hodgkin's lymphoma: Very low treatment-related mortality in 100 patients in sensitive relapse. J Clin Oncol 1990;8:784–791.

440. Freedman AS, Ritz J, Neuberg D, et al. Autologous bone marrow transplantation in 69 patients with a history of low-grade B-cell non-Hodgkin's lymphoma. Blood 1991;77:2524–2529.

441. Gribben JG, Freedman AS, Sunhee D, et al. All advanced stage non-Hodgkin's lymphomas with a polymerase chain reaction amplifiable breakpoint of bcl-2 have residual cells containing the bcl-2 rearrangement at evaluation and after treatment. Blood 1991;78:3275–3280.

442. Rohatiner AZS, Price CGA, Arnott S, et al. Myeloablative therapy with autologous bone marrow transplantation as consolidation of remission in patients with follicular lymphoma. Ann Oncol 1991;2(suppl 2):147–150.

443. Schouten LC, Bierman PJ, Vaughan WP, et al. Autologous bone marrow transplantation in follicular non-Hodgkin's lymphoma before and after histologic transformation. Blood 1989;74:2579–2584.

444. Longo DL. Biologic agents and approaches in the management of patients with lymphoma. A critical appraisal. Hematol Oncol Clin North Am 1991;5:1067–1087.

445. Gilewski TA, Richards JM. Biologic Response modifiers in non-Hodgkin's lymphomas. Semin Oncol 1990;17:74–87.

446. Gaynor ER, Fisher RI. Clinical trials of α-interferon in the treatment of non-Hodgkin's lymphoma. Semin Oncol 1991;18(suppl 7):12–17.

447. Urba WJ, Longo DL. Alpha-interferon in the treatment of nodular lymphomas. Semin Oncol 1986;13:40–47.

448. Hawkins MJ, O'Connell MJ, Schiller JH, et al. Phase I evaluation of recombinant A interferon alpha in combination with COPA chemotherapy. Proc Am Soc Clin Oncol 1985;4:229.

449. Rohatiner AZS, Richards MA, Barnett MJ, et al. Chlorambucil and interferon for low grade non-Hodgkin's lymphoma. Br J Cancer 1987;55:225–226.

450. Non-Hodgkin's Lymphoma Cooperative Study Group. Randomized study of chlorambucil (CB) compared to interferon (alfa-2b) combined with CB in low-grade non-Hodgkin's lymphoma: An interim report of a randomized study. Eur J Cancer 1991;27(suppl 4):31–33.

451. Price CGA, Rohatiner AZS, Steward W, et al. Interferon-α2b in the treatment of follicular lymphoma: Preliminary results of a trial in progress. Ann Oncol 1991;2(suppl 2):141–145.

452. Tourani J-M, Levy V, Briere J, et al. Interleukin-2 therapy for refractory and relapsing lymphomas. Eur J Cancer 1991;27:1676–1680.

453. Weber JS, Yang JC, Topalian SL, et al. The use of interleukin-2 and lymphokine-activated killer cells for the treatment of patients with non-Hodgkin's lymphoma. J Clin Oncol 1992;10:33–40.

454. Bernstein ZP, Vaickus L, Friedman N, et al. Interleukin-2 lymphokine-activated killer cell therapy of non-Hodgkin's lymphoma and Hodgkin's disease. J Immunotherapy 1991;10:141–146.

455. Margolin KA, Aronson FR, Sznol M, et al. Phase II trial of high-dose interleukin-2 and lymphokine activated killer cells in Hodgkin's disease and non-Hodgkin's lymphoma. J Immunotherapy 1991;10:214–220.

456. Meeker T, Lowder J, Maloney DG, et al. A clinical trial of anti-idiotype therapy for B cell lymphoma. Blood 1985;65:1349–1363.

457. Rankin EM, Hekman A, Somers R, et al. Treatment of two patients with B cell lymphoma with monoclonal anti-idiotype antibodies. Blood 1985;65:1373–1381.

458. Press OW, Appelbaum F, Ledbetter JA, et al. Monoclonal antibody 1F5 (anti-CD20) serotherapy of human B cell lymphomas. Blood 1987;69:584–591.

459. Dyer MJS, Hale G, Hayhoe FGJ, et al. Effects of CAMPATH-1 antibodies in vivo in patients with lymphoid malignancies: Influence of antibody isotype. Blood 1989;73:1431–1439.

460. Scheinberg SA, Straus DJ, Yeh SD, et al. A phase I toxicity, pharmacology, and dosimetry trial of monoclonal antibody OKB7 in patients with non-Hodgkin's lymphoma: Effects of tumor burden and antigen expression. J Clin Oncol 1990;8:792–803.

461. Meeker T, Lowder J, Cleary ML, et al. Emergence of idiotype variants during treatment of B-cell lymphoma with anti-idiotype antibodies. N Engl J Med 1985;312:1658–1665.

462. Raffeld M, Neckers L, Longo DL, et al. Spontaneous alteration of idiotype in a monoclonal B-cell lymphoma: Escape from detection by anti-idiotype. N Engl J Med 1985;312:1653–1658.

463. Zelenetz AD, Campbell MJ, Bahler DW, et al. Follicular lymphoma: A model of lymphoid progression in man. Ann Oncol 1991;2(suppl 2):115–122.

464. Nourigat C, Badger CC, Bernstein ID. Treatment of lymphoma with radiolabeled antibody: Elimination of tumor cells lacking target antigen. JNCI 1990;82:47–50.

465. Knox SJ, Levy R, Miller RA, et al. Determinants of the antitumor effect of radiolabeled monoclonal antibodies. Cancer Res 1990;50:4935–4940.

466. Press OW, Eary JF, Badger CC, et al. Treatment of refractory non-Hodgkin's lymphoma with radiolabeled MB-1 (anti-CD37) antibody. J Clin Oncol 1989;7:1027–1038.

467. DeNardo GL, DeNardo SJ, O'Grady LF, et al. Fractionated radioimmunotherapy of B-cell malignancies with ^{131}I-Lym-1. Cancer Res 1990;50:1014S–1016S.

468. O'Grady L, DeNardo S, Lewis J, et al. Radioimmunotherapy of lymphoma. Blood [Abstract 1452] 1990;76(suppl 1):365a.

469. Rosen ST, Zimmer AM, Goldman-Leikin R, et al. Radioimmunodetection and radioimmunotherapy of cutaneous T cell lymphomas using an ^{131}I-labeled monoclonal antibody: An Illinois Cancer Council study. J Clin Oncol 1987;5:562–573.

470. Stone M, Amlot P, Fay J, et al. Immunotoxin therapy of B cell lymphoma. Blood [Abstract 1488] 1990;76:374a.

471. Nadler L, Beitmeyer J, Grossbard M, et al. Anti-B4 blocked ricin immunotherapy for patients with B-cell malignancies: Phase I trial of 7 day continuous infusion. Blood [Abstract 1448] 1990;76:364a.

472. Cheson BD. The purine analogs—A therapeutic beauty contest. J Clin Oncol 1992;10:352–355.

473. Grever MR, Leiby JM, Kraut EH, et al. Low-dose deoxycoformycin in lymphoid malignancy. J Clin Oncol 1985;3:1196–1201.

474. Hochster HS, Kim K, Green MD, et al. Activity of fludarabine in previously treated non-Hodgkin's low-grade lymphoma: Results of an Eastern Cooperative Oncology Group study. J Clin Oncol 1992;10:28–32.

475. Whelan JS, Davis CL, Rule S, et al. Fludarabine phosphate for the treatment of low grade lymphoid malignancy. Br J Cancer 1991;64:120–123.

476. Kay AC, Saven A, Carrera CJ, et al. 2-Chlorodeoxyadenosine treatment of low-grade lymphomas. J Clin Oncol 1992;10:371–377.

477. Hainsworth JD, Johnson DH, Frazier SR, et al. Chronic daily administration of oral etoposide in refractory lymphoma. Eur J Cancer 1990;26:818–821.

478. Steward WP, Smith DB, Crowther D. Weekly oral 4-demethoxydaunorubicin in patients with relapsed low grade non-Hodgkin's lymphoma. Ann Oncol 1991;2:605–606.

479. Case DC Jr, Hayes DM, Gerber M, et al. Phase II study of oral idarubicin in favorable histology non-Hodgkin's lymphoma. Cancer Res 1990;50:6833–6835.

480. Greer JP, York JC, Cousar JB, et al. Peripheral T-cell lymphoma: A clinicopathologic study of 42 cases. J Clin Oncol 1984;2:788–798.

481. Pinkus GS, O'Hara CJ, Said JW. Peripheral/post-thymic T-cell lymphomas: A spectrum of disease. Clinical, pathologic, and immunologic features of 78 cases. Cancer 1990;65:971–998.

482. Lippman SM, Miller TP, Spier CM, et al. The prognostic significance of the immunotype in diffuse large-cell lymphoma: A comparative study of the T-cell and B-cell phenotype. Blood 1988;72:436–441.

483. Coiffier B, Brousse N, Peuchmaur M, et al. Peripheral T-cell lymphomas have a worse prognosis than B-cell lymphomas: A prospective study of 361 immunophenotyped patients treated with the LNH-84 regimen. Ann Oncol 1990;1:45–50.

484. Stein RS, Greer JP, Flexner JM, et al. Large cell lymphomas: Clinical and prognostic features. J Clin Oncol 1990;8:1370–1379.

485. Miller TP, Lippman SM, Spier CM, et al. HLA-DR (Ia) immune phenotype predicts outcome for patients with diffuse large cell lymphoma. J Clin Invest 1988;82:370–372.

486. O'Keane JC, Mack C, Lynch E, et al. Prognostic correlation of HLA-DR expression in large cell lymphoma as determined by LN3 antibody staining. An Eastern Cooperative Oncology Group (ECOG) study. Cancer 1990;66:1147–1153.

487. Hall PA, Richards MA, Gregory WM, et al. The prognostic value of Ki67 immunostaining in non-Hodgkin's lymphoma. J Pathol 1988;154:223–235.

488. Slymen DJ, Miller TP, Lippman SM, et al. Immunobiologic factors predictive of clinical outcome in diffuse large-cell lymphoma. J Clin Oncol 1990;8:986–993.

489. Brandt L, Johnson A, Olsson M. Mitotic activity and survival in advanced non-Hodgkin's lymphoma of unfavourable histology. Eur J Cancer 1990;26:227–230.

490. Jalkanen S, Joensuu H, Klemi P. Prognostic value of lymphocyte homing receptor and S phase fraction in non-Hodgkin's lymphoma. Blood 1990;75:1549–1556.

491. Jalkanen S, Joensuu H, Soderstrom K-O, et al. Lymphocyte homing and clinical behavior of non-Hodgkin's lymphoma. J Clin Invest 1991;87:1835–1840.

492. Horst E, Meijer CJLM, Radaszkiewica T, et al. Adhesion molecules in the prognosis of diffuse large-cell lymphoma: Expression of a lymphocyte homing receptor (CD44), LFA-1 (CD11a/18), and ICAM-1 (CD54). Leukemia 1990;4:595–599.

493. Levine EG, Arthur DC, Frizzera G, et al. Cytogenetic abnormalities predict clinical outcome in non-Hodgkin's lymphoma. Ann Intern Med 1988;108:14–20.

494. Cabanillas F, Pathak S, Grant G, et al. Refractoriness to chemotherapy and poor survival related to abnormalities of chromosomes 17 and 7 in lymphoma. Am J Med 1989;87:167–172.

495. Schouten HC, Sanger WG, Weisenburger DD, et al. Chromosomal abnormalities in untreated patients with non-Hodgkin's lymphoma: Associations with histology, clinical characteristics, and treatment outcome. Blood 1990;75:1841–1847.

496. Schouten HC, Sanger WG, Weisenburger DD, et al. Abnormalities involving chromosome 6 in newly diagnosed patients with non-Hodgkin's lymphoma. Nebraska Lymphoma Study Group. Cancer Genet Cytogenet 1990;47:73–82.

497. Fisher RI, Hubbard SM, DeVita VT Jr, et al. Factors predicting long-term survival in diffuse mixed, histiocytic or undifferentiated lymphoma. Blood 1981;58:45–51.

498. Danieu L, Wong G, Koziner B, et al. Predictive model for prognosis in advanced diffuse histiocytic lymphoma. Cancer Res 1986;46:5372–5379.

499. Velasquez WS, Jagannath S, Tucker SL, et al. Risk classification as the basis for clinical staging of diffuse large-cell lymphoma derived from 10-year survival data. Blood 1989;74:551–557.

500. Coiffier B, Lepage E. Prognosis of aggressive lymphomas: A study of five prognostic models with patients included in the LNH-84 regimen. Blood 1989;74:558–564.

501. Swan F Jr, Velasquez WS, Tucker S, et al. A new serologic staging system for large cell lymphomas based on initial beta₂-microglobulin and lactate dehydrogenase levels. J Clin Oncol 1989;7:1518–1527.

502. Harrington DS, Patil K, Lai PK, et al. Soluble interleukin 2 receptors in patients with malignant lymphoma. Arch Pathol Lab Med 1988;112:597–601.

503. Abate G, Coimella P, Marfella A, et al. Prognostic relevance of urinary neopterin in non-Hodgkin's lymphomas. Cancer 1989;63:484–489.

504. Sebban C, Lasne Y, Bernguer V, et al. CA 125 and malignant lymphomas. J Clin Oncol 1990;8:359–360.

505. Coiffier B, Shipp MA, Cabanillas F, et al. Report of the first workshop on prognostic factors in large-cell lymphoma. Ann Oncol 1991;2(suppl 2):213–217.

506. Cabanillas F, Bodey GP, Freireich EJ. Management with chemotherapy only of stage I and II malignant lymphoma of aggressive histologic types. Cancer 1980;46:2356–2361.

507. Miller TP, Jones SE. Initial chemotherapy for clinically localized lymphomas of unfavorable histology. Blood 1984;62:413–417.

508. Connors JM, Klimo P, Fairey RN, et al. Brief chemotherapy and involved field radiation therapy for limited-stage histologically aggressive lymphoma. Ann Intern Med 1987;107:25–29.

509. Longo DL, Glatstein E, Duffey PL, et al. Treatment of localized aggressive lymphomas with combination chemotherapy followed by involved-field radiation therapy. J Clin Oncol 1989;7:1295–1302.

510. Jones SE, Miller TP, Connors JM. Long-term follow-up and analysis for prognostic factors for patients with limited-stage diffuse large-cell lymphoma treated with initial chemotherapy with or without adjuvant radiotherapy. J Clin Oncol 1989;7:1186–1191.

511. Jones SE, Fuks Z, Kaplan HS, et al. Non-Hodgkin's lymphomas. V. Results of radiotherapy. Cancer 1973;32:682–691.

512. Reddy S, Saxena VS, Pelletiere EV, et al. Stage I and II non-Hodgkin's lymphomas: Long-term results of radiation therapy. Int J Radiat Oncol Biol Phys 1989;16:687–692.

513. Hagberg H, Pettersson U, Glimelius B, et al. Prognostic factors in non-Hodgkin lymphoma stage I treated with radiotherapy. Acta Oncol 1989;28:45–50.

514. Vokes EE, Ultmann JE, Golomb HM, et al. Long-term survival of patients with localized diffuse histiocytic lymphoma. J Clin Oncol 1985;3:1309–1317.

515. Hallahan DE, Farah R, Vokes EE, et al. The patterns of failure in patients with pathological stage I and II diffuse histiocytic lymphoma treated with radiation therapy alone. Int J Radiat Oncol Biol Phys 1989;17:767–771.

516. Kaminski MS, Coleman CN, Colby TV, et al. Factors predicting survival in adults with stage I and II large-cell lymphoma-treated with primary radiation therapy. Ann Intern Med 1986;104:747–756.

517. Prestidge BR, Horning SJ, Hoppe RT. Combined modality therapy for stage I–II large cell lymphoma. Int J Radiat Biol Oncol Phys 1988;15:633–639.

518. Armitage JO, Wen BC. Chemotherapy in patients who fail radiotherapy for diffuse aggressive non-Hodgkin's lymphoma. Int J Radiat Oncol Biol Phys 1987;13:1351–1354.

519. Shepherd FA, Evans WK, Kutas G, et al. Chemotherapy following surgery for stages IE and IIE non-Hodgkin's lymphoma of the gastrointestinal tract. J Clin Oncol 1988;6:253–260.

520. Azab MB, Henry-Amar M, Rougier P, et al. Prognostic factors in primary gastrointestinal non-Hodgkin's lymphoma. A multivariate analysis, report of 106 cases, and review of the literature. Cancer 1989;64:1208–1217.

521. Bellesi G, Alterini R, Messori A, et al. Combined surgery and chemotherapy for the treatment of primary gastrointestinal intermediate-or high-grade non-Hodgkin's lymphomas. Br J Cancer 1989;60:244–248.

522. Romaguera JE, Velasquez WS, Silvermintz KB, et al. Surgical debulking is associated with improved survival in stage I–II diffuse large cell lymphoma. Cancer 1990;66:267–272.

523. Burgers JMV, Taal BG, vanHeerde P, et al. Treatment results of primary stage I and II non-Hodgkin's lymphoma of the stomach. Radiother Oncol 1988;11:319–326.

524. Jones RE, Willis S, Innes DJ, et al. Primary gastric lymphoma. Problems in staging and management. Am J Surg 1988;155:118–122.

525. Mentzer SJ, Osteen RT, Pappas TN, et al. Surgical therapy of localized abdominal non-Hodgkin's lymphoma. Surgery 1988;103:609–614.

526. Kajanti M, Karkinen-Jaaskelainen M, Rissanen P. Primary gastrointestinal non-Hodgkin's lymphoma. A review of 36 cases. Acta Oncol 1988;27:51–55.

527. Tabbane F, Mourali N, Cammoun M, et al. Results of laparotomy in immunoproliferative small intestinal disease. Cancer 1988;61:1699–1706.

528. Rogers P, Hill I, Sinclair-Smith C, et al. Clinical and pathological evolution of alpha chain disease to immunoblastic lymphoma and response to COMP chemotherapy. Med Pediatr Oncol 1988;16:128–131.

529. Maor MH, Velasquez WS, Fuller LM, et al. Stomach conservation in stages IE and IIE gastric non-Hodgkin's lymphoma. J Clin Oncol 1990;8:266–271.

530. Schein PS, DeVita VT Jr, Hubbard SM, et al. Bleomycin, Adriamycin, cyclophosphamide, vincristine, and prednisone (BACOP) combination chemotherapy in the treatment of advanced diffuse histiocytic lymphoma. Ann Intern Med 1976;85:417–422.

531. Berd D, Cornog J, De Conti RC, et al. Long-term remission in diffuse histiocytic lymphoma treated with combination sequential chemotherapy. Cancer 1975;35:1050–1054.

532. Gaynor ER, Ultmann JE, Golomb HM, et al. Treatment of diffuse histiocytic lymphoma (DHL) with COMLA (cyclophosphamide, oncovin, methotrexate, leucovorin, cytosine arabinoside): A 10-year experience in a single institution. J Clin Oncol 1985;3:1596–1604.

533. McKelvey EM, Gottlieb JA, Wilson HE, et al. Hydroxydaunomycin (Adriamycin) combination chemotherapy in malignant lymphoma. Cancer 1976;38:1484–1493.

534. Coltman CA Jr, Dahlberg S, Jones SE, et al. CHOP is curative in 30 percent of patients with large cell lymphoma: A 12-year Southwest Oncology Group follow-up. In: Skarin AT, ed. Advances in cancer chemotherapy: Update on treatment for diffuse large cell lymphoma. New York: Park Row, 1986:71–77.

535. Skarin AT, Canellos GP, Rosenthal DS, et al. Improved prognosis of diffuse histiocytic and undifferentiated lymphoma by use of high-dose methotrexate alternating with standard agents (M-BACOD). J Clin Oncol 1983;1:91–98.

536. Shipp MA, Yeap BY, Harrington DP, et al. The m-BACOD combination chemotherapy regimen in large-cell lymphoma: Analysis of the completed trial and comparison with the M-BACOD regimen. J Clin Oncol 1990;8:84–93.

537. Laurence J, Coleman M, Allen SL, et al. Combination chemotherapy of advanced diffuse histiocytic lymphoma with the six-drug COP-BLAM regimen. Ann Intern Med 1982;97:190–195.

538. Coleman M, Gerstein G, Topilow A, et al. Advances in chemotherapy for large cell lymphoma. Semin Hematol 1987;24:8–20.

539. Todd M, Cadman E, Spiro P, et al. A follow-up of a randomized study comparing two chemotherapy treatments for advanced diffuse histiocytic lymphoma. J Clin Oncol 1984;2:986–993.

540. Fisher RI, DeVita VT Jr, Hubbard SM, et al. Diffuse aggressive lymphomas: Increased survival after alternating flexible sequences of ProMACE and MOPP chemotherapy. Ann Intern Med 1983;98:304–309.

541. Longo DL, DeVita VT Jr, Duffey PL, et al. Superiority of ProMACE-CytaBOM over ProMACE-MOPP in the treatment of advanced diffuse aggressive lymphoma: Results of a prospective randomized trial. J Clin Oncol 1991;9:25–28.

542. Boyd DB, Coleman M, Papish SW, et al. COPBLAM III: Infusional combination chemotherapy for diffuse large-cell lymphoma. J Clin Oncol 1988;6:425–433.

543. Baer MR, Stein RS, Greer JP, et al. Modified cyclophosphamide, vincristine, methotrexate, leucovorin, and cytarabine (COMLA) in intermediate-and high-grade lymphoma: An effective short course regimen. Cancer Treat Rep 1986;70:785–787.

544. Klimo P, Connors JM. MACOP-B chemotherapy for the treatment of diffuse large-cell lymphoma. Ann Intern Med 1985;102:596–602.

545. O'Reilly SE, Hoskins P, Klimo P, et al. MACOP-B and VACOP-B in diffuse large cell lymphomas and MOPP/ABV in Hodgkin's disease. Ann Oncol 1991;2(suppl 1):17–23.

546. Guglielmi C, Amadori S, Martelli M, et al. The F-MACHOP sequential combination chemotherapy regimen in advanced diffuse aggressive lymphomas: Long-term results. Ann Oncol 1991;2:365–371.

547. Coiffier B, Gisselbrecht C, Herbrecht R, et al. LNH-84 regimen: A multicenter study of intensive chemotherapy in 737 patients with aggressive malignant lymphoma. J Clin Oncol 1989;7:1018–1026.

548. Gulati SC, Shank B, Black P, et al. Autologous bone marrow transplantation for patients with poor-prognosis lymphoma. J Clin Oncol 1988;6:1303–1313.

549. Schneider AM, Straus DJ, Schluger AE, et al. Treatment results with an aggressive chemotherapeutic regimen (MACOP-B) for intermediate- and some high-grade non-Hodgkin's lymphomas. J Clin Oncol 1990;8:94–102.

550. Weick JK, Dahlberg S, Fisher RI, et al. Combination chemotherapy of intermediate-grade and high-grade non-Hodgkin's lymphoma with MACOP-B: A Southwest Oncology Group study. J Clin Oncol 1991;9:748–753.

551. Vitolo U, Bertini M, Brusamolino E, et al. MACOP-B treatment in diffuse large-cell lymphoma: Identification of prognostic groups in an Italian multicenter study. J Clin Oncol 1992;10:219–227.

552. Miller TP, Dahlberg S, Weick JK, et al. Unfavorable histologies of non-Hodgkin's lymphoma treated with ProMACE-CytaBOM: A group-wide Southwest Oncology Group study. J Clin Oncol 1990;8:1951–1958.

553. Longo DL, Duffey PL, DeVita VT Jr, et al. The calculation of actual or received dose intensity: A comparison of published methods. J Clin Oncol 1991;9:2042–2051.

554. Hryniuk WM, Goodyear M. The calculation of received dose intensity. J Clin Oncol 1990;8:1935–1937.

555. Fisher RI, Gaynor E, Dahlberg S, et al. A phase III comparison of CHOP vs. m-BACOD vs. ProMACE-CytaBOM vs. MACOP-B in patients with intermediate or high-grade non-Hodgkin's lymphoma: Preliminary results of SWOG-8516 (Intergroup 0067), the national high priority lymphoma study. Proc Am Soc Clin Oncol [Abstract 1067] 1992;11:315.

556. Meyer RM, Hryniuk WM, Goodyear MDE. The role of dose intensity in determining outcome in intermediate-grade non-Hodgkin's lymphoma. J Clin Oncol 1991;9:339–347.

557. DeVita VT Jr, Hubbard SM, Longo DL. The chemotherapy of lymphomas: Looking back, moving forward—The Richard and Linda Rosenthal Foundation Award lecture. Cancer Res 1987;47:5810–5824.

558. Kwak LW, Halpern J, Olshen RA, et al. Prognostic significance of actual dose intensity in diffuse large-cell lymphoma: Results of a tree-structured survival analysis. J Clin Oncol 1990;8:963–977.

559. Epelbaum R, Faraggi D, Ben-Arie Y, et al. Survival of diffuse large cell lymphoma. A multivariate analysis including dose intensity variables. Cancer 1990;66:1124–1129.

560. Banavali SD, Advani SH, Gopal R, et al. Continuous cyclophosphamide, doxorubicin, vincristine, and prednisolone. A new, innovative protocol for diffuse aggressive lymphomas. Cancer 1990;65:1704–1710.

561. Lee R, Cabanillas F, Bodey GP, et al. A 10-year update of CHOP-bleo in the treatment of diffuse large-cell lymphoma. J Clin Oncol 1986;4:1455–1461.

562. Goldie JH, Coldman AJ. The genetic origin of drug resistance in neoplasms: Implications for systemic therapy. Cancer Res 1984;44:3643–3653.

563. Carde P, Meerwaldt JH, van Glabbeke M, et al. Superiority of second over first generation chemotherapy in a randomized trial for stage II-IV intermediate and high-grade non-Hodgkin's lymphoma: The 1980–1985 EORTC trial. Ann Oncol 1991;2:431–435.

564. Browne MJ, Hubbard SM, Longo DL, et al. Excess prevalence of *Pneumocystis carinii* pneumonia in patients treated for lymphoma with combination chemotherapy. Ann Intern Med 1986;104:338–344.

565. Gherlinzoni F, Guglielmi C, Mazza P, et al. Phase III comparative trial (M-BACOD v M-BNCOD) in the treatment of stage II to IV non-Hodgkin's lymphomas with intermediate- or high-grade histology. Semin Oncol 1990;17(suppl 10):3–8.

566. Vose JM, Armitage JO, Weisenburger DD, et al. The importance of age in survival of patients treated with chemotherapy for aggressive non-Hodgkin's lymphoma. J Clin Oncol 1988;6:1838–1844.

567. Dixon DO, Neilan B, Jones SE, et al. Effect of age on therapeutic outcome in advanced diffuse histiocytic lymphoma: The Southwest Oncology Group experience. J Clin Oncol 1986;4:295–305.

568. O'Reilly SE, Klimo P, Connors JM. Low-dose ACOP-B and VABE weekly chemotherapy for elderly patients with advanced-stage diffuse large-cell lymphoma. J Clin Oncol 1991;9:741–747.

569. Sonneveld P, Michiels JJ. Full dose chemotherapy in elderly patients with non-Hodgkin's lymphoma: A feasibility study using a mitoxantrone containing regimen. Br J Cancer 1990;62:105–108.

570. Tokudome S, Tokunaga O, Shimamoto Y, et al. Incidence of adult T-cell leukemia/lymphoma among human T-lymphotropic virus type I carriers in Saga, Japan. Cancer Res 1989;49:226–228.

571. Yano T, van Krieken JHJM, Magrath IT, et al. Histogenetic correlations between subcategories of small noncleaved cell lymphomas. Blood 1992;79:1282–1290.

572. McMaster ML, Greer JP, Greco FA, et al. Effective treatment of small-noncleaved-cell lymphoma with high-intensity, brief duration chemotherapy. J Clin Oncol 1991;9:941–946.

573. Straus DJ, Wong GY, Liu J, et al. Small non-cleaved-cell lymphoma (undifferentiated lymphoma, Burkitt's type) in American adults: Results with treatment designed for acute lymphoblastic leukemia. Am J Med 1991;90:328–337.

574. Magrath IT, Janus C, Edwards BK, et al. An effective therapy for both undifferentiated (including Burkitt's) lymphomas and lymphoblastic lymphomas in children and young adults. Blood 1984;63:1102–1108.

575. Schwenn MR, Blattner SR, Lynch E, et al. HiC-COM: A 2-month intensive chemotherapy regimen for children with stage III and IV Burkitt's lymphoma and B-cell acute lymphoblastic leukemia. J Clin Oncol 1991;9:133–138.

576. Nathwani BN, Diamond LW, Winberg CD, et al. Lymphoblastic lymphoma: A clinicopathologic study of 95 patients. Cancer 1981;48:2347–2356.

577. Voakes JB, Jones SE, McKelvey EM. The chemotherapy of lymphoblastic lymphoma. Blood 1981;57:186–191.

578. Weinstein HJ, Cassady JR, Levey R. Long-term results of the APO protocol (vincristine, doxorubicin [Adriamycin], and prednisone) for the treatment of mediastinal lymphoblastic lymphoma. J Clin Oncol 1983;1:537–544.

579. Wollner N, Wachtel AE, Exelby PR, et al. Improved prognosis in children with intraabdominal non-Hodgkin's lymphoma following LSA$_2$-L$_2$ protocol chemotherapy. Cancer 1980;45:3034–3039.

580. Coleman CN, Picozzi VJ Jr, Cox RS, et al. Treatment of lymphoblastic lymphoma in adults. J Clin Oncol 1986;4:1628–1636.

581. Santini G, Coser P, Chisesi T, et al. Autologous bone marrow transplantation for advanced

stage adult lymphoblastic lymphoma in first complete remission. Report of the Non-Hodgkin's Lymphoma Cooperative Study Group. Ann Oncol 1991;2(suppl 2):181–185.

582. Shimamoto Y, Ono K, Sano M, et al. Difference in prognostic factors between leukemia and lymphoma type of adult T-cell leukemia. Cancer 1989;63:289–294.

583. Waldmann TA. Multichain interleukin-2 receptor: A target for immunotherapy in lymphoma. JNCI 1989;81:914–923.

584. Sirakawa F, Tanaka Y, Oda S, et al. Autocrine stimulation of interleukin-1α in the growth of adult human T-cell leukemia cells. Cancer Res 1989;49:1143–1147.

585. Eby NL, Grufferman S, Flannelly CM, et al. Increasing incidence of primary brain lymphoma in the US. Cancer 1988;62:2461–2465.

586. Jack CR Jr, Reese DF, Scheithauer BW. Radiographic findings in 32 cases of primary CNS lymphoma. AJR 1986;146:271–279.

587. Pollack IF, Lunsford LD, Flickinger JC, et al. Prognostic factors in the diagnosis and treatment of primary central nervous system lymphoma. Cancer 1989;63:939–947.

588. Shibamoto Y, Tsutsui K, Dodo Y, et al. Improved survival rate in primary intracranial lymphoma treated by high-dose radiation and systemic vincristine-doxorubicin-cyclophosphamide-prednisolone chemotherapy. Cancer 1990;65:1907–1912.

589. Gabbai AA, Hochberg FH, Linggood RM, et al. High-dose methotrexate for non-AIDS primary central nervous system lymphoma. Report of 13 cases. J Neurosurg 1989;70:190–194.

590. McLaughlin P, Velasquez WS, Redman JR, et al. Chemotherapy with dexamethasone, high-dose cytarabine, and cisplatin for parenchymal brain lymphoma. JNCI 1988;80:1408–1412.

591. Neuwelt EA, Dahlberg SA, Goldman D, et al. Significant prolongation of survival of primary CNS lymphoma patients by combination chemotherapy given in association with osmotic blood-brain barrier disruption. Proc Am Assoc Cancer Res [Abstract 1050] 1989;30:264.

592. Chamberlain MC, Levin VA. Adjuvant chemotherapy for primary lymphoma of the central nervous system. Arch Neurol 1990;47:1113–1116.

593. Giannone K, Greco FA, Hainsworth JD. Combination intraventricular chemotherapy for meningeal neoplasia. J Clin Oncol 1986;4:68–74.

594. Ziegler JL, Beckstead JA, Volberding PA, et al. Non-hodgkin's lymphoma in 90 homosexual men. Relation to generalized lymphadenopathy and the acquired immunodeficiency syndrome. N Engl J Med 1984;311:565–570.

595. Beral V, Peterman T, Berkelman R, et al. AIDS-associated non-Hodgkin lymphoma. Lancet 1991;337:805–809.

596. Pluda JM, Yarchoan R, Broder S. The occurrence of opportunistic non-Hodgkin's lymphomas in the setting of infection with the human immunodeficiency virus. Ann Oncol 1991;2(suppl 2):191–200.

597. Pluda JM, Yarchoan R, Jaffe ES, et al. Development of non-Hodgkin lymphoma in a cohort of patients with severe human immunodeficiency virus (HIV) infection on long-term antiretroviral therapy. Ann Intern Med 1990;113:276–282.

598. Gill PS, Levine AM, Krailo M, et al. AIDS-related malignant lymphoma: Results of prospective treatment trials. J Clin Oncol 1987;5:1322–1328.

599. Knowles, DM, Chamulak GA, Subar M, et al. Lymphoid neoplasia associated with the acquired immunodeficiency syndrome (AIDS). Ann Intern Med 1988;108:744–753.

600. Lowenthal DA, Straus DJ, Campbell SW, et al. AIDS-related lymphoid neoplasia. Cancer 1988;61:2325–2337.

601. Kaplan LD, Abrams DI, Feigal E, et al. AIDS-associated non-Hodgkin's lymphoma in San Francisco. JAMA 1989;261:719–724.

602. Bermudez MA, Grant KM, Rodvien R, et al. Non-Hodgkin's lymphoma in a population with or at risk for acquired immunodeficiency syndrome: Indications for intensive chemotherapy. Am J Med 1989;86:71–76.

603. Levine AM. Lymphoma in acquired immunodeficiency syndrome. Semin Oncol 1990;17:104–112.

604. Roithmann S, Toledano M, Tourani JM, et al. HIV-associated non-Hodgkin's lymphomas: Clinical characteristics and outcome. The experience of the French registry of HIV-associated tumors. Ann Oncol 1991;2:289–295.

605. Gill PS, Levine AM. HIV-related malignant lymphoma: Clinical aspects, treatment and pathogenesis. Cancer Invest 1988;6:413–416.

606. Freter CE. Acquired immunodeficiency syndrome-associated lymphomas. JNCI Monogr 1990;10:45–54.

607. Boyle MJ, Swanson CE, Turner JJ, et al. Definition of two distinct types of AIDS-associated non-Hodgkin lymphoma. Br J Haemtol 1990;76:506–512.

608. Shiramizu B, Herndier B, Meeker T, et al. Molecular and immunophenotypic characterization of AIDS-associated, Epstein-Barr virus-negative, polyclonal lymphoma. J Clin Oncol 1992;10:383–389.

609. Kaplan LD, Kahn JO, Crowe S, et al. Clinical and virologic effects of recombinant human granulocyte-macrophage colony-stimulating factor in patients receiving chemotherapy for human immunodeficiency virus-associated non-Hodgkin's lymphoma: Results of a randomized trial. J Clin Oncol 1991;9:929–940.

610. Levine AM, Wernz JC, Kaplan L, et al. Low-dose chemotherapy with central nervous system prophylaxis and zidovudine maintenance in AIDS-related lymphoma. A prospective multi-institutional trial. JAMA 1991;266:84–88.

611. Armitage JO. Bone marrow transplantation in the treatment of patients with lymphoma. Blood 1989;73:1749–1758.

612. Gribben JG, Goldstone AH, Linch DH, et al. Effectiveness of high-dose combination chemotherapy and autologous bone marrow transplantation for patients with non-Hodgkin's lymphomas who are still responsive to conventional-dose therapy. J Clin Oncol 1989;7:1621–1629.

613. Philip T, Chauvin F, Armitage J, et al. PARMA international protocol: Pilot study of DHAP followed by involved-field radiotherapy and BEAC with autologous bone marrow transplantation. Blood 1991;77:1587–1592.

614. Chao NJ, Rosenberg SA, Horning SJ. CEPP(B): An effective and well-tolerated regimen in poor-risk, aggressive non-Hodgkin's lymphoma. Blood 1990;76:1293–1298.

615. Longo DL, DeVita VT Jr. Lymphomas. Cancer Chemother Biol Response Modif 1992;13:349–403.

616. Philip T, Chauvin F, Bron D, et al. PARMA international protocol: Pilot study on 50 patients and preliminary analysis of the ongoing randomized study (62 patients). Ann Oncol 1991;2(suppl 1):57–64.

617. Moormeier JA, Williams SF, Kaminer LS, et al. High-dose tri-alkylator chemotherapy with autologous stem cell rescue in patients with refractory malignancies. JNCI 1990;82:29–34.

618. Glenn LD, Armitage JO, Bierman PH, et al. High-dose BCNU, etoposide, cytoxan and hydroxyurea (BECH) with autologous hematopoietic stem cell support for poor prognosis non-Hodgkin's lymphoma. Proc Am Assoc Cancer Res [Abstract 929] 1989;30:234.

619. Brandwein JM, Callum J, Sutcliffe SB, et al. Analysis of factors affecting hematopoietic recovery after autologous bone marrow transplantation for lymphoma. Bone Marrow Transplant 1990;6:292–294.

620. Kessinger A, Armitage JO, Smith DM, et al. High-dose therapy and autologous peripheral blood stem cell transplantation for patients with lymphoma. Blood 1989;74:1260–1265.

621. Gianni AM, Siena S, Bregni M, et al. Granulocyte-macrophage colony-stimulating factor to harvest circulating heamopoietic cells for autotransplantation. Lancet 1989;2:580–585.

622. Nemunaitis J, Rabinowe SN, Singer JW, et al. Recombinant granulocyte-macrophage colony-stimulating factor after autologous bone marrow transplantation for lymphoid cancer. N Engl J Med 1991;324:1773–1777.

623. Gianni AM, Bregni M, Siena S, et al. Recombinant human granulocyte-macrophage colony-stimulating factor reduces hematologic toxicity and widens clinical applicability of high-dose cyclophosphamide treatment in breast cancer and non-Hodgkin's lymphoma. J Clin Oncol 1990;8:768–778.

624. Ho AD, Del Valle F, Engelhard M, et al. Mitoxantrone/high-dose ara-C and recombinant human GM-CSF in the treatment of refractory non-Hodgkin's lymphoma. A pilot study. Cancer 1990;66:423–430.

625. Smith JW II, Longo DL, Alvord W, et al. Thrombopoietic effects of IL-1α in combination with high-dose carboplatin. Proc Am Soc Clin Oncol [Abstract 820] 1992;11:252.

626. Salmon SE, Grogan TM, Miller T, et al. Prediction of doxorubicin resistance in vitro in myeloma, lymphoma, and breast cancer by P-glycoprotein staining. JNCI 1989;81:696–701.

627. Miller TP, Grogan TM, Dalton WS, et al. P-glycoprotein expression in malignant lymphoma and reversal of clinical drug resistance with chemotherapy plus high-dose verapamil. J Clin Oncol 1991;9:17–24.

628. Wilson WH, Bryant G, Bates S, et al. Infusional etoposide (E), vincristine (O) and Adriamycin (H) with cyclophosphamide (C), prednisone (P) (EPOCH) and R-verapamil (RV) in relapsed lymphoma. Proc Am Soc Clin Oncol [Abstract 956] 1991;10:275.

629. Schauer PK, Straus DJ, Bagley DM Jr, et al. Angioimmunoblastic lymphadenopathy: Clinical spectrum of disease. Cancer 1981;48:2493–2498.

630. Steinberg AD, Seldin MF, Jaffe ES, et al. Angioimmunoblastic lymphoadenopathy with dysproteinemia. Ann Intern Med 1988;108:575–578.

631. Klinman DM, Steinberg AD, Mushinski JF. Effect of cyclophosphamide therapy on oncogene expression in angioimmunoblastic lymphadenopathy. Lancet 1986;2:1055–1057.

632. Repetto L, Jaiprakash MP, Selby PJ, et al. Aggressive angiofollicular lymph node hyperplasia (Castleman's disease) treated with high dose melphalan and autologous bone marrow transplantation. Hematol Oncol 1986;4:213–217.

633. Lipford EH Jr, Margolick JB, Longo DL, et al. Angiocentric immunoproliferative lesions: A clinicopathologic spectrum of post-thymic T-cell proliferations. Blood 1988;72:1674–1681.

Cancer: Principles & Practice of Oncology, Fourth Edition,
edited by Vincent T. DeVita, Jr., Samuel Hellman, Steven A. Rosenberg.
J.B. Lippincott Co., Philadelphia © 1993.

Paul A. Bunn, Jr
Richard T. Hoppe

CHAPTER **53**

Cutaneous Lymphomas

Investigating the functional, phenotypic, and genotypic properties of normal T lymphocytes and their malignant counterparts produced a better understanding of the biology and classification of T-cell lymphomas.[1-6] Advances in molecular biology and virology led to the discovery of a new T-cell lymphoma called acute T-cell leukemia-lymphoma (ATLL) caused by a type C retrovirus, human T-cell lymphotrophic virus-I (HTLV-I).[7,8] It is possible that other T-cell malignancies, including mycosis fungoides and the Sézary syndrome, are caused by related viruses. HTLV-V, a putative etiologic virus for the cutaneous T-cell lymphomas (CTCL), has been described.[9]

T-cell lymphomas in the United States are much less common than B-cell lymphomas. Peripheral T-cell lymphomas, T-cell chronic lymphocytic leukemia (CLL), and T-γ lymphoproliferative disorders are discussed in other chapters. The age-adjusted incidence of CTCL in the United States is about 4 cases per million persons annually, which is about double the rate from the early 1970s. There are approximately 800 to 1000 total new cases each year.[10-12] The peak incidence is in the sixth decade of life, and onset before age 30 is rare. The disease is slightly more common in men, and there is no racial predilection. Adult T-cell leukemia-lymphoma is rare in the United States. Less than 100 cases are reported in the literature. It is uncertain whether the incidence is rising due to an increased prevalence of HTLV-I infection or other environmental reasons.

Stem cells destined to become T lymphocytes originate in the bone marrow and migrate to the thymus, where they undergo differentiation under the influence of several thymic hormones.[13] During this differentiation, they undergo rearrangement of the T-cell receptor gene loci.[14,15] The exquisite specificity of T cells is a result of this cell surface receptor. The diversity with the ability to recognize millions of antigens is a result of the rearrangement of the gene. The human T-

cell receptor (Ti) has two major subunits, Ti-α and Ti-β, which are held together by disulfide bonds. The subunits are closely associated with the T3 molecule that consists of a 25-kd γ-chain and two 20-kd δ- and ϵ-chains (Fig. 53–1). The Ti subunits form a binding site for antigen and major histocompatibility complex molecules through interaction of their variable domains, and the T3 subunits serve a signal transduction function. The Ti subunit proteins are translated from genes that contain variable, diversity, joining, and constant regions (see Fig. 53–1). Southern analysis of DNA from patients' T cells can be used to determine whether malignant cells are T cells and whether there is monoclonal rearrangement of the T-cell receptor gene loci.[6]

Early T cells may express the 3A1 and T11 (CD2) antigens and intracellular terminal deoxyribonucleotide transferase (TdT) before rearrangement of the T-cell receptor gene.[14] The T11 antigen is the sheep erythrocyte receptor. This 50-kd surface glycoprotein facilitates interactions between T lymphocytes and target cells and activates resting T cells.[16] The ability of the T11 antigen to trigger T-cell activation independent of antigen and MHC molecules is important for amplification of the immune response. The T11 antigen is present on T cells throughout their differentiation. The function of the 3A1 antigen is unknown, and it is lost as the cells mature. The transcription of Ti-β precedes Ti-α; T3 transcription first occurs at about the same stage, but surface T3-Ti complex appears in the late thymocyte stage.[14]

The T4 (CD4) and T8 (CD8) surface glycoproteins appear during middle or late thymocyte development, and eventually cells retain or lose one of these antigens.[13] The CD4+ cells, called inducer or helper T cells, comprise approximately 67% of peripheral blood T cells and bind to invariant regions of class II MHC antigens. These cells facilitate the differentiation of B cells into antibody-producing plasma cells and facilitate the function of T8+ cytotoxic or suppressor T cells. The T4

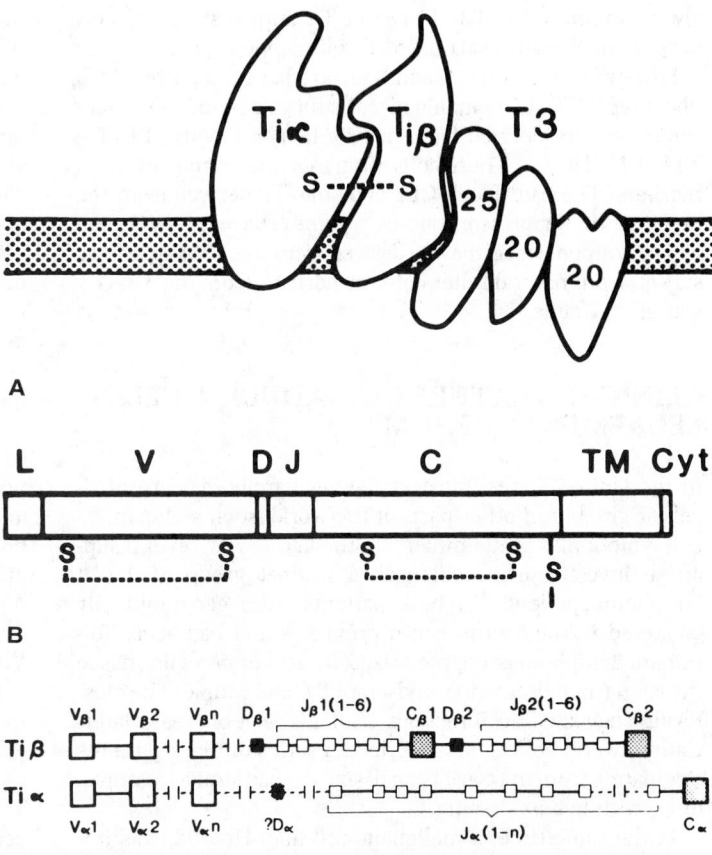

FIGURE 53–1. Structure of the human T-cell receptor and its subunits. **(A)** Subunit composition of the human T-cell receptor. The Ti α and Ti β subunits are held together by S-S bonds and are most closely associated with the 25-kd γ chain of the T3 molecule. The α and β subunits are anchored in the cell membrane with their transmembrane segments. The T3 complex consists of two additional subunits (δ and ϵ) with molecular weights of 20,000. Although not shown, a recently described 16-kd homodimer (32-kd nonreduced), called zeta, is also noncovalently associated with the T3-Ti complex. **(B)** Structure of the Ti subunits. The predicted primary structure of the β-chain subunit after translation from the cDNA sequence is depicted, as are the variable region leader (*L*), V, D, and J segments, a hydrophobic transmembrane segment (*TM*), and cytoplasmic part (*Cyt*) in the C region, potential intrachain sulfhydryl bonds (*S-S*), and the single SH group (*S*) that can form a sulfhydryl bond with the α subunit. **(C)** Scheme of the genomic organization of the human β- and α-chain genes. In the β locus, V indicates the V gene pool located at the 5' end, at an unknown distance from the $D_{\beta 1}$ element, the $J_{\beta 1}$ cluster, and the $C_{\beta 1}$ constant-region gene. Further downstream, a second $D_{\beta 2}$ element, $J_{\beta 2}$ cluster, and $C_{\beta 2}$ constant-region gene are indicated. A similar nomenclature is used for the Ti α locus in which only a single constant region is found. ?D indicates the uncertainty about the existence of a putative Ti α diversity element. (Reproduced with permission from Royer HD, Reinherz EL. T lymphocytes: Ontogeny. Function, and relevance to clinical disorders. N Engl J Med 1987;317:1136–1142)

molecule is also the receptor for the human immunodeficiency virus (HIV).[17] T8$^+$ cytotoxic T cells comprise approximately 33% of peripheral blood T cells and have specificity of antigen and class I MHC antigens. They are responsible for MHC-directed cytotoxicity of virus-infected and malignant cells, for graft rejection, for delayed hypersensitivity reactions and for inhibiting the differentiation of B cells into plasma cells.

T-cell proliferation results from events involving the T3-Ti complex and from binding of interleukin-2 (IL-2), a T-cell growth factor, to IL-2 receptors (IL-2R).[14,18,19] Resting T cells have no IL-2R. After antigen or MHC exposure, the number of surface antigen (Ti) receptors decreases, and the number of IL-2R increases. In contrast to resting lymphocytes and the low-grade T-cell lymphomas, the HTLV-I–infected malignant cells in ATLL constitutively express IL-2R. This may account for the rapid proliferation of these cells.

A small fraction of peripheral blood T cells lack T4 and T8 antigens and express the T3-Ti γ-δ receptor.[20] These cells have broad natural killer activity. Reports of target granular lymphocytic malignancies derived from this population of cells are now appearing.[21]

CLASSIFICATION OF T-CELL MALIGNANCIES

The Rappaport and Working Formulations were not developed for classifying T-cell malignancies.[22,23] Some T-cell malig-

nancies appear in these classifications, and others are omitted. The T-cell malignancies can be separated into low, intermediate, and high grades, as in the Working Formulation, and can be differentiated by their phenotypic properties.

The most immature T-cell malignancies are the lymphoblastic lymphomas and T-cell acute lymphoblastic leukemias.[24–26] The malignant cells in these disorders have prethymic or thymic markers and can be considered to be the leukemic or tissue phases of the same disease process, analogous to chronic lymphocytic leukemia and diffuse well-differentiated lymphocytic lymphoma. The malignant cells in these disorders usually have intracellular TdT and express the 3A1 antigen. Clinically, these disorders are often associated with mediastinal masses and a predilection for central nervous system (CNS) involvement. More detailed descriptions may be found elsewhere in this text. T-cell prolymphocytic leukemia is a rare leukemia derived from intermediate or mature thymocytes and may be T4$^+$T8$^+$ or T4$^+$T8$^-$.[27]

Malignancies of mature T cells may be low, intermediate, or high grade. ATLL is a high-grade T-cell leukemia-lymphoma with some distinct clinical features caused by the HTLV-I retrovirus.[1,7,8,28] The cells in ATLL have the helper phenotype and constitutively express IL-2R. All other T-cell lymphomas do not express IL-2R or have low-level expression. The peripheral T-cell lymphomas (including T-cell immunoblastic lymphoma, diffuse large noncleaved, and diffuse large noncleaved types) are intermediate or high grade. These lymphomas do not express immature T-cell markers, almost always express T1, T3, T11, and T4 antigens, and always have monoclonally rearranged T-cell receptor genes.[29]

Low-grade T-cell lymphomas always have a mature T-cell phenotype. CTCL, including mycosis fungoides and the Sézary syndrome, are derived from mature helper T cells (T1, T3, T11, T4$^+$, T8$^-$).[3-5] These cells often lose one or more of these markers. The true T-cell CLL cells may be derived from the helper or the suppressor subsets.[30,31] The cells in the syndrome of T-γ lymphocytosis may be derived from the T8$^+$ suppressor subset, from natural killer cells, or perhaps from the T3-Ti γ subset of T cells.[32-34]

CLINICAL FEATURES OF ADULT T-CELL LEUKEMIA-LYMPHOMA

In the United States, most malignant lymphomas are of B-cell origin, but in other parts of the world, such as Japan, T-cell lymphomas predominate.[1] In the late 1970s, several Japanese investigators recognized a distinct group of T-cell lymphoma patients.[35] These patients were geographically clustered in the southwestern provinces and had acute fulminant lymphomas characterized by leukemic cells, tissue invasion (including skin), and a rapidly fatal course. The clustering suggested an infectious etiology. Several years later, Catovsky and colleagues described a series of black patients originating from the Caribbean basin who had similar features, often with hypercalcemia.[36]

At the same time, a malignant cell line, Hut102, was initiated from a patient with an atypical CTLL at the National Cancer Institute (NCI).[37] This cell line, which grew without exogenous growth factors, produced IL-2, expressed high levels IL-2R, and was infected with HTLV-I.[1,7] Shortly thereafter, antibodies to this virus were detected in 100% of the patients with ATLL in Japan, the Caribbean, and the United States.[1,38] An identical virus was detected in Japanese patients and cell lines.

The HTLV-I retrovirus from Hut102 and other cell lines has been isolated and sequenced completely.[1] It contains 1096 nucleotides. There are long terminal repeats (LTR) positioned at the 5′ and 3′ ends that regulate transcription by providing sites for RNA polymerase attachment. The proviral RNA next contains *GAG*, *POL*, and *ENV* genes that encode for the structural proteins, the reverse transcriptase and the envelope proteins respectively. The most 3′ region termed pX contains a long open reading (LOR) frame that encodes for a protein that acts as a transcriptional activator of the LTR regions and perhaps as an activation for other genes.

There is overwhelming evidence that HTLV-I is the causative agent of ATLL.[1] ATLL occurs in areas endemic for HTLV-I, and ATLL patients have anti-HTLV-I antibodies in their serum. HTLV-I proviral genome is monoclonally integrated in malignant ATLL cells, and infection of normal T4 cells with HTLV-I causes alternations in morphology and independent growth properties characteristic of ATLL cells. Proviral integration into these cells and their descendants is monoclonal. However, the actual site of integration varies among patients and cell lines.

The clinical features of ATLL in the United States and the Caribbean have been described.[8,39] Most patients are from the southeastern United States or Hawaii or have emigrated from other endemic regions, such as Japan or the Caribbean basin. The disease has not been reported in children, and the median age at diagnosis is 35 to 55 years, with a slight male predominance. The disease tends to have a sudden onset, usually with hypercalcemia or rapidly developing skin lesions. The median interval between the onset of symptoms and a diagnosis of lymphoma is short (median, 2 months). Systemic "B" symptoms are common, and all patients are stage IV with involvement of at least one organ, usually the skin, gastrointestinal tract, pulmonary system, or CNS. Lymphadenopathy is invariably present; massive mediastinal node enlargement is uncommon. Opportunistic infections are extremely common because the patients are immunosuppressed.

Hypercalcemia or evidence of bone resorption are common in ATLL. The presence of hypercalcemia imparts a poor prognosis, and the hypercalcemia is difficult to manage without an excellent antitumor response. Osteolytic bone lesions, abnormal bone scans, and elevated alkaline phosphatase levels are other manifestations of the bone-resorbing features of ATLL. It appears that the malignant cells secrete an osteoclast-activating, bone-resorbing protein that is not yet characterized. Vitamin D and parathormone levels are normal.

Many patients with ATLL have T-cell leukemia in which the malignant circulating cells have a characteristic cloverleaf appearance.[28] The peripheral leukocyte count varies from normal to extremely high (>200,000/μl) in these patients. These cells allow a morphologic diagnosis to be more easily established. The histologic picture of different tissue sites varies. The lymphoma may be described as one of several in the Rappaport classification (*e.g.*, diffuse poorly differentiated lymphocytic, diffuse mixed, diffuse histiocytic), and the cell morphology may be quite pleomorphic.[28]

Few patients infected with HTLV-I develop ATLL. Many HTLV-I-infected patients never develop any disease. Some develop neurologic diseases, such as spastic paraparesis. Some HTLV-I-infected patients develop a chronic low-grade illness with abnormal, circulating cells, sometimes with adenopathy. This disease has been called chronic adult T-cell leukemia. It may persist many years without any sequelae, but it uncommonly may convert to classic ATLL.

CLINICAL FEATURES OF LOW-GRADE T-CELL LYMPHOMAS

CLINICAL FEATURES OF MYCOSIS FUNGOIDES AND THE SÉZARY SYNDROME

The diagnosis of mycosis fungoides (MF) is often preceded by a long (5–10 years) prediagnostic (premycotic) phase marked by the appearance of nonspecific patches, which may be pruritic. Biopsies during this phase are nonspecific. In its earliest diagnostic phase, scaling, erythematous patches or plaques with well-marginated borders but variable size and shape, are seen. They are often in a bathing trunk distribution, although any body surfaces may be affected. Occasionally, there may be a prominent component of poikiloderma, skin atrophy, associated alopecia, or follicular mucinosis.

Skin biopsies demonstrate an infiltrate of mononuclear cells in the epidermis and upper dermis. These mononuclear cells may form intraepidermal clusters, so-called Pautrier microabscesses. The nuclei of these cells are hyperconvoluted (or cerebriform).[55] Cell surface marker studies demonstrate them to be CD4+ (*i.e.*, helper T cells), although further evaluation often demonstrates that they have lost some mature T-cell antigens, such as Leu-8 and Leu-9 (CD7).[40] Eventually, patches may evolve into more numerous, infiltrated plaques, and patients with a long history of plaque disease may develop ulcerated or exophytic tumors. Some patients may present de novo with tumors (d'emblee).

Another variant of skin involvement is generalized erythroderma (l'homme rouge or the red-man syndrome), accompanied by atrophic or lichenified skin. Plaques and tumors may also occur. These patients are intensely symptomatic from pruritus and scaling. If there is peripheral blood involvement, they are considered to have the Sézary syndrome.

Most patients with MF never have any clinical evidence of disease other than skin involvement. However, 10% to 20% of patients eventually develop clinical manifestations of extracutaneous disease.[41] This often manifests initially as regional lymphadenopathy in areas draining extensive skin involvement. Later, visceral involvement may develop. Organs most frequently affected include the lungs, spleen, liver, and gastrointestinal tract. Autopsy studies indicate that involvement of any organ may occur in the final stages of disease.[11]

The Sézary syndrome is a variant of MF in which patients present with erythroderma and abnormal cells (>10%) circulating in the peripheral blood.[42] These cells are identical to the CD4+ helper T cells seen in the cutaneous infiltrates of MF. Lymphadenopathy and splenomegaly are often present.

In large cohorts of patients with long-term follow-up, the median survival after a diagnosis of MF is almost 10 years.[41] Among patients who present with patch or limited plaque disease, most die of unrelated causes, including cardiopulmonary disease or other cancers. However, for patients who present with tumorous involvement or the Sézary syndrome or who develop extracutaneous spread, the prognosis is more dismal. Most patients die of MF or complications related to the disease, such as infection and sepsis, with a median survival of less than 3 years.[11,43–45] Cytologic or histologic transformation into a high-grade lymphoma occurs in some patients and is associated with a poor prognosis.[53] Patients may develop other malignancies, including skin cancers, Hodgkin's disease, and myeloid leukemias.[1,3]

OTHER CUTANEOUS LYMPHOMAS AND LYMPHOMA-LIKE LESIONS

B-cell lymphomas may involve the skin as a primary site of disease or as a manifestation of systemic involvement. Histologically, these can usually be differentiated readily from MF, because the neoplastic infiltrate is usually limited to the dermis, sparing the epidermis and dermal-epidermal junction (Grenz zone) until rather late in the course of disease, when secondary ulceration may occur. Immunophenotyping can confirm the B-cell origin of these lymphomas. These lymphomas may be classified according to the criteria of the Working Formulation, and prognosis is related to histology and stage of disease.[46]

Pagetoid reticulosis (*i.e.*, Woringer-Kolopp disease) is a hyperkeratotic, verrucous form of MF, which presents with limited involvement of a single site, usually an extremity.[47] It has an indolent course, but it may become locally invasive and destructive. It is a monoclonal T-cell lymphoproliferative disease, documented by clonal rearrangements of the T-cell receptor in biopsied tissue.[48]

Lymphomatoid papulosis is a T-cell disease characterized clinically by waxing and waning nodular lesions. Histologic examination reveals atypical cells that resemble Reed-Sternberg cells or hyperconvoluted MF cells. Studies of T-cell receptor gene rearrangements indicate that lymphomatoid papulosis is often a monoclonal T-cell proliferation.[49] There is an increased risk for the development of lymphomatoid papulosis among patients with MF, and patients with lymphomatoid papulosis may later develop frank MF. The relation between these diseases is not clearly understood. Treatment should be symptomatic until a confirmed diagnosis of MF or other lymphoma is clearly established.

STAGING

A staging classification system for MF was proposed at the NCI Workshop on Cutaneous T-Cell Lymphomas in 1978.[50] Table 53–1 summarizes this TNMB system. In large series, approximately 21% of patients present with limited plaque (<10% of the skin surface involved; T1), 36% with generalized plaque (>10% of the skin surface involved; T2), 24% with tumorous involvement (T3), and 19% with erythroderma (T4). The extent of skin involvement has major prognostic importance. The 5- and 10-year survivals for patients with MF, based on the extent of skin involvement, are shown in Table 53–2.

Stage groupings are based on the TNMB criteria. Clinical groupings based on this staging system clearly define patients with a good prognosis (*i.e.*, limited or generalized plaque disease only, with no evidence of extracutaneous spread), who have a median survival greater than 12 years; an intermediate prognosis (*i.e.*, cutaneous tumors, erythroderma, or lymph node involvement), with a median survival of about 5 years; or a poor prognosis (*i.e.*, extracutaneous disease involving viscera), with a median survival less than 3 years.[45] Circulating abnormal cells in the peripheral blood may have little independent effect on prognosis, but this condition is strongly correlated with T stage (usually T4) and extracutaneous disease.

The staging procedures should always include a careful examination of the skin, including the scalp, palms, soles, and perineum. A complete blood count, Sézary cell preparation, screening chemistries, and baseline chest radiograph are reasonable screening studies. Lymph node biopsies should be obtained if there is lymphadenopathy, because lymph node involvement and the lymph node histology affect the stage and prognosis. Visceral biopsies should be considered if there are unexplained clinical findings, such as abnormal liver function studies or an infiltrate on the chest radiograph. Histologically, lymph node biopsies may only reveal nonspecific changes of dermatopathic lymphadenitis. However, even these lymph nodes may show evidence of minimal involvement by MF if DNA content analysis, electron microscopy, or T-cell receptor rearrangements are used.[51,52] The microscopic se-

TABLE 53–1. National Cutaneous T-Cell Lymphoma Workshop Staging Classification

T	Skin	N	Lymph Nodes	M	Visceral Organs*
T1	Limited plaques (<10% BSA)†	N0	No adenopathy; histology negative	M0	No involvement
T2	Generalized plaques	N1	Adenopathy; histology negative	M1	Visceral involvement
T3	Cutaneous tumors	N2	No adenopathy; histology positive		
T4	Generalized erythroderma	N3	Adenopathy; histology positive		

Stage

I Limited (IA) or generalized plaques (IB) without adenopathy or histologic involvement of lymph nodes or viscera (T1N0M0 or T2N0M0)

II Limited or generalized plaques with adenopathy (IIA) or cutaneous tumors with or without adenopathy (IIB); without histologic involvement of lymph nodes or viscera (T1–2N1M0, T2N0–1M0)

III Generalized erythroderma with or without adenopathy; without histologic involvement of lymph nodes or viscera (T4N0–1M0)

IV Histologic involvement of lymph nodes (IVA) or viscera (IVB) with any skin lesion and with or without adenopathy (T1–4N2–3M0 for IVA; T1–4N0–3M1 for IVB)

* Blood involvement should be recorded as absent (B0) or present (B1) but is not currently used to determine final stage.
† BSA, body surface area.

verity of lymph node involvement may be defined using a "lymph node staging system" that correlates with prognosis.[53] Patients with lymph node biopsies showing dermatopathic changes or small numbers of malignant cells (*i.e.*, LN1 or LN2) had a 5-year survival rate of 80%, those with dermatopathic changes and large clusters of paracortical malignant cells (LN3) had a 5-year survival rate of 30%, and those with effaced nodes had a 5-year survival rate of only 15%.

TREATMENT

THERAPY FOR ADULT T-CELL LEUKEMIA

Therapy for adult T-cell leukemia is unsatisfactory, and patients have a poor prognosis. Complete remissions have been observed in about 50% of patients given intensive combination chemotherapy regimens such as PROMACE/CYTOBOM or M-BACOD.[8] These regimens generally alleviate symptoms such as hypercalcemia and skin lesions, but long-term remissions are not observed. Opportunistic infections, spread to the CNS, and relapse are major problems. Numerous biologic agents have been evaluated. Unlabeled monoclonal antibodies (*e.g.*, T101, anti-Tac), deoxycoformycin, and interferons have not been useful. Antibody conjugates are being evaluated as are antiviral agents.[54] For the rare patients with an indolent asymptomatic course, observation is reasonable.

THERAPY FOR MYCOSIS FUNGOIDES

The essential ingredient for successful management of MF is effective treatment of the skin. Nonspecific topical treatments such as emollients, antipruritics, and antiinflammatories, including hydrocortisone, may provide some relief of symptoms, especially in patients with minimal disease. More effective management demands the use of intensive topical photochemotherapy, nitrogen mustard, or irradiation. With all of these topical therapies, patients may experience an apparent exacerbation of disease at the outset, which is probably related to stimulation of an inflammatory reaction in areas of minimal disease. With continuation of therapy, the skin disease usually responds.

Topical Photochemotherapy

Topical photochemotherapy (*i.e.*, PUVA) includes the oral administration of 8-methoxypsoralen (0.4–0.6 mg/kg) followed 2 hours later by exposure to light in the UVA spectrum.

TABLE 53–2. Survival of 459 Patients With Mycosis Fungoides at Stanford University

T Stage	Characteristic	No. of Patients	5-Year Survival (%)	10-Year Survival (%)
T1	Limited plaque	95	91	82
T2	Generalized plaque	167	72	52
T3	Tumorous	112	35	19
T4	Erythroderma	85	46	28

(Hoppe RT, Wood GS, Abel EA. Mycosis fungoides and the Sézary syndrome: Pathology, staging, and treatment. Curr Probl Cancer 1990;14:295–361)

The psoralens intercalate with DNA, and on exposure to ultraviolet light in the 360-nm range, they form monofunctional and bifunctional adducts, which interfere with DNA replication.[55] The UVA does not penetrate beyond the epidermis and upper dermis. Patients receive timed exposure to the UVA (1.5–15 J/cm^2) in a phototherapy unit (PUVA box). Only the eyes are shielded. All other body surfaces may be treated, but certain areas such as the perineum, axillae, and other skin-fold areas may not receive adequate exposure. In the initial clearing phase of treatment, patients are treated two to three times each week. After the skin has cleared, a maintenance program of gradually decreasing frequency is employed. The average time to clearance is 2 to 6 months, with the likelihood of clearance related to the extent of skin involvement. Patients with minimal patch disease achieve complete response rates as high as 90%. Patients with more infiltrated plaques achieve complete response rates of 60% to 80%.[56–60] Maintenance therapy is continued 1 to 4 times per month after the skin has cleared, and if discontinued, most patients relapse. However, resumption of treatment is often associated with a secondary response.

Acute complications of PUVA treatment include mild erythema, pruritus, skin dryness, and nausea. Potential long-term complications include increased risk of cataracts, necessitating the use of UVA-opaque goggles during therapy. Some patients who undergo long-term continuous treatment with PUVA risk developing secondary cutaneous squamoproliferative lesions, including basal cell and squamous carcinomas.[61] Among patients treated for MF, this risk appears to be greatest if multiple topical therapies are used sequentially.[62]

Topical Chemotherapy

The most commonly used topical chemotherapy for MF is nitrogen mustard (HN$_2$). HN$_2$ may be prepared in an aqueous solution or in an ointment base, such as aquaphor. The mechanism of action after being applied topically is uncertain.[63] It is not likely that the alkylating agent activity that HN$_2$ demonstrates when administered systemically is the important factor, because the delay between preparation of the solution and application to the skin far exceeds the half-life of the active ethyleneimonium ion that forms after the HN$_2$ is put into solution. It is possible that one of the degradation products serves as the active agent or that one or more of these products stimulates an immune response, affecting the disease directly or by some interaction with the epidermal cell–Langerhans' cell–T-cell axis.

Nitrogen mustard is initially applied daily. When the aqueous preparation is used, patients prepare the solution themselves in a 10 to 20 mg per 100 ml solution and apply it to the skin with a cloth or brush. Nitrogen mustard in aquaphor is prepared by the pharmacist in a concentration of 10 to 20 mg per 100 g of aquaphor. The skin may be treated in its entirety, with the exception of the eyelids, lips, and vaginal and anal orifices. Skin-fold areas may be treated intermittently to avoid irritation. The aqueous and aquaphor preparations have similar efficacy, although a randomized trial has not been performed.[64] The choice often depends on convenience or patient preference. Complete response rates from 30% to 60% overall, with the likelihood of response depending on initial extent of skin involvement: about 50% for limited plaque and 25% for generalized plaque disease.[64–66] The median time to skin clearance is about 8 months. Maintenance treatment is continued for 1 to 2 years after skin clearance; the schedule varies. After treatment is discontinued, more than half of patients experience skin relapses, but most respond to resumption of therapy. The overall proportion of patients treated with topical HN$_2$ who have durable complete responses is about 20%.

The primary complication of topical HN$_2$ therapy is an acute or delayed hypersensitivity reaction. This may occur in as many as 30% of people treated with the aqueous preparation, but in less than 5% of patients treated with the ointment preparation.[64] Desensitization may be achieved with a variety of topical or systemic desensitization programs. Some patients treated with topical HN$_2$ have developed secondary squamoproliferative lesions of the skin.[66] This was a problem primarily among patients who were treated with multiple sequential topical therapies for the control of active disease and was observed only occasionally among patients treated with topical HN$_2$ alone. There is no systemic absorption of topically applied nitrogen mustard, and systemic complications such as hematologic depression or sterility are not potential toxicities.

Another chemotherapeutic agent that has been used topically is carmustine (BCNU).[67] The efficacy of BCNU is similar to topical HN$_2$, but because of the systemic absorption of BCNU, the potential hematologic complications are greater, and the duration of treatment is limited.

Irradiation

Irradiation has been used in the management of MF for almost a century. Mycosis fungoides is an exquisitely radiosensitive neoplasm, and rather modest doses are capable of achieving long-term control.[68] The responsiveness of MF is related to the intrinsic radiosensitivity of the infiltrating neoplastic lymphocytes. The D$_0$ of human lymphocytes is less than 100 cGy.

Spot treatment with orthovoltage x-rays (150–250 kV) or low-energy electron-beam therapy (6–9 MeV) may be used in the management of individual plaques or tumors. Fractionated doses of 1500 to 2500 cGy are often adequate for local control. The more important challenge is the effective treatment of large surfaces of skin, as are often involved in patients with the generalized plaque or tumorous phase of skin involvement. Several techniques of total-skin electron-beam therapy (EBT) have been developed. Commonly, patients are treated in the standing position at a distance of 3 to 4 m from a linear accelerator, which is set in the electron mode. This distance enables treatment of large surfaces. Patients stand on a rotating platform or assume several different positions during treatment to treat their entire circumference.[69] The dosimetry of this technique reveals a superficial depth of penetration, which depends on the energy of the incident electrons.[70] For example, using 6-MeV electrons, the 80% depth dose is at 0.3 cm, and the 50% depth dose is at 0.6 cm. For 9-MeV electrons, the corresponding values are 0.7 cm and 1.25 cm.[41] This provides adequate treatment to the depth of most MF patches and plaques, but exophytic or more deeply infiltrating tumors require supplemental boost treatment to achieve local control. The soles of the feet, perineum, and areas under skin folds are treated in a supplementary fashion with orthovoltage x-rays or electrons.

Using total-skin EBT, the usual dose is 2400 to 3600 cGy given in 6 to 12 weeks. In large series, the complete response rate for patients with patch or plaque disease ranges from 71% to 98%.[41,71] The complete response rate for patients who present with tumorous involvement is 60% to 70%. As many as 50% of patients with limited plaque disease and 25% of patients with generalized plaque disease who achieve a complete response enjoy long-term freedom from relapse after the completion of therapy. Relapses usually occur in the skin. Treatment with topical HN_2 at that time can achieve a similar response rate as the de novo use of HN_2. A comparison of response and survival for patients treated with topical HN_2 or EBT is shown in Table 53–3.

The acute complications of EBT include erythema, temporary epilation, temporary loss of fingernails and toenails, and impaired ability to sweat.[41] Chronic complications include dry skin and the development of telangiectasia, which is usually minimal if the techniques of treatment have been appropriate. Cutaneous carcinogenesis is another potential hazard, which is amplified in these patients by the use of multiple sequential therapies.[62]

Radiation may also provide an important palliative benefit for patients with localized extracutaneous disease. Megavoltage photons ($\geq$4 MeV) can be used to treat symptomatic adenopathy or visceral sites of disease, with techniques similar to those used for other lymphomas. The dose should be titrated to the response, but typically it is limited to 2400 to 3600 cGy.

PUVA therapy is highly effective in clearing skin lesions, and approximately 60% of treated patients in all T stages achieve responses.[67–70] However, maintenance therapy is required in all completely responding patients, because its discontinuation results in a prompt relapse. With maintenance therapy, durable remissions are observed with a mean duration after skin clearing of 6 to 16 months.

SYSTEMIC THERAPY FOR CUTANEOUS T-CELL LYMPHOMAS

Chemotherapeutic principles in treating CTCL are similar to those employed for the low-grade B-cell lymphomas.[1,3] Objective responses producing palliation of symptoms produced by refractory cutaneous lesions or extracutaneous disease are frequent (70% response rates), but chemotherapy is not curative. The most active agents include methotrexate, alkylating agents (*e.g.*, cyclophosphamide, chlorambucil) etoposide (VP-16), and cisplatin.[1,3,72] Combination chemotherapy produces higher complete response rates but is not curative. Regimens commonly used are similar to those employed for B-cell lymphomas, including chlorambucil plus prednisone, cyclophosphamide plus vincristine plus prednisone (CVP), or similar regimens.[2,3,73,74] No randomized studies have proven the superiority of combinations over single agents. Chemotherapy is often combined with one of the topical therapies previously discussed because of the bulk disease within the skin.[74]

Recombinant interferons are active agents against CTCL, with response rates of about 50% for patients with advanced disease refractory to other treatments and 90% for early-stage untreated patients.[75,76] Whether interferons should be combined with other effective therapies and whether they should be used initially can only be determined by future trials. Initial studies used extremely high doses, but similar response rates were found with lower, more tolerable doses such as 3 to 10 million units every other day or three times weekly.

COMBINED-MODALITY THERAPY

Combined-modality therapy may be considered in the context of combined topical therapies or as combined topical and systemic treatment. Because of the reliably high complete response rate to total-skin EBT and the high risk for relapse after completion of that treatment, combined treatment with EBT and a topical cutaneous adjuvant therapy is a common approach for aggressive initial treatment of the skin. Adjuvant therapies have included topical HN_2 and PUVA.[77,78] Either of these adjuvants may prolong the duration of the disease-free interval, but it is not clear that the long-term rate of relapse is altered.

Topical and systemic therapies have been combined to achieve a better outcome. Phase II reports of successful treatment with combined EBT and systemic chemotherapy led to a randomized trial at the NCI.[79] Patients with all stages of disease were randomized to conservative therapy (*i.e.*, sequential treatment with topical HN_2, PUVA, total-skin EBT, oral methotrexate, and systemic combination chemotherapy) or combined therapy (*i.e.*, total-skin EBT combined with cyclophosphamide, doxorubicin, etoposide, and vincristine) at the outset. The overall response rate was significantly higher in the combined-therapy group (90% versus 65%; p=0.003).

TABLE 53–3. Results of Topical Therapy for Myocosis Fungoides With Nitrogen Mustard or Electron Beam at Stanford University

T Stage	Treatment	CR (%)	PR (%)	10-Year FFR (%) (n = 123)	10-Year Survival (%) (n = 226)
T1	HN_2	51	37	30	83
	EBT	98	2	50	80
T2	HN_2	26	43	0	42
	EBT	71	29	25	45
T3	HN_2		33		
	EBT	36	64		25
T4	HN_2	22	44		
	EBT	64	36		

HN_2, topical nitrogen mustard; EBT, total-skin electron-beam therapy; CR, complete response; PR: partial response; FFR, freedom from relapse.
(Hoppe RT, Abel EA, Deneau DG, Price NM. Mycosis fungoides: Management with topical nitrogen mustard. J Clin Oncol 1987;5: 1796–1803 and Hoppe RT, Wood GS, Abel EA. Mycosis fungoides and the Sézary syndrome: Pathology, staging, and treatment. Curr Probl Cancer 1990;14:295–361)

However, actuarial plots of disease-free and overall survival rates were similar for either approach. The median survival after combined therapy was 91 months, compared with more than 76 months (median not yet reached) after conservative therapy. Combined chemotherapy and EBT is not recommended as initial therapy unless there is advanced systemic disease or cytologic transformation.

More effective systemic management is needed to improve the efficacy of combined-modality therapy. An innovative approach with excellent preliminary results is the combination of PUVA with interferon.[80] The complete response rate with this combination was higher than reported for PUVA alone, interferon alone, and combined chemotherapy and EBT, and the response duration was longer than with other therapies.[81] Randomized trials comparing this combination with PUVA alone are indicated. Other combinations recently evaluated in small numbers of patients are described under investigational therapies.

BIOLOGIC AND EXPERIMENTAL THERAPIES

Antithymocyte globulin (ATG) and monoclonal antibodies that react with T-cell antigens produced responses, but the therapy was limited by toxicity (especially with ATG) and the brief duration of the responses.[82–85] A chimeric antibody produced less immunotoxicity, but the response rate and duration were still suboptimal.[86] Radiolabeled antibodies in high doses can produce substantial remissions compared with unlabeled antibody.[85] This approach is still highly experimental because of the myelosuppression caused by free radioisotope. Toxin-conjugated antibodies are being evaluated, but their use remains experimental.[87]

Fludarabine is a newly approved chemotherapeutic agent for the treatment of CLL that is also active in CTCL. In a phase II trial using advanced refractory patients, a response rate of 20% was reported.[88] This agent requires additional study for use in CTCL. Deoxycoformycin is a potent inhibitor of adenosine deaminase and has been evaluated in several chronic lymphoid neoplasms. It is active against hairy cell leukemia and CTCL.[89,90] In one series, a 50% response rate and long duration was reported for refractory patients.[90] It is being evaluated in combination with interferon for treatment of both of these disorders, but its use remains investigational. Retinoic acid derivatives such as 13-*cis*-retinoic acid (Accutane), etretinate, and arotinoid-ethylester produce responses in about 50% of patients with advanced disease.[91–93] Like deoxycoformycin, they are being evaluated in combination with interferon. In a trial combining a retinoid with bleomycin, cyclophosphamide, and prednisone, a complete response rate of 80% lasting 8 months was reported.[94] Retinoids have also been combined with PUVA.[95] High response rates were reported, but it is not clear whether the response rates or duration are superior to PUVA alone.

There have been anecdotal reports of responses to acyclovir and cyclosporine.[96–99] The responses observed after acyclovir have been used to support a viral cause for CTCL. These agents remain investigational until larger controlled trials document their value.

Patients with the Sézary syndrome often have many circulating cells that migrate between the skin, peripheral blood, and lymph nodes.[100] Leukophoresis with removal of large numbers of circulating cells causes transient remissions in some cases.[101] After the development of PUVA therapy, Edelson and coworkers evaluated extracorporeal photophoresis by administering oral methoxsalen 2 hours before leukophoresis.[102] The peripheral blood cells were exposed to UVA light during the leukophoresis. Objective responses were observed in 64% of 37 evaluable patients. As with the agents listed earlier, the exact mechanism of action is unknown and further trials are necessary to define the ultimate role of this modality.

The combined use of total-skin electron irradiation combined with wide-field "systemic" irradiation was evaluated in several investigational studies. The Philadelphia group used total-nodal irradiation with skin electron irradiation.[103] Complete responses were observed in most cases. Remission duration was longest in patients with disease confined to the skin. A group in France employed 125 cGy of total-body irradiation (12.5 cGy twice daily three times weekly) before and after 2400 cGy of total-skin electron irradiation.[104] There was considerable myelosuppression, but 8 of 18 patients survived a median of 30+ months without evidence of disease.

REFERENCES

1. Broder S, Bunn PA Jr. Neoplasms of T-cell origin: Immunological aspects and therapy. Semin Oncol 1980;7:310–331.
2. Broder S, Bunn PA Jr, Jaffe ES, et al. T-cell lymphoproliferative syndrome associated with human T-cell leukemia-lymphoma virus. Ann Intern Med 1984;100:543–557.
3. Sausville EA, Bunn PA Jr. Biologic and clinical spectrum of T-cell neoplasms. In: Harrison's principles of internal medicine, update VII, oncology. 1986:159–189.
4. Broder S, Edelson RL, Lutzner M, et al. The Sézary syndrome. A malignant proliferation of helper T cells. J Clin Invest 1976;58:1297–1306.
5. Haynes BR, Metzger RS, Minna JD, Bunn PA Jr. Phenotypic characterization of cutaneous T-cell lymphoma. N Engl J Med 1981;304:1319–1323.
6. Bertness V, Kirsch I, Hollis G, Johnson B, Bunn PA Jr. T-cell receptor gene rearrangements as clinical markers of human T-cell lymphomas. N Engl J Med 1985;313:534–538.
7. Poixsz BJ, Ruscetti FM, Gazdar AF, et al. Detection and isolation of type-c retrovirus particles from fresh and cultured lymphocytes of a patients with cutaneous T-cell lymphoma. Proc Natl Acad Sci USA 1980;77:7415–7419.
8. Bunn PA Jr, Schechter GP, Blayney D, et al. Clinical course of retrovirus-associated adult T-cell lymphoma in the United States. N Engl J Med 1983;309:257–264.
9. Manzari V, Gismondi A, Barillari G, et al. HTLV-V: A new human retrovirus in Tac-negative T cell lymphoma/leukemia. Science 1987;238:1581–1583.
10. Greene MH, Dalager NA, Lamberg SI, et al. Mycosis fungoides. Epidemiologic observations. Cancer Treat Rep 1979;63:596–606.
11. Epstein EH, Levine DL, Croft JD, et al. Mycosis fungoides. Survival prognostic features, response to therapy, and autopsy findings. Medicine (Baltimore) 1972;51:61–72.
12. Weinstock MA, Holm JW. Mycosis fungoides in the United States: Increasing incidence and descriptive epidemiology. JAMA 1988;260:42–46.
13. Reinherz EL, Schlossman SF. Regulation of the immune response: Inducer and suppressor T lymphocyte subsets in human beings. N Engl J Med 1980;303:370–373.
14. Royer HD, Reinherz EL. T lymphocytes: Ontogeny, function, and relevance to clinical disorders. N Engl J Med 1987;317:1136–1142.
15. Davis MM, Chin Y-H, Gascoigne NRJ, Hedrick SM. A murine T cell receptor gene complex: Isolation, structure, and rearrangement. Immunol Rev 1984;81:235–258.
16. Yang SY, Chowaif S, Dont B. A common pathway for T lymphocyte activation involving both CD3-Ti complex and CD2 sheep erythrocyte receptor determinants. J Immunol 1986;137:1097–1100.
17. McDougal JS, Kennedy MS, Sligh JM, et al. Binding of HTL VIII/LAV to T4 and T cells by a complex of the 11K viral protein and the T4 molecule. Science 1986;231:382–385.
18. Smith KA, Baker PE, Gillis S, Ruscetti FW. Functional and molecular characteristics of T cell growth factor. Mol Immunol 1980;17:579–589.
19. Waldmann TA. The structure, function, and expression of interleukin-2 receptors on normal and malignant lymphocytes. Science 1986;232:727–732.
20. Moingeon P, Ythier A, Goubin G, et al. A unique T cell receptor complex expressed on human fetal lymphocytes displaying natural-killer-like activity. Nature 1986;323:638–640.
21. Oshimi K, Hoshino S, Takahashi M, et al. Ti(WT31)-negative, CD3-positive, large granular lymphocyte leukemia with nonspecific cytotoxicity. Blood 1988;71:923–931.
22. Rappaport H. Tumors of the hematopoietic system. In: Atlas of tumor pathology, Sec. III, fasc. 8. Washington, DC: Armed Forces Institute of Pathology, 1966.

23. Rosenberg S, Non-Hodgkin's Lymphoma Pathologic Classification Project. National Cancer Institute sponsored study of non-Hodgkin's lymphoma. Cancer 1982;49:2112–2135.
24. Nathwani BN, Kim H, Rappaport H. Malignant lymphoma, lymphoblastic. Cancer 1976;38:964–983.
25. Catovsky D, Goldman JM, Okos A, et al. T-lymphoblastic leukemia, a distinct variant of acute leukemia. Br Med J 1974;2:643–646.
26. Weiss LM, Bindl J, Picozzi VJ, et al. Lymphoblastic lymphoma, an immunophenotypic study of 26 cases with comparison to T cell acute lymphoblastic leukemia. Blood 1986;67:474–478.
27. Catovsky D, Okos A, Willt-Shaw E, et al. Prolymphocytic leukemia of B and T cell type. Lancet 1973;2:232–235.
28. Jaffe ES, Blattner WA, Blayney DW, Bunn PA, Robert-Guroff M, Gallo RC. The pathologic spectrum of HTLV associated leukemia/lymphoma in the United States. Am J Surg Pathol 1984;8:263–275.
29. Greer JP, York JC, Cousar JB, et al. Peripheral T-cell lymphoma. A clinicopathologic study of 42 cases. J Clin Oncol 1984;2:788.
30. Pandolfi F, De Roossi G, Semenzato G, et al. Immunologic evaluation of T chronic lymphocyte leukemia cells. Correlations among phenotype, functional activities, and morphology. Blood 1982;59:688–695.
31. Reinherz EL, Nadler LM, Rosenthal DS, et al. T-cell subset characterization of human T-CLL Blood 1979;53:1066–1074.
32. Aisenberg AC, Wilkes BM, Harris N, et al. Chronic T-cell lymphocytosis with neutropenia. Report of a case studied with monoclonal antibody. Blood 1981;58:818–822.
33. Kruskall, MS, Weitzman SA, Stossel TP, et al. Lymphoma with autoimmune neutropenia and hepatic sinusoidal infiltration: A syndrome. Ann Intern Med 1982;97:202–206.
34. Rumke HC, Miedema F, Ten Berge IJM, et al. Functional properties of T cells in patients with chronic TG lymphocytosis and chronic T-cell neoplasia. J Immunol 1982;129:419–426.
35. Uchiyama T, Yodoi J, Sagawa K, Takatsuki K, Uchimo H. Adult T cell leukemia: Clinical and hematological features of 16 cases. Blood 1977;50:481–492.
36. Catovsky D, Rose M, Goolden AWG, et al. Adult T cell lymphoma-leukemia in blacks from the West Indies. Lancet 1982;1:639–643.
37. Gazdar AF, Carney DN, Bunn PA, et al. Mitogen requirements for the in vitro propagation of cutaneous T cell lymphomas. Blood 1980;55:409–417.
38. Gallo RC, Kalyanaraman VS, Sarngadharan MG, et al. Association of the human type C retrovirus with a subset of adult T cell cancers. Cancer Res 1983;43:3892–3899.
39. Gibbs WN, Lofters WS, Campbell M, et al. Non-Hodgkin lymphoma in Jamaica and its relation to adult T cell leukemia-lymphoma. Ann Intern Med 1987;106:361–368.
40. Wood GS, Abel EA, Hoppe RT, Warnke RA. Leu-8 and Leu-9 antigen phenotypes. Immunologic criteria for the distinction of mycosis fungoides from cutaneous inflammations. J Am Acad Dermatol 1986;14:1006–1013.
41. Hoppe RT, Wood GS, Abel EA. Mycosis fungoides and the Sézary syndrome: Pathology, staging, and treatment. Curr Probl Cancer 1990;14:295–361.
42. Wieselthier JS, Koh HK. Sézary syndrome: Diagnosis, prognosis, and critical review of treatment options. J Am Acad Dermatol 1990;22:381–401.
43. Posner LE, Fossieck BE, Eddy JL, et al. Septicemic complications of the cutaneous T-cell lymphomas. Am J Med 1981;71:210–216.
44. Merlo CJ, Hoppe RT, Abel E, et al. Extracutaneous mycosis fungoides. Cancer 1987;60:397–402.
45. Sausville EA, Eddy JL, Makuch RW, et al. Histopathologic staging at initial diagnosis of mycosis fungoides and the Sézary syndrome: Definition of three distinctive prognostic groups. Ann Intern Med 1988;109:372–382.
46. Burke JS, Hoppe RT, Cibull ML, Dorfman RF. Cutaneous malignant lymphoma: A pathologic study of 50 cases with clinical analysis of 37. Cancer 1981;47:300–310.
47. Deneau DG, Wood GS, Beckstead J, Hoppe RT, Price NM. Woringer-Kolopp disease (pagetoid reticulosis). Four cases with histopathologic, ultra-structural, and immunohistologic observations. Arch Dermatol 1984;120:1045–1051.
48. Wood GS, Weiss LM, Hu C-H, et al. T-cell antigen deficiencies and clonal T-cell receptor gene rearrangements in pagetoid reticulosis (Woringer-Kolopp disease). N Engl J Med 1988;318:164–167.
49. Weiss LM, Wood GS, Trela M, et al. Clonal T-cell populations in lymphomatoid papulosis. Evidence for a lymphoproliferative etiology in a clinically benign disease. N Engl J Med 1986;315:475–479.
50. Bunn PA, Lamberg SI. Report of the committee on staging and classification of cutaneous T-cell lymphomas. Cancer Treat Rep 1979;63:725–728.
51. Bunn PA, Huberman MS, Whang-Peng J, et al. Prospective staging evaluation of patients with cutaneous T-cell lymphomas. Demonstration of a high frequency of extracutaneous dissemination. Ann Intern Med 1980;93:223–230.
52. Weiss LM, Hu E, Wood GS, Moulds C, et al. Clonal rearrangements of the T-cell receptor gene in mycosis fungoides and dermatopathic lymphadenopathy. N Engl J Med 1985;313:539–544.
53. Sausville EA, Worsham GF, Matthews MJ, et al. Histologic assessment of lymph nodes in mycosis fungoides/Sézary syndrome (cutaneous T-cell lymphoma): Clinical correlation and prognostic import of a new classification system. Hum Pathol 1985;16:841–849.
54. Kronke M, Pepper JM, Leonard WJ, Vitetta ES, Waldmann TA, Greene WC. Adult T cell leukemia: A potential target for ricin A chain immunotoxins. Blood 1985;65:1416–1421.
55. Gilchrest BA. Methoxsalen photochemotherapy for mycosis fungoides. Cancer Treat Rep 1979;63:663–667.
56. Vella Briffa D, Warin AP, Harrington CI, et al. Photochemotherapy in mycosis fungoides. A study of 73 patients. Lancet 1980;2:49–53.
57. Molin L, Thomsen K, Volden G, et al. Photochemotherapy (PUVA) in the pretumour stage of mycosis fungoides: A report from the Scandinavian mycosis fungoides study group. Acta Dermatol Venereal 1980;61:47–51.
58. Honigsmann H, Brenner W, Rauschmeier W, et al. Photochemotherapy for cutaneous T-cell lymphoma. J Am Acad Dermatol 1984;10:238–245.
59. Rosenbaum MM, Roenigk HH, Carol WA, et al. Photochemotherapy in cutaneous T-cell lymphoma and parapsoriasis en plaques. Long-term follow-up in forty-three patients. J Am Acad Dermatol 1985;13:613–622.
60. Abel EA, Sendagorta E, Hoppe RT, Huch M. PUVA treatment of erythrodermic and plaque type mycosis fungoides. Ten-year follow-up. Arch Dermatol 1987;123:897–901.
61. Stern RS, Laird N, Melski J, et al. Cutaneous squamous cell carcinoma in patients treated with PUVA. N Engl J Med 1984;310:1156–1161.
62. Abel EA, Sendagorta E, Hoppe RT. Cutaneous malignancies and metastatic squamous cell carcinoma following therapies for mycosis fungoides. J Am Acad Dermatol 1986;14:1029–1038.
63. Vonderheid EC. Topical mechlorethamine chemotherapy: Considerations on its use in mycosis fungoides. Int J Dermatol 1984;23:180–186.
64. Hoppe RT, Abel EA, Deneau DG, Price NM. Mycosis fungoides: Management with topical nitrogen mustard. J Clin Oncol 1987;5:1796–1803.
65. Ramsay DL, Halperin PS, Zeleniuch-Jacquotte A. Topical mechlorethamine therapy for early stage mycosis fungoides. J Am Acad Dermatol 1988;19:684–691.
66. Vonderheid EC, Tan ET, Kantor AF, et al. Long-term efficacy, curative potential and carcinogenicity of topical mechlorethamine chemotherapy in cutaneous T-cell lymphoma. Am Acad Dermatol 1989;20:416–428.
67. Zackheim HS, Epstein EH, JR, Crain WR. Tropical carmustine (BCNU) for cutaneous T-cell lymphoma. A 15-year experience in 143 patients. J Am Acad Dermatol 1990;22:802–810.
68. Kim JH, Nisce LZ, D'Anglo GJ. Dose-time fractionation study in patients with mycosis fungoides and lymphoma cutis. Radiology 1976;119:439–442.
69. Hoppe RT, Fuks Z, Bagshaw MA. Radiation therapy in the management of cutaneous T-cell lymphomas. Cancer Treat Rep 1979;63:625–632.
70. Cox RS, Heck RJ, Fessenden P, et al. Development of total-skin electron therapy at two energies. Int J Radiat Oncol Biol Phys 1990;18:659–669.
71. Tadros AAM, Tepperman BS, Hryniuk WM, et al. Total skin electron irradiation for mycosis fungoides. Failure analysis and prognostic factors. Int J Radiat Oncol Biol Phys 1983;9:1279–1287.
72. McDonald CJ, Bertino JR. Treatment of mycosis fungoides lymphoma: Effectiveness of infusions of methotrexate followed by oral citrovorum factor. Cancer Treat Rep 1978;62:1009–1011.
73. Grozea PN, Jones SE, McKelvey EM, et al. Combination chemotherapy for mycosis fungoides: A Southwest Oncology Group study. Cancer Treat Rep 1979;63:647–652.
74. Zakem MH, Davis BR, Adelstein DJ, Hines JD. Treatment of advanced stage mycosis fungoides with bleomycin, doxorubicin and methotrexate with topical nitrogen mustard (BAM-M). Cancer 1987;58:2611–2619.
75. Bunn PA Jr, Foon KA, Ihde DC, et al. Recombinant leukocyte A interferon: An active agent in advanced refractory cutaneous T-cell lymphomas (mycosis fungoides and Sézary syndrome). Ann Intern Med 1984;101:484–488.
76. Covielli A, Cavalieri R, Coppola G, et al. Recombinant leukocyte A interferon as initial therapy in mycosis fungoides and Sézary syndrome. Proc Am Soc Clin Oncol 1987;6:189.
77. Price NM, Hoppe RT, Constantine FS, et al. The treatment of mycosis fungoides: Adjuvant topical mechlorethamine after electron-beam therapy. Cancer 1977;40:2851–2853.
78. Spittle MF. Electron-beam therapy in England. Cancer Treat Rep 1979;63:639–641.
79. Kaye FJ, Bunn PA Jr, Steinberg SM, et al. A randomized trial comparing combination electron-beam radiation and chemotherapy with topical therapy in the initial treatment of mycosis fungoides. N Engl J Med 1989;321:1784–1790.
80. Kuzel TM, Gilyon K, Springer E, et al. Interferon alfa-2a combined with phototherapy in the treatment of cutaneous T-cell lymphoma. JNCI 1990;82:203–207.
81. Kuzel TM, Roenigk H Jr, Samuelson E, et al. Therapy of mycosis fungoides with interferon alfa-2a combined with phototherapy: Phase I and II trial long-term follow-up. Proc Am Soc Clin Oncol 1991;10:271.
82. Foon KA, Schroff RW, Bunn PA Jr. Monoclonal antibody therapy for patients with leukemia and lymphoma. In: Foon KA, Morgan AC Jr, eds. Monoclonal antibody therapy for human cancer. Hingham, MA: Martinus Nijhoff, 1985:85–101.
83. Dillman RO, Shawler DL, Dillman JB, et al. Therapy of chronic lymphocytic leukemia and cutaneous T-cell lymphoma with T101 monoclonal antibody. J Clin Oncol 1984;2:881.
84. Carrasquillo JA, Bunn PA Jr, Keenan AM, et al. Radioimmunodetection of cutaneous T-cell lymphoma with ^{111}In-T101 monoclonal antibody. N Engl J Med 1986;315:673.
85. Rosen ST, Zimmer AM, Goldman-Leiken R, et al. Radioimmunodetection and radioimmunotherapy of cutaneous T-cell lymphomas using an ^{131}I-labeled monoclonal antibody: An Illinois Cancer Council study. J Clin Oncol 1987;5:562.
86. Knox SJ, Levy R, Hodgkinson S, et al. Observations on the effect of chimeric anti-CD4 monoclonal antibody in patients with mycosis fungoides. Blood 1991;77:20–30.
87. Le Maistre CF, Rosen S, Frankel A, et al. Phase I trial of H-65-RTA immunoconjugates in patients with cutaneous T-cell lymphoma. Blood 1991;78:1173–1182.
88. Von Hoff DD, Cahlberg S, Hartstock RJ, et al. Activity of fludarabine monophosphate in patients with advanced mycosis fungoides: A Southwest Oncology Group study. JNCI 1990;82:1353–1355.
89. Grever MR, Leiby JM, Kraut EH, et al. Low-dose deoxycoformycin in lymphoid malignancy. J Clin Oncol 1985;3:1196–1201.

90. Cummings FJ, Kyungmann K, Nieman RS, et al. Phase II trial of pentostatin in refractory lymphomas and cutaneous T-cell disease. J Clin Oncol 1991;9:565–571.

91. Kessler JF, Meyskens FL, Levine N, et al. Treatment of cutaneous T-cell lymphoma (mycosis fungoides) with 13-*cis*-retinoic acid. Lancet 1983;1:1345–1347.

92. Molin L, Thomsen K, Volden G, et al. Oral retinoids in mycosis fungoides and Sézary syndrome. A comparison of isoretinoin and etretinate. Acta Dermatol Venereol (Stockh) 1987;67:232–236.

93. Hoting E, Meissner K. Arotinoid-ethylester: Effectiveness in refractory cutaneous T-cell lymphoma. Cancer 1988;62:1044–1048.

94. Zachariae H, Thestrup-Pedersen K. Combination chemotherapy with bleomycin, cyclophosphamide, prednisone and etretinate (BCPE) in advanced mycosis fungoides. A six-year experience. Acta Dermatol Venereol (Stockh) 1987;67:433–437.

95. Thomsen K, Hammar H, Molin L, et al. Retinoids plus PUVA (RePUVA) and PUVA in mycosis fungoides, plaque stage: A report from the Scandinavian Mycosis Fungoides Group. Acta Dermatol Venereol (Stockh) 1989;69:536–538.

96. Scheman AJ, Steinberg I, Taddeini, L. Abatement of Sézary syndrome lesions following treatment with acyclovir. Am J Med 1986;80:1199–1202.

97. Resnick L, Schleider-Kushner N, Horwitz SN, Prost P. Remission of tumor stage mycosis fungoides following intravenously administered acyclovir. JAMA 1984;251:1571–1573.

98. Jensen JR, Thestrup-Pedersen K, Zachariae H, Sogaard H. Cyclosporin A therapy for mycosis fungoides. Arch Dermatol 1987;123:160–167.

99. Puttick L, Pollock A, Fairburn E. Treatment of Sézary syndrome with cyclosporin. J R Soc Med 1983;76:1063–1069.

100. Bunn PA Jr, Edelson RL, Ford SS, Shackney SE. Patterns of cell proliferation and migration in patients with Sézary syndrome. Blood 1981;57:452–463.

101. Edelson RL, Facktor M, Andrews A, et al. Successful management of the Sézary syndrome. Mobilization and removal of extravascular neoplastic T-cell by leukapheresis. N Engl J Med 1974;291:293–297.

102. Edelson R, Berger C, Gasparro F, et al. Treatment of cutaneous T-cell lymphoma by extracorporeal photochemotherapy. N Engl J Med 1987;316:297–300.

103. Micaily B, Vonderheid EC, Brady L, et al. Total electron beam and total nodal irradiation for treatment of patients with cutaneous T-cell lymphoma. Int J Radiat Oncol Biol Phys 1985;11:1111–1119.

104. Hariot JC. Personal communication.

Cancer: Principles & Practice of Oncology, Fourth Edition,
edited by Vincent T. DeVita, Jr., Samuel Hellman, Steven A. Rosenberg.
J.B. Lippincott Co., Philadelphia © 1993.

Michael J. Keating

Elihu Estey

Hagop Kantarjian

CHAPTER **54**

Acute Leukemia

Acute leukemia is an uncommon form of malignancy affecting approximately 5 persons per 100,000 in the United States annually.[1] The disproportionate interest in acute leukemia compared with other malignancies over the years is a consequence of the devastating nature of untreated disease, with a 90% mortality rate within 1 year of diagnosis, and the valuable biologic and therapeutic lessons learned from the study of this disease.[2] Many new drugs with proven activity in malignant disease have been discovered initially in treatment of patients with acute leukemia, and the principles of combination chemotherapy were developed in the management of childhood acute lymphocytic leukemia (ALL).

Acute myelogenous leukemia (AML), also called acute nonlymphocytic leukemia, is five times more common than ALL, although the ratio of patients referred to tertiary centers may vary (Table 54–1).[1] AML is proportionately more common in patients older than 50 years of age, as demonstrated by patients referred to the M.D. Anderson Cancer Center (MDACC). Many of the older patients present with a preceding myelodysplastic phase.

Although the prognosis for adults with leukemia improved dramatically during the 1970s, progress was less impressive in the 1980s. However, there were major insights into the biology of acute leukemia. Although formerly the classification of acute leukemia relied entirely on morphology and histochemical stains, there has been a recent explosion of information on the cytogenetic patterns of acute leukemia and correlations with immunophenotype, oncogene expression, and gene mutations. The transformation of acute leukemia from a universally fatal disease to one that is curable in certain subsets of patients is one of the major accomplishments of cancer chemotherapy.

ETIOLOGY

The causes of most acute leukemias, especially adult ALL, are unknown. Epidemiologic studies have concentrated on the usually small variability in the incidence in different countries and within countries.[3,4] The incidence of AML and ALL is consistently higher in men than women, and this sex difference is more striking in older patients, causing speculation about the role of increased exposure to leukemogenic agents in male patients with AML (see Table 54–1). Although the incidence of leukemia overall has been stable for the last 30 years, the increasing age of our population will presumably result in a greater number of cases being reported.[3,5] There are minor ethnic differences. Acute leukemia is less common in blacks than whites, and the incidence for Jews is higher than for non-Jews.[6,7] Acute leukemia is more common in higher socioeconomic settings.

The contribution of heredity to leukemia has been focused on in the last few years as a result of increasing awareness of the importance of genetic rearrangements in acute leukemia. Several families with a clustering of leukemia have been reported, but siblings of patients with leukemia are only twice as likely as others to develop the disease.[8,9] The exception to this is in childhood leukemia, with concordance in identical twins of approximately one in four.[10,11] Parental consanguinity is a common feature in families with genetically related leukemias.[12]

The strongest association of heredity with leukemia is in Down's syndrome (*i.e.*, constitutional trisomy of chromosome 21), for which there is a 20-fold risk of leukemia.[13] Hereditary disorders with a tendency to chromosome breakage, such as Fanconi's anemia and Bloom's syndrome, are associated with

TABLE 54-1.   Distribution of Patients

Age (y)*	AML		ALL	
	Total	% Male	Total	% Male
<20	19	58	45	60
20–29	88	56	70	60
30–39	94	56	44	75
40–49	83	41	35	66
50–59	95	63	34	53
60–69	104	54	31	61
≥70	60	48	11	64
Total	543	54	270	63

AML, acute myelogenous leukemia; ALL, acute lymphocytic leukemia.
* Patients with leukemia seen at M.D. Anderson Cancer Center, 1980–1990.

an increased risk of AML.[14] Patients with Bruton type X-linked agammaglobulinemia and hereditary ataxia-telangiectasia have an increased risk of lymphoid neoplasms, including leukemia.[4] This increased risk is also associated with congenital agammaglobulinemia, severe combined immune deficiency, and Wiscott-Aldrich syndrome.[15,16]

The dominant piece of evidence for the causal association of radiation with AML and ALL is the markedly increased incidence of these diseases in survivors of the atomic bomb explosions in Japan. The overall incidence increased 10-fold to 15-fold and was greater for ALL than AML. The increased risk was first manifested 1 to 2 years after the explosions, peaked 5 to 6 years later, and then declined to baseline levels over the next 15 years.[17,18] There was no shift in age distribution. No increase in incidence could be demonstrated in patients estimated to be exposed to less than 100 cGy.[19] A possible association of increased risk of leukemia in military personnel present at nuclear bomb tests in Nevada has been reported.[20]

The strongest association of therapeutic irradiation with leukemia is in patients with ankylosing spondylitis who received x-ray therapy between 1935 and 1954, after which there was an overall fivefold increase in cases.[3,21] The time course was similar to that for the atomic bomb explosions. The use of therapeutic irradiation for menorrhagia and thymic enlargement, thorium dioxide (Thorotrast) in radiologic examinations, and ^{32}P for polycythemia vera are associated with an increased risk of AML.[22–25] Workers exposed to radium and U.S. radiologists working in the early part of this century had an increased risk of leukemia.[26,27] The risk of leukemia in children may be increased by parental preconceptual irradiation exposure and by exposure to extremely low-frequency nonionizing radiation.[28,29] Diagnostic radiologic procedures and the use of ^{131}I treatment of thyrotoxicosis and localized radiation for cancer of the cervix have not been associated with an increase incidence of leukemia.[30,31] The role of radiation treatment for other malignancies as a leukemogenic factor is discussed later.

There is substantial evidence for the leukemogenicity of benzene.[32–35] Benzene causes aplastic anemia. Many patients develop leukemia after a protracted period of cytopenia. Most patients developed leukemia within 5 years, but the increased likelihood may persist for 20 years.[35] Most cases have been a variant of AML. Erythroleukemia (M6) appears to be more frequent than expected. The level of exposure of most of these patients had been high for prolonged periods.[33,35] There have been reports of a geographic association of radon levels in homes with the incidence of AML, and investigators from Great Britain suggest that as many as 25% of cases of AML may be caused by radon exposure.[53] A recent report of an excess of radiation exposure in fathers of children with leukemia has not been validated.[54,55]

Little evidence supports the association of leukemia in adults with exposure to phenylbutazone or chloramphenicol, which can cause aplastic anemia, although an increased risk of childhood ALL in China was associated with chloramphenicol use.[30] There have been reports of an increased risk of AML with cigarette smoking, perhaps with a predisposition to certain cytogenetic subgroups.[36,37] Studies seeking an association with the use of pesticides by farmers have not provided strong evidence for increased risk.[38]

The viral cause of leukemia has been strengthened by data demonstrating integration of human T-cell leukemia virus-I (HTLV-I) into the genome of the leukemic cells in patients with adult T-cell leukemia-lymphoma and is supported by several seroepidemiologic studies.[39–42] HTLV-I is a retrovirus with reverse-transcriptase activity that enables the integration of DNA synthesized from the viral RNA template into the human genome. Missense or silent point mutations of the p53 gene were found in 5 of 10 patients with adult T-cell leukemia.[43] Adult T-cell leukemia-lymphoma is associated with mature-looking CD4-positive T cells that commonly invade the skin and is not a typical acute leukemia.[44] Retroviruses can cause acute leukemia in animals, such as the feline leukemia virus.[45] This common cause of leukemia (usually lymphoid) in cats has caused concern that pet owners and veterinarians may have an increased incidence of leukemia, but this has not been supported.[46,47] Leukemia did not increase in incidence after inoculation with polio myelitis and yellow fever vaccines, which contained SV40 viruses and avian leukosis virus, respectively.[48,49] No association of leukemia with the Epstein-Barr virus, which causes infectious mononucleosis, has been found.[50] Although one study associated ALL in Iowa farmers with cattle density and distribution of bovine lymphocytoma in herds, this may be related to other factors, such as the use of agricultural chemicals.[51,52]

SECONDARY LEUKEMIAS

Leukemia occurring after treatment of another malignancy is called secondary acute leukemia (SAL) or treatment-related leukemia. Most cases are AML or myelodysplastic syndrome (MDS).[56–59] Hodgkin's disease, lymphomas, myeloma, ovarian, and breast carcinomas are associated with an increased risk of secondary AML.[57–59] The peak time of development is 4 to 5 years after diagnosis of the initial malignancy.[58] Several factors, such as the causative agent(s) for the original neoplasm, radiation therapy, chemotherapy, immune status, and age of the patient, may affect the risk. Many chemotherapeutic agents, such as alkylating agents and procarbazine, are leukemogenic in animals and cause chromosome damage.[60,61]

The most intensively studied malignancy associated with a secondary AML is Hodgkin's disease.[62-64] Untreated Hodgkin's disease was not associated with secondary AML.[62] Most patients develop AML with their Hodgkin's disease still in remission after treatment.[65] The more intensive the treatment for the Hodgkin's disease, the shorter is the latent period to the second malignancy.[63] The incidence of AML after irradiation alone appears to be low.[65,66] Chemotherapy is more strongly associated with secondary AML in combined-modality therapy with chemotherapy preceding irradiation.[63] Most patients received MOPP chemotherapy (*i.e.*, nitrogen mustard, vincristine, procarbazine, prednisone), with a lower incidence seen with regimens such as ABVD (*i.e.*, doxorubicin, bleomycin, vinblastine, dacarbazine).[67] Older patients with Hodgkin's disease are more likely to develop secondary AML.[57,68] Most cases of secondary AML after myeloma have received melphalan and a disproportionate number have M4 or M5 morphology.[58,70] Most patients with lymphoma and myeloma reported with secondary AML have received chemotherapy and radiation therapy.[58,69,70] A report from the polycythemia vera study group showed that 1% of patients treated with phlebotomy alone developed acute leukemia, compared with 6% for the patients in the ^{32}P group and 11% in the chlorambucil group, within 6 years of initiation of treatment.[71] Morphologically, most patients with secondary AML have myeloblastic subtypes (*i.e.*, M1, M2) with a lower frequency of monocytic forms of leukemia (*i.e.*, M4, M5). Acute promyelocytic leukemia (APL, M3) is rarely seen as a secondary leukemia.[58] AML after chronic lymphocytic leukemia is an uncommon event.[72] Although an acute myeloid transformation is common in chronic myelogenous leukemia, it is considered as an evolutionary step in the disease process rather than a secondary AML.

A 21-fold elevated risk of developing secondary AML after treatment for ovarian cancer has been reported.[73] Alkylating agents are considered far more potent causative factors than irradiation. The only solid tumor associated with secondary AML is breast cancer.[74,75] Several of these patients have been diagnosed simultaneously as having leukemia and breast cancer, an event that is less common in the other associated malignancies. Most of the reported chemotherapeutic agents associated with the development second leukemias are immunosuppressive and cause DNA damage.

The karyotype of the abnormal cells in secondary AML is strikingly different from de novo AML.[58,76] More than 90% of patients with secondary AML have clonal cytogenetic abnormalities. Three quarters of the patients have lost all or part of chromosome 5 or 7. The modal chromosome number is often hypodiploid (<46). Deletion in the leukemic cells in chromosome 7 is from band 3;4 at the end of the long arm of the chromosome. Loss or deletion of chromosomes involving 5q31 appear to be the critical factor in secondary leukemias involving chromosome 5, suggesting that there may be loss of a tumor suppressor gene from this area. Administration of epidophyllotoxins (*i.e.*, etoposide, teniposide) is associated with a secondary AML and chromosome abnormalities involving 11q23.[77,78] For patients referred to the MDACC, classic cytogenetic abnormalities, such as translocation between or within chromosomes, especially t(8;21), t(15;17), and inv(16), are uncommon in secondary AML or in patients who present with prior MDS (Table 54–2).[58,76] The prognosis for response to treatment and survival of secondary AML and secondary MDS is determined by the cytogenetic pattern, patient age, and percentage of blast cells in the bone marrow.[76] The survival of the few patients with secondary AML with a favorable karyotype is good, survival of those with diploid patterns is intermediate, and those with -5/-7 abnormalities have the shortest survival (Fig. 54–1).

DIAGNOSIS AND CLASSIFICATION

CLINICAL FEATURES

Most patients with AML present with nonspecific symptoms of fatigue and malaise.[79,80] The degree of anemia is not closely correlated with the symptoms of fatigue. Only one fourth of the patients have had symptoms for more than 3 months before diagnosis. The relative distribution of clinical characteristics, symptoms, and laboratory findings in patients with AML, ALL, and acute undifferentiated leukemia (AUL) presenting at the MDACC between 1980 and 1990 are illustrated in Table 54–3.

TABLE 54–2. Cytogenetic Abnormalities in AML and MDS

Cytogenetics	De Novo AML (%)			Secondary AML (%) (101)	AML After MDS (%) (219)	MDS (%) (536)
	(<60 y, 322)*	(≥60 y, 127)	(Total, 449)			
t(8;21)	8	2	7	5	4	1
t(15;17)	13	2	10	2	1	0
Inv(16)	8	1	6	3	3	<1
Diploid	38	50	41	21	37	34
+8	4	7	5	9	12	7
−5, −7	8	15	10	26	19	31
Miscellaneous	14	14	14	25	12	12
Insufficient	6	8	7	8	10	10

AML, acute myelogenous leukemia; MDS, myelodysplastic syndrome.
* Patients seen at M.D. Anderson Cancer Center.

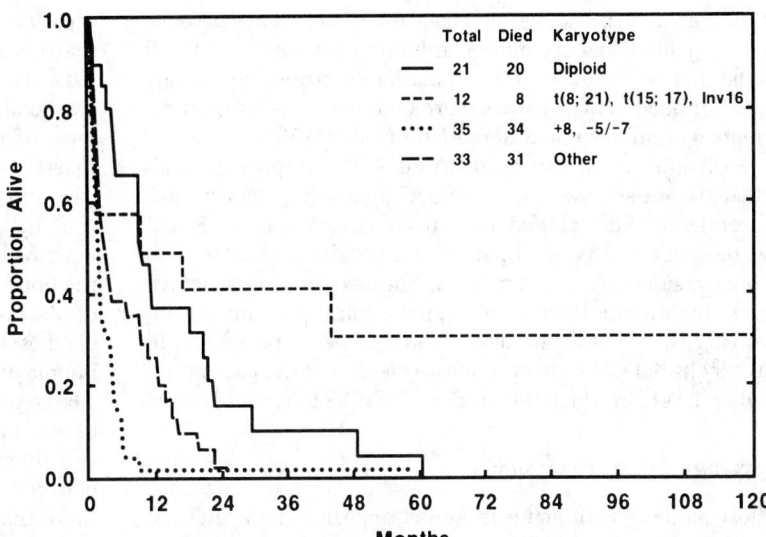

	Total	Died	Karyotype
—	21	20	Diploid
---	12	8	t(8; 21), t(15; 17), Inv16
····	35	34	+8, −5/−7
– –	33	31	Other

FIGURE 54–1. Survival by cytogenetic pattern of secondary acute myelogenous leukemia patients treated at the M.D. Anderson Cancer Center from 1980 to 1990.

TABLE 54–3. Clinical and Laboratory Features of Adults With AML, ALL, or AUL

	Percentage With Features*		
Characteristics	*AML*	*ALL*	*AUL*
Male	54	63	65
Age			
<30 y	20	43	14
≥50 y	48	48	51
Presenting symptoms			
Hemorrhage	28	23	16
Bone pain	7	13	6
Infection	30	18	26
Weight loss > 4.5 kg	8	14	14
Presenting signs			
Hepatomegaly	17	26	17
Splenomegaly	11	34	22
Lymphadenopathy	17	37	13
Mediastinal nodes	3	9	0
Gum infiltration	5	2	2
Blood findings			
WBC > 25,000/mm³	42	36	28
Platelets < 50,000/mm³	46	49	45
Special stains			
Peroxidase (>3%)	95	0	0
Nonspecific esterase	37	9	11
TdT	15	86	8
Chloroacetate esterase	74	1	9
Acid phosphatase	5	41	17
Auer rods	41	0	0

AML, acute myelogenous leukemia; ALL, acute lymphocytic leukemia; AUL, acute undifferentiated leukemia.
* Patients seen at M.D. Anderson Cancer Center, 1980–1990.

Symptoms of dyspnea, infection, and bleeding are relatively common. The most common infections were relatively minor upper respiratory tract infections or vague flu-like illnesses. Pneumonia was relatively common (~5%) but septicemia was uncommon (<1%) at the time of diagnosis. Many patients who are febrile at the time of presentation have no documented cause of fever. Symptoms of petechiae and ecchymoses are more common in patients with AML. Bleeding symptoms are far more common in patients with APL. Ecchymoses are common only in patients with APL and are associated with the coagulation disturbance rather than the platelet count. The incidence of petechiae correlates well with platelet count but is more common at platelet counts higher than 20,000μl than in other causes of thrombocytopenia, presumably due to impaired platelet function. Anorexia and significant weight loss are relatively uncommon. Bone pain is more common in patients with ALL. Bleeding manifestations and palpable lymph nodes are the only strong features suggesting a diagnosis of leukemia. Many other illnesses can be associated with the nonspecific presenting symptoms observed in most patients.

PHYSICAL FINDINGS

The most common physical finding in leukemia is pallor, and the associated tachycardia is proportionate to the degree of anemia.[79,80] Ecchymoses commonly occur on limbs and are spontaneous or often associated with minor trauma. Petechiae are more common in the lower limbs, presumably because of the hypostatic pressure of dependency. Clinical features of infection are often not striking, because the low neutrophil count and impaired neutrophil function do not allow development of abscesses in many circumstances or consolidation of the lung in patients with pneumonia.[81,82] Throat and gingival infections are relatively common and are often associated with hemorrhagic features. Perianal infections and other soft tissue infections are seldom associated with abscess formation. Hepatomegaly and splenomegaly, uncommon in AML, are more common in ALL (see Table 54–3). Palpable lymph node enlargement is also more prominent in patients with ALL.

Enlarged mediastinal lymph nodes are seen in a few patients on x-ray films and are more common in patients with T-cell leukemia. Within the AML population, hepatosplenomegaly and lymphadenopathy were more common (15–20%) in patients with monocytic differentiation (M4, M5).

Skin infiltration can occur in all AML morphologies, although some series suggest an association with monocytic differentiation. Sternal tenderness occurs in approximately half of the patients. Skeletal pain is not usually associated with abnormalities on x-ray films but can be associated with marked abnormalities on bone scans. Initial clinical presentation involving the central nervous system (CNS) is rare, even in ALL.[83] Initial CNS involvement suggests that the patient has a B-cell ALL, in which the incidence of CNS leukemia is high.

DIFFERENTIAL DIAGNOSIS

Most patients with acute leukemia appear to be acutely or chronically ill, with pallor and often with fever. A complete blood count, differential leukocyte and platelet counts, and blood smear can disclose marked abnormalities in most parameters (Table 54–4). Anemia, thrombocytopenia, elevated leukocyte count with a substantial number of blast cells is almost pathognomonic of acute leukemia. More difficulty is experienced in patients who have pancytopenia without circulating blast cells. Even ALL patients with low leukocyte counts often have a small proportion of circulating blast cells in the peripheral blood. Auer rods in the circulating leukemic cells is almost pathognomonic of AML (see Table 54–3). Auer rods can also be present in some mature cells.

Abnormalities in hematologic counts and the presence of atypical cells should prompt a bone marrow examination. Bone marrow aspiration and biopsy should be performed. In some patients, packing of the marrow with a high proportion of blast cells or development of a reticulin reaction to the presence of the abnormal cells can prevent an adequate bone marrow aspirate.[84] Some patients have hypoplastic bone marrows in association with an increased proportion of blast cells (*i.e.*, hypoplastic acute leukemia) and have inadequate bone marrow aspirates, necessitating a biopsy. In AML and ALL, the bone marrows are usually hypercellular. The proportion of blast cells is usually high (>50%). The major differential diagnosis is between other infiltrative diseases such as lymphoma or other solid tumors such as breast cancer. However, a large proportion of blast cells strongly suggests the diagnosis of acute leukemia.

If there is an increase in the proportion of blast cells to between 5% and 30%, a diagnosis of MDS is suggested.[85] If more than 30% blast cells are present, a diagnosis of acute leukemia is made, with the differential diagnosis among AML, ALL, AUL, or mixed-lineage leukemia. If more than 3% of the blast cells are positive on myeloperoxidase staining, a diagnosis of AML is made.[85,86] If fewer than 3% of the blast cells are peroxidase positive, a terminal deoxynucleotidyl transferase (TdT) stain is performed. If the cells are peroxidase negative and TdT positive, a diagnosis of ALL is likely. Some patients have negative peroxidase and TdT stains, and they are classified as having AUL.

Patients with fever, cytopenia, and a small proportion of circulating blast cells or a minor increase in blast cells in the bone marrow can be difficult to differentiate. Such reactions occasionally occur in tuberculosis, systemic lupus erythe-

TABLE 54–4. Hematologic Values at the Time of Initial Presentation With AML

Characteristics*	Value	AML (%)	ALL (%)	AUL (%)
Hemoglobin (g/dl)	<8	21	15	35
	8–12	71	71	58
	>12	7	14	6
Leukocytes (× 10³/µl)	<10,000	44	48	59
	10–24.9	15	16	14
	25–99.9	29	24	26
	≥100	13	12	2
Platelet count (× 10³/µl)	<25	23	19	24
	25–49	26	23	22
	50–100	27	25	20
	>100	25	29	35
Blasts + promyelocytes (% blood)	0	9	14	20
	1–24	23	25	28
	25–49	15	9	16
	≥50	53	52	37
Neutrophil count (× 10³/µl)	<0.25	33	23	28
	0.25–0.99	21	22	28
	1.0–5.0	27	40	31
	>5.0	19	15	14

AML, acute myelogenous leukemia; ALL, acute lymphocytic leukemia; AUL, acute undifferentiated leukemia.
* Patients (305) seen at M.D. Anderson Cancer Center, 1980–1990.

matosus, paroxysmal nocturnal hemoglobinuria, megaloblastic anemia due to folic acid or vitamin B_{12} deficiency, and aplastic anemia. Patients recovering from the effects of drug-induced marrow suppression often have a transient increase in blast cells during the recovery phase, and differentiation from AML in such patients requires only a repeat bone marrow evaluation after recovery is complete.

Most patients with cytopenias and modest increases in blast cells (5–30%) have features of dysplasia of the erythrocyte, leukocyte, or megakaryocytic series and are classified as MDS patients. These patients often have anemia, neutropenia, monocytopenia, or thrombocytopenia as single or multiple abnormalities. Although the cellularity of the bone marrow is usually increased, it is occasionally decreased. Megaloblastic changes are often prominent in the erythroid series, and care should be taken to separate these patients from folate and vitamin B_{12} deficiency syndromes. Cytogenetic analysis is the single most definitive test to separate MDS from other differential diagnoses. A cytogenetic abnormality occurs in three quarters of MDS patients (see Table 54–2). The finding of the abnormal cytogenetic population supports a strong presumptive diagnosis of a malignant process. The finding of a normal karyotype or insufficient metaphases does not negate the diagnosis of MDS.

The major differential diagnosis for ALL is lymphomas. Most transient viral infections (*e.g.*, infectious mononucleosis) can be sorted out using surface antigen studies, bone marrow aspiration and biopsy, and serologic studies. The differential diagnosis between ALL and lymphoma depends on the clinical pattern of presentation, whether the bone marrow and peripheral blood are involved, and the surface antigen expression. Lymphoblastic lymphoma and ALL appear to be part of the same spectrum of disease, and in adults, they are treated with similar regimens and have similar prognoses. The differential diagnosis between these two categories is less important. If more than one third of the bone marrow is involved, most investigators classify the patients as having ALL.

Difficult morphologic cases can be clarified by the use of electron microscopy. Patients whose cells are undifferentiated on light microscopy can have peroxidase granules detected using electron microscopy. In difficult cases, particularly if a megakaryocytic lineage is involved, electron microscopy studies to identify platelet peroxidase-positive cells is useful to confirm the diagnosis of megakaryocytic leukemia (M7).[87] Other useful stains are the Sudan black stain, the activity of which closely parallels the activity of the myeloperoxidase stain.[86] Cells with acute monocytic leukemia (M5) can be differentiated from AML using a nonspecific esterase stain,

such as naphthyl acetate.[88] The esterase activity is inhibited by sodium fluoride in acute monocytic leukemia but not in ALL or other AML subcategories. The periodic acid-Shiff (PAS) reaction is now less commonly used in the diagnosis of acute leukemia. PAS staining is positive in the blast cells of many patients with ALL, in whom blocks of positive staining material are found. The PAS stain is often positive in AML, but the staining pattern is usually more granular than in blocks.[89] TdT staining is not specific for ALL, because the TdT stain is positive (in 5% to 20% of patients with AML; see Table 54–3).

IMMUNOPHENOTYPING

A large literature documents monoclonal antibodies that react with surface antigens expressed on leukemia cell membranes. International workshops have evaluated leukocyte surface antigens and grouped them into 78 cluster designations.[90] The antibodies are useful for confirming the morphologic diagnosis and separating difficult cases. They have limited usefulness in allocating treatment or assessing prognosis. The most commonly used antigens for diagnosing AML are CD11, CD13, CD33, CD14, HLA-DR, CD41, and CD42. CD33 is positive in approximately three quarters of cases, CD13 in two thirds of cases, and CD14 in one third overall and in more than one half of M4 and M5 FAB subtypes. CD11 is positive in half of the cases of monocytic differentiation (Table 54–5). Approximately 20% of cases of AML express lymphoid markers of T-cell lineage.

In T-cell ALL, the most sensitive marker is CD7. CD1, CD2, CD3, and CD5 are other useful confirmatory markers. CD4 and CD8, which identify the helper and suppressor immunophenotypes, are positive in subsets of patients with T-cell ALL. The non-T-cell ALLs react in almost all cases with CD19 and commonly with CD20 and CD22. Most cases are HLA-DR positive. The most mature B cells (L3, Burkitt-type ALL) express surface membrane immunoglobulin of the kappa or lambda phenotype. CD10 (*i.e.*, common acute lymphocytic leukemia antigen or CALLA) is present on most cases of pre-B-cell ALL. The differential diagnosis of the different morphologies can be completed with a relatively defined range of surface antigens. A representative panel of surface markers that can be used to diagnose subtypes of acute leukemia is shown in Table 54–5. In addition, CD41 and CD42 are useful for diagnosing megakaryocytic leukemia and glycophorin, which is specific to red cells, is useful for diagnosing erythroleukemia.

Surface antigens characteristic of T cells exist in approxi-

TABLE 54–5. Surface Markers Useful in the Differential Diagnosis of Acute Leukemias

Leukemia	HLA-DR	CD33	CD11	CD13	CD14	CD3	CD5	CD7	TdT	CD15	CD22	CIg	SIg
AML	+*	+	+	+	+†	−	−	+	±	−	−	−	−
T-cell ALL	−	−	−	−	−	+	+	+	++	−	−	−	−
Non-T-cell ALL	+	−	−	−	−	−	−	−	+	+	+	+	+‡

* Except M3.
† M4 or M5.
‡ Mature B cell.

mately 20% of patients with AML, and myeloid antigens occur in 20% of patients with T-cell ALL.[91-93] A combination of morphologic evaluation, special stains, electron microscopy, and surface marker studies can establish the diagnosis of AML or ALL in more than 90% of patients. Other subsets express myeloid and lymphoid characteristics and are often called mixed-lineage leukemias.[94,95] Associations among surface antigen expression, cytogenetic pattern, clinical features, and response are emerging.[95] One study correlated surface antigen expression and response with therapy in AML.[97] Some truly undifferentiated leukemias exist.[96] Many of the undifferentiated leukemias are found to be acute megakaryocytic leukemias if electron microscopy is performed or if studies to detect platelet-specific surface antigens are performed.

Immunoglobulin (Ig) gene rearrangement and T-cell receptor rearrangement studies have been undertaken to separate different types of leukemia. However, 10% to 15% of patients with AML have Ig heavy chain (IgH) gene rearrangements and fewer than 5% have Ig kappa light chain rearrangements. Rearrangement of T-cell receptor genes (*i.e.,* TCR-β, TCR-γ, and TCR-δ genes) are found in 5% to 10% of patients with AML.[98] Ten percent to 15% of patients with T-cell ALL have rearrangements of IgH genes, but TCR-β, TCR-γ, and TCR-δ gene rearrangements or deletions have been found in 33%, 55%, and 80%, respectively, of precursor B-cell ALL.[99-101] The proliferation of methods to delineate lineage has not clarified the area, and few clinical decisions are made on the basis of these sophisticated tests.

LABORATORY FINDINGS

Anemia is found in most patients at the time of initial diagnosis. The erythrocyte morphology is usually normochromic and normocytic in AML and ALL. In AML, moderate macrocytosis can occur. Iron deficiency at the time of diagnosis is rare. Two percent to 5% of patients with AML have nucleated red cells in the peripheral blood smears. Marked anemia is more common in patients with erythroleukemia.

The proportion of patients with high leukocyte counts is similar in AML and ALL (see Table 54-4). Although absence of circulating blast cells are found on routine examination of peripheral blood counts in approximately 10% of patients, close scrutiny often can demonstrate some abnormal blast cells. Within the category of AML, low leukocyte counts are common in APL (M3) and higher counts are observed in monocytic forms (M4, M5) of AML (Table 54-6). Life-threatening thrombocytopenia (<25,000/μl) exists in one fourth of the patients at presentation and is more common in the M3 and M6 varieties of AML. Granulocyte and monocyte morphology is abnormal only in AML cases. Giant platelets or circulating micromegakaryocytes can occasionally be seen in AML. A variety of abnormalities in neutrophil and platelet functions have been described in AML but not in ALL.

BONE MARROW FINDINGS

The cellularity of the bone marrow is best evaluated using the bone marrow biopsy. A bone marrow aspirate with smears evaluates the morphologic type of leukemia better than biopsies. If inadequate aspirates are obtained for smears, a touch preparation of the biopsy material is often useful to allow good morphologic analysis. The causes of difficulty in aspirating marrow are extreme hypercellularity or hypocellularity, increased reticulin or collagen fibrosis, or marrow necrosis. Marrow necrosis is rare in AML and is more common in patients with ALL. Cellularity of the bone marrow is usually higher than 90% in two thirds of patients with AML and 75% of patients with ALL. Hypocellular (<30%) bone marrows are rare (<5%). More than 50% of the nucleated cells are blast cells in 80% to 90% of patients with AML and ALL. Megakaryocytes are usually decreased in number and may have an abnormal morphology in AML.

CLASSIFICATION

In 1976, the French-American British Cooperative Group established classification systems for acute leukemias and MDS.[102] They classified ALL into three morphologic subtypes:

TABLE 54-6. Percentage of Leukemic Patients With Clinical or Laboratory Characteristics According to Morphology

Characteristics*	M1 or M2 (n = 53)	M3 (n = 62)	M4 (n = 107)	M5 (n = 40)	M6 (n = 5)	L1 (n = 47)	L2 (n = 153)	L3 (n = 18)
>50 y	53	27	47	48	60	15	28	44
Male	59	55	48	35	60	72	61	78
AHD*	38	10	30	21	45	4	8	6
WBC > 25,000/mm³	38	11	66	57		34	39	22
Hepatomegaly	16	8	16	20	20	34	22	39
Splenomegaly	9	5	10	20	20	47	37	44
Lymphadenopathy	13	8	30	25	0	40	36	29
Gum infiltration	4	5	8	14	0	4	1	0
Fibrinogen < 150 mg/dl	2	40	3	11	0	4	3	6
Platelets < 25,000/mm³	22	45	20	7	40	21	18	11
Hyperuricemia	14	10	25	39	40	26	33	83
Creatinine ≥ 1.4 mg/dl	11	8	21	30	12	6	10	28

* Patients seen at the M.D. Anderson Cancer Center, 1980–1990.
† Antecedent Hematologic Disorder for ≥1 month.

L1, L2, and L3. AML was categorized as M1 through M6.[85] Subsequent modifications of the classification has broadened the AML categorization to include M0 (undifferentiated) and M7 (megakaryocytic) and subclassified M5 into M5a and M5b.[89,96,103] Acute myelomonocytic leukemia (AMML, M4) has been subclassified into M4e (*i.e.*, a subset of patients with dysplastic eosinophils).[85,89]

In ALL, the blast cells are usually round with amphophilic cytoplasm.[104] Granules are rarely present in the cytoplasm. The nucleus is usually round and has an open homogenous chromatin network. There are usually one or two small nucleoli. The AML cells are usually larger than in those of ALL, with more variation in the size and shape and with more cytoplasm. Granulation is usually seen. Auer rods are in the cytoplasm of the blasts and sometimes in more differentiated cells (40–45% of patients). Nuclear chromatin is usually reticulated with multiple nucleoli within the nucleus. Sole reliance on morphology and the appearance on Wright-Giemsa stain is inadequate, and ancillary aids such as special stains, immunophenotyping, and cytogenetics are used to establish the cell lineage.

In ALL, the reproducibility of the FAB system has been improved by the addition of a scoring system.[104] Approximately one third of adult patients are L1 type, and most of the others are L2 type. L3 morphology occurs in fewer than 5% of all adults with ALL. The scoring system for separating FAB L1 and L2 relies on the nuclear-cytoplasmic ratio, which tends to be high in L1 (with 0 or 1 nucleoli and small size in L1), the regularity of the nuclear membrane, and the size of the cells.

In AML, the FAB classification runs from M0 to M7. M0 shows minimal evidence of maturation. These cells are peroxidase negative by light microscopy but are often peroxidase positive by transmission electron microscopy, and they have myeloid surface antigens. In FAB M1, the cells tend to have some fine azurophil granules and may have a few Auer rods. There is minimal evidence of differentiation along the rest of the granulocytic or monocytic lineages. In FAB M2, the proportion of blast cells is greater than 30%, and the proportion of monocytic precursors is less than 20%. The cells have abundant cytoplasm and moderate to marked granularity. In FAB M3, otherwise known as APL, the predominant cell is heavily granulated with azurophil granulation. At least some and usually many cells have bundles of Auer rods. The nucleus is often bilobed or kidney shaped. Some cases have less extensive granulation (*i.e.*, microgranular variant). In FAB M4 (formerly AMML), the myeloid precursors (*i.e.*, myeloblast, promyelocytes, myelocytes) and other granulocytic precursors are between 20% to 80% of the nonerythroid nucleated cells. The monocytic cells comprise 20% or more of the nonerythroid nucleated cells. A proportion of these patients have dysplastic eosinophils, and these have been called M4e. In M5 (acute monocytic leukemia), the proportion of granulocyte precursors is less than 20%. In M5a, the blast cells are large with abundant cytoplasm and vacuolated basophilic cytoplasm. In M5b, the cells are more differentiated, and 20% or more of the abnormal cells are recognizable promonocytes or more mature with twisted, folded nuclei. In M6 (acute erythroleukemia), less than 30% of the cells are of myeloid or monocytic lineage, and more than 50% are megaloblastic erythroid precursors. M7 (acute megakaryocytic leukemia) is often asso-

ciated with extensive marrow fibrosis, with an increase in reticulin or collagen. The bone marrow biopsy often shows clusters of micromegakaryoblasts and other abnormal megakaryoblasts.

In the FAB classification subtypes, M1 and M2 usually stain strongly with peroxidase and chloroacetate esterase. M4 stains with PAS stain and α-naphthyl esterase. M5 stains strongly with PAS, α-naphthyl esterase, and acid phosphatase.

The reproducibility of the FAB myeloclassification is still not high (67%).[105,106] Some subtypes, especially M3, are easily recognized by most cytopathologists. Separation of the other subtypes remains difficult. The approximate distribution of the FAB subgroups in AML are M0<5%, M1=20%, M2=30%, M3=10%, M4=15% to 20%, M4e=5% to 10%, M5a=5%, M5b=5%, M6<5%, and M7<5%. There is little correlation between the FAB subclassification system and the response to treatment or survival.

DIFFICULTIES IN CLASSIFICATION OF ACUTE LEUKEMIA

Acute leukemia is a clonal disease involving stem cells. Supporting evidence for this is obtained from morphologic, cytogenetic, and in vitro growth data and surface antigen expression. The first decisions for the hemopoietic stem cell is whether to differentiate along lymphoid or myeloid lines. Subsequently, the myeloid lineage diverts along erythroid, megakaryocytic, or granulocyte lineages, including monocytic, neutrophilic, eosinophilic, or basophilic lines. Biphenotypic leukemia, in which some cells appear myeloid and others appear lymphoid, presumably arise from pluripotent stem cells. Later steps in the decision-making hierarchy are presumably decided at a nuclear level or under the influence of humoral factors (possibly autoregulatory) that direct the cells to grow along a particular lineage. The cell population can be predominantly eosinophilic, basophilic, monocytic, erythroid, megakaryocytic, neutrophilic, or a combination of these in myeloblastic leukemia. Single cells can demonstrate lineage infidelity, with surface antigens indicating commitments to multiple lines, such as erythroid, granulocytic, megakaryocytic, or even lymphoid lineage.[107-109] The presence of rearranged immunoglobulin genes and T-cell receptor genes in many cases of myelogenous leukemia and expression of myeloid surface antigens in 15% to 20% of cases of ALL emphasize the difficulties in categorizing many of these cases.[98-101]

Acute megakaryocytic leukemia is an uncommon form of leukemia strongly associated with myelofibrosis.[103,110] Detection of platelet peroxidase using transmission electron microscopy, immunohistochemical stains, and monoclonal antibodies against platelet antigens such as CD41 and CD42 have demonstrated that perhaps 5% of patients with AML have megakaryocytic involvement. Megakaryocytic leukemia is characteristically associated with secondary AML and has a high incidence of unfavorable cytogenetic abnormalities. The prognosis is poor.[110] Megakaryocytic hyperplasia often causes myelofibrosis as a reactive process not directly involved in the malignancy, and a normal karyotype has been found in the fibroblasts of these patients.[111]

Eosinophilic leukemia is rare.[112] The eosinophilia may be manifest in the peripheral blood or the bone marrow. There is often infiltration of cardiac, pulmonary, and central nervous systems, as observed in the benign hypereosinophilia syndrome. Most patients with AML with eosinophils in the blood or marrow have M4e associated with inversion of chromosome 16. Eosinophilia can be associated with a diploid karyotype or t(8q;21q) and other chromosomal abnormalities.[113] Reactive eosinophilia can occur in patients with ALL or lymphoma sometimes associated with a hypereosinophilic syndrome, presumably as a result of cytokine production by the lymphoid lineage.[114]

Chronic myelogenous leukemia (CML) presenting de novo in myeloid or lymphoid blast crisis can have substantial eosinophilia. Cytogenetic analysis is important in the evaluation of such patients. Acute basophilic or mast cell leukemia is rare, and most patients have variants of CML in blast crisis. Markedly abnormal basophilic staining can occur in patients with M3 and M4e in association with t(15;17) and inv(16).

MYELODYSPLASTIC SYNDROME

Patients who have cytopenias and persistently abnormal marrows with dysplasia of one or multiple lineages are classified as having MDS.[115] In refractory anemia (RA), there is predominant dysplasia in the erythroid series with less than 5% blast cells in the bone marrow, and less than 1% blast cells in the peripheral blood. In some of these patients, more than 15% of the nucleated erythroid cells are ring-sideroblasts (RASA). Patients with refractory anemia with excess blasts (RAEB) have marked dysplasia of the granulocytes and erythrocytes. The marrow blast cells comprise 5% to 20%. Refractory anemia with excess blasts in transformation (RAEBT) is diagnosed if patients have 20%% to 30% blasts cells in the marrow and sometimes more than 5% blasts in the peripheral blood. Auer rods in MDS patients places them in the RAEBT group. Some patients with MDS have an absolute monocytosis in the peripheral blood of at least 1,000/μl, a condition called chronic myelomonocytic leukemia (CMML). Otherwise, these patients resemble the other MDS groups, and the monocyte count has no prognostic significance.

BIOCHEMICAL AND GENETIC IRREGULARITIES

BIOCHEMICAL ABNORMALITIES

Many patients with leukemia present with abnormalities in a variety of biochemical parameters. The serum uric acid is elevated in 20% of patients with AML, especially M4 and M5 types, and 30% with ALL. It is markedly elevated (>10 mg/dl) in 5% to 10% of patients. Uric acid urinary excretion is almost always increased.[116] Renal impairment due to urate nephropathy is uncommon until treatment is initiated. At that point, rapid lysis of tumor cells can cause a sudden uric acid load for excretion.[117] Tumor lysis syndrome is more common in ALL than AML. A high serum uric acid level is more common in patients with high leukocyte counts, large tumor burden, and monocytic morphology in AML patients. Elevation of the blood urea nitrogen (BUN or serum creatinine) occurs in 10% to 15% of patients at diagnosis. Renal impairment is more common in patients who are elderly or who present with fever or documented infection. Serum muramidase levels

are elevated in AML but not ALL and are more strikingly elevated in M4 or M5 patients.[118]

The serum lactate dehydrogenase (LDH) level is elevated in most patients.[118] The most striking elevations appear to occur in patients with ALL, especially B-cell ALL. The serum LDH is an important prognostic factor for remission duration and CNS leukemia in adult ALL.[83,119] The elevated LDH correlates with large tumor burden and a high labeling index in the blast cells.[120]

Mild hepatic dysfunction occurs in a small proportion of patients with acute leukemia. Hypoalbuminemia is common (30–40%) and is an adverse prognostic factor for survival in AML and ALL. The serum calcium level correlates with the serum albumin level and is therefore modestly decreased in a substantial number of patients.

Hypercalcemia rarely occurs in acute leukemia, and if present, suggests ALL, possibly acute T-cell leukemia. The vitamin B_{12}-binding proteins and folic acid-binding proteins are commonly elevated in AML and correlate with the height of the leukocyte count.[121,122] Hypokalemia is commonly found in AML and less commonly in ALL.[123] It is more common in cases with monocytic differentiation. Hypofibrinogenia (<150 mg/dl) occurs in 40% of patients with M3 morphology, 10% of those with M5, and 2% to 5% of other cases of AML and ALL who present to the MDACC (see Table 54–6).

CYTOGENETIC ABNORMALITIES

Most patients with acute leukemia studied with Giemsa or quinacrine banding techniques have an abnormal karyotype in their leukemic cells.[124] High-resolution banding techniques suggest that almost all patients have cytogenetic abnormalities.[125] The changes in chromosome number and structure are not random. Several well-defined clinical syndromes have been described in AML and ALL. The commonest translocations that have been described in AML (5–10% of cases in each) are translocations between chromosomes 8 and 21, t(8q;21q), and between chromosomes 15 and 17, t(15q;17q). Pericentric inversions or translocations of chromosome number 16 also occur in 5% to 10% of patients with AML (see Table 54–2). These three specific translocations occur only in AML and more common in young patients, and overall, they occur in 25% of all patients with de novo AML (see Table 54–2).[124,126] There is a strong association of t(8q;21q) with M2 morphology, presence of Auer rods, and loss of an X or Y chromosome in one half of cases, t(15q;17q) with M3 morphology, and inv(16) in M4e patients.[124]

The breakpoint on chromosome 15 in APL occurs at the PML transcription unit and the retinoic acid receptor-alpha gene is involved in chromosome number 17.[127–130] This generates a chimeric PML-RARA gene product. This chromosome abnormality is associated with a dramatic response of M3 patients to treatment with all-*trans*-retinoic acid.

Trisomy of chromosome 8 or deletions or losses of chromosomes 5 or 7, alone or with additional changes, are common in patients with MDS or secondary AML, are more common in older patients, and are rarely Auer rod positive (see Table 54–2).[126] A small group of male patients with AML demonstrate loss of the Y chromosome in their leukemic cells. These patients tend to behave as if they had no chromosome abnormality.[131]

Two thirds of adults with AML have cytogenetic abnormalities. Abnormalities in chromosome 11 with a breakpoint at 11q23 occur in several cases of monocytic differentiation and biphenotypic cases.[95] The other chromosomes involved in the translocations with chromosome 11 vary but include chromosomes 8, 4, and 9. Inversion in chromosome 3 occurs in a small proportion of patients, and translocation between chromosomes 6 and 9 also occurs in a few patients.[132] Abnormalities in chromosome 20q- are somewhat common in AML and are more common in MDS.[133] The Philadelphia chromosome has been described in a variety of patients with AML.[134] It is described less commonly now in AML than previously for unknown reasons. Several studies confirm the consistent clinical usefulness of the cytogenetic pattern as a prognostic factor in AML.[135-138]

Approximately 10% to 15% of adults with ALL have insufficient metaphases for cytogenetic analysis. Great attention to technique in childhood ALL has been associated with improved ability to document clonal abnormalities, now observed in more than 90% of patients with ALL.[139] The specific cytogenetic abnormalities commonly observed in adult ALL are t(4;11), t(9;22) or t(8;14), t(2;8), and t(8;22).[140,141] Other abnormalities include 14q+ and 6q−. The marked hyperdiploidy (>50 chromosomes) that is common in good-prognosis childhood ALL is rare in adults (<5%).[141] Twenty-five percent of adults have the Philadelphia chromosome present. The abnormality, t(9;22)(q34;q11), has a chromosome break at the breakpoint cluster region (*BCR*) gene in chromosome 22, and the *ABL* protooncogene from chromosome 9 is translocated to the breakpoint in the *BCR* gene. This creates a chimeric *BCR-ABL* gene. In one half of the patients, the chimeric gene ultimately gives rise to the formation of a 210-kd protein (p210) and the other half to a 190-kd protein (p190) in adults. It does not appear that there is a difference in response or survival for the p210 or p190 protein patients.[142]

The t(8;14), t(2;8), and t(8;22) are important although uncommon abnormalities.[141, 143-145] They occur in L3 morphology ALL or Burkitt-type leukemia. In this disease, the *MYC* oncogene on chromosome 8 is brought into apposition with the heavy or light chain regions of the immunoglobulin genes. The t(4;11) is often associated with a biphenotypic leukemia, with features of ALL and monocytic differentiation.[146] All of these cytogenetic abnormalities are associated with a poor prognosis in adult ALL. The t(1;19) that is common in childhood pre-B ALL is uncommon in adults.[147]

GENE REARRANGEMENTS IN LEUKEMIA-ASSOCIATED CHROMOSOMAL TRANSLOCATIONS

Molecular biology has enabled the delineation of specific abnormalities in identified genes. Many of these have been observed in ALL. The *MYC* involvement in t(8;14), t(2;8), and t(8;22) has been well described, as has been the situation with t(15;17) with *PML* and *RARA*. The t(1;19) translocation involves genes *PBX1* on chromosome 1 and *E2A* on chromosome 19. The Philadelphia chromosome abnormality of *ABL* and *BCR* is also well known. Common involvement of chromosome 14q11 in T-cell ALL involves the T-cell receptor genes *TCR-α* and *TCR-δ*. Several other protooncogenes are involved in human malignancies (*e.g.*, *ETS1* oncogene in t(4;11) ALL, *ETS2* in t(8;21) AML (M2), *TCL2* and *TCL3* in

T-cell ALL, *PRL* in pre-B t(1;19) ALL, and *CAN* in t(6;9). These specific changes in association with clinical syndromes suggest that they are crucial components in the pathophysiology of some cases of AML and ALL.[148] The specific breakpoints suggest that therapeutic interventions targeted to these abnormalities can be useful.[149]

Structural alterations in protooncogenes and tumor suppressor genes are an area of active exploration. A mutation of the *RAS* genes occurred in 15% to 25% of cases in acute leukemia, more commonly in AML M4 or M5 (33%), and is most common in CMML.[150-152] Fifteen percent to 20% of patients with myelodysplasia and AML have mutations in the *FMS* protooncogene.[153,154] Mutations of the p53 gene have been described in AML and ALL, as have abnormalities in the retinoblastoma (*RB1*) tumor suppressor gene.[155-158] The exact roles of these abnormalities in leukemogenesis require further exploration.

There are additional roles for oncogenes. Qualitative alterations in oncogene expressions, such as mutations, deletions, or rearrangements, and quantitative alterations, such as gene amplification, occur in human leukemia. Because the expression of several of these oncogene products depends on the cell cycle, normal or exaggerated levels of the protein do not necessarily indicate involvement in the disease process. Further work in this area is certain to lead to major advances in our understanding of acute leukemia.

BIOLOGIC FEATURES OF ACUTE LEUKEMIA

AML is characterized not by rapid cell proliferation but a gradual accumulation in the bone marrow or in other organs of undifferentiated cells. The proportion of blast cells in S phase (*i.e.*, undergoing DNA synthesis) or in mitosis in leukemia is lower than in normal bone marrow blasts.[159-162] Considerable heterogeneity exists in the proportion of cells in each cell cycle. Small blast cells tend to have low labeling indices (*i.e.*, percent of cells in S phase), but larger cells are more commonly in S phase.[163] Some cells are considered to be dormant (G_0) but can be recruited into the cycle. Blast cells can recirculate from the peripheral blood to the bone marrow.[164] The proportion of cells in the cell cycle is higher at the time of relapse than at initial presentation.[159,165]

Most antineoplastic agents are more effective on cells participating in the cell cycle. Several agents, such as vincristine, corticosteroids, alkylating agents, and L-asparaginase, appear to cause direct cell lysis of leukemic cells.[166-169] Several drugs, such as cytosine arabinoside (ara-C), amsacrine, 5-azacytidine, and purine analogs, inhibit DNA synthesis, and the anthracyclines arrest cells at the G_2-M interface.[170-175] Vincristine, VP-16, and VM-26 affect cells in mitosis.[176]

Initial attempts at recruiting leukemic cells into the cycle to make them more susceptible to chemotherapy used agents such as ara-C and hydroxyurea.[170,177-180] Growth factors such as (granulocyte-macrophage colony-stimulating factor (GM-CSF) and interleukin-3 (IL-3) stimulate growth and differentiation of leukemic cells.[181-185] Clinical trials have attempted to synchronize the cells into S phase using GM-CSF.[186-190] The results of these trials are equivocal, with some reporting promising results, but others demonstrated a negative impact.[189,190] The clinical concern is that the stimulation of growth of leukemic cells may have a deleterious effect on the patient's outcome.[190]

The prognostic impact of measurements of the cell cycle, such as the percentage of cells in S phase, using flow cytometry or tritiated thymidine labeling indexes has not been reproducible. Some studies correlated a high S-phase percentage with a high complete remission rate, but others have not found this result.[178,179,191,192] A high S-phase percentage has been associated with shorter remission duration.[192] One study demonstrated a discordance of the prognostic impact of S phase on response according to age, with high S-phase percentage associated with a good response in younger patients but a poor response in older patients.[193] The proportion of cells in S phase is higher in bone marrow biopsy specimens than aspirates, because aspirates are diluted with peripheral blood in which a smaller proportion of the blast cells are in the cycle.[194,195] AML appears to be a disease in which cells with limited ability to differentiate accumulate in the bone marrow. Ten percent to 25% of these cells appear to be in G_0 and less susceptible to the effect of chemotherapeutic agents.

Fewer cell cycle studies have been conducted using adults with ALL. Using flow cytometry, the ALL cells show considerable heterogeneity. A high proportion of cells in S phase occurs in B-cell ALL (L3). The mean percentage of cells in S phase is the same as in AML, but there are more cells with high proportions of cells in S phase. The RNA index is lower in ALL than in AML. The results of cell cycle kinetics and the RNA index did not affect outcome for ALL or AML patients in one study.[196]

GROWTH IN CULTURE

Several investigators have attempted to grow leukemic cells in a variety of media. Most studies have used semisolid culture media, such as agar. Normal bone marrow reproducibly grows in agar with colonies of cells (>40 cells) and clusters that are smaller groups of cells.[197] There is no widely used reproducible method of growing ALL cells.[198] A variety of growth stimuli have been applied, such as phytohemaglutinin or placenta conditioned media. GM-CSF has been added alone or with other growth factors to enhance the growth of leukemic cells.[185,199] Similar actions are observed with IL-3.[183] Growth is enhanced with combinations of growth factors compared with the use of single growth factors.[200] The cells that grow from patients with AML can be replated and in some circumstances continue to form colonies and clusters. This is called secondary plating efficiency or the self-renewal capacity and is reported to be a prognostic factor in obtaining a complete remission with chemotherapy. The pattern of growth in agar is reported to indicate a poor prognosis for remission for patients whose cells grow large clusters.[201]

DIFFERENTIATION

Several factors can cause differentiation of AML cells. These include dimethyl sulfoxide, hexamethyl bis-acetamide, and vitamin A and vitamin D analogs.[202–204] G-CSF and GM-CSF caused differentiation of AML cells, and drugs such as ara-C, 5-azacytidine, and aclacinomycin in low doses induced dif-

ferentiation in some cell lines.[205–209] The most potent evidence for differentiation appears to be with the application of *trans*-retinoic acid to HL60 cells, other cell lines, and patient samples, which translated into therapy to induce complete remissions in APL.[210–213] Few data are available on differentiation of ALL cells in adults.

TREATMENT

Treatment of AML and ALL involves remission induction and postremission therapy. Complications occurring during induction that may be fatal are infection, hemorrhage, and organ failure. Remission is usually obtained by causing severe marrow hypoplasia with high doses of chemotherapy and allowing the normal residual stem cells the opportunity to regrow faster than the leukemic cells, restoring normal neutrophil and platelet counts and the hemoglobin level.

Meticulous surveillance for infection and institution of early vigorous antimicrobial treatment is paramount. The prevention of bleeding from severe thrombocytopenia and coagulation disturbances is crucial. The evaluation of the patient initially should include an estimate of the hemoglobin level, neutrophil count and platelet count, fibrinogen level, and renal and hepatic function. If the patient is febrile and neutropenic, immediate initiation of broad-spectrum antibiotic therapy is mandatory. The risk of dying within 24 hours of untreated gram-negative septicemia is about 20% to 30%.[214] Leukemia alone is seldom a cause of fever at initial diagnosis, and the fever is almost always associated with occult or overt infection. Common sites of infection are the oropharynx, lungs, bloodstream, perirectal areas, and the urinary tract. Chest x-ray films and cultures of the throat, urine, blood, and any obvious lesions must be performed immediately.[214]

If the platelet count is less than 20,000/μl, the patient should receive prophylactic platelet transfusions, and these should be continued as needed (even 1–2 times a day) until the patient achieves complete remission.[215] Most patients need to be transfused with platelets two or three times each week during the remission-induction phase. Approximately 15% to 20% of patients are relatively or absolutely refractory to platelet transfusions at the time of diagnosis. HLA-matched platelets or transfusions from parents, siblings, or children may overcome this resistance.[216]

Disseminated intravascular coagulation (DIC) occurs at the time of presentation, predominantly in patients with APL or those with monocytic morphologies (see Table 54–6). Vigorous treatment with fresh frozen plasma or cryoprecipitate to maintain a fibrinogen level of more than 100 μg/dl and a platelet count above 50,000/μl in patients with evidence of DIC is essential. The role of heparin therapy in DIC in AML is uncertain and has been recently addressed.[217]

Leukostasis occurs in a significant number of patients with high circulating leukemic cell counts (>100,000/μl) and is more common in AML.[218,219] It occurs in 10% to 20% of patients at diagnosis.[220] The most effective way to decrease clinical leukostasis that involves the brain and the lungs is to commence chemotherapy immediately to decrease the cell count and to prevent proliferation of cells that have invaded vessel walls and then grown to form colonies of leukemic cells. Approximately 10% of patients with a leukocyte count of more than 100,000/μl die within the first 10 days of therapy of cerebral or pulmonary hemorrhage.[220] Leukapheresis is also useful in decreasing the circulating blast counts but does not prevent the growth of leukemic cells that have already left the vessel wall and invaded tissues.

Other features requiring effective medical treatment include hepatic and renal insufficiency, which can occur as a result of infiltrating leukemic cells but are more often associated with the presence of infection, hyperuricemia, and dehydration. Organ dysfunction due to proliferation of leukemic cells is an indication for immediate chemotherapy. Hypokalemia occurs frequently and hypocalcemia and hypomagnesemia less frequently, and they should be corrected to prevent arrhythmias, especially if amsacrine is being used.[221] Hyperuricemia should be managed with allopurinol and alkalinization of the urine, particularly in patients with ALL, because tumor lysis is more common in this disease.

CHEMOTHERAPY FOR ACUTE LEUKEMIA

The early treatment of AML and ALL in adults used corticosteroids, methotrexate, 6-mercaptopurine, and vincristine, initially as single agents and subsequently in combinations.[222-224] The emergence of ara-C as the major single agent

in the management of AML in the late 1960s converted this incurable disease to a potentially curable condition.[225-227] The subsequent development of the anthracyclines, such as daunorubicin, doxorubicin (Adriamycin), rubidazone, and idarubicin, allowed new combinations with these agents to be developed.[228-232] Representative results of chemotherapy regimens such as the 3/7 regimen, ara-C plus thioguanine, TAD or DAT (daunorubicin, ara-C, thioguanine), and idarubicin plus ara-C regimens are shown in Table 54-7.[233-240]

A study of daunorubicin plus ara-C compared with doxorubicin plus ara-C demonstrated no significant difference in response rate with these regimens.[241] Several studies have substituted mitoxantrone and amsacrine for the anthracycline combination with ara-C.[242,243] Higher doses of ara-C have been studied to overcome pharmacokinetic resistance. The vinca alkaloids, alone or in combination with corticosteroids, and the epidophyllotoxins, methotrexate, 6-mercaptopurine, cyclophosphamide, and L-asparaginase have only minor activity in adult AML, despite marked activity in ALL.

Most regimens in adult ALL incorporate vincristine, corticosteroids, prednisone or dexamethasone, anthracyclines, or L-asparaginase in the initial remission induction phase (see Table 54-7).[248-252] Most remission maintenance therapies rely heavily on 6-mercaptopurine and methotrexate, which are

TABLE 54-7. Commonly Used Remission Induction Regimens for Acute Myelogenous and Lymphocytic Leukemia

Regimen	Drugs	Dose Plus Schedule	No. of Patients	References	Complete Response (%)	Comments
AML						
3/7	Ara-C	100 mg/m²/d × 7 CIVI				
D 3/7	+ Daunorubicin	45 mg/m²/d × 3	646	238, 239, 242, 244, 245	358 (55)	Various studies
I 3/7	+ Idarubicin	12–13 mg/m²/d × 3	161	238, 239	116 (72)	Two randomized studies vs D 3/7
M 3/7	+ (Mitoxantrone)	12 mg/m²/d × 3	98	242	62 (63)	Randomized study vs D 3/7
TAD	Thioiguanine		216	244	123 (57)	Randomized vs 3/7
	ARA-C		576	246	374 (65)	TAD 9
	Daunorubicin		1127	247	757 (67)	D 1/5
ALL						
VAD	Vincristine	0.4 mg/d × 4 CIVI	105	248	(84)	38% CCR at 14 y
	Doxorubicin	12 mg/m²/d × 4 CIVI				
	Dexamethasone	40 mg/d, days 1–4, 9–12, 17–20				
Gimena	Prednisone	40 mg/m²/d × 6 wk	358	249	284 (79)	25% CCR at 4 y, consolidation not helpful
	Vincristine	1.5 mg/m² q w × 6				
	L-Asparaginase	10,000 I.V./m² q wk × 3 (wk 1,2,3)				
	Daunorubicin	40 mg/m² q wk × 3 (wk 3,4,5)				
German	Prednisone	60 mg/m²/d × 28 d	368	250	272 (74)	40% CCR at 4 y
	Vincristine	1.5 mg/m² q wk × 4				
	Daunorubicin	25 mg/m² q wk × 4				
	L-Asparaginase	5000 I.V./m²/d × 14 d				
Linker	Prednisone	60 mg/m²/d × 28 d	109	251	96 (88)	~45% CCR at 4 y for all <50 y of age, 4% induction mortality
	Vincristine	2 mg q wk × 4				
	Daunorubicin	50 mg/m²/d × 3				
	L-Asparaginase	6000 I.V./m²/d × 12 (d 17–28)				

active in adult ALL. Mitoxantrone, amsacrine, and alkylating agents have some activity in salvage therapy of ALL and have been incorporated into combination regimens. VM-26 has been used in children in combination with ara-C as salvage therapy.[253] The clinical pharmacology of these chemotherapeutic agents was discussed in an earlier chapter. Because the regimens used in the management of AML and ALL are different, they are discussed separately.

MANAGEMENT OF ACUTE MYELOGENOUS LEUKEMIA

Most remission induction regimens for AML incorporate a combination of ara-C and an anthracycline. Ara-C is usually given by a 7-day continuous infusion at a dose of 100 to 200 mg/m² per day. No advantage was found for the higher dose.[245] Traditionally, daunorubicin at a dose of 45 mg/m² per day for 3 days has been added to ara-C to form the traditional 3/7 regimen (see Table 54–7). Attempts to enhance the complete remission rate by extending the duration of infusion to 10 days or adding thioguanine to the regimen has not enhanced the response rate in comparative clinical trials.[244] Subsequently, the 3/7 regimen has become the "gold standard" against which other regimens are compared.

Idarubicin plus ara-C was compared with daunorubicin plus ara-C, with ara-C being maintained at the same schedule and dose.[238–240] One study demonstrated a significantly higher complete remission rate in the idarubicin plus ara-C arm compared with the daunorubicin plus ara-C arm.[238] Two other comparative trials suggested that idarubicin plus ara-C was equivalent or slightly superior to daunorubicin plus ara-C.[239,240] Idarubicin differs from daunorubicin in that its major metabolite (*i.e.*, idarubicinol) has antileukemic activity, but daunorubicinol has no significant antileukemic activity and is still toxic.[238] Idarubicin may be less susceptible to the effect of a multidrug resistance (*MDR1*) gene in terms of accumulation and retention of the drug in cell lines.[238] There is no evidence that doxorubicin or rubidazone have superior activity to daunorubicin. Bishop and colleagues reported that the addition of etoposide to the standard daunorubicin plus ara-C 3/7 regimen is associated with a significantly better remission duration in younger patients.[254]

Mitoxantrone was compared with daunorubicin. There is no significant difference in the complete remission rate in the studies of this agent combined with ara-C.[242]

Ara-C is given by continuous infusion, because there is good evidence for schedule dependency in animal and human clinical studies.[225–227] Ara-C requires uptake by the leukemic cells and activation by an enzyme called deoxycytidine kinase to the triphosphate form.[255] Cytidine deaminase deaminates ara-CMP to ara-UMP and ara-C to ara-U.[255] The triphosphate form of ara-C inhibits DNA synthesis by competitive inhibition of DNA polymerases and by incorporation into DNA.[256–258] It is thought that cells can become resistant to ara-C by lack of an effective level of deoxycytidine kinase, having increased d-CTP to compete for inhibition of DNA polymerase, and rapid egress from the cell of ara-CTP.[259–261] High-dose ara-C regimens are expected to overcome partially the second and third postulated components of resistance. The proposed mechanisms of actions of the various drugs used in the management of AML are discussed in the chapter on pharmacology. The activities of these drugs as single agents are described largely in relapsed patients.

The standard remission induction regimen for treatment of AML can include an anthracycline plus conventional-dose ara-C given by continuous infusion. A complete remission rate of 70% to 80% can be obtained in typical protocol patients. These patients are usually younger than 60 to 65 years of age, with no preceding MDS, no prior malignancy, normal or near-normal hepatic and renal function, and good performance status. Unfortunately, these patients are a minority of patients who present to physicians. Substantially lower response rates are obtained at MDACC in older patients with poor performance status, impaired renal function, MDS, or treatment-associated or secondary AML (Table 54–8 and Fig. 54–2).

The major cause of failure to achieve remission induction is death from infection and hemorrhage (Table 54–9). Ten percent to 20% of patients fail to achieve remission because they are refractory to the chemotherapy administered. Causes of failure to achieve complete remission in patients presenting with de novo acute leukemia, those with secondary AML or a history of MDS, and those with impaired hepatic or renal functional or poor performance status are illustrated in Table 54–9. Nonprotocol patients (groups 2–4) are more likely to fail to achieve remission because of infection (especially fungal), hemorrhage, or organ failure, which occurs during the induction course. Resistance also appears to be more common in these subsets of patients. Questions still remain about the wisdom of treating some nonprotocol-eligible elderly patients with vigorous chemotherapy regimens. There is little evidence

TABLE 54–8. Outcome of Remission Induction Treatment According to Age and Protocol Eligibility Status

Age (y)	Protocol Eligibility*	No. of Patients†	Complete Response (%)	Resistant (%)	Death (%)
<60	Yes	315	81	9	10
<60	No	173	47	19	34
≥60	Yes	101	55	16	29
≥60	Yes	193	36	19	44

* Eligibility criteria: performance status, 0–2 (Zubrod); serum creatinine < 2 mg/dl; bilirubin < 2 mg/dl; no prior myelodysplastic syndrome or secondary acute myelogenous leukemia.
† Patients seen at the M.D. Anderson Cancer Center, 1980–1990.

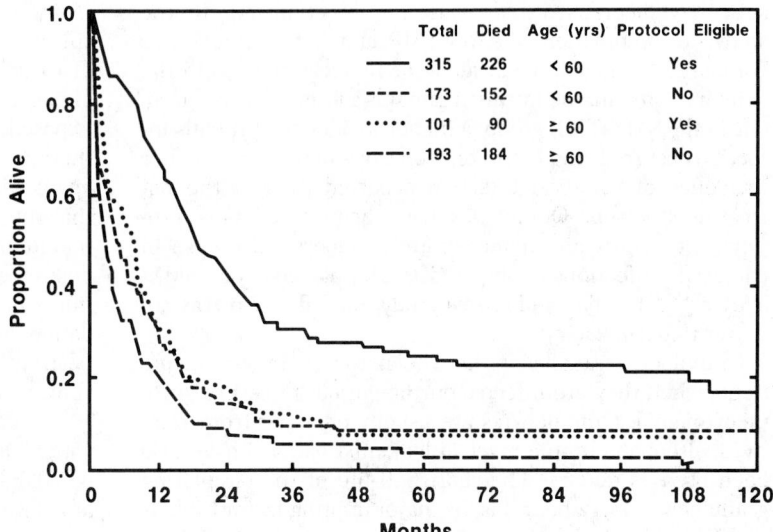

Total	Died	Age (yrs)	Protocol Eligible
315	226	< 60	Yes
173	152	< 60	No
101	90	≥ 60	Yes
193	184	≥ 60	No

FIGURE 54–2. Survival by age and protocol eligibility groups of patients with acute myelogenous leukemia (AML) patients treated at the M.D. Anderson Cancer Center from 1980 to 1990.

that there is a substantial cure fraction in this group of patients (see Fig. 54–2). However, some patients with advanced age and no prior MDS (group 3) have a smooth remission induction course and a satisfying remission duration. The proportion of patients older than 70 who are cured with chemotherapy is small.[262]

Preisler defined the causes of failure as type 1 or drug resistance with persistence of leukemia after treatment; type 2 or drug resistance with regrowth of leukemia after aplasia; type 3 or regeneration failure with death after prolonged aplasia (>40 days); type 4 or aplastic death with death from hypoplasia (<40 days); and type 5 or early death within 7 days after a course of chemotherapy.[263] Partial remission is defined as type 2 resistance.

The morbidity of induction therapy is predominantly associated with the intensity of the myelosuppression that occurs. Most patients have a period of 3 to 4 weeks of severe neutropenia and thrombocytopenia. Virtually no patient goes through remission induction therapy without having an episode of fever. Organ failure is usually associated with severe infection. Most patients require vigorous support with erythrocyte and platelet transfusions. Hair loss is usually significant because of the doses of anthracyclines that are used.

With the advent of more effective antibacterial agents, the number of patients dying during remission induction from gram-negative bacterial infections is decreasing. However,

gram-positive organisms such as methicillin-resistant *Staphylococcus aureus* and *Enterococcus fecalis* are emerging as more frequent contributors to morbidity and mortality.[264-266] The major emerging problem is the development of fungus infections.[267] *Aspergillus* infections are increasing, and many fungal infections that were formerly caused by *Candida albicans* are now associated with a variety of other *Candida* species.[268] The most common site of fatal infections remains the lungs. Most pulmonary infections in which no pathogenic source can be identified are eventually identified at autopsy as fungal infections. Opportunistic infections such as *Pneumocystis carinii*, cytomegalovirus, and herpes simplex are uncommon causes of fatal pneumonias.

Infection Prevention

Early attempts at prevention of death by decreasing infection focused on management in protected environments (PE). Two of three randomized studies demonstrated a higher complete remission rate for patients who were treated in a protected environment.[269-271] The optimal antibiotic regimen to decrease the probability of infection used in conjunction with PEs has not been demonstrated. A variety of regimens incorporating nonabsorbable antibiotics and systemic antibiotics have been used. Oral sulfamethoxazole plus trimethoprim (SMX-TMP) and the quinolones (*e.g.*, ciprofloxacin, norflox-

TABLE 54–9. Factors Contributing to Death During Remission Induction for Acute Myelogenous Leukemia

No. of Patients*	Infections (%)			Hemorrhage (%)	Organ Failure (%)†
	Bacterial	Fungal	Unknown		
315	3.2	1.6	1.9	6.0	5.7
173	4.4	14.5	7.5	15.6	25.4
101	6.9	14.9	5.9	14.9	22.8
193	12.4	17.1	12.4	12.4	33.7

* Patients seen at the M.D. Anderson Cancer Center, 1980–1990.

acin) have been used to decrease the infection rate. In one study, a combination of SMX-TMP and ketoconazole was compared with each agent alone or no treatment.[272] In the combination arm, the infection rate was substantially reduced, but in the SMX-TMP group, a higher incidence of fungus infection occurred, and in the ketaconazole-alone arm, a higher incidence of bacterial infection occurred than in the no-treatment group. Quinolones have been studied as prophylactic agents and demonstrated a superior decrease in bacterial infections compared with placebo or SMX-TMP.[273,274] In one randomized study, ciprofloxacin was superior to norfloxacin.[275]

Granulocyte transfusions have been used to support the patients when they are infected during periods of severe granulocytopenia. Granulocytes are usually obtained from relatives, although chronic myeloid leukemia patients have also been used as donors. The short half-life of the circulating granulocytes (<12 hours) is the major limiting factor in their use. It is difficult to harvest enough granulocytes to be useful in sustaining a circulating neutrophil count over a 24-hour period. The prospects of using agents such as G-CSF and GM-CSF to increase the circulating granulocyte count in normal donors is attractive. Randomized trials confirm the beneficial effect of granulocyte transfusions in severe infections in neutropenic patients.[276-278]

The cornerstone of management of infectious complications is to initiate empiric broad-spectrum antibacterial therapy that covers *Pseudomonas* spp., *Klebsiella* spp., and *E. coli.* Although gram-positive infections are becoming more common, they are seldom fatal within the first 48 hours. Fungus infections seldom cause precipitous demise of the patient. Therefore, broad-spectrum gram-negative coverage using a third- or fourth-generation cephalosporin alone or combined with a semisynthetic penicillin or aminoglycoside is satisfactory.[279-282] Regimens incorporating vancomycin to cover gram-positive organisms have been successfully used.[283] If the fever persists for 2 to 4 days and there is evidence of pneumonia, the addition of antifungal therapy with fluconazole, fluorocytosine, or amphotericin-B is recommended.[284] Positive blood cultures for methicillin-resistant *Staphylococcus aureus* or α- or γ-hemolytic streptococci with no response to initial therapy suggests that vancomycin should be added to the regimen.[283]

Fungal infections are more common in older and poor-prognosis patients.[267] *Aspergillus* should be considered in any patient developing a nodular or cavitating pneumonia or a pneumonia associated with a pleural friction rub or sinusitis.[285] Unfortunately, the response to amphotericin-B in fungal infections in the presence of severe neutropenia is poor. Fluconazole has good clinical activity against *Candida* spp. but not against *Aspergillus.*[286]

Postremission Therapy

Many terms have been used to described postremission therapy. These include consolidation, intensification, and maintenance therapy. Consolidation or intensification therapy regimens use doses of chemotherapy that cause severe and often prolonged neutropenia and thrombocytopenia, as occur during remission induction, but maintenance regimens produce low neutrophil counts of the order of 250 to 500/μl and platelet counts of approximately 50,000 to 100,000/μl. Initially,

maintenance therapy was continued indefinitely. Late intensification procedures were introduced to decrease the duration of therapy and to eliminate any residual leukemic cells by giving agents to which the patient had not been previously exposed and they demonstrated the ability to discontinue therapy.[287,288] The question of duration of maintenance therapy is still unresolved. Most studies of no maintenance show that the remission duration is usually slightly longer in the maintenance group of patients.[246,289,290] Studies have demonstrated a slight improvement in complete remission duration when maintenance has been given after early consolidation or intensification.[246,291] No significant advantage of postremission therapy for more than 1 year compared with shorter times has been demonstrated.[292,293]

CONSOLIDATION THERAPY. Several studies have evaluated the use of one or two courses of high-dose ara-C, usually at a dose of 3 g/m^2 over 1 to 2 hours every 12 hours for 8 to 12 doses, usually combined with daunorubicin or amsacrine. These are single-arm studies with no comparison with conventional therapy. These strategies have been applied predominantly to patients with AML who were younger than 50 years of age. The probability of being alive and in remission at 3 to 8 years (*i.e.,* potentially cured) varies from 32% to 49%.[294-299] The intensification regimens are associated with considerable morbidity and mortality. One study failed to find an advantage for adding high-dose ara-C to postremission therapy.[295] This was the only comparative study, and there were no differences observed in patients receiving conventional high-dose ara-C regimens. The most popular approach to postremission therapy is to give one or two courses of an intensive postremission regimen incorporating high-dose ara-C. No comparative trials or historically controlled trials have demonstrated convincingly the optimal approach to postremission therapy.

ALLOGENEIC BONE MARROW TRANSPLANTATION AND INTENSIFICATION THERAPY. Several studies of allogeneic transplantation during first remission have been conducted. In one large study from Seattle, the long-term survival rates were 45% to 50%.[300] Similar results were obtained by the International Bone Marrow Transplant Registry (IBMTR).[301] Other studies compared transplantation with intensive chemotherapy. A UCLA study found a significant difference in the probability of remaining in remission at 5 years but no significant difference in survival.[301] A Seattle study compared allogeneic transplant with two consolidation courses of TAD.[302] Some patients in that study elected not to undergo transplantation; 43 patients received chemotherapy because they did not have a donor, and 33 patients received a transplant. There was a higher likelihood of the transplant patients being alive and in remission at 5 years than in the chemotherapy group. There was a slight increase in the 5-year survival rate of 40% in the transplant plus the "assigned to transplant" group compared with 30% in the chemotherapy group, but this was not statistically significant. A subsequent study from UCLA compared 28 adult patients who had a histocompatible transplantation for AML during first remission, with 54 consecutive age-matched adult patients treated with one or more cycles of high-dose ara-C-based consolidation therapy.[297] The relapse rate was significantly lower in the transplant group, but the treatment-related mortality was much higher in the group treated with bone marrow transplantation. There was no significant difference in survival at 5 years for the two groups.

In all reports, it appears that the relapse rate in the transplant population is less, the mortality associated with the transplant is greater, and there is a 5% to 10% higher 5-year survival in the allogeneic transplant group than in the intensive chemotherapy group. The use of partially mismatched related donors and matched unrelated donors is being actively explored.[303]

AUTOLOGOUS BONE MARROW TRANSPLANTATION. Because of the lack of HLA-compatible siblings for allogeneic transplant, there has been considerable interest in the use of autologous bone marrow transplantations in patients during first remission of AML. Several single-arm noncomparative trials show disease-free survival rate of 25% to 60%.[304-308] The largest experience reported suggests that chemopurging is beneficial.[308] The time from complete remission to bone marrow transplantation was usually 3 to 6 months. For this reason, patients at risk of early relapse were excluded from these studies. Not all studies, particularly two from Holland, have demonstrated an improved disease-free survival; in the Holland studies, the proportion of disease-free patients is approximately one in three.[304,307] Comparative trials are underway to document the usefulness of autologous bone marrow transplantation during first remission compared with intensive chemotherapy. The usefulness of bone marrow purging with chemotherapy or monoclonal antibodies and the optimal methodology for purging remain questionable.

MANAGEMENT OF ADULT ALL

As with AML, the phases of treatment of ALL include remission induction and postremission phases. The principles of supportive care apply equally to management of ALL and AML. One difference is that the likelihood of tumor lysis syndrome is higher in patients with ALL, and greater attention should be paid to adequate hydration and monitoring of serum uric acid, phosphate, and potassium levels in the first 3 to 5

days after commencing chemotherapy. Allopurinol should be given prophylactically and the urine alkalinized before chemotherapy. Allopurinol can be given safely except for regimens including 6-mercaptopurine. (Allopurinol markedly increases the serum levels of 6-mercaptopurine.) The tumor lysis syndrome is most frequently observed in patients with B-cell ALL and T-cell ALL and can occasionally occur in non-T, non-B cases with a large tumor burden.

Regimens that incorporate L-asparaginase should have the fibrinogen level monitored, because it can decrease after L-asparaginase therapy. Fibrinogen replacement should be considered if the level falls below 100 mg/dl.

Most regimens are based on the use of vincristine and prednisone or dexamethasone, and most include daunorubicin or doxorubicin (see Table 54–7). Many regimens include L-asparaginase. The usefulness of the addition of L-asparaginase to regimens that use vincristine, prednisone, and an anthracyclines is uncertain. The complete remission rate after chemotherapy is 60% to 85%. The most recent MDACC studies including the VAD regimen report remission rates between 70% and 85% (see Table 54–7).[248-251]

The largest experiences are from the cooperative groups coordinated by Mandelli in Italy and Hoelzer in Germany. In three of these studies, the complete remission rates were 79%, 74%, and 75%. The median remission durations in various studies range from 19 to 27 months, with 22% to 41% of patients predicted to be in complete remission at 5 years. Clarkson and colleagues reported the L10/L10M and L17/L17M protocols in 1985 and obtained complete remission rates of 82% to 85%, with long remission durations and 45% of patients predicted to be in complete remission at 5 years.[309] The remission duration curve and the survival curve of the MDACC VAD regimen patients by age are shown in Figures 54–3 and 54–4.

Of the 20% to 30% of adult ALL patients who do not achieve remission, approximately 10% die during the first 8 weeks of treatment.[250] Most of these patients die of infection, especially fungal infection. The remainder are resistant to chemotherapy, and although some can achieve a remission on salvage therapy, the prospect of cure for this group of patients with chemotherapy is extremely small.

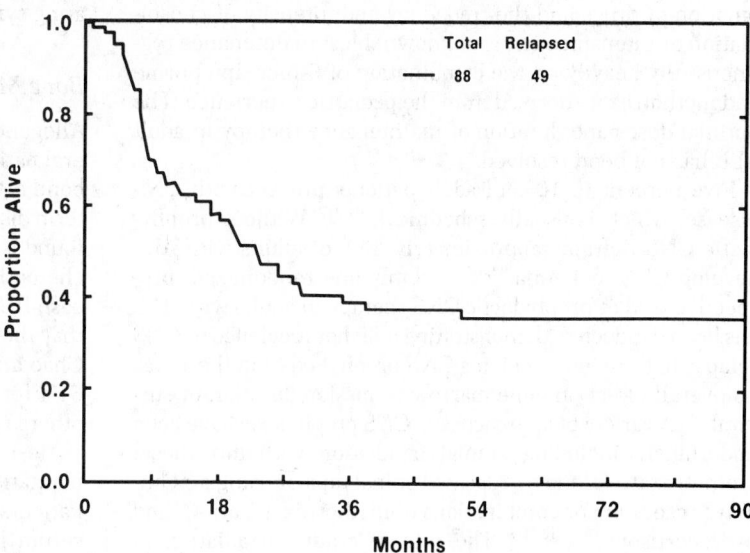

FIGURE 54–3.   Remission duration curve for adults with acute lymphocytic leukemia treated with vincristine, doxorubicin, and dexamethasone (VAD) at the M.D. Anderson Cancer Center.

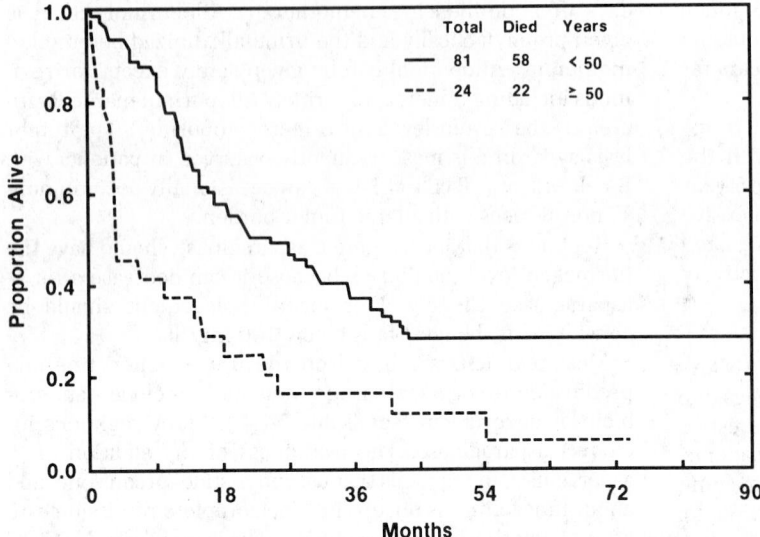

FIGURE 54–4. Survival duration curves for adults with acute lymphocytic leukemia treated with vincristine, doxorubicin, and dexamethasone (VAD) at the M.D. Anderson Cancer Center.

High-dose chemotherapy studies adding methotrexate or rubidazone for treating adult ALL did not improve the complete remission rate in a variety of studies.[310,311] High-dose ara-C has been administered to several patients as the initial therapy.[311–315] The response rate overall is approximately 75%. The median remission duration and proportion of patients in continued complete remissions is not superior to conventional regimens.

Postremission Therapy

Postremission treatment of ALL uses the same terminology as in AML (*i.e.*, intensification, consolidation, maintenance). The regimens are complicated and described in several publications.[248–251,309,312] Intensification strategies using L-asparaginase or ara-C plus cyclophosphamide or ara-C plus daunorubicin have prolonged complete remission durations but have usually not improved overall survival. Two studies of intensification demonstrated prolongation of the median remission duration, and one showed a superior survival for patients receiving consolidation therapy.[311,312] The best combination of drugs and the frequency and intensity of consolidation or intensification is unknown. Most maintenance regimens rely heavily on the combination of 6-mercaptopurine and methotrexate derived from the pediatric experience. The optimal doses and duration of maintenance therapy in adult ALL has not been resolved.

Five percent to 10% of adult patients present with CNS disease, which is usually subclinical.[309,319] Without prophylactic CNS therapy, approximately 40% of adults with ALL develop CNS leukemia.[83,316–318] Only one randomized, prospective trial of prophylactic CNS therapy in adults with ALL has been conducted, demonstrating a higher incidence of CNS relapse in those not receiving CNS prophylaxis, but there was no overall effect on bone marrow remission duration or survival.[318] A variety of approaches to CNS prophylaxis have been undertaken, including cranial irradiation with intrathecal methotrexate (alone by repeated spinal taps or using an Ommaya reservoir) or combinations of methotrexate, ara-C, and hydrocortisone.[309,316–318] The role of cranial irradiation in

preventing adult CNS disease has not been prospectively addressed. Different risk features have been identified for the probability of developing CNS disease. A high serum LDH level, high leukocyte count, high percent of cells in S phase in the bone marrow, and B-cell morphology are associated with a high probability of CNS disease.[83,248,250]

If CNS leukemia occurs, treatment is usually undertaken with intrathecal therapy with methotrexate alone or combined with ara-C or hydrocortisone.[249] Many investigators use cranial irradiation, and this is certainly indicated in patients who have cranial nerve or peripheral nerve palsies, because it is likely that there is infiltration of the nerve roots deeper within the nerve than can be reached by topical application of chemotherapeutic agents.[83] CNS therapy is not without side effects.[319,322] Cranial irradiation is associated with somnolence and can aggravate myelosuppression associated with systemic therapy. Repeated spinal taps are associated with the development of arachnoiditis in a small percentage of patients, causing pain in the lumbosacral area, fever, and occasionally meningism. This is less likely if preservative-free saline, Ringers' solution, or Elliot's B solution are used. Demyelinating syndromes have been reported.

Bone Marrow Transplantation

Allogeneic bone marrow transplantation is being used in several patients with ALL.[323] A major Seattle study of allogeneic bone marrow transplantation in ALL found only a 21% long-term disease-free survival.[324] The IBMTR data on 251 patients found a disease-free survival rate of 44%.[325] Comparison of chemotherapy and the IBMTR data suggests that overall disease-free survival was comparable for the two treatments and that the same prognostic factors for failure applied to both. Chao and colleagues reported a disease-free survival rate of 61% for 53 high-risk patients with ALL in first remission, and others reported 40% to 50% disease-free survival rates.[326,327]

Most investigators recommend that bone marrow transplantation be offered during first remission for high-risk adult patients, such as those with high initial leukocyte counts, high serum LDH levels, B-cell ALL, Philadelphia chromosome-positive ALL, and those who take a long time to achieve complete remission.[326,327] The better-risk group of patients have an excellent survival on conventional chemotherapy, and it is recommended that allogeneic transplant be conducted in patients in second remission if necessary.

Autologous bone marrow transplantation is being investigated in adult ALL. Data for second or later remissions have not been promising, with long-term survival rates of less than 20%.[323] There are several difficulties preventing ALL and AML patients from eventually receiving autologous transplants, and these are illustrated by Berman and colleagues.[328]

SALVAGE THERAPY

The prognosis of patients who failed to achieve remissions with their initial therapy (primary refractory) or who relapse after achieving remission (relapsed) remains poor. Overall, only 1 of 3 patients can achieve a second remission, and for most patients, the second remission is shorter than the first. The main prognostic factor associated with the probability of achieving complete remission on the first salvage therapy is response to initial therapy. Patients who have failed initial therapy or relapsed in less than 1 year have a response rate for initial salvage therapy of 25% to 35%.[329,330] Patients whose first complete remission lasted 18 months or longer appear to have a similar prognosis to de novo AML patients. Younger patients with normal organ function, no prior malignancy or MDS, and good performance status have a superior prognosis, as in the initial therapy of AML (Fig. 54–5).[329]

The median survival after initiating salvage therapy is only 14 weeks because of the high mortality during remission induction, and only 15% survived for 1 year. Patients with favorable cytogenetic parameters, such as t(8;21), t(15;17), and inv(16), have the highest probability of obtaining second complete remissions. The second remissions in this subset of patients with long first remissions (particularly >18 months) or favorable karyotypes is associated with a long-term continuous complete remission fraction of 15% to 20%.[330] There is a strong correlation between the duration of first remission and karyotype. Patients with favorable karyotypes of t(8;21), t(15;17), and inv(16) tend to have the longest remissions.

Several regimens have been tried to improve the complete remission rate.[329,330] High-dose cytosine arabinoside, alone or combined with amsacrine or mitoxantrone, has been used.[331-336] New drugs that have activity in AML include idarubicin, mitoxantrone, amsacrine, and diaziquone.[337-341] 5-Azacytidine has modest activity as salvage therapy. Mitoxantrone and VP-16 are commonly used together as a salvage regimen.[343-344] The complete remission rate for amsacrine as a single agent is 20% to 30%. Patients who have Auer rods in their leukemic cells have a markedly high complete remission rate with amsacrine therapy.[345] Mitoxantrone as a single agent has complete remission rates of 10% to 33%.[338-339]

The initial reports on high-dose ara-C (2–3 g/m^2 over 1 to 3 hours for 9 to 12 doses every 12 hours) claimed to have complete remission rates of 50% to 60%.[332-334] More experience with the regimen applied to a nonselected patient population suggests that the first salvage complete remission rate in unselected patients is closer to 33%.[331] Several schedules using lower doses of ara-C with or without asparaginase have produced complete remission rates equivalent to the more toxic high-dose schedules.[333,346] Intermediate doses of ara-C are less toxic and as effective as higher doses when combined with mitoxantrone in relapsed patients with AML.[347] In one of the few randomized studies of salvage therapy for AML, high-dose ara-C and amsacrine were equally disappointing.[348]

Allogeneic transplantation for patients who have disease that is primary refractory or who relapse is an attractive approach, because it is associated with a complete remission rate of approximately 50% to 60% and with 10% to 20% of patients who are long-term survivors.[349] Autologous bone marrow transplantation using bone marrow that has been cryopreserved during first remission has resulted in complete remissions in approximately 50% of patients. Most of these patients relapsed.[350,351] The use of autologous bone marrow transplantation as an intensification strategy for second remissions has been associated with long-term survival for a few patients.[352]

Relatively few salvage regimens have been developed for adult ALL. A variety of programs incorporating high-dose ara-C, alone or with L-asparaginase, amsacrine, mitoxantrone, or idarubicin, have been studied.[353] Great variability in complete

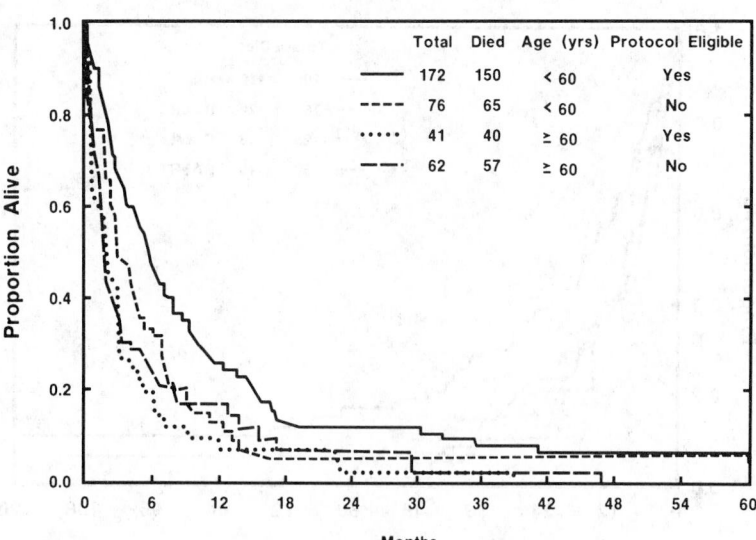

FIGURE 54–5. Survival by age and protocol eligibility status of patients with acute myelogenous leukemia after the first salvage therapy.

remission rates (21–86%) has been reported using these regimens, suggesting a high degree of patient selection. The best results have been reported with a combination of high-dose ara-C with mitoxantrone, idarubicin, or amsacrine.[355–358] Using high-dose ara-C alone, approximately one third of patients achieve remission, but in published series, a combination of high-dose ara-C with mitoxantrone or amsacrine produces a complete remission rate of 50% or greater. The use of GM-CSF after treatment with mitoxantrone and high dose ara-C has decreased the mortality rate but has not increased the complete remission rate.[359]

MANAGEMENT OF ACUTE LEUKEMIA IN THE ELDERLY

Most clinical protocols, particularly those from cooperative groups, address the treatment of AML patients younger than 60. Early trials of chemotherapy failed to achieve remissions in most older patients. The major cause of an adverse outcome was death during remission induction. The complete remission rate with agents such as ara-C and daunorubicin with or without corticosteroids was only 10% to 22%.[360–362] Combinations of ara-C and anthracyclines yielded complete remission rates of approximately 30% in such patients.[363] The 3/7 regimen improved the complete remission rate to 46%, and a combination of rubidizone, ara-C, vincristine, and prednisone achieved a complete remission rate of 48% in patients older than 50 years of age.[241,364,365] The major cause of failure is death during induction due to infection or hemorrhage. Patients older than 60 have a higher likelihood of having a previous MDS, previous malignancy, adverse cytogenetic pattern, reduced performance status, and impaired renal function. All these factors correlate with probability of failure to achieve complete remission in this elderly population.

MANAGEMENT OF MYELODYSPLASTIC SYNDROME

Management of this frustrating group of disorders is limited by the fact that these patients are predominantly elderly and have unfavorable karyotypes (see Table 54–2). Early attempts at chemotherapy resulted in low response rates, primarily because of high mortality during remission induction therapy. This led to attempts at treatment with low-dose cytosine arabinoside, differentiating factors such as *cis*-retinoic acid, and therapeutic strategies using growth factors such as G-CSF, GM-CSF, and erythropoietin.[366–368] The response rate from ara-C has been reported between 20% to 60% but is generally considered to be 20%.[366] The degree of patient selection in these clinical trials presumably explains the variability in complete remission rates.

Although ara-C was thought to function in low doses as a differentiating agent, most of the patients who achieved complete remission developed hypoplastic bone marrows before obtaining complete remissions. None of the differentiation strategies has proven effective in achieving complete remissions in clinical trials with substantial numbers of patients.[368]

G-CSF and GM-CSF can reproducibly improve the neutrophil count in 80% to 90% of patients.[369–372] However, trilineage response involving improvement in hemoglobulin and platelet count are uncommon (<20%). Approximately 20% of patients, usually those with RAEB and RAEBT, have documented leukemia progression when receiving GM-CSF. This has not been observed in patients to whom G-CSF have been administered. G-CSF is usually better tolerated than GM-CSF, which can be associated with fever, lethargy, bone pain, and fluid retention. Trials of IL-3 in MDS results in increase of bone marrow cellularity and increases in neutrophil, eosinophil, basophil, lymphocyte, and monocyte counts. Leukemia progression was not observed. Platelet counts improved in several patients, but erythrocyte production was not increased.[373,374] There is no clinical trial demonstrating a survival advantage for patients treated with growth factors.

One study demonstrated that the survival of patients with MDS when stratified according to karyotype is similar to that of AML.[375] The overall survival of MDS patients at the MDACC according to FAB group is shown in Figure 54–6. Studies were initiated to treat patients with MDS with chemotherapy. Patients with favorable karyotypes have been treated with anthracycline and ara-C combinations.[376–378] More than half of the patients treated on these regimens achieved complete re-

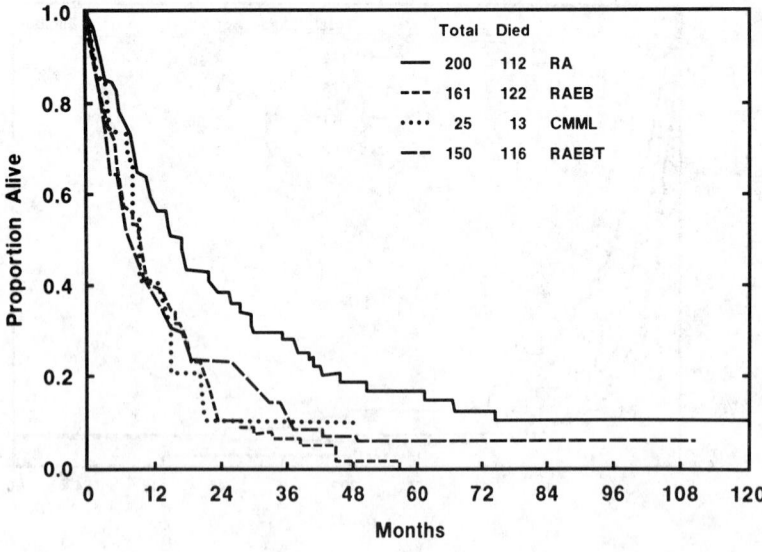

FIGURE 54–6. Survival by FAB group of patients with myelodysplastic syndrome treated at the M.D. Anderson Cancer Center between 1980 and 1990.

missions, suggesting that chemotherapy is an effective strategy in some patients with improved supportive care. Responses after chemotherapy are typical trilineage improvements, with normalization of hemoglobin and of the neutrophil, platelet, and bone marrow differential counts.

USE OF GROWTH FACTORS AS SUPPORTIVE THERAPY

Because of the severe myelosuppression that occurs after intensive chemotherapy in acute leukemia, efforts have been undertaken to increase the speed of recovery of the neutrophil count. High-risk patients have received GM-CSF to enhance recovery of neutrophils.[379] No differences in response rate, duration of neutropenia, or complications were found compared with historic controls. One study administered GM-CSF to poor-prognosis or relapsed AML patients who had hypoplasia after intensive chemotherapy.[380] The 50% complete remission rate compared favorably with a 32% remission rate in historic controls. Two patients had evidence of leukemia regrowth that appeared related to the GM-CSF. A randomized study of G-CSF was conducted by Ohno and colleagues.[381] Patients with refractory or relapsed acute leukemia received chemotherapy and were randomly assigned to receive G-CSF or placebo. The G-CSF-treated group had fewer infectious complications and tolerated higher dose of antileukemic therapy. Recovery of granulocytes was more rapid in the G-CSF group. The complete remission rate was somewhat higher in the G-CSF group (50% versus 36%). No influence on leukemia cell growth was observed.

PROGNOSTIC FACTORS

A variety of prognostic factor analyses have been undertaken for AML and ALL. The patterns have some similarities in the two diseases and distinct differences. Advancing age is an adverse prognostic factor, with patients older than 50 years with either disease faring worse than younger patients.[249,250,382-384]

For each disease, the importance of genetic determination is illustrated by the powerful impact of the cytogenetic profile on probability of outcome.[385] In AML, patients with t(8;21) or inv(16) have an excellent response to therapy (>90% complete remission rate) and a probability of long-term survival of 30% to 40%. Patients with t(15;17) have a complete remission rate of approximately 75%, and if they achieve complete remission have a 30% to 40% probability of long-term survival. Patients who are diploid (*i.e.*, no abnormality detected on cytogenetic analysis) or whose only abnormality is the loss of the Y chromosome have a complete remission rate of 65% to 70%, and approximately 20% of patients remain in complete remission. Patients who have lost part or all of chromosome 5 or 7 or have an additional chromosome 8 as a single chromosome abnormality or combined with other features have response rates of less than 50%, and few of these patients (<5%) remain in complete remission for 3 to 5 years.

A history of MDS is an adverse prognostic factor, as are features of poor performance status or impaired organ function. A low serum albumin level appears to be an adverse prognostic factor in all leukemias.[384,385] Several predictive models have been developed to determine the probability of response based on these variables.

In adult ALL, the major factors predicting response are age, with younger patients having a superior probability of responding, and cytogenetic pattern.[249-251,386] Patients who have the Philadelphia chromosome or have B-cell ALL have a lower complete remission rate. Diploid patients with ALL and those with insufficient metaphases have superior outcomes to those with other abnormalities. There has been no favorable karyotype identified in patients with adult ALL. The favorable karyotype of hyperdiploidy (>50 chromosomes) determined in children is uncommon in adults (<5%). A low serum albumin level and myeloid markers on the blast cells are unfavorable factors for complete remission. L3 morphology (B-cell ALL) is a known adverse factor. Patients with L1 morphology have a higher complete remission rate than patients with L2 morphology. It appears that patients with T-cell ALL may have the best prognosis, with patients with B-cell having the worst prognosis for survival. Prognostic factors for probability of relapse in ALL are dominated by the leukocyte count, serum LDH level, and time to achieving complete remission. All patients with the Philadelphia chromosome eventually relapse.[381,383]

DIFFERENTIATION THERAPY FOR ACUTE PROMYELOCYTIC LEUKEMIA

The use of all-*trans*-retinoic acid in treating promyelocytic leukemia provides a paradigm of differentiation therapy. APL occurs in 5% to 10% of newly diagnosed patients with AML. Huang and colleagues documented the ability to achieve complete remissions in patients with APL, a finding that was subsequently confirmed.[387-389]

Administration of all-*trans*-retinoic acid (ATRA) rapidly corrects coagulation disorders in APL. The leukocyte count increases for the first 3 weeks, and over a period of 2 to 3 months, the bone marrow and blood shows evidence of progressive differentiation into complete remission. No episode of marrow hypoplasia occurs. The response appears to be optimal in previously treated patients with APL.[389] Nineteen of 20 complete remissions were reported in one study.

Use of ATRA as second or third salvage is not as beneficial as for initial salvage therapy. The major complication occurring with this agent is an increase in the circulating leukocyte count, which is more common in patients who commence with elevated leukocyte counts.[390] Some patients develop complications of pulmonary insufficiency, and if the leukocyte count rises above 20,000/μl, treatment with chemotherapy or leukapheresis is recommended. Patients who achieve a complete remission on ATRA relapse if the drug is used alone as maintenance. It is thought that this is, in part, a result of a lowering of plasma ATRA levels with continued therapy. Eventually, the ATRA level becomes too low to have an effect on differentiation.[391]

It is now known that on chromosome 15 is a breakpoint in the *PML* gene (formerly called *MYL*), and the breakpoint on chromosome 17 involves the *RARA* gene, causing a chimeric gene product of PML-RARA.[127-130] The interaction of TRA with the the α, β, and γ receptors for retinoic acid and nuclear retinol binding factors are areas of intense research.

Approximately 75% of patients with newly diagnosed APL

achieve complete remission. Because some patients have been dying of complications of the leukostasis syndrome, combination chemotherapy approaches should be explored. This sequence of investigations demonstrates the need to coordinate clinical observations based on differentiation of cell lines in the laboratory with the molecular genetic findings of specific receptor disturbance. It is hoped that similar observations can be made for other translocations, such as t(8;21), inv(16), t(1;19), and t(9;22).

TRENDS IN THE MANAGEMENT OF LEUKEMIA

The predominant treatments for acute leukemia have been in place for 5 to 15 years. No major new class of drugs for the management of acute leukemia has been discovered. The allogeneic and autologous marrow transplant programs with monoclonal purging and chemotherapy purging have been applied with no major difference in response or survival rates. Development of new drugs that are selected for particular subsets of leukemia patients is of the highest priority.

The availability of hemopoietic tissue growth factors, such as G-CSF, GM-CSF, IL-3, IL-4, IL-6, and stem cell factor, suggests that leukemia cells may be able to be induced into proliferation or differentiation. Explorations of these combinations may lead to new conceptual and therapeutic advances. The ability of the investigators to deliver chemotherapy at maximal doses is enhanced by the availability of the growth factors to accelerate recovery of normal elements. This should enable peripheral blood cells to be collected before intensive chemotherapy for autologous peripheral blood support for chemotherapy.

The discovery that all-*trans*-retinoic acid can achieve complete remissions in APL and the discovery that the *RARA* gene is involved in the specific translocation associated with APL suggests that increased knowledge of the genetic abnormalities observed in leukemia should enhance our ability to delivery specific therapies tailored to the genetic derangement. Further conceptual advances require the dissection of the dysregulation of growth involving growth stimulatory and inhibitory factors. Delineation of risk groups would enable those who are already being cured with conventional treatment to be identified, so that they could be spared aggressive high-dose therapies.

Applications of techniques such as polymerase chain reaction to identify genetic abnormalities should enable selection of patients with minimal residual disease. If subclinical leukemia cell burden under the influence of treatment can be detected before relapse occurs, new treatments can be initiated before the patient has evidence of clinical relapse. Gene therapy or introduction of specific antisense nucleotides into leukemic cells require more refined analysis of the genetic aberrations involved in leukemogenesis.

REFERENCES

1. National Cancer Institute. 1987 Annual cancer statistics review. NIH publication no. 88-2789. Washington, DC: U.S. Department of Health and Human Services, 1988.
2. Tivey H. The natural history of untreated acute leukemia. Ann NY Acad Sci 1954;60:322.
3. Alderson M. The epidemiology of leukemia. Adv Cancer Res 1980;31:1.
4. Heath CW Jr. The leukemias. In: Schottenfeld D, Fraumeni JF Jr, eds. Cancer epidemiology and prevention.
5. Lund E, Lie SO. Incidence of acute leukemia in Norway 1957–1981. Report from the Norwegian Cancer Registry and Pediatric Research Institute, National Hospital of Norway, Oslo, Norway. Scand J Haematol 1983;31:488.
6. McPhedran P, Heath CW Jr, Garcia JS. Racial variations in leukemia incidence among the elderly. JNCI 1970;45:25.
7. Graham S, Gibson R, Lilienfeld A, et al. Religion and ethnicity in leukemia. Am J Public Health 1970;60:266.
8. Gunz FW, Gunz JP, Veale AMO, et al. Familial leukemia: A study of 909 families. Scand J Hematol 1975;15:117.
9. Gunz FW, Gunz JP, Vincent PC, et al. Thirteen cases of leukemia in a family. JNCI 1978;60:1243.
10. Jackson EW, Norris FD, Klauber MR. Childhood leukemia in California-born twins. Cancer 1969;23:913.
11. MacMahon B, Levy MA. Prenatal origin of childhood leukemia. Evidence from twins. N Engl J Med 1964;270:1082.
12. Steinberg A. The genetics of acute leukemia in children. Cancer 1960;13:985.
13. Fraumeni JF Jr, Miller RW. Epidemiology of human leukemia: Recent observations. JNCI 1967;38:593.
14. Miller RW. Radiation, chromosomes and viruses in the etiology of leukemia. N Engl J Med 1964;271:30.
15. Kirkpatrick CH. Cancer in immunodeficiency disease. Birth Defects 1976;12:61.
16. Spector BD, Perry GS, III, Kersey JH. Genetically determined immunodeficiency disease and malignancy. Report from the Immunodeficiency Cancer Registry. Clin Immunol Immunopathol 1978;11:12.
17. Beebe GW, Kato H, Land CE. Studies of the mortality of A-bomb survivors. 6. Mortality and radiation dose, 1950–1974. Radiat Res 1978;75:138.
18. Stewart AM. Delayed effects of A-bomb radiation: A review of recent mortality rates and risk estimates for five-year survivors. J Epidemiol Community Health 1982;36:80.
19. Land CE. Estimating cancer risks from low doses of ionizing radiation. Science 1980;209:1197.
20. Caldwell GG, Kelley D, Zack M, et al. Mortality and cancer frequency among military nuclear test (Smoky) participants, 1957 through 1979. JAMA 1983;250:620.
21. Smith PG, Doll R. Mortality among patients with ankylosing spondylitis after a single treatment course with x-rays. Br Med J 1982;284:449.
22. Smith PG. Leukemia and other cancers following radiation treatment of pelvic disease. Cancer 1977;39:1901.
23. Murray R, Heckel P, Hempelmann LH. Leukemia in children exposed to ionizing radiation. N Engl J Med 1959;261:585.
24. Da Silva Horta J, da Motta LC, Tavares MH. Thorium dioxide effects in man. Environ Res 1974;8:131.
25. Modan B, Lilienfeld AM. Polycythemia vera and leukemia—the role of radiation treatment. Medicine (Baltimore) 1965;44:305.
26. Polednak AP, Stehney AF, Rowland RE. Mortality among women first employed before 1930 in the U.S. radium dialpainting industry. Am J Epidemiol 1978;107:179.
27. March HC. Leukemia in radiologists. Radiology 1944;43:275.
28. Fulton JP, Cobb S, Preble L, et al. Electrical wiring configurations and childhood leukemia in Rhode Island. Am J Epidemiol 1980;111:292.
29. Savitz DA, Wachtel H, Barnes FA, et al. Case-control study of childhood cancer and exposure to 60-Hz magnetic fields. Am J Epidemiol 1988;128:21.
30. Pochin EE. Leukemia following radioiodine treatment of thyrotoxicosis. Br Med J 1960;2:1545.
31. Boice JD, Hutchison GB. Leukemia in women following radiotherapy for cervical cancer: Ten-year follow-up of an international study. JNCI 1980;65:115.
32. Austin H, Delzell E, Cole P. Benzene and leukemia. Am J Epidemiol 1988;127:419.
33. Aksoy M, Dincol K, Erdem S, Dincol G. Acute leukemia due to chronic exposure to benzene. Am J Med 1972;52:160.
34. Vigliani EC, Forni A. Benzene and leukemia. Environ Res 1976;11:122.
35. Rinsky RA, Smith AB, Hornung R, et al. Benzene and leukemia. N Engl J Med 1987;316:1044.
36. Shu XO, Gao YT, Linet MS, et al. Chloramphenicol use and childhood leukemia in Shanghai. Lancet 1987;2:934.
37. Crane MM, Keating MJ, Trujillo JM, et al. Environmental exposures in cytogenetically defined subsets of acute nonlymphocytic leukemia. JAMA 1989;262:634.
38. Severson RK. Cigarette smoking and leukemia. Cancer 1987;60:141.
39. Yoshida M, Seiki M, Hattori S, et al. Monoclonal integration of human T-cell leukemia provirus in all primary tumors of adult T-cell leukemia suggests causative role of HTLV in disease. Proc Natl Acad Sci USA 1984;81:2534.
40. Robert-Guroff M, Nakao Y, Notake K, et al. Natural antibodies to human retrovirus HTLV in a cluster of Japanese patients with adult T-cell leukemia. Science 1982;215:975.
41. Hinuma H, Komoda H, Chosa T, et al. Antibodies to adult T-cell leukemia virus-associated antigen in sera from patients with ATL and controls in Japan: A nationwide seroepidemiologic study. Int J Cancer 1982;29:631.
42. Blattner WA, Blayney DW, Robert-Guroff M, et al. Epidemiology of human T-cell leukemia/lymphoma virus. J Infect Dis 1983;147:406.
43. Sakashita A, Hattori T, Miller CW, et al. Mutations of the p53 gene in adult T-cell leukemia. Blood 1992;79:477.
44. Yamada Y. Phenotypic and functional analysis of leukemic cells from 16 patients with adult T-cell leukemia/lymphoma. Blood 1983;61:192.
45. Essex M. Feline leukemia and sarcoma viruses. In: Klein G, ed. Viral oncology. 1980:205.
46. Blair A, Hayes HM, JR. Cancer and other causes of death among U.S. veterinarians, 1966–1977. Int J Cancer 1980;25:181.

47. Heath CW Jr. The epidemiology of leukemia. In: Schottenfeld D, ed. Cancer and epidemiology and prevention. 1975:316.

48. Fraumeni JF, Ederer F, Miller RW. An elevation of the carcinogenicity of simian virus 40 in man. JAMA 1963;185:713.

49. Waters TD, Anderson PS Jr, Beebe GW, et al. Yellow fever vaccination, avian leukosis virus, and cancer risk in man. Science 1972;177:76.

50. Miller G, Shope T, Heston L, et al. Prospective study of Epstein-Barr virus infections in acute lymphoblastic leukemia of children. J Pediatr 1972;80:932.

51. Blair A, Thomas TL. Leukemia among Nebraska farmers: A death certificate study. Am J Epidemiol 1979;110:264.

52. Blair A, White DW. Death certificate study of leukemia among farmers from Wisconsin. JNCI 1981;66:1027.

53. Henshaw DL, Eatough JP, Richardson RB. Radon as a causative factor in induction of myeloid leukaemia and other cancers. Lancet 1990:1008.

54. Gardner MJ, Snee MP, Hall AJ, et al. Results of case-control study of leukaemia and lymphoma among young people near Sellafield nuclear plant in West Cumbria. Br Med J 1990;300:423.

55. Neel JV. Update on the genetic effects of ionizing radiation. JAMA 1991;266:698.

56. Albain K, LeBeau M, Rowley J, et al. Secondary acute nonlymphocytic leukemia (ANNL) and dysmyelopoietic syndrome (DMPS) in 46 patients: Clinical and cytogenetic correlations. Cancer Genet Cytogenet 1983;8:107.

57. Coltman C Jr. Treatment related leukemias. In: Bloomfield CD, ed. Adult leukemias, vol. 1. 1982:62.

58. Ross HJ, Rowley JD, Koeffler HP. Therapy-related acute nonlymphocytic leukemia. In: Wiernik PH, Canellos GP, Kyle RA, Schiffer CA, eds. Neoplastic diseases of the blood. 1991:303.

59. Kantarjian HM, Estey EH, Keating MJ. Treatment of therapy-related leukemia and myelodysplastic syndrome. Hematol Oncol Clin North Am (in press).

60. Sieber SM, Adamson RH. Toxicity of antineoplastic agents in man: Chromosomal aberrations, antifertility effects, congenital malformations and carcinogenic potential. Adv Cancer Res 1975;22:57.

61. Wantzin GL, Jensen MK. The induction of chromosome abnormalities by melphalan in rat bone marrow cells. Scand J Haematol 1973;11:135.

62. Cadman EC, Capizzi RL, Bertino JR. Acute non-lymphocytic leukemia—a delayed complication of Hodgkin's disease therapy: Analysis of 109 cases. Cancer 1977;40:1280.

63. Valagussa P, Santoro A, Kenda RE, et al. Second malignancies in Hodgkin's disease: A complication of certain forms of treatment. Br Med J 1980;1:216.

64. Kaldor JM, Day NE, Clarke A, et al. Leukemia following Hodgkin's disease. N Engl J Med 1990;322:7.

65. Toland DM, Coltman CA Jr, Moon TE. Second malignancies complicating Hodgkin's disease: The Southwest Oncology Group experience. Cancer Clin Trials 1978;1:21.

66. Coleman CN, Williams CJ, Flint A, et al. Hematologic neoplasia in patients treated for Hodgkin's disease. N Engl J Med 1977;297:1249.

67. Valagussa P, Santoro A, Bellani F, et al. Absence of treatment-induced second neoplasms after ABVD in Hodgkin's disease. Blood 1982;59:488.

68. Pedersen-Bjergaard J, Philip P, Mortensen B, et al. Acute nonlymphocytic leukemia, preleukemia and acute myeloproliferative syndrome secondary to treatment of other malignant disease. Clinical and cytogenetic characteristics and results of in vitro culture of bone marrow and HLA typing. Blood 1981;57:712.

69. Travis LB, Curtis RE, Boice JD Jr, et al. Second cancers following non-Hodgkin's lymphoma. Cancer 1991;67:2002.

70. Bergsagel D, Bailey A, Langley G. The chemotherapy of plasma-cell myeloma and the incidence of acute leukemia. N Engl J Med 1979;300:743.

71. Berk P, Goldberg J, Silverstein M. Increased incidence of acute leukemia in polycythemia vera associated with chlorambucil therapy. N Engl J Med 1981;304:441.

72. McPhedran P, Heath CW. Acute leukemia occurring during chronic lymphocytic leukemia. Blood 1970;35:7.

73. Reimer RR, Hoover R, Fraumeni JF Jr, et al. Secondary primary neoplasms following ovarian cancer. JNCI 1978;61:1195.

74. Rosner F, Carey RW, Zarrabi NH. Breast cancer and acute leukemia: Report of 24 cases and review of the literature. Am J Hematol 1978;4:151.

75. Curtis RE, Boice JD, Moloney WC, et al. Leukemia following chemotherapy for breast cancer. Cancer Res 1990;50:2741.

76. Kantarjian HM, Keating MJ, Walters RS, et al. Therapy-related leukemia and myelodysplastic syndrome: Clinical, cytogenetic, and prognostic features. J Clin Oncol 1986;4:1748.

77. Whitlock JA, Greer JP, Lukens JN. Epipodophyllotoxin-related leukemia. Cancer 1991;68:600.

78. Pin C, Behn F, Raimondi S, et al. Secondary acute myeloid leukemia in children treated for acute lymphoid leukemia. N Engl J Med 1989;321:136.

79. Boggs DR, Sofferman SA, Wintrobe MM, et al. The acute leukemias. Medicine (Baltimore) 1962;41:163.

80. Roath S, Israels MCG, Wilkinson JF. The acute leukemias: A study of 580 patients. Q J Med 1964;33:257.

81. Bodey GP, Buckley M, Sathe YS, et al. Quantitative relationships between circulating leukocytes and infection in patients with acute leukemia. Ann Intern Med 1966;64:328.

82. Suda T, Onai T, Mekawa T. Studies on abnormal polymorphonuclear neutrophils in acute myelogenous leukemia: Clinical significance and changes after chemotherapy. Am J Hematol 1983;15:45.

83. Stewart DJ, Keating MJ, McCredie KB, et al. Natural history of central nervous system acute leukemia in adults. Cancer 1981;47:184.

84. Manoharan A, Horsley R, Ptiney WR. The reticulin content of bone marrow in acute leukaemia in adults. Br J Haematol 1979;43:185.

85. Bennett JM, Catovsky D, Daniel MT, et al. Proposed revised criteria for the classification of acute myeloid leukemia. Ann Intern Med 1985;103:626.

86. Bennett JM, Reed CE. Acute leukemia cytochemical profile: Diagnosis and clinical implications. Blood Cells 1975;1:101.

87. El-Mohandes E, Hayhoe FGJ. 5'-nucleotidase activity of megakaryoblasts in a case of acute megakaryoblastic leukemia. Br J Haematol 1983;53:523.

88. Daniel MT, Flandrin G, Le Jeune F, et al. Les esterases, specifiques moncytaire. Utilization des leucemies, aigues. Nouv Rev Fr Hematol 1971;11:233.

89. Bennett JM. Classification of the acute leukemias: Cytochemical and morphologic considerations. In: Wiernik PH, ed. Neoplastic diseases of the blood. 1991:172.

90. Knapp W, Rieber P, Dorken B, et al. Towards a better definition of human leukocyte surface molecules. Immunol Today 1989;10:253.

91. Rovigatti U, Mirro J, Kitchingman G, et al. Heavy chain immunoglobulin gene rearrangement in acute nonlymphocytic leukemia. Blood 1984;63:1023.

92. Fontenay M, Flandrin G, Baurman H, et al. T cell receptor delta gene rearrangement occurs predominantly in immature myeloid leukemia exhibiting lineage promiscuity. Leukemia 1990;4:100.

93. Sobol RE, Mick R, Royston I, et al. Clinical importance of myeloid antigen expression in adult acute lymphoblastic leukemia. N Engl J Med 1987;316:1111.

94. Mirro J, Zipf TF, Pui C-H, et al. Acute mixed lineage leukemia: Clinicopathologic correlations and prognostic significance. Blood 1985;66:1115.

95. Cuneo A, Michaux J-L, Ferrant A, et al. Correlation of cytogenetic patterns and clinicobiological features in adult acute myeloid leukemia expressing lymphoid markers. Blood 1992;79:720.

96. Lee EJ, Pollak A, Leavitt RD, et al. Minimally differentiated acute nonlymphocytic leukemia: A distinct entity. Blood 1987;70:1400.

97. Griffin JD, Davis R, Nelson DA, et al. Use of surface marker analysis to predict outcome of acute myelogenous leukemia. Blood 1986;68:1232.

98. Adriaansen HJ, Soeting PWC, Wolvers-Tettero ILM, et al. Immunoglobulin and T-cell receptor gene rearrangements in acute non-lymphocytic leukemias. Analysis of 54 cases and a review of the literature. Leukemia 1991;5:744.

99. Kitchingman GR, Rovigatti U, Mauer AM, et al. Rearrangement of immunoglobulin heavy chain genes in T cell acute lymphoblastic leukemia. Blood 1985;65:725.

100. Felix CA, Wright JJ, Poplack DG, et al. T cell receptor α-, β-, and γ-genes in T cell and pre-B cell acute lymphoblastic leukemia. J Clin Invest 1987;80:545.

101. Hara J, Benedict SH, Champagne E, et al. Relationship between rearrangement and transcription of the T-cell receptor α, β, and γ genes in B-precursor acute lymphoblastic leukemia. Blood 1989;73:500.

102. Bennett JM, Catovsky D, Daniel MT, et al. Proposals for the classification of the acute leukaemias. Br J Haematol 1976;33:451.

103. Bennett JM, Catovsky D, Daniel M-T, et al. Criteria for the diagnosis of acute leukemia of megakaryocytic lineage (M7). A report of the French-American-British Cooperative Group. Ann Intern Med 1985;103:460.

104. Bennett JM, Catovsky D, Daniel MT, et al. The morphologic classification of acute lymphoblastic leukaemia: Concordance among observers and clinical correlations. Br J Haematol 1981;47:553.

105. Bennett JM, Begg CB. ECOG study of cytochemistry of acute myeloid leukemia by correlation or subtypes with response and survival. Cancer Res 1981;41:4833.

106. Head DR, Savage RA, Cerezo L, et al. Reproducibility of the French-American-British classification of acute leukemia: The Southwest Oncology Group experience. Am J Hematol 1985;18:47.

107. Cross AH, Goorha RM, Nuss R, et al. Acute myeloid leukemia with T-lymphoid features: A distinct biologic and clinical entity. Blood 1988;72:579.

108. Smith LJ, Curtis JE, Messner HA, et al. Lineage infidelity in acute leukemia. Blood 1983;61:1138.

109. Pui C-H, Dahl GV, Melvin S, et al. Acute leukaemia with mixed lymphoid and myeloid phenotype. Br J Haematol 1984;56:121.

110. Cuneo A, Mecucci C, Kerim S, et al. Multipotent stem cell involvement in megakaryoblastic leukemia: Cytologic and cytogenetic evidence in 15 patients. Blood 1989;74:1781.

111. Van Slyck EJ, Weiss L, Dully M. Chromosomal evidence for the secondary role of fibroblastic proliferation in acute myelofibrosis. Blood 1970;36:729.

112. Benvenisti DS, Ultmann JE. Eosinophilic leukemia. Ann Intern Med 1969;71:731.

113. Holmes R, Keating MJ, Cork A, et al. A unique pattern of central nervous system in acute myelomonocytic leukemia associated with inv(16)(p13a22). Blood 1985;65:1017.

114. Wimmer RS, Raney RB Jr, Naiman JL. Hypereosinophilia with acute lymphocytic and acute myelocytic leukemia in childhood. J Pediatr 1978;92:244.

115. Bennett JM, Catovsky D, Daniel MT, et al. Proposals for the classification of the myelodysplastic syndromes. Br J Haematol 1982;51:189.

116. Hickling RA. Leukaemia and related conditions and the blood-uric-acid. Lancet 1958;1:175.

117. Krakoff IH. Use of allopurinol in preventing hyperuricemia in leukemia and lymphoma. Cancer 1966;19:1489.

118. Levi JA, Speden JB, Vincent PC, et al. Studies on muramidase in hematologic disorders. I. Serum muramidase and serum lactic dehydrogenase in leukemia. Cancer 1973;31:939.

119. Kantarjian HM, Walters RS, Keating MJ, et al. Results of the vincristine, doxorubicin and dexamethasone regimen in adults with standard- and high-risk acute lymphocytic leukemia. J Clin Oncol 1990;8:994.

120. Keating MJ, Smith TL, Gehan EA, et al. A prognostic factor analysis for use in development of predictive models for response in adult acute leukemia. Cancer 1982;50:457.

121. Rachmilewitz D, Rachmilewitz EA, Polliack A, et al. Acute promyelocytic leukemia: A report of five cases on the diagnostic significance of serum vitamin B$_{12}$ determination. Br J Haematol 1972;22:87.

122. Gorst DW, Courtis M, Delamore IW. Folic acid binding protein in acute myeloid leukemia. J Clin Pathol 1976;29:60.

123. Mir MA, Brabin B, Tang OT, et al. Hypokalaemia in acute myeloid leukaemia. Ann Intern Med 1975;82:54.

124. The Fourth International Workshop on Chromosomes in Leukemia, Chicago, IL, September 2–7, 1982. A prospective study of acute nonlymphocytic leukemia. Cancer Genet Cytogenet 1984;11:251.

125. Yunis JJ, Brunning RD, Howe RB, et al. High-resolution chromosome as an independent prognostic indicator in adult acute nonlymphocytic leukemia. N Engl J Med 1984;311:812.

126. Keating MJ, Cork A, Broach Y, et al. Toward a clinically relevant cytogenetic classification of acute myelogenous leukemia. Leuk Res 1987;11:119.

127. Borrow J, Goddard AD, Sheer D, et al. Molecular analysis of acute promyelocytic leukemia breakpoint cluster region on chromosome 17. Science 1990;249:1577.

128. de The H, Chomienne C, Lanotte M, et al. The t(15;17) translocation of acute promyelocytic leukemia fuses the retinoic acid receptor a gene to a novel transcribed locus. Nature 1990;347:558.

129. Alcalay M, Zangrilli D, Paolo P, et al. Translocation breakpoint of acute promyelocytic leukemia lies within the retinoic acid receptor α locus. Proc Natl Acad Sci USA 1991;88:1977.

130. Chang K-S, Trjillo JM, Ogura T, et al. Rearrangement of the retinoic acid receptor gene in acute promyelocytic leukemia. Leukemia 1991;5:200.

131. Holmes RI, Keating MJ, Cork A, et al. Loss of the Y chromosome in acute myelogenous leukemia: A report of 13 patients. Cancer Genet Cytogenet 1985;694:10.

132. Vermaelen K, Michaux JL, Louwagie A, et al. Reciprocal translocation t(6;9)(p21;q3): A new characteristic chromosome anomaly in myeloid leukemias. Cancer Genet Cytogenet 1983;10:125.

133. Davis MP, Dewald GW, Pierre RV, et al. Hematologic manifestations associated with deletions of the long arm of chromosome 20. Cancer Genet Cytogenet 1984;12:63.

134. Maddox A-M, Keating MJ, Trujillo J, et al. Philadelphia chromosome-positive adult acute leukemia with monosomy of chromosome number seven: A subgroup with poor response to therapy. Leuk Res 1983;7:509.

135. Bloomfield CD, Secker-Walker LM, Goldman AI, et al. Six-year follow-up of the clinical significance of karyotype in acute lymphoblastic leukemia. Cancer Genet Cytogenet 1989;40:171.

136. Machnicki JL, Bloomfield CD. Clinical significance of the cytogenetics of acute leukemias. Oncology 1990;4:23.

137. Arthur DC, Berger R, Golomb HM, et al. The clinical significance of karyotype in acute myelogenous leukemia. Cancer Genet Cytogenet 1989;40:203.

138. Schiffer CA, Lee EJ, Tomiyasu T, et al. Prognostic impact of cytogenetic abnormalities in patients with de novo acute nonlymphocytic leukemia. Blood 1989;73:263.

139. Williams DL, Raimondi SC, Rivera G, et al. Presence of clonal chromosome abnormalities in virtually all cases of acute lymphoblastic leukemia. N Engl J Med 1985;313:640.

140. Machnicki JL, Bloomfield CD. Clinical significance of the cytogenetics of acute leukemias. Oncology 1990;4:23.

141. Third International Workshop on Chromosomes in Leukemia. Chromosomal abnormalities and their clinical significance in acute lymphoblastic leukemia. Cancer Res 1983;43:868.

142. Kantarjian HM, Talpaz M, Dhingra K, et al. Significance of the p210 versus p190 molecular abnormalities in adults with Philadelphia chromosome-positive acute leukemia. Blood 1991;78:2411.

143. Kaiser-McCaw B, Epstein AL, Kaplan HS, et al. Chromosome 14 translocation in African and North American Burkitt's lymphoma. Int J Cancer 1977;19:482.

144. Miyoshi I, Hiraki S, Kimura I, et al. 2/8 Translocation in a Japanese Burkitt's lymphoma. Experientia 1979;35:742.

145. Berger R, Bernheim A, Weh HJ, et al. A new translocation in Burkitt's tumor cells. Hum Genet 1979;53:111.

146. Mirro J, Kitchingman G, Williams D, et al. Clinical and laboratory characteristics of acute leukemia with the 4;11 translocation. Blood 1986;67:689.

147. Michael PM, Levin MD, Garson OM. Translocation 1;19—a new cytogenetic abnormality in acute lymphocytic leukemia. Cancer Genet Cytogenet 1984;12:133.

148. Cline MJ, Ahuja H. Oncogenes and anti-oncogenes in the evolution of human leukemia/lymphoma. Leukemia Lymphoma 1991;4:153.

149. Clarkson B. New pharmacologic approaches to treatment of leukemia. Semin Hematol 1991;28:99.

150. Radich JP, Kopecky KY, William CL, et al. N-ras mutations in adult de novo acute myelogenous leukemia: Prevalence and clinical significance. Blood 1990;76:801.

151. Needleman SW. Ras protooncogene activation in acute myeloid leukemia and related disorders. Leukemia Lymphoma 1991;5:85.

152. Hirsch-Ginsberg C, Le Maistre AC, Kantarjian H, et al. RAS mutations are rare even in Philadelphia chromosome-negative/bcr gene rearrangement-negative chronic myelogenous leukemia, but are prevalent in chronic myelomonocytic leukemia. Blood 1990;76:1214.

153. Ridge SA, Worwood M, Oscier D, et al. FMS mutations in myelodysplastic, leukemic, and normal subjects. Proc Natl Acad Sci USA 1990;87:1377.

154. Tobal K, Pagliuca A, Bhatt B, et al. Mutation of the human FMS gene (M-CSF receptor) in myelodysplastic syndromes and acute myeloid leukemia. Leukemia 1990;4:486.

155. Slingerland JM, Minden MD, Benchimol S. Mutation of the p53 gene in human acute myelogenous leukemia. Blood 1991;77:1500.

156. Fenaux P, Jonveaux P, Quiquandon I, et al. P53 gene mutations in acute myeloid leukemia with 17p monosomy. Blood 1991;78:1652.

157. Gaidano G, Ballerini P, Gong JZ, et al. P53 mutations in human lymphoid malignancies: Association with Burkitt lymphoma and chronic lymphocytic leukemia. Proc Natl Acad Sci USA 1991;88:5413.

158. Ahuja HG, Jat PS, Foti A, et al. Abnormalities of the retinoblastoma gene in the pathogenesis of acute leukemia. Blood 1991;78:3259.

159. Clarkson BD. Review of recent studies of cellular proliferation in acute leukemia. NCI Monogr 1969;30:81.

160. Cronkite EP. Kinetics of leukemic cell proliferation. In: Dameshek W, Dutcher RM, eds. Perspectives in leukemia. New York: Grune & Stratton, 1968.

161. Greenberg ML, Chanana AD, Cronkite EP, et al. The generation time of human leukemic myeloblasts. Lab Invest 1972;26:245.

162. Sjogren U. Mitotic activity in myeloid leukaemias. A study of 277 cases. Scand J Haematol 1977;19:309.

163. Killmann S-A. Acute leukemia: Development, remission/relapse pattern, relationship between normal and leukemic hemopoiesis, and the "sleeper-to-feeder" stem cell hypothesis. Semin Hematol 1968;1:103.

164. Killmann S-A, Karle H, Ernst P, et al. Return of human leukemic myeloblasts from blood to bone marrow. Acta Med Scand 1971;189:137.

165. Dosik G, Barlogie B, Smith TL, et al. Pretreatment flow cytometry of DNA content in adult acute leukemia. Blood 1980;55:474.

166. Hill BT, Baserga R. The cell cycle and its significance for cancer treatment. Cancer Treat Rev 1975;2:159.

167. Stryckmans PA, Lurie PM, Manaster J, et al. Mode of action of chemotherapy in vivo on human acute leukemia. II. Vincristine. Eur J Cancer 1973;9:613.

168. Ernst P, Killman S-A. Perturbation of generation cycle of human leukemic blast cells by cytostatic therapy in vivo: Effect of corticosteroids. Blood 1970;36:689.

169. Ernst P. Perturbation of generation cycle of human leukaemic lymphoblasts in vivo by L-asparaginase. Br J Haematol 1973;25:33.

170. Ernst P, Faille A, Killman S-A. Perturbation of cell cycle of human leukaemic myeloblasts in vivo by cytosine arabinoside. Scand J Haematol 1973;10:209.

171. Furlong NB, Sato J, Brown T, et al. Induction of limited DNA damage by the antitumor agent Cain's acridine. Cancer Res 1978;38:1329.

172. Stryckmans PA, Manaster J, Lachapelle F, et al. Mode of action of chemotherapy in vivo on human acute leukemia. I. Daunomycin. J Clin Invest 1973;52:126.

173. Li LH, Olin EJ, Fraser TJ, et al. Phase specificity of 5-azacytidine against mammalian cells in tissue culture. Cancer Res 1970;30:2770.

174. Le Page GA. Basic biochemical effects and mechanism of action of 6-thioguanine. Cancer Res 1963;23:1202.

175. Ernst P. Perturbation of generation cycle of human leukaemic blast cells in vivo by daunomycin. Scand J Haematol 1973;11:13.

176. Krishan A, Paika K, Frei E. Cytofluorometric studies on the action of podophyllotoxin and epipodophyllotoxins (VM-26, VP-16-213) on the cell cycle traverse of human lymphoblasts. J Cell Biol 1975;66:521.

177. Buchanan JG, Matthews JRD, Postlewaight BF, et al. The proliferative activity of leukaemic myeloblasts following the intravenous infusion of cytarabine. Pathology 1979;11:349.

178. Vogler WR, Kremer WB, Knospe WH, et al. Synchronization with phase-specific agents in leukemia and correlation with clinical response to chemotherapy. Cancer Treat Rep 1976;60:1845.

179. Vincent PC, Gunz FW, Levi JA, et al. Prognostic value of cytokinetic studies in adult acute leukemia. In: Fliedner TM, Perry S, eds. Workshops in prognostic factors in human acute leukemia. Advances in the Biosciences, vol 14. 1975:345.

180. Smets LA, Taminiau J, Hahlen K, et al. Cell kinetic responses in childhood acute nonlymphocytic leukemia during high-dose therapy with cytosine arabinoside. Blood 1983;61:79.

181. Cannistra SA, Groshek P, Griffin JD. Granulocyte-macrophage colony-stimulating factor enhances the cytotoxic effects of cytosine arabinoside in acute myeloblastic leukemia and in the myeloid blast crisis of chronic myeloid leukemia. Leukemia 1989;3:328.

182. Tafuri A, Andreeff M. Kinetic rationale for cytokine-induced recruitment of myeloblastic leukemia followed by cycle-specific chemotherapy in vitro. Leukemia 1990;4:826.

183. Brach MA, Henschler R, Mertelsmann R, et al. To overcome pharmacologic and cytokinetic resistance to cytarabine in the treatment of acute myelogenous leukemia by using recombinant interleukin-3? Semin Hematol 1991;28:39.

184. Lista P, Brizzi MF, Rossi M, et al. Different sensitivity of normal and leukaemic progenitor cells to ara-C and IL-3 combined treatment. Br J Haematol 1990;76:21.

185. Hoang T, Nara N, Wong G, et al. Effects of recombinant GM-CSF on the blast cells of acute myeloblastic leukemia. Blood 1986;68:313.

186. Cannistra SA, DiCarlo J, Groshek P, et al. Simultaneous administration of granulocyte-macrophage colony-stimulating factor and cytosine arabinoside for the treatment of relapsed acute myeloid leukemia. Leukemia 1991;5:230.

187. Bettelheim P, Valent P, Andreeff M, et al. Recombinant human granulocyte-macrophage colony-stimulating factor in combination with standard induction chemotherapy in de novo acute myeloid leukemia. Blood 1991;77:700.

188. Estey EH, Dixon D, Kantarjian HM, et al. Treatment of poor-prognosis, newly diagnosed acute myeloid leukemia with ara-C and recombinant human granulocyte-macrophage colony-stimulating factor. Blood 1990;75:1766.

189. Maschmeyer G, Ludwig W-D, Sauerland M-C, et al. Recombinant human granulocyte-macrophage colony-stimulating factor after chemotherapy in patients with acute myeloid leukemia at higher age or after relapse. Blood 1991;78:1190.

190. Estey E, Thal PF, Kantarjian H, et al. Treatment of newly diagnosed acute myelogenous leukemia with GM-CSF prior to and during continuous-infusion high-dose ara-C

(CHDAC) + daunorubicin: Comparison to patients treated without GM-CSF. Blood (in press).

191. Hart JS, George SL, Frei E III, et al. Prognostic significance of pretreatment proliferative activity in adult acute leukemia. Cancer 1977;39:1603.

192. Crowther D, Beard MEJ, Bateman CJT, et al. Factors influencing prognosis in adults with acute myelogenous leukaemia. Br J Cancer 1975;32:456.

193. Kantarjian HM, Barlogie B, Keating MJ, et al. Pretreatment cytokinetics in acute myelogenous leukemia: Age-related prognostic implications. J Clin Invest 1985;76:319.

194. Dosik G, Barlogie B, Gohde W, et al. Flow cytometry of DNA content in human bone marrow—a critical reappraisal. Blood 1980;55:734.

195. Hiddemann W, Buchner T, Andreeff M, et al. Cell kinetics in acute leukemia—a critical reevaluation based on new data. Cancer 1982;50:250.

196. Walters RS, Johnston DA, Dixon DO, et al. Nucleic acid flow cytometry—an aid to diagnosis and prognosis in acute leukemia in adults. In: Stass, ed. The acute leukemias—Biologic, diagnostic, and therapeutic determinants. , 1987:203.

197. Moore MAS, Spitzer G, William N, et al. Agar culture studies in 127 cases of untreated acute leukemia: The prognostic value of reclassification of leukemia according to in vitro growth characteristics. Blood 1974;44:1.

198. Estrov Z, Freedman MH. Growth requirements for human acute lymphoblastic leukemia cells: Refinement of a clonogenic assay. Cancer Res 1988;48:5901.

199. Griffin JD, Young D, Herrmann F, et al. Effects of recombinant human GM-CSF on proliferation of clonogenic cells in acute myeloblastic leukemia. Blood 1986;67:1448.

200. Herrmann F, Vellenga E. The role of colony stimulating factors in acute leukemia. J Cancer Clin Oncol 1990;116:275.

201. McCulloch EA, Curtis JE, Messner HA, et al. The contribution of blast cell properties to outcome variation in acute myeloblastic leukemia (AML). Blood 1982;59:601.

202. Sachs L. The differentiation of myeloid leukemia cells: New possibility for therapy. Br J Haematol 1978;40:509.

203. Pegoraro L. Abraham J, Cooper RA, et al. Differentiation of human leukemias in response to 12-O-tetradecanoyl-phorbol-13-acetate in vitro. Blood 1980;55:859.

204. Moore MAS, Gabrilove J, Sheridan AP. Myeloid leukemic cell differentiation induced by human postendotoxin serum and vitamin analogues. In: Neth R, Gallo RC, Greaves MF, Moore MAS, Winkler K, eds. Modern trends in human leukemia. 1983:327.

205. Tomonaga M, Golde DW, Gasson JC. Biosynthetic (recombinant) human granulocyte-macrophage colony-stimulating factor: Effects on normal bone marrow and leukemia cell lines. Blood 1986;67:31.

206. Kelleher C, Miyauchi J, Wong G, et al. Synergism between recombinant growth factors, GM-CSF and G-CSF, acting on the blast cells of acute myeloblastic leukemia. Blood 1987;69:1498.

207. Pinto A, Attadia V, Fusco A, et al. 5-aza-2'-deoxycytidine induces terminal differentiation of leukemic blasts from patients with acute myeloid leukemias. Blood 1984;64:922.

208. Castaigne S, Daniel MT, Tilly H, et al. Does treatment with ara-C in low dosage cause differentiation of leukemic cells? Blood 1983;62:85.

209. Sakurai M, Sampi K, Hozumi M. Possible differentiation of human acute myeloblastic leukemia cells by daily intermittent administration of aclacinomycin A. Leuk Res 1983;7:139.

210. Koeffler HP. Induction of differentiation of human acute myelogenous leukemia cells: Therapeutic implications. Blood 1983;62:709.

211. Breitman TR, Collins SJ, Keen BR. Terminal differentiation of human promyelocytic leukemia cells in primary culture in response to retinoic acid. Blood 1981;57:1000.

212. Chen ZX, Wang W, Wu WL. Heterogenous response of primarily cultured bone marrow cells of patients with variety of leukemias to differentiation inducers. Clin Med J 1989;102:174.

213. Chen ZX, Xue YQ, Zhang R, et al. A clinical and experimental study on all-*trans* retinoic acid-treated acute promyelocytic leukemia patients. Blood 1991;78:1413.

214. Bodey GP, Bolivar R, Fainstein V. Infectious complications in leukemia patients. Semin Hematol 1982;19:193.

215. Gaydos LA, Freireich EJ, Mantel N. The quantitative relation between platelet count and hemorrhage in patients with acute leukemia. N Engl J Med 1962;266:905.

216. Hester JP, Ventura GJ. Characteristics of refractoriness (R) to platelet concentrate transfusions (PC-TX) in newly diagnosed acute myeloid leukemia patients (AML) (PT). Blood 1988;72:278.

217. Tallman MS, Kwaan HC. Reassessing the hemostatic disorder associated with acute promyelocytic leukemia. Blood 1992;79:543.

218. McKee Jr LC, Collins RD. Intravascular leukocyte thrombi and aggregates as a cause of morbidity and mortality in leukemia. Medicine (Baltimore) 1974;53:463.

219. Freireich EJ, Thomas LB, Frei E III, et al. A distinctive type of intracerebral hemorrhage associated with "blastic crisis" in patients with leukemia. Cancer 1960;13:146.

220. Hug V, Keating MJ, McCredie KB, et al. Clinical course and response to treatment of patients with acute myelogenous leukemia presenting with a high white cell count. Cancer 1983;52:773.

221. Legha SS, Latreille J, McCredie KB, et al. Neurologic and cardiac rhythm abnormalities associated with 4'-(9-acridinylamino) methanesulfon-*m*-anisidide (AMSA) therapy. Cancer Treat Rep 1979;63:11.

222. Freireich EJ, Gehan EA, Sulman D, et al. The effect of chemotherapy on acute leukemia in the human. J Chron Dis 1961;14:593.

223. Freireich EJ, Karon M, Frei E III. Quadruple combination therapy (VAMP) for acute lymphocytic leukemia in childhood. Proc Am Assoc Clin Res [Abstract] 1964;5:20.

224. Freireich EJ, Henderson ES, Karon MR, et al. The treatment of acute leukemia considered with respect to cell population kinetics. 21st Annual Symposium on Fundamental Cancer Research: The proliferation and spread of neoplastic cells. 1967:441.

225. Ellison RR, Holland JF, Weil M, et al. Arabinosyl cytosine: A useful agent in the treatment of acute leukemia in adults. Blood 1968;32:507.

226. Bodey GP, Freireich EJ, Monto RW, et al. Cytosine arabinoside (NSC 63878) therapy for acute leukemia in adults. Cancer Chemother Rep 1969;53:59.

227. Bodey GP, Coltman CA, Hewlett JS, et al. Progress in the treatment of adults with acute leukemia: Review of regimens containing cytarabine studied by the Southwest Oncology Group. Arch Intern Med 1976;136:1383.

228. Jacquillat CL, Boiron M, Weil M, et al. Rubidomycin, a new agent active in the treatment of acute leukemia. Lancet 1966;2:27.

229. Weil M, Glidewell OJ, Jacquillat C, et al. Daunorubicin in the therapy of acute granulocytic leukemia. Cancer Res 1973;33:921.

230. Wilson HE, Bodey GP, Moon TE. Adriamycin therapy in previously treated adult acute leukemia. Cancer Treat Rep 1977;61:905.

231. Jacquillat CL, Weil M, Gemon-Auclerc MF, et al. Clinical study of rubidazone (22 040 R.P.), a new daunorubicin-derived compound, in 170 patients with acute leukemias and other malignancies. Cancer 1976;37:653.

232. Daghestani A, Arlin ZA, Leyland-Jones, et al. Phase I and II clinical and pharmaceutical study of 4-demethoxydaunorubicin (idarubicin) in adult patients with acute leukemia. Cancer Res 1985;45:1408.

233. Yates JW, Wallace HJ Jr, Ellison RR, et al. Cytosine arabinoside and daunorubicin therapy in acute nonlymphocytic leukemia. Cancer Chemother Rep 1983;57:485.

234. Clarkson BD, Dowling MD, Gee TS, et al. Treatment of acute leukemia in adults. Cancer 1975;36:775.

235. Rees JKH, Sandler RM, Challener J, et al. Treatment of acute myeloid leukemia with a triple cytotoxic regimen: DAT. Br J Cancer 1977;36:770.

236. Wiernik PH, Glidewell OJ, Hoagland HC, et al. A comparative trial of daunorubicin, cytosine arabinoside, and thioguanine and a combination of the three agents for the treatment of acute myelocytic leukemia. Med Pediatr Oncol 1979;6:261.

237. Finnish Leukemia Group. The effect of thioguanine in a combination of daunorubicine (sic), cytarabine and prednisone in the treatment of acute leukemia in adults. Scand J Haematol 1979;23:124.

238. Berman E, Heller G, Santorsa J, et al. Results of randomized trial comparing idarubicin and cytosine arabinoside with daunorubicin and cytosine arabinoside in adult patients with newly diagnosed acute myelogenous leukemia. Blood 1991;77:1666.

239. Wiernik PH, Banks PLC, Case DC Jr, et al. Cytarabine plus idarubicin or daunorubicin as induction and consolidation therapy for previously untreated adult patients with acute myeloid leukemia. Blood 1992;79:313.

240. Vogler WR, Velez-Garcia E, Omura G, et al. A phase III tiral comparing daunorubicin or idarubicin combined with cytosine arabinoside in acute myelogenous leukemia. Semin Oncol 1989;16:21.

241. Yates J, Glidewell OJ, Wiernik PH, et al. Cytosine arabinoside with daunorubicin or Adriamycin for therapy of acute myelocytic leukemia: A CALGB study. Blood 1982;60:454.

242. Arlin Z, Case DC Jr, Moore J, et al. Randomized multicenter trial of cytosine arabinoside with mitoxantrone or daunorubicin in previously untreated adult patients with acute nonlymphocytic leukemia (ANLL). Leukemia 1990;4:177.

243. Keating M, Gehan E, Smith T, et al. A strategy for evaluation of new treatments in untreated patients: Application to a clinical trial of AMSA for acute leukemia. J Clin Oncol 1987;5:710.

244. Preisler H, Davis RB, Kirshner J, et al. Comparison of three remission induction regimens and two postinduction strategies for the treatment of acute nonlymphocytic leukemia: A cancer and leukemia group B study. Blood 1987;69:1441.

245. Dillman RO, Davis RB, Green MR, et al. A comparative study of two different doses of cytarabine for acute myeloid leukemia: A phase II trial of cancer and leukemia group B. Blood 1991;78:2520.

246. Buchner T, Urbanitz D, Hiddemann W, et al. Intensified induction and consolidation with or without maintenance chemotherapy for acute myeloid leukemia (AML): Two multicenter studies of the German AML Cooperative Group. J Clin Oncol 1985;3:1583.

247. Rees JKH, Swirsky D, Gray RG, et al. Principal results of the Medical Research Council's 8th acute myeloid leukaemia trial. Lancet 1986;2:1236.

248. Kantarjian HM, Walters RS, Keating MJ, et al. Results of the vincristine, doxorubicin, and dexamethasone regimen in adults with standard- and high-risk acute lymphocytic leukemia. J Clin Oncol 1990;8:994.

249. GIMENA Cooperative Group. GIMENA ALL 0183: A multicentric study on adult acute lymphoblastic leukaemia in Italy. Br J Haematol 1989;71:377.

250. Hoelzer D, Thiel E, Loffler H, et al. Prognostic factors in a multicenter study for treatment of acute lymphoblastic leukemia in adults. Blood 1988;71:123.

251. Linker CA, Levitt LJ, O'Donnell M, et al. Treatment of adult acute lymphoblastic leukemia with intensive cyclical chemotherapy: A follow-up report. Blood 1991;78:2814.

252. Schauer P, Arlin ZA, Mertelsmann R, et al. Treatment of acute lymphoblastic leukemia in adults—Results of the L-10 and L-10M protocols. J Clin Oncol 1983;1:462.

253. Rivera GK, Dahl GV, Bowman WP, et al. VM-26 and cytosine arabinoside combination chemotherapy for the initial induction failures in childhood lymphocytic leukemia. Cancer 1980;46:1727.

254. Bishop JF, Lowenthal RM, Joshua D, et al. Etoposide in acute nonlymphocytic leukemia. Blood 1990;75:27.

255. Monparler RL. A model for the chemotherapy of acute leukemia with 1-β-D-arabinofuranosylcytosine. Cancer Res 1974;34:1775.

256. Iwagaki A, Nakamura T, Wakisaka G. Studies on the mechanism of action of 1-β-D-arabinofuranosylcytosine as an inhibitor of DNA synthesis in human leukemic leukocytes. Cancer Res 1969;29:2169.

257. Chu MY, Fisher GA. A proposed mechanism of action of 1-β-D-arabinofuranosylcytosine as an inhibitor of the growth of leukemic cells. Biochem Pharmacol 1962;11:423.

258. Major PP, Egan EW, Beardsley GP, et al. Lethality of human myeloblasts correlated with the incorporation of arabinosylcytosine into DNA. Proc Natl Acad Sci USA 1981;78: 3235.

259. Chu MY, Fisher GA. Comparative studies of leukemic cells sensitive and resistant to cytosine arabinoside. Biochem Pharmacol 1965;14:333.

260. Harris AW, Reynolds EC, Finch LR. Effect of thymidine on the sensitivity of cultured mouse tumor cells to 1-β-D-arabinofuranosylcytosine. Cancer Res 1979;39:538.

261. Rustum YM, Preisler H. Metabolism and intracellular retention of ³H-arabinosylcytosine as predictors of response of animal tumors. Cancer Res 1978;38:543.

262. Walters RS, Kantarjian HM, Keating MJ, et al. Intensive treatment of acute leukemia in adults 70 years of age and older. Cancer 1987;60:149.

263. Preisler HD. Failure of remission induction in acute myelocytic leukemia. Med Pediatr Oncol 1978;4:275.

264. Pizzo PA, Ladisch S, Simon RM, et al. Increasing incidence of gram-positive sepsis in cancer patients. Med Pediatr Oncol 1978;5:241.

265. Wade JC, Schimpff SC, Newman KA, et al. *Staphylococcus epidermidis:* An increasing cause of infection in patients with granulocytopenia. Ann Intern Med 1982;97:503.

266. Pizzo PA, Ladisch S, Witebsky FG. Alpha-hemolytic streptococci: Clinical significance in the cancer patient. Med Pediatr Oncol 1978;4:367.

267. Estey EH, Keating MJ, McCredie KB, et al. Causes of initial remission induction failure in acute myelogenous leukemia. Blood 1982;60:309.

268. Gerson SL, Talbot GH, Hurwitz S, et al. Prolonged granulocytopenia: The major risk factor for invasive pulmonary aspergillosis in patients with acute leukemia. Ann Intern Med 1984;100:345.

269. Schimpff SC, Green WH, Young VM, et al. Infection prevention in acute nonlymphocytic leukemia. Laminar air flow room reverse isolation with oral, nonabsorbable antibiotic prophylaxis. Ann Intern Med 1975;82:351.

270. Bodey GP, Keating MJ, McCredie KB, et al. Prospective randomized trial of antibiotic prophylaxis in acute leukemia. Am J Med 1985;78:407.

271. Rodriguez V, Bodey GP, Freireich EJ, et al. Randomized trial of protected environment-prophylactic antibiotics in 145 adults with acute leukemia. Medicine (Baltimore) 1978;57:253.

272. Estey EH, Maksymiuk A, Smith TL, et al. Infection prophylaxis in acute leukemia: Comparative effectiveness of sulfamethoxazole and trimethoprim, ketoconazole, and a combination of the two. Arch Intern Med 1984;144:1562.

273. Karp JE, Merz WG, Hendricksen C, et al. Oral norfloxacin for prevention of gram-negative bacterial infections in patients with acute leukemia and granulocytopenia. A randomized, double-blind, placebo-controlled trial. Ann Intern Med 1987;106:1.

274. Bow EJ, Rayner E, Louie TJ. Comparison of norfloxacin with cotrimoxazole for infection prophylaxis in acute leukemia. The tradeoff for reduced gram-negative sepsis. Am J Med 1988;84:847.

275. The GIMEMA Infection Program. Prevention of bacterial infection in neutropenic patients with hematologic malignancies—A randomized, multicenter trial comparing norfloxacin with ciprofloxacin. Ann Intern Med 1991;115:7.

276. Vallejos C, McCredie KB, Bodey GP, et al. White blood cell transfusions for control of infections in neutropenic patients. Transfusion 1975;15:28.

277. Vogler WR, Winton EF. A controlled study of the efficacy of granulocyte transfusions in patients with neutropenia. Am J Med 1977;63:548.

278. Alavi JB, Root RK, Djerassi I, et al. A randomized clinical trial of granulocyte transfusions for infection in acute leukemia. N Engl J Med 1977;296:706.

279. Winston DJ, Ho WG, Bruckner DA, et al. Beta-lactam antibiotic therapy in febrile granulocytopenic patients—A randomized trial comparing cefoperazone plus piperacillin, ceftazidime plus piperacillin, and imipenem alone. Ann Intern Med 1991;115: 849.

280. Bodey GP, Elting L, Jones P, et al. Imipenem/cilastatin therapy of infections in cancer patients. Cancer 1987;60:255.

281. Love LJ, Schimpff SC, Hahn DM, et al. Randomized trial of empiric antibiotic therapy with ticarcillin in combination with gentamicin, amikacin or netilmicin in febrile patients with granulocytopenia and cancer. Am J Med 1979;66:603.

282. Bodey GP, Ketchel SJ, Rodriquez V. A randomized study of carbenicillin plus cefamandole or tobramycin in the treatment of febrile episodes in cancer patients. Am J Med 1979;67: 608.

283. Karp JE, Dick JD, Angelopulos C, et al. Empiric use of vancomycin during prolonged treatment-induced granulocytopenia. Am J Med 1986;81:237.

284. Hiddemann W, Essink ME, Fegeler W, et al. Antifungal treatment by amphotericin B and 5-fluorocytosine delays the recovery of normal hematopoietic cells after intensive cytostatic therapy for acute myeloid leukemia. Cancer 1991;68:9.

285. Fisher BD, Armstrong D, Yu B, et al. Invasive aspergillosis: Progress in early diagnosis and treatment. Am J Med 1981;71:571.

286. Grant SM, Clissold SP. Fluconazole—A review of its pharmacodynamic and pharmacokinetic properties, and therapeutic potential in superficial and system mycoses. Drugs 1990;39:877.

287. Bodey GP, Freireich EJ, Gehan EA, et al. Late intensification therapy for acute leukemia in remission. JAMA 1976;235:1021.

288. Bodey GP, Freireich EJ, McCredie KB, et al. Prolonged remissions in adults with acute leukemia following late intensification chemotherapy and immunotherapy. Cancer 1981;47:1937.

289. Embury SH, Elias L, Heller PH, et al. Remission maintenance therapy in acute myelogenous leukemia. West J Med 1977;126:267.

290. Vogler WR, Winton EF, Gordon DS, et al. A randomized comparison of postremission therapy in acute myelogenous leukemia: A southeastern cancer study group trial. Blood 1984;63:1039.

291. Cassileth PA, Begg CB, Bennett JM, et al. A randomized study of the efficacy of consolidation therapy in adult acute nonlymphocytic leukemia. Blood 1984;63:843.

292. Preisler H, Davis R, Kirshner J, et al. Comparison of three remission induction regimens and two postinduction strategies for the treatment of acute nonlymphocytic leukemia: A Cancer and Leukemia Group B study. Blood 1987;69:1441.

293. Kantarjian HM, Keating MJ, Walters RS, et al. Early intensification and short-term maintenance chemotherapy does not prolong survival in acute myelogenous leukemia. Cancer 1986;58:1603.

294. Wolff SN, Herzig RH, Fay JW, et al. High-dose cytarabine and daunorubicin as consolidation therapy for acute myeloid leukemia in first remission: Long-term follow-up and results. J Clin Oncol 1989;7:1260.

295. Preisler HD, Raza A, Early A, et al. Intensive remission consolidation therapy in the treatment of acute nonlymphocytic leukemia. J Clin Oncol 1987;5:722.

296. Phillips GL, Reece DE, Shepherd JD, et al. High-dose cytarabine and daunorubicin induction and postremission chemotherapy for the treatment of acute myelogenous leukemia in adults. Blood 1991;77:1429.

297. Schiller GJ, Nimer SD, Territo MC, et al. Bone marrow transplantation versus high-dose cytarabine-based consolidation chemotherapy for acute myelogenous leukemia in first remission. J Clin Oncol 1992;10:41.

298. Buchner T, Hiddemann W, Loffler G, et al. Improved cure rate by very early intensification combined with prolonged maintenance chemotherapy in patients with acute myeloid leukemia: Data from the AML cooperative group. Semin Hematol 1991;28: 76.

299. Harousseau JL, Milpied N, Briere J, et al. Double intensive consolidation chemotherapy in adult acute myeloid leukemia. J Clin Oncol 1991;9:1432.

300. Clift R, Buckner C, Thomas E, et al. The treatment of acute non-lymphoblastic leukemia by allogeneic marrow transplantation. Bone Marrow Transplant 1987;2:243.

301. Champlin R, Advisory Committee of the International Bone Marrow Transplant Registry. Bone marrow transplantation for acute leukemia: A preliminary report from the International Bone Marrow Transplant Registry. Transplant Proc 1987;19:2626.

302. Champlin R, Ho W, Gale R. Treatment of acute myelogenous leukemia: A prospective controlled trial of bone marrow transplantation versus consolidation chemotherapy. Ann Intern Med 1985;102:285.

303. Beatty PG, Hansen JA, Longton GM, et al. Marrow transplantation from HLA-matched unrelated donors for treatment of hematologic malignancies. Transplantation 1991;51: 443.

304. Lowenberg B, Verdonck LJ, Dekker AW, et al. Autologous bone marrow transplantation and acute myeloid leukemia in first remission: Results of a Dutch prospective study. J Clin Oncol 1990;8:287.

305. Korbling M, Hunstein W, Fliedner TM, et al. Disease-free survival after autologous transplantation in patients with acute myelogenous leukemia. Blood 1989;74:1898.

306. McMillan AK, Goldstone AH, Linch DC, et al. High dose chemotherapy and autologous bone marrow transplantation in acute myeloid leukemia. Blood 1990;76:480.

307. Ferrant A, Doyen C, Delannoy A, et al. Allogeneic or autologous bone marrow transplantation for acute nonlymphocytic leukemia in first remission. Bone Marrow Transplant 1991;7:303.

308. Gorin NC, Labopin M, Meloni G, et al. Autologous bone marrow transplantation for acute myeloblastic leukemia in Europe: Further evidence of the role of marrow purging by mafosfamide. Leukemia 1991;5:896.

309. Clarkson B, Ellis S, Little C, et al. Acute lymphoblastic leukemia in adults. Semin Oncol 1985;12:160.

310. Esterhay RJ, Wiernik PH, Grove WR, et al. Moderate dose methotrexate, vincristine, asparaginase, and dexamethasone for treatment of adult acute lymphocytic leukemia. Blood 1982;59:334.

311. Fiere D, Extra JM, David B, et al. Treatment of 218 adult acute lymphoblastic leukemias. Semin Oncol 1987;14(suppl 1):64.

312. Stryckmans P, de Witte T, Bitar N, et al. Cytosine arabinoside for induction, salvage, and consolidation therapy of adult acute lymphoblastic leukemia. Semin Oncol 1987;14(suppl 1):67.

313. Lister TA, Barnett MJ, Rohatiner AZS, et al. Intensive chemotherapy including high dose cytosine arabinoside for acute lymphoblastic leukemia (ALL). [Abstract] Presented at the 4th International Symposium on Therapy of Acute Leukemias, Rome, 1987: 150.

314. Cassileth P, Anderson J, Hoagland H, et al. Efficacy of high-dose cytarabine in initial therapy of adult acute lymphocytic leukemia (ALL). Proc Am Soc Clin Oncol 1987;6: 158.

315. Boogaerts MA, Emonds MP, Kennes C, et al. Intensive consolidation and maintenance therapy for acute lymphoblastic leukemia in adults. [Abstract] Presented at the 4th International Symposium on Therapy of Acute Leukemias, Rome, 1987:442.

316. Woodruff RK. The management of adult acute lymphoblastic leukemia. Cancer Treat Rev 1978;5:95.

317. Willemze R, Drenthe-Schonk AM, van Rossum J, et al. Treatment of acute lymphoblastic leukaemia in adolescents and adults. Comparison of two schedules for CNS leukaemia prophylaxis. Scand J Haematol 1980;24:421.

318. Omura GA, Moffitt S, Vogler WR, et al. Combination chemotherapy of adult acute lymphoblastic leukaemia with randomised central nervous system prophylaxis. Blood 1980;55:199.

319. Kantarjian HM, Walters RS, Smith TL, et al. Identification of risk groups for development of central nervous system leukemia in adults with acute lymphoblastic leukemia. Blood 1988;72:1784.

320. Pochedly C. Neurotoxicity due to CNS therapy for leukemia. Med Pediatr Oncol 1977;3: 101.

321. Radford JE, Burns CP, Jones MP, et al. Adult acute lymphoblastic leukemia: Results of the Iowa HOP-L protocol. J Clin Oncol 1989;7:58.

322. Stewart DJ, Smith TL, Keating MJ, et al. Remission from central nervous system involvement in adults with acute leukemia—Effect of intensive therapy and prognostic factors. Cancer 1985;56:632.

323. Ramsay NKC, Kersey JH. Indications for marrow transplantation in acute lymphoblastic leukemia. Blood 1990;75:815.

324. Doney K, Fisher LD, Appelbaum FR, et al. Treatment of adult acute lymphoblastic leukemia with allogeneic bone marrow transplantation: Multivariate analysis of factors affecting acute graft vs. host disease relapse and relapse-free survival. Bone Marrow Transplant 1991;7:453.

325. Horowitz MM, Messerer D, Hoelzer D, et al. Chemotherapy compared with bone marrow transplantation for adults with acute lymphoblastic leukemia in first remission. Ann Intern Med 1991;115:13.

326. Chao NJ, Forman SJ, Schmidt GM, et al. Allogeneic bone marrow transplantation for high-risk acute lymphoblastic leukemia during first complete remission. Blood 1991;78:1923.

327. Wingard JR, Piantadosi S, Santos GW, et al. Allogeneic bone marrow transplantation for patients with high risk acute lymphoblastic leukemia. J Clin Oncol 1990;8:820.

328. Berman E, Little C, Gee T, et al. Reasons that patients with acute myelogenous leukemia do not undergo allogeneic bone marrow transplantation. N Engl J Med 1992;326:156.

329. Keating MJ, Kantarjian H, Smith TL, et al. Response to salvage therapy and survival after relapse in acute myelogenous leukemia. J Clin Oncol 1989;7:1071.

330. Kantarjian HM, Keating MJ, Walters RS, et al. The characteristics and outcome of patients with late relapse acute myelogenous leukemia. J Clin Oncol 1988;6:232.

331. Keating MJ, Estey EH, Plunkett W, et al. Evolution of clinical studies with high-dose cytosine arabinoside (ara-C) at the M.D. Anderson Hospital. Semin Oncol 1985;12(suppl 3):98.

332. Herzig RH, Wolff SN, Lazarus HM, et al. High-dose cytosine arabinoside therapy for refractory leukemia. Blood 1983;62:361.

333. Capizzi RL, Poole M, Cooper MR, et al. Treatment of poor-risk acute leukemia with sequential high-dose ara-C and asparaginase. Blood 1984;63:694.

334. Preisler HD, Epstein J, Barcos M, et al. Prediction of response of acute nonlymphocytic leukaemia to therapy with "high-dose" cytosine arabinoside. Br J Haematol 1984;58:19.

335. Hines JD, Oken MM, Mazza JJ, et al. High-dose cytosine arabinoside and m-AMSA is effective therapy in relapsed acute nonlymphocytic leukemia. J Clin Oncol 1984;2:545.

336. Hiddemann W, Kreutzmann H, Straif K, et al. High-dose cytosine arabinoside and mitoxantrone: A highly effective regimen in refractory acute myeloid leukemia. Blood 1987;69:744.

337. Carella AM, Santini G, Martinengo M, et al. 4-Demethoxydaunorubicin (idarubicin) in refractory or relapsed acute leukemias—A pilot study. Cancer 1985;55:1452.

338. Larson RA, Daly KM, Choi KE, et al. A clinical and pharmacokinetic study of mitoxantrone in acute nonlymphocytic leukemia. J Clin Oncol 1987;5:391.

339. Koeller J, Eble M. Mitoxantrone: A novel anthracycline derivative. Clin Pharm 1988;7:574.

340. Legha SS, Keating MJ, Zander AR, et al. 4'-(9-acridinylamino) methanesulfon-*m*-anisidide (AMSA): A new drug effective in the treatment of adult acute leukemia. Ann Intern Med 1980;93:17.

341. Lee EJ, Van Echo DA, Egorin MJ, et al. Diaziquone given as a continuous infusion is an active agent for relapsed adult acute nonlymphocytic leukemia. Blood 1986;67:182.

342. Schiffer CA, Lee EJ. Approaches to the therapy of relapsed acute myeloid leukemia. Oncology 1989;3:23.

343. Archimbaud E, Leblond V, Michallet M, et al. Intensive sequential chemotherapy with mitoxantrone and continuous infusion etoposide and cytarabine for previously treated acute myelogenous leukemia. Blood 1991;77:1894.

344. Ho AD, Lipp T, Ehninger G, et al. Combination of mitoxantrone and etoposide in refractory acute myelogenous leukemia—An active and well-tolerated regimen. J Clin Oncol 1988;6:213.

345. Estey EH, Keating MJ, Smith TL, et al. Prediction of complete remission in patients with refractory acute leukemia treated with AMSA. J Clin Oncol 1984;2:102.

346. Plunkett W, Iacoboni S, Estey EH, et al. Pharmacologically directed ara-C therapy for refractory leukemia. Semin Oncol 1985;12:20.

347. Hiddemann W, Schleyer E, Uhrmeister C, et al. High-dose versus intermediate-dose cytosine arabinoside in combination with mitoxantrone for the treatment of relapsed and refractory acute myeloid leukemia—Preliminary clinical and pharmacological data of a randomized comparison. Cancer Treat Rev 1990;17:279.

348. Vogler WR, Preisler HD, Winton EF, et al. Randomized trial of high-dose cytarabine versus amsacrine in acute myelogenous leukemia in relapse: A leukemia intergroup study. Cancer Treat Rep 1986;70:455.

349. Thomas ED, Buckner CD, Rudolph RH, et al. Allogeneic marrow grafting for hematologic malignancy using HLA-matched donor recipient sibling pairs. Blood 1971;38:267.

350. Zander AR, Culbert S, Jagannath S, et al. High dose cyclophosphamide, BCNU, and VP-16 (CBV) as a conditioning regimen for allogeneic bone marrow transplantation for patients with acute leukemia. Cancer 1987;59:1083.

351. Maraninchi D, Abecasis M, Gastaut JA, et al. High-dose melphalan and autologous bone marrow transplant for relapsed acute leukaemia. Cancer Chemother Pharmacol 1983;10:109.

352. Yeager AM, Kaizer H, Santos GW, et al. Autologous bone marrow transplantation in patients with acute nonlymphocytic leukemia using ex vivo marrow treatment with 4-hydroperoxycyclophosphamide. N Engl J Med 1986;315:141.

353. Hoelzer D. High-dose chemotherapy in adult acute lymphoblastic leukemia. Semin Hematol 1991;28:84.

354. Capizzi RL, Pool M, Cooper MR, et al. Treatment of poor risk acute leukemia with sequential high-dose ara-C and asparaginase. Blood 1984;63:694.

355. Arlin ZA, Feldman E, Kempin S, et al. Amsacrine with high-dose cytarabine is highly effective therapy for refractory and relapsed acute lymphoblastic leukemia in adults. Blood 1988;72:433.

356. Keating MJ, Kantarjian H, O'Brien S, et al. The M.D. Anderson Cancer Center Experience with mitoxantrone in acute leukemia. Ann Hematol 1991;62:A3.

357. Milpied N, Gisselbrecht C, Harousseau JL, et al. Successful treatment of adult, acute lymphoblastic leukemia after relapse with prednisone, intermediate-dose cytarabine, mitoxantrone, and etoposide (PAME) chemotherapy. Cancer 1990;66:627.

358. Arcese W, Amadori S, Meloni G, et al. Allogeneic or autologous bone marrow transplantation for intensification of salvage therapy in patients with high-risk advanced acute lymphoblastic leukemia. Semin Hematol 1991;28:116.

359. Kantarjian HM, Estey EH, O'Brien S, et al. Intensive chemotherapy with mitoxantrone and high-dose cytosine arabinoside followed by granulocyte-macrophage colony-stimulating factor in the treatment of patients with acute lymphocytic leukemia. Blood 1992;79:876.

360. Bodey GP, Coltman CA, Freireich EJ, et al. Chemotherapy of acute leukemia. Comparison of cytarabine alone and in combination with vincristine, prednisone, and cyclophosphamide. Arch Intern Med 1974;133:260.

361. Wiernik PH, Schimpff SC, Schiffer CA, et al. Randomized clinical comparison of daunorubicin (NSC-82151) alone with a combination of daunorubicin, cytosine arabinoside (NSC-63878), 6-thioguanine (NSC-752), and pyrimethamine (NSC-3061) for the treatment of acute nonlymphocytic leukemia. Cancer Treat Rep 1976;60:41.

362. Peterson BA, Bloomfield CD, Theologides A, et al. Daunorubicin-prednisone in the treatment of acute nonlymphocytic leukemia. Cancer Treat Rep 1981;65:29.

363. Beguin Y, Bury J, Fillet G, et al. Treatment of acute nonlymphocytic leukemia in young and elderly patients. Cancer 1985;56:2587.

364. Rai KR, Holland JF, Glidewell OJ, et al. Treatment of acute myelocytic leukemia: A study by Cancer and Leukemia Group B. Blood 1981;58:1203.

365. Keating MJ, McCredie KB, Benjamin RS, et al. Treatment of patients over 50 years of age with acute leukemia with a combination of rubidazone and cytosine arabinoside, vincristine, and prednisone (ROAP). Blood 1981;58:584.

366. Cheson BD, Simon R. Low-dose ara-C in acute nonlymphocytic leukemia and myelodysplastic syndromes: A review of 20 years' experience. Semin Oncol 1987;14(suppl 1):126.

367. Kizaki M, Koeffler HP. Differentiation-inducing agents in the treatment of myelodysplastic syndromes. Semin Oncol 1992;19:95.

368. Greenberg PL. Treatment of myelodysplastic syndromes with hemopoietic growth factors. Semin Oncol 1992;19:106.

369. Vadhan-Raj S, Keating M, LeMaistre A, et al. Effects of recombinant human granulocyte-macrophage colony stimulating factor in patients with myelodysplastic syndromes. N Engl J Med 1987;317:1545.

370. Ganser A, Volkers B, Greher J, et al. Recombinant human granulocyte-macrophage colony-stimulating factor in patients with myelodysplastic syndromes—A phase I/II trial. Blood 1989;73:31.

371. Thompson JA, Lee DJ, Kidd P, et al. Subcutaneous granulocyte-macrophage colony-stimulating factor in patients with myelodysplastic syndrome: Toxicity, pharmacokinetics, and hematological effects. J Clin Oncol 1989;7:629.

372. Negrin RS, Haeuber DH, Nagler A, et al. Treatment of myelodysplastic syndromes with recombinant human granulocyte colony stimulating factor. Ann Intern Med 1989;110:976.

373. Ganser A, Seipelt G, Lindemann A, et al. Effects of recombinant human interleukin-3 in patients with myelodysplastic syndromes. Blood 1990;76:455.

374. Kurzrock R, Talpaz M, Estrov Z, et al. Phase I study of recombinant human interleukin-3 in patients with bone marrow failure. J Clin Oncol 1991;9:1241.

375. Estey EH, Keating MJ, Dixon DO, et al. Karyotype is prognostically more important than the FAB system's distinction between myelodysplastic syndrome and acute myelogenous leukemia. Hemato Path 1987;1:203.

376. Tricot G, Boogaerts MA. The role of aggressive chemotherapy in the treatment of myelodysplastic syndromes. Br J Haematol 1986;63:477.

377. Fenaux P, Lai JL, Jouet JP, et al. Aggressive chemotherapy in adult primary myelodysplastic syndromes. Blut 1988;57:297.

378. Aul C, Schneider W. The role of low-dose cytosine arabinoside and aggressive chemotherapy in advanced myelodysplastic syndromes. Cancer 1989;64:1812.

379. Estey EH, Dixon D, Kantarjian HM, et al. Treatment of poor-prognosis, newly diagnosed acute myeloid leukemia with ara-C and recombinant human granulocyte-macrophage colony stimulating factor. Blood 1990;75:1766.

380. Buchner T, Hiddemann W, Koenigsmann M, et al. Recombinant human granulocyte-macrophage colony-stimulating factor after chemotherapy in patients with acute myeloid leukemia at higher age or after relapse. Blood 1991;78:1190.

381. Ohno R, Tomonaga M, Kobayashi T, et al. Effect of granulocyte colony-stimulating factor after intensive induction therapy in relapsed or refractory acute leukemia. N Engl J Med 1990;323:871.

382. Keating MJ, Smith TL, Gehan EA, et al. A prognostic factor analysis for use in development of predictive models for response in adult acute leukemia. Cancer 1982;50:457.

383. Smith TL, Gehan EA, Keating MJ, et al. Prediction of remission in adult acute leukemia: Development and testing of predictive models. Cancer 1982;50:466.

384. Gaynor J, Chapman D, Little C, et al. A cause-specific hazard rate analysis of prognostic

factors among 199 adults with acute lymphoblastic leukemia: The Memorial Hospital experience since 1969. J Clin Oncol 1988;6:1014.

385. Keating MJ, Smith TL, Kantarjian H, et al. Cytogenetic pattern in acute myelogenous leukemia: A major reproducible determinant of outcome. Leukemia 1988;2:403.

386. Bloomfield CD, Goldman AI, Alimena G, et al. Chromosomal abnormalities identify high-risk and low-risk patients with acute lymphoblastic leukemia. Blood 1986;67: 415.

387. Huang ME, Ye YC, Chai JR, et al. Use of all *trans* retinoic acid in the treatment of acute promyelocytic leukemia. Blood 1988;72:567.

388. Castaigne S, Chomienne C, Daniel MT, et al. All *trans* retinoic acid as a differentiation therapy for acute promyelocytic leukemia: I. Clinical results. Blood 1990;76:1704.

389. Degos L, Chomienne C, Daniel MT, et al. Treatment of first relapse in acute promyelocytic leukemia with all *trans* retinoic acid. Lancet 1990;:1440.

390. Warrel RM, Frankel SR, Miller WH, et al. Differentiation therapy of acute promyelocytic leukemia with tretinoin (all *trans* retinoic acid). N Engl J Med 1991;324:1385.

391. Muindi J, Frankel SR, Miller WH Jr, et al. Continuous treatment with all *trans* retinoic acid causes a progressive reduction in plasma drug concentrations: Implication for relapse and retinoid "resistance" in patients with acute promyelocytic leukemia. Blood 1992;79:299.

Cancer: Principles & Practice of Oncology, Fourth Edition,
edited by Vincent T. DeVita, Jr., Samuel Hellman, Steven A. Rosenberg.
J.B. Lippincott Co., Philadelphia © 1993.

Albert B. Deisseroth   Michael J. Keating

Michael Andreeff   Hagop Kantarjian

Richard Champlin   Issa F. Khouri

Moshe Talpaz

CHAPTER **55**

Chronic Leukemias

During the past 50 years, a major problem facing those responsible for the design and implementation of therapy of the chronic leukemias has been the dose limitations that the nonhematopoietic toxicities of chemotherapy have imposed on therapy. This situation arose in part from the narrow margin of selectivity that conventional chemotherapeutic agents exhibit with respect to chronic leukemia cells, which are often less rapidly proliferating and therefore less sensitive to phase-specific and cycle-dependent chemotherapy than acute leukemia cells. During the 1970s, dose intensification with exogenous hematopoietic reconstitution was used as a means of increasing the safety and effectiveness of therapy. The use of autologous and allogeneic bone marrow transplantation permitted the safe delivery of effective doses of therapy for these diseases. The utility of this approach was limited in part by the medical factors that limit eligibility for this type of therapy in chronic leukemia patients due to their advanced chronologic and physiologic age. During the 1980s, recombinant growth factors were produced in quantities sufficient for therapy. Although these agents were useful adjuncts in limiting the hematopoietic toxicity of conventional-dose therapy, there was no detectable incremental impact of this support modality on survival.

New drugs and molecular approaches to diagnosis are contributing to more selective therapy. It is now possible to define the molecular defects that create leukemic hematopoietic cells, and a new level of selectivity is possible because therapy can be directed to the basic biologic changes that lead to the disease. The ultimate extension of this trend is genetic therapy, which involves the replacement of missing sequences within abnormal cells to correct their defects. In this chapter we review the developments that are permitting the integration of molecular and genetic approaches to therapy with more conventional modalities of chemotherapy, biologic therapy, and molecular and genetic therapy with bone marrow transplantation in the chronic leukemias.

CHRONIC LYMPHOCYTIC LEUKEMIA

Chronic lymphocytic leukemia (CLL) is a monoclonal hematopoietic disorder with expansion of small lymphocytes of B-cell (95%) or T cell lineage (5%). (Other sources provide a more extensive review of this process than can be offered in this chapter.[1,2]) CLL cells accumulate in blood, bone marrow, lymph nodes, and spleen, resulting in enlargement of these organs and decreased bone marrow function.

In 1924, Minot and Isaacs reported the natural history of CLL and described the effects of radiation therapy.[3] In 1975, Rai and colleagues described a clinical staging system and documented the adverse effects of anemia and thrombocytopenia on survival.[4] Another staging system was suggested by Binet.[5]

The monoclonal nature of CLL has been confirmed by surface marker analysis: restriction of light-chain type on the surface of B cells, expression of a single isoenzyme in the lymphocytes of female patients who are heterozygous for glucose-6-phosphate dehydrogenase, immunoglobulin (Ig) gene rearrangements showing single V_L and V_H regions, and by cytogenetic analysis.[6-8]

ETIOLOGY AND INCIDENCE

CLL is the most common leukemia, with an annual incidence of 1.8 to 3.0 per 100,000 population in the United States.[9] Incidence is age related, with 5.2 per 100,000 persons between 35 and 59 years of age and 30.4 per 100,000 persons between 80 and 84 years of age. It affects twice as many men as women.

CLL is less common in Japanese and other Asian populations. Clusters of CLL in families have been reported, and first-degree relatives of patients with CLL have a threefold increased risk for CLL and other lymphoid neoplasms compared with the general population.[10-12] There is no increased incidence after exposure to radiation, and there is no evidence for retroviral initiation of the disease.

CYTOGENETIC ABNORMALITIES

The paucity of metaphases in fresh preparations of CLL cells, which are characterized by a very low mitotic index, makes cytogenetic analysis difficult. B-cell mitogens such as lipopolysaccharide from *E. coli*, 12-0-tetradecanoylphorbol-13-acetate, cytochalasin B, pokeweed mitogen, phytohemagglutinin, and Epstein-Barr virus allow the preparation of metaphases in 90% of cases.[13-16] Using conventional banding techniques, 30% to 50% of patients with CLL have detectable chromosomal abnormalities.[17-21] Patients with clonal chromosomal abnormalities have a poorer prognosis than patients with diploid karyotypes.[16] The most frequent abnormalities involve chromosomes 12 or 14.[22-25] Other changes include −8, iso(2p), 6q−, iso(7p), t(13;21), 14q−, trisomy 18, and −X. At M.D. Anderson Cancer Center, 475 CLL samples were studied with conventional cytogenetic techniques (G-banding) after short-term culture, and abnormal karyotypes were identified in 31% of cases. Of those, 22.8% had trisomy 12 alone or in combination with other abnormalities, and 1.9% had structural abnormalities of chromosome 12. Other abnormalities were 11q− (16.7% of abnormal karyotypes), 14q+ (7.9%), 13q− (7%), t(11;14) (6.1%), 6q− (4.4%), −17 (4.3%), ±19 (4.3%), ±18 (3.5%), ±21 (2.6%), −16 (2.6%), and iso(17q) (1.8%).

The technique of interphase cytogenetics with fluorescence in situ hybridization (FISH) using repetitive DNA sequences as specific probes for the centromeric regions of individual chromosomes is independent of cell division and the presence of metaphases (Fig. 55–1).[26] FISH identified trisomy 12 in 30 (28.6%) of 104 patients.[27] In this study with a short follow-up, there was a significant correlation between the percentage of CD19+ or CD20+ cells and the percentage of cells showing trisomy 12 (R = 0.46, $p < 0.05$). Trisomy 12 was not found in FACS-sorted T cells in B-cell CLL. There was no difference in overall survival between trisomy 12 and diploid patients, but the time to progression of the disease after fludarabine therapy was significantly shorter in patients who had trisomy 12.[27] Trisomy 12 is thought to be associated with early-stage disease, and other abnormalities are acquired in advanced stages.[24,28]

Abnormalities of chromosome 14 include translocations (t[11;14]), deletions (14q−), and inversions (inv[14q]).[29] The presence of 14q+ is associated with a high leukocyte count and poor response to therapy. The genes for the Ig heavy chain (14q32) and for the α-chain of the human T-cell receptor (14q11.2) are localized on chromosome 14.[30] The chromosome 11 segment translocated to the J segment of the heavy chain locus at 14q32 contains the *BCL1* oncogene and results in the production of a novel protein.

Survival of patients with abnormal cytogenetics is significantly shorter than in patients with normal karyotypes. In a study from Roswell Park, there was no correlation of chro-

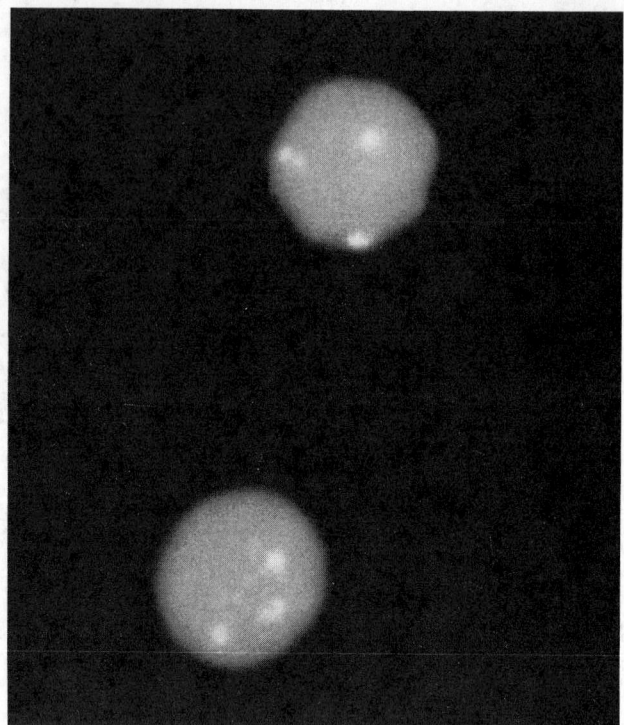

FIGURE 55–1. Detection of trisomy of chromosome 12 in chronic lymphocytic leukemia.

mosomal abnormalities with age, sex, treatment status, or disease duration, but the 10-year survival rate was 86% for patients with normal karyotypes and 57% for those with abnormal karyotypes.[13] In a study by Juliusson and coworkers of 433 patients with B-cell CLL, 391 patients could be evaluated, and 218 had clonal chromosomal changes.[16] Trisomy of chromosome 12 was found in 30.7% of those with abnormal karyotypes, structural abnormalities of chromosome 13 in 23.4%, and abnormalities of chromosome 14 in 18.8%. Translocations or interstitial deletions involving 13q14, the retinoblastoma gene locus, existed in 35 of 51 patients with abnormalities of chromosome 13. The presence of any clonal abnormalities carried a poor prognosis: survival of these patients was 7.7 years, compared with longer than 15 years for patients with normal karyotypes. Patients with abnormalities of 14q had a poorer survival than those with 13q abnormalities (Fig. 55–2). A high percentage of cells in metaphase with chromosomal abnormalities, perhaps indicating high proliferative activity of leukemic cells, was associated with poor survival ($p < 0.0058$) in multivariate analysis.

IMMUNOLOGIC PHENOTYPING

B-cell CLL is characterized by clonal B cells carrying only a single Ig light-chain type and single antibody specificity (*i.e.,* idiotype).[31] Cells of most patients have a low number of surface membrane IgM molecules, but serum IgM is found in only a small fraction of samples tested with standard protein electrophoresis techniques. CLL cells have C′3 and Fc receptors and express CD19, CD20, CD21, CD5, and HLA-DR.[32-33] In many patients, CD5, an antigen found on normal adult and fetal B cells but not on mature B lymphocytes, is coexpressed.

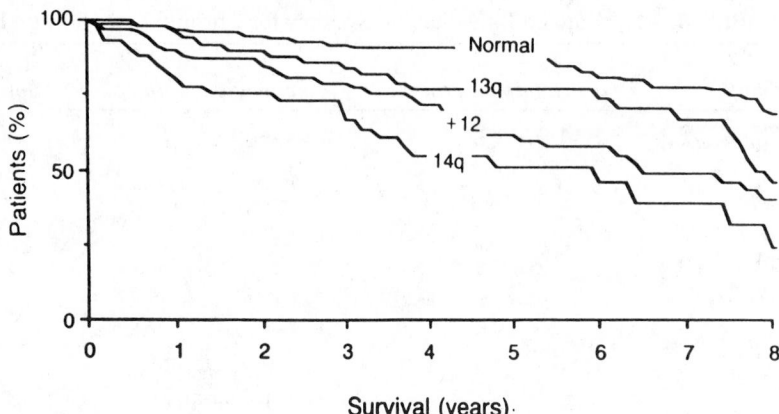

FIGURE 55–2. Survival by karyotype. (Juliusson G, Oscher DG, Fitchett M, et al. Prognostic subgroups in B-cell chronic lymphocytic leukemia defined by specific chromosomal abnormalities. N Engl J Med 1990;323:720)

The monoclonality observed by immunologic phenotyping was confirmed by studies of glucose 6-phosphate dehydrogenase. Although myeloid and T cells are not clonally involved, functional and numeric T-cell abnormalities have been reported in patients with CLL.[34–36] The number of T cells may be increased in absolute numbers, the T4:T8 ratio is decreased, possibly because of an absolute increase in T8 cells. Suppressor T cells may infiltrate the marrow and therefore directly suppress erythropoiesis.[37] The response of circulating T cells to IL-2 is diminished, reflecting functional abnormalities.[38] Lymphokine-activated killer (LAK) cell generation is defective, as is the susceptibility to allogeneic and autologous LAK cells.[39] Clonogenic cells in CLL appear to depend on yet undefined factors provided by activated T cells and conditioned media.[40–41] The complex role of the T-cell compartment in B-cell CLL is not yet fully understood.

Approximately 10% of cases with B-cell CLL show a clonal rearrangement of T-cell receptor consistent with the occurrence of immature B cells.

In half of the patients with CLL, hypogammaglobulinemia is significant and contributes to an increased risk of infection.[42] Decreases in IgM precede deficiencies in IgG and IgA.

The coexpression of CD19, CD20, CD21, or CD24 with CD5 is a useful marker for the detection of minimal disease in B-cell CLL.[43] Patients with no detectable disease by flow cytometry who responded to fludarabine and prednisone therapy with complete remissions had a 2-year disease-free survival rate of 83%, compared with 28% for patients with detectable residual disease ($p < 0.001$).

The cell kinetics of CLL are characterized by a low, almost undetectable number of cells in S phase in peripheral blood and bone marrow (0.2%).[44–45] In one report, however, the labeling index was as high as 60% in CLL lymph nodes.[46] In studies of continuous infusion of ^{3}H-labeled thymidine over 7 days, about 95% of small peripheral blood lymphocytes were long lived, with turnover times of more than 1 year, and CLL can therefore be considered to have an accumulative type of growth. The malignant transformation may protect CLL cells from programmed cell death (*i.e.*, apoptosis), as found for the *BCL2* gene in lymphomas. The notion that most CLL cells are in G_0 may not be correct. Flow cytometric measurements of chromatin structure in intact cells using the acridine orange technique revealed T-α values varying over a large range from "G_0" to G_1. The high expression of the cell cycle-related protooncogene *p53* and high expression of the proliferating cell nuclear antigen (PCNA) suggests that CLL cells are not entirely quiescent.[47–49] Clinically, the determination of lymphocyte-doubling times may provide a measure of net increase in cell mass and may inform the decision about when to initiate treatment.[50]

Expression of the *MDR1* and *MDR3* multidrug-resistance genes have been reported often. Herweijer and colleagues reported *MDR1* positivity in 17 of 17 B-cell CLL patients but in none of 7 B-cell prolymphocytic leukemia (PLL) patients.[51] *MDR3* expression was detected in B-cell CLL (17 of 17), B-cell PLL (7 of 7), and hairy cell leukemia (2 of 2). In these cases, steady-state accumulation of daunorubicin was significantly increased by cyclosporine, an inhibitor of the P-glycoprotein efflux pump, an observation that may be useful for the development of novel therapeutic modalities.

CLINICAL FEATURES AND STAGING

The approach to management of CLL differs from the approach taken in most malignant diseases. The treatment has been palliative, because of the assumption that older patients (most are >60 years) cannot tolerate aggressive chemotherapy. An additional cause for concern was the immunosuppression and myelosuppression associated with CLL, as well as the development of associated hypogammaglobulinemia, T-cell immunodeficiency, neutropenia, and thrombocytopenia. Available treatment (predominantly with alkylating agents such as chlorambucil or cyclophosphamide with or without corticosteroids) seldom achieved complete remissions, and there was no evidence of a cure fraction in CLL.

A major reason for selecting conservative therapy was the observation that many patients with CLL live for long periods without requiring therapeutic intervention. The ability to identify these patients has improved in recent years. The Rai and Binet classifications (Table 55–1) have proven useful in identifying different risk categories.[52,53] Both classifications are based on the presence of marrow compromise (*e.g.*, anemia, thrombocytopenia) in advanced stages and increasing tumor burden in the earlier stages. When applied prospectively, both staging systems yield good prognostic information. Patients who have Rai stage 0 disease at diagnosis have approximately two chances in three of surviving for 20 years or more. In early-stage disease (Rai 0—II, Binet stage A), a group of patients with "smoldering" chronic lymphocytic leukemia have been determined whose hemoglobin is more than 13 g/

TABLE 55–1. Rai and Binet Staging Systems for Chronic Lymphocytic Leukemia

Stage	Lymphocytosis	Lymphadenopathy	Hepatomegaly or Splenomegaly	Hemoglobin (g/dl)	Platelets × $10^3/\mu l$
Rai System					
0	+	−	−	≥11	≥100
I	+	+	−	≥11	≥100
II	+	±	+	≥11	≥100
III	+	±	±	<11	≥100
IV	+	±	±	Any	<100
Binet System					
A	+	± (<3 lymphatic groups* positive)	±	≥10	≥100
B	+	± (≥3 lymphatic groups* positive)	±	≥10	≥100
C	+	±	±	<10	<100

* Cervical, axillary, inguinal nodes; liver; and spleen are each considered one group whether unilateral or bilateral.

dl, platelet count is greater than 150,000, and lymphocyte count is less than 30,000/μl, with a doubling time of peripheral lymphocytes of longer than 1 year and with a nondiffuse bone marrow histology.[54] These patients have a survival equivalent to an age- and sex-matched healthy population.

Overall, the survival of patients seen at the M.D. Anderson Cancer Center before the initiation of any treatment was a median of approximately 6 years. The survival strongly correlates with Rai and Binet stages. Attempts have been made to combine the Rai and Binet stages into a hybrid staging system.[55] Most clinical trials in the United States use the Rai staging system, and those in Europe use the Binet staging system. Important prognostic variables for survival in CLL in addition to stage include the age of the patient, doubling time of the peripheral blood lymphocyte count, and the pattern of bone marrow involvement. The influence of karyotype on survival is uncertain. It appears that patients who have residual normal metaphases or those that are diploid have a better survival than patients who have 100% abnormal metaphases. Different subsets of abnormal cytogenetic patterns are associated with various prognoses.[16]

TREATMENT

Indications

Clinical trials in CLL have been marked by wide diversity of entry criteria and response criteria. Most clinicians treat patients with Rai stage III or IV or Binet stage C at diagnosis, because anemia and thrombocytopenia are adverse prognostic factors (median survival, 18 months to 4 years). Clinicians usually do not treat Rai stage 0 patients. The approach to treatment for patients with adenopathy or hepatosplenomegaly has varied. An National Cancer Institute (NCI) Working Group has come up with indications for treatment in NCI-sponsored clinical trials.[56] In addition to advanced stage, massive adenopathy or massive hepatomegaly or splenomegaly, evidence of progressive enlargement of lymph nodes, liver, or spleen and a doubling time of peripheral blood lymphocytes

of less than 6 months are indications for treatment. Development of anemia or thrombocytopenia, which are thought not to be immune mediated, are indications for initiation of treatment. Development of antibody-induced anemia and thrombocytopenia usually triggers treatment with corticosteroids. Most patients responded well to this modality of treatment, but most do not remain stable for long periods, and treatment of the leukemia after correction of the anemia or thrombocytopenia is recommended. Hypogammaglobulinemia or monoclonal gammopathy without symptoms related to these conditions are not considered adequate indications for initiation of treatment.

In addition, the NCI Working Group and the International Working Group for CLL have developed criteria for response to therapy.[57] Many early clinical trials evaluated only clinical examination and peripheral blood findings to evaluate response. In the last decade, increasing emphasis has been placed on the bone marrow as a criterion for remission. The NCI Working Group and International Working Group on CLL require restoration of relatively normal hemoglobin levels and neutrophil and platelet counts, with a decrease in the lymphocyte count to less than 4,000/μl and bone marrow infiltration to lower than 30% lymphocytes for the patient to be considered in complete remission. Both schemes allow persistent lymphoid nodules or aggregates in the bone marrow, because it is uncertain whether these are normal residual lymphoid aggregates or pathologic aggregates. Widespread adoption of these criteria for response should make comparison of clinical trials more reliable.

Conventional Treatment

The workhorse of treatment of CLL has been chlorambucil. Chlorambucil, used in the management of malignant lymphoproliferative disease since the mid-1950s, is available in tablet form and is rapidly and almost completely absorbed from the gastrointestinal tract, with a peak plasma concentration occurring within 1 hour.[58,59] The liver is a predominant metabolic site, and the principal metabolite (*i.e.,* phenylacetic acid mustard) is active against CLL.[60] Fifty percent to 65% of a single oral dose is excreted in the urine within 24 hours. Early studies by Galton and Ezdinli demonstrated that approximately three quarters of patients achieved some response, with two thirds of patients responding to second and subsequent courses.[59,60] The interval between courses of treatment became shorter with a lesser response as the disease progressed. Knospe introduced the concept of intermittent therapy with a single dose of 0.4 mg/kg chlorambucil every 2 weeks.[61] He concluded that biweekly oral administration was effective for CLL, producing less myelosuppression than daily treatment. Before this approach, most patients were treated with a continuous oral dose of 0.1 to 0.4 mg/kg per day for 4 to 8 weeks until response or myelosuppression was observed.

Cyclophosphamide has had minimal evaluation as a single agent but is often combined with vincristine and prednisone in the CVP regimen if chlorambucil fails.[62,63] In single-arm studies of the CVP regimen, the response rates varied from 44% to 77%, with a higher response rate found for patients who had never received previous treatment than for the previously treated group of patients.[62,63]

Corticosteroids have been evaluated over the last 30 years as single agents in doses of 20 to 80 mg per day. Complete responses are rare.[64,65] Decrease in node, liver, and spleen enlargement commonly occur, and improvements in anemia and thrombocytopenia can result. Studies evaluating corticosteroids as single agents focused attention on the incidence of infection with prolonged administration of corticosteroids.[59,64,65]

Since the early 1970s, most investigators have used a combination of chlorambucil and prednisone. This is based on a single small study by Han with 15 patients receiving the combination of chlorambucil and prednisone compared with 11 patients treated with chlorambucil alone.[66] A higher response rate was observed in the combination arm than in the single-agent arm. No significant survival advantage was detected. Prednisone was compared with chlorambucil plus prednisone by the Cancer and Leukemia Group B (CALGB), with chlorambucil given to one group of patients intermittently and to the other group by continuous daily administration.[64] The combination protocols were superior to the prednisone-alone arm, but no difference in the response rate was found for the two schedules of chlorambucil. No survival advantage was found in any arm of the study. Subsequently, most investigators have compared chlorambucil plus prednisone to other regimens. Chlorambucil plus prednisone produced response rates of 64% to 74% in several studies.[67–70] Higher response rates were observed for patients with indolent disease than for patients with active disease defined as those having marrow compromise, constitutional symptoms, bulky disease, or progressive and painful enlargement of lymph nodes or spleen. The median survival in most of these studies is approximately 5 years, with most studies demonstrating better survival for responders than for nonresponders.

Comparative Trials

Several trials have been conducted in which chlorambucil and prednisone were compared with several other regimens.

Monserrat compared chlorambucil and prednisone with CVP (see Table 55–1).[68] A higher response rate was observed for chlorambucil and prednisone than for CVP treatment. The same group compared chlorambucil and prednisone with a combination regimen including cyclophosphamide, melphalan, and prednisone (CMP).[69] No superiority was found for the CMP study. The Eastern Cooperative Group in 1991 published comparison of chlorambucil and prednisone with CVP.[70] No significant difference in survival was observed; median values were 4.8 years for chlorambucil and prednisone and 3.9 years for the CVP patients. Complete response rates were 25% and 23% in the two arms of the study. Median survival reported in this study for Rai stage III and IV patients was 4.1 years, which is better than the 18 to 24 months reported in older studies.[52]

The combination of chlorambucil and prednisone has emerged as the gold standard of treatment of CLL. There is no evidence that vincristine has any activity in this disease. The question of dose intensity has been raised by a comparative trial conducted by Jaksic and colleagues.[71] Chlorambucil and prednisone were compared with single-agent continuous chlorambucil at a dose of 15 mg per day. This latter regimen was administered until complete remission or myelosuppression dictated discontinuation of therapy. There was a significant difference in survival between the two groups; the chlorambucil-alone arm produced a median survival of 6 years, and the combination of chlorambucil plus prednisone produced a median survival of 3 years. The intensity of the chlorambucil dose in the single-agent arm was five to six times that used in the combination arm. This study raises the question of a dose-response relation in the treatment of CLL, which has not previously been addressed.

French Cooperative Group Studies

Dr. Binet and his colleagues in the French Cooperative Group for CLL conducted several comparative trials using the Binet staging system.[72–74] For Binet stage A patients, a study of immediate versus delayed continuous oral chlorambucil was conducted.[72] Six hundred twelve patients were randomized. Survival was slightly superior in the 309 patients randomized to delayed treatment. A significantly higher number of epithelial cancers was observed in the group receiving immediate treatment with chlorambucil. Other groups have conducted studies of early and delayed treatment for stage A patients and showed no advantage for earlier treatment.[75] Time to development of progressive disease (stages B and C) is delayed in the immediate-treatment arm, but survival after progression is less, and overall survival was not been influenced. Other trials have not found the increase in incidence of epithelial cancers.[75] For Binet stage B, patients receiving continuous oral chlorambucil were compared with those on the CVP regimen. The study enrolled 191 patients. No difference in survival between the two arms was found before and after adjusting for differences in prognostic factors. The median survival was approximately 5 years.[75]

A surprising outcome was observed in the comparative study conducted using Binet stage C patients.[74] The COP regimen was compared with the CHOP regimen; the COP regimen was fixed and doxorubicin added at a dose of 25 mg/m² on day 1 in the CHOP arm. Seventy stage C patients were randomized between the treatments. The overall survival was significantly better for the CHOP group. The median survival was 62 months for the CHOP group and 22 months for the COP group. This well-conducted clinical trial has been criticized because the COP arm had inferior results to those reported in more recent studies of Binet stage C patients.[70] In addition, anthracyclines as single agents do not have marked activity in CLL, and the addition of such a modest dose to COP surprised investigators with the significance of the outcome. Ongoing studies compare CHOP in various dosage regimens to chlorambucil and prednisone in Binet stages B and C.[76,77] Higher remission rates were observed in the CHOP arms, but there were no survival advantages.

Other clinical trials have been conducted with anthracyclines. Two studies from the M.D. Anderson Cancer Center of CAP (cyclophosphamide, doxorubicin [Adriamycin], and prednisone) resulted in 43% of patients achieving complete responses and 23% achieving partial responses, for a total response rate of 66%.[78] The response criteria included bone marrow biopsy. The POACH study, which used the same three drugs with vincristine and cytosine arabinoside, was conducted using 34 previously untreated patients.[79] Fifty-six percent of the patients responded, with 21% obtaining complete remissions. This regimen was also administered to 31 previously treated patients using the same criteria, and 26% of these patients responded, and only 2 patients achieved complete remissions. Median survival of the previously treated patients was 15 months. Chemotherapy regimens including the anthracyclines were well tolerated in both studies.

Multiple Alkylating Agents

Multiple alkylating agents have been combined in the M2 protocol from the Memorial Sloan-Kettering Cancer Center. The regimen uses vincristine, cyclophosphamide, BCNU, melphalan, and prednisone.[80] Of 63 patients studied, 17% obtained complete remissions, and 44% achieved partial responses. The complete response rate was significantly higher for untreated patients than previously treated (11 of 37 versus 0 of 26).

New Agents

Nucleoside analogs are being increasingly studied for the treatment of CLL. Fludarabine and 2-chlorodeoxyadenosine, which are analogs of ara-adenine and pentostatin (an adenosine deaminase inhibitor) have been studied. The most widely studied is fludarabine, which was first evaluated in CLL by Grever and colleagues in 22 patients.[81] In this phase II trial, all patients had received extensive prior treatment. One patient achieved a complete response, 3 patients had excellent partial responses, and 15 had some evidence of response. Larger studies of this agent were conducted at the M.D. Anderson Cancer Center.[82,83] Fludarabine was used as a single agent to treat 68 patients with previously treated CLL. Ten patients (14%) achieved complete responses, and 44% achieved partial responses. Response was higher in the Rai stage O–II patients than for Rai stages III and IV. Using the NCI criteria for complete remission, which allows persistence of residual nodules in the bone marrow, the complete response rate was 29%, and 28% of patients fulfilled the NCI criteria

for partial response. The major toxic effects associated with fludarabine were fever and infection. These were much more common in patients with advanced Rai stage and hypoalbuminemia. Myelosuppression was the most common toxic effect. Fifty-six percent of chemotherapy courses were associated with neutropenia and 25% with significant thrombocytopenia. Neurotoxicity, a marked feature of high doses used in the management of acute leukemia, was not observed in these and subsequent studies.

Fludarabine was used to treat 33 previously untreated patients with CLL.[83] The complete remission rate was 75%. Half of these complete responders had residual lymphoid nodules in the bone marrow as the only evidence of disease. Fludarabine is the most effective single agent that has been evaluated in the management of CLL. It is not possible to assess the impact of response on survival at this time. Fludarabine was combined with prednisone in the treatment of 101 previously treated patients.[84] Thirty-six percent of patients achieved complete responses, and 19% achieved partial responses, for a total response rate of 55%. The addition of prednisone did not increase the response rate nor improve survival when compared retrospectively with the fludarabine single-agent study. In the corticosteroid-treated group, *Pneumocystis carinii* and *Listeria* infections occurred, but they did not develop in the single-agent study. Another study using a lower total dose of fludarabine with a continuous infusion reported a response rate above 50%, with no complete remissions reported.[85]

Pentostatin has been studied by several groups, using doses of 4 mg/m² every 2 weeks in most studies.[86,87] The response rate with this agent is between 20% and 25%, with few patients achieving complete remissions. A higher response rate was observed in previously untreated patients in a small study conducted by CALGB.[87] Infections were the most common adverse effect in the pentostatin-treated group of patients.

2-Chlorodeoxyadenosine, which is structurally similar to fludarabine, was used to treat 90 patients with refractory CLL.[88] The usual dose was 0.1 mg/kg per day by continuous infusion for 7 days. The median number of cycles was two. All patients had failed prior therapy. It is uncertain whether they were resistant or not. Eighty-seven of the 90 patients had stage C disease. Four patients obtained complete remissions, and 36 patients had partial responses. The median duration of response was 4 months. Thrombocytopenia was dose limiting, and 10 of the 90 patients developed pulmonary infiltrates. Other modalities, total-body irradiation, and splenic irradiation are being studied in the treatment of CLL, with no evidence of a substantial response rate or improvement in survival.

Changing Criteria of Response to Therapy

There are now defined criteria for response to therapy, and increasing emphasis is being given to the documentation of residual disease. Two-parameter flow cytometry is being used to detect residual abnormal cells that coexpress CD5 and CD19 or 20 or 21 surface antigens. Normalization of $\kappa:\lambda$ ratio is being studied, as is the prognostic impact of persistent lymphoid aggregates. Lymphoid aggregates may be nodular, interstitial, or mixed nodular and interstitial patterns. Return to a germline pattern for immunoglobulin gene rearrangement is also being studied in several patients.[89] Using the strict criteria, several patients with CLL are achieving true complete remissions.

The ability of a large number of CLL patients to achieve complete responses raises the prospect of conducting autologous bone marrow transplantation, with bone marrows being purged by a variety of monoclonal antibodies against B-cell antigens. These studies are ongoing. Allogeneic bone marrow transplantation has been conducted in a series of patients with CLL.[90] Seventeen patients received an allogeneic transplant. Approximately 45% of the patients are alive and free of disease for as long as 4 years. Fifteen of the 17 patients engrafted. Two patients had early deaths, 4 of the 15 with complete responses died, and 2 relapsed; 9 of 17 patients are alive and in complete remission.

Treatment Prospects

The addition of the nucleoside analogs to the therapeutic armamentarium raises the prospect of achieving complete remissions in most previously untreated patients with CLL. Comparative trials are being conducted under the auspices of the NCI of chlorambucil versus fludarabine versus fludarabine plus chlorambucil to evaluate the role of fludarabine in this disease. The duration of chemotherapy is an unresolved issue. It appears that most patients who achieve complete remission still have significant immunosuppression. Research on immunorestoration in this group is needed.

PROLYMPHOCYTIC LEUKEMIA

PLL is characterized by massive splenomegaly and extremely high circulating lymphocyte counts with B- or T-cell phenotypes.[91] Lymphadenopathy is unusual, and median survival is less than 3 years.[92] The B cells in PLL have abundant surface immunoglobulin. A serum monoclonal protein is seen in 30% of cases, and reactivity with the monoclonal antibody FMC-7 is considered evidence for the relative maturity of PLL cells compared with those of B-cell CLL. PLL B cells do not express CD5 and frequently have a cytogenetic abnormality involving chromosome 14. Other abnormalities involve chromosomes 1, 12, and a specific translocation, t(6;12)(q15;p13).[93] In 20% of PLL patients, T-cell markers are expressed, and the cells also have positivity for α-naphthyl acetate esterase. Splenectomy and chemotherapy with CHOP are effective, but responses are short. Encouraging results have been reported for fludarabine (30 mg/m^2 over 30 minutes daily $\times$ 5 days every 4 weeks with or without prednisone); 35% of patients had complete or partial remissions.[94] These results require longer follow-up.

HAIRY CELL LEUKEMIA

The clinical features of hairy cell leukemia include pancytopenia, splenomegaly, and only infrequent lymphadenopathy.[95] Immunoglobulin genes are rearranged.[96,97] The "hairy" morphology of hairy cell leukemia cell is best appreciated by scanning electron microscopy and positivity for tartrate-resistant acid phosphatase. Hairy cell features can be induced in CLL cells exposed to phorbol esters in vitro.[98]

Historically, splenectomy was the standard approach to therapy. This measure was designed to correct the neutropenia associated with this disease. Interferon-α (INF-α) and 2-deoxycoformycin (pentostatin) supplemented splenectomy because these two therapies reduced the total leukemia cell burden.[99,100] Two groups initiated the use of 2-chlorodeoxyadenosine in the treatment of hairy cell leukemia, one from San Diego and one from Houston, with a complete remission frequency of 11 of 12 (San Diego) and 36 of 46 patients (Houston).[101,102] A dose of 0.1 mg/kg was administered by continuous intravenous infusion for 7 days. Remissions are long lasting, but fever, sepsis, and a reduced CD4:CD8 ratio may be consequences of this therapy. Although it is not possible at this time to ascertain which of the four therapeutic options is most effective for this disease, it is clear that splenectomy has now been supplemented by one type of biologic therapy (INF-α) and two excellent chemotherapeutic options (2-chlorodeoxyadenosine and 2-deoxycoformycin).

T-CELL CHRONIC LYMPHOCYTIC LEUKEMIA

Two percent of cases of CLL have lymphocytes that form rosettes with sheep red blood cells and are classified T-cell CLL.[103–107] Rearrangement of the T-cell receptor β-chain genes reflects clonality, and the phenotypes include CD4 and CD8 forms. CD4 positive CLL patients are characterized by young age, adenopathy, frequent skin involvement, hyperlymphocytosis, and diffuse marrow infiltration. Survival is less than 2 years.

The large granular lymphocytosis syndrome (CD8-positive CLL) is characterized by lymphoid cells with abundant cytoplasms containing azurophilic granules.[107] The neoplastic cells originate from natural killer cells, and patients frequently have neutropenia and less frequently have pure red cell aplasia. Most cases have a rather benign course.[108–111]

The CLL can transform into PLL, acute lymphoblastic leukemia, or diffuse large cell lymphoma (Richter syndrome).[112–116] These transformations are associated with poor survival. The pronounced neutropenia found in T-cell CLL can be treated with corticosteroids and splenectomy, with limited success. The role of cytokines (*e.g.*, rhGM-CSF, rhG-CSF) to stimulate granulopoiesis has not yet been established. The combination chemotherapy used in B-cell CLL is not effective, but new compounds like 2-chlorodeoxyadenosine are promising. Infections require antibiotic therapy, and patients with recurrent infections can be considered. The CD4-positive T-cell CLL patients respond poorly to cytotoxic agents but are amenable to leukapheresis when leukocytosis develops.

CHRONIC MYELOGENOUS LEUKEMIA

Chronic myelogenous leukemia (CML) starts with the acquisition of the Philadelphia chromosome translocation, which generates a chimeric tyrosine-specific protein kinase gene. This gene arises from a chromosomal translocation breakpoint between the second exon of the *BCR* gene on chromosome 22 and the second exon of the *ABL* gene on chromosome 9 or between the third exon of the *BCR* gene and the second exon of the *ABL* gene. The protein product of this chimeric gene, the P210 protein, makes the cell independent of extracellular growth factor stimulation, perhaps due to transcriptional activation of genes that rescue the cell from programmed cell death (*i.e.*, apoptosis), such as *BCL2*.

The *BCR-ABL* rearrangement may be detected by fluorescent in situ hybridization, Southern blot, and by the polymerase chain reaction (PCR)-induced amplification of the reverse transcript generated from the RNA of the CML cells. Although most patients contain a Philadelphia chromosome in all of their CML cells, patients whose disease features suggest CML but in whose cells no Philadelphia chromosome is detectable should be studied by Southern blot analysis for a rearranged *BCR* gene or by the PCR for *BCR-ABL*-encoded mRNA. The latter assay is also useful in following the course of the response to allogeneic bone marrow transplantation. At least 30% of patients have a positive PCR result for several months after an allograft, but most of these eventually convert to a negative assay. Reconversion from the Philadelphia-negative to Philadelphia-positive status is a grave prognostic sign, if it is not due to a contamination of the assay. Rarely, patients with a cytogenetically detectable Philadelphia chromosome but without *BCR-ABL*-encoded mRNA have been detected.

The disease is characterized by a progressive replacement of the normal diploid elements of the marrow with mature myeloid cells that are insensitive to the mechanisms that govern proliferation of normal myeloid cells. This results, in the beginning of the disease, in an ever-increasing ratio of leukemic to normal cells. Because the normal cells are still sensitive to the suppressive effect of an increased level of a circulating myeloid cell mass, without treatment, the disease evolves to greater and greater levels of abnormal cells.

The acquisition of somatic mutations and additional chromosomal abnormalities, such as an extra Philadelphia chromosome, trisomy 8, 17p-, or 22-, decreases the capability of maturation, which terminates in blastic crisis (*i.e.*, blast count in the marrow greater than 30%, severe anemia, and severe thrombocytopenia), often accompanied by basophilia. At this stage, all of the organs of the body are invaded by these blasts, the circulating count can reach several hundred thousand blasts per cubic millimeter, and the patient dies of bleeding, infection, or CNS hemorrhage or thrombosis in organs such as the brain. This process usually evolves in a median of 4 years, and the probability for a given patient for evolving into blastic phase is increased if the following are found at diagnosis: basophilia, additional chromosomal abnormalities, and a blast count that is above 5% in the peripheral blood. There is a 25% probability for blastic conversion for each year of the chronic phase. The phenotype of the blastic conversion is usually myeloid (60%), lymphoid (20%), and smaller percentages of erythroid and megakaryocyte phenotypes.

TREATMENT

Therapy for Chronic-Phase Chronic Myelogenous Leukemia

The criteria for assignment of response are summarized in Table 55–2. Radiation therapy of the spleen and radioactive phosphorous treatment for CML were instituted at the beginning of the century.[117-119] These treatments induced symptomatic relief and improved the quality of life in the chronic phase. Chemotherapeutic agents for the management of CML were introduced in 1952 with busulfan (Myleran or 1,4-dimethanesulfonyloxybutane), a sulfonic acid alkylating agent, and hydroxyurea, a ribonucleotidase inhibitor of DNA synthesis that was evaluated a decade later.[120,121] Both maintained the chronic phase by lowering leukocyte counts, reducing symptoms, and reversing splenomegaly. Although busulfan acts on early progenitor cells, and therefore its effect is prolonged, hydroxyurea induces rapid disease control but shorter remission duration.[122-127] Busulfan is occasionally associated with serious side effects, such as severe myelosuppression in 5% to 10% of patients, pulmonary, endocardial and marrow fibrosis, and an Addison-like wasting syndrome.[128] Survival of CML patients was not affected by either type of therapy, even at higher doses, and only rare cytogenetic remissions were reported after prolonged busulfan, ara-C, or hydroxyurea therapy.[129-141]

Intensive combination chemotherapy did not result in durable suppression of Philadelphia-positive cells.[142-145] Although different programs produced a significant Philadelphia chromosome suppression to less than 35% Philadelphia-positive metaphases in 30% to 50% of patients, these were predominantly transient, lasting for a median of 3 to 9 months.[142,144,146]

TABLE 55–2. Response Criteria for Interferon Therapy for Chronic Myelogenous Leukemia

Cytogenetic or Hematologic Remission	Leukocyte Count	Splenomegaly	Bone Marrow With Philadelphia Chromosome (%)
Complete	<9 × 10³/μl Normal morphology	None	0
Partial	<20 × 10³/μl	Persistence	≤35
Minor			35–95
Failure or none	>20 × 10³/μl	Persistence	100

(Talpaz M, McCredie KB, Mavligit GM, Gutterman JU. Leukocyte interferon-induced myeloid cytoreduction in chronic myelogenous leukemia. Blood 1983;62:689–692)

Other treatment modalities such as leukapheresis and splenectomy have been used to achieve disease control. Leukapheresis did not alter the course of the disease, and it is used today as an initial measure to prevent leukostasis-related complications and in pregnant patients to avoid fetal teratogenic effects of chemotherapy.[147-150] Splenectomy was added after several studies had demonstrated disease progression in the spleen preceding other disease sites.[151-156] However, controlled studies failed to substantiate an advantageous effect of splenectomy on the onset of blastic phase or on survival.[158,159] Prior splenectomy did not alter the prognosis of blastic crisis patients.[160] Though reported to result in faster recovery after bone marrow transplantation, splenectomy had no effect on posttransplant survival.[161,162] Splenectomy or intraarterial cytarabine perfusion in nonsurgical candidates are now reserved for symptomatic relief in unresponsive patients.[163]

Interferons

Since the discovery of interferon in 1957, it has been learned that interferons are a complex group of naturally occurring proteins produced by eukaryotic cells in response to various stimuli.[164,165] These proteins have pleiotropic biologic activities, among which are antiproliferative, immunomodulatory, antiviral, and differentiation-inducing effects.[166] The interferons consist of three distinct groups of peptides: IFN-α, IFN-β, and IFN-γ. IFN-α and IFN-β are acid stable, bind to the same receptor, and are produced primarily by leukocytes and fibroblasts respectively. IFN-γ is an acid-labile, structurally distinct molecule that binds to a different receptor and is produced mainly by T lymphocytes.[167]

The clinical activity of interferons in CML was first demonstrated with partially pure IFN-α (Finnish Red Cross, Hensinki), given at doses of 3 to 9×10^6 U/day to early-chronic-phase patients. A larger study revealed that laboratory indices of disease activity, such as elevated lactate dehydrogenase and B_{12} levels and increased bone marrow cellularity, normalized among responding patients (70%). Subsequently, cytogenetic responses with various degrees of Philadelphia chromosome suppression were found in 41% of the patients.[168,169]

Studies with the recombinant molecule rIFN-α-2a (Roferon; Hoffman-LaRoche, Nutley, NJ) at a dose of 5×10^6 U/m^2 administered intramuscularly daily demonstrated a 75% response rate (33 of 45 patients) with early Philadelphia-positive CML.[170,171] Eleven patients (23%) achieved complete cytogenetic responses on at least one test. Partial cytogenetic responses were seen in 3 additional patients.[171,172]

Studies with rIFN-α-2b (Intron; Schering, Kenilworth, NJ) demonstrated similar activities to those of rIFN-α2a.[169-172] Niederle and colleagues reported responses for 40 of 59 Philadelphia-positive CML patients treated with rIFN-α-2b with a dose of 4×10^6 U/m^2/day. Thirty-three percent of these patients had cytogenetic responses.[173] Alimena and associates reported a 68% hematologic remission rate and 56% rate of cytogenetic improvements among 63 Philadelphia-positive CML patients administered doses of 2 to 5×10^6 U/m^2 of rIFN-α-2b intramuscularly daily.[174] Similar results were seen by a large cooperative study conducted by the CALGB. Of 47 evaluable patients treated with 5×10^6 U/m^2/day of rIFN-α-2b, 27 (57%) achieved complete hematologic remissions; 40% of the patients had cytogenetic improvements.[175,176]

The relation between response and dose intensity was addressed in the Italian study. Patients were treated with 2×10^6 U/m^2 daily or 5×10^6 U/m^2 daily of rIFN-α-2b, and the results indicated a higher response rate with the higher dose and frequent responses among patients initially assigned to the lower dose and subsequently switched to the higher one.[174] However, there is no evidence that further escalation beyond 5×10^6 U/m^2 can increase response rate. The feasibility of further dose escalation is also questionable because of dose-limiting toxicity. Certain prognostic factors influenced the degree of response. When patients were evaluated according to the multivariate regression model, hematologic and cytogenetic responses were more common in low-risk patients.[169] Time from diagnosis influenced therapy outcome as well; patients who were treated within less than 1 year from diagnosis demonstrated approximately 70% hematologic response rate, in sharp contrast to patients with long-standing disease who exhibited a dramatic decline in the hematologic response rate and for whom complete and partial cytogenetic responses were absent (Table 55-3).[171]

Randomized studies of the course and survival of previously untreated patients assigned to conventional chemotherapy or to interferon therapy are ongoing in different centers.[177,178] Preliminary results of 220 patients randomized to 3 to 9×10^6 U/day of IFN-α-2a versus 102 randomized to conventional chemotherapy demonstrated that after 8, 14, and 24 months, a cytogenetic response occurred in 45%, 47% and 50% of the IFN arm and in 20%, 19% and 0%, respectively, of the conventional chemotherapy arm.[177] Another randomized study that accrued 600 patients failed to show any advantage for interferon over busulfan or hydroxyurea.[183] However, interferon was introduced late in the study. Interferon doses were lower than those in single-arm studies, which may clearly affect incidence and duration of responses.[178,183]

Only one study provides sufficient follow-up to assess re-

TABLE 55–3. Hematologic and Cytogenetic Responses Among Philadelphia-Positive CML Patients Treated With rINF-α2a

Characteristics	Disease Duration	
	≤1 Year	>1 Year
Number of patients studied	45	16
Complete hematologic remission	34 (75%)*	4 (25%)
Philadelphia-chromosome status:		
No cytogenetic response	11 } (44%)	1 } (25%)
>35% to 95%	9	3
>5% to <35%	3 }	
0%	} (31%)	(0%)
Partial hematologic remission	11 }	
Resistant disease	2 (4%)	1 (6%)
	9 (21%)	11 (69%)

* Rate of response is given in parentheses.
(Talpaz M, Kantarjian HM, McCredie KB, Keating MJ, Trujillo J, Gutterman J. Clinical investigation of human alpha interferon in chronic myelogenous leukemia. Blood 1987;69:1280–1288)

mission duration and survival.[172] The overall duration of complete hematologic remission was 41 months. However, the remissions lasted significantly longer in patients who had achieved complete or partial cytogenetic remission compared with patients who achieved minor or no cytogenetic response ($p = 0.02$ by the log rank test; Fig. 55–3).

Lasting complete cytogenetic remission was demonstrated in a group of patients with early Philadelphia-positive CML. Eighteen of 96 patients treated with partially pure IFN-α obtained a complete cytogenetic response. Of these, 11 patients had durable ongoing complete cytogenetic responses from 6 to more than 45 months, as shown in Table 55–3.[172]

Southern blot analysis of DNA extracted from CML patients in complete cytogenetic remission did not reveal any improved sensitivity in detecting residual disease over that of standard cytogenetic analysis.[179] However, a PCR assay provides a means of detecting one Philadelphia-positive cell in 10^5 to 10^6 cells.[180] Eighteen patients in complete cytogenetic remission after therapy with IFN-α were subjected to PCR analysis, revealing that 17 of the patients had evidence of residual disease and 1 patient had no residual disease.[181] However, another laboratory has reported that all patients in cytogenetic remission are PCR positive. The significance of this finding for assessing the risk of relapse in these patients and changes in the residual disease over time is not clear, and the results must be matched to clinical outcome.

The overall survival outlook for IFN-treated CML patients was examined in one study by Talpaz and colleagues.[172] This group found a median survival of 63 months, which is significantly longer than for its matched historic controls. However, factors such as earlier diagnosis and change in the natural history of the disease may have influenced this outcome. The projected survival is excellent for complete and partial cytogenetic responders, and the median survival for this group of patients has not been reached (Fig. 55–4). It is already significantly longer than that of the other responders and the nonresponders.

Toxicities to IFN-α can be divided into those observed early in the course of therapy and those developing during the maintenance of the remission.[172] Initially, patients develop fever, chills, malaise, myalgias, fatigue, and headaches, described as an influenza-like syndrome. Acetaminophen or indomethacin can relieve many of these symptoms. Tachyphylaxis usually develops after 1 or 2 weeks of continuous IFN-α administration. Musculoskeletal effects, such as myalgias and arthralgias, are common and transient. However, approximately 10% of the patients develop severe bone pain requiring bed rest. This toxicity was aborted completely with the addition of hydroxyurea, which lowers the initial cell counts (M. Talpaz, unpublished results).

Gastrointestinal toxic effects include elevation of liver transaminase levels to two to three times above baseline values and occasional nausea and diarrhea. Renal toxicity occurs in about 15% of patients and usually manifests as proteinuria. Reversible hair thinning is seen occasionally. Immunomediated hemolysis or thrombocytopenia have been rarely observed.

Perhaps the most significant side effects are neurologic, including impairment of concentration, short-term memory, and other cognitive functions. More serious neurotoxicity with frontal lobe and Parkinsonian syndromes, depression, and psychotic reactions have been observed and mandate discontinuation of therapy.

Late autoimmune side effects such as hypothyroidism and generalized autoimmune phenomena were documented (M. Talpaz, unpublished data). The development of systemic lupus erythematosus in a patient with CML after 45 months of therapy with IFN was reported.[183]

INTERFERON COMBINED WITH OTHER TREATMENT MODALITIES. Combination therapies were initiated to improve the response rate. Maintenance therapy with IFN-α-2b with a dose 2×10^6 U/m² three times weekly after remission induction with busulfan was evaluated by Bergsagel and coworkers.[184] With low-dose therapy, these investigators were able to maintain remission in 6 of 8 patients studied for 3+ to 24+ months. Another approach included intensive chemotherapy induction followed by IFN-α.[185] Intensive chemotherapy consisted of three cycles of daunorubicin (120 mg/m² on day 1), cytarabine (80 mg/m² daily for 10 days), vincristine (2 mg on day 1), and prednisone (100 mg daily for 5 days). Maintenance therapy with IFN-α at doses of 3×10^6 to 5×10^6 U/m² daily was adjusted according to cell counts and toxicity. Of the 32 patients studied in the benign phase of the disease, 28 (86%) had Philadelphia chromosome suppression with intensive chemotherapy; 21 (66%) of them had major or complete Philadelphia chromosome suppression. The effect was transient in most the patients, but cytogenetic remission was maintained in 8 patients (31%) for 12+ months, for a range of 22+ to 42+ months.

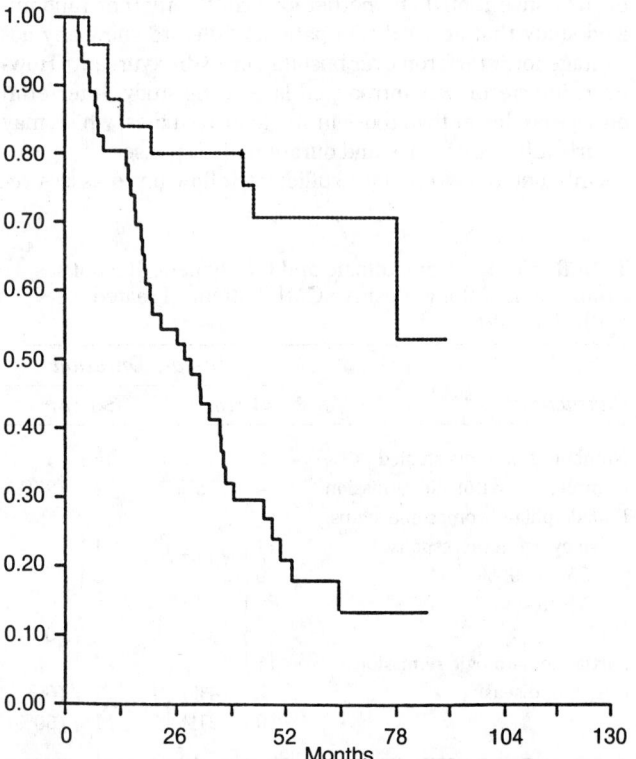

FIGURE 55–3. Kaplan-Meier estimate of the probability of relapse-free survival in patients achieving complete and partial cytogenetic remissions (*dotted line*) compared with that of patients with hematologic remission associated with minor or no cytogenetic response (*solid line*) ($p < 0.001$).

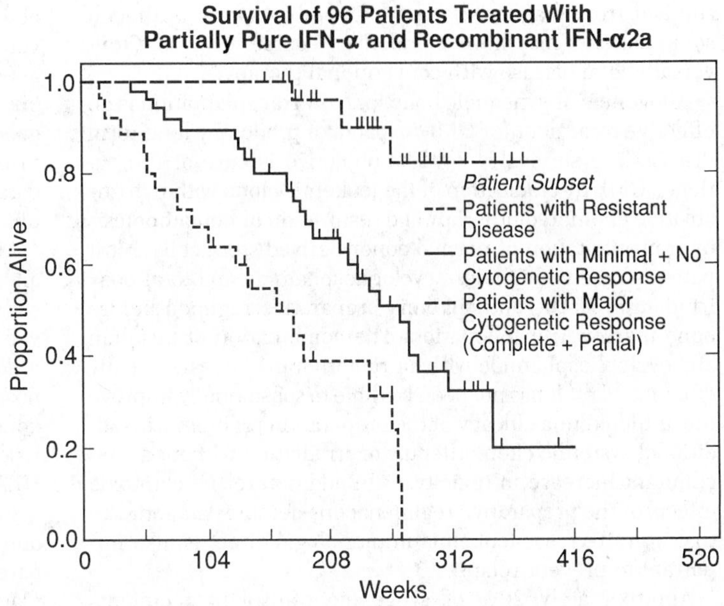

**Survival of 96 Patients Treated With
Partially Pure IFN-α and Recombinant IFN-α2a**

FIGURE 55–4. Survival of complete and partial cytogenetic responders, minor or no cytogenetic responders, and CML patients resistant to interferon therapy.

Concomitant administration of IFN-α with various drugs was studied by several investigators. The combination of IFN-α and low-dose cytarabine or hydroxyurea compares favorably with the results of IFN-α alone. However, the combination-therapy studies have not accrued a sufficient number of patients nor have they been followed long enough to draw conclusions about improvement in the survival rate or the incidence of durable cytogenetic response.[186–188]

IFN-γ suppresses in vitro hematopoietic progenitors in a fashion similar to IFN-α and induces differentiation of leukemia cells.[189–192] A study of IFN-γ (Genentech, South San Francisco, CA) at doses of 0.25 to 0.5 mg/m² given intramuscularly daily was conducted in CML Philadelphia-positive patients.[193] Six of 26 patients have achieved a complete hematologic remission; 4 had partial hematologic remissions. Five patients had minor cytogenetic improvements, with emergence of 5% to 45% diploid cells in the bone marrow. Control of thrombocytosis was achieved in all 4 patients with a baseline platelet count of more than $1 \times 10^6/\mu l$. Fever and flu-like symptoms were the most common side effects. The study of combined INF-α and INF-γ in the treatment of CML was prompted by the in vitro synergistic effect of the two molecules.[194,195] Recombinant IFN-α and rIFN-γ were administered on alternating weeks, each at doses ranging from 2 to 10×10^6 U/m² given intramuscularly daily. Eleven (41%) of 27 patients achieved complete hematologic remissions, and 3 (11%) achieved partial hematologic remissions. Cytogenetic responses were seen in 6 patients. Niederle and associates found similar results; hematologic responses could be induced in 12 (23%) of 23 patients, with durations of 8+ to 20+ months, and partial hematologic remissions were achieved by another 8 patients.[196] Two patients achieved complete cytogenetic remissions. We and others failed to demonstrate improved response rates with the combination of INF-α and INF-γ, although the schedule used may not have been optimal.

MECHANISMS OF INTERFERON ACTION. The cause of IFN resistance among CML patients is poorly understood. IFN binds to a specific receptor on the cell surface. However, no discernible defects were detected in receptor binding affinity and receptor down regulation after therapy with IFN.[197]

IFN induces multiple genes, commonly known as IFN-stimulated genes (ISG), some with defined function (*e.g.*, 2′,5′-oligoadenylate synthetase [2′,5′A], interferon-associated protein kinase P67; major histocompatibility complex class I; metallothionein II), others with still unknown functions (*e.g.*, ISG-15, ISG-54; genes denoted 6-16, 6-26, and 9-27).[198–202] Studies of cell lines sensitive and resistant to IFN-α have demonstrated a spectrum of defects in induction of 2′,5′A, ISG-15, ISG-54, or 6-16 mRNA in IFN-resistant CML patients.[203–206]

A different approach evaluated the interaction between CML progenitor cells and bone marrow stroma layers.[207] It was suggested that the clinical efficacy of IFN in CML may be due in part to its ability to counteract the defect in attachment of CML progenitor cells to stroma, bringing them under more normal regulatory control. However, no report is available on the changes in IFN-resistant disease. IFN was also shown to interfere with the effect of various growth factors by modulating the receptor to these cytokines or by altering the growth factor-induced cellular signal transduction.[208–210] These studies suggested that resistance may be due to the autonomous production of cytokines by the malignant clone during the progression of CML.[211,212]

Bone Marrow Transplantation

ALLOGENEIC BONE MARROW TRANSPLANTATION. CML is a hematologic malignancy characterized by excessive proliferation of a single clone myeloid cells and their progenitors. The disease can be divided into two phases, an initial chronic phase in which cell maturation is normal, followed by transformation to the acute phase (*i.e.*, blast crisis), characterized by maturation arrest at the level of the myeloblast or lymphoblast.[213] Some patients develop a transient accelerated phase before development of overt blast crisis. Median survival from diagnosis is approximately 4 years. Although some patients may have a prolonged course, CML is a universally fatal disease with conventional therapy.

Allogeneic or syngeneic bone marrow transplantation is an effective treatment for CML, capable of producing long-term disease-free survival.[214,215] The objective is cure of the patient's CML by eradication of the leukemic clone with marrow ablative chemoradiotherapy and restoration of hematopoiesis by transplantation of normal donor-derived stem cells. Most patients receive high-dose cyclophosphamide and total-body irradiation as the antileukemia preparative regimen before bone marrow transplantation. The combination of busulfan and cyclophosphamide without radiotherapy appears equally effective.[216,217] It has not been possible to substantially improve the antileukemia efficacy of the preparation regimen with additional systemic chemotherapy or irradiation without a concomitant increase in toxicity.[218] In addition to the cytotoxic effects of the preparative regimen, considerable data indicate that a graft-versus-leukemia immunologic effect is also important to prevent relapse.[219]

Approximately 20% of syngeneic transplant recipients transplanted in blast crisis have survived free of disease longer than 5 years, demonstrating that the intensive marrow ablative therapy can eradicate even far advanced disease in some patients.[200] Better results have been reported for patients receiving syngeneic bone marrow transplantation while in chronic phase; the actuarial continuous remission rate and survival rate are each approximately 65% at longer than 5 years.

Over 2000 patients with CML have received allogeneic marrow transplantation from an HLA-identical donor.[221–225] For patients transplanted in acute phase, 10% to 20% survive over 5 years in continuous remission; the major cause of treatment failure is leukemia relapse; the actuarial relapse rate is approximately 60%. Patients transplanted while in an accelerated phase or a second chronic phase after blast crisis have had somewhat better results; the actuarial relapse rate is approximately 40%, and the 5-year survival rate is 30%. The best results have been reported with allogeneic bone marrow transplantation for patients in the chronic phase; the actuarial disease-free survival rate is approximately 50% to 60% at 5 years, and fewer than 20% of patients have relapsed. The best results are reported for young patients and those transplanted within 1 year of diagnosis.[226]

Several conclusions can be drawn from these data. Patients with CML in blast crisis or the accelerated phase have a poor prognosis with conventional treatment; median survival is less than 3 months, and few patients survive 1 year. Allogeneic and syngeneic bone marrow transplantations are generally unsuccessful in these patients, but a small proportion may achieve long-term disease-free survival. Results have been better in patients transplanted in chronic phase. The optimal timing of transplantation in chronic-phase patients is controversial. The risks and potential benefits of early bone marrow transplantation must be balanced against the risk of delaying the treatment (*i.e.*, transformation of the leukemia). For patients who are clinically stable, there is a relatively constant risk of transformation to the acute phase; approximately 25% of patients surviving at any point develop acute-phase disease during the ensuing year and die of their disease. Several investigators have reported prognostic factors that may identify

good-, average-, and poor-risk groups when treated with conventional treatment.[227,228] Early bone marrow transplantation appears justified in patients with an average or poor prognosis, but a conservative approach may advisable for patients with good prognostic features. This recommendation may need to be reexamined because of the encouraging preliminary data for using INF-α in some patients with early chronic-phase CML.[229]

Most patients who are otherwise appropriate candidates for allogeneic bone marrow transplantation lack an HLA-identical sibling donor. An alternative approach for transplantation involves the use of HLA-nonidentical relatives or unrelated HLA-matched donors. There is a greater risk of acute graft-versus-host disease and graft failure with mismatched or unrelated donor transplants and a higher risk of early mortality. The risk of chronic graft-versus-host disease is also increased with HLA nongenotypically matched transplants.[230–235]

Related donor-recipient pairs that are mismatched for only one A, B, or D HLA locus or HLA phenotypically identical parent-child pairs have survival indistinguishable from transplantation between HLA-identical siblings.[230] Patients mismatched for 2 or more loci have poorer results with a high risk of graft rejection, graft-versus-host disease, and other complications. The development of large registries of potential unrelated donors has allowed evaluation of allogeneic bone marrow transplantation from unrelated HLA phenotypically identical or closely matched donors.[232–235] Approximately 45% of patients transplanted in CML in chronic phase or acute leukemia in remission and 30% with more advanced disease have achieved disease-free survivals of longer than 2 years.[236–237] The higher risks associated with transplants from unrelated or HLA-nonidentical donors have led many centers to reserve this approach for patients who fail to respond to interferon or other more conservative initial therapy.

GRAFT-VERSUS-LEUKEMIA. Allogeneic bone marrow transplantation was originally proposed as a means to escalate the doses of myelotoxic chemoradiotherapy to supralethal levels, using marrow transplantation to restore hematopoiesis. Considerable evidence indicates that the preparative regimen does not usually eradicate the malignancy and an additional immunomediated graft-versus-leukemia effect is important to prevent relapse.

Graft-versus-leukemia is closely associated with the presence of graft-versus-host disease.[238,239] This antileukemic effect correlates best with chronic graft-versus-host disease. The impact of acute graft-versus-host disease is uncertain, but the lowest rate of relapse occurs in patients with acute and chronic graft-versus-host disease. These data suggest that the graft-versus-leukemia effect occurs over many months to years.

Patients receiving transplants from identical twin donors do not develop graft-versus-host disease; these patients have at least twice the risk of relapse of CML as transplant recipients from HLA-identical siblings.[219,224] Conversely, patients transplanted from unrelated donors have a significantly higher rate of graft-versus-host disease; these patients appear to have a lower risk of leukemia relapse than those with transplants from HLA-identical siblings.[235] T-cell depletion of donor bone marrow is the most effective means of preventing acute and chronic graft-versus-host disease, but this benefit has been offset by the substantial increase in the risk of leukemia relapse.[215,234,240–242] The net effect is no change or worsening of disease-free survival.[243] The increase in leukemia relapse is most striking for patients with CML than other forms of leukemia.[243] In a study of the International Bone Marrow Transplant Registry, 12% of patients with CML in chronic phase receiving unmodified HLA-identical bone marrow transplants relapsed, compared with a relapse rate of more than 50% with T-cell-depleted transplants.[244] This marked increase in the rate of relapse is seen in comparing T-cell-depleted recipients who develop graft-versus-host disease with unmodified allograft recipients without graft-versus-host disease. This strongly suggests an effect of T lymphocytes independent of graft-versus-host disease. The high relapse rate for T-cell-depleted transplants indicates that viable leukemia cells survive the preparative regimen and are capable of reestablishing the disease in most patients. Consistent with these data is the observation that after transplantation of unmodified bone marrow, Philadelphia-positive metaphases can be detected intermittently in many patients, even though most never experience a hematologic relapse; growth of these leukemic cells is presumably controlled by the graft-versus-leukemia effect that must be operative over an extended period.[244] It may still be possible to successfully employ T-cell depletion to prevent graft-versus-host disease; several centers are evaluating the use of higher doses of total-body irradiation or the addition of thiotepa or other drugs to the preparative regimen to enhance engraftment and improve the cytotoxicity against leukemia cells.

The recognition and effector mechanisms that mediate graft-versus-leukemia and the cell populations involved are incompletely understood. CD4- and CD8-positive T-cell clones reactive with leukemia cells have been described, and cytotoxic T lymphocytes are likely to be the primary effector cells. LAK and natural killer cells may also be important in this process, and IL-2 may enhance the antileukemic activity.[245–247]

It is uncertain whether the graft-versus-leukemia reaction can be differentiated from graft-versus-host disease in humans or whether the same or different cell populations mediate each process. After allogeneic marrow transplants, stable chimerism with donor-derived hematopoiesis is the rule, although mixed chimerism occurs in some cases. The graft-versus-leukemia effect may result from reactivity directed against host hematopoietic tissue in general. Such an effect would prevent competitive repopulation by normal and leukemic host-derived hematopoietic cells, and this potential mechanism would not require recognition of leukemia-specific antigens.

It is conceivable that different cellular subsets are responsible for graft-versus-host disease and the graft-versus-leukemia effect. CD4-positive T cells recognize antigens presented with class II MHC antigens. CD8-positive lymphocytes recognize antigens presented in the context of class I loci. CD4-positive cells mediate acute graft-versus-host disease in MHC class II disparate recipients, and CD8-positive cells are primarily responsible with class I disparate transplants in mice.[246] Depletion of the CD8-positive suppressor T cells is sufficient to reduce or prevent graft-versus-host disease in most donor-recipient murine strain combinations that are MHC compatible but mismatched for minor histocompatibility loci. We reported that selective depletion of CD8-positive cells

in combination with posttransplant cyclosporine resulted in a significantly reduced rate of acute graft-versus-host disease and an increase in the risk of leukemia relapse.[247] Improved methods to selectively enhance the graft-versus-leukemia effect may be possible.

AUTOLOGOUS BONE MARROW TRANSPLANTATION. For the past 2.5 years, patients at the M.D. Anderson Cancer Center who are ineligible for interferon or allograft therapy have been allocated to intensive therapy followed by autologous bone marrow transplantation without purging in an attempt to decrease the evolution of the disease from the early indolent phase to the more aggressive fulminant acute leukemic transformation, which results in death from bleeding and infection. Kantarjian first exposed patients to conventional-dose chemotherapy (*i.e.*, daunomycin, high-dose ara-C), which is designed to reduce the total leukemia cell burden and to permit the regrowth of normal cells in the marrow. In 50% of patients, some degree of cytogenetic remission was achieved. After recovery from this conventional-dose chemotherapy, peripheral blood cells were collected during the stages of early recovery (total leukocyte count between $300/mm^3$ and $800/mm^3$), because it had been shown by Carella and his colleagues that the probability of collecting circulating diploid early progenitor cells in the peripheral blood was high at this time of early hematopoietic recovery.

The patients then were exposed to total-body irradiation, cyclophosphamide, and VP-16 in doses that would totally ablate endogenous hematopoietic activity. Marrow function was regenerated through infusion of an engrafting dose of the autologous marrow. After recovery of hematopoietic function, interferon maintenance therapy was used. This last stage was designed to provide biologic maintenance therapy that would serve the function associated with the graft-versus-leukemia effect in allograft patients. These patients were treated at a median of 2.5 years from diagnosis. The median follow-up was 800 days for this group of patients. The patients who were given the autologous transplants in first chronic phase with this regimen had a survival rate that was equivalent to patients treated with allografts with the same preparative regimen.

In contrast to the favorable survival (70%) of the first chronic-phase patients, the survival rate of the second chronic-phase accelerated or blast crisis patients given autografts was in the 35% range. There are at least two possible explanations for the adverse lower survival of the second group. First, an overall increase in resistance in advanced disease patients results in persisting systemic disease after delivery of the preparative regimen. Second, the small number of neoplastic cells that are infused in the autologous marrow may have more significant impact on the natural history of the disease in advanced chronic patients.

There are two possible responses to this data: deliver more intensive systemic preparative therapy or increase the stringency of purging. Unfortunately, an increase in treatment-related mortality may accompany the use of more stringent preparative regimens due to an increase in nonextramedullary toxicity. Increasing the stringency of the marrow-cleansing procedures may remove too many reconstituting progenitor cells, delaying recovery and increasing the mortality from infections during neutropenia. It is important to have an assay that can differentiate between a relapse that arose from residual systemic disease or insufficient stringency of bone marrow purging.

RETROVIRAL MARKING TO IDENTIFY ORIGIN OF RELAPSE AFTER MARROW TRANSPLANTATION. As shown in Figure 55–5, retroviral marking is a procedure that can differentiate the origin of relapse in autologous bone marrow transplantation. In this procedure, autologous cells are collected after recovery from conventional-dose therapy that is designed to promote repopulation of the marrow by normal autologous stem cells. The cells are then concentrated and fractionated with monoclonal antibodies that recognize antigens specific for normal or leukemia cells, and the resulting marrow is exposed to a safety-modified retrovirus to mark the leukemia and normal cells in the autologous marrow. The marrow is reinfused, and the patient followed.

If relapse occurs, the cells are assayed for the presence of leukemia cells that contain the viral marker using a PCR assay. The leukemia cells that are marked can be identified by a PCR assay for *BCR-ABL*-encoded mRNA. If the leukemia cells contain the viral marker, we conclude that the relapse arose from residual cells left in the autologous marrow after the purging of the autologous marrow. In that case, we would focus on increasing the stringency of the marrow purging

procedure. Our algorithm for this program is summarized in Table 55–4.

GENETIC THERAPY

A natural extension of the marking program in autologous transplantation is the use of autologous transplants for genetic therapy. Genetic therapy involves the replacement of the missing or nonfunctional molecular elements in the DNA of living cells or the introduction of additional genetic elements into these cells. This therapy is designed to correct alterations within living cells that lead to disease in man.

Several steps are required to implement such therapy. The oncologist must have the capability for isolating the progenitor cells, which when modified can contribute to the repopulation of marrow after intensive therapy and which dominate that tissue and the population of cells that arise within it for prolonged periods. The genetic information and introducing the genetic information must not result in undesirable changes within these populations of living cells. The genetic changes introduced must confer a selective advantage for the cell or at least are subject to selective techniques that have limited potential for generating toxicity and at the same time can suppress the unmodified population of cells. The genetic change must involve a single genetic defect that is dominant

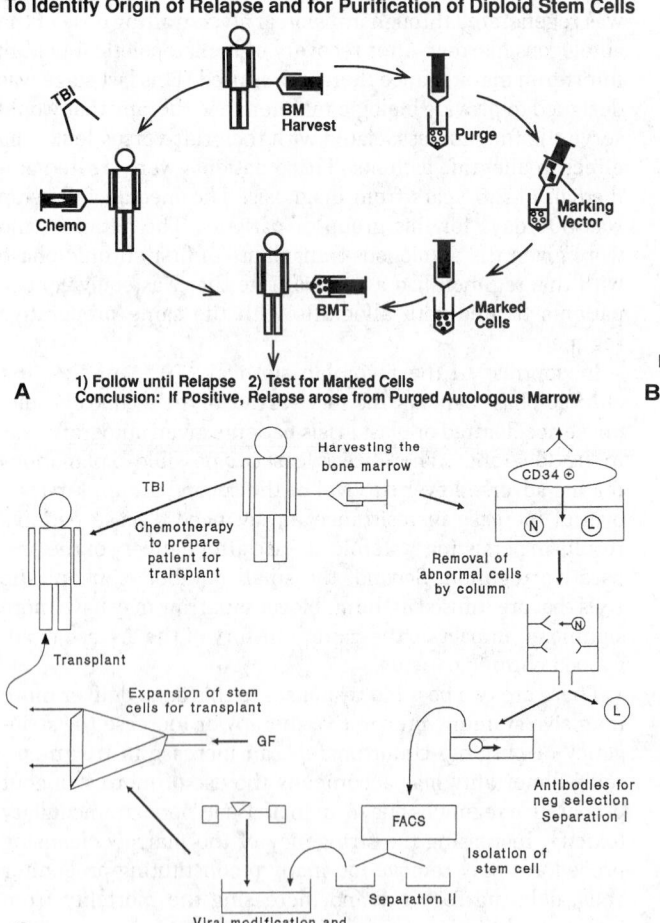

FIGURE 55–5. **(A)** Molecular marking with safety-modified retroviruses in CML. **(B)** Transfer of chemotherapy resistance genes using safety modified retroviruses. **(C)** Transfer of therapeutic molecules to normal and leukemic cells using safety modified retroviruses. The therapeutic molecule, a stretch of antisense mRNA homologous to a functional region of the *BCR-ABL*-encoded mRNA of CML cells, is embedded in the 3′ untranslated region of the multidrug chemotherapy resistant cDNA. All cells without the virus are killed by chemotherapy. The normal cells transduced by the virus are protected from chemotherapy. Although the transduced leukemia cells can acquire drug resistance, they will be suppressed by the antisense ribozyme sequence.

TABLE 55–4. Molecular Marking Program

   I. Daunomycin-high dose cytosine arabinoside to induce second chronic phase or cytogenetic remission
  II. Harvesting of autologous marrow
 III. CD34-positive selection of early progenitor cells
 IV. Negative selection
  V. Marking with safety-modified retrovirus
 VI. Preparative therapy with total-body irradiation, VP-16, and cyclophosphamide
VII. Infusion with marked marrow
VIII. Interferon maintenance therapy after hematopoietic recovery

---

in the population of hematopoietic cells under consideration for therapy.

CML, because it arises from a single chromosomal translocation that produces a known genetic change within the hematopoietic population of progenitor cells, has been studied as a possible model for this molecular targeting approach. The fact that a single genetic change has occurred within the population of abnormal cells permits the use of molecular assays that are totally specific and unusually sensitive to measure the impact of the genetic therapy on the phenotype of the cell, to optimize the conditions that result in genetic modification, and to evaluate immediately the impact of therapy.

This marking program could be the first stage of a three-step program to use bone marrow transplantation and retroviral marking to develop populations of hematopoietic cells that are enriched in the early pluripotent hematopoietic stem cell and to then genetically modify these cells before autologous transplantation as corrective therapy for the disease:

1. Use of safety-modified retroviruses to mark the autologous cells used for transplant after purging (see Figure 55–5A). This helps identify the origin of relapse, differentiating between residual systemic disease and the neoplastic cells left in the autologous cells after purging and the degree to which the fractionation procedures are enriching the early progenitor cells by the percentage of cells that contain the retroviral transgenome.
2. Use of safety-modified retroviruses to introduce into normal early progenitor cells chemotherapy-resistance genes (see Figure 55–5B). This helps to decrease hematopoietic toxicity after chemotherapy and to establish methods for in vivo selection of genetically modified hematopoietic cells. This would be done in solid tumor patients whose marrow is not involved with cancer.
3. Use of safety-modified retroviruses that contain chemotherapy-resistance genes and therapeutic molecules (see Figure 55–5C) that can be used to control a disease.

The use of fractionation of hematopoietic cells with monoclonal antibodies for purging of leukemia cells and the use of retroviruses in the transplantation setting provide opportunities to develop populations of autologous marrow that are enriched in normal early progenitor cells.

It is possible that investigators will be able to use the percentage of diploid cells that are positive for the retroviral transgenome and the lineage distribution of such cells to monitor the efficiency of fractionation in enriching the hematopoietic stem cell. After fractions of autologous marrow that are sufficiently enriched in early normal progenitor cells

are developed by this method, genetic correction models that have shown promise in preclinical or in vitro models will be tested.

CONCLUSION

Major advances are occurring in the therapy for the chronic leukemias. It is likely that these diseases will be a major proving ground for the development of genetic and molecular approaches to therapy, as they have for the established modalities of radiation therapy, chemotherapy, biologic therapy, and bone marrow transplantation during the past 40 years.

REFERENCES

1. Polliack A, Catovsky D, eds. Chronic lymphocytic leukemia. Jerusalem, Israel: Harwood Academic Publishers, 1988.
2. Silber R, Stahl R. Chronic lymphocytic leukemia and related diseases. In: Williams W, Beutler E, Erslev AJ, Lichtman MA, eds. Hematology. New York: McGraw-Hill, 1990:1005.
3. Minot GR, Isaacs R. Lymphatic leukemia: Age incidence, duration and benefit derived from irradiation. Boston Med Surg 1924;191:1.
4. Rai KR, Sawitsky A, Cronkite EP, et al. Clinical staging of chronic lymphocytic leukemia. Blood 1975;46:219.
5. Binet JL, LePorrier M, Dighiero G, et al. A clinical staging system for chronic lymphocytic leukemia. Cancer 1977;40:855.
6. Preud'homme JL, Seligmann M. Surface-bound immunoglobulins as a cell marker in human lymphoproliferative diseases. Blood 1972;40:777.
7. Korsmeyer SJ. Hierarchy of immunoglobulin gene rearrangements in B-cell leukemias. In: Waldman TA, ed. Molecular genetic analyses of human lymphoid neoplasms: Immunoglobulin genes and the c-*myc* oncogene. Ann Intern Med 1985;102:497.
8. Gahrton G, Robert K-H, Friberg K, et al. Nonrandom chromosomal aberrations in chronic lymphocytic leukemia revealed by polyclonal B-cell-mitogen stimulation. Blood 1980;56:640.
9. Surveillance Epidemiology End Results Incidence and Mortality Data: 1973–1977. NCI monograph 57. Bethesda, MD: National Cancer Institute, 1981:10.
10. Gunz FW, Dameshek W. Chronic lymphocytic leukemia in a family including twin brothers and a son. JAMA 1957;164:1323.
11. Reilly EB, Rappaport SI, Karr NW, et al. Familial chronic lymphatic leukemia. Arch Intern Med 1952;90:87.
12. Conley CL, Misiti J, Laster AJ. Genetic factors predisposing to chronic lymphocytic leukemia and to autoimmune disease. Medicine (Baltimore) 1980;5:323.
13. Han T, Ozer H, Sadamori N, et al. Prognostic importance of cytogenetic abnormalities in patients with chronic lymphocytic leukemia. N Engl J Med 1984;310:288.
14. Gahrton G, Robert K-H, Friberg K, Zech L, Bird AG. Nonrandom chromosomal aberrations in chronic lymphocytic leukemia revealed by polyclonal B-cell-mitogen stimulation. Blood 1980;56:640.
15. Hurley JN, Fu SM, Kunkel HG, Chaganti RSK, German J. Chromosome abnormalities of leukaemic B lymphocytes in chronic lymphocytic leukaemia. Nature 1980;283:76.
16. Juliusson G, Oscher DG, Fitchett M, et al. Prognostic subgroups in B-cell chronic lymphocytic leukemia defined by specific chromosomal abnormalities. N Engl J Med 1990;323:720.
17. Han T, Ozer H, Sadamori N, et al. Prognostic importance of cytogenetic abnormalities in patients with CLL. N Engl J Med 1984;310:288.
18. Vahdati M, Graafland H, Emberger JM. Isochromosome 17q in cell lines of two cases of B cell chronic lymphocytic leukemia. Cancer Genet Cytogenet 1983;9:227.
19. Han T, Henderson ES, Emrich LJ, et al. Prognostic significance of karyotypic abnormalities in B-cell chronic lymphocytic leukemia: An update. Semin Hematol 1987;24:257.
20. Callen DF, Ford JH. Chromosome abnormalities in chronic lymphocytic leukemia revealed by TPA as a mitogen. Cancer Genet Cytogenet 1983;10:87.
21. Morita M, Minowada J, Sandberg AA. Chromosomes and causation of human cancer and leukemia. XLV: Chromosome patterns in stimulated lymphocytes of chronic lymphocytic leukemia. Cancer Genet Cytogenet 1981;3:293.
22. O'Donnell PV, Nowinski RC, Stockert E. Amplified expression of murine leukemia virus (MuLV)-coded antigens on thymocytes and leukemia cells of AKR mice after infection by dualtropic (MCF) MuLV. Virology 1982;119:450.
23. Gahrton G, Robert KH, Friberg K, et al. Extra chromosome 12 in chronic lymphocytic leukemia. Lancet 1980;1:146.
24. Knuutila S, Elonen E, Teerenhovi L, et al. Trisomy 12 in B-cells of patients with B-cell chronic lymphocytic leukemia. N Engl J Med 1986;314:865.
25. Erikson J, Finan J, Tsujimoto Y, et al. The chromosome 14 breakpoint in neoplastic B cells with the t(11;14) translocation involves the immunoglobulin heavy chain locus. Proc Natl Acad Sci USA 1984;81:4144.
26. Jones GT, Abramson N. Gastrointestinal necrosis in acute leukemia: A complication of induction therapy. Cancer Invest 1983;1:315.

27. Escudier SM, Pereira-Leahy JM, Goodacre AM, et al. Fluorescence in situ hybridization (FISH) and cytogenetic studies of trisomy 12 in chronic lymphocytic leukemia (CLL). Blood 1991;78(suppl 1):329A.

28. Han T, Emrich LJ, Ozer H, Sandberg AA. Prognostic implications of trisomy 12 and non-trisomy 12 karyotypes in B-cell chronic lymphocytic leukemia. Blood 1985;65:470.

29. Zech L. Inversion of chromosome 14 marks human T-cell chronic lymphocytic leukaemia. Nature 1984;308:858.

30. Croce CM, Isobe M, Palumbo A, et al. Gene for alpha-chain of human T-cell receptor location on chromosome 14 region involved in T-cell neoplasms. Science 1985;227:1044.

31. Freedman AS, Boyd AW, Bierber FR. Normal cellular counterparts of B cell chronic lymphocytic leukemia. Blood 1987;70:418.

32. Martin PJ, Hansen JA, Stadak AW, Nowinski RC. Monoclonal antibody recognizing normal human T lymphocytes and malignant human B lymphocytes: A comparative study. J Immunol 1981;127:1920.

33. Perri RT, Royston I, LeBien T, Kay NE. Chronic lymphocytic leukemia progenitor cells carry the antigens T65, BA-1 and Ia. Blood 1983;61:871.

34. Kay NE, Oken MM, Perri RT. The influential T cell in B-cell neoplasms. J Clin Oncol 1983;1:810.

35. Kay NE, Kaplan ME. Defective T cell responsiveness in chronic lymphocytic leukemia: Analysis of activation events. Blood 1986;67:578.

36. Davis S. The variable pattern of circulating lymphocyte subpopulations in chronic lymphocytic leukemia. N Engl J Med 1974;294:1150.

37. Mangan KF, D'Alessandro L. Hypoplastic anemia in B cell chronic lymphocytic leukemia: Evolution of T cell-mediated suppression of erythropoiesis in early-stage and late-stage disease. Blood 1986;66:533.

38. Ayanlar-Bateman O, Ebert E, Hauptman SP. Defective IL-2 production and responsiveness by T cells in patients with chronic lymphocytic leukemia of B cell variety. Blood 1986;67:279.

39. Foa R, Fierro MT, Raspadori D, et al. Lymphokine-activated killer (LAK) cell activity in B and T chronic lymphoid leukemia: Defective LAK generation and reduced susceptibility of the leukemic cells to allogeneic and autologous LAK effectors. Blood 1990;76:1349.

40. Perri RT. Impaired expression of cell surface receptors for B-cell growth factor by chronic lymphocytic leukemia cells. Blood 1986;67:943.

41. Dadmarz R, Rabinowe SN, Cannistra SA, Anderson JW, Freedman AS, Nadler LM. Association between clonogenic cell growth and clinical risk group in B-cell chronic lymphocytic leukemia. Blood 1990;76:142.

42. Rai KR, Sawitsky A. Studies in clinical staging, lymphocyte function, and markers as an approach to the treatment of CLL. In: Silber R, Gordon AS, Lobue J, Muggia FM, eds. Contemporary hematology/oncology. New York: Plenum, 1981:227.

43. Robertson LE, Huh Y, Hirsch-Ginsberg C, et al. Clinical, immunophenotypic and molecular analysis of the completeness of response in chronic lymphocytic leukemia after fludarabine. Blood [Abstract] 1990;76(suppl 1):314A.

44. Andreeff M. Cell kinetics of leukemia. Semin Hematol 1986;23:300.

45. Andreeff M. Flow cytometry of leukemia. In: Melamed MR, Mendelsohn ML, eds. Flow cytometry and cell sorting. New York: Alan R. Liss, 1990:697.

46. Theml H, Trepel G, Schick P, et al. Kinetics of lymphocytes in chronic lymphocytic leukemia: Studies using continuous ³H-thymidine infusion in two patients. Blood 1973;42:623.

47. Squires J, Redner A, Andreeff M. P53 expression in human leukemia: Restriction to lymphoid cell lineage and potential prognostic importance in acute lymphoblastic leukemia. Proc Am Assoc Cancer Res [Abstract] 1988;29:454.

48. del Giglio A, Zhang W, O'Brien S, et al. Relationship of elevated intranuclear p53 levels in chronic lymphocytic leukemia to marrow architecture and PCNA antigen expression. Proc Am Assoc Cancer Res 1991;32:290.

49. del Giglio A, O'Brien S, Ford R, et al. The prognostic value of proliferating cell nuclear antigen expression in chronic lymphoid leukemia. Blood (in press).

50. Montserrat E, Sanchez-Bisono J, Vinolas N, Rozman C. Lymphocyte doubling time in chronic lymphocytic leukaemia: Analysis of its prognostic significance. Br J Haematol 1986;62:567.

51. Herweijer H, Sonneveld P, Baas F, Nooter K. Expression of mdr1 and mdr3 multidrug resistance genes in human acute and chronic leukemias and association with stimulation of drug accumulation by cyclosporine. JNCI 1990;82:1133.

52. Rai KR, Sawitsky A, Cronkit EP, Chanana AD, Levy RN, Pasternack BS. Clinical staging of chronic lymphocytic leukemia. Blood 1975;46:219.

53. Binet J, Auquier A, Dighiero G, et al. A new prognostic classification of chronic lymphocytic leukemia derived from a multivariate survival analysis. Cancer 1981;48:198.

54. Montserrat E, Vinolas N, Reverter JC, Rozman C. Natural history of chronic lymphocytic leukemia: On the progression and prognosis of early clinical stages. Nouv Rev Fr Hematol 1988;30:359.

55. Binet JL, Catovsky D, Chandra P, et al. Chronic lymphocytic leukaemia: Proposals for a revised prognostic staging system, Report from the International Workshop on CLL. Br J Haematol 1981;48:365.

56. Cheson BD, Bennett JM, Rai KR, et al. Guidelines for clinical protocols for chronic lymphocytic leukemia: Recommendations of the National Cancer Institute-sponsored Working Group. Am J Hematol 1988;29:152.

57. International Workshop on Chronic Lymphocytic Leukemia. Chronic lymphocytic leukemia: Recommendations for diagnosis, staging and response criteria. Ann Intern Med 1989;110:236.

58. Galton DAG, Wiltshaw E, Szur L, Dacie JV. The use of chlorambucil and steroids in the treatment of chronic lymphocytic leukemia. Br J Haematol 1961;7:73.

59. Ezdinli EZ, Stutzman L. Chlorambucil therapy for lymphomas and chronic lymphocytic leukemia. JAMA 1965;191:444.

60. Alberts DS, Chang SY, Chen HSG, Larcom BJ, Jones SE. Pharmacokinetics and metabolism of chlorambucil in man: A preliminary report. Cancer Treat Rev 1979;6:9.

61. Knospe WH, Loeb V Jr, Huguley CM Jr. Bi-weekly chlorambucil treatment of chronic lymphocytic leukemia. Cancer 1974;33:555.

62. Liepman M, Votaw ML. The treatment of chronic lymphocytic leukemia with COP chemotherapy. Cancer 1978;41:1664.

63. Oken MM, Kaplan ME. Combination chemotherapy with cyclophosphamide, vincristine, and prednisone in the treatment of refractory chronic lymphocytic leukemia. Cancer Treat Rep 1979;63:441.

64. Sawitsky A, Rai KR, Glidewell O, Silver RT, and participating members of the Cancer and Leukemia Group B. Comparison of daily versus intermittent chlorambucil and prednisone therapy in the treatment of patients with chronic lymphocytic leukemia. Blood 1977;50:1049.

65. Ezdinli EZ, Stutzman L, Aungst CW, Firat D. Corticosteroid therapy for lymphomas and chronic lymphocytic leukemia. Cancer 1969;23:900.

66. Han T, Ezdinli EZ, Shimaoka K, Desai DV. Chlorambucil vs. combined chlorambucil-corticosteroid therapy in chronic lymphocytic leukemia. Cancer 1973;31:502.

67. Keller JW, WH Knospe, Raney M, et al. Treatment of chronic lymphocytic leukemia using chlorambucil and prednisone with or without cycle-active consolidation chemotherapy. Cancer 1986;58:1185.

68. Montserrat E, Alcala A, Parody R, and participating members of Pethema, Spanish Cooperative Group for Hematological Malignancies Treatment, Spanish Society of Hematology. Treatment of chronic lymphocytic leukemia in advanced stages. Cancer 1985;56:2369.

69. Montserrat E, Alcala A, Alonso C, and participating members of Pethema, Spanish Society of Hematology. A randomized trial comparing chlorambucil plus prednisone vs cyclophosphamide, melphalan, and prednisone in the treatment of chronic lymphocytic leukemia stages B and C. Nouv Rev Fr Hematol 1988;30:429.

70. Raphael B, Andersen JW, Silber R, et al. Comparison of chlorambucil and prednisone versus cyclophosphamide, vincristine, and prednisone as initial treatment for chronic lymphocytic leukemia: Long-term follow-up of an Eastern Cooperative Oncology Group randomized clinical trial. J Clin Oncol 1991;9:770.

71. Jaksic B, Brugiatelli M. High dose chlorambucil for the treatment of B-chronic lymphocytic leukemia (CLL). Update of I.G.C.I. CLL trials, Proceedings of the 5th International Workshop on CLL—Sitges, Barcelona, 1991:62.

72. The French Cooperative Group on Chronic Lymphocytic Leukemia. Effects of chlorambucil and therapeutic decision in initial forms of chronic lymphocytic leukemia (stage A): Results of a randomized clinical trial on 612 patients. Blood 1990;75:1414.

73. The French Cooperative Group on Chronic Lymphocytic Leukaemia. A randomized clinical trial of chlorambucil versus COP in stage B chronic lymphocytic leukemia. Blood 1990;75:1422.

74. The French Cooperative Group on Chronic Lymphocytic Leukaemia. Effectiveness of "CHOP" regimen in advanced untreated chronic lymphocytic leukaemia. Lancet 1986:1346.

75. Catovsky D, Richards S, Fooks J, Hamblin TJ. CLL trials in the United Kingdom—The medical research council CLL trials 1, 2 and 3. Leuk Lymphoma 1991;5:105.

76. Hansen MM, Andersen E, Birgens H, et al. CHOP versus chlorambucil + prednisolone in chronic lymphocytic leukemia. Leuk Lymphoma 1991;5:97.

77. Kimby E, Mellstedt H. Chlorambucil/prednisone versus CHOP in symptomatic chronic lymphocytic leukemias of B-cell type. A randomized trial. Leuk Lymphoma 1991;5:93.

78. Keating MJ, Hester JP, McCredie KB, Burgess MA, Murphy WK, Freireich EJ. Long-term results of CAP therapy in chronic lymphocytic leukemia. Leuk Lymphoma 1990;2:391.

79. Keating MJ, Scouros M, Murphy S, et al. Multiple agent chemotherapy (POACH) in previously treated and untreated patients with chronic lymphocytic leukemia. Leukemia 1988;2:157.

80. Kempin S, Lee BH III, Thaler HT, et al. Combination chemotherapy of advanced chronic lymphocytic leukemia: The M-2 protocol (vincristine, BCNU, cyclophosphamide, melphalan and prednisone). Blood 1982;60:1110.

81. Grever MR, Kopecky KJ, Coltman CA, et al. Fludarabine monophosphate: A potentially useful agent in chronic lymphocytic leukemia. Nouv Rev Fr Hematol 1988;30:457.

82. Keating MJ, Kantarjian H, Talpaz M, et al. Fludarabine: A new agent with major activity against chronic lymphocytic leukemia. Blood 1989;74:19.

83. Keating MJ, Kantarjian H, O'Brien S, et al. Fludarabine: A new agent with marked cytoreductive activity in untreated chronic lymphocytic leukemia. J Clin Oncol 1991;9:44.

84. Keating MJ, Kantarjian H, O'Brien S, Redman J, Childs C, McCredie K. Fludarabine (FLU)–prednisone (PRED): A safe, effective combination in refractory chronic lymphocytic leukemia. Proceedings of the American Society of Clinical Oncology, San Francisco, 1989:210.

85. Puccio CA, Mittelman A, Lichtman SM, et al. A loading dose/continuous infusion schedule of fludarabine phosphate in chronic lymphocytic leukemia. J Clin Oncol 1991;9:1562.

86. Grever MR, Leiby JM, Kraut EH, Wilson HE, Neidhart JA, Wall RL, Balcerzak SP. Low-dose deoxycoformycin in lymphoid malignancy. J Clin Oncol 1985;3:1196.

87. Dillman RO, Mick R, McIntyre OR. Pentostatin in chronic lymphocytic leukemia: A phase II trial of cancer and leukemia group B. J Clin Oncol 1989;7:433.

88. Saven A, Carrera CJ, Carson DA, Beutler E, Piro LD. 2-Chlorodeoxyadenosine treatment of refractory chronic lymphocytic leukemia. Leuk Lymphoma 1991;5:133.

89. Robertson LE, Huh Y, Hirsch-Ginsberg C, et al. Clinical, immunophenotypic, and

molecular analysis of the completeness of response in chronic lymphocytic leukemia after fludarabine. Blood 1990;76:314A.

90. Michallet M, Corront B, Molina L, et al. Allogeneic bone marrow transplantation in chronic lymphocytic leukemia: 17 cases. Report of the EBMT. Leuk Lymphoma 1991;5:127.

91. Jansen J, Schutt HRE, Zwet TL van, Meifer CJLM, Hijmans W. Hairy-cell leukaemia: A B-lymphocytic disorder. Br J Haematol 1979;42:21.

92. Galton DAG, Goldman JM, Wiltshaw E, et al. Prolymphocytic leukemia. Br J Haematol 1974;27:7.

93. Sadamori N, Han T, Minowada J, et al. Possible specific chromosome change in prolymphocytic leukemia. Blood 1983;62:729.

94. Kantarjian H, Childs C, O'Brien S, et al. Efficacy of fludarabine, a new adenine nucleoside analogue in patients with prolymphocytic leukemia and the prolymphocytoid variant of chronic lymphocytic leukemia. Am J Med 1991;90:223.

95. Golomb HM, Catovsky D, Golde DW. Hairy cell leukemia: A clinical review based on 71 cases. Ann Intern Med 1978;89:677.

96. Cleary ML, Good GS, Warnke R, et al. Immunoglobulin gene rearrangements in hairy cell leukemia. Blood 1984;64:99.

97. Golomb HM, Vardiman JW. Response to splenectomy in 65 patients with hairy cell leukemia: An evaluation of spleen weight and bone marrow involvement. Blood 1983;61:349.

98. Caligaris-Cappio F, Pizzolo G, Chilosi M, et al. Phorbol ester induces abnormal chronic lymphocytic leukemia cells to express features of hairy cell leukemia. Blood 1985;66:1035.

99. Quesada JR, Hersh EM, Manning J, et al. Treatment of hairy cell leukemia with recombinant alpha interferon. Blood 1985;68:493.

100. Spiers ASD, Moore D, Cassileth P, et al. Remission in hairy cell leukemia with pentostatin. N Engl J Med 1987;316:825.

101. Piro LD, Carrera CJ, Carson DA, Beutler E. Lasting remissions in hairy cell leukemia induced by a single infusion of 2-chlorodeoxyadenosine. N Engl J Med 1990;322:117.

102. Estey E, Kurzrock R, Kantarjian H, et al. Treatment of hairy cell leukemia with 2-chlorodeoxyadenosine (2-CdA). Blood 1992;79:882.

103. Hoffman R, Kopel S, Hsu SD, Dainiak N, Zanjani ED. T cell chronic lymphocytic leukemia: Presence in bone marrow and peripheral blood of cells that suppress erythropoiesis in vitro. Blood 1978;52:255.

104. Aisenberg AC, Krontiris TG, Mak TW, et al. Rearrangement of the gene for the beta chain of the T-cell receptor in T-cell chronic lymphocytic leukemia and related disorders. N Engl J Med 1985;313:529.

105. Brouet JC, Flandrin G, Sasportes M, et al. CLL of T-cell origin: Immunologic and clinical evaluation in 11 patients. Lancet 1973;2:890.

106. Foa R, Pelicci P-G, Mignone N, et al. Analysis of T-cell receptor beta chain (T-beta) gene rearrangements demonstrates the monoclonal nature of T-cell chronic lymphoproliferative disorders. Blood 1986;67:247.

107. Chan WC, Link S, Mawle A, et al. Heterogeneity of large granular lymphocyte proliferations-delineation of two major subtypes with distinct origins, immunophenotypes, functional and clinical characteristics. Blood 1986;68:1142.

108. Palutke M, Eisenberg L, Kaplan J, et al. Natural killer and suppressor T-cell chronic lymphocytic leukemia. Blood 1983;62:627.

109. Melo JV, Catovsky D, Galton DAG. The relationship between chronic lymphocytic leukaemia and prolymphocytic leukaemia. II. Patterns of evolution of prolymphocytoid transformation. Br J Haematol 1986;64:77.

110. Melo JV, Catovsky D, Galton DAG. The relationship between chronic lymphocytic leukaemia and prolymphocytic leukaemia. IV: Analysis of survival and prognostic features. Br J Haematol 1987;65:23.

111. Zarrabi MH, Grunwald HW, Rosner F. Chronic lymphocytic leukemia terminating in acute leukemia. Arch Intern Med 1977;137:1059.

112. Brouet JC, Preud'homme JL, Seligmann M, et al. Blast cells with monoclonal surface immunoglobulin in two cases of acute blast crisis supervening on chronic lymphocytic leukaemia. Br Med J 1973;4:23.

113. McPhedran P, Heath CW. Acute leukemia occurring during chronic lymphocytic leukemia. Blood 1970;35:7.

114. Januszewicz E, Cooper IA, Pilkington G, et al. Blastic transformation of chronic lymphocytic leukemia. Am J Hematol 1983;15:399.

115. Richter MN. Genealized reticular cell sarcoma of lymph nodes associated with lymphocytic leukemia. Am J Pathol 1928;4:285.

116. Foucar K, Rydell RE. Richter's syndrome in chronic lymphocytic leukemia. Cancer 1980;46:118.

117. Minot GR, Buckman TE, Isaacs R. Chronic myelogenous leukemia: Age, incidence, duration and benefit derived from irradiation. JAMA 1924;82:1489–1494.

118. Reinhard EH, Neely L, Samples DM. Radioactive phosphorus in the treatment of chronic leukemias: Long-term results over a period of 15 years. Ann Intern Med 1959;50:942.

119. Barrett AJ, Longhurst P, Humble JG, Newton KA. Effect of splenic irradiation on circulating colony-forming cells in chronic granulocytic leukaemia. Br Med J 1977;14:1259.

120. Galton DAG. Myleran in chronic myeloid leukemia. Lancet 1953;1:208.

121. Fishbein WN, Carbone PP, Freireich EJ. Clinical trials of hydroxyurea in patients with cancer and leukemia. Clin Pharmacol Ther 1964;5:574.

122. Haut A, Abbott WS, Wintrobe MM, Cartwright GE. Busulfan in the treatment of chronic myelocytic leukemia: The effect of long-term intermittent therapy. Blood 1961;17:1.

123. Sokal JE. Evaluation of survival data from chronic myelocytic leukemia. Am J Hematol 1979;1:493–500.

124. Kennedy BJ, Yarbro JW. Metabolic and therapeutic effects of hydroxyurea in chronic myeloid leukemia. JAMA 1966;195:1038–1043.

125. Kennedy BJ. Hydroxyurea therapy in chronic myelogenous leukemia. Cancer 1972;29:1052–1056.

126. Tanzer J, Briere J, Aucleic A, et al. Long term results for 47 patients with Ph¹+ chronic myelocytic leukemia given hydroxyurea as major treatment. Blood 1979;54:212A.

127. Schwartz JH, Canellos GP. Hydroxyurea in the management of hematologic complications of chronic granulocytic leukemia. Blood 1975;46:11–16.

128. Feingold ML, Koss LG. Effects of long-term administration of busulfan. Arch Intern Med 1969;124:66–71.

129. Bolin RW, Robinson WA, Sutherland J, Hamman R. Busulfan vs hydroxyurea in long-term therapy of chronic myelogenous leukemia. Cancer 1982;50:1683–1686.

130. Rushing D, Goldman A, Gibbs G, Howe R, Kennedy BJ. Hydroxyurea versus busulfan in the treatment of chronic granulocytic leukemia. Am J Clin Oncol 1982;5:307–313.

131. Sullivan JR, Hurley, Bolton JH. Treatment of chronic myeloid leukemia with repeated single doses of busulfan. Cancer Treat Rev 1977;61:43–45.

132. Vicariot M, Goldman JM, Catovsky D, Galton DAG. Treatment of chronic granulocytic leukaemia with repeated single doses of busulfan. Eur J Cancer 1979;15:559–563.

133. Schwarzenberg L, Mathe G, Pouillart P, et al. Hydroxyurea, leucopheresis, and splenectomy in chronic myeloid leukemia at the problastic phase. Br Med J 1973;1:700–703.

134. Djaldetti M, Padeh B, Pinkhas J, Deries A. Prolonged remission in chronic myeloid leukemia after one course of busulfan. Blood 1966;27:103–109.

135. Finney R, McDonald GA, Baikie AG, Douglas AS. Chronic granulocytic leukaemia with Ph¹ negative cells in hypoplasia. Br J Haematol 1972;23:283–288.

136. Golde DW, Bersch NL, Sparkes RS. Chromosomal mosaicism associated with prolonged remission in chronic myelogenous leukemia. Cancer 1976;37:1849–1852.

137. Brandt L, Mitelman F, Panani A, Lenner HC. Extremely long duration of chronic myeloid leukaemia with Ph¹ negative and Ph¹ positive bone marrow cells. Scand J Haematol 1976;16:321–325.

138. Singer CRJ, McDonald GA, Douglas AS. Twenty-five year survival of chronic granulocytic leukemia with spontaneous karyotype conversion. Br J Haematol 1984;57:309–313.

139. Zago MA, Costa FF, Bottura C. Cytogenetic remission in a Ph¹-positive case of chronic myelogenous leukaemia. Scand J Haematol 1977;22:91–95.

140. Sokal JE, Leong SS, Gomez GA. Preferential inhibition by cytarabine of CFU-GM from patients with chronic granulocytic leukemia. Cancer 1987;59:197–202.

141. Spiers ASD, Lorch CA, Harrison BA. Chronic granulocytic leukemia (CGL) in chronic phase with two Ph+ cell lines and suppression of one line by hydroxyurea. Blood Suppl 1986;1:233a.

142. Cunningham I, Gee T, Dowling M, et al. Results of treatment of Ph¹+ chronic myelogenous leukemia with an intensive treatment regimen (L-5 protocol). Blood 1979;53:375–396.

143. Hester JP, Waddell CC, Coltman CA Jr, et al. Response of chronic myelogeneous leukemia patients to COAP-splenectomy. Cancer 1984;54:1977–1982.

144. Kantarjian HM, Vellekoop L, McCredie KB, et al. Intensive combination chemotherapy (ROAP) and splenectomy in the management of chronic myelogenous leukemia. J Clin Oncol 1985;3:192–300.

145. Brodsky L, Fuscaldo KE, Kahn SB, Conroy JF, Lamping CG. Chronic myelogenous leukemia: A clinical and experimental evaluation of splenectomy and intensive chemotherapy. Semin Hematol 1975;8:143.

146. Got T, Nishikori M, Arlin Z. Growth characteristics of leukemia and normal hematopoietic cells in Ph+ chronic myelogenous leukemia and effects of intensive treatment. Blood 1982;59:793–803.

147. Fitzgerald D, Rowe JM, Heal J. Leukapheresis for control of chronic myelogenous leukemia during pregnancy. Am J Hematol 1986;22:213–218.

148. Lowenthal RM, Buskard NA, Goldman JM, et al. Intensive leukapheresis as initial therapy for chronic granulocytic leukemia. Blood 1975;46:835–844.

149. Vallejos CS, McCredie KB, Brittin GM, Freireich EJ. Biological effects of repeated leukapheresis of patients with chronic myelogenous leukemia. Blood 1973;42:925–933.

150. Goldman JM, Lowenthal RM, Buskard NA, Spiers ASD, Th'ng KH, Park DS. Chronic granulocytic leukemia-selective removal of immature granulocytic cells by leukapheresis. Semin Hematol 1975;8:28–40.

151. Neiman F, Brandt L, Nilsson PG. Cytogenetic evidence for splenic origin of blast transformation in chronic myelogenous leukemia. Scand J Haematol 1974;13:87–90.

152. Baccarani M, Zaccaria A, Santucci AM, et al. A simultaneous study of bone marrow, spleen, and liver in chronic myeloid leukemia: Evidence for differences in cell composition and karyotypes. Semin Hematol 1975;8:81–112.

153. Mitelman F. Comparative cytogenetic studies of bone marrow and extramedullary tissues in chronic myeloid leukemia. Semin Hematol 1975;8:113–117.

154. Sharp JC, Joyner MV, Wayne AW, et al. Karyotypic conversion in Ph¹-positive chronic myeloid leukaemia with combination chemotherapy. Lancet 1979;1:1370–1372.

155. Smalley RV, Vogel J, Huguley CM, et al. Chronic granulocytic leukemia: Cytogenetic conversion of the bone marrow with cycle-specific chemotherapy. Blood 1977;50:107–113.

156. Ihde DC, Canellos GP, Schwartz JH, DeVita VT. Splenectomy in the chronic phase of chronic granulocytic leukemia. Effects in 32 patients. Ann Intern Med 1976;84:17–21.

157. Spiers ASD, Ermidou-Szeidis C, Richards HGH. Chronic granulocytic leukaemia: Clinical course, blood and bone marrow changes after chemotherapy and splenectomy. Haematologica 1979;64:616–634.

158. Medical Research Council's Working Party for Therapeutic Trials in Leukemia. Ran-

domized trial of splenectomy in Ph¹ positive chronic granulocytic leukaemia, including an analysis of prognostic factor. Br J Haematol 1983;54:415–430.

159. The Italian Cooperative Study Group on Chronic Myeloid Leukemia. Results of a prospective randomized trial of early splenectomy in chronic myeloid leukemia. Cancer 1984;54:333–338.

160. Kantarjian HM, Keating MJ, Talpaz M, et al. Chronic myelogenous leukemia in blast crisis: An analysis of 242 patients. Am J Med 1987;83:445–454.

161. Goldman JM, Johnson SA, Islam A, Catovsky D, Galton DAG. Haematological reconstitution after autografting for chronic granulocytic leukaemia in transformation: The influence of previous splenectomy. Br J Haematol 1980;45:223–231.

162. Gratwohl A, Goldman J, Gluckman E, Zwann F. Effect of splenectomy before bonemarrow transplantation on survival in chronic granulocytic leukaemia. Lancet 1985;2: 1290–1291.

163. Canellos GP, Sutliffe SB, DeVita VT, Lister TA. Treatment of refractory splenomegaly in myeloproliferative disease by splenic artery infusion. Blood 1979;53:1014–1017.

164. Isaacs A, Lindemann J. Virus interference. 1. The interferons. Proc R Soc Lond (Biol) 1957;147:258–267.

165. Stewart WEI, ed. The interferon system. New York: Springer-Verlag, 1979.

166. Borden EC, Fall LA. Interferons: Biochemical, cell growth, inhibitory, and immunological effects. Prog Hematol 1981;12:299–339.

167. Vilcek J, Gray PW, Rinderknecht E, et al. Interferon-gamma: A lymphokine for all seasons. In: Rick E, ed. Lymphokines, vol 12. Orlando: Academic Press, 1985:1.

168. Talpaz M, McCredie KB, Mavligit GM, Gutterman JU. Leukocyte interferon-induced myeloid cytoreduction in chronic myelogenous leukemia. Blood 1983;62:689–692.

169. Talpaz M, Kantarjian HM, McCredie KB, Keating MJ, Trujillo J, Gutterman J. Clinical investigation of human alpha interferon in chronic myelogenous leukemia. Blood 1987;69:1280–1288.

170. Talpaz M, Kantarjian HM, McCredie KB, Trujillo JM, Keating MJ, Gutterman JU. Hematologic remission and cytogenetic involvement induced by recombinant human interferon alpha in chronic myelogenous leukemia. N Engl J Med 1986;314:1065–1069.

171. Talpaz M, Kurzrock R, Kantarjian H, Gutterman JU. Recent advances in the therapy of chronic myelogenous leukemia. In: DeVita V, ed. Important advances in oncology. Philadelphia: JB Lippincott, 1988:297.

172. Talpaz M, Kantarjian H, Kurzrock R, Trujillo JM, Gutterman JU. Interferon-alpha produces sustained cytogenetic responses in chronic myelogenous leukemia. Philadelphia chromosome-positive patients. Ann Intern Med 1991;114:532–538.

173. Niederle N, Doberauer C, Kloke O, Osieka R, Schweers C, Schmidt CG. Treatment of chronic myelogenous leukemia with recombinant interferon alpha (IFN-α2b). Proc Am Soc Clin Oncol 1986;5:236.

174. Alimena G, Morra E, Lazzarino M, et al. Interferon alpha-2b as therapy for Ph1-positive chronic myelogenous leukemia: A study of 82 patients treated with intermittent or daily administration. Blood 1988;72:642–647.

175. Ozer H, Mick R, Testa J, et al. Subcutaneous α-interferon (α-IFN) shows substantial activity in untreated chronic phase Philadelphia chromosome positive (Ph¹) chronic myelogenous leukemia (CML). Proc Am Soc Clin Oncol 1988;7:A684.

176. Ozer H. Biotherapy of chronic myelogenous leukemia with interferon. Semin Oncol 1988;15:14–20.

177. Tura S, Russo D, Zuffa E, Fiacchini M. A prospective comparison of human recombinant interferon α-2A (Roferon-A) and convential chemotherapy in chronic myeloid leukemia (CML). Interim report of the Italian Study. Blood 1990;76(suppl 1):329A.

178. Hehlmann R, Manneheim, Heimpel H, et al. Prospective controlled comparison of busulfan vs hydroxyurea vs interferon alpha in chronic myelogenous leukemia (CML). Blood 1990;76(suppl 1):279A.

179. Yoffe G, Blick M, Kantarjian H, Spitzer G, Gutterman J, Talpaz M. Molecular analysis of interferon-induced suppression of Philadelphia chromosome in patients with chronic myeloid leukemia. Blood 1987;69:961–963.

180. Lee MS, Chang KS, Freireich EJ, et al. Detection of minimal residual bcr/abl transcripts by a modified polymerase chain reaction. Blood 1988;72:893–897.

181. Dhingra K, Kurzrock R, Kantarjian H, et al. Polymerase chain reaction (PCR) for minimal residual disease in 20 CML patients in complete cytogenetic response induced by interferon therapy. Blood 1989;74:235A.

182. Kurzrock R, Gutterman JU, Kantarjian H, Talpaz M. Therapy of chronic myelogenous leukemia with interferon. Cancer Invest 1989;7:83–91.

183. Schilling PJ, Kurzrock R, Kantarjian H, Gutterman JU, Talpaz M. Development of systemic lupus erythematosus after interferon therapy for chronic myelogenous leukemia. Cancer 1991;68:1536–1537.

184. Bergsagel DE, Haas RH, Messner HA. Interferon alpha 2 in treatment of chronic granulocytic leukemia. Semin Oncol 1986;13:29–34.

185. Kantarjian HM, Talpaz M, Keating MJ, et al. Intensive chemotherapy induction followed by interferon-alpha maintenance in patients with Philadelphia chromosome-positive chronic myelogenous leukemia. Cancer 1991;68:1201–1207.

186. Ma DDF, Arthur CK. Treatment of chronic myeloid leukemia (CML) using alpha-interferon (IFN), and low dose cytosine arabinoside (ara-C). Blood 1989;74:363A.

187. Guilhot F, Tanzer J, Brizard A, Huret JL, Dreyfus B. Combination of alpha-2a interferon and chemotherapy in Ph⁺ chronic myelogenous leukemia (CML) updated results. Proc Am Soc Clin Oncol 1989;8:A788.

188. Kantarjian H, Keating M, McCredie K, et al. Treatment of advanced stages of Philadelphia-chromosome (Ph)-positive chronic myelogenous leukemia (CML) with alpha interferon (IFN-A) and low-dose cytosine arabinoside (ara-C). Blood 1989;7:235A.

189. Klimpel GR, Fleischmann WF Jr, Klimpel KD. Gamma interferon (IFN-gamma) and IFN-alpha/beta suppress murine myeloid colony formation (CFUOC): Magnitude of suppression is dependent upon level of colony-stimulating factor (CSF). J Immunol 1982;129:76–80.

190. Raefsky EL, Platanias LC, Zoumbos NC, Young NS. Studies of interferon as a regulator of hematopoietic cell proliferation. J Immunol 1982;135:2507–2512.

191. Broxmeyer HE, Williams DE, Lu L, et al. The suppressive influences of human tumor necrosis factor on bone marrow hematopoietic progenitor cells from normal donors and patients with leukemia: Synergism of tumor necrosis factor and interferon-gamma. J Immunol 1986;136:4487–4495.

192. Ball ED, Guyre PM, Shen L, et al. Gamma-interferon induces monocytoid differentiation in the HL-60 cell line. J Clin Invest 1984;73:1072–1077.

193. Kurzrock R, Talpaz M, Kantarjian H, et al. Therapy of chronic myelogenous leukemia with recombinant interferon-γ. Blood 1987;70:943–947.

194. Talpaz M, Kurzrock R, Kantarjian H, et al. A phase II study of alternating alpha-2a-interferon and gamma-interferon therapy in patients with chronic myelogenous leukemia. Cancer 1991;68:2125–2130.

195. Czarniecki CW, Fennie CW, Powers DB, Estell DA. Synergistic antiviral and antiproliferative activities of E. coli derived human alpha, beta, and gamma interferons. J Virol 1984;49:490–496.

196. Niederle N, Wandl U, Kloke O, et al. Efficacy of interferon alpha (IFN alpha-2b) and IFN gamma in chronic myelogenous leukemia (CML). Proc Am Soc Clin Oncol 1989;8: 185.

197. Maxwell B, Talpaz M, Gutterman JU. Down-regulation of peripheral blood cell interferon receptors in chronic myelogenous leukemia patients undergoing human interferon (HuIFN) therapy. Int J Cancer 1985;36:23–28.

198. Levy D, Larner A, Chaudhuri A, Babiss LE, Darnell JE Jr. Interferon-stimulated transcription: Isolation of an inducible gene and identification of its regulatory region. Proc Natl Acad Sci USA 1986;83:8929–8933.

199. Larner AC, Chaudhuri A, Darnell JE Jr. Transcriptional induction by interferon. New protein(s) determine the extent and length of the induction. J Biol Chem 1986;261: 453–459.

200. Kelly JM, Porter ACG, Chernajovsky Y, Gilbert CS, Stark GR, Kerr IM. Characterization of a human gene inducible by α- and γ-interferons and its expression in mouse cells. EMBO J 1986;5:1601–1606.

201. Rutherford MN, Hannigan GE, Williams BRG. Interferon-induced binding of nuclear factors to promoter elements of the 2-5A synthetase gene. EMBO J 1988;7:751–759.

202. Rice AP, Kerr SM, Roberts WK, Brown RE, Kerr IM. Novel 2′,5′-oligoadenylates synthesized in interferon-treated, vaccinia virus-infected cells. J Virol 1985;56:1041–1044.

203. Dron M, Tovey MG, Eid P. Isolation of Daudi cells with reduced sensitivity to interferon. III. Interferon-induced proteins in relation to the phenotype of interferon resistance. J Genet Virol 1985;66:787–795.

204. Reid TR, Race ER, Wolff BH, Friedman RM, Merigan TC, Basham TY. Enhanced in vivo therapeutic response to interferon in mice with an in vitro interferon-resistant B-cell lymphoma. Cancer Res 1989;49:4163–4169.

205. Affabris E, Romeo G, Belardelli F, et al. 2-5A synthetase activity does not increase in interferon-resistant Friend leukemia cell variants treated with α/β interferon despite the presence of high-affinity interferon receptor sites. Virology 1983;125:508–512.

206. Talpaz M, Chernajovsky Y, Troutman-Worden K, et al. Interferon stimulated genes in interferon-sensitive and resistant chronic myelogenous leukemia (CML) patients. Cancer Res (in press).

207. Dowding C, Guo A-P, Osterholz J, Siczkowski M, Goldman J, Gordon M. Interferon-α overrides the deficient adhesion of chronic myeloid leukemia primitive progenitor cells to bone marrow stromal cells. Blood 1991;78:499–505.

208. Pfeffer LM, Donner DB, Tamm I. Interferon-alpha down-regulates insulin receptors in lymphoblastoid (Daudi) cells. Relationship to inhibition of cell proliferation. J Biol Chem 1987;262:3665–3670.

209. Fish EN, Banerjee K. Growth control: Characterizations of the antagonism between growth factors and interferon. J Interferon Res 1989;9:2–7.

210. Pfeffer LM, Tamm I. Interferon-beta inhibition of concanavalin A-stimulated calcium uptake and exchange in HeLa cells. J Interferon Res 1986;6:551–556.

211. Estrov Z, Kurzrock R, Wetzler M, et al. Suppression of chronic myelogenous leukemia colony growth by IL-1 receptor antagonist and soluble IL-1 receptors: A novel application for inhibitors of IL-1 activity. Blood 1991;78:1476–1484.

212. Wetzler M, Kurzrock R, Lowe DG, Kantarjian H, Gutterman JU, Talpaz M. Alteration in bone marrow stromal growth factor expression: A novel mechanism of disease progression in chronic myelogenous leukemia. Blood 1991;78:2400–2406.

213. Champlin RE, Golde DW. Chronic myelogenous leukemia: Recent advances. Blood 1985;65:1039–1047.

214. Thomas ED, Storb R, Clift RA, et al. Bone marrow transplantation. N Engl J Med 1975;292:832–843, 895–902.

215. Champlin RE, Goldman JM, Gale RP. Bone marrow transplantation in chronic myelogenous leukemia. Semin Hematol 1988;25:74–80.

216. Santos GW, Tutschka PJ, Brookmeyer R, et al. Marrow transplantation for acute non-lymphocytic leukemia after treatment with busulfan and cyclophosphamide. N Engl J Med 1983;309:1347.

217. Copelan EA, Grever MR, Kapoor N, Tutschka PJ. Marrow transplantation following busulfan and cyclophosphamide for chronic myelogenous leukaemia in accelerated or blastic phase. Br J Haematol 1989;71:487–491.

218. Clift RA, Buckner CD, Appelbaum FR, et al. Allogeneic marrow transplantation in patients with chronic myeloid leukemia in the chronic phase: A randomized trial of two irradiation regimens. Blood 1991;77:1660–1665.

219. Gale RP, Champlin RE. How does bone marrow transplantation cure leukemia? Lancet 1984;2:28.

220. Fefer A, Cheever MA, Greenberg PD, et al. Treatment of chronic granulocytic leukemia with chemoradiotherapy and transplantation of marrow from identical twins. N Engl J Med 1982;306:63–68.

221. Champlin R, Ho W, Arenson E, Gale RP. Allogeneic bone marrow transplantation in chronic myelogenous leukemia in chronic or accelerated phase. Blood 1982;60:1038–1041.

222. McGlave PB, Arthur DC, Weisdorf D, et al. Allogeneic bone marrow transplantation as treatment for accelerating chronic myelogenous leukemia. Blood 1984;63:219–222.

223. Thomas ED, Clift RA, Fefer A, et al. Marrow transplantation for the treatment of chronic myelogenous leukemia. Ann Intern Med 1986;104:155–163.

224. Goldman JM, Gale RP, Bortin MM, et al. Bone marrow transplantation for chronic myelogenous leukemia in chronic phase: Increased risk of relapse associate with T-cell depletion. Ann Intern Med 1988;108:806–814.

225. Speck B, Bortin MM, Champlin R, et al. Allogeneic bone marrow transplantation for chronic myelogenous leukemia. Lancet 1984;1:665–668.

226. Thomas ED, Clift RA. Indications for marrow transplantation in chronic myelogenous leukemia. Blood 1989;73:861–864.

227. Sokal JE. Evaluation of survival data for chronic myelocytic leukemia. Am J Hematol 1976;1:493–500.

228. Tura S, Baccarni M, Corbelli G, et al. Staging of chronic myeloid leukemia. Br J Haematol 1981;47:105–109.

229. Talpaz M, Kantarjian H, Kurzrock R, Trujillo JM, Gutterman JU. Interferon-alpha produces sustained cytogenetic responses in chronic myelogenous leukemia. Philadelphia chromosome-positive patients. Ann Intern Med 1991;114:532–538.

230. Beatty PG, Clift RA, Mickelson EM, et al. Marrow transplantation from related donors other than HLA-identical siblings. N Engl J Med 1985;313:765.

231. Anasetti C, Amos D, Beatty PG, et al. Effect of HLA compatibility on engraftment of bone marrow transplants in patients with leukemia or lymphoma. N Engl J Med 1989;320:197–204.

232. Beatty PG, Hansen JA, Longton GM, et al. Marrow transplantation from HLA-matched unrelated donors for treatment of hematologic malignancies. Transplantation 1991;51:443–447.

233. Gajewski JL, Ho WG, Feig SA, Hunt L, Kaufman N, Champlin RE. Bone marrow transplantation using unrelated donors for patients with advanced leukemia or bone marrow failure. Transplantation 1990;50:244–249.

234. McGlave PB, Beatty P, Ash R, Hows JM. Therapy for chronic myelogenous leukemia with unrelated donor bone marrow transplantation: Results in 102 cases. Blood 1990;75:1728–1732.

235. Ash RC, Casper JT, Chitambar CR, et al. Successful allogeneic transplantation of T-cell-depleted bone marrow from closely HLA-matched unrelated donors. N Engl J Med 1990;322:485–494.

236. Weiden PL, Sullivan KM, Flournoy N, Storb R, Thomas ED. Antileukemic effect of chronic graft-versus-host disease: Contribution to improved survival after allogeneic marrow transplantation. N Engl J Med 1981;304:1529–1532.

237. Sullivan KM, Weiden PL, Storb R, et al. Influence of acute and chronic graft-versus-host disease on relapse and survival after bone marrow transplantation from HLA-identical siblings as treatment of acute and chronic leukemia. Blood 1989;73:1720–1728.

238. Sullivan KM, Storb R, Buckner CD, et al. Graft-versus-host disease as adoptive immunotherapy in patients with advanced hematologic neoplasms. N Engl J Med 1989;320:828–834.

239. Horowitz MM, Gale RP, Sondel PM, et al. Graft-versus-leukemia reactions after bone marrow transplantation. Blood 1990;75:555–562.

240. Champlin R. T-cell depletion to prevent graft-versus-host disease after bone marrow transplantation. Hematol Oncol Clin North Am 1990;4:687–698.

241. Marmont AM, Horowitz MM, Gale RP, et al. T-cell depletion of HLA-identical transplants in leukemia. Blood 1991;78:2120–2130.

242. Arthur CK, Apperley JF, Guo AP, et al. Cytogenetic events after bone marrow transplantation for chronic myeloid leukemia in chronic phase. Blood 1988;71:1179–1186.

243. Sosman JA, Oettel KR, Smith SD, Hank JA, Fisch P, Sondel PM. Specific recognition of human leukemic cells by allogeneic T-cells: II. Evidence for HLA-D restricted determinants on leukemic cells that are crossreactive with determinants present on unrelated nonleukemic cells. Blood 1990;75:2005–2016.

244. Delmon L, Ythier A, Moingeon P, et al. Characterization of antileukemia cells' cytotoxic effector function. Implications for monitoring natural killer responses following allogeneic bone marrow transplantation. Transplantation 1986;42:252.

245. Hauch M, Gazzola MV, Small T, et al. Anti-leukemia potential of interleukin-2 activated natural killer cells after bone marrow transplantation for chronic myelogenous leukemia. Blood 1990;75:2250–2262.

246. Korngold R, Sprent J. T cell subsets and graft-versus-host disease. Transplantation 1987;44:335–339.

247. Champlin R, Ho W, Gajewski J, et al. Selective depletion of CD8+ T-lymphocytes for prevention of graft-versus-host disease after allogeneic bone marrow transplantation. Blood 1990;76:418–423.

Cancer: Principles & Practice of Oncology, Fourth Edition,
edited by Vincent T. DeVita, Jr., Samuel Hellman, Steven A. Rosenberg.
J.B. Lippincott Co., Philadelphia © 1993.

Sydney E. Salmon
J. Robert Cassady

CHAPTER **56**

Plasma Cell Neoplasms

Plasma cell neoplasms are a group of related disorders, each of which is associated with proliferation and accumulation of immunoglobulin-secreting cells that are derived from the B-cell series of immunocytes. Tumor cells in these neoplasms retain the cytoplasmic differentiation of normal plasma cells and are adapted to high rates of synthesis and secretion of immunoglobulin (Ig). In the normal immune response, individual plasma cells can synthesize and secrete antibody immunoglobulin at rates up to 100,000 molecules each minute.

On the basis of synthesis and secretion of an electrophoretically homogenous immunoglobulin (*i.e.,* M-component or M-protein), plasma cell neoplasms appear to be monoclonal, derived from a single transformed B lymphocyte or plasma cell. Current laboratory data support the concept of the monoclonal origin of B-cell neoplasms. Several synonyms have been applied to plasma cell neoplasms: dysproteinemias, gammopathies, immunoglobulinopathies, monoclonal gammopathies, paraproteinemias, and plasma cell dyscrasias. In terms of incidence and severity, the most important malignant plasma cell neoplasm is multiple myeloma.

The plasma cell neoplasms can be characterized by their monoclonal immunoglobulin products. M-components are seen in the malignant plasma cell disorders (*e.g.,* multiple myeloma, Waldenström's macroglobulinemia) and in clinically ambiguous or idiopathic circumstances, and these products may be associated with benign, premalignant, or early malignant disorders. Idiopathic M-proteins are best described clinically as monoclonal gammopathies of unknown significance (MGUS).[1] Transient M-components have been observed in patients recovering from pneumonia, hepatitis, and other infections; after drug reactions; after other illnesses; or after bone marrow transplantation. The monoclonal immunoglobulins secreted in malignant plasma cell disorders are the equivalent of homogenous normal antibody molecules.

The few identified antibody arrangements of M-components appear to be random designs not focused on any specific or tumor-associated antigenic stimulus. An M-component can be detected and differentiated from normal immunoglobulins by serum electrophoresis if the concentration is approximately 0.5 g/dl or higher. Detection of a serum M-component is of major diagnostic value in plasma cell disorders. Quantities of Ig in the range of 0.5 g/dl are the product of approximately 10^9 to 10^{10} monoclonal immunoglobulin-secreting cells in the body.[2] A classification of diseases associated with M-component secretion appears in Table 56–1.

There are five major classes of immunoglobulins synthesized by B lymphocytes and plasma cells: IgG, IgA, IgM, IgD, and IgE. Antibody protein molecules in each of these classes have common monomeric structures. Any one antibody molecule has a monomeric structure composed of two identical heavy (H) chains and two identical light (L) chains, each of which has constant (c) and variable (v) regions of amino acid sequence. The constant regions of the heavy chains for the various classes are γ, α, μ, δ, or ϵ, respectively. There are two types of L chains, κ or λ, and both types are associated with all five immunoglobulin classes.

The constant regions of the molecule define its class specificity and several other biologic characteristics (*e.g.,* the ability to fix complement). Separate genes code for the constant regions of the H and L chains for each H chain class and L chain type. The *variable regions* of H and L chains are considered to be structurally related to the region of the specific antigen-binding site of the molecule and are unique to each specific antibody. A large set of *v* genes code for the variable portions of the Ig molecule, which create the wide variety of antibody specificities in the normal immune response. The variable region of an M-component can be identified immunologically as having a specific *idiotype,* or unique structural region, that

TABLE 56–1. Classification of Disorders Associated With Monoclonal Immunoglobulin (M-Component) Secretion

Disorder	M-Component	
Plasma Cell Neoplasms		
Multiple myeloma	IgG > IgA > IgD > IgE; ±free L chain or L chain alone ($\kappa > \lambda$); rarely biclonal or without detectable Ig abnormality	
"Solitary" myeloma of bone		
Extramedullary plasmacytoma		
Macroglobulinemia	IgM ± free L chain ($\kappa > \lambda$)	
Heavy-chain disease	γ, α, or μ chain or fragment; δ, or ϵ	
Primary amyloidosis	Free L chain ($\lambda > \kappa$) or L chain fragment alone or plus IgG, IgA, IgM, or IgD	
Monoclonal gammopathy of unknown significance	IgG, IgM, IgA, or IgD usually without urinary L chain secretion	
Other B-Cell Neoplasms		
Chronic lymphocytic leukemia	M-component (occasionally secreted) IgM > IgG	
B-cell non-Hodgkin's lymphomas (any morphologic pattern or lymphoid cell types)		
Nonlymphoid Neoplasms		
Chronic myelogenous leukemia	No consistent patterns	
Carcinoma of colon, breast, prostate, or other sites		
"Autoimmune" or Autoreactive Disorders	M-component	Antibody activity of M-component
Cold agglutinin disease (some characteristics of Waldenström's)	IgMκ most common	Anti-I antigen of RBC membrane
	IgM	Anti-IgG
Mixed cryoglobulinemia	IgG	Anti-IgG
Hypergammaglobulinemia	IgM	?
Sjögren's syndrome		
Miscellaneous Inflammatory Storage, or Infectious Disorders		
Lichen myxedematosus	IgGλ	
Gaucher's disease	IgG	
Cirrhosis, sarcoid, parasitic diseases, renal acidosis	No consistent pattern	

(Modified from Salmon SE. Plasma cell disorders. In: Wingaarden JB, Smith LH Jr, eds. Cecil textbook of medicine. 18th ed. 1988:1026–1036)

differentiates it from virtually all other immunoglobulin antibody molecules. Table 56–2 summarizes structural and functional properties of normal immunoglobulins. These properties are generally shared by M-proteins.

Although not clinically practical, radioimmunoassay for the idiotype on a serum M-component could detect as few as 10^3 to 10^4 neoplastic cells in the body.[2] For all Ig classes other than IgM, the monomeric form of the Ig is secreted and has a molecular mass (M_r) of approximately 150,000 to 190,000. Immunoglobulin is secreted as a pentameric unit with a M_r of 900,000. As with several other proteins, immunoglobulins are secreted with various amounts of attached carbohydrate; this also applies to M-components. Although myeloma can be diagnosed in patients with any of the Ig types previously summarized, IgM M-components are usually associated with other malignant or benign plasma cell disorders. The synthesis of

H and L chains is usually well balanced in normal antibody-producing clones. However, in neoplastic clones, biosynthesis of intracellular H and L chains is sometimes "unbalanced," with an excess synthesis of free L chains that are secreted by the cell as dimers of M_r 60,000. Because of their relatively low molecular mass, L chain dimers are normally filtered by the renal glomerulus, partially reabsorbed and catabolized in the renal tubules, and partially excreted in the urine. Detection of substantial quantities of free light chains in the urine serves as a useful diagnostic test in myeloma and related disorders.

Serum M-components are usually observed as a sharp peak or "spike" in the β- or γ-globulin regions on electrophoresis. Urinary M-components are usually detected in concentrates of 24-hour urine collections, and they migrate similarly on electrophoresis. Definition of an M-component as monoclonal requires H and L chain typing. This is done with immuno-

TABLE 56–2.   Properties of Normal Immunoglobulins

Characteristics	IgG	IgA	IgM	IgD	IgE
Molecular mass	150,000	160,000	900,000	180,000	200,000
Subclasses	4	2	1	2(?)	1
Serum concentration (mg/dl; mean)	1140	180	100	3	0.03
Fixes complement	+	+	+	–	+
Carbohydrate (%)	2.6	5–10	10	10–12	11
$T_{1/2}$ (days)	23.6*	5.8	5.1	2.8	2.3

* Half-life varies proportionally to total serum IgG concentration.

electrophoresis or immunofixation techniques. Examples of serum and urine protein electrophoresis and H and L chain typing by immunofixation in a myeloma case are depicted in Figure 56–1.

HISTORY

Although skeletal evidence for the existence of myeloma in earlier millennia has been obtained from Egyptian mummies and other anthropologic remains, the first published descriptions of major clinical features of a patient with multiple myeloma were made in about 1850 in England. A well-respected tradesman, Thomas Alexander McBean, was seen by Dr. William Macintyre of London in 1845. The patient's symptoms included episodes of fatigue, diffuse bone pain, and urinary frequency. Macintyre treated McBean during the course of that year, and from urinalysis tests, Macintyre detected a urinary protein with the heat properties often observed for urinary L chains. He diagnosed "mollities and fragilitas ossium" based on the patient's bony symptoms and consulted with Dr. Thomas Watson concerning therapy for his patient.[4] Later that year, Dr. Henry Bence Jones also tested urine specimens provided by Macintyre and Watson and corroborated the heat properties of urinary L chains (*i.e.*, now called Bence Jones proteins). Bence Jones thought that the protein was the "hydrated deuteroxide of albumin" and published his findings several years before Macintyre published his case report.[5] Bence Jones also emphasized the potential importance of looking for this urinary protein in other cases with mollities ossium. After the patient died in 1846, a surgeon, Dr. John Dalrymple, examined several bones and made gross and microscopic observations. His drawings are consistent with the morphology of myeloma cells.[6]

In 1873, Rustizky independently described a similar patient and employed the term *multiple myeloma* for the first time to focus on the multiple bone tumors that were present.[7] In 1889, Kahler published a major view on multiple myeloma, and the disease became known, particularly in Europe, as Kahler's disease.[8] Ellinger, in 1899, identified the increased serum proteins and sedimentation rate in myeloma.[9] In 1900, Wright published a case report in which he indicated that myeloma did not arise from the red marrow but was a neoplasm comprising specifically plasma cells.[10] Wright's case was probably the first in which x-ray films were used to show diagnostic abnormalities in the patient's ribs.

Other developments that enhanced the diagnosis or understanding of myeloma included the development of bone marrow aspiration in 1929 and of electrophoresis to separate serum proteins in 1937.[11,12] Within several years after the development of electrophoresis, the tall narrow-based spike in the γ-globulin zone was identified in myeloma.[13] In 1938, Magnus-Levy[14] described amyloidosis as a complication of multiple myeloma, and in 1953, Grabar and Williams[15] developed immunoelectrophoresis, which enabled the precise immunologic identification of the H and L chains in a monoclonal immunoglobulin, enhancing the diagnosis of monoclonality of an Ig. In the 1970s, structural evidence for the relation of amyloid in myeloma to the variable component of L chains was subsequently achieved by Glenner and his colleagues by studying the amino acid sequence of solubilized amyloid fibrils.[16] Other developments included quantitation

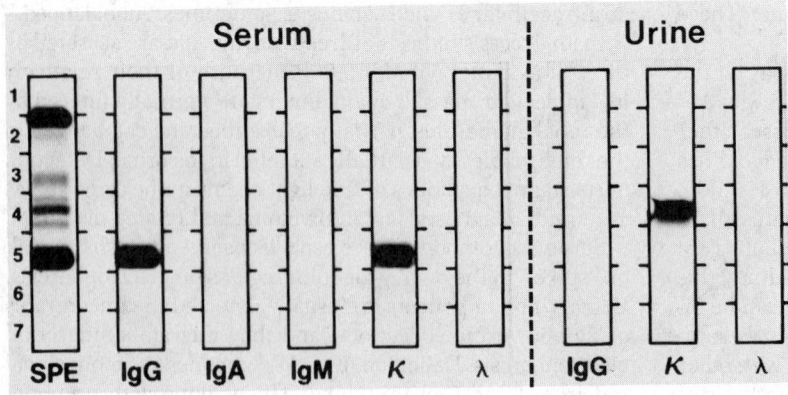

FIGURE 56–1. Identification of serum and urine M-components by the immunofixation technique. The labels indicate the specificity of the antiserum used in developing the immunofixation pattern. In this case, the patient has an IgGκ serum M-component and κ Bence Jones proteinuria.

of the total body burden of tumor cells in myeloma and development of a useful staging system.[17] Several cytokines or interleukins (IL), such as IL-1 and IL-6, have been implicated in myeloma pathophysiology.

Systemic treatment was essentially without effect until 1947, when initial results with urethan in a few patients provided evidence that chemotherapeutic approaches might be of value.[18] A subsequent randomized trial indicated that the survival of patients receiving urethan was inferior to that observed with a placebo.[19] Several other drugs, including nitrogen mustard, 6-mercaptopurine, and 5-fluorouracil, were tried and appeared to be of no value.[20] In 1958, the use of a racemic mixture of D- and L-phenylalanine mustards (Sarcolysine) was reported to be of use in myeloma by Blokhin and colleagues.[21] Subsequently, the D- and L-isomers of phenylalanine mustard were tested separately, and the antimyeloma activity was found to reside in the L-isomer, melphalan. In 1962, Bergsagel and colleagues of the Southwest Oncology Group (SWOG) reported that melphalan could induce remissions in about one third of myeloma patients.[19] Several years later, similar activity was observed with cyclophosphamide.[22] Administration of high doses of the glucocorticoid, prednisone, alone on alternate days, was first reported to induce remissions in relapsing or refractory myeloma in 1967.[23] The use of melphalan in combination with prednisone was then studied extensively.[24,25] A few other single agents with definite activity in myeloma have subsequently been reported, including carmustine (BCNU), doxorubicin (Adriamycin), and interferon-α (INF-α).[26-28]

INCIDENCE AND MORTALITY

Incidence data in the United States as reported by the Surveillance, Epidemiology, and End Result (SEER) program of the National Cancer Institute (NCI) for the period 1973 to 1977 indicate that multiple myeloma accounts for 1.1% of all malignancies in whites and 2.1% in blacks.[29] The average age-adjusted annual incidence for myeloma in whites is 4.3 of 100,000 males and 3.0 of 100,000 females.[29] In blacks, the incidence is higher: 9.6 of 100,000 males and 6.7 of 100,000 females.[29] Myeloma is the most common lymphoid malignancy in blacks and the second most common in whites, for whom non-Hodgkin's lymphoma ranks first. Incidence and mortality rates for myeloma in whites analyzed by SEER rose considerably for both sexes from the late 1940s to the late 1970s, with net increases of 145% or more.[30] In 1983 and 1984, the incidence for whites with myeloma in the United States was 2.8 of 100,000 males and 2.1 of every 100,000 females. Rates for multiple myeloma in Western European countries are similar to those for the American white population, and the incidence is estimated at 2.6 of 100,000 in England and 3.3 of 100,000 in Sweden.[31,32]

The incidence of myeloma in whites and blacks increases with increasing age. Fewer than 2% of the patients are younger than 40 years of age at diagnosis, but the disease has occurred in young adults and children.[33] In the United States, the median age of onset is 68 for men and 70 for women.[28] The mortality patterns closely parallel the incidence curves; the median age at death is 70 years for men and 71 for women.[34] In 1983 and 1984, the mortality rate for the United States

white population with multiple myeloma was 8.7 of 100,000 men and 5.1 of 100,000 women.[30] Incidence and mortality appear to be rising, but the data supporting this trend suggest that the apparent increases in myeloma may reflect prior underdiagnosis, rather than a true increase in incidence.[30,35]

A similar age distribution is also observed in the related plasma cell disorders of MGUS and Waldenström's macroglobulinemia.[36] MGUS occurs much more frequently than multiple myeloma, but it can be detected only with specific screening examinations for monoclonal immunoglobulins. Axelsson and colleagues screened for serum M-components in 6995 asymptomatic adults older than 25 who composed most of the adult population in four parishes in Sweden.[37] Sera from 1% of these persons contained M-components. The prevalence of MGUS in this population increased with age, from 2% of those in the eighth decade to almost 6% of those in the ninth decade. Use of more sensitive screening tests for M-components appears to increase the frequency with which MGUS is detected.[38] Because MGUS has a long natural history and cases tend to accumulate over time, the annual age-related incidence is unknown.

PATHOGENESIS

Myeloma occurs in humans and in mice, rats, hamsters, cats, and dogs.[39-45] In rodents, increased susceptibility to plasma cell tumors has been selected fortuitously in some strains as a result of nonrandom breeding patterns used to create genetic uniformity. An additional factor in various domesticated species, which is probably important, is the prevalence of endogenous retroviruses. Retroviruses are associated with the development of B-lymphoid neoplasms through mutagenicity resulting from insertion of viral genomes into cellular DNA and as a result of the transforming ability of certain recombinant retroviruses.[46]

MURINE MODELS OF DISORDERS ASSOCIATED WITH M-COMPONENTS

Study of inbred mouse strains has yielded substantial information on the occurrence of asymptomatic monoclonal gammopathies without obvious tumor formation (perhaps the equivalent of MGUS) and on mechanisms of induction of plasma cell neoplasms.[47] Monoclonal gammopathies (usually IgG) without tumor formation occur spontaneously in approximately 60% of mice of the inbred C57BL/Ka strain within 24 months, but BALB/c and CBA/Rij mice have a low spontaneous incidence of monoclonal gammopathies.[48] Spontaneous plasmacytomas are infrequent findings in old mice, and they are usually encountered as an incidental finding.[48] Unlike the low spontaneous susceptibility of BALB/c mice to monoclonal gammopathy or spontaneous plasma cell tumors, peritoneal plasmacytomas can be readily induced in inbred strains.[49-51] However, the C57BL/Ka strain, which expresses spontaneous monoclonal gammopathies, is relatively resistant to plasmacytoma induction.[52] Plasmacytomas can be induced in BALB/c mice with the intraperitoneal injection of mineral oils or by implantation of solid plastic materials such as Lucite.[53-55] The plasmacytomas develop within oil or foreign-body granulomas in the peritoneum or mesentery, and each plasmacytoma produces a unique M-component. Chemically defined mineral oil alkane components, such as pristane, also induce plasmacytomas, and this process can be facilitated by subsequent infection of the mice with the Abelson virus.[56]

The murine plasmacytomas lead to the production of a growth factor in the peritoneal fluid that sustains the growth of the neoplasm.[57,58] Plasmacytoma growth factors that support the growth of human myeloma cells in culture have been isolated from the splenic macrophages of oil-treated BALB/c mice and from several other sources.[59-62] A human B-cell growth factor, IL-6, has been isolated from Epstein-Barr virus (EBV)-infected B cells or monocytes.[63] IL-6 has been produced by recombinant DNA methods and has been identified as a plasmacytoma growth factor. IL-6 is a 184-amino acid glycoprotein that stimulates the growth of EBV-infected human B cells and mouse and rat plasmacytomas. Another factor that is probably also produced by BALB/c splenic macrophages in plasmacytoma-bearing mice and that inhibits the normal humoral antibody response has been identified.[64]

Antigenic stimulation by normal bacterial flora has a direct or an indirect effect on plasmacytoma formation; there is a marked reduction in the incidence of myeloma in pristane-treated BALB/c mice that have been raised in a germ-free environment, although other lymphoid neoplasms may arise. Germ-free mice have a less-stimulated or less-developed immune apparatus and may lack the B-cell populations most susceptible to myeloma induction.[65] BALB/c mice are known to harbor oncogenic retroviruses, which may play a role in myeloma induction. Mouse plasmacytomas contain large numbers of intracisternal A particles that are not seen in normal plasma cells.[66] These particles are thought to represent a distinct group of retroviruses.[67]

Nonrandom chromosomal translocations and the expression or alteration of specific oncogenes have been observed in murine plasmacytomas. The distal part of chromosome 15 is translocated to chromosome 12 (where the heavy chain genes reside) in several long-term transplanted plasmacytomas.[68,69] A similar phenomenon has been reported in human Burkitt's lymphoma, in which translocations between the long arm of chromosome 8 (band 24) and the bands on chromosomes 14, 2, and 22 that contain the genetic loci for heavy chain, κ light chain, and λ light chain, respectively.[70]

The finding that the translocated component of chromosome 15 in the mouse and of chromosome 8 in man transfers the *MYC* oncogene to the locus of an immunoglobulin gene suggests that the control of *MYC* expression is enhanced by this translocation and leads to increased cell proliferation and tumor formation. Abnormal expression and alterations in *MYC* have been reported in human myeloma.[71,72] However, this gene was detected in about one fourth of the patients studied.[71] These data suggest that the *MYC* oncogene may have some pathologic role in the evolution of myeloma in humans.[71]

ETIOLOGIC CONSIDERATIONS IN HUMANS

Although the cause of multiple myeloma and related plasma cell disorders remains unknown, several factors have been implicated in the pathogenesis. Several lines of evidence suggest that genetic factors may play a role in predisposing persons to developing myeloma or related disorders. One factor that may implicate genetics is race, because of the increased

prevalence of the disease in U.S. blacks, but this could also indicate environmental differences.[73,74]

Genetic marker studies have yielded only minimal information on the gammopathies. The frequency of HLA antigens of the 4C group appears to be slightly increased in myeloma.[75-78] The incidence of myeloma appears to be increased in first-degree relatives, and familial myeloma has been the subject of several case reports. At the Mayo Clinic, during one 6-year period, myeloma was diagnosed in 8 siblings of 440 patients with myeloma, an incidence that far exceeds that generally reported.[79] In another study, the median age and sex ratio of 75 reported familial cases resembled those of nonfamilial cases.[80] Because related cases usually have been observed in siblings and only rarely in spouses, it appears that transmission is vertical rather than horizontal.[81,82] Within a given family, the heavy chain types of M-components differ; however, there is concordance in light chain types in 80% of the patients.[80]

Idiopathic monoclonal peaks (*i.e.*, MGUS) have been reported sporadically in relatives of patients with myeloma.[79,83-85] Genetic factors in MGUS are suggested by its relation to selected HLA types, the predominance of the IgG1 subclass, and by reports of the familial occurrence of myeloma and macroglobulinemia.[86-92] At the Mayo Clinic, where 241 patients with MGUS were followed for at least 10 years, MGUS was evaluated as a precursor to myeloma.[1] During this period, 38% of patients had no change in the concentration of the M-component and remained asymptomatic. An additional 35% of the patients died without developing myeloma or any other B-cell neoplasm. In 9%, the M-component increased significantly, but myeloma or a related disorder was not diagnosed. Most importantly, 17% of the 44 patients had a diagnosis of myeloma, macroglobulinemia, amyloidosis, or lymphoma. Multiple myeloma was the diagnosis in 30 (68%) of these patients. This report and anecdotal observations in the literature implicate MGUS as a premalignant condition. In one fascinating case, a patient received passive serotherapy with horse antiserum to tetanus in the 1930s and subsequently developed a serum M-component that persisted for more than 3 decades before overt myeloma developed. After the diagnosis was made, it was determined that the serum IgG M-component exhibited antibody activity with specificity directed toward horse α_2-macroglobulin.[93]

These findings and others have given rise to a "two-hit hypothesis," in which antigenic stimulation in a susceptible host is the first hit, giving rise to a benign monoclone. The second hit is postulated to be a mutagenic or transforming event that gives rise to myeloma from the expanded monoclonal B-cell population.[94]

Environmental or occupational factors in myeloma have been examined in large occupational studies, but these data must be interpreted cautiously because some associations may have occurred by chance alone. A large British case-control study involved 399 myeloma patients and an equal number of matched controls evaluated for a variety of occupational and environmental exposures and for immunization, infection, and immune defects.[95] A strong risk of myeloma (relative risk of 1.8) was associated with agriculture, food processing, and exposure to chemicals. Another case-control study involved 100 white myeloma patients and 100 matched controls in the Baltimore area.[96] Positive associations were documented for a history of occupational exposure to petroleum products, with an observed rate of myeloma that was 3.7 times the expected rate (range, 1.3–10.3), and to asbestos, with an observed rate of 3.5 (range, 1.0–12.0). Among a large number of medications assessed, the use of laxatives appeared to elevate risk of myeloma to 3.5 times the expected rate.

The finding of increased risk with exposure to petroleum products in this study confirms earlier reports of an excessive number of cases of myeloma in workers exposed to petroleum.[1,97] The increased risk of myeloma in petroleum workers correlates well with the mineral oil-induced model for plasma cell neoplasms in BALB/c mice. One patient developed a plasmacytoma in the cutaneous pocket in which a Silastic-covered cardiac pacemaker was installed.[98]

Prior reports of 61 patients with asbestosis have documented the occurrence of four cases of myeloma, one of macroglobulinemia, and one of chronic lymphocytic leukemia (CLL), suggesting that this known carcinogen may be involved in the induction B-cell neoplasms.[99] Although chronic antigenic stimulation in disorders such as cholecystitis, osteomyelitis, and reactions to allergen hyposensitization injections has been suggested as a predisposing factor for human plasma cell neoplasms, data from various studies are inconclusive.[100–117]

As in other hematologic malignancies, a significant association has been observed between radiation exposure and the subsequent development of myeloma. This has been documented in the studies of survivors of the atomic bombs in Hiroshima and Nagasaki.[118,119] Among 109,000 survivors, 29 myeloma deaths were identified between 1950 and 1976. For persons exposed to 100 cGy, the observed rate of myeloma was approximately 4.7 times greater than controls, with the excess risk in this high-dose exposure group becoming apparent after a latent period of about 20 years. Associations between myeloma and low-dose irradiation exposure are more controversial than the atomic bomb casualty reports.[118] However, studies of radiologists have shown excessive mortality resulting from myeloma, as for workers in nuclear plants.[120–123] In an epidemiologic study, there was evidence of an increase in myeloma risk (but not leukemia or lymphoma) with increasing numbers of diagnostic radiographs, but the overall myeloma risk was not high.[124] These findings support the view that even low-level radiation may be a risk factor for myeloma.

PATHOLOGY

The morphologic appearance of plasma cells in malignant and benign disorders are often similar. Plasma cells are at least two to three times the size of peripheral lymphocytes and are round or egg shaped, with one or more eccentrically placed nuclei containing diffuse or clumped chromatin (Fig. 56–2). The light microscopic appearance was first drawn by Dalrymple and published from a woodcut in 1846.[6] Plasma cells contain a highly differentiated cytoplasm that is rich in rough-surfaced endoplasmic reticulum specialized for Ig synthesis. The cytoplasm normally stains blue or blue-purple with Romanovsky-type stains, but some myeloma cells stain red-orange and have been called thesaurocytes or flame cells.[125,126] Once thought to be diagnostic of IgA myeloma, flame cells are now recognized in any plasma cell proliferation in which

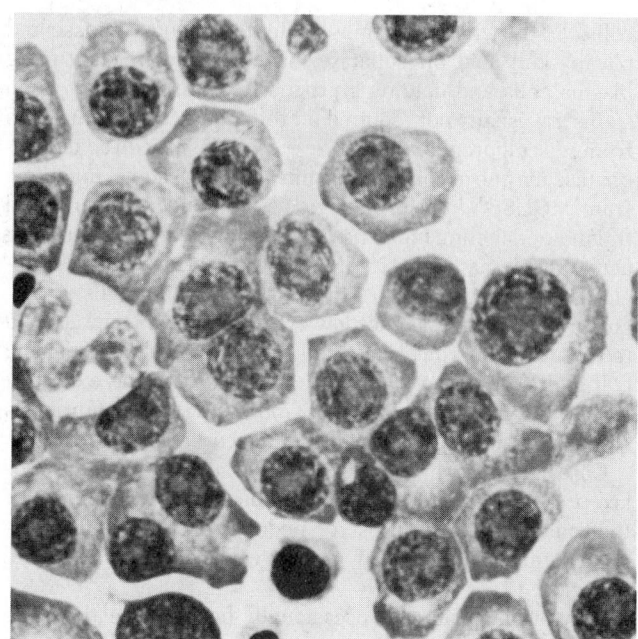

FIGURE 56–2. Bone marrow plasma cell in a patient with IgG myeloma. With the exception of a single cell in the neutrophilic series, the remaining cells are neoplastic plasma cells at various stages of differentiation.

the M-component has a high carbohydrate content.[126,127] A perinuclear clear zone is usually present in plasma cells and is the site of the Golgi apparatus, wherein Ig is packaged and glycosylated for secretion.[128] Other cytoplasmic findings can include numerous vacuoles (*e.g.*, Mott cells, cells with Russell bodies, grape cells, morula cells).[129] Electron microscopy reveals protein-filled secretion vacuoles or dilated cisternae in the endoplasmic reticulum. Although the cytoplasm is well differentiated, the nucleus in malignant plasma cell disorders can be relatively less differentiated, often has diffuse chromatin, and may have several nucleoli and intranuclear inclusions. None of these features absolutely differentiates benign from malignant plasma cell proliferations.

Myeloma patients with large numbers of plasmablasts in their marrow may have a poorer prognosis than those with predominantly mature plasma cells. In macroglobulinemia, cells may have a "lymphoplasmacytic" appearance, with morphologic variations in size and characteristics of those of small lymphocytes to large plasma cells. This pattern is occasionally observed in myeloma. When lymphoplasmacytic cells are examined with immunofluorescence, most contain large amounts of cytoplasmic M-component. Cell surface Ig usually cannot be demonstrated on plasma cells.

In addition to the conventional morphologic assessments of plasma cells, use of monoclonal antibody reagents, histochemical analyses, and other morphologic approaches have been useful in analyzing plasma cells. Several plasma cell-associated antigens have been identified with specific monoclonal antibodies. Some patients' cells react strongly with antibodies to the common acute lymphocytic leukemia antigen (CALLA); these patients may have a poorer prognosis.[130] Immunologic and cytogenetic markers have been used to identify a series of characteristics associated with myeloma stem cells.[131] Histochemical stains, including β-glucuronidase and plasma cell acid phosphatase, have assisted in identifying plasma cells and obtaining prognostic information.[132] Such stains are usually not required for differentiating plasma cells from red cell progenitors; however, the plasma cell acid phosphatase may be of some use in differentiating active myeloma from MGUS.[133,134] Morphologic assessment of the tritiated thymidine-labeling index has been valuable in differentiating active myeloma from MGUS and other entities.[135,136] Monoclonal antibody reagents capable of evaluating cells undergoing DNA synthesis and flow cytometry have been applied to the evaluation of plasma cell disorders.[137,138] The plasma cell β-glucuronidase has been correlated with the extent of disease. With some exceptions, increasing tumor burden is associated with higher plasma cell glucuronidase levels.[139]

Core bone marrow biopsies demonstrate that myeloma cells are present in cords in a reticular network. Involvement of the marrow can be diffuse or nodular, although diffuse involvement with sheets of plasma cells is somewhat more common.

Amyloid deposits can occasionally be found in the bone marrow in the vicinity of myeloma cells or in biopsies of soft-tissue plasmacytomas. Other biopsy sites, such as the abdominal fat and rectal mucosa, have a higher likelihood of demonstrating the presence of amyloid.[140]

The symptoms and signs of multiple myeloma and its effects on the patient result from the secreted products from the myeloma cells, which have a variety of hormonal, immunologic, and physicochemical effects and from the growth kinetics and total-body tumor burden of malignant plasma cells. Several cytokines may play roles in the pathophysiology of myeloma. IL-6 is a major growth factor for myeloma, particularly in the terminal phase of the disease.[141] IL-6 may support myeloma growth through a paracrine mechanism, with its production provided by adherent cells in the monocyte-macrophage series rather than the myeloma cells themselves.[142] In a study using IL-6 antisense oligonucleotides, growth inhibition was observed in human myeloma cells lines, suggesting that IL-6 autocrine mechanisms may also be involved.[141]

HYPERCALCEMIA

In the clinical phase of myeloma, hematogenous dissemination to various skeletal sites is usually extensive and leads to bone pain and hypercalcemia. Radiographic findings of skeletal destruction are depicted in Figure 56–3. In areas of bone resorption, it appears that the cells adjacent to the bony matrix in the resorption lacunae are osteoclasts, which are separated from the myeloma cells by a membrane. This morphologic finding and those of functional studies using myeloma cell secretion products provided the basis for the concept that myeloma cells liberated an osteoclast-activating factor responsible for bone destruction.[143,144] The production of osteoclast-activating factor by a patient's myeloma cells correlates with the extent of skeletal involvement.[145] Several bone-resorbing cytokines have been identified, including lymphotoxin, tumor necrosis factor (TNF) produced by myeloma cells, and IL-1.[146] Antibodies to IL-6 but not to TNF or lymphotoxin partially blocked myeloma osteoclast-activating factor activity,

suggesting that IL-1 may play a role in the development of bone lesions.[147]

ANEMIA

Marrow involvement results in the development of a normochromic, normocytic anemia, heralding the symptoms of fatigue and weakness. Reduced erythrocyte production and increased destruction have been observed. High concentrations of serum M-component in the blood lead to rouleaux formation and may lead to blood sludging, which further increases hemolysis.

RENAL FAILURE

Renal failure is a common complication of myeloma that can be significant at the time of clinical presentation. It is an adverse prognostic factor that has a negative impact on overall survival. The renal failure appears to be multifactorial and is most frequently correlated with Bence Jones proteinuria, hypercalcemia, or both. The presence of λ light chains in the urine is more strongly correlated with renal failure than is the excretion of κ chains, suggesting that they often are more nephrotoxic. Light chains normally pass the glomerulus and are reabsorbed and catabolized in the proximal tubules.[148–150] An assay system has been developed to assess the intrinsic nephrotoxic potential of Bence Jones proteins.[151] The excretion of dense (often laminated) tubular casts is a characteristic finding in patients with myeloma kidney.[151] The casts contain albumin, intact Ig molecules, or Bence Jones proteins.[151–161] The proteinuria comprises monoclonal light chains and some albumin. Infection, hyperuricemia, and amyloidosis also contributing to renal failure. Amyloid deposition in the kidney usually appears in the blood vessels, basement membranes of the tubules, interstitium, and occasionally in glomeruli. Proteinuria in patients with renal amyloid is often generalized, and this can provide a clue for differentiating the syndrome from myeloma kidney.

IMMUNODEFICIENCY

Increased susceptibility to bacterial infections, particularly before treatment, is principally due to an acquired hyporesponsiveness to antigenic stimulation. Reduced serum levels of normal serum antibody immunoglobulins are observed in almost all patients with multiple myeloma and in many MGUS patients.[162] The normal pre-B-cell and B-cell compartments are reduced in myeloma.[163] Studies using mice indicate that myeloma cells produce a humoral PC-factor that stimulates monocytes and macrophages to produce a second factor, PIMS, which inhibits normal antigen-stimulated B-cell proliferation after antibody production.[164] Mixing experiments using peripheral blood mononuclear cells from patients with myeloma and those from normal persons indicates that monocytic cells in the myeloma patient's blood can inhibit normal B-cell Ig synthesis induced with pokeweed mitogen.[165] The precise molecular nature of these immunosuppressive cytokines is not established.

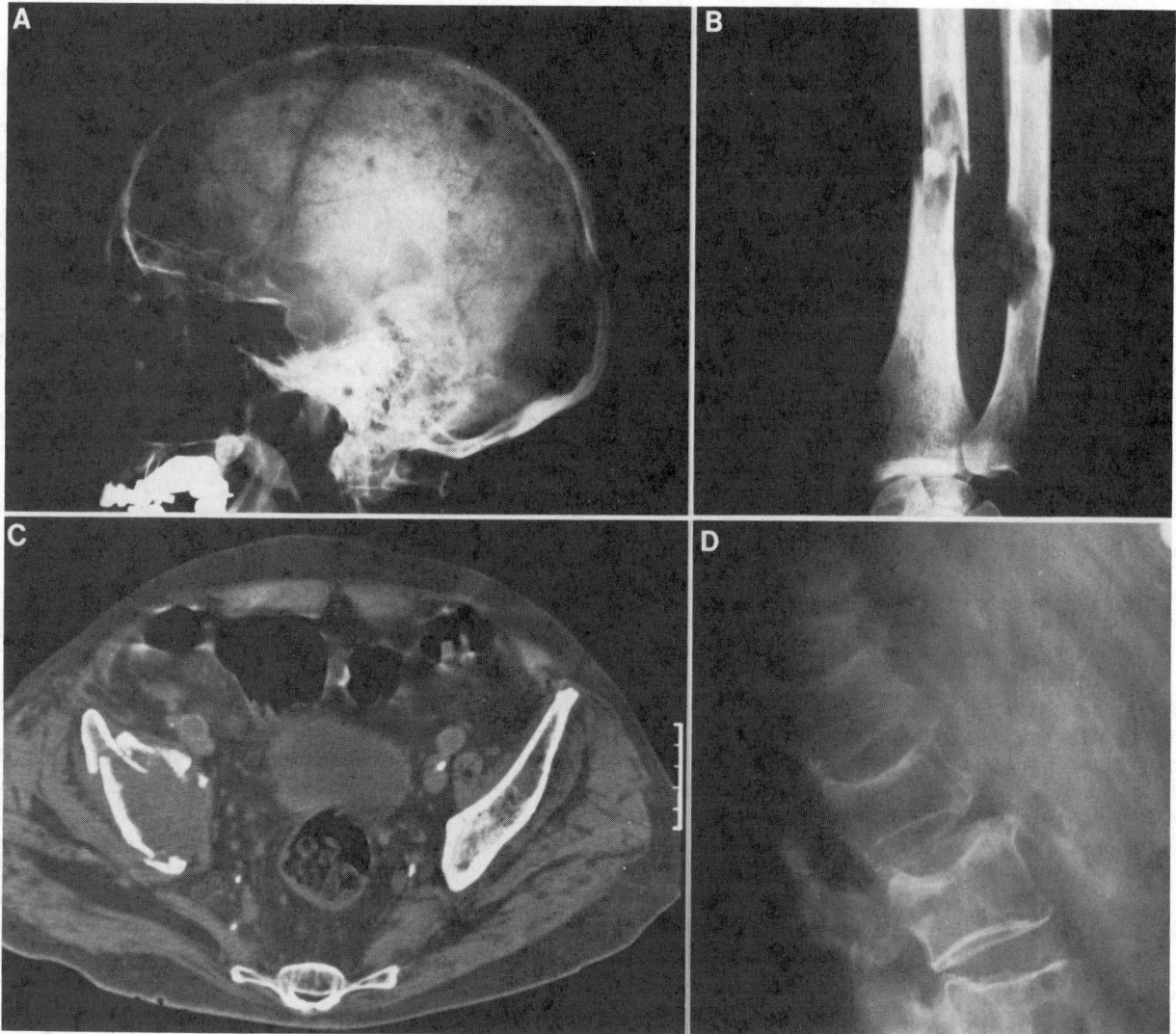

FIGURE 56–3. Typical radiographic evidence of bone involvement in myeloma. **(A)** Punched-out lesions in the skull. **(B)** Intramedullary expansile lesions in a forearm with fracture. **(C)** Pelvic plasmacytoma with a fracture and associated soft tissue mass seen on a computed tomography scan. **(D)** Vertebral compression fractures in the spine.

PHYSICOCHEMICAL OR IMMUNOLOGIC EFFECTS OF M-COMPONENTS

M-components in myeloma and related disorders can cause clinically significant abnormalities in blood flow and function.[166] The most common of these phenomena is the hyperviscosity syndrome. Although more common in macroglobulinemia than in myeloma, it results from a sufficient concentration of an M-protein with a high molecular mass or with a tendency to self-aggregation and a resultant increase in intrinsic viscosity. The hyperviscosity syndrome is rarely seen until the serum viscosity exceeds 4.0 cp units, relative to normal saline, and it is usually manifested by the occurrence of neurologic findings and by spontaneous bleeding phenomena in the absence of thrombocytopenia. In other instances, an M-component exhibits antibody activity, leading to clinical syndromes such as acquired deficiency of factor VIII, with bleeding phenomena and hyperlipidemia.[167–169]

GROWTH KINETICS AND TUMOR BURDEN

Myeloma is a low-growth-fraction tumor, with only a small percentage of tumor cells in the cell cycle at any given time. It is thought to arise from a single transformed cell (10^0 cell). Tritiated thymidine-labeling indices for myeloma cells in patients with active disease usually are in the range of 1% to 3%.[136] Studies of the generation time indicate that the cell cycle time of actively proliferating cells is approximately 1 to 3 days.[170,171] In IgG myeloma, tumor burden ranges from 0.5×10^{12} cells in early asymptomatic cases to 5×10^{12} cells or more in patients with widespread bone destruction.[17]

Studies of growth kinetics have been carried out by measuring the doubling time of serum M-components of patients not actively receiving treatment and by use of mathematical modeling for measurements of progressive tumor growth in patients who have had their total-body tumor burden determined.[170] Using serum M-component doubling times of 4 to

6 months in untreated patients and assuming exponential growth, it was initially proposed that the natural history of myeloma might require 20 to 30 years to evolve from a single malignant plasma cell to clinically evident disease.[172] In some instances, this model would predict that myeloma was initiated before conception! However, subsequent studies using measurements of M-component metabolism and more precise mathematical modeling techniques determined that the growth of myeloma followed Gompertzian kinetics and that the subclinical phase of malignant tumor cell proliferation was about 1 to 3 years before clinical diagnosis.[171] A typical myeloma growth curve is depicted in Figure 56–4.

The phase of myeloma after diagnosis can be viewed as a chronic phase, not dissimilar to that in chronic myeloid leukemia. This chronic phase in myeloma may last from 1 to 10 or more years, during which time treatment is usually beneficial. Late in the course of myeloma, the doubling time (as determined from serum M-component levels) may progressively shorten; this may be analogous to the blast crisis phase of chronic myeloid leukemia.[173] Integration of tritiated thymidine-labeling index and tumor-burden studies defined these patients as having high-growth-fraction, high-tumor-burden myeloma.[136] This patient group has a poor prognosis, with rapid myeloma growth and early death.[136,174] Patients whose myelomas have more rapid growth kinetics have a propensity for extramedullary tumor growth, including soft-tissue plasmacytomas and central nervous system (CNS) involvement. In some instances, the neoplasm takes on a less-differentiated morphologic appearance, similar to that of a large cell lymphoma, with a cell surface Ig that usually corresponds with the prior serum Ig.[94,175,176]

In earlier phases of disease, the quantity of M-component synthesis as determined from serum or urine measurements corresponds with the amount of tumor in the body. However, in the terminal phase, the M-component synthesis rate per tumor may decline or qualitatively change as the tumor progresses, suggesting the development of a mutant clone. Some patients who previously had only a serum M-component switch to primarily urinary light chains, reflecting additional biochemical abnormalities in Ig synthesis and assembly.[177]

Unlike the aggressive forms of the disease, another subset of patients have indolent or smoldering myeloma in which, despite evidence of bone lesions, the disease progresses slowly even without treatment. These patients previously could be identified only from their clinical course; however, the use of tritiated thymidine-labeling studies usually identifies these patients as having hypoproliferative myeloma cells, with fewer than 0.5% of the tumor cells labeling and in a range similar to that of MGUS.[135,136]

DIAGNOSIS AND CLINICAL STAGING OF MYELOMA

Presenting symptoms and signs of myeloma usually include bone pain, which may be associated with compression fractures of the spine or pathologic fractures of long bones; weakness and anemia; and infection, usually due to pneumococcal or other gram-positive bacteria. Hypercalcemia, renal failure, spinal cord compression, or a mixture of these findings may be present. Punched-out osteolytic bone lesions are commonly seen on skeletal x-ray films (see Fig. 56–3). A complete skeletal x-ray series, including the axial and appendicular skeleton, should always be obtained at the time of diagnosis. Only in this way can the number and location of lesions be identified to determine if any potentially unstable osteolytic lesions are present.

Studies using magnetic resonance imaging (MRI) scanning suggest that this approach can provide greater detail on myelomatous abnormalities in the vertebral column than conventional radiographs (Fig. 56–5). However, because this procedure is expensive and takes several hours to acquire the imaging information on the entire spine of a single patient, this technique must be used selectively. Bone scans are of no value in the assessment of skeletal involvement in myeloma, because the bone disease is almost purely osteolytic and the nuclear medicine isotopes are taken up only in areas of osteoblastic activity.

An increase in the number of plasma cells is usually demonstrable in the bone marrow or in a biopsy of a plasmacytoma. A serum or urinary M-component can be demonstrated in 99% of the patients. However, in some instances, not all criteria are present, and a mixture of criteria is needed to establish a diagnosis of multiple myeloma and to differentiate it from other plasma cell disorders. Useful diagnostic criteria are summarized in Table 56–3.

A clinical staging system for multiple myeloma was developed at the Arizona Cancer Center by Durie and Salmon by analyzing the presenting features of a series of patients with multiple myeloma who had their tumor burden directly measured using the metabolic techniques.[177] On the basis of these clinical correlations, multiple myeloma was divided into three tumor burden groups: stage I (low), II (intermediate), and III (high). Tumor mass stage alone was predictive of survival.

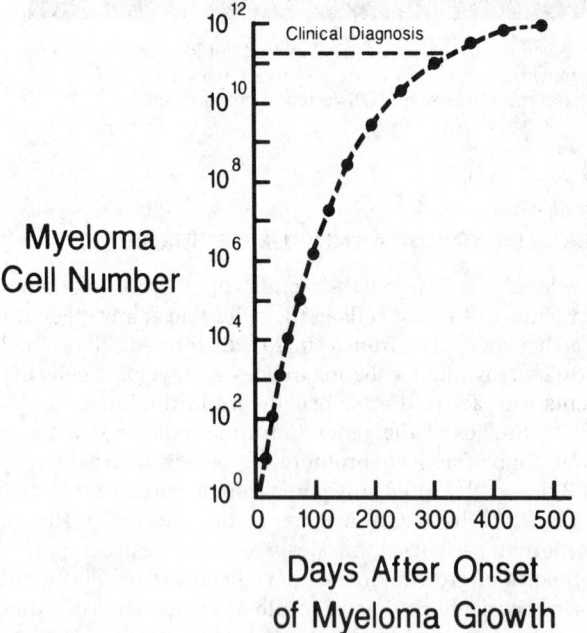

FIGURE 56–4. Gompertzian growth curve in multiple myeloma. In this untreated patient with IgG myeloma, serial measurements of M-component production were used to extrapolate the preclinical phase of myeloma cell proliferation of approximately 1 year.

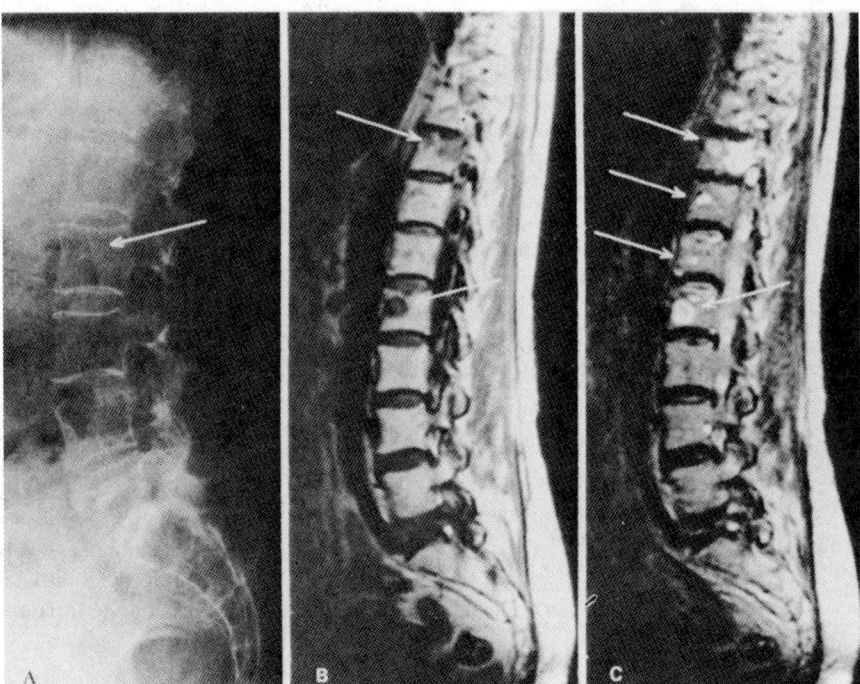

FIGURE 56–5. **(A)** Radiograph of lower spine compared with **(B, C)** magnetic resonance images. The osteolytic lesions in the vertebral bodies of T10–12 and L1 that were poorly visualized on plain films were much more visible on the **(B)** T1-weighted and **(C)** T2-weighted MR images. (Ludwig M, Tscholakoff D, Neuhold A, et al. Magnetic resonance imaging of the spine in multiple melanoma. Lancet 1987;2:364–366)

An additional prognostic factor, renal function, independently impinged on survival and was included in the staging system, with normal renal function (*i.e.*, serum creatinine <2.0 or blood urea nitrogen <30) as substage A and higher values as substage B (Table 56–4).

Several other investigations applied the Durie-Salmon myeloma staging system to evaluate survival by stage in myeloma (Table 56–5). In studies of response to treatment and survival, the clinical features that correlated with a given stage in terms of tumor burden predicted survival in the original patient set and in subsequent reports by other investigative groups.[183,189,190] Figure 56–6 depicts the influence of clinical stage and renal function on the survival of patients with multiple myeloma. In the original study used in developing the Durie-Salmon myeloma staging system, the percentage of bone marrow plasma cells was an important factor, but it was not included in the staging system because it could be replaced by other clinical features and was potentially susceptible to sampling errors. Bone marrow involvement was deleted from the staging criteria after consideration of the potential difficulties that might be encountered in accurately and reproducibly counting plasma cells in the bone marrow differential at different centers. Patients with Bence Jones-only myeloma have been assessed for measured tumor cell burden, and they appear to represent a higher-risk subgroup with a higher tumor cell mass and shorter survival.[192]

DIFFERENTIAL DIAGNOSIS

The criteria shown in Table 56–3 provide the basis for differentiating myeloma from other major plasma cell disorders with M-component secretions other than IgM. The IgM M-components are usually attributable to Waldenström's macroglobulinemia and occasionally to MGUS or other entities. Multiple myeloma with IgM secretion has rarely been reported, and it should be diagnosed only if the patient has multiple osteolytic bone lesions that contain monoclonal plasma cells.[94] Marrow plasmacytosis is observed in several chronic infectious or inflammatory diseases and in hypersensitivity reactions, autoimmune disease, unrelated neoplasms, and occasionally in other conditions; it is not associated with secretion of an M-component, but it is associated with polyclonal hyperglobulinemia.

The major differential diagnosis is usually between myeloma and MGUS. There is an overlap between the findings for patients with MGUS and those with stage I myeloma (or macroglobulinemia) that can often be recognized only by serial follow-up of the patient for at least 1 year without any form of treatment. In MGUS, the M-component level remains constant over many years, but in the malignant plasma cell disorders, the M-component gradually rises, and other symptoms and signs of the disease develop. A policy of watch and wait is completely justifiable, because there is no evidence that treatment improves the outcome in stage I myeloma or MGUS, and the use of chemotherapy has potential hazards that should be avoided if the patient does not have an invasive, progressive plasma cell malignancy. If, after a year's follow-up of the patient's M-component and symptoms and signs at 1- to 2-month intervals, there is no evidence of progression, the most likely diagnosis is MGUS, and follow-up examinations should be done at least annually because approximately 2% of these patients progress to a diagnosis of B-cell neoplasm each year.[1]

Patients presenting with only Bence Jones proteinuria usually have myeloma alone or with amyloidosis.[193,194] It has been stated that its excretion has "sinister significance."[195] However, Bence Jones MGUS has been reported and followed without specific therapy for several years in a few patients.[160,196] It is nonetheless reasonable to have a higher index of suspicion when patients present with idiopathic Bence Jones proteinuria, because it usually progresses within 6 months to 1 year to clearly diagnosed myeloma, which should be treated

TABLE 56–3. Diagnostic Criteria for Multiple Myeloma, Myeloma Variants, and Monoclonal Gammopathy of Unknown Significance (MGUS)

A. Multiple myeloma
  Major criteria
    I. Plasmacytoma on tissue biopsy
    II. Bone marrow plasmacytosis with >30% plasma cells
    III. Monoclonal globulin spike on serum electrophoresis exceeding 3.5 g/dl for G peaks or 2.0 g/dl for A peaks, ≥1.0 g/24 h of κ- or λ-light chain excretion on urine electrophoresis in the presence of amyloidosis
  Minor criteria
    a. Bone marrow plasmacytosis 10% to 30% plasma cells
    b. Monoclonal globulin spike present but less than the level defined above
    c. Lytic bone lesions
    d. Residual normal IgM < 50 mg/dl, IgA < 100 mg/dl, or IgG < 600 mg/dl*
    Diagnosis will be confirmed when any of the following features are documented in symptomatic patients with clearly progressive disease. The diagnosis of myeloma requires a minimum of one major + one minor criterion or three minor criteria that must include a + b, *i.e.*:
      1. I + b, I + c, I + d (I + a not sufficient)
      2. II + b, II + c, II + d
      3. III + a, III + c, III + d
      4. a + b + c, a + b + d
B. Indolent myeloma (same as myeloma except)
    I. No bone lesions or only limited bone lesions (≤3 lytic lesions); no compression fractures
    II. M-component levels: (a) IgG < 7 g/dl; (b) IgA < 5/dl
    III. No symptoms or associated disease features, *i.e.*:
    a. Performance status > 70%
    b. Hemoglobin > 10 g/dl
    c. Serum calcium normal
    d. Serum creatinine < 2.0 mg/dl
    e. No infections
C. Smoldering myeloma (same as indolent myeloma except)
    I. No bone lesions
    II. Bone marrow plasma cells ≤ 30%
D. MGUS
    I. Monoclonal gammopathy
    II. M-component level
      IgG ≤ 3.5 g/dl
      IgA ≤ 2.0 g/dl
      BJ protein ≤ 1.0 g/24 h
    III. Bone marrow plasma cells < 10%
    IV. No bone lesions
    V. No symptoms

* IgA, immunoglobulin A; IgG, immunoglobulin G; IgM, immunoglobulin M; BJ, Bence Jones light chain.
(From references 135, 160, 179, 180)

β₂-MICROGLOBULIN

β_2-microglobulin is an important prognostic factor in multiple myeloma.[197] It is a low-molecular-mass protein, which is the light chain of the HLA antigen and is synthesized by all nucleated cells.[198] It falls in the class of tubular proteins that pass the glomerulus and are excreted in the urine, but renal functional impairment elevates the serum level of β_2-microglobulin. β_2-Microglobulin can be measured by radioimmunoassay. If corrected for renal function, serum β_2-microglobulin levels correlate strongly with tumor burden in multiple myeloma.[197,199–203] Because the serum levels are a function of myeloma cell mass and renal function, measurement of β_2-microglobulin may provide an alternative to clinical staging for predicting survival.[204] The relation of β_2-microglobulin to survival in myeloma is depicted in Figure 56–7. β_2-Microglobulin can serve as a pretreatment prognostic factor in clinical trials because it permits a more direct comparison of risk factors among the various cooperative groups and institutions interested in myeloma therapy.[205,206] Although it has been proposed that β_2-microglobulin can be used to differentiate between MGUS and myeloma, significant overlap prevents this.[197,200,207] Serial β_2-microglobulin levels have not proven to be as useful as M-component measurements after response to treatment of myeloma. INF-α is reported to raise β_2-microglobulin levels in myeloma.[208] In our own experience, β_2-microglobulin has not proved useful in patients lacking an M-component (nonsecretory myeloma).

TREATMENT

PRINCIPLES

The diagnosis of a monoclonal gammopathy does not represent an immediate mandate for treatment, and patients with MGUS, stage I myeloma, and indolent or smoldering myeloma are often best followed without treatment until it is warranted by the development of clear-cut progression of the disease.

Because multiple myeloma is a disseminated plasma cell neoplasm, the primary approach to treatment is systemic antineoplastic therapy. Symptoms and signs that warrant immediate institution of therapy include the development of bone pain, hypercalcemia, renal failure, severe suppression of bone marrow functions, or spinal cord compression. If the patient has spinal cord compression, completion of local therapy (usually with radiation therapy) should normally precede the initiation of systemic chemotherapy unless other serious complications mandate simultaneous systemic treatment and radiation therapy. Patients presenting with long-bone fractures should have them internally fixed orthopedically before the initiation of chemotherapy. Presentation with constellations of findings, such as marked anemia plus the presence of lytic bone lesions, bacterial sepsis, or Bence Jones proteinuria, provide reasons for initiation of therapy. If there is significant infection, initiation of treatment should usually be delayed until the infection has been controlled. If the clinical findings are ambiguous, a period of observation that includes serial M-component measurements is usually warranted.

Doubling in the M-component in less than 1 year with other clinical findings of myeloma can also be used as a basis for treatment. For example, patients with rising M-component levels or progressive bone lesions are candidates for treatment even if they are asymptomatic. Useful adjuncts to systemic treatment include management of local problems with radiation therapy and a variety of supportive care measures.

Beneficial effects of systemic therapy can be obtained in most patients with newly diagnosed progressive myeloma in

appropriately. Patients with unrelated metastatic neoplasms occasionally have MGUS, and a series of diagnostic studies and biopsies are required to establish that the patient does not have myeloma. Myeloma and an unrelated metastatic neoplasm may be diagnosed.

TABLE 56-4. Myeloma Staging System

Criteria	Measured Myeloma Cell Mass (Cells × $10^{12}/m^2$)
Stage I	
All of the following:	
Hemoglobin value > 10 g/dl	
Serum calcium value normal (<12 mg/dl)	
On roentgenogram, normal bone structure (scale 0) or solitary bone plasmacytoma only	
Low M-component production rates	<0.6 (low)
IgG value < 5 g/dl*	
IgA value < 3 g/dl	
Urine light chain M-component on electrophoresis < 4 g/24 h	
Stage II	
Overall data not as minimally abnormal as shown for stage I and no single value as abnormal as defined for stage II.	0.6–1.20 (intermediate)
Stage III	
One or more of the following	
Hemoglobin value < 8.5 d/gl	
Serum calcium value > 12 mg/dl	
Advanced lytic bone lesions (scale 3)	
High M-component production rates	>1.20 (high)
IgG value > 7 d/gl	
IgA value > 5 g/dl	
Urine light chain M-component on electrophoresis > 12 g/24 h	
Subclassification	
A = relatively normal renal function (serum creatinine value > 2.0 mg/dl)	
B = abnormal renal function (serum creatinine value ≥ 2.0 gm/dl)	
Examples	
Stage IA = low cell mass with normal renal function	
Stage IIIB = high cell mass with abnormal renal function	

* IgA, immunoglobulin A; IgG, immunoglobulin G.
(Alexanian R, Balcerzak S, Bonnet JD, et al. Prognostic factors in multiple myeloma. Cancer 1975;36: 1192–1201)

TABLE 56-5. Median Survival in Relation to Stage at Diagnosis

Investigations	No. of Patients	Median Survival (mo)				
		Stage				
		I	II	III	A	B
Durie and Salmon[181]	71	>60	50	26		
Alexanian et al[182]	343	39	27	17		
Woodruff et al[183]	237	64	32	6	21	2
Merlini et al[184]	123	76	41	12		
Belpomme et al[185]	118	>60	28	7	>60	12
Gobbi et al[186]	91	>79	51	33		
Santoro et al[187]	81	48	41	23	35	7
Bergsagel et al[188]	364	46	32	23	32	11
Summary	1428	>60	41	23		

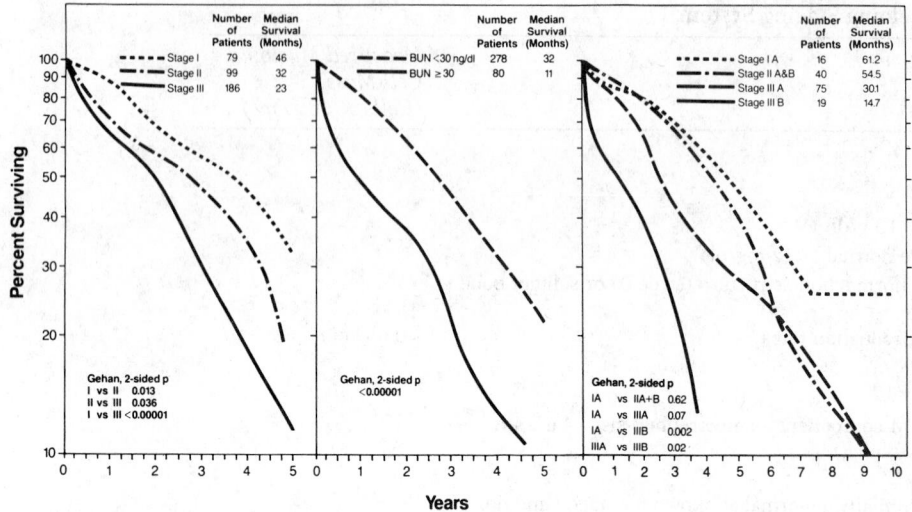

FIGURE 56–6. Influence of clinical stage and renal function on survival of patients with plasma cell myeloma as redrawn from published illustrations. The left two panels are from a Canadian NCI study[189] and show the separate effects of clinical stage and renal function, respectively. The right panel depicts an Arizona Cancer Center study,[191] and the survival curves are shown with clinical stage and renal function integrated with the use of the clinical staging system shown in Table 56-4. Statistical comparisons of survival outcome for the various stages and risk groups in the studies appear in each panel.

clinical stages II or III. The best improvement in survival of patients with myeloma has been obtained for those with stage III disease. The clinical phases of myeloma under treatment include an initial drug sensitive phase, which is observed in most patients; a plateau phase, during which tumor burden is reduced and appears to be stable during maintained or unmaintained remission; and an eventual drug-resistant phase, during which the neoplasm may exhibit altered growth kinetics and resistance to conventional cytotoxic drugs.[2,209] About 15% to 20% of patients manifest resistance even to aggressive parenteral chemotherapy at the time of initial presentation with progressive myeloma.

Systemic therapy usually relieves bone pain relatively promptly, but many other aspects of the disease improve gradually and may require other supportive measures initially. Even with prompt institution of systemic treatment, the drug-

sensitive phase of disease usually lasts only 2 to 3 years for most patients before drug resistance manifests. Although the median survival before the era of effective systemic therapy was less than 1 year, it is now in the range of 3 to 4 years. In a few patients, sensitivity to systemic therapy may persist for 5 to 10 years or longer.

Care must include maximal efforts to relieve pain, hypercalcemia, severe anemia, and various local complications promptly to keep the patient from being bedridden, minimizing bone demineralization and superinfections. Patients should be encouraged to drink several liters of fluid daily to avoid dehydration and enhance urinary excretion of light chains and calcium.

EVALUATION OF RESPONSE TO TREATMENT

Because myeloma has a variety of clinical manifestations, a series of initial and follow-up studies are needed to assess the response to systemic treatment. These include a thorough history, physical examination, and following laboratory studies, which include the complete blood count with differential and platelet counts; M-component levels in the serum, 24-hour urine, or both; serum calcium, creatinine, or blood urea nitrogen levels; and skeletal radiographs. Although serum electrophoresis is extremely useful in the initial diagnostic workup, baseline and follow-up quantitation of the serum M-components is most reliably measured using laser nephelometry of the involved immunoglobulin. Serum electrophoresis is sometimes a useful alternative, particularly as the M-component level approaches the normal range for the involved Ig. The radial immunodiffusion test should not be used to measure myeloma immunoglobulins, because it has not proved reliable. Quantitation of urinary Bence Jones protein is best determined by protein electrophoresis using a 24-hour concentrate. The relative value of β_2-microglobulin useful for following the course of myeloma has not been established, but β_2-microglobulin is not as specific as M-component measurements, because its serum concentration is affected by tumor burden and renal function.

In the absence of specific symptoms, follow-up radiographs should be obtained every 6 to 12 months. The initial skeletal

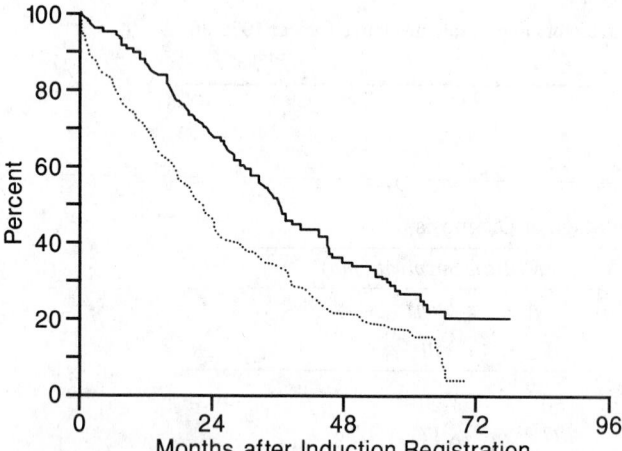

FIGURE 56–7. Life table survival curves in multiple myeloma in relation to serum β_2-microglobulin (β_2M) concentration. The upper curve (*solid line*) is for 324 patients with a serum concentration of less than 6 g/ml (median survival, 36 months). The lower curve (*dotted line*) is for 224 patients with higher serum levels (median survival, 22 months; $p < 0.0001$). (Salmon SE, Tesh D, Crowley J, et al. Chemotherapy is superior to sequential hemibody irradiation for remission consolidation in multiple myeloma: A Southwest Oncology study. J Clin Oncol 1990;8:1575–1584)

x-ray evaluation before therapy should include a complete metastatic survey, because myelomatous involvement can be located in any area of the axial or appendicular skeleton. Isotopic bone scans are of little or no value for myeloma and are not recommended. Bone marrow involvement should be assessed initially with an aspirate and a core bone marrow biopsy. Caution is needed to avoid excessive pressure on the needle when the needle is inserted, because in some myeloma patients, the bone matrix is extremely fragile. Follow-up bone marrow specimens are obtained to confirm remission status after therapy and to explain an unexpected pancytopenia. Marrow involvement with myeloma is usually diffuse, but occasionally it is spotty and may be subject to sampling error for needle aspiration but usually not for core biopsy. "Dry taps" on aspirates can be due to needle placement within a plasmacytoma. Table 56–6 summarizes a useful schedule for obtaining initial and follow-up studies in myeloma patients.

M-component production usually correlates with tumor burden in myeloma patients, and its serial assessment usually provides an excellent guide to the response to treatment or disease progression. Objective response criteria should identify patients who have achieved significant tumor regression and separate them from patients who have only stabilized or who have had symptomatic improvement without having achieved remission status. In 1973, the Leukemia-Myeloma Task Force of the NCI published the criteria for response in myeloma, which required a 50% reduction in the serum or urinary levels of an M-component to define remission.[210] Although the task force criteria were created to identify groups of patients responsive to treatment, they were developed before the acquisition of detailed knowledge of Ig metabolism. Analysis of Ig metabolism led to the recognition that for the major classes of IgG (IgG1, IgG2, and IgG4, which comprise 90% of serum IgG), metabolism is not linear with the serum concentration.[211] With a relatively high serum IgG M-component value, the half-life of IgG may be as short as 8 to 10 days, but with a low value, the half-life may be 40 days or longer. This concentration-dependent phenomenon applies to IgG M-component levels in 90% of patients with IgG myeloma or approximately 50% of all myeloma cases. Comparisons of serum levels in these patients underestimate the degree of change, depending on the initial and follow-up serum M-protein values.[2] Correction can be made for changes in the metabolic rate for IgG through the calculation of a synthetic index from the serum values.[212] A useful nomogram for this purpose has been derived from the metabolic equations.[2] A nomogram with an extended scale for IgG values appears in Figure 56–8.

Assessment of urinary light chain excretion is affected significantly by the degree of catabolism that takes place in the kidney, which is a function of the absolute levels of light chains passing the glomerulus and the degree of renal functional impairment.[192] To avoid difficulties in assessment, criteria for improvement in Bence Jones proteinuria must be quite stringent. The response criteria adopted by SWOG are summarized in Table 56–7. Response in accord with the SWOG criteria is strongly correlated with improvement in survival. When these criteria are applied, reduction in the synthetic index of serum M-proteins to less than 10% of control levels is associated with a better survival than if reduction is 10% to 24%, which is better than a reduction to 24% to 50% of control

TABLE 56–6. Checklist of Laboratory Studies for Patients With Multiple Myeloma

Routine Pretreatment Evaluation

Complete blood count, differential, and platelets
Serum protein electrophoresis
Serum immunoglobulins (nephelometry)
Serum β_2-microglobulin
24-h urine for total protein and electrophoresis
Antigenic typing of serum and urine monoclonal Igs by immunofixation or immunoelectrophoresis
Bone marrow aspiration and biopsy
Serum creatinine
Serum calcium
Serum electrolytes
Serum uric acid
Liver functions
Chest radiograph
Skeletal x-ray survey (entire skeleton)
Electrocardiogram

Specialized Studies for Selected Patients

Abdominal fat pad or rectal biopsy for amyloid (also tap joint effusions for amyloid)
Solitary lytic lesion, soft tissue or lymph node biopsy
Serum viscosity if IgM component present or if any serum M-component > 7.0 g/dl
Plasma volume if serum relative viscosity > 4.0
Myelogram (or in some instances MRI) if paraspinal mass or symptoms and signs of spinal cord or nerve root compression. (Spinal fluid should be sent for cell count, cytospin differential, glucose, and protein.)

Routine Follow-Up Studies

Before every course of treatment
  CBC, differential, platelets (should be repeated to check nadirs on first few courses)
At least every 3 months (and on completion of induction or change to alternative therapy for refractory patients)
  Serum monoclonal Ig by nephelometry or electrophoresis
  24-h urine protein electrophoresis (if Bence Jones protein present)
  Serum chemistry panel
At least annually
  Skeletal x-ray survey (entire skeleton), chest film, serum β_2-microglobulin
  Bone marrow aspiration if any significant abnormality in blood counts, Igs, or new symptoms
  Serum Igs (nephelometry)

values. Lesser degrees of reduction in tumor burden are not associated with improvement in survival. Patients whose hemoglobin, renal function, and albumin levels improve have a better outcome than if the clinical variables remain unchanged or worsen. Responsive patients have improvement in general well-being and in ambulation, and they have marked relief of symptoms of bone pain. However, recalcification of osteolytic bone lesions is observed in fewer than 5% of patients who respond to chemotherapy.

A retrospective analysis of 69 stage II and 80 stage III myeloma patients treated at a single institution was evaluated with Myeloma Task Force and SWOG response criteria.[213] In

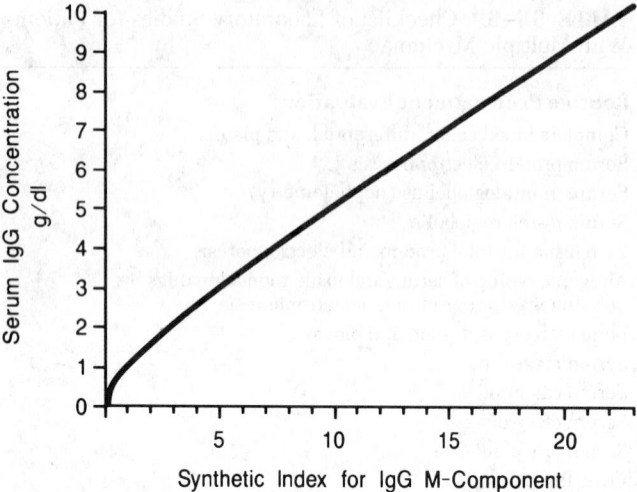

FIGURE 56–8. Nomogram for determining the synthetic index for IgG M-components of subclasses IgG1, IgG2, and IgG4, which comprise 90% of IgG myelomas. Using the patient's initial serum IgG concentration (g/dl) on the vertical axis, read down from the line to the horizontal axis to determine the synthetic index for that IgG value (Syn1). The same procedure is followed for the follow-up value (Syn2). Syn2/Syn1 × 100 = % of baseline synthetic index and tumor burden. This nomogram corrects for concentration-dependent changes in M-component synthesis and myeloma cell mass and gives a more accurate assessment of changes in tumor burden in IgG myeloma than can be calculated directly from the serum levels. The nomogram is not required for IgG3, IgA, IgD, or IgM serum M components, and changes in serum values for these Igs can be used directly to determine the percent change in tumor burden. The equation used to develop this nomogram has been incorporated into a program for a pocket calculator to calculate tumor cell mass. (Salmon SE, Wampler SE. Multiple myeloma: Quantitative staging and assessment of response with a programmable pocket calculator. Blood 1977;49:379–389)

TABLE 56–7. SWOG Myeloma Response Criteria

A. Responsive patients who satisfy all of the following criteria are considered to have achieved definite objective improvement.

A sustained decrease in the synthesis index of serum M protein to 25%, or less, of the pretreatment value on at least two measurements separated by 4 wk. For IgA and IgG3 M-proteins, the synthetic index is the same as the serum concentration. For IgG M-proteins of subclasses 1, 2, and 4, the synthetic index must be estimated using the nomogram shown in Figure 47-6.

A sustained decrease in 24-h urine globulin to 10%, or less, of the pretreatment value, and to less than 0.2 g/24 h on at least two occasions separated by 4 wk.

In all responsive patients the size and number of lytic skull lesions must not increase, and the serum calcium must remain normal. Correction of anemia (hematocrit > 27 vol. %) and hypoalbuminemia (>3.0 g/dl) is required if they are considered to be secondary to myeloma.

With equivocal data (*e.g.*, nonsecretors, L chain producers for whom the pretreatment urine collection was lost), the following support the conclusion that an objective response has occurred:

Recalcification of lytic skull lesions.

Significant increments in depressed normal immunoglobulins (*e.g.*, increments >200 mg/dl IgM, >400 mg/dl IgA, and >4000 mg/dl IgG).

B. Improved patients show a decline in the serum M-protein synthesis rate to less than 50%, but not less than 25% of the pretreatment value.

C. Unresponsive patients fail to satisfy the criteria for responsive or improved patients.

(Alexanian R, Bonnet J, Gehan E, et al. Combination chemotherapy for multiple myeloma. Cancer 1972;30:382–389)

carrying out this analysis, 2 stage II patients and 9 stage III patients who failed to live 3 months were censored to minimize the "guarantee time" inherent in including early deaths as nonresponders by usual statistical methods. The researchers concluded from this analysis of a relatively small series of patients that the Myeloma Task Force criteria of response may have similar predictive value to that of the SWOG for stage II patients. They found that the SWOG criteria had greater predictive value for stage III patients but believed that the latter difference was of questionable significance. Further analysis of significantly larger patient populations is warranted to authenticate the association of M-component reduction and tumor regression in multiple myeloma.

RADIATION THERAPY

Palliation for Bone Pain and Soft Tissue Masses

Radiation therapy has been recognized for many years as a rapid and highly effective palliative agent in the treatment of multiple myeloma.[225–229] Despite advances in the systemic treatment of this disease, radiation therapy continues to be important. It has been estimated that almost 70% of all patients eventually require and potentially benefit from treatment with irradiation.[230]

Treatment of painful, disabling bony sites is usually rapidly successful because of the radioresponsive nature of myeloma.

In addition to rapid relief of pain, with accompanying decrease in narcotic requirements, pain relief allows patients to maintain much more normal activity, reducing the structural weakness in bone caused by calcium loss from bedrest. Because treatment is often rapidly effective at relatively modest doses, irradiation can arrest local tumor progression in bone and prevent pathologic fractures, minimizing the morbidity of more invasive therapeutic interventions for these patients. These positive features of irradiation enable a much more normal functional existence for patients.[225–228]

Myeloma is usually quite responsive to radiation therapy, and tumor doses of approximately 2000 to 2400 cGy in five to seven fractions over 1 to 1.5 weeks are usually sufficient.[226,228] Relief of pain is obtained in more than 90% of treated patients.[230,231] From 30% to 65% of responses are complete.[230] An analysis of 100 patients treated at the University of Arizona demonstrated no increase in response probability with doses greater than 1500 cGy. Limited numbers of sites were treated with lower doses. Neither the probability of recurrent symptoms nor the time to relapse at the treated site was influenced by the radiation dose. Except for solitary disease, higher doses have not been advantageous, and because of the generalized nature of the disease and its relatively long natural history, higher doses may preclude a necessary second course of treatment to a site caused by tumor reseeding, extension, or regrowth.

Careful treatment planning is necessary to ensure inclusion

of the entire lesion(s) responsible to the localized problem, and imaging studies such as computed tomography (CT) scans may be helpful in delineating the extent of tumor.

Judgment and experience are necessary in determining when radiation therapy is appropriate (versus systemic treatment), especially early in the course of this often chronic condition. Although irradiation relieves the most disabling symptom(s), a similar result often can be achieved by chemotherapy, especially early in the course of myeloma, with no resultant compromise in future delivery of chemotherapy because of myelosuppression. This is particularly true in the treatment of sites containing considerable bone marrow, such as the pelvis. A Cancer and Leukemia Group B (CALGB) study that attempted "total bone marrow" treatment by sequential irradiation in combination with chemotherapy was not beneficial.[232] Recirculation of myeloma into previously treated sites may partially explain the negative study.[233] Ideal management requires close coordination with the physician administering the patient's systemic chemotherapy.

Structural changes brought about by tumor involvement may, by nerve compression or orthopedic instability, be responsible for a substantial portion of a patient's pain. It is usually a mistake to treat a patient with multiple myeloma to progressively higher doses than those previously used if some level of pain persists, assuming that careful prior imaging studies and treatment planning have been accomplished.

Special Indications for Radiation Therapy

Several other localized manifestations of myeloma may be indications for palliative irradiation, especially in the patient who has proved resistant to most conventional systemic agents. Included are patients who present with proptosis caused by sphenoid or orbital bone involvement, those who present with dental or facial abnormalities caused by maxillary or mandibular involvement, or those who present with CNS symptoms caused by extensive calvarial or base of the skull involvement. A treatment philosophy and approach similar to that for palliation of bone pain is appropriate.

CHEMOTHERAPY

Systemic Chemotherapy

The initial approach to treatment for most patients with symptoms and signs of progressive disease is with systemic chemotherapy. Cycle-nonspecific cytotoxic drugs, particularly alkylating agents, represent the current mainstay of standard therapy.

Bifunctional alkylating agents, particularly melphalan and cyclophosphamide; nitrosoureas, including carmustine and lomustine (CCNU); doxorubicin; and glucocorticoids represent the major active agents used in systemic therapy for multiple myeloma.[23,26,27,214,215] Vincristine has been used in several treatment programs; although there is evidence it can reduce tumor burden somewhat, there is no indication that its addition to other drugs increases survival.[216–218] INF-α has antitumor activity in myeloma and is currently under investigation to determine whether it can play a role with other systemic agents in the drug-sensitive phase of disease.[219–224] All of these agents have been subjected to clinical trials as single agents

in myeloma and have been incorporated into various drug combinations for evaluation in previously untreated patients.

Remission-Induction Chemotherapy

ALKYLATING AGENTS WITH OR WITHOUT PREDNISONE. A variety of simple alkylating agent—prednisone combinations and more complex regimens have been used for remission induction for patients with multiple myeloma. Overall objective response rates in various series using single alkylating agents alone or in combination with prednisone usually are 20% to 70%, and the rates are influenced by the response criteria used and the aggressiveness with which the regimens can be administered because of their myelosuppressive effects. Prednisone and other glucocorticoids have been combined with alkylating agents because of their single-agent activity, lack of overlapping toxicity, and the suggestion that they may potentiate the action of other agents. In most instances, patients in these trials received maintenance chemotherapy after remission induction.

Many studies used a variety of schedules of oral administration of melphalan or cyclophosphamide alone or in combination with prednisone, with generally similar therapeutic results. Useful dosage schedules for the commonly used alkylating agents appear in Table 56–8. Dosage adjustments for myelosuppression are commonly employed, but dose escalation in the absence of myelosuppression is not usually followed satisfactorily. Inadequate dose escalation (particularly with melphalan) can produce significant underdosing. Melphalan has variable absorption by the oral route, and the drug is best absorbed when ingested on an empty stomach.[234] Although oral absorption is not usually a problem with oral cyclophosphamide or CCNU, regular monitoring of the leukocyte count and differential count can detect patients with compliance problems with the self-administration of oral agents. Nadir absolute granulocyte counts below 2000/μl should be achieved between intermittent courses of therapy, but with continuous courses, the dosage should be adjusted to

TABLE 56–8. Selected Schedules Using Intermittent or Continuous Schedules of Alkylating Agents for Treatment of Myeloma Alone or in Combination With Prednisone

---

Intermittent Schedules

Cyclophosphamide
- I.V. 1000 mg/m² (27 mg/kg) q 3 weeks
  (Significantly higher doses now being evaluated)
- Oral 250 mg/m² per d × 4d q 3 wk

Melphalan
- I.V. 16 mg/m² q 2 wk × 4 then q 4 wk
  Reduce initial dosing by 50% if serum creatinine > 2.0 mg/dl (BUN > 30 mg/dl)
- Oral 8 mg/m² q 3 wk or 9 mg/m² q 4 wk
  (Because of varying bioavailability of oral melphalan, the dose must be increased to induce hematologic toxicity or significant underdosing may occur.)

Carmustine (BCNU)
- I.V. 100–150 mg/m² q 4–6 wk

Lomustine (CCNU)
- Oral 130 mg/m² q 4–6 wk

---

maintain the leukocyte count between 2000 and 3500/μl. Although intravenous schedules provide more predictable dose delivery, the largest experience has been with oral regimens.

Regardless of the dosage schedules or objective response rates in major clinical trials, the median survival time of patients receiving oral melphalan or cyclophosphamide alone or in combination with prednisone have ranged from 18 to 35 months, with an overall median of about 24 months (Table 56–9). Some "response rates" have varied because different criteria were used to determine objective response in the reported studies. Similar results have been observed with the nitrosoureas, although these agents have not been studied extensively.[26]

The survival outcome in myeloma patients is now clearly superior to that observed before the introduction of alkylating agents, when median survival times from diagnosis were in the range of 3.5 to 11.5 months.[235-237] The improvement in survival that occurred in myeloma after the introduction of the alkylating agents is due to these drugs, rather than to changes in earlier diagnosis or changes in supportive care. Equivalent therapeutic effects have been reported with intermittent and continuous schedules. An initial loading dose followed by a subsequent continuous dose, as used by the CALGB, produced similar results.[25] Intermittent schedules may have advantages in terms of assuring regular monitoring of the patient's progress and avoiding cumulative toxicity.

MULTIAGENT COMBINATION CHEMOTHERAPY. An area of continuing controversy for myeloma therapy is the comparative effectiveness of the simple oral melphalan plus prednisone (MP) or cyclophosphamide plus prednisone (CP) combinations with more complex regimens. Several institutions and cooperative groups have explored a variety of multiagent combinations, with a subset of these studies reporting significantly better survival results than have been observed with the simple combinations; however, this is far from uniform. Multiagent combinations incorporate agents with different mechanisms of action, little or no cross-resistance, and reduced overlapping toxicities, enabling greater cytoreduction of the myeloma cell burden. Some experimental evidence suggests that combinations of alkylating agents may be potentiating because there are different mechanisms of membrane uptake and other potential differences in their mode of action and cellular cytotoxicity.[245]

Some of the most widely used multiagent combinations include the M2 protocol developed at Memorial Sloan-Kettering Cancer Center[246] and the alternating combination chemotherapy regimens developed by SWOG.[190] In the initial SWOG report of alternating combinations, vincristine, melphalan, carmustine, and prednisone (VMCP) was alternated with vincristine, carmustine, doxorubicin, and prednisone (VBAP) or vincristine, cyclophosphamide, doxorubicin, and prednisone (VCAP).[190] In subsequent trials, the alternation has been limited to VMCP and VBAP, because VBAP can reinduce remission in myeloma patients who have previously responded and relapsed from therapy with melphalan or cyclophosphamide combinations.[247] The dosage schedules for these Memorial Sloan-Kettering and SWOG combination programs are summarized in Table 56–10. The fifth Medical Research Council's (MRC5) trial of alternating combination chemotherapy used

TABLE 56–9. Effects of Some Major Trials of Single Alkylating Agents Alone or in Combination With Prednisone on Survival in Multiple Myeloma

Investigations	Treatment* (Alkylating Agent Scheduled)	No. of Patients	Response Rate†	Median Survival From Start of Therapy (mo)
Alexanian et al[238]	Melphalan (i)	82	49–59	23
Alexanian et al[239]	Melphalan (d)	35	17–19	18
	Melphalan, prednisone (i)	79	~65	24
Bergsagel et al[21]	Melphalan (d)	165	14	25
Bergsagel et al[189]	Melphalan, prednisone (i)	100	72	28
Costa et al[25]	Melphalan (d)	60	~25	26
	Melphalan, prednisone (d)	71	~48	35
	Melphalan, prednisone + testosterone (d)	58	~54	24
Hoogstraten et al[240]	Melphalan (d)	64	45	23
Hoogstraten et al[241]	Melphalan (i)	48	45	26
Korst et al[22]	Cyclophosphamide (d)	165	~48	24.5
McArthur et al[237]	Melphalan (d)	39	41	28
MRC 1st study[242]	Melphalan (d)	133	NR	18
	Cyclophosphamide (d)	141	NR	18
MRC 2nd study[243]	Melphalan, prednisone (d)	128	NR	20
	Cyclophosphamide (d)	124	NR	20
MRC 3rd study[244]	Melphalan (i)	179	NR	20
	Cyclophosphamide (i) (intravenous)	174	NR	26

* d, daily; i, intermittent; NR, not reported.
† Response rates shown with Myeloma Task Force Criteria or approximated from published data.

TABLE 56–10. Dosage Schedules for the M2, VMCP–VBAP, and ABCM Regimens

Drug Regimen	Vincristine	Melphalan	Cyclophosphamide	BCNU	Doxorubicin	Prednisone
M2 regimen[246]	0.03 mg/kg day 1	0.25 mg/kg days 1–7	10 mg/kg day 1	0.5 mg/kg day 1		1 mg/kg days 1–7
VMCP[190]	1.0 mg day 1	6 mg/m²/d days 1–4	125 mg/m²/d days 1–4			60 mg/m²/d days 1–4
VBAP[190]	1.0 mg day 1			30 mg/m² day 1	30 mg/m² day 1	
ABCM[248]		6 mg/m²/d days 1–4	100 mg/m²/d days 1–4	30 mg/m² day 1	30 mg/m² day 1	days 1–4

As currently used, the M2 protocol is usually repeated at 4- to 5-wk intervals. The VMCP–VBAP program repeats courses of chemotherapy in 21-day cycles using either a direct alternation of the two regimens or a syncopated alternation wherein VMCP is used for three cycles followed by VBAP for three cycles with similar therapeutic results by either of these schedules. Currently an every-3-week alternation is used. The MRC has used an almost identical schedule to VMCP–VBAP in their alternating program, except that vincristine and prednisone have been deleted. Alternations are also at 3-wk intervals in the MRC's ABCM program.

drug dosages that were essentially identical with that of SWOG, with the deletion of vincristine and prednisone (see Table 56–10).[248]

Slight changes in dosages of the M2 regimen have been used in various series.[206] With the M2 regimen, improved survival has been reported in a nonrandomized study, in which survival was calculated from the date of diagnosis rather than from the onset of therapy.[246] Subsequent randomized studies carried out by the Eastern Cooperative Group (ECOG) in the United States and by a multihospital group from Denmark compared the M2 regimen to melphalan and prednisone.[249,250] Both studies failed to show a survival advantage with the M2 regimen, although good-risk subsets in the ECOG study had improved survival.[249] An update on the ECOG study reported improved survival for stage III patients.[247]

Two successive studies carried out by SWOG compared the alternating combination regimens to a simpler regimen of MP or vincristine, cyclophosphamide, plus prednisone (VCP). In both studies (evaluated by different study coordinators), quite similar advantages in terms of improved response rate and improved median survival were observed with the alternating combination compared with the simpler regimen.[190,251] Results of the first of these studies were reanalyzed in 1985, again demonstrating a survival advantage of alternating combination chemotherapy over MP.[190,251] The second of SWOG's evaluations of alternating combinations demonstrated remarkably similar survival plots for the VMCP plus VBAP compared with the simpler VCP regimen. Analysis of pretreatment prognostic factors showed that the treatment groups were quite comparable. A significantly larger proportion of patients responded to the alternating combinations, suggesting that the additional responsive patients may have required combination therapy to reach remission status and could be anticipated to have had a poorer prognosis and below average remission duration. Analysis of the data on high-risk stage III patients in some studies supports this interpretation and is consistent with the overall remission duration in the VMCP-VBAP group being diluted with the addition of poor-risk patients "recruited into" the responsive category with the aggressive combina-

tions who would not have achieved remission with the simple regimens.[246]

A similar interpretation may apply to studies from ECOG and the CALGB, who found improved response rates, survival time, or both in specific subsets of patients with multiagent combinations compared with the MP regimen.[249,252] In these two studies, overall survival for all patients was not improved, suggesting that the increased toxicity of the aggressive regimens may have a detrimental effect on survival of subsets of patients. The MRC study made a similar observation to that by SWOG. In the MRC study, 627 patients were randomized to receive almost identical schedules of the cytotoxic agents used in the SWOG VMCP-VBAP studies, except that vincristine and prednisone were omitted. The MRC study compared alternating MC and BA to M in a study begun in 1982 and closed in 1986. In the MRC's study, the survival advantage for the 314 patients receiving the alternating combinations was significantly superior ($p=0.0003$) to that obtained with M alone.[248] Curves for the MRC5 study are similar to the SWOG results despite the omission of vincristine and prednisone. The MRC's comparison of ABCM to M is significantly larger than the SWOG study or other studies comparing multiagent chemotherapy to M or MP.[248] A summary of results from these studies appear in Table 56–11.

Other multicenter randomized trials using VMCP-VBAP or variants of the M2 protocol (VBMCP) failed to show better results than simpler regimens (Table 56–12).[253] Comparison of the different trials is difficult because of different prognostic factors, differences in the treatments used, and differences in dose modifications and other factors. Several studies compared sequential administration of various alkylating agents with simultaneous combinations or MP (data not shown). These studies showed inferiority or no advantage for the sequential regimens.[188,252] Although there are discrepancies between multiagent and simpler regimens in various trials, none of these regimens are curative or control the disease for 4 years or longer. Therefore newer therapeutic approaches are needed.

Although INF-α is known to have some activity in mye-

TABLE 56–11. Results of Recent Alternating Combination Chemotherapy Regimens Used for Remission Induction in Multiple Myeloma in Multicenter Randomized Trials

Investigations*	Treatment	No. of Patients	% Responding† (mo)	Median Survival
SWOG Alternating Combinations vs MP or VCP				
Study 7704[190,251]	VMCP + VBAP or VCAP	160	54	42
	MP	77	32	23
Study 7927[251]	VMCP + VBAP	93	54	48
	VCP	107	28	29
MRC Alternating Combination vs M				
Myelomatosis V[248]	ABCM	314	61	32
	M	316	59	24

* In these studies, patients had a statistically significant improvement in survival with alternating combination chemotherapy as compared with melphalan or MP therapy.
† Response criteria varied between SWOG and the MRC groups but were consistent within each group's trial.

loma patients in relapse, the recombinant forms of IFN-α have had only limited study in previously untreated patients.[219–222,259–261] In an initial report, 7 of 14 patients with previously untreated myeloma with stages I or II myeloma responded to treatment.[223] The response was associated with an increase in residual polyclonal immunoglobulins. However, two randomized trials comparing initial therapy with IFN-α to chemotherapy have shown IFN-α monotherapy to be less active than standard chemotherapy.[262,263] Recombinant IFN-α has also been integrated into combination chemotherapy with alkylating agent and prednisone combinations.[224] On the basis of the initial experience with this approach, the CALGB

TABLE 56–12. Results With Combination Chemotherapy Regimens Used for Remission Induction in Multiple Myeloma in Multicenter Randomized Trials That Failed to Show a Survival Advantage With Multiagent Chemotherapy Compared With Simple Alkylating Agent Regimens

Investigations	Treatment	No. of Patients	% Response (mo)	Median Survival
Argentine[255]	MeCCMVP	105	46	41
	MP	129	38	39
CALGB[254]	MCBP (I.V.)	156	56	29
	MCBPA (I.V.)	157	44	26
	MP (I.V.)	146	47	33
Canadian[189]	MCBP	116	47*	31
	MP	125	31*	28
Danish[250]	M2	31	45	21
	VMP	32	73	30
	MP	33	58	21
ECOG[256]	M2	134	74	~31
	MP	131	53	~30
Finnish[257]	MOCCA	64	75	41
	MP	66	54	45
Norwegian[258]	M2	33	74	33
	MP	34	67	33
SECSG[256]	BCP	186	49	36
	MP	187	52	36
Italian[253]	VMCP-VBAP	158	77	32
	MP	146	64	37

MeC, methyl-CCNU; B, BCNU; C, cyclophosphamide; V, vincristine; P, prednisone; A, doxorubicin (Adriamycin); MOCCA, melphalan, vincristine, CCNU, cyclophosphamide, doxorubicin.
* SWOG response criteria (all others reported by Myeloma Task Force Criteria).

initiated a randomized trial comparing the effectiveness of MP to MP plus recombinant IFN-α2.[261] There appears to be no advantage to using aggressive regimens in treatment of stage I patients. The major issue is whether any therapy should be employed until clear evidence of symptomatic disease progression occurs. Application of additional prognostic factors, such as the pretreatment β_2-microglobulin level or evaluation of the proliferative index of myeloma cells, may assist in better identifying the patient groups most likely to benefit from aggressive systemic therapy.

TUMOR CELL REDUCTION WITH INDUCTION CHEMOTHERAPY. The magnitude of tumor cell reduction with chemotherapy can be assessed using the quantitative methods to determine response in terms of the degree of cytoreduction achieved. For myeloma, this was first achieved using a computer-based method in which serial measurements of the amount of M-component produced per cell in vitro, intravascular mass of M-components, and catabolic rate were integrated.[2,170] For the current standard treatment programs and magnitude of cell death determined from M-component-derived measurements, the maximal degree of cytoreduction observed in patients treated with conventional chemotherapy rarely exceeds 90% to 99%. Despite continued treatment, the tumor burden appears to plateau in most cases.[170] Kinetic analysis of the plateau-phase population suggests that the residual tumor cells behave differently from those present before treatment, and they are comparatively hypoproliferative and perhaps less responsive to cytotoxic chemotherapy.[209]

With a total tumor burden in most patients in the range of 10^{12} myeloma cells or more, it is not surprising that there is not a strong correlation between the exact magnitude of cytoreduction (*e.g.,* 75%, 90%, 99%) and overall survival. However, remission durations after induction chemotherapy can vary substantially in comparably staged patients with similar degrees of apparent cytoreduction and the presence of a clearly measurable residual M-component peak in the serum. Although the median duration of unmaintained remission is 11 months, unmaintained remissions after induction chemotherapy in some patients with stage III myeloma may last for 5 years or longer.[264,265] This suggests that there is an alteration in the residual myeloma cell population or in the tumor-host relation. Such observations provide the basis for seriously questioning whether the residual cell mass determined from M-component levels in remission reflects the initial population of malignant plasma cells or a less malignant population more akin to that in patients with MGUS. However, patients regularly relapse with overt myeloma from unmaintained remissions, indicating that an underlying highly malignant monoclone persists but may be submerged under a population of less highly proliferative M-component-secreting cells.

Analysis of the myeloma regrowth rate based on M-component doubling times has been carried out for patients studied sequentially after a series of unmaintained remissions.[169] Even in the presence of continued chemosensitivity (as reflected by cytoreduction after reinstitution of chemotherapy), some patients studied developed a progressive shortening of the M-component doubling time during subsequent unmaintained remissions. Such observations suggest progressive loss of growth control with the emergence of a kinetically more aggressive tumor cell population.

Remission Maintenance Versus Unmaintained Remission

Therapeutic approaches in myeloma have usually been developed in an analogous fashion to those for other advanced neoplasms and have included remission-induction phase and remission-maintenance phase treatments. Myeloma patients who exhibit drug sensitivity and achieve remission usually have been maintained on a similar form of chemotherapy until the time of relapse.

The usefulness of maintenance therapy with cytotoxic drugs has been examined in several studies with similar results.[264,266–268] Patients achieving remission with chemotherapy were randomized to maintenance chemotherapy with MP or to no maintenance therapy. Patients randomized to no maintenance received alkylating agent chemotherapy again at the earliest evidence of relapse as manifested by a rise in M-component levels or recurrent symptoms and signs of active myeloma. There was no overall survival advantage for patients receiving maintenance chemotherapy. Continuation of conventional alkylating agent therapy for patients achieving remission appears to offer no obvious advantage over unmaintained remission, as long as patients are followed closely and have treatment reinstituted when there is laboratory or clinical evidence of reactivation of myeloma. In general, patients followed in unmaintained remission should be followed monthly, with regular monitoring of serum and urine M-components to detect the first signs of relapse. Patients presenting initially with stage III myeloma with heavy Bence Jones proteinuria or amyloidosis must be followed closely, because fulminant relapse from unmaintained remission can lead to irreversible complications unless treatment is reinstituted promptly at the first sign of disease reactivation.

An approach to remission maintenance that used recombinant IFN-α was reported by the Italian Multiple Myeloma Study Group.[269,270] In this study, 70 patients with remissions induced with MP or VMCP-VBAP (on a randomized induction) were re-randomized to maintenance therapy with recombinant IFN-α2 or to no treatment. The IFN-α2 was administered at a dosage of 3×10^6 IU/m^2 subcutaneously three times weekly. After 27 months of follow-up, 8 (24%) of 33 of evaluable patients receiving IFN-α2 and 22 (59%) of 37 patients with no maintenance had relapsed, with a significant difference ($p<0.01$) in the actuarial curves of remission duration in the two groups.[270] A larger study of IFN maintenance conducted by the SWOG with over 200 patients randomized to interferon maintenance or observation using 3×10^6 of IFNα2 given intravenously with the same schedule showed no advantage of IFNα2 over unmaintained remission for remission duration or survival.[271] Further follow-up of these two studies and several other interferon maintenance studies are required before the role for IFN maintenance can be established.

SOLITARY PLASMACYTOMA OF BONE AND EXTRAMEDULLARY PLASMACYTOMA

About 7% of all patients with plasma cell malignancies present with solitary lesions in bone or soft tissues, with bone marrow examinations demonstrating fewer than 5% plasmacytes. Several factors differentiate patients with solitary lesions from those with multiple myeloma. Age at presentation tends to be younger, and a higher percentage are male (70% versus 55%). A smaller fraction (30% versus 97%) present with serum or urinary M-components.

The demonstration that an elevation in M-component may persist after high-dose local irradiation, but may return to normal with subsequent long-term disease-free survival after nonradical surgical excision of Waldeyer's ring material, suggests two alternative possibilities for the response of certain malignant plasma cells to irradiation. One alternative is that a substantial population of cells in certain patients is highly resistant to irradiation. However, several factors mitigate against this explanation, especially the long disease-free survival after a nonradical surgical approach. Because of the monoclonal nature of the disease in these patients and their generally excellent response to irradiation, it seems more likely that these persistent cells represent clonogenically nonviable foci that fail to manifest radiation damage because they divide slowly or not at all. Such behavior is somewhat analogous to functioning pituitary adenomas in which elevated hormone levels may be observed for months or years after radiation therapy without evidence of ultimate progression.

Several studies have shown a relatively favorable course for both these groups of patients, but many long-term studies have demonstrated the distinct difference in ultimate prognosis between patients with solitary lesions in bone and those with extramedullary lesions.[272–275,277] Although they experience significantly longer survivals than patients with classic multiple myeloma, virtually all patients with solitary bone lesions develop systemic disease if followed for sufficient periods.[272–275] In one study, although almost 35% of patients were progression-free at 10 years, by 13 years, more than 90% of patients experienced widespread evidence of disease.[274] The report by Chak and coworkers is slightly more optimistic.[276] More than 80% of patients treated for extramedullary lesions are progression free at periods exceeding 10 years after treatment.[272–274,277]

Despite this difference in ultimate prognosis, long-term survival is observed in substantial numbers in both groups and suggests the desirability for long-term local control. Radiation doses of 3500 to 5000 cGy have been proposed, with doses at the lower end of this spectrum usually applied with shortened treatment times and increased daily radiation fractions. We favor a total dose of 4500 to 5000 cGy in 4.5 to 5 weeks,

using megavoltage fields that adequately encompass necessary soft tissue and bony structures. In primary bony lesions, the entire medullary cavity of the bone must be encompassed, as in patients with Ewing's tumor because of the possibility of medullary cavity spread.

Few data are available on the probability of regional lymph node spread, and treatment of nodal sites, in addition to adequately encompassing of the primary lesion, usually is not recommended. The report of Knowling and associates suggests that treatment may be of value in selected patients.[273] Typical survival curves after radiation treatment for these two groups of patients appear in Figure 56–9.[272–274,276,277]

IN VITRO TESTING OF CLONOGENIC MYELOMA CELLS

In vitro methods have been developed to support the growth of colony-forming neoplastic plasma cells from the bone marrows of some patients with multiple myeloma and to assess the response of the clonogenic myeloma cells to a variety of anticancer drugs.[59,278–281] Clonogenic growth of myeloma cells has been applied to in vitro drug testing by several laboratories.[278,279,281,282] At the Arizona Cancer Center, true-positive correlations between in vitro sensitivity and clinical response were obtained in 22 (79%) of 28 instances in which in vitro sensitivity was observed, and true-negative correlations with in vitro drug resistance were observed in 35 (99%) of 37 instances.[281] Although such findings suggest that this assay may have potentially broad application, it is still applicable to only a few of the patients tested, because of inadequate colony growth in many instances. Due to technical limitations, it is currently impractical to routinely test patients' myeloma cells for drug sensitivity. However, in the research setting, we continue to find this approach an aid in the discovery of new drugs with activity against myeloma cells and in identifying potentially active drugs for a selected subset of patients whose cells can be cultivated in vitro. New information on cytokines that support the growth of plasmacytoma cells and the use of more sensitive assays may increase the applicability of this approach to myeloma in the future.[61,63,283–285]

TREATMENT OF REFRACTORY MYELOMA

Patients who relapse after unmaintained remission can often be reinduced into remission with a regimen similar to that used initially and are not considered to be refractory to therapy

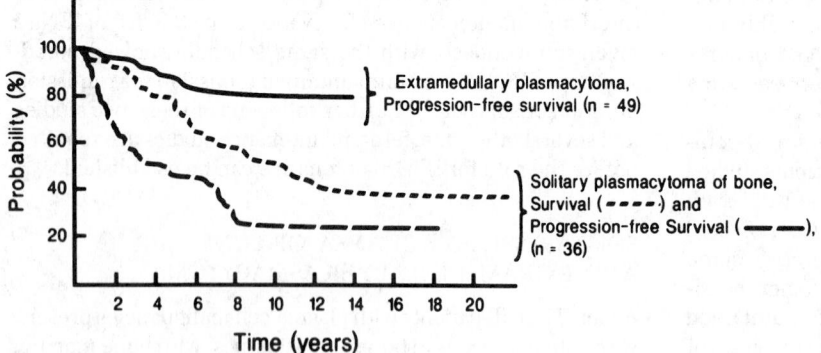

FIGURE 56–9. Survival and disease-free survival for patients with solitary plasmacytoma of bone and disease-free survival of those with solitary soft-tissue disease. Notice the significant advantage for those with soft tissue disease and low disease-free survival (in time) for those with bone disease.

unless they fail to achieve remission on reinduction.[264,286] However, at least one third of patients with multiple myeloma fail to respond to induction chemotherapy, and those who initially achieve remission eventually relapse and require additional treatment. Standard and new agents and approaches have been evaluated in refractory patients.[287,288] Therapeutic agents used for treatment of refractory patients usually include the same drugs used in initial remission-induction therapy (*e.g.*, anthracyclines, glucocorticoids, vinca alkaloids, alkylating agents, nitrosoureas), often given in alternative dosages, schedules, and combinations to those used initially. INF-α has activity as a phase II agent, but remissions are usually short, and IFN-α has yet to be integrated effectively into combination therapy for second-line therapy.[221,222,289-291]

It is important to differentiate between the two subsets of patients who are usually classified as refractory, because their prognoses differ substantially. For simplicity, refractory myeloma patients are usually divided into drug-resistant and relapsing groups. Patients who fail to respond to induction chemotherapy and are drug-resistant have the poorest overall prognosis, and only a few respond to alternate treatments. The second major category comprises relapsing patients who respond to induction chemotherapy but then relapse while still receiving chemotherapy or within a few months thereafter. They have a higher probability of responding to second-line therapy than do the drug-resistant patients.

High-Dose Glucocorticoids

The antitumor activity of single-agent prednisone for a high-dose, alternate-day schedule for resistant and relapsing patients was first reported over 20 years ago.[23] This single-agent activity of high doses of glucocorticoids has been confirmed and extended using prednisone and dexamethasone in alternate-day or pulse schedules.[214,287,292,293] High-dose dexamethasone recently has been studied in previously untreated patients with myeloma and has been found to be active when used as monotherapy.[293a] A P-glycoprotein-expressing multidrug-resistant myeloma cell line was reported to develop collateral sensitivity to glucocorticoids, suggesting that there may be some specificity of steroids for drug-resistant cells.[294] Overall, approximately 40% of resistant and relapsing myeloma patients achieve second remissions with glucocorticoids. Because glucocorticoids are nonmyelosuppressive, they are particularly useful in refractory patients with poor bone marrow reserves. In our experience, some pancytopenic patients have remissions of myeloma for several years with alternate-day prednisone alone. Efforts have been made to quantitate glucocorticoid receptors in myeloma, and these measurements may aid in identifying patients potentially sensitive to glucocorticoids.[295]

Combination Chemotherapy Regimens

Although there were a few initial favorable reports on combination regimens that included primarily alkylating agents, most reports have been less promising, with response rates in the range of 8% for resistant and 22% for refractory patients.[246,297-302] These regimens are far more active for reinducing remissions in patients who have disease reactivation from unmaintained remission.[264,286,303-305]

More favorable results have been obtained with doxorubicin-based combinations. Although doxorubicin alone exhibits activity in only 10% of patients, when combined with BCNU or with BCNU, vincristine, and prednisone (VBAP) or cyclophosphamide instead of vincristine, somewhat better results are obtained.[27,306-310] Approximately 30% of relapsing patients respond to these regimens, but only 10% of resistant patients respond. Although not all studies report the remission durations of responders or overall survival, the remission duration is usually less than 1 year. Significantly better results have been obtained by using the vincristine, doxorubicin, and dexamethasone (VAD) regimen developed at the M.D. Anderson Cancer Center.[311] Vincristine and doxorubicin are administered by continuous infusion over 4 days through an indwelling venous catheter, and dexamethasone is given orally (Table 56–13).

In an initial report, 14 (70%) of 20 patients with refractory myeloma responded to VAD, with a projected survival in excess of 1 year for responders.[311] Although granulocytopenia was only moderate, infection represented the most frequent complication, perhaps because of the large doses of dexamethasone used. In a follow-up report, VAD or dexamethasone were administered on a nonrandom basis to 85 refractory patients.[214] Among relapsing patients, 65% responded to VAD, but only 21% responded to dexamethasone alone. Among resistant patients, only 32% responded to VAD, a result quite similar to the 27% response rate observed with dexamethasone alone. This suggests that response to the VAD regimen in initially unresponsive patients is primarily due to the glucocorticoid in the regimen.[214] Similar therapeutic results have been confirmed with the VAD regimen by other investigators.[312-314] Toxicity has been the major limitation of the VAD regimen, with serious infection attributed primarily to the steroid program. Serious gastrointestinal toxicity, including gastric perforations, and steroid psychoses have been observed. Overall, approximately one third of patients receiving VAD develop moderate to severe toxic effects. Nonetheless, it appears to be the most effective treatment for myeloma relapses.

For patients with primary drug resistance, steroid alone is preferable to VAD. The multidrug resistance mechanism associated with P-glycoprotein expression appears to be frequently expressed by myeloma cells from patients with drug-resistant disease.[329-331] A novel means for reversing resistance to VAD has been reported for relapsing patients who previously

TABLE 56–13. Dosage Schedule for VAD Regimen

Vincristine	0.4 mg/d I.V. for 4 d
Doxorubicin	9 mg/m^2/d I.V. for 4 d
Dexamethasone	40 mg/d orally for 4 d beginning on days 1, 9, and 17 of the first 28-d cycle and on alternate cycles thereafter. On the other cycles dexamethasone is given only on days 1–4.

All patients also received cimetidine for antacid prophylaxis and trimethoprim—sulfamethoxazole as antiinfective prophylaxis.

(Barlogie B, Smith L, Alexanian R. Effective treatment of advanced multiple myeloma refractory to alkylating agents. N Engl J Med 1984;310:1353–1356)

responded to the VAD regimen and subsequently developed multidrug resistance associated with expression of the P-glycoprotein.[315] The P-glycoprotein was detected using a murine monoclonal antibody and by mRNA dot blot analysis. Five refractory myeloma patients were first treated with the VAD regimen, and at the time of relapse or failure to respond to VAD, the calcium channel blocker verapamil was administered at high dosage by continuous infusion along with VAD. Resistance was at least partially reversed in 2 patients, with improvement in M-component and hematologic values. In one patient whose myeloma cells were tested in vitro, verapamil exposure significantly increased intracellular accumulation of doxorubicin, suggesting a possible mechanism by which the verapamil effect was mediated. In a subsequent expansion of this trial, 5 (23%) of 22 VAD-refractory patients achieved remission again after high-dose intravenous verapamil was added to the VAD regimen.[316] However, verapamil is not a good agent to use as a chemosensitizer in myeloma patients, because it induces hypotension that can further compromise renal function in patients with Bence Jones proteinuria and impaired renal function. These studies provide proof that multidrug resistance can be circumvented, but better chemosensitizers are needed. Recently, cyclosporin also has been reported to reverse multidrug resistance when combined with the VAD regimen for use in VAD-resistant myeloma patients.[331a]

SYSTEMIC RADIATION THERAPY

Rider, Bergsagel, and colleagues were instrumental in pioneering wide-field or hemibody irradiation for systemic illness.[317,318] A variety of treatment schemes have been used, but in most, a radiation dose of 750 to 850 cGy in 150-cGy fractions (dose rate of ≥50 cGy/minute) is given to the hemibody (umbilicus used as midpoint) after pretreatment preparation with corticosteroids and antiemetics. Total-body approaches have also been used.[233] Patients have usually been a a poor-prognosis group with stage III disease, who have usually relapsed after first-line chemotherapy.[206] In most patients, the lower hemibody was treated initially. Approximately 50% to 75% of patients complete treatment to hemibody segments in most series.[317,318,320–325]

Because of the incidence of radiation pneumonitis in patients treated initially, cumulative lung doses have been reduced to 600 to 650 cGy (usually not corrected for air transmission) in more recently treated patients.[326] Although laboratory evidence of hematologic toxicity exists for most patients who have received treatment to the whole body, with some patients requiring platelet or erythrocyte transfusions, major clinical morbidity from hematologic toxicity has been moderate. In some instances, it can be prolonged. By using this irradiation approach, approximately half of all treated patients have experienced significant subjective relief.

Median survivals in irradiated patients have averaged 6 months, with mean survival times averaging 12 months. Some patients from this group have survived more than 18 months, and two reports documented more than 24 months of survival in several patients.[327,328]

In an attempt to use this treatment modality for better-prognosis patients, the SWOG carried out a phase III prospectively randomized trial (SWOG 8229/8230) in which previously untreated patients who achieved remission (≥75% tumor mass regression) randomized to maintenance chemotherapy or to sequential hemibody irradiation (750 cGy per five fields for 1 week) with 4 to 6 weeks or more elapsing between the two irradiation courses, depending on the severity and duration of hematologic toxicity.[206]

In the SWOG study, the survival outcome for patients receiving hemibody irradiation was significantly inferior to that of patients receiving maintenance chemotherapy. The difference in survival could be attributed to a shorter relapse-free survival with irradiation. Survival time from relapse to death was identical in both groups.[206,319] Myelosuppression was significantly more severe in patients receiving hemibody radiation therapy than those receiving maintenance chemotherapy. The primary toxicity was prolonged thrombocytopenia. These findings indicate that chemotherapy maintenance is more effective than hemibody irradiation for remission consolidation in myeloma patients who respond to induction chemotherapy.

HIGH-DOSE THERAPY ALONE OR WITH BONE MARROW TRANSPLANTATION

More aggressive approaches to the therapy of multiple myeloma use high-dose chemotherapy alone or high-dose chemotherapy with total-body irradiation and autologous or allogeneic bone marrow transplantation to overcome drug resistance to conventional-dose therapy.[332–346] The drug most commonly used in high doses has been melphalan, administered intravenously in doses ranging from 80 to 140 mg/m^2, without or with bone marrow or peripheral blood stem cell support. With high-dose melphalan alone, a high response rate is observed, including complete remissions associated with complete disappearance of the M-component and normalization of the bone marrow.[338] Unfortunately, the responses to high-dose melphalan alone among relapse patients have usually lasted only 3 months to 1 year. Toxicity has included profound myelosuppression, mucositis, diarrhea, nausea, and vomiting. Treatment-related deaths are not uncommon and are associated with host failure and severe hematologic toxicity. However, because the use of high-dose melphalan is still relatively new, further experience may provide a means to enhance efficacy and reduce toxicity (*e.g.*, with the use of myeloid colony-stimulating factors or by limitation of high-dose melphalan administration to patients with good performance status).

Prognostic factors associated with better outcome with autologous bone marrow transplantation in myeloma include the presence of drug-sensitive disease.[347] The addition of autologous bone marrow transplantation with or without purging has reduced the severity of myelosuppression. When total-body irradiation (usually 200 cGy twice daily for 3 days; total dose, 1200 cGy) delivered at a reduced dose rate (5–50 cGy/minute)) was combined with high-dose melphalan and autologous bone marrow transplantation, significantly longer remissions were observed.[339] In many instances, evidence of a residual M-component was still detected with immunofixation. Efforts to develop purging techniques to remove residual myeloma from the marrow are being attempted to enhance the potential of autologous transplantation. As an alternative to purging, autologous blood stem cells have been used for hematopoietic reconstitution.[348–353] The main limitation appears to be the difficulty of eradicating myeloma with the available preparative regimens for transplantation.

A promising study of 90 patients was published by the European Cooperative Group for Bone Marrow Transplantation.[354] This study showed good outcome for a significant fraction of patients receiving HLA-matched sibling donor marrow. The complete remission rate after marrow transplantation was 43% for all patients and 58% for patients with engraftment. The actuarial survival rate at 76 months was 76% (Fig. 56–10). Of 90 patients undergoing allogeneic bone marrow transplantation, 43% of all patients and 58% of patients who engrafted achieved complete remission. The median duration of relapse-free survival for complete remission patients was 48 months, and overall survival at 76 months was 40% (see Fig. 56–10). Allogeneic transplantation should be considered for selected patients younger than 55 who have an HLA-matched sibling donor.

ACTIVITY OF AGENTS IN PHASE II TRIALS

A few other antitumor agents have induced remissions in 10% or more of myeloma patients in relapse in phase II trials. These include pentostatin,[356] epirubicin, poly (I,C)-LC (an interferon inducer), peptichemio, and teniposide.[355,357-360] Except for the interferon inducer, these agents warrant additional investigation in refractory cases to better define their activity.

Other chemotherapeutic agents that have been subjected to phase II clinical trials in myeloma and found to have minimal activity (with less than a 10% response rate in refractory patients) include aclarubicin, acronine, amsacrine, bleomycin, cisplatin, chlorozotocin, cytarabine, diaziquone, etoposide, hexamethylmelamine, mitoxantrone, prednimustine, procarbazine, pyrazofurin, urethane, vindesine, fludarabine, or amonafide.[19,361-380] Although hexamethylmelamine appeared to exhibit greater than 10% activity, this was probably attributable to the concomitant use of glucocorticoids in the protocol.[381]

COMPLICATIONS AND SPECIAL PROBLEMS

RENAL FAILURE

In most studies, approximately 20% of patients with multiple myeloma present with renal failure, which adversely affects survival.[382] In one report, patients with stage IIIB myeloma had a median survival of only 4 months.[383] For patients who have normal or minimally impaired renal function, it is important to take actions that minimize the likelihood of subsequent development of renal failure. Myeloma patients should have a high fluid intake (*e.g.*, at least 2 L/day) to facilitate the excretion of calcium, Bence Jones proteins, uric acid, and other nephrotoxic excretory products. Patients with Bence Jones proteinuria and evidence of advanced or progressive myeloma should promptly be started on a chemotherapy regimen.

Adequate chemotherapy and hydration are important in managing myeloma patients with renal failure.[382] Administration of allopurinol with chemotherapy is a worthwhile precaution in stage III patients, at least for the first few courses of therapy. Patients with known myeloma should not be dehydrated for intravenous pyelography, and hypercalcemia and urinary tract infections should be treated promptly. The use of antibiotics with known nephrotoxicity (*e.g.*, the aminoglycosides) should be avoided if possible. Agents causing sustained hypotension and reduced renal blood flow should also be avoided. When melphalan is administered intravenously to patients in renal failure, increased myelosuppression has been observed.[384] Pharmacokinetic studies of intravenous melphalan in dogs and of oral administration in myeloma patients established that melphalan elimination is reduced by renal insufficiency.[385,386] Dose reductions are often needed for melphalan when it is administered intravenously, but because of the varying bioavailability of oral melphalan, dose reductions for renal failure may further compromise its therapeutic activity.

In the fourth MRC myeloma chemotherapy trial, management of renal failure was studied prospectively.[387] Of the 522 patients admitted to the trial, 80 had evidence of renal failure that persisted after an initial 24-hours of rehydration. Seventy-three of the 80 patients who had renal failure were maintained with a fluid intake of at least 3 L/day in addition to receiving chemotherapy. These patients were randomized to receive sodium bicarbonate or no supplement to render the urine pH neutral. The remaining 7 patients had congestive heart failure or required continued dialysis for oliguric renal failure and were not eligible for evaluation of oral fluid supplementation. Of 49 patients who survived more than 100 days, 39 achieved reversal of renal failure (18 complete, 21 partial). Death of 14 of the patients was directly attributable to renal failure rather than other complications or manifestations of myeloma. Patients who received bicarbonate did marginally better than those who did not. The survival outcome of patients with renal failure in the MRC's third myeloma trial appeared to be inferior to that obtained in the fourth trial, in which high fluid

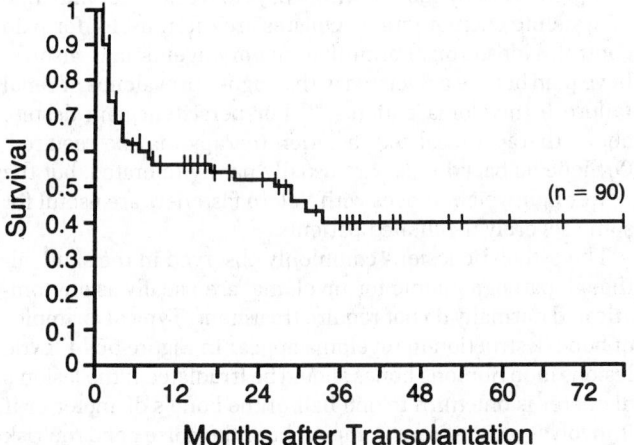

FIGURE 56–10. Actuarial survival after bone marrow transplantation for all 90 patients reported from the European Group for Bone Marrow Transplantation Registry as having allogeneic transplants performed for multiple myeloma. The actuarial survival at 76 months was 40%. The median duration of relapse-free survival among patients who were in complete remission after their transplants was 48 months. (Gahrton G, Sante T, Per L, et al. Allogeneic bone marrow transplantation in multiple myeloma. N Engl J Med 1992;325:1267–1273)

intake was mandated. This study showed that, in many cases, renal failure in myeloma can be reversed completely or partially by simple fluid administration, but in oliguric renal failure of myeloma, the glomeruli may open up after a period of dialysis.

Several of the patients who had improvement in renal function with these measures were subsequently able to lead more active lives. However, prolonged survival is not likely unless renal failure can be reversed rapidly.[388] For patients who have myeloma and signs of acute renal failure, dialysis is indicated.[389] Peritoneal and hemodialysis have been used successfully, but continued dialysis is not indicated for patients who have evidence of progressive myeloma while receiving chemotherapy.[390-392] Plasmapheresis can be of temporary benefit to myeloma patients who develop acute renal failure because of an inability to adequately excrete light chains. Plasmapheresis is tenfold more effective than peritoneal dialysis for this acute complication.[393-396] Renal transplantation has been carried out successfully for a patient responsive to chemotherapy.[397] Before considering renal transplantation, the patient's presenting stage, age, response to treatment, and prognosis must be considered in view of the eventual fatal outcome of the disease and the added morbidity and complexities of management associated with transplantation.

HYPERCALCEMIA

About one forth of multiple myeloma patients have hypercalcemia with a serum calcium concentration in excess of 11.5 mg/dl (after correction for the serum albumin), and a significant fraction of patients develop hypercalcemia in the refractory phase of myeloma.[398] The serum calcium concentration should be measured routinely as part of staging evaluation in the initial workup of all patients with myeloma. The physicians should suspect hypercalcemia if the patient complains of polyuria, constipation, nausea or vomiting, lethargy, or mental confusion or has signs of dehydration or coma. The symptoms and signs of hypercalcemia correlate well with the level of ionized calcium rather than with the total calcium level, although the ionized level usually cannot be conveniently measured. Patients with bone pain or fractures who are bedridden or immobilized are also prone to hypercalcemia, and every effort should be made to mobilize them as quickly as possible.

As in other settings of malignant disease in which hypercalcemia occurs, vigorous hydration and diuresis should be used as soon as hypercalcemia is recognized, and the patient should be started promptly on corticosteroid therapy (*e.g.*, 50–100 mg of prednisone per day), because steroids have a direct affect on myeloma cells and in blocking osteoclastic activity and reducing negative calcium balance. Hypercalcemia in newly diagnosed patients and those relapsing from unmaintained remission usually comes promptly under control with institution of systemic chemotherapy for myeloma. Additional useful agents to control severe hypercalcemia (*i.e.*, serum calcium >13.5 mg/dl) or to use for patients in whom fluids, diuretics, and steroids prove inadequate over several days include parenteral mithramycin, gallium nitrate, Pamidronate or other diphosphonates, and calcitonin. For severe hypercalcemia, Pamidronate is administered in a dose of 90 mg as a 24-hour infusion and is more effective than multiple daily doses of etidronate.[399] A dose of 60 mg of Pamidronate is usually sufficient for moderate hypercalcemia, but it must be given by 24-hour infusion. Treatments can be repeated at 7-day intervals if needed. For chronic hypercalcemia, oral phosphates are usually administered in a dosage of 1 to 3 g/day. Phosphate enemas can be used as an alternative to oral phosphate for patients with nausea and vomiting. Phosphates should not be used in patients in renal failure with an elevated serum phosphorus level. When needed, these supplementary agents represent additions to hydration and steroid therapy. When treatment is effective at normalizing the serum calcium, patients usually experience reduction in bone pain and in hypercalciuria and hydroxyproline excretion.

Although calcium binding is primarily attributable to serum albumin, in some myeloma patients, the M-component firmly binds calcium, leading to an asymptomatic elevation in the serum calcium concentration without an increase in the ionized calcium level.[400-402] Myeloma patients who are asymptomatic but have a chronically elevated serum calcium concentration should have the serum level of ionized calcium determined by a reference laboratory.

BONE PAIN

Bone pain is the most common symptom of myeloma and usually results from pathologic fractures. Bone disease in myeloma is the result of increased bone resorption associated with myeloma cell infiltration and osteoclast activation.[403] Skeletal damage in myeloma manifests as generalized osteoporosis or as focal punched-out osteolytic lesions without the rim of new bone formation often observed with metastatic carcinomas. One common bone manifestation of myeloma consists of compression fractures in the thoracic or lumbar spine. Bone density is reduced, resulting in gradual or sudden compression of the vertebral plates, which often results in a "fish-mouth" deformity. Pain is often radicular and lancinating to one or both sides, is aggravated by movement, and probably is related to instability of the weak bone substance. Symptoms usually subside within days to weeks after initiation of systemic chemotherapy. Opiates are often useful for pain control. Nonsteroidal antiinflammatory agents may also relieve pain but are associated with a higher prevalence of renal failure in myeloma patients.[404] For persistent pain despite chemotherapy, localized radiation therapy may be required. Orthopedic back braces are usually poorly tolerated, but the newer lightweight braces with Velcro fasteners are useful for some severely debilitated patients.

The osteolytic lesions commonly observed in the skull, although pathognomonic for myeloma, are usually asymptomatic and normally do not require treatment. Typical examples of bone destruction in myeloma appear in Figure 56–4. Lytic lesions in major long bones should be irradiated if the lesion's diameter is one third to one half of the bone's diameter or if it involves a significant component of the cortex and the risk of pathologic fracture is high. Systemic chemotherapy infrequently leads to significant recalcification of large lesions, and they remain susceptible to pathologic fracture, even after achieving remission with systemic therapy.

Skeletal strength is enhanced by ambulation, which should be encouraged as soon as it is feasible. Internal fixation of a pathologic fracture of the femur should be carried out promptly, because the myeloma patient's general condition usually deteriorates rapidly if they are maintained at bedrest in skeletal traction. Intramedullary fixation of fractures of long bones should be followed with local radiation therapy. Administration of sodium fluoride (50 mg twice daily) with calcium carbonate (1.0 g four times daily) can enhance bone density as determined by quantitative studies on bone biopsies.[405] The addition of 50,000 units of vitamin D twice weekly and of androgens may be beneficial.[406,407] However, in a large randomized chemotherapy trial, fluoride, calcium, and vitamin D did not significantly improve outcome after a trial of chemotherapy alone but were thought to contribute to morbidity.[258] The effects of the oral diphosphonate etidronate were evaluated in a double blind study in newly diagnosed myeloma patients in conjunction with chemotherapy. Unfortunately, etidronate failed to have significant impact on bone disease in myeloma.[408] Several of the newer diphosphonate derivatives that are much more potent than etidronate may enhance bone density, but they are still undergoing clinical trials.

SPINAL CORD COMPRESSION AND OTHER NEUROLOGIC SYNDROMES

Spinal cord compression is a serious complication of multiple myeloma that occurs in 10% to 15% of patients and is usually observed early in the patient's course or in the late relapse phase of the disease. As with other neoplastic causes of spinal cord compression, back pain is usually the initial symptom. The presence of a paraspinal mass suggests that this complication may be imminent. Compression of the spinal cord usually results from ingrowth of the tumor through an intervertebral foramina or by direct extension from a heavily involved vertebra. If initial skeletal x-ray studies obtained for staging indicate a paraspinal mass, follow-up evaluation with an MRI scan or CT scan is warranted to exclude invasion of the spinal canal. The earliest symptom of spinal cord compression often is radicular pain, which is accentuated by coughing or sneezing; motor or sensory loss or abnormality in bowel or bladder function are signs of more extensive compression. Paraplegia is a late and usually irreversible finding.

Any of the symptoms or signs demand imaging of the spinal cord by MRI or CT scanning or myelography. We continue to be impressed with the value and accuracy of myelography, even though lumbar and cisternal introduction of contrast are frequently necessary. Currently available data suggest that noninvasive MRI scanning may provide information that is equally useful, but in some instances, MRI fails to provide the needed information. Controlled studies comparing myelography, CT, and MRI are currently underway. If permanent cord damage has not yet occurred, initiation of emergency radiation therapy and high-dose steroid therapy usually results in marked improvement or complete resolution of the patient's symptoms. If paralysis has occurred, emergency treatment usually only prevents further worsening of the patient's disability. If myelography is performed and demonstrates a partial or complete block, the contrast medium should be left in place to assist in treatment planning and for following the response to treatment.

Steroid dosage for myeloma patients with spinal cord compression should initially be in the range of 16 mg of dexamethasone per day in divided doses, with tapering starting after the completion of radiation therapy. For radiation therapy, wide margins are necessary to encompass the disease, but treatment of the entire vertebral column is rarely indicated because of the palliative treatment philosophy and the need to resume myelosuppressive chemotherapy. Decompression laminectomy is usually not required in the diagnosis or treatment of spinal cord compression syndromes in myeloma, because plasma cell tumors are usually quite radiation sensitive. The acute debilitation resulting from this form of surgery presents a special problem for myeloma patients because of the protracted period of complete bedrest after surgery, which further increases the likelihood of developing infection or hypercalcemia. Nerve root compression syndromes and the few instances of cerebral compression by a cranial or dural plasmacytoma can usually be treated successfully with radiation therapy.[409-416] Because plasmacytomas in the skull are normally chemosensitive and rarely cause substantial cerebral compression, specialized imaging studies and radiation therapy are indicated only if the patient develops localized CNS symptoms and signs of involvement during the course of systemic treatment.

Other neurologic syndromes encountered in myeloma patients include an acute encephalopathy associated with hypercalcemia, hyperviscosity, uremia, or meningitis. A variety of peripheral neuropathies are also encountered, most commonly caused by amyloidosis.[417] In fewer than 1% of patients, a mixed sensory-motor neuropathy develops, usually involving the extremities. It does not appear to be the result of amyloid or direct tumor infiltrate and usually improves after the initiation of chemotherapy.[418-423] The neuropathy can be painful and debilitating. In some instances, the neuropathy may be the result of a direct binding between the M-component and peripheral nerve constituents. It has commonly been reported in patients with macroglobulinemia, but it has also been observed in patients with multiple myeloma, including in some with osteosclerotic myeloma.[419,424-428] The antigen binding in sural nerve biopsies has been seen with myelin-associated glycoprotein and associated with demyelination and, in other cases, with binding to endoneurial constituents.[429] Nerve binding of IgM in patients has been passively transferred to mice with purified IgM fractions, with evidence of specificity.[430]

Another rare neuropathy sometimes associated with myeloma is the POEMS syndrome composed of polyneuropathy organomegaly, endocrinopathy, monoclonal gammopathy, and skin changes.[431] The pathophysiology of this disorder is not understood.

HEMATOLOGIC COMPLICATIONS

Anemia

Anemia is the most common hematologic complication of myeloma, with a hemoglobin level of less than 12 g/dl in 62% of patients at the time of presentation.[432] Severe anemia with a hemoglobin level of less than 8.5 g/dl and a marked reduction in erythrocytes are observed in approximately 25% of patients. The degree of anemia correlates with total-body tumor burden.[181] In patients with the hyperviscosity syndrome, expansion of the plasma volume and its resulting hemodilution can exaggerate the reduction in hemoglobin out of proportion to the reduction in erythrocyte mass.

The anemia of myeloma usually improves significantly with response to chemotherapy unless the patient has persistent renal failure. Severe symptomatic anemia requires transfusion of packed erythrocytes, because the recovery of adequate hemoglobin values usually does not occur until the patient has been receiving chemotherapy for at least 3 months. Recovery of an adequate level of circulating erythrocytes is not enhanced by administration of folic acid, vitamin B_{12}, or iron unless a factor deficiency can be documented. In some instances, folate deficiency may be due to excessive folate use by the myeloma cells.[433]

Some patients whose hemoglobin level does not improve sufficiently with chemotherapy improve after receiving a potent androgen (*e.g.*, testosterone enanthate, 600 mg intramuscularly every 4–6 weeks; fluoxymesterone, 15–30 mg orally daily). Androgen therapy often needs to be continued for 3 to 6 months to see benefit. Recombinant erythropoietin has substantial effect on increasing the erythrocyte mass in noncancer patients with the anemia of renal failure.[434,435] Several reports indicate that it can be useful in correcting anemia in some myeloma patients, even in the absence of renal failure.[436,437]

Granulocytopenia and Thrombocytopenia

Although mild granulocytopenia (<3000 granulocytes/μl) is common in myeloma, moderate to severe granulocytopenia or thrombocytopenia is uncommon, but if present, it is usually attributable to extensive bone marrow involvement with myeloma. If detected at diagnosis, marked granulocytopenia or thrombocytopenia should not lead to reduction in the dosage of induction chemotherapy. Patients should be treated aggressively with myeloma chemotherapy, blood components, and supportive care in a fashion analogous to the management of acute leukemia. Recombinant granulocyte colony-stimulating factor or granulocyte-macrophage colony-stimulating factor can help to normalize the absolute granulocyte count in neutropenic myeloma patients.

Acute Leukemia and Myelodysplastic Syndromes

An association between multiple myeloma and acute leukemia was first reported in 1965, and it has been confirmed extensively since then.[438,439] In the first myeloma trial conducted by the Clinical Trials Group of the NCI of Canada, 15 cases of acute leukemia were observed among 365 myeloma patients treated with combinations of alkylating agents and prednisone.[189,438] The incidence of leukemia in that study was 230 times higher than expected in the normal population.[438] On an actuarial basis, the risk of acute leukemia was projected to be 19.6% at 50 months after the start of treatment. Although it appears that acute leukemia was a more frequent complication in this study than in other reported myeloma trials, it nonetheless underscores the importance of this potential complication. The actual number of cases is significantly less than the actuarial incidence predicted.

There has been much speculation about the cause of acute leukemia in myeloma patients, and the predominant view is that it is a complication of the alkylating agents or radiation therapy.[439,440] However, there also are reports of acute leukemia in patients with myeloma before the general use of

alkylating agents for treatment, and myelodysplastic changes have occasionally been observed in the marrow of myeloma patients before treatment.[441,442] Acute leukemia has also been observed in untreated patients with macroglobulinemia or MGUS. Although the actual incidence of acute nonlymphocytic leukemia in untreated myeloma patients is unknown, some researchers have speculated that there may be an intrinsic increased susceptibility to acute leukemia in patients with plasma cell neoplasia.[438]

Analyses of incidence of acute leukemia in cancer trials for myeloma or ovarian cancer in which patients received melphalan or cyclophosphamide therapy strongly incriminate melphalan as a leukemogenic agent. In the MRC's first two trials for myeloma, 12 of 648 patients developed a myelodysplastic syndrome (considered to be preleukemic) or acute leukemia.[443] This corresponds to a 5-year actuarial prevalence of 3% and an 8-year prevalence of 10%. In these two MRC studies, patients were randomized to receive melphalan or cyclophosphamide. A significant association was found with the length of melphalan treatment ($p=0.0001$) but none for cyclophosphamide. In this analysis, the risk of a secondary hematopoietic neoplasm in myeloma patients after 10 years of follow-up was approximately 3% for each year of melphalan treatment, with much of the risk occurring within 3 years of the last melphalan treatment.[443] It was the the researchers' view that if there was an intrinsic element of increased risk for secondary hematologic neoplasms in myeloma, it would be difficult to explain the association they found with melphalan exposure.

A similar conclusion about the leukemogenicity of melphalan was reached in an analysis of 1794 1-year survivors of ovarian cancer treated with chemotherapy.[444] In the ovarian cancer study, there was a 93-fold increase in the incidence of acute nonlymphocytic leukemia overall, with the greatest risk in the first 5 years after chemotherapy. The 10-year accumulated risk of acquiring leukemia was 11.2% after receiving melphalan and 5.4% after cyclophosphamide. Moreover, there was a definite dose-response relation for melphalan therapy, and women receiving melphalan were two to three times more likely to develop leukemia than those receiving cyclophosphamide.[444]

The results of these studies indicate that the choice of alkylating agent and dose administered may significantly influence the risk for late complications of chemotherapy in myeloma. The effect of melphalan dosage in these studies also suggests that the current trials using high-dose intravenous melphalan in myeloma may be associated with a significant incidence of leukemia as a therapy-related complication.

The acute nonlymphocytic leukemias that evolve in myeloma patients often evolve after a period of bone marrow injury with an associated pancytopenia or morphologic evidence of myelodysplasia. As for other secondary acute leukemias (*e.g.*, in Hodgkin's disease), treatment of the leukemia is difficult because of the preexisting impaired bone marrow reserve resulting from the disease or treatment. In myeloma, advanced age, immunodeficiency, and impaired renal function may further compromise the treatment of acute leukemia. Nonetheless, worthwhile hematologic remissions of secondary leukemia are sometimes achieved in myeloma patients using standard induction chemotherapy regimens incorporating an anthracycline and cytarabine (cytosine arabinoside).

Coagulopathy

Coagulation disorders in the absence of thrombocytopenia occur commonly in patients with macroglobulinemia or cryoglobulinemia and somewhat less often in patients with myeloma. Purpura, epistaxis, and ecchymosis, and retinal hemorrhages or mucosal bleeding caused by coagulopathies may be observed in patients with monoclonal gammopathy. In the syndromes discussed later, the functional abnormality of the bleeding disorder appears related to the presence of the M-component. There are many mechanisms of coagulopathy in patients with M-components. In several case reports, inhibitors of individual coagulation factors have been observed, including inhibitors of factors V, VII, VIII, and X and of the prothrombin complex.[445] In some instances, patients have reductions in multiple coagulation factors, including factors II, V, VII, and VIII and fibrinogen.

The mechanism of multifactor depression is obscure, but it has been suggested that the M-component binds to or coprecipitates with coagulation complexes.[446] In macroglobulinemia, specific M-components appear to interact with or bind to fibrin during the clotting process and inhibit the polymerization of the fibrin monomer. This can be detected as a prolongation in the thrombin time.[447] However, this abnormality usually does not cause clinical bleeding, unless platelet function is also impaired. In some instances, the hemostatic defect is associated with impaired platelet function. Prolonged bleeding time, impaired clot retraction, prolongation of the thromboplastin generation time with the patient's platelets, and defective platelet aggregation are indicators of impaired platelet function.[448,449] In some instances, the M-component appears to coat the platelets, leading to the release of platelet factor III and impaired aggregation.[450–452] A patient with plasma cell leukemia had a circulating heparin sulfate proteoglycan anticoagulant.[453] Fibrinolysis with severe bleeding was reported in a patient with myeloma and amyloidosis who had an associated deficiency of α_2-plasmin inhibitor. Treatment with ϵ-aminocaproic acid reduced bleeding and was associated with recovery of the plasmin inhibitor level.[454]

SYNDROMES RESULTING FROM PHYSICOCHEMICAL PROPERTIES OF M-COMPONENTS

Hyperviscosity

The hyperviscosity syndrome occurs in approximately 50% of patients with macroglobulinemia but in fewer than 5% of patients with multiple myeloma.[455–461] Hyperviscosity results from the protein-protein interactions of large, long molecules with high intrinsic viscosity (*e.g.*, IgM M-components) or from high concentrations of specific IgG or IgA M-components, which have a tendency to form multimolecular aggregates.[455–460] It rarely or never occurs in patients with light-chain-only myeloma because of the small molecular size of Bence Jones proteins. Although plasma viscosity rises with increasing concentration of an M-component, beyond a critical point, viscosity rises much more steeply, even with relatively small additional increments in serum M-component concentration. Variations among patients in the relation of M-component concentration to viscosity make prediction of plasma viscosity difficult without direct measurement.[462]

As a result of poorly understood homeostatic mechanisms,

increases in plasma viscosity lead to expansion of the plasma volume.[463] The hemodilution resulting from plasma volume expansion can dilute the circulating erythrocytes, giving the appearance of an anemia. To clarify this situation, use of nuclear medicine techniques to directly measure the plasma volume (with radioiodinated albumin) and the erythrocyte mass (with radiochromate-labeled erythrocytes) are of value. The intrinsic viscosity of serum or plasma can be measured by noting the time necessary for a given volume of serum to pass a constriction in a glass tube (Ostwald viscometer or a leukocyte pipette) and relating the time to that of a normal saline control.

Symptoms and signs of the hyperviscosity syndrome are usually not seen unless the serum relative viscosity is greater than 4.0 cp, and the full-blown classic syndrome is usually not seen unless the viscosity is greater than 5.0 cp (normal human serum relative viscosity is in the range of 1.4–1.8 cp). Clinical symptoms and signs of the hyperviscosity syndrome include bleeding disorders, retinopathy, neurologic findings, and evidence of hypervolemia. Hemorrhagic complications include bruising, purpura, and mucosal bleeding that is often manifest as severe or recurrent bleeding from the nose or uterus. Characteristic ocular findings include marked dilatation and segmentation of the retinal veins (giving the appearance of a line of boxcars or sausage links), retinal hemorrhages, or papilledema. Neurologic abnormalities range from fatigue, weakness, headache, vertigo, nystagmus, and confusion, to transient paralysis and frank coma. Findings of hypervolemia include distension of peripheral blood vessels and symptoms and signs of heart failure.

Therapeutically, the initial approach to patients with the hyperviscosity syndrome is to perform plasmapheresis. Plasmapheresis is performed most effectively with a continuous or a discontinuous flow blood cell separator. Another high-efficiency method uses plasma cascade filtration through a cellulose diacetate membrane that selectively removes the high-molecular-mass M-components while permitting return of the patient's albumin with reasonable efficiency.[463–465] However, if the needed equipment for high-efficiency plasmapheresis or filtration is not available, conventional double-double plasma separation packs can be used with centrifugation.[466] Patients who have acute hyperviscosity usually need treatment of at least 2 to 3 L daily for 4 to 5 days or as long as needed until the viscosity falls below 4.0 cp. Although plasmapheresis relieves the hyperviscosity syndrome on a temporary basis, for long-term control, systemic chemotherapy, as used for multiple myeloma or macroglobulinemia, should be initiated to reduce M-component production and tumor burden. In some drug-resistant cases of macroglobulinemia, satisfactory long-term control of hyperviscosity can be maintained with intermittent plasmapheresis alone at 2- to 3-week intervals.

Cryoglobulinemia

Cryoglobulinemia should be suspected in patients with acrocyanosis or Raynaud's phenomenon alone or with purpura, particularly after cold exposure. Cryoglobulins in macroglobulinemia or myeloma are M-components with low thermal amplitude, which can be readily demonstrated by drawing blood in a warm syringe and allowing it to clot and retract in a 37°C water bath. The serum is then transferred to a clean tube and placed in a refrigerator for 1 to 2 days, after which time the cryoglobulin has formed a flocculent white precipitate or a gel in the bottom of the tube. Cryoglobulins can usually be quantitated by carrying out the cold exposure in hematocrit tubes and centrifuging them to determine a "cryocrit." Cryoglobulins in B-cell neoplasms are usually IgM or IgG M-components; however, IgA M-components and mixed cryoglobulins have also been reported.[467–471]

Treatment with alkylating agents and steroids usually relieves most symptoms of cryoglobulinemia, although some patients continue to need gloves and earmuffs or a move to a warmer climate in the winter. Patients with cryoglobulinemia who present with purpura and other bleeding manifestations or evidence of renal failure should be treated initially with plasmapheresis before the start of chemotherapy.

Anomalous Serum Chemistries

Several abnormalities in serum chemistries are commonly observed in myeloma patients who have high concentrations of serum M-components. These can be confused with abnormalities of clinical significance, but they are usually of little or no clinical importance. These include apparent hyponatremia, hypoglycemia, and the "anion gap."[472–474] The apparent reductions in serum sodium and glucose are attributed to the displacement of the water-based solutes and electrolytes in serum by the large physical mass of the M-component solute, which does not contain sodium or glucose and displaces water in the serum. The reduced serum sodium has been described as "isotonic hyponatremia."[475] An apparent low anion gap has been attributed to the fact that M-components are cationic (*i.e.*, net positive charge). To balance such unmeasured protein cations, chloride and bicarbonate are retained to neutralize the protein's charge. A low anion gap has also been observed in MGUS.[476] The finding of a low anion gap in a patient not known to have an M-component should lead the physician to order appropriate diagnostic studies to look for a monoclonal protein. For patients with known monoclonal gammopathies, saline infusions should not be given for hyponatremia unless there is additional documentation that the patient is sodium and volume depleted. Hyponatremia associated with inappropriate secretion of antidiuretic hormone has been reported in patients with macroglobulinemia.[475]

BACTERIAL SEPSIS

Humoral immunodeficiency is the principal underlying cause for bacterial sepsis in patients with myeloma.[477–482] *Streptococcus pneumoniae* and *Hemophilus influenzae* are the most common pathogens in previously untreated myeloma patients and those nonneutropenic patients responding to chemotherapy. However, in neutropenic patients and in those with refractory disease, *Staphylococcus aureus* and gram-negative bacteria are the preponderant organisms.[483] Patients with fever, productive cough, or other symptoms of bacterial infection should have bacterial culture and appropriate x-ray studies performed as quickly as possible, and bactericidal antibiotic therapy should be started.

If patients present with signs of sinopulmonary infection and are in suitable condition to be treated on an outpatient basis, the combination of amoxicillin and clavulanate usually suffices because its spectrum is broad enough to cover most common organisms. For neutropenic patients or for those whose overall condition requires hospitalization, the use of vancomycin plus a third-generation cephalosporin (*e.g.*, ceftazidime) or an aminoglycoside plus an antipseudomonal penicillin (*e.g.*, ticarcillin) is usually indicated. If an aminoglycoside regimen is used, special attention must be paid to renal function, and the frequency of follow-up doses of the aminoglycoside should be judged based on serum assays and renal function. Patients who have repeated episodes of sinopulmonary infections often benefit from being provided with a supply of a suitable oral cephalosporin (*e.g.*, cefaclor) or the amoxicillin-clavulanate combination or ciprofloxacin so that they can start therapy at the time of initial symptoms. For patients who have difficulties with compliance, prophylactic treatment with benzathine penicillin G should be considered if there has been a history of prior pneumococcal or meningococcal infection.

In a controlled study, intramuscular injection of 20 ml of γ-globulin every 2 weeks did not reduce the frequency of bacterial infections, and it is not indicated for infection prophylaxis in myeloma.[484] Although far larger doses of γ-globulin can be given intravenously, patients with IgG myeloma still catabolize this formulation rapidly. This form of supportive therapy is expensive and has yet to be proven useful in controlled clinical trials in myeloma. Use of pneumococcal vaccination may be worth trying.[485] However, most myeloma patients respond poorly to bacterial antigenic stimulation. Vaccines containing live organisms (*e.g.*, varicella) are contraindicated in patients with myeloma because their immunodeficiencies permit infection to disseminate.

AMYLOIDOSIS

Systemic amyloidosis is a complication that occurs in approximately 15% of patients with multiple myeloma. The fibrillar amyloid protein deposited in myeloma has a pattern of tissue distribution characteristically observed in "primary amyloidosis," a condition with bone marrow plasmacytosis, Bence Jones proteinuria, or a serum M-component but no osteolytic bone lesions. Differentiation of the amyloid associated with myeloma from that of primary amyloidosis is artificial because the amyloid is of similar genesis and tissue distribution, and the conditions are more appropriately considered to be parts of the spectrum of the same basic disease process.[490]

There is a clear structural relation between amyloid fibril deposits and Bence Jones proteins. Amyloid fibrils from primary amyloidosis and amyloidosis associated with myeloma are homogenous and homologous to the variable region fragment of κ or λ light chains, as defined by amino acid sequence analysis of purified amyloid proteins.[486,487] Primary amyloidosis and the amyloidosis associated with myeloma, other monoclonal gammopathies, and agammaglobulinemia have immunoglobulin amyloid fibrils or amyloid L-chain proteins. Most monoclonal L chains do not appear to be amyloidogenic, suggesting that specific structural properties must be present to undergo fibrillar deposition. Although κ-type L chains are more frequent than the λ-type L chains on M-components or as Bence Jones proteins, amyloidogenic L chains of the λ type are significantly more frequent than those of the κ type.[488] Amyloid fibrils are at best sparingly soluble in physiologic saline or plasma, but they can be solubilized in distilled water or low ionic strength media; therefore, it is not surprising that they tend to deposit in tissues. Serum amyloid P component (SAP) has been radioiodinated and its clearance studied in normal persons and patients with systemic amyloid. In these studies, SAP was cleared more rapidly in amyloid patients and accumulated and persisted in their amyloid deposits.[489]

The presenting symptoms of amyloidosis (with or without myeloma) include weakness, weight loss, ankle edema dyspnea, paresthesias, light-headedness, or syncope.[490] Aching in the hands (particularly at night) can be symptomatic of median nerve compression associated with the carpal tunnel syndrome caused by amyloid infiltration of the transverse carpal ligament. Physical findings include enlargement of the tongue and liver, purpura, and ankle edema. Ankle edema is usually due to congestive heart failure or a nephrotic syndrome. A peripheral neuropathy may also be present.[417] Macroglossia occurs in approximately 20% of patients. The tongue frequently shows indentations from the teeth and may prevent closure of the mouth. Splenomegaly (usually slight) affects fewer than 10% of patients. The tissues most subject to amyloid deposition in myeloma include the tongue, gastrointestinal tract, heart, skin, and skeletal muscle. Although macroglossia or periorbital purpura in a myeloma patient should suggest the diagnosis, a knowledgeable and alert physician is needed in most instances. Purpura of the eyelids is characteristic of amyloid, and unilateral or bilateral periorbital purpura ("raccoon eyes") may appear suddenly after placing the head in a dependent position, as during proctoscopy; it has been called postproctoscopic purpura or PPP.[489,491] Other skin manifestations include plaques, papules, or nodules. Joint involvement with amyloid can result in an appearance similar to rheumatoid arthritis.[490,492] Involvement of the glenohumeral joints can give a "shoulder pad" appearance. Low voltage on the electrocardiogram can be suggestive of cardiac involvement. More specific is two-dimensional echocardiographic evidence of amyloidosis involving the heart, with thickening of ventricular walls, septum, papillary muscles, and pericardial effusion, and a characteristic "granular sparkling" appearance of the thickened cardiac walls.[493]

A rectal biopsy has been the classic method of establishing the diagnosis of amyloidosis, and it is positive in more than 60% of patients.[490] Another study showed that abdominal fat aspiration, using a 19-gauge needle, can yield positive results in more than 70% of patients. This procedure can be done at the bedside and is probably the simplest way to diagnose amyloidosis.[140] Resected carpal ligaments should be examined for the presence of amyloid, and the specimens can be evaluated retrospectively from tissue blocks from previously resected ligaments. Amyloid can be demonstrated in needle biopsies of the liver or kidney, but these procedures are more hazardous because of the increased risk of bleeding from vascular wall involvement or from deficiency of factor X. Cracking or rupture of the liver after biopsy has been observed when there is heavy infiltration with amyloid. Amyloid stains pink with hematoxylin and eosin and has metachromatic staining properties with methyl or crystal violet. Congo red stain produces an apple-green birefringence under polarized light and is the most specific stain for amyloid under the light

microscope. Electron microscopy may be somewhat more sensitive and has shown the presence of amyloid fibrils even when Congo red staining has not revealed amyloid.[490] Serum β_2-microglobulin levels appear to predict survival in patients with systemic amyloidosis without associated myeloma.[494]

Treatment for amyloidosis with myeloma is essentially the same as the treatment for multiple myeloma, but it usually does not have as great an impact on resolving amyloid deposits as it does in causing tumor regression. However, treatment may stop or slow further amyloid deposition, and this can be important for patients with early cardiac involvement.[495] The authors of a retrospective analysis concluded that a trial of chemotherapy was warranted in patients with myeloma and amyloidosis and that patients with objective response of the myeloma had a better survival than those that did not. Although there were no absolute predictors of response, patients who achieved remission were much less likely to have cardiac amyloid but were more likely to have high β_2-microglobulin or κ L-chain M-component levels.[496] In a double-blind study of primary amyloidosis (without overt myeloma), patients given melphalan and prednisone were able to continue treatment longer than those given placebo, and improvement in nephrotic syndrome or proteinuria was observed, but survival did not differ significantly between the two groups.[497] Detection of a high plasma cell labeling index was reported to be useful for identifying patients with amyloidosis who were responsive to chemotherapy, but their overall survival was still poor (14 months).[498] Colchicine, dimethylsulfoxide, and penicillamine have been tried in treating L-chain amyloid without success. Congestive heart failure caused by amyloid represents a poor prognostic feature of the disease and usually does not respond to cardiac glycosides.[499] Diuretics are useful for relief of edema.

OTHER PLASMA CELL NEOPLASMS

MACROGLOBULINEMIA

In 1944, Waldenström raised the question of whether a new syndrome that differed from multiple myeloma could be identified in the setting of a high-molecular-mass M-component and a bleeding syndrome of the type associated with hyperviscosity.[500] Development of immunodiagnostic techniques, such as immunoelectrophoresis, led to the recognition that a serum IgM M-component was a common feature in patients with the syndrome described by Waldenström.[501] Although the disease was initially thought to occur predominantly in men, later reports suggested an approximately equal sex prevalence.[461,502–505]

Macroglobulinemia is far less common than multiple myeloma.[107,506–508] Pathogenetic mechanisms similar to those in myeloma may be involved, but there is considerable literature indicating an element of familial susceptibility that is more significant than that for myeloma, including families with multiple cases of macroglobulinemia or IgM MGUS in first-degree relatives.[89,509–511] Macroglobulinemia in a pair of monozygotic twins was reported.[512] The case for environmental factors was made for a canary breeder who developed pulmonary symptoms and was found to have a pulmonary infiltrate with IgM-containing cells, Waldenström's macroglobulinemia, and an M-component that exhibited antibody activity against an antigen in canary droppings.[513]

Patients with macroglobulinemia are usually first seen with findings analogous to those of advanced non-Hodgkin's lymphomas: hepatosplenomegaly and lymphadenopathy. The patients often develop the hyperviscosity syndrome, with attendant bleeding manifestations (Table 56–14). The fundi of patients with macroglobulinemia should be examined routinely with an ophthalmoscope for evidence of hyperviscosity. The fundic changes can revert rapidly in response to plasmapheresis.

The presence of a serum IgM M-component is not tantamount to a diagnosis of macroglobulinemia because there are other B-cell neoplasms in which serum IgM M-components exist, but with the exception of macroglobulinemia and myeloma, the levels are usually lower than 1.0 g/dl and almost always lower than 2.0 g/dl. Only 25% of patients with IgM M-components have Waldenström's macroglobulinemia; other entities with IgM secretion include subsets of patients with CLL, non-Hodgkin's lymphomas, the cold hemagglutinin syndrome, and MGUS. Patients with osteolytic bone lesions in addition to an IgM serum M-component are rare, but they are usually classified as having IgM multiple myeloma, rather than macroglobulinemia.[514] Lacking definitive causal agents or other markers to differentiate these entities, this spectrum of neoplasms should be considered as representing various expressions of B-cell lymphoplasmacytic tumors, with their morphology "frozen" at different stages of differentiation and with clinical manifestations that vary as a function of M-component production, tumor cell proliferation, and invasiveness.[94] Supporting that concept is the report on the cytogenetics in a case of Waldenström's macroglobulinemia with an 8:14 translocation with breakpoints (q24;p32) similar to those found in Burkitt's lymphoma.[515]

Hematologic manifestations of macroglobulinemia include anemia in at least 70% of patients (often partially dilutional because of the expanded plasma volume) and some degree of thrombocytopenia in approximately 30% of patients. Bone marrow involvement is common in macroglobulinemia, and

TABLE 56–14. Clinical Manifestations in 260 Patients With Macroglobulinema

Mean age (y)	
At onset of symptoms	63
At diagnosis	65 (range, 18–92)
Symptoms, % of patients with	
Severe fatigue	85
Bleeding	60
Neurologic	17
Bone pain	10
Signs, % of patients with	
Lymphadenopathy	40
Hepatomegaly	30
Splenomegaly	30
Hepatosplenomegaly	25

(Modified from MacKenzie MR. Macroglobulinemia. In: Wiernik PH, Canelloa GP, Kyle RA, Schiffer CA, eds. Neoplastic diseases of the blood, vol. 2. New York: Churchill-Livingstone, 1985:575–592)

the morphologic appearance of the plasma cells is pleomorphic, with a range of light microscopic appearances from small lymphoid cells to mature plasma cells. Immunofluorescent studies have shown that most of the lymphoid cells have cell-surface IgM but lack cytoplasmic Ig, and the plasma cells contain cytoplasmic IgM. In a flow cytometry study, patients with macroglobulinemia usually had circulating lymphoid cells that contained intracytoplasmic μ chains and cell-surface expression of the B-cell-specific antigens B1, B2, and B4 and the plasma cell antigen PCA-1.[516]

As with myeloma, quantitation of the IgM M-component should be performed by laser nephelometry or electrophoresis and not with immunodiffusion methods. Serum viscosity determinations should be performed in all patients at the time of diagnosis and serially in patients who have a serum relative viscosity higher than 3.0 cp. Residual normal immunoglobulins are often depressed, but less severely than in myeloma.[517] In contrast to the high percentage of myeloma patients with urinary light chain excretion, only about 10% of macroglobulinemic patients have Bence Jones proteins detectable in the urine by standard techniques, and tubular casts are absent.[518] Renal disease is seen only infrequently in macroglobulinemia and is markedly different from that seen in myeloma, taking on the appearance of an immunologically mediated glomerulonephritis or nephrotic syndrome.[518–521]

Neurologic syndromes observed in patients with macroglobulinemia include the neurologic entities discussed as myeloma complications, and they are usually due to the hyperviscosity syndrome or occur as peripheral neuropathies. Peripheral neuropathies are seen in approximately 20% of patients with macroglobulinemia.

The treatment of macroglobulinemia is similar to that of other indolent B-cell neoplasms. Oral alkylating agents (*e.g.*, chlorambucil, melphalan, cyclophosphamide) are the mainstays of therapy and are usually used alone or in combination with prednisone, administered with the same dosage schedules as those used in multiple myeloma or CLL.[502,504,505,522–527] Plasmapheresis is often needed initially to treat hyperviscosity. Systemic treatment is normally continued until the serum IgM level plateaus. At that point, treatment can be discontinued until there is evidence of a rising serum viscosity or other evidence of relapse. Although complete remission is rarely achieved, responsive patients have been reported to have median survivals in the range of 50 months, and nonresponsive patients have survivals about half that long.[461,505] Some patients have indolent macroglobulinemia (analogous to indolent myeloma) survive for more than 2 decades.

A case has been made for continuing the use of plasmapheresis and the cytotoxic agents, so that the dose required of the cytotoxic agent or the frequency of plasma exchange can be reduced.[528] Sequential hemibody irradiation has been used with some benefit, but it did not eliminate the patient's requirement for intermittent plasmapheresis.[529] Because of the relative rarity of the disease, comparative evaluations of treatment programs for macroglobulinemia have not been reported, and it is best to use one of the standard regimens for CLL or myeloma. Patients who become refractory to alkylating agents can be maintained effectively on long-term plasmapheresis if the IgM production rate is not too high. One macroglobulinemic patient with alkylating agent resistance has been maintained on plasmapheresis every 2 weeks for the past 12 years. On the basis of our experience and unpublished and published reports by others, patients with refractory macroglobulinemia may achieve drug-induced remissions with fludarabine, doxorubicin, the M2 protocol, VBAP, INF-α, or pentostatin.[530-533] Patients with macroglobulinemia treated with alkylating agents have developed acute leukemia in a fashion analogous to that seen after treatment with melphalan or chlorambucil in myeloma or polycythemia vera.[523,533-537]

LICHEN MYXEDEMATOSUS

Lichen myxedematosus (*i.e.*, papular mucinosis or scleromyxedema) is a rare skin disorder that is usually associated with the presence of a serum IgGλ M-component that is basic and has a marked cathodal electrophoretic mobility.[538] Some cases have been reported with IgA or IgM M-components, usually also with λ L chains. However, osteolytic bone lesions, marrow plasmacytosis, or Bence Jones proteinuria are found only rarely.[539] This dermatologic condition is manifested as raised papules or plaques containing a mucinous material mainly composed of hyaluronic acid. Skin fibroblasts from a patient with typical skin lesions and an IgGμ M-component grew to a lower cell density in culture but produced more glycosaminoglycans (with a higher ratio of hyaluronic acid to sulfated glycosaminoglycans) and less collagen than did normal fibroblasts.[540] Compared with the effect of normal serum, serum from a patient with lichen myxedematosus was found to stimulate hyaluronic acid and prostaglandin E production by normal foreskin or synovial fibroblasts.[541] These data suggest that the serum M-component is acting directly on the skin fibroblasts, altering their metabolism and inducing the skin lesions. Striking cutaneous and systemic improvements have been observed when patients have been treated with melphalan or cyclophosphamide.[542-544] The presence of the monoclonal M-component and the response to alkylating agent therapy suggest that lichen myxedematosus is an unusual plasma cell neoplasm. Isotretinoin therapy was tried in several patients.[545]

HEAVY-CHAIN DISEASES

The heavy-chain diseases are rare lymphoplasmacytic neoplasms in which a fragment of an Ig heavy chain is secreted by the tumor cells and is detected in the serum or in the urine. The heavy-chain fragments have an intact Fc portion but a deletion in the Fd region. The first report on a heavy-chain disease was on γ-heavy-chain disease in 1964 by Franklin and associates, who predicted that α- and μ-chain diseases would also be discovered.[546] This prediction was validated with the subsequent identification of unique syndromes associated with α- and μ-chain fragment secretion. Analysis of the structure of fragments secreted in the heavy-chain diseases has shed some light on normal Ig structure and immunogenetics.[547-550]

γ-Heavy-Chain Disease

Since the initial description of γ-heavy-chain disease (γ-HCD), more than 90 additional cases have been reported, mostly as individual case reports.[551] The world literature on this entity was reviewed.[552] In most cases, the clinical de-

scription is similar to that of non-Hodgkin's lymphoma, with nodal or external involvement, and in 4 patients, a picture somewhat more like that of multiple myeloma, with osteolytic bone lesions, was reported.[553] γ-HCD is not a specific pathologic process; it is a mutant molecular expression in the spectrum of B-cell neoplasia.[552] In 4 patients, chromosome abnormalities have been reported, but a unique abnormality has yet to be identified.[554] The median age at diagnosis of γ-HCD is 60, but it appears in some patients before the age of 20, and the disease is slightly more common in men than women.[555]

Most patients present with fever, anemia, weakness, and lymphadenopathy, often accompanied with hepatosplenomegaly. Involvement of Waldeyer's ring is relatively common. Leukopenia, eosinophilia, and thrombocytopenia are often present, and atypical lymphocytes and plasma cells may be found in the blood smears. The bone marrow aspirate and biopsy specimens usually show an increase in the lymphoplasmacytic series and occasionally some degree of eosinophilia. Immunofluorescent studies have shown that the cells throughout the lymphoplasmacytic spectrum contain γ chains.[556] However, in some instances, the bone marrow findings are normal.

The γ chain in γ-HCD is incomplete, and because of the major deletions, the molecular mass of the protein is between one half and three quarters that of a normal γ chain.[557] The pattern on serum protein electrophoresis varies, with broad-based increases in γ-globulin, a discrete M-component spike, or a normal or hypogammaglobulinemic pattern. Immunoelectrophoresis has been used to identify most γ-HCD cases, and it is likely that the frequency of this disorder may be underreported because the test is not routinely used in the workup of patients with diffuse lymphomas. Proteinuria may be undetectable or may range up to 20 g/day. Electrophoresis usually shows the presence of an M-component or γ-globulin band that is negative on the heat test for Bence Jones proteins and can be demonstrated antigenically to have γ-type H-chain characteristics but is totally devoid of L-chain antigens. Most patients have less than 1 g/day of urinary protein excretion, and renal failure is uncommon.[546,555,558]

The clinical course of γ-HCD is highly variable, with some patients succumbing to a rapidly progressing neoplasm within weeks to others who survive 5 years or more.[559-561] The median survival for 49 patients for whom data was available was 12 months (range, 1–264 months).[555] Because of the diffuse nature of the disease, most patients are treated with programs similar to those used for patients with non-Hodgkin's lymphomas (*e.g.*, CVP, CHOP). Local radiation therapy may be useful for symptomatic relief of palatal edema and respiratory distress in patients with Waldeyer's ring involvement.

α-Heavy-Chain Disease

α-Heavy-chain disease (α-HCD) was first described by Seligmann and associates in an Arab woman with a severe malabsorption syndrome resulting from a lymphoplasmacytic infiltrate in the small bowel and monoclonal α chains in the serum.[562] This disease is the most common of the heavy-chain diseases, and there were more than 150 cases in the literature, including several detailed reviews of this syndrome.[563-568] α-HCD is also known as Mediterranean lymphoma and immunoproliferative small intestinal disease, with several articles appearing in the gastroenterologic and the oncologic literature. Most reports on α-HCD have been of Arab or Jewish patients from the Mediterranean area, including North Africa and the Middle East. However, the disease is not limited to Semitic peoples or to a given geographic area; one case was reported from Taiwan.[569]

In some instances, α-HCD appears to be premalignant, with a complete reversal of the syndrome after antibiotic therapy.[570–573] Often the disease relapses despite antibiotics and takes on a more malignant form.[574] The prevalence is slightly higher in males than in females, and the peak age of incidence is distinctly lower than that for myeloma or macroglobulinemia, with most patients in their twenties or thirties, but with a few children as young as 10 years of age.[575] Most patients with α-HCD are from undernourished populations with poor hygiene and infestation with intestinal parasites. Compared with normal persons and patients with other malabsorption syndromes, patients with α-HCD have a greater association of HLA-AW19 and HLA-B12 antigens, suggesting a genetic element in the disease.[576]

Characteristic symptoms of α-HCD include diarrhea, steatorrhea, weight loss, and abdominal pain. Abdominal masses may be palpable, although hepatosplenomegaly and peripheral lymphadenopathy are uncommon.[577] Clubbing of the fingers and growth retardation (including secondary sex characteristics) may occur.[578] Hypocalcemia and other electrolyte disturbances occur as a result of the diarrhea in this syndrome. X-ray studies and intestinal biopsy specimens demonstrate extensive infiltration and thickening of the mucosa with tumor. On biopsy, the infiltrate is lymphoplasmacytic, and the neoplastic cells usually contain α chains. The lamina propria is infiltrated with plasma cells, and the infiltrate may involve the submucosa and the mesenteric lymph nodes. Chromosomal analysis of mesenteric lymph nodes was reported for 4 patients with α-HCD, and abnormalities were found in 3 of them.[579] In 2 of these patients, there were rearrangements of chromosome 14 (band q32) resulting from translocations that differ from those observed in most other non-Hodgkin's lymphomas. In one prior case, a closely related abnormality in chromosome 14 (14q+) was reported in a patient with α-HCD.[580]

Unlike other monoclonal gammopathies, an M-component spike is normally not seen on electrophoresis in α-HCD. For about one half of the patients, a diffusely increased band is seen in the $α_2$- or β-globulin zones, but for the remaining patients, there was no overt abnormality on serum electrophoresis. Presumptive diagnosis of α-HCD based on serum protein analysis requires that the α-H chain be identified with anti-α-chain antisera on immunoelectrophoresis or immunofixation without a reaction to anti-L-chain antisera. However, because not all L-chain antisera detect L chains on IgA globulins, definitive diagnosis requires isolation and purification of the protein, followed by reduction and alkylation and demonstration that the reduced monoclonal protein constituents do not contain light chains.[581]

All reported cases of α-HCD have been of the $α_1$ subtype rather than the $α_2$ subtype. The molecular mass of the α-HCD proteins is about one half to three quarters that of the intact α chain and appears to result from an internal deletion of most of the variable region in the H chain and the C1α do-

mains.[555] The α chains have a tendency to polymerize to variously sized molecules with different net charges; this property probably accounts for the presence of a diffuse band rather than a characteristic monoclonal spike on electrophoresis. The abnormal α chains have also been found in modest quantities in the patients' urine in the absence of Bence Jones proteinuria.

Treatment of some patients with antibiotics alone (*e.g.*, tetracycline) has resulted in resolution of the syndrome, and α-HCD has therefore been considered a potential example of "immune escalation" from benign monoclonal immunoproliferation to frank neoplastic transformation.[94] In most patients, aggressive therapy with melphalan or cyclophosphamide plus prednisone or multiagent combinations has been required.[582] In some patients, complete remissions have been obtained, primarily for those with stage A disease (*i.e.*, mature plasmacytic or lymphoplasmacytic infiltration limited to the lamina propria).[581,583] Usually the tumor is at a more advanced stage, with involvement of the submucosa or muscularis (stage B), or has undergone conversion to an immunoblastic sarcoma with involvement of the mesenteric nodes and bowel (stage C), for which remissions are only transient, and the disease progresses to a fatal outcome associated with cachexia or sepsis.

μ-Heavy-Chain Disease

The first patient with μ-heavy-chain disease (μ-HCD) was reported by several groups in 1970 and had a clinical picture of CLL.[584,585] In 1975, Franklin reported a series of 7 patients, all but one of whom had CLL.[586] Since that time, most additional reports of cases of μ-HCD have been of CLL. Almost all of the patients with μ-HCD have a clinical picture of CLL, but there is one clearly documented case with a clinical syndrome of myeloma with amyloid and osteolytic bone lesions with a μ-H chain in the serum, and one patient with an apparent μ-chain MGUS has also been identified.[555,587] Although μ-HCD patients usually have a CLL-like picture, the converse is not true. In a detailed immunologic analysis of 120 patients with CLL, none proved to have μ-HCD.[588] A common finding in the bone marrow of patients with μ-HCD is the presence of vacuolated plasma cells, and this finding should lead to a search for this entity. The diagnosis is established by demonstrating the presence of a μ-H chain in the serum by immunoelectrophoresis or immunofixation. Approximately two thirds of patients with μ-HCD have free L chains in the urine (Bence Jones proteins), usually of the κ-type.[588]

Molecular studies of the purified μ chains from these patients have been difficult because of the small amounts usually present and difficulty in isolation, but as with γ-HCD and α-HCD, μ chains in μ-HCD commonly have large deletions in the variable region.[589] In one patient with a leukemic picture, μ-HCD, and free L-chain production, the tumor cells produced a shortened μ chain that lacked the entire variable region.[549] The deletion was further localized to a defect at the level of the Ig gene structure and assembly that deletes coding information and results in aberrant RNA processing, which yields a truncated μ-chain protein that lacks a variable region and cannot assemble with light chains.[550]

The clinical course of patients with μ-HCD is varied but usually follows the course of CLL. When treatment is indicated, patients are usually treated with alkylating agents and prednisone in a fashion similar to that used in the treatment of CLL and with some benefit.

δ-Heavy-Chain Disease

In a single patient who presented with osteolytic bone lesions and renal failure, the serum M-component comprised closed tetramers of δ chains.[590] Monoclonal L chains were not detected with standard immunologic techniques. At autopsy, the patient also had subendothelial deposits on the basement membranes of the renal glomeruli, and the patient was reported as having δ-HCD.[590] The patient's clinical syndrome was consistent with multiple myeloma.

PERSPECTIVE

There has been a substantial advancement in our understanding of multiple myeloma and related plasma cell neoplasms since 1970. This has been the result of increased research efforts in the basic and clinical areas and the major impact of advances in immunobiology. At the clinical level, the development of a useful staging system, the identification of serum β_2-microglobulin as a major pretreatment prognostic factor, and the incorporation of anthracyclines into combination treatment regimens for remission induction in advanced stage and refractory patients offer evidence of progress. Current combination chemotherapy regimens for patients with active disease have achieved better results than the simpler regimens brought into use in the 1960s. However, intrinsic drug sensitivity in plasma cell neoplasms is not as marked as in some of the less-well-differentiated B-cell neoplasms, and kinetic and drug-resistance phenomena appear responsible for the inability to achieve true complete remissions. Higher-dosage alkylating agent regimens with myeloid growth factor support or with bone marrow transplantation may change this picture for good-risk patients. Recent results with allogeneic bone marrow transplants from HLA-matched siblings are encouraging, but this approach is only applicable to younger patients (≤55), and the median age at the time of diagnosis is 62 in most series. The procedure is therefore relevant to 10% or fewer myeloma patients.

The potential role of INF-α for remission maintenance after cytoreduction requires thorough investigation. Because there is now substantial clinical and preclinical evidence that melphalan is more leukemogenic than cyclophosphamide, selection of chemotherapeutic drugs should be guided by the goal of reducing the frequency of late side effects of treatment.

The use of monoclonal antibodies for identification of plasma cell and B-cell-associated cell-surface antigens provides a new approach to classification of patients with plasma cell neoplasms and the basis for developing new therapeutic agents capable of purging marrow of myeloma cells for autologous transplantation and for targeted cytotoxic destruction of residual myeloma-associated antigen-bearing cells in remission patients.

The role of drug-resistance mechanisms in blunting the effectiveness of chemotherapy is only now beginning to be understood at a cellular and molecular level in myeloma. With a better understanding of these mechanisms, development of pharmacologic means to abrogate drug resistance appears to be a realistic possibility that may have a major impact on future management of multiple myeloma. The clinical introduction of recombinant growth factors that stimulate the proliferation of normal progenitor populations in the bone marrow offers the promise that the anemia of myeloma and the granulocytopenia associated with its treatment may prove amenable to therapy for patients entering the next generation of clinical trials. Identification of IL-6 as a major plasmacytoma growth factor opens new avenues of therapy through the development of agents that inhibit the production of IL-6 or block its receptor-mediated effects on myeloma progenitor cells.[141]

REFERENCES

1. Kyle RA. Monoclonal gammopathy of undetermined significance (MGUS): A review. In: Hoffbrand AV, Lasch HG, Nathan DG, Salmon SE, eds. Clinics in Hematology. Eastbourne: WB Saunders, 1982:123–150.
2. Salmon SE. Immunoglobulin synthesis and tumor kinetics of multiple myeloma. Semin Hematol 1973;10:136–147.
3. Salmon SE. Plasma cell disorders. In: Wingaarden JB, Smith LH Jr, eds. Cecil textbook of medicine. 18th ed. 1988:1026–1036.
4. Macintyre W. Case of mollities and fragilitas ossium, accompanied with urine strongly charged with animal matter. Med Chir Trans Lond 1859;33:211.
5. Bence Jones H. On a new substance occurring in the urine of a patient with mollities and fragilitas ossium. Phil Trans R Soc Lond 1848;55:673.
6. Dalrymple J. On the microscopical character of mollities ossium. Dublin Q J Med Sci 1846;2:85.
7. Rustizky J. Multiple myeloma. Deutsch Z Chir 1972;3:162–172.
8. Kahler O. Zur Symptomatologie des multiplen Myeloma: Beobachtung von Albumosurie. Prog Med Wochnschr 1889;14:33–45.
9. Ellinger A. Das Vorkommen des Bence Jones' schen Korpers in Harn bei Tumoren des Knochenmarks und seine diagnostische Bedeutung. Deutsch Arch Klin Med 1899;62:266–278.
10. Wright JH. A case of multiple myeloma. Bull Johns Hopkins Hosp 1933;52:156.
11. Arinkin MI. Die intravitale Untersuchungs—Methodik des Knochenmarks. Folia Haematol (Leipz) 1929;38:233.
12. Tiselius A. Electrophoresis of serum globulin. II. Electrophoretic analysis of normal and immune sera. Biochem J 1937;31:1464.
13. Longsworth LG. Shedlovsky T, MacInnes DA. Electrophoretic patterns of normal and pathological human blood serum and plasma. J Exp Med 1939;70:399.
14. Magnus-Levy A. Multiple myeloma. Acta Med Scand 1938;95:217–280.
15. Grabar P. Williams CA. Methode permettant l'etude conjuguee des proprietes electrophoretiques et immunochimiques d'un melange de proteines. Application au serum sanguin. Biochim Biophys Acta 1953;10:193.
16. Glenner GG, Terry W, Harada M, et al. Amyloid fibril proteins: Proof of homology with immunoglobulin light chains by sequence analysis. Science 1971;172:1150–1151.
17. Salmon SE, Smith BA. Immunoglobulin synthesis and total body tumor cell number in IgG multiple myeloma. J Clin Invest 1970;49:1114.
18. Alwall N. Urethane and stilbamidine in multiple myeloma: Report on 2 cases. Lancet 1947;2:388–389.
19. Holland JF, Hosley H, Scharlau C, et al. A controlled trial of urethane treatment in myeloma. Blood 1966;27:328–342.
20. Bergsagel DE, Griffith KM, Haut A, et al. The treatment of plasma cell myeloma. Adv Cancer Res 1967;10:311–359.
21. Bergsagel DE, Sprague CC, Austin C, et al. Evaluation of new chemotherapeutic agents in the treatment of multiple myeloma. IV. L-phenylalanine mustard (NSC-8806). Cancer Chemother Rep 1962;21:87–99.
22. Korst DR, Clifford GO, Fowler WM, et al. Multiple myeloma. II. Analysis of cyclophosphamide in 165 patients. JAMA 1964;189:758–762.
23. Salmon SE, Shadduck RK, Schilling A. Intermittent high-dose prednisone therapy for multiple myeloma. Cancer Chemother Rep 1967;51:179.
24. Alexanian R, Bonnet J, Gehan E, et al. Combination chemotherapy for multiple myeloma. Cancer 1972;30:382–389.
25. Costa G, Engle RL Jr, Schilling A, et al. Melphalan and prednisone: An effective combination for the treatment of multiple myeloma. Am J Med 1973;54:589–599.
26. Salmon SE. Nitrosoureas in multiple myeloma. Cancer Treat Rep 1976;60:789–794.
27. Alberts DS, Salmon SE. Adriamycin (NSC-123127) in the treatment of alkylator-resistant multiple myeloma: A pilot study. Cancer Chemother Rep 1975;59:345–350.
28. Mellstedt A, Aahre A, Bjorkholm M, et al. Interferon therapy in myelomatosis. Lancet 1979;1:245–247.
29. Young JL, Percy CL, Asire AJ. Surveillance, epidemiology, and end results: Incidence and mortality data, 1973–1977. NCI Monograph 57. Bethesda: Department of Health and Human Services, NIH, 1981;81–2330.

30. Devesa SS, Silverman DT, Young JL Jr, et al. Cancer incidence and mortality trends among whites in the United States, 1947–84. JNCI 1987;79:701–770.
31. Martin NH. The incidence of myelomatosis. Lancet 1961;1:237–239.
32. Malignant neoplasms of lymphatic and haematopoietic tissues: Multiple myeloma. WHO Epidemiol Vital Stat Rep 1965;18:414–415.
33. Hewell GM, Alexanian R. Myeloma in young persons. Ann Intern Med 1976;84:441–443.
34. Blattner WA, Blair A, Mason TJ. Multiple myeloma in the United States, 1950–75. Cancer 1981;48:2547.
35. Linos A, Kyle RA, O'Fallon MW, et al. Incidence and secular trend of multiple myeloma in Olmstead County, Minnesota: 1965–77. JNCI 1981;66:17.
36. Blattner WA. Multiple myeloma and macroglobulinemia. In: Schottenfeld D, Fraumeni JF Jr, eds. Cancer epidemiology and prevention. Philadelphia: WB Saunders, 1982: 722.
37. Axelsson U, Bachmann R, Hallen J. Frequency of pathological proteins (M-components) in 6995 sera from an adult population. Acta Med Scand 1966;179:235–247.
38. Englisova M, Englis M, Kyral V, et al. Changes of immunoglobulin synthesis in old people. Exp Gerontol 1968;3:125–127.
39. Bazin H, Deckers C, Beckers A, et al. Transplantable immunoglobulin-secreting tumors in rats. I. General features of Lou/Wsl strain rat immunocytomas and their monoclonal proteins. Int J Cancer 1972;10:568–580.
40. Bazin H, Beckers A, Deckers C, et al. Transplantable immunoglobulin-secreting tumors in rats. V. Monoclonal immunoglobulins secreted by 250 ileocecal immunocytomas in Lou/Wsl rats. JNCI 1973;51:1359–1361.
41. Cotran RS, Fortner JG. Serum-protein abnormality in a transplantable plasmacytoma of the Syrian golden hamster. JNCI 1962;28:1193–1205.
42. Farrow BRH, Penny R. Multiple myeloma in a cat. J Am Vet Assoc 1971;158:606–611.
43. Kehoe JM, Hurvitz AI, Capra JD. Characterization of three feline paraproteins. J Immunol 1972;109:511–516.
44. Osborne CA, Perman V, Sautter JH, et al. Multiple myeloma in the dog. J Am Vet Assoc 1968;153:1300–1319.
45. Hurvitz AI. Animal model for human disease: Canine monoclonal gammopathies/immunoglobulins. Comp Pathol Bull 1971;3:4.
46. Payne GS, Bishop JM, Varmus HE. Multiple arrangements of viral DNA and an activated host oncogene in bursal lymphomas. Nature 1982;295:209.
47. Potter M. Concepts of pathogenesis and experimental models of immunoglobulin-secreting tumors in animals. In: Weirnick PH, Canellos GP, Kyle RA, Schiffer CA, eds. Neoplastic diseases of the blood, vol. 1. New York: Churchill-Livingstone, 1985: 393–412.
48. Radl J. Hollander CF, Van Den Berg P, et al. Idiopathic paraproteinemia. I. Studies in an animal model—the aging C57BL/KaLWRij mouse. Clin Exp Immunol 1978;33: 395.
49. Dunn TB. Plasma cell neoplasms beginning in the ileocecal area in strain 3CH mice. JNCI 1957;19:371.
50. Potter M, Wax JS. Genetics of susceptibility to pristane induced plasmacytomas in BALB/cAN. Reduced susceptibility in BALB/cJ with a brief description of pristane-induced arthritis. J Immunol 1981;127:1591.
51. Potter M, Wax JS. Peritoneal plasmacytomas—genesis in mice. A comparison of three pristane dose regimens. JNCI 1983;71:391.
52. Potter M, Pumphrey JG, Bailey DW. Genetics of susceptibility of plasmacytoma induction. I. BALB/cAnN(C), C57BL/6N(B6), C57BL/Ka(BK), (C × B6)F₁ (C × BK)F₁ and C × B recombinant inbred strains. JNCI 1975;54:1413.
53. Potter M. Pathogenesis of plasmacytomas in mice. In: Becker FF, ed. Cancer: A comprehensive treatise. New York: Plenum Press, 1982.
54. Potter M, Boyce C. Induction of plasma cell neoplasms in strain BALB/c mice with mineral oil and mineral oil adjuvants. Nature 1962;193:1086.
55. Merwin RM, Redman LW. Induction of plasma cell tumors and sarcomas in mice by diffusion chambers placed in the peritoneal cavity. JNCI 1963;31:998–1007.
56. Anderson PN. Plasma cell tumor induction in BALB/c mice. Proc Am Assoc Cancer Res [Abstract] 1970;11:3.
57. Potter M, Pumphrey JG, Walters JL. Brief communication: Growth of primary plasmacytomas in the mineral oil-conditioned environment. JNCI 1972;49:305–308.
58. Potter M, Walters JL. Effect of intraperitoneal pristane on established immunity to the Adj-PC-5 plasmacytoma. JNCI 1973;51:875–881.
59. Hamburger AW, Salmon SE. Primary bioassay of human myeloma stem cell. J Clin Invest 1977;60:846–854.
60. Namb Y, Hanaoka M. Immunocytology of cultured IgM-forming cells of mouse. I. Requirement of phagocytic cell factor for the growth of IgM-forming tumor cells in tissue culture. J Immunol 1972;109:1193–1200.
61. Nordan RP, Potter M. A macrophage-derived factor required by plasmacytomas for survival and proliferation in vitro. Science 1986;233:566–568.
62. Metcalf D. The serum factor stimulating colony formation in vitro by murine plasmacytoma cells: Response to antigens and mineral oil. J Immunol 1974;113:235–243.
63. Tosato G, Seamon KB, Goldman ND, et al. Monocyte-derived human B-cell growth factor identified as interferon-β₂ (BSF-2, IL-6). Science 1988;239:502–504.
64. Hamburger AW. Inhibition of B lymphocyte clonal proliferation by spleen cells from plasmacytoma-bearing mice. JNCI 1980;65:1337–1343.
65. McIntire KR, Princler GL. Prolonged adjuvant stimulation in germfree BALB/c mice: Development of plasma cell neoplasia. Immunology 1969;17:481–487.
66. Dalton AJ, Potter M, Merwin RM. Some ultrastructural characteristics of a series of primary and transplanted plasma cell tumors of the mouse. JNCI 1961;26:1221–1267.

67. Kuff EL, Smith LA, Lueders KK. Intracisternal A particle genes in *Mus musculus*. A conserved family of retrovirus-like elements. Mol Cell Biol 1981;1:216.
68. Shepard JS, Pettengill OS, Wurster-Hill DH, et al. A specific chromosome breakpoint associated with mouse plasmacytomas. JNCI 1978;61:225.
69. Yosida MC, Moriwaki K, Migita S. Specificity of the deletion of chromosome no. 15 in mouse plasmacytoma. JNCI 1978;60:235–238.
70. Dickman SH, Goldstein M, Kahn T, et al. Amyloidosis: An unusual complication of Gaucher's disease. Arch Pathol Lab Med 1978;102:460–462.
71. Selvaney P, Block M, Narni R, et al. Alteration and abnormal expression of the c-*myc* oncogene in human multiple myeloma. Blood 1988;71:30–35.
72. Palumbo AP, Boccadero M, Battaglo S, et al. Human homologue of Moloney leukemia virus integration-4 locus (MLVI-4) located 20 kilobases 3' of the *myc* gene, is rearranged in multiple myelomas. Cancer Res 1990;50:6478–6482.
73. MacMahon B, Clark DW. The incidence of multiple myeloma. J Chron Dis 1956;4: 508–515.
74. McPhedran P, Heath CW Jr, Garcia J. Multiple myeloma incidence in metropolitan Atlanta, Georgia: Racial and seasonal variations. Blood 1972;39:866.
75. Bertrams J, Kuwert E, Bohme U, et al. HL-A antigens in Hodgkin's disease and multiple myeloma—increased frequency of W18 in both diseases. Tissue Antigens 1972;2: 41.
76. Jeannet M, Magnin C. HL-A antigens in haematological malignant diseases. Eur J Clin Invest 1971;2:39.
77. Mason DY, Cullen P. HL-A antigen frequencies in myeloma. Tissue Antigens 1975;5: 238.
78. McDevitt HO, Bodner WF. Histocompatibility antigens, immune responsiveness and susceptibility to disease. Am J Med 1972;52:1.
79. Maldonado JE, Kyle RA. Familial myeloma. Report of eight families and a study of serum proteins in their relatives. Am J Med 1974;57:875–884.
80. Blattner WA. Epidemiology of multiple myeloma and related plasma cell disorders: An analytic review. In: Potter M, ed. Progress in myeloma: Biology of myeloma. New York: Elsevier North-Holland, 1980:1.
81. Kyle RA, Heath CW Jr, Carbone P. Multiple myeloma in spouses. Arch Intern Med 1971;127:944–946.
82. Pietruszka M, Rabin BS, Srodes G. Multiple myeloma in husband and wife. Lancet 1976;1:314.
83. Kyle RA. Monoclonal gammopathy of undetermined significance: Natural history in 241 cases. Am J Med 1978;64:814.
84. Meijers KAE, Leeuw B, Voormolen-Kalova M. The multiple occurrence of myeloma and asymptomatic paraproteinaemia within one family. Clin Exp Immunol 1972;12: 185.
85. Youinou P. Genetic propensity to benignity in monoclonal gammopathy. Acta Haematol (Basel) 1979;62:173.
86. Axelsson U, Hallen J. Familial occurrence of pathological serum proteins of different gammaglobulin groups. Lancet 1965;2:369.
87. Williams RC, Erickson JL, Polesky HF, et al. Studies of monoclonal immunoglobulins (M-components) in various kindreds. Ann Intern Med 1967;67:309.
88. Blattner WA, Garber J, Mann DL, et al. Waldenström's macroglobulinemia and autoimmune disease in a family. Ann Intern Med 1980;93:830.
89. Björnsson OG, Arnason A, Gudmundsson S, et al. Macroglobulinema in an Icelandic family. Acta Med Scand 1978;203:283.
90. Fine JM, Lambin P, Valentin L, et al. IgG monoclonal gammopathy in the sister of a patient with Waldenström's macroglobulinemia. Biomedicine 1973;19:117.
91. Fraumeni JF Jr, Wertelecki W, Blattner WA, et al. Varied manifestations of a familial lymphoproliferative disorder. Am J Med 1975;59:145.
92. Kalff MW, Hijmans W. Immunoglobulin analysis in families of macroglobulinemia patients. Clin Exp Immunol 1969;5:479.
93. Seligmann M, Sassy C, Chevalier A. A human IgG myeloma protein with anti-alpha₂-macroglobulin antibody activity. J Immunol 1973;110:85.
94. Salmon SE, Seligmann M. B-cell neoplasia in man. Lancet 1974;2:1230.
95. Cuzick J, De Stavola B. Multiple myeloma. A case control study. Br J Cancer 1988;57: 516–520.
96. Linet MS, Sioban DH, McLaughlin JK. A case-control study of multiple myeloma in whites: Chronic antigenic stimulation, occupation and drug use. Cancer Res 1987;47: 2978–2981.
97. Hamaker WR, Lindell ME, Gomez AC. Plasmacytoma arising in a pacemaker pocket. Ann Thorac Surg 1976;21:354.
98. Gerber MA. Asbestosis and neoplastic disorders of the hematopoietic system. Am J Clin Pathol 1970;53:204–208.
99. Kagan E, Jacobson RJ, Yeung K-Y, et al. Asbestosis-associated neoplasms of B cell lineage. Am J Med 1979;67:325–330.
100. Osserman EF, Takatsuki L. Considerations regarding the pathogenesis of the plasmacytic dyscrasias. Semin Hematol 1965;4:28–49.
101. Pratt PW, Estren S, Kochwa S. Immunoglobulin abnormalities in Gaucher's disease: Report of 16 cases. Blood 1968;31:633–640.
102. Wolf P. Monoclonal gammopathy in Gaucher's disease. Lab Med 1973;4:28–29.
103. MacDonald M, McCathie M, Faed MJW, et al. Gaucher's disease with bronchial gammopathy. J Clin Pathol 1975;28:757.
104. Turesson I, Rausing A. Gaucher's disease and benign monoclonal gammopathy. Acta Med Scand 1975;197:507–512.
105. Penny R, Hughes S. Repeated stimulation of the reticuloendothelial system and the development of plasma cell dyscrasias. Lancet 1970;1:77–78.
106. Rosenblatt J, Hall CA. Plasma-cell dyscrasia following prolonged stimulation of reticuloendothelial system. Lancet 1970;1:301–302.

107. Isobe T, Osserman EF. Pathologic conditions associated with plasma cell dyscrasias: A study of 806 cases. Ann N Y Acad Sci 1971;90:507–518.

108. Goldenberg GJ, Paraskevas F, Israels LG. The association of rheumatoid arthritis with plasma cell and lymphocytic neoplasms. Arthritis Rheum 1969;12:569–579.

109. Wegelius O, Skrifvars B. Rheumatoid arthritis terminating in plasmacytoma. Acta Med Scand 1970;187:133–138.

110. Wohlenberg H. Osteomyelitis and plasmacytoma. N Engl J Med 1970;283:822–823.

111. Isomaki HA, Hakulmen T, Joutsenlahti U. Excess risk of lymphomas, leukemias and myelomas in patients with rheumatoid arthritis. J Chron Dis 1978;31:691–699.

112. Imahori S, Moore GE. Multiple myeloma and prolonged stimulation of reticuloendothelial system. N Y State J Med 1972;72:1625.

113. Jancelewicz Z, Takatsuki K, Sugai S, et al. IgD multiple myeloma. Review of 133 cases. Arch Intern Med 1975;135:87.

114. Schafer AI, Miller JB. Association of IgA multiple myeloma with preexisting disease. Br J Haematol 1979;41:19–24.

115. Schafer AI, Miller JB, Lester EP, et al. Monoclonal gammopathy in hereditary spherocytosis: A possible pathogenetic relation. Ann Intern Med 1978;88:45–46.

116. Waldbaum B, Gelfand M. Myelomatosis in the Rhodesian African. Trop Geogr Med 1974;26:26.

117. Krause RM. Factors controlling the occurrence of antibodies with uniform properties. Fed Proc 1970;29:59.

118. Ichimaru M, Ishimaru T, Mikami M, et al. Multiple myeloma among atomic bomb survivors, Hiroshima and Nagasaki, 1950–1976. Radiation effects research foundation technical report no. 9–79. Hiroshima: Radiation Effects Research Foundation, 1979.

119. Cuzik J. Radiation-induced myelomatosis. N Engl J Med 1981;304:204–210.

120. Lewis EB. Leukemia, multiple myeloma, and aplastic anemia in American radiologists. Science 1963;142:1492.

121. Matanoski GM. Risk of cancer associated with occupational exposure in radiologists and other radiation workers. In: Burchenal JH, Oettgen HF, eds. Cancer, achievements, challenges, and prospects for the 1980s. New York: Grune & Stratton, 1982:241.

122. Matanoski GM, Seltzer R, Santwell RE, et al. The current mortality rates of radiologists and other physician specialists: Specific causes of death. Am J Epidemiol 1975;101:199.

123. Mancuso TE, Stewart A, Kneale G. Radiation exposures of Hanford workers dying from cancer and other causes. Health Phys 1977;33:369.

124. Boice JD Jr, Morin MM, Glass AG, et al. Diagnostic x-ray procedures and risk of leukemia, lymphoma and multiple myeloma. JAMA 1991;265:1290–1294.

125. Hayhoe FGJ, Neuman Z. Cytology of myeloma cells. J Clin Pathol 1976;29:916.

126. Paraskevas F, Heremans J, Waldenström J. Cytology and electrophoretic pattern in γ,A (B₂A) myeloma. Acta Med Scand 1961;170:575–589.

127. Maldonado JE, Bayrd ED, Brown AL. The flaming cell in multiple myeloma: A light and electron microscopy study. Am J Clin Pathol 1965;44:605.

128. Farquhar MG, Palade GE. The Golgi apparatus (1954–1981) from artifact to center stage. J Cell Biol 1981;91:77–103.

129. Blom J, Mansa B, Wiik A. A study of Russell bodies in human monoclonal plasma cell by means of immunofluorescence and electron microscopy. Acta Pathol Microbiol Scand [A] 1976;84:335.

130. Durie B, Grogan T. CALLA positive myeloma an aggressive subtype with poor survival. Blood 1985;66:229–232.

131. Grogan TM, Durie BGM, Lomen C, et al. Delineation of a novel pre-B cell component in plasma cell myeloma: Immunochemical, immunophenotypic, genotypic, cytologic, cell culture, and kinetic features. Blood 1987;70:932–942.

132. Bataille R, Durie BGM, Sany J, Salmon SE. Myeloma bone marrow acid phosphatase staining: A correlative study of 38 patients. Blood 1980;55:802.

133. Cassuto JP, Hammou JC, Pastorelli E, et al. Plasma acid cell phosphatase, a discriminative test for benign and malignant monoclonal gammopathies. Biomedicine 1977;27:197.

134. Tortarolo M, Cantore N, Grande M, et al. Plasma cell acid phosphatase an adjunct in the differential diagnosis of monoclonal immunoglobulinemias. Acta Haematol 1981;65:103.

135. Kyle KA, Greipp PR. Smoldering multiple myeloma. N Engl J Med 1980;302:1347–1349.

136. Durie BGM, Salmon SE, Moon TE. Pretreatment tumor mass, cell kinetics, and prognosis in multiple myeloma. Blood 1980;55:364–372.

137. Greipp PR, Witzig TE, Gonchoroff NJ, et al. Immunofluorescence labeling indices in myeloma and related monoclonal gammopathies. Mayo Clin Proc 1987;62:969–977.

138. Barlogie B, Latreille J, Alexanian R, et al. Quantitative cytology in myeloma research. In: Hoffbrand AV, Lasch HG, Nathan DG, Salmon SE, eds. Clinics in Hematology. Eastbourne: WB Saunders, 1982:19–46.

139. Seigneurin D, David J, Sotto JJ, et al. β-Glucuronidases plasmocytaires dans les dysglobulinemias. Interet diagnostique de leur mise en evidence. Pathol Biol 1979;27:467.

140. Duston MA, Skinner M, Shirahama T, et al. Diagnosis of amyloidosis by abdominal fat aspiration. Am J Med 1987;82:412–414.

141. Levy Y, Tsapis A, Brovet JC. Interleukin-6 antisense oligonucleotides inhibit the growth of human myeloma cell lines. J Clin Invest 1991;88:696–699.

142. Klein B, Zhang XG, Jourdan M, et al. Paracrine rather than autocrine regulation of myeloma-cell growth and differentiation by Interleukin-6. Blood 1989;73:517–526.

143. Mundy GR, Raisz LG, Cooper RA, et al. Evidence for the secretion of an osteoclast stimulating factor in myeloma. N Engl J Med 1974;291:1041–1046.

144. Valentin-Opran A. Charhon SA. Meunier PJ, et al. Quantitative histology of myeloma-induced bone changes. Br J Haematol 1982;52:602–610.

145. Durie BGM, Salmon SE, Mundy GR. Relation of osteoclast activating factor production to the extent of bone disease in multiple myeloma. Br J Haematol 1981;47:21–30.

146. Garret IR, Durie BGM, Nedwin GE, et al. Production of lymphotoxin, a bone-resorbing cytokine by cultured human myeloma cells. N Engl J Med 1987;317:526–532.

147. Cozzolino F, Torcia M, Aldinucci D, et al. Production of interleukin-1 by bone marrow myeloma cells. Blood 1989;74:380–387.

148. Solomon A, Waldmann TA, Fahey JL, et al. Metabolism of Bence Jones proteins. J Clin Invest 1964;43:103–117.

149. Waldmann TA, Strober W, Mogielnicki RP. The renal handling of low-molecular-weight proteins. II. Disorders of serum protein catabolism in patients with tubular proteinuria, the nephrotic syndrome, or uremia. J Clin Invest 1964;51:2162–2174.

150. Wochner RD, Strober W, Waldmann TA. The role of catabolism of Bence Jones proteins and immunoglobulin fragments. J Exp Med 1967;126:207–221.

151. Solomon A, Weiss DT, Kattine AA. Nephro-toxic potential of Bence Jones proteins. N Engl J Med 1991;324:1845–1851.

152. Levi DF, Williams RC Jr, Lindstrom FD. Immunofluorescent studies of the myeloma kidney with special reference to light chain disease. Am J Med 1968;33:92–933.

153. Costanza DJ, Smoller M. Multiple myeloma with the Fanconi syndrome. Study of a case, with electron microscopy of the kidney. Am J Med 1963;34:125–133.

154. Engle RL Jr, Wallis LA. Multiple myeloma and the adult Fanconi syndrome. I. Report of a case with crystal-like deposits in the tumor cells and in the epithelial cells of the kidney. Am J Med 1957;22:5–12.

155. Finkel PN, Kronenberg K, Pesce AJ, et al. Adult Fanconi syndrome, amyloidosis, and marked kappa light chain proteinuria. Nephron 1973;10:1–24.

156. Sirtoa JH, Hamerman D. Renal function studies in an adult subject with the Fanconi syndrome. Am J Med 1954;16:138–152.

157. Preuss HG, Hammack WJ, Murdaugh HV. The effect of Bence Jones protein on the in vitro function of rabbit renal cortex. Nephron 1967;5:210–216.

158. Preuss HG, Weiss FR, Iammarino RM, et al. Effect on rat kidney slice function in vitro of proteins from the urines of patients with myelomatosis and nephrosis. Clin Sci Mol Med 1974;46:283–294.

159. Maldonado JE, Velosa JA, Kyle RA, et al. Fanconi syndrome in adults. A manifestation of a latent form of myeloma. Am J Med 1975;58:354–364.

160. Kyle RA, Greipp PR. "Idiopathic" Bence Jones proteinuria. Long-term follow-up in seven patients. N Engl J Med 1982;306:564–567.

161. Pruzanski W, Ogryzlo MA. Abnormal proteinuria in malignant diseases. Adv Clin Chem 1970;13:335–382.

162. Pruzanski W, Gidon MS, Roy A. Suppression of polyclonal immunoglobulins in multiple myeloma: Relationship to the staging and other manifestations at diagnosis. Clin Immunol Immunopathol 1980;17:280.

163. Duperray C, Bataille R, Boiron JM, et al. No expansion of the pre-B and B cell compartments of the bone marrow in patients with multiple myeloma. Cancer Res 1991;51:3224–3228.

164. Ullrich S, Zolla-Pazner S. Immunoregulatory circuits in myeloma. In: Hoffbrand AV, Lasch HG, Nathan DG, Salmon SE, eds. Clinics in Hematology. Eastbourne: WB Saunders, 1982:87–111.

165. Broder S, Humphrey R, Durm M, et al. Impaired synthesis of polyclonal (non-paraprotein) immunoglobulin by circulating lymphocytes from patients with multiple myeloma: Role of suppressor cells. N Engl J Med 1975;293:887–892.

166. Salmon SE. Paraneoplastic syndromes associated with monoclonal lymphocyte and plasma cell proliferation. Ann N Y Acad Sci 1974;230:228–239.

167. Bovill EG, Ershler WB, Golden EA, et al. A human myeloma-produced monoclonal protein directed against the active subpopulation von Willebrand factor. Am J Clin Pathol 1986;85:115–123.

168. Merlini G, Farhangi M, Osserman EF. Monoclonal immunoglobulins with antibody activity in myeloma, macroglobulinemia and related plasma cell dyscrasias. Semin Oncol 1986;13:350–365.

169. Kilgore LL, Patterson BW, Parenti DM, et al. Immune complex hyperlipidemia induced by an apolipoprotein-reactive immunoglobulin A paraprotein from a patient with multiple myeloma. J Clin Invest 1985;76:225–232.

170. Sullivan PW, Salmon SE. Kinetics of tumor growth and regression in IgG myeloma. J Clin Invest 1972;51:1597.

171. Drewinko B, Alexanian R, Boyer H, et al. The growth fraction of human myeloma cells. Blood 1981;57:333.

172. Hobbs JR. Growth rates and response to treatment in human myelomatosis. Br J Haematol 1969;16:607.

173. Bergsagel DE. Assessment of the response of mouse and human myeloma to chemotherapy and radiotherapy. In: Drewinko B, Humphreya RM, eds. Growth kinetics and biochemical regulation of normal and malignant cells. University of Texas Cancer Center, M.D. Anderson Hospital and Tumor Institute, 29th Annual Symposium on Fundamental Cancer Research. Baltimore: Williams & Wilkins, 1977:705–717.

174. Bergsagel DE, Pruzanski W. Treatment of plasma cell myeloma with cytotoxic agents. Arch Intern Med 1975;135:172–176.

175. Suchman AL, Coleman M, Mouradian JA, et al. Aggressive plasma cell myeloma: A terminal phase. Arch Intern Med 1981;141:1315–1320.

176. Falini B, DeSolas I, Levine AM, et al. Emergence of B-immunoblastic sarcoma in patients with multiple myeloma: a clinicopathologic study of 10 cases. Blood 1982;59:923–933.

177. Hobbs JR. Immunocytoma o' mice an' men. Br Med J 1971;2:67.

178. Ludwig H, Tscholakoff D, Neuhold, et al. Magnetic resonance imaging of the spine in multiple myeloma. Lancet 1987;2:364–366.

179. Alexanian R. Localized and indolent myeloma. Blood 1980;56:521.

180. Durie BGM, Salmon SE. Multiple myeloma, macroglobulinaemia and monoclonal

gammopathies. In: Hoffbrand AV, Brain MC, Hirsh J, eds. Recent advances in haematology. Edinburgh: Churchill-Livingstone, 1977:243.

181. Durie BGM, Salmon SE. A clinical staging system for multiple myeloma. Correlation of measured myeloma cell mass with presenting clinical features, response to treatment and survival. Cancer 1975;36:842–852.

182. Alexanian R, Balcerzak S, Bonnet JD, et al. Prognostic factors in multiple myeloma. Cancer 1975;36:1192–1201.

183. Woodruff RK, Wadworth J, Malpas JS, et al. Clinical staging in multiple myeloma. Br J Haematol 1979;42:199–205.

184. Merlini G, Waldenström JC, Jayakar SD. A new improved clinical staging system for multiple myeloma based on analysis of 123 treated patients. Blood 1980;55:1011–1019.

185. Belpomme D, Simon F, Pouillart P, et al. Prognostic factors and treatment of multiple myeloma: Interest of a cyclic sequential chemohormonotherapy combining cyclophosphamide, melphalan and prednisone. Recent Results Cancer Res 1978;65:28–40.

186. Gobbi M, Cavo M, Savelli G, et al. Prognostic factors and survival in multiple myeloma. Analysis of 91 cases treated by melphalan and prednisone. Haematology 1980;65:437–445.

187. Santoro A. Schieppati G, Franchi F, et al. Clinical staging and therapeutic results in multiple myeloma. Eur J Cancer Clin Oncol 1983;19:1353–1359.

188. Bergsagel DE, Phil D, Bailey AJ, et al. The chemotherapy of plasma cell myeloma and the incidence of acute leukemia. N Engl J Med 1979;301:743.

189. Bergsagel DE, Bailey AJ, Langley GR, et al. The chemotherapy of plasma cell myeloma and the incidence of acute leukemia. N Engl J Med 1979;301:743.

190. Salmon SE, Haut A, Bonnet J, et al. Alternating combination chemotherapy improves survival in multiple myeloma. A Southwest Oncology Group study. J Clin Oncol 1983;1:453.

191. Durie BGM. Staging and kinetics of multiple myeloma. In: Hoffbrand AV, Lasch HG, Nathan DG, Salmon SE, eds. Clinics in Hematology. Eastbourne: WB Saunders, 1982:3–18.

192. Durie BGM, Cole PW, Chen HSG, et al. Synthesis and metabolism of Bence Jones protein and calculation of tumour burden in patients with Bence Jones myeloma. Br J Haematol 1981;47:7.

193. Waldenström J. Diagnosis and treatment of multiple myeloma. New York: Grune & Stratton, 1970.

194. Seligmann M, Basch A. The clinical significance of pathological immunoglobulins. In: XII International Congress of Hematology (plenary session papers). New York: International Society of Hematology, 1968:21–31.

195. Hobbs JR. Paraproteins, benign or malignant? Br Med J 1967;3:699–704.

196. Kyle RA, Maldonado JE, Bayrd ED. Idiopathic Bence Jones proteinuria—a distinct entity? Am J Med 1973;55:222–226.

197. Norfolk D, Child JA, Cooper EH, et al. Serum β_2-microglobulin in myelomatosis: Potential value in stratification and monitoring. Br J Cancer 1980;42:510–515.

198. Karlsson FA, Groth T, Sege K, et al. Turnover in humans of β_2-microglobulin: The constant chain of HLA-antigens. Eur J Clin Invest 1980;10:293–300.

199. Cassuto JP, Krebs BJ, Viot G, et al. β_2-microglobulin, a tumour marker of lymphoproliferative disorders. Lancet 1978;2:108.

200. Bataille R, Magullo M, Greinier J, et al. Serum beta-2-microglobulin in multiple myeloma: Relation to presenting factors and clinical status. Eur J Cancer Clin Oncol 1982;18:59–66.

201. Scarffe JH, Anderson H, Palmer MK, et al. Prognostic significant of pretreatment serum β-2-microglobulin levels in multiple myeloma. Eur J Cancer Clin Oncol 1983;19:1361–1364.

202. Bataille R, Magulo M, Greinier J, et al. Serum beta-2-microglobulin in multiple myeloma: A simple, reliable marker for staging. Br J Haematol 1983;55:439.

203. Bataille R, Grenier J. Serum beta-2 microglobulin in multiple myeloma—A critical review. Eur J Cancer 1987;23:1829–1832.

204. Bataille R, Durie BGM, Grenier J, et al. Prognostic factors and staging in multiple myeloma: A reappraisal. J Clin Oncol 1986;4:80–87.

205. Durie BGM, Stock-Novack D, Salmon SE, et al. Prognostic value of pretreatment serum β_2-microglobulin in myeloma: A Southwest Oncology Group study. Blood 1990;75:823–830.

206. Salmon SE, Tesh D, Crowley J, et al. Chemotherapy is superior to sequential hemibody irradiation for remission consolidation in multiple myeloma: A Southwest Oncology study. J Clin Oncol 1990;8:1575–1584.

207. Karlsson FA, Wibell L, Evrin PE. β_2-microglobulin in clinical medicine. Scand J Clin Lab Invest 1980;40(suppl 154):27.

208. Tienharra A, Remes K, Pelliniemi TT. Alpha interferon raises serum beta-2-microglobulin in patients with multiple myeloma. Br J Haematol 1991;77:335–338.

209. Durie BGM, Russell DH, Salmon SE. Reappraisal of plateau phase in myeloma. Lancet 1980;2:65–68.

210. Chronic Leukemia-Myeloma Task Force, National Cancer Institute. Proposed guidelines for protocol studies. II. Plasma cell myeloma. Cancer Chemother Rep 1973;4:145–158.

211. Waldmann TA, Strober W. Metabolism of immunoglobulins. Prog Allergy 1969;13:1.

212. Salmon SE, Wampler SE. Multiple myeloma: Quantitative staging and assessment of response with a programmable pocket calculator. Blood 1977;49:379–389.

213. Palmer M, Belch A, Brox L, et al. Are the current criteria for response useful in the management of multiple myeloma? J Clin Oncol 1987;5:1373–1377.

214. Alexanian R, Barlogie B, Dixon D. High-dose glucocorticoid treatment of resistant myeloma. Ann Intern Med 1983;105:8–11.

215. Sporn JR, McIntyre OR. Chemotherapy of previously untreated multiple myeloma patients: An analysis of recent treatment results. Semin Oncol 1986;13:318–325.

216. Salmon SE. Expansion of the growth fraction in multiple myeloma with alkylating agents. Blood 1975;45:119–129.

217. Jackson DV, Case LD, Pope EK, et al. Single agent vincristine by infusion in refractory multiple myeloma. J Clin Oncol 1985;3:1508–1512.

218. MacLennan IC, Cusick J. Objective evaluation of the role of vincristine in induction and maintenance therapy for myelomatosis. Medical Research Council Working Party on Leukaemia in Adults. Br J Cancer 1985;52:153–158.

219. Mellstedt H, Bjorkholm M, Johansson B. Interferon therapy in myelomatosis. Lancet 1979;1:245–248.

220. Gutterman JU, Blumenschein GR, Alexanian R. Leucocyte interferon-induced tumor regression in human metastatic breast cancer, multiple myeloma, and malignant lymphoma. Ann Intern Med 1980;93:399–406.

221. Costanzi JJ, Cooper MR, Scarffe JH, et al. Phase II study of recombinant alpha-2 interferon in resistant multiple myeloma. J Clin Oncol 1985;3:654–659.

222. Oken MM, Kyle RA, Kay NE, et al. A phase II trial of interferon alpha$_2$ (rIFN$_2$) in the treatment of resistant multiple myeloma. Proc Am Soc Clin Oncol [Abstract 837] 1985;4:215.

223. Quesada JR, Alexanian R, Hawkins M, et al. Treatment of multiple myeloma with recombinant β-interferon. Blood 1986;67:275–278.

224. Cooper MR, Fefer A, Thompson J, et al. Alpha-2-interferon/melphalan/prednisone in previously untreated patients with multiple myeloma: A phase I-II trial. Cancer Treat Rep 1986;70:473–476.

225. Benson WJ, Scarffe JH, Todd IDH, et al. Spinal cord compression in myeloma. Br Med J 1979;1:1541–1544.

226. Mill WB, Griffith R. The role of radiation therapy in the management of plasma cell tumors. Cancer 1980;45:647–652.

227. Mill WB. Radiation therapy in multiple myeloma. Radiology 1975;115:175–178.

228. Garrett MJ. Spinal myeloma and cord compression—diagnosis and management. Clin Radiol 1970;21:42–46.

229. Garland LH, Kennedy BR. Roentgen treatment of multiple myeloma. Radiology 1948;50:297–316.

230. Bosch A, Frias Z. Radiotherapy in the treatment of multiple myeloma. Int J Radiat Oncol Biol Phys 1988;15:1363–1369.

231. Rostom AY. A review of the place of radiotherapy in myeloma with emphasis in whole body irradiation. Hematol Oncol 1988;6:193–198.

232. McIntyre OR, Tefft M, Propert R, et al. Melphalan and prednisone plus total bone marrow irradiation as initial treatment for multiple myeloma. Int J Radiat Oncol Biol Phys 1988;15:1007–1012.

233. Ellwanger FR. Controlling multiple myeloma. Int J Radiat Oncol Biol Phys 1989;16:909.

234. Alberts DS, Chang FY, Chen HSG, et al. Oral melphalan kinetics. Clin Pharmacol Ther 1979;6:737–745.

235. Feinleib M, MacMahon B. Duration of survival in multiple myeloma. JNCI 1960;24:1259–1269.

236. Osgood EE. The survival time of patients with plasmocytic myeloma. Cancer Chemother Rep 1960;9:1–10.

237. McArthur JR, Athens JW, Wintrobe MM, et al. Melphalan and myeloma. Experience with a low-dose continuous regimen. Ann Intern Med 1970;72:665–670.

238. Alexanian R, Bergsagel DE, Migliore PJ, et al. Melphalan therapy for plasma cell myeloma. Blood 1968;31:1–10.

239. Alexanian R, Haut A, Khan AU, et al. Treatment for multiple myeloma. JAMA 1969;208:1680–1685.

240. Hoogstraten B, Sheehe PR, Cuttner J, et al. Melphalan in multiple myeloma. Blood 1967;30:74–83.

241. Hoogstraten B, Costa J. Intermittent melphalan therapy in multiple myeloma. JAMA 1969;209:251–253.

242. Medical Research Council. Myelomatosis: Comparison of melphalan and cyclophosphamide therapy. Br Med J 1971;1:640–641.

243. Medical Research Council. Report on the second myelomatosis trial after five years of follow-up. Br J Cancer 1980;42:813–822.

244. Medical Research Council. Treatment comparisons in the third MRC myelomatosis trial. Br J Cancer 1980;42:823–830.

245. Ogawa M, Bergsagel D, McCulloch E. Chemotherapy of mouse myeloma: Quantitative cell cultures predictive of response in vivo. Blood 1973;41:7–15.

246. Case DC, Lee BJ III, Clarkson BD. Improved survival times in multiple myeloma treated with melphalan, prednisone, cyclophosphamide, vincristine and BCNU: M2 protocol. Am J Med 1977;63:897–903.

247. Bonnet J, Alexanian R, Salmon S, et al. Vincristine-BCNU-Adriamycin-prednisone (VBAP) combination in the treatment of relapsing or resistant multiple myeloma. A Southwest Oncology Group study. Cancer Treat Rep 1982;66:1267–1271.

248. MacLennan IC, Chapman C, Dunn J, Kelly K. Combined chemotherapy with ABCM versus melphalan for treatment of myelomatosis. Lancet 1992;340:433–438.

249. Oken MM, Tsiatis A, Abramson N, et al. Comparison of MP with intensive VBMCP therapy for the treatment of multiple myeloma (MM). Proc Am Soc Clin Oncol [Abstract] 1984;3:270.

250. Hansen OP, Clausen NT, Drivsholm A, et al. Phase II study of intermittent 5-drug regimen (VBCMP) versus intermittent 3-drug regimen (VMP), versus intermittent melphalan and prednisone (MP) in myelomatosis. Scand J Haematol 1985;35:518–524.

251. Durie BGM, Dixon B, Carter S, et al. Improved survival duration with combination chemotherapy induction for multiple myeloma: A Southwest Oncology Group study. J Clin Oncol 1986;4:1127–1237.

252. Harley JB, Pajak TF, McIntyre OR, et al. Improved survival of increased-risk myeloma patients on combined triple alkylating agent therapy: A study of the CALGB. Blood 1979;54:13–22.

253. Boccadero M, Marmont F, Tribalto M, et al. Multiple myeloma: VMCP/VBAP alternating melphalan and prednisone even in high risk patients. J Clin Oncol 1991;9: 444–448.

254. Cooper MR, McIntyre OR, Propert KJ, et al. Single, sequential, and multiple alkylating agent therapy for multiple myeloma: A CALGB study. J Clin Oncol 1986;4:1331–1339.

255. Pavlovsky S, Saslavsky J, Tezanos Pinto M, et al. A randomized trial of melphalan and prednisone versus melphalan, prednisone, cyclophosphamide, MeCCNU, and vincristine in untreated multiple myeloma. J Clin Oncol 1984;2:836–840.

256. Palva IP, Ahrenberg A, Almquist K, et al. Aggressive combination chemotherapy in multiple myeloma. A multicentre trial. Scand J Haematol 1985;35:205–209.

257. Kildahl-Anderson P, Bjark P, Bondevik A, et al. Multiple myeloma in central Norway 1981–1982: A randomized clinical trial of 5-drug combination therapy versus standard therapy. Scand J Haematol 1986;37:243–248.

258. Cohen HJ, Silberman HR, Tornyos K, et al. Comparison of two long-term chemotherapy regimens, with or without agents to modify skeletal repair, in multiple myeloma. Blood 1984;63:639–648.

259. Mettstedt H, Aahre A. Bjorkholm M. Interferon therapy of patients with myeloma. In: Terry WD, Rosenberg SA, eds. Immunotherapy of human cancer. New York: Elsevier, 1982:387–391.

260. Case DC, Sonneborn HL, Paul SD, et al. Phase II study of rDNA alpha-2 interferon (intron A) in patients with multiple myeloma utilizing an escalating induction phase. Cancer Treat Rep 1986;70:1251–1254.

261. Cooper MR, Welander CE. Interferons in the treatment of multiple myeloma. Semin Oncol 1986;13:334–340.

262. Ludwig H, Cortelezzi A, Van Camp BGK, et al. Treatment with recombinant-alpha-2C. Multiple myeloma and thrombocythaemia in myeloproliferative diseases. Oncology 1985;42(suppl 1):19–25.

263. Ahre A, Bjorkholm M, Mellstedt H, et al. Human leukocyte interferon and intermittent high-dose melphalan-prednisone administration in the treatment of multiple myeloma: A randomized clinical trial from the Myeloma Group of Central Sweden. Cancer Treat Rep 1984;68:1331–1338.

264. Alexanian R, Gehan E, Haut A, et al. Unmaintained remissions in multiple myeloma. Blood 1978;51:1005–1011.

265. Alexanian R. Long unmaintained remission in multiple myeloma. Am J Clin Oncol 1986;9:458–460.

266. Southwest Oncology Group study. Remission maintenance therapy for multiple myeloma. Arch Intern Med 1975;135:147.

267. Belch A. White D, Bergsagel D, et al. The role of maintenance chemotherapy for multiple myeloma. Proc Am Soc Clin Oncol [Abstract c1050] 1984;3:268 1984.

268. Cohen JH, Bartolucci AA, Forman WB, et al. Consolidation and maintenance therapy in multiple myeloma: Randomized comparison of a new approach to therapy after initial response to treatment. J Clin Oncol 1986;5:888–899.

269. Tribalto M, Mandelli F, Cantonetti M, et al. In: Bernasconi C, ed. New trends in the therapy of leukemia and lymphoma. Pavia, Italy: Edizione Medic Scientifiche, 1987: 61–68.

270. Mandell F, Tribalto M, Cantonetti M, et al. Recombinant alpha 2β interferon as maintenance therapy in responding multiple myeloma patients. Blood 1987;70(suppl 1):247a.

271. Salmon SE, Crowley J. Impact of glucocorticoids and interferon on outcome in multiple myeloma. Proc Am Soc Clin Oncol [Abstract] 1992;11:316.

272. Crowin J, Lindberg RD. Solitary plasmacytoma of bone vs extramedullary plasmacytoma and their relationship to multiple myeloma. Cancer 1979;43:1007–1013.

273. Knowling M, Harwood A, Bergsagel DE. A comparison of extramedullary plasmacytoma with multiple and solitary plasma cell tumors of bone. J Clin Oncol 1983;1:255–262.

274. Wiltshaw E. The natural history of extramedullary plasmacytoma and its relation to solitary myeloma of bone and myelomatosis. Medicine (Baltimore) 1976;55:217–238.

275. Woodruff RK, Malpas JS, White FE. Solitary plasmacytoma. II. Solitary plasmacytoma of bone. Cancer 1979;43:2344–2347.

276. Chak LY, Cox S, Bostwick DG, et al. Solitary plasmacytoma of bone: Treatment, progression, and survival. J Clin Oncol 1987;5:1811–1815.

277. Woodruff RK, Whittle JM, Malpas JS. Solitary plasmacytoma. I. Extramedullary soft tissue plasmacytoma. Cancer 1979;43:2340–2343.

278. Hamburger AW, Salmon SE. Primary bioassay of human tumor stem cells. Science 1977;197:461–463.

279. Otsuka T, Okamura S, Niho Y. Colony assay in patients with multiple myeloma—relationship between colony growth and clinical stage. Acta Haematol Jpn 1986;49: 1792–1799.

280. Salmon SE, Hamburger AW, Soehnlen BJ, et al. Quantitation of differential sensitivity of human tumor stem cells to anticancer drugs. N Engl J Med 1978;298:1321–1327.

281. Salmon SE. In vitro cloning and chemosensitivity of human myeloma stem cells. In: Hoffbrand AV, Lasch HG, Nathan DG, Salmon SE, eds. Clinics in Hematology. Eastbourne: WB Saunders, 1982:47–64.

282. Ludwig H, Fritz E. Individualized chemotherapy in multiple myeloma by cytostatic drug sensitivity testing of colony-forming stem cells. Anticancer Res 1981;1:329–334.

283. Nordan RP, Pumphrey JG, Rudikoff S. Purification and NH₂-terminal sequence of a plasmacytoma growth factor derived from the murine macrophage cell line P388D1. J Immunol 1987;139:813–817.

284. Van Snick J, Cayphas S, Vink A, et al. Purification and NH₂-terminal amino acid sequence of a T-cell derived lymphokine with growth factor activity for B-cell hybridomas. Proc Natl Acad Sci USA 1986;83:9679–9683.

285. Tanigawa N, Kern DH, Hikasa Y, et al. Rapid assay for evaluating the chemosensitivity of human tumors in soft agar culture. Cancer Res 1982;42:2159–2164.

286. Alexanian R, Salmon S, Gutterman J, et al. Chemoimmunotherapy of multiple myeloma. Cancer 1981;47:1923–1929.

287. Buzaid AC, Durie BGM. Management of refractory myeloma: A review. J Clin Oncol 1988;6:889–905.

288. Kyle RA, Greipp PR, Gertz MA. Treatment of refractory multiple myeloma and considerations for future therapy. Semin Oncol 1986;13:326–333.

289. Medenica R, Slack N. Clinical results of leucocyte interferon-induced tumor regression in resistant human metastatic cancer resistant to chemotherapy and/or radio-therapy-pulse therapy schedule. Cancer Drug Deliv 1985;2:53–76.

290. Wagstaff A, Loynds R, Scarffe JH. Phase II study of rDNA human alpha-2 interferon in multiple myeloma. Cancer Treat Rep 1985;69:495–498.

291. Ohno R, Kimura K, Amaki I, et al. Treatment of multiple myeloma with recombinant human leucocyte α interferon. Cancer Treat Rep 1985;69:1433–1435.

292. Alexanian R, Yap BS, Bodey GP. Prednisone pulse therapy for refractory myeloma. Blood 1983;62:572–577.

293. Alexanian R, Dimopoulos M, Barlogie B. Intermittent dexamethasone as initial chemotherapy for multiple myeloma. Blood 1991;78:174a.

293a. Alexanian R, Dimopoulos MA, Barlogie B. Primary dexamethasone treatment of multiple myeloma. Blood 1992;80:887–890.

294. Dalton WS, Durie BGM, Alberts DS, et al. Characterization of a new drug resistant human myeloma cell line which expresses P-glycoprotein. Cancer Res 1986;45:5125–5130.

295. Murakami T, Togawa A, Satch H, et al. Glucocorticoid receptor in myeloma. Eur J Haematol 1987;39:54–59.

296. Bergsagel DE, Cowan DH, Hasselbach R. Plasma cell myeloma: Response of melphalan-resistant patients to high-dose intermittent cyclophosphamide. Can Med Assoc J 1972;107:851–855.

297. Kyle RA, Sligman BR, Wallace J, et al. Multiple myeloma resistant to melphalan (NSC-8806) treated with cyclophosphamide (NSC-26271), prednisone (NSC-10023), and chloroquine (NSC-187208). Cancer Chemother Rep 1975;59:557–562.

298. Tornyos K, Silberman H, Soloman A. Phase II study of oral methyl-CCNU and prednisone in previously treated alkylating agent-resistant multiple myeloma. Cancer Treat Rep 1977;61:785–787.

299. Buonanno G, Tortarolo M, Valente A, et al. Drug-resistant multiple myeloma. A trial with the M₂ cyclic alkylating agent polychemotherapy. Haematologica (Pavia) 1978;63: 45–55.

300. Kyle RA, Gailani S, Seligman BR, et al. Multiple myeloma resistant to melphalan: Treatment with cyclophosphamide, prednisone, and BCNU. Cancer Treat Rep 1979;63: 1265–1269.

301. Blade J, Feliu E. Rozman C, et al. Cross-resistance to alkylating agents in multiple myeloma. Cancer 1983;52:786–789.

302. Steinke B, Busch FW, Becherer C, et al. Cancer Chemother Pharmacol 1985;14: 279–281.

303. Paccagnella A, Salvagno L, Bolzonella S, et al. Second and third response to M₂ (BCNU, VCR, CTX, PRED) in multiple myeloma. Am Soc Clin Oncol [Abstract] 1985;4:217.

304. Paccagnella A, Cartel G, Fosser V, et al. Treatment of multiple myeloma with M₂ protocol and without maintenance therapy. Eur J Cancer Clin Oncol 1982;19:1345–1351.

305. Belch A, Shelley W, Bergsagel D, et al. A randomized trial of maintenance versus no maintenance melphalan and prednisone in responding multiple myeloma patients. Br J Cancer 1988;57:94–99.

306. Alberts DS, Durie BGM, Salmon SE. Doxorubicin/BCNU chemotherapy for multiple myeloma in relapse. Lancet 1976;1:926–928.

307. Bonnet JD, Alexanian R, Salmon SE, et al. Addition of cisplatin and bleomycin to vincristine-doxorubicin-prednisone (VBAP) combination in the treatment of relapsing or resistant multiple myeloma: A Southwest Oncology Group study. Cancer Treat Rep 1984;68:481–485.

308. Blade J, Rozman C, Montserrat E, et al. Treatment of alkylating resistant multiple myeloma with vincristine, BCNU, doxorubicin and prednisone (VBAP). Eur J Cancer Clin Oncol 1986;22:1193–1197.

309. Present CA, Klahr C. Adriamycin, 1,3-bis-(2-chloroethyl)-1-nitrosourea (BCNU, NSC #409962), cyclophosphamide plus prednisone (ABC-P) in melphalan-resistant multiple myeloma. Cancer 1978;42:1222–1227.

310. Kyle RA, Pajak TF, Henderson ES, et al. Multiple myeloma resistant to melphalan: Treatment with doxorubicin, cyclophosphamide, carmustine (BCNU), and prednisone. Cancer Treat Rep 1982;66:451–456.

311. Barlogie B, Smith L, Alexanian R. Effective treatment of advanced multiple myeloma refractory to alkylating agents. N Engl J Med 1984;310:1353–1356.

312. Sheehan T, Judge M, Parker AC. The efficacy and toxicity of VAD in the treatment of myeloma and related disorders. Scand J Hematol 1986;37:425–428.

313. Monconduit M, Le Loet X, Bernard JF, et al. Combination chemotherapy with vincristine, doxorubicin, dexamethasone for refractory or relapsing multiple myeloma. Br J Haematol 1986;63:599–601.

314. Monconduit M, Bauters F, Najman A. Evaluation of the association vincristine-Adriamycin plus high-dose dexamethasone (VAD) in severe previously treated myeloma. Blood 1986;68(suppl 1):240a.

315. Dalton WS, Grogan TM, Meltzer PS, et al. Resistance in multiple myeloma and non-Hodgkin's lymphoma: Detection of P-glycoprotein and potential circumvention by addition of verapamil to chemotherapy. J Clin Oncol 1989;7:415–424.

316. Salmon SE, Dalton WS, Grogan TM, et al. Multidrug-resistant myeloma: Laboratory and clinical effects of verapamil as a chemosensitizer. Blood 1991;78:44–50.
317. Fitzpatrick PJ, Rider WD. Half-body radiotherapy. Int J Radiat Oncol Biol Phys 1976;1:197–207.
318. Rider WB. Half-body radiotherapy, an update. Int J Radiat Oncol Biol Phys 1978;4(suppl 2):69–70.
319. Salmon SE, Crowley J, Tesh D. Chemotherapy is sequential to hemibody irradiation for remission consolidation in multiple myeloma. J Clin Oncol [Letter to the editor] 1991;9:2234–2235.
320. Jaffe JP, Bosch A, Raich PC. Sequential hemi-body radiotherapy in advanced multiple myeloma. Cancer 1979;43:124–128.
321. Qasim MM. Techniques and results of half-body irradiation (HBI) in metastatic carcinoma and myeloma. Clin Oncol 1979;5:65–68.
322. Rowland CG, Garrett MJ, Crowley, et al. Half-body radiation in plasma cell myeloma. Clin Radiol 1983;34:507–510.
323. Coleman M, Soletan S, Wolf D, et al. Whole bone marrow irradiation for the treatment of multiple myeloma. Cancer 1982;49:1328–1333.
324. Richards JDM, Coates PB, Closs SP, et al. Case of macroglobulinemia treated with hemibody irradiation. Lancet [Letter] 1983;2:844.
325. Tobias JS, Richards JDM, Blackman GM, et al. Hemibody irradiation in multiple myeloma. Radiother Oncol 1985;3:11–16.
326. Prato FS, Kurdyak R, Saibil EA, et al. The incidence of radiation pneumonitis as a result of single fraction, upper half-body irradiation. Cancer 1976;39:71–78.
327. Jacobs P, LeRoux I, King HS. Sequential half-body irradiation as salvage therapy in chemotherapy-resistant multiple myeloma. Am J Clin Oncol 1988;11:104–109.
328. Singer CRJ, Tobias JS, Giles F, et al. Hemibody irradiation: An effective second line therapy in drug resistant multiple myeloma. Cancer 1989;63:2446–2451.
329. Kartner N, Everndaleporelle D, Bradley G, et al. Detection of P-glycoprotein in multidrug-resistant cell lines by monoclonal antibodies. Nature 1985;316:820–823.
330. Dalton WS, Grogan TM, Rybski JA, et al. Immunohistochemical detection and quantitation of P-glycoprotein in multiple drug resistant human myeloma cells: Association with level of drug resistance and drug accumulation. Blood 1989;73:747–752.
331. Salmon SE, Grogan TM, Miller TP, et al. Prediction of doxorubicin resistance in vitro in myeloma, lymphoma and breast cancer by P-glycoprotein staining. JNCI 1989;81:696–701.
331a. Sonneveld P, Durie BG, Lokhorst HM, et al. Modulation of multidrug-resistant multiple myeloma by cyclosporin. Lancet 1992;340(8814):255–259.
332. Perren TJ, Selby PJ, Mbidde EK, et al. High dose chemotherapy of multiple myeloma (MM) with melphalan (HDM) and with methylprednisolone (HDMP). Am Soc Clin Oncol [Abstract] 1986;5:158.
333. McElwain TJ, Powles RL. High-dose intravenous melphalan for plasma-cell leukaemia and myeloma. Lancet 1983;2:822–824.
334. Lenhard RE, Oken MM, Barnes JM, et al. High-dose cyclophosphamide. An effective treatment for advanced refractory multiple myeloma. Cancer 1984;53:1456–1460.
335. Lenhard RE, Tsiatis AA, Oken MM, et al. Time sequential high-dose cyclophosphamide (CY) and vincristine (VCR) treatment of multiple myeloma (MM). Proc Am Soc Clin Oncol [Abstract] 1985;4:217.
336. Barlogie B, Hall R, Zander A, et al. High-dose melphalan with autologous bone marrow transplantation for multiple myeloma. Blood 1986;67:1298–1301.
337. Barlogie B, Alexanian R, Dicke KA, et al. High-dose melphalan (HDM) + total body irradiation (TBI) and bone marrow transplantation (BMT) for refractory myeloma. Blood 1986;68(suppl 1):240a.
338. Selby PJ, McElwain TJ, Nandi AC, et al. Multiple myeloma treated with high dose intravenous melphalan. Br J Haematol 1987;66:55–62.
339. Barlogie B, Alexanian R, Dicke K, et al. High-dose chemoradiotherapy and autologous bone marrow transplantation for resistant myeloma. Blood 1987;70:869–872.
340. Osserman EF, DiRe Lb, DiRe J, et al. Identical twin marrow transplantation in multiple myeloma. Acta Haematol (Basel) 1982;68:215–223.
341. Ozer H, Han T, Nussbaum-Blumenson A, et al. Allogenic bone marrow transplantation and idiotype (ID) monitoring in multiple myeloma. Clin Invest [Abstract] 1984;25:161.
342. Gahrton G, Tura S, Flesch M, et al. Bone marrow transplantation in multiple myeloma: Report from the European Cooperative Group for Bone Marrow Transplantation. Blood 1987;69:1262–1264.
343. Gallamini A, Buffa F, Bacigalupo A, et al. Allogeneic bone marrow transplantation in multiple myeloma. Acta Haematol 1987;77:111–114.
344. Feffer A. Personal communication, 1987.
345. Tura S. Bone marrow transplantation in multiple myeloma: Current status and future perspectives. Bone Marrow Transplant 1986;1:17–20.
346. Gahrton G, Ringden O, Lonnqvist B. Bone marrow transplantation in multiple myeloma. Acta Med Scand 1986;219:523–527.
347. Jagannoth S, Barlogie B, Dicke K, et al. Autologous bone marrow transplantation in multiple myeloma: Identification of prognostic factors. Blood 1990;76:1860–1866.
348. Tong AM, Lee JC, Fay JW, et al. Elimination of clonogenic stem-cells from human multiple myeloma cell lines by a plasma cell-reactive monoclonal antibody and complement. Blood 1987;70:1482–1489.
349. Rhodes EG, Baker P, Rhodes JM, et al. Peanut agglutinin in combination with CD19 monoclonal antibody has potential as a purging agent in myeloma. Exp Hematol 1991;19:833–837.
350. Anderson KC, Barut BA, Ritz J, et al. Monoclonal antibody-purged autologous bone marrow transplantation therapy for multiple myeloma. Blood 1991;77:712–720.
351. Dinota A, Barbieri L, Gobbi M, et al. An immunotoxin containing momordin suitable for bone marrow purging in multiple myeloma patients. Br J Cancer 1989;60:315–319.
352. Shimazaki C, Wisniewski D, Scheinberg DA, et al. Elimination of myeloma cells from bone marrow by using monoclonal antibodies and magnetic immunobeads. Blood 1988;72:1248–1254.
353. Fermand JP, Levy Y, Gerota J, et al. Treatment of aggressive multiple myeloma by high-dose chemotherapy and total body irradiation followed by blood stem cells autologous graft. Blood 1989;73:20–23.
354. Gahrtner G, Tura S, Ljungman P, et al. Allogeneic bone marrow transplantation in multiple myeloma. N Engl J Med 1991;325:1267–1272.
355. Belch AR, Henderson JF, Brox LW. Treatment of multiple myeloma with deoxycoformycin. Cancer Chemother Pharmacol 1985;14:49–52.
356. Grever MR, McGee RA, Kraut ER, et al. Deoxycoformycin in refractory myeloma. Blood 1987;70(suppl 1):246a.
357. Case DC Jr, Oldham F, Ervin T, et al. Phase I–II study of epirubicin in multiple myeloma. Am Soc Clin Oncol [Abstract] 1987;6:146.
358. Durie BGM, Levy HB, Voakes J, et al. Poly (I,C)-LC as an interferon inducer in refractory multiple myeloma. J Biol Response Mod 1985;4:518–524.
359. Paccagnella A, Salvagno L, Chiarion-Sileni V, et al. Peptichemio in pretreated patient with plasma cell neoplasms. Eur J Cancer Clin Oncol 1986;22:1053–1058.
360. Tirelli U, Carbone A, Zagonei V, et al. Phase II study of teniposide (VM-26) in multiple myeloma. Am J Clin Oncol 1985;8:329–331.
361. Gockerman JP, Silberman H, Bartolucci AA. Phase II evaluation of aclarubicin in refractory multiple myeloma: A Southeastern Cancer Study Group trial. Cancer Treat Rep 1987;71:773–774.
362. Scarffe JH, Beaumont AR, Crowther D. Phase I–II evaluation of acronine in patients with multiple myeloma. Cancer Treat Rep 1983;67:93–94.
363. Ahmann FR, Meyskens FL, Jones SE, et al. Phase II evaluation of amsacrine (m-AMSA) in solid tumors, myeloma, and lymphoma: A University of Arizona and Southwest Oncology Group study. Cancer Treat Rep 1983;67:697–700.
364. Blum RH, Carter SK, Agre K. A clinical review of bleomycin, a new anti-neoplastic agent. Cancer 1973;31:903–913.
365. Bennett JM, Silber R, Ezdinli E, et al. Phase II study of Adriamycin and bleomycin in patients with multiple myeloma. Cancer Treat Rep 1978;62:1367–1369.
366. Corder MP, Elliot TE, Bell SJ. Dose limiting myelotoxicity and absence of significant nephrotoxicity with the weekly outpatient schedule of cis-platinum (II) diammine-dichloride. J Clin Hematol Oncol 1977;7:645–651.
367. Cornell CJ Jr, Pajak TF, McIntyre OR. Chlorozotocin: Phase II evaluation in patients with myeloma. Cancer Treat Rep 1984;68:685–686.
368. Forman WB, Cohen HJ, Bartolucci AA. Phase II evaluation of chlorozotocin in refractory multiple myeloma. Cancer Treat Rep 1984;68:1409–1410.
369. Kantarjian H, Dreicer R, Barlogie B, et al. High-dose cytosine arabinoside in multiple myeloma. Eur J Cancer Clin Oncol 1984;20:227–231.
370. Vinciguerra V, Anderson K, McIntyre OR. Diaziquone for resistant multiple myeloma. Cancer Treat Rep 1985;69:331–332.
371. Stuckey WJ, Crowley J, Baker LH, et al. Phase II trial of diaziquone in patients with refractory and relapsing multiple myeloma: A Southwest Oncology Group study. Cancer Treat Rep 1987;71:1095–1096.
372. Gockerman JP, Bartolucci AA, Nelson MO, et al. Phase II evaluation of etoposide in refractory multiple myeloma: A Southeastern Cancer Study Group trial. Cancer Treat Rep 1986;70:801–802.
373. Cohen HJ, Bartolucci AA. Hexamethylmelamine and prednisone in the treatment of refractory multiple myeloma. Am J Clin Oncol 1982;5:21–27.
374. Alberts DS, Balcerzak SP, Bonnet JP, et al. Phase II trials of mitoxantrone in multiple myeloma: A Southwest Oncology Group study. Cancer Treat Rep 1985;69:1321–1323.
375. Tirelli U, Sorio R, Magri MD, et al. Prednimustine in elderly patients with multiple myeloma: A phase II study. Cancer Treat Rep 1986;70:537–538.
376. Moon JH, Edmonson JH. Procarbazine (NSC-77213) and multiple myeloma. Cancer Chemother Rep 1970;54:245–248.
377. Lake-Lewin D, Myers J, Lee BL, et al. Phase II trial of pyrazofurin in patients with multiple myeloma refractory to standard cytotoxic therapy. Cancer Treat Rep 1979;63:1403–1404.
378. Houwen B, Ockhuizen T, Marrink J, et al. Vindesine therapy in melphalan-resistant myeloma. Eur J Cancer 1981;17:227–232.
379. Kraut EH, Crowley JJ, Gever MR, et al. Phase II study of fludarabine phosphate in multiple myeloma. A Southwest Oncology Group study. Invest New Drugs 1990;8:199–200.
380. Hanson KH, Crowley J, Salmon SE, et al. Evaluation of amonafide in refractory and relapsing multiple-myeloma—A Southwest Oncology Group study. Anticancer Drug Des 1991;2:247–250.
381. Oken MM, Lenhard RE, Tslatis AA, et al. Contribution of prednisone to the effectiveness of hexamethylmelamine in refractory multiple myeloma. Cancer Treat Rep 1987;71:807–811.
382. Alexanian R, Barlogie B, Dixon D. Renal failure in multiple myeloma. Ann Intern Med 1990;150:1693–1695.
383. Cavo M, Baccarani M, Galieni P, et al. Renal failure in multiple myeloma. A study of the presenting findings, response to treatment and prognosis in 26 patients. Nouv Rev Fr Hematol 1986;28:147–152.
384. Cornwell CG, Pajak TF, McIntyre OR, et al. Influence of renal failure on the myelosuppressive effects of melphalan: Cancer and Leukemia Group B experience. Cancer Treat Rep 1982;66:475–481.
385. Alberts DS, Chen H-SY, Berg D, et al. Effects of renal dysfunction in dogs on the disposition and marrow toxicity of melphalan. Br J Cancer 1981;43:330–334.
386. Adair CG, Bridges JM, Desai ZR. Renal function in the elimination of oral mephalan in patients with multiple myeloma. Cancer Chemother Pharmacol 1986;17:185–188.

387. MRC Working Party on Leukemia in Adults. Analysis and management of renal failure in fourth MRC myelomatosis trial. Br Med J 1984;288:1411–1416.

388. Bernstein SP, Humes DH. Reversible renal insufficiency in multiple myeloma. Arch Intern Med 1982;142:2083–2086.

389. Coward RA, Mallick NP, Delamore IW. Should patients with acute renal failure associated with myeloma be dialysed? Br Med J 1983;287:1575–1578.

390. Iggo N, Palmer AB, Severn A, et al. Chronic dialysis in patients with multiple myeloma and renal failure: A worthwhile treatment. Q J Med 1989;270:903–910.

391. Johnson WJ, Kyle RA, Pineda AA, et al. Treatment of renal failure associated with multiple myeloma. Plasmapheresis, hemodialysis and chemotherapy. Arch Intern Med 1990;150:863–869.

392. Korzets A, Tam F, Russell G, et al. The role of continuous ambulatory peritoneal dialysis in end-stage renal failure due to multiple myeloma. Am J Kidney Dis 1990;16:216–223.

393. Russell JA, Fitzharris BM, Corringham R, et al. Plasma exchange vs peritoneal dialysis for removing Bence Jones protein. Br J Med J 1978;2:1397.

394. Feest TG, Burge PS, Cohen SL. Successful treatment of myeloma kidney by diuresis and plasmapheresis. Br J Med J 1976;1:503–505.

395. Misiani R, Remuzzi G, Bertani T, et al. Plasmapheresis is the treatment of acute renal failure in multiple myeloma. Am J Med 1979;66:684–688.

396. Pasquali S, Cagnoli L, Rovinetti C, et al. Plasma exchange therapy in rapidly progressive renal failure due to multiple myeloma. Int J Artif Organs 1984;8:27–30.

397. Humphrey RL, Wright JR, Zachary JB, et al. Renal transplantation in multiple myeloma. A case report. Ann Intern Med 1975;83:651–653.

398. Payne R, Little A, Williams R, et al. Interpretation of serum calcium in patients with abnormal serum proteins. Br Med J 1973;4:643.

399. Ralston SH, Gallacher SJ, Patel U, et al. Comparison of three intravenous biophosphonates in cancer-associated hypercelcemia. Lancet 1989;2:1180–1182.

400. Lingarde F, Zettervall O. Hypercalcemia and normal ionized serum calcium in a case of myelomatosis. Ann Intern Med 1973;78:396–399.

401. Soria J, Soria C, Dao C. Immunoglobulin bound calcium and ultrafilterable serum calcium in myeloma. Br J Haematol 1976;34:343–344.

402. Jaffe JP, Mosher DF. Calcium binding in a myeloma protein. Am J Med 1979;67:343–346.

403. Bataille R, Chappard D, Marcelli C, et al. Mechanisms of bone destruction in multiple myeloma. J Clin Oncol 1989;7:1909–1914.

404. Rota S, Mougenot B, Baudouin B, et al. Multiple myeloma and severe renal failure: A clinicopathologic study of outcome and prognosis in 34 patients. Medicine (Baltimore) 1987;66:126–137.

405. Kyle RA, Jowsey J, Kelly PJ, et al. Multiple myeloma bone disease. The comparative effect of sodium fluoride and calcium carbonate or placebo. N Engl J Med 1975;293:1334–1338.

406. Kyle RA, Jowsey J. Effect of sodium fluoride, calcium carbonate, and vitamin D on the skeleton in multiple myeloma. Cancer 1980;45:1669–1674.

407. Gardner FH. Fluorides for multiple myeloma. N Engl J Med 1972;287:1252–1253.

408. Belch AR, Bergsagel DE, Wilson K, et al. Effect of daily etidronate on the oesteolysis of myeloma. J Clin Oncol 1991;9:1397–1402.

409. Jakubowski J, Kendall BE, Symon L. Primary plasmacytoma of the cranial vault. Acta Neurochir 1980;55:117–134.

410. Stark RJ, Henson RA. Cerebral compression by myeloma. J Neurol Neurosurg Psychiatry 1981;44:833–836.

411. Kohli CM, Kawazu T. Solitary intracranial plasmacytoma. Surg Neurol 1982;17:307–312.

412. Atweh GF, Jabbour M. Intracranial solitary extraskeletal plasmacytoma resembling meningioma. Arch Neurol 1982;39:57–59.

413. Soffer D, Siegal T. Solitary dural plasmacytoma with conspicuous cytoplasmic inclusions. Cancer 1982;49:2500–2504.

414. Mancardi GL, Mandybur TI. Solitary intracranial plasmacytoma. Cancer 1983;51:2226–2233.

415. Coppeto JR, Monteiro MLR, Collias J, et al. Foster-Kennedy syndrome caused by solitary intracranial plasmacytoma. Surg Neurol 1983;19:267–272.

416. Pritchard PB III, Martinez RA, Hungerford GD, et al. Dural plasmacytoma. Neurosurgery 1983;12:576–579.

417. Benson MD, Brandt KD, Cohen AS, et al. Neuropathy, M components and amyloid. Lancet 1975;1:10–12.

418. Davis LE, Drachman DB. Myeloma neuropathy. Successful treatment of two patients and review of cases. Arch Neurol 1972;27:507–511.

419. Driedger H, Pruzanski W. Plasma cell neoplasia with peripheral neuropathy. A study of five cases and a review of the literature. Medicine (Baltimore) 1980;59:301–310.

420. Reitan JB, Pape E, Fossa SD, et al. Osteosclerotic myeloma with polyneuropathy. Acta Neurol Scand 1980;208:137–144.

421. Delauche MC, Clauvel JP, Seligmann M. Peripheral neuropathy and plasma cell neoplasias: A report of 10 cases. Br J Haematol 1981;48:384–392.

422. Osby E, Noring L, Hast R, et al. Benign monoclonal gammopathy and peripheral neuropathy. Br J Haematol 1982;51:531–539.

423. Kelly JJ Jr, Kyle RA, Miles JM, et al. Osteosclerotic myeloma and peripheral neuropathy. Neurology 1983;33:202–210.

424. Besinger UA, Toyka KV, Anzil AP, et al. Myeloma neuropathy: Passive transfer from man to mouse. Science 1981;213:1027–1030.

425. Lator N, Sherman WH, Nemni R, et al. Plasma cell dyscrasia and peripheral nerve myelin. N Engl J Med 1980;303:618–621.

426. Lamarca J, Casquero P, Pou A. Mononeuritis multiplex in Waldenström's macroglobulinemia. Ann Neurol 1987;22:268–272.

427. Vital C, Deminiere C, Bourgouin B, et al. Waldenström's macroglobulinemia and peripheral neuropathy: Deposition of M-component and kappa light chain in the endoneurium. Neurology 1985;35:603–606.

428. Ohi T, Kyle RA, Dyck PJ. Axonal attenuation and secondary segmental demyelination in myeloma neuropathies. Ann Neurol 1985;17:255–261.

429. Nobile-Orazio E, Marmiroli P, Baldini L, et al. Peripheral neuropathy in macroglobulinemia: Incidence and antigen-specificity of M-proteins. Neurology 1987;37:1506–1514.

430. Hoppe U, Drager HS, Patzold U, et al. Polyneuropathy in Waldenström's macroglobulinaemia. Passive transfer from man to mouse. Acta Neurol Scand 1987;75:112–116.

431. Schulz W, Domenico P, Nand S. The POEMS syndrome associated with polycythemia vera. Cancer 1989;63:1175–1178.

432. Kyle RA. Multiple myeloma. Review of 869 cases. Mayo Clin Proc 1975;50:29–40.

433. Hoffbrand AV, Hobbs JR, Kremenchuzky S, et al. Incidence and pathogenesis of megaloblastic erythropoiesis in multiple myeloma. J Clin Pathol 1967;20:699–705.

434. Winearls CG, Pippard MJ, Downing MR, et al. Effect of human erythropoietin derived from recombinant DNA on the anaemia of patients maintained by chronic haemodialysis. Lancet 1986;2:1175–1177.

435. Eschbach JW, Egrie JC, Downing MR, et al. Correction of the anemia of end-stage renal disease with recombinant human erythropoietin. Results of a combined phase I and II clinical trial. N Engl J Med 1987;316:73–78.

436. Ludwig H, Fritz E, Kotzmann H, et al. Erythropoietin treatment of anemia associated with multiple myeloma. N Engl J Med 1990;322:1693–1699.

437. Oster W, Herrmann F, Gamm H, et al. Erythropoietin for the treatment of anemia of malignancy associated with neoplastic bone marrow infiltration. J Clin Oncol 1990;8:956–962.

438. Bergsagel DE. Plasma cell neoplasms and acute leukaemia. In: Hoffbrand AV, Lasch HG, Nathan DG, Salmon SE, eds. Clinics in Hematology. Eastbourne: WB Saunders, 1982:221–234.

439. Holland D, Muller JM, Leger J, et al. Association myeloma, leucose myeloide et lymphosarcome. Reflexions nosologiques. Lyon Med 1965;213:967–974.

440. Kyle RA, Robert MD, Pierre RV, et al. Multiple myeloma and acute myelomonocytic leukemia. N Engl J Med 1970;283:1121–1125.

441. Nordenson NG. Myelomatosis: A clinical review of 30 cases. Acta Med Scand (Suppl) 1966;445:178–186.

442. Mufti GJ, Hamblin TJ, Clein GP, et al. Coexistent myelodysplasia and plasma cell neoplasia. Br J Haematol 1983;54:91–96.

443. Cuzick J, Erskine S, Edelman D, et al. A comparison of the incidence of the myelodysplastic syndrome and acute myeloid leukaemia following melphalan and cyclophosphamide treatment for myelomatosis. Br J Cancer 1987;55:523–529.

444. Green MH, Harris EL, Gershensen DM, et al. Melphalan may be a more potent leukemogen than cyclophosphamide. Ann Intern Med 1986;105:360–367.

445. Lackner H. Hemostatic abnormalities associated with dysproteinemias. Semin Hematol 1973;10:125–133.

446. Henstell HH, Kligerman M. A new theory of interference with the clotting mechanism: The complexing of euglobulin with factor V, factor VII, and prothrombin. Ann Intern Med 1958;49:371–387.

447. Lackner H. Hemostatic abnormalities associated with dysproteinemias. Semin Hematol 1973;10:125–133.

448. Godal HC, Borchgrevink CF. The effect of plasmapheresis on the hemostatic function in patients with macroglobulinemia Waldenström and multiple myeloma. Scand J Clin Lab Invest 1965;17(suppl 84):133–137.

449. Doumenc J, Prost RJ, Samama M, et al. Anomalie de l'agregation plaquettaire au cours de la maladie de Waldenstrom (a propos de 3 cas). Nouv Rev Fr Hematol 1966;6:734–738.

450. Penny R, Castaldi PA, Whitsed HM. Inflammation and hemostasis in paraproteinemias. Br J Haematol 1971;20:35–44.

451. Pachter MR, Johnson SA, Neblett TR, et al. Bleeding, platelets, and macroglobulinemia. Am J Clin Pathol 1959;31:467–482.

452. Pachter MR. Johnson SA. Basinski DH. The effect of macroglobulins and their dissociation units on release of platelet factor 3. Thromb Diath Haemorrh 1959;3:501–509.

453. Khoory MS, Nesheim ME, Bowie EJW, et al. Circulating heparin sulfate proteoglycan anticoagulant from a patient with a plasma cell disorder. J Clin Invest 1980;65:666–674.

454. Meyer K, Williams EC. Fibrinolysis and acquired alpha-2 plasmin inhibitor deficiency in amyloidosis. Am J Med 1985;79:394–396.

455. Somer T. Hyperviscosity syndrome in plasma cell dyscrasias. Adv Microcirc 1975;6:1–55.

456. Fahey JL. Serum protein disorders causing clinical symptoms in malignant neoplastic disease. J Chron Dis 1963;16:703–712.

457. Fahey JL, Barth WF, Soloman A. Serum hyperviscosity syndrome. JAMA 1965;192:464–467.

458. Bloch KJ, Maki DG. Hyperviscosity syndromes associated with immunoglobulin abnormalities. Semin Hematol 1973;10:113–124.

459. McGrath MA, Penny R. Paraproteinemia: Blood hyperviscosity and clinical manifestations. J Clin Invest 1976;58:1158–1162.

460. MacKenzie MR, Lee TK. Blood viscosity in Waldenström macroglobulinemia. Blood 1977;49:507–510.

461. MacKenzie MR, Fudenberg HH. Macroglobulinemia: An analysis for forty patients. Blood 1972;39:874.

462. Crawford J, Cox EB, Cohen HJ. Evaluation of hyperviscosity in monoclonal gammopathies. Am J Med 1985;79:13–22.

463. MacKenzie MR, Brown E, Fudenberg HH, et al. Waldenström's macroglobulinemia

correlation between expanded plasma volume and increased serum viscosity. Blood 1970;35:934.

464. Valbonesi M, Tarantino M, Montani F, et al. Biochemical and clinical evaluation of a new cellulose diacetate secondary filter for cascade filtration. Int J Artif Organs 1985;8:105–108.

465. Valbonesi M, Monani F, Guzzini F, et al. Efficacy of discontinuous flow centrifugation compared with cascade filtration in Waldenström's macroglobulinemia: A pilot study. Int J Artif Organs 1985;8:165–168.

466. Avnstorp C, Nielson H, Drachman O, et al. Plasmapheresis in hyperviscosity syndrome. Acta Med Scand 1985;217:133–137.

467. Whittaker JA, Tuddenham EGD, Bradley J. Hyperviscosity syndrome in IgA multiple myeloma. Lancet 1973;2:572.

468. Pruzanski W, Jancelewicz Z, Underdown B. Immunological and physiochemical studies of IgA (λ) cryogelglobulinemia. Clin Exp Immunol 1973;15:181–191.

469. Meltzer M, Franklin EC. Cryoglobulinemia: A study of twenty-nine patients. I. IgG and IgM cryoglobulins and factors affecting cryoprecipitability. Am J Med 1966;40:828–836.

470. MacKay IR, Erikson N, Motulsky AG, et al. Cryo- and macroglobulinemia: Electrophoretic, ultracentrifugal, and clinical studies. Am J Med 1956;20:564–587.

471. Liss M, Fudenberg HH, Kritzman J. A Bence Jones cryoglobulin: Clinical, physical, and immunological properties. Clin Exp Immunol 1967;2:467–475.

472. Bloth B. Christensson T, Mellstedt H. Extreme hyponatremia in patients with myelomatosis. An effect of cationic paraproteins. Acta Med Scand 1978;203:273–275.

473. Emmett ME, Narins RG. Clinical use of the anion gap. Medicine (Baltimore) 1977;56:38–54.

474. Murray T, Long W, Narins RG. Multiple myeloma and the anion gap. N Engl J Med 1976;292:574–575.

475. Braden GL, Mikolich DJ, White CF, et al. Syndrome of inappropriate antidiuresis in Waldenström's macroglobulinemia. Am J Med 1986;80:1242–1244.

476. Schnur MJ, Appel GB, Karp G, et al. The anion gap in asymptomatic plasma cell dyscrasia. Ann Intern Med 1977;86:304–305.

477. Jacobson DR, Zolla-Pazner S. Immunosuppression and infection in multiple myeloma. Semin Oncol 1986;13:282–290.

478. Zinneman HH, Wall WH. Recurrent pneumonia in multiple myeloma and some observations on immunologic response. Ann Intern Med 1954;41:1152–1163.

479. Fahey JR, Scoggins R, Utz JP, et al. Infections, antibody response and γ globulin components in multiple myeloma and macroglobulinemia. Am J Med 1963;35:698–707.

480. Meyers BR, Hirschman SZ, Axelrod JA. Current patterns of infection in multiple myeloma. Am J Med 1972;52:87–92.

481. Twomey JJ. Infections complicating multiple myeloma and chronic lymphocytic leukemia. Arch Intern Med 1973;132:562–565.

482. Norden CW. Infections in patients with multiple myeloma. Arch Intern Med [Editorial] 1980;140:1150–1151.

483. Savage DG, Lindenbaum J, Garret TJ. Biphasic pattern of bacterial infection in multiple myeloma. Ann Intern Med 1982;96:47–50.

484. Salmon SE, Samai BA, Hayes DM, et al. Role of gamma globulin for immunoprophylaxis in multiple myeloma. N Engl J Med 1967;227:1336–1340.

485. Nolan CM, Baxley PJ, Frasch CE. Antibody response to infection in multiple myeloma. Implications for vaccination. Am J Med 1979;67:331–334.

486. Glenner GG, Ein D, Eanes ED, et al. The creation of "amyloid" fibrils from Bence Jones protein in vitro. Science 1971;174:712–714.

487. Glenner GG. Amyloid deposits and amyloidosis: The β-fibrilloses. N Engl J Med 1980;302:1283–1292.

488. Cathcart ES, Ritchie RF, Cohen AS, et al. Immunoglobulins and amyloidosis. An immunologic study of sixty-two patients with biopsy-proven disease. Am J Med 1972;52:93–101.

489. Hawkins PN, Wootton R, Pepys MB. Metabolic studies of radioiodinated serum amyloid P component in normal subjects and patients with systemic amyloidosis. J Clin Invest 1990;86:1862–1869.

490. Kyle RA. Amyloidosis. In: Hoffbrand AV, Lasch HG, Nathan DG, Salmon SE, eds. Clinics in Hematology. Eastbourne: WB Saunders, 1982:151–180.

491. Kyle RA, Bayrd ED. Amyloidosis: Review of 236 cases. Medicine (Baltimore) 1975;54:271–299.

492. Gordon DA, Pruzanski W, Ogryzlo MA, et al. Amyloid arthritis simulating rheumatoid disease in five patients with multiple myeloma. Am J Med 1973;55:142–154.

493. Siqeria-Filho AG, Cunha CLP, Tajik AJ, et al. M-mode and two dimensional echocardiographic features in cardiac amyloidosis. Circulation 1981;63:188–196.

494. Gertz MA, Kyle RA, Greipp PR. Beta-2-microglobulin predicts survival in primary systemic amyloidosis. Am J Med 1990;89:609–614.

495. Buxbaum JN, Hurley ME, Chuba J, Spira T. Amyloidosis of the AL type: Clinical, morphologic, and biochemical aspects of the response to therapy with alkylating agents and prednisone. Am J Med 1979;67:867–878.

496. Fielder K, Durie BG. Primary amyloidosis associated with multiple myeloma. Predictors of successful therapy. Am J Med 1986;80:413–419.

497. Kyle RA, Greipp PR. Primary systemic amyloidosis: Comparison of melphalan and prednisone versus placebo. Blood 1978;52:818–827.

498. Gertz MA, Kyle RA, Greipp PR. The plasma cell labeling index: A valuable tool in primary amyloidosis. Blood 1989;74:1108–1111.

499. Kyle RA, Greipp PR, O'Fallon WM. Primary systemic amyloidosis: Multivariate analysis for prognostic factors in 168 cases. Blood 1986;68:220–224.

500. Waldenström J. Incipient myelomatosis or "essential" hyperglobulinemia with fibrogenopenia—A new syndrome? Acta Med Scand 1944;117:216–222.

501. Waldenström J. Macroglobulinemia. Adv Metab Dis 1965;2:115.

502. Carter P, Koval JJ, Hobbs JR. The relation of clinical and laboratory findings to the survival of patients with macroglobulinaemia. Clin Exp Immunol 1977;28:241–249.

503. Stein RS, Ellman L, Bloch KJ. The clinical correlates of IgM M-components: An analysis of thirty-four patients. Am J Med Sci 1975;269:209–216.

504. McCallister BD, Bayrd ED, Harrison EG Jr, et al. Primary macroglobulinemia. Review with a report on thirty-one cases and notes on the value of continuous chlorambucil therapy. Am J Med 1967;43:394–434.

505. Krajny M, Pruzanski W. Waldenström's macroglobulinemia: Review of 45 cases. Can Med Assoc J 1976;114:899–905.

506. Ameis A, Ko HS, Pruzanski W. M components: A review of 1242 cases. Can Med Assoc J 1976;114:889.

507. Benbassat J, Fluman N, Zlotnick A. Monoclonal immunoglobulin disorders: A report of 154 cases. Am J Med Sci 1976;271:325.

508. Peltonen S, Wasastjerna C, Wager O. Clinical features of patients with a serum M component. Acta Med Scand 1978;203:257.

509. Massari R, Find JM, Metais R. Waldenström's macroglobulinaemia observed in two brothers. Nature 1962;196:176.

510. Seligmann M. A genetic predisposition to Waldenström's macroglobulinaemia. Acta Med Scand 1966;445:140.

511. Fine JM, Lambin P, Massari M, et al. Malignant evolution of asymptomatic monoclonal IgM after seven and fifteen years in two siblings of a patients with Waldenström's macroglobulinaemia. Acta Med Scand 1982;211:237.

512. Fine JM, Muller JY, Rochu D, et al. Waldenström's macroglobulinemia in monozygotic twins. Acta Med Scand 1986;220:368–373.

513. James JM, Brouet JC, Orvoenfrija E, et al. Waldenström's macroglobulinemia in a bird breeder: A case history with pulmonary involvement and antibody activity of the monoclonal IgM to canary's droppings. Clin Exp Immunol 1987;68:397–401.

514. Takahashi K, Yamamura F, Motoyama H. IgM multiple myeloma—its distinction from Waldenström's macroglobulinemia. Acta Pathol Jpn 1986;36:1553–1563.

515. San Roman C, Ferro T, Guzman M, et al. Clonal abnormalities in patients with Waldenström's macroglobulinemia with special reference to a Burkitt-type t(8;14). Cancer Genet Gytogenet 1985;18:155–158.

516. Kucharska-Pulczynska M, Ellegaard J, Hokland P. Analysis of leukocyte differentiation antigens in blood and bone marrow from patients with Waldenström's macroglobulinemia. Br J Haematol 1987;65:395–399.

517. MacKenzie MR. Macroglobulinemia. In: Wiernik PH, Canelloa GP, Kyle RA, Schiffer CA, eds. Neoplastic diseases of the blood, vol. 2. New York: Churchill-Livingstone, 1985:575–592.

518. Morel-Maroger L, Basch A, Danon F, et al. Pathology of the kidney in Waldenström's macroglobulinemia: Study of 16 cases. N Engl J Med 1970;283:123–129.

519. Martelo OJ, Schultz DR, Pardo V, et al. Immunologically mediated renal disease in Waldenström's macroglobulinemia. Am J Med 1975;58:567–575.

520. Lindstrome FD, Hed J, Enestrom S. Renal pathology of Waldenström's macroglobulinemia with monoclonal antiglomerular antibodies and the nephrotic syndrome. Clin Exp Immunol 1980;41:196–204.

521. Hory B, Saunier F, Wolff R, et al. Waldenström's macroglobulinemia and nephrotic syndrome with minimal change lesion. Nephron 1987;45:68–70.

522. Bayrd ED. Continuous chlorambucil therapy in primary macroglobulinemia of Waldenström: Report of 4 cases. Proc Mayo Clin 1963;36:40.

523. Bierling P, Rochant H, Brum B, et al. Macroglobulinemie de Waldenström a forme pancytopenique. Remission complete apres polychimiotherapie avec recul de 26 mois. Ann Med Interne (Paris) 1979;130:443.

524. Cass RM, Anderson BR, Vaughan JH. Waldenström's macroglobulinemia with increased serum IgG levels treated with low doses of cyclophosphamide. Ann Intern Med 1969;71:971.

525. Cohen RJ, Bohannon RA, Wallerstein RO. Waldenström's macroglobulinemia: A study of ten cases. Am J Med 1966;41:274.

526. Heading RC, Girdwood RH, Eastwood MA. Macroglobulinemia treated with prednisone, azathioprine, and folic acid. Br Med J 1970;3:750.

527. Sokalova A, Gazova A, Hrubisko M, et al. Clinical utilization of plasmapheresis and cyclophosphamide in the treatment of malignant lymphoproliferative processes. Neoplasma 1973;20:335.

528. Busnach G, Dal Col A, Brando B, et al. Efficacy of a combined treatment with plasma exchange and cytostatics in macroglobulinemia. Int J Artif Organs 1986;9:267–270.

529. Jacobs P, Wood L, Le Roux I, et al. Waldenström's macroglobulinemia treated with sequential hemibody irradiation. J Clin Apheresis 1987;3:181–184.

530. Kantarjian HM, Alexanian R, Koller CA, et al. Fludarabine therapy in microglobulinemic lymphoma. Blood 1990;75:1928–1931.

531. Clamon GH, Corder MP, Burns CP. Successful doxorubicin therapy of primary macroglobulinemia resistant to alkylating agents. Am J Hematol 1980;9:21.

532. Case DC Jr. Combination chemotherapy (M-2 protocol) (BCNU, cyclophosphamide, vincristine, melphalan and prednisone) for Waldenström's macroglobulinemia. Blood 1982;59:934.

533. Riddell S, Johnston JB, Rayner HL, et al. Response of Waldenström's macroglobulinemia to pentostatin (2'-deoxycoformycin) Cancer Treat Rep 1986;70:546–548.

534. Allen EL, Metz EN, Balcerzak SP. Acute myelomonocytic leukemia with macroglobulinemia, Bence Jones proteinuria, and hypercalcemia. Cancer 1973;32:121.

535. Martelli MF, Falini B, Firenze A, et al. Acute leukemia complicating Waldenström's macroglobulinemia. Haematologica 1981;66:303.

536. Rosner F, Grunwald HW. Multiple myeloma and Waldenström's macroglobulinemia terminating in acute leukemia. N Y State J Med 1980;80:558.

537. Sondergaard Peterson H. Erythroleukaemia in a melphalan-treated patients with primary macroglobulinaemia. Scand J Haematol 1973;10:5.

538. James K, Fudenberg H, Epstein WL, et al. Studies on a unique diagnostic serum globulin in papular mucinosis (lichen myxedematosus). Clin Exp Immunol 1967;2: 153.

539. Cream JJ. Pyoderma gangrenosum with a monoclonal IgM red cell agglomerating factor. Br J Dermatol 1971;84:223–226.

540. Turakainen H, Valimaki M, Penttinen R. Synthesis of glycosaminoglycans and collagen in skin fibroblasts cultured from a patient with lichen myxedematosus. Arch Dermatol Res 1985;277:55–59.

541. Yaron M, Yaron I, Yust I, et al. Lichen myxedematosus (scleromyxedema) serum stimulates hyaluronic acid and prostaglandin E production by human fibroblasts. J Rheumatol 1985;12:171–175.

542. Feldman P, Shapiro L, Pick Al, et al. Scleromyxedema. A dramatic response to melphalan. Arch Dermatol 1969;99:51–56.

543. Degos R, Civatte J, Clauvel JP, et al. Anomalies globuliniques dans les mucinoses cutanees. Bull Soc Fr Dermatol Syphiligr 1970;77:579–591.

544. Truhan AP, Roenigk HH Jr. Lichen myxedematosus. An unusual case with rapid progression and possible internal involvement. Int J Dermatol 1987;26:91–95.

545. Milam CP, Cohen LE, Fenske NA, Ling NS. Schleromyxedema: Therapeutic response to isotretinoin in three patients. J Am Acad Dermatol 1988;19:469–477.

546. Franklin EC, Lowenstein J, Bigelow B, et al. Heavy chain disease: A new disorder of serum γ-globulins. Report of the first case. Am J Med 1964;37:332–350.

547. Frangione B, Franklin EC. Heavy-chain diseases: Clinical features and molecular significance of the disordered immunoglobulin structure. Semin Hematol 1973;10: 53–64.

548. Franklin EC, Kyle R, Seligmann M. Correlation of protein structure and immunoglobulin gene organization in the light of two new deleted heavy chain disease proteins. Mol Immunol 1979;16:919.

549. Bakhshi A, Guglielmi P, Coligan JE. A pre-translational defect in a case of human mu heavy chain disease. Mol Immunol 1986;23:725–732.

550. Bakhshi A, Guglielmi P, Siebenlist U, et al. A DNA insertion/deletion necessitates an aberrant RNA splice accounting for a mu heavy chain disease protein. Proc Natl Acad Sci USA 1986;83:2689–2693.

551. Kyle RA, Greipp PR, Banks PM. The diverse picture of gamma heavy-chain disease: Report of seven cases and review of literature. Mayo Clin Proc 1981;56:439.

552. Fermand JP, Brovet JC, Danon F, Seligmann M. Gamma heavy chain "disease": heterogeneity of the clinico-pathologic features. Report of 16 cases and review of the literature. Medicine (Baltimore) 1989;68:321–335.

553. Kanoh T, Nakasato H. Osteolytic gamma chain disease. Eur J Haematol 1987;39: 60–65.

554. O'Connor GT Jr, Wrandt HE, Innes DJ, et al. Gamma heavy chain disease: Report of a case associated with a trisomy of chromosome 7. Cancer Genet Cytogenet 1985;15: 1–5.

555. Kyle RA. The heavy-chain diseases. In: Wiernik PH, Canelloa GP, Kyle RA, Schiffer CA, eds. Neoplastic diseases of the blood, vol. 2. New York: Churchill-Livingstone, 1985:593–605.

556. Buxbaum JN, Preud'homme JL. Alpha and gamma heavy chain disease in man: Intracellular origin of the aberrant polypeptides. J Immunol 1972;109:1131.

557. Seligmann M, Mihaesco E, Preud'homme JL, et al. Heavy chain diseases: Current findings and concepts. Immunol Rev 1979;48:145–167.

558. Zamadzki ZA, Benedek TG, Ein D, et al. Rheumatoid arthritis terminating in heavy-chain disease. Ann Intern Med 1969;70:335.

559. Block KJ, Lee L, Mills JA, et al. Gamma heavy chain disease—an expanding clinical and laboratory spectrum. Am J Med 1973;55:61.

560. Shirakura T, Kobayshi Y, Murai Y, et al. A case of gamma heavy chain disease associated with autoimmune haemolytic anaemia: Clinical haematological, immunological and pathological details. Scand J Haematol 1976;16:387.

561. Westin J, Eyrich R, Falsen, et al. Gamma heavy chain disease: Reports of three patients. Acta Med Scand 1972;192:281.

562. Seligmann M, Danon F, Hurez D, et al. Alpha-chain disease: A new immunoglobulin abnormality. Science 1968;162:1396.

563. Rambaud JC, Galian A, Matuchansky C, et al. Natural history of alpha-chain disease and the so-called Mediterranean lymphoma. Recent Results Cancer Res 1978;64: 271.

564. Roth S, Riecken EO. Alpha-chain disease: Mediterranean lymphoma and primary intestinal lymphoma in Western countries; a review of the cases in the literature. Ergeb Inn Med Kinderheilkd 1977;39:79.

565. Seligmann M. Immunobiology and pathogenesis of alpha chain disease. Ciba Found Symp 1977;46:263.

566. Selzer G, Sherman G, Callihan TR, et al. Primary small intestinal lymphomas and α-heavy-chain disease: A study of 43 cases from a pathology department of Israel. Isr J Med Sci 1979;15:111.

567. Haghighi P, Wolf PL. Alpha-heavy chain disease. Clin Lab Med 1986;6:477–489.

568. Isaacson PG. Middle Eastern intestinal lymphoma. Semin Diagn Pathol 1985;2:210–223.

569. Shi LY, Liaw SJ, Hsueh S, et al. Alpha-chain disease. Report of a case from Taiwan. Cancer 1987;59:545–548.

570. Monges H, Aubert L, Chamlian A, et al. Maladie des chaines alpha a forme intestinale: Preventation d'un cas traite par antibiotherapie avec remission clinique, histologique et immunologique. Arch Fr Mal Appar Dign 1975;64:223.

571. Roge J, Druet P, Marche C. Lymphome Mediterranean avec maladie des chaines alpha: Triple remission clinique, anatomique et immunologique. Pathol Biol (Paris) 1970;18:851.

572. Roge J, Druet P, Marche C, et al. Alpha-chain disease cured with antibiotics. [Letter] Br Med J 1975;4:225.

573. O'Keefe SJ, Winter TA, Newton KA, et al. Severe malnutrition associated with alpha heavy chain disease: Response to tetracycline and intensive nutritional support. Am J Gastroenterol 1988;83:995–1001.

574. Mir-Madjlessi SH, Mir-Ahmadian M. Alpha-chain disease—A report of eleven patients from Iran. J Trop Med Hyg 1979;82:229.

575. Savilahi E, Brandtzaeg P, Kuitunen P. Atypical intestinal alpha-chain disease evolving into selective immunoglobulin: A deficiency in a Finnish boy. Gastroenterology 1980;79:1303.

576. Nikbin B, Banisadre M, Ala F, et al. HLA AW19, B12 in immunoproliferative small intestinal disease. Gut 1976;20:226.

577. Al-Bahrani Z, Al-Saleem T, Al-Mondiry M, et al. Alpha heavy chain disease (report of 18 cases from Iraq). Gut 1978;19:627.

578. Tabbane S, Tabbane F, Cammoun M, et al. Mediterranean lymphomas with alpha heavy chain monoclonal gammopathy. Cancer 1989;1976;38:1989.

579. Berger R, Bernheim A, Tsapis A, et al. Cytogenetic studies in four cases of alpha chain disease. Cancer Genet Cytogenet 1986;22:219–223.

580. Gafter U, Kessler E, Shabtay F, et al. Abnormal chromosomal marker (D14q+) in a patient with alpha heavy chain disease. J Clin Pathol 1980;33:136.

581. Seligmann M. Immunochemical, clinical, and pathological features of α-heavy chain disease. Arch Intern Med 1975;135:78–82.

582. Doe WF. Alpha chain disease: Clinicopathological features and relationship to so-called Mediterranean lymphoma. Br J Cancer 1975;31(suppl 2):350.

583. Galian A, Lecestre M-J, Scotto J, et al. Pathological study of alpha-chain disease with special emphasis on evolution. Cancer 1977;39:2081.

584. Ballard HS, Hamilton LM, Marcus AJ, et al. A new variant of heavy-chain disease (μ-chain disease). N Engl J Med 1970;282:1060.

585. Forte FA, Prelli F, Yount WJ, et al. Heavy chain disease of the μ (γM) type: Report of the first case. Blood 1970;36:137.

586. Franklin EC. μ-Chain disease. Arch Intern Med 1975;135:71.

587. Pruzanski W, Hasselback R, Ratz A, et al. Multiple myeloma (light chain disease) with rheumatoid-like amyloid arthropathy and μ-heavy chain fragment in the serum. Am J Med 1978;65:334.

588. Brouet J-C, Seligmann M, Danon F, et al. μ-Chain disease: Report of two new cases. Arch Intern Med 1979;139:672.

589. Levo Y, Recht B, Michaelsen T, et al. The interaction of immunoglobulin heavy and light chains in the absence of the V_H domain. J Immunol 1977;119:635.

590. Vilpo JA, Irjala K, Viljanen MK, et al. δ-Heavy chain disease: A study of a case. Clin Immunol Immunopathol 1980;17:584.

Cancer: Principles & Practice of Oncology, Fourth Edition,
edited by Vincent T. DeVita, Jr., Samuel Hellman, Steven A. Rosenberg.
J.B. Lippincott Co., Philadelphia © 1993.

Paul A. Bunn, Jr

E. Chester Ridgway

CHAPTER **57**

Paraneoplastic Syndromes

Tumors produce signs and symptoms in the patient by invasion, obstruction, and bulk mass at the primary tumor site and in regional and distant deposits. Tumors can produce signs and symptoms at a distance from the tumor or its metastases. These are collectively referred to as "paraneoplastic syndromes" or "remote effects" of malignancy.[1-4] By definition, these syndromes are not produced directly by the tumor or its metastases. The best characterized paraneoplastic syndromes are those produced by tumors secreting a polypeptide hormone (*e.g.,* adrenocorticotropin [ACTH] or parathormone [PTH]) that is distributed by the circulation and acts on target organ(s) at a distance from the tumor. In these instances, the course of the paraneoplastic syndrome runs parallel to the course of the underlying malignancy, and removal or destruction of the tumor halts production of the hormone. A thorough review of the response of paraneoplastic syndromes to various therapies was published.[5]

Various nonendocrine paraneoplastic syndromes were thought to be produced by unidentified tumor-secreted proteins. During the past decade, many of these new tumor-secreted proteins were described. Previously described paraneoplastic syndromes can be attributed to these proteins, and new syndromes are being recognized. Newly described tumor-derived proteins responsible for paraneoplastic syndromes include growth factors and cytokines. Many of the hematologic paraneoplastic syndromes are caused by tumor secretion of colony-stimulating factors.[6,7] Tumor secretion of transforming growth factor-α (and possibly epidermal growth factor) by malignant melanoma cells was shown to produce acanthosis nigricans, the sign of Leser-Trelat, and multiple acrochordons.[8]

Paraneoplastic syndromes may also be caused by proteins produced by normal cells in response to the tumor. Molecular studies demonstrated that the monokines, tumor necrosis factor, and cachectin, are identical proteins.[9-11] Cachectin may

be responsible for the cachexia syndrome in some patients with malignancy. Antibodies produced in response to malignancy are responsible for many of the neurologic paraneoplastic syndromes, including cerebellar degeneration, the Eaton-Lambert syndrome, paraneoplastic retinopathy, and sensory neuronopathy.[12-15] There are many paraneoplastic syndromes of unknown cause that may be produced by tumor-secreted proteins. Some of these syndromes may be caused by nonparaneoplastic factors.

Progressive multifocal leukoencephalopathy (PML) was initially described as a neurologic paraneoplastic syndrome.[16] PML is caused by a virus, and although patients with malignancy may be prone to develop this viral syndrome, PML is not truly paraneoplastic.[17]

Endocrine tumors can be functional, and their hormonal products (*e.g.,* polypeptide, catecholamines, iodothyronine, steroids) give symptoms at a distance from the primary tumor, but for practical purposes, this chapter deals only with syndromes produced by tumors arising in sites other than the pituitary, adrenals, endocrine pancreas, endocrine cells of the gastrointestinal tract, and endocrine cells of the ovaries and testes and all forms of the carcinoid syndrome. These are discussed in other chapters.

Paraneoplastic syndromes develop in a minority of cancer patients. Their exact frequency is difficult to determine for a variety of reasons, including various definitions, unknown causes, and lack of systematic case-control studies. For example, in an uncontrolled study, Croft and Wilkinson reported that 7% of cancer patients have neurologic paraneoplastic syndromes, but in a case-control study, Brody found no difference in the frequency of neurologic syndromes in patients with lung cancer and controls with benign chronic lung disease.[18,19] The frequency figures given in this chapter are usually from uncontrolled studies.

The importance of the paraneoplastic syndromes (including

hormones detected by immunoassay) and the elucidation of their mechanisms are important for many reasons. Their appearance may be the first sign of a malignancy, which allows its early detection in a curable state. They may simulate metastatic disease and prevent patients from having curative therapy. Conversely, treatable complications of malignancy (*e.g.*, metastatic disease, infection) may be ascribed to a paraneoplastic syndrome, leading to the withholding of appropriate therapy. They can be used as tumor markers in previously treated patients to detect early recurrence or in patients undergoing adjuvant therapy to guide further therapy. In patients with metastatic disease, their syndromes can be disabling, and appropriate treatment of the paraneoplasia may be the best means of palliating patients. The hormones released by tumors may be required for tumor growth (*i.e.*, the tumor may produce its own growth factors and "autostimulate"), and appropriate identification of such hormones may allow a new rational therapeutic approach to treatment of the neoplasms.[20]

Because of their importance, numerous articles and reviews describing paraneoplastic syndromes have been published in the past 20 years.[1–4,21,22]

ETIOLOGY AND PATHOGENESIS OF PARANEOPLASTIC SYNDROMES

Paraneoplastic syndromes can arise in several ways:

1. Tumor-produced biologically active proteins or polypeptides, including peptide hormones, their precursors, growth factors, interleukins, cytokines, prostaglandins, fetal proteins such as carcinoembryonic antigen (CEA) or α-fetoprotein (AFP), other proteins such as immunoglobulins, and enzymes produced and released by tumors
2. Autoimmunity or immune complex production and immune suppression
3. Ectopic receptor production or a competitive blockade of normal hormone action by tumor-produced biologically inactive hormones
4. "Forbidden contact" in which there is release of enzymes (*e.g.*, placental alkaline phosphatase) or other products that normally are not circulated but that takes place because of abnormal tumor vasculature or disrupted basement membranes, allowing antigenic reactions, inappropriate initiation of normal physiologic functions, and other toxic manifestations to occur
5. Unknown causes.

DIFFERENTIAL DIAGNOSIS

The importance and frequency of paraneoplastic syndromes make it imperative to establish the appropriate diagnosis. If the cause of the paraneoplastic syndrome is unknown, this may mean excluding all other known causes of the syndrome. Each section of this chapter includes a listing of the differential diagnoses. In general, paraneoplastic syndromes must be differentiated from

1. Direct invasion by the primary tumor or its metastases
2. Obstruction caused by tumor or tumor products

3. Vascular abnormalities
4. Infections
5. Fluid and electrolyte abnormalities
6. Toxicity of cancer therapy, including cytotoxic chemotherapy, radiation therapy, immunotherapy, or antibiotic therapy.

ENDOCRINOLOGIC MANIFESTATIONS OF MALIGNANCY

Paraneoplastic syndromes caused by the production of polypeptide hormones are the most frequent and best understood paraneoplastic syndromes. To establish a paraneoplastic cause for alterations in hormone production, conclusive evidence that the hormone is produced by the tumor must be established. The differential diagnosis of endocrinologic abnormalities in the cancer patient is shown in Table 57–1.

The laboratory evaluation begins after a complete history and physical examination. Abnormal levels of the hormone in question should be documented, usually by radioimmunoassay. Paraneoplastic hormone production usually is independent of the normal regulatory mechanisms. There is other direct evidence that a tumor produces a hormone causing the paraneoplastic syndrome:

1. Fall in hormone levels after removal or treatment of the tumor
2. Maintenance of elevated hormone levels after extirpation of the "normal" gland of origin of the hormone
3. Demonstration of an arteriovenous gradient of hormone levels across the tumor
4. Demonstration of synthesis and secretion of the hormone by tumor tissue in vitro
5. Demonstration of hormone synthesis and secretion by in vitro clonal tissue culture isolates of the tumor cells.

Secretion of polypeptide hormones by tumors has been known for most of this century to cause recognized paraneoplastic syndromes. In the past 10 years, many previously unknown polypeptide hormones have been discovered. Most of these peptides have been identified within the central nervous system (CNS) or the gastrointestinal tract.[24,25] Table 57–2 lists the categories of mammalian polypeptide hormones; some cause known paraneoplastic syndromes, and some are produced by human tumor cells. The function of many of the hormones, such as neurophysin, bombesin, and physalaemin, is unknown. However, they are produced by human tumors,

TABLE 57–1. Endocrinologic Manifestations of Malignancy: Differential Diagnosis

1. Hormone production by benign cells (*e.g.*, parathyroid adenoma)
2. Hormone production by a malignancy of an endocrine organ (*e.g.*, MEN)
3. Alterations in hormone production as a direct result of infiltration of an endocrine gland by a primary tumor or its metastases
4. Alterations in hormone production by therapy
5. Alterations in hormone production by infection
6. Paraneoplastic

TABLE 57–2. Categories of Mammalian Brain Peptides Producing Proven or Potential Paraneoplastic Syndromes

Hypothalamic-Releasing Hormones

Thyrotropin-releasing hormone
Gonadotropin-releasing hormone
Somatostatin
Corticotropin-releasing hormone
Growth hormone-releasing hormone

Neurohypophyseal Hormones

Vasopressin*†
Oxytocin
Neurophysin(s)†

Pituitary Peptides

Adrenocorticotropic hormone*†
β-Endorphin†
Melanocyte-stimulating hormone*†
Prolactin
Luteinizing hormone
Growth hormone†
Thyrotropin

Invertebrate Peptides

FM RT amide
Hydra head activator

Nonbrain Hormones

Parathormone*†
β-hCG*†
T₃

Gastrointestinal Peptides

Vasoactive intestinal peptide*†
Cholecystokinin
Gastrin
Substance P
Neurotensin†
Met-enkephalin
Leu-enkephalin
Insulin
Glucagon†
Bombesin†
Gastrin-releasing peptide†
Secretin
Somatostatin†
Thyrotropin-releasing hormone
Motilin

Others

Angiotensin II
Bradykinin
Carosine
Sleep peptide(s)
Calcitonin†
CGRP
Neuropeptide Y
Physalaemin†
Neuron-specific enolase†

* Produces a proven paraneoplastic syndrome.
† Produced by small cell lung cancer or carcinoid tumors.
(Kreiger DT, Martin JB. Brain peptides. N Engl J Med 1981;304:876–885; Kreiger DT. Brain peptides: What, where, and why? Science 1983;222:975–985)

such as small cell lung cancer.[26–28] Some of the paraneoplastic syndromes for which the cause is unknown and perhaps some unrecognized paraneoplastic syndromes will probably be ascribed to these hormones after more is learned of their function.

The endocrine paraneoplastic syndromes, the responsible hormone, the most frequently associated tumor types, and incidence are shown in Table 57–3.[23,29] With the development of radioimmunoassays and screening of cancer patients, it was found that hormone production in cancer patients (presumably from their tumors) was much more frequent than previously realized.[3,23] Table 57–4 lists screening studies of lung cancer patients or tumor extracts for the presence of various hormones using radioimmunoassays.[30–35] These frequencies are much higher than those of the clinically recognized paraneoplastic syndromes related to these hormones because the large-molecular-weight hormone precursors, fragments, or subunits secreted by tumors are often biologically inactive. Other factors that obscure the true frequency of hormone secretion by tumors include inadequate clinical follow-up (*e.g.,* spot-checks of patients rather than observation throughout the clinical course); production of a hormone that does not have easily recognizable clinical effect (*e.g.,* acromegalic effects of growth hormone, which may take years to manifest); operation of normal physiologic feedback mech-

anisms, which suppress normal hormone production; secretion of multiple hormones (*e.g.,* secretion of ACTH obscuring the clinical effect of simultaneous arginine vasopressin [AVP] secretion); and investigator and laboratory facility bias.

ACTH AND CUSHING'S SYNDROME

Evidence from analysis of cultured tumor cells, pituitary extracts, and recombinant DNA work demonstrates that the prohormone (*i.e.,* stem hormone) molecule of ACTH contains the following in sequence from the NH_2-terminal to the COOH-terminal end (Fig. 57–1).[24,25,36–38]

1. A putative signal peptide (amino acid position −141 to −110)
2. A NH_2-terminal region with unknown function (position −110 to −53)
3. γ-MSH (position −53 to −48)
4. A region with unknown function (position −48 to −1)
5. ACTH (position 1 to 39) or "classic" ACTH, which contains within it α-MSH (position 1 to 13) and corticotropin-like intermediate lobe peptide (position 18 to 39)
6. β-Lipotropin hormone (β-LPH; position 42 to 134), which contains within it γ-LPH (position 42 to 101) and β-MSH (position 84 to 101)

TABLE 57–3. Endocrine Paraneoplastic Syndromes

Syndrome	Hormone	Tumor	Incidence (%)
Cushing's syndrome	ACTH	Lung cancer—all types	0–2.0
		Small cell lung cancer	6
Inappropriate antidiuresis	AVP	Lung cancer—all types	0.9–2.0
	ANP	Small cell lung cancer	9
Nonmetastatic hypercalcemia	PTH	Lung cancer—all types	1.0–7.5
		Squamous cell lung cancer	15
		Other tumors	14
Gynecomastia		Lung cancer—all types	0.5–0.9
		Small cell lung cancer	2.0
Hyperthyroidism		Lung cancer	0–1.4
Calcitonin		Medullary carcinoma of the thyroid	
		Small cell lung cancer	
		Other lung cancer types	
		Breast cancer	
Acromegaly	GHRH	Carcinoids, pheochomocytoma—rare	
		Pancreatic cancer	

(Lees LH. The biosynthesis of hormones by nonendocrine tumours—A review. J Endocrinol 1975;67: 143–175; Richardson RL, Greco FA, Oldhan RK, Liddle GW. Tumor products and potential markers in small cell lung cancer. Semin Oncol 1978;5:253–262)

7. Met-enkephalin (position 104 to 108)
8. β-Endorphin (position 104 to 134)

The prohormone molecule has been called "big ACTH" or proopiocortin and contains four repetitive sequences based on the ACTH-MSH core, with these sequences separated by paired basic residues. The importance of the promolecule is that it can be split into many biologically active fragments. These activities include adrenal gland stimulation to make corticosteroids and androgens (*e.g.*, by ACTH); melanocyte stimulation-hyperpigmentation activity (*e.g.*, by MSH-containing peptides); and opiate-like activity (*e.g.*, β-LPH, β-endorphin, met-enkephalin). There has been an explosion of knowledge concerning the biologic activity of fragments of this molecule, particularly the opioid peptides (*e.g.*, β-LPH, β-endorphin, met-enkephalin), which mimic morphine in their action.[39-41] The paired basic residues flank the biologically active sequences. Proteolytic processing takes place at these sites that determines the biologic activities and the paraneoplastic syndromes seen in humans. The regulation of cleavage of the promolecule in neoplastic states is important. The cleavage patterns change during development and may

TABLE 57–4. Frequency of Peptide Hormone Elevation in the Blood of Lung Cancer Patients

Hormone	Patients With Significantly Elevated Levels (%)*			
	Small Cell	Epidermoid	Adenocarcinoma	Large Cell
ACTH	30–69	0–80	17–75	26
LPH	54	33	20	Not done
Calcitonin	48–64	9	0	11
ADH	32			
PTH	27	32	0	17
β-hCG	1–32	19	17	26
GH	0	3	0	0
GRP	74	17	20	7
SLI	27	11	Not done	Not done
NSE	69	Not done	Not done	Not done
Neurophysins	65	14	29	20

* Not all studies were done in all patients.
(Data from references 30–35)

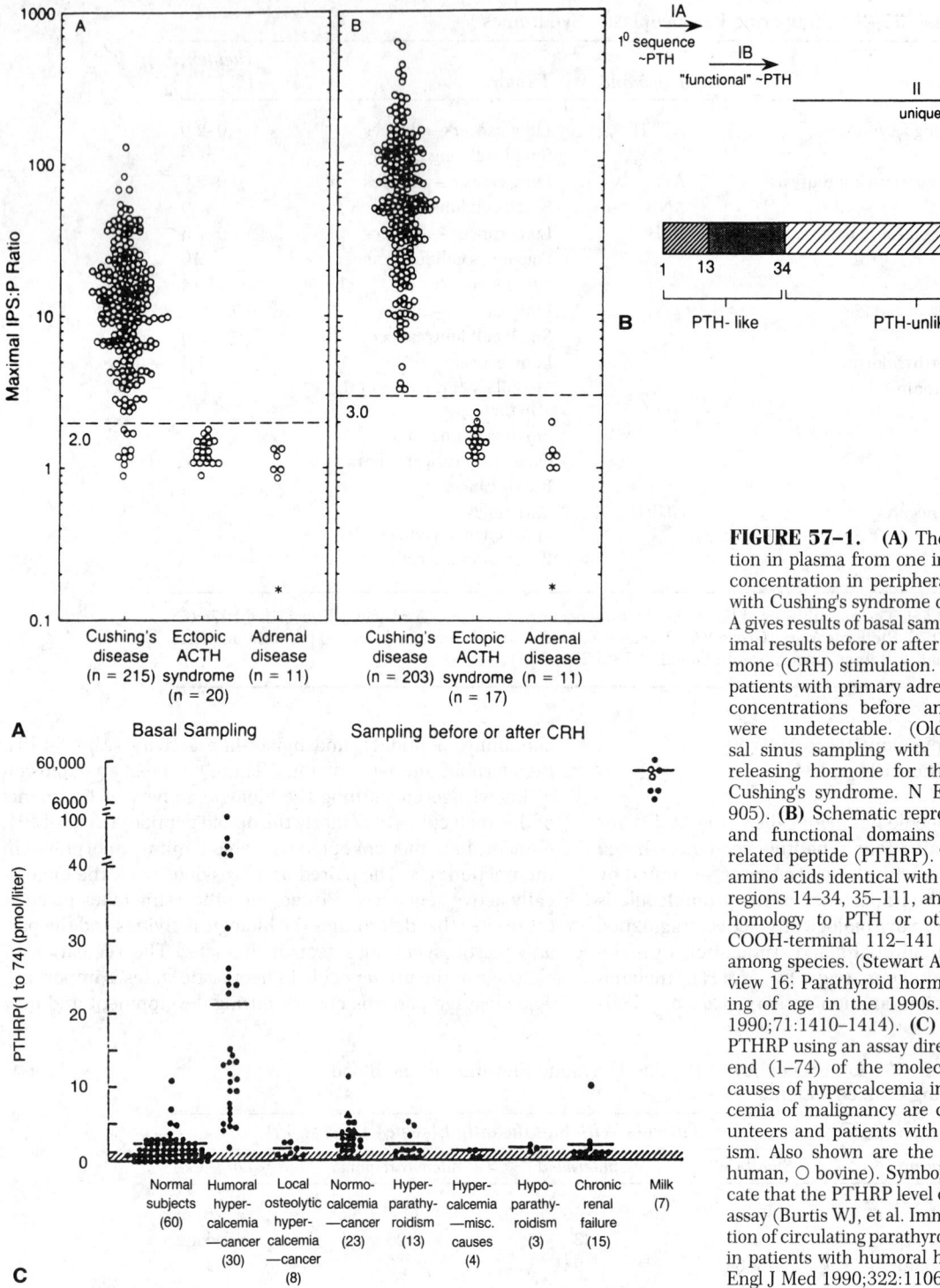

FIGURE 57–1. **(A)** The ratio of ACTH concentration in plasma from one inferior petrosal sinus to the concentration in peripheral blood (IPS:P) in patients with Cushing's syndrome due to various causes. Panel A gives results of basal samples, and Panel B gives maximal results before or after corticotropin-releasing hormone (CRH) stimulation. The asterisks represent five patients with primary adrenal disease in whom ACTH concentrations before and after CRH stimulation were undetectable. (Oldfield EH, et al. Petrosal sinus sampling with and without corticotropin-releasing hormone for the differential diagnosis of Cushing's syndrome. N Engl J Med 1991;325:897–905). **(B)** Schematic representation of the structural and functional domains of parathyroid hormone-related peptide (PTHRP). The 1–13 region contains 8 amino acids identical with the PTH sequence, but the regions 14–34, 35–111, and 112–141 bear little or no homology to PTH or other known peptides. The COOH-terminal 112–141 region is poorly conserved among species. (Stewart AF, Broadus AE. Clinical review 16: Parathyroid hormone related proteins: Coming of age in the 1990s. J Clin Endocrinol Metab 1990;71:1410–1414). **(C)** Plasma concentrations of PTHRP using an assay directed to the amino-terminal end (1–74) of the molecule. Patients with various causes of hypercalcemia including humeral hypercalcemia of malignancy are compared with healthy volunteers and patients with primary hyperparathyroidism. Also shown are the PTHRP levels in milk (● human, ○ bovine). Symbols in the hatched area indicate that the PTHRP level could not be detected in the assay (Burtis WJ, et al. Immunochemical characterization of circulating parathyroid hormone-related protein in patients with humoral hypercalcemia of Cancer. N Engl J Med 1990;322:1106–1112)

be different in tumors than in adult pituitary tissue.[41] Proopiocortin is a glycosylated peptide, and glycosylation may play an important role in proteolysis, packaging, and storage. Classically, ectopic ACTH production is thought to be unregulated, but some tumor tissues studied in vitro continue to show some control over ACTH secretion by means of a cyclic AMP-dependent mechanism.[42]

Clinical Features of Ectopic Proopiocortin Excess

The clinical features of the ectopic ACTH syndrome include hypokalemia, hyperglycemia, edema, muscle weakness or atrophy, hypertension, and weight loss. Other features seen in pituitary Cushing's disease or exogenous corticosteroid excess (*e.g.*, centripetal obesity, cutaneous striae, moon facies, buffalo hump, pigmentation) are uncommonly seen in highly malignant tumors (*e.g.*, oat cell lung cancer) but are more frequent in the indolent carcinoids, thymomas, and pheochromocytomas. Although the cases first reported involved men, the increased prevalence of lung cancer in women may be associated with more features seen in women, including hirsutism, which was seen in Brown's original patient.[43]

FREQUENCY OF ECTOPIC PROOPIOCORTIN PRODUCTION BY TUMORS. The major clinical association of ectopic ACTH production is with lung cancer, particularly of the small cell histologic type.[3,23,38] Clinically apparent Cushing's syndrome is found in 0.4% to 2% of patients with lung cancer of all histologic types (see Table 57–3).[23,29,44,45] In small cell lung cancer, 5.5% of 473 patients in several large series had clinical manifestations of Cushing's syndrome.[46–48] Lung cancer represents more than 50% of the clinically obvious cases, carcinoids and neural crest tumors (*e.g.*, pheochromocytomas, neuroblastomas, medullary carcinomas of the thyroid) amount to 15% each, and bronchial carcinoid and thymomas represent 10% each. The frequency of significantly elevated levels of ACTH by radioimmunoassay (RIA) in the blood and tumor extracts of lung cancer patients (Table 57–5) is much higher than the frequency of the ectopic Cushing's syndrome.[49–57] Similarly, the frequency of increased fasting morning cortisol levels with dexamethasone suppression (49–71%) or without dexamethasone suppression (38%) is higher than the frequency of the ectopic syndrome.[23,31,57–59] Although these differences could be due to the presence of inactive proACTH or stress, Bondy and Gilby suggest that the tumors secrete only small amounts of excess hormone.[57]

The ectopic ACTH is not secreted under feedback control, enters the plasma without normal diurnal variations, and is not suppressed normally by exogenous dexamethasone, but it is not sufficient to cause clinical abnormalities. The clinical syndrome occurs only in the uncommon tumors that secrete large excesses of active hormone. Most extracts of small cell lung cancer tumors have increased levels of ACTH and LPH detected by RIA. The other histologic types vary in positivity between 6% and 40%. Although non-small cell lung cancer types have increased cortisol levels, the mechanism of this is unknown.[22,23,49] The frequency of ectopic ACTH-associated clinical syndromes and adrenal function is not well described for other tumor types.[38]

HISTOLOGY OF ACTH-PRODUCING TUMORS. Azzopardi and Williams reviewed the world's literature on the ectopic syndrome and found that 112 of 130 cases arose in the lung, pancreas, or thymus.[60] The most frequent histologic finding was a small cell cancer or a carcinoid structure. Other tumors included pheochromocytomas, related tumors, and certain ovarian tumors. Ten years later, Skrabanek and Powell continued the literature review of cases with ectopic ACTH and Cushing's syndrome and found that all such tumors with clinically apparent ACTH excess could be grouped into a carcinoid-oat cell (small cell) group and a pheochromocytoma-neuroblastoma class based on histologic appearance.[61] They thought that tumors found in organs other than the lung (*e.g.*, thymus, all thymic carcinoids rather than epithelial thymoma), thyroid (*e.g.*, medullary carcinoma), esophagus, stomach, pancreas, small intestine, appendix, salivary gland, ovary, testis, uterine cervix, and prostate had a carcinoid or a small cell lung cancer-type tissue structure.[62,63] They and others postulated that these tumors arose only where normal Kulchitsky-type cells occur and could potentially have a common origin.

If a histologic type other than these described is suggested (*e.g.*, adenocarcinoma), the finding should be viewed with skepticism and carefully documented. The histologic material should be reviewed and more obtained, if necessary. The extrapulmonary cancers with small cell structure should be treated as if they were small cell carcinoma of the lung, and

TABLE 57–5. Frequency of ACTH Elevation in Blood and Tumor Extracts Detected by RIA in Lung Cancer Patients Without Clinically Evident Ectopic ACTH Syndrome

Source of Material Tumor Type	Patients (n)	Positive (%)	References
Patient's Blood			
All histologic types	290	19, 41, 42, 88	49, 50, 51, 52
Epidermoid	88	0–50	49, 51
Adenocarcinoma	25	17–26	49, 51
Large cell carcinoma	28	26–49	49, 51
Small cell carcinoma	49, 51	11, 29–30	49, 51
Chronic obstructive pulmonary disease	101	25*	49, 50, 52
Tumor Extracts (Surgical Specimens)			
All histologic types	127	31, 58, 93, 100	49, 50, 53, 54
Epidermoid	49	49	49
Adenocarcinoma	17	6	49
Large cell carcinoma	8	25	49
Small cell carcinoma and carcinoid	12	100	55, 56

* Seventeen percent of patients with elevated ACTH levels developed lung cancer within 2 years.
(Data from references 49–57)

those with a carcinoid tissue structure should be dealt with as carcinoids.[64,65] It is important to obtain more studies on the efficacy of chemotherapy on tumors producing ACTH that do not have typical small cell or carcinoid tissues.

DIAGNOSIS OF ECTOPIC CUSHING'S SYNDROME. About 40% of patients presenting with overt Cushing's syndrome have pituitary Cushing's with an obvious tumor, 28% have pituitary Cushing's syndrome without tumors (both of these usually occur in women of childbearing age), 17% have adrenal Cushing's (usually in children), and 15% have the ectopic Cushing's syndrome (usually in adult men). Although the production of proopiocorticoid molecule may have unrecognized clinical effects, the diagnosis of clinically significant ectopic ACTH excess begins with thinking about the possibility in the appropriate clinical setting, such as an older man with small cell lung cancer or a patient with unexplained hypokalemic alkalosis, particularly if it is accompanied by edema, hypertension, profound muscular weakness or atrophy, mental changes, or glucose intolerance. Patients with ectopic ACTH from thymic tumors and bronchial carcinoids are usually younger and present with more classic features of Cushing's syndrome, primarily because of the more indolent course of the neoplasms. When clinical features are present, a plasma ACTH value of over 200 pg/ml suggests ectopic ACTH production.

The biochemical diagnosis of Cushing's syndrome that results from ectopic ACTH production involves the demonstration of excessive cortisol production by measuring a 24-hour urinary free cortisol. Abnormal values are higher than 100 µg/day, and values as high as 1000 µg/day may be seen. A simultaneous plasma ACTH value of over 200 pg/ml suggests ectopic ACTH production. However, many cases of ectopic ACTH production due to a bronchial or thymic carcinoid may have ACTH values between 20 and 200 pg/ml. Abnormal suppression of elevated cortisol production is documented by showing that plasma cortisol levels do not suppress after administering dexamethasone, 2 mg every 6 hours for 48 hours, or after giving a single 8-mg dose of dexamethasone at midnight before obtaining a sample to test the plasma cortisol level at 8:00 A.M. the next morning. Elevations in the 24-hour urinary free cortisol, elevations in the plasma ACTH concentration, and abnormal dexamethasone suppressibility are highly suggestive of the ectopic ACTH syndrome. Unfortunately, these diagnostic criteria are not perfect in making the diagnosis of ectopic ACTH production. For example, a high-dose dexamethasone suppression test suppresses cortisol production in almost half the patients with ectopic ACTH tumors caused by bronchial carcinoids.[66,67] A high-dose dexamethasone suppression test fails to suppress cortisol production in about 20% of patients with Cushing's disease due to a pituitary tumor.[67a]

To improve the precision in diagnosing ectopic ACTH production and differentiating it from pituitary-dependent Cushing's disease, the simultaneous sampling of ACTH from the inferior petrosal sinuses has provided a major advance.[68,69,69a] If the source of ACTH is from a pituitary tumor, plasma ACTH levels in the petrosal venous sinuses should be much higher than peripheral levels. If the ACTH source is from a tumor distant from the pituitary, ACTH levels in petrosal venous sinuses and peripheral venous blood should be similar. This

procedure has been validated in a large group of patients at the National Institute of Health for whom ACTH levels measured in the inferior petrosal sinuses (IPS) are related to ACTH levels in peripheral blood plasma (P) and expressed as an IPS:P ratio.[69a] An IPS:P ratio of 2 or more in basal samples correctly identified the source of ACTH in patients with Cushing's disease with a sensitivity of 95% and no false-positive results. Results were improved if the sampling was performed after the administration of corticotropin-releasing hormone (CRH) in which a peak IPS:P ratio of 3 or more identified the source of ACTH in 100% of Cushing's disease with no false-positive results. Patients with ectopic ACTH syndrome uniformly had IPS:P ratios less than 2 in basal samples and less than 3 in CRH-stimulated samples (see Fig. 57–1A). In patients with benign or malignant adrenal tumors, the ACTH levels in plasma are low or undetectable, and the cortisol levels are not suppressed with dexamethasone. The IPS:P ratio in these cases is always below 2 or 3 in basal or CRH-stimulated samples.

Other sources of difficulty in the correct diagnosis of ectopic Cushing's syndrome can occur with the simultaneous production of two hormones (*e.g.*, ACTH and AVP) or of a peptide hormone or amine product.[23,70] Multiple hormone secretion indicates a nonpituitary tumor. Other cases of dexamethasone suppression of ectopic ACTH production have been linked to secretion of CRH itself by the tumor.[71,72] Well-defined cases of Cushing's syndrome resulting from tumor production of CRH have been documented.[73-75] The CRH is postulated to act on the pituitary to stimulate pituitary ACTH release or at the tumor level to stimulate tumor cell ACTH production.

Treatment of Ectopic ACTH and Related Syndromes

The treatment of ectopic proopiocorticoid syndromes should be directed primarily at the tumor. In carcinoids, this can involve surgery, and with thymomas, surgery or radiotherapy. With appropriate therapy, the syndrome is usually cured, and the high levels of ACTH are reduced in most patients.[76] Although previous reviews have stated that a prognosis of less than 4 months is expected for the ectopic ACTH syndrome with small cell lung cancer, these predated the substantial gains in treatment and potential cure of some patients with small cell carcinoma. (The principles of the treatment of small cell lung carcinomas with combination chemotherapy is discussed in detail in Chap. 23). If the histologic appearance of any mediastinal or extrathoracic tumor is compatible with a small cell tumor, we favor treating the patient as though he had small cell lung cancer. The data on response to therapy of Cushing's syndrome in small cell cancer patients are anecdotal, but reports of a fall in ACTH levels after combination chemotherapy, with or without radiotherapy, have appeared.[30,48] If treatment of the tumor fails, drugs that inhibit adrenal corticoid production may be used, such as aminoglutethimide, metyrapone, or mitotane.[68,77-79] (The reader should review appropriate endocrinology sources for directions in using these adrenal suppressants.) After drug treatment, patients should be treated with supplemental steroids to avoid hypoadrenalism. Because of the increasing use of aminoglutethimide in breast cancer patients, this drug is probably the first choice. Another possibility is combining aminoglutethimide and metyrapone to lower the dose-related toxicity of both agents with dexamethasone and fludrocortisone.[80] In rare cases, with chronic ectopic ACTH excess and indolent tumors, bilateral adrenalectomy can be considered.

Use of proACTH and β-Lipotropin Hormone for Early Cancer Detection

Odell and associates found significant blood elevations of proACTH in 92% of pancreatic cancers, 72% of lung cancers, 54% of gastric or esophagus cancers, 41% of breast cancers, and 27% of colon cancers, and the corresponding values for elevated LPH were 25%, 36%, 14%, 0%, and 10%, respectively, for these tumor types.[32] In general, the quantitative levels of proACTH-ACTH and LPH were correlated. Some 20% of patients with chronic obstructive pulmonary disease had blood elevations of proACTH, whereas 13% had elevations of LPH. Other studies found proACTH elevations in chronic lung disease, suggesting that the lung may produce or bind proACTH or LPH in response to injury.[50–52] Five of 20 of the patients with elevated proACTH in chronic obstructive pulmonary disease eventually developed lung cancer, but only 2 of 81 of the patients with normal plasma levels of ACTH developed lung cancer.[45]

When ACTH, calcitonin, and hCG were measured simultaneously, significant elevated levels were found in 65% of 109 lung cancer patients and 78% of small cell cancer patients, suggesting the usefulness of several markers in concert to detect lung cancer.[31] More studies are needed to know if the proACTH-LPH or other peptide hormone assays are predictors of the development of lung cancer and if they can be useful in following the course of the disease. Extracts of tumors other than lung cancer showed significant elevations (>1 ng/g tissue) of proACTH or LPH: 6 of 16 colon cancers, 3 of 4 breast cancers, and 22 of 31 miscellaneous tumors and metastatic lesions. Although elevated levels of immunoreactive material were found, there is no direct evidence that the tumors produced the peptides. Many tumors may make preopiocorticoid, but only some have the ability to cleave it appropriately into biologically active forms. The expression of the syndromes may depend more on the promolecule processing than the presence of the ectopic prohormone itself.[2]

With the development and use of RIAs for measuring lipotropin and β-endorphin and receptor assays for measuring endogenous opiate peptides in human cerebrospinal fluid and plasma, it may become possible to correlate unusual neurologic syndromes and mental behavior directly with fragments derived from the proopiocorticoid molecule.[32,39,81] It is reasonable to start applying these assays to patients with such symptoms and appropriate tumor settings (*e.g.,* lung cancer). Circulating immune complexes of ACTH and human immunoglobulins have been reported.[82] ACTH also may be involved in an immune complex paraneoplastic syndrome. A portion of the ACTH promolecule with opioid activity undergoes a striking increase in the pituitary of newborn monkeys. This increase in endogenous opioid may help the fetus withstand the stress of parturition.[41] Likewise, tumor production of an analgesic-like material such as β-endorphin may allow the cancer patient a measure of relief from tumor-related symptoms. Additional work quantitating the amount and nature of such endogenous analgesics is necessary.

SYNDROME OF INAPPROPRIATE SECRETION OF ANTIDIURETIC HORMONE

Hyponatremia was first associated with lung cancer in 1938; the syndrome of "inappropriate secretion" of antidiuretic hormone (SIADH; ADH = arginine vasopressin [AVP]) was postulated by Schwartz and coworkers in 1957 to be caused by stimulation of the posterior pituitary to secrete AVP by a thoracic tumor.[83,84] In 1963, Amatruda and coworkers showed it to be related to tumor production of AVP.[85] AVP, oxytocin, and neurophysins have been found by RIA in tumors, and the AVP is bioactive and immunoreactive.[23,86] The neurophysins normally are synthesized, stored, and secreted in parallel with AVP and oxytocin.[87] These polypeptides function as binding proteins for AVP and oxytocin; there are different neurophysins for AVP and oxytocin.[88] Whether AVP and oxytocin actually form a promolecule with their respective neurophysins is under investigation.[23] Currently, there are no recognized syndromes related to tumor production of neurophysins or oxytocin, but tumor production of AVP results in hyponatremia.

Clinical Findings and Pathophysiology

Continuous tumor production, exogenous administration, and posterior pituitary production of AVP all result in a syndrome of hyponatremia, urine inappropriately higher in osmolality than the plasma, and high urinary sodium concentrations in the face of serum hyponatremia.[2,3,23] This is thought to result from the action of AVP on the renal tubule with resultant water retention. The hyponatremia comes from renal sodium loss and dilution by water retention. The mechanism of the natriuresis is not defined but could include an increased filtered sodium load, a decreased aldosterone secretion, or a decreased tubular reabsorption of sodium. The major clinical symptoms are caused by water intoxication (*i.e.,* hypoosmality and hyponatremia) and manifested by altered mental status, confusion, lethargy, psychotic behavior, seizures, coma, or occasionally death.[2,3,23,89] Focal neurologic findings can be associated with water intoxication from SIADH alone without brain metastases.[89] Because of the predominant occurrence of SIADH with small cell lung cancer and the frequent presence of brain metastases in this cancer, all patients with neurologic syndromes in small cell lung cancer should have serum sodium levels checked for hyponatremia, and all small cell cancer patients with hyponatremia and neurologic syndromes should be evaluated for brain metastases.

Diagnosis of Ectopic Arginine Vasopressin Production

Hyponatremia is the usual mode of presentation of SIADH because of the routine use of serum electrolytes in patient evaluation (Table 57–6). Some patients present with neurologic symptoms. The first major problem is to differentiate SIADH from the multiple other causes of hyponatremia, such as diuretic use; cardiac, hepatic, and renal failure; dilutional causes; diminished function of adrenals, anterior pituitary, or thyroid. Various drugs can impair free water excretion by acting on the renal tubule or by inducing pituitary AVP, including chlorpropamide, thiazide diuretics, cyclophosphamide, vincristine, and morphine.[90–92] To separate these causes of hy-

TABLE 57–6. Differential Diagnosis for the Syndrome of Inappropriate Antidiuretic Hormone

Tumors
  Small cell lung cancer
  Other types
Pulmonary, chest conditions
  Infection (tuberculosis, abscess, pneumonia—viral or bacterial),
    mitral stenosis (status after surgical correction)
Central nervous system
  Trauma (skull fracture, subdural, concussion, subarachnoid
    hemorrhage, thrombosis)
  Intracranial space-occupying lesions (primary and metastatic
    tumor)
  Infections (meningitis, encephalitis, lues)
  Vasculitis (lupus)
  Guillian-Barré
  Acute intermittent porphyria
  Pain and emotional stress
Drugs
  Chlorpropamide
  Morphine
  Nicotine
  Ethanol
  Cyclophosphamide
  Vincristine
  Idiopathic

ponatremia from SIADH, it is mandatory to demonstrate the following:

1. Hypoosmolality (usually <280 mOsm/kg)
2. Urinary osmolality greater than the plasma (≥500 mOsm/kg)
3. Continued urinary excretion of sodium (>20 mEq/L) although taking no diuretics
4. Absence of signs of volume depletion
5. Normal renal function
6. Normal adrenal and thyroid function.

Fichman and Bethune studied 86 patients with SIADH and found serum sodium levels of 88 to 126 mEq/L, urine sodium levels of 35 to 175 mEq/24 hours, serum osmolalities of 190 to 273 mOsm/kg, and urine osmolalities of 332 to 780 mOsm/kg.[92] The most common mistake in diagnosis of SIADH is failing to notice the previous administration of a diuretic or of occult volume depletion with resulting dilutional hyponatremia. Repeat clinical examinations can exclude these causes. Although AVP can be measured by RIA, this is not routinely available, and many conditions can be associated with the "appropriate" and the "inappropriate" secretion of AVP.

The most common disorders associated with SIADH besides small cell lung cancer include CNS diseases (*e.g.*, CNS infection, head trauma, intracranial space-occupying lesions, subarachnoid hemorrhage, acute intermittent porphyria, pain, emotional stress) and pulmonary infections (see Table 57–6). If any of these affect patients with SIADH and malignant disease (including small cell cancer), they should be treated in an effort to control the SIADH. Water loading can elicit clinically occult SIADH but can be dangerous in patients with

hyponatremia and probably should not be done if the serum sodium concentration is 125 mEq/L or less.[90]

In studies of lung cancer patients with SIADH and high levels of AVP by RIA, fluid restriction further increased the already elevated AVP level, probably from stimulation of the pituitary to release AVP.[93] The other causes of SIADH (particularly drugs) account for some of the SIADH seen in tumor patients without small cell lung cancer or carcinoid histologic findings and stress the need for biosynthetic studies of AVP by cultured tumor cells to prove the source of the AVP. Other complications (*e.g.*, pneumonia) usually occur because of the cancer, and the development of SIADH represents a "secondary" paraneoplastic syndrome. For example, cyclophosphamide and vincristine are used to treat small cell lung cancer. When cyclophosphamide is given in high doses and the patient is hydrated to prevent cystitis, the combined effect of cyclophosphamide to decrease free water clearance and the water load can lead to SIADH.[92,94,95] Whether this represents release of pituitary AVP or a direct effect of cyclophosphamide metabolites on the renal tubules is unknown.[94]

If the histology of the tumor-associated SIADH is small cell cancer, the cancer is treated and correlation is made between the tumor response and the SIADH. If the tumor's histologic structure is other than small cell or carcinoid, the physician should be skeptical about tumor production of AVP until all causes of the SIADH are sought. If no other causes of SIADH are apparent, the physician should consider obtaining more tumor tissue, because a component of small cell carcinoma may be present. This dictates a more aggressive chemoradiotherapy approach than that for an "unresponsive" non-small cell tumor type.

If a patient presents with idiopathic SIADH, a careful search and follow-up for small cell tumor must be maintained; although cases like this are uncommon, the workup probably should include a full staging evaluation for small cell cancer, including fiberoptic bronchoscopy and computed tomography (CT) scans of the chest and abdomen to locate small tumor masses. The tumor should declare itself within a few months. In comparing tumor-related SIADH and SIADH resulting from other causes, serum and urinary sodium levels, osmolality, blood urea nitrogen, plasma AVP, and renin levels all failed to differentiate neoplastic from nonneoplastic causes.[94] The speed of rise in serum sodium concentration with water restriction supposedly is faster (3 days versus 7–10 days) for nonneoplastic causes than for neoplastic causes of SIADH.[96] However, this distinction may not be clear enough to be useful clinically.

Frequency and Tumor Types

Almost all of the tumors that produce AVP are small cell carcinomas of the lung.[2,3,23,29] However, SIADH has been seen with other tumor types, including carcinomas of the prostate, adrenal cortex, esophagus, pancreas, duodenum, colon, bronchial carcinoids, thymomas, head and neck, Hodgkin's disease, and non-Hodgkin's lymphomas.[2,3,23] At least some of these may have had a nonpulmonary small cell or carcinoid histologic structure. Small cell lung cancer lines grown in tissue culture make immunologically detectable AVP.[97,98] There have been no clear biosynthetic studies of cultured tumor cells of other histologic types.

Collected series show that 9% of 523 small cell lung cancer patients have clinically evident SIADH with hyponatremia.[23,46,59,99,100] Like ACTH, measurement of blood AVP by RIA has shown significant elevations in an even larger fraction of cases (32–44%).[31,100] Evidence of SIADH by water loading of patients showed that 53% to 68% had subclinical but evocable SIADH.[31,100] Odell and associates found 41% of lung cancer patients of all histologic types and 43% of colon cancer patients to have significantly elevated blood AVP levels without clinically evident SIADH.[2] North's group studied neurophysins in 72 small cell cancer patients and found significantly elevated levels of one or both (AVP or oxytocin) neurophysins in 65%.[88]

Treatment

The fundamental principle of the treatment of tumor-associated SIADH involves successful treatment of the underlying cancer (see Chap. 23).[99] If chemotherapy is not effective, radiotherapy of bulk tumor mass or, in selected cases of non-small cell lung cancer limited to the chest, surgical removal of the tumor may be considered. There are several major decisions that are influenced by antitumor treatment:

1. The problem of water restriction and high-dose chemotherapy
2. Management of severely symptomatic hyponatremia
3. The problem of differentiating SIADH that develops during treatment from other causes and true tumor relapse
4. Treatment of recurrent SIADH with tumor progression on primary therapy.

For symptomatic hyponatremia and serum sodium levels of less than 130 mEq/L, fluid restriction to less than 500 ml/24 hours allows patients to increase their plasma osmolality slowly over 7 to 10 days. If chemotherapy requires hydration and the chemotherapy could induce more hyponatremia (*e.g.*, cyclophosphamide in high doses), this usually can be handled by careful monitoring of body weight, input and output, daily or more frequent serum sodium determinations, and urine sodium and potassium measurements while giving normal saline with furosemide diuretics and electrolyte replacement.[95,101,102] If the patient is severely hyponatremic or symptomatic (*e.g.*, serum sodium <125 mEq/L), correction of this over several days may be required before instituting chemotherapy. An excellent correlation of antitumor response to chemoradiotherapy and disappearance of SIADH was reported by the National Cancer Institute group for 7 of 7 patients and by the Vanderbilt group for 16 of 17 newly diagnosed small cell cancer patients.[102] North and coworkers studied 18 patients with elevated neurophysins (some of which represent elevated AVP) by RIA and found complete agreement between tumor and neurophysin levels and response to chemotherapy (reduction of neurophysin levels in 12 patients with complete or partial remissions and rise in 6 patients with progressive tumor).[103] Because these latter markers occur in 65% of small cell cancer patients initially, the neurophysins may prove to be excellent tumor markers.

When a patient presents severely symptomatic from SIADH (*e.g.*, comatose), more acute measures are needed. The procedure of Hantman and associates involves using 3% hypertonic saline and intravenous furosemide to increase the net free water clearance.[104] Furosemide (1 mg/kg body weight) is given intravenously and subsequent doses are given as needed to obtain the desired negative fluid balance. Besides routine vital signs, urinary losses of sodium and potassium are measured hourly and replaced by an infusion of appropriate amounts of hypertonic sodium chloride solution, to which appropriate amounts of potassium chloride are added. Using an estimated total-body water content of 60% of female body weight and 70% of male body weight, the negative fluid balance necessary to raise the plasma osmolality to 270 mOsm/kg water is calculated for an individual patient by the following formula:

$$\text{Desired negative water balance in liters}$$
$$= \text{total body water (TBW)}$$
$$= \text{weight in kg}$$
$$\times 0.6 \text{ or } 0.7 - \frac{\text{TBW} \times \text{plasma osmolality}^{104}}{270}$$

This approach resulted in the serum sodium concentrations rising from 120 to 133 mEq/L in 6 to 8 hours.[104] Although none of these patients had small cell carcinoma, the Johns Hopkins group has used this regimen successfully in small cell cancer.[89] This procedure also could be used to prepare patients for chemotherapy.

In patients who have relapsed and who have recurrent SIADH with no or only minimally effective chemotherapy available, therapy with demeclocycline or urea can be tried. Demeclocycline is more effective in treating SIADH than lithium carbonate.[105-107] Demeclocycline blocks AVP action at the level of the renal tubule by inhibiting AVP-induced cAMP formation and blocking the effect of any cAMP generated with more reproducibility than lithium carbonate. A positive correlation between serum sodium and blood urea was found in patients with SIADH, suggesting the use of urea therapy to correct SIADH. Urea given in dosages of 30 g/day corrected the salt-losing tendency of SIADH in 2 patients with small cell cancer and in normal persons given exogenous AVP.[108] Because it induces an osmotic diuresis, urea therapy allows a normal daily intake of water despite continued SIADH. Thirty grams of urea (99% pure crystalline material) is dissolved in 100 ml of water with 15 g of magnesium and aluminum hydroxide (Maalox) and is taken at noon; this has been maintained for as long as 11 weeks without water restriction.[108] The urea is taken orally because of good gastrointestinal absorption and because cells are freely permeable to urea. There is no risk of cardiac failure from rapid shifts of water, as is possible in a mannitol-induced diuresis.

Although hyponatremia and SIADH are the classic presenting features of tumor secretion of AVP, other paraneoplastic syndromes may occur, because at much higher concentrations, AVP acts on the cardiovascular system and other smooth muscles throughout the body.[91]

Hyponatremia Secondary to Ectopic Atrial Natriuretic Peptide Secretion

Atrial natriuretic peptide (ANP), produced by human atrial tissue has potent natriuretic activity. Several series demonstrated that it may be a circulating hormone producing hyponatremia and SIADH.[109] Kamoi and coworkers described a patient with small cell lung cancer and hyponatremia who had sustained high plasma levels of ANP, but normal levels of AVP, suggesting the ANP produced the hyponatremia.[110] In this case, evaluation of tumor tissue showed no ANP, indicating an increased secretion by atrial tissue. The overall frequency of ANP-induced hyponatremia in cancer patients is unknown.

HYPERCALCEMIA

Hypercalcemia is common in cancer patients; about 10% of patients with cancer have hypercalcemia, and 10% to 15% of these do not have associated bone metastases.[111,112] The most common tumor types associated with hypercalcemia are breast cancer (15%, usually associated with bone metastases), lung cancer (10%), and multiple myeloma (>50%, usually associated with bone involvement). Although most breast cancer patients with hypercalcemia have bone metastases, a prospective series showed that 24% had no bone metastases and a purely hormonal mechanism was postulated.[113] Patients with squamous cell carcinomas, especially of lung, head, neck, and esophagus have a high frequency of paraneoplastic hypercalcemia.[114,115] This is rare in small cell lung cancer. Hypercalcemia with or without bone metastases is seen in most patients with adult T-cell leukemia, and it occurs in lower frequency in other lymphomas.[116]

There are several documented mechanisms of hypercalcemia in cancer patients, including bone metastases, the simultaneous occurrence of primary hyperparathyroidism, ectopic tumor-produced parathormone-like substances, tumor-produced prostaglandins (*e.g.*, PGE$_1$,PGE$_2$), tumor-produced osteoclast-activating factor, tumor growth factor-α, 1,25-dihydroxyvitamin D, and other osteolytic factors.[23,111,115,117-119] In normal persons, calcium is maintained by a series of control mechanisms that govern bone resorption and osteolysis, which are stimulated by PGE, PTH, osteoclast-activating factor, thyroxine (T$_4$), and a monocyte-derived osteolytic factor and are inhibited by calcitonin and estrogen. Absorption of calcium from the gastrointestinal and renal tubular tracts is stimulated by PTH, growth hormone, and vitamin D.[111] Production by tumors of any of these materials could cause hypercalcemia. Although paraneoplastic syndromes usually are considered to be those humorally mediated at a distance from the primary tumor or its metastases, in hypercalcemia the mediators released by the tumor cells may act locally, as with PGE and osteoclast-activating factor.

The most frequent cause of paraneoplastic hypercalcemia is tumor secretion of a parathyroid hormone-related peptide (PTHRP).[120-122] This fascinating protein is derived from a gene that has been identified in multiple species. The gene for PTHRP is different from that of PTH. They reside on different chromosomes, and the two genes may have developed by an evolutionary duplication. The human gene expresses three mRNAs that encode three distinct peptides, all different at the COOH-terminal region of the molecule consisting of amino acids of 139, 141, and 173 residues. However, 8 of the first 13 amino acids are the same as PTH (see Fig. 55–1B). The PTHRP gene is expressed in many normal tissues, including the keratinocyte, the pancreas islet cells, nor-

mal parathyroid cells, cells of pituitary, adrenal, ovarian, testicular, and brain origin, and the placenta and lactating breast. In normal persons, the PTHRP protein is low or not detected in the circulation, suggesting that expression of the gene gives rise to a protein that serves an autocrine or paracrine role in local calcium homeostasis. For example, the highest levels of PTHRP protein reported in normal humans is in breast milk, and its concentration there is presumably a reflection of important calcium-modulating roles related to breast milk. High circulating levels of PTHRP in humans are found in the syndrome of humeral hypercalcemia of malignancy. In these circumstances, the circulating levels of PTHRP are similar to those of PTH. This is reported most often in squamous cell carcinoma of the head, neck, and lung and for a variety of adenocarcinomas, including breast cancer (see Fig. 57–1C). Approximately 50% to 80% of cases of humeral hypercalcemia of malignancy have abnormal levels of PTHRP in the serum, depending on the specific assay. These patients have increased levels of cAMP, increased serum levels of calcium, and low serum levels of phosphorous. The level of intact PTH measured by new immunoradiometric assays is low or undetectable in these cases, unlike patients having primary hyperparathyroidism, in which high levels of intact PTH are found. The development of new assays for PTHRP and PTH have facilitated the diagnosis of primary hyperparathyroidism and humeral hypercalcemia of malignancy.

The hypercalcemia in multiple myeloma and lymphomas is usually ascribed to osteoclast-activating factors.[116,123-127] These cases have normal or low levels of PTH, cAMP, 1,25-dihydroxyvitamin D, and evidence of osteoclast activation on bone biopsy. The osteoclast-activating factor appears to be a locally secreted lymphokine. It is not clear whether the lymphokine is the same or is different in various lymphomas and myelomas. Interleukin-1β (IL-1β) may also be a bone-resorbing lymphokine secreted by some of the lymphoproliferative malignancies.

Tumor secretion of PGE is rare and is associated with normal or low PTH, cAMP, and vitamin D levels. Such secretion has been reported in hypernephomas and rarely in other tumor types.[117,118,128-133] It is important to recognize because prostaglandin inhibitors, such as indomethacin (Indocin), may be successful therapeutically.

Active metabolites of vitamin D have also been produced by some malignancies including lymphoma, small cell lung cancer, and melanoma. In general, these cases show hypercalcemia, elevated 1,25-dihydroxyvitamin D levels, low PTH, and low urinary and AMP excretion.[134-136] Treatment of the tumors surgically or by chemotherapy usually reverses the chemical abnormalities. In some instances, vitamin D metabolites have been purified from tumor cells or shown to be synthesized in vitro by the tumor cells.

Transforming growth factors α and β have also been associated with hypercalcemia of malignancy.[120] Transforming growth factor α has been isolated from squamous cell carcinomas of the lung, head and neck, kidney, and breast. It is a 5000 Da protein with 50 amino acids. It mediates its effect predominantly through the EGF receptor and antibodies; the EGF receptors can block the bone-resorbing activity.

All of the mechanisms of hypercalcemia should be considered in cancer patients, and determining the cause of the hypercalcemia is important because of the therapeutic implications. The pathophysiology, clinical manifestations, and treatment are discussed in Chapter 60.

HYPOCALCEMIA

In patients with bone metastases, hypocalcemia occurs in 16% and hypercalcemia only in 9%.[137-140] Hypocalcemia commonly occurs with osteoblastic metastases of the breast, prostate, and lung.[138,141] Only rarely is tetanic hypocalcemia seen with these osteoblastic metastases.[142] However, with more refined studies of nerve, muscle, or other physiologic function testing, hypocalcemia may be found to impair a patient's neuromuscular function. Hypocalcemia may be mediated by way of tumor-secreted calcitonin, although there is no direct evidence for this. No specific therapy is indicated, except in the rare case of tetany, for which calcium can be given.

HYPOPHOSPHATEMIC OSTEOMALACIA ASSOCIATED WITH BENIGN MESENCHYMAL TUMORS

An acquired, adult-onset, vitamin D-resistant rickets with bone pain, severe phosphaturia, renal glycosuria, hypophosphatemia, normocalcemia (normal PTH levels), low 1,25-dihydroxyvitamin D levels, and increased alkaline phosphatase levels is associated with benign mesenchymal tumors that occur in soft tissues or bone (*i.e.*, tumoral osteomalacia, oncogenic osteomalacia).[143-146] They are also called ossifying mesenchymal tumors, giant cell tumors of bone, sclerosing hemangioma, cavernous hemangioma, or reparative giant cell granuloma.[147] The syndrome often precedes the discovery of the tumor by several years.[25] The basis of treatment is resection of the mesenchymal tumor, which results in resolution of the syndrome.[143,144,148] Otherwise, treatment requires large doses of vitamin D and phosphate. The proposed mechanisms include inhibition of the conversion of 25-hydroxyvitamin D to 1,25-dihydroxyvitamin D and a tumor-secreted "phosphaturic substance." It is possible that a single protein produces both of these effects. Active osteoclastic bone resorption has been reported. Rarely, this syndrome has been reported with lung and prostate cancers.[149,150] The importance of recognizing this syndrome is its cure with surgical resection. Sometimes multiple osteolytic lesions or osteoblastic-like lesions are seen in sclerosing hemangiomas of bone. These require treatment with oral phosphate and vitamin D, which give relief of bone pain and weakness.[145] These bone lesions can resemble diffuse metastases on a roentgenogram, and careful pathologic examination is required.

CALCITONIN PRODUCTION BY TUMORS

The polypeptide hormone calcitonin normally is produced by the C cells of the thyroid. It prevents calcium release from bone and causes an increase in renal excretion of calcium, sodium, and phosphate.[151] However, no described clinical syndromes are associated with tumor production of calcitonin, although one small cell cancer patient with high calcitonin levels had hypocalcemia.[30] The major clinical use of calcitonin assay is in monitoring patients with medullary carcinoma of the thyroid. This tumor produces large amounts of calcitonin without clinical signs or symptoms.[151] Calcitonin is an ex-

tremely sensitive indicator of residual tumor after surgery.[89] It is useful in identifying patients with type II multiple endocrine neoplasia, a familial disorder involving an association of medullary carcinoma of the thyroid, pheochromocytoma, and parathyroid adenomas. These are described in detail in Chapter 41. Because of the excellent clinical correlation of calcitonin with medullary thyroid cancer, the hormone has been studied in other tumor types.

Elevated plasma calcitonin levels are consistently found in 48% to 64% of patients with small cell lung cancer and at other rates with the other lung cancer cell types (see Table 57–4).[22,30,31,152] Urinary calcitonin is elevated in 75% of lung cancer patients: 53% of epidermoid, 45% of adenocarcinomas, 20% of large cell cancers, but surprisingly only 17% of small cell cancers.[153] When antiserum detecting the COOH-terminal end and midportion of the calcitonin molecule was used on serum and urine samples, more than 90% of lung cancer patients had abnormal values.[153] Calcitonin levels mirrored clinical tumor status 67% of the time in lung cancer patients, but selective venous sampling showed tumoral and thyroidal production of the elevated calcitonin levels.[152] Its usefulness as a marker of lung cancer is not yet established. Other tumor types associated with increased plasma calcitonin levels include carcinoids, breast cancer (in some studies, up to 100%), colon cancer (24%), and gastric cancer (38%). High calcitonin levels do not correlate with bone metastases.[152] However, a variety of nonneoplastic conditions are associated with elevated calcitonin levels, including hypercalcemia, chronic renal failure, pregnancy, pernicious anemia, Zollinger-Ellison syndrome, and pancreatitis.[22,152] Its use as a screen for the early detection of cancer is problematic.

Because of the several possible sources of calcitonin, biosynthetic studies would be useful. Immunoreactive calcitonin has been found in many tumor extracts, including small cell cancer, pheochromocytomas, malignant carcinoids, other types of lung cancer, breast, melanoma, colon, gastric, esophagus, and pancreatic cancer.[97,154,155] These studies failed to show that calcitonin and ACTH were on a common precursor molecule, as predicted by some, but they did show a high-molecular-mass form of calcitonin.[156,157] The nature of the calcitonin precursor molecule is unknown. Calcitonin is a polypeptide hormone, apparently produced by many cancers, waiting for definition of a clinically evident paraneoplastic syndrome and prospective documentation as a marker of response to therapy.

CHROMOGRANIN A PRODUCED BY TUMORS

Chromogranin A is a 48,000-d acidic glycoprotein, which may account for as much as 10% of the weight of cells of the neuroendocrine system.[158] It is secreted by several neuroendocrine tumors, especially small cell lung cancer.[158-160] It is stored in vesicles of chromaffin cells and released with catecholamines after splanchnic stimulation. It may act in neuroendocrine secretion by binding intravesicular calcium. Its sequence is almost identical to pancreastatin, which inhibits insulin and somatostatin secretion from the pancreas.[161,162] Pancreastatin may be generated from chromogranin A or from a chromogranin A-like precursor. Like calcitonin, it is unknown whether there is an associated paraneoplastic syndrome.

HUMAN PLACENTAL AND PITUITARY GLYCOPROTEIN HORMONES PRODUCED BY TUMORS

Gonadotropins

Precocious puberty in children, gynecomastia in men, and oligomenorrhea in premenopausal women may result from excessive gonadotropin production by tumors.[2,3,23,163] Very high levels of gonadotropin secretion may result in thyroid stimulation and hyperthyroidism.[164,165] Gonadotropin secretion may occur in pituitary tumors, gestational trophoblastic tumors (*e.g.*, choriocarcinoma, hydatidiform mole), germ cell tumors of testis and ovary, germ cell tumors arising or presenting in extragonadal primary sites, or hepatoblastomas in children and large cell and adenocarcinoma of the lung in adults.[2,3,23,163,166,167]

The tumors arising in gestational tissue, testis, ovary, and endocrine organs are discussed in other chapters, in which the great value of gonadotropin measurement as a marker in the treatment of gestational trophoblastic tumors and testicular cancer is discussed.[168,169] Their usefulness as a marker in these tumors stimulated intense study of gonadotropin expression in other tumors to see if they could be used as markers for early diagnosis or monitoring of subsequent treatment.[170]

The human hormones with gonadotrophic properties are follicle stimulating hormone (FSH), luteinizing hormone (LH), and human chorionic gonadotropin (hCG).[163] These three hormones are composed of two polypeptide chains, α- and a β-subunits. The α-subunit is common to all the hormones, and the β-subunit confers immunologic and biologic specificity. Both subunits are required for bioactivity.[163] Radioimmunoassay can differentiate between the various types of β-subunits.[163] In normal persons, FSH and LH are produced by the pituitary and are normally present in serum, but biologically active hCG is produced by the placenta and usually is found only in pregnant women. Because levels of FSH and LH vary widely under normal physiologic conditions, the assay for β-hCG is theoretically the best hormone to use for following patients with suspected paraneoplastic production of gonadotropin excess. An hCG-like material has been found in extracts of all normal tissue by RIA and radioreceptor assay, calling into question the use of hCG in cancer patients. However, this hCG is carbohydrate-free, and that produced by the placenta and many tumors contains carbohydrate. Carbohydrate-free hCG is cleared rapidly from the circulation and has marked loss of bioactivity.[163,171]

Many studies have looked at "elevations" of hCG, β-hCG, and α-hCG (Table 57–7). Many of the common tumors (*e.g.*, lung, colorectum, breast) had frequent elevations of these markers. However, 5% to 10% of patients with nonmalignant chronic disease also had hormone elevations, calling the specificity of the findings in tumor patients into doubt. In pursuing this, Blackman and coworkers conducted a detailed study of human placental and pituitary glycopeptide hormones and their subunits in the sera of patients with lung cancer, gastrointestinal cancer, malignant carcinoid, and malignant islet cell tumors and compared their results with 579 appropriately matched controls (Table 57–8).[170,173,174] Values for the α- and β-subunit of hCG were significantly higher in the cancer patients, and elevations of FSH-β, TSH-β, and LH-β were not

TABLE 57–7. Elevations of Human Chorionic Gonadotropin or its β-Subunit and the α-Subunit of Placental and Pituitary Glycoprotein Hormones in Various Tumors

Tumor Type	% Elevated	
	hCG or β-hCG	α-Subunit
Lung*	0–12	3–30
Colorectal	0–20	20–26
Breast	7–50	30
Pancreatic adenocarcinoma	11–50	
Gastric carcinoma	0–24	
Prostate cancer	1	0
Islet cell carcinoma	22–50	52
Carcinoid of gut and lung		16
Small intestine	13	
Hepatoma	17–20	
Nonmalignant lung disease	7	
Nonmalignant GI disease	9	
Nonmalignant breast disease	4	

* Within lung, there were 32% epidermoid cancers; 27% small cell lung cancers; 13% large cell lung cancers; 11% adenocarcinoma; and 17% miscellaneous and undetermined histologic malignant diseases. Within GI cancer, there were 13% pancreatic adenocarcinomas; 8% gastric cancers; 4% hepatomas; 10% other types of upper GI cancer; and 65% lower GI cancers. Carcinoid lesions included 80% of GI origin; malignant islet cell neoplasms included 28% insulinomas and 40% gastrinomas. Normal controls included 299 healthy subjects, 123 patients with chronic lung disease, 110 with benign GI disease, and 47 with benign endocrine diseases.
(Winkler WA, Crankshaw OF. Chloride depletion in conditions other than Addison's disease. J Clin Invest 1938;17:1–6; Thomas TH, Morgan DB, Swaminathan R, et al. Severe hyponatremia. Lancet 1978;1: 621–624)

observed. The sensitivity of detection of cancer patients increased by combining the results from the two tests. They and others found differences in the ratio of α-hCG/β-hCG positivity between sexes and among cancer groups, a finding that is unexplained.

Because of the frequency of elevation in common tumors, such as lung and gastrointestinal cancers, and because of the correlation with response in trophoblastic disease and testicular tumors, it is important to test prospectively the roles of α-hCG and β-hCG in monitoring the therapy of common tumors. In some nontrophoblastic tumors, these markers have been valuable in monitoring therapy.[172,176] However, these reports are still anecdotal. For example, Broder and associates reported a patient with prostatic cancer and elevated hCG whose serum hCG levels mirrored the clinical course more reliably than the concomitant acid phosphatase levels.[175] Muggia and coworkers reported 4 patients with metastatic cancer, and in seven of nine episodes, clinical remission was associated with marker decrease or exacerbation associated with marker increase.[172] Metz and coworkers reported a patient with an hCG-secreting large cell carcinoma of the lung with painful gynecomastia and testicular atrophy.[176] Investigation revealed elevated levels of β-hCG subunits and elevated

TABLE 57–8. Elevations of the β-Subunits of Chorionic Gonadotropin or the α-Subunit of Glycoprotein Hormones in Patients With Lung and Gastrointestinal Cancer

Tumor Type*	Patients (n)	% of Tumor Patients With Hormone Elevations Over 95th Percentile of Normal Controls		
		α-Subunit	β-hCG	α-Subunit or BhCG
Lung cancer				
Men	269	11	41	45
Women	31	16	16	29
Gastrointestinal cancer				
Men	92	32	28	48
Women	71	18	34	41
Carcinoid				
Men	25	50	0	50
Women		13	50	50
Malignant islet cell				
Men	40	61	6	61
Women		38	19	43

* Within lung cancer 32% were epidermoid.
(Blackman MR, Weintraub BD, Rosen SW, et al. Human placental and pituitary glycoprotein hormones and their subunits as tumor markers: A quantitative assessment. JNCI 1980;65:81–93)

α-subunits, normal estradiol levels, low-normal testosterone levels, and abnormal (delayed) pituitary response to LHRH. These abnormal findings reverted to normal after surgical resection of the tumor (shown to contain high levels of hCG), recurred with tumor regrowth, and regressed again with the addition of combination chemotherapy, which produced a complete clinical remission of the tumor and the biochemical parameters.[176] The β-hCG level was more sensitive than gynecomastia in predicting recurrence. This was an important case because it demonstrated the usefulness of the β-hCG marker in a common solid tumor to monitor therapy and achieve potential cure with the use of chemotherapy in a semiadjuvant setting.

Studies of tumor lines in vitro agree with these studies of serum samples. The β- and α-subunits of hCG are produced by human tumor cell lines in vitro.[170,177,178] Unbalanced synthesis of α- and β-subunits is seen, but no evidence of production of FSH-β or TSH-β existed, and only rarely and at low levels was LH-β found.

Although tumor-produced α- and β-hCG are found frequently, there are no definitive reports of tumor-produced FSH, TSH, or LH.[3,23] Patients with suspected tumor production of these hormones should be carefully documented and reported. Some elevations of LH and FSH may occur in cancer patients, probably as the result of gonadal failure related to age, stress, chronic illness, or treatment.[170] Blackman and associates showed that 50% to 59% of men with malignant lung disease, 28% to 32% of men with benign lung disease, but only 10% of normal persons had evidence of hypogonadism when assessed with serum testosterone, LH, and FSH.[179] Obviously other causes of elevated hormones, such as those seen in physiologic causes of hypergonadotropinemia, hyper-

thyrotropinemia, pituitary adenomas, pregnancy, and uremia, must be excluded.[170]

DIFFERENTIAL DIAGNOSIS. The exact frequency of symptoms associated with tumor-produced gonadotropin is unknown, although an intact hormone (both subunits) and an appropriate host (*i.e.*, child for precocious puberty, man for gynecomastia, premenopausal women for oligomenorrhea) are required simultaneously for clinical expression. A detailed discussion of the differential diagnosis of these conditions is beyond the scope of this chapter. However, the most common problem is a male patient presenting with unexplained gynecomastia. In this situation, a β-hCG determination should be performed and a careful examination of the testes and radiographic examination of the chest and mediastinum should be done. It is important to use an RIA, because routine urinary pregnancy tests are not sensitive enough to detect many hCG secretory neoplasms.[176] Germ cell tumors of the testis or extragonadal sites and lung cancers are the most frequent cause of the combination of gynecomastia and hCG elevation, and these men should be persistently and thoroughly evaluated, because this syndrome can present before a clinically evident cancer is found.[179a]

Other tumors associated with biologically active hCG are rare. Skrabanek and associates found only 44 extragonadal cases in the world's literature, and these involved the lung, adrenal gland, liver, gastrointestinal tract, and nongonadal portions of the genitourinary tract.[180] Analysis of the histologic specimens revealed that all contained syncytial giant cells or frankly choriocarcinomatous elements similar to classic trophoblastic germ cell tumors. Greco and associates found that 40% of patients with extragonadal germ cell tumors, "masquerading" as poorly differentiated carcinomas, had immunochemical tumor staining for β-hCG and AFP without serum elevations of the markers.[181] Many patients responded to combination chemotherapy. These results suggest that immunohistochemistry and a chemotherapy approach similar to that for histologically classic germ cell tumors are warranted for the potentially curable poorly differentiated midline carcinomas in young adults.

Precocious puberty has been found in children with hepatoma or hepatoblastomas. In these children, secondary sexual characteristics developed prematurely, with advanced skeletal maturation and hyperplasia of prostatic and testicular interstitial cells.[23,182–184] Abnormal endocrine manifestations consisting of precocious puberty, irregular bleeding, amenorrhea, and hirsutism occurred in 9 (60%) of 15 patients with tumors of the ovary, and biopsy specimens stained immunohistochemically for hCG in syncytiotrophoblast-like cells and for AFP in embryonal carcinoma cells.[185]

TUMOR-PRODUCED HUMAN PLACENTAL LACTOGEN, GROWTH HORMONE, GROWTH HORMONE-RELEASING HORMONE, PROLACTIN, AND THYROTROPIC SUBSTANCE

Human placental lactogen (hPL) was detected in the sera of 5% to 8% of patients with nontrophoblastic nongonadal tumors.[186,187] Many of these patients with elevated hPL also had elevated levels of estrogens and had gynecomastia. Some of these patients also have elevated hCG levels. When hPL is found in nonpregnant women, it is a specific indication of malignancy.[187]

Elevated growth hormone levels have been reported in patients with lung cancer and gastric cancer, but that may be uncommon. Although patients with these neoplasms may not live long enough to develop acromegaly, it has been speculated that growth hormone may cause hypertrophic pulmonary osteoarthropathy, and the syndrome has been reversed by resection of lung tumors.[187a] However, a study of patients with and without osteoarthropathy failed to reveal any relation between the syndrome and elevated plasma growth hormone levels, and none were acromegalic.[188]

Acromegaly has been produced by tumor secretion of growth hormone-releasing hormone (GHRH).[189–193] The GHRH is a 44-amino acid peptide that has been isolated from two GHRH-secreting pancreatic tumors. A GHRH-induced acromegaly was reported with bronchial carcinoids. The clinical symptoms of acromegaly decreased after surgical resection. The secretion of GHRH can also be controlled by administration of long-acting somatostatin analogs.

Three patients with elevated prolactin levels (*i.e.*, undifferentiated lung cancer, small cell lung cancer, and hypernephroma) were reported, only one of whom had associated galactorrhea.[3,23] Resection or irradiation decreased the levels of prolactin in all patients. Cases of nonpituitary prolactin-secreting tumors are rare, and any suspected cases should be differentiated carefully from pituitary lesions and reported.

Cancer patients frequently have a "hypermetabolic state" that may resemble hyperthyroidism, and 1.4% of lung cancer patients reportedly are hyperthyroid, but documentation of tumor-caused syndromes is uncommon.[194] Four substances that could stimulate the thyroid gland are pituitary-like TSH, chorionic thyrotropin, hCG, and long-activating thyroid-stimulating substances (LATS). Documented examples of hyperthyroidism produced by TSH, LATS, and chorionic thyrotropin probably do not exist. Isolated reports of tumor-associated TSH without thyrotoxicosis have been made.[195] However, a definite association is found between hyperthyroidism and gestational trophoblastic disease (*e.g.*, choriocarcinoma, hydatidiform mole), in which 8% of cases can have biochemical evidence of hyperthyroidism. This is also seen in testicular tumors.[23,196] In all cases, the relation seems to be between trophoblastic tumors and very high levels of hCG, in which the thyroid-stimulating substance occasionally was hCG.[164,165,197]

HYPOGLYCEMIA

Hypoglycemia frequently is caused by insulinomas. Hypoglycemia associated with non-islet cell tumors is an uncommon and poorly characterized paraneoplastic syndrome. Other types of neoplasms associated with hypoglycemia are mesenchymal (64%), including mesothelioma, fibrosarcoma, neurofibrosarcoma, and hemangiopericytoma; hepatomas (21%); adrenal carcinomas (6%); gastrointestinal tumors (5%); and miscellaneous (5%), including anaplastic carcinomas of unknown primary, pseudomyxoma, hypernephromas, lymphomas, pheochromocytomas.[2,3,78,198]

The tumors usually are quite large (1–10 kg; average, 2.4

kg), often invade the liver, and often have protracted courses over many years.[2,3] Hypoglycemia may be the presenting symptom of a tumor.[2] Mesotheliomas are the most common cause of hypoglycemia, and about 50% of these occur in the abdomen, and the remainder occur in the chest. The signs and symptoms are those of hypoglycemia with neurologic findings (*e.g.*, stupor, coma, focal findings, agitated behavior) predominating until the hypoglycemia is discovered.[89]

Tumors can cause hypoglycemia by ectopic insulin production, production of nonsuppressible insulin-like activity (NSILA) or insulin-like growth factors I and II, overuse of glucose, production of a material stimulating ectopic insulin release, massive infiltration of the liver or production of an inhibitor of hepatic glucose output, insulin binding by an M-protein in myeloma, or insulin receptor proliferation.[199,200]

Tumor use of glucose to a degree that causes hypoglycemia has not been substantiated, and only rarely is liver infiltration by tumor massive enough to cause hypoglycemia.[2,3,201] There are rare reports of insulin production by non-islet cell tumors but no definitive biosynthetic studies to prove this.[202] A massive thoracic mesothelioma associated with hypoglycemia and very low glucagon levels was postulated as the source of a factor that suppresses glucagon secretion.[203] Artifactual hypoglycemia may occur in acute leukemia if the high number of circulating leukemia cells metabolizes the plasma glucose while standing in the collection tube.[204]

The most likely mechanism is tumor production of somatomedins, also called NSILA, and insulin-like growth factors.[2,3,89,205–207] Somatomedins are a family of peptide hormones normally produced by the liver under growth hormone regulation.[208] By current definitions, substances with identical bioassay properties of insulin in the rat diaphragm or epididymal fat pad and that also react in insulin radioreceptor assays (RRA) but do not react in insulin RIA, are somatomedins. Approximately half of the 200 μU of biologically active insulin and insulin-like activity in normal human serum is related to NSILA-somatomedin activity.[209] Hypoglycemia associated with cancer generally occurs after fasting and physical exertion, but reactive postprandial hypoglycemia usually is not part of the paraneoplastic syndrome.[89] Some cancer patients with hypoglycemia have elevated tumor extract levels of biologically active insulin-like activity that is not suppressed or reactive with antiinsulin antibodies but is reactive in the RRA.[209,210] These patients appear to have tumors producing NSILA, and it is important to study tissue culture lines of tumors from them to see if they produce this substance. The evaluation of these patients is experimental after the common causes of severe hypoglycemia (*e.g.*, exogenous insulin or sulfonylureas, insulinoma, islet cell tumor, adrenal or pituitary insufficiency, ethanol abuse, poor nutrition) have been excluded.

Initially, the treatment of paraneoplastic hypoglycemia involves glucose infusion to control the acute symptoms. Reduction of tumor bulk, usually by surgical resection, should then be carried out. However, there are no good data on the long-term effectiveness of any surgical, radiotherapy, or chemotherapy approach. If tumor treatment is not possible or is inadequate, other possibilities include the use of intermittent subcutaneous or long-acting intramuscular glucagon or high-dose corticosteroids.[89] However, there are few data on the long-term effectiveness of these agents in controlling hypoglycemia.

NEUROGASTROINTESTINAL PEPTIDES UNASSOCIATED WITH KNOWN PARANEOPLASTIC SYNDROMES

Neurogastrointestinal peptides have important roles in the perception of pain; in memory, learning, and behavior, in psychiatric diseases; and in temperature and blood pressure regulation.[24,25] Changes in levels of somatostatin, cholecystokinin, substance P, VIP, and enkephalin have been reported in two major idiopathic neurologic diseases: Alzheimer's disease and Huntington's disease.[211-215] In a patient with subacute necrotizing encephalopathy, naloxone administration reversed the symptoms of apnea, unconsciousness, hypothermia, and restlessness.[216] Analysis of spinal fluid showed an increased level of an uncharacterized opioid-like activity, and autopsy examination revealed increased concentrations of met- and leu-enkephalin in the cortex. Ectopic tumor production of these hormones may produce previously described neurologic paraneoplastic syndromes of unknown cause such as limbic encephalitis or other previously undescribed syndromes.

NEUROLOGIC MANIFESTATIONS OF MALIGNANCY

Neurologic problems occur frequently in patients with cancer. In the experiences of Posner and coworkers at Memorial Hospital, 17% of all patients at admission have neurologic symptoms and signs requiring neurologic consultation.[217] In patients with established cancer, true paraneoplastic syndromes account for a minority of neurologic problems, and the diagnosis of paraneoplastic syndrome can be established only after other diagnoses are excluded. The differential diagnosis of the cancer patient with neurologic signs and symptoms is provided in Table 57–9. Most frequently, neurologic complications are caused directly by the tumor or its metastases. For example, 40% to 65% of lung cancers metastasize to the brain, and overall Posner and Chernick reported that intracranial metastases were found in 24% of autopsies at Memorial Sloan-Kettering Cancer Center.[219-220]

Neurologic syndromes caused by endocrine, fluid, and electrolyte abnormalities are the second most common cause of neurologic symptoms and signs in cancer patients. Hepatic encephalopathy and hypercalcemia are the most frequent of

TABLE 57–9. Differential Diagnosis of Neurologic Syndromes

Syndromes due to effects of primary or metastatic tumor

Syndromes due to endocrine or metabolic tumor products (*e.g.*, ADH, calcium, glucose, electrolytes)

Syndromes due to cerebral and spinal vascular disease

Syndromes due to toxicity of primary treatment (chemotherapy, radiotherapy)

Syndromes due to CNS infections

Paraneoplastic syndromes associated with malignancy with unknown mechanisms

TABLE 57–10. Causes of Stroke in Cancer Patients

Cause	Frequency (%)
Embolic infarction	27
Septic	13
Marantic	12
Tumor	2
Thrombotic infarction	19
Atherosclerotic	10
Disseminated intravascular coagulation	9
Miscellaneous infarction	6
Intraparenchymal hemorrhage	32.5
Spontaneous	13
Tumor related	13
Hypertension	5
Unknown	1.5
Subdural hemorrhage	8.5
Subarachnoid hemorrhage	3
Superior sagittal sinus occlusion	4
Total	100

(From studies by Allen,[217] Rosen,[221] Collins,[222] and Sigsbee[223])

these. Cerebral and spinal vascular disease are common in cancer patients and are found in 13% of autopsied cancer patients.[217] The causes of the vascular problems in these autopsied patients are shown in Table 57–10. Clearly the causes of stroke in these patients are strikingly dissimilar from those in the general population. Marantic and septic emboli, disseminated intravascular coagulation, tumor-related hemorrhage, superior sagittal sinus occlusion, and many of the cases of subarachnoid hemorrhage were directly tumor related and account for more than 50% of strokes.[220-224] Risk factors for the general population, including hypertension, atherosclerotic heart disease, and diabetes, are less important in the cancer patient.

Several associations of cancer and neurologic vascular disease are noteworthy. Marantic endocarditis with emboli (*i.e.*, nonbacterial thrombotic endocarditis) occurs predominantly in patients with adenocarcinoma, especially of the lung, and may present neurologically as multifocal abnormalities, focal abnormalities or progressive encephalopathy without any focal deficits.[221,224] Hemorrhage is seen most often in the leukemias, especially acute nonlymphocytic leukemia.[222] Fungi are the most frequent cause of septic emboli. Paraneoplastic thrombosis of cerebral venous structures, a part of the hypercoagulable state associated with malignancy, produces headaches, followed by the abrupt onset of CNS dysfunction.[225] This may include motor abnormalities, sensory complaints, vision and speech abnormalities, rapid mental deterioration, and seizures. The diagnosis is made by angiography. Angioendotheliosis may be another neurologic paraneoplastic syndrome associated with vascular disease produced by endothelial cell proliferation and causing silent strokes and dementia.[226-229]

Paraneoplastic syndromes or remote effects of tumors on the CNS are uncommon, although the incidence varies considerably in different reports. Croft and Wilkinson found neuromyopathies in 7% of 1476 cancer patients; lung cancers were the most frequent.[18] Brody, however, found no difference in the frequency of neurologic syndromes between patients with lung cancer and controls with chronic lung disease.[19] Some specific neurologic syndromes occur exclusively or with much higher frequency in cancer patients. The patient with no known cancer who develops one of these syndromes should alert the physician to suspect an occult cancer, and a full evaluation for cancer is warranted. These syndromes include subacute cerebellar degeneration, subacute motor neuropathy, dermatomyositis in older men, Eaton-Lambert syndrome, and dorsal root ganglionitis. If a patient not known to have cancer develops a neurologic syndrome less often associated with malignancy, a careful history and physical examination should be performed, but exhaustive laboratory and radiologic searches for tumor are not indicated (Table 57–11). In these instances and for a highly suspect syndrome with negative evaluation result, careful patient follow-up is required.

Most paraneoplastic syndromes run a course parallel to the underlying tumor. This is less often the case in neurologic paraneoplastic syndrome, in which the course of the neurologic abnormalities is frequently independent of the underlying tumor. In many instances, this can be attributed to the inability of the nervous tissue to divide and repair damage. In some instances, such as the myasthenic syndrome and polymyositis, cases of a parallel course of tumor and syndrome have been documented.

Many neurologic paraneoplastic syndromes are produced by "autoimmune" immunologic reactions, in which the tumor shares antigens with normal nervous tissue.[230–232] The host immune response to the tumor then produces immunologic damage of the nervous system. Evidence suggests that subacute cerebellar degeneration, optic neuritis, sensory carcinomatous neuropathy, and the Eaton-Lambert syndrome may be caused by immunologic cross-reactions.[12–15,233,238,245,272] The antineuronal antibodies may have diagnostic and therapeutic implications. In a large series, Moll and colleagues reported finding antineuronal antibodies in 38% of patients with paraneoplastic syndromes with a high specificity (98.6%).[233a] The sensitivity may increase as other antibody-antigen reagents are used. Plasmapheresis has been used to remove the antibodies from the serum or cerebrospinal fluid.[233b] Only limited success was reported, and treatment of the tumor remains the primary approach.

Numerous neurologic syndromes have been described. For convenience they are listed in Table 57–11, which is divided by area within the nervous system.

REMOTE EFFECTS ON THE CEREBRUM AND CRANIAL NERVES

Remote paraneoplastic syndromes involving the brain and cranial nerves are less common than those involving other areas of the neuraxis. In one large series involving 1476 cancer patients, only 162 had neurologic abnormalities, and of these, only 15 had lesions of the brain.[18] These 15 had subacute cerebellar degeneration, which is one of the syndromes with a strong association with malignancy.

Subacute cerebellar degeneration is commonly associated with lung cancer, but many other tumor types have been described. It is characterized by a subacute and progressive, bilateral, symmetric cerebellar failure with ataxia, dysarthria,

hypotonia, and pendular reflexes.[234–238e] Dementia may occur. Frequently present are a cerebrospinal fluid lymphocytosis and elevated protein levels. Pathologically, there is atrophy with loss of Purkinje cells.

Paraneoplastic cerebellar degeneration is one of the neurologic syndromes caused by antineuronal antibodies.[12,238a–d] These antibodies were reported to be specific for Purkinje cells, but they may react with other neurons. The anti-Yo antibody described in patients with gynecologic cancers reacts with antigens of 62-kd and 34-kd. The gene encoding the 34-kd antigen was cloned and shown to be a leucine-zipper DNA-binding protein, which may play a role in gene expression. Another antibody was shown to react with a 51-kd antigen whose gene was cloned and was unique and separate from the anti-Yo 34-kd protein. Another group isolated an antibody that reacts with the repeat hexapepticle Phe-Leu-Glu-Asp-Val-Asp. This hexapepticle is almost identical to the sequence in α_2-macroglobulin and α_1-trypsin inhibitor. This led to speculation that the presence of these antibodies may confer a better outcome. Improvement in paraneoplastic cerebellar degeneration was observed after removal of the primary tumor, corticosteroid administration, plasmapheresis, and effective therapy of Hodgkin's disease.

Dementia is probably the most frequent cerebral abnormality in cancer patients. Because it is also frequent in the general population, its association with malignancy is attenuated. Dementia is often associated with abnormalities in other areas of the nervous system. The electroencephalograph shows generalized slowing, and a cerebrospinal fluid pleocytosis may exist. In some instances, rapid-onset dementia may be caused by angioendotheliomatosis. This syndrome is a proliferative disorder of endothelial cells of blood vessels and may produce a clinical picture of multiple infarct dementia with edema.[226–228] It has been described as a primary endothelial disorder, perhaps even malignant. More likely, it is produced by tumor secretion of an angiogenic peptide.[228,229] Angiogenic peptides include fibroblast growth factors (acidic and basic), tumor necrosis factor, transforming growth factors-α and -β, and IL-1β. Acidic fibroblast growth factor and IL-1β are quite homologous. The syndrome has responded to high-dose steroids, chemotherapeutic agents, and radiation.

Limbic encephalitis is characterized by a progressive dementia associated with degenerative changes in the hippocampus and amygdaloid nuclei. Pathologically, there are inflammatory and degenerative changes. The cerebrospinal fluid may be normal or show a pleocytosis. In one case, magnetic resonance (MR) imaging showed signal abnormalities in the medial portions of both temporal lobes, the amygdaloid nuclei, and the hypothalamus. An MR-guided biopsy confirmed the presence of encephalitis.[243a] The syndrome does not appear to improve with removal of the primary tumor and did not improve after resection of primary lung tumors; it has been reported to improve after successful chemotherapy for small cell lung cancer, Hodgkin's disease, and testicular cancer.[241–243] Viral and immunologic causes have been postulated.

Optic neuritis is characterized by scotomas, decreased vision, and papilledema, which may be unilateral or bilateral. Pathologically, demyelination is found. This syndrome is related to the visual paraneoplastic syndrome characterized by binocular loss of vision in patients with small cell lung cancer.[13,245,246] The triad of photosensitivity, ring scotomatous

TABLE 57–11. Paraneoplastic Syndromes of the Nervous System

Site	Syndrome	Investigations	Clinical Features	Associated Neoplasms	Comments
Brain	Subacute cerebellar degeneration*	Brain[234] Paone[235] Victor[236] Steven[237] Greenlee[12] Dropcho[238] Furneaux[238a] Shaykh[238b] Duncan[238c] Sakai[238d]	Subacute, progressive, bilateral, symmetric, cerebellar failure often with dementia, dysarthria, CSF lymphocytosis, and elevated protein	Lung Prostate Colorectal Ovary Cervix Hodgkin's Other	Some reports of improvements with removal of primary tumor; no other known treatment; caused by specific anti-Purkinje cell antibodies
	Dementia	Shapiro[239] Dorfman[240]	Variable presentation, acute to slowly progressive; often associated with abnormalities in other areas of the neuraxis; EEG shows slowing; CSF pleocytosis sometimes seen	Lung	Relatively common (30–40%)
	Limbic encephalitis	Corsellis[241] Dorfman[240] Brennan[242] Carr[293] Lacomis[243a] Burton[243b]	Dementia with degenerative changes in the hippocampus and amygdaloid nuclei; often associated with inflammatory and degenerative lesions in other areas of the neuraxis	Lung Hodgkin's Testicular Other	May or may not improve with removal of primary tumor (Ophelia syndrome); MRI may be useful for diagnosis
	Optic neuritis/visual retinopathy	Sawyer[244] Grunwald[13,245] Pillay[246] Thirkill[246a] Jacobson[246b]	Decrease in vision, photosensitivity, ring scotomatous field loss, attenuated retinal arteriole caliber, papilledema; unilateral or bilateral	Small-cell lung cancer	Rare; produced by antiretinal antibodies; improves after immunosuppressive therapy
	Opsoclonus/ataxia	Lugue[246c]	Eye movement disorder (opsoclonus) and ataxia	Breast Gynecologic	Produced by anti-Ri antibody
	Progressive multifocal leukoencephalopathy	Padgett[247] Richardson[16] Weiner[17]	Dementia, paralysis, aphasia, ataxia, dysarthria, visual field defects, blindness, coma, seizures; demyelination of white matter; CSF often normal; death usually rapid	Leukemias, lymphomas, sarcomas, other	Caused by papova viruses of 2 types: JC virus or SV-40-like virus
	Angioendotheliosis	Petito[227] Person[226] Gallego[228] Folkman[229]	Rapid onset of multiple infarct dementia; CT/MRI findings consistent with multiple strokes	Lymphomas, other	Not proved; may be caused by angiogenic peptides
Spinal cord	Amyotropic lateral sclerosis (ALS)	Norris and Engel[248]	Upper and lower motoneuron disease with spasticity, extensor plantar responses, wasting, and fasciculations		Syndrome similar to that in patients without cancer but sometimes progresses more slowly; cancer found in 10% of ALS patients in one report, but others find cancer less frequently
	Subacute necrotic myelopathy	Mancall[249] Handforth[250] Dansey[250a]	Rapid ascending motor and sensory paralysis to thoracic level; elevated CSF protein	Lung Kidney Hodgkin's	Severe tissue destruction of grey and white matter

(continued)

TABLE 57-11. *(Continued)*

Site	Syndrome	Investigations	Clinical Features	Associated Neoplasms	Comments
	Subacute motor neuropathy*	Walton[251]	Slowly developing lower motoneuron weakness without sensory changes; most often in irradiated patients with lymphoma	Lymphoma	No known treatment; occasional spontaneous recovery; ? viral origin
Peripheral nerves	Sensory neuropathy*	Horwich[252] Henson[253] Graus[14]	Subacute onset of sensory loss including deep tendon reflexes, with normal strength and normal motor conduction velocity; elevated CSF protein	Lung Other	Uncommon, also called dorsal root ganglionitis may be caused by antineuronal antibody
	Sensorimotor peripheral neuropathy	Croft[254] Dayan[255] Newman[256] Victor[257] Forman[257a]	Distal weakness and wasting, areflexia, distal sensory loss; elevated CSF protein; single-fiber electromyography may help in diagnosis	Lung GI Breast Other	Quite common; recovery rare even with removal of primary tumor
	Ascending acute polyneuropathy (Guillian–Barré)	Lisak[258]	Bilateral, usually symmetric weakness (flaccid), usually beginning in lower extremities and ascending; sensory symptoms and signs usually develop as well; elevated CSF protein	Lymphoma	Association not definite
	Autonomic and gastrointestinal neuropathy	Schuffer[259] Siemsen[260] Park[261] Ahmed[262] Ogilvie[263]	Orthostatic hypotension; neurogenic bladder; intestinal pseudo-obstruction	Lung (small cell)	Many cases of Ogilvie's syndrome (colonic pseudo-obstruction) may be paraneoplastic
Muscle and neuromuscular junction	Dermatomyositis and polymyositis*	DeVere[264] Barnes[265] Williams[266] Sigurgeirsson[266a]	Progressive muscle weakness developing gradually over weeks to months (proximal > distal); usually not disabling; elevated muscle enzymes and sedimentation rate	Lung Stomach Ovary Other	Stringent association in older males; less frequent in colorectal tumors
	Myasthenic syndrome* (Eaton-Lambert syndrome)	Lambert[267,268] Simpson[269] Cherrington[270] Jenkyn[271] Fukunaga[15] Login[272] McEvoy[272a]	Weakness and fatigability of proximal muscles, especially pelvic girdle and thigh; dryness of mouth; dyspagia, dysarthria, and peripheral paresthesias common; EMGs show a facilitated response in active muscles	Lung (small cell) Stomach Ovary Other	Poor response to Tensilon; should respond to therapy of primary tumor; guanidine and 3,4-diaminopyridine may also be useful
	Myasthenia gravis	Tyler[273]	Weakness with predilection for ocular and cranial muscles, tendency for fluctuation and partial reversibility by cholinergic drugs	Thymoma Lymphomas Breast Other	Except for thymoma, association not proved

* These syndromes are so strongly associated with malignancy that a thorough investigation for malignancy is indicated when they develop in patients not known to have cancer.

visual field loss, and attenuated arteriole caliber were reported.[246a] There is specific loss of retinal ganglion cells and their processes due to immune deposits of antibodies that react with antigens shared by normal retinal and small cell lung cancer cells.[246d]

A syndrome of opsoclonus (eye movement disorder) and ataxia in patients with breast cancer and gynecologic cancers was reported.[246c] Opsoclonus can be diagnosed at the bedside by the presence of spontaneous, large amplitude conjugate saccades occurring in all directions of gaze without a saccadic interval. An antibody called anti-Ri was found in these patients.

Progressive multifocal leukoencephalopathy is included in this section, although multiple areas of the neuraxis are involved and it is not a true paraneoplastic syndrome because a viral cause has been established. The syndrome is characterized by dementia, paralysis, aphasia, ataxia, dysarthria, visual field defects, blindness, and sometimes coma or seizures. It usually is rapidly progressive, with death occurring within 6 months. The cerebrospinal fluid is usually normal. This syndrome occurs most often in malignancies associated with impaired immunity (*e.g.*, leukemias, lymphomas) but also occurs in many benign conditions with altered immunity (*e.g.*, sarcoidosis, steroid therapy). Pathologically, demyelination of white matter is found throughout the nervous system. Evidence suggests the illness is caused by one or two types of papovavirus.[17,247]

REMOTE EFFECTS INVOLVING THE SPINAL CORD

In the large series of Croft and Wilkinson, paraneoplastic syndromes primarily involving the spinal cord accounted for only 9% of all nervous system syndromes.[18] From a different perspective, Norris and Engel reported that 10% of 130 patients with amyotrophic lateral sclerosis (ALS) had underlying malignancies.[248]

ALS is characterized by widespread lower motor neuron muscle weakness, atrophy, spasticity, hyperreflexia, extensor plantar responses, and fasciculations. If associated with cancer, the sex distribution is predominantly male, and the age is older. The course of ALS may progress more slowly in cancer patients. Despite the report of Norris and Engel, many observers feel that far fewer than 10% of ALS patients have underlying cancers.[248]

Subacute necrotic myelopathy is characterized by a rapidly ascending motor and sensory paralysis, which is most severe in the thoracic region. It usually terminates in death in a matter of days or weeks. There are often degenerative lesions in other areas of gray and white matter. The cerebrospinal fluid protein level usually is elevated. In one case of Hodgkin's disease, an elevated cerebrospinal fluid level of B_2-microglobulin was reported. The syndrome improved, and the cerebrospinal fluid B_2-microglobulin level decreased after treatment with intrathecal corticosteroids.[250a] The syndrome is most often associated with lung cancer, but other tumors have been reported.

Subacute motor neuropathy is strongly associated with malignancy, particularly the lymphomas. It is characterized by slowly developing but progressive lower motor weakness without sensory changes. It occurs most often in irradiated patients. Although the course often progresses slowly, it may wax and wane, and there may be spontaneous recovery. A viral cause has been speculated.

REMOTE EFFECTS ON THE PERIPHERAL NERVOUS SYSTEM

Paraneoplastic syndromes involving the peripheral nerves are the most frequent site in the nervous system. The association was first reported in the late 1800s, and several reports appeared in the late 1940s and early 1950s. A large series was reported by Croft and Wilkinson in 1965, who divided these neuropathies into two groups: a symmetric sensory peripheral neuropathy that usually developed late in the course of the neoplasm and an acute or subacute severe sensory motor neuropathy that often progresses to paralysis before other signs of malignancy.[18] The cerebrospinal fluid protein often is elevated in these syndromes. Single-fiber electromyography may be useful for diagnosis.[257a] The neurologic abnormalities may wax and wane, and steroids are occasionally associated with clinical improvement. In one small cell lung cancer patient for whom combined therapy with chemoradiotherapy and plasma exchange was used, neurologic recovery occurred.[257b] However, surgical removal of the tumor rarely leads to improvement. The syndrome has been reported with a wide variety of neoplasms, most commonly lung cancer.[273]

Pure sensory neuropathy associated with degeneration of dorsal root ganglia (*i.e.*, dorsal root ganglionitis) is strongly associated with malignancy. In most instances, the tumor is located in the chest (*e.g.*, lung cancer, thymoma, lymphomas involving the mediastinum, laryngeal or esophageal carcinomas). The syndrome is characterized by the subacute development of distal sensory loss, especially proprioception, and loss of deep tendon reflexes with normal muscle strength. Motor nerve conduction velocities are normal. The cerebrospinal fluid protein often is elevated. The illness usually precedes the development of cancer, leaves the patient severely disabled, and rarely improves. An immunologic mechanism has been postulated for these sensory neuropathies because organ-specific antibrain antibodies have been reported in sera and cerebrospinal fluid.[14] In 1 patient with a plasma cell dyscrasia and peripheral neuropathy, pathologic and immunologic studies indicated that an IgM κ-antibody directed against peripheral nerve myelin produced the neuropathy.[274]

Ascending acute polyneuropathy (*i.e.*, Guillain-Barré syndrome) has been reported in some patients with malignancy, particularly Hodgkin's disease and malignant lymphomas.[233] The syndrome has been clinically similar to that found in patients without malignancy. Because both are relatively common and parallel clinical courses have not been demonstrated, the association may be coincidental. Autonomic neuropathy has been associated most commonly with lung cancer, usually small cell lung cancer.[259,263] The most frequently reported syndrome has been orthostatic hypotension. Neurogenic bladder, disordered peristalsis of the esophagus, stomach, and intestine, and intestinal pseudo-obstruction (*i.e.*, Olgivie's syndrome) have been reported. The neuropathologic findings in these cases have resembled those in other neurologic paraneoplastic syndromes with neuronal and axonal degeneration associated with infiltration by lymphocytes, plasma cells, and histiocytes.[259]

Peripheral nerve abnormalities may be found as a result of other phenomena associated with the cancer. For example, patients with multiple myeloma may have neuropathies secondary to amyloid deposition. Johnson and coworkers reported 3 patients who developed peripheral neuropathy (*i.e.*, mononeuritis multiplex) as a result of tumor-related vasculitis limited to the peripheral nervous system.[275] Neuropathies secondary to hemorrhage into the nerves have been reported in leukemic patients.

REMOTE EFFECTS ON MUSCLE AND NEUROMUSCULAR FUNCTION

Dermatomyositis and Polymyositis

In large series, 7% to 34% of patients with dermatomyositis or polymyositis also have cancer. The patients with these disorders have five to seven times the incidence of malignancy as the general population.[264,266] In a Swedish population-based study, the relative risk of cancer was 1.75 in patients with polymyositis and 2.9 in patients with dermatomyositis compared with the normal population.[266a] Both were statistically significant increases. It appears from these retrospective series that the association is most striking in men older than 50, of whom more than 70% have developed cancer.

The syndrome is characterized by gradually progressive muscle weakness occurring over weeks to months. The weakness eventually stabilizes and usually is not disabling. The weakness involves the proximal musculature. Reflexes usually are present but diminished. Muscle enzymes and sedimentation rate usually are elevated. The electromyogram tracing is abnormal, and muscle biopsies show muscle fiber necrosis with minimal inflammatory changes.

In most instances, the myopathy and cancer appear within 1 year of each other. In one long-term follow-up study, patients with dermatomyositis continued at risk for developing cancer for longer than 5 years.[266a] Most reported cases do not relate the temporal cause of the tumor and the dermatomyositis. Barnes was able to find 29 reports of improvement in tumor and dermatomyositis and seven reports of worsening of both in a review of 258 cases.[265] Steroids have been useful, although this is controversial, and there are no well-controlled therapeutic studies.

Myasthenic Syndrome

The myasthenic syndrome (*i.e.*, Eaton-Lambert syndrome) is uncommon but strongly associated with small cell undifferentiated bronchogenic carcinoma. The syndrome is characterized by muscle weakness and fatigue, which are most pronounced in the pelvic girdle and thigh, making it difficult to climb stairs or get out of a chair. Other features include dryness of mouth, dysarthria, dysphagia, blurred vision or diplopia, ptosis, paresthesias, and muscle pain. In contrast to true myasthenia gravis, muscle strength improves with exercise, and there is poor response to edrophonium (Tensilon). The electromyogram confirms the increase in muscle action potential with repeated nerve stimulation at rates faster than 10 per second. Most patients have lung cancer, particularly small cell lung cancer. Lambert and associates reported that fewer than 1% of all lung cancer patients, but 6% of all small cell lung cancer patients, have this syndrome.[267,268] In the authors' experience, these syndromes are infrequent in lung cancer patients. There are a few reports of the relation between response to antitumor therapy and improvement in the syndrome.[271] Recovery from the syndrome has been observed

in patients with small cell lung cancer treated with combination chemotherapy. Because more than 90% of patients with small cell lung cancer respond to combination chemotherapy, this should be tried as a first measure. For patients failing chemotherapy or having no improvement in muscle strength with response to chemotherapy, guanidine and 3,4-diaminopyridine have been reported to be useful.[270] There are accumulating data that the Eaton-Lambert syndrome is an autoimmune condition. This is supported by the ability to transfer the syndrome to mice by the administration of immunoglobulin or purified IgG from patients' serum.[15] Studies suggest that IgG autoantibody inhibits acetylcholine release through a functional blockade of calcium channels.[272] Alternatively, the autoantibodies may induce excess production of acetylcholinesterase.[269]

Myasthenia Gravis

The association of myasthenia gravis and thymoma is well established. Several tumors including lymphomas, pancreas, breast, prostate, ovary, thyroid, cervix, kidney, rectum, and palate have been associated with myasthenia gravis, but many researchers conclude that the incidence is no greater than that expected in the normal population.[273]

HEMATOLOGIC MANIFESTATIONS OF MALIGNANCY

Abnormalities in all the hematopoietic cell lines and in the clotting proteins have been reported in cancer patients. As with the other paraneoplastic syndromes, these abnormalities are most often produced as a direct result of marrow infiltration by the tumor or its metastases. Infection and the toxic effects of cancer therapies are more common than true paraneoplastic effects. As our understanding of hormones and protein factors regulating hematopoiesis has increased in recent years with newer in vitro cell culture techniques, the mechanisms for hematologic paraneoplastic syndromes, particularly increases in cell numbers, appear to be caused by aberrant production of hematopoietic colony-stimulating factors.[6,7,270,276]

ERYTHROCYTOSIS

Common Forms

Tumor-associated erythrocytosis is well documented in the literature. In a review of 340 cases of tumor-associated erythrocytosis, 35% were hypernephromas, 14% were benign renal problems (*e.g.*, cystic kidneys, hydronephrosis), 3% were other tumors involving the kidney (*e.g.*, Wilms' tumor, hemangioma, adenomas, sarcomas), 19% were hepatomas, 15% were cerebellar hemangioblastomas, 7% were uterine fibroids (often aldosterone-secreting adenomas), 3% were adrenal (often aldosterone-secreting adenomas) tumors and pheochromocytomas, and 3% were miscellaneous tumors (*e.g.*, ovary, lung, thymus).[277] Overall, 53% of cases had some renal involvement. About 1% to 5% of patients with renal tumors and 9% to 20% of patients with cerebellar hemangioblastomas have erythrocytosis.[278] The erythrocytosis usually regresses with removal of the primary tumor and recurs with tumor progression.[277]

Increased erythropoietin levels were found in 64% of the tumor extracts of cystic fluids tested, but no erythropoietin was detected in normal tissues. Elevated serum erythropoietin levels were found in 53% of patients. Although Wilms' tumor usually is not associated with erythrocytosis, elevated plasma erythropoietin levels have been found in patients without erythrocytosis, but the exact frequency of this is unknown.[277] All of this suggests that about half of certain tumors associated with erythrocytosis make erythropoietin.[277]

Erythropoietin normally is produced by the kidney but may be produced by the liver in anephric persons.[23] It is not surprising that certain renal and liver tumors may produce erythropoietin. Direct production of erythropoietin activity by human renal cell carcinomas in vitro has been demonstrated.[279] There are various mechanisms by which tumors could cause elevated erythropoietin levels: tumor production of erythropoietin; induction of local kidney or systemic hypoxia by tumor mass effect, vascular obstruction, or hypoxia; secretion by the tumor of a factor that stimulates the release of ectopic erythropoietin; and change in the metabolism of erythropoietin by the tumor.[277]

With renal cysts, local renal hypoxia is a likely cause, but most cases are probably a result of tumor production of erythropoietin.[277]

Other Mechanisms Generating Erythrocytosis in Cancer Patients

Because not all cancer patients with erythrocytosis have elevated tumor levels of erythropoietin, other mechanisms that cause erythrocytosis must exist. Adrenal cortical tumors and virilizing ovarian tumors can produce androgenic hormones with erythropoietic effects.[23] This may be the mechanism of erythrocytosis associated with Cushing's syndrome. Although pheochromocytomas and aldosterone-producing adrenal adenomas may cause erythrocytosis by this mechanism, the exact hormonal basis has not been defined.[277]

Another possible mechanism is tumor-produced prostaglandins, because prostaglandins enhance the effects of erythropoietin on erythroid differentiation.[23] This is likely because elevated prostaglandin levels associated with hypercalcemia usually were found in patients with renal tumors.[129,130] It would be interesting to consider a trial of indomethacin for cancer-associated erythrocytosis in patients without elevated erythropoietin levels.

By convention, erythrocytosis is diagnosed if there is increased red cell mass, usually associated with hematocrit values over 55% for a man and over 50% for a woman.[280] Elevated but lower hematocrits in the setting of appropriate tumors (*e.g.*, hypernephromas, hepatomas, CNS tumors) should alert suspicion of a paraneoplastic syndrome. The differential diagnosis of erythrocytosis includes the panmyelosis (all blood elements) and splenomegaly of polycythemia vera, stress polycythemia, arterial desaturation from many causes, a hemoglobinopathy with aberrant oxygen-binding features, and dehydration with hemoconcentration.[280] A physical examination, arterial Po_2 determination, a hemoglobin electropho-

resis, and family history can resolve most of these. Demonstration of elevated erythropoietin in the blood would confirm the diagnosis, but this test is usually not performed because of the difficulty bioassay. If a tumor is evident, it is probably wise to rule out other causes of erythrocytosis; an intravenous pyelogram (looking for cysts or other benign abnormalities), careful pelvic examination (looking for fibroids), and neurologic examination for cerebellar signs should always be performed.

The erythrocytosis usually does not need treatment, and phlebotomy is rarely used.[277] Tumor resection is successful in controlling the erythrocytosis in more than 97% of resectable cases; this should be the primary approach.[277] There are no good data on the response of erythrocytosis to chemotherapy (*e.g.*, of a hepatoma). Because only half of the patients with resectable tumors had increased serum or tumor extract erythropoietin levels before surgery and because the erythrocytosis corrected with resection, nonerythropoietin-mediated tumor erythrocytosis should be treated primarily with resection, if possible.

ANEMIA ASSOCIATED WITH CANCER

Anemia occurs frequently in cancer patients. Various mechanisms may explain the anemias, including the anemia of chronic disease; bone marrow invasion; blood loss; marrow suppression by chemoradiotherapy; hypersplenism; immune hemolysis of warm and cold antibody types; megaloblastic anemia; vitamin and iron deficiency; microangiopathic hemolytic anemia; and pure red cell aplasia.[281–303] The reader is referred to other general hematologic sources for the general evaluation of anemia in cancer patients, but the mechanisms of anemia associated with cancer usually have not been elucidated.[281,282]

Anemia found in leukemias probably is not explained by "crowding out" of normal marrow.[281] For many patients, a good explanation of anemia cannot be found, and the diagnosis of anemia of chronic disease is given. Although this is easy to treat with transfusions, the cause is unknown and probably represents a remote effect of the tumor on bone marrow function, red cell metabolism, or cell kinetics. The anemia of chronic malignancy has no associated cancer types and is usually normocytic and normochromic or hypochromic states, with normal iron stores (but low serum iron levels and low total iron-binding capacity), normal reticulocyte count, normal red cell maturation, moderately increased erythropoiesis, and slightly shorter red cell survival.[281,283,284] New approaches to finding the mechanisms include study of red cell production in nude mice bearing human tumors associated with malignancy or cocultivation of in vitro erythropoiesis systems with human tumor cells.

Pure red aplasia with a severe anemia is associated with a variety of tumors, with about one half having thymomas.[285–287] A selective absence of marrow erythropoiesis occurs, and hypogammaglobulinemia may occur.[285,286] Reports of pure red cell aplasia associated with carcinomas have included gastric and breast adenocarcinomas, adenocarcinomas of unknown primary site, lung and skin squamous cell carcinomas, anaplastic lung cancers, and T-γ lymphoproliferative diseases.[288] In the latter cases, T-cell-mediated suppression of erythropoiesis was demonstrated, and the anemia improved after cyclophosphamide therapy. Many patients with and without thymomas have responded to cyclophosphamide therapy, and the mechanism of the aplasia may be through some T-lymphocyte-mediated system.

Megaloblastic anemia without folate or vitamin B_{12} deficiency is seen in the bone marrow of cancer patients before chemotherapy; this is unexplained. A macrocytic anemia of unknown origin occasionally is associated with multiple myeloma. The marrow is megaloblastic and the serum vitamin B_{12} levels low, but the patients fail to respond to B_{12}.[289]

Hypersplenic anemia with shortened erythrocyte survival probably is not a paraneoplastic syndrome because it usually occurs with myelofibrosis or, rarely, with a chronic granulocytic leukemia.[280] However, the cause of the fibrosis in the marrow and the spleen may be a humoral factor.

Autoimmune hemolytic anemias (AHA) associated with tumors usually are found with B-cell lymphoproliferative neoplasms.[290,292] The mechanisms by which the B-cell neoplasms upset the normal immunoregulatory circuits are unidentified. However, the monoclonal immunoglobulins produced by the B-cell neoplasms on their surface membranes probably are not themselves responsible for the hemolysis.

Rarely, AHA are associated with solid tumors. In a review of a large series of patients with AHA, only 2% had associated solid tumors.[296–298] In these cases, the mean age is 10 years older than in patients presenting with idiopathic AHA.[295] When AHA presents in the elderly, it is important to consider the possibility of an underlying carcinoma. A wide variety of tumor types are reported to be associated with AHA, including lung cancer of all histologic types, hypernephromas, ovarian, breast, stomach, uterine cervix, colon, and cecal cancer, seminoma, dermoid cysts of the ovary, and microcysts in adenomas of the pancreas.

In tumor-associated AHA, anemia is often the presenting symptom, with mean hemoglobin levels of 7.4 g/dl and frequent reticulocytosis. Splenomegaly is common. Response to corticosteroids is infrequent, in contrast to the high response seen in idiopathic AHA. However, successful treatment of the primary tumor with resection, radiation therapy, or chemotherapy usually leads to improvement or cure of the AHA.[295,300] In some cases, recurrent tumor was associated with recurrent AHA. Definitive tumor treatment should be the first approach, rather than corticosteroids or splenectomy. If this fails, splenectomy can be tried and does work in some patients. The two most likely causes are immune response to antigens shared by the tumor with erythrocytes (but exposed on the erythrocyte in a nonstimulating form) or attachment of immune complexes to erythrocytes. Evans' syndrome is characterized by the simultaneous occurrence of AHA and immune thrombocytopenia (ITP).[298,299] It occurs less often than AHA or ITP alone and has been observed with various carcinomas and lymphomas. The syndrome could be caused by cross-reacting antibodies, tumor production of autoantibodies, or tumor production of a substance altering erythrocytes and platelets, rendering them immunogenic to the host immune system.

Microangiopathic hemolytic anemia (MAHA) has been associated with 55 cancer patients in a comprehensive review.[301]

By definition, the peripheral blood smear in MAHA contains fragmented erythrocyte forms.[302] Severe MAHA is rare in cancer patients, in one series occurring in only 8 of 3200 patients.[303] However, Antman and associates postulate that a careful search of the peripheral blood film for signs of microangiopathy (*e.g.*, schistocytosis) may uncover many more cases of a milder nature.[301] In the reported MAHA patients, the hemolysis was abrupt and severe, requiring several units of transfused blood daily to maintain a 20% hematocrit. The mean hemoglobin level was 7 g/dl, the mean percentage of nucleated erythrocytes was 30%, elevated bilirubin levels were found in 93%, and a leukoerythroblastic blood film was found in 35% of patients. The mean number of days from diagnosis of MAHA to death was 21 (range, 2–90 days). The Coombs' test result was always negative. Associated laboratory findings of disseminated intravascular coagulation (DIC) were found in 50% to 60%, and some of the patients had migratory thrombophlebitis. However, some of the patients with MAHA did not have signs of DIC.

Most of the tumors were mucin-producing adenocarcinomas; 55% were gastric cancer, 10% were of unknown primary (possibly gastric), and breast and lung accounted for 13% and 7%, respectively. The remainder were divided among prostate, ovary, pancreas, colon, hepatoma, cholangiocarcinoma, and seminal vesicle tumors.[301] Several of the gastric primaries were occult and found only at autopsy.

MAHA is easily diagnosed by the presence of a severe hemolytic anemia, with fragmented erythrocyte forms on the peripheral blood smear and a negative Coombs' test result. The causes of the MAHA syndrome represent various diseases associated with lesions of small blood vessels, including thrombotic thrombocytopenic purpura (TTP); congenital vascular abnormalities, such as the Kasabach-Merritt syndrome; hemolytic-uremic syndrome; DIC; malfunction at an aortic valve prosthesis; and neoplastic disease. The differentiating MAHA caused by neoplastic diseases from TTP or DIC may be impossible because TTP and DIC have been reported in association with malignancy.[304,305] The renal function of patients with MAHA associated with malignancy was not indicated but supposedly was not unusual.

Although heparin has been used to treat other causes of MAHA, particularly the hemolytic uremic syndrome, it appears ineffective when given alone in MAHA of neoplastic disease. In contrast, in 7 of 9 patients, the MAHA syndrome responded to hormonal anticancer therapy (for breast and prostate cancer) or chemotherapy.[301] However, if DIC is associated with MAHA, it would appear reasonable to treat with heparin to control the immediate DIC problem while instituting appropriate anticancer therapy, as is done in acute promyelocytic leukemia.[305]

The pathophysiology of MAHA associated with cancer may represent various causes of erythrocyte shearing, including fibrin strands from DIC; pulmonary intraluminal tumor emboli (31% of MAHA patients); and narrowing of pulmonary arterioles by intimal proliferation or a side effect of chemotherapy.[301] The presence of tumor emboli diffusely involving pulmonary arterioles occurs in about 1% of cancer patients.[301] Association of MAHA with gastric cancer may be explained by its tendency for widespread vascular metastasis and mucin production. Mucin can act as a procoagulant and potentially cause DIC. The occurrence of intimal proliferation is thought to cause pulmonary hypertension and increase the shearing force on the erythrocyte.[301]

GRANULOCYTOSIS ASSOCIATED WITH NONHEMATOLOGIC MALIGNANCIES

Elevation in the peripheral granulocyte count to more than 20,000/μl without overt infection or leukemia occurs in association with several neoplasms.[6,280,306–309] Monocyte elevation may be seen.[310] Neoplasms associated with a granulocytosis syndrome are gastric, lung, pancreas, melanoma, and brain tumors; Hodgkin's disease; and diffuse histiocytic lymphoma (*i.e.*, reticulum cell sarcoma).[280,311] The exact frequency in each histologic type is unknown, but many cases have been reported during the past 50 years.[280] The granulocytosis usually is asymptomatic and consists of mature neutrophils.[282]

Although there are many potential causes of neutrophilia in cancer patients (*e.g.*, infection, inflammatory disorders, drugs, metabolic disorders, physical and emotional stimuli), the major diagnostic problem for a persistently high neutrophil count is to differentiate it from coexistent chronic myelogenous leukemia (CML).[280] The major features differentiating a paraneoplastic "leukemoid reaction" in the cancer patient from CML are a leukocyte count less than 100,000/μl; no left shift to blast or progranulocytic forms; normal platelet and basophil levels; absent splenomegaly; elevated leukocyte alkaline phosphatase levels; normal serum B_{12} levels; and no Philadelphia chromosome.[282] After other disorders and coexistent CML are ruled out in cancer patients, a paraneoplastic granulocytosis is likely.

The mechanism behind tumor-associated granulocytosis is most often tumor production of a colony-stimulating factor (CSF).[282a] The colony-stimulating factors include granulocyte CSF (G-CSF), granulocyte-macrophage CSF (GM-CSF), macrophage CSF (M-CSF; CSF-1), interleukin-3 (IL-3), and interleukin-1 (IL-1).[276] The genes for these proteins have been cloned, and probes for DNA and RNA expression are available, as are antibodies to the factors. Future studies will establish exactly which protein is responsible for these syndromes. Prior studies were concluded before these tools were available. For example, Robinson tested the serum and urine of 12 patients with cancer and unexplained sustained granulocytosis for CSF activity using in vitro bone marrow culture assays.[306] In his series, there were five lung cancers (type unspecified), two melanomas, two adrenal cancers, an unknown primary, hepatoma, and multiple myeloma. He found elevated CSF levels in all of these patients, and the levels correlated with the degree of elevation of the peripheral neutrophil count. The two adrenal tumors did not make CSF in culture; the other tumors were not tested. Several laboratories have reported establishing cultures of human tumor cell lines of lung cancer (squamous), oral cavity (squamous), and fibrous histiocytoma, which produce large amounts of a CSF-like factor.[312–314] The activity can be demonstrated in marrow cultures in vitro, and after the human tumors are heterotransplanted, they cause neutrophilia in athymic nude mice.[312,313] Neutrophilia is frequent in Sweet's syndrome, characterized by pyrexia, neutrophilia, and painful cutaneous plaques.[315] It is likely that this syndrome is also caused by tumor production of a CSF, perhaps IL-1. There is no specific therapy for the granulocytosis other

than to treat the underlying malignancy.[282] Paraneoplastic syndromes with hypercalcemia and granulocytosis were attributed to tumor production of IL-1, G-CSF, and parathyroid hormone-related protein.[315a]

GRANULOCYTOPENIA AS A PARANEOPLASTIC SYNDROME

Granulocytopenia associated with cancer usually is the result of chemotherapy, radiotherapy, other drugs, or severe infection.[311] Granulocytopenia rarely has been reported with thymomas and may have the same immunologic basis as pure red cell aplasia.[311] Neutropenia alone may develop with marrow involvement by carcinoma, lymphoma, myeloma, or leukemia, but a pancytopenia is more common.[371] With the exception of leukemia, the neutropenia usually is not life threatening. Despite the frequent involvement of the bone marrow with cancer, significant granulocytopenia unrelated to therapy must be uncommon in cancer patients. However, experimental evidence suggests that a paraneoplastic syndrome involving granulopoiesis may exist. When 10^5 normal bone marrow cells are plated in semisolid medium with CSF, 20 to 100 hematopoietic colonies (containing 40 or more cells) and five to ten times that number of "cluster" (aggregates of 3–40 cells) are found.[316] In contrast, when marrow from patients with acute leukemia, preleukemic states, and CML in blast transformation are plated, mainly clusters and only rare colonies are found, suggesting that the leukemic process may inhibit the activity of the exogenously added CSF in some unknown way. Similar findings occur with solid tumors.

McCarthy and coworkers studied 9 small cell lung cancer patients for bone marrow colony formation with CSF.[316] The marrows of 2 of these patients (1 with and 1 without small cell cancer marrow involvement) were not able to form colonies in agar but had large numbers of clusters with or without CSF. The patient with marrow involvement had neutrophilia, and the one without marrow involvement had neutropenia.[316] It is likely that some tumors may suppress granulopoiesis by interfering with the action of CSF on marrow progenitor cells. Neutropenia is associated with T-γ lymphoproliferative diseases.[317] It is thought that the abnormal T cells interfere directly with granulocyte production. Corticosteroids and alkylating agents have led to improvement in some patients.

EOSINOPHILIA AND BASOPHILIA ASSOCIATED WITH NEOPLASMS

Eosinophilia is associated with nonleukemic neoplasms, particularly Hodgkin's disease (in as many as 20% of cases) and mycosis fungoides, but it has been found with other lymphomas, melanoma, brain tumors, and other cancers. The exact frequency in these tumors is not documented.[280,311,318]

It is possible that the eosinophilia itself may be symptomatic if the cell count is sufficiently high and an allergic or Loeffler's-like syndrome (*i.e.*, fleeting nodular pulmonary infiltrates with eosinophilia [PIE syndrome], with mild cough, lassitude, and low-grade fever) is produced in cancer patients. A small peptide that acts as an eosinophilopoietin has been described, and the tumor cells may be producing or stimulating the secretion of this factor.[319] Slungaard and associates found that serum and tumor extracts from a patient with large cell bronchogenic carcinoma and eosinophilia markedly stimulated the growth of eosinophil colonies from human bone marrow.[320] The tumor-associated eosinophilopoietic factor was found to be a glycoprotein of M_r 45 kd.

Therapy should be directed against the tumor, particularly in cases of the malignant lymphomas that are potentially curable. If this does not work or if pulmonary symptoms are troublesome, a trial of corticosteroids could be given because this sometimes gives dramatic results in other forms of the PIE syndrome, but data for cancer patients are lacking.[318]

Eosinopenia as a tertiary result of tumor secretion of ACTH or other hormones is possible but should give no clinical symptoms. Basophilia commonly is associated with CML, myelofibrosis, and polycythemia vera, but it has not been reported with other malignancies, and there now is no recognized basophilic paraneoplastic syndrome.[280]

THROMBOCYTOSIS ASSOCIATED WITH CANCER

Thrombocytosis (platelet count $>400,000/\mu l$) is said to occur in as many as 30% to 40% of cancer patients.[321-323] The differential diagnosis of thrombocytosis in the cancer patient includes myeloproliferative disorders (which may represent a paraneoplastic syndrome); acute and chronic inflammatory disorders; acute hemorrhage, iron deficiency; hemolytic anemias; postsplenectomy and other surgical procedures; and responses to vincristine or epinephrine.[321] Thrombocytosis has been seen with carcinomas, leukemias, Hodgkin's disease, and non-Hodgkin's lymphomas; a fall in the platelet count is associated with a response to therapy.[282] Although not characterized, there is a "thrombopoietin" that regulates normal megakaryocyte production and maturation.[324] Patients with neoplasms and thrombocytosis should have serum and tumor levels of thrombopoietin assayed. Although platelet counts above 1×10^6 cells/μl may lead to thrombosis or hemorrhage, these are rarely seen associated with malignancy, and such symptoms do not appear to occur with any regularity with the thrombocytosis of malignancy. No specific treatment of the thrombocytosis is indicated, except to treat the underlying malignancy.

UNEXPLAINED THROMBOCYTOPENIA IN CANCER PATIENTS

Thrombocytopenia commonly is seen in cancer patients and usually is related to chemotherapy, radiotherapy, acute leukemia, or DIC. A syndrome resembling ITP occasionally is seen associated with malignancy.[325-330] This association is uncommon, and in one study of ITP, it represented 4% of 381 patients with otherwise unexplained thrombocytopenia; all of these patients had lymphomas.[326] In another evaluation of patients with ITP, 9 of 52 had cancer.[325]

The diagnosis of an ITP-like syndrome is made by finding thrombocytopenia without anemia and with normal or increased numbers of normal erythrocytes on a peripheral smear; no evidence of DIC; and no evidence of a drug-induced thrombocytopenia.[325] The types of neoplasms associated with this syndrome are Hodgkin's disease; chronic lymphocytic leukemia; non-Hodgkin's lymphoma; acute lymphoblastic

leukemia; immunoblastic sarcomas; and carcinomas of the lung, breast, rectum, gallbladder, and testis.[283,284] The association with chronic lymphocytic leukemia and Hodgkin's disease is widely known, and the syndrome occurs in approximately 30% of patients with immunoblastic lymphadenopathy.[328-330] However, the association with other tumors is less widely recognized. The mean age of patients is older (54 years) than the mean age of patients with ITP alone. About 80% of patients are symptomatic, with bleeding, petechiae, or purpura. Most have platelet counts under $30,000/\mu l$.[325] Response of platelet counts to high-dose (60 mg/day) prednisone is common but transient. However, 6 of 10 patients had a complete and apparently permanent response to splenectomy.[325]

The syndrome is called ITP-like because the course is much like classic ITP, but an immune mechanism has not been demonstrated. In the future, studies of antiplatelet antibodies will have to be done with tests of antibody cross-reactivity with tumor cells. Most patients have been treated with splenectomy in addition to various antineoplastic therapies; the effect of tumor treatment alone on the thrombocytopenia is unknown.[325] Other causes of thrombocytopenia need to be excluded, particularly the use of thiazide diuretics and quinidine or the presence of DIC or severe infection. In thrombocytopenic patients receiving antineoplastic therapy, ITP-like syndromes should be considered. The clues are thrombocytopenia disproportionate to granulocytopenia, normal or increased numbers of marrow megakaryocytes, and a rapid fall in transfused platelets. This diagnosis should be remembered particularly in lymphoproliferative disorders. Therapy consists of platelet transfusions, initial corticosteroids, and then splenectomy. Because of the poor response to steroids and inconsistent response to treatment of the underlying malignancy, a reasonable approach is to take the patient directly to splenectomy after other causes of thrombocytopenia have been excluded.

Abnormalities of platelet function sometimes are associated with plasma cell dyscrasias and are thought to result from the interference of the monoclonal protein with platelet function.[292]

MIGRATORY THROMBOPHLEBITIS, DISSEMINATED INTRAVASCULAR COAGULATION, AND NONBACTERIAL THROMBOTIC ENDOCARDITIS

Hemorrhage, thrombotic, and embolic complications occur frequently in cancer patients.[304,305,331] These may arise from a variety of specific mechanisms, including treatment-related thrombocytopenia, local tissue disruption from tumor or therapy, infection, vitamin deficiency, liver disease, circulating anticoagulants, and DIC. Usually, there is no specific cause, and successful therapy of the underlying malignancy alleviates the problem. The clinical association between cancer and thrombophlebitis was first observed by Trousseau.[332] In 1949, Marder and colleagues reported afibrinogenemia in metastatic prostate cancer.[333] Other abnormalities in clotting characteristics, frank DIC, and nonbacterial thrombotic endocarditis (NBTE) were later recognized to occur with greater than expected frequency in patients with cancer.[334-352] Sack and coworkers recognized that thrombophlebitis, DIC, coagulation abnormalities, and NBTE often occurred in the same patient and that each was part of a spectrum of the hypercoagulable state in cancer.[304] Many theories on mechanisms of activation of the coagulation system have been postulated and are reviewed by Rickles and Edwards.[349]

Thrombophlebitis

The incidence of clinical episodes of thrombophlebitis in cancer patients varies from 1% to 11%, and the incidence has been even higher in autopsy studies.[334] Many years ago, Trousseau recognized that cancer patients frequently have multiple episodes of thrombophlebitis and that these often occurred in veins in which deep venous thromboses were uncommon.[332] This syndrome of migratory thrombophlebitis is referred to as Trousseau's syndrome, a syndrome that he developed after its description. Migratory thrombophlebitis may occur before or after malignancy is documented. Like many paraneoplastic syndromes, its presence should lead to an investigation for occult cancer. For patients presenting with a deep venous thrombosis, one series showed that patients subsequently shown to have cancer were older, had lower hemoglobin levels, and had higher eosinophil counts than patients who did not develop cancer.[352] These factors can be used to select patients for a workup for occult cancer.

Mucin-secreting adenocarcinomas of the gastrointestinal tract most frequently are associated with migratory thrombophlebitis, but lung, breast, ovarian, prostate, and other tumors also are associated.[349] Although the greatest risk may be associated with pancreatic cancer (a prevalence of up to 57% or 50 times higher than control subjects with chronic pancreatitis), lung cancer is the most common association because of its greater prevalence. The treatment of migratory thrombophlebitis usually is difficult; acute episodes require heparin therapy. Long-term therapy with warfarin generally is unsuccessful, and extended subcutaneous heparin therapy has met with only limited success.[304,353] Treatment of the underlying malignancy is the mainstay of treatment.

Coagulation Abnormalities and Disseminated Intravascular Coagulation

DIC may present as a chronic coagulation disorder, usually of a thrombotic nature as an acute hemorrhage diathesis, or as a coagulation abnormality detected by laboratory tests alone (Table 57–12).[304,305,331–342,354] Abnormalities of routine blood coagulation tests have been reported in as many as 92% of cancer patients.[349] The most common abnormalities are elevated levels of fibrin or fibrinogen degradation products, thrombocytosis, and hyperfibrinogenemia.[349] These abnormalities are consistent with overcompensated intravascular coagulation with fibrinolysis. The low-grade coagulation with accelerated factor use may be accompanied by increased synthesis rates for fibrinogen, clotting factors, and platelets, resulting in actual increases in their circulating levels. Overt DIC with consumption of platelets and clotting factors and resultant bleeding is rare. The most commonly associated neoplasms are acute promyelocytic leukemia and adenocarcinomas.[349] The DIC may be exacerbated in patients with acute promyelocytic leukemia after treatment with cytotoxic agents.

For cancer patients suspected of having DIC or other

TABLE 57–12. Frequency of Different Cancer Types Associated With Disseminated Intravascular Coagulopathy

Tumor Type	Chronic DIC (n = 213)[304]	% of Tumors Making Up Various DIC Series* Bleeding Disorder (n = 134)[305]	Coagulation Abnormality (n = 86)[354]
Pancreas	24	2	0
Lung	20	1.5	12
Prostate	13	18	8
Stomach	12	4	0
Acute leukemia	9	64	19
Colon	5	0.7	6
Unknown primary	5	0	0
Ovary	4	0.7	1
Gallbladder (cholangiocarcinoma)	4	0.7	2
Lymphomas	1	1.5	16
Breast	0.5	0	10
Melanomas	0.5	0	3
Miscellaneous others	3	3	10

* Some of the cases in refs. 304 and 305 may overlap. The data in ref. 304 were obtained from a literature review from 1960–1970 looking for the association of malignancy and thrombophlebitis, hemorrhagic diathesis, DIC, arterial embolism, or nonbacterial thrombotic endocarditis. The data in ref. 305 are based on a literature review to find cases to permit a tentative diagnosis of DIC. The data in ref. 354 come from review of the coagulation laboratory and medical records from 1971–1974 at the Memorial Sloan-Kettering Cancer Center looking for laboratory evidence of DIC.

thrombotic or hemorrhagic phenomena, Sack and coworkers stressed the need for sequential monitoring of coagulation tests and the striking decreases that occurred in fibrinogen and platelet levels associated with the acute vascular events.[304] They postulated that this was due to a shift from a "compensated" to a "decompensated" coagulation status engendered by the tumor.[304] Although the thrombotic events of chronic DIC are clearly related to the coagulation disorder, the relation is not so clear for the multiple organ system dysfunction seen in acute (often hemorrhagic) DIC.[305] The situations that appear most related to DIC are the adult respiratory distress syndrome; oliguric renal insufficiency with gram-negative sepsis, and the hemolytic-uremic syndrome; neurologic syndromes related to intracranial bleeding and thrombosis; pulmonary hemorrhage syndrome; and the infarcted skin of purpura fulminans.[305] Autopsy studies show DIC usually contributes strongly to patient morbidity and mortality, particularly with thrombosis or bleeding in the lung, CNS, or gastrointestinal tract.[305]

MANAGEMENT OF DISSEMINATED INTRAVASCULAR COAGULATION IN MALIGNANCY. There is universal agreement that identification and treatment of all precipitating factors is the keystone to DIC management.[260,293] This should include not only treatment of cancer, but evaluation of patients with DIC for other precipitating factors (*e.g.*, sepsis, volume deficit, hypotension, hypoxemia, acidosis, fungus infection, transfusion reactions, vessel manipulation). Other hemostatic deficits should be identified and corrected. A response of the malignancy to tumor treatment often is associated with response of the DIC, and the long-term goal is appropriate antineoplastic therapy.[304,347]

A major controversy is whether heparin should be used.[305,335] There is a tendency to use heparin more in DIC with thrombotic, thromboembolic, or necrotizing complications, as is often seen in the chronic DIC of malignancy.[305,306] However, randomized trials of heparin therapy in the DIC of malignancy have not been conducted. After the association between DIC and acute promyelocytic leukemia (APL) was established, Gralnick and associates showed that heparin could improve the coagulation abnormalities.[336] Subsequently, nonrandomized trials suggested that heparin should be used prophylactically in all APL patients.[341,342] Later studies suggest heparin need not be given to all patients.[343] The liberal use

of fresh-frozen plasma and platelets was suggested by the researchers. Until randomized trials are conducted, coagulation values should be monitored closely in APL patients. Heparin should be considered if there is overt bleeding or a change in laboratory evaluations.

Sack and associates, in their review of the literature on chronic DIC in malignancy, found positive responses to anticoagulant therapy (defined as cessation of signs or symptoms of thrombophlebitis, hemorrhage, or arterial emboli) in 65% of 55 patients treated with heparin initially and 33% of 26 patients treated with heparin after failing warfarin therapy.[304] Only 19% of 32 patients treated with warfarin alone responded. In addition, 53% of 36 patients had recurrence of symptoms of the thrombotic-hemorrhage disorder after the heparin was stopped, suggesting a therapeutic role of heparin in control of the DIC. Table 57–13 summarizes the results of anticoagulant and antineoplastic therapy in the treatment of the chronic DIC of malignancy. All combinations of antineoplastic and anticoagulant therapy were associated with response of the DIC symptoms in more than half of the cases, but only 10% to 20% of patients had long-term control, presumably reflecting the lack of control of the underlying tumor. Although in many patients the temporal correlation of heparin therapy with cessation of DIC is persuasive, spontaneous remission of DIC occurring with persistent cancer has been reported.[348]

After DIC associated with malignancy is diagnosed and other factors corrected, it is wise to establish the tempo of the DIC. If the DIC is acute with life-threatening symptoms (*e.g.*, uncontrolled bleeding) or if it is chronic and the symptoms debilitating (*e.g.*, recurrent thromboembolic lesions), a trial of heparin therapy should be given. The doses used in the literature range from 300 to 600 U/kg per 4 hours. Bell and associates showed that heparin prevented thrombotic events in several patients and that sudden catastrophic events occurred when it was discontinued.[353] They recommended continuous intravenous heparin (administered by an external pump connected to an indwelling catheter) if the heparin requirements (to maintain the PTT at 1.5 to 2 times normal) exceed 40,000 U/day. Otherwise, intermittent subcutaneous or intravenous (every 6–8 hours) heparin was satisfactory. After heparin therapy has begun, the repletion of coagulation factors with platelets, cryoprecipitates, and whole blood can be used, particularly in highly symptomatic, hemorrhagic,

TABLE 57–13. Treatment of Chronic Disseminated Intravascular Coagulopathy in Malignancy

Treatment Given		No. of Patients	% Response*	
Antineoplastic	Anticoagulant†		Short-Term	Long-Term
+	+	27	52	15
+	–	22	55	18
–	+	48	60	10
+	+	12‡	75	?

* Data from ref. 304. Response is defined as cessation of signs or symptoms of thrombophlebitis, hemorrhage, or arterial emboli. Long-term indicates for over 250 days or until death.
† In most cases, the anticoagulant therapy was heparin; 81 of 87 patients reported for anticoagulant response received heparin.
‡ Patients with recurrent DIC after stopping heparin therapy were again given heparin.

acute DIC.[305] Although heparin treatment may be maintained for weeks, it is only a temporary measure, and control of the underlying malignancy affords the only long-term control of chronic DIC.

NONBACTERIAL THROMBOTIC ENDOCARDITIS

NBTE, another cause of thrombotic or hemorrhagic complications, may occur with or without DIC and is characterized by the presence of sterile verrucous, bland, fibrin-platelet lesions in the left-side heart valves.[221,304,344-346] Patients often present with emboli to the brain and to other organs. The brain emboli may have an abrupt or a gradual onset of neurologic symptoms with development of focal neurologic deficits or diffuse abnormalities such as confusion, disorientation, generalized seizure, or disturbances in consciousness. Neurologic signs are often the only evidence of thromboembolism.[224] For these patients cerebral angiography showing multiple arterial occlusions is the definitive diagnostic test.[224] Only one third or fewer of the patients have heart murmurs, usually systolic. Patients are usually afebrile, but all patients should have blood cultures if emboli are suspected. Echocardiography may be of diagnostic use for vegetations larger than 2 mm, but most lesions are smaller and are not detected by echocardiography. Arterial emboli can go to the CNS, heart, spleen, kidneys, and peripheral sites. Occlusion of large and small vessels is detected pathologically in the brain. Myocardial infarction can result from emboli to coronary arteries.[344,345] Paraneoplastic endocarditis can present with early malignancy or in later stages and does not mean incurability.[346]

In Rosen's series, the autopsy incidence of NBTE in patients with adenocarcinoma of the lung (7.5%) was twice that of adenocarcinomas of the prostate or pancreas (3–4%) and more than seven times that of other solid tumors, lymphomas, or leukemias.[350] In Goodnight's review of NBTE, bleeding frequently was found in the skin (77–100%), CNS (22–49%), genitourinary tract (38–42%), eye, ear, nose, and mouth (31–47%), and gastrointestinal (24–56%) and respiratory (20–31%) tracts in leukemias and solid tumor patients, respectively.[334] Of the leukemias and solid tumor patients, 37% had autopsy evidence of fibrin thrombi, but only 1% had evidence of NBTE.

The principles of treating NBTE are similar to those in treating other aspects of the hypercoagulable state. Treatment of the underlying malignancy is the primary therapy. In anecdotal cases, warfarin has been unsuccessful; heparin has been used with limited success. There are no studies reporting the use of antiplatelet drugs or fibrinolytic agents.

RENAL MANIFESTATIONS OF MALIGNANCY

Numerous problems involving the kidneys develop in patients with malignancies. The causes of these complications are listed in Table 57–14. In most instances, the renal abnormalities are not paraneoplastic in origin. Only the glomerular lesions and obstruction by tumor products can be considered to be true paraneoplastic syndromes.

Massive proteinuria with the nephrotic syndrome is the major consequence of these paraneoplastic glomerular lesions,

TABLE 57–14. Differential Diagnosis of Renal Abnormalities in Patients With Malignancy

Direct infiltration of the kidney by tumor
Obstruction of the urinary tract by tumor
Electrolyte imbalances, many of which are caused by the tumor or its treatment (*e.g.,* calcium, uric acid, potassium)
Fluid imbalances induced by the tumor or its treatment (prerenal)
Infection
Toxicity of therapy (chemotherapy, radiotherapy, immunotherapy, antibiotics)
Glomerular lesions of uncertain cause (usually associated with nephrotic syndrome), paraneoplastic
Obstruction by tumor products

although renal failure may develop later. In patients with malignancy, the nephrotic syndrome may develop as a result of neoplastic infiltration of the kidneys, renal vein thrombosis, or amyloid infiltration. Besides these established causes of the nephrotic syndrome, there does seem to be a true paraneoplastic syndrome. Until 1966, there were only a few scattered case reports of an association between idiopathic nephrotic syndrome and malignancy. In 1966, Lee and associates reported that among 101 patients with the nephrotic syndrome of unknown cause, 11 were found to have cancer.[355] The neoplastic syndrome preceded discovery of the cancer in 7 of these 11 patients, who were all over the age of 40. Since that time, the nephrotic syndrome has been associated with several cancers, although recent studies suggest the incidence is lower than that reported by Lee and associates.[356]

Clinical and immunologic evidence supports the true paraneoplastic nature of this syndrome.[355-362] The nephrotic syndrome may precede the development of neoplastic disease.[358] Surgical removal of tumor or response to radiotherapy or chemotherapy usually is associated with dramatic diminution in proteinuria, but recurrence of the neoplasm is followed by increased proteinuria.[357,359,360] Tumor-specific antigens and antibodies and carcinoembryonic antigen have been found in the glomeruli of some patients.[361-363]

The most frequently reported associated neoplasm is Hodgkin's disease.[357,358,360,364-366] In patients with Hodgkin's disease, the most common (80%) renal lesion is lipoid nephrosis (minimal glomerular changes).[364-367] In most of these instances, the renal findings have been similar to those seen in idiopathic lipoid nephrosis, including an absence of electron-dense deposits on electron microscopy and an absence of immunoglobulin deposits.[364] In the remaining 20% of cases, lesions typical of membranous glomerulopathy, focal sclerosis, or a membranoproliferative glomerulonephritis have been observed.[357,360,365]

In the non-Hodgkin's lymphomas (*i.e.,* Burkitt's lymphomas, lymphocytic and histiocytic lymphomas), the frequency of the nephrotic syndrome appears to be lower than that in Hodgkin's disease and some other carcinomas, although there are numerous case reports.[369,374] In 35 patients in the literature, 5 had minimal-change lesions, 7 had membranous, and 7 had membranoproliferative lesions.[369] In several of the patients with non-Hodgkin's lymphomas, immunoglobulin deposits have been identified, suggesting an immune complex as the cause of the syndrome.[373,374]

There is a striking difference in the type of renal lesions described in patients with carcinomas when compared with Hodgkin's disease. The most frequently observed glomerular lesion in patients with carcinomas is membranous glomerulonephritis.[368,370-372,375,376] Membranous glomerulonephritis is characterized by subepithelial electron-dense deposits and granular peripheral capillary deposits of IgG with or without C3.[357] It occurs in 80% to 90% of patients with carcinoma and nephrotic syndrome. The remaining patients have lipoid nephrosis or proliferative glomerulonephritis.[357,368,372] Patients with neoplasia account for 5% to 10% of all patients with membranous glomerulonephritis.[377,378]

There is a similarity between the immunopathologic features of the membranous glomerulonephritis associated with carcinomas and experimentally induced immune complex nephritis in animals. It has been suggested that there is a common pathophysiologic mechanism with glomerular deposition of circulating antigen-antibody complexes.[357,370] Tumor-specific antibodies have been eluted from the kidneys of 2 patients with lung cancer and the nephrotic syndrome, and a tumor-specific antigen was demonstrated in the glomeruli of a patient with colonic carcinoma.[357,362,370] In another patient with colon cancer, carcinoembryonic antigen-antibody complexes were found in the glomeruli, and a patient with prostate cancer had positive immunoperoxidase staining for prostate-specific acid phosphate, prostate-specific antigen, and immune deposits detected by electron microscopy in the glomerulus.[363,363a]

The pathogenesis of lipoid nephrosis in patients with Hodgkin's disease seems to have a different mechanism. There is some evidence that lipoid nephrosis may be a result of deficient T-cell function, and abnormalities of T-cell function are common in Hodgkin's disease.[379]

Other renal abnormalities caused directly or indirectly by tumor products include renal dysfunction in patients with multiple myeloma amyloidosis; renal potassium wasting and hypocalcemia related to lysozyme in acute monocytic or myelomonocytic leukemia; intrarenal obstruction by mucoprotein in pancreatic carcinoma; and nephrogenic diabetes insipidus with leiomyosarcoma.[380-399]

The renal problems of myeloma are discussed in Chapter 60.

PARANEOPLASTIC LESIONS INVOLVING THE SKIN

A long list of fascinating cutaneous syndromes have been reported with malignancies.[399] The salient features of these syndromes are outlined in Tables 57–15 through 57–20. There is great variation in the associations among the cutaneous lesions and the malignancies. In some instances (*e.g.*, acanthosis nigricans, tripe palms, erythema gyratum repens) the cutaneous syndrome is uncommon but usually associated with cancer. In other instances the cutaneous lesions may be common (*e.g.*, bullous lesions, exfoliative dermatitis, erythema multiforme) and be associated with benign disorders or cancers. In some instances (*e.g.*, bullous lesions), the association of the skin lesions and cancer may not be proved. The cutaneous syndrome may always be associated with a particular tumor (*e.g.*, esophageal cancer, tylosis), or the cutaneous le-

sions may be associated with various neoplasms (*e.g.*, dermatomyositis). The cause of the cutaneous lesion is well known in some instances (*e.g.*, hirsutism in adrenal or ovarian tumors or flushing in carcinoid tumors), but in most, the mechanism is unknown.

Because many cutaneous paraneoplastic syndromes are proliferative, a causal role for tumor-secreted growth factors has been suggested. Ellis and coworkers demonstrated that malignant melanoma cells secreted transforming growth factor-α (TGF-α). This growth factor bound to normal epidermal growth factor receptor-bearing epidermal cells, producing acanthosis nigricans, the sign of Leser-Trelat, and multiple acrochordons.[8] As with some neurologic paraneoplastic syndromes, there may be an immunologic mechanism, as described with paraneoplastic pemphigus.

PATIENT EVALUATION

The evaluation of cutaneous lesions suspected of being paraneoplastic begins with the clinical history, with particular emphasis on drug and other exposures, associated medical conditions, and family history. An evaluation for an underlying cancer should be undertaken only if there is no evidence of drug exposure. Many of the cutaneous syndromes are hereditary. The onset of symptoms in the paraneoplastic cutaneous lesions often is more rapid than in other benign conditions (*e.g.*, dermatomyositis, malignant down, or erythema gyratum repens). The physical examination is of critical importance. For example, while café au lait spots are not always associated with von Recklinghausen's disease, the finding of six or more café au lait spots greater than 1.5 cm in diameter or the presence of axillary freckling are diagnostic aids for the earlier recognition of neurofibromatosis.[402]

Laboratory evaluations are helpful for cutaneous lesions suspected of being metabolic (*e.g.*, hyperpigmentation in Cushing's and Addison's disease). Skin biopsy is the most important procedure for establishing the correct diagnosis and should be performed in most instances; it may provide important information. For example, exfoliative dermatitis in patients with mycosis fungoides may be associated with infiltration of the skin, as in the Sézary syndrome, but may occur in patients with uninvolved skin areas. It may occur in these patients as a result of treatment with chemotherapy or electron-beam radiotherapy.

The differential diagnosis for cutaneous lesions of possible paraneoplastic origin includes benign, nonrelated skin conditions, cutaneous lesions resulting from a primary tumor or its metastases, cutaneous infections, and toxicity from anticancer therapy (particularly cytotoxic chemotherapy or radiotherapy). Numerous cytotoxic chemotherapeutic agents have mucocutaneous toxicities. Although a detailed discussion is beyond the scope of this chapter, an excellent review is available.[403]

Pigmented Lesions

Of special interest is acanthosis nigricans.[8,404-406] This skin lesion is characterized by the presence of symmetric brown areas of hyperpigmentation with hyperkeratosis, exaggerated skin markings, and warty lesions, particularly in the intertriginous and flexural areas such as the axilla, neck, anogenital

TABLE 57–15. Pigmented Lesions and Keratoses

Disorder	Investigations	Description	Predominant Malignancy	Cause	Comments
Acanthosis nigricans*	Brown[404] Curth[405] Ellis[8] Matsuoka[406]	Hyperkeratosis and pigmentation, especially of axillae, neck, flexures, and anogenital region	Gastric 60%; abdominal 90%; other	Unknown	Important to differentiate benign forms present from birth and benign forms associated with various syndromes
Tripe palms	Cohen[406a]	Exaggerated ridges and tumors on palms	Lung; gastric	Unknown	Often associated with acanthosis nigricans. Strongly associated with comar (94%).
Leser-Trelat*	Dantzig[408] Ronchese[409] Snedden[407] Holdiness[410] Curry[411]	Sudden showing of large numbers of seborrheic (wart-like) keratoses	NHL; miscellaneous GI adenocarcinomas	Unknown	Must be differentiated from multiple seborrheic keratoses, which are common and may not be associated with malignancy; occasionally associated with acanthosis nigricans
Bowen's disease	Graham[412] Anderson[413]	A persistent, progressive, nonelevated red, scaly, or crusted plaque caused by an intraepidermal neoplasm	Lung; GI; GU; skin	Generally unknown; arsenic exposure in some cases	25% developed systemic cancers an average of 5 years after initial skin lesions, but significance of association has been questioned
Chronic arsenism	Minkowsky[414]	A corn-like, punctate keratosis more profuse on the extremities and characteristically affecting the palms and feet	Lung; miscellaneous	Chronic exposure to arsenic	Not a true paraneoplastic lesion
Generalized melanosis	Fitzpatrick[415] Helm[400]	A diffuse darkening of the skin with a ruddy gray color secondary to chronic liver disease; generalized blue-gray appearance	Lymphoma; hepatoma; metastatic liver tumors, melanoma	Melanin deposits in dermis	Also seen in a variety of benign conditions; may be rapid at onset
Paget's disease	Ashikari[416]	Erythematous keratotic patch over areola, nipple, or accessory breast tissue	Breast	Paget cells are either migrants from the carcinoma or Langerhans' cells	Occurs in fewer than 3% of breast cancers
Bazex's disease*	Braverman[401] Witkowski[417] Wishart[418] Bolognia[418a]	Erythema hyperkeratosis with scales and pruritus predominantly on palms and soles.	Head and neck, esophagus, lung, especially squamous histology, GI	Unknown, may be immunologic	Males only; responds to removal of primary tumor and may respond to etretinate (Tegason)
Sweet's syndrome*	Cohen[315]	Fever, neutrophilia, multiple painful cutaneous plaques and neutrophilic dermal infiltrate	Hematologic malignancies, various carcinomas	Section of a lymphokine such as IL-1 (?)	Rapid response to steroids; 10–15% associated with cancer

* True paraneoplastic syndromes.[315]

TABLE 57–16. Erythemas

Disorder	Investigations	Description	Predominant Malignancy	Cause	Comments
Erythema gyratum repens*	Purdy[420] Gammell[419] Summerly[421] Appell[421a]	Rapidly changing and advancing gyri with scaling and pruritus; wood grain appearance	Breast, lung, other	Unknown	Almost always associated with malignancy
Erythema annulare centrifugum	Lazar[422]	Slowly migrating annular and configurate erythematous lesions	Prostate, myeloma, other	Unknown	Occurs also with infections and other disorders
Necrolytic migratory erythema (glucagonoma)*	Wilkinson[423] Church[424]	Circinate and gyrate areas of blistering and erosive erythema on limbs; stomatitis	Islet cell on pancreas	Glucagonoma or other metabolic product	See chapter on islet cell tumors
Flushing*	Sjoerdsma[425] Mason[426]	Episodic flushing of face and neck	Carcinoids, medullary carcinoma of thyroid	Serotonin or other vasoactive peptides	See chapter on carcinoids
Exfoliative dermatitis†	Abrahams[427] Nicolis[428] Helm[400]	Progressive erythema followed by scaling	Cutaneous T-cell lymphomas, NHL, Hodgkin's disease, non-Hodgkin's lymphoma	Unknown	Account for 10–20% of all exfoliative dermatitis
Erythema multiforme	Elias[429]	Distinctive target lesions in symmetric distribution, sometimes with plaques or bullae			

* True paraneoplastic syndromes.
† True neoplastic syndrome only in some instances.

TABLE 57–17. Endocrine and Metabolic Lesions

Disorder	Investigations	Description	Predominant Malignancy	Cause	Comments
Systemic nodular pannicutitis* (nodular relapsing fat necrosis; Weber-Christian disease*)	Fitzpatrick[430]	Recurrent crops of tender erythematous subcutaneous nodules; may be accompanied by abdominal pain, fat necrosis in bone marrow, lungs, and other organs	Adenocarcinoma of pancreas	Effect of pancreatic enzymes released into circulation on fatty tissues	Usually associated with pancreatic disease but may be benign pancreatic disease
Porphyria cutanea tarda*	Weddington[431] Thompson[432]	Photosensitive skin lesions, often painful or pruritic	Liver	Increased porphyrins in skin tissues	Rare
Cushing's syndrome		Broad purple striae, atrophy, hyperpigmentation (uncommon), plethora, telangiectasia, mild hirsutism	Ectopic lung (small cell), thyroid, testes, ovary, adrenal tumors; pancreatic islet cell, pituitary, other	Increased ACTH	
Addison's syndrome		Generalized hyperpigmentation, especially scars, pressure points, points of friction; increased amounts of hair	Adrenal gland invasion, lymphomas or carcinomas	Decreased glucocorticoids	Rarely caused by tumors invading the adrenal
Hirsutism			Adrenal tumors, ovarian tumors	Increased glucocorticoid, increased testosterone	Associated with virilism

* True paraneoplastic syndrome.

TABLE 57–18. Bullous and Urticarial Lesions

Disorders	Investigations	Description	Predominant Malignancy	Cause	Comments
Pemphigoid	Stone[433] Anhalt[433a]	Large tense bullae with histologically absent acantholysis	Lymphomas, miscellaneous	Autoantibodies that react with an antigen complex composed of desmoplakin I, the bullous pemphigoid antigens and two unidentified antigens	Although the clinical association of bullous pemphigoid and malignancy was once accepted, recent age-matched studies have failed to support the association
Dermatitis herpetiformis	Tobias[434] Helm[400]	Pleomorphic symmetric subepidermal bullae particularly with scarring	Lymphomas, miscellaneous	Related to autoantibodies	

region, umbilicus, and areola. The salient features are shown in Table 57–15. The lesions of Leser-Trelat with multiple seborrheic keratoses have been described in patients with acanthosis nigricans (see Table 57–15), and both may be produced by tumor secretion of TGF-α.[8,407] There is a strong association between acanthosis nigricans and malignancy, with more than half of all reported cases having cancer. However, the acanthosis nigricans may precede, occur simultaneously with, or occur after the diagnosis of malignancy has been made. There are several documented cases of regression after surgical tumor removal. The most frequent association is with adenocarcinomas of the gastrointestinal tract (92%), particularly of the stomach (50–60%). However, the lesions have been reported in a variety of other tumors, including breast cancer, lymphomas, and squamous carcinomas.[404,405]

The most important part of the differential diagnosis is to differentiate between true acanthosis nigricans associated with malignancy, benign acanthosis, and pseudoacanthosis. Benign acanthosis is a nevoid condition present at birth or beginning in childhood and associated with several benign syndromes. Pseudoacanthosis occurs in obese persons, especially those with dark complexions. It may occur in patients with gigantism, acromegaly, Stein-Leventhal syndrome, or diabetes mellitus. It may develop after prolonged administration of corticosteroids, diethylstilbestrol, or nicotinic acid. Insulin resistance is common in these patients. However, insulin resistance caused by the development of antibodies against the insulin receptor has been reported in acanthosis nigricans associated with malignancy (e.g., pheochromocytoma).[406] Because of the strong association of acanthosis and cancer, patients developing true acanthosis nigricans after the age of 40 should be evaluated for malignancy, including a thorough evaluation of the gastrointestinal tract, lymph nodes, and breasts. Tripe palms is the appearance of exaggerated dermatoglyphics on the palmar surfaces of the palms and fingers.[406a] The palms may have a thickened velvety appearance, exaggeration of ridges and furrows and brown hyperpigmentation. In a review of the world's literature, 94% of cases occurred in patients with cancer.[406a] Tripe palms occurred with acanthosis nigricans in 77% of patients and alone in 23%. The common malignancies were lung and gastric cancers in

about half the cases. Trip palms were the presenting feature of a previously undiagnosed cancer in 40% of cases.[406a]

Although more rare than acanthosis nigricans, the sudden development and rapid increase in size of seborrheic keratoses (sign of Leser-Trelat) are strongly associated with malignancy, particularly of the gastrointestinal tract.[407,408] As with many cutaneous paraneoplastic syndromes, the most important feature is the rapid change, because multiple seborrheic keratoses may be common, especially in older age groups.

Salient features of other pigmented or proliferative lesions are summarized in Table 57–15.

Erythemas

The major features of erythemas associated with malignancy are summarized in Table 57–16. Erythema gyratum repens is usually associated with malignancy, and necrolytic migratory erythema is pathognomonic of glucagonoma. Exfoliative dermatitis can be caused by a variety of malignancies, drug reactions, or unknown causes.[400,427,428] Various studies report that 10% to 20% of cases may be associated with malignancy, particularly lymphomas. In some instances, the skin lesions are not paraneoplastic, because cutaneous infiltration of the skin can be documented by skin biopsy. In some instances, there is no demonstrable cutaneous tumor, and the condition may improve after therapy, and the skin condition appears to be a true paraneoplastic syndrome. Although the mechanism is unknown, some have speculated that there is an immunologic response to some antigenic material derived from the tumor.[400]

Endocrine and Metabolic Lesions and Bullous and Urticarial Lesions

Important skin lesions associated with endocrine and metabolic tumors (Table 57–17) are systemic nodular panniculitis, with adenocarcinoma of the pancreas, and porphyria cutanea tarda, with hepatomas. The associations of malignancy with bullous and urticarial lesions are not completely proven (Table 57–18). However, Anhalt and colleagues described 5 patients with cancer who had a novel acantholytic skin disease char-

TABLE 57–19. Miscellaneous Lesions

Disorder	Investigations	Description	Predominant Malignancy	Cause	Comments
Dermatomyositis*	Williams[465] Arundell[435] DeVere[264] Barnes[265]	Purplish pink erythema, especially of eyelids, neck, and hands	Miscellaneous	Unknown	Malignant disease reported in 7–50%; precedes carcinoma by days to years with an average of 6 mo
Hypertrichosis languginosa* (malignant down)	Lyell[436] Hegedus[437]	Rapid development of fine, long, silky hair, especially on ears and forehead and may involve the entire body	Lung, colon, bladder, uterus, gall bladder	Unknown	High association with cancer
Acquired ichthyosis*	VanDijk[438] Flint[439]	Generalized dry, crackling skin, hyperkeratotic palms and soles, rhomboidal scales	Hodgkin's disease, other lymphomas, multiple myeloma, other	Unknown	Should be differentiated from hereditary form, which occurs before age 20
Pachydermoperi- ostosis*	Vogl[440]	Thickening of skin and creation of new folds; thickened lips, ears, and lids; macroglossia; thick forehead and scalp; clubbing; excessive sweating	Lung (uterus)	Unknown	Occurs also in lung abscess and benign tumors
Pruritus*	Rajka[441] Cormia[442]	Failure to determine an overt or covert cutaneous cause of generalized pruritus necessitates evaluation for a possible underlying systemic disease	Lymphomas, leukemias, multiple myelomas, CNS tumors, abdominal tumors	Unknown	Also associated with many benign diseases
Amyloid deposits		Macroglossia, pinch purpura, superficial waxy yellow and pink elevated nodules	Multiple myeloma, Waldenström's macroglobulinemia	Amyloid deposition in blood vessels and dermis	Also associated with primary systemic amyloid and other benign conditions
Herpes zoster	Schimpff[443] Dolin[444] Huberman[445]	Vesicular eruption in a dermatomal distribution	Hodgkin's disease, non-Hodgkin's lymphomas, chronic lymphocytic leukemia, small cell lung cancer	Immunosuppression	Increased incidence in cancers associated with immunosuppression and after severely immunosuppressive therapy
Caput medusa Thrombophlebitis Gynecomastia					

* True paraneoplastic syndrome.

acterized by autoantibodies that were pathogenic after passive transfer to mice.[433a] The autoantibodies reacted with an antigen complex composed of desmoplakin I, a 230-kd antigen of bullous pamphizoid, and two unidentified epithelial antigens (Table 57–18).

Miscellaneous Lesions

The cutaneous lesions in dermatomyositis are characterized by purple-pink heliotrope erythema of the face with edema of the eyelids, with spread to the neck and arms (Table 57–19). Erythematous purplish papules and plaques over the knuckles and interphalangeal joints (*i.e.*, Grotton's sign) may be characteristic but usually occur late. All types of malignancies have been reported.[264–266,435] Overall, cancers are reported in 7% to 52% of patients with dermatomyositis. There are reports of dramatic improvement in dermatomyositis after antitumor therapy, supporting its identification as a true paraneoplastic syndrome.[266,435]

An important feature of paraneoplastic acquired ichthyosis

TABLE 57–20. Hereditary Disorders

Disorders	Investigations	Description	Predominant Malignancy	Heredity	Comments
Gardner's syndrome	Gardner[446] Bussey[447] Jones[448]	Epidermal cysts, sebaceous cysts, dermoid tumors, lipomas, fibromas	Adenocarcinoma of large or small bowel	Autosomal dominant	Associated with polyposis of colon and bony exostoses
Peutz-Jeghers syndrome	Jeghers[449] Riley[450]	Pigmentation of lips, face, oral mucosa, and digits	GI adenocarcinomas	Autosomal dominant	Low (2–3%) incidence
Tylosis (palmaris and plantaris)	Howel-Evans[451]	Hyperkeratosis of palms and soles after age 10	Esophageal carcinoma	Autosomal dominant	95% incidence of carcinoma by age 65
Multiple mucosal neuromas	Williams[452]	Neuromas of eyelids, lips, tongue, and oral mucosa	Pheochromocytoma, medullary carcinoma of thyroid (MEN II)	Autosomal dominant	Parathyroid adenomas, hypertension common
Cowden's disease—multiple harmartoma syndrome	Lloyd[435]	Fibromas of oral mucosa, acral verucous papulas, trichilemmomas of the face	Thyroid, breast carcinomas	Autosomal dominant	Associated with multiple hamartomas, lipomas, neuromas, hemangiomas, thyroid adenomas
Multiple basal cell neuromas syndrome	Solomon[454]	Multiple basal cell carcinomas, pits on soles and palms	Medulloblastoma, fibrosarcoma (jaw)	Autosomal dominant	Infrequent association with internal malignancy
Neurofibromatosis (von Recklinghausen)	Crowe[402]	Neurofibromas, café au lait spots	Pheochromocytoma	Autosomal dominant	Malignancies develop in a minority of patients
Tuberous sclerosis (Bourneville)	Butterworth[455]	Lipopigmented macules, adenomas, fibromas	Neurologic malignancies	Autosomal dominant	Malignancies develop in a minority of patients
Cerebelloretinal hemangioblastoma (von Hippel-Lindau)	Christoferson[456]	Retinal malformation, papilledema	Neurologic malignancies	Autosomal dominant	Malignancies develop in a minority of patients
Encephalotrigeminal syndrome (Sturge-Weber)	Doll[457]	Capillary or cavernous hemangiomas within the cutaneous distribution of the trigeminal nerve	Neurologic malignancies	Autosomal dominant	Malignancies develop in a minority of patients
Ataxia-telangiectasia	Doll[457] Frizzera[458]	Telangiectasias	Lymphomas, leukemias	Autosomal recessive	IgA ± IgE deficiency; sinopulmonary infections, tumors in <10%
Bloom's syndrome	Helm[402]	Photosensitivity, telangiectasias, erythema of face	Leukemia	Autosomal recessive	Stunted growth, high incidence
Fanconi's anemia	Helm[400]	Patchy hyperpigmentation	Leukemias	Autosomal recessive	High incidence
Chédiak-Higashi syndrome	Doll[456]	Recurrent pyoderma, giant melanosomes, dilution of skin and hair color	Lymphomas	Autosomal recessive	High incidence
Werner's syndrome (adult progeria)	Epstein[459]	Scleroderma-like changes, premature aging, leg ulcers, short stature	Sarcomas, meningiomas, others	Autosomal recessive	Cancers in about 10%
Wiskott-Aldrich syndrome	Doll[457] Frizzeria[458]	Eczematous dermatitis, pyroderma	Lymphomas	Sex linked (males)	>10% incidence
Bruton's sex-linked agammaglobulinemia	Helm[400]	Recurrent infections	Lymphoma, leukemias	Sex linked	>5% incidence

is the rapid development of the lesions. The lesions are characterized by generalized dry cracking skin with hyperkeratotic palms and soles. The acquired forms are associated most often with Hodgkin's disease and other malignant lymphomas, although associations with solid tumors have been reported.[438,439] The acquired forms can be differentiated from genetic forms by the fact that the latter arise usually before the age of 20. A parallel course of the malignant lymphoma and acquired ichthyosis has been reported for many patients.[439]

Hereditary Disorders

Many hereditary disorders associated with malignant disease and skin lesions of presumed paraneoplastic nature are summarized in Table 57–20.

GASTROINTESTINAL PARANEOPLASTIC SYNDROMES

The Zollinger-Ellison, carcinoid, and other syndromes resulting from hormone-producing endocrine tumors are discussed in Chapter 41. One of the most frequent of all the paraneoplastic syndromes is the malignancy associated anorexia and cachexia. It may be caused by a tumor-secreted cytokine, TNF-α.[8-11]

PROTEIN-LOSING ENTEROPATHIES ASSOCIATED WITH MALIGNANCY

More than 90% of cancer patients have low serum albumin levels.[412] Metabolic studies show that this can be due to decreased albumin synthesis, abnormal distribution of albumin in effusions, or increased loss of protein into the gastrointestinal tract (*e.g.*, protein-losing enteropathy).[460] The most common mechanism is decreased albumin synthesis, but why this is so is unknown.[460] Although patients usually present with other signs of malignancy, unexplained edema and hypoproteinemia were the initial manifestations of malignancy in a few patients.

The mechanisms of protein-losing enteropathy include inflammation and ulceration of the gastrointestinal mucosa and exudative loss of proteins; disorders of the intestinal lymphatic channels from neoplastic obstruction (*e.g.*, with lymphomas); congestive failure (*e.g.*, in patients with carcinoid or pericardial construction) with resultant loss of protein and lymphocytes rich in lymph into the gastrointestinal lumen; and a group of undefined mechanisms. The resulting hypoalbuminemia leads to edema, and the lymphopenia decreases cellular immunity with impaired skin test reactivity.[460] Although these syndromes may not fulfill all of the criteria for paraneoplasia (*i.e.*, acting at a distance from the tumor), anecdotal case reports indicate that protein-losing enteropathy can be reversed by appropriate treatment of the underlying tumor. Profuse watery diarrhea, hypokalemia, and hypochlorhydria usually are associated with pancreatic non-β-islet cell tumors or villous adenomas of the rectum. This syndrome can be found in patients with lung cancer, but the mechanism is unknown.[461]

MALABSORPTION

Malabsorption syndromes for several or specific substances may occur by a variety of mechanisms in cancer patients, including side effects of surgery, irradiation, and chemotherapy. Malabsorption often is associated with lymphoma involving the small bowel or with gastric, hepatic, or biliary tract tumors, particularly if biliary obstruction exists. These examples are not remote effects of the tumor. However, some malabsorption syndromes may be paraneoplastic, as suggested by finding histologic abnormalities of the small bowel in as many as 62% of various cancers in some studies.[462-464] Although the exact frequency of the histologic types is unknown, the abnormalities include "flat" mucosa with simple or partial villous atrophy. Subtotal villous atrophy is less common. However, the severity of associated malabsorption does not correlate with the severity of the small bowel histologic changes.[462] The tumors associated with small bowel abnormalities are colon, lung, prostate, and pancreatic cancers and lymphomas. The mechanisms behind the loss of villous height are unknown. Treatment should be directed at the underlying tumor plus administration of exogenous nutrients and vitamins to bypass the malabsorption.

HEPATOPATHY AS A PARANEOPLASTIC SYNDROME

An elevated hepatic alkaline phosphatase level has occurred with a malignant schwannoma and disappeared with surgical resection.[465] This also occurs in hypernephroma, in which there can be reversible abnormalities of liver function not associated with liver metastases.[465-468] Decreased albumin synthesis rises to normal after resection of the renal tumor. Biochemical abnormalities, such as elevated alkaline phosphatase levels or hyperglobulinemia, hypocholesterolemia, and prolonged prothrombin time, and hepatosplenomegaly, have disappeared after primary tumor removal in 4 of 6 patients.[466,468] The mechanisms for the hepatopathy associated with hypernephroma are unknown, but they may include hepatic amyloid or be related to the generalized hepatic hypervascularity seen on angiography or the nonspecific focal periportal inflammation seen on biopsy.[466,467,469] It is important to recognize the hepatopathy syndrome so that these signs are not confused with metastases to the liver. Biopsy confirmation of liver metastases from renal carcinoma is highly desirable if this metastatic site alone would preclude resection of the primary renal tumor for cure.

ANOREXIA, CACHEXIA, AND TASTE ABNORMALITIES AS PARANEOPLASTIC MANIFESTATIONS

Problems with anorexia, taste, weight loss, and cachexia are common in cancer patients.[470,476] One third or more of cancer patients are in negative nitrogen balance; they can even be in positive nitrogen balance and still maintain a caloric deficit.[472] The syndrome comprises anorexia, cachexia, asthenia, loss of body tissue, and inability to conserve normal regulatory functions of metabolism and bears no correlation to the amount, type, or site of neoplastic tissue.[473] It can occur as an early symptom of disease or appear in the presence of bulk neoplasms. The best evidence of the paraneoplastic nature of the anorexia-cachexia syndrome comes when it appears before the malignancy is discovered and disappears with the resection or control of the tumor.[472] Obviously, cancer patients can have these symptoms as a result of therapy toxicity, gross invasion, or obstruction of structures by tumor. Cachexia may result from decreased caloric intake, malabsorption, loss of material from the body (*e.g.*, from effusions, hemorrhage, ulcers), or a change in the body metabolism. Anorexia and taste changes may result in decreased caloric intake. However, a variety of experimental evidence suggests that malnutrition alone cannot explain the cachexia of malignancy.[472] In malignancy and cachexia, the caloric expenditure remains high, and the basal metabolic rate is increased despite the reduced dietary intake, indicating a profound systemic derangement of host metabolism.[472] These findings are in contrast to the lower metabolic rates and adaptation that normal subjects make after starvation.[473] With starvation in normal persons, the caloric expenditure is lowered, amino acids cease being used for gluconeogenesis, and exogenous glucose is readily oxidized, but it is not in malignancy. Protein synthesis is maintained in malignancy rather than reduced as in starvation.

Studies demonstrated that circulatory factors could produce cancer anorexia-cachexia.[474] Other studies demonstrated that the cytokines, TNF-α and IL-1β, could produce a similar syndrome in animals.[475] TNF-α was shown to be identical with cachectin.[8-11] This cytokine inhibits lipoprotein lipase activity in peripheral tissues and may orchestrate the metabolic changes leading to tumor cachexia-anorexia.[457a] Other hypolytic factors produced by tumor cells may be responsible for cancer cachexia in some patients.[475b]

Aversion to meats and other protein-containing food frequently occurs in cancer patients. DeWys found that 16 of 50 cancer patients of various types had an aversion to meat; this was correlated with a lowered threshold for bitter taste (*i.e.*, urea).[471] These patients had elevated thresholds for sweet (*i.e.*, sucrose) substances. The taste abnormalities were correlated with a patient's body burden of tumor and then normalized after response to treatment.[471]

The regulation of hunger and satiety is complex and involves a CNS ''satiety'' center in the ventromedial nuclei of the hypothalamus and a ''feeding'' center in the lateral hypothalamic nuclei.[472] Alimentary tract regulation; glucostatic, lipostatic, thermostatic, and osmotic regulation; hormone regulation by insulin; regulation of growth hormone, glucagon, enterogastrone, adrenal corticosteroids, amino acid levels, and of an as yet unidentified anorexigenic pituitary polypeptides take place.[479] It appears likely that mechanisms underlying the paraneoplastic anorexia-cachexia syndrome involve molecules produced by the tumor that impinge on one or more of the regulatory mechanisms of hunger, satiety, metabolism, or taste and cause the organism to falsely disrupt these patterns and enter into a metabolically chaotic state.[472] The treatment of the underlying tumor appears to be the best general approach to reversing the state of cancer cachexia. The progestin megace may be used in symptomatic patients.

MISCELLANEOUS PARANEOPLASTIC SYNDROMES

FEVER AS A PARANEOPLASTIC SYNDROME

Fever occurs frequently in cancer patients and usually is caused by infection. Although other noninfectious causes (*e.g.*,

drug toxicity, adrenal insufficiency) exist, certain tumors are associated with fever.[477] Of 351 cancer patients, Petersdorf found that 30% developed fever and 5% had fever that could be related only to their cancer.[494] The major associations are with Hodgkin's disease, myxomas, hypernephromas, osteogenic sarcomas, and a variety of other tumors.[478,479] Tumor-associated fever usually is defined as unexplained fever that coincides with tumor growth, disappears promptly on tumor removal or control, and reappears with tumor regrowth. Alternatively, when the fever persists with uncontrolled tumor without any other reasonable cause, the tumor is a likely cause of the fever.[477] In Hodgkin's disease, fever as a systemic symptom suggests a worse prognosis stage-by-stage, and its disappearance is required to document remission of tumor and subsequent cure. There are no data about the influence on prognosis of fever associated with other tumors.

The cause of the tumor-associated fever may be release of pyrogen from tumor cells, normal leukocytes, or a variety of other normal cells that have endogenous pyrogen. For example, the Kupffer cells of the liver contain endogenous pyrogen that could cause fever with hepatoma or with metastases to the liver from other tumors.[480] The pyrogen acts on the hypothalamus to cause some reset of temperature regulation. Tumor cells can produce pyrogen. Bodel showed that five of six hypernephromas placed in vitro released pyrogen into the supernatant medium (detected by injection into a rabbit).[477] Similarly, spleen and lymph node tissue from Hodgkin's disease patients produce pyrogen when cultured into the medium in vitro. However, pyrogen production, although correlated with lymph node involvement, did not correlate with histologic involvement of the spleen or with fever in the patient.[477] It is still unknown whether tumor cells themselves or other normal cells mixed in the incubated specimens produce the pyrogen. IL-6 has been implicated as the pyrogen in some cases and was shown to be released by tumor cells.[477a] Treatment should be directed at the underlying tumor, and the most dramatic remissions of paraneoplastic fever come in successfully treated patients with Hodgkin's disease or hypernephroma.

LACTIC ACIDOSIS

Lactic acidosis usually is associated with acute lymphatic or myelogenous leukemia, Hodgkin's disease, and other lymphomas and responds in parallel with tumor regression to therapy.[481-483] Bicarbonate therapy is often needed.

HYPERLIPIDEMIA

Hyperlipidemia frequently is seen in lymphoma-bearing hamsters and normalizes after tumor treatment.[480] Hyperlipidemias have been seen in multiple myeloma, hepatoma, and colon cancer.[484-486] Total lipid levels of 2 g/dl, cholesterol levels above 500 mg/dl, and triglyceride levels of 580 mg/dl have been found. However, no associated vascular abnormalities have been reported. With myeloma, monoclonal proteins sometimes have reacted with α- or β-lipoproteins or with lipolytic enzymes. The mechanism in the other tumor types is obscure but may involve invasion by tumor.

HYPERTENSION AND HYPOTENSION

Malignant hypertension and hypokalemia associated with apparent tumor production of renin have been reported with lung cancer, hypernephroma, and Wilms' tumor.[487–490] Hypertension recedes with control of the tumor. Endothelin-1 is a potent vasoconstrictor peptide produced by endothelial cells. It has been implicated in the hypertension produced by some cases of hemangioendothelioma, a malignant vascular neoplasm.[490a]

An antihypertension syndrome has been seen with a PGA-secreting renal cell tumor, and abnormally low baroreceptor pressure responses have been seen with intrathoracic carcinomas.[491,492] The latter syndrome appears related to interference of transmission of impulses from intrathoracic stretch receptors, resulting in orthostatic hypotension and abnormalities of sodium excretion.

AMYLASE ELEVATION

Synthesis and secretion of amylase by tumors are uncommon; the tumors have all been lung cancer, usually adenocarcinoma.[493] These tumors make the salivary type of amylase, which allows differentiation from a pancreatic source of the amylase evaluation. The tumor-produced amylase itself apparently does not cause symptoms, but its appearance can lead to great concern and medical evaluation for the presence of pancreatitis or various types of pancreatic fistulas.[493]

HYPERTROPHIC PULMONARY OSTEOARTHROPATHY

Hypertrophic pulmonary osteoarthropathy (HPO) is a paraneoplastic syndrome comprising clubbing of the fingers and toes, periostitis of the long bones, and sometimes a polyarthritis resembling rheumatoid arthritis.[494–497] Periostitis-arthritis produces pain in the knees, wrists, and ankles with tenderness and swelling of the affected bones. Involved bones usually include the distal ends of the tibia, fibula, humerus, radius, or ulna. Hyperemia of the affected joints or hands and feet is seen.[494] The syndrome may precede the discovery of the neoplasm by several months and usually has a fairly defined onset. Patients often do not present with clubbing but appear with joint pain or polyarthritis, and in adult patients presenting with unexplained polyarthritis or joint pain, the HPO syndrome should be kept in mind.[494] Pathologic examination of the joints may show pannus formation; however, most joints show only hyperemia.[494] If polyarthritis is present, joint effusions, particularly of the knees, with noninflammatory synovial fluid and good mucin clot are present. Ossifying periostitis is seen on roentgenogram at the distal end of the shafts of long bones as a thin opaque line of new bone formation, separated from the underlying denser cortex by a narrow radiolucent band. Radionuclide bone scans often are positive over the bones involved with periostitis before the other radiologic changes appear.[498] In advanced cases, other bones (*e.g.*, the ribs, clavicle, iliac crests, vertebral column) may be involved.

Hypertrophic pulmonary osteoarthropathy is encountered most frequently in lung cancer, occurring in 12% of patients with adenocarcinoma and less frequently in other cell types; HPO is almost nonexistent in small cell lung cancer.[499,500] Of interest, the HPO syndrome occurs often with benign mesothelioma and the rare neurolemmomas of the diaphragm, but malignant mesotheliomas are thought never to produce HPO.[494] Other tumors metastatic to the chest can cause HPO, including metastases from renal cancer, thymoma, leiomyoma of the esophagus, intrathoracic Hodgkin's disease, osteogenic sarcoma, fibrosarcoma, and the undifferentiated nasopharyngeal tumors of young people after the tumors metastasize to mediastinal lymph nodes.[501–507]

The diagnosis is made by physical findings, radionuclide bone scan, and radiographic appearance of the bones. Although benign causes should be considered, the bone changes of hyperparathyroidism can simulate HPO and should be ruled out, although it is possible for HPO and ectopic PTH to coexist. The cause is unknown, although estrogens, circulatory factors, neurogenic factors, and growth hormone have been postulated to play a role.[452,457,508–510] Other arthropathies associated with cancer include secondary gout and carcinoma polyarthritis.[507a]

AMYLOIDOSIS

Amyloid deposition (*i.e.*, paraneoplastic β-fibrils) is a pathologic process whose manifestations depend on the formation of a specific, unique protein conformation—the twisted β-pleated sheet fibril.[511] Histochemically, these fibrils have green polarization color after Congo red staining. This structure normally is not found in mammalian tissues and can occur with a variety of proteins produced by several different pathogenic mechanisms. Immunoglobulin fragments produced by plasma cell dyscrasias are the most common neoplastic mechanism. Because of the β-pleated structure, the fibrils are resistant to normal proteolytic digestion under physiologic conditions and accumulate as inert fibrils in tissues. This causes pressure atrophy, morbidity, and death from interference of normal physiologic processes of the affected vital organs (*e.g.*, heart, kidneys, nerves, joints).

Although amyloidosis may have several nonmalignant causes, 15% of cases occur with malignant disease, including multiple myeloma, lymphomas, and carcinomas.[511,513] Amyloid occurs in 6% to 15% of multiple myeloma and Waldenström's macroglobulinemia, in 4% of Hodgkin's disease, and 1% of other lymphomas, and probably all B-cell lymphomas can give rise to amyloidosis. Carcinomas associated with amyloidosis are hypernephromas, bladder and renal pelvic cancer, uterine cervix cancer, and biliary tract cancer.[512] Hypernephroma is reported to represent more than 25% of all tumors associated with amyloidosis, but the nature of the protein in the amyloid deposit of hypernephromas is unknown.[511,512]

The "amyloidogenic" protein can be monoclonal light chains (designated AL) or other proteins (designated AA).[511] Amyloid fibrils from medullary carcinoma of the thyroid contain part of the calcitonin molecule; peptides produced by several tumors, if they contain sequences that can form β-pleated sheets, may cause amyloid.[511] In amyloidosis with multiple myeloma, Bence Jones proteinuria is usually present, and the occurrence is higher in free light-chain myeloma.[511]

The signs and symptoms of amyloidosis of malignancy, particularly with myeloma, are a peripheral neuropathy (*e.g.*, painful stocking-glove condition), autonomic nervous symptoms of sexual impotence, gastrointestinal motility disturbances, orthostatic hypotension, and dyshidrosis.[511] Motor function is impaired from median nerve entrapment, and weight loss is frequent. A restrictive cardiomyopathy, with signs and symptoms of right heart failure with only minimal radiographic evidence of cardiomegaly, occurs. Low-voltage electrocardiographic changes, arrhythmias, conduction disturbances, and electrocardiographic pattern-simulating myocardial infarction may occur. The patients are extremely sensitive to digitalis, and several toxic deaths from this have been reported. Pinch purpura, periorbital purpura after procedures, macroglossia, waxy cutaneous papules, subcutaneous nodules, alopecia, and scleroderma-like skin infiltration may occur. Joint infiltration often produces painless limitation of the range of motion. The large joints are affected in amyloid arthropathy, and the "shoulder pad" sign develops, with massive infiltration of the glenohumeral articulation. Carpal and tarsal tunnel syndromes occur with infiltration of these regions.

The diagnosis of amyloid is made by the demonstration of the characteristic emerald-green birefringence of tissue specimens stained by Congo red and examined by polarization microscopy.[511] Biopsies of infiltrated lesions, gingiva, skin, bone marrow, or rectum can be used. The prognosis of clinically evident amyloidosis with malignancy is poor, and in myeloma, median survival from diagnosis is 14 months or less.[511] There is not good evidence that treatment of myeloma or other neoplastic disorders can reverse the amyloid already deposited, but it probably halts amyloid progression. Supportive care problems abound because the congestive heart failure from amyloid does not respond to digitalis. (Amyloid patients started on digitalis therapy should be hospitalized because of potential toxicity.) Diuretics can cause dehydration and cardiovascular collapse because of concurrent renal damage, postural hypotension, adrenal insufficiency, autonomic neuropathy, and low cardiac output. Mineralocorticoids, elastic stockings, broad-spectrum antibiotics for bacterial overgrowth in bowel with disturbed motility, gastrostomy and tracheostomy for macroglossia, hemodialysis, and surgical decompression of carpal tunnel syndrome have been used.[511]

PALMAR FASCIITIS AND ARTHRITIS

The shoulder-hand syndrome, a variant of reflex sympathetic dystrophy has been reported with malignancy.[514-516] Brain and lung cancers were reported most often, although cancers of the bladder, uterus, breast, and esophagus were described. Palmar fasciitis and arthritis associated with ovarian carcinoma have more dramatic and progressive findings with complete loss of upper-extremity function and contracture. The severe syndrome has been reported in patients with small cell lung cancer, adenocarcinoma of the pancreas, CML, and Hodgkin's disease. The cause is unknown, but immunoglobulin deposits were found in the fascial tissue of a patient, suggesting an immunologic cause. The syndrome often preceded the diagnosis of malignancy and improved after successful antitumor therapy.

ARTHRITIS, POLYMYALGIA RHEUMATICA, SYSTEMIC LUPUS ERYTHEMATOSUS, VASCULITIS

Rheumatoid arthritis or asymmetric polyarthritis may occur with malignancy or may be related by chance.[4,517-519] Joint manifestations regress on removal or control of the underlying malignancy in 48% of patients. About 80% of female patients with asymmetric polyarthritis and malignancy had breast cancer. Some 83% of patients with polymyalgia rheumatica are said to develop a malignancy within 3 months, and some of these cases may represent arterial emboli to muscle from

nonbacterial thrombotic endocarditis. Lymphomas may be associated with systemic rheumatic disease.[519,520] In Sjögren's syndrome, a spectrum of benign to malignant lymphoproliferations can be seen, but whether this is "at a distance from the tumor" remains to be determined.[521] Metastases to joints can simulate rheumatoid arthritis, and cytologic studies should be done on joint effusions in cancer patients.[522,523]

Systemic lupus erythematosus (SLE) is associated with lymphomas, lymphoblastic leukemia, thymomas, testicular and ovarian tumors, and lung cancer, and remission of the SLE often occurs with tumor treatment.[521,524] The syndrome may be caused by an antinuclear antibody recognizing a novel antigen.[575]

In a study of 222 patients with vasculitis, 11 were found to have an associated malignancy.[526] Hematologic malignancies were most common in this and other similar series. The cause of the vasculitis is uncertain but may have an immunologic basis.

REFERENCES

1. Hall TC, ed. Paraneoplastic syndromes. Ann N Y Acad Sci 1974;230:1–577.
2. Odell WD, Wolfsen AR. Humoral syndromes associated with cancer. Ann Rev Med 1978;29:379–406.
3. Blackman MR, Rosen SW, Weintraub BD. Ectopic hormones. Adv Intern Med 1978;23:85–113.
4. Shneider BS, Manalo A. Paraneoplastic syndromes. Unusual manifestations of malignant disease. Dis Month 1979;Feb:1–60.
5. Markman M. Response of paraneoplastic syndromes to antineoplastic therapy. West J Med 1986;144:580–585.
6. Ascensao JL, Oken MM, Ewing SL, et al. Leukocytosis and large cell lung cancer. A frequent association. Cancer 1987;60:903–905.
7. Hocking W, Goodman J, Golde D. Granulocytosis associated with tumor cell production of colony stimulating activity. Blood 1983;61:600–603.
8. Ellis DL, Kafka SP, Chow JC, et al. Melanoma, growth factors, acanthosis nigricans, the sign of Leser-Trelat, and multiple acrochordons. A possible role of alpha-transforming growth factor in cutaneous paraneoplastic syndromes. N Engl J Med 1987;317:1582–1587.
9. Beutler B, Greenwald D, Hulmes JD, et al. Identity of tumor necrosis factor and the macrophage-secreted factor cachectin. Nature 1985;316:552–554.
10. Torti FM, Dieckmann B, Beutler B, et al. A macrophage factor inhibits adipocyte gene expression: An in vitro model of cachexia. Science 1985;229:867–870.
11. Theologides A. Anorexins, asthenins, and cachectins in cancer. Am J Med 1986;81:696–698.
12. Greenlee JE, Lipton HL. Anticerebellar antibodies in serum and cerebrospinal fluid of a patient with oat cell carcinoma of the lung and paraneoplastic cerebellar degeneration. Ann Neurol 1986;19:82–85.
13. Grunwald GB, Kornguth SE, Towfighi J, et al. Autoimmune basis for visual paraneoplastic syndrome in patients with small cell lung carcinoma. Cancer 1987;60:780–786.
14. Graus F, Elkon KB, Cordon-Cardo C, Posner J. Sensory neuronopathy and small cell lung cancer. Antineuronal antibody that also reacts with the tumor. Am J Med 1986;80:45–52.
15. Fukunaga H, Engel AG, Lang B, et al. Passive transfer of Eaton-Lambert myasthenic syndrome with IgG from man to mouse depletes the presynaptic membrane active zones. Proc Natl Acad Sci USA 1983;80:7636–7640.
16. Richardson EP. Progressive multifocal leukoencephalopathy. In: Vinken PJ, Bruryn GW, eds. Handbook of clinical neurology. Amsterdam: Elsevier North-Holland, 1970:485–499.
17. Wiener LP, Henden RM, Narayan O, et al. Virus related to SV40 in patients with progressive multifocal leukoencephalopathy. N Engl J Med 1972;286:385–390.
18. Croft P, Wilkinson M. The incidence of carcinomatous neuromyopathy in patients with various types of carcinoma. Brain 1965;88:427–434.
19. Wilner EC, Brody JA. An evaluation of the remote effects of cancer on the nervous system. Neurology 1967;18:1120–1124.
20. De Larco JE, Todaro GJ. Growth factors from murine sarcoma virus-transformed cells. Proc Natl Acad Sci USA 1978;75:4001–4005.
21. Waldenström JG. Paraneoplasia, biological signals in diagnosis of cancer. New York: John Wiley & Sons, 1978.
22. Odell WD, Wolfsen AR. Hormones from tumors: Are they ubiquitous? Am J Med 1980;68:317–318.
23. Lees LH. The biosynthesis of hormones by nonendocrine tumours—A review. J Endocrinol 1975;67:143–175.
24. Kreiger DT, Martin JB. Brain peptides. N Engl J Med 1981;304:876–885.

25. Kreiger DT. Brain peptides: What, where, and why? Science 1983;222:975–985.
26. Moody TW, Pert CS, Gazdar AF, et al. High levels of intracellular bombesin characterize human small-cell lung carcinoma. Science 1981;214:1246–1248.
27. Maurer LH, O'Donnell JF, Kennedy S, et al. Human neurophysins in carcinoma of the lung. Relation to histology, disease stage, response rate, survival and syndrome of inappropriate antidiuretic hormone secretion. Cancer Treat Rep 1983;67:971–976.
28. Lazarus LH, Di Augustine RP, Jahnke CD, Hernandez O. Physalaemin: An amphibian tachykinin in human lung small cell carcinoma. Science 1983;219:79–81.
29. Richardson RL, Greco FA, Oldhan RK, Liddle GW. Tumor products and potential markers in small cell lung cancer. Semin Oncol 1978;5:253–262.
30. Gropp C, Havemann K, Scheuer A. Ectopic hormones in lung cancer patients at diagnosis and during therapy. Cancer 1980;46:347–354.
31. Hansen M, Hansen HH, Hirsch FR, et al. Hormonal polypeptides and amine metabolites in small cell carcinoma of the lung, with special reference to stage and subtypes. Cancer 1980;45:1432–1437.
32. Odell WD, Wolfsen AR, Bachelot I, Hirose FM. Ectopic production of lipotropin by cancer. Am J Med 1979;66:631–638.
33. Roos BA, Lindall AW, Ells J, et al. Increased plasma and tumor somatostatin-like immunoreactivity in medullary thyroid carcinoma and small cell lung cancer. J Clin Endocrinol Metab 1981;52:187–194.
34. Yamaguchi K, Abe K, Kameya T, et al. Production and molecular size heterogeneity of immunoreactive gastrin-releasing peptide in fetal and adult lungs and primary lung tumors. Cancer Res 1983;43:3932–3939.
35. Carney DN, Ihde DC, Cohen MH, et al. Serum neuron-specific enolase: A marker for disease extent and response to therapy of small cell lung cancer. Lancet 1982;1:583–585.
36. Nakanishi S, Inoue A, Kita T, et al. Nucleotide sequence of cloned cDNA for bovine corticotropin-β-lipotropin precursor. Nature 1979;278:423–427.
37. Bertagna XY, Nicholson WE, Pettengill OS, et al. Corticotropin, lipotropin, and β-endorphin production by a human nonpituitary tumor in culture: Evidence for a common precursor. Proc Natl Acad Sci USA 1978;75:5160–5164.
38. Jeffcoate WJ, Rees LH. Adrenocorticotropin and related peptides in nonendocrine tumors. Curr Top Exp Endocrinol 1978;3:57–74.
39. Guillemin R. Endorphins, brain peptides that act like opiates, N Engl J Med 1977;296:226–228.
40. Huges J. Opioid peptides and their relatives. Nature 1979;278:394–395.
41. Silman RE, Holland D, Chard T, et al. The ACTH "family tree" of the rheusus monkey changes with development. Nature 1978;276:526–528.
42. Hirata Y, Yamamoto H, Matsukura S, Imura H. In vitro release and biosynthesis of tumor ACTH in ectopic ACTH producing tumors. J Clin Endocrinol Metab 1975;41:106–114.
43. Brown WH. A case of pluriglandular syndrome: Diabetes of bearded women. Lancet 1928;2:1022–1023.
44. Rassam JW, Anderson G. Incidence of paramalignant disorders in bronchogenic carcinoma. Thorax 1975;30:86–90.
45. Ross EJ. Endocrine syndromes of non-endocrine origin: Cancer and the adrenal cortex. Proc R Soc Med 1966;59:335–338.
46. Lokich JJ. The frequency and clinical biology of the ectopic hormone syndromes of small cell carcinoma. Cancer 1982;50:2111–2114.
47. Singer W, Kovacs K, Ryan N, Horvath E. Ectopic ACTH syndrome. Clinicopathological correlation. J Clin Pathol 1978;31:591–598.
48. Abeloff MD, Trump DL, Baylin SB. Ectopic adrenocorticotrophic (ACTH) syndrome and small cell carcinoma of the lung: Assessment of clinical implications in patients on combination chemotherapy. Cancer 1981;48:1082–1087.
49. Yallow RS, Eastridge CE, Higgins G Jr, Wolf J. Plasma and tumor ACTH in carcinoma of the lung. Cancer 1979;44:1789–1792.
50. Wolfsen AR, Odell WD. ProACTH. Use for early detection of lung cancer. Am J Med 1979;66:765–772.
51. Liddle GW, Island D, Meador CK. Normal and abnormal regulation of corticotropin secretion in man. Recent Prog Horm Res 1962;18:125–166.
52. Ayvazian LF, Schneider B, Gewirtz G, Yalow RS. Ectopic production of big ACTH in carcinoma of the lung. Its clinical usefulness as a biologic marker. Am Rev Respir Dis 1975;3:279–287.
53. Ratcliff JG, Knight RA, Besser GM. Tumour and plasma ACTH concentrations in patients with and without the ectopic ACTH syndrome. Clin Endocrinol 1972;1:27–44.
54. Gewirtz G, Yalow RS. Ectopic ACTH production in carcinoma of the lung. J Clin Invest 1974;53:1022–1032.
55. Abe K, Adachi I, Miyakawa S, et al. Production of calcitonin, adrenocorticotropic hormone, and β-melanocyte stimulating hormone in tumors derived from amine precursors uptake and decarboxylation cells. Cancer Res 1977;37:4100–4194.
56. Bloomfield GA, Holdaway IM, Corrin B, et al. Lung tumours and ACTH production. Clin Endocrinol 1977;6:95–104.
57. Gilby ED, Rees LH, Bondy PK. Ectopic hormones as markers of response to therapy in cancer. In: Proceedings of the Sixth International Symposium of Biological Characterizations of Human Tumors. New York: American Elsevier, 1976:132–138.
58. Amatruda TT, Upton GV. Hyperadrenocorticism and ACTH-releasing factor. Ann N Y Acad Sci 1974;230:168–180.
59. Eagan RT, Maurer LH, Forcier RJ, Tulloh M. Small cell carcinoma of the lung: Staging, paraneoplastic syndromes, treatment and survival. Cancer 1974;33:527–532.
60. Azzopardi JG, Williams ED. Pathology of "nonendocrine" tumors associated with Cushing's syndrome. Cancer 1968;22:273–286.

61. Skrabanek P, Powell D. Unifying concept of non-pituitary ACTH secreting tumors: Evidence of common origin of neural-crest tumors, carcinoids, and oat-cell carcinomas. Cancer 1978;42:1263–1269.
62. Lojek MA, Fer MF, Kasselberg AG, et al. Cushing's syndrome with small cell carcinoma of the uterine cervix. Am J Med 1980;69:140–144.
63. Matsuyama M, Inoue T, Ariyoshi Y, et al. Argyrophil cell carcinoma of the uterine cervix with ectopic production of ACTH, β-MSH, serotonin, histamine, and amylase. Cancer 1979;44:1813–1823.
64. Levenson RM, Ihde DC, Matthews MJ, et al. Small cell carcinoma presenting as an extrapulmonary neoplasm: Sites of origin and response to chemotherapy. J Natl Cancer Inst 1981;67:607–612.
65. Remick SC, Ruckdiscel JC. Extrapulmonary and pulmonary small cell carcinoma: Tumor biology, therapy and outcome. Med Pediatr Oncol 1992;20:89–99.
66. Rees LH, Ratcliffe JG. Ectopic hormone production by nonendocrine tumors. Clin Endocrinol 1974;3:263–299.
67. Bailey RE. Periodic "hormonogenesis"—a new phenomenon. Periodicity in function of a hormone-producing tumor in man. Clin Endocrinol 1971;32:317–327.
67a. Nieman LK, Chrousos GP, Oldfield EH, et al. The ovine corticotropin-releasing hormone stimulation test and the dexamethasone suppression test in the differential diagnosis of Cushing's syndrome. Ann Intern Med 1986;105:862–867.
68. Gold EM. The Cushing syndromes: Changing views of diagnosis and treatment. Ann Intern Med 1979;90:829–844.
69. Howlett TA, Perry L, Rees LH, et al. Diagnosis and management of ACTH dependent Cushing's syndrome: Comparison of the features in ectopic and pituitary ACTH production. Clin Endocrinol 1986;24:699–713.
69a. Oldfield EH, Deppman JL, Nieman LK, et al. Petrosal sinus sampling with and without corticotropin-releasing hormone for the differential diagnosis of Cushing's syndrome. N Engl J Med 1991;325:897–905.
70. Hattori M, Imura H, Matsukura S, et al. Multiple hormone-producing lung carcinoma. Cancer 1979;43:2429–2437.
71. Mason AMS, Ratcliffe JA, Buckly RM, Mason AS. ACTH secretion by bronchial carcinoid tumors. Clin Endocrinol 1972;1:3–25.
72. Imura H, Matsukura S, Yamamoto H, et al. Studies on ectopic ACTH-producing tumors. II. Clinical and biochemical features of 30 cases. Cancer 1975;35:1430–1437.
73. Corey RM, Varma SK, Drake CR, et al. Ectopic secretion of corticotropin-releasing factor as a cause of Cushing's syndrome. A clinical, morphologic and biochemical study. N Engl J Med 1984;311:13.
74. Belsky JL, Cuello B, Swanson LW, et al. Cushing's syndrome due to ectopic production of corticotropin-releasing factor. J Clin Endocrinol Metab 1985;60:496.
75. Schleingart DE, Lloyd RV, Akil H, et al. Cushing's syndrome secondary to ectopic corticotropin-releasing hormone—adrenocorticotropin secretion. J Clin Endocrinol Metab 1986;63:770.
76. Orth DN, Liddle GW. Results of treatment of 108 patients with Cushing's syndrome. N Engl J Med 1971;285:243–247.
77. Gordon P, Becker CE, Levey GS, Roth J. Efficacy of aminoglutethimide in the ectopic ACTH syndrome. J Clin Endocrinol Metab 1968;28:921–923.
78. Carey RM, Orth DN, Hartmann WH. Malignant melanoma with ectopic production of adrenocorticotrophic hormone: Palliative treatment with inhibitors of adrenal steroid biosynthesis. J Clin Endocrinol Metab 1973;36:482–487.
79. Vaughn CB, Pearson S, Chapman J, et al. The treatment of ACTH paraneoplastic syndrome with aminoglutethimide. J Natl Med Assoc 1979;71:21–23.
80. Child DF, Burke CW, Burley DM, et al. Drug control of Cushing's syndrome. Combined aminoglutethiamide and metapyrone therapy. Acta Endocrinol 1976;82:330–341.
81. Naber D, Pickar D, Dionne RA, et al. Assay of endogenous opiate receptor ligands in human CSF and plasma. Subst Alcohol Actions Misuse 1980;1:83–91.
82. Gropp C, Havemann K, Scharfe T, Ax W. Incidence of circulating immune complexes in patients with lung cancer and their effect on antibody dependent cytotoxicity. Oncology 1980;37:71–76.
83. Winkler WA, Crankshaw OF. Chloride depletion in conditions other than Addison's disease. J Clin Invest 1938;17:1–6.
84. Schwartz WDF, Bennett W, Curelop S, Bartter F. A syndrome of renal sodium loss and hyponatremia probably resulting from inappropriate secretion of antidiuretic hormone. Am J Med 1957;23:529–542.
85. Amatruda TT, Mulrow PJ, Gallagher JC, Sawyer WH. Carcinoma of the lung with inappropriate antidiuresis. N Engl J Med 1963;269:544–549.
86. Hamilton BPM, Upton GV, Amatruda TT. Evidence for the presence of neurophysins in tumors producing the syndrome of inappropriate antidiuresis. J Clin Endocrinol Metab 1972;35:764–767.
87. Cheng KW, Friesen HG. Physiological factors regulating secretion of neurophysin. Metabolism 1970;19:876–890.
88. Maurer LH, O'Donnell JF, Kennedy S, et al. Human neurophysins in carcinoma of the lung: Relation to histology, disease stage, response rate, survival and syndrome of inappropriate anti-diuretic hormone secretion. Cancer Treat Rep 1983;67:970–976.
89. Trump DL, Baylin SB. Ectopic hormone syndromes. In: Abeloff MD, ed. Complications of cancer: Diagnosis and management. Baltimore: Johns Hopkins University Press, 1979:211–241.
90. Moses AM, Miller M, Streeten DHP. Pathophysiologic and pharmacologic alterations in the release and action of ADH. Metabolism 1976;25:697–721.
91. Goodman LS, Gilman A, Gilman AG, Koelle GB. The Pharmacological basis of therapeutics. 5th ed. New York: MacMillan, 1975.
92. Fichman M, Bethune J. Effects of neoplasms on renal electrolyte function. Ann N Y Acad Sci 1974;230:448–472.

93. Padfield PL, Morton JJ, Brown JJ, et al. Plasma arginine vasopressin in the syndrome of antidiuretic hormone excess associated with bronchogenic carcinoma. Am J Med 1976;61:825–831.

94. Harlow PJ, DeClerck YA, Shore NA, et al. A fatal case of inappropriate ADH secretion induced by cyclophosphamide therapy. Cancer 1979;44:896–898.

95. DeFronzo RA, Braine H, Colvin OM, Davis PJ. Water intoxication in man after cyclophosphamide therapy: Time course and relation to drug activation. Ann Intern Med 1973;78:861–869.

96. Thomas TH, Morgan DB, Swaminathan R, et al. Severe hyponatremia. Lancet 1978;1: 621–624.

97. Radice PA, Dermody WC. Clonal heterogeneity of hormone produced by continuous cultures of small cell carcinoma of the lung. Proceedings of the American Association for Cancer Research and American Society of Clinical Oncology 1980;21:41.

98. Pettengill OS, Caulkner CS, Wurster-Hill DH, et al. Isolation and characterization of a hormone-producing cell line from human small cell anaplastic carcinoma of the lung. JNCI 1977;58:511–518.

99. Hainsworth JD, Workman R, Greco FA. Management of the syndrome of inappropriate antidiuretic hormone secretion in small cell lung cancer. Cancer 1983;51:161–165.

100. Comis RL, Miller M, Ginsberg SJ. Abnormalities in water homeostasis in small cell anaplastic lung cancer. Cancer 1980;45:2414–2421.

101. Munro AHG, Crompton GK. Inappropriate antidiuretic hormone secretion in oat cell carcinoma of bronchus: Aggravation of hyponatremia by intravenous cyclophosphamide. Thorax 1972;27:640–642.

102. Cohen MH, Bunn PA Jr, Ihde DC, et al. Chemotherapy rather than demeclocycline for inappropriate secretion of antidiuretic hormone. N Engl J Med 1978;298:1423.

103. North WG, Maurer H, O'Donnell JF. Human neurophysins and small cell carcinoma. Clin Res 1979;27:390A.

104. Hantman D, Rossier B, Zohlman R, Schrier R. Rapid correction of hyponatremia in the syndrome of inappropriate secretion of antidiuretic hormone. An alternative treatment to hypertonic saline. Ann Intern Med 1973;78:870–875.

105. Forrest JN Jr, Cox M, Hong C, et al. Superiority of demeclocycline over lithium in the treatment of chronic syndrome of inappropriate secretion of antidiuretic hormone. N Engl J Med 1978;298:173–177.

106. DeTroyer A. Demeclocycline treatment for syndrome of inappropriate antidiuretic hormone secretion. JAMA 1977;237:2823–2826.

107. White MG, Fetner DC. Treatment of the syndrome of inappropriate secretion of antidiuretic hormone with lithium carbonate. N Engl J Med 1975;292:390–392.

108. Decaux G, Brimioulle S, Genette F, Mockel J. Treatment of the syndrome of inappropriate secretion of antidiuretic hormone by urea. Am J Med 1980;69:99–106.

109. Cogan E, Debieve M-F, Philipart I, et al. High plasma levels of atrial natriuretic factor in SIADH. Lancet 1986;2:1258–1259.

110. Kamoi K, Ebe T, Hasegawa A, et al. Hyponatremia in small cell lung cancer. Mechanisms not involving inappropriate ADH secretion. Cancer 1987;60:1089–1093.

111. Trump DL. Abnormalities of bone and mineral metabolism. In: Abeloff MD, ed. Complications of cancer. Diagnosis and management. Baltimore: Johns Hopkins University Press, 1979:263–281.

112. Myers WPL. Differential diagnosis of hypercalcemia and cancer. CA 1977;27:258–272.

113. Isales C, Carcangiu ML, Stewart AF. Hypercalcemia in breast cancer. Reassessment of the mechanism. Am J Med 1987;82:1143–1147.

114. Holtz G, Johnson TR Jr, Schrock ME. Paraneoplastic hypercalcemia in ovarian tumors. Obstet Gynecol 1979;54:483–487.

115. Cryer PE, Kissane JM. Clinicopathologic conference. Malignant hypercalcemia. Am J Med 1979;65:486–494.

116. Bunn PA, Schechter GP, Blayney DP, et al. Clinical course of retrovirus-associated adult T-cell lymphoma in the United States. N Engl J Med 1983;309:257–262.

117. Moseley JM, Kubota M, Diefenbach-Jagger H, et al. Parathyroid hormone related protein purified from a human lung cancer cell line. Proc Natl Acad Sci USA 1987;84: 5048–5052.

118. Tashjian AH, Voelkel EF, Levine L. Evidence that the bone resorption-stimulating factor produced by mouse fibrosarcoma cells is prostaglandin E₂: A new model for the hypercalcemia of cancer. J Exp Med 1972;135:1329–1343.

119. Voelkel EF, Tashjian AH Jr, Franklin R, et al. Hypercalcemia and tumor-prostaglandins: The VX2 carcinoma model in the rabbit. Metabolism 1975;24:973–986.

120. Budayr WJ, Nissenson RA, Klein RF, et al. Increased serum levels of a parathyroid hormone-like protein in malignancy-associated hypercalcemia. Ann Intern Med 1989;111:807–812.

121. Stewart AF, Broadus AE. Clinical review 16: Parathyroid related proteins: Coming of age in the 1990s. J Clin Endocrinol Metab 1990;71:1410–1414.

122. Burtis WJ, Brady TG, Orloff JJ, et al. Immunochemical characterization of circulating parathyroid hormone-related protein in patients with humoral hypercalcemia of malignancy. N Engl J Med 1990;322:1106–1112.

123. Horton JE, Raisz LG, Simmons HA, et al. Bone resorbing activity in supernatant fluid from cultured human peripheral blood leukocytes. Science 1972;177:793–795.

124. Luben RA, Mundy GR, Trummel CL, Raisz LG. Partial purification of osteoclast-activating factor from phytohemagglutinin-stimulated human leukocytes. J Clin Invest 1974;53:1473–1480.

125. Mundy GR, Raisz LG, Cooper RA, et al. Evidence for the secretion of an osteoclast stimulating factor in myeloma. N Engl J Med 1974;291:1041–1046.

126. Elion G, Mundy GR. Direct resorption of bone by human breast cancer cells in vitro. Nature 1978;276:726–728.

127. Koeffler HP, Mundy GR, Golde DW, Cline MJ. Production of bone-resorbing activity in poorly differentiated monocytic malignancy. Cancer 1978;41:2438–2443.

128. Seyberth HW. Prostaglandin-mediated hypercalcemia: A paraneoplastic syndrome. Klin Wochenschr 1978;56:373–387.

129. Brereton HD, Halushka PV, Alexander RW, et al. Indomethacin-responsive hypercalcemia in a patient with renal-cell adenocarcinoma. N Engl J Med 1975;29:83–85.

130. Robertson RP, Baylink DJ, Marini JJ, Adkison HW. Elevated prostaglandins and suppressed parathyroid hormone associated with hypercalcemia and renal cell carcinoma. J Clin Endocrinol Metab 1975;41:164–167.

131. Ito H, Sanada T, Katayama T, Shimazaki J. Indomethacin-responsive hypercalcemia. N Engl J Med 1975;293:558–559.

132. Seyberth HW, Segre GV, Morgan JL, et al. Prostaglandins as mediators of hypercalcemia associated with certain types of cancer. N Engl J Med 1975;293:1278–1283.

133. Tashjian AH Jr. Prostaglandins, hypercalcemia and cancer. N Engl J Med 1975;293: 1317–1318.

134. Shigeno C, Yamamoto I, Dokoh S, et al. Identification of 1,24-dihydroxyvitamin D₃-like bone-resorbing lipid in a patient with cancer-associated hypercalcemia. J Clin Endocrinol Metab 1985;61:761–768.

135. Rosenthal N, Insogua KL, Godsall JW, et al. Elevations in circulating 1,25-dihydroxy-vitamin D in three patients with lymphoma-associated hypercalcemia. J Clin Endocrinol Metab 1985;60:29–33.

136. Frankel TL, Mason RS, Hersey P, et al. The synthesis of vitamin D metabolites by human melanoma cells. J Clin Endocrinol Metab 1983;57:627–630.

137. Raskin P, McClain CJ, Medsger TA. Hypocalcemia associated with metastatic bone disease. Arch Intern Med 1973;132:539–543.

138. Sackner MA, Spivak AP, Balian LJ. Hypocalcemia in the presence of osteoblastic metastases. N Engl J Med 1960;262:173–176.

139. Hall TC, Griffiths CT, Petranek JR. Hypocalcemia: An unusual metabolic complication of breast cancer. N Engl J Med 1966;275:1474–1477.

140. Jackson HJ, Taylor FHL. Calcium, potassium, and inorganic phosphate content of the serum in cancer patients. Effect of roentgen ray radiation on the level of these substances in the blood of cancer patients. Am J Cancer 1933;19:379–388.

141. Ehrlich M, Goldsten M, Heinemann HO. Hypocalcemia, hypoparathyroidism and osteoblastic metastases. Metabolism 1963;12:516–526.

142. Gordon GS. Hyper-and hypocalcemia: Pathogenesis and treatments. Ann N Y Acad Sci 1974;230:181–186.

143. Salassa RM, Jowsey J, Arnaud C. Hypophosphatemia osteomalacia associated with "nonendocrine" tumors. N Engl J Med 1970;283:65–69.

144. Stanbury W. Tumor-associated hypophosphatemia, osteomalacia and rickets. Clin Endocrinol Metabol 1972;1:256–259.

145. Daniels RA, Weisenfeld I. Tumorous phosphaturic osteomalacia. Report of a case associated with multiple hemangiomas of bone. Am J Med 1979;67:155–159.

146. Siris ES, Clemens TL, Dempster DW, et al. Tumor-induced osteomalacia. Kinetics of calcium, phosphorus, and vitamin D metabolism and characteristics of bone histomorphometry. Am J Med 1987;82:307–312.

147. Olefsky J, Compson R, Jones H, Reaven G. "Tertiary" hyperparathyroidism, and apparent "cure" of vitamin D resistant rickets after removal of an ossifying mesenchymal tumor of the pharynx. N Engl J Med 1972;286:740–746.

148. Evans DJ, Azzopardi JG. Distinctive tumours of bone and soft tissue causing acquired vitamin-D-resistant osteomalacia. Lancet 1972;1:353–354.

149. Taylor HC, Velasco ME, Fallan MD. Oncogenic osteomalacia and inappropriate antidiuretic hormone secretion due to oat cell carcinoma. Ann Intern Med 1984;101: 786–788.

150. Ryan EA, Reiss E. Oncogenous osteomalacia. Review of the world literature of 42 cases and report of two new cases. Am J Med 1984;77:501–512.

151. Tashjian AH, Wolfe HJ, Voelkel EF. Human calcitonin: Immunologic assay, cytologic localization and studies of medullary thyroid carcinoma. Am J Med 1974;56:840–849.

152. Silva OL, Broder LE, Doppman JL, et al. Calcitonin as a marker for bronchogenic cancer: A prospective study. Cancer 1979;44:680–684.

153. Becker KL, Nash DR, Silva OL, et al. Urine calcitonin levels in patients with bronchogenic carcinoma. JAMA 1980;243:670–672.

154. Ellison M, Woodhouse D, Hillyard C, et al. Immunoreactive calcitonin production by human lung carcinoma cells in culture. Br J Cancer 1975;32:373–379.

155. Bertagna XY, Nicholson WE, Pettengill OS, et al. Ectopic production of high molecular weight calcitonin and corticotropin by human small cell carcinoma cells in tissue culture: Evidence for separate precursors. J Clin Endocrinol Metab 1978;47:1390–1393.

156. Lips CJ, Vander Sluys V, Van Der Donk JA, Van Dam RH. Common precursor molecule as origin for the ectopic-hormone-producing tumor syndrome. Lancet 1978;1:16–18.

157. Hillyard V, Coombes RC, Greenberg PB, et al. Calcitonin in breast and lung cancer. Clin Endocrinol 1976;5:1–8.

158. Iacangelo A, Affolter HV, Eiden LE, et al. Bovine chromogranin A sequence and distribution of its messenger RNA in endocrine tissues. Nature 1986;323:82–86.

159. Sobol RE, O'Connor DT, Addison J, et al. Elevated serum chromogranin A concentrations in small cell lung cancer. Ann Intern Med 1986;105:698–700.

160. O'Connor DT, Deftos LI. Secretion of chromogranin A by peptide producing endocrine neoplasms. N Engl J Med 1986;314:1145–1151.

161. Huttner WB, Benedum UM. Chromogranin A and pancreastatin. Nature 1987;325: 305.

162. Eiden LE. Is chromagranin a prohormone? Nature 1987;325:301.

163. Vaitukaitis JL, Ross GT, Braunstein GD, Rayford PL. Gonadotropins and their subunits: Basic and clinical studies. Recent Prog Horm Res 1976;32:289–321.

164. Kenimer JG, Hershman JM, Higgins HP. The thyrotropin in hydatidiform moles is human chorionic gonadotropin. J Clin Endocrinol Metab 1975;40:481–491.

165. Nisula BC, Ketelslegers JM. Thyroid-stimulating activity and chorionic gonadotropin. J Clin Invest 1974;54:494–499.

166. Faiman C, Colwell JA, Ryan RJ, et al. Gonadotropin secretion from a bronchogenic carcinoma. N Engl J Med 1967;277:1395–1399.

167. Fusco FD, Rosen SW. Gonadotropin-producing anaplastic large-cell carcinomas of the lung. N Engl J Med 1966;275:507–515.

168. Anderson T, Waldmann TA, Glatstein E. Testicular germ-cell neoplasms: Recent advances in diagnosis and therapy. Ann Intern Med 1979;90:373–385.

169. Lewis JL. Chemotherapy of gestational choriocarcinoma. Cancer 1972;30:1517–1521.

170. Blackman MR, Weintraub BD, Rosen SW, et al. Human placental and pituitary glycoprotein hormones and their subunits as tumor markers: A quantitative assessment. JNCI 1980;65:81–93.

171. Tsuruhara T, Dufau ML, Hickman J, Catt KJ. Biological properties of hCG after removal of terminal sialic acid and galactose residues. Endocrinology 1972;91:296–301.

172. Muggia FM, Rosen SW, Weintraub BD, Hansen HH. Ectopic placental proteins in nontrophoblastic tumors: Serial measurements following chemotherapy. Cancer 1975;36:1327–1337.

173. Kahn CR, Rosen SW, Weintraub BD, et al. Ectopic production of chorionic gonadotropin and its subunits by islet cell tumors: A specific marker for malignancy. N Engl J Med 1977;197:565–569.

174. Bender RA, Weintraub BD, Rosen SW. Prospective evaluation of two tumor-associated proteins in pancreatic adenocarcinoma. Cancer 1979;45:591–595.

175. Broder LE, Weintraub BD, Rosen SW, et al. Placental proteins and their subunits as tumor markers in prostatic carcinoma. Cancer 1977;40:211–216.

176. Metz SA, Weintraub B, Rosen SW, et al. Ectopic secretion of chorionic gonadotropin by a lung carcinoma. Pituitary gonadotropin and subunit secretion and prolonged chemotherapeutic remission. Am J Med 1978;65:325–333.

177. Tashjian AH Jr, Weintraub BD, Barowksy NJ, et al. Subunits of human chorionic gonadotropin: Unbalanced synthesis and secretion by clonal cell strains derived from a bronchogenic carcinoma. Proc Natl Acad Sci USA 1973;70:1419–1422.

178. Rosen SW, Weintraub BD, Aaronson SA. Nonrandom ectopic protein production by malignant cells: Direct evidence in vitro. J Clin Endocrinol Metab 1980;50:834–841.

179. Blackman MR, Weintraub BD, Rosen SW, Harmen SM. Comparison of the effects of lung cancer, benign lung disease, and normal aging on pituitary—gonadal function in men. J Clin Endocrinol Metab 1988;66:88–95.

179a. Rudnick P, Odell WD. In search of a cancer. N Engl J Med 1971;284:405–408.

180. Skrabanek P, Kirrane J, Powell D. A unifying concept of chorionic gonadotropin production in malignancy. Invest Cell Pathol 1979;2:75–85.

181. Greco FA, Fer MF, Oldham RD, et al. Intracytoplasmic localization of ectopic β-human chorionic gonadotropin and α-fetoprotein in suspected extragonadal germ cell cancers by immunohistochemical methods. Clin Res 1980;28:415A.

182. Novarro C, Sancho A, Morales L, et al. Paraneoplastic precocious puberty. Report of a new case with hepatoblastoma and review of the literature. Cancer 1985;56:1725–1729.

183. Root AW, Bongiovanni AM, Eberlein WR. A testicular-interstitial-cell stimulating gonadotropin in a child with hepatoblastoma and sexual precocity. J Clin Endocrinol Metab 1968;28:1317–1322.

184. McArthur J, Toll GD, Russfield AB, et al. Sexual precocity attributable to ectopic gonadtropin secretion by hepatoblastoma. Am J Med 1973;54:390–403.

185. Kurman RJ, Norris HJ. Embryonal carcinoma of the ovary: A clinicopathologic entity distinct from endodermal sinus tumor resembling embryonal carcinoma of the adult testes. Cancer 1976;38:2420–2433.

186. Weintraub BD, Rosen SW. Ectopic production of human chorionic somatomammotrophin by nontrophoblastic cancers. J Clin Endocrinol Metab 1971;32:94–101.

187. Rosen SW, Weintraub BD, Vaitukaitis JL, et al. Placental proteins and their subunits as tumor markers. Ann Intern Med 1975;82:71–83.

187a. Steiner H, Dahlback O, Waldenstrom J. Ecotpic growth-hormone production and osteoarthropathy in carcinoma of the bronchus. Lancet 1968;1:783–785.

188. Ennis CG, Cameron DP, Burger HG. On the etiology of hypertrophic pulmonary osteoarthropathy in bronchogenic carcinoma: Lack of relationship to elevated growth hormone levels. Aust N Z J Med 1973;3:157–161.

189. Sonksen PH, Ayres AB, Braimbridge M, et al. Acromegaly caused by pulmonary carcinoid tumors. Clin Endocrinol 1976;5:505–513.

190. Scheithauer BW, Bloch B, Carpenter PC, Brazeau P. Ectopic secretion of a growth hormone-releasing factor. Report of a case of acromegaly with bronchial carcinoid tumor. Am J Med 1984;76:605–616.

191. Thorner MO, Vance ML, Kovacs K. Ectopic growth hormone-releasing hormone (GHRH) syndrome and significance. Proc Int Chemother Cong [Abstract] 1986:5051.

192. Boizel R, Labat F, Bachelot I, et al. Acromegaly due to a growth hormone releasing hormone secreting bronchial carcinoid tumor. Further information on the abnormal responsiveness of the somatotroph cells and their recovery after successful treatment. J Clin Endocrinol Metab 1987;64:304–308.

193. Roth KA, Eberwine J, Kovacs K, et al. Acromegaly and pheochromocytoma: A multiple endocrine syndrome caused by a plurihormonal adrenal medullary tumor. J Clin Endocrinol Metab 1986;63:1421–1464.

194. Anderson G. The incidence of paramalignant syndromes. In: Anderson G, ed. Paramalignant syndromes in lung cancer. London: William Heinemann, 1973:4.

195. Hennen G. Characterization of a thyroid-stimulating factor in human cancer tissue. J Clin Endocrinol Metab 1967;27:610–614.

196. Odell WD, Bates RW, Rivlin RS, et al. Increased thyroid function without clinical hyperthyroidism in patients with choriocarcinoma. J Clin Endocrinol Metab 1963;23:658–668.

197. Cave WT Jr, Dunn JT. Choriocarcinoma with hyperthyroidism: Probable identity of the thyrotropin with human chorionic gonadotropin. Ann Intern Med 1976;85:60–63.

198. Bommer G, Altenahr E, Kuhnau J Jr, Kloppel G. Ultrastructure of hemangiopericytoma associated with paraneoplastic hypoglycemia. Z Krebsforsh 1976;85:231–241.

199. Sluiter WJ, Marrink J, Houwen B. Monoclonal gammopathy with an insulin binding IgG(κ) M-component associated with severe hypoglycemia. Br J Haematol 1986;62:679–687.

200. Stuart CA, Prince MJ, Peters EJ, et al. Insulin receptor proliferation: A mechanism for tumor-associated hypoglycemia. J Clin Endocrinol Metab 1986;63:879–885.

201. Younus S, Soterakis J, Sossi AJ, et al. Hypoglycemia secondary to metastases to the liver. A case report and review of the literature. Gastroenterology 1977;72:334–337.

202. Kiang DT, Bauer GE, Kennedy BJ. Immunoassayable insulin in carcinoma of the cervix associated with hypoglycemia. Cancer 1973;31:801–805.

203. Silvert CK, Rossini AA, Ghazvinian S, et al. Tumor hypoglycemia: Deficient splanchnic glucose output and deficient glucagon secretion. Diabetes 1976;25:202–206.

204. Solomon J. Case report: Spurious hypoglycemia and hypperkalemia in myelomonocytic leukemia. Am J Med Sci 1974;267:359–363.

205. Zapf J, Walter H, Froesch ER. Radioimmunological determination of insulin-like growth factors I and II in normal subjects and in patients with growth disorders and extrapancreatic tumor hypoglycemia. J Clin Invest 1981;68:1321–1330.

206. Gorden P, Hendricks CM, Kahn CR, et al. Hypoglycemia associated with non-islet cell tumor and insulin like growth factors. N Engl J Med 1981;305:1452–1455.

207. Li TCM, Reed C, Stubenbard WT, et al. Surgical cure of hypoglycemia associated with cystosarcoma phylloides and elevated NSILP. Am J Med 1983;74:1080–1084.

208. Van Wyk JJ, Underwood LE, Hintz RL, et al. The somatomedins: A family of insulin-like hormones under growth hormone control. Recent Prog Horm Res 1974;30:259–318.

209. Chandalia HB, Boshell BR. Hypoglycemia in association with extrapancreatic tumors. Arch Intern Med 1972;129:447–456.

210. Megyesi K, Kahn CR, Roth J, Gorden P. Hypoglycemia in association with extrapancreatic tumors: Demonstration of elevated plasma NSILA-S by a new radioreceptor assay. J Clin Endocrinol Metab 1974;38:931–934.

211. Farsang C, Ramirez-Gonzalez MD, Mucci L, Kunos G. Possible role of an endogenous opiate in the cardiovascular effects of central α-adrenoceptor stimulation in spontaneously hypertensive rats. J Pharmacol Exp Ther 1980;214:203–208.

212. Davies P, Joseph J, Thompson A. Anterior to posterior variations in the concentration of somatostatin-like immunoreactivity in human basal ganglia. Brain Res Bull 1981;7:365–368.

213. Perry RH, Dockray GJ, Dimaline R, et al. Neuropeptides in Alzheimer's disease, depression and schizophrenia. J Neurol Sci 1981;51:465–472.

214. Emson PC, Arregui A, Clement-Jones V, et al. Regional distribution of methionine-enkephalin and substance P-like immunoreactivity in normal brain and in Huntington's disease. Brain Res 1980;199:147–160.

215. Aronin N, Cooper PE, Lorenz LJ, et al. Somatostatin is increased in the basal ganglia in Huntington disease. Ann Neurol 1983;13:519–526.

216. Brandt NJ, Teremius L, Jacobsen BB, et al. Hyper-endorphin syndrome in a child with necrotizing encephalomyelopathy. N Engl J Med 1980;303:914–916.

217. Allen JC, Deck MDF, Foley KM, et al. Neuro-oncology, vol 2. New York: Memorial Sloan-Kettering Cancer Center, 1979.

218. Newman SJ, Hansen HH. Frequency, diagnosis, and treatment of brain metastases in 247 consecutive patients with bronchogenic carcinoma. Cancer 1974;33:492–496.

219. Nugent JL, Bunn PA Jr, Matthews MJ, et al. CNS metastases in small cell bronchogenic carcinoma. Increasing frequency and changing pattern with lengthening survival. Cancer 1979;44:1855–1893.

220. Posner JB, Chernik NL. Intracranial metastasis from systemic cancer. Adv Neurol 1978;19:575–587.

221. Rosen P, Armstrong D. Nonbacterial thrombotic endocarditis in patients with malignant neoplastic disease. Am J Med 1973;54:23–29.

222. Collins RC, Al-Mondhiry H, Chernik NL, Posner JB. Neurologic manifestations of intravascular coagulation in patients with cancer: A clinical-pathological analysis of 12 cases. Neurology 1975;25:795–806.

223. Sigsbee B, Deck MDF, Posner JB. Non-metastatic superior saggital sinus thrombosis complicating systemic cancer. Neurology 1979;29:139–146.

224. Rogers LR, Cho ES, Kempin S, Posner JB. Cerebral infarction from nonbacterial thrombotic endocarditis. Clinical and pathologic study including effects of anticoagulation. Am J Med 1987;83:746–756.

225. Hickey WF, Garnick MB, Henderson IC, Dawson DM. Primary cerebral venous thrombosis in patients with cancer—A rarely diagnosed paraneoplastic syndrome. Am J Med 1982;73:740–750.

226. Persen JR. Systemic angioendotheliosis: A possible disorder of a circulating angiogenic factor. Br J Dermatol 1977;96:329–331.

227. Petito CK, Gottlieb GJ, Dougherty JH, Petito FH. Neoplastic angioendotheliosis: Ultrastructural study and review of the literature. Ann Neurol 1978;3:393–399.

228. Gimenez-Gallego G, Rodkey J, Bennett C, et al. Brain derived acidic fibroblast growth factor: Complete amino acid sequence and homologies. Science 1985;230:1385–1833.

229. Folkman J. A family of angiogenic peptides. Nature 1987;329:671–672.

230. Bell CE Jr, Seetharam S. Expression of endodermally derived and neural crest-derived differentiation antigens by human lung and colon tumors. Cancer 1979;44:12–18.

231. Bunn PA, Gazdar AF, Carney DN, Minna JD. Small cell lung carcinoma and natural killer cells share an antigen determinant, Leu-7. Clin Res 1984;32:413A.

232. Schuller-Petrovic S, Gebhart W, Lassmann H, Rumpold H, Kraft D. A shared antigenic determinant between natural killer cells and nervous tissue. Nature 1983;306:179–181.

233. Wilkinson PC, Zeroniski J. Immunofluorescent detection of antibodies against neurones in sensory carcinomatoms neuropathy. Brain 1965;88:529–538.

233a. Moll JWB, Henzen-Logmans SC, Splinter TAW, van der Burg MEL, Vecht CJ. Diagnostic value of anti-neuronal antibodies for paraneoplastic disorders of the nervous system. J Neurol Neurosurg Psychiatry 1990;53:940–943.

233b. Grause F, Abos J, Roquer J, Mazzara R, Pereira A. Effect of plasmapheresis on serum and CSF auto-antibody levels in CNS paraneoplastic syndromes. Neurology 1990;40: 1621–1623.

234. Brain WR, Wilkinson M. Subacute cerebellar degeneration associated with neoplasms. Brain 1965;88:465.

235. Paone JF, Jeyasingham K. Remission of cerebellar dysfunction after pneumonectomy for bronchogenic carcinoma. N Engl J Med 1980;302:156–157.

236. Victor M, Adams RD, Mancall EL. A restricted form of cerebellar cortical degeneration occurring in alcoholic patients. Arch Neurol 1959;1:579–688.

237. Steven MM, Carnegie PR, Mackay IR, et al. Cerebellar cortical degeneration with ovarian carcinoma. Postgrad Med J 1982;58:47–51.

238. Dropcho EJ, Chen Y-T, Posner JB, Old LB. Cloning of a brain protein identified by autoantibodies from a patient with paraneoplastic cerebellar degeneration. Proc Natl Acad Sci USA 1987;84:4552–4556.

238a. Furneaux HM, Rosenblum MK, Dalmau J, et al. Selective expression of purkinje-cell antigens in tumor tissue from patients with paraneoplastic cerebellar degeneration. N Engl J Med 1990;322:1844–1851.

238b. Fathallah-Shaykh H, Wolfs, Wang E, Posner JB, Furneaux HM. Cloning of a leucine-zipper protein recognized by the sera of patients with antibody-associated paraneoplastic cerebellar degeneration. Proc Natl Acad Sci USA 1991;88:3451–3454.

238c. Duncan MB, Cobos E, Maccario M. Paraneoplastic cerebellar degeneration due to Hodgkin's Disease. West J Med 1989;150:463–465.

238d. Sakai K, Mitchell DJ, Tsudamoto T, Steinman L. Isolation of a complementary DNA clone encoding an autoantigen recognized by an anti-neuronal cell antibody from a patient with paraneoplastic cerebellar degeneration. Ann Neurol 1990;28:692–698.

238e. Komguth SE. Neuronal proteins and paraneoplastic syndromes. N Engl J Med 1989;321:1607–1608.

239. Shapiro WR. Remote effects of neoplasm on the central nervous system: Encephalopathy. Adv Neurol 1976;15:101–117.

240. Dorfman LH, Forno LS. Paraneoplastic encephalomyelitis. Acta Neurol Scand 1972;48: 556–574.

241. Corsellis JAN, Goldberg GJ, Norton AR. "Limbic encephalitis" and its association with carcinoma. Brain 1968;91:481–497.

242. Brennan LV, Craddock PR. Limbic encephalopathy as a nonmetastatic complication of oat cell lung cancer. Am J Med 1983;75:518–520.

243. Carr I. The Ophelia syndrome: Memory loss in Hodgkin's disease. Lancet 1982;1: 844–845.

243a. Lacomis D, Khoshbin S, Schick RM. MR imaging of paraneoplastic limbic encephalitis. J Comput Assist Tomogr 1990;14:115–117.

243b. Burton GV, Bullard DE, Walther PJ, Burger PC. Paraneoplastic limbic encephalopathy with testicular carcinoma. A reversible neurologic syndrome. Cancer 1988;62:2248–2251.

244. Sawyer RA. Blindness caused by photoreceptor degeneration as a remote effect of cancer. Am J Ophthalmol 1976;81:606–613.

245. Grunwald GB, Simmonds MA, Klein R, Kornguth SE. Autoimmune basis for visual paraneoplastic syndrome in patients with small cell lung carcinoma. Lancet 1985;1: 658–661.

246. Pillary N, Ebers GC, Gilbert JJ, Brown JD. Internuclear opthalmoplegia and "optic neuritis": Paraneoplastic effects of bronchial carcinoma. Neurology 1984;34:788–791.

246a. Thirkill CE, FitzGerald P, Sergott RC, et al. Cancer-associated retinopathy (CAR syndrome) with antibodies reacting with retinal, optic nerve, and cancer cells. N Engl J Med 1989;321:1589–1594.

246b. Jacobson DM, Thirkill CE, Tipping SJ. A chemical triad to diagnose paraneoplastic retinopathy. Ann Neurol 1990;28:162–167.

246c. Luque FA, Furneaux HM, Ferziger R, et al. Anti-Ri: An antibody associated with paraneoplastic opsoclenus and breast cancer. Ann Neurol 1991;29:241–251.

247. Padgett BL. JC papovavirus in progressive multifocal leukoencephalopathy. J Infect Dis 1976;133:686–690.

248. Norris FH Jr, Engel WK. Carcinomatous amyotrophic lateral sclerosis. In: Brain WR, Norris FH Jr, eds. The remote effects of cancer on the nervous system. New York: Grune & Stratton, 1965.

249. Mancall EL, Rosales RK. Necrotizing myelopathy associated with visceral carcinoma. Brain 1964;87:636–639.

250. Handforth A, Nag S, Sharp D, Robertson DM. Paraneoplastic subacute necrotic myelopathy. Can J Neurol Sci 1983;10:204–207.

250a. Dansey RD, Hammond-Tooke GD, Lai K, Bergwoda WR. Subacute myelopathy: An unusual paraneoplastic complication of Hodgkin's disease. Med Pediatr Oncol 1988;16: 284–286.

251. Walton JN, Tomlinson BE, Pearce GW. Subacute "poliomyelitis" and Hodgkin's disease. J Neurol Sci 1968;6:435–445.

252. Horwich MS, Cho L, Porro RS, Posner JB. Subacute sensory neuropathy: A remote effect of carcinoma. Ann Neurol 1977;1:7–19.

253. Henson RA, Hoffman HL, Urich H. Encephalomyelitis with carcinoma. Brain 1965;88: 449–464.

254. Croft PB, Urich H, Wilkinson M. Peripheral neuropathy of sensorimotor type associated with malignant disease. Brain 1967;90:31–66.

255. Dayan AD, Croft PB, Wilkinson M. Association of carcinomatous neuromyopathy with different histological types of carcinoma of the lung. Brain 1965;88:435–448.

256. Newman MK, Gugino RJ. Neuropathies and myopathies associated with occult malignancies. JAMA 1964;190:575–577.

257. Victor M, Banker BQ, Adams RD. The neuropathy of multiple myeloma. J Neurol Neurosurg Psychiatry 1958;21:73–88.

257a. Founan A. Peripheral neuropathy in cancer patients: Incidence, features, and pathophysiology. Oncology 1990;4:57–62, 85–89.

257b. Weissman DE, Gottshall JL. Complete remission of paraneoplastic sensorimotor neuropathy: A case associated with small cell lung cancer responsive to chemotherapy, plasma exchange and radiotherapy. J Clin Apheresis 1989;5:3–5.

258. Lisak RP. Gullain-Barre syndrome and Hodgkin's disease: Three cases with immunological studies. Ann Neurol 1977;1:72–78.

259. Schuffer MD, Baird HW, Fleming CR, et al. Intestinal pseudo-obstruction as the presenting manifestation of small cell carcinoma of the lung. Ann Intern Med 1983;98: 129–134.

260. Siemsen JK, Meister L. Bronchogenic carcinoma associated with severe orthostatic hypotension. Ann Intern Med 1963;58:669–676.

261. Park DM, Johnson RH, Crean GP, Robinson JF. Orthostatic hypotension in bronchial carcinoma. Br Med J 1972;3:510–511.

262. Ahmed MN, Carpenter S. Autonomic neuropathy and carcinoma of the lung. Can Med Assoc J 1975;113:410–412.

263. Ogilvie H. Large intestine colic due to sympathetic deprivation. Br Med J 1948;2: 671–673.

264. DeVere R, Bradley WG. Polymyositis: Its presentation, morbidity and mortality. Brain 1976;98:637–666.

265. Barnes BE. Dermatomyositis and malignancy. A review of the literature. Ann Intern Med 1976;84:68–76.

266. Williams RC Jr. Dermatomyositis and malignancy: A review of the literature. Ann Intern Med 1959;50:1174–1181.

266a. Sigurgeirsson B, Lindelof B, Edhag O, Allander E. Risk of cancer in patients with dermatomyositis or plymyositis. A population-based study. N Engl J Med 1992;326: 363–367.

267. Lambert EH, Eaton LM, Rooke ED. Defect of neuromuscular conduction associated with malignant neoplasms. Am J Physiol 1956;187:612.

268. Lambert EH, Rooke ED. Myasthenic state and lung cancer. In: Brain WR, Norris FH Jr, eds. The remote effects of cancer on the nervous system. New York: Grune & Stratton, 1965:67–80.

269. Simpson JA. The myasthenic (Eaton-Lambert) syndrome associated with carcinoma: Enzyme induction as a possible mechanism of paraneoplastic syndromes. Scott Med J 1982;27:220–228.

270. Cherington M. Guanidine and germline in Eaton-Lambert syndrome. Neurology 1976;26:944–946.

271. Jenkyn LR, Brooks PL, Forcier RJ, et al. Remission of the Lambert-Eaton syndrome and small cell anaplastic carcinoma of the lung induced by chemotherapy and radiotherapy. Cancer 1980;46:1123–1127.

272. Login IS, Kim YI, Judd AM, et al. Immunoglobulins of Lambert-Eaton myasthenic syndrome inhibit rat pituitary hormone release. Ann Neurol 1987;22:610–614.

272a. McEvoy KM, Windebank AS, Draube JR, Low PSA. 3,4-Diaminopyricline in the treatment of Lambert-Eaton myasthenic syndrome. N Engl J Med 1989;321:1567–1571.

273. Tyler HR. Paraneoplastic syndromes of nerve, muscle, and neuromuscular junction. Ann N Y Acad Sci 1974;230:348–357.

274. Latov N, Sherman WH, Nemni R, et al. Plasma cell dyscrasia and peripheral neuropathy with a monoclonal antibody to peripheral-nerve myelin. N Engl J Med 1980;303: 618–621.

275. Johnson PC, Rolak LA, Hamilton RH, Laguna JF. Paraneoplastic vasculitis of nerve: A remote effect of cancer. Ann Neurol 1979;5:437–444.

276. Clark SC, Kamen R. The human hematopoietic colony stimulating factors. Science 1987;236:1229–1237.

277. Hammond D, Winnick S. Paraneoplastic erythrocytosis and ectopic erythropoietins. Ann N Y Acad Sci 1974;230:219–227.

278. Valentine WN, Hennessy TG, Lang E, et al. Polycythemia: Erythrocytosis and erythremia. Ann Intern Med 1968;69:587–606.

279. Sytkowski AJ, Richie JP, Bicknell KA. New human renal carcinoma cell line established from a patient with erythrocytosis. Cancer Res 1983;43:1415–1419.

279a. Da Silva JL, Lacombe C, Bruneval P, et al. Tumor cells are the site of erythropoietin synthesis in human renal cancers associated with polycythemia. Blood 1990;75:577–582.

280. Williams WJ, Beutler E, Erslev AJ, Rundles RW. Hematology. 2nd ed. New York: McGraw-Hill, 1977.

281. Berlin NI. Anemia of cancer. Ann N Y Acad Sci 1974;230:209–211.

282. Waterbury L. Hematologic problems. In: Abeloff MD, ed. Complications of cancer: Diagnosis and management. Baltimore: Johns Hopkins Press, 1979:121–145.

282a. Hocking W, Goodman J, Golde D. Gramulocytosis associated with tumor production of colony stimulating factor. Blood 1983;61:600–609.

283. Cartwright GE, Lee GR. The anemia of chronic disorders. Br J Haematol 1971;21: 147–152.

284. Crowthers D, Bateman CJT. Hematological aspects of systemic disease-malignant disease. Clin Haematol 1972;1:447–455.

285. Jacobs EM, Hutter RVP, Pool JL, Ley AB. Benign thymoma and selective erythroid aplasia of the bone marrow. Cancer 1959;12:47–57.

286. Vasavada PJ, Bournigal LJ, Reynolds RW. Thymoma associated with pure red cell aplasia and hypogammaglobulinemias. Postgrad Med 1973;54:93–98.

287. Guthrie TH, Thornton RM. Pure red cell aplasia obscured by a diagnosis of carcinoma. South Med J 1983;76:632–634.
288. Akard LP, Brandt J, Lee L, et al. Chronic T cell lymphoproliferative disorder and pure red cell aplasia. Am J Med 1987;83:1069–1074.
289. Hoffbrand AV, Hobbs JR, Kremenchuzky S, Mallin DL. Incidence and pathogenesis of megaloblastic erythropoiesis in multiple myeloma. J Clin Pathol 1967;20:699–705.
290. Pirofsky B. Clinical aspects of autoimmune hemolytic anemia. Semin Hematol 1976;13:251–265.
291. Ludwin D, Sacks P, Lynch S, et al. Autoimmune hematological complications occurring during the treatment of malignant lymphoproliferative diseases. S Afr Med J 1974;48:2143–2145.
292. Lackner H. Hemostatic abnormalities associated with dysproteinemias. Semin Hematol 1973;10:125–133.
293. Burkert L, Becker G, Pisciotta AV. Ovarian malignancy and hemolytic anemia. Ann Intern Med 1970;73:91–93.
294. Dawson MA, Tolbert W, Yarbro JW. Hemolytic anemia associated with an ovarian tumor. Ann J Med 1971;50:552–556.
295. Spira MA, Lynch EC. Autoimmune hemolytic anemia and carcinoma: An unusual association. Am J Med 1979;67:753–758.
296. Dacie JV. The hemolytic anemias: Congenital and acquired. Part III: Secondary and symptomatic hemolytic anemias. New York: Grune & Stratton, 1967.
297. Pirofsky B. Autoimmunization and the autoimmune hemolytic anemias. Baltimore: Williams & Wilkins, 1968.
298. Evans RS, Takahasi K, Duane RT, et al. Primary thrombocytopenic purpura and acquired hemolytic anemia. Evidence for a common etiology. Arch Intern Med 1957;87:48–65.
299. Doll DC, List AF, Yarbro JW. Evans' syndrome associated with microcystic adenoma of the pancreas. Cancer 1987;59:1366–1368.
300. Barry KG, Crosby WH. Autoimmune hemolytic anemia arrested by removal of an ovarian teratoma: Review of the literature and report of a case. Ann Intern Med 1957;47:1002–1007.
301. Antman KH, Skarin AT, Mayer RJ, et al. Microangiopathic hemolytic anemia and cancer: A review. Medicine (Baltimore) 1979;58:377–384.
302. Brain MC, Dacie JV, Hourihane OB. Microangiopathic hemolytic anemia: The possible role of vascular lesions in pathogenesis. Br J Haematol 1962;8:358–374.
303. Lohrmann HP, Adam W, Heymer B, Kubanek B. Microangiopathic hemolytic anemia in metastatic carcinoma: Report of eight cases. Ann Intern Med 1973;79:368–375.
304. Sack GH, Levin J, Bell WR. Trousseau's syndrome and other manifestations of chronic disseminate coagulopathy in patients with neoplasms. Medicine (Baltimore) 1977;56:1–37.
305. Colman RW, Robboy SJ, Minna JD. Disseminated intravascular coagulation: A reappraisal. Ann Rev Med 1979;30:359–374.
306. Robinson WA. Granulocytosis in neoplasia. Ann N Y Acad Sci 1974;230:212–218.
307. Meyer LM, Rotter SD. Leukemoid reaction (hyperleukocytosis) in malignancy. Am J Clin Pathol 1942;12:218–222.
308. Fahey RJ. Unusual leukocyte response in primary carcinoma of the lung. Cancer 19521;4:930–935.
309. Hughes WF, Highley CS. Marked leukocytosis resulting from carcinomatosis. Ann Intern Med 1952;37:1095–1098.
310. Barrett O Jr. Monocytosis in malignant disease. Ann Intern Med 1970;73:991–992.
311. Finch SC. Granulocytopenia and granulocytosis. In: Williams WJ, Beutler E, Erslev AJ, Rundles RW, eds. Hematology. 2nd ed. New York: McGraw-Hill, 1977.
312. Asano S, Urabe A, Okabe T, et al. Demonstration of granulopoietic factor(s) in the plasma of nude mice transplanted with a human lung cancer and in the tumor tissue. Blood 1977;49:845–852.
313. Okabe T, Sato N, Kondo Y, Asano S, Ohsawa N, Kosaka K, Ueyama Y. Establishment and characterization of a human cancer cell line that produces human colony-stimulating factor. Cancer Res 1978;38:3910–3917.
314. Di Persio JF, Brennan JK, Lichtman MA, Speiser BL. Human cell lines that elaborate colony-stimulating activity for the marrow cells of man and other species. Blood 1978;51:507–519.
315. Cohen PR, Kurzrock R. Sweet's syndrome and malignancy. Am J Med 1987;82:1220–1226.
315a. Sato K, Fujii Y, Kakiuchi T, et al. Paraneoplastic syndrome of hypercalcemia and leukocytosis caused by squamous carcinoma cells (T3M-1) producing parathyroid hormone-related protein, interleukin 2, and granulocyte colony stimulating factor. Cancer Res 1989;49:4740–4746.
316. McCarthy JH, Sullivan JR, Ungar B, Metcalf D. Two cases of carcinoma of the lung characterized by a bone marrow agar culture pattern resembling acute myeloid leukemia. Blood 1979;54:530–533.
317. Aisenberg AC, Wilkes BM, Harris N, et al. Chronic T-cell lymphocytosis with neutropenia: Report of a case studied with monoclonal antibody. Blood 1981;58:818–823.
318. Knowles JH. Miscellaneous disorders of the lung. In: Harrison TR, Adams RD, Bennett IL, et al, eds. Harrison's principles of internal medicine. 5th ed. New York: McGraw-Hill, 1966:955–957.
319. Liddle GW, Nicholson WE, Island DP, et al. Clinical and laboratory studies of ectopic humoral syndromes. Recent Prog Horm Res 1969;25:283–314.
320. Slungaard A, Ascensao J, Zanjani E, Jacob HS. Pulmonary carcinoma with eosinophilia: Demonstration of a tumor-derived eosinophilopoietic factor. N Engl J Med 1983;309:778–781.
321. Williams WJ. Thrombocytosis. In: Williams WJ, Beutler E, Erslev AJ, Rundles RW, eds. Hematology. 2nd ed. New York: McGraw-Hill, 1977.
322. Levin J, Conley CL. Thrombocytosis associated with malignant disease. Arch Intern Med 1964;114:497–500.
323. Davis RB, Theologides A, Kennedy BJ. Comparative studies of blood coagulation and platelet aggregation in patients with cancer and nonmalignant disease. Ann Intern Med 1967;71:67–80.
324. Aster RH. Control of platelet production. In: Williams WJ, Beutler E, Erslev AJ, Rundles RW, eds. Hematology. 2nd ed. New York: McGraw-Hill, 1977.
325. Kim HD, Boggs DR. A syndrome resembling idiopathic thrombocytopenic purpura in 10 patients with diverse forms of cancer. Am J Med 1979;67:371–377.
326. Doan C, Bouroncle BA, Wiseman BK. Idiopathic and secondary thrombocytopenic purpura. Clinical study and evaluation of 381 cases over a period of 28 years. Ann Intern Med 1960;53:861–876.
327. Bellone JD, Kunicki TS, Aster RH. Immune thrombocytopenia associated with carcinoma. Ann Intern Med 1983;99:470–472.
328. Kaden BR, Rosse WF, Hauch TW. Immune thrombocytopenia in lympho proliferative diseases. Blood 1979;53:545–551.
329. Khilanani P, Al-Sarraf M. The association of autoimmune thrombocytopenia and Hodgkin's disease. Oncology 1973;28:238–245.
330. Jones SE. Autoimmune disorders and malignant lymphoma. Cancer 1973;31:1092–1098.
331. Bowie EJW, Owen CA Jr. Hemostatic failure in clinical medicine. Semin Hematol 1977;14:341–364.
332. Trousseau A. Phlegmasia alba dolens. Clinique medicale de l'Hotel-Dieu de Paris. London. N Sydenham Soc 3:94, 1865.
333. Marder M, Weiner M, Shulman P, Shapiro S. Afibrinogenemia occurring in a case of malignancy of the prostate with bone metastases. N Y State J Med 1949;49:1197–1198.
334. Goodnight SH Jr. Bleeding and intravascular clotting in malignancy: A review. Ann N Y Acad Sci 1974;230:271–288.
335. Sharp AA. Diagnosis and management of disseminated intravascular coagulation. Br Med Bull 1977;33:265–272.
336. Gralnick HR, Abrell E. Studies of the procoagulant and fibrinolytic activity of promyelocytes in acute promyelocytic leukemia. Br J Hematol 1973;24:59–99.
337. Colman RW, Robby SJ, Minna JD. Disseminated intravascular coagulation (DIC): An approach. Am J Med 1972;52:679–689.
338. Siegal T, Seligsohn U, Aghai E, Modan M. Clinical and laboratory aspects of dessem-inated intravascular coagulation (DIC): A study of 118 cases. Thromb Haemost 1978;39:122–134.
339. Merskey C, Johnson AJ, Kleiner GJ, Wohl H. The defibrination syndrome: Clinical features and laboratory diagnosis. Br J Haematol 1967;13:528–549.
340. Owen CA Jr, Bowie EJ. Chronic intravascular coagulation syndromes: A summary. Mayo Clin Proc 1974;49:673–679.
341. Drapkin RL, Gee TS, Dowling MD, et al. Prophylactic heparin therapy in acute promyelocytic leukemia. Cancer 1978;41:2484–2490.
342. Gralnick HR, Sultan C. Acute prolmyelocytic leukemia: Haemorrhagic manifestation and morphologic criteria. Br J Haematol 1975;29:333–336.
343. Goldberg MA, Ginsberg D, Mayer RJ, et al. Is heparin administration necessary during induction chemotherapy for patients with acute promyelocytic leukemia? Blood 1987;69:187–191.
344. Fayemi AO, Deppisch LM. Nonbacterial thrombotic endocarditis and myocardial infarction. Am Heart J 1979;97:405–406.
345. MacDonald RA, Robbins SL. The significance of nonbacterial thrombotic endocarditis: Autopsy and clinical study of 78 patients. Ann Intern Med 1957;46:255–273.
346. Studdy P, Wiloughby JMT. Non-bacterial thrombotic endocarditis in early cancer. Br J Med 1976;1:752.
347. Susens GP, Hendrickson C, Barto DA, Sams BJ. Disseminated intravascular coagulation syndrome with metastatic melanoma: Remission after treatment with 5-(3,3-dimethyl-l-traizeno)-imidazole-4-carboxamide (DTIC). Ann Intern Med 1976;84:175.
348. Alving BM, Abeloff MD, Bell W. Spontaneous remission of recurring disseminated intravascular coagulation associated with prostatic carcinoma. Cancer 1976;37:928–930.
349. Rickles FR, Edwards RL. Activation of blood coagulation in cancer: Trousseau's syndrome revisited. Blood 1983;63:14–31.
350. Rosen P, Armstrong D. Nonbacterial thrombotic endocarditis in patients with malignant neoplastic disease. Am J Med 1973;54:23–29.
351. Sun NC, McAfee WM, Hum GJ, Weiner JM. Hemostatic abnormalities in malignancy: A prospective study in one hundred eight patients: I. Coagulation studies. Am J Clin Pathol 1979;71:10–16.
352. Aderka D, Brown A, Zelikovski A, Pinkhas J. Idiopathic deep vein thrombosis in an apparently healthy patient as a premonitory sign of occult cancer. Cancer 1986;57:1846–1849.
353. Bell WR, Starksen NF, Tang S, Porterfield JK. Trousseau's syndrome. Devastating coagulopathy in the absence of heparin. Am J Med 1985;79:423–430.
354. Al-Mondhiry H. Disseminated intravascular coagulation: Experience in a major cancer center. Thromb Diathes Haemorrh 1975;34:181–193.
355. Lee JC, Yamuchi H, Hopper J Jr. The association of cancer and the nephrotic syndrome. Ann Intern Med 1966;64:51.
356. Alpers CE, Cotran RS. Neoplasia and glomerular injury. Kidney Int 1986;30:465–473.
357. Glassock RJ, Friedler RM, Massry SG. Kidney and electrolyte disturbances in neoplastic diseases. Contrib Nephrol 1977;7:2–41.
358. Ghosh L, Meuhrhe RC. The nephrotic syndrome: A prodrome to lymphoma. Ann Intern Med 1970;72:379–382.

359. Cantrell EG. Nephrotic syndrome cured by removal of gastric carcinoma. Br Med J 1969;2:739.

360. Plager J, Stutzman L. Acute nephrotic syndrome as a manifestation of active Hodgkin's disease. Am J Med 1971;50:56–66.

361. Lewis MG, Loughridge LW, Phillips TM. Immunological studies in nephrotic syndrome associated with extrarenal malignant disease. Lancet 1971;2:134–185.

362. Couser WG, Wagonfeld JB, Spargo BH, Lewis EJ. Glomerular deposition of tumor antigen in membranous nephropathy associated with colonic carcinoma. Am J Med 1974;57:962–970.

363. Costanza ME, Perin V, Schwartz RS, Nathansen L. Carcinoembryonic antigen-antibody complexes in a patient with colonic carcinoma and nephrotic syndrome. N Engl J Med 1973;289:520–522.

363a. Haskell LP, Fusco MJ, Wadler S, Sablay LB, Mennemeyer RP. Crescentic glomerulonephritis associated with prostatic carcinoma: Evidence of immune-mediated glomerular injury. Am J Med 1990;88:189–192.

364. Sherman RL, Susin M, Weksler ME, Becker EL. Lipoid nephrosis in Hodgkin's disease. Am J Med 1972;52:699–706.

365. Lokich JJ, Galvanek EG, Moloney WC. Nephrosis of Hodgkin's disease. Arch Intern Med 1973;132:597–600.

366. Moorthy AV, Zimmerman SW, Burkholder PM. Nephrotic syndrome in Hodgkin's disease. Am J Med 1976;61:471–477.

367. Carpenter CB. Case records of the Massachusetts General Hospital. N Engl J Med 1973;289:1241–1247.

368. Richard-Mendes da Costa C, Dupont E, Hamers R, et al. Nephrotic syndrome in bronchogenic carcinoma: Report of two cases with immunochemical studies. Clin Nephrol 1974;2:245–251.

369. Dobbs DJ, Striker LM, Mignon F, Striker G. Glomerular lesions in lymphomas and leukemias. Am J Med 1986;80:63–70.

370. Gagliano RG, Costanzi JJ, Beathard GA, et al. The nephrotic syndrome associated with neoplasia: An unusual paraneoplastic syndrome: Report of a case and review of the literature. Am J Med 1976;60:1026–1031.

371. Moorthy AV. Minimal change glomerular disease: A paraneoplastic syndrome in 2 patients with bronchogenic carcinoma. Am J Kidney Dis 1983;3:58–62.

372. Jermanovich NB, Glammarco R, Ginsberg SJ, et al. Small cell anaplastic carcinoma of the lung with mesangial proliferative glomerulonephritis. Arch Intern Med 1982;142:397–399.

373. Cameron JS. Nephrotic syndrome in chronic lymphatic leukemia. Br Med J 1974;4:164–167.

374. Hyman LR, Burkholder PM, Joo PA, Segar WE. Malignant lymphoma and the nephrotic syndrome: A clinicopathologic analysis with light immunofluorescence and electron microscopy of the renal lesions. J Pediatr 1973;82:207–217.

375. Higgins MR, Randall RE, Still WJS. Nephrotic syndrome with oat-cell carcinoma. Br Med J 1974;3:450.

376. Karpen HO, Bhat JG, Feiner HD, Baldwin DS. Membranous nephropathy associated with renal cell carcinoma: Evidence against a role of renal tubular or tumor antibodies in pathogenesis. Am J Med 1978;64:864–867.

377. Hopper JH Jr. Tumor related renal lesions. Ann Intern Med 1974;81:550–551.

378. Row PG, Cameron JS, Turner DR, et al. Membranous nephropathy: Long-term follow-up and association with neoplasia. Q J Med 1975;44:207–239.

379. Shalhoub RJ. Pathogenesis of lipoid nephrosis: A disorder of T-cell function. Lancet 1974;2:556–558.

380. Osserman EF, Lawlor DP. Serum and urinary lysozyme (muramidase) in monocyte and monomyelocytic leukemia. J Exp Med 1966;124:921–951.

381. Pruzanki W, Platts MF. Serum and urinary proteins, lysozyme (muramidase) and renal dysfunction in mono- and myelomonocytic leukemia. J Clin Invest 1970;49:1694–1707.

382. Hobbs JR, Evans DJ, Wrong OM. Renal tubular obstruction by mucoprotein from adenocarcinoma of pancreas. Br Med J 1974;2:87–89.

383. Freibusch J, Barbosa-Saldivar JL, Bernstein RS, Robertson GL. Tumor-associated nephrogenic diabetes insipidus. Ann Intern Med 1980;92:797–798.

384. Kyle RA. Multiple myeloma: Review of 869 cases. Mayo Clin Proc 1975;50:29–40.

385. DeFronzo RA, Cooke CR, Wright JR, Humphrey RL. Renal function in patients with multiple myeloma. Medicine (Baltimore) 1978;57:151–161.

386. Zlotnick A, Rosenmann E. Renal pathologic findings associated with monoclonal gammopathies. Arch Intern Med 1975;135:40–45.

387. Schubert GE, Viegel J, Lennert K. Structure and function of the kidney in multiple myeloma. Virchows Arch [A] 1972;355:135–137.

388. Brown WW, Herbert LA, Piering WF, et al. Reversal of chronic and stage renal failure due to myeloma kidney. Ann Intern Med 1979;90:793–794.

389. Leech SH, Polesky HF, Shapiro FL. Chronic hemodialysis in myelomatosis. Ann Intern Med 1972;77:239–242.

390. Richmond J, Sherman RS, Diamond HD, Craver LF. Renal lesions associated with malignant lymphomas. Am J Med 1962;32:184–207.

391. Martinez-Maldonado M, Ramirez de Arellano GA. Renal involvement in malignant lymphomas: A survey of 49 cases. J Urol 1966;95:485–488.

392. Matthews MJ. Problems in morphology and behavior of monchopulmonary malignant disease. In: Israel L, Chanimian P, eds. Lung cancer, facts, problems and perspectives. New York: Academic Press, 1976:23–46.

393. Brin EN, Schiff M Jr, Weiss RM. Palliative urinary diversion for malignancy. J Urol 1975;113:619–622.

394. Fichman M, Bethune J. Effects of neoplasms on renal electrolyte function in paraneoplastic syndromes. Ann N Y Acad Sci 1974;230:448–472.

395. Garnic MB, Mayer RJ. Acute renal failure associated with neoplastic disease and its treatment. Semin Oncol 1976;5:155–165.

396. Keane WF, Crosson JT, Staley NA, et al. Radiation-induced renal disease: A clinicopathologic study. Am J Med 1967;60:127–137.

397. Dosik GM, Gutterman JE, Hersh EM, et al. Nephrotoxicity from cancer immunotherapy. Ann Intern Med 1978;89:41–46.

398. Bennett WM, Muther RS, Parker RA, et al. Drug therapy in renal failure: Dosing guidelines for adults. Ann Intern Med 1980;93:286–325.

399. Kierland RR. Cutaneous signs of internal malignancy. South Med J 1972;65:563–568.

400. Helm F, Helm J. Cutaneous markers of internal malignancies. In: Helm F, ed. Cancer dermatology. Philadelphia: Lea & Febiger, 1979:247–283.

401. Braverman IM. Skin signs of systemic disease. Philadelphia: WB Saunders, 1970.

402. Crowe FW. Axillary freckling as a diagnostic aid in neurofibromatosis. Ann Intern Med 1964;61:1142–1143.

403. Levine N, Greenwald ES. Mucocutaneous side effects of cancer chemotherapy. Cancer Treat Rev 1978;5:67–84.

404. Brown J, Winkelmann RK. Acanthosis nigricans: A study of 90 cases. Medicine (Baltimore) 1968;47:33–51.

405. Curth HO. Classification of acanthosis nigricans. Int J Dermatol 1976;15:592.

406. Matsuoka MY, Goldman J, Wortsman J, et al. Antibodies against the insulin receptor in paraneoplastic acanthosis nigricans. Am J Med 1987;82:1253–1256.

406a. Cohen PR, Grossman ME, Almeida L, Kurzrock R. Tripe palms and malignancy. J Clin Oncol 1989;7:669–678.

407. Sneddon IB, Roberts JBM. An incomplete form of acanthosis nigricans. Gut 1962;3:269–272.

408. Dantzig PI. Sign of Leser-Trelat. Arch Dermatol 1973;108:700–701.

409. Ronchese F. Keratoses, cancer and "the sign of Leser-Trelat." Cancer 1965;18:1003–1006.

410. Holdiness MR. The sign of Leser-Trelat. Int J Dematol 1986;25:564–572.

411. Curry SS, King LE. The sign of Leser-Trelat. Arch Dermatol 1980;116:1059–1060.

412. Graham JH, Helwig EB. Bowen's disease and its relationship to systemic cancer. Arch Dermatol 1961;83:738–758.

413. Anderson SL, Nielsen A, Reymann F. Relationship between Bowen's disease and internal malignancy. Arch Dermatol 1973;108:367–370.

414. Minkowsky S. Multiple carcinomata following the ingestion of medicinal arsenic. Ann Intern Med 1964;61:296–299.

415. Fitzpatrick TB, Montgomery H, Lerner AB. Pathogenesis of generalized dermal pigmentation secondary to malignant melanoma and melanuria. J Invest Dermatol 1954;22:163–172.

416. Ashikari R, Park K, Huvos AG, Urban JA. Paget's disease of the breast. Cancer 1970;26:680–685.

417. Witkowski JA, Parish LC. Bazex's syndrome: Paraneoplastic acrokeratosis. JAMA 1983;248:2883–2884.

418. Wishart JM. Bazex paraneoplastic acrokeratosis: A case report and response to Tagason. Br J Dermatol 1986;115:595–599.

418a. Bolognia JL, Brewer YP, Cooper DL. Bazex syndrome (acroheratosis paraneoplastica): An analytical review. Medicine (Baltimore) 1991;70:269–280.

419. Gammel JA. Erythema gyratum repens: Skin manifestations of patients with carcinoma of breast. Arch Dermatol 1952;66:494–505.

420. Purdy MJ. Erythema gyratum repens: Report of a case. Arch Dermatol 1959;80:590–591.

421. Summerly R. The figurate erythemas and neoplasia. Br J Dermatol 1964;80:370–373.

421a. Appell ML, Ward W, Tyring SK. Erythema gyratum repens. A cutaneous marker of malignancy. Cancer 1988;62:548–550.

422. Lazar P. Cancer, erythema annulare centrifugum and autoimmunity. Arch Dermatol 1963;87:246–253.

423. Wilkinson DS. Necrolytic migrating erythema with pancreatic carcinoma. Proc R Soc Med 1971;64:1197–1198.

424. Church RE, Crane WAJ. A cutaneous syndrome associated with islet cell carcinoma of the pancreas. Br J Dermatol 1967;79:284–286.

425. Sjoerdsma A, Weissbach H, Udenfriend S. A clinical, physiologic, and biochemical study of patients with malignant carcinoid (argentaffinoma). Am J Med 1956;21:520–532.

426. Mason DT, Melmon KL. New understanding of the mechanism of the carcinoid flush. Ann Intern Med 1966;65:1334–1339.

427. Abrahams F, McCarthy JT, Sanders SL. 101 Cases of exfoliative dermatitis. Arch Dermatol 1963;87:96–103.

428. Nicolis GD, Helwig EB. Exfoliative dermatitis: A clinicopathologic study of 135 cases. Arch Dermatol 1973;108:788–979.

429. Elias PM, Fritsch PO. Erythema multiforme. In: Fitzpatrick TB, Eisen AZ, Wolf K, et al, eds. Dermatology in general medicine. 2nd ed. New York: McGraw-Hill, 1979:295–303.

430. Fitzpatrick TB, Clark WH Jr. Recurrent attacks of abdominal pain and cutaneous lesions. N Engl J Med 1964;270:1248–1251.

431. Waddington RT. A case of primary liver tumor associated with porphyria. Br J Surg 1972;59:653–654.

432. Thompson RPH, Nicholson DC, Farman T, et al. Cutaneous porphyria due to a malignant primary hepatoma. Gastroenterology 1970;59:779–783.

433. Stone SP, Schroeder AL. Bullous pemphigoid and associated malignant neoplasms. Arch Dermatol 1975;111:991–994.

433a. Anhalt GJ, Kim SC, Stanley JR, et al. Paraneoplastic pemphigus. An autoimmune microcutaneous disease associated with neoplasia. N Engl J Med 1990;323:1729–1735.

434. Tobias N. Dermatitis herpetiformis associated with visceral malignancy. Urol Cutan Rev 1951;55:352.
435. Arundell FD, Wilkinson RD, Haserick Jr. Dermatomyositis and malignant neoplasm in adults. Arch Dermatol 1960;82:772–775.
436. Lyell A, Whittle CH. Hypertrichosis languinosa acquired type. Br J Dermatol 1951;63: 411–413.
437. Hegedus SI, Schorr WF. Acquired hypertrichosis lanquinosa and malignancy. Arch Dermatol 1972;106:84–88.
438. Van Dijk E. Ichthyosiform atrophy of the skin with internal malignant diseases. Dermatologica 1963;127:413–428.
439. Flint GL, Flam M, Soter NA. Acquired ichthyosis. Arch Dermatol 1975;111:1446–1447.
440. Vogl A, Goldfischer S. Pachydermoperiostosis. Primary or idiopathic hypertrophic osteoarthropathy. Am J Med 1962;33:166–187.
441. Rajka G. Investigation of patients suffering from generalized pruritus, with special references to systemic diseases. Acta Dermato-Venereol 1966;46:190–194.
442. Cormia FE. Pruritus, an uncommon but important symptom of systemic cancer. Arch Dermatol 1965;92:36–39.
443. Schimpff S, Serpick A, Stoler B, et al. Varicella-zoster infection in patients with cancer. Ann Intern Med 1972;76:241–254.
444. Dolin R, Reichman RC, Mazur MH, Whitley RJ. Herpes zoster-varicella infections in immunosuppressed patients. Ann Intern Med 1978;89:375–388.
445. Huberman M, Fossieck BE Jr, Bunn PA Jr, et al. Herpes zoster and small cell bronchogenic carcinoma. Am J Med 1980;68:214–218.
446. Gardner EJ. Follow-up study of a family group exhibiting dominant inheritance for a syndrome including intestinal polyps, osteomas, fibromas, and epidermal cysts. Am J Hum Genet 1962;16:376–390.
447. Bussey HJR. Gastrointestinal polyposis. Gut 1970;11:970–978.
448. Jones EL, Cornell WP. Garnder's syndrome: Review of the literature and report on a family. Arch Surg 1966;92:287–300.
449. Jeghers H, McKusick VA, Katz KH. Generalized intestinal polyposis and melanin spots of the oral mucosa, lips and digits: A syndrome of diagnostic significance. N Engl J Med 1949;241:933–1005, 1031–1036.
450. Riley E, Swift M. A family with Peutz-Jeghers syndrome and bilateral breast cancer. Cancer 1980;46:815–817.
451. Howel-Evans W, McConnell RR, Clarke CA, Sheppard PM. Carcinoma of the esophagus with keratosis palmaris et plantaris (tylosis). Q J Med 1958;27:413–429.
452. Williams ED, Pollock DJ. Multiple mucosal neuromata with endocrine tumors: A syndrome allied to Von Recklinghausen's disease. J Pathol Bacteriol 1966;91:71–80.
453. Lloyd KM, Dennis M. Cowden's disease, a possible new symptom complex with multiple system involvement. Ann Intern Med 1963;58:136–142.
454. Solomon LM, Fretzin DF, Dewald RL. The epidermal nevus syndrome. Arch Dermatol 1968;97:273–285.
455. Butterworth T, Wilson M Jr. Dermatologic aspects of tuberous sclerosis. Arch Dermatol Syph 1941;43:1–41.
456. Christoferson LA, Gustafson MB, Petersen AG. Von Hippel-Lindau's disease. JAMA 1961;178:280–282.
457. Doll R, Kinlen L. Immunosurveillance and cancer: Epidemiologic evidence. Br Med J 1970;4:420–422.
458. Frizzera G, Rosai J, Dehner LP, et al. Lymphoreticular disorders in primary immunodeficiencies: New findings based on an up-to-date histologic classification of 35 cases. Cancer 1980;46:692–699.
459. Epstein CJ, Martin GM, Schultz AL, Motulsky AG. Werner's syndrome: A review of the symptomatology, natural history, pathologic features, genetics, and relationship to the natural aging process. Medicine (Baltimore) 1966;45:177–221.
460. Waldman TA, Broder S, Strober W. Protein-losing enteropathies in malignancy. Ann N Y Acad Sci 1974;230:306–317.
461. Lucy K, Scobie BA. Watery diarrhoea (WDHA) syndrome associated with carcinoma of the lung. Aust N Z J Med 1976;6:490–491.
462. Troncale FJ. Distant manifestations of colonic carcinoma. Ann N Y Acad Sci 1974;230: 332–347.
463. Klipstein FA, Smorth G. Intestinal structure and function in neoplastic disease. Am J Dig Dis 1969;14:887–889.
464. Gilat T, Fischel B, Danon J, Lowewnthal M. Morphology of small bowel mucosa and malignancy. Digestion 1972;12:147–155.
465. Henderson AR, Grace DM. Liver-originating isoenzymes of alkaline phosphatase in the serum: A paraneoplastic manifestation of a malignant schwannoma of the sciatic nerve. J Clin Pathol 1976;29:237–240.
466. Walsh PN, Kissane JM. Nonmetastatic hypernephroma with reversible hepatic dysfunction. Arch Intern Med 1968;122:214–222.
467. Utz DC, Warren MM, Gregg JA, et al. Reversible hepatic dysfunction associated with hypernephroma. Mayo Clin Proc 1970;45:161–169.
468. Cronin RE, Kaehny WD, Miller PD, et al. Renal cell carcinoma: Unusual systemic manifestations. Medicine (Baltimore) 1976;55:291–311.
469. Mena E, Bull FE, Bookstein JJ, et al. Angiography of the nephrogenic hepatic dysfunction syndrome. Radiology 1974;111:65–68.
470. DeWys WD. Working conference on anorexia and cachexia of neoplastic disease. Cancer Res 1970;30:2816–2818.
471. De Wys WD. Abnormalities of taste as a remote effect of a neoplasm. Ann N Y Acad Sci 1974;230:427–434.
472. Theologides A. The anorexia-cachexia syndrome: A new hypothesis. Ann N Y Acad Sci 1974;230:14–22.
473. Waterhouse C. How tumors affect host metabolism. Ann N Y Acad Sci 1974;230:86–93.

474. Beck SA, Tisdale MJ. Production of lipolytic and proteolytic factors by a murine tumor producing cachexia in the host. Cancer Res 1987;47:5919–5923.
475. Ternell M, Moldawer LC, Lonnroth C, et al. Plasma protein synthesis in experimental cancer compared to paraneoplastic conditions, including monokine administration. Cancer Res 1987;47:5825–5830.
475a. Yoneda T, Alsina MA, Chavez JB, et al. Evidence that tumor necrosis factor plays a role in the paraneoplastic syndromes of cachexia, hypercalcemia, and leukocytosis in a human tumor in nude mice. J Clin Invest 1991;87:977–985.
475b. Beck SA, Mulligan HD, Tisdale MJ. Lipolytic factors associated with murine and human cancer cachexia. JNCI 1990;82:1922–1926.
476. Gold J. Cancer cachexia and gluconeogenesis. Ann N Y Acad Sci 1974;230:103–110.
477. Bodel P. Tumors and fever. Ann N Y Acad Sci 1974;230:6–13.
477a. Fukumoto s, Matsumoto T, Harada S, et al. Pheochromocytoma with pyrexia and marked inflammatory signs: A paraneoplastic syndrome with possible relation to interleukin-6 production. J Clin Endocrinol Metab 1991;73:877–881.
478. Petersdorf RG. Fever and cancer. Hosp Med 1965;1:2–10.
479. Lobell M, Boggs DR, Wintrobe MM. The clinical significance of fever in Hodgkin's disease. Arch Intern Med 1966;117:335–342.
480. Gluckman JB, Turner MD. Systemic manifestations of tumors of the small gut and liver. Ann N Y Acad Sci 1974;230:318–331.
481. Block JB. Lactic acidosis in malignancy and observations on its possible pathogenesis. Ann N Y Acad Sci 1974;230:94–102.
482. Nadiminti Y, Wang JC, Chou S, et al. Lactic acidosis associated with Hodgkin's disease: Response of chemotherapy. N Engl J Med 1980;303:15–17.
483. Spechler SJ, Esposito AL, Koff RS, Hong WK. Lactic acidosis in oat cell carcinoma with extensive hepatic metastases. Arch Intern Med 1978;138:1663–1664.
484. Eridani S, Burdick L, Periti M, Arosio A, Libretti A. Primary carcinoma of the colon and hyperlipemia: A paraneoplastic syndrome. Biomedicine 1976;25:324–326.
485. Glueck HL, MacKenzie M, Glueck CJ. Crystalline IgG protein in multiple myeloma: Identification of effects on coagulation and on lipoprotein metabolism. J Lab Clin Med 1972;79:731–744.
486. Santer MA, Waldmann TA, Fallon HJ. Erythrocytosis and hyperlipemia as manifestations of hepatic carcinoma. Arch Intern Med 1967;120:735–739.
487. Gangulu A, Gribble J, Tune B, et al. Renin-secreting Wilms' tumor with severe hypertension: Report of a case and brief review of renin-secreting tumors. Ann Intern Med 1973;79:835–837.
488. Genest J, Rojo-Ortega JM, Kuchel O, et al. Malignant hypertension with hypokalemia in a patient with renin-producing pulmonary carcinoma. Trans Assoc Am Physicians 1975;88:192–201.
489. Aurell M, Rudin A, Tisell LE, et al. Captopril effort on hypertension in patient with renin-producing tumor. Lancet 1979;2:149–150.
490. Hollifield JW, Page DL, Smith C, et al. Renin-secreting clear cell carcinoma of the kidney. Arch Intern Med 1975;135:859–864.
490a. Yokokawa K, Tahara H, Kohno M, et al. Hypertension associated with endothelin-secreting malignant hemangioendothelioma. Ann Int Med 1991;114:213–215.
491. Zusman RM, Snider JJ, Cline A, et al. Antihypertensive function of renal-cell carcinoma: Evidence for a prostaglandin A secreting tumor. N Engl J Med 1974;290: 843–845.
492. Boasberg PD, Henry JP, Rosenbloom AA, et al. Case reports and studies of paraneoplastic hypotension: Abnormal low pressure baroreceptor responses. Med Pediatr Oncol 1977;3:59–66.
493. Braganza JM, Butler EB, Fox H, et al. Ectopic production of salivary type amylase by a pseudomesotheliomatous carcinoma of the lung. Cancer 1978;41:1522–1525.
494. Mills JA. A spectrum of organ systems that respond to cancer: The joints and connective tissue. Ann N Y Acad Sci 1974;230:443–447.
495. Greenfield GB, Schorsch HA, Shkolnik A. The various roentgen appearance of pulmonary hypertrophic osteoarthropathy. Am J Roentgenol Radium Ther Nucl Med 1967;101:927–931.
496. LeRoux BT. Bronchial carcinoma with hypertrophic pulmonary osteoarthropathy. S Afr Med J 1968;42:1074–1075.
497. Jao JY, Barlow JJ, Krant MKJ. Pulmonary hypertrophic osteoarthropathy, spider angiomata and estrogen hypersecretion in neoplasms. Ann Intern Med 1969;70:580–584.
498. Donnelly B, Johnson PM. Detection of hypertrophic pulmonary osteoarthropathy by skeletal imaging with ^{99m}Tc-labeled diphosphonate. Radiology 1975;114:389–391.
499. Green N, Kurohara SS, George FW III, Crews QE Jr. The biologic behavior of lung cancer according to histologic type. Radiol Clin Biol 1972;41:160–170.
500. Yesner R. Spectrum of lung cancer and ectopic hormones. In: Sommers SC, Rosen PP, eds. Pathology annual, vol 12. New York: Appleton-Century-Crofts, 1978:217–240.
501. Goldstraw P, Walbraun PR. Hypertrophic pulmonary osteoarthropathy and its occurrence with pulmonary metastases from renal carcinoma. Thorax 1976;31:205–211.
502. Miller ER. Carcinoma of the thymus with marked pulmonary osteoarthropathy. Radiology 1939;32:651–660.
503. Ullal SR. Hypertrophic osteoarthropathy and leiomyoma of the oesophagus. Am J Surg 1972;123:356–358.
504. Shapiro RF, Zvaifler NJ. Concurrent intrathoracic Hodgkin's disease and hypertrophic osteoarthropathy. Chest 1973;63:912–916.
505. Howard CP, Telander RL, Hoffman AD, Burgert EO Jr. Hypertrophic osteoarthropathy in association with pulmonary metastasis from osteogenic sarcoma. Mayo Clin Proc 1978;53:538–541.
506. Papavasiliou C, Pavlatou M, Pappas J. Nasopharyngeal cancer in patients under the age of thirty years. Cancer 1977;40:2312–2316.
507. Ellouz R, Cammoun M, Attia RB, Bahi J. Clinical aspects: Nasopharyngeal carcinoma

in children and adolescents in Tunisia: Clinical aspects and the paraneoplastic syndrome. IARC Sci Pub 1978;20:115–129.

507a. Thomas CR Jr, Rest EB, Brown CR Jr. Rheumatologic manifestations of malignancy. Med Pediatr Oncol 1988;18:146–158.

508. Cudkowicz L, Armstrong JB. Finger clubbing and changes in the bronchial circulation: Arterio-venous shunts in hypertrophic pulmonary osteoarthropathy. Br J Tuberc 1953;47:227–232.

509. Carroll KB, Doyle L. A common factor in hypertrophic osteoarthropathy. Thorax 1974;29:262–264.

510. Riyami AM, Anderson EG. Hypertrophic pulmonary osteoarthropathy: A clinical and biochemical study. Br J Dis Chest 1974;68:193–196.

511. Glenner GC. Amyloid deposits and amyloidosis: The β-fibriloses. N Engl J Med 1980;303:1283–1292, 1333–1347.

512. Azzopardi JG, Lehner T. Systemic amyloidosis and malignant disease. J Clin Pathol 1966;19:539–548.

513. Kyle RA, Bayrd ED. Amyloidosis: Review of 236 cases. Medicine (Baltimore) 1975;54: 271–547.

514. Shiel WC, Prete PE, Jason M, Andrews BS. Palmar fasciitis and arthritis with ovarian and non-ovarian carcinomas. Am J Med 1985;79:640–644.

515. Pfinsgraff J, Buckingham RB, Killian PJ, et al. Palmar fasciitis and arthritis with malignant neoplasms: A paraneoplastic syndrome. Semin Arthritis Rheum 1986;16: 118–125.

516. Michaels RM, Sorber JA. Reflex sympathetic dystrophy as a probable paraneoplastic syndrome: Case report and literature review. Arthritis Rheum 1984;27:1183–1185.

517. Mills JA. Connective tissue disease associated with malignant neoplastic disease. J Chron Disi 1963;16:797–811.

518. Calabro J. Cancer and arthritis. Arthritis Rheum 1967;10:553–567.

519. Cammarata R, Rodnan GP, Jensen WM. Systemic rheumatic disease and malignant lymphoma. Arch Intern Med 1963;111:112–119.

520. Miller D. The association of immune disease and malignant lymphoma. Ann Intern Med 1967;66:507–521.

521. Anderson LG, Talal N. The spectrum of benign to malignant lymphoproliferation in Sjögrens syndrome. Clin Exp Immunol 1971;9:199–221.

522. Murray GC, Persellin RH. Metastatic carcinoma presenting as nonarticular arthritis: A case report and review of the literature. Arthritis Rheum 1980;23:95–100.

523. Karten I, Bartfield H. Bronchogenic carcinoma simulating early rheumatoid arthritis. JAMA 1962;179:160–161.

524. Tumulty PA. Systemic lupus erythematosus. In: Wintrobe MM, Thorn GW, Adams RD, Brauwald E, Isselbacher KJ, Petersdorf RG, eds. Harrison's principles of internal medicine. 6th ed. New York: McGraw-Hill, 1971:1962–1967.

525. Freundlich B, Makover D, Maul GG. A novel antinuclear antibody associated with a lupuslike paraneoplastic syndrome. Ann Intern Med 1988;109:295–297.

526. Sanchez-Guerro J, Gutierrez-Vrena S, Vidaller A, et al. Vasculitis as a paraneoplastic syndrome. Report of 11 cases and review of the literature. J Rheumatol 1990;17: 1458–1462.

Cancer: Principles & Practice of Oncology, Fourth Edition,
edited by Vincent T. DeVita, Jr., Samuel Hellman, Steven A. Rosenberg.
J.B. Lippincott Co., Philadelphia © 1993.

F. Anthony Greco

John D. Hainsworth

CHAPTER **58**

Cancer of Unknown Primary Site

Patients with cancer of unknown primary site are common, representing 5% to 10% of all cancer patients. Within this heterogenous patient group there are several clinical presentations and histologic tumor types. The largest group of patients have metastatic carcinoma of unknown primary site. Others have equivocal histologic diagnoses and tumors that are difficult to classify using the time-honored method of light microscopic examination. Specialized pathologic studies are essential in delineating the type of neoplasm present in many of these patients, and at times may suggest the site of origin. Extreme heterogeneity in clinical presentations, histologic appearances, and natural histories has made systematic evaluation of these patients difficult, and an established base of knowledge has developed slowly. Only a few investigators have been interested in detailed studies of these patients. Therefore, past information suffers from many generalizations and is not representative of the entire patient population. These data are derived from grouping all patients and deal primarily with results of various chemotherapeutic regimens.

Over the past few decades several important issues have changed in oncology. Combination chemotherapy, often used with surgery or radiation therapy, has proved to be potentially curative for several metastatic tumors of known primary site. In addition, palliation and prolongation of survival has been demonstrated with systemic therapy for many other tumor types. These therapeutic improvements have relevance for patients with cancers of unknown primary site, because some have these responsive neoplasms (*i.e.,* with occult primaries or atypical histologies).

Diagnostic pathology has improved remarkably. The more routine use of electron microscopy and the emerging fields of immunohistochemistry and molecular genetics are con-

tributing to the more precise diagnosis of neoplasms. It is possible to define more reliably the histology and, at least in selected patients, the origin and biology of their neoplasms. In concert with the evolving diagnostic techniques, several clinical syndromes and features are being recognized and are helping physicians to better understand and manage these patients. Oncologists are rethinking the issues with respect to patients with cancers of unknown primary site.

Appropriate patient management requires an understanding of several clinicopathologic features that help to identify patients with responsive tumors. A patient with cancer of unknown primary site typically develops symptoms or signs at a metastatic site, and the diagnosis is made by biopsy of a metastatic lesion. History, physical examination, chest radiograph, and laboratory studies fail to identify the primary site. The initial biopsy should be generous because many studies may be required. Routine light microscopic histology establishes the neoplastic process and provides a practical classification system on which the patient can be subsequently evaluated and managed. In the broad category of cancers of unknown primary site, there are four major light microscopic diagnoses:

1. Poorly differentiated neoplasms
2. Well-differentiated and moderately well-differentiated adenocarcinoma
3. Squamous cell carcinoma
4. Poorly differentiated carcinoma and poorly differentiated adenocarcinoma

These diagnoses vary with respect to clinical characteristics, recommended diagnostic evaluation, treatment, and prognosis.

POORLY DIFFERENTIATED NEOPLASMS OF UNKNOWN PRIMARY SITE

If the pathologist is confident of a cancer but cannot differentiate a general category of neoplasm (*e.g.*, carcinoma, lymphoma, melanoma, sarcoma), it is designated a poorly differentiated neoplasm of unknown primary site. A more precise diagnosis is essential in this group of patients because many have responsive tumors. About 5% of all patients with cancers of unknown primary site present with this diagnosis. The number will decrease as specialized pathology is more widely used. The most frequent tumor for which specific effective therapy is available is non-Hodgkin's lymphoma. In reported series, 35% to 65% of poorly differentiated neoplasms were found to be lymphomas after further pathologic study.[1-4] Most of the remaining tumors in this group are carcinomas. Melanoma and sarcoma together account for less than 15% of all patients.

The evaluation of poorly differentiated tumors requires specialized pathologic studies. Immunoperoxidase tumor staining, electron microscopy, and genetic analysis can be helpful in the differential diagnosis. The most common cause of a nonspecific light microscopic diagnosis is an inadequate biopsy specimen. Fine-needle aspiration biopsy should not be performed in these patients as an *initial* diagnostic procedure, because the histology is poorly preserved and the ability to perform special studies is limited. Frequently, a definitive diagnosis can be made by obtaining a larger biopsy. Communication with the pathologist is important if repeat biopsy is performed, because some pathologic studies require special tissue processing. Some neoplasms remain unclassifiable by light microscopy, even with an adequate biopsy specimen. Additional pathologic study is always indicated in these tumors.

IMMUNOPEROXIDASE TUMOR STAINING

Immunoperoxidase staining is the most widely available specialized technique for the classification of neoplasms. Immunoperoxidase staining often can be done on formalin-fixed, paraffinized tissue, which broadens its applicability, making repeat biopsy unnecessary in some patients. Immunoperoxidase antibodies are either monoclonal or polyclonal and are directed at cell components or products, which can include enzymes (*e.g.*, prostatic acid phosphatase, neuron-specific enolase [NSE]), normal tissue components (*e.g.*, keratin, desmin, vimentin, neurofilaments, common leukocyte antigen [CLA]), hormones and hormone receptors (*e.g.*, estrogen receptor), oncofetal antigens (*e.g.*, α-fetoprotein [AFP], carcinoembryonic antigen [CEA]), and other substances (*e.g.*, S-100 protein, chromogranin). Many new antibodies are being developed and appear almost monthly, making this area of diagnostic pathology a dynamic and evolving field. Specific diagnoses usually cannot be made on the basis of immunoperoxidase staining alone, because none of these reagents is directed at tumor-specific antigens. Therefore, results must be interpreted in conjunction with the light microscopic appearance and the clinical picture. Immunoperoxidase staining patterns that are useful in the differential diagnosis of poorly differentiated neoplasms are outlined in Table 58–1.

Several important questions can usually be answered by

TABLE 58–1. Immunoperoxidase Tumor Staining Patterns Useful in the Differential Diagnosis of Poorly Differentiated Neoplasms

Tumor Type	Immunoperoxidase Staining
Carcinoma	Epithelial stains (*e.g.*, cytokeratin, EMA; +)
	CLA, S-100, vimentin (−)
Lymphoma	CLA (+)
	EMA occasionally (+)
	All other stains (−)
Sarcoma	
Mesenchymal	Vimentin (+)
	Epithelial stains usually (−)
Rhabdomyosarcoma	Desmin (+)
Angiosarcoma	Factor VIII antigen (+)
Melanoma	S-100, vimentin (+)
	NSE often (+)
	Epithelial stains (−)
	HMB-45 (+)
Neuroendocrine tumor	NSE, chromogranin (+)
	Epithelial stains (+)
Germ cell tumor	HCG, AFP (+)
	Epithelial stains (+)
Prostate cancer	PSA (+)
	Epithelial stains (+)
Breast cancer	ER, PR (+)
	Epithelial stains (+)

+, positive result; −, negative result; AFP, α-fetoprotein; CLA, common leukocyte antigen; EMA, epithelial membrane antigen; ER, estrogen receptor; HCG, human chorionic gonadotropin; NSE, neuron-specific enolase; PR, progesterone receptor; PSA, prostate-specific antigen.

immunoperoxidase staining (see Table 58–1). The CLA stain usually can be used to make the important distinction between lymphoma and carcinoma.[5-6] Staining for NSE and chromogranin can suggest a neuroendocrine carcinoma (*e.g.*, small cell lung cancer, carcinoid, islet cell tumor).[7-8] Staining for prostate-specific antigen (PSA) strongly suggests prostate carcinoma in a male with metastatic adenocarcinoma.[9] Certain staining characteristics can suggest amelanotic melanoma (*e.g.*, positive staining for S-100 protein, vimentin, HMB-45) or sarcoma (*e.g.*, positive staining for desmin, vimentin, factor VIII antigen).[10-13] Staining for human chorionic gonadotropin (HCG) or AFP can suggest the diagnosis of a germ cell tumor in an appropriate clinical situation.[14,15]

Several problems are associated with immunoperoxidase stains. Technical expertise is required to perform these tests accurately and reproducibly, and proper interpretation requires an experienced pathologist. Appropriate control slides are stained and examined concurrently because nonspecific staining occasionally is a problem. Care must be taken to avoid overinterpretation, because no staining pattern is entirely specific. Certain stains, particularly CLA and PSA are specific; however, false-positive and false-negative results can occur with any of these stains. For example, some carcinomas stain with vimentin, some sarcomas stain with keratin, and a wide variety of carcinomas (other than neuroendocrine and germ cell tumors) stain with NSE and HCG, respectively.

In some circumstances, diagnoses based on immunoperoxidase staining in patients with poorly differentiated neoplasms of unknown primary site can be used to plan therapy and predict outcome. Undifferentiated neoplasms identified as lymphoma on the basis of positive CLA staining respond well to the combination chemotherapy used for non-Hodgkin's lymphoma.[1] In 35 patients with equivocal routine light microscopic histology and positive CLA staining, treatment with a variety of standard lymphoma regimens resulted in an actuarial disease-free survival of 45% at 30 months. Their outcome was similar to a group of concurrently treated patients who had non-Hodgkin's lymphomas with typical light microscopic histology. In patients diagnosed on the basis of immunoperoxidase staining with tumors other than lymphoma, only limited data exist concerning treatment outcome. These data are discussed later concerning patients with poorly differentiated carcinoma.

ELECTRON MICROSCOPY

A diagnosis can be made by electron microscopy in some poorly differentiated neoplasms. Electron microscopy is not widely available, requires special tissue fixation, is relatively expensive, and should be reserved for the study of neoplasms whose lineage is unclear after routine light microscopy and immunoperoxidase staining. Like immunoperoxidase staining, electron microscopy is reliable in differentiating lymphoma from carcinoma. It may be superior to immunoperoxidase staining for the identification of poorly differentiated sarcoma. Other specific structures such as neurosecretory granules (neuroendocrine tumors) or premelanosomes (melanoma) can suggest a particular tumor. Undifferentiated tumors often have nonspecific ultrastructural features; therefore, the absence of a particular ultrastructural finding cannot be used to rule out a specific diagnosis. Some neoplasms defy further classification despite specialized pathologic study.

In some instances, electron microscopy provides evidence for adenocarcinoma or squamous cell carcinoma. Features of adenocarcinoma include intercellular and intracellular lumina and surface microvilli. Squamous carcinomas are characterized by frequent and prominent desmosomes and by prominent bundles of prekeratin filaments in the adjacent cytoplasm. It usually is not possible to determine the origin of poorly differentiated adenocarcinoma or squamous carcinoma by electron microscopic features. Treatment implications for adenocarcinoma and squamous carcinoma recognized only by ultrastructural features are unclear (see the section on poorly differentiated carcinoma).

GENETIC ANALYSIS

The identification of chromosomal abnormalities and genetic changes associated with neoplasms is becoming increasingly important in predicting prognosis. The use of tumor-specific chromosomal abnormalities in diagnosis is still limited, but it is likely that future research will identify many additional specific genetic abnormalities.

Chromosomal abnormalities have been best studied in hematopoietic neoplasms. Most B cell non-Hodgkin's lymphomas are associated with tumor-specific immunoglobulin gene rearrangements, and typical chromosomal changes have been identified in some B cell and T cell lymphomas and in Hodgkin's disease.[16-17] In the rare instance when the diagnosis of lymphoma cannot be definitively established with either immunoperoxidase staining or electron microscopy, detection of chromosomal translocations t(14:18); t(8:14) or the presence of an immunoglobulin gene rearrangement provides definitive diagnostic information.

Two specific chromosomal rearrangements associated with nonlymphoid tumors have been identified. A specific chromosomal translocation, t(11:22), has been found in peripheral neuroepitheliomas and frequently in Ewing's tumor.[18,19] An isochromosome of the short arm of chromosome 12 (i12p) and other chromosome 12 abnormalities are found in a large percentage of testicular and extragonadal germ cell tumors in men.[20-22] Because these tumor types are poorly differentiated and are often metastatic at the time of diagnosis, identification of these chromosomal abnormalities may provide a specific diagnosis. Genetic analysis has been applied successfully to a subset of patients with carcinoma of unknown primary site (see the section on poorly differentiated carcinoma).

ADENOCARCINOMA OF UNKNOWN PRIMARY SITE

CLINICAL CHARACTERISTICS

Well-differentiated or moderately well-differentiated adenocarcinoma is the most frequent light microscopic diagnosis in patients with carcinoma of unknown primary site, accounting for about 60% of patients. Typically, patients with this diagnosis are elderly and have metastatic tumors at multiple sites. The sites of tumor involvement frequently determine the clinical presentation; common metastatic sites include liver, lung, and bone.

The clinical course is often dominated by symptoms and signs related to the metastases. The primary site becomes obvious in only 15% to 20% of patients during life.[23] At autopsy, however, 70% to 80% of patients have a primary site detected. The most common primaries identified at autopsy are the lung and pancreas, accounting for about 40%.[24] Other gastrointestinal sites (*e.g.*, stomach, colon, liver) are frequent, although adenocarcinomas from a wide variety of other primary sites are encountered occasionally. Adenocarcinomas of the breast, prostate, and ovary are rare in this group of patients.[24]

As a group, patients with metastatic adenocarcinoma of unknown primary site have a poor prognosis, with inexorable progression and a median survival of only 3 to 4 months. Many patients in this group have widespread metastases and poor performance status at the time of diagnosis. However, it is an error to stereotype *all* patients with carcinoma of unknown primary site, because within this large group are subsets of patients with more favorable prognoses. These patients often can be identified, as is discussed later in this chapter.

PATHOLOGY

The diagnosis of well-differentiated or moderately well-differentiated adenocarcinoma is based on light microscopic features, particularly the formation of glandular structures by neoplastic cells. We have considered patients with well-differentiated or moderately well-differentiated adenocarcinoma as one group. These histologic features are shared by all adenocarcinomas, and the site of the primary tumor usually cannot be determined by histologic examination. Certain histologic features typically are associated with a particular tumor type (*e.g.*, papillary features with ovarian cancer, and signet ring cells with gastric cancer). However, these characteristics are not specific enough to be used as definitive evidence of the primary site. Immunoperoxidase stains and electron microscopy are of limited use in identifying the site of origin of most well-differentiated or moderately well-differentiated adenocarcinomas. The stain for PSA is an exception because it is specific for prostate cancer, and it should be used in men with suggestive clinical findings. Positive immunoperoxidase staining for estrogen receptor suggests metastatic breast cancer in women with metastatic adenocarcinoma. Rarely, neuroendocrine stains (*e.g.*, NSE, chromogranin) can identify an unsuspected neuroendocrine neoplasm.

The diagnosis of poorly differentiated adenocarcinoma should be viewed differently, because some of these patients may be distinctive in tumor biology and responsiveness to systemic therapy (see the section on poorly differentiated carcinoma). This diagnosis is usually made when only minimal glandular formation is seen on histologic examination or, on occasion, when tumors exhibit positive staining for mucin but have no glandular features. Well-differentiated adenocarcinoma, poorly differentiated adenocarcinoma, and poorly differentiated carcinoma are diagnoses that probably represent parts of a spectrum of tumor differentiation rather than specific, sharply demarcated entities. These histologies represent a heterogenous group of tumors with various biologic properties. Different pathologists may use slightly different criteria for making each of these three diagnoses. It is therefore appropriate to perform additional study with immunoperoxidase staining or electron microscopy in all poorly differentiated adenocarcinomas. Guidelines for the evaluation and treatment of patients with poorly differentiated adenocarcinoma are provided later in this chapter.

DIAGNOSTIC EVALUATION

An exhaustive search for the primary site is not indicated because it rarely can be found. Therefore, the clinical evaluation should be performed to evaluate any suspicious clinical symptoms or signs and to determine the extent of metastatic disease. Routine initial evaluation should include a thorough history and physical examination, standard laboratory screening tests (*i.e.*, complete blood count, liver function tests, serum creatinine, urinalysis), and chest radiography. All men should have a serum PSA or acid phosphatase determination, and all women should undergo mammography. Computed tomographic (CT) scans of the abdomen can identify a primary site in 10% to 35% of patients and frequently are useful in identifying additional sites of metastatic disease.[25,26] Additional

symptoms, signs, or abnormal physical and laboratory findings should be evaluated with appropriate diagnostic studies. Extensive radiologic evaluation of asymptomatic areas is rarely useful in identifying a primary site, is expensive, and often results in confusing or false-positive results.

TREATMENT

The group of patients with adenocarcinoma of unknown primary site contains several clinically defined subgroups for which useful therapy can be given. Effective therapy does not exist for most patients who do not fall into one of these subgroups, although some patients benefit from empiric hormonal therapy or chemotherapy.

Peritoneal Carcinomatosis in Women

Adenocarcinoma causing diffuse peritoneal involvement is typical of ovarian carcinoma, although carcinomas from the gastrointestinal tract or breast can occasionally produce this clinical picture. Several women have been described with diffuse peritoneal carcinomatosis who had no primary site found in the ovaries or elsewhere in the abdomen at the time of laparotomy.[27-33] These patients frequently had histologic features typical of ovarian carcinoma, such as papillary configuration or psammoma bodies. This syndrome has been termed "multifocal extraovarian serous carcinoma" or "peritoneal papillary serous carcinoma." In the early 1980s, several anecdotal case reports documented excellent responses to cisplatin-based chemotherapy in women with this syndrome.[27-30]

Recently, larger series of patients have been described (Table 58-2).[31-33] Eighteen women with abdominal carcinomatosis and no primary site documented at laparotomy were reported from Vanderbilt University.[32] The clinical features in these patients were similar to those seen in patients with advanced ovarian carcinoma. Metastases outside the peritoneal cavity were unusual. The histologic features were similar to ovarian carcinoma; however, only 7 of 18 patients had serous adenocarcinoma. Patients were managed as if they had advanced ovarian cancer, using initial surgical cytoreduction followed by cisplatin-based combination chemotherapy. The median survival for the entire group was 23 months. Seven of 18 patients had complete clinical response to chemotherapy, and 3 have remained continuously disease free for more than 4 years after completing treatment.

A second group of 31 patients with extraovarian peritoneal serous papillary carcinoma was reported recently.[31] All these patients underwent initial surgical cytoreduction followed by chemotherapy. Most patients in this group received single-agent chemotherapy with chlorambucil or cisplatin or both. Ten of 31 patients responded to treatment; 3 had complete response and 2 are long-term disease-free survivors.

A third series by Ransom and colleagues described 33 patients with papillary adenocarcinoma of the peritoneum.[33] All but 2 patients had debulking surgical procedures. All received cisplatin-based combination chemotherapy. Several patients responded, and 2 had a negative second look laparotomy. Three patients remain alive 7 years after therapy, and the median survival of the entire group was 17 months.

TABLE 58–2.   Therapy for Women With Peritoneal Adenocarcinomatosis of Unknown Primary Site

Investigations	No. of Patients	Therapy	Complete Response Rate (%)	Long-Term Survival (%)	Median Survival (mo)
Strand et al, 1989[32] (Vanderbilt)	18	Surgical cytoreduction and cisplatin-based chemotherapy	39	17	23
Dalrymple et al, 1989[31] (King George Hospital)	31	Surgical cytoreduction and chemotherapy*	10	6	11
Ransom et al, 1990[33] (Mayo Clinic)	33	Surgical cytoreduction and cisplatin-based chemotherapy	13†	9	17

* Single-agent chlorambucil or cisplatin-based chemotherapy.
† Sixteen of 33 patients had laparotomy to evaluate response; 2 of these patients had complete response.

Women with metastatic adenocarcinoma involving the peritoneal surface and no obvious primary site have tumors that are distinct in biology and are often responsive to chemotherapy. Many of these patients have elevations of serum CA 125 levels. The site of origin of these carcinomas is unknown, but some may arise from the peritoneal surface. Because ovarian epithelium is in part an extension of the mesothelial surface, some carcinomas arising from the peritoneal (mesothelial) surface may share a similar lineage (müllerian derivation) and biology with ovarian carcinoma. There is some question whether men can develop this tumor. Certainly, this possibility should be considered and would not be surprising (*e.g.*, papillary mesothelioma). Optimal management of these patients includes aggressive surgical cytoreduction followed by postoperative chemotherapy. The intensive cisplatin-based regimens considered optimal for the treatment of advanced ovarian cancer would seem a reasonable choice for initial chemotherapy. Some patients in this group have complete responses to therapy, and a small percentage have prolonged disease-free survival.

Women With Axillary Lymph Node Metastases

Breast cancer should be suspected in women who have axillary lymph node involvement with adenocarcinoma. Men with occult breast cancer could present in this fashion but would be rare. The initial lymph node biopsy should include measurement of estrogen and progesterone receptors. Elevated levels provide strong evidence for the diagnosis of breast cancer.[34] If no other metastases are identified, these patients may have stage II breast cancer with an occult primary, which is potentially curable with appropriate therapy. Modified radical mastectomy has been recommended in such patients, even when physical examination and mammography are normal. An occult breast primary has been identified after mastectomy in 44% to 68% of patients.[35,36] Primary tumors are usually less than 2 cm in diameter; in occasional patients, only noninvasive tumor is identified in the breast.[37] Prognosis after primary therapy is similar to that of other patients with stage II breast cancer.[35–37] Radiation therapy to the breast after axillary lymph node dissection may be an effective alternative primary therapy. Adjuvant systemic chemotherapy after primary therapy appears indicated in this setting.

Women with metastatic sites in addition to the axillary lymph nodes may have metastatic breast cancer with an occult primary. These women should be managed as if they have metastatic breast cancer. Elevated serum levels of CA 15-3 suggest the possibility of breast cancer. Estrogen and progesterone receptor status is of particular importance in these patients, because those with positive hormone receptors may derive major palliative benefit from hormonal therapy or chemotherapy or both.

Men With Skeletal Metastases

Metastatic prostate carcinoma should be suspected with adenocarcinoma involving predominantly bone, particularly if the metastases are blastic. In this setting, elevated levels of serum acid phosphatase of PSA or tumor staining with PSA provides confirmatory evidence of prostate cancer. Hormonal therapy may provide effective palliation.

Chemotherapy for Metastatic Adenocarcinoma of Unknown Primary Site

Most patients with well-differentiated or moderately differentiated adenocarcinoma of unknown primary site are not in one of the three clinical subgroups outlined above. Chemotherapy has been ineffective in most of these patients, producing low response rates and few complete responses. The results of chemotherapy in reported series of 10 or more patients are summarized in Table 58–3. Some patients with poorly differentiated carcinomas of unknown primary site were included in some of these series. Most of these patients did not receive cisplatin-based chemotherapy. The only drug that has been studied adequately as a single agent is 5-fluorouracil (5-FU); response rates ranged from 0% to 16%.[23,38,39] The FAM regimen (5-FU, doxorubicin, mitomycin C) and various modifications have been used frequently, based on the demonstrated activity of these regimens against some gastrointestinal cancers.[40–46] Response rates varied from 7% to 39%, median survival remained in the 4 to 11 month range,

TABLE 58–3. Empiric Chemotherapy Results in Series of Patients
With Adenocarcinoma of Unknown Primary Site

Investigations	Chemotherapy Regimen	No. of Patients	Response Rate (%)	Median Survival (mo)
Single-Agent Trials				
Schildt et al, 1983[23]	F	20	0	3.5
Johnson et al, 1964[38]	F	65	6	—
Moertel et al, 1972[39]	F	88	16	4
Combination Chemotherapy				
Woods et al, 1980[42]	AM	25	36	4.2
Eagan et al, 1987[43]	AM	28	7	5.5
Milliken et al, 1987[40]	AM	51	39	4.5
McKeen et al, 1980[41]	FAM	28	21	8+
Goldberg et al, 1986[44]	FAM	43	30	11
Fiore et al, 1985[46]	A + vindesine	38	13	8+
Kambhus et al, 1986[45]	AM + vindesine	55	26	6
Woods et al, 1980[42]	CMeF	22	5	3
Schildt et al, 1983[23]	CAF	16	0	3
Anderson et al, 1983[63]	CAV	20	50	8
Eagan et al, 1987[42]	AMP	27	19	5
Pasterz et al, 1986[64]	CAFP	47	28	7
Milliken et al, 1987[40]	PVeB	50	39	5

A, doxorubicin (Adriamycin); B, bleomycin; C, cyclophosphamide; F, 5-fluorouracil; M, mitomycin C; Me, methotrexate; P, cisplatin, V, vincristine; Ve, vinblastine; —, no data.

and long-term disease-free survivors were not reported. Cisplatin does not appear to have a major role in the treatment of well-differentiated adenocarcinoma of unknown primary site. In two randomized studies comparing a cisplatin-containing regimen to doxorubicin plus mitomycin C, no difference in median survival was observed, and increased toxicity occurred in the cisplatin-containing arm.[40,43] The combination of cisplatin and etoposide has not been evaluated adequately in patients with adenocarcinoma of unknown primary site, nor has the combination of 5-FU and leucovorin.

Patients with good performance status should be considered for a trial of chemotherapy. Regimens containing doxorubicin and mitomycin C have usually produced partial responses in 20% to 40% of patients. Complete responses are rare. No compelling evidence exists to include cisplatin in these regimens unless the histology is poorly differentiated (see the section on poorly differentiated carcinoma). Cisplatin-containing regimens have been studied in too few patients to make firm conclusions. In patients with widespread metastases and poor performance status, systemic chemotherapy is unlikely to be of benefit. In these patients it has been our policy to administer tamoxifen (for women) and megestrol acetate (for women and men) as a therapeutic trial.

SQUAMOUS CARCINOMA OF UNKNOWN PRIMARY SITE

Squamous carcinoma at a metastatic site represents about 5% of all patients with unknown primary carcinomas. Effective treatment is available for patients with certain clinical syndromes, and appropriate evaluation of these patients is important.

SQUAMOUS CARCINOMA INVOLVING CERVICAL AND SUPRACLAVICULAR LYMPH NODES

The cervical lymph nodes are the most common metastatic site. Patients are usually middle-aged or elderly, and frequently they have abused tobacco or alcohol. When the upper or middle cervical lymph nodes are involved, a primary tumor in the head and neck region should be suspected. Clinical evaluation should include an examination of the oropharynx, hypopharynx, nasopharynx, larynx, and upper esophagus by direct endoscopy, with biopsy of any suspicious areas. When the lower cervical or supraclavicular lymph nodes are involved, a primary lung cancer should be suspected. Fiberoptic bronchoscopy should be performed if the chest radiograph and head and neck examination are normal. Of patients presenting with squamous carcinoma in cervical lymph nodes, 20% to 40% will subsequently have a primary site documented during the clinical course. In these patients, most primary sites become manifest in the head and neck region.

When no primary site is identified, local treatment should be given to the involved neck. The reported results involve retrospective, single-institution experiences, often using a variety of treatment modalities (Table 58–4). In most reports, a substantial percentage of patients achieved long-term disease-free survival after local treatment modalities. The results obtained using radical neck dissection, high-dose radiation

TABLE 58–4. Squamous Carcinoma of Unknown Primary Site Involving Cervical Lymph Nodes: Summary of Results, 1970–1990

Investigations	No. of Patients	Treatment	5-Year Survival (%)
Barrie et al, 1970[47]	104	Surger ± RT	31
Jessie et al, 1973[48]	184*	Surgery, RT, surgery + RT	43
Coker et al, 1977[49]	39	Surgery + RT	54
Jose et al, 1979[50]	54*	RT ± surgery	29
Nordstrom et al, 1979[51]	51*	Surgery, RT, surgery + RT	29
Fermont et al, 1980[52]	139*	RT	5
Leipzig et al, 1981[53]	32	Surgery, RT, surgery + RT	32 (3-y)
Pacini et al, 1981[54]	42	RT	23
Spiro et al, 1983[55]	79	Surgery, RT, surgery + RT	29
Mobit-Tabatabasi et al, 1986[56]	46	Surgery, RT, surgery + RT	18
Yang et al, 1983[57]	80	RT	37
Yang et al, 1983[57]	33	Chemotherapy	5
Carlson et al, 1986[58]	93†	RT ± surgery	70
McCunniff et al, 1986[59]	25	RT ± surgery	48
Bataini et al, 1987[60]	138	RT ± surgery	35
De Braud et al, 1989[61]	25	Surgery, RT, surgery + RT	44
De Braud et al, 1989[61]	16	Chemotherapy + RT + surgery	69 (3-y)

RT, radiation therapy.
* Includes patients with poorly differentiated carcinoma and adenocarcinoma.
† Excludes patients with massive neck involvement (*i.e.,* "incurable" patients).

therapy, or a combination of these modalities have been similar. The volume of tumor in the involved neck influences outcome, with N1 or N2 disease having a significantly higher cure rate than N3 or massive neck involvement. When resection alone is used as the primary treatment modality, a primary tumor in the head and neck subsequently becomes obvious in 20% to 40% of patients. Primary tumors surface less commonly when radiation therapy is used, presumably due to the eradication of occult head and neck primary sites within the radiation field. Radiation therapy dosages and techniques should be similar to those used in patients with primary head and neck cancer,[58] and the nasopharynx, oropharynx, and hypopharynx should be included in the irradiated field.

Patients with low cervical and supraclavicular nodes do not do as well because lung cancer is a frequent site of occult primary tumors. Patients with no detectable disease below the clavicle should be treated with aggressive local therapy because 10% to 15% of these patients will have long-term disease-free survival.

The role of chemotherapy for metastatic squamous carcinoma in cervical lymph nodes is undefined. One small nonrandomized comparison of patients treated with local modalities alone or with local modalities combined with chemotherapy (cisplatin and 5-FU) showed a higher complete response rate (81% versus 60%) and longer median survival time (>37 months versus 24 months) in patients also receiving chemotherapy.[61] Larger, randomized studies are necessary to verify the role of chemotherapy. The role of neoadjuvant chemotherapy in locally advanced head and neck carcinoma re-

mains unproved; the role in this more unusual patient group is unlikely to be clarified soon.

SQUAMOUS CARCINOMA INVOLVING INGUINAL LYMPH NODES

Most patients with a tumor in inguinal lymph nodes have a detectable primary site in the genital or anorectal areas. Careful examination of vulva, vagina, cervix, penis, and scrotum is important, with biopsy of any suspicious areas. Digital examination and anoscopy should be performed to exclude lesions in the anorectal area. Identification of a primary site in these patients is important, because curative therapy is available for carcinomas of the vulva, vagina, cervix, and anus, even after spread to regional lymph nodes. For the patient in whom no primary site is identified, surgical resection with or without radiation therapy to the inguinal area sometimes results in long-term survival.[62]

SQUAMOUS CARCINOMA METASTATIC TO OTHER SITES

Metastatic tumor in areas other than the cervical or inguinal lymph nodes usually represents metastasis from an occult primary lung cancer. CT scans of the chest and fiberoptic bronchoscopy should be considered. Chemotherapy with regimens employed in the treatment of non-small cell lung cancer may be considered in patients with good performance status.

Patients with the diagnosis of poorly differentiated squamous carcinoma should be evaluated carefully, particularly if other clinical features are atypical for lung cancer (*i.e.*, young patient, nonsmoker, unusual metastatic sites). Occasionally, adenocarcinomas, particularly in the breast, undergo squamous differentiation at metastatic sites. As with the diagnosis of poorly differentiated adenocarcinoma, this histologic diagnosis is sometimes based on minimal histologic findings. Additional pathologic evaluation with immunoperoxidase stains or electron microscopy should be considered. When the diagnosis remains unclear, such patients should be considered for a trial of therapy for poorly differentiated carcinoma as discussed later in this chapter.

POORLY DIFFERENTIATED CARCINOMA AND ADENOCARCINOMA OF UNKNOWN PRIMARY SITE

Patients with poorly differentiated carcinoma or adenocarcinoma of unknown primary site appear to represent distinctive subgroups with specific therapeutic implications. They account for about 30% of all patients with carcinoma of unknown primary site; about 20% have poorly differentiated carcinoma, and 10% have poorly differentiated adenocarcinoma. Chemotherapy trials in the past often included these patients along with the more common patients with well-differentiated adenocarcinoma of unknown primary. All these patients were assumed to be similar, and they experienced a poor response to 5-FU-based chemotherapy and a short survival (see Table 58–3).[23,38–46,63,64] These chemotherapy trials included drugs likely to be useful in a palliative sense for patients with gastrointestinal and breast carcinomas. Some patients with poorly differentiated carcinomas have responsive neoplasms, and some are curable with cisplatin-based combination chemotherapy.[65–72] Clinical and pathologic evaluation is therefore crucial in patients with poorly differentiated carcinoma.

CLINICAL CHARACTERISTICS

The clinical characteristics in this diverse group of patients appears to differ substantially from the characteristics of patients with well-differentiated adenocarcinoma. The median age of this patient group is younger, although both groups have a wide age range. Patients with poorly differentiated carcinoma often give a history of rapid progression of symptoms (often <30 days) and have objective evidence of rapid tumor growth.[24,65,73] Most importantly, the location of metastases differs, and the predominant sites of involvement are frequently lymph nodes, mediastinum, and retroperitoneum, occurring much more commonly than in well-differentiated adenocarcinoma.

PATHOLOGIC EVALUATION

Light microscopic features that can differentiate chemotherapy-responsive tumors from nonresponsive tumors have not been identified.[66] Even with careful retrospective review of these tumors, responsive tumors of well-defined types (*e.g.*, germ cell tumor, lymphoma) are only rarely identified.

These tumors should undergo additional pathologic study with immunoperoxidase staining, electron microscopy, and genetic analysis. The use of routine light microscopy alone is not adequate to assess these tumors. The information provided by these additional pathologic studies has been summarized previously (see the section on poorly differentiated neoplasms). The frequency of more specific diagnoses, particularly lymphoma, is much lower in the carcinoma group than in the group initially diagnosed by routine light microscopy as poorly differentiated neoplasm. This is not surprising because carcinoma is a more specific diagnosis. Other diagnoses may still be suggested.

To assess the clinical utility of immunoperoxidase tumor-cell staining in patients with poorly differentiated carcinoma of unknown primary site, we retrospectively performed a battery of stains on archival tumors in 1989 from 87 patients treated between 1978 and 1983.[67] Poorly differentiated carcinoma or poorly differentiated adenocarcinoma was diagnosed on the basis of routine light microscopic examination, and all patients were treated before the technology of immunoperoxidase staining was routinely used. Therefore, results of immunoperoxidase staining could be correlated with clinical outcome in this group of similarly treated patients with a long median follow-up. Immunoperoxidase staining confirmed the diagnoses of poorly differentiated carcinoma in 49 patients (56%) and yielded other diagnoses in 14 patients (16%): melanoma (in 8 patients), lymphoma (4), prostatic carcinoma (1), and yolk sac carcinoma (1). In 24 patients (28%), the immunoperoxidase staining pattern was inconclusive; electron microscopy was occasionally helpful in clarifying the diagnosis in these patients. Seventy-five patients (86%) received combination chemotherapy with a cisplatin-based regimen, and 24 patients (28%) had a complete response. Nine of these patients were later given specific diagnoses by immunoperoxidase staining; lymphoma was diagnosed in 4 patients, melanoma in 4 patients, and yolk sac tumor in 1 patient. All patients with an immunoperoxidase diagnosis of lymphoma had clinical features compatible with lymphoma and are long-term survivors. Patients with immunoperoxidase features suggesting melanoma were surprisingly responsive to chemotherapy, with 3 of 7 complete responses and 2 long-term survivors. Patients with melanoma diagnosed by immunoperoxidase staining alone should not be excluded from a trial of cisplatin-based therapy. Immunoperoxidase staining is useful in the routine evaluation of metastatic poorly differentiated carcinoma of unknown primary site, as it can occasionally suggest the lineage of the tumor and have specific therapeutic implications.

Immunoperoxidase staining should be used in the evaluation of poorly differentiated carcinomas to do the following:

1. Confirm the diagnosis of carcinoma
2. Identify a primary site of a recognized carcinoma (*e.g.*, prostate)
3. Identify patients who may have other neoplasms, such as lymphoma or melanoma (although therapeutic recommendations for neoplasms other than lymphoma identified in this manner remain to be established)
4. Identify a group of patients in whom electron microscopy may provide important additional information

Electron microscopy can be useful for a small minority of these carcinomas. In general, electron microscopy should be reserved for those tumors not diagnosed by immunoperoxidase stains. Lymphoma can be diagnosed reliably in most instances in those tumors mistakenly believed to be carcinoma. In addition, sarcoma, melanoma, mesothelioma, and neuroendocrine tumors occasionally are defined by subcellular features. Neuroendocrine differentiation is particularly important and is discussed later in this chapter.

Chromosomal analysis is becoming an increasingly important method of diagnosis. Specific abnormalities have been identified in some leukemias, lymphomas, germ cell tumors, peripheral neuroepithelioma, and Ewing's sarcoma.[16–22,74] Evaluation for these specific abnormalities may be useful in patients with poorly differentiated carcinoma of unknown primary site. In reference to germ cell tumors, Motzer and colleagues performed genetic analysis (cytogenetic study and Southern blot analyses) on tumors in 8 patients with midline carcinomas of uncertain histology.[22] In 4 of the 8 patients with poorly differentiated carcinoma, abnormalities of chromosome 12 (*e.g.*, i[12p]; del [12 q]; multiple copies of 12 p) were diagnostic of germ cell tumor. Three of the 4 patients diagnosed on basis of genetic analysis achieved a complete response to cisplatin-based chemotherapy. This confirms the previously formulated hypothesis that some of these patients have histologically atypical germ cell tumors.[69] These genetic findings can be diagnostic in these patients. Additional specific chromosomal abnormalities in other solid tumors probably will be identified in the future, further improving the ability to establish tumor lineage.

Autopsy data looking specifically at patients with poorly differentiated carcinoma of unknown primary site are limited. Unfortunately, the number of postmortem examinations in medicine in general is declining. Based on the limited necropsy data we have accumulated, it appears that primary sites are found only occasionally in these patients (<35%). These findings are contrary to those for well-differentiated adenocarcinoma of unknown primary site, in which the primary site is found in most patients (>75%) at autopsy.[24]

DIAGNOSTIC EVALUATION

The clinical evaluation of these patients is similar to that described for patients with well-differentiated adenocarcinoma of unknown primary site. A history, physical examination, routine laboratory testing, and chest radiograph should be obtained in each patient. Any clues are followed with appropriate diagnostic testing. CT scans of the chest and abdomen should be performed in all patients in this group, due to the frequency of mediastinal and retroperitoneal involvement. Serum levels of HCG and AFP should be measured because substantial elevations of these markers suggest the diagnosis of germ cell tumor. The correlation of other serum tumor markers, such as CEA, CA 125, CA 19-9, and CA 15-3 with response to chemotherapy has not been established.

TREATMENT

When additional pathologic studies identify a specific neoplasm (*e.g.*, lymphoma, sarcoma), appropriate therapy can be administered. Patients with elevated serum levels of HCG or AFP and clinical features suggestive of extragonadal germ cell tumor (*e.g.*, mediastinal or retroperitoneal mass) should be treated with chemotherapy effective for germ cell tumors, even when pathologic examination is not diagnostic.

Most patients have multiple metastases and only the nonspecific diagnoses of poorly differentiated carcinoma or poorly differentiated adenocarcinoma despite additional pathologic study. The first reports showing that some of these patients (a small subset) have highly responsive tumors appeared about a decade ago.[68–71] Most of these patients were young men with mediastinal tumors; serum levels of HCG or AFP were frequently elevated. These patients initially were thought to have histologically atypical extragonadal germ cell tumors.

Further evidence for the responsiveness of other tumors in patients with poorly differentiated carcinoma of unknown primary site has accumulated during the last decade. The large prospectively collected group of patients from Vanderbilt University Medical Center will be discussed in detail because this group of patients is by far the largest group evaluated and treated in a similar fashion. Many recommendations for management are derived from this experience. Several other smaller patient groups have been reported recently and will be discussed briefly.

Prospective Series of Patients Compiled at Vanderbilt University Medical Center

Between 1978 and 1989, a series of 220 patients with poorly differentiated carcinoma of unknown primary site was prospectively compiled. Of these patients, 170 were initially seen and evaluated at Vanderbilt Medical Center. One hundred forty-two patients received their entire course of chemotherapy at Vanderbilt, and 28 patients were treated elsewhere according to our initial recommendations. After consultation, these patients were treated according to our recommendations, and detailed treatment records were obtained. Because of our ongoing interest in these patients, we frequently receive telephone consultations from oncologists practicing elsewhere. We have included 50 such patients from various regions of the United States in this series. These patients represent all telephone consultation patients during the years of this study who met entrance criteria and were treated (at our recommendation) with cisplatin-based chemotherapy. Therefore, the group of 220 patients includes all patients with poorly differentiated carcinoma or poorly differentiated adenocarcinoma of unknown primary site seen at Vanderbilt and all similar patients made known to us by telephone consultation during this 12-year period. Sixty-four of these 220 patients were evaluated and treated between 1978 and 1982 and were reported thereafter.[65]

Patients were included in this series if they had metastatic tumor at one or more sites and had one of the following light microscopic diagnoses: poorly differentiated carcinoma, poorly differentiated adenocarcinoma, poorly differentiated squamous carcinoma, or poorly differentiated small cell (questionable neuroendocrine) carcinoma. A few patients with the initial light microscopic diagnosis of poorly differentiated malignant neoplasm were included; in each of these tumors, specialized pathologic testing had confirmed the diagnosis of carcinoma. Between 1978 and 1982, at least one of the following clinical features was also required for inclusion: patient younger than 50 years, tumor involving primarily midline structures, elevated serum levels of HCG or AFP, clinical evidence of rapid tumor growth, or tumor responsive to previously administered radiation therapy or chemotherapy. After 1982, patients were included on the basis of histologic diagnosis alone, and no additional clinical feature was required.

PRETREATMENT EVALUATION. Because of the great variability in clinical presentation, diagnostic and staging procedures in these patients varied. All patients had a thorough history and physical examination, routine laboratory studies (complete blood counts, electrolytes, urinalysis, SMA12), and chest roentgenograms. Most patients also had CT scans of the chest and abdomen, and most had pretreatment determinations of serum HCG and AFP. Specific abnormalities identified by history, physical examination, or routine laboratory tests were investigated with further diagnostic studies in an attempt to identify a primary site. Fiberoptic bronchoscopy was performed in patients with radiographic evidence suggesting a lung cancer; patients with endobronchial lesions compatible with lung cancer were excluded from this series. In general, patients did not undergo an exhaustive radiologic search for a primary site in the absence of specific signs and symptoms, because this approach has not been found useful.

Biopsy specimens from all patients were examined at Vanderbilt University Medical Center. The initial diagnosis was always made on the basis of either an excisional biopsy or a core needle biopsy. Cytologic analysis alone (*e.g.*, fine-needle aspiration) was not used for diagnosis in any patient. Histochemical staining from mucin (or mucicarmine) was performed in 187 patients (85%). Most biopsies were evaluated further with immunoperoxidase staining or electron microscopy or both. A few tumors were studied by genetic analysis. During the first several years of this study, immunoperoxidase staining was not a standard part of the evaluation of poorly differentiated tumors because the antibodies were not available. Immunoperoxidase stains were subsequently performed on paraffin-fixed tumor specimens from many patients in this series, as part of a separate retrospective study.[67] Most of the patients in whom neither electron microscopy nor immunoperoxidase staining was performed had poorly differentiated adenocarcinoma by light microscopy; in these patients, the pathologist believed that further study was unlikely to result in additional useful information. Subsequently, several of these tumors were better defined by specialized pathology (see the summary of pathology studies below).

The light microscopic diagnosis of poorly differentiated carcinoma was based on the finding of a pleomorphic population of large cohesive malignant cells growing with no definable histologic pattern. Poorly differentiated adenocarcinoma was diagnosed if any adenomatous differentiation occurred, such as rudimentary gland formation or polarity of cells. In addition, some tumors with histologic features of poorly differentiated carcinoma were called poorly differentiated adenocarcinoma if the histochemical staining for mucin was strongly positive. All tumors with features of well-differentiated or moderately well-differentiated adenocarcinoma (*i.e.*, well-formed glandular structures, ducts with lumina, and mucin evident from hematoxylin-eosin staining) were excluded from this series. Poorly differentiated small cell carcinomas (questionable neuroendocrine) had a cohesive, homogenous population of small cells, with a high nucleus-to-cytoplasm ratio and dispersed chromatin in the nucleus.

CLINICAL CHARACTERISTICS. The clinical characteristics of the 220 patients are summarized in Table 58–5. The median age was 39 years, and 76% of the patients were younger than 50 years. Males outnumbered females by about 3 to 1. There were only 9 blacks (4%), which may reflect patterns of patient referral or rarity in blacks. One hundred seventeen patients (53%) had a history of tobacco use (more than 10 pack-years). Most patients were ambulatory and had only mild to moderate symptoms at the time of diagnosis.

Serum levels of HCG, AFP, and lactic dehydrogenase (LDH) were measured in most patients. HCG and AFP levels were infrequently elevated. Serum LDH levels were elevated in 48% of patients; however, 32 of 96 patients (33%) with elevated levels also had liver metastases as a possible source for LDH. Serum CEA levels were measured in 127 patients and were elevated in 47 (37%). Other more recently available markers (*e.g.*, CA 125, CA 15-3, CA 19-9) were measured in only a few patients.

Staging evaluation revealed metastases in two or more sites in 74% of patients. Many of the patients with metastases in only one site also had extensive tumor; for example, patients with multiple liver metastases or multiple bone metastases as the only site of tumor involvement were included in this group. In none of these patients was the single site of tumor believed to be a primary site, and in only 4 of the 57 patients in this group could a complete resection be accomplished. These 4 patients had tumor involving a single peripheral lymph node area.

Patients were categorized according to their predominant site of tumor involvement (see Table 58–5). Because most patients had two or more sites of metastases, assignment of a dominant site was sometimes arbitrary but was based on the site containing the greatest bulk of tumor. For example, a patient with a large retroperitoneal mass and several small liver defects on CT scan was classified as having predominant disease in the retroperitoneum. One hundred five patients (48%) had predominant tumor involvement in the mediastinum, retroperitoneum, or other peripheral lymph node groups. Patients with predominant lung involvement usually had multiple lung masses, and most had normal fiberoptic bronchoscopy. Fifty patients had tumor involving multiple metastatic sites, without an identifiable dominant site of involvement.

SUMMARY OF PATHOLOGY STUDIES. Based on initial routine light microscopic evaluation, 193 patients (88%) were given the diagnoses of poorly differentiated carcinoma (142 patients) or poorly differentiated adenocarcinoma (51 patients). Histochemical staining for mucin or mucicarmine was performed in 187 patients as a part of the initial evaluation. This test was positive in 47 patients (25%); most tumors with positive staining were called poorly differentiated adenocarcinomas. The remaining 27 patients were given the following diagnoses by light microscopy: poorly differentiated small cell carcinoma or poorly differentiated carcinoma with neuroendocrine features (12 patients), poorly differentiated malignant

TABLE 58–5. Clinical Characteristics of 220 Patients
With Poorly Differentiated Carcinoma of Unknown Primary
Site Treated at Vanderbilt University Medical Center

Characteristics	No. of Patients (%)
Sex	
Female/male	54/166
Race	
White	209
Black	9
Asian	2
Performance Status	
ECOG 0, 1	188
ECOG 2, 3	32
Dominant Metastatic Site	
Mediastinum	43 (20)
Retroperitoneum	42 (19)
Lung	29 (13)
Lymph nodes (cervical, axillary, inguinal)	20 (9)
Liver	11 (5)
Pleura/peritoneum	6
Bone	5
Pelvic mass	4
Pancreas	3
Soft tissue	2
Brain	2
Other (1 each)	3
Multiple sites (no dominant site)	50 (23)
Serum Tumor Markers	
HCG (N = 206)	
• Normal	174
• Elevated	32 (16)
AFP (N = 201)	
• Normal	190
• Elevated	11 (5)
LDH (N = 199)*	
• Normal	103
• Elevated	96 (48)
CEA (N = 127)	
• Normal	80
• Elevated	47 (37)
No. of Metastatic Sites	
1	57 (26)
2	67 (31)
3	60 (27)
>3	36 (16)

AFP, α-fetoprotein; CEA, carcinoembryonic antigen; ECOG, Eastern
Cooperative Oncology Group; HCG, human chorionic gonadotropin;
LDH, lactic dehydrogenase.
* Thirty-two of 96 patients had liver metastases as possible source
for elevated LDH.

neoplasm (11 patients), and poorly differentiated squamous
carcinoma (4 patients).

In most patients, other specialized pathologic studies were
performed in addition to light microscopy. Immunoperoxidase
studies were performed on 147 tumors and electron microscopy on 96 tumors. In only 46 cases was the final diagnosis
based on light microscopic appearance alone. Immunoperoxidase studies in 32 patients were performed later (retrospectively) when the technology become available,[67] long after
these patients had been treated. Patients in whom specialized
pathologic evaluation before therapy resulted in a tumor diagnosis with specific therapeutic implications (e.g., lymphoma) were not included in the series and received appropriate tumor-specific therapy.

In only 30 patients (13%) was the primary site or tumor
type eventually identified (Table 58–6). In 17 of these 30
patients, the definitive diagnosis was made at repeat biopsy
later during the course of the disease or at autopsy. In the
remainder, retrospective specialized pathology studies provided the basis for diagnosis. All six lymphomas were identified
retrospectively: 4 by immunoperoxidase staining, 1 by repeat
biopsy at the time of tumor relapse, and 1 by genetic analysis
(detection of an immunoglobulin gene rearrangement). Unfortunately, only 26 autopsies were done, and in only 9 (34%)
was a primary site identified. In the remainder, metastatic
poorly differentiated carcinoma or poorly differentiated adenocarcinoma with no primary site was found. In addition, 9
patients were thought to have melanoma on the basis of
pathologic review or special pathologic studies; however, none
of these patients had a known primary site, and none had
typical light microscopic findings of melanoma.

THERAPY. At the time of identification, 198 patients had
received no previous treatment for their cancer, whereas 22
patients had received radiation therapy (10 patients), chemotherapy (10 patients), or both (2 patients). In addition, 2
patients had a distant history of a previous neoplasm for which
they had received radiation therapy (1 patient) or chemotherapy (1 patient).

All patients were treated with cisplatin-based combination
chemotherapy (Table 58–7). One hundred sixteen patients
treated between 1978 and 1984 received the cisplatin,
vinblastine, bleomycin regimen (PVB) or a doxorubicin-
containing modification of the PVB regimen. In 1985, etoposide was substituted for vinblastine in the treatment regimen, due to the synergy of etoposide with cisplatin and the
demonstration of reduced toxicity and at least equivalent results.[75] Since 1985, 104 patients have received regimens including cisplatin and etoposide. In most patients, cisplatin
and etoposide were administered for 5 days (cisplatin 20 mg/
m^2 intravenously daily for 5 days, and etoposide 100 mg/m^2
intravenously daily for 5 days). In 55 patients, bleomycin (30
units weekly) was added to cisplatin and etoposide. Nine patients received regimens that included other agents in addition
to cisplatin and etoposide.

Patients received two courses of therapy at 3-week intervals
and were then evaluated for response. All patients showing
any evidence of response after two courses received a total
of four courses of therapy. Patients who failed to show any
initial response were treated with alternative therapy.

TABLE 58–6. Specific Pathologic Diagnoses Confirmed

Diagnosis	Autopsy	Rebiopsy (After Initial Therapy)	Review of Light Microscopy	Electron Microscopy	Immunoperoxidase Staining	Genetic Analysis	Total
			Method of Diagnosis				
Lymphoma		1			4	1	6
Sarcoma (no primary site)		1		5			6
Lung							
Adenocarcinoma	5						5
Mixed adenocarcinoma and small cell carcinoma		1					1
Germ cell tumor							
Extragonadal		2	1				3
Testis		1					1
Carcinoid tumor*	2	1					3
Peripheral neuroepithelioma						1	1
Kidney carcinoma	1						1
Pancreatic carcinoma	1						1
Prostatic carcinoma					1		1
Breast carcinoma		1					1
Total	9	8	1	5	5	2	30

* Primary sites identified in 2 of 3 patients (rectum 1, lung 1).

Complete reevaluation was performed after completion of four courses of chemotherapy. All previously abnormal radiographic studies were repeated, and some patients had exploratory surgery for resection or biopsy of residual masses to better define tumor response. Patients were considered complete responders if no residual evidence of malignancy was found at reevaluation (*i.e.*, normalization of all previously abnormal physical or radiographic findings and normalization of biochemical findings). Partial response was defined as an objective decrease of 50% or greater in tumor size (product of perpendicular diameters), without interval appearance of any new lesions. All remaining patients were considered nonresponders. Duration of survival was calculated from the first day of treatment.

TABLE 58–7. Combination Chemotherapy in 220 Patients With Poorly Differentiated Carcinoma/Adenocarcinoma

Chemotherapy	No. of Patients
Cisplatin, vinblastine, bleomycin (PVB regimen)	107
PVB + doxorubicin	9
Cisplatin, etoposide, bleomycin	55
Cisplatin, etoposide	40
Cisplatin, etoposide, vinblastine	3
Cisplatin, etoposide, bleomycin, vinblastine	2
Cisplatin, etoposide, ifosfamide	2
Cisplatin, etoposide, cyclophosphamide, vincristine, methotrexate	2

TREATMENT RESULTS. Two hundred nine patients received at least two courses of treatment and were evaluable for response to therapy. Eleven patients were inevaluable for response, for the following reasons: 6 died of treatment-related complications before the second course, 3 died of unrelated intercurrent illnesses during chemotherapy, and 2 refused treatment after only one course. These patients are all considered treatment failures in calculating the actuarial survival curve.

Fifty-eight patients (26%) had complete response to cisplatin-based therapy, whereas 80 patients (36%) had a partial response. An additional 4 patients were treated after surgical excision of their metastatic lesion, at a time when they had no evaluable tumor. Three of these 4 patients had tumor at the margins of the resection and therefore were known to have residual local disease. These patients were not assessed for response to chemotherapy but are included in the overall survival curve. Thirty-six patients (16% of the entire group) were free of disease at a median of 61 months following therapy (range 11 to 142 months). Thirty-two of these patients have been continuously disease free since completion of chemotherapy. Three patients relapsed after an initial complete response and are in a second complete response after salvage chemotherapy. One patient had a partial response to initial cisplatin-based chemotherapy but achieved complete response with subsequent resection of residual tumor followed by local radiation therapy. In addition to the 36 patients known to be disease free, 2 patients were lost to follow-up while in complete remission 28 and 42 months after completion of therapy. Twenty-four of 27 patients (89%) who relapsed after achieving complete remission did so during the first 12 months after treatment; only 1 patient has relapsed more than 24 months after completing therapy.

The actuarial survival curves for the entire group of patients and for the subset of patients who achieved complete remission are shown in Figures 58–1 and 58–2. Median survival for the entire group is 12 months, with an actuarial 16% 12-year survival. The actuarial survival at 12 years for patients achieving complete response is 62%. Treatment results do not differ significantly after deletion of the 30 patients in whom specific diagnoses were eventually made. In the remaining 190 patients, 49 (26%) had complete response, 70 (37%) had partial response, and 30 (16%) are long-term disease-free survivors.

Results in the 170 patients seen or treated at Vanderbilt were compared with the 50 patients seen and treated elsewhere. The complete response rate was significantly higher in patients treated elsewhere (21 of 50 [42%] versus 41 of 170 [24%], $p<0.05$). The percentage of long-term survivors was higher in the group treated elsewhere but did not attain statistical significance at the $p<0.05$ level (13 of 50 [26%] versus 24 of 170 [14%]). These results further clarify that these patients are being seen and managed appropriately in the community.

Treatment Results From Other Recent Series

Other investigators have demonstrated the responsiveness of these tumors.[73, 76–78] Van der Gaast and colleagues from Holland treated 40 patients with either poorly differentiated carcinoma or poorly differentiated adenocarcinoma; combination chemotherapy included bleomycin, etoposide, and cisplatin.[73] Eighteen of 34 patients (53%) responded, with 4 (12%) complete responses and 2 long-term disease-free survivors.

In the report of Raber and colleagues at the M.D. Anderson Cancer Center, 36 evaluable patients (21 patients with adenocarcinoma, 14 with undifferentiated carcinoma, and 1 with squamous cell carcinoma) received cisplatin, 5-FU, and etoposide.[76] Eight patients (22%) responded, but 4 (11%) had complete responses with durations of 19, 19, 24+ and 37+ months. Briassoulis and colleagues from Greece treated 42 patients (31 patients with poorly differentiated carcinoma and 11 with adenocarcinoma) with either cisplatin-based or carboplatin-based combination regimens. Nine of 42 (21%) responded with 3 (7%) complete responders.[77] Zarba and col-

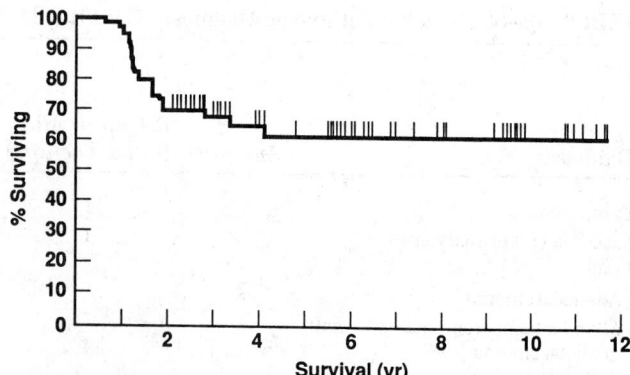

FIGURE 58–2. Actuarial survival curve of complete responders (62%). Tick marks indicate patients free of tumor.

leagues from France reported 22 evaluable patients (all adenocarcinoma) treated with 5-FU, mitomycin C, epirubicin, and cisplatin.[78] Nine patients (40%) responded with 2 (10%) complete responders. In each of these series, with the exception of the series by van der Gaast and colleagues, some patients had well-differentiated or moderately well-differentiated adenocarcinoma.

The achievement of complete remissions in a minority of these patients is reproducible, as is a small cohort (5% to 15%) of long-term disease-free survivors. Combination chemotherapy should include cisplatin and etoposide with or without bleomycin. Results for this combination are at least as good as previous results using cisplatin, vinblastine, and bleomycin and are achieved with less toxicity. A therapeutic trial of two courses should be given. Responders should complete a total of four treatment courses. No evidence exists that more prolonged treatment will improve results, and nearly all long-term survivors have received only four treatment courses. In patients with residual palpable or radiographic abnormalities, surgical resection should be contemplated.

Although these results represent marked improvement when compared with the dismal historical results, this group of patients is heterogenous, and there are many patients with unresponsive tumors. Many of these patients should be considered for investigational trials of newer approaches. Several responsive subsets can be identified using clinical and pathologic features.

CLINICAL AND PATHOLOGIC CHARACTERISTICS PREDICTIVE OF RESPONSIVE TUMORS

A detailed analysis of the series of 220 patients compiled at Vanderbilt has revealed several important features. Table 58–8 shows the relation of response and long-term survival to the site of dominant tumor involvement. Most groups of patients had high overall response rates. Tumor responses usually correlate with good palliation and prolongation of survival. Complete responses and long-term survival were more frequent when tumor involved predominantly the retroperitoneum or peripheral lymph node areas (*e.g.*, cervical, axillary, or inguinal). Patients with multiple visceral sites of involvement had only a small chance of long-term disease-free survival.

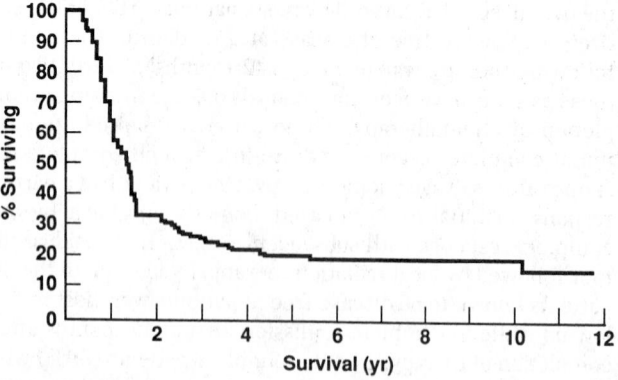

FIGURE 58–1. Twelve-year actuarial survival curve for all 220 patients with poorly differentiated carcinoma of unknown primary site (16% at 12 years).

TABLE 58–8. Chemotherapy Response, Survival, and Predominant Site of Tumor

Dominant Tumor Site	No. of Patients	Overall Response Rate (CR + PR) (%)	No. of Complete Responders (%)	No. of Disease-Free Survivors (%)
Retroperitoneum	42	35 (83)	21 (50)	13 (31)
Peripheral lymph nodes (cervical, axillary, inguinal)	20	14 (70)	11 (55)	9 (45)
Mediastinum	43	29 (67)	13 (30)	7 (16)
Bone	5	3 (60)	1 (20)	1 (20)
Pelvic mass	4	4 (100)	1 (25)	1 (25)
Lung	29	21 (72)	6 (21)	2 (7)
Liver	11	5 (45)	1 (9)	1 (9)
Pleura/peritoneum	6	2 (33)	1 (17)	0
Multiple sites (no dominant site)	50	25 (50)	5 (10)	2 (4)
Other sites*	10	4 (40)	2 (20)	1 (10)
Total	220	142 (65)	62 (28)	37 (17)

* Sites include pancreas (3 patients), brain (2), subcutaneous tissue (2), stomach (1), parotid (1), and nasopharynx (1).

The chance for complete response and long-term survival depends on several clinical and pathologic characteristics (Table 58–9). The following clinical features are highly predictive of an excellent therapeutic outcome, as determined by univariate analysis:

1. Predominant tumor location in the retroperitoneum or peripheral lymph nodes
2. Tumor limited to one or two metastatic sites
3. Normal serum CEA level
4. Normal serum LDH level
5. No history of cigarette use

Other characteristics, including age, sex, light microscopic histology, and cisplatin-based regimen had no significant influence on treatment outcome.

A Cox multivariate regression analysis was performed using the following prognostic factors: age, sex, smoking history, light microscopic histology (poorly differentiated carcinoma versus poorly differentiated adenocarcinoma), predominant tumor location (retroperitoneum or peripheral lymph nodes versus all other sites), number of metastatic sites (1 or 2 versus >2), LDH level, CEA level, and tumor marker (HCG, AFP) levels. The following factors were shown to have favorable prognostic significance: predominant tumor location in the retroperitoneum or peripheral lymph nodes ($p<0.001$), limited (1 or 2) metastatic sites ($p<0.001$), negative smoking history ($p=0.003$), and younger age ($p=0.028$).

Finally, a group of patients with clinical features highly suggestive of extragonadal germ cell tumors was analyzed for response to therapy and long-term survival. This group included 34 men younger than 45 years who had predominant disease in the mediastinum or retroperitoneum. Six of these men had elevated serum levels of AFP, HCG, or both. The histologic features of all tumors in this group were re-reviewed, and only one had typical features of a germ cell tumor (yolk sac tumor).[66] In this group, 29 of 34 patients (85%) responded to therapy, with 17 patients (50%) having complete response.

Ten patients in this group (29%) remain disease free. Therefore, selection of patients with *clinical features* suggestive of extragonadal germ cell tumor, despite the nondiagnostic histology, defines a subgroup with a higher complete response rate and long-term survival than the group as a whole (see the section on special issues in cancer of unknown primary site).

Neuroendocrine Carcinomas of Unknown Primary Site

Electron microscopic examination of poorly differentiated carcinomas identifies neurosecretory granules in about 10% of tumors. These tumors are called "poorly differentiated neuroendocrine tumors" or "primitive neuroectodermal tumors" on this basis. Neuroendocrine features are suggested occasionally by light microscopic examination in some of these tumors. In most tumors, however, the light microscopic diagnosis is poorly differentiated carcinoma. A group of 29 patients with poorly differentiated neuroendocrine tumors was reported from Vanderbilt University (Table 58–10).[72] Most patients had clinical evidence of a high-grade tumor, and most had metastases in multiple sites. The retroperitoneum, lymph nodes, and mediastinum were frequently involved. Eighteen of 23 evaluable patients responded to chemotherapy with either a cisplatin-based combination or a combination regimen useful for patients with small cell lung cancer. Six patients had complete responses, and 3 patients remain continuously disease free more than 2 years after completion of therapy. Four other patients with limited involvement at only one site were treated with local modalities only (surgical excision in 3 patients and radiation therapy in 1 patient). All 4 patients have had long-term disease-free survival.

The nature and lineage of these tumors in most patients remains unclear. In 4 patients, specific diagnoses were made later in their clinical course or at autopsy. Two patients were found to have carcinoid tumors with undifferentiated growth pattern (both presented with abdominal carcinomatosis), 1

TABLE 58–9. Clinical and Pathologic Characteristics Predictive of Chemotherapy Responsiveness

Clinical/Pathologic Characteristics	No. of Patients	No. of Complete Responders (%)	p Value	No. of Disease-Free Survivors (%)	p Value
Age					
≤35 y	81	28 (35)	NS	18 (22)	
>35 y	139	34 (24)		19 (14)	NS
Sex					
Male	166	48 (29)	NS	29 (17)	NS
Female	54	14 (26)		8 (15)	
Dominant Tumor Location					
Retroperitoneum/peripheral nodes	62	32 (52)	<0.001	22 (35)	<0.001
All others	158	30 (19)		15 (9)	
Smoking History					
>10 pack-years	117	24 (21)	0.007	14 (12)	0.038
≤10 pack-years	103	38 (37)		23 (22)	
Light Microscopic Histology					
PDC	142	43 (30)	NS	28 (20)	NS
PDA	51	9 (18)		5 (10)	
No. of Metastatic Sites					
1 or 2	124	46 (37)	<0.001	32 (26)	<0.001
>2	96	16 (17)		5 (5)	
Chemotherapy					
PVB ± A	116	29 (25)		15 (13)	NS
Cisplatin/etoposide	104	33 (32)	NS	22 (21)	
Serum Markers					
LDH: Normal	103	36 (35)	0.01	25 (24)	0.018
Elevated	96	18 (18)		11 (11)	
CEA: Normal	80	26 (33)	<0.001	17 (21)	0.003
Elevated	47	2 (4)		1 (6)	

A, doxorubicin (Adriamycin); CEA, carcinoembryonic antigen; LDH, lactic dehydrogenase; NS, not significant; PDA, poorly differentiated adenocarcinoma; PDC, poorly differentiated carcinoma; PVB, cisplatin, vinblastine, and bleomycin.

patient had small cell lung cancer, and 1 patient had an extragonadal germ cell tumor with predominant neuroendocrine differentiation. A few similar patients, some with long-term survival after chemotherapy, have been reported and classified as "extrapulmonary small cell carcinoma."[79,80] The histology of these tumors was always small cell carcinoma and most of these patients had a recognized primary site (*e.g.,* head and neck, salivary gland, esophagus, bladder). Because most of our patients did not have small cell carcinoma histology and primary sites were not identified, it is unlikely their tumors represent this entity. Similarly, it is possible that some patients had unrecognized small cell lung cancer with an occult primary. The histology was usually not typical, and almost half of the patients had no smoking history. This finding, coupled with the lack of pulmonary involvement, makes this possibility unlikely. The clinical and biologic behavior of these poorly

differentiated tumors is not typical of most of the other known types of neuroendocrine tumors in adults (*e.g.,* carcinoid tumors, islet cell tumors, medullary carcinoma of the thyroid, paraganglioma), which are well-defined clinical entities with typical histologic appearance and often indolent biology.

Perhaps some of these tumors represent an undifferentiated form of a well-recognized type of neuroendocrine tumor (*e.g.,* carcinoid, peripheral neuroepithelioma), albeit without a recognizable primary site. In the undifferentiated form, the clinical and pathologic characteristics no longer resemble the characteristics of the more differentiated counterpart. Some of these neoplasms may represent a newly defined (previously unrecognized) type of neuroendocrine tumor. It is likely, but not confirmed, that most of these tumors may be recognized by immunoperoxidase staining with chromogranin and NSE.

Although the nature of these tumors remains undefined,

TABLE 58–10. Poorly Differentiated Neuroendocrine Tumors of Unknown Primary Site in 29 Patients

	No. of Patients
Clinical Characteristics	
Male/female	21/8
Smoking (>10 pack-years)	17
Dominant Tumor Site	
Retroperitoneum	8
Lymph nodes	7
Mediastinum	3
Bone	2
Liver	2
Other	4
Multiple sites without dominant site	3
Treatment	
Cisplatin-based combinations	19
Cyclophosphamide, doxorubicin, vincristine ± etoposide	6
Surgical excision	3
Radiation therapy	1
Response to Chemotherapy	
Complete response	6
Partial response	12
No response or inevaluable	7
Continuously disease-free	3

(Data from Hainsworth JD, Johnson DH, Greco FA. Poorly differentiated neuroendocrine carcinoma of unknown primary site: A newly recognized clinicopathologic entity. Ann Intern Med 1988;109:364–371)

the presence of neuroendocrine differentiation (as determined by electron microscopy or immune staining) identifies a highly treatable subgroup. Chromosome studies of these tumors may be helpful if an 11:22 translocation is found, because this would support a diagnosis of peripheral neuroepithelioma or soft tissue Ewing's sarcoma. All of these patients should be considered for a trial of cisplatin-based chemotherapy. Some patients with limited single-site involvement may be curable with local treatment modalities alone.

SUMMARY OF DATA
ON POORLY DIFFERENTIATED CARCINOMA

These treatment results provide evidence that patients with poorly differentiated carcinoma or poorly differentiated adenocarcinoma of unknown primary site are distinct from other patients with carcinoma of unknown primary site. In these data collected prospectively over 12 years from the group of 220 patients at Vanderbilt, an overall response rate of 62% with intensive cisplatin-based chemotherapy was achieved. More importantly, 26% of patients had complete response to therapy, and the 12-year actuarial survival is 16%. Many of the complete responders have been continuously disease free for more than 5 years and are undoubtedly cured. Long-term

survivors were included in the groups treated at Vanderbilt and elsewhere, and somewhat better results were achieved in patients in the outside group, who were treated by oncologists from various regions of the United States. Similar results have been reported in small groups of patients identified prospectively using similar criteria and treated with cisplatin-based regimens.[73,76–78] Results in all these groups of patients contrast sharply with those previously reported for adenocarcinoma of unknown primary site, where the overall response rate was less than 30%, with rare complete responses and no long-term survivors.

The initial light microscopic diagnosis can reliably define this patient subgroup. About 60% of patients with carcinoma of unknown primary site have carcinomas with easily identified glandular features; these well-differentiated adenocarcinomas were excluded from our series, but some of these patients were included in other recent reports of cisplatin-based therapy.[76–78] Patients with only minimal histologic features of adenocarcinoma, or those with positive mucin stains as the only evidence of adenocarcinoma (poorly differentiated adenocarcinoma) have been included. Patients with the initial diagnosis of poorly differentiated neoplasm were excluded, unless additional pathologic studies provided evidence of carcinoma. Therefore, the identification of patients has relied primarily on well-defined, traditional histologic criteria, and consequently should be generally applicable and reproducible.

Despite detailed and specialized pathologic study, few tumors previously known to be potentially curable with chemotherapy can be defined. Only 4 patients with germ cell tumors and 1 patient with peripheral neuroepithelioma were eventually identified. Five patients with lymphoma are free of disease; however, the other 31 disease-free patients in this series had no well-defined tumor type.

The clinical characteristics of patients with poorly differentiated carcinoma differ from those previously described in the literature for patients with carcinoma of unknown primary site. This may be explained by the fact that the groups previously analyzed were comprised largely of patients with well-differentiated adenocarcinoma. The median age of patients in the Vanderbilt series was 39 years, substantially younger than reported for patients with adenocarcinoma of unknown primary site. The dominant site of metastatic tumor was frequently the mediastinum, retroperitoneum, or peripheral lymph nodes (50% of patients). These are uncommon sites of tumor involvement in patients with well-differentiated adenocarcinoma of unknown primary site, who usually have metastases involving liver, lungs, or bone. Considerable overlap exists between these two patient groups, and about 25% of the poorly differentiated carcinomas had metastases at multiple visceral sites.

Because most of the highly responsive tumors cannot be identified despite extensive pathologic evaluation, a variety of clinical features have been found to be useful as prognostic indicators (see Tables 58–8 and 58–9). Although evaluation of these clinical features enables the identification of patients with a higher chance of complete response, none of these indicators is specific enough to be able to exclude a patient from a therapeutic trial reliably.

Twelve years ago, we hypothesized that the highly responsive carcinomas probably were unrecognized or histologically atypical extragonadal germ cell tumors. We still believe that some of the highly responsive tumors are germ cell tumors that are marker negative and are not identifiable using all available pathologic methods. Strong support for this hypothesis has been provided by Motzer and colleagues, who demonstrated chromosome 12 abnormalities diagnostic of germ cell tumors in several young men with poorly differentiated midline carcinomas.[22] The excellent response to treatment and survival (50% complete responders, 29% disease-free survival) for patients with clinical features highly suggestive of extragonadal germ cell tumor suggests that these are germ cell tumors, albeit histologically atypical. These treatment results do not differ greatly from those in patients with known extragonadal germ cell tumors treated with standard cisplatin-based therapy.[81,82] If feasible, chromosomal analysis on tumor tissue should be done as a diagnostic test for selected patients with carcinoma of unknown primary site.

The responsive tumors in this patient group are heterogenous in their origin, and probably only a small subset of patients have histologically atypical germ cell tumors. A few of the patients have non-Hodgkin's lymphoma. Certain lymphomas are recognized to be confused with anaplastic carcinomas; some lymphomas, notably the Ki-1 lymphomas, also can stain positively with epithelial membrane antigen, further complicating their differentiation from carcinomas.[83] Hopefully, this confusion will be minimized or eliminated with the routine use of immunoperoxidase staining for CLA. A second group of highly responsive patients have poorly differentiated neuroendocrine tumors. The origin of such tumors remains speculative but may be an anaplastic variant of occult primary carcinoid. Metastatic poorly differentiated neuroendocrine carcinomas with known gastrointestinal or pancreatic primary sites have demonstrated marked sensitivity to chemotherapy with cisplatin and etoposide.[84]

The nature of the other responsive tumors in this heterogenous group of patients remains even more speculative. Malignant thymoma is a tumor recently recognized to be responsive to cisplatin-based therapy, with some patients experiencing long-term complete remissions.[85] Some patients with poorly differentiated carcinoma located predominantly in the mediastinum may have thymoma. A few patients in the Vanderbilt series who were long-term survivors were identified as having melanoma on the basis of immunoperoxidase stains. This diagnosis seems unusual because melanoma is a tumor that is usually unresponsive to chemotherapy. It is possible that melanomas identifiable only by immunoperoxidase staining or electron microscopy represent a uniquely chemotherapy-sensitive subset. Finally, it is possible that some responsive tumors represent a heretofore undefined tumor type. Alternatively, some may represent highly undifferentiated, and therefore perhaps chemotherapy-sensitive, epithelial tumors from occult primary sites, which are usually much less responsive to systemic therapy. It is likely that future knowledge and refinements in genetic diagnosis will establish the identity of many of these tumors.

The large series of patients compiled at Vanderbilt and smaller recent series provide firm evidence that patients with poorly differentiated carcinoma or poorly differentiated adenocarcinoma of unknown primary site require specific evaluation and treatment. Most of these patients have a major

tumor response to cisplatin-based therapy, and a few are cured with such treatment. The fact that 220 patients with poorly differentiated carcinoma were collected in a 12-year period at a single institution indicates these tumors are not rare. Many such patients continue to be treated with supportive care only, with local radiation therapy, or with 5-FU-based regimens, as a result of previous pessimism and data concerning patients with adenocarcinoma of unknown primary site. Patients evaluated and treated by several oncologists from around the United States (compiled at Vanderbilt) did as well as those patients treated at a single institution. This confirms that these patients can be identified appropriately and treated successfully outside an academic setting. Multivariate analysis of a large group of patients has identified important prognostic factors. The lack of importance of other factors (*i.e.*, sex, light microscopic histology, serum HCG and AFP levels) has been documented. Poorly differentiated carcinomas evaluated with state-of-the-art pathologic techniques have shown that *most* responsive tumors in this group are *not* misdiagnosed or poorly diagnosed but are truly of unknown origin and biology.

It is imperative to consider the large group of patients with well-differentiated or moderately well-differentiated adenocarcinoma as clinically distinct from those with poorly differentiated carcinomas. All patients with poorly differentiated carcinoma should be considered for a therapeutic trial with cisplatin-based chemotherapy. Those with favorable prognostic features are likely to respond well. Although treatment results appear similar with the cisplatin-based regimens, the combination of cisplatin, etoposide, and bleomycin has been shown to have less toxicity than the cisplatin, vinblastine, and bleomycin regimen and is therefore preferred. The usefulness of cisplatin-based therapy for patients with no favorable prognostic features is less certain. Responses are frequent, and a few long-term survivors have been seen even in poor prognostic groups (see Tables 58–8 and 58–9). Responses usually occur rapidly, and a brief therapeutic trial should be considered. If no response is observed after one or two courses, therapy should be discontinued and alternate approaches considered. Poorly differentiated carcinoma of unknown primary site should be viewed as a highly responsive tumor to appropriate combination chemotherapy. Many patients can enjoy substantial clinical benefit, prolongation of survival, and, at times, cure.

SPECIAL ISSUES IN CARCINOMA OF UNKNOWN PRIMARY ORIGIN

EXTRAGONADAL GERM CELL CANCER SYNDROME

Selected patients with poorly differentiated carcinoma almost certainly have germ cell tumors, although the histologic features are atypical, even when generous pathologic specimens are available for study. Chromosomal analysis may provide a definitive diagnosis in some of these patients, particularly if their tumor cells contain specific chromosome 12 abnormalities. Even if not found or in the absence of tumor karyotypic study, young people who have mediastinal or retroperitoneal masses with or without elevated serum levels of HCG or AFP should be suspected of harboring a germ cell tumor. Lymphoma should be ruled out by immunoperoxidase stains, electron microscopy, or, if necessary, cytogenetic studies (*e.g.,* chromosome analysis and immunoglobulin gene rearrangement evaluation). The clinical extragonadal germ cell cancer syndrome was described in 1979.[68,69] The full syndrome has the following features:

1. The syndrome usually occurs in young men (<50 years).
2. Tumors are predominantly located in the midline (mediastinum, retroperitoneum) or multiple pulmonary nodules.
3. The symptom interval is short (<3 months), and there is a history of rapid tumor growth.
4. Serum levels of HCG, AFP, or both are elevated.
5. There is a good response to previously administered radiation therapy or chemotherapy.

Few patients have all elements of this syndrome. These clinical features are those of extranodal germ cell tumors, but without definitive histology the diagnosis is not unequivocal. In rare cases, women can have these tumors, and the other features are not absolute. Any one feature suggests the possibility of a germ cell tumor. It is prudent to treat patients having these atypical germ cell tumors with cisplatin-based therapy.

A SINGLE SITE OF NEOPLASM

In the unusual situation where only one site of neoplasm is identified (*e.g.,* one node group or one large mass), the possibility of an unusual primary tumor mimicking metastatic disease should be considered. Several unusual tumors could present in this fashion, including Merkel's cell tumors, skin adnexal tumors (*e.g.,* apocrine, eccrine, and sebaceous carcinomas), and even sarcomas or melanomas that are mistakenly interpreted as metastatic carcinoma (pathologically and clinically). Patients with one site of involvement usually have metastatic carcinoma, and many other sites are present but are not detectable. In the absence of any other documented metastatic disease, these patients should be treated with aggressive local therapy (*i.e.,* resection, radiation therapy, or both) because a minority will enjoy long-term disease-free survival. If a definitive diagnosis cannot be established, and the neoplasm is poorly differentiated, we believe these patients should receive adjuvant cisplatin-based chemotherapy, but it is difficult to know if this treatment is superior to local therapy alone.

On occasion, patients will present with apparent solitary metastasis of adenocarcinoma or poorly differentiated carcinoma in the brain, liver, subcutaneous tissue, lymph nodes, or other areas. In most instances, other metastases will become clinically apparent with time. There are certainly examples of resection or radiation of these single areas and of patients doing well with no evidence of recurrence. At times, the resection may be planned as palliative, particularly with a brain metastases. The method of choice in managing these patients is to resect the single lesion. After resection and depending on the other clinical circumstances, patients may be candidates for chemotherapy, particularly if their histology is poorly differentiated carcinoma. In those patients with single metastases (*i.e.,* brain), it would be prudent to consider radiation

therapy after surgical resection. Isolated axillary adenocarcinoma in women often arises from an occult breast cancer (see the section on adenocarcinoma).

PROSTATE CANCER WITH ATYPICAL METASTASES

There have been patients with clinical presentations atypical for prostate cancer in whom the diagnosis was suggested only by tumor staining for PSA.[86,87] These patients usually presented with adenocarcinoma metastases to the lung, mediastinal lymph nodes, or upper abdominal lymph nodes, with no obvious involvement of bone or pelvic lymph nodes. Some of these patients respond to therapy for metastatic prostate cancer.

UNSUSPECTED GESTATIONAL CHORIOCARCINOMA

In young women with poorly differentiated carcinoma or anaplastic neoplasms, particularly with lung nodules, be aware of the possibility of metastatic gestational choriocarcinoma. The history of recent pregnancy, spontaneous abortion, or missed menstrual periods should suggest the possibility. In this group of patients, serum HCG levels are invariably elevated. On occasion, biopsy specimens do not show the classic appearance of choriocarcinoma but simply that of metastatic carcinoma, usually poorly differentiated. Ultrasound or CT scan of the abdomen may show an enlarged uterus, and a dilation and curettage may be indicated in these patients. Most of these patients are curable with single-agent methotrexate.

ISOLATED PLEURAL EFFUSION

An isolated pleural effusion containing carcinoma in women will occasionally represent metastatic disease from occult ovarian carcinoma or be accompanied by peritoneal carcinomatosis. Even when the patient has no symptoms or signs and an abdominopelvic CT scan is normal, the primary may reside in the abdomen or pelvis. These occult abdominal neoplasms may arise from the ovary or the peritoneal surface and most characteristically cause a right pleural effusion. Should there be no clue of neoplasm in the abdomen, an elevated plasma CA 125 level suggests the possibility of this phenomena. In the absence of clinical findings in the abdomen, laparoscopy or exploratory laparotomy might be diagnostic, but these procedures are not therapeutic in this setting. Some of these tumors are particularly responsive to cisplatin-based treatment.

An isolated pleural effusion can be a manifestation of a peripheral lung carcinoma (usually adenocarcinoma) or a mesothelioma. Diagnosis may be difficult; at times the primary is not apparent even after chest tube drainage. Cytology usually shows adenocarcinoma. Electron microscopy may reveal ultrastructural features diagnostic of mesothelioma. The therapy of these patients is difficult. In those with poor performance status or advanced age, a trial of tamoxifen or megestrol acetate is reasonable. In fit patients, a trial of cisplatin-based chemotherapy should be considered.

TABLE 58–11. Carcinoma of Unknown Primary Site: Summary of Evaluation and Therapy of Responsive Subsets

	Clinical Evaluation*	Special Pathologic Studies	Subsets	Therapy	Prognosis
Adenocarcinoma (well-differentiated or moderately differentiated)	Abdominal CT scan Men: Serum PSA Women: Mammogram Serum CA 15-3 Serum CA 125 Additional studies to evaluate symptoms, signs	Men: PSA stain Women: ER, PR	1. Women, axillary node involvement 2. Women, peritoneal carcinomatosis 3. Men, blastic bone metastases, high serum PSA, or PSA tumor staining 4. Single peripheral nodal site of involvement	Treat as primary breast cancer Surgical cytoreduction + chemotherapy effective in ovarian cancer Hormonal therapy for prostate cancer Lymph node dissection ± radiotherapy	Poor for entire group (median survival: 4 mo); better for subgroups
Squamous carcinoma	Cervical node presentation Panedoscopy Supraclavicular presentation Bronchoscopy Inguinal presentation Pelvic, rectal exams, anoscopy	None	Cervical adenopathy Supraclavicular Inguinal adenopathy	Radiation therapy ± neck dissection Radiation therapy Inguinal node dissection ± radiation therapy	25–50% 5-y survival 5–15% 5-y survival Potential long-term survival
Poorly differentiated carcinoma, poorly differentiated adenocarcinoma	Chest, abdominal CT scans; serum HCG, AFP; additional studies to evaluate symptoms, signs	Immunoperoxidase staining Electron microscopy Genetic analysis	1. Atypical germ cell tumors (identified by chromosomal abnormalities only) 2. Neuroendocrine tumors 3. Predominant tumor location in retroperitoneum, peripheral nodes	Treatment for germ cell tumor Cisplatin-based therapy Cisplatin/etoposide/bleomycin	40–50% cure rate High response rate 50% prolongation of survival; 10–20% cured

AFP, α-fetoprotein; ER, estrogen receptor; HCG, human chorionic gonadotropin; PR, progesterone receptor; PSA, prostate-specific antigen.
* In addition to history, physical examination, routine laboratory tests, and chest x-ray films.

GERM CELL TUMORS WITH METASTASES OF OTHER HISTOLOGIES

On occasion, patients with germ cell tumors, particularly extragonadal primaries, may have a metastatic lesion that consists of only somatic tumor cells. This is particularly true for neuroendocrine or sarcomatous differentiation. Patients therefore may be diagnosed as having a neuroendocrine tumor or sarcoma. In these rare instances, a primary germ cell tumor (usually extragonadal) is present elsewhere and subsequently will be clinically apparent. It is difficult to make the diagnosis initially. An elevated plasma AFP or HCG level is suggestive. The presence of a mediastinal, retroperitoneal, or testicular mass support this possibility. Chromosomal analysis of tumor tissue may be diagnostic if a specific chromosome 12 abnormality is found. If the patient has metastatic germ cell tumor with metastases of other histologies, the treatment of choice is cisplatin-based chemotherapy. These patients appear to have a worse prognosis than those with typical germ cell tumors because the somatic cell tumors are less sensitive to chemotherapy.

CARCINOID TUMORS OF UNKNOWN PRIMARY SITE

In rare instances, patients have metastatic typical carcinoid tumors but with an unknown primary site. This is more likely to manifest as multiple liver metastasis with an occult primary in the intestinal tract, usually in the ileum or rectum. These patients should be managed no differently than those with known primaries. In the event of a solitary lesion in a node, bone, liver, lung, or elsewhere, aggressive local therapy (*i.e.*, resection and radiation therapy) is indicated because there is a possibility of long-term control. If the histology is poorly differentiated, cisplatin-based chemotherapy is likely to be beneficial. Most of these patients with typical carcinoids (well-differentiated pattern) have indolent tumors, and recurrence over years is likely. The primary never becomes apparent in some patients, but the bronchus and gastrointestinal tract eventually reveal the primary in most cases.

SMALL CELL CARCINOMAS OF UNKNOWN PRIMARY SITE

Tumors with typical histologic features of small cell carcinomas of unknown primary site are not rare. These patients usually have an occult primary in the lung (bronchus), and CT chest scan or bronchoscopy may find the primary. Postmortem examination has disclosed clinically undetectable primaries in some patients. In rare instances, the occult primary arises from extrapulmonary sites (*e.g.*, salivary gland, esophagus, bladder). Poorly differentiated or atypical carcinoid tumors can mimic these tumors, as can other anaplastic neuroendocrine lesions. A poorly differentiated neuroendocrine carcinoma subset has been defined by electron microscopy and immunoperoxidase stains (see the section on poorly differentiated carcinoma). These patients usually do *not* have the classic or typical histologic features of small cell carcinomas. Patients with small cell carcinoma of unknown primary site should receive aggressive local therapy with resection or radiation therapy or both, followed by chemotherapy known to be useful in small cell lung cancer.

SUMMARY

The recognition of subsets of responsive tumors in patients within the large heterogenous population of cancers of unknown primary site represents an improvement in the management of these patients. These patients with responsive tumors can often be defined with appropriate clinical and pathologic evaluation. A summary of several subsets and an outline of the evaluation necessary for their identification is given in Table 58–11. A therapeutic trial is the only absolute method to determine if a patient has a responsive tumor, and some patients who do not conform to a defined subset do respond to chemotherapy. Even for responsive carcinomas, the tumor biology and lineage continue to be an enigma. Unfortunately, a large group of patients with insensitive tumors remains. Improved therapy for these patients will probably follow advances in the treatment of non-small cell lung cancer, pancreatic cancer, and the other gastrointestinal cancers, because most insensitive adenocarcinomas probably arise from these occult primary sites.

A registry has been established at Vanderbilt, and an attempt is being made to collect and catalog patients from other physicians around the country. Pathologic material, clinical summaries, and follow-up data on all such patients are being requested. A bank of unstained slides currently exists, and special stains developed in the future may be evaluated rapidly. These data eventually may provide a better assessment of the frequency and spectrum of these neoplasms and allow for more specific diagnoses and therapy.

REFERENCES

1. Horning SJ, Carrier EK, Rouse RV, et al. Lymphomas presenting as histologically unclassified neoplasms: Characteristics and response to treatment. J Clin Oncol 1989;7: 1281–1287.
2. Hales SA, Gatter KC, Heryet A, Mason DY. The value of immunocytochemistry in differentiating high-grade lymphoma from other anaplastic tumours: A study of anaplastic tumours from 1940 to 1960. Leuk Lymphoma 1989;1:59–63.
3. Gatter KC, Alcock C, Heryet A, Mason DY. Clinical importance of analysing malignant tumours of uncertain origin with immunohistochemical techniques. Lancet 1985;2: 1302–1305.
4. Azar HA, Espinoza CG, Richman AV et al. "Undifferentiated" large cell malignancies: An ultrastructural and immunocytochemical study. Hum Pathol 1982;13:323–333.
5. Warnke RA, Gatter KC, Falini B, et al. Diagnosis of human lymphoma with monoclonal antileukocyte antibodies. N Engl J Med 1983;209:1275–1281.
6. Battifora H, Trowbridge IS. A monoclonal antibody useful for the differential diagnosis between malignant lymphoma and nonhematopoietic neoplasms. Cancer 1983;51:816–821.
7. Tapra FJ, Polak JM, Barbosa AJA, et al. Neuron-specific enolase is produced by neuroendocrine tumors. Lancet 1981;1:808–811.
8. O'Connor DT, Burton D, Deftos LJ. Immunoreactive human chromogranin A in diverse polypeptide hormone producing human tumors and normal endocrine tissues. J Clin Endocrinol Metab 1983;57:1084–1086.
9. Allhof EP, Proppe KH, Chapman CM. Evaluation of prostate-specific acid phosphatase and prostate-specific antigen. J Urol 1983;129:316–319.
10. Denk H, Knepler R, Artlieb U, et al. Proteins of intermediate filaments: An immunohistochemical and biochemical approach to the classification of soft tissue tumors. Am J Pathol 1983;110:193–208.
11. Osborn M, Weber K. Biology of disease: Tumor diagnosis by intermediate filament type—a novel tool for surgical pathology. Lab Invest 1983;48:372–394.
12. Kahn HJ, Marks A, Thom H, et al. Role of antibody to S-100 protein in diagnostic pathology. Am J Clin Pathol 1983;79:341–347.
13. Gown AM, Vogel AM, Hoak D, et al. Monoclonal antibodies specific for melanocytic tumors distinguish subpopulations of melanocytes. Am J Pathol 1986;123:195–203.
14. Bosman FT, Giard RWM, Nieuwenhuijen-Kruseman AC, et al. Human chorionic gonadotrophin and alpha fetoprotein in testicular germ cell tumors: A retrospective immunohistochemical study. Histopathology 1980;4:673–684.
15. Kurman KJ, Scardino PT, McIntire KR, et al. Cellular localization of alpha fetoprotein and human chorionic gonadotropin in germ cell tumors of the testis using an indirect immunoperoxidase technique: A new approach to classification utilizing tumor markers. Cancer 1977;40:2136–2151.

16. Arnold A, Cossman J, Bakhshi A, et al. Immunoglobulin-gene rearrangements as unique clonal markers in human lymphoid neoplasms. N Engl J Med 1983;309:1593–1599.

17. Rowley JD. Recurring chromosome abnormalities in leukemic and lymphoma. Semin Hematol 1990;27:122–130.

18. Turc-Carel C, Philip I, Berger MP, et al. Chromosomal translocation in Ewing's sarcoma. N Engl J Med 1983;309:497–498.

19. Whang-Peng J, Triche TJ, Knutsen T, et al. Chromosome translocation in peripheral neuroepithelioma. N Engl J Med 1984;311:584–585.

20. Bosl GJ, Dmitrovsky E, Reuter V, et al. i(12p): A specific karyotypic abnormality in germ cell tumors. Proc Am Soc Clin Oncol [Abstract] 1989;8:131.

21. Atkin NB, Baker MC. Specific chromosome change, i(12p), in testicular tumors. Lancet 1982;2:1349–1356.

22. Motzer RJ, Rodriguez E, Reuter VE, et al. Genetic analysis as an aid in diagnosis for patients with midline carcinomas of uncertain histologies. JNCI 1991;83:341–346.

23. Schildt RA, Kennedy PS, Chen TT, et al. Management of patients with metastatic adenocarcinoma of unknown origin: A Southwest Oncology Group study. Cancer Treat Rep 1983;67:77–79.

24. Nystrom JS, Weiner JM, et al. Metastatic and histologic presentations in unknown primary cancer. Semin Oncol 1977;4:53–58.

25. McMillan JH, Levine E, Stephens RH. Computed tomography in the evaluation of metastatic adenocarcinoma from an unknown primary site. Radiology 1982;143:143–146.

26. Karsell PR, Sheedy PF, O'Connell MJ. Computerized tomography in search of cancer of unknown origin. JAMA 1982;248:340–343.

27. Hochster H, Wernz JC, Muggia FM. Intra-abdominal carcinomatosis with histologically normal ovaries. Cancer Treat Rep [Letter] 1984;68:931–932.

28. Gooneratne S, Sassone M, Blaustein A, Talerman A. Serous surface papillary carcinoma of the ovary: A clinicopathologic study of 26 cases. Int J Gynecol Pathol 1982;1:258–269.

29. Chen KT, Flam MS. Peritoneal papillary serous carcinoma with long-term survival. Cancer 1986;58:1371–1373.

30. August CZ, Murad TM, Newton M. Multiple focal extraovarian serous carcinoma. Int J Gynecol Pathol 1985;4:11–23.

31. Dalrymple JC, Bannatyne P, Russell P, et al. Extraovarian peritoneal serous papillary carcinoma: A clinicopathologic study of 31 cases. Cancer 1989;64:110–115.

32. Strnad CM, Grosh WW, Baxter J, et al. Peritoneal carcinomatosis of unknown primary site in women. Ann Intern Med 1989;111:213–217.

33. Ransom DT, Patel SR, Keeney GL, et al. Papillary serous carcinoma of the peritoneum: A review of 33 cases treated with cisplatin-based chemotherapy. Cancer 1990;66:1091–1094.

34. Bhatia SK, Saclarides TJ, Witt TR, et al. Hormone receptor studies in axillary metastases from occult breast cancers. Cancer 1987;59:1170–1172.

35. Ashikari R, Rosen PP, Urban JA, Senoo T. Breast cancer presenting as an axillary mass. Ann Surg 1976;183:415–417.

36. Patel J, Nemoto T, Rosner D, et al. Axillary lymph node metastases from an occult breast cancer. Cancer 1981;47:2923–2927.

37. Rosen PP. Axillary lymph node metastases in patients with occult noninvasive breast carcinoma. Cancer 1980;46:1298–1306.

38. Johnson RO, Castro R, Ansfield FJ. Response of primary unknown cancers to treatment with 5-fluorouracil. Cancer Chemother Rep 1964;38:63–64.

39. Moertel CG, Reitemeier RJ, Schutt AJ, Hahn RG. Treatment of the patient with adenocarcinoma of unknown origin. Cancer 1972;30:1469–1472.

40. Milliken ST, Tattersall MHN, Woods RL, et al. Metastatic adenocarcinoma of unknown primary site: A randomized study of two combination chemotherapy regimens. Eur J Cancer Clin Oncol 1987;23:1645–1648.

41. McKeen E, Smith F, Haidak D, et al. Fluorouracil, adriamycin and mitomycin-C for adenocarcinoma of unknown origin. Proc Am Assoc Cancer Res [Abstract] 1980;21:358.

42. Woods RL, Fox RM, Tattersall MHN, et al. Metastatic adenocarcinomas of unknown primary: A randomized study of two combination-chemotherapy regimens. N Engl J Med 1980;303:87–89.

43. Eagan RT, Thernean TM, Rubin J, et al. Lack of value for cisplatin added to mitomycin-doxorubicin combination chemotherapy for carcinoma of unknown primary site. Am J Clin Oncol 1987;10:82–85.

44. Goldberg RM, Smith FP, Ueno W, et al. Fluorouracil, adriamycin and mitomycin in the treatment of adenocarcinoma of unknown primary. J Clin Oncol 1986;4:395–399.

45. Kambhus, Kelsen D, Niedzwiecki D, et al. Phase II trial of mitomycin C, vindesine, and adriamycin and predictive variables in the treatment of patients with adenocarcinoma of unknown primary site. Proc Am Assoc Cancer Res [Abstract] 1986;27:734.

46. Fiore JJ, Kelsen DP, Gralla RJ, et al. Adenocarcinoma of unknown primary origin: Treatment with vindesine and doxorubicin. Cancer Treat Rep 1985;69:591–594.

47. Barrie JR, Knapper WH, Strong EW. Cervical nodal metastases of unknown origin. Am J Surg 1970;120:466–470.

48. Jesse RH, Perez CA, Fletcher GH. Cervical lymph node metastasis: Unknown primary cancer. Cancer 1973;31:854–859.

49. Coker DD, Casterline PF, Chambers RG, Jacques DA. Metastases to lymph nodes of the head and neck from an unknown primary site. Am J Surg 1977;134:517–522.

50. Jose B. Bosch A, Caldwell WL, Frias Z. Metastasis to neck from unknown primary tumor. Acta Radiol Oncol 1979;18:161–170.

51. Nordstrom DG, Tewfik HH, Latourette HB. Cervical lymph node metastases from an unknown primary. Int J Radiat Oncol Biol Phys 1979;5:73–76.

52. Fermont AC. Malignant cervical lymphadenopathy due to an unknown primary. Clin Radiol 1980;31:355–358.

53. Leipzig B, Winter ML, Hokanson JA. Cervical nodal metastases of unknown origin. Laryngoscope 1981;91:593–598.

54. Pacini P, Olmi P, Cellai E, Chiavacci A. Cervical lymph node metastases from an unknown primary tumour. Acta Radiol Oncol 1981;20:311–314.

55. Spiro RH, DeRose G, Strong EW. Cervical node metastasis of occult origin. Am J Surg 1983;146:441–446.

56. Mobit-Tabatabasi MA, Dasmaphapatra KS, Rush BF Jr, Ohanian M. Management of squamous cell carcinoma of unknown origin in cervical lymph nodes. Am Surg 1986;52:152–154.

57. Yang ZY, Hu YH, Yan JH, et al. Lymph node metastases in the neck from an unknown primary: Report on 113 patients. Acta Radiol Oncol 1983;22:17–22.

58. Carlson LS, Fletcher GH, Oswald MJ. Guidelines for the radiotherapeutic techniques for cervical metastases from an unknown primary. Int J Radiat Oncol Biol Phys 1986;12:2101–2110.

59. McCunniff AJ, Raber M. Metastatic carcinoma of the neck from an unknown primary. Int J Radiat Oncol Biol Phys 1986;12:1849–1852.

60. Bataini JP, Rodriguez J, Jaulerry C, et al. Treatment of metastatic neck nodes secondary to an occult epidermoid carcinoma of the head and neck. Laryngoscope 1987;97:1080–1084.

61. De Braud F, Heilbrun LK, Ahmed K, et al. Metastatic squamous cell carcinoma of an unknown primary localized to the neck: Advantages of an aggressive treatment. Cancer 1989;64:510–515.

62. Guarischi A, Keane TJ, Elhakim T. Metastatic inguinal nodes from an unknown primary neoplasm: A review of 56 cases. Cancer 1987;59:572–577.

63. Anderson H, Thatcher N, Rankin E, et al. VAC (vincristine, Adriamycin and cyclophosphamide) chemotherapy for metastatic carcinoma from an unknown primary site. Eur J Cancer Clin Oncol 1983;19:49–52.

64. Pasterz R, Savoraj N, Burgess M. Prognostic factors in metastatic carcinoma of unknown primary. J Clin Oncol 1986;4:1652–1657.

65. Greco FA, Vaughn WK, Hainsworth JD. Advanced poorly differentiated carcinoma of unknown primary site: Recognition of a treatable syndrome. Ann Intern Med 1986;104:547–556.

66. Hainsworth JD, Wright EP, Gray GF Jr, Greco FA. Poorly differentiated carcinoma of unknown primary site: Correlation of light microscopic findings with response to cisplatin-based combination chemotherapy. J Clin Oncol 1987;5:1275–1280.

67. Hainsworth JD, Wright E, Davis B, Johnson D, Greco FA. Immunoperoxidase staining in the evaluation of poorly differentiated carcinoma of unknown primary site. Proc Am Soc Clin Oncol [Abstract] 1989;8:11.

68. Richardson RL, Greco FA, Wolff S, et al. Extragonadal germ cell malignancy: Value of tumor markers in metastatic carcinoma in young males. Proc Am Assoc Cancer Res [Abstract] 1979;20:204.

69. Richardson RL, Schoumacher RA, Fer MF, et al. The unrecognized extragonadal germ cell cancer syndrome. Ann Intern Med 1981;94:181–186.

70. Hainsworth JD, Greco FA. Poorly differentiated carcinoma of unknown primary site. In: Fer MF, Greco FA, Oldham R, eds. Poorly differentiated neoplasms and tumors of unknown origin. Orlando: Grune & Stratton, 1986:189–202.

71. Fox RM, Woods RL, Tattersall MHN. Undifferentiated carcinoma in young men: The atypical teratoma syndrome. Lancet 1979;1:1316–1318.

72. Hainsworth JD, Johnson DH, Greco FA. Poorly differentiated neuroendocrine carcinoma of unknown primary site: A newly recognized clinicopathologic entity. Ann Intern Med 1988;109:364–371.

73. Van der Gaast A, Verweij J, Henzen-Logmans SC, et al. Carcinoma of unknown primary: Identification of a treatable subset. Ann Oncol 1990;1:119–123.

74. Kurzrock R, Gutterman JU, Talpazm P. The molecular genetics of Philadelphia chromosome-positive leukemias. N Engl J Med 1988;319:990–998.

75. Williams SD, Birch R, Einhorn LH, et al. Treatment of disseminated germ-cell tumors with cisplatin, bleomycin, and either vinblastine or etoposide. N Engl J Med 1987;316:1435–1440.

76. Raber MN, Faintuch J, Abbruzzese J, et al. Continuous infusion 5-fluorouracil, etoposide and cis-diamminedichloroplatinum in patients with metastatic carcinoma of unknown primary site. Ann Oncol 1991;2:519–520.

77. Briassoulis E, Foutzilas G, Theoharis D, et al. The role of platinum-containing chemotherapy in carcinoma of unknown primary: A Hellenic Cooperative Oncology Group study. Eur J Cancer [Abstract] 1991;27(Suppl 2):1347.

78. Zarba J, Izzo J, Hahjoubi R, et al. Treatment of unknown primary adenocarcinoma with fluorouracil, mitomycin, epirubicin and platinum. Eur J Cancer [Abstract] 1991;27(Suppl 2):1350.

79. Van der Gaast A, Verwey J, Prins E, Splinter TAW. Chemotherapy as treatment of choice in extrapulmonary undifferentiated small cell carcinomas. Cancer 1990;65:422–424.

80. Kasimis BS, Wuerker RB, Malefatto JP, Moran EM. Prolonged survival of patients with extrapulmonary small cell carcinoma arising in the neck. Med Pediatr Oncol 1983;11:27–32.

81. Hainsworth JD, Einhorn LH, Williams SD, et al. Advanced extragonadal germ-cell tumors: Successful treatment with combination chemotherapy. Ann Intern Med 1982;97:7–11.

82. Israel A, Bosl GJ, Golbey RB, et al. The results of chemotherapy for extragonadal germ-cell tumors in the cisplatin era: The Memorial Sloan Kettering Cancer Center experience (1975–1982). J Clin Oncol 1985;3:1073–1078.

83. Agnarsson BA, Kadin ME. Ki-1 positive large cell lymphoma: A morphologic and immunologic study of 19 cases. Am J Surg Pathol 1988;12:264–274.

84. Moertel CG, Kovals LK, O'Connell MJ, et al. Treatment of neuroendocrine carcinomas with combined etoposide and cisplatin: Evidence of major therapeutic activity in the anaplastic variants of these neoplasms. Cancer 1991;68:227–233.

85. Loehrer PJ, Perez CA, Roth LM, et al. Chemotherapy for advanced thymoma: Preliminary results of an intergroup study. Ann Intern Med 1990;113:520–524.

86. Tell DT, Khoury JM, Taylor HG, et al. Atypical metastasis from prostate cancer: Clinical utility of the immunoperoxidase technique for prostate-specific antigen. JAMA 1985;253:3574–3575.

87. Gentile PS, Carloss HW, Huang T-Y, et al. Disseminated prostatic carcinoma simulating primary lung cancer. Cancer 1988;62:711–715.

Cancer: Principles & Practice of Oncology, Fourth Edition,
edited by Vincent T. DeVita, Jr., Samuel Hellman, Steven A. Rosenberg.
J.B. Lippincott Co., Philadelphia © 1993.

Judith E. Karp
Jerome E. Groopman
Samuel Broder

CHAPTER **59**

Cancer in AIDS

The relation between immunodeficiency and cancer has been well documented for several decades. The predisposition to develop neoplasia was perhaps first clearly detected in patients with genetically determined disorders of cellular and humoral immunity, in particular ataxia-telangiectasia and Wiskott-Aldrich syndrome, and then, not surprisingly, in patients receiving immunosuppressive therapies for autoimmune disorders or transplantation. The malignancies arising in the context of insufficient immune function are frequently of lymphoid origin, most commonly B-cell, but epithelial and endothelial-related cancers (in particular, Kaposi's sarcoma [KS]) occur as well. The common themes underlying the emergence and perpetuation of the diverse cancers in these heterogenous immunocompromised states include three major factors: the absence of protective immune surveillance to recognize and eradicate abnormal clones; disruption of the normal balance between cell proliferation and differentiation that, in part, may be augmented by abnormal growth-factor expression; and chronic antigenic stimulation, sometimes accompanied by infection with "oncogenic" viruses, that leads to expansion of one or more cell cohorts. The uncovering of the molecular lesions that cause immune dysfunction, whether inherited or acquired, and the elucidation of mechanisms that permit malignant transformation in this setting will lead to the development of targeted molecular strategies that may be applicable to the therapy and prevention of cancers in general.

This association is being detected in patients with acquired immunodeficiency syndrome (AIDS), caused by infection with the pathogenic retrovirus known as human immunodeficiency virus (HIV). The multiple factors that operate to promote or permit the emergence of cancers in other immunodeficiency disorders also operate in AIDS. Further, the types of malignancies and their incidence rates are increasing in AIDS as the development of effective antiretroviral therapies and pro-

phylaxis against opportunistic infections leads to prolonged survival in what would otherwise be a lethal immunocompromised state.

Although there is not yet a cure for HIV infection, there are now a number of therapies, the dideoxynucleoside zidovudine (azidothymidine; AZT) being the first and dideoxyinosine (ddI) being the second of several antiretroviral agents capable of suppressing viral replication and consequently prolonging survival for AIDS patients. Before 1986 (before the wide availability of AZT), the median survival of AIDS patients was less than 1 year.[1-3] With the use of AZT in conjunction with prophylaxis against *Pneumocystis carinii* and herpesvirus suppressive therapy, the duration of survival has more than doubled[2-7] and is likely to lengthen dramatically in the near future. Moreover, Rosenberg and colleagues[8] found that starting between 1987 and 1988 (the first year after AZT was approved by the Food and Drug Administration), there has been a sharp decrease in the quarterly incidence of new AIDS cases (but not in HIV seropositivity) in white gay men, for whom the incidence has fallen by nearly 30%. This decrease likely reflects the ability of AZT and other medical interventions to delay progression of HIV infection to AIDS. In early disease, AZT also delays the loss of CD4-positive cells.

It is, however, the net prolongation of survival in the face of impaired immunity that may drive the increasing incidence of malignancies in the AIDS population. For example, the risk for development of non-Hodgkin's lymphoma (NHL) is not uniform over time but, rather, appears to increase at around 2 years after AZT institution for full-blown AIDS.[7,9,10] This is worth noting because studies that do not provide follow-up data for more than 2 years will not detect this association accurately. Recent projections estimate that about 4700 new cases of AIDS lymphomas (range, 2900–9800) will occur annually in the near future, and some projections suggest that

10% to 20% of all new NHL cases may eventually be related to AIDS in the United States.[3]

We will discuss the major opportunistic malignancies associated with HIV infection in the approximate order in which each has been recognized as a significant and related complication: KS, human papillomavirus (HPV)-associated anogenital carcinoma, and AIDS-related NHL (AIDS-NHL).

AIDS-RELATED KAPOSI'S SARCOMA

Kaposi's sarcoma was initially described in 1872 by Moricz Kaposi[11] (a pseudonym) as "idiopathic, multiple pigmented sarcomas of the skin." The classic KS is a rare tumor with an indolent clinical course that occurs in elderly men (usually of Mediterranean or Ashkenazi Jewish descent) and is characterized by lower-extremity skin nodules caused by blood vessel proliferation. An endemic KS variant is prevalent in Central Africa (mainly Kenya, Tanzania, and Zaire) and accounts for 10% of all neoplasms in that region, with striking male predominance. In contrast to classic KS, the endemic form occurs mainly in younger black male adults and has a clinical spectrum that ranges from a benign, localized, nodular disease to an aggressive, locally invasive malignancy. The lymphadenopathic variant of endemic KS occurs in black African children of both sexes as a highly aggressive, widely disseminated tumor with extensive lymph node and deep visceral involvement that has a rapidly progressive and ultimately fatal course.[12] The epidemiologic and clinical features of these and other KS variants are summarized in Table 59–1.

The etiologic linkage between KS and immunodeficiency was first recognized in settings of iatrogenic immunosuppression, including organ transplantation, where the incidence of KS is about 200 to 400 times higher than expected in the general population. In addition, KS can arise in the presence of other malignancies that compromise the integrity of immunologic function, for example, B-cell malignancies such as NHL and multiple myeloma or adult T-cell leukemia caused by the human T-cell leukemia type 1 retrovirus.[13,14] In the milieu of immunocompromise, the clinical presentation can resemble the indolent classic KS or the highly malignant lymphadenopathic KS variant. With the AIDS epidemic, KS has risen from an interesting but unusual neoplasm to a prominent challenge, occurring in about 20% of all AIDS patients. Until recently, KS was the first manifestation of AIDS in 30% to 40% of patients; now, KS is the AIDS-defining illness in only about 10%.[12,15] The decrease in KS as the presenting feature of AIDS may relate to several factors, including a change in sexual practices that have been associated with KS development, changing demographics, increasing numbers of HIV-positive women, the increasing ability to detect HIV infection before immune impairment, and the advent of effective antiretroviral therapies, which can delay HIV disease progression. However, although the incidence of KS as the initial, AIDS-defining opportunistic event is declining, KS remains a prevalent and life-threatening complication of AIDS.

ETIOLOGY AND PATHOGENESIS

A number of genetic factors and environmental cofactors have been examined for their relative contributions to KS development in HIV-infected patients, which occurs almost exclusively (at least 95%) in homosexual males.[15,16] There appear a few predisposing genetic factors, including race (black) and ethnicity (Haitian).[17] The original suggestion, however, that HLA-DR5 conferred heightened susceptibility and an increased severity of classic KS[18] and epidemic AIDS-related KS (AIDS-KS) has not been substantiated as the number of affected people has increased over time. Behavioral cofactors associated with the development of AIDS-KS include homosexuality (as opposed to intravenous drug use) and specific sexual practices (including anal-receptive intercourse and the use of various inhaled nitrate aphrodisiacs).[15,19]

The role of cytomegalovirus (CMV) as a critical cofactor in the emergence and perpetuation of KS in HIV-infected men is controversial. All KS variants are associated with a high incidence of CMV seropositivity.[20,21] It is also likely that CMV, like other DNA viruses of the herpesvirus family, encodes transcriptional activators capable of enhancing HIV gene expression and increasing HIV-related immunosuppression.[20,22] On the other hand, the presence or absence of anti-CMV antibodies in HIV-positive homosexual men does not usefully discriminate among those who will or will not develop AIDS-KS. Furthermore, molecular studies have not detected the presence of CMV DNA sequences in AIDS-KS or endemic (African) KS tumor tissue.[23] Although it is intriguing to postulate that CMV infection enhances HIV disease progression and facilitates the development of KS through that route, the direct role of CMV in the pathogenesis of KS remains undetermined.

AIDS-RELATED KAPOSI'S SYNDROME AS A PARADIGM OF NEOPLASIA DRIVEN BY GROWTH FACTORS

One of the most intriguing aspects of AIDS-KS pathogenesis is the sensitivity of this malignancy to numerous growth factors. The origin of the AIDS-KS cell, specifically the transformed spindle cell, is as yet undetermined, but likely candidates are endothelial cells (vascular or lymphatic) and pluripotent mesenchymal cells (Schwann cells). A major pathophysiologic component of AIDS-KS is angiogenesis and the production of multiple growth factors that promote new blood vessel formation. The transformed spindle cell, whatever its origin, is a potent source for such factors.

The initial polyclonal expansion of multiple interactive cell types—namely, T cells, monocytes, and vascular endothelial cells—is likely driven by the diverse cytokines produced by host cells (neoplastic and virus-infected) and by HIV. In addition to the potpourri of cytokines produced by HIV-infected T cells and monocytes (in particular, interleukin-6 [IL-6]),[24,25] AIDS-KS cells, when exposed to soluble factors liberated from activated CD4-positive T cells, produce at least eight growth factors that induce autocrine and paracrine growth stimulation. These growth factors include the basic and a unique KS-derived fibroblast growth factor (FGF), platelet-derived growth factor (PDGF), endothelial growth factor (which is identical to acidic-FGF), transforming growth factor-β, IL-1, IL-6, and granulocyte-macrophage colony-stimulating factor (GM-CSF).[26–29] Many of these are angiogenesis factors, which stimulate vascular endothelial cell proliferation and new blood vessel formation, and lymphohematopoietic stimulators.

TABLE 59–1. Distinctive Clinical Features of Classic, Endemic, Iatrogenic, and Epidemic Variants of Kaposi's Sarcoma

Type	Epidemiology			Clinical Manifestations			Clinical Course	
	Major Population Affected	Age (y)	Male/ Female Ratio	Mucocutaneous	Lymph Node	Visceral	Behavior	Survival (y)
Classic	Mediterranean Ashkenazi Jewish	50–80	10–15:1	Patches, plaques and nodules, localized to lower extremities	Rare (late-onset)	Occasional (late-onset)	Indolent	10–15—up to one third develop lymphoma
Endemic	Black men in Central Africa	25–40	13–17:1	Nodules localized to lower extremities	Rare	Rare	Indolent	8–10
				Aggressive exophytic lesions with underlying bone invasion	Rare	Occasional	Progressive	5–8
				Florid, widely disseminated nodular lesions	Occasional	Common	Rapidly progressive	3–5
	Children (lymphadenopathic variant)	2–13	3:1	Minimal	Generalized	Common	Virulent and rapidly progressive	1–3
Iatrogenic	Patients receiving immunosuppressive therapy (e.g., renal transplantation, autoimmune disorders)	20–60	2.3:1	Patches, plaques and nodules, usually localized but can disseminate	Rare	Common	Indolent or rapidly progressive; may reverse with reduction or discontinuation of immunosuppression	30% fatal within 2–3
Epidemic AIDS	Homosexual men	18–65	>100:1	Irregular fusiform plaques and nodules; multifocal	Common	Common (gastrointestinal, lung)	Fulminant	<2

AIDS-KS cells respond to corticosteroids by expressing cytokines that induce proliferation and vascular permeability and also express angiogenic activity in chicken chorioallantoic membrane, nude mouse, and guinea pig in vivo assay systems.[30] Corticosteroids may predispose to the development of AIDS-KS by two distinct mechanisms: growth perturbation (by growth-factor induction) and immunosuppression (*e.g.*, by direct lymphocytolysis).

Of particular interest is the KS-specific FGF (K-FGF), a member of the heparin-binding FGF cytokine family that shares partial homology with basic and acidic FGF and has related angiogenic activities. K-FGF is encoded by the KS oncogene, which is identical to the *HST* oncogene (found in human stomach cancers) located on chromosome 11q12-13 and to the mouse *INT*2 oncogene (the site of mouse mammary tumor virus integration).[26] The KS oncogene is constitutively expressed in AIDS-KS, and its K-FGF product may contribute to an autocrine mechanism of tumor proliferation.[27] K-FGF is also secreted extracellularly, where it may stimulate capillary endothelial cell proliferation in paracrine fashion. When the K-FGF gene is transfected into cultured human adrenocortical carcinoma cells, and the gene-transfected cells are then transplanted into athymic nude mice, the transplanted cells secrete large amounts of K-FGF and undergo KS-like cell growth, with development of rapidly growing, highly vascularized tumors (rather than growth typical of the parent tumor cell line).[31] These findings lend credence to the hypothesis that the KS oncogene and its K-FGF gene product might play important roles in the growth dysregulation, malignant transformation, and pathogenesis of AIDS-KS.

Like K-FGF, the gene encoding basic FGF (b-FGF) is expressed at high levels in AIDS-KS cells, resulting in synthesis of large quantities of b-FGF, which is then secreted extracellularly and can induce autocrine effects on tumor cells and paracrine effects on endothelial cells.[28] It has been shown that b-FGF can stimulate the gene expression and secretion of macrophage CSF (M-CSF or CSF-1) from bone marrow stromal cells, which, in turn, may serve as a positive feedback mediator for the production of several "inflammatory" cytokines.[32] M-CSF also enhances replication of a monocytotropic strain of HIV-1 in infected bone marrow stem cells that are undergoing macrophage differentiation.[33] This may be a key mechanism of action for many of the heparin-binding growth factors, and as such, it may contribute to autocrine and paracrine aspects of proliferation in AIDS-KS and to the progression of HIV disease activity.

Similarly, IL-1 (mainly the IL-1β form) is expressed in high amounts in AIDS-KS cells[28] and may also induce a cascade of cytokines in multiple cell types involved in the pathogenesis and progression of AIDS-KS. IL-1 stimulates the synthesis and release of many growth-modulating cytokines (*e.g.*, PDGF, GM-CSF, M-CSF, and IL-6) in a variety of cell types, including vascular endothelial cells, mesenchymal cells, and fibroblasts from several sources (notably bone marrow and skin). IL-1 also increases the expression of adhesion molecules by endothelial cells.[34] Studies demonstrate the expression of functional IL-1 receptors of the type expressed on T cells and fibroblasts on human vascular endothelial and smooth muscle cells.[35] It is logical to surmise that these receptors mediate the autocrine and paracrine growth-promoting effects of IL-1 on vascular cells. The discovery and recombinant production of an IL-1 receptor antagonist (IL-1ra) that competitively inhibits IL-1 binding to its receptors (especially the receptors found on T cells and fibroblasts)[34] offers a potential therapeutic tool for diseases such as AIDS-KS in which IL-1 may play a pathogenic role, and is worthy of further exploration. Some patients with HIV-associated KS have extensive edema and tissue swelling, and it is thought that such sequelae are mediated by IL-1.

Of the many other cytokines produced by AIDS-KS, HIV-infected, fibroblastic, and endothelial cells, IL-6 is secreted by all such cell types (in some instances, induced by IL-1) and is autostimulatory for AIDS-KS cells, monocytes, and HIV replication.[24,29] Of particular relevance is the mechanism for the positive feedback loop in AIDS-KS, namely the IL-6-induced upregulation of the IL-6 receptor.[29] This mechanism is perhaps similar to the one detected for multiple myeloma, in which IL-6 is constitutively expressed by the dysregulated plasma cells, acts as an autocrine growth factor, and likely facilitates eventual transformation or expansion of neoplastic clones.[36–38]

AIDS-KS cells may also proliferate in response to HIV regulatory proteins. Specifically, AIDS-KS cells respond to the HIV TAT protein.[39] The HIV transactivating gene, *TAT*, and its protein product (TAT) are essential for viral gene expression and replication and may contribute to immunodeficiency by modulating host cell gene expression and T-cell antigenic response. In addition, and perhaps more important for the growth of AIDS-KS, HIV-infected CD4 cells and monocytes may release biologically active TAT. This extracellular TAT can then be taken up by cells in close proximity. After uptake, extracellular TAT localizes in the nucleus and transactivates HIV-1 long-terminal-repeat-directed gene expression, can stimulate growth of AIDS-KS and mesenchymal cell types, and mediates cell attachment to culture plates through binding to cell surface integrins expressed by mesenchymal cells and other cell types.[39] This latter activity may be especially important to the proliferation of AIDS-KS cells. Therefore, the HIV-1 TAT protein may have a pivotal role in the pathogenesis and clonal expansion of AIDS-KS, particularly as an extracellular product. By stimulating proliferation of AIDS-KS cells and normal mesenchymal cells and by inducing HIV-1 viral replication, extracellular TAT may act as a promoting or progression factor in KS development and in the immunodeficiency occurring in HIV-1 infected patients. These are interesting possibilities, but they cannot be taken as clinical facts because further research is needed.

HISTOPATHOLOGY

The microscopic appearances of the cutaneous lesions from the classic, endemic, and epidemic forms of KS are remarkably similar. The clinical spectrum of cutaneous and mucosal lesions is paralleled histologically in terms of features connoting aggressiveness. Histopathology of early macular patches, with involvement limited to the upper portion of the reticular dermis, demonstrates irregular and dilated vascular spaces as a result of blood vessel proliferation but not much evidence for angiogenesis, inflammation, or cellular dysplasia. Progression to papules and plaques that extend into the subcutis is accompanied by increasing numbers and aggregates of spindle cells (the presumptive AIDS-KS cell), erythrocyte extravasation, and intense inflammatory cell infiltration. Ultimately, these lesions develop into deeply invasive nodules that, on histologic examination, evince significant nuclear atypia, dense infiltration and active proliferation of spindle cells, intense inflammation and erythrophagocytosis, exuberant neoangiogenesis, and obliteration of vascular spaces.

CLINICAL MANIFESTATIONS AND STAGING

As noted previously, AIDS-KS commonly presents as an aggressive and widely disseminated neoplasm, arising in multiple foci from vascular endothelium or lymphatic tissue in skin, mucosal surfaces, lymph nodes, and visceral organs, including liver, spleen, gastrointestinal (GI) tract, and lung. In some patients, KS is confined to the skin and may not require therapy per se. In many cases, however, the tumor parallels the clinical course seen in the lymphadenopathic variant of endemic KS and aggressive variants of KS emerging from the background of immunosuppression. Lesions at all sites (skin and viscera) commonly progress from macules to plaques and nodules, often coalesce, and ultimately develop into fungating or ulcerated masses (Fig. 59-1).

Multiorgan involvement occurs in most AIDS-KS patients at initial clinical presentation. Although virtually any organ can be involved by KS, the most common (and most life-threatening) are the GI tract and the lung. GI tract lesions, submucosal or nodal, have been detected in 50% to 70% of KS patients and are frequently associated with enteropathic and hemorrhagic symptoms;[40] however, they can also be clinically silent. Pulmonary involvement, a particularly ominous development, has been reported in 20% to 50% of patients and often mimics (and can occur concomitantly with) opportunistic infections on clinical grounds.[41] The definitive diagnosis of pulmonary KS is further complicated by recurrent episodes of hemorrhage that can acutely exacerbate pulmonary compromise. The discrimination of pulmonary KS from infectious complications has been facilitated by lung computed tomography (Fig. 59-2) and may obviate the need to pursue invasive diagnostic techniques in some patients.[42] Pulmonary KS is exceedingly difficult to treat with any modality.

Because AIDS-KS appears to arise from multiple foci, classic oncologic staging criteria have not adequately characterized the extent of the disease process in an entirely satisfactory way.[43] Furthermore, any staging classification of AIDS-KS, if it is going to be relevant to overall prognosis and therapeutic outcome, should incorporate measurements of immunologic function and other parameters of virus activity and extent of tumor involvement.[44] Krown and colleagues[43] developed a system for uniform staging and evaluation of clinical trials outcomes for AIDS-KS patients based on the three broad stratification criteria: extent of tumor involvement, immunologic status, and systemic illness (including other opportunistic infections or HIV-related malignancies; Table 59-2). Such standardization will facilitate the interpretation of clinical results, the evaluation of innovative anti-KS therapies, and the appropriate application of specific therapies, such as interferon (detailed later), on the basis of clearly defined prognostic criteria.

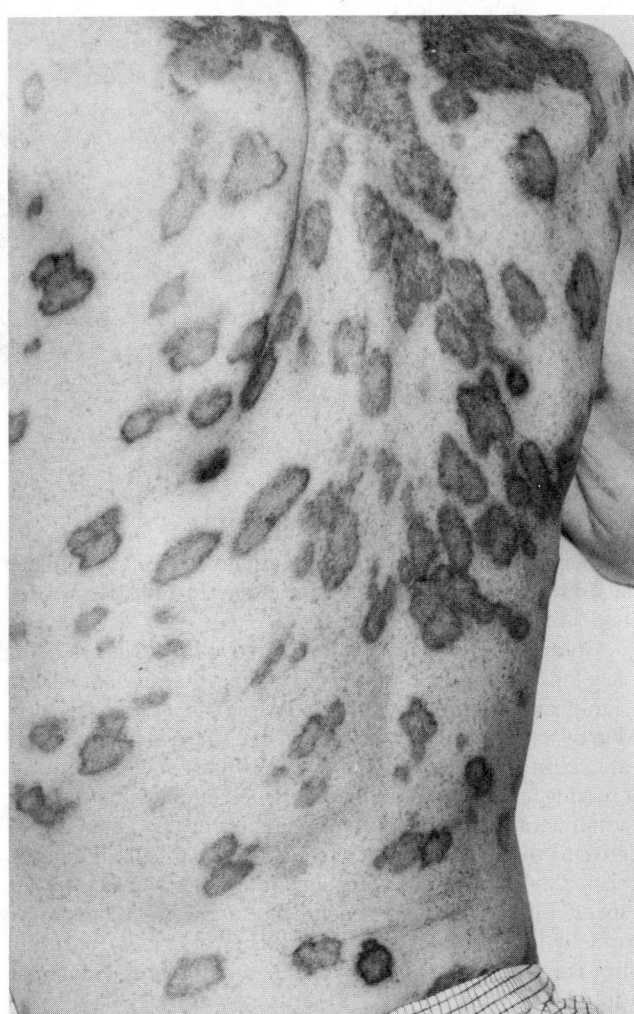

FIGURE 59-1. Extensive cutaneous plaques on the trunk of a patient with HIV-associated Kaposi's sarcoma. Several plaques have coalesced and are irregular and fusiform in shape. Notice the bilateral symmetry and the prominence at sites of skin cleavage. (Courtesy of James M. Pluda, MD)

LOCAL AND SYSTEMIC THERAPEUTIC APPROACHES

Like other malignancies arising in the immunocompromised host, the therapy of AIDS-KS is a multifaceted challenge. The complexity of this challenge is conferred by the multiple levels of dysregulation exerted by the interactions between HIV and the host. The net result in many patients is aggressive tumor behavior and increased host cell toxicity in response to chemotherapy- or radiation therapy-induced cell damage. Some of the local and systemic therapeutic approaches to AIDS-KS are delineated in Table 59-3.

Local therapies have been useful for palliation of localized cutaneous or mucosal lesions or for mass lesions producing obstructive findings such as lymphedema.[44,45] Radiation therapy (1500–2200 cGy) for all such lesions and carbon dioxide and neodymium:yttrium-aluminum-garnet laser therapy for more isolated lesions (*e.g.*, oral or urethral meatus) bring about significant but often incomplete and temporary resolution. Local recurrence is common. Whole-lung irradiation also

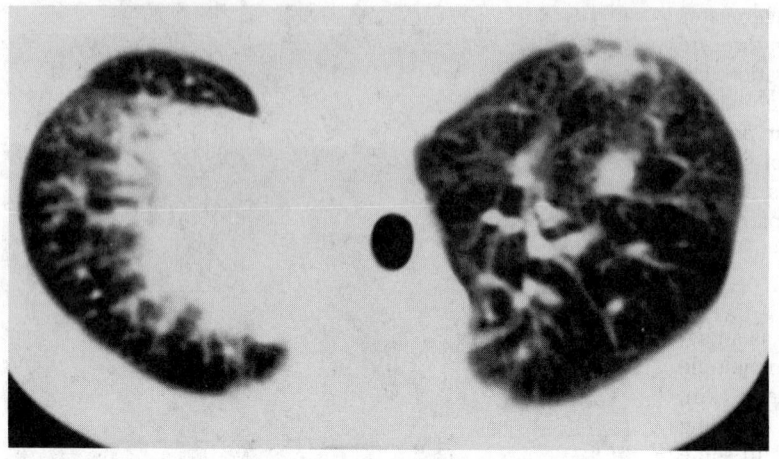

FIGURE 59–2. Chest CT scan of a patient with HIV-associated pulmonary Kaposi's sarcoma, demonstrating massive hilar involvement with extension into the pulmonary parenchyma and multiple pulmonary nodules. (Courtesy of James M. Pluda, MD)

provides palliation but not long-term control for pulmonary KS lesions. Radiation therapy is complicated by a heightened susceptibility of uninvolved host tissue to radiation-related toxicities.

A number of novel radiation-related approaches are being developed for AIDS-KS. Photodynamic therapy has shown significant antitumor activity in diverse cancers such as bladder, ovary, esophagus, and lung cancers. This modality, aimed at maximizing toxicity to tumor foci while concomitantly decreasing toxicity to nontumorous tissues, employs the systemic administration of a photosensitizing agent (*e.g.*, hematoporphyrin) that is selectively retained by tumor cells and not by normal host cells. The compound is activated on exposure to specific light wavelengths delivered to a well-circumscribed area by laser and, when activated, is cytotoxic. Early results from preliminary trials demonstrate tumor regression in multiple KS nodules.

An important form of local therapy for cutaneous and mucosal KS involves intralesional drug administration.[44,45] Local injection of cytotoxic agents (*e.g.*, vinblastine or bleomycin) or biomodulatory agents, such as interferon or tumor necrosis factor (TNF), have met with tumor regression and minimal systemic toxicity. Other agents that might be experimental candidates for this innovative approach to mucocutaneous tumor suppression could be targeted to the autocrine and paracrine growth factors operating in AIDS-KS. Examples include IL-1 receptor antagonists[34]; various derivatives of retinoic acid, which, as discussed in more detail later, may interdict IL-6-mediated autostimulation[46]; immunotoxin molecules, for instance, b-FGF conjugated to a *Pseudomonas* exotoxin (b-FGF-PE-40); or monoclonal antibodies directed against stimulatory factors, such as anti-IL-6.[47] Such compounds have potential to effect significant local tumor control, perhaps with additional salutary effects on involved accessory cell types near

TABLE 59–2. Staging Classification for AIDS-Related Kaposi's Sarcoma

	Good Risk (0) (all *the parameters listed*)	Poor Risk (1) (any *of the parameters listed*)
Tumor (T)	Small tumor burden with limited involvement of one or more: Skin, Lymph nodes, Oral*	Large tumor burden: Oral, Gastrointestinal, Pulmonary, Other visceral involvement. Tumor-associated edema or ulceration
Immune system (I)	CD4+ cells ≥ 200/mm³	CD4+ cells < 200/mm³
Systemic illness (S)	No opportunistic infection (including thrush) or B symptoms†	History of opportunistic infection or thrush. B symptoms. Other HIV-related illness (*e.g.*, NHL or other malignancy, neurologic disease, wasting syndrome)

* Limited oral disease is confined to the palate and is not nodular.
† B symptoms are unexplained fever, night sweats, weight loss of more than 10% body weight, or diarrhea persisting for longer than 2 weeks.
(Modified from Krown SE, Metroka C, Wernz JC. Kaposi's sarcoma in the acquired immunodeficiency syndrome: A proposal for uniform evaluation, response, and staging criteria. J Clin Oncol 1989;7: 1201)

TABLE 59–3. Promising Therapeutic Strategies for AIDS-Related Kaposi's Sarcoma

Therapeutic Strategy	*Specific Modality*
Current Approaches	
Local interventions	Radiation therapies
	Fractionated radiation
	Whole-body electron beam
	Laser (including photodynamic therapy)
	Intralesional therapies
	Cytotoxic drugs (vinblastine, bleomycin)
	Biomodulators (IFN-α, tumor necrosis factor)
	Topical
	Liquid nitrogen
Systemic chemotherapies	
Cytotoxic chemotherapies	Single-agent
	Vinca alkaloids, VP-16, anthracyclines, cisplatin, bleomycin; response rate 40–50% (complete responses up to 25%)
	Combination
	Doxorubicin + bleomycin + vincas or VP-16 ± methotrexate; response rate 60–85% (complete responses up to 40%)
Antiviral therapies	Single-agent
	IFN-$\alpha \geq 20 \times 10^6$ U/m^2/d; response rate 25–40% (complete responses up to 25%)
	Combination
	IFN-α 9–18 $\times 10^6$ U/m^2/d + AZT 600 mg/d; response rate 45–55% (complete responses up to 40%)
Biomodulation	
Marrow protection during systemic therapies	Granulocyte-macrophage or granulocyte colony-stimulating factors
Antiangiogenesis and growth-factor inhibition	IFN-α, heparin analogs (suramin, pentosan)
Future Approaches	
Local interventions	Growth-factor inhibition
	IL-1 receptor antagonists
	Anti-IL-6 (monoclonal antibodies, retinoids)
	Immunotoxins (*e.g.*, b-FGF-PE-40, IL-6-PE-40)
Systemic interventions	
New antiretrovirals	Dideoxynucleosides (AZT, ddI, ddC) in combination with IFN-α or other antivirals
	TAT gene or TAT protein inhibitors
Antiangiogenesis and growth-factor inhibition	Angioinhibins (fumagillin analogs)
	Tissue inhibitor of metalloproteinase-2
	IL-1 receptor antagonists
	Anti-IL-6 (retinoids, pentoxifylline)
	Immunotoxins

IFN-α, interferon-α; PE, *pseudomonas* exotoxin.

tumor mass (endothelial or stromal cells, as examples) and are worthy of further clinical investigation.

AIDS-KS, like KS arising in other settings of immunodeficiency and in contrast to the classic KS of elderly Mediterranean or Ashkenazi Jewish men, is characterized by extensive mucocutaneous involvement and is frequently associated with deep tissue involvement, in particular the lung and the GI tract. Although local modalities can confer local disease control for a limited tumor burden, AIDS-KS patients usually require systemic therapy for widespread superficial or tissue-invasive tumor at some point in the clinical course. Systemic treatment of disseminated KS has evolved from initial trials of single cytotoxic or antiviral agents to the development of non-cross-resistant drug combinations and antiviral combinations (*i.e.*, anti-HIV and interferon).

Several individual antitumor agents (especially vinca alkaloids, epipodophyllins such as VP-16, anthracyclines, cisplatin, and bleomycin) have demonstrated anti-KS activity, each inducing tumor responses in 40% to 50% of patients. Combinations of these active agents—most commonly, doxorubicin, bleomycin, a vinca alkaloid (vincristine or vinblastine), and VP-16, with or without methotrexate—have led to responses in 60% to 85% of patients with widespread KS. Gill and coinvestigators[48] demonstrated remarkable efficacy of low-dose combination chemotherapy with doxorubicin (Adriamycin), bleomycin, and VP-16 (ABV). This regimen yields complete responses in almost 40% of patients (including patients with pulmonary involvement) and has an overall response rate of more than 80%. Further, in their randomized, prospectively stratified clinical trial comparing ABV with doxorubicin alone, disease-free survival in the ABV-treated patients was significantly prolonged (median 9 months versus 3.5 months, $p = 0.004$). To date, however, ABV has not had a major impact on overall survival in these heterogenous AIDS patients with extensive KS. As with all other regimens, the overriding determinants of clinical response and survival are the manifestations of deep immunocompromise and HIV activity, namely the extent of CD4 cell destruction and the prior history of opportunistic infections.

With respect to antiviral therapy, the use of interferon-α (IFN-α) as a single agent has produced clinically significant responses in about 30% of AIDS-KS patients (range, 20–50%), especially in those patients treated with at least 20×10^6 U/m^2/d and in those with less extensive immunosuppression.[49] Other IFN species (IFN-β and IFN-γ preparations) have not yielded clinically meaningful antitumor responses, although IFN-β has shown some suppression of HIV activity (decreases in HIV p24 antigenemia) in patients with relatively early HIV disease.[50] In a trial conducted by Lane and colleagues,[51] high-dose IFN-α (35×10^6 U/d) induced complete remissions in 24% and partial remissions in another 14% of patients, for an overall response rate of 38%. All patients with CD4 counts higher than 400/mm^3, but none with CD4 counts lower than 150/mm^3, had a meaningful response. In addition, there was evidence of HIV suppression in clinical responders, as manifested by at least a 75% decrease in HIV p24 antigenemia.

The relation between CD4 count and probability of response to IFN is noteworthy. In all trials using adequate dosage, it was clear that IFN-α possesses antitumor and anti-HIV activity, particularly in those patients whose immune function is relatively well preserved (*i.e.*, CD4 count higher than 400/mm^3).[49,52] Tumor responses may not occur before 1 to 2 months of therapy, and maximal responses require 6 or more months. In general, the parameters associated with clinical refractoriness to IFN therapy parallel those that determine a poor response to cytotoxic therapies, namely, visceral tumor, deep HIV-related immunosuppression, and features of progressive HIV activity (constitutional symptoms and high levels of serologic markers such as β_2-microglobulin, neopterin, and endogenous IFN levels). Side effects of IFN therapy include constitutional influenza-like symptoms (malaise, fever, chills, myalgia, arthralgia) and transient hypotension, which frequently occur when IFN is initiated, are partly dose-related, and subside with continued IFN administration.[44,49] The development of tachyphylaxis allows patients to tolerate gradual increases in IFN dosage. Myelosuppression (mainly neutrophils and platelets) and hepatic enzyme elevations (transaminases in particular) are commonly transient and reversible with attenuation of IFN dose.[49,52,53]

IFN antiretroviral activity differs from that of AZT or other dideoxynucleosides such as ddI and dideoxycytidine (ddC). IFN appears to act late in the HIV life cycle, specifically on viral packaging and budding of infectious particles from the host cell membrane. By contrast, the dideoxynucleosides act early in the process of HIV replication by inhibiting the HIV reverse-transcriptase enzyme.[2,4] In contrast to IFN-α, the antiretroviral drug AZT has not shown any antitumor effect against AIDS-KS when used as a single agent, despite suppression of HIV activity. When AZT is combined with IFN-α, however, there is evidence of synergy with respect to anti-KS and anti-HIV effects. Krown and colleagues[52] and Fischl[53] documented significant tumor regression in 45% to 55% of patients, which occurred within 3 to 4 months of combination therapy (3 to 6 months earlier than with IFN-α alone), a notably sustained (longer than 40 weeks) increase in CD4 cell counts with a concomitant heightened skin test reactivity, sustained suppression of HIV p24 antigenemia in a high proportion of patients, and prevention of emergence of AZT resistance. Major dose-limiting toxicities, namely, AZT-related neutropenia and IFN-related hepatotoxicity, were effectively abrogated by using attenuated doses of both agents without compromising antitumor, immunologic, or virologic effects. The regimen based on these trials to provide an optimal therapeutic ratio is AZT 600 mg/d plus IFN-α 9 to 18×10^6 U/d.

Scadden and colleagues[54] added the hematopoietic stimulator GM-CSF to AZT 1200 mg/d plus IFN-α 9 $\times$ 10^6 U/d. GM-CSF permitted the administration of full-dose AZT. With this approach, tumor responses occurred in half of patients receiving GM-CSF (80% of whom were poor-risk), without an obvious negative impact on immunologic or virologic modulation. As in all other clinical therapy trials in AIDS-KS, the most salutary results are achieved in patients with less HIV-related immune impairment (*i.e.*, CD4 counts higher than 200/mm^3). Overall, these results are encouraging and support the need for early therapeutic intervention at a time when tumor burden is low and some immune function persists. Future trials of other hematopoietic stimulators or reverse-transcriptase inhibitors associated with less myelosuppression, specifically ddI and ddC, may be used in combination or alternating with AZT.[2,4] Such approaches are unproved and should be undertaken only in an approved protocol. The use of multiple antiretroviral agents may permit the administration of higher doses of IFN-α, perhaps with cycles of cytotoxic combinations such as ABV. The potential improved tolerance for therapy and non-cross-resistant HIV suppression might facilitate the implementation of multimodal regimens aimed at curing AIDS-KS.

BIOMODULATION AND ANTIANGIOGENESIS APPROACHES

Theoretically, the multiple diverse pathogenic factors that may contribute to the emergence and perpetuation of KS in AIDS patients can serve as targets for therapy. Some of these factors are being addressed through combined antiviral therapies aimed at the control of HIV replication and the replication of potential viral cofactors, such as Epstein-Barr virus (EBV) or CMV. Other targets, such as the enhancement of immune function, inhibition of angiogenic factors such as FGF, inhibition of stimulatory cytokines such as IL-1 and IL-6, inhibition of viral proteins such as TAT, and hormonal manipulations, are or will become the focus of innovative anti-KS therapy and prevention measures.

The striking production of autostimulatory and angiogenic growth factors by KS cells suggests that these factors should be an important target for therapy. To this end, pentosan (a heparin analog related to the growth-factor inhibitor suramin) inhibits angiogenesis and the proliferative effects of KS-specific FGF on the autocrine growth of AIDS-KS cells and has anti-HIV activity that is synergistic with AZT in vitro.[55] Although early clinical trials have not demonstrated an antitumor activity, second- and third-generation compounds are worth exploring. Fumagillin, a unique angiogenesis inhibitor derived from the fungus *Aspergillus fumigatus*, and its synthetic analogs ("angioinhibins") block endothelial cell proliferation, tumor-induced neovascularization, and in vivo growth of diverse tumors in mice.[56,57] The human protein known as tissue inhibitor of metalloproteinase-2 (TIMP-2) blocks tumor cell invasion by complexing with and blocking the action of collagenase enzymes.[58] TIMP-2 also inhibits angiogenesis in an in vitro assay and in animal models, apparently by a direct action on human endothelial cells. Each of these novel biomodulators provides important approaches for future development.

One cytokine that likely has a pivotal role in autocrine stimulation of host cell proliferation and viral expression is IL-6. IL-6 may be a critical factor in the genesis and clonal expansion of AIDS-KS and B-cell malignancies, in particular NHL. The role of IL-6 in lymphomagenesis and the possible clinical application of IL-6 inhibitors to antilymphoma therapy are addressed later in this chapter. IL-6 inhibitors may have potential therapeutic value in AIDS-KS as well. For example, studies by Sidell and colleagues[46] of multiple myeloma cells demonstrate that retinoic acid can down-regulate IL-6 receptors and inhibit IL-6-mediated autocrine growth stimulation. This mechanism of inhibition may also apply to AIDS-KS, which, like multiple myeloma, appears to be driven by IL-6 in an autostimulatory fashion through upregulation of tumor cell IL-6 receptors. Along similar lines, the methylxanthine pentoxifylline (Trental) inhibits intracellular HIV replication by inhibiting TNF-α synthesis.[59] Since IL-6 expression is linked to TNF production through an autocrine loop, it is intriguing to speculate that pentoxifylline might provide anti-retroviral and anti-IL-6 effects in AIDS-KS (and perhaps in AIDS-lymphomas).

AIDS-RELATED ANOGENITAL CANCERS

Anogenital tumors, in particular those associated with HPV, have a notably aggressive course in patients infected with HIV.[60-62]. At least two mechanisms may operate, in theory, to predispose HIV-infected patients to HPV-induced malignant transformation. The HPV oncoproteins E6 and E7, especially those from the transforming HPV types 16 and 18, bind to or degrade the tumor suppressor proteins p53 and RB.[63,64] The potential importance of the loss of normal tumor suppressor mechanisms to the pathogenesis of AIDS lymphomas is discussed later. Further, HPV and HIV act synergistically through their respective transactivating factors (*i.e.*, products of the E2 and TAT genes) to increase cellular transcription and to augment each other's gene expressions.[20] The enhanced expression of viral proteins that increase viral replication, abrogate host tumor suppressor functions, and further exacerbate cellular immunodeficiency contribute to the high incidence of advanced-stage disease that is rapidly progressive and refractory to therapy.

Kiviat and colleagues[60] and Palefsky and colleagues[62] detected the presence of anal HPV, in particular the oncogenic strains 16 and 18, in more than half of HIV-seropositive gay men. Moreover, abnormal anal cytology occurs in about 40% and anal intraepithelial neoplasia in 15% of these men, particularly in those with CD4 counts lower than 200/mm^3 and with severe HIV infection.[60] The presence of DNA from a single HPV strain confers about a fivefold increased risk for developing preneoplastic cytopathology; however, infection with multiple strains, a common finding in this patient cohort, confers a dramatically increased (up to 40-fold) risk of detecting cytologic abnormalities, which, in turn, are directly associated with the development of an intraanal neoplastic lesion. The presence and magnitude of the constellation of findings related to HPV-induced anal squamous cell cancer is linked to the presence and severity of HIV infection.

Similarly, advanced cervical cancer is emerging as a major complication as HIV affects increasing numbers of women.[61] In this regard, cervical cancer is an opportunistic cancer, much like KS, NHL, and the related HPV-associated anal squamous cell cancers in HIV-infected men. HPV coinfection is common in women with HIV; in fact, 60% of HIV-infected women have cervical dysplasia noted on Papanicolaou tests (similar to anal epithelial dysplasia in men). Studies to define the true incidence and natural history of concomitant HPV and HIV infections, cervical intraepithelial neoplasia (an early or premalignant lesion), and cervical cancer will lay the groundwork for effective strategies aimed at early detection and prevention.

AIDS-RELATED NON-HODGKIN'S LYMPHOMAS

Even before AIDS, NHL was an increasing problem. The National Cancer Institute Surveillance, Epidemiology, and End Results (SEER) data base is informative.[65] The incidence of NHL in the United States and other Western countries has risen steadily over the past decade and is still largely unexplained. This increase in NHL has not been accompanied by an increased incidence of Hodgkin's disease (Fig. 59–3). Hodgkin's disease can occur in the setting of HIV infection, however, specifically in intravenous drug users. Predominant histologic subtypes are mixed cellularity and lymphocyte depletion, and more than 80% of Hodgkin's disease patients present with advanced-stage disease.[66] The apparent propensity of HIV-infected patients who use drugs to develop Hodgkin's disease, in contrast to gay men who acquire AIDS by sexual transmission (and who seem to preferentially develop NHL) is unexplained and is a topic for future investigation.

EPIDEMIOLOGY AND CLINICAL MANIFESTATIONS

In the United States, there has been about a 50% increase in incidence and a 22% increase in the death rate of NHL since

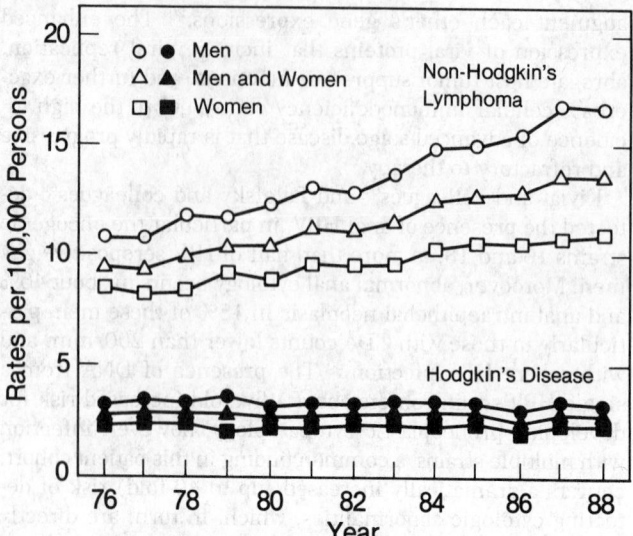

FIGURE 59–3. Incidence rates for non-Hodgkin's lymphoma (NHL) and Hodgkin's disease (HD) in men and women of all ages from 1976 to 1988. The incidence of NHL increased by about 50% during this period, substantially due to an increased incidence in men, and is still not explained. This increase antedated the AIDS pandemic, but AIDS has aggravated these statistics (see Fig. 59–5). In contrast, no such increase was detected in the incidence of HD for either men or women during this time frame. (Courtesy of Edward J. Sondik, PhD)

the early 1970s.[65] About 38,000 cases of NHL are reported per year in the United States alone, and this disease entity can no longer be considered minor or rare. In more recent years, a significant new component of this increase reflects the emergence of lymphomas associated with AIDS.[9,10,67,68] The SEER program has been able to track the unexpected increase in incidence of specific types of NHL.[65] The connection between AIDS and NHL was first reported in 1982. Beginning in 1983, a sharp rise in the incidence of NHL has been detected exclusively for men aged 20 to 54 years (Fig. 59–4). In an analysis of almost 100,000 unselected AIDS patients from 1981 to 1989, about 3% had NHL, a 60-fold increase over that expected for the general population.[69] Further, in an autopsy series of 101 AIDS patients from 1981 to 1987, lymphomas were detected in 20 patients: five tumors were located in the brain, and eight (including four of the brain tumors) were detected only at autopsy.[70]

The increase in AIDS-NHL has occurred predominantly in high-grade B-cell types, with large cell immunoblastic and small noncleaved lymphomas comprising about 70% of AIDS-NHL and with the intermediate-grade diffuse large cell lymphomas making up the remaining 30%.[9,67] Frequently, AIDS-related lymphomas have the histology and cytogenic pattern characteristic of Burkitt's lymphoma.[67,69]

AIDS lymphomas resemble NHL occurring in other severely immunocompromised settings by their frequent involvement of extranodal sites (particularly GI tract and brain) and by the high incidence of stage IV disease, especially in Burkitt's lymphoma (in which bone marrow infiltration is common).[9,67,68] In particular, primary central nervous system (CNS) lymphoma may occur with striking frequency in large cell immunoblastic or small noncleaved cell types, usually as

mass lesions (Fig. 59–5) but on occasion as a more diffuse leptomeningeal process.[71] Pluda and colleagues[9] described 5 of 8 AIDS patients with NHL at the National Cancer Institute who had primary CNS involvement, and Moore and colleagues[72] described 10 of 24 AIDS patients with NHL from a multicenter study who had primary CNS involvement. Like NHL that arises from a background of chronic immunosuppression and unlike NHL that occurs outside a known immunosuppressed state, AIDS lymphomas demonstrate a high frequency of multiclonality. A 2-year (1987–1989) prospective multicenter study of over 1000 patients with advanced HIV who received AZT detected an overall 2.3% prevalence of NHL, rising to 3.2% after 2 years of antiretroviral therapy.[72] The median CD4 cell count at the start of AZT therapy was 104/mm³, and, as in other series of AIDS patients undergoing AZT treatment, the probability of survival at 2 years was 50%.[2,4,9] In this group, risk factors for NHL development can be explained by immunosuppression and infection with other viruses, namely the presence of prior KS, CMV infection, and oral hairy leukoplakia (an EBV-related lesion). The modest overall proportion of NHL cases in this patient cohort may relate to two factors: (1) the median observation period of 600 days with a maximum of 2 years, which is when NHL occurrence in AZT-treated patients began to escalate in the studies by Pluda and colleagues[9]; and (2) the relative preservation of CD4 count (higher than 100/mm³) at study entry. Analyses by Yarchoan and colleagues[7] and the Centers for Disease Control[10] suggest that the greatest risk for NHL development and death from any cause occurs when there is a substantial impairment of cellular immunity, represented by CD4 counts less than 50/mm³.

NHL is likely to be a particular problem for patients with CD4-positive lymphocyte counts less than 50/mm³.[7,10] In the analysis by Pluda and colleagues[9], 8 of 55 (14.5%) AIDS patients undergoing antiretroviral therapy at the National Cancer

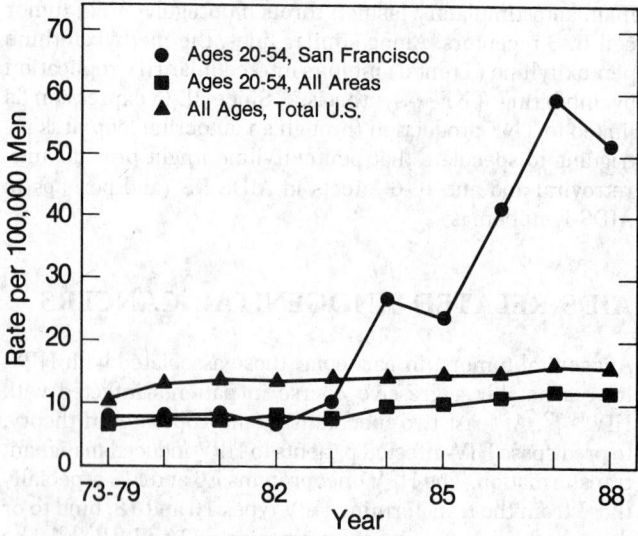

FIGURE 59–4. The increasing incidence of non-Hodgkin's lymphoma in men 20 to 54 years old since 1983. The incidence is particularly striking for men of this age group in San Francisco and is clearly associated with the AIDS pandemic. (Courtesy of Edward J. Sondik, PhD)

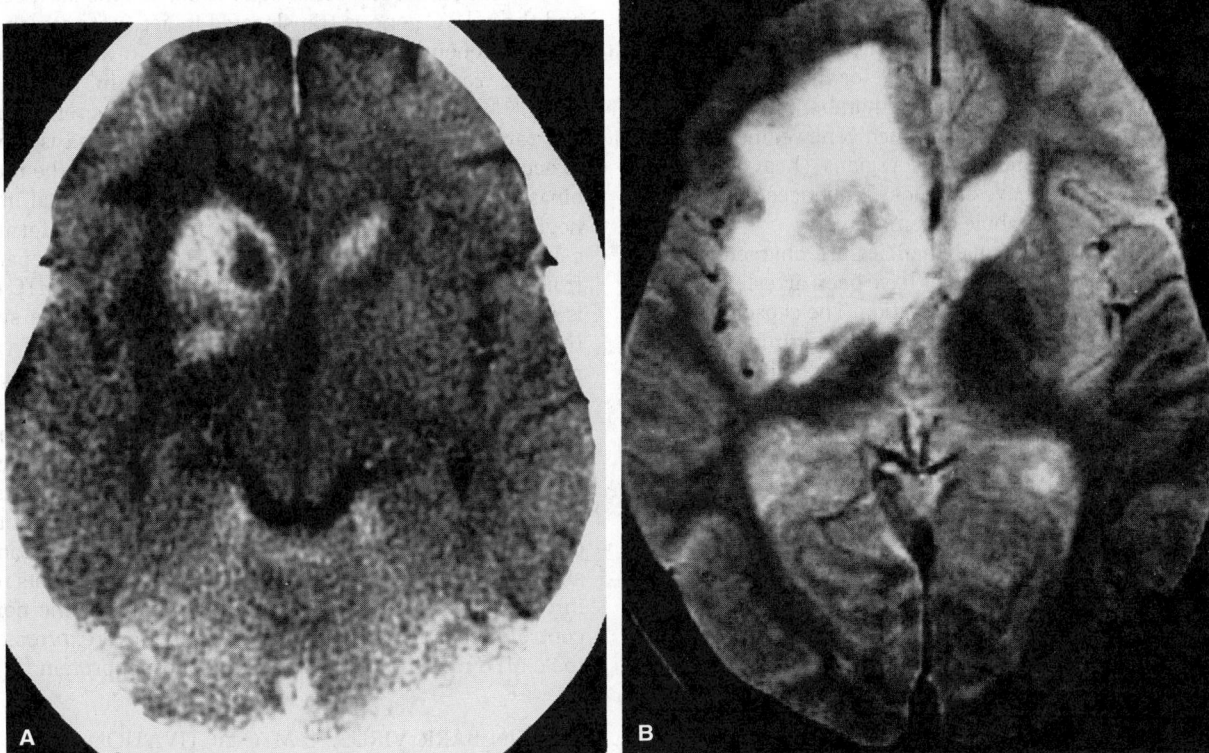

FIGURE 59–5. **(A)** CT scan of the brain (with intravenous contrast dye injection) of an AIDS patient with primary central nervous system lymphoma, small noncleaved cell morphology. **(B)** T2-weighted spin echo magnetic resonance image of the same patient. (Courtesy of Irwin Feuerstein, MD)

Institute developed aggressive B-cell NHL (extranodal involvement, especially CNS) an average of 2 years after beginning AZT therapy, with the estimated actuarial probability of developing NHL rising to about 30% after 3 years of antiretroviral therapy. The median CD4 count at the onset of AZT therapy was 74/mm³, and at the time of NHL development it was 6/mm³. All eight patients had serologic evidence of EBV infection, and two patients developed primary CNS lymphoma in the setting of prior toxoplasmosis; it is reasonable to speculate that these infections led to polyclonal B-cell activation, a prelude to malignant transformation (discussed later). In this closely followed cohort of patients, where consistent and frequent observations were made over an extended period, virtually all who developed NHL did so with CD4 counts higher than 50/mm³ for 12 months or more (median 18 months) before NHL emerged. The depth of immunocompromise—as specifically reflected by a CD4 cell count higher than 50/mm³—appears to be a critical factor in the emergence of opportunistic NHL in the setting of AIDS.[7,9,10] Lymphomas can and do occur with CD4 counts higher than 50/mm³; however, the risk is significantly elevated once this threshold is crossed. Ultimately, prevention of NHL development may hinge on an ability to restore immune function or at least maintain it at a critical protective level.

A primate model in cynomolgus monkeys infected with simian immunodeficiency virus (SIV) may provide a close parallel to human AIDS.[73] In this model, high-grade B-cell NHL develops 5 to 15 months after SIV inoculation, in conjunction with severe immunodeficiency. Median CD4 counts at the time of NHL onset are 80/mm³, similar to the AZT-treated patient cohort from the National Cancer Institute series.[9] As with humans, there is a disproportionate incidence of Burkitt's lymphomas with wide dissemination, and some tumors demonstrate integration of the EBV genome in tumor cell DNA. The primate model validates the association of retrovirus-induced profound immunosuppression and a propensity for NHL development and is important for future studies of pathogenesis, treatment, and prevention that may extrapolate to HIV-infected humans.

GENE REARRANGEMENTS IN NORMAL AND MALIGNANT B-CELL DEVELOPMENT

Normal B- and T-lymphocyte differentiation is accomplished through rearrangements of gene sequences that encode antigen receptors, namely immunoglobulin and T-cell-receptor genes, respectively. The process of gene rearrangements in these antigen receptor genes, accomplished through DNA breakage and rejoining and mediated by recombinase enzymes, confers diversity in the repertoire of specialized immune responses to a variety of antigens. Focusing specifically on B-lineage development, molecular rearrangement of the three gene segments encoding the variable regions of the immunoglobulin heavy chain—variable (V), diversity (D), and joining (J)—takes place in early precursors, namely pre-B and immature B cells.[74,75] The three gene segments, located on discontinuous portions of the long arm of chromosome 14 (14q32), are joined in a specific pattern (V_H-D-J_H). The sequence of recombination events is orderly, but juxtaposition of specific molecular sequences within each region is random, providing the first element of diversity in the generation of an antibody response. The capacity for diversity is further increased by variation in nucleotide number and type within the joining regions of the recombined gene segments. In addition, all immunoglobulin gene regions (heavy and light chains, both κ and λ) have enhancer sequences that activate transcription over the whole chromosome.

Lymphohematopoietic malignancies are characterized by the clonal expansion of cells that have been arrested at a specific developmental stage of maturation. The capacity for self-renewal is preserved, but the capacity for terminal differentiation is blocked. In this regard, the finding by Berberian and colleagues[76] of a clonal deficit in rearrangements of a specific subfamily of the genes encoding the variable region of the immunoglobulin heavy chain, specifically the VH3L subfamily, in B cells of HIV-infected patients is provocative. The clonal defect reflects B-cell maturation arrest within lymph node germinal centers and results in a deficit in memory B cells.[77] This impaired B-cell differentiation is accompanied by an increase in circulating levels of IL-6,[78] which may provide a chronic proliferative stimulus for the arrested B-cell clone and thereby drive expansion of certain B-cell clones.

One pathogenic mechanism underlying the malignant transformation of lymphoid precursors in general and of B cells specifically is the translocation of a normal growth-promoting gene (or *protooncogene*) to the lineage-specific antigen receptor genes (in the case of B cells, the immunoglobulin genes). The juxtaposition of the protooncogene segment with the immunoglobulin gene, in particular its transcriptionally active enhancer sequences, results in deregulation of the translocated growth-promoting gene, which (by virtue of overexpression) now functions as a true oncogene. This process does not require literal proximity. In addition, aberrant recombinase function may contribute to the pathogenesis of lymphoid malignancies by catalyzing chromosomal breaks and translocations that involve 14q32 (the locus of the heavy-chain gene), especially those occurring at the 5' region of the J_H segment of the gene.[75,79]

A classic example of oncogene activation resulting from this type of chromosomal rearrangement occurs in Burkitt's lymphoma, in which the c-*MYC* gene, located on the long arm of chromosome 8 (8q24),[80] participates in a translocation to the immunoglobulin gene heavy-chain locus on 14q32. There are a number of mechanisms by which *MYC* activation can ensue, all of which may operate to some degree in t(8;14).[81–83] Transcriptional activation of c-*MYC* can occur from juxtaposition to immunoglobulin gene enhancer sequences or from the action of long-range enhancers on chromosome 14. Inactivation of the 5' regulatory sequences of the c-*MYC* gene locus can occur through point mutations or truncation of the 5' region or by separation of the regulatory region from the rest of the gene. The translocated portion of c-*MYC* can be rearranged, for example, by inverting itself on insertion into the breakpoint on 14q32. All these mechanisms permit *MYC* overexpression.

The translocation and recombination of 8q24 and 14q32 typify Burkitt's lymphoma in its endemic (African) and sporadic (American) forms; however, the c-*MYC* gene may behave differently in the two variants.[79,82,83] In the endemic form, the breakpoint on chromosome 8q24 is outside the *MYC* region, and the c-*MYC* gene is translocated intact (not rearranged), albeit frequently with point mutations, to a break in the V_H-D-J_H recombination, most commonly in the J_H segment.[75,82] This translocation occurs in a nonsecretory pre-B-cell (an early stage of B-cell differentiation) and is thought to occur in conjunction with aberrant function of the recombinase enzyme in the process of completing normal immunoglobulin gene rearrangement.[79,84] In the sporadic form, the c-*MYC* gene is disrupted within its 5' portion and separated from its regulatory (or *repressor*) region. The first *MYC* exon is translocated in some instances to a break in the switch region of the heavy-chain gene (S_μ) and is inverted (rearranged) on translocation.[81–85] The breakpoint on 14q32 results from an error in the action of isotype-switching enzymes in a more mature B cell that is capable of immunoglobulin secretion. The net result of c-*MYC* translocation to the immunoglobulin gene locus for the endemic or sporadic type is the abrogation of the effects of negative regulatory elements on c-*MYC* transcription. More than transcriptional activation or amplification of *MYC* per se, these gene rearrangements result in constitutive *MYC* expression and a failure of the normal control mechanisms, which leads to a net overexpression of the c-*MYC* mRNA-and DNA-binding phosphoprotein.[75,80]

EPSTEIN-BARR VIRUS, C-*MYC* ACTIVATION, AND B-CELL LYMPHOMAGENESIS

The role of EBV in B-cell lymphomagenesis has been established for endemic (African) Burkitt's lymphoma and postulated for many of the B-cell malignancies that arise in the setting of chronic immunosuppression. In the case of EBV-associated endemic Burkitt's lymphoma, c-*MYC* breakpoints occur outside the 5' regulatory region, and the c-*MYC* gene is altered mainly through mutations within its first exon (most commonly at Pvu site II) rather than through truncation or rearrangement on translocation.[83] In the absence of EBV DNA, in the sporadic form, c-*MYC* breakpoints occur within the 5' region of the gene and commonly result in truncation of the gene when it is translocated. Translocation to the nonswitch region of 14q32 results in transcription activation by immunoglobulin gene enhancer sequences; alternatively, translocation of the disrupted c-*MYC* gene to the switch region of 14q32 is accompanied by c-*MYC* gene inversion or true rearrangement, which results in direct oncogene overexpression. Nonetheless, for EBV-related Burkitt's lymphomas, c-*MYC* deregulation must involve other mechanisms. In this regard, EBV latent genes encode viral nuclear antigens (EBNAs) that act as transcriptional activators to enhance the survival and self-renewal capacities of EBV-infected host cells and viral genome.[86] EBNAs may also interact with the c-*MYC* regulatory region to effect gene overexpression and may further augment the effects of any point mutations occurring within the 5' regulatory region.

Yet another mechanism of EBV-induced B-cell stimulation may operate through BCRF-1, an EBV-encoded protein that shares remarkable structural and functional homology with IL-10.[87,88] BCRF-1 causes a decrease in T-cell (and possibly natural killer-cell) synthesis of IFN-γ and perhaps IL-2, the net result of which is functional suppression of T-cell antiviral activity. Consequently, viral survival is enhanced as the by-product of BCRF-1-related immunomodulation. B-cell activation and polyclonal B-cell expansion are promoted as a result of ongoing EBV propagation.

EBV has also been implicated in the cause of non-Burkitt's B-cell lymphomas, most commonly those that occur in the setting of chronic, profound immunosuppression. In contrast to Burkitt's lymphomas, these lymphoproliferative malignancies are often characterized by the presence of multiple neoplastic clones and by an immunoblastic large cell morphology with plasmacytoid features.[89-91] In this situation, EBV may provoke polyclonal B-cell activation, which, in the absence of normal T-cell controls, permits unopposed B-cell expansion with increased numbers of cells susceptible to destabilizing genetic events such as chromosomal breaks and recombinations. The etiologic effects of EBV have been demonstrated by inducing lymphomas in mice with severe combined immunodeficiency disease (SCID) that have been reconstituted with EBV-negative human peripheral or nodal lymphocytes (SCID/hu chimeric mice) and subsequently infected with EBV[92] or with peripheral blood lymphocytes from EBV-seropositive donors.[93] Of note is the absence of c-*MYC* and *BCL2* translocations or rearrangements. This animal model parallels the large cell immunoblastic B lymphomas that occur in humans with severe immunodeficiency (*e.g.*, after organ transplantation)[89,91,94] and in primary CNS lymphomas (now recognized as an AIDS-associated lesion).[20,71,90] In the human tumors, as in the SCID/hu mouse model, EBV genome is present in tumor cells, and the tumors (often with multiclonal origin) develop from a background polyclonal activation that is likely a consequence of EBV infection.

The mechanisms by which EBV may induce B-cell malignant transformation in the setting of AIDS are reminiscent of the mechanisms that operate in other states of chronic immunosuppression. Despite these similarities, however, the direct etiologic role of EBV in AIDS-related lymphomas remains a focus of investigation. It is likely that EBV is but one of many possible inducers of malignant transformation. Other DNA viruses of the herpesvirus family—most notably, CMV and human herpesvirus type 6 (HHV-6)—may also enhance B-cell activation and promote B-cell clonal expansion. These potential cofactors interact with HIV in ways that may enhance transcriptional activation and HIV replication.[20,22,95] Herpesviruses, like HIV, upregulate the expression of several cytokines by virus-infected lymphocytes and monocytes. These cytokines can induce host cell proliferation and viral replication through a positive feedback mechanism and, in this way, may provide a chronic stimulus for B-cell proliferation and activation.

Cells from about half (up to as many as 80%, in some series) of AIDS-NHL contain EBV DNA sequences.[20,96] Studies examining EBV genomic termini as clonal markers of infection have demonstrated the presence of the monoclonal episomes of EBV DNA, usually in the form of closed circles.[97] Of eight peripheral (nonprimary CNS) AIDS-associated lymphomas at the National Cancer Institute, seven were shown to contain EBV genomic sequences in the configuration of monoclonal episomes.[97a] Nevertheless, at least in selected human Burkitt's lymphoma and other B-lymphoblastoid cell lines, the EBV genome has been found to be integrated into host DNA, preferentially being inserted into segments of numerous chromosomes (in particular, 1, 5, and 13).[98] Whatever the structural particulars, all these findings are consistent with the hypothesis that EBV precedes and probably causes clonal expansions in AIDS-NHL and in endemic and some cases of sporadic Burkitt's lymphomas.[97] In addition, when EBV DNA and EBNAs are detected in nodes from HIV-positive patients with generalized lymphadenopathy, their presence signifies the likely emergence of NHL (with persistence of the EBV genome in the malignant clones); in contrast, cells from patients with EBV-negative lymphadenopathy do not appear to undergo malignant transformation,[99] supporting the notion that EBV has a direct etiologic role in NHL development in at least some AIDS patients.

In most cases in which NHL cells from AIDS patients contain the EBV genome or its protein products, there is concomitant alteration and deregulation of the c-*MYC* gene. However, there is not an inextricable linkage between EBV and c-*MYC* perturbations in AIDS-NHL.[100-102] In a few cases of phenotypically unusual B-lineage AIDS-NHL, EBV DNA sequences, gene products, and virus-induced surface antigens (*e.g.*, Ki-24) are detectable without associated c-*MYC* alterations.[101] More commonly, when there is dissociation of EBV and c-*MYC*, c-*MYC* mutations or rearrangements (present in about 70% of all large cell AIDS-NHL) occur in the absence of detectable EBV DNA or EBNAs.[100,102] Most cases of non-EBV, non-Burkitt's NHL have c-*MYC* rearrangements and 14q32 switch region breaks that mimic the sporadic Burkitt-type; but endemic-type breakpoints in c-*MYC* and 14q32 occur in about one fourth of cases of non-EBV AIDS-NHL and are accompanied by similar point mutations in the first *MYC* exon.[81] In terms of c-*MYC* breakpoints and the sites of c-*MYC* translocation to the heavy-chain gene (J_H versus S_u), AIDS lymphomas show both patterns. Overall, the prevalence of abnormalities in c-*MYC* structure and function is consistent with the notion that c-*MYC* has a central role in the malignant transformation and clonal expansion of B-cell lymphomas in AIDS.

POTENTIAL ROLE OF ABERRANT TUMOR SUPPRESSION IN THE PATHOGENESIS OF AIDS LYMPHOMAS

The loss of normal tumor suppressor gene and gene product function is thought to be a critical step in the pathogenesis and progression of diverse epithelial and lymphohematopoietic cancers.[103] Investigations have uncovered losses or mutations in specific tumor suppressor genes, particularly the retinoblastoma (*RB*) gene on chromosome 13q14 and the *p53* gene on chromosome 17p13, in myeloid and lymphoid leukemias and lymphomas.[103-105] The presence of *RB* and *p53* abnormalities is associated with clonal evolution and increasing aggressiveness of these malignancies, and there is a suggestion that the altered tumor suppressor genes may act in concert with activated oncogenes to effect the full transformation process.

The interaction between viral proteins and tumor suppressor proteins has been documented for several oncogenic DNA viruses and for RB and p53, the nuclear phosphoprotein products of the *RB* and *p53* genes.[106,107] In fact, the roles that tumor suppressors play in cell cycle regulation—in particular, their inhibition of movement from G1 into S phase—have been defined by the binding of viral proteins, such as SV40 large T antigen (for RB and p53) and adenovirus E1A (for RB) or E1B (for p53) to suppressor proteins and inactivation of their antiproliferative effects.[106,108] The blocking effects of HPV oncoproteins on RB and p53 activity may be important to the induction of anogenital cancers by HPV.[63,64] Studies of herpes simplex virus type 1 suggest that the virus may induce relocation of RB and p53 from their usual nuclear compartments to the sites of viral DNA replication, thereby facilitating host cell and virus replication.[107] Abrogation of tumor suppression may be a common mechanism by which any or all herpesviruses (including EBV) could operate in the pathogenesis of AIDS lymphomas and other AIDS-related cancers.

The sequential acquisition of aberrant oncogene and tumor suppressor gene and gene product function may be especially relevant to the process of viral tumorigenesis. In such cases, viruses might enhance the process of transformation and growth dysregulation through any one of several mechanisms: chromosomal breakage and translocation, leading to c-*MYC* or other oncogene activation; or production of viral proteins that bind to and alter the function of tumor suppressors that normally control transition through the cell cycle. These interactions may contribute to the pathogenesis of AIDS lymphomas through a direct effect of HIV or through other viruses, such as EBV, CMV, or HHV-6. Along these lines, the finding that exogenous HIV infection of EBV-seropositive, HIV-seronegative human peripheral blood B lymphocytes enhance EBV and endogenous c-*MYC* gene expression, in association with in vitro transformation of a subpopulation of those B cells to a malignant phenotype capable of B-lymphoma formation in SCID mice,[109] is provocative but requires confirmation. Theoretically, under some conditions that could have clinical relevance, HIV might act synergistically with EBV to exert a direct transforming effect, perhaps through transcriptional activation.

INTERLEUKINS AND THE DEVELOPMENT OF AIDS LYMPHOMAS

The proliferation and differentiation of lymphohematopoietic elements from pluripotent stem cells into mature end-stage cells is directed by a "family" of interactive glycoproteins, the *hematopoietic growth factors*, or *cytokines*. More than 20 cytokines—interleukins, colony-stimulating factors, interferons, and other growth factors—have been identified and characterized with respect to molecular and mechanistic features. Heightened cytokine production in response to HIV infection (and perhaps to other viruses) may contribute to the development of lymphomas in AIDS. The major cellular sources of production are T cells, monocytes, and bone marrow stromal cells of mesenchymal origin (namely fibroblasts), which can be infected by HIV and respond to HIV or other virus infection by increasing cytokine production.[24,25] Of the many lymphohematopoietic growth factors liberated under normal and virus-perturbed conditions, IL-6 may be especially relevant to pre-malignant polyclonal B-cell expansion and to eventual malignant transformation in AIDS-NHL. IL-6 promotes the growth and differentiation of B cells, particularly the induction of immunoglobulin gene expression and the final differentiation from immature B-cell precursors to plasma cells.[36,110] IL-6 also plays a role in the recruitment of resting T cells to the proliferative state and their differentiation along

the cytotoxic T-lymphocyte pathway. IL-6 has major effects on the proliferation, differentiation, and net expression of multiple arms of the immune response. The increase in serum IL-6 levels that accompanies the HIV-associated clonal VH3L defect in B-cell maturation[76,78] may represent an attempt (albeit abortive) to drive the differentiation of the arrested B-cell clone. The B-cell maturation arrest occurs early in HIV infection, even before subclinical evidence for cellular immune impairment,[76] suggesting that the compensatory increase in circulating IL-6 levels also occurs early in HIV infection and can drive B-cell proliferation chronically over a long period of time. Further, IL-6 may augment HIV replication (and hence disease progression) in an autocrine loop through its enhancement of T-cell and monocyte growth.[24] Similar autocrine growth may exist in other tissues, such as brain. The production of IL-6 by brain tissue, particularly virus-infected tissue, is intriguing in light of the proclivity of AIDS-NHL to involve the CNS. Additionally, the production of IL-6 from HIV-infected monocytes promotes the proliferation of activated B cells (*e.g.*, by EBV), thereby driving immunoglobulin synthesis and causing the nonspecific hyperimmunoglobulinemia commonly seen in early HIV infection.[24,111]

In addition to mechanisms that directly stimulate B-cell expansion, suppression of helper T-cell antiviral or cytotoxic surveillance activities can permit the establishment of malignant clones. The recently described IL-10, called *cytokine synthesis inhibitory factor,* is such a suppressor of T-cell function.[87,88] IL-10 shares significant homology with the EBV protein BCRF-1 and likewise impairs T-cell synthesis of IFN-γ and IL-2. Besides their antiviral activities, IFN-γ and IL-2 upregulate major histocompatibility complex II surface antigen expression (which provokes the generation of cytotoxic T lymphocytes, a major effector of antitumor immune surveillance) and support the clonal expansion of immune-activated T cells in autocrine fashion. Excess IL-10 may permit viral replication (particularly EBV and possibly HIV) to go unchecked, which promotes the cascade of events that culminates in the establishment of clonal B-cell malignancy.

OPPORTUNITIES FOR THERAPEUTIC INNOVATION

Like other lymphomas arising in immunodeficient hosts, AIDS-NHL is a resilient, clinically aggressive therapeutic challenge. AIDS lymphomas are histologically high-grade tumors that usually present with multiorgan involvement and a substantial tumor burden. CNS tumor is especially common and, partly because it is protected as a sanctuary site, a frequent site of relapse. HIV-related bone marrow suppression (likely a consequence of direct progenitor cell infection or stromal cell infection with attendant suppression of hematopoietic growth factors)[25] and the presence of multiple chronic opportunistic infections act in concert to limit the host's ability to tolerate full cytotoxic therapy. Moreover, the absence of any antitumor immunity permits the expansion of tumor cells remaining after therapy to proceed unchecked.

As a result, multidrug regimens effective in de novo NHL—for example, ProMACE-MOPP (prednisone, methotrexate, doxorubicin [Adriamycin], cyclophosphamide [Cytoxan], etoposide–mechlorethamine, vincristine, procarbazine, prednisone) or variants containing bleomycin (MACOP-B, M-BACOD) and cytosine arabinoside (ProMACE-CytaBOM)

TABLE 59–4. Hematopoietic Growth Factors in the Therapy of AIDS and AIDS-Related Malignancies

	Erythropoietin	Granulocyte-CSF	GM-CSF	Macrophage-CSF	IL-3
Hematopoietic target cell	Erythrocyte	Granulocyte	Granulocyte, eosinophil, monocyte	Monocyte	Granulocyte, eosinophil, monocyte, platelets?
Amelioration of AZT-induced myelosuppression (in vivo)	+	+	+	?	?
Enhanced viral replication in monocyte/macrophage target cells	–	–	+	+	+
Enhanced AZT antiretroviral activity		+	–	+	
Marrow-protective effects demonstrated during antitumor chemotherapy		+ (KS)	+ (KS, NHL)		

—have met with variable results in AIDS lymphomas. Such combinations of alternating non-cross-resistant agents that reproducibly achieve complete remission rates of 70% to 90%, median disease-free survivals longer than 3 to 5 years, and median overall survivals exceeding 5 to 7 years in patients with advanced-stage aggressive NHL[112] have yielded remission rates of 20% to 50%, with overall survivals far less than 1 year for AIDS-associated lymphomas.[113] A potentially significant factor in the poor responses for AIDS-NHL is the attenuation or complete omission of therapy cycles on the basis of functionally impaired marrow reserve or uncontrollable opportunistic infection. The roles of marrow-protective hematopoietic growth factors in antiretroviral therapies for HIV infection and in antitumor therapies for AIDS-related malignancies are being defined through integrated laboratory and clinical investigations[33,54,114-118] (Table 59–4). Multiagent chemotherapy regimens combined with CNS therapy, antiretroviral therapy, anti-*Pneumocystis* prophylaxis, and marrow-protective colony-stimulating factors[114,116] are being tested in clinical trials (Table 59–5). A clinical trial by McMaster and colleagues[119] employing two cycles of intensive, multiagent non-cross-resistant cytoreductive therapy (including CNS therapy) to patients with high-grade, extensive small noncleaved cell lymphomas yielded promising results. Each of three HIV-infected patients in this trial achieved complete remission, and two were alive and well 2 to 3 years after therapy; however, none of these patients had full-blown preexisting AIDS.

A multimodality approach combines intensive cytotoxic antilymphoma therapy, antiretroviral therapy, and allogeneic or syngeneic bone marrow transplantation aimed at hematopoietic and immune reconstitution.[120] The net effects of allogeneic transplantation on immunocompetence are complex, but the ability to reinitiate some capacity for immune responsiveness seems crucial to the achievement of long-lasting antitumor effects. In this respect, transplantation of pluripotent stem cells offers the potential for long-term control of HIV infection and AIDS-NHL. Such approaches would likely require antiretroviral coverage.

For AIDS-NHL, it is likely that IL-6, alone or in concert with other B-stimulatory and T-suppressing lymphokines, chronically drives B-cell clonal expansion.[4,24] As discussed for AIDS-KS, it is logical to search for therapeutic agents that might inhibit net IL-6 activity, such as retinoic acid, pentoxifylline, anti-IL-6 antibodies, or for other molecular modifications that might block IL-6 binding and signaling. The ability to target and modify the activity of specific overexpressed genes with antisense oligodeoxynucleotides offers a novel approach to anti-HIV[121,122] and anticancer therapies.[123-125] At least in theory, this form of gene-directed therapy suppresses

TABLE 59–5. National Cancer Institute Protocol Therapy for AIDS-Related Non-Hodgkin's Lymphoma

I. Cyclic Chemotherapy (Cycles Repeated Every 21 Days)

Day One
  Cyclophosphamide, 500 mg/m²
  VP-16, 100 mg/m²
  Doxorubicin, 15 mg/m²
Day Eight
  Vincristine, 1.4 mg/m²
  Methotrexate, 120 mg/m²
  Leucovorin, 25 mg/m² q6h × four doses (beginning 24 h after methotrexate)

All drugs are given intravenously.

II. Prophylaxis and Therapy for CNS Lymphoma

Intrathecal methotrexate, 12.5 mg, and cytosine arabinoside, 70 mg, are given weekly × 6.
For lymphomatous meningitis, intrathecal therapy is given twice weekly until clear, then weekly × 6. In addition, whole-brain irradiation, 3600 cGy, is administered daily in 180 cGy fractions.

III. Marrow-Protective Therapy

Granulocyte-macrophage colony-stimulating factor (GM-CSF), 10 μg/kg/d, is administered subcutaneously on days 2 through 7 and 9 through 14 of each cycle.

IV. Antiretroviral Therapy

AZT 500 mg PO, is administered daily

V. Anti-*Pneumocystic Carinii* Pneumonia Prophylaxis

Aerosolized pentamidine inhalation therapy is given monthly.

TABLE 59–6. Potential Factors Involved in the Pathogenesis of AIDS-Related Lymphomas

Pathogenic Factor	Specific Host or Virus Effector	Mechanism for Malignant Transformation	Mechanism for (Poly) Clonal Expansion
Oncogene activation	c-MYC	Chromosomal translocation	Deregulated (constitutive?) gene expression
			Blockade of apoptosis
Tumor suppressor inactivation	RB, p53	Gene loss or mutation	Loss of cell cycle regulation at G_1 and S boundary
		Binding inactivation by viral oncoproteins	
HIV	VH3L gene	Maturation arrest in germinal center B cells	(Compensatory) increase in IL-6 production
	Transcriptional activation?	c-MYC	EBV gene expression
Oncogenic viral cofactors	DNA viruses (e.g., EBV, CMV, HHV-6)	c-MYC breakage, mutation, translocation, and deregulation	Transcriptional activation
			Blockage of T-cell antiviral lymphokines
			Synergy with HIV
			Growth-factor induction
			Chronic antigenic stimulation
Lymphokines	IL-6	Enhanced gene expression	Autocrine growth stimulation
		Genetic instability?	
	IL-10	Enhanced viral replication or expression	Inhibition of T-cell synthesis of IFN-γ and IL-2
DNA damage or repair	Aberrant recombinase activity	Maturational arrest?	?
	HIV	Replication of damaged or abnormally rearranged DNA	?

the malignant clone while sparing normal host tissues. Antisense oligomers can be made complementary to a specific aberrant mRNA transcribed from aberrant gene segments, for example, the fusion BCR-ABL gene that typifies chronic myelogenous leukemia[125] or the first intron of a translocated c-MYC gene present in a Burkitt's lymphoma cell line.[123] In both instances, the antisense constructs selectively inhibit the net expression of the targeted tumor cell gene, tumor cell proliferation, and survival without affecting normal cell counterparts. The development of diffusible phosphodiester and phosphorothioate oligodeoxynucleotides complementary to specific sequences in the BCL2 protooncogene and the demonstration that incubation of these antisense compounds with leukemic lymphoblasts results in growth inhibition and eventual cytotoxicity is a template for future gene-targeted therapies.[124] BCL2, however, is discussed only as a model since it is not known to be abnormally expressed in AIDS-related lymphomas.

FUTURE DIRECTIONS: PREVENTION

As with all malignancies, the most effective strategies are those targeted to prevention. The ability, early in the course of active HIV infection, to interfere with mechanisms that promulgate B-cell hyperproliferation and clonal expansion—especially growth factors (IL-6, in particular) and concomitant viral infections (mainly EBV, but also CMV and HHV-6)—might decrease the occurrence or prolong the time to development of AIDS-related malignancies. Ultimately, however, the key strategies will be those directed toward maintaining

the CD4 cell count at a level that prevents the establishment and perpetuation of transformed clones. From the studies of Yarchoan and colleagues,[7] the critical level for NHL development appears to be a CD4 count of about 50/mm³. The identification of factors that portend a significant risk of cancer development for an HIV-infected patient (Table 59–6) and the development of antiretroviral strategies that confer long-term suppression of HIV activity and relative preservation of immune function (perhaps in combination with specific antigrowth-factor or other antiviral therapies) are essential to the ultimate prevention of all malignancies that arise as a consequence of HIV-induced immunosuppression. Although much remains to be done, we have a strong foundation to build new approaches for preventing and treating these important neoplastic complications of AIDS.

REFERENCES

1. Siegal B, Levinton-Kriss S, Schiffer A, et al. Kaposi's sarcoma in immunosuppression. Cancer 1990;65:492.
2. Broder S, Mitsuya H, Yarchoan R, et al. Antiretroviral therapy in AIDS. Ann Intern Med 1990;113:604
3. Gail MH, Pluda JM, Rabkin CS, et al. Projections of the incidence of non-Hodgkin's lymphoma related to acquired immunodeficiency syndrome. J Natl Cancer Inst 1991;83:695
4. Yarchoan R, Pluda JM, Perno C-F, et al. Antiretroviral therapy of HIV infection: Current strategies and challenges for the future. Blood 1991;78:859.
5. McKinney RE, Maha MA, Connor EM, et al. A multicenter trial of oral zidovudine in children with advanced human immunodeficiency virus disease. N Engl J Med 1991;324:1018.
6. Moore RD, Hidalgo J, Sugland BW, et al. Zidovudine and the natural history of the acquired immunodeficiency syndrome. N Engl J Med 1991;324:1412.
7. Yarchoan R, Venzon DJ, Pluda JM, et al. CD4 count as a mortality risk indicator in human immunodeficiency virus (HIV)-infected patients receiving antiretroviral therapy: Experience in a research hospital. Ann Intern Med 1991;115:184.

8. Rosenberg PS, Gail MH, Schrager LK, et al. National AIDS incidence trends and the extent of zidovudine therapy in selected demographic and transmission groups. J AIDS 1991;4:392.

9. Pluda JM, Yarchoan R, Jaffe ES, et al. Development of non-Hodgkin's lymphoma in a cohort of patients with severe immunodeficiency virus (HIV) infection on long-term antiretroviral therapy. Ann Intern Med 1990;113:276.

10. Centers for Disease Control. Current trends: Opportunistic non-Hodgkin's lymphomas among severely immunocompromised HIV-infected patients surviving for prolonged periods on antiretroviral therapy—United States. MMWR 1991;40:591.

11. Kaposi M. Idiopathisches multiples pigmentsarkom der haut. Arch Dermatol Syph 1872;4:265.

12. Friedman-Kien AE, Saltzman BR. Clinical manifestations of classical, endemic African, and epidemic AIDS-associated Kaposi's sarcoma. J Am Acad Dermatol 1990;22:1237.

13. Greenberg SJ, Jaffe ES, Ehrlich GD. Kaposi's sarcoma in human T-cell leukemia virus type I-associated adult T-cell leukemia. Blood 1990;76:971.

14. Lind SE, Gross PL, Andiman WA, et al. Malignant lymphoma presenting as Kaposi's sarcoma in a homosexual man with the acquired immunodeficiency syndrome. Ann Intern Med 1985;102:338.

15. Haverkos HW, Friedman-Kien AE. The changing incidence of Kaposi's sarcoma among patients with AIDS. J Am Acad Dermatol 1990;22:1250.

16. Krigel RL, Friedman-Kien AE. Epidemic Kaposi's sarcoma. Semin Oncol 1990;17:350.

17. Pitchenik AE, Fischl MA, Dickinson GM, et al. Opportunistic infections and Kaposi's sarcoma among Haitians: Evidence of a new acquired immunodeficiency state. Ann Intern Med 1983;98:277.

18. Marmor M, Friedman-Kien AE, Zolla-Pazner S, et al. Kaposi's sarcoma in homosexual men. Ann Intern Med 1984;100:809–819.

19. Jaffe HW, Choi K, Thomas PA, et al. National case-control study of Kaposi's sarcoma and *Pneumocystis carinii* pneumonia in homosexual men: Part 1, epidemiologic results. Ann Intern Med 1983;99:145.

20. Cremer KJ, Spring SB, Gruber J. Role of human immunodeficiency virus type I and other viruses in malignancies associated with acquired immunodeficiency disease syndrome. J Natl Cancer Inst 1990;82:1016.

21. Rogers MF, Morens DM, Steward JA, et al. National case-control study of Kaposi's sarcoma and *Pneumocystis carinii* pneumonia in homosexual men: Part 2, laboratory results. Ann Intern Med 1983;99:151.

22. Laurence J. Molecular interactions among herpesviruses and human immunodeficiency virus. J Infect Dis 1990;162:338.

23. Ambinder RF, Newman C, Hayward GS, et al. Lack of association of cytomegalovirus with endemic African Kaposi's sarcoma. J Infect Dis 1987;156:193.

24. Birx DL, Redfield RR, Tencer K, et al. Induction of interleukin-6 during human immunodeficiency virus infection. Blood 1990;76:2303.

25. Scadden DT, Zeira M, Woon A, et al. Human immunodeficiency virus infection of human bone marrow stromal fibroblasts. Blood 1990;76:317.

26. Delli Bovi P, Curatola AM, Kern FG, et al. An oncogene isolated by transfection of Kaposi's sarcoma DNA encodes a growth factor that is a member of the FGF family. Cell 1987;50:729.

27. Delli-Bovi P, Curatola AM, Newman KM, et al. Processing, secretion, and biologic properties of a novel growth factor of the fibroblast growth factor family with oncogenic potential. Mol Cell Biol 1988;8:2933.

28. Ensoli B, Nakamura S, Salahuddin SZ, et al. AIDS-Kaposi's sarcoma-derived cells express cytokines with autocrine and paracrine growth effects. Science 1989;243:223.

29. Miles SA, Rezai AR, Salazar-Gonzalez JF, et al. AIDS Kaposi sarcoma-derived cells produce and respond to interleukin 6. Proc Natl Acad Sci USA 1990;87:4068.

30. Salahuddin SZ, Nakamura S, Biberfeld P, et al. Angiogenic properties of Kaposi's sarcoma-derived cells after long-term culture in vitro. Science 1988;242:430.

31. Wellstein A, Lupu R, Zugmaier G, et al. Autocrine growth stimulation by secreted Kaposi fibroblast growth factor but not by endogenous basic fibroblast growth factor. Cell Growth Differ 1990;1:63.

32. Abboud SL, Pinzani M. Peptide growth factors stimulate macrophage colony-stimulating factor in murine stromal cells. Blood 1991;78:103.

33. Kitano K, Abboud CN, Ryan DH, et al. Macrophage-active colony-stimulating factors enhance human immunodeficiency virus type I infection in bone marrow stem cells. Blood 1991;77:1699.

34. Dinarello CA. Interleukin-1 and interleukin-1 antagonism. Blood 1991;77:1627.

35. Boraschi D, Rambaldi A, Sica A, et al. Endothelial cells express the interleukin-1 receptor type I. Blood 1991;78:1262.

36. Hirano T. Interleukin 6 (IL-6) and its receptor: Their role in plasma cell neoplasias. Int J Cell Cloning 1991;9:166.

37. Schwab G, Siegall CB, Aarden LA, et al. Characterization of an interleukin-6-mediated autocrine growth loop in the human multiple myeloma cell line U266. Blood 1991;72:587.

38. Zhang XG, Klein B, Bataille R. Interleukin-6 is a potent myeloma-cell growth factor in patients with aggressive multiple myeloma. Blood 1989;73:11.

39. Ensoli B, Barillari G, Salahuddin SZ, et al. Tat protein of HIV-1 stimulates growth of cells derived from Kaposi's sarcoma lesions of AIDS patients. Nature 1990;345:84.

40. Friedman SL. Kaposi's sarcoma and lymphoma of the gut in AIDS. Bailliere's Clin Gastroenterol 1990;4:455.

41. Ognibene FP, Steis RG, Macher AM, et al. Kaposi's sarcoma causing pulmonary infiltrates and respiratory failure in the acquired immunodeficiency syndrome. Ann Intern Med 1985;102:471.

42. Heitzman ER. Pulmonary neoplastic and lymphoproliferative disease in AIDS: A review. Radiology 1990;177:347.

43. Krown SE, Metroka C, Wernz JC. Kaposi's sarcoma in the acquired immune deficiency syndrome: A proposal for uniform evaluation, response, and staging criteria. J Clin Oncol 1989;7:1201.

44. Pluda JM, Brawley OW, Yarchoan R, et al. Neoplasms associated with AIDS. In: Calabresi P, Schein PS, eds. Medical oncology: Basic principles and clinical management of cancer. Elmsford, UK: Pergamon Press, 1992 (in press).

45. Northfelt DW, Kahn JO, Volberding PA. Treatment of AIDS-related Kaposi's sarcoma. Hematol Oncol Clin North Am 1991;5:297.

46. Sidell N, Taga T, Hirano T, et al. Retinoic acid-induced growth inhibition of a human myeloma cell line via down-regulation of IL-6 receptors. J Immunol 1991;146:3809.

47. Waldmann TA. Monoclonal antibodies in diagnosis and therapy. Science 1991;252:1657.

48. Gill PS, Rarick M, McCutchan JA, et al. Systemic treatment of AIDS-related Kaposi's sarcoma: Results of a randomized trial. Am J Med 1991;90:427.

49. Krown SE. Interferon and other biologic agents for the treatment of Kaposi's sarcoma. Hematol Oncol Clin North Am 1991;5:311.

50. Miles SA, Wang H, Cortes E, et al. Beta-interferon therapy in patients with poor-prognosis Kaposi sarcoma related to the acquired immunodeficiency syndrome (AIDS): A phase II trial with preliminary evidence of antiviral activity and low incidence of opportunistic infections. Ann Intern Med 1990;112:582.

51. Lane HC, Kovacs JA, Feinberg J, et al. Antiretroviral effects of interferon-alpha in AIDS-associated Kaposi's sarcoma. Lancet 1988;ii:1218.

52. Krown SE, Gold JWM, Niedzwiecki D, et al. Interferon-a with zidovudine: Safety, tolerance, and clinical and virologic effects in patients with Kaposi sarcoma associated with the acquired immunodeficiency syndrome (AIDS). Ann Intern Med 1990;112:812.

53. Fischl MA. Antiretroviral therapy in combination with interferon for AIDS-related Kaposi's sarcoma. Am J Med 1991;90:2S.

54. Scadden DT, Bering HA, Levine JD, et al. Granulocyte-macrophage colony-stimulating factor mitigates the neutropenia of combined interferon alfa and zidovudine treatment of acquired immune deficiency syndrome-associated Kaposi's sarcoma. J Clin Oncol 1991;9:802.

55. Wellstein A, Zugmaier G, Califano JA III, et al. Tumor growth dependent on Kaposi's sarcoma-derived fibroblast growth factor inhibited by pentosan polysulfate. J Natl Cancer Inst 1991;83:716.

56. Folkman J, Weisz PB, Joullie MM, et al. Control of angiogenesis with synthetic heparin substitutes. Science 1989;243:1490.

57. Ingber D, Fujita T, Kishimoto S, et al. Synthetic analogues of fumagillin that inhibit angiogenesis and suppress tumor growth. Nature 1990;348:555.

58. Albini A, Melchiori A, Santi L, et al. Tumor cell invasion inhibited by TIMP-2. J Natl Cancer Inst 1991;83:775.

59. Fazely F, Dezube BJ, Allen-Ryan J, et al. Pentoxifylline (Trental) decreases the replication of the human immunodeficiency virus type I in human peripheral blood mononuclear cells and in cultured T cells. Blood 1991;77:1653.

60. Kiviat N, Rompalo A, Bowden R, et al. Anal human papilloma-virus infection among human immunodeficiency virus-seropositive and -seronegative men. J Infect Dis 1990;162:358.

61. Maiman M, Fruchter RG, Serur E, et al. Human immunodeficiency virus infection and cervical neoplasia. Gynecol Oncol 1990;38:377.

62. Palefsky JM, Gonzales J, Greenblatt RM, et al. Anal intraepithelial neoplasia and anal papillomavirus infection among homosexual males with group IV HIV disease. JAMA 1990;263:2911.

63. Dyson N, Howley PM, Munger K, et al. The human papilloma virus-16 E7 oncoprotein is able to bind to the retinoblastoma gene product. Science 1989;248:934.

64. Werness BA, Levine AJ, Howley PM. Association of human papillomavirus types 16 and 18 E6 proteins with p53. Science 1990;248:76.

65. Cancer Statistics Review 1973-1988. National Cancer Institute, Division of Cancer Prevention and Control. NIH publication No. 91-2789, 1991.

66. Monfardini S, Tirelli U, Vaccher E, et al. Hodgkin's disease in 63 intravenous drug users with human immunodeficiency virus. Ann Oncol (Supplement) 1991;2:201.

67. Knowles DM, Chamulak GA, Subar M, et al. Lymphoid neoplasia associated with the acquired immunodeficiency syndrome (AIDS). Ann Intern Med 1988;108:744.

68. Ziegler JL, Beckstead JA, Volberding PA, et al. Non-Hodgkin's lymphoma in 90 homosexual men: Relation to generalized lymphadenopathy and the acquired immunodeficiency syndrome. N Engl J Med 1984;211:565.

69. Beral V, Peterman T, Berkelman R, et al. AIDS-associated non-Hodgkin lymphoma. Lancet 1991;337:805.

70. Wilkes MS, Fortin AH, Felix JC, et al. Value of necropsy in acquired immunodeficiency syndrome. Lancet 1988;ii:85.

71. Gill PS, Levine AM, Meyer PR, et al. Primary central nervous system lymphoma in homosexual men: Clinical, immunologic and pathologic features. Am J Med 1985;78:742.

72. Moore RD, Kessler H, Richman DD, et al. Non-Hodgkin's lymphoma in patients with advanced HIV infection treated with zidovudine. JAMA 1991;265:2208.

73. Feichtinger H, Putkonen P, Parravicini C, et al. Malignant lymphomas in cynomolgus monkeys infected with simian immunodeficiency virus. Am J Pathol 1990;137:1311.

74. Waldmann TA, Korsmeyer SJ, Bakhshi A, et al. Molecular genetic analysis of human lymphoid neoplasms: Immunoglobulin genes and the *c-myc* oncogene. Ann Intern Med 1985;102:497.

75. Croce CM, Nowell PC. Molecular basis of human B cell neoplasia. Blood 1985;65:1.

76. Berberian L, Valles-Ayoub Y, Sun N, et al. A VH clonal deficit in human immunodeficiency virus-positive individuals reflects a B-cell maturational arrest. Blood 1991;78:175.

77. Braun J, Galbraith L, Valles-Ayoub Y, Saxon A. Human immunodeficiency resulting from maturational arrest of germinal center B cells. Immunol Lett 1991;27:205.

78. Breen EC, Rezai AR, Nakajima K, et al. Infection with HIV is associated with elevated IL-6 levels and production. J Immunol 1990;144:480.

79. Haluska FG, Tsujimoto Y, Croce CM. Mechanisms of chromosome translocation in B- and T-cell neoplasia. Trends Genet 1987;3:11.

80. Dalla-Favera R, Bregni M, Erikson J, et al. Human c-myc oncogene is located on the region of chromosome 8 that is translocated in Burkitt lymphoma cells. Proc Natl Acad Sci USA 1982;79:7824.

81. Ladanyi M, Offitt K, Jhanwar SC, et al. MYC rearrangement and translocations involving band 8q24 in diffuse large cell lymphomas. Blood 1991;77:1057.

82. Pellici PG, Knowles DM, Magrath I, et al. Chromosomal breakpoints and structural alterations of the c-myc locus differ in endemic and sporadic forms of Burkitt lymphoma. Proc Natl Acad Sci USA 1986;83:2984.

83. Shiramizu B, Barriga F, Neequaye J, et al. Patterns of chromosomal breakpoint locations in Burkitt's lymphoma: Relevance to geography and Epstein-Barr virus association. Blood 1991;77:1516.

84. Klein G. Multiple phenotypic consequences of the Ig/Myc translocation in B-cell-derived tumors. Genes Chromosomes Cancer 1989;1:3.

85. Gauwerky CE, Croce CM. Molecular biology of leukemias and lymphomas. In: Broder S, ed. Molecular foundations of oncology. Baltimore, MD: Williams and Wilkins, 1991:295–310.

86. Gregory CD, Dive C, Henderson S, et al. Activation of Epstein-Barr virus latent genes protects human B cells from death by apoptosis. Nature 1991;349:612.

87. Hsu D-H, Malefyt RD, Fiorentino DF, et al. Expression of interleukin-10 activity by Epstein-Barr virus protein BCRF1. Science 1990;250:830.

88. Moore KW, Vieira P, Fiorentino DF, et al. Homology of cytokine synthesis inhibitory factor (IL-10) to the Epstein-Barr virus gene BCRF1. Science 1990;248:1230.

89. Hanto DW, Frizzera G, Gajl-Peczalska KJ, et al. Epstein-Barr virus-induced B-cell lymphoma after renal transplantation: Acyclovir therapy and transition from polyclonal to monoclonal B-cell proliferation. N Engl J Med 1982;306:913.

90. Hochberg FH, Miller G, Schooley RT, et al. Central-nervous-system lymphoma related to Epstein-Barr virus. N Engl J Med 1983;309:745.

91. Shearer WT, Ritz J, Finegold MJ, et al. Epstein-Barr virus associated B-cell proliferations of diverse clonal origins after bone marrow transplantation in a 12-year-old patient with severe combined immunodeficiency. N Engl J Med 1985;312:1151.

92. Cannon MJ, Pisa P, Fox RI, et al. Epstein-Barr virus induces aggressive lymphoproliferative disorders of human B cell origin in SCID/hu chimeric mice. J Clin Invest 1990;85:1333.

93. Rowe M, Young LS, Crocker J, et al. Epstein-Barr Virus (EBV)-associated lymphoproliferative disease in the SCID mouse model: Implications for the pathogenesis of EBV-positive lymphomas in man. J Exp Med 1991;173:147.

94. Penn I. Tumors arising in organ transplant recipients. Adv Cancer Res 1978;28:31.

95. Lusso P, De Maria A, Malnati M, et al. Induction of CD4 and susceptibility to HIV-1 infection in human CD8+ T lymphocytes by human herpesvirus 6. Nature 1991;349:533.

96. Hamilton-Dutoit SJ, Pallesen G, Karkov J, et al. Identification of EBV-DNA in tumour cells of AIDS-related lymphomas by in-situ hybridisation. Lancet 1989;i:554.

97. Neri A, Barriga F, Inghirami G, et al. Epstein-Barr virus infection precedes clonal expansion in Burkitt's and acquired immunodeficiency syndrome-associated lymphomas. Blood 1991;77:1092.

97a. Raffeld M. Personal communication. National Cancer Institute, January 1992.

98. Trescol-Biemont MC, Biemont C, Daillie J. Localization polymorphism of EBV DNA genomes in the chromosomes of Burkitt lymphoma cell lines. Chromosoma 1987;95:144.

99. Shibata D, Weiss LM, Nathwani BN, et al. Epstein-Barr virus in benign lymph node biopsies from individuals infected with the human immunodeficiency virus is associated with concurrent or subsequent development of non-Hodgkin's lymphoma. Blood 1991;77:1527.

100. Groopman JE, Sullivan JL, Mulder C, et al. Pathogenesis of B cell lymphoma in a patient with AIDS. Blood 1986;67:612.

101. Knowles DM, Inghirami G, Ubriaco A, et al. Molecular genetic analysis of three AIDS-associated neoplasms of uncertain lineage demonstrates their B-cell derivation and the possible pathogenetic role of the Epstein-Barr virus. Blood 1989;73:792.

102. Subar M, Neri A, Inghirami G, et al. Frequent c-myc oncogene activation and infrequent presence of Epstein-Barr virus genome in AIDS-associated lymphoma. Blood 1988;72:667.

103. Stanbridge EJ, Nowell PC. Origins of human cancer revisited. Cell 1990;63:867.

104. Ginsberg AM, Raffeld M, Cossman J. Inactivation of the retinoblastoma gene in human lymphoid neoplasms. Blood 1991;77:833.

105. Hollstein M, Sidransky D, Vogelstein B, Harris CC. p53 Mutations in human cancers. Science 1991;253:49.

106. Hollingsworth RE, Lee WH. Tumor suppressor genes: New prospects for cancer research. J Natl Cancer Inst 1991;83:91.

107. Wilcock D, Lane DP. Localization of p53, retinoblastoma and host replication proteins at sites of viral replication in herpes-infected cells. Nature 1991;349:429.

108. DeCaprio JA, Ludlow JW, Lynch D, et al. The product of the retinoblastoma susceptibility gene has properties of a cell cycle regulatory element. Cell 1989;58:1085.

109. Laurence J, Astrin SM. Human immunodeficiency virus induction of malignant transformation in human B lymphocytes. Proc Natl Acad Sci 1991;88:7635.

110. Kishimoto T. The biology of interleukin-6. Blood 1989;74:1.

111. Yarchoan R, Redfield RR, Broder S. Mechanisms of B cell activation in patients with acquired immunodeficiency syndrome and related disorders. J Clin Invest 1986;78:439.

112. Longo DL, DeVita VT, Duffey PL, et al. Superiority of ProMACE-CytaBOM over ProMACE-MOPP in the treatment of advanced diffuse aggressive lymphoma: Results of a prospective randomized trial. J Clin Oncol 1991;9:25.

113. Raphael BG, Knowles DM. Acquired immunodeficiency syndrome-associated non-Hodgkin's lymphoma. Semin Oncol 1990;17:361.

114. Kaplan LD, Kahn JO, Crowe S, et al. Clinical and virologic effects of recombinant granulocyte-macrophage colony stimulating factor in patients receiving chemotherapy for human immunodeficiency virus-associated non-Hodgkin's lymphoma: Results of a randomized trial. J Clin Oncol 1991;9:929.

115. Koyanagi Y, O'Brien WA, Zhao JQ, et al. Cytokines alter production of HIV-1 from primary mononuclear phagocytes. Science 1988;241:1673.

116. Perno CF, Cooney DA, Currens MJ, et al. Ability of anti-HIV agents to inhibit HIV replication in monocyte/macrophages or U937 monocytoid cells under conditions of enhancement by GM-CSF or anti-HIV antibody. AIDS Res Hum Retroviruses 1990;6:1051.

117. Pluda JM, Yarchoan R, Smith PD, et al. Subcutaneous recombinant granulocyte-macrophage colony-stimulating factor used as a single agent and in an alternating regimen with azidothymidine in leukopenic patients with severe human immunodeficiency virus infection. Blood 1990;76:463.

118. Schuitemaker H, Kootstra NA, van Oers MHJ, et al. Induction of monocyte proliferation and HIV expression by IL-3 does not interfere with anti-viral activity of zidovudine. Blood 1990;76:1490.

119. McMaster ML, Greer JP, Greco A, et al. Effective treatment of small-non-cleaved-cell lymphoma with high-intensity, brief-duration chemotherapy. J Clin Oncol 1991;9:941.

120. Holland HK, Saral R, Rossi JJ, et al. Allogeneic bone marrow transplantation, zidovudine, and human immunodeficiency virus type 1 (HIV-1) infection: Studies in a patient with non-Hodgkin's lymphoma. Ann Intern Med 1989;111:973.

121. Stein CA, Ranajit P, DeVico AL, et al. Mode of action of 5'-linked cholesteryl phosphorothioate oligodeoxy-nucleotides in inhibiting syncytia formation and infection by HIV-1 and HIV-2 in vitro. Biochemistry 1991;30:2439–2444.

122. Sullenger BA, Gallardo HF, Ungers GE, et al. Overexpression of TAR sequences renders cells resistant to human immunodeficiency virus replication. Cell 1990;63:601.

123. McManaway ME, Neckers LM, Loke SL, et al. Tumour-specific inhibition of lymphoma growth by an antisense oligodeoxynucleotide. Lancet 1990;335:808.

124. Reed JC, Stein C, Subasinghe C, et al. Antisense-mediated inhibition of BCL-2 protooncogene expression and leukemic cell growth and survival: Comparisons of phosphodiester and phosphorothioate oligodeoxynucleotides. Cancer Res 1990;50:6565.

125. Szczylik C, Skorski T, Nicolaides NC, et al. Selective inhibition of leukemic cell proliferation by BCR-ABL antisense oligodeoxynucleotides. Science 1991;253:562.

Cancer: Principles & Practice of Oncology, Fourth Edition,
edited by Vincent T. DeVita, Jr., Samuel Hellman, Steven A. Rosenberg.
J.B. Lippincott Co., Philadelphia © 1993.

CHAPTER **60**

Oncologic Emergencies

SECTION **1**

JOACHIM YAHALOM

Superior Vena Cava Syndrome

Superior vena cava syndrome (SVCS) is the clinical expression of obstruction of blood flow through the superior vena cava (SVC). Characteristic symptoms and signs may develop quickly or gradually when this thin-walled vessel is compressed, invaded, or thrombosed by processes in the superior mediastinum. The first pathologic description of SVC obstruction in a patient with syphilitic aortic aneurysm appeared in 1757.[1] In 1954, Schechter reviewed 274 well-documented cases of SVCS reported in the literature; 40% of them were due to syphilitic aneurysms or tuberculosis mediastinitis.[2] These entities have since virtually disappeared, and cancer of the lung is now the underlying process in approximately 70% of the patients with SVCS.

ANATOMY AND PATHOPHYSIOLOGY

The SVC is the major vessel for drainage of venous blood from the head, neck, upper extremities, and upper thorax. It is located in the middle mediastinum and is surrounded by relatively rigid structures such as the sternum, trachea, right bronchus, aorta, pulmonary artery, and the perihilar and paratracheal lymph nodes. The SVC extends from the junction of the right and left innominate veins to the right atrium for a distance of 6 to 8 cm. The distal 2 cm of the SVC is within the pericardial sac, with a point of relative fixation of the vena cava at the pericardial reflection. The azygos vein, the main auxiliary vessel, enters the SVC posteriorly, just above the

pericardial reflection. The SVC maintains blood at a low pressure. It is large but thin-walled, compliant, and easily compressible, and it is vulnerable to any space-occupying process in its vicinity. The SVC is completely encircled by chains of lymph nodes that drain all the structures of the right thoracic cavity and the lower part of the left thorax. The auxiliary azygos vein is also threatened by enlargement of paratracheal nodes. Other critical structures in the mediastinum, such as the main bronchi, esophagus, and the spinal cord, may be involved by the same process that led to obstruction of the SVC.[3–5]

When the SVC is fully or partially obstructed, an extensive venous collateral circulation may develop. The azygos venous system is the most important alternative pathway. Carlson found that dogs could not survive sudden ligation of the SVC below the level of the azygos vein, but they tolerated well ligation of the SVC above it.[6] He could, however, successfully obstruct the SVC and the azygos vein in operations performed in two stages, presumably by allowing time for collaterals to form. Other collateral systems are the internal mammary veins, lateral thoracic veins, paraspinous veins, and the esophageal venous network. The subcutaneous veins are important pathways, and their engorgement in the neck and thorax is a typical physical finding in SVCS. Despite these collateral pathways, venous pressure is almost always elevated in the upper compartment if there is obstruction of the SVC. Venous pressures have been recorded as high as 200 to 500 cm H_2O in severe SVCS.[7]

ETIOLOGY AND NATURAL HISTORY

The syndrome usually has an insidious onset and progresses to typical symptoms and signs. Review of the data from three

2111

TABLE 60–1. Common Symptoms and Physical Findings of Superior Vena Cava Syndrome

Symptoms	Patients Affected* (%)	Physical Findings	Patients Affected (%)
Dyspnea	63	Venous distention of neck	66
Facial swelling or head fullness	50	Venous distention of chest wall	54
Cough	24	Facial edema	46
Arm swelling	18	Cyanosis	20
Chest pain	15	Plethora of face	19
Dysphagia	9	Edema of arms	14

* Analysis based on data from 370 patients.[8–10]

recent series (Table 60–1) shows dyspnea to be the most common symptom.[8–10] Dyspnea occurred in 63% of the patients with SVCS. A sensation of fullness in the head and facial swelling was reported by 50% of the patients. Other complaints were cough (24%), arm swelling (18%), chest pain (15%), and dysphagia (9%). The characteristic physical findings were venous distention of the neck (66%) and chest wall (54%), facial edema (46%), plethora (19%), and cyanosis (19%). These symptoms and signs may be aggravated by bending forward, stooping, or by lying down.

Malignant disease is the most common cause of SVCS. The percentage of patients in different series with a confirmed diagnosis of malignancy varies from 78% to 86% (Table 60–2).[3,9–11] Lung cancer was diagnosed in 65% of 415 patients analyzed in these series.[3,9–11] Armstrong and Perez did a retrospective review of 4100 cases treated for bronchogenic carcinoma between 1965 and 1984, and identified 99 patients (2.4%) with SVCS.[8] Salsali observed SVCS in 4.2% of 4960 patients with lung cancer; 80% of the tumors inducing SVCS were of the right lung.[12] Small cell lung cancer is the most common histologic subtype (Table 60–3), and it was found in 38% of the patients who had lung cancer and SVCS. Among 225 consecutive patients with small cell cancer, 26 (11.5%) had SVCS when the malignancy was diagnosed.[13] The second most common histologic subtype is squamous cell carcinoma, found in 26% of lung cancer patients with SVCS.

Lymphoma involving the mediastinum was the cause of SVCS in 8% of the patients reported in the series (see Table 60–2). Armstrong and Perez found SVCS in 1.9% of 952 lymphoma patients.[8] Perez-Soler identified 36 cases (4%) of SVCS among 915 patients with non-Hodgkin's lymphoma (NHL)

treated at the M.D. Anderson Cancer Center.[14] Twenty-three patients (64%) had diffuse large cell lymphoma, 12 (33%) had lymphoblastic lymphoma, and 1 patient had follicular large cell lymphoma. Of their patients with diffuse large cell lymphoma and lymphoblastic lymphoma, 7% and 21% had SVCS, respectively. Hodgkin's lymphoma commonly involves the mediastinum, but it rarely causes SVCS. Other primary mediastinal malignancies that cause SVCS are thymoma and germ cell tumors. Breast cancer is the most common metastatic disease that causes SVCS.[3,9,11]

Nonmalignant conditions causing SVCS are not as rare as previously reported.[8,15] When the data were collected from general hospitals, as many as 22% of the patients had noncancerous causes of SVCS.[3,9,11] Parish[9] reported 19 patients with benign causes of SVCS, and Schraufnagel[3] included 16 such patients in his series. Fifty percent of the patients in both reports had a diagnosis of mediastinal fibrosis, which was probably due to histoplasmosis. Parish reported 6 patients with thrombosis of SVC, and in 5, thrombosis developed in the presence of central vein catheters or pacemakers.[9] Sculier reviewed 24 cases of central venous catheter-induced SVC.[16] Of these, 18 were caused by pacemaker catheters. LeVeen shunts, Swan-Ganz catheters, and hyperalimentation catheters were also involved. The increasing use of these devices for the delivery of chemotherapy agents or for hyperalimentation contributes to the development of SVCS in the cancer patient.[17]

Obstruction of SVC in the pediatric age group is rare and has a different etiologic spectrum. The causative factors are mainly iatrogenic, secondary to cardiovascular surgery for congenital heart disease, ventriculoatrial shunt for hydro-

TABLE 60–2. Primary Pathologic Diagnoses for Superior Vena Cava Syndrome

Histologic Diagnosis	Bell[10] 159 Patients (%)	Schraufnagel[3] 107 Patients (%)	Parish[9] 86 Patients (%)	Yellin[11] 63 Patients (%)	Total 415 Patients (%)
Lung cancer	129 (81)	67 (63)	45 (52)	30 (48)	271 (65)
Lymphoma	3 (2)	10 (9)	8 (9)	13 (21)	34 (8)
Other malignancies (primary or metastatic)	4 (3)	14 (13)	14 (16)	8 (13)	40 (10)
Nonneoplastic	2 (1)	16 (15)	19 (22)	11 (18)	50 (12)
Undiagnosed	21 (13)				21 (5)

TABLE 60–3. Lung Cancer Subtypes Associated With Superior Vena Cava Syndrome

Histology	No. of Patients (%)
Small cell	142 (38)
Squamous cell	97 (26)
Adenocarcinoma	52 (14)
Large cell	43 (12)
Unclassified	34 (9)
Total	370 (100)

TABLE 60–4. Chest Radiographic Findings for 86 Patients With Superior Vena Cava Syndrome

Finding	No. of Patients (%)
Superior mediastinal widening	55 (64)
Pleural effusion	22 (26)
Right hilar mass	10 (12)
Bilateral diffuse infiltrates	6 (7)
Cardiomegaly	5 (6)
Calcified paratracheal nodes	4 (5)
Mediastinal (anterior) mass	3 (3)
Normal	14 (16)

(Parish JM, et al. Etiologic considerations in SVCS. Mayo Clin Proc 1981;56:407–413)

cephalus, and SVC catheterization for parenteral nutrition.[18] In a report of 175 children with SVCS, 70% were iatrogenic. Of the remaining 53 cases, 37 (70%) were caused by mediastinal tumors, 8 (15%) were caused by benign granuloma, and 4 (7.5%) by congenital anomalies of the cardiovascular system. Two thirds of the tumors causing SVCS in childhood are lymphomas.[18,19] Of 16 children reported from St. Jude Children's Research Hospital with SVCS at presentation, 8 were diagnosed with NHL, 4 had acute lymphoblastic leukemia, 2 had Hodgkin's disease, 1 had neuroblastoma, and 1 had a yolk sac tumor.[20] Most children who developed SVCS late in the course of their malignancy had recurrent solid tumors.[20] Issa reported that mediastinal fibrosis secondary to histoplasmosis caused SVCS in 7 (5%) of the 150 patients reviewed.[18]

DIAGNOSTIC PROCEDURES

The SVCS has long been considered to be a potentially life-threatening medical emergency.[4,15,21] It was common practice to immediately apply radiation therapy with initial high-dose fractions, sometimes even before the histologic diagnosis of the primary lesion was established.[15,21,22] Diagnostic procedures, such as bronchoscopy, mediastinoscopy, thoracotomy, or supraclavicular lymph node biopsy, were often avoided because they were considered to be hazardous in the presence of SVCS.[4,15] The traditional therapeutic philosophy was recently challenged.[3,23,24] The reported clinical experience was reassessed, and the safety and importance of diagnostic procedures were reevaluated. Multidrug chemotherapy, sometimes combined with radiation therapy, is potentially curative for small cell carcinoma of the lung and non-Hodgkin's lymphoma even when presented as SVCS. The current practice of using different modalities for different primary causes of SVCS makes the accurate histologic diagnosis of SVCS invaluable. Mediastinal irradiation before biopsy precludes proper interpretation of the specimen in almost half of the patients.[25]

The clinical identification of SVCS is simple, because the symptoms and signs are typical and unmistakable. The chest film shows a mass in most patients. Only 16% of the patients studied by Parish had normal chest films.[9] The most common radiographic abnormalities are superior mediastinal widening and pleural effusion (Table 60–4). A computed tomography (CT) scan provides more detailed information about the SVCS, its tributaries, and other critical structures, such as the bronchi

and the cord.[26] The additional information is necessary because involvement of these structures requires prompt action for relief of pressure. Moncada outlined the advantages of combining a CT scan with CT digital phlebography in SVCS[27]:

1. Detailed resolution of the intrathoracic structures and musculoskeletal anatomy
2. Accurate identification of the site and extent of obstructing thrombus in the SVC and of external compression or invasion by a mediastinal mass
3. Contrast opacification of the venous trunks and collateral circulation sufficient to make confident surgical decisions and to determine late graft patency
4. Accurate guidance for percutaneous biopsy techniques
5. Guidance for radiation therapy to ensure that radiation ports fully encompass the disease
6. Monitoring the effect of therapy.

The role of magnetic resonance imaging (MRI) has been insufficiently investigated but appears promising, especially because this modality is totally noninvasive.[28]

Contrast venography is controversial.[5,29] It provides important information for determining if the vena cava is completely obstructed or remains patent and extrinsically compressed.[29] Dyet and Moghissi demonstrated by venography that 41% of patients with SVCS have patent SVCs that are displaced or involved but not obstructed by tumor.[30] Another 19% have SVC obstruction below the azygos vein, for which collateral venous compression should be adequate. Venography is valuable if surgical bypass is considered for the obstructed vena cava.[31] Lokich stated that venograms are relatively contraindicated because interruption of the integrity of the vessel wall, in the presence of increased intraluminal pressures, may result in excessive bleeding from the puncture site.[15] However, there is no evidence of this complication. Although venography can confirm the clinical diagnosis and outline the anatomy, priority should still be given to procedures that help establish the histolytic diagnosis. Radionuclide technetium 99m venography is an alternate, minimally invasive method of imaging the venous system.[32,33] Although images that are obtained by this method are not as well defined as those that are achieved with contrast venography, they demonstrate patency and flow patterns. Collateral circulation can be evaluated in a general manner and quantified to some degree by radionuclide venography.

In 58% of 107 patients reported by Schraufnagel, SVCS developed before the primary diagnosis was established.[3] The diagnostic procedures that were employed in different studies are summarized in Table 60–5. Sputum cytology established the diagnosis for almost half of the patients. Cytologic diagnosis is as accurate as tissue diagnosis in small cell carcinoma.[35] Bronchoscopy supplies the malignant cells for cytologic evaluation in most cases of small cell disease.[36] In the presence of pleural effusion, thoracocentesis established the diagnosis of malignancy in 71% of the patients. Biopsy of a supraclavicular node, especially if there was a suspicious palpatory finding, was rewarding in two thirds of the reported attempts. Small cell carcinoma of the lung and non-Hodgkin's lymphoma often involve the bone marrow. A biopsy of the bone marrow may provide the diagnosis and stage for these patients.

Mediastinoscopy has a high success rate in providing a diagnosis, but Painter reported complications in five of nine procedures attempted.[34] In 2 patients, the procedure had to be terminated before completion. In 3 patients, complications occurred after the mediastinoscopy, but these complications were managed successfully, and the procedure was diagnostic in each case. Lewis and associates reported their experience in performing cervical mediastinoscopies in 15 patients with SVCS.[37] All mediastinoscopies were diagnostic, and no complications were observed.

Percutaneous transthoracic (CT-guided fine-needle biopsy) is emerging as an effective and safe alternative to an open biopsy or mediastinoscopy.[38] Successful diagnostic transluminal atherectomy has also been reported.[39] A thoracotomy is diagnostic if all other procedures have failed.

Ahmann examined the traditional opinion that diagnostic procedures carry with them significant hazard, primarily excessive bleeding.[15,21,23] He reviewed 843 invasive and semiinvasive diagnostic procedures and found only 10 reported complications, none of them fatal. Ahmann and others found minimal evidence to suggest that diagnostic procedures such as venographies, thoracotomies, bronchoscopies, mediastinoscopies, and lymph node biopsies carry an excessive risk in patients with SVCS.[11,24]

TREATMENT

The goals of treatment of SVCS are to relieve the symptoms and to attempt the cure of the primary malignant process. Small cell carcinoma of the lung, non-Hodgkin's lymphoma, and germ cell tumors constitute almost half of the malignant causes of SVCS. These disorders are potentially curable, even in the presence of SVCS. The treatment of SVCS should be selected according to the histologic disorder and stage of the primary process. The prognosis of patients with SVCS strongly correlates with the prognosis of the underlying disease.

SMALL CELL LUNG CANCER

Combination chemotherapy alone or in conjunction with radiation therapy is considered to be the standard treatment for small cell lung cancer. Dombernowsky reported the results

TABLE 60–5. Positive Yield of Diagnostic Procedures for Patients With Superior Vena Cava Syndrome

Procedure	No. of Procedures	No. Positive	Percent Positive
Sputum cytology	59	29	49
Thoracocentesis	14	10	71
Bone marrow biopsy	13	3	23
Lymph node biopsy	95	64	67
Bronchoscopy	124	65	52
Mediastinoscopy	54	44	81
Thoracotomy	49	48	98

of the treatment of 26 patients with small cell carcinoma of the lung presenting with SVCS.[13] Of these 26 patients, 22 were initially treated with combination chemotherapy alone and, in all these patients, the resolution of the SVCS was prompt (median, 7 days). Maddox reported on 56 patients with small cell lung cancer who presented with SVCS.[40] Correction of SVCS was obtained in 64% (9 of 16) of patients treated with radiation alone, in 100% (23 of 23) of those given chemotherapy, and in 83% (5 of 6) of patients receiving combined therapy. The type of treatment did not substantially influence survival.

Among 643 patients with small cell lung cancer, Sculier identified 55 patients (8.5%) with SVCS.[41] One half of the patients developed the manifestations of SVCS before the histologic diagnosis was established. In the rest of the patients, the syndrome developed after the pathologic diagnosis of small cell lung cancer was made but before specific treatment was started. Symptomatic relief of SVCS was obtained in 35 (73%) of 48 patients initially treated with chemotherapy and in 3 (43%) of 7 patients who were initially treated with radiation. Relief of SVCS occurred within 7 to 10 days after initiation of therapy. Fourteen patients had recurrent SVCS after initial treatment. Improvement of recurrent SVCS was obtain in 8 of 12 patients treated with radiation, one of two patients treated with chemotherapy, and three of four patients treated with combined modality.

Spiro analyzed 37 patients with SVCS who, after initial chemotherapy for small cell lung cancer, were randomized to receive chemotherapy alone or radiation therapy followed by more chemotherapy.[42] The addition of a radiation dose of 4000 cGy to the mediastinum did not increase the protection from local recurrence or improve the survival. In several reports, SVCS was not found to be an adverse prognostic for patients with small cell lung cancer.[13,41–43]

Three randomized trials have shown that there is an advantage for combining radiation therapy with chemotherapy over chemotherapy alone in the treatment of limited-disease small cell cancer of the lung.[44–46] The optimal sequence of the two modalities and the dose and fractionation of radiotherapy have not been established. However, the use of combination chemotherapy as the initial modality, with subsequent rapid shrinkage of the tumor, may eliminate the necessity of irradiating a large volume of lung tissue. When chemotherapy is administered, the arm veins should be avoided. Veins of the lower extremities provide an alternative simple venous access.

NON-HODGKIN'S LYMPHOMA

The most extensive experience of treating SVCS secondary to non-Hodgkin's lymphoma is reported from the M. D. Anderson Cancer Center.[14] Twenty-two patients with diffuse large cell lymphoma, and 8 patients with lymphoblastic lymphoma were evaluated for the results of treatment. The patients were treated with chemotherapy alone, chemotherapy combined with irradiation, or with radiotherapy alone. All patients achieved complete relief of SVCS symptoms within 2 weeks of the onset of any type of treatment. No treatment modality appeared to be superior in achieving clinical improvement. The presence of dysphagia, hoarseness, or stridor was a major adverse prognostic factor for patients with lymphoma presenting with SVCS. Eighteen (81%) of 22 patients with large cell lymphoma achieved complete response. Relapse occurred in all 6 patients treated with irradiation alone, in 4 of 7 patients treated with chemotherapy alone, and in 5 of 9 patients treated with chemotherapy and radiotherapy. The median survival was 21 months. All 8 patients with lymphoblastic lymphoma achieved complete response. Six relapses occurred in this group, and all were in sites not initially involved. Median survival was 19 months.

From these results, the researchers concluded that SVCS secondary to lymphoma is rarely an emergency that requires treatment before a histologic diagnosis is made. They recommended that the choice of treatment should be based on the histologic diagnosis and that the patients should undergo, if possible, a complete staging workup before therapy. However, lymphangiography should be avoided to prevent embolization of contrast material that could result in respiratory failure. They advocated chemotherapy as the treatment of choice, because it provides both local and systemic therapeutic activity. They suggested that local consolidation with radiation therapy may be beneficial in patients with large cell lymphoma with mediastinal masses larger than 10 cm.

NONMALIGNANT CAUSES

Patients with nonmalignant causes of SVCS differ significantly from patients with malignant disease. If the cause is not malignant, the patients often have symptoms long before they seek medical advice, it takes more time to establish the diagnosis, and their survival is markedly longer.[3] Schraufnagel reported that the average survival was 9 years if the primary process was benign, compared with an average survival of 5 months for patients with lung cancer.[3] Mahajan reviewed the literature of benign SVCS and reported 16 new cases.[47] Twelve (75%) of these 16 patients had a mediastinal granuloma that was attributed to histoplasmosis. Most patients had an insidious onset of SVCS and were relatively young. Ten patients who were available for a follow-up of 1 to 11 years were all doing well at the time of the report. It was suggested that the good prognosis of patients with benign SVCS caused by fibrosing mediastinitis does not provide a role for SVC bypass surgery.[47,48] However, Nieto and Doty advocate surgery for SVCS caused by benign disorders if the syndrome develops suddenly, progresses, or persists after 6 to 12 months of observation for possible collateral vessel development.[29] In patients whose histoplasmosis complement fixation titers suggest active disease, ketoconazole treatment may prevent recurrent SVCS.[49]

CATHETER-INDUCED OBSTRUCTION

In catheter-induced SVCS, the mechanism of obstruction is usually thrombosis. Streptokinase, urokinase, or recombinant tissue-type plasminogen activator may cause lysis of the thrombus early in its formation.[16,50–53] Heparin and oral anticoagulants may reduce the extent of the thrombus and prevent its progression. Removal of the catheter, if possible, is another option and should be combined with anticoagulation to avoid embolization. In patients for whom electrodes of a pacemaker must be changed, the broken wire should be removed to prevent the risk of developing SVCS.[16,50,54] Percutaneous transluminal angioplasty with or without thrombolytic therapy has been successfully used to open catheter-induced SVC obstructions.[50,55,56]

RADIATION THERAPY

In patients with SVCS as a result of non-small cell carcinoma of the lung, radiotherapy is the primary treatment. The likelihood of relieving the symptoms and signs of SVCS is high, but the overall prognosis for these patients is poor.[3,4,8,23] In Armstrong's series, the 1-year survival for these patients was 17%, and the survival at 2 years declined to 2%.[8]

Radiotherapy has been advocated as standard treatment for most patients with SVCS.[15,21,22] It is employed as the initial treatment if a histologic diagnosis cannot be established and the clinical status of the patient is deteriorating. However, recent reviews suggest that SVC obstruction alone rarely represents an absolute emergency that requires treatment without a specific diagnosis.[11,23,24] The syndrome may be the earliest manifestation of invasive involvement of additional critical structures in the thorax (Table 60-6), such as the bronchi. Under such circumstances, prompt treatment with irradiation may be required without any delay.

TABLE 60-6. Complications of Malignant Invasion

Complication	No. of Patients* (%)
Esophagus	
Symptoms of dysphagia or esophageal dysfunction	26 (24)
Anatomic evidence of esophageal invasion	6 (6)
Trachea	
Displaced on examination or roentgenogram	7 (7)
Compressed or invaded by lesion	14 (13)
Vocal cord paralysis	
Unilateral	6 (6)
Bilateral	3 (3)
Pericardium	
Tamponade	3 (3)
Neoplastic invasion at necropsy	6 (6)

* Some patients may have had more than one complication.
(Schraufnagel DE, et al. Superior vena caval obstruction. Am J Med 1981;70:1169–1174)

The fractionation schedule of radiation usually includes two to four large initial fractions of 300 to 400 cGy, followed by conventional fractionation to a total dose of 3000 to 5000 cGy.[4,15,21] Patients treated with initial high-dose fractions showed a slightly faster symptomatic improvement than patients receiving conventional-dose radiation.[8] Improvement within 2 weeks or less was observed in 70% of those treated with initial high-dose fractions and in 56% of patients receiving conventional-dose therapy. This difference was not statistically significant. Serial venograms and autopsies suggest that the symptomatic improvement achieved by radiotherapy is not always due to improvement of flow through the SVC, but it is probably also a result of the development of collaterals after the pressure in the mediastinum is eased.[23]

The field of radiation for SVCS induced by lung cancer should encompass the gross tumors with appropriate margins and the mediastinal, hilar, and supraclavicular lymph nodes. In Armstrong's series, supraclavicular failures occurred in 8 (9%) of 91 patients receiving radiation therapy to the supraclavicular fossae, and 2 (33%) of 6 patients not receiving therapy to these lymph nodes failed at this site.[8]

TRANSLUMINAL ANGIOPLASTY

Percutaneous transluminal angioplasty using balloon technique or insertion of expandable wire stents has been successfully used to open and maintain the patency of the SVC even after maximal-tolerance radiation therapy.[55-60] In two cases, percutaneous atherectomy was used for establishing the histologic diagnosis of SVCS and treatment of the obstruction.[39] In catheter-induced SVCS, administering a thrombolytic agent through the angioplasty device may be therapeutically beneficial.[56]

SURGERY

The experience with successful direct bypass graft for SVC obstruction is limited. It was recommended that autologous grafts of almost the same size as the SVC should be used.[61] Doty used a composite spiral graft, which was constructed from the patient's saphenous vein.[62] He reported 15 years of experience with this procedure in 9 patients with benign obstruction of SVC. Seven maintained patent SVCs, and all patients were relieved of symptoms of SVCS. Avashti reported four successful bypasses of obstructed SVCs using Dacron prostheses.[63]

The preferred bypass route is between an innominate or jugular vein on the left side and the right atrial appendage, using an end-to-end anastomosis.[29] Piccione used the autologous pericardium to reconstruct the SVC after resection for malignant obstruction.[64] In a patient with malignancy-induced SVCS, surgical intervention should be considered only after other therapeutic maneuvers with irradiation and chemotherapy have been exhausted. Most patients with SVCS of benign origin have long survivals without surgical intervention.[47,48] However, if the process progresses rapidly or if there is a retrosternal goiter or aortic aneurysm, surgical intervention may relieve the obstruction.

THROMBOLYTIC THERAPY

Successful experience with thrombolytic agents is limited to the treatment of catheter-induced SVCS.[16,53,65] A review of the response of SVCS to thrombolytic therapy from the Cleveland Clinic showed that the thrombus was effectively lysed in 8 (73%) of 11 patients with a central venous catheter, compared with only 1 of 5 patients who responded to thrombolytic therapy in the absence of a central catheter.[53,66] The higher yield of thrombolytic therapy in patients with catheters is probably related to the mechanism of obstruction, the ability to deliver the agent directly to the thrombus, and to earlier recognition of SVCS in patients with malfunctioning catheters. In the Cleveland Clinic experience, urokinase was more effective than streptokinase, and a delay administering therapy beyond 5 days of symptoms onset was associated with a treatment failure.[53] Favorable experience with recombinant tissue-type plasminogen activator as a thrombolytic agent for catheter-induced SVCS has been reported.[51,52]

GENERAL MEASURES

Medical measures other than specific chemotherapy may be beneficial in temporarily relieving the symptoms of SVCS. Bed rest with the head elevated and oxygen administration can reduce the cardiac output and venous pressure. Diuretic therapy and a reduced-salt diet to reduce edema may have an immediate palliative effect, but the risk of thrombosis enhanced by dehydration should not be ignored. Steroids are commonly used, but their effectiveness has never been properly evaluated. They may improve obstruction by decreasing a possible inflammatory reaction associated with tumor or with irradiation. However, Green and Rubin demonstrated the lack of inflammatory reaction and edema after radiotherapy for experimental SVCS, but documentation in a controlled fashion is lacking.[67] Thrombolytic therapy with urokinase, streptokinase, and recombinant tissue-type plasminogen activator was effective in catheter-induced SVCS.[51-53,65,66]

MANAGEMENT RECOMMENDATIONS

In patients without a clear cause of SVCS, an efficient diagnostic effort should be attempted before any specific treatment. Three deep-cough sputum specimens should be obtained for cytologic analysis. A positive cytologic evaluation provides reliable pathologic information, particularly in the diagnosis of small cell lung carcinoma.[35] If there is pleural effusion, thoracocentesis should be performed and the centrifuge-prepared specimen examined for the presence of malignant cells. If a suspicious lymph node is palpable, particularly in the supraclavicular area, a needle or an open biopsy should be the next diagnostic step. In the absence of positive sputum results, pleural effusion, or accessible suspicious lymph node analysis, a bronchoscopy should be performed, and brushing, washing, and biopsy samples should be obtained for cytologic and histologic analysis. If these efforts do not provide the histologic diagnosis of the primary process, percutaneous transthoracic fine-needle biopsy under CT or fluoroscopic guidance is safe and highly effective.[38,39] In the rare patient for whom less-invasive procedures have failed to establish the diagnosis, the location of the suspicious lesion in the chest and the experience of the surgical team should determine whether mediastinoscopy or thoracotomy be performed.

During the diagnostic process, the patient can benefit from bed rest with the head elevated and with oxygen administration. Some clinicians advocate the use of diuretics and steroids (*e.g.*, 6–10 mg of dexamethasone given orally or intravenously every 6 hours) as a temporary palliative measure if the patient is uncomfortably symptomatic. Anticoagulation is of no proven benefit and may interfere with diagnostic procedures. After the cause of SVCS has been established, treatment of the primary process should promptly follow. Combination chemotherapy with an appropriate regimen is the treatment of choice for small cell lung cancer or non-Hodgkin's lymphoma. Radiation therapy of the lesion and adjacent nodal areas may enhance control after initial response to chemotherapy. Non-small cell lung cancer causing SVCS is best treated with radiation therapy. The incorporation of CT scan information into a carefully designed treatment plan may enable the administration of a total radiation dose above 5000 cGy, which may provide long-term local control for some patients.

Most patients with nonmalignant causes for SVCS have an indolent course and a good prognosis. Percutaneous transluminal angioplasty should be considered an effective alternative to surgery. Surgery is indicated only when the process is rapidly progressing or caused by a retrosternal goiter or an aortic aneurysm. If SVCS is induced by a catheter, the catheter should be removed if possible. Heparin should be administered during the removal of the catheter to prevent embolization. In catheter-induced SVCS, urokinase, streptokinase, or recombinant tissue-type plasminogen activator are of value if used early in the thrombotic process.[51-53,65]

The clinical course of SVCS rarely represents an absolute emergency. In these situations, the bronchus is likely to be obstructed by the same basic process, and irradiation may have to be started immediately, even before the histologic diagnosis is established.

REFERENCES

1. Hunter W. The history of an aneurysm of the aorta, with some remarks on aneurysms in general. Med Observ Inq 1757;1:323–357.
2. Schechter MM. The superior vena cava syndrome. Am J Med Sci 1954;227:46–56.
3. Schraufnagel DE, Hill R, Leech JA, Pare JAP. Superior vena caval obstruction. Is it an emergency? Am J Med 1981;70:1169–1174.
4. Davenport D, Ferree C, Blake D, Raben M. Radiation therapy in the treatment of superior vena caval obstruction. Cancer 1978;42:2600–2603.
5. Rubin P, Hicks GL. Biassociation of superior vena caval obstruction and spinal-cord compression. N Y State J Med 1973;73:2176–2182.
6. Carlson HA. Obstruction of the superior vena cava: An experimental study. Arch Surg 1934;29:669–677.
7. Roswit B, Kaplan G, Jacobson HG. The superior vena cava syndrome in bronchogenic carcinoma. Radiology 1953;61:722–737.
8. Armstrong BA, Perez CA, Simpson JR, Hederman MA. Role of irradiation in the management of superior vena cava syndrome. Int J Radiat Oncol Biol Phys 1987;13:531–539.
9. Parish JM, Marschke RF, Dines DE, Lee RE. Etiologic considerations in superior vena cava syndrome. Mayo Clin Proc 1981;56:407–413.
10. Bell DR, Woods RL, Levi JA. Superior vena caval obstruction: A 10-year experience. Med J Aust 1986;145:566–568.
11. Yellin A, Rosen A, Reichert N, Lieberman Y. Superior vena cava syndrome. The myth—the facts. Am Rev Respir Dis 1990;141:1114–1118.
12. Salsali M, Cliffton EE. Superior vena caval obstruction in carcinoma of lung. N Y State J Med 1969;69:2875–2880.
13. Dombernowsky P, Hansen HH. Combination chemotherapy in the management of superior vena caval obstruction in small-cell anaplastic of the lung. Acta Med Scand 1978;204:513–516.
14. Perez-Soler R, McLaughlin P, Velasquez WS, et al. Clinical features and results of management of superior vena cava syndrome secondary to lymphoma. J Clin Oncol 1984;2:260–266.
15. Lokich JJ, Goodman R. Superior vena cava syndrome: Clinical management. JAMA 1975;231:58–61.
16. Sculier JP, Feld R. Superior vena cava obstruction system: Recommendation for management. Cancer Treat Rev 1985;12:209–218.
17. Bertrand M, Presant CA, Klein L, Scott E. Iatrogenic superior vena cava syndrome. A new entity. Cancer 1984;54:376–378.
18. Janin Y, Becker J, Wise L, et al. Superior vena cava syndrome in childhood and adolescence: A review of the literature and report of three cases. J Pediatr Surg 1982;17:290–295.
19. Issa PY, Brihi ER, Janin Y, Slim MS. Superior vena cava syndrome in childhood: Report of ten cases and review of the literature. Pediatrics 1983;71:337–341.
20. Ingram L, Rivera GK, Shapiro DN. Superior vena cava syndrome associated with childhood malignancy: Analysis of 24 cases. Med Pediatr Oncol 1990;18:476–481.
21. Perez CA, Presant CA, Van Amburg AL III. Management of superior vena cava syndrome. Semin Oncol 1978;5:123–134.
22. Scarantino, C, Salazar OM, Rubin R, et al. The optimum radiation schedule in the treatment of superior vena caval obstruction: Importance of ^{99m}Tc scintinangiograms. Int J Radiat Oncol Biol Phys 1979;5:1987–1995.
23. Ahmann FR. A reassessment of the clinical implications of the superior vena cava syndrome. J Clin Oncol 1984;2:961–969.
24. Shimm DS, Lugue GL, Tigsby LC. Evaluating the superior vena cava syndrome. JAMA 1981;245:951–953.
25. Loeffler JS, Leopold KA, Recht A, et al. Emergency prebiopsy radiation for mediastinal masses: Impact on subsequent pathologic diagnosis and outcome. J Clin Oncol 1986;4:716–721.
26. Yedlicka JW, Schultz K, Moncada R, Flisak M. CT findings in superior vena cava obstruction. Semin Roentgenol 1989;24:84–90.
27. Moncada R, Cardella R, Demos TC, et al. Evaluation of superior vena cava syndrome by axial CT and CT phlebography. AJR 1984;143:731–736.
28. Hansen ME, Spritzer CE, Sostman HD. Assessing the patency of mediastinal and thoracic inlet veins: Value of MR imaging. AJR 1990;155:1177–1182.
29. Nieto AF, Doty DB. Superior vena cava obstruction: Clinical syndrome, etiology and treatment. Curr Probl Cancer 1986;10:442–484.
30. Dyet JF, Moghissi K. Role of venography in assessing patients with superior vena cava obstruction caused by bronchial carcinoma for bypass operations. Thorax 1980;35:628–630.
31. Stanford W, Jolles H, Ell S, Chiu LC. Superior vena cava obstruction: A venographic classification. AJR 1987;148:259–262.
32. Son YH, Wetzel RA, Wilson WA. ^{99m}Tc pertechnetate scintiphotography as diagnostic and follow-up aids in major vascular obstruction due to malignant neoplasm. Radiology 1968;91:349–375.
33. Van Houtte P, Fruhling J. Radionuclide venography in the evaluation of superior vena cava syndrome. Clin Nucl Med 1981;6:177–183.
34. Painter TD, Karpf M. Superior vena cava syndrome: Diagnostic procedures. Am J Med Sci 1983;285:2–6.
35. Yesner R, Gersti B, Auerbach O. Application of the World Health Organization classification of lung carcinoma to biopsy material. Ann Thorac Surg 1965;1:33–49.
36. Ihde DC, Cohen MH, Bernath AM, et al. Serial fiberoptic bronchoscopy during chemotherapy of small cell carcinoma of the lung. Chest 1978;74:531–536.
37. Lewis RJ, Sisler GE, Mackenzie JW. Mediastinoscopy in advanced superior cava obstruction. Ann Thorac Surg 1981;32:458–462.
38. Cosmos L, Haponik EF, Dariak JJ, Summer WR. Neoplastic superior vena caval obstruction: Diagnosis with percutaneous needle aspiration. Am J Med Sci 1987;293:99–102.
39. Dake MD, Zemel G, Dolmatch BL, Katzen BT. The cause of superior vena cava syndrome diagnosis with percutaneous atherectomy. Radiology 1990;174:957–959.
40. Maddox AM, Valdivieso M, Lukeman J, et al. Superior vena cava obstruction in small cell bronchogenic carcinoma. Cancer 1983;52:2165–2172.
41. Sculier JP, Evans WK, Feld R, et al. Superior vena caval obstruction in small cell lung cancer. Cancer 1986;57:847–851.
42. Spiro SG, Shah S., Harper PG, et al. Treatment of obstruction of the superior vena cava by combination chemotherapy with and without irradiation in small-cell carcinoma of the bronchus. Thorax 1983;38:501–505.
43. Van Houtte P, De Jager R, Lustman-Marechal J, Kenis Y. Prognostic value of the superior vena cava syndrome as the presenting sign of small-cell anaplastic carcinoma of the lung. Eur J Cancer 1980;16:1447–1450.
44. Perez CA, Einhorn LH, Oldham RK, et al. Randomized trial of radiotherapy to the thorax in limited small cell carcinoma of the lung treated with multiagent chemotherapy and elective brain irradiation: A preliminary report. J Clin Oncol 1984;2:1200–1208.
45. Perry MC, Eaton WL, Chahinian P, et al. Chemotherapy with or without radiation therapy in limited small cell cancer of the lung. Proc Am Soc Clin Oncol 1986;5:173.
46. Bunn P, Cohen M, Lichter A, et al. Randomized trial of chemotherapy versus chemotherapy plus radiotherapy in limited stage small cell lung cancer. Proc Am Soc Clin Oncol 1983;2:200.
47. Mahajan V, Strimlan V, Van Ordstrand HS, Loop FD. Benign superior cava syndrome. Chest 1975;68:32–35.

48. Effler DB, Groves LK. Superior vena caval obstruction. J Thorac Cardiovasc Surg 1962;43: 574–584.

49. Urshel HC Jr, Razzuk MA, Netto GJ, Disiere J, Chung SY. Sclerosing mediastinitis: Improved management with histoplasmosis titer and ketoconazole. Ann Thorac Surg 1990;50:215–221.

50. Goudevonos JA, Reid PG, Adams PC, Holden MP, Williams DO. Pacemaker-induced superior vena cava syndrome: Report of four cases and review of the literature. PACE 1989;12:1890–1895.

51. Fine DG, Shepherd RF, Welch TJ. Thrombolytic therapy for superior vena cava syndrome. Lancet [Letter] 1989;1:1200–1201.

52. Greenberg S, Kosinski R, Daniels J. Treatment of superior vena cava thrombosis with recombinant tissue type plasminogen activator. Chest 1991;99:1298–1301.

53. Gray BH, Olin JW, Grador RA, Young JR, Bartholomew JR, Ruschhaupt WF. Safety and efficacy of thrombolytic therapy for superior vena cava syndrome. Chest 1991;99: 54–59.

54. Blackburn T, Dunn M. Pacemaker-induced superior vena cava syndrome: Consideration of management. Am Heart J 1988;116:893–896.

55. Grace AA, Sutters M, Schofield PM. Balloon dilation of pacemaker-induced stenosis of the superior vena cava. Br Heart J 1991;65:225–226.

56. Montgomery JH, D'Souza VJ, Dyer RB, et al. Non-surgical treatment of the superior vena cava syndrome. Am J Cardiol 1985;56:829–830.

57. Ali MK, Ewer MS, Balakrishnan PV, et al. Balloon angioplasty for superior vena cava obstruction. Ann Intern Med 1987;107:856–857.

58. Walpole HT Jr, Lovett KE, Chuang VP, West R, Clements SD Jr. Superior vena cava syndrome treated by percutaneous transluminal balloon angioplasty. Am Heart J 1988;115:1303–1304.

59. Capek P, Cope C. Percutaneous treatment of superior vena cava syndrome. AJR 1989;152: 183–184.

60. Putnam JS, Uchida BT, Antonovic R, Rosch J. Superior vena cava syndrome associated with massive thrombosis: Treatment with expandable wire stents. Radiology 1988;167: 727–728.

61. Scherck JP, Kerstein MD, Stansel HC. The current status of vena caval replacement. Surgery 1974;76:209–233.

62. Doty DB, Doty JR, Jones KW. Bypass of superior vena cava. Fifteen years' experience with spiral vein graft for obstruction of superior vena cava caused by benign disease. J Thorac Cardiovasc Surg 1990;99:889–896.

63. Avashti RB, Moghissi K. Malignant obstruction of the superior vena cava and its palliation. J Thorac Cardiovasc Surg 1977;74:244–248.

64. Piccione W Jr, Faber LP, Warren WH. Superior vena caval reconstruction using autologous pericardium. Ann Thorac Surg 1990;50:417–419.

65. Meister FL, McLaughlin TF, Tenney RD, Sholkoff SD. Urokinase. A cost-effective alternative treatment of superior vena cava thrombosis and obstruction. Arch Intern Med 1989;149:1209–1210.

66. Comerota AJ. Safety and efficacy of thrombolytic therapy for superior vena caval syndrome. Chest [Editorial comment] 1991;99:3–4.

67. Green J, Rubin P, Holzwasser G. The experimental production of superior vena cava obstruction. Radiology 1963;81:406–414.

SECTION **2**

Spinal Cord Compression

THOMAS F. DELANEY
EDWARD H. OLDFIELD

Spinal cord or cauda equina compression frequently complicates uncontrolled cancer. It is the second most common neurologic complication of cancer after brain metastasis. At autopsy, its occurrence is documented in approximately 5% of patients with malignancies.[1] Black estimated an annual incidence of 18,000 new cases in the United States.[2] The incidence of spinal cord compression will increase as palliative, noncurative therapies evolve and the population continues to age. Patients rarely die of spinal cord compression, but it is a medical emergency, because delay in treatment often results in irreversible paralysis and loss of sphincter control.

The neurologic status at initiation of treatment is the most significant factor influencing neurologic outcome. This is true despite the tumor type, level of spinal axis involved, degree of systemic tumor involvement, or treatment by radiotherapy or by surgery and radiotherapy. Because successful treatment is much more likely in ambulatory patients who retain intact bowel and bladder control at the start of treatment, early recognition of the problem and initiation of therapy is essential.[3–5] Fortunately, most patients with spinal metastasis have pain and characteristic physical and diagnostic findings that prompt early diagnosis by the astute clinician before significant and irreversible loss of neurologic function occurs. Patients who receive treatment while they are still ambulatory remain ambulatory. Despite this understanding, as many as 80% of patients treated in the last half of the 1980s could not walk at presentation.[6] Patients with a diagnosis of cancer must be advised that the development of back pain is a potentially ominous symptom that should be brought to the attention of their doctors without delay.

PATHOPHYSIOLOGY

Although compression of the spinal cord or the cauda equina can arise from intradural metastases, the spinal involvement is usually extradural.[7,8] Compression usually results from tumor involvement of the vertebral column, affecting a vertebral body or a neural arch.[85] Most often, tumor in the vertebral body presses on the anterior aspect of the dural sac (Fig. 60–1). Progressive tumor expansion posteriorly compresses the spinal cord (or the cauda equina in lesions below the L1–L2 vertebral level) and produces neurologic impairment. Tumor occasionally metastasizes to the epidural space without bone involvement.[9] Paraspinal tumors, such as malignant lymphoma or neuroblastoma, may invade through the intervertebral foramen and compress the cord without bony involvement. No difference in treatment or functional outcome has been reported for lesions involving the cauda equina, and they are discussed with spinal cord compression.[9]

Several models have been used to study the pathophysiology of neurologic dysfunction from compression of the spinal cord by tumor. Tarlov related neurologic recovery after release of mechanically induced cord compression in dogs to the rate of induction and the duration of compression.[10–12] After gradual induction, decompression could be delayed and neurologic function still return. Rapid compression required rapid decompression if paralysis was to be reversed. The recovery of neurologic function was greatly enhanced with incomplete cord compression. Ushio and colleagues induced spinal cord compression by transplanting Walker 256 carcinoma cells into the paravertebral area of rats.[13] They found vasogenic edema in the compressed cord and histologic evidence of neuronal injury. Spinal cord edema and neurologic signs were transiently improved by treating symptomatic animals with dexamethasone.

Siegal and associates demonstrated in rats with neoplastic spinal cord compression that edema in compressed spinal cord segments was associated with a consistent increase in prostaglandin estradiol (PGE_2) production.[14–16] Increased PGE_2 production also occurred in rats with early neurologic dysfunction before development of cord edema.[14] PGE_2 is a

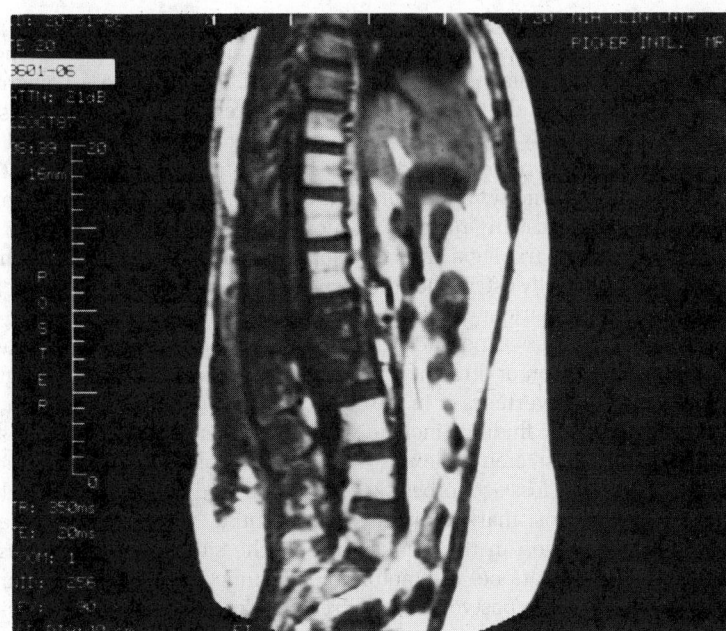

FIGURE 60–1. T1-weighted, sagittal magnetic resonance image of a 21-year-old woman with a Ewing's sarcoma involving the first and second lumbar vertebrae, which appear darker than the uninvolved spine. Tumor has produced structural deformities in the involved vertebral bodies and is compressing the dural sac.

mediator of inflammation and edema.[17] The researchers found that spinal cord specific gravity was higher in untreated rats than in normal controls and that it appeared to be the sum expression of multiple tissue changes.[16] They reported that dexamethasone and indomethacin corrected specific gravity abnormalities and delayed onset of paraplegia.[16] Methylprednisolone, which decreases edema but does not normalize tissue specific gravity, failed to delay the onset of paraplegia.[18]

CLINICAL PRESENTATION

The most common tumors causing spinal cord compression are listed in Table 60–7.[19] Depending on the institution, 8% to 47% of patients present with spinal cord compression as the initial clinical manifestation of malignancy.[1,3,7] More commonly, spinal cord compression occurs in patients with previously diagnosed cancer. The interval from primary diagnosis to epidural cord compression from metastatic disease varies widely with different tumors. Patients with lung cancer usually develop epidural cord compression within a few months after the diagnosis of the primary lesion (average, 6 months).[7] Patients with breast cancer manifest spinal cord

compression as long as 20 years (average, 4 years) after presentation of the primary tumor.[3]

The segment of spine involved—approximately 10% cervical, 70% thoracic, and 20% lumbosacral—reflects the number and volume of vertebral bodies in each anatomic segment.[1,3,19–21] Epidural cord compression at one site frequently accompanies spinal involvement elsewhere, which may also threaten the cord. This is particularly true with widely disseminated breast and prostate cancer and with myeloma. Many patients with spinal epidural metastases subsequently develop a second site of epidural metastases. Reported frequencies of second epidural metastases range from 8% to 37%.[22–24] More than 90% of patients present with pain, which is often localized to the spine.[9,80]

Pain, which is usually from involved bone, may be exacerbated by movement, recumbency, cough, sneeze, or strain. The distribution of pain may be radicular.[3,78] Radicular pain localizes the lesion to within one or two vertebral segments. Most patients have pain for weeks to months before the onset of neurologic symptoms.[83] The development of neck or back pain in a patient with cancer should be considered an ominous symptom that requires prompt investigation. Without treatment, the next symptom is usually weakness. This is often accompanied or occasionally preceded by sensory loss.

TABLE 60–7. Relation Between Tumor Type and Spinal Cord Compression

Patients With Cord Compression	Lung	Breast	Unknown Primary	Lymphoma	Myeloma	Sarcoma	Prostate	Kidney	Gastro-intestinal	Thyroid	Other Tumors
Number	129	94	91	86	68	65	52	44	34	24	116
Percent	16	12	11	11	9	8	7	6	4	3	15

(Adapted from Bruckman JE, Bloomer WD. Management of spinal cord compression. Semin Oncol 1978;5:135–140)

Numbness usually begins in the toes and gradually ascends to the level of cord compression. Weakness combined with sensory loss, particularly loss of proprioception, may produce ataxia. Autonomic dysfunction with urinary retention and constipation usually appears late. Although pain usually precedes the other symptoms by days or weeks, after sensory, motor, or autonomic symptoms or signs develop, progression of myelopathy is usually rapid. Without treatment, complete and irreversible paraplegia often develops over hours to days. Examination usually establishes the level of cord compression and, in a cancer patient, the likely diagnosis.

Signs include tenderness to percussion over the involved spine. Neck flexion or straight leg raising may produce pain over the involved vertebra or in the distribution of an involved nerve root. Motor findings include weakness, spasticity, abnormal muscle stretch reflexes, and extensor plantar responses. Sensory loss occurs below the involved cord segment and is usually most marked distally. If present, a "level" of decreased sensation in the trunk indicates the site of cord compression. In patients with autonomic dysfunction, a palpable bladder, large postvoid urinary residual, or diminished anal tone may be present.

DIAGNOSTIC EVALUATION

The patient's neurologic status influences the nature and tempo of the diagnostic evaluation. Patients with signs or symptoms of spinal cord compression, such as motor impairment, urinary urgency or retention, or ascending numbness, require emergent evaluation and treatment. Patients should be seen by the oncologist, neurologist, radiation oncologist, and neurosurgeon. Dexamethasone should be administered immediately if the history and neurologic examination suggest cord compression.[25] High-dose intravenous dexamethasone (10 mg intravenously followed by 4 mg every 6 hours) may rapidly relieve pain and improve function.[3,21] Animal studies demonstrate reduction in cord edema and a diminished rate of loss of neurologic function with high-dose steroids.[26] The optimal steroid dose in patients has not been established.[86] A small, randomized study found no difference in pain relief and neurologic improvement between a single high-dose intravenous dexamethasone bolus of 10 or 100 mg if followed by 4 mg every 6 hours after the initial bolus.[27] The steroid dosage is tapered after radiation therapy or surgery, as soon as clinical circumstances permit. The serious complications of high-dose steroids (*e.g.*, infection, myopathy, ulcer) can be avoided if the duration of use is not prolonged.[28]

More than two thirds of patients with cord compression have bony abnormalities seen on plain radiographs of the spine.[20,29–31] Spine radiographs are accurate in detecting spinal epidural metastases in as many as 83% of patients with back pain.[22] Findings diagnostic of spinal tumor include erosion and loss of pedicles, partial or complete collapse of vertebral bodies, and paraspinous soft tissue masses. Normal spine films, however, do not exclude epidural metastases. In patients with lymphoma, more than 60% of patients with epidural tumor may have normal spine radiographs.[22]

Although the myelogram has been the standard for diagnosis and localization of epidural cord compression, magnetic resonance imaging (MRI) is increasingly used as the primary study to diagnose and localize spinal metastases.[22,25,32–37] Although several early studies suggested that myelography is slightly more sensitive than MRI (especially if small epidural masses or root compressions are responsible for symptoms), MRI has several advantages over myelography that have led most investigators to recommend MRI as the initial study, to be followed by myelography and computed tomography (CT) only if the MRI is nondiagnostic.[35–39,77]

There are other advantages for MRI.[35,37] Lumbar puncture, which is required for myelogram, is associated with a 16% to 24% rate of rapid neurologic deterioration requiring surgery in patients with complete subarachnoid block.[40] Patients with coagulopathies may experience local bleeding complications with myelography. MRI is noninvasive, less uncomfortable, and safer. MR examinations require 60 to 90 minutes, compared with 90 to 120 minutes for myelography or CT plus myelography.

Identification of paravertebral tumor extension by MRI can be used in designing the fields for radiation therapy and in planning surgery. Because MR images the entire spine and is sensitive in demonstrating bone metastases, it provides important information for designing radiation therapy fields. MRI allows visualization of areas of spinal cord compression that occur between sites of myelographic blocks. In patients with a complete myelographic block, routine myelography after lumbar injection fails to demonstrate the upper extent of the lesion that blocks the flow of contrast and additional rostral lesions that compromise the subarachnoid space, which are present in about 15% of patients. Because such information is important for treatment planning, myelographic demonstration of such lesions requires that contrast be introduced from above through a C1–C2 puncture to demarcate the upper border of the myelographic block and define any other lesions. An alternative approach is CT after metrizamide myelography to define the extent of epidural compressions in patients with complete blocks.[33] Although this approach is less uncomfortable than performing a C1–C2 puncture, it is often less satisfactory in the patient with another spinal lesion above the block.[41]

MRI can differentiate extradural from extramedullary and intramedullary intradural lesions. MRI for suspected epidural cord compression can generally be performed without gadolinium (Gd-DTPA) contrast, although gadolinium enhancement helps differentiate disk herniation, indicates regions of more active tumor for biopsy, and delineates response to therapy.[42] Gadolinium is an essential component of the imaging process for intramedullary and extramedullary intradural lesions. If the MRI is diagnostic, no further imaging is required. If it is negative or equivocal in the face of neurologic signs or symptoms, myelography, with or without CT scanning, is recommended.

Although MRI and CT have eliminated the need for myelography in most patients, myelography is occasionally employed according to the previously outlined guidelines. A spinal needle with a small diameter, 22 gauge or smaller, is used for myelography. Just before instillation of the contrast agent, a small cerebrospinal fluid sample (<2 ml) should be drawn for cytologic, protein, and glucose evaluations. Because of its low viscosity and water solubility, Metrizamide (Amipaque), a nonirritant water-soluble agent, mixes readily with cerebrospinal fluid, travels freely in the subarachnoid space, and provides homogenous diffusion in the cerebrospinal fluid that can be used for CT imaging of the spine after conventional myelography.

For patients with back pain but no neurologic signs the diagnostic evaluation can be performed on an outpatient basis in an expedient manner. Patients with abnormalities on plain films should undergo MRI, because as many as 81% of these patients have epidural tumors.[22] If bone films are normal, bone scintigraphy is indicated, because it is more sensitive than plain films in detecting bony involvement by tumor. Although epidural metastases are uncommon with an abnormal bone scan and normal plain radiographs, the information that the bone scan provides about other bony areas involved by the tumor are helpful in planning and assessing the results of treatment.[22]

TREATMENT

The goals of therapy for patients with epidural spinal neoplasms are recovery or preservation of normal neural function, local tumor control, spinal stability, and pain relief. Because cure is currently not possible for most patients with advanced cancer, palliation is a reasonable objective in the management of spinal metastases.

Several important points about the anticipated response to treatment merit emphasis. Approximately 40% to 60% of all patients treated for epidural cord compression by radiotherapy alone or combined laminectomy and irradiation are ambulatory after treatment.[3,28,21,29-31,43,44,87] The outcome after treatment closely correlates with the degree of neurologic impairment before therapy (Table 60–8). Most ambulatory patients treated with irradiation alone or surgery followed by postoperative irradiation remain ambulatory after treatment.[4-6,28] Paraplegia is a grave prognostic feature; fewer than 10% of adult patients with no voluntary movement in their lower extremities become ambulatory after treatment.[28,30,31] Early diagnosis and initiation of treatment is essential.

For many years, treatment for spinal metastases implied decompressive laminectomy. Laminectomy entails removal of the spinous processes and laminae overlying and one level above and below the site of cord compression (Fig. 60–2). If the tumor involves the posterior bony elements or the tumor is visible in the spinal canal, it is removed. The theoretical basis of the universal application of this procedure, regardless of whether the patient had tumor anterior or posterior to the spinal cord, was that it permitted the cord to move dorsally

away from compression by anterior lesions or allowed removal of the offending tumor mass for lesions located posteriorly. However, the results of laminectomy were disappointing. Approximately 30% of patients improved (*i.e.*, ambulatory after treatment), and operative mortality averaged 9%, 11% had nonfatal complications, and 12% were worse after surgery (Table 60–9).[2]

By the early 1980s, several retrospective reviews that compared laminectomy with radiation therapy had demonstrated that irradiation alone produces similar or superior results and less morbidity and mortality than treatments that included laminectomy.[2,3,43,45,46] If all patients are considered, radiotherapy was shown by Gilbert and colleagues[3] and by Black[2] (in a review of reports before 1979) to provide benefit comparable to surgery plus radiation therapy, and irradiation alone and surgery followed by irradiation were superior to surgery alone (see Table 60–9). This finding also applied when patients were analyzed according to the degree of neurologic deficit before treatment. The better the neurologic status of the patient before treatment, the better was the outcome, despite the choice of treatment (see Table 60–8).

As a result of these studies, radiation therapy combined with steroids became the treatment used for most patients. Surgery was recommended only for patients with no previous tissue diagnosis, progressive neurologic dysfunction during irradiation, or recurrent cord compression after previous radiation therapy. However, that surgical management should be limited to decompressive laminectomy to relieve cord compression, regardless of the site of pressure at the circumference of the cord, has been questioned.[47-50] Surgery selected on the basis of the site of tumor involvement in the spinal column (see Fig. 60–2), such as anterior or anterolateral resection of the tumor and involved vertebral body for tumor anterior to the cord and laminectomy only for tumor posterior to the cord, yields results greatly superior to those obtained previously with laminectomy alone.[47-56] For these reasons, the role of surgery in patients with epidural cord compression and metastatic tumor is being reconsidered.

Because there is no definitive prospective study that compares current treatments under similar conditions, absolute recommendations for management of patients with spinal metastases cannot be made. Clinical experience and published reports indicate that radiotherapy and surgery are effective treatments to be used alone or in combination as required by the circumstances of the patients. Chemotherapy is effective treatment for selected patients. The choice of treatment depends on the clinical presentation, the availability of a his-

TABLE 60–8. Effect of Pretreatment Motor Function on Treatment Outcome

Pretreatment Condition	Laminectomy and Irradiation		Irradiation Only	
	No. Ambulatory/ No. Treated	Percent Ambulatory	No. Ambulatory/ No. Treated	Percent Ambulatory
Ambulatory	14/22	64	46/58	79
Paraparetic	15/33	45	37/83	45
Paraplegic	1/10	10	1/29	3

(Adapted from Gilbert RW, Kim JH, Posner JB. Epidural spinal cord compression from metastatic tumor: Diagnosis and treatment. Ann Neurol 1978;3:40)

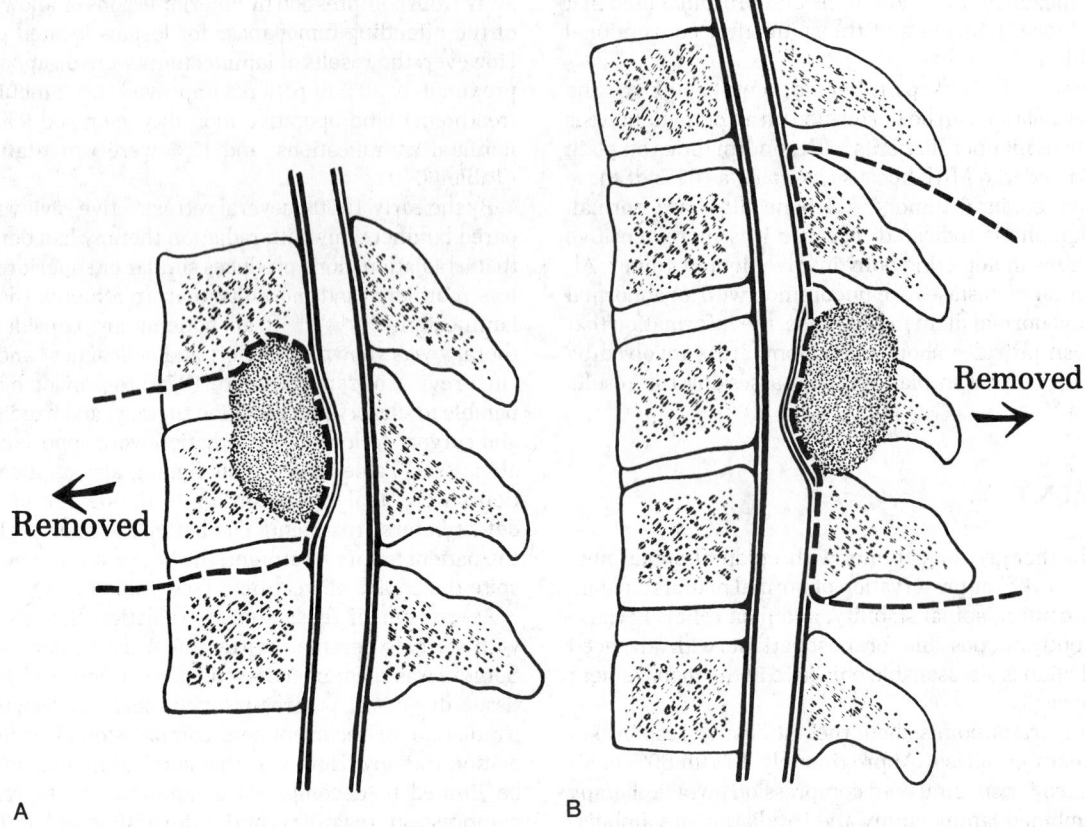

A   B

FIGURE 60–2. **(A)** Most spinal metastases occur in the vertebral column anterior to the spinal canal. If surgery is indicated for tumors anterior to the spinal canal, surgical excision of the tumor and involved vertebral body with immediate stabilization of the spinal column effectively reverses compression of the spinal cord. **(B)** Spinal cord compression by tumors posterior to the spinal canal can be successfully relieved by laminectomy (*i.e.,* removal of the laminae and spinous processes one level above and one level below the site of tumor) and tumor excision.

tologic diagnosis, the rapidity of the clinical course, the tumor type, the site of spinal involvement, the stability of the spine, and the nature of any previous treatment. However, it is reasonably clear when irradiation or surgery should be used, and definite recommendations can be made for the management of most patients.

SURGERY

Although epidural tumors located lateral or posterior to the spinal canal in the laminae or pedicles can be readily removed by laminectomy, tumor involvement of the vertebral body limits the potential for improvement after laminectomy. This was observed by Wright as early as 1963.[30] In 81 patients with metastatic spinal tumor treated with laminectomy, 38% of the patients with lateral or posterior compartment tumor had a satisfactory outcome, but only 19% with vertebral involvement were improved. Correlation of tumor location with outcome after laminectomy was studied by Hall and McKay, who found that 35% to 39% of patients with tumors in the posterior elements of the spinal canal (*i.e.,* removable by laminectomy) improved compared with only 9% with tumors anterior to the spinal canal.[57]

Laminectomy frequently fails to relieve neurologic deficits or myelographic block in patients with ventral compression

of the spinal cord due to tumor in a vertebral body or due to pathologic collapse of a vertebra with posterior migration of the bony elements into the anterior aspect of the spinal canal. Many patients with radiosensitive tumors with associated structural changes in the spine and cord compression cannot be relieved, even if the local tumor is effectively treated by irradiation. Removal of the neural arches at laminectomy can produce spinal instability and increase neurologic deficits.[58] In patients with structural instability of the spinal column as a result of metastatic tumor, restoration and maintenance of spinal stability represents an important goal of therapy and one that can only be successfully accomplished with surgery.[79] The overall unsatisfactory results with laminectomy may not reflect the potential results of surgery, but those produced by an unselective surgical strategy.

Several reports indicate the importance of selecting the surgical approach on the basis of location of the tumor mass or bone encroachment on the spinal canal.[47–56,59,82] Because 85% of epidural tumors arise in a vertebral body and remain largely anterior to the spinal cord, the focus of the surgical procedure for most patients should be the involved vertebral body. A posterolateral approach is used for thoracic lesions and for many lumbar lesions. For cervical and certain lumbar lesions, a more direct anterior approach is used. The intervertebral disks and the vertebral body are removed. All tumor

TABLE 60–9. Results of Therapies
for Spinal Cord Compression

Treatment	No. of Patients	Ambulatory Patients After Treatment	
		No.	Mean %
Laminectomy*	275	85	31
Radiotherapy*	387	176	45
Laminectomy plus radiotherapy*	216	111	51
Vertebral body resection†‡	101	78	78
Selective surgery†§	140	117	84
Vertebral body resection for anterior tumor	108	101	94
Laminectomy for posterior tumor	32	16	50

* Cumulative data from several published series. Each series consisted of a heterogenous group of metastatic tumors. (Adapted from Black P. Spinal metastasis: Current status and recommended guidelines for management. Neurosurgery 1979;5:726)
† Radiotherapy in addition to surgery in most patients.
‡ Includes only patients with vertebral body involvement with tumor. (Data from Sundaresan N, Galicich JH, Lane JM, et al. Treatment of neoplastic epidural cord compression by vertebral body resection and stabilization. J Neurosurg 1985;63:676)
§ Treatment selected on basis of site of spinal involvement—whether the vertebral body or the neural arch was involved by tumor. (Data combined from Siegal T, Siegal T. Surgical decompression of anterior and posterior malignant epidural tumors compressing the spinal cord: A prospective study. Neurosurgery 1985;17:424 and Sundaresan N, Digiacinto GV, Hughes JEO, et al. Treatment of neoplastic spinal cord compression: Results of a prospective study. Neurosurgery 1991;29:645)

and devitalized bone are removed down to the dura. Various techniques for spinal stabilization permit tumor excision and structural stabilization of the spine during the same operation and with one operative approach.[47–56,59,60]

Sundaresan and associates treated 101 consecutive patients with epidural cord compression by vertebral body resection, tumor excision, and immediate stabilization.[50] Patients received surgery who had a pathologic compression fracture as the presenting feature of malignancy, a solitary site of tumor relapse, destruction of the spine by a paraspinous tumor, a known radioresistant tumor (*e.g.*, melanoma, sarcoma, kidney tumor), a structural abnormality of the spine producing compression of the spinal cord, or segmental instability of the spine after previous local treatment with irradiation. Of the 101 patients, 78 (78%) left the hospital walking (including 51 patients who had local tumor relapse after a full course of radiation therapy). Thirty-two (70%) of 46 patients who were nonambulatory before treatment were ambulatory, with or without support, at hospital discharge. Pain relief was achieved in 85% of the patients with significant back or radicular pain. The incidence of complications—8 patients died within 30 days and 10% had nonfatal complications—was considered acceptable. The median survival of all patients was 8 months, and 37% lived longer than 1 year after treatment. Similar results were reported by Harrington.[47]

Siegal and Siegal treated 167 episodes of cord compression prospectively by a standard protocol in which the selection

of the surgical approach, when surgery was indicated, depended on the tumor location.[70] This was the first study in which selection of the appropriate surgical approach (*i.e.*, anterior versus posterior based on the site of neoplastic cord compression) was carried out according to strict criteria. Because most tumors arise anteriorly, most patients received vertebral body resection. Irradiation was the primary therapy for patients who had poor general medical status, had multiple myelographic blocks, were paraplegic for longer than 72 hours, or had previously diagnosed radiosensitive tumors without previous radiation treatment. Of the 18 patients with radiosensitive tumors who were treated only with irradiation, 13 (72%) were ambulatory after treatment. Surgical treatment was assigned primarily to 86 patients who had no previous histologic diagnosis of their tumor, who received previous treatment with irradiation at the involved site, who had a known radioresistant tumor (*e.g.*, osteogenic sarcoma, melanoma, giant cell tumor of bone), or who developed neurologic deterioration during radiation treatment. Twenty-five patients had posterior or posterolateral tumor and received laminectomy for tumor removal, decompression of the spinal cord, and if indicated, spinal fixation with spinal rods and bone cement for instability. Although 25% of this group deteriorated as a direct result of surgery, 40% were ambulatory after surgery (92% of this group were nonambulatory before surgery), and normal sphincter control was achieved in 57% (76% were incontinent preoperatively).

Sixty-one patients had anterior tumors and received vertebral body resections; 55 (91%) had spinal instability and received immediate internal spinal fixation using acrylic replacement of the involved vertebral body. The 30-day mortality rate for this group was 7%, 80% were ambulatory within 30 days (72% of this group were nonambulatory preoperatively), 93% had normal sphincter control (41% were incontinent preoperatively), and although 97% had persistent pain before treatment, complete pain relief was obtained in 56% after surgery. The median survival of these patients was 16 months. The high ambulation rate, which was superior to that generally reported for irradiation alone, occurred although more than half of the patients treated by vertebral body resection had relapsed after receiving previous irradiation.

In a study of 54 patients who prospectively received surgery with a approach based on the tumor site, all patients were ambulatory after surgery, including the 24 patients who could not walk before surgery (completely paraplegic patients were excluded from the study prospectively).[51] Twenty-three of the 25 patients who survived at 2 years continued to be ambulatory.

These studies indicate that proper patient selection and the choice of surgical approach based on the tumor location are prerequisites for successful surgery. Laminectomy, which is the generally accepted surgical approach to the treatment of metastatic epidural mass lesions, is ineffective and can be harmful when the pathologic process is anterior to the spinal cord. The outcome of a selective surgical approach (*i.e.*, 80% ambulation and 93% sphincter control) is superior to results obtained by irradiation alone or irradiation combined with laminectomy (see Tables 60–8 and 60–9). It remains to be determined if similar results can be achieved in the unselected population of cancer patients seen at most general hospitals, where most patients are treated.

If surgical decompression is to be used, excision of the tumor, adequate decompression of the spinal cord, and correction of any significant spinal deformity must be accomplished. To ensure optimal exposure for tumor removal and decompression at the site of direct pressure on the spinal cord, posterior lesions are approached posteriorly by a wide laminectomy, and anterior and anterolateral lesions receive anterior or anterolateral resection of the tumor and the involved vertebral body. Complete tumor removal should be attempted, because early relapse of myelopathy after radiotherapy usually occurs in the same region from regrowth of residual tumor.[23] For instability of the spine, fusion should be performed during the same procedure by instrumentation with or without methylmethacrylate reconstruction, which produce immediate stability. Neurologic improvement is due to correctly directed and efficient decompression of the spinal cord and to immediate stabilization of the spinal column. Local pain in patients with spinal metastases often results from segmental spinal instability. This is suggested by demonstration of a collapsed vertebra and by pain that is relieved by immobilization, bed rest, or traction. Immediate spinal stability enhances rehabilitation by permitting immediate ambulation, if neurologic recovery allows, and eliminates pain from segmental instability.

Children with metastatic sarcoma (*e.g.*, Ewing's sarcoma, soft tissue sarcoma, osteogenic sarcoma, rhabdomyosarcoma) seem to be an exception to the previously described recommendations. Pediatric tumors frequently enter the spinal canal by the intervertebral foramen and compress the cord circumferentially, which permits laminectomy to accomplish decompression. In one large series, 66% of children (all tumor types) with no motor or sensory function below the level of compression became ambulatory after laminectomy combined with irradiation or medical therapy.[61]

RADIATION THERAPY

Response to treatment with irradiation alone is well established. An early report by Mones and colleagues described a favorable response, defined as the ability to ambulate, in 14 (34%) of 41 patients with epidural cord compression treated only with radiation therapy.[45] Response to treatment was excellent in their patients with radioresponsive tumors, such as lymphoma, Ewing's sarcoma, and neuroblastoma, less satisfactory in patients with metastatic breast cancer and poor in patients with lung cancer.[45] Complete or partial reversal of neurologic deficits occurred in 41% of 82 additional patients treated similarly at the same hospital.[62] Paraplegic patients had limited responses, with only 16% improved compared with 58% of patients with some initial motor function.

Gilbert and associates at Memorial Hospital retrospectively reviewed the clinical findings and results of treatment in 130 consecutive patients who were treated for epidural spinal cord compression by irradiation alone or laminectomy followed by irradiation.[3] No significant differences in treatment outcomes were seen. After treatment, 49% of patients who received irradiation alone walked, compared with 46% of those who received surgery and postoperative irradiation. The duration of improvement in the two treatment groups was similar, with approximately 75% of patients ambulatory after treatment remaining so for 6 months or longer. Patients with radiore-

sponsive tumors generally received irradiation, as did most who were paraplegic at presentation and felt to have little chance to recover after laminectomy. Patients without prior histologic diagnosis, those who had previously received spinal irradiation, and patients with rapidly progressing myelopathy usually received surgery. Regardless of the treatment chosen, 73% of ambulatory patients remained so, 36% of the paraparetic patients (*i.e.*, nonambulatory but able to lift the legs) regained ambulation, but only 1 of 39 paraplegic patients improved. Tumors considered radioresponsive (*e.g.*, seminoma, lymphoma myeloma, Ewing's sarcoma, neuroblastoma) responded better to either therapy than less radioresponsive tumors (*e.g.*, carcinomas, melanoma, soft tissue sarcomas). Patients with rapid progression of spinal cord dysfunction, formerly considered an indication for surgery, improved more often with irradiation alone than with decompressive laminectomy followed by irradiation. Of the 9 patients with weakness that developed over less than 48 hours who underwent surgical decompression, none improved, but 7 of 13 patients irradiated without surgery improved. Autonomic dysfunction predisposed to a worse outcome after treatment. Of 65 patients with urinary incontinence or retention before treatment, 43 (66%) were or became nonambulatory, but inability to walk occurred in fewer than 50% of patients without autonomic dysfunction.

Recovery of motor function and ambulation in patients presenting with complete paralysis may be delayed for some time after irradiation. Helweg-Larsen reported recovery of ambulation in 5 patients and recovery of motor function in a sixth among 15 patients who presented with total leg paralysis and underwent irradiation.[63] Recovery in these patients occurred 3 to 18 months after treatment. The duration of paralysis before treatment ranged from 1 to 10 days. The median time from initial motor symptoms to total paralysis was longer (45 days) in the 6 patients who recovered than the 9 who remained paralyzed (9 days). This observation is consistent with the experimental observations of Tarlov for mechanically induced cord compressions in dogs.[10–12]

Greenberg and colleagues administered high-dose dexamethasone (100 mg) at diagnosis and began radiation therapy within several hours.[21] After daily doses of 500 cGy for the first 3 days of treatment, 300 cGy/day were given to a total dose of 3000 cGy. Dexamethasone was continued at 96 mg daily in divided doses for 3 days and then tapered during the course of radiation therapy if symptoms permitted. They compared their results with those from the same institution by Gilbert and associates and reported no differences in outcome with the new treatment program.[3] They did, however, find a substantial reduction in pain in 64% of patients in the first day of treatment, which they attributed to dexamethasone, because improvement occurred even before the initiation of irradiation in 6 patients. The optimal steroid regimen is not established.

Cobb and colleagues reported the retrospective analysis of 44 patients with epidural cord compression from metastatic breast cancer, 26 of whom received initial laminectomy and 18 of whom received initial radiotherapy.[43] No significant difference in treatment outcome occurred, with 75% of ambulatory patients remaining so. Deterioration of neurologic function developed in 6 patients undergoing initial radiation therapy. Two of these patients underwent decompressive laminectomy, with a favorable outcome for 1 patient. The researchers highlight the need for close neurologic examination during radiotherapy and recommend surgery in patients who show evidence of neurologic deterioration during irradiation.

Although the number of patients is small, one randomized, prospective study compared the outcome in 16 patients who underwent decompressive laminectomy plus radiotherapy with 13 patients who received irradiation only.[46] There were no significant differences in outcome between the two groups.

The effect of the type of tumor on outcome of treatment with irradiation is difficult to assess, because of the relatively small numbers of patients with each specific histologic diagnosis in any single series. Pooled data may not account for difference in ambulatory status, treatment techniques, and dose. Nevertheless, the results reported suggest excellent outcomes after irradiation with lymphomas and myelomas, good results in patients with prostate, breast, and renal cancers and generally disappointing results in patients with lung carcinomas.[3,19,21,28,43,45,46,64,65] Herbert and associates reported that a treatment program of radiation therapy with or without laminectomy was effective in palliating the symptoms of epidural cord compression caused by metastatic melanoma.[66] Improvement was seen in 86% of treated sites and was complete in 30%. A radiation dose of more than 3000 cGy was significantly associated with the probability of a complete response.

Radiation therapy portals are designed using information from the history and physical examination, spine radiographs, MRI or myelography, bone scan if available, and CT scans if indicated. MRI scans or myelograms are mandatory for radiation therapy treatment planning for patients with neurologic symptoms or signs. Calkins and colleagues showed that myelography influenced field size in 69% of patients.[32] Even in patients with discrete bony lesions, results of myelography affected treatment 45% of the time.

After the diagnosis of spinal cord compression is established, high-dose steroid therapy should be started. Patients who are to undergo irradiation should start treatment immediately after diagnosis. The radiation portal includes the site of the epidural disease and in addition should extend two vertebral bodies above and below.[3,23] Because in one series all second subsequent sites of epidural metastasis occurring within 7 months of initial treatment appeared within two vertebral bodies of the original site of disease, these guidelines appear prudent.[23] Modification may be necessary, depending on previous radiation portals and other sites of tumor seen on bone radiographs or scans. Paravertebral tumor should be included if possible in the treatment field. For cervical spine lesions, parallel-opposed lateral portals are usually employed. Most thoracic lesions can be treated with a single posterior field, generally prescribing to a depth of 6 cm.[84] Because the anterior edge of the lumbar spine is near the midline, lesions of the lumbar spine generally require parallel-opposed anteroposterior fields. This technique avoids overdosage to the spinal cord from a single posterior field.

The optimal radiation dose and fractionation scheme have not been established, but several guidelines are available. Spinal cord tolerance to irradiation cannot be exceeded. The radiation therapy should be delivered such that the rapidity of tumor regression and the probability of disease control in the irradiated volume is maximized. Friedman and associates demonstrated a good response in 71% of patients who received more than than 2500 cGy for epidural cord compression from malignant lymphoma, compared with 34% in the group that received 2500 cGy or less.[67] No clear dose-response relation has been demonstrated for other histologies except melanoma, although higher doses (time-dose fraction >60.5) appear to reduce the rate of recurrence within the original treatment field.[24] Commonly employed doses are 3000 to 4000 cGy over 2 to 4 weeks.

Experimental data for rats with epidural cord compression secondary to lymphoma or carcinoma demonstrate more rapid neurologic recovery after large daily fractions of radiation (500 cGy) than after smaller daily doses (100–200 cGy).[26,68] Fractionated doses provide more prolonged functional improvement than large single-dose treatment in rats.[26] Large initial fractions (300–400) cGy are advocated for the first 3 days of therapy, which are followed by smaller daily doses (150–300 cGy).[21,69] Despite concerns about irradiation-induced edema from large fractions, experimental evidence fails to confirm its development.[68,71,81]

CHEMOTHERAPY

Several reports describe successful chemotherapy for epidural cord compression for tumors known to be responsive to chemotherapy (*e.g.*, lymphomas, germ cell neoplasms, neuroblastoma, Ewing's sarcoma).[70,72–74] Experiments with the Walker 256 carcinoma cell line in the rat show that cyclophosphamide is more effective for relieving the neurologic signs of cord compression than laminectomy or 1500 cGy of irradiation delivered in three fractions.[26] Hayes and colleagues reported 9 children with neuroblastoma and 5 children with Ewing's sarcoma who had epidural cord compression by tumor.[70] Five children received laminectomy before referral, but only 1 had neurologic recovery. The other 9 patients did not undergo surgery. All 14 patients received chemotherapy with rapid regression of tumor and neurologic deficits.

Chemotherapy is a feasible alternative to laminectomy and irradiation in the management of certain types of epidural tumors. In infants and children, in whom growth inhibition from irradiation may be significant, it seems reasonable to consider chemotherapy for sensitive tumors, as long as the patients are closely monitored by the oncologist, radiation oncologist, and neurosurgeon so that other interventions may be quickly undertaken if needed. Children with severe canal encroachment by tumor (near complete or complete) demonstrated by myelography or filling more than 50% of the spinal canal on MR scans should be considered for laminectomy. Twenty-five of 26 such patients undergoing laminectomy improved or stabilized, compared with 4 of 7 patients who were treated without surgery in one report.[75]

Friedman and associates reported 2 adult patients with testicular cancers who had neurologic recovery after successful decompression of an epidural cord compression by chemotherapy with cyclophosphamide, bleomycin, vinblastine, and cisplatin.[73] In the adult patient with epidural cord compression from metastatic tumor that is responsive to chemotherapy, the physician should consider adding chemotherapy to surgery or irradiation or using chemotherapy if surgery or irradiation are not tenable.

CONCLUSION

Epidural spinal cord compression is an oncologic emergency that requires prompt evaluation and treatment. Because the best results of treatment of spinal metastases are obtained if there is minimal loss of neurologic function, early diagnosis and treatment are the most important elements of successful treatment. Evaluation should include a careful physical examination, complete spine radiographs, spinal MRI or complete myelography (including cervical myelography in cases of complete block), and if indicated, bone scintigraphy or CT. Patients should be assessed at presentation by the medical or pediatric oncologist, neurologist, radiation oncologist, and neurosurgeon. Corticosteroids should be started after the diagnosis is established.

Although there is no definitive prospective study that compares current treatments under similar conditions, it is reasonably clear when irradiation or surgery should be used, and recommendations can be made for the management of most patients as outlined in Table 60–10. Radiation therapy is recommended as initial treatment for patients with cord compression who have radiation-sensitive tumors that are not associated with spinal instability. Patients who have spinal involvement by tumor that is neither causing neurologic symptoms nor spinal instability should be treated initially with radiation therapy. Patients whose neurologic status deteriorates during radiation therapy and patients who relapse at the site of previous irradiation should undergo surgery. Surgery should be the initial treatment for patients with a pathologic fracture resulting in spinal instability or compression of the spinal cord by bone and in patients with radiation-resistant tumors. Surgery has traditionally been the initial treatment in patients without a previous tissue diagnosis. The use of percutaneous needle biopsy to determine the histology has been proposed as a reliable and logical approach to deciding on the treatment modality.[76] If surgery is indicated, the surgical procedure should be based on the site of tumor involvement by using the appropriate anterior or posterior approach. Because of the difficulty of completely resecting tumor adjacent to the spinal cord, surgery should be followed by postoperative radiation therapy as long as the spinal cord tolerance is not exceeded.

Chemotherapy may be used as an adjuvant in adult patients with tumors responsive to chemotherapy or as primary therapy if irradiation or surgery are not tenable. In selected pediatric patients with chemosensitive tumors, chemotherapy may be considered for initial treatment if the patients are closely monitored for any signs of progressive neurologic dysfunction during chemotherapy. We emphasize that the most appropriate treatment in each case is also the most effective if instituted before major neurologic dysfunction develops.

TABLE 60–10. Recommendations for Management of Patients With Spinal Metastases*

Radiation Therapy Only

Known radiation-sensitive tumor and no spinal instability (regardless of rate of progression or neurologic condition)
Spinal involvement without spinal instability or neurologic deficit

Surgery† Followed by Radiation

Pathologic fracture with spinal instability or compression of the spinal cord by bone
Radiation-resistant tumor with neurologic deficit
Unknown tissue diagnosis (if a radiosensitive tumor is suspected, needle biopsy can provide the diagnosis)

Surgery† Only

Relapse at the site of previous irradiation
Failure to respond to radiation therapy

Chemotherapy

Pediatric patients with responsive tumors
Adjuvant treatment in adult patients with responsive tumors
Relapse of a responsive tumor at site of previous irradiation and surgery

* Steroid therapy should be used in the early phases of therapy with radiation, surgery, or chemotherapy.
† Surgery should be based on the site of tumor (anterior versus posterior).

REFERENCES

1. Barrons KD, Hirano A, Araki S, Terry RD. Experiences with metastatic neoplasms involving the spinal cord. Neurology (Minn) 1959;9:91.
2. Black P. Spinal metastasis: Current status and recommended guidelines for management. Neurosurgery 1979;5:726.
3. Gilbert RW, Kim JH, Posner JB. Epidural spinal cord compression from metastatic tumor: Diagnosis and treatment. Ann Neurol 1978;3:40.
4. Sorensen PS, Borgensen SE, Rohde K, et al. Metastatic epidural spinal cord compression: Results of treatment and survival. Cancer 1990;65:1502.
5. Maranzano E, Latini P, Checcaglini F, et al. Radiation therapy in metastatic cord compression. A prospective analysis of 105 consecutive patients. Cancer 1991;67:1311.
6. Kim RY, Spencer SA, Meredith RF, et al. Extradural spinal cord compression: Analysis of factors determining functional prognosis. Radiology 1990;176:279.
7. Stark RJ, Henson RA, Evans SJW. Spinal metastases. A retrospective survey from a general hospital. Brain 1982;105:189.
8. Meyer PC, Reah TG. Secondary neoplasms of the central nervous system and meninges. Br J Cancer 1953;7:438.
9. Posner JB. Spinal cord compression: A neurologic emergency. Clin Bull 1971;1:65.
10. Tarlov IM, Klinger H, Vitale S. Spinal cord compression studies. I. Experimental techniques to produce acute and gradual compression. Arch Neurol Psychiatry 1957;70:813.
11. Tarlov IM, Klinger H. Spinal cord compression studies. II. Time limits for recovery after acute compression in dogs. Arch Neurol Psychiatry 1954;71:271.
12. Tarlov IM. Spinal cord compression studies. III. Time limits for recovery after gradual compression in dogs. Arch Neurol Psychiatry 1954;71:588.
13. Ushio Y, Posner R, Posner JB, Shapiro WR. Experimental spinal cord compression by epidural neoplasms. Neurology 1977;27:422.
14. Siegal T, Shohami E, Siegal TZ. Indomethacin and dexamethasone treatment in experimental spinal cord compression. Part II. Effect on edema and prostaglandin synthesis. Neurosurgery 1988;22:334–339.
15. Siegal T, Siegal TZ, Shapira Y, et al. Experimental neoplastic spinal cord compression. Evoked potentials, edema, prostaglandins, and light and electron microscopy. Spine 1987;12:440.
16. Siegal T, Siegal TZ, Sandbank U, et al. Indomethacin and dexamethasone treatment in experimental spinal cord compression. Part I. Effect on water content and specific gravity. Neurosurgery 1988;22:328.
17. Johnson M, Corey F, McMillan RM. Alternative pathways of arachidonate metabolism: Prostaglandins, thromboxane, and leukotrienes. Essays Biochem 1983;19:41.
18. Siegal T, Siegal TZ. Current considerations in the management of neoplastic spinal cord compression. Spine 1989;14:223.
19. Bruckman JE, Bloomer WD. Management of spinal cord compression. Semin Oncol 1978;5:135.
20. Torma T. Malignant tumors of the spine and the spinal epidural space. A study based on 250 histologically verified cases. Acta Chir Scand 1957;225:1.
21. Greenberg HS, Kim JH, Posner JB. Epidural spinal cord compression from metastatic tumor: Results with a new treatment protocol. Ann Neurol 1980;8:361.
22. Rodichok LD, Harper GR, Ruckdeschel JC, et al. Early diagnosis of spinal epidural metastases. Am J Med 1981;70:1181.
23. Kaminski HJ, Diwan VG, Ruff RC. Second occurrence of spinal epidural metastases. Neurology 1991;41:744.
24. Loeffler JS, Glicksman AS, Tefft M, Gelch M. Treatment of spinal cord compression: A retrospective analysis. Med Pediatr Oncol 1983;11:347.

25. Portenoy RK. Lipton RB, Foley KM. Back pain in the cancer patient: An algorithm for evaluation and management. Neurology 1987;37:134.
26. Ushio Y, Posner R, Kim J, et al. Treatment of experimental spinal cord compression caused by extradural neoplasms. J Neurosurg 1977;47:380.
27. Vecht CJ, Haaxma-Reiche H, Van Putten WLJ, et al. Initial bolus of conventional versus high-dose dexamethasone in metastatic spinal cord compression. Neurology 1989;39: 1255.
28. Martenson JA Jr, Evans RG, Lie MR, et al. Treatment outcome and complications in patients treated for malignant epidural spinal cord compression (SCC). J Neurol Oncol 1985;3:77.
29. Wild WO, Porter RW. Metastatic epidural tumor of the spine. A study of 45 cases. Arch Surg 1963;87:137.
30. Wright RL. Malignant tumors in the spinal extradural space: Results of surgical treatment. Ann Surg 1963;157:227.
31. White WA, Patterson RH, Bergland RM. Role of surgery in the treatment of spinal cord compression by metastatic neoplasm. Cancer 1971;27:55B.
32. Calkins AR, Olson MA, Ellis JH. Impact of myelography on the radiotherapeutic management of malignant spinal cord compression. Neurosurgery 1986;19:614.
33. Fink IJ, Garra BS, Zabell A, Doppman JL. Computed tomography with metrizamide myelography to define the extent of spinal canal block due to tumor. J Comput Assist Tomogr 1984;8:1072.
34. Aichner F, Poewe W, Rogalsky W, et al. Magnetic resonance imaging in the diagnosis of spinal cord diseases. J Neurol Neurosurg Psychiatry 1985;48:1220.
35. Harnsberger HR, Dillon WP. The radiologic role in diagnosis, staging and follow-up of neoplasia of the brain, spine, and head and neck. Semin Ultrasound CT MR 1989;10: 431.
36. Smoker WRK, Godersky JC, Knutzon RK, et al. The role of MR imaging in evaluating metastatic spinal disease. AJNR 1987;8:901.
37. Sarpel S, Sarpel G, Yu E, et al. Early diagnosis of spinal-epidural metastasis by magnetic resonance imaging. Cancer 1987;59:1112.
38. Hagenau C, Grosh W, Currie M, et al. Comparison of spinal magnetic resonance imaging and myelography in cancer patients. J Clin Oncol 1987;5:1663.
39. McAfee PC, Bohlman HH, Han JS, Salvagno RT. Comparison of nuclear magnetic resonance imaging and computed tomography in the diagnosis of upper cervical spinal cord compression. Spine 1986;11:295.
40. Hollis PH, Malis LI, Zappullo RA. Neurological deterioration after lumber puncture below complete spinal subarachnoid block. J Neurosurg 1986;64:253.
41. Johansen JG, Orrison WW, Amundsen P. Lateral C1–2 puncture for cervical myelography. Part 1: Report of a complication. Radiology 1983;146:391.
42. Sze G, Krol G, Zimmerman RD, et al. Malignant extradural spinal tumors: MR imaging with Gd-DTPA. Radiology 1988;167:217.
43. Cobb CA III, Leavens ME, Eckles N. Indications for nonoperative treatment of spinal cord compression due to breast cancer. J Neurosurg 1977;47:653.
44. Raichle ME, Posner JB. The treatment of extradural spinal cord compression. Neurology 1970;20:391.
45. Mones RJ, Dozier D, Berrett A. Analysis of medical treatment of malignant extradural spinal cord tumors. Cancer 1966;19:1842.
46. Young RF, Post EM, King GA. Treatment of spinal epidural metastases: Randomized prospective comparison of laminectomy and radiotherapy. J Neurosurg 1980;53:741.
47. Harrington KD. Anterior cord decompression and spinal stabilization for patients with metastatic lesions of the spine. J Neurosurg 1984;61:107.
48. Sundaresan N, Galicich JH. Treatment of spinal metastases by vertebral body resection. Cancer Invest 1984;2:383.
49. Siegal T, Siegal T. Surgical decompression of anterior and posterior malignant epidural tumors compressing the spinal cord: A prospective study. Neurosurgery 1985;17: 424.
50. Sundaresan N, Galicich JH, Lane JM, et al. Treatment of neoplastic epidural cord compression by vertebral body resection and stabilization. J Neurosurg 1985;63:676.
51. Sundaresan N, Digiacinto GV, Hughes JEO, Cafferty M, Vallejo A. Treatment of neoplastic spinal cord compression: Results of a prospective study. Neurosurgery 1991;29:645.
52. Shaw B, Mansfield FL, Borges L. One-stage posterolateral decompression and stabilization for primary and metastatic vertebral tumors in the thoracic and lumbar spine. J Neurosurg 1989;70:405.
53. Cybulski GR, Stone JL, Opesanmi O. Spinal decompression via a modified costotransversectomy approach combined with posterior instrumentation for management of metastatic neoplasms of the thoracic spine. Surg Neurol 1991;35:280.
54. Johnston FG, Uttley D, Marsh HT. Synchronous vertebral decompression and posterior stabilization in the treatment of spinal malignancy. Neurosurgery 1989;25:872.
55. Moore AJ, Uttley D. Anterior decompression and stabilization of the spine in malignant disease. Neurosurgery 1989;24:713.
56. Manabe S, Tateishi A, Abe M, Ohno T. Surgical treatment of metastatic tumors of the spine. Spine 1989;14:41.
57. Hall AJ, MacKay NNS. The results of laminectomy for compression of the cord and cauda equina by extradural malignant tumor. J Bone Joint Surg [Br] 1973;55:497.
58. Findlay GF. Adverse effects of the management of malignant spinal cord compression. J Neurol Neurosurg Psychiatry 1984;47:761.
59. Hall DJ, Webb JK. Anterior plate fixation in spine tumor surgery: Indications, technique, and results. Spine 1991;16:S80.
60. Haid RW Jr, Carter RL, MacMillan M. Cotrel-Dubousset instrumentation for spinal neoplasms. J Neurosurg 1990;72:350A.
61. Klein SL, Sanford RA, Muhlbauer MS. Pediatric spinal epidural metastases. J Neurosurg 1991;74:70.
62. Zevallos M, Chan PYM, Munoz L, et al. Epidural spinal cord compression from metastatic tumor. Int J Radiat Oncol Biol Phys 1981;13:875.
63. Helweg-Larsen S, Rasmusson B, Sorensen PS. Recovery of gait after radiotherapy in paralytic patients with metastatic epidural spinal cord compression. Neurology 1990;40: 1234.
64. Haddad P, Thael JF, Kiely JM, et al. Lymphoma of the spinal extradural space. Cancer 1976;38:1862.
65. Khan FR, Glicksman AS, Chu FCH, Nickson JJ. Treatment by radiotherapy of spinal cord compression due to extradural metastases. Radiology 1967;89:495.
66. Herbert SH, Solin LJ, Rate WR, et al. The effect of palliative radiation therapy on epidural compression due to metastatic malignant melanoma. Cancer 1991;678:2472.
67. Friedman M, Kim TM, Panahon AM. Spinal cord compression in malignant lymphoma. Cancer 1976;37:1485.
68. Rubin P. Extradural spinal cord compression by tumor. Part I. Experimental production and treatment trials. Radiology 1969;93:1243.
69. Rubin P, Mayer E, Poutter C. Exrtradural spinal cord compression by tumor. Part II. High daily dose experience without laminectomy. Radiology 1969;93:1243.
70. Hayes FA, Thompson EL, Avizdala E, et al. Chemotherapy as an alternative to laminectomy and radiation in the management of epidural tumor. J Pediatr 1984;104:221.
71. Redmond H. Effects of whole-brain irradiation. Presented at the Work in Progress Session of the 52nd Scientific Assembly and Meeting of the Radiological Society of North America, Chicago, 1966.
72. Silverberg IJ, Jacobs EM. Treatment of spinal cord compression in Hodgkin's disease. Cancer 1971;27:308.
73. Friedman HM, Sheetz S, Levine HC, et al, eds. Combination chemotherapy and radiation therapy. The medical management of epidural spinal cord compression from testicular cancer. Arch Intern Med 1986;146:509.
74. Gale GB, O'Connor DM, Chu J-Y, et al. Successful chemotherapeutic decompression of epidural malignant germ cell tumor. Med Pediatr Oncol 1986;14:97.
75. Raffel C, Neave VCD, Lavine S, McComb JG. Treatment of spinal cord compression by epidural malignancy in childhood. Neurosurgery 1991;28:349.
76. Findlay GFG, Sandeman DR, Buxton P. The role of needle biopsy in the management of malignant spinal compression. Br J Neurosurg 1988;2: 479.
77. Bosley TM, Cohen DA, Schatz NJ, et al. Comparison of metrizamide computed tomography and magnetic resonance imaging in the evaluation of lesions at the cervicomedullary junction. Neurology 1985;35:485.
78. Brady LW, Asbell SO, Antoniades J, et al. The treatment of metastatic disease of the nervous system by radiation therapy. In: Seydel HG, ed. Tumors of the nervous system. New York; John Wiley & Sons, 1975:177–188.
79. Cybulski GR. Methods of surgical stabilization for metastatic disease of the spine. Neurosurgery 1989;25:240.
80. Elsberg CA. Surgical diseases of the spinal cord membranes and nerve roots: Symptoms, diagnosis, and treatment. New York: Hueber, 1941:501.
81. Gregersen MI, Pallavicini C, Chien S. Studies on the chemical composition of the central nervous system in relation to the effects of x-irradiation and of disturbances in water and salt balance. Radiat Res 1967;17:209.
82. Kostiuk JP. Anterior spinal cord decompression for lesions of the thoracic and lumber spine, techniques, new methods of internal fixation, results. Spine 1983;8:512.
83. Livingston KE, Perrin RG. The neurosurgical management of spinal metastases causing cord and cauda equina compression. J Neurosurg 1978;49:839.
84. Millburn L, Hibbs GG, Hendrickson FR. Treatment of spinal cord compression from metastatic carcinoma. Cancer 1969;21:447.
85. Mullan J, Evans JP. Neoplastic disease of the spinal extradural space. Arch Surg 1957;74: 900.
86. Renaudin J, Fewer D, Wilson CB, et al. Dose dependence of Decadron in patients with partially excised brain tumors. J Neurosurg 1973;39:302.
87. Smith R. An evaluation of surgical treatment of spinal cord compression due to metastatic carcinoma. J Neurol Neurosurg Psychiatry 1965;28:152.

SECTION **3** RAYMOND P. WARRELL, JR

Metabolic Emergencies

Patients with cancer present a microcosm of the metabolic and endocrinologic problems encountered in internal medicine, albeit frequently to an extreme degree. Grouped among the paraneoplastic syndromes are metabolic disorders associated with cancer or its treatment that require urgent medical therapy for treatment or prevention.

HYPERCALCEMIA

EPIDEMIOLOGY

Hypercalcemia is the most common life-threatening metabolic disorder associated with cancer. The most reasonable estimates of the prevalence of this disorder in the United States and Western Europe range from 15 to 20 cases per 100,000 persons.[1,2] The incidence of hypercalcemia varies with the underlying cancer diagnosis; it is highest in myeloma and breast cancer (40–50%), intermediate in non-small cell lung cancer, and rare in small cell carcinoma of the lung and colon cancer.[3–6]

DIFFERENTIAL DIAGNOSIS

Hypercalcemia is associated with a wide variety of pathologic states (Table 60–11). Several excellent reviews discuss the diagnostic evaluation and differential diagnosis of patients with hypercalcemia.[7–10] Primary hyperparathyroidism and cancer are the two most common causes of hypercalcemia, and both diseases are prevalent.[11,12] The differential diagnosis of hypercalcemia in cancer and hyperparathyroidism has been linked to changes in serum chloride, phosphorus, "nephrogenous" cyclic adenosine monophosphate (cAMP), immunoreactive parathyroid hormone (PTH), and the results of steroid suppression tests.[13–15] A patient who presents with a recent onset of symptomatic hypercalcemia and weight loss is more likely to have a malignant disorder. In hypercalcemic patients who require hospitalization, cancer has been previously diagnosed or becomes apparent after minimal diagnostic evaluation in most cases.[1] Asymptomatic hypercalcemia and chronic symptoms are the most common presentations of primary hyperparathyroidism.[2] With current assays, a low or normal serum immunoreactive PTH level, especially when combined with elevated serum PTH-related protein, can reliably exclude the diagnosis of primary hyperparathyroidism.[16,17]

Serum calcium is highly bound to albumin, and measurements of total serum calcium fluctuate with changes in serum protein concentrations. Some patients with myeloma present with striking elevations of total serum calcium due solely to an increase in serum proteins that bind calcium.[18–20] Measurements of ionized calcium by ion-specific electrode are essential in such cases. However, for most patients, an approximate estimate of the severity of hypercalcemia can be made by using one of several formulas that adjust serum calcium levels for serum albumin concentration, as follows:

$$\text{Corrected [calcium] (mg/dl)} = \text{measured [calcium] (mg/dl)}$$
$$- \text{[albumin] (g/dl)} + 4.0 \ (20)$$

In this equation, concentrations in mg/dl can be converted to SI units by multiplication with 0.2495, yielding concentrations expressed in mmol/L.

CLINICAL MANIFESTATIONS

Patients with hypercalcemia can present with a wide variety of symptoms affecting multiple organs (Table 60–12). The severity of the presentation is not exclusively related to the degree of elevation of serum calcium. Patients with slight or moderate elevations (12–13 mg/dl) may become obtunded if the increase occurs acutely. Conversely, patients with long-standing hypercalcemia (*e.g.*, those with parathyroid carcinoma) may tolerate a serum calcium level of more than 14 mg/dl with few symptoms. Other factors, especially age, performance status, sites of metastases, and hepatic or renal dysfunction, contribute to the severity of symptoms.

TABLE 60–11. Diseases Associated With Hypercalcemia

Endocrine or metabolic diseases:
  Primary hyperparathyroidism
  Hyperthyroidism
  Pheochromocytoma
  Osteopetrosis
  Infantile hyperphosphatasia
  Familial hypercalcemia with hypercalciuria
Cancer
Infectious diseases:
  Tuberculosis
  Coccidioidomycosis
  HIV infection
Renal insufficiency
Granulomatous diseases:
  Sarcoidosis
  Berylliosis
Dietary or drug-related:
  Vitamin D intoxication
  Vitamin A intoxication
  Calcium supplements
  Lithium
  Milk-alkali syndrome

TABLE 60–12. Clinical Manifestations of Cancer-Related Hypercalcemia

General: dehydration, weight loss, anorexia, pruritus, polydipsia
Neuromuscular: fatigue, lethargy, muscle weakness, hyporeflexia, confusion, psychosis, seizure, obtundation, coma
Gastrointestinal: nausea, vomiting, constipation, obstipation, ileus
Genitorenal: polyuria, renal insufficiency
Cardiac: bradycardia, prolonged P-R interval, shortened Q-T interval, wide T-wave, atrial or ventricular arrhythmias

In patients with evolving hypercalcemia, fatigue, lethargy, constipation, nausea, and polyuria are the most common initial complaints. It is important to evaluate the serum calcium of patients who have these relatively nonspecific complaints, because the combination of polyuria and nausea can lead to rapid dehydration and substantial worsening of the hypercalcemic state. Patients in late stages may present in stupor or coma, and the condition is easily mistaken for diabetic ketoacidosis or drug overdose.

PATHOPHYSIOLOGY

In the past, cancer-related hypercalcemia was conveniently categorized according to the presence or absence of bone involvement. Hypercalcemia in the former group was believed to be associated with direct bone destruction by cancer cells, and the second group was characterized by various humorally mediated mechanisms. It is now evident that hypercalcemia— even in patients with extensive osteolysis—is probably mediated by factors released from or induced by malignant cells that ultimately act to resorb calcium from bone.

Parathyroid Hormone and the PTH-Related Protein

Some patients with cancer-related hypercalcemia have biochemical characteristics suggesting PTH stimulation, including increased tubular reabsorption of calcium, hypophosphatemia with phosphaturia, and elevated levels of nephrogenous cAMP.[21-23] However, most studies of ectopic hyperparathyroidism have been based on bioassays or measurements of immunoreactive material that do not satisfy current criteria of proof for ectopic hormone production.[24] Studies examining PTH-specific mRNA in tumors have confirmed that ectopic PTH production is not a common cause of hypercalcemia.[25] Convincing evidence for tumor secretion of authentic PTH has been presented in only two case reports.[26,27] True ectopic hyperparathyroidism is an exceptionally rare event.

In the mid-1980s, a PTH-related protein was isolated, and this factor has been fully characterized.[28-34] PTH-related protein and authentic human PTH are homologous for only 8 of the first 13 amino acids in the amino-terminal portion. Like the recently cloned receptor for PTH, screening studies have shown that PTH-related protein is widely distributed in normal tissues, such as brain, kidney, parathyroid, skin, uterus, and breast.[35-40] The specific function of the this factor in normal physiology remains uncertain, but it appears likely that the protein is involved only in local signaling and that it probably is not released into the general circulation under normal conditions.

PTH-related protein appears to be the most common mediator of cancer-related hypercalcemia.[41-45] In a study using immunoassay detection of PTH-related protein (Fig. 60–3), the factor was strikingly elevated in patients with solid tumors, particularly patients with squamous (epidermoid) carcinomas.[43] The factor is not associated with most hematologic cancers, such as myeloma or lymphoma, although high levels have been reported in HTLV-I associated T-cell lymphoma and non-Hodgkin's lymphomas associated with human immunodeficiency virus infection. Elevated serum PTH-related protein levels have been found in 30% to 50% of hypercalcemic patients with breast cancer.[41-43,46] The factor is elaborated at sites of bone metastases.[47,48] These data have clearly indicated that previous classifications of hypercalcemic syndromes based on the presence or absence of bone metastases were erroneous.

Prostaglandins

Prostaglandins have long been implicated as circulating mediators of cancer-related hypercalcemia, and certain prostaglandins, especially the E series, have potent bone-resorptive activity in vitro.[49-52] Although occasional hormonally induced flares of hypercalcemia in breast cancer have been linked to prostaglandin release, hypercalcemia rarely responds to cyclooxygenase inhibition, and circulating levels of prostaglandin E in hypercalcemic patients are far too low to account for the observed degree of accelerated bone resorption.[53-56] Prostaglandins may have an important role in cancer-related osteolysis but one that is distinctly time-dependent and highly focal.[57,58]

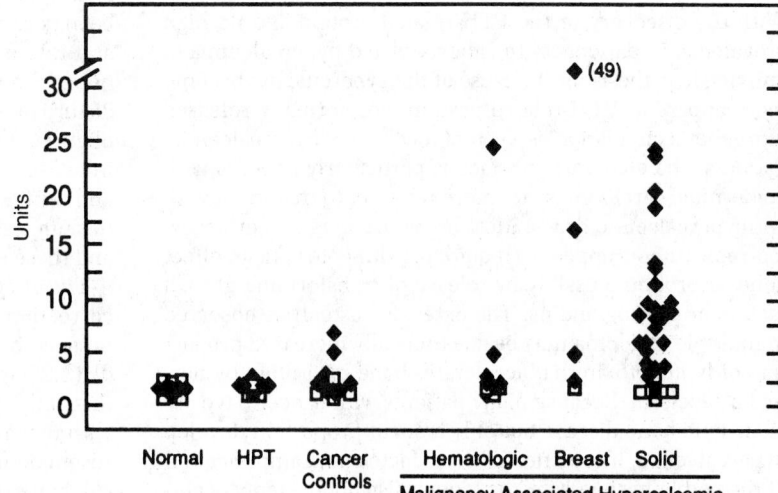

FIGURE 60–3. Serum levels of parathyroid hormone-related protein in normal controls, patients with primary hyperparathyroidism, and patients with diseases associated with cancer-related hypercalcemia. (Budayr AA, Nissenson RA, Klein RF, et al. Increased serum levels of a parathyroid hormone-like protein in malignancy-associated hypercalcemia. Ann Intern Med 1989;111: 807–812)

Cytokines

Factors with osteoclast-activating activity were originally isolated from lymphoid cells.[59,60] This activity is now understood to be associated with a wide variety of cytokines. The transforming growth factors (TGFs) are released in an autocrine manner by a variety of cancer cells and appear to be important regulatory factors for normal bone resorption and formation.[61] TGF-α shares partial similarity of amino acid sequence with epidermal growth factor (EGF), binds to the EGF receptor, and is a potent inducer of bone resorption in vitro.[62–64] Conversely, TGF-β is secreted by osteoblasts and may regulate osteoblast growth and differentiation.[65,66] Dysregulated TGF secretion may lead to uncoupling of bone resorption and formation and could partially account for the mixed lytic and blastic appearance of skeletal metastases in diseases such as carcinoma of the breast and prostate. Other cytokines, including interleukin-1, platelet-derived growth factor, tumor-derived hematopoietic colony-stimulating factors, tumor necrosis factor (TNF), particularly TNF-β (lymphotoxin), are potent inducers of bone resorption in vitro.[67–74] Although the local interaction of these factors in vivo is complex, there is little evidence that circulating cytokines are important mediators of cancer-related hypercalcemia.

Vitamin D

Elevated serum 1,25-dihydroxy vitamin D_3 levels have been reported in patients with Hodgkin's disease, non-Hodgkin's lymphoma, myeloma, and some patients with solid tumors.[75–80] These effects may result from increased enzymatic conversion of 25-OH-vitamin D by 1-α-vitamin D-hydroxylase, similar to patients with granulomatous disease. However, these observation do not prove an etiologic association; the observed elevations in serum vitamin D have generally been well below levels that are known to cause hypercalcemia in patients with vitamin D intoxication. Whether vitamin D plays an important physiologic role or acts merely as a marker of tumor burden is unknown. Normalization of serum vitamin D levels and resolution of hypercalcemia occurs with control of the underlying disease.

Mechanism of Cancer-Related Hypercalcemia

With the discovery of the PTH-related protein and its high prevalence in patients with cancer-related hypercalcemia, a unifying hypothesis for the cause of this syndrome has become more apparent. PTH-related protein, not normally released into general circulation, is a potent mediator of hypercalcemia. Patients who elaborate this factor, particularly patients with epidermoid carcinomas, are more resistant to treatment with antihypercalcemic drugs. Most breast cancers and other osteotropic tumors appear to require proximity to bone to effect bone resorption, possibly by release of transforming growth factors or prostaglandins. The extensive osteolysis observed in multiple myeloma may be due to focally increased production of lymphotoxin that accelerates bone resorption by normal osteoclasts. Because many patients with cancer have obvious lytic bone disease but only a small proportion develop hypercalcemia, interaction of these factors and amplification of the pathophysiology by the kidney also undoubtedly occur.

TREATMENT

General Measures

Although the best treatment for cancer-related hypercalcemia is therapy directed at the underlying disease, hypercalcemia most commonly occurs in patients with advanced disease who have failed prior therapy. The usual therapies for hypercalcemia are directed at decreasing serum calcium by increasing urinary calcium excretion or decreasing bone resorption by inhibition of osteoclast function. For practical purposes, increased intestinal absorption of calcium does not make an important contribution to hypercalcemia in patients with cancer; thus, low-calcium diets are ineffective.

Immobilization should be minimized because inactivity tends to aggravate hypercalcemia. Drugs that inhibit urinary calcium excretion (especially thiazides) should be discontinued.[81] Nonsteroidal antiinflammatory drugs and H_2-receptor antagonists (*e.g.*, cimetidine, ranitidine) decrease renal blood flow and should be avoided if possible. The patient should be carefully interviewed with respect to dietary aberrations. Medications containing calcium, vitamin D, vitamin A, and retinoids should be stopped.[82–84]

Specific Measures

The literature on the treatment of cancer-related hypercalcemia contains few controlled studies. Interpretation of clinical trial results has been confounded by tremendous variability in patient selection, underlying diagnoses, severity of hypercalcemia, and unique methods of reporting results.[85] Table 60–13 summarizes current therapies and provides an estimate of the relative potency of particular therapies.

INTRAVENOUS FLUIDS AND DIURETICS. Hypercalcemic patients frequently present with loss of intravascular volume because of vomiting and obligate water losses associated with calciuresis. Intravenous rehydration, preferably with isotonic saline, is the mainstay of acute therapy for hypercalcemia. Volume expansion and natriuresis increase renal blood flow and enhance calcium excretion due to ionic exchange of calcium for sodium in the distal tubule.[86–88] The rate of fluid administration depends on a clinical estimate of the extent of dehydration, cardiovascular function, and renal excretory capacity. Assuming renal function has previously been normal and cardiac reserves are adequate, saline infusion at a rate of 300 to 400 ml/hour is recommended for 3 to 4 hours. Slower hydration is indicated for less severe metabolic disturbances or in the settings of congestive heart failure or oliguria. After several hours, serum levels of calcium, creatinine, and electrolytes should be reassessed, and urinary output and cardiac status should be reevaluated. Potassium and magnesium losses frequently occur with hydration and diuretics, and these should be replaced as needed.

The effectiveness of hydration with or without diuretics for correction of clinically significant hypercalcemia is low. In a prospective study of patients with serum calcium of 13.0 mg/dl (3.25 mmol/L) or more, Hosking and colleagues found that only 5 of 16 patients (31%) achieved normocalcemia with normal saline (4000 ml/day for 2 days).[89] Although furosemide-induced natriuresis theoretically enhances urinary calcium excretion, no controlled studies have been conducted

TABLE 60–13.   Therapy for the Treatment of Cancer-Related Hypercalcemia

Treatment Characteristics	Normal Saline	Oral Phosphorus	Corticosteroids	Calcitonin	Etidronate	Plicamycin	Gallium Nitrate	Pamidronate
Dose	200–400(+) ml/h	1–3 g/d orally, divided doses	40–100 mg/d prednisone or equivalent	2–8 U/kg SC or IM every 6–12 h	7.5 mg/kg I.V. over 4 h daily for 3–5 d	10–50 (usually 25) micrograms/kg I.V. by brief infusion	100–200 mg/m²/day by continuous I.V. infusion up to 5 d	60–90 mg I.V. over 24 h
Indications	Hypovolemia, dehydration	Mild or moderate hypercalcemia, hypophosphatemia	Hypercalcemia from myeloma, lymphoma, hormonal flare	Mild or moderate hypercalcemia; acute control	Mild or moderate hypercalcemia	Moderate or severe hypercalcemia	Moderate or severe hypercalcemia	Moderate or severe hypercalcemia
Onset of action	12–24 h	24–48 h	3–5 d	1–4 h	48 h	24–48 h	24–48 h	24–48 h
Relative potency*	20%	30%	0–40%, depending on disease	30%	30–40%	80%	80%	70–80%
Advantages	Corrects dehydration	Orally available; minimal toxicity	Orally available	Minimal toxicity	Usually well tolerated; decreases bone resorption	Highly effective	Highly effective, decreases bone resorption	Highly effective, decreases bone resorption
Disadvantages/ toxicity	Pulmonary edema, hypernatremia, fluid overload	Nausea, diarrhea, extraosseous calcification	Hyperglycemia, gastritis, osteopenia	Nausea, hypersensitivity	Occasional nephrotoxicity	Nausea, nephrotoxicity, hepatotoxicity, thrombocytopenia, coagulopathy	Prolonged infusion, nephrotoxicity, hypophosphatemia	Fever, venous irritation

* Potency is defined as the expected proportion of patients with a serum calcium ≥12.0 mg/dl who will achieve normocalcemia.

to indicate that hypercalcemic patients benefit from routine furosemide treatment. The drug also increases the risk for developing hypovolemia; the resultant decrease in glomerular filtration may actually stimulate renal calcium reabsorption.[90]

The heroic degrees of saline hydration and forced diuresis that comprised past therapy for cancer-related hypercalcemia are no longer indicated.[91] Such treatment frequently results in problems with fluid overload, including life-threatening pulmonary edema and massive weight gain, that are exceptionally difficult to resolve. Except in uncomplicated patients with mild hypercalcemia, fluid administration with or without diuretics should not be solely relied on unless early intervention with systemic anticancer treatment is also contemplated. Treatment with antiresorptive drugs should be initiated promptly after rehydration for control of hypercalcemia in most hospitalized patients.

PHOSPHATES. An increase in serum phosphorus concentration decreases osteoclastic activity, inhibits calcium resorption from bone, and causes a significant reduction in urinary calcium excretion.[92–94] However, administration of exogenous phosphate to hypercalcemic patients also shifts calcium from blood to other tissues, which can result in severe toxicity. Oral phosphate (0.5–3 g/day) may be highly effective, particularly in mild forms of hypercalcemia.[95–98] Principal side effects are diarrhea and nausea, which may lead to noncompliance. For patients with nausea or impaired mental status, phosphate can be administered rectally by retention enema at a dose of 1.5 g twice per day. Serum phosphorus concentrations should be monitored in all patients who receive oral phosphorus, especially patients with decreased renal function or preexisting hyperphosphatemia.[99] Serum creatinine should be regularly monitored to avoid renal insufficiency. When the calcium × phosphorus product (expressed in mg/dl) exceeds 60, phosphates are usually discontinued.

Intravenous phosphate is highly effective, and the onset of hypocalcemic action occurs more rapidly than with any other hypocalcemic therapy.[100,101] However, renal failure, hypotension, extraskeletal calcification, and severe hypocalcemia are common sequelae of parenteral phosphate therapy, and the use of intravenous phosphate has largely been abandoned.[102–106] Although uncommon, these effects have occasionally been seen with oral phosphates.

PROSTAGLANDIN INHIBITORS. Inhibitors of prostaglandin synthesis may reduce serum calcium in some patients, but fewer than 5% of unselected patients with cancer-related hypercalcemia respond to such drugs, and it is not possible to predict which patients will respond based on clinical findings.[107–109] Because most nonsteroidal antiinflammatory drugs decrease renal blood flow, the use of these drugs for treatment of hospitalized patients or those with compromised renal function is not recommended.[110,111]

SULFATE, CITRATE, AND EDTA. Sodium sulfate and sodium citrate have been used to increase natriuresis and to complex with calcium in urine.[112] However, these therapies are associated with substantial toxicity, including hypervolemia, pulmonary edema, and renal failure.[113,114] EDTA (ethanediamine tetraacetate), a calcium chelating agent, has been

associated with a particularly high incidence of renal failure when used in patients with hypercalcemia.[115] These agents are of historical interest only, and their use is no longer recommended.

CORTICOSTEROIDS. Steroids acutely inhibit osteoclast-mediated bone resorption in vitro and decrease gastrointestinal calcium resorption.[116–118] Corticosteroids are most useful in patients whose underlying tumor is responsive to the cytostatic action of these drugs. This group includes patients with myeloma, lymphoma, leukemia, and some patients with carcinoma of the breast, particularly those who have a hypercalcemic flare due to treatment with hormones.[119,120] Steroids do not have consistent hypocalcemic activity in other diseases, and the use of steroids is associated with a variety of undesirable consequences, such as hyperglycemia, hyperosmolar states, gastrointestinal hemorrhage, and osteopenia.[121–123] Prednisone (40–100 mg/day or equivalent) is usually effective in controlling hypercalcemia due to hematologic cancers. Lower doses (15–30 mg/day) may suffice for patients with hypercalcemic flares due to breast cancer.

CALCITONIN. Pharmacologic doses of calcitonin reduce serum calcium by increasing renal calcium excretion and inhibiting bone resorption.[124,125] Calcitonin is especially advantageous due to its rapid onset of action (2–4 hours) and its lack of serious toxicity other than rare hypersensitivity reactions.[126–129] The hypocalcemic effect of calcitonin is relatively weak; the acute response peaks at 48 hours and diminishes thereafter despite continued treatment (*i.e.,* "escape").[130,131] Fewer than 30% of hypercalcemic patients treated with calcitonin as a single agent achieve a normal serum calcium value. Maximally recommended doses of calcitonin (8 IU/kg every 6 hours) should be employed for acute treatment of hypercalcemia. If there is no thrombocytopenia, the drug should be administered intramuscularly rather than subcutaneously to ensure complete absorption. For chronic use, lower doses (4 IU/kg) can be injected subcutaneously once or twice per day on an ambulatory basis. Corticosteroids do not appear to enhance the hypocalcemic effects of calcitonin in patients whose underlying disease is not steroid responsive.[130] Due to its rapid action, calcitonin has been increasingly used in combination with more potent antiresorptive drugs such as gallium nitrate and the bisphosphonates. These combinations may represent optimal treatment of patients with acute severe hypercalcemia.

BISPHOSPHONATES. Bisphosphonates (formerly diphosphonates) are chemical analogs of pyrophosphate. These compounds are not susceptible to hydrolysis by pyrophosphatase and are stable for long periods in vivo. Bisphosphonates adsorb to the surface of crystalline hydroxyapatite and directly inhibit calcium release from bone.[132,133] The main compounds in clinical use are etidronate, clodronate, pamidronate, and alendronate.[134,135]

Oral etidronate has been used for the treatment of Paget's disease of bone and postmenopausal osteoporosis; the drug has also been approved for intravenous therapy of cancer-related hypercalcemia.[136] Reports of the effectiveness of etidronate have varied.[137,138] In a randomized study against saline placebo, normocalcemia was achieved in 27% of patients treated with intravenous etidronate—a degree of potency comparable to calcitonin.[130,139] Etidronate has been compared with gallium nitrate and pamidronate in randomized, double-blind studies; the response to high doses of etidronate in both studies was similar: 43% and 42%, respectively (Fig. 60–4).[140,141] Etidronate is administered intravenously at a maximal dose of 7.5 mg/kg/day for 3 to 5 days. The drug should be given as a slow infusion over 4 hours to avoid renal insufficiency.[142] Similar to all antiresorptive drugs except calcitonin, the drug should not be given until hydration has been initiated and adequate urinary output has been established. Despite the activity of oral etidronate in Paget's disease and osteoporosis, controlled studies do not suggest the oral formulation is useful for prolonging the duration of normocalcemia.[143]

Pamidronate and alendronate are the most potent bisphosphonates currently available. Like etidronate, both of these agents are generally well tolerated. Acute side effects are limited to infusion-site irritation and fever that occurs after the first infusion in approximately 20% of patients. Multiple doses and schedules of pamidronate were employed during its clinical development.[144–147] The recommended dose schedule for pamidronate is 60 mg infused over 24 hours for patients with mild or moderate hypercalcemia. A dose of 90 mg has been recommended for patients with more severe hypercalcemia (total calcium >13.0 mg/dl).[147] The recommended dose of alendronate is 10 or 15 mg, depending on the initial level of serum calcium.[148] Both agents have been used in clinical studies that employed shorter infusion times (2–6 hours) without excessive toxicity.

GALLIUM NITRATE. Gallium nitrate is another potent inhibitor of bone resorption.[149–153] Elemental gallium is incorporated into bone and renders hydroxyapatite less soluble and more resistant to cell-mediated resorption.[154,155] The agent impairs osteoclast acidification of bone matrix by decreasing proton transport across the cell membrane; it may also enhance bone formation by stimulation of bone collagen synthesis and by increasing calcium accretion into bone.[155–157] Two randomized, double-blind studies have demonstrated superiority of gallium nitrate compared with calcitonin and etidronate (see Fig. 60–4B) for acute treatment of resistant hypercalcemia.[130,140] After administration as a continuous intravenous infusion (100–200 mg/m²/day over 24 hours for up to 5 days), gallium nitrate induces normocalcemia in approximately 80% to 90% of patients.[130,140,158] The maximal hypocalcemic effect may occur several days after the drug has been discontinued. In studies using high doses of gallium nitrate for cancer treatment, nephrotoxicity was dose limiting, but the incidence of renal toxicity in studies of hypercalcemia was similar to etidronate and calcitonin and was not appreciably different from the background incidence of renal insufficiency in this disorder.[130,140] Like the bisphosphonates, gallium nitrate should be administered after the patient has been rehydrated. A daily urinary output of 2000 ml should be maintained during the infusion, and highly nephrotoxic drugs such as aminoglycosides and cisplatin should not be administered concurrently.

PLICAMYCIN. Plicamycin (mithramycin) is an antitumor antibiotic with substantial activity in testicular cancer.[159] Hypocalcemia was observed as an unexpected side effect and current use of this agent is limited to treatment of resistant Paget's disease and hypercalcemia.[160–165] Plicamycin acts directly by killing osteoclasts, thereby decreasing cell-mediated bone resorption.[166–168] Plicamycin is administered at doses ranging from 10 to 50 μg per kilogram of body weight. The usual dose is 25 μg/kg or a total dose of 1.5 to 2.0 mg given

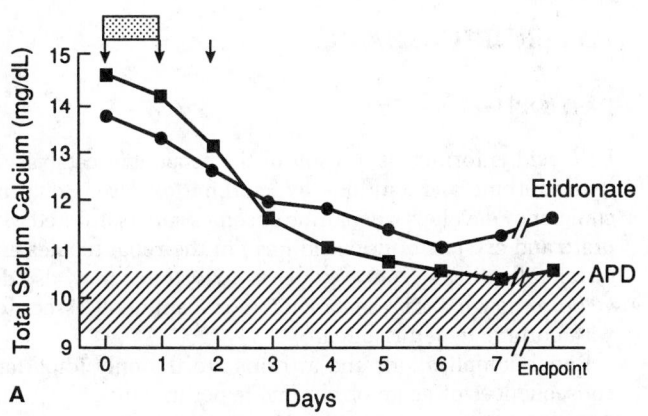
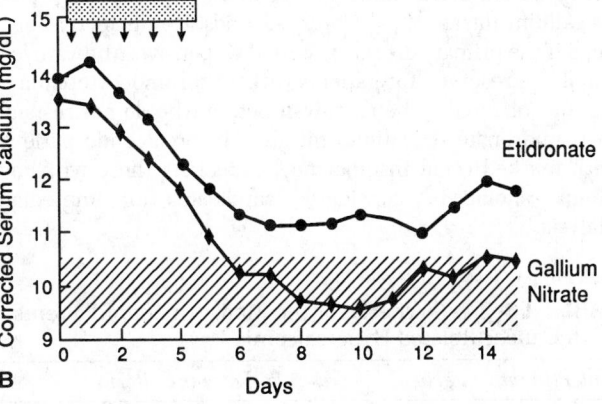

FIGURE 60–4. (A) The top graph shows the relative hypocalcemic effects of pamidronate (APD) compared with etidronate in a randomized, double-blind study. Solid squares represent mean daily concentrations of serum calcium for patients receiving APD; solid circles represent data for patients receiving etidronate. Duration or frequency of infusion times are indicated at the top left; APD was administered as a single 24-hour infusion, and etidronate was administered as a 4-hour infusion daily for 3 days. The normal range for total serum calcium is indicated by the shaded area. (Gucalp R, Ritch P, Wiernik PH, et al. Comparative study of pamidronate disodium and etidronate disodium in the treatment of cancer-related hypercalcemia. J Clin Oncol 1992;10:134–142). (B) The bottom graph shows the relative hypocalcemic effects of gallium nitrate compared with etidronate in a randomized, double-blind study. (Warrell RP Jr, Heller G, Murphy WP, Schulman P, O'Dwyer P. A randomized double-blind study of gallium nitrate compared to etidronate for acute control of cancer-related hypercalcemia. J Clin Oncol 1991;9:1467–1475)

as a brief infusion. Because the onset of action occurs after 24 to 48 hours, doses should not be repeated more frequently than every 2 days. Except for nausea, single injections are generally well tolerated; the incidence of adverse effects (*e.g.*, renal insufficiency, hepatotoxicity, thrombocytopenia, hemorrhagic diathesis) increase with multiple injections.[169]

Management Approach

Patients with hypercalcemia can be grouped according to those who require urgent in-hospital therapy and those for whom out-patient therapy can be considered. Table 60–14 presents a list of considerations that influence this decision. Hospitalization should be considered for any patient with a serum calcium level greater than 12.0 mg/dl or for any patient who is symptomatic. Hospitalization is especially indicated for patients who are dehydrated or who have a significant degree of nausea that precludes increased oral hydration. Hypercalcemia that has evolved slowly may rapidly progress after a patient begins vomiting or if mentation is impaired.

EMERGENCY TREATMENT OF HOSPITALIZED PATIENTS. Intravenous hydration is the initial treatment of choice for all patients who require hospitalization. Furosemide should be given only if diuresis is inadequate or to treat problems related to fluid retention. Most patients with significant hypercalcemia (total calcium ≥12.0 mg/dl) do not respond satisfactorily if acute treatment is limited to intravenous fluids and diuretics, no matter how aggressive. Given the toxicity of aggressive hydration, the use of other newly available antiresorptive drugs should be considered after hydration has been started and satisfactory urinary output established. Calcitonin (4–8 U/kg as an intramuscular injection every 6–8 hours) can be given immediately to provide an immediate but short-lived and incomplete hypocalcemic effect. However, optimal treatment probably combines hydration, calcitonin, with a potent bisphosphonate (pamidronate or alendronate) or gallium nitrate.[170,171] Corticosteroids are distinctly beneficial if the primary disease is steroid responsive. Mithramycin should be reserved for patients without thrombocytopenia or significant renal or hepatic dysfunction who do not respond to pamidronate or gallium nitrate. Hypercalcemic patients with marked renal insufficiency, especially those with myeloma, should be considered candidates for immediate dialysis.[172]

TABLE 60–14. Criteria for the Management of Patients With Cancer-Related Hypercalcemia

Out-Patient Criteria	In-Patient Criteria
Serum calcium <12.0 mg/dl	Serum calcium ≥12.0 mg/dl
No significant nausea	Nausea or vomiting
Able to ingest fluids	Dehydration
Fatigue	Altered mental status
Normal renal function	Renal insufficiency
Stable cardiac rhythm	Cardiac arrhythmia
Mild constipation	Obstipation, ileus
Companion for supervision	Lives alone
Access to emergency care	Limited access to medical care

AMBULATORY MANAGEMENT OF HYPERCALCEMIC PATIENTS. Treatment of ambulatory patients is preferably undertaken in conjunction with specific cytotoxic therapy, such as irradiation or chemotherapy. Certain anticancer drugs (*e.g.*, dactinomycin, doxorubicin, cisplatin) have hypocalcemic actions independent of demonstrable effects on the primary tumor.[173] The hypocalcemic mechanism is the same as with mithramycin: lethal toxicity to bone cells.[174]

Ambulatory patients must receive clear instructions regarding increased oral fluid intake. The amount of fluid should be stated in terms that the patient and family can understand. It is imperative that a family member or companion attend the patient to ensure that nausea due to worsening hypercalcemia does not lead to further dehydration. Diuretics such as furosemide should not be added because the risk of dehydration outweighs theoretical benefits in ambulatory patients who are not edematous. Oral phosphate can be an extremely useful adjunct. One to 3 g/day of oral phosphorus in divided doses are usually well tolerated. Patients who receive phosphorus must not have preexisting hyperphosphatemia nor any significant degree of renal impairment (*e.g.*, creatinine clearance <30 ml/minute). Corticosteroids are helpful if the underlying disease is responsive. Subcutaneous injections of calcitonin (100–200 U/day) may be useful for mild forms of hypercalcemia. Although oral etidronate is probably not effective, intermittent infusions (once per week) of pamidronate or alendronate may be useful for out-patient treatment. Low doses of gallium nitrate (20 mg/m²/day) have been administered with some success after acute normalization with intravenous therapy. Plicamycin can be administered in doses of 10 to 25 μg/kg once or twice weekly. Patients who receive plicamycin therapy as outpatients must be closely monitored for evidence of myelosuppression and for changes in renal or hepatic function.

HYPERURICEMIA

PATHOPHYSIOLOGY

Uric acid is formed as a result of the sequential catalysis of hypoxanthine and xanthine by xanthine oxidase. Renal insufficiency develops when urine becomes supersaturated with urate and crystals of uric acid form in the renal tubules and distal collecting system.[175,176] Uric acid stones may also develop, although this presentation is more commonly associated with chronic hyperuricemia.

Renal complications and arthritis are the only important consequences of acute or chronic hyperuricemia.[177–181] The disorder occurs most commonly in hematologic neoplasms, particularly the leukemias, high-grade lymphomas, and myeloproliferative diseases such as polycythemia vera.[178–181] Acute urate nephropathy has been reported after chemotherapy for solid tumors.[182] Patients at highest risk include those with bulky high-grade lymphomas, patients with high leukocyte counts undergoing remission-induction chemotherapy for acute or chronic leukemia, and persons with preexisting renal impairment, especially those with ureteral obstruction. Hyperuricemia is a side effect of certain agents, notably diuretics (*e.g.*, thiazides, furosemide), antituberculosis drugs (*e.g.*, pyrazinamide, ethambutol, and nicotinic acid), and the cytotoxic agent tiazofurin.[183]

TREATMENT

Recognition of patients at risk is essential for proper therapy. It is essential that prophylactic measures be undertaken *before* cytotoxic therapy is initiated. Drugs that tend to elevate serum urate or that produce an acidic urine (*e.g.*, thiazides, salicylates) should be withdrawn. All patients should receive intravenous hydration to correct preexisting deficits of intravascular volume and to ensure continued urinary output. Increased urinary volume decreases the concentration of urate in urine and minimizes problems with respect to urate solubility.[184] Although furosemide theoretically promotes increased tubular urate reabsorption, this effect is outweighed by its acute diuretic action; the drug can be used to maintain satisfactory urine output if urine volume and electrolytes are monitored and replaced. Alkalinization of the urine should be initiated to maintain a urine pH of 7.0 or higher. Although oral sodium bicarbonate can be used, it is usually simpler to add sodium bicarbonate solution (50–100 mmol/L) to intravenous fluids and adjust the admixture so that an alkaline urine pH is maintained. Acetazolamide, an inhibitor of carbonic anhydrase, may be used to increase the effects of alkalinization. However, it should be recognized that alkalinization is secondary to the overall goal of decreasing urinary uric acid concentration by increasing urinary volume.[230]

The mainstay of current drug therapy is allopurinol.[185,186] Initially developed as a method of cancer treatment, allopurinol was incidentally found to cause hypouricemia, and this indication represents its principal current use.[187,188] Allopurinol inhibits xanthine oxidase and consequently increases plasma and urinary concentrations of xanthine and hypoxanthine. Although xanthine is somewhat more soluble than uric acid, allopurinol has occasionally been associated with renal failure due to xanthine nephropathy.[189,190]

Allopurinol is generally well tolerated. The most common adverse reaction is a blanching, erythematous skin rash that indicates hypersensitivity. The onset of this reaction is usually delayed for several days after initial administration, and the drug can usually be continued throughout periods of greatest risk in patients who have not had prior exposure. In acute situations, the drug is administered orally once or twice daily in total daily doses ranging from 300 to 900 mg. Intravenous allopurinol is available on an investigational basis.[191] The dose of certain drugs (*e.g.*, 6-mercaptopurine) that are metabolized by xanthine oxidase must be substantially reduced during treatment with allopurinol.

Patients in renal failure and allopurinol-sensitive persons represent uncommon but difficult management problems.[192] Azapropazone, merbarone, and benzbromarone are effective hypouricemic drugs that are available on an investigational basis.[193–195] Intravenous administration of uricase has also been useful in certain circumstances.[196] In the face of acute oliguria, ultrasonography or computed tomography (CT) scanning should be used to evaluate possible ureteral obstruction by urate calculi. Administration of intravenous contrast agents for pyelography should be avoided because of an increased risk of acute tubular necrosis.[197] Peritoneal dialysis or hemodialysis are effective in reversing renal failure due to urate deposition.[198]

TUMOR LYSIS SYNDROME

PATHOPHYSIOLOGY

The tumor lysis syndrome occurs as a result of the rapid release of intracellular contents into the bloodstream, which may then increase to life-threatening concentrations. The syndrome is characterized by hyperuricemia, hyperkalemia, hyperphosphatemia, and hypocalcemia. Lethal cardiac arrhythmias are the most serious consequences of hyperkalemia. Hyperphosphatemia may result in acute renal failure.[199–201] Elevated serum phosphorus may decrease renal function, which can further reduce urinary potassium and phosphate excretion. Hypocalcemia—a result of hyperphosphatemia—may cause muscle cramps, cardiac arrhythmias, and tetany.

The tumor lysis syndrome occurs most commonly in diseases with large tumor burdens and high proliferative fractions that are exquisitely sensitive to cytotoxic treatment. These disorders include high-grade lymphomas, leukemias with high leukocyte counts, and much less commonly, solid tumors.[202–209] The syndrome has been observed with agents that have potent myelosuppressive activity and with drugs such as interferon-α, tamoxifen, and intrathecal methotrexate.[210–212] Although technically not related to tumor lysis, severe hypocalcemia has been associated with cisplatin treatment, estrogenic treatment of prostate cancer, and accelerated bone formation in patients with leukemia.[213–215]

TREATMENT

Recognition of risk and prevention are essential to management. Patients at risk should be identified before the initiation of chemotherapy. If possible, intravenous hydration should be started 24 to 48 hours before the administration of chemotherapy. Any acid-base or electrolyte disorders should be corrected, although intravenous administration of sodium bicarbonate may aggravate symptoms of hypocalcemia. Treatment with allopurinol should be undertaken with other measures to minimize hyperuricemia as described previously. Serum electrolytes, uric acid, phosphorus, calcium, and creatinine should be checked repeatedly for 3 to 4 days after initiating cytotoxic treatment. The frequency of monitoring depends on the clinical condition of the patient. If hyperkalemia or hypocalcemia become evident, an electrocardiogram should be obtained, and the cardiac rhythm should be monitored while these abnormalities are corrected. Hypocalcemia can be corrected with intravenous administration of calcium gluconate, but hypocalcemia may persist for several days despite continued therapy. Hyperkalemia (serum $[K^+] \geq 5.0$ mg/dl) should be treated with an oral sodium-potassium exchange resin (*e.g.*, 15 g of Kayexalate given orally every 6 hours) or with combined insulin and glucose therapy.

In the face of acutely worsening renal function after administration of chemotherapy, consideration should be given to *early* initiation of renal dialysis to rapidly control serum concentrations of potassium, calcium, phosphate, and uric acid and other problems related to uremia. The dose of many drugs, especially antineoplastics, requires substantial modification for renal insufficiency.[216]

HYPOGLYCEMIA

Insulin-producing islet cell tumors are the most frequent cause of hypoglycemia in patients with cancer, but more than 250 cases of hypoglycemia associated with non-islet cell tumors have been reported.[217,218] Non-islet cell tumors associated with hypoglycemia tend to be large. Mesenchymal tumors (*e.g.*, fibrosarcomas, leiomyomas, rhabdomyosarcomas, liposarcomas, mesotheliomas) comprise approximately 50% of cases; another 25% are hepatomas.[217] Classic symptoms of hypoglycemia (*e.g.*, weakness, dizziness, diaphoresis, nausea) are nonspecific and may develop slowly. In the initial phases, symptoms tend to be worse in the early morning due to overnight fasting and improve after ingestion of food. However, patients may present with seizures, coma, and focal or diffuse neurologic deficits.

PATHOPHYSIOLOGY

Several etiologic mechanisms for cancer-related hypoglycemia have been proposed: secretion of insulin-like substances; excessive glucose use by the tumor that exceeds hepatic production; and failure of counter-regulatory mechanisms that usually prevent hypoglycemia. Substances with nonsuppressible insulin-like activities (NSILAs) have been detected in serum from patients with hypoglycemia. These factors are composed of two general classes: relatively low-molecular-weight substances that are soluble in acid and ethanol, and high-molecular-weight substances that are acid-ethanol precipitable. The low-molecular-weight compounds consist of four peptides, the insulin-like growth factors (*e.g.*, IGF-I, IGF-II, somatomedin A, somatomedin C).[219–221] IGF-I and II share a high degree of amino acid similarity with proinsulin, but they do not react with antiinsulin antibodies, and they have only 1% to 2% of the specific metabolic activity of insulin.[220] The NSILAs with high molecular weights are less well characterized.[222] Approximately 40% of cancer patients with symptomatic hypoglycemia have elevated plasma levels of low-molecular-weight NSILAs.[218,223] These observations suggested that humoral mechanisms (*i.e.*, tumor production of IGFs) might be responsible for hypoglycemia in a significant proportion of patients.

Accelerated glucose use by large tumors could account for cancer-related hypoglycemia. It has been estimated that a 1 kg tumor may use 50 to 200 g of glucose daily.[224] Because the liver can produce approximately 700 g of glucose daily, hepatic production should theoretically be sufficient to prevent hypoglycemia. However, many patients with hypoglycemia have primary tumors that weigh several kilograms and extensive hepatic metastases; the combination of accelerated glucose use with impaired production may lead to hypoglycemia.

Failure of the usual counter-regulatory mechanisms in patients with large tumors may induce hypoglycemia.[225] Impaired liver function can decrease glycogenolysis and gluconeogenesis. Certain patients with cancer have a depressed hyperglycemic response to the administration of glucagon; depressed secretion of counter-regulatory hormones such as glucagon, ACTH, glucocorticoids, and growth hormone has been reported. Insufficient data currently exist to establish the importance of these mechanisms as independent causes of hypoglycemia.

TREATMENT

The therapy for hypoglycemia should match the severity of the condition. As with most paraneoplastic syndromes, specific antitumor therapy is the preferred treatment. Chemotherapeutic agents that are cytotoxic for islet cells or that block insulin release or activity have had little effect on production, release, or activity of NSILAs. Mild hypoglycemia can usually be managed by increasing the frequency of meals. In patients with more severe or unpredictable symptoms, the administration of corticosteroids and glucagon may afford symptomatic relief. Intravenous infusions of glucose provide temporary support while other specific treatment (*e.g.*, surgery, chemotherapy, irradiation) is administered. Under certain circumstances, continuous infusions of glucagon using portable pumps have been used with some success.[226]

ADRENAL FAILURE

Symptomatic adrenocortical insufficiency due to destruction of cortical tissue by metastatic carcinoma is uncommon. More common are iatrogenic causes, such as surgical adrenalectomy, treatment with mitotane and inhibitors of steroid synthesis like aminoglutethimide, and chronic corticosteroid therapy.[227,228] Nonetheless, technical improvements in CT and magnetic resonance imaging have increased the likelihood of making an antemortem diagnosis of adrenal metastases. In one study, 19% of patients with metastatic cancer and enlargement of the adrenal glands detected by CT scans developed symptoms of adrenal insufficiency.[229] In a separate study in which 15 patients with metastatic cancer and adrenal enlargement on CT scan were evaluated by ACTH stimulation, one third were judged to have adrenal insufficiency. Further clinical study revealed symptoms of nausea, anorexia, and orthostatic hypotension in all of these patients.[230] Adrenal insufficiency may develop insidiously in patients with adrenal metastasis, and CT scans and ACTH testing may be useful diagnostic tools.

CLINICAL MANIFESTATIONS

Classic signs and symptoms of adrenal insufficiency include weakness, weight loss, anorexia, hyperpigmentation, and postural hypotension. At least one of these symptoms is evident in most patients, but the onset of symptoms is frequently insidious. Circulatory collapse and shock are uncommon but may develop with the onset of infection. Biochemical evaluation frequently reveals a mild acidosis without an anion gap, hyponatremia, and hypokalemia.

EVALUATION AND TREATMENT

Because an ACTH-stimulation test is a benign procedure, this test is recommended when symptoms suggestive of adrenal insufficiency are evident. Typically, patients receive Cosyntropin (0.25 mg intravenously), and serum cortisol is monitored at baseline, 30 minutes, and 1 hour. An increase in serum cortisol of 5 to 7 μg/dl over baseline levels (to a minimum of 15 μg/ml) is considered normal. If adrenal insufficiency is strongly suspected on clinical grounds, steroid replacement or stress doses of steroids should be started immediately, and subsequent therapy can be reevaluated after results of the ACTH test become available.

Physiologic glucocorticoid replacement is attained by administration of cortisone acetate (25 mg in the morning and 12.5 mg in the early evening). During periods of stress (*e.g.*, operative procedures, infection), these doses may need to be doubled or tripled. Occasionally, mineralocorticoid replacement (*e.g.*, 0.05–0.1 mg of fludrocortisone) is required in addition to cortisone acetate. In patients with no adrenocortical function whatsoever, maintenance doses of dexamethasone or prednisone do not provide adequate mineralocorticoid coverage, and fludrocortisone must be given. Pharmacologic doses of parenteral glucocorticoids are required in the setting of acute adrenal failure and circulatory collapse. Typically, aqueous-soluble forms of hydrocortisone (*e.g.*, sodium succinate salt) at doses of 100 mg intravenously every 8 hours are required. Thereafter, the patient should be monitored for evidence of hyperglycemia, hypokalemia, or hypernatremia.

LACTIC ACIDOSIS

Lactic acidosis is a rare but potentially severe metabolic complication in patients with cancer. Type A lactic acidosis is due to impaired delivery of oxygen to peripheral tissue and is commonly seen with shock and septicemia. Type B lactic acidosis is associated with a variety of diseases, including diabetes, renal failure, liver disease, infection, and cancer, and with drugs, toxins, and hereditary conditions.[231–234] Lactic acidosis is characterized by decreased arterial pH (<7.37) secondary to accumulation of blood lactate (>2 mEq/L). The disorder is a consequence of increased lactate production and impaired use. Lactate is a metabolite of pyruvate and is produced in a cytosolic reaction catalyzed by lactic dehydrogenase—an enzyme with an absolute requirement for nicotinamide adenine dinucleotide (NAD). Consequently, the concentrations of pyruvate, hydrogen ion, and NAD regulate lactate metabolism. Accelerated glycogenolysis increases pyruvate production and decreases tissue oxygen, which decreases levels of NAD. As NAD is depleted, gluconeogenesis is halted and pyruvate increases. Anaerobic metabolism of pyruvate to lactate is increased, which leads to accumulation of NADH and hydrogen ions.

Sculier and colleagues reviewed 25 cases of lactic acidosis in which the underlying tumor was believed to represent the primary etiologic factor.[235] More than two thirds of these cases were associated with leukemia or lymphoma, and the remainder were associated with various solid tumors. The development of lactic acidosis coincided with the onset of progressive disease, and most patients with solid tumors had extensive liver metastases. Typically, the patient with lactic acidosis presents with hyperventilation and hypotension. Nonspecific clinical symptoms such as tachycardia, weakness, nausea, and stupor may proceed to frank shock as the acidosis worsens. Laboratory studies show decreased blood pH, a widened anion gap, and a low serum bicarbonate level.

The prognosis for patients with a serum lactate concentration greater than 4 mEq/L is exceedingly poor, but the outcome is largely determined by the underlying disease and not the acidosis. Several reports suggested that administration of sodium bicarbonate increases production of lactate and

CO_2 and impairs oxygen delivery without improving survival.[236–239] Detrimental effects of severe acidemia on cardiovascular function can probably be ameliorated by bicarbonate administration, and this temporizing measure may be useful while effective anticancer therapy is attempted.[240–244]

REFERENCES

1. Fisken RA, Heath DA, Bold AM. Hypercalcemia—a hospital survey. Q J Med 1980;49:405–418.
2. Mundy GR. Primary hyperparathyroidism: Changes in the pattern of clinical presentation. Lancet 1980;1:1317–1320.
3. Brada M, Rowley M, Grant DJ, Ashley S, Powles TJ. Hypercalcemia in patients with disseminated breast cancer. Acta Oncol 1990;29:577–580.
4. Bender RA, Hanson H. Hypercalcemia in bronchogenic carcinoma: A prospective study of 200 patients. Ann Intern Med 1974;80:205–208.
5. Coggeshall J, Merrill W, Hande K, Des Prez R. Implications of hypercalcemia with respect to diagnosis and treatment of lung cancer. Am J Med 1986;80:325–328.
6. Hayward ML Jr, Howell DA, O'Donnell JF, Maurer LH. Hypercalcemia complicating small cell carcinoma. Cancer 1981;48:1643–1646.
7. Strewler GJ, Nissenson RA. Nonparathyroid hypercalcemia. Adv Intern Med 1987;32:235–258.
8. Insogna KL, Broadus AE. Hypercalcemia of malignancy. Annu Rev Med 1987;38:241–256.
9. Boyd JC, Ladenson JH. Value of laboratory tests in the differential diagnosis of hypercalcemia. Am J Med 1984;77:863–872.
10. Lafferty FW. Differential diagnosis of hypercalcemia. J Bone Miner Res 1991;6(suppl 2):S51–S59.
11. Heath HH III, Hodgson SF, Kenedy MA. Primary hyperparathyroidism: Incidence, morbidity, and potential economic impact on the community. N Engl J Med 1980;302:189–193.
12. Axelrod DM, Bockman RS, Wong GY, Osborne MP, Kinne DW, Brennan MF. Distinguishing features of primary hyperparathyroidism in patients with breast cancer Cancer 1987;60:60:1620–1624.
13. Wills MR. Value of plasma chloride concentration and acid-base status in the differential diagnosis of hyperparathyroidism from other causes of hypercalcaemia. J Clin Pathol 1971;24:219–227.
14. Lufkin EG, Kao PC, Heath H. Parathyroid hormone radioimmunoassays in the differential diagnosis of hypercalcemia due to primary hyperparathyroidism or malignancy. Ann Intern Med 1987;106:559–560.
15. Watson L, Moxham J, Fraser P. Hydrocortisone suppression test and discriminant analysis in differential diagnosis of hypercalcemia. Lancet 1980;1:1320–1325.
16. Ratcliffe WA, Hutcheson ACJ, Bundred NJ, Ratcliffe JG. Role of assays for parathyroid hormone-related protein in investigation of hypercalcaemia. Lancet 1992;339:164–167.
17. Nussbaum SR, Potts JT Jr. Immunoassays for parathyroid hormone 1-84 in the diagnosis of hyperparathyroidism. J Bone Miner Res 1991;6(suppl 2):S43–S50.
18. Hazani A, Silvian I, Tatarsky I, Spira G. Non-symptomatic hypercalcemia in a myeloma patient. Am J Med Sci 1982;283:169–273.
19. Annesley TM, Burritt MF, Kyle RA. Artifactual hypercalcemia in multiple myeloma. Mayo Clin Proc 1982;57:572–575.
20. Payne RB, Carver ME, Morgan DB. Interpretation of serum total calcium: Effects of adjustment for albumin concentration on frequency of abnormal values and on detection of change in the individual. J Clin Pathol 1979;32:56–60.
21. Rizzoli R, Caverzasia J, Fleisch H, Bonjour JP. Parathyroid hormone-like changes in renal calcium and phosphate reabsorption induced by Leydig cell tumor in thyroparathyroidectomized rats. Endocrinology 1986;119:1004–1009.
22. Stewart AF, Horst R, Deftos LJ, Cadman EC, Lang R, Broadus AE. Biochemical evaluation of patients with cancer-associated hypercalcemia: Evidence for humoral and non-humoral groups. N Engl J Med 1980;303:1377–1383.
23. Kukreja SC, Shemerdiak WP, Lad TE, et al. Elevated nephrogenous cyclic AMP with normal serum parathyroid hormone levels in patients with lung cancer. J Clin Endocrinol Metab 1980;52:765–771.
24. Skrabanek P, McPartlin J, Powell D. Tumor hypercalcemia and "ectopic hyperparathyroidism." Medicine (Baltimore) 1980;59:262–282.
25. Simpson EL, Mundy GR, D'Souza SM, Ibbotson KJ, Bockman RS, Jacobs JW. Absence of parathyroid messenger RNA in nonparathyroid tumors associated with hypercalcemia. N Engl J Med 1983;309:325–330.
26. Nussbaum SR, Gaz RD, Arnold A. Hypercalcemia and ectopic secretion of parathyroid hormone by an ovarian carcinoma with rearrangement of the gene for parathyroid hormone. N Engl J Med 1990;323:1324–1328.
27. Strewler GJ, Budayr AA, Bruce RJ, Clark OH, Nissenson RA. Secretion of authentic parathyroid hormone by a malignant tumor. Clin Res 1990;38:462A.
28. Broadus AC, Goltzman D, Webb AC, Kronenberg HM. Messenger ribonucleic acid from tumors associated with humoral hypercalcemia of malignancy directs the synthesis of a secretory parathyroid hormone-like peptide. Endocrinology 1985;117:1661–1666.
29. Strewler GJ, Williams RJ, Nissenson RA. Human renal carcinoma cells produce hypercalcemia in the nude mouse and a novel protein recognized by parathyroid hormone receptors. J Clin Invest 1983;71:769–774.
30. Burtis WJ, Wu T, Bunch C, et al. Identification of a novel 17,000-dalton parathyroid

hormone-like adenylate cyclase-stimulating protein from a tumor associated with humoral hypercalcemia of malignancy. J Biol Chem 1987;262:7151–7156.

31. Moseley JM, Kubota M, Dieffenbach-Jagger H, et al. Parathyroid hormone-related protein purified from a human lung cancer cell line. Proc Natl Acad Sci USA 1987;84:5048–5052.

32. Suva LJ, Winslow GA, Wettenhall REH, et al. A parathyroid hormone-related protein implicated in malignant hypercalcemia: Cloning and expression. Science 1987;237:894–897.

33. Mangin M, Webb AC, Dreyer BE, et al. Identification of a cDNA encoding a parathyroid hormone-like peptide from a human tumor associated with humoral hypercalcemia of malignancy. Proc Natl Acad Sci USA 1988;85:597–601.

34. Mangin M, Ikeda K, Dreyer BE, Broadus AE. Isolation and characterization of the human parathyroid hormone-like peptide gene. Proc Natl Acad Sci USA 1989;86:2408–2412.

35. Abou-Samra AB, Jueppner H, Freeman MW, et al. Expression and cloning of the parathyroid hormone (PTH) bone receptor cDNA. Clin Res 1991;39:342A.

36. Merendino JJ Jr, Insogna KL, Milstone LM, Broadus AC, Stewart AF. A parathyroid hormone-like protein from cultured human keratinocytes. Science 1986;231:288–290.

37. Weir EC, Brines ML, Ikeda K, Burtis WJ, Broadus AE, Robbins RJ. Parathyroid hormone-related peptide gene is expressed in the mammalian central nervous system. Proc Natl Acad Sci USA 1990;87:108–112.

38. Broadus AE, Mangin M, Ikeda K, et al. Humoral hypercalcemia of cancer. Identification of a novel parathyroid hormone-like peptide. N Engl J Med 1988;319:556–562.

39. Thiede MA, Rodan GA. Expression of a calcium-mobilizing parathyroid hormone-like peptide in lactating mammary tissue. Science 1988;242:278–280.

40. Thiede MA, Daifotis AG, Weir EC, et al. Intrauterine occupancy controls expression of the parathyroid hormone-related peptide gene in preterm rat myometrium. Proc Natl Acad Sci USA 1990;87:6969–6973.

41. Burtis WJ, Brady TG, Orloff JJ, et al. Immunochemical characterization of circulating parathyroid hormone-related protein in patients with humoral hypercalcemia of cancer. N Engl J Med 1990;322:1106–1112.

42. Budayr AA, Nissenson RA, Klein RF, et al. Increased serum levels of a parathyroid hormone-like protein in malignancy-associated hypercalcemia. Ann Intern Med 1989;111:807–812.

43. Henderson JE, Shustic C, Kremer R, Rabbani SA, Hendy GN, Goltzman D. Circulating concentrations of parathyroid hormone-like peptide in malignancy and hyperparathyroidism. J Bone Miner Res 1990;5:105–113.

44. Insogna KL. Humoral hypercalcemia of malignancy. The role of parathyroid hormone-related protein. Endocr Metab Clin North Am 1989;18:779–794.

45. Kao PC, Klee GG, Taylor RL, Heath H. Parathyroid hormone-related peptide in plasma of patients with hypercalcemia and malignant lesions. Mayo Clin Proc 1990;65:1399–1407.

46. Motokura T, Fukumoto S, Matsumoto T, et al. Parathyroid hormone-related protein in adult T-cell leukemia-lymphoma. Ann Intern Med 1989;111:484–488.

47. Southby J, Kissin MW, Danks JA, et al. Immunohistochemical localization of parathyroid hormone-related protein in human breast cancer. Cancer Res 1990;50:7710–7716.

48. Powell GJ, Southby J, Danks JA, et al. Localization of parathyroid hormone-related protein in breast cancer metastases: Increased incidence in bone compared with other sites. Cancer Res 1991;51:3059–3061.

49. Seyberth HW, Segre GV, Morgan JL, Sweetman BJ, Potts JT Jr, Oates JA. Prostaglandins as mediators of hypercalcemia associated with certain types of cancer. N Engl J Med 1975;293:1278–1283.

50. Tashjian AH Jr. Prostaglandins, hypercalcemia and cancer. N Engl J Med 1975;293:1317–1318.

51. Tashjian AH Jr, Tice JE, Sides R. Biological activities of prostaglandin analogues and metabolites on bone resorption in vitro. Nature 1977;266:645–647.

52. Raisz LG, Dietrich JW, Simmons HA, et al. Effects of prostaglandin endoperoxides and metabolites on bone resorption in vitro. Nature 1977;267:532–535.

53. Valentin-Opran A, Eilon G, Saez S, et al. Estrogens and antiestrogens stimulate release of bone-resorbing activity by cultured human breast cancer cells. J Clin Invest 1985;75:726.

54. Brenner BE, Harvey HA, Lipton A, Demers L. A study of prostaglandin E₂, parathormone, and response to indomethacin in patients with hypercalcemia of malignancy. Cancer 1982;49:556–561.

55. Metz SA, McRae JR, Robertson RP. Prostaglandins as mediators of paraneoplastic syndromes: Review and update. Metabolism 1981;30:299–316.

56. Robertson RB, Baylink DJ, Metz SA, Cummings KB. Plasma prostaglandin E in patients with cancer with and without hypercalcemia. J Clin Endocrinol Metab 1976;43:1330–1335.

57. Lau K-HW, Lee MY, Linkhart TA, et al. A mouse tumor-derived osteolytic factor stimulates bone resorption by a mechanism involving local prostaglandins production in bone. Biochim Biophys Acta 1985;840:56–68.

58. Bringhurst FR, Bierer BE, Godeau F, Neyhard N, Varner V, Segre GV. Humoral hypercalcemia of malignancy: Release of a prostaglandin-stimulating bone resorbing factor in vitro by human transitional-cell carcinoma cells. J Clin Invest 1986;77:456–464.

59. Mundy RR, Raisz LG, Cooper RA, Schechter GP, Salmon SE. Evidence for the secretion of an osteoclast stimulating factor in myeloma. N Engl J Med 1974;291:1041–1046.

60. Mundy GR, Luben RA, Raisz LG, Oppenheim JJ, Buell DN. Bone-resorbing activity in supernatants from lymphoid cell lines. N Engl J Med 1974;290:867–871.

61. Sporn MB, Roberts AB. Autocrine growth factors and cancer. Nature 1985;313:745–747.

62. Todaro GJ, Fryling C, De Larco JE. Transforming growth factors produced by certain human tumor cells: Polypeptides that interact with epidermal growth factor receptors. Proc Natl Acad Sci USA 1980;77:5258–5262.

63. Ibbotson KJ, Twardzik DR, D'Souza SM, et al. Stimulation of bone resorption in vitro by synthetic transforming growth factor-alpha. Science 1985;228:1007–1009.

64. Stern PH, Krieger NS, Nissenson RA, et al. Human transforming growth factor-alpha stimulates bone resorption in vitro. J Clin Invest 1985;76:2016–2019.

65. Sporn MB, Roberts AB, Wakefield LM, de Crombrugghe B. Some recent advances in the chemistry and biology of transforming growth factor-beta. J Cell Biol 1987;105:1039–1045.

66. Robey PG, Young MF, Flanders KC, et al. Osteoblasts synthesize and respond to TGF-beta in vitro. J Cell Biol 1987;105:457–463.

67. Gowen G, Wood DD, Ihrie EJ, McGuire MKB, Russell RGG. An interleukin 1-like factor stimulates bone resorption in vitro. Nature 1983;306:378–380.

68. Dewhirst FE, Stashenko PP, Mole JE, et al. Purification and partial sequence of human osteoclast activating factor: Identity with interleukin-1 beta. J Immunol 1985;135:2562–2568.

69. Stashenko P, Dewhirst FE, Peros WJ, Kent RL, Ago JM. Synergistic interactions between interleukin-1, tumor necrosis factor, and lymphotoxin in bone resorption. J Immunol 1987;138:1464–1468.

70. Mundy GR, Ibbotson KJ, D'Souza DM. Tumor products and the hypercalcemia of malignancy. J Clin Invest 1985;76:391–394.

71. Lee MY, Liu CC, Lottsfeldt JL, Judkins SA, Howard GA. Production of granulocyte-stimulating and bone cell-modulating activities from a neutrophilia hypercalcemia-inducing murine mammary cancer cell line. Cancer Res 1987;47:4059–4065.

72. Sato K, Mimura H, Han DC, et al. Production of bone-resorbing activity and colony-stimulating activity in vivo and in vitro by a human squamous cell carcinoma associated with hypercalcemia and leukocytosis. J Clin Invest 1986;78:145–154.

73. Bertolini DR, Nedwin GE, Bringman TS, Smith DD, Mundy GR. Stimulation of bone resorption and inhibition of bone formation in vitro by human tumor necrosis factors. Nature 1986;319:516–518.

74. Garrett IR, Durie BGM, Nedwin GE, et al. Production of lymphotoxin, a bone-resorbing cytokine, by cultured human myeloma cells. N Engl J Med 1987;317:526–532.

75. Davies M, Mawer EB, Hayes ME, Lumb GA. Abnormal vitamin D metabolism in Hodgkin's lymphoma. Lancet 1985;1:1186–1188.

76. Rieke JW, Donaldson SS, Horning SJ. Hypercalcemia and vitamin D metabolism in Hodgkin's disease. Is there an underlying immunoregulatory relationship? Cancer 1989;63:1700–1707.

77. Breslau NA, McGuire JL Zerwekh JE, Frenkel EP, Pak CYC. Hypercalcemia associated with increased serum calcitriol levels in three patients with lymphoma. Ann Intern Med 1984;100:1–7.

78. Adams JS, Fernandez M, Gacad MA, et al. Hypercalcemia and hypercalciuria associated elevated serum 1,25-dihydroxyvitamin D concentrations in patients with AIDS and non-AIDS-related lymphoma. Blood 1989;73:235–239.

79. Helikson MA, Harvey AD, Zerwekh JE, Breslau NA, Gardner DW. Plasma cell granuloma producing calcitriol and hypercalcemia. Ann Intern Med 1986;105:379–381.

80. Shigeno H, Yamamoto I, Dokoh S, et al. Identification of 1,24-(R)-dihydroxyvitamin D₃-like-bone-resorbing lipid in a patient with cancer-associated hypercalcemia. J Clin Endocrinol Metab 1985;61:761–768.

81. Stote RM, Smith LH, Wilson DM, et al. Hydrochlorothiazide effects on serum calcium and immunoreactive parathyroid hormone concentration: Studies in normal subjects. Ann Intern Med 1972;77:587–591.

82. Mawer EB, Hann JT, Berry JL, et al. Vitamin D metabolism in patients intoxicated with ergocalciferol. Clin Sci 1985;68:135–141.

83. Katz CM, Tzagournis M. Chronic adult hypervitaminosis A with hypercalcemia. Metabolism 1972;21:1171–1176.

84. Valentic JP, Elias AN, Weinstein GD. Hypercalcemia associated with oral isotretinoin in the treatment of severe acne. JAMA 1983;250:1899–1900.

85. Warrell RP Jr. Questions about clinical trials in hypercalcemia. J Clin Oncol [Editorial] 1988;6:759–761.

86. Blythe WB, Gitelman HJ, Welt LG. Effect of expansion of the extracellular space on the rate of urinary excretion of calcium. Am J Physiol 1968;214:52–57.

87. Massry SG, Coburn JW, Chapman LW, et al. Effect of NaCl infusions on urinary Ca⁺⁺ and Mg⁺⁺ during reduction in their filtered loads. Am J Physiol 1967;213:1218–1224.

88. Massry SG, Friedler RM, Coburn JW Excretion of phosphate and calcium: Physiology of their renal handling and relation to clinical medicine. Arch Intern Med 1973;131:828–836.

89. Hosking DJ, Cowley A, Bucknall CA. Rehydration in the treatment of severe hypercalcemia. Q J Med 1981;200:473–481.

90. Suki WN, Hull HR, Rector FC Jr, et al. Mechanism of the effect of thiazide diuretics on calcium and uric acid. J Clin Invest 1967;46:1121.

91. Suki WN, Yium JJ, Von Minden M, et al. Acute treatment of hypercalcemia with furosemide. N Engl J Med 1970;283:836–840.

92. Yates AJ, Oreffo ROC, Mayor K, Mundy GR. Inhibition of bone resorption by inorganic phosphate is mediated by both reduced osteoclast formation and decreased activity of mature osteoclasts. J Bone Miner Res 1991;6:473–478.

93. Herbert LA, Lemann J, Peterson JR, et al. Studies of the mechanism by which phosphate infusion lowers serum calcium concentration. J Clin Invest 1966;45:1886–1894.

94. Eisenberg E. Effect of intravenous phosphate on serum strontium and calcium. N Engl J Med 1970;282:889–892.

95. Spaulding SW, Walser M. Treatment of experimental hypercalcemia with oral phosphate. J Clin Endocrinol 1970;31:531–538.

96. Mundy GR, Wilkinson R, Heath DA. Comparative study of available medical therapy for hypercalcemia of malignancy. Am J Med 1983;74:421–432.

97. Heath DA. The use of inorganic phosphate in the management of hypercalcemia. Metab Bone Dis Rel Res 1980;2:213–215.

98. Thalassinos N, Joplin GF. Phosphate treatment of hypercalcemia due to carcinoma. Br Med J 1968;4:14–19.

99. Ayala G, Chertow BS, Shah JH, et al. Acute hyperphosphatemia and acute persistent renal insufficiency induced by oral phosphate therapy. Ann Intern Med 1975;83:520–521.

100. Goldsmith RS, Ingbar SH. Inorganic phosphate in the treatment of hypercalcemia of diverse etiologies. N Engl J Med 1966;274:1–7.

101. Massry SG, Mueller E, Silverman AG, et al. Inorganic phosphate treatment of hypercalcemia. Arch Intern Med 1968;121:307–312.

102. Shackney S, Hasson J. Precipitous fall in serum calcium, hypotension, and acute renal failure after intravenous phosphate therapy for hypercalcemia: Report of two cases. Ann Intern Med 1967;66:906–916.

103. Carey RW, Schmott GW, Kopald HH, et al. Massive extraskeletal calcification during phosphate treatment of hypercalcemia. Arch Intern Med 1968;122:150–155.

104. Dudley FJ, Blackburn CRB. Extraskeletal calcification complicating oral neutral phosphate therapy. Lancet 1970;2:628–630.

105. Laflamme GH, Jowsey J. Bone and soft tissue changes with oral phosphate supplements. J Clin Invest 1972;51:2834–2840.

106. Breuer RI, LeBauer J. Caution in the use of phosphates in the treatment of severe hypercalcemia. J Clin Endocrinol Metab 1967;27:695–698.

107. Seyberth HW, Segre GV, Hamet P, Sweetman BJ, Potts JT Jr, Oates JA. Characterization of the group of patients with the hypercalcemia of cancer who respond to treatment with prostaglandin synthesis inhibitors. Trans Assoc Am Physicians 1976;89:92–104.

108. Brenner DE, Harvey HA, Lipton A. A study of prostaglandin E₂, parathormone, and response to indomethacin in patients with hypercalcemia. Cancer 1982;49:556–561.

109. Coombes RC, Neville AM, Bondy PK, et al. Failure of indomethacin to reduce hydroxyproline excretion or hypercalcemia in patients with breast cancer. Prostaglandins 1976;12:1027–1035.

110. Sandler DP, Burr R, Weinberg CR. Nonsteroidal anti-inflammatory drugs and the risk for chronic renal disease. Ann Intern Med 1991;115:165–172.

111. Whelton A, Stout RL, Spilman PS, Klassen DK. Renal effects of ibuprofen, piroxicam, and sulindac in patients with asymptomatic renal failure. A prospective, randomized, crossover comparison. Ann Intern Med 1990;112:568–576.

112. Chakmajian ZH, Bethune JE. Sodium sulfate treatment of hypercalcemia. N Engl J Med 1966;275:862–869.

113. Heckman BA, Walsh JH. Hypernatremia complicating sodium sulfate therapy for hypercalcemic crisis. N Engl J Med 1967;276:1082–1083.

114. Kahill M, Orman B, Gyorkey F, Brown H. Hypercalcemia—experience with phosphate and sulphate therapy. JAMA 1967;201:721–724.

115. Spencer H, Greenberg J, Berger E, Perrone M, Laszlo D. Studies on the effect of ethylenediaminetetraacetic acid in hypercalcemia. J Lab Clin Med 1956;47:29–41.

116. Raisz LG, Trummel CL, Wener JA, et al. Effect of glucocorticoids on bone resorption in tissue culture. Endocrinology 1972;90:961–967.

117. Bentzel CJ, Carbone PP, Rosenberg L. The effect of prednisone on calcium metabolism and ⁴⁷Ca kinetics in patients with multiple myeloma and hypercalcemia. J Clin Invest 1964;43:2132–2145.

118. Kimberg DB, Baerg RD, Gershon E, et al. Effect of cortisone treatment on the active transport of calcium by the small intestine. J Clin Invest 1971;50:1309–1321.

119. Muggia FM, Heinemann HO. Hypercalcemia associated with malignant disease. Ann Intern Med 1970;73:281–290.

120. Myers WPL. Cortisone in the treatment of hypercalcemia in neoplastic disease. Cancer 1958;11:83–88.

121. Percival RC, Yates AJP, Grey RES, et al. Role of glucocorticoids in the management of malignant hypercalcemia. Br Med J 1984;289:287.

122. Ashkar FS, Miller R, Katins RB. Effect of corticosteroids on the hypercalcemia of malignant disease. Lancet 1971;1:41.

123. Thalassinos NC, Joplin G. Failure of corticosteroid therapy to direct the hypercalcemia of malignant disease. Lancet 1970;2:537–538.

124. Austin LA, Heath H III. Calcitonin: Physiology and pathophysiology. N Engl J Med 1981;304:269–278.

125. Krane SM, Harris ED Jr, Singer FR, et al. Acute effects of calcitonin on bone formation in man. Metabolism 1973;22:51–58.

126. Vaughn CB, Vaitkevicius K. The effects of calcitonin in hypercalcemia in patients with malignancy. Cancer 1974;34:1268–1271.

127. Hosking DJ. Treatment of severe hypercalcemia with calcitonin. Metab Bone Dis Rel Res 1980;2:207–212.

128. Wisneski LA, Groom WP, Silva DL, Becker KL. Salmon calcitonin in hypercalcemia. Clin Pharmacol Ther 1978;23:219–222.

129. Wisneski LA. Salmon calcitonin in the acute management of hypercalcemia. Calcif Tissue Int 1990;46:S26–S30.

130. Warrell RP Jr, Israel R, Frisone M, Snyder T, Gaynor JJ, Bockman RS. A randomized double-blind study of gallium nitrate versus calcitonin for acute treatment of cancer-related hypercalcemia. Ann Intern Med 1988;108:669–674.

131. Wener JA, Gorton SJ, Raisz LG. Escape from inhibition of resorption in cultures of fetal bone treated with calcitonin and parathyroid hormone. Endocrinology 1978;90:752–759.

132. Reitsma PH, Teitelbaum SL, Bijvoet OLM, Kahn AJ. Differential action of the bisphosphonates (3-amino-1-hydroxypropylidene)-1,1-biphosphonate (APD) and disodium dichloromethylidene biphosphonate (Cl₂MDP) on rat macrophage-mediated bone resorption in vitro. J Clin Invest 1982;70:927–933.

133. Carano A, Teitelbaum SL, Konsek JD, Schlesinger PH, Blair HC. Bisphosphonates directly inhibit the bone resorption activity of isolated avian osteoclasts in vitro. J Clin Invest 1990;85:456–461.

134. Witte RS, Koeller J, Davis TE, et al. Clodronate: A randomized study in the treatment of cancer-related hypercalcemia. Arch Intern Med 1987;147:937–939.

135. Bonjour J-P, Rizzoli R. Clodronate in hypercalcemia of malignancy. Calcif Tissue Int 1990;46:S20–S25.

136. Storm T, Thamsborg G, Steiniche T, Genant HK, Sorensen OH. Effect of intermittent cyclical etidronate therapy on bone mass and fracture rate in women with postmenopausal osteoporosis. N Engl J Med 1990;322:1265–1271.

137. Hasling C, Charles P, Mosekilde L. Etidronate disodium for treating hypercalcaemia of malignancy: A double blind, placebo-controlled study. Eur J Clin Invest 1986;16:433–437.

138. Ryzen E, Martodam RR, Troxell M, et al. Intravenous etidronate in the management of malignant hypercalcemia. Arch Intern Med 1985;145:449–452.

139. Singer FR, Ritch PS, Lad TE, et al. Treatment of hypercalcemia with intravenous etidronate: A controlled multicenter study. Arch Intern Med 1991;151:471–476.

140. Warrell RP Jr, Heller G, Murphy WP, Schulman P, O'Dwyer P. A randomized double-blind study of gallium nitrate compared to etidronate for acute control of cancer-related hypercalcemia. J Clin Oncol 1991;9:1467–1475.

141. Gucalp R, Ritch P, Wiernik PH, et al. Comparative study of pamidronate disodium and etidronate disodium in the treatment of cancer-related hypercalcemia. J Clin Oncol 1992;10:134–142.

142. Bounameaux HM, Schifferli J, Monatni J-P, Chatelanat F. Renal failure associated with intravenous diphosphonates. Lancet 1983;1:471.

143. Schiller JM, Rasmussen P, Benson AB, et al. Maintenance etidronate in the prevention of malignancy-associated hypercalcemia. Arch. Intern Med 1987;147:963–966.

144. Thiebaud D, Jaeger P, Jacquet AF, et al. Dose response in the treatment of hypercalcemia of malignancy by a single infusion of the bisphosphonate AHPrBP J Clin Oncol 1988;6:762–768.

145. Body JJ, Magritte A, Seraj F, Sculier JP, Borkowski A. Aminohydroxypropylidene bisphosphonate (APD) treatment for tumor-associated hypercalcemia: A randomized comparison between a 3-day treatment and single 24-hour infusions. J Bone Miner Res 1989;4:923–928.

146. Body JJ, Pot M, Borkowski A, Sculier JP, Klastersky J. Dose-response study of aminohydroxypropylidene bisphosphonate in tumor-associated hypercalcemia. Am J Med 1987;82:957–963.

147. Nussbaum SR, Mallette L, Gagel R, et al. Single dose treatment of hypercalcemia of malignancy with aminohydroxypropylidene bisphosphonate (APD). J Bone Miner Res 1989;4:S313.

148. Adami S, Bolzicco GP, Rizzo A, et al. The use of dichloromethylene bisphosphonate and aminobutane bisphosphonate in hypercalcemia of malignancy. Bone Miner 1987;2:395–404.

149. Warrell RP Jr, Bockman RS, Coonley CJ, Isaacs M, Staszewski H. Gallium nitrate inhibits calcium resorption from bone and is effective treatment for cancer-related hypercalcemia. J Clin Invest 1984;73:1487–1490.

150. Bockman RS, Boskey A, Alcock N, Bullough P, Warrell R. Gallium nitrate inhibits bone resorption, increases bone calcium content, but is not cytotoxic to bone cells. J Bone Miner Res 1985;1:65.

151. Cournot-Witmer G, Bourdeau A, Lieberherr M, et al. Bone modeling in gallium-nitrate-treated rats. Calcif Tissue Int 1987;40:270–275.

152. Hall TJ, Chambers TJ. Gallium inhibits bone resorption by a direct effect on osteoclasts. Bone Miner 1990;8:211–216.

153. Warrell RP Jr, Alcock NW, Skelos A, Bockman RS. Gallium nitrate inhibits accelerated bone turnover in patients with bone metastases. J Clin Oncol 1987;5:292–298.

154. Bockman RS, Repo MA, Warrell RP, et al. Distribution of trace levels of therapeutic gallium in bone as mapped by synchrotron x-ray microscopy. Proc Natl Acad Sci USA 1990;87:4149–4153.

155. Bockman RS, Bosley A, Blumenthal NC, Alcock NW, Warrell RP. Gallium increases bone calcium and crystallite perfection of hydroxyapatite. Calcif Tissue Int 1986;39:376–381.

156. Schlesinger PH, Teitelbaum SL, Blair HC. Osteoclast inhibition by Ga³⁺ contrasts with bisphosphonate metabolic suppression: Competitive inhibition of H⁺ ATPase by bone-bound gallium. J Bone Miner Res 1991;6(suppl 1):S127.

157. Bockman RS, Israel R, Alcock N, Ferguson R, Warrell RP. Gallium nitrate stimulates bone collagen synthesis. Clin Res 1987;35:620A.

158. Warrell RP Jr, Skelos A, Alcock NW, Bockman RS. Gallium nitrate for acute treatment of cancer-related hypercalcemia: Clinicopharmacologic and dose-response analysis. Cancer Res 1986;46:4208–4212.

159. Brown JH, Kennedy BJ. Mithramycin in the treatment of disseminated testicular neoplasms. N Engl J Med 1965;272:111–118.

160. Kennedy BJ. Metabolic and toxic effects during mithramycin therapy. Am J Med 1970;49:494–503.

161. Lebbin D, Ryan WG, Schwartz TB. Outpatient treatment of Paget's disease of bone with mithramycin. Ann Intern Med 1974;81:635–637.

162. Perlia CP, Gubisch NJ, Wolter J, et al. Mithramycin treatment of hypercalcemia. Cancer 1970;25:389–394.

163. Elias EG, Evans JT. Hypercalcemic crisis in neoplastic diseases: Management with mithramycin. Surgery 1972;71:631–635.

164. Stapleton FB, Linshaw MA. Treatment of hypercalcemia associated with osseous metastases. J Pediatr 1976;89:1209–1030.

165. Coombes RC, Dady P, Parsons C, et al. Mithramycin therapy: An adjunct to conventional treatment of hypercalcemia and bone metastases in breast cancer. Metab Bone Dis Rel Res 1980;2:199–202.

166. Kiang DT, Loken MK, Kennedy BJ. Mechanism of the hypocalcemic effect of mithramycin. J Clin Endocrinol Metab 1979;48:341–344.

167. Minkin C. Inhibition of parathyroid hormone stimulated bone resorption in vitro by the antibiotic mithramycin. Calcif Tissue Int 1973;13:249–257.

168. Parsons DM, Baum M, Self M. Effect of mithramycin on calcium and hydroxyproline metabolism in patients with malignant disease. Br Med J 1967;1:474–477.

169. Green L, Donehower RC. Hepatic toxicity of low doses of mithramycin in hypercalcemia. Cancer Treat Rep 1984;68:1379–1381.

170. Ralston SH, Gardner MD, Dryburgh FJ, Jenkins AS, Cowan RA, Boyle IT. Comparison of aminohydroxypropylidene diphosphonate, mithramycin, and corticosteroids/calcitonin in treatment of cancer-associated hypercalcemia. Lancet 1985;2:907–910.

171. Thiebaud D, Jacquet AF, Burckhardt P. Fast and effective treatment of malignant hypercalcemia: Combination of suppositories of calcitonin and a single infusion of 3-amino-1-hydroxypropylidene-1-bisphosphonate. Arch Intern Med 1990;150:2125–2128.

172. Miach PJ, Dawborn JK, Martin TJ, et al. Management of the hypercalcemia of malignancy by peritoneal dialysis. Med J Aust 1975;1:782–784.

173. Lad TE, Mishoulam HM, Shevrin DH, Kukla LJ, Abramson EC, Kukreja SC. Treatment of cancer-associated hypercalcemia with cisplatin. Arch Intern Med 1987;147:329–332.

174. Bockman RS, Bohnsack R, Warrell RP. Effect of metal-based compounds on bone resorption. Clin Res 1986;34:390A.

175. Robinson RR, Yarger WE. Acute uric acid nephropathy. Arch Intern Med 1977;137:839–840.

176. Klinenberg JR, Kippen I, Bluestone R. Hyperuricemic nephropathy: Pathophysiologic features and factors influencing urate deposition. Nephron 1975;14:88–98.

177. Crittendon DR, Ackerman GL. Hyperuricemic acute renal failure in disseminated carcinoma. Arch Intern Med 1977;137:97–99.

178. Maidemont CG, Greaves MF, Black AJ. T-cell leukemia presenting with hyperuricaemia, acute renal failure, and gout. Clin Lab Haematol 1983;5:423–426.

179. Cohen LF, Balow JE, Magrath IT, Poplack DG, Ziegler JL. Acute tumor lysis syndrome. A review of 37 patients with Burkitt's lymphoma. Am J Med 1980;68:486–491.

180. Garnick MB, Mayer RB. Acute renal failure associated with neoplastic disease and its treatment. Semin Oncol 1978;5:155–165.

181. Yu T-F. Secondary gout associated with myeloproliferative diseases. Arthitis Rheum 1965;8:765–771.

182. Ultmann J. Hyperuricemia in disseminated neoplastic disease other than lymphomas or leukemias. Cancer 1962;15:122–129.

183. Melink TJ, Von Hoff DD, Kuhn JG, et al. Phase I evaluation and pharmacokinetics of tiazofurin (2-beta-D-ribofuranosylthiazole-4-carboxamide, NSC 286193). Cancer Res 1985;45:2859–2865.

184. Conger JD, Falk SA. Intrarenal dynamics in the pathogenesis and prevention of acute urate nephropathy. J Clin Invest 1977;59:786–793.

185. Muggia FM, Ball TJ Jr, Ultmann JE. Allopurinol in the treatment of neoplastic disease complicated by hyperuricemia. Arch Intern Med 1967;120:12–18.

186. Krakoff IH, Meyer RL. Prevention of hyperuricemia in leukemia and lymphoma. JAMA 1965;193:1–6.

187. Skipper HE, Robins RK, Thomson JR, et al. Structure-activity relationships observed on screening a series of pyrazolopyrimidines against experimental neoplasms. Cancer Res 1957;17:579–596.

188. Rundles RW, Wyngaarden JB, Hithcings GH, Elion GB, Silberman HR. Effects of a xanthine oxidase inhibitor on thiopurine metabolism, hyperuricemia, and gout. Trans Assoc Am Physicians 1963;76:126–140.

189. Band PR, Silberberg DS, Henderson JF, et al. Xanthine nephropathy in a patient with lymphosarcoma treated with allopurinol. N Engl J Med 1970;283:354–357.

190. Hande KR, Hixson CV, Chabner BA. Postchemotherapy purine excretion in lymphoma patients receiving allopurinol. Cancer Res 1981;41:2273–2279.

191. Ortega JA, Ruccione K, Weinberg K, Sato J, Lammers P. Use of an investigational form of intravenous (IV) allopurinol for the treatment of hyperuricemia in children with malignancy. Proc Am Soc Clin Oncol 1985;4:257.

192. Simmons HA, Cameron JS, Morris GS, Davies PM. Allopurinol in renal failure and the tumor lysis syndrome. Clin Chim Acta 1986;160:189–195.

193. Templeton JS. Azapropazone or allopurinol in the treatment of chronic gout and/or hyperuricemia. A preliminary report. Br J Clin Pract 1982;36:353–358.

194. Gibson T, Simmonds HA, Armstrong RD, Fairbanks LD, Rodgers AV. Azapropazone—a treatment for hyperuricaemia and gout? Br J Rheumatol 1984;23:44–51.

195. Warrell RP Jr, Muindi J, Stevens Y-W, Isaacs M, Young CW. Induction of profound hypouricemia by a non-sedating C-5 monosubstituted thiobarbiturate. Metabolism 1989;38:550–554.

196. Jankovic M, Zurlo MG, Rossi E, et al. Urate-oxidase as hypouricemic agent in a case of acute tumor lysis syndrome. Am J Pediatr Hematol Oncol 1985;7:202–204.

197. Mandell GA, Swacus JR, Rosenstock J, Buck BE. Danger of urography in hyperuricemic children with Burkitt's lymphoma. J Can Assoc Radiol 1983;34:273–277.

198. Steinberg SM, Galen MA, Lazarus JM. Hemodialysis for acute uric acid nephropathy. Am J Dis Child 1975;129:956–958.

199. Monballyou J, Zachee P, Verherckmoes R, Boogaerts MA. Transient acute renal failure due to tumor lysis-induced severe phosphate load in a patient with Burkitt's lymphoma. Clin Nephrol 1984;22:47–50.

200. Wollner A, Shalit M, Brezis M. Tumor genesis syndrome. Hypophosphatemia accompanying Burkitt's lymphoma cell leukemia. Miner Electrolyte Metab 1986;12:173–175.

201. Boles JM, Dutel JL, Briere J, et al. Acute renal failure caused by extreme hyperphosphatemia after chemotherapy of an acute lymphoblastic leukemia. Cancer 1984;53:2425–2429.

202. Tsokos GC, Balow JE, Speigel RJ, et al. Renal and metabolic complications of undifferentiated and lymphoblastic lymphomas. Medicine (Baltimore) 1981;60:218–229.

203. Cervantes F, Ribera JM, Granena A, et al. Tumor lysis syndrome with hypocalcemia in chronic granulocytic leukemia. Acta Haematol 1982;68:157–159.

204. Boccia RV, Longo DL, Lieher ML, Jaffe ES, Fisher RI. Multiple recurrences of acute tumor lysis syndrome in an indolent non-Hodgkin's lymphoma. Cancer 1985;56:2295–2297.

205. Zusman J, Brown DM, Nesbit ME. Hyperphosphatemia, hyperphosphaturia, and hypocalcemia in acute lymphoblastic leukemia. N Engl J Med 1973;289:1335–1340.

206. Ettinger DS, Harker WG, Gerry HW, Sanders RC, Saral R. Hyperphosphatemia, hypocalcemia, and transient renal failure: Results of cytotoxic treatment of acute lymphoblastic leukemia. JAMA 1978;239:2472–2474.

207. Gomez GA, Han T. Acute tumor lysis syndrome in prolymphocytic leukemia. Arch Intern Med 1987;147:375–376.

208. Vogelzang NJ, Nelimark RA, Nath KA. Tumor lysis syndrome after induction chemotherapy of small cell bronchogenic carcinoma. JAMA 1983;249:513–514.

209. Stark ME, Dyer MC, Coonley CJ. Fatal acute tumor lysis syndrome with metastatic breast carcinoma. Cancer 1987;60:762–764.

210. Fer MF, Bottino GC, Sherwin SA, et al. Atypical tumor lysis syndrome in a patients with T-cell lymphoma treated with recombinant leukocyte interferon. Am J Med 1984;77:953–956.

211. Cech P, Block JB, Cone IA, Stone R. Tumor lysis syndrome after tamoxifen flare. N Engl J Med 1986;315:263–264.

212. Simmons ED, Somberg KA. Acute tumor lysis syndrome after intrathecal methotrexate administration. Cancer 1991;67:2062–2065.

213. Gonzalez C, Villasanta U. Life-threatening hypocalcemia and hypomagnesemia associated with cisplatin chemotherapy. Obstet Gynecol 1982;59:732–734.

214. Harley HA, Mason R, Phillips PJ. Profound hypocalcemia associated with oestrogen treatment of carcinoma of the prostate. Med J Aust 1983;2:41–41.

215. Schenkein DP, O'Neill WC, Shapiro J, Miller KB. Accelerated bone formation causing profound hypocalcemia in acute leukemia. Ann Intern Med 1986;105:375–378.

216. Schilsky RL. Renal and metabolic complications of cancer chemotherapy. Semin Oncol 1982;9:75–83.

217. Papaioannou AN. Tumors other than insulinoma associated with hypoglycemia. Surg Gynecol Obstet 1966;123:1093–1109.

218. Daughaday WH. Hypoglycemia in patients with non-islet cell tumors. Endocrinol Metab Clin North Am 1988;18:91–101.

219. Hall K, Takano K, Fryklund L, Sievertsson H. Somatomedins. Adv Metab Disorders 1975;8:19–46.

220. Rinderknecht E, Humbel RE. The amino acid sequence of human insulin-like growth factor I and its structural homology with proinsulin. J Biol Chem 1978;253:2769–2776.

221. Zapf J, Schmid C, Guler HP, et al. Regulation of binding proteins for insulin-like growth factors (IGF) in humans. Increased expression of IGF binding protein 2 during IGF I treatment of healthy adults and in patients with extrapancreatic tumor hypoglycemia. J Clin Invest 1990;86:952–961.

222. Shapiro ET, Bell GI, Polonsky KS, Rubenstein AH, Kew MC, Tager HS. Tumor hypoglycemia: Relationship to high molecular weight insulin-like growth factor-II J Clin Invest 1990;85:1672–1679.

223. Axelrod L, Ron D. Insulin-like growth factor II and the riddle of tumor-induced hypoglycemia. N Engl J Med 1988;319:1477–1479.

224. Tisdale MJ, Brennan RA. Metabolic substrate utilization by a tumour cell line which induces cachexia in vivo. Br J Cancer 1986;54:601–606.

225. Davis MR, Shamoon H. Deficient counterregulatory hormone responses during hypoglycemia in a patient with insulinoma. J Clin Endocrinol Metab 1991;72:788–792.

226. Samaan NA, Pham FK, Sellin RV, Fernandez JF, Benjamin RS. Successful treatment of hypoglycemia using glucagon in a patient with and extreapancreatic tumor. Ann Intern Med 1990;113:404–406.

227. Hoffken K, Kemf H, Miller AA, et al. Aminoglutethimide without hydrocortisone in the treatment of postmenopausal patients with advanced breast cancer. Cancer Treat Rep 1986;70:1153–1157.

228. Spiegel RJ, Oliff AI, Bruton J, et al. Adrenal suppression after short-term corticosteroid therapy. Lancet 1979;1:630–633.

229. Seidenwurm DJ, Elmer EB, Kaplan LM, Williams EK, Morris DG, Hoffman AR. Metastases to the adrenal glands and the development of Addison's disease. Cancer 1984;54:552–557.

230. Redman DG, Pazdur R, Zingas AP, Loredo R. Prospective evaluation of adrenal insufficiency in patients with adrenal metastasis. Cancer 1987;60:103–107.

231. Frommer JP. Lactic acidosis. Med Clin North Am 1983;67:815–829.

232. Mizock BA. Controversies in lactic acidosis. Implications in critically ill patients. JAMA 1987;258:497–501.

233. Doolittle GC, Wurster MW, Rosenfeld CS, Bodensteiner DC. Malignancy-induced lactic acidosis. South Med J 1988;81:533–536.

234. Madias NE. Lactic acidosis. Kidney Int 1986;29:752–754.

235. Sculier JP, Nicaise C, Klastersky J. Lactic acidosis: A metabolic complications of extensive metastatic cancer. Eur J Clin Oncol 1983;19:597–601.

236. Fraley, DS, Adler, R, Bruns, FJ, Zetts, B. Stimulation of lactate production by administration of bicarbonate in a patient with a solid neoplasm and lactic acidosis. N Engl J Med 1980;303:1100–1102.

237. Cooper DJ, Walley KR, Wiggs BR, Russell JA. Bicarbonate does not improve hemodynamics in critically ill patients who have lactic acidosis. A prospective controlled clinical study. Ann Intern Med 1990;112:492–498.

238. Stacpoole PW. Lactic acidosis: The case against bicarbonate therapy. Ann Intern Med [Editorial] 1986;105:276–279.

239. Ritter JM, Doktor HS, Benjamin N. Paradoxical effect of bicarbonate on cytoplasmic pH. Lancet 1990;335:1243–1246.

240. Androgue HJ, Brensilver J, Cohen JJ, et al. Influence of steady-state alterations in acid-base equilibrium on the fate of administered bicarbonate in the dog. J Clin Invest 1983;71:867–879.

241. Graf L, Leach WJ, Arieff AI. Metabolic effects of sodium bicarbonate in hypoxic lactic acidosis in dogs. Am J Physiol 1985;249:F630–F635.

242. Narins RC, Cohen JJ. Bicarbonate therapy for organic acidosis: The case for its continued use. Ann Intern Med 1987;106:615–618.

243. Narins RG, Jones ER, Dornfield LP. Alkali therapy of the organic acidoses: A critical assessment of the data and the case for judicious use of sodium bicarbonate. In: Narins RG, ed. Controversies in nephrology and hypertension. New York: Churchill-Livingstone, 1984:359.

244. Stacpoole PW, Wright EC, Baumgartner TG, et al. A controlled clinical trial of dichloroacetate for treatment of lactic acidosis in adults. N Engl J Med 1992;327:1564–1569.

SECTION 4

ALAN R. BAKER

Surgical Emergencies

The patient with cancer is potentially susceptible to a constellation of physical insults. Some arise as a direct consequence of the primary tumor or its metastatic sequelae; some appear in the aftermath of treatment and are toxicity related. Still others arise completely independent of the malignancy. For the surgeon called on to evaluate an emergency in a patient with cancer, a thorough understanding of the natural history of the specific tumor and an appreciation of where he or she intercepts the patient in the course of that neoplastic encounter help to clarify problems that otherwise can be quite perplexing. No effort is made in this chapter to summarize general surgery or physical diagnosis, because good references abound for these topics.[1-3] The natural histories of the many different tumor types are discussed in the chapters on specific diseases in this text. This chapter examines the clinically pressing circumstances that arise in the context of successful or failed treatment of the tumor. Diagnostic manipulations and therapeutic maneuvers that have proven useful adjuncts to difficult judgment making at the bedside are presented. Although there exist few texts covering these topics, three good references should be reviewed.[4-6]

DIAGNOSIS AND CONSULTATION

Pain, tenderness, fever, chills, nausea, vomiting, diarrhea, obstipation, distension, and blood, whether occult or frank, issuing from mouth or anus are the often cited problems that invite surgical consultation. These symptoms and signs must be taken with utmost seriousness and should prompt the surgeon to a thorough understanding of the patient's total problem. A meticulous history must be elicited from the patient and the family, and the patient's records must be queried for specific information. This is the time to read the pertinent prior operative notes and pathology reports and examine the details of recent and remote treatment measures. How much radiation therapy has the patient received and to what portals? Which antineoplastic agents has the patient been given in the past 6 weeks? What other drugs, with particular emphasis on narcotics, steroids, and diuretics, has the patient been taking?

With the chart in hand, the patient's recent laboratory data are reviewed to determine the impact of treatment and the extent of aberration caused by acutely deranged physiology. Bone marrow reserve and response are assessed through determinations of hemoglobin or hematocrit, leukocyte count and differential, and platelet count. Serum electrolytes, particularly potassium and magnesium, amylase, BUN, creatinine, and liver function tests including prothrombin time and, if pertinent, serum tumor marker levels are observed. Recent data from the microbiology laboratory are reviewed with particular reference to positive blood cultures and possibly stool *Clostridium difficile* titers.

A diligent but directed physical examination, usually coupled with rectal and, for women, pelvic assessment should be performed. Extra time spent in eliciting evidence of peritoneal irritation, as manifested by cough or shake tenderness and truly absent bowel sounds, is well spent.

Although the data afforded by the history, physical examination, and laboratory studies frequently does not completely reveal the problem, they can provide direction about which more elaborate, more expensive, and often more invasive additional studies should be obtained. They provide important baseline information, because changes in the patient's clinical condition over time measured in hours often weigh heavily in making the decision about whether to proceed to operation. Alternatively, changes sometimes proceed more slowly than expected, and fully appreciating them requires once or twice daily visits, stretched over a couple of weeks, as host defenses recover and homeostatic integrity is restored.

For most problems, it is usual to obtain initial plain roentgenograms of the chest (posteroanterior [PA] and lateral views) and abdomen (supine and upright views). When these x-ray films are examined, it is always profitable to take the extra time to compare them with prior similar films and review all contrast-enhanced fluoroscopic studies and CT and MR scans.

The complexity of the cancer patient's clinical story creates and contributes to uncertainty and confusion. Determining whether the apparent urgent situation is a consequence of the tumor or the therapy directed at it can be quite difficult. Leukemic or lymphomatous organ infiltration can simulate the pain that results from a myriad of other causes of the acute surgical abdomen.[7-12] Steroids occasionally mask the usual response to peritoneal soilage and make the most sinister of circumstances seemingly serene.[13] The fever, chills, and rigors associated with severe chemotherapy-induced neutropenia can deceptively mimic the sepsis picture of bowel perforation or undrained accumulations of pus.[14] Some paraneoplastic factors and certain antineoplastic agents can produce a profound degree of gut neuropathy that simulates mechanical intestinal obstruction.[15,16] Resolving these kinds of ambiguity can prove a significant clinical challenge but must be done to determine whether the urgent circumstance warrants or demands surgical intervention. Additional diagnostic tests are usually needed.

The past two decades have witnessed a technologic explosion in the number, kind, and complexity of tests available for sorting out difficult problems. The astute clinician must decide which tests to do, when to obtain them, and reckon the cost of the information derived in terms of time, effort, dollars, and potential morbidity. Subtle problems in communication among the subspecialists involved can make this task more difficult. Every test or study ordered should be directed at answering a question. Couched in these terms, the consultant diagnostic or invasive radiologist, nuclear medicine specialist, or endoscopist can better understand the problem and nature of the help sought and be better able to assist in the determination of which of the available options can most expeditiously provide the needed information.

DECIDING TO OPERATE

Many cancer patients, particularly those in therapy, are significantly depleted, immunologically compromised hosts with exceedingly limited reserves. Compound their chronic illness with an acute, catabolic, and occasionally catastrophic insult, and the stage is set for significant morbidity and high mortality rate outcomes.

In a survey by Turnbull and Starnes at Memorial Sloan-Kettering Cancer Center, one third (66 of 200) of the urgent procedures were done to manage the cancer or a complication of chemotherapy.[5] Forty-four percent (88 of 200) were performed to manage a complication of the prior cancer surgery, and 21% (42 of 200) of the laparotomies were necessitated by nonneoplastic or antineoplastic treatment related diagnoses. In fact, 13 of these 42 procedures were done in patients without evidence of cancer. Laparotomy failed to reveal an urgent problem in the remaining 2% (4 of 200).

Salvage after surgery to manage these urgent problems was disappointing, although not unexpectedly so. In 36% (72 of 200) of the cases, the patient died before discharge from the hospital. If postprocedure recovery led to discharge, survival was less than 3 months for roughly 10% (19 of 200) of procedures, between 3 and 6 months for 11% (22 of 200) of procedures, between 6 and 12 months for 11% (22 of 200) of procedures, and exceeded 1 year for the remaining 32% (65 of 200).

That cancer patients receiving chemotherapy are acutely vulnerable to insults that necessitate operation is highlighted by the fact that 45% (64 of 140) of the procedures had to be done in this setting. That their expectation for survival is poor is additionally reflected in the experience reported by Ferrara.[17] Of 21 patients actively in treatment who suffered catastrophic perforative (15) or hemorrhagic (6) complications, 17 died (81%) after operation. An additional 2 patients died within 1 month of hospital discharge: 1 patient survived 5 months, and the last remained alive and disease free 9 months after discharge at the time of the report. Nineteen of these 21 patients suffered a total of 51 postoperative complications that included pneumonia or respiratory failure (15), septicemia (9), hemorrhage (7), hepatic failure (3), bone marrow failure (3), wound infection (5), and nonspecified problems (5). The four second operations were categorized as complications.

Because oncologic patients can ill afford a procedure that creates more problems than it solves, the surgeon before proceeding to operation must clarify or resolve several important questions.[18] What is the exact nature of the problem? What surgically, in specific terms, must be done to provide remedy? Are there any less invasive, equally suitable alternatives to operation available? In this setting, I think the role of the purely exploratory laparotomy is of questionable value.

URGENT CONDITIONS

The urgent problems surgeons most often confront in cancer patients can be grouped as obstruction, perforation, hemorrhage, and infection. Some overlap syndromes are seen, but usually one of these four clinical features becomes dominant and compelling. Table 60–15 summarizes the results reported by Turnbull and Starnes of the urgent reasons for which cancer patients required surgery.[5] Instructive representative clinical examples within each category are examined later in this section.

PERFORATION

A perforated intestinal viscus and the attendant peritonitis it causes almost always produces a clinically dramatic picture. Severe, constant abdominal pain with associated diffuse tenderness, guarding, and often rigidity, profound ileus with consequent distension and quiet to absent bowel sounds, fever and the hemodynamic sequelae of third space fluid accumulation, and bacteremia with resultant tachycardia, hypotension, and oliguria contribute to an appropriate sense of bedside urgency. The upright chest x-ray film or left-side-down lateral decubitus view, which usually demonstrates free intraabdominal air, strongly favors colonic or gastroduodenal perforation and usually demands urgent exploration.[19] I have never regretted making some preoperative effort to determine the site of perforation. Moderate or severely edematous bowel, covered by a fibrinopurulent exudate in the setting of multiple adhesions from the usual prior abdominal procedure, can make finding the site of perforation quite difficult. Being able to proceed directly to the sigmoid colon or to an initial look at the distal stomach and duodenum permits the physician to make the optimal incision, saves operative time, and minimizes the chance for unintended injury to structures encountered during a tedious, otherwise undirected exploration.

TABLE 60–15. Gastrointestinal or Intraabdominal Problems Requiring Operation in 310 Patients With Cancer

Problem	No. of Patients (%)
Obstruction	89 (29)
Perforation	66 (21)
Hemorrhage	85 (28)
Infection	47 (15)
Other	23 (7)
Total	310 (100)

(Turnbull ADM. Surgical emergencies in the cancer patient. Chicago: Year Book Medical Publishers, 1987:157;195)

If the clinical history favors gastroduodenal perforation (*e.g.*, steroids, prior ulcer disease, hematemesis or occult blood in the stool), it is wise to proceed with a Gastrografin study by mouth or through the nasogastric tube that had initially been placed. If the findings favor a colonic lesion (*e.g.*, prior diverticular disease, antecedent crampy lower abdominal pain), it is better to start with a Gastrografin enema. With a positive initial study, the surgeon can proceed directly to operation. If the initial study is negative and the patient's clinical condition permits, the alternative examination is done. During the 2 hours required and after blood cultures have been obtained, broad-spectrum antibiotics (*e.g.*, gentamycin, ampicillin, clindamycin) are instituted and energetic intravascular volume resuscitation initiated.

Alternatively, the perforation may not be into the free peritoneal cavity. If it occurs into another hollow viscus, it produces an enteroenteric, enterovessical, enterovaginal, or enteroureteral fistula.[20] If the leak tracks to an external surface, an enterocutaneous fistula results. Perforation into the vascular tree produces an arterioenteric fistula with clinical manifestations of intermittent sepsis and episodes of sentinel or massive hemorrhage.[21] Retroperitoneal tumors can on occasion erode into the gut.[22] The clinical picture in this circumstance is similar to that seen if the leak from an intestinal segment is contained or walled off by surrounding structures, and it heralds itself as an abscess with septic features.

Clinically significant acute pancreatitis can mimic the acute abdomen seen with bowel infarction and impending or frank nonfree gut perforation. Although most often idiopathic, alcohol, or gallstone related, it can be seen after the administration of chemotherapeutic agents, most notably L-asparaginase.[23,24] Because it is usually desirable to avoid operation for patients with acute pancreatitis, it is helpful to obtain a serum amylase and lipase preoperatively. Normal values virtually exclude acute pancreatitis, and significantly elevated values make the diagnosis likely. Because some amylase can be released from infarcting intestine, the minimally elevated value leaves the physician in a diagnostic quandary. If intraperitoneal fluid is present, it can be helpful to tap it by paracentesis or culdocentesis; measure amylase, lipase, glucose, and lactic acid dehydrogenase levels in it; examine the fluid by Gram's stain; and culture for organisms and quantitate the numbers of leukocytes and erythrocytes. The laboratory profile is usually diagnostic.

Most perforations occur through a portion of bowel wall involved by a clinically known or undiagnosed tumor. Mural involvement by lymphoma at the level of the colon, small intestine, or stomach can perforate spontaneously or in the wake of effective antitumor chemotherapy.[25-27] Several nongut primary tumors, including lung, breast, melanoma, and kidney, can metastasize to bowel wall, undergo necrosis, and produce perforative sequelae.[28] Primary gastric and colon cancer can present as gut perforations. The site of the perforation is usually at the tumor, although sometimes a more distally located colon tumor produces sufficient closed-loop obstructive difficulty (in the presence of a competent ileocecal valve) and distension to lead to cecal perforation.

A host of other etiologic factors may play a role, particularly if the site of perforation is through bowel wall uninvolved by tumor. Included among these are acid-peptic, diverticular, and benign gastric ulcer disease associated with or without concomitant steroids.[13,29] Toxic colitis or typhlitis, often seen in the context of drug-related (*e.g.*, cytarabine, vinca alkaloids, taxol) profound neutropenia, can lead to appendiceal or colonic perforation.[30-33] Similarly, cytomegalovirus infection associated with human immunodeficiency virus infection or with tumor- or drug-induced immunocompromise can produce incipient or frank gut perforation as can severe *C. difficile* toxin-associated enterocolitis.[34,35] Immunotherapy with interleukin-2 has produced this complication.[36] On occasion, a suture line leak or disruption at the site of enterotomy closure or formal anastomosis, particularly if the bowel has been subjected to significant prior irradiation, can produce the clinical picture of bowel perforation.[37,38] A summary of the complex constellation of etiologically associated factors is provided in Table 60–16.

Perforative problems and their sequelae can be dire clinical events in cancer patients, with an associated mortality rate in excess of 50%.[13,17,39-42] Because these hosts often exhibit a diminished capacity to provide hemostasis, resist microbial attack, and repair injured tissue, several principles of management must be remembered. These are summarized in Table 60–17. The surgeon must remember that the surgical procedure does not have to solve all the patient's problems at once. It should instead strive to eradicate only the most life-threatening problems identified and restore the patient to a condition that permits continued attention to and therapy for the primary disease. Liberal provision of blood and blood product support, nutritional supplementation, and aggressive antimicrobial drug administration are critical elements in bolstering weakened host defenses.

The following cases and pertinent associated diagnostic studies illustrate several features and issues encountered in relation to the patient with perforative pathology.

Patient No. 1

Six years earlier, a 49-year-old woman had undergone a complete hysterectomy for a high-grade uterine leiomyosarcoma. A large, left-sided malignant pleural effusion and pulmonary metastases were proven at diagnostic thoracotomy 2 months before referral. After receiving a hematoporphyrin photosensitizer on April 23, 1991, she underwent median sternotomy, left pneumonectomy, right middle lobe nodule wedge excision, and photodynamic therapy to the

TABLE 60–16. Etiologic Factors in Gut Perforation

Tumor at Site of Perforation	*Perforation Through Noninvolved Gut Wall*
Primary colon	Cecal perforation with distal obstructing colon cancer
Primary stomach	Acid-peptic, diverticular disease (±steroids)
Lymphoma	Colitis
Leukemia	Neutropenic enterocolitis (drug)
	Viral (CMV)
	Bacterial (*C. difficile*)
	Interleukin-2
Primary small bowel	Gastric ulcer
Metastatic cancer from lung, breast, melanoma, kidney	Failure of anastomosis or enterotomy closure (±irradiation)

TABLE 60–17. Surgical Principles in the Management of Gut Perforations in Cancer Patients

1. Eliminate the source of continued septic insult by resecting the site of perforation. Exteriorization/resection, particularly for colonic perforation, is preferred. Suture plication should be used for benign duodenal ulcer, benign gastric ulcer, and traumatic perforation only.
2. Be conservative in immediately restoring bowel continuity. Stomas (*e.g.*, colostomy, ileostomy, mucous fistula) are recommended. Anastomotic leaks should be avoided.
3. Copiously irrigate the peritoneal cavity with antibiotic solutions to reduce the burden of contamination.
4. Place drains so that enteric leaks can be comfortably converted to controlled fistulas.
5. Achieve adequate hemostatis using electrocautery, sutures, hemoclips, and topical thrombin or Gelfoam as needed.
6. Minimize wound complications by delayed primary closure techniques and the use of retention sutures.
7. Use liberal tube decompression to avoid adverse impact of distension on healing bowel or abdominal incision. These tubes can later be used for enteral feeding.

chest cavity. On her third postoperative day, she developed severe abdominal pain. A chest x-ray film (Fig. 60–5A,B) showed new, free intraperitoneal air, and a Gastrografin swallow (see Fig. 60–5C,D) revealed contrast extravasation through a perforated duodenal ulcer. The problem was managed at laparotomy with plication and an omental patch graft. Her subsequent recovery proved uneventful, and she was discharged home on the 13th postlaparotomy day. She remained well until 8 months later, when recurrent chest, axillary,and neck nodal metastatic disease developed.

Patient No. 2
An 11-year-old boy with an abdominal mass underwent right colectomy for mural and mesenteric nodal involvement by diffuse histiocytic lymphoma. He received 2100 cGy of postoperative abdominal radiotherapy and multidrug chemotherapy consisting of cyclophosphamide, vincristine, methotrexate, and prednisone. One week after the administration of cycle three, he developed severe abdominal pain, nausea, and vomiting. A chest x-ray film and Gastrografin swallow revealed free intraperitoneal air and contrast agent extravasation similar to that seen in patient #1. A gastric perforation through an area of lymphomatous involvement (Fig. 60–6) was found at laparotomy and handled with resection by partial gastrectomy and splenectomy. On recovery from surgery, two additional cycles of chemotherapy were administered, followed by autologous bone marrow transplantation. Despite this approach, his lymphoma progressed, and he died 5 months after the gastric perforative catastrophe.

OBSTRUCTION

The patient with intestinal obstruction suffers symptoms of spectral severity ranging from "can't eat to can't drink to can't handle endogenous secretions, swallowed air, or gut elaborated gases." Partial or complete deprivation of oral intake imposes a significant quality of life debit and leaves the patient anywhere from mildly distressed to deeply miserable. The accompanying, usually crampy abdominal pain, nausea, vomiting, obstipation, absent flatus, distension, and usually hyperactive (with rushes and tinkles) or dystonic (amphoric and resonant) bowel sounds invite surgical consultation and force the need to pose and methodically answer the following questions. Is there a mechanical impediment or problem present? At what and how many sites is it located? To what functional degree is the lumen compromised? Is bowel viability threatened as a consequence of distension? What is or are the causes of the blockage? What is the likelihood of spontaneous resolution?

Plain films of the abdomen (supine and upright) and chest (PA and lateral) should demonstrate the absence of free air and usually show luminal distension which, depending on degree, distribution, and the presence of differential air-fluid levels, permit inferences about whether the obstruction is partial or complete, its site, and its mechanism. Unless early in its evolution, gas seen in the rectum and rectosigmoid colon strongly suggest an incomplete blockage. Extensive colonic and small bowel dilation suggest a distal colonic site, and differential air-fluid levels favor a mechanical rather than a metabolic cause.

Significant hypokalemia, hypomagnesemia, and hypocalcemia and the recent intake of narcotics or administration of vinca alkaloids can severely impair neuromuscular function and produce profound and ubiquitous gut distension. These kinds of drug-associated toxicity represent an often seen constellation in the cancer patient and can contribute significantly to what may prove a multifactor basis for an obstructive picture. A normal serum amylase or lipase reassuringly rules out pancreatitis with its attendant ileus.

Unless there is fever, focal tenderness, and significant leukocytosis, any of which create a sense of urgency by provoking concern about gut ischemia and infarction, the passage of a nasogastric tube usually provides some degree of decompression, buys time, and permits repletion of third space fluid losses and a decision about which additional diagnostic studies or procedures to perform.[43] Serial plain films of the abdomen are quite useful and provide a sense about whether the situation is getting better or worse.

A colonic component in any obstructive picture significantly complicates the workup and management of the problem and must be appreciated before surgery. For the cancer patient, if time and circumstances permit, the colon should be "prepped" before any operation directed at relieving obstruction. Meaningfully obstructed colon is difficult to prepare well for surgery. Cathartics like GoLytely, castor oil, or magnesium citrate are contraindicated. Depending on how proximal the obstruction is and its degree, enemas may be inefficient in evacuating feces upstream of it. Nonabsorbable antibiotics given by mouth may never reach the colon. Dealing with an unprepared colon at surgery is a major hazard. Obstipated feces themselves can compound the mechanical obstructive problem and potentially threaten the integrity of a proximal anastomosis or enterotomy closures and provide significant peritoneal contamination if the colon is inadvertently entered. Colonic pathology in the unprepared colon is usually managed with a colostomy, the surgical alternative that virtually every patient dreads.

Because primary colonic inflammatory pathology, such as diverticulitis, focal ischemic colitis, Crohn's disease, or a walled-off perforative neoplasm, often deceptively mimics pure small bowel obstruction, it is usually wise to rule out a large bowel component to the obstructive picture. Sigmoid-

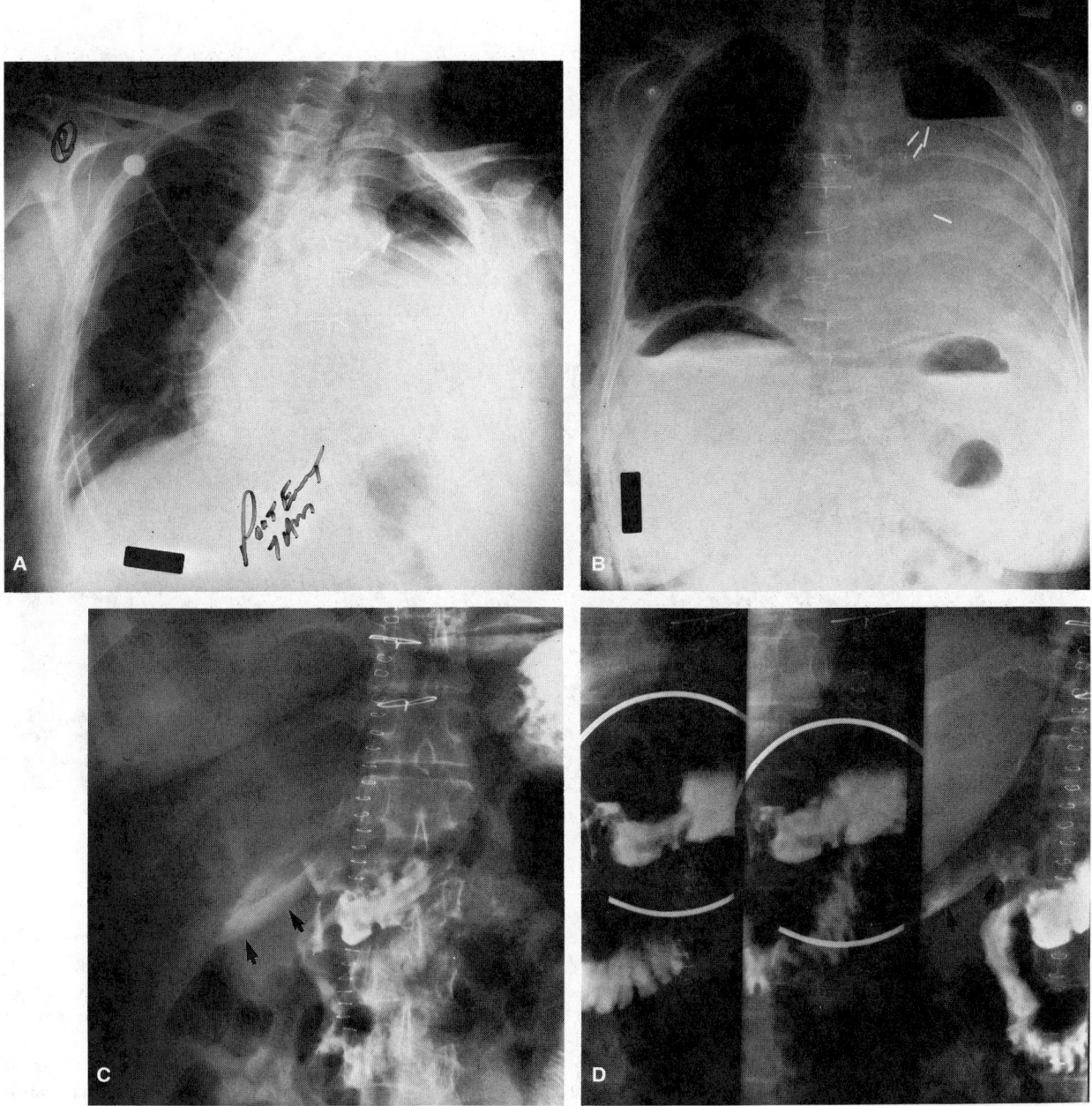

FIGURE 60–5.   **(A)** Poststernotomy chest x-ray film that shows no free intraperitoneal air. **(B)** B) Radiograph taken 2 days later, shortly after the abdominal pain developed, shows free intraperitoneal air. **(C, D)** Extravasation of contrast agent (*arrows*) through the perforated duodenal ulcer.

oscopy followed by barium enema suitably accomplishes this objective. If on fluoroscopy a significant obstructive colonic process is seen, the radiologist must terminate the study and try to minimize the quantity of barium sulfate permitted to go proximal to it. Water absorbed by the colon from the barium sulfate suspension proximal to an even partially obstructive colonic problem will make it impossible to adequately prepare the bowel.

If the barium enema acquits the colon of playing any pathogenetic role in the obstructive picture, it becomes safe and often useful to later perform an upper gastrointestinal series with small bowel follow through or a similar prograde study done through a long gastrointestinal tube (*e.g.*, Miller-Abbott,

Cantor). The long tube minimizes the amount of information-obscuring barium sulfate required and makes it easier to delineate the areas of obstructive pathology. In this instance, barium sulfate is much preferred to a water-soluble contrast agent like Gastrografin, which tends to become progressively more dilute, with resultant loss of information, as it flows distally into fluid filled loops. Unlike the colon, the small intestine is unable to absorb significant water from the barium sulfate suspension used. Even if it remains upstream of a complete block for a significant period, barium concretions never form, and no iatrogenic compounding of the problem ensues. The upper gastrointestinal series (Fig. 60–7), done in error as the initial study for presumptive small bowel ob-

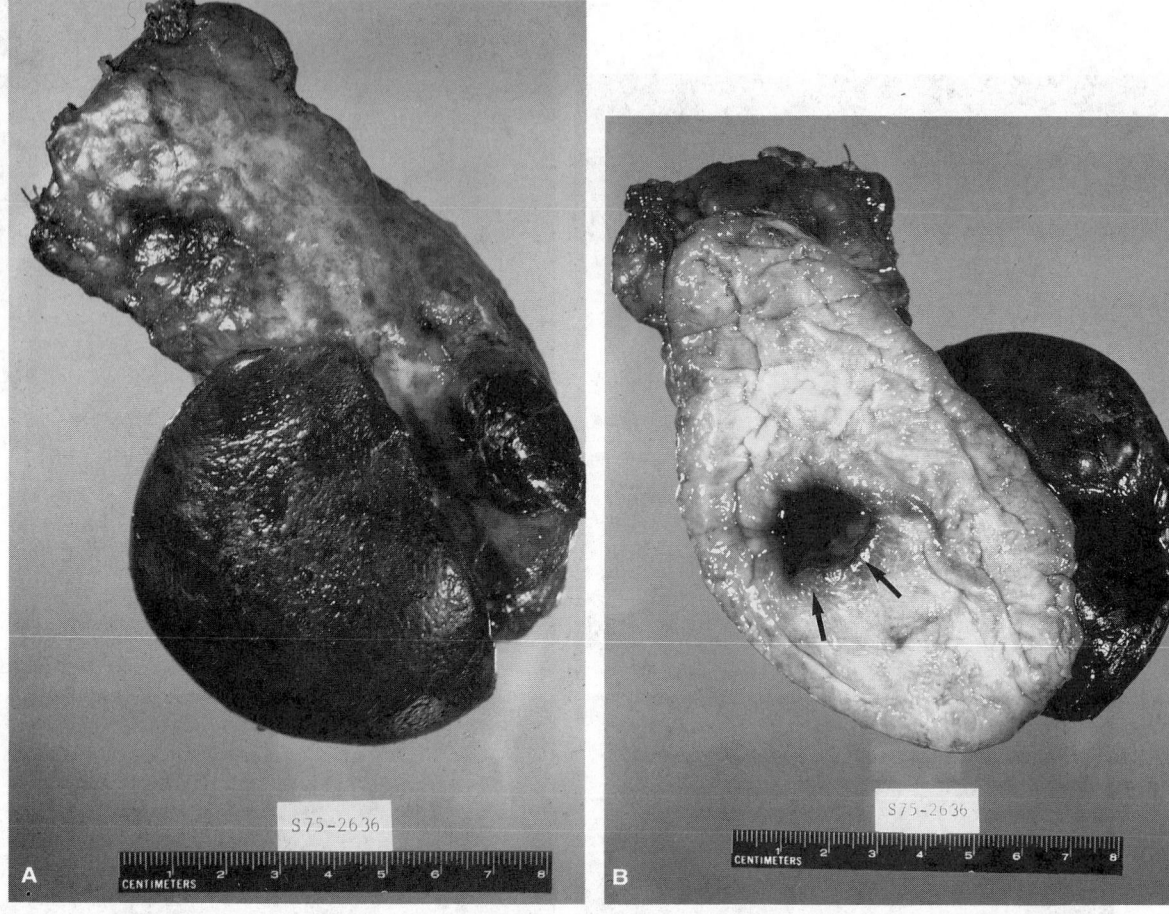

FIGURE 60–6.   (A) Photograph of the resected specimen, consisting of a portion of the greater curvature of stomach and spleen. (B) The stomach has been opened, and the lymphomatous ulcer (*arrows*) is readily seen.

struction, illustrates the problem created when barium sulfate irretrievably impacts in a markedly distended cecum just proximal to an obstructing primary colon cancer.

Somewhat perversely, a swallowed barium sulfate meal often passes through and clears the gut of a patient who is intermittently vomiting and unable to adequately aliment. Regrettably, the barium meal, a not quite stringent enough test for the problem, neither pleases the palate nor has any nutritional value. The fluoroscopist may be unable to identify one or more focal points of obstruction. He should however, provide qualitative information about the amount and coherence of peristaltic activity and provide a measure of gut transit time. In this situation, it can be particularly helpful to pass a long gastrointestinal tube. The Miller-Abbott or Cantor tube is an almost too stringent test for mechanical obstruction. Although it may hang up prematurely in a proximal small bowel loop, it often proceeds quite a distance into the jejunum. Every loop the tube does traverse is a functionally unobstructed loop. At later operation, when virtually unrecognizable, matted, and plastered bowel loops can create much confusion and consternation, the palpable presence of the tube helps to identify the location in the gut and permits bypass of the obstructive problem by performing an anastomosis between the most distal tube-containing (*i.e.*, unobstructed) small bowel loop and some anatomically convenient portion of the colon,

previously shown to be unobstructed by barium enema. I have no preference for the long tube over the nasogastric tube, aside from its unique utility in the just described situation. Both fairly efficiently decompress the gut, but the nasogastric tube is easier to place and maintain.

The information summarized in Table 60–18, garnered from nine reports spanning the past 2 decades that examined populations of cancer patients who developed intestinal obstruction, helps to put any given patient in clinical perspective.[44–52] Although the number of patients reported in each series is modest, a total of 583 patients were tracked. In most instances, the percentage of patients falling within each subgroup is provided; notice that these percentages do not always sum to 100% due to using denominators in subgroup calculations that differ from the total number of patients in the actual series.

The history of a prior malignancy or the presence of recurrent tumor, even if at sites outside the abdomen, substantially increase the probability that a bout of intestinal obstruction is due to tumor. The proportion with malignant causes for their obstructions is between 59% and 97% (mean, 78%).[44,45,47,48,50–52] This figure contrasts strikingly to the roughly 10% of patients with a malignant cause for the problem reported in nonselective series of patients with gut obstruction, for whom the far more frequent cause is benign

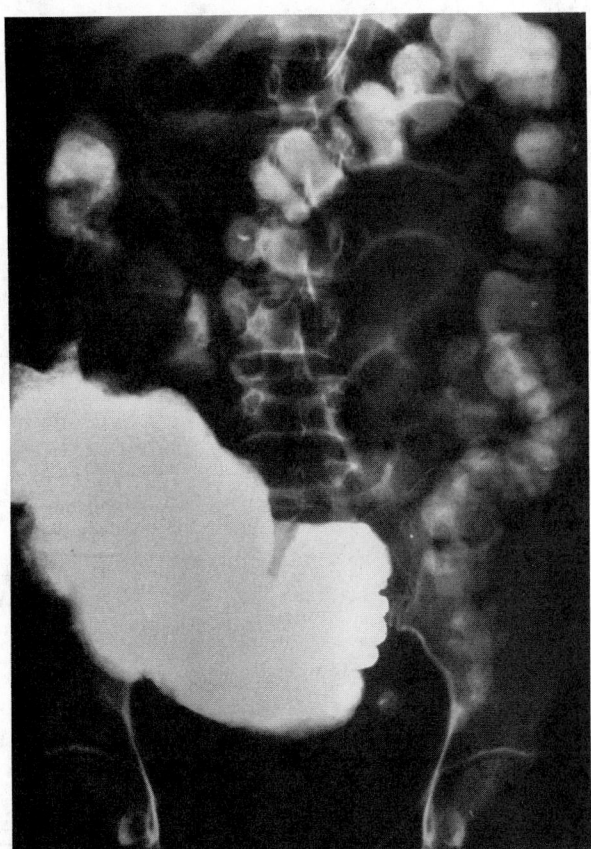

FIGURE 60–7. Irretrievable, orally administered barium sulfate is impacted in the cecum and ascending colon of a patient with an obstructing colonic cancer.

postoperative adhesions.[49,53] Cancer patients can have benign causes for their intestinal obstructions; between 3% and 38% (mean, 23%) were in this group.[44–48,50–52] If radiation therapy had been employed, radiation enteritis was more often implicated as a cause.[44,47]

The primary tumors most commonly predisposing to obstruction were of colorectal, ovarian, gastric pancreatic, uterine, and bladder lesions. Lymphoma was frequently found, as were tumors arising outside the abdominal cavity, such as breast, melanoma, and sarcoma.

Clinically appreciated persistent or recurrent cancer and a short free interval between treatment for the primary lesion and the presentation of the obstructive problem seem to increase the likelihood of a malignant cause for the blockage.[45,50,51]

Reliable differentiation before operation of patients with ischemic or infarcted gut can be exceedingly difficult.[54] Experienced clinical judgment is at best faulty. None of our tests are adequately sensitive or specific. Because the morbidity and mortality of operations complicated by this finding are higher than for those that deal with simple obstruction, the expectant or nonoperative management of the obstructed patient is somewhat anxiety provoking. Fortunately and reassuringly, most series of bowel obstruction in cancer patients report a relatively small proportion of patients, usually between 0% and 5%, with strangulation.[49–52] The highest figure, an anomalous 19%, was reported by Butler.[44]

Between 12% and 28% of cancer patients spontaneously resolve their obstructive difficulties.[44,46,49,50] Even those who seemingly resolve on gut decompression and intravenous fluid support can develop a recurrent bout, often soon after the initial episode that necessitated surgery.[44,46,50]

Probably little is lost with conservative management for 3 to 10 days. During that interval, the patient's anatomic problem can be better defined and initial efforts made at physiologically and psychologically preparing him for what lies ahead.

If surgery becomes necessary, the technical options include lysis of adhesions, gut bypass, bowel resection, or fashioning of a colostomy, ileostomy, or jejunostomy. A combination of these alternatives is often required by the anatomic sites and etiologic circumstances of blockage. Often difficult to detect preoperatively is extensive carcinomatosis, with multiple sites of obstruction, foreshortened mesentery, and presumed neural plexus infiltration. In this context, the meaningful options are exceedingly limited. When nothing can apparently be done to relieve the obstruction, placement of a palliative gastrostomy can be helpful.

For the cancer patient with intestinal obstruction, the realistic prospects for surgical intervention are rather grim. Operative mortality is high, 9% to 35% (average, 19%), as is the corresponding operative morbidity rate of 15% to 49%.[44–52] Between 4% and 45% (average, 15%) of the operations fail to resolve the obstructive problem, or it recurs soon after surgery. Repeated operations, although occasionally done, rapidly approach diminishing returns.[50–52] Unless a benign cause for the obstruction is found, survival for these patients is on the order of several months.[45,46,48,50] A small proportion of patients do survive for prolonged periods, and those fortunate enough to be relieved of their obstructive distress enjoy far better quality of life. Baines and coworkers at St. Christopher's Hospice, London, in an enlightening report, detailed the "aggressive medical measures" that can be done to optimize the quality of a patient's remaining life if surgery fails or is not undertaken.[55] Pharmacologic manipulations with a variety of agents, often administered by patient-controlled, continuous, parenteral infusion, permit comfortable nasogastric tube-free existence for periods ranging between 1 and 12 months.

The previous comments do not apply to intestinal obstruction in the cancer patient in the perioperative context. In this setting, most bouts of apparent bowel obstruction respond to conservative measures and often need to be patiently waited out. Without clinical findings to suggest causes such as bowel suture line leak, volvulus, retention suture bowel loop entrapment, or incarcerated gut with an internal hernia, I have let periods as long as 21 days go by, awaiting spontaneous lysis of these presumed perioperative, filmy adhesions. The judicious use of parenteral, centrally, or peripherally administered hyperalimentation ensures minimal further loss of nutritional ground during this period.

Pseudo-obstruction involving the small or large intestine is a pathogenetically, poorly understood entity that has been reported with increasing frequency in the recent literature.[56–58] Although it occasionally is seen in cancer patients, it more commonly afflicts those with collagen-vascular and metabolic diseases. Affection of the small bowel can often be satisfactorily managed with long tube decompression, and

TABLE 60–18. Experiences With Intestinal Obstruction in Cancer Patients

Characteristics	Butler, 1991[44] (n = 54)	Clarke, 1987[45] (n = 49)	Gallick, 1986[46] (n = 84)	Walsh, 1984[47] (n = 53)	Aabo, 1984[48] (n = 41)	Bizer, 1981[49] (n = 35)	Osteen, 1980[50] (n = 66)	Annest, 1979[51] (n = 34)	Ketcham, 1970[52] (n = 117)
Known or recurrent cancer (%)	48	92					59	100	
Benign cause of obstruction (%)	32	14	26	32	17		38	3	18
Malignant cause of obstruction (%)	68	86		68	83		59	97	82
Gut strangulation (%)	19		Rare			3	2	0	5
Spontaneous resolution (%)	28		12			14	24		Seldom, temporary
Subsequently recurred (%)	45		41				41		
Recurrent or persistent obstruction after surgical treatment (%)	32	27	45	4	33	13	20	38	33
Operative mortality (%)	22	14	35	14	24		9	18	14
Operative morbidity (%)	49	49				20	15 wound	44	
Survival for all patients (mo)		5.7 (7 pts >1 y)	2.5	11 (15 pts >1 y)	4.5			4	(13% >3 y)
Survival with benign cause (mo)	49				36		5.5		(38% >3 y)
Survival with malignant cause (mo)	4.9				3		3 (6 pts >6 mo)		11 (4% >3 y)

similar, viability-threatening colonic involvement can usually be therapeutically decompressed with the colonoscope. Figure 60–8 illustrates an example of what was thought to be a severe case of vincristine-induced gut neuropathy.

A case is presented to illustrate the obstructive picture complex.

Patient No. 3

Eighteen years earlier, this 80-year-old man underwent abdominoperineal resection for adenocarcinoma of the rectum. A diagnosis of Wegener's granulomatosis was made 5 years ago on open lung biopsy; the hospital course was complicated by sepsis and pulmonary insufficiency that required a lengthy intensive care unit stay. Three years ago, the patient developed prostate cancer with extensive bony metastases treated with 7200 cGy to the prostate, 5400 cGy to pelvic lymph nodes, and bilateral orchiectomy. His disease remained stable for the next 3 years until he developed gross hematuria. At cystoscopy, bullous edema was found, and a mass was seen elevating the floor of the bladder. Biopsies revealed adenocarcinoma that stained immunohistochemically positive for carcinoembryonic antigen (CEA). Serum CEA was elevated to 144 ng/ml, and serum prostate specific antigen and acid phosphatase levels were normal. Chest x-ray films showed about 20 new pulmonary nodules. After suffering several weeks of intermittent abdominal distension and crampy pain, the patient developed frank small bowel obstruction confirmed on flat and upright abdominal films (Fig. 60–9A,B). A Gastrografin enema revealed no obstructive colonic component, refluxed the ileocecal valve, and showed a critically stenotic segment of distal ileum (see Fig. 60–9C,D). This finding was corroborated on abdominal CT scan (see Fig. 60–9E). At explor-

atory laparotomy numerous adhesions were lysed, a 6 × 8 cm pelvic mass identified, and a segment of strictured distal small bowel, presumably secondary to prior radiation therapy, bypassed with an ileoascending colostomy. Meaningful palliation was achieved when gastrointestinal integrity and function resumed uneventfully after operation. The patient died about 4 months later with progressive pulmonary metastatic disease and inanition.

HEMORRHAGE

Spontaneous hemorrhage of massive proportions from neoplastic lesions is a relatively uncommon problem. It can arise from a tumor, usually metastatic in nature and involving the mucosa of some portion of the gastrointestinal tract; from an extraluminal site, usually a hepatoma or hepatic adenoma; or more rarely a hepatic metastasis.[59–64] Occasionally, lymphomatous or leukemic gut infiltrative disease can produce this same problem.[25,65,66]

Far more common are episodes of hemorrhage that occur in an iatrogenically flavored context: postoperative bleeding after surgery for the primary lesion, a metastasis, or a treatment-related complication; spontaneous hemorrhage from an intercurrent benign lesion in the setting of chemotherapy-associated thrombocytopenia or clotting factor coagulopathy; or after percutaneous liver biopsy or central access line placement.[67]

The thought process triggered by most of these situations addresses several critical questions. What is the specific site of the hemorrhage? Point-source hemorrhage is far easier to control than diffuse bleeding. Ligatures are effective only when

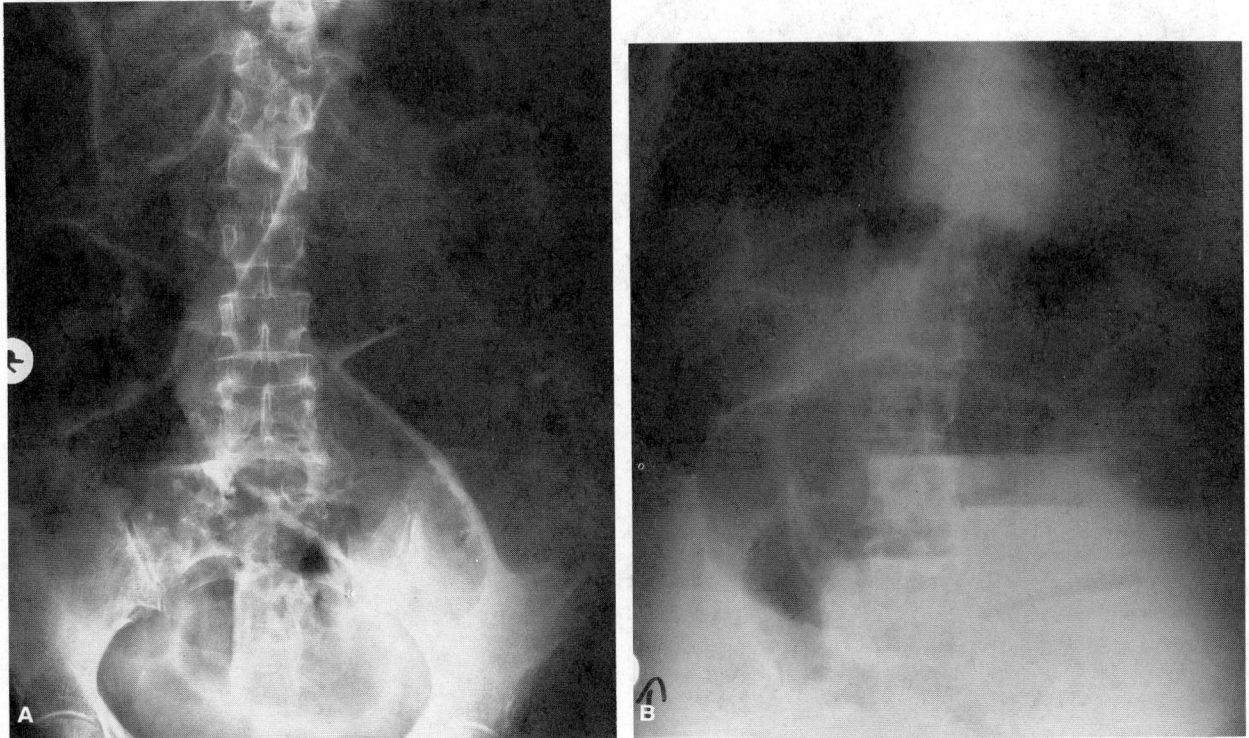

FIGURE 60–8.   (A, B) Plain abdominal films illustrate a severe vincristine-induced ileus that persisted for several weeks.

thrown about the bleeding vessel rather than in rough proximity to it. Are coagulopathic problems identifiable and will correction of them result in cessation of the hemorrhage? Is the bleeding of sufficient magnitude that specific therapeutic measures should be initiated to control it?

The stigmata of hemorrhage are tempo driven. Hemodynamic instability, ranging from tachycardia, mild weakness, and orthostatic pressure changes to frank shock with profound hypotension, is seen. Intravascular volume and erythrocyte support must be expeditiously provided. A useful approach to the patient suffering a bout of hemorrhage is summarized in Table 60–19. Several points deserve emphasis and elaboration. Although listed serially, the enumerated maneuvers are usually made concomitantly.

In a gratifying proportion of instances, with volume support and coagulopathy correction, the bleeding spontaneously remits. If it does not and its site can be determined, the less invasive alternatives usually undertaken to define the site often control or stop the hemorrhage.

In experienced hands, endoscopically performed injection, electrocoagulation, or photocoagulation of bleeding gastroduodenal lesions provides definitive control of hemorrhage in about 75% of the patients.[68–70] Forceps or brush biopsy of suspicious looking lesions can provide additional information about benign, neoplastic, fungal, or viral causes.

Continuing hemorrhage, at a rate of about 1 ml per minute in the colon or small intestine is best evaluated by angiography. The more actively bleeding the lesion, the easier it is to angiographically demonstrate. Unwisely administered gut contrast agents, until cleared, preclude this option. Patients who are hemodynamically unstable, particularly if oliguric because

of the contrast dye load needed, are stressful to study. The overall complexity of the effort required makes multiple studies difficult to accomplish and probably unwise and unreasonable to attempt. Because of these practical limitations, the timing of the study is critical, and this decision should be shared by surgeon and angiographer. Because a complete study may require several hours for runs of the inferior mesenteric artery, superior mesenteric artery, and celiac axis and a substantial administered dye load, it is wise to evaluate first the site most likely to be bleeding. If a diagnostic angiographic blush is identified, judgments can then be made about vasopressin infusion therapy (Athanasoulis) or transcatheter instillation of materials capable of producing vessel occlusion. Autogenous clot, Gelfoam torpedoes, Ivalon sponge, and metallic coils have been used with various degrees of success.[72,73] End-artery occlusion can produce significant organ ischemia and lead to complicating bowel infarction and perforation.

The importance of the invasive radiologist's technical virtuosity and judgmental expertise cannot be overstated. The former permits him to catheterize successfully and selectively the bleed vessel at a most distal or peripheral site, and the latter dictates which vessels can be successfully occluded without organ infarction.

If the less invasive therapeutic alternatives are not successful or not recommended, at least prior identification of the bleeding site lets the surgeon operate with the intent to suture-ligate or resect the affected tissues.

Hemorrhage into the free abdominal cavity, into the liver, or from the retroperitoneum or rectus sheaths is best evaluated by an abdominopelvic CT scan.[74] Spontaneous bleeding into the psoas or rectus muscles usually tamponades itself, can be

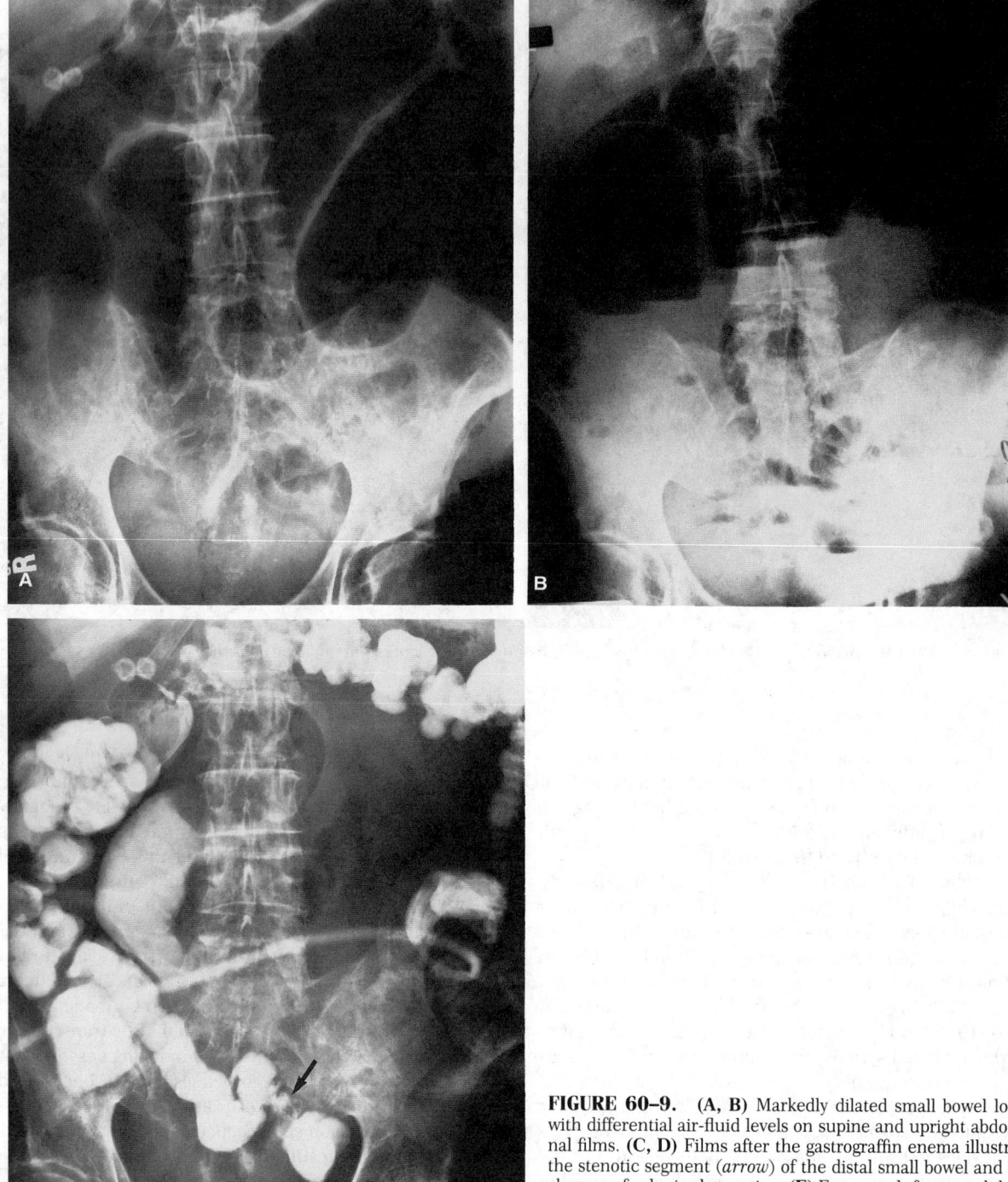

FIGURE 60–9. **(A, B)** Markedly dilated small bowel loops with differential air-fluid levels on supine and upright abdominal films. **(C, D)** Films after the gastrograffin enema illustrate the stenotic segment (*arrow*) of the distal small bowel and the absence of colonic obstruction. **(E)** Four panels from an abdominal CT scan, demonstrate the narrowed distal ileal segment (*arrow*).

managed expectantly, and resorbs in time. After needle biopsy, liver hemorrhage usually remits, but it occasionally becomes a hemodynamic threat. Angiographic approaches, as previously described, can permit the patient to escape surgical intervention. Figure 60–10A illustrates a contrast-enhanced abdominal CT scan obtained hours after percutaneous needle biopsy of the liver and shows a large right lobe hematoma. Figure 60–10B is a cut from an arteriogram done several hours later because of persistent hemorrhage. A dye blush shows

the site of continued active bleeding, which was satisfactorily controlled by instillation of multiple Gelfoam torpedoes into the right hepatic artery.

The cancer patient deserves the time-tested surgical approaches to control free intraperitoneal hemorrhage from spleen, liver, aorta, or other sources. Fibrin glue, delivered as an aerosolized spray at surgery, has helped to control diffuse surface hemorrhage from the liver, spleen, and retroperitoneum.[75]

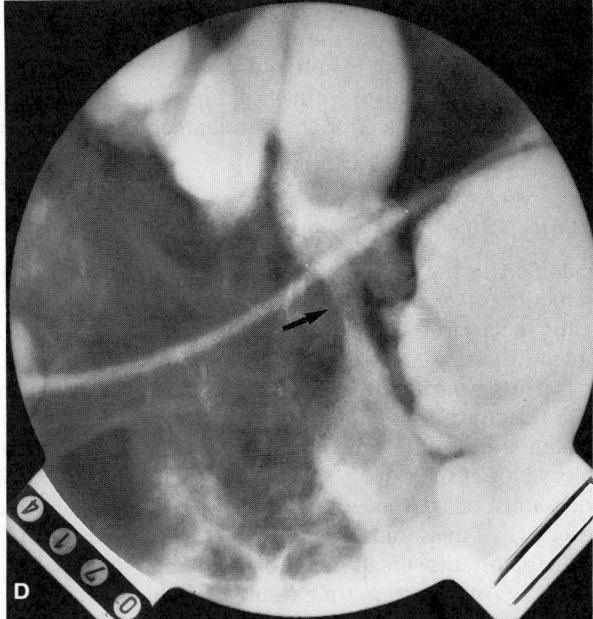
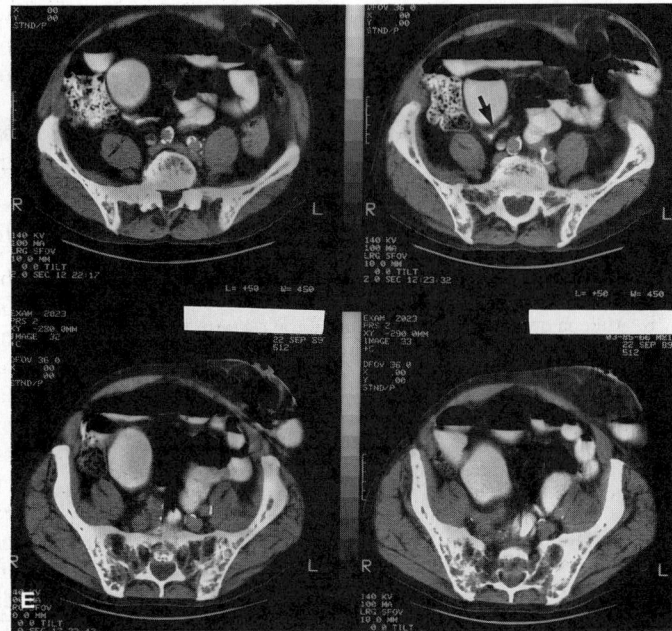

FIGURE 60–9. *(Continued)*

Anemia with subtly presenting symptoms of lassitude, fatigue, weakness, palpitations, and breathlessness is the result of slow chronic gut blood loss secondary to mucosal involvement by primary or metastatic tumor. Melanoma, metastatic to the bowel, often produces this sinister symptomatic picture and, after anatomic localization, can be palliated by segmental resection of the involved site.[76]

The following case presentation and accompanying studies reinforce several important points in regard to the urgent situation heralded by hemorrhage.

Patient No. 4
A 58-year-old man underwent subtotal gastrectomy for adenocarcinoma of the stomach in 1979. He observed bright red blood from the rectum 7 months earlier, and 4 weeks before the National Institutes of Health (NIH) referral, a large rectal cancer, fixed to the left pelvic sidewall was biopsied. Cystoscopy showed no bladder invasion, and the patient was treated with from 3600 cGy of preoperative pelvic irradiation complicated by urinary retention, proctitis, and severe perianal inflammation. In December of 1984, abdominoperineal resection was done in conjunction with placement of afterloading catheters and a silicone-gel-filled pelvic prosthesis, the latter to displace small bowel out of the pelvis and protect it from further radiation injury. Four months later, an upper gastrointestinal series suggested partial small bowel obstruction, and an abdominal CT scan showed a hydronephrotic left kidney (Fig. 60–11A). The patient was admitted to the hospital, where he suffered a massive (18 units of blood) lower gastrointestinal hemorrhage. An arteriogram revealed an arterioenteric fistula from the left internal iliac artery to small bowel (see Fig. 60–11B–D). Exsanguinating hemorrhage was controlled with transient balloon inflation and methylmethacrylate instillation into the internal iliac artery (see Fig. 60–11E). One day later, the patient developed a cold, pulseless, insensate foot and required Fogarty catheter thrombectomy. Spiking temperatures ensued, and three blood cultures positive for *Streptococcus fecalis* were ob-

tained. Three days after methylmethacrylate occlusion, the patient rebled, and an urgent laparotomy was performed. Takedown of the internal iliac artery to small bowel fistula was accomplished by ligating the internal iliac artery and resecting the involved small bowel segment. The silicone gel pelvic prosthesis was removed, a left nephrostomy performed, and the severely damaged, obstructed, distal left ureter ligated. Five weeks later, a recurrent, severe, acute left foot and ischemic leg was managed with a femorofemoral Gortex bypass graft. In November 1985, 5 months later, cystoscopy revealed a fibrotic, small, nonfunctional bladder, and the patient underwent jejunal loop diversion. In April 1986, he developed multiple pulmonary metastases and progressive cachexia. He died several months later.

INFECTION

Sepsis represents a constant threat to the patient with a malignancy. This often older population frequently has a host of chronic problems that can include malnutrition, diabetes, relatively asymptomatic periodontal disease, sinusitis, cholelithiasis, diverticulosis, and anorectal pathology. Although capable of erupting at any time, the patient is at greatest risk for a clinically problematic episode of infection during periods of treatment related vulnerability.

Febrile Neutropenia

Empiric antibiotic therapy has become the standard management approach to the common episodes of febrile granulocytopenia in cancer patients undergoing intensive chemotherapy.[77,78] Antifungal agents are often added to the therapy regimen if the patient fails to initially respond to treatment.[79] These patients can appear systemically quite ill with a paucity of focal findings, and surgical consultation is often sought. Infectious agents are frequently identified and presumably often arise from endogenous sources. Handled in this fashion,

TABLE 60–19. Evaluation and Treatment of Cancer Patients With Hemorrhage

1. Define the site, source, and cause. Consider the less invasive therapeutic alternatives.
   A. Hematemesis is almost always from the stomach, duodenum, or proximal-most jejunum. Pass nasogastric or larger bore orogastric tube to evacuate clot. Perform upper gastrointestinal endoscopy. Consider injection, electrocoagulation, photocoagulation for lesions of acid-peptic disease, gastritis, Mallory-Weiss tear, or sclerotherapy for varices.
   B. Melena or bright red blood around the rectum. Perform sigmoidoscopy to rule out source in distal 25 cm of colon if no blood is found in nasogastric aspirate. Consider angiogram. If actively bleeding lesion is seen in small bowel or colon consider infusional or occlusional therapy. Consider radionuclide-labeled erythrocyte scan as a diagnostic alternative to angiogram. Consider colonoscopy, which is occasionally helpful if the rate of bleeding permits cleansing of the colon for adequate inspection.
   C. Extraluminal hemorrhage. CT scan of abdomen or pelvis to rule out intraperitoneal, retroperitoneal, or rectus sheath bleeds.
2. Determine and correct all coagulopathic problems: platelet count, prothrombin time, partial thromboplastin time, bleeding time, other coagulation factor level assessment. Consider platelet transfusion, vitamin K, fresh frozen plasma, or factor concentrates as appropriate.
3. Eliminate the chemical offenders: aspirin, nonsteroidal antiinflammatory agents, heparin (sometimes only by line flush), Coumadin, alcohol, and caffeine.
4. Initiate the surface protective agents (for gastroduodenal bleeding): H_2-receptor blockers or sucralfate.
5. Surgical intervention for recalcitrant bleeding. Use suture ligation or resection as appropriate for the site or cause.

with bone marrow recovery and the restoration of more normal neutrophil numbers, most episodes remit, and there is no need for surgical intervention.

Persistent fever with or without continued neutropenia, the appearance of jaundice, or the development of focal signs invite further diagnostic study.

Jaundice

In addition to the more common specific causes of biliary obstruction secondary to tumor or stone disease, extensive hepatic metastases, cirrhosis, hepatitis, or hepatotoxic drugs, jaundice occurs as a poorly understood consequence of sepsis. Pancreatitis can produce sufficient gland edema to impede bile drainage and cause mild to modest elevation in the serum bilirubin and must be ruled out. The diagnostic question of cholecystitis of the calculous or more treacherous acalculous variety must be addressed. An ultrasound of the biliary tree, particularly if the serum bilirubin has reached the level of 10 mg/dl, usually answers the question of whether there is ductal dilation, the often unremitting result of mechanical blockage. The study is the best test for the presence of gallstones, the inciter of cholecystitis and, if causing common ductal obstruction, cholangitis. Even without stones, if the gallbladder appears to be thick walled, enlarged, and full of sludge, the possibility of acalculous infection exists and can often be addressed with a radionuclide HIDA (*N*-[2,6-diethylacetanilido]-iminodiacetic acid) scan. Nondilated ducts and a normal HIDA scan reassuringly eliminate the need to contemplate cholecystectomy or a biliary drainage procedure. A CT scan of the liver makes useful complementary comments on the gallbladder and biliary ductal tree.

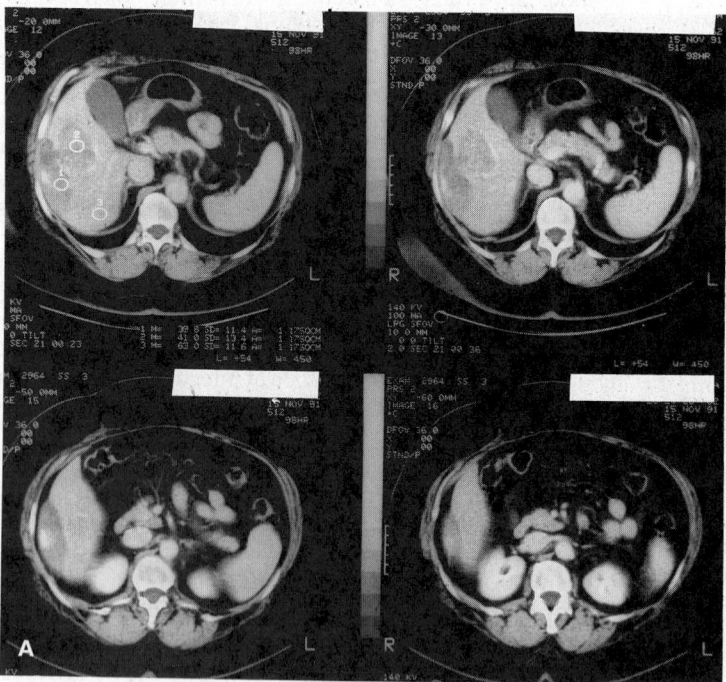
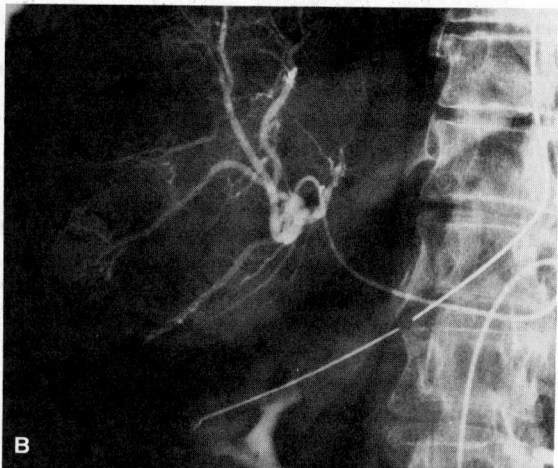

FIGURE 60–10. **(A)** Four panels from a contrast-enhanced abdominal CT scan illustrate the large right lobar hepatic hemorrhage. **(B)** A cut from the hepatic arteriogram demonstrates a dye blush (*arrow*), representing continued bleeding.

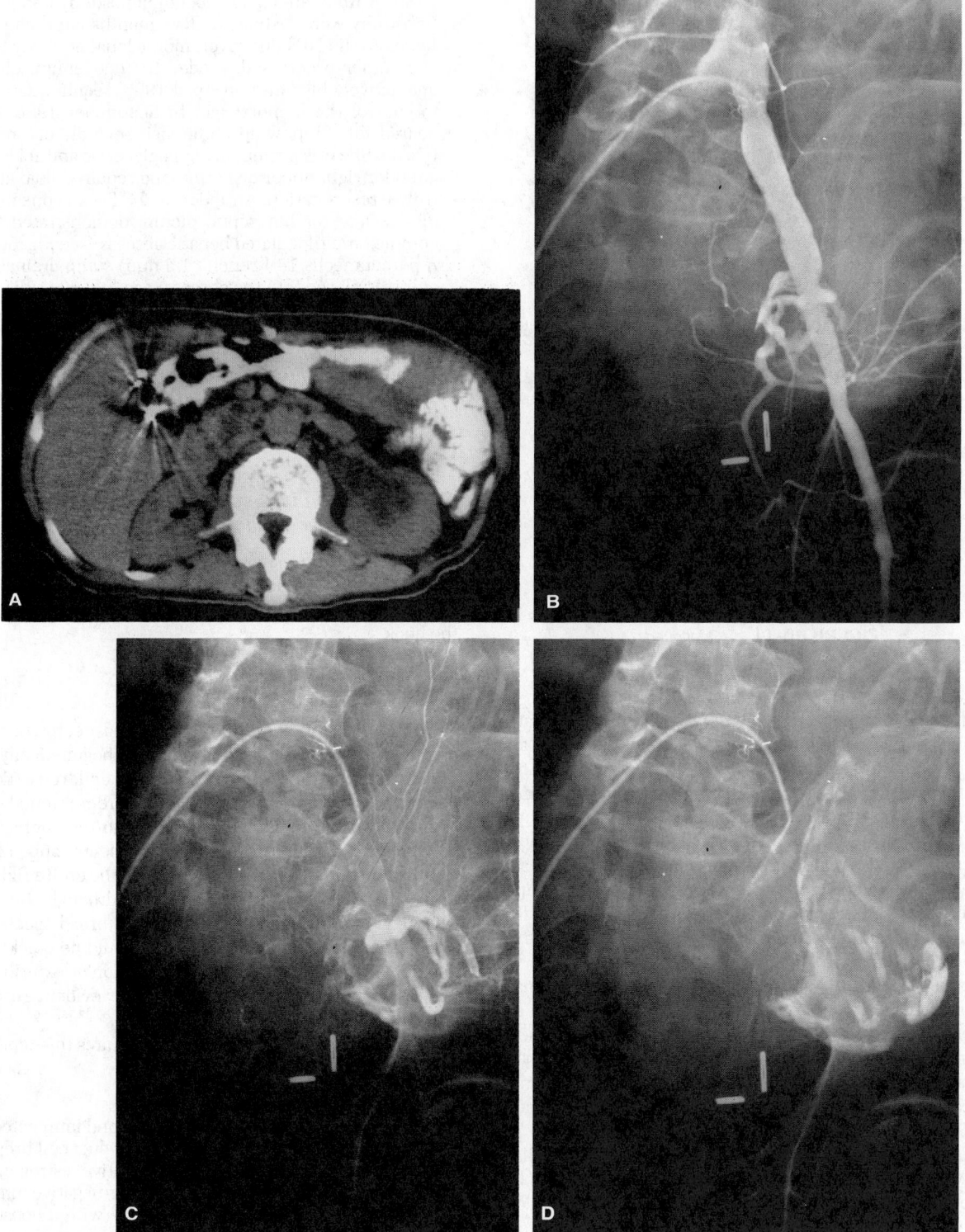

FIGURE 60–11. (A) A panel from the abdominal CT scan illustrates the left hydronephrosis. (B–D) Arteriographic cuts demonstrate arteriovenous shunting and the arterioenteric fistula. (E) The angiogram balloon occludes the left internal iliac artery before methylmethacrylate instillation.   *(continued)*

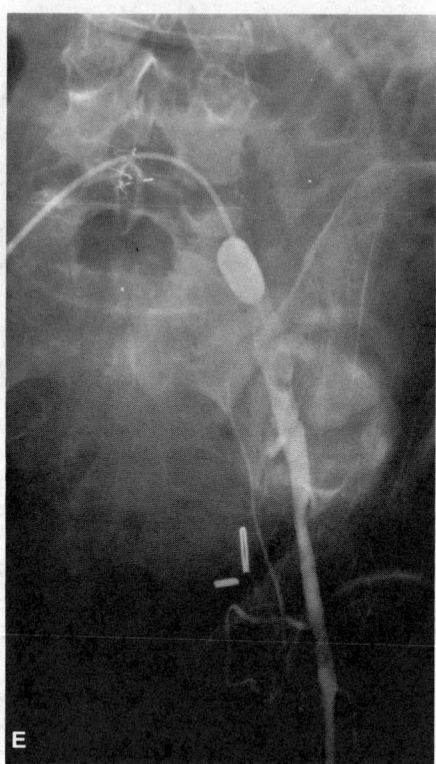

FIGURE 60-11. *(Continued)*

Gallbladder or biliary tree infection, particularly associated with stones, that does not quickly respond to antibiotics and supportive therapy requires drainage. Percutaneous cholecystostomy with or without an endoscopic retrograde common duct drainage procedure can, particularly in the high-risk patient, represent a salutary alternative to laparotomy, cholecystectomy, and possibly common duct exploration and drainage.[80–82] Malignant biliary obstructive problems, even if complicated by infection, can often be satisfactorily handled by the interventional radiologist with a percutaneous transhepatic approach.[83,84]

Like ultrasound, the abdominal CT scan can detect mass lesions, such as abscess or tumor, in the liver. Hepatic abscesses caused by bacterial or fungal infection are being seen with increasing frequency in patients with leukemia or lymphoma and gastrointestinal malignancy.[85] For one to four abscesses, the patient, can often be well managed by percutaneous drainage and escape laparotomy.[86,87]

If the initial assessments of the hepatobiliary tree fail to provide an explanation for the jaundice, a more thorough CT scan of the abdomen and pelvis, particularly in the patient recovering from a laparotomy classified as contaminated, can prove useful. An otherwise occult intraabdominal or pelvic abscess is being sought, and if found, it can often be handled by percutaneous drainage.[88–93]

A case illustrates the diagnostic utility of the CT scan and salutary problem resolution through invasive percutaneous radiologic intervention.

Patient No. 5
A 62-year-old woman with obstructive jaundice underwent laparotomy for unresectable pancreas cancer in August 1985. A Roux-en-Y choledochojejunostomy and gastroenterostomy were fashioned. Two months later, she was referred to the NIH and given monoclonal antibody therapy. Her tumor progressed, eroded the duodenum, ulcerated, and actively bled and, in April 1986, required laparotomy to control the hemorrhage. In September 1986, she appeared for a follow-up clinic visit severely obtunded and febrile. She was profoundly hypoglycemic and acidotic, had a tender right upper quadrant, and required fluid and electrolyte resuscitation. An abdominal CT scan done in pursuit of a source for her septic picture demonstrated a large, complex multiloculated hepatic abscess (see Fig. 60–12A). A percutaneous 14 French (4.6 mm) sump drainage catheter was placed into the abscess (see Fig. 60–12B) and 2.1 L of pus evacuated, which on culture grew *E. coli, Klebsiella pneumoniae, Streptococcus fecalis,* and *Bacteroides melanogenicus.* The patient's postdrainage course was complicated by the development of adult respiratory distress syndrome and coagulopathy. She recovered after a 2-week stay in the intensive care unit and was discharged home for continued supportive care.

Central Access Line Sepsis and Suppurative Thrombophlebitis

The diagnosis and management of central access line sepsis and suppurative thrombophlebitis, an increasingly common surgical emergency, are thoroughly discussed elsewhere in the book.

Enterocolitis

Typhlitis, neutropenic enterocolitis, and necrotizing enteropathy are terms used to describe a pathogenetically poorly understood syndrome seen most often in children undergoing chemotherapy for leukemia, but the disorder is found in some adults with solid malignancies. Although the edematous involvement can be limited to the distal ileum, appendix, and cecum alone, it often extends to involve the entire right colon and sometimes the transverse colon. Although the process often remits on supportive therapy and broad-spectrum antibiotics, the conservative approach should be quickly abandoned in favor of laparotomy and resection or exteriorization and resection of the afflicted tissues if any evidence of further clinical deterioration becomes apparent.[30,32,33,94,95]

The following case presentation illustrates this septic complication of treatment.

Patient No. 6
A 36-year-old women was 2 years beyond lumpectomy and axillary adenectomy for an infiltrating duct cell breast cancer. After operation for her node-negative, estrogen receptor-negative, and progesterone receptor-negative tumor, she received breast irradiation (4500 cGy with a boost to the tumor bed to 5940 cGy) and six cycles of adjuvant therapy with cyclophosphamide, methotrexate, and 5-fluorouracil (CMF). Two months earlier, a chest CT scan showed bilateral pulmonary nodules, one of which proved cytologically positive for breast cancer on fine-needle aspiration. Eight days after starting taxol, doxorubicin, and granulocyte colony-stimulating factor therapy, she developed crampy abdominal pain, distension, diarrhea, and severe febrile neutropenia. Broad-spectrum antibiotics were started, and because of marked lower abdominal tenderness, an abdominal CT scan was obtained (Fig. 60–13A) which suggested

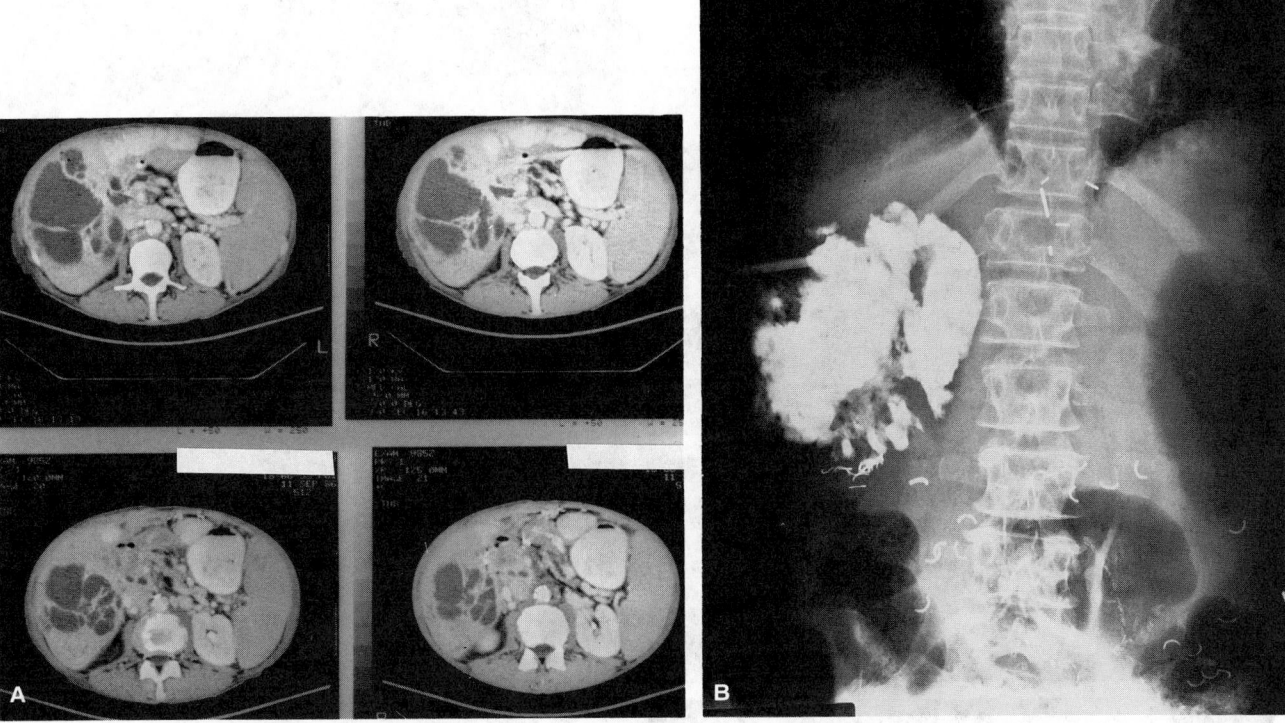

FIGURE 60–12. (A) Four panels from an abdominal CT scan demonstrate the large, complex, multiloculated hepatic abscess. (B) X-ray film illustrates the drainage catheter in the abscess that was filled with contrast material.

an inflammatory process involving bowel in the right lower quadrant. Because insufficient orally ingested contrast opacified these bowel loops, dilute gastrograffin was administered by enema and fluoroscopy and additional CT images obtained (see Fig. 60–13B–D). A phlegmonous, ulcerated process involving the cecum was clearly delineated that, on continued supportive care, slowly resolved clinically and roentgenographically over the next 3 weeks.

Perirectal Infection

Anorectal symptoms are common among cancer patients; pain, with or without bowel movements is the most frequent complaint. Hemorrhoidal pathology is exceedingly common and often made more problematic by the bouts of diarrhea and constipation that complicate chemotherapy and the use of narcotic pain medication. Anal fissuring, probably secondary to constipation, is slow to heal in the catabolic patient. Although underreported in the literature, anal gland inflammation in the neutropenic patient can rapidly progress to extensive perirectal cellulitis or frank abscess formation.[96]

Perirectal infection, particularly when the patient is febrile and neutropenic, can be quite difficult to sort out. Inspection, facilitated by buttock cheek retraction and a Valsalva maneuver, and gentle external palpation sometimes reveals a thrombosed or ulcerative internal hemorrhoid, a fissure, point tenderness, or an indurated bulge. Often nothing is appreciated on this kind of limited assessment. A pelvic CT scan that permits evaluation of the perirectal spaces and fat pyramids for symmetry, inflammatory streaking, edematous

change, or frank abscess formation can be helpful. Ambiguous findings often dictate whether to proceed immediately with a digital rectal examination and anoscopy. These assessments usually cannot be made without giving the patient an anesthetic.

An initial period of conservative local management is usually tried. Warm Sitz baths, Tucks to promote local hygiene, stool softeners, or antidiarrheal agents as indicated and analgesics are helpful. If stability or slight clinical improvement is not seen after 24 to 48 hours, the more invasive diagnostic efforts can be made.

Perianal cellulitis, particularly in the face of neutropenia and thrombocytopenia, is initially best managed with intravenously administered, high-dose, broad-spectrum antibiotics. Abscesses characterized by frank fluctuance require incision and drainage by standard surgical approaches. Infrequently, the infection becomes so locally and systemically aggressive that fecal diversion becomes necessary.

Soft Tissue Infection

In addition to the usual array of soft tissue infections that include acne-like pustules, furuncles, carbuncles, paronychia, felons, foreign-body-related infections, and cellulitis, which are handled in standard surgical fashion, several unusual circumstances merit consideration.

After axillary or groin lymphadenectomy, the extremity becomes particularly susceptible to an aggressive, virulent streptococcal (often mixed streptococcal and staphylococcal)

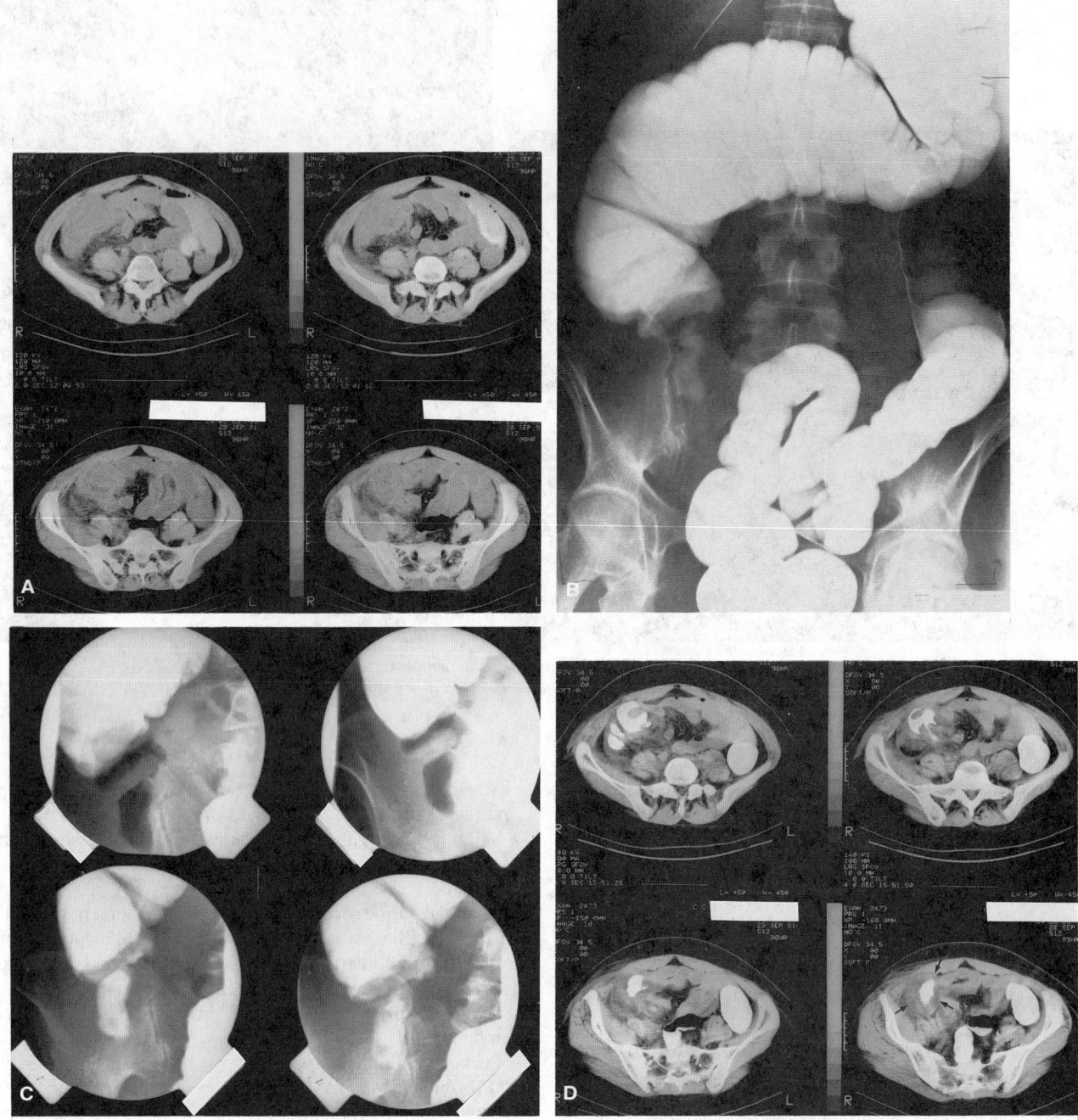

FIGURE 60–13. **(A)** Four panels from the initial abdominal CT scan that demonstrates only dilated, fluid-filled bowel loops and suggest an edematous, inflammatory process involving bowel in the right lower quadrant. **(B, C)** X-ray films obtained after a gastrograffin enema show a large, ulcerated area involving the cecum. **(D)** Abdominal CT scan cuts obtained after a gastrograffin enema corroborate the markedly edematous, thick-walled, ulcerated cecum (*arrows*) seen in typhlitis.

cellulitis called erysipelas. An initial innocuous-appearing patch of cutaneous erythema, sometimes after an otherwise harmless scratch, can progress in several hours with significant swelling to involve the entire extremity and leave the patient markedly febrile, prostrate, and systemically toxic. No portal of entry for the bacteria is identified for many cases, although the cutaneous cracks consequent to preventable foot fungal infection can admit the organisms. Successful treatment rests on early recognition of the infection's virulent po-

tential. Intravenous administration of high-dose antibiotics directed at both potentially offending organisms, extremity elevation, and rest are the therapy cornerstones. Due to the adenectomy-imposed compromise to lymphatic fluid return, I usually omit warm compresses or soaks, which encourage increased blood flow into the tissues and contribute to potentially problematic edema formation.

The chronic and intermittently acute immunocompromised nature of the cancer patient makes him susceptible to an additional group of gangrene-producing, exceedingly virulent soft tissue infections that, depending on the organisms involved and tissues affected, go by the names of necrotizing fasciitis, anaerobic cellulitis, gas gangrene, bacterial synergistic gangrene, or necrotizing cutaneous mucormycosis. These entities are thoroughly considered in a text by Howard and Simmons.[97] The infection commonly follows a contaminated surgical procedure and usually involves the wound. This life-threatening infection characteristically produces extensive tissue necrosis, potentially involving skin, fat, fascia, and muscle. Prompt, aggressive, and wide surgical incision, drainage, and debridement coupled with broad-spectrum antibiotics that include anaerobic coverage is imperative. Hyperbaric oxygen administration can probably help if clostridial myonecrosis is involved.

Because of their heightened susceptibility to the unusual and the usually identified organisms, it is essential to pursue infections in these hosts with energetic efforts to culture and identify the offender. An unsuspected but treatable fungus, like *Aspergillus,* is sometimes found.

DECIDING ON AGGRESSIVE OR CONSERVATIVE MANAGEMENT

Regrettably, cancer patients often succumb to medically recalcitrant progressive disease. This circumstance is understandably trying, tension provoking, and frustrating for the patient, the family, and the physician. If inanition, pulmonary infection, and metabolic derangement are the terminal issues, the surgeon remains uninvolved, but if obstruction, hemorrhage, or the consequences of a progressive mass are the insults provoking a sense of urgency, the surgeon will be asked to intervene. This situation, perhaps more than any other, tests the judgmental acumen of the surgeon and demands from him or her an honest assessment of what a surgical undertaking potentially affords. If the expectations for serious-minded palliation are realistic and not insubstantial, proceeding to operation is reasonable, but if the likelihood of minimally deferring the inevitable while protracting the burden of suffering at ever increasing cost is more likely, than alternative, pain-alleviating measures should be liberally instituted.

NUTRITION AND OTHER SUPPORT

Cancer and the treatments we direct at it invariably represent a catabolic insult. Resultant malnutrition, poor wound healing, and immunocompromise are the almost inescapable consequences. "Food is medicine" is the message that must be tirelessly preached to patient and family alike. The liberal use of high-calorie enteral supplements and a multivitamin preparation should be regularly encouraged.

Constipation, often associated with narcotic usage and poor fluid intake, contributes to the development of symptomatic anorectal difficulty and should be anticipated and prevented through the use of stool softeners and bulk-restoring agents. The conscientious physician must provide the patient with a mild cathartic to facilitate elimination of the barium burden administered with fluoroscopic gastrointestinal studies. Obstipation, impaction, and painful and unpleasant digitally as-

sisted evacuation or stercoral colonic ulceration and perforation are preventable.

Stress-related anxiety and depression are associated with cancer. Anxiety contributes to erosive, acid-peptic gastroduodenal bleeding and can be managed effectively with mucosal surface-protective agents, like sucralfate or the H_2-receptor blockers, and depression adversely affects the patient and the family's quality of life and saps strength that might otherwise be marshaled in the struggle to survive.[98] Group support systems, professional psychiatric help, and mood-impacting medicines can be quite helpful and should not be forgotten.

Treatment-complicating intercurrent problems or issues like symptomatic gallstones, diverticular disease, anorectal pathology, or the threat of an unwanted pregnancy should be anticipated. Often the nonvulnerable period before treatment or the quiescent intervals between treatments can be use to surgically address and prevent problems that may later erupt in far more morbid, unmanageable forms. The advent of less invasive, safer surgical procedures, like laparoscopic cholecystectomy, with rapid postprocedure recovery, will doubtless encourage these preventive considerations.[99]

REFERENCES

1. Botsford TW, Wilson RE. The acute abdomen: An approach to diagnosis and management. 2nd ed. Philadelphia: WB Saunders, 1977.
2. Dunphy RE, Botsford TW. Physical examination of the surgical patient: An introduction to clinical surgery. 4th ed. Philadelphia: WB Saunders, 1975.
3. Schwartz SI, Shires GT, Spencer FC, eds. Principles of surgery. 5th ed. New York: McGraw-Hill, 1989.
4. Shiloni E, Weiss CM, Baker AR. Surgical management of the critically ill immunocompromised patient. In: Parillo JE, Masur H, eds. The critically ill immunocompromised patient: Diagnosis and management. Bethesda, MD: Aspen Publication, 1987:557–584.
5. Turnbull ADM, Starnes HF Jr. Surgical emergencies in the cancer patient. Chicago: Year Book Medical Publishers, 1987.
6. Wilson RE. Surgical problems in immuno-depressed patients. In: Major problems in clinical surgery, vol 30. Philadelphia: WB Saunders, 1984.
7. Sherlock P. The gastrointestinal manifestations and complications of malignant lymphoma. Schweiz Med Wochenschr 1980;110:1031–1037.
8. Herrmann R, Panahon AM, Barcos MP, et al. Gastrointestinal involvement in non-Hodgkin's lymphoma. Cancer 1980;46:215–222.
9. Lewin KJ, Ranchod M, Dorfman RF. Lymphomas of the gastrointestinal tract—a study of 117 cases presenting with gastrointestinal disease. Cancer 1978;42:693–707.
10. Sherman NJ, Wooley MM. The ileocecal syndrome in acute childhood leukemia. Arch Surg 1973;107:39–42.
11. Klener P, Donner L, Bocanova M, et al. Gastrointestinal lesions and complications in hemoblastoses. Folia Haematol (Leipz) 1973;100:57–66.
12. Lee JR, Gray SW, Brown BC, et al. Diffuse histiocytic lymphomas of the gastrointestinal tract in the adult. Surg Gynecol Obstet 1983;157:286–300.
13. Remine SG, McIlrath DC. Bowel perforation in steroid treated patients. Ann Surg 1980;192:581–586.
14. Pizzo PA. Granulocytopenia and cancer therapy—past problems, current solutions, future challenges. Cancer 1984;54:2649–2661.
15. Shuffler MD, Baird HW, Fleming CR, et al. Intestinal pseudoobstruction as the presenting manifestation of small cell carcinoma of the lung. A paraneoplastic neuropathy of the gastrointestinal tract. Ann Intern Med 1983;98:129–134.
16. Rosenthal S, Kaufman S. Vincristine neurotoxicity. Ann Intern Med 1974;80:733–737.
17. Ferrara JJ, Martin EW, Carey LC. Morbidity of emergency operations in patients with metastatic cancer receiving chemotherapy. Surgery 1982;92:605–609.
18. Pauker SG, Kopelman RI. Clinical problem solving—Trapped by an incidental finding. N Engl J Med 1992;326:40–43.
19. Roh JJ, Thompson JS, Harned RK, et al. Value of pneumoperitoneum in the diagnosis of visceral perforation. Am J Surg 1983;146:830–833.
20. Zer M, Wolloch Y, Lombrozo MD, et al. Palliative treatment of duodenoenteric fistulas. World J Surg 1980;4:131–135.
21. Vetto JT, Culp SC, Smythe TB, et al. Iliac aterial-enteric fistulas occurring after pelvic irradiation. Surgery 1987;101:643–647.
22. Kostroff KM, Turnbull AD, Rotstein LE, et al. Duodenojejunostomy and stapled occlusion for distal duodenal perforation from malignant retroperitoneal tumors. J Surg Oncol 1984;26:252–255.
23. Bertolone SJ, Fuenfer MM, Groff DB, et al. Delayed pancreatic pseudocyst formation—Long-term complication of L-asparaginase treatment. Cancer 1982;50:2964–2966.
24. Puckett JB, Butler WM, McFarland JA. Pancreatitis and cancer chemotherapy. Ann Intern Med [Letter] 1982;97:453.

25. Hande KR, Fisher RI, DeVita VT, et al. Diffuse histiocytic lymphoma involving the gastrointestinal tract. Cancer 1978;41:1984–1989.

26. Weingrad DN, DeCosse JJ, Sherlock P, et al. Primary gastrointestinal lymphoma: A 30-year review. Cancer 1982;49:1258–1265.

27. Rajagopalan AE, Pickleman J. Free perforation of the small intestine. Ann Surg 1982;196:576–579.

28. Leidich RB, Rudolf LE. Small bowel perforation secondary to metastatic lung carcinoma. Ann Surg 1981;193:67–69.

29. Perkins JD, Shield CF III, Chang FC, et al. Acute diverticulitis—Comparison of treatment in immunocompromised and nonimmunocompromised patients. Am J Surg 1984;148:745–748.

30. Shamberger RC, Weinstein HJ, Delorey RN, et al. The medical and surgical management of typhlitis in children with acute nonlymphocytic (myelogenous) leukemia. Cancer 1986;57:603–609.

31. Sauter ER, Vauthey JN, Bolton, et al. Selective management of patients with neutropenic enterocolitis using peritoneal lavage. J Surg Oncol 1990;45:63–67.

32. Wade DS, Douglas H Jr, Nava HR, et al. Abdominal pain in neutropenic patients. Arch Surg 1990;125:1119–1127.

33. Starnes HF, Moore FD, Mentzer S, et al. Abdominal pain in neutropenic cancer patients. Cancer 1986;57:616–621.

34. Frank D, Raicht RF. Intestinal perforation associated with cytomegalovirus infection in patients with acquired immune deficiency syndrome. Am J Gastroenterol 1984;79:201–205.

35. Rosenberg JM, Walker M, Welch JP, Mullany L. *Clostridium difficile* colitis in surgical patients. Am J Surg 1984;147:486–491.

36. Schwartzentruber D, Lotze MT, Rosenberg SA. Colon perforation—An unusual complication of therapy with high-dose interleukin-2. Cancer 1988;62:2350–2353.

37. Galland RB, Spencer MS. Surgical management of radiation enteritis. Surgery 1986;99:133–138.

38. Morganstern L, Hart M, Lugo D, Friedman NB. Changing aspects of radiation enteropathy. Arch Surg 1985;120:1225–1228.

39. Lundy J, Sherlock P, Kurtz R, et al. Spontaneous perforation of the gastrointestinal tract in patients with cancer. Am J Gastroenterol 1975;63:447–450.

40. Isabella V, Marotta E, Bianchi F. Ischemic necrosis of proximal gastric remnant following subtotal gastrectomy with splenectomy. J Surg Oncol 1984;25:124–132.

41. Koretz MJ, Neifeld JP. Emergency surgical treatment for patients with leukemia. Surg Gynecol Obstet 1985;161:149–151.

42. Vaughn EA, Key CR, Sterling WA Jr. Intraabdominal operations in patients with leukemia. Am J Surg 1988;156:51–53.

43. Dunn JT, Halls JM, Berne TV. Roentgenographic contrast studies in acute small bowel obstruction. Arch Surg 1984;119:1305–1308.

44. Butler JA, Brian CL, Morrow M, Kahng K, et al. Small bowel obstruction in patients with a prior history of cancer. Am J Surg 1991;162:624–628.

45. Clarke-Pearson DL, Chin NO, DeLong ER, et al. Surgical management of intestinal obstruction in ovarian cancer. 1. Clinical features, postoperative complications and survival. Gynecol Oncol 1987;26:11–18.

46. Gallick HL, Weaver DW, Sachs RJ, Bouwman DL. Intestinal obstruction in cancer patients: An assessment of risk factors and outcomes. Am Surg 1986;52:434–437.

47. Walsh HPJ, Schofield PF. Is laparotomy for small bowel obstruction justified in patients with previously treated malignancy. Br J Surg 1984;71:933–935.

48. Aabo K, Pedersen H, Bach F, Knudsen J. Surgical management of intestinal obstruction in the late course of malignant disease. Acta Chir Scand 1984;150:173–176.

49. Bizer LS, Liebling RW, Delany HM, Gleidman ML. Small bowel obstruction. Surgery 1981;89:407–413.

50. Osteen RT, Guyton S, Steele G Jr, Wilson RE. Malignant intestinal obstruction. Surgery 1980;87:611–615.

51. Annest LS, Jolly PC. The results of surgical treatment of bowel obstruction caused by peritoneal carcinomatosis. Am Surg 1979;45:718–721.

52. Ketcham AS, Hoye RC, Pilch YH, Morton DL. Delayed intestinal obstruction following treatment for cancer. Cancer 1970;25:406–410.

53. Stewardson RH, Bombeck T, Nyhus LM. Critical operative management of small bowel obstruction. Ann Surg 1978;187:189–193.

54. Sarr MG, Bulkley GB, Zuidema GD. Preoperative recognition of intestinal strangulation obstruction: Prospective evaluation diagnostic capability. Am J Surg 1983;145:176–182.

55. Baines M, Oliver DJ, Carter RL. Medical management of intestinal obstruction in patients with advanced malignant disease. Lancet 1985;2:990–993.

56. Richards WO, Williams LF Jr. Obstruction of the large and small intestine. Surg Clin North Am 1988;68:355–376.

57. Geelhoed GW. Colonic pseudo-obstruction in surgical patients. Am J Surg 1985;149:258–265.

58. Nivatvongs S, Vermeulen FD, Fang DT. Colonic decompression of acute pseudo-obstruction. Ann Surg 1982;196:598–600.

59. Gordon B, Lossef SV, Jelinger E, et al. Embolotherapy for small bowel hemorrhage from Metastatic renal cell carcinoma: Case report. Cardiovasc Intervent Radiol 1991;14:311–313.

60. Plukker JT, Koops HS, Sleijfer DT, et al. Intestinal hemorrhages in patients with a nonseminomatous testicular tumor. Cancer 1991;68:2630–2632.

61. Harris MN. Massive gastrointestinal hemorrhage. Arch Surg 1964;88:1049–1051.

62. Okasaki M, Higashihara H, Koganemaru F, Nakamura T. Intraperitoneal hemorrhage from hepatocellular carcinoma: Emergency chemoemboliztion or embolization. Radiology 1991;180:647–651.

63. Foster JH, Berman MM, eds. Solid liver tumors. In: Major problems in clinical surgery, vol XXII. Philadelphia: WB Saunders, 1977:79, 155.

64. Erb RE, Gibler WB. Massive hemoperitoneum following rupture of hepatic metastases from unsuspected choriocarcinoma. Am J Emerg Med 1989;7:196–198.

65. Rosenfelt F, Rosenberg SA. Diffuse histiocytic lymphoma presenting with gastrointestinal tract lesions: The Stanford experience. Cancer 1980;45:2188–2193.

66. Schaller RT, Schaller JF. The acute abdomen in the immunologically compromised child. J Pediatr Surg 1983;18:937–944.

67. McGill DB, Rakela J, Zinmeister AR, Ott BJ. A 21-year experience with major hemorrhage ager percutaneous liver biopsy. Gastroenterology 1990;99:1396–1400.

68. Cook DJ, Guyatt GH, Salena BJ, Laine LA. Endoscopic therapy for acute nonvariceal upper gastrointestinal hemorrhage: A meta-analysis. Gastroenterology 1992;102:139–148.

69. Waring JP, Sanowski RA, Sawyer RL, et al. A randomized comparison of monopolar electrocoagulation and injection sclerosis for the treatment of bleeding peptic ulcer. Gastrointest Endosc 1991;37:295–298.

70. Hui WM, Ng MMT, Lok ASF, Lai CL. A randomized comparative study of laser photocoagulation, heater probe, and bipolar electrocoagulation in the treatment of actively bleeding ulcers. Gastrointest Endosc 1991;37:299–304.

71. Athanasoulis CA, Baum S, Waltman AC, et al. Control of acute gastric mucosal hemorrhage. N Engl J Med 1974;290:597–603.

72. Pisco JM, Martins JM, Correia MG. Internal iliac artery: Emobolization to control hemorrhage from neoplasms. Radiology 1989;172:337–339.

73. Chuang VP, Wallace S, Gianturco C. A new improved coil for tapered-tip catheter for arterial occlusion. Radiology 1980;135:507–509.

74. Jeffrey RB Jr, Cardoza JD, Olcott EW. Detection of active intraabdominal arterial hemorrhage: Value of dynamic contrast-enhanced CT. AJR 1991;156:725–729.

75. Kram HB, Shoemaker WC, Clark SR, Macabee JR. Spraying of aerosolized fibrin glue in the treatment of nonsuturable hemorrhage. Am Surg 1991;57:381–384.

76. Das Gupta TK, Brasfield RD. Metastatic melanoma of the gastrointestinal tract. Arch Surg 1964;88:969–973.

77. Gucalp R. Management of the febrile neutropenic patient with cancer. Oncology 1991;5:137–147.

78. Pizzo PA, Hathorn JW, Hiemenz J, et al. A randomized trial comparing ceftazidime alone with combination antibiotic therapy in cancer patients with fever and neutropenia. N Engl J Med 1986;315:552–558.

79. Pizzo PA, Robichaud KJ, Wesley R, Commers JR. Fever in the pediatric and young adult patient with cancer. Medicine (Baltimore) 1982;61:153–165.

80. Klimberg S, Hawkins I, Vogel SB. Percutaneous cholecystostomy for acute cholecystitis in high-risk patients. Am J Surg 1987;153:125–129.

81. van Sonnenberg E, Wittich GR, Casola G, et al. Diagnostic and therapeutic gallbladder procedures. Radiology 1986;160:23–26.

82. Frazee RC, Nagorney DM, Mucha P Jr. Acute acalculous cholecystitis. Mayo Clin Proc 1989;64:163–167.

83. Ring EJ. Radiologic approach to malignant biliary obstruction: Review and commentary. Cardiovasc Intervent Radiol 1990;13:217–222.

84. Walta DC, Fausel CS, Brant B. Endoscopic biliary stents and obstructive jaundice. Am J Surg 1987;153:444–447.

85. Thaler M, Pastakia B, Shawker TH, et al. Hepatic candidiasis in cancer patients: The evolving picture of the syndrome. Ann Intern Med 1988;108:88–100.

86. Haaga JR. Imaging intraabdominal abscesses and nonoperative drainage. World J Surg 1990;14:204–209.

87. Pruett TL, Simmons RL. Status of percutaneous catheter drainage of abscesses. Surg Clin North Am 1988;68:89–105.

88. Olak J, Christou NV, Stein LA, et al. Operative vs percutaneous drainage of intra-abdominal abscesses: Comparison of morbidity and mortality. Arch Surg 1986;121:141–146.

89. Johnson WC, Gerzof SG, Robbins AH, Nabseth DC. Treatment of abdominal abscesses: Comparative evaluation of operative versus percutaneous catheter drainage by guided computed tomography or ultrasound. Ann Surg 1981;194:510–552.

90. Lurie K, Plzak L, Deveney CW. Intra-abdominal abscessess in the 1980s. Surg Clin North Am 1987;67:621–632.

91. Flancbaum L, Nosher JL, Brolin RE. Percutaneous catheter drainage of abdominal abscesses associated with perforated viscus. Am Surg 1990;56:52–56.

92. Lent WM, Goldman MJ, Bizer LS. An objective appraisal of the role of computed tomographic (CT) guided drainage of intraabdominal abscesses. Am Surg 1990;56:688–690.

93. Stabile BE, Puccio E, van Sonnenberg E, Neff CC. Preoperative percutaneous drainage of diverticular abscesses. Am J Surg 1990;159:99–105.

94. Alt B, Glass NR, Sollinger H. Neutropenic enterocolitis in adults. Am J Surg 1985;149:405–408.

95. Villar HV, Warneke JA, Peck MD, et al. Role of surgical treatment in the management of complications of the gastrointestinal tract in patients with leukemia. Surg Gynecol Obstet 1987;165:217–222.

96. Sehdev MK, Dowling MD Jr, Seal SH, Stearns MW Jr. Perianal and anorectal complications in leukemia. Cancer 1973;31:149–152.

97. Howard RJ, Simmons RL, eds: Surgical infectious disease. 2nd ed. Norwalk, CT: Appleton & Lange, 1988:377–442.

98. McCarthy DM. Sucralfate. N Engl J Med 1991;235:1017–1025.

99. Southern Surgeons Club: A prospective analysis of 1518 laparoscopic cholecystectomies. N Engl J Med 1991;324:1074–1078.

PAUL RUSSO

SECTION **5**

Urologic Emergencies

Urologic emergencies are common in the cancer patient and are related mainly to complications of bladder hemorrhage, upper or lower urinary tract obstruction, urinary tract infection, and priapism. The causes, clinical presentations, and management of these emergencies are the focus of this chapter.

BLADDER HEMORRHAGE

Urinary tract hemorrhage can occur in a variety of clinical settings in the cancer patient and can rapidly evolve into a life-threatening emergency. Gross hematuria is often the presenting sign of a urologic malignancy (*e.g.*, kidney, urothelial, prostatic) or may be secondary to direct invasion of colonic and gynecologic cancers or pelvic sarcomas into the urinary tract. Occasionally, a benign process, such as a renal angiomyolipoma or arteriovenous malformation, bleeds massively into the urinary tract. Hemorrhagic cystitis after chemotherapy or radiation therapy or secondary to viral infection in an immunocompromised host can also cause life-threatening hemorrhage. Disorders in hemostasis due to the systemic manifestations of cancer (*e.g.*, thrombocytopenia, disseminated intravascular coagulation) can cause occult tumors or damaged urothelium to bleed. More than one etiologic factor may be responsible for the bleeding.

PATHOPHYSIOLOGY AND ETIOLOGY

Drug-Induced Hemorrhagic Cystitis

Hemorrhagic cystitis is defined as an acute or insidious diffuse bladder inflammation with hemorrhage that can be caused by numerous toxic agents. Metabolites of chemotherapeutic agents, bladder injury secondary to radiation therapy, and viral infection account for most cases of hemorrhagic cystitis encountered in cancer patients.[1,2]

In the early experience with cyclophosphamide used as a chemotherapeutic agent or in preparation for bone marrow transplantation, the incidence of hemorrhagic cystitis was as high as 40% to 68%.[3,4] When massive bladder hemorrhage occurred in the bone marrow transplant population, a mortality rate as high as 75% was reported.[5]

There are no clinical predictors to indicate which patient will experience this complication. Acute hemorrhage usually occurs during or shortly after treatment, and delayed hemorrhage is most common in patients on chronic long-term oral cyclophosphamide.[1] With acute hemorrhage, the patient may complain of dysuria and urinary frequency. Microscopic hematuria due to a hyperemic, edematous, and ulcerated bladder mucosa may precede serious bladder hemorrhage.[6] Of 100 patients treated with cyclophosphamide at the Mayo Clinic who developed hemorrhagic cystitis, bleeding sufficient enough to require transfusion occurred in 20%. Hemorrhagic cystitis developed after a mean cumulative oral dose of 90 g

and a mean cumulative intravenous dose of 18 g of cyclophosphamide. Three patients developed hemorrhagic cystitis after a single intravenous dose. Although most of the patients recovered, cystectomy with urinary diversion was performed as a lifesaving measure in 9 patients, and death secondary to exsanguinating bladder hemorrhage or complications of hemorrhage occurred in 10 patients.[6]

Liver metabolites of cyclophosphamide and its analog ifosfamide, are phosphoramide mustard and acrolein. Acrolein is the urinary metabolite that has been implicated as the urotoxic substance, but the exact mechanism by which it damages the urothelium is unknown.[7] Overhydration to dilute urinary acrolein is successful in reducing the incidence of major bladder hemorrhage associated with cyclophosphamide.[5] Sodium 2-mercaptoethane sulfonate (mesna) is an effective uroprotectant that does not interfere with the chemotherapeutic efficacy of cyclophosphamide.[8,9] Within minutes of its intravenous administration, mesna is oxidized in the serum to a stable, inactive disulfide that is activated in the kidney and binds to urinary acrolein to form an inert thioether. Mesna slows the degradation of the 4-hydroxy-metabolites of ifosfamide and cyclophosphamide, further inhibiting their breakdown and the release of acrolein. The only side effects associated with its administration are mild nausea and occasional vomiting.[1] The serum half-life of mesna is 90 minutes, and that of cyclophosphamide is 6 hours.[1,10] To be effective, mesna must be present in the bladder at the time the acrolein comes into contact with the urothelium. Mesna must be administered before the first dose of cyclophosphamide and continued after the last dose, using one of several schedules that employ continuous infusion or intravenous bolus methods.[11–13] The use of mesna has dramatically reduced the incidence of hematuria and hemorrhagic cystitis after cyclophosphamide-based chemotherapy to less than 5%, has reduced cyclophosphamide-induced complications of bone marrow transplantation, and has obviated the need for chemotherapy dose reductions.[11–16]

Radiation-Induced Cystitis

Approximately 20% of patients receiving definitive radiation therapy for gynecologic, genitourinary, and rectal cancers experience bladder complications.[17,18] Although symptoms of urinary urgency, frequency, and urinary retention may occur after pelvic irradiation, serious bladder hemorrhage is an unusual acute event.[1] The small vessel injury caused by irradiation leads to interstitial bladder wall fibrosis, reduced bladder capacity, and the formation of friable, telangiectatic blood vessels that course the bladder mucosa and can spontaneously rupture leading to massive hemorrhage.

Although there are no specific measures to prevent radiation-induced cystitis, acute symptoms of urgency, dysuria, and frequency may be relieved by topical analgesics (*e.g.*, phenazopyridine hydrochloride) and antispasmodics (*e.g.*, oxybutynin chloride). A period of bladder catheterization may be necessary to relieve symptoms of bladder irritability or treat acute urinary retention. Currently under clinical investigation for the treatment of radiation-induced hemorrhagic cystitis are sodium pentosulfanpolysulfate, hyperbaric oxygen, and conjugated estrogen—each of which attempts to stabilize the damaged urothelium and promote healing.[19–21]

Virus-Induced Hemorrhagic Cystitis

Efforts to understand the late onset of hemorrhagic cystitis in bone marrow patients focused on a possible viral infection. Although hemorrhagic cystitis secondary to adenovirus type 11 was reported in immunologically competent children, this virus was infrequently detected in the urine of bone marrow transplant patients.[22-24] Rice and colleagues identified the BK type of human polyomavirus in the urine of 5 of 6 bone marrow recipients, 2 of whom had hemorrhagic cystitis.[25] The BK virus in healthy people is ubiquitous, persists in the kidney after primary infection, and is only occasionally associated with a mild respiratory illness.[26] The BK virus is activated during periods of immunosuppression (*e.g.*, organ and marrow transplantation) and is recoverable in the urine.[27] A prospective study of 53 bone marrow recipients demonstrated BK virus in the urine of 47%.[28] Hemorrhagic cystitis lasting longer than 7 days occurred four times as frequently in patients who excreted BK virus than in those who did not. Urinary BK virus was identified in 55% of patients during episodes of hemorrhagic cystitis but in only 11% of patients who were cystitis free. Despite the use of mesna and overhydration during bone marrow transplantation, BK virus activation remains a major factor in the evolution of hemorrhagic cystitis in this group of cancer patients.

TREATMENT

If bladder hemorrhage is massive and intractable, the patients develop clot urinary retention and complain of severe suprapubic and flank pain. The urologist must reestablish urinary outflow quickly by inserting a large diameter, multiple hole urethral catheter into the bladder and initiate a saline lavage and clot evacuation. Often the hemorrhage slows or ceases after removing the clots and decompressing the bladder. When the lavage has a clear or pink-tinged return, continuous bladder irrigation using a three-way Foley catheter can be effective in removing any residual small clots and maintaining free bladder drainage.

Bedside lavage is not always effective in evacuating all clots, especially if they have been present for many hours. Continued irrigation in this setting may increase intravesical pressure and cause bladder rupture (Fig. 60–14A,B). Instead, the patient should be taken to the operating room for an endoscopic clot evacuation under anesthesia. Under direct vision, the urologist can mechanically disrupt the clots, inspect the bladder for a controllable source of bleeding, and fulgurate any bleeding vessels or tumor.

Diffuse bleeding from any cause that persists despite clot evacuation and fulguration is an indication for intravesical instillation of a hemostatic agent such as formalin, which acts

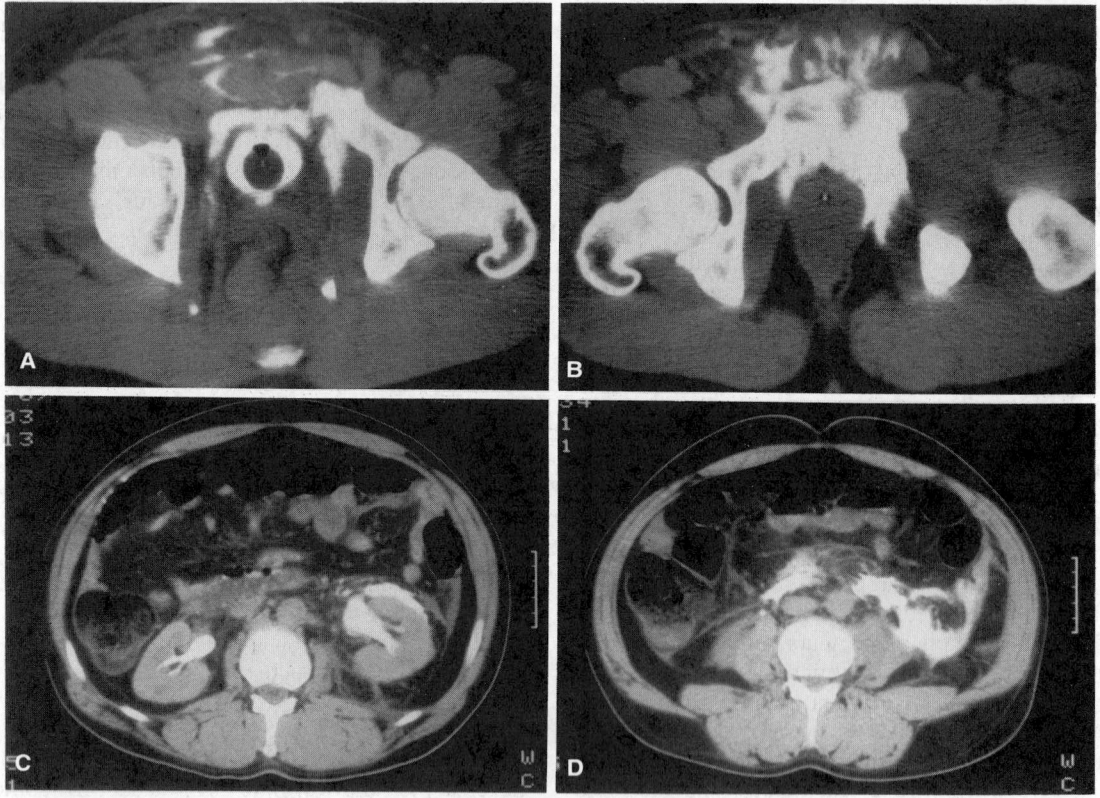

FIGURE 60–14. **(A, B)** Pelvic CT scans demonstrate extraperitoneal bladder rupture with urinary extravasation into the retropubic space and abdominal wall soft tissues after unsuccessful bedside lavage for a patient with clot urinary retention. **(C, D)** Abdominal CT scans demonstrate rupture of the renal calyceal fornix from acute distal ureteral obstruction, leading to extravasation of urine into perinephric fat and retroperitoneal soft tissues. (Courtesy of Dr. Susan Hilton, Department of Radiology, Memorial Sloan-Kettering Cancer Center, New York, NY)

as chemical cautery to control bleeding from submucosal and mucosal vessels.[1,2] In 1969, the use of a 10% formalin instillation was reported effective in controlling intractable bladder hemorrhage in 24 patients treated with radiation therapy for bladder cancer.[29] Complications of renal papillary necrosis, renal failure, ureteral stenosis, bladder contracture, and bladder rupture with fatal intraperitoneal extravasation tempered the initial enthusiasm for the use of 10% formalin.[2,30] In 1974, Fair reported the use of a 1% to 2% formalin solution to treat hemorrhagic cystitis and found it to be effective without the toxicity of 10% formalin.[31] Complications of formalin appear infrequently if concentrations of 4% or less are used. More than 75% of patients with hemorrhagic cystitis have their bleeding controlled by this method.[32] The technique of formalin instillation currently used at our institution is as follows:

1. Spinal or general anesthesia is required because formalin is caustic to sensory nerves within the bladder. Cystoendoscopy is performed to evacuate clots and fulgurate bleeding vessels.

2. A cystogram is performed to identify vesicoureteral reflux or evidence of bladder perforation. If reflux is documented, the involved ureteral orifice(s) must be occluded with a Fogarty balloon-tip catheter before formalin instillation. Any evidence of bladder perforation is an absolute contraindication to formalin instillation.

3. Formalin and formaldehyde are not equivalent compounds. Formalin is a 37% solution of formaldehyde. The stock solution is diluted with sterile water to the desired concentration as follows: 10% formalin is 3.7% formaldehyde and 1% formalin is a 0.37% formaldehyde solution. The order to the pharmacy for the preparation of the desired formalin solution must be explicitly written and the solutions checked by the operating team to avoid serious error.

4. An 18 French (6 mm) Foley catheter is used to catheterize the bladder, and a 1% solution of formalin (500–1000 ml) is instilled under gravity at no higher than 15 cm above the pubis for an overall contact time of approximately 10 to 15 minutes. During the instillation, the catheter should not be clamped, because formalin induced bladder contraction may occur increasing the likelihood of reflux or intravascular absorption. In the female patient, the perineum should be painted with petroleum jelly and the vagina packed with petroleum gauze to prevent skin irritation from formalin.

5. After the formalin instillation, the bladder is thoroughly irrigated with at least 1 L of distilled water, and a Foley catheter is left indwelling for 24 to 48 hours.

6. The instillation of 2.0%, 4%, and rarely 10% formalin using the steps outlined may be necessary to control persistent hemorrhage. Retreatment with formalin should be avoided for at least 48 hours, because its favorable effects may not be apparent for that time. Concentrations of greater than 10% formalin should not be administered.[32]

Other methods of controlling bleeding in hemorrhagic cystitis, including intravesical alum, prostaglandins, phenol, intravesical silver nitrate, hydrostatic distention, iced saline lavage, and parenteral or oral aminocaproic acid have been used with various degrees of success.[1,2] Of these agents, intravesical 1% alum and prostaglandin E_2 and F_2, each of which can be instilled without anesthesia, are the most effective. A 1% alum solution (*i.e.*, the ammonium or potassium salt dissolved in water) delivered by continuous bladder irrigation causes protein precipitation, vasoconstriction, and decreased capillary permeability.[33–35] During instillation, bladder spasms may occur but are usually well controlled by antispasmodic medication. The principal advantage to alum in the treatment of hemorrhagic cystitis is that it can be delivered at the bedside using a three-way indwelling catheter without the need for anesthesia. Some urologists recommend the initial use of alum for massive bladder hemorrhage with formalin as second line treatment. A significant disadvantage of alum irrigation is that it may take as long as 7 days to effectively control the bleeding. Serum aluminum levels should be monitored as rare cases of alum-induced encephalopathy have been reported.[36]

Prostaglandin E_2 and F_2 can also be instilled intravesically without anesthesia and have been reported to be effective in controlling intractable hemorrhagic cystitis, possibly by protecting the microvasculature and epithelium and inhibiting the development of tissue edema.[37,38] Prostaglandin induced severe bladder spasms may limit their overall utility.

Despite all conservative efforts, exsanguinating hemorrhage from the bladder may persist, necessitating open surgical attempts to control the bleeding. Control of the bleeding may require open cystotomy with bladder packing, cutaneous ureterostomy, hypogastric artery embolization, or cystectomy with urinary diversion.[6,39–41] Surgical intervention in these already critically ill patients should be performed only if conservative measures have failed. Surgical control of hemorrhage may still not be possible.

OBSTRUCTIVE UROPATHY

UPPER TRACT OBSTRUCTION

Obstruction of one or both ureters in the cancer patient may be secondary to direct tumor invasion, compression of the ureter by a retroperitoneal tumor, encasement of the ureter by retroperitoneal or pelvic lymph nodes involved with metastatic disease, or rarely by direct metastases to the ureter. Seventy percent of tumors causing ureteral obstruction are genitourinary (*e.g.*, cervical, bladder, prostate) in origin (Fig. 60–15), with breast, gastrointestinal, and lymphoma comprising most of the remainder (Fig. 60–16).[42,43] Ureteral obstruction may be secondary to retroperitoneal fibrosis after combinations of surgery, chemotherapy, or pelvic radiation therapy.[44] Acute ureteral obstruction usually causes flank pain and colic typical of the symptoms of urolithiasis. In contrast, chronic unilateral obstruction is usually a silent event—often detected incidentally as hydronephrosis with renal cortical atrophy on upper abdominal imaging studies (Fig. 60–17).

Acute or chronic bilateral ureteral obstruction is associated with decreased urine output and symptoms of uremia. In one study of 50 patients with acute renal failure secondary to bilateral ureteral obstruction, 76% of the patients had malignant disease as the cause of the obstruction, and half of these patients had uremia as the presenting sign of their cancer.[45] Increased renal pelvic pressure may cause rupture of the renal calyceal fornix, leading to extravasation of urine into the renal

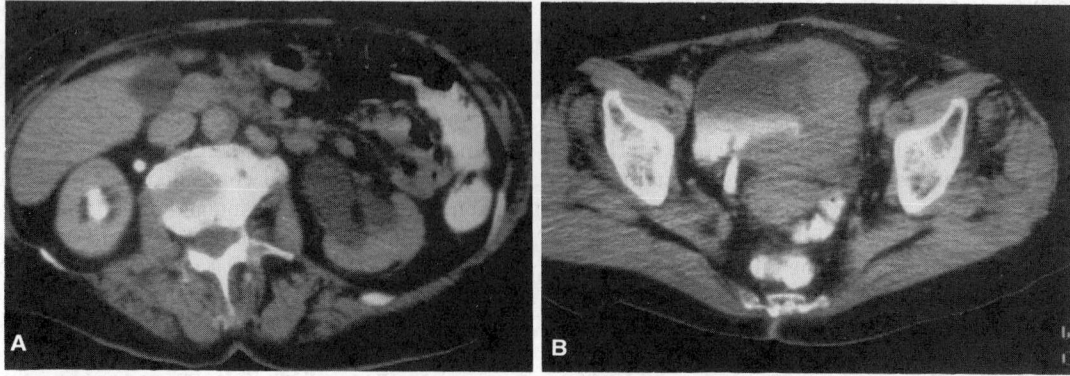

FIGURE 60–15. **(A)** Abdominal CT scan demonstrates the lack of function of the left kidney with hydro-nephrosis. **(B)** Pelvic CT demonstrates a large, invasive bladder tumor with extravesical extension responsible for distal left ureteral obstruction.

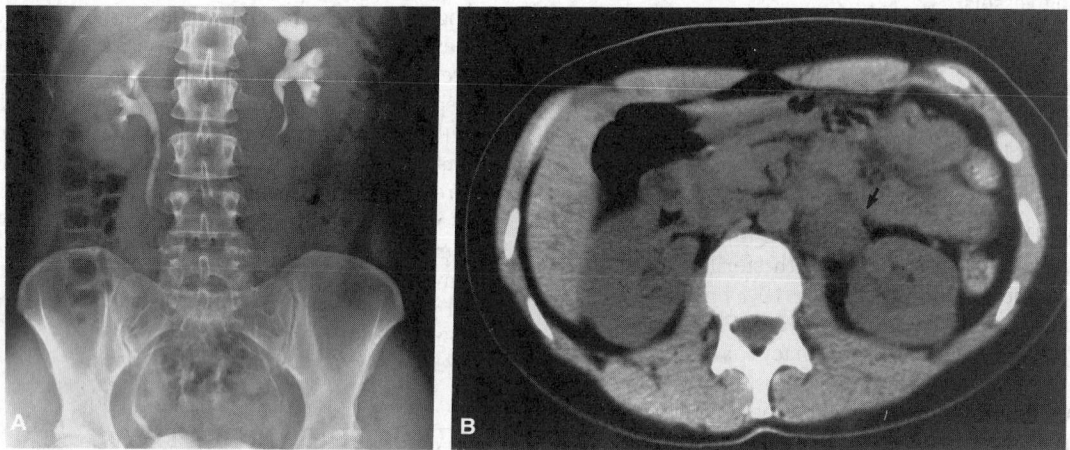

FIGURE 60–16. **(A)** Intravenous urogram of a 30-year-old woman with a history of invasive breast cancer demonstrates left hydronephrosis. **(B)** Abdominal CT scan demonstrates a metastatic deposit (*arrow*) in the area of the left proximal ureter that is responsible for obstruction.

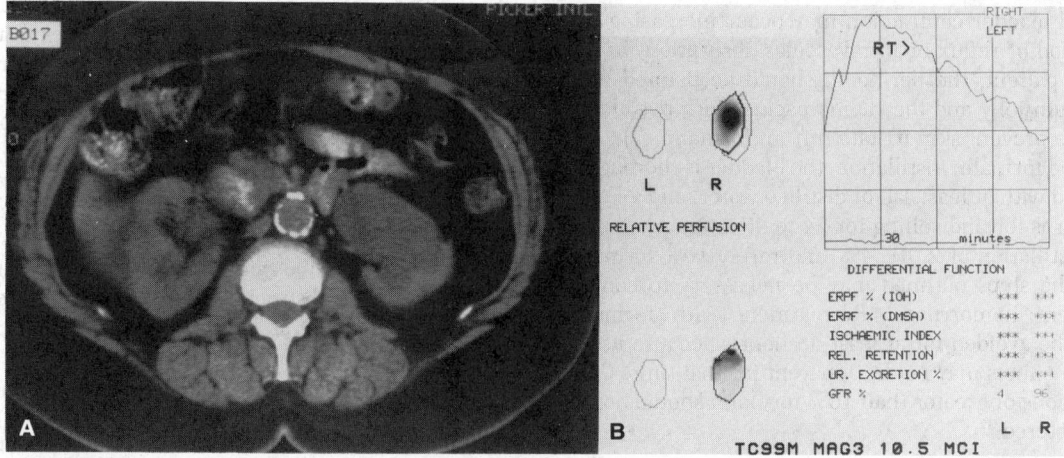

FIGURE 60–17. **(A)** CT scan of the abdomen demonstrates left hydronephrosis with cortical atrophy secondary to a pelvic recurrence of cervical cancer in a 58-year-old woman. **(B)** Radionuclide renogram (DMSA) demonstrates a nonfunctioning left kidney and normal function of the right. Because of the documented lack of function in the left kidney, decompression was not advised.

sinus with the formation of a perinephric urinoma (Figure 60–14C,D).[46] If infected urine exists in the obstructed system, fever, chills, and eventual urosepsis may ensue, requiring emergency urologic decompression. The diagnosis of ureteral obstruction may be made by intravenous urogram, computed tomography (CT) scan, renal ultrasound, retrograde pyelogram, or radionuclide renography.[47] Of these, abdominal CT has the advantage of better defining any extrarenal pathology that may account for the obstruction.

A difficult ethical question arises with the diagnosis of ureteral obstruction in the patient with an incurable malignancy. Is decompression going to facilitate treatment with chemotherapy and palliate symptoms or will it merely address a short-term problem and prolong the patient's suffering? Palliative urinary diversion or decompression with ureteral stents is justified if improvement in renal function facilitates the use of chemotherapy or if symptoms of ureteral obstruction (*e.g.*, pain, urosepsis) can be alleviated.

Malignant ureteral obstruction was previously managed by open surgical placement of a nephrostomy tube, a procedure associated with a major complication rate of up to 45%.[42] Approximately 25% of patients undergoing open nephrostomy died within 30 days of operation, and the average survival after the procedure was approximately 6 months. In the last 10 years, techniques have evolved using percutaneous and endoscopic techniques to decompress the obstructed urinary tract. Using these "endourologic" techniques, decompression of obstructed kidneys, removal of obstructing ureteral stones, and dilation of ureteral strictures can be performed without an open operation. The percutaneous tubes and stents are composed of flexible synthetic materials (*e.g.*, polyurethane) that minimize migration within the urinary tract due to the "double J" configuration of the stents (*i.e.*, one end coiled in the bladder and the second end coiled in the renal pelvis) (Fig. 60–18). Stents of this type cause less encrustation and are easy to change.[48] Flexible guidewires can negotiate narrowed ureteral lumens and sharp bends in the obstructed ureter and aid in the placement of the stents during retrograde cystoscopic or antegrade percutaneous procedures. Recent reports of experience with endourologic decompression of ureteral obstruction in prostate cancer, gynecologic tumors, colorectal cancer, and breast cancer confirm the value of these techniques.[49–52] A mean survival in the range of 10 months

can be obtained after diversion or stenting in patients with advanced malignancy and ureteral obstruction. In patients with bilateral ureteral obstruction, significant palliation and return of near-normal renal function is possible after decompression of the obstructed kidney, with more substantial remaining cortex as determined by CT or ultrasound examination.

Endourologists can incise or balloon dilate and stent benign ureteral strictures or ureteral enteric stenoses after urinary diversion (Fig. 60–19).[53,54] After a ureteral stent or percutaneous nephrostomy is placed, subsequent management requires meticulous follow-up, including periodic monitoring of renal function, upper tract imaging (*e.g.*, CT, renal ultrasound), frequent urine cultures, and periodic stent or tube replacement (every 4–6 months). If chemotherapy or radiation therapy directed at the primary tumor successfully eliminates the lesion responsible for the ureteral obstruction, such as retroperitoneal adenopathy from breast cancer or leukemic infiltrates of the ureter (Fig. 60–20), removal of the percutaneous nephrostomy or ureteral stents can be done if imaging studies document the restoration of normal urinary drainage from the involved kidney.[52,55]

Complications of endourologic procedures include gross hematuria with perinephric hematoma, splenic or bowel injury, and hemothorax or pneumothorax.[56] Indwelling ureteral stents can migrate, obstruct with proteinaceous encrustations, become infected, fragment, cause uncomfortable vesicoureteral reflux, and erode through the urinary tract.[48] Patients may complain of bladder spasm from irritation of the trigone, which generally subsides within several weeks of stent placement. Open nephrostomy, cutaneous ureterostomy, or operative urinary diversion should be reserved for unusual cases in which endourologic techniques are not successful, the patients are in satisfactory medical condition, and for patients with life expectancies that do not preclude major surgical procedures.[57] Major operative reconstruction (*e.g.*, revision of ileal ureteral anastomosis, ureteral reimplantation, ileal ureter interposition) may be considered in this setting.

BLADDER OUTLET OBSTRUCTION AND URINARY RETENTION

Acute urinary retention and bladder outlet obstruction (*e.g.*, hesitancy, dribbling, incomplete bladder emptying, overflow

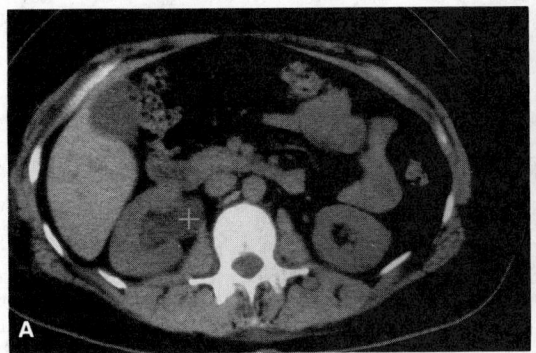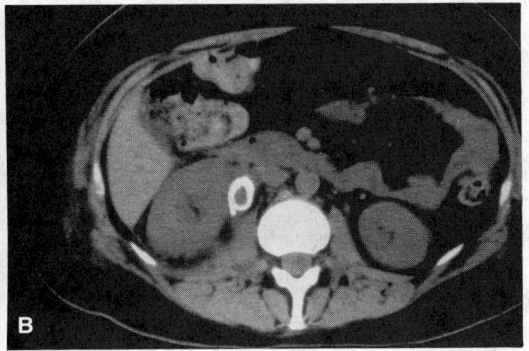

FIGURE 60–18. **(A)** CT scan of the abdomen demonstrates right hydronephrosis in a 48-year-old women with pelvic recurrence of cervical cancer. **(B)** CT scan of the abdomen demonstrates decompression of an obstructed kidney with a cystoscopically placed double J ureteral stent, which is seen coiled in the right renal pelvis.

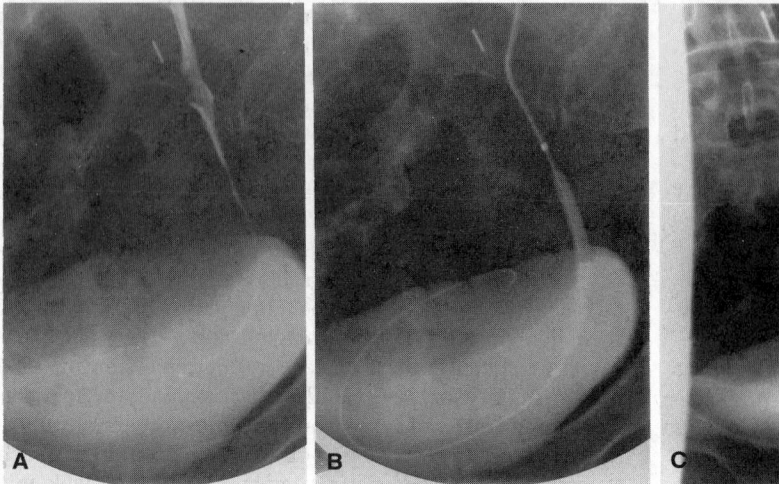
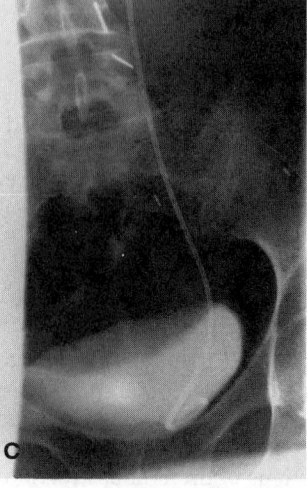

FIGURE 60–19. **(A)** Antegrade ureterogram demonstrates a benign stricture of the distal left ureter in a 54-year-old woman treated with pelvic irradiation for cervical cancer. **(B)** Balloon dilation of a ureteral stricture is performed over a flexible guidewire, which is coiled in the bladder. **(C)** Antegrade placement of double J stent through a previous ureteral stricture.

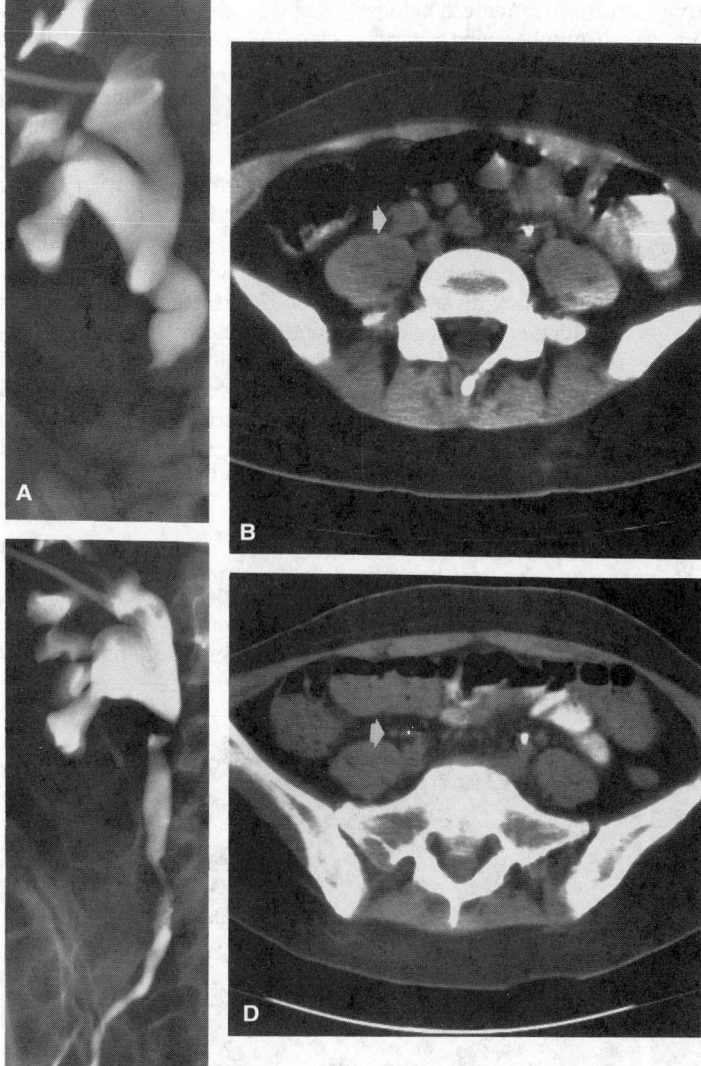

FIGURE 60–20. **(A)** Right hydronephrosis with complete distal ureteral obstruction. The kidney is decompressed with percutaneous nephrostomy. **(B)** Abdominal CT scan demonstrates a leukemic infiltrate (*arrow*) in the area of the proximal ureter that is responsible for the obstruction. **(C)** Antegrade nephrostogram demonstrates the patency of the distal ureter after systemic chemotherapy. **(D)** Complete resolution of the infiltrate responsible for the obstruction after chemotherapy.

incontinence, decrease in the force of the voided stream) can be caused by mechanical or neurophysiologic factors. These factors may be primary manifestations of the malignancy, secondary to treatment, or due to preexisting benign conditions involving the lower urinary tract. A patient with urinary retention complains of severe suprapubic pain and has a palpable suprapubic fullness secondary to a distended bladder. Pelvic and rectal examination may reveal a genitourinary or rectal tumor that is responsible for obstructing the bladder outlet. Complete bladder outlet obstruction can lead rapidly to bilateral hydroureteronephrosis with renal insufficiency and should be treated emergently.

If a malignant cause of bladder outlet obstruction is excluded, a preexisting benign mechanical condition, such as benign prostatic hyperplasia (BPH) or urethral stricture, may be the cause. Less likely causes of retention include constipation and neurologic disorders.[58] It is estimated that 5% to 10% of men at age 40 and 80% of men at age 80 have BPH, although the symptoms vary widely and do not correlate directly with prostate size by digital rectal examination.[59] Many patients have significant obstructive symptoms and may compensate by limiting their fluid intake. During chemotherapy, the combination of antiemetic medication and hydration may precipitate urinary retention in patients with preexisting prostatism.

Improved understanding of the neurophysiology of micturition has allowed us to more precisely diagnose and treat acute nonmechanical causes of bladder outlet obstruction. Urodynamic evaluation, including uroflow, cystometrogram, and perineal sphincter electromyography, are useful in assessing the micturition reflex, which includes sensory nerves in the bladder wall, voluntary cerebral control over the pontine micturition center, sacral parasympathetic nerves (S2–S3), cholinergic nerves to the external sphincter, and sympathetic nerves to the bladder neck.[60–62] Anatomic or neuropharmacologic interference with the micturition reflex occurs frequently in the cancer patient and can lead to acute urinary retention. For example, postoperative urinary retention, often attributed to prostatism, can be caused by the use of certain anticholinergic anesthetic agents that depress detrusor contractility, pain and stress-induced sympathetic activity that increase tone in the bladder neck and proximal urethral muscles, and perioperative pain medications (*e.g.*, opiates) that directly inhibit the pontine micturitional center and depress the urge to void.[63]

Tumors arising in or metastasizing to the brain and or spinal cord can directly interfere with the central voluntary control of micturition and the coordination of bladder emptying and sphincter muscle relaxation. This condition, detrusor external sphincter dyssynergia, can lead to a functional bladder outlet obstruction characterized by bladder wall hypertonicity and hypertrophy with reduced capacity, vesicoureteral reflux, and incomplete bladder emptying. Hypotonic bladder dysfunction may occur in as many as 50% of patients undergoing abdominoperineal resection for rectal carcinoma or radical hysterectomy in which extensive pelvic dissection can disrupt the pelvic parasympathetic nerves necessary for normal detrusor muscle contraction.[64] This effect is usually permanent in only 10% of patients. Viral radiculomyelitis secondary to herpes simplex in an immunocompromised host can cause a flaccid neurogenic bladder, which is usually self-limiting, with the

return of normal bladder function expected in approximately 2 weeks.[65]

The first step in the management of urinary retention is the passage of a small (14 French or 4.6 mm) urethral catheter into the bladder. In a male patient, distal urethral obstruction from preexisting stricture disease may be encountered. The urologist may dilate the stricture using filiforms and followers—a procedure that should be rapidly terminated if blood appears at the urethral meatus. A curved urethral catheter (Coudé tip) may be required to pass an enlarged benign or malignant prostate. In the male patient, a Foley catheter should be passed to its hub, with urine return observed before inflating the balloon. This maneuver avoids the inadvertent inflation of the catheter balloon in the prostatic urethra and subsequent brisk bleeding. Forcing a catheter that is not passing easily may cause urethral lacerations and create false passages beneath the prostatic capsule, allowing blood and urine to extravasate into the pelvis and perineum. Should infected urine extravasate, a case of urinary retention can rapidly be converted iatrogenically into urosepsis and soft tissue infection. If transurethral catheterization is not easily accomplished, a percutaneous suprapubic cystotomy tube should be placed, allowing a more orderly approach to the diagnosis and treatment of the underlying obstruction.

In the case of long-standing and complete urinary retention, elevations in ureteral pressure can cause a secondary decrease in renal blood flow, a decrease in glomerular filtration rate, renal tubular dysfunction, and cellular atrophy. The abrupt relief of lower urinary obstruction can initiate a postobstructive diuresis, during which the urine output can be as great as 200 ml/hour for 6 to 12 hours. This initial diuresis is a normal physiologic response to the relief of bladder outlet obstruction, with the kidneys appropriately excreting retained urea, salt, and water. Excessive supplementary intravenous fluids should be avoided, because this tends to prolong the period of diuresis. A pathologic response can occur in patients with more extensive renal tubular damage and nephrogenic diabetes insipidus can develop. In these patients, excessive water loss continues even after the retained water and solutes have been eliminated. The urine remains dilute with low osmolality, and the administration of antidiuretic hormone is ineffective. Normally, the conscious patient retains a normal thirst mechanism and is able to avoid dehydration until renal tubular function normalizes. Rarely, a salt-losing nephropathy occurs, leading to hypotension and hyponatremia. Close monitoring and fluid resuscitation with normal or hypertonic saline must be undertaken until tubular function normalizes.[66]

Treatment of the cancer patient in urinary retention should be conservative. Patients are often debilitated from the effects of the primary tumors and treatment, and they are further frustrated by the new inability to urinate. Many patients, when given another chance to void after a period of catheter decompression, are able to urinate normally and may be spared any invasive procedures.[67]

After bladder decompression is accomplished, the decision about when to give the patient another voiding trial should be based on the patient's clinical status. In the postoperative patient in urinary retention, it is prudent to wait for some recovery from the operation, a decrease in the requirement for pain medication, and the ability to ambulate before another voiding trial is initiated. In the chemotherapy patient in urinary retention, the voiding trial should be delayed until the period of hydration is passed and the need for antiemetic medication is lessened. There is no role for "bladder training" (*i.e.*, clamping and unclamping of the catheter to give the bladder more tone), which was previously advocated by some for patients in retention.

During periods of bladder catheterization, urine cultures should be obtained every 3 days. If colonization of the urine occurs, an appropriate antibiotic to which the organism is sensitive can be administered at the time of the voiding trial. The use of continuous antibiotics in the catheterized patient should be avoided because this will lead to colonization by resistant organisms. If the colonizing organism is urease-producing (*e.g.*, *Proteus mirabilis*), the urine can become alkaline, and magnesium ammonium phosphate (struvite) calculi can form. To prevent this, a short course of an appropriate antibiotic should be administered.[68]

The male patient with a significant antecedent history of prostatism may remain in urinary retention despite voiding trials. Radiologic imaging of the upper urinary tract with intravenous urography, ultrasound, or CT scan can determine if hydronephrosis or renal cortical atrophy exist.[69] Ultrasound has emerged as the most cost effective means of evaluating the urinary tract and has the added appeal of avoiding the use of iodinated contrast materials, which can occasionally cause nephrotoxicity.[70,71] Most patients can have their bladder outlet obstructions relieved by transurethral resection of the prostate (TURP) with acceptable morbidity, although complications of bleeding, clot retention, infection, and persistent failure to void make careful case selection in the cancer patient population important.[72–74] Alternatives to prostatectomy under clinical investigation include luteinizing hormone-releasing hormone analogs, inhibition of 5α-reductase and androgen ablation, α-adrenergic blockers, urethral stents, local microwave hyperthermia, and balloon dilation.[75–80] Although select patients may benefit from these techniques alone or in combination, their overall efficacy appears to be less than standard prostatectomy in the short term, and long-term follow-up data is unavailable.

After a neurologic cause for urinary retention is diagnosed, the mainstay of treatment is clean intermittent self-catheterization, which is performed every 4 to 6 hours.[81] This method of alleviating urinary retention can preserve kidney function, reduce infection rates, reduce stone formation, and improve the quality of patients' lives compared with chronic indwelling Foley catheters. In a report of 75 patients with neurogenic bladders followed for a mean of 7 years, all patients had preservation of upper urinary tract function. Complications occurred in 20% and included urethral injury or stenosis (13), epididymitis (6), bladder calculi (3), and pyelonephritis (1).[82] Antibiotics are not given prophylactically to patients on intermittent self-catheterization, because they have not been shown to lower the incidence of clinical urinary tract infection.[83]

URINARY TRACT INFECTION

Urinary tract infections occur in the cancer patient when normal defense barriers are disrupted during hospitalization.[84] These barriers include normal perineal flora (*e.g.*, lactobacilli, streptococci, coagulase-negative staphylococcus) and an anatomically intact urinary tract with normal micturitional reflexes. Most urinary tract infections are ascending, with the presence of an indwelling bladder catheter the principal portal of entry.[85] The approximately 5% incidence of urinary tract infection in neutropenic and bone marrow transplant patients is directly related to the frequency and duration of bladder catheterization.[84] The bladder catheterization procedure may introduce bacteria into the bladder at rates as high as 20% in the hospitalized patient.[86] Closed catheter drainage systems have reduced bacteriuria, but hospital-acquired bacteria still gain access to the system. After periurethral colonization, pathogenic bacteria can track along the catheter causing urethritis and eventual bladder infection. The risk of bacteriuria increases 5% to 10% for each day of catheterization, a fact that should provide the impetus for early catheter removal or the institution of intermittent catheterization.[87] Cancer patients receiving systemic antibiotics have alterations in periurethral flora favoring colonization with enteric organisms and resistant organisms prevalent in the hospital environment, such as *Pseudomonas aeruginosa* and *Candida albicans*.

The most common pathogens causing urinary tract infection are gram-negative bacteria, with *E. coli* responsible for 50% to 75% of cases of clinical pyelonephritis.[88] Bacteria can adhere to mucosal and catheter surfaces in a biofilm (*e.g.*, glycocalyx), which protects them from the mechanical flow of urine, inflammatory defenses, and antibiotics.[89] Bacterial bladder infection causes an initial inflammatory response that results in acute and chronic cystitis but is usually not associated with fever or an elevated leukocyte count. With longer catheterization, bacteria can ascend into the ureters and invade the renal epithelium causing inflammatory infiltrates in the kidneys. Acute pyelonephritis is marked by fever, flank pain, bacteremia, and an elevated leukocyte count.[90] Upper tract infection can lead to stone formation due to urea-splitting organisms such as *Proteus mirabilis*, xanthogranulomatous pyelonephritis (Fig. 60–21A), renal cortical abscess (Fig. 60–21B), perinephric abscess, renal carbuncle, emphysematous pyelonephritis, and urosepsis.[91]

The diagnostic approach to the patient with renal infection should begin with a plain film radiograph of the abdomen to detect calculi or abnormal gas collections overlying the kidney. Contrast-enhanced CT scans and renal ultrasound can precisely identify cortical or perinephric abscess or acute focal bacterial nephritis and have supplanted ^{67}Ga citrate or ^{111}In-labeled white blood cell scans in the diagnosis of kidney abscess.[92]

The prevention of urinary tract infection in the cancer patient begins with the selective use of indwelling catheters for the treatment of urinary retention, the assessment of hourly urine output when critical, or in the immediate postoperative period. The catheter should be removed as soon as possible to limit the chances of bacterial colonization. Systemic antibiotics should be avoided during periods of indwelling catheterization to prevent the emergence of resistant organisms. At the end of a long period of urinary catheterization, a urine culture should be obtained and a short course (3–5 days) of an appropriate oral antibiotic prescribed to sterilized the urine.

A common complication of long-term bladder catheterization in the presence of systemic antibiotics is candiduria.[90] This form of bladder colonization is usually asymptomatic

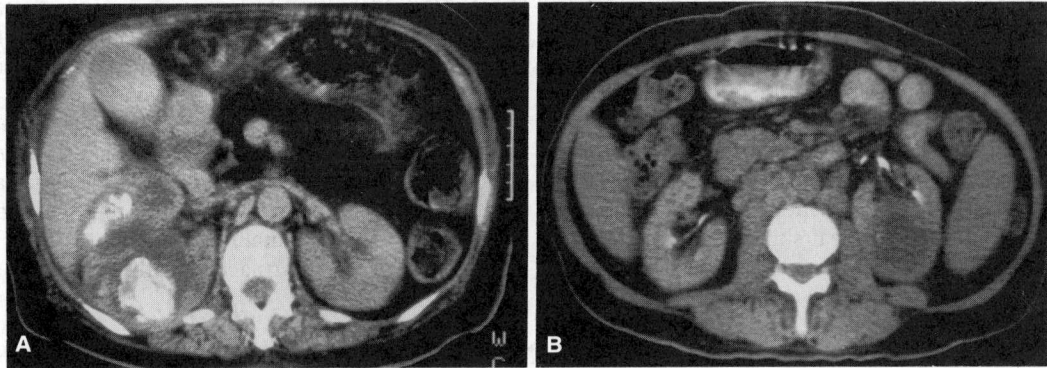

FIGURE 60–21. **(A)** CT scan of the abdomen demonstrates right xanthogranulomatous pyelonephritis with several large struvite calculi in a patient with a long-standing foley catheter. **(B)** CT scan of the abdomen demonstrates a left renal cortical abscess.

and resolves on removal of the catheter. If prolonged catheterization is required and candiduria is persistent, continuous bladder irrigation through a three-way catheter using amphotericin B (50 mg dissolved in 1 L of sterile water) usually eradicates the infection. Persistent candiduria with budding yeast forms should prompt upper tract imaging studies and cystoendoscopy to rule out the presence of fungal balls that would require urgent surgical removal.

If acute pyelonephritis occurs, a 10-day course of parenteral antibiotics should be administered—a treatment duration effective in curing 90% of uncomplicated cases.[93] Before blood and urine culture data are available, a combination of an aminoglycoside to cover enteric gram-negative rods and *Pseudomonas* and ampicillin to cover enterococcus should be started. When the antibiotic sensitivities are known, the choice of antibiotic should be made based on degree of effectiveness, potential nephrotoxicity, allergic history, and cost.[88] Failure to respond to appropriate antibiotics within 48 hours should raise the possibility of septic ureteral obstruction, renal cortical abscess, perinephric abscess, or renal carbuncle. An ultrasound or CT scan of the kidney should be performed to rule out these conditions. If an abscess is diagnosed, prompt open

surgical drainage or CT-guided percutaneous drainage is required.[94] If a septic course is prolonged and imaging studies reveal a nonfunctional kidney without abscess formation consistent with a renal carbuncle, emergency nephrectomy may be required to eliminate the infection.

Secondary infections of the prostate and epididymis can occur as urethral or bladder pathogens pass through the vas deferens and prostatic ducts, causing acute epididymitis or acute prostatitis. These infections can cause painful febrile illnesses that can result in abscess formation requiring emergency surgical drainage or orchiectomy (Fig. 60–22A).[95,96] It is often difficult to culture the offending pathogen, and empiric antibiotic treatment for 10 to 14 days and local measures (*e.g.*, scrotal elevation, warm sitz baths, antiinflammatory agents) are often effective in alleviating symptoms. The most common urologic manifestation of acquired immunodeficiency syndrome-related tuberculosis is an epididymo-orchitis with abscess formation and a draining scrotal sinus (Fig. 60–22B). The involved testicle is usually completely destroyed by tuberculous granulomas, and orchiectomy in conjunction with systemic antituberculous therapy is the treatment of choice.[97]

Rarely, extravasation of infected urine from the anterior

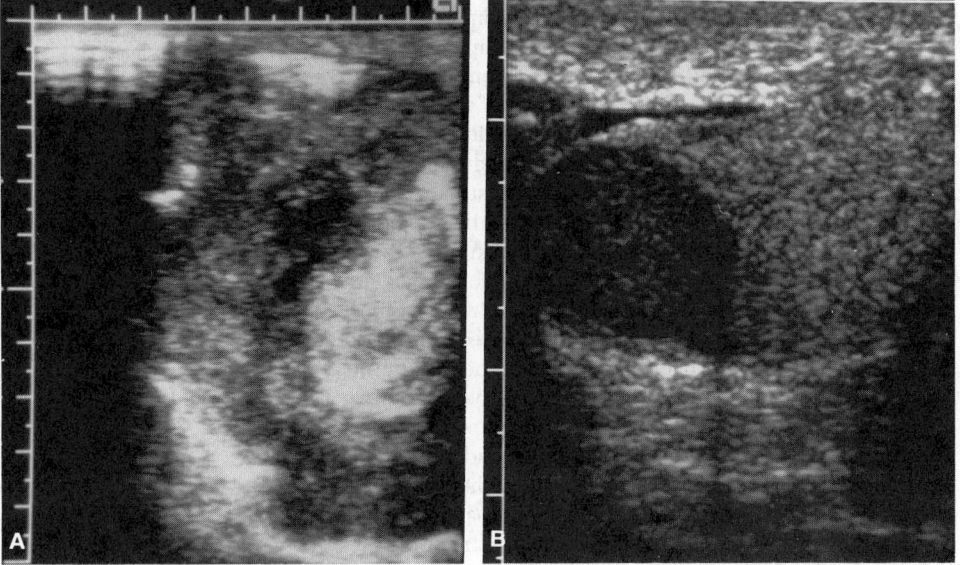

FIGURE 60–22. **(A)** Scrotal ultrasound, transverse section, demonstrates a testicular abscess after an episode of epididymal orchitis. **(B)** Scrotal ultrasound, longitudinal section, demonstrates a tuberculous abscess in the right testicle of a 26-year-old man with AIDS.

urethra into perineal soft tissues (*e.g.*, after traumatic dilation of a urethral stricture or infection of periurethral glands) or the perineal extension of a perirectal abscess can cause a polymicrobial infection involving enteric gram-negative and gram-positive anaerobes. This synergistic infection, marked by early fever, chills, and genital discomfort out of proportion to physical findings, causes an obliterating end-arteritis, which can lead rapidly to subcutaneous ischemia, evolving necrosis of the penile, scrotal, and perineal skin with the anaerobic production of hydrogen and nitrogen gas. The gas is clinically detectable as subcutaneous crepitus and plain x-ray films of the pelvis show air in the soft tissues. Aggressive medical and surgical management must be instituted as soon as the diagnosis of scrotal (Fournier's) gangrene is entertained. Triple antibiotic therapy, including an aminoglycoside, high dose-penicillin, and clindamycin, covers aerobic and anaerobic components of the infection. All nonvital genital tissue must be widely debrided and, depending on the source of the infection, urinary or fecal stream diversion should be performed. Aggressive wound debridement, often requiring repeated operations, can be followed later by skin grafts or myocutaneous flaps for skin coverage. Despite early recognition and aggressive treatment of Fournier's gangrene, mortality rates as high as 33% are reported. In immunocompromised and neutropenic patients, the mortality rate is higher.[98,99]

PRIAPISM

Priapism is defined as a persistent state of painful erection associated with elevated intracavernous pressures not due to sexual stimulation. If left untreated, priapism can cause endothelial damage, thrombosis, and fibrosis leading to impotency. Most cases of priapism have no discernible cause. In the United States, however, sickle cell anemia accounts for approximately 20% of adult cases and 60% of pediatric cases.[100] In the cancer patient, priapism may be due to a primary hematologic malignancy (*e.g.*, leukemia, myeloma), metastatic disease to the corporal bodies of the penis, disruption of venous outflow from the penis secondary to a pelvic tumor, or intracavernous drug therapies used in the treatment of impotence.

Schreibman and colleagues reported priapism in 4 patients with chronic granulocytic leukemia; the priapism resolved after the institution of effective systemic chemotherapy for their underlying disease and normalization of the leukocyte count.[101] Metastatic disease to the corporal bodies of the penis has been reported in cases of clinically advanced genitourinary (*e.g.*, bladder, prostate, kidney) or gastrointestinal (*e.g.*, colorectal) cancer.[102] Although the exact mechanism whereby the metastatic deposits cause priapism is unknown, thrombosis, perhaps in conjunction with a malignancy-associated hypercoagulable state, occurs, and venous drainage from the corporal bodies is blocked. Treatment directed toward the primary tumor (*e.g.*, androgen deprivation in the case of metastatic prostate cancer) may improve or resolve the state of priapism. Occasionally, radiation therapy to the corporal bodies can be effective. In cases of priapism secondary to malignancy, corporal shunting procedures used in idiopathic cases are usually ineffective; treatment should be palliative, with relief of pain and urinary obstruction the primary objectives.

Urologists treating patients who are impotent after radical pelvic surgery with intracavernous injections of papaverine or prostaglandin E_1 face an 8% incidence of pharmacologically induced priapism.[103] When this occurs, corporal aspiration to reduce intracavernous pressures and remove excess vasoactive agent in conjunction with the injection of an α-adrenergic agent (*e.g.*, phenylephrine hydrochloride) is usually effective treatment. Shantha and colleagues reported the use of a 5-mg oral dose of terbutaline, a β_2-agonist, to be effective in rapidly reversing pharmacologically induced priapism.[104]

REFERENCES

1. DeVries CR, Freiha FS. Hemorrhagic cystitis: A review. J Urol 1990;143:1–9.
2. Levine LA, Richie JP. Urologic complications of cyclophosphamide. J Urol 1989;141:1063–1069.
3. Watson NA, Noteley RG. Urologic complications of cyclophosphamide. Br J Urol 1973;45:606.
4. Texter JH, Koontz WW, McWilliams NB. Hemorrhagic cystitis as a complication of the management of pediatric neoplasm. Urol Surv 1979;29:47.
5. Droller MJ, Saral S, Santos, G. Prevention of cyclophosphamide-induced hemorrhagic cystitis. Urology 1982;20:256.
6. Stillwell TJ, Benson RC. Cyclophosphamide induced hemorrhagic cystitis. A review of 100 patients. Cancer 1988;61:451–457.
7. Cox PJ. Cyclophosphamide-induced cystitis-identification of acrolein as the causative agent. Biochem Pharmacol 1979;28:2045.
8. Freedman A, Ehrlich RM, Ljung BM. Prevention of cyclophosphamide cystitis with 2-mercaptoethane sodium sulfonate: A histologic study. J Urol 1984;132:580.
9. Ehrlich RM, Freedman A, Goldsobel AB, et al. The use of sodium 2 mercaptoethane sulfonate to prevent cyclophosphamide cystitis. J Urol 1984;131:960.
10. Jardine I, Ferselau C, Appler M, et al. Quantification by gas chromatography, chemical ionization, mass spectrometry of cyclophosphamide, phosphoramide mustard and nitrogen mustard in the plasma and urine of patients cyclophosphamide therapy. Cancer Res 1978;38:408–415.
11. Antman KH, Ryan L, Elias A, et al. Response to ifosamide and mesna: 124 previously treated patients with metastatic or unresectable sarcoma. J Clin Oncol 1989;7:126–131.
12. Pratt CB, Horowitz ME, Meyer WH, et al. Phase 2 trial of ifosfamide in children with malignant solid tumors. Cancer Treat Rep 1987;71:131.
13. Williams SD, Munshi, N, Einhorn LH, et al. Cyclophosphamide and ifosfamide: Role of uroprotective agents. Cancer Invest 1990;8:269.
14. Andriole GL, Sandlund JT, Miser JS, et al. The efficacy of mesna (2-mercaptoethane sodium sulfonate) as a uroprotectant in patients with hemorrhagic cystitis receiving further oxazaphosphorine chemotherapy. J Clin Oncol 1987;5:799–803.
15. Brugieres L, Hartmann JP, Travagli E, et al. Hemorrhagic cystitis following high-dose chemotherapy and bone marrow transplantation in children with malignancies: Incidence, clinical course, and outcome. J Clin Oncol 1989;7:194–199.
16. Shepherd JD, Pringle LE, Barnett MJ, et al. Mesna versus hyperhydration for the prevention of cyclophosphamide-induced hemorrhagic cystitis in bone marrow transplantation. J Clin Oncol 1991;9:2016–2020.
17. Dean RJ, Lytton B. Urologic complications of pelvic irradiation. J Urol 1978;119:64.
18. Schellhammer PF, Jordan GH, El-Mahdi AM. Pelvic complications after interstitial and external beam irradiation of urologic and gynecologic malignancy. World J Surg 1986;10:259–268.
19. Parsons CL. Successful management of radiation cystitis with sodium pentosanpolysulfate. J Urol 1986;136:813.
20. Weiss JP, Boland FP, Mori H, et al. Treatment of radiation induced cystitis with hyperbaric oxygen. J Urol 1986;134:352–354.
21. Liu YK, Harty JI, Steinbock GS, et al. Treatment of radiation or cyclophosphamide induced cystitis using conjugated estrogen. J Urol 1990;144:41–43.
22. Numazaki Y, Shigeta S, Kumaska T, et al. Acute hemorrhagic cystitis in children: Isolation of adenovirus type 11. N Engl J Med 1968;278:700–704.
23. Mufson MA, Belshe RB. A review of adenoviruses in the etiology of acute hemorrhagic cystitis. J Urol 1976;115:191–194.
24. Ambinder RF, Burns W, Forman M, et al. Hemorrhagic cystitis associated with adenovirus infection in bone marrow transplantation. Arch Intern Med 1986;146:1400–1401.
25. Rice SJ, Bishop JA, Apperley J, et al. BK virus as cause of hemorrhagic cystitis after bone marrow transplantation. Lancet 1985;2:844–845.
26. Shah KV, Daniel RW, Warszawski RM. High prevalence of antibodies to BK virus, an SV40-related papovavirus, in residents of Maryland. J Infect Dis 1973;128:784–787.
27. Heritage J, Chesters PM, McCance DJ. The persistence of papovavirus BK DNA sequences in normal human renal tissue. J Med Virol 1981;8:143–150.
28. Arthur RR, Shah KV, Baust SJ, et al. Association of BK viuruia with hemorrhagic cystitis in recipients of bone marrow transplants. N Engl J Med 1986;315:230–234.
29. Brown RB. A method of management of inoperable carcinoma of the bladder. Med J Aust 1969;1:23.
30. Donahue LA, Frank IN. Intravesical formalin of hemorrhagic cystitis: Analysis of therapy. J Urol 1989;141:809.

31. Fair WR. Formalin in the treatment of massive bladder hemorrhage. Techniques, results, and complications. Urology 1974;3:573.

32. Godec CJ, Gleich P. Intractable hematuria and formalin. J Urol 1983;130:688.

33. Ostroff EB, Chenault OW. Alum irrigation for the control of massive bladder hemorrhage. J Urol 1982;128:929–930.

34. Goel AK, Rao MS, Bhagwat AG, et al. Intravesical irrigation with alum for the control of massive bladder hemorrhage. J Urol 1984;133:956–957.

35. Arrizabalga M, Extramiana JL, Parra JL, et al. Treatment of massive hematuria with aluminous salts. Br J Urol 1987;60:223–226.

36. Kavoussi LR, Gelstein LD, Andriole GL. Encephalopathy and an elevated serum aluminum level in a patient receiving intravesical alum irrigation for severe urinary hemorrhage. J Urol 1986;136:665.

37. Mohuiddin J, Prentice HG, Schey S, et al. Treatment of cyclophosphamide-induced cystitis with prostaglandin E_2. Ann Intern Med 1984;101:142.

38. Shurafa M, Shumaker E, Cronin S. Prostaglandin F_2-alpha bladder irrigation for control of intractable cyclophosphamide-induced hemorrhagic cystitis. J Urol 1987;137:1230.

39. Andriole GL, Yuan JJ, Catalona WJ. Cystotomy, temporary urinary diversion and bladder packing in the management of severe cyclophosphamide-induced hemorrhagic cystitis. J Urol 1990;143:1006.

40. Pomer S, Karcher G, Simon W. Cutaneous ureterostomy as last resort treatment of intractable hemorrhagic cystitis following radiation. Br J Urol 1983;55:392.

41. Golin AI, Benson RC. Cyclophosphamide hemorrhagic cystitis requiring urinary diversion. J Urol 1977;118:110.

42. Holden S, McPhee M, Grabstald H. The rationale of urinary diversion in the cancer patient. J Urol 1979;121:19.

43. Zadra JA, Jewett, MA, Keresteci AG, et al. Nonoperative urinary diversion for malignant ureteral obstruction. Cancer 1987;60:1353.

44. Montana GS, Fowler WC. Carcinoma of the cervix: Analysis of bladder and rectal radiation dose and complications. Int J Radiat Oncol Biol Phys 1989;16:95.

45. Norman RW, Mack FG, Awad SA, et al. Acute renal failure secondary to bilateral ureteral obstruction: Review of 50 cases. Can Med Assoc J 1982;127:601.

46. Rose BS, Ragosin R, La Rosa JL, et al. Pyelosinus extravasation and urinoma associated with malignancy. Urology 1988;31:349.

47. Cronan JJ. Contemporary concepts in imaging urinary obstruction. Radiol Clin North Am 1991;29:527.

48. Saltzman B. Ureteral stents: Indications, variations, and complications. Urol Clin North Am 1988;15:481.

49. Chiou RK, Chang WY, Horan J. Ureteral obstruction associated with prostate cancer. The outcome after percutaneous nephrostomy. J Urol 1990;143:957.

50. Soper JT, Blaszczyk TM, Oke E, et al. Percutaneous nephrostomy in gynecologic oncology patients. Am J Obstet Gynecol 1988;158:1126.

51. Lee PH, Khauli RB, Baker S, et al. Prognostic and therapeutic observations of manifestations in the genitourinary tract of adenocarcinoma of the colon and rectum. Surg Gynecol Obstet 1989;169:511.

52. Reloux P, Weiser M, Piccart M, et al. Ureteral obstruction in patients with breast cancer. Cancer 1988;61:1904.

53. Meretyk S, Albala DM, Kavoussi LR. Endosurgery: Noncalculus application in the upper urinary tract. Monogr Urol 1991;12:67.

54. Meretyk S, Clayman RV, Kavoussi LR, et al. Endourologic treatment of ureteroenteric anastomotic strictures: Long-term follow-up. J Urol 1991;145:723.

55. Blumenthal D, Russo P, Orr J. Unilateral ureteral obstruction in a patient with acute leukemia. Urol Radiol 1990;12:61.

56. Brannen GE, Bush WH. Complications of endourology. AUA Update Series 9, Lesson 3. Houston: American Urological Association, 1985.

57. MacGregor PS, Montie JE, Straffon RA. Cutaneous ureterostomy as palliative diversion in adults with malignancy. Urology 1987;30:31.

58. Murray K, Massey A, Feneley RCL. Acute urinary retention—A urodynamic assessment. Br J Urol 1984;56:468.

59. Christensen MM, Bruskewitz RC. Clinical manifestations of benign prostatic hyperplasia and indications for therapeutic intervention. Urol Clin North Am 1990;17:509.

60. Chancellor MB, Blaivis JG, Kaplan SA, et al. Bladder outlet obstruction versus impaired detrusor contractility: The role of uroflow. J Urol 1991;145:810.

61. Blaivas JG. Multichannel urodynamic studies in men with benign prostatic hyperplasia. Urol Clin North Am 1990;17:543.

62. Blaivas JG. The neurophysiology of micturition. A clinical study of 550 patients. J Urol 1982;127:958.

63. Anderson JB, Grant JBF. Postoperative retention of urine: A prospective urodynamic study. Br Med J 1991;302:894.

64. Eickenberg HU, Amin M, Klompus W, et al. Urologic complications following abdominoperineal resection. J Urol 1976;115:180.

65. Steinberg J, Rukstalis DB, Vickers MA. Acute urinary retention secondary to herpes simplex meningitis. J Urol 1991;145:359.

66. Loo MH, Vaughan ED. Obstructive nephropathy and postobstructive diuresis. AUA Update Series 4, Lesson 9. Houston: American Urological Association, 1985.

67. Taube M, Gajraj H. Trial without catheter following acute retention. Br J Urol 1989;63:180.

68. Russo P, Packer MG, Fair WR. Prophylactic antibiotics in urological surgery. Semin Urol 1983;1:155.

69. McClennan BL. Diagnostic imaging evaluation of benign prostatic hyperplasia. Urol Clin North Am 1990;17:517.

70. Reisman ME, Kennedy TJ, Roehrborn CG, et al. A prospective study of urologist-performed sonographic evaluation of the urinary tract in patients with prostatism. J Urol 1991;145:1186.

71. Bryd L, Sherman RL. Radiocontrast induced acute renal failure. Medicine (Baltimore) 1979;58:270.

72. Mebust WK. Transurethral prostatectomy. Urol Clin North Am 1990;17:575.

73. Mebust WK, Holtgrewe HL, Cockett ATK, et al. Transurethral prostatectomy: Immediate and postoperative complications. A cooperative study of 13 participating institutions evaluating 3885 patients. J Urol 1989;141:243.

74. Meyerhoff HH, Gleason DM, Bottaccini MR. The effects of transurethral resection on the urodynamics of prostatism. J Urol 1989;142:785.

75. Keane PF, Timoney AG, Kiely E, et al. Response of benign hypertrophied prostate to treatment with LHRH analogue. Br J Urol 1988;62:163.

76. McConnell JD. Androgen ablation and blockade in the treatment of benign prostatic hyperplasia. Urol Clin North Am 1990;17:661.

77. Caine M. The present role of alpha adrenergic blockers in treatment of benign prostatic hypertrophy. J Urol 1986;136:1.

78. Nissenkorn I. Experience with a new self-retaining intraurethral catheter in patients with urinary retention: A preliminary report. J Urol 1989;142:942.

79. Strohmaier WL, Bichler KH, Flucter SH, et al. Local microwave hyperthermia of benign prostatic hyperplasia. J Urol 1990;144:913.

80. Dowd JB, Smith JJ. Balloon dilation of the prostate. Urol Clin North Am 1990;17:671.

81. Lapides J, Diokno AC, Silber S, et al. Clean intermittent self-catheterization in the treatment of urinary tract disease. J Urol 1972;107:458.

82. Wyndaele JJ, Maes D. Clean intermittent self-catheterization: A 12-year follow-up. J Urol 1990;143:906.

83. Maynard F, Diokno A. Urinary infection and complications during clean intermittent catheterization following spinal cord injury. J Urol 1984;132:943.

84. Korzeniowski OM. Urinary tract infection in the impaired host. Med Clin North Am 1991;75:391.

85. Warren JW. The catheter and urinary tract infection. Med Clin North Am 1991;75:481.

86. Garibaldi RA, Burke JP, Dickman ML, et al. Factors predisposing to bacteriuria during indwelling urethral catheterization. N Engl J Med 1974;291:215.

87. Stamm WE. Nosocomial infections: Etiologic changes, therapeutic challenges. Hosp Pract 1981;16:75.

88. Fierer J. Acute pyelonephritis. Urol Clin North Am 1987;14:251.

89. Nickel JC, Ruseska I, Wright JB, et al. Tobramycin resistance of *Pseudomonas aeruginosa* cells growing as a biofilm on urinary catheter material. Antimicrob Agents Chemother 1985;27:619.

90. Warren JW, Muncie HL, Hall-Craggs M. Acute pyelonephritis associated with bacteriuria of long-term catheterization: A prospective clinico-pathological study. J Infect Dis 1988;158:1341.

91. Roberts JA. Pyelonephritis, cortical abscess, perinephric abscess. Urol Clin North Am 1986;13:637.

92. Merenich WM, Popky GL. Radiology of renal infection. Med Clin North Am 1991;75:425.

93. Sheenan G, Harding G, et al. Advances in the treatment of urinary tract infection. Am J Med 1984;15:141.

94. Kuligowska E, Newman B, White SJ, et al. Interventional ultrasound in detection and treatment of renal inflammatory disease. Radiology 1983;147:521.

95. Berger RE. Acute epididymitis: Etiology and therapy. Semin Urol 1991;9:28.

96. Pfau A. Prostatitis: A continuing enigma. Urol Clin North Am 1986;13:695.

97. Vapnek JM. Urologic disease in HIV infection. Infect Urol 1991;4:104.

98. Cohen MS. Fournier's gangrene. AUA Update Series 5, Lesson 6. Houston: American Urological Association, 1986.

99. Jones RB, Hirschmann JV, Brown GS, et al. Fournier's syndrome: Necrotizing subcutaneous infection of the male genitalia. J Urol 1979;122:279.

100. Nelson JH, Winter CC. Priapism: Evolution of management in 48 patients in a 22-year series. J Urol 1977;117:455.

101. Schreibman SM, Gee TS, Grabstaldt H. Management of priapism in patients with chronic granulocytic leukemia. J Urol 1974;111:786.

102. Powell BL, Craig JB, Muss HB. Secondary malignancies of the penis and epididymis: A case report and review of the literature. J Clin Oncol 1985;3:110.

103. Nolens RE, Ells L, Crammer-Levied D. pharmacologic erection: Diagnosis and treatment applications in 69 patients. J Urol 1987;138:52.

104. Shantha TR, Finnerty DP, Rodriquez AP. Treatment of persistent penile erection and priapism using terbutaline. J Urol 1989;141:1427.

Cancer: Principles & Practice of Oncology, Fourth Edition,
edited by Vincent T. DeVita, Jr., Samuel Hellman, Steven A. Rosenberg.
J.B. Lippincott Co., Philadelphia © 1993.

CHAPTER **61**

Treatment of Metastatic Cancer

SECTION **1**

DONALD C. WRIGHT
THOMAS F. DELANEY
JAN C. BUCKNER

Treatment of Metastatic Cancer to the Brain

Physicians caring for patients with oncologic disease face a daunting challenge when invasion of the nervous system by generalized cancers becomes evident. The appearance of neurologic symptoms in this setting evokes a feeling of dread in patients and in their families and occasionally prompts a concealed nihilism among the treating physicians. Successful, appropriate management of cerebral metastatic spread requires rapid diagnosis and institution of therapy to minimize neurologic injury and maximize the duration and quality of survival. Selected patients derive tremendous benefit from combined treatment approaches, and careful management limits the neurologic impairment in many others. Extending this success to the majority of patients with brain metastases, however, remains an elusive goal.

Metastases to the central nervous system (CNS), a favored site for metastatic spread among the more common cancers affecting the U.S. population, occur in 25% to 35%[1] of all cancer patients. This chapter focuses on the treatment of *parenchymal* metastases to the nervous system, the more common mode of CNS involvement by cancer. Epidemiologic estimates of CNS involvement by cancer in the 1992 U.S. population (Table 61–1)[2] forecast that more than 152,600 patients, or 13.5% of the total U.S. cancer population, will develop symptomatic metastasis to the brain.[1–6]

CLASSIFICATION AND EPIDEMIOLOGY OF CEREBRAL METASTASES

ANATOMIC DISTRIBUTION

The specific anatomic site(s) or "compartments" involved in a metastatic process, as well as the primary histologic type, temporal profile, and clinical status of the patient at the time of diagnosis, are useful criteria in determining prognosis and the most efficacious therapy. The anatomic cerebral compartments commonly involved by metastasis (Fig. 61–1) are the skull, dura, leptomeninges (arachnoid and pia), and parenchymal substance of the brain (pituitary and extracranial sites are omitted in this chapter). Central nervous system involvement in cancer ranges from 20% to 30%, reflecting the difference between clinical detection during life and careful necropsy examination.[1,5,7] *Intracranial* involvement is estimated as 25%, with *intradural* (parenchymal and leptomeningeal) deposits affecting 20% and *parenchymal* involvement only present in 10% of patients.[5,8]

Clinical series indicate that multiple deposits are present in 53% of patients. Autopsy examination and increasingly sensitive diagnostic studies suggest that the frequency of multiple tumors is higher.[4,5,8,9] Certain tumor types are typically associated with single (renal, ovarian, osteogenic sarcoma, breast) and multiple (lung, melanoma, seminoma) metastases.[5] The detection of multiple metastatic deposits plays a critical role in the choice of therapy, because most authors restrict surgery to single metastases.

HISTOPATHOLOGY: FREQUENCY OF METASTASES BY TUMOR TYPE

Parenchymal patterns of metastases are determined by the general incidence of a specific cancer and the relative ten-

TABLE 61–1. Epidemiologic Estimates of Brain Metastases—1992

Site or Type	Systemic Cancer 1992: New Cases	Frequency of Symptomatic Metastases*	New Cases: Symptomatic Metastases†	1992 Deaths	Deaths With Symptomatic Metastases‡
All sites	1,130,000	0.135	152,600	520,000	70,200
Lung	168,000	0.263	44,200	146,000	38,400
Breast	181,000	0.158	28,600	45,300	7200
Colon and rectum	156,000	0.045	7000	58,300	2600
Urinary organs	78,100	0.128	10,000	20,200	2600
Melanoma	32,000	0.37	11,800	6700	2500
Prostate	132,000	0.053	7000	34,000	1800
Pancreas	28,300	0.04	1100	25,000	1000
Leukemia	28,200	0.06	1700	19,200	1200
Lymphoma§	44,400	0.038	1800	20,900	800
Liver	15,400	0.04	600	12,300	500
Female genital	71,500	0.015	1100	24,000	400

* Symptomatic parenchymal location only (does not include skull, dura, or leptomeninges).
† Estimated by (new 1992 cases) × (metastatic frequency).
‡ Estimated by (1992 cancer deaths) × (metastatic frequency of symptomatic parenchymal metastases).
§ Includes all lymphoma (Hodgkin's and non-Hodgkin's types).
(Boring CC, Squires TS, Tong R. Cancer statistics, 1992. CA 1992;42:19–38; Hildebrand J. Lesions of the nervous system in cancer patients. Monograph series of the European Organization for Research on Treatment of Cancer. Vol 5. New York: Raven Press, 1978; Takakura K, Sano K, Hoho S, et al. Metastatic tumors of the central nervous system. Tokyo: Igaku-Shoin, 1982; Galicich JH, Sundaresan N. Metastatic brain tumors. In: Wilkins RH, Rengachary SS, eds. Neurosurgery. New York: McGraw-Hill, 1985:597–610)

dency for cerebral spread. Table 61–2 indicates the parenchymal metastatic patterns for the most common cancers in a large autopsy series.[5] Lung, gastrointestinal, and urinary tract primary tumors account for 80% of metastases in men, whereas breast, lung, gastrointestinal tract, and melanoma account for 80% of metastases in women.

Lung carcinoma, by virtue of its relative frequency, is the most common metastasis, accounting for 40% to 60% of all parenchymal deposits in the U.S. population.[5,6,10] Melanoma has the highest likelihood of cerebral spread, with 65% of patients developing this complication during the course of the disease. The relative metastatic attack rates for breast (51%) and lung (41%) are lower, but they contribute a greater number of patients by virtue of their greater overall prevalence.

TEMPORAL PATTERNS OF PRESENTATION

Brain metastasis may present in three distinct temporal profiles: *precocious* (occult primary), *synchronous* (simultaneous primary), and *metachronous* (antecedent primary).[7] Lung, melanoma, and renal tumors tend to have brief intervals from the time of initial diagnosis to evolution of a brain metastasis, whereas breast, colon, and sarcomas have long intervals. The majority of patients (81%) present with an antecedent (*metachronous*) primary tumor before development of cerebral spread.

Other clinical classification approaches are useful (see section on Clinical Aspects of Brain Metastases) for prognosis and as an aid in choosing the most efficacious treatment modality for a given patient.

PATHOGENESIS AND PATHOPHYSIOLOGY OF CEREBRAL METASTASES

The general concepts of tumor metastasis are germane to cerebral metastasis[11]; the brain, however, has a unique anatomic, physiologic, and immunologic organization that influences the localization, growth pattern, and spread of metastases.[12,13] Cerebral metastases are generally a "tertiary" phenomenon of metastatic spread more commonly arising after secondary metastatic sites (*e.g.*, lung, liver) have developed.[14] Brain metastases arise either from hematogenous dissemination of circulating tumor cells or, less commonly, by contiguous spread from adjacent sites (skull, basal foraminae, and soft tissues of the head and neck). Hematogenous spread occurs when tumor cells are passively disseminated into the bloodstream.[5,7,15–17] The distribution patterns for parenchymal metastases (Fig. 61–2) generally correlate with the regional brain weight and blood flow, with approximately 80% of metastases occurring in the supratentorial compartment.[3] A preferential distribution by metastases for the superficial distal arterial fields (watershed areas) was noted in an antemortem study[13] that also demonstrated a posterior fossa predilection by metastases from pelvic and gastrointestinal primary tumors. Another explanation for nonrandom or preferential involvement of the brain by certain primary tumors (*e.g.*, melanoma and small cell carcinoma of the lung) is the observation that primary tumors have metastatic cell subpopulations with "site-specific" characteristics that favor the brain as a preferential site for metastatic spread.[18–21]

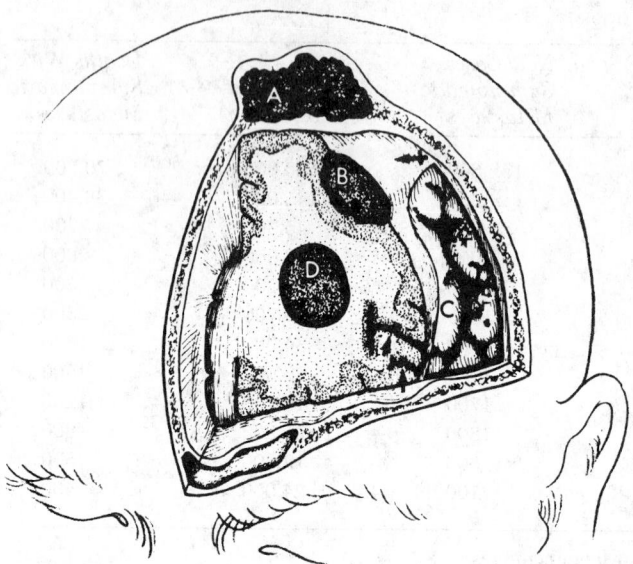

FIGURE 61–1. Anatomic classification of brain metastases. Three-quarter view of left frontal cranium, showing **(A)** a large metastasis to the skull diploë; **(B)** a dural metastasis; **(C)** superficial leptomeningeal invasion; and **(D)** a parenchymal metastasis (revealed by a coronal cut made at the posterior border of the frontal lobe). Open arrows indicate areas of leptomeningeal spread. Crossed arrow indicates the convex surface of the brain with dura intact. Solid arrows indicate leptomeningeal spread into several sulci. (Courtesy of Pat Kenny, Medical Illustration Section, National Institutes of Health, Bethesda, MD) (Wright DC. Surgical treatment of brain metastases. In: Rosenberg SA, ed. Surgical treatment of metastatic cancer. Philadelphia: JB Lippincott, 1987:165–222)

CEREBRAL PATHOPHYSIOLOGY IN METASTASIS

Clinical symptoms from brain metastases arise by impairment of the homeostatic mechanisms necessary for maintenance of normal brain function. Mechanical distortion and displacement (herniations) by a progressively increasing neoplastic mass; increases in intracranial pressure (ICP) and decreases in cerebral blood flow (CBF); propagation of vasogenic cerebral edema; and derangement of metabolic energy processes represent the major pathophysiologic changes that can occur.

Brain swelling occurs as a result of mass lesions (*e.g.*, neoplasm, hematoma), obstruction of cerebrospinal fluid (CSF) pathways (hydrocephalus), alterations in cerebrovascular regulation (*e.g.*, hyperemia, local dysregulation of vascular tone or blood flow), and propagation of cerebral edema.

Rapid changes in the intracranial volume-pressure relation by progressive neoplastic growth result in elevated intracranial pressure if the normal buffering system of the brain cannot compensate by reciprocal reductions in CSF and vascular and extracellular volumes.[22–25] Various stereotypical clinical herniation syndromes[26] arise when severe mechanical distortions occur and frequently result in permanent neurologic injury or death of the patient.

Brain edema is an increase in brain water and ions (primarily sodium)[27] arising either by direct injury to cells (cytotoxic edema) or from injury to the vascular endothelium (vasogenic edema).[27,28] Direct injury to the endothelium by compressing or invading tumor, dysplastic vascular structures present within tumors,[29] and biochemically mediated alterations of capillary permeability[30–33] contribute to the development of vasogenic edema. Water and ions passively diffuse into the brain extracellular space in areas of increased vascular permeability, primarily affecting the cerebral white matter. Edema fluid may travel along longitudinally oriented white

TABLE 61–2. Brain Metastases by Histologic Type*

Site of Primary Neoplasm	No. of Patients	No. of Metastases*	% Total†	Relative Frequency (%)‡
Lung	774	266	7.9	48
Breast	526	111	3.3	20
Gastrointestinal	773	43	1.3	8
Urinary	199	34	1.0	6
Melanoma	69	34	1.0	6
Prostate	140	10	0.3	2
Liver & pancreas	293	14	0.4	3
Other	585	43	1.3	8
Total	3359	555	16.5	100

* Parenchymal metastases only.

† Expressed as $\dfrac{\text{number (parenchymal) metastases}}{\text{total number of cancer autopsies}}$

‡ Relative frequency = $\dfrac{\text{number (parenchymal) metastases by tumor type}}{\text{total number of parenchymal metastases}} \times 100$

(Modified from Takakura K, Sano K, Hoho S, et al. Metastatic tumors of the central nervous system. Tokyo: Igaku-Shoin, 1982)

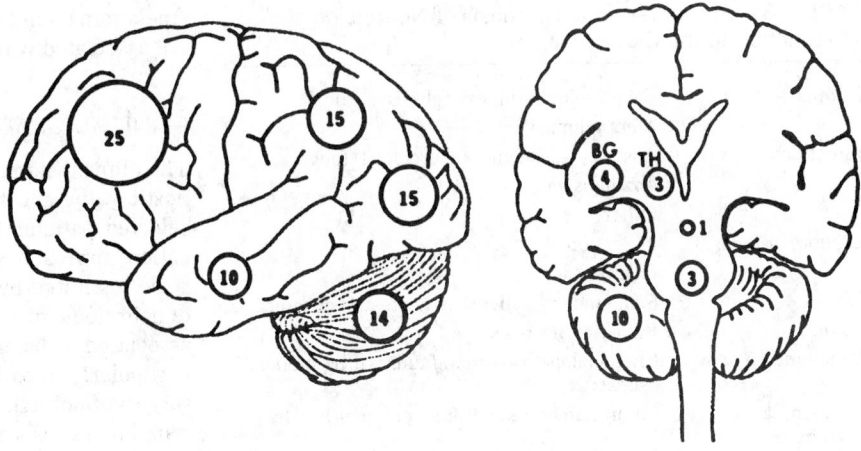

FIGURE 61–2. Parenchymal distribution of brain metastases. The distribution and relative frequency (%) are diagrammed according to metastatic site. The subcortical gray structures (BG, basal ganglia; Th, thalamus) receive 7% of metastases, and cerebellar hemispheres receive 10% of metastases. (Adapted from Takakura K, Sana K, Hoho S, et al. Metastatic tumors of the central nervous system. Tokyo: Igaku-Shoin, 1982. Reproduced from Wright DC. Surgical treatment of brain metastases. In: Rosenberg SA, ed. Surgical treatment of metastatic cancer. Philadelphia, JB Lippincott, 1987:165–222)

matter tracts at great distances (Fig. 61–3) from the focal "source" of increased capillary permeability[34] with ultimate deterioration in neurologic function.

CLINICAL ASPECTS OF BRAIN METASTASES

The definitive diagnosis of brain metastasis cannot be made solely on the basis of the clinical examination,[6] because the presenting symptoms and signs are not distinct from those of other intracranial mass lesions (Table 61–3). Various disease processes mimic brain metastases both clinically and by diagnostic studies. Benign, treatable conditions simulating a metastasis must be identified (even in the patient with an established diagnosis of cancer) to avoid inappropriate or dangerous therapy.[9,35,36] Those patients without a prior diagnosis of cancer require an unequivocal pathologic diagnosis. Complications of disease or iatrogenic injuries (infectious, cerebrovascular, toxic) are common in the cancer patient and frequently account for neurologic symptoms rather than the

primary disease process and require specific evaluation and treatment.

PRESENTATION: SYMPTOMS AND SIGNS

The presenting neurologic symptoms and signs (Table 61–4) of brain metastases are headache, weakness, cognitive or affective disturbance, and seizures.[4,10,37–42] The pathogenesis of neural injury previously discussed can be aligned with presenting symptoms in a general way: focal symptoms and signs (unilateral headache, weakness, seizures) generally result from direct parenchymal injury by neoplasm, whereas diffuse symptoms and signs (generalized headache, cognitive or behavioral changes, papilledema) reflect the global effects of cerebral edema, metabolic dysfunction, or CSF obstruction.

Headaches, the most common (≥50%) presenting symptom, arise as a result of either direct injury, such as traction or distortion of pain-sensitive structures (dura, dural venous sinuses, large blood vessels, cranial nerves), or indirect mechanisms (edema, CSF obstruction). The headache is usually remitting, occurring in the morning or early hours and

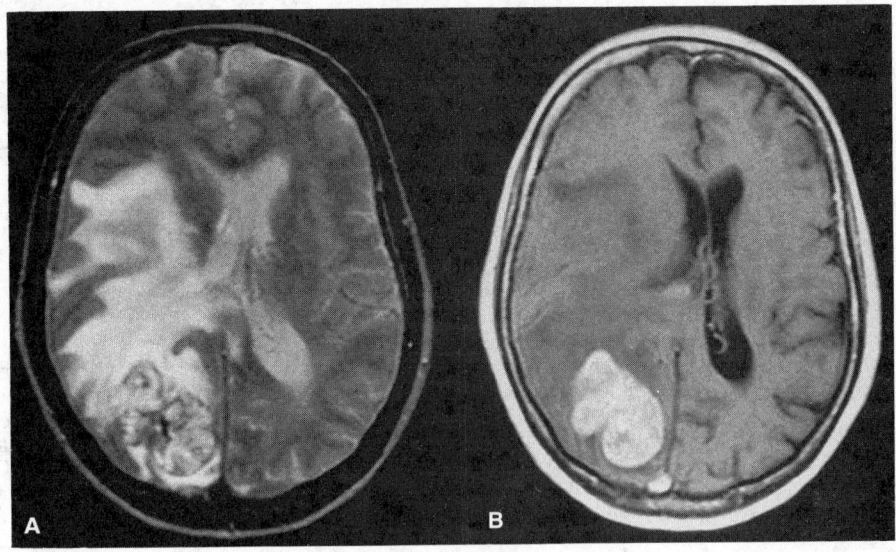

FIGURE 61–3. Parenchymal metastasis to the right parietooccipital lobe. **(A)** A T2-weighted scan illustrating distant spread of vasogenic cerebral edema along the subcortical white matter tracts. Note the mass effect on the lateral ventricle. **(B)** Localized enhancement of tumor by gadolinium-DTPA using T1-weighting techniques. The superior sagittal sinus is also enhancing (not indicative of tumor) just posterior and medial to the tumor mass.

TABLE 61–3. Differential Diagnosis of Neurologic Dysfunction in the Cancer Patient

Neoplastic*	Primary brain tumors (glial series)
	Meningioma
Infectious	Abscess—pyogenic, tuberculous, fungal
	Toxoplasma
	Other
Cerebrovascular	Infarction
	Hemorrhage
	Sub, epidural collection; acute and chronic
Toxic	Radiation necrosis
Metabolic	Encephalopathy (organ failure, drug-induced, sepsis)
Paraneoplastic syndromes	Eaton-Lambert syndrome, polyneuropathy

* Partial listing; not intended to serve as complete differential diagnostic list.
(Modified from Weiss HD. Neoplasms. In: Samuels MA, ed. Manual of neurologic therapeutics. Boston: Little, Brown, 1986)

gradually increasing in duration and frequency until associated with symptoms and signs of increased intracranial pressure (ICP). Paroxysmal headache, when present, is occasionally accompanied by fluctuating neurologic signs (*e.g.,* hemiparesis) and reflects abnormalities of intracranial pressure dynamics (plateau waves).[37] Unilateral headaches, when present, are of localizing value in the majority of patients.[10]

Weakness, the most common focal sign, is symptomatic in 40% of patients and elicitable on examination in 65%.[37] Ataxia may be present in patients with CSF obstruction and is associated with cerebellar deposits. Disturbances in mental functions (changes in behavior, memory, speech, and cognitive skills) appear in a third of patients as presenting symptoms and are demonstrated on psychological testing in 50% to 75% of patients.[37,43]

Seizures account for the most common acute onset of symptoms and, if focal, are of localizing value. Certain tumors

(melanoma) and tumor patterns (leptomeningeal deposits) are associated with a high incidence of seizures.[37,44]

CLINICAL GRADING

The clinical status of patients at initial treatment is of prognostic value and has a positive correlation with outcome in selected patients subjected to surgery.[6,38,45,46] Most classification approaches employ the long-standing performance scale instituted by Karnofsky[47] supplemented by a measure of neurologic function.[1,48] The extent of disseminated disease associated with cerebral metastasis also has prognostic value, particularly in patients subjected to the physiologic stress of surgery. Such clinical grading of patients at the time of cerebral metastasis greatly facilitates risk evaluation and guides the clinician in choosing a rational approach to treatment; likewise, the comparison of various treatment modalities in matched patient groups is facilitated by this clinical classification.

SPECIALIZED NEURODIAGNOSTIC EVALUATION

In addition to standard screening diagnostic and laboratory studies routinely performed for patients with cancer, neurodiagnostic studies are increasingly employed in routine evaluation because of the high incidence of cerebral metastases in the more common cancers affecting the U.S. populations. Computed tomographic (CT) scanning, magnetic resonance imaging (MRI), and arteriography constitute the primary studies currently employed in neurodiagnostic evaluation for cerebral metastases. These imaging studies provide diagnostic information and, more important, anatomic localization of the mass lesion(s). This localization is critical to the radiation therapist for treatment planning and to the surgeon for accurate placement of scalp flaps, bone openings, and cortical incisions.[6,25]

Contrast CT scanning has, until recently, been the single most important neurodiagnostic study in patients with suspected brain metastases. Contrast (gadolinium-DTPA) MRI scanning, now widely available, is currently the most sensitive

TABLE 61–4. Symptoms and Signs of Cerebral Metastases

Symptoms	*Frequency (%)*	*Signs*	*Frequency (%)*
Headache	53	Hemiparesis	66
Weakness, focal	40	Impaired cognition	77
Mental disturbance	31	Sensory loss, unilateral	27
Seizures	15	Papilledema	26
Gait disorder	20	Ataxia	24
Visual disturbance	12	Aphasia	19
Language disturbance	10		

(Data from Takakura K, Sano K, Hoho S, et al. Metastatic tumors of the central nervous system. Tokyo: Igaku-Shoin, 1982; Posner JB. Diagnosis and treatment of metastases to the brain. Clin Bull 1974;4:47–57; Gamache FW Jr, Posner JB, Galicich JH. Treatment of brain metastases by surgical extirpation. In: Weiss L, Gilbert H, Posner J, eds. Brain metastases. Boston: GK Hall, 1980:390–414; Order SE, Hellman S, Von Essen CF, et al. Improvement in quality of survival following whole-brain irradiation for whole-brain metastasis. Radiology 1968;91:149–153)

study for detection of metastases,[49] although CT scanning is still preferred by many radiation therapists and surgeons because of the superior diagnostic specificity and depiction of bone (localization) detail. Parenchymal metastases are typically spheroidal, with peritumoral edema formation, and located in the gray matter-white matter junction (see Fig. 61–3).[13] Enhancement (both CT and MRI) occurs because of permeability changes in the "blood-brain" and "blood-tumor" vascular endothelium[50,51] and because of the increased vascular volumes (neovascularity) characteristically found in metastatic tumors, which prolong the transit times for water-soluble conjugates (meglumine–iodine and gadolinium-DTPA) used clinically as contrast agents. The value of CT or MRI scanning extends beyond the initial evaluation; serial scanning is a very effective means to monitor tumor development, progression, response to therapy, and detection of secondary complications.

Arteriography provides neoplastic and normal vascular detail, such as the origin of arterial supply, routes of venous drainage, and degree of neovascularity. Because of the wide availability of CT and MRI scanners, arteriography is generally reserved for the patient in whom tumor vascular characteristics play an important role in surgical planning.

Emphasis should be made regarding caution in the performance of lumbar puncture in the setting of cerebral metastasis. This procedure is hazardous in any patient with increased intracranial pressure, particularly where focal masses produce regional transients of increased tissue pressure, a common situation in brain metastasis. Lumbar puncture has diagnostic value in situations where infectious or neoplastic involvement of the CSF space is suspected. These represent the only entities where a *specific* diagnosis can be inferred from examination of the cerebrospinal fluid. Neurologic consultation and CT scanning should be performed in a patient with known or suspected cancer before performance of a lumbar puncture.

Specialized neurodiagnostic studies have dramatically altered the immediate hazards of therapy by minimizing the morbidity of neoplastic and treatment-related complications. This ability has vastly improved selection of the most appropriate therapy by localizing lesions to the specific anatomic compartment(s) involved, and it has allowed identification of metastatic complications (hemorrhage, hydrocephalus, edema, infection) arising from treatment (surgical complications, radiation necrosis).

PRINCIPLES OF MANAGEMENT

THERAPEUTIC GOALS

Secondary spread of a generalized cancer to the brain places the patient in a precarious situation demanding urgent treatment to prevent or minimize progressive neurologic injury. Neurologic dysfunction arising from cerebral metastases, particularly of cognitive and motor systems, has a disproportionate impact on the functional performance of the patient when compared with the disability arising from systemic metastases elsewhere. The principal therapeutic goals for patients with brain metastasis are to maximize and maintain the highest neurologic function attainable; the quality of survival for

most patients is dramatically improved if control of intracranial metastases is achieved.

The principal treatment regimens applied specifically toward cerebral metastasis are radiation therapy alone or surgery combined with adjunctive postoperative radiation therapy. The therapeutic approach varies for a given patient with cerebral metastases depending on the tumor type and clinical setting. All patients should receive general supportive care, steroids, and radiation therapy; selected patients should undergo surgical resection followed by radiation therapy. Surgery may be employed as primary treatment for attempted total resection of a single metastasis or as a secondary procedure for diagnostic biopsy. Adjunctive chemotherapy is indicated in selected patients and specific tumor types. Seizure prophylaxis is indicated for patients who present with seizures[52] and those patients subjected to surgery.

PHARMACOLOGIC THERAPY OF ELEVATED INTRACRANIAL PRESSURE

Effective treatment of the various causes of elevated intracranial pressure (ICP) associated with cerebral metastases contributes to the emergent palliation of neurologic dysfunction and reduces the morbidity associated with definitive treatment (surgery or radiation therapy). Specifically, the means to control vasogenic cerebral edema guided the progressive advances in therapy since the introduction of glucocorticoids and other agents in this role.[53–55] Steroids (dexamethasone, methylprednisolone, prednisone) exert rapid clinical responses (6–24 hours)[56,57] benefiting 60% to 80% of patients in resolving or reducing clinical symptoms.[9,53,58] Steroids are used empirically because their optimal dose is unknown and their mechanism of action only partially understood.[25] Typically, starting doses (Table 61–5) for dexamethasone (or equivalent doses of other steroids) of 16–24 mg/day are used[59] (with or without a bolus loading dose), and higher doses (100 mg/day) are sometimes effective in patients without benefit at lower doses.[58] Steroids are used for both acute and chronic relief of generalized symptoms of increased ICP (headache, papilledema, confusion), but benefit is usually transient if no additional therapy is employed.

Osmotherapy, commonly used in the emergent control of ICP, reduces brain extracellular water and total body water. ICP is lowered by a reduction of brain extracellular volume, which also promotes movement of edema fluid out of the brain.[60] Diuretics (*e.g.*, furosemide, acetazolamide) and hyperosmolar solutions (mannitol, urea) are used acutely to lower ICP by reducing brain extracellular volume in areas with intact blood–brain barrier. Mannitol also has direct rheologic effects that increase local cerebral blood flow. Clinical dosages (see Table 61–5) for mannitol are 1.0 to 1.5 g/kg intravenous bolus, or intermittent intravenous administration to maintain serum osmolality between 295 and 320 mOsm. Furosemide is given in intermittent intravenous doses of 10 to 20 mg (40–80 mg/day) to achieve a brisk diuresis.

NEUROLOGIC EMERGENCIES IN CEREBRAL METASTASES

Patients with cerebral metastases may develop neurologic deficits acutely (seizure, cerebral hemorrhage, CSF outflow ob-

TABLE 61–5. Common Pharmacologic Measures in Cerebral Metastases

Drug	Use or Indications	Mode of Administration	Dose*	Therapeutic Range Comments
Dexamethasone	Vasogenic cerebral edema	I.V. or PO	16–24 mg	Empiric
Prednisolone	Vasogenic cerebral edema	I.V. or PO	105–160 mg	Empiric
Mannitol	Cerebral edema mass effect	I.V	1.0–1.5 g/kg	Maintain serum osmolality > 295 < 320
Furosemide	Cerebral edema mass effect	I.V. or PO	40–80 mg/d	Empiric; maintain osmolality > 295 < 320
Acetazolamide	Cerebral edema mass effect	I.V. or PO	500–1000 mg/d	Empiric; maintain osmolality > 295 < 320
Phenytoin	Anticonvulsant	I.V. or PO	200–400 mg/d (5 mg/kg/d)	5–20 μg/ml; loading dose is 15 mg/kg
Carbamazepine	Anticonvulsant	PO	600–800 mg/d (7–15 mg/kg/d)	3–12 μg/ml

(Samuels MA, ed. Manual of neurologic therapeutics. Boston: Little, Brown, 1986:1–424)

struction)[61,62] or manifest a deteriorating neurologic syndrome (cerebral edema, rapidly expanding neoplasm, communicating hydrocephalus). The former situation generally arises in patients with unsuspected or occult cerebral lesions, whereas the latter is a common feature of patients with relapsing tumors in whom initial therapeutic measures are ineffective. In either setting, rapid diagnostic evaluation and initiation of therapy is paramount. Examination of the patient (general and neurologic systems), diagnostic imaging (CT or MRI), and other specialized diagnostic studies (*e.g.*, electroencephalogram [EEG]) are required to identify the etiology of the deterioration. Focal neurologic symptoms and signs generally arise from intracranial pressure shifts that result in various herniation syndromes. Global, nonspecific alterations in neurologic function (headache, nausea and vomiting, impaired mental status, cognitive dysfunction, and so forth) usually result from a generalized increase in intracranial pressure or an encephalopathic process (metabolic disturbances of electrolytes, hepatic/renal dysfunction, CNS infection). Treatment is directed toward correction of the underlying cause and may require medical care, surgical intervention, or both.

Immediate, nonspecific measures[61] may be necessary to stabilize neurologic function in a patient before clinical evaluation until a specific diagnosis and appropriate therapy can be formulated. Such maneuvers include hyperventilation (decreases pCO_2), osmotherapy, steroids, and seizure control (see Table 61–5), if indicated. Occasionally, neurologic resuscitation for severely ill or rapidly deteriorating patients requires airway protection (intubation) and ventilatory support. Neurosurgical intervention may be required for neurologic monitoring (ventricular catheter for drainage; placement of ICP monitoring devices) or, more common, to correct underlying treatable causes of increased ICP (tumoral hemorrhage, ventricular obstruction, and so forth). Rational therapy requires a specific diagnosis as well as knowledge of the extent of systemic disease processes. Surgical indications and the results of emergent surgery are discussed in the following sections.

RADIATION THERAPY APPROACHES IN CEREBRAL METASTASES

Radiation is employed in nearly all patients with cerebral metastases, either as primary therapy or as an adjunct to surgical excision of a neoplastic mass. Numerous studies[42,63–68] have established the efficacy of radiation therapy and have identified specific factors influencing the radiation response for a given histologic tumor type and patient profile.[69]

Randomized prospective clinical trials[70] have investigated the optimal time-dose schedules for patients with cerebral metastases stratified according to histology of the primary site and the presence or absence of metastases to sites other than the brain. While no differences were seen in the randomized groups with respect to response or median survival, the shorter time-dose fractionation schemes had equal efficacy and less expense over longer treatment schedules. A program of 30 Gy/2 weeks (1 Gy = 100 rads) to the entire cranial cavity is generally well tolerated and can be followed by a boost of 9 Gy in three additional fractions to areas of gross disease as defined by diagnostic images.

These initial studies suggested significantly longer survivals in both ambulatory and nonambulatory patients when the brain was the only site of metastases or when the primary lesion was controlled, and they prompted an additional trial to investigate higher radiation doses. Patients with brain metastases and no evidence of other sites of disseminated disease were randomized to receive 50 Gy/4 weeks or 30 Gy/2 weeks. This study group was predominated by patients with aggressive cancers (80% had lung cancer) and demonstrated no statistically significant advantage of one treatment over the other for symptom relief, median survival, or prevention of death by brain metastases.[71]

Very rapid fractionation programs (*e.g.*, 10 Gy in one fraction) have also been tested for palliation of brain metastases. Response rates, promptness of neurologic improvement, treatment morbidity, and median survival were comparable to those of patients receiving higher doses in multiple fractions. However, the duration of improvement, time to deterioration of neurologic status, and rate of complete disappearance of neurologic symptoms were generally less for those patients who received 10 or 12 Gy, suggesting that ultra-rapid, high-dose irradiation schedules might not be as effective as conventionally fractionated higher dose schedules in the palliation of brain metastases.[70,72] A high complication rate has been associated with this strategy, especially in moribund patients with evidence of increased intracranial pressure, who should be considered unsuitable for rapid, high-dose schedules.[65,73]

Specialized Radiation Approaches to Brain Metastases

Because 30% to 50% of patients treated with conventional external radiation therapy for brain metastases will develop progressive intracranial disease, there has been considerable interest in combination therapy (surgery plus radiation therapy) and innovative radiation approaches. Normal tissue (brain) irradiation tolerance limits the dose (55–70 Gy) that can be safely delivered with conventional external radiation techniques. *Focal* radiation delivered either by tightly collimated, multiple trajectory ports (stereotactic radiosurgery) or by image-directed brachytherapy (interstitial radiation) increases the tumor dose without exceeding normal tissue tolerance. Brachytherapy allows local application of continuous radiation exposure during the treatment interval (typically between 7 and 60 days), which is analogous to delivering the radiation dose in a large number of very small fractions. Radiation sources are surgically implanted within the tumor borders and configured to deliver doses (80–150 Gy) higher than those possible with conventional external radiation techniques.[74] The physical characteristic of the isotope used determines such factors as the dose rate and distance the emitted radiation travels in tissue, permitting relative control over the dose distribution. This strategy aims to achieve a high-dose "local boost" to the tumor, creating a focal area of radiation necrosis within the borders of the neoplasm while minimizing radiation exposure to normal tissues. Response is determined by such factors as tumor size and geometry, ability to accurately image the tumor-brain interface, and tumor radiosensitivity.

This approach has been used for reirradiation in a small number of patients with recurrent metastases[74–76] or to deliver "boost" treatment in addition to external cranial irradiation in selected patients with brain metastases at presentation.[75] Some patients with recurrent disease have been noted to remain free of progressive intracranial tumor for over a year and up to 4 years after brachytherapy.[75,76] Neurologic function is generally preserved, but there is a risk of focal radiation necrosis when implants are used in this setting.

Recently, stereotactic external irradiation ("stereotactic radiosurgery," Gamma knife, linear accelerator [LINAC], and so forth) has been used to treat patients with brain metastases.[77–79] This technique uses single high doses of irradiation from a specially designed cobalt source or from a modified linear accelerator. Multiple, nonplanar, narrow beams are stereotactically directed to the site of metastatic disease by use of sophisticated radiation dosimetry techniques. Because the whole-brain dose of irradiation increases rapidly with increases in the target volume, the technique is limited to small, circumscribed lesions, generally ≤3.5 cm in diameter. A recent analysis indicated that radiosurgery of intracranial tumors is associated with a low risk of complications for lesions <10 ml treated with a single isocenter to maximum tumor doses <25 Gy with a tumor dose inhomogeneity <10 Gy.[80] Clinical experience with this technique, although limited, demonstrated that the majority of patients improved neurologically and could be withdrawn from corticosteroid therapy. Patients with adenocarcinomas demonstrated radiographic regression of treated lesions. The procedure was well tolerated, and no patients developed symptomatic radiation necrosis.

While these reports hold promise, the technical demands of such approaches will probably limit application to selected patients with a single recurrent or unresectable, isolated brain metastasis (<3.5 cm in size and not involving the corpus callosum) in the setting of controlled systemic disease.

CHEMOTHERAPY FOR CEREBRAL METASTASES

The role of chemotherapy in the treatment of brain metastases has not been clearly defined. In the past, the assumption that the blood–brain barrier prevents the passage of most chemotherapeutic agents into cerebral tumors discouraged clinical investigation. Recently, clinical studies have demonstrated tumor regressions with intravenous administration of conventional chemotherapeutic agents. The extent to which tumor regression influences overall control of brain metastases remains uncertain.

Microcirculation and Drug Delivery

The microcirculation of cerebral metastases differs substantially from that of the normal blood–brain barrier. Capillaries within brain metastases contain membrane fenestrations, gap junctions, and open endothelial junctions.[81] The clinical correlation of the ultrastructural anatomy is illustrated by the passage of CT and MRI scan contrast media into cerebral metastases and by laboratory studies that have demonstrated the presence of chemotherapeutic agents within resected and autopsy specimens of patients with metastatic and primary brain tumors. Clinical drug uptake studies in patients with primary and metastatic tumors[82] show variable biodistribution of drug (*e.g.*, cisplatin) to tumor and cerebrospinal fluid. Significant regional variation of drug concentration within tumor was also demonstrated, suggesting a variable degree of disruption of the normal cerebral vasculature. Other preliminary studies suggest that various chemotherapeutic agents (etoposide,[83] teniposide,[84] pentamethylmelamine,[85] 3-deazauridine,[86] AZQ,[87] MGBG,[88] vinblastine,[89] PALA,[90] ANCU,[91] and TCNU[92]) can reach sufficient concentrations in tumor tissue to be cytotoxic.

Tumor Response: Inherent and Acquired Chemoresistance

Apart from issues of drug delivery, there are two other factors that may prevent successful treatment of brain metastases with chemotherapy. First, the histologic types of primary malignancies that most frequently metastasize to brain are themselves chemoresistant. Almost half of all cases of brain metastases result from lung primaries, and the non-small cell histologic forms will predominate. Because only 20% to 40% of primary non-small cell lung cancer patients respond to current chemotherapy regimens,[93] the likelihood of response in the brain is also low. Although breast carcinoma, the second most common source of brain metastases, is relatively responsive to chemotherapy, 25% to 50% of patients will not respond.[94] The third, fourth, and fifth most common sources of brain metastases are gastrointestinal carcinomas, urinary (particularly renal) malignancies, and melanoma. Colorectal carcinoma, by far the most common gastrointestinal cancer, responds to current regimens in approximately 20% to 40% of cases.[95] Both renal cell carcinoma and melanoma are notably chemoresistant, usually responding to chemotherapy or immunotherapy in less than 20% of patients.[96–98] Given the limited success of chemotherapy for the primary malignancies that most commonly spread to the brain, one would expect limited success in treating brain metastases with chemotherapy.

Second, most patients (81%) develop brain metastases after diagnosis and treatment of the primary tumor.[46] Metastases that appear despite prior drug therapy are likely to be more resistant to subsequent chemotherapy. Relapse in the brain is most commonly part of widespread drug-resistant systemic relapse rather than an isolated phenomenon. The majority of patients with brain metastases die of systemic manifestations of disease rather than the brain metastases.[63]

SURGICAL MANAGEMENT OF CEREBRAL METASTASES

Perioperative Care

The most important prognostic factor influencing the results for patients subjected to surgery is the preoperative state.[6,38,45,46,48,99] Morbidity, 30-day mortality, and the postoperative neurologic functional level are directly related to the preoperative classification of patients[6]; maximal benefit is achieved for surgically treated patients when preoperative steps to optimize the general condition and neurologic performance are taken. Careful preoperative assessment of cardiopulmonary function and other potential medical problems (coagulopathy, abnormalities of electrolytes and water balance, malnutrition, infectious hazards) and management of vasogenic cerebral edema are necessary preludes to successful surgery. Measures to resist brain swelling in the perioperative period are begun before surgery (24–48 hours) and reduce the morbidity substantially (see Table 61–5). Stabilizing decompensated patients medically has superior results compared with emergent surgical decompression in unstable, post-herniated, or moribund patients.[38,100]

Surgical Indications, Goals, Benefits

Surgery, when appropriate, is generally employed to achieve an accurate diagnosis based on pathologic examination of tissue, to remove or reduce a mass lesion, or to relieve CSF

TABLE 61–6. Selection Criteria for Surgical Therapy of Brain Metastases*

Diagnostic uncertainty
Solitary metastasis
Life-threatening or critically located multiple metastases
Recurrent or persistent symptoms after nonsurgical therapy
Clinically resistant tumors
Treatment of metastatic complications—hemorrhagic, infectious, CSF obstruction
Placement of delivery devices for intrathecal access (Ommaya reservoir)

* Criteria are suggested guidelines rather than absolute indications; see text.

obstruction (Table 61–6). The indications for surgery are related to the therapeutic goals and are dependent on the clinical setting. Gross total removal of a metastasis is achieved in 80% or more of selected patients,[5,6,45] with this as a preoperative goal, and has superior benefit over subtotal removal or biopsy.[48,99,101–103]

Technical Aspects: Application of Microsurgical Technique

Consistent application of advanced surgical technique and use of available technical aids are not always routinely considered. Most metastases are sizable "macroscopic" lesions (≥ 3 cm) and have historically been resected without sophisticated techniques. Preservation of the normal brain and microcirculation adjacent to metastasis is routinely possible and should be the technical goal in all surgical patients.[25] Precise preoperative and intraoperative localization (CT, MRI, stereotaxis, ultrasound) allows accurately placed scalp, bone, and cortical incisions, and use of standard microsurgical techniques to preserve local microcirculation (*e.g.*, longitudinal rather than transverse gyral incisions)[6,25,104] minimizes morbidity from the surgical procedure. Gross total removal in selected patients with such techniques has superseded the era when regional surgical procedures with sacrifice of normal tissue (wide tumor margins, lobectomy) were required to control postoperative edema. Surgical biopsy for diagnosis (*e.g.*, precocious presentation) and clinical staging has achieved impressive levels of safety and diagnostic accuracy since the introduction of various image-guided stereotactic systems.[25]

CEREBRAL METASTASES: RESULTS OF THERAPY

Modern-era expectations for patients with cerebral metastatic disease have gradually translated into modest benefit for the majority of patients and guarded optimism for selected patients with favorable prognostic factors. Treatment modalities (surgery, radiation therapy) have changed only marginally, but advances in perioperative care, application of microsurgical technique, and highly accurate diagnostic imaging devices have had a significant impact on management. Relatively few definitive conclusions can be drawn as to the effectiveness of a particular treatment approach for cerebral metastases, despite the existing literature since 1960. With several notable exceptions,[36] these studies lack comparable matched treatment groups and differ in defining such variables as clinical–anatomic classification, response to therapy, quality of survival, relapse rates, morbidity, mortality, and cause of death (neurologic versus systemic disease). Despite these difficulties, several generalizations can be drawn from these clinical reports (Tables 61–7 and 61–8). The natural history of untreated cerebral metastases is one of progressive neurologic deterioration, with a median survival of 1 to 2 months.[5,41,63,105] Steroids sustain neurologic performance and extend median survival to 2.5 months,[106] and the use of radiation therapy further increases median survival to 3 to 6 months. Selected patients treated with surgery, radiation therapy, and steroids[36,38] have a median survival exceeding 6 months.

RADIATION THERAPY

Although the majority of patients (80%) treated with radiation therapy have an initial response, a surprisingly modest gain in survival ensues when they are compared with untreated and steroid groups. Morbidity and mortality (5%) during the course of radiation further reduce benefit, because 10% to 20% of patients fail to complete the prescribed course of therapy.[36,70,107] A strict interpretation of these reports (see Table 61–8) can be misleading, because this group tends to have unselected patients with poor prognostic factors and high mortality from uncontrolled systemic disease. Improvement in functional neurologic performance was noted in 50% to 60% of patients treated with whole-brain irradiation, and, not surprisingly, those patients with mild deficits had the greatest benefit. Sustained neurologic performance was relatively brief in those responders surviving to 6 months after therapy, illustrating a failure to control intracranial disease in a substantial proportion of patients treated.[70]

A favorable subgroup of patients irradiated for brain metastases has been identified by the Radiation Therapy Oncology Group (RTOG).[69] The favorable prognostic factors include: Karnofsky performance status of 70 to 100, an absent/controlled primary tumor, age <60 years, and metastatic spread limited to the brain. Patients with all four favorable factors had a 52% predicted probability of 6-month survival from the start of treatment. Patients with three of the four characteristics had a 33% to 40% probability of 6-month survival, and patients with none of the four had only an 8% chance of surviving 6 months. Fifty-three percent of patients were in a poor prognostic group with a median survival of 3.1 months. Radiation alone in this setting fails to permanently control intracranial disease in a substantial proportion of treated patients.

Two trials of radiation sensitizers have failed to demonstrate either improved local control or improved survival in patients with brain metastases undergoing cranial irradiation. The RTOG studied misonidazole and found no improvement over radiation therapy alone.[108] Lonidamine, an indazole carboxylic acid shown to be synergistic with radiotherapy in tissue culture and animal models, failed to improve response rate or survival.[109]

Because of the high frequency of uncontrolled tumor in the brain (50–70%), the issue of retreatment with irradiation will arise in many patients with brain metastases. The use of stereotactic radiosurgery in this role has been discussed above. Several reports[42,64,110,111] describe neurologic improvement in

TABLE 61–7. Treatment for Selected Combined Therapy* Series of Brain Metastases

Investigations	Collection Interval	Cases	Mortality (%)†	Survival Median‡	Survival 1-Year (%)
Stortebecker, 1954[39]	1922–1951	125	25	3.6	21
Richards and McKissock, 1963[103]	1946–1960	108	32	5.0	17
Lang and Slater, 1964[41]	1933–1963	208	22	4.0	20
Vieth and Odom, 1965[116]	1938–1962	155	15	6.0	13
Raskind et al, 1971[149]	1959–1968	51	12	6.0	30
Haar and Paterson, 1972[102]	1933–1968	167	11	6.0	22
Ransohoff, 1975[120]	1970–1973	100	10	6.0	28
Winston et al, 1980[45]	1967–1977	79	10	6.0	22
Gamache et al, 1980[46]	1968–1977	94	8.5	6.0	25
Galicich, 1981[104]	1977–1980	75	9	9.0	45
Takakura et al, 1982[5]	1960–1981	259	14§	9.1	26
Smalley et al, 1987[140]	1972–1982	85	—	13.5‖	59‖

* The majority of patients in combined therapy series were treated with surgery and postoperative radiation therapy.
† Reported as 30-day mortality, except Stortebeck (20 days), Vieth (14 days), and Raskind (14 days).
‡ Median survival is given in months.
§ All mortality occurred before 1976 (prior use of CT scanning for patient selection).
‖ Overall results: results of surgery plus adjuvant radiation therapy (34 patients) were superior to those of surgery alone (51 patients), 21 months versus 11.5 months median survival.

TABLE 61–8.   Treatment for Selected Radiation Therapy Series* of Brain Metastases

Investigations	Collection Interval	Cases	Mortality (%)	Survival Median (mo)	Survival Mean (mo)	Survival 1-Year (%)
Order et al, 1968[107]	1958–1966	108	—	3–6.0	6.3	9
Deeley and Edwards, 1968[147]	Not given	88	—	<6.0	—	14
Hindo et al, 1970[65]	Not given	54	—		5.6	9
Nisce et al, 1971[42]	Not given	560	—	6.0	—	16
Montana et al, 1972[121]	1966–1971	47	—	3.0	—	10
Young et al, 1974[73]	1967–1972	162	4.3	3.0	3.4	
Deutsch et al, 1974[66]	1962–1971	88	36†	3–6.0		10
Berry et al, 1974[67]	1964–1973	124	—	4		9
Hendrickson, 1977[68]	1971–1976	1001	—	5.8		15
Cairncross et al, 1980[63]	1977–1978	183	4.0	4.0		8
Kurtz et al, 1981[71]	1976–1979	309	4.0	4.5		—

* Majority of patients treated by radiation therapy only, except Order (26), Deeley (7), Nisce (376), Young (89), Deutsch (17), and Berry (29), where parentheses indicate total cases subjected to surgery before radiation.
† Includes patients unable to complete therapy.

patients retreated by external-beam irradiation, with an average remission of 4 months. Others are less sanguine about the prospects of retreatment,[72] citing a risk of radiation necrosis and only transient benefit, with a median survival after retreatment of only 8 weeks.[112] Selection of patients probably accounts for the difference in reported results of reirradiation. Cooper and colleagues selected patients for reirradiation who had remained in good general condition for at least 4 months after their initial course of radiation therapy and had then experienced neurologic deterioration from recurrent brain metastases.[113] Forty-two percent of treated patients experienced improvement in neurologic function, and the survival after retreatment averaged 5 months. The benefits of reirradiation appear modest, but it may be appropriate for selected patients who remain in good general condition for some months after initial irradiation and who have limited extracranial disease.

SURGERY

Surgery for cerebral metastases was generally regarded as a futile endeavor in the era before modern-day diagnostic and perioperative management methods.[114,115] As morbidity and mortality declined for neurosurgical procedures, it became evident that meaningful benefit and prolongation of survival were possible for selected patients.[10,39,41,103,116–119]

Over the last 30 years, clinical investigators have established the efficacy of various treatment approaches and clarified the role of surgery for this group of patients. The principal surgical gains during this period have been dramatic reductions in operative morbidity and mortality, largely by improved selection of patients and advances in tumor localization, neuroanesthesia, surgical technique, and perioperative care. The overall 30-day mortality associated with surgery for cerebral metastasis has fallen tenfold during this period from approximately 30%[103] to 3%,[5,6,36,46] with similar progress in associated morbidity.

A small, uncontrolled group of patients subjected to surgery alone for metastases, as well as surgery combined with radiation therapy, gradually led clinical investigators to a general recognition that surgical therapy, when indicated, had a modest advantage over irradiation alone, particularly with respect to long-term survival.[5,9,38,46,100,107,120–122]

CHEMOTHERAPY TRIALS IN CEREBRAL METASTASES: PRELIMINARY RESULTS

Despite obstacles to successful treatment of brain metastases with chemotherapy, there are several reports of favorable results.[123–130] As one might expect, combination regimens effective for diffuse systemic metastases yield the greatest benefit for patients harboring chemosensitive tumors or malignancies with brain metastases present at the time of diagnosis of the primary disease. Small cell carcinomas of the lung are particularly responsive to combination chemotherapy,[123–125] with response rates of 64% to 78% in patients with metastatic disease to the brain and extracerebral sites. These reported response rates in the brain and periphery are quite similar to the expected response rates for first-line and salvage-treatment regimens for small cell lung carcinoma in general.[131] Notable successes have also been achieved in germ cell tumors[126] and gestational choriocarcinoma.[127]

Each of the studies involving very chemosensitive malignancies, such as small cell lung carcinoma, germ cell tumors, and gestational choriocarcinoma, reported favorable outcome when the patients were treated at presentation with agents known to be effective against the primary tumor. Salvage chemotherapy, on the other hand, was much less effective. Studies reporting results of chemotherapy for less chemosensitive tumors follow a similar pattern.

Breast carcinoma is considered to be relatively chemosensitive, with approximately 50% to 75% of patients with metastatic breast carcinoma expected to respond to first-line combination chemotherapy regimens. Rosner and colleagues reported the results of treating 100 breast cancer patients with brain metastases who had received no prior chemotherapy.[128] Although the results have not been confirmed by other investigators, there were 10 complete and 40 partial responders (N = 100), the best responses (52%) occurring in the group treated with cyclophosphamide, fluorouracil, and prednisone (CFP). All but 6 of the 100 patients treated with first-line chemotherapy received prednisone as part of the regimen, and the degree to which corticosteroid use affected interpretation of response is unknown. Recently, Cocconi and colleagues reported an overall response rate of 55% (5 complete and 7 partial responses) in 22 consecutive patients with brain metastases from breast carcinoma treated with etoposide and cisplatin.[129] Responses in the brain paralleled responses of systemic metastases, and all responses occurred while patients remained on stable or decreased corticosteroid doses.

Results of chemotherapy for brain metastases in less chemosensitive tumors are difficult to assess. Most reports include a few cases of various histologic types of malignancies treated with a single type of chemotherapy in previously treated patients.[130,132–139] The majority of patients had non-small cell lung or breast carcinomas, and responses were infrequent in those malignancies known to be chemoresistant. Jacquillat and colleagues, in a large phase II trial of fotemustine (an investigational nitrosourea) for patients with disseminated melanoma and no prior therapy, demonstrated parallel response rates in brain compared with other organs (cerebral metastatic response, 25%; visceral metastatic response, 19.2%).[130]

Based on the limited information currently available in the literature, chemotherapy can effect regression of brain metastases if regimens known to be effective in the treatment of chemosensitive malignancies are used before the development of widespread drug-resistant disease. Significant neurologic deterioration during chemotherapy and before radiotherapy has not been reported under these circumstances. Studies comparing cranial irradiation with chemotherapy alone or chemotherapy followed by radiation therapy have not been performed. It would appear that such studies could be performed safely in chemosensitive tumors. The contribution of chemotherapy toward reducing morbidity and prolonging survival in patients with brain metastases remains to be defined.

COMBINED THERAPY

The decline of morbidity associated with surgery and the relatively high rate of uncontrolled cerebral deposits after radiation therapy alone form the basis for a combined treatment approach in suitable patients. Retrospective studies[45,99,101,140,141] have strongly supported a combined approach, and a recent randomized study[36] lends further support.

As alluded to previously, comparison of nonrandomized studies lacking comparable treatment groups has long been recognized[9,38,63] to be of limited value; fortunately, preliminary results of controlled trials[36,142–144] are becoming available to supplement the existing literature regarding the respective roles of surgery, radiation therapy, and chemotherapy. Careful evaluation of selected clinical studies (see Tables 61–7 and 61–8) and newly available randomized trials provides some reliable conclusions regarding the expected results of therapy for brain metastases.

The Patchell study consisted of patients with a single metastasis randomly assigned to a surgical group (treated by surgical removal and postoperative radiation therapy) and a radiation group (treated with diagnostic biopsy and radiation therapy).[36] The study group included 48 adult patients with Karnofsky performance status ≥70 and excluded patients with tumors that were highly radiosensitive (small cell lung cancer, germ cell tumors, lymphoma, myeloma). All patients on study were biopsied before randomization. Six patients (11% of total) with solitary brain lesions and a prior cancer diagnosis were in fact noted on biopsy *not* to have a metastatic lesion (and were excluded from the study). The six nonmetastatic lesions included two glioblastomas, one low-grade astrocytoma, two abscesses, and one nonspecific inflammatory reaction, emphasizing the importance of biopsy in this setting.

Survival was longer in the surgery group (median, 40 weeks) compared with the radiation group (median, 15 weeks), and recurrence at the site of the original metastasis was less frequent (Fig. 61–4) in the surgery group (20%) compared with the radiation group (52%). Patients treated with surgery remained functionally independent longer (median, 38 weeks) compared with the radiation group (median, 8 weeks). Only surgical treatment and the absence of other systemic metastases were associated with a decreased risk of recurrence of the original brain metastasis. Fifty percent of radiation patients died from neurologic causes, compared with 29% of surgery patients, although this was not significant. Operative mortality was 4% and morbidity 8%, which was similar to the 30-day mortality and morbidity rates of 4% and 17% in the radiation group. Multivariate analysis showed that surgical treatment was associated with longer survival in patients with a long interval between the primary diagnosis and the development of the brain metastasis. The presence of disseminated cancer and older age were associated with declining survival. Nevertheless, survival was still less than 10% in both the surgery and radiation groups by 90 weeks after treatment, underlining the guarded prognosis in these patients, even with aggressive treatment.

Several retrospective studies have examined the role of postoperative radiation after surgical resection of solitary brain metastatic lesions. All but one demonstrate improved control of intracranial disease with the combination of surgery and radiation therapy compared with surgery alone. In the one negative study, Dosoretz and colleagues found no significant difference in survival or local recurrence rate in the brain when comparing patients receiving adjuvant whole-brain irradiation with those patients who were observed (no radiation) after complete resection of tumor.[145] A larger retrospective review (85 patients, 1972–1982) of a similar patient group rendered clinically disease-free by the resection of a solitary cerebral metastasis demonstrated a significant reduction of brain relapse in the 34 patients who received adjuvant whole-brain radiotherapy compared with the surgery-only group (21% versus 85%, respectively).[140] The median survival in the group receiving adjuvant radiotherapy (21 months) exceeded that of the surgery-only group (11.5 months). Those patients who received adjuvant radiation doses ≥39 Gy had an 11% rate of subsequent brain failure, as contrasted with a 31% relapse rate seen in patients receiving <39 Gy, suggesting that higher doses may be appropriate for these prognostically favored patients with solitary brain metastases and no other clinical evidence of systemic disease.

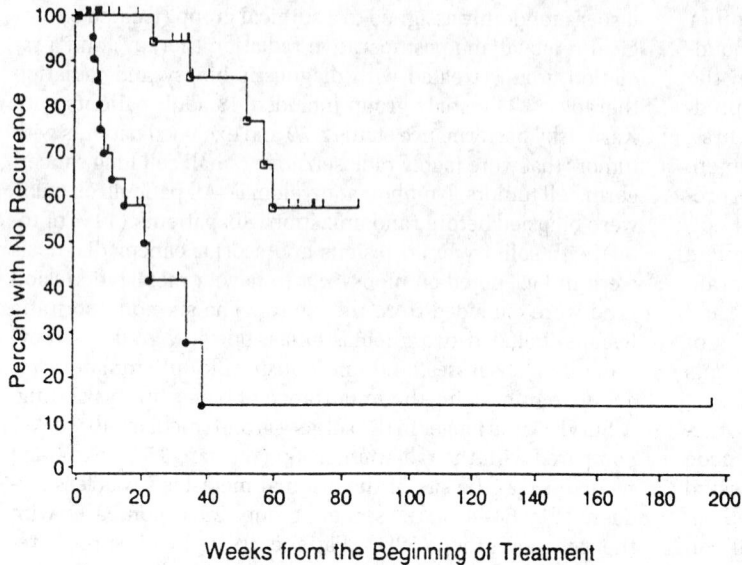

FIGURE 61–4. Length of time to local recurrence by treatment group. Open circles represent patients treated with surgery and postoperative radiation. Solid circles represent patients treated with diagnostic biopsy and radiation alone. Median time to recurrence was longer than 59 weeks (surgery) versus 21 weeks (radiation). Recurrence was defined as the reappearance of a metastasis at the same site as the initial cerebral deposit. (Patchell RA, Tibbs PA, Walsh JW, et al. A randomized trial of surgery in the treatment of single metastases to the brain. N Engl J Med 1990;322:494–500)

DeAngelis and associates found that postoperative whole-brain irradiation after resection of a solitary brain metastasis significantly prolonged the time to neurologic relapse, with a 1-year recurrence rate of 22% in the irradiated group and 46% in the surgery-alone patients.[109] Radiation appeared to decrease the likelihood of recurrence at the site of the resected metastasis but did not seem to affect the relapse rate elsewhere in the brain. The median survival in the irradiated group was 20.6 months compared with 14.4 months in the surgery-alone group, but this was not statistically significant. Eleven percent of the irradiated patients developed severe radiation-induced neurologic toxicity, with dementia, ataxia, and urinary incontinence. This was seen only with large-fraction (4–6 Gy), short-course radiation programs.

Hagen and colleagues reported a reduction in death from neurologic causes and a longer interval to CNS relapse in patients receiving postoperative whole-brain irradiation after resection of a single brain metastasis from melanoma.[146] Eighty-five percent of the surgery-only group died of neurologic causes, whereas 24% of the surgery-plus-radiation therapy patients died of neurologic causes. Neurologic relapse also occurred earlier in the operative group, but overall survival was no different, because patients in the combined group would continue to die from uncontrolled systemic disease.

In spite of the encouraging results with a combined therapeutic approach, the majority (≥60%) of patients are unsuited for surgery and undergo irradiation (with or without steroids) as the primary treatment for intracranial metastatic disease. This direction in patient management is influenced by the clinical profile of the patients with brain metastases. Although approximately 50% of patients harbor solitary brain metastases,[8] nearly one half of this group with solitary deposits will not be candidates for operation because of widespread systemic disease, major neurologic dysfunction, poor performance status, or other factors.[36] In addition, the lack of effective systemic therapy for many malignancies limits an aggressive surgical and radiotherapeutic approach for those patients with the combination of brain metastases and uncontrolled systemic disease.

PROGNOSTIC FACTORS: EXTENDED SURVIVAL IN BRAIN METASTASES

The *preoperative neurologic condition* and *extent of systemic disease* are the two most important prognostic factors influencing the short-term results for combined treatment (surgery, radiation therapy, and steroids) and also correlate with the long-term survival. Figures 61–5 and 61–6 reflect the influence of these two prognostic variables in the results for combined therapy. Patient age and the interval from the detection of a primary tumor to the development of a symptomatic metastasis also have a strong correlation with survival.

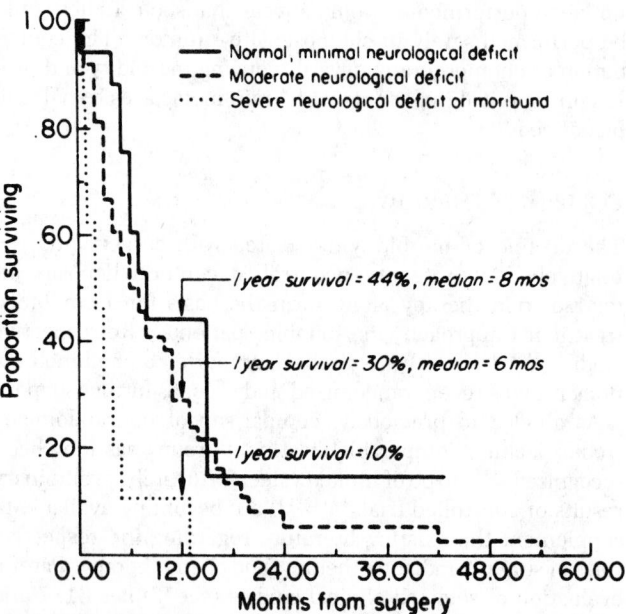

FIGURE 61–5. Survival curve for patients treated with surgery and irradiation according to preoperative patient status. (Galicich JG, Sundaresan N, Arbit E, et al. Surgical treatment of single brain metastasis: Factors associated with survival. Cancer 1980;45:381–386)

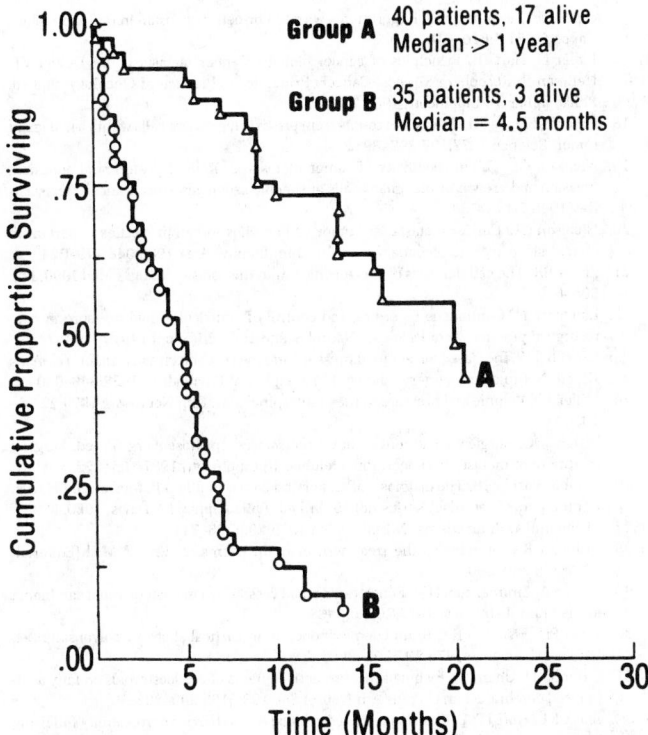

FIGURE 61–6. Survival plot according to extent of disease. Group A represents patients without evidence of extra-CNS disease. Group B had evidence of disseminated disease outside the CNS. All patients were treated with surgery and irradiation. CNS, central nervous system. (Galicich JH, Sundaresan N. Metastatic brain tumors. In: Wilkins RH, Rengachary SS, eds. Neurosurgery New York: McGraw-Hill, 1985:597–610)

Extended survival (greater than 2 years)[5,10,41,45,63,99,102,118,122,140,147,148] is an occasional feature of clinical reports, and the majority of long survivors have been subjected to various forms of combined therapy (surgery, radiation therapy, steroids, chemotherapy), although numerous anecdotal reports document long survival with surgery as the only therapy.[41,45,116,140,145,149] The more indolent tumors constitute the largest group of extended survivors (*e.g.*, breast carcinoma has a 38% 2-year survival rate). Long-term survival (≥5 years), however, is not exclusively restricted to patients with less malignant tumors. A precocious presentation with an occult systemic primary tumor and no evidence of extraneural metastases is associated with long survivals in a fraction of patients.[45,99] Definitive identification of prognostic factors for extended survival beyond 3 to 5 years is not currently possible, but subjecting patients with favorable clinical profiles to aggressive combined therapy may provide further insight to this occasional phenomenon.

RELATIVE INDICATIONS
FOR SURGICAL INTERVENTION

Surgical indications (see Table 61–6) have been previously discussed, and these general guidelines serve for most clinical settings, with only occasional exceptions. Emergent situations sometimes arise where rapid neurologic compromise has occurred because of progressive tumor growth in patients in whom maximal medical therapy has failed or metastatic complications (*e.g.*, hemorrhage, abscess formation, CSF obstruction) arise. In such situations, urgent surgical intervention is only occasionally appropriate for patients in poor neurologic condition and multiple medical problems arising from uncontrolled or widespread systemic metastases. Such patients are best managed with aggressive neurologic and medical resuscitation measures when appropriate, and they should be subjected to surgery only when they are stabilized and their preoperative state improves.[6] Metastatic complications should be promptly treated as if metastases were a secondary problem, unless severe risks attend a surgical approach. Dramatic benefit can be realized from correction of CSF obstruction (external/internal shunting) or drainage of hemorrhagic and infectious (abscess) complications.

Patients with multiple metastases who progressively deteriorate (neurologically) despite the best available nonsurgical therapy, or after completion of medical therapy, represent an unsolved problem in the management of metastases. If favorable prognostic factors are present (*e.g.*, good neurologic status, minimal or controlled extra-CNS disease), surgery may represent the only treatment option. Surgery is generally not indicated for multiple metastases or leptomeningeal spread, other than diagnostic biopsy, because mortality is significantly increased. Critically located deposits (*e.g.*, posterior fossa mass obstructing CSF pathways) are occasionally appropriate for resection despite the increased risk if other (supratentorial) deposits are small or clinically silent.

Lastly, surgical resection of dominant hemispheric masses in critically functional brain areas is not necessarily associated with increased morbidity.[6,48] The preoperative neurologic performance largely determines the risk in these patients; if careful microtechnique with precise localization and intraoperative monitoring is used, the discrete nature of most metastases allows gross total removal with minimal morbidity in such locations.

CEREBRAL METASTASES: SUMMARY

The potentially severe consequences of brain involvement by cancer is a common problem confronting the oncologic specialties. Symptomatic parenchymal lesions are projected to afflict 152,600 patients in the United States annually, with lung, breast, gastrointestinal, renal, and melanoma contributing the majority of lesions coming to clinical attention. Timely, effective therapy for brain metastases can restore neurologic function or prevent the neurologic complications of cancer for the duration of survival. Limiting the disability of metastases is difficult, and available therapy is not fully effective.

Since the previous edition of this text, important contributions have been made in regard to the role of surgery in selected patients,[36] advances in radiation techniques,[69,75,79,109] and preliminary results of chemotherapy trials.[144,150] The surgery plus radiation group reported by Patchell and colleagues had advantages over radiation alone in neurologic relapse, length and quality of survival, and deaths by neurologic cause (uncontrolled brain metastases).[36] The optimal radiation time-dose regimen has been further developed, and progress in more effective control (combination chemotherapy) of both systemic and metastatic sites has been noted.

Rational selection of the appropriate therapy for patients with brain metastases requires accurate diagnosis, localization, and determination of prognostic criteria. The major prognostic variables for this group are the pretreatment neurologic state, the metastatic interval, and the extent of systemic disease.

Surgery combined with adjuvant radiation therapy for selected patients achieves the best results in therapy of resistant malignancies of the lung, kidney, thyroid, colon, and skin, as well as many soft tissue sarcomas. The indications for surgery are well established; the most suitable surgical patients have a single lesion with minimal neurologic impairment, limited extra-CNS disease, a prolonged antecedent (metachronous) tumor history before cerebral metastasis, or a precocious presentation with occult systemic disease. The risks of surgery are generally determined by the preoperative state and the extent of systemic disease. Superior results are realized when the dual goals of total gross resection and minimal brain injury are achieved. Surgery for brain metastases is applicable to only 10% to 30% of patients, with the use of conservative selection criteria; the majority have unfavorable neurologic impairment, uncontrolled systemic tumor, and other factors increasing the risk and reducing the potential benefit of a combined approach.

Patients with prohibitive risk factors should have maximal medical management including radiation therapy delivered with one of the shorter treatment programs. Consideration of the novel radiation therapy approaches recently described[75,79] may be warranted, but experience in the use of these approaches is limited. Chemotherapy, particularly for sensitive tumors without prior drug therapy, offers increasing efficacy and safety.

A multidisciplinary approach in this patient population is mandatory, with cooperating specialists fully cognizant of the limitations of their respective therapeutic measures.

REFERENCES

1. Posner JB. Brain metastases: A clinician's view. In: Weiss L, Gilbert HA, Posner JB, eds. Brain metastases. Boston: GK Hall, 1980:2–29
2. Boring CC, Squires TS, Tong T. Cancer statistics, 1992. CA 1992;42:19–38.
3. Walker AE, Robins M, Weinfeld FD. Epidemiology of brain tumors: The national survey of intracranial neoplasms. Neurology 1985;35:219–226.
4. Hildebrand J. Lesions of the nervous system in cancer patients. Monograph series of the European Organization for Research on Treatment of Cancer. Vol 5. New York: Raven Press, 1978.
5. Takakura K, Sano K, Hoho S, et al. Metastatic tumors of the central nervous system. Tokyo: Igaku-Shoin, 1982.
6. Galicich JH, Sundaresan N. Metastatic brain tumors. In: Wilkins RH, Rengachary SS, eds. Neurosurgery. New York: McGraw-Hill, 1985:597–610.
7. Rubin R, Green J. Solitary metastases. Springfield, IL: Charles C Thomas, 1968.
8. Posner JB, Chernik NL. Intracranial metastases from systemic cancer. Adv Neurol 1978;19:575–587.
9. Posner JB. Diagnosis and treatment of metastases to the brain. Clin Bull 1974;4:47–57.
10. Simionescu MD. Metastatic tumors of the brain. A follow-up study of 195 patients with neurosurgical considerations. J Neurosurg 1960;17:361–373.
11. Liotta LA, Kohn E. Cancer invasion and metastasis. JAMA 1990;263:1123–1126.
12. Katz DA, Liotta LA. Tumor invasion and metastasis in the central nervous system. In: Zimmerman HM, ed. Progress in neuropathology. Vol 6. New York: Raven Press, 1986:119–131.
13. Delattre JY, Krol G, Thaler HT, Posner JB. Distribution of brain metastases. Arch Neurol 1988;45:741–744.
14. Weiss L. Metastatic brain tumors. Factors that govern the metastatic process. In: Wilkins RH, Rengachary SS, eds. Neurosurgery. New York: McGraw-Hill, 1985:591–596.
15. Warren BA. Arrest and extravasation of cancer cells with special reference to brain metastases and the microinjury hypothesis. In: Weiss L, Gilbert HA, Posner JB, eds. Brain metastases. Boston: GK Hall, 1980:81–99.
16. Coman D, DeLong R. The role of the vertebral venous system in the metastasis of cancer to the spinal cord: Experiments with tumor-cell suspension in rats and rabbits. Cancer 1951;4:610–618.
17. Fidler IJ, Hart IR. Principles of cancer biology: Cancer metastasis. In: DeVita VT, Hellman S, Rosenberg SA, eds. Cancer. Principles & Practice of Oncology. 2nd ed. Philadelphia: JB Lippincott, 1985:113–124.
18. Fidler IJ, Kripke ML. Metastasis results from pre-existing variant cells within a malignant tumor. Science 1977;197:893–895.
19. Nicolson GL. Organ specificity of tumor metastasis: Role of preferential adhesion, invasion and growth of malignant cells at specific secondary sites. Cancer Metastasis Rev 1988;7:143–188.
20. Nicolson GL. Cancer metastasis: Tumor cell and host organ properties important in metastasis to specific secondary sites. Biochim Biophys Acta 1988;948:175–224.
21. Zetter BR. The cellular basis of site-specific tumor metastasis. N Engl J Med 1990;322:605–612.
22. Lundberg N. Continuous recording and control of ventricular fluid pressure in neurosurgical practice. Acta Psychiatr Neurol Scand 1960;36(Suppl 149):1–193.
23. Langfitt TW. Increased intracranial pressure and the cerebral circulation. In: Youmans JR, ed. Neurological surgery. 2nd ed. Philadelphia: WB Saunders, 1982:846–930.
24. Miller JD. Volume and pressure in the craniospinal axis. Clin Neurosurg 1975;22:76–105.
25. Wright DC. Surgical treatment of brain metastases. In: Rosenberg SA, ed. Surgical treatment of metastatic cancer. Philadelphia: JB Lippincott, 1987:165–222.
26. Plum F, Posner JB. The diagnosis of stupor and coma. In: Plum F, McDowell FH, eds. Contemporary neurology series no. 19. 3rd ed. Philadelphia: FA Davis, 1980.
27. Fishman RA. Brain edema. N Engl J Med 1975;293:706–711.
28. Fishman RA. Steroids in the treatment of brain edema. N Engl J Med [Editorial] 1982;306:359–360.
29. Hirano A, Zimmerman HM. Fenestrated blood vessels in a metastatic renal carcinoma in the brain. Lab Invest 1972;26:465–468.
30. Chan PH, Fishman RA. Brain edema: Induction in cortical slices by polyunsaturated fatty acids. Science 1978;201:358–360.
31. Caronna JJ, Chan PH, Fishman RA. Protective effects of corticosteroids on fatty acid-induced cerebral edema. Trans Am Neurol Soc 1980;105:200–202.
32. Black KL, Hoff JT. Leukotrienes increase blood–brain barrier permeability following intraparenchymal injections in rats. Ann Neurol 1985;18:349–351.
33. Senger DR, Galli SJ, Dvorak AM, et al. Tumor cells secrete a vascular permeability factor that promotes accumulation of ascites fluid. Science 1983;219:983–985.
34. Blasberg RG, Gazendam J, Patlak CS, Fenstermacher JD. Quantitative autoradiographic studies of brain edema and a comparison of multi-isotope autoradiographic techniques. Adv Neurol 1980;28:255–270.
35. Raskind R, Weiss SR. Conditions simulating metastatic lesions of the brain. Report of eight cases. Int Surg 1970;43:40–42.
36. Patchell RA, Tibbs RP, Walsh JW, et al. A randomized trial of surgery in the treatment of single metastases to the brain. N Engl J Med 1990;322:494–500.
37. Posner JB. Clinical manifestations of brain metastasis. In: Weiss LGH, Posner JB, eds. Brain metastasis. Boston: GK Hall, 1980:189–207.
38. Gamache FW Jr, Posner JB, Patterson RH. Metastatic brain tumors. In: Youmans JR, ed. Neurological surgery. 2nd ed. Vol 4. Philadelphia: WB Saunders, 1982:2872–2898.
39. Stortebecker TP. Metastatic tumors of the brain from a neurosurgical point of view: A follow-up study of 158 cases. J Neurosurg 1954;11:84–111.
40. Paillas JE, Pellet W. Brain metastases. In: Vinken PJ, Bruyn GW, eds. Handbook of clinical neurology. Vol 18. Amsterdam: North-Holland Publishing Co., 1975:201–232.
41. Lang EF Jr, Slater J. Metastatic brain tumors. Results of surgical and non-surgical treatment. Surg Clin North Am 1964;44:865–872.
42. Nisce IZ, Hilaris BS, Chu FCH. A review of experience with irradiation of brain metastasis. AJR 1971;111:329–333.
43. Strub RL, Black RW. The mental status examination in neurology. Philadelphia: FA Davis, 1977.
44. Hayward RD. Secondary malignant melanoma of the brain. Clin Oncol 1976;2:227–232.
45. Winston KR, Walsh JW, Fischer EG. Results of operative treatment of intracranial metastatic tumors. Cancer 1980;45:2639–2645.
46. Gamache FW Jr, Posner JB, Galicich JH. Treatment of brain metastases by surgical extirpation. In: Weiss L, Gilbert H, Posner JB, eds. Brain metastases. Boston: GK Hall, 1980:390–414.
47. Karnofsky DA, Burchenol JH. The clinical evaluation of chemotherapeutic agents in cancer. In: McLeod CN, ed. Evaluation of chemotherapeutic agents. New York: Columbia University Press, 1949:191–205.
48. Galicich JH, Sundaresan N, Arbit E, Pase A. Surgical treatment of single brain metastasis: Factors associated with survival. Cancer 1980;45:381–386.
49. Sze G, Milano E, Johnson C, Heier L. Detection of brain metastases: Comparison of contrast-enhanced MR with unenhanced MR and enhanced CT. Am J Neuroradiol 1990;11:785–791.
50. Gado MH, Phelps ME, Coleman RE. An extravascular component of contrast enhancement in cranial computed tomography (parts I and II). Radiology 1975;117:589–597.
51. Takeda N, Tanaka R, Nakai O. Dynamics of contrast enhancement in delayed computed tomography of brain tumors: Tissue-blood ratio and differential diagnosis. Radiology 1982;142:663–668.
52. Cohen N, Strauss G, Lew R, Silver D, Recht L. Should prophylactic anticonvulsants be administered to patients with newly-diagnosed cerebral metastases: A retrospective analysis. J Clin Oncol 1988;6:1621–1624.
53. Galicich JH, French LA, Ueki K, Melby JC. Use of dexamethasone in the treatment of cerebral edema associated with brain tumors. Lancet 1961;81:46–53.

54. French LA. The use of steroids in the treatment of cerebral edema. Bull NY Acad Med 1966;42:301–311.

55. Renaudin J, Fewer D, Wilson CB, et al. Dose dependency of Decadron in patients with partially excised brain tumors. J Neurosurg 1973;39:302–305.

56. Gutin PH. Corticosteroid therapy in patients with cerebral tumor: Benefits, mechanisms, problems, practicalities. Semin Oncol 1975;2:49–56.

57. Ransohoff J. The effects of steroids on brain edema in man. In: Reulen HJ, Schurmann K, eds. Steroids and brain edema. Berlin: Springer-Verlag, 1972:211–221.

58. Ehrenkranz JRL, Posner JB. Adrenocorticosteroid hormones. In: Weiss L, Gilbert H, Posner JB, eds. Brain metastasis. Boston: GK Hall, 1980:340–363.

59. Samuels MA, ed. Manual of neurologic therapeutics: With essentials of diagnosis. 3rd ed. Boston: Little, Brown and Co., 1986:1–424.

60. Fenstermacher JD. Volume regulation of the central nervous system. In: Staub NC, Taylor AE, eds. Edema. New York: Raven Press, 1984:383–404.

61. Weiss HD. Neoplasms. In: Samuels MA, ed. Manual of neurologic therapeutics: With essentials of diagnosis. 3rd ed. Boston: Little, Brown and Co., 1986.

62. Quest DO. Increased intracranial pressure, brain herniation, and their control. In: Wilkins RH, Rengachary SS, eds. Neurosurgery. New York: McGraw-Hill, 1985:332–342.

63. Cairncross JG, Kim J-H, Posner JB. Radiation therapy for brain metastases. Ann Neurol 1980;7:529–541.

64. Chu FCH, Hilaris BB. Value of radiation therapy in the management of intracranial metastasis. Cancer 1961;14:577–581.

65. Hindo WA, DeTrana FA, Lee MS, et al. Large dose increment irradiation in treatment of cerebral metastases. Cancer 1970;26:138–141.

66. Deutsch M, Parsons JA, Mercado R Jr. Radiotherapy for intracranial metastases. Cancer 1974;34:1607.

67. Berry HC, Parke RG, Gerdes AJ. Irradiation of brain metastases. Acta Radiol Ther 1974;13:535–544.

68. Hendrickson FR. The optimum schedule for palliative radiotherapy for metastatic brain cancer. Int J Radiat Oncol Biol Phys 1977;2:165–168.

69. Diener-West M, Dobbins TW, Phillips TL, Nelson DF. Identification of an optimal subgroup for treatment evaluation of patients with brain metastases using RTOG study 7916. Int J Radiat Oncol Biol Phys 1991;16:669–673.

70. Borgelt B, Gelber R, Kramer S, et al. The palliation of brain metastases: Final results of the first two studies by the Radiation Therapy Oncology Group. Int J Radiat Oncol Biol Phys 1980;6:1–9.

71. Kurtz JM, Gelber R, Brady LW, et al. The palliation of brain metastases in a favorable patient population: A randomized clinical trial by the Radiation Therapy Oncology Group. Int J Radiat Oncol Biol Phys 1981;7:891–895.

72. Harwood AR, Simpson WF. Radiation therapy of cerebral metastases. A randomized prospective clinical trial. Int J Radiat Oncol Biol Phys 1977;2:1091–1094.

73. Young DF, Posner JB, Chu FCH, et al. Rapid-course radiation therapy of cerebral metastases: Results and complications. Cancer 1974;34:1069–1076.

74. Gutin PH, Phillips TL, Hosobuchi Y, et al. Permanent and removable implants for the brachytherapy of brain tumors. Int J Radiat Oncol Biol Phys 1981;7:1371–1381.

75. Prados M, Leibel S, Barnett CM, Gutin PH. Interstitial brachytherapy for metastatic brain tumors. Cancer 1989;63:657–660.

76. Heros DO, Kasdon DL, Chun M. Brachytherapy in the treatment of recurrent solitary brain metastases. Neurosurgery 1988;23:733–737.

77. Sturm V, Kober B, Hover KH, et al. Stereotactic percutaneous single dose irradiation of brain metastases with a linear accelerator. Int J Radiat Oncol Biol Phys 1987;13:279–282.

78. Loeffler JS, Kooy HM, Wen PY, et al. The treatment of recurrent brain metastases with stereotactic radiosurgery. J Clin Oncol 1990;8:576–582.

79. Coffey RJ, Flickinger JC, Bissonette DJ, Lunsford LD. Radiosurgery for solitary brain metastases using the cobalt-60 gamma unit: Methods and results in 24 patients. Int J Radiat Oncol Biol Phys 1991;20:1287–1295.

80. Nedzi LA, Kooy H, Alexander E III, et al. Variables associated with the development of complications from radiosurgery of intracranial tumors. Int J Radiat Oncol Biol Phys 1991;21:591–599.

81. Long DM. Capillary ultrastructure in human metastatic brain tumours. J Neurosurg 1979;51:53–58.

82. Stewart DJ, Leavens M, Maor M, et al. Human central nervous system distribution of cis-diamminedichloroplatinum and use as a radiosensitizer in malignant brain tumors. Cancer Res 1982;42:2472–2479.

83. Stewart DJ, Richard MR, Hugenholtz H, et al. Penetration of VP-16 (etoposide) into human intracerebral and extracerebral tumors. J Neurooncol 1984;2:133–139.

84. Stewart DJ, Richard MR, Hugenholtz H, et al. Penetration of teniposide (VM-26) into human intracerebral tumors. J Neurooncol 1984;2:315–324.

85. Stewart DJ, Benvenuto JA, Leavens M, et al. Human central nervous system pharmacology of pentamethylmelamine and its metabolites. J Neurooncol 1983;1:357–364.

86. Stewart DJ, Benvenuto J, Leavens M, et al. Penetration of 3-deazauridine in human brain, intracerebral tumor, and cerebrospinal fluid. Cancer Res 1979;39:4119–4122.

87. Savaraj N, Lu K, Feun LF, et al. Intracerebral penetration and tissue distribution of 2,5-diaziridinyl 3,6-bis (carboethoxyamino) 1,4-benzoquinone, (9AZQ NSC 182986). J Neurooncol 1983;1:15–20.

88. Rosenblum M, Stewart DJ, Yap BS, et al. Penetration of methylglyoxal bis-(guanylhydrazone) into intracerebral tumor in humans. Cancer Res 1981;41:459–462.

89. Stewart DJ, Lu K, Benjamin RS, et al. Concentrations of vinblastine in human intracerebral tumor and other tissues. J Neurooncol 1983;1:139–144.

90. Stewart DJ, Leavens M, Friedman J, et al. Penetration of N-(phosphyonacetyl)-L-aspartate into human central nervous system and intracerebral tumor. Cancer Res 1980;40:3163–3166.

91. Hori T, Muraoka K, Yoshikazu S, et al. Influence of modes of ACNU administration on tissue and blood drug concentration in malignant brain tumors. J Neurosurg 1987;66:372–378.

92. Whittle IR, MacPherson JS, Miller JD, et al. The disposition of TCNU (tauromustine) in human malignant glioma: Pharmacokinetic studies and clinical implications. J Neurosurg 1990;72:721–725.

93. Mulshine J, Ruckdeschel JC. The role of chemotherapy in the management of disseminated non-small cell lung cancer. In: Roth J, Ruckdeschel J, Weisenburger T, eds. Thoracic oncology. Philadelphia: WB Saunders, 1989:220–228.

94. Henderson IC. Chemotherapy of breast cancer. A general overview. Cancer 1983;51:2553–2559.

95. Poon MA, O'Connell MJ, Moertel CG, et al. Biochemical modulation of fluorouracil: Evidence of significant improvement of survival and quality of life in patients with advanced colorectal carcinoma. J Clin Oncol 1989;7:1407–1417.

96. Creagan ET. Regional and systemic strategies for metastatic malignant melanoma. Mayo Clin Proc 1989;64:852–860.

97. Harris DT. Hormonal therapy and chemotherapy for renal cell carcinoma. Semin Oncol 1983;10:422–430.

98. Muss HB. The role of biological response modifiers in metastatic renal cell carcinoma. Semin Oncol 1988;15(Suppl 5):30–34.

99. Ransohoff J. Surgical therapy of brain metastases. In: Weiss L, Gilbert HA, Posner JB, eds. Brain metastases. Boston: GK Hall, 1980:380–389.

100. Posner JB. Management of central nervous system metastases. Semin Oncol 1977;4:81–91.

101. Galicich JH, Sundaresan N, Thaler HT. Surgical treatment of single brain metastasis: Evaluation of results by computerized tomography scanning. J Neurosurg 1980;53:63–67.

102. Haar F, Paterson R Jr. Surgery for metastatic intracranial neoplasm. Cancer 1972;30:1241–1245.

103. Richards P, McKissock W. Intracranial metastases. Br Med J 1963;1:15–18.

104. Galicich JH. Surgery of malignant brain tumors. In: Vick NA, ed. Seminars in neurology. Vol 1. New York: Thieme-Stratton, 1981:159–168.

105. Posner JB. Neurological complications of systemic cancer. Med Clin North Am 1971;55:625–646.

106. Horton J, Baxter DD, Olson DB, et al. The management of metastases to the brain by irradiation and corticosteroids. AJR 1971;111:334–336.

107. Order SE, Hellman S, Von Essen CF, et al. Improvement in quality of survival following whole-brain irradiation for whole brain metastasis. Radiology 1968;91:149–153.

108. Kamarnicky LT, Phillips TL, Martz K, et al. A randomized phase III protocol for the evaluation of misonidazole combined with radiation in the treatment of patients with brain metastases (RTOG-7916). Int J Radiat Oncol Biol Phys 1991;20:53–58.

109. DeAngelis LM, Mandell LR, Thaler HT, et al. The role of postoperative radiotherapy after resection of single brain metastases. Neurosurgery 1989;24:798–805.

110. Shehata WM, Hendrickson FR, Hindo WA. Rapid fractionation technique and retreatment of cerebral metastases by irradiation. Cancer 1974;34:257–261.

111. Kurup P, Reddy S, Hendrickson FR. Results of re-irradiation for cerebral metastases. Cancer 1980;46:2587–2589.

112. Hazuka MB, Kinzie JJ. Brain metastases: Results and effects of re-irradiation. Int J Radiat Oncol Biol Phys 1988;15:433–437.

113. Cooper JS, Steinfeld R, Lerch IA. Cerebral metastases: Value of reirradiation in selected patients. Radiology 1990;174:883–885.

114. Grant FC. Concerning intracranial malignant metastases; their frequency and the value of surgery in their treatment. Ann Surg 1926;84:635–646.

115. Dandy WE. Brain tumors—General diagnosis and treatment. In: Lewis JR, ed. Practice of surgery. Vol 12. New York: Harper & Row, 1932:443–674.

116. Vieth R, Odom G. Intracranial metastases and their neurosurgical treatment. J Neurosurg 1965;23:375–383.

117. Bakay L. Results of surgical treatment of intracranial metastasis from pulmonary cancer. Report of a case with five-year survival. J Neurosurg 1958;15:338–341.

118. Lang EF Jr. Neurosurgical management of intracranial metastatic malignancy. Surg Clin North Am 1967;47:737–742.

119. Olivecrona H. The metastatic tumors. In: Olivecrona HTW, ed. Handbuch der Neurochirurgie. Berlin: Springer-Verlag, 1967:292–298.

120. Ransohoff J. Surgical management of metastatic tumor. Semin Oncol 1975;2:23–27.

121. Montana GS, Meacham WF, Caldwell WL. Brain irradiation for metastatic disease of lung origin. Cancer 1972;29:1477–1480.

122. Modesti LM, Feldman RA. Solitary cerebral metastasis from pulmonary cancer. Prolonged survival after surgery. JAMA 1975;231:1064.

123. Lee JS, Murphy WK, Glisson BS, et al. Primary chemotherapy of brain metastasis in small-cell lung cancer. J Clin Oncol 1989;7:916–922.

124. Twelves CJ, Souhami RL, Harper PG, et al. The response of cerebral metastases in small cell lung cancer to systemic chemotherapy. Br J Cancer 1989;61:147–150.

125. Postmus PE, Haaxma-Reiche H, Sleijfer DT, et al. High dose etoposide for brain metastases of small cell lung cancer. A phase II study. Br J Cancer 1989;59:254–256.

126. Rustin GJS, Newlands ES, Bagshawe KD, et al. Successful management of metastatic and primary germ cell tumors in the brain. Cancer 1986;57:2108–2113.

127. Rustin GJS, Newlands ES, Begent RHJ, et al. Weekly alternating etoposide, methotrexate, and actinomycin/vincristine and cyclophosphamide chemotherapy for the treatment of CNS metastases for choriocarcinoma. J Clin Oncol 1989;7:900–903.

128. Rosner D, Nemoto T, Lane WW. Chemotherapy induces regression of brain metastases in breast carcinoma. Cancer 1986;58:832–839.
129. Cocconi G, Lottici R, Bisagni G, et al. Combination therapy with platinum and etoposide for brain metastases from breast carcinoma. Cancer Invest 1990;8:327–334.
130. Jacquillat C, Khayat D, Banzet P, et al. Chemotherapy by fotemustine in cerebral metastases of disseminated malignant melanoma. Cancer Chemother Pharmacol 1990;25:263–266.
131. Bunn PA. Recent advances in the biology and treatment of small cell lung cancer. Adv Oncol 1986;2:9–15.
132. Cascino TL, Bryn TN, Deck MDF, et al. Intra-arterial BCNU in the treatment of metastatic brain tumors. J Neurooncol 1983;1:211–218.
133. Madajewicz S, West CR, Park HC, et al. Phase II study: Intra-arterial BCNU therapy for metastatic brain tumors. Cancer 1981;47:653–657.
134. Feun LG, Wallace S, Stewart DJ, et al. Intracarotid infusion of cis-diamminedichloroplatinum in the treatment of recurrent malignant brain tumors. Cancer 1984;54: 794–799.
135. Stewart DJ, Grahovac Z, Hugenholtz H, et al. Intraarterial mitomycin-C for recurrent brain metastases. Am J Clin Oncol 1987;10:432–436.
136. Feun LG, Lee Y, Yung WKA, et al. Intracarotid VP-16 in malignant brain tumors. J Neurooncol 1987;4:397–401.
137. Kolaric K, Roth A, Jelicic I, et al. Phase II clinical trial of cis-dichlorodiammine platinum (cis-DDP) in metastatic brain tumours—A preliminary report. In: Davis W, Maltoni C, Tanneberger S, eds. The control of tumour growth and its biological bases. Boston: Martinus Nijhoff Publishers, 1983:287–291.
138. Neuwelt EA, Dahlborg SA. Chemotherapy administered in conjunction with osmotic blood–brain barrier modification in patients with brain metastases. J Neurooncol 1987;4: 195–207.
139. Conte PF, Giaccone G, Musella R, et al. Combination chemotherapy for metastatic brain tumors. Tumori 1981;67:559–562.
140. Smalley SR, Schray MF, Laws ER, O'Fallon JR. Adjuvant radiation therapy after surgical resection of solitary brain metastasis: Association with patterns of failure and survival. Int J Radiat Oncol Biol Phys 1987;13:1611–1616.
141. Sause WT, Crowley JJ, Morantz R, et al. Solitary brain metastasis: Results of an RTOG/SWOG protocol evaluation: Surgery + RT versus RT alone. Am J Clin Oncol 1990;13: 427–432.
142. Otter R, Hermans J, Brand R, et al. Solitary brain metastasis treatment: A randomized trial. Neurology 1988;38(Suppl 1):393.
143. Posner JB. Surgery for metastases to the brain. N Engl J Med 1990;322:544–545.
144. Ushio Y, Arita N, Hayakawa T, et al. Chemotherapy of brain metastases from lung carcinoma: A controlled randomized study. Neurosurgery 1991;28:201–205.
145. Dosoretz DE, Blitzer PH, Russell AH, et al. Management of solitary metastasis to the brain: The role of elective brain irradiation following complete surgical resection. Int J Radiat Oncol Biol Phys 1980;6:1727–1730.
146. Hagen NA, Cirrincione C, Thaler HT, DeAngelis LM. The role of radiation therapy following resection of single brain metastasis from melanoma. Neurology 1990;40: 158–160.
147. Deeley TJ, Edwards JM. Radiotherapy in the management of cerebral secondaries from bronchial carcinoma. Lancet 1968;1:1209–1213.
148. Dayes LA, Rouhe SA, Barnes RW. Excision of multiple intracranial metastatic hypernephroma: Report of a case with a 7-year survival. J Neurosurg 1977;46:533–535.
149. Raskind R, Weiss RS, Manning JJ, et al. Survival after surgical excision of single metastatic brain tumors. Am J Roentgenol Rad Ther Nucl Med 1971;111:323–328.
150. Siegers HP. Chemotherapy for brain metastases: Recent developments and clinical considerations. Cancer Treat Rev 1990;17:63–76.

SECTION **2**   HARVEY I. PASS

Treatment of Metastatic Cancer to the Lung

There have been numerous reports regarding an aggressive approach for the management of metastases to the lung. The value of complete resection of isolated pulmonary metastases from soft tissue sarcoma and osteogenic sarcoma has been documented with improved survival compared with patients whose disease could not be totally extirpated. The magnitude of the problem of pulmonary metastases can be appreciated when one considers that the lungs are the second most common site of metastases for all histologies[1] and that the lungs serve as the most common site of first recurrence in patients with sarcomas.[2] Moreover, up to 20% of cases with pulmonary metastases at autopsy have no other detectable tumor in other sites.[3]

HISTORY

Weinlechner is credited with the first removal of a pulmonary metastasis in 1882, with the resection accomplished en bloc during a chest wall sarcoma excision.[4] Concomitant excision of a lung nodule at the time of resection of a chest wall sarcoma was reported by Krolein shortly thereafter in 1884. Divis in 1926 removed a right lower lobe metastasis at a separate procedure. In 1939, Barney and Churchill resected a solitary renal adenosarcoma pulmonary metastasis.[5] The long duration of survival (23 years) coupled with the patient's death from unrelated causes (coronary artery disease) gave credibility to the concept of metastasectomy. In 1947, Alexander and Haight

reported apparent cures in 3 of 6 patients after resection of metastases.[6]

Although these efforts clearly intimated a survival benefit from pulmonary metastasectomy, it was not until the maturation of techniques in thoracic surgery and anesthesia in the 1950s and 1960s that efforts to treat large numbers of patients began. Thomford and colleagues found comparable postthoracotomy survival rates for patients with excision of a solitary or multiple carcinomas and sarcoma lung metastases, justifying a more aggressive approach to resection.[7] Martini and colleagues[8] and Morton and associates[9] confirmed these observations by reporting comparable survival rates after resection of solitary or bilateral multiple metastases.

PATHOPHYSIOLOGY

ROUTES OF PRODUCTION

The most common pathway for true pulmonary metastatic disease is by way of *hematogenously disseminated malignant emboli* arising from invasion of thin-walled capillaries,[10] with transportation through the pulmonary artery. Most of these cells are destroyed in the bloodstream, and the number of tumor emboli correlate not only with the primary tumor duration and size but also with the probability of producing pulmonary metastases.[11] Other pathways include *endobronchial metastases* by way of a parenchymal or mediastinal nodal mass with secondary bronchial invasion, direct *lymphatic* spread, transbronchial *aspiration*, and *bronchial arterial* spread.[12–14] *Lymphangitic spread*, also by way of hematogenous dissemination, can occur by retrograde lymphatic spread through involved abdominal lymph nodes to hilar and mediastinal nodes.[12,15,16] *Pleural fluid* associated with parietal pleural metastases may be due to increased capillary permeability due to obstructive pneumonitis, decreased absorption, or erosion of vessels.[17]

MORPHOLOGIC CHARACTERISTICS

The number and morphology of nodules are important considerations in the evaluation of the etiology of pulmonary metastases. A solitary nodule in a patient with known extracellular malignancies is usually a second primary tumor if the original cancer was a squamous carcinoma. It is a metastasis or a second primary tumor if the original lesion was adenocarcinoma, but it is virtually always a metastasis if the original was melanoma or sarcoma.[18]

There is no predilection for laterality of pulmonary metastases,[19] and tumor distribution is usually greater at the bases, reflecting the flow characteristics of the pulmonary circulation.[2] The exception to this is choriocarcinoma, which, because of trophoblastic dissemination at the time of curettage, is posteriorly distributed to the upper lobes.[20,21]

The size of the metastasis is related to its detection during its natural history, and virtually 80% to 90% of these metastases are found in the periphery or outer third of the lung in a subpleural position.[22,23] Large peripheral lesions can actually assume a plaque-like shape that conforms to the shape of the chest wall and visceral pleura.

SIGNS AND SYMPTOMS

Because of the peripheral, subpleural, or parenchymal location of metastases, 85% to 95% of patients with metastases are asymptomatic.[24-26] Slow development of *dyspnea* may be due to airway obstruction, pleural effusion, or parenchymal replacement by innumerable lesions. Sudden shortness of breath may be due to hemorrhage into a lesion with space occupation or pleural effusion, or due to the development of a pneumothorax. The nature of the metastatic pneumothorax is unexplainable but may be due to rupture of subpleural blebs by growth of the lesion.[27-29] *Hemoptysis* demands bronchoscopic examination to rule out endobronchial tumor. Patients with increasing dyspnea, with diminished diffusing capacity and arterial desaturation in the absence of radiographic findings, may have lymphangitic spread of tumor.[30,31] The appearance of *chest pain* usually portends an ominous situation with discontinuous parietal pleural metastases.

ROENTGENOGRAPHIC APPEARANCE

Most pulmonary metastases, independent of histology, present as nodules (*i.e.*, increased densities that are roughly spherical in shape, are not associated with linear densities, and are sharply demarcated).[2] Pulmonary lesions with an irregular border usually imply primary lung cancer or infection,[12] but lesion age, hemorrhage, and previous treatment (see below) may influence the appearance of the metastases.

Cavitation may occur in approximately 5% of metastases, chiefly with sarcoma or squamous histologies due to central necrosis with liquefaction from rapid growth or treatment.[12] *Bleb formation* can be associated with testicular metastases.[32] *Calcification* may also be noted in metastases; therefore, calcification in a lesion must not be dismissed as a benign occurrence. Osteogenic sarcoma, chondrosarcoma, and synovial sarcoma are all associated with calcification, and infrequently calcified lung metastases are seen in thyroid, ovarian, and mucinous gastrointestinal malignancies and breast tumors.

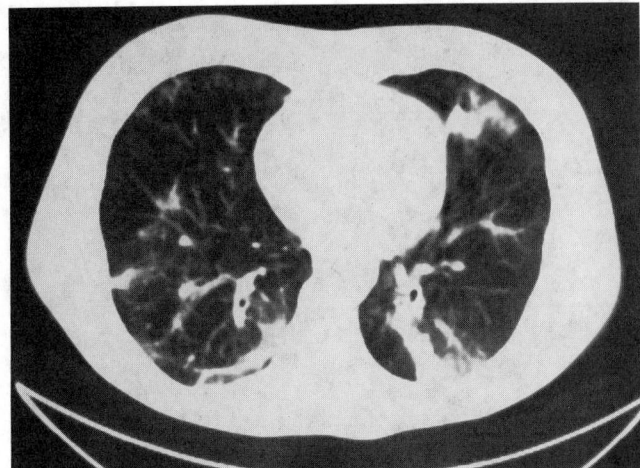

FIGURE 61–7. Computed tomographic scan of a patient with lymphangitic metastases from breast cancer. Notice the patchy, linear densities extending toward the hilum.

Postchemotherapeutic or postradiotherapeutic manipulation causing degeneration of metastases may result in calcification in a variety of pulmonary metastases.[33-38]

Lymphangitic carcinomatosis from lung, gastric, breast, pancreatic, or prostatic cancer may have minimal chest radiographic findings.[11,15] In the late stages there will be linear markings and possibly enlarged hilar nodes. Computed tomographic (CT) findings are much more specific for lymphangitic spread than are the plain radiographic findings (Figs. 61–7 and 61–8).

Lobar or total collapse is usually associated with endobronchial metastases from kidney, breast, colon, rectum, female genital tract, thyroid, or melanoma (Figs. 61–9 and 61–10). The frequency of metastatic involvement of the bronchus is approximately 2% to 28% of cancer patients.[39-41]

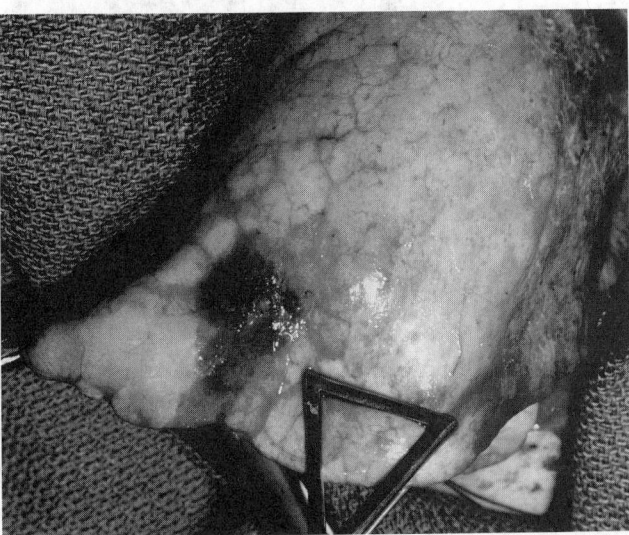

FIGURE 61–8. Operative photograph of patient with chest computed tomographic scan seen in Figure 61–7. The darkened area on the visceral pleura is a confluence of lymphatic channels plugged with tumor.

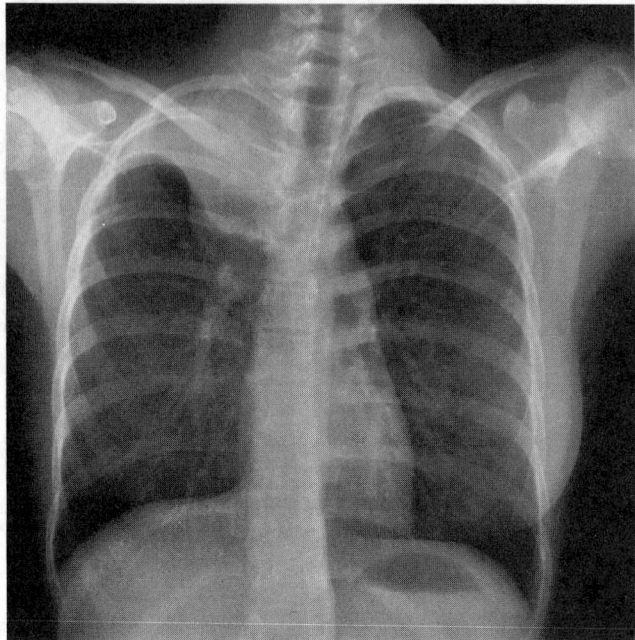

FIGURE 61–9. Right upper lobe collapse in a child with osteogenic sarcoma metastatic to the bronchus. The lesion was visible on bronchoscopy.

ROENTGENOGRAPHIC EXAMINATION

In any patient with extrathoracic malignant disease, either at the time of primary resection or during follow-up in the surveillance for pulmonary metastases, posteroanterior and lateral chest radiography is mandatory. In the initial evaluation of a patient, the chest radiograph serves as a useful baseline and also indicates coexisting benign cardiopulmonary disease.

An abnormality on chest radiography in the initial examination demands the diligent examination of previous chest radiographs to define the morphologic characteristics of the abnormality and to document any change in the appearance of the lesion over time. Nevertheless, *computed tomography* (CT) of the chest has become the standard of care for the detection, operative planning, and follow-up of patients at risk for the development of pulmonary metastases. The ideal CT should be able to detect the smallest of abnormalities, be specific enough to pinpoint malignancy either on initial nodule examination or on follow-up, and be cost-effective so it can be repeated at frequent intervals without subjecting the patient to excessive irradiation. Unfortunately, such a standard does not exist at this time; however, more recent developments with the "fast CT" scanners may impart greater nodule differentiation with less distortion because of volume averaging. Certainly, CT has surpassed the use of conventional linear tomograms in the documentation of pulmonary metastases[42] because of the elimination of structural overlap and shadows by the cross-sectional depiction in CT scanning (Figs. 61–11 and 61–12). Subpleural abnormalities are easily detected, and contrast resolution exceeds conventional techniques by at least a factor of 10.[2] More lesions can be detected on CT, and lesions as small as 3 mm can be detected.[2] Partial volume averaging, in which a lesion is not fully in the CT volume and is not shown as an area of increased attenuation because of abutting of aerated lung, usually underestimates the number of lesions. Moreover, small nodules close to vessels are sometimes difficult to identify, but this has been improved with contrast enhancement.[43–48]

The real use of CT is its ability to take small nodules and define their natural history over a short time interval. The temporal pattern of appearance of hematogenous pulmonary metastases is variable. The appearance of the lung at any particular time is a cumulative phenomenon depending on

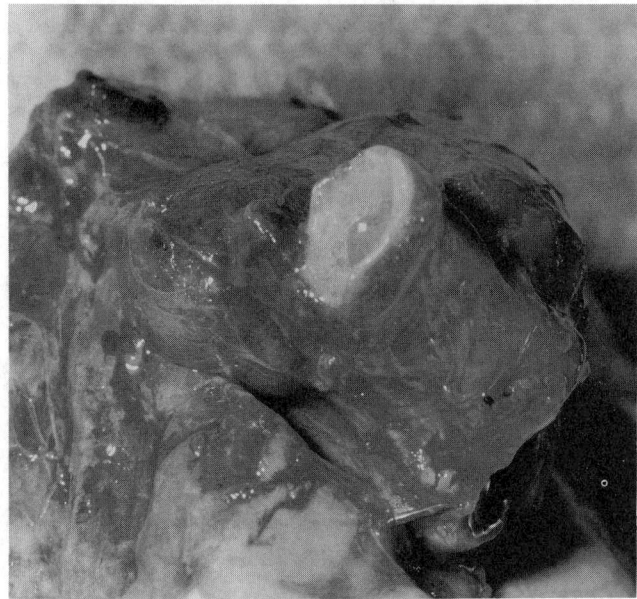

FIGURE 61–10. Operative photograph of the resected bronchus as a sleeve lobectomy (sparing the middle and lower lobe) in the patient with the chest radiograph seen in Figure 61–9. The bulbous lesion is seen just inside the superior cut end of the bronchus.

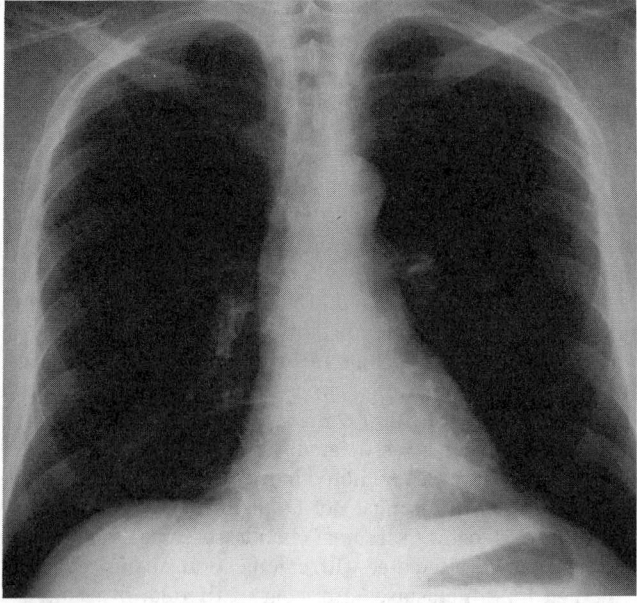

FIGURE 61–11. Routine surveillance chest radiograph in a patient with soft tissue sarcoma. No abnormality was detected.

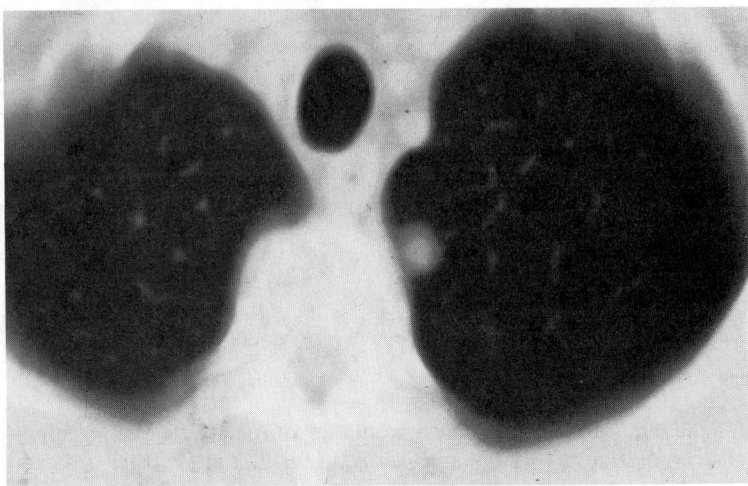

FIGURE 61–12.   Computed tomographic scan reveals a lesion in the left upper lobe in the patient with the normal-appearing radiograph in Figure 61–11.

the frequency and intensity of the embolic showers, the capacity of the metastases to colonize, and the duration of the patient's disease. In the surveillance of pulmonary metastases, the problem is essentially to distinguish between benign and malignant processes. Usually the benign nodule is static in growth. Serial CT scanning can determine the dynamic properties of the pulmonary lesions, specifically in a homogenous patient population. Nodules can be classified as *stable, developing, or growing.* The predictive value of CT in defining a nodule as a malignancy is not as high in stable nodules on sequential scans.[2] The development of a new CT abnormality, however, in the sarcoma population or growth of a previous nodule will be histologically documented as malignant with a 90% confidence level. Questionable abnormalities demand repeat CTs at 2- to 3-month intervals to document any biologic change that would justify exploration.

USE OF CT IN MONITORING SPECIFIC HISTOLOGIES

If a nodule appears questionable on conventional studies, CT should be performed not only to verify the finding but also to document other possible lesions. In patients known to have an extrathoracic tumor that is likely to metastasize first to the lung (*i.e.,* testicular carcinoma, soft tissue sarcoma, or choriocarcinoma), chest CT should be performed initially as a baseline. This is especially true if an aggressive approach to the resection of metastases from these histologic types is to be maintained. In patients who present with extrathoracic tumors and multiple nodules on chest radiography, CT is of questionable usefulness except for the documentation of response to therapies. Chest radiography can probably suffice for more frequent examinations in these patients.

If CT of the liver is negative and there is no clinical or laboratory evidence of hepatic metastases in patients with cancers whose first metastases would be to the liver (*i.e.,* cancers of the colon, rectum, pancreas, or stomach), pulmonary metastases are unlikely. In this setting, a negative chest radiograph is probably most likely a true negative finding.[49] Similarly, if a bone scan is negative in patients with a high probability of first metastases to bone (*i.e.,* those with prostate cancer), CT of the thorax should be reserved for evaluation of abnormalities seen on the chest radiograph.

Surveillance intervals for the detection of pulmonary metastases depend on the probability that a given histologic type will metastasize to the lung. For lesions such as soft tissue sarcoma and osteogenic sarcomas, which are most likely to metastasize within the first 2 years of diagnosis, 3-month intervals are usually recommended.

NEWER ROENTGENOGRAPHIC METHODS

Because a considerable amount of radiation is delivered to patients in an attempt to detect pulmonary metastases, a sensitive screening modality free of ionizing radiation would be of value, especially in young persons. *Magnetic resonance imaging* (MRI) has made considerable diagnostic strides for the diagnosis of chest diseases, yet few studies have addressed its use in the detection of pulmonary metastases. A prospective trial was recently completed at the National Cancer Institute (NCI), where MRI, chest radiography, computed tomography, and surgical verification of disease were all obtained in 12 patients.[50] All images were interpreted in a blinded fashion (Fig. 61–13). For individual nodules, MRI was at least as sensitive as CT for nodules greater than 5 mm, and significantly more sensitive than chest radiographs. The sequences of the MRI could be changed for added sensitivity, as was the addition of contrast enhancement with gadopentetate dimeglumine. Future studies with higher generation MRI scanners will be needed, however, to displace CT as the "gold standard" for detection and surveillance of pulmonary metastases.

INVASIVE DIAGNOSTIC MEANS EXCLUSIVE OF THORACOTOMY

The pursuit of a histologic diagnosis of the undiagnosed chest nodule will depend on the equivocality of the radiographic studies, the physiologic reserve of the patient, the location of the lesions, the histology of the primary focus, and whether the surgeon feels the patient could be rendered free of disease. Certainly any pleural effusion associated with nodules in the chest demands cytologic verification of malignancy, and possibly pleural biopsy. Patients with poor performance status who cannot tolerate thoracotomy but need histologic verification of disease for further management may require his-

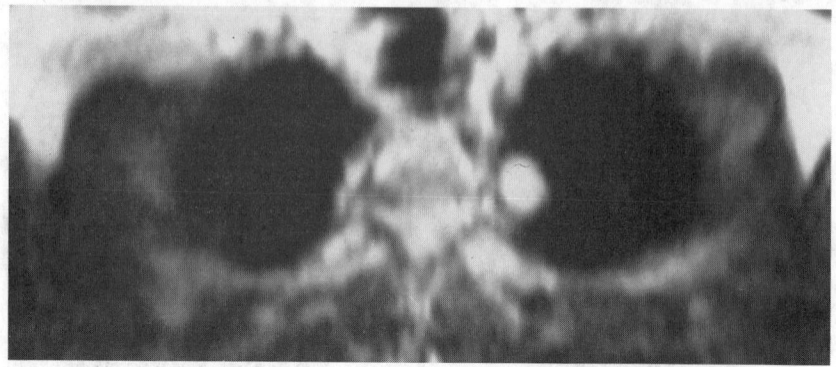

FIGURE 61–13. Magnetic resonance image reveals the lesion seen in the computed tomographic scan of Figure 61–12. The T2-weighted image highlights the lesion. (Photograph courtesy of Dr. Irwin Feuerstein, Department of Diagnostic Radiology Clinical Center, National Institutes of Health, Bethesda, MD)

tologic inquiries. Finally, if documentation of metastatic disease would have a major impact on the magnitude of the primary operation (limb salvage versus amputation for cure in the patient with multiple pulmonary nodules), verification of diagnosis as well as feasibility of complete resection need to be documented.

Diagnostic studies that are useful in other thoracic neoplasms are of limited value in the diagnosis of pulmonary metastases. In one series, *sputum cytologic examination* revealed malignant cells in only 5% of patients, and *bronchoscopy* provided notable findings in only 10% of patients with documented pulmonary metastases.[51] Bronchoscopies *should* be performed, however, to verify endobronchial metastases to define whether operative intervention is possible. In the case of an isolated metastasis seen by bronchoscopy, lobectomy or sleeve lobectomy may be performed with favorable survival. If resection is not possible, endobronchial management with or without laser ablation may be of great palliative interest (see later).

In general, there are few indications for *fine-needle aspiration biopsies (FNAB)* to avoid open thoracotomy for diagnosis, for if the primary lesion is favorable for resection, there is no reason for fine-needle aspiration biopsy. If the patient is unable to undergo thoracotomy, and histologic verification is necessary to guide treatment options, fine-needle aspiration is a reasonable alternative.[52] High sensitivity (88%) of FNAB for melanoma,[53] breast cancer, gastrointestinal cancer, germinal tumors,[53,54] and soft tissue sarcomas[55–57] has been reported in those series in which the aspirate can be compared with the primary tumor. Major complications include a 4% chance of a pneumothorax requiring chest tube treatment,[58] transient hemoptysis (2–4%), and, rarely, air embolism. Needle track implantations are rare.[59]

THORACOSCOPY

The use of thoracoscopy to diagnose pleural effusions and pulmonary metastases has increased and is now combined with video monitoring for documentation and ease of exploration. The multiple trocar technique and newly designed instruments for endoscopic surgery, including instruments to accomplish wedge resection of lung, have made this technique very popular for thoracic diseases. Certainly, for lesions on the surface of the visceral pleura, resection can be performed, although the length of time that these endoscopic resections require seems to be minimized in the literature. The ability of video thoracoscopy to ensure a complete resection of pulmonary metastases, however, remains to be demonstrated, because, as described in the following sections, deeper parenchymal lesions must be palpated in order to be found, and the technology of the endoscopic instruments for resection at this time is applicable for only the most superficial of lesions.[60–63]

SURGICAL RESECTION OF PULMONARY METASTASES

ELIGIBILITY FOR SURGICAL RESECTION

The selection of patients for thoracotomy for pulmonary metastasectomy must fulfill basic criteria, because only a portion of the patients will derive a survival benefit, and fewer will be cured of their disease. These criteria include: (1) local control of the primary tumor or the ability to gain local control if pulmonary exploration is performed first; (2) absence of metastatic lesions in nonpulmonary sites; (3) radiologic findings consistent with metastases; (4) potential for operative resection to preserve adequate functioning lung tissue; (5) ability of the pulmonary metastatic disease to be completely resected; and (6) lack of any other effective antitumor therapy. Occasionally, if a patient presents with synchronous pulmonary lesions and a lesion that could be handled by amputation or marginal limb-sparing option, it is preferable to determine complete resectability in the chest before committing the patient to an amputation in the face of unresectable pulmonary disease. Of the 30% of patients with malignant disease who develop pulmonary metastases, only one third will meet the defined basic treatment criteria of primary disease control and lack of metastases in other sites.[41]

In order to satisfy the above criteria, an extensive functional and staging workup is usually required. Computed tomography, magnetic resonance imaging, or appropriate endoscopic or barium studies must be performed to rule out evidence of disease at the primary site. *Sarcomas* will usually metastasize to the lungs in preference to other sites, so the primary site evaluation and radionuclide bone scans are all that are needed in these patients before the resection. *Carcinomas* and *melanomas* require a more extensive evaluation of peripheral sites, including the liver, adrenal glands, and brain.

A thorough functional evaluation must also be performed to determine whether the patient can safely withstand thoracotomy with low cardiopulmonary risk. Patients with carcinoma will tend to be older than sarcoma patients, necessitating a workup directed toward the cardiovascular/renal/pulmonary axis. Patients who have had cytotoxic chemotherapy must have recovery of their marrow to ensure the absence of bleeding, and it is necessary to search for clinical and subclinical evidence of cardiomyopathy or congestive heart failure in sarcoma patients and other patients who have had doxorubicin (Adriamycin),[64] particularly if the dose exceeds 500 mg/m².[65] Such assessment can be accomplished by measurement of ejection fraction at rest and during exercise.[66]

The majority of patients will simply require wedge resections for their lesions, but in the occasional patient who requires lobectomy or multiple wedge resections, a thorough evaluation of respiratory reserve must be performed by pulmonary function testing. In general, a patient must have postoperative FEV_1 of 800 to 1000 ml to avoid prolonged respiratory management after resection. The use of quantitative ventilation perfusion scanning may assist in determining residual FEV_1 after resection.[67] Diligent workup of a patient's pulmonary function should also be routine in patients who are having repeated thoracotomies for metastasis resection, or who have been previously exposed to pulmonary fibrotic inducing agents under high inspired oxygen conditions, such as bleomycin. Preexposure to bleomycin will dictate low inspired oxygen concentrations during and after the resection.

PROGNOSTIC FACTORS FOR THE RESECTION OF PULMONARY METASTASES

In the ideal situation, independent of histology, there would be a number of factors that would define preoperatively or intraoperatively who the best candidates would be for long-term survival after pulmonary metastasectomy. Unfortunately, despite a significant number of publications that have attempted to define such parameters, there is no uniform agreement as to which are the most important factors that predict a successful (*i.e.*, long-term survival) outcome. Many of the factors are based on biologic characteristics of the tumor, including disease-free interval and tumor doubling time, whereas other factors are based on the sensitivity of present radiographic studies, which will detect only 50% of the metastases found at operation. Moreover, different histologies seem to have varying factors that may prognosticate survival, and, unfortunately, uniform agreement does not appear in the literature, even with the same histology. The following discussion of prognostic factors, therefore, must serve only as a *superficial guide* to the practitioner to advise his patient regarding the possible outcome of metastasectomy before operation.

RESECTABILITY

There is almost uniform agreement that the ability to completely resect all nodules that are metastases (as opposed to an incomplete or unresectable situation) will be associated with an improved outcome compared with patients who remain with disease. This has been confirmed for carcinoma,[68] sarcoma,[25,69,70] osteogenic sarcoma[24,70] and other histologies.[71,72] Unfortunately, because of the limited sensitivity of the present radiographic studies, as well as the differing phi-

losophies among different thoracic surgeons regarding how many nodules to remove, such a factor cannot be predicted unless the patient undergoes exploration. One must, therefore, define what *is* resectability in this situation. Any disease outside the confines of the visceral envelope (*i.e.*, pleural metastases, diaphragmatic involvement, discontinuous pericardial involvement, presence of pleural effusion histologically positive for malignancy, and tumor involvement of lymph nodes) must be considered unresectable disease and must be recorded as such. Moreover, if the patient's pulmonary functions are limiting and one cannot remove all disease for fear of irreversible pulmonary compromise, this is also an unresectable situation.

NUMBER OF METASTASES RESECTED

It would seem logical that the presence of a large number of metastases would have a more grave prognosis for patients undergoing metastasectomy than for those with few metastases. Indeed, in the early studies from the National Cancer Institute, longer postthoracotomy survival time was associated with fewer metastases.[25] Patients with resectable disease and 15 or fewer metastases had a longer postthoracotomy survival than did patients with 16 or more. Unfortunately, only 3 patients had 16 or more nodules. In a more recent study of 74 patients over a more modern era (1982–1987), however, no differences in long-term survival were found in completely resected patients who had one to four metastases as opposed to five or more metastases (Fig. 61–14).[69] The absence of correlation with number of metastases removed at operation, at least for the sarcoma patient, has also been pointed out in other more recent studies.[70] In osteogenic sarcoma[24] and Ewing's sarcoma,[71] if four or more nodules are resected there will likely be increased survival with less burden of disease. In colon cancer, a poor prognosis has been noted when there is more than one metastasis.[73] In patients with breast carcinoma, however, there does not seem to be a correlation with survival and number of metastases resected.[74] No correlation between solitary or multiple metastases and survival has been reported in other series with varying histologies (Table 61–9).[75]

The survival of patients after pulmonary metastasectomy *may* be more influenced by the completeness of resection, regardless of the number of nodules, in the face of extrathoracic disease control. Such an aggressive approach, however, still needs to be tempered by the biology of the metastasis kinetics, as seen with disease-free interval.

DISEASE-FREE INTERVAL

With the exception of the report by Pastorini,[70] there is general agreement that the resection of pulmonary metastases from osteogenic and soft tissue sarcoma is influenced by the disease-free interval from the time of the primary tumor resection to the removal of the pulmonary metastases (see Table 61–9). An original series of 93 patients with soft tissue sarcoma metastases from 1974 to 1982[25] and a second series resected from 1982 to 1987 both confirmed that a disease-free interval of less than a year was associated with a poor survival after metastasectomy (Fig. 61–15).[69] Other studies have confirmed this finding.[68,76] The importance of the disease-free interval was not seen in Ewing's sarcoma,[71] or most recently in me-

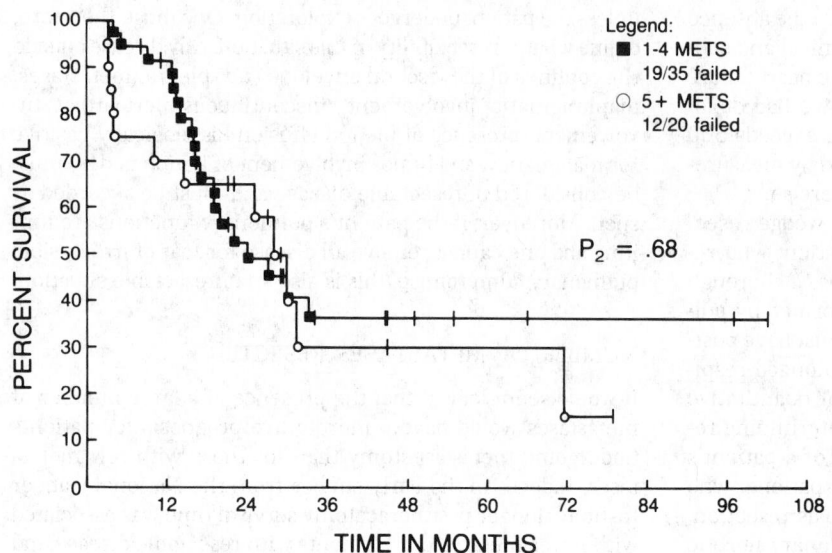

FIGURE 61–14. Survival rates of sarcoma patients. No difference in survival was noted in patients who were completely resected of pulmonary metastases from soft tissue sarcoma at the National Cancer Institute (NCI) from 1982 to 1987. (Reproduced with permission from Jablons D, Steinberg SM, Roth J, Pittaluga S, Rosenberg SA, Pass HI. Metastasectomy for soft tissue sarcoma. J Thorac Cardiovasc Surg 1989;97:695–705)

tastasectomy for colon cancer.[73] Breast cancer metastases that occurred less than 1 year after the primary resection were associated with a decreased survival after metastasectomy.[74]

One of the more intriguing subcategories of biologic factors involves patients with *synchronous lung metastases* at the time of the primary tumor resection. Putnam found that only 46% of such patients with synchronous pulmonary metastases in primary tumors could have their pulmonary metastases resected.[25] However, those patients with synchronous presentation who were completely resected had the same survival as patients with metachronous metastases. Such a finding has been documented in Ewing's sarcoma[71] and carcinoma,[68] as well as in renal cell cancer metastases.[77]

TUMOR DOUBLING TIME

There has been much effort to document that tumor doubling time correlates positively with prognosis after resection (*i.e.,* the shorter the doubling time, the shorter the survival). One must consider whether it is wise to measure tumor doubling

TABLE 61–9. Prognostic Factors for Pulmonary Metastasectomy

Histology	Investigations	No. of Patients	Correlation With Survival
Disease-Free Interval			
Carcinoma–Sarcoma	Vogt-Moykopf[68]	368	Negative ≤3 y vs >3 y
Sarcoma	Liennard[76]	19	Negative ≤1 y vs >1 y
Sarcoma	Jablons[69]	74	Negative ≤1 y vs >1 y
Sarcoma	Pastorini[87]	56	None
Ewing's sarcoma	Lanza[71]	19	None
Melanoma	Pogrebniak[106]	33	None
Colon	McAfee[73]	139	None
Breast	Lanza[74]	44	Negative ≤1 y vs >1 y
Renal cell	Pogrebniak[77]	23	None
Number of Metastases Resected			
Carcinoma–Sarcoma	Vogt-Moykopf[68]	386	None
Carcinoma–Sarcoma	Venn[75]	118	None
Sarcoma	Jablons[69]	74	None
Sarcoma	Pastorini[87]	56	None
Ewing's sarcoma	Lanza[71]	19	Negative >4 y
Melanoma	Pogrebniak[106]	33	None
Colon	McAfee[73]	139	Negative >1 y
Breast	Lanza[74]	44	None
Renal cell	Pogrebniak[77]	23	None

SARCOMA PATIENTS – SURVIVAL

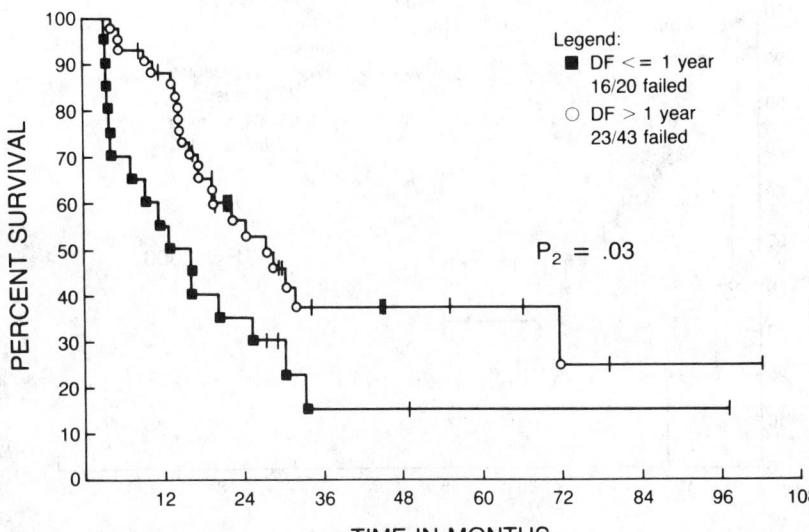

FIGURE 61–15. Survival rates of sarcoma patients. A disease-free interval of less than 1 year correlated with shorter long-term survival in patients resected for metastatic soft tissue sarcoma. (Reproduced with permission from Jablons D, Steinberg SM, Roth J, Pittaluga S, Rosenberg SA, Pass HI. Metastasectomy for soft tissue sarcoma. J Thorac Cardiovasc Surg 1989;97:695–705)

time in these patients, especially if the patient has a resectable number of metastases on preoperative studies, is able to tolerate thoracotomy, and has a substantial disease-free interval. Without denying that there is probably prognostic significance for a rapidly doubling tumor,[25,78,79] it is probably safe to say that serial examination of CT scans in patients with a known or developing abnormality should be reserved only for those rare instances when the nodule is not distinct, or where there is a history (*i.e.*, pneumonitis, septic emboli) that would suggest that the abnormality may resolve within a period of 1 or 2 months. In most patients considered for metastasectomy, the nodule will be of new onset, no other standard therapies will be available, and the procedure will be possible if the patient has the physiologic reserve and his peripheral workup is negative. Therefore, delaying the surgery (especially with a risk of mortality of less than 1%) in order to document a tumor doubling time seems unnecessary. An examination of the recent literature also reveals this "deemphasis" on the tumor doubling time as a useful prognostic factor.[80]

PREOPERATIVE RADIOGRAPHIC STUDIES

It seems pointless to use the preoperative number of nodules as a prognostic factor because the absolute number of metastases resected may not correlate with long-term survival as long as the patient can be rendered completely free of disease. At the time the preoperative studies are performed, however, it is not known with 100% certainty that the patient is, indeed, resectable. Moreover, the number of nodules seen on the preoperative studies will always underestimate the number of nodules resected by as much as a factor of 2.[2] Unfortunately, a systematic analysis of the number of nodules on preoperative studies has been performed only in the osteogenic and soft tissue sarcoma situation. Putnam found, in his analysis on the number of nodules on preoperative conventional lung tomograms, that survival was significantly prolonged in patients with osteogenic and soft tissue sarcoma if there were four or fewer nodules.[25] Jablons noted in a follow-up report that when computed tomography was adopted as standard for roentgen-

ographic surveillance at the National Cancer Institute, patients with six or more CT nodules had a significantly decreased survival (Fig. 61–16).[69] One must remember, however, that these numbers are somewhat artificial because they include patients who were found to be unresectable at the time of thoracotomy.

OTHER PROGNOSTIC VARIABLES EXAMINED

NODAL STATUS

It is rare that the nodal status of patients with resection of pulmonary metastases is noted, because if they are deemed to have mediastinal disease on preoperative studies, they are not offered surgery. Nevertheless, the survival of patients with soft tissue sarcoma found to have hilar or mediastinal involvement is significantly poorer than that of patients not found to have nodal involvement.[25,69,79]

UNILATERAL VERSUS BILATERAL METASTASES

No correlation of unilaterality or bilaterality with survival is noted if the patients are completely resected.[25]

AGE/SEX

Neither age nor sex correlates with survival after metastasectomy.

ADJUVANT CHEMOTHERAPY

There are no randomized studies to compare survival of patients who receive postoperative or preoperative adjunctive chemotherapy along with metastasectomy with survival of those who do not receive this treatment. Nevertheless, in a subset of 32 patients from the National Cancer Institute who did not receive chemotherapy after their primary sarcoma

SARCOMA PATIENTS – SURVIVAL

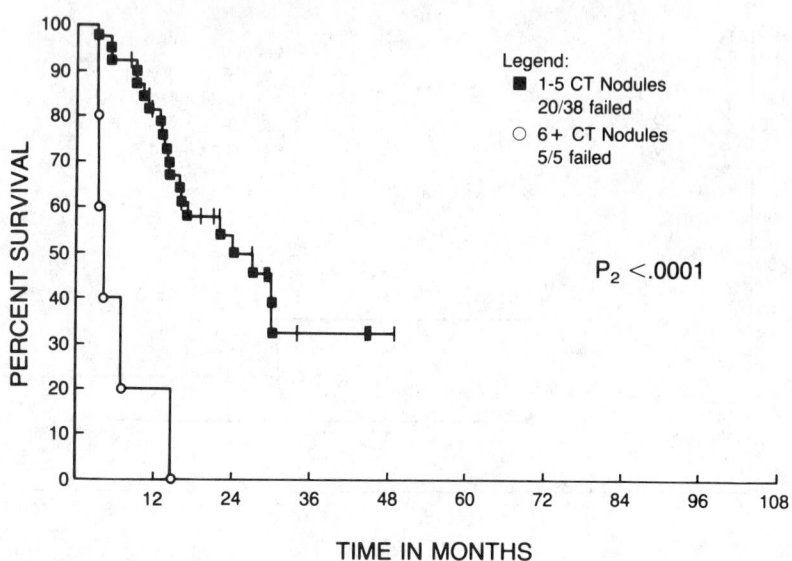

Legend:
■ 1-5 CT Nodules
  20/38 failed
○ 6+ CT Nodules
  5/5 failed

$P_2 < .0001$

FIGURE 61–16. Survival rates of sarcoma patients. Patients with six or more nodules from metastatic soft tissue sarcoma to the lungs have decreased survival compared with patients with five or fewer nodules noted by computed tomography. (Reproduced with permission from Jablons D, Steinberg SM, Roth J, Pittaluga S, Rosenberg SA, Pass HI. Metastasectomy for soft tissue sarcoma. J Thorac Cardiovasc Surg 1989;97:695–705)

was resected, 15 received chemotherapy after the metastases and 17 did not. No survival differences were noted between the two groups.[69] Similarly, in a study from the M.D. Anderson Cancer Center, the survival after resection of pulmonary metastases from soft tissue sarcoma could not be accurately predicted based on the clinical response to the preoperative chemotherapy.[81]

TECHNIQUE OF PULMONARY METASTASECTOMY

The technique of pulmonary metastasectomy has been standardized and essentially involves the median sternotomy or lateral thoracotomy approach. Double-lumen endotracheal tubes (Fig. 61–17) are used to totally collapse the lung for a thorough exploration. The thoracic cavity, including the me-

diastinum, the chest wall, and the hilar nodes are thoroughly explored. Palpable abnormalities that do not appear to be obvious granulomas or intrapulmonary lymph nodes are excised with the automatic stapling device (Fig. 61–18). For peripheral lesions, a Duval lung clamp can be positioned on either side of the nodule, and for small nodules, the nodule can be positioned in the cutout portion of the clamp. The 30-, 55-, or 90-mm automatic stapling device is then placed across the base of the lesion depending on its size. Deeper lung lesions may require use of the GIA (gastrointestinal anastomosis) stapler, which simultaneously cuts and staples. Resection of metastases with the lung inflated will prevent removal of excessive lung tissue and still provide an adequate margin. For lesions that cannot be removed by wedge resection without ensuring a negative margin, lobectomy or segmentectomy can be performed if the patient's pulmonary reserve is adequate to support such anatomic resection.

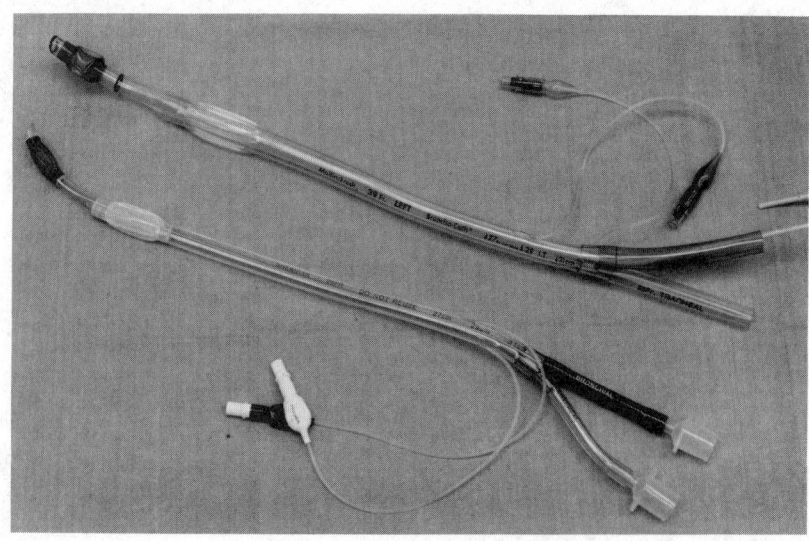

FIGURE 61–17. Double-lumen endotracheal tubes, both adult and child size, are a prerequisite to the proper performance of pulmonary metastasectomy. Other bronchial blockade methods can be used; however, these tubes are the most convenient technique for one-lung anesthesia.

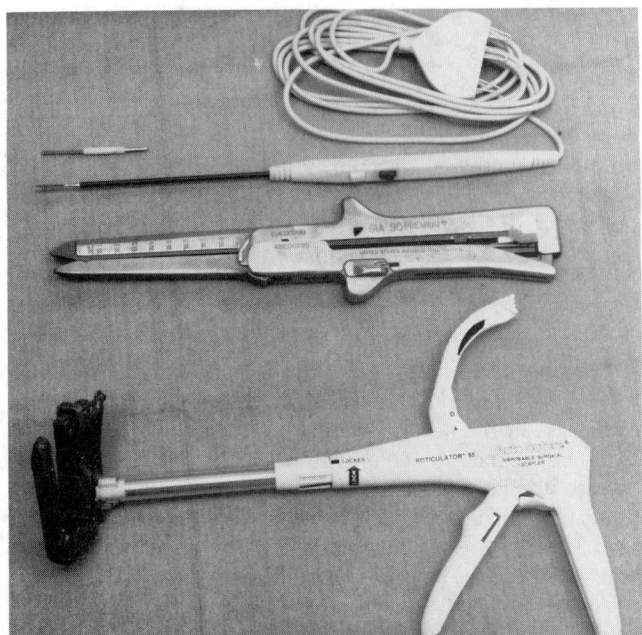

FIGURE 61–18. The long-handled electrocautery, the gastrointestinal anastomosis stapling device, and the standard or roticulated stapling machines are the surgeon's primary tools for accomplishing metastasectomy.

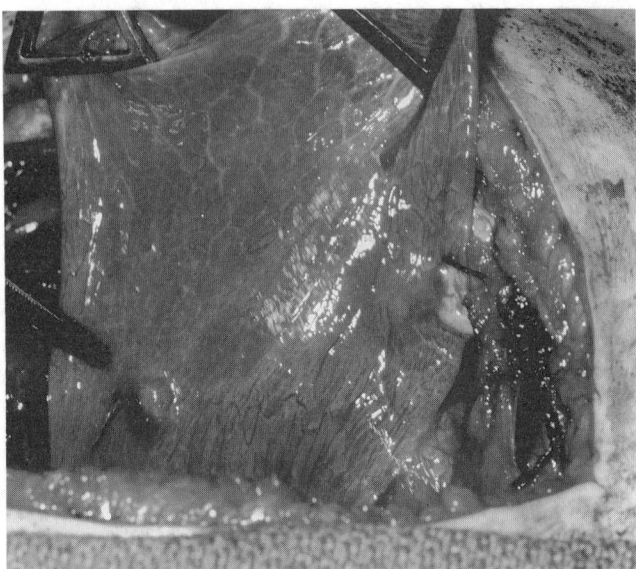

FIGURE 61–20. Typical appearance, by the use of double-lumen anesthesia, of a nodular pulmonary metastasis in a lung that is collapsed.

MEDIAN STERNOTOMY OR THORACOTOMY?

The desired approach, if feasible, for the removal of pulmonary metastases is the use of the median sternotomy.[69,70,72] Both lungs can be palpated simultaneously, and frequently unsuspected metastases not detected by radiographic methods will be found (Fig. 61–19). There are no differences, however, with regard to long-term survival advantage, morbidity, or mortality when comparing median sternotomy with lateral thoracotomy.[19] The avoidance of a second procedure (because of the necessity for staged thoracotomies for patients with bilateral disease), however, is probably advantageous. Moreover, with few exceptions, any procedure related to the eradication of pulmonary metastatic disease can be performed by sternotomy once the surgeon becomes comfortable with the approach. Wide mediastinal exposure, complete lung collapse, placement of posterior packs and elevation of the lung with lung clamps, and release of the inferior pulmonary ligament are all maneuvers to facilitate the operation. The anesthesiologist must be alerted when the surgeon is placing traction on the pulmonary vein so that he can carefully monitor blood pressure and rhythm changes. Early decisions should be made regarding the necessity for a formal resection, and if there are ten or more nodules on one side, or a lesion requires anatomic lobectomy or segmentectomy, the contralateral lung should be explored for location, size, and number of nodules before resecting the first side, to rule out an unresectable situation (Fig. 61–20). Concomitant procedures, such as chest wall resection (Fig. 61–21), can be performed through the

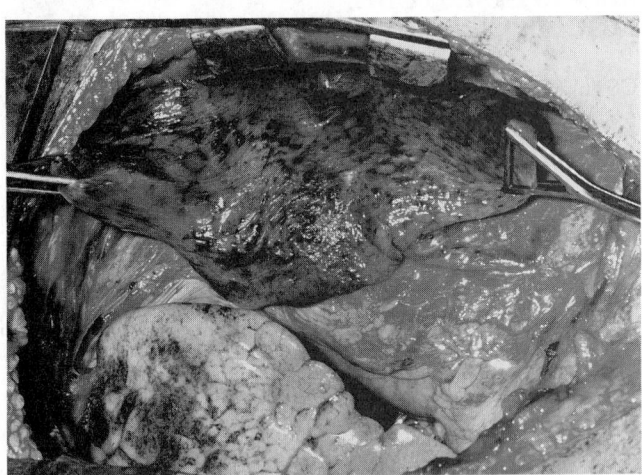

FIGURE 61–19. Wide exposure by way of the median sternotomy. The patient's head is to the left; the left upper lobe is collapsed and grasped with lung clamps. Inferiorly and to the right, the right lung is expanded, as seen through the widely opened pleura.

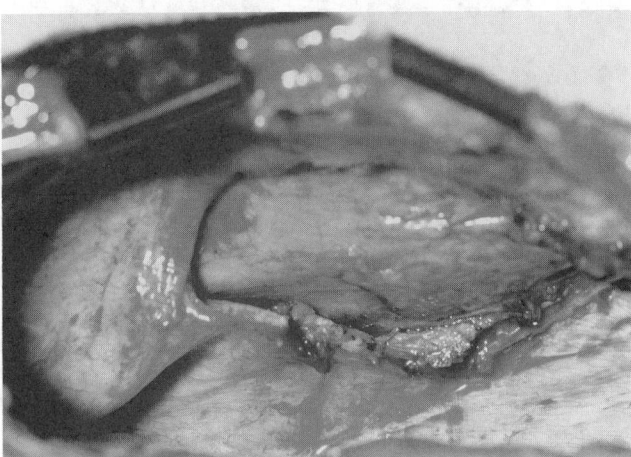

FIGURE 61–21. View from the median sternotomy to the left chest. A chest wall resection has been accomplished completely through the sternotomy, and just above the resected pleura is the posterior fascia of the pectoralis major.

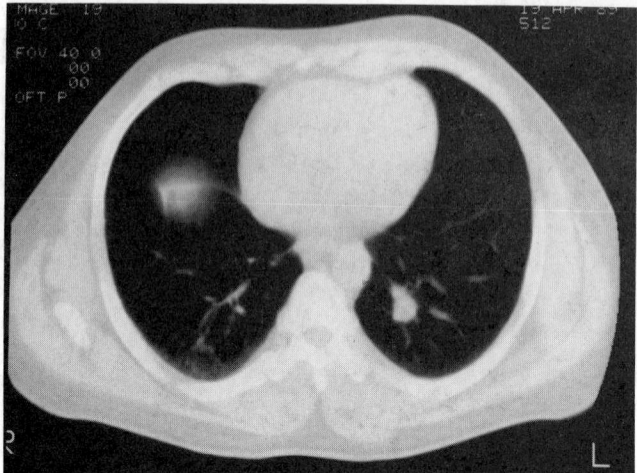

FIGURE 61–22. Computed tomographic scan of a parenchymal renal cell metastasis in the basilar segment of the left lower lobe.

median sternotomy approach. The most difficult resection by this technique, of course, is a left lower lobectomy, but even this can be performed in most patients without difficulty (Figs. 61–22 and 61–23).

There are a few preoperative hints, however, that may make lateral thoracotomy preferable to median sternotomy. Very large posterior or central lesions, specifically in the left lower lobe, may force one to abandon the median sternotomy approach and perform initial or concomitant left lateral thoracotomy. Previous sternal irradiation should probably be an absolute contraindication to the midline approach because of poor wound healing. Central staple line recurrences, posteromedial chest wall disease, and the preoperative assessment of the necessity for a sleeve-type resection also usually dictate a lateral thoracotomy approach. Finally, exposure of the mediastinum becomes difficult in obese individuals with a large heart and a narrow retrosternal space, and these patients should probably be explored through a lateral thoracotomy.

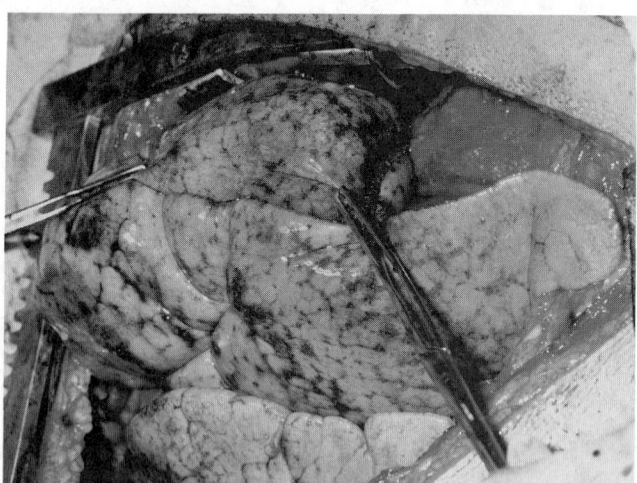

FIGURE 61–23. Operative photograph of the completed resection of the basilar segment of the left lower lobe of the patient whose computed tomographic scan is depicted in Figure 61–22. The lung clamps are holding the superior segment of the left lower lobe, just medial to which is the left upper lobe. The right lung is seen inferiorly.

REOPERATIVE METASTASECTOMY

Some institutions have attempted to define an aggressive approach for the management of patients who present with recurrent pulmonary metastases.[82-84] In most histologies, it is unknown whether reresection of pulmonary metastases is associated with a long-term survival benefit. There are data, however, that support the reresection of pulmonary metastases in metastatic soft tissue sarcoma. At the National Cancer Institute since 1976, 43 patients have had two or more thoracic explorations for the purpose of resecting pulmonary metastases by way of 89 reexplorations through either a median sternotomy or a lateral thoracotomy. There was an operative mortality of 0%, and 31 of the 43 patients were rendered free of disease at the second thoracotomy. The median survival from the second thoracotomy for the patients with resectable disease was 25 months, whereas the median survival of patients who had unresectable disease was 10 months (Fig. 61–24). There were no fixed guidelines with regard to the operative approach; however, after four median sternotomies, subsequent resections were performed by the lateral thoracotomy. The majority of these resections, despite reexploration, were wedge resections. A disease-free interval of more than 18 months between the first and second thoracotomies was associated with prolonged survival after the second thoracotomy. Other than resectability and disease-free interval (Fig. 61–25), no other factors in an unvaried analysis could foretell the long-term survival benefit.[83] A similar series of patients from the M.D. Anderson Cancer Center with adult soft tissue sarcoma have also been analyzed with regard to reoperative pulmonary metastasectomy. In the series of 39 patients undergoing two or more metastasectomies, a significantly longer median survival was found for the 34 patients whose recurrent metastases could be completely resected.[84] In that particular series, the only factor predicting longer postthoracotomy survival was the resection of a solitary metastatic nodule. Patients who had two or more recurrent nodules resected had a median survival of 14 months only.

METASTASECTOMY FOR SPECIFIC HISTOLOGIES

OSTEOGENIC SARCOMA

Before the use of aggressive resection of pulmonary metastases from osteogenic sarcoma, the survival of amputated patients was poor, with 5-year disease-free survival rates of 17% (Table 61–10).[85] The development of pulmonary metastases in 80% of these patients within the first year was associated with a 50% death rate in that first year after the primary resection. When resection was coupled with neoadjuvant or adjuvant programs including methotrexate, vincristine, and doxorubicin, a significant increase in salvage of these patients was documented by Telander at the Mayo Clinic (1946–1974: 5-year survival, 23%; versus 1974–1977: 5-year survival, 57%)[86] and Pastorini (1970–1983: 3-year survival, 20%; versus 1984–1988: 3-year survival, 46%).[87] It is impossible, however, to sort out the relative contribution of the intensive chemotherapeutic approach or the aggressive surgical resection to the prolongation of survival in these patients. The gen-

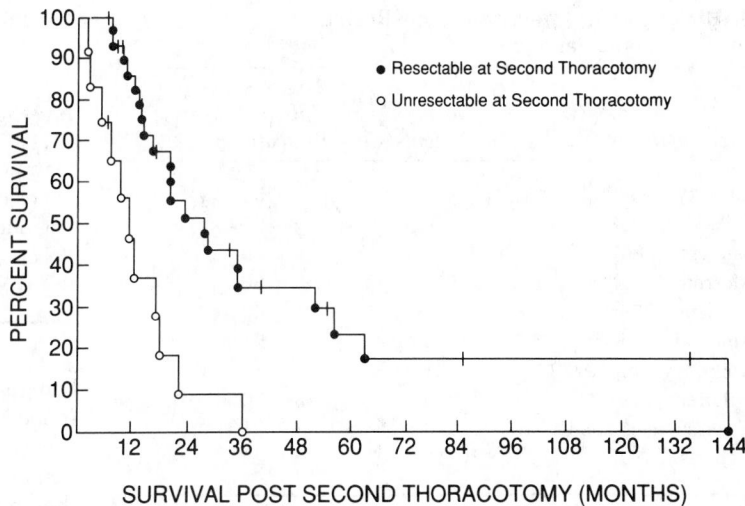

FIGURE 61–24.   Reoperative metastasectomy in patients with soft tissue sarcoma can provide long-term survival in completely resected individuals.

erally accepted 5-year salvage rate for osteogenic sarcoma is now 35% to 40%, justifying initial and repeated metastasectomies in this patient population.[24,68,88–95]

SOFT TISSUE SARCOMA

Metastases from soft tissue sarcomas occur within the first 2 years of the primary tumor management and are confined to the lung in the majority of patients. Multiple series have now documented that approximately a 33% salvage rate with aggressive or repeated metastasectomies can be accomplished (Table 61–11).[25,68,69,95–97] At the National Cancer Institute, two time periods with separate groups of patients have confirmed a 32% and 35% 3-year survival rate from the initial thoracotomy in the soft tissue sarcoma population.[25,69] The disease-free interval, the ability to render patients free of disease, and possibly the number of nodules in preoperative studies seem to correlate with survival. No correlation with the number of metastases resected has been seen in the most recent study of patients rendered free of disease with soft tissue sarcoma; therefore, there are no guidelines regarding an unresectable number of nodules as long as the patient has

been left with sufficient pulmonary reserve at the completion of the resection.

URINARY TRACT CANCER

Approximately half of all patients with renal cell cancer will present with or develop pulmonary metastases.[77] There have been multiple reports of the efficacy of resection of renal cell pulmonary metastases, with 5-year survival ranging from 13% to 50% and median survival ranging from 23 to 33 months (Table 61–12).[68,77,90,92,93] Unfortunately, however, in addition to analyzing patients having resection of pulmonary metastases, the majority of these studies also include patients who underwent resection of isolated extrapulmonary metastases in the brain, in bone, or in adrenal, subcutaneous, or other sites. Pogrebniak analyzed the results of metastasectomy in 23 patients who underwent resection of pulmonary metastases from renal cell carcinoma between 1985 and 1991.[77] Mean survival from exploration was 43 months, and survival after resection did not correlate with the number of nodules on preoperative tomograms, the number of nodules resected, or the disease-free interval. Patients who underwent complete

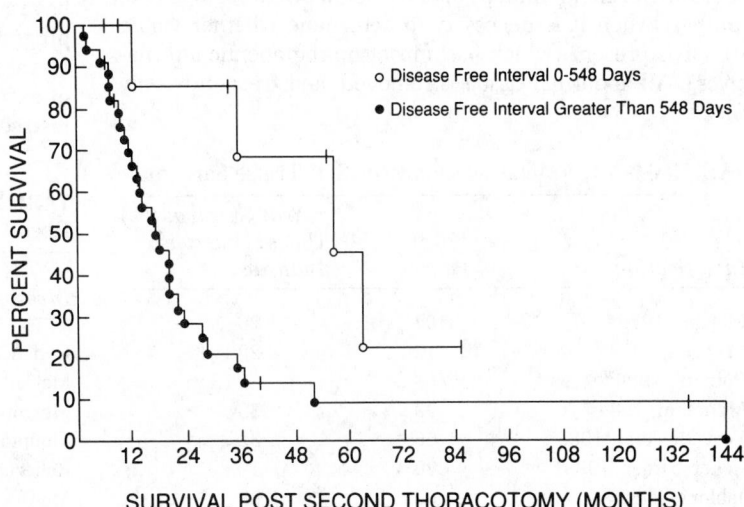

FIGURE 61–25.   A disease-free interval of more than 1.5 years between thoracotomies is associated with longer survivals in patients having re-resection of soft tissue sarcoma pulmonary metastases.

TABLE 61-10. Metastasectomy Results for Osteogenic Sarcoma

Investigations	No. of Patients	5-Year Survival (%) Unless Otherwise Indicated
Giritsky, 1986[88]	12	58 (3 y)
Telander, 1978[86]	28	57 (4 y)
Burgess, 1980[89]	6	60
Morrow, 1981[90]	11	36
Putnam, 1983[24]	39	40
Mountain, 1984[26]	56	51
Vogt-Moykopf, 1988[68]	41	33 (3 y)
DiLorenzo, 1988[94]	10	50
Eckersberger, 1988[95]	6	31
Roberts, 1989[93]	16	23

resection of metastatic disease had a significantly longer survival (mean of 49 months) than did patients who were incompletely resected (median of 16 months). There is no general agreement in other studies regarding the importance of synchronous versus metachronous lesions, number of nodules on preoperative studies, or number of nodules resected. The number of metastases resected in Pogrebniak's study did not correlate with survival as long as the patient could be rendered free of disease at exploration. The majority of the patients in Pogrebniak's studies received biologic modifiers (*i.e.*, interleukin-2 [IL-2]). The contribution of this therapy to long-term survival cannot be sorted out at this time, but future studies, specifically in renal cell cancer patients who receive immunotherapy, may point to synergistic benefits of treatment with immunotherapy and metastatic pulmonary resection.[98]

TESTICULAR CANCER

Nonseminomatous germ cell tumors of the testis are characterized by wide dissemination, including pulmonary metastases and extreme sensitivity to chemotherapy. Indications for thoracotomy in these patients are: (1) when there is no response to chemotherapy, (2) when there is partial response followed by recurrence while on chemotherapy, (3) when there are no chemotherapy options, but markers begin to rise, and (4) when it is necessary to determine whether viable tumor is present (which has impact on therapeutic alternatives). All abnormal tissue is removed, and frequently only

TABLE 61-11. Metastasectomy for Soft Tissue Sarcoma

Investigations	No. of Patients	5-Year Survival (%) Unless Otherwise Indicated
Martini, 1978[96]	102	26
Creagen, 1979[97]	112	29
Putnam, 1984[25]	63	30 (3 y)
Mountain, 1984[26]	49	33
Vogt-Moykopf, 1988[68]	56	33
Eckersberger, 1988[95]	29	18
Jablons, 1989[69]	68	33

TABLE 61-12. Metastasectomy for Urinary Tract Cancer

Investigations	No. of Patients	5-Year Survival (%) Unless Otherwise Indicated
Morrow, 1981[90]	30	24
Mountain, 1984[26]	20	54
Vogt-Moykopf, 1988[68]	42	42
Roberts, 1989[93]	33	24
Pogrebniak, 1991[77]	23	43 mo (mean)

benign teratomas (because of successful chemotherapy) are found.[68,75,90,92] In a recent report, 24 patients with both retroperitoneal disease and metastatic pulmonary disease of testicular germ cell cancer who received preoperative chemotherapy had synchronous sternotomy and retroperitoneal lymph node dissection.[99] Overall, chemotherapy altered metastases to mature teratomas in the majority of patients, and among 22 patients with necrotic masses, 19 were long-term survivors. The overall cure rate for patients with this disseminated testicular cancer was approximately 80%, and that of the entire thoracic surgical group was 74%.

HEAD AND NECK

With the exception of the lip, tonsil, and adenoid, the lung is the first site of recurrence for head and neck cancer including the nose, nasopharynx, larynx, mouth, tongue, salivary glands, and oropharynx. In these patients, there is a high prevalence for second primary lung cancers. Resection is indicated to rule out either the possibility of a new primary tumor or metastases, with 5-year salvage rates of close to 44%.[68,92,100]

COLORECTAL CANCER

A minority of patients with colorectal cancer (1%) will present with isolated pulmonary metastases (as opposed to the liver) as the first site of recurrence. Although certain authors have stressed a difference in survival when comparing resection of colon with resection of rectal metastases, most series have not separated their results, and survival rates are 13% to 61% (Table 61-13).[73,90,92,93,100,101] The largest series of patients has recently demonstrated a 5-year survival of 31%.[73] Poor prognostic indicators include more than one metastasis and elevated carcinoembryonic antigen. Aggressive management of extrapulmonary disease, in addition to the pulmonary metastases, also results in equal 5-year survival rates.

TABLE 61-13. Metastasectomy for Colon and Rectal Cancer

Invesigations	No. of Patients	5-Year Survival (%)
Cahan, 1974[101]	31	31
McCormack, 1979[103]	40	15
Morrow, 1981[90]	16	13
Mountain, 1984[26]	28	28
Roberts, 1989[93]	13	23
McAfee, 1991[73]	139	30

BREAST

Approximately 21% of breast cancer patients will die of isolated metastases to the lung that were potentially resectable during the course of the disease, and despite the large number of cases of breast cancer, there are few reports concerning the efficacy of metastasis resection. Mountain and colleagues originally reported a 5-year survival rate of 27%,[92] while Wright[102] and McCormack[103] had 5-year survival rates of 27% and 30%, respectively. A recent series from the M.D. Anderson Cancer Center reports a 50% 5-year survival in 37 patients after complete resection of their metastatic breast cancer.[74] A disease-free interval of more than 1 year correlated with enhanced survival. Such increases in survival may also relate to improved and more intensive chemotherapy regimens, yet the individual contributions of surgery and chemotherapy cannot be separated.

MELANOMA

As seen in Table 61–14, metastasectomy for malignant melanoma has been generally unrewarding.[90,92,104,105] This has been recently documented at the National Cancer Institute, where 49 patients had resection of presumed pulmonary metastases from melanoma between 1970 and 1986.[106] Median survival for all patients with malignant disease was 13 months, and survival after resection did not correlate with Clark level, lymph node status, disease-free interval, or number of nodules on preoperative tomogram. Two of 10 patients with one nodule

TABLE 61–14. Metastasectomy for Other Histologies

Investigations	No. of Patients	5-Year Survival (%) Unless Otherwise Indicated
Testicular Cancer		
Morrow, 1981[90]	6	30
Mountain, 1984[26]	20	54
Venn, 1989[75]	42	84
Vogt-Moykopf, 1988[68]	42	82 (2 y)
Head and Neck Cancers		
McCormack, 1979[103]	25	44
Mountain, 1984[26]	48	41
Vogt-Moykopf, 1988[68]	12	44
Uterine–Cervical Cancer		
Morrow, 1981[90]	22	8
Mountain, 1984[26]	34	24
Breast Cancer		
McCormack, 1979[103]	34	30
Mountain, 1984[26]	30	27
Wright, 1982[102]	18	27
Lanza, 1991[74]	37	50
Melanoma		
Morrow, 1981[90]	12	12
Dahlback, 1980[104]	8	7-mo median
Cahan, 1973[105]	12	33
Mountain, 1984[26]	58	13-mo median
Pogrebniak, 1988[106]	33	13-mo median

resected were long-term survivors. Nevertheless, 16 patients were found to have only benign disease, despite the appearance of a new nodule in 13. Hence, exploration in patients with presumed metastases from melanoma may be justified simply to rule out benign disease, even if a new solitary nodule is detected. In general, however, the multiplicity of nodules, as well as the unfavorable natural history independent of pulmonary disease, rules out melanoma as a favorable histology for metastasectomy.

REFERENCES

1. Willis RA. Secondary tumors of the lung. In: The spread of tumors in the human body. London: Butterworths, 1973:167–174.
2. Pass HI, Dwyer A, Makuch R, Roth JA. Detection of pulmonary metastases in patients with osteogenic and soft tissue sarcoma: The superiority of CT scan compared with conventional linear tomograms using dynamic analyses. J Clin Oncol 1985;3:1261–1265.
3. Viadana E, Irwin D, Bross J, Pickren JW. Cascade spread of blood-borne metastases in solid and non-solid cancers of humans. In: Weiss L, Gilbert H, eds. Pulmonary metastasis. Boston: GK Hall, 1978:143–167.
4. van Dongen JA, van Slooten EA. The surgical treatment of pulmonary metastases. Cancer Treat Rep 1978;5:29–48.
5. Barney JD, Churchill ED. Adeno-carcinoma of the kidney with metastasis to the lungs treated by pulmonary resection. J Urol 1939;42:269–276.
6. Alexander J, Haight C. Pulmonary resection for solitary metastatic sarcomas and carcinomas. Surg Gynecol Obstet 1947;85:129–135.
7. Thomford NR, Wodner LB, Clagett OT. The surgical treatment of metastatic tumors in the lungs. J Thorac Cardiovasc Surg 1965;49:357–363.
8. Martini N, Huvos AG, Mike V, et al. Multiple pulmonary resections in the treatment of osteogenic sarcoma. Ann Thorac Surg 1971;12:271–280.
9. Morton DL, Joseph WL, Ketcham AS, et al. Surgical resection and adjunctive immunotherapy for selected patients with multiple pulmonary metastases. Ann Surg 1973;178:360–365.
10. Liotta LA, Kleinerman J, Saidel FM. The significance of hematogenous tumor cell clumps in the metastatic process. Cancer Res 1976;36:889.
11. Dwyer AJ, Reichert CM, Woltering EA, et al. Diffuse pulmonary metastasis in melanoma: Radiographic pathologic correlation. AJR 1984;143:983.
12. Libshitz HI, North LB. Pulmonary metastases. Radiol Clin North Am 1982;20:437.
13. Berg HK, Petrelli NJ, Herrera L, et al. Endobronchial metastasis from colorectal carcinoma. Dis Colon Rectum 1984;27:745.
14. Shapshay SM, Strong MS. Tracheobronchial obstruction from metastatic distant malignancies. Ann Otol Rhinol Laryngol 1982;91:648.
15. Janower ML, Blennerhassett HJB. Lymphangitic spread of metastatic cancer to the lung. Radiology 1971;101:267.
16. Heitzman ER, Markarian B, Raasch BN, et al. Pathways of tumor spread through the lung: Radiologic correlations with anatomy and pathology. Radiology 1982;144:3.
17. Naidich DP, Zerhouni EA, Siegelman SS. Pleura and chest wall. In: Naidich DP, Zerhouni EA, Siegelman SS, eds. New York: Raven Press, 1984:261.
18. Cahan WG, Shah JP, Castro ELB. Benign solitary lung lesions in patients with cancer. Ann Surg 1978;187:241.
19. Roth JA, Pass HI, Wesley MN, et al. Comparison of median sternotomy and thoracotomy for resection of pulmonary metastases in patients with adult soft tissue sarcomas. Ann Thorac Surg 1986;42:134.
20. Hendin AS. Gestational trophoblastic tumors metastatic to the lung. Cancer 1984;53:58.
21. Wagner D. Trophoblastic cells in the blood stream in normal and abnormal pregnancy. Acta Cytol 1968;12:137.
22. Crow J, Slavin G, Kreel L. Pulmonary metastasis: A pathologic and radiologic study. Cancer 1981;47:2595.
23. Scholten ET, Kreel L. Distribution of lung metastases in the axial plane. Radiol Clin North Am 1977;46:248.
24. Putnam JB, Roth JA, Wesley MN, et al. Survival following aggressive resection of pulmonary metastases from osteogenic sarcoma: Analysis of prognostic factors. Ann Thorac Surg 1983;36:516.
25. Putnam JB, Roth JA, Wesley MN, et al. Analysis of prognostic factors in patients undergoing resection of pulmonary metastasis from soft tissue sarcomas. J Thorac Cardiovasc Surg 1984;87:260.
26. Mountain C. Surgery for pulmonary metastasis. Ann Thorac Surg 1984;38:323.
27. D'Angio GJ, Iannoccone G. Spontaneous pneumothorax as a complication of pulmonary metastases in malignant tumors of childhood. AJR 1961;86:1092.
28. Lodmell EA, Capps SC. Spontaneous pneumothorax associated with metastatic sarcoma: Report of three cases. Radiology 1949;52:88.
29. Macklin MT, Macklin CC. Malignant interstitial emphysema of the lungs and mediastinum as an important occult complication in many respiratory diseases and other conditions. Medicine 1944;23:281.
30. Lome LG, John T. Pulmonary manifestations of prostatic carcinoma. J Urol 1973;109:680.
31. Schwarz MI, Waddell LC, Dombeck DH, et al. Prolonged survival in lymphangitic carcinomatosis. Ann Intern Med 1969;71:779.

32. Sarno RC, Carter BL. Bullous change by CT heralding metastatic sarcoma. Comput Radiol 1985;9:115.

33. Morse D, Reed JO, Bernstein J. Sclerosing osteogenic sarcoma. AJR 1963;88:491.

34. Fraser RG, Pare JAP. Neoplastic disease of the lung. In: Fraser RG, Pare JAP, eds. Diagnosis of diseases of the chest. Philadelphia: WB Saunders, 1989:1630.

35. Zollikofer C, Castaneda-Zuniga W, Stenlund R, et al. Lung metastases from synovial sarcoma simulating granulomas. AJR 1980;135:161.

36. Rosenfield AT, Sanders RC, Custer LE. Widespread calcified metastases from adenocarcinoma of the jejunum. Am J Dig Dis 1975;20:990.

37. Fraley EE, Lange PH, Kennedy BJ. Germ cell testicular cancer in adults. N Engl J Med 1979;301:1370.

38. Panella J, Mintzer RA. Multiple calcified pulmonary nodules in an elderly man. JAMA 1980;244:2559.

39. King DS, Castleman B. Bronchial involvement in metastatic pulmonary malignancy. J Thorac Surg 1943;12:305.

40. Braman SS, Whitcomb ME. Endobronchial metastases. Arch Intern Med 1975;135:543.

41. Shepherd MP. Endobronchial metastatic disease. Thorax 1982;37:362.

42. Pass HI, Roth JA. Diagnosis of pulmonary metastases. In: Rosenberg SA, ed. Surgical treatment of metastatic cancer. Philadelphia: JB Lippincott, 1987:37–67.

43. Cohen M, Grosfeld J, Baehner R, et al. Lung CT for detection of metastases: Solid tissue neoplasms in children. AJR 1982;139:895.

44. Piekarski JD, Schlumberger M, Leclere J, et al. Chest computed tomography (CT) in patients with micronodular lung metastases of differentiated thyroid carcinoma. Int J Radiat Oncol Biol Phys 1985;11:1023.

45. Lund G, Heilo A. Computed tomography of pulmonary metastases. Acta Radiol 1982;23:617.

46. Sones PJ, Torres WE, Colvin RS, et al. Effectiveness of CT in evaluating intrathoracic masses. AJR 1982;139:469.

47. Krudy AG, Doppman JL, Herdt JR. Failure to detect a 1.5 cm lung nodule by chest computed tomography. J Comput Assist Tomogr 1982;6:1178.

48. Kuhns LR, Borlaza G. The "twinkling star" sign. An aid in differentiating pulmonary vessels from pulmonary nodules on computed tomograms. Radiology 1980;135:763.

49. Chiles C, Ravin CE. Intrathoracic metastasis from an extrathoracic malignancy: A radiographic approach to patient evaluation. Radiol Clin North Am 1985;23:427.

50. Feuerstein I, Jicha D, Pass HI, et al. A comparison of computerized tomography and magnetic resonance imaging for diagnosis of pulmonary metastases. Radiology 1992;182:123–129.

51. Vincent RG, Choksi LB, Takita H, et al. Surgical resection of the solitary pulmonary metastasis. In: Weiss L, Gilbert HA, eds. Pulmonary metastases. Boston: GK Hall, 1978:224.

52. Johnston WW. Percutaneous fine needle aspiration biopsy of the lung: A study of 1,015 patients. Acta Cytol 1984;28:218.

53. Poellein S, Rothenberg J, Penkava RR. Metastatic malignant melanoma in the lung: Diagnosis by thin-needle aspiration biopsy. Arch Pathol Lab Med 1982;106:119.

54. Pilotti S, Rilke F, Gribaudi G, et al. Transthoracic fine needle aspiration biopsy in pulmonary lesions, updated results. Acta Cytol 1984;28:225.

55. Silverman JF, Weaver MD, Gardner EW, et al. Aspiration biopsy cytology of malignant schwannoma metastatic to the lung. Acta Cytol 1984;29:15.

56. Nieberg RK. Fine needle aspiration cytology of alveolar soft-part sarcoma. Acta Cytol 1984;228:198.

57. Nguyen GK, Jeannot A. Cytopathologic aspects of pulmonary metastasis of malignant fibrous histiocytoma, myxoid variant. Acta Cytol 1982;26:349.

58. Crosby JH, Hager B, Hoeg K. Transthoracic fine-needle aspiration. Cancer 1985;56:2504.

59. Nordenstrom BEW. Technical aspects of obtaining cellular material from lesions deep in the lung. Acta Cytol 1984;28:233.

60. Page RD, Jeffrey RR, Donnelly RJ. Thoracoscopy: A review of 121 consecutive surgical procedures. Ann Thorac Surg 1989;48:66–68.

61. Bonniot JP, Homasson JF, Roden SL, Angebault ML, Renault PC. Pleural and lung cryobiopsies during thoracoscopy. Chest 1989;95:492–493.

62. Lewis RJ, Caccavale RJ, Sisler GE. Special report: Video-endoscopic thoracic surgery. N J Med 1991;88:473–475.

63. Inderbitzi R, Molnar J. Experiences in the diagnostic and surgical video-endoscopy of the thoracic cavity. Schweiz Med Wochenschr 1990;120:51–52.

64. Dresdale A, Bonow RO, Wesley R, et al. Prospective evaluation of doxorubicin-induced cardiomyopathy resulting from post-surgical adjuvant treatment of patients with soft tissue sarcomas. Cancer 1983;52:51–60.

65. Gottindiener JS, Mathisen DJ, Borer JS, et al. Doxorubicin cardiotoxicity: Assessment of late left ventricular dysfunction by radionuclide cineangiography. Ann Intern Med 1981;94:430–435.

66. Mason JW, Bristow MR, Billingham ME, et al. Invasive and noninvasive methods of assessing Adriamycin cardiotoxic effects in man: Superiority of histopathologic assessment using endomyocardial biopsy. Cancer Treat Rep 1978;62:857–864.

67. Boysen PG, Block AJ, Olsen GN, et al. Prospective evaluation for pneumonectomy using the 99m technetium quantitative perfusion lung scan. Chest 1977;72:422–425.

68. Vogt-Moykopf I, Bulzebruck H, Merkle NM, Probst G. Results of surgical treatment of pulmonary metastases. Eur J Cardiothorac Surg 1988;2:224–232.

69. Jablons D, Steinberg SM, Roth J, Pittaluga S, Rosenberg SA, Pass HI. Metastasectomy for soft tissue sarcoma. J Thorac Cardiovasc Surg 1989;97:695–705.

70. Pastorini U, Valente M, Gasparini M, et al. Median sternotomy and multiple lung resections for metastatic sarcomas. Eur J Cardiothorac Surg 1990;4:477–481.

71. Lanza LA, Miser JS, Pass HI, Roth JA. The role of resection in the treatment of pulmonary metastases from Ewing's sarcoma. J Thorac Cardiovasc Surg 1987;94:181–187.

72. Regal A-M, Reese P, Antkowiak J, Hart T, Takita H. Median sternotomy for metastatic lung lesions in 131 patients. Cancer 1985;55:1334–1339.

73. McAfee MK, Allen MS, Trastek VF, Ilstrup DM, Deschamps C, Pairolero PC. Colorectal lung metastases: Results of surgical excision. Ann Thorac Surg 1992;53:780–786.

74. Lanza LA, Natarajan G, Roth JA, Putnam JB Jr. Long-term survival following resection of pulmonary metastases from carcinoma of the breast. Ann Thorac Surg 1992;54:244–247.

75. Venn GE, Sarin S, Goldstraw P. Survival following pulmonary metastasectomy. Eur J Cardiothorac Surg 1989;3:105–110.

76. Linard D, Rocmans P, Lejeune FJ. Resection of lung metastases from sarcomas. Eur J Surg Oncol 1989;15:530–534.

77. Pogrebniak HW, Haas G, Linehan WM, Rosenberg SA, Pass HI. Renal cell carcinoma: Resection of solitary and multiple metastases. Ann Thorac Surg 1992;54:33–38.

78. Joseph WL, Morton DL, Adkins PC. Prognostic significance of smear tumor time in evaluating operability in pulmonary metastatic disease. J Thorac Cardiovasc Surg 1971;61:23–32.

79. Takita H, Edgerton F, Karakousis C, et al. Surgical management of metastases to the lung. Surg Gynecol Obstet 1981;152:191–194.

80. Yellin A, Lieberman Y. Surgery for pulmonary metastases: Review of literature and experience at the Shaba Medical Center. In: Martini N, Vogt-Moykopf I, eds. Thoracic surgery: Frontiers and uncommon neoplasms. St. Louis: CV Mosby, 1989:275–284.

81. Lanza LA, Putnam JB Jr, Benjamin RS, Roth JA. Response to chemotherapy does not predict survival after resection of sarcomatous pulmonary metastases. Ann Thorac Surg 1991;51:219–224.

82. Rizzoni WE, Pass HI, Wesley MN, et al. Reoperative pulmonary metastasectomies in patients with adult soft-tissue sarcomas. Ann Thorac Surg 1986;121:1248–1252.

83. Pogrebniak HW, Roth JA, Steinberg SM, Rosenberg SA, Pass HI. Reoperative pulmonary resection in patients with metastatic soft tissue sarcoma. Ann Thorac Surg 1991;52:197–203.

84. Casson AG, Putnam JB, Natarajan G, et al. Efficacy of pulmonary metastasectomy for recurrent soft tissue sarcoma. J Surg Oncol 1991;47:1–4.

85. Marcove RC, Mike V, Hajek JV, et al. Osteogenic sarcoma under the age of 21: A review of 145 operative cases. J Bone Joint Surg 1970;52:411–421.

86. Telander RL, Pairolero PC, Pritchard DJ. Resection of pulmonary metastatic osteogenic sarcoma in children. Surgery 1978;84:335–341.

87. Pastorini U, Valente M, Santoro A, et al. Results of salvage surgery for metastatic sarcomas. Annals of Oncology 1990;1:269–273.

88. Gritsky AS, Etcubanas E, Mark JBD. Pulmonary resection in children with metastatic osteogenic sarcoma. J Thorac Surg 1986;75:354–362.

89. Burgers JMV, Breur K, Van Dobbenburgh OA, et al. Role of metastasectomy without chemotherapy in the management of osteosarcoma in children. Cancer 1980;45:1664–1668.

90. Morrow CE, Vassilopoulos P, Grage TB. Surgical resection for metastatic neoplasms of the lung. Cancer 1981;45:2981–2985.

91. Meyer WH, Schell MJ, Kumar AP, et al. Thoracotomy for pulmonary metastatic osteosarcoma: An analysis of prognostic indicators of survival. Cancer 1987;59:374–379.

92. Mountain CF, McMurtrey MJ, Hermes KE. Surgery for pulmonary metastases: A 20-year experience. Ann Thorac Surg 1984;38:323.

93. Roberts DG, Lepore V, Cardillo G, Dernevik L, et al. Long-term follow-up of operative treatment for pulmonary metastases. Eur J Cardiothorac Surg 1989;3:292–296.

94. DiLorenzo M, Collin PP. Pulmonary metastases in children: Results of surgical treatment. J Pediatr Surg 1988;23:762–765.

95. Eckersberger F, Moritz E, Wolner E. Results and prognostic factors after resection of pulmonary metastases. Eur J Cardiothorac Surg 1988;2:433–437.

96. Martini N, McCormack PM, Bains MS, et al. Surgery for solitary and multiple pulmonary metastasis. N Y State J Med 1978;78:1711–1713.

97. Creagan ET, Fleming TR, Edmonson JH, Pairolero PC. Pulmonary resection for metastatic nonosteogenic sarcoma. Cancer 1979;44:1908–1912.

98. Sherry RM, Pass HI, Rosenberg SA, Yang JC. Surgical resection of metastatic renal cell carcinoma and melanoma after response to interleukin-2 based immunotherapy. Cancer 1992;69:1850–1855.

99. Mandelbaum I, Yaw PB, Einhorn LH, Williams SD, et al. The importance of one-stage median sternotomy and retroperitoneal node dissection in disseminated testicular cancer. Ann Thorac Surg 1983;36:524–528.

100. McCormack PM, Attiyeh FF. Resection of pulmonary metastases from colorectal cancer. Dis Colon Rectum 1979;22:553–556.

101. Cahan WG, Castro EB, Hajdu SI. The significance of a solitary lung shadow in patients with colon carcinoma. Cancer 1974;33:414–421.

102. Wright JO, Brandt B, Ehrenhaft JL. Results of pulmonary resection for metastatic lesions. J Thorac Cardiovasc Surg 1982;83:94–99.

103. McCormack PM, Martini N. The changing role of surgery for pulmonary metastases. Ann Thorac Surg 1979;41:833–840.

104. Dahlback O, Hafstrom L, Johnsson PE, et al. Lung resection for metastatic melanoma. Clin Oncol 1980;6:15–20.

105. Cahan WG. Excision of melanoma metastases to lung: Problems in diagnosis and management. Ann Surg 1973;178:703–709.

106. Pogrebniak HW, Stovroff M, Roth JsA, Pass HI. Resection of pulmonary metastases from malignant melanoma: Results of a 16-year experience. Ann Thorac Surg 1988;46:20–23.

JOHN E. NIEDERHUBER
WILLIAM D. ENSMINGER

SECTION **3**

Treatment of Metastatic Cancer to the Liver

The spread of malignant cells from a primary tumor to the liver and their growth therein carry a grave prognosis for the patient. While these metastatic liver tumors may be the first evidence of the progression of a patient's cancer, and often—especially in colorectal cancer—are the only tumors detected, they almost always signal widespread dissemination of the malignancy. Despite improvements in early detection of liver metastases, new drug development, improved surgical techniques for resection, and innovative targeted therapies, most patients will not survive.

In spite of the gravity of the diagnosis of liver metastases, those responsible for treating such patients know of the occasional success of surgical resection with resultant long-term survival. It is this observation more than any other that has suggested the existence of at least a subset of patients whose metastases reach biologic significance only in their liver. The existence of such a subset of patients has been essentially the exclusive property of colorectal cancer. As such, it has been the rationale behind much of the effort to provide long-term survival and even cure for patients with isolated liver metastases by aggressive resection of their metastases and by innovative regional infusion of active agents.

An extensive literature documents the history of these efforts now spanning several decades. The task here is to provide a meaningful and timely review.

LIVER METASTASES FROM COLORECTAL CANCER

INCIDENCE

In 1992, more than 150,000 Americans will be diagnosed with colorectal cancer, and over 60,000 will die from this tumor. The incidence of colorectal cancer remains quite constant and is exceeded only by cancers of the breast, lung, and prostate.[1] At the time of diagnosis, 15% to 25% will have hepatic metastases, and another 20% to 30% will develop metastatic lesions subsequent to resection of their primary tumors. Ultimately, at least 50% of these 150,000 patients will die secondary to metastatic disease, and for many, progressive involvement of the liver will be a major determinant, or the only determinant, of their survival.[1-4] Although the overall mortality from colorectal cancer has decreased in recent years, patients with metastatic disease continue to face a grim prognosis.

NATURAL HISTORY

Metastatic tumors to the liver develop a rich blood supply and tend to grow rapidly. The natural progression of these lesions depends on a number of factors, including primary histologic type, extent of hepatic involvement, physiologic status of the liver parenchyma, and growth properties of the tumor cells. In addition, the extent of the primary lesion and whether local recurrences can be prevented (especially for rectal cancer) affect the overall survival of the patient.[5-9] Left untreated, metastatic lesions to the liver from colorectal cancers are associated with survival of 3 to 24 months.

Hepatic resection of colorectal metastases may be the only hope for "cure" in a select subgroup of patients. As a result, it has been difficult to subject patients with potentially "curable" hepatic metastases to prospective randomized trials where these lesions are left untreated in order to determine the natural progression of the disease and the ultimate survival benefit of resection. Historically, high operative mortality and morbidity rates associated with hepatic resections discouraged many physicians and surgeons from offering resection as a treatment option. Retrospective reviews, therefore, have provided some insight into the natural history of these lesions by analyzing groups of patients with tumors that would now be deemed "resectable" (Table 61–15).[2,7-19]

Table 61–15 summarizes multiple reports illustrating the poor clinical outcome in patients with intrahepatic metastases from colorectal cancers not surgically resected. It is important to note that these collective data are not categorized by extent of the primary lesions or extent of hepatic involvement. In some reports, patients with extensive metastatic disease (both intrahepatic and extrahepatic) were included. Although there are anecdotal reports of long-term survivors with hepatic lesions left untreated, it is clear from these reports that most patients die within 2 years of diagnosis—median survival for cited reviews is 6 months.[2,7-20] It is of interest to note that the recently published series have patients with longer median length of survival. This most likely reflects earlier detection of metastatic lesions secondary to the use of newer diagnostic modalities, and more aggressive monitoring of patients after resection of their primary tumor.

TABLE 61–15. Survival of Patients With Intrahepatic Colorectal Metastases

Investigations	No. of Patients	Median Survival (mo)	5-Year Survivors
Steele, 1991[7]	47	16.5	NA
Scheele, 1990[10]	983	6.9–14.2	0
Finan, 1985[11]	86	8–15.5	0
Wagner, 1984[12]	252	11–21	<5%
Lahr, 1983[13]	147	4.5–12	1
Goslin, 1982[9]	125	10–24	0
Boey, 1981[14]	73	6–9	0
Bengtsson, 1981[15]	25	3–6	0
Wood, 1976[2]	113	3–17	1
Baden, 1975[16]	105	10	1
Abrams, 1971[17]	58	7	0
Cady, 1970[8]	241	13	2
Bengmark, 1970[18]	38	6 (mean)	0
Sterns, 1954[19]	22	11	1

NA, not available.

DIAGNOSIS

The largest solid organ in the human body is the liver, and it is the most common site for many hematogenously disseminated tumors, with gastrointestinal tumors being the most frequent.[21-27] Modern modalities have aided early detection of colonic lesions, but until recently, secondary hepatic tumors were frequently diagnosed at advanced stages.

Physical findings and clinical symptoms are, perhaps, the least accurate means of diagnosing liver involvement by metastatic tumors. Clinical symptoms such as ascites, jaundice, and pain associated with large or rapidly growing hepatic tumors are a late and ominous sign. Other physical signs of metastatic disease, such as palpable nodularity at the liver edge or an audible bruit, are also late findings, and all carry a dismal prognosis, with most patients dying soon after diagnosis.[2,12,18,21]

Laboratory measurements of various tumor markers and liver enzymes are easily obtainable, and many patients can be screened with little expense and relative ease. Among those most commonly used are γ-glutamyl transpeptidase, aspartate aminotransferase, alkaline phosphatase, and carcinoembryonic antigen (CEA). Even though Wanebo and colleagues reported elevated CEA levels in approximately 90% of patients with metastases from colorectal cancer, most authors have been unable to correlate the extent of CEA elevation with prognosis.[7,28-30] Although there is some controversy as to the prognostic significance of these various laboratory values, CEA levels can be especially helpful when tracking patients after primary tumor resection and may be the first indication of potential recurrence of metastasis.

Preoperative assessment of liver function is often difficult when clinical evidence of cirrhosis is absent. Many authors have studied liver enzyme tests in an attempt to quantitate parenchymal reserve; however, it remains difficult to correlate these laboratory tests with capacity of the liver parenchyma to regenerate after resection. A multivariate regression analysis by Lahr and colleagues showed that abnormal liver function tests are independent factors that may predict median survival of patients with colorectal metastases to the liver.[13] They found that hyperbilirubinemia (1–5 mg/dl) was associated with a median survival of 2.5 months and a 1-year survival rate of 7%. Elevated alkaline phosphatase levels also predicted a poor prognosis, with a median survival of 2.5 months compared with 9.2 months in patients with normal values.[13,29] A commonly used assessment of liver function in selecting patients and assessing operative risk relies on Child's classification, and patients judged as Child's class A or B (Table 61–16) have a better prognosis.[64-66]

Improvements in radiographic studies of the liver, such as preoperative and intraoperative ultrasonography, contrast-enhanced computed tomography (CT), magnetic resonance imaging (MRI), and arteriography, have helped define the extent of metastatic disease and have aided the surgeon in planning resection of potentially "curable" lesions.

Ultrasound is the least expensive noninvasive radiologic test available to aid in the diagnosis of intrahepatic disease. Ultrasonic examination is highly dependent on the sophistication of the equipment used and the experience of the clinician interpreting the findings. In addition, results may vary in relation to patient obesity, amount of "bowel gas," and inability to detect lesions in anatomic regions of the liver that may be

TABLE 61–16. Assessment of Liver Function With the Modified Child Classification

Parameter	Score		
	1	2	3
Serum bilirubin (mg/100 ml)	1–2	2–3	>3
Albumin (g/L)	>35	28–35	<28
Prothrombin time (seconds prolonged)	1–4	4–6	>6
Encephalopathy (grade)	—	1–2	3–4
Ascites	Absent	Slight	Moderate

Child group equivalents: A, 5–6 points; B, 7–9 points; C, 10–15 points. (Pugh RNH, Murray-Lyon IM, Danson JL, Pietroni MC, Williams R. Transsection of esophagus for bleeding varices. Br J Surg 1973;60: 646)

difficult to image. Nonetheless, preoperative ultrasound is very effective in detecting tumors 1 to 2 cm in size and in distinguishing solid from cystic (possibly benign) lesions.

Ultrasonic guidance is frequently used for directing percutaneous needle biopsies to obtain histologic diagnosis before operation. Intraoperative ultrasound can be extremely helpful in guiding the surgeon through segmental resections and can often identify metastases 2 to 4 mm in size deep within the liver parenchyma that would be missed by palpation. Recent experience with intraoperative ultrasound has supported the importance of this modality as the definitive step in assessing resectability.[22,31,36,70-72]

The early-generation CT scanners and many present scanners can detect intrahepatic lesions approximately 1 to 2 cm in diameter, but it is not uncommon for metastases to be missed on routine scanning. Enhancement of intraabdominal CT scans with intravenous contrast agents improves these results, and smaller liver tumors (0.5 cm) may be reliably detected.[32,67] Caution must be used when employing intravenous dyes because they can be associated with severe allergic reactions. CT scan also allows for assessment of other potential sites of metastases (i.e., celiac, perihepatic, paraaortic lymph nodes, etc.) that may preclude or alter the possibility of a "curative" resection.

Magnetic resonance imaging can be very useful in visualizing hepatic tumors, and, as with CT, these images can be enhanced with specific contrast agents.[33-35] The role of MRI in the screening and staging of metastatic lesions in the liver is an evolving one, and determining surgical resectability of limited hepatic metastases by preoperative radiographic studies is an area of intense research. Several investigators have compared the sensitivity and specificity of CT versus MRI scans.[35,67-69] For example, Sitzmann and colleagues compared MRI, arteriographically enhanced CT, and routine CT screening of 100 patients with suspected hepatic metastases.[34] Enhanced CT (with portal arteriography) detected 94% of lesions, compared with 70% by MRI and 66% by routine CT. In particular, the sensitivity of enhanced CT was significantly greater than the sensitivity of MRI for lesions ≤1 cm (82% versus 20%). MRI, however, was significantly more accurate than CT in demonstrating vascular involvement.[67]

Some authors recommend MRI in the initial evaluation of hepatic lesions when trying to distinguish benign cysts or hemangiomas from malignant disease. There are several advantages to MRI in this setting: (1) intravenous contrast agents are not always needed, and (2) MRI can distinguish between benign and malignant tumors with a high degree of specificity (93%) and sensitivity (89%).[67,68] New techniques using superparamagnetic particulate iron oxide contrast agents are being studied to increase the accuracy of MRI scanning in detecting small metastatic hepatic lesions.[35,69]

The role of scintigraphy and angiography in the preoperative evaluation of hepatic tumors has changed dramatically because of the improvements in CT, MRI, and ultrasound. The present and future focus of research with scintigraphy is to develop immunologic markers that can be used to aid in the clinical staging of patients with metastatic disease.[37,38] A recent multicenter study demonstrated that radiolabeled antibody imaging may be helpful as an adjunct in the preoperative assessment of patients with colorectal cancer. Immunoscintigraphy was used in 116 patients and correlated with the pathologic diagnoses in 70% of patients with metastases and 90% of patients who were disease free.[38] Although these new techniques have limited clinical significance at this time, they may soon serve as a useful tool in the preoperative workup of patients with malignant disease.

Knowledge of arterial and venous structures before hepatic resection is most helpful when embarking on segmental or anatomic resections, whereas wedge resection of peripheral lesions does not necessarily require preoperative angiography. Preoperative angiography continues to be the best method of determining arterial anatomy and assessing tumor involvement of hepatic vein(s) or the portal venous system.

Although these radiologic tests are extremely useful in determining the stage and extent of disease, they should be used selectively. In most situations it will not be necessary to use multiple imaging techniques for the accurate evaluation of patients with colonic tumors or with metastases to the liver.

The imaging methods described are critical to the decision of recommending operative exploration, but the most accurate assessment of hepatic metastases occurs at the time of laparotomy when the surgeon can palpate all areas of the liver. An experienced surgeon can palpate most superficial lesions and some deeper lesions (particularly those in the left lobe). Intraoperative ultrasonography can detect lesions 2 to 4 mm in diameter within the liver parenchyma.[71] Intraoperative ultrasonic evaluation of hepatic tumors can delineate the extent of tumor invasion, can illustrate relations to vital vascular and biliary structures, and can be used to direct needle biopsies of intrahepatic lesions.

Use of an appropriate combination of imaging techniques provides the best opportunity for early detection and subsequent resection of small metastatic tumors. Earlier surgical intervention combined with second-line adjuvant therapy could increase overall survival of these patients.

TREATMENT OPTIONS

Treatment options for hepatic metastases include aggressive surgical resection of all gross tumor, administration of regional chemotherapeutic agents, arterial embolization, systemic chemotherapy, radiotherapy, or other palliative and investigational procedures.[53,73–80] To date, the only means shown to prolong survival in patients with limited metastatic disease from colorectal cancer (potential for "cure") is surgical re-

section.[7] Future combinations of treatment modalities may ultimately define other options as well. Unfortunately, fewer than 10% of patients with metastatic colorectal cancers are candidates for surgical resection.[4] To determine the feasibility and potential benefit from hepatic resection of secondary tumors, a thorough preoperative evaluation is essential. Systemic treatment of liver metastases and other locoregional therapeutic options are addressed in subsequent sections of this chapter.

LIVER METASTASES FROM NONCOLORECTAL TUMORS

A clear understanding of the properties that allow tumor cells to become blood borne and establish a new nest of tumor cells (metastasize) does not exist. There is, however, no doubt that many tumors have a propensity for implantation and growth within the liver. Although primary tumors arising from the gastrointestinal tract are the ones most likely to invade the liver, many other secondary tumors are detected as isolated liver metastases or as part of disseminated tumor. Once diagnosis of these lesions is established, the natural history of these tumors lends an equally grim or worse prognosis than

TABLE 61–17. Histology of Hepatic Metastases Resected in 153 Patients

Type of Lesion	No. of Patients
Secondary hepatic malignancy	153
Colorectal cancer	118
Intestinal cancer	6
Carcinoid	4
Spindle cell sarcoma	1
Leiomyosarcoma	1
Kidney cancer	5
Renal cell cancer	3
Wilms' tumor	2
Adrenal cancer	5
Adrenocortical carcinoma	4
Neuroblastoma	1
Breast cancer	4
Adenocarcinoma	2
Comedocarcinoma	1
Angiosarcoma	1
Gastric leiomyosarcoma	2
Ovarian adenocarcinoma	2
Uterus cancer	2
Squamous cell cancer	1
Endometrial sarcoma	1
Melanoma	2
Glucagonoma, pancreas	1
Leiomyosarcoma, rectum	1
Thyroid medullary carcinoma	1
Ewing's sarcoma	1
Mesothelioma	1
Rhabdomyosarcoma, colon	1
Adenocarcinoma, stomach	1

(Iwatsuki S, Sheahan DG, Starzl TE. The changing face of hepatic resection. Curr Probl Surg 1989;26[5]:283–379)

TABLE 61–18. Survival After Liver Resection of Noncolorectal, Nonendocrine Liver Metastases

Cancer Type	Postoperative Survivors	5-Year Survivors	Died of Recurrence After 5 Years
Wilms' tumor[12,13,16,18]	20	6 (14, 17 y)	?
Renal cell cancer[12,13,15–17]	11	3 (5 y, 7 y, and 12 y)	0
Adrenal carcinoma[12,16,19]	4	2 (6 y and 7 y)	0
Leiomyosarcoma[12,13,16–19]	16	2 (12 y)	1
Melanoma[12,18]	13	1	1
Pancreatic cancer[12,16,17]	8	1	1
Stomach cancer[12,15–17]	23	0	—
Other adult sarcomas[12,17,18]	9	0	—
Breast cancer[6,12,15,17]	7	0	—
Ovarian cancer[12,15,18]	5	0	—
Uterine and cervical cancer[12,13,18]	7	0	—
Lung cancer[12,15]	2	0	—
Esophageal cancer[15,16,74]	3	1 (13 y)[74]	—
Rhabdomyosarcoma[16]	1	0	—
Neuroblastoma[12]	1	0	—
Thyroid cancer[12]	1	0	—
Choriocarcinoma[13]	1	0	—
Periampullary cancer[17]	1	0	—

(Sugarbaker PH, Reinig JW, Hughes KS. Diagnosis of hepatic metastases. In: Rosenberg SA, ed. Surgical treatment of metastatic cancer. Philadelphia: JB Lippincott, 1987)

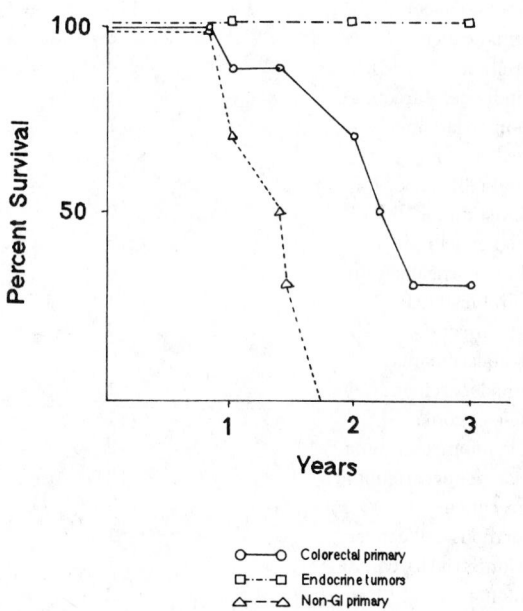

Percent Survival Following Resection of Intrahepatic Metastases

*Adapted from: Gozetti and Mazziotti (1989)

FIGURE 61–26. Percent survival after resection of intrahepatic metastases. (Adapted from Gozetti G, Mazziotti A. Expectations and possibilities of liver resection in the management of secondary liver tumors. In: Lygidakis NJ, Tytgat GNJ, eds. Hepatobiliary and pancreatic malignancies. Diagnosis, medical and surgical management. New York: Georg Thieme Verlag Stuttgart, Thieme Medical Publishers, 1989:183–190)

that of metastatic colorectal cancer. An exception appears to be metastatic neuroendocrine tumors, and a few anecdotal reports exist regarding long-term survivors after resection of liver metastases arising from neuroendocrine primaries.

There are limited reports in the literature regarding survival after resection of non-gastrointestinal-tract metastatic tumors to the liver. Unlike the reports for metastatic colorectal cancer, most reports collecting information regarding other liver metastases do not give a favorable outcome. Table 61–17, summarizing 153 hepatic tumors that were resected, is a representative sampling of the frequency with which secondary tumors from other sites occur.[40] Table 61–18 shows the poor results seen in patients after resection of noncolorectal, nonendocrine metastases, and Figures 61–26 and 61–27 illustrate similar findings.[2,7–20,41,81] In general, patients with neuroendocrine tumors (*i.e.,* carcinoid) that are resected have the best long-term survival rates, even if gross tumor is left unresected. In contrast, although the data are not conclusive, most studies indicate poor prognosis and lack of survival benefit after resection of secondary tumors originating from noncolorectal primaries[6,20,41]

HEPATIC RESECTION OF SECONDARY TUMORS

HISTORICAL PERSPECTIVES

The earliest surgical experiences with hepatic surgery dealt with traumatic injuries. Later, surgeons attempted elective hepatic resections, and Langenbruch is credited with the first

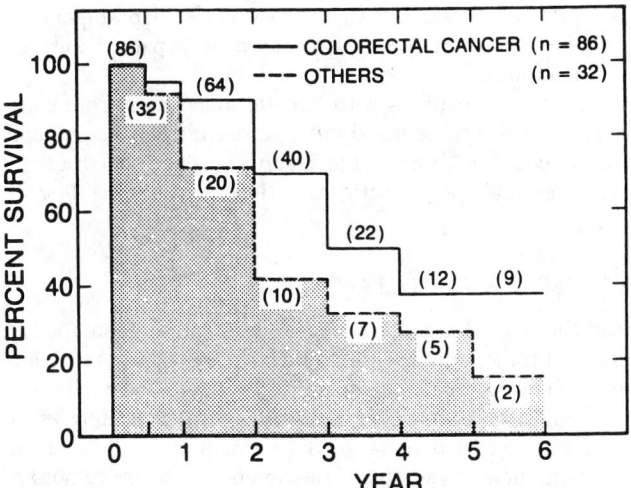

FIGURE 61–27. Actuarial survival after resection of intrahepatic metastases. (Iwatsuki S, Sheahan DG, Starzl TE. The changing face of hepatic resection. Curr Probl Surg 1989;26[5]:283–379. Reproduced with permission)

successful hepatic resection for tumor in 1888.[21,42] Several reports by Keen, Wendell, and others followed in later years, but with little knowledge of the segmental anatomy and physiology of the liver, results were not optimal. Hemorrhage was one of the greatest obstacles facing these surgical pioneers, as is evident by Keen's remark, ". . . the whole question of the operative surgery of the liver practically is one of haemostasis."[21,42,43] A major contribution to hepatic surgery was made by Couinauld with his description of the "segmental" anatomy of the liver (Fig. 61–28). He described anatomically distinct areas, each supplied by a separate arterial branch and biliary radical, each with a venous tributary of the right, middle, or left hepatic vein.[44–46] This allowed for control of these major structures during segmental/anatomic resections, thereby decreasing blood loss and postoperative complications.

In recent years, the number of hepatic resections has markedly increased because of advances in surgical and anesthetic techniques, the use of intraoperative autotransfusion devices, and the extensive preoperative evaluation and careful selection of surgical candidates. In addition, operative techniques and experience with postoperative care used in the management of patients undergoing orthotopic liver transplantation have contributed greatly to improvements in surgical outcome after major liver resections. As a result, the operative morbidity and mortality associated with hepatic surgery has significantly decreased, with most current studies reporting operative mortality rates between 2% and 7%.[3–8,10,20,39–41,60,62] Although operative mortality is low, liver resections are major undertakings for the patients and their families. Surgical intervention for metastatic disease should be offered only when the potential to extend the patient's disease-free survival exists. A thorough evaluation will aid in selecting those patients who will gain maximum benefit from resection of metastatic lesions.

PREOPERATIVE EVALUATION

Before any major abdominal surgery, a careful diagnostic workup, with particular attention to the patient's general health and cardiovascular and pulmonary status, is essential. The patient's age is of consideration in relation to the above; however, advanced age itself has not been shown to increase operative mortality after liver resection.[6,20] An extensive search for extrahepatic metastases is mandatory because this may contraindicate hepatic resection or the option of regional infusion therapy. Preoperative evaluation should include laboratory tests to determine hepatic reserve and renal function, and radiographic studies to determine the extent of intrahepatic and extrahepatic metastases. As mentioned earlier, arteriography, including a venous phase depicted on subtraction films, is helpful in delineating the vascular anatomy of the tumor as well as the native vascular anatomy of the liver, because anatomic variants are common (Table 61–19 and Fig. 61–29).[73,74]

Liver resection in the face of compromised hepatic function can be disastrous. One of the most important factors influencing major hepatic resection is the underlying physiologic

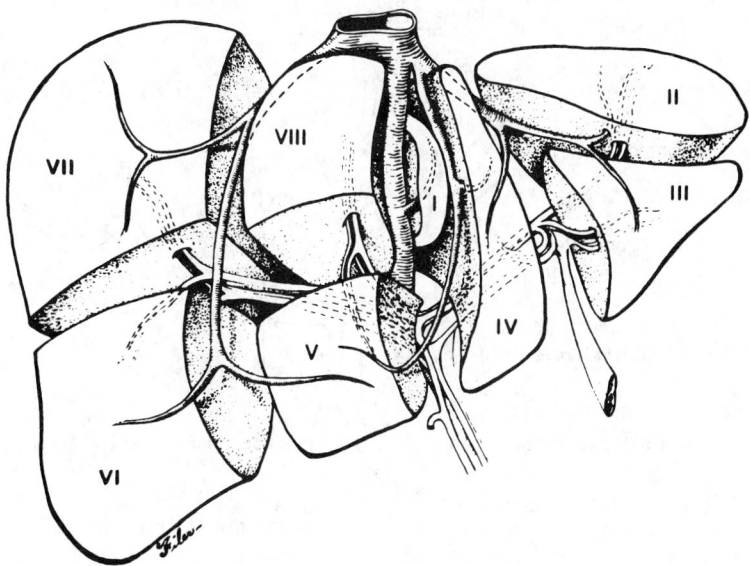

FIGURE 61–28. Segmental anatomy of the liver as described by Couinauld. There are eight segments numbered I through VIII. (Iwatsuki S, Sheahan DG, Starzl TE. The changing face of hepatic resection. Curr Probl Surg 1989;26[5]:283–379. Reproduced with permission)

TABLE 61–19. Hepatic Artery Anatomy in 232 Patients (University of Michigan)

Anatomy	No. of Patients
Standard	137 (59%)
Trifurcation	38 (16%)
RRHA*	36 (16%)
LHA replaced to LGA†	15 (6%)
Other‡	6 (3%)

* Right hepatic artery replaced to superior mesenteric artery. This includes one RRHA originating from the aorta.
† Left hepatic artery (LHA) replaced to the left gastric artery (LGA).
‡ A variety of anomalous origins of right and left hepatic arteries. (Niederhuber JE. Colorectal cancer metastatic to the liver: Hepatic artery chemotherapy. In: Cameron JL, ed. Current surgical therapy. 3rd ed. Toronto, Philadelphia: BC Decker, 1989:222–233)

state of the normal liver parenchyma and its capacity to regenerate and function after surgery. Patients with significant hepatic impairment face increased morbidity secondary to hemorrhage, poor nutritional status, compromised immune and renal function, and poor regenerative capacity of the liver, all of which will affect their intraoperative or postoperative course. It is difficult to quantitate hepatic reserve with the use of liver enzyme studies. Most surgeons are willing to undertake hepatic resection in patients assessed as Child's class A or B. Prolongation of prothrombin time that does not correct with administration of vitamin K suggests poor synthetic capacity of the liver and may be suggestive of cirrhosis. These patients have significantly higher mortality rates, and most authors agree that major hepatic resections should be avoided in the face of poor hepatic function.[21] In contrast, a recent study that examined 123 cirrhotic patients with hepatocellular carcinoma indicates that limited resection of small, peripherally located tumors in this select group of patients may be appropriate. Overall operative mortality rate was 13%, 1-year survival 77%, and 5-year survival 49%. As expected, postoperative mortality was most frequently caused by hepatic failure or sepsis, or both.[47]

In summary, patients with hepatic metastases from colorectal tumors, and selected other tumor histologies, in good general health with favorable prognostic signs should be offered the option of hepatic resection as their first line of therapy.

DETERMINING RESECTABILITY

After thorough evaluation by an experienced surgeon, the extent of intrahepatic disease and timing of hepatic resection must be determined. Many factors considered in determining resectability of secondary hepatic tumors will ultimately affect prognosis, and vice versa. In this section, we will focus on factors influencing surgical resection of secondary tumors.

When hepatic metastases are found at the time of initial resection of a colorectal primary tumor, the lesions should be carefully examined, their size and location should be noted, and intraoperative biopsy should be performed. It should be stressed that all patients diagnosed as having a resectable primary tumor should be completely staged preoperatively. There should rarely be the surprise of finding an unexpected liver metastasis. In such instances, however, intraoperative ultrasonic evaluation should be considered to determine the full extent of hepatic involvement. Although many surgeons will delay resection of hepatic metastases until a later date, a well-prepared experienced surgeon can easily and safely accomplish resection of the primary as well as the secondary liver metastasis. If resection of liver metastases is deferred, it appears that a short period of delay will not affect prognosis.[6,20,41,48,49] Certainly when a single small peripheral tumor, confirmed by frozen section, is noted, it should be resected at the time of initial laparotomy. Experience with patients who present with synchronous metastases in the liver indicates that they have a worse overall prognosis. However, this prognosis does not appear to be related to surgical resection of these lesions but rather to the properties of the underlying disease.[6,20,39,61,82]

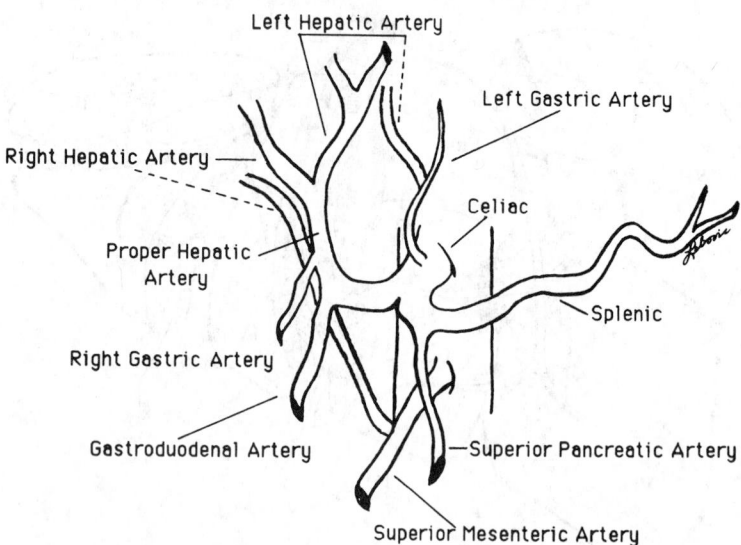

FIGURE 61–29. Schematic drawing of hepatic arterial blood supply and common aberrant origins of the right and left hepatic arteries (indicated by dotted line).

Patients being evaluated for resection of secondary hepatic tumors that become evident months to years after resection of their primary tumors should undergo a comprehensive workup to ensure that the liver is the only site of metastasis. If deemed resectable, surgical strategy for excision of the hepatic lesions is planned, and exploratory laparotomy with careful examination for evidence of extrahepatic metastases is performed. Particular attention is given to the primary site of the colorectal tumor, as well as to regional, mesenteric, celiac, and perihepatic lymph nodes. Any suspicious tissue is examined by frozen section. The presence of extrahepatic disease has been associated with early recurrence and may affect the overall length of survival after resection of hepatic metastases.

It should be emphasized that the presence of extrahepatic disease is not an absolute contraindication to hepatic resection.[6,10,20,39,49,50] Once abdominal exploration is complete, the liver is thoroughly examined, and the results are compared with the preoperative radiographic studies. Intraoperative ultrasound is used to visualize deep parenchymal lesions, to define the relation of the tumor(s) to vascular and biliary structures, and to rule out the presence of other metastases not detected before surgery. Present information, primarily from the prospective evaluation conducted by the Gastrointestinal Tumor Study Group (GITSG), suggests that it is possible to resect up to four lesions, even if they are bilobar.[7] When dealing with a healthy, noncirrhotic liver, as much as 50% to 80% of the liver can be removed with a large tumor mass while maintaining acceptable liver function and parenchymal regeneration. Taking all of this information into account, the surgeon determines the extent of, feasibility of, and technical approach to resection.

TECHNICAL ASPECTS OF RESECTION

There are many excellent surgical atlases, well-written manuscripts, and monographs that can provide the reader with an in-depth description on how to perform hepatic resections. Such a discussion is beyond the scope of this chapter, and the reader is referred to the following sources for additional information: references 20, 21, 23, 24, 40, 42, and 44. Some comments here regarding the segmental anatomy of the liver, and special surgical techniques that allow safe surgical intervention in the treatment of hepatic metastases, may, however, be of value.

The surgical anatomy of the liver has been described by many authors, and there are some discrepancies in the nomenclature as it pertains to surgical resection. For the purposes of this discussion, we will use terminology most frequently used in the United States.

On gross examination, it is tempting to divide the liver into right and left lobes along the falciform ligament; however, the true anatomic division of the right and left lobes is defined along "Cantlie's" line, a sagittal plane passing through the gallbladder bed posteriorly toward the vena cava.[51] To the right of this line lies the entire right lobe of the liver. The portion of tissue between Cantlie's line and the falciform ligament is the medial segment of the left lobe, and all tissue to the left of the falciform ligament constitutes the lateral segment of the left lobe. The right lobe can be further divided

into an anterior and posterior segment by a coronal plane, and Couinauld's further division of both lobes into four subsegments creates a total of eight distinct anatomic segments of the liver (see Figs. 61–28 and 61–30).[4]

Identifying and controlling the arterial and venous structures within the liver parenchyma are crucial to minimizing blood loss, and the surgeon must be well versed in normal as well as variant anatomy. Most metastatic tumors derive 90% to 95% of their blood supply from the hepatic artery and only a small fraction from the portal venous system.[52–57] In over 59% of cases, the common hepatic artery arises from the celiac axis, traverses the upper border of the antrum of the stomach in the lesser omentum where it gives rise to the right gastric and gastroduodenal arteries, and then becomes known as the proper hepatic artery.[73,74] The proper hepatic artery lies medial to the common bile duct and anterior to the portal vein within the hepatoduodenal ligament. Later, it branches into the right and left hepatic arteries, each of which gives rise to terminal segmental arteries. A number of anatomic variants exist. In roughly 16% to 20% of cases, the right hepatic artery arises directly from the superior mesenteric artery and courses anteriorly and to the right of the portal vein in the hepatoduodenal ligament.[21,58,73,74] The most common aberrant site of origin of the left hepatic artery is the left gastric artery (see Fig. 61–29). Preoperative angiography can be most useful in defining the vascular anatomy so that the surgeon may plan appropriately for resection. The venous phase of the arteriogram is even more valuable in delineating both the portal and hepatic venous structures.

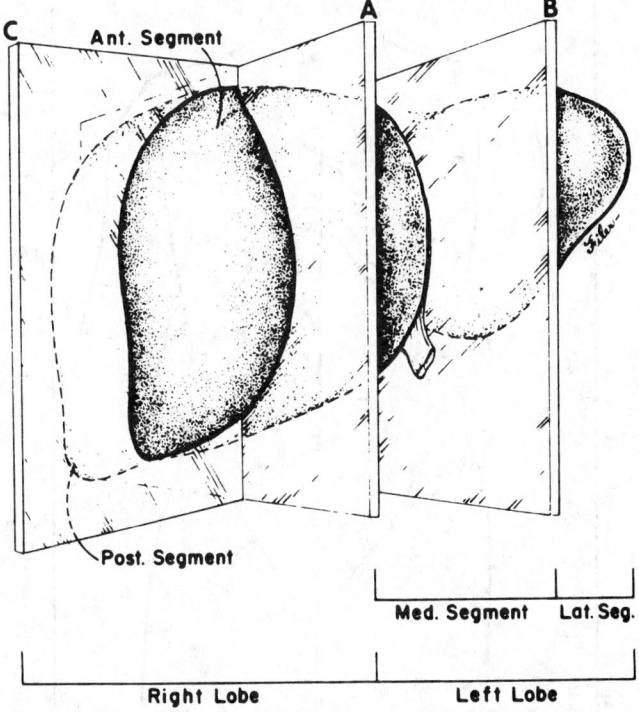

FIGURE 61–30. Anatomic divisions of the liver. **(A)** Cantlie's line divides the right and left lobe. **(B)** Left lobe subdivided into medial and lateral segments. **(C)** Right lobe divided into anterior and posterior segments by a coronal plane. (Iwatsuki S, Sheahan DG, Starzl TE. The changing face of hepatic resection. Curr Probl Surg 1989;26[5]:283–379. Reproduced with permission)

In preparation for hepatic resection, the patient is positioned in the supine position with slight extension of the torso. It is prudent to prep the entire chest and abdomen in the event that greater exposure becomes necessary. Most hepatic resections can be achieved through a generous midline incision, although some surgeons use an extended right subcostal approach. Additional exposure can be obtained by extension of the incision superiorly in the midline, splitting the sternum, or extension into the right thoracic cavity (Fig. 61–31).[21] After abdominal exploration, the liver is mobilized by detachment of its ligamentous reflections to the diaphragm. The anterior and posterior coronary ligaments, present on both the right and left sides, are divided. Attention is then directed toward dissection and identification of all structures within the hepatoduodenal ligament, with complete exposure of the hepatic arteries, the right and left bile ducts, and the right and left portal veins.

A formal lobectomy or trisegmentectomy will require careful bisection of the liver from the inferior vena cava. Each small branch is meticulously ligated in continuity and then divided. A second figure-of-eight 5-0 proline suture is placed in the inferior vena cava to secure these vessels. At this point, the major hepatic veins are exposed and enough of the vena cava is isolated above and below the liver to ensure rapid control if the situation requires. If possible, it is much safer to take the major hepatic veins just within the liver parenchyma.

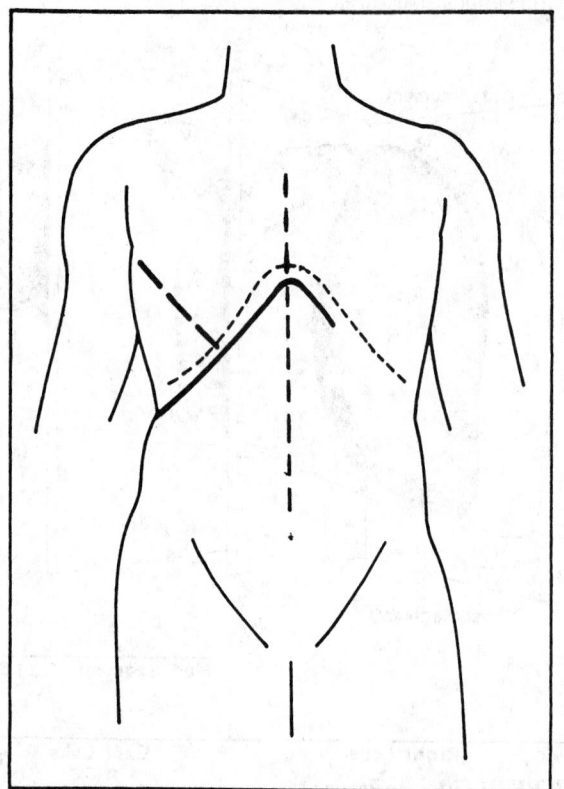

FIGURE 61–31. Extended right subcostal incision. Also shown are incisions into chest, which may be used for additional exposure as needed. (Schwartz SI. Primary and metastatic hepatic malignant tumors, and hepatic resection. In: Seymour I, Schwartz SI, Ellis H, eds. Maingot's abdominal operations. 9th ed. Norwalk, CT: Appleton & Lange, 1989:1253–1290. Reproduced with permission)

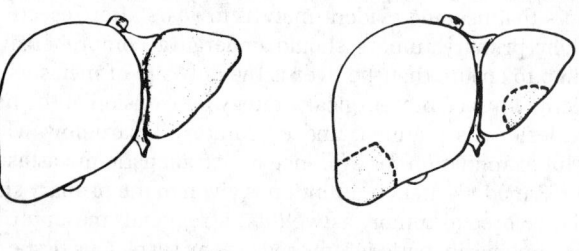

LATERAL SEGMENTECTOMY   NON-ANATOMICAL RESECTION

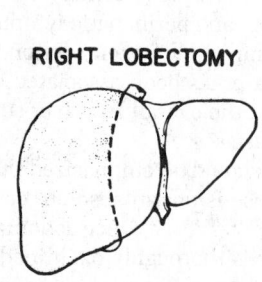

LEFT LOBECTOMY   **RIGHT LOBECTOMY**

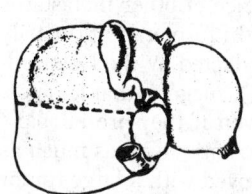   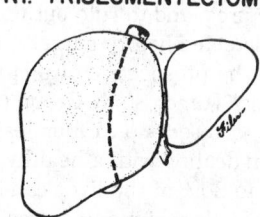

LT. TRISEGMENTECTOMY   **RT. TRISEGMENTECTOMY**

FIGURE 61–32. Anatomic hepatic resections commonly performed (right trisegmentectomy = extended right lobectomy/hepatectomy). (Iwatsuki S, Sheahan DG, Starzl TE. The changing face of hepatic resection. Curr Probl Surg 1989;26[5]:283–379. Reproduced with permission)

More limited resections such as nonanatomic wedge excisions do not require this degree of dissection and isolation of the structures cited above.

Depending on the type of resection to be performed, the surgeon uses a number of special techniques designed to allow for disruption of the liver parenchyma while permitting controlled dissection, ligation, and transection of vascular and biliary radicals. Finger fracture is a useful technique that permits isolated ligation of critical structures after manually disrupting the surrounding liver tissue.[21] More sophisticated devices, such as the Cavitron ultrasonic aspirator (CUSA; Valleylab, Boulder, CO) ultrasonic dissector, use this same principle. The metal tip vibrates at an ultrasonic frequency that shatters the hepatocytes because of the relatively high water content and aspirates the debris, leaving vascular and biliary structures intact to be properly ligated and divided.[59] Electrocautery and the argon-beam laser coagulator are also helpful in controlling bleeding from the raw surfaces of the transected liver tissue.

Figure 61–32 illustrates several anatomic and segmental hepatic resections commonly performed. The choice of resection is dependent on the extent of tumor involvement, as described in earlier sections. Evidence supports the conclusion that modest resection affecting a margin of 1 to 2 cm of normal liver provides results similar to those of more extensive resections.[7]

TABLE 61–20.   Survival After Resection of Intrahepatic Colorectal Metastases

Investigations	No. of Patients	5-Year Survival	Operative Mortality (%)
Steel, 1991[7]	87	Median survival 29 mo	2.7
Scheele, 1990[10]	183	40/27% at 5/10 y	5.5
Lise, 1990[3]	39	32%	5
Iwatsuki, 1989[40]	86	38%	0
Hughes, 1989[6]	800	32%	NA
Gozzetti, 1989[41]	45	30% (3 y)	2.2
Butler, 1986[200]	62	34%	10
Gennari, 1986[5]	48	Median survival 30 mo	2
Coppa, 1985[201]	25	25%	4
Adson, 1984[39]	141	25%	4
August, 1985[4]	33	35%	0
Cady, 1970[8]	23	40%	0
Fortner, 1984[60]	65	40%	0–9 (0 since 1980)
Foster, 1981[62]	231	23%	6

NA, not available.

RESULTS

Surgical resection of colorectal metastases to the liver improves overall survival as well as disease-free survival and may provide a significant chance for "cure" in carefully selected patients. Many series have consistently reported these findings with acceptable operative morbidity and mortality rates. Table 61–20 summarizes the results of studies published during the past decade. These data indicate that 5-year actuarial survival rates after hepatic resection for colorectal metastases range from 23% to 40%, with operative mortality between 0% and 10%. This contrasts sharply with the data in Table 61–15, which reflects the dismal outcome of these patients when hepatic metastases are not resected.

Many factors may affect a patient's outcome after resection of hepatic metastases, but perhaps the most important is the clinician's judgment in properly selecting appropriate surgical candidates. Large retrospective studies have provided information regarding metastatic tumors to the liver that can be used to identify appropriate patients for resection. Much of these data were gathered and entered into the multiinstitutional "Registry of Hepatic Metastases." Hughes, Scheele, and Sugarbaker have made a significant contribution by analyzing this large body of information.[6,20,22] In addition, an extensive review of the literature suggests that the following factors may affect the prognosis (5-year survival and disease-free interval) of patients with metastatic lesions to the liver undergoing resection.

Stage of Primary Tumor. Most studies suggest that patients with Dukes' B carcinomas have a significantly improved 5-year survival when compared with patients with Dukes' C primary lesions (Fig. 61–33).[20,39,60,61]

Number of Metastases. Data suggest that patients with one or two metastases have the same 5-year survival. Those with three or four lesions, even if bilobar, have a slightly worse prognosis, but there is no clear cutoff. Most authors agree that resection of up to four metastases is reasonable.[4,6,8,20,25,39,62]

Size of Metastases. Size of metastatic lesions has been considered an important variable, and some studies have shown that patients with large (>5 cm) solitary metastases appear to have a worse prognosis.[5,6,20,25,62] This should not preclude surgical resection if technically feasible, and in some cases, resection of large symptomatic lesions may be considered as a means of palliation.

Extrahepatic Metastases. Though controversial, there appears to be no significant difference in overall survival when limited "nonnodal" extrahepatic metastases are resected at the time of hepatic resection (*i.e.,* a solitary pulmonary nodule). However, the *disease-free* 5-year survival rates of these patients are significantly decreased compared with those of patients free of

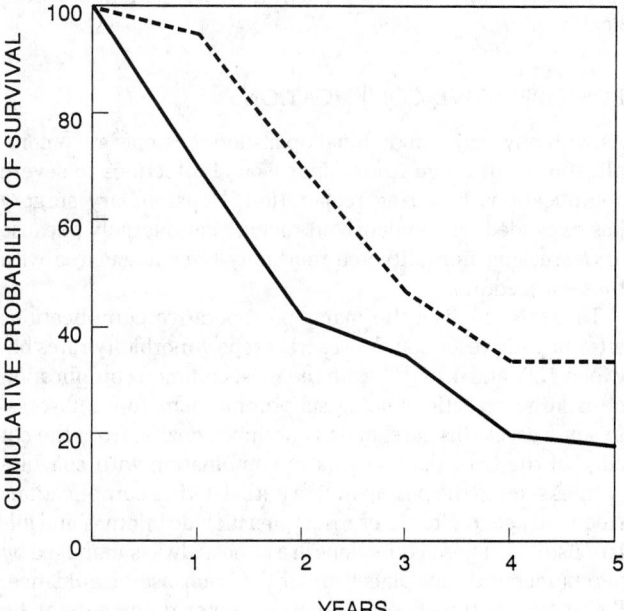

FIGURE 61–33.   Survival curves for patients after hepatic resection. *Dashed line,* Dukes' stage B; *solid line,* Dukes' stage C.

extrahepatic disease at the time of hepatic resection.[6,10,20,39,49,50,85]

Surgical Resection. Several authors have noted that clear pathologic margins surrounding resected metastases significantly improve patients' survival. A margin of at least 1 cm of normal liver parenchyma should be excised with the specimen. The specific type of surgical resection (anatomic versus segmental or wedge resection) does not appear to affect survival when treating lesions <4 cm in diameter. Anatomic lobectomy for larger lesions has been associated with improved outcome, which may relate to obtaining adequate surgical margins.[4,6,8,20]

Disease-Free Interval. Studies have shown that patients who present with metastatic disease more than 1 year after resection of the primary tumor have a better prognosis than those who present with synchronous lesions or develop metastases during the 12 months after resection of a primary tumor. This most likely reflects the biologic properties of the tumor, and rapid growth or obvious spread that occurs after resection of a primary colorectal tumor may preclude resection.[6,20,39,61,82]

Nodal Status. Patients with tumor involvement of the celiac or hepatic nodes have a significantly decreased 5-year survival rate, even when all gross tumor is removed at the time of hepatic resection.[6,20]

Cirrhosis. Many studies have shown that patients with poor hepatic function have a higher morbidity and mortality rate after hepatic resection. Useful indicators of acceptable parenchymal function are patients classified as Child's (modified classes A and B) and a minimum rate of urea-nitrogen synthesis of 6 g/day. Patients with normal liver function may present with evidence of portal hypertension and ascites secondary to compression from a large tumor mass, and this does not necessarily contraindicate resection.[47,64–66]

Other Factors. Patients with CEA levels <5 ng/ml may have a better overall prognosis; however, these findings are inconsistent throughout the literature. Chronologic age does not appear to affect prognosis in patients with good general health.

Most series indicate that in carefully selected patients, 5-year survival rates of 20% to 40% are attainable, and the experienced surgeon should aggressively pursue resection of secondary tumors from colorectal cancers unless deemed technically impossible or prohibited by the patient's overall health status.

POSTOPERATIVE COMPLICATIONS

As with any major abdominal operation, postoperative complications can range from minor wound infections to severe complications requiring reoperation. Hepatobiliary surgery has expanded tremendously in recent years, largely because of decreasing mortality and morbidity rates associated with these procedures.

Table 61–21 lists the major postoperative complications after hepatic resection. Most series report morbidity rates between 15% and 43%,[20,84] with the most common complication after large resections being subphrenic hematoma/abscess. In some cases this is related to continued oozing from the cut edge of the liver parenchyma in combination with coagulopathies seen in the postoperative period. Other complications frequently seen after liver resections include bilomas and biliary fistulae. These collections are almost always managed by percutaneous drains placed under CT or ultrasonic guidance. Percutaneous transhepatic biliary catheter drainage may be necessary.

Intraoperative blood loss can be significant with major hepatic resections, and some authors have suggested a direct

TABLE 61–21. Postoperative Complications Commonly Seen After Hepatic Resections

Subphrenic abscess
Intraabdominal hemorrhage at operative site
Bile leak (bilomas and biliary fistulae)
Hepatic failure
Coagulopathies
Transfusion reaction
Pulmonary complications/pleural effusion
Renal failure
Cardiac arrhythmias/myocardial infarction
Gastrointestinal bleeding
Small-bowel obstruction
Wound infection
Wound dehiscence
Deep venous thrombosis

(Hughes KS, Sugarbaker PH. Resection of the liver for metastatic solid tumors. In: Rosenberg S, ed. Surgical treatment of metastatic cancer. Philadelphia: JB Lippincott, 1987; Iwatsuki S, Sheahan DG, Starzl TE. The changing face of hepatic resection. Curr Probl Surg 1989; 26[5]:283–379; Vetto JT, Hughes KS, Rosenstein R, Sugarbaker PH. Morbidity and mortality of hepatic resection for metastatic colorectal carcinoma. Dis Colon Rectum 1990;33[5]:409–413)

relation between intraoperative blood loss and postoperative morbidity.[5,64,83,84] The use of new operative techniques and equipment, such as the argon-beam coagulator and CUSA ultrasonic dissector, have helped to decrease intraoperative blood loss substantially, thereby decreasing operative morbidity.

Most patients are monitored in the intensive care unit postoperatively, and coagulopathies are aggressively treated. Hepatic failure due to inadequate functioning of the remaining parenchyma is another cause for postoperative morbidity, and this is often accompanied by renal failure. It is essential to avoid renal failure in these patients, because their mortality rates are very high when this complication occurs.

PATTERNS OF FAILURE

Unfortunately, the natural progression of colorectal cancer will ultimately lead to recurrence of disease, and even after removal of all grossly visible hepatic metastases, most patients will return with metastatic disease again in the liver. There are many reports of resection of these recurrent tumors as well, but the majority of these patients will again return with liver metastases. The length of time before recurrence, the site of recurrence, and the extent of recurrence are intimately linked to the biologic behavior of the primary tumor. Patients with stage I lesions appear to have a better disease-free interval.[50]

Close follow-up of patients with colorectal cancers is essential. Most clinicians recommend colonoscopy every 6 to 12 months, frequent CEA levels, and close monitoring of hepatic function tests. Detection of recurrent disease in these patients is most reliably found by a persistent clinician looking for signs of recurrence long before the patient becomes symptomatic. Rising CEA levels may be the first indication of a recurrence, and follow-up studies, such as CT scans, should be pursued without hesitation.

CONCLUSIONS

Hepatic resection for metastatic colorectal cancer has become a widely accepted procedure with the ability to prolong overall and disease-free survival in patients who would otherwise face a grim prognosis. In properly selected patients, 5-year actuarial survival rates range from 20% to 40%, with very acceptable mortality and morbidity rates. Nonetheless, many of these patients remain daunted by the ultimate return of their tumors and will face death secondary to recurrent disseminated disease. There is little doubt that surgical management of metastatic colorectal cancer affects the natural course of disease significantly; however, surgery alone is not enough. It is important to note an intergroup study currently in progress (ECOG-9288, INT-0103). This study has been designed to prospectively evaluate: (1) resection of limited hepatic metastases from colon cancer alone versus (2) resection in combination with continuous hepatic arterial infusion of FUDR (floxuridine) plus systemic infusion of 5-FU (5-fluorouracil). Continued research will hopefully define a role for innovative adjuvant treatment options and aggressive systemic therapy of disseminated disease that can be combined with surgical management to provide optimal curative treatment of primary and metastatic cancers.

SYSTEMIC CHEMOTHERAPY

For several reasons, systemic chemotherapy represents the modality most frequently used in the treatment of hepatic metastases. Although hepatic metastases are often predominant in the generation of morbidity, the liver is rarely the sole site of metastatic disease. Liver involvement with breast cancer, lung cancer, melanoma, and even pancreatic and gastric cancer either occurs with or heralds the subsequent development of tumor in multiple metastatic sites. Application of systemic chemotherapy has the potential to reach all sites of disease. In addition, for those tumors that are responsive to systemic chemotherapy, intravenous drug treatment represents the most convenient, cost-effective, and efficient approach. The relative ease with which hepatic metastases can be evaluated with modern radiologic techniques makes liver tumor nodules useful as indicator lesions for response evaluation with systemic therapies.

Colorectal cancer frequently metastasizes to the liver. As demonstrated by surgical resection for cure, the liver may truly represent the sole site of metastatic disease in a minority of patients. The majority of patients with hepatic metastases from colorectal cancer either have or will develop extrahepatic tumor and therefore are reasonable candidates for systemic chemotherapy. The standard chemotherapeutic agent for advanced colorectal cancer has been 5-FU, which generates a response rate of about 20% as a single agent when used intensively (Table 61–22). Prolonged continuous infusions of 5-FU have been shown to generate a higher response rate (30%) when compared with an equitoxic bolus regimen (7%).[104]

A variety of combination chemotherapy regimens based on 5-FU have been evaluated in advanced colorectal cancer. Table 61–22 illustrates that hepatic metastases from colorectal cancer respond to systemic therapy with rates similar to those found in general with each specific regimen. Drug treatments

using biochemical modulation of 5-FU with leucovorin (LV) have become standard in practice based on multiple phase III studies demonstrating superiority in response rate of 5-FU plus LV over 5-FU alone.[97,105–107] More important, the regimen of 5-FU plus low-dose LV has been shown to produce a significant improvement in median survival (12 months) over that resulting from 5-FU alone (7.7 months).[108]

Pancreatic and gastric adenocarcinomas represent the two other common gastrointestinal malignancies that frequently metastasize to the liver as well as to multiple other sites. Response rates to systemic chemotherapy for hepatic metastases in these diseases are low (~25%) and are associated with a short survival of 3 to 4 months.[109]

Carcinoid tumors and islet cell carcinomas frequently metastasize to the liver. Compared with other neoplasms of the gastrointestinal tract, these neuroendocrine tumors are rare yet notable for their relative indolence and production of hormone-related symptoms. Combination chemotherapy for carcinoid tumors produces response rates of approximately 30% with durations of response of less than 9 months.[110,111] The octapeptide somatostatin analog, octreotide acetate (Sandostatin), has become standard therapy for symptomatic control of the carcinoid syndrome, such as occurs with liver metastases. Islet cell tumors appear to be more responsive to systemic chemotherapy, with responses of up to 60% and response durations of up to several years.[110,111]

Systemically administered chemotherapy used to treat hepatic metastases is limited by and generates the customary systemic toxicities of the agents applied. Usually mucositis, diarrhea, and myelosuppression are dose-limiting, with little or no limitation of therapy due to liver toxicity.

Most patients developing liver metastases from gastrointestinal cancers will ultimately die in a manner causally related to the disease within the liver. In other cancers such as breast cancer, lung cancer, and melanoma, progression in multiple sites generates morbidity and mortality coincidental to hepatic progression.

After initial systemic therapy has failed to control growth of liver metastases, second-line therapeutic options are determined by the type of cancer and the extent of extrahepatic disease. For nongastrointestinal cancers, systemic chemotherapy options should be foremost and should be selected from historical experience or available research regimens. For colorectal cancer, carcinoid, and islet cell hepatic metastases, regional treatment options as discussed below may be of benefit.

REGIONAL CHEMOTHERAPY

RATIONALE AND PHARMACOLOGY

The direct injection of chemotherapeutic agents into the blood supply of the liver has received much attention over the years. The goal of such regional chemotherapy has been to provide higher drug exposures to tumor within the liver with concurrently lower systemic exposures. Based on dose-response effects, improved selectivity of drug exposure should increase the regression of hepatic cancer while decreasing systemic toxicities.[112,113] In the last 15 years, application of regional chemotherapy to the treatment of metastatic disease within the liver has been spurred on by developments in pharmacokinetics, drug delivery, and methods of tumor evaluation.

TABLE 61–22. Response of Liver Metastases From Colorectal Carcinoma to Systemic Chemotherapy

Investigations	No. of Patients	Response (%)	No. With Liver Metastases	Response (%)
FU				
Moertel, 1969[87]	144	15	118	24
Baker, 1976[88]	42	10	11	0
Siefert, 1975[89]	36	17	5	20
Grage, 1979[90]	31	23	31	23
FU + MeCCNU ± VCR				
MacDonald, 1976[91]	25	40	14	43
Baker, 1976[88]	152	32	41	31
Buroker, 1978[92]	133	16	93	18
Kemeny, 1979[93]	69	11	41	11
FU + MeCCNU + VCR + strep				
Kemeny, 1983[94]	35	34	29	30
Kemeny, 1980[95]	74	32	58	45
FU + LV				
Machover, 1986[96]	86	39	73	30
Petrelli, 1989[97]	109	30	85	27
Ardalan, 1991[98]	22	45	18	44
FU + MTX				
Kemeny, 1984[99]	43	32	33	31
FU + MTX + LV				
Nordic Group, 1989[100]	119	17	84	18
FU + Mito + DDP + VCR				
Pandya, 1986[101]	23	48	15	30
FU + DDP				
Leohrer, 1985[102]	38	29	22	16
Kemeny, 1987[103]	105	28	77	20

FU, 5-fluorouracil; LV, leucovorin; DDP, cisplatin; Mito, mitomycin C; strep, streptozotocin; MTX, methotrexate; MeCCNU, methylcyclohexylnitrosurea; VCR, vincristine.

Although the liver receives most of its nutrient blood flow by way of the portal vein, there is considerable evidence that macroscopically detectable cancers derive their blood supply directly from the hepatic artery.[56–58,114] Based on such evidence, the administration of continuous hepatic arterial chemotherapy was introduced by Sullivan and associates in the early 1960s.[115] Considering the diseases in question, the response rates achieved exceeded rates with standard intravenous chemotherapy by twofold to threefold. Over the subsequent two decades, many reports demonstrated that, for colorectal cancer in particular, higher response rates could be achieved by hepatic arterial therapy than were found with standard intravenous therapy with 5-FU (Table 61–23).

Interest in hepatic arterial chemotherapy was rekindled and broadened during the late 1970s for a variety of reasons. The disease most frequently metastatic to the liver, colorectal cancer, was found to be extremely refractory, with a lack of success in the development of new agents. Clearly, any ap-

TABLE 61–23. Intraarterial Therapy of Hepatic Metastases With Use of External Pumps in Patients With Colorectal Cancer

Investigations	Drugs Used	No. of Evaluable Patients	Response Rate (%)
Sullivan, 1965[116]	Multiple regimens	39	62
Watkins, 1970[117]	FUDR	82	73
Cady, 1974[118]	FUDR	51	57
Buroker, 1976[119]	FUDR	21	35
Grage, 1979[90]	FU	30	34
Oberfield, 1979[120]	FU/FUDR	48	75
Patt, 1979[121]	Mitomycin/FUDR	12	83
Reed, 1981[122]	FUDR	77	76

FUDR, floxuridine; FU, 5-fluorouracil.

proach having higher activity than was achievable with intravenous therapy was felt to have a role in the treatment of colorectal liver metastases.

Other developments during the late 1970s provided added impetus to hepatic arterial chemotherapy. Pharmacologic studies were carried out with a variety of antineoplastic drugs (Table 61–24). Clinical pharmacologic investigation of 5-fluoro-2'-deoxyuridine (5-FUDR) and 5-FU demonstrated that high hepatic extraction could lead to reduced systemic drug levels, validating the rationale for the use of these agents.[123] 5-FUDR was found to be 97% to 99% extracted by the liver when given by the hepatic artery, whereas hepatic extraction of 5-FU was less efficient at 25% to 30%. These data suggested that 5-FUDR was the more selective of the two agents for regional chemotherapy by the hepatic artery.

Important refinements in pharmacokinetic theory were subsequently defined.[124,125] It was shown that the relative advantage (R_d) of hepatic arterial infusion (in terms of regional drug exposure to tumor fed by the hepatic artery) versus an intravenous infusion of a given drug is determined by the drug's total body clearance (CL_{TB}), the arterial blood flow (Q), and the fraction of drug extracted across the liver (E_H). The relation was shown to be:

$$R_d = 1 + \frac{CL_{TB}}{Q(1 - E_H)}$$

Table 61–24 illustrates the estimated exposure advantage for a number of agents. It should be noted that the high hepatic extraction of 5-FUDR generates negligible systemic exposure, particularly in comparison to the related, but much less effectively extracted drug, 5-FU. In light of these pharmacologic studies, the earlier reports of high response rates with hepatic arterial chemotherapy could be viewed as a logical extension of dose-response effects for the fluorinated pyrimidines. However, when considering the increased exposures possible with hepatic arterial infusion, it must be recognized that there is not likely to be a linear pharmacodynamic relation between target organ effect (or response) and concentration.[124] For example, preclinical studies of 5-bromo-2'-deoxyuridine (5-BUDR), an agent similar to 5-FUDR in some respects, have demonstrated that incorporation of the 5-BUDR into DNA is nonlinear and levels off at higher concentrations.[126] Extension

of such investigations into hepatic arterial 5-BUDR infusions with the VX-2 tumor grown in rabbit liver demonstrates a marked decline in regional selectivity with increasing rates of drug infusion.[127]

Developments in nuclear medicine have affected hepatic arterial therapy as well. During the late 1970s, nuclide angiography was developed as a technique to define and mimic drug flow distribution patterns during the slow fluid infusion rates used in hepatic arterial chemotherapy.[128] Radioactively labeled, γ-emitting particles (^{99m}Tc-macroaggregated albumin, TcMAA) were injected at slow flow rates through the hepatic artery. It was found that the pattern of flow distribution, as seen by the entrapment of these microparticulates within the first capillary bed of the liver, correlated with the pattern of regression of tumor. Nuclide flow to a particular region of the liver was correlated with a high probability of response for tumors in that region, whereas a lack of direct drug flow was found to correlate with a lack of response. This raised the possibility that response rates would actually be higher if catheters were always positioned within the hepatic artery such that there was direct drug infusion to the entire tumor-bearing liver. Recognition of the important roles of catheter position and infusion patterns meant that more attention had to be paid to these variables during surgical and radiologic catheter placement (see below). Recent studies have suggested that the intensity of tumor uptake of TcMAA with arterial nuclide flow scans can be predictive of tumor response: 16 of 31 patients with increased TcMAA uptake relative to liver responded to arterial chemotherapy, whereas only 1 of 16 responded to arterial chemotherapy when there was decreased TcMAA uptake.[129]

A recent important nuclear medicine study performed by the Memorial Sloan Kettering group in patients with colorectal liver metastases used radioactive (tritiated) 5-FUDR.[130] Tumor uptake of the agent was determined after hepatic arterial or portal venous administration. Liver and tumor biopsies demonstrated that the mean tumor 5-FUDR level after hepatic arterial infusion was 12.4 mmol/g, whereas the mean level after portal venous infusion of a similar 5-FUDR dose was 0.8 mmol/g. This crucial study validated the choice of the hepatic arterial route for chemotherapy with 5-FUDR for macroscopic liver metastases. It is noteworthy that radiola-

TABLE 61–24. Pharmacokinetically Rational Agents for Hepatic Arterial Infusion

Drug	Estimated Increased Hepatic Exposure With Hepatic Arterial Infusion	Retained Systemic Exposure Relative to Intravenous Use (%)	Dose-Limiting Toxicity of Hepatic Arterial Therapy
Fluorouracil (5-FU)	50–100-fold	60–70	Mucositis/diarrhea
Floxuridine (5-fluoro-2'-deoxyuridine; 5-FUDR)	100–400-fold	<5	Hepatobiliary
Carmustine (bischlorethyl-nitrosourea; BCNU)	7–13-fold	~100	Myelosuppression
Mitomycin	3–5-fold	80–90	Myelosuppression
Cisplatin	2–4-fold	~100	Renal

(Adapted from Ensminger WD, Gyves JW. Regional cancer chemotherapy. Cancer Treat Rep 1984;68: 101–115)

beled TcMAA was administered in the same solution with 5-FUDR in this study and that tumor uptake of 5-FUDR correlated directly and significantly with TcMAA retention by tumor.

CLINICAL THERAPEUTICS

External Drug Delivery Systems

Until the early 1980s, hepatic arterial infusions used externalized catheters and external pumps (see Table 61–23). However, the use of externalized catheters placed either at operation or by the Seldinger radiologic technique resulted in high complication rates, including catheter displacement, sepsis, and gastrointestinal hemorrhage. For example, Oberfield and colleagues reported complications in 80% of cases, with complete or partial hepatic artery thrombosis in 39% and catheter displacement in 33% of patients.[120] Reed and colleagues reported on 109 patients who had hepatic artery catheters either placed with the Seldinger technique or directly inserted at laparotomy.[122] Complications resulting in interruption of therapy occurred in 35% of patients, with catheter or arterial thrombosis and catheter displacement accounting for most of the complications. Although published data suggested that direct hepatic arterial infusion could generate improved tumor response rates, difficulties in achieving and sustaining hepatic arterial infusions with the available options in externalized systems prevented widespread use of such therapy.

Implanted Drug Delivery Systems

In the late 1970s and early 1980s, interest in hepatic arterial infusions was stimulated by the development of an implantable pump that, when attached to a surgically implanted catheter, constituted a totally implanted system.[131] In 1980, Buchwald and associates at the University of Minnesota reported on the application of an implantable pump they had invented for heparin infusion for hepatic arterial therapy of 5 patients with 5-FUDR.[132] In 1981, investigators at the University of Michigan described their results in 13 patients using the commercial variant of the Minnesota pump, denoted the model 400 Infusaid pump.[133] The model 400 INFUSAID pump (INFUSAID, Norwood, MA) had a SIDEPORT that bypassed the

pumping mechanism and allowed direct injection into the catheter for nuclide angiography with TcMAA, for bolus drug administration, and for clearing of obstruction in the catheter. The limiting toxicities of continuous-infusion 5-FUDR were defined in this initial study and were found to be gastrointestinal and hepatic. Infusion system problems were minimal compared with prior external systems. The response rate in the 13 patients, with the use of physical examination and nuclide liver scans, was found to be 85% when mitomycin was given by the Sideport on failure of single-agent 5-FUDR.

Interest stirred by the initial, albeit limited, positive results with use of the implanted drug delivery system generated additional phase II studies focused on colorectal cancer (Table 61–25). Subsequent phase II studies used more restrictive and defined criteria of response, leading to lower response rates that were, nonetheless, considerably higher than those described for most studies of systemic chemotherapy (see Table 61–22). Unfortunately, survival impact and the role of patient selection in achieving improved response rates could not be distinguished in these phase II studies.

Prospective, randomized trials were developed to compare hepatic arterial FUDR with systemic chemotherapy in the treatment of liver metastases from colorectal cancer. The results of the four major published studies are noted in Table 61–26. It should be pointed out that mitomycin was not used in any of these randomized studies, whereas most of the earlier phase II studies used hepatic arterial mitomycin in addition to 5-FUDR. The results of these four studies define a significant and greater than twofold improvement in response rate with hepatic arterial 5-FUDR as compared with intravenous infusions of 5-FUDR or 5-FU. The NCI and Mayo Consortium trials examined survival in the two treatment groups and found no significant difference.[143,144] The NCI trial enrolled patients both with and without hepatic lymph nodes positive for tumor. When survival of the subset of patients with negative hepatic lymph nodes was examined, the 2-year actuarial survival for the arterial group (47%) was improved over that for the intravenous group (13%) ($p = 0.03$). The Mayo consortium trial included 5 patients who did not receive hepatic arterial therapy and 7 patients with documented extrahepatic intraabdominal cancer in the hepatic arterial group (33 patients) for survival analysis comparison. It was noted that the 7 patients with extrahepatic disease had a significantly shorter

TABLE 61–25. Phase II Studies With Use of an Implanted Drug Delivery System for Hepatic Metastases From Colorectal Cancer

Investigations	No. of Patients	Drugs Used	Response Rate (%)
Balch, 1983[134]	81	FUDR/Mito	88
Niederhuber, 1984[135]	93	FUDR/Mito	78
Kemeny, 1984[136]	41	FUDR/Mito	44
Shepard, 1985[137]	40	FUDR/Mito	20
	13	FUDR/DichloroMTX	69
Kemeny, 1985[138]	24	FUDR	73
Patt, 1986[139]	29	FUDR/Mito/Cisplatin	52
Cohen, 1986[140]	36	FUDR/Mito/BCNU	70

FUDR, floxuridine; Mito, mitomycin C; MTX, methotrexate; BCNU, carmustine.

TABLE 61–26. Randomized Studies of Intrahepatic Chemotherapy Versus Systemic Chemotherapy for Hepatic Metastases From Colorectal Cancer

Group	No. of Patients	Intrahepatic		Systemic		
		Drug	Response (%)	Drug	Response (%)	
MSKCC[141]	99	FUDR	50	FUDR	20	$p = 0.001$
NCOG[142]	115	FUDR	42	FUDR	10	$p = 0.001$
NCI[143]	64	FUDR	62	FUDR	17	$p = 0.003$
Mayo consortium[144]	60	FUDR	48	FU	21	$p = 0.02$

MSKCC, Memorial Sloan-Kettering Cancer Center; NCOG, Northern California Oncology Group; NCI, National Cancer Institute; FUDR, floxuridine; FU, 5-fluorouracil.

survival ($p = 0.04$) and shorter time to overall (any site) progression ($p = 0.01$) than did patients without extrahepatic disease. The Mayo investigators noted that the significantly higher response rate of hepatic tumor to hepatic arterial therapy provided a rationale for further studies combining hepatic arterial and systemic chemotherapy to provide control of both hepatic and extrahepatic disease. In this regard, the efficient hepatic extraction of 5-FUDR would be expected to lead to negligible systemic effects on extrahepatic tumor when the agent is given into the hepatic artery (see Table 61–24).

Technical Considerations for Establishing Arterial Access

Hepatic arterial infusions may be accomplished with either percutaneous angiographic placement or surgical placement at laparotomy. Angiographic catheters are of necessity stiffer than the silicone rubber catheters used in operative placement. In general, the stiffness of the angiographic catheter and the motion of the tip of the catheter have made radiologic placement most suitable for short-duration (up to 2 weeks) infusions. Repeated angiographic insertions for repeated courses of therapy generate a progressive probability for arterial thrombosis and intimal damage. In addition, although blood flow distribution can be changed from an unfavorable to a favorable pattern (*i.e.*, one where a single catheter infuses the entire liver and nothing outside of the liver) with angiographic embolic techniques, the skills involved are considerable.[145] As described below, surgical techniques for achieving protracted hepatic arterial access are much more refined at present.

Proper placement of the hepatic arterial catheter is critical to ensure equal distribution of chemotherapeutic agents to the right and left lobes of the liver and to minimize the extent of extrahepatic perfusion. This procedure may seem straightforward; however, the operation can be much more difficult than is generally appreciated. The liver may be increased in size, making exposure difficult; there may be extensive adhesions from previous operations; and the arterial blood supply may be complex and difficult to define.

Preoperative preparation includes a complete workup to determine the extent of metastatic disease, hepatic angiography, a complete bowel prep, and administration of intravenous antibiotics. This brief section will describe the basic principles for catheter placement in the patient with "standard" hepatic arterial anatomy. Several anatomic variants are

illustrated in Figures 61–34 through 61–37, and for further details the reader is referred to previous reports.[146,147]

Abdominal exploration is performed through a standard midline incision. Careful exposure of the portal triad with definition of the hepatic arterial anatomy is essential, because placement of the perfusion catheter will vary depending on the patient's particular anatomy. Elective cholecystectomy is routinely done at the beginning of the operation. This facilitates exposure of the hepatic arteries and will eliminate the problem of chemical cholecystitis in the postoperative period. After cholecystectomy, attention is directed toward proper placement of the silicon catheter. In general, the gastroduodenal artery is the vessel used for catheter placement, and it is ligated distal to the point of insertion (see Fig. 61–34). To

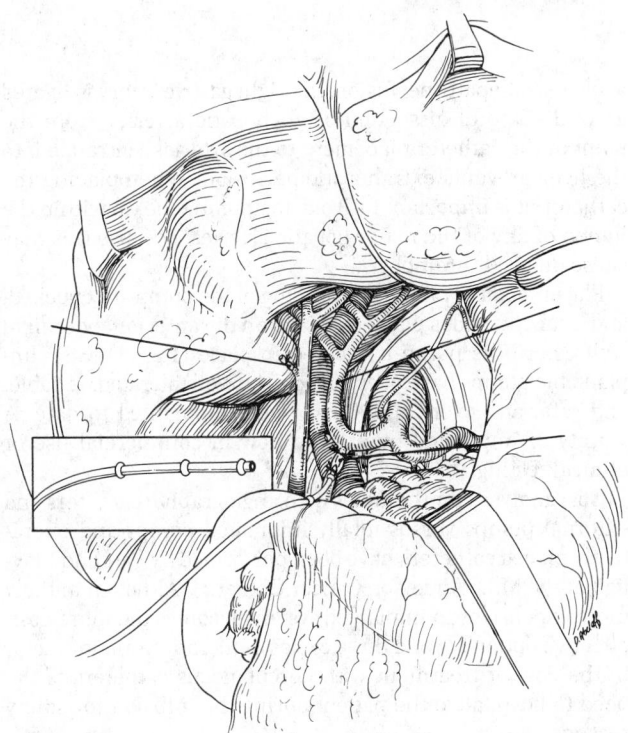

FIGURE 61–34. The patient has "standard" hepatic arterial anatomy permitting the catheter to be placed in the gastroduodenal artery. Note that the tip of the catheter is positioned just at the junction of the gastroduodenal artery with the hepatic artery. A close-up view of the beaded catheter is shown in the inset. The silicone rubber catheter has an outer diameter of 2.3 mm and an inner diameter of 0.63 mm.

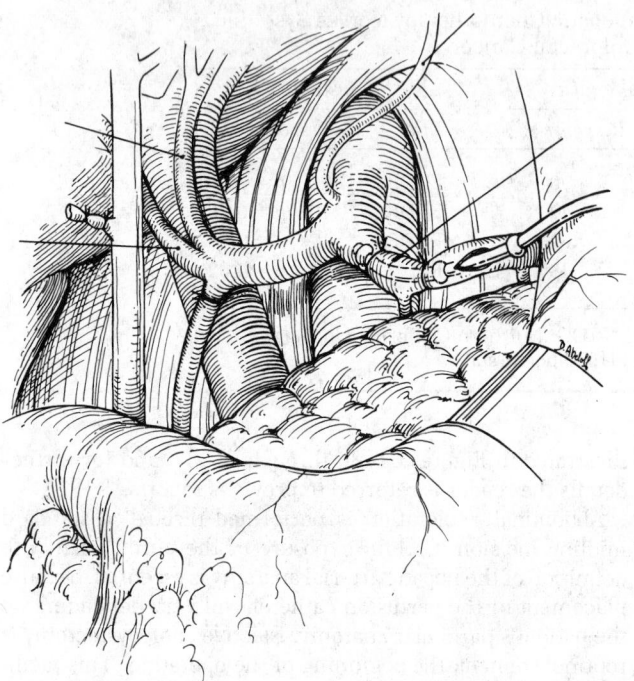

FIGURE 61–35. In this patient, the right and left hepatic arteries originate too close to the gastroduodenal artery to allow its use for the catheter placement. A catheter placed in the gastroduodenal artery would not permit adequate mixing of the drug in the arterial blood to provide equal distribution to right and left lobes of the liver. Thus, the splenic artery has been isolated and ligated for catheter placement. The gastroduodenal artery and all other branches have been carefully identified and ligated to prevent extrahepatic distribution of drug.

avoid extrahepatic perfusion, the right gastric artery is ligated as well. Careful dissection of all hepatic arteries from the point of the catheter placement to the arteries' entrance into the liver prevents extrahepatic perfusion. When placing the catheter, it is important to avoid positioning the tip within the lumen of any of the major hepatic arteries, because this may cause delayed thrombosis.

Placement and proper functioning of the pump are checked, and a subcutaneous pocket is made on the anterior abdominal wall where the pump is secured in place (Fig. 61–38). Implantable pumps have been found to be well tolerated, reliable, and safe, and over 25,000 have been implanted to date. A variety of implanted pumps are now in commercial use or clinical testing.[148]

Cost analyses for therapies with angiographic catheters and external pumps versus totally implanted pumps and operatively placed catheters have been performed by Patt and Mavligit at the M.D. Anderson Cancer Center.[149] Although initially more expensive, an implanted system becomes the more cost-effective option beyond three cycles of therapy. A major factor in the cost of treatment with percutaneous catheters is the need to hospitalize the patient during the infusion for safety reasons.

Toxicities

Hepatic arterial therapy has a number of toxicities or complications not seen with conventional intravenous therapy.[148]

These include thrombosis of the hepatic artery or other visceral arteries with resultant pain and inability to use further arterial therapy. Placement (radiologically) and maintenance of a transbrachial or transfemoral percutaneous catheter are associated with the risk of thrombosis of the vessels through which the catheter passes and of embolic damage to the extremity with the insertion site. Embolic injury from fibrin sheaths or clots forming on the catheter can involve varied internal organs and the brain, causing temporary ischemia or infarction. Thrombosis related to entrance into the brachial or femoral artery may cause ischemia of the extremity and may necessitate thrombectomy. Infection initiated at the entrance site can also occur, usually with *Staphylococcus aureus*. For implanted systems, additional complications include permanent occlusions of the implanted catheter, catheter rupture when attempting to clear such occlusions, and pump pocket seromas, hematomas, and infections. The risk and severity of complications bear some relation to the experience, skill, and dedication of the radiologists, surgeons, and medical oncologists involved in such treatment.

The lowered risks associated with totally implanted systems for hepatic arterial 5-FUDR infusion made it possible for a large number of centers to administer chronic, protracted therapy, which had not been possible with externalized systems. In contrast to the toxicity of systemically administered chemotherapy, which is frequently myelosuppression, the toxicity of chronic hepatic arterial chemotherapy was found

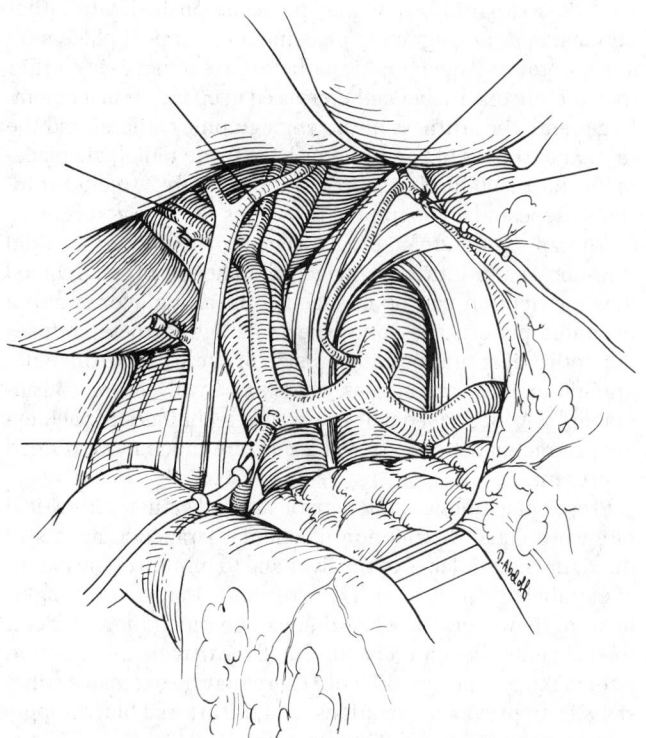

FIGURE 61–36. The left hepatic artery in this patient arises from the left gastric artery. The middle and right hepatic arteries have their normal origins from the proper hepatic artery. This situation requires a dual-catheter pump. One catheter is positioned in the left gastric artery and inserted so the tip is just at the left hepatic artery, with care being taken not to obstruct flow. The right lobe is perfused by way of a second catheter positioned in the gastroduodenal artery.

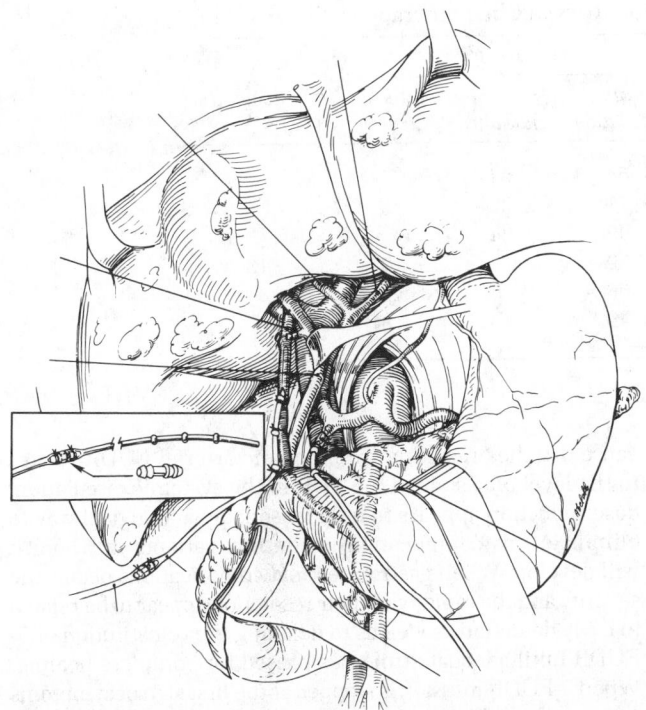

FIGURE 61–37.   Two catheters are also required in patients with a right hepatic artery replaced to the superior mesenteric artery. There are no significant accessible branches of the RRHA, making it necessary to introduce a special thin-walled catheter directly into the lumen. The introduction of the catheter is accomplished by inserting an 18-gauge needle into the lateral wall of the exposed vessel. A guide wire is passed through the needle. The needle is removed and a beaded catheter is passed over the wire and threaded for a short distance into the lumen of the artery until the first catheter bead rests against the adventitia. A silk stitch is placed through the adventitia of the artery just behind the first catheter bead and is used to secure the catheter alongside the RRHA. This special thin-walled catheter is connected to one of the two pump catheters.

to relate primarily to the regionally high (and protracted) exposure to 5-FUDR or 5-FU. In early studies, the incidence of symptomatic gastric injury and of hepatobiliary damage, the major regional toxicities associated with hepatic arterial infusion of 5-FUDR, was approximately 50% for each (Table 61–27).

The primary mechanism for gastric toxicity with hepatic arterial infusion appears to be direct blood flow to the stomach through vessels distal to the site of drug entrance into the hepatic artery (*i.e.,* distal to the catheter tip). Gastric toxicity was described earlier for hepatic arterial infusion that used percutaneous angiographically placed hepatic arterial catheters. One study described the development of gastric ulcers in 8 of 251 patients who received intrahepatic infusion of 5-FU by way of a catheter inserted percutaneously and positioned in the hepatic artery.[151] None of these patients had a history of ulcers. Four of the patients developed bleeding, and there was gastric perforation in 1 patient. In every patient with ulceration, the catheter tip had become dislodged and was found to be either directly infusing the left gastric artery or proximal to the right gastric artery or to the gastroduodenal artery, allowing direct flow of 5-FU to the stomach. Each of the patients was symptomatic for several days before the doc-

umentation of the diagnosis of gastric ulcer. A subsequent study documented the development of severe dyspepsia in 18 of 124 patients receiving hepatic arterial chemotherapy through percutaneous, angiographically positioned catheters.[152] Ten of the 18 patients had documented gastrointestinal pathology: 6 had gastric ulcers and gastritis, 2 had duodenal ulcers, 1 had pyloroduodenitis, and 1 had pancreatitis. Investigators in the study noted that endoscopically defined ulceration and gastritis caused by hepatic arterial infusion chemotherapy were confined to the distribution of the infused arteries. Nine of the 10 patients with toxicity had received 5-FUDR as well as mitomycin C through the hepatic artery catheter.

Initial results with the totally implanted drug delivery system showed significant gastrointestinal (GI) toxicity (see Table 61–27). Fortunately, however, the report by Hohn and associates, describing their experience with 35 patients who received hepatic arterial FUDR administered with the implanted infusion pump, demonstrated that gastric ulceration could be prevented.[153] These investigators found that none of the 35 patients in their study developed signs or symptoms of gastritis or ulcer attributable to chemotherapy because particular care was taken at surgery to identify and divide those vessels arising from the hepatic artery (distal to the point of cannulation) that supplied the superior border of the distal stomach and proximal duodenum. They found that, despite the standard approach of meticulous devascularization of the upper border of the distal stomach and proximal duodenum, infusion of fluorescein intraoperatively into the pump Sideport demonstrated residual gastroduodenal perfusion requiring further dissection and ligation of previously unrecognized

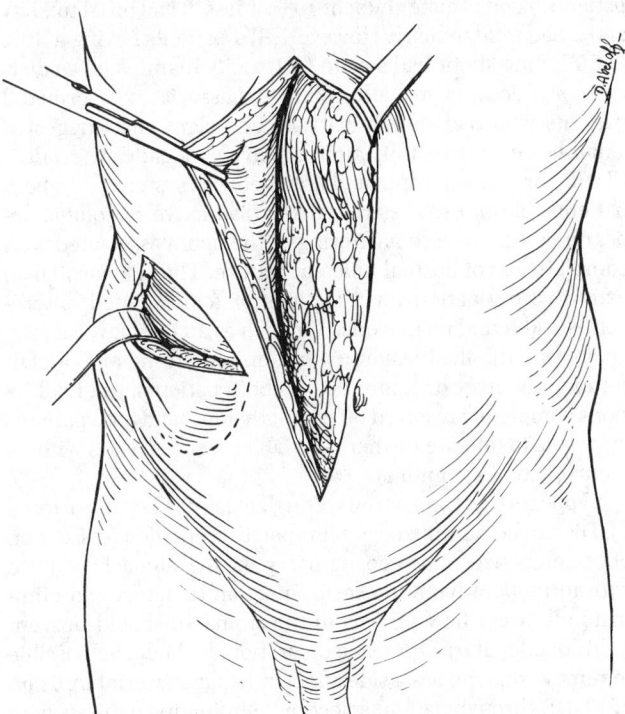

FIGURE 61–38.   A midline incision with a subcutaneous pocket for the implanted pump positioned in the right lower quadrant of the abdomen.

TABLE 61–27.   Toxicities of Chronic Hepatic Arterial Chemotherapy

	Gastric (%)		Hepatic (%)			Cholecystitis (%)
Investigations	Symptoms	Ulcers	Enzyme Elevation	Jaundice	Biliary Stenosis	
Niederhuber, 1984[135]	56		54	24		
Kemeny, 1984[136]	46	29	71	22		
Shepard, 1985[137]		18	49	24		
Kemeny, 1985[138]	15	4	59		17	13
Hohn, 1986[150]	0	0	56	5	29	
Kemeny, 1987[141]		17	42	19	8	

blood vessels in 7 patients. Residual vessels were most commonly identified adjacent to the common bile duct and portal vein. As will be described below, it is noteworthy that these same investigators describe a relatively high incidence of biliary sclerosis, perhaps related, in part, to a more efficient devascularization of proximal parts of the biliary tree.

It is probable that the maintenance of a low level of 5-FUDR in the systemic circulation can, by itself, inflict a different form of gastrointestinal toxicity, namely, diarrhea. Studies in which 5-FUDR has been administered intravenously for 14 days have described a high incidence of significant diarrhea.[141,142] Although the efficiency of hepatic extraction of 5-FUDR exceeds 95%, this holds true only when there is a low percentage of arteriovenous (AV) shunting. Using hepatic arterial angiography with TcMAA, Kaplan and associates found a correlation between lung shunting (*i.e.,* the percentage of a dose of hepatic arterial TcMAA that goes through AV shunts in the liver and is trapped in the lung) and diarrhea.[154] In 10 patients having a lung shunt of 15% or less, 8 had no GI toxicity and 2 had mild toxicity. However, all 4 patients having a 30% to 50% lung shunt had severe GI toxicity manifested as diarrhea or mucositis, or both. Gluck and associates described 2 patients who had severe diarrhea and signs that suggested small-bowel obstruction after receiving hepatic arterial 5-FUDR through an implanted drug delivery system.[155] In both patients, barium studies revealed a distinctive radiologic appearance with severe narrowing of the ileum associated with complete loss of normal mucosal pattern. They performed an extensive evaluation for infectious or toxin-related enterocolitis and found no evidence for such as an etiology, thereby attributing the ileal lesions to systemic shunting of 5-FUDR through the liver or tumor bed. In both patients, the ileal lesions completely resolved off chemotherapy, and both patients were able to tolerate further 5-FUDR at reduced doses without recurrence of symptoms.

It appears that the gastrointestinal toxicity of hepatic arterial FUDR can be minimized or eliminated. Meticulous dissection of vessels between the hepatic artery and the stomach, coupled with intraoperative fluorescein injection to detect and eliminate all direct flow of drug to the stomach, should prevent gastroduodenal irritation and ulceration. It should be possible to remove diarrhea as a side effect of hepatic arterial infusion of FUDR through patient selection, eliminating patients with AV shunts through the liver that are of such magnitude that 20% or more of TcMAA injected into the hepatic artery flows directly through the liver into the pulmonary circulation. Because diarrhea resulting from hepatic arterial FUDR relates to the level of sustained 5-FUDR in the systemic circulation, dose reduction appears to be a reasonable and logical way to eliminate this complication in the few patients in whom it will develop. When gastrointestinal complications occur, the severity and the rapidity of their resolution appear to be related to early detection as well as to delaying the reinstitution of 5-FUDR until adequate time has passed for complete healing. When 5-FUDR infusion is stopped at the first sign of symptoms that may be related to gastrointestinal irritation, such symptoms tend to rapidly resolve. Further administration of drug in the face of the development of such symptoms tends to make the symptoms much more intense and their resolution much more protracted. Avoiding the reinstitution of 5-FUDR for at least a month after resolution of symptoms and then reinstituting infusion at a lower dose or for a shorter duration appears to be prudent. Any severe symptoms or protracted symptoms mandate the use of endoscopy to document gastrointestinal pathology.

The major and most severe toxicity of chronic hepatic arterial FUDR is hepatobiliary damage. There are three elements to hepatobiliary damage: cholecystitis, biliary stricture/sclerosis, and hepatitis.[147,156] The incidence of hepatobiliary toxicity appears relatively uniform from study to study and seems to affect approximately 50% of patients (see Table 61–27). Cholecystitis, previously noted to occur with hepatic arterial chemotherapy with 5-FUDR and mitomycin C administered through percutaneous angiographic catheters,[154] may develop in as many as 33% of patients receiving chronic FUDR treatment with the implanted drug delivery system.[138] The symptoms generated by a chemically induced cholecystitis can become quite confusing in the care of patients who have metastatic cancer within the liver. The relatively high incidence of cholecystitis and associated morbidity have led to the recommendation for a prophylactic cholecystectomy at the time of hepatic arterial catheter implantation.

The gallbladder and the biliary tree are thought to receive their total blood supply directly from the hepatic artery, whereas hepatocytes receive a mixed blood supply, with about 33% from the hepatic artery and 66% from the portal vein.[157] Hence, with hepatic arterial chemotherapy, the gallbladder and biliary tree will be exposed to protracted drug levels that are some threefold higher than those of the hepatocytes. Removal of the gallbladder is a reasonable solution to the problem of chemical cholecystitis. On the other hand, toxicity of 5-FUDR to the biliary tree is a much more serious problem.

During initial studies with the implanted drug delivery system for hepatic arterial chemotherapy, it was noted that approximately 25% of patients would become jaundiced during treatment and that generally jaundice would resolve when there was a protracted drug-free period.[133] In some patients, however, jaundice did not resolve. Kemeny and associates reported that 8 of 46 (17.4%) patients treated with continuous hepatic arterial infusion of FUDR developed biliary strictures.[158] They noted that the lesions were clinically, radiographically, and pathologically identical to the idiopathic sclerosing cholangitis frequently seen in association with inflammatory bowel disease. Two of their 8 patients died of the complication. All 35 patients receiving intraarterial 5-FUDR in the study of Hohn and associates developed significant increases in alkaline phosphatase, and 7 of the patients who were studied cholangiographically had sclerosis of the intrahepatic or extrahepatic bile ducts, or both.[159] Liver biopsies done on these patients showed cholestasis and pericholangitis with minimal hepatocyte damage.

Although Hohn and colleagues suggest that "biliary sclerosis" rather than "chemical hepatitis" is the predominant toxicity associated with hepatic arterial infusions of 5-FUDR,[159] Doria and associates describe additional liver histopathology and clinical features of 8 patients who developed hepatitis while receiving hepatic arterial chemotherapy.[160] All 8 patients who developed hepatitis had responded to the treatment. Clinical findings included nausea, vomiting, abdominal pain, and jaundice. Serum transaminases, alkaline phosphatase, and bilirubin levels were increased. Pathologic examination of biopsies revealed hepatocyte necrosis, steatosis, cholestasis, central vein sclerosis, and alterations in the portal triad (primarily fibrosis). In addition, central vein lesions like those accompanying venoocclusive disease and micronodular sclerosis as induced by alcohol were encountered. These latter investigators noted that the degree of damage appeared to be related to the dose and duration of hepatic arterial infusion.

Biliary sclerosis is a serious toxicity that may greatly compromise the life of patients who otherwise may have benefited from significant tumor reduction. The development of biliary sclerosis is uniformly preceded by an elevation in liver function tests, particularly alkaline phosphatase. Careful monitoring of the liver function tests over cycles of therapy can sort out those patients who are most susceptible to this toxicity. The manipulation that is available to the physician to deal with hepatobiliary toxicity is an alteration of dose-schedule. For example, 1 week of 5-FUDR instead of 2 weeks of 5-FUDR with longer drug-free intervals between the infusions may be more tolerable in susceptible patients. Reductions in the dose rate of 5-FUDR to levels of 0.1 or 0.05 mg/kg/day may lower the incidence of hepatobiliary toxicity.

In an effort to study the effect of altering dose schedule on biliary toxicity and in an attempt to increase cumulative drug tolerated, a phase I and II clinical trial was initiated at Johns Hopkins Oncology Center under the direction of Louise Grochow.[53] This trial has studied weekly 48-hour infusions of FUDR using an implanted drug delivery system. This initial infusion dose was 0.2 mg/kg/day for 48 hours each week. Doses were escalated in cohorts of 3 new patients. At 0.5 mg/kg/day, 2 of 2 patients had grade IV hepatic toxicity. At 0.4 mg/kg/day, no patient had dose-limiting hepatic toxicity. Two of 35 patients experienced complete response and 51% had

partial response. The median duration of response was greater than 20 months. As experience has accumulated, it has become clear that patients treated less aggressively and monitored more closely tend to do better in the long run. Although the overall incidence of hepatobiliary toxicity may not be decreasing, the severity of the toxicity appears to be declining to a more tolerable level with accumulating experience.[141,142] Studies in a dog model may ultimately define the mechanism of this toxicity and how to control it more effectively.[161] A recent clinical study suggests that dexamethasone may play a role in decreasing such toxicity as well.[162]

Patterns of Failure

Colorectal cancer represents the only type of metastatic liver disease consistently treated in a defined manner, with hepatic arterial therapy making it possible to evaluate for sites of disease control and failure. Aggressive hepatic arterial therapy can generate hepatic tumor control such that extrahepatic tumor progression is the cause of death in ~75% of patients.[135] The lung is the most frequent site of extrahepatic disease at death in patients initially presenting with metastatic colorectal cancer confined to the liver. Patients with evidence for extrahepatic disease at the time of pump implantation have a high incidence of progressive disease in the lung and in extrahepatic abdominal sites at time of death. In the Memorial Sloan Kettering study of hepatic arterial versus intravenous 5-FUDR, failure within the liver occurred in only 37% of patients on arterial treatment as compared with 82% of patients on intravenous treatment.[140] Extrahepatic failure was found to occur in 56% of patients on arterial therapy and 37% of patients on the intravenous arm. In this regard, it is relevant that the high hepatic extraction of over 95% of 5-FUDR means that little drug goes into the systemic circulation with hepatic arterial infusion.

It is interesting to compare hepatic arterial therapy for colorectal cancer with surgical resection in terms of sites of failure. In the largest multiinstitutional study of resection, 55% of patients had extrahepatic failure either alone or with failure in the liver.[163] Of total failures, 78% were extrahepatic. It is reasonable to assume that patients undergoing hepatic resection of colorectal metastases have disease of decreased metastatic potential. It is likely that such patients should have less propensity to develop extrahepatic disease as compared with patients receiving hepatic arterial therapy alone. In summary, the data on sites of failure with regional treatments indicate that the achievement of survival benefit in the majority of patients with colorectal liver metastases will require the application of more effective systemic therapies to control extrahepatic disease.

Hepatic Arterial Therapy Plus Systemic Chemotherapy

Extrahepatic tumor growth occurring frequently in the setting where intrahepatic tumor is controlled by hepatic arterial FUDR has led to several clinical trials in which additional systemic therapy was added. In one study, dual-catheter implanted pumps were used to simultaneously deliver hepatic arterial and intravenous 5-FUDR.[164] Although extrahepatic spread of tumor during therapy occurred less frequently with combined treatment (33%) than with hepatic arterial treatment (61%) in this randomized study, survival was the same for both treatment groups. In a small phase I trial, the addition of a 5-day infusion of systemic 5-FU immediately after a standard 14-day infusion of hepatic arterial 5-FUDR was shown to be feasible, although systemic toxicities (mucositis, diarrhea) appeared to be moderately increased.[165] A shortened duration (7 days) of hepatic arterial 5-FUDR combined with bolus injections of hepatic arterial 5-FU by way of the Sideport of the Infusaid pump (days 15, 22, and 29 of a 35-day cycle) was found to produce less hepatobiliary toxicity while retaining a high response rate (50%) and a prolonged survival (26.6 months).[166] In this latter study, the first evidence of disease progression occurred in the liver in 50% of patients, in an extrahepatic site in 35% of patients, and in the liver plus an extrahepatic site in 15% of patients. The less efficient hepatic extraction of 5-FU means that more systemic effect will occur with this agent than with the highly extracted agent 5-FUDR. Unfortunately, the solubility and potency of 5-FU necessitate use of an external pump for high-volume infusions of 5-FU through either surgically placed port-catheter systems or radiologically placed catheters.[148,167] One such study using 5-FU with leucovorin and mitomycin C reported a 58% response rate.[168] Yet, despite the potential of this regimen to produce systemic effects, extrahepatic tumor, primarily in the lung and peritoneum, developed during treatment in 58% of patients.

SUMMARY OF CURRENT HEPATIC ARTERIAL THERAPY FOR COLORECTAL HEPATIC METASTASES

There is recognition, supported by the phase II and III studies described above, that the response rate for regression of colorectal cancer within the liver is greater for hepatic arterial 5-FUDR than for systemically administered 5-FU or 5-FUDR. A survival benefit for hepatic arterial 5-FUDR has not been demonstrated because of limitations imposed on hepatic arterial therapy by hepatobiliary toxicity and because of a lack of control of systemic disease with such regionally focal treatment. The technology for hepatic arterial therapy has been refined with improved drug delivery systems and mechanisms for ensuring and defining infusion such that all hepatic tumor sees the higher drug exposures generated thereby. It is anticipated that progress will be made in terms of understanding and controlling hepatobiliary toxicity and in combining systemic with regional treatment to control all sites of disease. Further additions to the therapeutic armamentarium are likely to be created out of attempts to develop innovative second-line treatments as described below.

CURRENT HEPATIC ARTERIAL THERAPY FOR NONCOLORECTAL LIVER METASTASES

There are no randomized, controlled studies of hepatic arterial therapy in diseases other than colorectal cancer. The number of patients with liver metastases as the sole site of disease with other tumor types is extremely small. In actual practice, such patients are often considered together with colorectal patients in phase II studies and treated in the same manner. Nonetheless, for centers skilled in the delivery of hepatic arterial therapy, other agents such as doxorubicin (Adriamycin) and cisplatin have been used in addition to 5-FUDR, 5-FU, and mitomycin C.[139,169] Although of low incidence, hepatic involvement with carcinoid and nonfunctional islet cell neuroendocrine tumors represents a situation where hepatic arterial therapy is applicable. Infusional hepatic arterial chemotherapy with agents such as 5-FU and streptozocin can produce responses.[110,111,170,171] The relative hypervascularity of neuroendocrine tumors within the liver appears to make them especially susceptible to vascular occlusion with use of hepatic arterial embolization with Gelfoam or polyvinyl alcohol particles.[172–175] The majority of patients treated with embolization are reported to have symptomatic improvement as well as evidence of reduction in bulk hepatic tumor.

SECOND-LINE THERAPEUTIC OPTIONS

Radiation Therapy Combined With Hepatic Arterial Therapy

Although it has long been recognized that 5-FU has radiosensitizing properties, only recently has it been demonstrated that 5-FUDR is also capable of producing radiosensitization at clinically achievable concentrations.[176] A variety of studies have been conducted using primarily hepatic arterial 5-FU or 5-FUDR with external beam radiotherapy (Table 61–28). Generally, these treatment schemes have used total radiation doses of less than 3000 cGy to limit the potential for radiation hepatitis such as occurs with larger doses.[184,185] Recently, the development of computer-assisted three-dimensional (3D) radiotherapy planning has made it possible to exceed the 3000 cGy dose by giving focal radiotherapy to tumor-bearing partial liver volumes.[183,186] With the sparing of volumes of normal liver, as is made possible by dose-volume histogram analyses, Lawrence and associates found no hepatic toxicity with the delivery of up to 6000 cGy to localized hepatic tumors despite concurrent hepatic arterial 5-FUDR (Fig. 61–39).[186–188] The delivery of such high doses of radiotherapy to focal hepatic tumor nodules is a step in developing a radiotherapy equivalent to surgical metastasectomy. It is highly likely that the more effective radiosensitizers, 5-iodo-2'-deoxyuridine (5-IUDR) and 5-bromo-2'-deoxyuridine (5-BUDR), can be administered in hepatic arterial therapy combined with high-dose, three-dimensionally planned focal radiotherapy for improved therapeutic potential.[189–191]

Hepatic Arterial Microsphere Therapy

Several less conventional forms of hepatic arterial therapy have used microspheres to deliver either radiotherapy or chemotherapy to hepatic tumors. Most neuroendocrine hepatic metastases and some colorectal metastases can be relatively hypervascular when evaluated through use of tracer microparticles such as TcMAA.[52,129]

Yttrium 90 (^{90}Y) incorporated into microspheres has been used as a radiotherapeutic agent for hepatic arterial therapy of metastatic tumors.[192,193] It is not yet understood why liver tolerance to ^{90}Y microsphere therapy is such that doses of 10,000 cGy and higher produce little or no hepatic damage. Y-90 microsphere therapy has received approval for use as a conventional therapy in Canada.

TABLE 61–28. Hepatic Irradiation and Infusional Chemotherapy

Investigations	Drug	Total Radiation Dose	No. of Patients	Response (%)	Hepatic Toxicity (%)
Barone, 1982[177]	FUDR or FU	3000 cGy	18	56	20
Herbsman, 1978[178]	FUDR	2500–3000 cGy	13	46	30
Webber, 1978[179]	FUDR	2500 cGy	25	33	1
Lokich, 1982[180]	FU	2500–3000 cGy	15	75	
Raju, 1987[181]	FUDR or FU	2100 cGy	12	83	
Friedman, 1979[182]	FU, Ad	1350–2100 cGy	22	55	0
Lawrence, 1991[183]	FUDR	3300 cGy	20	39	
		4500–6000 cGy (by DVH)	13	64	

FU, fluorouracil; FUDR, floxuridine; Ad, doxorubicin (Adriamycin); DVH, dose determined by dose-volume histogram.

Biodegradable starch microspheres were investigated as a means to deliver more chemotherapy to hepatic tumor in the early 1980s in the United States, and investigations still continue outside of the United States.[194–196] Pharmacologic studies demonstrated the ability of hepatic arterial injection of starch microspheres within a chemotherapeutic drug solution (a form of chemoembolization) to reduce systemic drug exposure and to increase drug delivery to hepatic tumor.[196]

The use of hepatic arterial microsphere therapy as described above carries with it an even greater need for precise delivery of agent than that seen with fluoropyrimidine infusions. The therapeutic agent is administered in a very short time period (several minutes) in a highly potent suspension. Maldistribution in the delivery pattern could lead to high concentrations of the cytotoxic agent directly reaching the stomach or duodenum and inflicting severe damage. Alternatively, if the flow distribution is such that all of the hepatic tumor is not directly infused, essentially no therapeutic effect can be expected.

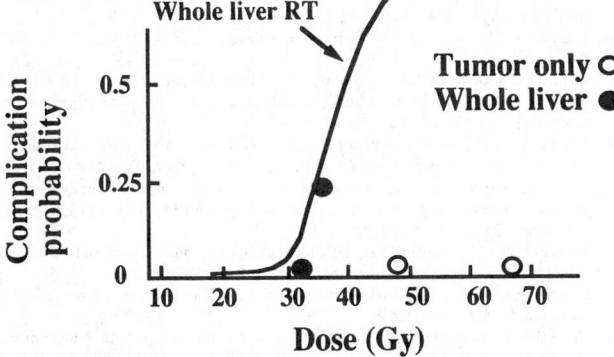

FIGURE 61–39. Ability to deliver high doses of radiation to intrahepatic tumors using three-dimensionally planned radiation therapy based on dose volume histogram analysis. Solid symbols represent observed complication probability for patients who received whole-liver irradiation; open symbols show data from patients receiving focal irradiation to tumor with sparing of 33% (48 Gy) and 66% (66 Gy) of normal liver.[185] Solid line represents compilation of complication probabilities derived from the literature.[186]

Focal Treatments for Hepatic Tumors

Treatments that are applicable when there are small numbers of hepatic metastases include surgical resection and focal external beam radiotherapy as described previously. The delivery of tissue-destroying agents to intrahepatic tumors localized by direct observation, ultrasound, or CT by way of needles inserted into such lesions extends the concept of metastasectomy to nodules not amenable to resection and to patients unable to tolerate major surgery. Radioactive seeds can be positioned for interstitial, focal radiotherapy.[197] Alternatively, direct instillation of absolute alcohol or liquid nitrogen into tumor nodules can be used to achieve focal destruction through fixation and freeze-thawing, respectively.[198,199] Although abscess formation is a possible concern, a major limitation of such approaches is that such debulking treatment does not address the subclinical presence of other metastatic tumor. With focal treatments, it is especially important that adjunctive chemotherapy regimens be considered to deal with occult metastatic tumor likely to be present elsewhere in the liver and in extrahepatic sites.

CONCLUSIONS

The importance of hepatic metastases transcends even the high frequency of morbidity and mortality associated with the disease. The fact that, under defined circumstances, the resection of metastatic nodules leads to a cure in an appreciable proportion of patients (30% in colorectal cancer) has provided hope for patients, an impetus for aggressive surgical resection, and some insight into relevant tumor biology. The unique ability to deliver therapeutic agents in high concentrations directly to the metastatic tumor using the hepatic artery has validated concepts in regional pharmacokinetics and dose-response effects. In addition, hepatic arterial chemotherapy has been pivotal in the technologic development of implantable drug delivery pumps and ports for vascular access. Distinguishing aspects of tumor blood supply have proved useful in tumor detection and in various forms of embolic therapies. The circumscribed and often isolated nature of hepatic tumor nodules, which makes them sometimes resectable, also makes them amenable to attack with direct implantation of therapeutic agents as well as with high-dose, focal external beam radiotherapy. It is likely that future integration of these regional technologies will increase the potential for cure (in some patients) or, at least, for significant palliation (in most patients).

Unfortunately, the subsequent development of extrahepatic tumor continues to frustrate cure in most instances. Nonetheless, recent advances in the adjuvant therapy of colorectal cancer suggest that the debulking induced by hepatic tumor removal or sterilization might be reasonably combined with adjunctive systemic therapy. In such efforts, progress will require the cooperation of surgical, medical, and radiation therapists working together, driven by a dissatisfaction with current outcomes that is coupled with optimism from successes to date.

REFERENCES

1. NIH Consensus Conference. Adjuvant therapy for patients with colon and rectal cancer. JAMA 1990;264(11):1444–1450.
2. Wood CB, Gillis CR, Blumgart LH. A retrospective study of patients with liver metastases from colorectal cancer. Clin Oncol 1976;2:285–288.
3. Lise M, Dabian PP, Nitti D, et al. Colorectal metastases to the liver: Present status of management. Dis Colon Rectum 1990;35(8):688–694.
4. August DA, Sugarbaker PH, Ottow RT. Hepatic resection of colorectal metastases. Ann Surg 1985;201:210–218.
5. Gennari L, Doi R, Bignami P, Bozzetti F. Surgical treatment of hepatic metastases from colorectal cancer. Ann Surg 1986;203(1):49–54.
6. Hughes K, Scheele J, Sugarbaker PH. Surgery for colorectal cancer metastatic to the liver. Surg Clin North Am 1989;69(2):339–359.
7. Steele G Jr, Bleday R, Mayer RJ, et al. A prospective evaluation of hepatic resection for colorectal carcinoma metastases to the liver: Gastrointestinal Tumor Study Group Protocol, 6584. J Clin Oncol 1991;9(7):1105–1112.
8. Cady B, Monson DO, Swinton NW. Survival of patients after colonic resection for carcinoma with simultaneous liver metastases. Surg Gynecol Obstet 1970;131:697–700.
9. Goslin R, Steele G Jr, Zamcheck N, et al. Factors influencing survival in patients with hepatic metastases from adenocarcinoma of the colon and rectum. Dis Colon Rectum 1982;25:749–754.
10. Scheele J, Stangl R, Altendorf-Hofmann A. Hepatic metastases from colorectal carcinoma: Impact of surgical resection on the natural history. Br J Surg 1990;77(11):1241–1246.
11. Finan PJ, Marshall RJ, Cooper EH, et al. Factors affecting survival in patients with synchronous hepatic metastases from colorectal cancer: A clinical and computer analysis. Br J Surg 1985;72:373–377.
12. Wagner JS, Adson MA, vanHeerden JA, et al. The natural history of hepatic metastases from colorectal cancer. Ann Surg 1984;199:502.
13. Lahr CJ, Scong SJ, Cloud G, et al. A multifactorial analysis of prognostic factors in patients with liver metastases from colorectal carcinoma. J Clin Oncol 1983;1:720–726.
14. Boey J, Choi TK, Wong J, et al. Carcinoma of the colon and rectum with liver involvement. Surg Gynecol Obstet 1981;153:864–868.
15. Bengtsson G, Carlson G, Hofstrom L, et al. Natural history of patients with untreated liver metastases from colorectal cancer. Am J Surg 1981;141:586–589.
16. Baden H, Anderson B. Survival of patients with untreated liver metastases from colorectal cancer. Scand J Gastroenterol 1975;10:221–223.
17. Abrams MS, Lerner HJ. Survival of patients at Pennsylvania Hospital with hepatic metastases from carcinoma of the colon and rectum. Dis Colon Rectum 1971;14:431–434.
18. Bengmark S, Hofstrom L. The natural history of primary and secondary malignant tumors of the liver: I. The prognosis for patients with hepatic metastases from colonic and rectal carcinoma by laparotomy. Cancer 1970;23:198–202.
19. Sterns MW, Binkley GE. Palliative surgery for cancer of the rectum and colon. Cancer 1954;7:1016–1019.
20. Hughes KS, Sugarbaker PH. Resection of the liver for metastatic solid tumors. In: Rosenberg SA, ed. Surgical treatment of metastatic cancer. Philadelphia: JB Lippincott, 1987.
21. Schwartz SI. Primary and metastatic hepatic malignant tumors, and hepatic resection. In: Schwartz SI, Ellis H, eds. Maingot's abdominal operations. 9th ed. Norwalk, CT: Appleton & Lange, 1989:1253–1290.
22. Sugarbaker PH, Reinig JW, Hughes KS. Diagnosis of hepatic metastases. In: Rosenberg SA, ed. Surgical treatment of metastatic cancer. Philadelphia: JB Lippincott, 1987.
23. Foster JH, Ensminger WF. Treatment of metastatic cancer to the liver. In: DeVita VT Jr, Hellman S, Rosenberg S, eds. Cancer principles and practice of oncology. 2nd ed. Philadelphia: JB Lippincott, 1985.
24. Kemeny N, Sugarbaker PH. Treatment of metastatic cancer to the liver. In: DeVita VT Jr, Hellman S, Rosenberg S, eds. Cancer principles and practice of oncology. 3rd ed. Philadelphia: JB Lippincott, 1989.
25. Foster JH. Surgical treatment of metastatic liver tumors. Hepatogastroenterology 1990;37:182–187.
26. Weiss L, Grundman E, Torkorst J, et al. Hematogenous metastatic patterns in colonic carcinoma: An analysis of 1541 necropsies. J Pathol 1986;150:195–203.
27. Welch JP, Donaldson GA. The clinical correlation of an autopsy study of recurrent colorectal cancer. Ann Surg 1979;189:496.
28. Wanebo JH, Rao B, Pinsky CM, et al. Preoperative carcinoembryonic antigen level as a prognostic indicator in colorectal cancer. N Engl J Med 1978;299:448–451.
29. Roh MS. Hepatic resection for colorectal liver metastases. Hematol Oncol Clin North Am 1989;3(1):171–181.
30. Klose G, Schmiegel W. Laboratory investigations in hepatobiliary and pancreatic malignancies: The role of tumor markers. In: Lygidakis NJ, Tytgat GNJ, eds. Hepatobiliary and pancreatic malignancies. Diagnosis, medical and surgical management. New York: Georg Thieme Verlag Stuttgart, Thieme Medical Publishers, 1989:157–161.
31. Rosenbusch G, Smits NJ, Reeders JWAJ. Ultrasonography in hepatobiliary and pancreatic malignancies. In: Lygidakis NJ, Tytgat GNJ, eds. Hepatobiliary and pancreatic malignancies. Diagnosis, medical and surgical management. New York: Georg Thieme Verlag Stuttgart, Thieme Medical Publishers, 1989:51–65.
32. Strake LTE, Reeders JWAJ. Computed tomography in hepatobiliary and pancreatic malignancies. In: Lygidakis NJ, Tytgat GNJ, eds. Hepatobiliary and pancreatic malignancies. Diagnosis, medical and surgical management. New York: Georg Thieme Verlag Stuttgart, Thieme Medical Publishers, 1989:79–89.
33. Engelholem L, Mathieu D, Segebarth C, et al. Magnetic resonance imaging (MRI) in hepatobiliary and pancreatic malignancies. In: Lygidakis NJ, Tytgat GNJ, eds. Hepatobiliary and pancreatic malignancies. Diagnosis, medical and surgical management. New York: Georg Thieme Verlag Stuttgart, Thieme Medical Publishers, 1989:90–99.
34. Sitzmann JV, Coleman JA, Pitt HA, et al. Preoperative assessment of malignant hepatic tumors. Am J Surg 1990;159:137–142.
35. Laufer I, Braffman B, Gefter W. Diagnosis and imaging of gastrointestinal tract cancers. Curr Opin Oncol 1991;3(4):730–736.
36. Castaing D, Edmond J, Kunstlinger F, Bismuth H. Utility of operative ultrasound in the surgical management of liver tumors. Ann Surg 1986;204:600–605.
37. Takahashi H, Carlson R, Ozturk M, Sun S, et al. Radioimmunolocation of hepatic and pulmonary metastasis of human colon adenocarcinoma. Gastroenterology 1989;96:1317–1329.
38. Doerr RJ, Abdel-Nabi H, Kray D, Mitchell E. Radiolabelled antibody imaging in the management of colorectal cancer. Ann Surg 1991;214(2):118–124.
39. Adson MA, vanHeerden JA, Adson MH, Wagner JS, Ilstrup DM. Resection of hepatic metastases from colorectal cancer. Arch Surg 1984;119:647.
40. Iwatsuki S, Sheahan DG, Starzl TE. The changing face of hepatic resection. Curr Probl Surg 1989;26(5):283–379.
41. Gozzetti G, Mazziotti A. Expectations and possibilities of liver resection in the management of secondary liver tumors. In: Lygidakis NJ, Tytgat GNJ, eds. Hepatobiliary and pancreatic malignancies. Diagnosis, medical and surgical management. New York: Georg Thieme Verlag Stuttgart, Thieme Medical Publishers, 1989:183–190.
42. Meyers WC. Neoplasms of the liver. In: Sabiston D Jr, ed. Textbook of surgery. The biological basis of modern surgical practice. 13th ed. Philadelphia: WB Saunders, 1986:1079–1092.
43. Ravitch MM. Chapter 22. In: Ravitch MM, ed. A century of surgery. Philadelphia: JB Lippincott, 1982:318–319.
44. Kremer B, Henne-Burns D. Surgical techniques. In: Lygidakis NJ, Tytgat GNJ, eds. Hepatobiliary and pancreatic malignancies. Diagnosis, medical and surgical management. New York: Georg Thieme Verlag Stuttgart, Thieme Medical Publishers, 1989:195–218.
45. Couinauld C. Bases anatomiques des hepatectomies gauche et droit reglees: Techniques qui en decoulent. J Chir (Paris) 1954:70:933.
46. Couinauld C. Le foie: Etudes anatomiques et chirugicales. Paris: Masson & Cis, 1957:3–9.
47. Paquet KJ, Koussouris P, Mercado MA, et al. Limited hepatic resection for selected cirrhotic patients with hepatocellular or cholangiocellular carcinoma: A prospective study. Br J Surg 1991;78:459–462.
48. Sitzmann JV. Colorectal cancer metastatic to the liver: Resection. In: Cameron JL, ed. Current surgical therapy. 3rd ed. Philadelphia: BC Decker, 1989:220–225.
49. Nordlinger B, Parc R, Delva E, et al. Hepatic resection for colorectal liver metastases. Influence on survival of preoperative factors and surgery for recurrences in 80 patients. Ann Surg 1986;305(3):256–263.
50. Bozzetti F, Doci R, Bignami P, et al. Patterns of failure following surgical resection of colorectal cancer liver metastases. Ann Surg 1986;305(3):264–270.
51. Cantlie J. On a new arrangement of the right and left lobes of the liver. Proc Anat Soc Gr Britain Ireland 1898:32:4–9.
52. Gyves JW, Ziessman HA, Ensminger WD, et al. Definition of hepatic tumor microcirculation by single photon emission computerized tomography (SPECT). J Nucl Med 1984;25:972.
53. Niederhuber JE, Grochow LB. Status of infusion chemotherapy for the treatment of liver metastases. Principles and Practices of Oncology (Updates) 1989;3(3):1–9.
54. Breedes C, Young G. The blood supply of neoplasms in the liver. Am J Pathol 1954;30:227.
55. Hesly JE. Vascular patterns in human metastatic liver tumors. Surg Gynecol Obstet 1965;120:1187.
56. Lin B, Lunderquist A, Hogersteand L, et al. Postmortem examination of the blood supply and vascular pattern of small liver metastases in man. Surgery 1984;96:517.

57. Ridge JA, Bading JR, Gelbard AS, et al. Perfusion of colorectal hepatic metastases: Relative distribution of flow from the hepatic artery and portal vein. Cancer 1987;59:1547.

58. Schuur KH, Reeders JWAJ. Angiography in the preoperative staging of hepatobiliary and pancreatic malignancies. In: Lygidakis NJ, Tytgat GNJ, eds. Hepatobiliary and pancreatic malignancies. Diagnosis, medical and surgical management. New York: Georg Thieme Verlag Stuttgart, Thieme Medical Publishers, 1989:136–146.

59. Putnam CW. Techniques of ultrasonic dissection in resection of the liver. Surg Gynecol Obstet 1982;157:475.

60. Fortner JG, Silva JS, Golbey RB, et al. Multi-variate analysis of a personal series of 247 consecutive patients with liver metastases from colorectal cancer. Ann Surg 1984;199:306.

61. Attiyeh FF, Wanebo HJ, Stearns MW. Hepatic resection for metastasis from colorectal cancer. Dis Colon Rectum 1978;21:160.

62. Foster JH, Lundy J. Pathology of liver metastasis. Curr Probl Surg 1981;18:157.

63. Tomas-de la Vega JE, Donahue EJ, Doolas A, et al. A ten year experience with hepatic resection. Surg Gynecol Obstet 1984;159:223–228.

64. Bismuth H, Houssin D, Ornowski J, Meriggi F. Liver resections in cirrhotic patients: A Western experience. World J Surg 1986;10:311–317.

65. Kanematsu T, Takenake K, Matsumata T, et al. Limited hepatic resection effective for selected cirrhotic patients with primary liver cancer. Ann Surg 1984;199:51–56.

66. Yomanaka N, Okamoto E, Kuwata K, Tanaka N. A multiple regression equation for prediction of posthepatectomy liver failure. Ann Surg 1984;200:658–663.

67. Sitzmann JV, Coleman JA, Pitt HA, et al. Preoperative assessment of malignant hepatic tumors. Am J Surg 1990:159:137–142.

68. Egglin TK, Rummeny E, Stark DD, et al. Hepatic tumors: Quantitative tissue characterization with MR imaging. Radiology 1990;176:107–110.

69. Hahn PF, Stark DD, Weissleder R, et al. Clinical application of superparamagnetic iron oxide in MR imaging of tissue perfusion in vascular liver tumors. Radiology 1990;174:361–366.

70. Charnley RM, Morris DL, Dennison AR, et al. Detection of colorectal liver metastases using intraoperative ultrasonography. Br J Surg 1991;78(1):45–48.

71. Steele G Jr, Ravikumar TS. Resection of hepatic metastases from colorectal cancer. Ann Surg 1989;210(2):127–138.

72. Brower ST, Dumistrescu O, Rubinoff S, et al. Operative ultrasound establishes resectability of metastases by major hepatic resection. World J Surg 1989;13(5):649–657.

73. Niederhuber JE. Surgical aspects of intrahepatic artery therapy. In: Bottino JC, Opfell RW, Muggia FM, eds. Liver cancer. Boston: Martinus Nijhoff Publishing, 1985:179–194.

74. Niederhuber JE. Colorectal cancer metastatic to the liver: Hepatic artery chemotherapy. In: Cameron JL, ed. Current surgical therapy. 3rd ed. Philadelphia: BC Decker, 1989:222–233.

75. Szakacs JG, Szakacs JE, Karl RC. Surgical resection versus perfusion in the treatment of metastatic and primary liver tumors. Ann Clin Lab Sci 1990;20(4):245–257.

76. Kuroda C, Sakurai M, Monden M, et al. Transcatheter arterial embolization for metastatic liver tumors: A study in resected cases. Cardiovasc Intervent Radiol 1989;12:72–75.

77. Akuta K, Ahe M, Kondo M, et al. Combined effects of hepatic arterial embolization using degradable starch microspheres in hyperthermia for liver cancer. Int J Hyperthermia 1991;7(2):231–242.

78. Vetter D, Wenger JJ, Bergier JM, et al. Transcatheter oily chemoembolization in the management of advanced hepatocellular carcinoma in cirrhosis: Results of a Western comparative study in 60 patients. Hepatology 1991;13(3):427–433.

79. Livraghi T, Vettori C, Lazzaroni S. Liver metastasis: Results of percutaneous ethanol injection in 14 patients. Radiology 1991;179:709–712.

80. Onik G, Rubinsky B, Zemel R, et al. Ultrasound-guided hepatic cryosurgery in the treatment of metastatic colon carcinoma. Cancer 1991;67(4):901–907.

81. Iwatsuki S, Starzl TE. Hepatic resection for metastatic tumor. In: Lygidakis NJ, Tytgat GNJ, eds. Hepatobiliary and pancreatic malignancies. Diagnosis, medical and surgical management. New York: Georg Thieme Verlag Stuttgart, Thieme Medical Publishers, 1989:191–194.

82. Schlag P, Hohenberger P, Herfath C. Resection of liver metastases in colorectal cancer—Competitive analysis of treatment results in synchronous versus metachronous metastases. Eur J Surg Oncol 1990;16:360–365.

83. Brown DA, Pomnier RF, Woltering EA, et al. Nonanatomic hepatic resection for secondary hepatic tumors with special reference to hemostatic technique. Arch Surg 1988;123:1063.

84. Vetto JT, Hughes KS, Rosenstein R, Sugarbaker PH. Morbidity and mortality of hepatic resection for metastatic colorectal carcinoma. Dis Colon Rectum 1990;33(5):409–413.

85. Murray KD. Excision of pulmonary metastasis of colorectal cancer. Semin Surg Oncol 1991;7:157–161.

86. Pugh RNH, Murray-Lyon IM, Danson JL, Pietroni MC, Williams R. Transsection of esophagus for bleeding varices. Br J Surg 1973;60:646.

87. Moertel CG, Reitemeier RJ. Advanced gastrointestinal cancer—Clinical management and chemotherapy. New York: Harper & Row, 1969.

88. Baker LH, Talley RW, Maiter R, et al. Phase III comparison of the treatment of advanced gastrointestinal cancer with bolus weekly 5-FU vs methyl-CCNU plus bolus weekly 5-FU. Cancer 1976;38:1–7.

89. Siefert P, Baker LH, Reed MD, et al. Comparison of continuously infused 5-fluorouracil with bolus injection in treatment of patients with colorectal adenocarcinoma. Cancer 1975;36:123–128.

90. Grage TG, Vassilopoulos P, Shingleton WW, et al. Results of a prospective randomized study of hepatic artery infusion with 5-fluorouracil vs intravenous 5-fluorouracil in patients with hepatic metastases from colorectal cancer. A Central Oncology Group study. Surgery 1979;86:550–555.

91. MacDonald JS, Kisner DF, Smythe T, et al. 5-Fluorouracil (5-FU), methyl-CCNU and vincristine in the treatment of advanced colorectal cancer. Phase II study utilizing weekly 5-FU. Cancer Treat Rep 1976;60:1597–1600.

92. Buroker J, Kim PN, Groppe C, et al. 5-FU infusion with methyl-CCNU in the treatment of advanced colon cancer. Cancer 1978;42:1228–1233.

93. Kemeny N, Yagoda A, Golbey RB. A randomized study of two different schedules of methyl-CCNU, 5-FU and vincristine for metastatic colorectal carcinoma. Cancer 1979;43:78–82.

94. Kemeny N, Yagoda A, Braun D. Metastatic colorectal carcinoma: A prospective randomized trial of methyl-CCNU, 5-fluorouracil (5-FU) and vincristine (MOF) versus MOF plus streptozotocin (MOF-strep). Cancer 1983;51:20–25.

95. Kemeny N, Yagoda A, Braun D. Therapy for metastatic colorectal carcinoma with a combination of methyl-CCNU, 5-fluorouracil, vincristine, and streptozotocin (MOF-strep). Cancer 1980;45:876–881.

96. Machover D, Goldschmidt E, Chollet P, et al. Treatment of advanced colorectal and gastric adenocarcinoma with 5-fluorouracil and high-dose folinic acid. J Clin Oncol 1986;4:685–696.

97. Petrelli N, Douglass HO Jr, Herrera L, et al. The modulation of fluorouracil with leucovorin in metastatic colorectal carcinoma: A prospective randomized phase III trial. J Clin Oncol 1989;7:1419–1426.

98. Ardalan B, Chua L, Tian EM, et al. A phase II study of weekly 24-hour infusion with high-dose fluorouracil with leucovorin in colorectal carcinoma. J Clin Oncol 1991;9:625–630.

99. Kemeny N, Ahmed T, Michaelson R, et al. Activity of low dose methotrexate and fluorouracil in advanced colorectal carcinoma: Attempted correlation with tissue and blood levels of phosphoriboxylpyrophosphate. J Clin Oncol 1984;2:311–315.

100. Nordic Gastrointestinal Tumor Adjuvant Therapy Group. Superiority of sequential methotrexate, fluorouracil, and leucovorin to fluorouracil alone in advanced symptomatic colorectal carcinoma: A randomized trial. J Clin Oncol 1989;7:1437–1446.

101. Pandya KJ, Chan AYU, Qazi R, et al. Combination chemotherapy for advanced colorectal cancer. A pilot study. Am J Clin Oncol 1986;9:31–34.

102. Loehrer PJ Sr, Einhorn LH, Williams SD, et al. Cisplatin plus 5-FU for the treatment of adenocarcinoma of the colon. Cancer Treat Rep 1985;69:1359–1363.

103. Kemeny N, Reichman B, Botet J, et al. Continuous infusion 5-fluorouracil (FU) and bolus cisplatin (DDP) for metastatic colorectal cancer. Proc Am Soc Clin Oncol 1987;6:86.

104. Lokich JJ, Ahlgren JD, Gullo JJ, et al. A prospective randomized comparison of continuous infusion fluorouracil with a conventional bolus schedule in metastatic colorectal carcinoma: A Mid-Atlantic Oncology Program study. J Clin Oncol 1989;7:425–432.

105. Erlichman C, Fine S, Wong A, Elhakim T. A randomized trial of fluorouracil and folinic acid in patients with metastatic colorectal carcinoma J Clin Oncol 1988;6:469–475.

106. Doroshow JH, Multhauf P, Leong L, et al. Prospective randomized comparison of fluorouracil versus fluorouracil and high-dose continuous infusion leucovorin calcium for the treatment of advanced measurable colorectal cancer in patients previously unexposed to chemotherapy. J Clin Oncol 1990;8:491–501.

107. Bruckner HW, Motwani BT. Chemotherapy of advanced cancer of the colon and rectum. Semin Oncol 1991;18:443–461.

108. Poon MA, O'Connell MJ, Moertel CG, et al. Biochemical modulation of fluorouracil: Evidence of significant improvement of survival and quality of life in patients with advanced colorectal carcinoma. J Clin Oncol 1989;7:1407–1417.

109. Kemeny N. The systemic chemotherapy of hepatic metastases. Semin Oncol 1983;10:148–159.

110. Kvols LK, Buck M. Chemotherapy of endocrine malignancies: A review. Semin Oncol 1987;14:343–353.

111. Ajani JA, Carrasco CH, Samaan NA, Wallace S. Therapeutic options for patients with advanced islet cell and carcinoid tumors. Reg Cancer Treat 1991;3:235–242.

112. Ensminger WD, Gyves JW. Regional cancer chemotherapy. Cancer Treat Rep 1984;68:101–115.

113. Frei E III, Canellos GP. Dose: A critical factor in cancer chemotherapy. Am J Med 1980;69:585–594.

114. Bierman HR, Byron RL, Kelly KH, Grady A. Studies on the blood supply of tumors in man III. Vascular patterns of the liver by hepatic arteriography in vivo. JNCI 1951;12:107–117.

115. Sullivan RD, Norcross JW, Watkins E. Chemotherapy of metastatic liver cancer by prolonged hepatic-artery infusion. N Engl J Med 1964;270:321–327.

116. Sullivan RD, Zurek WZ. Chemotherapy for liver cancer by protracted ambulatory infusion. JAMA 1965;194:481–486.

117. Watkins E, Khazei AM, Nahra KS. Surgical basis for arterial infusion chemotherapy of disseminated carcinoma of the liver. Surg Gynecol Obstet 1970;130:581–605.

118. Cady B, Overfield RA. Regional infusion chemotherapy of hepatic metastases from carcinoma of the colon. Am J Surg 1974;127:220–227.

119. Buroker T, Samson M, Correa J, et al. Hepatic artery infusion of 5-FUDR after prior systemic 5-fluorouracil. Cancer Treat Rep 1976;60:1277–1279.

120. Oberfield RA, McCaffrey JA, Polio J, et al. Prolonged and continuous percutaneous intra-arterial hepatic infusion chemotherapy in advanced metastatic liver adenocarcinoma from colorectal primary. Cancer 1979;44:414–423.

121. Patt YZ, Mavligit GM, Chuang VP, et al. Percutaneous hepatic arterial infusion (HAI) of mitomycin C and floxuridine (FUDR): An effective treatment for metastatic colorectal carcinoma in the liver. Cancer 1979;46:261–265.

122. Reed ML, Vaitkevicius VK, Al-Sarraf M, et al. The practicality of chronic hepatic artery

infusion therapy of primary and metastatic hepatic malignancies; ten-year results of 124 patients in a prospective protocol. Cancer 1981;47:402–409.

123. Ensminger WD, Rosowsky A, Raso V, et al. A clinical-pharmacological evaluation of hepatic arterial infusions of 5-fluoro-2'-deoxyuridine and 5-fluorouracil. Cancer Res 1978;38:3784–3792.

124. Collins JM. Pharmacologic rationale for regional drug delivery. J Clin Oncol 1984;2: 498–504.

125. Collins JM. Pharmacokinetics and clinical monitoring. In: Chabner BA, Collins JM, eds. Cancer chemotherapy principles & practice. Philadelphia: JB Lippincott, 1990.

126. Stetson PL, Maybaum J, Wagner JW, et al. Tissue-specific pharmacodynamics of 5-bromo-2'-deoxyuridine incorporation into DNA in VX 2 tumor-bearing rabbits. Cancer Res 1988;48:6900–6905.

127. Knol JA, Stetson PL, Wagner JG, et al. 5-Bromo-2'-deoxyuridine incorporation into DNA in hepatic VX2 tumor-bearing rabbits. J Surg Res 1989;47:112–116.

128. Kaplan WD, Ensminger WD, Come SE, et al. Radionuclide angiography to predict patient response to hepatic artery chemotherapy. Cancer Treat Rep 1980;64:1217–1222.

129. Daly JM, Butler J, Kemeny N, et al. Predicting tumor response in patients with colorectal hepatic metastases. Ann Surg 1985;202:384–393.

130. Sigurdson ER, Ridge JA, Kemeny N, Daly JM. Tumor and liver drug uptake following hepatic artery and portal vein infusion. J Clin Oncol 1987;5:1836–1840.

131. Blackshear PJ, Dorman FD, Blackshear PL Jr, et al. The design and initial testing of an implantable infusion pump. Surg Gynecol Obstet 1972;134:51–56.

132. Buchwald H, Grage TB, Vassilopoulos PP, et al. Intra-arterial infusion chemotherapy for hepatic carcinoma using a totally implantable infusion pump. Cancer 1980;45: 866–869.

133. Ensminger WD, Niederhuber J, Dakhil S, et al. Totally implanted drug delivery system for hepatic arterial chemotherapy. Cancer Treat Rep 1981;65:393–400.

134. Balch CM, Urist MM, Soong SJ, McGregor M. A prospective phase II clinical trial of continuous FUDR regional chemotherapy for colorectal metastases to the liver using a totally implantable drug infusion pump. Ann Surg 1983;198:567–573.

135. Niederhuber JE, Ensminger WD, Gyves J, et al. Regional chemotherapy of colorectal cancer metastatic to the liver. Cancer 1984;53:1336–1343.

136. Kemeny N, Daly J, Oderman P, et al. Hepatic artery pump infusion: Toxicity and results in patients with metastatic colorectal carcinoma. J Clin Oncol 1984;2:595–600.

137. Shepard KV, Levin B, Karl RC, et al. Therapy for metastatic colorectal cancer with hepatic artery infusion chemotherapy using a subcutaneous implanted pump. J Clin Oncol 1985;3:161–169.

138. Kemeny MM, Goldberg DA, Browning S, et al. Experience with continuous regional chemotherapy and hepatic resection as treatment of hepatic metastases from colorectal primaries. Cancer 1985;55:1265–1270.

139. Patt YZ, Boddie AW Jr, Charnsangavej C, et al. Hepatic arterial infusion with floxuridine and cisplatin: Overriding importance of antitumor effect versus degree of tumor burden as determinants of survival among patients with colorectal cancer. J Clin Oncol 1986;4: 1356–1364.

140. Cohen AM, Schaeffer N, Higgins J. Treatment of metastatic colorectal cancer with hepatic artery combination chemotherapy. Cancer 1986;57:1115–1117.

141. Kemeny N, Daly J, Reichman B, et al. Intrahepatic or systemic infusion of fluoro-deoxyuridine in patients with liver metastases from colorectal carcinoma. Ann Intern Med 1987;107:459–465.

142. Hohn DC, Stagg RJ, Friedman MA, et al. A randomized trial of continuous intravenous versus hepatic intraarterial floxuridine in patients with colorectal cancer metastatic to the liver: The Northern California Oncology Group trial. J Clin Oncol 1989;7:1646–1654.

143. Chang AE, Schneider PD, Sugarbaker PH, et al. A prospective randomized trial of regional versus systemic continuous 5-fluorodeoxyuridine chemotherapy in the treatment of colorectal liver metastases. Ann Surg 1987;206:685–693.

144. Martin JK, O'Connell MJ, Wieand HS, et al. Intra-arterial floxuridine vs systemic fluorouracil for hepatic metastases from colorectal cancer. Arch Surg 1990;125:1022–1027.

145. Chuang VP, Wallace S. Hepatic arterial redistribution for intraarterial infusion of hepatic neoplasms. Radiology 1980;135:295–299.

146. Daly JM, Kemeny N. Therapy of colorectal hepatic metastases. In: DeVita VT Jr, Hellman S, Rosenberg SA, eds. Important advances in oncology. Philadelphia: JB Lippincott, 1986.

147. Niederhuber JE, Ensminger WD. Surgical considerations in the management of hepatic neoplasia. Semin Oncol 1983;10:135–147.

148. Ensminger WD. Intraarterial therapy. In: Perry MC, ed. The chemotherapy sourcebook. Baltimore: Williams & Wilkins, 1992.

149. Patt YZ, Mavligit GM. Arterial chemotherapy in the management of colorectal cancer: An overview. Semin Oncol 1991;18:478–490.

150. Hohn DC, Rayner AA, Economou JS, et al. Toxicities and complications of implanted pump hepatic arterial and intravenous floxuridine infusion. Cancer 1986;57:465–470.

151. Narsete T, Ansfield F, Wirtanen G, et al. Gastric ulceration in patients receiving intrahepatic infusion of 5-fluorouracil. Ann Surg 1977;186:734–736.

152. Chuang VP, Wallace S, Stroehlein J, et al. Hepatic artery infusion chemotherapy: Gastroduodenal complications. Am J Radiol 1981;137:347.

153. Hohn DC, Stagg RJ, Price DC, et al. Avoidance of gastroduodenal toxicity in patients receiving hepatic arterial 5-fluoro-2'-deoxyuridine. J Clin Oncol 1985;3:1257–1260.

154. Kaplan WD, Come SE, Takvorian RW, et al. Pulmonary uptake of technetium 99m macroaggregated albumin: A predictor of gastrointestinal toxicity during hepatic artery perfusion. J Clin Oncol 1984;2:1266–1269.

155. Gluck WL, Akwari OE, Kelvin FM, et al. A reversible enteropathy complicating continuous hepatic artery infusion chemotherapy with 5-fluoro-2'-deoxyuridine. Cancer 1985;56:2424–2427.

156. Carrasco CH, Freeny PC, Chuang VP, et al. Chemical cholecystitis associated with hepatic artery infusion chemotherapy. AJR 1983;141:703–706.

157. Northover JMA, Terblanche J. A new look at the arterial supply of the bile duct in man and its surgical implications. Br J Surg 1979;66:379–384.

158. Kemeny MM, Battifora H, Blayney DW, et al. Sclerosing cholangitis after continuous hepatic artery infusion of FUDR. Ann Surg 1985;202:176–181.

159. Hohn D, Melnick J, Stagg R, et al. Biliary sclerosis in patients receiving hepatic arterial infusions of floxuridine. J Clin Oncol 1985;3:98–102.

160. Doria MI Jr, Shepard KV, Levin B, et al. Liver pathology following hepatic arterial infusion chemotherapy. Cancer 1986;58:855–861.

161. Andrews JC, Knol J, Wollner I, et al. Floxuridine-associated sclerosing cholangitis. A dog model. Invest Radiol 1989;24:47–51.

162. Kemeny N, Seiter K, Niedzwiecki D, et al. A randomized trial of intrahepatic infusion of fluorodeoxyuridine with dexamethasone versus fluorodeoxyuridine alone in the treatment of metastatic colorectal cancer. Cancer 1992;69:327–334.

163. Hughes KS, Simon R, Songhorabodi S, et al. Resection of the liver for colorectal carcinoma metastases: A multi-institutional study of patterns of recurrence. Surgery 1986;100:278–284.

164. Safi F, Bittner R, Roscher R, et al. Regional chemotherapy for hepatic metastases of colorectal carcinoma (continuous intraarterial versus continuous intraarterial/intravenous therapy). Cancer 1989;64:379–387.

165. Seiter K, Kemeny N, Sigurdson E, et al. A phase I trial of hepatic artery fluorodeoxyuridine combined with systemic 5-fluorouracil for the treatment of metastases from colorectal cancer. Reg Cancer Treat 1991;3:293–297.

166. Stagg RJ, Venook AP, Chase JL, et al. Alternating hepatic intra-arterial floxuridine and fluorouracil: A less toxic regimen for treatment of liver metastases from colorectal cancer. JNCI 1991;83:423–428.

167. Sheen MC, Wang YW. Complications of port-catheter systems in intra-arterial infusion chemotherapy. Reg Cancer Treat 1991;4:92–97.

168. Walther H, Kahle M, Filler RD. Hepatic artery infusion via an implantable catheter system using the 5-fluorouracil, leucovorin, mitomycin C regimen. Reg Cancer Treat 1991;4:136–139.

169. Khayat D, Le Cesne A, Weil M, et al. Intra-arterial treatment of hepatic metastases using the 5-fluorouracil, adriamycin, mitomycin C (FAM) chemotherapeutic regimen. Reg Cancer Treat 1988;1:62–64.

170. Gyves JW, Stetson P, Ensminger WD, et al. Hepatic arterial streptozocin: A clinical pharmacologic study in patients with liver tumors. Cancer Drug Delivery 1983;1:63–68.

171. Reed ML, Kuipers FM, Vaitkevicius VK, et al. Treatment of disseminated carcinoid tumors including hepatic-artery catheterization. Treat Carcinoid Tumors 1963;269: 1005–1010.

172. Ajani JA, Carrasco CH, Charnsangavej C, et al. Islet cell tumor metastatic to the liver: Effective palliation by sequential hepatic artery embolization. Ann Intern Med 1988;108: 340–344.

173. Mitty HA, Warner RRP, Newman LH, et al. Control of carcinoid syndrome with hepatic artery embolization. Radiology 1985;155:623–626.

174. Allison DJ, Modlin IM, Jenkins WJ. Treatment of carcinoid liver metastases by hepatic artery embolisation. Lancet 1977;2:1323–1325.

175. Carrasco CH, Chuang VP, Wallace S. Apudomas metastatic to the liver: Treatment by hepatic artery embolization. Radiology 1983;149:79–83.

176. Bruso CE, Shewach DS, Lawrence TS. Fluorodeoxyuridine-induced radiosensitization and inhibition of DNA double strand break repair in human colon cancer cells. Int J Radiat Oncol Biol Phys 1990;19:1411–1417.

177. Barone RM, Byfield JE, Goldfarb PB, et al. Intra-arterial chemotherapy using an implantable infusion pump and liver irradiation for the treatment of hepatic metastases. Cancer 1982;50:850–862.

178. Herbsman H, Gardner B, Harshaw D, et al. Treatment of hepatic metastases with a combination of hepatic artery infusion chemotherapy and external radiotherapy. Surg Gynecol Obstet 1978;147:13–17.

179. Webber BM, Soderberg CH, Leone LA, et al. A combined treatment approach to management of hepatic metastases. Cancer 1978;42:1087–1095.

180. Lokich JJ, Kinsella T, Perri J, et al. Concomitant hepatic radiation and intra-arterial fluorinated pyrimidine therapy: Correlation of liver scan, liver function tests, and plasma CEA with tumor response. Cancer 1982;48:2569–2574.

181. Raju PI, Maruyama Y, DeSimone P, MacDonald J. Treatment of liver metastases with a combination of chemotherapy and hyperfractionated external radiation therapy. Am J Clin Oncol 1987;10:41–43.

182. Friedman M, Cassidy M, Levine M, et al. Combined modality therapy of hepatic metastasis. Cancer 1979;44:906–913.

183. Lawrence TS, Dworzian LM, Walker-Andrews S, et al. Treatment of cancers involving the liver and porta hepatis with external beam irradiation and intraarterial hepatic fluorodeoxyuridine. Int J Radiat Oncol Biol Phys 1991;20:555–561.

184. Ingold JA, Reed GB, Kaplan HS, Bagshaw MA. Radiation hepatitis. Am J Roentgenol 1965;93:200–208.

185. Wharton JT, Declos L, Gallager W, Smith JP. Radiation hepatitis induced by abdominal irradiation with cobalt 60 moving strip technique. AJR 1973;117:73–80.

186. Lawrence TS, Kessler ML, Lavigne ML, et al. The use of 3-D dose volume analysis to predict radiation hepatitis. Proceedings of the American Society for Therapeutic Radiology and Oncology 1991;21:187.

187. Lawrence TS, TenHaken RK, Kessler ML, et al. The use of 3-D volume analysis to predict radiation hepatitis. Int J Radiat Oncol Biol Phys 1992;23(4):781–788.
188. Emani B, Lyman J, Brown A, et al. Tolerance of normal tissue to therapeutic irradiation. Int J Radiat Oncol Biol Phys 1991;21:109–122.
189. Chang AE, Collins JM, Speth PAJ, et al. A phase I study of intraarterial iododeoxyuridine in patients with colorectal liver metastases. J Clin Oncol 1989;7:662–668.
190. Speth PAJ, Kinsella TJ, Chang AE, et al. Selective incorporation of iododeoxyuridine into DNA of hepatic metastases versus normal human liver. Clin Pharmacol Ther 1988;44:369–375.
191. Ensminger WD, Andrews JC, Walker-Andrews S, et al. Clinical pharmacology of hepatic arterial 5-bromo-2'-deoxyuridine (BUDR). In: Ensminger WD, Selam JL, eds. Update in drug delivery systems. New York: Futura, 1989.
192. Herba MJ, Illescas FF, Thirlwell MP, et al. Hepatic malignancies: Improved treatment with intraarterial Y-90. Radiology 1988;169:311–314.
193. Andrews JC, Shapiro B, Walker-Andrews SC, Ensminger WD. Hepatic radioembolization with Y-90 microspheres: Initial results. Radiology 1990;177:257–258.
194. Gyves JW, Ensminger WD, VanHarken D, et al. Improved regional selectivity of hepatic arterial BCNU with degradable microspheres. Clin Pharmacol Ther 1983;34:259–265.

195. Lorenz M, Herrmann G, Kirkowa-Reimann M, et al. Temporary chemoembolization of colorectal liver metastases with degradable starch microspheres. Eur J Surg Oncol 1989;15:453–462.
196. Civalleri D, Esposito M, Fulco RA, et al. Liver and tumor uptake and plasma pharmacokinetics of arterial cisplatin administered with and without starch microspheres in patients with liver metastases. Cancer 1991;68:988–994.
197. Dritschilo A, Grant EG, Harter KW, et al. Interstitial radiation therapy for hepatic metastases: Sonographic guidance for applicator placement. AJR 1986;147:275–278.
198. Livraghi T, Festi D, Monti F, et al. US-guided percutaneous alcohol injection of small hepatic and abdominal tumors. Radiology 1986;161:309–312.
199. Ravikumar TS, Kane R, Cady B, et al. Hepatic cryosurgery with intraoperative ultrasound monitoring for metastatic colon carcinoma. Arch Surg 1987;122:403–409.
200. Butler J, Attiyeh FF, Daly JM. Hepatic resection for metastases of the colon and rectum. Surg Gynecol Obstet 1986;162:109–113.
201. Coppa GF, Eng K, Ranson JHC, et al. Hepatic resection for metastatic colon and rectal cancer: An evaluation of preoperative and postoperative factors. Ann Surg 1985;202:203–208.

SECTION **4**

MARTIN M. MALAWER
THOMAS F. DELANEY

Treatment of Metastatic Cancer to Bone

Metastatic cancer is the most common neoplasm involving the skeletal system. Of approximately 965,000 new cancer patients per year in the United States, about 30% to 70% will develop involvement.[1–3] Like primary bone tumors, metastatic skeletal cancer is best treated with a multimodality approach that involves the combined expertise of the medical, surgical, and radiation oncologist. Major advances have been made in the early detection, diagnosis, and surgical/radiotherapeutic treatment of metastatic bone disease. The use of bone scintigraphy, computed tomography (CT), and magnetic resonance imaging (MRI) permits extremely early detection and localization of bony lesions and aids in treatment and preoperative planning.[4–9] During the early 1970s, paralleling the development of joint replacements and the use of a bone cement, polymethylmethacrylate (PMMA), orthopedic surgeons for the first time had a relatively simple and reliable method of treating patients with pathologic fractures.[10,11] The use of PMMA and prosthetic replacements allowed reconstruction of large tumor defects without having to depend on bone healing. This permitted immediate and reliable stabilization of tumor defects and increased early function and ambulation. As these techniques have developed, so has an interest in identifying patients at high risk for pathologic fracture, and thereby the concept of prophylactic fixation has developed. Similarly, improved techniques of spinal surgery have been applied to the treatment of metastatic cancer of the spine, resulting in marked improvement in the ability to decompress and stabilize the spine involved by tumor, with resultant improvement of neurologic status.[12,13]

Most patients do not require surgery; radiation therapy and medical management generally suffice. Megavoltage irradiation, along with radioisotopes for specific tumor types, is permitting a significant number of patients to be treated successfully.[14–20]

This chapter concentrates on the metastatic carcinoma. Sarcomas, melanomas, and the hematogenous malignancies are described briefly. Radiographic imaging techniques, mechanisms of bony metastases and biomechanical effects, biopsy/histologic techniques, and surgical/radiotherapeutic management are described. Specific emphasis is placed on the unique considerations of the different carcinomas and the different anatomic sites.

INCIDENCE AND ANATOMIC SITES OF SKELETAL METASTASES

Bony metastases occur primarily to the axial skeletal and lower extremities. Abrams and colleagues analyzed 1000 consecutive autopsies of patients who died of neoplasms of epithelial origin and reported bone metastasis in 272 cases.[2] The sites of the primary tumors associated with bony metastasis were breast (73.1%), lung (32.5%), kidney (24%), rectum (13%), pancreas (13%), stomach (10.9%), colon (9.3%), and ovary (9%). Clain analyzed 2000 patients who died of cancer with bone metastasis and reported involvement of the following sites: vertebra (69%), pelvis (41%), femur (especially the hip) (25%), and skull (14%).[20] The upper extremity is much less commonly involved; approximately 10% to 15% of bony metastasis occur at this site.[2] The pattern of involvement is similar for most carcinomas, although some tumors show a predilection for specific skeletal sites (*e.g.*, prostate tumors for the pelvic bones).

Pathologic fractures requiring surgical intervention occur in approximately 9% of patients with metastatic bone disease.[21] Higinbotham and Marcove reported that 165 of 1800 patients with solitary or multiple metastatic cancer to bone treated at the Bone Tumor Service at Memorial Sloan-Kettering Hospital between 1931 and 1965 required surgery for fracture; 150 had metastatic carcinoma, and 15 had metastatic sarcoma or myeloma.[21] Most of these fractures were of the femur, humerus, or both. Four types of tumors accounted for nearly 80% of the fractures: breast (53%), kidney (11%), lung (8%), and thyroid (5%). Many studies have shown a similar distribution.[2,10,11,22,23]

GENERAL CONSIDERATIONS

CLINICAL CHARACTERISTICS

The hallmark of skeletal metastases, irrespective of histogenesis, is localized pain. The pain pattern is similar to that of primary bone tumors (*i.e.*, initially intermittent, unrelated to activity, and eventually becoming continuous and unrelenting). Many metastatic lesions, however, are not painful and are detected only by radiographic or bone scintigraphy.[9,24] Additional characteristics are related to the specific sites involved. Shoulder girdle metastases often present as a "frozen" shoulder, whereas thoracic and vertebral body involvement may cause referred pain to the chest wall and the lower extremities, respectively. Lumbar vertebral disease often presents as "low back pain," sciatica, or both. The most serious complication of vertebral metastases is secondary epidural compression of the spinal cord or cauda equina. Early cord compression is heralded by increasing back pain, and the patient must be immediately evaluated for this complication. Any cancer patient who develops skeletal pain should undergo plain radiography of the affected area and bone scintigraphy.

LABORATORY EVALUATION

Laboratory evaluation for the detection of skeletal disease includes serum calcium/phosphorus, alkaline and acid phosphatase, and carcinoembryonic antigen (CEA) assays. None of these tests is specific for bony metastases. Hypercalcemia is not directly related to the extent of bony disease, although patients with bony metastases often have high serum calcium levels.[3,25,26]

DIAGNOSIS

The clinical presentation, plain radiography, and bone scintigraphy findings are usually typical of metastatic disease. A confirmatory pathologic evaluation is performed by simple needle or aspiration biopsy in most anatomic sites.[7,27] In the adult, entities that may be confused with metastatic cancer are the hematologic malignancies (myeloma, leukemia, lymphoma) and Paget's disease of bone. A primary sarcoma of bone may occasionally be mistaken for a metastatic cancer; therefore, solitary metastases must be appropriately staged and biopsied. Radiation-induced sarcomas should also be considered if a bony lesion arises in a previous radiation therapy field after an appropriate latency period.

GOALS AND TYPES OF TREATMENT

Most skeletal metastases do not require surgery. Radiation therapy, chemotherapy, and hormonal manipulation provide good symptomatic relief. A pending or actual pathologic fracture requires operative fixation, because fractures through a tumor-bearing bone rarely heal without such intervention.

The goals of fixation are to relieve pain, to improve function and ambulation, to facilitate medical and nursing care, and to improve psychologic well-being.[28] This requires a surgical approach different from that used for nonneoplastic lesions. Immediate fixation must be provided. A variety of techniques are in use, including replacement by a prosthesis (especially about the hip) or a combination of internal fixation and

PMMA.[10,22,23,28] Both provide immediate stability. In general, radiation therapy is used after wound healing to arrest local tumor growth, permit bony repair, and prevent regrowth of tumor around the fixation device.

MECHANISM AND PATHOGENESIS OF SKELETAL METASTASIS

The way in which tumor cells travel to the skeletal system and establish metastases, their relation to the primary tumor, and the way in which they destroy normal bone are poorly understood. Attempts to explain the phenomenon have focused on the unique nature of the venous system, the bony microvascular structure, and, recently, the relation of tumor cell to bone, termed the microenvironment.[29–31]

VASCULAR AND MICROVASCULAR CONSIDERATIONS

Normal bone does not contain lymphatic channels. Skeletal metastases occur hematogenously.[29,32] The peculiarities of the venous system[33–40] are considered the main pathway of mechanical transport of cancer cells to the skeletal system.

Batson initially emphasized the significant role of a complex network of vertebral, epidural, and perivertebral veins, a system heretofore not appreciated or named, in the transport of cancer cells to the skeleton (Fig. 61–40).[31,33,41,42] This system parallels, joins, and also *bypasses* the other three venous systems. External pressure, not valves, determines the flow within this system. Blood within this system flows in different directions, depending on the pressure exerted by physiologic activity. This network partially explains the frequency and distribution of metastases along the vertebral column, in the

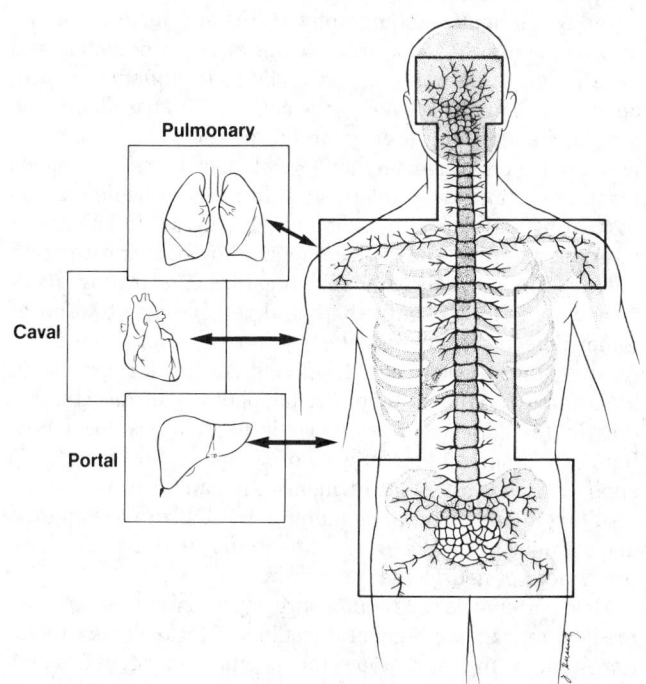

FIGURE 61–40. Batson's plexus. (Modified from Batson OV. The function of the vertebral veins and their role in the spread of metastases. Ann Surg 1940;112:138–149)

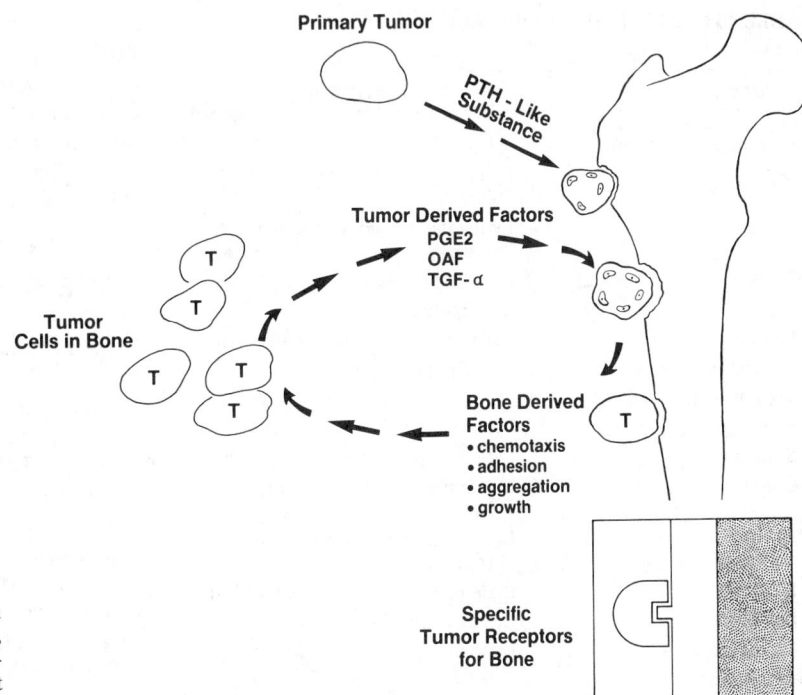

FIGURE 61–41. Mechanisms of tumor cell growth and bone destruction. (Modified from Manishen WJ, Sivananthan K, Orr WF. Resorbing bone stimulates tumor cell growth. A role for the host microenvironment in bone metastasis. Am J Pathol 1986;123:39–45)

pelvic and shoulder girdle, and in apparent "aberrant" sites. In addition, the increased susceptibility of red marrow is related to the special hemodynamic and microanatomic aspects of its vasculature.[4,29] Its unique cellular structure contributes to the propensity of tumor cell extravasation and to the formation of foci of tumor cells within the red marrow.[43]

TUMOR CELL-HOST BONE RELATION

Tumor cells may destroy bone directly, produce mediators that stimulate resorption by osteoclasts, or produce other newly described mediators such as transforming growth factor (TGF) and prostaglandins (PGE₁ and PGE₂) (Fig. 61–41).[3,30,44] Much of this information comes from studies of patients with malignant hypercalcemia. Prostaglandins in bone act similarly to parathormone (*i.e.*, they stimulate cAMP, activate collagenase synthesis, and increase osteoclast number and activity).[32] Galasko demonstrated that osteoclastic proliferation and subsequent bony resorption occurred quite soon after tumor invasion.[3] An osteoclast-activating factor (OAF) has been identified (from lymphoma and myeloma cells) that might be dependent on prostaglandins.[45] It has been suggested that tumor cells may have specific receptors for bone marrow.[46] Another possibility is that resorbing bone itself can release chemoattractants that will cause tumor cell adherence and migration.[47]

RADIOGRAPHIC DIAGNOSIS AND EVALUATION OF METASTASES

The diagnosis of metastatic cancer to the skeletal system is based on one of several radiographic imaging studies, followed by a definitive biopsy. The skeletal system can be easily and accurately imaged by several imaging modalities. The choice, indications, and advantages of each are summarized.

RADIOGRAPHY

Plain radiographs are highly accurate in differentiating metastatic carcinoma from other benign or malignant lesions of bone. In many cases, no other tests may be required. Wilner described the general characteristics of these lesions.[48]

Location

The most common sites of metastasis are the spine, hip, and femur. When long bones are involved, the metaphyseal area and, less commonly, the middiaphyseal area are affected. Tumor generally reaches the medullary area before invading the cortex; primary cortical metastases are rare.

Size, Shape, and Number

Multiple bony lesions are the hallmark of metastatic disease. Solitary metastases occur occasionally and are difficult to differentiate from a primary bone tumor. In general, metastatic carcinomas are small (1–3 cm) and well defined. Lesions of the hip and pelvis may be larger. Appreciation of tumor size and shape, in conjunction with multiplicity, usually enables one to diagnose metastatic cancer with confidence. Extraosseous extension (*i.e.*, a soft tissue component) rarely occurs with metastatic cancer; it is largely a characteristic of primary sarcomas of bone. Among the primary multiple tumors of bone that might be confused with metastatic carcinoma are histiocytosis, enchondromatosis, and fibrous dysplasia. Each of these tends to occur in the younger patient.

Radiographic Pattern

Bone that is invaded by metastatic cancer typically exhibits three patterns: osteolytic, osteoblastic, and, less commonly, mixed (Table 61–29). A given patient may demonstrate a

TABLE 61–29. Radiographic Appearance
of Skeletal Metastases

Primary Tumor	Radiographic Appearance
Common primary cancer	
Breast	Lytic; also mixed; frequently blastic
Lung	Lytic; also mixed; occasionally blastic
Kidney	Invariably lytic
Thyroid	Invariably lytic
Prostate	Usually blastic; occasionally lytic
Head and neck	Usually lytic
Gastrointestinal tract	
Esophagus	Lytic or mixed
Stomach	Lytic or mixed; occasionally blastic
Colon	Lytic or mixed; infrequently blastic
Rectum	Lytic or mixed; infrequently blastic
Pancreas	Lytic or mixed; occasionally blastic
Liver	Lytic or mixed
Gallbladder	Lytic or mixed
Genitourinary tract	
Urinary bladder	Lytic; infrequently blastic
Adrenal	Lytic
Reproductive system	
Uterine cervix	Lytic or mixed; occasionally blastic
Uterine corpus	Lytic
Skin	
Squamous and basal cell carcinoma	Lytic
Malignant melanoma	Lytic
Carcinoid tumors	
Bronchial and abdominal	Blastic; frequently mixed

(Modified from Wilner D. Cancer metastasis to bone. In: Wilner D,
ed. Radiology of bone tumors and allied disorders. Philadelphia: WB
Saunders, 1982:3646)

combination of patterns, often even within one bone. There
are three types of osteolytic patterns: (1) moth-eaten (multiple, small-to-medium-sized lesions that may coalesce to form
large defects such as those often seen with breast cancer);
(2) diffuse infiltrative (often seen with round cell tumors such
as lymphoma, neuroblastoma, and Ewing's sarcoma); and
(3) large, expansile lesions (thyroid, hypernephroma)
(Fig. 61–42).

Osteoblastic metastases, which are less common, are frequently seen in conjunction with cancers of the prostate and
breast. They tend to be smaller than osteolytic lesions. There
are three types of osteoblastic patterns: (1) rounded, discrete
(well-circumscribed, uniform density); (2) mottled (irregular
areas with varying sclerosis); and (3) diffuse (large lesions).
The osteoblastic component is *not* neoplastic osteoid tissue
but rather represents the reaction of normal bone to the metastatic cancer. The amount and pattern of sclerosis indicate
the growth rate of tumor: the denser the pattern, the slower
the growth. If growth is fast, a mixed dense and lytic pattern
is seen. Increasing sclerosis is a sign of repair.

Involvement of the cortex adjacent to metastatic cancer
rarely causes periosteal elevation; when it does, one should
consider cancer of the prostate or lung. In general, periosteal
elevation is associated with primary bony neoplasms. In addition, primary tumors such as Paget's sarcoma, malignant
fibrous histiocytoma (MFH) of bone, or primary fibrosarcoma
should be considered if periosteal elevation is present.

BONE SCINTIGRAPHY

Radionuclide imaging of the skeletal system is extremely useful in the diagnosis and management of the patient with skeletal metastasis.[2,8,9,24,49–51] With the development of whole-body
imaging, the Gamma camera, and a reliable bone imaging
agent (^{99m}Tc-diphosphonate), bone scanning has become a
routine method of evaluating the skeletal system for metastatic
disease. It is used for detection and staging, for following the
response of a bone lesion to treatment, and as a guide in performing needle biopsies for difficult lesions.[2,7–9,50,51]

In general, bone scans will detect metastatic lesions before
they are evident on plain radiographs (Fig. 61–43). Wilner
estimates that bone scans will detect lesions about 3 months
earlier than plain radiographs.[48] Galasko reported a range of
2 months to 18 months, with 75% of breast cancer patients
developing corresponding changes within 6 months.[32] Bone
scans are most reliable for tumors of the breast, prostate,
lung, and kidney. They are least accurate for the diagnosis of
round cell tumors, myeloma, lymphoma, and the leukemias.[32]
Areas of *decreased* uptake ("photopenic" areas) are often observed with myeloma and, occasionally, with breast and lung
cancers.

THE SOLITARY LESION

A unique problem with bone scintigraphy in following patients
with a known cancer is the appearance of a solitary lesion.
This occurs in 6% to 8% of all patients.[9] McNeil reviewed
273 reports of such cases and reported that 55% represented
metastatic disease.[9] Trauma (25%), infection (10%), and
miscellaneous factors (10%) accounted for the nonmalignant
causes. McNeil emphasized that anatomic site is important
in this differentiation; 80% of the vertebral lesions, compared
with 18% of the rib lesions, proved to be metastatic in patients
with a known primary tumor. If scintigraphy reveals a solitary
lesion, additional evaluation, including high-resolution plain
radiographs, CT, and possibly biopsy, is recommended.

BONE SCAN-GUIDED NEEDLE BIOPSY

Within the past few years, several reports[3,4] have described
the use of bone scintigraphy as an aid to biopsy.[7,8] The scan
may be used to mark an area of abnormality before biopsy or
may confirm that the correct area has been biopsied intraoperatively. These techniques have enhanced the accuracy of
the biopsy in cases in which other modalities have not demonstrated a lesion. Zegel and colleagues described a technique
of localizing "hot" rib lesions with nuclear medicine guidance
by the use of a lead ring.[7] Percutaneous biopsies reported in
conjunction with positive scans revealed that 13 of 14 patients
had metastatic tumor. Little and associates described a tech-

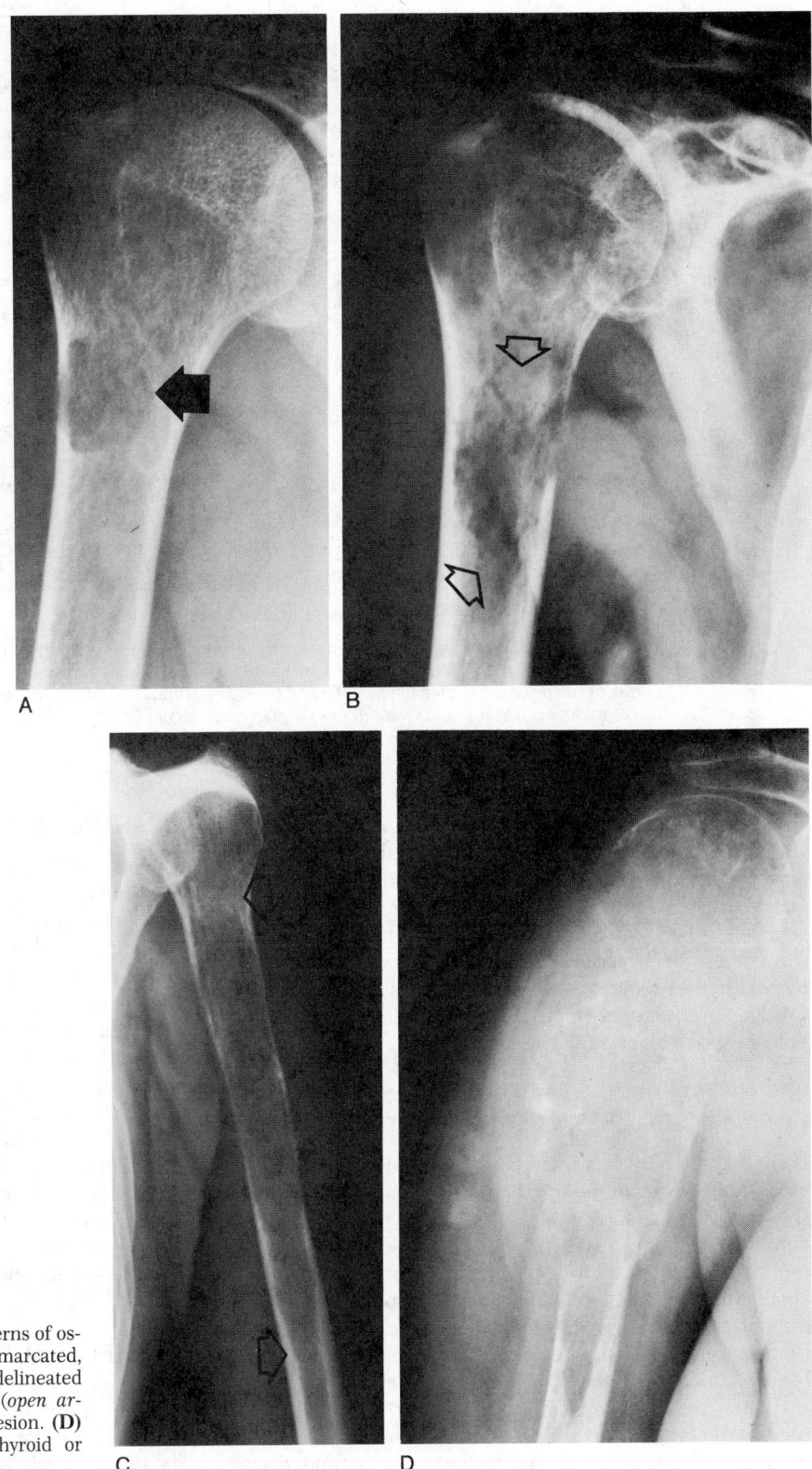

FIGURE 61–42. Different radiographic patterns of osteolytic metastatic cancer. **(A)** Sharply demarcated, punched-out defect (*solid arrow*) with well-delineated borders. **(B)** Diffuse but well-localized lesion (*open arrows*). **(C)** Large, diffuse, extensive osteolytic lesion. **(D)** Large, expansile lesion, usually seen with thyroid or hypernephroma.

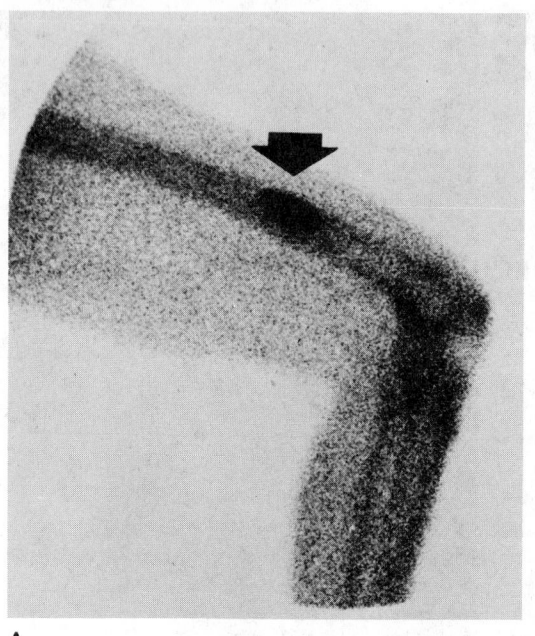

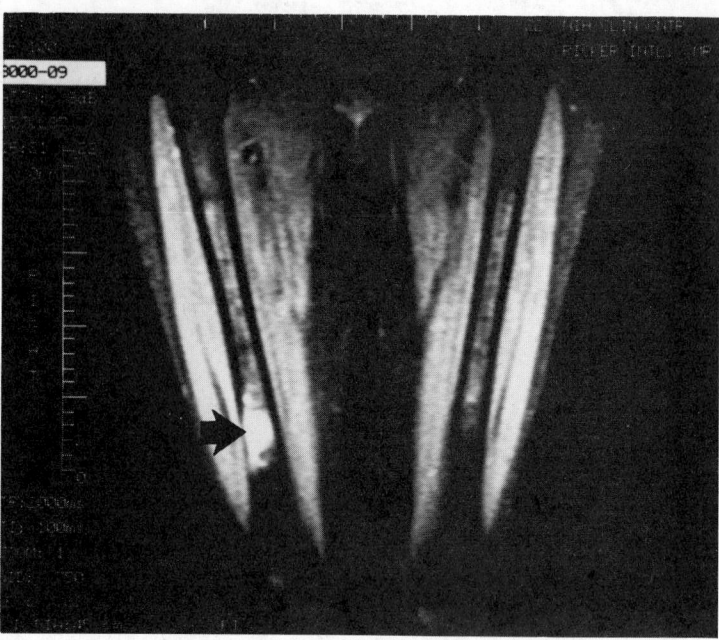

FIGURE 61–43.   Radiographic imaging for metastatic cancer. Plain radiograph of the femur failed to demonstrate a metastatic lesion. **(A)** Bone scintigraphy (lateral view) showing increased uptake in the anterior cortex of the distal femoral diaphysis. **(B)** A T2-weighted image that demonstrates an area of medullary tumor involvement seen as an area (*solid arrow*) of increased signal (*white*).

nique of marking the suspected rib under scintigraphic control with methylene blue and surgically excising the marked area.[8] None of their 15 patients had a grossly identifiable lesion, yet 10 patients had metastatic disease. Abnormal scans in the remainder had nonneoplastic causes. A portable Gamma camera has been used in the operating room to localize a lesion after a preoperative injection of ^{99m}Tc-diphosphonate for deeper structures (hip, femur, acetabulum). It prevents false-negative biopsies for these lesions.

EVALUATION OF RESPONSE TO TREATMENT

Bone scan activity of a metastatic bony lesion generally decreases after chemotherapy/hormone therapy or radiation therapy if a response is obtained.[9] Plain radiographs may demonstrate bone healing and reossification within a few months. The limitation of plain radiographs is that only a small percentage will show reossification, and changes in the osteoblastic lesions are difficult to determine. With bone scintigraphy, one can compare the activity. Most experience has been obtained with breast cancer patients. Healing is indicated as a decrease in activity. Approximately 10% to 15% of patients will demonstrate a "flare" phenomenon (*i.e.,* a period of increased uptake is presumably due to new, nonneoplastic reparative bone attempting to heal the tumor defect). Occasionally, this response is associated with pain. After this period, a repeat bone scan will show decreased uptake with no new lesions. In rare cases, previously unappreciated lesions will ossify, suggesting a new lesion; in retrospect, these can usually be identified as old lesions.

QUANTITATIVE BONE SCANNING

Quantitative bone scanning (QBS) is a technique used to measure changes in bone scans to avoid the variations obtained in routine scintigraphy. The proportion of increased uptake in the diseased region is compared with the average uptake in the normal regions.[6] It gives an objective measurement of the change of activity in any region relative to normal for a given patient. This technique has been used for comparing response to treatment in patients with metastatic and other diseases. Drelichman and colleagues described 10 patients with prostate carcinoma in whom sequential QBS was performed.[6] Those patients with more than a 50% average decrease had a partial remission, as defined by their criteria. All patients had an increase within the first month (corresponding to the "flare" phenomenon), and no significant decrease occurred until 3 months. Similar results have been obtained with patients with breast carcinoma.[9]

COMPUTED TOMOGRAPHY

Computed tomography has not been used in the evaluation of metastatic skeletal cancer as commonly as it has in other organ systems, although the literature on the usefulness of CT for malignant and benign primary bone neoplasms is extensive. Recently, CT has proved useful in evaluating "hot" spots to confirm the presence of metastatic or other disease.[5] During and associates evaluated 44 breast cancer patients with positive bone scans and negative radiographs; 25 of these patients presented with solitary hot spots on bone scans, and 19 became positive after definitive treatment of their primary disease. Seventy-six percent (19/25) of those presenting with a positive bone scan and a normal radiograph had a benign cause identified by CT. Similar to surgical staging for primary bone tumors, CT is used in the preoperative evaluation of metastatic spinal disease and tumors of the pelvis.[52]

MAGNETIC RESONANCE IMAGING

Magnetic resonance imaging (MRI) accurately images the medullary (marrow) component of bone and is therefore ideal for the early detection of metastatic cancer, especially primary infiltrative neoplasms such as leukemia, lymphoma, and multiple myeloma (see Fig. 61–43).[4,5] Its ability to detect such lesions is due to the high signal intensity (brightness) of normal marrow, which is mostly fat. Because of increased cellularity and therefore a higher water content, infiltrating neoplasms will appear as a darker area on T1-weighted images. Lesions within the skeletal system that are most difficult to image by other modalities (*e.g.*, round cell tumors) are accurately detected by MRI. Daffner and colleagues reported a prospective study of 80 patients with known malignancies; 50 had suspected metastases and 30 had multiple myeloma.[5] All patients who were evaluated with plain radiographs and bone scintigraphy (80%) were shown to have disease.[40] Ten (20%) had no evidence of metastasis, and the abnormalities on bone scintigraphy were shown to be due to other causes. Of the 30 patients with multiple myeloma, 6 (20%) had positive scans, 20 (67%) had abnormal radiographs, and 11 (37%) had abnormal CT scans. MRI demonstrated abnormalities in all 30 patients; these were confirmed by needle aspiration. These authors emphasize the importance of correlating MRI with other studies, because infection, infarction, and other entities can also yield a decreased signal. In general, they recommend that MRI studies of the coronal sections of the pelvis and hips and sagittal sections of the spine (*i.e.*, the hematopoietic-active sites) be performed when evaluating for metastatic cancer.

ANGIOGRAPHY

Angiography is rarely used for diagnosis of metastases to bone. Its main use is for preoperative assessment of large lesions and for embolization of vascular tumor (see Preoperative Evaluation).[53–56]

BIOMECHANICAL AND HEALING CONSIDERATIONS OF TUMOR DEFECTS AND PATHOLOGIC FRACTURES

BIOMECHANICAL CONSIDERATIONS

The strength of normal bone depends on the continuity of the cortex and the underlying medullary/metaphyseal trabecular structure.[57,58] The torsional (rotational), compressive, and bending forces are transmitted and absorbed by both components. A typical metastatic lesion of a long bone destroys a segment of the medullary structure and the corresponding cortical bone (Fig. 61–44). Cortical defects greatly weaken a bone to torsional forces. A defect whose length is less than the diameter of the bone (termed a "stress riser") decreases torsional strength by 70%, whereas a defect larger than the diameter of the bone (termed an "open section," and the most common defect encountered clinically) effects a 90% reduction in strength.[57,58] The aim of an orthopedic procedure is to convert an open section to a closed section so as to allow significant axial and torsional loads to be carried.

HEALING CONSIDERATIONS

The determinants of bony union after a pathologic fracture are quite different from those associated with nonneoplastic fracture. Bony union almost never occurs without surgical or radiotherapeutic treatment. Although pathologic fractures are quite common, few investigators have evaluated the rate and determinants of union. Gainor and Buchert reviewed 129 fractures of long bones in 123 patients treated between 1955

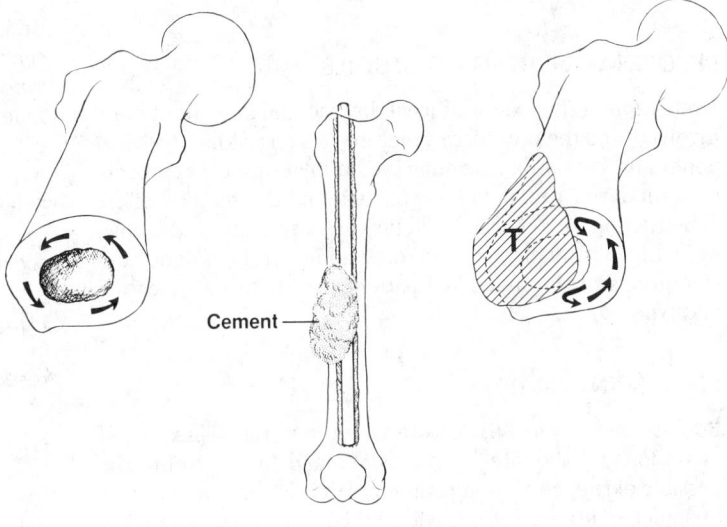

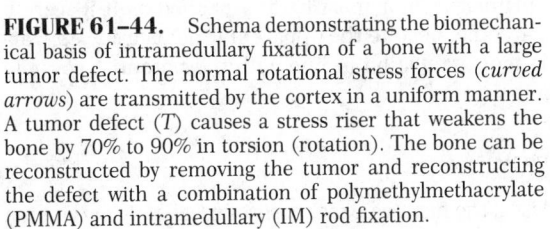

FIGURE 61–44. Schema demonstrating the biomechanical basis of intramedullary fixation of a bone with a large tumor defect. The normal rotational stress forces (*curved arrows*) are transmitted by the cortex in a uniform manner. A tumor defect (*T*) causes a stress riser that weakens the bone by 70% to 90% in torsion (rotation). The bone can be reconstructed by removing the tumor and reconstructing the defect with a combination of polymethylmethacrylate (PMMA) and intramedullary (IM) rod fixation.

Cement

and 1979.[59] The overall healing rate was 36% (45 of 129 fractures). Individual healing rates were: multiple myeloma (67%), hypernephroma (44%), and breast cancer (37%). None of the patients with lung cancer healed. The length of patient survival was the main determinant of fracture healing. Fracture healing was found to be multifactorial. Determinants of bony union of pathologic fractures are summarized[59]:

1. *Type of Tumor:* Lung and colorectal tumors and melanomas tend not to heal. Multiple myelomas, tumors of the breast, and hypernephromas have the highest rate of healing.
2. *Type of Fixation:* Internal fixation combined with PMMA significantly increases the chance of osseous union.
3. *Duration of Survival:* Longer survival (greater than 6 months) increases the rate of union.
4. *Amount of Postoperative Radiation Therapy:* High-dose postoperative radiation therapy (greater than 3000–3500 rads) is associated with poorer healing.
5. *Effects of Chemotherapy:* There is little evidence regarding the impact of chemotherapy on bony repair.

PREOPERATIVE EVALUATION, LOCAL STAGING, AND BIOPSY CONSIDERATIONS

PREOPERATIVE CONSIDERATIONS

Special preoperative considerations are needed in cases of metastasis to bone because these patients often have extensive underlying metabolic, hematologic, and nutritional deficits. The risk of infection is increased because of multiple sources of possible sepsis (*e.g.*, colostomy, urinary tract infection), neutropenia from chemotherapy or other adjuvant modalities, and poor local skin condition from prior radiation therapy or other procedures. Perioperative antibiotics are recommended for all patients. All patients should have hematologic and clotting evaluation. Adequate blood replacement should be available, because curettage of many carcinomas, especially myeloma, thyroid tumor, and renal cell carcinoma, often leads to significant blood loss. Thrombocytopenia occasionally occurs intraoperatively and should be monitored. Disseminated intravascular coagulation may occur.[60]

PREOPERATIVE STAGING STUDIES

Evaluation of the extent of local disease, the amount of bone involved, and the presence of multiple lesions within the same bone is necessary to determine the optimal surgical approach, the amount of tumor to be removed, and the method of reconstruction. In general, the following studies are used; however, there is much variation, depending on the unique considerations of the individual patient and the tumor location and type.

BONE SCINTIGRAPHY

Bone scans are used to demonstrate the intraosseous extent of tumor and the site of the lesions and to determine the possible existence of multiple tumors. It is extremely common to detect additional lesions within the same bone. In general,

all lesions within the same bone require simultaneous treatment; usually this requires placement of an intramedullary (IM) rod.

CT/MRI

Computed tomography is usually required for lesions of the pelvis and spine; it is rarely required for extremity lesions. Tumors of the bony pelvis often have large soft tissue components that may bleed excessively or lead to mechanical failure of reconstruction if they are not recognized preoperatively. Vertebral body lesions are best evaluated by CT, MRI, or both. The amount of destruction and extent of epidural disease are best estimated with these studies.[13,52,61] Soft tissue components rarely occur with carcinomas of the extremities; however, they are common with metastatic sarcoma (*e.g.*, primary sarcomas), some hypernephromas, and melanomas.

ANGIOGRAPHY

Angiography is not routinely performed; specific indications are pelvic tumors with large extraosseous components and lesions in which preoperative embolization is considered. Patients with metastatic hypernephroma should undergo angiography with embolization.[53–55,62,63]

BIOPSY: TECHNIQUE AND CONSIDERATIONS

There are three situations in which a biopsy is warranted: (1) to confirm metastatic disease in a patient with a known primary tumor; (2) to evaluate a "suspicious" radiographic lesion; and (3) to obtain tissue for hormonal/immunohistochemical evaluation. The technique of biopsy varies, depending on the tumor location and the specific answers sought.

In general, needle aspiration and cytologic evaluation can reliably confirm the diagnosis of cancer.[8,60,64–64B] If the radiograph demonstrates a lesion, biopsy should be performed under fluoroscopic guidance. Permanent x-ray films should be obtained to document that the correct area has been sampled. Several aspirations or cores should be obtained. The material should routinely be sent for culture, because indolent infections occasionally can present as metastatic lesions. Frozen sections or touch preps should be obtained to determine the types of cells present. If the primary tumor is unknown, sufficient tissue should be obtained for special stains (see later), especially immunohistochemical studies. This may require a large sample. If there is excessive bleeding, an absorbable gelatin sponge (Gelfoam) or PMMA should be packed into the defect. One must not assume that all "solitary" lesions in the adult are metastatic. A solitary lesion in the adult without a known primary tumor must be approached as if it were a primary sarcoma, despite the apparent "metastatic" appearance. The biopsy must be in line with the potential possible resection incision.

HISTOLOGY

In most cases, the histologic diagnosis of metastatic carcinoma to bone is easily established. This depends on the recognition of squamous patterns of glandular structures, the features of which are highly typical of the carcinomas that most frequently metastasize to bone. This diagnosis is further facilitated when representative microscopic slides from the primary neoplasm are available for comparison.

Metastatic poorly differentiated carcinomas, and some melanomas (particularly those containing abundant spindled and pleomorphic cells), can closely mimic primary bone sarcomas such as fibrosarcoma or MFH. This pitfall is most often encountered with renal cell carcinoma. The application of selected histochemical studies to demonstrate cellular products has been helpful to confirm the presumption of metastatic carcinoma and to aid in determining the source of an unknown primary lesion. Alcian blue and mucicarmine stains will reveal the presence of epithelial mucins in some adenocarcinomas of the breast, lung, and gastrointestinal tract. Abundant cytoplasmic glycogen typically occurs in renal cell carcinoma and in some clear cell neoplasms from other organs. The demonstration of cytoplasmic melanin granules with the Fontana stain supports the diagnosis of melanoma.

The recent development of immunohistochemical techniques that can be applied to paraffin-embedded tissues has created a powerful diagnostic tool.[65,66] With this procedure, peroxidase-conjugated antibodies, directed against a variety of known antigenic markers, are detected at antibody-antigen reaction sites by the addition of peroxidase-sensitive chromogens. For example, an epithelial tumor (carcinoma) can contain a variety of cytokeratins, epithelial membrane antigen, or carcinoembryonic antigen. The application of an appropriately selected panel of antibodies will produce a recognizable pattern of positive staining of tumor cells that confirms the presence of carcinoma.[67] Similarly, there are antibodies available to identify specific markers of neuroendocrine tumors and melanoma (anti-S-100 protein and anti-melanoma-specific antigens).[68] Metastatic carcinoma and adenocarcinoma of the prostate and metastatic follicular carcinoma of the thyroid can appear quite similar. Immunohistochemical studies to detect prostatic-specific acid phosphatase or thyroglobulin will usually resolve this problem in differential diagnosis.[69] It must be noted, however, that immunohistochemical techniques require meticulous methodology and are fraught with numerous artifacts and interpretive pitfalls.[70]

PRINCIPLES OF SURGICAL TREATMENT FOR SKELETAL METASTASIS

Within the past 20 years, the surgical treatment of metastatic cancer involving the skeletal system has undergone dramatic change as a result of the development of techniques to replace and stabilize large segments of abnormal bone.[11,19,21,22,28,33,61,71a] These techniques have been paralleled by developments in total joint replacements and by procedures developed by the orthopedic oncologist in the treatment of primary bone tumors. Prosthetic replacements now permit the removal and immediate reconstruction of destroyed bone.[23] PMMA, when combined with various metallic rods or prostheses, or both, permits immediate filling and reconstruction of large defects and immediate stabilization.

The common local surgical procedures for metastatic tumors of the extremities are:

1. *Composite Osteosynthesis:* curettage of tumor combined with internal fixation, either bone plates and screws (composite osteosynthesis) or intramedullary fixation with IM rods. This technique is most often used for the shaft (diaphysis) of long bones, most commonly the humerus and femur.[22,28,71a]
2. *Hemijoint Replacement:* resection of a joint with reconstruction by an endoprosthesis combined with PMMA. This technique is most often used for tumors of the hip (Fig. 61-45).[23]
3. *Segmental Resection:* resection of a large segment of bone combined with custom segmental prosthetic replacement and PMMA. This technique is less common and involves substantially more surgical morbidity. It is most often used when no significant bone remains that can be reconstructed by the techniques mentioned above.
4. *Cryosurgery:* Cryosurgery may be combined with any of the above procedures in order to increase local tumor control and control hemorrhage.[71b,72]
5. *Amputations:* Amputations are occasionally necessary to control serious complications of extremity lesions, usually after inadequate tumor control.[73]

The general principles of management of pathologic or pending fractures are:

1. Preoperative embolization for suspected vascular lesions
2. Perioperative antibiotics
3. Adequate hematologic evaluation and blood and component replacement
4. Modification of standard incisions, if necessary, to avoid prior radiation fields and to provide adequate soft tissue coverage and adequate closure to ensure healing
5. Curettage and removal of all gross disease, if possible
6. Composite reconstruction with internal fixation or prosthetic replacement and PMMA. Assurance that PMMA fills the defect and extends proximal and distal to the abnormal area
7. Postoperative radiation therapy for local control

AMPUTATIONS

Amputations are rarely required today for metastatic cancer. Occasionally, radical amputation is indicated when advanced cancer of an extremity results in uncontrollable, intractable pain, a necrotic or functionless extremity, fungation and sepsis, or erosion and hemorrhage of a major vessel at the tumor site. These complications occur after inadequate tumor con114trol. Elimination of pain and sepsis with restoration of function may be achieved by amputation.[73]

CRYOSURGERY

Cryosurgery is the use of liquid nitrogen as a surgical adjunct to tumor curettage to freeze (cryonecrosis) any residual tumor cells. The aim is to enhance local control.[71,72,74] Necrosis is obtained by a double or triple freeze-thaw cycle requiring temperatures between $-20°$ and $-40°C$. Marcove at Memorial Sloan-Kettering Hospital has treated several hundred patients with this technique since 1964.[71,72] It is useful for tumors that have recurred despite radiation therapy and those in difficult anatomic locations, and in the treatment of hypernephromas.

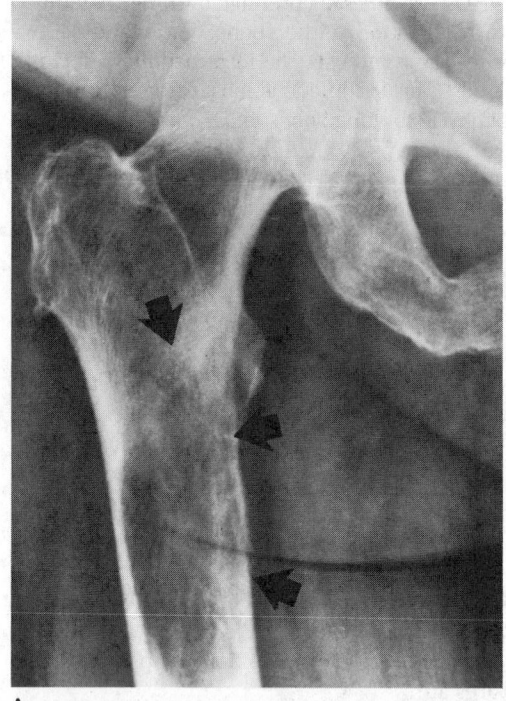

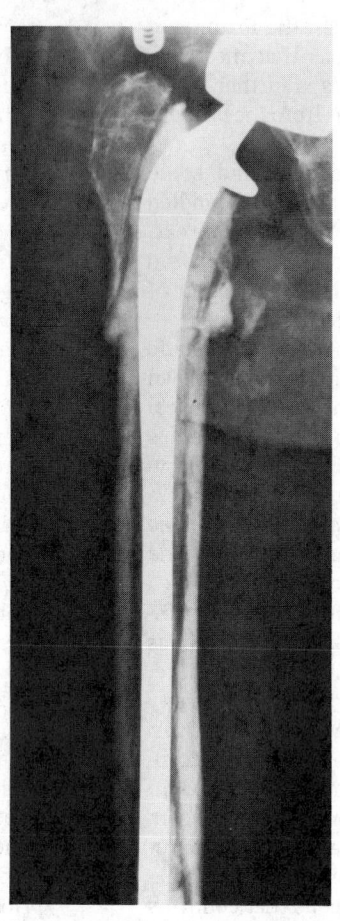

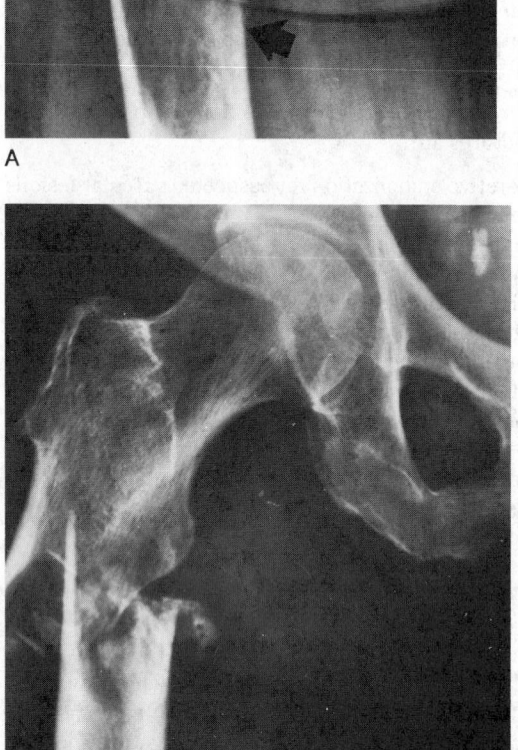

FIGURE 61–45.   Typical pathologic hip fracture. **(A)** Large subtrochanteric lesion (*solid arrows*) with medial cortical destruction from a metastatic breast cancer. **(B)** A subtrochanteric fracture occurred during administration of radiation therapy. **(C)** The tumor was curetted and a long-stem endoprosthesis was used with PMMA for fixation. The patient was allowed to ambulate several days after surgery. Postoperative radiation therapy to the entire femur is routinely recommended. A long-stem prosthesis with PMMA is recommended for all pathologic fractures of the hip.

GENERAL PRINCIPLES OF RADIATION THERAPY FOR SKELETAL METASTASIS

Radiation is an effective treatment for cancer that has metastasized to bone. Aims of treatment include pain relief, elimination or reduction of the need for narcotics, improvement in ambulation, and arrest of local tumor growth that might otherwise lead to intractable pain, cord compression, or pathologic fracture. With thoughtful treatment planning and appropriate high-energy equipment, localized treatment can usually be delivered to symptomatic sites with minimal morbidity. The efforts of the radiation oncologist should be closely coordinated with those of other physicians and health care personnel. Careful consideration of the nature of the patient's disease is important in determining the most appropriate radiation therapy strategy and technique.

Eighty to ninety percent of patients with a limited number of sites of disease can be effectively treated with external-beam irradiation.[75–82] If there is a single site of bony metastatic disease, high-dose radiation therapy may render the patient disease free for an extended period of time. For patients with symptoms of disease at multiple sites, systemic therapy with chemotherapy or endocrine therapy should be instituted. If symptoms persist, several approaches should be considered. These include localized external radiation therapy to the most symptomatic areas or, for patients with widely disseminated disease, hemibody irradiation or internally administered radionuclide treatment.

TREATMENT PLANNING

The radiation fields should be planned with the use of data from the history and physical examination, the bone scan, plain skeletal films, and, where indicated, myelograms, CT scans, and MRI (see Preoperative Staging Studies, earlier). Soft tissue masses, most often associated with bony metastases to the vertebral bodies or pelvis, must be included in the radiation therapy fields. The distribution of bone marrow is an important consideration, because irradiation for bony metastases will suppress hematopoiesis in the treatment field (Table 61–30). Bone marrow suppression secondary to irradiation is more significant in patients who have received or are receiving myelosuppressive chemotherapy. Blood counts should be monitored closely during treatment. All previous radiation treatment portals must be reviewed. Damage to normal tissue can result from improperly matched or overlapping fields.

Lesions not responding to treatment should prompt another review of the diagnostic studies, particularly in a patient with multiple metastases in whom a lesion not in the treatment field might in fact be causing persistent symptoms. Another possibility is that a soft tissue mass adjacent to the bony lesion being radiated is not completely encompassed by the treatment field.

TABLE 61–30. Marrow Distribution in the Adult

Anatomic Site	% of Total Red Marrow
Head	13.1
Cranium	12.0
Mandible	1.1
Upper limbs	8.3
2 humeri	2.0
2 scapulae	4.8
2 clavicles	1.5
Sternum	2.3
Ribs	7.9
Vertebrae	42.3
Cervical	3.4
Thoracic	14.1
Lumbar	10.9
Sacrum	13.9
Lower limb girdle	26.1
2 os coxae	22
Femoral head and neck	4

(Extracted from Ellis RE. The distribution of active bone marrow in the adult. Phys Med Biol 1961;5:255)

PAIN RELIEF

Approximately 80% to 90% of patients undergoing radiation therapy for pain from osseous metastases will have partial pain relief.[75–82] Most patients will begin to experience some pain relief 10 to 14 days after the start of therapy. In one study, 70% of patients had pain relief by 2 weeks after the completion of treatment; 90% had relief within 1 to 3 months.[81] A sudden increase in pain during treatment should raise concern about a pathologic fracture, and appropriate films and orthopedic evaluation should be done. In a recent study, 70% of patients experiencing pain relief did not develop recurrent pain in the treatment field.[75] Another study noted sustained relief of pain in 55% to 65% of patients during the first year after treatment.[83]

In spite of the clinical impression that painful osseous metastases from the thyroid, lung, and kidney are more difficult to palliate with radiation, several small studies have failed to document any clear differences in overall response rates among different histologies.[81,83,84] It has been observed, however, that the time to achieve pain relief after treatment was longer with slowly proliferating tumors such as prostate cancer.[84] The final report from the large, randomized study by the Radiation Therapy Oncology Group (RTOG) indicated that a significantly higher percentage of patients with metastases from breast and prostate primary tumors achieved complete pain relief when compared with patients with lung and other primary tumors.[75] The sites of metastases have not been shown to correlate with the degree of pain relief.[18,75] Severe and frequent pain has been shown to be a poor prognostic feature.[75]

BONE HEALING

Radiation affects both tumor and adjacent bone. The presence of tumor, however, is a significant threat to the structural integrity of bone, and this is worse than the adverse effects of radiation on bone healing. Bone reossification will often occur after tumor eradication. Seventy-eight percent of osteolytic lesions treated in one study recalcified, and another 15% showed no further progression after radiation therapy.[80,85,86] In a study of bone reformation at the base of the skull after irradiation for carcinoma of the nasopharynx, 11 patients showed apparent bone reformation within 4 to 6 months of treatment.[87] These patients received treatment with doses of 5000 to 7000 cGy, which are higher than those used in patients treated for metastatic lesions to the bone.

DOSE, FRACTIONATION, AND TYPES OF RADIATION

There is considerable debate among radiation oncologists about the optimal dose and fractionation scheme for delivering radiation therapy to metastatic lesions in bone. Total dose, fraction size, and duration of treatment are the major issues. In patients with metastatic cancer in whom life expectancy is limited, one would like to deliver effective treatment with minimal morbidity over as short a time span as possible. The RTOG studied pain relief in 759 patients randomized to a variety of dose-fractionation schedules: 270 cGy $\times$ 15 fractions, 300 $\times$ 10, 300 $\times$ 5, 400 $\times$ 5, and 500 $\times$ 5. No significant difference in response was seen, although an independent reanalysis of the data suggested that the protracted fractionation schemes (270 × 15 or 300 × 10) were more likely to provide complete pain relief with cessation of the use of narcotics.[88]

Several other reported randomized trials do not indicate a clear advantage for the longer, multiple-fraction regimens when compared with shorter or single-course regimens.[89-91] In a study at the Royal Marsden Hospital, 288 patients with painful bony metastases were randomized to receive either 800 cGy in one fraction or 3000 cGy in ten fractions.[79,92] There was no difference in the percentage of patients responding to treatment (80%), the rapidity of response, or the duration of pain relief between the two regimens. A larger number of patients who received the single treatment were subsequently retreated with irradiation to the same site. This was also noted in the RTOG trial, where substantially more patients in the short-course regimens were reirradiated. This, however, may only reflect the reluctance of radiation oncologists to reirradiate areas that received prior high-dose, multifractionated regimens. No late normal tissue complications were seen in the single-fraction group. Other trials have shown equivalent pain relief when comparing 400 cGy × 6 fractions with 1000 cGy × 2, 400 cGy × 6 with 800 cGy × 1, and 200 cGy × 15 with 450 cGy × 5.[121-123] Four retrospective studies of single (400–1500 cGy) versus multiple (2000–4000 cGy) treatment regimens have not shown any striking differences between the two.[16,17,80,93]

While it has been supposed that tumor shrinkage is responsible for pain relief in this setting, the very rapid pain relief associated with orchiectomy or hemibody irradiation for prostate cancer and hypophysectomy for breast cancer does raise the possibility that pain relief might in fact be due to a cytotoxic effect on host cells secreting chemical mediators of the pain response.[89] Even lower doses of single-fraction irradiation for palliation of pain relief are also currently being studied. Single fractions of 400 cGy were recently reported to produce partial pain relief in 9 of 21 (43%) evaluable patients and complete relief in 1 of 21 (5%), with responses occurring within 3 weeks.[94] Seven of the ten responders, however, subsequently developed recurrent pain at the irradiated site.

It might be expedient to give single-fraction irradiation to a debilitated patient for whom repeated, daily trips for treatment would be burdensome. Single large fractions, however, to the abdomen and brain may not be well tolerated acutely. Therefore, each radiation oncologist must consider the site of disease, the patient's performance status and social situation, and any normal tissue in the treatment field when deciding on a treatment regimen. Patients with one or few sites of metastases who have a good performance status and a primary disease that responds well to systemic therapy may live for many years after irradiation for bony pain. Therefore, large fractions that are known to produce more late effects in normal tissue must be used with considerable caution, especially when radiation fields include the brain, spinal cord, kidneys, or significant portions of the liver or bowel. Such patients may also survive long enough to have problems with recurrent tumor in bones that have not been irradiated to high doses. Patients with bony metastases producing spinal cord compression are not suitable for single-fraction treatment because of the obvious neurologic risks of recurrent tumor at this site.

It has been difficult to demonstrate a clear dose-response relation in the treatment of bone metastases, often because the groups studied have been heterogenous, with different histologies and survival times after treatment. Arcangeli reported a higher frequency of complete pain relief when doses of ≥4000 cGy were employed.[95] In patients with good performance status, limited metastatic disease, and long expected survival after palliative irradiation, doses of ≥4000 cGy with conventional fractionation are recommended. For patients whose expected survival is short, a high dose is probably less important because they will not live long enough to manifest recurrent tumor.

HEMIBODY IRRADIATION

Sequential hemibody irradiation has been used as an alternative to localized radiation therapy directed at specific sites of metastatic disease for patients with widely disseminated bony metastases.[15,18] It is designed to avoid repeated trips to the hospital for multiple courses of irradiation in such patients. One study reported complete relief of pain in 21% and partial relief in 77% of patients, most of whom had breast, prostate, or lung cancer.[15] Pain control was achieved rapidly, with improvement noted within 2 days among half of the patients experiencing pain relief. Patients received 600 to 800 cGy of irradiation to either the upper, middle, or lower portions of the body. Patients treated for metastases of the upper body were hospitalized for a day, hydrated, and premedicated with antiemetics and corticosteroids: those undergoing midbody and lower body therapy were premedicated as outpatients to minimize nausea and vomiting. Treatment to the lower body and midbody was tolerated relatively well, with severe or life-threatening nausea and vomiting, diarrhea, and hematologic toxicity occurring in 2%, 6%, and 8% of patients, respectively. Upper body treatment induced severe or life-threatening nausea and vomiting, fever, and hematologic toxicity in 15%, 4%, and 32% of the patients, respectively. Hematologic complications were worse in patients who had received prior intensive courses of chemotherapy and had started treatment with low peripheral blood counts. There were no fatalities related to treatment, yet side effects as described above were prominent, especially with the upper body treatment. Kuban reported good palliation with hemibody irradiation in patients with disseminated prostate cancer.[96] Palliative effects were maintained until death in 82% of the patients treated in the upper half of the body and 67% of the patients treated in the lower half of the body. Doses of 600 to 800 cGy to the upper and 800 cGy to the lower hemibody were well tolerated. Fractionated hemibody irradiation has been reported to yield more durable pain relief by a group from Memorial Sloan-Kettering Cancer Center without any increase in complications.[97]

SYSTEMIC RADIONUCLIDES

Systemically administered isotopes have been used to palliate pain caused by widespread osseous metastases. Iodine 131 (^{131}I) can provide pain relief in patients with well-differentiated thyroid carcinoma, and radioactive phosphorus (^{32}P) and subsequently strontium 89 (^{89}Sr) and ^{131}I-diphosphonates have been used to treat patients with other histologies. ^{32}P-orthophosphate has been the most commonly administered form of ^{32}P. Localization studies show that it is primarily taken up in bone spicules adjacent to the site of metastatic cancer cells.[98] Pain relief responses of varying durations in the range of 60% to 90% have been reported, which is similar to that noted for sequential hemibody irradiation.[99] [32]P tends to cause worse bone marrow suppression but does not have the concomitant risk of nausea, vomiting, pneumonitis, and alopecia seen with hemibody irradiation.[93,99] Some have advocated the use of priming with testosterone to increase uptake in prostate tumor, or parathyroid hormone to increase uptake in bone.[19,102-105] Response rates with endocrine priming do not appear substantially different from those with ^{32}P alone. Moreover, testosterone priming followed by ^{32}P therapy has been reported to cause transient exacerbation of pain, irreversible morbidity such as spinal cord compression, or even death.[103,105] Most investigators currently do not advocate endocrine priming.[99]

Recently, several groups have employed ^{89}Sr, a bone-seeking radionuclide with a lower energy beta emission than [32]P. Two groups reported favorable response rates ranging from 72% to 91%, while a third institution noted improvement in 51% of patients so treated.[106-108] Less bone marrow toxicity has been reported in these patients. Therefore, this isotope may prove to be a useful therapy for patients with widespread bony metastases. A recent phase I study of ^{131}I-diphosphonates, which also have a high affinity for bone, showed complete pain relief in 44% of patients, substantial pain relief in 6%, minimal improvement in 22%, and no change in 28%. Systemic toxicity and marrow toxicity were minimal.[19A] Other new isotopes under investigation include rhenium 185 (tin) and hydroxyethylidene diphosphonate ([153]Sm-EDTMP).[109,110] Both are bone seekers, emit gammas that permit imaging, have favorable beta emissions for therapy, and have favorable half-lives for radiation safety purposes. Early studies show responses in the 65% to 80% range. Controlled trials will be needed to determine the optimal role for these newer radionuclides in the treatment of patients with symptomatic, advanced bony metastatic disease.

SPECIFIC TUMORS: UNIQUE CLINICAL AND MANAGEMENT CONSIDERATIONS

In general, the medical management of bony metastases is similar to that of disseminated disease for each individual tumor type.[108] The unique clinical characteristics and surgical and radiotherapeutic aspects of management of bony metastases are summarized for the most common tumors.

BREAST CANCER

Between 50% and 85% of all breast cancer patients will develop bony metastases.[2,9,32,50,51,111] In general, bony lesions respond well to radiation therapy, hormonal therapy, or chemotherapy, or all three.[75,108]

Radiation therapy is recommended for lesions not responding to endocrine therapy or chemotherapy, for sites of pathologic fracture after fixation, and for areas such as the femoral neck and vertebral bodies, which are prone to complication in the event of tumor progression. The intent of radiation therapy should be to provide long-term control of symptomatic sites and to prevent late complications in normal tissue. This generally means fractionated, high-dose treatment to appro-

priately planned fields with megavoltage machines. To avoid any injury to normal tissue, one should be aware of any overlap with previous radiation fields involving the breast or draining nodal areas. Early (prophylactic) surgery is recommended for large lesions of the hip or femur, or both, to avoid fracture (see Indications for Prophylactic Fixation, later), especially for those who remain symptomatic despite radiation therapy. Pathologic fractures of the long bones are treated by a combination of intramedullary rod fixation and PMMA. A subgroup of breast cancer patients (with skeletal metastases only) has been been recently described.[14,112,113] Because of their prolonged survival, it is recommended that these patients undergo aggressive management of skeletal metastases.[14]

RENAL CELL CARCINOMA (HYPERNEPHROMA)

Approximately 25% of patients with hypernephroma develop bony metastases.[115-117] One significant surgical consideration of metastatic hypernephromas is that they are extremely vascular; life-threatening hemorrhage can easily occur from a small incision. A second consideration is that, unlike other metastatic carcinomas, hypernephromas are often associated with a large extraosseous component. Therefore, before any surgical intervention, CT and angiography are recommended. Biopsy of a suspected hypernephroma should be undertaken only after careful planning; a needle biopsy is recommended. If an open biopsy is required, preoperative embolization should be performed. The need for surgery is indicated by large lesions, progressive bony destruction, instability, or pending fracture. Preoperative embolization and proximal vascular control are mandatory to avoid extensive hemorrhage.[46,63] Cryosurgery has been used as a surgical adjuvant in decreasing bleeding and in increasing local tumor control.[118,119] Palliative embolization alone (without surgery) for large tumors, especially those of the pelvis, has been reported to effect good pain relief.[63] Transient increases in pain and fever may occur as a postinfarction syndrome.

Many radiation oncologists believe that pain from renal call carcinoma metastatic to bone is difficult to palliate. Arcangeli reported a lower rate of complete pain relief in patients with this histology.[95] Improved results were seen with doses of 4000 cGy or more.[120] Other authors do not describe a significant impact of histology on response rate.[92,114]

COLORECTAL CARCINOMA

Skeletal metastases (4%) occur infrequently from colorectal cancer; when they do, it is usually late in the course of the disease.[121] The most common sites of metastases are the lumbar spine and sacrum. Radiation therapy is the most effective mode of palliation in these anatomic sites.[121,122] Long-bone fractures are rare.

LUNG CARCINOMA

Metastatic bony disease occurs in 20% to 40% of lung cancer patients.[115,123] Palliative radiation therapy is usually successful in 60% to 80% of patients.[92,95] A dose of 3000 rads in ten fractions is frequently employed. Fractures are less common in these patients than in others with osteolytic lesions, probably because the bony lesions do not have time to grow. When fractures do occur, treatment is similar to that of the other carcinomas.[22]

THYROID CANCER

McCormack reported bone metastases in 33 of 259 patients (12.7%) with thyroid cancer.[124] Most metastatic bony lesions can be treated with radioisotopes or external irradiation, or both.

Well-differentiated thyroid tumors, follicular carcinomas, and some papillary tumors often retain their affinity for iodine. It is therefore possible to deliver localized radioactive ^{131}I to these lesions when they have metastasized to bone after appropriate surgical ablation of normal thyroid.[19,20] Effective treatment with ^{131}I usually requires several doses given at 3-month intervals. Therefore, sites of severe bone pain should be managed with local external-beam irradiation to achieve early pain relief.[33] For thyroid lesions that do not take up iodine, external-beam irradiation usually provides relief. Pathologic fracture is rare. If surgery is required, bleeding may be excessive. Preoperative angiography and embolization may be useful. For the rare situation of a solitary bone metastasis, Niederle and colleagues have recommended surgical removal in lieu of radioiodine, especially for follicular or papillary carcinoma.[125]

MELANOMA

Stewart and associates reported an overall incidence of bony involvement in melanoma of 6.9%.[126,127] The authors emphasized that these patients may not go through the sequential stage devised for the characterization of melanomas; approximately half of the patients they studied were clinically stage I before the detection of a bony lesion. Bone involvement is a grave prognosis; mean survival was only 3.6 months.[127] They strongly recommended nonoperative management unless the fracture was unstable, because radiation therapy provided good symptomatic relief and expected survival was short.

PROSTATE CANCER

Metastatic prostate cancer most often involves the axial skeleton and pelvis. Typically, bony metastases are osteoblastic (dense), multiple, and small. Occasionally, difficulty arises in distinguishing Paget's disease from metastatic lesions, and solitary metastases from a primary sarcoma. Acid phosphatase is almost always elevated in the presence of bony metastases and is helpful in these differentiations. Pathologic fractures tend not to occur because of the osteoblastic reaction. Despite the frequency of prostate cancer, only 4% of patients in most large series of pathologic fractures have prostate cancer.[9,10,22,23] Prophylactic surgery is rarely required.[19,102,104,105] Localized external irradiation will palliate most sites of bony metastatic disease.[95] Hemibody irradiation or radioisotopes should be considered for patients with multiple sites of symptomatic bony metastases.[97]

LEUKEMIA, LYMPHOMA, AND MYELOMA

The leukemias and lymphomas, while exquisitely sensitive to irradiation, are usually managed with systemic chemotherapy when metastases are present. Pathologic fractures are uncommon, except with multiple myeloma. If surgery is required, the major problem is excessive bleeding due to

thrombocytopenia, unexpected coagulopathy, and, rarely, disseminated intravascular coagulopathy. Multiple myeloma tends to be notoriously vascular.

Should a metastasis involve a vertebral body with potential compromise of the spinal cord or nerve roots, localized radiation is recommended. Sites refractory to drug therapy can also be irradiated. For the indolent lymphomas and the leukemias, 2000 to 2500 cGy should provide excellent palliation. For the aggressive lymphomas, doses in the range of 3000 to 4000 cGy should be used. Radiation treatment can provide excellent palliation for patients with symptomatic bony diseases from multiple myeloma.[75-77]

SARCOMAS

Pathologic fracture through a primary sarcoma of bone is rare. In general, a pathologic fracture through a spindle cell sarcoma requires an amputation (see Bone Sarcomas). Radiation therapy generally offers good palliation for metastatic sarcomas to bone.[100] If surgery is required, a primary prosthetic replacement is preferred to internal fixation to avoid progressive local disease.

SPECIFIC ANATOMIC SITES: CLINICAL, SURGICAL, AND RADIOTHERAPEUTIC CONSIDERATIONS

The surgical and radiotherapeutic considerations for metastatic tumors of the most common anatomic sites are discussed.

PROXIMAL FEMUR (HIP)

The hip is the most common site of pathologic fracture (see Fig. 61-4).[10,22,23,32] The aim of treatment is to reduce pain and to keep the patient ambulatory. In general, all pathologic fractures of the hip require surgical reconstruction followed by postoperative radiation therapy. Even in the weakened, nonambulatory patient, surgery is often warranted to relieve pain, to permit simple nursing care, and to enable the patient to sit in a chair.

Indications for Prophylactic Fixation

Firm indications for pending fracture of the hip have not been established; criteria for operative repair based on the experience at Memorial Sloan-Kettering Hospital are summarized here.[23] These authors noted that whenever one of the following three circumstances was present, significant loss of bone substance and continuity was found at surgery:

1. A painful intramedullary lytic lesion equal to or greater than 50% of the cross-sectional diameter of the bone
2. A painful lytic lesion involving a length of cortex equal to or greater than the cross-sectional diameter of the bone or larger than 2.5 cm in axial length
3. A lesion of bone in which pain was unrelieved after radiation therapy

Several investigators have described similar radiographic criteria for the high-risk fracture.[10,128,129] In the largest study to date, Keene and colleagues attempted to identify the clinical and radiographic risk factors for pathologic fracture of the femur.[129] The authors reviewed the skeletal surveys of 2673 patients with breast cancer. Eleven percent (293) of the patients had proximal femoral metastases; 203 of these patients were evaluable. Overall, only 11% of these patients sustained pathologic fracture. There was no difference in the average age, height, weight, pain pattern, or response to radiation therapy between those sustaining fracture and those who did not. These authors were unable to identify either a specific percent involvement of the bone or a critical diameter for metastasis to fracture. The 12 measurable lesions that fractured had the same degree of involvement as the 208 measurable lesions that did not fracture. There are no accurate criteria to select the patient at risk. Keene and colleagues concluded that radiographic measurements alone cannot identify the high-risk patient. To date, exact criteria for prophylactic fixation have not been determined.

Because of this difficulty in predicting which patients might fracture through a long-bone metastasis, Mirels and associates developed a weighted scoring system to quantify the risk of fracture.[130] This system analyzes and combines four roentgenographic and clinical factors into a single score (range, 3–12). The four clinical factors are: anatomic site, pain pattern, type of lesion, and size (Table 61–31).

Seventy-eight lesions were analyzed. Fifty-one lesions did not fracture in the subsequent 6 months and 27 lesions did fracture. The nonfracture group had a mean score of 7 versus a mean score of 10 for the fracture group. As the score increased above 7, so did the risk of fracture. The authors concluded that the lesions of long bones with scores below 7 could safely be irradiated, whereas those with a score of 8 or higher should be treated by internal fixation before irradiation (see Table 61–31). They noted that a score of 9 had a 33% fracture rate and a score of 10 had an 82% fracture rate. Analysis of their results shows that the rate of fracture was small (5%) when the size of the lesion was less than two thirds of the diameter of the bone but increased to 81% for lesions larger than two thirds. They emphasized the difficulty of using standard roentgenograms and recommended the use of CT in difficult cases. They also noted that pain alone was not a major determinant, but if it were "functional" pain (*i.e.*, made worse by use of the extremity), almost all went on to fracture. Importantly, these lesions measured greater than two thirds of the diameters of the involved bones. The probability of fracture with nonfunctional pain was 10%. This system is the first attempt to score and predict potential fractures.

Radiographs and bone scans of the entire femur and acetabulum must be obtained before surgery. It is not uncommon to detect other lesions farther down the shaft, a situation that indicates the need for simultaneous fixation. In general, a long-stem prosthesis will treat both the femoral neck and the diaphyseal lesion. The acetabulum must be evaluated. If there is substantial disease, surgery should include curettage of that lesion and total replacement of the hip and acetabulum. Harrington emphasizes the need for removal of all gross disease and replacement with PMMA and internal fixation (see next section).[11,61] Significant bleeding may occur, especially in patients with myelomas, thyroid tumors, and hypernephromas. Preoperative angiography and embolization of the profundus femoris artery should be considered.

Surgical Treatment

Metastatic fractures of the hip may be intracapsular, intertrochanteric, or subtrochanteric (see Fig. 61–45). Surgical treatment of intracapsular fractures entails endoprosthetic replacement (usually long stem) or total hip replacement. The treatment of intertrochanteric and subtrochanteric fractures varies; plate and screw fixation (with PMMA) and Zickel rods (Howmedica, Rutherford, NJ), respectively, have been described with good success. Recently, Lane has recommended long-stem prostheses with PMMA for any of these three areas.[23] Endoprosthetic replacement has many advantages. It is reliable and simple, avoids late failure or fixation seen with other devices, simultaneously treats lesions more distal in the shaft, and permits early mobilization. Lane reported no instances of loosening or dislocation and only two infections in 167 patients (1.2%). A bicentric device is now preferred in lieu of a fixed-head endoprosthesis.[23]

Similarly, Rinkes and colleagues evaluated the treatment of manifest and pending fractures of the femoral neck in 34 patients.[131] They emphasized the use of cemented hemiarthroplasty for immediate fixation and early mobilization (average, 9 days). All patients experienced pain relief. Mean survival was 17.6 months (12 months for manifest and 40 months for impending fracture). They emphasized the necessity for complete tumor curettage and filling of the defect with PMMA. It is important to note that segmental resections were not required. PMMA was used to fill large tumor defects. We agree with the authors that proximal femoral lesions should be treated aggressively to improve function, ambulation, nursing management, and pain relief.

Technique

A standard posterolateral approach is used. The trochanter should not be osteotomized. The head and neck are removed and the canal is reamed with *flexible* reamers; solid reamers may perforate abnormally thin bone. The length of the stem of the prosthesis should be at least to the isthmus or distal to any shaft lesions, or both. The incision may be extended to curette all gross tumor. Any absent bone can be reconstructed

TABLE 61–31. Scoring System for Pathologic Fractures

| Variable | Score | | |
	1	2	3
Site	Upper limb	Lower limb	Peritrochanter
Pain	Mild	Moderate	Functional
Lesion	Blastic	Mixed	Lytic
Size*	<⅓	⅓–⅔	>⅔

* In relation to the diamter of the bone.
(Mirels H. Metastatic disease in long bones. A proposed scoring system. Clin Orthop 1989;249:256–265)

with PMMA. It is extremely important to obtain a good cement mantle around the stem of the prosthesis and distal to the tip. The PMMA should be cooled before injection to increase the time of polymerization. The patient is mobilized within 2 to 3 days. If there is extensive loss of proximal bone, a segmental prosthesis is used. This technique is associated with significant operative morbidity and is not routinely performed. When required, however, it can successfully reconstruct large proximal defects.

Radiation Therapy

Radiation portals should encompass the involved area of the proximal femur and extend distally to any sites of involvement of the femoral shaft. If surgery has been performed, radiation therapy should be started after the surgical wound has healed. Intramedullary or other fixation devices are generally included in the radiation field to encompass any microscopic tumor that might be dislodged by the surgery. Radiation fields should spare the knee joint unless there is frank tumor involvement of the adjacent distal femur. As is customary in other extremity sites, a strip of soft tissue should be left unirradiated to preserve lymphatic drainage.

FEMORAL SHAFT

Fractures of the femoral shaft should be treated by IM fixation and PMMA (Fig. 61–46). Combined osteosynthesis (*i.e.*, plate and screw fixation and PMMA) may be successful; however, it is not preferred because of the risk of fracture proximal and distal to the plate, increased operative time, and the need for a more extensive surgical exposure. In general, IM rod fixation is performed by the "open" method: the tumor/fracture site is exposed, the tumor is curetted, PMMA is injected proximal and distal, and the IM rod is inserted. The proximal and distal fragments should be carefully reamed of all gross disease to permit easy insertion of the PMMA and rod. A uniform cement mantle should be obtained around the rod. Immediate ambulation with full weight bearing is permitted a few days after surgery.

Prophylactic Femoral Shaft Fixation

Small lesions of the femoral shaft may be treated before fracture by the "closed" method (*i.e.*, fluoroscopically inserting an IM rod from a small incision at the tip of the greater trochanter and passing through the lesion to obtain good distal fixation). When using this procedure, it is difficult to insert PMMA. This method is indicated only for small lesions of the femoral shaft with normal bone proximal. Interlocking the rod is useful. Careful preoperative evaluation of the hip is required, because progression and subsequent treatment of an undetected hip lesion would be extremely difficult with an IM rod in place.

Supracondylar Femoral Fixation

Healy and Lane evaluated the Zickel supracondylar device for patients with difficult metastatic lesions of the distal femoral diaphysis (Fig. 61–47).[132] They reported good functional and symptomatic relief in 11 of 14 patients. They emphasized that both medial and lateral incisions were necessary. They also stressed that no matter what the size of the defect, PMMA was used to obtain immediate fixation and stability in all cases. This device is not indicated for distal femoral metaphyseal lesions. This situation is best treated by a custom distal femoral replacement.

PELVIS AND ACETABULUM

Metastatic tumors of the pelvis usually present with progressive pain; fractures are rare. The pelvis can be successfully treated nonoperatively with radiation therapy. Fortunately, marked bony destruction is uncommon; when it occurs, surgery can provide pain relief and enable the patient to walk again. Harrington classified and described the surgical management of 58 patients with severe acetabular insufficiency (classes I, II, III).[11,61] This classification is based on the amount and location of bony destruction and the surgical procedure required for stabilization.

Extensive preoperative evaluation of the bony pelvis, ex-

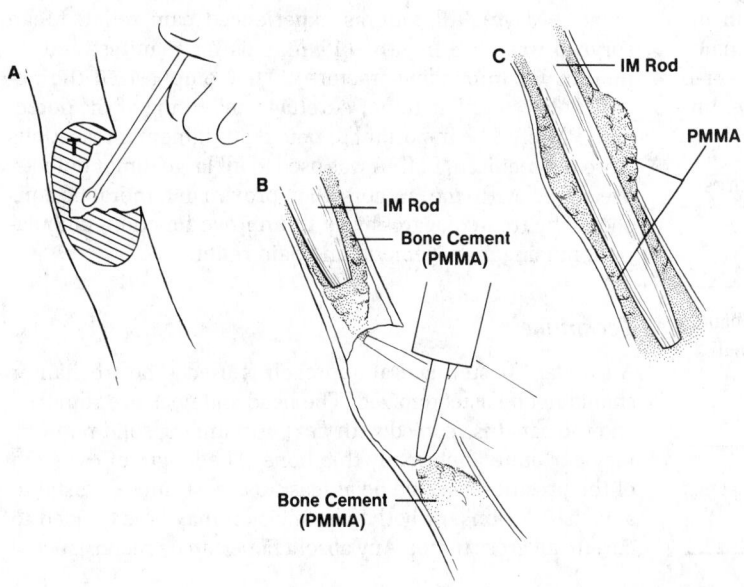

FIGURE 61–46. Diaphyseal reconstruction for metastatic cancer. Long bones (femur and humerus) with metastatic tumors of the shafts (diaphysis) are reconstructed by intramedullary (IM) rod fixation combined with polymethylmethacrylate (PMMA). **(A)** Curettage of the tumor. **(B)** It is important to get the PMMA proximal and distal to the site of the tumor or fracture site, or both, in addition to filling the tumor defect. **(C)** Stable fixation depends on this combined fixation. Small diaphyseal tumors may be treated prophylactically without opening the fracture site by using fluoroscopic control.

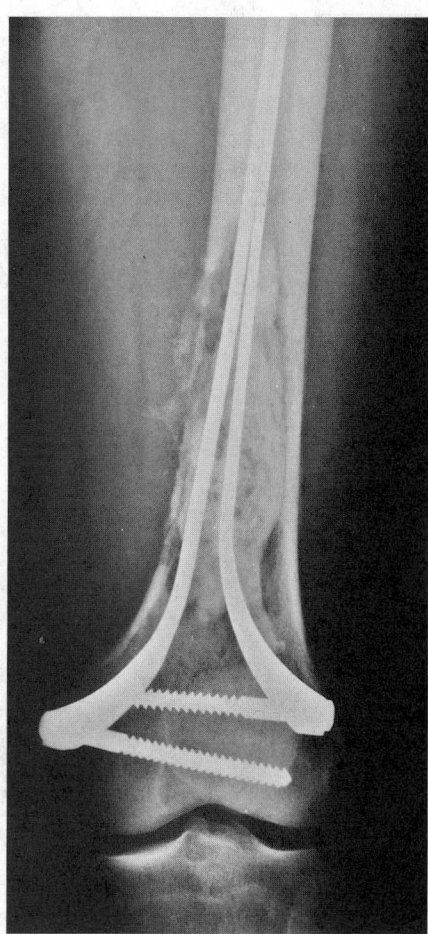

FIGURE 61–47. Zickel (Howmedica, Rutherford, NJ) supracondylar rod fixation of a distal femoral metastatic lesion.

traosseous tumor extension, and tumor vascularity is required. CT/MRI is more reliable than bone scintigraphy for evaluating pelvic tumor extent and is recommended for all patients. Angiography should be performed on all patients before surgery, with embolization of the vascular tumors. Significant blood loss must be anticipated; Harrington reported a mean blood loss of 1800 ml each for classes I and II and a loss of 2790 ml for class III (range, 1125–8550 ml).[61] He emphasized that these procedures are indicated only in a *highly* select group of patients with a predictive long-term survival. For this select group, results are quite good. Sixty-seven percent of the patients reported excellent or good pain relief at 6 months, and 43% at 2 years. Eighty percent were ambulatory at 6 months.

Surgical Treatment

The surgical solution for overcoming the insufficiency of the roof or bony rim is to transmit the forces away from the local periacetabular bone into the superior part of the ilium and sacrum, which is still structurally intact. A standard anterior approach is used. It is unnecessary to enter the retroperitoneal space unless there is a large extraosseous component. All gross disease must be curetted. Hemostasis can be obtained by rapid tumor curettage and PMMA. Reconstruction is accomplished with a combination of Steinmann pins (Howmedica, Ruth-

erford, NJ), protrusio cups, and wire mesh. The trochanter should not be osteotomized. Close intraoperative monitoring of blood loss and hematologic parameters is required.

Malawer and colleagues recently reported a new technique for the treatment of large acetabular lesions that require surgery. This technique curettes out gross tumor and reconstructs the defect with a Saddle prosthesis (Waldermar-Link, Hamburg, Germany), which articulates with the remaining ilium. No other reconstruction is required (Fig. 61–48).[133] This technique avoids the difficult reconstructions using PMMA, screws, and special acetabular components. Reported operative time and surgical blood loss for the Saddle prosthesis have been less than those reported by Harrington for acetabular reconstruction.[61,133]

Pelvic Radiation Therapy

Radiation therapy is recommended for all symptomatic pelvic and acetabular lesions after surgical procedures. Radiation therapy fields must encompass the area of bone involved by tumor and yet spare bone not grossly infiltrated by tumor to minimize irradiation of the marrow. Consideration of the effect of irradiation on bone marrow will be particularly important in patients receiving chemotherapy. If only a portion of the pelvis is treated, field edges should be designed to facilitate matching, in case treatment elsewhere in the pelvis is required at a later date. Pelvis fields will necessarily include some small bowel; the dose and fractionation must be within the limits of small bowel tolerance.

SPINE

The vertebral bodies are most often affected by metastatic cancer (Fig. 61–49). Pain may be secondary to intraosseous disease, instability, collapse or pathologic fracture, or epidural compression, with or without nerve root involvement. Most vertebral pain can be treated with nonoperative modalities such as chemotherapy, radiation therapy, and an external orthosis. The "radiosensitive" solid tumors, lymphomas, and myelomas will respond with decreased pain and reossification. Indications for surgery include progressive neurologic symptoms, intractable pain, and progressive deformity. The traditional aim of such treatment has been decompression of the spinal canal by a posterior laminectomy and, occasionally, posterior stabilization with Harrington rods and PMMA. Recently, significant disagreement has arisen regarding the efficacy of posterior decompression.[12,13,134,135] It is based on the fact that the site of metastatic disease to the spine is anterior, primarily involving the vertebral body. Several reports have described an anterior approach to the affected vertebrae, with removal of all gross disease, that permits decompression of the spinal cord and nerve roots and immediate stabilization by use of PMMA for vertebral body reconstruction.[12,13,134]

Computed tomography, MRI, and myelography are required before surgery. The CT scan demonstrates the amount of bony destruction, while the MRI and myelogram localize the level and extent of epidural disease. The indications for anterior decompression are progressive neurologic deficit after surgery or radiation therapy, and kyphosis with significant deformity (especially of the cervical spine).[12,13] All authors emphasize that this procedure is technically demanding, with significant

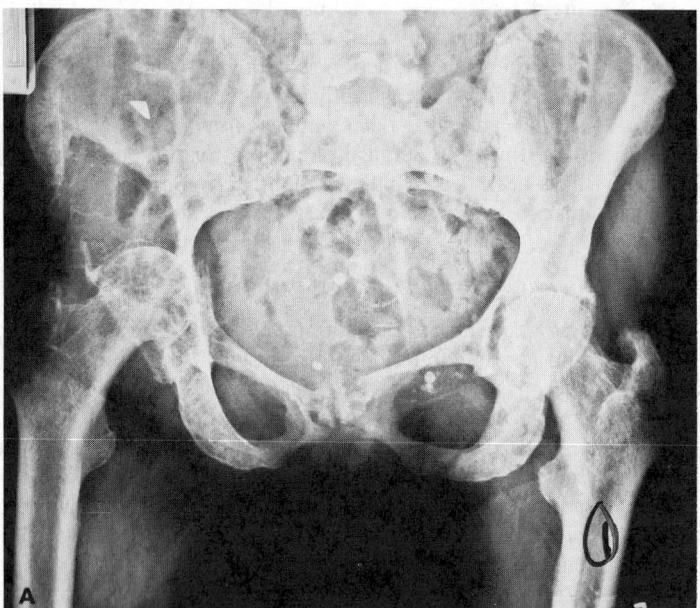
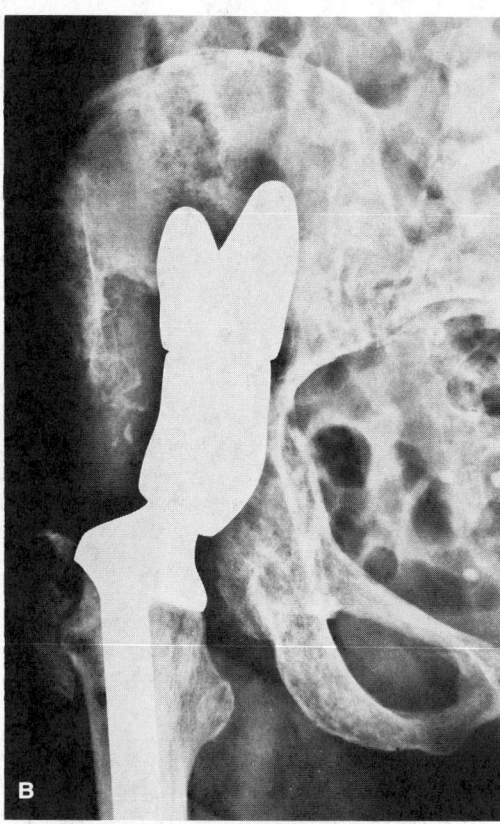

FIGURE 61–48. **(A)** Multiple myeloma of the pelvis with marked destruction of the right acetabulum. This represents a difficult reconstructive problem. **(B)** A saddle prosthesis is used to reconstruct the hip after curettage of the tumor.

morbidity and blood loss. It should be used only in highly selected patients by skilled surgeons. Harrington initially reported 14 patients treated by vertebral body resection and PMMA replacement; 9 of 12 patients with major preoperative neurologic impairment recovered completely, 2 recovered partially, and 1 had no change.[12] Thirteen of the 14 patients had excellent pain relief. Average blood replacements for the cervical/thoracic and lumbar procedures were 200 and 1200 ml, respectively. Sundaresan and associates have performed 100 vertebral body resections and stabilizations for spinal metastases.[13] Eighty percent of these patients had significant pain relief immediately. Complications were related to previous treatment with intensive chemotherapy or radiation therapy. Minimal morbidity occurred in the de novo case.

Recently, Rosenthal and associates (1991) reviewed their experience with anterior corpectomy for metastatic cancer at Memorial Sloan-Kettering Cancer Center.[136] They evaluated 53 patients and concluded that, in addition to anterior decompression, posterior stabilization is required in all patients undergoing decompression, except patients with thoracic lesions. They noted a loss in neurologic and functional status due to tumor progression or collapse of the anterior reconstruction between 7.1 and 8.2 months, whereas the average patient survival was 16 months (range, 1–47 months). They emphasized that these procedures were difficult, with an overall mortality of 5% to 10%.

Surgical Technique

A thoracic or thoracolumbar approach is used. The lumbar vertebrae are approached from the left side, and the aorta is mobilized and retracted. Care must be taken not to injure the segmental vessels, which must be carefully ligated. All gross disease is removed from the affected vertebral body, and the adjacent disks are removed (Fig. 61–50). Gelfoam and continuous irrigation are used to protect the dura from the heat of polymerization before placing the PMMA. Steinmann pins or short distraction rods are placed as vertical supports between the vertebral bodies and then embedded within the PMMA.[12,134] The adjacent bodies are undercut to permit snug PMMA fixation. Care must be taken not to put pressure on the cord.

Newer techniques and concepts of metastatic disease of the spine continue to evolve. Techniques based on advances in spinal surgery, instrumentation, and prosthetic design have permitted various radical methods of vertebral body resection to be performed for selected patients with vertebral body metastases. It must be emphasized that these procedures are performed in highly selected spinal treatment and cancer centers.[137] The overall goals of surgical treatment are:

1. To decompress the spinal cord
2. To leave the patient with a stable spine
3. To leave the patient with a painless spine

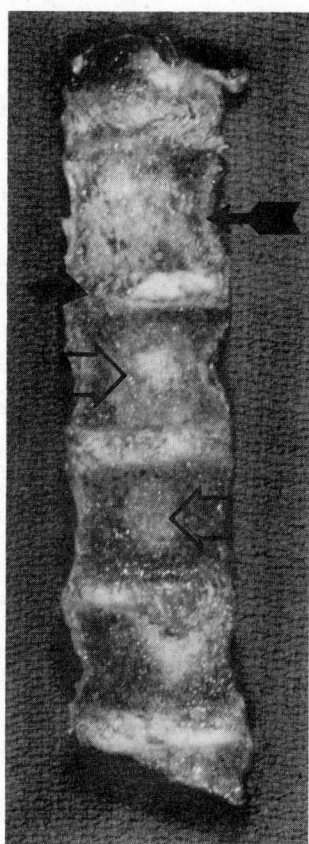

FIGURE 61–49. Metastatic spinal disease. The spine is the most common site of metastatic disease. Metastatic cancer characteristically involves the anterior portion (vertebral body) of the spine. Shown is a gross specimen of the lumbar vertebra with characteristic metastatic tumor deposits within the vertebral bodies (*arrows*). The top vertebra (*straight solid arrow*) is almost completely replaced by tumor, and the adjacent disk space is being destroyed (*short curved arrow*). The lower two vertebrae show small, rounded central deposits of metastatic cancer (*open arrows*).

Cochran and colleagues described a single posterior approach for total vertebrectomy with vertebral body replacement.[137] They reported the largest series to date with 13 patients. This technique permits complete spinal cord decompression with immediate stability. Significant pain relief and preservation of neurologic function were reported.

Radiation Therapy

Radiation therapy is recommended for symptomatic lesions and after surgical decompression. Radiation portals should include sites of symptomatic vertebral disease and other involved vertebrae that can be conveniently included without undue morbidity. Spinal cord tolerance must not be exceeded. Treatment of a portion of a vertebral body is not recommended because of the inherent danger of matching later treatment fields over the spinal cord should disease recur in the untreated portion of the vertebra. Paravertebral soft tissue masses should be included in the treatment field.

HUMERUS

Small lesions can be treated nonoperatively with radiation therapy and sling immobilization. Large lesions or those with a pathologic fracture are best treated by curettage, intramedullary fixation, and PMMA.[28] Proximal humeral lesions are approached through the standard deltopectoral interval. Tumors of the shaft require two incisions: one should be proximal, over the greater tuberosity, and the second should be over the tumor. Lesions of the supracondylar area are best treated by two rods inserted through the epicondyles. If the patient also has lower extremity lesions, early surgery for the humerus is recommended to permit crutch use and protect the lower extremities.

LESIONS DISTAL TO THE KNEE AND ELBOW

Leeson reported that 7% (57/827) of patients with metastatic cancer had distal extremity involvement.[138] The most common primary cancers associated with distal metastases are lung, breast, kidney, and gastrointestinal tract. Tumors of the forearm or tibia are best treated by intramedullary fixation with PMMA. A recent poll of 163 hand surgeons showed that amputation of the digit was recommended in lieu of complicated surgical procedures and difficult radiation. Tumors of the hand may require amputation for local control and palliation, although substantial experience with extremity preservation has been accumulated with combined modality therapy for primary sarcomas of the hand and foot.[139] Patients with metastatic disease to the hand or foot should undergo irradiation for attempted palliation. Amputation can be used for patients not palliated with irradiation.

FIGURE 61–50. Technique of vertebral body reconstruction. The anterior aspect of the spine (vertebral bodies) can be approached successfully with reliable tumor removal, decompression of the spinal cord, and reconstruction in carefully selected patients. Significant morbidity and bleeding must be anticipated.

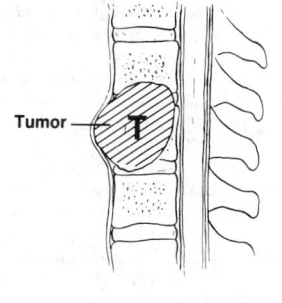

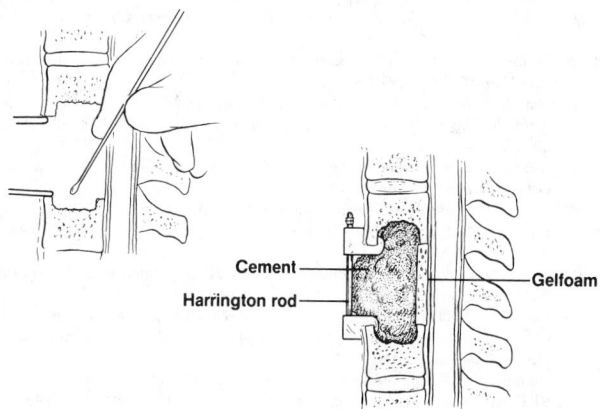

REFERENCES

1. Silverberg E, Lubera J. Cancer statistics, 1987. CA 1987;37:2–20.
2. Abrams HL, Spiro R, Goldstein N. Metastases in carcinoma. Analysis of 1000 autopsied cases. Cancer 1950;23:74–85.
3. Galasko CSB. Mechanisms of lytic and blastic metastatic disease of bone. Clin Orthop 1982;169:20–27.
4. Porter BA, Sheilds AF, Olson DO. Magnetic resonance imaging of bone marrow disorders. Radiol Clin North Am 1986;24:269–288.
5. Daffner RH, Lupetin AR, Dash N, Sefczek RJ, Schapiro RL. MRI in the detection of malignant infiltration of bone marrow. Am J Radiol 1986;146:353–358.
6. Drelichman A, Decker DA, Al-Sarraf M, et al. Computerized bone scan. A potential useful technique to measure response in prostatic carcinoma. Cancer 1984;53:1061–1065.
7. Zegel HG, Turner M, VelchiK MG, et al. Percutaneous osseous needle aspiration biopsy with nuclear medicine guidance. Clin Nucl Med 1984;9:89–91.
8. Little AG, DeMeester TR, Kirchner PT, et al. Guided biopsies of abnormalities on nuclear bone scans. Technique and indications. J Thorac Cardiovasc Surg 1983;85:396–403.
9. McNeil BJ. Value of bone scanning in neoplastic disease. Semin Nucl Med 1984;14:277–286.
10. Harrington KD, Johnston JJ, Turner RH, Green DL. The use of methylmethacrylate as an adjunct in the internal fixation of malignant neoplastic fractures. J Bone Joint Surg [Am] 1972;54:1665–1676.
11. Harrington KD. New trends in the management of lower extremity metastasis. Clin Orthop 1982;169:53–61.
12. Harrington KD. The use of methylmethacrylate for vertebral-body replacement and anterior stabilization of pathological fracture-dislocations of the spine due to metastatic malignant disease. J Bone Joint Surg [Am] 1981;63:36–46.
13. Sundaresan N, Galicich JH, Lane JM, et al. Treatment of neoplastic epidural cord compression by vertebral body resection and stabilization. J Neurosurg 1985;63:676–684.
14. Sherry MM, Greco FA, Johnson DH, Hainsworth JD. Metastatic breast cancer confined to the skeletal system, an indolent disease. Am J Med 1986;81(3):381–386.
15. Salazar OM, Rubin P, Hendrickson FR, et al. Single-dose half-body irradiation for palliation of multiple bone metastases from solid tumors: Final Radiation Therapy Oncology Group report. Cancer 1986;58:29.
16. Vargha ZO, Glicksman AS, Boland J. Single-dose radiation therapy in the palliation of metastatic disease. Radiology 1969;93:1180.
17. Penn CRH. Single dose and fractionated palliative irradiation for osseous metastases. Clin Radiol 1976;27:405.
18. Fitzpatrick PJ, Rider WD. Half-body radiotherapy. Int J Radiat Oncol Biol Phys 1976;1:197.
19. Lawrence JH, Tobias CA. Radioactive isotopes and nuclear radiations in the treatment of cancer. Cancer Res 1956;16:185.
19a. Eisenhut M, Berberich R, Kimming B, Oberhausen E. Iodine-131-labelled diphosphonates for palliative treatment of bone metastases: II. Preliminary clinical results with iodine-131 BDP3. J Nucl Med 1986;27:1255.
20. Clain A. Secondary malignant disease of bone. Br J Cancer 1965;19:15.
21. Higinbotham NL, Marcove RC. The management of pathological fractures. J Trauma 1965;5:792–798.
22. Haberman ET, Sachs R, Stern RE, et al. The pathology and treatment of metastatic disease of the femur. Clin Orthop 1982;169:70–82.
23. Lane JM, Sculco TP, Zolan S. Treatment of pathological fractures of the hip by endoprosthetic replacement. J Bone Joint Surg [Am] 1980;62:954–959.
24. Goris ML, Bretille J. Skeletal scintigraphy for the diagnosis of malignant metastatic diseases of bone. Radiother 1985;4:319–329.
25. Mundy GR, Ibbotson KJ, D'Souza SM. Tumor products and hypercalcemia of malignancy. J Clin Invest 1985;76:391–394.
26. Beard DB, Haskell CM. Carcinoembryonic antigen in breast cancer. Clinical review. Am J Med 1986;80:241–245.
27. El-Khoury GY, Terepka RH, Mickelson MR, et al. Fine-needle aspiration biopsy of bone. J Bone Joint Surg [Am] 1983;65:522–525.
28. Sim F, Pritchard D. Metastatic disease of the upper extremity. Clin Orthop 1982;169:83–94.
29. Berrettoni BA, Carter JR. Mechanisms of cancer metastasis to bone. J Bone Joint Surg [Am] 1986;68:308–311.
30. Manishen WJ, Sivananthan K, Orr FW. Resorbing bone stimulates tumor cell growth. A role for the host microenvironment in bone metastasis. Am J Pathol 1986;123:39–45.
31. Batson OV. The function of the vertebral veins and their role in the spread of metastases. Ann Surg 1940;112:138–149.
32. Galasko CSB. Skeletal metastases. Clin Orthop 1986;210:18–30.
33. Batson OV. Role of vertebral veins in metastatic processes. Ann Intern Med 1942;16:38–45.
34. Coman DR. Mechanisms responsible for origin and distribution of blood-borne tumor metastases. Review. Cancer Res 1953;13:397–404.
35. Coman DR, DeLong RP. The role of the vertebral venous system in the metastasis of cancer to the spinal column. Experiment of tumor-cell suspension in rats and rabbits. Cancer 1951;4:610–618.
36. Turner JW, Jaffe HL. Metastatic neoplasms. AJR 1940;43:479–494.
37. Clark RL. Systemic cancer and the metastatic process. Cancer 1979;43:790.
38. Hollinshead WH, McFarlane JA. A collateral venous drainage system from kidney following occlusion of renal vein in dog. Surg Gynecol Obstet 1953;97:213–219.
39. Brookes M. Blood vessels in bone marrow. In: The blood supply of bone. An approach to bone biology. London: Butterworths, 1971:67–91.
40. Enneking WF. Metastatic carcinoma. In: Enneking WF, ed. Musculoskeletal tumor surgery. vol 2. New York: Churchill Livingstone, 1983:1541.
41. Dodds PR, Cardie VJ, Lytton B. The role of the vertebral veins in the dissemination of prostatic carcinoma. J Urol 1981;126:753–755.
42. del Regato JA. Pathways of metastatic spread of malignant tumors. Semin Oncol 1977;4:33–38.
43. Brookes M. Blood vessels in bone marrow. In: The blood supply of bone. An approach to bone biology. London: Butterworths, 1971:67–91.
44. Gephardt M, et al. Prostaglandins. Clin Oreth and Rel Res
45. Mundy GR, Raisz LG, Cooper RA, et al. Evidence for the secretion of an osteoclast-stimulating factor in myeloma. N Engl J Med 1974;291:1041–1046.
46. Kamenov B, Kiernan MW, Barrington-Leight, et al. Homing receptors as functional markers for classification, prognosis and therapy of leukemias and lymphomas. Proc Soc Exp Biol Med 1984;177:211–219.
47. Lam WC, Delikatny JE, Orr FW, et al. The chemotactic response of tumor cells. A model of cancer metastasis. Am J Pathol 1981;104:69–76.
48. Wilner D. Cancer metastasis to bone. In: Wilner D, ed. Radiology of bone tumors and allied disorders. Philadelphia: WB Saunders, 1982:3641–3908.
49. Pollne JJ, Witztum KF, Ashburn WL. The flare phenomenon of radionuclide bone scan in metastatic prostate cancer. Am J Radiol 1984;142:773–776.
50. Hortobagyi GN, Lipshitz HI, Seabod JE. Osseous metastases of breast cancer. Clinical, biochemical, radiographic, and scintigraphic evaluation of response to therapy. Cancer 1984;53:577–582.
51. Hayward RB, Frazier TG. A re-evaluation of bone scans in breast cancer. J Surg Oncol 1985;28:111–113.
52. Weissman DE, Gilbert M, Wang H, Grossman SA. The use of computed tomography of the spine to identify patients at high risk for epidural metastases. J Clin Oncol 1985;3:1541–1544.
53. Wallace S, Granmayeh M, DeSantos LA, et al. Arterial occlusion of pelvic bone tumors. Cancer 1979;43:322–328.
54. Wallace S, Charnsangavej C, Carrasco H, Bechtel W. Infusion-embolization. Cancer 1984;54:2751–2765.
55. Jonsson K, Johnell O. Preoperative angiography in patients with bone metastases. Acta Radiol Diagn 1982;23:485–489.
56. Bowers TA, Murray JA, Charnsangavej C, Soo C, et al. Bone metastases from renal carcinoma, the preoperative use of transcatheter arterial occlusion. J Bone Joint Surg [Am] 1982;64:749–754.
57. Pugh J, Sherry H, Futterman B, et al. Biomechanics of pathologic fractures. Clin Orthop 1982;169:109–114.
58. Ryan JR, Begeman PC. The effects of filling experimental large cortical defects with methylmethacrylate. Clin Orthop 1984;185:306–310.
59. Gainor BJ, Buchert P. Fracture healing in metastatic bone disease. Clin Orthop 1983;178:297–302.
60. Unger AS, Boothe RE. Disseminated intravascular coagulopathy in a patient undergoing total hip arthroplasty. A case report. Clin Orthop 1984;183:76–78.
61. Harrington KD. The management of acetabular insufficiency secondary to metastatic malignant disease. J Bone Joint Surg [Am] 1981;63:653–663.
62. Schobinger R. The arteriographic picture of metastatic bone disease. Cancer 1958;11:1265–1268.
63. Varm J, Huben RP, Wajsman Z, Pontes JE. Therapeutic embolization of pelvic metastases of renal cell carcinoma. J Urol 1984;131:647–649.
64. Mink J. Percutaneous bone biopsy in the patient with known or suspected osseous metastases. Radiology 1986;161:191–194.
64a. Michele AA, Krueger FJ. Surgical approach to the vertebral body. J Bone Joint Surg [Am] 1949;31:873–878.
64b. Schajowicz F, Derequic JC. Puncture biopsy in lesions of the locomotor system. Review of results in 4050 cases, including 941 vertebral punctures. Cancer 1968;21:531–548.
65. Taylor CR, Kledzik G. Immunohistologic techniques in surgical pathology—A spectrum of "new" special stains. Hum Pathol 1981;12:590–596.
66. Pinkus GS. Diagnostic immunocytochemistry of paraffin-embedded tissues. Hum Pathol 1982;13:411–415.
67. Pinkus GS, Kurtin PJ. Epithelial membrane antigen—A diagnostic discriminant in surgical pathology. Hum Pathol 1985;16:929–940.
68. Kahn HJ, Marks A, Thom H, Baumal R. Role of antibody to S100 protein in diagnostic pathology. Am J Clin Pathol 1983;79:341–347.
69. Nadji M, Tabei SZ, Castro A, Chu TM, Morales AR. Prostatic origin of tumors. An immunohistochemical study. Am J Clin Pathol 1980;73:735–739.
70. Nadji M. Immunoperoxidase techniques I. Facts and artifacts. Am J Dermatopathol 1986;8:32–36.
71a. Sangeorzan BJ, Ryan JR, Salciccioli GG. Prophylactic femoral stabilization with the Zickel nail by closed technique. J Bone Joint Surg [Am] 1986;68:991–999.
71b. Marcove RC, Miller TR. Treatment of primary and metastatic bone tumors by cryosurgery. JAMA 1969;207:1890.
72. Marcove RC. A 17-year review of cryosurgery in the treatment of bone tumors. Clin Orthop 1982;163:231.
73. Malawer MM, Baker A. Amputations for tumors. In: Evarts CM, ed. Surgery of the musculoskeletal system. 2nd ed. New York: Churchill Livingstone, 1990.
74. Malawer MM, Marks MR, McChecney D, et al. The effect of cryosurgery and polymethylmethacrylate (PMMA) in dogs with experimental bone defects comparable to tumor defects. Clin Orthop 1988;226:229–310.

75. Tong D, Gillick L, Hendrickson FR. The palliation of symptomatic osseous metastases: Final results of the Radiation Therapy Oncology Group. Cancer 1982;50:893.

76. Delclos L. New and old concepts in radiotherapeutic treatment. Int J Radiat Oncol Biol Phys 1976;1:1217.

77. Hendrickson FR, Sheinkop MB. Management of osseous metastases. Semin Oncol 1975;2:399.

78. Weber DA. The quantitative measurement of the response to treatment. Int J Radiat Oncol Biol Phys 1976;1:1221.

79. Yarnold JR. Role of radiotherapy in the management of bone metastases from breast cancer. J R Soc Med 1985;78(Suppl):23.

80. Garmatis CJ, Chu FCH. The effectiveness of radiation therapy in the treatment of bone metastases from breast cancer. Radiology 1978;126:235.

81. Allen KL, Johnson TW, Hibbs GG. Effective bone radiation as related to various treatment regimens. Cancer 1976;37:984.

82. Twycross RG. Analgesics and relief of pain. In: Stoll BA, Parbhoo S, eds. Bone metastasis: Monitoring and treatment. New York: Raven Press, 1983.

83. Gilbert HA, Kagan HR, Nussbaum H, et al. Evaluation of radiation therapy for bone metastases: Pain relief and quality of life. AJR 1977;129:1095–1096.

84. Hendrickson FR, Shehata WM, Kirchner AR. Radiation therapy for osseous metastasis. Int J Radiat Oncol Biol Phys 1976;1(3–4):275–278.

85. Bhadrwaj S, Holland JF. Chemotherapy of metastatic cancer to bone. Clin Orthop 1982;169:28–37.

86. Greenberg EJ, Chu FCH, Dwyer AJ, et al. Effects of radiation therapy on bone lesions as measured by 47-Ca and 85-Sr local kinetics. J Nucl Med 1972;13:747.

87. Unger JD, Chiang LC, Unger GF. Apparent reformation of the base of the skull following radiotherapy for nasopharyngeal carcinoma. Radiology 1978;126:779.

88. Blitzer PH. Reanalysis of the RTOG study of the palliation of symptomatic osseous metastasis. Cancer 1985;55:1468.

89. Madsen EL. Painful bone metastasis: Efficacy of radiotherapy assessed by the patients: A randomized trial comparing 4 Gy × 6 versus 10 Gy × 2. Int J Radiat Oncol Biol Phys 1983;9:1775–1779.

90. Cole DJ. A randomized trial of a single treatment versus conventional fractionation in the palliative radiotherapy of painful bone metastases. Clin Oncol 1989;1:59–62.

91. Okawa T, Kita M, Goto M, et al. Randomized prospective clinical study of small, large and twice-a-day fraction radiotherapy for painful bone metastases. Radiother Oncol 1988;13:99–104.

92. Price P, Hoskin PJ, Easton D, et al. Prospective randomised trial of single and multifraction radiotherapy schedules in the treatment of painful bony metastases. Radiother Oncol 1986;6:247–255.

93. Qasim MM. Single dose palliative irradiation for bony metastases. Strahlentherapie 1977;153:531.

94. Price P, Hoskin PJ, Easton D, et al. Low dose single fraction radiotherapy in the treatment of metastatic bone pain: A pilot study. Radiother Oncol 1988;12:297–300.

95. Arcangeli G, Micheli A, Arcangeli G, et al. The responsiveness of bone metastases to radiotherapy: The effect of site, histology and radiation dose on pain relief. Radiother Oncol 1989;14:95–101.

96. Kuban DA, Delbridge T, El-Mahdi AM, Schellhammer PF. Half-body irradiation for treatment of widely metastatic adenocarcinoma of the prostate. J Urol 1989;141:572–574.

97. Zelefsky MJ, Scher HI, Forman JD, et al. Palliative hemiskeletal irradiation for widespread metastatic prostate cancer: A comparison of single dose and fractionated regimens. Int J Radiat Oncol Biol Phys 1989;17:1281–1285.

98. Kaplan E, Miree J, Hirsh E, et al. Autoradiographic localization of 32P phosphate in metastatic carcinoma of the breast to bone. Int J Appl Radiat Isot 1959;5:94–98.

99. Montebello JF, Hartson-Eaton M. The palliation of osseous metastasis with 32P and 89Sr compared with external beam and hemibody irradiation. Cancer Invest 1989;7(2):139–160.

100. McKenna WG, Barnes MM, Kinsella TJ, et al. Combined modality treatment of adult soft tissue sarcomas of the head and neck. Int J Radiat Oncol Biol Phys 1987;13:1127.

101. Ellis RE. The distribution of active bone marrow in the adult. Phys Med Biol 1961;5:255.

102. Maxfield JR, Maxfield JJG, Maxfield WS. The use of radioactive phosphorus and testosterone in metastatic bone lesions from breast and prostate. South Med J 1958;51:320.

103. Ariel IM, Hassouna H. Carcinoma of the prostate: The treatment of bone metastases by radioactive phosphorus (32P). Int Surg 1985;70:63.

104. Aziz H, Choi K, Sohn C, et al. Comparison of 32P therapy and sequential hemibody irradiation (HBI) for bony metastases as methods of whole body irradiation. Am J Clin Oncol 1986;9:264.

105. Fowler JE Jr, Whitmore WF Jr. Considerations for the use of testosterone with systemic chemotherapy in prostatic cancer. Cancer 1982;49:1373.

106. Firusian N, Mellin P, Schmidt CG. Results of 89 strontium therapy in patients with carcinoma of the prostate and incurable pain from bone metastases: A preliminary report. J Urol 1976;116:764.

107. Reddy EK, Robinson RG, Mansfield CM. Strontium-89 therapy for palliation of bone metastases. J Natl Med Assoc 1986;78:27.

108. Bhadrwaj S, Holland JF. Chemotherapy of metastatic cancer to bone. Clin Orthop 1982;169:28–37.

109. Maxon HR III, Schroeder LE, Thomas SR, et al. Re-186(Sn) HEDP for treatment of painful osseous metastases: Initial clinical experience in 20 patients with hormone-resistant prostate cancer. Radiology 1990;176:155–159.

110. Turner JH, Claringbold PG, Hetherington EL, et al. A phase I study of samarium-153 ethylenediaminetetramethylene phosphonate therapy for disseminated skeletal metastases. J Clin Oncol 1989;7:1926–1931.

111. Miller F, Whitehill R. Carcinoma of the breast metastatic to the skeleton. Clin Orthop 1984;184:121–127.

112. Sherry MM, Greco A, Johnson DH, Hainsworth JD. Breast cancer with skeletal metastases at initial diagnosis. Cancer 1986;58:178–182.

113. Scheid V, Buzdar AU, Smith TL, et al. Clinical course of breast cancer patients with osseous metastasis treated with combination chemotherapy. Cancer 1986;58:2589–2593.

114. Arkless R. Renal carcinoma: How it metastasizes. Cancer 1965;84:496–501.

115. Garfield DH, Kennedy BJ. Regression of metastatic renal cell carcinoma following nephrectomy. Cancer 1972;30:190–196.

116. Dorn W, Gladden MP, Rankin EA. Regression of a renal-cell metastatic osseous lesion following treatment. J Bone Joint Surg [Am] 1975;57:869–870.

117. Chute R, Houghton JD. Solitary distant metastases from unsuspected renal carcinomas. J Urol 1958;80:420–424.

118. Marcove RC, Sadrieh J, Huvos AG, et al. Cryosurgery in the treatment of solitary or multiple bone metastases form renal cell carcinoma. J Urol 1972;108:540.

119. Marcove RC, Searfoss RC, Whitmore WF, et al. Cryosurgery in the treatment of bone metastases from renal cell carcinoma. Clin Orthop 1972;127:220.

120. Delaney TF. Personal experience.

121. Bonnheim DC, Petrelli NJ, Herrera L, Walsh D, Mittelman A. Osseous metastases from colorectal carcinoma. Am J Surg 1986;151:457–459.

122. Seife B. Osseous metastases from carcinoma of the large bowel. Cancer 1973;119:414–418.

123. Napoli LD, Hansen HH, Muggia FM, et al. The incidence of osseous involvement in lung cancer, with special reference to the development of osteoblastic changes. Radiology 1973;108:17–21.

124. McCormack KR. Bone metastases from thyroid carcinoma. Cancer 1966;19:181–184.

125. Niederle B, Roka R, Schemper M, et al. Surgical treatment of distant metastases in differentiated thyroid cancer: Indications and results. Surgery 1986;100:1088–1097.

126. Wilner D, Breckenridge RL. Bone metastasis in malignant melanoma. 1949;62:388–394.

127. Stewart WR, Gelerman RH, Harrelson JM, et al. Skeletal metastases of melanoma. J Bone Joint Surg [Am] 1978;60:645–649.

128. Beals RK, Lawton GD, Snell WE. Prophylactic internal fixation of the femur in metastatic breast cancer. Cancer 1971;28:1350–1354.

129. Keene JS, Sellinger DS, McBeath AA, Engber WD. Metastatic breast cancer in the femur. A search for the lesion at risk of fracture. Clin Orthop 1986;203:282–288.

130. Mirels H. Metastatic disease in long bones, a proposed scoring system. Clin Orthop 1989;249:256–265.

131. Rinkes IHB, Wiggers T, Bouma WH, Van Geel AN, Boxma H. Treatment of manifest and impending pathological fractures of the femoral neck by cemented hemiarthroplasty. Clin Orthop 1990;260:220–223.

132. Healy JH, Lane JM. Treatment of pathological fractures of the distal femur with the supracondylar nail. Clin Orthop 1990;250:216–220.

133. Aboulafia AJ, Faulks W, Li W, Buch R, Matthews J, Malawer MM. Reconstruction using the Saddle prosthesis following excision of malignant periacetabular tumors. In: Brown KLB, ed. Complications of limb salvage: Prevention, management and outcome. Montreal: International Society of Limb-Sparing Surgery, 1991.

134. Siegal T. Vertebral body resection of epidural compression by malignant tumors. Results of forty-seven consecutive operative procedures. J Bone Joint Surg [Am] 1985;67:375–382.

135. Harrison KM, Muss HB, Ball MR, et al. Spinal cord compression in breast cancer. Cancer 1985;55:2839–2844.

136. Rosenthal HG, Healy JH, Peterson M, et al. Outcome analysis of corpectomy without posterior instrumentation. In: Brown KLB, ed. Complications of limb salvage: Prevention, management and outcome. Montreal: International Society of Limb-Sparing Surgery, 1991.

137. Cochran JM, Keppler L, Biscup RS, Brantigan JW, Enker P, Steffee AD. Total posterior vertebrectomy with vertebral body replacement. In: Brown KLB, ed. Complications of limb salvage: Prevention, management and outcome. Montreal: International Society of Limb-Sparing Surgery, 1991.

138. Leeson MC, Makley JT, Carter JR. Metastatic disease distal to the elbow and knee. Clin Orthop 1986;206:94–99.

139. Kinsella TJ, Miser JS, Waller B. Extremity preservation by combined modality therapy in sarcomas of the hand and foot: An analysis of local control, disease free survival and functional results. Int J Radiat Oncol Biol Phys 1983;9:1115–1119.

SECTION **5** HARVEY I. PASS

Treatment of Malignant Pleural and Pericardial Effusions

The occurrence of a new pleural or pericardial effusion in a cancer patient merits complete investigation by the oncologist. The degree of symptoms attending such effusions is variable, and the cause may not be due to malignancy. Appropriate therapy, however, must be dictated by objective documentation of a cause, especially when treatment may involve operative intervention or innovative therapy.

PLEURAL EFFUSIONS

PATHOPHYSIOLOGY

Five to 10 L of fluid move through the pleural space in 24 hours, of which 35% to 75% is turned over each hour, leaving 5 to 20 ml of fluid with a protein content of less than 2 g/dl.[1] Eighty percent to 90% of the fluid is reabsorbed, and abnormal fluid collections result from increased capillary permeability, increased hydrostatic pressure (congestive heart failure), increased negative intrapleural pressure (atelectasis), decreased oncotic pressure (hypoalbuminemia), or increased pleural fluid oncotic pressure (pleural tumor growth).[2] Processes that impair pleural lymphatic drainage also lead to effusion. There is a strong relation between carcinomatous infiltration of mediastinal lymph nodes and pleural effusion; however, the extent of direct pleural involvement by metastases bears no relation to the development of pleural effusion.[3] Therefore, the key elements in *malignant* pleural effusions include increased capillary permeability through inflammation or disruption of the capillary endothelium or impaired lymphatic drainage secondary to obstruction by tumor.[2] Although cancer patients may have transudative effusions on the basis of hypoalbuminemia, heart failure, or liver disease, malignant effusions are classically described as exudative with a protein content of >3 g/dl, specific gravity >1.015, pleural protein/serum protein ratio >0.5, and pleural lactate dehydrogenase (LDH)/serum LDH ratio >0.6. As protein concentration in the pleura increases, pleural osmotic pressure increases, which impedes efflux of pleural fluid. Pleural tumor involvement leads to mesothelial shedding and subsequently pleural thickening. Capillary engorgement and lymphocyte infiltration of the pleura commonly lead to a lymphocyte-abundant, bloody pleural effusion from tumor directly invading the blood vessels, from occlusion of venules, or from capillary dilation by vasoactive substances. A bloody effusion is the single strongest positive predictive element of malignancy.[4,5]

SYMPTOMS AND SIGNS

Twenty-three percent of patients are asymptomatic at the time of presentation, and 50% to 90% of patients with primary or metastatic pleural malignancy will have pleural effusion as their initial presenting manifestation.[6] Most (90%) will have effusions of more than 500 ml, and approximately 33% will have bilateral effusions at the time of presentation.

Dyspnea, cough, and *chest pain* are the common presenting complaints. The degree of symptom severity is related to the rapidity with which the fluid develops rather than the amount of fluid present.[7] Dyspnea is related to pulmonary compression. Pleuritic chest wall pain occurs with parietal pleural inflammation, whereas dull continuous pain is usually associated with parietal pleural metastases.[1] Diaphragmatic pleural irritation may be referred to the ipsilateral shoulder. Cough is usually dry and nonproductive and is due to compression of bronchial walls by fluid.[7]

Objective findings include tachypnea, labored breathing, and restricted chest wall expansion. Dullness to percussion, decreased fremitus, increased intercostal fullness, and undetectable diaphragmatic excursion may be present. Massive effusions may cause contralateral tracheal deviation.

DIAGNOSTIC TECHNIQUES

Radiography

Blunting of the costophrenic angle seen in the upright posteroanterior (PA) x-ray film will be observed with as little as 175 to 525 ml of fluid, and a lateral decubitus film will detect as little as 100 ml.[8–11] Fluid can be loculated within pulmonary fissures (pseudotumors) or between the lung and the diaphragm (Fig. 61–51).

An opacified hemithorax with mediastinal shift usually indicates massive effusion (>1500 ml). Opacification without shift should alert one to the possibility of mainstem bronchial obstruction, mediastinal fixation with malignant lymph nodes, or malignant mesothelioma.[3]

Small pleural effusions can be detected on computed tomography (CT), and CT can sometimes delineate an underlying pleural malignancy. The use of CT attenuation numbers (Hounsfield units) for the differentiation of pleural fluid from pleural tumors is controversial.[12] The usual place for CT in

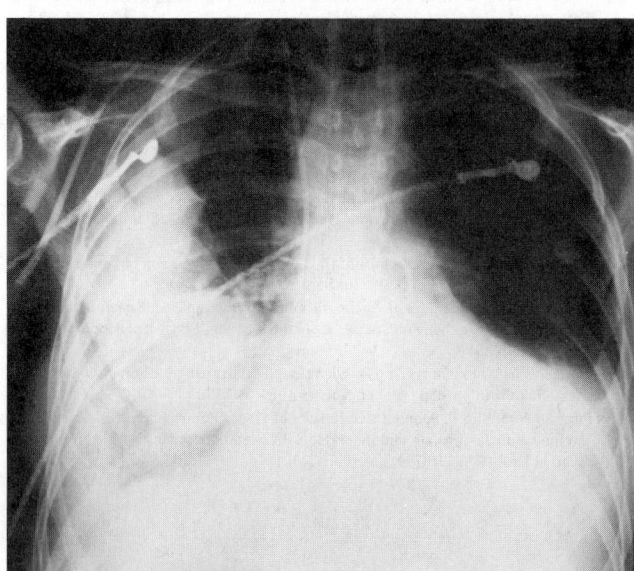

FIGURE 61–51. Patient with right-side pseudotumor, pleural effusion, and large pericardial effusion from breast cancer.

the management of malignant pleural effusions is *after* pleural drainage, which then allows the radiologist to evaluate subtle changes in pleural structure, new parenchymal infiltrates or masses, or enlargement of mediastinal lymph nodes. This is especially useful if previous chest tomograms are available from before the development of the effusion. Ultrasound techniques with the use of both A- and B-mode scans have been widely used to detect and sample pleural effusions.[13] Ultrasonography can identify pleural fluid and can differentiate between pleural thickening and pleural fluid.[5] The use of ultrasonic guidance to determine the proper site for thoracentesis and establish the depth of the fluid decreases the risk of complications, especially in small effusions demonstrated by radiographic techniques.[5,14]

Cytology

Demonstration of malignant cells in pleural fluid is the sine qua non of a malignant pleural effusion. Samples prepared for examination of pleural fluid include wet mounts stained with toluidine blue; smears fixed in 95% alcohol or air dried; membrane-filtered, cytocentrifuge preparations; and cell blocks for paraffin embedding and sectioning. Staining is by the modified Papanicolaou method, cytocentrifuge specimens by Wright-Giemsa, and paraffin sections by hematoxylin-eosin.

The rate of positivity for pleural cytologic specimens varies among large series. Sears,[15] Lopes-Cardozo,[16] and Johnston[17] have reported positive pleural cytologic appearances in 44%, 29% and 9%, respectively, of all pleural specimens submitted. The results of the cytologic examination vary according to the site of the effusion, the type and site of the primary neoplasm, and the method of processing the specimen.[15,16,18-20] Cytologic specimens from patients *known to have neoplasms* have given positive results in 42% to 96% of patients, whereas the false-positive rates have ranged from 0% to 3%.[16,18,19,21,22]

Recognition of cancer cells by cytopathologic techniques has become highly accurate when performed by an experienced clinical morphologist. Difficulties arise when trying to differentiate cancer cells from reactive mesothelial cells or when trying to classify the organ of origin. The use of immunocytochemical techniques as an adjunct to the diagnosis of malignant pleural effusions has, until recently, been limited by the availability, sensitivity, and specificity of the assays using polyclonal sera or monoclonal antibodies. Immunochemical techniques are now routinely performed in the diagnosis of malignancy. Anti-carcinoembryonic antigen (anti-CEA) heteroantisera has demonstrated reactivity with approximately 50% of cancer cells, whereas no reactivity is noted with mesothelial cells or benign effusions.[23] Polyclonal antisera to epithelial membrane antigen has demonstrated reactivity with 54% of carcinomatous effusions and no reactivity with benign effusions.[24-26] B72.3, an IgG1 monoclonal antibody, has recently been shown to recognize 100% of adenocarcinomas in patients with effusions from cancers of breast, ovary, and lung, and when additional metastatic adenocarcinomas from other sites are considered, overall recognition is 95%, including poorly differentiated squamous cell lung cancer.[27,28] Cytochemical staining with acid phosphatase, α-naphthylacetate esterase, and periodic acid-Schiff, as well as sheep erythrocyte rosetting, is useful in recognizing malignant lymphocytes.[29]

Cytogenetic analysis of pleural effusions combining cytologic and chromosome analyses of pleural effusions has correctly diagnosed 83% to 91% of malignant effusions, a result that was better than that with either technique alone[30]; however, the false-positive rate is higher in chromosome analysis than in ordinary cytology.[5] Other studies[31,32] have yielded nearly a 90% positive diagnosis of malignancy, with a 3% false-negative rate. Pleural cytogenetics, however, is limited by expense and time consumption.

Biochemical Analysis

The CEA levels in pleural fluid may be useful in detecting malignancy,[5] with a pleural fluid level of >20 ng/ml having a 91% sensitivity and 92% specificity in effusions caused by adenocarcinoma. In patients with metastatic bronchogenic adenocarcinoma in the pleura, the CEA level is higher than 10 ng/ml in 90% of the patients. Reported sensitivities in malignant effusion range from 25% to 57%, with cutoff values between 10 and 20 ng/ml.[33-35] The CEA level assays are expensive, are time-consuming, and lack sensitivity and specificity for malignancy in general. Hyaluronic acid levels have been noted to be elevated in patients with mesothelioma[15]; however, this assay lacks sensitivity and will not provide a definitive diagnosis.[36]

Thoracentesis

Thoracentesis of suspected malignant pleural effusions can be both diagnostic and therapeutic, although the symptomatic relief of fluid removal is usually short-lived without other adjuvant measures. Bleeding, pneumothorax with peripheral bronchopleural fistula, and "pleural shock," an exaggerated vagal response as the needle passes through the parietal pleura, causing bradycardia, are possible complications. The latter is easily reversed with intravenous fluids, atropine, and Trendelenberg positioning. Oxygen therapy and narcotics may be necessary because of the pain of reexpansion. Thoracentesis of volumes larger than 1500 ml may cause reexpansion pulmonary edema.[37-39]

The fluid withdrawn is sent for cytologic and bacteriologic determinations, and for levels of protein, LDH, glucose, specific gravity, and cell count to determine the transudative or exudative nature of the fluid.

Pleural Biopsy

Closed pleural biopsy is a relatively easy technique that can be coordinated with CT guidance to try to decrease sampling error. The pleural biopsy should be done before fluid aspiration to avoid pulmonary injury. Cytologic examination of pleural fluid alone has a higher sensitivity than needle biopsy,[40,41] and the yield of diagnosis of pleural neoplasm by needle biopsy alone ranges from 40% to 69%.[42-46] When pleural biopsy is combined with cytology, however, the diagnostic yield is increased from 81% to 90%.[47,48]

The morbidity of pleural biopsy is 0.6%,[49] with the most commonly reported complications being pneumothorax, pleural shock, hemothorax, subcutaneous emphysema, and inadequate biopsy. Cancer implantation, associated with the use of larger needles and hematoma formation, occurs in 4.1% of patients.[50]

Thoracoscopy

In undiagnosed suspected malignant pleural effusions with persistently negative cytologic results, thoracoscopy has been useful in establishing the diagnosis in 93% to 96% of the patients (Fig. 61–52).[51–53] Recently, video thoracoscopy, employing television monitoring of the procedure and transthoracic trocars to aid in lung manipulation, has been used to enhance the efficacy of malignant effusion treatment. With the use of lateral decubitus positioning and double-lumen endotracheal intubation with ipsilateral lung collapse, the videoscope, retractors, and instruments are introduced through separate 10-mm incisions. Greater documentation of disease extent, and the ability to perform pleurectomy for increased sclerosis efficacy, may make this rapidly developing technique invaluable in the future. Synchronous sclerosis of malignant pleural effusions at the time of thoracoscopy has been reported with good success.[54,55]

Thoracotomy

The need for open thoracotomy in the management of malignant pleural effusion is reserved for the rare case of nondiagnostic studies and continued suspicion of malignant disease. Even after thoracotomy, a significant number of patients will be found not to have malignant disease.[2,5]

PROGNOSIS AND TREATMENT

The prognosis of patients who develop malignant pleural effusions varies with the histologic type of the primary tumor. When one considers all effusions regardless of the histologic type, 65% of the patients will be dead within 3 months and 80% within 6 months. Patients with breast cancer will have a mean survival of 7 to 15 months posteffusion[15,56] and a 3-year survival of 20%.[57] Mean survival time in patients with lung cancer has been reported to be as low as 2 months from

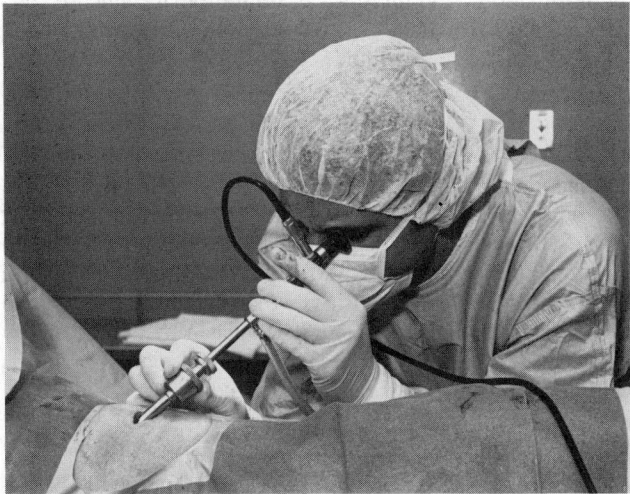

FIGURE 61–52. Thoracoscopy with the rigid thoracoscope permits visualization of pleural abnormalities and direct biopsy.

the time of diagnosis of malignant pleural effusion,[56] and 66% of the patients will be dead by 3 months. Thirty-three percent of patients with ovarian cancer will die within a mean time of 10 months after the diagnosis of malignant effusion, and the mean survival time is 3 months.[15]

Treatment should palliate symptoms in the most reliable, least complicated, and, hopefully, most durable manner. In selected instances, local treatment can be combined with systemic regimens (*i.e.*, testicular carcinoma, lymphoma, breast cancer), depending on the efficacy of the systemic agents for a given malignant histologic type. In most cases of solid tumors with malignant effusions, only local therapy is considered, to control reaccumulation of pleural fluid and diminish or eliminate the need for repeated thoracenteses required by repeated bouts of respiratory compromise.

From the literature, it is difficult to objectively evaluate composites of large series for the success of treatment of malignant pleural effusions because of the differing criteria used to denote responsivity. Moreover, time endpoints for evaluation differ among studies. The most useful criterion has been a failure of the effusion to recur at 4 to 6 weeks, because patients treated by simple thoracentesis and followed for 1 month have a 97% recurrence rate. Some of the newer strategies (*e.g.*, the use of bacillus Calmette-Guérin [BCG] vaccine and *Corynebacterium parvum*), which do not employ tube thoracostomy, define a complete response as no reaccumulation after one thoracentesis employing intrapleural treatment.

METHODS OF TREATMENT

Sclerotherapy

The management of malignant pleural effusions involves the proper technique of sclerotherapy after space obliteration by placement of a large-bore thoracostomy tube. Initial removal of the effusion allows the visceral pleura to come into contact with the chest wall parietal pleura and thereby obliterates, by continuous, underwater-seal suction drainage, the space occupied by the effusion. A sclerosing agent (*i.e.*, antibiotic, antineoplastic, or radioactive) can then be delivered intrapleurally to produce mesothelial fibrosis and obliterate small pleural blood vessels, rather than produce specific antineoplastic activity.[58] Table 61–32 represents a survey of the available literature on the efficacy of intrapleural sclerotherapy. Some groups have attempted to relate the outcome of sclerosis (specifically with talc) to alterations in pleural fluid chemistry.[50] Glucose levels less than 60 mg/dl in the pleural fluid seem to correlate with the extent of pleural disease, and the cytology yield will be positive for malignancy in 87% of such neoplastic pleural effusions. Moreover, patients with a low glucose level or a low pH (*i.e.*, less than 7.3) had significantly worse results with regard to achieving pleural symphysis with successful effusion management, with a 50% failure rate. These findings, although interesting, require verification in larger numbers of patients.

TECHNIQUE OF PLEURAL SCLEROTHERAPY. The intrapleural instillation of agents in patients with neoplastic pleural disease has been fairly standardized. The first order of business is a careful examination of the available roent-

TABLE 61–32. Management of Malignant Pleural Effusions*

Treatment	Histologic Type					
	Lung	Breast	Lymphoma	Ovary	Other	Overall (%)
Chest tube alone	1/6	18/38	—	—	1/10	20/54 (37)
Tetracycline	17/28	24/44	0/1	0/1	20/40	61/114 (54)
Quinacrine	30/37	39/49	7/9	5/8	19/26	100/129 (78)
Bleomycin	7/11	33/38	4/6	5/6	32/55	81/116 (70)
Nitrogen mustard	35/53	109/225	7/19	8/11	24/50	183/358 (51)
5-FU						23/35 (66)
Thiotepa	0/1	11/21		2/2	0/2	14/26 (54)
Talc	54/59	71/75	4/4	8/9	71/90	208/237 (88)
Irradiation	8/10	2/3	9/10	—	11/15	30/38 (79)
Isotopes	102/190	234/413	22/44	32/54	85/177	475/878 (54)
BCG						5/9 (56)
Corynebacterium parvum						57/70 (81)

BCG, bacillus Calmette-Guérin vaccine.
* Number successful/number reported.

genographic studies, including lateral decubitus films, upright PA films, lateral chest films, and chest CT scans (if available). One must first determine whether or not this is a free-flowing pleural effusion without loculations, which may have developed because of initial multiple thoracenteses. The development of loculations in such a situation makes it difficult for a single chest tube placement to obtain adequate evacuation of the fluid. Fortunately, however, most patients have free-flowing pleural effusions without loculations.

Placement of the chest tube should be done by an experienced physician to minimize the patient's discomfort. The chest tube can usually be placed laterally in the sixth or seventh interspace, in a position lying in the anterior axillary line, such that the patient will not be lying on the chest tube when he is supine. Premedication with 75 to 100 mg of meperidine (Demerol) or 6 to 8 mg of morphine, subcutaneously, will relax the patient and decrease discomfort. The appropriate chest is sterilely prepared with an iodine-based cleansing solution, and sterile towels are placed. The skin is infiltrated locally with 1% lidocaine (Xylocaine) at the appropriate site for chest tube placement. Usually 10 to 30 ml of 1% lidocaine, placed intradermally and subdermally and down to the chest wall, will provide a satisfactory local block. Once the skin and chest wall are anesthetized, a quick thoracentesis is performed to document good flow of effusion in this designated area. If free flow of fluid is not obtained, another site that will guarantee good flow of fluid should be chosen for chest tube placement. A short 1- to 3-cm incision is then made in the skin and carried down to the subcutaneous tissues. A curved scissors is then used to create a tunnel through the chest wall musculature, directly down to the interspace of choice. The more care that is taken with the development of this subcutaneous tunnel down to the intercostal muscles over the appropriate rib, the less discomfort the patient will have when the chest tube is placed. Some physicians prefer the use of a trocar chest tube; however, the use of a surgical clamp to open into the pleural space under controlled conditions will allow the finger to be placed into the chest to assure that there are no

adhesions that could be violated by chest tube placement. An appropriate-sized chest tube, either 28 or 32 French, is then placed through the subcutaneous tunnel into the pleural cavity and directed cephalad by having a clamp on the introducing end of the chest tube and a clamp at the end of the chest tube, closing it off to prevent open pneumothorax and a rush of fluid out of the chest tube. The chest tube is then connected to an underwater-seal drainage system, using any of a variety of systems. A stitch of heavy silk is used to anchor the chest tube to the skin, and sterile dressings are applied. A chest x-ray film is then obtained and viewed for proper tube placement. We repeat chest radiographs daily after chest tube placement and subsequent sclerosis therapy.

For the first 24 hours, the chest tube should be connected to underwater-seal drainage with negative suction (approximately 15–20 cm H_2O) applied to the device. This will ensure maximum expansion of the compressed, underlying lung and total evacuation of the fluid. Because the use of a chest tube alone is associated with a low success rate (see Table 61–32), we always approach the patient who has a chest tube placed for neoplastic pleural disease as a candidate for intrapleural therapy. If the chest x-ray film, taken 24 hours after the placement of the chest tube, shows total evacuation of fluid with good lung expansion, the sclerotherapy can be started. Sclerotherapy should not be performed if the patient has a large volume of residual fluid left in the chest. Doing this will doom the treatment to failure because of dilution of the sclerosing medium and the insufficient expansion of the underlying lung.

When the decision is made to give sclerotherapy, the patient is medicated 30 minutes before treatment with a narcotic agent. The sclerosing drug is then instilled directly through the chest tube with an irrigating catheter, followed by clamping of the chest tube and connection of the end of the chest tube back to the drainage system. Essentially, the sclerosing agent remains in the chest cavity because the chest tube is clamped, and the patient is instructed to change positions every 15 minutes for 4 hours (*i.e.*, lying flat, right-side-up, left-side-up, head-down, and head-up) to equally distribute this 100 ml throughout the pleural cavity. At the end of this 4 hours, the chest tube clamp is removed and the fluid is allowed to drain, with suction for another 24 hours.

Twenty-four hours after the sclerotherapy, the patient is disconnected from suction and the chest is allowed to drain by gravity. The patient is maintained connected to this underwater-seal system, with daily monitoring of the amount of effluent. When the drainage has decreased substantially (*e.g.,* to 50–100 ml/24 hours) and the lung remains reexpanded (as seen on x-ray films) with the chest tube in, the tube is removed and the site is closed with a stitch of 3-0 silk or with gauze. We prefer suture closure of the chest tube site to ensure the absence of continued drainage onto the skin or a sucking chest wound. Twenty-four hours after chest tube removal, the patient should have a chest radiograph that reveals no further accumulation of fluid and total lung expansion, at which point the patient can be considered for discharge. A follow-up radiographic examination should be performed 1 month later.

Specific Sclerosing Agents

TETRACYCLINE. Intrapleural tetracycline (TCN) has gained popularity because of its overall efficiency, convenience, low cost, and minimal morbidity. Prospective trials comparing TCN with quinacrine,[59] with a comparable pH placebo,[60] or with tube thoracostomy alone[61] show consistently better results with intrapleural TCN, with significantly less fever and pleuritic chest pain. Premedication of the patient with a narcotic, and the addition of lidocaine (150 mg) to the sclerosis medium,[62] may abate the pleurisy. Experimental models reveal that TCN increases pleural capillary permeability, allowing an accumulation of clotting factors in the pleural space and inactivation of the common fibrinolytic mechanism of pleural fluid. The fibrin matrix allows fibroblast attachment.[63] The effusion recurrence rate after TCN sclerosis is related to progression of the underlying malignancy, and the optimum dose of tetracycline for instillation is not clear.[64] In a 10-year retrospective review with only 59% of the patients classified as a treatment success, the authors commented that the dose of tetracycline was an important factor in predicting outcome, with a significantly higher complete response rate noted. No recurrence of effusion at 30 days was noted for the patients who were treated with more than 1 g of tetracycline.[65] Patients may be successfully retreated with TCN sclerosis.

The era of tetracycline sclerosis, however, may be completed, because the availability of intravenous tetracycline will be severely limited in the future. In the absence of randomized trials, it is difficult to recommend a viable alternative; nevertheless, the chief contenders for comparable sclerotherapy efficacy are sterilized (baked) talc, bleomycin, and doxycycline.

TALC. The administration of intrapleural talc, either at the time of thoracoscopy under general anesthesia or by aerosolization through a chest tube, has been a popular means of controlling malignant pleural effusions in Great Britain and Europe, despite the absence of randomized trials.[53,66–70] In selected studies, talc sclerotherapy has proved more effective than tetracycline in patients with pleural effusion from breast cancer.[71] An insufflation catheter is introduced through the thoracoscope. The talc should be free of asbestos and incubated in a dry-heat oven at 125°C for 12 hours and then cultured; it should show no bacterial or fungal contamination over a 7-day period before it is released for operative use. No more than 10.5 g of the talc is routinely used in adult patients. When performed under general anesthesia at the time of thoracotomy or thoracoscopy, talc administration is 85% to 100% effective if there is complete expansion of the underlying lung.[72]

ANTINEOPLASTIC AGENTS. Cytotoxic drugs most likely are effective by inducing inflammatory pleurodesis in the pleural space. Nitrogen mustard, thiotepa, bleomycin, doxorubicin, and 5-fluorouracil have been used for intrapleural management of malignant effusions, with the major side effects being bone marrow depression and leukopenia. Bleomycin seems to be the most successful. It has the fewest side effects at an instillation dose of 60 mg[73] and has minimal myelosuppressive problems and minimal fever and pain. An older randomized study comparing bleomycin with TCN revealed equal response rates.[74] Fortunately, with the limited availability of TCN in the future, a recent trial compared 85 patients with documented malignant pleural effusion who were randomized to treatment with either intrapleural bleomycin (60 U; 44 patients) or intrapleural tetracycline (1 g; 41 patients) after the pleural cavity was drained of accumulated fluid.[75] Sixty-seven percent of the tetracycline patients had recurrent effusion within 30 days, compared with 36% who received bleomycin. Unfortunately, not all patients were restudied in the first 30 days. At 90 days, 19/36 tetracycline patients had recurrent effusion compared with 11/37 bleomycin patients ($p = 0.047$). These data imply, at least, that bleomycin will be a viable alternative to tetracycline for sclerotherapy on a consistent basis in the future, despite the cost considerations that at one time made this agent a less desirable therapy than TCN.

A more aggressive approach with combination intrapleural agents, including cisplatin and cytarabine, has been used by some groups (overall response rate at 3 weeks = 49%).[76]

BIOLOGIC AGENTS. Intrapleural instillation of *C. parvum*, 5 to 10 mg, streptococcal preparation OK432, and BCG cell wall skeleton have demonstrated promising results in the management of malignant effusion. Recently, however, a randomized trial of *C. parvum* versus bleomycin revealed a higher but not statistically significant percentage of responses in the bleomycin group (74% versus 43%).[77] The *C. parvum* effect is not associated with evidence of enhancement of local cell-mediated immunity.[78]

The most recent developments in the use of biologic therapies for pleural effusions involve the use of the interferons or interleukins for intracavitary treatment. Five to 20 million units of interferon-β for a maximum administration of three doses was delivered by way of an intracavitary route in 32 patients with recurrent pleural effusions. Eleven (28%) showed complete remission and three (10%) showed partial remission.[79] Small effusion size (<1000 ml) correlated with treatment efficacy. Intrapleural infusion of interferon-γ twice a week over 2 months in stage I patients with diffuse pleural mesotheliomas yielded four thoracoscopic histopathologic responses and one partial response (56%).[80] Patients with higher-stage disease had minimal responses.

Recent reports from China demonstrate disappearance of effusion in 9 of 15 patients with malignant pleurisy, with significant decreases in the other 6 patients with the use of lymphokine-activated killer cells combined with recombinant interleukin-2 (rIL-2) or rIL-2 alone.[81] No serious side effects were found except for transient fever in 7 patients. In a series of 11 patients with malignant pleurisy due to lung cancer, pleural effusions and cancer cells disappeared after intrapleural instillations of recombinant IL-2.[82] Such studies require verification in larger numbers of patients.

External Radiation

Only lymphomatous pleural effusions seem to respond favorably to external-beam irradiation. Close to 90%[1,83] of malignant lymphoma effusions were controlled in a small series of patients with the use of mediastinal and hemithorax irradiation (1.4–2.3 Gy). Systemic chemotherapy is also used.[84]

Surgical Interventions

PLEURECTOMY. Stripping of the parietal pleura from the rib cage and mediastinum, essentially removing 90% of the pleura, is infrequently used because of the modern-day success of sclerotherapy. Its limited reported applications[85–87] include highly selected patients who have failed all other approaches, usually because of the presence of trapped or nonexpansile lung. A 23% complication rate and a 9% mortality are reported. Control of effusion is reported to be 87% to 100%.

PLEUROPERITONEAL SHUNTING. Internal drainage of malignant pleural effusions to the abdomen was first described in 1984. The valved, pumping chamber of a Denver shunt (Denver Biomaterials, Evergreen, CO) was placed subcutaneously with a proximal limb in the pleural effusion and a distal limb in the abdomen (Fig. 61–53). The pleuroperitoneal shunt can be used in instances for which sclerotherapy has failed, particularly when the failure is due to inability of the lung to expand. The procedure can be performed under local anesthesia, and complications are minimal. Patients must be sufficiently strong to pump the device, or the family must be taught to do this.

PERICARDIAL EFFUSIONS

INCIDENCE

Malignant involvement of the heart or pericardium is not uncommon in patients with advanced cancer, and its prevalence has been described in a number of autopsy studies. The prevalence of combined metastasis to the pericardium and heart has ranged from 0.1% to 21%.[88–91] In a series of 3327 autopsies, tumor lesions of the heart were detected in 5.1% of the cases.[92] When such data are available from autopsy series,[89,92–94] the pericardium is solely involved in 45% of the cases, the myocardium alone in 32%, and the myocardium and pericardium in 22%.

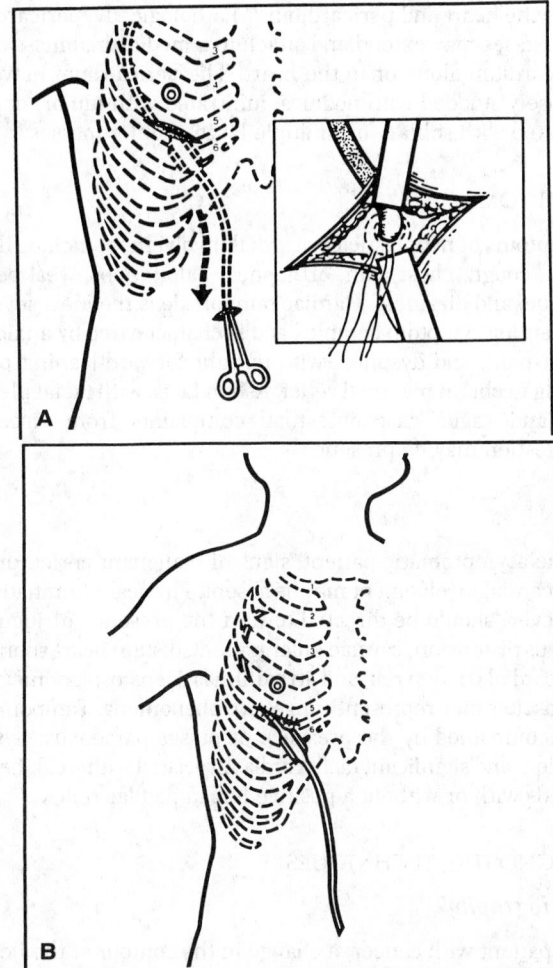

FIGURE 61–53. **(A)** Placement of pleuroperitoneal shunt for drainage of intractable pleural effusions from chest to abdominal cavity. (**Insert**) A small pursestring suture seals the entry site into the peritoneum. **(B)** View of the completed procedure. (Reprinted with permission of Denver Biomaterials, Evergreen, CO)

The most common malignancies involving the heart or pericardium include lung, breast, leukemia, Hodgkin's and non-Hodgkin's lymphoma, melanoma, gastrointestinal primaries, and sarcomas. Lung and breast predominate all autopsy series as the most likely neoplasms to cause myopericardial metastases, and it is estimated that 35% of patients with lung cancer will be found to have pericardial metastases at autopsy,[95] whereas as many as 25% of patients with breast cancer will have pericardial involvement at autopsy.[96–98]

PATHOPHYSIOLOGY

In the pericardial sac there is usually no more than 50 ml of pericardial fluid, which serves as a lubricant. The increase in pericardial fluid seen in malignant pericardial effusions is due to obstruction of lymphatic and venous drainage of the heart, and this disturbs the level of intrapericardial pressure, depending on the rate of fluid accumulation, pericardial compliance, ventricular mass, and intravascular volume. Mediastinal nodal involvement, frequently seen with lung and breast cancer, disturbs lymphatic drainage through the cardiac nodes from the heart and pericardium.[99] Pathologically, pericardial metastases may extend and attach to a mediastinal mass and pericardium alone or to the heart. The pericardium may be diffusely studded with nodules, infiltrated with tumor, or associated with solitary or multiple large nodular masses.[92]

SYMPTOMS

Symptoms of neoplastic pericardial involvement include dyspnea, cough, chest pain, orthopnea, palpitations, weakness, fatigue, and dizziness. Cardiac tamponade is the most severe presenting symptom complex and is characterized by anxiety, chest pain, and dyspnea, with upright forward-leaning posturing to obtain maximal relief. Ashen faces with facial plethora and vague gastrointestinal complaints from visceral congestion may be present.[94]

SIGNS

In the asymptomatic patient, signs of malignant pericardial/myocardial involvement may be absent. Physical examination, however, should be directed toward the presence of jugular venous distension, cardiac enlargement, distant heart sounds, pericardial friction rub, and arrhythmias. Hepatosplenomegaly and ascites may represent congestive phenomena. Tamponade is accompanied by the presence of pulsus paradoxus, hypotension, and significant tachycardia associated with weak heart sounds with or without a positive hepatojugular reflex.

DIAGNOSTIC TECHNIQUES

Radiography

In a patient with cancer, a change in the contour of the heart shadow on an upright AP x-ray film of the chest, in association with the aforementioned symptoms, should alert the clinician to the possibility of neoplastic pericarditis. A normal chest roentgenogram, however, does not exclude the possibility of effusion.[100] Classically, there is an enlargement of the cardiopericardial silhouette, described as a water-bottle heart, with bulging and loss of the normal contours of the pericardial reflection. The regular use of CT in diagnosing and staging lymphoma demonstrates pericardial involvement earlier and with greater accuracy than conventional radiography.[101] Effusions that are difficult to detect, such as those distorted by pneumonectomy for lung cancer, are more readily detected by CT.[102] Malignant pericardial disease is suspected by CT criteria, including: (1) pericardial effusion with high CT density, (2) localized or diffuse pericardial thickening, (3) masses from or contiguous with the pericardium, and (4) obliteration of normal tissue planes between a paracardiac mass and the heart or pericardium.[103,104]

Echocardiography (ECHO) represents the least invasive, least time-consuming, and most precise method for rapid demonstration and quantitation of malignant pleural effusion. Precise bedside confirmation of placement of pericardial catheters can also be accomplished with ECHO.

ELECTROCARDIOGRAPHIC ABNORMALITIES

The electrocardiogram (ECG) changes seen with neoplastic pericarditis include tachycardia, premature contractions, low QRS voltage, and nonspecific ST-segment and T-wave changes.[1] The alternans pattern will disappear with appropriate therapy for the effusion.[94]

Pericardiocentesis

TECHNIQUE AND USE IN DIAGNOSIS. The use of percutaneous pericardiocentesis guided by two-dimensional echocardiography is associated with a high diagnostic yield, a low frequency of complications, and rapid amelioration of symptoms of tamponade in patients with malignant pericardial effusions.[105] The risk of pericardiocentesis is dependent on the amount and location of the fluid. Patients with loculated effusion in a posterior position usually cannot be drained by the routine approaches. The use of fluoroscopy or ECHO guidance decreases, to a minimum, the previously reported risk of cardiac chamber puncture, ventricular tachycardia, and tension pneumothorax.[106,107]

USE OF PERICARDIOCENTESIS FOR CYTOLOGIC DIAGNOSIS. Hemorrhagic fluid is usually associated with positive pericardial cytologic results, especially in lung cancer, and cytologic examination will demonstrate malignant cells in 80% to 90% of the patients with neoplastic pericarditis. There is, however, a significant percentage of false-negative cytologic results observed, and a negative report does not eliminate cancer from the differential diagnosis.[108,109] There is a definite frequency of late effusive constructive pericarditis that is seen in patients with lymphoma who have received mediastinal irradiation. A frequency of radiation-related pericardial effusion of 31% has been reported after upper-mantle radiation therapy for Hodgkin's disease.[110] These patients will usually present with negative cytologic evaluations yet will require management of the effusion and the possible constrictive symptoms.

TREATMENT

The ultimate outcome for patients with malignant pericardial disease will depend on the performance status of the patients, the presence of metastatic disease, the availability of adjuvant systemic therapy, and the local management of the pericardial effusion for the long-term abolition of tamponade-like symptoms. Despite the prevalence of this manifestation of malignant disease, there are no prospective randomized trials comparing methods of local therapy to evaluate long-term effectiveness or survival.

Catheter Drainage Alone

The use of pericardial drainage alone has met with equivocal success in a small number of patients, as reported in the literature. Of 6 patients having a single pericardiocentesis or 24 to 48 hours of pericardial drainage, 4 had effusion control for 1 month or longer.[111] Of 16 patients with malignant effusions in another study,[106] only 2 required subsequent pericardiectomy for recurrence. Nine of the 16, however, had other nonsurgical therapy. In a more recent study of patients with histologically confirmed neoplastic (breast) pericarditis, all 3 patients treated by pericardiocentesis alone relapsed, at 11, 40, and 1462 days, respectively, after the tap. One of these patients died, in relapse or tamponade, and the other two required surgery.

Instillational Local Therapy

Nitrogen mustard, thiotepa, and quinacrine were all used for intrapericardial instillation in the 1970s, but they were associated with severe pain and bone marrow toxicity. Treatment with TCN instillation usually requires multiple instillations for it to be effective. Of the 28 patients described, each treated with a mean TCN instillation of 500 mg/instillation, a success rate of longer than 1 month was seen in 75%, with a mean of 120 days without recurrence.[111,112] Complications included mild fever, arrhythmias, and pain. Bleomycin (4 patients),[113] cisplatin (1 patient),[114] and vinblastine (1 patient)[115] have also been used for local instillation. These studies further verify that the pericardial catheter can be successfully left in place longer than 72 hours without infection and that catheter occlusion is more prevalent with continuous drainage as opposed to intermittent flushing.[106]

Radiation Therapy

Although formerly used for pericardial effusions related to various histologic types of carcinoma, pericardial radiation is most suited for the management of pericardial effusions from lymphoma.[116] Recommended dosages are 2.0 to 3.0 Gy, fractionated over a 2- to 3-week period.

Surgery

Most of the patients will be able to have emergent placement of a pericardial catheter to relieve tamponade symptoms and be more favorable surgical-anesthetic candidates. It is generally agreed that surgical intervention should be considered in those medically fit patients whose effusive pericarditis is unresponsive to radiation therapy or to intrapericardial therapy, or who have required repeated pericardiocentesis. Finally, patients with constrictive pericarditis caused by radiation or neoplastic pericardial constriction, documented hemodynamically by catheterization, and who would be expected to have a reasonable long-term survival, should have pericardial resection.

The subxiphoid approach has received many enthusiastic commendations in the literature, from a number of institutions, as being the procedure of choice in the management of malignant effusions. The use of local anesthesia; direct exposure of the pericardium; complete drainage of the pericardial space by chest tubes, allowing pericardial and epicardial symphysis; and the avoidance of a thoracotomy have all been expounded as the advantages of this technique. When one examines the reports in the literature and defines the subset of patients with malignant effusions who had subxiphoid drainage (Table 61–33), it is difficult to label this procedure as the "cure all to end all" for neoplastic pericarditis. Ideally, the minimum mortality in cancer patients is 8%, and the ideal described recurrence rate is 7%. This procedure is probably superior to simple window formation by a left thoracotomy, relative to mortality and recurrence. Moreover, the type of pericardiectomy does not seem to have any influence on the postoperative survival in patients with malignant disease. Survival in patients with malignant disease is affected by the tumor cell type, with lung cancer having a mean survival of 3.5 months; breast cancer, after surgical intervention, having a survival of 9.3 to 18.5 months; and lymphoma having a

TABLE 61–33. Subxiphoid Approach for Malignant Pericardial Effusion

Investigations	No. of Patients	Mortality	Recurrence
Ghosh, 1985[117]	20	0	1
Hankins, 1980[118]	13	0	0
Raza, 1980[118]	49	0	3
Williams, 1980[118]	26	0	3
Osuch, 1985[119]	12	1	0
Berman, 1984[120]	3	0	0
Little, 1984[121]	19	6	0
Piehler, 1985[122]	10	1	3
Miller, 1985[122]	3	2	—
Prager, 1982[123]	6	3	—
Total	161	13 (8%)	10 (7%)

survival of approximately 10 months. The amount of pericardium remaining after surgical drainage, however, does impinge directly on the development of late postoperative complications (*e.g.*, recurrence of effusion). Patients who have a complete pericardiectomy have significantly fewer late failures than those who have a window pericardiectomy. Therefore, in patients who have other salvage therapies, either radiation or chemotherapy, or those expected to have a longer survival (*e.g.*, lymphoma or breast cancer), the widest pericardial resection should be considered to prevent future recurrence. Moreover, radiation-induced effusions should not be managed by a subxiphoid window because of a high late-failure rate.

REFERENCES

1. McKenna RJ, Ali MK, Ewer MS, et al. Pleural and pericardial effusions in cancer patients. Curr Probl Cancer 1985;9:1.
2. Hausheer FH, Yarbro JW. Diagnosis and treatment of malignant pleural effusion. Semin Oncol 1985;12:54.
3. Sahn SA. Malignant pleural effusions. Clin Chest Med 1985;6:113.
4. Martensson G, Pettersson K, Thiringer G. Differentiation between malignant and non-malignant pleural effusion. Eur J Respir Dis 1985;67:326.
5. Dhillon DP, Spiro SG. Malignant pleural effusions. Br J Hosp Med 1983;29:506.
6. Chernow B, Sahn SA. Carcinomatous involvement of the pleura: An analysis of 96 patients. Am J Med 1977;63:695.
7. Zehner LC, Hoogstraten B. Malignant effusions and their management. Semin Oncol Nurs 1985;1:259.
8. Austin EH, Flye MW. The treatment of recurrent malignant pleural effusion. Ann Thorac Surg 1979;28:190.
9. Kaunitz J. Landmarks in simple pleural effusions. JAMA 1939;113:1312.
10. Peterson JA. Recognition of infrapulmonary pleural effusion. Radiology 1960;74:34.
11. Woodring JH. Recognition of pleural effusion on supine radiographs: How much fluid is required? AJR 1984;142:59.
12. Salonen O, Kivisaari L, Nordenstam G, et al. Computed tomography of pleural lesions with special reference to the mediastinal pleura. Acta Radiol Diagn 1986;27:527.
13. Doust BD, Baum JK, Maklad NF, et al. Ultrasonic evaluation of pleural opacities. Radiology 1975;114:135.
14. Ravin CE. Thoracentesis of loculated pleural effusions using grey scale ultrasonic guidance. Chest 1977;71:666.
15. Sears D, Hajdu SI. The cytologic diagnosis of malignant neoplasm in pleural and peritoneal effusions. Acta Cytol 1987;31:85.
16. Lopes-Cardozo PL. A critical evaluation of 3000 cytologic analyses of pleural fluid, ascitic fluid, and peritoneal fluid. Acta Cytol 1966;10:455.
17. Johnston WW. The malignant pleural effusion: A review of cytopathologic diagnosis of 584 specimens from 472 consecutive patients. Cancer 1985;56:905.
18. Jarvi OH, Kunnas RJ, Laitio MT, et al. The accuracy and significance of cytologic cancer diagnoses in pleural effusions. Acta Cytol 1972;16:152.
19. Johnson WD. The cytologic diagnosis of cancer in serous effusions. Acta Cytol 1966;10:161.
20. Melamed MR. The cytologic preparation of malignant lymphomas and related disease in effusions. Cancer 1963;16:413.

21. Ceelen GH. The cytologic diagnosis of ascitic fluid. Acta Cytol 1964;8:175.
22. Spriggs AL. Br Med J [Letter] 1981;282:1972.
23. Schested M, Ralfkiaer E, Rasmussen J. Immunoperoxidase demonstration of carcinoembryonic antigen in pleural and peritoneal effusions. Acta Cytol 1983;27:124.
24. To A, Coleman V, Dearnaley DP, et al. Use of antisera to epithelial membrane antigen for the cytodiagnosis of malignancy in serous effusions. J Clin Pathol 1981;24:1326.
25. To A, Dearnaley DP, Ormerod G, et al. Epithelial membrane antigen: Its use in the cytodiagnosis of malignancy in serous effusions. Am J Clin Pathol 1982;77:214.
26. Walts AE, Said JW, Banks-Schlegel S. Keratin and carcinoembryonic antigen in exfoliated mesothelial and malignant cells: An immunoperoxidase study. Am J Clin Pathol 1983;80:671.
27. Johnston WW, Szpak CA, Lottich SC, et al. Use of a monoclonal antibody (B72.3) as an immunocytochemical adjunct to diagnosis of adenocarcinoma in human effusions. Cancer Res 1985;45:1894.
28. Martin SE, Moshiri S, Thor A, et al. Identification of adenocarcinoma in cytospin preparations of effusions using monoclonal antibody B72.3. Am J Clin Pathol 1986;86:10.
29. Das DK, Gupta SK, Ayzagari S, et al. Pleural effusions in non-Hodgkin's lymphoma: A cytomorphologic, cytochemical, and immunologic study. Acta Cytol 1987;31:119.
30. Musilova J, Michalova K. Cytogenetic study of cancer cells in effusions. Cancer Genet Cytogenet 1986;19:271.
31. Carlevaro C, Rossi GA, Cerri E, et al. Cytogenetic study of pleural effusions. Tumori 1978;64:335.
32. Fraisse J, Brizard CO, Emonot A, et al. Diagnosis of malignancy by cytogenetic means in effusions. Clin Genet 1978;14:288.
33. McKenna JM, Chandraesekhar AJ, Henkin RE. Diagnostic value of carcinoembryonic antigen in exudative pleural effusion. Chest 1980;78:587.
34. Rutgers RA, Loewenstein MS, Feinerman AE, et al. Carcinoembryonic antigen levels in benign and malignant pleural effusions. Ann Intern Med 1978;88:631.
35. Vladutin AO, Brason FW, Adler RH. Differential diagnosis of pleural effusions: Clinical usefulness of cell marker quantitation. Chest 1981;79:297.
36. Rasmussen KN, Faher V. Hyaluronic acid in 247 pleural fluids. Scand J Respir Dis 1967;48:366.
37. Ratliff JL, Chavez CM, Hamchuk A, et al. Reexpansion pulmonary edema. Chest 1973;64:654.
38. Trapnell DH, Thurston JGB. Unilateral pulmonary edema after pleural aspiration. Lancet 1970;1:1367.
39. Yamazaki S, Ogawa J, Shohyu A, et al. Pulmonary blood flow to rapidly re-expanded lung on spontaneous pneumothorax. Chest 1982;81:118.
40. Prakash UBS. Malignant pleural effusions. Postgrad Med 1986;80:201.
41. Prakash UBS, Reiman HM. Comparison of needle biopsy with cytologic analysis for the evaluation of pleural effusion: Analysis of 414 cases. Mayo Clin Proc 1985;60:158.
42. Hanson G, Philips T. Pleural biopsy in diagnosis of thoracic disease. Br Med J 1962;2:300.
43. Sisson BS, Weiss W. Needle biopsy of the parietal pleura in patients with pleural effusion. Br Med J 1962;2:298.
44. Scerbo J, Keltz H, Stone DJ. A prospective study of closed pleural biopsies. JAMA 1971;218:377.
45. Liss HP. Cope needle biopsy. South Med J 1984;77:837.
46. Bevelaque FA, Aranda C, Leon W. The role of closed pleural biopsy in suspected malignant effusions. N Y State J Med 1984;84:229.
47. Salyer WR, Eggleston JC, Eroyan YS. Efficacy of pleural needle biopsy and pleural fluid cytopathology in the diagnosis of malignant neoplasm involving the pleura. Chest 1975;67:536.
48. Winkelman M, Pfitzer P. Blind pleural biopsy in combination with cytology of pleural effusions. Acta Cytol 1981;25:373.
49. Schools GS. Needle biopsy of parietal pleura: Current status. Tex State J Med 1963;59:1056.
50. Jones FL. Subcutaneous implantation of cancer: A rare complication of pleural biopsy. Chest 1970;57:189.
51. Boutin C, Cargrino P, Viallat JR. Thoracoscopy in the early diagnosis of malignant pleural effusions. Endoscopy 1980;12:155.
52. Weissburg D, Kaufman M, Zurkowski Z. Pleuroscopy in patients with pleural effusions and pleural masses. Ann Thorac Surg 1980;29:205.
53. Weissburg D, Kaufman M. Diagnostic and therapeutic pleuroscopy: Experience with 127 patients. Chest 1980;78:732.
54. Oakes DD, Sherck JP, Brodsky JB, et al. Therapeutic thoracoscopy. J Thorac Cardiovasc Surg 1984;87:269.
55. Weissburg D. Diagnostic and therapeutic pleuroscopy. Chest 1980;5:732–735.
56. Chernow B, Sahn SA. Carcinomatous involvement of the pleura. Am J Med 1977;37:291.
57. Roy RH, Can DT, Payne WS. The problem of chylothorax. Mayo Clin Proc 1967;42:457.
58. Leff A, Honeywell PC, Costello J. Pleural effusion from malignancy. Ann Intern Med 1978;88:532.
59. Bayly TC, Kisner DL, Sybert A, et al. Tetracycline and quinacrine in the control of malignant pleural effusions: A randomized trial. Cancer 1978;41:1188.
60. Zaloanek AJ, Oswald SG, Langin M. Intrapleural tetracycline in malignant pleural effusions: A randomized study. Cancer 1983;51:752.
61. O'Neill W, Spurr C, Muss H, et al. A prospective study of chest tube drainage and tetracycline sclerosis versus chest tube drainage in the treatment of malignant pleural effusion. Proc Am Soc Clin Oncol 1979;21:349.
62. Wallach H. Chest [Letter] 1978;73:246.
63. Sahn SA, Good JT. The effect of common sclerosing agents on the rabbit pleural space. Am Rev Respir Dis 1981;124:65.
64. Dunkel TB. Intrapleural tetracycline in the treatment of malignant pleural effusions. Minn Med 1986;69:717.
65. Gravelyn TR, Michelson MK, Gross BH, Sitrin RG. Tetracycline pleurodesis for malignant pleural effusions. Cancer 1987;59:1973–1977.
66. Sorensen PG, Svendsen TL, Enk B. Treatment of malignant pleural effusion with drainage, with and without instillation of talc. Eur J Respir Dis 1984;65:131.
67. Adler RH, Sayek I. Treatment of malignant pleural effusion: A method using tube thoracostomy and talc. Ann Thorac Surg 1976;22:8.
68. Starkey GW. Recurrent malignant pleural effusions. N Engl J Med 1964;270:436.
69. Jones GR. Treatment of malignant pleural effusion by iodized talc pleurodesis. Thorax 1969;24:69.
70. Shedbalker AR, Head JM, Head LR, et al. Evaluation of talc pleural symphysis in management of malignant pleural effusion. J Thorac Cardiovasc Surg 1971;61:492.
71. Fentiman IS, Rubens RD, Hayward JI. A comparison of intracavitary talcum and tetracycline for the control of pleural effusion secondary to breast cancer. Eur J Cancer Clin Oncol 1986;22:1079.
72. Daniel TM, Tribble CG, Rodgers BM. Thoracoscopy and talc poudrage for pneumothoraces and effusions. Ann Thorac Surg 1990;50:186–189.
73. Ostrowski M. An assessment of the long term results of controlling the reaccumulation of malignant effusions using intracavitary bleomycin. Cancer 1986;57:721.
74. Gupta N, Opfell RW, Padova C, et al. Intrapleural bleomycin vs tetracycline for control of malignant pleural effusions. A randomized study. Am Soc Clin Oncol [Abstract] 1980;C-189:366.
75. Moores DWO. Malignant pleural effusion. Semin Oncol 1991;18:59–61.
76. Rusch VW, Figlin R, Godwin D, Piantadosi S. Intrapleural cisplatin and cytarabine in the management of malignant pleural effusions: A Lung Cancer Study Group trial. J Clin Oncol 1991;9:313–319.
77. Ostrowski MJ, Priestman TJ, Houston RF, Martin WMC. A randomized trial of intracavitary bleomycin and *Corynebacterium parvum* in the control of malignant pleural effusions. Radiother Oncol 1989;14:19–26.
78. Rossi GA, Felletti R, Balbi R, et al. Symptomatic treatment of recurrent malignant pleural effusions with intrapleurally administered *Corynebacterium parvum*. Am Rev Respir Dis 1987;135:885.
79. Rosso R, Rimoldi R, Salvati F, et al. Intrapleural natural beta interferon in the treatment of malignant pleural effusions. Oncology 1988;45:253–256.
80. Boutin C, Viallat JR, Van Zandwijk N, et al. Activity of intrapleural recombinant gamma-interferon in malignant mesothelioma. Cancer 1991;67:2033–2037.
81. Dianjun L, Yaorong W, Ziaodong Y, Jie S, Yunfu C, Denian B. Treatment of patients with malignant pleural effusions due to advanced lung cancer by transfer to autologous LAK cells combined with rIL-2 or rIL-2 alone. Proc Chin Acad Med Sci Peking Union Med Coll 1990;5:51–55.
82. Yasumoto K, Miyazaki K, Nagashima A, et al. Induction of lymphokine-activated killer cells by intrapleural instillations of recombinant interleukin-2 in patients with malignant pleurisy due to lung cancer. Cancer Res 1987;47:2184–2187.
83. Weick JK, Killy JM, Harison EG, et al. Pleural effusion in lymphoma. Cancer 1973;31:848.
84. Xaubet A, Duimenjo MC, Maren A, et al. Characteristics and prognostic value of pleural effusion in non-Hodgkin's lymphoma. Eur J Respir Dis 1985;66:135.
85. Martini N, Bains M, Beattie EJ. Indications for pleurectomy in malignant effusion. Cancer 1975;35:734.
86. Jensik R, Cagle JE, Melloy F, et al. Pleurectomy in the treatment of pleural effusion due to metastatic malignancy. J Thorac Cardiovasc Surg 1963;46:322.
87. Anderson CB, Philpott GW, Ferguson TB. The treatment of malignant pleural effusions. Cancer 1974;33:916.
88. Yates WM. Tumors of the heart and pericardium. Arch Intern Med 1931;48:627.
89. Scott RW, Garvin CF. Tumors of the heart and pericardium. Am Heart J 1939;17:431.
90. Bisel HF, Wroblewski F, LaDue JS. Incidence and clinical manifestations of cardiac metastases. JAMA 1953;153:712.
91. Thurber DL, Edwards JE, Achor RWP. Secondary malignant tumors of the pericardium. Circulation 1962;26:228.
92. Skhvatsabaju LV. Secondary malignant lesions of the heart and pericardium in neoplastic disease. Oncology 1986;43:103.
93. Goudie RB. Secondary tumors of the heart and pericardium. Br Heart J 1955;17:183.
94. Theologides A. Neoplastic cardiac tamponade. Semin Oncol 1978;5:181.
95. Shenkai T, Tomenagu K, Saijo N, et al. The incidence of cardiac metastases in primary lung cancer and the management of malignant pericardial effusion. Jpn J Clin Oncol 1982;12:23.
96. Buck M, Ingle JN, Guilani ER, et al. Pericardial effusion in women with breast cancer. Cancer 1987;60:263.
97. Hagemeister FB, Buydan AU, Luna MA, et al. Causes of death in breast cancer. Cancer 1980;46:162.
98. Nakayama R, Yoneyama T, Takatani O, et al. A study of metastatic tumors to the heart, pericardium and great vessels. Jpn Heart J 1966;7:227.
99. Oruigbo WIB. The spread of lung cancer to the heart, pericardium, and great vessels. Jpn Heart J 1974;15:234.
100. Pories WJ, Gaudiani VA. Cardiac tamponade. Surg Clin North Am 1975;55:573.
101. Jochelson MS, Balikian JP, Mauch P, et al. Peri- and paracardial involvement in lymphoma: A radiographic study of 11 cases. AJR 1983;140:483.
102. Dighton DH, Golding R, de Feytes PJ. Post-pneumonectomy pericardial effusion. Chest 1982;82:389.

103. Golding RD, Zanten TEG. Computed tomography in malignant conditions affecting the pericardium. J Belge Radiol 1984;67:371.

104. Johnson FE, Wolverson MIL, Sundaram M, et al. Unsuspected malignant pericardial effusion causing cardiac tamponade. Chest 1982;82:501.

105. Callahan JA, Seward JB, Nishimura RA, et al. Two-dimensional echocardiographically guided pericardiocentesis: Experience in 117 consecutive patients. Am J Cardiol 1985;55:476.

106. Kopecky SL, Callahan JA, Tajek AJ, et al. Percutaneous pericardial catheter drainage: Report of 42 consecutive cases. Am J Cardiol 1986;58:633.

107. Wong B, Murphy J, Chang CJ, et al. The risk of pericardiocentesis. Am J Cardiol 1979;44:1110.

108. Zepf RE, Johnston WW. The role of cytology in the evaluation of pericardial effusions. Chest 1972;62:593.

109. Reyes CV, Strinden C, Banerji M. The role of cytology in neoplastic tamponade. Acta Cytol 1982;26:299.

110. Applefeld MM, Cole JF, Pollock SH, et al. The late appearance of chronic pericardial disease in patients treated by radiotherapy for Hodgkin's disease. Ann Intern Med 1981;94:338.

111. Pavis S, Sharma SM, Blumberg ED, et al. Intrapericardial tetracycline for the management of cardiac tamponade secondary to malignant pericardial effusion. N Engl J Med 1978;299:1113.

112. Shephard FA, Ginsberg JS, Evans WR, et al. Tetracycline sclerosis in the management of malignant pericardial effusion. J Clin Oncol 1985;3:1678.

113. Maher FR, Buckman R. Intrapericardial instillation of bleomycin in malignant pericardial effusion. Am Heart J 1986;111:613.

114. Markman M, Howell SB. Intrapericardial instillation of cisplatin in a patient with a large malignant effusion. Cancer Drug Deliv 1985;2:49.

115. Primrose WR, Clee MD, Johnston RN. Malignant pericardial effusion managed with vinblastine. Clin Oncol 1983;9:67.

116. Terry LN, Klegerman MM. Pericardial and myocardial involvement by lymphomas and leukemias: The role of radiotherapy. Cancer 1970;25:1003.

117. Ghosh SC, Larrieu A, Ablaza S, et al. Clinical experience with subxyphoid pericardial decompression. Int Surg 1985;70:5.

118. Hankins JR, Sattersfield JR, Aisner J, et al. Pericardial window for malignant pericardial effusion. Ann Thorac Surg 1980;30:465.

119. Osuch JR, Khandehar JN, Fry WA. Emergency subxyphoid pericardial decompression for malignant pericardial effusion. Am Surg 1985;51:298.

120. Berman K, Fielding MB, Richi AA. Diagnosis and treatment of malignant pericardial effusion: The subxyphoid approach. Conn Med 1984;48:701.

121. Little AG, Krimser PC, Wade JL, et al. Operation for diagnosis and treatment of pericardial effusions. Surgery 1984;96:738.

122. Piehler JM, Pluth JR, Schaff HV, et al. Surgical management of effusive pericardial disease. J Thorac Cardiovasc Surg 1985;90:506.

123. Prager PL, Wilson CH, Bender AW. The subxyphoid approach to pericardial disease. Ann Thorac Surg 1982;34:6.

SECTION **6**

ALAN R. BAKER
JEFFREY S. WEBER

Treatment of Malignant Ascites

MALIGNANT ASCITES

The development of a malignant peritoneal effusion or disseminated peritoneal carcinomatosis is a prognostically adverse event in the natural history of a number of tumors, particularly ovarian, colorectal, gastric, and uterine cancer. Anorexia, early satiety, difficulty with ambulation, and respiratory compromise are associated with significant intraperitoneal disease or ascites. Although the median survival is about several months (Table 61–34), mechanical intervention to drain ascitic fluid can provide good palliation, and newer therapeutic approaches with the use of intracavitary chemotherapy and aggressive surgery have resulted in prolonged survival for selected patients in small phase I and II studies. Numerous therapies have historically been tested in patients with malignant ascites and intraperitoneal disease,[1] such as systemic and intraperitoneal chemotherapy, external-beam and intracavitary radiocolloid instillation, intraperitoneal instillation of biologic response modifiers with and without lymphokine-activated killer (LAK) cells, and internal ascitic fluid shunting. However, internal peritoneovenous shunting is still the standard of care for patients with malignant ascites, and promising initial results with local instillation of chemotherapy or immunotherapeutic reagents need to be tested in expanded phase II and III studies.

The pathogenesis of malignant ascites is multifactorial. Tumor cells can be shown to invade the subdiaphragmatic lymphatic channels and plexuses as shown by Feldman[2,3] and others,[4,5] and this can compromise drainage of the peritoneal cavity. Although excess fluid generation is probably a more important factor in the genesis of cirrhotic ascites, Hirabayashi[6] has demonstrated that it occurs in the setting of ovarian cancer, and Garrison and colleagues[7] have suggested that tu-

mors can elaborate humoral factors that cause increased capillary leakage, even across normal peritoneal surfaces and omentum. The hydrodynamic disequilibria caused by hypoalbuminemia, portal venous obstruction, or hepatic venous obstruction, noted when the liver is extensively replaced by metastatic tumor, probably promotes the formation of ascitic fluid as well.

DIAGNOSIS AND WORKUP

Ascites and increasing abdominal girth from bulky intraperitoneal tumor are often presenting signs of advanced ovarian cancer but more often are harbingers of relapse and metastatic disease in patients with ovarian, uterine, colorectal, or gastric carcinoma. Nonneoplastic causes for ascites, such as congestive heart failure, cirrhosis, or nephrosis with protein wasting, and, less frequently, complications of radiation therapy or chemotherapy can occur and should be ruled out.

Abdominal paracentesis should be performed in cancer patients with ascites to assess the chemistry profile of the fluid and its cell count, differential, cytology, Gram's stain, and culture. Removal of as much fluid as possible will temporarily reduce symptoms and give an opportunity to assess the time for reaccumulation. To prevent infrequently seen orthostatic changes from rapid intravascular fluid shifts, or electrolyte aberrations that follow removal of a large volume of ascitic fluid, an intravenous line should be in place, or the patient should be encouraged to take fluids liberally. Patients should also be cautioned about dizziness or lightheadedness, reflecting intravascular depletion after a paracentesis.

The character of the aspirated fluid can offer clues to its etiology. Malignant collections are often bloody or serosanguineous; serous fluid is consistent with a cirrhotic, nephrotic, pancreatic, or cardiac origin; turbid or cloudy fluid can be indicative of infectious peritonitis; and chylous fluid suggests lymphoma, gut lymphatic injury, or thoracic duct injury.

No single feature in the biochemical profile of ascitic fluid is diagnostic for a malignant etiology, although the presence of an elevated ascitic/serum protein ratio (>0.4), increased ascitic/serum lactic dehydrogenase (LDH) ratio (>1.0), in-

TABLE 61–34. Reported Experience With Peritoneovenous Shunt Management of Malignant Ascites

Investigations	Underlying Malignancy					Comments	Patient Survival	
	Ovary	GI	Breast	Unknown Adenocarcinoma	Other		Median (wk)	% Alive at 1 y
Straus, 1979[56]	13	10	3	2	9	27/37 (73%) Good shunt function and palliation	8	
Osterlee, 1980[57]	6	7	2	1	4	13/20 (65%) Good shunt function and palliation	7	5
Raaf, 1980[58]		2	1	1	1	5/5 (100%) Ascites controlled	5	0
Lokich, 1980[59]	3		3	1	1	6/8 (75%) Ascites controlled and meaningful palliation	8	12
Lund, 1982[61]	14	9	5		7	Excellent initial and long-term therapy for ascites	16	11
Qazi, 1982[62]	28	4	8			28/40 (70%) Effective palliation		
Cheung, 1982[63]	2	7	4		9		5	10
Reinhold, 1983[64]	6	3	6		4	6/19 (32%) Excellent symptomatic relief	6	
Souter, 1983[65]	9	4	4	4	5	23/26 (88%) Satisfactory palliation	16	12
Gough, 1984[66]	4	4	2		7	13/17 (76%) Ascites controlled, worthwhile palliation	13	6
Downing, 1984[60]		2	3	1	1	4/7 (57%) Good shunt function and palliation	13	0
Kostroff, 1985[67]	11	8	5		7		8	0
Campioni, 1986[68]	8	14	7	7	6	Safe and effective way to improve quality of life	7	7
Sonnenfeld, 1986[69]		16		5	6	19/27 (70%) Good palliation	8	0
Roussel, 1986[70]	12	10	11		3	Effective palliation for most patients	13	0
Soderlund, 1986[71]	7	15			2	No benefit for patients with GI malignancy	7	4
Shepherd, 1988[72]	2	8	1		3	Majority of patients got little benefit	6	7
Edney, 1989[73]	8	24	8		5	75% experience relief of symptoms	33	13+
Smith, 1989[74]	3	23	9	5	10	36/50 (72%) Adequate palliation	22	4+
Total	136	170	82	27	90		5–33	0–12

GI, gastrointestinal (colon, stomach, pancreas, hepatobiliary).

creased carcinoembryonic antigen (CEA) (>10), OC-125 or other tumor markers favor neoplasia.[7-10] Greater than 10,000 erythrocytes/μL, and more than 1000 leukocytes/μL, in the absence of bacteria or fungus on Gram stain and a sterile fluid culture characterize a malignant effusion. Papanicolaou stain of the ascitic cells from a spun pellet or cell block will show malignant cells on cytology 50% or more of the time, and this will confirm the diagnosis. The information in Table 61–35 summarizes important features in the workup of a patient with suspected malignant peritoneal effusion.

TREATMENT

To date, no well-controlled, randomized trials have been performed in cancer patients comparing the alternative methods of managing malignant ascites. In many studies, the reported median survival for patients with newly diagnosed malignant ascites is approximately 2 months (see Table 61–34), suggesting that for most patients it is an indicator of end-stage disease. Therefore, therapy for malignant ascites, and for patients diagnosed with diffuse intraperitoneal carcinomatosis, has focused on palliation of symptoms as opposed to attempts

at achieving a long-term regression of bulky tumor masses and large peritoneal effusions. While it is true that efforts in these patients should be directed at maximizing ambulatory out-of-hospital time and minimizing treatment-induced morbidity, newer, more experimental approaches to malignant ascites and intraperitoneal disease will also be discussed in this section. With these considerations in mind, we will describe the current therapeutic options, proceeding from the less invasive to the more invasive and more morbid alternatives.

DIET AND DIURESIS

Although a useful maneuver in the management of cirrhotic ascites, dietary salt restriction, aldosterone-inhibiting diuretics, and loop diuretics have little impact on malignant ascites. Sodium retention is less important as a pathologic factor than increased fluid elaborated from the tumor-involved peritoneal surface and lymphatic obstruction that inhibits fluid resorption. However, Greenway and colleagues[11] have reported decreased malignant peritoneal effusions in 13 of 15 patients treated with high doses of spironolactone (150–450 mg/day).

TABLE 61–35.   Assessment of the Patient
With a Peritoneal Effusion

Diagnosis/Workup
  History
    Increasing abdominal girth—"clothes don't fit"
    Indigestion and early satiety
    Ankle swelling
    Easy fatigability
    Shortness of breath
  Physical examination
    Fluid wave
    Shifting dullness
  Radiographic studies
    Abdominal flat plate: generalized ground-glass appearance; air-filled small bowel loops occupy central position and are separated by fluid between loops; psoas shadows obscured
  Ultrasound, abdominal CT: both are sensitive tests that definitively diagnose small amounts of ascites
  Paracentesis
    Gross character on inspection: bloody, serous, milky, turbid
    Cell count and differential
    Chemistries: Total protein, LDH, CEA, OC-125, amylase
    Cytology
    Microbiology: Gram's stain and culture

CT, computed tomography; LDH, lactic dehydrogenase; CEA, carcinoembryonic antigen.

The only treatment-related toxicity noted was nausea in 2 of 15 patients. Baseline elevated plasma renin levels were measured in 5 of 5 patients, with elevated aldosterone levels noted in 3 of the 5 tested.

REPEATED PARACENTESIS AND EXTERNAL DRAINS

Frequently reported abdominal taps, while a commonly used technique to palliate the discomfort, bloating, and shortness of breath caused by malignant ascites,[12,13] can lead to protein depletion, postural hypotension, and electrolyte abnormalities. In addition, the frequent insertion of a catheter into the sterile intraperitoneal space can lead to visceral injury and bleeding, as well as bacterial inoculation and subsequent peritonitis.

A newer approach to external drainage of ascites is a permanently implanted abdominal drain.[14] In one small series, 17 patients with intractable ascites had a Silastic catheter permanently implanted in the peritoneal space; relief of symptoms was obtained in the 15 patients who had patent catheter function, although bacterial growth was eventually seen in the peritoneal fluid of 8. In addition, there have been isolated case reports of the use of implanted Tenckoff catheters (Davol, Cranston, RI) to drain malignant ascites.[15]

INTRACAVITARY THERAPY

Intraperitoneal therapy to treat malignant ascites or diffuse peritoneal tumor was initially described over 40 years ago by Muller,[16] who used radioactive ^{63}Zn. ^{198}Au later became the instilled isotope of choice,[17] but colloidal suspensions of ^{32}CrPO$_4$ have been used mainly in the last decade or two. At least two series of patients have been studied,[18,19] suggesting that half of those treated with radiocolloid ^{32}P derive palliative benefit from this approach while suffering minimal treatment-related toxicity.

Chemotherapeutic agents were initially studied as long ago as 1955, when Weisberger reported the results of intraperitoneal nitrogen mustard treatment of 7 patients with ovarian cancer.[20] Diminution of ascites was seen in all patients, albeit with a significant amount of toxicity—mainly abdominal pain. Further interest in direct intracavitary instillation of chemotherapy drugs was generated at the National Cancer Institute (NCI) by Dedrick and colleagues,[21] who hypothesized that a 2 to 3 log higher local concentration of drug could be achieved by intraperitoneal rather than systemic administration, without causing unacceptable systemic toxicity from high serum levels. This theory was initially tested by Ozols and colleagues at the NCI[22]; they demonstrated that in patients with ovarian cancer who had ascites or diffuse intraperitoneal disease, or both, there was a significant pharmacokinetic advantage over the intravenous route for chemotherapy agents instilled intraperitoneally. There was a significant and large ratio of the "area under the curve" (AUC) or drug concentration versus time for the peritoneal cavity as opposed to plasma. Agents known to be metabolized during first passage through the liver, such as doxorubicin or 5-FU, or drugs that have limited systemic clearance, such as mitoxantrone, can have mean peritoneal to plasma AUC ratios of up to 1400, suggesting a significant advantage to the intraperitoneal route.[23,24] The development of the indwelling Port-A-Cath system (Pharmacia, St. Paul, MN) has led to minimal discomfort and increased compliance by patients receiving intraperitoneal therapy,[25] but there is still potential for bleeding, infection, or chemical peritonitis as a significant source of morbidity.[26]

A large number of phase I and II studies have demonstrated that single agents, particularly cisplatin,[27] as well as others[28,29] and combinations of up to three[30,31] drugs, can be given safely to patients with advanced ovarian and colorectal cancer who have diffuse intraperitoneal disease. With cisplatin, the single most active agent in ovarian cancer, several groups have performed phase II studies and have demonstrated a 30% pathologically confirmed complete response rate in patients with small-volume residual disease (<2 cm) who had failed first-line platinum-containing systemic regimens.[32] It is likely, however, that patients with bulky disease (defined as >2 cm), after a second- or third-look laparotomy, will not respond to intraperitoneal therapy. In one study by Howell and colleagues, a group of 25 patients with microscopic residual (<0.5 cm) disease after first-line chemotherapy were treated with intraperitoneal instillation of cisplatin and achieved a median survival of greater than 49 months, with 74% having a 4-year survival.[33] In the most recent platinum combination intraperitoneal trials, patients who fail first-line chemotherapy but have microscopic residual disease (<0.5 cm) at laparotomy can achieve 45% to 50% pathologic complete response rates. However, these encouraging results should be interpreted with caution, because randomized phase III studies to compare survival in patients treated with systemic or intraperitoneal second-line therapies have not matured. In addition, other phase III studies are currently in progress comparing intraperitoneal chemotherapy in previously untreated patients with advanced ovarian cancer with standard systemic therapy.[34] Other studies to evaluate the use of intraperitoneal chemotherapy as an adjuvant in early- or late-stage disease after definitive surgical or systemic chemotherapeutic management are being performed. Some investigators have recommended that intraperitoneal chemotherapy be a standard treatment option in patients with persistent microscopic residual disease (<0.5 cm) after cisplatin- or carboplatinum-based chemotherapy who have shown a response to the initial systemic therapy.[35] Certainly, no established therapy has shown superior results in this scenario, but a randomized phase III trial is needed to demonstrate that a survival advantage exists for the intraperitoneal option.

A number of biologic response modifiers such as interferon-α (INF-α)[36,37] and interleukin-2 (IL-2) with or without LAK cells have been administered intraperitoneally to patients with ascites or disseminated carcinomatosis, or both, caused by ovarian or colorectal cancer. Interferon-α2b was administered to 13 patients with ovarian carcinoma and ascites, and there was a significant decrease in ascites in 5 of the 13 who had microscopic disease.[36] Berek and colleagues treated 14 patients with residual disease after first-line chemotherapy and second-look laparotomy with escalating doses of intraperitoneal INF-α and achieved a 45% pathologically confirmed response rate (4 complete and 1 partial); all patients had less than 0.5 cm of disease.[37]

Both allogeneic and syngeneic LAK cells have been employed with intraperitoneal IL-2 to treat patients with ovarian and colorectal cancer. Steis and colleagues[38] treated 24 patients who had diffuse peritoneal carcinomatosis, mostly from ovarian, colorectal, or uterine cancer, with IL-2 and LAK cells instilled intraperitoneally by way of a Tenckoff catheter. Seven of 24 patients had pathologically confirmed partial responses, albeit with significant morbidity that limited therapy, including peritoneal fibrosis in 10 patients and significant abdominal pain in 22 patients.[37,38]

Finally, while interferon-γ (INF-γ) has been instilled intraperitoneally in a phase I trial[39] and has been shown to have no significant antitumor activity, it may have clinical utility in immunotherapy for its ability to locally upregulate major histocompatibility complex (MHC) and tumor antigen expression on ascites tumor cells from patients exposed to the drug intraperitoneally. Subsequent therapy with tumor-specific T cells administered into the peritoneum may allow increased recognition and killing of tumor cells.

RADICAL SURGERY

Sugarbaker and colleagues have studied small numbers of patients with disseminated carcinomatosis from colorectal and gastric cancer who received aggressive debulking surgery followed by early postoperative intraperitoneal chemotherapy and, in some cases, abdominal radiation.[40,41] They claim that the majority of patients receiving intraperitoneal chemotherapy and aggressive debulking with use of a ball-type electrocautery device have disease-free survival of greater than 3 years. Although these results may be impressive for patients with uniformly lethal gastrointestinal malignancies, they need to be confirmed in larger follow-up phase III studies. The same group has studied 50 patients with cystadenocarcinoma limited to peritoneal surfaces; 26 had massive ascites. All were treated with radical debulking surgery and early (within 72 hours of surgery) intraperitoneal chemotherapy; 36 are alive 1 to 8 years after therapy.

PERITONEOVENOUS SHUNTING

Although the concept of returning an ascitic fluid collection to the intravascular space is over 75 years old,[42,43] the technology to accomplish this objective in a minimally cumbersome fashion with continuous reinfusion has evolved significantly over the past 25 years.[44-47] The availability of several relatively simple, reasonably effective peritoneovenous (PV) shunt devices (LeVeen, Becton-Dickenson and Leveen, Rutherford, NJ and Denver; Johnson and Johnson, Evergreen, CO) has led to their fairly widespread use. The devices consist of (1) a length of multiply perforated tubing to be implanted in the free peritoneal cavity, (2) a length of tubing to be inserted into the superior vena cava or right atrium, and (3) a unidirectional flow valve connecting the two limbs.

The principal difference between the LeVeen and Denver shunts is that the one-way valve in the Denver shunt can be manually pumped by physician or patient to flush it clear of possibly accumulating debris at periodic intervals. Despite this potentially theoretic advantage, the literature fails to demonstrate functional superiority for one or the other of these devices; either may be chosen on the basis of personal preference. This approach, with substantial pathophysiologic rationale,[48] was initially applied to the management of intractable ascites from cirrhosis.[49-55] Numerous series that address its applicability in the management of malignant ascites have been recently published.[56-74]

In principle, the PV shunt takes advantage of the fact that a 5- to 15-cm H_2O pressure head exists between the ascites-laden peritoneal cavity and the central venous circulation. On inspiration, when intrathoracic pressure becomes more negative, the pressure differential further increases. Whenever the pressure gradient exceeds about 3 to 5 cm H_2O, the unidirectional flow valve opens, and ascitic fluid moves through the tubing from peritoneal cavity to central circulation. Several excellent reports that describe details of shunt placement are available[46,47,50,75-77] and might profitably be perused by the uninitiated in an effort to avoid any one of the numerous technical pitfalls responsible for early shunt malfunction.

Figure 61–54 represents a schematic illustration of the shunt in place. In brief, the operation may be performed under general anesthesia or under local anesthesia supplemented with sedation. Prophylactic antibiotics are used. The peritoneal limb of the shunt is placed first through a roughly 7.6-cm-long, muscle-splitting, subcostal incision. A nonabsorbable pursestring suture, which includes some transversus abdominus muscle, secures this limb in a watertight fashion. If the Denver shunt is used, a subcutaneous pocket overlying the lower rib cage is made for the pump device, and it is secured in position. Free flow of ascitic fluid is demonstrated by holding the open end of the venous limb several inches below heart level. Most surgeons remove about 50% of the patient's ascitic fluid burden at this point, submitting some for culture and perhaps the rest for cytologic analysis. A cervical incision is then made exposing the internal jugular vein, and a fine Prolene pursestring suture (Ethicon, Somerville, NJ) is placed in its anterior wall. A uterine sound can then be used to make

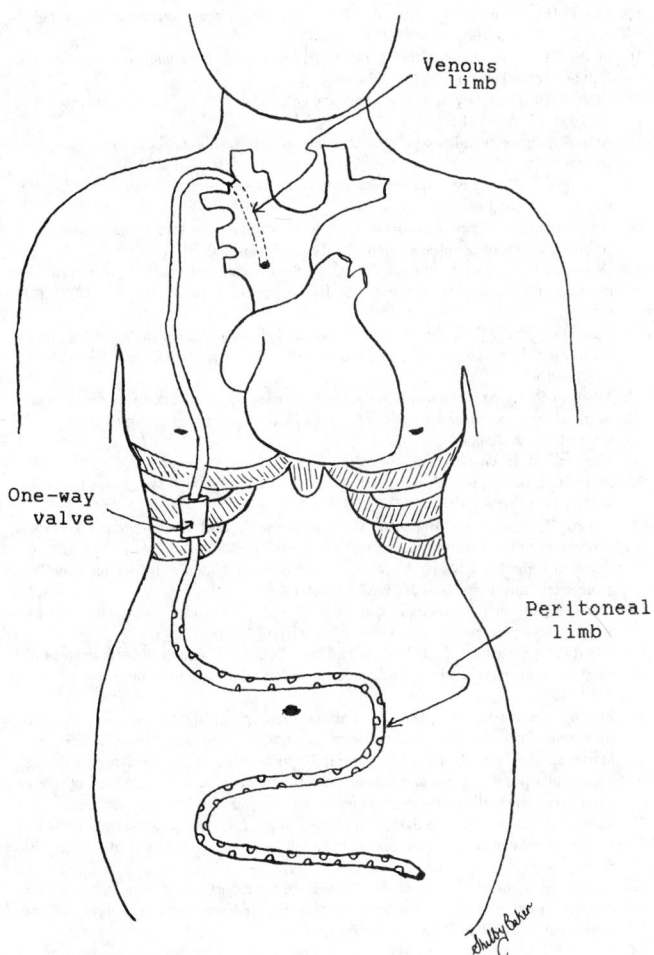

Venous
limb

One-way
valve

Peritoneal
limb

FIGURE 61–54.   The peritoneovenous shunt in situ.

a graceful subcutaneous tunnel linking the abdominal and neck incisions such that all tubing will lie in a kink-free manner. The venous limb is then passed through the tunnel, exiting into the cervical incision. After free flow of ascitic fluid is again demonstrated and the venous limb is cut to permit its tip to lie in the superior vena cava or right atrium, the venous limb is placed through a stab wound in the internal jugular vein and advanced centrally. It is useful to confirm the position of the PV shunt at this point, either fluoroscopically or with portable chest and abdominal x-ray films. The wounds are then irrigated with antibiotic solution and inspected, perfect hemostasis is assured, and the wounds are closed.

Although able to afford palliation, PV shunting is no panacea. Before a PV shunt procedure is attempted, the patient's ascites, at the very least, should have proved refractory to first-line treatment for the underlying malignant condition. This is particularly true in the setting of ovarian cancer, for which ascites can be a component of relatively early stage (IC or IIC) disease and can come under control with hysterectomy-salpingo-oophorectomy alone. Furthermore, multidrug regimens have proved quite successful, at least initially, in controlling the manifestations of much more extensive intra-abdominal dissemination and may significantly impinge on the ascitic fluid component of the tumor-imposed burden.

The data in Table 61–34 summarize the results of 19 reported studies of patients managed by placement of a PV shunt to control malignant ascites. Although each includes only a modest number of patients, 505 patients in all are reported, with the majority suffering cancer of the gastrointestinal tract (34%), ovary (27%), and breast (16%). The fact that end-stage illness is an apt characterization of the patient population's clinical condition is attested to by the median survivals of about 2 to 6 months and the 1-year survivals of about 10%. Although, for the most part, the authors emphasize that patients derive significant symptomatic relief and improvement in qualitative existence, this regrettably translates into substantial quantitative postshunt survival only anecdotally.

COMPLICATIONS

Although the litany of potential and reported complications is long, with the exception of shunt malfunction, they tend to occur infrequently and, on occasion, are preventable.

Shunt occlusion with flow cessation can occur at any time after insertion. Ten percent to 42% of shunts placed stop functioning before the patient's death.[56–61,66,67,69,70,77,78] Immediate malfunction often is due to technical factors, such as tube kinking or tip malposition. Later failures may be secondary to fibrin clot formation and debris accumulation at the valve. Heavily blood-tinged ascites, particularly rich in protein with a somewhat viscous character, portend this complication. Valve chamber pumping (Denver) and shunt flushing with thrombolytic agents[61] can, on occasion, restore flow, but revision or replacement, if clinically indicated, is usually required. Late occlusion may also reflect thrombosis of the venous system around that limb of the PV shunt.

Ascitic fluid leakage at the peritoneal insertion site predisposes to infection, and it is perhaps best prevented by using a double-pursestring suture buttressed by transversus abdominus muscle and fascia at this location.[50,69]

Acute postinsertion problems with fluid overload, pulmonary congestion, and respiratory insufficiency occur infrequently.[61,67] To help avoid this problem, most authors recommend removing about 50% of the ascitic fluid accumulation at the time of shunt placement. Careful postoperative monitoring is required and includes central venous pressure assessment, input-output determination, daily weight, and abdominal girth measurement. A Foley catheter facilitates management of the often brisk, post-PV shunt insertion, diuretic-abetted diuresis and can help to more accurately monitor fluid fluxes. Judicious intravenous fluid support and the liberal use of diuretics and potassium replacement are often necessary to prevent intravascular volume overload and hypokalemia. Because shunt flow volume is hydrostatically determined, simply raising or lowering the head of the patient's bed will alter significantly the flow pressure gradient. Need for this maneuver can be monitored by central venous pressure determination, and change can be made accordingly.

Although disseminated intravascular coagulation (DIC) and bleeding diatheses occur often[79–81] after PV shunt management of cirrhotic ascites, they are rarely a clinical problem when shunts are placed in the neoplastic ascites context.[56,62,79] Laboratory evidence for the ongoing process at a subclinical level is readily demonstrable. Mild decreases in platelet count, slight prolongation in prothrombin and partial thromboplastin time, and measurable increases in fibrin degradation products have been reported.[62,81,82] Significant preshunt hepatic dysfunction, particularly as evidenced by a serum bilirubin level higher than 3 mg/dl, may well presage clinical coagulopathy and probably will contraindicate the procedure.[80,83]

Although shunt-induced tumor dissemination is a potentially adverse complication, it appears more of a theoretic consideration than a clinical contraindication. Although several reports, particularly in the setting of ovarian malignancy, suggest that this can occur and can produce serious consequences,[57,59,78,84,85] in most instances this problem has not occurred. Tarin and colleagues prospectively studied a series of 29 PV shunt recipients, 15 of whom came to autopsy.[86,87] All had large numbers of viable malignant cells ($8-600 \times 10^6$/ 100 ml ascites—95+% viable) in their ascitic fluid. Most formed colonies when grown in soft agar. Postshunt peripheral blood samples often revealed bizarre multinucleated cells, morphologically suggestive of tumor. Eight of the 15 patients had no evidence of hematologic dissemination at postmortem examination. The longest survivor, a patient with an ovarian primary lesion, lived 27 months after initial shunt placement. The 7 patients with evidence of hematogenous spread survived 1 to 9 months after shunt placement; 6 of the 7 had evidence of multiple, uniform-sized, small pulmonary nodules, possibly of iatrogenic origin but clinically not felt to have caused the patient's death. It may well be that the otherwise limited longevity of the PV shunt recipient precludes this theoretic difficulty from becoming a problematic clinical reality. Not unexpectedly, tumor growth along the subcutaneous shunt tunnel[58,88] and at the venotomy site of the venous limb[49,62] has been reported.

Although fever in the immediate postoperative period has been noted by most authors,[66,67] it usually remits spontaneously and is only rarely the harbinger of serious sepsis.[51,63]

REFERENCES

1. Lacy JH, Wieman TJ, Shively EH. Management of malignant ascites. Surg Gynecol Obstet 1984;159:397–412.
2. Feldman GB, Knapp RC, Order SE, Hellman S. The role of lymphatic obstruction in the formation of ascites in a murine ovarian carcinoma. Cancer Res 1972;32:1663–1666.
3. Feldman GB, Knapp RC. Lymphatic drainage of the peritoneal cavity and its significance in ovarian cancer. Am J Obstet Gynecol 1974;119:991–994.
4. Coates G, Bush RS, Aspin N. A study of ascites using lymphoscintigraphy with 99 Tc sulfur colloid. Radiology 1973;107:577–583.
5. Bronskill MJ, Bush RS, Ege GN. A quantitative measurement of peritoneal drainage in malignant ascites. Cancer 1977;40:2375–2380.
6. Hirabayashi K, Graham J. Genesis of ascites in ovarian cancer. Am J Obstet Gynecol 1970;106:492–497.
7. Garrison RN, Kaelin LD, Heusser LS, Galloway RH. Malignant ascites. Ann Surg 1986;203:644–651.
8. Greene LS, Levine R, Gross MJ, Gordon S. Distinguishing between malignant and cirrhotic ascites by computerized step-wise discriminant functional analysis of its biochemistry. Am J Gastroenterol 1978;70:448–454.
9. Nystrom JS, Dyce B, Wada J, et al. Carcinoembryonic antigen titers on effusion fluid. Arch Intern Med 1977;137:875–879.
10. Lowenstein MS, Rittgers RA, Kupchik HZ, et al. Improved detection of malignant ascites and pleural effusions by combined assay of fluid CEA and cytology. Clin Res 1975;23:596A.
11. Greenway B, Johnson PJ, Williams R. Control of malignant ascites with spironolactone. Br J Surg 1982;69:441–442.
12. Appleqvist P, Silvo J, Salmela L, Kostiainen S. J Surg Oncol 1982;20:238–242.
13. Lifshitz S. Ascites, pathophysiology and control measures. Int J Radiat Oncol Biol Phys 1982;8:1423–1426.
14. Belfort MA, Stevens RJ, DeHaek K, Soeters R, et al. A new approach to the management of malignant ascites. A permanently implanted abdominal drain. Eur J Surg Oncol 1990;16:47–53.
15. Lomas DA, Willis PJ, Stockley RA. Palliation of malignant ascites with a Tenckoff catheter. Thorax 1989;44:828–831.
16. Muller JH. Zur medizinisch-therapoeutischen verwendung der kunstlichen radioaktivitat. Bull Schweiz Akad Wiss 1949;5:584.
17. Rose RG. Intracavitary radioactive colloidal gold: Results in 257 cancer patients. J Nucl Med 1962;3:323–331.
18. Ariel IM, Oropeza R, Pack GT. Intracavitary administration of radioactive isotopes in the control of effusions due to cancer. Cancer 1966;19:1096–1102.
19. Jackson GL, Blosser NM. Intracavitary chromic phosphate (32-P) colloidal suspension therapy. Cancer 1981;48:2596–2598.
20. Weisberger AS, Levine B, Storasli JP. Use of nitrogen mustard in the treatment of serous effusions of neoplastic origin. JAMA 1955;159:1704–1707.
21. Dedrick RL, Myers CE, Bungay PM, et al. Pharmacokinetic rationale for peritoneal drug administration in the treatment of ovarian cancer. Cancer Treat Rep 1978;62:1–9.
22. Ozols RF, Young RC, Speyer JL, et al. Phase I and pharmacological studies of Adriamycin administered intraperitoneally to patients with ovarian cancer. Cancer Res 1982;42:4265–4269.
23. Alberts DS, Young L, Mason N, et al. In vitro evaluation of anticancer drugs against ovarian cancer at concentrations achievable by intraperitoneal administration. Semin Oncol 1985;12(Suppl 4):38–42.
24. Markman M. Intracavitary chemotherapy. Crit Rev Oncol Hematol 1985;3:205–233.
25. Pfeifle CE, Howell SB, Markman M, et al. Totally implantable system for peritoneal access. J Clin Oncol 1984;2:1277–1280.
26. Piccart MJ, Speyer JL, Markman M, et al. Intraperitoneal chemotherapy: Technical experience at five institutions. Semin Oncol 1985;12:90–96.
27. Howell SB, Pfeifle CE, Wang WE, et al. Intraperitoneal cisplatin with systemic thiosulfate protection. Ann Intern Med 1982;97:845–851.
28. Ozols RF, Speyer JL, Jenkins J, et al. Phase II trial of 5-FU administered IP to patients with refractory ovarian cancer. Cancer Treat Rep 1984;68:1229–1232.
29. Alberts DS, Surwit EA, Peng Y-M, et al. Phase I clinical pharmacokinetic study of mitoxantrone given to patients by intraperitoneal administration. Cancer Res 1988;48:5874–5877.
30. Reichman B, Markman M, Hake T, et al. Intraperitoneal cisplatin and etoposide in the treatment of refractory recurrent ovarian carcinoma. J Clin Oncol 1989;7:1327–1332.
31. Markman M, Cleary S, Lucas WE, Howell SB. Intraperitoneal chemotherapy with high dose cisplatin and cytosine arabinoside for refractory ovarian carcinoma and other malignancies principally involving the peritoneal cavity. J Clin Oncol 1985;3:925–931.
32. Kirmani S, Lucas WE, Kim S, et al. A phase II trial of IP cis platinum and etoposide as salvage treatment for minimal residual ovarian carcinoma. J Clin Oncol 1991;9:649–657.
33. Howell SB, Zimm S, Markman M, et al. Long term survival of advanced refractory ovarian carcinoma patients with small-volume disease treated with intraperitoneal chemotherapy. J Clin Oncol 1987;5:1607–1612.
34. Howell SB, Kirmani S, Lucas WE, et al. A phase II trial of intraperitoneal cisplatin and etoposide for primary treatment of ovarian epithelial cancer. J Clin Oncol 1990;8:137–145.
35. Markman M. Intraperitoneal chemotherapy. Semin Oncol 1991;18:248–254.
36. Bezwoda WR, Seymour L, Dansey R. Intraperitoneal recombinant interferon-alpha 2b for recurrent malignant ascites due to ovarian cancer. Cancer 1989;64:1029–1033.
37. Berek JS, Hacker HF, Lichtenstein A, et al. Intraperitoneal recombinant alpha-interferon for "salvage" immunotherapy in stage III epithelial ovarian cancer. A Gynecologic Oncology Group study. Cancer Res 1985;45:4447–4453.
38. Steis RG, Urba WJ, Vander Molan LA, et al. Intraperitoneal lymphokine-activated killer cell and interleukin-2 therapy for malignancies limited to the peritoneal cavity. J Clin Oncol 1990;8:1618–1629.
39. D'Acquisto R, Markman M, Hakes T, et al. A phase I trial of intraperitoneal recombinant gamma-interferon in advanced ovarian carcinoma. J Clin Oncol 1988;6:689–695.
40. Sugarbaker PH. Surgical treatment of peritoneal carcinomatosis: 1988 DuPont Lecture. Can J Surg 1989;32:164–170.
41. Sugarbaker PH. Mechanisms of relapse for colorectal cancer: Implications for intraperitoneal therapy. J Surg Oncol 1991;52:36–41.
42. Routte M. De l'abouchement des veines saphenes internes au peritoine abdominal dans certains cas d'ascite a reproduction. Lyon Med 1910;114:911–921.
43. Evler T. Autoserotherapie bei bauchfelltuberculose durch dauerdrainage des Aszites unter die haut. Med Klin 1910;16:627–628.
44. Hyde GL, Eisman B. Peritoneal atrial shunt for intractable ascites. Arch Surg 1967;95:369–373.
45. Pollock AV. The treatment of resistant malignant ascites by insertion of a peritoneo-atrial Holter valve. Br J Surg 1975;62:104–107.
46. LeVeen HH, Christoudias G, Ip M. Peritoneo-venous shunting for ascites. Ann Surg 1974;180:580–591.
47. Lund RH, Newkirk JB. Peritoneo-venous shunting system for surgical management of ascites. Contemp Surg 1979;14:31–45.
48. Stanley MM. Treatment of intractable ascites in patients with alcoholic cirrhosis by peritoneovenous shunting (LeVeen). Med Clin North Am 1979;63:523–536.
49. LeVeen HH, Wapnick S, Grosberg S, et al. Further experiences with peritoneo-venous shunt for ascites. Ann Surg 1976;184:574–581.
50. Reinhardt GF, Stanley MM. Peritoneovenous shunting for ascites. Surg Gynecol Obstet 1977;145:419–424.
51. Greig PD, Langer B, Blendis LM, et al. Complications after peritoneovenous shunting for ascites. Am J Surg 1980;139:125–131.
52. Greenlee HB, Stanley MM, Reinhardt GF. Intractable ascites treated with peritoneovenous shunts (LeVeen). Arch Surg 1981;116:518–524.

53. Bernhoft RA, Pelligrini CA, Way LW. Peritoneovenous shunts for refractory ascites. Arch Surg 1982;117:631–635.

54. Stanley MM, Shigeru O, Lee KK, Nemchausky BA, et al. Peritoneovenous shunting as compared with medical treatment in patients with alcoholic cirrhosis and massive ascites. N Engl J Med 1989;321:1632–1638.

55. Gines P, Arroyo V, Vargas V, Planas R, et al. Paracentesis with intravenous infusion of albumin as compared with peritoneovenous shunting in cirrhosis with refractory ascites. N Engl J Med 1991;325:829–835.

56. Straus AK, Roseman DL, Shapiro RM. Peritoneovenous shunting in the management of malignant ascites. Arch Surg 1979;114:489–491.

57. Osterlee J. Peritoneovenous shunting for ascites in cancer patients. Br J Surg 1980;67:633–666.

58. Raaf JH, Stroehlein JR. Palliation of malignant ascites by the LeVeen peritoneo-venous shunt. Cancer 1980;45:1019–1024.

59. Lokich J, Reinhold R, Silverman M, et al. Complications of peritoneovenous shunt for malignant ascites. Cancer Treat Rep 1980;64:305–309.

60. Downing R, Black J, Windsor CW. Palliation of malignant ascites by the Denver peritoneovenous shunt. Ann R Coll Surg Engl 1984;66:340–343.

61. Lund RH, Moritz MW. Complications of Denver peritoneovenous shunting. Arch Surg 1982;117:924–928.

62. Qazi R, Savlov ED. Peritoneovenous shunt for palliation of malignant ascites. Cancer 1982;49:600–602.

63. Cheung DK, Raaf JH. Selection of patients with malignant ascites for a peritoneovenous shunt. Cancer 1982;50:1204–1209.

64. Reinhold RB, Lokich JJ, Tamashefski J, et al. Management of malignant ascites with peritoneovenous shunting. Am J Surg 1983;145:455–457.

65. Souter RG, Tarin D, Kettlewell MGW. Peritoneovenous shunts in the management of malignant ascites. Br J Surg 1983;70:478–481.

66. Gough IR. Control of malignant ascites by peritoneovenous shunting. Cancer 1984;54:2226–2230.

67. Kostroff KM, Ross DW, Davis JM. Peritoneovenous shunting for cirrhotic versus malignant ascites. Surg Gynecol Obstet 1985;161:204–208.

68. Campioni N, Pasquali, Lasagni RP, Vitucci C, et al. Peritoneovenous shunt and neoplastic ascites: A 5 year experience report. J Surg Oncol 1986;33:31–35.

69. Sonnenfeld T, Tyden G. Peritoneovenous shunts for malignant ascites. Acta Chir Scand 1986;152:117–121.

70. Roussel JGJ, Kroon BBR, Hart GAM. The Denver type for peritoneovenous shunting of malignant ascites. Surg Gynecol Obstet 1986;162:235–240.

71. Soderlund C. Denver peritoneovenous shunting for malignant or cirrhotic ascites. Scand J Gastroenterol 1986;21:1161–1172.

72. Shepherd KE, Miller BJ. Peritoneovenous shunts—Devices of last resort. Can J Surg 1988;31:444–447.

73. Edney JA, Hill A, Armstrong D. Peritoneovenous shunts palliate malignant ascites. Am J Surg 1989;158:598–601.

74. Smith DAP, Weaver DW, Bouman DL. Peritoneovenous shunts (PVS) for malignant ascites: An analysis of outcome. Am Surg 1989;55:445–449.

75. Hyde GL, Dillon M, Bivins BA. Peritoneal venous shunting for ascites: A 15 year perspective. Am Surg 1982;48:123–127.

76. Holman JM, Albo D Jr. Peritoneovenous shunting in patients with malignant ascites. Am J Surg 1981;142:774–776.

77. LeVeen HH, Vujic I, D'Ovidio NG, Hutto RB. Peritoneovenous shunt occlusion—Etiology, diagnosis and therapy. Ann Surg 1984;200:212–223.

78. Souter RG, Wells C, Tarin D, et al. Surgical and pathologic complications associated with peritoneovenous shunting in the management of malignant ascites. Cancer 1985;55:1973–1978.

79. Ragni MV, Lewis JH, Spero JA. Ascites-induced LeVeen shunt coagulopathy. Ann Surg 1983;198:91–95.

80. Schwartz ML, Swaim WR, Vogel SB. Coagulopathy following peritoneovenous shunting. Surgery 1979;85:671–676.

81. Harmon DC, Demirjian Z, Ellman L, Fischer JE. Disseminated intravascular coagulation with the peritoneovenous shunt. Ann Intern Med 1979;90:774–776.

82. Glysteen JJ, Hussey CV, Heckman MG. The cause of coagulopathy after peritoneovenous shunt for malignant ascites. Arch Surg 1990;125:474–477.

83. Tempero MA, Davis RB, Reed E, et al. Thrombocytopenia and laboratory evidence of disseminated intravascular coagulation after shunts for ascites in malignant disease. Cancer 1985;55:2718–2721.

84. Maat B, Osterlee J, Sapps JAJ, et al. Dissemination of tumor cells via LeVeen shunt. Lancet 1979;1:988.

85. Smith RRL, Sternberg SS, Paglia MA, et al. Fatal pulmonary tumor embolization following peritoneovenous shunting for malignant ascites. J Surg Oncol 1981;16:27–35.

86. Tarin D, Price JE, Kettlewell MGW, et al. Mechanisms of human tumor metastasis studied in patients with peritoneovenous shunts. Cancer Res 1984;44:3584–3592.

87. Tarin D, Vass ACR, Kettlewell MGW, et al. Absence of metastatic sequellae during long term treatment of malignant ascites by peritoneo-venous shunting. Invasion Metastasis 1984;4:1–12.

88. Berger A, Goldberg MI. Subcutaneous cancer growth complicating the peritoneovenous shunting of malignant ascites. Surgery 1983;93:374–376.

Cancer: Principles & Practice of Oncology, Fourth Edition,
edited by Vincent T. DeVita, Jr., Samuel Hellman, Steven A. Rosenberg.
J.B. Lippincott Co., Philadelphia © 1993.

CHAPTER **62**

Bone Marrow Dysfunction in the Cancer Patient

SECTION **1**

RALPH O. WALLERSTEIN, JR
ALBERT B. DEISSEROTH

Use of Blood and Blood Products

As the intensity of cancer chemotherapy has increased, the need for skilled use of blood and blood products has increased. The improved technologies for leukocyte depletion, testing of blood products for infectious agents and for preventing their transmission, and for the collection and manipulation of bone marrow and peripheral blood stem cells must be understood by the practicing oncologist.

ERYTHROCYTE TRANSFUSION

INDICATIONS

The indications for erythrocyte transfusion depend on the physiologic status of the host, the cause of anemia, and the rate of development of the anemia. Before ordering a transfusion, it is useful to recall that anemia is a laboratory finding (*i.e.*, hemoglobin <2 SD below normal for the population group being studied) for which an explanation should be sought and not a diagnosis. It is not sufficient to attribute the anemia to cancer. A minimal evaluation should include review of the mean corpuscular volume, the reticulocyte count, and the morphology of the peripheral smear and determination

of the platelet count, leukocyte count, and differential count.[1] A systematic approach to the laboratory evaluation of anemia ensures appropriate specific therapy and prevents serious morbidity due to delayed diagnosis, such as autoimmune hemolytic anemia complicating lymphoma or chronic lymphocytic leukemia or hemolytic-uremic syndrome after bone marrow transplantation or administration of mitomycin C.

Most patients tolerate a hemoglobin level of 10 g/dl. Because cardiac output begins to increase as the hemoglobin drops below 10 g/dl, patients with cardiopulmonary, renal, hepatic, or cerebral vascular disease should be maintained at or above this level. Younger patients may tolerate a hemoglobin as low as 6 or 7 g/dl, but most cancer patients are transfused when their hemoglobin is 8 g/dl or less.

For most transfusions, the physician should order packed cells. The use of specific blood components rather than whole blood limits the volume of the transfusion and allows the plasma and platelets to be used for other patients. In patients who are expected to have a chronic transfusion requirement over many years, such as those with myelodysplasia of the refractory anemia or refractory anemia with ringed sideroblasts subtypes, prophylactic desferrioxamine therapy should be considered.

ADVERSE REACTIONS

The most common reactions after transfusion of erythrocytes are fever and chills (Table 62–1). Most fevers are caused by febrile nonhemolytic transfusion reactions (FNHTRs) due to antibodies in the recipient directed against granulocyte-specific and HLA antigens on leukocytes in the donor blood.[2]

TABLE 62–1. Differential Diagnosis
of Acute Transfusion Reactions

Symptoms	Possible Diagnosis
Fever and chills	Major hemolytic transfusion reaction
	Reaction to foreign HLA and granulocyte-specific antigens on transfused leukocytes and platelets
Dyspnea	Fluid overload
	Major hemolytic transfusion reaction
	Contaminated blood
	Air embolism
	Anaphylactic reaction due to transfusion of IgA-containing plasma to IgA-deficient recipient with anti-IgA
Bleeding	Disseminated intravascular coagulation due to major hemolytic transfusion reaction or contaminated blood
	Thrombocytopenia due to massive transfusion of packed erythrocytes
	Washout of coagulation factors due to massive transfusion of packed erythrocytes
Arrhythmia	Circulatory overload
	Hyperkalemia
	Hyperthermia
	Hypocalcemia
	Major hemolytic transfusion reaction
	Contaminated blood
	Air embolism
Hypotension	Major hemolytic transfusion reaction
	Contaminated blood
	Anaphylaxis due to IgA deficiency
Hemoglobinuria	Major hemolytic transfusion reaction
	Excessive infusion pressure through small-bore needle
	Overheating with blood warmer
	Contaminated blood

In most cases, the chills do not start until at least 30 minutes into the transfusion and often not until 1 to 2 hours into the transfusion. These FNHTRs are uncommon in children but may occur in 20% of multiparous females due to prior sensitization and in as many as 79% of multiply transfused patients. Although these reactions can be treated or in some cases prevented by the use of acetaminophen before transfusion, some patients still experience recurrent severe chills and fever with packed erythrocytes. For these patients, the use of leukocyte-poor or leukocyte-depletion methods is indicated.

A unit of packed cells contains about 1 to 3×10^9 leukocytes, depending on the donor's white count. If leukocyte contamination is reduced to less than 5×10^8 per unit, the incidence of chill or fever reactions is markedly reduced.[3] This one-log reduction of leukocytes may be accomplished by several means, including differential centrifugation, freezing with glycerol as a cryoprotectant (which appears to protect only the erythrocytes so that the leukocytes are lysed) followed by washing to remove the leukocyte debris, or use of leukocyte depletion filters. Leukocyte depletion filters may be employed at the time of collection, in the blood bank before issuing, or

at the bedside. By preventing granulocyte disintegration, which occurs during the first 2 days of storage, depletion at the time of collection may decrease the amount of soluble granulocyte membrane antigens in the plasma. It is possible that these soluble antigens account for some of the chill and fever reactions that continue to occur despite leukocyte filtration at the time of administration. The current generation of leukocyte depletion filters result in a 99.3% to 99.5% depletion (2 logs) with 87.4% to 92.2% erythrocyte recovery.[4] For patients who still experience severe chill or fever reactions with leukocyte-depleted erythrocytes, a trial of frozen deglycerolized erythrocytes should be considered.

The physician must always consider the possibility of a major hemolytic transfusion reaction in the differential diagnosis of chill and fever reactions, particularly if the chills occur in the first 30 minutes, if the patient is nulliparous and has never been transfused, or if there are other associated systemic symptoms like low back pain, chest pain, restlessness, dyspnea, and pain at the site of transfusion. Signs include tachycardia, hypotension, oliguria, hemoglobinuria, tachypnea, and generalized bleeding (if disseminated intravascular coagulation [DIC] has developed). Most major hemolytic transfusion reactions result from human error, particularly at the time the clot is drawn for type and crossmatch tests if the specimen is mislabelled.

Bacterial contamination is another cause for chill and fever reactions, and the onset may be acute or delayed, depending on the amount of contamination and whether the bacteria have produced a toxin. Contamination of packed erythrocytes is uncommon because of the rigorous antiseptic techniques used in blood collection, the storage of blood at 4°C, and the natural antibacterial properties of blood. Bacterial contamination is more of a problem with platelets, because they are stored at room temperature. Nevertheless, certain cryopathic organisms, mostly gram-negative organisms, can proliferate at 4°C. Several cases of *Yersinia enterocolitica* (which can cause minimal symptoms in the donor even when bacteremic and which can proliferate at 4°C) sepsis transmitted by transfusion have been reported, some of which were fatal.[5–6] Aber recommended excluding donors with gastrointestinal symptoms in the 4 weeks before donation and minimizing the period of storage at 4°C as a means of risk reduction, although others have been concerned that this would exclude many potential donors.[7] It does seem prudent to consider bacterial contamination in the differential diagnosis of severe chill and fever reactions, to obtain blood cultures of the patient and the unit of blood, and to consider empiric antibiotic coverage pending the results of culture.

Allergic reactions, including urticaria and hives, may occur in 3% to 5% of transfused patients. Some of these reactions are due to recipient antibodies against immunoglobulin components or other soluble proteins in the plasma. The best defined of these reactions occurs in patients with congenital deficiency of IgA (1 of 800 people). Some of these patients develop IgG or IgE antibodies against IgA, and when transfused with any blood product containing even small amounts of plasma, they may develop severe allergic or even fatal anaphylactic reactions. These patients should receive extensively washed erythrocytes or preferably blood from IgA-deficient donors. Most urticarial reactions, however, occur in non-IgA-deficient recipients and are rarely life threatening. The transfusion is temporarily stopped, the patient is treated with intravenous diphenhydramine, and the transfusion is resumed in 30 minutes. If the allergic reactions recur or increase, transfusion of that unit should be discontinued and further use of that donor for that patient stopped. Such urticarial reactions generally do not recur. For the few patients who experience recurrent or severe urticarial reactions, the physician should measure the quantitative immunoglobulins to exclude IgA deficiency and order washed erythrocytes from which virtually all of the plasma has been removed (Table 62–2).

TRANSFUSION-INDUCED GRAFT-VERSUS-HOST DISEASE

All blood products given to severely immunocompromised patients should be treated with 1500 cGy of gamma radiation to prevent viable T lymphocytes from causing transfusion-induced graft-versus-host disease (GVHD) in the recipient.[8,9] The clinical manifestations of GVHD when caused by transfusion include the rash, diarrhea, and abnormal liver function seen after allogeneic bone marrow transplant. In addition,

TABLE 62–2. Blood Component Therapy Indications and Complications

Component	Indications	Complications
Packed erythrocytes	Anemia	Fever, volume overload, hepatitis and other infections
		Urticaria, hemolytic transfusion reaction
Leukocyte-poor packed erythrocytes	Prior febrile reactions to packed erythrocytes	Increased viscosity
	May delay alloimmunization	
Washed or plasma-poor packed erythrocytes	Prior urticarial reactions, IgA deficiency, need to avoid complement transfusion	
Frozen packed erythrocytes	Rare blood types, autologous donations, process also removes leukocytes and plasma	
Whole blood	None	
Random-donor platelets	Bleeding with platelet count <100,000/mm³, bleeding and qualitative platelet dysfunction	Fever
	Elective surgery and thrombocytopenia	Urticaria
	Prophylactic for platelets <10,000–20,000/mm³	Hepatitis
		Bacterial contamination
Single-donor platelets	May delay alloimmunization	
	Lower risk of infection because exposed to one donor	
Leukoctye-poor platelets	Prior febrile reactions to packed erythrocytes or platelets	
HLA-matched single-donor platelets	Poor response to platelet transfusion due to alloimmunization	
Autologous frozen platelets	Refractoriness to HLA-matched platelets	
Granulocytes	Documented bacterial infection not responding to appropriate antibiotics, with severe neutropenia not expected to recover for several days.	Fever
Respiratory distress		
Alloimmunization		
Fresh-frozen plasma	Coagulation factor deficiency, including rapid warfarin reversal with plasmapheresis for TTP	Hepatitis and other infections
Volume overload		Hypernatremia
Cryoprecipitate	Severe von Willebrand's disease	Hypocalcemia
Hepatitis and other infections	Hypofibrinogenemia	
	Uremic bleeding	
Intravenous immunoglobulin	Hypogammaglobulinemia	Systemic reactions
	Idiopathic thrombocytopenic purpura	Local venous reaction
	Bleeding and alloimmunization, even to HLA-matched platelets	Anaphylaxis
	Passive immunization	
	Prevention of GVH	
Heat-treated lyophilized factor VIII	Hemophilia A	
Non-A, non-B hepatitis		
Heat-treated lyophilized prothrombin	Hemophilia B	
Non-A, non-B hepatitis complex	Factor VIII inhibitor	Thrombosis
Albumin	Volume expansion	

pancytopenia occurs because the hematopoietic cells are foreign to the attacking lymphocytes, but in allogeneic transplant the attacking lymphocytes and marrow are both of donor origin. There is no effective treatment, and the mortality is 85% to 90% after a median of 21 days.

Lymphocyte proliferation in response to allogeneic cells is completely abolished after 500 cGy. After 1500 cGy, there was a 90% reduction in mitogen-stimulated ^{14}C-thymidine incorporation in one study and an 85% reduction in mitogen-induced blast transformation in another. A dose of 5000 cGy decreased these to 97% and 98.5%, respectively.

Other cells are less sensitive than lymphocytes to irradiation. Erythrocytes are unaffected by doses up to 20,000 cGy, but platelets may suffer after exposure to 5000 cGy. Granulocyte function may be affected above 2000 to 5000 cGy. Although 500 cGy may be sufficient to inhibit some lymphocyte functions, a dose of 1500 cGy provides a safe and effective dose, and there have been no documented transfusion-related GVHD cases reported from large centers using this dose. Although there have been no adverse reactions reported from the use of irradiated blood products, their use is associated with additional expense, because the cost of the irradiator and the radiation source is $50,000. Irradiated pluripotent stem cells may survive with sublethal damage, which may allow mutated stem cells to survive. Although the likelihood of harm is remote, because of theoretical concerns and real cost concerns, irradiated blood products should only be used for the specific indications mentioned.

Patients at risk of GVHD include those with profound immunosuppression due to cancer and its treatment, such as allogeneic and autologous (especially with total-body irradiation [TBI] in the preparative regimen) transplant recipients, those undergoing combined modality treatment for Hodgkin's and non-Hodgkin's lymphoma, patients with acute lymphocytic leukemia, those with congenital immunodeficiency, and neonatal patients receiving large volume exchange transfusions. GVHD has occurred in patients with Hodgkin's disease receiving chemotherapy alone. Fatal transfusion-induced graft-versus-host disease may occur in nonimmunocompromised patients, if the blood donor is homozygous for one of the HLA haplotypes of the recipient. This situation is most likely to occur with designated donor transfusions from first-degree relatives or in geographic areas with less genetic diversity.

Other possible complications of transfusions are listed in Table 62–3. The signs and symptoms of a major hemolytic transfusion reaction have been discussed. If the reaction is suspected, the physician should stop the blood transfusion immediately and notify the blood bank. Verification of the identification on the blood unit and the patient should be sought. Remaining blood in the bag should be returned to the blood bank, and repeat blood samples should be drawn from the recipient to repeat the type and crossmatch and to determine if there is pink or brown plasma that would indicate hemoglobinemia. A urine sample should be tested for hemoglobinuria. If the plasma is pink or brown, suggesting intravascular hemolysis has occurred, the physician should order tests for DIC, including partial thromboplastin time (PTT), platelet count, fibrinogen, fibrin monomer, and fibrin-split products. If the patient is bleeding and has DIC, replace clotting factors and platelets if a significant deficiency is documented. Blood pressure should be maintained with intravenous fluids and

TABLE 62–3. Complications of Transfusion

Fever or chills
Allergy
    Urticaria
    Anaphylaxis
Infection
    Hepatitis
    Human immunodeficiency virus
    Cytomegalovirus
    Bacterial contamination
    Parasites
Volume overload
Major hemolytic transfusion reaction
Delayed hemolytic transfusion reaction
Graft-versus-host disease
Posttransfusion purpura
Hypocalcemia
Hyperkalemia
Hypothermia
Respiratory distress
Iron overload
Air embolism
Alloimmunization

pressors, and a urine output greater than 100 ml/hour should be maintained with intravenous fluids. If needed, mannitol or Lasix should be used to prevent oliguric acute tubular necrosis. The physician should monitor input, output, and serum electrolytes, blood urea nitrogen (BUN), and creatinine. A nephrologist should be consulted if renal failure occurs. Most major hemolytic transfusion reactions are due to a clerical error, which occurs at the time the initial blood type and crossmatch sample is drawn and labeled.

Delayed hemolytic transfusion reactions occasionally occur if the recipient has a titer of alloantibody that is too low to be detected in the antibody screen and crossmatching procedure but develops a strong anamnestic antibody response that causes a fall in hemoglobin and an increase in bilirubin and lactate dehydrogenase (LDH) 5 to 10 days after transfusion. This is particularly common for alloantibodies to antigens of the Kidd blood group system.[10]

Patients who develop profound thrombocytopenia 5 to 8 days after transfusion should be suspected of having posttransfusion purpura. Two percent of people lack the platelet antigen P1^{A1}. P1^{A1}-negative patients, when transfused with blood containing platelets or soluble platelet antigen, particularly if they have been previously immunized by prior transplacental contamination from a P1^{A1}-positive fetus or by prior transfusion, may develop severe thrombocytopenia. The intriguing aspect is that the patient's own P1^{A1}-negative platelets are destroyed as well, a process that may continue for several weeks if untreated. Suspected cases of posttransfusion purpura are confirmed by measuring antibody to P1^{A1} in the recipient's serum. Plasmapheresis is the treatment of choice for this problem. The cause of the destruction of the patient's own platelets is unclear. Some investigators suspect that the P1^{A1} antigen is soluble and circulates and binds to the patient's own platelets, causing their destruction. Other investigators feel that the development of the alloantibody to P1[A1] causes the simultaneous development of an autoantibody.

Although massive transfusions (>10 units in 1–6 hours) have been associated with hypocalcemia, hyperkalemia, hypothermia, and bleeding due to coagulation factor and platelet washout, these reactions are relatively uncommon in patients with cancer. Low levels of ionized calcium are due to the citrate in the anticoagulated packed erythrocytes. Except in severe liver dysfunction, citrate usually is rapidly metabolized. Although stored erythrocytes progressively increase the extracellular potassium concentration, it is unusual to see clinical hyperkalemia, except with renal failure. Coagulation factor washout has occurred in patients with trauma, in whom accelerated consumption due to DIC is probably more of a factor than dilution. Prophylactic transfusion of fresh-frozen plasma is not indicated, but the decision should be guided by the PT and activated PTT. Platelet washout is a potential problem with massive transfusion, but the physician should follow the specific platelet count as a guide to platelet repletion.

TRANSMISSION OF INFECTIOUS AGENTS

Bacterial contamination has already been discussed. Other infections that may be transmitted through blood include human immunodeficiency virus (HIV); hepatitis A, B, or C; cytomegalovirus (CMV); human T-cell lymphotropic virus type I (HTLV-I); and parasites.

The risk of HIV infection in a recipient of blood from an infected donor is substantial. Perkins and colleagues identified patients with newly diagnosed acquired immunodeficiency syndrome (AIDS) reported to the San Francisco Public Health Department who had donated blood before the diagnosis of AIDS.[11] Sixty-two percent of the recipients of blood from these donors showed evidence of infection, including recipients of whole blood, erythrocytes, platelet concentrates, and fresh-frozen plasma. The closer the donation was given before the diagnosis of AIDS in the donor, the higher the risk of infection. Nine of 10 recipients from donations given in the 12 months immediately before AIDS diagnoses became infected. Recipients younger than 11 years of age or older than 79 were more likely to have developed AIDS or AIDS-related complex (ARC) at the time of follow-up.[12] Other investigators reported an 89% incidence of infection after transfusion of HIV-seropositive blood. A recent projection by Medley suggests that the mean incubation period for transfusion associated with AIDS is 1.97 years for children younger than 5 and 8.23 years for persons 5 to 59 years old.[13]

HIV infection from blood transfusion has been significantly reduced because blood banks excluded high-risk groups from donating in March 1983 and began screening donated blood for antibody to HIV in the spring of 1985. The physician must be alert for the development of HIV-related disorders in patients transfused between 1976 and 1985, with the peak risk of transmission occurring in 1982 with an estimated risk of 1.1% per transfused unit.[14] Because some donors acutely infected with HIV may not develop an antibody response for a few weeks or months, the risk of acquiring HIV infection from blood products, although quite small (Table 62–4), is not zero.[15]

A recent report from the Centers for Disease Control found

TABLE 62–4. Risk of Viral Infection From Blood Products

Infection	Risk (%)
Human immunodeficiency virus	<0.001
Hepatitis C	0.1

(Herbert A. Perkins, MD, personal communication)

an overall prevalence of HIV positivity among blood donors of only 0.038%.[16] Improvements in methods to exclude persons at risk (*e.g.*, avoiding pressure to donate in blood drives) should reduce the number of persons who are infected but not yet antibody positive.[17] Improvements in the sensitivity of the enzyme immunoassay (EIA) are possible by detection of IgM or IgA to HIV in addition to the IgG that current kits detect.[18] In a report of 127 persons who were positive by EIA, 95 were positive on repeat EIA, and 32 were negative on repeat testing.[19] Of the 95 repeatedly positive, 9 were positive by Western blot, 31 were indeterminate, and 55 were negative. EIA was repeated 3 to 12 months later. All 32 who were negative on the initial repeat by EIA remained negative. All 55 who were HIV positive by EIA but negative by Western blot remained negative. Of the 31 indeterminate, 1 tested positive by polymerase chain reaction (PCR) amplification of conserved sequences of HIV specific nucleic acids (*i.e.*, *POL* gene) and subsequently converted to positive on Western blot when retested 3 to 12 months later. All 9 who were HIV positive by EIA and by Western blot were also positive by PCR amplification. Patients who are HIV positive but indeterminate by Western Blot should be periodically retested. PCR testing, although expensive and labor intensive, remains of interest in the evaluation of patients with equivocal results or those who may be passively antibody positive (*e.g.*, newborns of infected mothers).

The incidence of posttransfusion hepatitis depends on the effort taken to detect hepatitis, the adequacy of follow-up of patients, and the prevalence of the disease in the donor population. Before 1986, it was estimated that the incidence of posttransfusion hepatitis was 5% to 20%. At that time, many blood banks instituted a new policy of testing donated blood for elevations of alanine aminotransferase (ALT) and hepatitis B core antibody as "surrogate markers" for non-A, non-B hepatitis. In 1989, the hepatitis C virus (HCV) was isolated, and an enzyme linked immunoassay for a nonstructural antigen of HCV was approved by the FDA in May 1990. Because seroconversion to antibody positivity may take up to 1 year, the continued use of surrogate testing has been advocated. Recent estimates suggest that 91% of cases of posttransfusion non-A, non-B hepatitis are caused by HCV.[20]

HTLV-I is an RNA tumor virus that appears to cause adult T-cell leukemia-lymphoma and tropical spastic paraparesis.[21] The lifetime risk for HTLV-I-positive persons is estimated to be 2% to 5% for adult T-cell leukemia-lymphoma and 0.25% for the neurologic disorder.[22] In November 1988, a serologic test for HTLV-I was approved by the FDA. This test also detects HTLV-II, which has not been proven to cause any disease, although the ability to differentiate between the two viruses is fairly recent and more data are necessary to determine the effects of HTLV-II. Both viruses can be transmitted through transfusions. Erythrocytes stored for less than 4 days and platelets may be particularly infections due to the death of infected lymphocytes during prolonged refrigerator storage.[23] The ability of leukocyte depletion filters to prevent transmission is currently an area of research.

Because blood banks now routinely screen donors for HTLV-I and notify them of the results and because of the small but documented long-term risk of HTLV-I, three methods have been developed to differentiate HTLV-I from HTLV-II.[22] One method looks at the differential Western blot reactivity to specific viral antigens; reactivity to HTLV-I p19 antigen equal to or greater than to p24 favors HTLV-I, but if p24 is greater than p19, HTLV-II is favored. A second method uses an enzyme-linked immunoassay for HTLV-I gp46[env] or HTLV-II gp52[env]. The "gold standard" method uses PCR amplification in the viral regulatory genes with sequence-specific oligonucleotide hybridization to differentiate the two viruses.

The use of leukocyte filtration of blood products appears to decrease the transmissibility of CMV and possibly other viruses.[24-28] Although CMV primary infection and reactivation are of most concern in allogeneic transplantation, CMV interstitial pneumonitis does occur after autologous transplantation. It is likely that CMV contributes significantly to unexplained fevers, hepatitis, gastroenteritis, immunosuppression, and delayed hematopoietic recovery, which complicate intensive therapy. For CMV-negative recipients of allogeneic marrow from CMV-negative donors, the exclusive use of CMV-negative blood almost totally prevents CMV infection and pneumonitis. Even after CMV-negative patients receive allogeneic bone marrow transplants from CMV-positive donors, 25% do not seroconvert.[29]

Theoretically, a rationale for limiting CMV exposure through blood exists for this group. As high-dose therapy with autologous bone marrow transplantation (particularly when TBI is part of the preparative regimen) becomes more widely applied in the treatment of relapsed or refractory Hodgkin's and non-Hodgkin's lymphoma and solid tumors (*e.g.*, breast cancer, ovarian cancer), CMV infection and interstitial pneumonia are growing problems. Because the availability of exclusively CMV-negative blood products is limited, alternative strategies are necessary to support CMV-negative patients who are undergoing intensive therapy or who may undergo intensive therapy in the future. It is our policy to routinely leukocyte filter all blood products for these patients to decrease the likelihood or prevent primary CMV infection. We continue to provide CMV-negative blood products with intravenous IgG for CMV-negative allogeneic patients. Even in these patients, there may be a rationale for leukocyte depletion, depending on the rate of false-negative CMV serologies (reported sensitivities of the serologic tests are 89–93%) in the donor population.

Parasite transmission through blood transfusion is uncommon in the United States. As a result of excluding donors who have been in endemic malarial areas, only about 3 cases per year of transfusion-transmitted malaria occur in the United States.[30] Babesiosis transmission appears to be even less common. Travelers to the Middle East, including service personnel who served in Operation Desert Storm, are being excluded from donation because of the risk of leishmaniasis, which is transmitted by the bite of the sand fly. Transfusion-transmitted

Chagas' disease, particularly in immunocompromised patients, is of some concern, even though the documented cases are few, because of the increasing number of Central and South Americans emigrating to this country.[31] In areas with a high prevalence of at-risk donors, a combination of donor screening with questions and serologic evaluation has been implemented.

PLATELET TRANSFUSIONS

INDICATIONS

Platelet transfusions are indicated for prophylaxis or treatment of bleeding due to decreased number or function of platelets. As with anemia, it is important to have a systematic method for the laboratory evaluation of the bleeding patient to direct specific therapy and avoid missing factors contributing to the bleeding.[32]

The bleeding time increases linearly as the platelet count falls from 100,000 to 10,000, below which it tends to be prolonged indefinitely.[33] If the platelet count is greater than 100,000 and the bleeding time is prolonged, the patient has von Willebrand's disease or a qualitative platelet defect.[34,35] If von Willebrand's disease has been excluded by normal factor VIII antigen, factor VIII activity, ristocetin cofactor activity, and multimer analysis, the patient has a qualitative platelet defect. Patients with life-threatening bleeding due to a qualitative platelet defect should be given a platelet transfusion. For patients with qualitative platelet dysfunction due to uremia, transfused platelets will acquire the same qualitative defect, and the treatment of choice is vigorous hemodialysis. For patients already being dialyzed, desmopressin acetate (DDAVP) or cryoprecipitate may be useful. For patients with other than life-threatening bleeding due to qualitative platelet dysfunction, a trial of DDAVP is indicated because it is not associated with the risk of viral infection seen with cryoprecipitate and platelets.[36]

In 1962, Gaydos and coworkers documented a quantitative relation between platelet counts and hemorrhages in patients with acute leukemia (Fig. 62–1).[37] In these patients, the incidence of hemorrhage of any kind, including gross hemorrhage, rose dramatically as platelet counts declined, especially to levels less than 20,000/mm[3]. They also observed that bleeding episodes associated with thrombocytopenia frequently follow a decline in platelet count. They reported that of 8 patients with intracranial hemorrhage unassociated with high blast counts and intracerebral leukostasis, 7 patients had platelet counts of less than 5000/mm[3]. No intracranial bleeding was observed at a platelet count of 10,000/mm[3] or more.

Retrospective and prospective studies have shown a decreased incidence of bleeding episodes when platelets were transfused prophylactically for patients with platelet counts less than 20,000 to 30,000/mm[3] (Table 62–5).[38] At any given level, patients with thrombocytopenia due to decreased platelet production have a more prolonged bleeding time than patients with thrombocytopenia due to increased destruction, probably because with accelerated destruction there is usually accelerated production and release of young, hemostatically effective platelets. In the case of decreased production, the circulating platelets are several days old and less effective.

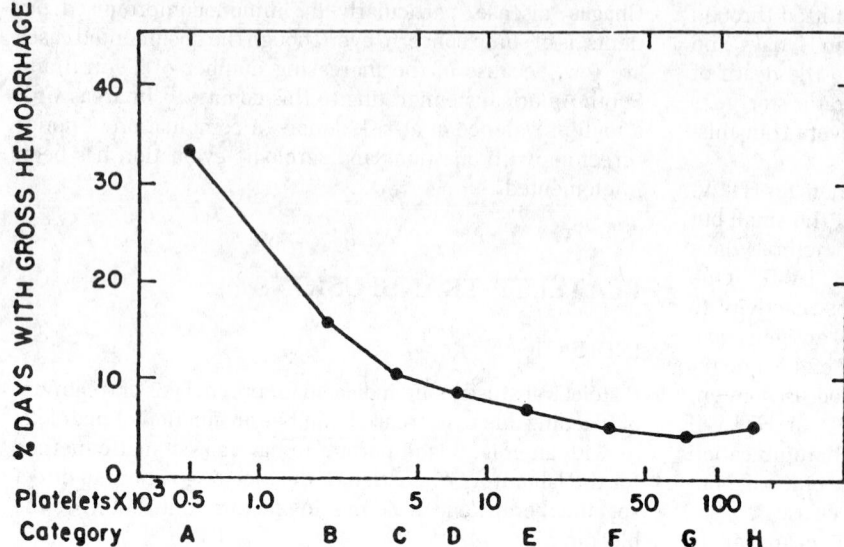

FIGURE 62–1. Relation between platelet counts and the number of days patients had grossly visible hemorrhage. Capital letters along the abscissa refer to the following categories of platelet counts: A, less than 1000/mm³; B, 1000–3000/mm³; C, 3000–5000/mm³; D, 5000–10,000/mm³; E, 10,000–20,000/mm³; F, 20,000–50,000/mm³; G, 50,000–100,000/mm³; H, >100,000/mm³.

The benefit of preventing bleeding by prophylactic platelet transfusions must be balanced against the risk of the patient developing alloantibodies to the transfused platelets, and if bleeding occurs in the future, transfused platelets may be less effective. In practice, when thrombocytopenia is expected to be limited (*e.g.*, induction chemotherapy for acute leukemia), prophylactic platelet transfusions are given to keep the platelet count above 10,000 to 20,000/mm³. For chronic thrombocytopenia (*e.g.*, myelodysplasia) most clinicians reserve platelet transfusions for bleeding episodes.

Platelets are prepared from differential centrifugation of donated whole blood or from platelet pheresis of single donors. Platelet concentrates can be administered through a standard blood bank filter (170 micropore size) during 10 to 20 minutes. Because platelets are stored at room temperature, small amounts of contaminating microorganisms present on day 1 may reach high titers by days 5 to 7.[39–41] At some major centers, platelet concentrates became the major source for transfusion-induced sepsis, and storage of platelets beyond 5 days is no longer permitted.[42]

ALLOIMMUNIZATION

A major limitation to the prevention of bleeding through the use of prophylactic platelet transfusions is the development of platelet alloimmunization. The likelihood of platelet alloimmunization may be decreased for diseases and treatments that decrease the immune response. For example, the incidence in acute lymphocytic leukemia and lymphoma patients undergoing intensive therapy is less than for patients with aplastic anemia or autotransplants for breast cancer.[43] HLA exposure through prior transfusions or pregnancy increases the incidence of alloimmunization. Individual immune response genes appear important, because the occurrence of alloimmunization has been reported to be independent of the number of transfusions and tends to occur within the first few weeks if it is going to occur at all.[44]

Development of alloimmunization requires the presence of class I antigens and class II antigens. Platelets alone do not result in the development of antibodies because they carry only class I HLA antigens and platelet-specific antigens. The class II antigens necessary for the development of alloimmunization are provided by monocytes, lymphocytes, and dendritic cells.[45,46] Although not rigorously proven, it appears that if the number of leukocytes can be reduced to less than 10⁶ per bag of platelets and erythrocytes, alloimmunization to platelets can be markedly delayed or prevented.[50–64] Another approach to preventing alloimmunization under investigation is ultraviolet irradiation.[65–70]

For patients who become refractory to random-donor platelets, single-donor platelets are used. For patients refractory to single-donor platelets, partial HLA matching may identify donors who will provide a better increment. In the absence of facilities for HLA typing, if several different single donors are tried and posttransfusion increments measured, a donor may be found empirically whose platelets are less rapidly destroyed. For allogeneic bone marrow transplantation, the marrow donor may be used as the source of HLA-identical platelet transfusions after the preparative regimen has begun. Some centers are developing methods for platelet crossmatching for alloimmunized patients.[71] After every platelet transfusion, a repeat platelet counts should be obtained within 10 to 60 minutes after transfusion and 24 hours later.[72] A poor increment (<10,000/μl/m² of body surface area per unit of platelets) at 1 hour is seen with splenomegaly or alloimmunization. A good 1-hour count that returns to baseline by 24 hours is much less specific and can be seen with bleeding, infection, poor-quality platelets, autoimmune or drug-induced immune thrombocytopenia, DIC, or any cause for accelerated platelet consumption.[47–49]

An alternative approach for patients who have recovered from a cycle of therapy during which they demonstrated platelet refractoriness is to collect and cryopreserve autologous platelets while in remission.[73,74] Over time, patients who have been previously refractory to random-donor or single-donor platelets may lose their alloimmunization, possibly as a result of disease progression, intensive therapy, or natural antibody decline with time, and it is worthwhile to periodically transfuse these patients and measure their 1-hour and 24-hour posttransfusion increments.

TABLE 62–5. Transfusion Guidelines for Commonly Encountered Hematologic Problems

Chronic Anemia

No significant cardiopulmonary compromise; stable patient.

No absolute indication for transfusion if hemoglobin is above 6 to 7 g/100 mg.

Consider transfusion for otherwise unexplained lassitude, malaise, tachycardia, dyspnea in association with hemoglobin less than 9 to 10 g/100 ml.

Cardiopulmonary disease; fever, surgery. Maintain hemoglobin level at 10 g/100 ml.

If management protracted (years), monitor for evidence of iron overload (secondary hemochromatosis).

Thrombocytopenia

Thrombocytopenia due to failure of platelet production.

Platelet count >20,000/mm³; stable patient without retinal hemorrhages.

Platelet transfusion probably not necessary.

Platelet count <20,000/mm³; patient not bleeding: Provide prophylactic platelet transfusion unless thrombocytopenia expected to be chronic, in which case transfuse only for bleeding.

Platelet count <50,000/mm³; patient bleeding or surgery anticipated: Use local measures to control bleeding; look for defects in coagulation pathways; maintain platelet counts at 50,000/mm³ or above with transfusion every 12 to 24 hours.

Platelet count <20,000/mm³; patient refractory to random platelet transfusion: Consider transfusion for evidence of bleeding, if retinal hemorrhages noted, or if platelet count is <10,000/mm³; use HLA-match platelets.

Granulocytopenia

Patient candidate for aggressive supportive care.

Granulocytes <500/mm³; afebrile, stable patient: No established indication for granulocyte transfusion.

Granulocytes <500/mm³; patient febrile, but cultures negative and no clinical evidence of infected area or tissue: No established indication for granulocyte transfusion.

Documented bacterial infection not improving after 48 hours of antibiotics to which the organism is sensitive in a patient with <500 neutrophils/mm³ and who is expected to have marrow aplasia for more than 1 week: Granulocyte transfusion indicated.

Some patients become refractory to HLA-matched platelets. Although this may be caused by antibodies to platelet-specific antigens, the physician should also consider the possibility of a drug-induced immune thrombocytopenia (*e.g.*, heparin or vancomycin) or the development of an autoantibody.[75] Although small randomized studies have not shown general benefit, high-dose intravenous immunoglobulin (400 mg/kg/day for 5 days) occasionally permits better platelet increments in platelet-refractory patients.[76-78] The patients who benefit possibly have a different mechanism of accelerated platelet destruction than the usual alloimmunized patient. Without a way to prospectively identify those who will benefit, given the minimal disadvantages of intravenous immunoglobulin other than cost, and because there are few alternative approaches,[79,80] an empiric trial of IgG seems reasonable for severely thrombocytopenic platelet refractory patients especially if they are bleeding.[112,113] For patients with no response to intravenous IgG, an empiric trial of plasmapheresis may be tried.

The physician must remain alert for DIC, thrombotic thrombocytopenia purpura (TTP), or hemolytic uremic syndrome (HUS) presenting as refractory thrombocytopenia. Particularly in advanced solid tumors (especially adenocarcinomas) DIC may present with thrombocytopenia, a normal or even short PT and PTT, and a normal or elevated fibrinogen, but the fibrin split products or D-dimer are usually elevated. A HUS-TTP-like syndrome may occur after allogeneic transplantation, possibly related to cyclosporine or TBI, and may mimic platelet refractoriness, but there is a concurrent microangiopathic hemolytic anemia with elevated LDH and schizocytes on the peripheral smear.

GRANULOCYTE TRANSFUSION

The frequency and severity of infection is inversely related to the number of circulating neutrophils and the duration of neutropenia. In 1966, Bodie and coworkers showed that, for patients with acute leukemia, the incidence of infection began to increase as the absolute neutrophil count fell below 1000/mm³.[81] For patients with breast cancer undergoing chemotherapy, the incidence of infection appears to increase below an absolute neutrophil count of 500/mm³.[82] It is likely that these differences are related to the immunosuppressive effect of the disease and to the concomitant mucositis often seen with induction therapy of acute leukemia, which increases the likelihood that intestinal bacteria will invade the bloodstream.

With the use of prophylactic platelet transfusions to prevent death due to bleeding, infection is the major cause of death for patients with acute leukemia, for whom pancytopenia lasts for several weeks.[83] There are no data that justify the use of prophylactic granulocyte transfusions. Several older prospective, randomized studies of the use of granulocyte transfusions reported an increase in survival rates, but the aggressive use of more potent antibiotics have markedly diminished the need for granulocyte transfusions.[84-87,99,100] However, for the severely neutropenic patient (<200/mm³), not expected to recover neutrophil counts for 1 week and with a documented bacterial or fungal infection not responding to appropriate antibiotics, granulocyte transfusions are still indicated. Profoundly neutropenic patients with progressive local infections such as cellulitis or perirectal infections may benefit from granulocyte transfusion.[88-96] For alloimmunized recipients, HLA-matched and granulocyte-compatible donors should be found.[97] CMV-seronegative donors should be used for seronegative recipients.[98] The granulocytes should be irradiated for severely immunosuppressed patients.

INTRAVENOUS IMMUNOGLOBULIN

Intravenous immunoglobulin is used to decrease the incidence of infection in cancer patients with hypogammaglobulinemia or impaired humoral immunity, to prevent and treat cytomegalovirus infection in bone marrow transplant patients, to treat several autoimmune disorders that may complicate particularly hematologic malignancies, and in some other selected situations.

The theoretical basis for the use of intravenous IgG in chronic lymphocytic leukemia, multiple myeloma, and low-grade lymphoma is the hypogammaglobulinemia, impaired antibody response to challenge even in the absence of lowered antibody levels, and possibly IgG subclass deficiency seen in these disorders and the high incidence of infection and death due to infection.[101,102] Because the major randomized study of intravenous IgG in chronic lymphocytic leukemia showed fewer moderate infections (*i.e.*, those requiring oral antibiotics) but not major infections (*e.g.*, those requiring intravenous antibiotics or hospitalization), and in view of the expense ($12,000–$16,000/year cost to the pharmacy) and inconvenience of prophylactic intravenous IgG, it would appear that the use of intravenous IgG should continue to be on a selective basis (*e.g.*, patients with recurrent sinopulmonary infections not responding to prophylactic oral antibiotics).

Another group of patients with apparently diminished B-cell reactivity are patients recovering from autologous or allogeneic bone marrow transplantation. After an uncomplicated allogeneic bone marrow transplantation, the total number of B cells return to normal in about 1 month, but the serum concentrations of IgG and IgM do not return to the normal range until 9 months, apparently due to delayed recovery of helper T cells.[103] Antibody production in response to antigenic stimulation is severely impaired in the first 3 months after allogeneic and syngeneic transplantation, indicating that it is not simply due to GVHD prophylaxis. Patients who develop acute or chronic GVHD experience substantial further delays in immune system reconstitution.

In a randomized prospective trial from Seattle, intravenous IgG (500 mg/kg weekly until day 90 and then monthly until day 360) reduced the incidence grade II through IV acute GVHD in patients older than 20 years of age, but no difference was observed in younger patients, possibly because of the low incidence in this group and the lack of adequate numbers to detect a difference; the results confirmed an earlier study of Winston and colleagues.[104,105] No increase in the rate of relapse or graft rejection was seen in the patients older than 20 in whom there was a reduction in GVHD. For those younger than 20 (in whom there had not been a reduction in GVHD), there was a 78% relapse rate compared with 47% for controls, but this difference appeared to be due to a larger number of advanced-stage patients in the immunoglobulin group. Determining whether the reduction in GVHD comes without an increase in graft rejection or relapse, as is the case with other measures that prevent GVHD, will need further confirmation. The incidence of gram-negative septicemia (positive culture with hypotension), but not bacteremia, was reduced. Overall, there was a reduction in the incidence of local infection from 144 (78%) in 185 control patients to 94 (51%) of 184 treated patients. No effect on the incidence of gram-positive or fungal septicemia was observed. In patients older than 20, there was a substantial reduction in the incidence of interstitial pneumonia (primarily due to CMV). Platelet recovery was accelerated (*i.e.*, median day of last platelet transfusion was 52 days in controls and 31 days in treated) and total platelet transfusion requirement reduced (*i.e.*, control patients required an average of 51 more units of platelets). This study is in line with most studies of intravenous IgG in the bone marrow transplantation setting in not finding a reduction of CMV infection but observing a modification of the severity of disease, primarily a reduced incidence of interstitial pneumonia and death.[106–108]

For CMV-seronegative recipients from CMV-seronegative donors, the exclusive use of CMV-negative blood products markedly reduces the incidence of CMV infection. For most transplants in which the donor or recipient is CMV positive, IgG is considered the standard of practice. There is great interest in the use of leukocyte-depleted blood products to decrease additional CMV exposure and the use of prophylactic ganciclovir to further reduce the incidence and severity of CMV infection. For the treatment of CMV pneumonia, intravenous immunoglobulin is generally given every other day concurrently with twice-daily full-dose ganciclovir. Prior studies had not shown a benefit for either agent alone. Although the ganciclovir prevents viral DNA replication, it does not prevent the host T-cell-mediated response to viral induced antigens on the surface of the lung cells. The IgG in this setting possibly coats the viral antigens or otherwise modifies the immunomediated lung parenchymal damage.

Intravenous immunoglobulin may be useful if autoimmune hemolytic anemia or thrombocytopenia complicate chronic lymphocytic leukemia, low-grade lymphoma, or other hematologic malignancies and for pure red cell aplasia due to persistent parvovirus B19.[109,110]

The consensus is that the current immunoglobulin preparations do not transmit HIV or hepatitis B or C.[114] Because of high levels of hepatitis B antibody, seronegative patients may become passively antibody positive for hepatitis B after infusion. A similar situation probably applies for hepatitis C, but this information is not yet available.

Adverse reactions to intravenous IgG are a function of the rate of infusion and the immunocompetence of the recipient. Overall, fewer than 1% of patients experience adverse reactions to IgG infusion, but approximately 10% of hypogammaglobulinemic patients who receive intravenous IgG for the first time or whose last treatment was over 6 to 8 weeks before infusion experience adverse reactions if the initial flow rate exceeds 1 ml per minute. Flushing of the face, chest tightness, chills, fever, nausea, vomiting, diarrhea, dizziness, wheezing, diaphoresis, and hypotension are the most common symptoms. When such symptoms occur, the infusion should be slowed or stopped. Pretreatment with steroids may be useful in the rare patient with recurrent symptoms. The explanation for the first dose effect is unknown, but it is thought that patients with low levels of immunoglobulin may build up an antigen load and that the first infusion of intravenous IgG results in the formation of a large number of antigen-antibody complexes and complement activation. With subsequent infusions, the rate can be increased, and for selected patients using 12% formulations and dissolving with water instead of saline, it may be possible to administer the IgG in 1 hour or less.[115] Because each lot of IgG is obtained from thousands of donors, any erythrocyte alloantibodies in the donors should be highly diluted, but occasionally, patients develop positive Coombs' tests or have frank hemolysis after IgG infusion.

APHERESIS

INDICATIONS

Apheresis, using the current generation of cell separators, has a limited but specific role to play in the management of malignant disease (Table 62–6).[116–128]

TABLE 62–6. Indications for Apheresis

Technique	Indications
Plasmaphersis	Hyperviscosity[114] syndrome in myeloma or Waldenstrom's with staph A column,[124–128] TTP/HUS
Leukapheresis	Hyperleukocytosis,[117] DIC in acute promyelocytic leukemia, CML in pregnancy,[121] to harvest lymphocytes for LAK cell production, for granulocyte transfusions
Platelet pheresis	Thrombocytosis with acute symptoms in polycythemia vera or essential thrombocytosis, for platelet transfusion
Photopheresis	Cutaneous T-cell lymphoma,[123] chronic graft-versus-host disease
Peripheral blood stem cell collection	Source of hematopoietic progenitor cells

In experienced hands, apheresis is a relatively safe procedure with minimal morbidity. Because citrate is used as an anticoagulant, hypocalcemia can develop, which usually manifests as paresthesias but can result in tetany or arrhythmias. Vasovagal reactions can result in hypotension, and this usually responds to volume infusion. If fresh-frozen plasma is used (*e.g.*, in the treatment of TTP), patients can have allergic reactions to the plasma and may acquire viral infections. Because of the catheters used for vascular access, complications may include thrombosis, bleeding, and infection. Overall, the incidence of minor morbidity is approximately 10%. Because at least 10 deaths have been reported with cytopheresis and more than 50 with plasmapheresis, this procedure should be reserved for specific, appropriate indications and only performed under the direction of physicians skilled in the use of this technique.[129,130]

PERIPHERAL BLOOD STEM CELLS

One of the newest and most exciting uses for apheresis is for the collection of peripheral blood stem cells (PBSC). Studies in the 1970s in mice, dogs, and humans demonstrated hematopoietic stem cells in the peripheral blood. It was subsequently observed that after moderate to high doses of chemotherapy, there was a rebound increase in the number of these hematopoietic stem cells in the peripheral blood for a few days. With the introduction of granulocyte-macrophage colony-stimulating factor (GM-CSF), granulocyte colony-stimulating factor, and interleukin-3 into clinical trials, it has been learned that these factors increase the number of stem cells in the peripheral blood. The combination of a stem cell-sparing chemotherapeutic agent (*e.g.*, cyclophosphamide) followed by growth factor in previously untreated patients dramatically increased PBSCs.[131]

PBSCs have been used primarily as a substitute for autologous marrow in patients with prior pelvic irradiation or for those with involvement of the marrow by tumor.[132] Many centers have reported engraftment rates similar to those obtained with autologous marrow. A second clinical use of major interest is the use of PBSCs to bone marrow and hematopoietic growth factors to accelerate neutrophil and platelet recovery after high-dose chemotherapy.[133,134]

The advantages of PBSCs over bone marrow include avoiding a general anesthetic, possibly accelerated hematopoietic recovery, the infusion of cryopreserved platelets with the stem cells, and the possible ability to exploit differences between peripheral blood and bone marrow stem cells with regard to cell number or function. Without chemotherapy or growth factor priming, 8 to 10 4-hour sessions are needed to collect an adequate number of cells. If chemotherapy priming is used, it generally must be intense enough to induce profound neutropenia, which may result in infection necessitating intravenous antibiotics and hospitalization. Heavily pretreated patients tend to show markedly diminished responses to growth factor priming. Some concern remains about the ability of PBSCs and particularly primed PBSCs to produce sustained engraftment of all cell lines after truly myeloablative preparative regimens.

BONE MARROW TRANSPLANTATION

AUTOLOGOUS BONE MARROW

The standard approach for autologous bone marrow harvesting is to perform multiple bone marrow aspirations from the posterior iliac crests in the prone position in the operating room under general anesthesia.[135] If one hemipelvis has been irradiated or the yield from the pelvis is poor, the patient can be turned and additional marrow aspirated from the anterior iliac crests and sternum. Generally, 1000 to 1200 ml of marrow are aspirated; 1500 to 2000 ml may be needed if the marrow will be purged because of loss of normal stem cells. The aspirated marrow is mixed with tissue culture medium and anticoagulated. A concentrate of mononuclear cells is often prepared by density-gradient centrifugation or by machine processing on a blood cell separator.[136–138] Next, purging is performed. In most cases, the marrow is then frozen using dimethyl sulfoxide (DMSO) or glycerol as a cryoprotectant and using a freezer that carefully controls the rate of freezing.[139] The marrow is stored in liquid nitrogen or in an electric freezer, but care must be taken with the latter to avoid power failure and accidental thawing. DMSO, in the concentrations used for cryopreservation, is toxic to normal stem cells at room temperature. Thawing should be accomplished rapidly at the patient's bedside and the marrow rapidly reinfused. Patients are routinely premedicated before autologous marrow infusion with hydrocortisone, diphenhydramine, and acetaminophen. Oxygen, intravenous fluids, and advanced cardiac life support medications are closely available.

Most patients experience some adverse reactions, which are thought to be due to the DMSO.[140,141] Most commonly, patients may have chills, fever, nausea, flushing, abdominal cramps, or vomiting. Dyspnea and a decrease in forced vital capacity may occur, which rarely results in respiratory failure. An increase in blood pressure and a decrease in heart rate are fairly common. Rarely, patients develop frank anaphylactic shock and death.[142] In patients who receive a double transplant, who develop urticarial or anaphylactic symptoms during the first transplant, consideration should be given to using glycerol as the cryoprotectant for subsequent harvests. Hematopoietic growth factors are now commonly given after autologous marrow infusion to accelerate neutrophil recovery.

MARROW PURGING

Most investigators think the primary reason for relapse after high-dose chemotherapy is the failure of the preparative regimen to eradicate disease in the patient and not due to reinfusion of a few malignant cells in the marrow. Nevertheless, marrow purging is an area of intense research interest and one that patients frequently focus on.

There are several ways to prevent reinfusion of malignant cells. One of the first methods used was monoclonal antibodies specific for antigens on the tumor cells but not on the pluripotent stem cells. These monoclonal antibodies are incubated with the mononuclear cell fraction in vitro before the addition of DMSO and freezing. In some cases, complement is added to causes cytolysis of the antibody coated cells; in others, the antibody is coupled to toxins (*e.g.*, ricin). The antibodies may be bound to magnetic spheres and the marrow subsequently passed through a strong magnetic field to extract the tumor cells. One of the limitations of negative purging is antigenic heterogeneity of the tumor cells and the possibility that the tumor stem cells may not express the antigens seen on the more differentiated cells, which are the primary cells represented when a tumor is screened.

Another method that uses monoclonal antibodies is called positive stem cell selection. In this approach, the antibodies are specific for antigens on the pluripotent stem cells but not on the tumor cells (*e.g.*, CD34). The antibodies may be attached to a column or bound to a specialized pan and the mononuclear cell fraction then poured in. Problems with this approach include nonspecific binding of tumor cells and the need to release the stem cells without damage. The magnetic bead approach can be adapted for positive stem cell collection. In this case, after separation of the normal stem cells in the magnetic field, a second monoclonal reagent is added that binds to the first near the Fab portion and alters its antigen binding site, releasing the stem cell unharmed.

Another strategy involves the in vitro incubation of the marrow with chemotherapy. The most commonly used agent has been 4-hydroperoxycyclophosphamide, which tends to spare the normal stem cells. In preclinical animal experiments, this approach eradicated leukemic cells in transplanted animals. One of the major problems with chemopurging is to ensure that the collateral damage to the normal stem cells is not so severe as to compromise hematopoietic recovery. The Seattle group reported that, if patients have graft failure after a chemopurged marrow autograft, GM-CSF frequently can not salvage the graft, presumably because there are not enough committed progenitors on which the growth factor can act.[143]

Although experience with autologous bone marrow transplantation after intensive therapy is improving with the advent of purging, relapses still occur. After relapse occurs, it is impossible to determine whether the origin of relapse arises from residual neoplastic cells in the purged bone marrow or from cells that escaped the cytotoxic effect of systemic preparative regimens. To resolve this problem and to provide a mechanism to monitor in vitro marrow manipulations, we and others have initiated the use of neutral safety-modified retroviruses for marking stem cells that are infused from purged autologous marrow. If the relapsed cells contain the genetic marker of the viral transgenome, relapse occurred from cells residual in the marrow after purging, suggesting that the methods used to purge the marrow were inadequate.

This marking procedure can be used to follow individual steps in the purging or positive stem cell selection process. Carried to its ultimate, this technique can lead to the purification of the hematopoietic progenitor cell if the infused marked populations are used for the transplantation after chemotherapy. By following the percentage of cells in each lineage and the lineage distribution of the retroviral transgenome, the researcher can identify the relative impact of a fractionation on the frequency representation of the hematopoietic progenitor cell.

ALLOGENEIC BONE MARROW

Another means for restoring marrow function in situations of marrow failure or after high-dose chemotherapy is the use of allogeneic bone marrow. The greatest experience has been using HLA-matched sibling marrow, although HLA-matched unrelated and HLA partially matched related (*e.g.*, from parent, child, or extended family) marrow are increasingly being used as techniques for preventing GVHD improve.

High-dose chemotherapy, with or without TBI, is given to the patient before the transplant to prevent graft rejection, to create space in the marrow, and to eradicate or cytoreduce the hematologic malignancy. The donor marrow is generally harvested as described for autologous transplantation about 1 week after the start of the high-dose chemoradiation preparative regimen, and the marrow is infused the same day as harvest without freezing. In some cases, the marrow is processed to partially deplete T cells or subsets of T cells to decrease the incidence and severity of GVHD. Immunosuppressive treatment, such as cyclosporine, methotrexate, or steroids, is usually given to the patient to prevent GVHD. The allogeneic marrow reconstitutes hematopoiesis, restoring leukocytes, platelets, and erythrocytes (often more quickly than with autologous transplant because the allogeneic marrow has not been exposed to cytotoxic agents), and provides a new immune system. It is this latter feature which differentiates allogeneic from autologous bone marrow transplantation, giving rise to the substantial morbidity and mortality of acute and chronic GVHD and to the graft-versus-leukemia (GVL) effect.

The cure rate with allogeneic bone marrow transplantation for severe aplastic anemia, leukemia, lymphoma, and other hematopoietic neoplasms is at least 50%. New methods of donor-recipient compatibility phenotyping (*e.g.*, polymorphism analysis with oligonucleotide and PCR or isoelective focusing analysis of HLA antigens) should reduce the incidence of GVHD as will new immunosuppressive drugs and tolerance induction regimens. Methods for stem cell fractionation using positive and negative selection procedures should decrease the morbidity and mortality of GVHD while preserving the GVL effect. Improvements in supportive care, such as new growth factors, ex vivo expansion of stem cells, and T-cell depletion, should improve the outcome of allogeneic bone marrow transplantation and expand its applicability.

CONCLUSION

An increasing number of patients will be eligible for intensive therapies in the future. Matched unrelated allogeneic transplantation is making transplant an option for patients without an HLA-matched sibling. Improved methods for the prevention and treatment of GVHD are increasing the upper age limit for this procedure. Autologous transplantation, which has established itself in the treatment of relapsed Hodgkin's and intermediate-grade non-Hodgkin's lymphoma, is increasingly applied in other hematologic malignancies and solid tumors. Conventional-dose chemotherapy is being intensified through the use of hematopoietic growth factors. For centers that deliver intensified therapies, the use of irradiated leukocyte-filtered blood products to prevent transfusion-induced GVHD decrease the incidence of chill and fever reactions, delay or prevent the development of platelet alloimmunization, and prevent the acquisition of CMV infection has become standard. It is essential for the initial treating physicians to be aware of these issues so that patients are not already CMV positive and alloimmunized by the time they are referred for more intensive therapies. Particularly for patients in whom prognostic variables at the time of diagnosis predict a high risk for relapse, consideration should be given early to the optimal timing for collection of bone marrow or peripheral blood stem cells and for employing all of the methods discussed to preserve the best opportunity for treatment with minimal morbidity and mortality.

It is anticipated that the next decade will bring tremendous technologic advances in our ability to collect, manipulate, and use stem cells, which undoubtedly represent the most pluripotent blood product.

REFERENCES

1. Wallerstein R Jr. Laboratory evaluation of the bleeding patient. West J Med 1989;150: 51–58.
2. Brubaker DB. Clinical significance of white cell antibodies in febrile nonhemolytic transfusion reactions. Transfusion 1990;30:733–737.
3. Perkins HA, Payne R, Ferguson J, et al. Nonhemolytic febrile transfusion reactions. Quantitative effects of blood components with emphasis on isoantigenic incompatibility of leukocytes. Vox Sang 1966;11:578–600.
4. Bodensteiner DC. Leukocyte depletion filters: A comparison of efficiency. Am J Hematol 1990;35:184–186.
5. Grossman BJ, Kollins P, Lau PM, et al. Screening blood donors for gastrointestinal illness: A strategy to eliminate carriers of *Yersinia enterocolitica*. Transfusion 1991;31: 500–501.
6. Tipple MA, Bland LA, Murphy JJ, et al. Sepsis associated with transfusion of red cells contaminated with *Yersinia enterocolitica*. Transfusion 1990;30:207–213.
7. Aber RC. Transfusion-associated *Yersinia enterocolitica*. Transfusion 1990;30:193–195.
8. Vogelsang GB. Transfusion-associated graft-versus-host disease in nonimmunocompromised hosts. Transfusion 1990;30:101–103.
9. Anderson KC, Weinstein HJ. Transfusion-associated graft-versus-host disease. N Engl J Med 1990;323:315–321.
10. Mollison PL. Blood transfusion in clinical medicine. Oxford: Blackwell Scientific, 1979: 578–583.
11. Perkins HA, Samson S, Garner J, et al. Risk of AIDS for recipients of blood components from donors who subsequently developed AIDS. Blood 1987;70:1604–1610.
12. Curran JW, Jaffe HW, Hardy AM, et al. Epidemiology of HIV infection and AIDS in the United States. Science 1988;239:610–616.
13. Medley GF, Anderson RM, Cox DR, et al. Incubation period of AIDS in patients infected via blood transfusion. Nature 1987;328:719–721.
14. Busch MP, Young MJ, Samson SM, et al. Risk of human immunodeficiency virus transmission by blood transfusions before the implementation of HIV-1 antibody screening. Transfusion 1991;31:4–11.
15. Busch MP, Eble BE, Khayam-Bashi H, et al. Evaluation of screened blood donations for human immunodeficiency virus type 1 infection by culture and DNA amplification of pooled cells. N Engl J Med 1991;325:1–5.
16. Petersen LR, Doll LS, et al. Human immunodeficiency virus type 1-infected blood donors: Epidemiologic, laboratory, and donation characteristics. Transfusion 1991;31: 698–703.
17. Doll LS, Peterson LR, White CR, et al. Human immunodeficiency virus type 1-infected blood donors: Behavioral characteristics and reasons for donation. Transfusion 1991;31: 704–709.
18. Epstein JS. Sensitivity and consistency of screening tests for antibodies to human immunodeficiency virus type 1. Transfusion 1991;31:388–389.
19. Perrin LH, Yerly S, Adami N, et al. Human immunodeficiency virus DNA amplification and serology in blood donors. Blood 1990;76:641–645.
20. Aach RD, Stevens CE, Hollinger FB, et al. Hepatitis C virus infection in post-transfusion hepatitis. N Engl J Med 1991;325:1325–1329.
21. Manns A, Blattner WA. The epidemiology of the human T-cell lymphotropic virus type I and type II. etiologic role in human disease. Transfusion 1991;31:67–75.
22. Hjelle B, Cyrus S, Swenson S, et al. Serologic distinction between human T-lymphotropic virus (HTLV) type I and HTLV type II. Transfusion 1991;31:731–736.
23. Donegan E, Busch MP, Galleshaw JA, et al. Transfusion of blood components from a donor with human T-lymphotropic virus type II (HTLV–II) infection. Ann Intern Med 1990;113:555–556.
24. Verdonck LF, Graan-Hentzen YC, Dekker AW, et al. Cytomegalovirus seronegative platelets and leukocyte poor red blood cells from random donors can prevent primary cytomegalovirus infection after bone marrow transplantation. Bone Marrow Transplant 1987;2:73–78.
25. Murphy MF, Metcalfe P, Thomas H, et al. Use of leukocyte-poor blood components to prevent primary cytomegalovirus (CMV) infection in patients with acute leukemia. Br J Haematol 1988;70:253–255.
26. De Gran-Hatzen YCE, Gratama JW, Mudde GC, et al. Prevention of primary cytomegalovirus infection in patients with hematologic malignancies by intensive white cell depletion of blood products. Transfusion 1989;29:757–760.
27. Gilbert GL, Hayes K, Hudson I, et al. Prevention of transfusion-acquired cytomegalovirus infection in infants by blood filtration to remove leukocytes. Lancet 1989;:1228–1231.
28. Bowden RA, Slichter SJ, Sayers MH, et al. Use of leukocyte-depleted platelets and cytomegalovirus-seronegative red blood cells for prevention of primary cytomegalovirus infection after marrow transplant. Blood 1991;78:246–250.
29. Hillyer CD, Snydman DR, Berkman EM. The risk of cytomegalovirus infection in solid organ and bone marrow transplant recipients: Transfusion of blood products. Transfusion 1990;30:659–666.
30. Shulman IA. Parasitic infections, an uncommon risk of blood transfusion in the United States. Transfusion 1991;31:479–480.
31. Schmuñis GA. Trypanosoma cruzi, the etiologic agent of Chagas' disease: Status of the blood supply in endemic and nonendemic countries. Transfusion 1991;31:547–557.
32. Wallerstein R Jr. Laboratory evaluation of the bleeding patient. West J Med 1989;150: 51–58.
33. Harker LA, Slichter SJ. The bleeding time as a screening test for evaluation of platelet function. N Engl J Med 1972;287:155–159.
34. Malpass TW, Harker LA. Acquired disorders of platelet function. Semin Hematol 1980;17:242–258.
35. Day HJ, Rao AK. Platelets and megakaryocytes: Semin Hematol 1986;23:89–101.
36. Kobrinsky NL, Gerrard JM, Watson CM, et al. Shortening of bleeding time by 1-deamino-8-D-arginine vasopressin in various bleeding disorders. Lancet 1984;1:1145–1148.
37. Gaydos LS, Freireich EJ, Mantel N. The quantitative relation between platelet count and hemorrhage in patients with acute leukemia. N Engl J Med 1962;266:905–909.
38. Menitove JE, Aster RH. Transfusion of platelets and plasma products. Clin Haematol 1983;12:239–266.
39. Gottschall JL, Rzad L, Aster RH. Studies of the minimum temperature at which human platelets can be stored with full maintenance of viability. Transfusion 1986;26:460–462.
40. Simon TL, Nelson EJ, Murphy S. Extension of platelet concentrate storage to 7 days in second-generation bags. Transfusion 1987;26:6–19.
41. Heal JM, Singal S, Sardisco E, et al. Bacterial proliferation in platelet concentrates. Transfusion 1986;26:388–390.
42. Braine HG, Kickler TS, Charache P, et al. Bacterial sepsis secondary to platelet transfusion: An adverse effect of extended storage at room temperature. Transfusion 1986;268:391–393.
43. Holohan TV, Terasaki P, Deisseroth A. Suppression of transfusion-related alloimmunization in intensively treated cancer patients. Blood 1981;58:122–128.
44. Dutcher JP, Schiffer CA, Aisner J, et al. Alloimmunization following platelet transfusion: The absence of a dose-response relationship. Blood 1981;57:395.
45. Claas FHJ, Smeenk RJT, Schmidt R, et al. Alloimmunization against the MHC antigens after platelet transfusions is due to contaminating leukocytes in the platelet suspension. Exp Hematol 1981;9:84–89.
46. Eernisee JG, Brand A. Prevention of platelet refractoriness due to HLA antibodies by administration of leukocyte-poor blood components. Exp Hematol 1981;9:77–83.
47. Daly PA, Schiffer CA, Aisner J, et al. Platelet transfusion therapy. One-hour post-transfusion increments are valuable in predicting the need for HLA-matched preparations. JAMA 1980;243:435–438.
48. Bishop JF, McGrath K, Wolf MM, et al. Clinical factors influencing the efficacy of pooled platelet transfusion. Blood 1988;71:383–387.
49. Schiffer CA. Prevention of alloimmunization against platelets. Blood [Editorial] 1991;77: 1–4.
50. Andreu G, Dewailly J, Leberre C, et al. Prevention of HLA immunization with leukocyte-poor packed red cells and platelet concentrates obtained by filtration. Blood 1988;72: 964–969.
51. Murphy MF, Metcalfe P, Thomas H, et al. Use of leukocyte-poor blood components and HLA-matched platelet donors to prevent HLA alloimmunization. Br J Haematol 1986;62:529–534.
52. Sniecinski I, O'Donnell MR, Nowicki B, et al. Prevention of refractoriness and HLA alloimmunization using filtered blood products. Blood 1988;71:1402–1407.
53. Saarinen UM, Kekomaki R, Siimes MA, et al. Effective prophylaxis against platelet

refractoriness in multitransfused patients by the use of leukocyte-free blood components. Blood 1990;75:512.

54. Van Marwijk Kooy M, van Prooijen C, Moes M, et al. Use of leukocyte-depleted platelet concentrates for the prevention of refractoriness and primary HLA alloimmunization: A prospective, randomized trial. Blood 1991;77:201–205.

55. Bock M, Wagner M, Knuppel W, et al. Preparation of white cell-depleted blood: Comparison of two bedside filter systems. Transfusion 1990;30:26–29.

56. Bodensteiner DC. Leukocyte depletion filters: A comparison of efficiency. Am J Hematol 1990;35:184–186.

57. Sirchia G, Wenz B, Rebulla P, et al. Removal of white cells from red cells by transfusion through a new filter. Transfusion 1990;30:30–33.

58. Van Marwijk Kooy M, van Prooijen HC, Borghuis L, et al. Filtration: A method of prepare white cell-poor platelet concentrates with optimal preservation of platelet viability. Transfusion 1990;30:34–38.

59. Steneker I, Biewenga J. Histologic and immunohistochemical studies on the preparation of white cell-poor red cell concentrates: The filtration process using three different polyester filters. Transfusion 1991;31:40–46.

60. Brecher ME, Pineda AA, Zylstra-Halling VW, et al. In vivo viability and functional integrity of filtered platelets. Transfusion 1990;30:718–721.

61. Rawal BD, Schwadron R, Busch MP, et al. Evaluation of leukocyte removal filters modelled by use of HIV-infected cells and DNA amplification. Blood 1990;76:2159–2161.

62. Sloand EM, Klein HG. Effect of white cells on platelets during storage. Transfusion 1990;30:333–338.

63. Högman CF, Gong J, Eriksson L, et al. White cells protect donor blood against bacteria contamination. Transfusion 1991;31:620–626.

64. Heal JM, Cohen HJ. Do white cells in stored blood components reduce the likelihood of post-transfusion bacterial sepsis? Transfusion [Editorial] 1991;31:581–583.

65. Capon SM, Sacher RA, Deeg HJ. Effective ultraviolet irradiation of platelet concentrates in Teflon bags. Transfusion 1990;30:678–681.

66. Deeg HJ. Ultraviolet irradiation in transplantation biology. Transplantation 1988;5:845–851.

67. Andreu G, Boccaccio C, Lecrubier C, et al. Ultraviolet irradiation of platelet concentrates: Feasibility in transfusion practice. Transfusion 1990;30:401.

68. Pamphilon DH, Potter M, Cutts M, et al. Platelet concentrates irradiated with ultraviolet light retain satisfactory in vitro storage characteristics and in vivo survival. Br J Hematol 1990;75:240.

69. Boccaccio C, Garcia I, Klaren J, et al. Ultraviolet irradiation of platelet concentrates: In vitro and in vivo preclinical evaluation. Transfus Sci 1990;11:141–147.

70. Pamphilon DH. Platelet concentrates and ultraviolet light. Transfus Sci 1990;11:149–152.

71. O'Connell BA, Schiffer CA. Donor selection for alloimmunized patients by platelet crossmatching of random-donor platelet concentrates. Transfusion 1990;30-4:314–317.

72. Daly PA, Schiffer CA, Aisner J, et al. Platelet transfusion therapy. One-hour post-transfusion increments are valuable in predicting the need for HLA-matched preparations. JAMA 1980;243:435–438.

73. Schiffer CA, Aisner J, Wiernik PH. Frozen autologous platelet transfusion for patients with leukemia. N Engl J Med 1978;299:7–12.

74. Dullemond AC, Prooijen HC, Riemens MI, et al. Cryo-preservation disturbs stimulus-response coupling in a platelet subpopulation. Br J Haematol 1987;67:325–333.

75. Christie DJ, Buren N, Lennon SS, Putnam JL. Vancomycin-dependent antibodies associated with thrombocytopenia and refractoriness to platelet transfusion in patients with leukemia. Blood 1990;75:518–523.

76. Berkman SA, Lee ML, Gale RP. Clinical uses of intravenous immunoglobulins. Ann Intern Med 1990;112:278–292.

77. Zeigler ZR, Shadduck RK, Rosenfeld CS, et al. High-dose intravenous gamma globulin improves responses to single-donor platelets in patients refractory to platelet transfusion. Blood 1987;70:1433–1436.

78. Lee EJ, Norris D, Schiffer CA. Intravenous immune globulin for patients alloimmunized to random-donor platelet transfusion. Transfusion 1987;27:245–247.

79. Sindet-Pederson S, Ramstrom G, Bernvil S, et al. Hemostatic effect of tranexamic acid mouthwash in anticoagulant-treated patients undergoing oral surgery. N Engl J Med 1989;320:840–843.

80. Mannucci PM. Desmopressin: A non-transfusional form of treatment for congenital and acquired bleeding disorders. Blood 1988;72:1449–1455.

81. Bodey GP, Buckley M, Sathe YS, et al. Quantitative relationships between circulating leukocytes and infection in patients with acute leukemia. Ann Intern Med 1966;64:328–340.

82. Esparza L, Yap HY, Smith T, et al. Quantitative relationship between degree of myelosuppression and infection in patients with metastatic breast cancer (MBC). Proc Am Soc Clin Oncol [Abstract C-348] 1983;2:39.

83. Bodey GP. Infection in cancer patients: A continuing association. Am J Med 1986;81:11–26.

84. Clift RA, Buckner CD. Granulocyte transfusions. Am J Med 1984;76:631–636.

85. Wright DG. Leukocyte transfusions: Thinking twice. Am J Med 1984;76:637–644.

86. Young LS. The role of granulocyte transfusions in treating and preventing infection. Cancer Treat Rep 1983;67:109–111.

87. Winston DJ, Ho WG, Gale RP. Therapeutic granulocyte transfusions for documented infections. Ann Intern Med 1982;97:509–515.

88. Strauss RG, Hester JP, Vogler WR, et al. A multicenter trial to document the efficacy and safety of a rapidly excreted analog of hydroxyethyl starch for leukapheresis with a note on steroid stimulation of granulocyte donors. Transfusion 1986;26:258–264.

89. Strauss RG, Goeken JA, Eckermann I, et al. Effects of intensive granulocyte donation on donors and yields. Transfusion 1986;26:441–445.

90. Robinson EAE. Single donor granulocytes and platelets. Clin Haematol 1984;13:186–216.

91. Strauss RG, Goeken JA, Imig KM. Effects on immunity of multiple leukapheresis using a rapidly excreted analog of hydroxyethyl starch. Transfusion 1986;26:265–268.

92. Hersman J, Meyers JD, Thomas E, et al. The effect of granulocyte transfusions on the incidence of cytomegalovirus infection after allogeneic marrow transplantation. Ann Intern Med 1982;96:149–152.

93. Dutcher JP, Schiffer CA, Johnson GS, et al. Alloimmunization prevents the migration of transfused indium-111-labeled granulocytes to sites of infection. Blood 1983;62:354–360.

94. Wright DG, Robichaum KJ, Pizzo PA, et al. Lethal pulmonary reactions associated with the combined use of amphotericin B and leukocyte transfusions. N Engl J Med 1981;304:1185–1189.

95. Dana BW, Durie GBM, White RF, et al. Concomitant administration of granulocyte transfusions and amphotericin B in neutropenic patients: Absence of significant pulmonary toxicity. Blood 1981;57:90–94.

96. Schiffer CA. Granulocyte transfusion therapy. Cancer Treat Rep 1983;67:113–119.

97. Buckner CD, Clift RA. Prophylaxis and treatment of infection of the immunocompromised host by granulocyte transfusions. Clin Haematol 1984;13:557–572.

98. Bowden RA, Sayers M, Flournoy N, et al. Cytomegalovirus immune globulin and seronegative blood products to prevent primary cytomegalovirus infection after marrow transplantation. N Engl J Med 1986;314:1006–1010.

99. Herzig RH, Herzig GP, Graw RG, et al. Successful granulocyte transfusion therapy from gram-negative septicemia. N Engl J Med 1977;296:701–705.

100. Alavi JB, Root RK, Djerassi I, et al. A randomized clinical trial of granulocyte transfusions for infection in acute leukemia. N Engl J Med 1977;296:706–711.

101. Berkman SA, Lee ML, Gale RP. Clinical uses of intravenous immunoglobulins. Ann Intern Med 1990;112:278–292.

102. Cooperative Group for the Study of Immunoglobulin in Chronic Lymphocytic Leukemia. Intravenous immunoglobulin for the prevention of infection in chronic lymphocytic leukemia. N Engl J Med 1988;319:902–907.

103. Atkinson K. Reconstruction of the haemopoietic and immune systems after marrow transplantation. Bone Marrow Transplant 1990;5:209–226.

104. Sullivan KM, Kopecky KJ, Jocom J, et al. Immunomodulatory and antimicrobial efficacy of intravenous immunoglobulin in bone marrow transplantation. N Engl J Med 1990;323:705–712.

105. Winston DJ, Ho WG, Lin C-H, et al. Intravenous immune globulin for prevention of cytomegalovirus infection and interstitial pneumonia after bone marrow transplantation. Ann Intern Med 1987;106:12–18.

106. Bowden RA, Sayers M, Flournoy, N, et al. Cytomegalovirus immune globulin and seronegative blood products to prevent primary cytomegalovirus infection after marrow transplantation. N Engl J Med 1986;314:1006–1010.

107. Verdonch LF, Middeldorp JM, Kreeft HAJG, et al. Primary cytomegalovirus infection and its prevention after autologous bone marrow transplantation. Transplantation 1985;39:455–457.

108. Levin MJ, Zaia JA, Spector SA, et al. Current approaches to the prevention and treatment of cytomegalovirus disease after bone marrow transplantation: An overview. Semin Hematol 1990(suppl 1);27:2.

109. Anderson LJ. Human parvoviruses. J Infect Dis 1990;161:603–608.

110. Frickhofen N, Abkowitz JL, Safford M, et al. Persistent B19 parovirus infection in patients infected with human immunodeficiency virus type I (HIV-I): A treatable cause of anemia in AIDS. Ann Intern Med 1990;113:926–933.

111. Berkman SA, Lee ML, Gale RP. Clinical uses of intravenous immunoglobulins. Ann Intern Med 1990;112:278–292.

112. Zeigler ZR, Shadduck RK, Rosenfeld CS, et al. High-dose intravenous gamma globulin improves responses to single-donor platelets in patients refractory to platelet transfusion. Blood 1987;70:1433–1436.

113. Lee EJ, Norris D, Schiffer CA. Intravenous immunoglobulin for patients alloimmunized to random-donor platelet transfusion. Transfusion 1987;27:245–247.

114. Wells MA, Wittek AE, Epstein JS, et al. Inactivation and partition of human T-cell lymphotropic virus, type III, during ethanol fractionation of plasma. Transfusion 1986;26:210–213.

115. Schiff RI, Sedlak D, Buckley RH. Rapid infusion of Sandoglobulin in patients with primary humoral immunodeficiency. J Allergy Clin Immunol 1991;88:61–67.

116. Linker CL. Plasmapheresis in clinical medicine. West J Med 1983;138:60–69.

117. Bunin NJ, Pui CH. Differing complications of hyperleukocytosis in children with acute lymphoblastic or acute nonlymphoblastic leukemia. J Clin Oncol 1985;3:1590–1595.

118. Gale RP, Foon KA. Chronic lymphocytic Leukemia. Ann Intern Med 1985;103:101–120.

119. Yam LT, Klock JC, Mielke CH. Therapeutic leukapheresis in hairy cell leukemia: Review of literature and personal experience. Semin Oncol 1984;11:493–501.

120. Golomb HM. The treatment of hairy cell leukemia. Blood 1987;69:979–983.

121. Fitzgerald D, Rowe JM, Heal J. Leukapheresis for control of chronic myelogenous leukemia during pregnancy. Am J Hematol 1986;22:213–218.

122. Rosenberg SA, Lotze MT, Muul LM, et al. A progress report on the treatment of 157 patients with advanced cancer using lymphokine-activated killer cells and interleukin-2 or high-dose interleukin-2 alone. N Engl J Med 1987;316:889–897.

123. Edelson R, Berger C, Gasparro F, et al. Treatment of cutaneous T-cell lymphoma by extracorporeal photochemotherapy. N Engl J Med 1987;316:297–303.

124. Ventura GJ, Buzdar AU, Kau S, et al. Clinical trail of plasma perfusion over immobilized staphylococcal protein A in metastatic breast cancer. Cancer Treat Rep 1987;71:411–413.

125. MacKintosh FR, Bennett K, Schiff S, et al. Treatment of advanced malignancy with plasma perfused over staphylococcal protein A. West J Med 1983;139:36–40.

126. Messerschmidt GL, Henry DH, Snyder HW, et al. Protein A immunoadsorption in the treatment of malignant disease. J Clin Oncol 1988;6:203–212.

127. Murgo AJ. Thrombotic microangiopathy in the cancer patient including those induced by chemotherapeutic agents. Semin Hematol 1987;24:161–177.

128. Korec S, Schein PS, Smith FP, et al. Treatment of cancer-associated hemolytic syndrome with staphylococcal protein A immunoperfusion. J Clin Oncol 1986;4:210–215.

129. Hazards of apheresis. Lancet 1982;2:1025–1026.

130. Council on Scientific Affairs. Current status of therapeutic plasmapheresis and related techniques: Report of the AMA panel on therapeutic plasmapheresis. JAMA 1985;253: 819–825.

131. Siena S, Bregni M, Brando B, et al. Circulation of CD34⁺ hematopoietic stem cells in the peripheral blood of high-dose cyclophosphamide-treated patients: Enhancement by intravenous recombinant human granulocyte-macrophage colony-stimulating factor. Blood 1989;74:1905–1914.

132. Kessinger A, Armitage JO. The evolving role of autologous peripheral stem cell transplantation following high-dose therapy for malignancies. Blood 1991;77:211–213.

133. Gianni AM, Bregni M, Siena S, et al. Rapid and complete hemopoietic reconstitution following combined transplantation of autologous blood and bone marrow cells. A changing role for high-dose chemo-radiotherapy? Hematol Oncol 1989;7:139–148.

134. Siena S, Bregni M, Brando B, et al. Flow cytometry for clinical estimation of circulating hematopoietic progenitors for autologous transplantation in cancer patients. Blood 1991;77:400–409.

135. Thomas ED, Storb R. Technique for human marrow grafting. Blood 1970;36:507–515.

136. Beaujean F, Gourdin MF, Farcet JP, et al. Separation of large quantities of mononuclear cells from human blood using a blood processor. Transfusion 1985;25:152–154.

137. English D, Lamberson R, Graves V. Semiautomated processing of bone marrow grafts for transplantation. Transfusion 1989;29:12–16.

138. Areman EM, Cullis H, Spitzer T, et al. Automated processing of human bone marrow can result in a population of mononuclear cells capable of achieving engraftment following transplantation. Transfusion 1991;31:724–730.

139. Gorin NC. Collection, manipulation and freezing of haemopoietic stem cells. Clin Haematol 1986;15:19–48.

140. Davis JM, Rowley SD, Braine HG, et al. Clinical toxicity of cryopreserved bone marrow graft infusion. Blood 1990;75:781–786.

141. Stroncek DF, Fautsch SK, Lasky LC, et al. Adverse reactions in patients transfused with cryopreserved marrow. Transfusion 1991;31:521–526.

142. Rapoport AP, Rowe JM, Packman CH, et al. Case report: Cardiac arrest after autologous marrow infusion. Bone Marrow Transplant 1991;7:401–403.

143. Nemunaitis J, Singer JW, Buckner CD, et al. Use of recombinant human granulocyte-macrophage colony-stimulating factor in graft failure after bone marrow transplantation. Blood 1990;76:245–253.

SECTION **2**

JANICE L. GABRILOVE
DAVID W. GOLDE

Hematopoietic Growth Factors

The cellular elements of the blood are essential to life and may be viewed as operating centrally in host defense. The erythrocytes protect against hypoxia and function solely to deliver oxygen to the tissues. Erythrocytes are anucleate and survive for about 120 days in the peripheral blood. Platelets defend against bleeding and play a primary role in the initiation of hemostasis and clotting; they circulate in the blood for approximately 8 days.

Neutrophils are primarily concerned with defense against microorganisms, particularly bacteria and fungi and they have a half-life in the peripheral blood of only about 8 hours. The other granulocytes include the eosinophils and basophils whose role in host defense is not clearly defined although the eosinophils function importantly in extracellular killing of large parasites.

The monocytes are the blood form of the mononuclear phagocyte system and are important in antimicrobial function and the removal of organic and inorganic debris. The tissue component of the mononuclear phagocyte system comprises the resident macrophages in most tissues and organs, including the Kupffer cell of the liver, the alveolar macrophage of the lung, and the Langerhans cell of skin. Tissue macrophage populations can be self-sustaining and are not critically dependent on an influx of precursor cells from the bone marrow.

The circulating T and B lymphocytes respectively comprise the cell-mediated and humoral arms of the immune system. Some T and B cells may live for many years, perhaps for the person's life span.

Surprisingly, this diverse and highly specialized array of blood cells originates from a common stem cell in the bone marrow. A stem cell may be defined as a cell with extensive ability to reproduce itself and to differentiate along several lineages.[1] The totipotent hematopoietic stem cell is normally quiescent but is capable of giving rise to all hematopoietic lineages and repopulating lethally irradiated recipients. This repopulating property of stem cells is critical to the success of bone marrow transplantation. The mouse hematopoietic stem cell has been enriched to high purity, and human stem cells thought to have pluripotent repopulating capability have been isolated.[2] The ability to isolate and cryopreserve human stem cells will have considerable impact on autotransplantation for cancer and for allogeneic procedures. Positive selection of stem cells may be a potent means of purging bone marrow of malignant cells and reducing the incidence of graft-versus-host disease in the allogeneic situation.

As pluripotent stem cells differentiate, they become restricted to one or more hematopoietic lineages. Ultimately, commitment to a single lineage occurs, such as for the erythroid lineage. The process of stem cell differentiation is poorly understood, although the "decision" along which lineage to differentiate is thought to be stochastic (*i.e.*, random). However, the microenvironment can influence this decision, and environmental influences probably play an important role in initiating stem cell replication. The important manifestation of lineage commitment is the expression of receptors for specific hematopoietic hormones. The expression of receptors allows the cell to respond to hormonal signals in the environment and ultimately produce mature cells in appropriate numbers for the specific function required.

HUMORAL REGULATION OF HEMATOPOIESIS

Mature blood cells are produced at a prodigious rate. Approximately 10 billion erythrocytes, neutrophils, and platelets are produced in the average person every hour, and this baseline production can be increased many fold in times of need. Most of the regulation of mature blood cell production occurs in the morphologically identifiable pools in the bone marrow, and under stable conditions, it is thought that few stem cells enter the active cell cycle.

The various hormones that regulate hematopoiesis are known as hematopoietic growth factors or hematopoietins, and considerable information has been obtained about their molecular biology, biochemistry, and therapeutic use. Substantially less is known about the physiology of the hematopoietic growth factors, particularly their function in daily regulation of hematopoiesis. Erythropoietin is clearly identified as the major regulator of erythrocyte production, but relatively little is known about the specific hormones regulating the production of platelets.

PRINCIPLES OF THERAPY WITH HEMATOPOIETIC GROWTH FACTORS

Because the blood cells are concerned with host defense, the primary reason for giving growth factors is to improve or optimize the patient's host defense capabilities. Although most clinicians are comfortable with the concept of replacement therapy, such an approach does not play a major role in hematopoietic growth factor treatment in cancer. For growth factors other than erythropoietin, serum levels may be difficult to measure, or the hormone may not circulate, and measurement may provide little guide to therapy. The clinician must think in terms of regulating blood cell production in the face of complex circumstances, frequently involving the administration of chemotherapy, infection, and bone marrow failure.

Physiologic responses, although normal, are seldom optimal. The erythropoietic response to an important change in altitude occurs over time and not with sufficient rapidity to be optimal. Adaptation to altitude could be optimized by erythropoietin administration, and similarly, host defense against microorganisms and tumors must aim at an optimal response. Such principles may be difficult to put into practice because the ideal blood counts for a patient at a given time can be difficult to ascertain. A normal neutrophil count may be inadequate in some circumstances. Despite incomplete information, the physician must decide the appropriate level of circulating mature cells for a given situation. Using the hematopoietic growth factors, we can regulate the production of erythrocytes, neutrophils, eosinophils, and monocytes, but we still do not have a growth factor to regulate thrombopoietin, although interleukin-3 (IL-3) shows some potential in this regard. Because the hematopoietic growth factors also regulate mature cell function, the therapist must consider the number of effector cells and their level of activation. The identification of functional defects usually requires special testing, but the oncologist should be aware of the specific alterations in mature cell function induced by administration of the hematopoietic growth factors.

Because the host defense system marshals cellular defenses against a biologically hostile environment, recognition becomes the crucial element in directing effector cell function. In autoimmunity, recognition is confused, and the host defense system may be subverted to attack normal tissue. Because several hematopoietic growth factors play a crucial role in inflammation, the possibility of host defense cell damage to normal tissues is an important complicating issue that should be considered. Activated mature host defense cells may cause appropriate inflammation, and hematopoietic growth factors may have effects on nonhematopoietic tissues that could be therapeutically deleterious. To be effective, the hematopoietic hormones must have target cells expressing appropriate receptors, and if they are absent due to bone marrow aplasia, therapeutic intervention is ineffective. The clinician must decide with incomplete information how the use of hemato-

poietic growth factors can optimize the cancer patient's ability to fight infection, transport oxygen, and prevent bleeding. Ultimately, strategies for using hematopoietic growth factors to treat cancer itself will depend on appropriately directing the immune system and the various effector cells.

ERYTHROPOIETIN

Erythropoietin is the circulating hormone primarily responsible for regulating the rate of red blood cell production in the bone marrow (Fig. 62–2).[3] Erythropoietin is a glycoprotein hormone, approximately 90% of which is produced in the kidneys and 10% in the liver. The hormone was purified in 1977 from human urine, and its molecular mass was about 34 kd.[4] In 1985, the gene for human erythropoietin and its cDNA was molecularly cloned. The gene is single copy and consists of five exons. The cDNA sequence predicts a molecule of 18,398 d, and the most highly purified protein has a specific activity approaching 200,000 units per milligram of protein. Erythropoietin for clinical use is produced in Chinese hamster ovary cells and is glycosylated with a total molecular weight of about 29,900 and a specific activity of 120,000 units per milligram of protein.

Erythropoietin interacts with precursor cells in the bone marrow expressing the erythropoietin receptor. The erythropoietin receptor has been molecularly cloned and is part of the hemopoietin receptor superfamily. It has an extracellular ligand binding domain, a transmembrane region, and an intracellular portion that lacks an intrinsic tyrosine kinase domain. The erythropoietin receptor is expressed by cells committed to erythroid differentiation under control of specific transcription factors. Erythroid precursors respond to erythropoietin by replication and maturation, and erythropoietin is necessary for cellular development to the mature erythrocyte. Under conditions of maximal erythropoietin stimulation, erythropoiesis can be expanded approximately tenfold.

Erythropoietin produced in the kidney is synthesized and elaborated largely in response to the need for oxygen-carrying capacity. The oxygen "sensor" links erythropoietin synthesis to oxygen-carrying demand. If a normal person moves to a higher altitude, relative hypoxemia is sensed, and erythropoietin elaboration is increased, which leads to increased erythrocyte production and homeostasis being achieved at the higher hematocrit necessary for normal oxygen-carrying capacity. After the person returns to sea level, erythropoietin elaboration is decreased in response to excess oxygen-carrying capacity, and the hematocrit drops appropriately. The relation between the hematocrit and plasma erythropoietin concentration is shown in Figure 62–3. Physiologic responses tend to be suboptimal, and in disease states, compensatory mechanisms are often inadequate. In the anemia of chronic inflammation, for example, plasma erythropoietin levels are low relative to the degree of anemia.[5–7]

Anemia in cancer patients is common, and the specific causes should be determined by careful investigation. Blood loss, iron deficiency, vitamin B_{12} or folate deficiency, hemolysis, chemotherapy, drug toxicity, hypersplenism, and tumor involvement of the bone marrow may occur in various combinations. There is an entity known as the anemia of cancer. Although this may not be a specific process, careful study of

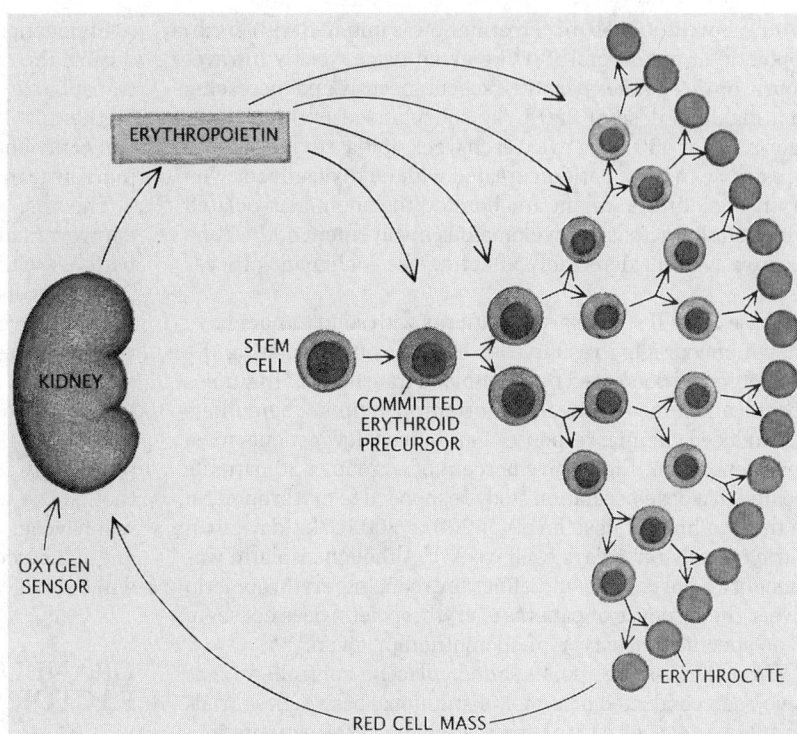

FIGURE 62–2. Regulation of red cell mass by erythropoiesis. (Golde DW. Hormones that stimulate the growth of blood cells. Sci Am 1988;259:62–70)

these patients has shown that they have an inadequate erythropoietin response for a given degree of anemia.[7] Relative erythropoietin deficiency may exist in otherwise hematologically uncomplicated tumors. Malignancies of hematopoietic tissue clearly interfere with normal erythrocyte production, but pharmacologic doses of erythropoietin can be effective. A central element in considering the potential benefit of erythropoietin therapy is the adequacy of the endogenous erythropoietin response, which is best evaluated by a plasma erythropoietin concentration interpreted with regard to the hematocrit.

In addition to impaired erythropoietin response to anemia in cancer patients, there may be a diminished responsiveness of bone marrow erythroid precursors to erythropoietin. The cause of this reduced responsiveness of the bone marrow to erythropoietin is uncertain, but inflammatory cytokines such as interleukin-1 (IL-1) and tumor necrosis factor (TNF) elaborated in association with malignant disease can impair erythropoiesis. Erythropoietic impairment may be due to decreased responsiveness and decreasing elaboration of erythropoietin.[8] The anemia of cancer is pathophysiologically similar to the anemia of chronic inflammation, as occurs in active rheumatoid arthritis. The cancer patient may have reduced hematopoietic progenitors because of cytotoxic chemotherapy, radiation therapy, or disruption of the marrow architecture by invasion of malignant cells.

Recombinant erythropoietin is cleared from the circulation in an exponential fashion with a half-life of 9.3 ± 3.2 hours. After seven treatments with erythropoietin, the half-life tends to decrease by about 30%. In normal persons, the mean half-life is 4 to 6 hours after intravenous injection. Subcutaneous delivery results in peak serum levels of about 5% of those achieved after an equivalent intravenous dose, and the time necessary to reach peak serum levels is 5 to 24 hours. Peak levels after intravenous administration are achieved in 0.5 hour. The disposal of erythropoietin is poorly understood. Less than 10% is excreted by the kidneys, and small amounts are cleared by the liver. No dose modifications are recommended for renal or hepatic failure.

Early trials of erythropoietin in cancer involved patients with anemia associated with marrow infiltration with non-Hodgkin's lymphoma and multiple myeloma.[8–11] These patients had modestly elevated endogenous erythropoietin levels

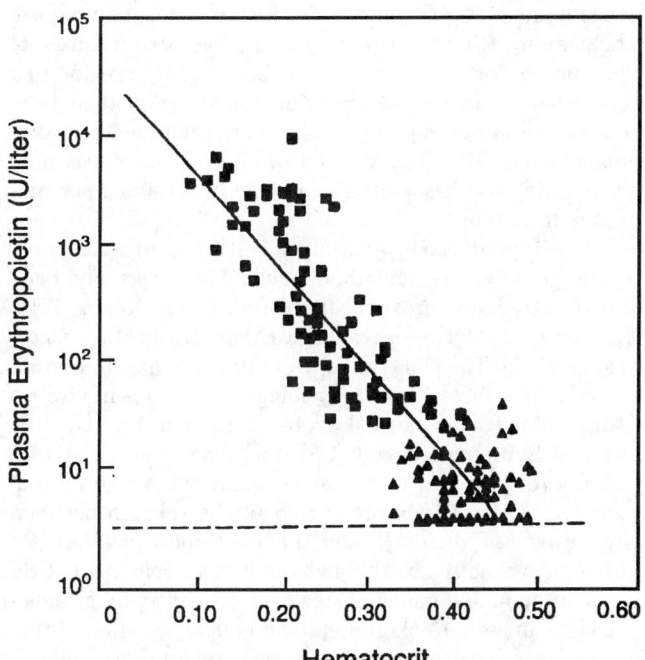

FIGURE 62–3. Relation of plasma erythropoietin concentration to hematocrit in 175 persons. (Erslev AJ. Erythropoietin. N Engl J Med 1991;324:1339–1344)

rarely above 200 mU/ml. Treatment was initiated with erythropoietin at a dose of 150 U/kg given twice weekly intravenously or three times per week subcutaneously and increasing to a maximal dose of 250 U/kg subcutaneously three times each week or 450 U/kg twice each week. Initial studies showed a response in most patients treated with no toxic effects. The erythropoietin treatment ameliorated the anemia associated with lymphomatous or myelomatous involvement of the bone marrow without detectably affecting the malignant process itself.

Phase I and II studies using patients with solid tumors have shown encouraging results with increases in circulating hemoglobin and decreased need for blood transfusion.[8] In studies specifically aimed at the use of erythropoietin in chemotherapy-induced anemia, responses in relatively few patients were dose dependent. Eighty-five percent of a group of 30 patients treated in a dose-escalation study responded to erythropoietin in the two highest dose levels of 200 to 300 IU/kg/day given intravenously for 5 days each week.[12] Although cisplatin was thought to have a specific effect on reducing erythropoietin levels, the response of patients to erythropoietin does not seem to be specific to the type of chemotherapy given.[13]

Three large-scale, double-blind, placebo-controlled trials have been conducted on a multiinstitutional basis. These trials enrolled a total of 413 patients, including 124 patients in a no-chemotherapy group, 157 patients in a no-cisplatin group, and 132 patients in a cisplatin-receiving group of patients. In each of these trials, patients randomized to erythropoietin treatment had a significantly greater increase in hematocrit than patients receiving placebo. In analyzing the two chemotherapy trials, there was a significantly lower transfusion requirement in the erythropoietin-treated patients during the second or third month of the trial. Quality of life parameters were improved for patients receiving erythropoietin whose hematocrit increased by 6% or more.[8]

The studies indicate that erythropoietin treatment can ameliorate the anemia associated with cancer and chemotherapy, reduce the need for transfusions, and possibly enhance the quality of life. The reduced need for transfusion is the major objective of erythropoietin therapy, reducing the cost, inconvenience, and potential toxicity of blood transfusions.

The question of dose is problematic because efficacy depends in part on the relative impairment of erythropoietin elaboration with respect to the degree of anemia and in part on the level of impaired responsiveness of the bone marrow.[14] A reasonable starting point is 150 U/kg subcutaneously thee times each week. This amounts to approximately 10,000 U for a 70-kg person. Patients with lower plasma erythropoietin concentrations may respond to lower doses of erythropoietin, and higher doses may be needed in patients with apparent bone marrow resistance to erythropoietin. The timing of erythropoietin administration with respect to chemotherapy or radiation therapy has not been sufficiently studied. Most investigations have involved erythropoietin administration concomitantly with chemotherapy. Given our current understanding of the physiology and pathophysiology of erythropoietin responses, this approach does not appear to be ideal. Subsequent investigations may show high-dose administration of erythropoietin for a limited time after chemotherapy to be more efficacious and cost effective.

Endogenous erythropoietin responses tend to be blunted during the 2 or 3 weeks immediately after bone marrow transplantation preceded by intensive chemotherapy and radiotherapy, suggesting that impaired erythropoietin response can contribute to the delayed erythrocyte recovery after bone marrow transplantation.

The role of erythropoietin therapy in myelodysplasia is controversial, with some studies showing responses only in patients with the lowest pretreatment endogenous erythropoietin levels.[15-18] Intensive, high-dose erythropoietin therapy has shown responses in a higher percentage of patients with myelodysplasia. One study showed responses in 24% of patients receiving erythropoietin at a dose of 1200 to 1600 U/kg intravenously twice weekly.[19]

None of the studies of erythropoietin in cancer have reported any significant toxicity due to the erythropoietin, although the cost is significant. It appears that erythropoietin will have an important role in ameliorating the multifactorial anemia associated with cancer, and ultimately, this efficacy will be judged by the decreased need for transfusion.

GRANULOCYTE COLONY-STIMULATING FACTOR

Granulocyte colony-stimulating factor (G-CSF) is a glycoprotein that regulates the production and function of neutrophil granulocytes. G-CSF was originally identified as a leukemia differentiation factor that could be detected in murine serum or lung-conditioned medium after endotoxin administration.[20] Purification revealed that this leukemia differentiation activity was identical to a colony-stimulating factor that exclusively supported the growth of neutrophil granulocyte precursors. Human G-CSF was first purified to homogeneity from the human bladder carcinoma cell line, 5637; subsequently, the gene for human G-CSF and its cDNA were molecularly cloned. The gene for G-CSF is single copy and has been localized to the long arm of chromosome 17 (17q11–q23), a region that contains other genes previously demonstrated or thought to be involved in neutrophil granulocyte development. Recombinant human G-CSF, produced in *Escherichia coli*, is nonglycosylated and has a specific activity of 10^8 units per milligram of protein.[21]

G-CSF is produced by a variety of cell types, including neutrophil granulocytes, endothelial cells, fibroblasts, and bone marrow stromal cells after stimulation by endotoxin, TNF, IL-1, or granulocyte-macrophage colony-stimulating factor (Table 62–7). The cell type representing the most important source of this factor under physiologic conditions in vivo remains unknown. In normal adults (>20 years), circulating levels of immunoreactive G-CSF range between 20 and 95 pg/ml, are unrelated to age or sex, and exhibit no diurnal variation. There is controversy about the relation between circulating G-CSF levels and the neutrophil count under physiologic conditions. Although the precise role that G-CSF plays in the maintenance of steady-state neutrophil granulopoiesis is uncertain, Hammond and colleagues showed that normal dogs can develop neutralizing antibodies to canine G-CSF after administration of human recombinant G-CSF, and they develop profound neutropenia.[22] This result suggests that G-CSF is critical for the regulation and production of neutro-

TABLE 62–7. Sources of Colony-Stimulating Factors

Cell Type	Stimulus	G-CSF	GM-CSF	IL-3	M-CSF
T-lymphocytes	Antigen, lectin IL-1		+	+	
			+		
B-lymphocytes	LPS, TPA		+		
Natural killer cells	IL-2/CD16 phorbol diester, calcium ionophore		+		+
				+	
Macrophages	LPS, IL-3, γIFN, GM-CSF	+*			+
		+			
		+			+
Mast cells	IgE, calcium ionophore		+		
Osteoblasts	PTH, LPS		+		
Mesothelial cells	EGF, TNF		+		
Endothelial cells	IL-1	+	+		
Fibroblasts	TNF	+			
	IL-1		+		
Neutrophils	γIFN, GM-CSF	+			
Bone marrow stroma	IL-1	+	+		+

G-CSF, granulocyte colony-stimulating factor; GM-CSF, granulocyte-macrophage colony-stimulating factor; IL-3, interleukin-3; M-macrophage colony-stimulating factor; LPS, lipopolysaccharide; TPA, 12 tetradecanoylphorbol 13 acetate; IL-1, interleukin-1; IL-2, interleukin-2; γIFN, gamma interferon; PTH, parathyroid hormone; EGF, endothelial growth factor; TNF, tumor necrosis factor.
* +, possesses this biologic activity.

phil granulocytes. In bacteremia, in which the characteristic leukocytosis is neutrophilic, G-CSF levels have exceeded 2000 pg/ml, providing additional evidence that G-CSF is systemic regulator of neutrophil production.[23]

G-CSF promotes the survival and stimulates the growth and expansion of immature neutrophil granulocyte precursor cells, enriched promyelocytes, and myelocytes. G-CSF enhances the effector cell capability of the neutrophil granulocyte (Table 62–8) and functions as a weak chemoattractant for these same terminally differentiated cells. G-CSF induces human vascular endothelial cells to proliferate and migrate.

Low numbers of high-affinity receptors for G-CSF exist on normal and malignant myeloid cells and on endothelial cells, placenta, and certain nonhematopoietic tumor cell lines.[24]

TABLE 62–8. Effects of Colony-Stimulating Factors on Myeloid Cells

Factor	Progenitors	Mature Cells			
		Neutrophil	Eosinophil	Basophil	Monocyte
GM-CSF	Stimualtes CFU-GEMM, CFU-GM, and BFU-E	ADCC, phagocytosis, degranulation, superoxide production, viability, arachidonic acid release, Mo1 expression, cytokine production, changes in cell surface receptor (FMLP) expression, leukotriene and PAF synthesis chemoattractant migration inhibition	ADCC, phagocytosis, viability, cytotoxicity, leukotriene production	Histamine release	ADCC, cytotoxicity, cytokine production, oxidative metabolism, adherence, chemoattractant
G-CSF	Stimulates CFU-G and pre-CFU	ADCC, enhances migration, changes in cell surface receptors for FMLP, weak chemoattractant			
IL-3	Stimulates CFU-GEMM, CFU-GM, BFU-E, CFU-blast		ADCC, cytotoxicity, phagocytosis	Histamine release	ADCC, cytotoxicity
M-CSF	Stimulates CFU-M				ADCC, cytotoxicity

CFU-GEMM, colony-forming unit granulocyte erythroid, megakaryocyte monocyte macrophage; CFU-GM, colony-forming unit granulocyte macrophage; BFU-E, burst forming unit erythroid; CFU-G, colony-forming unit granulocyte; CFU, colony-forming unit; CFU-M, colony forming unit monocyte macrophage; ADCC, antibody-dependent cellular cytotoxicity; FMLP, F-MET-LEU-PHE; PAF, platelet-activating factor.

The molecular mass of the receptor observed in cross-linking experiments is about 150 kd. The high-affinity receptor for human G-CSF has been cloned and found to have an amino-terminal immunoglobulin domain, three fibronectin type III regions, and four conserved cysteine residues characteristic of the cytokine receptor superfamily. A portion of the extracellular domain of the G-CSF receptor exhibits a striking similarity to the prolactin receptor and some similarity to the NCAM family of adhesion molecules. A G-CSF receptor molecule with a deleted transmembrane domain has been cloned, suggesting that it is secreted and can function as a soluble binding protein.[24]

Preclinical studies demonstrated the ability of G-CSF to augment the number of functionally normal neutrophil granulocytes in normal and tumor-bearing mice, hamsters, and cynomolgus monkeys. This neutrophil granulocytosis results from an augmentation in the number of divisions and a reduction (from 96 to 24 hours) in the time required for maturing neutrophil granulocyte precursors to develop into terminally differentiated cells released into the circulation.[25] G-CSF reduced the period of neutropenia in cynomolgus primates treated with high-dose cyclophosphamide, busulfan, or total-body irradiation with autologous marrow reinfusion and in dogs given DLA-identical littermate transplants. G-CSF is radioprotective and can augment survival in murine and canine models of supralethal irradiation without bone marrow rescue.[26]

Three initial human studies revealed that an intravenous bolus, continuous intravenous infusion, subcutaneous injection, or continuous subcutaneous infusion of G-CSF resulted in a dose-dependent increase in the circulating neutrophil granulocyte count.[27-29] This increase in absolute neutrophil count was due primarily to an increase in mature segmented polymorphonuclear leukocytes and was associated with an expansion of the bone marrow myeloid compartment. Morphologic changes (*e.g.*, Döhle bodies, toxic granulations, decreased nuclear lobulation) observed in neutrophil granulocytes after G-CSF are consistent with the marked reduction in the bone marrow transit time of neutrophil precursors mediated by G-CSF. Neutrophil granulocytes produced in response to G-CSF have been shown to be functionally normal, as measured by phagocytic, in vitro, or in vivo migration assays, or to be activated, as evidenced by an increase in leukocyte alkaline phosphatase. An intravenous dose of G-CSF results in an initial decline in the circulating neutrophil count followed by a subsequent rise, with a peak value achieved 4 to 6 hours after G-CSF treatment. After a subcutaneous injection, no initial decline in the neutrophil count is observed, and the maximal neutrophil count achieved is observed 10 to 12 hours after the administered dose of G-CSF. The time at which a blood count is drawn must be taken into account when evaluating a patient's neutrophil response to G-CSF treatment. On discontinuation of G-CSF, neutrophil counts decrease by one half daily and generally return to baseline within 4 days of discontinuing treatment.

Other hematopoietic cell lineages are unaffected by the administration of G-CSF except at higher doses (>60 μg/kg/day, intravenously), for which an increase in circulating monocytes has been reported.[27]

Intravenous and subcutaneous administration of G-CSF is effective for rapidly elevating G-CSF levels in serum. After a single intravenous injection, the peak serum concentration achieved and area under the concentration-time curve are dose dependent. The elimination half-life is about 3.5 hours.[27] After subcutaneous injection, peak levels are achieved within 4 to 6 hours, and levels of more than 10 ng/ml are maintained for 10 to 16 hours thereafter.[30] The mode of G-CSF clearance is unknown.

Neutropenia in cancer patients is a major cause of morbidity and mortality and results from malignant disease and its treatment. Phase I and II studies using a broad spectrum of commonly employed chemotherapeutic regimens demonstrated the ability of G-CSF to accelerate recovery from chemotherapy-induced neutropenia (Table 62–9). In all of these studies, G-CSF was administered 24 hours after cessation of chemotherapy. Optimization of timing and duration of G-CSF treatment has been investigated in patients receiving high-dose melphalan.[31] This study demonstrated accelerated recovery from neutropenia even when G-CSF treatment was begun 8 days after chemotherapy. The ability to delay the use of G-CSF, but not GM-CSF, and commence treatment closer to the time of expected nadir most likely results from the ability of G-CSF to rapidly mobilize neutrophil granulocytes from the bone marrow mitotic compartment. These data suggest that the rate limiting step for G-CSF-mediated recovery from neutropenia is the availability of G-CSF-responsive progenitors.

Based on the phase I and II trials, a randomized, double-blind, placebo-controlled trial of G-CSF was designed to definitively evaluate the incidence of infection as manifested by fever with neutropenia (absolute neutrophil count <1000 cells/μl at 38.2°C).[32] A total of 211 patients were randomly assigned to receive placebo (110) or G-CSF (101), of which 199 were evaluable for efficacy. At least one episode of fever with neutropenia occurred in 77% of placebo group and 40% of the G-CSF-treated group. Over all cycles of chemotherapy, the median duration of severe neutropenia (<500 cells/μl) was 6 days with placebo and 1 day with G-CSF. During cycles of blinded treatment, the days of intravenous antibiotic use, hospitalization, and the incidence of confirmed infections were reduced by 50% with G-CSF administration compared with placebo.

This pivotal phase III trial and earlier studies led to the approval of G-CSF in the United States, Europe, and Japan to reduce the incidence of infection manifested by febrile neutropenia in adult and pediatric patients with nonmyeloid malignancies receiving myelosuppressive chemotherapy. Although only limited data exist for the use of G-CSF for myelosuppressive chemotherapy in the pediatric population, considerable data show a comparable safety profile of G-CSF for children and adults. The recommended starting dose is 5 μg/kg/day subcutaneously to begin after the cessation of chemotherapy, with careful monitoring of blood counts thereafter to avoid leukocytosis. Treatment should be discontinued when the absolute neutrophil count is more than 10,000 cells/μl, after the expected chemotherapy-induced nadir.

Although G-CSF has been of clinical benefit in the treatment of chemotherapy-induced myelosuppression, the use of G-CSF after myeloablative chemotherapy for acute myelogenous leukemia is more controversial. Ohno and colleagues conducted a prospective randomized trial of G-CSF in patients with de novo acute myelogenous leukemia, leukemic trans-

TABLE 62–9. Clinical Trials of G-CSF in Cancer Treatment

Investigations	Phase	G-CSF Dose + Route	Tumor Type	Chemotherapy	No. of Patients	Major Findings
Chemotherapy						
Bronchud[29]	I–II	1–40 µg/kg I.V. 14 days	Small cell lung cancer	Doxorubicin (50 mg/m²), Ifosfamide (5 g/m²), Mesna (8 g/m²) day 1; Etoposide (120 mg/m²/d) days 1–3; repeat q 21 days	12	Decrease in the days of neutropenia, decrease in febrile neutropenia, decrease antibiotic use
Gabrilove[27]	I–II	1–60 µg/kg/d I.V. 8 days (d 4–11)	Transitional cell urothelial carcinoma	Methotrexate (30 mg/m²) days 0, 14, 21; Vinblastine (3 mg/m²) days 1, 14, 21; Doxorubicin (30 mg/m²) and Cisplatin (70 mg/m²) day 1; repeat q 28 days	40	Decrease in days of neutropenia, decrease in febrile neutropenia, decrease antibiotic use, decrease mucositis, increase in patients qualified to receive full dose chemotherapy on schedule
Morstyn[28]	I–II	0.3, 1 or 3 µg SC or 3–10 µg/kg CSCl	Metastatic malignancies day 1	Melphalan (25 mg/m²)	15	Decreased leukopenia
Morstyn[31]	I–II	0.3–10 µg/kg/d SC 5 schedules 1) d 2–13 2) d 8–13 3) d 2–18 4) d 8–18 5) −9 to −2 + d 2–13	Metastatic malignancies	Melphalan (25 mg/m²) day 1	31	Decreased leukopenia
Crawford[32]	III double-blind, randomized, placebo-controlled trial	5 µg/kg/day	Small cell lung cancer	Cyclophosphamide (1 g/m²); Etoposide (120 mg/m² d 1–3) Doxorubacin (50 mg/m²d 1)	210	Statistically significant decrease in days of neutropenia, statistically significant decrease in febrile neutropenia, statistically significant decrease in documented infections
Dose-Intensified Chemotherapy						
Bronchud[37]	I–II	5 µg/kg/day C1 × 11 d	Ovarian and breast carcinoma	Doxorubacin 75, 100, 125, or 150 mg/m² q 14 days	21	Dose escalation of doxorubicin to 100 mg/m² q 2 weeks
Neidhart[38]	I–II	23–69 µg/kg I.V. d 8–28	Refractory malignancy	Cisplatin (105 mg/m²) Etoposide (1500 mg/m²) Cyclophosphamide (5 g/m²)	18	Dose intensity able to be delivered
Bone Marrow Transplantation						
Sheridan[34]	I–II	20 µg/kg/d SC: scheduled dose reductions: 5 µg/kg/d ANC >1000 × 3 days; 1 µg/kg/d if ANC >1000 × 3 days on 5 µg/kg/d 28 days total treatment	Hodgkin's/non-Hodgkin's lymphoma, germ cell, ALL, ANLL	Busulfan (4 mg/kg/d) days −7 to −4; Cyclophosphamide (60 mg/kg/d) days −3 and −2	15	Reduction in days of neutropenia compared to historic controls

(continued)

TABLE 62–9. *(Continued)*

Investigations	Phase	G-CSF Dose + Route	Tumor Type	Chemotherapy	No. of Patients	Major Findings
Taylor[35]	I–II	60 μg/kg/d scheduled dose reductions: 30 μg/kg/d if ANC >2500 × 3 days, 8 μg/kg/d if ANC increase further on 30 μg/kg/d 28 days (max)	Hodgkin's disease	Cyclophosphamide (1.5 g/m^2/d) days −6 to −3; carmustine (300 mg/ m^2); day −6; etoposide (125 mg/m^2 q 12 h) days −6 to −4	18	Reduction in days of severe neutropenia (<200 cells/μl and <500 cells/μl)
Peters[36]	I–II	16–64 μg/kg C1 × 14 days	Breast cancer or melanoma	Cyclophosphamide (5625 mg/m^2), cisplatin (165 mg/m^2), carmustine (600 mg/m^2)	15	Reduction in days of neutropenia

formation from myelodysplastic syndrome (MDS), acute lymphocytic leukemia, or blastic phase of chronic myelogenous leukemia after mitoxantrone, etoposide, and bentenoyl-cytosine arabinoside therapy.[33] G-CSF significantly accelerated the recovery of neutrophils, reduced the incidence of documented infection, and did not preferentially promote the regrowth of leukemic cells.

G-CSF has been used in patients with breast carcinoma, Hodgkin's disease, and non-Hodgkin's lymphoma undergoing autologous bone marrow transplantation.[34–36] The G-CSF administered after ablative therapy was effective in augmenting recovery from neutropenia compared with historic controls.

Although treatment with G-CSF has rendered standard cancer treatment more tolerable with respect to neutropenia and its complications, a larger question remains about whether it will permit significant intensified therapy and whether such therapy will contribute to improved survival for cancer patients. Bronchud and colleagues demonstrated that G-CSF allowed administration of dose-intensified doxorubicin (100 mg/m^2 every 2 weeks) for three cycles to patients with ovarian or breast carcinoma refractory to standard-dose chemotherapy.[37] Treatment resulted in a response rate of 80%. Neidhart and coworkers demonstrated the ability of G-CSF to reduce grade IV neutropenia and antibiotic requirements in patients treated with dose-intensified cisplatin (150 mg/m^2), etoposide (150 mg/m^2), and cyclophosphamide (5 g/m^2).[38] These two studies show that dose-intensified chemotherapy is feasible, but a significant period of neutropenia was observed despite concomitant treatment with G-CSF. The use of earlier-acting hematopoietic growth factors or specific progenitor populations harvested from the peripheral blood will probably be required to provide greater protection from myelosuppression and permit safe study of dose-intensified regimens.

Neutropenia is an important problem in hematopoietic malignancies, pancytopenic states, acquired immunodeficiency syndrome (AIDS), and genetic disorders of granulocyte production. Pilot studies of G-CSF in patients with hairy cell leukemia, myelodysplastic syndrome, and aplastic anemia have demonstrated improvements in circulating neutrophil counts associated in some instances with a decrease in the incidence of or enhanced recovery from active infection.[39–41] No evidence of treatment-induced proliferation of the malignant clone has been observed. G-CSF, administered alone or in combination with erythropoietin, can ameliorate zidovudine-induced myelotoxicity in patients with AIDS without stimulating p24 antigen expression.[42] Initial pilot studies of G-CSF in patients with primary neutropenic disorders (*e.g.*, cyclic neutropenia, congenital neutropenia, idiopathic neutropenia) demonstrated the ability of G-CSF to augment circulating neutrophil counts, reduce the incidence of infection and mucositis, and improve quality of life parameters.[43–45] These preliminary findings have been confirmed by a phase III randomized trial of G-CSF in patients with severe chronic neutropenia, suggesting that this hematopoietic growth factor can play an important role in the management and treatment of these disorders.

Treatment with G-CSF is generally well tolerated, with the most consistent and significant clinical side effect being "medullary" bone pain. This bone discomfort is felt most in the lower back, pelvis, and sternum and is usually experienced within a 24-hour period as the neutrophil count begins to recover. It is observed most commonly after intravenous administration. Chronic G-CSF administration in patients with primary neutropenia has been associated with the detection of clinically inapparent splenomegaly as measured by magnetic resonance imaging or computed tomography scanning in 13% of patients. This effect of G-CSF is more commonly seen in children. Other unusual side effects, reported in single patients, have included a flare in psoriasis, recurrence of Sweet's syndrome (*i.e.*, cutaneous neutrophilic vasculitis) and cutaneous vasculitis.

GRANULOCYTE-MACROPHAGE COLONY-STIMULATING FACTOR

Granulocyte macrophage colony-stimulating factor (GM-CSF) is one of a family of glycoproteins that have potent effects in stimulating the proliferation and function of hematopoietic cells. Human GM-CSF was purified by Gasson and colleagues from a human T-cell leukemia virus (HTLV-II)-infected T-lymphoblastoid cell line.[46] The purified protein was identical to the previously described T-lymphocyte-derived lymphokine referred to as neutrophil-migration inhibition factor. Human GM-CSF is highly and variably N- and O-glycosylated, accounting for a wide range in reported molecular weights (14–35 kd). The complementary cDNA encoding the human GM-CSF protein was molecularly cloned by Wong and coworkers.[47] The gene for human GM-CSF is single copy and has been mapped by in situ hybridization to the long arm of chromosome 5 (5q23–31). This region contains a number of growth factors and receptors that are involved in the regulation of hematopoiesis and the inflammatory response. Complementary DNA encoding GM-CSF has been expressed in Chinese hamster ovary cells (CHO cells), yeast, and *E. coli*. The three forms of recombinant GM-CSF, which have been produced for clinical use, have specific acclivies of 4.4×10^6 units, 5×10^7 units, and 2×10^8 units per milligram of protein, respectively.

GM-CSF is produced by activated T lymphocytes, B lymphocytes, endothelial cells, mast cells, fibroblasts, macrophages, mesothelial cells, and osteoblasts in response to specific activating agents (see Table 62–7). GM-CSF is also constitutively produced by a number of tumor cell lines and placenta. Unlike G-CSF, GM-CSF is not detectable in serum under physiologic conditions, suggesting that GM-CSF normally acts in a paracrine fashion. Analogous to IL-1, GM-CSF has been detected in synovial fluid from patients with inflammatory arthropathies, suggesting that it might play a role in the tissue damage associated with the inflammatory process.

GM-CSF supports the in vitro growth of uncommitted multilineage precursors (in the presence of erythropoietin) and committed cells (*i.e.*, granulocyte, monocyte) precursor cells (see Table 62–8). In addition to its effects on bone marrow progenitors, GM-CSF enhances the function of mature neutrophil and eosinophil granulocytes and monocytes and macrophages. The effects of GM-CSF on mature effector cells of several lineages, in contrast to G-CSF, may reflect the wide role of this cytokine in host defense and the inflammatory response (see Table 62–8). GM-CSF directly affects neutrophil expression of cellular adhesion molecules, locomotion, responsiveness to chemotactic factors, biosynthetic function, and tumoricidal and phagocytic activity. Priming effects of GM-CSF on neutrophils include stimulation of the respiratory burst, degranulation and enhanced synthesis of mediators of inflammation such as leukotrienes, platelet-activating factor, and elaboration of cytokines such as TNF, M-CSF, IL-1, and G-CSF. In the presence of GM-CSF, mature eosinophils and macrophages demonstrate enhanced tumoricidal and phagocytic activity. In contrast to M-CSF, GM-CSF is a more potent inducer of secondary cytokines secreted by monocytes, such as IL-1 and TNF-α, perhaps accounting for the difference in side effects reported in vivo with these two molecules. GM-CSF has enhanced the replication of human immunodeficiency virus (HIV) in normal monocytes and macrophages and potentiated the anti-HIV activity of zidovudine by facilitating drug entry and subsequent phosphorylation.

Similar to G-CSF, M-CSF, and IL-3, GM-CSF was produced by some blasts obtained from patients with acute myelogenous leukemia. Controversy exists about whether this represents constitutive production or induction secondary to in vitro cell manipulation. GM-CSF has also been shown, as have G-CSF and IL-3 but not M-CSF, to augment the proliferation of myeloid leukemic cells. Progenitors derived from patients with

juvenile chronic myelogenous leukemia exhibit an enhanced sensitivity to the stimulatory effects of GM-CSF.[48] Overexpression of GM-CSF in murine bone marrow results in a myeloproliferative syndrome that is fatal but nonneoplastic.[49] A comparable model employing G-CSF results in sustained neutrophilia and organ infiltration by neutrophilic granulocytes without organ damage or premature death.[50] A role for GM-CSF in the pathogenesis of myeloid leukemias is uncertain.

Receptors for GM-CSF exist on normal neutrophils and their precursors, eosinophils, and monocytes and macrophages.[24,51] These cells normally express a low number of high-affinity binding sites with dissociation constants of 30 to 100 pM. High-affinity receptors have been found on cell lines derived from small cell carcinoma, malignant myeloid (HL-60 and KG-1), and monocytoid (U937) leukemias and on nonhematopoietic tissue, such as placenta and endothelial cells.[24] Low-affinity binding sites have been identified on malignant hematopoietic cells and on COS cells, human melanoma, osteogenic sarcoma, and breast carcinoma cell lines and primary melanoma.[24] Controversy exists about whether these low-affinity receptors mediate proliferation in all cells in which it is expressed. The low-affinity human GM-CSF receptor (α subunit) has been cloned and sequenced and localized to the pseudoautosomal region of the sex chromosomes. Hayashida and colleagues isolated a human homolog of the murine IL-3 receptor cDNA, which encodes a 120-kd transmembrane adapter protein (β subunit) that confers high-affinity binding to the low-affinity (α) GM-CSF receptor.[51] Specific α subunits exist for GM-CSF, IL-5, and IL-3 receptors, but they share and may compete for the same B subunit.

In preclinical studies, the administration of human GM-CSF to normal rhesus monkeys resulted in a dramatic leukocytosis consisting initially of only neutrophil granulocytes and monocytes followed by an additional substantial increase in eosinophil granulocytes.[52] Treatment was associated with significant reticulocytosis, but no changes in hemoglobin or hematocrit were observed. A model of pancytopenia induced by simian type D retrovirus in rhesus monkeys provided data supporting the clinical application of GM-CSF in patients with AIDS, bone marrow failure states, and infectious disease.[52] Models investigating the utility of GM-CSF after total-body irradiation and autologous bone marrow reinfusion demonstrated the myelorestorative effect of GM-CSF in the transplant setting and provided the framework for designing clinical trials with humans.

The initial clinical investigation of GM-CSF, which was the first clinical study of a hematopoietic growth factor in humans, was conducted using 16 relatively well patients with AIDS and leukopenia.[53] Continuous intravenous infusion of CHO cell-derived recombinant GM-CSF (0.3–4.5 μg/kg/day for 14 days) resulted in a dramatic augmentation in circulating granulocytes and with a lesser increase in monocytes. Neutrophils produced in 6 of these patients exhibited improved phagocytosis and antibody-dependent cellular cytotoxicity. Additional studies evaluating the safety of *E. coli*-derived GM-CSF and the chronic subcutaneous administration of CHO cell-derived GM-CSF showed improved leukocyte counts and enhanced monocyte function in treated patients with AIDS; however, treatment has been associated with an increase in serum HIV p24 antigen in some cases, suggesting stimulation of HIV replication.[54] In patients randomized to receive GM-CSF after chemotherapy for HIV-associated non-Hodgkin's lymphoma, there was a more than twofold increase in HIV p24 compared with controls.[55] In contrast, the subcutaneous administration of nonglycosylated GM-CSF to HIV patients receiving ganciclovir or yeast-derived GM-CSF to patients with AIDS-associated Kaposi's sarcoma receiving zidovudine and interferon-α has not been associated with any discernible stimulation of HIV replication and has resulted in the abrogation of therapy-associated neutropenia.[56] Similarly, the administration of zidovudine alternating with GM-CSF in patients previously treated with GM-CSF alone is associated with a return to baseline of serum HIV p24 values, permitting patients to receive zidovudine who otherwise could not tolerate conventional doses of antiviral medication. These data suggest that, although GM-CSF holds promise for use in AIDS in combination with antiviral agents, there are a number of complex interactions that still require investigation. The impressive leukocyte responses observed in these studies also underscores the remarkable sensitivity of leukopenic AIDS patients to low doses of GM-CSF. Although these patients are highly responsive to GM-CSF, they also seem to be more sensitive to toxic effects and often do not tolerate chronic administration well.

In hematologically normal and leukopenic cancer patients, a dose-dependent increase in neutrophils is observed after short or continuous intravenous infusion and subcutaneous injection of CHO cell, yeast, and bacterially derived GM-CSF; intravenous bolus of nonglycosylated GM-CSF appears to be less efficacious. Patients who have received extensive prior chemotherapy or radiotherapy exhibit the smallest elevations in circulating leukocytes in response to GM-CSF treatment. The neutrophils produced in response to GM-CSF appear to function normally, as measured by phagocytosis and generation of superoxide; however, impaired migration in vivo has been reported in patients receiving continuous intravenous infusions of CHO cell-derived GM-CSF but not bacterially derived GM-CSF administered as a 4-hour infusion.[57,58]

After the administration of CHO cell or bacterially derived GM-CSF (given as a short or continuous intravenous infusion), there is an immediate transient neutropenia, eosinopenia, and monocytopenia. The time of maximal nadir is 30 minutes, with a rebound in leukocyte count to baseline or above baseline by 2 hours. Radionucleotide labeling studies show that this leukopenia is due primarily to sequestration within the lungs.[59] After subcutaneous administration, the nadir occurs 60 minutes after treatment and can persist for up to 4 hours.

In addition to neutrophilia, treatment with GM-CSF results in an augmentation of circulating monocytes with, in some instances, enhanced tumoricidal activity. The ability to stimulate monocyte-macrophage number and function may be responsible for the reported serum cholesterol lowering activity of GM-CSF. Eosinophils also increase after 7 days of treatment with GM-CSF. No consistent effects on hemoglobin, reticulocyte, or platelet counts have been found after treatment with GM-CSF; however, the occurrence of thrombocytopenia secondary to reactivation of idiopathic thrombocytopenic purpura has been reported.

The augmentation in circulating leukocyte counts after glycosylated and nonglycosylated GM-CSF administration is associated with an 18-fold and eightfold increase in circulating myeloid and erythroid hematopoietic precursor cells, respec-

tively.[60] Additional studies in chemotherapy-naive patients demonstrated impressive mobilization of peripheral blood progenitors (up to 1000-fold) when GM-CSF is administered after myelosuppressive chemotherapy.[61] No comparable changes in bone marrow progenitors have been reported, although marrow cellularity and myeloid-to-erythroid cell ratios are increased; however, an increase in the percentage of bone marrow-derived myeloid and erythroid progenitors, myeloblasts, promyelocytes and myelocytes in S phase has been observed in patients receiving 3 and 6 days of yeast-derived GM-CSF.[62] An increase in the rate of hematopoietic cells entering the cell cycle, a decrease in the actual cell cycle time, and a decrease in the duration of the S-phase portion of the cell cycle has also been reported. After discontinuation of GM-CSF, the proportion of cells in S phase decreases to values below that observed before treatment. These findings suggest a period where hematopoietic cells may exhibit relative refractoriness to cell-cycle-specific antineoplastic agents.

The pharmacokinetics of glycosylated GM-CSF and nonglycosylated GM-CSF have been extensively studied. A two-compartment model has been determined for both with comparable elimination times: $T_{1/2}\alpha$ of 10 ± 3 minutes and a $T_{1/2}\beta$ of 85 ± 35 minutes for yeast-derived GM-CSF; $T_{1/2}\alpha$ of 5 minutes and $T_{1/2}\beta$ of 150 minutes for bacterially derived GM-CSF.[30] In contrast, a rise in detectable GM-CSF levels occurs within 1 hour, peaks in 2 to 4 hours, and declines 2 to 12 hours after subcutaneous administration of nonglycosylated GM-CSF. The time during which nonglycosylated GM-CSF remains detectable is dose dependent. After the injection of 10 μg/kg nonglycosylated GM-CSF, plasma levels of GM-CSF equivalent to the maximal activity required to stimulate progenitor cell development and granulocyte-monocyte function are achieved and are detectable for 12 hours.

Several studies have explored the role of glycosylated and nonglycosylated GM-CSF in ameliorating the myelosuppression associated with autologous bone marrow transplantation for breast carcinoma, melanoma, lymphoid malignancies, and non-Hodgkin's lymphoma (Table 62–10).[63–65] The first trial in this clinical setting demonstrated that CHO cell-derived GM-CSF, administered as a continuous intravenous infusion beginning 3 hours after autologous marrow infusion, resulted in accelerated recovery of circulating leukocyte counts and reduced bacteremia, hepatotoxicity, and nephrotoxicity compared with historic controls.[63] A second historically controlled trial of yeast-derived GM-CSF administered as a daily 2-hour infusion for 14 days, beginning 1 hour after completion of autologous or allogeneic bone marrow transplantation, demonstrated that treatment (at doses >60 μg/m^2) resulted in fewer days of neutropenia (neutrophil count <500 cells/μl), fever, and required platelet transfusions.[64] No enhancement of graft-versus-host disease was found in the few patients receiving allogeneic transplants.

A randomized, double-blind, placebo-controlled trial of yeast-derived GM-CSF after autologous bone marrow transplantation for lymphoid cancer was later completed.[65] Sixty-three patients received daily 2-hour infusions of GM-CSF for 21 days, beginning within 4 hours of marrow infusion, and 63 patients received placebo. The patients treated with GM-CSF had a recovery of neutrophils to 500 cells/μl 7 days earlier than patients who received placebo, 3 fewer days of antibiotics,

(text continues on page 2288)

TABLE 62–10. Clinical Trials of GM-CSF in Cancer Treatment

Investigations	Phase	GM Prep	GM Dose + Route	Tumor Type	Chemotherapy	No. of Patients	Results
Chemotherapy							
Antman[63]	I–II	Glycosylated CHO cell	CI	Sarcoma	Isofamide, doxorubicin, dacarbazine	16	Less severe and shorter neutropenia: no difference in febrile neutropenia
Gianni[65]	I–II	Glycosylated (CHO)	CI 5.5 μg/kg/d d 1–14	Breast, non-Hodgkin's lymphoma	Cyclophosphamide (7 g/m^2)	15	Reduction in the duration of neutropenia, decrease in infections complications
De Vries[67]	II	Glycosylated (CHO)	SC 0.25–0.75 μg/m^2	Ovarian carcinoma	Carboplatin, cyclophosphamide	15	Improved hematologic (neutrophil and platelet count) recovery after successive cycles of chemotherapy
Morstyn[64]	I–II	Nonglycosylated	SC 5–15 μg/kg/d d 7–21	Small Cell Lung carcinoma	CBDCA Etoposide	18	Improved neutrophil counts
Hermann[67]	II	Nonglycosylated	SC 6.1 μg/kg/d 10 days	Various	Several regimens	22	Reduction in duration neutropenia earlier neutrophil nadir improved delivery of chemotherapy on schedule reduction in infectious episodes
Barloggie[66]	I–II	Nonglycosylated	SC 0.25–0.75 mg/m^2	Multiple myeloma	Melphalan	23	Reduction in duration of neutropenia in younger patients with adequate hematopoietic reserve
Logethetis[69]	I	Nonglycosylated	SC or CI d 3–13 120–500 μg/m^2	Bladder carcinoma	Methotrexate, vinblastine	32	Reduction in severity and duration of granulocytopenia
Bone Marrow Transplantation							
Nemunaitis[61]	I	Glycosylated (yeast)	I.V. (2h) 1–250 μg/m^2 × 21 days	Lymphoid cancers	Cyclophosphamide and total-body irradiation	15	In patients receiving ≥60 μg/m^2, the following was observed: enhanced neutrophil count recovery, decrease in episodes of infection, reduction in days of hospitalization, and decrease in the number of days to become platelet transfusion independent
Brandt[60]	I	Glycosylated (CHO)	Continuous I.V.	Breast carcinoma and melanoma	Cyclophosphamide, cisplatin, carmustine	19	Enhanced recovery of neutrophil count, decrease in transplant-associated morbidity with decrease in elevations of creatinine and bilirubin and decrease in bacteremia
Nemunaitis[62]	III (randomized, double blind)	Glycosylated (yeast)	250 μg/m^2 2-h I.V. infusion × 21 days	Lymphoid cancers		126	Decrease in neutropenic (<500 cells/μl) days, decrease in infectious episodes, decrease in antibiotic requirements, decrease in the days of hospitalization

TABLE 62–11. Clinical Trials of Hematopoietic Growth Factors in Myelodysplastic Syndrome

Investigations	Growth Factor	Dose	Route and Schedule	No. of Patients	Prior Therapy	MDS Subtype	Blasts in Bone Marrow (%)	Blasts in Blood (%)	Results: Decreased RBC TX	Decreased Platelets TX	Other Findings	POD to AML
Vadhan-Raj	Glycosylated GM (yeast)	30–500 μg/m²	Continuous infusion (CI) × 14 d every 2 wk	8	2 hormonal/ vitamin 4 Dauna/Ara-C	1 RA 3 RAEB 3 RAEBIT 1 Hypoplasia after Chemo RX	>10% (6)	0/8 with circulating blasts	2/4 (1 who had hypoplasia p RX)	2/8 (1 had hypoplasia p RX)	Increase WBC and ANC	0
Rifkin	Glycosylated GM (yeast)	30–480 μg/m²	Subcutaneous 4 wk	11	NA	RA RAEB + RAEBT	NA	NA		1	Increase in ANC (10/11) Increase in retics (2/11) 2 patients progressed to acute leukemia	
Antin	Glycosylated GM (yeast)	15–480 μg/m²	Short intravenous infusion 7 or 14 d	7	NA	2 RA 4 RAEB	NA	NA	No change	No change	Increase in ANC, monocytes and reticulocytes (6/ 7) increase in eosinophils (2/ 7) increase in blasts (2/7)	0
Ganser	Nonglycosylated GM (E. coli)	15–50 μg/m²	Intravenous (I.V.) bolus day 1: 8 hour infusion, thereafter ×	11	1 LDAra-C	3 RA 4 RAEB 2 CMMOL	>14% (4)	4/11	No change	No change	Increase WBC and ANC (8/ 11), increase bone marrow and circulating blasts in 1 patient with no prior circulating blasts: increase circulating blasts in 1 patient with prior circulating blasts	5
Thompson	Nonglycosylated GM (E. coli)	0.3–10 μg/kg/d	Subcutaneous (SC) daily × 28 d	16	7 hormonal/ vitamin 1 LDAra-C	7 RA 8 RAEB 1 RAEBIT	≥10% (8)	NA	No change	No change	Increase ANC (12/16), increase monos/ eos (10/16), transient increase in retics (2).	1

				N	Prior RX	Diagnosis					Comments
Estey	Glycosylated GM	120 µg/m²	CI	22	NA	17 RAEBT	NA	NA	NA	2	Increase in bone marrow blasts (5) decrease bone marrow blasts (4); Increase in ANC in all patients; Increase bone marrow blasts (4/22); increase platelets (2/22)
Hermann	Nonglycosylated GM and yeast-derived GM (E. coli)	5–750 µg/m² × 5	I.V. q 5 h q 10 d × 11	4	1 HDAra-C 3 LDAra-C 1 Mithramycin	1 RAEB 1 RAEBT 2 CMML	17–29%	NA	No change		Increase in ANC with >500 µg/m² yeast GM or >250 E. coli GM; Increase × >2-fold in circulating blasts
Kobaychi	G-CSF nonglycosylated (E. coli)	50–1600 µg/m²	I.V.	5	NA	RAEB	0–67% before treatment	NA	NA	NA	Increase in bone marrow blasts; Increase in ANC
Negrin	G-CSF nonglycosylated	0.1–3.0 µg/kg/d	SC × 6–8 wk	13	Retinoic Acid Danozol	2 RA 8 RAEBT	≥21%	0–13% peripheral blood myeloblasts	2/9 transfusion dependent	0	Increase ANC (11/13); Increase retics (5/13)
Ganser	IL-3 nonglycosylated	250–500 µg/m²	SC daily × 15 d	9	GM-CSF (2) Steroids (2) Ara-C (1) Androgens (1)	6 RA 3 RAEB	NA	>10% (1)	1	2	Increase WBC 1.3- to 3.6-fold; Increase platelets in 7/9; Decrease platelets transiently 2/9

Dauna/Ara-C, Daunorubicin, cytosine arabinoside; NA, not available; HD, high dose; RX, treatment; RA, refractory anemia; RAEB, refractory anemia with excess blasts; CMMOL, chronic myelomonocytic leukemia; Ara-C, cytosine arabinoside; LD, low dose; RAEBT, refractory anemia with excess blasts in transformation; Chemo RX, chemotherapy; ANC, absolute neutrophil count; WBC, white blood cell count; retics, reticulocyte count; GM, granulocyte macrophage colony-stimulating factor; G-CSF, granulocyte colony-stimulating factor; IL-3, interleukin-3; TX, transfusion; POD, progression of disease.

and 6 fewer days of initial hospitalization; however, no difference in survival was observed at 100 days after transplantation. Based on these data, yeast-derived GM-CSF was approved in the United States to reduce infection in the setting of autologous bone marrow transplantation.

The therapeutic utility of glycosylated and nonglycosylated GM-CSF in ameliorating myelosuppressive toxicity of chemotherapy, in the absence of marrow reinfusion, has been investigated in patients with sarcoma, small cell carcinoma of the lung, non-Hodgkin's lymphoma, myeloma, ovarian carcinoma, other advanced solid tumors, and acute myelogenous leukemia (see Table 62–10).[66–72] The results of these nonrandomized trials suggest that treatment with GM-CSF hastens the recovery of granulocytes but not platelets or erythrocytes.

GM-CSF used after chemotherapy for acute nonlymphocytic leukemia has not been associated with an increased incidence of relapse or induction failure. In these trials, GM-CSF was begun immediately after the administration of chemotherapy. Gianni and coworkers compared the granulocyte recovery observed when CHO cell-derived GM-CSF was administered 1 day or 5 days after high-dose cyclophosphamide (7 g/m²). In this study, no accelerated leukocyte recovery was observed when GM-CSF treatment was delayed, suggesting that the immediate administration of GM-CSF after completion of chemotherapy is critical if a therapeutic benefit is to be preserved. Three additional studies examined the therapeutic contribution of GM-CSF to the successful implementation of dose-intensified chemotherapeutic regimens, with conflicting results.[73–75] Although the administration of nonglycosylated GM-CSF permitted dose-intensified M-VAC regimen to be safely administered, resulting in significant tumor responses in previously unresponsive patients, the coadministration of this same preparation of GM-CSF did not maintain the initial hematologic improvement observed over multiple 21-day cycles of doxorubicin (75 mg/m²) plus cyclophosphamide (750 mg/m²) therapy in patients with advanced breast carcinoma.[73,74] GM-CSF did not permit additional dose escalation of these two agents. Similarly, treatment with GM-CSF (125 μg/m² over 6 hours on days 6 through 21) resulted in significantly more erythrocyte and platelet transfusions and infectious episodes in patients treated with high-dose etoposide (800 mg/m² continuous infusion × 96 hours), cisplatin (100 mg/m² by continuous infusion × 96 hours), Solu-Medrol (500 mg by intravenous bolus on days 1–5), and cytosine arabinoside (1.5 g/m² on day 5), compared with the prophylactic antibiotics ketoconazole (200 mg/day) and ciprofloxacin (750 mg orally twice daily on days 6 through 21).

Clinical investigations of GM-CSF in aplastic anemia indicate that treatment results in augmentation of circulating monocytes and granulocytes, in patients with some evidence of residual myelopoiesis but does not affect consistent changes in platelet count, erythrocytes, or transfusion requirements.[76–79] Prior treatment has no effect on therapeutic response, and most patients require continued treatment to maintain the desired hematologic effect. Discontinuation of treatment is associated with a return to baseline peripheral blood counts and bone marrow cellularity.

Nonrandomized clinical trials investigating the role of yeast and bacterially derived GM-CSF in patients with myelodysplastic syndrome reported similar increases in granulocyte counts, without consistent improvements in other hematopoietic lineages (Table 62–11).[80–84] In patients with more advanced disease (*e.g.*, refractory anemia with excess blasts or refractory anemia with excess blasts in transformation) or chronic myelomonocytic leukemia, treatment is associated with an increase in circulating and bone marrow blasts, although in most cases, the blast count returned toward pretreatment values after discontinuation of treatment. Initial results from a phase III randomized trial in patients with refractory anemia and severe neutropenia, receiving 6 months of GM-CSF or no treatment demonstrate that GM-CSF does accelerate transformation to acute leukemia within the time frame studied and augments neutrophil counts. Whether treatment results in a significant reduction in serious infection in this category of patients remains to be determined.

Several side effects have been reported in patients receiving glycosylated and nonglycosylated GM-CSF. Fever and bone pain are the most common side effects observed in patients treated with nonglycosylated GM-CSF. Pericarditis was dose limiting in patients treated with 20 to 30 μg/kg/day, but this side effect was not observed in 16 patients treated with lower doses. In patients receiving nonglycosylated GM-CSF, a peculiar first-dose reaction including flushing, hypotension, transient hypoxia, and tachycardia has been described.[85] Subsequent doses do not elicit this response; however, if treatment is discontinued for 10 or more days and GM-CSF is reintroduced, the first dose again may produce this reaction. Morstyn and colleagues reported that the reaction appears to occur predominantly in patients receiving short infusions and perhaps more commonly in patients with active pulmonary disease.[85]

The major side effects associated with glycosylated GM-CSF appear to be fever, bone pain, myalgia, and constitutional symptoms. The fever observed secondary to CHO cell-derived GM-CSF can be abrogated by the concomitant administration of indomethacin, suggesting that it is mediated by prostaglandins. Short intravenous infusion of yeast-derived GM-CSF has been associated with dose-limiting epigastric distress, nausea, and vomiting. In two studies, higher doses (>32 μg/kg/day) of CHO cell-derived GM-CSF used before chemotherapy or after autologous bone marrow transplantation resulted in generalized edema, thrombophlebitis, hypotension, and acute renal failure. Comparable side effects with yeast-derived GM-CSF have not been reported, but comparable doses have not been explored in equivalent clinical settings. The side effects have been minimal for yeast-derived GM-CSF used in the setting of autologous bone marrow transplantation for lymphoid malignancies. Treatment with glycosylated and nonglycosylated GM-CSF has been associated with a transient decline in platelet count and with reactivation of idiopathic thrombocytopenic purpura.

MACROPHAGE COLONY-STIMULATING FACTOR

Macrophage colony-stimulating factor (M-CSF or CSF-1) is a mononuclear phagocyte-specific growth factor first identified and purified from mouse L cells and human urine.[86] M-CSF is a heavily glycosylated disulfide-linked homodimer biochemically related to the insulin-relaxin family of hormones. Complementary cDNAs have been cloned that encode two different biologically active forms of M-CSF, resulting from differential splicing. The larger M-CSF precursor (mRNA,

4.0 kb) encodes a protein that is proteolytically cleaved within the cell; the resulting 70,000-kd glycoprotein product is secreted from the cell. This M-CSF is the major form excreted in human urine. The smaller precursor (mRNA, 2.0 kb) encodes a membrane-bound protein from which multiple forms of soluble extracellular M-CSF are generated by proteolytic cleavage. Removal of carbohydrate does not affect the biologic function of M-CSF, but treatment with disulfide-reducing agents abolishes activity. Human M-CSF is coded for by a single gene, which was initially localized to the long arm of chromosome 5 (5q33.1), but which recently has been reassigned to the short arm of chromosome 1 (1p13–21). Recombinant human M-CSF for clinical use is produced in *E. coli* and CHO cells and has a specific activity 1×10^7 units and 0.8×10^6 units per milligram of protein, respectively.

M-CSF is constitutively produced by fibroblasts and bone marrow stromal cells. Monocyte-macrophages and endothelial cells also synthesize M-CSF in response to activators involved in the inflammatory response. Uterine glandular epithelial cells express M-CSF in response to ovarian hormones, suggesting that M-CSF may be of importance in placental development or function.[86] M-CSF is normally detected in human serum and appears to be increased in patients with myeloproliferative disorders.

Radiolabeled M-CSF-binding studies demonstrate a single class of high-affinity receptors on the surface of mononuclear phagocytes and trophoblasts.[24] This cell-surface receptor is now known to be the *CSF1R* (formerly *FMS*) protooncogene product, an integral transmembrane glycoprotein with ligand stimulated protein-tyrosine kinase activity. Binding of M-CSF to its receptor activates the kinase resulting in autophosphorylation of the receptor and phosphorylation of other cellular proteins on tyrosine residues. The physiologic substrates for the receptor kinase activity have not been identified.

In vitro, M-CSF stimulates the growth and maturation of monocyte and macrophages. M-CSF also enhances macrophage migration, expression of Fc receptors and adhesion molecules, cytotoxicity and respiratory burst activity, and bacterial and fungal killing in vitro. M-CSF primes but does not directly induce monocytes to secrete cytokines such as TNF and IL-1. M-CSF has been implicated in the growth, maturation, and function of osteoclasts, and alterations in the M-CSF gene are responsible for congenital osteopetrosis in op/op mutant mice.[87]

In vivo, M-CSF increases circulating monocytes that are functionally activated and exhibit enhanced tumoricidal cytotoxicity.[88] There is an associated expansion of bone marrow monocytic elements. M-CSF protects mice from lethal infection after challenge with *Candida albicans*.

The first clinical trials of M-CSF employed highly purified human urinary CSF and demonstrated some myelorestorative activity.[89] The administration of recombinant glycosylated and nonglycosylated M-CSF in cancer patients stimulates a prominent increase in the number of circulating monocytes.[90,91] Monocytes induced by M-CSF display enhanced antibody-dependent cellular cytotoxicity, respiratory burst activity, migration, and degranulation and ingestion of *Candida*. The ability of M-CSF to augment intracellular killing of fungal organisms prompted a trial designed to evaluate the ability of M-CSF to enhance recovery from invasive fungal infection in marrow transplant recipients receiving conventional antifungal therapy. The results suggest that M-CSF may be useful

in this setting, but further investigation is needed to establish its therapeutic benefit. In these initial clinical investigations, adverse events included bone pain and thrombocytopenia due presumably to peripheral destruction of platelets. Administration of glycosylated M-CSF has also been associated with a marked reduction in serum cholesterol. Additional studies designed to explore this biologic property should prove informative.

INTERLEUKIN-3

IL-3 (multi-CSF) is a glycoprotein hormone related to GM-CSF that supports the growth of multilineage colonies in vitro. Murine IL-3 was identified and characterized by Ihle and associates, and the human IL-3 cDNA was isolated by expression cloning of mRNA from a Gibbon T-cell line.[92] Human IL-3 exists as a single copy gene mapped to the long arm of chromosome 5 (5q23–31) within 9 kb of the gene for GM-CSF. IL-3 and GM-CSF share conserved regions in their promoter sequences, suggesting a common regulatory mechanism for their expression. Recombinant human IL-3 for clinical use is produced in *E. coli* and yeast and has a specific activity of 4.3×10^6 units and $0.9–6.7 \times 10^8$ units per milligram of protein, respectively.

IL-3 is a lymphokine and is produced primarily by activated T lymphocytes and natural killer cells. IL-3 supports the growth of early hematopoietic progenitors in vitro. IL-3 augments the functional activity of monocytes, macrophages, and eosinophils, and it stimulates the growth of basophils and the production of intracellular histamine.

IL-3 administration to normal primates results in a modest and delayed leukocytosis with increases in neutrophil, eosinophil, and basophil granulocytes and a dose-dependent increase in intracellular and plasma histamine levels.[93] Increases in corrected reticulocyte counts and variable increases in platelets have been observed. The administration of IL-3 to cynomolgus monkeys after treatment with cyclophosphamide or 5-fluorouracil significantly reduced the duration of severe neutropenia (neutrophil count <500 cells/μl). Platelet recovery appears to occur earlier in animals treated with IL-3.

The ability of glycosylated and nonglycosylated IL-3 to abrogate chemotherapy-induced myelosuppression, alone or in combination with more lineage-specific factors, is under investigation in humans. Several trials exploring the therapeutic utility of IL-3 in correcting the pancytopenia associated with aplastic anemia or myelodysplastic syndrome have been conducted (see Table 62–11).[94,95] In these studies, IL-3 administration resulted in an increase in neutrophil and eosinophil granulocyte counts, with increases in basophil granulocytes, erythrocytes, and platelets being more variable. Studies in humans have shown relatively modest toxicities including fever, headaches, and flushing, but the toxicity profile has not been determined at high doses.

HEMATOPOIETIC GROWTH FACTORS IN COMBINATION

It is clear that the regulation of hematopoietic cell development is sensitivity controlled by an intricate network of positive and negative influences. To optimally enhance host defense and to effect more complete hematopoietic reconstitution, we will probably need to employ a combination of regulatory factors that act at different levels along the pathway of blood cell development. Considerable in vitro evidence suggests that synergism is achieved when certain hematopoietic growth factors are employed in combination. IL-3, an early-acting factor, synergizes with GM-CSF and G-CSF to enhance the proliferation and differentiation of myeloid committed progenitors, suggesting that combinations of early-acting and lineage-restricted regulatory molecules may have clinical utility in patients with iatrogenic or disease-related myelosuppression. Because individual CSFs enhance monocyte and neutrophil effector cell function, combinations may better augment host defenses.

Preclinical studies exploring the combination of GM-CSF or G-CSF plus IL-3 have demonstrated that IL-3 potentiates the myeloid responsiveness of the host to subsequent administration of the lineage specific growth factor. Combinations of low concentrations of IL-3 and M-CSF, which by themselves were inactive, increased the percentage and cycle status of macrophage high-proliferative and low-proliferative potential colony-forming cells. The combination of IL-1 and G-CSF enhanced neutrophil recovery in murine and primate nontumor-bearing and tumor-bearing models of chemotherapy-induced myelosuppression compared with the administration of each growth factor alone.[96,97]

Colony-stimulating factors have reduced treatment-related neutropenia and infectious morbidity, but thrombocytopenia remains a significant clinical problem. It is likely that the clinical application of hematopoietic growth factors, which stimulate uncommitted progenitors and promote megakaryocyte formation, such as stem cell factor and IL-1, -4, -6 and -11, will reduce this complication. The use of these newer regulatory molecules in combination with colon-stimulating factors and "primed" progenitors harvested from the peripheral blood should enable more complete hematopoietic reconstitution and permit the successful implementation of dose-intensified regimens designed to cure malignant disease.

REFERENCES

1. Golde DW. The stem cell. Sci Am 1991;265:86–93.
2. Spangrude GJ, Smith L, Uchida N, et al. Mouse hematopoietic stem cells. Blood 1991;78:1395–1402.
3. Krantz SB. Erythropoietin. Blood 1991;77:419–434.
4. Miyake T, Kung CKH, Goldwasser E. Purification of human erythropoietin. J Biol Chem 1977;252:5558.
5. Boyd HK, Lappin TRJ. Erythropoietin deficiency in the anaemia of chronic disorders. Eur J Haematol 1991;46:198–201.
6. Schilling RF. Anemia of chronic disease: A misnomer. Ann Intern Med 1991;115:572–573.
7. Miller CB, Jones RJ, Piantadosi S, et al. Decreased erythropoietin response in patients with the anemia of cancer. N Engl J Med 1990;322:1689–1992.
8. Doweiko JP, Goldberg MA. Erythropoietin therapy in cancer patients. Oncology 1991;5:31–37.
9. Abels RI, Rudnick SA. Erythropoietin: Evolving clinical applications. Exp Hematol 1991;19:842–850.
10. Ludwig H, Fritz E, Kotzmann H, et al. Erythropoietin treatment of anemia associated with multiple myeloma. N Engl J Med 1990;322:1693–1699.
11. Oster W, Herrmann F, Gamm H, et al. Erythropoietin for the treatment of anemia of malignancy associated with neoplastic bone marrow infiltration. J Clin Oncol 1990;8:956–962.
12. Platanias LC, Miller CB, Mick R, et al. Treatment of chemotherapy-induced anemia with recombinant human erythropoietin in cancer patients. J Clin Oncol 1991;9:2021–2026.
13. Smith DH, Goldwasser E, Vokes EE. Serum immunoerythropoietin levels in patients with cancer receiving cisplatin-based chemotherapy. Cancer 1991;68:1101–1105.
14. Abels RI, Larholt KM, Krantz KD, Bryant EC. Recombinant human erythropoietin (r-HuEPO) for the treatment of the anemia of cancer. Data on file: RW Johnson Pharmaceutical Research Institute, Raritan, NJ.
15. Bowen D, Culligan D, Jacobs A. The treatment of anaemia in the myelodysplastic syndromes with recombinant human erythropoietin. Br J Haematol 1991;77:419–423.
16. Hirashima K, Bessho M, Susaki K, et al. Improvement of anemia by intravenous injections of recombinant erythropoietin in patients with myelodysplastic syndromes and aplastic anemia. Exp Hematol 1989;17:657.
17. Van Kamp H, Prinsze-Postema TC, Kluin PM, et al. Effect of subcutaneously administered human recombinant erythropoietin on erythropoiesis in patients with myelodysplasia. Br J Haematol 1991;78:488–493.
18. Hellström E, Birgegård G, Lockner D, et al. Treatment of myelodysplastic syndromes with recombinant human erythropoietin. Eur J Haematol 1991;47:355–360.
19. Stein RS, Abels RI, Krantz SB. Pharmacologic doses of recombinant human erythropoietin in the treatment of myelodysplastic syndromes. Blood 1991;78:1658–1663.
20. Burgess A, Metcalf D. Characterization of a serum factor stimulating the differentiation of myelomonocytic leukemic cells. Int J Cancer 1980;26:647–654.
21. Souza LM, Boone TC, Gabrilove J, et al. Recombinant pluripotent human granulocyte colony stimulating factor: Effects on normal and leukemic myeloid cells. Science 1986;232:61–65.
22. Hammond WP, Boone TC, Donahue RE, Souza LM, et al. A comparison of treatment of canine cyclic hematopoiesis with recombinant human granulocyte-macrophage colony-stimulating factor (GM-CSF), G-CSF, interleukin-3, and canine G-CSF. Blood 1990;76:523–532.
23. Kawakami M, Tsutsumi H, Kumakawa T, et al. Levels of serum granulocyte colony-stimulating factor in patients with infections. Blood 1990;76:1962–1964.
24. Kaczmarski RS, Mufti GJ. The cytokine receptor superfamily. Blood Rev 1991;5:193–203.
25. Lord BI, Molineux G, Pojda Z, et al. Myeloid cell kinetics in mice treated with recombinant interleukin-3, granulocyte colony-stimulating factor (CSF), or granulocyte-macrophage CSF in vivo. Blood 1991;77:2154–2159.
26. Schuening FG, Storb R, Goehle S, et al. Recombinant human granulocyte colony-stimulating factor accelerates hematopoietic recovery after DLA-identical littermate marrow transplants in dogs. Blood 1990;76:636–640.
27. Gabrilove JL, Jakubowski A, Fain K, et al. Phase I study of granulocyte colony-stimulating factor in patients with transitional cell carcinoma of the urothelium. J Clin Invest 1988;82:1454–1461.
28. Morstyn G, Souza LM, Keech J, et al. Effect of granulocyte colony stimulating factor on neutropenia induced by cytotoxic chemotherapy. Lancet 1988;1:667–672.
29. Bronchud MH, Scarffe JH, Thatcher N, et al. Phase I/II study of recombinant human granulocyte colony-stimulating factor in patients receiving intensive chemotherapy for small cell lung cancer. Br J Cancer 1987;56:809–813.
30. Layton JE, Hockman H, Sheridan WP. Evidence for a novel in vivo control mechanism of granulopoiesis: Mature cell-related control of a regulatory growth factor. Blood 1989;74:1303–1307.
31. Morstyn G, Campbell L, Lieschke G, et al. Treatment of chemotherapy-induced neutropenia by subcutaneously administered granulocyte colony-stimulating factor with optimization of dose and duration of therapy. J Clin Oncol 1989;7:1554–1562.
32. Crawford J, Ozer H, Stoller R, et al. Reduction by granulocyte colony-stimulating factor of fever and neutropenia induced by chemotherapy in patients with small-cell lung cancer. N Engl J Med 1991;325:164–170.
33. Ohno R, Tomonaga M, Kobayashi T, et al. Effect of granulocyte colony-stimulating factor after intensive induction therapy in relapsed or refractory acute leukemia. N Engl J Med 1990;323:871–877.
34. Sheridan WP, Wolf M, Lusk J, et al. Granulocyte colony-stimulating factor and neutrophil recovery after high-dose chemotherapy and autologous bone marrow transplantation. Lancet 1989;1:891–894.
35. Taylor KM, Jagannath S, Spitzer G, et al. Recombinant human granulocyte colony-stimulating factor hastens granulocyte recovery after high-dose chemotherapy and autologous bone marrow transplantation in Hodgkin's Disease. J Clin Oncol 1989;7:1791–1799.
36. Petros W, Rabinowitz J, Stuart A, et al. Comparative pharmacokinetics of granulocyte colony-stimulating factor (rHuGM-CSF) in patients receiving high-dose chemotherapy and autologous bone marrow support. Proc Am Assoc Clin Oncol 1991;10:97.
37. Bronchud MH, Howell A, Crowther D, et al. The use of granulocyte colony-stimulating factor to increase the intensity of treatment with doxorubicin in patients with advanced breast and ovarian cancer. Br J Cancer 1989;60:121–125.
38. Neidhart J, Mangalik A, Kohler W, et al. Granulocyte colony-stimulating factor stimulates recovery of granulocytes in patients receiving dose-intensive chemotherapy without bone marrow transplantation. J Clin Oncol 1989;7:1685–1692.
39. Glaspy JA, Baldwin GC, Robertson PA, et al. Therapy for neutropenia in hairy cell leukemia with recombinant human granulocyte colony-stimulating factor. Ann Intern Med 1988;109:789.
40. Greenberg P, Negrin R, Nagler A, et al. Effects of prolonged treatment of myelodysplastic syndromes with recombinant human granulocyte colony-stimulating factor. Int J Cell Cloning 1990;8:293–302.
41. Kojima S, Fukuda M, Miyajima Y, et al. Cyclosporine and recombinant granulocyte colony-stimulating factor in severe aplastic anemia. N Engl J Med 1990;323:920–921.
42. Miles SA, Mitsuyasu RT, Lee K, et al. Recombinant human granulocyte colony-stimulating factor increases circulating burst forming unit-erythron and red blood cell production in patients with severe human immunodeficiency virus infection. Blood 1990;75:2137–2142.
43. Hammond WP, Price TH, Souza LM, et al. Treatment of cyclic neutropenia with granulocyte colony-stimulating factor. N Engl J Med 1989;320:1306–1311.
44. Bonilla MA, Gillio AP, Ruggeiro M, et al. Effects of recombinant human granulocyte

colony-stimulating factor on neutropenia in patients with congenital agranulocytosis. N Engl J Med 1989;320:1574–1580.

45. Jakubowski AA, Souza L, Kelly F, et al. Effects of human granulocyte colony-stimulating factor in a patient with idiopathic neutropenia. N Engl J Med 1989;320:38–42.

46. Gasson JC, Weisbart RH, Kaufman S, et al. Purified human granulocyte macrophage colony stimulating factor: Direct action on neutrophils. Science 1984;226:1339–1349.

47. Wong GG, Witek JS, Temple PA, et al. Human GM-CSF. molecular cloning of complementary DNA and purification of the natural and recombinant proteins. Science 1985;228:810–815.

48. Emanuel PD, Bates LJ, Castleberry RP, et al. Selective hypersensitivity to granulocyte-macrophage colony-stimulating factor by juvenile chronic myeloid leukemia hematopoietic progenitors. Blood 1991;77:925–929.

49. Johnson GR, Gonda TJ, Metcalf D, et al. A lethal myeloproliferative syndrome in mice transplanted with bone marrow cells infected with a retrovirus expressing granulocyte-macrophage colony stimulating factor. EMBO J 1989;8:441.

50. Chang JM, Metcalf D, Gonda TJ, et al. Long-term exposure to retrovirally expressed granulocyte-colony-stimulating factor induces a nonneoplastic granulocytic and progenitor cell hyperplasia without tissue damage in mice. J Clin Invest 1989;84:1488.

51. Hayashida K, Kitamura T, Gorman DM, et al. Molecular cloning of a second subunit of the receptor for human granulocyte-macrophage colony-stimulating factor (GM-CSF): Reconstitution of a high-affinity GM-CSF receptor. Proc Natl Acad Sci USA 1990;87: 9655–9659.

52. Donahue RE, Wang EA, Stone DK, et al. Stimulation of haematopoiesis in primates by continuous infusion of recombinant human GM-CSF. Nature 1986;321:872–875.

53. Groopman JE, Mitsuyasu RT, De Leo MJ, et al. Effect of recombinant human granulocyte-macrophage colony-stimulating factor on myelopoiesis in the acquired immunodeficiency syndrome. N Engl J Med 1987;317:593–598.

54. Pluda JM, Yarchoan R, Smith PD, et al. Subcutaneous recombinant granulocyte-macrophage colony-stimulating factor used as a single agent and in an alternating regimen with azidothymidine in leukopenic patients with severe human immunodeficiency virus infection. Blood 1990;76:463–472.

55. Kaplan LD, Kahn JO, Crowe S, et al. Clinical and virologic effects of recombinant human granulocyte-macrophage colony-stimulating factor in patients receiving chemotherapy for human immunodeficiency virus-associated non-Hodgkin's lymphoma: Results of a randomized trial. J Clin Oncol 1991;9:929–940.

56. Scadden DT, Bering HA, Levine JD, et al. Granulocyte-macrophage colony-stimulating factor mitigates the neutropenia of combined interferon alfa and zidovudine treatment of acquired immune deficiency syndrome-associated Kaposi's sarcoma. J Clin Oncol 1991;9:802–808.

57. Peters WP, Stuart A, Affronti ML, et al. Neutrophil migration is defective during recombinant human granulocyte-macrophage colony-stimulating factor infusion after autologous bone marrow transplantation in humans. Blood 1988;72:1310–1315.

58. Toner GC, Gabrilove JL, Gordon M, et al. Phase I/II study of intraperitoneal and intravenous granulocyte-macrophage colony stimulating factor. Proc Am Assoc Cancer Res 1990;31:1042.

59. Devereux S, Linch DC, Campos Costa D, et al. Transient leukopenia induced by granulocyte-macrophage colony-stimulating factor. Lancet 1987;1:1523–1524.

60. Socinski MA, Elias A, Schnipper L, et al. Granulocyte-macrophage colony stimulating factor expands the circulating haemopoietic progenitor cell compartment in man. Lancet 1988;1:1194–1198.

61. Gianni AM, Bregni M, Stern AC, et al. Granulocyte-macrophage colony-stimulating factor to harvest circulating hematopoietic stem cells for autotransplantation. Lancet 1989;1:580–584.

62. Aglietta M, Piacibello W, Sanavio F, et al. Kinetics of human hemopoietic cells after in vivo administration of granulocyte-macrophage colony-stimulating factor. J Clin Invest 1989;83:551–557.

63. Brandt SJ, Peters WP, Atwater SK, et al. Effect of recombinant human granulocyte-macrophage colony-stimulating factor on hematopoietic reconstitution after high-dose chemotherapy and autologous bone marrow transplantation. N Engl J Med 1988;318: 869–876.

64. Nemunaitis J, Singer JW, Buckner CD, et al. Use of recombinant human granulocyte-macrophage colony-stimulating factor in autologous marrow transplantation for lymphoid malignancies. Blood 1988;72:834–836.

65. Nemunaitis J, Rabinowe SN, Singer JW, et al. Recombinant granulocyte-macrophage colony-stimulating factor after autologous bone marrow transplantation for lymphoid cancer. N Engl J Med 1991;324:1773–1778.

66. Antman KS, Griffin JD, Elias A, et al. Effect of recombinant human granulocyte-macrophage colony-stimulating factor on chemotherapy-induced myelosuppression. N Engl J Med 1988;319:593–598.

67. Morstyn G, Stuart-Harris R, Bishop J, et al. Optimal scheduling of granulocyte macrophage colony stimulating factor (GM-CSF) for the abrogation of chemotherapy induced neutropenia in small cell lung cancer (SCLC). Proc Am Soc Clin Oncol 1989;8:850.

68. Gianni AM, Bregni M, Siena S, et al. Recombinant human granulocyte-macrophage colony-stimulating factor reduces hematologic toxicity and widens clinical applicability of high-dose cyclophosphamide treatment in breast cancer and non-Hodgkin's lymphoma. J Clin Oncol 1990;8:768–778.

69. Barlogie B, Jagamath S, Dixon DO, et al. High dose melphalan and granulocyte-macrophage colony stimulating factor for refractory multiple myeloma. Blood 1990;76: 677.

70. De Vries EGE, Biesma B, Willemse PHB, et al. A double-blind placebo controlled study with granulocyte-macrophage colony stimulating factor during chemotherapy for ovarian carcinoma. Cancer Res 1991;51:116–122.

71. Herrmann F, Schulz G, Wieser M, et al. Effect of granulocyte-macrophage colony-stimulating factor on neutropenia and related morbidity induced by myelotoxic chemotherapy. Am J Med 1990;88:619–624.

72. Buchner T, Hiddemann W, Koenigsmann M, et al. Recombinant human granulocyte-macrophage colony stimulating factor after chemotherapy in patients with acute myeloid leukemia at higher age or after relapse. Blood 1991;78:1190–1197.

73. Logothelis L, Dexeus F, Sella A, et al. Escalated (ESC) M-VAC (MTX 30 μg/m², Adriamycin 60 μg/m², vinblastine 4 μg/m², cisplatin 100 μg/m²) with recombinant human granulocyte macrophage stimulating factor (rhGM-CSF) for patients with advanced and chemotherapy refractory urothelium tumors: A phase I study. Proc Am Soc Clin Oncol 1989;8:514.

74. Hoekman K, Wagstaff J, van Groeningen CJ, et al. Effects if recombinant human granulocyte-macrophage colony-stimulating factor on myelosuppression induced by multiple cycles of high-dose chemotherapy in patients with advanced breast cancer. JNCI 1991;83:1546–1533.

75. Rodriquez MA, Swan F, Hagemeister F, et al. High-dose ESHAP with GM-CSF vs. prophylactic antibiotics. Blood 1990;76(suppl 1):10.

76. Champlin RE, Nimer SD, Ireland P, et al. Treatment of refractory aplastic anemia with recombinant human granulocyte-macrophage-colony-stimulating factor. Blood 1989;73: 694–699.

77. Antin JH, Smith BR, Holmes W, et al. Phase I/II study of recombinant human granulocyte-macrophage colony-stimulating factor in aplastic anemia and myelodysplastic syndrome. Blood 1988;72:705–713.

78. Vadhan-Raj S, Buescher S, Broxmeyer HE, et al. Stimulation of myelopoiesis in patients with aplastic anemia by recombinant human granulocyte-macrophage colony-stimulating factor. N Engl J Med 1988;319:1628–1634.

79. Guinan EC, Sieff CA, Oette DH, et al. A phase I/II trial of recombinant granulocyte-macrophage colony-stimulating factor for children with aplastic anemia. Blood 1990;76: 1077–1082.

80. Vadhan-Raj S, Keating M, LeMaistre A, et al. Effects of recombinant human granulocyte-macrophage colony-stimulating factor in patients with myelodysplastic syndromes. N Engl J Med 1987;317:1545–1551.

81. Ganser A, Völkers B, Greher J, et al. Recombinant human granulocyte-macrophage colony-stimulating factor in patients with myelodysplastic syndromes—A phase I/II trial. Blood 1989;73:31–37.

82. Rifkin RM, Hersh EM, Hultquist KN, et al. Therapy of the myelodysplastic syndrome (MDS) with subcutaeously (SC) administered recombinant human granulocyte-macrophage colony-stimulating factor. Proc Am Soc Clin Oncol 1989;8:178.

83. Thompson JA, Lee DJ, Kidd P, et al. Subcutaneous granulocyte-macrophage colony-stimulating factor in patients with myelodysplastic syndrome: Toxicity, pharmacokinetics, and hematological effects. J Clin Oncol 1989;7:629–637.

84. Herrmann F, Lindemann A, Klein H, et al. Effect of recombinant human granulocyte-macrophage colony-stimulating factor in patients with myelodysplastic syndrome with excess blasts. Leukemia 1989;3:335–338.

85. Lieschke GJ, Maher D, Cebon J, et al. Effects of bacterially synthesized recombinant human granulocyte-macrophage colony-stimulating factor in patients with advanced malignancy. Ann Intern Med 1989;110:357–364.

86. Rettenmier CW, Sherr C. The mononuclear phagocyte colony-stimulating factor (CSF-1, M-CSF). Hematol Oncol Clin North Am 1989;3:479–493.

87. Wiktor-Jedrzejczak W, Bartocci A, Ferrante AW Jr, et al. Total absence of CSF-1 in macrophage deficient osteopetrolic (op/op) mice. Proc Natl Acad Sci USA 1987;87: 4828–4832.

88. Munn DH, Garnick MB, Cheung NKV. Effects of parenteral macrophage colony-stimulating factor (M-CSF) on circulating monocyte number, immunophenotype and anti-tumor activity in cynomolgus monkeys. Blood 1988;72:127a.

89. Motoyoshi K, Takaku F, Miura Y. High serum colony-stimulating activity of leukocytopenic patients after intravenous infusions of human urinary colony-stimulating factor. Blood 1983;62:685–688.

90. Bajorin DF, Jakubowski A, Cody B, et al. Phase I trial of recombinant macrophage colony stimulating factor (rhM-CSF) in patients (pts) with melanoma (MEL). Blood 1989;74:1222.

91. Nemunaitis J, Meyers J, Buckner CD, et al. Phase I/II trial of recombinant human macrophage-colony stimulating factor (M-CSF) in patients with invasive fungal infection. Blood 1990;76:2065.

92. Ihle JN, Keller J, Henderson L, et al. Procedures for the purification of interleukin-3 to homogeneity. J Immunol 1982;129:2431.

93. Donahue RE, Seehra J, Metzger M, et al. Human IL-3 and GM-CSF act synergistically in stimulating hematopoiesis in primates. Science 1988;241:1820–1823.

94. Ganser A, Seipelt G, Lindemann A, et al. Effects of recombinant human interleukin-3 in patients with myelodysplastic syndromes. Blood 1990;76:455–462.

95. Ganser A, Lindmann A, Seipelt G, et al. Effects of recombinant human interleukin-3 in aplastic anemia. Blood 1990;76:1297–1292.

96. Warren DJ, Moore MAS. Synergism among interleukin-1, interleukin-3, and interleukin-5 in the production of eosinophils from primitive hemopoietic stem cells. J Immunol 1988;140:94–99.

97. Moore MAS, Stolfi RL, Martin DS. Hematologic effects of interleukin-1β, granulocyte colony-stimulating factor, and granulocyte-macrophage colony-stimulating factor in tumor-bearing mice treated with fluorouracil. Exp Hematol 1990;82:1031–1037.

PHILIP A. PIZZO
JOEL MEYERS
ALISON G. FREIFELD
THOMAS WALSH

SECTION **3**

Infections in the Cancer Patient

The associations among malignancy, immunocompromise, and infectious morbidity and mortality are established.[1-4] More intensive treatment regimens have produced more patients with cancer who are immunocompromised. The life-threatening infectious complications can limit the benefits of antineoplastic therapy. The oncologist must be familiar with the risk factors contributing to infection and knowledgeable about the infectious syndromes and the available therapies.

The patient with cancer may be immunocompromised because of the underlying malignancy or the antineoplastic therapy. Specific malignancies may be associated with immune deficits that predispose to infection with particular pathogens. For example, patients with Hodgkin's or non-Hodgkin's lymphomas tend to have abnormalities of the cellular immune system that heighten their risk for viral and fungal infections. Therapeutic modalities such as corticosteroids, cytotoxic chemotherapy, and localized or widespread irradiation result in additional deficiencies of host defense. The consequence of these interrelated abnormalities of immune function is the immunocompromised cancer patient.

IMPAIRED HOST DEFENSES OF THE CANCER PATIENT

INTEGUMENTARY AND MUCOSAL BARRIERS

The skin and mucosal surfaces constitute the primary host defense against invasion by endogenous and acquired microorganisms. The integrity of this physical barrier can be disrupted by the patient's tumor or by its treatment. Mucosal and epithelial cells contain specific and nonspecific receptors for the attachment or adherence of microorganisms.[5,6] These receptors can be altered by disease and by certain therapies, particularly antibiotics, permitting colonization of the immunosuppressed cancer patient with new pathogens.[6-8] Colonization is influenced by suppression of the host's anaerobic microflora, because these organisms can resist colonization by aerobic pathogens.[9] The anaerobic flora are suppressed by many antibiotics, particularly the β-lactams. The mucosal changes provide a nidus for microbial colonization, a focus for local infection, and a portal for systemic invasion.

PHAGOCYTIC DEFENSES

The neutrophil and the monocyte-macrophage are the major cellular defenses against most bacteria and fungi.[10] Whether

disease related or as a consequence of therapy, the degree of severe neutropenia is inversely related to the risk of serious infection (Table 62–12).[11] To meet rapidly changing needs, there is normally a large bone marrow granulocyte reserve that exceeds the circulating pool of neutrophils that is distributed equally between the blood stream and a marginating pool. The half-life of cells in the circulating granulocyte pool is 6 to 7 hours, after which the cells marginate along the vascular endothelial surfaces or move into extravascular spaces. If granulopoiesis is depressed by disease or treatment, the granulocyte reserves are rapidly depleted, with severe granulocytopenia ensuing within 5 to 7 days.

Several glycoprotein hormonal growth factors integral to granulopoiesis have been characterized, their genes cloned, and recombinant proteins purified. It has become apparent that various cells, including T and B lymphocytes, monocytes, fibroblasts, and endothelial cells, produce cytokines that are integral to hematopoiesis. The colony-stimulating factors (CSF) include the granulocyte-macrophage CSF (GM-CSF), granulocyte CSF (G-CSF), macrophage CSF (M-CSF), and multiprotein CSF (*i.e.*, IL-3).[12,13] These hematopoietic growth factors affect many target cells, and some (*e.g.*, IL-3, GM-CSF) stimulate several blood cell lineages. Cloned GM-CSF and G-CSF can shorten the recovery of neutrophils after chemotherapy-induced or radiation-induced myelosuppression. In addition to accelerating neutrophil recovery, these cytokines can enhance phagocyte activity, including superoxide generation, phagocytosis, and antibacterial activity.[15-18]

Several cytokines appear to be interlinked in generating GM-CSF or in initiating cell reactivity. Included among these are tumor necrosis factor (TNF or cachectin), interleukin-1 (IL-1), interleukin-2, and interferon.[19-28] A variety of cytokines play an integral role in host defense and cell regulation. The characterization, purification, cloning, and production of these growth factors offer new prospects for studying the biology of hematopoiesis and for bolstering host defenses that are altered in patients undergoing treatment for cancer.[29]

In addition to quantitative defects, qualitative abnormalities of neutrophil function have been described in patients with hematologic malignancies. These include defects in chemotaxis, phagocytosis, bactericidal capacity, and the absence of the respiratory burst that usually accompanies phagocytosis.[30] Although phagocytic capacity remains normal, decreased spontaneous migratory and chemotactic leukocyte functions have been described in untreated patients with lymphoma and carcinoma, suggesting the presence of a circulating inhibitor in the sera of these patients.[31,32]

Cancer chemotherapy may produce defects of neutrophil function. Corticosteroids, for example, can decrease phagocytosis and neutrophil migration. The combination of prednisone with vincristine and asparaginase or 6-mercaptopurine and methotrexate can produce a significant decrease in the phagocytic and killing capability.[33] Although the mechanism is not understood, bactericidal activity may be transiently impaired within the 3 months after craniospinal irradiation in patients with leukemia, which may contribute to the infectious complications that occur during that period.[34] Analgesic narcotics such as morphine can cause a dose-dependent suppression of granulocytes and can exacerbate infections in experimental animals.[35]

The mature macrophage is more resistant to cytotoxic che-

This chapter is dedicated in memory of Joel Meyers (deceased, October 1991), who contributed so much to the prevention and management of infectious complications in cancer patients, especially those undergoing bone marrow transplantation.

TABLE 62–12. Percentage of Cancer Patients Who Develop Serious Infections With Granulocytopenia and the Cumulative Risk of Infection With Prolonged Granulocytopenia

Granulocyte Level (per mm³)		Percentage of Serious Infections (duration of granulocytopenia in weeks)							
Initial	Change	1	2	3	4	6	10	12	14
Any level	Any fall	12							
Any level	Fall to 2000	2							
Any level	Fall to 1500	5							
Any level	Fall to 1000	10	30	45	50	65	70	85	100
Any level	Fall to 500	19							
Any level	Fall to <100	28	50	72	85	100			

(Adapted from Bodey GP, Buckley M, Sathe YS, et al. Quantitative relationships between circulating leukocytes and infection in patients with acute leukemia. Ann Intern Med 1966;61:328–340)

motherapy than the granulocyte and provides some residual phagocytic capacity during periods of severe neutropenia. The activated macrophage is an important defense against mycobacteria, *Listeria*, *Brucella*, and several fungi, protozoans, and viruses. Macrophages are important in the initiation of the immune responses, because they are triggered into a metabolically active state by antigenic stimuli and subsequently process and present these antigens to T and B lymphocytes. Macrophages produce a variety of low-molecular-weight polypeptide hormones (*i.e.*, monokines) that regulate lymphocyte function and CSFs that are important in granulopoiesis.[12,13] If macrophage function is altered, as with steroids, the primary defense against fungal pathogens is altered, further aggravating the altered host defense of the neutropenic host.[36]

CELLULAR AND HUMORAL IMMUNITY

Patients with lymphoid malignancies, especially Hodgkin's disease, may have abnormalities of cell-mediated immunity, such as anergy and decreased phytohemagglutinin responsiveness, which may persist even after the underlying malignancy has been treated.[37] These defects are aggravated by chemotherapy with glucocorticosteroids and by infections like disseminated histoplasmosis, making patients susceptible to viral (*e.g.*, herpes zoster) or fungal (*e.g.*, *Cryptococcus*) infections.[38]

Cytotoxic chemotherapy adversely affects B-cell and T-cell functions, resulting in diminished opsonizing activity, inadequate agglutination and lysis of bacteria, and deficient neutralization of bacterial toxins.[39] Impaired antibody production has been described in untreated patients with chronic lymphocytic leukemia, multiple myeloma, or Hodgkin's disease.[40] Suppressor lymphocytes may contribute to impaired antibody production in patients with multiple myeloma and Hodgkin's disease and may relate to the fungal infections that occur in some of these patients.[41] In animal studies, the glucocorticoid-induced defects in lymphocyte function and decreased neutralizing-antibody formation contribute to the increased lethality of fungal, protozoan, and viral infections.

The importance of humoral defenses in the cancer patient has become apparent from several lines of evidence.[42–46] First, patients with defective antibody production (*e.g.*, chronic lymphocytic leukemia and multiple myeloma) have an increased frequency of pyogenic infections, even if they are not neutropenic. Patients with acute leukemia have lower levels of antibody to the core glycolipid of the Enterobacteriaceae than noncancer patients, and the antibody level falls in patients receiving cytotoxic therapy.[47] The protective role of this antibody is based on the fact that gram-negative bacteria share in common a core glycolipid composed of 2-keto-3-deoxy-octonate (KDO) and lipid A (endotoxin). A rough mutant of *Escherichia coli* 0111 exposes this core glycolipid and has been used to prepare a vaccine and antisera, known as the J5 antisera, which has protected rabbits challenged with endotoxin and has improved survival in nonneutropenic patients with gram-negative sepsis.[48,49] Monoclonal antibodies to J5 have been developed and evaluated in the clinic.

RETICULOENDOTHELIAL SYSTEM AND SPLENECTOMY

The spleen serves as a mechanical filter and an early source of opsonizing activity. Splenectomized patients manifest diminished antibody production when challenged with particulate antigens, are deficient in tuftsin (phagocytosis-promoting peptide), and have decreased levels of IgM and properdin.[50] Consequently, splenectomized patients are at increased risk for septicemia with encapsulated bacteria, particularly *Streptococcus pneumoniae*, *Neisseria meningitis*, and *Hemophilus influenzae*, and with *Babesia microti*.[51] Septicemia in these patients is characteristically fulminant, with large numbers of organisms in the blood stream. Although the incidence of postsplenectomy septicemia is especially significant in children and adolescents (1.4–20%) receiving chemotherapy, bacteremia with *S. pneumoniae* or *H. influenzae* can occur even when patients are not granulocytopenic, suggesting that splenectomy is an important independent risk factor for cancer patients.[52–54] Splenectomy does not appear to enhance the risk for most nonbacterial infections.[55]

NUTRITION

Malnutrition is a frequent complication of cancer, and its treatment contributes to the loss in integrity of the integumentary and mucosal barrier, to impaired phagocytic capacity, to decreased macrophage mobilization, and to depressed lymphocyte function.[56] Total parenteral nutrition to attenuate drug-induced bone marrow suppression or decrease mucosal cell damage has produced mixed results in clinical trials.[57]

EXOGENOUS AND ENDOGENOUS MICROBIAL FLORA

Unperturbed, the endogenous microbial flora exists as a carefully balanced, synergistic microenvironment within the host. However, more than 80% of the infections that occur in cancer patients arise from endogenous microbial flora, almost half of which are acquired by the patient during hospitalization. The most frequent isolates are gram-negative and gram-positive bacteria and *C. albicans*.[58–62] Numerous sources contribute to the colonization of the hospitalized patient, including transmissions from staff to patient and from patient to patient; contamination of food, air, water, special equipment such as catheters, respirators, or humidifiers; and medical or surgical procedures (Fig. 62–4).[63,64] These inanimate reservoirs of microorganisms require human vectors for transmission, particularly furnished by poor hand-washing techniques.[65] Fewer than 30% of physicians caring for seriously ill patients wash their hands between patient contacts.[66] This emphasizes the need for continued education and reinforcement of this important infection-control practice.

Current technology has provided new routes for the transmission of microorganisms, particularly the increased use of indwelling catheters, hyperalimentation lines, and hemodynamic monitoring devices.[67,68] Even the disinfectants and antiseptics used to cleanse the skin before an invasive procedure are occasionally contaminated.[69]

Interface of Colonization and Infection

Contact with microorganisms does not necessarily result in colonization or infection; hospital workers or psychiatric patients rarely become colonized with gram-negative organisms.[70] However, more than 80% of seriously ill noncancer patients eventually become colonized in the oropharynx with gram-negative bacteria, presumably due to alterations in the epithelial adherence of these organisms.[5] Attachment is mediated by a specific lock-and-key mechanism, in which ligand molecules (adhesions) on the surface of the microbe interact with complementary molecules (receptors) on the epithelial cell surface. The biochemical structures of adhesions include proteins (*e.g., E. coli, Neisseria gonorrhoeae*), the lipid protein of a glycolipid (*e.g., S. pyogenes*), and carbohydrates (*e.g.*, many cariogenic streptococci). In healthy persons, integumentary and mucosal attachment sites are populated with relatively innocuous normal flora, consisting predominantly of aerobic gram-positive and a variety of anaerobic organisms.[5,6]

In cancer patients, a decrease in the normal aerobic gram-positive flora and colonization of the oropharynx and stool with aerobic gram-negative organisms is observed soon after hospitalization, even before the patient receives antibiotics, although antibiotics enhance colonization.[8] Endogenous properties of the microorganisms are important for colonization and infection. For example, certain biotypes of Enterobacteriaceae are more capable of colonizing the host than others, and certain colonizing organisms are more likely to result in infection, presumably because of their inherent virulence.[59,60] Although *E. coli* is the most frequently isolated organism, few of the patients who become colonized develop infections. In contrast, 40% to 68% of patients who are colonized with or who acquire *Pseudomonas aeruginosa* while in the hospital develop serious infections with this organism during subsequent periods of granulocytopenia.[60,61] Antibiotic regimens can influence colonization and infection, as evidenced by the increase in streptococcal infections in patients receiving quinolone antibiotics (*e.g.*, cyprofloxacin) for prophylaxis.

The relation between colonization and infection also applies to nonbacterial organisms. For example, *Candida albicans* is ubiquitous and can be cultured from the oropharynx and stool of more than 80% patients who have received broad-spectrum antibiotics.[62] Although *C. tropicalis* is less frequently isolated

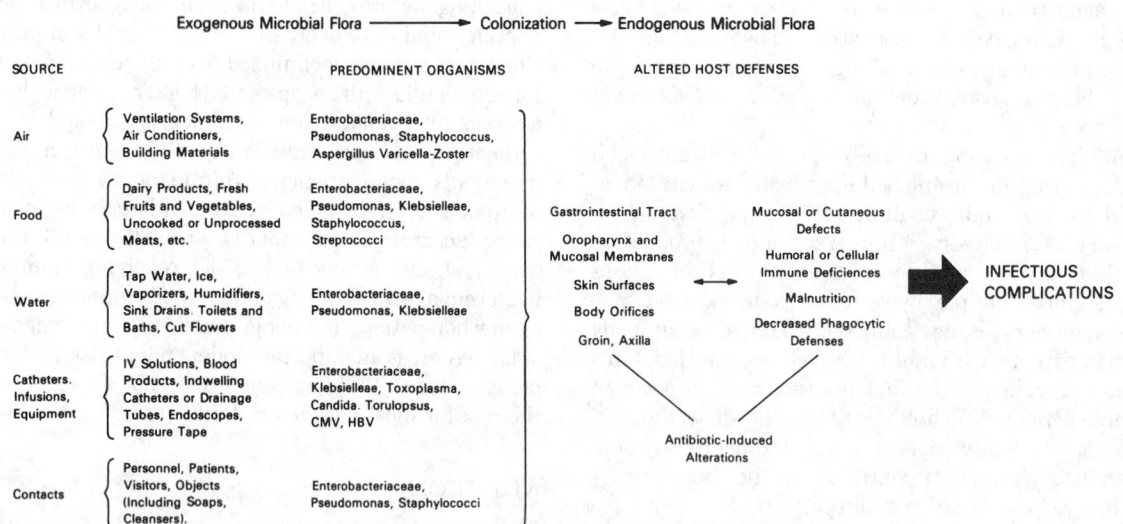

FIGURE 62–4.   Sources of nosocomial infection in high-risk patients and interactions between colonization and infection.

and causes fewer overall infections, it appears to be more pathogenic, because 14 of the 25 patients colonized by *C. tropicalis* in the series reported by Wingard and colleagues developed an infection with this organism.[71] The reservoir for organisms may vary among institutions and can be influenced by changes in antimicrobial practice. For example, *Candida krusei* has been observed in cancer patients receiving fluconazole for antifungal prophylaxis.[72]

Interactions among different components of the host's endogenous microflora (*e.g.*, viruses with bacteria or protozoa) may result in alterations of the microenvironment and consequent infectious complications, such as the increase in α-streptococcal infections in cancer patient with oral herpes simplex virus (HSV) who are also receiving cytotoxic therapy with cytosine arabinoside. Viruses can suppress or alter immune functions, which has been appreciated since the advent of the acquired immunodeficiency syndrome (AIDS) and its etiologic agent, the human immunodeficiency virus (HIV). Other human viruses, including parvoviruses and herpesviruses (*e.g.*, HSV, Epstein-Barr virus, cytomegalovirus), can be immunosuppressive. This can result from destruction of a specific lymphocyte or macrophage target or from the release of soluble factors or activated suppressor cells that alter host immunity while responding to the viral infection.[73]

Predominant Pathogens in the Cancer Patient

The spectrum of infecting organisms has changed during the last 3 decades. During the 1950s and early 1960s, *Staphylococcus aureus* was the most frequent bacterial isolate in immunosuppressed patients. When the β-lactamase-resistant antistaphylococcal penicillins were introduced and provided effective therapy for *S. aureus,* gram-negative bacillary organisms became the predominant bacterial pathogens (especially *E. coli, Klebsiella* species, and *P. aeruginosa*).[1–4] During the 1980s, infections with *P. aeruginosa* have inexplicably decreased in many institutions, a phenomenon that affects the selection and the probable success of initial empiric antibiotics. Increased infections due to nonaeruginosa pseudomonads (*e.g.*, *P. maltophilia, P. cepacia, P. stutzeri*) have been observed in cancer patients as nosocomial infections or as a consequence of antibiotic resistance.[74] In some centers, an increase in multiply-resistant gram-negative bacterial isolates (*e.g.*, *Enterobacter* species, *Citrobacter* species, *Acinetobacter* species, *S. marcescens*) are presumably a consequence of antibiotic use and misuse.

In most centers, gram-positive bacteria became the common isolates during the 1980s.[75] *S. aureus* and the coagulase-negative staphylococci were the predominant isolates, especially in patients with indwelling intravenous catheters.[76–78] Although some centers experienced major problems with methicillin-resistant *S. aureus*, most were able to contain the spread of the isolates with careful infection control practices, especially hand washing.[79–81] During the last decade, the coagulase-negative staphylococci became increasingly resistant to all β-lactam antibiotics, making vancomycin the drug of choice. There was a report of a coagulase-negative staphylococcal isolate that was resistant to vancomycin.[82] Although some investigators reported serious infectious complications, including pneumonia, endocarditis, meningitis, with coagu-

lase-negative staphylococci, most found this organism to be less virulent and only rarely associated with serious sequelae.[83–86]

Alpha-hemolytic, viridans streptococci, and corynebacteria, some of which are multiply-antibiotic-resistant diphtheroids (CDC group JK), can result in serious infections, particularly in patients with prolonged granulocytopenia.[87–92]

Although anaerobes play a lesser role than aerobes in primary infections in cancer patients, they are responsible for approximately 5% of bacteremias and are responsible for mixed infections in the mouth and perianal area. *Clostridia perfringens* and *C. septicum* are well-described isolates, but *C. tertium*, previously considered a contaminant, has been associated with serious infection.[93] Only half of the isolates of *C. tertium* are sensitive to standard antianaerobic agents (*e.g.*, clindamycin, metronidazole), but most are sensitive to vancomycin. *Bacillus* species have been associated with infection in cancer patients and are difficult to eradicate in patients who have indwelling Silastic catheters, unless the venous access device is removed.[94]

Mycobacterial infections are uncommon in cancer patients, although *M. avium-intracellulare* has become a highly prevalent pathogen in patients with AIDS.[95,96] Infections with rapid growers (*e.g.*, *M. chelonei, M. fortuitum*) have been observed in patients with indwelling catheters.[97]

Fungi are major pathogens, especially in immunosuppressed patients who have prolonged granulocytopenia and who receive protracted courses of antibiotics.[98] The predominant fungal pathogens are *Candida* species, *Aspergillus* species, *Cryptococcus neoformans*, and the *Phycomycetes*. There is considerable institutional variation in the predominant fungal pathogens, although in many centers, *Aspergillus* infections have increased in frequency.[98] Although their incidence is less common, the *Mucoraceae* (*Mucor, Absidia,* and *Rhizopus* species) can cause pulmonary disease or invade the sinuses, causing rhinocerebral syndrome. *Cryptococcus* is a noteworthy pathogen for patients with lymphoma, and it is responsible for disseminated infection in AIDS patients.[99] *Trichosporon* species, an arthrospore-forming yeast, can cause local skin lesions and invasive disease.[100] Infections due to *Fusarium* species, *Dreschlera, Pseudoallescheria boydii*, and *Malassezia furfur* have been described in cancer patients.[98] Although geographic mycoses such as *Histoplasma, Coccidioides*, and *Blastomyces* have not increased in frequency, there is an increase in their severity and invasiveness when infection occurs.

In addition to bacteria and fungi, parasitic and viral infections are important primary or secondary complications. *P. carinii* is an important cause of pneumonia, particularly in patients on corticosteroids or with AIDS. Viral infections represent a considerable source of morbidity in immunosuppressed hosts. The herpesviruses HSV, varicella-zoster virus (VZV), and CMV are particularly important. Rodents infected with CMV have a higher mortality rate when challenged with *P. aeruginosa* or *Candida* species than noninfected controls; the clinical corollary of this is that patients who become infected with CMV have a higher incidence of bacterial superinfections.[101,102]

The immunosuppressed host is at risk for a staggering array of infectious complications. Often, the same patients have multiple infections, further confounding their management.

EVALUATION AND MANAGEMENT OF THE FEBRILE CANCER PATIENT

FEVER AND GRANULOCYTOPENIA

Fever is common in cancer patients and can result from tumor necrosis, inflammation, transfusions, and chemotherapeutic or antimicrobial drugs. Although the patient's underlying malignancy can cause fever, 55% to 70% of the fevers that occur in cancer patients are caused by infections, especially in patients who are granulocytopenic, defined as having fewer than 500 polymorphonuclear leukocytes and bandforms per 1 mm[3].[103] The activated monocyte-macrophage is thought to be the most important source of physiologically relevant IL-1, but other phagocytic cells, including polymorphonuclear leukocytes, fixed tissue cells of the reticuloendothelial system, keratinocytes, gingival and corneal epithelial cells, renal mesangial cells, and astrocytes, are capable of producing IL-1-like molecules.[28] IL-1 and TNF mediate an array of metabolic, endocrinologic, neurologic, and immunologic functions common to the acute-phase inflammatory response, the effect of which is a unified host response against an infectious insult. Directly or indirectly, these include the production of fever, polymorphonuclear leukocytosis, hepatic synthesis of acute-phase reactants, activation of T and B lymphocytes, and the metabolic changes (*e.g.*, mobilization of amino acids, decreased serum iron and zinc, increased serum copper) that inhibit bacterial replication.

The initial evaluation and management of the febrile patient depends on the underlying malignancy and the degree of treatment-induced host compromise. For example, altered cellular immunity places the patient with Hodgkin's disease at increased risk for *H. zoster* infection or cryptococcal meningitis; patients who have undergone allogeneic bone marrow transplantation are at risk for severe interstitial pneumonia, especially with CMV.[104–106]

Although evaluation of the nonimmunosuppressed febrile cancer patient can proceed according to general medical principles, the detection of infection and the management of the febrile granulocytopenic patient is complicated by two important factors. First, granulocytopenia markedly alters the host's inflammatory response, making it difficult to detect the presence of infection. Second, an undetected and untreated infection can be rapidly fatal in the granulocytopenic cancer patient.[107]

Because the classic signs and symptoms of infection often are missing in the granulocytopenic cancer patient (*e.g.*, pyuria may be detectable in only 11% of patients with a urinary tract infection or purulent sputum in only 8% of patients with pneumonia), the physician must take a careful history and perform a scrupulous physical examination, being especially attentive to subtle signs of inflammation.[108] The physical examination may need to be repeated frequently, especially if an initial source of infection is not discernible.

All granulocytopenic cancer patients deserve prompt empiric antibiotic management when they become febrile. Adults with solid tumors are at risk for fever when rendered neutropenic and appear to do well when treated empirically with antibiotics.[109] In a survey of 1001 consecutive episodes of fever in 324 pediatric and young adult cancer patients treated at the National Cancer Institute (NCI), 39.5% had at least one febrile episode while they were granulocytopenic. There was no apparent difference in the incidence, pattern, or severity of infectious complications that occurred, regardless of the patient's underlying malignancy, after they became granulocytopenic. All granulocytopenic patients should be considered to be at risk for infection and, once febrile, should be considered as candidates for early empiric therapy.

Although some investigators recommend starting antibiotics if the granulocyte count falls below 1000/mm[3], the Consensus Conference of the Infectious Diseases Society of America and the Immunocompromised Host Society have agreed that the risk is really increased if the granulocyte count is less than 500/mm[3].[110a,110b] The incidence of bacteremia is particularly increased if the granulocyte count is less than 100/mm[3]. Perhaps more important than the absolute nadir is the rate at which the counts are falling.

The level of fever that should prompt therapy has been defined. In general, two or three low-grade elevations above 38°C (taken orally) or a single elevation above 38.5°C in concert with a granulocyte count of less than 500/mm[3] are sufficient criteria to begin empiric therapy. Fever should not be caused by blood products, cancer, or medications, and the physician should ascertain if the patient is receiving drugs that mask a febrile response (*e.g.*, steroids, antipyretic-containing analgesics). Institutional criteria for fever and granulocytopenia should be defined and rigidly adhered to. Such a policy plays an important role in reducing infection-related morbidity and mortality.

PREANTIBIOTIC EVALUATION

In a prospective evaluation of 140 febrile granulocytopenic patients, it was not possible to differentiate patients with bacteremia-induced fever from those with unexplained fever by their age, sex, underlying malignancy, or the types of therapeutic modalities or invasive diagnostic procedures they had received.[110] The absence of physical findings suggesting infection did not exclude a potentially life-threatening bacteremia, because more than half of the bacteremic patients in this study lacked any specific physical findings.

Patients about to receive empiric therapy should have a baseline chest radiograph, urinalysis, at least two sets of preantibiotic blood cultures, and aspirate or biopsy cultures from any accessible sites suggesting infection. If blood cultures are obtained from an indwelling Silastic catheter, it is essential to obtain additional cultures from a peripheral vein. It is important to obtain blood cultures from each port in patients with multilumen catheters.

Even with a comprehensive evaluation, an infectious cause is demonstrated in only 30% to 40% of febrile granulocytopenic patients.[111,112] Moreover, definitive diagnosis may take days, presumably because of the low microbial inoculum. This probably reflects the short period that elapses between the onset of fever and evaluation and initiation of empiric therapy. Even subtle indications of inflammation must be considered as sites of infection in the context of granulocytopenia. For example, minimal perirectal erythema and tenderness may be the harbinger of a perirectal cellulitis. Minimal erythema and serious discharge at the site of a Hickman catheter exit may herald a tunnel or exit site infection. Accordingly, any clinically suspicious and accessible site of infection in the neutropenic patient should be aspirated for culture and tested with Gram's stain. It is generally not possible to differentiate granulocytopenic patients who have a bacteremia from those with unexplained fever (FUO).[110]

Because the patients' colonizing flora frequently can be implicated as the cause of infection, some have advocated surveillance cultures as an aid to diagnosis and antibiotic management. To assess this approach, we evaluated serial surveillance cultures of the nose, throat, urine, and stool from 271 patients at the NCI during 652 episodes of fever and neutropenia.[62] Sixty-two percent of these patients were colonized with the organism ultimately found to be responsible for the infection. However, the clinical usefulness of these surveillance cultures was limited, because there was not any one body site that was consistently predictive, and invariably other potential pathogens were isolated, making it difficult to differentiate prospectively the true pathogen. By the time the results from a routine surveillance culture (stool) were known, the true pathogens had been found in pure growth in blood cultures. The cost of routine surveillance is enormous. Even knowing the colonizing flora is unlikely to have a tremendous impact on initial antibiotic management, because most clinicians routinely employ broad-spectrum antibiotics for empiric treatment of febrile granulocytopenic patients. Routine surveillance cultures should not be part of the patients' evaluations. Exceptions to this may be patients in protected isolation, where stool cultures may be of use, or centers with a high incidence of *Aspergillus* infections, where nasal swabs may be helpful in identifying high-risk patients.[64]

Nuclear scanning with indium 111 has been used to define occult sites of infection.[113,114] Rubin described a method for linking ^{111}In to IgG, increasing its sensitivity in detecting sites of inflammation or infection.[115] The use of this technique for patients with fever and neutropenia must be further explored.

Although rapid diagnostic assays, such as the limulus assay for endotoxin, the enzyme-linked immunosorbent assay, and latex particle agglutination, have been successfully employed in certain common infections, they have had little impact on the rapid diagnosis of the bacterial and fungal infections that occur in cancer patients. This is primarily a consequence of the many antigenically diverse pathogens that can infect the cancer patient. Because of the difficulty in diagnosing fungal infections in cancer patients, several nonculture-dependent, rapid diagnostic techniques have been investigated. The detection of *Candida* enolase, especially if coupled with blood cultures, provides high specificity and sensitivity for detecting invasive candidiasis.[116] Sensitive methods for detecting *Aspergillus* are critically needed.[98]

EMPIRIC ANTIBIOTIC THERAPY

The prompt initiation of empiric antibiotics when the neutropenic cancer patient becomes febrile has been the single most important advance in the management of the immunocompromised host (Fig. 62–5).[108] Before this policy, the mortality of gram-negative infections, especially with *P. aeruginosa*, *E. coli*, and *K. pneumoniae*, approached 80%.[117,118] Since the widespread use of effective empiric antibiotics, the overall survival rate is between 60% and 90%.[119,120]

What are the criteria for an empiric antibiotic regimen? Between 85% and 90% of pathogens proven or associated

with new fevers in the immunosuppressed patients are bacteria.[110,120] However, because gram-positive and gram-negative bacteria can be responsible for these initial infections, the empiric regimen must be broad, achieve high bactericidal levels, and be as nontoxic and as simple to administer as possible. This has usually necessitated the combination of two or more antibiotics. The availability of third-generation cephalosporins and carbapenems offers an alternative to combination regimens, because many of these single-agent antibiotics provide an exceedingly broad range of activity and high bactericidal levels (see Table 62–12).[121-123] Unlike the aminoglycosides, these newer β-lactam antibiotics do not require monitoring of serum levels and have minimal toxicity.

No particular combination has been shown to be clearly superior, and the regimen that is chosen at a given institution should reflect specific epidemiologic considerations (*e.g.*, local resistance patterns) and cost.[124-127]

Despite the proven efficacy of combination therapy, the potential of a single antibiotic for the empiric management of the febrile neutropenic patient is attractive for its ease of administration, cost, and lack of toxicity. To assess the efficacy of a monotherapeutic regimen, a prospective randomized trial was initiated at the NCI that compared monotherapy using ceftazidime with combination therapy using cephalothin, carbenicillin, and gentamicin for the initial empiric management of 550 episodes of fever and neutropenia.[112] The early evaluation at 72 hours was performed to assess the efficacy of the antibiotics during the period when they were used in an empiric manner (*i.e.*, before definitive microbiologic data). The overall evaluation was performed at the resolution of the neutropenic episode. The responses were categorized as "successes" (with or without modification of the initial regimen) if the patients survived the episode of neutropenia and as "failures" if the patients died while neutropenic. The importance of including additions to or modifications of the initial antibiotic regimen in the analysis of studies evaluating empiric antibiotic therapy has been underscored by the Immunocompromised Host Society's Consensus conference.[110b]

In the NCI study, there was no significant difference in terms of success for patients randomized to ceftazidime or the combination regimen among patients classified as FUO or as having a clinically or microbiologically documented infections. A significantly greater number of modifications were required among the patients randomized to ceftazidime: 58 (21%) of 282, compared with 29 (11%) of 268 (p^2=0.002 by chi-square).[115] This increased need for antibiotic modifications at the early evaluation reflected the need for anaerobic coverage in patients randomized to ceftazidime who developed necrotizing gingivitis or perirectal cellulitis and the greater need for vancomycin in patients with documented gram-positive infections, especially those due to *S. epidermidis*.

The result at the overall evaluation demonstrated equivalent success rates for the two regimens for patients with FUO or with documented infections. The percentage of patients treated successfully without modification of the initial antimicrobial therapy was predictably less than that at the early evaluation (Table 62–13). Patients with documented infections required changes in antimicrobial therapy more often than FUO patients, but the need for modifications of the initial therapy for patients randomized to monotherapy (59%) and those randomized to combination therapy (59%). In terms of

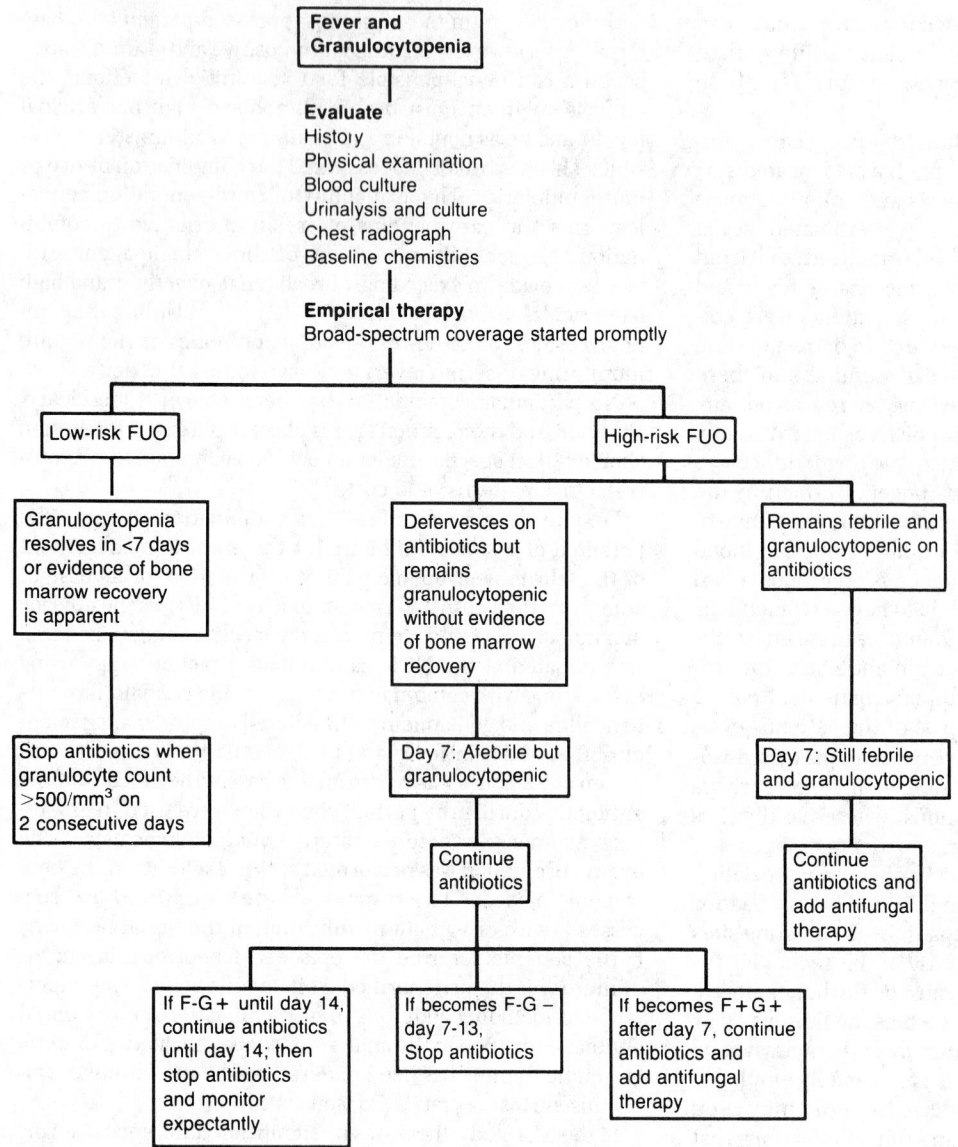

FIGURE 62–5. Algorithm for the initial management of the patient who has unexplained fever and neutropenia.

the overall outcome and the frequency with which modifications of the initial empiric regimen were necessary, monotherapy with ceftazidime was as effective as combination therapy with cephalothin (Keflin), carbenicillin, and gentamicin for these patients.

Other antibiotics are being evaluated for use as monotherapy in patients with neutropenia. Among the most important is imipenem, a member of the carbapenem class of antibiotics, that provides activity against most gram-positive bacteria (including the enterococci), the Enterobacteriaceae, P. aeruginosa (but not not *Pseudomonas maltophilia*), and anaerobes.[122] Overall, it has the broadest spectrum of activity of any available antibiotic. Early results of a randomized study comparing ceftazidime with imipenem at the NCI demonstrate to corroborate is efficacy in this setting. More than 500 episodes of fever and neutropenia have been enrolled in an NCI study that randomly assigned pediatric and adult patients to receive monotherapy with ceftazidime or imipenem and cilastatin; the data suggest that the overall outcome is comparable. More gram-positive infections have been observed in patients ran-

domly assigned to receive ceftazidime and a significantly higher incidence of *Clostridium difficile* colitis occurred in patients randomly assigned to receive imipenem. Despite its broad spectrum of activity, imipenem has several potential drawbacks, including the emergence of resistant strains of *P. aeruginosa* (caused by alterations of the organism's porin channels), the risk for breakthrough infections with *Pseudomonas (Xanthomonas) maltophilia* resistant to imipenem, and the potential for imipenem to decrease the seizure threshold in patients with central nervous system abnormalities. We have observed unexpectedly frequent nausea and vomiting in patients receiving imipenem, despite a slow rate of infusion.

Because of the increasing incidence of gram-positive infections in patients with cancer during the 1980s and because of the increased resistance to β-lactam antibiotics, several groups suggested that vancomycin or teicoplanin (a new glycopeptide antibiotic with activity similar to that of vancomycin) be included in initial empiric regimens.[128–130] Conversely, it has been argued that many of these bacteria are relatively low in virulence and that vancomycin may be safely withheld until the gram-positive isolate has been identified microbiologically.

Although two randomized studies have demonstrated a reduction in gram-positive infections in patients receiving a vancomycin regimen, no significant differences in survival were observed in patients who received vancomycin in a pathogen-directed manner. A retrospective analysis from the NCI of 550 patient episodes indicated that no excess morbidity occurred as a result of delaying the institution of vancomycin to wait for a microbiologic or clinical indication for its use (*i.e.*, a positive culture for a resistant gram-positive organism, or a clinical infection developing during other antibiotic therapy).[131] A study by the European Organization for Research and Treatment of Cancer and the National Cancer Institute of Canada evaluated data on 747 febrile patients with granulocytopenia and failed to demonstrate a benefit derived from empiric vancomycin therapy.[132] Comparable results were obtained in children with fever and neutropenia. Moreover, a study of teicoplanin as an alternative to vancomycin failed to demonstrate a significant benefit when teicoplanin was administered empirically.[133]

It seems reasonable not to include vancomycin routinely in all empiric antibiotic regimens. Its use should be guided by institutional experience and sensitivity patterns. Patterns of infecting microorganisms may fluctuate. For example, penicillin-resistant α-hemolytic streptococci are particularly virulent pathogens in some centers, perhaps related to the use of high-dose cytosine arabinoside therapy or to alteration of the oral mucosa by infection with HSV.[134] Centers with a high frequency of infection with methicillin-resistant *S. aureus* should routinely use vancomycin empirically. The emergence of new pathogens or of pathogens with altered sensitivity profiles may force changes in our use of antibiotics.

NEWER ANTIBIOTICS FOR THE COMPROMISED HOST

The monobactams are another novel group of antibiotics, of which aztreonam is the prototype.[135,136] Susceptible organisms include most enteric gram-negative rods, including *P. aeruginosa*. Aztreonam has no significant activity against any of the clinically important gram-positive aerobic organisms or against anaerobes. A particularly useful feature of aztreonam is its apparent lack of cross-reactivity to the other β-lactams in patients who have penicillin or β-lactam allergies. It may be most useful for the treatment of the patient with a significant allergy to β-lactams for whom therapy with an anti-*Pseudomonas* β-lactam antibiotic is still desirable or who requires a bacterial agent

β-Lactams are combined with β-lactamase inhibitors (*e.g.*, clavulanic acid and sulbactam). Three preparations are now available: amoxicillin plus clavulanic acid (oral formulations only), ticarcillin plus clavulanic acid, and ampicillin plus sulbactam. Others, such as piperacillin plus sulbactam, are under development.

The quinolones represent a group of structurally distinct synthetic synthetic antibiotics with a broad spectrum of activity and a unique mechanism of action characterized by the inhibition of DNA gyrase.[137] The spectrum of activity of the fluoroquinolones includes most gram-negative organisms encountered in neutropenic hosts. However, the currently available quinolones have only moderate activity against many species of streptococci, including *Enterococcus* species and *Streptococcus pneumoniae*, and are virtually devoid of activity against the clinically important anaerobic bacteria.[138,139]

The appropriate role for the quinolones in the patient with neutropenia has yet to be defined. Because of their relatively limited activity against certain gram-positive organisms, they should not be used alone for empiric therapy. They may be useful for the completion of therapy in patients who initially responded to intravenously administered antibiotics and who have had a fever of undetermined origin or a susceptible bacterial isolate, an issue that is currently under study at the NCI. However, with expanded use the resistant isolates have emerged. Moreover, the quinolones are not approved for use in the pediatric population because of articular abnormalities observed in the weight-bearing joints in the young of some experimental animals, although phase I and II trials are in progress in children with cancer and cystic fibrosis.

MANAGEMENT APPROACHES

Prolonged Granulocytopenia

The question of the duration of empiric antibiotic therapy in patients with persistent neutropenia is a matter of practical significance. This can be approached by placing patients in one of two categories: those whose initial examination (at the time of presentation with fever and neutropenia) did not reveal a source of infection and those whose initial studies revealed a documented infection to account for the fever (*i.e.*, positive culture, clinically infected site) At most centers, the majority of patients are in the unexplained-fever category, although this proportion varies with the institution, the therapy, and the patient population.

UNEXPLAINED FEVER. For patients whose granulocytopenia is of short duration (<1 week), stopping antibiotic therapy after recovery of the leukocyte count can be practical and effective. Some studies suggest that afebrile patients recovering from their neutropenia (but whose absolute granulocyte count remains below 500/mm^3) can have their antibiotics discontinued with adverse sequelae.[140] However, a problem arises in the population with more prolonged granulocytopenia. In a study from the NCI, patients with unexplained fever and persistent granulocytopenia were randomly selected to discontinue the use of antibiotics on day 7 of therapy or to continue under the resolution of the neutropenia. Almost 40% of afebrile patients who stopped antibiotic therapy had recurrent fever subsequently, and 38% of febrile patients whose antibiotic therapy was discontinued had hypotensive episodes. It was concluded that day 7 was too early to discontinue antibiotic treatment in this group.

A subsequent study conducted at the NCI randomly selected afebrile patients with persistent neutropenia to continue or discontinue antibiotic therapy on day 14. Analysis showed no difference between the two groups; approximately one third of patients became afebrile again regardless of whether they stopped or continued treatment with antibiotics.[142] However, those whose fevers recurred after discontinuation of antibiotic therapy responded to reinstitution of their initial regimens, but those continuing to receive antibiotics required the addition of amphotericin B. On this basis, it seems reasonable to discontinue antibiotic therapy on day 14 in patients who

(text continues on page 2308)

TABLE 62-13. Antimicrobial Agents Commonly Used in Cancer Patients

Antimicrobial Agent	Trade Name	Major Indications	Usual Daily Dosage (I.V.)	Daily Dosage Schedule	Usual Maximal Adult Dose per Day
Penicillins					
Penicillin G	Benzathin Permapen Bicillin	S. pneumoniae, S. pyogenes, S. viridens, S. bovis, Neisseria, most anaerobes (except B. fragilis)	25–500,000 units/kg	q 4 h	20 g
Penicillinase resistant					
Methicillin	Straphcillin, celbenin	S. aureus, streptococci	1–300 mg/kg	q 4 h	12 g
Nafcillin	Unipen		1–300 mg/kg	q 4 h	12 g
Oxacillin	Prostaphin, bactocill		1–300 mg/kg	q 4 h	12 g
Aminopencillin					
Ampicillin	Omipen Prinipen Polycillin Penbritin	S. fecalis, L. monocytogenes, Hemophilus, E. coli, Salmonella, Proteus	2–400 mg/kg	q 4 h	12 g
Ampicillin/ sulbactam	Unasyn	Same as ampicillin but with more reliable gram-negative activity and broader anaerobic activity	100–400 mg/kg	q 6 h	12 g
Carboxy penicillins					
Carbenicillin	Pyopen, Geopen	P. aeruginosa, Enterobacter, Proteus, Serrata, Acinetobacter, Providentia.	500 mg/kg	q 4 h	36 g
Ticarcillin	Ticar	Anaerobes including some Bacteroides sp., some Clostridium sp. Peptostreptococcus, Fusobacterium	300 mg/kg	q 4 h	21 g
Extended-spectrum					
Mezlocillin	Mezlin	Same as carboxy penicillin plus Klebsiella sp.	300 mg/kg	q 4 h	21 g
Piperacillin	Pipercil	Same as mezlocillin plus increased activity against P. aeruginosa	300 mg/kg	q 4 h	21 g
Azlocillin	Azlin	Same as piperacillin	300 mg/kg	q 4 h	21 g
Cephalosporins					
First generation:					
Cephalothin	Keflin	E. coli, Klebsiella, Proteus, Hemophilus, S. aureus, S. epidermidis, streptococci	170 mg/kg	q 4 h	12 g
Cefazolin	Kefzol, Ancef	Similar to cephalothin, more active against Klebsiella, E. coli	50 mg/kg	q 6 h	2–6 g
Second generation:					
Cephamandole	Mandol	More active against Hemophilus, Klebsiella, E. coli, Enterobacter sp., Proteus; less active against gram-positive cocci	100–200 mg/kg	q 4 h	6–12 g
Cefoxitin	Mefoxitin	Same as cephalothin plus Proteus sp., and anaerobes, including B. fragilis	200 mg/kg	q 4 h	6–12 g

Peak Serum Level (μg/ml)	$T_{1/2}$ (h)		Modifications for Renal Failure (adults)		Comments
	Normal	Renal Failure	Moderate C_{CR} 10–50 ml/min	Severe C_{CR} <10 ml/min	
2	0.5	2.5	NC	1,600,000 units q 6 h	
40	0.5	4	NC	2 g q 8 h	Rare nephritis
6	0.5	1.5	NC	NC	Rare SGOT elevation
2.6	0.5	1.0	NC	NC	Rare neutropenia, hepatotoxicity
3.5	1.0	8	NC	0.5–1 g q 8 h	Diarrhea common Synergistic with aminoglycoside for *Enterococcus*
Same as ampicillin	1.0	9	C_{CR} 15–29: 1.5–3.0 g q 12 h	C_{CR} 5–14: 1.5–3.0 q 24 h	
200	1.1	15	3 g q 4 h	2 g q 8 h	Synergistic with gentamicin for *Pseudomonas* Higher sodium load (carbticar)—hypokalemia
140	1.2	15	2 g q 4 h	2 g q 8 h	Rare platelet dysfunction Should never be mixed in same bottle with aminoglycosides
100–110	0.8	1.6	NC	25 mg/kg/dose q 6 h	Similar to carboxy penicillins Bleeding reactions not described
100–110	1.0	3.1	NC	25 mg/kg/dose q 6 h	The extended-spectrum penicillins have a lower sodium content (1.8–2.0 mEq g)
100–110	0.8	4	NC	45 mg/kg/dose q 12 h	They have a lower protein binding and higher biliary excretion than the carboxy penicillins.
80	0.5–0.8	2	1 g q 4–6 h	1 g q 8 h	Most gram-positive activity among cephalosporins
135	1.5	20–40	0.5 g q 6–12 h	0.5 g q 24–48 h	Longer half-life than cephalothin
36	0.9–1.5		1.2 g q 6–8 h	0.5 g q 8–12 h	Cefuroxime (Zinacef) provides comparable coverage with a slightly longer half-life
20–23	0.75	22	15–30 mg/kg/dose q 12–24 h	15 mg/kg/dose q 24 h	Cefoxitin can induce production of β-lactamases which can hydrolyze other β-lactam antibodies used in combination

(continued)

TABLE 62–13. *(Continued)*

Antimicrobial Agent	Trade Name	Major Indications	Usual Daily Dosage (I.V.)	Daily Dosage Schedule	Usual Maximal Adult Dose per Day
Cefuroxime	Zinacef	Similar to cefamandole, penetrates into CSF	0.75–1.5 g	q 8 h	5–9 g
Third generation:					
Cefotaxime	Claforan	Same as cephalothin plus *Enterobacter* sp., indole positive *Proteus*, *H. influenzae*, *Citrobacter* sp., *Serratia* sp., and some *P. aeruginosa* and *Bacteroides* sp.	200 mg/kg	q 4 h	12 g
Ceftriaxone	Rocephin	Similar to cefotaxime	1–2 g	q 12–24 h	2 g
Cefoperazone	Cefaloid	Same as cefotaxime but with better *P. aeruginosa* activity	200 mg/kg	q 8 h	12 g
Ceftizoxime	Cefizox	Same as cefotaxime	200 mg/kg	q 8 h	12 g
Ceftazidime	Fortaz	Same as cefoperazone but with less anaerobic activity. Most active agent against *P. aeruginosa*	100 mg/kg	q 8 h	6 g
Carbapenems					
Imipenem/cilastatin	Primaxin	In addition to the Enterobacteriaceae and *P. aeruginosa*, primaxin has efficacy against *S. aureus*, group D streptococci, many coagulase-negative staphylococci, listeria, and anaerobes. Only *P. maltophilia* and *P. cepacia* are not covered.	50–60	q 6 h	3–4
Monobactams					
Monobactems					
Aztreonam	Azactam	Broad gram-negative but no gram-positive coverage. Is not cross-reactive with other β-lactams so can be used in penicillin or cephalosporin allergic patients	100–150	q 6 h	4–6
Aminoglycosides					
Gentamicin	Garamycin	*P. aeruginosa*, Enterobacteriaceae, Enterococcus (with ampicillin)	3–6 mg/kg	q 6–8 h	

Peak Serum Level (µg/ml)	$T_{1/2}$ (h)		Modifications for Renal Failure (adults)		Comments
	Normal	Renal Failure	Moderate C_{CR} 10–50 ml/min	Severe C_{CR} <10 ml/min	
100	1–2	15	0.75–1.5 g q 8–12 h	0.75–1.5 q 24 h	Cefuroxime also is dispensed in an oral formulation
125–175	1.3–1.6	27	NC	30 mg/kg q 12 h	All third-generation cephalosporins have less gram-positive activity than first-generation agents. None are effective against enterococci or *Listeria*. They have variable coverage against pseudomonads and anaerobes
270	8	11.9–15.4	0.5–1 g q 12–24 h	0.5–1 g q 12–24 h	Longest half-life of third-generation cephalosporins, permits once- or twice-daily dosing. Also has activity against *N. gonorrhoeae*
175–225	1.6–2.1	4.2	NC	20 mg/kg dose q 12 h	Highest biliary excretion of the third generation group. It contains the methylthiotetrazole group and may cause serious bleeding
150–200	2.1–2.8	19.3	1 g q 12	0.5 g q 24 h	
150–200	1.6–2.1		C_{CR}31–50: 1 g q 12 h C_{CR}16–30: 1 g q 24 h	C_{CR}6–15: 0.5 mg q 24 h C_{CR}5: 0.5 mg q 48 h	Best activity against *P. aeruginosa*
43–78	1	4	0.5–1 g q 6–12 h	0.5–1 g q 12–24 h	Can cause seizures in patients with preexisting CNS disease or in patients with altered renal functions. Higher doses can cause nausea and vomiting
125	1.7–2	6–8.7	0.5–2 g q 12–24 h	0.5–2 g q 12–24 h	Not cross-rective with β-lactams and can be used in the penicillin or cephalosporin allergic patient.
4–8	2.3	45–55	Monitor serum levels		All aminoglycosides synergistic or additive with penicillins or cephalosporins against *Pseudomonas*, enterococcus, staph., strep., Enterobacteriaceae

(continued)

TABLE 62–13. *(Continued)*

Antimicrobial Agent	Trade Name	Major Indications	Usual Daily Dosage (I.V.)	Daily Dosage Schedule	Usual Maximal Adult Dose per Day
Tobramycin	Nebicin	Similar to gentamicin (except not as active against enterococcus with ampicillin)	3–6 mg/kg	q 6–8 h	
Amikacin	Amikin	*Serratia, Proteus, Pseudomonas,* Enterobacteriaceae, *Providentia*	15 mg/kg	q 8–12 h	
Miscellaneous					
Chloramphenicol	Chloromycetin	*Hemophilus, B. fragilis, S. pneumoniae, Neisseriae, Salmonella, Klebsiella,* most anaerobes, *Rickettsia*	50–100 mg/kg	q 6 h	3–6 g
Erythromycin	Ilotycin Gluceptate	*Legionella Mycoplasma*	30–50 mg/kg	q 6 h	6 g
Clindamycin	Cleocin	*B. fragilis, Clostridia, S. pneumoniae, S. viridens, S. pyogenes, S. aureus*	30 mg/kg	q 6 h	2400 mg
Vancomycin	Vancocin	*C. difficile, S. aureus, S. epidermidis, S. fecalis,* multiply resistant *Corynebacteria, S. bovis*	25–40 mg/kg	q 8–12 h	3 g
Trimethoprim-Sulfamethoxazole (1:5 ratio)	Bactrim Septra	*P. carinii, S. aureus, S. pneumoniae, S. pyogenes, Salmonella, Listeria, E. coli, Proteus, Serratia, Hemophilus, Neisseria*	10–20 mg/kg as trimethoprim	q 8–12 h	960 g
Ciprofloxacin	Cinoxacin	Gram negatives including Enterobacteriaceae, *P. aeruginosa, Hemophilus, Branhamella,* gonococci. Also active against *Chlamydia,* some mycoplasma, *Legionella.* Less active against gram-positive bacteria, especially streptococci	250–500 mg	q 6–12 h	1.5 g
Antiparasitics					
Pentamidine Isethionate	Lomidine	*P. carinii*	4 mg/kg IM	Once/day	
Thiabendazole	Mintezol	*Strongyloides,* visceral larva migrans	50 mg/kg 2 days	q 12 h	3 g
Antifungal Agents					
Amphotericin B	Fungizone	*Candida, Aspergillus, Zygomycetes, Torulopsis, Cryptococcus, Histoplasma*	0.5–1.0 mg/kg	Once/day	

| Peak Serum Level ($\mu g/ml$) | $T_{1/2}$ (h) | | Modifications for Renal Failure (adults) | | Comments |
	Normal	Renal Failure	Moderate C_{CR} 10–50 ml/min	Severe C_{CR} <10 ml/min	
4–8	2.3	45–55	Monitor serum levels		All have renal and ototoxicity
15–25	2.3	50–80	Monitor serum levels		
12	4.1	4.2	NC	NC	Both idiosyncratic and dose-related bone marrow toxicity
					Dosage must be reduced with hepatotoxicity
0.4–1.8	1.4	5	NC	NC	Burning and phlebitis intravenously
10	2.4	6	NC	NC	Risk for pseudomembranous enterocolitis
					(Treat with vancomycin or metronidazole)
25–50	6	9 d	1 g q 36 h	1 g q 10–14 d	Drug of choice for antibiotic (C. difficile) induced colitis but must be given orally (125 mg PO q 6 h). Also drug of choice for S. epid. and methicillin-resistant staph (I.V.)
1.6–3.2 trimethoprim	7½	25	10 mg/kg q 12 h	5 mg/kg q 12 h	May be useful for prophylaxis against P. carinii
					May result in myelosuppression, particularly in AIDS
2.4	3.9	5–10	250 mg q 12–24 h	Not recommended	Both oral and parenteral formulations available. Accumulates in cartilage and not approved for children
0.2	Very short		q 36 h	q 48 h	Very toxic: hypotension, renal damage, sterile abscesses, hypo- and hyperglycemia
					Available only through CDC
	1				Rare hepatoxicity. May cause nausea, vomiting, headache, dizziness
0.5–2.0	24	NC	NC	0.5 mg/kg/q 36 h	Dose modification necessary for patients with hepatic abnormalities
					Major toxicities are fever, electrolyte disturbances. May be combined with 5-FC to treat cryptococcal meningitis

(continued)

TABLE 62–13. *(Continued)*

Antimicrobial Agent	Trade Name	Major Indications	Usual Daily Dosage (I.V.)	Daily Dosage Schedule	Usual Maximal Adult Dose per Day
5-Fluorocytosine	Flucytosine Ancobon	*Cryptococcus, Candida, Torulopsis, Chromomycosis*	50–150 mg/kg	q 6 h	
Clotrimazole	Lotrimin	*Candida* sp., dermatophytes	50 mg (troche)	q 6 h	
Miconazole	Monistat	*Candida* sp., *Aspergillus* sp., *Zygomycetes, Torulopsis, Cryptococcus, Petriellidium, Blastomyces, Coccidioides, Histoplasma, Paracoccidiides, Sporothrix*	1500–3600 mg/d		
Ketoconazole	Nizoral	Similar to miconazole	2–400 mg/d	q d	400 (higher doses are being investigated)
Fluconazole	Diflucan	*Candida, Crytococcus, Histoplasma, Blastomyces, Coccidioides*	100–400 mg/d (oral or I.V.)	q d	Excellent penetration into CSF
Antiviral Agents Adenosine arabinoside	Vidarabine	H. simplex varicella-zoster	10–15 mg/kg/d	12-h infusion	
Acycloguanosine	Acyclovir	H. simplex, varicella-zoster	750 mg/m²/d (H. simplex) 1500 mg/m²/d (VZV)	q 8 h	
Ganciclovir	Cytovene	Cytomegalovirus reninitis, pneumonia, colitis	5 mg/kg q 12 h × 14–21 day induction then 5 mg/kg q d or 6 mg/kg 5 d/wk for maintenance.	Induction	
Interferons (α, β, γ)		H. simplex, VZV	1×10^4 5×10^5 units/kg/d	q d	

NC, no change.

Peak Serum Level (μg/ml)	$T_{1/2}$ (h) Normal	$T_{1/2}$ (h) Renal Failure	Modifications for Renal Failure (adults) Moderate C_{CR} 10–50 ml/min	Modifications for Renal Failure (adults) Severe C_{CR} <10 ml/min	Comments
30	3.4	200	12–25 mg/kg once	Not given	Rapid resistance develops when used alone
					Normal use is in conjunction with amphotericin
					Parenteral form investigational
					For topical use only (e.g., oral troche). If systemically absorbed, is inactivated by hepatic enzymes
2–8 μg	0.4, 2.1, 24.2 h (3 compartments)		NC	NC	No proven efficacy in invasive fungal infections in immunocompromised hosts
					Can cause hyponatremia, anemia, thrombocytosis, nausea, vomiting, cardiac arrhythmias. Less than 1% excreted in urine. 50% excreted in feces
2–13 μg	2–8 h (biphasic)		NC	NC	No proven value in immunocompromised hosts. May cause nausea, vomiting, hepatic enzyme elevation, dizziness, gynecomastia, adrenal insufficiency. Antacids and cimetidine impede absorption
4–8 μg/ml	3–5 h		No established guidelines. Reduce by 25% in severe renal failure and monitor metabolites		No activity against CMV
					Anorexia, nausea, vomiting, diarrhea. Rare myelosuppression, neurotoxicity. Excessive fluid requirements
30–50 μM	2.2–5 h		5–10 mg/kg q 12 h for C_{CR} 25–50.; 5–10 mg/kg q 24 h for C_{CR} 10–25	2.5–5 mg/kg q 24 h	Twice maintenance fluids necessary with higher doses to avoid renal toxicity
					Neurotoxicity (at high doses)
					Thymidine kinase resistant mutants have been described
8–11 μg/ml	3–4 h		28–5 h	Dose adjustments necessary	Poace and bioavailabiilty require maintenance in HIV patients, can cause marrow suppression
					Local pain, fever, alopecia, fatigue, anorexia, bone marrow suppression

have remained consistently afebrile during empiric therapy, recognizing that when the antibiotics are withdrawn, these patients must be closely monitored for recurrent fever or infection until the resolution of their granulocytopenia. The question of whether the antibiotic therapy could be delivered orally for these patients is being explored by the NCI Pediatric Branch. The results of this study will help to define the safety of ciprofloxacin in children and its utility for simplifying continuation of therapy for patients with prolonged neutropenia.

DOCUMENTED INFECTIONS AT PRESENTATION. For patients with persistent neutropenia who have had clinical and microbiologic resolution of their infection, and who are afebrile at day 14 (for a minimum of 7 days), antibiotic therapy may be discontinued. The ultimate decision of whether to continue or discontinue antibiotic therapy depends on potential antibiotic toxicity, the predicted duration of neutropenia, the seriousness of the initial infection, and the presence or absence of other factors predisposing the patient to subsequent infection. Antibiotics are usually administered for 10 to 14 days unless there is a residual site of infection (*e.g.*, perianal cellulitis) and the neutropenia persists. In such cases, antibiotic therapy should be continued until resolution of the signs of infection or recovery from neutropenia.

The question of whether the spectrum of antibiotics can be narrowed when a specific isolate is determined is of practical relevance.[143] Although a primary infection caused by an identified organism can be treated successfully with a broad-spectrum or a pathogen-specific antibiotic, the risk of second (or breakthrough) infections is increased in patients with prolonged neutropenia (>7 days) who receive a narrow-spectrum antibiotic.

Therapy Modifications During the Granulocytopenic Course

Empiric antibiotic therapy has its greatest impact early in the course of neutropenia. It should not be assumed that a regimen demonstrating initial efficacy will suffice as the sole antimicrobial therapy throughout a protracted course of neutropenia. During a prolonged granulocytopenic episode, the patient is at increased risk for secondary infections or superinfections; this risk increases the longer that the neutropenia persists. Throughout the course of the patient's disease, the persistence of fever and changing clinical findings may dictate that modifications be made to ensure a successful outcome. Few of these new infections represent a failure of the initial therapy. Most should be viewed as part of the "natural history" of patients with prolonged neutropenia, and needed modifications of the initial regimens should be expected and planned, with the goal of maximizing the patient's chance for survival.

Bacterial isolates that are resistant or that become resistant to the initial empiric regimen are invariably encountered in patients with neutropenia. Some of them can be anticipated; others emerge sporadically. For example, at most centers, the majority of coagulase-negative staphylococci are resistant to β-lactams, and breakthrough infections with these organisms should be anticipated if a regimen not containing vancomycin is employed. Fortunately, coagulase-negative staphylococci are relatively low in virulence. For patients with evidence of gram-positive infection during therapy with one or more β-lactam antibiotics or for those with evidence of a catheter-site infection, vancomycin should usually be added to the initial antibiotic regimen.

Breakthrough bacteremia with gram-negative organisms, particularly *Enterobacter*, *Serratia*, and *Citrobacter*, are of concern, especially if a β-lactam antibiotic is used alone. Many of the organisms likely to break through an antibiotic regimen can often be predicted from an understanding of the defined limitations of the antibiotic.

The appearance of a new site of infection (*e.g.*, cellulitis, pneumonia) and the progression of infection at a previously documented site are additional reasons for modifications of the antimicrobial regimen.

Empiric Antifungal Therapy

Patients who have prolonged periods of profound neutropenia after intensive cytotoxic chemotherapy or ablative irradiation are at increased risk of acquiring invasive fungal infections.[144] The early diagnosis of invasive fungal infections in children with granulocytopenia can be difficult, and fever may be the only manifestation of infection. Moreover, withholding antifungal therapy until infection is proved by culture or histologic examination increases the likelihood of disseminated infection. This has led to the concept of employing empiric antifungal therapy to prevent fungal overgrowth in patients with prolonged granulocytopenia and to provide early treatment of clinically occult infection.[145] Two randomized clinical trials demonstrated that the use of empirically administered amphotericin B in persistently or recurrently febrile patients with granulocytopenia decreases the frequency, morbidity, and mortality rates for invasive fungal infections, especially in patients with profound granulocytopenia who are not receiving antifungal prophylaxis.[146,147] The morbidity and mortality rates for untreated or undertreated invasive fungal infections in patients with granulocytopenia usually supersede the toxic effects of amphotericin B, which are usually reversible.

Treatment with amphotericin B (0.5 mg/kg/day) should be instituted in patients with granulocytopenia who remain persistently or recurrently febrile after 7 days. Nonetheless, because of the side effects associated with amphotericin administration, less toxic alternatives are highly desirable. Orally administered ketoconazole is comparable to amphotericin B in preventing the onset of a fungal disease, but after infection does arise, it invariably progresses unless the patient is given amphotericin B.[148] Fluconazole, a new antifungal triazole with significant activity against *Candida*, is currently being evaluated for empiric antifungal therapy in children.[149,150] However, the absence of activity against *Aspergillus* is likely to limit the value of fluconazole. This limitation underscores the need for newer antifungal agents with broader profiles.

Even empiric amphotericin B therapy does not completely prevent the development of fungal infections; invasive infection with organisms more resistant to amphotericin B (*e.g.*, *Aspergillus*, *Pseudallescheria*, *Trichosporon*, *Fusarium*) has been reported in patients who were receiving the drug at dosages of 0.5 to 0.6 mg/kg per day.[151] Higher dosages of empiric amphotericin (1.0–1.5 mg/kg/day) may be necessary for patients with more prolonged neutropenia or who develop recurrent fever and pulmonary signs and symptoms while receiving standard dosages of amphotericin B.

TREATMENT OF INFECTIOUS COMPLICATIONS

BACTEREMIA

Approximately 10% to 20% of febrile neutropenic cancer patients have bacteremia at the time of presentation. Among immunocompromised patients, the respiratory tract is the most common initial site of sepsis (25%), followed by a perianal and perioral cellulitis, the gastrointestinal tract, and the genitourinary tract (each approximately 10%). Indwelling intravascular devices have become a common source of bacteremias. Unfortunately, there is no clinically reliable method for prospectively identifying febrile neutropenic patients who are bacteremic.[62,110]

Until the late 1970s, gram-negative aerobic organisms were the most frequently isolated pathogens. The pattern of infections has shifted, and gram-positive bacteria now are isolated as often as gram-negative bacteria at most cancer centers. Among the gram-positive pathogens, *S. aureus, S. epidermidis,* and *Streptococcus* species (including the viridans and group D) are the most commonly isolated. Documented septicemia with *S. bovis,* although uncommon, is important because of its close association with carcinoma of the colon and should heighten the clinician's suspicion of an undetected neoplasm.[152] Species of *Corynebacterium* (*e.g.,* CDC group JK, *C. diphtheriae, C. equi*) and *Bacillus* are less frequently isolated and tend to occur in patients with prolonged episodes of granulocytopenia or indwelling vascular access devices, respectively. *E. coli, K. pneumoniae,* and *P. aeruginosa* are the most frequently isolated gram-negative bacilli, although more resistant species (*e.g.,* nonaeruginosa Pseudomonades, *Serratia marcescens, Enterobacter* species, *Citrobacter* species) are also found.

Primary bacteremia due to anaerobic organisms are uncommon, accounting for less than 5% of the septicemia in cancer patients. For reasons that are unclear, the incidence of infections due to *P. aeruginosa* has been decreasing in recent years. The morbidity and mortality rates due to gram-positive bacteria, especially the coagulase-negative staphylococci, are less than those due to gram-negative pathogens.

The most important therapeutic intervention for patients ultimately shown to be bacteremic is the prompt initiation of empiric antibiotics when fever and neutropenia occur. Modifications of the regimen should be based on the microbiologic sensitivity pattern of the bloodstream isolate (Table 62–14). The minimal duration of therapy for bacteremic patients is 10 to 14 days, although patients with persistent neutropenia or a persistent site of infection are likely to require longer treatment.

Catheter-Associated Bacteremias

Catheter-related bacteremias have become increasingly important during the past several years, largely because of the increased use of indwelling right atrial Hickman-Broviac catheters.[68] Although the benefit of these catheters in providing venous access to patients is enormous, the frequency of catheter-associated bacteremia and other problems is significant. Complication rates have been between 3% and 60%, which may be caused by different techniques of catheter in-

TABLE 62–14. Modification of Therapy

Clinical Event	Possible Modifications of Therapy
Breakthrough bacteremia	If gram-positive isolate (*e.g.,* S. *epidermidis*), add vancomycin
	If gram-negative isolate (*i.e.,* presumably resistant), switch to regimen containing noncross-resistant antibiotics (*e.g.,* aminoglycoside plus a carbapenem or extended-spectrum penicillin).
Catheter-associated infection	Add vancomycin (and gram-negative coverage if not already being given).
Severe oral mucositis or necrotizing gingivitis	Add specific antianaerobic agent (*e.g.,* clindamycin or metronidazole)
Esophagitis	Trial of oral clotrimazole, ketoconazole, or I.V. amphotericin B.
Pneumonitis	
Diffuse or interstitial	Trial of trimethoprim-sulfamethoxazole and erythromycin (plus broad-spectrum antibiotics if the patient is granulocytopenic).
New infiltrate in a granulocytopenic patient also receiving antibiotics	If granulocyte count is rising, watch and wait.
	If granulocyte count is not recovering, biopsy to establish diagnosis; if biopsy cannot be done, add amphotericin B empirically.
Perianal tenderness	If patient is already receiving broad-spectrum antibiotics, add a specific antianaerobic agent.
	If patient is not on antibiotics, begin broad-spectrum therapy with anaerobic coverage.
Persistent fever and neutropenia	Continue antibiotics after 1 week of persistent fever and neutropenia; add systemic antifungal therapy empirically.

sertion, care, and maintenance. Differences in patient populations, their therapies, degree of catheter use, and definition of catheter-related infection and complications also influence the rates of complications.

The diagnosis of a catheter-related bacteremia is made by documenting positive blood cultures from the catheter lumen(s) and a peripheral venous site. The colony count from the lumen sample is ordinarily greater than that from the peripheral site. Most catheter-associated infections are caused by the coagulase-positive staphylococci, but other gram-positive bacteria (*e.g.*, *S. aureus*, streptococci), gram-negative organisms (*Acinetobacter* species, *P. aeruginosa*, *Bacillus* species, *Corynebacterium* species), and *Candida* can cause infection. *Malassezia furfur* has been isolated in compromised hosts, particularly where hyperalimentation and intralipids were being delivered. Polymicrobial infections occur in rare cases. An outbreak of catheter-exit site infections due to *Aspergillus flavus* was described in association with air contamination in an operating room.[153] Local skin infections due to mycobacteria, particularly *M. fortuitum* and *M. chelonei*, also were described, although these were geographically distributed.[97]

It is important to obtain blood cultures from all ports and from peripheral sites. Careful inspection of the catheter exit site and the subcutaneous tunnel for Hickman-Broviac catheters or the subcutaneous reservoir for implanted Port-a-Cath and Med-I-Port catheters is imperative in management of infections.

If bacteremia occurs in a patient with a foreign body, the device or catheter usually should be removed to ensure eradication of the infection. However, it has become apparent that more than 80% of catheter-associated bacteremias caused by coagulase-negative staphylococci can be treated without removing the catheter if a 10-day course of vancomycin is infused through the catheter (Fig. 62–6). If the patient has a multilumen catheter, the antibiotic infusion should be rotated to include all ports and lumens. Catheter and peripheral venous samples must be obtained after therapy is started. If the cultures remain positive despite 24 hours of appropriate therapy, the catheter should be removed and vancomycin continued; the possibility of endocarditis should be considered for patients with persistent positive blood cultures, and a cardiac echo should be performed. If there is evidence of tenderness or induration along the subcutaneous track of the catheter from its exit to its insertion into the subclavian or jugular vein ("tunnel infection"), the catheter should be removed because these infections are not otherwise treatable.

Not all organisms are as treatable as the coagulase-negative staphylococci. For example, catheter-associated bacteremia caused by *Bacillus* species or by *Candida* usually necessitates catheter removal, even if the organisms are sensitive to the antibiotics being administered.[94] To determine if the type of catheter influences the incidence of infection or ease of the treatment, we compared the incidence of infectious complications in patients randomized to receive Hickman-Broviac or subcutaneously implanted Port-a-Caths. No differences in the incidence of infectious or noninfectious catheter-related complications were observed.

The presence of an indwelling catheter influences the use of antibiotics for a febrile cancer patient. Data for nonneutropenic patients with catheters are lacking, but because of the morbidity associated with untreated gram-negative infection, we recommend that these patients should have cultures obtained and then receive a 48-hour trial of antibiotics (we use ceftraxone because of its ease of administration until it is determined that the fever was not due to a catheter-associated infection. If the cultures are negative, the antibiotics are discontinued; if positive, a full course of treatment is administered.

If the patient is neutropenic and has a catheter and becomes febrile, the empirical use of vancomycin would seem appro-priate. We reviewed our experiences at the NCI and found that, although gram-positive and gram-negative bacteremias are more common in patients with indwelling catheters than without, there was no apparent advantage from the addition of vancomycin to the broad-spectrum regimen. We treat neutropenic patients who become febrile without empiric vancomycin, regardless of whether they have an indwelling catheter.

Antibiotic Considerations for the Septicemia Patient

The optimal management of the neutropenic patient with a defined infection poses a dilemma. Should the patient continue to receive a broad-spectrum antibiotic regimen or can the antibiotics be narrowed to a pathogen-directed therapy? Continuing broad-spectrum therapy maintains antimicrobial activity against a wide range of gram-positive and gram-negative pathogens and may effectively eradicate or suppress second bacterial infections. However, this approach may allow the proliferation of resistant bacteria and fungi and result in secondary bacteremias or disseminated mycoses. The advantage of pathogen-directed therapy is less disturbance of the patient's microbial flora, potentially decreasing the risk of infection with multiply-resistant bacteria or fungi.

A study conducted at the NCI reviewed 78 neutropenic patients with gram-positive (primarily *S. aureus*) bacteremia who received specific therapy with nafcillin or oxacillin or continued broad-spectrum therapy. Patients who remained granulocytopenic for less than 1 week did well regardless of the therapy chosen. Among patients with more prolonged granulocytopenia, 47% of those who received specific therapy developed a second infection due to a gram-negative aerobe.[154]

A prospectively randomized trial revealed no significant difference between patients treated with narrow- or broad-spectrum coverage with respect to second infections, new fevers, or mortality. However, many patients treated with a narrowed antibiotic regimen required subsequent modification of the therapy.[143]

Current recommendations for the management of immunosuppressed and neutropenic patients with documented bacterial infections can be summarized as follows. For patients whose neutropenia is expected to last less than 7 days, a narrowed antimicrobial regimen may be safely employed. For patients with more prolonged neutropenia, there seems to be no advantage to narrowing the initial empiric antibiotic regimen. If the empiric regimen is narrowed (*e.g.*, simplification of fluid administration, cost constraints), the patient's course must be carefully monitored for evidence of recrudescent fever, progression of an infection, or clinical deterioration. Any change should immediately prompt the reexpansion of antimicrobial coverage.

As a supplement to antimicrobial therapy, high doses of corticosteroid have been administered to patients with shock or with the adult respiratory distress syndrome associated with sepsis. Controlled clinical trials, however, have failed to demonstrate the benefit of high-dose steroids in either of these clinical settings.[155,156] Monoclonal antibodies (HA-1A) against the J5 core glycolipid have reduced mortality among patients with documented gram-negative bacteria. Whether these benefits will apply to neutropenic patients is unknown. Monoclonal antibody against TNF will soon be available with other

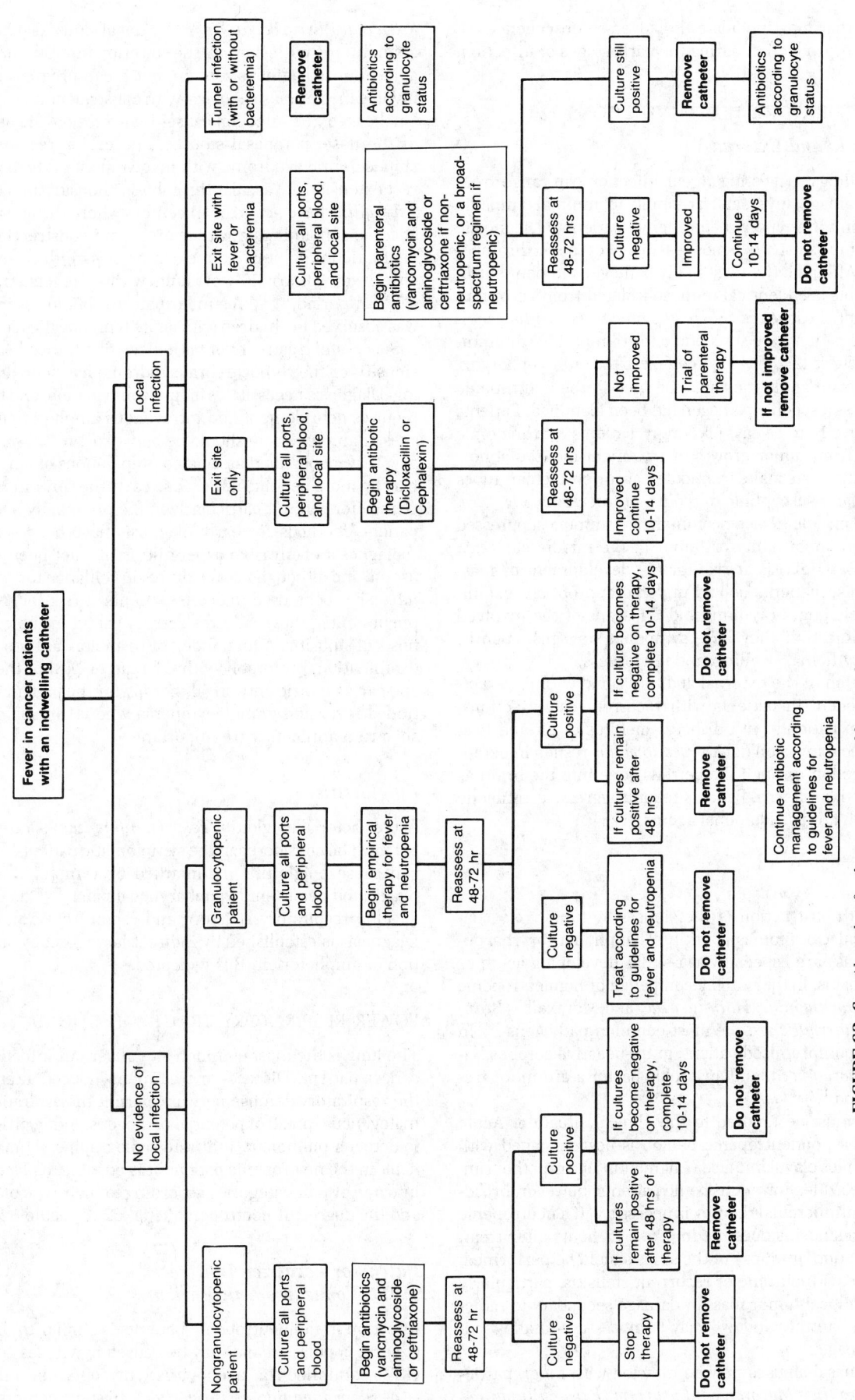

FIGURE 62–6. Algorithm for the management of fever in the cancer patient with an indwelling intravenous catheter.

biologicals that may modulate the adverse consequences of cytokine overproduction during the early stages of infection.

UPPER RESPIRATORY TRACT INFECTIONS

Otitis Media and Externa

Clinical findings suggesting an ear infection can range from ear pain, drainage, fever, and irritability to minimal tympanic erythema in profoundly neutropenic patients. Diagnostic tympanocentesis usually is not feasible because of thrombocytopenia. Although the most likely pathogens in nonneutropenic patients are identical to those isolated from an immunocompetent host (*i.e., S. pneumoniae, H. influenzae*), neutropenic patients are susceptible to gram-positive or gram-negative bacteria that may have colonized the oronasopharynx. Broad-spectrum antibiotics must be used in the neutropenic patient unless a specific pathogen has been identified. Patients should receive 10 to 14 days of therapy. Patients with anatomic alterations from tumor growth or treatment-induced abnormalities of the external ear, middle ear, or eustachian tubes are particularly susceptible to recurrent infections.

Although mastoiditis is uncommon, the immunosuppressed host with an abnormality or tumor of the middle ear (*e.g.,* rhabdomyosarcoma) is at risk for the development of mastoiditis. These patients should undergo appropriate examinations, including x-ray films and CT scans of the involved area, particularly if they have symptoms or signs, such as localized erythema, swelling, and tenderness.

Colonization of the external auditory canal with *P. aeruginosa* is frequent in patients with recurrent ear infections. However, in patients with diabetes mellitus or altered host defenses, local invasion due to *Pseudomonas* results in extension of infection through the petrous bone into the brain as malignant otitis externa. Patients require aggressive antibiotic therapy with antipseudomonal agents.

Sinusitis

Patients with obstruction of the sinuses by tumor (*e.g.,* nasopharyngeal carcinomas, Burkitt's lymphoma, or rhabdomyosarcomas) are especially at risk for developing acute or chronic sinusitis. In the immunocompetent or nonneutropenic patient, *S. pneumoniae, H. influenzae,* and Moraxella (*Branhamella*) *catarrhalis* are the most common pathogens.[182] In an immunocompromised patient, gram-negative aerobes, including *P. aeruginosa,* and anaerobic bacteria are more frequently found.[157–159]

Therapy must be tailored to the clinical situation. Acute sinusitis in a nonneutropenic person is best managed with amoxicillin plus clavulanic acid (Augmentin) or trimethoprim-sulfamethoxazole. For neutropenic patients, however, broad-spectrum antimicrobial therapy is necessary. If a neutropenic patient with sinusitis does not improve 72 hours after treatment, aspiration or biopsy of the sinus should be performed. For patients with chronic or recurrent sinusitis, particularly those with a local tumor mass or damage secondary to radiotherapy, an "antral window" may be necessary to allow adequate drainage.

The paranasal sinuses may be infected with fungi, particularly *Aspergillus, Mucoraceae, Fusarium, Exserohilum,* and

Pseudoalescheria boydii.[98,160–163] Fungal sinusitis may begin as a small crusted lesion on the anterior inferior turbinate or adjacent cartilaginous septum, but it can progress rapidly to involve the paranasal sinuses with consequent facial swelling. Unchecked, the infection causes bony erosion and destruction of the nose, paranasal sinuses, and orbits, resulting in the rhinocerebral syndrome with involvement of the brain by direct extension or vascular thrombosis. Sinusitis infections with *Aspergillus* have occurred in centers where the air supply has become contaminated with spores from construction dust or ventilation problems. At one center, *Aspergillus* sinusitis was observed in almost 20% of adults with acute leukemia during a 5-year period.[163,164] A similar pattern (but lower incidence) was observed in children with acute lymphocytic leukemia.[165]

Successful treatment of patients with advanced *Aspergillus* sinusitis or the rhinocerebral syndrome has been disappointing. Diagnosis necessitates biopsy confirmation, and treatment requires debridement and intravenous amphotericin B. Dosages of amphotericin should be between 1 to 1.5 mg/kg each day. If available, lipid-associated preparations of amphotericin may be more beneficial. Because early therapy offers the best chance for control, particularly in the profoundly neutropenic patient, methods for early diagnosis have been sought. Serodiagnosis of invasive aspergillosis has not been clinically useful, and although nasal culture surveillance for *Aspergillus flavus* has been used to detect patients at risk for *Aspergillus* pneumonitis, these cultures are not useful in the early diagnosis of sinusitis. A high index of suspicion, a thorough nasal examination, preferably with CT scan or MRI of the sinuses, and early empiric antifungal therapy for the patient with continued fever and granulocytopenia who is already on broad-spectrum antibiotics are important.

Epiglottitis

Acute bacterial epiglottitis (*e.g., H. influenzae*) is rare in adults but must be considered in the symptomatic patient.[166] *Candida* can cause epiglottitis, hallmarked by symptoms of odynophagia and persistent hypopharyngeal pain.[167,168] Patients can develop respiratory stricture and require close monitoring. Diagnosis is established by indirect laryngoscopy, and initiation of amphotericin B is indicated.

LOWER RESPIRATORY TRACT INFECTIONS

The lung is the most common site of serious infection in the cancer patient. Disease- or treatment-induced alterations of the respiratory defense network permit the aspiration or hematogenous spread of potential pathogens. Although the ability to detect a pulmonary infiltrate radiographically may be difficult in the neutropenic patient, it is possible to place patients into one of four categories according to their type of infiltrate and the degree of neutropenia (Fig. 62–7, Table 62–15).

Patchy or Localized Infiltrate in the Nonneutropenic Patient

Infection in nonneutropenic patients is similar to that in the general population and may be caused by viruses (*e.g.,* RSV, HSV, parainfluenza, adenovirus), mycoplasma, or bacteria (*e.g., S. pneumoniae, H. influenzae*). In some centers, *Legion-*

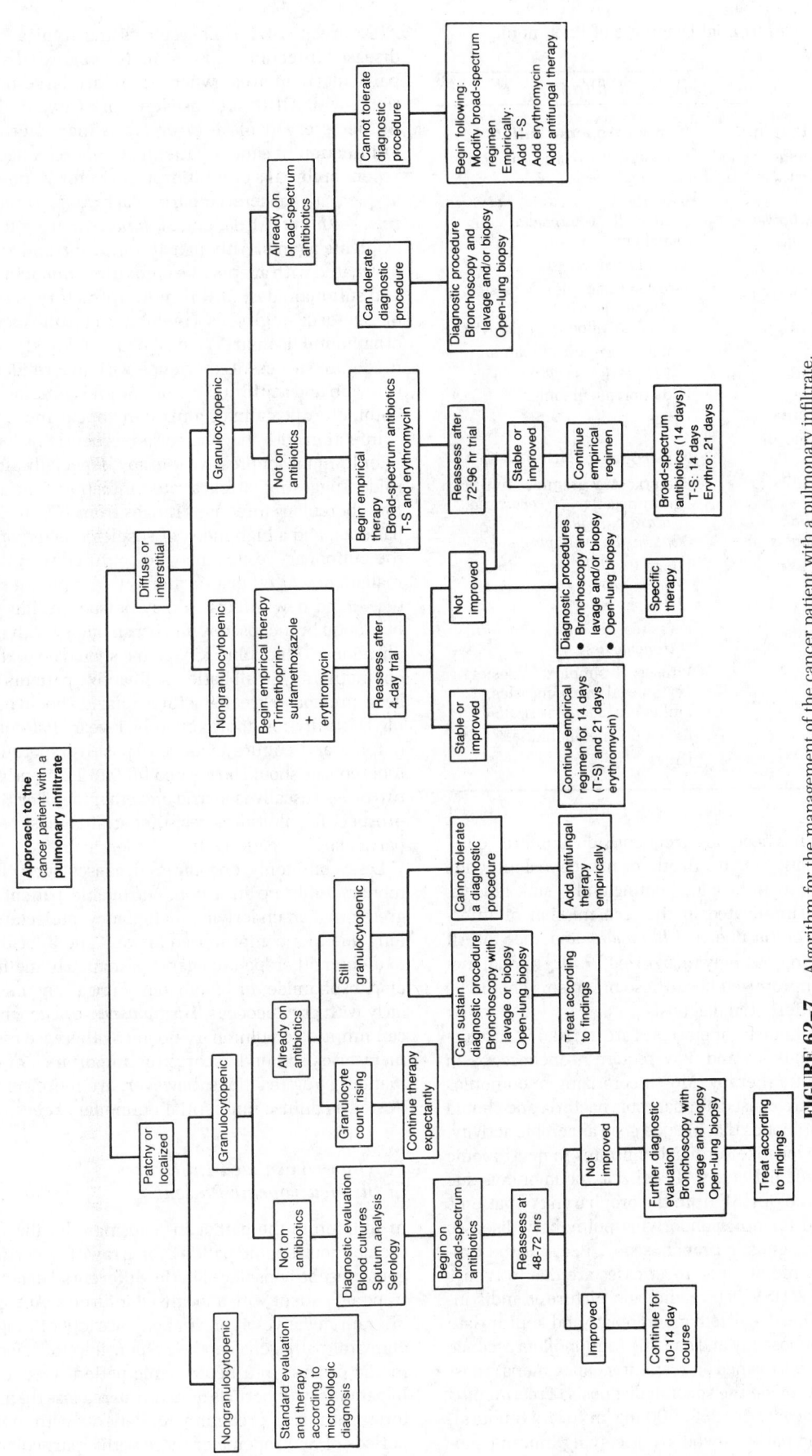

FIGURE 62-7. Algorithm for the management of the cancer patient with a pulmonary infiltrate.

TABLE 62–15. Differential Diagnosis of Pneumonia in Cancer Patients

Localized Infiltrate	Diffuse Infiltrate
Nonneutropenic Patients	**Nonneutropenic Patients**
Bacteria: *S. pneumoniae, Hemophilus, Mycobacteria*	Parasites: *P. carinii, T. gondii, Strongyloides*
Fungi: *Cryptococcus, Histoplasma, Coccidioides*	Bacteria: *Mycobacteria, Nocardia, Legionella, Chlamydia* (including TWAR)
Viruses: RSV, adenovirus	*Mycoplasma*
Underlying tumor	Viruses: H. simplex, V. zoster, cytomegalovirus, measles, influenza, adenovirus
Drugs: busulfan, bleomycin, cyclophosphamide, methotrexate, cytosine arabinoside	Fungi: *Aspergillus, Candida, Zygomycetes, Cryptococcus*
Radiation pneumonitis	Radiation pneumonitis
	Drugs
Neutropenic Patients	**Neutropenic Patients**
Bacteria: Any gram-positive or gram-negative, *Mycobacteria, Nocardia*	Bacteria: Any gram-positive or gram-negative, *Mycobacteria, Nocardia, Legionella, Chlamydia, Mycoplasma*
Fungi: *Aspergillus, Zygomycetes, Candida, Cryptococcus, Histoplasma*	Fungi: *Candida, Aspergillus, Zygomycetes, Cryptococcus, Histoplasma*
Viruses: H. simplex, V. zoster	Parasites: *P. carinii, T. gondii, Strongyloides*
Drugs (see above)	Viruses: H. simplex, V. zoster, cytomegalovirus, measles, influenza, adenovirus, RSV
Radiation pneumonitis	Radiation pneumonitis
	Drugs

ella pneumophila has become a frequently encountered community-acquired pathogen, but in others, nosocomial infection has been observed, with hospital cooling tanks, sink faucets, and showerheads implicated in the transmission of infection.[169,170] Pneumonitis due to *Chlamydia* and the TWAR strain, have been increasingly recognized.[171,172] Although not unique to the compromised host, these organisms should be included in the differential diagnosis.

Patients with pulmonary metastases are at risk for obstructive bronchopneumonias and may require bronchoscopy in addition to antibiotic therapy. Most necrotizing pneumonias or lung abscesses are caused by anaerobic bacteria and should be treated with antibiotics that include good anaerobic activity.

HSV may cause localized or focal infiltrates in neutropenic and nonneutropenic patients.[173] Localized pneumonia is due to contiguous spread of HSV from the oropharynx of patients who are intubated for other underlying pulmonary diseases or who undergo diagnostic bronchoscopy. Because the oropharynx is the source of virus, most cases are due to type 1 rather than type 2 HSV. The radiologic picture is indistinguishable from other localized pneumonias, and appropriate studies (*e.g.*, bronchoscopy and specific immunofluorescence and virus cultures performed on respiratory specimens) must be carried out to provide the specific diagnosis. Treatment is with intravenous acyclovir (250–500 mg/m² every 8 hours).

Nonneutropenic patients who are receiving immunosuppressive therapy (including corticosteroids) and patients with

AIDS are at risk for tuberculosis and atypical mycobacterial disease. Infections due to *M. tuberculosis* have increased, particularly in areas where there are large numbers of patients with AIDS, such as New York City.[174,175] This change in the reservoir of *M. tuberculosis* may alter the incidence of infection in cancer patients. Of more concern have been recent outbreaks of multidrug-resistant *M. tuberculosis*. The atypical mycobacteria, particularly *M. fortuitum, M. avium-intracellulare* (MAI), and *M. kansasii*, are often resistant to available agents. Although *M. fortuitum* and *M. chelonei* can be treated with agents like cefoxitin, amikacin, tetracycline, and sulfonamides, MAI is more refractory to therapy. Four- or five-drug regimens (including ciprofloxacin, amikacin, ethambutol, isoniazid) have been employed with minimal to moderate success. Experience with macrolides like clarithromycin and azithromycin, alone and combined with ethambutol, ciprofloxacin or amikacin appear more promising.

Infection with mycobacteria frequently becomes apparent after immunosuppressive therapy, especially after corticosteroids, suggesting a reactivated infection. The mortality rate for tuberculous infections ranges from 17% to 50% in cancer patients, and a high index of suspicion is important, because the pulmonary lesions may be confused with the underlying malignancy or other infections.[176,177] Sputum should be cultured, and new infiltrates may be successfully diagnosed by fiberoptic bronchoscopy and brush biopsy with minimal complications. Tuberculin skin testing should be performed before chemotherapy in all patients. Reactive patients who have not been previously treated with isoniazid should be treated prophylactically for approximately 1 year. Patients with radiographic and culture evidence (positive sputum) for typical tuberculosis should be treated for 9 to 12 months with at least two drugs (usually isoniazid and ethambutol or rifampin). The prospect for multidrug resistant strains must be entertained, particularly in patients from endemic areas.

Less commonly encountered causes for a localized pulmonary infiltrate in a nonneutropenic patient include progression of an underlying malignancy, atelectatic segment of lung due to a compromised airway, and a localized reaction to a chemotherapeutic agent, particularly methotrexate, cyclophosphamide, or bleomycin. Fungal pneumonia, particularly with cryptococcus, *Histoplasma*, or coccidioidomycosis, can mimic the pulmonary nodules otherwise associated with metastases and underscores the importance of tissue confirmation. Drug reactions, however, are more commonly manifested as diffuse, interstitial pulmonary processes.

Patchy or Localized Infiltrates in the Neutropenic Patient

In addition to the pathogens causing a localized infiltrate in the nonneutropenic patient, an array of opportunistic pathogens must be considered in the differential diagnosis of a neutropenic patient with a localized infiltrate. Any gram-positive or gram-negative organism and a variety of fungal, parasitic, and viral pathogens can be responsible for a localized pneumonic process in a neutropenic patient (see Table 62–15). In patients with periods of neutropenia less than 14 days, bacterial pathogens predominate. Patients with more prolonged periods of neutropenia or those with a particular clinical pattern (*e.g.*, after allogeneic bone marrow transplantation) are more prone to develop a fungal (*Candida* or *Aspergillus*) or viral infection (CMV).

Unless the clinical presentation suggests otherwise, it is appropriate to initiate 48 to 72 hours of broad-spectrum antibiotic therapy before proceeding to an invasive diagnostic procedure (see Fig. 62–7). If the patient has stabilized or improved by 72 hours, continuing treatment for 10 to 14 days is necessary. If the patient has not stabilized or improved after broad-spectrum antibiotics, further evaluation is mandatory to exclude other potentially treatable organisms. Although diagnostic material occasionally can be obtained with transtracheal aspiration, bronchoscopy, or percutaneous needle biopsy, the yield with these procedures rarely approaches 50%.

The bronchoalveolar lavage (BAL) has come into vogue because it has a low morbidity and can be safely performed by experienced hands in neutropenic patients with platelet counts as low as 30,000/mm³.[178–181] A transbronchial biopsy, however, should not be performed during the BAL in patients whose platelet count is less than 50,000/mm³.

If the diagnosis cannot be established with BAL, the next procedure to consider is the open lung biopsy. Unlike the minithoracotomy, which can be performed for the patient with a diffuse infiltrate, a more complete thoracotomy is often necessary for the patient with a localized infiltrate.[208] It is important that the biopsy be obtained from the center of the lesion and from its outer borders to decrease the chance for a false-negative biopsy. Biopsy or tissue samples, touch preps, ground material, and sections should be comprehensively analyzed microscopically by Gram's stain, wet mount, toluidine blue, modified methylene blue, acid-fast, methenamine silver, Dieterle or Gimenez, and if necessary, *Legionella*-direct immunofluorescent antibody and electron microscopy. Routine aerobic, anaerobic, acid-fast, fungal, and supplemented charcoal-yeast extract cultures should be made. After a comprehensive analysis, the diagnostic yield from an open lung biopsy is very high, unless the patient is already receiving multiple antimicrobial therapies.

LEGIONELLA. Although not common at most centers, an important pathogen to consider as the cause of localized pneumonia in an immunosuppressed host is *Legionella*.[182] *Legionella* species are ubiquitous and usually found in water, including air conditioning cooling towers and hospital shower heads.[4] Aerosolization of contaminated water is probably the most common mechanism of transmission, and nosocomial infections have been described.

Although legionellosis is a multisystem disease, the lung represents the primary target organ. Incubation ranges from 2 to 10 days (median, 4 days), although immunosuppressed patients tend to have shorter incubation periods and a more abrupt onset of symptoms. The initial symptoms are generally nonspecific and include malaise, anorexia, lethargy, and headache. A nonproductive cough develops in 90% of patients, although it usually follows the initial symptoms by 2 to 3 days. Diarrhea, which occurs in approximately 50% of patients, may proceed or follow the respiratory symptoms.

Fever is usually the initial sign of *Legionella* and is normally unremitting until institution of effective therapy. Two-thirds of patients manifest a pulse deficit (*i.e.*, relative bradycardia) and one third have some degree of neurologic dysfunction, ranging from disorientation, depression, hallucinations, and

seizures to lethargy, stupor, and coma. Physical examination may reveal hyperreactive or hyporeactive deep tendon reflexes, nystagmus, peripheral sensory or motor neuropathies, and rarely, signs of meningeal irritation.

The initial radiographic abnormality is a patchy, alveolar infiltrate involving a single lobe. If translobar consolidation occurs, it usually involves contiguous segments. Cavitary lesions or abscess formation is unusual except for *L. micdadei*.

The most rapid and accurate means of diagnosis is a direct fluorescent antibody (DFA) or DNA probe test performed on respiratory tract secretions, pulmonary tissue from biopsy specimens, pleural fluid, or pus or urine antigen test. However, not all serotypes are detectable, and a negative DFA does not eliminate *Legionella* as a diagnostic consideration. Culturing of the organism on a charcoal-yeast extract medium requires 2 to 7 days.

Erythromycin (40–50 mg/kg/day, with a maximum of 4 g in four divided doses for 3 weeks) is the treatment of choice. Therapy should be administered intravenously for the first several days in seriously ill patients; subsequent therapy may be oral. Patients unable to tolerate erythromycin should receive doxycycline (5 mg/kg/day in two divided doses). Rifampin (20 mg/kg/day in two divided doses) may be given in addition to erythromycin or doxycycline for seriously ill patients. Response to therapy is normally prompt, with a resolution of fever and subjective improvement within 24 to 48 hours.

Nocardia asteroides and *N. brasiliensis* may present as localized pulmonary infiltrates, although miliary and microcavitary patterns have been described in cancer patients.[21,183] Approximately 30% of patients with a pulmonary infection due to *N. asteroides* have associated cutaneous and central nervous system (CNS) infection, usually brain abscesses. Diagnosis depends on positive cultures or histopathologic demonstration of tissue invasion by the organisms. Microscopically, the gram-positive organisms are irregularly stained, beaded or branching, and partially acid-fast staining and filamentous. Skin lesions, usually subcutaneous abscesses, are associated with *Nocardia*. Sulfonamides (*e.g.*, sulfadiazine, 4–6 g/day for 4–6 months) provide the most effective therapy for this infection, but mortality is significant (30%) after the infection has become disseminated. Favorable responses have been observed with ampicillin plus erythromycin or with minocycline. Trimethoprim-sulfamethoxazol has in vitro activity and has been used clinically, although late relapses have been reported.

FUNGI. Fungal infections constitute the greatest threat for the neutropenic patient who develops a new or progressive pulmonary infiltrate while receiving broad-spectrum antibiotic therapy, often occurring as part of a disseminated infection (see Table 62–15).[184] Two groups can be identified patients who developed a new infiltrate while the granulocyte count was rising and patients who developed a new infiltrate while they were granulocytopenic.[185] Patients who developed infiltrates in conjunction with bone marrow recovery did well without therapeutic modifications. In contrast, the patients who developed a new and progressive infiltrate while on antibiotics and while still granulocytopenic were likely to have a fungal cause for their new infiltrates. Ideally, an open lung biopsy should be performed in these patients to establish the diagnosis and guide the therapy. If a biopsy cannot be performed, amphotericin B should be instituted empirically, because a significant survival advantage can be observed for patients who received early, empiric antifungal therapy. In such cases, higher doses of amphotericin B (1–1.5 mg/kg/day) should be administered.

The presence of *Candida* in the sputum correlates poorly with overt infection. Although a positive blood culture for *Candida* is highly correlated with invasive or disseminated infection in the immunocompromised patient, negative blood cultures are not infrequent. Measurement of the *Candida* enolase may provide a means for early diagnosis of invasive candidiasis. Isolation of *C. tropicalis* from multiple body sites (*e.g.*, sputum, urine, and stool) has been correlated with invasive disease.[71] Definitive diagnosis usually requires histopathologic confirmation.

Endophthalmitis, characterized by focal, white, fluffy, mound-like retinal lesions that can extend rapidly into the vitreous, has been associated with disseminated candidiasis.[186]

In many treatment centers, the incidence of aspergillosis in cancer patients from *A. fumigatus, A. flavus, A. niger,* and *A. terreus* has increased over the last decade. The upper airway is the most frequent route of entry of these organisms, and clusters of nosocomial aspergillosis have occurred in hospitals in which construction materials have been contaminated with *Aspergillus* spores. The pathologic hallmark of aspergillosis is blood vessel invasion, with consequent thrombosis and infarction. *Aspergillus* pneumonia in the immunocompromised host is a rapidly invasive, necrotizing bronchopneumonia or a hemorrhagic infection with thrombosis of the pulmonary arteries and veins, with a possibility for life-threatening hemoptysis. Approximately half of the patients are also infected with other organisms, especially *Pseudomonas*.

A characteristic radiographic appearance for *Aspergillus* pneumonia has not been described, but the development of a new pulmonary infiltrate in a neutropenic patient who is receiving broad-spectrum antibiotics, especially if accompanied by new or persistent fever despite antibiotics, chest pain, or hemoptysis, should raise suspicion. Patients receiving low-dose empiric amphotericin B (0.5 mg/kg/day) may break through with pulmonary aspergillosis. Blood cultures are rarely positive, even though disseminated infection occurs in 30% of patients. Extrapulmonary sites include the sinuses, CNS, liver, kidney, skin, and heart valves. Diagnosis of aspergillosis by noninvasive measures is suboptimal, although reports suggest that positive sputum or BAL cultures in a patient with prolonged fever, neutropenia, and a progressive infiltrate is highly correlated with a diagnosis of *Aspergillus* pneumonia.[187] Despite initially optimistic reports, antigen and antibody methods of detection have not been as sensitive as had been hoped and are associated with too many false-negative results. Studies with mannitol offer some encouragement, but definitive confirmatory data are still lacking. A definitive diagnosis still requires histologic confirmation or a positive BAL culture obtained in a clinically relevant setting.

Treatment of *Aspergillus* pneumonia requires an early diagnosis and prompt intervention. Optimal therapy is amphotericin B. Although standard dosages of amphotericin B have ranged between 0.5 and 1.0 mg/kg/day, 14 patients treated with high-dose amphotericin (1–1.5 mg/kg/day) had an exceptional survival rate.[188] Controlled clinical trials are needed to test this approach and to test amphotericin B encapsulated into liposomes because of the encouraging results obtained in preclinical models and early clinical trials. Although not proven, the addition of 100 to 150 mg/kg/day of 5-fluorocytosine (5-FC) in three divided doses to amphotericin B may be helpful. If 5-FC is given, blood levels should be measured. Even with appropriate pharmacologic intervention, the most important prognosticator of a successful outcome is the return of adequate levels of granulocytes. Infrequently, *Aspergillus* causes a mycetoma or fungus ball in immunocompromised patients, and resection is usually recommended.

The *Phycomycetes* (especially *Mucor* and *Rhizopus*) are the third most frequent cause of invasive fungal infection in cancer patients.[184] Like *Aspergillus,* the *Phycomycetes* are acquired by way of the respiratory tract and cause a necrotizing bronchopneumonia or infarction after vascular invasion and thrombosis. Dissemination to the kidney, gastrointestinal tract, CNS, liver, pancreas or heart may occur in 50% of patients with *Phycomycetes* infections. Early biopsy of suspicious lesions and aggressive therapy with amphotericin B and surgical debridement are essential.

Histoplasmosis can cause serious pneumonia in the cancer patient, usually manifested as a military infiltrate.[190] Infection is usually disseminated, and the reticuloendothelial system is generally so heavily infected that the resultant adenopathy, hepatosplenomegaly, and bone marrow involvement can sometimes be confused with the underlying malignancy. Consequently, careful histologic examination of biopsies from the nodes, liver, or bone marrow for the intracellular yeast forms, using Giemsa or methenamine-silver staining, is extremely important in evaluating suspected patients or those from endemic areas.

Coccidioides immitis and *Cryptococcus neoformans* can result in serious pneumonia and disseminated infections in cancer patients and can mimic nodules that appear to be tumor metastases. *Torulopsis* (or *Candida*) *glabrata* has been isolated increasingly from cancer patients and associated with serious fungal infections. Infection with *T. glabrata* occurs predominantly in debilitated, neutropenic patients, but it has also been associated with a foreign body (*e.g.*, hyperalimentation catheter, urinary catheter). The most common sites of infection are lung, kidney, and gastrointestinal tract. Fungemia with this organism may occasionally produce an endotoxin-like shock syndrome. Because of its similarity to *Candida,* diagnosis of *T. glabrata* is difficult, and differentiation rests on its smaller size and lack of pseudomycelia. *Trichosporon* species, an arthrospore-forming yeast, can cause local skin lesions and invasive disease in cancer patients.[98] *T. beigelii* is the cause of white piedra in noncompromised hosts but can involve the lungs, kidneys, skin, and eyes in immunocompromised patients. The serum from patients with trichosporosis can react with the cryptococcal latex agglutination test due to shared antigens between *T. beigelii* and *C. neoformans.* Successful therapy depends on the early initiation of amphotericin B and, most importantly, recovery from neutropenia. Although rare, serious pulmonary infection can result from *Fusarium* and *Pseudoallecheria boydii,* both of which can mimic *Aspergillus.*

Treatment options for the patient with serious fungal disease are currently limited to a few drugs, the most reliable of which is still amphotericin B (see Table 62–12). Although amphotericin achieves a concentration in excess of the minimum inhibitory concentration of most major fungal pathogens, it is associated with significant acute and delayed toxicity, and there is a spectrum of sensitivity. For example, some isolates of *Candida* appear tolerant to amphotericin B, and all isolates of *Pseudoallescheria boydii* are resistant to amphotericin B, although sensitive to miconazole.

Most patients receiving amphotericin B experience fever, chills (sometimes with rigors), nausea, and vomiting. Less commonly, hypotension, bronchospasm, or seizures may occur. With continued administration, nephrotoxicity, including azotemia, elevated creatinine, renal tubular acidosis, and cylindruria, and electrolyte disturbances, especially hypokalemia, occur. Particular attention should be paid to hydration and salt loading, because this can decrease the nephrotoxicity. A decreased erythrocyte production and thrombocytopenia may occur after 22 to 35 days of amphotericin B therapy. Because most immunosuppressed patients who become candidates for amphotericin are already receiving nephrotoxic antibiotics, the decision to initiate therapy is often difficult.

When therapy is instituted in the cancer patient, it is important to achieve an effective serum concentration of amphotericin as rapidly as possible. We initially administer a test dose of 1 mg; if tolerated, the remaining dose of 0.5 mg/kg/day is given within 2 to 4 hours. Premedication with acetaminophen and the addition of hydrocortisone sodium succinate (25–50 mg) to the infusion bottle may reduce toxicity. The dose of 0.5 mg/kg (therapeutic range, 0.4–0.6 mg/kg) is administered over 2 to 3 hours daily for routine empiric therapy. Patients with lesions suggesting (or confirmed to be) aspergillosis or mucormycosis should receive 1 to 1.5 mg/kg/day. The infusion should not be interrupted because of fever and chills, because this is a self-limited reaction. Meperidine (Demerol, 0.5–1 mg/kg intravenously) is helpful in controlling the rigors, although the mechanism of action is unknown. Potassium supplementation is important with hydration and NaCl loading, and if toxicity is excessive, an every-other-day amphotericin schedule may help.

The total dose for disseminated infection often averages 1.5 to 2 g (30–40 mg/kg). Recommended doses of amphotericin B are not based on controlled clinical trials and depend on the site and nature of infection. For example, a short course (5–7 days) of low-dose amphotericin B (0.1–0.3 mg/kg) may be adequate for patients with oral or esophageal mucosal candidiasis.[191] For uncomplicated candidemia, a course of 500 mg/kg (10 mg/kg total dose) is successful in treating the fungemia and preventing endophthalmitis. More protracted and higher doses of amphotericin B (*e.g.*, 5–7 g) may be necessary for the treatment of hepatic candidiasis. The combination of amphotericin B with other agents, such as rifampin or 5-FC, is frequently considered, but demonstrable efficacy with amphotericin B plus 5-FC has been shown only for the treatment of patients with cryptococcal meningitis.[192–194] The therapeutic index in experimental candidiasis was improved when amphotericin B was encapsulated into liposomes, and preliminary reports suggest enhanced clinical efficacy, particularly in hepatic candidiasis.[163,164] Unfortunately, difficulties in formulating a standard liposomal preparation have hampered controlled clinical trials, although multicenter studies are underway.

5-FC is an antimetabolite that has demonstrable in vitro efficacy against most fungi.[195] It can be administered orally (100–150 mg/kg/day every 6 hours) and is well absorbed. The data to support its efficacy as a single agent for the treatment of serious fungal infections in humans are meager. In vivo resistance to 5-FC develops rapidly, but 5-FC may be additive or synergistic with amphotericin B.[196] Toxic effects from 5-FC include nausea, vomiting, hepatotoxicity, and bone marrow depression.

Alternative antifungal drugs are the imidazoles and the azoles, a group of synthetic agents with in vitro activity against most fungi.[197] Clotrimazole has efficacy for the treatment of chronic mucocutaneous candidiasis, but it does not appear to be useful for systemic therapy.[198] Clotrimazole may be useful in preventing oral *Candida* infections, and we have found it helps some patients with esophagitis.

Miconazole has in vitro activity against almost all pathogenic fungi except *Mucor* and *Rhizopus*. The most extensive clinical experience with miconazole has been for patients with chronic or disseminated coccidioidomycoses. Miconazole has shown some efficacy against paracoccidioidomycosis, South American blastomycosis, chronic mucocutaneous candidiasis, esophageal candidiasis, and petriellidosis, although frequent relapse remains a problem.

The role of miconazole in cancer patients with invasive fungal infection has been limited. Toxic effects with miconazole has included nausea, phlebitis, anemia, hyponatremia, and pruritus; anaphylaxis and cardiac arrhythmia have also been observed during infusion. Miconazole is poorly absorbed, necessitating parenteral administration for prolonged periods. Coupled with its limited efficacy and high relapse rate, miconazole cannot be considered a first-line antifungal drug for cancer patients.

Ketoconazole has been evaluated in cancer patients. In vitro testing has documented sensitivity for a variety of fungi, including *Candida* species, *Paracoccidioides*, *Coccidioides*, *Cryptococcus*, and *Histoplasma*. Human trials have used ketoconazole has a single daily oral dose of 200 to 1200 mg and estimated the half-life range from 4 to 12 hours. However, ketoconazole is not effective against *Aspergillus* and *Mucor*, and its spectrum against *Candida* species is not complete. For example, *C. tropicalis* and *T. glabrata* are not covered by ketoconazole.

Despite the advantages of the oral preparation and although relatively nontoxic, a range of problems includes poor intestinal absorption, nausea and vomiting, dizziness, lethargy, headache, and confused states. Hepatic enzyme elevation is common, and one case of fatal hepatic necrosis has been reported. Prolonged use may result in gynecomastia, azoospermia, depressed adrenal and testosterone synthesis, and decreased libido.

Although ketoconazole appears useful for the treatment of patients with mucosal infections (*e.g.*, oral mucositis, esophagitis), its efficacy for immunosuppressed patients with invasive mycoses is unestablished. Studies suggest that ketoconazole should not be used for invasive mycoses and should be restricted to use in patients with superficial mycoses. Ketoconazole has been evaluated for antifungal prophylaxis, but its efficacy is limited.

Itraconazole is a triazole that inhibits steroid synthesis, is available with an oral formulation, and has a broad spectrum of antifungal activity that includes *Candida* and *Aspergillus*.

Although available in Europe, itraconazole has not yet been approved for use in the United States. Fluconazole has a narrower spectrum of activity that includes *Candida* and *Cryptococcus* but does not include *Aspergillus*. However, it has a long half-life and high bioavailability, and it crosses the blood-brain barrier avidly. Fluconazole has assumed an important role in the maintenance treatment of AIDS patients with cryptococcal meningitis and *Candida* esophagitis and severe oral mucositis. The role of fluconazole for the treatment of invasive candidiasis or hepatic candidiasis remains less well defined. As with other imidazoles, breakthrough infection (*e.g.,* *C. krusei*) has been observed when fluconazole was used for oral prophylaxis.

Interstitial Infiltrates in the Nonneutropenic Patient

Diffuse pulmonary infiltrates can be caused by bacterial, viral, fungal, and protozoal pathogens and are influenced by whether or not the patient is neutropenic (see Table 62–15).

PNEUMOCYSTIS PNEUMONIA. A nonneutropenic patient with diffuse pulmonary infiltrate is unlikely to have a bacterial or fungal process. Perhaps the most commonly encountered infection in this setting is *Pneumocystis carinii* pneumonia.[199] This infection is thought to result from a reactivation of latent cysts, because almost 100% of normal children possess detectable antibody to *P. carinii*.[200] Patient-to-patient transmission has been suggested by reports on nosocomial clusterings of cases.[201] The natural reservoir of *P. carinii* remains undefined.

Certain chemotherapeutic regimens may predispose patients to interstitial infiltrates caused by *P. carinii*.[202] For example, an increased prevalence of *P. carinii* pneumonia was observed at the NCI in a group of non-Hodgkin's lymphoma patients receiving combination chemotherapy. Patients had been randomized to one of two treatment arms, and only in the one containing cytosine arabinoside and bleomycin, in addition to drugs shared in common in both treatment arms, was the prevalence of *P. carinii* pneumonia increased. Whether this chemotherapy regimen enhanced reactivation of latent organisms or made patients more susceptible to reinfection from ambient organisms is unclear. This problem, however, has been abrogated by the prophylactic administration of trimethoprim-sulfamethoxazole to patients receiving this treatment regimen.

The most common clinical manifestations of *Pneumocystis* in cancer patients include fever, cough, and tachypnea, generally with intercostal retractions and the absence of detectable rales. A chest radiograph shows a hazy, bilateral alveolar infiltrate, which often begins at the hilus and spreads to the periphery. Arterial blood gases reflect a low PaO_2, normal $PaCO_2$, and alkaline pH. The clinical presentation can be indolent (1–2 months) but more often is fulminant (4–5 days). The chest roentgenographic findings may occasionally be atypical (*e.g.,* lobar consolidation, effusion, and even nodular) and, in rare cases, the radiograph may appear normal despite the presence of pneumocysts on biopsy. *P. carinii* pneumonia in cancer patients differs from that in AIDS patients by having a more smoldering and indolent course; the median duration of symptoms is 28 days in AIDS patients, but 5 days for non-AIDS patients.[203]

Diagnosis of *P. carinii* pneumonia requires demonstration of cysts or trophozoites in pulmonary material from patients with a clinically compatible course; cysts have been found in asymptomatic, previously healthy persons autopsied after traumatic deaths. In patients with AIDS, positive specimens may be obtained from sputum samples because the "cyst burden" is high.[204] In cancer patients, induced sputum can be positive, but cysts may be best demonstrated by BAL or open lung biopsy. The sensitivity of these examinations is enhanced by the use of special strains and monoclonal antibodies with indirect immunofluorescence. Serologic confirmation is of questionable value.

If the likelihood of *P. carinii* pneumonia is great, the choice is to proceed with diagnostic procedure or to administer an empiric course of therapy with trimethoprim-sulfamethoxazole (see Fig. 62–7). If induced sputum or BAL is readily available, it is the procedure of choice for establishing the diagnosis. However, if induced sputum or BAL is not available or if the patient's clinical or hematologic status does not permit a BAL, an empiric trial of trimethoprim-sulfamethoxazole (20 mg/kg/day of trimethoprim) plus erythromycin (for *Legionella*) is recommended, rather than proceeding directly to open lung biopsy. This is based on the results of a randomized NCI trial demonstrating that in nonneutropenic patients with diffuse infiltrates, empiric therapy is as safe and effective an open lung biopsy.[205] However, a response may not be apparent for 4 to 5 days, although stabilization or slight improvement in alveolar air exchange generally occurs within 72 to 96 hours.[206] Failure to improve (*e.g.,* continued fever, depressed PaO_2, progressive infiltrates) after 4 days of therapy serves as an indication to modify therapy, usually with the addition of pentamidine (4 mg/kg/day as a 1–2-hour infusion). The early use of steroids has been shown to improve the outcome of AIDS patients with moderate to severe *P. carinii* pneumonia (as evidenced by a room air arterial PO_2 of 75 mm Hg or less on presentation).[207,208] Whether early steroid use will benefit cancer patients with *P. carinii* pneumonia is unknown, but many advocate its use for cancer patients.

If a histologic diagnosis is necessary and not achievable by BAL, not all procedures, such as transtracheal aspirate, transbronchial biopsy or aspirate, or open lung biopsy, are of comparable diagnostic accuracy. Burt and colleagues examined each of 17 patients having an open lung biopsy for the diagnosis of a diffuse interstitial infiltrate with a transthoracic needle aspirate and a transbronchial brush and biopsy.[209] The patients in this unique study served as their own controls. A diagnosis was established from only 30% of the aspirates and from 59% of the transbronchial biopsy samples; it suggests that the open lung biopsy is the procedure of choice. Open lung biopsy provides the best guidance for patient management, especially if the patient is neutropenic and requires multiple antimicrobial agents. The role of open lung biopsy for neutropenic patients already receiving antibiotic and antifungal therapy appears less defined because the diagnostic yield is low and therapeutic modifications are minimal.[210]

Because the patients who are candidates for open lung biopsy are often thrombocytopenic, appropriate hematologic preparation for surgery is vital. Elevation of the platelet count to a surgically safe level of 30,000/mm³ or greater can usually be accomplished by the infusion of 4 to 8 units of platelet concentrates 1 hour before surgery. Maintenance of the platelet count at this level for 24 hours after surgery with additional platelet concentrates minimizes any postoperative bleeding complications.

Because of the importance the *P. carinii* has assumed in patients with AIDS, the search for new therapeutic agents has intensified. Other agents that have been explored include trimetrexate, primaquine plus clindamycin, and the quinone, 566C80, which has shown promising activity in adults with AIDS.

The appropriate course of treatment in the cancer patient with proved or putative *P. carinii* pneumonia is to begin with trimethoprim-sulfamethoxazole and, if the patients has not stabilized or improved by day 4 of therapy, to add pentamidine. If there is no improvement after 4 days of pentamidine, trimetrexate should be substituted.

VIRAL PNEUMONIAS. CMV has been a cause of severe interstitial pneumonia, especially among patients receiving allogeneic marrow transplants for hematologic malignancies. Renal, cardiac, and liver allograft recipients and patients with lymphoma or leukemia are also at risk, albeit at a lower incidence. Although the pathogenesis of CMV pneumonia is incompletely defined, several risk factors for CMV pneumonia after allogeneic marrow transplant have been identified.[211,212] These include being seropositive for antibody to CMV before transplant, undergoing allogeneic or autologous transplantation, receiving total-body irradiation as part of the conditioning regimen, and developing acute graft-versus-host disease (GVHD) after transplant.

In addition to active CMV infection, disordered immune function undoubtedly underlies the development of CMV pneumonia. For example, the lack of GVHD, which is as immunosuppressive as its treatment, is the putative explanation for the paucity of CMV pneumonia after syngeneic or autologous transplantation. However, whether it is the lack of specific immune responsiveness to CMV or an immunopathologic immune response directed at CMV antigens in pulmonary tissue is undefined. Investigation of pulmonary immune responses may clarify the pathogenesis of this syndrome.

Depending on the various risk factors, as many as 50% of marrow allograft recipients develop interstitial pneumonia, 70% of which is associated with CMV. CMV pneumonia characteristically occurs within the first 3 months after transplantation, with a median onset of 50 to 70 days. Late cases developing after 100 days occur among patients with chronic GVHD. Diffuse infiltrates are most common, but localized and nodular infiltrates have been described. However, patients with apparently localized disease have diffuse involvement when other portions of lung are examined by sensitive virologic techniques. Pleural effusions are rare.

CMV pneumonia is clinically indistinguishable from other causes of diffuse infiltrates in the compromised host, especially *Pneumocystis carinii*, and specific virologic studies must be done to provide the diagnosis. Rising antibody titers to CMV or excretion of virus in throat, urine, or blood are not of sufficient to obviate the need for direct examination of pulmonary specimens.[213] Open lung biopsy was previously considered the necessary diagnostic procedure, but BAL has shown high sensitivity among marrow transplant patients with pulmonary infiltrates.[212] Specificity and negative predictive value are of

concerns, and results in marrow transplant patients cannot necessarily be extrapolated to other immunocompromised patients, especially those with AIDS. If BAL is not diagnostic, open lung biopsy should be performed. Specimens obtained by open biopsy or BAL should be examined by rapid virologic techniques because conventional cultures usually do not become positive for CMV for 2 to 3 weeks, and 4 to 5 weeks is sometimes required. Direct examination of specimens by specific immunofluorescence using murine monoclonal antibodies is rapid (2–4 hours), but has a sensitivity of only about 60% depending on the quality of the specimen. Inoculation of viral cultures by centrifugation followed by immunofluorescent staining for immediate or early CMV antigens (centrifugation or "shell vial" cultures) is extremely sensitive (>95%), specific, and rapid, with results available within 24 hours; some specimens may be positive as soon as 4 hours.[214] Other techniques include standard histologic staining for intranuclear inclusions and cytomegalic cells. Nucleic acid hybridization remains investigational and may not be more sensitive than centrifugation cultures.

CMV may involve other organs, including the liver, spleen, kidney, adrenal, gastrointestinal tract, heart, CNS, and the eye. Enteritis and retinitis have been particularly common among patients with AIDS, but they also occur in organ allograft recipients. CMV has been associated with other organisms including *P. carinii*, bacteria, fungi, and other viruses.

Therapy for CMV pneumonia after marrow transplant combines ganciclovir and intravenous CMV immunoglobulin, with survival rates of 50% to 70% reported for a previously virtually untreatable infection.[215,216] Foscarnet has entered the antiviral armamentarium and has demonstrated benefit for patients with CMV retinitis alone or, in a few cases, in combination with ganciclovir. The specific role of these agents for cancer patients with CMV pneumonitis is less well defined, but they appear to add to the therapeutic options.

The sole use of seronegative blood products can eliminate primary CMV infection in seronegative marrow transplant recipients who have seronegative marrow donors.[278] Similar observations have been made after cardiac and renal transplants. Although passive immunoprophylaxis with intravenous immunoglobulins continues to be studied in seronegative patients, results of clinical trials have been conflicting, and this modality should not be used in place of seronegative blood products. Other approaches to prophylaxis, such as use of interferon, have not been successful after marrow transplantation. Effective prophylaxis has been observed with high doses of acyclovir and with ganciclovir.[217,218]

Other viruses may cause severe, diffuse pneumonias. HSV can cause diffuse pulmonary infiltrates. The pathogenesis includes viremia and involvement of other organs, including liver or brain; type 1 and type 2 HSV have been implicated. Because of clinical similarity to other viral pneumonias like CMV, bronchoscopy or open biopsy is needed for diagnosis. VZV can cause severe, diffuse pneumonia, although this is rare in the absence of cutaneous manifestations of disseminated VZV infection. Treatment of HSV and VZV pneumonia is with intravenous acyclovir (500 mg/m^2 every 8 hours).

The measles virus can cause severe pneumonia in immunocompromised patients. The incidence of measles in young children and adolescents has increased sharply in recent years throughout the United States because of the failure to vaccinate young infants or the loss of vaccine protection among teenagers and young adults. The oncologist must be aware that measles may be more likely now than during the past 20 years. It may occur concomitantly with the initial illness with fever, coryza, and rash, or it may develop as long as 6 months after initial infection.[281] Diagnosis may require open lung biopsy for specific immunofluorescence and culture. Immunosuppressed patients who have never received measles vaccine and are seronegative for antibody to measles and who have contact with measles should receive prophylactic γ-globulin (0.5 ml/kg, maximal dose of 15 ml) as soon after exposure as possible. Treatment of measles is supportive. Live virus vaccines should not be used in immunocompromised patients.[282]

Although the incidence of influenza and other common respiratory viruses (*e.g.*, parainfluenza 1 and 3, respiratory syncytial virus, rhinoviruses) does not appear to be increased in the cancer patient, infection due to these viruses may be severe.[219] Both primary viral pneumonias and secondary bacterial infections may occur. With adenoviruses, increased severity and an increased incidence due to reactivation of latent viruses may occur. Disseminated adenovirus infection commonly involves lung, liver, and kidney, although hemorrhagic cystitis with or without nephritis may occur without other manifestations. Specific immunofluorescence performed on respiratory specimens and virus cultures are necessary for diagnosis. Respiratory syncytial virus (RSV) pneumonia in immunocompromised patients occurs in children and adults with severe clinical courses and high mortality rates.

The synthetic nucleoside, ribavirin, given by aerosol, has been used for treatment of RSV, influenza, and parainfluenza infections and should be given to children or adults with cancer who develop symptomatic infection.[220] Amantadine (or rimantadine) has prophylactic efficacy against influenza A and may have some therapeutic efficacy as well. Some centers routinely use the killed influenza vaccine for cancer patients, although the antibody response to this vaccine may be diminished in patients receiving chemotherapy.[288,289]

Interstitial Infiltrate in the Neutropenic Patient

In addition to *P. carinii* and CMV, gram-positive and gram-negative bacteria and several fungi can cause interstitial infiltrates in neutropenic patients. Broad-spectrum antibiotics and trimethoprim-sulfamethoxazole are necessary for empiric therapy in these patients. Failure of the patient to improve necessitates lung biopsy and consideration of antifungal therapy.

CARDIOVASCULAR INFECTIONS

Cardiovascular infections are relatively uncommon among cancer patients, probably because of the early institution of broad-spectrum antimicrobial therapy. However, cancer patients who have predisposing factors for cardiovascular infections (*e.g.*, dental abscesses, intravenous drug abuse, congenital cardiac anomalies) are at risk. Guidelines for dental prophylaxis should be followed, and procedures should be avoided in patients who are neutropenic. If however, dental work is essential in a patient who is neutropenic, broad-spectrum antibiotic prophylaxis should be used.

Endovascular infections are more likely with the increased use of indwelling venous access catheters. Although gram-positive bacteria (*e.g.*, enterococcus, viridans streptococci, β-hemolytic streptococci, and S. aureus) most commonly cause endovascular infections, aerobic gram-negative bacilli (*e.g.*, P. aeruginosa) and fungal organisms (Candida, Aspergillus) may also cause disease. Diagnosis can be difficult and can be enhanced by using esophageal probes for ultrasonography. These pathogens are particularly difficult to eradicate, and morbidity and mortality rates are discouragingly high. Myocardial microabscesses occur more frequently (Candida), and myocarditis may be associated with viruses and protozoa (*Toxoplasma*). Endocarditis may suggest an underlying malignancy (*e.g.*, association of S. bovis with colon cancer).

The clinical manifestations of endocarditis in the immunosuppressed patient are similar to those in an immunocompetent patient. Nonspecific complaints of fever, chills, malaise, fatigue, night sweats, and weight loss are common. Unfortunately, these complaints are not diagnostically specific. In most instances, the diagnosis of an endovascular infection in an immunocompromised patient must be made based on physical and laboratory evaluation. The numerous physical stigmata of endocarditis should be sought (*e.g.*, heart murmurs, splinter hemorrhages, Roth's spots, splenomegaly), but the diagnosis is confirmed by the isolation of an organism from multiple blood cultures. The complications of endovascular infections are similar to those described for noncancer patients. Valvular insufficiency resulting in congestive heart failure, embolic phenomenon, and renal failure are the most serious complications. Fungal endocarditis is particularly likely to cause large vessel embolization. Patients with *Candida* or *Aspergillus* endocarditis are candidates for valve replacement.

Therapy must be directed at the specific pathogen. The isolation of *S. aureus* or *S. epidermidis* from multiple blood samples, even if the patient has an indwelling catheter, is not sufficient criteria for prolonged antibiotic therapy unless confirmation of a valvular infection can be made. Standard therapy of 10 to 14 days suffices for these patients.[221]

GASTROINTESTINAL TRACT INFECTIONS

The gastrointestinal tract is a major reservoir of microorganisms, is associated with several characteristic infectious complications, and serves as a major portal for systemic infection during periods of host compromise.

Oral Mucositis

Ulceration of the oral mucosa frequently occurs with chemotherapy. Colonization of drug-induced lessons by the indigenous aerobic or anaerobic oral flora may result in local infection and may provide portal for septicemia in the neutropenic patient. Mucositis, gingivitis, and other dental-related problems may occur in as many as 85% of leukemic patients during the course of their disease.

Measures have been sought to lower the risk of oral gingivitis and mucositis. Peterson and coworkers evaluated 38 febrile patients undergoing treatment for acute nonlymphocytic leukemia and found a 32% incidence of local oral infections, more than half of which were thought to cause the patients' fevers.[222] The periodontium was the most common site of infection, cultures of which usually revealed mixed flora, including many of the organisms associated with systemic infection in cancer patients (*e.g., S. aureus, S. epidermidis, C. albicans, P. aeruginosa*). In adults, preexisting periodontitis is common (>90%) and is exacerbated with immunosuppression. The presence of marginal or necrotizing gingivitis, characterized by an erythematous periapical gingiva, is caused by mouth anaerobes and should be treated with specific antianaerobic agents (*e.g.,* clindamycin or metronidazole). The vigorous use of mouth cleansing salts and solutions (*e.g.,* equal parts of a nonirritating mouth wash, hydrogen peroxide, and water swished every 2 hours) may decrease or control the mucositis.

The oral mucosa is a difficult site to decontaminate fully, and several organisms, such as *C. albicans,* are especially problematic. Although oral candidiasis (thrush) is predominantly a superficial infection, it may serve as a portal for systemic invasion in severely neutropenic patients. Oral nystatin is of only minimal benefit. Oral clotrimazole troches (10 mg, 5 troches daily) has been used successfully in patients with mild to moderate infection. Patients with more extensive oral candidiasis, may benefit from fluconazole at dosages of 200 to 400 mg/day or from a short course of amphotericin B (0.1–0.5 mg/kg/day for 7 days).

HSV may cause significant oral disease. Oral HSV infection may not manifest with typical cutaneous or intraoral vesicles and may not be distinguishable from radiation-induced or chemotherapy-induced mucositis. Viral cultures or immunofluorescence or both must be performed for diagnosis. Intravenous acyclovir and vidarabine have demonstrated efficacy in the treatment of immunosuppressed patients with proven mucocutaneous HSV infection.[223,224] Results are better with acyclovir. Treatment with intravenous acyclovir (250 mg/m^2 every 8 hours for 7 days) shortened the period of virus shedding by almost 2 weeks and the period of healing by 1 week.[225] Orally administered acyclovir (400 mg 5 times daily for 7–10 days) appears comparable to intravenous acyclovir among patients who can comply with oral drugs. Topical acyclovir ointment is beneficial, but it is only effective against external lesions and is less effective than oral or intravenous acyclovir.[226] Patients who are seropositive for antibody to HSV have a 70% to 80% incidence of HSV reactivation during leukemic induction therapy or after organ allografting.[227] They may be protected against virus reactivation with intravenous (250 mg/m^2 every 8–12 hours) or oral (400 mg 4–5 times daily or 800 mg every 12 hours) acyclovir given during the period of major risk, usually defined as the period of leukopenia.[228,229] Reduction in streptococcal superinfection and bacteremia has been reported among patients receiving prophylaxis.[230]

Esophagitis

Clinically significant esophagitis may be the result of infectious and noninfectious causes. For example, a syndrome clinically identical to an infectious esophagitis occurs in patients who have received extensive chest wall or mediastinal irradiation. An infectious esophagitis most commonly occurs among patients who have been granulocytopenic and receiving antibiotics for several days. Patients most often present with a subacute onset of retrosternal, burning chest pain and odyn-

ophagia. Fungal, viral, and bacterial organisms can all cause an infectious esophagitis in the immunocompromised host.[231,232]

The occurrence of an infectious esophagitis in the nonneutropenic person is rare. In nonneutropenic patients, esophagitis is most commonly due to chemical irritation of the distal esophagus by refluxed gastric contents (*e.g.,* chemotherapy-induced emesis). These patients are best managed with judicious use of antacids or histamine antagonists. If the nonneutropenic patient has persistent esophageal discomfort, esophagoscopy with brushings for culture and a biopsy should be done. In nonneutropenic patients with AIDS, herpetic or candidal esophagitis are common.

For the neutropenic patient who is already receiving broad-spectrum antibiotic therapy, *Candida* is the most likely cause of esophagitis, but severe esophagitis with fatal hematemesis has been reported with *Aspergillus*. HSV, alone or with *Candida*, and bacteria also deserve careful consideration. CMV has emerged as a frequent cause of esophagitis in AIDS patients or marrow allograft recipients. A common dilemma is whether endoscopy and biopsy should be performed to establish the diagnosis. Although barium swallow or simple fiber-optic esophagoscopy can demonstrate cobblestoning or the putative "white curtain" associated with *Candida*, both are nonspecific and are associated with false-positive and false-negative results. The only definitive way to establish the diagnosis is with biopsy, culture, and histologic examination. For example, when patients with acute nonlymphocytic leukemia with symptomatic esophagitis were endoscoped, 3 of 7 cases that appeared to be *Candida* were shown by biopsy to be nonfungal.

It is not always possible or safe to biopsy the patient with esophagitis, particularly if the patient is profoundly thrombocytopenic. An alternative to biopsy is a short course of empiric therapy. Patients with esophageal candidiasis usually respond within 48 hours to oral clotrimazole, ketoconazole, or fluconazole. If patients have persistence or worsening of the esophageal complaints after 48 hours of therapy, they should be given a trial of low-dose amphotericin B (0.1–0.5 mg/kg/day for 5 days). If the patient has persistent symptoms after 48 hours of intravenous amphotericin B, it is unlikely that *Candida* is the cause. Although some physicians advocate esophagoscopy at this point, an alterative is an empiric course of acyclovir (750 mg/m^2/day, at 8-hour intervals), because the second most likely pathogen or copathogen is HSV. If the patient responds, acyclovir should be given for 5 to 7 days.

Intraabdominal Infections

The clinical presentation of even common intraabdominal processes (*e.g.,* appendicitis, infectious diarrheal syndromes) can be altered by granulocytopenia and compounded by complications of cancer or its treatment. For example, obstructive lesions may be due to primary or metastatic cancer (*e.g.,* lymphoma); cholangitis or a conjugated hyperbilirubinemia may be due to extrahepatic biliary obstruction by tumor (*e.g.,* rhabdomyosarcoma); and chronic abdominal pain or diarrheal syndromes may be caused by bowel wall infiltration by malignant disease or infection.

Intraabdominal complaints must be expeditiously evaluated with a thorough abdominal and pulmonary examination, including a judiciously performed rectal examination. Repetitive rectal examinations must not be performed in the neutropenic patient, because bacteremia and local infection may result. Appropriate laboratory studies include routine hematologic and serum chemistry values, tests for amylase and total and direct bilirubin, and flat and upright abdominal radiographs. Additional diagnostic procedures (*e.g.*, abdominal or pelvic ultrasound, CT scans) should be pursued if appropriate. As a general rule, invasive diagnostic or radiographic procedures (*e.g.*, barium enema, endoscopy) should be avoided in the neutropenic patient unless absolutely required.

Foremost among the intraabdominal infections that are unique to the cancer patient is typhlitis (*i.e.*, necrotizing enterocolitis), an inflammatory cellulitis involving the cecum.[233,234] Typhlitis most commonly occurs in association with prolonged episodes of granulocytopenia and broad-spectrum antimicrobial therapy in patients with acute leukemia, although any granulocytopenic patient is at risk. Patients normally present with subacute or acute onset of right lower quadrant abdominal pain, which frequently becomes generalized over several hours with the development of fever, diarrhea, and prostration. The agents responsible for typhlitis include gram-negative bacteria, especially *P. aeruginosa*. Abdominal ultrasonography reveals bowel wall thickening and ascites and can help in the differential diagnoses. Optimal management includes supportive care, including appropriate hydration, nasogastric suction, adjustments of antimicrobial therapy to cover resistant gram-negative and anaerobic species, and if necessary, aggressive surgical intervention to resect a necrotic bowel. Proposed indications for surgery include evidence of persistent gastrointestinal bleeding despite resolution of hematologic abnormalities; evidence of an intraperitoneal perforation; clinical deterioration suggesting uncontrolled sepsis (*e.g.*, need for vasopressors, large fluid volume replacement); or development of symptoms compatible with an acute abdomen that would otherwise indicate a need for surgery. Despite aggressive measures, mortality rates are 30% to 50%.

An infrequently encountered clinical syndrome is peritonitis and bacteremia due to *Clostridia*. Patients with clostridial peritonitis classically have a fulminant clinical course with fever, tachycardia, abdominal wall ecchymoses and crepitance, and significant hemolysis. *C. perfringens* and *C. septicum* are the two most frequently isolated organisms. A less fulminant bacteremic syndrome due to *C. tertium* has been described.[93] Most patients have been granulocytopenic children with acute leukemia maintained on broad-spectrum antimicrobial therapy for prolonged periods (*e.g.*, 17 days). The gastrointestinal tract has most often implicated as the source of infection. Most patients with *C. tertium* have been relatively resistant to the penicillins, cephalosporins, and clindamycin, and they require the use of vancomycin for successful therapy.

Antibiotic-associated colitis (AAC) has long been associated with the administration of clindamycin, ampicillin, and broad-spectrum β-lactam antibiotics. *Clostridium difficile* has been isolated in most cases.[235] The symptomatic disease is related to toxin production by the organism. In cancer patients, antineoplastic agents and antibiotics increase the risk for AAC. Patients with AAC classically present with acute, generalized abdominal pain, fever, leukocytosis, and watery or mucoid, foul-smelling diarrhea. A high index of suspicion is necessary

because of similar abdominal symptoms in cancer patients receiving chemotherapy or periabdominal radiation therapy. Cancer patients with diarrhea should be evaluated with stool cultures for *C. difficile* and with toxin assays. Toxin production, not just a positive culture for *C. difficile*, is necessary for diagnosis of ACC, because as many as 42% of hospitalized patients receiving antibiotics will be culture positive, but not toxin positive, for *C. difficile*.

Treatment of documented *C. difficile*-associated colitis requires oral vancomycin (125 mg four times daily for 10–14 days) or metronidazole (250 mg four times daily for 10 days). There is a 10% to 20% rate of relapse, although most patients respond to a second course with the same or alternative therapy. *C. difficile* may be nosocomially transmitted, and patients who are culture and toxin positive for *C. difficile* should be placed on enteric precautions.

Hyperinfection syndrome is an infrequently encountered clinical problem. It is caused by the intestinal nematode, *Strongyloides stercoralis*.[235,236] The clinical syndrome of fever, nausea, vomiting, diarrhea, and abdominal pain is caused by the invasion and ulceration of the gastrointestinal mucosa by the filariform larvae. Chemotherapy promotes the maturation of these filariform larvae from a quiescent rhabditiform stage. Polymicrobial sepsis may accompany the stage of intestinal invasion, presumably as a result of the ulcerated intestinal mucosa. Overwhelming pulmonary and meningeal involvement has been described in immunocompromised patients. Diagnosis requires demonstration of the larvae in feces or duodenal fluid and should be sought in patients who have resided in subtropical climates or endemic regions. Treatment of asymptomatic infestation is accomplished with the administration of thiabendazole (25 mg/kg twice daily for 2 days). Immunocompromised patients with the hyperinfection syndrome should be treated for 2 to 3 weeks, although the mortality rate is high despite long-term treatment.

Hepatitis may be caused by a variety of infectious agents, including those that infect the liver primarily (*e.g.*, hepatitis A, B, C and the delta agent) and secondarily (*e.g.*, HSV, CMV, EBV, coxsackievirus B, adenoviruses, toxoplasmosis). Hepatitis C (HCV), previously referred to as non-A, non-B hepatitis, is a small single-stranded RNA virus that is the most commonly encountered cause of blood-bone hepatitis in cancer patients.[237] Antibody to HCV has been found in 80% to 100% of persons who develop histologically confirmed non-A, non-B hepatitis. Clinically, hepatitis C closely resembles hepatitis B, with an insidious onset and a prolonged, relapsing course. There is substantial evidence for a chronic carrier state, and chronic sequelae may occur in as many as 50% of infected persons. The development of antibody after infection with hepatitis C is usually delayed, with an average interval of 20 or more weeks, making serologic testing late during the clinical course important. Interferon-α has been effective in patients with hepatitis C, with dosages of 3 million units three times per week resulting in normalization of amino transferases and improvement in histologic findings in almost 50% of the treated patients.[238]

Hepatitis B infection (HBV) may result in acute and chronic infections, including chronic active, chronic persistent, and an asymptomatic carrier state. Diagnosis is aided by detection of specific viral antigens in the serum of infected patients, especially hepatitis B surface antigens (HBsAg), DNA polymerase, and the hepatitis Be antigen, all of which are present before and at the onset of clinical symptoms. HBsAg may be detected in the serum as early as 6 days after infection with HBV, although it is usually observed 29 to 43 days after parenteral exposure and 67 to 82 days after oral exposure. In patients with self-limited HBV infection, the DNA polymerase titer falls early, and the HBsAg titer falls later in the clinical disease course, eventually being replaced by antibody to HBsAg and HBeAg.

HBV may result in acute infection, chronic infection, or a symptomatic carrier state, with or without hepatic disease. Although the frequency of HBsAg is approximately 0.1% in the general population of the United States, it has been detected in 10% to 20% of children or adults with cancer.[239,240] This is a consequence of multiple transfusions, although currently available sensitive screening tests have reduced this risk dramatically. Nonparenteral transmission (*e.g.*, saliva, urine, feces, semen, effusions, cerebrospinal fluid) constitutes an important vector. Immunosuppressive therapy may increase the risk of hepatitis, and enhance the development of a chronic carrier state and can reactivate HBV infections in asymptomatic chronic carriers.[241,242]

Because many of the chemotherapeutic agents currently used in cancer treatment are metabolized or excreted by the liver, altered hepatic function caused by HBV hepatitis can seriously compromise the pharmacokinetics of administered chemotherapy. This is most pronounced for patients with chronic hepatitis, in whom even reduced dosages of chemotherapy may permit the maintenance of the viral carrier state and aggravate drug-induced hepatic injury.

The delta agent, an incomplete RNA virus, requires existing or co-infection with the hepatitis B virus for clinical expression. Hepatitis due to the delta agent only occurs in three circumstances: as a superimposed infection in a patient with active hepatitis B; as an acute delta hepatitis in a chronic hepatitis B carrier; and as a chronic delta infection in a chronic hepatitis B carrier. Although hepatitis due to the delta agent has been noticed among multiply-transfused patients, its incidence should decrease as the prevalence of hepatitis B diminishes.

Treatment of the patient with chronic active hepatitis is controversial. The current recommendation is that immunosuppressive therapy be restricted to patients who are symptomatic and who have subacute hepatitis with multilobular necrosis and active cirrhosis. Encouraging therapeutic results have been observed using human leukocyte and fibroblast interferon for patients with chronic hepatitis.[243] A short course (10–14 days) of interferon leads to a decreased serum levels of DNA polymerase, HBsAg, and anti-HBsAg; HBeAg remains unchanged; and all virologic markers again become elevated after the termination of the interferon therapy. However, with 4 to 5 months of continuous interferon therapy, HBsAg may be eliminated in some patients without rebound after discontinuing therapy. Further study of the dose and schedule of interferon may enhance this therapy.

Because of the morbidity of HBV, trials using standard serum immunoglobulin have been compared with serum globulin containing a high titer or an intermediate titer of antibody to HBsAg for patients or medical staff who have been potentially inoculated with HBV. Although earlier studies suggested that the high-titer globulin was effective, subsequent observations suggest that it may merely delay the onset of hepatitis as long as 9 months, with the incidence of hepatitis remaining unchanged at 7%. High-titer globulin (0.07 mg/kg) is, however, currently recommended for patients or staff who have had a significant inoculation or ingestion of HBV and who are also negative for anti-HBsAg. Hepatitis B vaccine produced by recombinant technology (Recombivax) is strongly recommended for seronegative hospital personnel at high risk for hepatitis B.

Several viruses may secondarily affect the liver as part of a more widespread systemic infection. EBV, CMV, HSV, rubella, rubeola, mumps, adenovirus, and coxsackie virus B have been associated with hepatic enzyme elevation. The hepatic dysfunction with these secondary infections is generally self-limited and less severe than that associated with primary viral hepatitis. However, fulminant hepatic necrosis, coma, and death have been described with several of these agents, especially the herpesvirus group, in the immunocompromised host.

All cancer patients with clinical or biochemical evidence of hepatitis should undergo a serologic evaluation to characterize the cause. Serum tests for anti-HAV (IgM), HBsAg, and anti-HBC (IgM) can identify patients with hepatitis A or B. Patients who test negative for hepatitis A or B should be evaluated repeatedly for anti-HCV, because it can take months antibody to develop.[244] Patients who remain negative to all of these viruses may have non-A, non-B, non-C hepatitis and may have a delta virus infection or hepatitis due to some other infectious or noninfectious cause. Hepatitis enzyme elevation or hyperbilirubinemia can occur with bacterial sepsis, fungal infection of the liver (especially *Candida* or *Aspergillus*), or toxoplasmosis.

In addition to the morbidity and mortality directly attributable to the hepatitis, significant alteration in hepatic function can affect the pharmacokinetics of antineoplastic agents, especially those metabolized or excreted by the liver (*e.g.*, methotrexate, doxorubicin).

Therapy for patients with hepatitis is primarily supportive, with bed rest and avoidance of further hepatic insult. Patients with hepatitis due to HSV should receive acyclovir. Chronic B or C hepatitis can be treated with interferon-α.

Hepatic candidiasis is increasingly diagnosed and is characterized by the presence of "bull's eye" lesions in the liver on ultrasound or CT scans (Fig. 62–8).[245,246] These lesions are not apparent in patients who are neutropenic but become recognizable at the time of neutrophil recovery. The MRI scan may be the most sensitive imaging technique, but variations among patients determines which imaging study is best. It is important to recognize that hepatic lesions may be smaller than the degree of resolution of current imaging techniques and in high-risk patients with a negative abdominal ultrasound or CT scans, a biopsy may still be necessary to confirm or rule out hepatic candidiasis. Patients are characterized by the persistence of fever at the time of recovery from an episode of neutropenia, frequently with right upper quadrant discomfort, nausea, and an elevated level of alkaline phosphatase and a leukocytosis. The lesions are granulomas, consisting of an inner core of central necrosis (where the yeast and pseudohyphae can be found), surrounded by a ring of inflammatory cells and an outer ring of fibrosis. To confirm the diagnosis, a liver biopsy is necessary. Because of the focality of the le-

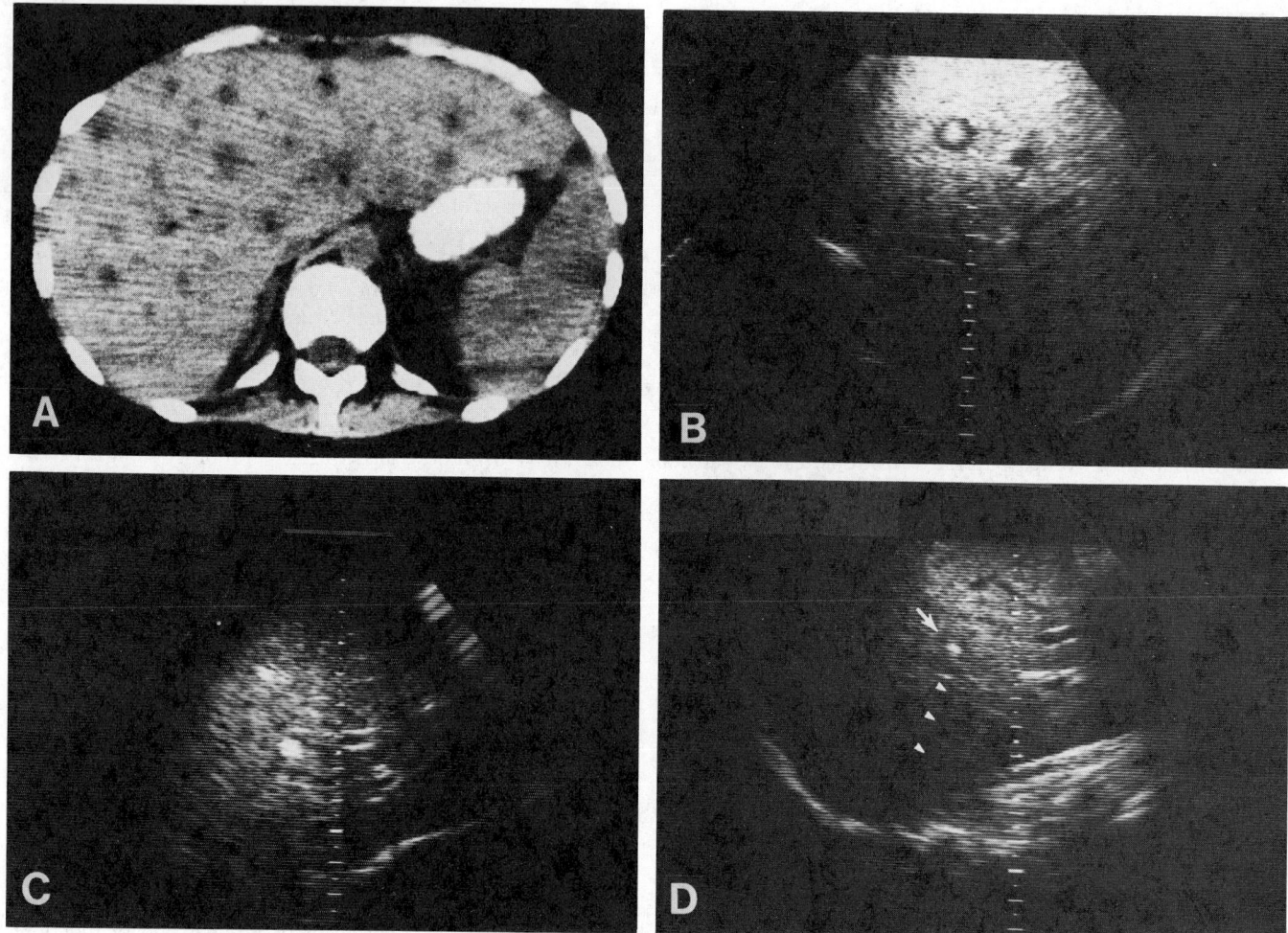

FIGURE 62–8. **(A)** CT scan of the liver shows numerous rounded areas of decreased attenuation compatible with the diagnosis of hepatic candidiasis. This is a nonspecific finding. **(B)** Ultrasound examination in the same patient shows the typical bull's eye lesion of candidiasis, characterized by a central echogenic nidus surrounded by a radiolucent halo. This is seen early in the natural history of the disease. **(C)** The radiolucent halo is now less obvious than in B. This illustrates the variable appearances of *Candida* abscesses on ultrasound studies at different times in the same patient. **(D)** Late in the course of the disease, the microabscesses become denser (*arrow*). The acoustic shadow posterior to the lesion was caused by attenuation of the sound beam (*arrow heads*). (Thaler M, Pastakia B, Shawker TM, et al. Hepatic candidiasis in cancer patients: The evolving picture of the syndrome. Ann Intern Med 1988;108:88–100)

sions, an open biopsy or peritoneoscopy guarded procedure is preferable. Cultures of the lesions are likely to be negative, and diagnosis requires demonstration of yeast forms or pseudohyphae. Serial sections of the biopsy may be necessary to confirm the presence of yeasts. These imaged lesions change over time and with treatment; on resolution, they become calcified, an important endpoint of therapy.

Hepatic candidiasis poses a therapeutic challenge because long courses of treatment are necessary, and the average dose of amphotericin B is 5 g. Experimental data suggest that the combination of amphotericin B with 5-FC is preferable. Serial biopsy may be necessary to confirm the resolution of infection. Although experience is limited, several investigators have suggested that lipid associated complexes or liposomal amphotericin B may be more effective and less toxic than deoxycholate amphotericin. The total dosage of amphotericin can be delivered much more rapidly. Although experience is limited, fluconazole has been given to patients who have failed

to respond to amphotericin B and has been used for combination therapy in patients who have received short courses of amphotericin B.[247,248]

Perirectal Cellulitis

The overall incidence of perirectal cellulitis has decreased in recent years, presumably due to the early use of empiric antibiotic therapy when granulocytopenic patients become febrile. Nonetheless, there is still a risk for perianal cellulitis, especially for patients with prolonged (>7 days) and profound degrees (<100/mm^3) of granulocytopenia. Predisposing factors include perirectal mucositis due to chemotherapy or localized radiotherapy, hemorrhoids, anal fissures, and any type of rectal manipulation (*e.g.,* barium enema, anoscopy, sigmoidoscopy). Constipation should be avoided with stool softeners because passage of hard stool promotes the formation of anal fissures and increases the risk for perianal infections.

The most common pathogens in perirectal cellulitis are aerobic gram-negative bacilli (*e.g.*, *P. aeruginosa*, *K. pneumoniae*, *E. coli*), the group D streptococci, and bowel anaerobes.[249] Because of the involvement and anaerobic organisms, antibiotic coverage must include a specific antianaerobic agent (*e.g.*, clindamycin or metronidazole) in addition to the broad-spectrum aerobic coverage. Therapy should commence at the time of the first complaints of tenderness, ideally before florid symptoms of cellulitis develop. Additional supportive measures include the use of sitz baths three or four times daily, stool softeners, a low-bulk diet, and avoidance of unnecessary rectal manipulation, especially repetitive digital examinations. Surgical intervention should be restricted to patients who demonstrate persistence of erythema or induration or progressive involvement of ischiorectal fossa despite optimal antimicrobial therapy.[249,250]

GENITOURINARY TRACT INFECTIONS

The genitourinary tract is infrequently the source of infection in the immunocompromised child. However, local obstruction due to tumor, neurologic dysfunction mediated by spinal cord compression or medications (*e.g.*, vincristine, narcotics), and local therapeutic maneuvers (*e.g.*, radiotherapy, surgery, bladder catheterization) can predispose cancer patients to genitourinary infections. Most commonly, gram-negative aerobic bacilli (*e.g.*, *E. coli*, *Klebsiella* species, *Proteus* species, *P. aeruginosa*) and enterococci are the causative agents.

An important distinction must be made between a pathogen and colonizing organism when interpreting the results of the urine cultures obtained from an immunocompromised patient. In a nonneutropenic patient, a single organism colony count of greater than 10^5/ml is considered diagnostic of a urinary tract infection in a symptomatic person. In neutropenic patients, a colony count greater than 10^3/ml of a single organism may be considered diagnostic of a urinary tract infection if the patient is symptomatic (*e.g.*, dysuria, urgency, frequency, fever), and a colony count greater than 10^5/ml of a single organism should prompt antibiotic intervention whether or not the patient is symptomatic. Leukocytes in the urine must not be relied on as a diagnostic criterion in the neutropenic patient.

The distinction between colonization and tissue invasion is particularly difficult for fungal pathogens. Fungal colonization is especially prevalent among patients with indwelling urinary catheters or in patients receiving broad-spectrum antimicrobial therapy. Unlike the typical situation with bacterial pathogens, in which clinical signs and symptoms are present, fungal invasion of the genitourinary tract may be insidious. The repetitive isolation of a particular fungal species (usually *C. albicans*, *C. tropicalis*, or *T. glabrata*) in association with fever, deteriorating renal function, or flank pain should prompt the institution of systemic amphotericin B. Heavily colonized or superficial bladder infections, manifested by the persistence of positive urine cultures despite removal of predisposing factors, may be effectively treated with a single dose of amphotericin B and fluconazole or, in refractory cases, with instillation of amphotericin B (50 mg in 1 L D5W daily) into the bladder.

CUTANEOUS INFECTIONS

The integrity of this primary physical defense barrier is frequently disrupted in the cancer patient (*e.g.*, needle punctures, biopsies, surgery, irradiation, chemotherapy). Local cutaneous infections with bacteria or fungi are common and may result in disseminated infection during periods of immunosuppression. Vigilant skin cleansing with iodophor solutions is essential before any procedure that may permit pathogens. Careful attention to the physical examination of the skin in febrile cancer patients may yield a lesion from which a specific diagnosis can be made.[251]

The skin can become infected during bacteremia (*e.g.*, *P. aeruginosa*, *A. hydrophilia*, *C. equi*, *S. marcescens*); fungemia (*e.g.*, *Aspergillus*, *Candida*, *Mucor*, *C. neoformans*, *H. capsulatum*); or viremia (*e.g.*, HSV, VZV). There are noninfectious processes that mimic infection (*e.g.*, pyoderma gangrenosa, Sweet's syndrome). Skin lesions may permit the early diagnosis of generalized infection, and fresh lesions should be aspirated or biopsied and the material cultured and examined with Gram's stain, potassium hydroxide, methylene blue, and modified acid-fast stain.

If a viral infection is suspected, the base of several fresh vesicles should be scrapped with a Dacron swab, which should then be used to prepare microscope slides and placed into appropriate viral transport media for subsequent virus culture. The microscope slides should be examined by specific immunofluorescence for HSV and VZV. Immunofluorescence performed on appropriately prepared slides remains the most sensitive (approximately 85%) diagnostic test for varicella or herpes zoster. Viral cultures are useful for diagnosis if immunofluorescence is negative or if the slides are not adequate for examination, although cultures may not be positive for 2 to 4 weeks in the case of VZV. Wright-Giemsa staining (Tzanck test) of the microscope slides for detection of multinucleated giant cells may be performed, but the process does not differentiate between HSV and VZV infections. The diagnosis of vesicular lesions in the cancer patient is important for appropriate patient management and permits the physician to decide if isolation is necessary for the protection of other patients and staff members.

Primary varicella (chicken pox) is the most serious vesicular eruption in pediatric cancer patients, with a mortality rate of 7%. The major complication is the visceral dissemination that occurs in 32% of patients. Pneumonia occurs in 79% of patients with visceral varicella, generally developing 3 to 7 days after the onset of skin lesions, usually presenting as bilateral, "fluffy," nodular infiltrates. Other target organs during disseminated VZV infection include the liver, spleen, CNS, gastrointestinal tract, bone marrow, and lymph nodes. Secondary bacterial infections account for the additional severity of varicella dissemination. The risk for visceral dissemination is increased in patients receiving chemotherapy at the time of infection, especially if they are also lymphopenic (<500/mm³). In children with AIDS, recurrent or chronic cutaneous varicella has been observed, in which lesions can range from verrucous to pyoderma gangrenosa and which can be a source of shedding virus.

Because of the severity of varicella infection in patients with cancer, attention has been directed at immunoprophylaxis. The most effective regimen is varicella-zoster immunoglobulin (VZIG), prepared from the sera of patients who have recently recovered from zoster and provided through the American Red Cross Blood Services. Administered within 72 hours of exposure, VZIG usually modifies the infection to a mild or subclinical form. If VZIG is not available, an alternative is one of the licensed intravenous immunoglobulins or zoster immune plasma (ZIP); the former is preferred.

Management of the seronegative patient exposed to varicella, commonly from a household or playmate contact, should include the discontinuation of all chemotherapy and the administration of VZIG, intravenous immunoglobulin, or ZIP within 72 hours of exposure. Chemotherapy should be withheld in patients with documented exposure until the end of the average incubation period, which is 21 days. In patients who develop overt varicella, immunosuppressive therapy should not be reinstituted until all the skin lesions have dried and scabbed.

Acyclovir, vidarabine, and interferon have been evaluated in the treatment of varicella and herpes zoster infections in immunocompromised patients. All have been effective compared with placebo.[252-255] Acyclovir (1500 mg/m^2/day in three divided doses) administered parenterally is the treatment of choice. Hydration should be maintained above baseline to avoid crystalluria. Therapy should be continued for a minimum of 7 of 10 days and potentially longer if the lesions have not become dry and scabbed. Orally administered acyclovir has been used for treatment of varicella in immunocompromised children, but it is poorly absorbed and produces plasma levels substantially lower than with intravenous acyclovir. Until controlled trials proving efficacy are available, oral acyclovir cannot be recommended for this purpose. Supportive management and early treatment of secondary bacterial infections are crucial for patients with established varicella.

Because varicella is highly contagious, there is a considerable risk for spread to other seronegative immunosuppressed patients. Varicella may be transmitted for 2 days before the appearance of rash. Extreme caution must be exercised in the management of potentially or overtly infected patients. Careful patient, parent, and staff education is essential. Absence from school where chicken pox has occurred may be necessary, usually for the 21-day incubation period. Parents should be alerted not to bring their children to the clinic waiting room area if chicken pox is suspected, and if hospitalization is required, reverse isolation should be undertaken, ideally on a hospital floor where immunosuppressed patients are not located.[342] Staff members should be checked for a history of chicken pox or tested serologically using the fluorescent antibody against membrane antigen or immune adherence hemagglutination technique to further minimize the possibility of nosocomial transmission.

A live attenuated chicken pox vaccine has been tested extensively in Japan, with demonstrable protection in normal and immunosuppressed children.[256] Although most active immunizations in patients receiving chemotherapy have been unsuccessful because of the inability to maintain effective antibody titers, current data suggest that children receiving maintenance chemotherapy can mount an antibody response if they can be vaccinated at a time when chemotherapy is stopped for 2 weeks.[257] Whether a similar response can be obtained in more intensively treated patients has not been established, and the consequences of administering a live

vaccine to seriously immunosuppressed patients must be carefully considered.

The incidence of reactivation infection with VZV (*i.e.*, herpes zoster or shingles) among patients with previous varicella infections ranges from 5% to 10% among patients with solid tumors to 35% to 50% among patients treated for Hodgkin's disease or who have received marrow allografts. Most cases occur within the first 2 years after treatment. Herpes zoster is due to reactivation of VZV that had been latent in dorsal root ganglia. The likelihood of reactivation increases with intensity of immunosuppression, with the suppression of cell-mediated immunity more important than humoral immunity. Local irradiation may have a role in reactivation of virus, with disease occurring in the irradiated dermatome. The most important complication of herpes zoster is dissemination outside of the original dermatome, which occurs 4 to 9 days after onset. Some patients with cutaneous dissemination develop manifestations of visceral dissemination, most commonly including pneumonia, hepatitis, and encephalitis. Cutaneous dissemination rates of 5% to 50% have been observed, with higher rates among patients with more severe immunosuppression. Some patients develop cutaneously disseminated disease without an initial dermatome infection (*i.e.*, atypical disseminated zoster), and they have higher mortality rates than patients with initial localization. The overall mortality of herpes zoster is lower than that of primary varicella, although mortality rates as high as 10% have been observed in some series. Death is usually due to VZV pneumonia, although encephalitis due to direct invasion of the CNS may occur.

The local morbidity of herpes zoster may be considerable, due to acute pain, secondary bacterial infection, or neurologic complications, including peripheral neuropathies, aseptic meningitis, or myelitis. Encephalitis may occur by direct involvement of the CNS by VZV or may be postinfectious. Zoster encephalitis usually appears within 2 weeks of the rash, although it may occur from 1 week before rash to 8 weeks after.

Ophthalmic zoster is associated with involvement of the nasociliary nerve and is suggested by lesions on the tip of the nose. A unique syndrome of ophthalmic zoster with contralateral hemiplegia has been described. Herpes zoster of the ophthalmic division of the trigeminal nerve may be especially troublesome because of acute pain and corneal involvement with scarring and subsequent blindness.

Another zoster syndrome is abdominal pain occurring before or without development of a rash. Because of obvious difficulties in diagnosis, these patients may have many diagnostic procedures performed, including laparotomy, before herpes zoster becomes apparent as the cause. The most common problem is postherpetic neuralgia, particularly in older patients; it has been reported in as many as 45% of patients in some treatment trials. Pain may last for months or years in some cases. Treatment of postherpetic neuralgia is often unsatisfactory, although some patients may derive benefit from phenytoin (Dilantin) or carbamazepine (Tegretol).

Diagnosis of varicella or herpes zoster is based on the characteristic appearance of the skin lesions, on the distribution of lesions, and on immunofluorescent staining of material from the base of the vesicles. HSV can cause localized cutaneous disease and dermatomal-appearing rashes, which may be mistaken for herpes zoster. Wright-Giemsa staining of vesicle scrapings or electron microscopy do not differentiate HSV from VZV, and specific immunofluorescence and viral cultures should be performed for diagnosis.

Local skin care and observation for secondary bacterial infections are important. Data about therapy with antiviral agents are similar to those for varicella. Although interferon, vidarabine, and acyclovir are effective when compared with placebo, acyclovir appears to be the agent of choice. A direct comparison of acyclovir (500 mg/m² every 8 hours) and vidarabine for treatment of herpes zoster, conducted primarily among marrow transplant recipients, showed acyclovir to be superior, with shorter durations of fever, new lesion formation, and acute pain and more rapid healing and elimination of cutaneous dissemination.[258] Acyclovir appears to be effective among patients in whom cutaneous dissemination has already occurred, although initiation of treatment within 48 to 72 hours of onset is highly desirable. VZV resistance to acyclovir has not been observed in vivo and continuation of new lesion formation and cutaneous dissemination occurring within the first 2 to 3 days after initiation of treatment should not be interpreted as treatment failure. Acyclovir treatment should be continued for 7 days or for 2 days after the last new lesion, whichever is longer. In severely immunosuppressed patients, acyclovir should be administered parenterally. In less immunosuppressed patients, oral acyclovir has been given, although validating clinical trials are lacking. Because of failure to develop adequate specific immune responses, some patients who have received acyclovir treatment for herpes zoster have "relapses" of herpes zoster within the succeeding 2 months; they should receive another treatment course. Attention must be paid to adequate hydration, because renal insufficiency and other side effects such as nausea have been observed more frequently among patients who become dehydrated during treatment.

Patients with lymphomas or leukemia or who have received marrow allografts, who are at highest risk of cutaneous and visceral dissemination, should be treated with intravenous acyclovir if they develop herpes zoster. Because of the potential for spread of VZV to other immunosuppressed patients, all patients with herpes zoster should be kept in single rooms, and glove and gown precautions should be used; strict isolation may be appropriate in some circumstances or institutions. Susceptible patients and hospital staff can acquire primary varicella after exposure to herpes zoster.

MUSCULOSKELETAL INFECTIONS

The musculoskeletal system is an uncommon primary site of infection in cancer patients. However, atypical infections such as deep pyomyositis due to *S. aureus* or gram-negative organisms or psoas muscle abscesses have been described in neutropenic and nonneutropenic leukemic patients. Treatment includes incision and drainage and appropriate antibiotic therapy.

Crepitance and soft tissue tenderness suggests an anaerobic infection with *Clostridia* or with the toxin-producing *Bacillus cereus*. Necrotizing fascitis due to *S. pyogenes* represents a potentially life-threatening infection, rarely caused by nonsteroidal antiinflammatory drugs.[259] Immediate intervention with debridement and antibiotics is essential, and hyperbaric oxygen may be used in some cases. Other gas-forming organisms (*e.g., E. coli*) may cause a similar clinical syndrome.

Septic arthritis or osteomyelitis in the cancer patient may be caused by gram-negative organisms (*e.g., Pseudomonas, Klebsiella, Salmonella, Eikenella*), fungi (*e.g., Candida*), or the more common gram-positive bacterial pathogens. Patients with local skeletal defects or who have undergone extensive surgery, such as amputation or soft tissue dissection, and patients with bacteremia or fungemia are considered to be at high risk. Occasionally, it may be difficult to differentiate osteomyelitis from Ewing's sarcoma or radionecrosis.

CENTRAL NERVOUS SYSTEM INFECTIONS

Infections of the CNS are surprisingly infrequent in patients with cancer, but patients who present with symptoms or signs suggesting CNS dysfunction must be expeditiously evaluated with the appropriate physical, laboratory, and radiographic examinations. Evaluation of cerebrospinal fluid from cancer patients should include aerobic culture and Gram's stain, cryptococcal antigen determination, fungal culture, and cytologic examination in addition to the routine cerebrospinal fluid tests. Potential infections include shunt (*e.g.*, Ommaya reservoir) infections, meningitis or meningoencephalitis, encephalitis, and brain abscesses.

Shunt Infections

Intraventricular shunts and Ommaya reservoirs are associated with an increased incidence of CNS infection. The responsible pathogens are most commonly those colonizing the adjacent skin: coagulase-positive and coagulase-negative staphylococci, *Propionibacterium acnes*, *Corynebacterium* species, enterococci, and gram-negative bacilli. Patients may be totally asymptomatic, or they may have fever, headache, increased intracranial pressure, and meningism. Most patients with Ommaya reservoir infections can be successfully treated without removing the device.

Meningitis

Meningitis or meningoencephalitis is most frequently encountered in patients with impaired cell-mediated immunity and is typically caused by *Cryptococcus neoformans* or *Listeria monocytogenes*. *C. neoformans* causes a meningoencephalitis that is typically indolent. The presenting complaints include headaches, altered mental status, low-grade, intermittent fevers, or meningism. Examination of the cerebrospinal fluid demonstrates a mild mononuclear pleocytosis (40–400 leukocytes/mm³) and minimally decreased glucose. Only 50% of patients have a detectable organism by an India ink preparation, and the most reliable means of diagnosis is documentation of cryptococcal antigen in serum or cerebrospinal fluid. Therapy for *C. neoformans* meningitis or meningoencephalitis includes the combination of amphotericin B (0.3–0.5 mg/kg/day) and oral 5-FC (150 mg/kg/day every 6 hours) for 4 to 6 weeks. Although a multicenter trial in adults with AIDS and cryptococcal meningitis found fluconazole to be comparable amphotericin B, the time to negative of cerebrospinal fluid cultures was longer for patients receiving fluconazole.

Listeria monocytogenes is a motile, gram-positive rod that causes several distinct clinical syndromes, including meningitis. Patients with impaired cell-mediated immunity and especially those with defects of T-cell-mediated immune function are susceptible. Although the organism can be isolated from soil, dust, water, sewage, and contaminated foods (especially cheese and dairy products), the exact mode transmission in most immunocompromised patients is unclear. Community outbreaks have occurred and hospital-associated clustering in immunosuppressed patients has been described. The most common presentation includes a subacute course of low-grade fevers and personality changes. Focal neurologic signs are occasionally present. Laboratory findings include a mild to moderate cerebrospinal fluid pleocytosis (6–12,000 cells/mm³) and may include a predominance of polymorphonuclear leukocytes or mononuclear cells. Protein levels are generally elevated (100–300 mg/100 ml), and cerebrospinal fluid glucose levels are usually decreased. Diagnosis depends on a high index of suspicion. Ampicillin or penicillin provide the optimal treatment and should be continued for 3 to 6 weeks, because relapses have been reported with shorter therapy. Third-generation cephalosporins are inactive against *Listeria*.

Encephalitis

HSV, VZV, and measles are the most likely causes of sporadic viral encephalitis. HSV encephalitis, which may present as a focal or generalized process, responds to acyclovir treatment; acyclovir is also appropriate treatment for VZV encephalitis.

Patients with encephalitis or encephalomyelitis commonly present with signs of meningeal irritation (*e.g.*, fever, headache, nuchal rigidity) and evidence of altered mentation. Confusion may progress to stupor and to coma. Focal neurologic signs and seizures are relatively common. Cerebrospinal fluid examination may demonstrate a pleocytosis (10–2000 cells/mm³), with a predominance of mononuclear cells. An increased number of cerebrospinal fluid red cells has been reported with HSV encephalitis. Cerebrospinal fluid protein levels are normally elevated, and the glucose characteristically remains within the normal range, except for a decreased level in mumps infection.

For the cancer patient with focal neurologic deficits or altered mentation, it is important to differentiate between an infectious, metabolic, toxic, or neoplastic causes. Unfortunately, diagnosis of the specific cause of encephalitis in an immunocompromised patient is difficult. Acute and convalescent serum antibody titers should be obtained, and specific cerebrospinal fluid antibody may be detected in cases of mumps, HSV, and varicella zoster. Although definitive diagnosis of HSV encephalitis requires a brain biopsy and because the clinician's therapeutic armamentarium against most causes of encephalitis is limited, empiric administration of acyclovir (500 mg/m² given every 8 hours) to the cancer patient with signs and symptoms suggesting of encephalitis seems warranted.

A treatable CNS infection that can present as an encephalitis in an immunosuppressed patient or as a mass lesion in the AIDS patient is due to the obligate intracellular parasite *Toxoplasma gondii*. Toxoplasmosis may represent newly acquired or reactivated infection and is rarely limited to the CNS, usually occurring in concert with fever, lymphadenopathy, hepatitis, pneumonitis, myocarditis, and pericarditis. The cerebrospinal fluid typically manifests a mononuclear pleocytosis, elevated protein levels, and a normal glucose concentration. A battery of serologic tests are available for the diagnosis of toxoplasmosis in the immunocompetent host, but most of these are limited in their applicability to the immunosuppressed patient due to suboptimal antibody responses. The definitive diagnosis requires demonstration of the parasite within tissue sections.

Treatment of active toxoplasmosis should include the combination of pyrimethamine and sulfadiazine or "triple sulfa" therapy—trisulfapyrimidines-sulfamerazine, sulfamethazine, and sulfadiazine. In immunodeficient patients, therapy should be continued for 4 to 6 weeks after the resolution of all clinical symptoms and signs. Clindamycin and pyrimethamine also benefit AIDS patients with central toxoplasmosis. The 566C80 quinone that has demonstrated activity against *P. carinii* also offers some benefit to patients with toxoplasmosis.

The important differential diagnosis in a cancer patient with evidence of a focal lesion (mass) within the CNS is between metastatic or primary malignancy and a brain abscess. Predisposing factors for brain abscesses include contiguous sites of infection (*e.g.*, otitis, sinusitis, dental abscesses), a history of penetrating cranial trauma, congenital cardiac disease, bacterial endocarditis, and pulmonary infections. In addition to the usual aerobic and anaerobic bacteria responsible for abscesses in immunocompetent patients, fungal and nocardial species are particularly prone to cause disease in an immunosuppressed patient. In patients with disseminated candidiasis, almost half may have CNS involvement, although this is usually unrecognized. In AIDS patients, CNS lesions may be caused by lymphoma or *T. gondii*. The association of pulmonary lesions with focal neurologic findings suggests *Nocardia, Aspergillus, Mucor,* or *Candida*.

Early evaluation and specific diagnosis are crucial in the management of brain abscesses, because effective antimicrobial or neurosurgical therapy is available. Diagnosis is commonly made by radiographic demonstration of a localized CNS mass, followed by an open or closed neurosurgical procedure to aspirate or resect the localized lesion.

Dementias

One of the disconcerting sequelae of modern chemotherapy has been the occurrence of leukoencephalopathy. Many of these dementing processes can be linked to intrathecal chemotherapy, especially the combination of irradiation and methotrexate. However, awareness that slow virus infections can produce CNS deterioration in humans has raised concern that some dementing processes may have a viral cause. Adults with lymphoma and symptoms of progressive mental and emotional deterioration, including decreased visual acuity, aphasia, and sensory and cerebellar signs, may have antibody to the human papillomavirus JC and isolation of virus from infected mononuclear cells, suggesting the diagnosis of progressive multifocal leukoencephalopathy.[260]

PREVENTING INFECTION IN CANCER PATIENTS

Despite a multitude of clinical trials investigating the efficacy of various measures to prevent or reduce the occurrence of infection, the most important antiinfective measure identified has been the simplest—careful hand-washing practices.[66] Several approaches have been taken to decrease the acquisition of new organisms or suppress those already colonizing the cancer patient (Table 62–16). Unfortunately, no method is singularly effective, each having promise and problems (Tables 62–17 and 62–18). As new preventive strategies are evaluated, they initially appear promising, but as additional studies are conducted, their beneficial results become less convincing.[261]

PREVENTING ACQUISITION OF NEW ORGANISMS

Because almost 85% of the organisms responsible for infections among patients with cancer are derived from the endogenous flora and almost half of these are acquired from the hospital environment, much attention has been directed toward preventing the acquisition of potential pathogens.

Inanimate objects within the hospital environment (*e.g.*, faucet aerators, shower heads, respirators, plants, floors) are reservoirs of pathogenic organisms. However, most epidemiologic studies suggest that transmission from such inanimate sources usually requires a human vector.[65] The simplest yet most efficacious intervention that can be performed is adherence to strict hand-washing precautions.[66] The easiest way to enforce such a policy is to educate the child and parents to disallow contact with anyone who has neglected to wash his hands.

A second maneuver to decrease the acquisition of new organisms is to maintain a cooked diet during periods of granulocytopenia, with avoidance of fresh fruits and vegetables and nonprocessed dairy products, because these foods are naturally contaminated with gram-negative bacteria, especially *K. pneumoniae*, *E. coli*, and *P. aeruginosa*. However, the true benefits of such a diet in reducing the acquisition of new organisms and the incidence of infection has not been proven.

Environmental sources can contribute to fungal (*e.g.*, *Aspergillus*) and bacterial (*e.g.*, *Legionella*) colonization and infection. In centers where *Aspergillus* is a significant problem, special air filtration systems (*e.g.*, high-efficiency particulate air filters) or water purification systems may help.

Although the technique of reverse isolation has often been used, it does not significantly reduce the acquisition of new organisms in an environment where hand-washing techniques are strictly followed.[262] There is no compelling reason to enforce this policy.

The total protective environment (TPE) is a comprehensive antiinfective regimen designed to reduce the patient's endogenous microbial burden while preventing the acquisition of new organisms (see Table 62–17). A sterile environment is created in a clean air room with constant positive air flow and is maintained by an aggressive program of surface decontamination, sterilization of all objects that enter the room, and an intensive regimen to disinfect the patient, including oral, nonabsorbable antibiotics, skin antiseptics, antibiotic sprays and ointments, and a low-microbial diet. Several studies have documented that the TPE can reduce infections in profoundly granulocytopenic patients. However, the TPE is expensive, and because of the improvement in treating established infections, it does not offer a survival advantage to patients. TPE is not necessary for the routine care of cancer patients and, with newer and less expensive modalities, is less frequently used in current clinical practice (see Table 62–18).

ANTIMICROBIAL PROPHYLAXIS

Antibacterial Prophylaxis

Many clinical trials have been conducted to investigate the utility of prophylactic antibiotic regimens in immunocompromised patients. Several strategies have been explored, including systemic prophylaxis, gastrointestinal decontamination, and selective gastrointestinal decontamination (*i.e.*, maintenance of "colonization resistance"). Unfortunately, the interpretation of many of these trials is difficult due to poor study design, nonuniform patient groupings, and failure to report or document compliance with the prophylactic regimens.[264]

Because the gastrointestinal tract is the source for many of the pathogens causing microbiologically defined infections, investigators have evaluated the efficacy of reducing the en-

TABLE 62–16. Methods for Preventing Infection in Cancer Patients

Prevent Acquisition and/or Suppress or Eliminate Microbial Flora	Improve or Modify Host Defenses
Isolation	**Immunization**
Simple or reverse isolation	Active
Isolation with HEPA air filtration	*Pseudomonas*
	Pneumococcus
Prophylactic Antibiotics	Passive
Nonabsorbable antibiotics	J-5 Core glycolipid
Trimethoprim-sulfamethoxazole	Pooled immunoglobulins
Selective decontamination	Specific monoclonal
Quinolones	
	Cell-Component Replacement
Prophylactic Antivirals	Leukocyte transfusions
Acycloguanosine (Acyclovir)	Accelerate granulocyte recovery
Gangciclovir	GM-CAF
Amantadine	G-CSF
	IL-3
Prophylactic Antifungals	Peripheral stem cells
Nystatin	
Imidazoles	
Prophylactic Antiparasitics	
Thiabendazole	
Trimethoprim-sulfamethoxazole	
Combination—Comprehensive	
Total protection isolation	

TABLE 62–17. Antimicrobial Activity of Various Prophylactic Regimens Against Exogenous and Endogenous Microorganisms

Sources	Total Protected Environment	Nonabsorbable Antibiotics	Trimethoprim-Sulfamethoxazole	Selective Decontamination	Quinolones
Exogenous Sources					
Air, food, water contacts	Yes	No	No	No	No
Endogenous Sources					
Nares	Yes	No	No	No	Yes
Oropharynx	Yes	+/–	No	Yes	Yes
Lower respiratory tract	+/–	No	+/–	+/–	Yes
Gastrointestinal tract	Yes	Yes	Yes	Yes	Yes
Perianal area	Yes	+/–	+/–	+/–	+/–
Skin	Yes	No	No	No	No
Central venous catheter	No	No	No	No	No
Peripheral catheters	No	No	No	No	No
Systemic effect	+/–	No	Yes	Yes	Yes

dogenous gastrointestinal flora by the administration of oral, nonabsorbable antibiotics. This technique has not been especially valuable and is fraught with problems. The antimicrobial agents used (*e.g.*, vancomycin, gentamicin, polymyxin B, nystatin, framycetin, colistin) are unpalatable and are generally poorly tolerated, making compliance difficult, especially among patients receiving emetogenic chemotherapy (see Table 62–17). Equally disturbing has been the emergence of

resistant bacterial strains when aminoglycoside-containing regimens have been used. Prophylactic regimens aimed solely at reducing the endogenous gastrointestinal flora cannot be recommended (see Table 62–18).

A modified technique is the "selective decontamination" of the gastrointestinal tract, employing antibiotics that preserve the anaerobic flora but reduce the aerobic bacteria. Data show that the preservation of the anaerobic flora of the gas-

TABLE 62–18. Effectiveness and Limitations of Various Strategies in Preventing Infection in Cancer Patients

Qualities Assessed	Total Protected Environment	Nonabsorbable Antibiotics	Trimethoprim-Sulfamethoxazole	Selective Decontamination	Quinolones
Efficacy					
Reduced infection	Yes	No	+/–	+/–	Yes
Decreased in fever	Yes	No	No	No	Yes
Decrease or shorten need for antibiotics and antifungals	No	No	No	+/–	Yes
Contributed to survival	No	No	No	No	No
Compliance					
Well tolerated?	No	No	+/–	+/–	Yes
Impact on efficacy	Yes	Yes	Yes	+/–	No
Liabilities					
Emergency of resistant organisms	Yes	Yes	Yes	Yes	Yes
Organ side effects:					
Interference with other drugs	Yes	Yes	Yes	No	No
BM suppression	No	No	Yes	Yes	No
Specific organ toxicity	No	No	Yes	Yes	Yes
Cost					
For the drugs or regimens	Yes	Yes	No	Yes	Yes
Surveillance or monitoring	Yes	Yes	Yes	Yes	Yes
Reducing need for hospitalization or need for drugs	No	No	No	+/–	+/–

trointestinal tract provides a colonization resistance against aerobic and fungal organisms.[265,266] Although initial clinical trials provided evidence of a reduction of infections in patients undergoing induction therapy for acute leukemia, clearly defined efficacy has not been established.[267,268] The most commonly investigated agent used for selective decontamination has been trimethoprim-sulfamethoxazole. Early trials investigating this antibiotic in children and adults demonstrated a reduction in all infections and in bacteremic episodes, but many follow-up clinical trials yielded conflicting results.[269-275] The reasons for the contradictory results are unclear, although factors such as variability in study design, nonuniform patient populations, and failure to properly monitor compliance have played a part. The potential for reduction in infectious morbidity and mortality must be balanced against the prolongation of granulocytopenia and emergence of resistant organisms.[276] Successful use of this approach requires close monitoring to properly adjust the antimicrobial regimen for resistant or newly emerging species, and this surveillance is expensive and time consuming.

Prophylactic antibiotic trials employing a derivative of nalidixic acid, the quinolone antibiotic norfloxacin, have shown promising results in a population of bone marrow transplant patients. Although fluoroquinolones such as ciprofloxacin can decrease the incidence of gram-negative bacteria, the use of these agents has not been associated with a reduction in infection-related mortality.

Although some investigators have suggested that the time the initiation of parenteral therapy is lengthened with the use of oral ciprofloxacin, two problems have been observed with prophylactic quinolones.[277,278] One is breakthrough infection with gram-positive organisms, a problem that can potentially be overcome with the addition of penicillin or amoxicillin with clavulanic acid. Of more concern is the increasing incidence of quinolone-resistant organisms.[263] The inappropriate use of these agents for prophylaxis can jeopardize the long-term benefits of this class of antibiotics. The quinolones cannot be used in children younger than 18 years of age because of putative joint toxicity, although studies evaluating their safety in pediatric patients are ongoing.

Antifungal Prophylaxis

Because of the increasing incidence of invasive mycoses in immunocompromised hosts, antifungal prophylaxis has been studied. The most frequently evaluated antifungal agents have included nystatin, amphotericin B, miconazole, clotrimazole, and ketoconazole. Most prophylactic regimens have been aimed at a reduction of invasive infections due to *Candida*, and by virtue of the antifungal activity of the agents employed, they would not be expected to have a significant impact against *Aspergillus* or *Mucormycoses*.

Interpretation of existing data is difficult, because studies suffer from different patient criteria, disparate dosage regimens, nonuniform response criteria, and lack of appropriate controls. An added problem is the inherent difficulty in the definitive diagnosis of a fungal infection in an immunocompromised patient.

Within the context of these limitations, several conclusions about antifungal prophylaxis can be offered. First, after an adequate dose of antifungal agent (*e.g.*, amphotericin B, ke-

toconazole, clotrimazole) has been administered, there has been a consistent decrease in fungal colonization.[279] However, decreased colonization has not clearly resulted in a decreased incidence of invasive mycotic disease, although a decrease in superficial infection has been found in some studies. Second, several studies employing prophylactic and empiric antifungal regimens have reported a shift in the colonization pattern of fungal organisms, mostly toward more resistant fungi. The prophylactic regimens may successfully eradicate the susceptible fungi (particularly *C. albicans*) but may permit the overgrowth and ultimate invasion by more resistant species, especially *Aspergillus*. This was recently observed with fluconazole, one of the newest antifungal agents to be introduced into clinical practice. Patients undergoing bone marrow transplantation and who received fluconazole prophylaxis had an increased incidence of infection with *Candida krusei*, a more resistant and difficult to treat organism. This trend must be closely monitored.

The potential benefits of prophylactic antifungal therapy must be balanced against the toxicities, epidemiologic considerations, and relative efficacy of the regimen employed. Until clear benefit can be proven, widespread chemoprophylaxis against fungi should not be attempted.

Antiviral Prophylaxis

Intravenous and oral formulations of acyclovir can prevent reactivation of HSV and resultant stomatitis among patients undergoing induction therapy for leukemia or lymphoma or marrow allografting.[280] Twice-daily administration of intravenous acyclovir appears to be almost as effective as use three times daily and is more convenient and less expensive. Prophylactic acyclovir may increase the development of acyclovir resistance. Prevention of CMV infection has been more problematic. Although primary CMV infection among seronegative patients can be prevented by use of screened seronegative blood products, use of CMV immunoglobulins or the licensed intravenous immunoglobulins remains controversial. Interferon-α has a prophylactic benefit in renal allograft patients, although this effect was not reproduced in one study among marrow allograft recipients. Intravenous acyclovir may have some effect against CMV if used prophylactically. Ganciclovir is beneficial if administered prophylactically in reducing the incidence of CMV pneumonitis.

Antiparasitic Prophylaxis

In centers where *P. carinii* occurs with some frequency, the administration of trimethoprim-sulfamethoxazole has convincingly reduced the incidence of infection. However, not all children undergoing cancer treatment require prophylactic treatment. It should be influenced by the patients underlying disease (*e.g.*, leukemia, solid tumors), the intensity or immunosuppression of the therapy being delivered, and the center where treatment is being administered. Current recommendations for children are for trimethoprim-sulfamethoxazole (150 mg/m^2) or trimethoprim in two divided doses on 3 consecutive days. In adults, two double-strength (check) tablets, twice daily on 3 consecutive days, is the recommended treatment. These schedules appear to be less associated with hematologic complications (*e.g.*, neutropenia) than daily therapy. Studies of adults with AIDS have demonstrated that trimethoprim-sulfamethoxazole is superior to aerosolized pentamidine in preventing *P. carinii* pneumonia. However, aerosolized pentamidine can be an alternative for patients unable to tolerate trimethoprim-sulfamethoxazole. Other alternatives include dapsone, and the reports of 566C80 suggest that it may be an important component of the anti-*P. carinii* repertoire.

Active and Passive Immunization and Biologicals

Fatal infections due to measles, polio, and vaccinia have occurred as a consequence of live virus immunizations in patients with impaired immune function. Although an initial antibody response may be elicited, the concurrent administration of cytotoxic chemotherapy is usually associated with a rapid decline of titers. Inactivated polio vaccine should be given to the immunologically deficient host and his or her siblings and other household contacts, because oral poliovirus vaccine strains are transmissible to the immunocompromised person. Live virus vaccines may be administered at least 3 months after all immunosuppressive therapy has ceased. An important exception to this rule appears to be the use of the live attenuated varicella vaccine that, despite a being associated with a relatively high incidence of adverse effects (primarily mild to moderate rash), appears to be effective in protecting children with cancer from severe natural varicella infection.

Inactivated vaccines may not yield protective immunity in immunosuppressed patients. Clinical trials have indicated that the efficacy of immunizations against influenza, pneumococcus, and *H. influenzae* type B given during the course of cancer chemotherapy are often impaired because of inadequate antibody responses.

Passive immunization with VZIG reduces the incidence of pneumonitis and encephalitis and decreases the mortality rate from between 5% and 7% to 0.5% in immunocompromised patients with primary varicella infection. Immunosuppressed persons who are seronegative or possess low-titer antivaricella antibody should receive 1 vial of globulin per 15 kg of body weight within 72 hours after exposure to a potentially infectious source.

Immunotherapy for gram-negative septic shock is a strategy based on the hypothesis that passive immunization with antibody against endotoxin, the lipopolysaccharide component of the gram-negative cell wall, can block the endotoxin-triggered release of factors that mediate shock and tissue damage. Initial studies employed high-titer human polyclonal antiserum directed against endotoxin core determinants of the J5 mutant of *E. coli* 0111:B4. Polyclonal J5 antiserum has decreased mortality in patients with documented gram-negative bacteremia and protected high-risk surgical patients from complications due to gram-negative infections.

A human monoclonal IgM antibody, HA-1A, binds specifically to the toxic moiety of endotoxin. In a large randomized, double-blind, placebo-controlled trial, HA-1A antibody significantly reduced mortality in patients who were ultimately proven to have gram-negative bacteremia.[281] However, the clinical criteria used to enroll patients in this study were only able to identify patients with a 30% to 40% probability of having gram-negative sepsis. Most patients in the study did not have gram-negative sepsis, and in those patients, HA-1A

antibody had no impact on mortality. Moreover, no benefit has yet been observed for neutropenic patients. Until better clinical criteria are developed to accurately predict gram-negative bacteremia, the widespread use of HA-1A antibody for all critically ill patients with presumed sepsis cannot be supported.

The therapeutic use of intravenous immunoglobulins is based on the observations that antibody deficiency and increased susceptibility to bacterial infections may occur in patients with hematologic cancers or in those who receive immunosuppressive therapies for cancer or in preparation for bone marrow transplantation. In a large, double-blind trial, intravenous immunoglobulin significantly decreased the number of bacterial infections in patients with chronic lymphocytic leukemia.[282] An extensive cost and benefit analysis of this study, however, revealed that this frequent administration of immunoglobulin over a long period did not improve the quality or length of life in patients with chronic lymphocytic leukemia and that it is an extremely expensive intervention compared with other generally accepted treatments.[283]

In the setting of allogeneic bone marrow transplantation, the prophylactic use intravenous immunoglobulins has significantly reduced the incidence and severity of acute GVHD and associated interstitial pneumonia related to cytomegalovirus and significantly decreased the frequency of sepsis and local infections. A decrease in transplant-related mortality was observed among patients older than 20 years of age who had received immunoglobulin.[284] These encouraging results suggest that the expense of intravenous immunoglobulin therapy in certain bone marrow transplant recipients may be justified. Further study is required to identify to the optimal dose, schedule and population for passive immunotherapy.

Perhaps the most exciting development is the cloning, purification, and clinical application of the hematopoietic growth factors, including the CSFs and several of the interleukins. These glycoproteins endogenously stimulate the proliferation and maturation of bone marrow progenitor cells into fully differentiated circulating blood cells. The two growth factors most intensively studied are G-CSF and GM-CSF. G-CSF specifically promotes the proliferation and maturation of neutrophilic precursors, and the function of mature neutrophils. GM-CSF additionally enhances the number and function of cells of the monocyte-macrophage lineage. The potential utility of the CSFs to attenuate the marrow toxic effects of cancer chemotherapy and radiotherapy has been assessed in several trials. Early, uncontrolled studies indicated that administration of recombinant human (rh)GM-CSF or rhG-CSF administration can decrease the duration and severity of neutropenia in patients after intensive chemotherapy for small cell lung cancer, bladder cancer, metastatic sarcomas, and other neoplasms and in those undergoing autologous bone marrow transplantation.[285–289] One trial showed a reduction in the number of days of neutropenia associated with rhG-CSF use during chemotherapy for relapsed or refractory acute myelogenous leukemia.

Data from several studies suggested that patients treated with CSFs experienced fewer infectious complications than historic controls. Two large, randomized, double-blind, placebo-controlled trials substantiated these results. Nemunaitis and colleagues observed that patients undergoing autologous bone marrow transplantation for lymphoid cancers who received rhGM-CSF had accelerated neutrophil recovery by 1 week, a reduced incidence of culture-proven infections, and a decreased duration of required antibiotic administration and hospitalization.[284] Similar findings were reported with the use of rhG-CSF in patients receiving chemotherapy for small cell lung cancer.[285] In these studies, rhGM- and G-CSF were well-tolerated, although others have reported significant toxicities associated with rhGM-CSF including fevers, rashes, malaise, arthralgias and myalgias, and a capillary leak syndrome, generally at high doses. Very few adverse effects have been seen with rhG-CSF. The encouraging results led to the licensing of G-CSF and GM-CSF as adjuncts to some of the highly marrow-suppressive cancer therapies.

These trials indicate that by minimizing the chemotherapy-induced toxicities of prolonged neutropenia and complicating infections, the CSFs may permit the delivery of chemotherapy in schedules and doses that maximize tumoricidal activity. With the identification and purification of an increasing array of immunomodulatory substances, (*e.g.*, interleukins, interferons, TNF) there is the potential for improving the altered host defenses of the cancer patient and reducing the complications and limitations of chemotherapy.[290]

REFERENCES

1. Bodey G. Infection in cancer patients: A continuing association. Am J Med 1986;81(suppl 1A):11–26.
2. Sculier JP, Weerts D, Klastersky J. Causes of death in febrile granulocytopenic cancer patients receiving empiric antibiotic therapy. Eur J Cancer Clin Oncol 1984;20:55–60.
3. Pizzo PA, Rubin M, Freifeld A, Walsh TJ. The child with cancer and infection. I. Empirical therapy for fever and neutropenia, and preventive strategies. J Pediatr 1991;119:676–694.
4. Pizzo PA, Rubin M, Freifeld A, Walsh TJ. The child with cancer and infection. II. Nonbacterial infections. J Pediatr 1991;119:845–857.
5. Beachey EH. Bacterial adherence: Adhesin-receptor interactions mediating the attachment of bacteria to mucosal surfaces. J Infect Dis 1981;143:325–345.
6. Schoolnik GK, Lark D, O'Hanley P. Bacterial adherence and anticolonization vaccines. In: Remington JS, Schwarz NM, eds. Current clinical topics in infectious diseases, vol 6. New York: McGraw Hill, 1985:85–102.
7. Johanson WG, Pierce AK, Sanford JP. Changing pharyngeal flora of hospitalized patients: Emergence of gram-negative bacilli. N Engl J Med 1969;281:1137–1140.
8. Fainstain V, Rodriguez V, Turk, et al. Patterns of oropharyngeal and fecal flora in patients with leukemia. J Infect Dis 1981;144:10–18.
9. Van der Waaij D. Gut resistance to colonization: Clinical usefulness of selective use of orally administered antimicrobial and antifungal drugs. In: Klastersky J, ed. Infection in cancer patients. New York: Raven Press, 1982:73–86.
10. Spitznagel JK, Shafer WM. Neutrophil killing of bacteria by oxygen-independent mechanism: A historical summary. Rev Infect Dis 1985;7:398–403.
11. Bodey GP, Buckley M, Sathe YS, et al. Quantitative relationships between circulating leukocytes and infection in patients with acute leukemia. Ann Intern Med 1966;64:328–340.
12. Sieff CA. Hematopoietic growth factors. J Clin Invest 1987;79:1549–1557.
13. Roilides E, Pizzo PA. Modulation of host defenses by cytokines. Evolving adjuncts in prevention and treatment of serious infection in immunocompromised hosts. Clin Infect Dis (in press).
14. Nienhuis AW, Donahue RE, Karisson S, et al. Recombinant human granulocyte-macrophage colony-stimulating factor (GM-CSF) shortens the period of neutropenia after autologous bone marrow transplantation in a primate model. J Clin Invest 1987;80:573–577.
15. Mayer P, Lam C, Obenaus H, et al. Recombinant human GM-CSF induces leukocytosis and activates peripheral blood polymorphonuclear neutrophils in nonhuman primates. Blood 1987;70:206–213.
16. Lopez AF, Williamson D, Gamble R, et al. Recombinant human granulocyte-macrophage colony-stimulating factor stimulates in vitro mature human neutrophil and eosinophil function, surface receptor expression, and survival. J Clin Invest 1986;78:1220–1228.
17. Weisbart RH, Kwan L, Golde DW, et al. Human GM-CSF primes neutrophils for enhanced oxidative metabolism in response to the major physiological chemoattractants. Blood 1987;69:18–21.
18. Glasson JC, Weisbard RH, Kaufman SE, et al. Purified human granulocyte-macrophage colony-stimulating factor: Direct action on neutrophils. Science 1984;226:1339–1342.
19. Lynch HT, Katz DA, Bogard PJ, Lynch JF. The sarcoma, breast cancer, lung cancer, and adrenocortical carcinoma syndrome revisited: Childhood Cancer. Am J Dis Child 1985;139:134–136.
20. Beutler B, Milsard IW, Cerami A. Passive immunization against cachectin/tumor necrosis factor protects mice from lethal effect of endotoxin. Science 1985;229:869–871.
21. Dinarello CA. Interleukin-1. Rev Infect Dis 1984;6:51–59.
22. Estrov Z, Roifman C, Mills G, et al. The regulatory role of interleukin-2 responsive T lymphocytes on human marrow granulopoiesis. Blood 1987;69:1161–1166.
23. Cannistra SA, Rambaldi A, Spriggs DR, et al. Human granulocyte-macrophage colony-stimulating factor induces expression of the tumor necrosis factor gene by the U937 cell line and by normal human monocytes. J Clin Invest 1987;79:1720–1720.
24. Zucali JR, Dinarello CA, Oblon DJ, et al. Interleukin-1 stimulates fibroblasts to produce granulocyte-macrophage colony-stimulating activity and prostaglandin E_2. J Clin Invest 1986;77:1857–1863.
25. Perfect JR, Granger DL, Durack DT. Effects of antifungal agents and γ-interferon on macrophage cytotoxicity for fungi and tumor cells. J Infect Dis 1987;156:316–323.
26. Wilson CB, Westall J. Activation of neonatal and adult human macrophages by alpha, beta, and gamma interferons. Infect Immunol 1985;49:351–356.
27. Dinarello CA, The proinflammatory cytokones interleukin 1 and tumor necrosis factor and treatment of nil septic shock syndrome. J Infect Dis 1991;163:1177–1184.
28. Dinarello CA, Mier JW. Lymphokines. N Engl J Med 1987;317:940–945.
29. Nathan DG. Hope for hematopoietic hormones. N Engl J Med 1987;317:626–628.
30. Curnette JT, Boxer LA. Clinically significant phagocytic cell defects. In: Remington J, Swartz M, eds. Current clinical topics in infectious diseases, vol 6. New York: McGraw Hill, 1985:103–156.
31. McCormack RT, Nelson RD, Bloomfield CD, et al. Neutrophilic function in lymphoreticular malignancy. Cancer 1979;44:920–926.
32. Snyderman R, Seigler HF, Meadows L. Abnormalities of monocyte chemotaxis in patients with melanoma. Effects of immunotherapy and tumor removal. JNCI 1977;58:37–41.
33. Pickering LK, Ericsson CD, Kohl S. Effect of chemotherapeutic agents on metabolic and bactericidal activity of polymorphonuclear leukocytes. Cancer 1978;42:1741–1746.
34. Baehner RL, Neiburger RG, Johnson DG, et al. Transient bactericidal defect of peripheral blood phagocytes from children with acute lymphoblastic leukemia receiving craniospinal irradiation. N Engl J Med 1973;289:1209–1213.
35. Tubaro E, Borelli G, Croce C, et al. Effect of morphine on resistance to infection. J Infect Dis 1983;148:656–666.
36. Schaffner A, Douglas H, Braude A. Selective protection against *Candidia* by mononuclear and against mycelia by polymorphonuclear phagocytes in resistance to *Aspergillus*. J Clin Invest 1982;69:617–631.
37. Fisher RI, DeVita VT, Bostick F. Persistent immunologic abnormalities in long term survivors of advanced Hodgkin's disease. Ann Intern Med 1980;92:595–599.
38. Dale DC, Petersdorf RG. Corticosteroids and infectious disease. Med Clin North Am 1973;57:1277–1287.
39. Nossai GJV. Current concepts: Immunology: The basic components of the immune system. N Engl J Med 1987;316:1320–1325.
40. Fahey JL, Scoggins R, Utz JP, et al. Infection, antibody response and gamma globulin components in multiple myeloma and macroglobulinemia. Am J Med 1973;35:698–707.
41. Stobo JD, Paul S, Von Scoy RE, et al. Suppressor thymus-derived lymphocytes in fungal infection. J Clin Invest 1976;57:319–328.
42. Zinner SH, McCabe WR. Effect of IgM and IgG antibody in patients with bacteremia due to gram-negative bacilli. J Infect Dis 1976;133:37–45.
43. Siber GR, Weitzman SA, Aisenberg AC, et al. Impaired antibody response to pneumococcal vaccine after treatment for Hodgkin's disease. N Engl J Med 1978;299:442–448.
44. Pier G, Thomas DM. Characterization of the human immune response to a polysaccharide vaccine from *Pseudomonas acruginosa*. J Infect Dis 1983;148:206–213.
45. Schildt RA, Boyd JF, McCracken JF, et al. Antibody response to pneumococcal vaccine in patients with solid tumors and lymphomas. Med Pediatr Oncol 1983;11:305–309.
46. Cooper M. B lymphocytes: Normal development and function. N Engl J Med 1987;317:1452–1456.
47. Peter G, Pizzo PA, Robichaud KR, et al. Possible protective effect of circulating antibodies to the shared glycolipid of enterobacteriaceae in children with malignancy. Pediatr Res 1979;13:466.
48. Braude AI, Douglas H, Davis CE. Treatment and prevention of intravascular coagulation with antiserum to endotoxin. J Infect Dis 1973;128:S157–S164.
49. Ziegler EJ, McCutchan JA, Fierer S, et al. Successful treatment of gram-negative bacteremia and shock with human antiserum to a UPD-GAL epimerase-deficient mutant *Escherichia coli*. N Engl J Med 1982;307:1225–1230.
50. Rosse WF. The spleen as a filter. N Engl J Med 1987;317:705–706.
51. Sun T, Tenenbaum MJ, Greenspan J, et al. Morphologic and clinical observations in human infection with *Babesia microti*. J Infect Dis 1983;148:239–248.
52. Donaldson SS, Glatstein E, Vosti KL. Bacterial infections in pediatric Hodgkin's disease. Relationship to radiation, chemotherapy and splenectomy. Cancer 1978;41:1949–1958.
53. Chilcote RR, Baehner RL, Hammond D, et al. Septicemia and meningitis in children splenectomized for Hodgkin's disease. N Engl J Med 1976;295:798–800.
54. Weitzman S, Aisenberg AC. Fulminant sepsis after the successful treatment of Hodgkin's disease. Am J Med 1977;62:47–50.

55. Schimpff SC, O'Connell MJ, Greene WH, et al. Infections in 92 splenectomized patients with Hodgkin's disease. A clinical review. Am J Med 1975;59:695–701.
56. Keusch GT. Nutrition and infection. In: Remington JS, Swartz NM, eds. Current clinical topics in infectious disease, vol 5. New York: McGraw-Hill, 1984:106–123.
57. Shamberger RC, Pizzo PA, Goodgame JT, et al. The effect of total parenteral nutrition on chemotherapy induced myelosuppression: A randomized study. Am J Med 1983;74:40–48.
58. Schimpff SC, Young VM, Greene WH, et al. Origin of infection in acute nonlymphocytic leukemia: Significance of hospital acquisition of potential pathogens. Ann Intern Med 1972;77:707–714.
59. Van der Waaij D, Tielemons-Speltie TM, de Houban-Roech AMJ. Infection by and distribution of biotypes of enterobacteriaceae species in leukaemic patients treated under ward conditions and in units for protective isolation in seven hospitals in Europe. Infection 1977;5:3–10.
60. Schimpff SC, Greene WH, Young VM, et al. Significance of Pseudomonas aeruginosa in the patient with leukemia or lymphoma. J Infect Dis 1974;130:S24–S31.
61. Kurrle E, Bhaduri S, Krieger D, et al. Risk factors for infections of the oropharynx and the respiratory tract in patients with acute leukemia. J Infect Dis 1981;144:128–136.
62. Kramer BK, Pizzo PA, Robichaud KJ, et al. Role of serial microbiological surveillance and clinical evaluation in the management of cancer patients with fever and granulocytopenia. Am J Med 1982;72:561–568.
63. Pizzo PA, Levine AS. The utility of protected environment regimens for the compromised host: A critical assessment. In: Progress in hematology, vol X. New York: Grune & Stratton, 1977:311–332.
64. Aisner J, Murillo J, Schimpff SC, et al. Invasive Aspergillus in acute leukemia: Correlation with nose cultures and antibiotic use. Ann Intern Med 1979;90:4–9.
65. Maki DG, Alvarado CJ, Hessewer CH, et al. Relation of the inanimate hospital environment to endemic nosocomial infection. N Engl J Med 1982;307:1562–1565.
66. Albert RK, Condie F. Handwashing patterns in medical intensive care units. N Engl J Med 1981;304:1465–1466.
67. Maki D. Infections associated with intravascular lines. In: Remington JS, Swartz M, eds. Current clinical topics in infectious disease. New York: McGraw Hill, 1982:309–363.
68. Hiemenz J, Skelton J, Pizzo PA. Perspective on the management of catheter related infections in cancer patients. Pediatr Infect Dis 1986;5:6–11.
69. Craven DE, Moody B, Connolly MG, et al. Pseudobacteremia caused by povidone-iodine solution contaminated with Pseudomonas cepacia. N Engl J Med 1981;305:621–623.
70. Johanson WG, Pierce AK, Sanford JP, et al. Nosocomial respiratory infections with gram-negative bacilli. The significance of colonization of the respiratory tract. Ann Intern Med 1972;77:701–706.
71. Wingard JR, Merz WG, Saral R. Candida tropicalis: A major pathogen in immunocompromised patients. Ann Intern Med 1979;91:539–543.
72. Wingard JR, Merz WG, Rinaldi MG, et al. Increase in Candida krusei infection among patients with bone marrow transplantation and neutropenia treated prophylactically with fluconazole. N Engl J Med 1991;325:1274–1277.
73. Rouse BT, Horohov DW. Immunosuppression in viral infections. Rev Infect Dis 1986;8:850–873.
74. Todeschini G, Rubin M, Gill V, et al. Non-aeruginosa bacteremias in cancer patients. Review of 10 years' experience at the National Cancer Institute. Proceedings of the 27th Interscience Conference on Antimicrobial Agents and Chemotherapy, New York: 1987:265.
75. Pizzo PA, Ladisch SL, Gill F, et al. Increasing incidence of gram-positive sepsis in cancer patients. Med Pediatr Oncol 1978;5:241–244.
76. Wade JC, Schimpff SC, Newman KA, et al. Staphylococcus epidermidis: An increasing cause of infection in patients with granulocytopenia. Ann Intern Med 1982;97:507–508.
77. Lowder JN, Lazarus HM, Herzig RH. Bacteremias and fungemias in oncologic patients with central venous catheters. Changing spectrum of infection. Ann Intern Med 1982;142:1456–1459.
78. Winston DJ, Dudnick FV, Chapin M, et al. Coagulase-negative staphylococcal bacteremia in patients receiving immunosuppressive therapy. Arch Intern Med 1983;143:32–36.
79. Myers JP, Linneman CC. Bacteremia due to methicillin-resistant Staphylococcus aureus. J Infect Dis 1982;145:532–536.
80. Haley RW, Hightower AW, Khabbaz RF, et al. The emergence of methicillin-resistant Staphylococcus aureus infections in United States' hospitals. Ann Intern Med 1982;97:297–308.
81. Walsh TJ, Vlahov D, Hansen SL, et al. Prospective surveillance in control of nosocomial methicillin-resistant Staphylococcus aureus. Infect Control 1987;8:7–14.
82. Schwabe RS, Stapleton JT, Gilligon PH. Emergence of vancomycin resistance in coagulase-negative staphylococci. N Engl J Med 1987;316:927–931.
83. Lowry FD, Hammer SM. Staphylococcus epidermidis infection. Ann Intern Med 1983;99:834–839.
84. Joshi J, Newman K, Tenny J, et al. Staphylococcus epidermidis pneumonia in granulocytopenic patients with acute leukemia. Proc Am Soc Clin Oncol 1983;2:90.
85. Thaler M, Gill V, Pizzo PA. Staphylococcal bacteremias in a cancer research hospital. Proceedings of the 26th Interscience Conference on Antimicrobial Agents and Chemotherapy, New Orleans, 1986.
86. Rubin M, Hathorn JW, Marshall D, et al. Gram-positive infections and the use of vancomycin in 550 episodes of fever and neutropenia. Ann Intern Med 1988;108:30–35.

87. Pizzo PA, Ladish SL, Witebsky F. Alpha-hemolytic streptococci: Clinical significance in cancer patients. Med Pediatr Oncol 1978;4:367–370.
88. Cohen J, Donnelly JP, Worsley AM, et al. Septicemia caused by viridans streptococci in neutropenic patients with leukaemia. Lancet 1983;2:1452–1454.
89. Von Etta LL, Filica GA, Ferguson RM, et al. Corynebacterium equi: A review of 12 cases of human infection. Rev Infect Dis 1983;5:1012–1018.
90. Hande KR, Witebsky FG, Brown MS, et al. Sepsis with a new species of Cornyebacterium. Ann Intern Med 1976;85:423–426.
91. Berg R, Chmel H, Mayo J, et al. Corynebacterium equi infection complicating neoplastic disease. Am J Clin Pathol 1977;68:73–77.
92. Gill VJ, Manning C, Lamson M, et al. Antibiotic-resistant group JK bacteria in hospitals. J Clin Microbiol 1981;13:472–477.
93. Thaler M, Gill V, Pizzo PA. Emergence of Clostridium tertium as a pathogen in neutropenic patients. Am J Med 1986;81:596–600.
94. Cotton DJ, Gu V, Hiemenz J, et al. Bacillus bacteremias in an immunocompromised patient population: Clinical features, therapeutic interventions, and relationship to chronic intravascular catheters in sixteen cases. J Clin Microbiol 1987;25:672–674.
95. Harsburg CR Jr. Mycobacaterium avium complex infection in the acquired immunodeficiency syndrome. N Engl J Med 1991;324:1332–1338.
96. Macher AM, Kovacs JA, Gill V, et al. Bacteremia due to Mycobacterium avium-intracellulare in the acquired immunodeficiency syndrome. Ann Intern Med 1983;99:782–785.
97. Hoy JF, Rolston KVI, Hopfer RL, et al. Mycobacterium fortuitum bacteremia in patients with cancer and long-term venous catheters. Am J Med 1987;83:213–217.
98. Walsh T, Pizzo PA. Nosocomial mycoses in immunocompromised patients. Annu Rev Microbiol (in press).
99. Macher AM. Infection in the acquired immunodeficiency syndrome. In: Fauci AJ, moderator. Acquired immunodeficiency syndrome: Epidemiologic, clinical, immunologic, and therapeutic considerations. Ann Intern Med 1984;100:92–106.
100. Walsh TJ, Newman KR, Moody M, et al. Trichosporonosis in patients with neoplastic disease. Medicine (Baltimore) 1986;65:268–279.
101. Hamilton JR, Overall JC, Glasgow LA. Synergistic effect on mortality in mice with murine cytomegalovirus and Pseudomonas aeruginosa, Staphylococcus aureus or Candida albicans infections. Infect Immunol 1976;14:982–989.
102. Rand KH, Pollard RB, Merigan TC. Increased pulmonary superinfections in cardiac transplant patients undergoing primary cytomegalovirus infection. N Engl J Med 1978;298:951–953.
103. Browder AA, Hoff JA, Petersdorf RG. The significance of fever in neoplastic disease. Ann Intern Med 1961;55:932–942.
104. Goodman R, Jaffe N, Filler R, et al. Herpes zoster in children with stage I–III Hodgkin's disease. Radiology 1976;118:429–431.
105. Kaplan MS, Rosen PP, Armstrong D. Cryptococcosis in a cancer hospital. Clinical and pathological correlates in forty-six patients. Cancer 1977;39:2265–2274.
106. Winston DJ, Gale RP, Meyer DV. Infectious complications of human bone marrow transplantation. Medicine (Baltimore) 1979;58:1–31.
107. Sickles EA, Green WH, Wiernik PH. Clinical presentation of infection in granulocytopenic patients. Arch Intern Med 1975;135:715–719.
108. Schimpff SC, Satterlee W, Young VM, et al. Empiric therapy with carbenicillin and gentamicin for febrile patients with cancer and granulocytopenia. N Engl J Med 1971;284:1061–1065.
109. Markman M, Abeloff M. Management of hematologic and infectious complications of intensive induction therapy for small cell carcinoma of the lung. Am J Med 1983;74:741–746.
110. Pizzo PA, Robichaud KJ, Wesley R, et al. Fever in the pediatric and young adult patient with cancer. A prospective study of 1001 episodes. Medicine (Baltimore) 1982;61:153–165.
110a. Hughes WT, Armstrong D, Bodey GP, et al. Guidelines for the use of antimicrobial agents in neutropenic patients with unexplained fever. A statement by The Infectious Disease Society of America. J Infect Dis 1990;161:381–396.
110b. Pizzo PA, Armstrong D, Bodey GP, et al. The design, analysis and reporting of clinical trials in the empirical antibiotic management of the neutropenic patient. J Infect Dis 1990;161:397–401.
111. The EORTC International Antimicrobial Therapy Project Group. Three antibiotic regimens in the treatment of infection in febrile granulocytopenic patients with cancer. J Infect Dis 1978;137:14–29.
112. Pizzo PA, Hathorn JW, Hiemenz JW, et al. A randomized trial comparing ceftazidime alone with combination antibiotic therapy in cancer patients with fever and neutropenia. N Engl J Med 1986;315:552–558.
113. Anstall HB, Coleman RE. Donor-leukocyte imaging in granulocytopenic patients with suspected abscesses: Concise communication. J Nucl Med 1978;23:319–321.
114. Dutcher JP, Schiffer CA, Johnston GS. Rapid migration of 111In-labelled granulocytes to sites of infection. N Engl J Med 1981;304:586–589.
115. Rubin E, Farber JL. Pathology. Philadelphia: JB Lippincott, 1988.
116. Walsh TJ, Hathorn JW, Sobel JD, et al. Antigenemia due to Candida enolase during invasive candidiasis in patients with neoplastic diseases: A prospective multicenter study. N Engl J Med 1991;324:1026–1031.
117. McCabe WR, Jackson GG. Gram-negative bacteremia. Arch Intern Med 1982;110:847–855.
118. Bryant RE, Hood AF, Hood CE, et al. Factors affecting mortality in gram-negative bacteremia. Arch Intern Med 1971;127:120–128.
119. Love LJ, Schimpff SC, Schiffer CA, et al. Improved prognosis for granulocytopenic patients with gram-negative bacteremia. Am J Med 1980;68:643–648.
120. Schimpff SC. Overview of empiric antibiotic therapy for the febrile neutropenic patient. Rev Infect Dis 1985;7(suppl 4):S734–S740.

121. Pizzo PA, Thaler M, Hathorn J, et al. New β-lactamase antibiotics in the granulocytopenic patient: New options and new questions. Am J Med 1985;79:75–82.

122. Huijgens PC, Ossenkoppele GJ, Weijers TF, et al. Imipenem-citastatin for empirical therapy in neutropenic patients with fever: An open study in patients with hematologic malignancies. Eur J Haematol 1991;46:42–46.

123. Neu HC. β-lactam antibiotics: Structural relationships affecting in vitro activity and pharmacologic properties. Rev Infect Dis 1986;8(suppl 3):S237–S259.

124. The EORTC International Antimicrobial Therapy Cooperative Group. Ceftazidime combined with a short or long course of amikacin for empirical therapy of gram-negative bacteremia in cancer patients with granulocytopenia. N Engl J Med 1987;317:1692–1698.

125. Pizzo PA. After empiric therapy. What to do until the granulocyte comes back. Rev Infect Dis 1987;9:214–219.

126. DePauw BE, Kauw F, Muytjens H, et al. Randomized study of ceftazidime versus gentamicin plus cefotaxime for infections in severely granulocytopenic patients. J Antimicrob Chemother 1983;12(suppl A):593–599.

127. Young L. Empirical antimicrobial therapy in the neutropenic host. N Engl J Med [Editorial] 1986;315:580–581.

128. Karp JE, Dick JD, Angelopoulos C, et al. Empiric use of vancomycin during prolonged treatment-induced granulocytopenia. Randomized, double-blind, placebo-controlled clinical trial in patients with acute leukemia. Am J Med 1986;81:237–242.

129. Kramer BJ, Ramphal R, Rand K. Randomized comparison between two ceftazidime containing regimens and cephalothin-gentamicin-carbenicillin in febrile granulocytopenic cancer patients. Antimicrob Agents Chemother 1986;30:64–68.

130. Shenep JL, Hughes WT, Roberson PK, et al. Vancomycin, ticarcillin and amikacin compared with ticarcillin-clavulanate and amikacin in the empirical treatment of febrile neutropenic children with cancer. N Engl J Med 1988;317:1053.

131. Rubin M, Hathorn JW, Marshall D, Gress J, Steinberg S, Pizzo PA. Gram-positive infections and the use of vancomycin in 550 episodes of fever and neutropenia. Ann Intern Med 1988;108:88–100.

132. European Organization for Research and Treatment of Cancer (EORTC), International Antimicrobial Therapy Cooperative Group and the National Cancer Institute of Canada-Clinical Trials Group. Vancomycin added to empirical combination therapy for fever in granulocytopenic cancer patients. J Infect Dis 1991;163:951–958.

133. Novakova I, Donnelly JP, DePauw B. Ceftazidime as monotherapy or combined with teicoplanin for initial empiric treatment of presumed bacteremia in febrile granulocytopenic patients. Antimicrob Agents Chemother 1991;35:672–678.

134. Dybedal I, Lomuik J. Respiratory insufficiency in acute leukemia following treatment with cytosine arabinoside and septicemia with *Streptococcus viridans*. Eur J Hematol 1989;42:405–406.

135. Sobel J. Imipenem and aztreonam. Infect Dis Clin North Am 1989;3:613–24.

136. Neu H. Aztreonam activity, pharmacology, and clinical uses. Am J Med 1990;88(suppl 3C):2S–6S.

137. Neu H. The quinolones. Infect Dis Clin North Am 1989;3:625–39.

138. Smith G, Leyland M, Farrell I, Geddes A. A clinical, microbiological and pharmacokinetic study of ciprofloxacin plus vancomycin as initial therapy of febrile episodes in neutropenic patients. J Antimicrob Chemother 1988;21:647–55.

140. Mullen CA, Buchanan GR. Early hospital discharge of children with cancer treated for fever and neutropenia: Identification and management of the low-risk patient. J Clin Oncol 1990; 8:12;1998–2004.

141. Pizzo PA, Robichaud KJ, Gill FA, et al. Duration of empiric antibiotic therapy in granulocytopenic cancer patients. Am J Med 1979;67:194–200.

142. Pizzo PA, Commers J, Cotton D, et al. Approaching the controversies in the antibacterial management of cancer patients. Am J Med 1984;76:436–449.

143. Cotton D, Marshall D, Gress J, et al. Pathogen-specific vs broad-spectrum antibiotics for granulocytopenic patients with proven infection. Proceedings of the 24th Interscience Conference on Antimicrobial Agents and Chemotherrapy, Washington, DC, 1984:158.

144. Walsh TJ, Pizzo PA. Fungal infections in granulocytopenic patients: Current approaches to classification, diagnosis, and treatment. In: Holmberg K, Meyer R, eds. Diagnosis and therapy of systemic fungal infections. New York: Raven Press, 1989:47–70.

145. Walsh TJ, Lee J, Lecciones J, et al. Empiric therapy with amphotericin B in febrile granulocytopenic patients. Rev Infect Dis 1991;13:496–503.

146. Pizzo PA, Robichaud RJ, Gill FA, et al. Empiric antibiotic and antifungal therapy for cancer patients with prolonged fever and granulocytopenia. Am J Med 1982;72:101–111.

147. EORTC International Antimicrobial Therapy Cooperative Group. Empiric Antifungal Therapy in Febrile Granulocytopenic Patients. Am J Med 1989;86:668–672.

148. Walsh TJ, Rubin M, Hathorn J, et al. Amphotericin B vs high-dose ketoconazole for empirical antifungal therapy among febrile, granulocytopenic cancer patients: A prospective, randomized study. Arch Intern Med 1991;151:765–770.

149. Fluconazole. Med Lett 1990;32:50–52.

150. Meunier F, Aoun M, Gerard M. Therapy for oropharyngeal candidiasis in the immunocompromised host: A randomized double-blind study of fluconazole vs. ketoconazole. Rev Infect Dis 1990;12(suppl 13):364–368.

151. Navarro E, Lecciones JA, Lee JW, et al. Invasive pulmonary aspergillosis developing during empirical antifungal therapy in febrile cancer patients (in press).

152. Klein RS, Catalona MT, Edberg SC, et al. *Streptococcus bovis* septicemia and carcinoma of the colon. Ann Intern Med 1979;91:560–562.

153. Mueller B, Skelton J, Callender D, et al. A prospective randomized trial comparing the infectious and non-infectious complications of externalized (Hickman-Broviac) versus subcutaneously implanted (Port-a-Cath) devices in cancer patients. J Clin Oncol 1992;10:1943–1948.

154. Pizzo PA, Ladisch SL, Robichaud K. Treatment of gram-positive septicemia in cancer patients. Cancer 1980;45:206–207.

155. Bone RC, Fisher CJ, Clemmer TP, et al. A controlled clinical trial of high-dose methylprednisolone in the treatment of severe sepsis and septic shock. N Engl J Med 1987;317:653–658.

156. Bernard GR, Luce JM, Sprung CL, et al. High-dose corticosteroids in patients with the adult respiratory distress syndrome. N Engl J Med 1987;317:1565–1570.

157. Frederick J, Braude AI. Anaerobic infection of the paranasal sinuses. N Engl J Med 1974;290:135–137.

158. Caplan ES, Hoyt NJ. Nosocomial sinusitis. JAMA 1982;247:639–641.

159. McGill TJ, Simpson G, Healy GB. Fulminant aspergillosis of the nose and paranasal sinuses: A new clinical entity. Laryngoscope 1980;90:748–754.

160. Meyer RD, Rosen P, Armstrong D. Phycomycosis complicating leukemia and lymphoma. Ann Intern Med 1972;77:871–879.

161. Eden OB, Santos J. Effective treatment for rhinopulmonary mucormycosis in a boy with leukemia. Arch Dis Child 1979;54:557–559.

162. Viollier AF, DeJongh C, Newman K, et al. *Aspergillus* sinusitis in cancer patients. Proceedings of the 21st Interscience Conference on Antimicrobial Agents and Chemotherapy, Chicago, Illinois, 1981:801.

163. Mahoney DH, Steuber CP, Starling KA, et al. An outbreak of aspergillosis in children with acute leukemia. J Pediatr 1979;95:70–71.

164. Berkow RL, Weisman SJ, Provisor AJ, et al. Invasive aspergillosis of paranasal tissues in children with malignancies. J Pediatr 1983;103:49–53.

165. Swerdlow B, Doresinski S. Development of *Aspergillus* sinusitis in a patient receiving amphotericin B. Treatment with granulocyte transfusions. Am J Med 1984;76:162–166.

166. Mayosmith MF, Hirsch PJ, Wodzinski SF, et al. Acute epiglottitis in adults. An eight-year experience in the state of Rhode Island. N Engl J Med 1986;314:1133–1139.

167. Cole S, Zawin M, Lundberg B, et al. *Candida* epiglottitis in an adult with acute non-lymphocytic leukemia. Am J Med 1987;82:662–663.

168. Walsh TJ, Gray W. *Candida* epiglottitis in immunocompromised patients. Chest 1987;9:482–485.

169. Arnow PM, Chou T, Weil D, et al. Nosocomial legionnaires: Disease caused by aero-solized tap water from respiratory devices. J Infect Dis 1982;146:460–467.

170. Helms CM, Massanari RM, Zeitter R, et al. Legionnaires' disease associated with a hospital water system: A cluster of 24 nosocomial cases. Ann Intern Med 1983;99:172–178.

171. Grayston TJ, Kuo CC, Wong SP, et al. A new *Chlamydia psittaci* strain, TWAR, isolated in acute respiratory tract infections. N Engl J Med 1986;315:161–168.

172. Marrie TJ, Grayston JT, Wong SP, et al. Pneumonia associated with the TWAR strain of *Chlamydia*. Ann Intern Med 1987;106:507–511.

173. Ramsey PG, Fife KH, Hackman RC, et al. Herpes simplex virus pneumonia: Clinical, virological and pathological features in 20 patients. Ann Intern Med 1982;97:813–820.

174. Barnes PF, Block AB, Davidson PT, Snider DE Jr. Tuberculosis in patients with human immunodeficiency virus infection. N Engl J Med 1991;324:1644–1650.

175. Daley CL, Small PM, Schecter GF, et al. An outbreak of tuberculosis with accelerated progression among persons infected with the human immunodeficiency virus. An analysis using restriction-fragment-length polymorphisms. N Engl J Med 1992;326:231–235.

176. Feld R, Bodey GP, Groschel D. Mycobacteriosis in patients with malignant disease. Arch Intern Med 1976;136:67–70.

177. Ludmerer KM, Kissnae JM. Fulminant pneumonia and death in an immunocompromised woman. Am J Med 1983;75:1043–1052.

178. Stover DE, Zamm MB, Hajdu SI, et al. Bronchoalveolar lavage in the diagnosis of diffuse pulmonary infiltrates in the immunocompromised host. Ann Intern Med 1984;101:1–6.

179. Thorpe JE, Baughman RP, Frame PT, et al. Bronchoalveolar lavage for diagnosing acute bacterial pneumonia. J Infect Dis 1987;155:855–861.

180. Kahn FW, Jones JM. Diagnosing bacterial respiratory infection by bronchoalveolar lavage. J Infect Dis 1987;155:862–869.

181. Levine SJ, Stover DE. Bronchoscopy and related techniques. In: Shelhamer J, Pizzo PA, Parrillo JR, Masur H, eds. Respiratory disease in the immunosuppressed host. Philadelphia: JB Lippincott, 1991:94–104.

182. Meyer RD, Ching WTW. *Legionella* pneumonia. In: Shelhamer J, Pizzo PA, Parrillo JR, Masur H, eds. Respiratory disease in the immunosuppressed host. Philadelphia: JB Lippincott, 1991:286–297.

183. Goldberg MB, Simm HB. Pneumonia due to *Nocardia* and *Actinomyces*. In: Shelhamer J, Pizzo PA, Parrillo JR, Masur H, eds. Respiratory disease in the immunosuppressed host. Philadelphia: JB Lippincott, 1991:330–337.

184. Jones JM. Pneumonia due to *Candida*, *Aspergillus* and *Mucaroles* species. In: Shelhamer J, Pizzo PA, Parrillo JR, Masur H, eds. Respiratory disease in the immunosuppressed host. Philadelphia: JB LIppincott, 1991:338–354.

185. Commers JC, Robichaud K, Pizzo PA. New pulmonary infiltrates in granulocytopenic patients being treated with antibiotics. Pediatr Infect Dis 1984;3:423–428.

186. Edwards JE. *Candida* endophthalmitis. In: Remington JS, Swartz MN, eds. Current clinical topics in infectious disease. New York: McGraw Hill, 1982:381–397.

187. Yu VL, Muder RR, Poorsattar A. Significance of isolation of *Aspergillus* from the respiratory tract in diagnosis of invasive pulmonary aspergillosis. Results from a three-year prospective study. Am J Med 1986;81:249–251.

188. Burch PA, Karp JE, Merz WG, et al. Favorable outcome of invasive aspergillosis in patients with acute leukemia. J Clin Oncol 1987;5:1985–1993.

189. Lopez-Berestein G, Bodey GP, Fainstein V, et al. Treatment of systemic fungal infections with liposomal amphotericin B. Arch Intern Med 1989;149:2533–2536.

190. Drutz DJ. Pneumonia due to endemic fungi. In: Shelhamer J, Pizzo PA, Parrillo JR, Masur H, eds. Respiratory disease in the immunosuppressed host. Philadelphia: JB Lippincott, 1991:355–385.

191. Medoff G. Controversial areas in antifungal chemotherapy: Short course and combination therapy with amphotericin B. Rev Infect Dis 1987;9:403–407.

192. Bennett JE, Dismukes WE, Duma RJ, et al. Amphotericin B flucytosine in cryptococcal meningitis. N Engl J Med 1979;301:126–131.

193. Dismukes WE, Cloud G, Gallis HA, et al. Treatment of cryptococcal meningitis with combination amphotericin B and flucytosine for four as compared with six weeks. N Engl J Med 1987;317:334–341.

194. Thaler M, Bacher J, O'Leary T, et al. Evaluation of single-drug and combination antifungal therapy in an experimental model of candidiasis in rabbits with prolonged neutropenia. J Infect Dis 1988;158:80–88.

195. Bennett JF. Flucytosine. Ann Intern Med 1977;86:319–322.

196. Stiller RL, Bennett JE, Scholer HJ, et al. Correlation of in vitro susceptibility test results with in vivo response: Flucytosine therapy in a systemic candidiasis model. J Infect Dis 1983;147:1070–1077.

197. Saag MS, Dismukes WE. Azole antifungal agents: Emphasis on new triazoles. Antimicrob Agents Chemother 1988;32:1–8.

198. Shechtman LB, Funaro L, Robin T, et al. Clotrimazole treatment of oral candidiasis in patients with neoplastic disease. Am J Med 1984;76:91–91.

199. Masur H. *Pneumocystis carinii* pneumonia. In: Shelhamer J, Pizzo PA, Parrillo JR, Masur H, eds. Respiratory disease in the immunosuppressed host. Philadelphia: JB Lippincott, 1991:409–427.

200. Meuwissen JH, Tauber I, Leewenberg AD, et al. Parasitologic and serologic observations of infection with *Pneumocystis* in humans. J Infect Dis 1977;136:4349.

201. Ruebush TK, Weinstein RA, Baehner RL, et al. An outbreak of *Pneumocystis* pneumonia in children with acute lymphocytic leukemia. Am J Dis Child 1978;132:143–148.

202. Browne M, Hubbard SM, Longo DL, et al. Excess prevalence of *Pneumocystis carinii* pneumonia in lymphoma patients with chemotherapy. Ann Intern Med 1986;104:338–344.

203. Kovacs JA, Hiemenz JW, Macher AM, et al. *Pneumocystis carinii* pneumonia: A comparison of clinical features in patients with the acquired immune deficiency syndrome and patients with other immune diseases. Ann Intern Med 1984;100:663–671.

204. Lipschik GY, Kovacs JA. Sputum evaluation and nonbronchoscopic lavage. In: Shelhamer J, Pizzo PA, Parrillo JR, Masur H, eds. Respiratory disease in the immunosuppressed host. Philadelphia: JB Lippincott, 1991:64–72.

205. Browne MJ, Potter D, Gress J, et al. A randomized trial of open lung biopsy versus empiric antimicrobial therapy in cancer patients with diffuse pullmonary infiltrates. J Clin Oncol 1990;8:222–229.

206. Masur H. Prevention and treatment of Pneumocystis pneumonia. N Engl J Med 1992;327:1853–1860.

207. Gagnon S, Boota AM, Fischl MA, et al. Corticosteroids as adjunctive therapy for severe *Pneumocystis carinii* pneumonia in the acquired immunodeficiency syndrome. N Engl J Med 1990;323:1444–1450.

208. Bozzette SA, Sattler FR, Chiu J, et al. A controlled trial of early adjunctive treatment with corticosteroids for *Pneumocystis carinii* pneumonia in the acquired immunodeficiency syndrome. N Engl J Med 1990;323:1451–1457.

209. Burt ME, Flye MW, Webber BL, et al. Prospective evaluation of aspiration needle, cutting needle, transbronchial and open lung biopsy in patients with pulmonary infiltrates. Ann Thorac Surg 1981;32:146–153.

210. McCabe RE, Remington JS. Open lung biopsy. In: Shelhamer J, Pizzo PA, Parrillo JR, Masur H, eds. Respiratory disease in the immunosuppressed host. Philadelphia: JB Lippincott, 1991:105–117.

211. Schooley RT. Pneumonia due to herpesviruses. In: Shelhamer J, Pizzo PA, Parrillo JR, Masur H, eds. Respiratory disease in the immunosuppressed host. Philadelphia: JB Lippincott, 1991:386–397.

212. Crawford JW, Meyers JD. Respiratory disease in bone marrow transplant patients. In: Shelhamer J, Pizzo PA, Parrillo JR, Masur H, eds. Respiratory disease in the immunosuppressed host. Philadelphia: JB Lippincott, 1991:595–623.

213. Meyers JD, Flournoy N, Thomas ED. Risk factors for cytomegalovirus infection after human marrow transplantation. J Infect Dis 1986;153:478–488.

214. Gleaves CA, Meyers JD. Rapid diagnosis of invasive cytomegalovirus infection by examination of tissue specimens in centrifugation culture. Am J Clin Pathol 1987;88:354–358.

215. Emanuel D, Cunningham I, Jules-Elysee K, et al. Cytomegalovirus pneumonia after bone marrow transplantation successfully treated with the combination of ganciclovir and high dose intravenous immune globulin. Ann Intern Med 1988;109:777–782.

216. Reed EC, Bowden RA, Dandliker PS, Lilleby KE, Meyers JD. Treatment of cytomegalovirus pneumonia with ganciclovir and intravenous cytomegalovirus immunoglobulin in patients with bone marrow transplantation. Ann Intern Med 1988;109:783–788.

217. Meyers JD, Reed EC, Shepp DH, et al. Acyclovir for prevention of cytomegalovirus infection and disease after allogeneic marrow tansplantation. N Engl J Med 1988;318:70–75.

218. Schmidt GM, Horak DA, Niland JC, et al. A randomized, controlled trial of prophylactic ganciclovir for cytomegalovirus pulmonary infection in recipients of allogeneic bone marrow transplants. N Engl J Med 1991;324:1005–1011.

219. Dolin R. Pneumonia caused by viruses other than herpes viruses. In: Shelhamer J, Pizzo PA, Parrillo JR, Masur H, eds. Respiratory disease in the immunosuppressed host. Philadelphia: JB Lippincott, 1991:398–408.

220. Smith DW, Frankel LR, Mathers LH, et al. A controlled trial of aerosolized ribavirin in infants receiving mechanical ventilation for severe respiratory syncytial virus infections. N Engl J Med 1991;325:24–29.

221. Ladisch S, Pizzo PA. S. aureus sepsis in children with cancer. Pediatrics 1978;61:231–234.

222. Peterson DE, Minah GE, Overholser CD, et al. Microbiology of acute periodontal infection in myelosuppressed cancer patients. J Clin Oncol 1987;5:1461–1468.

223. Meyers JD, Wade JC, Mitchell CD, et al. Multicenter collaborative trial of intravenous acyclovir for the treatment of mucocutaneous herpes simplex virus infection in the immunocompromised host. Am J Med 1982;73:229–235.

224. Whitley RJ, Spruance S, Hayden FC, et al (NIAID Collaborative Antiviral Study Group). Vidarabine therapy for mucocutaneous herpes simplex virus infection in the immunocompromised host. J Infect Dis 1984;149:1–8.

225. Shepp DH, Newton BA, Dandliker PS, et al. Oral acyclovir therapy for mucocutaneous herpes simplex virus infections in immunocompromised marrow transplant recipients. Ann Intern Med 1985;102:783–785.

226. Whitley RJ, Levin M, Barton N, et al. Infections caused by herpes simplex virus in the immunocompromised host: Natural history and topical acyclovir therapy. J Infect Dis 1984;150:323–329.

227. Meyers JD, Flournoy N, Thomas ED. Infection with herpes simplex virus and cell-mediated immunity after marrow transplant. J Infect Dis 1980;142:338–346.

228. Saral R, Ambinder RF, Burns WH, et al. Acyclovir prophylaxis against herpes simplex virus infection in patients with leukemia. Ann Intern Med 1983;99:773–776.

229. Wade JC, Newton B, Flournoy N, et al. Oral acyclovir for prevention of herpes simplex virus reactivation after marrow transplant. Ann Intern Med 1984;100:823–828.

230. Ringden O, Heimdahl A, Lonnqvist B, et al. Decreased incidence of viridans streptococcal septicaemia in allogeneic bone marrow transplant recipients after the introduction of acyclovir. Lancet [Letter] 1984;1:744.

231. McDonald GB, Sharma P, Hackman RC, et al. Esophageal infections in immunosuppressed patients after marrow transplant. Gastroenterology 1985;88:1111–1117.

232. Walsh TJ, Belitsos N, Hamiltol SR. Bacterial esophagitis in immunocompromised patients. Arch Intern Med 1986;146:1345–1348.

233. Varki AP, Armitage JO, Feagler JR. Typhlitis in acute leukemia: Successful treatment by early surgical intervention. Cancer 1979;43:695–697.

234. Skibber JM, Matler GJ, Lotze MT, et al. Right lower quadrant complications in young patients with leukemia: A surgical perspective. Ann Surg 1987;206:711–716.

235. McFarland LV, Mulligan ME, Kwok RYY, Stamm WE. Nosocomial acquisition of Clostridium difficile infection. N Engl J Med 1989;320:204–210.

236. Armstrong D, Paredes J. Strongyloidiasis. In: Shelhamer J, Pizzo PA, Parrillo JR, Masur H, eds. Respiratory disease in the immunosuppressed host. Philadelphia: JB Lippincott, 1991:428–432.

237. Choo Q-L, Kuo G, Weiner AM, et al. Isolation of a cDNA clone derived from a blood-borne non-A, non-B viral hepatitis genome. Science 1989;244:359–362.

238. Hoofnagle JH, Mullen KD, Jones B, et al. Treatment of chronic non-A, non-B hepatitis with recombinant human alpha interferon. A perliminary report. N Engl J Med 1986;315:1575–1578.

239. Tabor E, Gerety JR, Mott M, et al. Prevalence of hepatitis B in a high-risk setting: A serologic study of patients and staff in a pediatric oncology unit. Pediatrics 1978;61:711–715.

240. Wade JC, Gaffey M, Wiernik PH, et al. Hepatitis in patients with acute nonlymphocytic leukemia. Am J Med 1983;75:413–422.

241. Berk PD, Jones A, Plotz PH, et al. Corticosteroid therapy for chronic active hepatitis. Ann Intern Med 1976;85:523–524.

242. Hoofnagle JH, Dusheiko GM, Schafer DF, et al. Reactivation of chronic hepatitis B virus infection by cancer chemotherapy. Ann Intern Med 1982;96:447–449.

243. Davis GL, Balart LA, Schiff ER, et al. Treatment of chronic hepatitis C with interferon alpha. A multicenter randomized, controlled trial. N Engl J Med 1989;321:1501–1506.

244. After HJ, Purcell PH, Shih JW, et al. Detection of antibody to hepatitis C virus in prospectively followed transfusion recipients with acute and chronic non-A, non-B hepatitis. N Engl J Med 1989;321:1494–1500.

245. Haron E, Feld R. Tuffnell P, et al. Hepatic candidiasis: An increasing problem in immunocompromised patients. Am J Med 1987;83:17–26.

246. Thaler M, Pastakia B, Shawker TH, et al. Hepatic candidiasis in cancer patients: The evolving picture of the syndrome. Ann Intern Med 1988;108:88–100.

247. Kauffman CA, Bradley SF, Ross SC, Weber DR. Hepatosplenic candidiasis: Successful treatment with fluconazole. Am J Med 1991;91:137–141.

248. Anaissie E, Bodey GP, Kantarjian H, et al. Fluconazole therapy for chronic disseminated candidiasis in patients with leukemia and prior amphotericin B therapy. Am J Med 1991;91:142–150.

249. Glenn J, Cotton D, Wesley R, et al. Anorectal infections in patients with malignant diseases. Rev Infect Dis 1988;10:42–52.

250. Barnes SG, Sattler FR, Ballard JO. Improved survival after drainage of perirectal infections in patients with acute leukemia. Ann Intern Med 1984;100:515–518.

251. Kingston ME, Mackey D. Skin clues in the diagnosis of life-threatening infections. Rev Infect Dis 1986;8:1–11.

252. Whitley R, Hilty M, Haynes R, et al. Vidarabine therapy for varicella in immunosuppressed patients. J Pediatr 1982;101:125–131.

253. Prober CG, Kirk LE, Keeney RE. Acyclovir therapy of chickenpox in immunosuppressed children—a collaborative study. J Pediatr 1982;101:622–625.

254. Arvin AM, Feldman S, Merigan TC. Human leukocyte interferon in the treatment of varicella in children with cancer in preliminary controlled trial. Antimicrob Agents Chemother 1978;13:605–607.

255. Arvin AM, Kushner JH, Feldman S, et al. Human leukocyte interferon for the treatment of varicella in children with cancer. N Engl J Med 1985;306:761–765.

256. Takahashi M, Otsuka T, Okuno Y, et al. Live vaccine used to prevent the spread of varicella in children in the hospital. Lancet 1974;2:1288–1290.

257. Gershon A. Live attenuated varicella vaccine. J Pediatr 1987;110:154–157.

258. Shepp DH, Dandliker PS, Meyers JD. Treatment of varicella-zoster virus infection in severely immunocompromised patients: A randomized comparison of acyclovir and vidarabine. N Engl J Med 1986;314:208–212.

259. Rimailho A. Fulminant necrotizing fascitis and nonsteroidal anti-inflammatory drugs. J Infect Dis 1987;155:143–146.

260. Houff S, Major EO, Katz DA, et al. Involvement of JC virus-infected mononuclear cells from the bone marrow and spleen in the pathogenesis of progressive multifocal leukoencephalopathy. N Engl J Med 1988;318:301–305.

261. Pizzo PA. Considerations for preventing infectious complications in cancer patients. Rev Infect Dis 1989;11:S1551–S1563.

262. Nauseef WM, Maki DG. A study of the value of simple protective isolation in patients with granulocytopenia. N Engl J Med 1981;304:448–453.

263. Kotilainen P, Nikoskelainen J, Huovinen P. Emergence of ciprofloxacin-resistant coagulase-negative staphylococcal skin flora in immunocompromised patients receiving ciprofloxacin. J Infect Dis 1990; 161:41–44.

264. Pizzo PA. Antibiotic prophylaxis in the immunosuppressed patient with cancer. In: Remington JS, Swartz MN, eds. Current clinical topics in infectious Diseases. 4th ed. New York: McGraw Hill, 1983:153–167.

265. Van der Waaij D, Berghuis de Vries JN, Lekkerkerk van der Wees JEC, et al. Colonization resistance of the digestive tract in conventional and antibiotic treated mice. J Hyg (Lond) 1971;69:405–411.

266. Van der Waaij D, Berghuis de Vries JN. Selective elimination of enterobacteriae species from the digestive tract in mice and monkeys. J Hyg (Lond) 1974;72:205–211.

267. Guiot HFL, van der Brock PJ, van der Meer JWM, et al. Selective antimicrobial modulation of the intestinal flora of patients with acute nonlymphocytic leukemia. A double-blind placebo-controlled study. J Infect Dis 1983;147:615–623.

268. Sleijfer DT, Mulder NK, de Vries-Hospers HG, et al. Infection prevention in granulocytopenic patients by selective decontamination of the digestive tract. Eur J Cancer 1980;16:859–869.

269. Gurwith MJ, Brunton JL, Lank BA. A prospective controlled investigation of prophylactic trimethoprim-sulfamethoxazole in hospitalized granulocytopenic patients. Am J Med 1979;66:248–256.

270. Pizzo PA, Robichaud KJ, Edwards BK, et al. Oral antibiotic prophylaxis in patients with cancer: A double-blind randomized placebo-controlled trial. J Pediatr 1983;102:125–133.

271. Weiser B, Lange M, Fialkow MA, et al. Prophylactic trimethoprim-sulfamethaxozole during consolidated chemotherapy for acute leukemia: A controlled trial. Ann Intern Med 1981;95:436–438.

272. Dekker A, Rozenberg-Arska M, Sixma JJ, et al. Prevention of infection by trimethoprim-sulfamethoxazole plus amphotericin B in patients with acute nonlymphocytic leukemia. Ann Intern Med 1981;95:555–559.

273. Kauffman CA, Leipman MJ, Bergman AG, et al. Trimethoprim-sulfamethoxazole prophylaxis in neutropenic patients: Reduction of infections and effect on bacterial and fungal flora. Am J Med 1983;74:599–607.

274. Gaultieri RJ, Donowitz GR, Kaiser CE, et al. Double-blind randomized study of prophylactic trimethoprim-sulfamethaxozole in granulocytopenic patients with hematoloic malignancies. Am J Med 1983;74:934–940.

275. Wade JC, DeJongh CA, Newman KA, et al. Selective antimicrobial modulation as prophylaxis against infection during granulocytopenia: Trimethoprim-sulfamethoxazole versus nalidixic acid. J Infect Dis 1983;147:624–634.

276. Wilson JM, Guinery DG. Failure of oral trimethoprim-sulfamethoxazole prophylaxis in acute leukemia: Isolation of resistant plasmids from strains of enterobacteriaceae causing bacteremia. N Engl J Med 1982;306:16–20.

277. Karp JE, Merz WG, Hendricksen C, et al. Oral Norfloxacin for prevention of gram-negative bacterial infections in patients with acute leukemia and granulocytopenia. Ann Intern Med 1987;106:1–7.

278. Dekker AW, Rozenberg-Arska M, Verhoef J. Infection prophylaxis in acute leukemia: A comparison of cifrofloxacin with trimethoprim-sulfamethoxazole and colistin. Ann Intern Med 1987;106:7–12.

279. Meunier F. Prevention of mycoses in immunocompromised patients. Rev Infect Dis 1987;9:408–416.

280. Saral R, Bruns WH, Laskin OL, et al. Acyclovir prophylaxis of herpes simplex virus infections: A randomized, double-blind controlled trial in bone marrow transplant recipients. N Engl J Med 1981;305:63–67.

281. Zeigler EKJ, Fisher CJ, Sprung CL, et al. Treatment of gram-negative bacteremia and septic shock with HA-1A human monocular antibody against endotoxin. N Engl J Med 1991;324:429–436.

282. Cooperative Group for the Study of Immunoglobulin in Chronic Lymphocytic Leukemia. Intravenous immunoglobulin for the prevention of infection in chronic lymphocytic leukemia: A randomized, controlled clinical trial. N Engl J Med 1988;319:902–907.

283. Weeks JC, Tierney MR, Weinstein MC. Cost effectiveness of prophylactic intravenous immune globulin in chronic lymphocytic leukemia. N Engl J Med 1991;325:81–86.

284. Sullivan KM, Kopecky KJ, Jocom J, et al. Immunomodulatory and antimicrobial efficacy of intravenous immunoglobulin in bone marrow transplantation. N Engl J Med 1990;323:705–712.

285. Crawford J, Ozer H, Stoller R, et al. Reduction by granulocyte colony-stimulating factor of fever and neutropenia induced by chemotherapy in patients with small-cell lung cancer. N Engl J Med 1991;325:164–170.

286. Gabrilove J, Jakubowski A, Scher H, et al. Effect of granulocyte colony-stimulating factor on neutropenia and associated morbidity due to chemotherapy for transitional cell carcinoma of the urothelium. N Engl J Med 1988;318:1414–1422.

287. Brandt S, Peters W, Atwater S, et al. Effect of recombinant human granulocyte-macrophage colony-stimulating factor on hematopoietic reconstitution after high-dose chemotherapy and autologous bone marrow transplantation. N Engl J Med 1988;318:869–876.

288. Ohno R, Tomonaga M, Kobayashi T, et al. Effect of granulocyte colony-stimulating factor after intensive induction therapy in relapsed or refractory acute leukemia. N Engl J Med 1990;323:871–877.

289. Nemunaitis J, Rabinowe SN, Singer JW, et al. Recombinant granulocyte-macrophage colony-stimulating factor after autologous bone marrow transplantation for lymphoid cancer. N Engl J Med 1991;324:1773–1778.

290. Peters WP, Kurtzberg J, Kirkpatrick G, et al. GM-CSF primed peripheral blood progenitor cells coupled with autologous bone marrow transplantation will eliminate absolute leukopenia following high dose chemotherapy. Blood 1989;743(suppl 1):50a.

Cancer: Principles & Practice of Oncology, Fourth Edition,
edited by Vincent T. DeVita, Jr., Samuel Hellman, Steven A. Rosenberg.
J.B. Lippincott Co., Philadelphia © 1993.

CHAPTER **63**

Adverse Effects of Treatment

SECTION **1**

RICHARD J. GRALLA

Antiemetic Therapy

Control of chemotherapy-induced emesis is a standard of care; however, this represents a marked change that has occurred over the past 10 to 12 years. This change resulted from oncologists recognizing the increasing need for emetic control and developing a logical clinical research program emphasizing careful methodology. Interest and advances in related basic sciences were then stimulated by the clinical improvements. Increased knowledge in neuropharmacology has further enhanced the control of emesis.

With the potential to achieve complete control of nausea and vomiting in most patients comes the responsibility of the clinician to possess a deeper understanding of the problem. This increases the likelihood of controlling emesis and permits more appropriate and cost-effective approaches.

Progress has included the recognition of different emetic problems, the identification of effective agents, the establishment of appropriate doses and schedules for these agents, the testing of combination regimens of greater efficacy, the synthesis of newer agents with an improved therapeutic index, and the application of a useful study methodology.

PHYSIOLOGY AND PHARMACOLOGY IN CONTROLLING EMESIS

The mechanism by which chemotherapy induces emesis is not completely understood. Older studies of Borison and McCarthy[1] have had an important influence that has provided a framework for further research. Questions that remain include: Why is there a delay from the administration of chemotherapy to the onset of emesis? Is it the chemotherapy drug itself, a metabolite, or a neurotransmitter that stimulates a receptor and causes emesis? Why do different chemotherapy agents with similar intracellular effects have such varying potentials for inducing emesis?

Studies support the hypothesis that emesis is caused by stimulation of receptors in the central nervous system or in the gastrointestinal tract. Receptor areas have been identified in the medulla that are of particular interest. An area called the *vomiting* or *emetic center* is found in the lateral reticular formation. Once receptors in this region are stimulated, the complicated act of vomiting then follows. An important area also located in the medulla is the chemoreceptor trigger zone (CTZ), in the area postrema.[2] The CTZ is sensitive to chemical stimuli from both the blood and the cerebrospinal fluid.

Chemotherapeutic agents, their metabolites, or a neurotransmitter may stimulate receptors (such as dopamine or serotonin receptors) in the CTZ. Impulses generated in the CTZ and transmitted to the vomiting center may then lead to the initiation of emesis. Neuroreceptors in the gastrointestinal tract, which has afferents to the vomiting center, may also play a role in chemotherapy-induced nausea and vomiting.

The theory developed that drugs that bind to neurotransmitter receptors in the CTZ, the vomiting center, or the gastrointestinal tract have the potential to interrupt the process leading to emesis. Interest initially focused on agents that bind to dopamine receptors in that these receptors are found in high concentration in the CTZ. In the 1950s and 1960s, agents such as phenothiazines, butyrophenones, and substituted benzamides, which affect these receptors, became available.

Early trials with phenothiazines indicated some antiemetic

activity. As newer chemotherapy agents with emesis as a prominent side effect were introduced, the marked limitations of the phenothiazines became apparent. Unlike the phenothiazines, the substituted benzamide metoclopramide can be given in high intravenous doses without causing hypotension or other hazardous side effects.[3] This method of administration of metoclopramide demonstrated a high degree of efficacy with this agent known to block dopamine (D2) receptors.

Although the effectiveness of high-dose metoclopramide represented an important improvement in the control of chemotherapy-induced emesis, it was not clear why the elevated doses of the agent proved so effective. Metoclopramide binds avidly to dopamine receptors, and it was thought that even small doses of the drug would saturate the receptors, eliminating the need for very high doses. An important clue came with the investigation of serotonin (5-hydroxytryptamine, or 5-HT) receptors.[4,5] Metoclopramide blocks serotonin receptors (specifically the type 3, or 5-HT3, receptor) but with less affinity than it has for dopamine receptors or than the newer agents have for 5-HT3 receptors.[6] Therefore, very high doses of metoclopramide are required for it to prevent emesis as a 5-HT3 antagonist. It appears that metoclopramide may have served in a transitional role between the older dopamine-blocking agents and the newer, more selective 5-HT3 antiemetics. The antiemetic activity of metoclopramide may be exerted primarily through 5-HT3 receptors, while its side effects are the result of its interaction with dopamine receptors.

Does the importance of the role of serotonin receptors help answer some of the questions remaining in the neuropharmacology of chemotherapy-induced emesis? It has been suggested that this phenomenon may be mediated by serotonin itself; that is, a chemotherapeutic agent may have a direct effect on the small bowel, resulting in the liberation of a large amount of endogenous serotonin. This liberated serotonin then stimulates the 5-HT3 receptors in the central nervous system, resulting in emesis. The effect of the serotonin may be mediated through vagal nerves or through direct stimulation of the receptors by an elevated blood level of serotonin.

Cisplatin causes many rapid physiologic alterations, and one of those is an increased excretion of 5-HIAA, indicating a liberation of endogenous serotonin.[7,8] Certainly, the increased levels of serotonin and the association with cisplatin indicate the possibility that the hypothesis may be correct. Several arguments remain against the hypothesis that serotonin liberation mediates chemotherapy-induced emesis. These objections include the following:

1. Although 5-HIAA excretion is increased after cisplatin, the increase is generally only double that of baseline (often remaining in the normal range) and far less than levels frequently observed in carcinoid syndrome.[9]
2. Emesis is not a prominent finding in carcinoid syndrome.[9]
3. If the lack of emesis in carcinoid is due to a decreased sensitivity after prolonged exposure to serotonin, it is curious that patients with malignant carcinoid treated with cisplatin often are troubled by emesis.
4. The reflex may be mediated by vagal afferents from the gut, yet after the radical vagotomy involved in esophagectomy, emesis still results with cisplatin treatment.[10]

5. If the liberation of serotonin after cisplatin were sufficient to cause emesis, the full carcinoid syndrome would likely occur, especially in patients given 5-HT3-blocking agents, which do not inhibit serotonin release[7,8] and only affect the type 3 serotonin receptor.

Many questions remain concerning the mediation of chemotherapy-induced emesis and the neuropharmacology of the phenomenon.

EMETIC PROBLEMS

In patients receiving chemotherapy, three types of emetic problems have been identified. Careful attention to which problem is to be treated or prevented is significant since causes of and treatments for the various problems may differ. These emetic syndromes include acute chemotherapy-induced emesis, delayed emesis, and anticipatory emesis. An additional problem is that patients may have emesis for reasons other than their chemotherapy.

Patients with cancer have a variety of reasons for emesis that are not associated with chemotherapy. Prominent causes are medications. These particularly involve pain medications, bronchodilators (especially long-acting preparations), and antibiotics. Other common problems causing emesis include intestinal obstruction, brain metastases, ileus, and azotemia. In these instances, adjustment of medications or treatment of the complications of the tumor may be more important than the selection of the proper antiemetic drug.

Most antiemetic studies have investigated acute chemotherapy-induced emesis. This is the major topic of the subsequent discussion, with separate sections concerning delayed and anticipatory emesis.

ACUTE CHEMOTHERAPY-INDUCED EMESIS

The chemotherapeutic agent, its dose, and the route of administration can affect the incidence of nausea and vomiting (Table 63–1). With most agents, emesis begins between 1 and 2 hours after starting chemotherapy, in patients who have not previously received chemotherapy. Important exceptions to this pattern occur with cyclophosphamide and carboplatin, which can cause a late onset of emesis (a problem different than delayed emesis, which is discussed later). When cyclophosphamide is given intravenously in high doses, emesis often does not begin until 9 to 18 hours after chemotherapy.[11] Several studies have indicated that carboplatin also induces a late onset of emesis.[12] Although carboplatin is somewhat less emetic than cisplatin, it still can cause significant nausea and vomiting. A recent report concluded that a similar degree of good antiemetic control could be achieved with either of these platinum-containing drugs if appropriate antiemetic regimens are used.[13]

The late onset of emesis emphasizes two important principles. First, to be effective, an antiemetic regimen must consider the individual pattern and potential for causing emesis of the chemotherapeutic drug. Second, when combination chemotherapy is used, each of the drugs must be individually considered. Therefore, a regimen that is effective against cisplatin may not be well designed for the patient receiving cy-

TABLE 63–1. Emetic Potential of 25 Chemotherapeutic Agents

Most likely to result in emesis	Cisplatin
	Dacarbazine
	Dactinomycin
	Nitrogen mustard
	Hexamethylmelamine
	Cyclophosphamide*
	Carboplatin*
	Lomustine
	Carmustine
	Doxorubicin
	Daunorubicin
	Idarubicin
	Ifosfamide
	Cytosine arabinoside
	Vinorelbine
	Mitomycin C
	Etoposide
	Vindesine
	Bleomycin
	Methotrexate
	5-Fluorouracil
	Chlorambucil
	Vincristine
Least likely to result in emesis	Vinblastine
	Tamoxifen

* Associated with the late onset of emesis.

clophosphamide. Careful testing of antiemetic regimens for particular chemotherapeutic combinations is necessary before acceptance of a regimen as a standard. Activity of the antiemetic at the receptor is of greater importance than simply the blood level of the drug.

The differences in the likelihood of chemotherapeutic drugs to result in emesis are given in Table 63–1. In general, the agents most often associated with emesis also induce the greatest severity of this side effect. Differences occur among patients and even among treatment courses in the same patient.

Emesis and its control are best studied in patients given cisplatin. This has occurred for several reasons. First, cisplatin causes emesis in all patients if effective antiemetics are not given, and it results in a median of over ten episodes in those receiving this agent in high doses. Second, cisplatin is an important neoplastic agent in several malignancies. Third, antiemetics effective against cisplatin are useful with chemotherapeutic agents of lesser emetic potential. Therefore, cisplatin provides a model for the testing of antiemetics for all chemotherapy treatment regimens.

DELAYED EMESIS

Early into the use of cisplatin, it was clear that all patients experienced nausea and vomiting.[10,14,15] This emesis cleared after several hours in many patients; however, others continued to be troubled for many days. These were not considered to be separate events until after effective antiemetic regimens were introduced and carefully studied. Delayed emesis is now defined as nausea or vomiting beginning 24 hours or more after chemotherapy administration.

This problem is best described in patients treated with high total doses of cisplatin (100 mg/m^2, or more, given as a single dose or over several days). Whether other agents or lower doses of cisplatin cause this problem is unknown; consequently, statements made about this phenomenon that are not based on patients receiving these high doses of cisplatin may not be appropriate to generalize. The time of observation for the onset of emesis (24 hours after chemotherapy) is arbitrary. The phenomenon may begin earlier in some patients, and this may be important in planning for prevention of the phenomenon.

A natural history study observed that delayed emesis is less severe than acute chemotherapy-induced emesis and is not simply a deferral of the acute problem to a later period.[16] Nonetheless, delayed emesis still causes a great deal of discomfort as well as difficulties with hydration and nutrition. Although it occurs less often in those patients who have complete emetic control on the day of chemotherapy, delayed emesis is not necessarily eliminated, even in this most favorable group. Most patients treated with cisplatin at doses greater than 100 mg/m^2 experience some degree of delayed emesis. The onset is most frequent 48 to 72 hours after chemotherapy,[16] and the phenomenon gradually diminishes over the next 1 to 3 days. Although treatment is not ideal, appropriate regimens, as discussed later, can significantly reduce the incidence of delayed emesis.

ANTICIPATORY EMESIS

This problem is defined as nausea or vomiting beginning before the administration of chemotherapy.[17] It typically occurs in patients with poor control of emesis with past chemotherapy. This poor control can be with acute chemotherapy-induced emesis or with delayed emesis. Since this is a conditioned response, the hospital environment or other treatment-related associations may trigger the onset of emesis. The administration of the chemotherapy itself may bring on this response as a chemical stimulus or as a psychologic factor. The various contributing factors illustrate the difficulty with the definition of the problem and with determining the incidence of anticipatory emesis. Patients who have emesis before chemotherapy may have greater difficulty, but those who have conditioned emesis after chemotherapy administration are also troubled. The poorer control observed with subsequent cycles of chemotherapy may, at least in part, be related to conditioning. Anxiety or insomnia 1 or 2 days before a scheduled treatment may be a less dramatic expression of the same phenomenon. The stronger the likelihood of emesis and the poorer the control, the greater is the chance of developing anticipatory emesis.[17,18]

CONTROL OF EMESIS AND PATIENT CHARACTERISTICS

Several aspects of a patient's prior experience or characteristics may influence emetic outcome. Studies to date have indicated that alcohol intake history, prior experience with

TABLE 63–2. Factors Associated With Control of Emesis

Patients

Emesis with past chemotherapy
Chronic alcohol use history
Gender
Age

Chemotherapy

Agent
Dose
Schedule
Route

Antiemetic

Agent
Dose
Schedule

chemotherapy, age, and gender are important factors (Table 63–2).

ALCOHOL INTAKE HISTORY

Studies have indicated that emesis is more easily controlled in patients with chronic heavy alcohol use histories (more than 100 g/day, or about five mixed drinks) than in those without this past experience.[19,20] In a prospective evaluation in 52 patients receiving high-dose cisplatin and an appropriate combination antiemetic regimen, 93% of those with the high alcohol history had no emesis, as opposed to 61% ($p < 0.01$) of the other patients.[19] Subsequent trials examining this variable have confirmed the greater ease of controlling emesis in this population.[21] Patients do not have to continue to use alcohol to be considered as having a high chronic alcohol history and to be easier to treat. Also, patients with this history are at high risk of having emesis if the most effective antiemetic regimens are not used; however, their response to these regimens is enhanced. The alcohol usage history needs to be outlined for each treatment group in comparison trials.

PRIOR CHEMOTHERAPY EXPERIENCE

Poor control of emesis with past courses of chemotherapy predisposes a patient to unsatisfactory antiemetic results with subsequent similar chemotherapy. A report[3] of a trial in which patients received their initial treatment with the same antiemetic noted that major control was three times more likely in those who had not previously had chemotherapy. Whether this is due to the development of conditioned anticipatory emesis or to other possible factors is not clear.

AGE

Older age appears not to be a direct concern with the control of emesis; instead, younger age implies a predilection to experience acute dystonic reactions when receiving antiemetics with dopamine-receptor blocking as a mechanism of action.[22] This category of antiemetics includes such valuable agents as substituted benzamides, butyrophenones, and phenothiazines.

In a report[22] summarizing the experience of nearly 500 patients receiving metoclopramide, the incidence of trismus or torticollis was only 2% in those over 30 years of age; a 27% occurrence was reported in younger patients. In addition, when dopamine-blocking antiemetics are given on several consecutive days, dystonic reactions are also more common.[23] This can be especially important for younger patients in that several regimens for malignancies of this age group use chemotherapy on a daily schedule.

Many of the newer antiemetic agents exert their activity by blocking 5-HT3 receptors. Agents that are specific for this mechanism do not cause dystonic reactions. Although only a few pediatric studies with these agents have been conducted, the initial good results and lack of dystonic reactions already indicate that these are the drugs of choice for children receiving chemotherapy likely to result in emesis.

Formal antiemetic trials in older patients are unusual. Those patients over age 70 who have been treated with metoclopramide or ondansetron have generally tolerated the agents well at the same doses given to younger patients, and efficacy has been preserved. With the aging population in many continents and with the increasing incidence of many malignancies with age, formal analysis and testing of antiemetic regimens in the geriatric population is a mandatory objective for the near future.

GENDER

Several studies have suggested that it is more difficult to control emesis in women than in men. This is a complicated issue.[24] Women enlisted in antiemetic studies are more likely to be receiving two or more emetic agents given in combination (especially cisplatin plus cyclophosphamide) and are less likely to have histories of heavy alcohol usage. It is possible that factors other than gender are of greater importance in affecting the control of emesis. Multivariate analyses of large, well-conducted trials are needed to answer this question. One recent study suggests that gender is indeed an independent variable.[21]

NEW ANTIEMETIC AGENTS

Several agents have been synthesized that bind with greater affinity and specificity to 5-HT3 receptors than metoclopramide. As illustrated in Table 63–3, five agents (ondansetron, granisetron, tropisetron, dolasetron, and RG 12915) are at various stages of development. Factors varying among these agents include short (2- to 4-hour) versus moderate (9- to 16-hour) half-lives. Most of these drugs have good bioavailability, and studies only employing oral administration may prove useful.

Three of the agents are commercially available, and the remainder are in phase II or III trials. Research with this new class of antiemetic is directed toward preserving or improving the efficacy of metoclopramide and eliminating dopamine-related side effects.

Ondansetron has become widely available for the prevention of nausea and vomiting associated with emetic chemotherapy. In the United States, the dose and schedule recommended for ondansetron is 0.15 mg/kg intravenously for three doses, with

TABLE 63–3. Frequently Used Antiemetic Agents and Classes With Commonly Administered Doses

Antiemetic	Class	Dose and Schedule
Ondansetron	Serotonin-receptor antagonist	0.15 mg/kg I.V. × three doses every 2–4 h 8 mg I.V. × 1 32 mg I.V. × 1 Various oral regimens
Granisetron	Serotonin-receptor antagonist	10–40 µg/kg I.V. × 1 3 mg I.V. × 1
Tropisetron	Serotonin-receptor antagonist	5 or 10 mg I.V. × 1
Dolasetron	Serotonin-receptor antagonist	1.8–3.0 mg/kg I.V. × 1
RG 12915	Serotonin-receptor antagonist	5–25 mg PO × 1
Metoclopramide	Substituted benzamide	1–3 mg/kg I.V. × two to three doses every 2 h
Haloperidol	Butyrophenone	1–3 mg I.V. × two to three doses every 2–4 h
Prochlorperazine	Phenothiazine	10–20 mg PO every 3–6 h 25 mg PR every 4–6 h 10 mg I.V. every 4–6 h
Dexamethasone	Corticosteroid	10–20 mg I.V. × 1 given over 5 min
Dronabinol	Cannabinoid	2.5–5 mg PO every 3–6 h

the initial dose administered 30 minutes before chemotherapy and the two subsequent doses repeated every 4 hours thereafter. Somewhat different regimens are recommended in other countries. Of interest, studies have indicated that schedules of every 2 or 4 or 6 or 8 hours all have similar efficacy.[25,26] This flexibility allows patients to receive this agent in a variety of treatment settings where the length of treatment may be an important factor. This lack of schedule dependency supports preliminary studies indicating efficacy with 8 mg and 32 mg single-dose schedules. Because early clinical trials noted important dose-efficacy relations, it is surprising that the above two doses (8 mg and 32 mg) were chosen for further study. In particular, doses above or below the 0.15 mg/kg level (about 10–12 mg) either showed no advantage or were less effective.[27]

Trials comparing ondansetron with metoclopramide in patients receiving high doses of cisplatin have yielded similar results,[28-30] as outlined in Table 63–4. In an illustrative study, ondansetron was given at 0.15 mg/kg intravenously every 4 hours for a total of three doses, and metoclopramide was given at 2 mg/kg intravenously every 2 to 3 hours for a total of six doses.[29] The median number of emetic episodes was less with ondansetron (one versus two, $p = 0.005$). The difference in complete control did not reach significance (40% versus 30%); however, the major control rate difference (fewer than three episodes) of 65% versus 51% with metoclopramide was significant ($p = 0.016$) in the 307 patients. No akathisia or dystonic reactions occurred in those given ondansetron (versus 10% and 8%, respectively, in those receiving metoclopramide). Headache was more common on the ondansetron arm

TABLE 63–4. Random Assignment Trials With Ondansetron and Metoclopramide in Previously Untreated Patients Receiving Cisplatin

Investigations	No. of Evaluable Patients	Cisplatin Dose	Antiemetic Regimen	Major Control Rate (0–2 Episodes; $p < 0.02$)	
Hainsworth et al, 1991[29]	307	≥100 mg/m²	Ondansetron: 0.15 mg/kg I.V. q 4 h × 3 doses vs Metoclopramide: 2 mg/kg I.V. q 3 h × 6 doses	Ondansetron: Metoclopramide:	65% 51%
Marty et al, 1990[28]	76	80–100 mg/m²	Ondansetron: 8 mg I.V. followed by 1 mg/h × 24 h by continuous infusion vs	Ondansetron: Metoclopramide:	75% 42%
DeMulder et al, 1990[30]	95	50–100 mg/m²	Metoclopramide: 3 mg/kg I.V. followed by a continuous infusion of 5 mg/kg over 8 h	Ondansetron: Metoclopramide:	72% 42%

of the study (24% versus 11%, $p = 0.005$). This trial has been criticized for blinding only the patients and not the evaluating staff, for using an outdated metoclopramide regimen, and for having a somewhat better patient population for antiemetic control on the ondansetron arm (fewer women and more patients with a heavy alcohol history). All comparison studies, however, have yielded the same results favoring ondansetron.

The other agents listed in Table 63–5 are generally given in single-dose schedules. Granisetron has been registered in several countries and, after ondansetron, is the best studied agent. Several agents have been studied as both intravenous and oral agents, with the latter route emphasized in the development of RG 12915.

Antiemetic efficacy reported to date in patients receiving moderate to high doses of cisplatin and other emetic chemotherapy is similar among these agents, with complete control rates of 40% to 60% and major control rates of 60% to 80%.[31-36]

The side-effect profile of the serotonin antagonists provides a distinct advantage over the more conventional antiemetics. Extrapyramidal side effects, including acute dystonic reactions and akathisia, are not observed in patients receiving these serotonin antagonists. The lack of central nervous system effects with these agents is especially important for pediatric patients and young adults—those most prone to experience extrapyramidal side effects. Mild headaches and transient transaminase elevations have been characteristically yet inconsequentially associated with the serotonin antagonists.[25-37] Typically, the headache requires no treatment or the use of a mild analgesic, such as acetaminophen.

With efficacy clearly outlined for chemotherapy regimens containing high-dose cisplatin, patients receiving lesser emetic chemotherapy agents have even more favorable control of nausea and vomiting.[25,31,37]

The rationale for using combination antiemetic regimens as applied to conventional agents is being used with the 5-HT3 antagonists. Further improvement of response rates with serotonin antagonists can be accomplished with antiemetic combinations plus a corticosteroid. One report outlines a significant improvement in the complete control rate when 20 mg of dexamethasone was given intravenously in conjunction with 0.15 mg of ondansetron given intravenously three times over a 4-hour period.[37] Eighty-one percent of patients had complete control of both nausea and vomiting with the combination, as opposed to 56% who received ondansetron as a single agent.[37] Further combination antiemetic trials are confirming the results of safety and efficacy.[38,39] For use in current practice situations, the best results continue to be obtained by those who apply carefully established regimens in a precise manner.

STANDARD ANTIEMETIC AGENTS

Several antiemetic agents have been shown to be safe and effective (see Table 63–5). Among the best studied of the more effective agents are those that exert their activity by blocking dopamine receptors. These include such classes and agents as: (1) substituted benzamides (metoclopramide and alizapride), (2) butyrophenones (haloperidol and droperidol), and (3) phenothiazines (prochlorperazine and chlorproma-

TABLE 63–5. Metoclopramide Combination Regimens

Chemotherapy Indication	Antiemetic Regimen
Highly Emetogenic Agents	
Cisplatin, ≥70 mg/m² or	Metoclopramide, 3 mg/kg I.V. × 2 doses, every 2 h
Cyclophosphamide, 750 mg/m² or	plus
Carboplatin or dacarbazine	Dexamethasone, 20 mg I.V. × 1
	plus
	Lorazepam, 1–2 mg I.V × 1
Moderately Emetogenic Agents	
Cisplatin, ≤60 mg/m² or	Metoclopramide, 1–2 mg/kg I.V. × 2–3 doses, every 2 h
Cyclophosphamide, ≤600 mg/m² or	plus
Doxorubicin or ifosfamide	Dexamethasone, 20 mg I.V. × 1
	plus
	Lorazepam 1–2 mg I.V. × 1

zine). Additionally, corticosteroids (dexamethasone and methylprednisolone) are effective agents, and benzodiazepines and cannabinoids may also have a role.

SUBSTITUTED BENZAMIDES

The most commonly used and most effective drug of this class is metoclopramide. Although some controversy exists, a pharmacologic study demonstrated that efficacy was correlated with high blood levels (more than 850 ng/ml) of metoclopramide in patients receiving cisplatin.[40] Maintaining an adequate level of metoclopramide at the time of emetic vulnerability through the use of an appropriate dosing schedule may be important. In preventing emesis induced by cisplatin or by cyclophosphamide plus doxorubicin, metoclopramide administration every 2 hours (beginning shortly before chemotherapy) appears to be the most effective schedule. Unlike the selective 5-HT3 antagonists, metoclopramide is schedule-dependent. Doses and schedules of metoclopramide are outlined in Tables 63–5 and 63–6.

Random-assignment studies have shown metoclopramide to be superior to, or at least equivalent to, all other standard antiemetic agents that it has been compared with in cisplatin-

TABLE 63–6. Combination Antiemetic Regimens for High-Dose Cisplatin

Regimen A

Metoclopramide, 3 mg/kg I.V. every 2 h for 2 doses, plus
Dexamethasone, 20 mg I.V. × 1 dose (over 5 min), plus
Lorazepam, 1–2 mg I.V. × 1 dose

Regimen B

Serotonin-receptor antagonist (See Table 63–3 for dose and schedule), plus
Dexamethasone, 20 mg I.V. × 1 (over 5 min)

(Data from references 37, 48, and 64)

induced emesis.[10,14,15,41] Several reports have indicated useful activity against the emesis associated with a number of other chemotherapeutic agents.[44–46]

A recent study[47] explored markedly higher doses of metoclopramide (4 to 6 mg/kg) given only once in patients receiving cisplatin. Although the original antiemetic phase I trials did not exceed 3 mg/kg per dose, the total amount administered was as high as 15 mg/kg given over 10 hours.[3] The rationale behind the single very-high-dose study included several points: (1) a single dose of metoclopramide (in this case in combination with dexamethasone plus lorazepam) given before chemotherapy would be convenient and economical, with fewer administration charges, (2) a high peak level of the agent would be ensured, and a therapeutic level would likely be maintained throughout the period of emetic vulnerability, and (3) such high levels would be likely to saturate 5-HT3 receptors. The results of the trial indicated that these very-high-dose metoclopramide regimens are as safe and effective as lower-dose combinations and that the single prechemotherapy dose of each of the agents was convenient and cost-effective. These findings have been confirmed in a randomized comparison trial.[48] The recommended single-dose regimen is as follows: lorazepam, 1.5 mg/m² given intravenously 30 minutes before chemotherapy, plus dexamethasone, 20 mg given intravenously over 5 minutes at 25 minutes before chemotherapy, followed by a 20-minute intravenous infusion of metoclopramide, 4 mg/kg given immediately before chemotherapy.[47]

The side effects commonly associated with metoclopramide include mild sedation, dystonic reactions (age-related), akathisia (restlessness), and diarrhea (which may be an effect of specific chemotherapeutic agents, such as cisplatin).[49] In general, the side effects are easy to control or prevent. Akathisia is prevented or treated with a benzodiazepine; dystonic reactions can be dealt with similarly or with diphenhydramine. As is discussed in the section on combinations of antiemetics, dexamethasone, in addition to metoclopramide, improves efficacy and reduces diarrhea.[50]

BUTYROPHENONES

Haloperidol and droperidol were shown in initial trials to be active antiemetics.[51,52] Since substantial differences have not been demonstrated between these two butyrophenones, most of the subsequent comments refer to studies conducted with haloperidol. A formal study comparing haloperidol with metoclopramide in patients receiving cisplatin reported that both antiemetics are effective, although a trend toward greater activity was seen with metoclopramide.[42] Doses of 1 to 3 mg of haloperidol given intravenously every 2 to 6 hours are used most commonly (see Table 63–5); the higher doses and more frequent schedules more often are associated with better results. Toxicity commonly includes sedation, dystonic reactions, and akathisia, with hypotension occasionally observed.

PHENOTHIAZINES

The unsatisfactory results observed with oral and intramuscular phenothiazines encouraged the need for new studies to examine other classes of agents, different administration schedules, and higher dosage regimens. Structure-activity

studies indicated that variations of the side chain at position 10 of the phenothiazine ring affect the antiemetic properties of these drugs.[53] Agents such as prochlorperazine would be predicted to have greater activity than other commonly used phenothiazines, such as chlorpromazine. This predicted difference has not been established in patients receiving chemotherapy.

Prochlorperazine given in typical oral and intramuscular doses in random-assignment trials has been found to be less active than metoclopramide[10] or dexamethasone[54] and equivalent to or less active than tetrahydrocannabinol.[55–57] A study using intravenous prochlorperazine in comparison with metoclopramide has indicated more encouraging results.[58] Two problems with this trial should be considered: (1) an imbalance in the arms of the study (concerning additional cyclophosphamide with the late onset of emesis), and (2) failure to evaluate adequately the incidence of orthostatic blood pressure changes, which is an important side effect of phenothiazines with major implications for outpatient usage. Other side effects are similar to those listed for haloperidol.

CORTICOSTEROIDS

Although several theories exist, the antiemetic mechanism of action of corticosteroids remains unclear. Several open studies and random-assignment trials have confirmed their utility.[54,59–62] Dexamethasone doses generally have been in the range of 4 to 20 mg per dose. In most trials in which a corticosteroid was added to an effective agent of another class, improved antiemetic efficacy for the combination resulted. This improvement has been evident in trials combining corticosteroids with metoclopramide or butyrophenones or ondansetron.

Toxicity has generally been mild with short courses of dexamethasone or methylprednisolone. There has been no indication of a lessening of chemotherapeutic effect through the use of steroids as antiemetics. With the low degree of toxicity, the low cost of generic dexamethasone, and a different mechanism of action than other agents, corticosteroids are ideal candidates for use in combination antiemetic regimens.

BENZODIAZEPINES AND CANNABINOIDS

Benzodiazepines can be useful additions to antiemetic regimens. Trials with lorazepam have shown a high degree of patient acceptance with a marked decrease in akathisia and in anxiety.[63,64] Additionally, lorazepam may add a small degree of objective antiemetic efficacy.[64] In a phase I trial, only modest major antiemetic activity was observed, but the subjective benefits appeared to make it an agent worth considering for use in combination.[65] A major difficulty in evaluating this agent's true activity is that it produces a dose-related memory loss.[63,65]

Most cannabinoid trials have included δ9-tetrahydrocannabinol (THC)[14,55,66,67]; two synthetic cannabinoids, nabilone and levonantradol, have been tested clinically,[68–70] as has inhalant marijuana.[72] THC has been tried at many doses with differing schedules. Doses in the range of 5 to 10 mg/m² given orally every 3 to 4 hours appear to be among the most useful.[14,66,67] In general, THC has been found to be superior to placebo and equivalent to or superior to oral prochlorpera-zine.[55,57] Similar results have been reported with nabilone.[68,69] Side effects are frequent but generally manageable and include sedation, dry mouth, orthostatic hypotension, ataxia, dizziness, a "high," and euphoria or dysphoria.

The popular press has carried several stories extolling the properties of crude smoked marijuana for a variety of indications in patients with cancer or acquired immunodeficiency syndrome (AIDS). The most prominent of the indications is as an antiemetic. No cannabinoid has had efficacy close to that observed with the more effective agents (including those available for more than a decade) in patients given highly emetic chemotherapy.[14] Reputed benefits include the ability for the patient to titrate the dose independently, although no study has demonstrated this to be achievable.[72] Objections include the fact that marijuana includes dozens of chemicals without antiemetic properties, that microorganisms are found in the leaves and can be inhaled, and that there is no evidence to support efficacy superior to any other cannabinoid.[72]

The question of whether marijuana is superior to THC capsules was addressed in a double-blind, randomized, crossover trial.[72] Patients were given inhalant marijuana plus a placebo THC capsule, or THC plus an inhalant placebo cigarette, with their initial course of cisplatin or cyclophosphamide, and they were given the opposite with the next course. Overall, efficacy was poor on both arms of the trial.[72] There was a trend toward a patient preference for the THC in this blinded study; no superiority in blood levels or efficacy was seen for the patients titrating their own marijuana. The role of the cannabinoids remains unclear. It is apparent that such agents as ondansetron (as one of several effective and safe 5-HT3 antagonists), metoclopramide, and corticosteroids are superior antiemetics and have fewer side effects.[14,37,64]

ANTIEMETIC COMBINATIONS

Trials of single agents have indicated which are the most effective antiemetics and which are most likely to be compatible with other active drugs. Guidelines for effective combination regimens include the following:

1. Regimens should combine agents that have different mechanisms of activity without overlapping toxicities.
2. The drugs should be active as single agents, with the optimal doses, best route of administration, and proper schedules used in the combination.
3. Agents added to the combination may be useful if they lessen the side effects of the regimen or if they reduce other toxicities of the chemotherapy.

Studies have compared the activity of metoclopramide with the combination of metoclopramide plus a corticosteroid. In each of these studies, the combination of the two active antiemetics has been superior to the single agent.[50,73-75] In addition to improved antiemetic efficacy with the steroid plus metoclopramide, the incidence of diarrhea was significantly reduced.[50,73] An open study combining a butyrophenone with a corticosteroid also reported favorable results.[76] Recently, combination studies of ondansetron with dexamethasone have been completed.[37,39] In the larger of these studies, the combination was superior to ondansetron alone, with complete

TABLE 63–7. Regimens for Delayed Emesis in Patients Receiving High Cisplatin Doses

Recommended Regimen

To start 24 hours after cisplatin administration:

Metoclopramide, 0.5 mg/kg PO, 4 times per day for 2 days, plus

Dexamethasone, 8 mg PO, 2 times per day for 2 days, then 4 mg PO, 2 times per day for 2 additional days

Regimen for Consideration for Clinical Investigation

To start 16 hours after cisplatin administration:

Oral 5-HT3 receptor antagonist at full established dose for 2 days plus

Dexamethasone, 8 mg PO, 2 times per day for 2 days, then 4 mg PO, 2 times per day for 2 additional days

(Data from references 80 to 83)

control of both nausea and vomiting achieved in 81% of the cisplatin-treated patients[39] (see the section on new antiemetic agents for dosing details, or Table 63–7).

Regimens for patients receiving high doses of cisplatin (120 mg/m²) should generally include a corticosteroid plus either a selective 5-HT3 antagonist (such as ondansetron or granisetron) or metoclopramide, as outlined in Table 63–6.

Metoclopramide plus dexamethasone regimens benefit from the addition of a benzodiazepine such as lorazepam. The latter agent adds some subjective benefits, prevents akathisia and dystonic reactions, and appears to add a small amount of efficacy over similar combinations with diphenhydramine.[64] The recommended regimen is listed in Table 63–6. This table also outlines recommended regimens and alternatives for use with a variety of chemotherapeutic drugs. These regimens have all been tested, either in formal comparison studies or in open trials. It is clear from this table that in nearly all instances, unless an agent is contraindicated for a specific patient, combinations are recommended.

Chemotherapy regimens that involve several consecutive days of treatment present a special problem in controlling emesis. The antiemetics that block dopamine receptors appear to result in a greater incidence of dystonic reactions when given on multiple consecutive days.[23] When agents such as cisplatin or dacarbazine are given over several days without effective antiemetics, the emesis gradually lessens. Regimens with ondansetron have been tried in patients receiving chemotherapy in this setting. Paradoxically, efficacy is greatest over the first 1 or 2 days and then diminishes.[77] When ondansetron is given intravenously at 0.15 mg/kg for three doses per day, the agent is well tolerated with no change in its side-effect pattern.[25]

A regimen under investigation in patients over age 30, who are given cisplatin at 25 to 33 mg/m²/day for 3 to 4 days, gives gradually decreasing doses of antiemetics. Patients are given 20 mg of dexamethasone intravenously 30 minutes before chemotherapy on each day. Metoclopramide also is given at 2 mg/kg at 30 minutes before cisplatin administration. On the first and second treatment days, the same metoclopramide dose is repeated 90 minutes after cisplatin; on the third day, the metoclopramide dose is repeated, but only at 1 mg/kg, and no repeat dose is given on the fourth day. Diphenhydramine is given intravenously at 50 mg with the first metoclopramide dose each day. A recent multicenter study compared the ondansetron plus dexamethasone regimen (as in regimen B in Table 63-6) with a metoclopramide and dexamethasone combination (similar to regimen A in Table 63-6, but using diphenhydramine 50 mg intravenously instead of lorazepam). Overall, both regimens were effective in the previously untreated patients receiving cisplatin, who were the subjects in the trial. However, a significant advantage emerged for those patients assigned to the serotonin antagonist combination.[78]

CONTROLLING EMESIS IN SPECIAL SITUATIONS

Lessons learned in treating acute chemotherapy-induced emesis can be valuable when considering the approach to delayed or anticipatory emesis, as long as the differences are respected.

DELAYED EMESIS

Only a few facts are known about this phenomenon. First, it is associated with high total cisplatin doses (more than 100 mg/m^2); and second, the incidence peaks about 2 days after chemotherapy. The pathophysiology of delayed emesis remains unclear.

Two preliminary open trials indicated that steroids plus either metoclopramide or prochlorperazine can be useful in controlling this problem.[79,80] A random assignment comparison study was done in which all patients received cisplatin, 120 mg/m^2, as their initial chemotherapy and received high-dose intravenous metoclopramide plus dexamethasone for acute emesis on the day of cisplatin administration.[81] Beginning 24 hours after chemotherapy, patients were assigned to receive oral placebo, oral dexamethasone for 4 days, or the combination of the oral dexamethasone regimen plus oral metoclopramide. Significantly greater complete control over the 4-day period was observed for those receiving the oral combination (57%) over placebo (11%). Side effects were generally mild.[81] The recommended regimen for delayed emesis is given in Table 63-7.

Only a limited amount of experience in delayed emesis with selective 5-HT3 antagonists exists. As a single agent, given orally, ondansetron's activity has not been encouraging in this setting.[82,83] Little information can be found for the other 5-HT3 antagonists. There is no reason to expect that a single dose of these agents on the day of chemotherapy will protect against both acute and delayed emesis.

An important finding comes from the phase II studies in acute chemotherapy-induced emesis with the 5-HT3 antagonists. In most trials, the time of onset of emesis, in the 60% who vomit with high-dose cisplatin, is between 16 and 20 hours. This is not, however, the time defined as the beginning of delayed emesis. Rather, the definition of this phenomenon beginning at 24 hours after chemotherapy is solely an arbitrary one of convenience. The implication is that the delayed emesis prevention regimen, as outlined previously, should be started earlier. A trial comparing the start of delayed emesis medications at 24 hours versus 14 hours would be warranted to test this hypothesis and to try to improve on the 50% control

rate. An additional study of interest would be to test an oral regimen of dexamethasone plus a 5-HT3 antagonist versus the dexamethasone plus metoclopramide regimen shown in Table 63-6.

ANTICIPATORY EMESIS

Although treatment of this problem is important, prevention is imperative. The difficulties of anticipatory emesis underscore the importance of giving the most effective antiemetics with the initial course of emesis-producing chemotherapy.

Studies have indicated that behavior therapy can be helpful for patients with anticipatory emesis[84]; however, patients with this problem will need effective control of emesis with the next chemotherapy administration if further anticipatory emesis is to be avoided. In addition to behavior therapy, the use of antianxiety agents has been suggested. Benzodiazepines, especially lorazepam, may be helpful in patients with anticipatory emesis; however, formal trials have not carefully studied this question. When should these agents be started? Are they effective for patients who exhibit signs of anxiety a day or two before chemotherapy? Appropriate studies may allow a clearer approach to this problem.

COST OF TREATING EMESIS

Since effective antiemetics became available with high doses of metoclopramide, the question of the cost has been raised. Certainly, there is a great need to control this most disturbing and feared toxicity. It is important to reassure patients that helpful medicines are available. Chemotherapy patients should be reassured of the likelihood of control of nausea and vomiting.

A justification that has been given for high antiemetic costs has been that shortened hospital stays can result when effective agents are used. Additionally, convenient regimens with only single antiemetic doses can be cost-effective in that, for some agents, the cost of drug preparation and administration can exceed the actual cost of the drug.

Charges for drugs differ markedly among institutions, by reimbursement plans, and from country to country. This was illustrated in a recent survey showing a broad range of charges for the same doses of metoclopramide plus dexamethasone plus lorazepam among three different institutions in the United States.[85] The cost of an agent to the pharmacist or practice may vary by the market or nation but may be relatively constant within a market (especially when only a single supplier is available). When high-quality generic agents or competing agents are available, a variety of prices may be found.

Another factor of importance is the treatment regimen. When approval for marketing a drug is granted, the Food and Drug Administration typically approves the schedule and doses for the trials it has reviewed. If subsequent studies indicate that more practical schedules are available, these newer, more economical, and possibly more effective regimens are not necessarily indicated in the package labeling.

As seen in Table 63-8, several factors can influence the cost of antiemetic treatment. If the single low-dose serotonin antagonists plus steroid regimens prove to be as effective as multiple dose schemes, then the simpler regimen may be

TABLE 63–8. Factors Influencing the Cost
of Antiemetic Treatment

Factor	Comment
Hospitalization	Effective control can decrease or eliminate hospitalization.
Chemotherapy	Appropriate regimens (fewer days of treatment) can enhance antiemetic efficacy, lower costs, and maintain antitumor activity.
Antiemetic schedule	Single-dose schedules reduce nursing and pharmacy charges (which may exceed drug costs).
Cost of antiemetic agents	The lowest, equally effective dose should be used. Of the 5-HT3 antagonists (if of equal efficacy), a single-dose lower-unit cost agent should be the drug of choice. Generic drugs should be used.
Institutional markup	Markup often ranges between 50% and 300% and can exceed the cost of the antiemetic agent.

competitive with metoclopramide combinations. Knowledge of alternative regimens can result in substantial savings for patients, payers, and medical institutions.

CONCLUSION

The last 10 years have seen major improvements in the control of emesis. Effective antiemetic regimens have become part of a standard of care in most major cancer treatment hospitals and clinics. Efforts to control emesis have presented an ideal situation for the collaboration of physicians and nurses who are oncology specialists. More new agents are soon to be introduced and are likely to be helpful, and better application of available techniques can result in major improvements in patient care. The newer 5-HT3 inhibitors are contributing to the successful control of emesis. The goal of optimal control of emesis requires knowledge of the more active drugs, experience with their use in combination, and consideration of the emetic problem of each patient.

New studies, however, must be accurately interpreted. Precision in evaluation techniques is mandatory if accurate results are to be obtained. Additionally, attention to the differing patient characteristics and to specific emetic patterns of individual chemotherapeutic agents must be considered in the design of trials and in the planning of an individual patient's treatment regimen.

The control of emesis is one of many important topics in the supportive care of patients with cancer. The considerable research efforts of the past decade in this area have resulted in improvements; the application of these findings continues to be the responsibility of all of us in clinical oncology.

REFERENCES

1. Borison HL, McCarthy LE. Neuropharmacology of chemotherapy induced emesis. Drugs 1983;25:8–17.
2. Borison HL. Role of the area postrema in vomiting and related functions. Rev Pharmacol Clin Exp 1986;3:7–8.
3. Gralla RJ, Braun TJ, Squillante A, et al. Metoclopramide: Initial clinical studies of high dosage regimens in cisplatin-induced emesis. In: Poster D, ed. The treatment of nausea and vomiting induced by cancer chemotherapy. New York: Masson, 1981:167–176.
4. Fozard JR, Mobarok A. Blockade of neuronal tryptamine receptors by metoclopramide. Eur J Pharmacol 1978;49:109–112.
5. Ireland SJ, Straughan OW, Tyers MB. Influence of 5-HT uptake on the apparent 5-HT antagonist potency of metoclopramide on the rat isolated superior cervical ganglion. Br J Pharmacol 1987;90:151–160.
6. Miner WD, Sanger GJ, Turner DH. Evidence that 5-hydroxytryptamine 3 receptors mediate cytotoxic drug and radiation-evoked emesis. Br J Cancer 1987;56:159–162.
7. Cubbedu LX, Hoffman IS, Fuenmayor NT, et al. Efficacy of ondansetron (GR38032F) and the role of serotonin in cisplatin-induced nausea and vomiting. N Engl J Med 1990;327:810–816.
8. Gralla RJ, Clark RA, Lohman TP. Does serotonin mediate chemotherapy-induced emesis? Proc Am Soc Clin Oncol 1991;10:324.
9. Engelman K. Malignant carcinoid syndrome. In: DeGroot LG, Besser GM, Cahill GF, eds. Endocrinology. Philadelphia: WB Saunders, 1989:2649–2657.
10. Gralla RJ, Itri LM, Pisko SE, et al. Antiemetic efficacy of high-dose metoclopramide: Randomized trials with placebo and prochlorperazine in patients with chemotherapy-induced nausea and vomiting. N Engl J Med 1981;305:905–909.
11. Fetting JH, Grochow LB, Folstein MF, et al. The course of nausea and vomiting after high-dose cyclophosphamide. Cancer Treat Rep 1982;66:1487–1493.
12. Martin M, Diaz Rubio E, Sanchez A. The natural course of emesis after carboplatin treatment. Acta Oncol 1990;29:593–596.
13. Mangioni C, Bolis G, Pecorelli S, et al. Randomized trial in advanced ovarian cancer comparing cisplatin and carboplatin. J Natl Cancer Inst 1989;81:1464–1471.
14. Gralla RJ, Tyson LB, Borden LA, et al. Antiemetic therapy: A review of recent studies and a report of a random assignment trial comparing metoclopramide with delta-9-tetrahydrocannabinol. Cancer Treat Rep 1984;68:163–172.
15. Homesley HD, Gayney JM, Jobsen VN, et al. Double-blind placebo-controlled study of metoclopramide in cisplatin-induced emesis. N Engl J Med 1982;307:250–251.
16. Kris MG, Gralla RJ, Clark RA, et al. Incidence, course, and severity of delayed nausea and vomiting following the administration of high-dose cisplatin. J Clin Oncol 1985;3:1379–1384.
17. Morrow GR. Prevalence and correlates of anticipatory nausea and vomiting in chemotherapy patients. J Natl Cancer Inst 1982;68:585–588.
18. Wilcox PM, Fetting JH, Nettesheim KM, et al. Anticipatory vomiting in women receiving cyclophosphamide, methotrexate and 5-FU (CMF) adjuvant chemotherapy for breast carcinoma. Cancer Treat Rep 1982;66:1601–1604.
19. D'Acquisto RW, Tyson LB, Gralla RJ, et al. The influence of a chronic high alcohol intake on chemotherapy-induced nausea and vomiting. Proc Am Soc Clin Oncol 1986;5:257.
20. Sullivan JR, Leyten MJ, Bell R. Decreased cisplatin induced nausea and vomiting with alcohol ingestion. N Engl J Med 1983;309:13, 796.
21. Roila F, Tonato M, Basurto C, et al. Protection from nausea and vomiting in cisplatin-treated patients: High dose metoclopramide combined with methyl prednisolone versus metoclopramide combined with dexamethasone and diphenhydramine. A study of the Italian Oncology for Clinical Research. J Clin Oncol 1989;7:1693–1700.
22. Kris MG, Tyson LB, Gralla RJ, et al. Extrapyramidal reactions with high-dose metoclopramide. N Engl J Med 1983;309:433.
23. Allen JC, Gralla RJ, Reilly C, et al. Metoclopramide: Dose-related toxicity and preliminary antiemetic studies in children receiving cancer chemotherapy. J Clin Oncol 1985;3:1136–1141.
24. Gralla RJ, Clark RA, Kris MG, Tyson LB. Methodology in antiemetic trials. Eur J Cancer 1991;27:55–58.
25. Kris MG, Gralla RJ, Clark RA, et al. Phase II trials of the serotonin antagonist GR38032F for the control of vomiting caused by cisplatin. J Natl Cancer Inst 1989;81:42–46.
26. Hesketh PJ, Murphy WK, Lester RP, et al. GR38032F: A novel compound effective in the prevention of acute cisplatin-induced emesis. J Clin Oncol 1989;7:700–705.
27. Kris MG, Gralla RJ, Clark RA, et al. Dose ranging evaluation of the serotonin antagonist GR-C507/75 (GR38032F) when used as an antiemetic in patients receiving cancer chemotherapy. J Clin Oncol 1988;6:659–662.
28. Marty M, Pouillart P, Scholl S, et al. Comparison of the 5-hydroxytryptamine 3 (serotonin) receptor antagonist ondansetron (GR38032F) with high-dose metoclopramide in the control of cisplatin-induced emesis. N Engl J Med 1990;332:816–821.
29. Hainsworth J, Harvey W, Pendergrass K, et al. A single-blind comparison of intravenous ondansetron, a selective serotonin antagonist, with intravenous metoclopramide in the prevention of nausea and vomiting associated with high-dose cisplatin chemotherapy. J Clin Oncol 1991;9:721–728.
30. DeMulder PHM, Deynaere C, Vermorken JB, et al. Ondansetron compared with high-dose metoclopramide in prophylaxis of acute and delayed cisplatin-induced nausea and vomiting. Ann Intern Med 1990;113:834–840.
31. Baltzer L, Tyson LB, Kris MG, et al. Oral antiemetics for lung cancer chemotherapy: Studies with metoclopramide and RG12915. Proc 6th World Conf Lung Cancer 1991;7:148.
32. Clark RA, Gralla RJ, Tyson LB, et al. Controlling emesis with serotonin antagonists: Experience with 5 new agents in 109 patients. Proc 6th World Conf Lung Cancer 1991;7:148.
33. Grunberg SM, Kris MG, Gralla RJ, et al. High dose MDL 73, 147EF for the prevention of cisplatin-induced emesis. Proc 6th World Conf Lung Cancer 1991;7:148.
34. Kaplan HG, Jofthagen C. Use of granisetron to prevent platinol induced nausea and vomiting. Proc Am Soc Clin Oncol 1991;10:339.
35. Tyson LB, Gralla RJ, Kris MG, et al. Phase I antiemetic study of the serotonin antagonist ICS 205–930. Proc Am Soc Clin Oncol 1989;8:331.

36. Clark RA, Kris MG, Gralla RJ, et al. Serotonin antagonists demonstrate antiemetic effectiveness without extrapyramidal symptoms: Analysis of studies with 3 new agents in 155 patients. Proc Am Soc Clin Oncol 1990;9:332.

37. Roila F, Tonato M, Cognetti F, et al. Prevention of cisplatin-induced emesis: A double-blind multicenter randomized crossover study comparing ondansetron and ondansetron plus dexamethasone. J Clin Oncol 1991;9:674–678.

38. Tyson LB, Kris MG, Baltzer L, et al. Combining ondansetron with dexamethasone: A randomized antiemetic trial comparing two ondansetron schedules in patients receiving cisplatin. Proc Am Soc Clin Oncol 1991;10:341.

39. Smith DB, Newland ES, Rustin GJS, et al. Comparison of ondansetron and ondansetron plus dexamethasone as antiemetic prophylaxis during cisplatin-containing chemotherapy. Lancet 1991;338:487–498.

40. Meyer BR, Lewin M, Dreyer DE, et al. Optimizing metoclopramide control of cisplatin-induced emesis. Ann Intern Med 1984;100:393–395.

41. Frustacci S, Tumolo S, Tirell U, et al. High dose metoclopramide versus dexamethasone in the prevention of cisplatin induced vomiting. Proc Am Soc Clin Oncol 1983;2:87.

42. Grunberg Sm, Gala KV, Lampenfeld M, et al. Comparison of the antiemetic effect of high-dose intravenous haloperidol: A randomized double-blind crossover study. J Clin Oncol 1984;2:782–787.

43. Richards PD, Flaum MA, Bateman M, et al. The antiemetic efficacy of secobarbital and chlorpromazine compared to metoclopramide, diphenhydramine, and dexamethasone: A randomized trial. Cancer 1986;58:959–962.

44. Gralla RJ, Tyson LB, Clark RA, et al. An all oral combination antiemetic regimen for patients receiving Cytoxan + Adriamycin + vincristine. Proc Am Soc Clin Oncol 1985;4:267.

45. Strum SB, McDermed JE, Opfell RW, et al. Intravenous metoclopramide: An effective antiemetic in cancer chemotherapy. J Am Med Assoc 1982;247:2683–2686.

46. Tyson LB, Clark RA, Gralla, RJ. High dose metoclopramide: Control of dacarbazine-induced emesis in a preliminary trial. Cancer Treat Rep 1982;66:2108.

47. Clark RA, Gralla RJ, Kris MG, et al. Exploring very high doses of metoclopramide (4–6 mg/kg): Preservation of efficacy and safety with only a single dose in a combination regimen. Proc Am Soc Clin Oncol 1989;8:1286.

48. Basuto C, Roila F, Bracarda S, et al. Single vs divided dose of metoclopramide in a combined regimen of treatment of cisplatin induced emesis: A double-blind prospective comparative trial. Perugia International Cancer Conference III. In: Supportive therapy: Challenges for the '90s. 1990:109.

49. Von Hoff DD, Schilisky R, Reichert CM, et al. Toxic effects of disdichlorodiammine-platinum (II) in man. Cancer Treat Rep 1979;63:1527–1531.

50. Kris MG, Gralla RJ, Tyson LB, et al. Improved control of cisplatin-induced emesis with high-dose metoclopramide and with combinations of metoclopramide, dexamethasone, and diphenhydramine: Results of consecutive trials in 255 patients. Cancer 1985;55:527–534.

51. Grossman B, Lessen LS, Cohen P. Droperidol prevents nausea and vomiting from cisplatinum. N Engl J Med 1979;301:47.

52. Neidhart J, Gayen M, Metz E. Haldol and mustard induced vomiting when other agents fail. Proc Am Soc Clin Oncol 1980;21:365.

53. Wampler G. The pharmacology and clinical effectiveness of phenothiazines and related drugs for managing chemotherapy-induced emesis. Drugs 1983;25:31–51.

54. Markman M, Sheidler V, Ettinger DS, et al. Antiemetic efficacy of dexamethasone: Randomized, double-blind, crossover study with prochlorperazine in patients receiving cancer chemotherapy. N Engl J Med 1984;311:549–552.

55. Frytak S, Moertel CG, O'Fallon J, et al. Delta-9-tetrahydrocannabinol as an antiemetic in patients treated with cancer chemotherapy: A double-blind comparison with prochlorperazine and a placebo. Ann Intern Med 1979;91:825–830.

56. Orr LE, McKerman JF, Bloone B. Antiemetic effect of tetrahydrocannabinol. Arch Intern Med 1980;140:1431–1433.

57. Sallan SE, Cronin C, Zelen M, et al. Antiemetics in patients receiving chemotherapy for cancer: A randomized comparison of delta-9-tetrahydrocannabinol and prochlorperazine. N Engl J Med 1980;302:135–138.

58. Carr BI, Bertrand M, Browning S, et al. A comparison of the antiemetic efficacy of prochlorperazine and metoclopramide for the treatment of cisplatin-induced emesis: A prospective randomized double-blind study. J Clin Oncol 1985;3:1127–1132.

59. Aapro MS, Alberts DS. High dose dexamethasone for prevention of cisplatinum-induced vomiting. Cancer Chemother Pharmacol 1981;7:11–14.

60. Aapro MS, Plezia PM, Alberts DS, et al. Double-blind crossover study of the antiemetic efficacy of high-dose dexamethasone vs high-dose metoclopramide. Proc Am Soc Clin Oncol 1983;2:93.

61. Cassileth PA, Lusk EJ, Torri S, et al. Antiemetic efficacy of dexamethasone therapy in patients receiving cancer chemotherapy. Arch Intern Med 1983;143:1347–1349.

62. Lee BJ. Methylprednisolone as an antiemetic. N Engl J Med 1981;304:486.

63. Kris MG, Gralla RJ, Clark RA, et al. Consecutive dose-finding trials adding lorazepam to the combination of metoclopramide plus dexamethasone: Improved subjective effectiveness over the combination of diphenhydramine plus metoclopramide plus dexamethasone. Cancer Treat Rep 1985;69:1257–1262.

64. Kris MG, Gralla RJ, Clark RA, et al. Antiemetic control and prevention of side effects of anticancer therapy with lorazepam or diphenhydramine when used in conjunction with metoclopramide plus dexamethasone: A double-blind, randomized trial. Cancer 1987;69:1353–1357.

65. Laszlo J, Clark RA, Hanson DC, et al. Lorazepam in cancer patients treated with cisplatin: A drug having antiemetic, amnesic, and anxiolytic effects. J Clin Oncol 1985;3:864–869.

66. Chang AE, Shilling DJ, Stillman RC, et al. Delta-9-tetrahydrocannabinol as an antiemetic in patients receiving high-dose methotrexate: A prospective randomized evaluation. Ann Intern 1979;91:819–824.

67. Vincent BJ, McQuistion DJ, Einhorn LH, et al. Review of cannabinoids and their antiemetic effectiveness. Drugs 1983;25:52–62.

68. Herman TS, Einhorn LH, Jones SE. Superiority of nabilone over prochlorperazine as an antiemetic in patients receiving cancer chemotherapy. N Engl J Med 1979;300:1295–1297.

69. Steele N, Gralla RJ, Braun DW, et al. Double-blind comparison of the antiemetic effects of nabilone and prochlorperazine on chemotherapy-induced emesis. Cancer Treat Rep 1980;64:219–224.

70. Tyson LB, Gralla RJ, Clark RA, et al. Phase I trial of levonantradol in chemotherapy induced emesis. Am J Clin Oncol 1985;8:528–532.

71. Venner P, Bruera E, Diebrt D, et al. Intensive treatment scheduling of nabilone plus dexamethasone vs metoclopramide plus dexamethasone in cisplatinum-induced emesis. Proc Am Soc Clin Oncol 1986;5:253.

72. Levitt M, Faiman C, Hawks R, et al. Randomized double-blind comparison of delta-9-tetrahydrocannabinol (THC) and marijuana as chemotherapy antiemetics. Proc Am Soc Clin Oncol 1984;3:91.

73. Allan SG, Cornbleet MA, Warrington PS, et al. Dexamethasone and high-dose metoclopramide: Efficacy in controlling cisplatin-induced nausea and vomiting. Br Med J 1984;289:878–879.

74. Rosell R, Abad-Esteve A, Ribas-Mundo M, et al. Evaluation of a combination antiemetic regimen including IV high-dose metoclopramide, dexamethasone, and diphenhydramine in cisplatin-based chemotherapy regimens. Cancer Treat Rep 1985;69:909–910.

75. Grunberg SM, Akerley WL, Baker C, et al. Comparison of metoclopramide and metoclopramide + dexamethasone in complete prevention of cisplatinum induced emesis. Proc Am Soc Clin Oncol 1985;4:262.

76. Mason BA, Dambra J, Grossman B, et al. Effective control of cisplatin-induced nausea using high-dose steroids and droperidol. Cancer Treat Rep 1982;66:243–245.

77. Hainsworth JD, Omura GA, Khojasteba, et al. Ondansetron (GR 38032F): A novel antiemetic effective in patients receiving a multiple-day regimen of cisplatin chemotherapy. Am J Clin Oncol 1991;14:336–348.

78. Roila F, Tonato M, Favalli G, et al. A multi-center double-blind study comparing the antiemetic efficacy and safety of ondansetron (OND) plus dexamethasone (DEX) vs metoclopramide (MTC) plus DEX and diphenhydramine (DIP) in cisplatin (CDDP) treated cancer patients (PTS). Am Soc Clin Oncol 1992;11:394.

79. Clark RA, Kris MG, Tyson LB, et al. Antiemetic trials to control delayed vomiting following high-dose cisplatin. Proc Am Soc Clin Oncol 1986;5:257.

80. Strum S, McDermed J, Abrahano-Umali R, et al. Management of cisplatin-induced delayed-onset nausea and vomiting: Preliminary results with two drug regimens. Proc Soc Am Clin Oncol 1985;4:263.

81. Kris MG, Gralla RJ, Tyson LB, et al. Controlling delayed vomiting: Double-blind randomized trial comparing placebo, dexamethasone alone, and metoclopramide plus dexamethasone in patients receiving cisplatin. J Clin Oncol 1989;7:108–114.

82. Grunberg SM, Groshen S, Stevenson LI, et al. Double-blind randomized study of two doses of oral ondansetron for the prevention of cisplatin-induced delayed nausea and vomiting. Proc Am Soc Clin Oncol 1990;9:327.

83. Kris MG, Tyson LB, Clark RA, et al. Oral ondansetron for the control of delayed emesis after cisplatin: Report of a phase II study and a review of completed trials to manage delayed emesis. Cancer 1992;70:1012–1016.

84. Morrow GR, Morrell C. Behavioral treatment for the anticipatory nausea and vomiting induced by cancer chemotherapy. N Engl J Med 1982;307:1476–1480.

85. Muller RJ, Gralla RJ, Kris MG, et al. Administration of effective antiemetic regimens: Marked differences in patient changes among different institutions. Proc Am Soc Clin Oncol 1990;9:334.

RAYMOND B. WEISS
NICHOLAS J. VOGELZANG

SECTION **2**

Miscellaneous Toxicities

Chemotherapeutic agents can produce a variety of acute and chronic organ toxicities. Besides heart and lung toxicities, which are covered in other sections, damage to the kidneys, nerve tissue, liver, and blood vessels may occur. In addition, acute hypersensitivity reactions may produce immediate life-threatening problems, such as hypotension and respiratory distress. Such hypersensitivity reactions may necessitate cessation of treatment with the precipitating drug, or at least means must be found to minimize or prevent the problem. Acute hepatic, renal, or central nervous system toxicity may also be life-threatening but in a less immediate manner. If the offending drug is discontinued before irreversible damage occurs, the manifestations of toxicity usually wane. As patients live longer after receiving cancer chemotherapy, chronic toxicities such as Raynaud's phenomenon may become evident and sometimes debilitating and irreversible.

Antitumor drugs are often used in combination, and it may be difficult to determine which drug is most responsible for a particular form of tissue injury. Other medical conditions such as infections or the cancer itself may cause tissue injury during chemotherapy, and the antitumor agent may be blameless. Whether the toxicity is acute or chronic, awareness of the potential for toxicity with each agent in use is important, and appropriate monitoring (which may be simple patient questioning about symptoms or laboratory testing) must be accomplished. If not, severe and irreversible tissue injury may occur.

NEPHROTOXICITY

The kidneys are the elimination pathway of many drugs and their metabolites and therefore are vulnerable to injury. The entire anatomic renal pathway from glomerulus to distal tubule is at risk, depending on the drug involved. The symptoms vary from an asymptomatic rise in serum creatinine or mild proteinuria to acute renal failure with anuria requiring dialysis.

PLATINUM COMPOUNDS

The nephrotoxicity of cisplatin has been well known since it was first used in clinical trials in the early 1970s.[1,2] This obstacle to its use has been so profound that hundreds of cisplatin analogs have been synthesized in the hope of finding a less nephrotoxic compound of equal antitumor efficacy. Fortunately, a means was found to avoid nephrotoxicity from cisplatin by forcing diuresis and enhancing drug excretion.[3]

The renal toxicity is dose-related, cumulative, and manifested primarily by a rise in serum creatinine. Single doses under 40 mg/m^2 usually cause little renal injury, but higher doses require aggressive hydration, or abrupt irreversible renal failure may occur.[4] The hydration used most successfully is normal saline because the high chloride concentration possibly inhibits cisplatin hydrolysis in the tubules, providing a measure

of nephrotoxicity protection. Mannitol is also used to stimulate diuresis, but there is no evidence that mannitol is necessary. A urine output of at least 100 ml/hour for 2 to 4 hours before and 4 to 6 hours after cisplatin doses of 40 to 75 mg/m^2 reduces, but does not eliminate, nephrotoxicity. More intensive hydration schedules are necessary when higher cisplatin doses are used.

The pathologic lesion of cisplatin renal damage is primarily in the proximal and distal tubules but also may involve the collecting ducts,[5] while glomeruli are unaffected. This extensive area of tissue injury helps explain why electrolyte abnormalities, such as hyponatremia and hypomagnesemia, are so common after cisplatin administration.[6,7] The hypomagnesemia is usually asymptomatic, but it can last months to years.[8] The hyponatremia has been reported to cause persistent orthostatic hypotension.[7]

The precise mechanism of the tubular injury continues to be the subject of research. It is not simply the tubular handling of a heavy metal, because the *trans* isomer of cisplatin is not nephrotoxic.[9] Cisplatin produces DNA intrastrand crosslinks as one of its mechanisms of antitumor effect, and the same damage to DNA in tubular cells probably also occurs.

A variety of substances have been tested to minimize cisplatin nephrotoxicity, besides using the often inconvenient hydration and diuresis. These include probenecid, superoxide dismutase, amifostine (WR 2721), mesna, sodium thiosulfate, diethyldithiocarbamate, and hypertonic saline. None of these substances has achieved acceptance as a substitute for hydration. One simple technique for additional nephrotoxicity protection, besides hydration, is to administer cisplatin in the evening to take advantage of circadian rhythm effects that have been shown to reduce renal injury.[10]

A final measure of protection is to be certain that normal renal function is present initially by performing a pretreatment 24-hour urine creatinine clearance. A result of less than 70 ml/minute, especially in patients over age 60, probably precludes cisplatin administration without an inordinate risk of nephrotoxicity.[11] In addition, other renal tubular toxins, such as aminoglycoside antibiotics, should be avoided whenever possible to obviate additive tubular damage.

Carboplatin was synthesized as a cisplatin alternative with less nephrotoxicity. It is less nephrotoxic,[12] but it is not free of potential for renal injury, especially in patients who previously have received nephrotoxins or when given in high doses.[13,14] Usually, carboplatin-related dysfunction is detectable only by the sensitive means of measuring urine tubular enzyme excretion or glomerular filtration rate.[15] The serum creatinine and creatinine clearance are rarely affected.

MITOMYCIN

The capacity of mitomycin to produce renal toxicity has been known for over 20 years.[16] Renal effects from mitomycin are not as common as from the platinum compounds, but they can be immediately life-threatening in some cases.

The clinical manifestations vary from a chronic progressive rise in serum creatinine[17] without thrombocytopenia to microangiopathic hemolytic anemia (MAHA), which is usually fulminant in onset. MAHA has been reported in a large number of anecdotal cases,[18] but in one study[19] of adjuvant mitomycin, a 10.7% incidence occurred.

The MAHA toxicity is cumulative dose-related, but even one to three doses of mitomycin can initiate it. It also can develop a few months after mitomycin has been discontinued.[18,20] The incidence has been reported to rise to 25% to 30% if the cumulative mitomycin dose is over 70 mg/m^2.[20]

The clinical presentation of MAHA is an abrupt and often severe hemolytic anemia that usually precedes the renal dysfunction by 1 or 2 weeks. The peripheral blood smear shows schistocytes, and thrombocytopenia becomes apparent as renal failure develops. The thrombocytopenia is not part of a generalized coagulopathy because laboratory evidence of disseminated intravascular coagulation is usually not observed. Other accompanying abnormalities are rash, fever, arterial hypertension, central neurologic dysfunction, pericarditis, interstitial pneumonitis, hematuria, and proteinuria.[18,20] A high rate (65%) of patients have noncardiogenic pulmonary edema.[20] A prominent feature of this syndrome is the fact that it is often precipitated or worsened by blood transfusions, suggesting that blood product use should be avoided as much as possible when administering mitomycin. The outcome is often (over 50%) death, despite vigorous treatment.[19,20]

Treatment includes hemodialysis and plasmapheresis.[21] The most successful treatment has been plasma perfusion over filters containing staphylococcal protein A, a method of removing immune complexes from the blood.[20,22]

The pathogenesis of this acute form of nephrotoxicity is not certain. Cattell[23] showed that mitomycin caused glomerular endothelial damage when directly injected into the renal arteries of rats. Such vascular endothelial injury may activate platelets and lead to fibrin thrombi deposition in the microvasculature of the kidney, initiating renal dysfunction and hemolysis.

METHOTREXATE

When methotrexate is administered in conventional oral or intravenous doses, nephrotoxicity is only an occasional problem. If high doses are used, along with folinic acid rescue, acute nephrotoxicity can pose a greater danger.

Methotrexate is excreted rapidly in the urine whether it is administered orally or parenterally. Both parent compound and the main metabolite, 7-hydroxymethotrexate, are filtered by the glomeruli and actively secreted by the tubules. At physiologic pH, the drug is fully ionized, but in acidified form (pH less than 5.7), the parent drug and main metabolite are less ionized and may precipitate.[24] During urinary excretion, drug precipitation occurs as the urine is concentrated and acidified in the tubules. The solubility of 7-hydroxymethotrexate is only one fourth that of methotrexate, providing further potential for drug precipitation within the tubules and resulting in acute renal dysfunction.

Acute methotrexate nephrotoxicity produces abrupt renal insufficiency. The patient may complain of costovertebral angle pain while the serum creatinine and blood urea nitrogen rise rapidly. Dehydration, oliguria, and even anuria may occur.

Since methotrexate nephrotoxicity is largely a physical process of tubular drug precipitation, the incidence can be kept low by means of precipitation prevention. The two main methods are hydration and urine alkalinization.[25] Whenever a methotrexate dose high enough to require folinic acid rescue is being given, the urine should be kept alkaline (pH greater than 8) with sodium bicarbonate administration, and a urine output of over 100 ml/hour should be maintained. Serial serum methotrexate levels should be monitored until the concentration reaches 10^{-8} molar or less, 24 to 48 hours after administration.[25]

If renal clearance of methotrexate is impaired by renal dysfunction already present or by concurrently administered drugs, nephrotoxicity can be initiated or enhanced. Prior treatment with cisplatin may contribute to nephrotoxicity from methotrexate.[26] In addition, concurrent administration of nonsteroidal antiinflammatory drugs can provoke serious, and even fatal, methotrexate nephrotoxicity. Indomethacin,[27] ketoprofen,[28] diclofenac,[28] and naproxen[29] have been reported to increase the risk of such renal problems, whether the methotrexate is being given in a high dose[28] or low dose.[29] The mechanism of this drug interaction is not known, but it is probably mediated by a reduced methotrexate clearance through the kidney.

Treatment of acute nephrotoxicity from high methotrexate doses by hemodialysis and peritoneal dialysis has been minimally successful.[30] Charcoal hemofiltration by methods similar to those used to remove barbiturates from overdosed patients has been more effective.[31]

NITROSOUREAS

Streptozocin has the most potential for nephrotoxicity in this drug class, and this is its dose-limiting form of toxicity. The incidence rises with prolonged drug administration so that most patients eventually display it if therapy continues.

The kidneys are the major excretion pathway for both parent drug and metabolites, which may be the main factor in the pathogenesis of the renal toxicity. The sites of streptozocin injury are both the glomerulus and tubules (primarily the proximal) where histologic changes have been observed.[32] The mechanism of this injury, however, is not known. Hypophosphatemia and proteinuria are early indications of renal effect.[33] Renal tubular acidosis, with its characteristic abnormalities of glycosuria, acetonuria, hyperchloremia, and aminoaciduria, is seen frequently. If the drug is discontinued, these findings usually resolve. A rising serum creatinine is a later, and sometimes irreversible, finding. Hydration and diuresis have occasionally minimized renal dysfunction during therapy.[34]

The other two nitrosoureas in clinical use (carmustine and lomustine) are much less nephrotoxic. Carmustine usually causes problems of interstitial pneumonitis before it causes any renal toxicity. Lomustine has caused only rare instances of nephrotoxicity when large cumulative doses were administered.[35]

IFOSFAMIDE

Cyclophosphamide and ifosfamide are analogs with similar chemical structures. Both produce the metabolite acrolein, which causes hemorrhagic cystitis during urinary excretion. Despite similarities in structure, toxicity, and antitumor efficacy, they differ significantly in their ability to cause nephrotoxicity. Cyclophosphamide produces no kidney toxicity of clinical consequence, while ifosfamide produces a variety of renal abnormalities, some of which have been fatal.[36]

Early studies with ifosfamide showed that single high doses could result in acute tubular necrosis and renal failure within a few days of drug administration.[37] Such outcomes were one reason that a fractionated dose schedule was developed for this drug. Administration over five consecutive days reduced both renal and bladder toxicity. The most effective measure for reducing urinary tract toxicity was the development of mesna as a means of cystitis prevention. Mesna is now a standard accompaniment to ifosfamide use, but it does not obviate nephrotoxicity.[38]

The incidence of nephrotoxicity varies from several percent up to 33%, a level seen in young children.[39] Clinical manifestations include tubular dysfunction, Fanconi's syndrome, and a rising serum creatinine resulting in renal failure. The tubular injury is manifested by glycosuria, renal tubular acidosis, hypokalemia, proteinuria, and hypophosphatemia, which can even result in rickets in children.[40,41]

PLICAMYCIN

The first antitumor agent recognized to have nephrotoxicity potential was plicamycin (mithramycin).[42] Acute renal failure was a common toxicity when this drug was used for treating testicular cancer. Although it now is used only for its therapeutic effect in hypercalcemia, renal toxicity can still occur, even after only a single drug dose.[43] An acute rise in serum creatinine is the usual manifestation of such toxicity.

OTHER AGENTS

Table 63–9 lists antitumor agents that have been reported to cause renal injury. They are categorized by the risk of such toxicity from occasional anecdotal reports to high risk of severe damage.

Not only can individual drugs cause nephrotoxicity, but also

TABLE 63–9. Antitumor Agents That Cause Nephrotoxicity

High Potential for Nephrotoxicity

Azacitidine	Methotrexate (in high doses)
Cisplatin	Mitomycin
Diaziquone (in high doses)	Pentostatin
Gallium nitrate	Plicamycin
Ifosfamide	Streptozocin
Interleukin-2	

Azotemia Without Nephrotoxicity

Dacarbazine
L-Asparaginase

Occasional Irreversible Nephrotoxicity

Cisplatin	Mitomycin
Gallium nitrate	Streptozocin
Lomustine	

Low Potential for Nephrotoxicity

Azathioprine	Lomustine
Carboplatin	6-Mercaptopurine
Interferons	Methotrexate (in low doses)

combinations of agents can occasionally cause serious reactions, such as microangiopathic hemolytic anemia. The combination of cisplatin, bleomycin, and methotrexate or vincristine has initiated such toxicity in similar fashion to mitomycin.[44,45]

NEUROTOXICITY

VINCA ALKALOIDS

The first drug class to be recognized as having neurotoxicity was the vinca alkaloids, especially vincristine. Vincristine is unique among the antitumor agents in that neurotoxicity is dose-limiting. The neurologic injury can be to the peripheral, central, or autonomic nervous systems.[46,47]

The most common and initial manifestations of neurotoxicity are depression of the deep tendon reflexes and paresthesia of the distal extremities. The Achilles tendon reflexes and the fingertips are the respective initial sites of abnormalities. Loss of the Achilles tendon reflex is usually asymptomatic. The paresthesia commonly progresses proximally as vincristine therapy is continued and may involve the entire hands or feet. The hyporeflexia spreads to other sites, and areflexia develops next. Surprisingly, despite the presence of peripheral paresthesia, vibration sense, position sense, pinprick sensation, and two-point discrimination are generally unaffected.

Motor dysfunction and gait disorders are initially manifested as lower extremity weakness. Footdrop and a slapping gait may ensue, and if vincristine is continued, weakness to the point of paraparesis may develop. Severe bone pain and pain in the mandible region may occur acutely a few hours after vincristine administration. It usually subsides after a few days.

Cranial nerves may be affected and cause ophthamoplegia and facial palsy. Ataxia is seen rarely. The parasympathetic nervous system can be affected also, so that constipation and difficult micturation may develop. These symptoms can progress to paralytic ileus with obstipation and bladder atony. Autonomic neuropathy can manifest as orthostatic hypotension, which can be symptomatic or clinically silent.[48] Vocal cord paralysis producing hoarseness and dysphagia may occur. The risk of vincristine neurotoxicity is enhanced by certain underlying neuropathies, such as diabetic neuropathy and Charcot-Marie-Tooth disease.[49]

No effective treatment has been developed for the neurotoxicity except to stop vincristine therapy and wait for neurologic recovery. Depending on the severity of the neurologic dysfunction, recovery may take weeks or months to occur. Residual minor abnormalities sometimes persist indefinitely. Empiric vitamin therapy is ineffective. Intestinal dysfunction from autonomic neuropathy may be improved by metoclopramide use.[50]

Vincristine binds to the β-subunit of tubulin, causing disruption of microtubule function in neuronal axons. Electrophysiologic studies indicate distal axonal degeneration, and nerve conduction testing shows that sensory nerves are most affected with a reduced amplitude of nerve action potentials. Histologic changes are generally those of axonal degeneration.

The vincristine analog vinblastine also has potential for causing neurotoxicity, although it is less common, and the dose-limiting toxicity of vinblastine is myelosuppression, not neurotoxicity. The clinical manifestations are similar to those of vincristine. The degree of neurologic injury is related to both individual and cumulative doses.

CISPLATIN

Although nephrotoxicity is a major and cumulative dose-limiting toxicity for cisplatin, neurotoxicity is also a common toxicity and can be dose-limiting for both single and cumulative doses.[51-54] Cisplatin-induced neuropathy can be manifested as peripheral neuropathy, Lhermitte's sign,[55] autonomic neuropathy,[56] grand mal or focal seizures,[57] encephalopathy,[53] transient cortical blindness,[58] retrobulbar neuritis,[53] and retinal injury.[59]

The incidence ranges up to 50% but depends on individual and cumulative dose, duration of treatment, concomitant or prior neurotoxic drugs used, the presence of other medical conditions, and possibly gender (women being more sensitive).[51,52] If very high doses (200 mg/m^2 over 5 days) are used, the incidence rises to nearly 100%.[52] A cumulative cisplatin dose of 300 to 500 mg/m^2 raises the incidence significantly.[51,53]

Peripheral neuropathy similar to that induced by vincristine is the most common form of cisplatin neurotoxicity. Vincristine produces initial paresthesia in the fingers, while cisplatin most often affects the toes and feet.[54] Loss of the Achilles tendon reflexes is also an early sign, and continued treatment leads to loss of deep tendon reflexes at more proximal sites, loss of vibration sense, and sensory ataxia (from loss of sensation in the feet). Although muscle cramps are a common symptom, motor function is usually not affected.

The pathophysiology of the neurotoxicity is not known, but it may be related to the accumulation of inorganic platinum within neurons. Large sensory nerves are affected most and show axonal demyelination. Treatment is discontinuation of cisplatin, but the symptoms, particularly of the peripheral neuropathy, may take months to resolve, and may never resolve.[60] The symptoms and signs may even progress despite discontinuing treatment.[61] Because treatment of the neurotoxicity is of limited benefit, prevention has been explored using protective agents. Two investigational drugs, amifostine (WR 2721) and an adrenocorticotropic hormone analog called Org 2766, have demonstrated promise in delaying or preventing cisplatin neurotoxicity.[62,63]

CYTARABINE

This drug is administered both intravenously and intrathecally, and both routes produce neurotoxicity. The manifestations include cerebellar dysfunction, seizures, generalized encephalopathy, peripheral neuropathy, necrotizing leukoencephalopathy, spinal cord myelopathy, and pseudobulbar palsy.[64]

The highest incidence (15–37%) occurs in patients receiving high-dose therapy (*i.e.*, over 1 g/m^2 in multiple doses).[64,65] Generally, the toxicity is acute and not cumulative, in contrast to vincristine and cisplatin.

Cerebellar effects (dysarthria, ataxia, and dysmetria) are the most common form of neurotoxicity. These symptoms often occur within days of first treatment and are accompanied by somnolence, memory loss, altered mentation, and headache. Seizures have rarely occurred. These neurologic abnormalities can progress to coma and even death.

Peripheral neuropathy is rare. Symptoms range from a purely sensory neuropathy to sensorimotor polyneuropathies in a stocking-glove distribution.[64] Even this form of neurotoxicity can be severe and fatal,[66] by inducing a polyneuropathy causing flaccid paralysis and respiratory arrest.

Risk factors for neurotoxicity are age over 60, drug dose, prior cytarabine treatment, and renal dysfunction.[64,67] Although the risk for neurologic problems increases when high cytarabine doses are given to patients over age 60, it is not prohibitive, and older patients should be treated if indicated.[64]

Recovery from the neurologic effects usually occurs within a few days after discontinuing therapy. Most patients should probably not be retreated with cytarabine after recovery, unless special circumstances exist. There is no known therapy.

The mechanism of such neurologic toxicity is not known. Research suggests that cytarabine inhibits survival of neurons by blocking an essential deoxynucleoside[68] or by inducing production of large amounts of choline acetyltransferase enzyme.[69] Also unknown is why the cerebellum has a particular sensitivity to intravenous cytarabine. Intrathecal administration, which can cause myelopathy, spares the cerebellum in its toxic effect.

IFOSFAMIDE

Ifosfamide and cyclophosphamide have similar chemical structures, but ifosfamide induces neurotoxicity, while cyclophosphamide does not. Acute symptoms are hallucinations, vivid dreams, confusion, anxiety and restlessness, personality changes, seizures, cerebellar and cranial nerve dysfunction, hemiparesis, coma, and occasionally death.[70-72] The onset is a mean of 46 hours (and up to 5 days) after beginning ifosfamide,[70,71] and recovery usually occurs within a few days. Occasionally, memory and affect disorders may persist.[73] No cumulative-dose effects of ifosfamide on neural tissue have been reported.

The incidence has been reported to vary from 5% to 70%, depending on how carefully patients were monitored and results recorded.[70,71,73,74] The intensity of neurologic dysfunction is also variable, but an overall incidence of significant symptoms is 10% to 25%. The neurotoxicity is possibly due to high blood levels of a metabolite of ifosfamide, chloracetaldehyde.[75] It is not the uroprotective agent mesna.[70]

Factors that increase the risk of encephalopathy are low serum albumin, any degree of renal dysfunction, prior administration of cisplatin (resulting in subclinical renal abnormalities), and perhaps age. Giving ifosfamide in a 5-day continuous infusion appears to reduce the frequency of neurotoxicity.[76]

5-FLUOROURACIL

5-Fluorouracil (5-FU) has been known to cause neurotoxicity since the earliest clinical trials conducted with this drug.[77] Cerebellar dysfunction with findings of gait ataxia, nystagmus, dysmetria, and dysarthria is the most common form of neurotoxicity. Confusion and cerebral cognitive defects have also been reported.[78] A rare problem is optic neuropathy and decreased vision.[79]

The incidence is 5% to 10% and occurs with all schedules of administration in common use. This toxicity is acute in onset, and a cumulative-dose effect has not been observed.

The cause is not well understood. A 5-FU metabolite, fluorocitrate, was believed to induce the neurotoxicity,[80] but several patients have been reported who developed severe toxic symptoms due to an enzyme deficiency for metabolizing 5-FU.[81] This toxicity appears to be due to the parent compound and not metabolites. Patients with complete or partial deficiency of the enzyme, dihydropyrimidine dehydrogenase, appear particularly subject to 5-FU neurotoxicity.[81]

This neurotoxicity is usually reversible by discontinuing 5-FU. Since there is no cumulative effect, therapy can be resumed later if desired, usually with either a lower dose or a less frequent dosing schedule to prevent recurrence.

METHOTREXATE

Neurotoxicity from methotrexate drug can manifest as meningeal irritation, transient paraparesis, or encephalopathy.

When methotrexate is administered intrathecally, it can induce headache, nausea and vomiting, lethargy, nuchal rigidity, and other features of meningeal irritation.[82] A subacute set of abnormalities include paraparesis, cranial nerve palsies, and cerebellar symptoms, which can develop days to several weeks after therapy. If methotrexate is given repetitively, especially if it is administered through an intraventricular device, progressive necrotizing leukoencephalopathy may rarely develop. Symptoms include initial memory loss with later progression to severe dementia and seizures. Risk factors are cranial irradiation, presence of neoplastic cells in the spinal fluid, and cumulative dose.

Intravenous methotrexate also can produce encephalopathy, especially if cranial irradiation is used concomitantly or high methotrexate doses are given. The manifestations and risk factors are similar to those of intrathecal methotrexate. The neurologic dysfunction may be acute and transient with full recovery[83] or delayed in onset with personality changes.[84] The incidence varies from 5% to 15%. Neuroradiologic scans often show white matter abnormalities that are probably irreversible.[85]

The neurotoxic effect of methotrexate is probably a direct effect of high drug concentrations in the central nervous system. Neurotransmitter substance synthesis may be impeded by methotrexate.

PACLITAXEL (TAXOL)

This agent causes neurotoxicity similar to that of cisplatin and vincristine in the form of a peripheral neurotoxicity that can be a treatment-limiting effect.[86] The clinical manifestations are glove-stocking or perioral paresthesia, burning pain in the plantar surfaces of the feet, loss of vibration sense, loss of deep tendon reflexes, and orthostatic hypotension.[86,87] The symptoms may be greater than the degree of objective abnormalities found either on physical examination or by neurometric testing. Motor dysfunction is uncommon but has been severe when it occurs.[86] The onset of neurotoxicity can be rapid, with development of symptoms within a few days of receiving the drug.[87]

The neurotoxicity is both individual and cumulative dose-related.[86,88] Individual doses over 170 mg/m^2 and four or more courses are most often associated with neurotoxic manifestations. The incidence varies but has been reported to be as high as 25%.[87] Risk factors include the presence of preexisting alcoholic or diabetic neuropathy and the concomitant administration of cisplatin.[87,88] The mechanism of Taxol neurotoxicity is likely due to drug effect on neuronal and Schwann cell microtubules, causing axonal degeneration and demyelination. Neurometric testing demonstrates decreased nerve conduction velocities and absent sural nerve action potentials.[86,87] Sometimes abnormal test results are demonstrated in the absence of neurologic symptoms.

The only effective treatment, as with other neurotoxic drugs, is discontinuation of therapy. The symptoms usually resolve after a few months. Amitriptyline may help with symptomatic relief.

ALTRETAMINE (HEXAMETHYLMELAMINE)

This drug causes a variety of peripheral and central nervous system toxicities. Peripheral neuropathy is the most common form and manifests as paresthesia, hyperesthesia, hyporeflexia, and diminished proprioception.[89] Central nervous effects are confusion, dysphasia, personality changes, ataxia, somnolence, seizures, respiratory dyskinesia, and parkinsonian tremors.[89]

Neurotoxicity is related to both individual and cumulative doses. Intermittent dosing schedules help reduce this side effect. The incidence varies depending on the dose but can be as high as 40%.[89] Altretamine can be safely administered to patients who have been treated previously with cisplatin,[90] but not if significant cisplatin neuropathy is present.

Administration of pyridoxine has been used as neurotoxicity prophylaxis but has provided modest efficacy, and at least one study[91] suggested that pyridoxine can reduce antitumor effect. The most effective treatment is discontinuation of altretamine therapy. Symptoms, especially the severe ones, usually then resolve.

PROCARBAZINE

Neurotoxicity from this agent has been known since it was first used clinically.[92] Both central and peripheral neurotoxicity symptoms can occur. Cerebral symptoms predominate and consist of lethargy, depression, confusion, hallucinations, agitation, and rarely psychosis. Extremity paresthesia and depressed deep tendon reflexes are the manifestations of peripheral neuropathy.

Since this drug is most commonly used in combination with the vinca alkaloids, it is difficult to determine which agent is causing peripheral neuropathy symptoms. The incidence of neuropathy induced by procarbazine alone is 20% or less. It is much higher when procarbazine and vincristine are administered together.

Treatment is discontinuation of therapy. Cerebral symptoms usually resolve promptly, but peripheral neuropathy may last for weeks to months.

FLUDARABINE

When this agent was tested in phase I and II trials in acute leukemia, central nervous system toxicity was so severe that the studies had to be closed. Altered mental status, photophobia, amaurosis, generalized seizures, spastic or flaccid paralysis, quadriparesis, and coma occurred at doses over 90 mg/m² given for 5 to 7 days.[93,94] Despite discontinuing therapy, some patients had progressive neurologic abnormalities and died. Since such severe toxicity is clearly dose-related, the recommended fludarabine dose is 25 mg/m² daily for 5 days, monthly. Such doses usually cause no more than mild neurologic symptoms.[95] Even doses in this range, however, can occasionally cause severe, and even fatal, central nervous system toxicity.[94,96]

Fludarabine specifically affects the optic nerves and causes optic demyelination. It also can cause demyelination in the cerebral peduncles and pons.

OTHER AGENTS

Table 63–10 lists other drugs that can produce neurotoxicity and categorizes them based on the risk for this side effect. The manifestations are similar to those described for the individual drugs.

HEPATOTOXICITY

A number of antitumor agents cause hepatic injury (Table 63–11). This toxicity takes three main forms: hepatocellular dysfunction and chemical hepatitis, venoocclusive disease (VOD), and chronic fibrosis.

HEPATOCELLULAR DYSFUNCTION

This form of hepatic injury is usually due to a direct effect of either parent drug or a metabolite and is an acute event. Serum hepatic enzymes rise as cellular damage occurs. Fatty infil-

TABLE 63–10. Antitumor Agents That Cause Neurotoxicity

High Potential for Neurotoxicity

Altretamine	Interferons (in high doses)
L-Asparaginase	Methotrexate
Carboplatin	Pentostatin
Cisplatin	Procarbazine
Cytarabine	Suramin
Fludarabine	Taxol
5-Fluorouracil	Vincristine and vinblastine
Ifosfamide	

Occasional Irreversible Neurotoxicity

Cisplatin	Suramin
Cytarabine	Taxol
Ifosfamide	

Low Potential for Neurotoxicity

Amsacrine	Nitrosoureas
Dacarbazine	Teniposide
Etoposide	Thiotepa (intrathecal)
Interferons (in low doses)	

TABLE 63–11. Antitumor Agents That Cause Hepatotoxicity

High Potential for Hepatotoxicity

L-Asparaginase	Methotrexate (long-term therapy)
Cytarabine	Plicamycin (mithramycin)
Interferons (in high doses)	Streptozocin

High Potential for Hepatotoxicity With High Doses

Busulfan	Dactinomycin (in single doses)
Carmustine	Diaziquone
Cyclophosphamide	Methotrexate
Cytarabine	Mitomycin

Occasional Irreversible Hepatotoxicity

Azathioprine	Dacarbazine
Busulfan (in high doses)	Methotrexate
Carmustine (in high doses)	Mitomycin
Cytarabine	

Low Potential for Hepatotoxicity

Azathioprine	6-Mercaptopurine
Dacarbazine	Pentostatin
Hydroxyurea	6-Thioguanine
Interferons (in low doses)	Vincristine

tration and cholestasis may occur as the toxic effect progresses. Since hepatic metastases, viral hepatitis, and drugs administered for other therapeutic purposes (*e.g.*, antiemetics) can cause similar enzymatic abnormalities, the clinical picture, appropriate laboratory or radiologic studies, and the pattern of abnormal liver function tests must be analyzed to identify the cause of the hepatic changes.

The drugs most likely to cause enzymatic abnormalities are L-asparaginase, carmustine in high doses, cytarabine, dactinomycin, diaziquone, etoposide, azathioprine and 6-mercaptopurine, methotrexate in high doses, plicamycin (mithramycin), streptozocin, and vincristine. All these drugs can cause rises in the serum glutamic-oxaloacetic transaminase, serum glutamic pyruvate transaminase, and serum bilirubin, but the feature of azathioprine and 6-mercaptopurine toxicity is most often cholestatic jaundice.

L-Asparaginase causes the widest spectrum of liver abnormalities and has the highest incidence of toxicity. It produces changes in liver enzymes and in hepatic protein synthesis, resulting in low plasma levels of albumin, lipoproteins, and clotting factors.[97] Prolongation of the thrombin and prothrombin times occurs as a result. Fatty metamorphosis is commonly seen,[97] and these changes may persist for several months after discontinuing treatment.[98]

Cytarabine hepatotoxicity is a common event in the treatment of acute leukemia, especially when high doses are used.[99] Since patients with acute leukemia are subject to transfusion-related hepatitis and receive a variety of potentially hepatotoxic drugs, it is always difficult to establish cytarabine as the sole hepatotoxin. However, hyperbilirubinemia developing in temporal relation to cytarabine administration, accompanied by histologic abnormalities on liver biopsy, has demonstrated the hepatotoxicity potential of this agent.[100]

VENOOCCLUSIVE DISEASE

Venoocclusive liver disease results from blockage of venous outflow in the small centrilobular and sublobular hepatic vessels. Antitumor drugs known to produce this form of hepatotoxicity are azathioprine and 6-mercaptopurine, cytarabine, dacarbazine, and 6-thioguanine. In addition, busulfan, carmustine, cyclophosphamide, and mitomycin given in high doses can cause VOD.

Dactinomycin in combination with vincristine has been recognized to cause this severe hepatotoxicity, especially when dactinomycin is administered in single doses rather than over 5 days.[101] The clinical features are marked elevations in serum enzymes, ascites, hepatomegaly, and hepatic encephalopathy. The onset is often abrupt and the clinical course fulminant. In some cases, the histologic features are those of hepatic VOD, and in others, there is hepatocellular injury.[101]

Busulfan, carmustine, cyclophosphamide, and mitomycin all can produce hepatic VOD when they are administered in high doses for marrow transplantations. The incidence in transplantation settings is about 20%, and the mortality is high.[102,103] All the drugs reported to induce VOD at high doses have been alkylating agents. This may not be due to any unusual tendency of alkylating agents to cause VOD but rather to the fact that these are the drugs used in very large doses in marrow transplantation.

VOD is initiated by injury to hepatic venous endothelium, which then precipitates thrombosis and hepatocellular necrosis. There is probably also a component of hepatocellular injury directly related to the high-dose drug and not mediated by thrombosis.[103]

Conventional doses of certain antitumor agents (*e.g.*, dacarbazine, 6-mercaptopurine, 6-thioguanine) can also cause hepatic VOD. Dacarbazine has been recognized to have this toxicity most often, although only sporadic cases have been reported. Use of dacarbazine both alone and in combination with other drugs has been associated with hepatic VOD.[104] It is unknown why only some patients develop this life-threatening complication of dacarbazine, but a form of allergic or hypersensitivity reaction has been speculated as the mechanism.[105]

CHRONIC FIBROSIS

Methotrexate dosing schedules used for cancer treatment can produce acute and reversible hepatocellular injury and elevations of serum enzymes. Intermittent dosing seems to obviate chronic hepatic toxicity; however, long-term use of methotrexate for the treatment of nonmalignant disease (*e.g.*, psoriasis and rheumatoid arthritis) poses a greater hazard for development of hepatic fibrosis. Since patients with autoimmune diseases may already have underlying histologic abnormalities, there is controversy regarding how much hepatic damage methotrexate causes and whether periodic liver biopsies are necessary for patient monitoring.[106] It is clear, however, that a few patients suffer severe cirrhosis from this drug and require liver transplantation.[107]

HYPERSENSITIVITY REACTIONS

Most of the available antitumor drugs can produce hypersensitivity reactions, and a substantial minority cause such reactions in as many as 5% of patients treated. There are two agents for which hypersensitivity reactions are frequent enough to be a major treatment-limiting toxicity: L-asparaginase and Taxol. Most other agents produce such reactions only sporadically. The mechanism of these hypersensitivity reactions is often unknown or evaluated only in a single patient, and it is rarely possible to prevent them.

L-Asparaginase produces hypersensitivity reactions in 10% to 20% of patients, and it can be immediate and life-threatening with all the components of anaphylaxis. This high rate is undoubtedly related to the fact that L-asparaginase is a polypeptide of bacterial origin, displaying multiple antigenic sites.

The clinical manifestations are typical of type I reactions with acute onset of wheezing, pruritus, rash, angioedema, extremity pain, agitation, and hypotension.[97,108] A number of factors increase the risk for hypersensitivity reactions, including history of atopy or other drug allergy, prior L-asparaginase therapy (including even several years previously), high drug doses, and intravenous route of administration. Intramuscular administration often reduces the severity of reactions,[109] but they still can occur and may do so several hours after the drug is given. Concomitant treatment with prednisone and vincristine (for the acute leukemia being treated) also appears to reduce the risk of reactions.[108]

No reliable method has been developed to determine who is going to have a reaction with any dose of L-asparaginase. Intradermal skin testing can give both false-negative and false-positive results, and test doses of the drug are valueless.[108] Therefore, one must approach each dose of L-asparaginase as the one that could initiate a hypersensitivity reaction and be prepared to treat it. Antianaphylaxis medication must be close at hand, and the patient should be observed for about 1 hour after the drug is administered.

When a hypersensitivity reaction occurs with the *Escherichia coli* source of L-asparaginase, one can substitute the *Erwinia chrysanthemia* form and continue therapy. This form of drug is immunologically distinct[110] and appears to have a lower degree of immunogenicity. Patients may still sustain a hypersensitivity reaction from the *Erwinia* sp form, but most (75%) do not and can complete the planned therapy.[108] Precautions for treating anaphylaxis are as necessary for the *Erwinia* sp substitute as for the *E. coli* product. A third form of L-asparaginase has been developed that provides another alternative for the patient who is reactive to the other two forms and still needs L-asparaginase therapy. This form, a conjugate with polyethylene glycol (pegaspargase), may be the least immunogenic and has lower degrees of all toxicities.[111]

The mechanism of L-asparaginase reactions appears to be mediated by an immunoglobulin (Ig) E antibody in at least some cases.[112] There is also evidence that complement activation occurs, perhaps induced by specific IgG or IgM antibodies.[110]

Taxol is a newly approved drug that has high promise for being an effective addition to the oncologist's therapeutic arsenal. One of its toxicities has been hypersensitivity reactions, and it is standard procedure to administer drugs as prophylaxis for such reactions.[113]

The clinical manifestations are those of any type I hypersensitivity reaction and include bronchospasm and wheezing, rash, agitation, angioedema, and hypotension. These symptoms most often occur with the first or second drug exposure. The onset is usually within minutes of starting a drug infusion, and even very small drug doses are capable of initiating a hypersensitivity reaction.[113]

To prevent or assuage these reactions, Taxol is usually infused over 6 to 24 hours. In addition, premedication with corticosteroids and antihistamines is standard procedure. Such measures reduce the risk but do not fully prevent reactions.

It is unclear whether Taxol itself or the excipient, Cremophor EL, is the cause of hypersensitivity. Cremophor EL induces histamine release and could be responsible for acute reactions. The mechanism of these reactions has not been well studied, but the fact that they can occur with the first Taxol dose suggests a nonimmunologic one.

A number of other chemotherapeutic agents (Table 63–12) are known to produce hypersensitivity reactions in at least sporadic instances.[114] Most of these reactions have the features of a type I hypersensitivity, whether mediated by IgE or non-immunologically. Hemolytic anemia (type II reaction) is an uncommon form of toxicity.[18] Some drugs, such as procarbazine and methotrexate, produce acute episodes that are typical of a type III reaction and cause interstitial pneumonitis and vasculitis.[114] In most cases of hypersensitivity reactions from antitumor drugs, only isolated cases are studied adequately to define the cause of the reaction, and it is not possible to rule out the excipients used in drug formulation (*e.g.*, benzyl alcohol and dimethylacetamide) or other drugs used concomitantly (*e.g.*, mesna and mannitol) as the source of the reactivity.[114] When reactions occur from one drug, it is often possible to continue therapy by either substituting another drug in the same class or administering premedication as prophylaxis.

VASCULAR TOXICITY

Three main forms of vascular toxicity are produced by chemotherapeutic agents: VOD, venous or arterial thrombosis,

TABLE 63–12. Antitumor Agents That Cause Hypersensitivity Reactions

High Potential for Hypersensitivity Reactions

L-Asparaginase	Teniposide
Elliptinium	Taxol
Procarbazine	

Low Potential for Hypersensitivity Reactions

Anthracyclines	Ifosfamide
Azathioprine	Interferons
Bleomycin	Interleukin-2
Carboplatin	Mechlorethamine
Chlorambucil	Melphalan
Cisplatin	6-Mercaptopurine
Cyclophosphamide	Methotrexate
Cytarabine	Mitomycin
Dacarbazine	Mitoxantrone
Etoposide	Pentostatin
5-Fluorouracil	Vinca alkaloids
Hydroxyurea	

and vascular ischemia (involving cerebral, myocardial, or extremity arterial vessels).

VOD of the hepatic vein is discussed under the section on hepatotoxicity. This acute venous toxicity can also involve pulmonary vessels as a rare toxicity of chemotherapy.[115] It may be just one manifestation of pulmonary toxicity from such drugs as bleomycin and mitomycin.

Venous thrombosis in association with metastatic cancer has long been recognized (Trousseau's syndrome). Chemotherapeutic agents can also induce venous thrombosis in the form of extremity thromboses and pulmonary emboli, even in the absence of demonstrable metastatic cancer.[116,117] Although it is less common, thromboses of extremity arteries can also be initiated by chemotherapy, again in the absence of demonstrable cancer.[117,118] No one drug seems to be at fault, and the mechanism of thrombosis induction is unknown.

Arterial ischemia or thrombosis can be induced by chemotherapy in major coronary or cerebral vessels and in the small vessels of the extremities. Cerebrovascular accidents have been reported in association with the use of cisplatin and bleomycin in young men without other risk factors for such events.[119] In similar circumstances, acute myocardial infarction has occurred.[6,120] Myocardial ischemia and infarction occur in about 10% of patients who receive infusional 5-FU, and sudden death has occurred.[121] These events occur in patients who have no known underlying coronary vessel disease, and the pathogenesis seems to be coronary artery spasm. Anginal symptoms are often a precursor, which can be relieved by discontinuing the 5-FU therapy. Raynaud's phenomenon occurs as a chronic toxicity in about 40% of young men treated with cisplatin-based combination chemotherapy for testicular cancer.[6] Cigarette smoking increases the risk for this toxicity. Clinical manifestations are painful digits and paresthesia occurring a mean of 10 months after starting chemotherapy and lasting for 5 or more years. Patients often are unable to work outside in cold weather. The mechanism appears to be a vasospastic phenomenon, without any vascular obstruction, in the terminal arterioles due to impaired smooth muscle function.[122] It is not known which of the drugs used for testicular cancer is most involved in the cause of this toxicity, but bleomycin is the most likely candidate because it can cause Raynaud's phenomenon when used alone.[123]

REFERENCES

1. Rossof AH, Slayton RE, Perlia CP. Preliminary clinical experience with *cis*-diamminedichloroplatinum II (NSC 119875). Cancer 1972;30:1451–1456.
2. Talley RW, O'Bryan RM, Gutterman JU, et al. Clinical evaluation of toxic effects of *cis*-diamminedichloroplatinum (NSC-119875): Phase I clinical study. Cancer Chemother Rep 1973;57:465–471..
3. Hayes DM, Cvitkovic E, Golbey RB, et al. High dose cis-platinum diammine dichloride: Amelioration of renal toxicity by mannitol diuresis. Cancer 1977;39:1372–1381.
4. Hardaker WT, Stone RA, McCoy R. Platinum nephrotoxicity. Cancer 1974;34:1030–1032.
5. Tanaka H, Ishikawa E, Teshima S, et al. Histopathological study of human cisplatin nephropathy. Toxicol Pathol 1986;14:247–257.
6. Vogelzang NJ, Torkelson JL, Kennedy BJ. Hypomagnesemia, renal dysfunction, and Raynaud's phenomenon in patients treated with cisplatin, vinblastine, and bleomycin. Cancer 1985;56:2765–2770.
7. Hutchison FN, Perez EA, Gandara DR, et al. Renal salt wasting in patients treated with cisplatin. Ann Intern Med 1988;108:21–25.
8. Markman M, Rothman R, Reichman B, et al. Persistent hypomagnesemia following cisplatin chemotherapy in patients with ovarian cancer. J Cancer Res Clin Oncol 1991;117:89–90.
9. Leonard BJ, Eccleston E, Jones D, et al. Antileukaemic and nephrotoxic properties of platinum compounds. Nature 1971;234:43–45.

10. Hrushesky WJM. Circadian timing of cancer chemotherapy. Science 1985;228:73–74.

11. Hargis JB, Anderson JR, Propert KJ, et al. Predicting genitourinary toxicity in patients receiving cisplatin-based combination chemotherapy: A Cancer and Leukemia Group B study. Cancer Chemother Pharmacol 1992;30:291–296.

12. Mangioni C, Bolis G, Pecorelli S, et al. Randomized trial in advanced ovarian cancer comparing cisplatin and carboplatin. J Natl Cancer Inst 1989;81:1464–1471.

13. McDonald BR, Kirmani S, Vasquez M, et al. Acute renal failure associated with the use of intraperitoneal carboplatin: A report of two cases and review of the literature. Am J Med 1991;90:386–391.

14. Reed E, Jacob J. Carboplatin and renal dysfunction. Ann Intern Med 1989;110:409.

15. Sleijfer DT, Smit EF, Meijer S, et al. Acute and cumulative effects of carboplatin on renal function. Br J Cancer 1989;60:116–120.

16. Liu K, Mittelman A, Sproul EE, et al. Renal toxicity in man treated with mitomycin C. Cancer 1971;28:1314–1320.

17. Hanna WT, Krauss S, Regester RF, et al. Renal disease after mitomycin C therapy. Cancer 1981;48:2583–2588.

18. Doll DC, Weiss RB. Hemolytic anemia associated with antineoplastic agents. Cancer Treat Rep 1985;69:777–782.

19. Allum WH, Hallissey MT, Kelly KA for the British Stomach Cancer Group. Adjuvant chemotherapy in operable gastric cancer. Lancet 1989;1:571–574.

20. Lesesne JB, Rothschild N, Erickson B, et al. Cancer-associated hemolytic-uremic syndrome: Analysis of 85 cases from a national registry. J Clin Oncol 1989;7:781–789.

21. Chow S, Roscoe J, Cattran DC. Plasmapheresis and antiplatelet agents in the treatment of the hemolytic uremic syndrome secondary to mitomycin. Am J Kidney Dis 1986;7:407–412.

22. Korec S, Schein PS, Smith FP, et al. Treatment of cancer-associated hemolytic uremic syndrome with staphylococcal protein A immunoperfusion. J Clin Oncol 1986;4:210–215.

23. Cattell V. Mitomycin-induced hemolytic uremic kidney: An experimental model in the rat. Am J Pathol 1985;121:88–95.

24. Stoller RG, Jacobs SA, Drake JC, et al. Pharmacokinetics of high-dose methotrexate (NSC-740). Cancer Chemother Rep 1975;6:19–24, 1975.

25. Ackland SP, Schilsky RL: High-dose methotrexate: A critical reappraisal. J Clin Oncol 1987;5:2017–2031.

26. Goren MP, Wright RK, Horowitz ME, et al. Enhancement of methotrexate nephrotoxicity after cisplatin therapy. Cancer 1986;58:2617–2621.

27. Ellison NM, Servi RJ. Acute renal failure and death following sequential intermediate-dose methotrexate and 5-FU: A possible adverse effect due to concomitant indomethacin administration. Cancer Treat Rep 1985;69:342–343.

28. Thyss A, Kubar J, Milano G, et al. Clinical and pharmacokinetic evidence of a life-threatening interaction between methotrexate and ketoprofen. Lancet 1986;1:256–258.

29. Singh RR, Malaviya AN, Pandey JN, et al. Fatal interaction between methotrexate and naproxen. Lancet 1986;1:1390.

30. Thierry FX, Vernier I, Dueymes JM, et al. Acute renal failure after high-dose methotrexate therapy: Role of hemodialysis and plasma exchange in methotrexate removal. Nephron 1989;5:416–417.

31. Bouffet E, Frappaz D, Laville M, et al. Charcoal haemoperfusion and methotrexate toxicity. Lancet 1986;1:1497.

32. Loftus L, Cuppage FE, Hoogstraten B. Clinical and pathological effects of streptozotocin. J Lab Clin Med 1974;84:407–413.

33. Broder LE, Carter SK. Pancreatic islet cell carcinoma. II. Results of therapy with streptozotocin in 52 patients. Ann Intern Med 1973;79:108–118.

34. Tobin MV, Warenius HM, Morris AI. Forced diuresis to reduce nephrotoxicity of streptozotocin in the treatment of advanced metastatic insulinoma. Br Med J 1987;294:1128.

35. Ellis ME, Weiss RB, Kuperminc M. Nephrotoxicity of lomustine: A case report and literature review. Cancer Chemother Pharmacol 1985;15:174–175.

36. Focan C, Boossy J, Focan-Henrard D, et al. Phase II trial with high-dose ifosfamide and mesna given in a 24-h infusion for advanced GI tract cancer. Cancer Chemother Pharmacol 1989;23:192–193.

37. van Dyk JJ, Falkson HC, van der Merwe AM, et al. Unexpected toxicity in patients with iphosphamide. Cancer Res 1972;32:921–924.

38. Sangster G, Kaye SB, Calman KC, et al. Failure of 2-mercaptoethane sulphonate sodium (mesna) to protect against ifosfamide nephrotoxicity. Eur J Cancer Clin Oncol 1984;20:435–436.

39. Shore RW, Geary D, Koren G, et al. Iphosphamide (IP) related nephrotoxicity in children. Proc Am Soc Clin Oncol 1991;10:311.

40. Patterson WP, Khojasteh A. Ifosfamide-induced renal tubular defects. Cancer 1989;63:649–651.

41. Pratt CB, Meyer WH, Jenkins JJ, et al. Ifosfamide, Fanconi's syndrome, and rickets. J Clin Oncol 1991;9:1495–1499.

42. Parker GW, Wiltsie DS, Jackson CB. The clinical evaluation of PA-144 (mithramycin) in solid tumors of adults. Cancer Chemother Rep 1960;8:23–26.

43. Benedetti RG, Heilman KJ, Gabow PA. Nephrotoxicity following single dose mithramycin therapy. Am J Nephrol 1983;3:277–278.

44. Gradishar WJ, Vokes EE, Ni K. Chemotherapy-related hemolytic-uremic syndrome after the treatment of head and neck cancer: A case report. Cancer 1990;66:1914–1918.

45. Gardner G, Mesler D, Gitelman HJ. Hemolytic uremic syndrome following cisplatin, bleomycin, and vincristine chemotherapy: A report of a case and a review of the literature. Renal Failure 1989;11:133–137.

46. Weiden PL, Wright SE. Vincristine neurotoxicity. N Engl J Med 1972;286:1369–1370.

47. Weiss HD, Walker MD, Wiernik PH. Neurotoxicity of commonly used antineoplastic agents (second of two parts). N Engl J Med 1974;291:127–133.

48. Roca E, Bruera E, Politi PM, et al. Vinca alkaloid-induced cardiovascular autonomic neuropathy. Cancer Treat Rep 1985;69:149–151.

49. Griffiths JD, Stark RJ, Ding JC, et al. Vincristine neurotoxicity in Charcot-Marie-Tooth syndrome. Med J Aust 1985;143:305–306.

50. Garewal HS, Dalton WS. Metoclopramide in vincristine-induced ileus. Cancer Treat Rep 1985;69:1309–1311.

51. Gerritsen van der Hoop R, van der Burg MEL, ten Bokkel Huinink WW, et al. Incidence of neuropathy in 395 patients with ovarian cancer treated with or without cisplatin. Cancer 1990;66:1967–1702.

52. Legha SS, Dimery IW. High dose cisplatin administration without hypertonic saline: Observation of disabling neurotoxicity. J Clin Oncol 1985;3:1373–1378.

53. Cersosimo RJ. Cisplatin neurotoxicity. Cancer Treat Rev 1989;16:195–211.

54. Thompson SW, Davis LE, Kornfeld M, et al. Cisplatin neuropathy: Clinical, electro-physiologic, morphologic, and toxicologic studies. Cancer 1984;54:1269–1275.

55. Eeles R, Tait DM, Peckham MJ. Lhermitte's sign as a complication of cisplatin-containing chemotherapy for testicular cancer. Cancer Treat Rep 1986;70:905–907.

56. Cohen SC, Mollman JE. Cisplatin-induced gastric paresis. J Neurooncol 1987;5:237–240.

57. Mead GH, Arnold AM, Green JA, et al. Epileptic seizures associated with cisplatin administration. Cancer Treat Rep 1982;66:1719–1722.

58. Pippitt CH, Muss HB, Homesley HD, et al. Cisplatin-associated cortical blindness. Gynecol Oncol 1981;12:253–255.

59. Wilding G, Caruso R, Lawrence TS, et al. Retinal toxicity after high-dose cisplatin therapy. J Clin Oncol 1985;3:1683–1689.

60. Greenspan A, Treat J. Peripheral neuropathy and low dose cisplatin. Am J Clin Oncol (CCT) 1988;11:660–662.

61. Siegal T, Haim N. Cisplatin-induced peripheral neuropathy: Frequent off-therapy deterioration, demyelinating syndromes, and muscle cramps. Cancer 1990;66:1117–1123.

62. Mollman JE, Glover DJ, Hogan WM, et al. Cisplatin neuropathy: Risk factors, prognosis, and protection by WR 2721. Cancer 1988;61:2192–2195.

63. Gerritsen van der Hoop R, Vecht CJ, van der Burg MEL, et al. Prevention of cisplatin neurotoxicity with an ACTH (4–9) analogue in patients with ovarian cancer. N Engl J Med 1990;322:89–94.

64. Baker WJ, Royer GL, Weiss RB. Cytarabine and neurologic toxicity. J Clin Oncol 1991;9:679–693.

65. Graves T, Hooks MA. Drug-induced toxicities associated with high-dose cytosine arabinoside infusions. Pharmacotherapy 1989;9:23–28.

66. Nevill TJ, Benstead TJ, McCormick CW, et al. Horner's syndrome and demyelinating peripheral neuropathy caused by high-dose cytosine arabinoside. Am J Hematol 1989;32:314–315.

67. Damon LE, Mass R, Linker CA. The association between high-dose cytarabine neurotoxicity and renal insufficiency. J Clin Oncol 1989;7:1563–1568.

68. Wallace TL, Johnson EM. Cytosine arabinoside kills postmitotic neurons: Evidence that deoxycytidine may have a role in neuronal survival that is independent of DNA synthesis. J Neurosci 1989;9:115–124.

69. Patel AJ, Hunt A, Seaton P. The mechanism of cytosine arabinoside toxicity on quiescent astrocytes in vitro appears to be analogous to in vivo brain injury. Brain Res 1988;450:378–381.

70. Weiss RB. Ifosfamide vs cyclophosphamide in cancer therapy. Oncology (Williston Park) 1991;5:67–76.

71. Watkin SW, Husband DJ, Green JA, et al. Ifosfamide encephalopathy: A reappraisal. Eur J Cancer Clin Oncol 1989;25:1303–1310.

72. Merimsky O, Inbar M, Reider-Grosswasser I, et al. Ifosfamide-related acute encephalopathy: Clinical and radiological aspects. Eur J Cancer 1991;27:1188–1189.

73. Heim ME, Fiene R, Schick E, et al. Central nervous side effects following ifosfamide monotherapy of advanced renal carcinoma. J Cancer Res Clin Oncol 1981;10:113–116.

74. Pratt CB, Green AA, Horowitz ME, et al. Central nervous toxicity following treatment of pediatric patients with ifosfamide/mesna. J Clin Oncol 1986;4:1253–1261.

75. Goren MP, Wright RK, Pratt CB, et al. Dechloroethylation of ifosfamide and neurotoxicity. Lancet 1986;2:1219–1220.

76. Cerny T, Castiglione M, Brunner K, et al. Ifosfamide by continuous infusion to prevent encephalopathy. Lancet 1990;1:175.

77. Moertel CG, Reitemeier RJ, Bolton CF, et al. Cerebellar ataxia associated with fluorinated pyrimidine therapy. Cancer Chemother Rep 1964;41:15–18.

78. Lynch HT, Droszcz CP, Albano WA, et al. "Organic brain syndrome" secondary to 5-fluorouracil toxicity. Dis Colon Rectum 1981;24:130–131.

79. Adams JW, Bofenkamp TM, Kobrin J, et al. Recurrent acute toxic optic neuropathy secondary to 5-FU. Cancer Treat Rep 1984;68:565–566.

80. Koenig H, Patel A. Biochemical basis for fluorouracil neurotoxicity: The role of the Krebs cycle inhibition by fluoroacetate. Arch Neurol 1970;23:155–160.

81. Diasio RB, Beavers TL, Carpenter JT. Familial deficiency of dihydropyrimidine dehydrogenase: Biochemical basis for familial pyrimidinemia and severe 5-fluorouracil-induced toxicity. J Clin Invest 1988;81:47–51.

82. Nelson RW, Frank JT. Intrathecal methotrexate-induced neurotoxicities. Am J Hosp Pharm 1981;38:65–68.

83. Walker RW, Allen JC, Rosen G, et al. Transient cerebral dysfunction secondary to high-dose methotrexate. J Clin Oncol 1986;4:1845–1850.

84. Kramer ED, Lewis D, Raney B, et al. Neurologic complications in children with soft tissue and osseous sarcoma. Cancer 1989;64:2600–2603.

85. Lien HH, Blomlie V, Saeter G, et al. Osteogenic sarcoma: MR signal abnormalities of

the brain in asymptomatic patients treated with high-dose methotrexate. Radiology 1991;179:547–550.

86. Rowinsky EK, Cazenave LA, Donehower RC. Taxol: A novel investigational antimicrotubule agent. J Natl Cancer Inst 1990;82:1247–1259.

87. Lipton RB, Apfel SC, Dutcher JP, et al. Taxol produces a predominantly sensory neuropathy. Neurology 1989;39:368–373.

88. Rowinsky EK, Gilbert MR, McGuire WP, et al. Sequences of Taxol and cisplatin: A phase I and pharmacologic study. J Clin Oncol 1991;9:1692–1703.

89. Weiss RB. The role of hexamethylmelamine in advanced ovarian carcinoma treatment. Gynecol Oncol 1981;12:141–149.

90. Manetta A, MacNeill C, Lyter JA, et al. Hexamethylmelamine as a single second-line agent in ovarian cancer. Gynecol Oncol 1990;36:93–96.

91. Wiernik PH, Yeap B, Vogl E, et al. Hexamethylmelamine and low or moderate dose cisplatin with or without pyridoxine for treatment of advanced ovarian carcinoma: A study of the Eastern Cooperative Oncology Group. Cancer Invest 1992;10:1–9.

92. Brunner KW, Young CW. A methylhydrazine derivative in Hodgkin's disease and other malignant neoplasms: Therapeutic and toxic effects studied in 51 patients. Ann Intern Med 1965;63:69–86.

93. Warrell RP, Berman E. Phase I and II study of fludarabine phosphate in leukemia: Therapeutic efficacy with delayed central nervous system toxicity. J Clin Oncol 1986;4:74–79.

94. Chun HG, Leyland-Jones BR, Caryk SM, et al. Central nervous system toxicity of fludarabine phosphate. Cancer Treat Rep 1986;70:1225–1228.

95. Puccio CA, Mittelman A, Lichtman SM, et al. A loading/continuous infusion schedule of fludarabine phosphate in chronic lymphatic leukemia. J Clin Oncol 1991;9:1562–1569.

96. Merkel DE, Griffin NL, Kagen-Hallet K, et al. Central nervous system toxicity with fludarabine. Cancer Treat Rep 1986;70:1449–1450.

97. Oettgen HF, Stephenson PA, Schwartz MK, et al. Toxicity of E. coli L-asparaginase in man. Cancer 1970;25:253–278.

98. Pratt CB, Johnson WW. Duration and severity of fatty metamorphosis of the liver following L-asparaginase therapy. Cancer 1971;28:361–364.

99. Herzig RH, Wolff SN, Lazarus HM, et al. High-dose cytosine arabinoside therapy for refractory leukemia. Blood 1983;62:361–369.

100. Pizzuto J, Avilés A, Ramos E, et al. Cytosine arabinoside induced liver damage: Histopathologic demonstration. Med Pediatr Oncol 1983;11:287–290.

101. Green DM, Norkool P, Breslow NE, et al. Severe hepatic toxicity after treatment with vincristine and dactinomycin using single-dose or divided-dose schedules: A report from the National Wilms' Tumor Study. J Clin Oncol 1990;8:1525–1530.

102. Jones RJ, Lee KSK, Beschorner WE, et al. Venoocclusive disease of the liver following bone marrow transplantation. Transplantation 1987;44:778–783.

103. Rollins BJ. Hepatic veno-occlusive disease. Am J Med 1986;81:297–306.

104. Marsh JC. Hepatic vascular toxicity of dacarbazine (DTIC): Not a rare complication. Hepatology 1989;9:790–792.

105. Erichsen C, Jönsson PE. Veno-occlusive liver disease after dacarbazine therapy (DTIC) for melanoma. J Surg Oncol 1984;27:268–270.

106. Kaplan MM. Methotrexate hepatotoxicity and the premature reporting of Mark Twain's death: Both greatly exaggerated. Hepatology 1990;12:784–786.

107. Gilbert SC, Klintmaln G, Menter A, et al. Methotrexate-induced cirrhosis requiring liver transplantation in three patients with psoriasis. Arch Intern Med 1990;150:889–891.

108. Evans WE, Tsiatis A, Rivera G, et al. Anaphylactoid reactions of *Escherichia coli* and *Erwinia* asparaginase in children with leukemia and lymphoma. Cancer 1982;49:1378–1383.

109. Eden OB, Shaw MP, Lilleyman JS, et al. Non-randomized study comparing toxicity of *Escherichia coli* and *Erwinia* asparaginase in children with leukaemia. Med Pediatr Oncol 1990;18:497–502.

110. Fabry U, Körholz D, Jürgens H, et al. Anaphylaxis to L-asparaginase during treatment for acute lymphoblastic leukemia in children–evidence of a complement-mediated mechanism. Pediatr Res 1985;19:400–408.

111. Kurtzberg J, Friedman H, Asselin B, et al. The use of polyethylene glycol conjugated L-asparaginase (PEG-ASP) in pediatric patients with prior hypersensitivity to native L-asparaginase. Proc Am Soc Clin Oncol 1990;9:219.

112. Khan A, Hill JM. Atopic hypersensitivity to L-asparaginase: Resistance to immunosuppression. Int Arch Allergy 1971;40:463–469.

113. Weiss RB, Donehower RH, Wiernik PH, et al. Hypersensitivity reactions from Taxol. J Clin Oncol 1990;8:1263–1268.

114. Weiss RB. Hypersensitivity reactions. Semin Oncol 1992;19:458–477.

115. Joselson R, Warnock M. Pulmonary veno-occlusive disease after chemotherapy. Hum Pathol 1983;14:88–91.

116. Weiss RB, Tormey DC Holland JF, et al. Venous thrombosis during multimodal therapy of primary breast carcinoma. Cancer Treat Rep 1981;65:677–679.

117. Saphner T, Tormey DC, Gray R. Venous and arterial thrombosis in patients who received adjuvant therapy for breast cancer. J Clin Oncol 1991;9:286–294.

118. Wall JG, Weiss RB, Norton L, et al. Arterial thrombosis associated with adjuvant chemotherapy for breast carcinoma: A Cancer and Leukemia Group B study. Am J Med 1989;87:501–504.

119. Doll DC, List AF, Greco FA, et al. Acute arterial ischemic events following cisplatin-based combination chemotherapy for germ cell tumors of the testis. Ann Intern Med 1986;105:48–51.

120. Samuels BL, Vogelzang NJ, Kennedy BJ. Severe vascular toxicity associated with vinblastine, bleomycin, and cisplatin chemotherapy. Cancer Chemother Pharmacol 1987;19:253–256.

121. Gradishar WJ, Vokes EE. 5-fluorouracil cardiotoxicity: A critical review. Ann Oncol 1990;1:409–414.

122. Hansen SW, Olsen N, Rossing N, et al. Vascular toxicity and the mechanism underlying Raynaud's phenomenon in patients treated with cisplatin, vinblastine and bleomycin. Ann Oncol 1990;1:289–292.

123. Epstein E. Intralesional bleomycin and Raynaud's phenomenon. J Am Acad Dermatol 1991;24:785–786.

SECTION 3

McCLELLAN M. WALTHER

Cystitis

Cystitis, defined symptomatically as an irritation of the bladder, manifests itself with suprapubic discomfort, frequency, dysuria, and urgency. Severe cases may include urge incontinence and hematuria. The cause may be related to a chemical agent that is toxic to the bladder, radiation, thrombocytopenia with subsequent bleeding, or myelosuppression with associated infection. Patients may present with acute exsanguinating hematuria (discussed in Chapter 50, section 5) but more commonly develop milder symptoms and pathologic disease.

General measures taken in the initial evaluation of patients with cystitis should exclude urinary infection and the presence of malignancy. Symptomatic relief of discomfort on voiding can be obtained with urinary analgesics such as phenazopyridine hydrochloride (Pyridium). Suprapubic discomfort, frequency, urgency, and urge incontinence require antispasmodics to obtain relief. Oxybutynin chloride (Ditropan), propantheline bromide (Pro-banthine), hyoscyamine sulfate (Cysto-spaz, Levsin), and flavoxate hydrochloride (Urispas) are used for this purpose. Combinations of drugs, sometimes including antiseptics, are often helpful. These include methenamine, methylene blue, phenyl salicylate, benzoic acid, atropine sulfate, and hyoscyamine (Urised); phenazopyridine, hyoscyamine, and butabarbital (Pyridium Plus); and sulfisoxazole and phenazopyridine (Azo Gantrisin). Severe symptoms may require belladonna and opium rectal suppositories. Treatment measures unique to each cause are discussed next.

CHEMICAL CYSTITIS

OXAZAPHOSPHORINES

Cyclophosphamide (Cytoxan), the most commonly used oxazaphosphorine, is an alkylating agent first used in the treatment of malignant tumors in Europe in 1957. Cyclophosphamide has a role in the treatment of solid tumors and lymphomas as well as benign inflammatory states, most commonly Wegener's granulomatosis and rheumatoid arthritis. Other oxazaphosphorines—ifosfamide, trofosfamide, and sufosfamide—have been used since the 1970s for the treatment of solid malignancies and lymphomas. Dose-limiting toxicity with these compounds is usually urinary tract toxicity.

After treatment with these compounds, urinary symptoms (frequency, urgency, dysuria, and nocturia) develop in as many as 24% of patients treated with oral cyclophosphamide.[1] Microhematuria occurs in 7% to 53% of patients, and gross hematuria occurs in 0.6% to 15% of patients.[1-3] Gross hematuria can range from lightly stained urine to exsanguinating hemorrhage. Symptoms usually occur soon after cyclophosphamide is given but may occur years later.[2] Prolonged use can lead to chronic fibrosis or hemorrhage. Malignant lesions, usually transitional cell carcinoma, occur in 2% to 5% of patients who receive oral cyclophosphamide for nonmalignant disease.[1,4] The entire urothelium can be effected, but the bladder is the most frequently involved area.

Bladder pathology has been attributed to toxic metabolites of these compounds. Cyclophosphamide is broken down by hepatic microsomal cells to hydroxycyclophosphamide, then by target cells to aldophosphamide, and then to phosphoramide mustard, the active antineoplastic metabolite, and acrolein, which has no significant antitumor activity.[5-7] Similarly, ifosfamide is metabolized to ifosforamide mustard and acrolein.[6] Urinary excretion of acrolein is believed to be the major source of urothelial toxicity.[6] Most normal cells are able to break down the toxic metabolites and diminish their effect. Glutathione is a naturally occurring thiol that can confer such protection in most cells, but it is present in low levels in urine.[5] Oxazaphosphorine toxicity has been demonstrated in several animal models with systemic administration and by instillation of normal metabolic products directly into the bladder.[8,9] Urine from animals given these agents, when placed in other animal bladders, reproduces these findings, while instillation of cyclophosphamide does not.[9,10] Electron microscopy suggests that the initial toxic effect is disruption of the plasma membrane and cytoplasmic matrix.[11]

Bladder damage from these compounds is cumulative and is generally dose-related. Cyclophosphamide-induced cystitis occurs frequently and early after intravenous therapy, especially dose-intensive regimens. Cystitis usually takes weeks to develop after oral treatment but has been seen after as little as one dose.[12] Fibrosis has been found in as many as 25% of children receiving high-dose cyclophosphamide.[13] Severe hematuria and telangiectasia are more common in these patients.[13] Oxazaphosphorine-induced cystitis is potentiated by prior pelvic irradiation.[2,14]

Laboratory values reveal normal coagulation profiles, normal platelet count, and negative urine culture. Because these patients are at risk for developing urothelial malignancies, these episodes of cystitis and hematuria must be evaluated judiciously. Initial evaluation includes urinalysis and urine cytology. Patients receiving cyclophosphamide develop markedly abnormal urinary cytologic analyses demonstrating marked atypia, increased nuclear size, and bizarrely shaped cytoplasm, which frequently resolves with cessation of the drug.[15] These findings can be suggestive of malignancy and need to be interpreted with caution.[16] Patients who have abnormal urinary cytology that has not been investigated previously should undergo a thorough urologic evaluation. Cystoscopy may reveal a tumor or changes compatible with cyclophosphamide-induced cystitis. Acutely diffuse inflammation is seen. Chronic changes include a pale bladder mucosa with telangiectasia. Areas of edema can be present with patchy hemorrhagic areas that stain with methylene blue, an indicator of mucosal injury.[8] Biopsy specimens reveal hyperemia, hemorrhage, edema, mucosal thinning, and ulceration of the urothelium. Necrosis of mucosa, muscle, and small arterioles and telangiectasia can be present.[8,10,11] Atypia can be prominent, and abundant mitoses often occur.[10,11,15] These finding are similar to those seen after radiation therapy.

Hemorrhagic cystitis is managed by stopping or reducing the drug. Replacing the drug, usually with azathioprine, is necessary in as many as one third of patients who develop severe cystitis.[17] Hydration and diuresis are routinely used to dilute the metabolites in the urine and minimize their toxicity.[7] Because high-dose oxazaphosphorines cause accumulation of free water, patients can develop fluid overload with hyponatremia, seizures, or death if furosemide is not used.[18,19] Potassium levels need to be followed in patients on this regimen. The cystitis usually improves within several days after cessation of the drug but occasionally persists for months. Patients receiving high doses of oxazaphosphorines require additional measures to counter the effects.[19] Bladder irrigation is helpful in many of these patients.[20]

Development of drugs that can neutralize the toxic metabolites has been an important addition to treatment of cyclophosphamide-induced cystitis. Sodium 2-mercaptoethane sulfonate (mesna) was designed to function in the urinary tract to detoxify oxazaphosphorine metabolites with urothelial toxicity. Mesna is a sulfhydryl compound that is administered intravenously and rapidly excreted by the urinary tract. After intravenous administration, mesna undergoes oxidation, forming disulfide bonds and making an unreactive dimer (dimesna). One concern regarding such a class of drugs is that they might effect the antineoplastic properties of oxazaphosphorines. Mesna and dimesna are hydrophilic and do not normally penetrate cells, explaining their antineoplastic-sparing effect.[7] The unreactive form, dimesna, is filtered by the kidneys and undergoes tubular reabsorption, where one third of it is reduced to its active form, mesna, by glutathione reductase.[7] In the urinary tract, the sulfhydryl group of mesna complexes with the terminal methyl group of acrolein, joining the compound to the double bond of acrolein and forming a nontoxic thioether.[7] The presence of mesna also inhibits spontaneous breakdown of cyclophosphamide to acrolein in the urine.[21] In addition to decreasing chemical cystitis, the risk of bladder cancer is significantly reduced when mesna is used in the Sprague-Dawley rat model.[22] This is an important argument for its use whenever possible.

Oral mesna is well absorbed but slow to achieve adequate urinary concentrations. It has an unpleasant taste, which makes patient tolerance poor, particularly when there is concomitant administration of a chemotherapy that induces nausea.[5] Mesna is best given intravenously, and the manufacturer recommends three doses. A loading dose equivalent to 20% (wt/wt) of the ifosfamide dose, given 15 minutes before the ifosfamide, is followed by two similar doses 4 and 8 hours after the ifosfamide.[7] Doses as high as 60% to 120% (wt/wt) have been used with cyclophosphamide, given at a similar schedule. The timing of dosages of mesna is important because the half-life of mesna is 35 minutes, while that of cyclophosphamide is 4 hours.[7,23] Mesna toxicity is minimal, and its major side effects are diarrhea, headache, and limb pain.[5]

Another thiol compound, *N*-acetyl cysteine (NAC), has been used less extensively to ameliorate the effects of oxazaphosphorines. Animal data demonstrate that the bladder is protected when given at a dose of 1:1 (wt/wt) with cyclophosphamide in a similar schedule as mesna.[24] Problems with NAC include a wide distribution in the body, with low urinary levels. High intravenous doses or intravesical administration are required to reach effective concentrations.[25] Conflicting data concerning impairment of antitumor activity have not been resolved.

BONE MARROW TRANSPLANTATION

Hemorrhagic cystitis occurs in about 2% of conditioning regimens that do not contain cyclophosphamide and is frequently related to thrombocytopenia.[14] The incidence of hemorrhagic cystitis in regimens with cyclophosphamide is 13% to 56%.[14,26,27] Prior cyclophosphamide, radiation, urethral catheterization, infection (bacterial or previous viral), concurrent medication, or coagulation disorders (thrombocytopenia) can all contribute to the development of hemorrhagic cystitis in these patients. Prior administration of busulfan, an alkyl sulfonate, increases the risk of hemorrhagic cystitis to as high as 36%, compared with 4% in patients receiving the same regimen without prior exposure.[26] Concomitant use of these agents is associated with hemorrhagic cystitis in 0.5% to 50% of patients.[14,27,28]

Several viruses have been implicated in the cause of hemorrhagic cystitis in patients undergoing bone marrow transplantation, either as viral reactivation or a new infection. These include polyma (BK) virus[14,29]; adenovirus, especially adenovirus 11[29,30]; papovavirus; influenza A; and cytomegalovirus.[27,29] Patients in whom viral particles were recovered developed hematuria later after transplantation (55 days)[29] than did patients with so-called idiopathic hemorrhagic cystitis (25–27 days).[14] The viral type also had a longer duration than idiopathic cystitis.[29,30]

It has been recommended patients receiving the combination of cyclophosphamide and busulfan should receive continuous bladder irrigation during treatment.[27] Prophylactic treatment with mesna is efficacious and does not appear to effect engraftment.[31] A dose of 60% (wt/wt) has been adequate in children, but adults appear to require a higher dose (120–160% [wt/wt]).[31]

INTRAVESICAL CHEMOTHERAPY

Intravesical treatment of superficial bladder tumors with chemotherapeutic agents or biologic modifiers may cause chemical cystitis or an inflammatory response with marked symptoms. Several agents are commonly employed. Thiotepa is well tolerated, although 2% to 49% of patients experience cystitis[32,33] and about one third develop hematuria.[32] One third of patients receiving epodyl[33] and 26% to 50% of patients receiving doxorubicin develop cystitis.[33,34] Mitomycin C is best tolerated, with 6% to 33% of patients developing cystitis and one third developing hematuria.[32–34] Most hematuria is microscopic. Significant hemorrhagic cystitis is uncommon with any of these agents. Bladder contractures have rarely been reported in patients receiving thiotepa or mitomycin.

Most patients receiving bacillus Calmette-Guérin develop irritative voiding symptoms, which can be the most severe of all intravesical treatments. Biopsy specimens from these patients reveal acute and chronic inflammatory changes and granuloma formation. Urinary analgesics and antispasmodics are particularly helpful in this group. If symptoms are prolonged, isoniazid and acetaminophen or ibuprofen are given until symptoms resolve. It is uncommon for treatment regimens to be stopped because of toxicity.[35]

OTHER

Other chemotherapeutic regimens that do not include agents with known bladder toxicity appear to be able to induce cystitis and hematuria without associated thrombocytopenia.[36] The mechanism in these patients is not clear, although bleomycin has been suggested to be the culprit.[36,37]

Busulfan, an alkyl sulfonate used in the treatment of chronic granulocytic leukemia, has also been reported as a cause of hemorrhagic cystitis.[26,38] As many as 16% of patients in regimens with intravenous busulfan, and without cyclophosphamide, develop hemorrhagic cystitis.[14] Cystoscopy in these patients reveals generalized inflammation and edema. Biopsy specimens demonstrate metaplastic changes in the urothelium, submucosal inflammation, and telangiectasia.[38] Cystoscopic and histologic findings are similar to those for radiation or oxazaphosphorine cystitis. Bladder malignancies have not been associated with busulfan. Given orally, a cumulative dose of 2 to 5 kg appears necessary to induce these changes.[38,39] Stopping the drug and alleviation of irritative symptoms are the primary treatment.

INTRAVESICAL PHOTOTHERAPY

Treatment of superficial bladder tumors with phototherapy was first performed by Kelly and Snell in 1975. Treatment involves administration of an intravenous photosensitizer (usually a hematoporphyrin derivative), waiting 2 days, and then activation of the compound with light. The time lag allows preferential retention of sensitizer by tumor, with normal tissue levels decreasing, thus increasing the therapeutic index. An optical fiber placed in the bladder through a cystoscope transmits light to activate the sensitizer. Patients whose entire bladder mucosa is illuminated develop marked bladder irritation with suprapubic discomfort, urgency, and urge incontinence. Symptoms can be surprisingly mild the first day after activation but peak on the second or third day. Symptoms improve quickly and usually resolve after 4 to 6 weeks. Cystoscopy initially reveals exuberant local reaction and edema.[40] Biopsy specimens initially reveal coagulative necrosis and hemorrhage.[40] Later, acute and chronic inflammation and atypia are present.[41] The acute response can resolve with little residual effect visually apparent. Bladder fibrosis and reflux are unpredictable side effects of this therapy. Treatment of the acute symptoms includes drainage with a Foley catheter to put the bladder to rest and B&O suppositories to control bladder discomfort.

RADIATION

Patients undergoing primary radiation therapy of malignant pelvic tumors, most commonly uterine, bladder, and prostate neoplasms, can suffer direct or incidental damage to the bladder. The risk is increased when urinary infection is present or radiation therapy is repeated, when high-dose radiation therapy is given, or when surgery has been performed in the area. Cyclophosphamide, given systemically in combination with pelvic irradiation, greatly increases the risk for radiation cystitis.[42]

In the first 4 to 6 weeks after treatment, an acute inflammatory response with resultant irritative symptoms or hematuria develops. Mild symptoms occur in as many as 50% to 82% of patients and generally do not require medication.[43,44] Hemorrhagic cystitis can occur later, even years after successful treatment,[44] and frequently is associated with tumor recurrence.[45] The time between treatment and development of delayed symptoms (frequency, dysuria, and hematuria), is proportional to the dose received.[44] Patients with late cystitis develop bladder ulcers, bladder fibrosis, and ureteral strictures. These patients require thorough evaluation because they are at increased risk for developing transitional cell carcinoma of the bladder. Bladder biopsies should be done sparingly because the bladder mucosa heals poorly.

Some 3.7% of patients receiving intravaginal intracavitary irradiation alone (3200 cGy) for stage I endometrial carcinoma, after transabdominal hysterectomy and bilateral salpingo-oophorectomy, develop cystitis.[46] When external-beam irradiation (4000–5400 cGy) is added, 4% to 6.5% of patients develop cystitis.[46,47] Patients undergoing definitive radiation treatment of cervical carcinoma have a risk of cystitis that is dose-related.[45,48] At doses less than 6000 cGy, the development of cystitis has been strongly linked to recurrent tumor.[45] The incidence of cystitis in this group is 2.8% to 8%.[44,49,50] From 1.2% to 18% of patients receiving external-beam irradiation (3000–8500 cGy) for bladder cancer developed cystitis,[45,51,52] 8% hematuria,[45] and 5% a contracted bladder.[52] Chronic cystitis develops in 15% of patients. Radiation therapy to the prostate (5000–7200 cGy) and draining of the lymph nodes (5000 cGy) for cure of prostate cancer elicits dysuria and mild to moderate hematuria in 18% to 40% of patients.[53,54] Of these patients, 0.8% to 8.3% develop severe dysuria or hematuria, and 3.4% to 9% develop strictures or urethral obstruction as a delayed presentation.[53–55]

During the acute phase, cystoscopy reveals edema, erythema, and increased vascularity, which can be associated with a mild decrease in bladder capacity. Later, the bladder is pale, and telangiectasia is present. Focal areas of hyperemia and bullous edema may be present. Often, there is no focal area of bleeding. With extensive damage, necrosis and calcification can occur. Biopsy findings are dose- and time-dependent. In the first 24 hours, there is erythema due to hyperemia. This develops into a diffuse inflammatory response with hyperemia, edema, lymphocytic infiltration, and degeneration of the urothelium with atypia.[43,44,56] Shallow ulcers are occasionally seen but usually occur as a late response. This response lasts up to 4 months after therapy.[57] Later, sclerosing endarteritis, fibrosis, and atrophy occur. There may be edema and an inflammatory infiltrate. There can be ulceration, and healing is poor.[52,57,58] Treatment is symptomatic.

ANTIBIOTICS

Although most cystitis seen in the setting of oncologic care is related to antineoplastic agents, penicillins used in the treatment of chemotherapy-related infections represent another source. Methicillin, nafcillin, ticarcillin, piperacillin, carbenicillin, and penicillin G have all been implicated. The incidence of cystitis associated with the use of these agents is small, occurring in 4% to 8% of patients.[59] Symptoms are typical of cystitis. Laboratory investigation reveals eosinophilia, pyuria, hematuria, proteinuria, and negative urine cultures. The submucosal deposition of C3, IgG and IgM, and dimethoxyphenylpenicilloyl, a methicillin antigen, supports a hypersensitivity cause.[59–61] A diffuse hemorrhagic cystitis is seen at cystoscopy.[60] Biopsy specimens show an intense inflammatory reaction with erosion.[62] With repeated use, the time to development of symptoms shortens. Symptoms usually resolve promptly on cessation of the drug or substitution with an unrelated drug.[60,61]

REFERENCES

1. Stillwell TJ, Benson RC Jr, DeRemee RA, McDonald TJ, Weiland LH. Cyclophosphamide-induced bladder toxicity in Wegener's granulomatosis. Arthritis Rheum 1988;31:465–470.
2. Stillwell TJ, Benson RC Jr, Burgert EO Jr. Cyclophosphamide-induced hemorrhagic cystitis in Ewing's sarcoma. J Clin Oncol 1988;6:76–82.
3. Lawrence HJ, Simone J, Aur RJ. Cyclophosphamide-induced hemorrhagic cystitis in children with leukemia. Cancer 1975;36:1572–1576.
4. Fairchild WV, Spence CR, Solomon HD, Gangai MP. The incidence of bladder cancer after cyclophosphamide therapy. J Urol 1979;122:163–164.
5. Shaw IC, Graham MI. Mesna: A short review. Cancer Treat Rev 1987;14:67–86.
6. Cox PJ. Cyclophosphamide cystitis: Identification of acrolein as the causative agent. Biochem Pharmacol 1979;28:2045–2049.
7. Schoenike SE, Dana WJ. Ifosfamide and mesna. Clin Pharm 1990;9:179–191.
8. Chaviano AH, Gill WB, Ruggiero KJ, Vermeulen CW. Experimental Cytoxan cystitis and prevention by acetylcysteine. J Urol 1985;134:598–600.
9. Brock N, Pohl J, Stekar J. Detoxification of urotoxic oxazaphosphorines by sulfhydryl compounds. J Cancer Res Clin Oncol 1981;100:311–320.
10. Philips FS, Sternberg SS, Cronin AP, Vidal PM. Cyclophosphamide and urinary bladder toxicity. Cancer Res 1961;21:1577–1589.
11. Koss LG. A light and electron microscopic study of the effects of a single dose of cyclophosphamide on various organs in the rat. I. The urinary bladder. Lab Invest 1967;16:44–65.
12. Host H, Nissen-Meyer R. A preliminary clinical study of cyclophosphamide. Cancer Chemother Rep 1960;9:47–50.
13. Johnson WW, Meadows DC. Urinary-bladder fibrosis and telangiectasia associated with long-term cyclophosphamide therapy. N Engl J Med 1971;284:290–294.
14. Brugieres L, Hartmann O, Travagli JP, et al. Hemorrhagic cystitis following high-dose chemotherapy and bone marrow transplantation in children with malignancies: Incidence, clinical course, and outcome. J Clin Oncol 1989;7:194–199.
15. Forni AM, Koss LG, Geller W. Cytological study of the effect of cyclophosphamide on the epithelium of the urinary bladder in man. Cancer 1964;17:1348–1355.
16. Liedberg CF, Rausing A, Langeland P. Cyclophosphamide hemorrhagic cystitis. Scand J Urol Nephrol 1970;4:183–190.
17. Fauci AS, Haynes BF, Katz P, Wolff SM. Wegener's granulomatosis: Prospective clinical and therapeutic experience with 85 patients for 21 years. Ann Intern Med 1983;98:76–85.
18. Green TP, Mirkin BL. Prevention of cyclophosphamide-induced antidiuresis by furosemide infusion. Clin Pharmacol Ther 1981;29:634–642.
19. Droller MJ, Saral R, Santos G. Prevention of cyclophosphamide-induced hemorrhagic cystitis. Urology 1982;20:256–258.
20. Blume KG, Beutler E, Bross KJ, et al. Bone-marrow ablation and allogeneic marrow transplantation in acute leukemia. N Engl J Med 1980;302:1041–1046.
21. Brock N, Stekar J, Pohl J, Niemeyer U, Scheffler G. Acrolein, the causative factor of urotoxic side-effects of cyclophosphamide, ifosfamide, trofosfamide and sufosfamide. Arzneimittelforschung 1979;29:659–661.

22. Petru E, Schmahl D. Anticancer drugs: Second malignancies—risk reduction. Cancer Treat Rev 1987;14:337–343.

23. Schumacher MM, Dowd AL, eds. Physician's desk reference: Cytoxan. Oradell, NJ: ER Barnhart, 1991;723–725.

24. Tolley DA. The effect of N-acetyl cysteine on cyclophosphamide cystitis. Br J Urol 1977;49:659–661.

25. Ormstad K, Ohno Y. N-acetylcysteine and sodium 2-mercaptoethane sulfonate as sources of urinary thiol groups in the rat. Cancer Res 1984;44:3797–3800.

26. Thomas AE, Patterson J, Prentice HG, et al. Haemorrhagic cystitis in bone marrow transplantation patients: Possible increased risk associated with prior busulfan therapy. Bone Marrow Transplant 1987;1:347–355.

27. Atkinson K, Biggs J, Noble G, Ashby M, Concannon A, Dodds A. Preparative regimens for marrow transplantation containing busulfan are associated with haemorrhagic cystitis and hepatic veno-occlusive disease but a short duration of leucopenia and little oropharyngeal mucositis. Bone Marrow Transplant 1987;2:385–394.

28. Nevill TJ, Barnett MJ, Klingemann HG, Reece DE, Shepherd JD, Phillips GL. Regimen-related toxicity of a busulfan-cyclophosphamide conditioning regimen in 70 patients undergoing allogeneic bone marrow transplantation. J Clin Oncol 1991;9:1224–1232.

29. Arthur RR, Shah KV, Baust SJ, Santos GW, Saral R. Association of BK viruria with hemorrhagic cystitis in recipients of bone marrow transplants. N Engl J Med 1986;315:230–234.

30. Miyamura K, Takeyama K, Kojima S, et al. Hemorrhagic cystitis associated with urinary excretion of adenovirus type 11 following allogeneic bone marrow transplantation. Bone Marrow Transplant 1989;4:533–535.

31. Blacklock H, Ball L, Knight C, Schey S, Prentice G. Experience with mesna in patients receiving allogeneic bone marrow transplants for poor prognostic leukaemia. Cancer Treat Rev 1983;10:45–52.

32. Heney NM, Koontz WW, Barton B, et al. Intravesical thiotepa versus mitomycin C in patients with Ta, T1 and TIS transitional cell carcinoma of the bladder: A phase III prospective randomized study. J Urol 1988;140:1390–1393.

33. Lamm D. Intravesical therapy of superficial bladder cancer. AUA Update Series 1983;2:2–7.

34. Herr H, Laudone VP. Intravesical therapy for superficial bladder cancer. AUA Update Series 1989;8:90–95.

35. Lamm DL, Stogdill VD, Stogdill BJ, Crispen RG. Complications of bacillus Calmette-Guerin immunotherapy in 1,278 patients with bladder cancer. J Urol 1986;135:272–274.

36. Cantwell BM, Harris AL, Patrick D, Hall RR. Hemorrhagic cystitis after IV bleomycin, vinblastine, cisplatin, and etoposide for testicular cancer. Cancer Treat Rep 1985;70:548–549.

37. Creagan ET, Ahmann DL, Schutt AJ, Green SJ. Phase II study of the combination of vinblastine, bleomycin, and cisplatin in advanced malignant melanoma. Cancer Treat Rep 1982;66:567–569.

38. Pode D, Perlberg S, Steiner D. Busulfan-induced hemorrhagic cystitis. J Urol 1983;130:347–348.

39. Millard RJ. Busulfan-induced hemorrhagic cystitis. Urology 1981;18:143–144.

40. Benson RC, Kinsey JH, Cortese DA, Farrow GM, Utz DC. Treatment of transitional cell carcinoma of the bladder with hematoporphyrin derivative phototherapy. J Urol 1983;130:1090–1095.

41. Prout GR, Lin CW, Benson R, et al. Photodynamic therapy with hematoporphyrin derivative in the treatment of superficial transitional cell carcinoma of the bladder. N Engl J Med 1987;317:1251–1255.

42. Jayalakshmamma B, Pinkel D. Urinary-bladder toxicity following pelvic irradiation and simultaneous cyclophosphamide therapy. Cancer 1976;38:701–707.

43. Fajardo LF, Berthrong M. Radiation injury in surgical pathology: Part I. Am J Surg Pathol 1978;2:159–199.

44. Oration JP. Complications following radiation therapy in carcinoma of the cervix and their treatment. Am J Obstet Gynecol 1964;88:854–866.

45. Dean RJ, Lytton B. Urologic complications of pelvic irradiation. J Urol 1978;119:64–67.

46. Kucera H, Vavra N, Weghaupt K. Benefit of external irradiation in pathologic stage I endometrial carcinoma: A prospective clinical trial of 605 patients who received postoperative vaginal irradiation and additional pelvic irradiation in the presence of unfavorable prognostic factors. Gynecol Oncol 1990;38:99–104.

47. Jampolis S, Martin P, Schroder P, Horiot JC. Treatment tolerance and early complications with extended field irradiation in gynecological cancer. Br J Radiol 1977;50:195–199.

48. Montana GS, Fowler WC. Carcinoma of the cervix: Analysis of bladder and rectal radiation dose and complications. Int J Radiat Oncol Biol Phys 1989;16:95–100.

49. Montana GS, Fowler WC, Varia MA, Walton LA, Mack Y. Analysis of results of radiation therapy for stage II carcinoma of the cervix. Cancer 1985;55:956–962.

50. Buchler DA, Kline JC, Peckham BM, Boone ML, Carr WF. Radiation reactions in cervical cancer therapy. Am J Obstet Gynecol 1971;111:745–750.

51. Shiels RA, Nissenbaum MM, Mark SR, Browde S. Late radiation cystitis after treatment for carcinoma of the bladder. S Afr Med J 1986;70:727–728.

52. Ram MD. Visceral complications of supervoltage radiotherapy for carcinoma of the bladder. Br J Surg 1970;57:409–412.

53. Ray GR, Cassady JR, Bagshaw MA. Definitive radiation therapy of carcinoma of the prostate: A report on 15 years of experience. Radiology 1973;106:407–418.

54. Taylor WJ, Richardson RG, Hafermann MD. Radiation therapy for localized prostate cancer. Cancer 1979;43:1123–1127.

55. Harisiadis L, Veenema RJ, Senyszyn JJ, et al. Carcinoma of the prostate: Treatment with external radiotherapy. Cancer 1978;41:2131–2142.

56. Warren S VII. Effects of radiation on the urinary system. Arch Pathol 1942;34:1079–1084.

57. Haemorrhagic cystitis after radiotherapy. Lancet [Editorial] 1987;1:304–306.

58. Gowing NF III. Pathological changes in the bladder following irradiation. Br J Radiol 1960;33:484–487.

59. Relling MV, Schunk JE. Drug-induced hemorrhagic cystitis. Clin Pharm [Clinical Conference] 1986;5:590–597.

60. Bracis R, Sanders CV, Gilbert DN. Methicillin hemorrhagic cystitis. Antimicrob Agents Chemother 1977;12:438–439.

61. Marx CM, Alpert SE. Ticarcillin-induced cystitis: Cross-reactivity with related penicillins. Am J Dis Child 1984;138:670–672.

62. Cook FV, Farrar WE Jr, Kreutner A. Hemorrhagic cystitis and ureteritis, and interstitial nephritis associated with administration of penicillin G. J Urol 1979;122:110–111.

SECTION 4

DIANE E. STOVER

Pulmonary Toxicity

Pulmonary disease can be caused by a wide spectrum of pathogens in patients with cancer. These include a variety of infectious agents and neoplastic disorders as well as pulmonary hemorrhage, pulmonary edema (cardiogenic and noncardiogenic) and leukocyte agglutinin reactions. Pulmonary toxicity caused by antineoplastic agents is being recognized more frequently, and the number of drugs known or suspected to cause lung disease is steadily increasing. Because continuing the offending agent may cause death and because withholding the agent may result in resolution of the pulmonary toxicity, it is important to recognize radiation and drug-induced pulmonary disease. In this section, parenchymal lung disease caused by irradiation and chemotherapy is discussed. Mechanisms of lung injury, histopathologic findings, clinical and laboratory features, and diagnosis and treatment of the abnormality produced by these agents are reviewed.

RADIATION-INDUCED PULMONARY TOXICITY

MECHANISM OF LUNG INJURY

Radiation can affect dividing and nondividing cells and can cause genetic and nongenetic damage.[1,2] In the lung, a hypothetical reconstruction of radiation injury might be as follows. Therapeutic radiation may result in nongenetic damage that is apparent in all cells, but capillary endothelial and type I cells (epithelial lining cells) appear most susceptible.[3] Many of these cells, whether dividing or not, undergo early necrobiosis and slough. Over time, capillaries regenerate, and the alveolar epithelium is repopulated by type II cells (surfactant-producing cells) because type I pneumonocytes do not regenerate. Some of these type II cells redifferentiate into type I cells. If the injury is severe, damage to other nondividing materials of the lung, such as proteins and polysaccharides, takes place. This can impede reconstruction of tissue architecture and result in functional derangement and scar formation. Genetic damage to dividing cells, such as endothelial cells or type II pneumonocytes, can also occur. Depletion of these cells may result during successive mitoses, causing a loss of integrity of pulmonary capillaries and exudation of fluid into the alveoli. At the physiologic level, loss of compliance, abnormal gas exchange, and respiratory failure can occur due to leakage of plasma proteins onto the alveolar surface. This type of genetic damage also explains why pneumonitis can happen so late after radiation. One might speculate that some endothelial cells initially remain normal but that, in the course of the next four cell divisions, chromosomal aberrations prevent further reduplication, which leads to loss of integrity of the capillary.[1]

Certain factors are critical to the development of radiation pneumonitis. In general, damage to the lung increases as the volume of lung tissue irradiated increases. Also, the toxic effects of radiation as measured by symptoms and signs, radiographic changes, and physiologic tests are proportionate to the total amount delivered to the lung. Radiation pneumonitis seldom occurs with doses of less than 20 Gy but is highly likely when doses exceed 60 Gy.[4] Because local control of lung cancer is greater when higher doses are delivered to the tumor,[5] methods are being devised to give high doses to the target tissue while sparing normal surrounding lung. One such technique, called *three-dimensional treatment planning,* is being evaluated.[6,7] In addition, a cooperative, randomized trial is assessing the value of combined chemotherapy, which includes drugs that are toxic to the lungs and high-dose radiation therapy.[8] In the future, in situ isolated lung perfusion for the treatment of unresectable pulmonary tumors, preceded or followed by high-dose irradiation, may be clinically applicable as well.[9] Whether these treatment modalities will have a sparing effect on the lung or whether they will be associated with an increase in pulmonary toxicity is unknown.

Besides the total radiation dose, the number of fractions into which it is divided and, to a lesser extent, the time span over which it is delivered are important factors.[10] The greater the number of fractions in which the radiation is given, the lower is the damaging effect. Fractionation is different from dose rate, which refers to output of the machine during radiation therapy. Dose rate certainly has an effect on lung tolerance: radiation delivered as 5 cGy/minute is less damaging than radiation delivered at 30 cGy/minute, which in turn is less damaging than radiation delivered at 2 to 3 Gy/minute. In summary, the incidence and severity of radiation damage to the lungs are related principally to the volume of lung tissue irradiated, the total dose, the fractions into which the total dose is divided, and the quality of the radiation.

HISTOPATHOLOGY

The histopathologic changes of radiation-induced pulmonary toxicity can be divided into early, intermediate, and late stages based on the time, course, and intensity of the radiation injury.[11] Early radiation damage (0–2 months after radiation) is characterized by injury to small vessels and capillaries with the development of vascular congestion and increased capillary permeability.[12] At this stage, a fibrin-rich exudate is present in the alveolar spaces. Hyaline membranes form on the alveoli, probably from condensation of the intraalveolar fibrin. Abnormalities in the intermediate stage (2–9 months after radiation) are characterized by obstruction of pulmonary

capillaries by platelets, fibrin, and collagen. Alveolar-lining cells (primarily type II pneumonocytes) become hyperplastic, and the alveolar walls become infiltrated with fibroblasts. If the radiation injury is mild, these changes may subside entirely; however, when the injury is severe, a chronic phase (9 months or more after radiation) ensues that may persist or progress for months or years. The histopathologic appearance then is dominated by dense fibrosis, thickening of the alveolar walls, vascular subintimal fibrosis, and luminal narrowing. In some instances, the lung may shrink to less than half its original size with a thickened adherent pleura and scarred hilar structures.

CLINICAL FEATURES

Signs and Symptoms

The clinical syndrome of radiation pneumonitis develops in 5% to 15% of all irradiated patients. Factors that can add to the development of radiation pneumonitis include concomitant chemotherapy, previous irradiation, and withdrawal of steroids. There is not a significant difference in the incidence of radiation pneumonitis between the young and elderly, but the pneumonitis is inclined to be more severe in the latter.[13] Underlying chronic obstructive pulmonary disease does not appear to potentiate radiation damage.

Symptoms of acute radiation pneumonitis usually become evident 2 to 3 months after the completion of therapy; rarely, they occur within the first month and occasionally as late as 6 months after irradiation. In general, the early onset of symptoms implies a more serious and more protracted clinical course. The cardinal symptom of radiation pneumonitis is dyspnea.[11] It may be self-limited or may progress to severe respiratory distress depending on the extent and intensity of the injury. Patients may also have a nonproductive cough or a cough productive of small amounts of pinkish sputum. Frank hemoptysis early in the clinical course is distinctly uncommon; however, massive hemoptysis has been reported as a late complication of therapeutic pulmonary irradiation.[14] Fever is unusual but can be high and spiking; in severe cases, other constitutional symptoms may occur. Chest pain, which is rarely a prominent feature, may be due to fractured ribs, pleural changes, or coughing. Symptoms of airway obstruction can occur in the first few days of radiation therapy and are usually associated with swelling of a central bronchogenic carcinoma. Severe respiratory distress can result and may be prevented by the administration of steroids the day before and several days after the initiation of radiation therapy.

On physical examination, signs of pulmonary involvement are minimal. Occasionally, moist rales, a pleural friction rub, or evidence of pleural fluid may be heard over the area of irradiation. In severe cases, tachypnea and cyanosis may be present, and occasionally evidence of acute cor pulmonale appears, usually predicting a fatal outcome. Finger clubbing due to radiation is distinctly unusual and, if present, is most likely due to the underlying malignancy. Skin changes corresponding to the ports of irradiation are often present but provide no clue as to the presence or severity of the pulmonary reaction beneath.

Although patients with acute pneumonitis may show complete resolution of signs and symptoms, most develop gradual progressive fibrosis. In some cases, patients present with radiation fibrosis without a previous history of acute pneumonitis. The permanent changes of fibrosis take 6 to 24 months to evolve but usually remain stable after 2 years. Patients with fibrosis can be asymptomatic or can have varying degrees of dyspnea. The major complications of radiation pneumonitis occur late in the disease and are secondary to persistent fibrosis of a large volume of lung. These include cor pulmonale and respiratory failure.

Diagnostic Imaging

Although radiographic abnormalities are invariably found at the time clinical radiation pneumonitis is present, these changes may be seen in asymptomatic patients as well. Early radiographic changes include a ground-glass opacification, diffuse haziness, or indistinctness of the normal pulmonary markings over the irradiated area.[15] Later, the chest radiograph may show alveolar infiltrates or dense consolidation with or without air bronchograms. As the pneumonitis progresses to fibrosis, the radiographic appearance changes to that of linear streaks radiating from the area of pneumonitis and of contraction toward the hilar, the perimediastinal, or the apical areas. Pleural effusions, if present, are usually small and always coincident with the pneumonitis.[16] They can persist for long periods but often disappear spontaneously and never increase over a period of stability unless secondary complications occur, such as radiation-induced pericarditis. Mediastinal or hilar adenopathy and cavitation are almost always due to causes other than radiation pneumonitis.[2] Pneumothorax is occasionally associated with radiation fibrosis but not with acute pneumonitis.

One of the most characteristic features of radiation pneumonitis and fibrosis is that the radiologic changes are confined to the outlines of the field of radiation. In a few cases, extensive changes outside the field, even in the contralateral lung, have been observed. Obstruction of lymphatic flow from mediastinal irradiation,[17] hypersensitivity in response to radiation,[18] and absorption of x-rays by regions outside the irradiated ports are possible but poorly documented explanations of this phenomenon.[19]

Some data suggest that computed tomographic (CT) scans of the chest and gallium-67 citrate imaging are more sensitive than chest radiography in the detection of radiation changes.[20,21] Correlation of abnormalities seen in these tests with the development of physiologic dysfunction and clinical toxicity need clarification.

Pulmonary Function Tests

No gross physiologic changes occur in the lung until 4 to 8 weeks after completion of irradiation, usually coincident with the period of clinical pneumonitis. Then, one sees a decrease in lung volumes, which can progress.[22-25] These changes persist indefinitely with little evidence of recovery.[24] Gas exchange abnormalities, which include a decrease in diffusion capacity and arterial hypoxemia, especially with exercise, occur about the same time but show some tendency toward recovery after 6 to 12 months.[23-25] A fall in compliance coincidence with the clinical pneumonitis is usually seen in most

subjects.[23] Accordingly, the elastic work of breathing is increased, and dyspnea, resulting from the increased workload, ensues.[23] Air flow parameters remain close to normal in most studies.[22-25]

DIAGNOSIS

The diagnosis of radiation pneumonitis can sometimes be made clinically based on the timing of irradiation in relation to symptoms and the typical chest radiographic appearance (*i.e.*, infiltrates corresponding to the margins of the irradiated portal). Differentiation from recurrent malignancy or infection often poses a problem, and then lung biopsy is necessary. Although histopathologic changes are nonspecific for radiation pneumonitis, when elements of the acute stages of radiation pneumonia (fibrin exudate in the alveoli) are seen adjacent to the more chronic stages (alveolar fibrosis and subintimal sclerosis), this entity can be diagnosed with reasonable certainty.[26]

Biochemical markers that indicate radiation lung injury before the onset of clinical pathologic events would be valuable in the early diagnosis and management of patients with radiation toxicity. In irradiated animals, studies demonstrate that surfactant found in the serum may be a marker and predictor for later radiation pneumonitis.[27] Studies are needed in humans to identify the sensitivity and specificity of monitoring serum surfactant levels as an early means to diagnose clinical radiation toxicity. No standard tests are used to monitor patients for radiation pneumonitis because most methods are of no predictive value.

TREATMENT

Three modalities of therapy have been used prophylactically and therapeutically for radiation-induced pneumonitis: corticosteroids, antibiotics, and anticoagulants. Of these, corticosteroid therapy is the most important.

Corticosteroid administration during irradiation in mice markedly improved the physiologic abnormalities and decreased mortality, an effect that had been attributed to the stimulation of surfactant synthesis and secretion by type II alveolar epithelial cells.[28] Despite this study and other animal studies indicating that steroids reduce mortality from radiation pneumonitis,[29] no controlled clinical trials in humans are available on the efficacy of steroid therapy in radiation pneumonitis. Ruben and Casarett[2] collected data from eight studies on humans and categorized them according to whether corticosteroids were used prophylactically or therapeutically. Corticosteroids given prophylactically failed to prevent radiation pneumonitis, but when they were administered as clinical pneumonitis occurred, an objective response was seen. In other reports, steroid therapy failed to ameliorate severe pneumonitis. Nonetheless, it is our practice to begin prednisone 1 mg/kg as soon as the diagnosis is reasonably certain. The initial dose is maintained for several weeks and then reduced cautiously and slowly. It has been our experience that if steroids are tapered too rapidly, symptoms can be exacerbated, necessitating higher doses for longer periods of time. Similarly, if corticosteroids are part of a chemotherapeutic regimen, stopping them abruptly can precipitate clinically evident radiation pneumonitis in recently treated patients.

What parameters, if any, to follow during the tapering schedule are not known, and no studies are available. Generally, we follow symptoms. Most authors agree that corticosteroids have no place in the treatment of radiation fibrosis.

In experimental and clinical reports, antibiotic administration has no effect on the course or outcome of radiation pneumonitis.[2,30] Although there is some rationale for the use of anticoagulants in view of the effects of irradiation on the vascular system, neither heparin injections nor oral anticoagulants have been found to be beneficial.[30]

CHEMOTHERAPY-INDUCED PULMONARY TOXICITY

Nineteen chemotherapeutic agents have been reported to cause cytotoxic drug-induced lung disease (see Table 63–13). An overview of the potential mechanisms of lung damage, a summary of the pathologic findings, and common clinical features of pulmonary toxicity are discussed in this section. Characteristics of pulmonary disease caused by some of these drugs are presented.

MECHANISMS OF PULMONARY INJURY

Although details about the pathophysiology of specific chemotherapeutic agents are generally not known, several mechanisms of pulmonary toxicity mediated by these agents have been proposed. Certain cytotoxic drugs may induce pulmonary injury by triggering the formation of reactive oxygen metabolites, including the superoxide anion, hydrogen peroxide, and hydroxyl radicals. These substances can produce direct toxicity through participation in redox reactions and subsequent fatty acid oxidation, which leads to membrane instability.[31] Oxidants can cause other inflammatory reactions within the lung. For example, the oxidation of arachidonic acid is an initial step in the metabolic cascade that produces immunoreactive substances, including prostaglandins and leukotrienes.[32] Cytotoxic drugs may also effect the local immune system. Because the lung is exposed to so many substances that can activate its immune system, there appears to be a "pulmonary immune tolerance state" to avoid unnecessary over reactions.[33] This tolerance state in part may be a result of effector and suppressor cell balance. Cytotoxic drugs can alter the normal effector and suppressor balance, which may cause tissue damage.[34–36] Other balance systems within the lung can be affected as well, such as the balance between collagenesis and collagenolysis.[33] Through modulation of fibroblast proliferation, excessive collagen deposition may result in severe irreversible pulmonary fibrosis. Bleomycin is one cytotoxic agent that has this potential.[37,38] Imbalance between the protease and antiprotease system also has been implicated in a number of pulmonary disorders, including drug toxicities.[33] Bleomycin and cyclophosphamide produce substances that can inactivate the antiprotease system, enhancing the effects of proteolytic enzymes on the lung. Drugs may damage the lung through a variety of other mechanisms, and considerable investigation needs to be done to define and clarify the exact mechanism of lung injury for each chemotherapeutic drug.

HISTOPATHOLOGY

The histopathologic changes of drug-induced pulmonary toxicity show common features. Similar to radiation-induced damage, abnormalities are seen in endothelial and epithelial cells. The vascular damage is characterized by endothelial swelling with exudation of fluid into the interstitium and the intraalveolar spaces. There is destruction and desquamation of type I pneumonocytes with delamellation and proliferation of type II pneumonocytes. Mononuclear cell infiltration and fibroblast proliferation with fibrosis are common findings; the character of the inflammatory cellular infiltrate may be a feature that distinguishes the toxicity of one drug from another. Bronchoalveolar lavage studies in patients with methotrexate pulmonary toxicity have shown the presence of a T-lymphocytic alveolitis, while studies on some patients with bleomycin toxicity have revealed a polymorphonuclear alveolitis.[34,39] Eosinophil infiltration has been associated with drugs that cause apparent hypersensitivity reactions, such as methotrexate, procarbazine, and bleomycin.[33,34,40,41]

(text continues on page 2368)

TABLE 63–13. Chemotherapeutic Agents Associated With Pulmonary Parenchymal Disease

Alkylating Agents	Antimetabolites
Busulfan	Methotrexate
Cyclophosphamide	Azathioprine
Chlorambucil	Mercaptopurine
Melphalan	Cytosine arabinoside

Nitrosoureas	Miscellaneous
Carmustine (BCNU)	Procarbazine
Lomustine (CCNU)	Vinblastine
Semustine (methyl-CCNU)	Vindesine
Chlorozotocin (DCNU)	VM-26

Antibiotics
Bleomycin
Mitomycin
Neocarzinostatin (zinostatin)

TABLE 63–14. Factors Associated With Increased Risk of Drug-Induced Pneumonitis

Risk Factor	Drugs
Total dose	Bleomycin[42,43]; carmustine[42]
Age	Bleomycin[43]
Oxygen therapy	Bleomycin[44–46]; cyclophosphamide[45]; mitomycin[47]
Simultaneous or prior radiation therapy to lungs	Bleomycin[48,49]; busulfan[50]; mitomycin[51]
Increased toxicity when given with other drugs	Carmustine[52]; mitomycin[53]; cyclophosphamide[54,55]; bleomycin[55,56]; methotrexate[54]
Preexisting pulmonary disease	Carmustine[57]

TABLE 63–15. Clinical and Pathologic Features of Chemotherapy-Induced Toxicity

Drug	Mechanism of Injury	Histopathology	Clinical Features	Chest Roentgenogram	Diagnosis	Treatment
Alkylating Agents						
Busulfan (Myleran)[42,50,65,76–80]	No studies, but direct toxicity to epithelial lining cells is suggested	Pneumocyte dysplasia (degeneration of type I cells; atypical hyperplastic type II cells), atypical bronchial lining cells, mononuclear cell infiltration, fibrosis	4% incidence; no direct dose-dependent toxicity; may be threshold dose (>500 mg); radiation and other alkylating agents may enhance toxicity, insidious onset after 4 years (8 mo to 10 y). Dyspnea, cough, weight loss, weakness, fever; crepitant basilar rales, pigmentation is poor.	Most common bibasilar reticular pattern; rarely pleural effusion, pulmonary ossification, normal chest radiograph	Suggested by history and bizarre pneumocytes in sputum or lavage fluid. Definitive diagnosis by open lung biopsy	Withdrawal of the drug; anecdotal reports of improvement with high-dose steroids. Mean survival after diagnosis is 5 mo
Cyclophosphamide (Cytoxan)[42,45,74,81–84]	May be toxic through production of reactive oxygen species	Endothelial swelling, pneumocyte dysplasia, lymphocytic and histiocytic infiltration, fibrosis	Less than 1% incidence; does not appear dose-dependent, but synergy with oxygen and other agents possible. Subacute onset 3 w to 8 y after initiation of therapy, up to 8 y after stopping therapy. Cough, dyspnea, fever; basilar rales	Commonly, bibasilar reticular pattern; diffuse pulmonary edema pattern also reported	As above	Drug withdrawal; corticosteroids may hasten improvement but have no documented effect on mortality. Overall recovery about 65%
Chlorambucil[33,85]	Unknown	Similar to busulfan; fibrosis may predominate	Rare reports; subacute onset 6 mo to 3 y after therapy. Cough, dyspnea, anorexia; bibasilar rales	Bibasilar reticular pattern; rarely, normal radiograph; alveolar infiltrates not reported	As above	Half of reported patients died despite cessation of drug and administration of steroids. Anecdotal reports of response to steroids
Melphalan (Alkeran)[33,86,87]	Unknown	Similar to busulfan; pneumocyte dysplasia more common than fibrosis	Rare (five documented reports); appears 1 to 48 mo after therapy. Progressive dyspnea, productive cough, fever, malaise; bibasilar rales	Reticular and alveolar infiltrates	As above	Despite cessation of drug, 3 of 5 patients reported died of disease. In most cases, patients were receiving steroids for underlying disease
Antibiotics						
Bleomycin[33,37,38,69,70,88–95]	Several possible mechanisms: (a) direct toxicity through generation of reactive oxygen metabolites; (b) leukocyte influx and lung injury from release of proteases; (c) increased collagen synthesis and subsequent pulmonary fibrosis	Endothelial blebbing; interstitial edema, necrosis of type I cells and metaplastic type II cells; inflammation with polymorphonuclear cells; fibroblast proliferation and fibrosis; occasionally eosinophilic infiltration	Incidence 2–40%: age- and dose-related; synergy seen with oxygen therapy, radiation, and other agents. Occurs during and shortly after stopping therapy. Cough, dyspnea, fever; tachypnea, crepitant rales. Hypersensitivity pneumonitis variant	Bibasilar reticular pattern; multiple nodules similar to metastatic disease; acinar pattern, especially with hypersensitivity reaction; rarely, localized infiltrate and cavitary nodules	Bronchoalveolar lavage might suggest diagnosis (polymorphonuclear alveolitis). Transbronchial or open lung biopsy required for diagnosis, especially to rule out other causes.	Drug withdrawal. In bleomycin hypersensitivity reactions, definite role for steroids; in other forms of bleomycin toxicity, efficacy less clear. Mortality estimated at 50%.

Drug	Mechanism	Pathology	Clinical Features	Chest Radiograph	Diagnosis	Management/Prognosis
Mitomycin[33,51,53,73,96]	No studies, but probably similar to the alkylating agents	Similar to bleomycin; in patients with microangiopathic hemolytic anemia, prominent vascular changes are present.	3–12% incidence; does not appear dose-related, but possible synergy with oxygen, radiotherapy, and other agents. Dry cough and dyspnea; fever not seen; bibasilar rales	Diffuse reticular pattern; pleural effusions seen	Lung biopsy for definitive diagnosis; no bronchoalveolar lavage studies reported.	Drug withdrawal; steroids may alter outcome. Mortality approaches 50%.
Nitrosoureas*						
Carmustine (BCNU)[52,57,97-99]	Few studies; direct injury through generation of toxic oxidant molecules possible	Similar to bleomycin; fibrosis predominates.	20–30% incidence; dose-related; increased risk with preexisting lung disease and tobacco use; possible synergism with other agents; can be seen up to 17 y after drug stopped. Dry cough, dyspnea, bibasilar rales	Bibasilar reticular pattern; may be normal	As above	Early recognition and withdrawal of the drug; steroids not beneficial since most patients are on the drug for intracranial processes when toxicity develops. Mortality reported between 24% and 90%.
Antimetabolites						
Methotrexate[33,34,42,54,63,66]	Direct toxic effect may play a role but mechanism not known; hypersensitivity suggested by occurrence of eosinophils and presence of increased T lymphocytes in lavage fluid	Interstitial and alveolar infiltration of lymphocytes, eosinophils, and plasma cells; occasionally poorly formed, noncaseating granuloma; fibrosis unusual	8% incidence; synergism with other agents possible; occurs 12 d to 18 y after beginning therapy. Fever, chills, malaise, headache–a prodrome for days and weeks; cough, dyspnea, rales common. Skin rash in 17% and blood eosinophilia in 40%	Early interstitial infiltrates; later, alveolar infiltrates; hilar and mediastinal adenopathy, pleural effusions described; chest radiograph can be normal.	Clinical history suggestive; bronchoalveolar lavage might suggest diagnosis (increase T cells in fluid), but lung biopsy required for diagnosis.	Discontinue drug, but reports of reinstitution without recurrence of the abnormality. Dramatic responses to steroids reported. Mortality 1%; outlook favorable
Cytosine arabinoside[103,104]	Unknown	Pulmonary edema; proteinaceous exudate with extravasation of red blood cells, no inflammatory cells	If given within 30 days of death, high incidence of pulmonary edema. Abrupt onset of dyspnea; gastrointestinal toxicity coexists.	Diffuse interstitial and alveolar pattern	Clinical picture suggests diagnosis.	Supportive; no studies
Miscellaneous						
Procarbazine (Matulane)[40,67,105]	Hypersensitivity	Mononuclear cell infiltration and scattered foci of eosinophils; fibrosis in one case	Acute onset within hours to days of first dose. Nausea, fevers, chills, arthralgias, urticaria, dry cough, and dyspnea. Blood eosinophilia common.	Interstitial Infiltrates; pleural effusion	Clinical picture highly suggestive of diagnosis.	Rapid recovery following discontinuation of drug. Role of steroids not known.
Vinca alkaloids (vinblastine and vindesine)[53,73,106,107]	Unknown	Dysplasia of alveolar lining cells; interstitial and alveolar influx of inflammatory cells; fibrosis	Most common reports of pulmonary edema in association with mitomycin; some patients subsequently developed pulmonary fibrosis. Dyspnea and wheezing seen with vindesine.	Diffuse interstitial and alveolar infiltrates with combination drugs; normal chest radiograph with vinca alkaloid alone	Clinical history suggests diagnosis.	Drug withdrawal; steroids probably beneficial. Prognosis poor if pulmonary infiltrates develop.

* Pulmonary toxicity has been reported with all other nitrosoureas, including, lomustine (CCNU), semustine (methyl-CCNU), and chlorozotocin (DCNU).[100-102]

CLINICAL FEATURES

Table 63–14 lists predisposing factors associated with enhancement of drug-induced pneumonitis.[42-57] Because bleomycin toxicity is relatively common, it deserves special mention. Although toxicity drastically increases with doses in excess of 450 to 500 mg, it can occur with much lower doses, especially when other risk factors are present. These factors include age greater than 60 years; simultaneous or prior irradiation to the lungs; simultaneous or subsequent oxygen therapy, especially with inspired doses equal to or greater than 35%; and a decrease in creatinine clearance time during the period of administration of bleomycin. A recent study described 9 of 45 patients (20%) who developed lung toxicity when they received bleomycin after cisplatin infusion.[58] Renal damage after cisplatin administration, with subsequent accumulation of bleomycin, was a likely cause of the high pulmonary toxicity and mortality rate of 67%. Extreme caution is recommended in the administration of combined bleomycin and cisplatin chemotherapy, and if possible, bleomycin should precede cisplatin infusion to minimize the risk of lung toxicity. Some data suggest that continuous infusion of bleomycin may be associated with less pulmonary toxicity than bolus therapy[59]; however, these data are inconclusive, and further studies are warranted.

Long intervals between drug administration and onset of clinical toxicity have been described. Late-onset pulmonary fibrosis has been reported many years after discontinuing cyclophosphamide[60] and carmustine.[61]

Signs and Symptoms

The cardinal symptom of drug-induced pulmonary toxicity is dyspnea. Nonproductive cough, fatigue, and malaise are other commonly associated complaints. Although symptoms usually develop over a period of several weeks to months, hypersensitivity drug-induced lung disease can develop over hours. Fever may be a common finding with this type of toxicity. Chest pain has been reported during infusion of bleomycin[62] or immediately after therapy with methotrexate[63]; however, it is an unusual manifestation of toxicity. Because hemoptysis is an uncommon feature of drug-induced pulmonary toxicity, when it is present, other diagnoses should be considered. Physical examination of the lungs may be normal or may reveal end-inspiratory "Velcro rales." Finger clubbing is distinctly unusual, but it may be related to the underlying malignancy.

Diagnostic Imaging

The most common radiographic abnormality associated with drug-induced pulmonary toxicity is a reticulonodular pattern, which may be basilar or diffuse. Pleural effusions are uncommon but occasionally have been reported in association with mitomycin, busulfan, methotrexate, and procarbazine toxicity.[64-67] Hypersensitivity lung disease associated with methotrexate and procarbazine may present with bilateral acinar infiltrates that clear rapidly.[67] In some instances, the chest radiograph is normal, even in the presence of histologically proved pulmonary infiltration and fibrosis.[66,68] Most commonly, methotrexate and carmustine toxicity have been reported with normal chest radiograph findings. Hilar adenopathy is distinctly unusual and has been reported only with methotrexate toxicity.[66] Cavitating and noncavitating nodules, simulating metastatic disease, have been seen with bleomycin toxicity.[69,70]

Both high-resolution thin-section CT chest scans and gallium scintigraphy have been shown to be more sensitive techniques than chest radiography to detect pulmonary parenchymal changes in association with drug toxicity.[71] The full relation of these changes to the development of functional or physiologic impairment is unclear, and further studies are needed. Although magnetic resonance spectrometry of lung parenchyma is in the early stages of development, eventually it may be used clinically to noninvasively differentiate among fibrosis, edema, acute pneumonitis, and hemorrhage.[72]

Pulmonary Function Tests

The most common abnormalities associated with chemotherapy-induced pulmonary toxicity are a reduced diffusing capacity for carbon monoxide and a restrictive ventilatory defect.[33] Isolated gas transport abnormalities manifested by a decrease in the diffusing capacity and arterial hypoxemia, especially with exercise, have been seen.

Screening pulmonary function tests to predict which patients receiving chemotherapy are likely to develop toxicity would be helpful but have not been established.

DIAGNOSIS

Although one might have a high clinical suspicion of drug-induced pulmonary toxicity, lung biopsy is usually necessary for a definitive diagnosis. Because pathognomonic pathologic changes associated with drug-induced pneumonitis often are not present, a biopsy is necessary to eliminate other specific diagnoses, such as opportunistic infection and malignancy. Through the use of bronchoalveolar lavage, several studies reported the presence of a characteristic or predominant cell associated with particular drugs.[34,39] Although these data might be of value in understanding the pathogenesis of drug-induced lung disorders, their usefulness in diagnosing drug toxicity is limited.

TREATMENT

The most effective way to manage pulmonary toxicity associated with chemotherapeutic agents is to prevent it. If it occurs, withdrawal of the offending agent is the cornerstone of therapy. Although no control studies in humans have systematically examined the efficacy of corticosteroids, a trial of these agents is probably warranted in most cases. The optimal dose and duration of therapy are not known; however, 1 mg/kg is usually initiated with a slow and careful tapering schedule because clinical deterioration after tapering has been reported.[73,74] One report described the case of a 23-year-old male patient who underwent a single lung transplantation because of presumed drug-induced pulmonary fibrosis 12 years after undergoing chemotherapy for acute lymphocytic leukemia.[75] The use of lung transplantation in the treatment of drug-induced pulmonary fibrosis is exciting and needs further evaluation.

Table 63–15 lists the characteristics of pulmonary disease caused by the commonly used chemotherapeutic agents.

REFERENCES

1. Gross NJ. The pathogenesis of radiation-induced lung damage. Lung 1981;159:115.
2. Rubin P, Casarett GW. Clinical radiation pathology. Philadelphia: WB Saunders, 1968.
3. Adamson ILR, Bowden DH, Wyatt JP. A pathway to pulmonary fibrosis: An ultrastructural study of mouse and rat following radiation to the whole body and hemithorax. Am J Pathol 1970;58:481.
4. Jennings FL, Arden A. Development of radiation pneumonitis: Time and dose factors. Arch Pathol 1962;74:351.
5. Perez C, Stanley K, Grundy G, et al. Impact of irradiation technique and tumor extent in tumor control and survival of patients with unresectable non-oat cell carcinoma of the lung. Cancer 1982;50:1091.
6. Emami B, Purdy JA, Manolis J, et al. Three-dimensional treatment planning for lung cancer. Int J Radiat Oncol Biol Phys 1991;21:217.
7. Goitein M, Abrams M, Rowell D, et al. Multi-dimensional treatment planning. II. Beam's eye view back projection through CT sections. Int J Radiol Oncol Biol Phys 1983;9:789.
8. Arriagada R, Le Chevalier T, Quoix E, et al. Chemotherapy effect on locally advanced non-small cell lung carcinoma: A randomized study on 353 patients. Proceedings of the 32nd annual ASTRO meeting 1990. Int J Radiat Oncol Biol Phys 1990;19:195.
9. Minchin RF, Johnson MR, Schuller HM, et al. Pulmonary toxicity of doxorubicin administered by in situ siolated lung perfusion in dogs. Cancer 1988;61:1320.
10. Wara WM, Phillips TL, Margolis LW, et al. Radiation pneumonitis: A new approach to the deviation of time-dose factors. Cancer 1973;32:547.
11. Gross NJ. Pulmonary effects of radiation therapy. Ann Intern Med 1977;86:81.
12. Maisin JR. The ultrastructure of the lung of mice exposed to a supralethal dose of ionizing radiation on the thorax. Radiat Res 1970;44:545.
13. Koga K, Kusumoto S, Watanabe K, et al. Age factor relevant to the development of radiation pneumonitis in radiotherapy of lung cancer. Int J Radiat Oncol 1988;14:367.
14. Isaacs RD, Wallie WJ, Wells UE, et al. Massive hemoptysis as a late complication of pulmonary irradiation. Thorax 1987;42:77.
15. Bate D, Guttman RJ. Changes in lung and pleura following two-million-volt therapy for carcinoma of the breast. Radiology 1957;73:679.
16. Bachman AL, Macken K. Pleural effusions following supervoltage radiation for breast carcinoma. Radiology 1959;72:699.
17. Smith JC. Radiation pneumonitis: Case report of bilateral reaction after unilateral irradiation. Am Rev Respir Dis 1964;89:264.
18. Holt JAG. The acute radiation pneumonitis syndrome. J Coll Radiol Aust 1964;8:40.
19. Bennett DE, Million RR, Ackerman LV. Bilateral radiation pneumonitis, a complication of the radiotherapy of bronchogenic carcinoma. Cancer 1969;23:1001.
20. Ikezoe J, Takashima S, Morimoto S, et al. CT appearance of acute radiation-induced injury in the lung. Am J Roentgenol 1988;150:765.
21. Kataoka M. Gallium-67 imaging for the assessment of radiation pneumonitis. Ann Nucl Med 1989;3:73.
22. Brady LW, German PA, Cander L. The effects of radiation therapy on pulmonary function in carcinoma of the lung. Radiology 1965;85:130.
23. Emirgil C, Heinemann HO. Effects of radiation of the chest on pulmonary function in men. J Appl Physiol 1961;16:331.
24. Prato FS, Kurdyak R, Saibil EA, et al. Regional and total lung function in patients following pulmonary irradiation. Invest Radiol 1977;12:224.
25. Wohl MEB, Griscom NT, Traggis DG, et al. Effects of therapeutic irradiation delivered in early childhood upon subsequent lung function. Pediatrics 1975;55:507.
26. Warren S, Spencer J. Radiation reaction in the lung. AJR 1940;43:682.
27. Rubin P, McDonald S, Maasilta P, et al. Serum markers for prediction of pulmonary radiation syndromes. Int J Radiat Oncol Biol Phys 1989;17:553.
28. Gross NJ, Narine KR. Experimental radiation pneumonitis: Corticosteroids increase the replicative activity of avelolar type 2 cells. Radiat Res 1988;115:543.
29. Gross NJ, Narine KR, Wade R. Protective effect of corticosteroids on radiation pneumonitis. Radiat Res 1988;113:112.
30. Moss WT, Haddy FJ, Sweany SK. Some factors altering the severity of acute radiation pneumonitis: Variation with cortisone, heparin, and antibiotics. Radiology 1960;75:50.
31. Freeman BA, Crapo JD. Biology of disease: Free radicals and tissue injury. Lab Invest 1982;47:412.
32. Lewis RA, Austen KF. The biologically active leukotrienes: Biosynthesis, metabolism, receptors, functions and pharmacology. J Clin Invest 1984;73:889.
33. Cooper JAD, White DA, Matthay RA. Drug-induced pulmonary disease: Part I. Cytotoxic drugs. Am Rev Respir Dis 1986;133:321.
34. White DA, Rankin JR, Stover DE, et al. Methotrexate pneumonitis: Lavage findings suggest an immune mediated disorder. Am Rev Respir Dis 1989;139:18.
35. Askenase PW, Hayden BJ, Gershon RK. Augmentation of delayed-type hypersensitivity by doses of cyclophosphamide which do not affect antibody responses. J Exp Med 1974;141:697.
36. L'age-Stehr J, Diamanstein T. Induction of autoreactive T lymphocytes and their suppressor cells by cyclophosphamide. Nature 1978;27:1663.
37. Absher M, Hildebran J, Trombley L, et al. Characteristics of cultured lung fibroblasts from bleomycin-treated rats: Comparison with in vitro exposed normal fibroblasts. Am Rev Respir Dis 1984;129:125.
38. Clark JG, Kostal KM, Marino BA. Bleomycin induced pulmonary fibrosis in hamsters: An alveolar macrophage product increases fibroblast prostaglandin E2 and cyclic adenosine monophosphate and suppresses fibroblast proliferation and collagen production. J Clin Invest 1983;72:2082.
39. White DA, Kris MG, Stover DE. Bronchoalveolar lavage cell populations in bleomycin-induced pulmonary toxicity. Thorax 1987;42:551.
40. Jones Se, Moore M, Blank N, et al. Hypersensitivity to procarbazine (Matulane) manifested by fever and pleuropulmonary reaction. Cancer 1972;29:498.
41. Holoye PY, Luna MA, McKay B, et al. Bleomycin hypersensitivity pneumonitis. Ann Intern Med 1978;88:47.
42. Ginsberg SJ, Comis RL. The pulmonary toxicity of antineoplastic agents. Semin Oncol 1982;9:34.
43. Blum RH, Carter SK, Agre K. A clinical review of bleomycin: A new antineoplastic agent. Cancer 1973;31:903.
44. Goldiner PL, Carlon GC, Cvitkovic E, et al. Factors influencing postoperative morbidity and mortality in patients treated with bleomycin. Br Med J 1978;1:1664.
45. Hakkinen PJ, Whiteley JW, Witschi HR. Hyperoxia, but not thoracic x-irradiation, potentiates bleomycin and cyclophosphamide-induced lung damage in mice. Am Rev Respir Dis 1982;126:281.
46. Tryka AF, Godleski JJ, Brian JD. Differences in effects of immediate and delayed hyperoxia exposure on bleomycin-induced pulmonary injury. Cancer Treat Rep 1984;68:759.
47. Franklin R, Buroker TR, Vaishampayan W, et al. Combined therapies in esophageal squamous cell cancer. Proc Am Assoc Cancer Res [Abstract] 1979;20:223.
48. Einhorn L, Krause M, Hornback N, et al. Enhanced pulmonary toxicity with bleomycin and radiotherapy in oat cell cancer. Cancer 1976;37:2414.
49. Samuels ML, Johnson DE, Holoye PY, et al. Large-dose bleomycin therapy and pulmonary toxicity: A possible role of prior radiotherapy. JAMA 1976;235:1117.
50. Soble AR, Perry H. Fatal radiation pneumonia following subclinical busulfan injury. AJR 1977;128:15.
51. Buzdar AU, Legha SS, Luna MA, et al. Pulmonary toxicity of mitomycin. Cancer 1980;45:236.
52. Durant JR, Norgard MJ, Murad TM, et al. Pulmonary toxicity associated with bischloroethylnitrosourea (BCNU). Ann Intern Med 1979;90:191.
53. Luedke D, McLaughlin TT, Daughaday C, et al. Mitomycin C and vindesine associated pulmonary toxicity with variable clinical expression. Cancer 1985;55:542.
54. White DA, Orenstein M, Godwin TA, et al. Chemotherapy-associated pulmonary toxic reactions during treatment for beast cancer. Arch Intern Med 1984;144:953.
55. Skarin AT, Rosenthal DS, Maloney WC. The treatment of advanced non-Hodgkin's lymphoma (NHL) with bleomycin, Adriamycin, cyclophosphamide, vincristine and prednisone. Blood 1977;49:759.
56. Bauer KA, Skarin AT, Balikian JP, et al. Pulmonary complications associated with combination chemotherapy programs containing bleomycin. Am J Med 1983;74:557.
57. Aronin PA, Mahaley MS, Rudnick SA, et al. Prediction of BCNU pulmonary toxicity in patients with malignant gliomas: An assessment of risk factors. N Engl J Med 1980;303:1983.
58. Rabinowits M, Souhami L, Gil RA, et al. Increased pulmonary toxicity with bleomycin and cisplatin chemotherapy combinations. Am J Clin Oncol 1990;13:132.
59. Cooper KR, Hong WK. Prospective study of the pulmonary toxicity of continuously infused bleomycin. Cancer Treat Rep 1981;65:419.
60. Alvarado CS, Boat TF, Newman AJ. Late-onset pulmonary fibrosis and chest deformity in two children treated with cyclophosphamide. J Pediatr 1978;92:443.
61. O'Driscoll BR, Hasleton PS, Taylor PM. Active lung fibrosis up to 17 years after chemotherapy with carmustine (BCNU) in childhood. N Engl J Med 1990;323:378.
62. White DA, Schwartzberg L, Kris MG, et al. Acute chest pain during bleomycin infusions. Cancer 1987;59:1582.
63. Walden PAM, Mitchell-Heggs PF, Coppin C, et al. Pleurisy and methotrexate treatment. Br Med J 1977;2:867.
64. Orwoll ES, Kiessling P, Patterson R. Interstitial pneumonia from mitomycin. Ann Intern Med 1978;89:352.
65. Smalley RV, Wall RL. Two cases of busulfan toxicity. Ann Intern Med 1966;64:154.
66. Sostman HD, Matthay RA, Putnam CE. Methotrexate-induced pneumonitis. Medicine 1976;55:371.
67. Ecker MD, May B, Keohane MF. Procarbazine lung. AJR 1978;131:527.
68. Weiss RB, Poster DS, Penta JS. The nitrosoureas and pulmonary toxicity. Cancer Treat Rev 1981;8:111.
69. Glasier CM, Siegel MJ. Multiple pulmonary nodules: Unusual manifestations of bleomycin toxicity. AJR 1981;137:155.
70. Talcott JA, Garnick MB, Stomper PL, et al. Cavitary lung nodules associated with combination chemotherapy containing bleomycin. J Urol 1987;138:619.
71. Taylor CR. Diagnostic imaging techniques in the evaluation of drug-induced pulmonary disease. Clin Chest Med 1990;11:87.
72. Vinitski S, Pearson MG, Karlik ST, et al. Differentiation of parenchymal lung disorders with in vivo proton nuclear magnetic resonance. Magn Reson Med 1986;3:120.
73. Gunstream SR, Seidenfeld JJ, Sobonya RE, et al. Mitomycin-associated lung disease. Cancer Treat Rep 1983;67:301.
74. Spector JI, Zimbler H, Ross JS. Cyclophosphamide and interstitial pneumonitis. JAMA 1980;243:1133.
75. Grossman RF, Frost A, Zamel N, et al. Results of single lung transplantation for bilateral pulmonary fibrosis. N Engl J Med 1990;322:727.
76. Koss LG, Melamed MR, Mayer K. The effect of busulfan on human epithelia. Am J Clin Pathol 1965;44:385.
77. Stover DE, Zaman MB, Hajdu SI, et al. Bronchoalveolar lavage in the diagnosis of

diffuse pulmonary infiltrates in the immunosuppressed host. Ann Intern Med 1984;101: 1.

78. Kuplic JB, Higley CS, Niewoehner DE. Pulmonary ossification associated with long-term busulfan therapy in chronic myeloid leukemia. Am Rev Respir Dis 1972;106: 759.

79. Heard BE, Cooke RA. Busulfan lung. Thorax 1968;233:1987.

80. Burns WA, McFarland W, Matthews MJ. Busulfan-induced pulmonary disease: Report of a case and review of the literature. Am Rev Respir Dis 1970;101:408.

81. Collis CH. Lung damage from cytotoxic drugs. Cancer Chemother Pharmacol 1980;4: 17.

82. Mark GJ, Lehimgar-Zadeh A, Ragsdale BD. Cyclphosphamide pneumonitis. Thorax 1978;33:89.

83. Alvarado CS, Boat TF, Newman AJ. Late-onset pulmonary fibrosis and chest deformity in two children treated with cyclophosphamide. J Pediatr 1978;92:443.

84. Maxwell I. Reversible pulmonary edema following cyclophosphamide treatment. JAMA 1974;229:137.

85. Cole SR, Myers TJ, Klatsky AU. Pulmonary disease with chlorambucil therapy. Cancer 1978;41:455.

86. Taetle R, Dickman PS, Feldman PS. Pulmonary histopathologic changes associated with melphalan therapy. Cancer 1978;42:1239.

87. Goucher G, Rowland V, Hawkins J. Melphalan-induced pulmonary interstitial fibrosis. Chest 1980;77:805.

88. Berend N. Protective effect of hypoxia on bleomycin lung toxicity in the rat. Am Rev Respir Dis 1984;130:307.

89. Frank L. Protection from O_2 toxicity by pre-exposure to hypoxia: Lung antioxidant enzyme role. J Appl Physiol 1982;53:475.

90. Wesselius LJ, Catanzaro A, Wasserman SI. Neutrophil chemotactic activity generation by alveolar macrophages after bleomycin injury. Am Rev Respir Dis 1984;129:485.

91. Kelley J, Newman RA, Evans JN. Bleomycin-induced pulmonary fibrosis in the rat: Prevention with an inhibitor of collagen synthesis. J Lab Clin Med 1980;96:954.

92. White DA, Stover DE. Severe bleomycin-induced pneumonitis: Clinical features and response to corticosteroids. Chest 1984;86:723.

93. Luna MA, Bedrossian CWM, Lichtiger B, et al. Interstitial pneumonitis associated with bleomycin therapy. J Clin Pathol 1972;58:501.

94. DeLena M, Guzzon A, Monfardini S, et al. Clinical, radiologic and histopathologic studies on pulmonary toxicity induced by treatment with bleomycin (NSC-125066). Cancer Chemother Rep 1972;56:343.

95. Jules KJ, White DA. Bleomycin-induced pulmonary toxicity. Clin Chest Med 1990;11: 1.

96. Jolivet J, Giroux L, Laurin S, et al. Microangiopathic hemolytic anemia, renal failure, and noncardiogenic pulmonary edema: A chemotherapy-induced syndrome. Cancer Treat Rep 1983;67:429.

97. Nathan CF, Arrick BA, Murray HW, et al. Tumor cell antioxidant defenses: Inhibition of the glutathione redox cycle enhances macrophage-mediated cytolysis. J Exp Med 1981;153:766.

98. Reznil-Schuller HM, Smith AC, Thenot JP, et al. Pulmonary toxicity of the anticancer drug, bis-chloroethyl nitrosurea (BCNU) in rats. Toxicologist 1984;4:29.

99. Selker RG, Jacobs SA, Moore PB. BCNU (1,3-bis(2-chloroenthyl)-1-nitrosourea) introduced pulmonary fibrosis. Neurosurgery 1980;7:560.

100. Cordonnier C, Vernant J-P, Mital P, et al. Pulmonary fibrosis subsequent to high doses of CCNU for chronic leukemia. Cancer 1983;51:1814.

101. Lee W, Moore RP, Wampler GL. Interstitial pulmonary fibrosis as a complication of prolonged methyl-CCNU therapy. Cancer Treat Rep 1978;62:1355.

102. Sordillo EM, Sordillo PP, Stover DE, et al. Chlorozotocin (DCNU)-induced pulmonary toxicity. Cancer Clin Trials 1981;4:397.

103. Haupt HM, Hutchins GM, Moore GW. Ara-C lung: Noncardiogenic pulmonary edema complicating cytosine arabinoside therapy of leukemia. Am J Med 1981;70:256.

104. Hewlett RI, Wilson AF. Adult respiratory distress syndrome (ARDS) following aggressive management of extensive acute lymphoblastic leukemia. Cancer 1977;39:2422.

105. Lokich JJ, Moloney WC. Allergic reaction to procarbazine. Clin Pharmacol Ther 1972;13:573.

106. Kris MG, Pablo D, Gralla RJ, et al. Dyspnea following vinblastine or vindesine administration in patients receiving mitomycin plus vinca alkaloid combination therapy. Cancer Treat Rep 1984;68:1029.

107. Konits PH, Aisner J, Sutherland J, et al. Possible pulmonary toxicity secondary to vinblastine. Cancer 1982;50:2771.

SECTION **5**

LAUREL J. STEINHERZ
JOACHIM YAHALOM

Cardiac Complications of Cancer Therapy

The treatment of cancer has been improved by the expansion of chemotherapeutic agents and the refinement of radiation therapy over the past three decades. However, many of the most effective antineoplastic agents and mediastinal irradiation produce toxic effects on the heart. This section describes some of these problems and discusses attempts at prevention and management.

CHEMOTHERAPY

ANTHRACYCLINES

The anthracyclines have been associated with cardiomyopathy since their introduction in the late 1960s. Early reports included isolated cases of unexplained cardiac failure in patients undergoing treatment with daunorubicin[1-4] and, in the early 1970s, with doxorubicin.[5-10] In 1983, Lefrak and colleagues[11] reported a series of 399 patients treated with doxorubicin. He found a 30% incidence of cardiac failure in the patients who received more than 550 mg/m² of doxorubicin and a lower incidence in those who received less. This introduced the concept of increasing cardiotoxicity with cumulative doses above a "safe threshold" cumulative dose. In 1974, Halazen

and associates[12] reported a series of children with acute lymphoblastic leukemia in remission who were treated with two different maintenance protocols, one including and one excluding daunorubicin. There was a 10% incidence of cardiac failure in the children treated with daunorubicin and none in the other group. This report clearly demonstrated the relation of anthracycline treatment to the incidence of cardiac failure, and it excluded the influence of active malignancy or the stress of induction therapy as contributory factors. Von Hoff and colleagues demonstrated, in 5613 patients treated with daunorubicin[13] and in 4018 patients treated with doxorubicin,[14] a continuous exponential increase of incidence of cardiac failure with increasing cumulative dose. Subsequently, Bristow and colleagues[15,16] used endomyocardial biopsy to show that pathologic lesions progressively worsened in a linear relation to the increase in total cumulative dose, in contrast to the exponential increase in myocardial dysfunction. This contrast suggested a threshold of tolerable myocardial damage beyond which the administration of additional drug would result in clinical symptomatology. Both clinical and pathologic abnormalities increased at any dose level in patients who received mediastinal radiation therapy.[17]

Clinical Presentation

Anthracycline cardiomyopathy has been described as having three clinical presentations: acute, subacute, and late. The acute toxicity[18] presents as a myopericarditis and probably results from the combination of acute myocyte damage from drug exposure and the effects of the catecholamine and histamine[19,20] surge provoked by the administration of anthracyclines. This occurs within days of dose administration and includes transient arrhythmia,[21,22] pericardial effusion, and myocardial dysfunction, sometimes leading to transient cardiac failure and occasionally death.[15,18] Histologically, acute myocyte disruption and sometimes infiltration of the myocardium by granulocytes, lymphocytes, and histiocytes[23] are seen.

The classic subacute presentation has a more insidious onset and can appear immediately after the last dose or up to 30 months later,[24] with a peak onset of symptoms at 3 months from the last dose.[13] This insidious onset was duplicated by Jaenke[25] in rabbits treated with repeated sublethal doses of doxorubicin and then sacrificed at varying lengths of time after cessation of treatment. Rabbits treated with higher doses exhibited myocardial necrosis and lethal cardiac failure immediately after therapy, but the rabbits treated with low doses showed almost no myocardial damage when sacrificed immediately after treatment but showed increasing myocardial damage when sacrificed at increasingly later periods, even though no drug persisted in the blood or myocardium. The clinical picture presents with increasing tachycardia and fatigue, progressing in some to tachypnea, dyspnea, and finally pulmonary edema, right-sided congestive signs, and low cardiac output. The mortality of patients actually manifesting congestive heart failure in these early series ranged up to 60%, although some patients could be stabilized with intensive cardiac treatment,[26,27] and many showed remarkable improvement of cardiac function over the first few years after chemotherapy.[27-30] Evaluation of hemodynamics with exercise, however, has revealed significant underlying abnormalities even in asymptomatic patients with normal resting parameters.[31] The pathology noted on endomyocardial biopsy and autopsy within the first 2 years after completion of anthracyclines includes mitochondrial swelling, disruption and loss of myofibrils, and particularly swelling and distortion of the sarcoplasmic reticulum, producing intramyocyte vacuolization.[17,32,33] With mild toxicity, such damage is patchy; with higher doses and toxicity, it is found more extensively throughout the heart, with progression to myocyte necrosis and loss. Pathologic examination 41 to 47 months after chemotherapy reveals hypertrophy of the remaining myocytes without fibrosis and diminution of vacuolization, suggesting healing and compensation.[34]

The late presentation of anthracycline cardiomyopathy occurs 5 or more years after completion of anthracycline therapy (Table 63–16). It involves late clinical decompensation of patients who had recovered from subacute cardiac symptoms[35-37,39,40] (Fig 63–1) or the occurrence of de novo cardiac failure in patients with no previous symptoms 6 to 20 years after anthracycline therapy.[35-39,41] It has also been demonstrated subclinically as abnormal systolic cardiac function in 23%,[35-37] abnormal myocardial mass in 52%,[40,42] and abnormal diastolic function and exercise response in 80%[43,44] of patients. As with subacute toxicity, an increased incidence

TABLE 63–16. Late Cardiac Toxicity of Anthracyclines

Investigations	No. of Patients	Anthracycline (mg/m²) Range	Mean	Radiation Therapy	Follow-up (years) Range	Mean	No. of Abnormal Patients (%)	Methods of Evaluation	Types of Abnormalities Found
Steinherz et al, 1991[36,37]	201	200–1275	450	56	4–20	7	47 (23%)	ECHO, STI, Cath biopsy RNCA, 24 h ECG	47/201 ↓ FS, 9 ABN Biopsy 14 ABN 24 h ECG, 3 SD
Lipshultz et al, 1991[40]	115	45–550	334	No	1–15	6.4	66 (57%)	ECHO, FS, ESWS/VCF Exercise 24 h ECG	60/115 ↑ ESWS/ ↓ LV PW 32/115 ↓ FS 23/89 ABN 24 h ECG, 4VT
Hausdorf et al, 1988[42]	55	31–656	273	No	2–10	NS	NS	ECHO, carotid pulse Systolic/diastolic function ESWS, angiotensin II response	ABN diastolic function ↑ ESWS
Santoro et al, 1987[273]	26	NS	245	Yes	5–8	7	0	STI, ECHO, Rest RNCA	None
LaMonte et al, 1986[272]	19	83–229	176	Yes	1.3–5.9	3.25	5 (26%)	ECG, ECHO RNCA Rest and stress	2 ABN ECG 3 ABN EF rest 2 ABN EF stress
Weesner et al, 1991[43]	10	90–498	291	NS	4–13	7	NS	ECHO, Doppler, exercise, versus controls	Poor ↑ with stress of FS, aortic flow, and cardiac index
Larsen et al, 1992[45]	133	NS	219	51	NS	NS	≥110 (~90%)	ECG 24 h ECG	40 ABN ECG 110 ABN 24 h ECG 6 VPB pairs 4 VT
Jakacki et al, 1991[44]	57	≤350	263	16	2.1–20.7	5.4	≥40 (≥70%)	ECHO, ECG 24 h ECG RNCA Exercise	5 ABN FS, 18 ABN ECG ≥40 ABN 24 h ECG 9 ABN RNCA 25 ABN exercise

ABN, abnormal; Cath, cardiac catheterization; ECHO, echocardiogram; ECG, electrocardiogram; EF, ejection fraction; ESWS, end-systolic wall stress; FS, fractional shortening; LV, left ventricular; NS, not stated; PW, posterior wall thickening; RNCA, radionuclide cardiac angiography, SD, sudden death; STI, systolic time interval; VCF, velocity of circumferential fiber shortening; VPB, ventricular premature beats; VT, ventricular tachycardia.

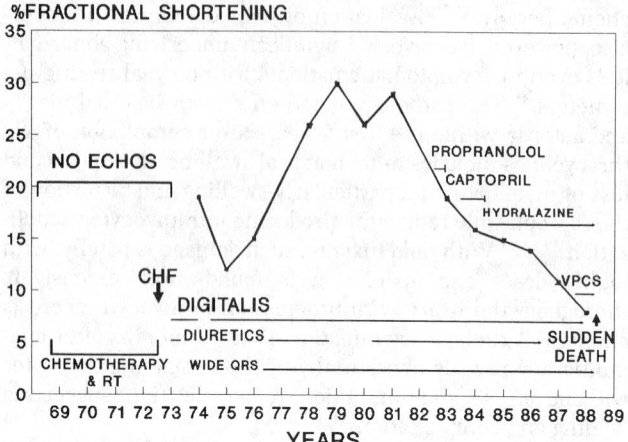

FIGURE 63–1. The clinical course of a patient after subclinical anthracycline cardiotoxicity. The initial increase and then progressive decrease of her fractional shortening (FS) on echocardiogram and increasing requirements for therapeutic support of cardiac function, can be seen. Despite an early FS of 11%, the patient gradually improved over the first 6 years. She discontinued diuretics, achieved modest exercise tolerance, and completed high school. The patient's FS on echocardiogram reached 30% 6 years after therapy. Eight years after doxorubicin therapy, however, she required increasing amounts of diuretics for recurrent edema. Ten years after chemotherapy, the patient had progressive deterioration of exercise tolerance and FS despite increasingly intensive medical management. During the last 2 years, she was found to have moderately frequent premature ventricular contractions but no syncope or runs of ectopic ventricular beats. She was deemed unsuitable for cardiac transplantation. Finally, 20 years after initial diagnosis and 17 years after her last anthracycline dose, the patient developed a tachy-brady arrhythmia that led to sudden syncope and cardiac arrest. CHF, congestive heart failure; VPCS, ventricular premature contractions; RT, radiotherapy.

of late abnormality correlates with increasing cumulative dose of anthracycline, and mediastinal irradiation is an additive risk factor.[36,37,40] Late abnormalities of resting echocardiograms, however, were found in patients treated with as little as 75 mg/m² of doxorubicin,[40] and late abnormalities of exercise response were seen in 55% of patients treated with low cumulative doses (median, 263 mg/m²).[44] Abnormalities of myocardial mass are said to be more pronounced in patients treated in early childhood, implying a negative effect on myocardial growth.[40] Abnormalities of systolic function do not correlate with age during chemotherapy.[36] Measurements of systolic function[36,37] and myocardial wall thickness[40] deteriorate progressively with time after anthracyclines (Fig 63–2). Serious arrhythmias have been identified in symptomatic and asymptomatic patients at late cardiac follow-up, including ventricular tachycardia and fibrillation and second-degree heart block.[36,37,40,44,45] Several young patients with late cardiomyopathy have died suddenly up to 15 years after chemotherapy.[36,37] The pathology found on biopsy and autopsy of patients with late cardiotoxicity is predominantly fibrosis and hypertrophy of remaining myocytes, with little remaining vacuolization.[36,37,41] Thus, even asymptomatic patients who have been treated with anthracyclines need long-term cardiac follow-up, and new symptoms suggestive of arrhythmia and especially syncope need vigorous investigation. Cardiac status on noninvasive testing during the year after completion of therapy predicts the likelihood of late abnormality (Fig. 63–3) and indicates the advisable frequency of follow-up.[36,37]

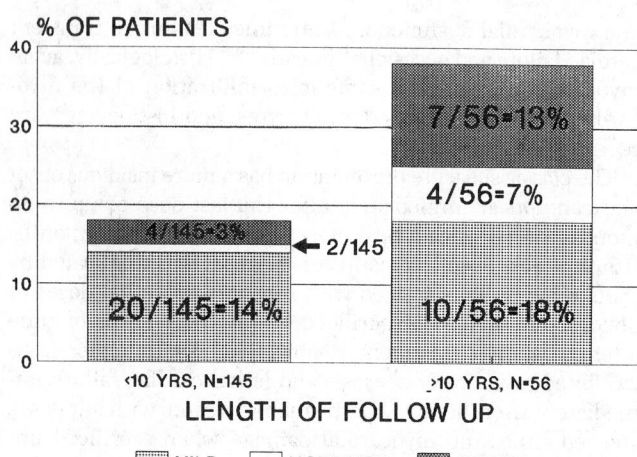

FIGURE 63–2. Percentage of patients found to have abnormal echocardiograms on long-term follow-up. Despite a similar cumulative anthracycline dose (495 versus 420 mg/m²), 38% of those followed for 10 years or longer had decreased fractional shortening (FS), compared with 18% of those followed for less than 10 years ($p < 0.004$). More than half of abnormalities (11/21) seen in the group followed for 10 or more years were moderate (FS = 21–24%), or severe (FS ≤ 20%), while the degree of abnormality was mild (FS = 25–28%) in 77% (20/26) of the abnormal patients followed for less than 10 years.

Mechanisms of Pathogenesis

An understanding of the mechanisms of cardiotoxicity is vital to attempts at prevention. There are many mechanisms proposed, and several may interact to cause the multiple sites of intracellular injury seen histologically. Doxorubicin is found to bind to cardiolipin in the inner mitochondrial membrane,[46,47] with two deleterious results. The electron transfer in the respiratory chain, which is dependent on the binding of cardiolipin to cytochrome *c* for its interaction with cyto-

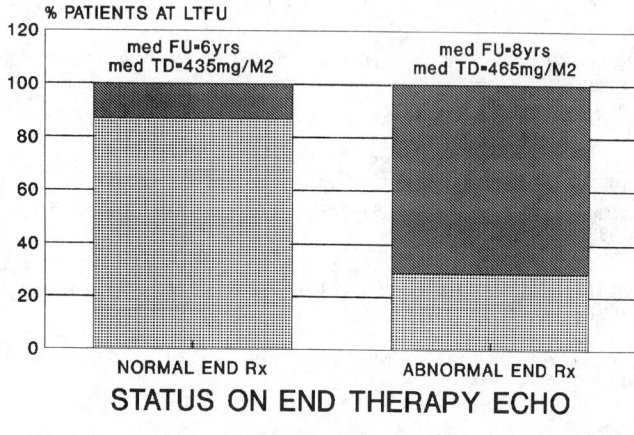

FIGURE 63–3. An echocardiogram taken after completion of anthracycline therapy has prognostic implications for cardiac function on late follow-up. Eighty-seven percent of patients who had normal fractional shortening on echocardiogram during the year after therapy remained normal at late follow-up, whereas only 29% of patients who were even mildly abnormal on end therapy echocardiogram were normal at late follow-up ($p < 0.0001$). ECHO, echocardiogram; LTFU, late follow-up.

chrome oxidase, and the activation by cardiolipin of the NADH-cytochrome *c* oxidoreductase complex (complex I–III), for the synthesis of adenosine triphosphate (ATP), are disrupted. This leads to depletion of ATP and phosphocreatine concentrations and depression of contractility.[48] In addition, the doxorubicin-cardiolipin complex promotes transfer of electrons through doxorubicin, forming a doxorubicin free radical that can reduce molecular oxygen, producing O_2^-.[46] This induces the generation of free hydroxyl radicals and H_2O_2, leading to mitochondrial membrane damage, further disruption of enzymatic respiration, and more extensive lipid peroxidation.[46,47] Oxidative damage is worsened by the concomitant decrease, during chemotherapy, of glutathione peroxidase, which normally serves as a free radical scavenger. Glutathione is especially important in myocytes, which lack catalase, which serves as a scavenger in other tissues. Free radical lipid peroxidation was identified[50] as an important mechanism of myocyte damage and has been found to depend, in the heart, on an iron-doxorubicin complex.[47,51,52] The resultant disruption of the sarcoplasmic reticulum and direct effects of the metabolite doxorubicinol have been shown to cause disturbances of Ca^{2+} transport,[47,53,54] which is critical to regulation of cardiac action potentials, contraction, and relaxation.[55] Chronically, there is alteration of contractile proteins and their enzymes with a shift in the ratio of prevalent isomyocin types and decreased production of α-myosin heavy chains, perhaps as an adaptation to chronic low-energy states.[56]

Prevention

MONITORING. Attempts at prevention of cardiomyopathy initially involved limitation of total cumulative dose below 450 to 550 mg/m[2]. This limit was chosen to avoid the rapid increase in prevalence of clinical cardiac dysfunction in excess of 30%, which occurs above that dose range. Arbitrary dose limitation was inadequate because of variability of individual tolerance. Therefore, therapy has been modified according to serial monitoring of cardiac status, by various means, to identify increasing risk of unacceptable toxicity. Monitoring of systolic time intervals and of electrocardiograms (ECGs) for QRS voltage loss[57] or ST-T changes was too nonspecific or showed changes too late to direct prevention. Serial echocardiography has been helpful in identifying changes in systolic and diastolic function, especially in children, where echo images are clear and more easily measurable.[58–61] The fractional shortening is the most frequent parameter followed, although some recent groups follow end systolic wall stress and the relation between wall stress and velocity of circumferential fiber shortening.[61] Radionuclide cardiac angiography has been used by many investigators to follow systolic[62–65] and diastolic function,[66] and specific guidelines for modification of chemotherapy on the basis of radionuclide ejection fraction in adults, proposed by Schwartz and colleagues,[62] has gained wide acceptance. Adherence to these guidelines reduced the incidence of cardiac failure from 21% to 3% in this study. The addition of measurements of contractility during exercise for comparison with those at rest adds sensitivity according to some authors[63–65] but is less helpful according to others.[67] Recommendations for monitoring, including radionuclide studies and quantitation of pathologic damage by endomyo-

cardial biopsy, have been offered by investigators from Stanford University Medical Center.[65] These recommendations, however, do not suggest monitoring until a cumulative dose of 450 mg/m[2] is reached, unless the baseline study is abnormal or unless the patient is over 70 years of age, has hypertension, has other cardiac disease, or was receiving mediastinal irradiation. Monitoring that follows these recommendations does not identify early sensitivity in patients without those particular risk factors. Another format for monitoring, using a combination of echocardiography and radionuclide studies, was formulated by the multiinstitutional Cardiology Discipline Committee of the Childrens Cancer Group.[58] These recommendations include cardiac evaluation before anthracycline administration and further monitoring before every other course until a cumulative dose of 300 mg/m[2] is reached and then for every course beyond this. Endomyocardial biopsy is suggested for abnormal or equivocal results. Although not yet included in routine monitoring, we hope that newer modalities, such as magnetic resonance imaging and indium-111-antimyosin scintigraphy,[68,69] will add to the efficacy of monitoring in the future.

SCHEDULE MODIFICATION. Other attempts to prevent cardiomyopathy involve decreasing the peak dose of anthracycline delivered to the heart by modification of schedules of delivery.[70–72] Legha and colleagues[70] demonstrated that patients receiving continuous infusions of doxorubicin developed lower peak plasma levels the longer the length of time of the infusion. Thus, levels with a 48-hour infusion were lower than with a 24-hour infusion, and a 96-hour infusion of the same dose per course produced still lower levels. Comparison of endomyocardial biopsy scores in patients receiving doxorubicin showed that patients receiving their dose by 48- or 96-hour infusion had significantly lower biopsy scores, indicating less cardiomyopathy than patients receiving the dose by 20-minute bolus. In addition, patients receiving 96-hour infusions had lower biopsy scores than those receiving 24-hour infusions. Infusions were administered through an indwelling intravenous line using a battery-powered, portable pump. Continuous infusion chemotherapy is usually given through a surgically implanted central venous catheter. A recent study by Shapira and colleagues[72] using radionuclide cardiac angiography to evaluate cardiotoxicity demonstrated a decline in left ventricular ejection fraction (LVEF) of only 6% after a total cumulative dose of 400 mg/m[2] administered by only 6-hour continuous infusion, compared with a drop of 21% in patients who received the same range of total doxorubicin dose by 20-minute bolus. More recently, Casper and colleagues[71] confirmed the cardioprotective effects of 72-hour infusion in a prospective randomized trial of 82 patients with soft tissue sarcoma. Schedules dividing the planned monthly doxorubicin dose into smaller weekly doses also decrease pathologic and physiologic abnormalities, allowing administration of higher cumulative doses.[73,74]

CARDIOPROTECTIVE AGENTS. Free radical scavengers, such as vitamin E,[75] N-acetylcysteine,[76] and other scavengers[77,78] have shown promise in animals but no clear benefit in patients. Similarly, trials of concomitant administration of coenzyme Q, verapamil,[79] prenylamine,[80,81] and other calcium-channel blockers; β-adrenergic and histamine blockers[82-84] to prevent the effects of excessive vasoactive agents; antiinflammatory agents, carnitine, digoxin,[85] and amrinone[86]; as well as encapsulation of the anthracycline in liposomes and binding to agarose[87] have not proved definitively useful in patients. The liposomes used during the patient trials of the last decade were highly unstable, and it is hoped that the new phase II trials with a more stable complex will show significant protection.[88] Attempts to exploit the importance of the iron-doxorubicin complex appear to be more successful. (+−)-1,2-bis(3,5-dioxopiperazinyl-1-yl)propane, known as ICRF-187 or ADR-529, is an iron chelator that has been shown to exhibit significant protection against anthracycline cardiotoxicity in various animal studies,[89,90] in a pilot study of 12 patients with various solid tumors,[91] and in a randomized therapeutic trial in women with breast cancer.[92,93] Patients were evaluated both by radionuclide ejection fraction and myocardial biopsy. Incidence of clinical toxicity, degree of decrease of ejection fraction, and biopsy score were significantly less in the ICRF arm of the studies. These results are being confirmed in a multicenter patient trial with similar monitoring. Recent animal studies have shown that there is no mediation of ICRF protection by changes of myocardial antioxidants[94] and that there is not merely a delay of appearance of the injury.[95] Examination of rabbits 3 months after discontinuation of therapy shows healing of lesions in those treated with ICRF.

NEW ANALOGS. Analogs of daunorubicin and doxorubicin have been studied in clinical trials. Many agents that appear to have decreased cardiotoxicity in animal studies and even in early clinical trials eventually have been found to have similar toxicity to the parent compound. Patients treated with zorubicin experienced cardiotoxicity, which was additive to prior anthracycline toxicity, and some developed cardiac failure.[96,97] 4'Epi-doxorubicin is another analog with cardiotoxicity similar to or possibly less than doxorubicin.[98-100] Incidents of atrioventricular block, ventricular fibrillation, decreased ejection fraction,[101] and decreased velocity of circumferential fiber shortening[102] have been reported in phase I and II trials with another analog, Aclarubicin. Demethoxy daunorubicin (idarubicin) has shown activity in patients whose malignancy has become resistant to daunorubicin, but it is also cardiotoxic.[103-105] The myelotoxicity of idarubicin is about four times that of daunorubicin. When given in amounts of equivalent myelotoxicity, the cardiotoxicity is also similar.[104,106] Thus, careful monitoring of this agent is warranted above a cumulative dose of 75 mg/m². Cardiac failure and subclinical decrease in ejection fraction occurred in patients treated with the analog esorubicin (DXDX). A 5% drop in mean LVEF was noted at 240 mg/m² and a 10% drop at 480 mg/m² of this agent.[107] Animal studies of 4'-deoxy-4'-iodo-doxorubicinol (I-DXR) indicate acute and chronic cardiotoxicity but possibly less than daunorubicin.[108] The ideal anthracycline has not been found.

Management

Clinical anthracycline cardiomyopathy needs to be managed with inotropic support and afterload reduction,[23] often initially by the intravenous route. Most patients can be stabilized and show clinical improvement. Patients who were refractory to treatment, had repeated bouts of pulmonary edema or increasing pulmonary resistance, and were free of malignancy benefited from cardiac transplantation.[109-111]

MITOXANTRONE

Mitoxantrone hydrochloride is an anthracenedione that is similar in structure to doxorubicin. Animal studies revealed conflicting findings in different species, including ECG abnormalities in treated monkeys, dose-related impairment of contractility in the rabbit heart,[112] and no ECG changes or progressive anthracycline-like lesions on endomyocardial biopsy specimens of beagle hearts.[113] Cases of cardiac failure and arrhythmia (mainly supraventricular) were reported from the early phase I and II trials of the National Cancer Institute.[114,115] The incidence of myocardial dysfunction and cardiac failure increased with increasing cumulative dose, as with doxorubicin.[114,116] Significant decrease in ejection fraction occurred in these trials around 110 mg/m²,[114] and a rapid increase in incidence of cardiac failure was noted at 160 mg/m².[116] Recent studies have continued to detect cardiomyopathy and cardiac failure in patients with[117] and without[118] prior anthracycline therapy; and conduction delay, with prolongation of PR, QRS, and QT intervals on ECG was also reported.[119] A British patient trial reported a 46% incidence of abnormal LVEF using radionuclide angiography during rest and cold pressor stress in patients who received a wide range of doses.[120] An Italian trial reported ECG abnormalities in 41%, echocardiographic abnormalities in 66%, and a 15% or more decrease in radionuclide LVEF in almost 25% of patients receiving a cumulative dose of 28 to 84 mg/m².[121] The overall incidence, reported by Lederle Laboratories, of subclinical moderate to serious decrement in LVEF was 13%; and the incidence of cardiac failure, up to a cumulative dose of 140 mg/m², was 2.6%.[122]

AMSACRINE

Amsacrine (AMSA) is an acridine derivative used mainly in patients with nonlymphoblastic leukemia. It has been associated with myocardial infarction[123] and ventricular arrhythmias, including fatal ventricular fibrillation.[124-126] These arrhythmias often have been attributed to coexisting electrolyte abnormalities, particularly hypokalemia. Recently, AMSA has been safely administered even to patients with preexisting atrial[127] and ventricular[128] arrhythmias. Noninvasive monitoring of cardiac function during a prospective study of AMSA revealed reversible abnormalities on serial echocardiograms in 18 of 27 patients and cardiac failure in 7 of 27 patients.[129,130] Echocardiographic abnormalities generally appeared within 1 week of AMSA therapy and resolved in most cases once therapy was discontinued. Four patients died with persistent cardiac failure. The incidence of echocardiographic abnormalities was related to total dose of AMSA, rate of AMSA administration, and total dose of anthracyclines previously received. No patient who received less than 200 mg/m² of AMSA in 48 hours, after having previously received less than 400 mg/m² of anthracyclines, had echocardiographic abnormalities. In contrast, all patients who received 200 mg/m² or more of AMSA within 48 hours after having previously received more than 400 mg/m² of anthracyclines exhibited echocardiographic abnormalities.[129] Arlin and colleagues[131] treated 24 patients with preexisting myocardial dysfunction with more than 200 mg/m² of AMSA over 48 hours and reported no occurrences of cardiac failure in this group. Nine of the patients had radionuclide ejection fractions determined after AMSA treatment and 2 of these patients showed a further decrease of ejection fraction by more than 10%. It was not stated how soon after treatment the radionuclide angiograms were obtained. Therefore, it is possible that there were additional transient deficits that were not detected in this study. The absence, however, of any clinical cardiac failure in these heavily treated patients is significant.

CYCLOPHOSPHAMIDE

Investigators disagree about whether cyclophosphamide in doses under 100 mg/kg/week contribute to cardiomyopathy.[15,28,73,132] In our experience, it does not. Higher doses used for cytoreduction and immunosuppression before bone marrow transplantation can cause an acute hemorrhagic pancarditis. This was initially described in case reports,[133-135] animal studies,[136] and autopsy series[137,138] as involving a serosanguineous pericardial effusion, mural thickening with edema, and endocardial, myocardial, and epicardial hemorrhage. This results from endothelial capillary damage that allows extravasation of fluid and red cells into cardiac and pulmonary tissues. Reports of patient series[139-142] described the acute course, with an onset during the first week after treatment, peak toxicity at 7 to 9 days, and improvement over the next 3 weeks. Abnormal findings of diastolic dysfunction, small to moderate pericardial effusion, restrictive cardiomyopathy (sometimes mimicking pericardial tamponade), and later systolic dysfunction were found described in more than half of patients.[140-142] Most patients remained asymptomatic; some had mild symptoms of fluid retention, edema, and tachypnea; and a few had an extremely fulminant course of cardiac failure and shock that was resistant to intensive treatment and resulted in death. Previous anthracycline therapy and previous abnormal cardiac function were identified as risk factors, and the importance of dose and rate of delivery was stressed.[140] A weekly dose of 170 mg/kg over 4 days without anthracyclines and 120 mg/kg over 2 days after anthracyclines predicted risk for at least subclinical changes. More rapid delivery of 120 mg/kg over 24 hours produced fulminant cardiomyopathy in 1 patient.[135,137] Mildly symptomatic patients responded to diuretics and, if necessary, transient digitalization or intravenous inotropic agents. Those with the more fulminant course required prolonged intravenous inotropic support, respiratory assistance, and hemofiltration.[142] Pericardial drainage has not been helpful, and the effusion can be managed conservatively and improves with time.[143] To avoid this clinical cardiotoxicity, patients have been screened during the past decade with echocardiography or radionuclide studies to identify abnormal cardiac function. The pretransplantation regimen can then be adjusted for higher risk patients by administering the cyclophosphamide over additional days or by using a preparatory regimen without cyclophosphamide. A pretreatment radionuclide LVEF of less than 50% has been correlated with increased risk of cardiotoxicity.[144,145] Recent studies suggested that giving the cyclophosphamide in smaller doses twice a day decreased the incidence of systolic

dysfunction, although changes in myocardial mass still occurred.[145] Children treated with anthracyclines for malignancy before transplantation who were evaluated during exercise at least 1 year after transplantation showed significant hemodynamic abnormalities. A small group of children with aplastic anemia who had not received anthracyclines, evaluated similarly, were normal.[146]

IFOSFAMIDE

Ifosfamide, an alkylating oxazaphosphorine related to cyclophosphamide, has been associated with atrial ectopy (including atrial fibrillation) and, less commonly, ST-T wave changes and bradycardia. These abnormalities were noted in patients who had received doses as high as 6.25 to 10 g/m² over 3 to 5 days.[147] ECG abnormalities, negative inotropic effects, and pathologic myocardial damage were also found in animals that received high doses of ifosfamide.[148,149]

RETINOIC ACID

Transretinoic acid is an agent that has proved effective for the treatment of acute promyelocytic leukemia. Its use is associated with RA syndrome in up to 25% of cases, characterized by fever, dyspnea, pleural and pericardial effusion, pulmonary infiltrates, peripheral edema, and transient myocardial dysfunction.[150] This is especially prevalent during the first 2 weeks of therapy and has responded to dexamethasone.

TAXOL

Taxol is a new antimicrotubule assembly inhibitor. It has activity against melanoma, refractory ovarian carcinoma, and non-small cell carcinoma of the lung through its induction of tubulin polymerization. Cases of significant disturbances of cardiac rhythm and conduction have been reported during phase I and II trials of this agent.[151] Significant sinus bradycardia (30–50 beats/minute) occurred in up to 29% of patients in the phase II trial for ovarian cancer.[152] Several patients exhibited progressive atrioventricular conduction delay from first-degree heart block, to complete heart block, to asystole[152] on continuous ECG monitoring during Taxol infusion as a single agent. The conduction delay reverted to normal with cessation of the infusion. Associated presyncope and syncope have been reported.[151] One patient required a demand pacemaker for further infusions. Episodes of sustained and nonsustained ventricular tachycardia have been reported with the combination of Taxol and cisplatin[153] during the Taxol infusion. Chest pain occurred in several patients receiving the combination, and a myocardial infarction, coincident with complete heart block, was documented in one man with coronary heart disease. It is not certain if the adverse effects on cardiac conduction relate to the Taxol itself or to its Cremophor EL vehicle. Preliminary experience with the synthetic analog Taxatere suggests a lesser potential for dysrhythmia. It has been recommended that continuous ECG monitoring accompany the use of these agents.[151]

HOMOHARRINGTONINE

Homoharringtonine is an alkaloid from the Chinese *cephalotaxus*. It is another drug that causes reversible atrioventricular block,[154] ventricular ectopy,[155] supraventricular tachycardia, and ST-T wave changes in animals[156] and patients.[154] It has also produced cardiac failure and hypotension, with vacuolar degeneration of the myocardium on pathologic examination.[154,156]

VINCRISTINE AND VINBLASTINE

Vincristine has been associated with cardiac autonomic dysfunction. One study demonstrated a loss of cyclic respiratory phase-related heart rate variation in 9 children during vincristine treatment.[157]

Vincristine[158] and vinblastine[159] have also been associated with myocardial infarction. Angina pectoris was reported in up to 38% of patients during treatment with vinblastine combined with cisplatin and bleomycin.[160] Another study of the same combination reported angina with infarct-like ECG changes and apical akinesia occurring repeatedly, during multiple courses, in a 47-year-old patient with normal coronary angiography.[161] This seemed to clearly implicate the chemotherapy as the cause.

MITOMYCIN C

Mitomycin C has been reported to increase the incidence of anthracycline cardiotoxicity when these agents are combined[162] due to enhancement of formation of superoxide and hydrogen peroxide.[163] It also has been described as a cause of acute congestive heart failure in a woman who received a cumulative dose of 225 mg/m^2 of mitomycin as a single agent[164] and in another patient when 30 mg/m^2 of mitomycin was added to treatment with 150 mg/m^2 doxorubicin.[165] The overall incidence of cardiotoxicity is said to be under 10% and limited to patients receiving a cumulative dose of at least 30 mg/m^2.[165,166]

5-FLUOROURACIL

The cardiotoxicity of 5-FU was first identified by Dent and McColl in 1975.[167] A survey of 1083 patients in 1982 reported cardiotoxicity in 1.1% of all patients and in 4.6% of patients with prior evidence of heart disease.[168] Since then, more frequent use of continuous-infusion 5-FU, increased awareness of the problem, and more sophisticated monitoring have increased the reported incidence. By 1990, there were more than 67 clinical cases described,[169] and an incidence ranging up to 68% of silent ischemic ECG changes was identified in patients monitored by continuous 24-hour ambulatory ECG during 5-FU infusion.[170] The clinical features of the cardiotoxicity included the following:

1. Precordial pain (both nonspecific and anginal)[169]
2. ECG ST-T wave changes (nonspecific and ischemic)[169,170]
3. Acute myocardial infarction (rare)[171,172]
4. Atrial arrhythmia (including atrial fibrillation) and, less frequently, ventricular ectopy (including refractory ventricular tachycardia and fibrillation)[170–173]
5. Ventricular dysfunction (usually global, less frequently segmental)

6. Cardiac failure, pulmonary edema, and cardiogenic shock (with and without ischemic symptoms)[172,174–177]
7. Sudden death[172,173]

In most cases, the arrhythmia was treatable and the ischemia-like symptoms and ECG changes disappeared (if the infusion was discontinued) or responded to nitrates, allowing the infusion to continue. The abnormalities of segmental and global ventricular function reverted to normal within days to weeks of cessation of infusion. Some patients needed intravenous inotropic and vasodilator support during the initial period.[174,175,177,178] In most cases with chest pain, with or without ECG changes, the CPK-MB fraction remained normal.[169,172,174,176] Most frequently, patients developed cardiac toxicity during the second or later course of treatment, but some experienced problems during the first course.[169] Those who developed cardiac toxicity and recovered usually had symptoms again when rechallenged with another infusion.[169,172] Some investigators reported success in preventing cardiotoxicity with calcium blockers such as nifedipine and diltiazem,[179] while others had less success.[176,180] There was no influence of age or sex on incidence.[169] Symptoms were reported in a 38-year-old man[177] and in several women in their 40s[169,174,175] with no prior cardiac history. Cardiac findings have occurred when 5-FU was given by infusion or bolus, as a single agent or with cisplatin and other drugs.[169] Although some felt that cardiac irradiation[181] and preexisting heart disease[168,170] were risk factors, others did not.[169,182] Several investigators documented normal coronary arteries in patients with severe symptoms.[172,175] One investigator excluded increased proclivity for coronary vasospasm by challenging a patient, who had previous angina, during 5-FU infusion with ergonovine during a posttreatment coronary study.[172] Findings on autopsy and endomyocardial biopsy have shown diffuse, interstitial edema, intracytoplasmic vacuolization of myocytes, and no inflammatory infiltrate.[183] Acute infarcts have been demonstrated pathologically in some, but not all, patients with clinical infarction.[169]

The ischemic-like pain and ECG findings, lack of CPK-MB fraction changes, and frequent response to nitrates and at times to calcium-channel blockers in the setting of anatomically normal coronary angiograms plus reversible contractility deficits suggest coronary vasospasm as a mechanism for 5-FU cardiotoxicity. The global dysfunction, however, possibly due to "stunned" myocardium, and the lack of universal response to coronary vasodilators leaves some questions about this hypothesis. Some investigators postulate a myocarditis or myocardiopathy pathogenesis.[184–186]

Although the mechanism is still uncertain, careful observation for cardiac symptoms and arrhythmia is warranted during drug infusion, especially in patients who were symptomatic in prior courses.

CISPLATIN

Cisplatin has been associated with arrhythmias such as atrial fibrillation[187] and with angina and ST-T wave changes on ECG.[188–191] These may be caused or exacerbated by electrolyte imbalances from the excessive hydration and forced diuresis required for the drug's administration.

INTERFERON

Cardiotoxicity has been identified in 44 of 432 patients from 15 phase I clinical trials of α-, α_2-, β-, and γ-interferon.[192] Significant abnormalities of cardiac rhythm and conduction,[192-195] ischemia and infarction,[192,196-198] and cardiomyopathy[192,199,200] were observed. These problems were identified with all types of interferon used except β-interferon, which was used in only a small subset of the patients.[192] No correlation with patient age, individual dose, or cumulative dose was identified, although some patients had less toxicity when retreated at doses lower than the dose that produced toxicity.[192,199] Cardiomyopathy was seen in patients after more prolonged treatment,[199] but the other forms of toxicity were seen frequently during the first 5 weeks of treatment, even within 1 to 7 days of initiation of therapy.[192] The occurrence of ischemia and infarction was definitely related to a prior history of ischemic heart disease and might have been related to increased myocardial oxygen demand, from the fever and stress of the influenza-like syndrome accompanying treatment, or to peripheral and coronary arterial constriction.[192] The arrhythmias were less clearly related to prior heart disease but might have been exacerbated by the features of this influenza-like syndrome as well. Arrhythmias and ischemic ECG changes were identified in mice treated with α-interferon with no myocardial lesions on necropsy, suggesting mediation by peripheral effects.[195] Arrhythmias have been seen in up to 20% of patients in clinical trials.[194] The arrhythmias observed include fatal[201] and reversible[202] ventricular fibrillation, ventricular tachycardia[193,194] atrial flutter and fibrillation, atrioventricular block, and less severe atrial and ventricular ectopy.[192] Sudden death occurred in 2 patients.[192] Cardiomyopathy, presenting as cardiac failure, with severe decrease in radionuclide ejection fraction to a range of 10% to 33%, was seen in 7 patients during prolonged administration of α- or α_2-interferon.[199,200,203,204] The cardiomyopathy was reversible in 4 of these patients after cessation of interferon, with and without inotropic, diuretic, and afterload reduction therapy. Congestive symptoms disappeared, and ejection fractions improved to a range of 29% to 46%. Two patients were retreated with lower doses of interferon without return of failure. Three of the patients with reversible cardiomyopathy had acquired immunodeficiency syndrome (AIDS) with Kaposi's sarcoma.[199] There is an AIDS-associated cardiomyopathy; however, this is not reversible. Two other patients had chronic myelogenous leukemia[203] and hairy cell leukemia,[200] and 2 more patients had other types of cancer.[204] Myocardial biopsy in 1 patient revealed only mild focal intramyocyte vacuolization.[199] The etiologic mechanism is unknown. In vitro studies have been conflicting. One study in isolated rat cardiac myocytes, incubated with interferon, showed inhibition of contractility and depletion of ATP,[205] while another similar study did not.[206] Some postulate an interaction between interferon and noradrenaline.[192,207] Cautious observation for cardiac symptoms and monitoring of rhythm appear to be warranted for these agents, with reduction in dose for significant abnormalities.

OTHER BIOLOGIC AGENTS

Interleukin-2 (IL-2) and tumor necrosis factor produced no reduction in ATP or decrease in contractility when incubated with isolated rat cardiac myocytes for 24 to 48 hours.[206] However, a major reduction in ventricular stroke work index was found in patients with a variety of solid tumors, who were monitored with indwelling arterial and pulmonary catheters during IL-2 treatment.[208] This resulted from a poor increase in cardiac index in comparison to the decrease in peripheral resistance. All patients developed a capillary leak syndrome requiring dopamine and crystaloid support. Deleterious effects on blood pressure, systemic resistance, and stroke work appeared to peak about 4 hours after individual doses and to worsen with subsequent doses.[208] In addition, there has been a significant (4–30% in various trials) incidence of apparent myocardial infarction with this agent.[208-213] One patient with elevated CPK-MB fraction, focal injury pattern on ECG, and segmental wall motion abnormality on radionuclide angiography underwent coronary angiography, which revealed normal coronary arteries.[214] This suggested a pathogenesis involving coronary vasospasm or focal myocarditis.

A new biologic agent, OK432, derived from *Streptococcus* sp was suspected of inducing an autoimmune cardiomyopathy; however, it was shown not to provoke the formation of anti-heart antibody or ECG changes in rabbits or patients.[215] Continued evidence of lack of cardiotoxicity should remove an obstacle to the development of OK432 as an active anticancer agent.

OTHER AGENTS

Case reports have attributed cardiotoxicity to several other agents. Melphalan,[216] bis(helenalinyl)malonate,[217] mithramycin,[218] bis[1,2-bis(diphenylphosphino)ethane]gold(I) chloride (a cytotoxic antineoplastic drug containing gold),[219] teniposide (VM26),[220] etoposide,[221] and busulfan[222] have been implicated in this respect.

RADIATION-INDUCED HEART DISEASE

Cardiac complications resulting from mediastinal irradiation were considered rare and insignificant for a long period in the history of radiation therapy.[223,224] Since the mid-1960s, when follow-up information on a large number of patients who had been cured of Hodgkin's disease with higher dose of radiation became available, the heart has no longer been considered radioresistant.[225] Radiation-induced heart disease (RIHD) has now been characterized[226,227] and investigated in experimental animals,[228-231] and the pathologic features of RIHD damage have been described with regard to the coronary arteries and all three layers of the heart.[232-235]

Pericarditis and pericardial effusion have been regarded as the most common side effects of cardiac irradiation.[226] Modern techniques of irradiation, dose fractionation, and reduction of the heart volume irradiated in most malignancies, however, have substantially reduced the frequency of this complication during the last decade.[236] At the same time, accumulated evidence suggests that ischemic heart disease resulting from radiation-induced coronary artery disease (CAD) is the most formidable potential long-term risk of cardiac irradiation.

The clinical spectrum of RIHD involves most structures of the heart and is summarized in Table 63–17. Although the

TABLE 63-17. Clinical Spectrum of Radiation-Induced Heart Disease

Pericardial disease
    Acute pericarditis during irradiation
    Delayed acute pericarditis
    Pericardial effusion
    Constrictive pericarditis
Myocardial dysfunction
Valvular heart disease
Electrical conduction abnormalities
Coronary artery disease

pathologic and clinical manifestations of RIHD may overlap in many patients, they are discussed separately in the following paragraphs.

PERICARDIAL DISEASE

Incidence

The risk of radiation-induced pericardial disease depends on both the dose given and on the volume of the heart irradiated.[226,237,238] Even when a large volume of the heart (60% or more) is irradiated at or below 4000 cGy, the risk for mild pericarditis is below 5%, and severe pericarditis is rare.[236] Smaller heart volumes (20–30%) may tolerate up to 6000 cGy, with an expected 2% risk of mild pericarditis. The importance of both volume and dose in the production of radiation pericarditis in Hodgkin's disease was demonstrated in an analysis of mantle field radiation therapy practices at Stanford.[239] In instances in which the whole pericardium was irradiated, the pericarditis incidence was 20%, but when most of the left ventricle was excluded, it was reduced to 7%. When an additional block was implemented to shield most of the heart after 3000 cGy, the incidence was reduced to only 2.5%. All series that showed a high risk for pericarditis[240–242] were of patients treated with a radiation technique, energy, and fractionation schedules that are no longer considered to be an acceptable standard of care in most centers.[238] With current radiation therapy techniques for Hodgkin's disease and breast cancer, pericarditis is an infrequent event.[238,243,244]

Pathology

Clinical and pathologic changes involving the pericardium are the most common abnormalities described after cardiac irradiation. The macroscopic abnormalities consist of pericardial thickening and effusion.[226] The parietal pericardium is more frequently and severely involved.[226] Collagen replaces the normal adipose tissue, fibrinous exudate is present on the surface and interstitially, and proliferation of small blood vessels can be observed microscopically.[226] The pericardial fluid is protein-rich and may contain strands of fibrin. The fluid ranges in appearance from serous to grossly sanguineous.[227] Over time, the fibrinous exudate may organize with the fibrotic pericardium and epicardium to develop into constrictive pericarditis. The mechanism for pericardial fibrosis and effusion is not clear. It may result from increased capillary permeability and inhibition of the local fibrinolytic mechanism.[226,245]

Radiation-induced hypothyroidism should also be considered as a cause of pericardial effusion after mediastinal irradiation.[246]

Acute Pericarditis During Radiation

Acute pericarditis during the course of radiation therapy is rare. It is almost always associated with massive mediastinal tumors adjacent to the heart. The signs and symptoms are of acute nonspecific pericarditis. It does not lead to a significant risk of late pericardial damage and is not an indication for interrupting the radiation course.[226]

Delayed Pericarditis

Radiation-induced pericarditis typically occurs within the first year after mediastinal irradiation. The common range is between 4 months to several years after treatment.[226,242,247–249] Pericardial disease presents either as an acute pericarditis, as a chronic pericardial effusion that may be asymptomatic, or as a combination of both. The symptoms of delayed acute pericarditis are indistinguishable from those of other types of pericarditis and usually consist of fever, pleuritic chest pain, pericardial friction rub, ST-T segment changes, and a decrease of the QRS voltage in the ECG.[226,227,242]

The differential diagnosis of pericardial effusion after radiation includes recurrent malignancy, idiopathic pericarditis, myxedema, and pericardial abscess.[227,250,251] It is estimated that 10% to 30% of patients with radiation-related pericardial effusion develop tamponade requiring pericardiocentesis.[241,252,253] Most cases of radiation-induced pericarditis and pericardial effusion resolve spontaneously, usually within 16 months.[253] About 20% of patients with delayed pericarditis progress within 5 to 10 years to develop symptomatic constriction requiring pericardiectomy.[254]

Treatment

Careful cardiac evaluation and monitoring with echocardiography and radionuclide ventriculography should be performed whenever RIHD is suspected.[247] Patients with mild symptoms and no hemodynamic compromise may be followed without treatment or receive symptomatic therapy with salicylates or other nonsteroidal antiinflammatory agents.[226,227] There are reports of a few patients who have received steroids with apparent improvement[255]; however, relapse of symptoms or unmasking of latent radiation injury after rapid withdrawal of steroid therapy has been reported.[256,257] Symptomatic pericardial effusion or clinical evidence for hemodynamic compromise warrants a drainage procedure. Pericardiocentesis with or without percutaneous placement of an indwelling catheter is successful in most patients.[251,258] Failure to relieve tamponade with pericardiocentesis, recurrence of effusion, or the presence of symptomatic constrictive pericarditis requires pericardiectomy.[229,242,259] The mortality of this procedure in patients with postirradiation pericarditis is high. Cameron and colleagues[260] reported a postoperative mortality of 21%, and a review by Ni and associates[261] showed an early mortality of 22% in patients operated for radiation-induced pericarditis and a late mortality (after more than 30 days) of 35%. The high rate of complication in previously irradiated patients is attributed to the existence of additional radiation injury to other cardiac and thoracic structures. Occult constrictive pericarditis requires no surgical intervention and usually has a good prognosis.[227]

MYOCARDIAL DYSFUNCTION

When myocardial dysfunction is detected after standard-dose mediastinal irradiation, it is typically mild or subclinical.[227,262,263] Impaired exercise capacity in asymptomatic patients after irradiation has been reported.[264,265] Noninvasive studies using echocardiography and radionuclide angiogram detected subtle left ventricular dysfunction in Hodgkin's disease patients evaluated a few years after mediastinal irradiation.[247,265,266] Most patients with abnormal ventricular function findings, however, do not have clinical heart failure.[263]

The magnitude of the potential contribution of cardiac irradiation to the risk of doxorubicin-induced cardiomyopathy is not well established, but some data suggest potentiation of anthracycline-induced cardiotoxicity when combined with radiation therapy.[13,17,26,267-269] The histopathologies of radiation heart disease and anthracycline heart disease are different,[270] and the combined effects are probably additive rather than synergistic.[226,270,271] Reducing the doxorubicin dose to 300 to 350 mg/m² in the setting of cardiac irradiation has been recommended.[13] In programs of combined modality therapy for Hodgkin's disease that included relatively low doses of doxorubicin (up to 250 mg/m²) and mediastinal irradiation of 2000 to 4000 cGy, no significant clinical myocardial dysfunction was detected.[272-274] Longer follow-up is required, however, to fully appreciate the potential risk of combined-modality cardiac toxicity.[36]

Symptomatic myocardial dysfunction after a radiation dose that does not exceed 6000 cGy is rare.[226] The few patients described with intractable heart failure had myocardial fibrosis as part of pancarditis, a generalized process with damage to all three layers of the heart. The hemodynamic pattern is usually of restrictive cardiomyopathy and is difficult to distinguish from constrictive pericarditis.[226,227,245] Its coexistence with pericarditis explains the poor outcome of pericardiectomy when attempted under these circumstances.[226,261]

VALVULAR DISEASE

Clinically significant valvular heart disease resulting from mediastinal irradiation is rare.[226,227,275] In a review of radiation-associated valvular disease, only 10 patients with symptomatic postirradiation valvular disease could be found.[275] When echocardiographic studies were performed in asymptomatic Hodgkin's disease patients more than 7 years after mediastinal irradiation, however, valvular abnormalities were detected in a third of the patients.[263,276] Most of the changes were found in the mitral or aortic valves and consisted of thickening or regurgitation.[263,275-277] In one series,[264] mild pulmonary stenosis was detected in 3 patients 6 to 12 years after radiation therapy. Surgical intervention for postirradiation valvular disease had been performed in 5 patients but was successful in only 3 of them.[275] Fibrous thickening of the valvular endocardium was found in 13 of 16 necropsies of young patients who received over 3500 cGy to the heart, but none had apparent valvular dysfunction.[232] The mean interval from irradiation to detection of valvular disease in 32 asymptomatic patients was 11.5 years.[275] In symptomatic patients, the interval was 16.5 years.[275] With longer follow-up, more patients may manifest symptoms related to radiation-induced valvular damage.[232,275]

ELECTRICAL ABNORMALITIES

Many ECG abnormalities were recorded years after mediastinal irradiation, the most common clinically significant abnormality being complete atrioventricular block.[247,264,278-284] Slama and associates[282] reported that radiation-related atrioventricular block was typically infranodal and occurred at long intervals (mean, 12 years), after radiation doses above 4000 cGy, most frequently in patients with abnormal conduction on ECG before the advent of complete block, and most frequently in patients who had other radiation-related cardiac abnormalities. At postmortem examination, fibrosis of the conduction system has been reported.[279,282]

CORONARY ARTERY DISEASE

Experiments in laboratory animals,[228-231,285-287] analysis of pathologic specimens,[232] clinical observations,[240,288-290] and long-term risk analyses in large series of patients treated for Hodgkin's disease[291-294] all indicate that mediastinal irradiation may facilitate the development of CAD.

Studies in rabbits on an atherogenic diet and exposed to radiation showed extensive atherosclerotic coronary damage to a degree that was disproportionately higher than what might have been expected from the summation of the changes induced by radiation alone and by high-cholesterol diet alone.[286] Similar observations have also been made in other experimental animals.[287,288]

An autopsy study in 16 young (aged 15 to 33 years) patients who received over 3500 cGy to the heart showed that 16 of 64 (25%) major coronary arteries had significant stenosis (more than 76% obstruction) compared with only one of 40 (2.5%) obstructed coronary arteries in a group of age- and sex-matched controls.[232] In this study, the proximal portion of the arteries had significantly more narrowing than the distal parts. McEniery and colleagues[290] described coronary angiograms of 15 patients with CAD after chest irradiation. Eight of these 15 had significant narrowing (more than 50% in diameter) of the left main coronary artery, and 4 had severe ostial stenosis of the right coronary artery. Stenosis at the origin of the coronary arteries appears to be a common finding for radiation-associated CAD.[295,296] After mediastinal irradiation, there is a greater likelihood for right coronary, left main, or left anterior descending coronary artery lesions as opposed to circumflex lesions, which may be due to the fact that the former vessels, particularly at their origin, receive more radiation.[297] Coronary spasm after radiation therapy has also been documented in patients who developed acute myocardial infarction with patent coronary arteries.[290,298]

Reports of CAD in young patients who received mediastinal irradiation for Hodgkin's disease have long implicated that radiation is a facilitating factor in this multifactorial disease process.[227,232,288-290,297] Only recently, however, analyses of large data bases of patients with Hodgkin's disease demonstrated a significantly increased risk of mortality from myo-

TABLE 63–18. Relative Risk of Mortality From Myocardial Infarction
After Mediastinal Irradiation for Hodgkin's Disease

Investigations	Center	No. of Patients	No. of Lethal MI Events	Relative Risk	95% Confidence Interval
Boivin et al, 1992[291]	Multiple	4665	68	2.6	1.1–5.9
Hancock et al, 1992[293]	Stanford	2060	45	3.2	1.5–5.8
Henry-Amar et al, 1991[292]	EORTC	1449	17	8.8	5.1–14.1
Tarbell et al, 1990[243]	JCRT	590	8	6.7	2.9–13.3

MI, myocardial infarction; EORTC, European Organization for Treatment and Research on Cancer;
JCRT, Joint Center for Radiation Therapy (Boston).

cardial infarction after mediastinal irradiation. These studies
are summarized in Table 63–18. Although only about 1% to
2% of Hodgkin's disease patients in these series died of myocardial infarction, the observed risk in all four series was still
higher than expected.[243,291–293] Boivin and colleagues[291] analyzed the risk of mortality from CAD in 4665 patients treated
for Hodgkin's disease and followed for an average period of
7 years. The age-adjusted relative risk of death with myocardial infarction after mediastinal irradiation was 2.6 and was
even higher (relative risk, 4) when myocardial infarction was
considered a direct cause of death. In this study, the onset of
increased risk was rapid, occurring within the first 5 years of
observation. None of the risk factors for CAD significantly
altered the relative risk estimates.

Mantle radiation therapy techniques, better fractionation
schemes, and modern equipment deliver smaller doses of radiation to the coronary arteries and may have a lower risk of
promoting CAD.[238] In Boivin's study,[291] the relative risk for
acute myocardial infarction was reduced from 6.33 for patients
treated during the years 1940 to 1966 to 1.97 (with no significant difference from unity) for patients irradiated from
1967 to 1985. Alternatively, data from Stanford[293] showed no
decrease in the risk of mortality from myocardial infarction
for patients treated after 1972, compared with patients treated
during earlier years.

Long-term mortality data from three trials that randomized
breast cancer patients to receive postmastectomy radiation therapy as opposed to no additional treatment demonstrated a higher incidence of cardiac death in the irradiated
group.[299–301] The excess in mortality did not appear until more
than 10 years after treatment.[300,301] In one study, the increase
in mortality risk was significant only in women who were
irradiated for tumors in the left breast.[301] It was also increased
in patients treated with orthovoltage irradiation as opposed
to those treated with more modern supervoltage equipment.[301]

These data demonstrate the risk associated with coronary
artery irradiation. The old breast irradiation techniques used
in these particular studies delivered high doses of radiation
to the heart.[238,302] These techniques are no longer in use in
most centers. Long-term follow-up of patients in similar randomized trials who were treated with heart-sparing techniques
did not show increased cardiovascular morbidity.[303,304] Prophylactic irradiation of the internal mammary nodes using a
single anterior photon beam ("hockey stick" technique),
which may deliver a high dose to the heart, is not indicated

in most patients irradiated for breast conservation or after
mastectomy.[305] Breast cancer patients irradiated with modern
techniques, energies, and fractionation schedules are unlikely
to receive a significant dose of radiation to the coronary
arteries.[302]

The radiation threshold for an increased risk of CAD has
not been determined. Lederman and associates[306] reported
that patients with seminoma who received a relatively low
dose of mediastinal irradiation (median, 2400 cGy) had more
ischemic heart disease than a similar group of patients whose
mediastinum was not irradiated. The observed cardiac risk in
the irradiated group, however, did not differ significantly from
the expected risk of a comparable normal population.

Monitoring and reduction of other contributing CAD factors
in patients who receive mediastinal irradiation should be part
of the follow-up of patients who undergo mediastinal irradiation. Early detection of CAD should be encouraged because
angioplastic or surgical intervention may be indicated in special anatomic or clinical situations. Successful treatment of
radiation-induced CAD with bypass surgery and with angioplasty has been reported.[290] In some cases, surgery may be
technically difficult because of mediastinal and pericardial
fibrosis.[290]

CONCLUSION

We look forward to the development of new chemotherapeutic
agents that are active against malignant cells but free of cardiotoxicity. We also hope that future modifications in techniques of radiation therapy will further decrease cardiotoxicity
from this mode of therapy. In the meantime, increased
awareness and knowledge about the potential cardiotoxicity
of these therapeutic modalities should enable physicians to
adequately monitor patients and modify therapy to minimize
serious acute and chronic cardiac sequelae. The increasing
information about late cardiac effects should facilitate early
diagnosis and therapeutic intervention for the benefit of previously treated patients.

REFERENCES

1. Tan CT, Tasaka H, Yu KP, et al. Daunomycin an antitumor antibiotic in the treatment
   of neoplastic disease. Cancer 1967;20:333–353.
2. Malpas JS, Scott RB. Rubidomycin in acute leukaemia in adults. Br Med J 1968;3:
   227–229.

3. Bonadonna G, Monfardini S. Cardiac toxicity of daunorubicin. Lancet 1969;1:837.

4. Marmont AM, Damasio E, Rossi F. Cardiac toxicity of daunorubicin. Lancet 1969;1: 837–838.

5. Bonadonna G, Monfardini S, De Lena M, et al. Phase I and preliminary phase II evaluation of adriamycin. Cancer Res 1970;30:2572–2582.

6. Tan C, Etcubanas E, Wollner N, et al. Adriamycin in children with acute leukemia and other neoplastic diseases. In: Carter SK, DiMarco A, Ghione M, Krakoff IH, Mathe G, eds. International symposium on Adriamycin. V. Clinical activity and side effects. Berlin, NY: Springer-Verlag, 1972:204–212.

7. Tan C, Etcubans E, Wollner N, et al. Adriamycin: an antitumor antibiotic in the treatment of neoplastic disease. Cancer 1973;32:9–17.

8. O'Bryan RM, Luce JK, Tally RW, et al. Phase II evaluation of adriamycin in human neoplasia. Cancer 1973;32:1–8.

9. Blum RH, Carter SK. Adriamycin: A new anticancer drug with significant clinical activity. Ann Intern Med 1974;80:249–259.

10. Gilladoga AC, Manuel C, Tan CT, et al. Cardiotoxicity of adriamycin in children. Cancer Chemother Rep 1975;6:75–80.

11. Lefrak EA, Pitha J, Rosenheim S, et al. A clinicopathologic analysis of Adriamycin cardiotoxicity. Cancer 1973;32:302–314.

12. Halazun JF, Wagner HR, Gaeta JF, et al. Daunorubicin cardiac toxicity in children with acute lymphocytic leukemia. Cancer 1974;33:545–554.

13. Von Hoff DD, Layard M, Basa P. Risk factors for doxorubicin induced congestive heart failure. Ann Intern Med 1979;91:701–717.

14. Von Hoff DD, Rozencweig M, Layard M, et al. Daunomycin-induced cardiotoxicity in children and adults. Am J Med 1977;62:200–208.

15. Bristow MR, Billingham ME, Mason JW, et al. Clinical spectrum of anthracycline cardiotoxicity. Cancer Treat Rep 1978;62:873–879.

16. Bristow MR. Pathophysiologic basis for cardiac monitoring in patients receiving anthracyclines. In: Crooke ST, Reich SD, eds. Anthracyclines: Current status and new developments. New York: Academic Press, 1988:255–270.

17. Billingham ME, Bristow MR, Glastein E, et al. Adriamycin cardiotoxicity: Endomyocardial biopsy evidence of enhancement by irradiation. Am J Surg Pathol 1977;1:17–23.

18. Bristow MR, Thompson PD, Martin RP, et al. Early anthracycline cardiotoxicity. Am J Med 1978;65:823–832.

19. Bristow MR, Minobe WA, Billingham ME, et al. Anthracycline-associated cardiac and renal damage in rabbits: Evidence for mediation by vasoactive substances. Lab Invest 1981;45:157–68.

20. Bristow MR, Billingham ME, Daniels JR. Histamine and catecholamines mediate Adriamycin cardiotoxicity. Proc Am Assoc Cancer Res 1979;20:118.

21. Wortman JE, Lucas VS, Schuster E, et al. Sudden death during doxorubicin administration. Cancer 1979;44:1588–1591.

22. Dindogru A, Barcos M, Henderson ES, et al. Electrocardiographic changes following Adriamycin treatment. Med Pediatr Oncol 1978;5:65–71.

23. Porembka DT, Lowder JN, Orlowski JP, Bastulli J, Lockrem J. Etiology and management of doxorubicin cardiotoxicity. Crit Care Med 1989;17:569–572.

24. Gottlieb SL, Edmiston WA, Haywood LJ. Late, late doxorubicin cardiotoxicity. Chest 1980;78:880–882.

25. Jaenke RS. Delayed and progressive myocardial lesions after Adriamycin administration in the rabbit. Cancer Res 1976;36:2958–2966.

26. Gilladoga AC, Manuel C, Tan CTC, et al. The cardiotoxicity of Adriamycin and Daunomycin in children. Cancer 1976;37:1070–1078.

27. Goorin AM, Borow KM, Goldman A, et al. Congestive heart failure due to Adriamycin cardiotoxicity: Its natural history in children. Cancer 1981;47:2810–2816.

28. Alexander J, Dainiak N, Berger HJ, et al. Serial assessment of doxorubicin cardiotoxicity with quantitative radionuclide angiocardiography. N Engl J Med 1979;300:278–283.

29. Cohen M, Kronzon I, Lebowitz A. Reversible doxorubicin-induced congestive heart failure. Arch Intern Med 1982;142:1570–1571.

30. Saini J, Rich MW, Lyss AP. Reversibility of severe left ventricular dysfunction due to doxorubicin cardiotoxicity. Ann Intern Med 1987;106:814–816.

31. Yeung ST, Yoong C, Spink J, Galbraith A, Smith PJ. Functional myocardial impairment in children treated with anthracyclines for cancer. Lancet 1991;337:816–818.

32. Bristow MR, Mason JW, Billingham ME, Daniels JR. Doxorubicin cardiomyopathy: Evaluation by phonocardiography, endomyocardial biopsy, and cardiac catheterization. Ann Intern Med 1978;88:168–175.

33. Billingham ME, Mason JW, Bristow MR, et al. Anthracycline cardiomyopathy monitored by morphologic changes. Cancer Treat Rep 1978;62:865.

34. Koh E, Imashuku S, Kiyosawa N, Sawada T. Anthracycline- induced congestive heart failure in two pediatric leukemia cases and long term follow-up. Pediatr Hematol Oncol 1988;5:245–251.

35. Steinherz L, Murphy ML, Steinherz P, et al. Long-term cardiac follow up 4–13 years post anthracycline therapy. In: Doyle E, Engle MA, Gersony W, Rashkin W, Talner N, eds. Pediatric cardiology. New York: Springer Verlag, 1986:1058–1061.

36. Steinherz LJ, Steinherz PG, Tan CTC, Heller G, Murphy ML. Cardiotoxicity 4–20 years after completing anthracycline therapy. JAMA 1991;266:1672–1677.

37. Steinherz LJ, Steinherz PG. Delayed anthracyclines cardiac toxicity. In: DeVita VT, Hellman S, Rosenberg SA, eds. Cancer: Principles and practice of oncology, PPO updates, 1991;5:1–15.

38. Steinherz L, Steinherz P. Cardiac failure more than six years post anthracyclines. Am J Cancer 1988;62:505.

39. Steinherz L, Steinherz P. Delayed cardiac toxicity from anthracycline therapy. Pediatrician 1991;18:49–52.

40. Lipshultz SE, Colan SD, Gelber RD, Perez-Atayde AR, Sallan SE, Sanders SP. Late cardiac effects of doxorubicin therapy for acute lymphoblastic leukemia in childhood. N Engl J Med 1991;324:808–815.

41. Goorin, AM, Chauvenet AR, Perez-Atayde AR, et al. Initial congestive heart failure, six to ten years after doxorubicin chemotherapy for childhood cancer. J Pediatr 1990;116:144–147.

42. Hausdorf G, Morf G, Beron G, et al. Long-term doxorubicin cardiotoxicity in childhood: Non-invasive evaluation of the contractile state and diastolic filling. Br Heart J 1988;60: 309–315.

43. Weesner KM, Bledsoe M, Chauvenet A, Wofford M. Exercise echocardiography in the detection of anthracycline cardiotoxicity. Cancer 1991;68:435–438.

44. Jakacki R, Silber J, Larsen R, Barber G, Goldwein J, Meadows A. Cardiac dysfunction following "Low risk" cardiotoxic treatment for childhood malignancy. Pediatr Res 1991;29:143A.

45. Larsen RL, Jakacki R, Vetter VL, Meadows AT, Silber J, Barber G. Electrocardiographic changes and arrythmias after cancer therapy in children and young adults. Am J Card 1992;70:73–77.

46. Goormaghtigh E, Huart P, Praet M, Brasseur R, Ruysschaert JM. Structure of the Adriamycin-Cardiolipin complex role in mitochondrial toxicity. Biophys Chem 1990;35: 247–257.

47. Fu LX, Waagstein F, Hjalmarson A. A new insight into Adriamycin-induced cardiotoxicity. Int J Cardiol 1990;29:15–20.

48. Kapelko VI, Saks VA, Novikova NA, Golikov MA, Kupriyanov VV, Popovich MI. Adaptation of cardiac contractile functions to conditions of chronic energy deficiency. J Mol Cell Cardiol 1989;21:79–83.

49. Myers CE, McGuire WP, Liss RH, Ifrim I, Grotzinger K, Young RC. Adriamycin: The role of lipid peroxidation in cardiac toxicity and tumor response. Science 1977;197: 165–167.

50. Rajagopalan S, Politi PM, Sinha BK, Myers CE. Adriamycin-induced free radical formation in the perfused rat heart: Implications for cardiotoxicity. Cancer Res 1988;48: 4766–4769.

51. Myers CE, Gianna L, Simone CB, Klecker R, Greene R. Oxidative destruction of erythrocyte ghost membranes catalyzed by the doxorubicin-iron complex. Biochemistry 1982;21:1707–1712.

52. Gutteridge JM. Lipid peroxidation and possible hydroxyl radical formation stimulated by the self-reduction of a doxorubicin-iron (III) complex. Biochem Pharmacol 1984;33: 1725–1728.

53. Olson RD, Mushlin PS, Brenner DE, et al. Doxorubicin cardiotoxicity may be caused by its metabolite doxorubicinol. Proc Natl Acad Sci USA 1988;85:3585–3589.

54. Pessah IN, Durie EL, Schiedt MJ, Zimanyi I. Anthraquinone-sensitized Ca2+ release channel from rat cardiac sarcoplasmic reticulum: Possible receptor-mediated mechanism of doxorubicin cardiomyopathy. Mol Pharmacol 1990;37:503–514.

55. Shenasa H, Calderone A, Vermeulen M, et al. Chronic doxorubicin induced cardiomyopathy in rabbits: Mechanical, intracellular action potential, and beta adrenergic characteristics of the falling myocardium. Cardiovasc Res 1990;24:591–604.

56. Cappelli V, Moggio R, Monti E, Paracchini L, Piccinini F, Reggiani C. Reduction of myofibrillar ATPase activity and isomyosin shift in delayed doxorubicin cardiotoxicity. J Mol Cell Cardiol 1989;21:93–101.

57. Minow RA, Benjamin RS, Lee ET, et al. QRS voltage change with Adriamycin administration. Cancer Treat Rep 1978;62:931–934.

58. Steinherz LJ, Graham T, Hurwitz R, et al. Guidelines for cardiac monitoring of children during and after anthracycline therapy: Report of the Cardiology Committee of the Childrens Cancer Study Group. Pediatrics 1992;89:942–949.

59. Bloom K, Bini R, Williams C, et al. Echocardiography in Adriamycin cardiotoxicity. 1978;Cancer 41:1265–1269.

60. Biancaniello T, Meyer RA, Wong KY, et al. Doxorubicin cardiotoxicity in children. J Pediatr 1980;97:45–50.

61. Borow K, Henderson I, Neuman A, et al. Assessment of left ventricular contractility in patients receiving doxorubicin. Ann Intern Med 1983;99:750–756.

62. Schwartz RG, McKenzie WB, Alexander J, et al. Congestive heart failure and left ventricular dysfunction complicating doxorubicin therapy: A seven year experience using serial radionuclide angiocardiography. Am J Med 1987;82:1109–1118.

63. Gottdiener JS, Mathisen DJ, Borer JS, et al. Doxorubicin cardiotoxicity: Assessment of late left ventricular dysfunction by radionuclide cineangiography. Ann Intern Med 1981;94:430–434.

64. Palmeri ST, Bonow RO, Myers CE, et al. Prospective evaluation of doxorubicin cardiotoxicity by rest and exercise radionuclide angiography. Am J Cardiol 1986;58:607–613.

65. McKillop JH, Bristow MR, Goris ML, et al. Sensitivity and specificity of radionuclide ejection fractions in doxorubicin cardiotoxicity. Am Heart J 1983;106:1048–56.

66. Lee BH, Goodenday LS, Muswick GJ, Yasnoff WA, Leighton RF, Skeel RT. Alterations in left ventricular diastolic function with doxorubicin therapy. J Am Coll Cardiol 1987;9: 184–188.

67. Bae JH, Schwaiger M, Mandelkern M, Lin A, Schelbert HR. Doxorubicin cardiotoxicity: Response of left ventricular ejection fraction to exercise and incidence of regional wall motion abnormalities. Int J Card Imaging 1989;3:193–201.

68. Estorch M, Carrio I, Berna L, et al. Indium-111-antimyosin scintigraphy after doxorubicin therapy in patients with advanced breast cancer. J Nucl Med 1990;31:1965–1969.

69. Jain D, Zaret BL. Antimyosin cardiac imaging: Will it play a role in the detection of doxorubicin cardiotoxicity? J Nucl Med 1990;31:1970–1974.

70. Legha SS, Benjamin RS, Mackay B, et al. Reduction of doxorubicin cardiotoxicity by prolonged continuous intravenous infusion. Ann Intern Med 1982;96:133–138.

71. Casper ES, Gaynor JJ, Hajdu SI, et al. A prospective randomized trial of adjuvant

chemotherapy with bolus versus continuous infusion of doxorubicin in patients with high-grade extremity soft tissue sarcoma and an analysis of prognostic factors. Cancer 1991;68:1221–1229.

72. Shapira J, Gotfried M, Lishner M, Ravid M. Reduced cardiotoxicity of doxorubicin by a 6-hour infusion regimen. Cancer 1990;65:870–873.

73. Torti FM, Bristow MR, Howes AE, et al. Reduced cardiotoxicity of doxorubicin delivered on a weekly schedule: Assessment by endomyocardial biopsy. Ann Intern Med 1983;99:745–749.

74. Weiss AT, Manthel RW. Experience with the use of Adriamycin in combination with other anti-cancer agents using a weekly schedule with particular reference to lack of cardiac toxicity. Cancer 1977;40:2046–2052.

75. Sonneveld P. Effect of α-tocopherol on the cardiotoxicity of Adriamycin in the rat. Cancer Treat Rep 1978;62:1033–1036.

76. Villani F, Galimberti M, Monti E, et al. Effect of glutathione and N-acetylcysteine on in vitro and in vivo cardiac toxicity of doxorubicin. Free Radic Res Commun 1990;11:145–151.

77. Perletti G, Monti E, Paracchini L, Piccinini F. Effect of trimetazidine on early and delayed doxorubicin myocardial toxicity. Arch Int Pharmacodyn Ther 1989;302:280–289.

78. Buc-Calderon P, Praet M, Ruysschaert JM, Roberfroid M. Increasing therapeutic effect and reducing toxicity of doxorubicin by N-acyl dehydroalanines. Eur J Cancer Clin Oncol 1989;25:679–685.

79. Kraft J, Grille W, Appelt M, et al. Effects of verapamil on anthracycline-induced cardiomyopathy: Preliminary results of a prospective multicenter trial. Hamatol Bluttransfus 1990;33:566–570.

80. Milei J, Marantz A, Ale J, Vazquez A, Buceta JE. Prevention of Adriamycin-induced cardiotoxicity by prenylamine: A pilot double blind study. Cancer Drug Deliv 1987;4:129–136.

81. Milei J, Vazquez A, Boveris A, et al. The role of prenylamine in the prevention of Adriamycin-induced cardiotoxicity: A review of experimental and clinical findings. J Int Med Res 1988;16:19–30.

82. Bartoli KF, Decorti G, Candussio L, et al. Effect of ketotifen on Adriamycin toxicity: Role of histamine. Cancer Lett 1988;39:145–152.

83. Harman GS, Craig JB, Kuhn JG, et al. Phase I and clinical pharmacology trial of crisnatol (BWA770u mesylate) using a monthly single-dose schedule. Cancer Res 1988;48:4706–4710.

84. Klugmann FB, Decorti G, Candussio L, et al. Amelioration of 4'epidoxorubicin-induced cardiotoxicity by sodium cromoglycate. Eur J Cancer Clin Oncol 1989;25:361–368.

85. Reeves WC, Griffith JW, Wood MA, Whitesell L. Exacerbation of doxorubicin cardiotoxicity by digoxin administration in an experimental rabbit model. Int J Cancer 1990;45:731–736.

86. Villani F, Manzotti C, Mella M, Monti E, Savi G, Zunino F. Effect of amrinone on anthracycline-induced lethal and cardiac toxicity in mice and rats. Med Oncol Tumor Pharmacother 1990;7:227–232.

87. Hacker MP, Lazo JS, Pritsos CA, Tritton TR. Immobilized Adriamycin: Toxic potential in vivo and in vitro. Sel Cancer Ther 1989;5:67–72.

88. Rahman A, Treat J, Roh JK, et al. A phase I clinical trial and pharmacokinetic evaluation of liposome-encapsulated doxorubicin. J Clin Oncol 1990;8:1093–1100.

89. Herman EH, Ferrans VJ. Reduction of chronic doxorubicin cardiotoxicity in dogs by pretreatment with (+) -1,2-bis(3,5-dioxopiperazinyl-l-yl) propane (ICRF-187). Cancer Res 1981;41:3436–3440.

90. Herman EH, Ferrans VJ, Jordan W, Ardalan B. Reduction of chronic daunorubicin cardiotoxicity by ICRF-187 in rabbits. Res Commun Chem Pathol Pharmacol 1981;31:85–97.

91. Belt RJ. Prevention of Adriamycin-induced cardiotoxicity by ICRF-187 (NSC-169780). Proc Am Soc Clin Oncol 1984;3:27.

92. Speyer JL, Green MD, Kramer E, et al. Protective effect of the bispiperazinedione ICRF-187 against doxorubicin-induced cardiac toxicity in women with advanced breast cancer. N Engl J Med 1988;319:745–752.

93. Speyer JL, Green MD, Sanger J, et al. A prospective randomized trial of ICRF-187 for prevention of cumulative doxorubicin-induced cardiac toxicity in women with breast cancer. Cancer Treat Rev 1990;17:161–163.

94. Alderto P, Gross J, Green MD. Role of (±)-1,2-bis(3,5-dioxopiperazinyl-1-yl) propane (ICRF-187) in modulating free radical scavenging enzymes in doxorubicin-induced cardiomyopathy. Cancer Res 1990;50:5136–5142.

95. Herman EH, Ferrans VJ. Examination of the potential long-lasting protective effect of ICRF-187 against anthracycline-induced chronic cardiomyopathy. Cancer Treat Rev 1990;17:155–160.

96. Tan C, Mitta SK, Steinherz L, Miller DR. Phase I trial of Rubidazone (NSC-164011) in children with cancer. Med Pediatr Oncol 1981;9:347–353.

97. Benjamin RS, Mason JW, Billingham ME. Cardiac toxicity of Adriamycin-DNA complex and Rubidazone: Evaluation by electrocardiogram and endomyocardial biopsy. Cancer Treat Rep 1978;62:935–939.

98. Tan CTC, Hancock C, Steinherz LJ. Preliminary results of epirubicin in children with acute leukemia. In: Bonadonna G, ed. Advances in anthracycline chemotherapy: Epirubicin. Milan: Masson Italia Editori 1984:129–132.

99. Nielsen D, Jensen JB, Dombernowsky P, et al. Epirubicin cardiotoxicity: A study of 135 patients with advanced breast cancer. J Clin Oncol 1990;8:1806–1810.

100. Neri B, Cini-Neri G, Bandinelli M, Pacini P, Bartalucci S, Ciapini A. Doxorubicin and epirubicin cardiotoxicity: Experimental and clinical aspects. Int J Clin Pharmacol Ther Toxicol 1989;27:217–221.

101. Mortensen SA. Aclarubicin: Preclinical and clinical data suggesting less chronic car-

diotoxicity compared with conventional anthracyclines. Eur J Haematol 1987;47(Suppl):21–31.

102. Wojnar J, Mandecki M, Wnuk-Wojnar AM, Holowiecki J. Clinical studies on aclacinomycin A cardiotoxicity in adult patients with acute non lymphoblastic leukemia. Folia Haematol (Leipz) 1989;116:297–303.

103. Carella AM, Berman E, Maraone MP, Ganzina F. Idarubicin in the treatment of acute leukemias: An overview of preclinical and clinical studies. Haematologica 1990;75:159–169.

104. Tan CT, Hancock C, Steinherz P, et al. Phase I and clinical pharmacological study of 4-demethoxydaunorubicin (Idarubicin) in children with advanced cancer. Cancer Res 1987;47:2990–2995.

105. Villani F, Galimberti M, Comazzi R, Crippa F. Evaluation of cardiac toxicity of idarubicin (4-demethoxydaunorubicin). Eur J Cancer Clin Oncol 1989;25:13–18.

106. Feig SA, Krailo MD, Harris RE, et al. Determination of the maximum tolerated dose of idarubicin when used in a combination chemotherapy program of reinduction of childhood ALL at first marrow relapse and a preliminary assessment of toxicity compared to that of daunorubicin: A report from the Children's Cancer Study Group. Med Pediatr Oncol 1992;20:124–129.

107. Ringenberg QS, Propert KJ, Muss HB, et al. Clinical cardiotoxicity of esorubicin (4'-deoxydoxorubicin,DxDx): Prospective studies with serial gated heart scans and reports of selected cases. A cancer and leukemia group B report. Invest New Drugs 1990;8:221–226.

108. Danesi R, Marchetti A, Bernardini N, La Rocca RV, Bevilacqua G, Del Tacca M. Cardiac toxicity and antitumor activity of 4'-deoxy-4'-iodo-doxorubicinol. Cancer Chemother Phamacol 1990;26:403–408.

109. Aldouri MA, Lopes ME, Yacoub M, et al. Cardiac transplantation for doxorubicin-induced cardiomyopathy in acute myeloid leukemia. Br J Haematol 1990;74:541.

110. Arico M, Nespoli L, Pedroni E, Bonetti F, Vigano M, Burgio GR. Heart transplantation in a child with doxorubicin-induced cardiomyopathy. N Engl J Med 1988;65:1353.

111. Edwards BS, Hunt SA, Fowler MB, Valantine HA, Stinson EB, Schroeder JS. Cardiac transplantation in patients with preexisting neoplastic diseases. Am J Cardiol 1990;65:501–504.

112. Tumminello FM, Leto G, Gebbia N, Gebbia V, Russo A, Rausa L. Acute myocardial effects of mitoxantrone in the rabbit. Cancer Treat Rep 1987;71:529–531.

113. Sparano BM, Gordon G, Hall C, Iatropoulos MJ, Noble FJ. Safety assessment of a new anticancer compound, mitoxantrone, in beagle dogs: Comparison with doxorubicin. II. Histologic and ultrastructural pathology. Cancer Treat Rep 1982;66:1145–1158.

114. Saletan S. Mitoxantrone: An active, new antitumor agent with an improved therapeutic index. Cancer Treat Rev 1987;14:297–303.

115. Shenkenberg TD, Von Hoff DD. Mitoxantrone: A new anticancer drug with significant clinical activity. Ann Intern Med 1986;105:67–81.

116. Posner LE, Dukart G, Goldberg J, Bernstein T, Cartwright K. Mitroxantrone: An overview of safety and toxicity. Invest New Drugs 1985;3:123–132.

117. Janmohammed R, Milligan DW. Mitoxantrone induced congestive heart failure in patients previously treated with anthracyclines. Br J Haematol 1989;71:292–293.

118. Pai GR, Reed NS, Ruddell WS. A case of mitoxantrone-associated cardiomyopathy without prior anthracycline therapy. Br J Radiol 1987;60:1125–1126.

119. Ewer MS, Ali MK, Abraham K, et al. Electrocardiographic (ECG) changes in patients receiving mitoxantrone previously treated with Adriamycin. Proc Am Soc Clin Oncol 1990;9:81.

120. Cassidy J, Merrick MV, Smyth JF, Leonard RC. Cardiotoxicity of mitozantrone assessed by stress and resting nuclear ventriculography. Eur J Cancer Clin Oncol 1988;24:935–938.

121. Villani F, Galimberti M, Crippa F. Evaluation of ventricular function by echocardiography and radionuclide angiography in patients treated with mitoxantrone. Drugs Exp Clin Res 1989;15:501–506.

122. Duffy M, ed. Physicians Desk Reference. 45th ed. Montvale, NJ, 1991;1195.

123. Lindpaintner K, Lindpaintner LS, Wentworth M, et al. Acute myocardial necrosis during administration of amsacrine. Cancer 1986;57:1284–1286.

124. Legha SS, Latreille J, McCredie KB, et al. Neurologic and cardiac rhythm abnormalities associated with 4'-(9-acridinylamino) methanesulfon-m-anisidide (AMSA) therapy. Cancer Treat Rep 1979;63:2001–2003.

125. Von Hoff DD, Elson D, Polk G, et al. Acute ventricular fibrillation and death during infusion of 4'-(9-acridinylamino)methanesulfon-m-anisidide (AMSA). Cancer Treat Rep [Letter] 1980;64:356–357.

126. Falkson G. Multiple ventricular extrasystoles following administration of 4'-(9-acridinylamino)methanesulfon-m-anisidide (AMSA). Cancer Treat Rep 1980;64:358.

127. Arlin Z, Mehta R, Feldman E, Sullivan P, Pucillo A. Amsacrine treatment of patients with supraventricular arrhythmias and acute leukemia. Cancer Chemother Pharmacol 1987;19:163–164.

128. Puccio CA, Feldman EJ, Arlin ZA. Amsacrine is safe in patients with ventricular ectopy. Am J Hematol 1988;28:197–198.

129. Steinherz LJ, Steinherz PG, Mangiacasale D, Tan C, Miller DR. Cardiac abnormalities after AMSA administration. Cancer Treat Rep 1982;66:483–488.

130. Tan CTC, Hancock C, Steinherz PG, et al. Phase II study of 4'-(9-Acridinylamino)methanesulfon-m-anisidide (NSC 249992) in children with acute leukemia and lymphoma. Cancer Res 1982;42:1579–1581.

131. Arlin ZA, Feldman EJ, Mittelman A, et al. Amsacrine is safe and effective therapy for patients with myocardial dysfunction and acute leukemia. Cancer 1991;68:1198–1200.

132. Praga C, Beretta G, Vigo PL, et al. Adriamycin cardiotoxicity: A survey of 1273 patients. Cancer Treat Rep 1979;63:827–834.

133. Santos GW, Sensenbrenner LL, Burke PJ, et al. Marrow transplants in man utilizing cyclophosphamide: Summary of Baltimore experience. Exp Hematol 1970;20:78–81.

134. Buckner CD, Rudolph RH, Fefer A, et al. High-dose cyclophosphamide therapy for malignant disease: Toxicity, tumor, response, and the effects of stored autologous marrow. Cancer 1972;29:357–365.

135. Mullins GM, Anderson PN, Santo GW. High dose cyclophosphamide therapy in solid tumors: Therapeutic, toxic and immunosuppressive effects. Cancer 1975;36:1950–1958.

136. Storb R, Buckner CS, Dillingham LA, et al. Cyclophosphamide regimens in rhesus monkeys with and without marrow infusion. Cancer Res 1970;30:2195–2202.

137. Slavin RE, Millan JC, Mullins GM. Pathology of high dose intermittent cyclophosphamide therapy. Hum Pathol 1975;6:693–709.

138. Buja LM, Ferrans VJ, Graw RG. Cardiac pathologic findings in patients treated with bone marrow transplantation. Hum Pathol 1976;7:17–44.

139. Applebaum FR, Strauchen JA, Graw RG, et al. Acute lethal carditis caused by high dose combination chemotherapy: A unique clinical and pathological entity. Lancet 1976;1:58–62.

140. Steinherz L, Steinherz P, Mangiacasale D, et al. Cardiac changes with cyclophosphamide. Med Pediatr Oncol 1981;9:417–422.

141. Gottdiener JS, Applebaum FR, Ferrans VJ, et al. Cardiotoxicity associated with high-dose cyclophosphamide therapy. Arch Intern Med 1981;141:758–763.

142. Steinherz LJ, Steinherz PG. Cyclophosphamide cardiotoxicity. Cancer Bull 1985;37:231–234.

143. Veys PA, McAvinchey R, Rothman MT, Mair GHM, Newland AC. Pericardial effusion following conditioning for bone marrow transplantation in acute leukemia. Bone Marrow Transplant 1987;2:213–216.

144. Bearman SI, Petersen FB, Schor RA, et al. Radionuclide ejection fractions in the evaluation of patients being considered for bone marrow transplantation: Risk for cardiac toxicity. Bone Marrow Transplant 1990;5:173–177.

145. Braverman AC, Antin JH, Plappert MT, Cook EF, Lee RT. Cyclophosphamide cardiotoxicity in bone marrow transplantation: A prospective evaluation of new dosing regimens. J Clin Oncol 1991;9:1215–1223.

146. Larsen RL, Barber G, Heise CT, August CS. Exercise assessment of cardiac function in children and young adults before and after bone marrow transplantation. Pediatrics 1992;89:722–729.

147. Kandylis K, Vassilomanolakis M, Tsoussis S, Efremidis AP. Ifosfamide cardiotoxicity in humans. Cancer Chemother Pharmacol 1989;24:395–396.

148. Herman EM, Mhatre RM, Warardekar VS, Lee IP. Comparison of the cardiovascular actions of NSC-109, 7824 (ifosfamide) and cyclophosphamide. Toxicol Appl Pharmacol 1972;23:178.

149. O'Connel TX, Berenbaum MC 1974 Cardiac and pulmonary effects of high doses of cyclophosphamide and isophosphamide. Cancer Res 1974;34:1586.

150. Frankel S, Weiss M, Warrell RP Jr. A "retinoic acid syndrome" in acute promyelocytic leukemia: Reversal by corticosteroids. Blood 1991;78:380a.

151. Rowinsky EK, McGuire WP, Guarnieri T, Fisherman JS, Christian MC, Donehower RC. Cardiac disturbances during the administration of Taxol. J Clin Oncol 1991;9:1704–1712.

152. McGuire WP, Rowinsky EK, Rosenshein NB, et al. Taxol: A unique antineoplastic agent with significant activity in advanced ovarian epithelial neoplasms. Ann Intern Med 1989;111:273–279.

153. Rowinsky EK, Gilbert MR, McGuire WP, et al. Sequences of Taxol and cisplatin: A phase 1 and pharmacologic study. J Clin Oncol 1991;9:1692–1703.

154. Tan CTC, Luks E, Bacha DM, Steinherz P, Steinherz L, Mondora A. Phase I trial of homoharringtonine (NSC 141633) in children with refractory leukemia. Cancer Treat Rep 1987;71:1245–1248.

155. Ajani JA, Dimery I, Chawla SP, et al. Phase II studies of homoharringtonine in patients with advanced malignant melanoma: Sarcoma and head and neck, breast and colorectal carcinomas. Cancer Treat Rep 1986;70:375–379.

156. Jongji L, Hui Y, Xueying L, et al. Experimental studies on the toxicity of harringtonine and homoharringtonine. Chin Med J 1979;92:175–180.

157. Hirvonen HE, Salmi TT, Heinonen E, Antila KJ, Valimaki IA. Vincristine treatment of acute lymphoblastic leukemia induces transient autonomic cardioneuropathy. Cancer 1989;64:801–805.

158. Mandel EM, Lewinski U, Djaldetti M. Vincristine-induced myocardial infarction. Cancer 1975;36:1979–1982.

159. Lejonc JL, Vernant JP, Macquin I, et al. Myocardial infarction following vinblastine treatment. Lancet 1980;2:692.

160. Stefenelli T, Kuzmits R, Ulrich W, Glogar D. Acute vascular toxicity after combination chemotherapy with cisplatin, vinblastine, and bleomycin for testicular cancer. Eur Heart J 1988;9:552–556.

161. Zeymer U, Neuhaus KL. Infarct-typical changes in the electrocardiogram following chemotherapy with vinblastine. Dtsch Med Wochenschr 1989;114:589–92.

162. Buzdar AR, Leghe SS, Tashimal CK, et al. Adriamycin and mitomycin C: Possible synergistic toxicity. Cancer Treat Rep 1978;62:1005–1008.

163. Doroshow JH. Mitomycin-C enhanced superoxide and hydrogen peroxide in the rat heart. J Pharmacol Exp Ther 1981;218:206–211.

164. Sivanesaratnam V. FRCOG Mitomycin-C cardiotoxicity. Med J Aust 1989;151:300.

165. Verweij J, Funke-Kupper AJ, Teule GJJ, Pinedo HM. A prospective study on the dose dependency of cardiotoxicity induced by mitomycin C. Med Oncol Tumor Pharmacother 1988;5:159–163.

166. Verweij J, Van Der Burg ME, Pinedo HM. Mitomycin C-induced hemolytic uremic syndrome: Six case reports and review of the literature on renal, pulmonary and cardiac side effects of the drug. Radiother Oncol 1987;8:33–41.

167. Dent R, McColl I. 5-Fluorouracil and angina. Lancet 1975;1:347–348.

168. Labianca R, Beretta G, Clerici M, Fraschini P, Luporini G. Cardiac toxicity of 5-fluorouracil: A study of 1083 patients. Tumori 1982;68:505–510.

169. Lomeo AM, Avolio C, Iacobellis G, Manzione L. 5-Fluorouracil cardiotoxicity. Eur J Gynaec Oncol 1990;3:237–241.

170. Rezkalla S, Kloner RA, Ensley J, et al. Continuous ambulatory ECG monitoring during fluorouracil therapy: A prospective Study. J Clin Oncol 1989;7:509–514.

171. Collins C, Weiden PL. Cardiotoxicity of 5-fluorouracil. Cancer Treat Rep 1987;71:733–736.

172. Freeman NJ, Costanza ME. 5-Fluorouracil-associated cardiotoxicity. Cancer 1988;61:36–45.

173. Eskilsson J, Albertsson M, Mercke C. Adverse cardiac effects during induction chemotherapy treatment with cis-platin and 5-fluorouracil. Radiother Oncol 1988;13:41–46.

174. Jakubowski AA, Kemeny N. Hypotension as a manifestation of cardiotoxicity in three patients receiving cisplatin and 5-fluorouracil. Cancer 1988;62:266–269.

175. McKendall GR, Shurman A, Anamur M, Most AS. Toxic cardiogenic shock associated with infusion of 5-fluorouracil. Am Heart J 1989;118:184–186.

176. Patel B, Kloner RA, Ensley J, Al-Sarraf M, Kish J, Wynne J. 5-Fluorouracil cardiotoxicity: Left ventricular dysfunction and effect of coronary vasodilators. Am J Med Sci 1987;294:238–243.

177. Misset B, Escudier B, Leclercq B, Rivara D, Rougier P, Nitenberg G. Acute myocardiotoxicity during 5-fluorouracil therapy. Intensive Care Med 1990;16:210–211.

178. Coronel B, Madonna O, Mercatello A, Caillette A, Moskovtchenko JF. Myocardiotoxicity of 5 fluorouracil. Intensive Care Med 1988;14:429–430.

179. Kleiman NS, Lehane DE, Geyer CE Jr, Pratt CM, Young JB. Prinzmetal's angina during 5-fluorouracil chemotherapy. Am J Med 1987;82:566–568.

180. Burger AJ, Mannino S. 5-Fluorouracil-induced coronary vasospasm. Am Heart J 1987;114:433–436.

181. Pottage A, Holt S, Ludgate S, Langlands A. Fluorouracil cardiotoxicity. Br Med J 1978;1:547.

182. Jeremic B, Jevremovic S, Djuric L, Mijatovic L. Cardiotoxicity during chemotherapy treatment with 5-fluorouracil and cisplatin. J Chemother 1990;2:264–267.

183. Martin M, Diaz-Rubio E, Furio V, Blazquez J, Almenarez J, Farina J. Lethal cardiac toxicity after cisplatin and 5-fluorouracil chemotherapy: Report of a case with necropsy study. Am J Clin Oncol 1989;12:229–234.

184. Liss RH, Chadwick M. Correlation of 5-fluorouracil distribution in rodents with toxicity and chemotherapy in man. Cancer Chemother Rep 1974;58:777–786.

185. Suzuki T, Nakanishi H, Hayashi A, Nakahata N, Takano S, Ito G. Cardiac toxicity of 5-fluorouracil in rabbits. Jpn J Pharmacol 1972;27(Suppl):137.

186. Matsubara I, Kamiya J, Imai S. Cardiotoxicity effects of 5-fluorouracil in the guinea pig. Jpn J Pharmacol 1980;30:871–879.

187. Menard O, Martinet Y, Lamy P. Cisplatin-induced atrial fibrillation. J Clin Oncol 1991;9:192–193.

188. Fassio T, Canobbio L, Gasparini G, Villani F. Paroxymal supraventricular tachycardia during treatment with cisplatin and etoposide combination. Oncology 1986;43:219–220.

189. Talley RW, O'Bryan RM, Gutterman JU, Brownlee RW, McCredie KB. Clinical evaluation of toxic effects of cis-diammine dichloroplatinum (NSC-119875). Phase I clinical study. Cancer Chemother Rep 1973;57:465–471.

190. Tomirotti M, Riundi R, Pulici S, et al. Ischemic cardiopathy from cis-diamminedichloroplatinum (CDDP). Tumori 1984;70:235–236.

191. Doll DC, List AF, Greco A, Hainsworth JD, Hande KR, Johnson DH. Acute vascular ischemic events after cisplatin-based combination chemotherapy for germ-cell tumors of the testis. Ann Intern Med 1986;105:48–51.

192. Sonnenblick M, Rosin A. Cardiotoxicity of interferon: A review of 44 cases. Chest 1991;99:557–561.

193. Friess GG, Brown TD, Wrenn RC. Cardiovascular rhythm effects of gamma recombinant DNA interferon. Invest New Drugs 1989;7:275–280.

194. Martino S, Ratanatharathorn V, Karanes C, Samal BA, Sohn YH, Rudnick SA. Reversible arrhythmias observed in patients treated with recombinant alpha 2 interferon. J Cancer Res Clin Oncol 1987;113:376–378.

195. Zbinden G. Effects of recombinant human alpha-interferon in a rodent cardiotoxicity model. Toxicol Lett 1990;50:25–35.

196. Dickson D. Death halts interferon trials in France. Science 1982;218:772.

197. Foon KA, Sherwin SA, Abrams PG, et al. Treatment of advanced non-Hodgkin's lymphoma with recombinant leukocyte A interferon. N Engl J Med 1984;311:1148–1152.

198. Brown TD, Koeller J, Beougher K, et al. A phase I clinical trial of recombinant DNA gamma interferon. J Clin Oncol 1987;5:790–798.

199. Deyton LR, Walker RE, Kovacs JA, et al. Reversible cardiac dysfunction associated with interferon alfa therapy in AIDS patients with Kaposi's sarcoma. N Engl J Med 1989;321:1246–1249.

200. Sonnenblick M, Rosenmann D, Rosin A. Reversible cardiomyopathy induced by interferon. Br Med J 1990;300:1174–1175.

201. Budd GT, Bukowski RM, Miketo L, Yen-Lieberman B, Proffitt MR. Phase I trial of ultrapure human leukocyte interferon in human malignancy. Cancer Chemother Pharmacol 1984;12:39–42.

202. Grunberg SM, Kempf RA, Itri LM, Venturi CL, Boswell WD, Mitchell MS. Phase II study of recombinant alpha interferon in the treatment of advanced non-small cell lung carcinoma. Cancer Treat Rep 1985;69:1031–1032.

203. Cohen MC, Huberman MS, Nesto RW. Recombinant alpha-2 interferon related cardiomyopathy. Am J Med 1988;85:549–550.

204. Sherwin SA. The interferons. Ann Intern Med 1987;106:425–426.

205. Lampidis TJ, Brouty-Boye D. Interferon inhibits cardiac cell function in vitro (41043). Proc Soc Exp Biol Med 1981;166:181–185.

206. Dorr Rt, Shipp NG. Effect of interferon, interleukin-2 and tumor necrosis factor on myocardial cell viability and doxorubicin cardiotoxicity in vitro. Immunopharmacology 1989;18:31–38.

207. Bialock JE, Stanton JD. Common pathways of interferon and hormonal action. Nature 1980;283:406–408.

208. Nora R, Abrams JS, Tait NS, Hiponia DJ, Silverman HJ. Myocardial toxic effects during recombinant interleukin-2 therapy. J Natl Cancer Inst 1989;81:59–63.

209. Rosenberg SA, Lotze MT, Muul LM, et al. A progress report on the treatment of 157 patients with advanced cancer using lymphokine-activated killer cell and interleukin-2 or high dose interleukin alone. N Engl J Med 1987;316:889–897.

210. Nora R, Belani C, Silverman H, et al. Immunotherapy of advanced cancer. N Engl J Med [Letter] 1987;316:275.

211. Nora R, Abrams J, Silverman HJ. Myocardial infarction (MI) in patients receiving high dose recombinant interleukin-2 (rIL-2). Proc Am Soc Clin Oncol 1987;6:245.

212. Fisher RI, Coltman CA, Doroshow JH, et al. Phase II clinical trial of interleukin-2 plus lymphokine-activated killer cells (IL2/LAK) in metastatic renal cell. Proc Am Soc Clin Oncol 1987;6:244.

213. Dutcher JP, Creekmore S, Weiss GR, et al. Phase II study of high dose interleukin-2 (IL-2) and lymphokine-activated killer (LAK) cells in patients (pts) with melanoma. Proc Am Soc Clin Oncol 1987;6:246.

214. Osanto S, Cluitmans FGM, Franks CR, et al. Myocardial injury after interleukin-2 therapy. Lancet 1988;2:48–49.

215. Torisu M, Goya T, Hayashi Y, Tanaka J, Sugisaki T, Yoshida T. Electrocardiogram studies on cancer patients treated with OK-432, a streptococcal preparation with potent biological response modifier activities. J Biol Response Mod 1989;8:665–75.

216. Sanz Manrique N, Valcarce Perez J, Broto Escapa P, et al. Enhancing factors in the cardiotoxicity of anthracyclines. An Esp Pediatr 1990;32:11–14.

217. Hall IH, Grippo AA, Holbrook DJ, et al. Renal, hepatic, cardiac and thymic acute toxicity afforded by bis(helenalinyl)malonate in BDF1 mice. Toxicity 1990;64:205–216.

218. Bashir Y, Tomson CR. Cardiac arrest associated with hypokalaemia in a patient receiving mithramycin. Postgrad Med J 1988;64:228–229.

219. Hoke GD, Macia RA, Meunier PC, et al. In vivo and in vitro cardiotoxicity of a gold-containing antineoplastic drug candidate in the rabbit. Toxicol Appl Pharmacol 1989;100:293–306.

220. Gebbia N, Flandina C, Leto G, et al. The role of histamine in doxorubicin and teniposide-induced cardiotoxicity in dog and mouse. Tumori 1987;73:279–287.

221. Schecter JP, Jones SE. Myocardial infarction in a 27 year old woman: Possible complication of treatment with VP-16-213 (NSC-141540), mediastinal irradiation or both. Cancer Chemother Rep 1975;59:887–888.

222. Winberger A, Pinkhas J, Sandbank U, et al. Endocardial fibrosis following busulfan treatment. JAMA 1975;231:495.

223. Desjardins AU. Action of roentgen rays and radium on the heart and lungs. AJR 1932;27:153–176, 303–335, 447–495.

224. Leach JEL. Effect of roentgen therapy on the heart: Clinical study. Arch Intern Med 1943;72:715–745.

225. Cohn KE, Stewart JR, Fajardo LF, et al. Heart disease following radiation. Medicine (Baltimore) 1967;46:281–298.

226. Stewart JR, Fajardo LF. Radiation-induced heart disease: An update. Prog Cardiovasc Dis 1984;27:3:173–194.

227. Arsenian MA. Cardiovascular sequelae of therapeutic thoracic radiation. Prog Cardiovasc Dis 1991;33:5:299–312.

228. Stewart JR, Fajardo LF, Cohn KE. Experimental radiation-induced heart disease in rabbits. Radiology 1968;91:814–817.

229. Fajardo LF, Stewart JR. Experimental radiation-induced heart disease. I. Light mircoscopic studies. Am J Pathol 1970;59:299–316.

230. Lauk S, Kiszel Z, Buschmann J, et al. Radiation-induced heart disease in rats. Int J Radiat Oncol Biol Phys 1985;II:801–808.

231. Gillette EL, McChesney SL, Hoopes PJ. Isoeffect curves for radiation-induced cardiomyopathy in the dog. Int J Radiat Oncol Phys 1985;II:2091–2097.

232. Brosius FC, Waller BF, Robert WG. Radiation heart disease: Analysis of 16 young (aged 15 to 33 years) necropsy patients who received over 3,500 rads to the heart. Am J Med 1981;70:519–530.

233. Fajardo LF, Stewart JR, Cohn KE. Morphology of radiation-induced heart disease. Arch Pathol 1968;86:512–519.

234. Fajardo LF, Stewart JR. Pathogenesis of radiation-induced myocardial fibrosis. Lab Invest 1973;29:244–257.

235. Fajardo LF. Radiation-induced heart disease. In: Sternberg S, ed. Pathology of radiation injury. New York: Masson Publishing USA, 1982.

236. Stewart JR. Normal tissue tolerance irradiation of the cardiovascular system. In: Vaeth JM, Meyer JL, eds. Radiation tolerance of normal tissues. Front Radiat Ther Oncol 1989;23:302–309.

237. Stewart JR, Fajardo LF. Dose response in human and experimental radiation-induced heart disease: Application of the nominal standard dose (NSD) concept. Radiology 1971;99:403–408.

238. Corn BW, Trock BJ, Goodman RL. Irradiation-related ischemic heart disease. J Clin Oncol 1990;8:741–750.

239. Carmel RJ, Kaplan HS. Mantle irradiation in Hodgkin's disease. Cancer 1976;37:2813–2815.

240. Appelfeld MM, Slawson RG, Spicer KM, et al. Long term cardiovascular evaluation of patients treated by thoracic mantle radiation therapy. Cancer Treat Rep 1982;66:1003–1013.

241. Appelfeld MM, Wiernik PH. Cardiac disease after radiation therapy for Hodgin's disease: Analysis of 48 patients. Am Heart J 1983;51:1679–1681.

242. Ruckdeschel JC, Chang P, Martin RG, et al. Radiation-related pericardial effusions in patients with Hodgkin's disease. Medicine 1975;54:245–259.

243. Tarbell NJ, Thompson L, Mauch P. Thoracic irradiation in Hodgkin's disease: Disease control and long-term complications. Int J Radiat Oncol Biol Phys 1990;18:275–281.

244. Harris JR, Recht A. Conservative surgery and radiotherapy. In: Harris JR, Hellman S, Henderson IC, Kinne DW, eds. Breast diseases. 2nd ed. Philadelphia: JB Lippincott, 1991:406.

245. Fleming WH, Szakacs TE, King ER. The effects of gamma radiation on the fibrinolytic system of the dog lung and its modification by certain drugs: Relationship to radiation pneumonitis and hyaline membrane formation in the lung. J Nucl Med 1962;3:34–351.

246. Blayney DW, Longo D. Radiation-induced pericarditis. N Engl J Med 1982;306:550–551.

247. Gottdeiner JS, Katin MJ, Borer JS, et al. Late cardiac effects of therapeutic mediastinal irradiation: Assessment by echocardiography and radionuclide angiography. N Engl J Med 1983;308:569–572.

248. Totterman KJ, Personen E, Siltanen P. Radiation-related chronic heart disease. Chest 1983;83:875–878.

249. Gomm SA, Stretton TB. Chronic pericardial effusion after mediastinal radiotherapy. Thorax 1981;36:149–150.

250. Posner MR, Cohen GI, Skarin AT. Pericardial disease in patients with cancer. Am J Med 1981;71:407–413.

251. Carey RW, Sawicka JM, Choi NC. Cytologically negative pericardial effusion complicating combined modality therapy for localized small-cell carcinoma of the lung. J Clin Oncol 1987;5:818–824.

252. Stewart JR, Fajardo LF. Radiation-induced heart disease. Radiol Clin North Am 1971;3:511–531.

253. Martin RG, Ruckdeschel JC, Chang P, et al. Radiation-related pericarditis. Am J Cardiol 1975;35:216–220.

254. Fajardo LF, Stewart JR. Radiation-induced heart disease. Human and experimental observations. In: Bristow MR, ed. Drug-induced heart disease. Amsterdam: Elsevier, North-Holland Biomedical Press, 1980:241–260.

255. Keelan MH, Rudders RA. Successful treatment of radiation pericarditis with corticosteroids. Arch Intern Med 1974;134:145–147.

256. Castellino RA, Glatstein E, Turbow MM, et al. Latent radiation injury of lungs or heart activated by steroid withdrawl. Ann Intern Med 1974;80:593–599.

257. Biran S. Corticosteroids in radiation-induced pericarditis. Chest 1978;74:96–98.

258. Krikorian JG, Hancock EW. Pericardiocentesis. Am J Med 1978;65:808–814.

259. Morton DL, Glancy L, Joseph WL, et al. Management of patients with radiation-induced pericarditis with effusion: A note on the development of aortic regurgitation in two of them. Chest 1973;64:291–297.

260. Cameron J, Osterle SN, Baldwin JC, et al. The etiologic spectrum of constrictive pericarditis. Am Heart J 1987;113:354–360.

261. Ni Y, von Segesser LK, Turina M. Futility of pericardiectomy for postirradiation constrictive pericarditis? Ann Thorac Surg 1990;49:445–448.

262. Savage DE, Constine LS, Schwartz RG, Rubin P. Radiation effects of left ventricular function and myocardial perfusion in long-term survivors of Hodgkin's disease. Int J Radiat Oncol Biol Phys 1990;19:721–727.

263. Perrault DJ, Levy M, Herman JD, et al. Echocardiographic abnormalities following cardiac radiation. J Clin Oncol 1985;3:546–551.

264. Pohjola-Sintonen S, Totterman KJ, Salmo M, et al. Late cardiac effects of mediastinal radiotherapy in patients with Hodgkin's disease. Cancer 1987;60:31–37.

265. Burns RJ, Bar-Shlomo B, Druck MN, et al. Detection of radiation cardiomyopathy by gated radionuclide angiography. Am J Med 1983;74:297–302.

266. Gomez GA, Park JJ, Panahon AM, et al. Heart size and function after radiation therapy to the mediastinum in patients with Hodgkin's disease. Cancer Treat Rep 1983;67:1099–1103.

267. Merrill J, Greco FA, Zimbler H, et al. Adriamycin and radiation: Synergistic cardiotoxicity. Ann Intern Med 1975;82:122.

268. Kinsella TJ, Ahmann DL, Giuliani ER, et al. Adriamycin cardiotoxibity in stage IV breast cancer: Possible enhancement with prior left chest radiation therapy. Int J Radiat Oncol Biol Phys 1979;5:1997–2002.

269. Mayer EG, Poulter CA, Aristizabal SA. Complications of irradiation related to apparent drug potentiation by Adriamycin. Int J Radiat Oncol Biol Phys 1976;1:1179–1188.

270. Eltringham JR, Fajardo LF, Stewart JR, et al. Investigation of cardiotoxicity in rabbits from Adriamycin and fractionated cardiac irradiation: Preliminary results. Front Radiat Ther Oncol 1979;13:21–35.

271. Petrovic D, Brown SM, Yatvin MB. Effects of Adriamycin and irradiation on beating of rat heart muscle cells in culture. Int J Radiat Oncol Biol Phys 1977;2:505–513.

272. LaMonte CS, Yeh SDJ, Straus DJ. Long-term follow-up of cardiac function in patients with Hodgkin's disease treated with mediastinal irradiation and combination chemotherapy including doxorubicin. Cancer Treat Rep 1986;70:439–444.

273. Santoro A, Bonadonna G, Valagusso P, et al. Long-term results of combined chemotherapy-radiotherapy approach in Hodgkin's disease: Superiority of ABVD plus radiotherapy versus MOPP plus radiotherapy. J Clin Oncol 1987;5:27–37.

274. Brice P, Tredaniel J, Monsuez JJ, et al. Cardiopulmonary toxicity after three courses of ABVD and mediastinal irradiation in favorable Hodgkin's disease. Ann Oncol 1991;2:73–76.

275. Carlson RG, Mayfield WR, Normann S, Alexander JA. Radiation-associated valvular disease. Chest 1991;99:538–545.

276. Kadota RP, Burgert EO Jr, Driscoll DJ, et al. Cardiopulmonary function in long-term survivors of childhood Hodgkin's lymphoma: A pilot study. Mayo Clin Proc 1988;63:362–367.

277. Warda M, Khan A, Massumi A, et al. Radiation-induced valvular dysfunction. J Am Coll Cardiol 1983;2:180–185.

278. Cohen SL, Bharati S, Glass J, et al. Radiotherapy as a cause of complete atrioventricular block in Hodgkin's disease. Arch Intern Med 1981;141:676–679.

279. Mary-Rabine L, Waleffe A, Kulbertius HE. Severe conduction disturbances and ventricular arrhythmias complicating mediastinal irradiation for Hodgkin's disease: A case report. PACE 1980;3:612–617.

280. Tzivoni D, Ratzkowski E, Biran S, et al. Complete heart block following therapeutic irradiation of the left side of the chest. Chest 1977;71:231–234.

281. Kereiakes DJ, Morady F, Ports TA. High degree atrioventricular block after radiation therapy. Am J Cardiol 1983;51:1233–1234.

282. Slama M-S, LeGuludec D, Sebag C, et al. Complete atrioventricular block following mediastinal irradiation: A report of six cases. PACE 1991;14:1112–1118.

283. Strender LE, Lindahl J, Larsson LE. Incidence of heart disease and functional significance of change in the electrocardiogram 10 years after radiotherapy for breast cancer. Cancer 1986;57:929–934.

284. Watchie J, Coleman CN, Raffin TA, et al. Minimal long-term cardiopulmonary dysfunction following treatment for Hodgkin's disease. Int J Radiat Oncol Biol Phys 1987;13:513–524.

285. Amronim GD, Solomon RD. Production of arteriosclerosis in the rabbit: A quantitative assessment. Arch Pathol 1965;75:219–227.

286. Gold H. Production of arteriosclerosis in the rat: Effect of x-ray and high-fat diet. Arch Pathol 1961;71:268–272.

287. Artom C, Lofton HB, Clarkson TB. Ionizing radiation atherosclerosis and lipid metabolism in pigeons. Radiat Res 1965;26:165–177.

288. Kopelson G, Herwig KJ. The etiologies of coronary artery disease in cancer patients. Int J Radiat Oncol Biol Phys 1978;4:895–906.

289. Yahalom J, Hasin Y, Fuks Z. Acute myocardial infarction with normal coronary arteriogram after mantle field radiation therapy for Hodgkin's disease. Cancer 1983;52:637–641.

290. McEniery PT, Dorosti K, Schiavone WA, et al. Clinical and angiographic features of coronary artery disease after chest irradiation. Am J Cardiol 1987;60:1020–1024.

291. Boivin JF, Hutchison GB, Lubin JH, Mauch P. Coronary artery disease mortality in patients treated for Hodgkin's disease. Cancer 1992;69:1241–1247.

292. Henry-Amar M, Hayat M, Meerwaldt JH. Causes of death after therapy for early stage Hodgkin's disease entered on EORTC protocols. Int J Radiat Oncol Biol Phys 1990;19:1155–1157.

293. Hancock SL, Cox RS, Rosenberg SA. Correction: Death after treatment of Hodgkin's disease. Ann Intern Med [Letter] 1992;114:810.

294. Cosset JM, Henry-Amar M, Meerwaldt JH. Long-term toxicity of early stages of Hodgkin's disease therapy: The EORTC experience. Am Oncol 1991;2:77–82.

295. Handler CE, Livesey S, Lawton PA. Coronary ostial stenosis after radiotherapy: Angioplasty or coronary artery surgery? Br Heart J 1989;61:208–211.

296. Grollier G, Commeau P, Mercier V, et al. Post-radiotherapeutic left main coronary ostial stenosis: Clinical and histiological study. Eur Heart J 1988;9:567–570.

297. Annest LS, Anderson RP, Li W, et al. Coronary artery disease following mediastinal radiation therapy. J Thorac Cardiovasc Surg 1983;85:257–263.

298. Miller DD, Waters DD, Dangoisse V, et al. Symptomatic coronary artery spasm following radiotherapy for Hodgkin's disease. Chest 1983;83:284–285.

299. Host H, Brennhoud IO, Loeb M. Post-operative radiotherapy in breast cancer: Long-term results from the Oslo study. Int J Radiat Oncol Biol Phys 1986;12:727–732.

300. Jones JM, Ribeiro GG. Mortality patterns over 34 years of breast cancer patients in a clinical trial of post-operative radiotherapy. Clin Radiol 1989;40:204–208.

301. Haybittle JL, Brinkley D, Houghton J, et al. Postoperative radiotherapy and late mortality: Evidence from the Cancer Research Campaign trial for early breast cancer. Br Med J 1989;298:1611–1614.

302. Levitt SH, Fletcher GH. Trials and tribulations: Do clinical trials prove that irradiation increases cardiac and secondary cancer mortality in the breast cancer patient? Int J Radiat Oncol Biol Phys 1991;20:523–527.

303. Wallgren A, Arner O, Bergstrom J, et al. Radiation therapy in operable breast cancer: Results from the Stockholm trial in adjuvant radiotherapy. Int J Radiat Oncol Biol Phys 1986;12:533–537.

304. Stender LE, Lindahl J, Larsson LE. Incidence of heart disease and functional significance of changes in the electrocardiogram 10 years after radiotherapy for breast cancer. Cancer 1986;57:929–934.

305. Harris JR, Hellman S. Put the "hockey stick" on ice. Int J Radiat Oncol Biol Phys 1988;15:497–499.

306. Lederman GS, Sheldon TA, Chaffey JT, et al. Cardiac disease after mediastinal irradiation for seminoma. Cancer 1987;60:772–776.

SECTION **6**   STEPHEN T. SONIS

Oral Complications of Cancer Therapy

The mouth is often a significant site of complications in the patient receiving therapy for cancer. Not only are patients with malignancies of the head and neck susceptible to such problems, but also affected are patients receiving treatment for more distant disease. Virtually all patients who receive radiation therapy to the head and neck develop oral side effects of their treatment, and about 40% of patients who are treated with chemotherapy develop oral complications. It has been demonstrated that aggressive oral evaluation before cancer therapy, intervention to eliminate potential sources of infection or irritation, and preventive measures taken during therapy result in a precipitous drop in the frequency of oral problems.[1]

In addition to affecting adversely the patient's ability to eat, speak, and control saliva, cancer therapy may have even more significant ramifications, especially relative to sepsis. Because of the mouth's vast bacterial and fungal flora, it is an important potential portal for these organisms in the myelosuppressed host; the mouth is the most frequently identifiable source of sepsis in the granulocytopenic cancer patient. Nevertheless, many of the oral problems associated with cancer therapy can be prevented or minimized with adequate pretherapy care and with aggressive preventive techniques during treatment.

ORAL COMPLICATIONS OF RADIATION THERAPY

For the most part, oral problems due to radiation therapy are the result of local tissue changes from direct irradiation. For this reason, implants tend to produce more problems than does beam irradiation. Radiation results in mucosal atrophy due to decreased cell renewal; fibrosis of the salivary glands, muscles, ligaments, and blood vessels; and damage to taste buds.[2]

Mucositis is the result of atrophic changes in the epithelium due to decreased cell renewal and usually is noted at a dose level of about 2000 cGy when therapy is administered at a rate of 200 cGy/day. Patients complain of generalized discomfort and drying of the mucosa; erythema is present; and any traumatized area may ulcerate. Generally, nonkeratinized epithelium of the cheeks, lips, soft palate, and ventral surface of the tongue is affected. Mucositis is extremely uncomfortable for the patient and may limit oral intake. Although it is self-limiting and usually resolves in 2 to 3 weeks after the termination of radiation treatment, severe mucositis may necessitate a temporary cessation of therapy. Ice chips or Popsicles are soothing. Patients should be instructed to avoid spicy or acidic foods. Unusually sharp teeth should be smoothed or eliminated. Removable prostheses should be used sparingly. Oral hygiene should be stressed.

Historically, treatment of mucositis has been palliative and aimed at minimizing mucosal trauma. Rinses such as Xylocaine Viscous, dyclonine hydrochloride (Dyclone), or Kaopectate and Benadryl provide varying degrees of relief.[3] Localized lesions can be treated with topical therapy using benzocaine in Orabase or benzocaine in a hydroxypropylcellulose base (Oratect gel). The latter purportedly provides lesion coverage for up to 4 hours.[4,5]

The successful use of sucralfate for the treatment of gastric ulcers has led to studies of its efficacy as a palliative rinse for the treatment of mucositis, but data are conflicting.[6-8] A number of studies have suggested that benzydamine HCl, a topical nonsteroidal antiinflammatory agent, can successfully soothe radiation- and chemotherapy-induced mucositis.[9-11] This drug is available in Europe and Canada, but not in the United States.

Biologically active treatments are also being studied for their potential efficacy in preventing or treating mucositis. The role of PGE2 in the development of or therapy for mucositis has been evaluated with mixed results. Data from early studies suggested that, although increases in plasma-extracted prostaglandin correlated with increases in mucositis, administration of moderate doses of prostaglandin inhibitors failed to affect the severity of lesions.[12] A later investigation, however, demonstrated that indomethacin administered orally at a dose of 25 mg four times a day delayed the onset and reduced the severity of mucositis induced by radiation therapy, compared with a placebo control.[13] Paradoxically, the administration of PGE2 by other investigators appeared to be beneficial in the treatment of mucositis.[14,15]

Another approach to the control of mucositis has been advocated by Spijkervet and colleagues.[16,17] They hypothesized that the selective elimination of gram-negative bacilli might have a favorable effect on mucositis since a shift to the latter was noted in patients receiving treatment for malignancies of the head and neck. Administration of lozenges of polymyxin E, tobramycin 1.8 mg, and amphotericin B 10 mg resulted in a reduced frequency of severe mucositis in response to radiation therapy.

Xerostomia is one of the most frequent side effects of irradiation to the head and neck and is due to changes in the salivary glands.[18-20] Generally, there is a direct relation between the dose of irradiation to the salivary glands and the extent of glandular changes.[21] Under 6000 cGy, changes in the salivary glands induced by irradiation, including edema and inflammation, are reversible. Over 6000 cGy, changes may be permanent, with fibrosis and glandular degeneration. Clinically, xerostomia has been reported with as little as two to three doses of 200 to 225 cGy.[21]

Xerostomia predisposes to increases in the number of oral bacteria because saliva is no longer available to help clear bacteria from the mouth, or as a source of IgA. The patient's ability to taste is altered.

The most consistent consequence of xerostomia is the development of radiation caries, which characteristically appears in the cervical regions or incisal edges of teeth a few months after the start of radiation therapy.[28] Left untreated, caries and decalcification may become so severe that the integrity of the tooth is compromised and fracture occurs. The causes of radiation caries include loss of salivary buffering capacity, lowered salivary pH, elimination of mechanical flushing, and decreased salivary IgA.

Treatment of xerostomia has four goals:

1. Stimulation of existing salivary flow
2. Replacement of lost secretions
3. Protection of the dentition
4. Reduction of sucrose intake

Stimulation of the patient's remaining salivary apparatus may be accomplished with sucrose-free lemon drops. Sugarfree chewing gum may satisfy the same objective; mint- and cinnamon-flavored gum should be avoided because it may irritate the mucosa. Saliva substitutes such as Xero-Lube or Salivart may be used before meals and at bedtime.[23]

Recent investigations by Fox and associates[25] and Greenspan and Daniels[24] indicate that relatively low doses of systemically administered pilocarpine may have a role in reducing radiation-induced xerostomia.

Prevention of radiation-induced caries is best accomplished by the aggressive use of fluorides.[26] Customized trays should be fabricated for patients so that they may deliver home fluoride treatments on a daily basis; this may be supplemented with fluoride rinses. Generally, acidulated fluorides are the most effective, although neutral fluorides may become necessary in patients with mucositis. Fluorides should be continued until full salivary function has returned. An alternative to fluoride-containing trays is the daily use of fluoride gel as a tooth brushing agent. Stannous fluoride 0.4% gel appears to be more effective than sodium fluoride 1.1% since it reduces detectable levels of caries-causing *Streptococcus mutans*.[7] In addition, scrupulous oral hygiene and aggressive professional maintenance are critical to minimizing the development of caries. Finally, the patient should be encouraged to avoid sucrose.

Loss of taste is a common sequela of radiation therapy. It usually is noted with a cumulative dose of between 1000 and 2000 cGy.[28] Most often, loss of the ability to differentiate sweet and salty is reported as often leading to an avoidance of foods with such tastes. Bitterness is common. Taste sensation usually returns 6 to 12 months after the completion of therapy.

The most serious local sequela of head and neck radiation therapy is osteoradionecrosis (ORN), which occurs when there is fibrotic thickening of blood vessels, replacement of bone marrow with connective tissue, subsequent lack of new bone formation, and bone death.[29] The bone becomes susceptible to infection, and its ability to heal is retarded. Patients develop open, foul-smelling wounds with areas of denuded bone. It is thought that ORN represents a defect in wound healing rather than a true osteomyelitis.[29] The reported incidence of ORN ranges from 4% to 44%; the actual frequency is about 15%. Ninety percent of cases occur in the mandible, which differs in vascularity and density compared with the maxilla. About 30% of cases occur spontaneously; the remainder are thought to be related to trauma, the most frequent form of which is tooth extraction. Most spontaneous cases of ORN occur within the first 6 to 24 months after treatment. By contrast, trauma-related osteonecrosis has two peaks of activity: the first peak typically occurs 3 months after radiation therapy, and the second peak occurs 2 to 5 years after treatment.[30,31]

Four major risk factors predispose to the development of ORN: (1) the anatomic site of the tumor, (2) the dose of radiation, (3) the dental status of the patient,[10] and (4) the type and source of radiation. Patients receiving radiation therapy to tumors anatomically related to the mandible develop ORN at five times the rate of patients with tumors at other sites. The risk of ORN is increased significantly at doses of 6000 cGy or more; the risk of developing ORN is increased twofold for patients receiving greater than 8000 cGy compared with patients receiving 5000 to 6000 cGy, and it is almost five times greater than for patients receiving 4000 to 5000 cGy. Dentulous patients are more likely to develop ORN than are edentulous patients. Furthermore, patients with dental disease are at twice the risk of developing ORN than patients without dental disease.[32] Therefore, meticulous oral hygiene, elimination of diseased teeth, aggressive prophylaxis, and follow-up should be stressed. Oral hygiene techniques for the patient receiving radiation therapy may include standard brushing and flossing. Water-irrigating devices (*e.g.*, Water-Pik) may be helpful for removal of food particles or other debris but are ineffective for the elimination of tooth-borne bacteria. Patients should be cautioned to use them at low pressure. Similarly, sucrose intake should be minimized, and topical fluorides should be used regularly. Patients receiving external-beam sources of radiation are at least twice as likely to develop ORN as those receiving radiation from implanted sources. Patients receiving supervoltage radiation therapy of 1 MeV or more are at significantly higher risk for osteonecrosis than are patients receiving particulate neutron beam therapy.[32]

For patients receiving interstitial radiation, a lead device may offer protection to the mandible and minimize the risk of ORN.[33]

Patients with poorly fitting prostheses are also at risk for ORN because breaks in the epithelium and pressure on supporting bone may cause infection and necrosis.

The issue of if and when dental extractions should be performed is unresolved.[31–32,34,35] At times when low-energy radiation was used, the common protocol was to extract all teeth in the path of the primary beam before the start of therapy to eliminate sources of infection and ORN. Improvements in the type of radiation used, more selective fields of radiation, increased concern for patient function and aesthetics, and the success of preventive dental protocols have modified this approach. An approach has evolved aimed at the elimination of actively infected teeth, with aggressive dental preventive techniques for the remaining dentition. It is important to note that sites of extractions performed before radiation therapy are also at increased risk for the development of ORN, although not at the same frequency as extraction sites created after the start of radiation therapy. Therefore, teeth demonstrating periapical pathology or active periodontal infection should be extracted as long as possible before the start of radiation therapy and at a minimum of 3 weeks before therapy. Nonrestorable teeth or teeth with deep caries and a significant risk of developing infection also should be eliminated. Teeth at marginal risk that are unlikely to become infected should be retained. When possible, extractions should be postponed until 1 year after the termination of radiation. Antibiotic prophylaxis is recommended. Endodontic therapy can be used as a temporary measure to "buy time" if a problem occurs during radiation therapy, although endodontics does not appear to have permanent efficacy in this group.[36]

Management of ORN depends on its severity. Most cases resolve spontaneously after about 6 months of conservative therapy consisting of local debridement and oral antibiotics. Hyperbaric oxygen therapy has been advocated for nonresolving cases.[37] In instances of intractable pain, severe trismus, orocutaneous fistulas, or persistent exposure of bone, surgical resection may be the only curative therapy available.

ORAL COMPLICATIONS OF CANCER CHEMOTHERAPY

Of all patients receiving chemotherapy, about 40% develop oral problems during each exposure to drug.[38] Although the spectrum of problems is wide, essentially all oral complications of chemotherapy occur through one of two major mechanisms: they are either a direct effect of the drug on the oral mucosa (direct stomatotoxicity) or an indirect result of myelosuppression (indirect stomatotoxicity; Fig. 63–4).

Not all patients are at equal risk of developing oral problems associated with their specific chemotherapy. Factors that influence the frequency and severity of these complications may be grouped into those that are related to the patient and those that are related to the drug. Patient-related factors include the types of malignancy, patient age, and the level of oral health before and during therapy.

Patients with hematologic malignancies (*e.g.*, leukemia, lymphoma) develop oral problems at two or three times the rate of patients with solid tumors.[39–41] This is probably because these patients are functionally myelosuppressed as a consequence of the malignancies.[42] Young patients tend to develop oral problems more frequently than older patients. Whereas 90% of patients between the ages of 1 and 20 years develop oral problems after chemotherapy, only 18% of patients over age 60 develop problems.[38] Part of the reason for this finding is attributable to the high incidence of hematologic malignancies in the younger age group. When oral problems are evaluated in patients with the same malignancy and the same chemotherapeutic regimen, however, this finding holds up. An explanation for this may be that cell renewal is decreased in older patients.[43] Additionally, the number of mitoses in the basal epithelium of younger patients is greater than in older patients. Patients in poor oral health, especially those with preexisting periodontal or pulpal disease, have a higher risk of developing oral infection in the face of chemotherapy-induced myelosuppression.[44–46] Similarly, patients with irritating prostheses or sharp or broken teeth are at increased risk for developing ulceration and mucositis. Patients in whom preexisting periodontal and dental disease is eliminated before therapy and who receive aggressive mouth care during treatment have a significant decrease in the frequency of oral problems associated with chemotherapy.[47–51]

Therapy-related variables also influence the frequency and severity with which patients develop problems. Probably the single most important factor in this area is choice of drug.[39,52–54] Although stomatotoxicity is a common side effect of many forms of chemotherapy, drugs differ significantly in the extent of the stomatotoxicity they cause. In many instances, stomatotoxicity is dose-related. This effect can be reduced by delivering an agent in divided doses rather than as a bolus.[53] Finally, concomitant therapy such as radiation increases the frequency and severity with which patients develop oral problems in response to chemotherapy.

DIRECT STOMATOTOXICITY

Direct stomatotoxicity is the consequence of the nonspecific effect of a drug on cells undergoing mitosis. Cells of the mouth undergo rapid renewal over a 7- to 14-day cycle. Chemotherapy causes a reduction in the renewal rate of the basal epi-

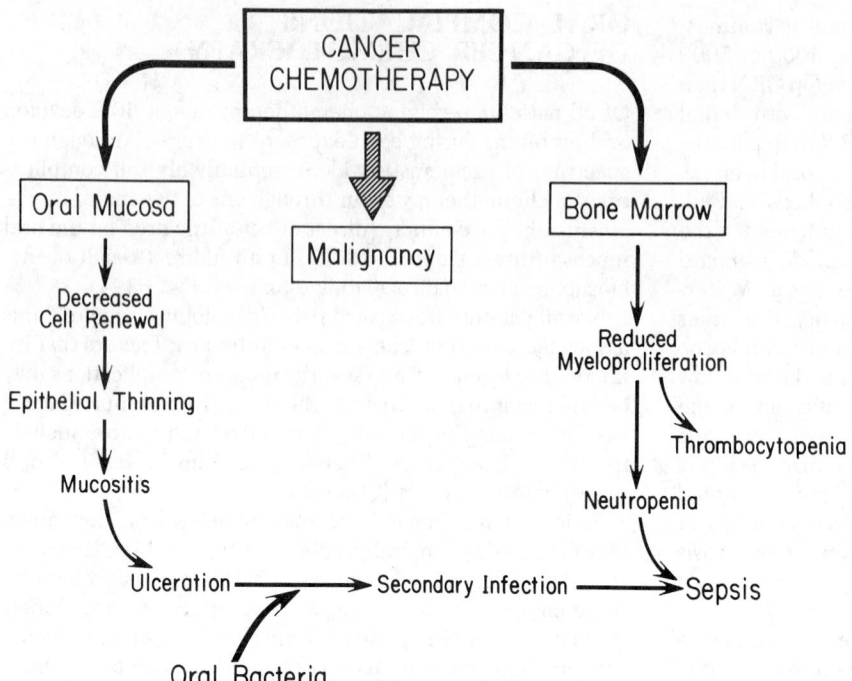

FIGURE 63–4.   Effects of cancer chemotherapy on both the oral basal epithelial cells and the bone marrow stem cells.

thelium, which results in mucosal atrophy.[55,56] Diminished nutritional intake secondary to mucositis[57] may compound the problem because there is an overall decrease in cell migration and renewal after starvation or protein deprivation. Clinically, patients experience pain from mucositis and ulceration. Lesions are generally discrete initially but often progress to produce confluent areas of ulceration (Fig. 63–5). Nonkeratinized mucosa is most often affected. The buccal, labial, and soft palatal mucosa, along with the ventral surface of the tongue and the floor of the mouth, are the most common sites. Lesions do not progress outside the mouth (Fig. 63–6). Direct stomatotoxicity is usually observed 5 to 7 days after

the administration of the drug. Left untreated, lesions generally heal without scarring within 2 to 3 weeks in the nonmyelosuppressed patient. A wide variety of agents may produce direct stomatotoxicity (Table 63–19).

The major clinical problem associated with direct stomatotoxicity is pain, with a consequent loss of function, especially ability to eat. Patients are miserable and are often unable to sleep because of oral pain. Treatment of direct stomatotoxicity is palliative (Table 63–20). A variety of agents are available, including Xylocaine viscous and Dyclone. A rinse of frequent benefit may be prepared by mixing equal proportions of elixir of Benadryl and Kaopectate. The use of milk of magnesia as

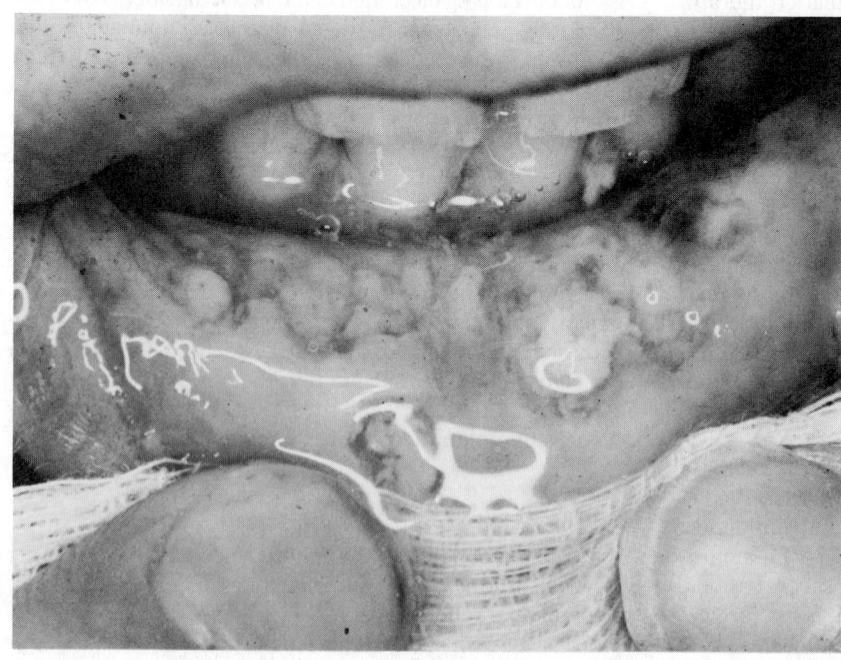

FIGURE 63–5.   Mucositis of the labial mucosa due to stomatotoxicity secondary to methotrexate. Notice the severe disruption of epithelial integrity. (Sonis S, Fazio R, Fang L. Principles and practice of oral medicine. Philadelphia: WB Saunders, 1984)

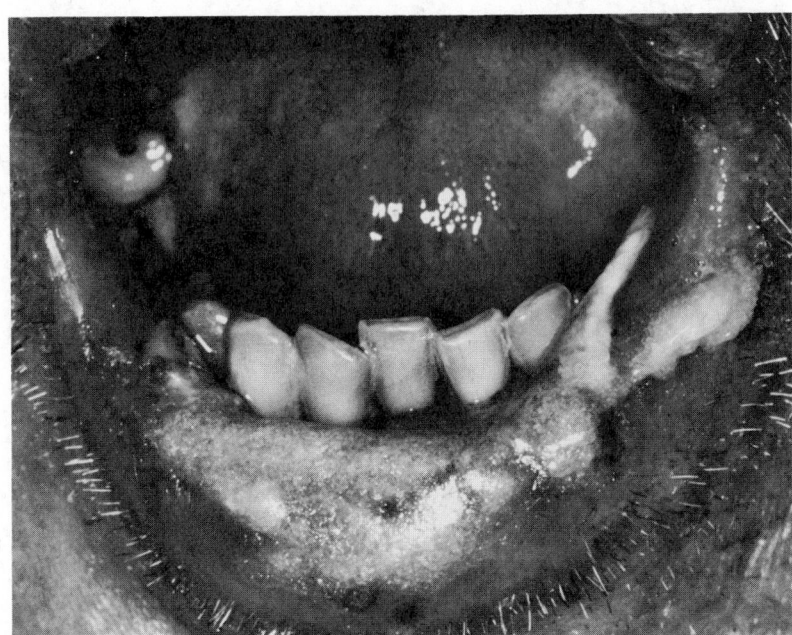

FIGURE 63–6. Severe breakdown of the labial mucosa as a result of direct stomatotoxicity. Notice the lack of involvement of nonmucosal surfaces. (Sonis S, Fazio R, Fang L. Principles and practice of oral medicine. Philadelphia: WB Saunders, 1984)

a vehicle for the delivery of palliative agents is to be avoided because of its desiccating effect on the mucosa. In severe cases, 2.5% to 5% cocaine rinses or spray may be used. The latter is recommended only in supervised inpatient settings because of the potential for neurotoxicity. In the case of discrete ulceration, ointments, such as benzocaine in Orabase, may be applied to the affected area after it is dried with a sponge. The use of systemic pain medication is often of value. Patients often find cold soothing; ice chips, Popsicles, and cold beverages may be helpful. Other approaches to the treatment of mucositis are discussed elsewhere in this section.

Cryotherapy reportedly has been helpful in marginally reducing the severity of chemotherapy-induced mucositis.[58] Additional controlled studies are required to confirm this observation.

The use of allopurinol, an inhibitor of orotidine-5'-phosphate decarboxylase, to prevent mucositis induced by 5-FU is unclear. Although two pilot studies suggested its efficacy, a larger, controlled investigation failed to substantiate its usefulness.[59–61] The vitamin A derivative, beta-carotene, may be beneficial in reducing the stomatotoxic effects of radiation therapy and chemotherapy, although large, well-controlled investigations are pending.[62]

Preliminary and anecdotal data suggest that some growth factors may have been positive modifiers of mucositis induced in myelosuppressed cancer patients.[63,64] Patients receiving human recombinant granulocyte colony-stimulating factor in conjunction with a stomatotoxic drug regimen for the treatment of transitional carcinoma of the bladder had an apparent reduction in mucositis. The effects of other growth factors on the development and course of mucositis is under investigation.[65]

Xerostomia is a common side effect of some forms of chemotherapy and accelerates the development of mucositis.[13] Management of xerostomia is discussed elsewhere in this section.

Plant alkaloids, particularly vincristine, may cause neurotoxicity that manifests as acute-onset dental pain, most frequently in the mandibular molar area, in the absence of odontogenic pathology.[66] The discomfort resolves after the drug is discontinued.

TABLE 63–19. Cancer Chemotherapeutic Drugs That Produce Direct Stomatotoxicity

Alkylating Agents	Natural Products
Mechlorethamine	Bleomycin
	Dactinomycin
Antimetabolites	Daunorubicin
Cytarabine hydrochloride	Doxorubicin
Floxuridine	Mithramycin
Fluorouracil	Mitomycin
Mercaptopurine	Vinblastine sulfate
Methotrexate	Vincristine sulfate
Thioguanine	
	Other Synthetic Agents
	Hydroxyurea
	Procarbazine hydrochloride

INDIRECT STOMATOTOXICITY

Indirect stomatotoxicity is the result of the effects of chemotherapy on a cell pool other than of the oral mucosa. The most significant target cells in this case are those of the bone marrow. Changes in the mouth that are associated with this action usually are noted at the patient's nadir and most often occur 12 to 14 days after drug administration.[20] The two most common forms of indirect stomatotoxicity are infection and hemorrhage.

The mouth is the most frequently identifiable source of sepsis in the granulocytopenic cancer patient.[64] Most often, oral infection is caused by bacteria, although fungal and viral infections also are relatively common. The degree and duration

TABLE 63-20. Formulary of Topical Medications for Specific Oral Problems

Problem	Medication	Use
General infection control	Chlorhexidine gluconate 0.12% oral rinse	Rinse twice daily after breakfast and at bedtime for 30 sec. Do not swallow.
	Povidone iodine rinse 0.5%	Rinse twice daily. Do not swallow.
Localized secondary topical lip infection	Neosporin	Apply to perioral lesions 2–5 times daily, depending on severity of lesion
Prevention of caries secondary to xerostomia	Acidulated fluoride rinse	Rinse daily for 1 min with 5 to 10 ml. Do not swallow. Switch to neutral fluoride if mucositis is present.*†
	Neutral fluoride rinse	Rinse daily for 1 min with 5 ml. Do not swallow. Switch back to acidulated fluoride rinse when mucositis resolves.
	Stannous fluoride gel 0.4%	Brush daily for 1 min, then hold in mouth and rinse for 30 sec. Do not swallow.†
	Sodium fluoride gel 1.1%	Brush daily at bedtime. Swish for 30 sec. Spit out and rinse.
Antifungal Agents		
Prevention and treatment of oral candidiasis	Nystatin oral suspension	Rinse and swallow 300,000 units 3–4 times daily. If intolerance to swallowing, rinse only.
	Clotrimazole troche 10 mg	Dissolve 1 tablet 5 times daily. The prophylactic use of clotrimazole for the prevention of candidiasis has not been adequately studied.
Treatment of candidiasis under dentures or at corners of mouth	Mycolog ointment	Apply to affected area 2 to 3 times daily or place under denture surface.
Palliation of mucositis (generalized)	Xylocaine viscous 2% solution	Swish 15 ml for 30 sec maximum every 3 h. Expectorate.
	Dyclonine hydrochloride 0.5% or 1% solution	Swish 15 ml for 30 sec every 2 to 3 h. Expectorate.
	Benadryl and Kaopectate mix solution of 50% each.	Swish 15 ml for 30 sec every 2 to 3 h. Expectorate.
Palliation of mucositis (localized)	Benzocaine in Orabase ointment	Apply to affected dried area every 2 to 3 h. Not to be used in presence of infection.
	Benzocaine 15% in Oratect gel.	Apply up to 4 times daily after drying mucosa.
Control of Local Bleeding		
Gingival	Topical thrombin solution	Apply to affected area with gauze sponge and hold in place with pressure for 30 min. Do not remove formed clots.
Mucosal surface bleeding	Microfibrillar collagen	Apply to dried site with dry sponge for 1 to 5 min. Do not use in closure of mucosal incisions.
Xerostomia		
Saliva substitutes	Salivart synthetic saliva spray	Spray as needed for xerostomia.
	Xerolube	Rinse as needed for xerostomia.
	Biotene chewing gum.	Use as needed.

* Fluoride gels in custom trays are preferred.
† Acidulated fluorides are contraindicated in patients with porcelain prostheses.

of granulocytopenia often determine the incidence and severity of infection. Although the normal flora is responsible for most infections, during myelosuppression, the oral flora changes to become primarily gram-negative (common isolated organisms include *Klebsiella, Serratia, Enterobacter, Escherichia coli, Pseudomonas,* and *Proteus*).[68] Most fungal infections are caused by *Candida albicans.*[69]

Bacterial infections may affect three sites in the mouth: the gingiva, the mucosa, and the teeth. Because the normal signs of inflammation and therefore infection are absent in the myelosuppressed patient, diagnosis is based on the presence of oral lesions in conjunction with fever and pain. Demonstration of a culturable local isolate in conjunction with a positive blood culture result confirms the diagnosis, although exotoxins and endotoxins from oral bacteria may produce fever in the absence of a positive blood culture.

Gingivae are a common site of infection, especially in the patient with preexisting periodontal disease.[70,71] Infection of this area presents as a necrotizing gingivitis that clinically resembles acute necrotizing ulcerative gingivitis (Vincent's disease). Patients develop painful necrosis of the marginal and papillary gingivae, usually beginning around one or two teeth and then spreading laterally. Fever and lymphadenopathy are present. The normal papillary architecture is eliminated, and a white, necrotic pseudomembrane is present. Treatment of necrotic gingivitis consists of parenteral antibiotics. Because spirochetes and fusiform organisms must be included in the spectrum of causative agents, coverage should include a penicillin as well as an agent specific for gram-negative organisms. The teeth should be gently debrided with cotton pellets soaked with 3% hydrogen peroxide. Frequent rinsing may be helpful.

Mucosal infection is usually due to secondary infection of ulcerations produced by direct stomatotoxicity or trauma (Fig. 63–7). Patients complain of pain and are febrile. Clinically, one observes ulceration, often deep, with a yellow-white necrotic center. The borders are often slightly raised and indurated. An erythematous border, usually associated with aphthous lesions, is conspicuously absent. Lesions are of variable size; the size of the lesion does not always relate directly to its potential to cause sepsis. The organisms causing these infections usually are mixed; therefore, isolation of organisms from the blood of septic patients is an important corroborating procedure in patients suspected of having an oral source.

It is often difficult to determine which mucosal lesions require antibiotic coverage. Patients with fever, neutropenia (fewer than 1000 leukocytes/mm^3), and an oral lesion must be presumed to have an oral source and should be appropriately treated until the leukocyte count recovers, the patient is afebrile, and the lesions begin to resolve.

Odontogenic infections in the myelosuppressed patient often present with confusing signs and symptoms because of the patient's inability to mount an inflammatory response.[52,72] Tooth pain and fever may be the only signs of odontogenic infection. Thorough dental examination, including radio-graphs, is often necessary to make a definitive diagnosis. Because many subacute odontogenic infections become symptomatic when the patient becomes myelosuppressed, the ideal treatment is elimination of questionable teeth before the initiation of chemotherapy. If this is not possible, and the patient develops a definite odontogenic infection, extraction to eliminate the source is the treatment of choice. This requires antibiotic and often platelet coverage. Extractions should be performed with as little trauma as possible, and block anesthesia should be avoided. Hemostatic gels should not be used because these may act as foci for bacterial infection. Primary closure of the wound with sutures is desirable.[73,74] Antibiotics should be continued for at least 1 week after extraction regardless of the patient's leukocyte count. Alternatively, if the patient is medically unstable, the necrotic pulp may be endodontically extricated and the tooth closed.

Oral fungal infections are common in the myelosuppressed cancer patient. Generally, these tend to be superficial infections of the oral mucosa caused by *C. albicans*, an organism present in about half of the normal population. Oral infection with *C. albicans* produces surface necrosis, which has a wide variety of clinical manifestations. Most frequently, lesions appear as raised, white curdy areas and can affect any of the oral soft tissues (Fig. 63–8). Angular cheilitis may also occur. Patients who wear removable prostheses may develop infections beneath their dentures that are broad, sensitive, erythematous macules. The major clinical significance of oral moniliasis is its potential regional or systemic spread. Patients are rarely febrile when *C. albicans* infections are limited to the mouth. Diagnosis is based on clinical appearance, the ability to scrape off the necrotic surface, and demonstration of the organism with potassium hydroxide smears.

The value of prophylactic antifungal medication is controversial.[74–78] One study concluded that patients whose leukocyte counts drop to 200 cells/mm^3 develop candidiasis despite topical medication. However, it appears that prophylactic use of topical antifungal agents begun simultaneously with chemo-

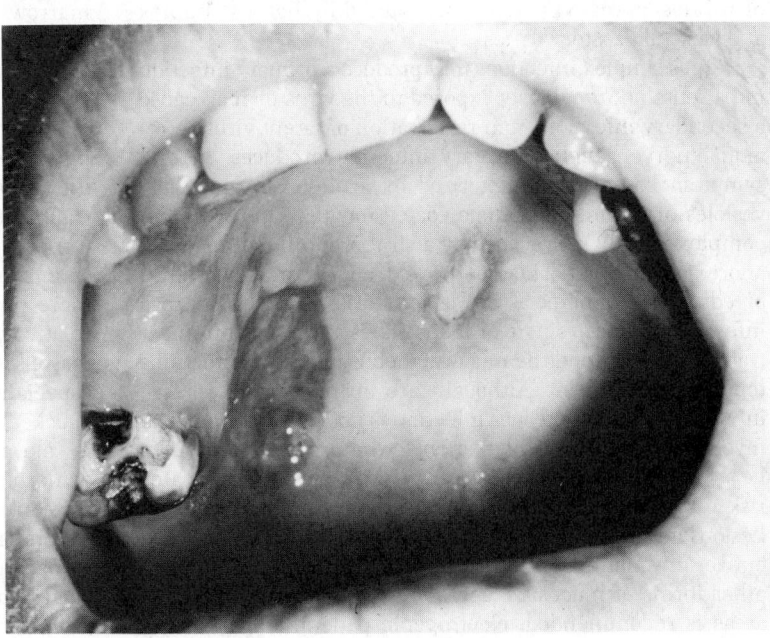

FIGURE 63–7. An unusual case of localized ulcerations of the hard palate in a patient hospitalized with fever of unknown origin. At the time of admission, the larger ulcer demonstrated evidence of infection. (Lockhart PB. Dental management of patients receiving chemotherapy. In: Peterson D, Sonis S, eds. Oral complications of cancer chemotherapy. Boston: Martinus Nijhoff, 1983)

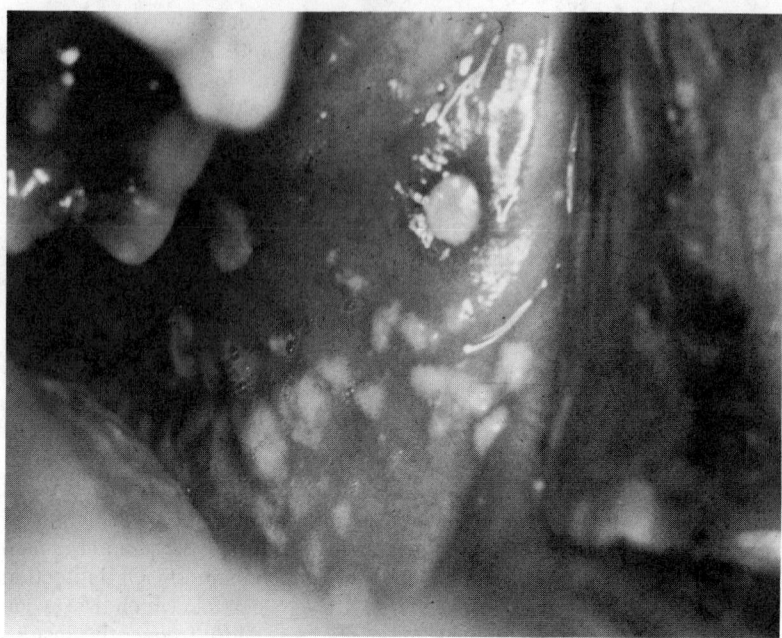

FIGURE 63–8.   Candidiasis of buccal mucosa in a 49-year-old woman with acute myelogenous leukemia. Notice raised, white croppy areas of fungae. A small ulcer is also present.

therapy reduces both the frequency and severity of infection. The polyene antibiotics (nystatin) are probably the most often used, usually as a suspension that is rinsed and swallowed. Popsicles made of nystatin diluted in water are often soothing and provide prolonged contact with the mucosa. Alternatively, the imidazole agents in trouche form may be preferred. It appears that their efficacy is comparable to nystatin.[79] Patients complaining of esophageal pain or dysphagia should be evaluated for spread of infection (see Chap. 64),[80] which should be treated early and aggressively with a systemic antifungal agent (*e.g.*, amphotericin B).

Other deep fungal infections may occur in the myelosuppressed patient. Fortunately, however, these are relatively rare.

The two most common viral infections affecting the mouths of myelosuppressed patients are caused by herpes simplex and varicella zoster viruses.

Herpes simplex infections may produce a primary infection in patients not previously exposed to the virus or may cause a secondary infection from reactivation of latent virus in regional nerve ganglia. Primary infection produces an oral symptom complex characterized by acute-onset gingivitis, vesicles of the mucosa, and a coated tongue. This symptom complex usually is preceded by a viral prodrome of malaise, anorexia, and fever. The mouth is extremely tender. Gingival bleeding may be noted as well as fetor oris. Secondary herpes infection produces single or crops of vesicles, most often extraoral, at or beyond the mucocutaneous junction. Infections tend to be recurrent. Although rare in the normal person, intraoral secondary herpes infection is not uncommon in the myelosuppressed patient. Patients who are seropositive to herpes simplex virus because of prior exposure are at greater risk of infection compared with seronegative patients.[80–82] Lesions may have a variety of appearances, including vesicles, bullae, or small or large ulcers. Since the latter resembles other forms of mucositis, aggressive culturing of suspicious areas is recommended. Neutropenic patients experiencing

herpes infections should be treated with acyclovir.[81–84] Extraoral lesions may become infected secondarily with bacteria. Healing often is helped by the presence of a lubricating ointment such as Neosporin.

The frequency of herpes simplex virus infections in patients receiving chemotherapy is not well resolved; the reported incidence ranges from about 11% to 48%. The differences in reported frequency are largely dependent on the method of diagnosis. In interpreting results, it must be remembered that herpes simplex virus is not an uncommon member of the normal oral flora and, in the absence of clinically detectable lesions, may not be of pathologic consequence.[85]

Chlorhexidine gluconate 0.12% may be efficacious in reducing the frequency and severity of mucositis and infection associated with chemotherapy and radiation therapy for bone marrow transplantations. The drug is used twice daily as a rinse. Side effects are minimal and include occasional burning, which may be reduced by dilution with water, and brown superficial tooth staining, which can be easily polished off.[86]

Thrombocytopenia predisposes to oral bleeding.[87,88] Bleeding may occur anywhere in the mouth but usually is provoked by trauma or preexisting periodontal disease. Minor mucosal trauma may result in hematoma formation or frank bleeding. Generally, hematoma formation is unusual with platelet counts greater than 25,000 cells/mm[3].[87] When patients are more profoundly thrombocytopenic, oral hematomas form relatively easily and are of clinical significance for two major reasons: (1) hematomas can act as sites of secondary infection, especially when there are breaks in the mucosa; and (2) unchecked submucosal bleeding in the sublingual area may result in elevation of the tongue and consequent respiratory compromise.

Spontaneous gingival bleeding is unusual with platelet counts greater than 10,000 cells/mm[3]. Patients with preexisting periodontal disease are more likely to demonstrate gingival hemorrhage than are patients in good gingival health. Therefore, dental prophylaxis and good oral hygiene are of significant benefit in reducing the likelihood of this problem. If gingival bleeding does occur, topical thrombin-soaked gauze held under pressure is often helpful. For open mucosal oozing, microcrystalline collagen may produce hemostasis. When local measures fail, patients may require platelet transfusion. The use of stints or surgical gingival packs should be avoided because the pressure of these often causes necrosis. Furthermore, these appliances harbor bacteria and are irritating to the gingiva.

REFERENCES

1. Sonis ST, Woods PD, White BA. Pretreatment oral assessment. J Natl Cancer Inst 1990;9:29–32.
2. Reynolds WR, Hickey AJ, Feldman MI. Dental management of the cancer patient receiving radiation therapy. Clin Prevent Dent 1980;2:5–9.
3. Miaskowski C. Management of mucositis during therapy. NCI Monograph 1990;9:95–98.
4. Rodu B, Russell CM, Ray KL. Treatment of oral ulcers with hydroxyprophycellulose film. Compend Contin Educ Dent 1988;9:420–422.
5. Rodu B, Russell CM. Performance of a hydroxyprophycellulose film former in normal and ulcerated mucosa. Oral Surg 1988;65:699–703.
6. Preiffer P, Madsen EL, Hansen O, et al. Effect of prophylactic sucralfate suspension on stomatitis induced by cancer chemotherapy. Acta Oncol 1990;29:171–173.
7. Shenep JL, Kalwinsky DK, Hutson PR, et al. Efficacy of oral sucralfate suspension in prevention and treatment of chemotherapy-induced mucositis. J Pediatr 1988;113:758–763.
8. Scherlacher A, Beaufort-Spontin F. Radiotherapy of head-neck neoplasms: Prevention of inflammation of the mucosa by sucralfate treatment. HNO 1990;38:24–28.
9. Samaranayake LP, Robertson AG, MacFarlane TW, et al. The effect of chlorhexidine and benzydamine mouthwashes on mucositis induced by therapeutic irradiation. Clin Radiol 1988;39:291–294.
10. Lever SA, Dupuis LL, Chan SL. Comparative evaluation of benzydamine oral rinse in children with antineoplastic-induced stomatitis. Drug Intell Clin Pharm 1987;21:359–361.
11. Epstein JB, Stevenson-Moore P, Jackson S, et al. Prevention of oral mucositis in radiation therapy: A controlled study with benzydamine hydrochloride rinse. Int J Oncol Biol Phys 1989;16:1571–1575.
12. Tanner NS, Stanford IF, Bennett A. Plasma prostaglandins in mucositis due to radiotherapy and chemotherapy for head and neck cancer. Br J Cancer 1981;43:767–771.
13. Pillsbury HC, Webster WP, Rosenman J. Prostaglandin inhibitor and radiotherapy in advanced head and neck cancer. Arch Otolaryngol Head Neck Surg 1986;112:552–553.
14. Portender H, Rausch E, Kment G, et al. Local prostaglandin E2 in patients with oral malignancies undergoing chemo- and radiotherapy. J Craniomaxillofac Surg 1988;16:371–374.
15. Matejka M, Nell A, Kment G, et al. Local benefit of prostaglandin E2 in radiochemotherapy-induced oral mucositis. J Craniomaxillofac Surg 1990;28:89–91.
16. Spijkervet FK, Van Saere HK, Van Saene JJ, et al. Effect of selective elimination of the oral flora on mucositis in irradiated head and neck cancer patients. J Surg Oncol 1991;46:167–173.
17. Spijkervet FK, Van Saere HK, Van Saene JJ, et al. Mucositis prevention by selective elimination of the oral flora in irradiated head and neck cancer patients. J Oral Pathol Med 1990;19:486–489.
18. Shannon IL, Starche EN, Wescott WB. Effect of radiotherapy on whole saliva flow. J Dent Res 1977;56:693.
19. Baker DG. The radiobiological basis for tissue reactions in the oral cavity following therapeutic x-irradiation. Arch Otolaryngol 1982;108:21–24.
20. Engelmeier RL, King GE. Complications of head and neck radiation therapy and their management. J Prosthet Dent 1983;49:514–522.
21. Eneroth Cm, Henrikson CO, Jakobson PA. Effects of fractionated radiotherapy on salivary gland function. Cancer 1972;30:1147–1153.
22. Karmiol M, Walsh RF. Dental caries after radiotherapy of the oral regions. J Am Dent Assoc 1975;91:838–845.
23. Shannon IL, Tordahl JN, Starcke EN. Remineralization of enamel by saliva substitute designed for use by irradiated patients. Cancer 1978;41:1746–1750.
24. Greenspan D, Daniels TE. Effectiveness of pilocarpine in postradiation xerostomia. Cancer 1987;59:1123–1125.
25. Fox PC, Vander Ven PF, Baum BJ, et al. Pilocarpine for the treatment of xerostomia associated with salivary gland dysfunction. Oral Surg Oral Med Oral Pathol 1986;61:243–248.
26. Keys HM, McCasland JP. Techniques and results of a comprehensive dental care program in head and neck cancer patients. Int J Radiat Oncol Biol Phys 1976;1:859–865.
27. Keene HJ, Fleming TJ. Prevalence of caries-associated microflora after radiotherapy in patients with cancer of the head and neck. Oral Surg 1987;64:421–426.
28. MacCarthy-Leventhal EM. Postradiation mouth-blindness. Lancet 1959;2:1138–1139.
29. Epstein JB, Wong FL, Stevenson-Moore P. Osteoradionecrosis: Clinical experience and a proposal for classification. J Oral Maxillofac Surg 1987;45:104–110.
30. Murray CG, Herson J, Daly TE, et al. Radiation necrosis of the mandible: A 10-year study. Part 1. Factors influencing the onset of necrosis. Int J Radiat Oncol Biol Phys 1980;6:543–548.
31. Marx RE, Johnson RP. Studies in the radiobiology of osteoradionecrosis and their clinical significance. Oral Surg 1987;64:379–390.
32. Murray CG, Daly TE, Zimmerman SO. The relationship between dental disease and radiation necrosis of the mandible. Oral Surg 1980;49:99–104.
33. Levendag PC, Visch LL, Driver N. A simple device to protect against osteoradionecrosis induced by interstitial irradiation. J Prosthet Dent 1990;63:665–670.
34. Murray CG, Herson J, Daly TE, et al. Radiation necrosis of the mandible: A 10-year study. Part II. Dental factors: Onset, duration and management of necrosis. Int J Radiat Oncol Biol Phys 1980;6:549–553.
35. Marciani RD, Plezia RA. Management of teeth in the irradiated patient. J Am Dent Assoc 1974;88:1021–1024.
36. Markitziu A, Heling I. Endodontic treatment of patients who have undergone irradiation of the head and neck. Oral Surg 1981;52:294–297.
37. Mansfield MJ, Saunders DW, Heimbadi RD, et al. Hyperbaric oxygen as an adjunct in the treatment of osteoradionecrosis of the mandible. J Oral Surg 1981;39:585–589.
38. Sonis ST, Sonis AL, Lieberman A. Oral complications in patients receiving treatment for malignancies other than of the head and neck. J Am Dent Assoc 1978;97:468–472.
39. Sonis AL, Sonis ST. Oral complications of cancer chemotherapy in pediatric patients. J Pedodontics 1979;3:122–128.
40. Dreizen S, McCredie KB, Bodey GPN, et al. Quantitative analysis of the oral complications of antileukemic chemotherapy. Oral Surg 1986;62:650–653.
41. Bodey GP. Oral manifestations of myeloproliferative diseases. Postgrad Med 1971;49:115–121.
42. Lockhart PB, Sonis ST. Relationship of oral complications to peripheral blood leukocyte and platelet counts in patients receiving cancer chemotherapy. Oral Surg 1979;48:21–28.
43. Baraket NJ, Toto PD, Choukas NC. Aging and cell renewal of oral epithelium. J Periodontol 1969;40:599–602.
44. Peterson DW, Overholser CD. Increased morbidity associated with oral infection in patients with acute leukemia. Oral Surg 1982;53:32–36.
45. Greenberg MS, Cohen SG, McKifrick JC, et al. The oral flora as a source of septicemia in patients with acute leukemia. Oral Surg 1982;53:32–36.
46. Overholser CD, Peterson DE, William SL, et al. Periodontal infection in patients with acute nonlymphocytic leukemia: Prevalence of acute exacerbations. Arch Intern Med 1982;14:551–554.
47. Beck S. Impact of a systemic oral care protocol on stomatitis after chemotherapy. Cancer News 1979;2:185–199.
48. Epstein JB. Infection prevention in bone marrow transplantation and radiation patients. NCI Monograph 1990;9:73–85.
49. Hickey AJ, Toth BB, Lindquist SB. Effect of intravenous hyperalimentation and oral care on the development of oral stomatitis during cancer chemotherapy. J Prosthet Dent 1982;47:188–193.
50. Dreizen S, Bodey GP, Rodriquez V. Oral complications of cancer chemotherapy. Postgrad Med 1975;58:95.
51. Sonis S, Kunz A. Impact of improved dental services on the frequency of oral complications for patients with non-head and neck malignancies. Oral Surg Oral Med Oral Pathol 1988;65:19–21.
52. Dreizen S. Stomatotoxic manifestations of cancer chemotherapy. J Prosthet Dent 1978;40:650–655.
53. Volger W, Huguley C, Kerr W. Toxicity and antitumor effect of divided doses of methotrexate. Arch Intern Med 1965;115:285–293.
54. Woo SB, Sonis ST, Sonis AL. Oral herpes simplex virus infection in bone marrow transplant recipients. Cancer 1990;66:2375–2379.
55. Guggenheimer J, Verbin RS, Appel BN, et al. Clinicopathologic effects of cancer chemotherapeutic agents on human buccal mucosa. Oral Surg 1977;44:58–63.
56. Lockhart PB, Sonis ST. Alterations in the oral mucosa caused by chemotherapeutic agents. J Dermatol Surg Oncol 1981;7:1019–1025.
57. Aker SN. Oral findings in the cancer patient. Cancer 1979;43:2102–2107.
58. Mahood D, Dose AM, Loprinzi C, et al. Inhibition of fluorouracil-induced stomatitis by oral cryotherapy. J Clin Oncol 1991;9:449–452.
60. Clark PI, Slevin ML. Allopurinol mouthwash and 5-fluorouracil induced oral toxicity. Eur J Surg Oncol 1985;11:267–268.
61. Tsavaris N, Caragiauris P, Kosmidis P. Reduction of oral toxicity of 5-fluorouracil by allopurinol mouthwashes. Eur J Surg Oncol 1988;14:405–406.
62. Mills EE. The modifying effect of beta-carotene on radiation and chemotherapy induced oral mucositis. Br J Cancer 1988;57:416–417.
63. Bonilla MA, Gillio AP, Ruggeiro M, et al. Effects of recombinant human granulocyte colony-stimulating factor on neutropenia in patients with congenital agranulocytosis. N Engl J Med 1989;320:1574–1580.
64. Gabrilove JL, Jakubowski A, Scher H, et al. Effect of granulocyte colony-stimulating factor on neutropenia and associated morbidity due to chemotherapy for transitional-cell carcinoma of the urothelium. N Engl J Med 1988;318:1414–1422.
65. Sonis ST. Personal communication, 1992.
66. Rosenthal S, Kaufman S. Vincristine neurotoxicity. Ann Intern Med 1974;80:733–734.
67. EORTC International Antimicrobial Therapy Project Group. Three antibiotic regimens in the treatment of infection in febrile granulocytopenic patients with cancer. J Infect Dis 1978;137:14–29.
68. Dreizen S, Brown LR. Oral microbial changes and infections during cancer chemotherapy. In: Peterson DE, Sonis ST, eds. Oral complications of cancer chemotherapy. Boston: Martinus-Nijhoff, 1983:41–47.
69. Bodey GP. Fungal infections complicating acute leukemia. J Chronic Dis 1966;19:667–687.

70. Peterson DE: Bacterial infections: Periodontal and dental disease. In: Peterson DE, Sonis ST, eds. Oral complications of cancer chemotherapy. Boston: Martinus-Nijhoff, 1983:113–149.

71. Peterson DE, Minah GE, Overholser CD, et al. Microbiology of acute periodontal infection in myelosuppressed cancer patients. Clin Oncol 1987;5:1461–1468.

72. Lockhart PB. Dental management of patients receiving chemotherapy. In: Peterson DE, Sonis ST, eds. Oral complications of cancer chemotherapy. Boston: Martinus-Nijhoff, 1983:113–149.

73. Overholser CD, Peterson DE, Bergman SA. Dental extractions in patients with leukemia. J Oral Surg 1982;40:296–298.

74. Williford SK, Salisbury PL, Peacock JE, et al. The safety of dental extractions in patients with hematologic malignancies. J Clin Oncol 1989;7:798–802.

75. Epstein JB, Pearsall NN, Truelove EL. Oral candidiasis: Effects of antifungal therapy upon clinical signs and symptoms, salivary antibody and mucosal adherence of Candida albicans. Oral Surg 1981;51:32–36.

76. Taschdjian CL, Kosinn PH, Toni EF. Opportunistic yeast infections with special reference to candidiasis. Ann NY Acad Sci 1970;174:606–622.

77. Pizzuto J, Conte G, Aviles A, et al. Nystatin prophylaxis in leukemia and lymphoma. N Engl J Med 1978;299:661–662.

78. Carpentieri U, Haggard ME, Lockhart LH, et al. Clinical experience in preventions of candidiasis by nystatin in children with acute leukemia. J Pediatr 1978;92:593–595.

79. Gombert ME, duBouchet L, Aulicino TM, et al. A comparative trial of clotrimazole troches and oral nystatin suspension in recipients of renal transplants: Use in prophylaxis of oropharyngeal candidiasis. JAMA 1987;258:2553–2555.

80. Jones JM. Necrotizing Candida esophagitis: Failure of symptoms and roentgenographic findings to reflect severity. JAMA 1980;244:2190–2191.

81. Saral R, Burns WH, Laskin OL, et al. Acyclovir prophylaxis of herpes simplex virus infections. N Engl J Med 1981;305:63–67.

82. Wade JC, Newton B, McLaren C, et al. Intravenous acyclovir to treat mucocutaneous herpes simplex virus infection after marrow transplantation: A double blind trial. Ann Intern Med 1982;96:265–269.

83. Wade JC, Day LM, Crowley JJ, et al. Recurrent infection with herpes simplex virus after marrow transplantation: Role of specific immune response and acyclovir treatment. J Infect Dis 1984;149:750–756.

84. Saral R, Burns WH, Prentice HG:.Herpes virus infections. Clinical manifestations and therapeutic strategies in immunocompromised patients. Clin Haematol 1984;13:645–660.

85. Montgomery MT, Redding SW, LeMaistre CF. The incidence of oral herpes simplex virus infection in patients undergoing cancer chemotherapy. Oral Surg 1986;61:238–242.

86. Ferretti GA, Ash RC, Brown AT, et al. Chlorhexidine in prophylaxis against oral infections and associated complications in patients receiving bone marrow transplantation. J Am Dent Assoc 1987;114:292–294.

87. Stafford R, Lockhart P, Sonis ST, et al. Hemotologic parameters as predictors of oral involvement in the presentation of acute leukemia. J Oral Med 1982;37:38–41.

88. Lynch MA, Ship II. Initial oral manifestations of leukemia. J Am Dent Assoc 1977;75:932–940.

SECTION 7

CLAUDIA A. SEIPP

Hair Loss

Alopecia is a psychologically distressing yet common side effect of many chemotherapeutic agents and radiation therapy. As patients embark on new therapies, hair loss can induce a negative body image, alter interpersonal relationships, and arouse enough anxiety to cause some patients to reject potentially curative treatment.

Frank discussion of the problem by clinicians and oncology nurses with recognition of the patient's stress is helpful in preparing the patient to confront this loss.[1] Although methods for the prevention of total-scalp hair loss and the use of wigs after hair loss are not entirely satisfactory for all patients, caregivers can offer psychological support and some practical suggestions. Often, the presence of a spouse, family member, or friend during this discussion helps the patient to place the problem in perspective.

The hair loss caused by scalp irradiation is unpredictable. Epilation can begin at doses of 500 cGy and generally progresses with spotty areas of baldness as the course of treatment continues. The prospects for hair regrowth diminish with increasing doses.[2] Radiation ports on extremities have been noted to be hair-free 10 years after radiation therapy and may never have hair regrowth. In lower-dose ranges, regrowth begins 8 to 9 weeks after cessation of therapy. Patients should be cautioned that the new hair may be different in character from the pretreatment hair.[3]

The extent of body hair loss by patients in any chemotherapeutic program is both drug- and dose-dependent and is related to the frequency of cycle repetition. Often, it is caused by more than one drug used in combination (Table 63–21).[4] Long-term therapy may result in loss of pubic, axillary, and facial hair in addition to scalp hair. It should be emphasized to patients that alopecia from chemotherapy is reversible, with hair regeneration beginning 1 to 2 months after therapy is discontinued. Alteration in color and texture of hair may occur;

hair may be a lighter or darker shade and is often curlier as it regrows.[5] Hair loss may begin 1 to 2 weeks after a single chemotherapeutic dose and reaches maximal loss within 2 months in most drug sequences. Doxorubicin and cyclophosphamide are common cytologic agents known to cause epilation after two cycles at doses of doxorubicin above 50 mg/m² and cyclophosphamide above 500 mg/m². Although agents differ in degree to which they cause hair loss, alopecia may be expected with other single-agent antibiotics, alkylating agents, nitrosoureas, and especially their combinations.[6]

HEAD COVERINGS

Most patients choose to cover their heads during periods of hair loss. Nurses and clinicians can suggest wigs or other head coverings such as stylish scarves, turbans, or hats. Wigs should be selected before hair loss begins so that the patient is prepared when alopecia occurs and so that hair color and style can be matched. Hairpieces are tax-deductible medical expenses and are covered by some medical insurance policies. Several small private businesses have been developed by former patients who distribute or sell head coverings of various designs. An American Cancer Society rehabilitation program called "Look Good, Feel Better" was developed specifically to assist women in compensating for hair loss and skin changes during cancer treatment.[7] Volunteer beauticians and cosmetologists help women look and feel more comfortable with changes in their appearance, such as dry, discolored, or blotching skin; discolored nails; and alopecia. Information is available through an American Cancer Society hotline (telephone number, 1-800-395-LOOK).

PREVENTION OF ALOPECIA

Since 1966, interventions have been proposed to prevent scalp hair loss from chemotherapy. The rationale for these procedures is to prevent drug circulation to the hair follicles by causing temporary vasoconstriction with either an occlusive

TABLE 63–21. Single Agents With Potential to Induce Reversible Alopecia*

Amsacrine	5-Fluorouracil
Bleomycin	Hydroxyurea
Cyclophosphamide	Ifosfamide
Dactinomycin	Methotrexate
Daunorubicin	Mitomycin
Doxorubicin	Melphalan
Epirubicin	Taxol
Etoposide	Vinblastine
Vincristine	

* The degree or onset of alopecia is dependent on dose, schedule of sequences, rate of delivery, route of delivery, and various combinations of agents.[4]

scalp tourniquet or localized hypothermia. The pharmacokinetics of the drugs to be used must be understood before either of these methods is considered. Occlusion of the superficial scalp veins must begin before the drugs are given and, to be effective, must be extended beyond the time of the peak plasma drug levels.[8–10]

Various types of scalp icing devices have been manufactured by several different U.S. companies. Although the Food and Drug Administration (FDA) had initially approved the marketing of cooling caps intended to cause localized scalp hypothermia, the FDA reviewed these applications early in 1990 and became concerned that the safety and efficacy of these devices had not been substantiated by adequate clinical data.[4,11–14] Regulatory action was initiated to address the following concerns:

1. The potential for scalp metastasis posed by the use of these devices
2. The potential for reducing drug circulation to other anatomic sites beyond the scalp, such as the skull and possibly the brain

3. The effectiveness of these devices in preventing hair loss and how specific cytologic doses and other variables affected the results achieved

The FDA halted the commercial distribution of these devices, and a year after their withdrawal, no company had come forward with supporting clinical evidence of reasonable safety and effectiveness.[15]

The safety limitations and inconclusive and conflicting reports of the usefulness of scalp hypothermia should be discussed with patients seeking information about these devices and hair preservation techniques.[16]

REFERENCES

1. Wagner L, Bye MG. Body image and patients experiencing alopecia as a result of cancer chemotherapy. Cancer Nurs 1979;2(5):365–369.
2. Moss WT, Brand WN, Battiford H. Radiation oncology: Rationale, techniques, results. 5th ed. St. Louis: CV Mosby, 1979:57–58.
3. Nordstrom RE, Holsti LR. Hair transplantation in alopecia due to radiation. Plast Reconstr Surg 1983;72:454–458.
4. Keller JF, Blausey LA. Nursing issues and management in chemotherapy-induced alopecia. Oncol Nurs Forum 1988;15:5, 603–607.
5. Cancer, cancer therapy, and hair. Lancet [Editorial] 1983;2:1177–1178.
6. Cline BW. Prevention of chemotherapy-induced alopecia: A review of the literature. Cancer Nurs 1984;7:221–228.
7. American Cancer Society Hotline. Personal communication, telephone 1-800-395-LOOK.
8. Dean JC, Salmon SE, Griffith KS. Prevention of doxorubicin-induced hair loss with scalp hypothermia. N Engl J Med 1979;302:1427–1429.
9. Satterwaite B, Zimm S. The use of scalp hypothermia in the prevention of doxorubicin-induced hair loss. Cancer 1984;54:34–37.
10. Robinson MH, Jones AC, Durant KD. Effectiveness of scalp cooling in reducing scalp alopecia caused by epirubicin treatment in breast cancer. Cancer Treat Rep 1987;71: 913–914.
11. Middleton J, Franks D, Buchanan RB, et al. Failure of scalp hypothermia to prevent hair loss when cyclophosphamide is added to doxorubicin and vincristine. Cancer Treat Rep 1985;69:373–375.
12. Wheelock JB, Myers MB, Krebs HB, et al. Ineffectiveness of scalp hypothermia in the prevention of alopecia in patients treated with doxorubicin and cis-platin combinations. Cancer Treat Rep 1984;68:1387–1388.
13. Seipp CA. Scalp hypothermia: Indicators for precaution. Oncol Nurs Forum [Letter] 1983;10:12.
14. Whitman G, Cadman E, Chen M. Misuse of scalp hypothermia. Cancer Treat Rep 1981;65:507–508.
15. Harson C. Personal communication. November 1991.
16. Camp-Sorrell D. Scalp hypothermia devices: Current status. ONS News 1991;7:1.

SECTION **8**   RICHARD J. SHERINS

Gonadal Dysfunction

Accompanying the success of cytotoxic chemotherapy in the treatment of cancer and nonmalignant disorders are new concerns for the long-term toxic effects of these therapies on normal host tissues. Although many of the acute and chronic toxicities of antineoplastic drugs have been well defined, comparatively little attention has been paid to gonadal dysfunction resulting from antitumor therapy. In part, this lack of attention has stemmed from the absence of any immediate or life-threatening symptoms resulting from gonadal injury; and, until recently, it has reflected the absence of a group of long-term cancer survivors who are concerned about their reproductive potential.

Neoplastic disease and its treatment can potentially interfere with any of the cellular, anatomic, physiologic, behavioral, or social processes that contribute to normal sexual and reproductive function. The tumor may directly involve the gonad, and cancer surgery itself may require incidental gonadectomy. For the male, genital mutilation or retroperitoneal lymph node dissection can result in failure of emission, retrograde ejaculation, loss of orgasm, and impotence (Table 63–22). Many drugs used in the treatment of cancer have profound and lasting effects on gonadal function. Both germ cell production and endocrine function may be affected. The magnitude of the effect varies with the drug class, the total dose administered, and the age and pubertal status of the patient at the time of therapy. Radiation therapy can also result in germ cell depletion and clinical hypogonadism, and, as with chemotherapeutic drugs, can induce mutagenic effects in the germ cell and teratogenic effects in the fetus. Recent evidence from rodent studies suggests that direct drug effects on sperm, as well as seminal transmission to the female of drugs administered to the male, may have adverse effects on the developing fetus and embryo without affecting male fer-

TABLE 63–22. Reproductive Consequences of Cancer and Cancer Therapy

Tumor	Direct gonadal involvement
	Hypothalamic and pituitary involvement
Surgery	Removal of gonad
	Neurogenic dysfunction
	Failure of emission
	Retrograde ejaculation
	Loss of orgasm
	Impotence
	Genital mutilation
Therapy	Germ cell depletion
	Clinical hypogonadism
	Mutagenic changes in germ cell
	Teratogenic effects on fetus
	Seminal transmission of drug

tility.[1,2] The reproductive consequences of cancer chemotherapy are drug-specific, dose-dependent, age-related, sex-dependent, and species-specific.

A separate category of effects concerns social and behavioral responses to the disruptions of cancer and its therapy. The nature of the patient's illness, the extent of necessary surgery, chemotherapy, or radiation therapy, and the patient's relationship with spouse and family all may play an important role in reestablishing normal sexual interest and function after treatment for cancer. Detailed reviews of the reproductive consequences of cancer and cancer therapy are available.[3-8]

CHEMOTHERAPY EFFECTS IN ADULT MEN

CLINICAL PATHOPHYSIOLOGY

Testicular function in adult men is particularly susceptible to injury by many chemotherapeutic agents. The primary histopathologic lesion produced by the drugs is one of progressive, dose-related depletion of the germinal epithelium lining the seminiferous tubule.[9-15] Frequently, the germinal tissue disappears completely, and only the supporting Sertoli cells remain lining the tubular lumen, a state described as *germinal aplasia*. The Leydig cells remain morphologically intact, although they may be functionally abnormal.

The clinical manifestations of germinal depletion (Table 63–23) are a marked reduction in testicular volume (atrophy), reduction in sperm count (oligospermia or azoospermia), and infertility. Because the gonad regulates pituitary gonadotropin secretion, serum follicle-stimulating hormone (FSH) and luteinizing hormone (LH) levels reflect the state of the seminiferous epithelium (Fig. 63–9). Germinal aplasia results in a fivefold increase in serum FSH levels (Fig. 63–10); and partial germinal depletion results in a lesser increase in FSH concentration.[16] By contrast, serum LH and testosterone levels tend to remain within normal limits in the presence of germinal depletion. The serum FSH level serves as a convenient marker for testicular germ cell loss. The changes in FSH are attributed to loss of inhibin, a peptide released from the Sertoli cells lining the seminiferous tubules of the testis, which normally inhibits FSH release from the pituitary.[7] Administration of hypothalamic gonadotropin-releasing hormone to patients with germinal aplasia results in an exaggerated LH response, however, suggestive of subtle Leydig's cell failure.[17] Furthermore, men with germinal aplasia, who maintain normal plasma LH and total testosterone concentrations, have been shown to have a 50% reduction in the amount of testosterone produced and in the level of circulating free testosterone[18] (see Table 63–23). This decrease in Leydig's cell function may account for the "selective" increase in plasma FSH level since, in steroid-replaced castrated male rats, it has been shown that high FSH levels accompanied by normal LH levels can be induced when testosterone is replaced at subphysiologic levels in association with high estradiol administration.[19]

SINGLE AGENTS

The anticancer agents most commonly associated with testicular germ cell depletion are listed in Table 63–24. Studies

TABLE 63–23. Evaluation of Gonadal Function in Men After Cancer Therapy

A. Sexual History
   1. Pretreatment fertility history of both partners
   2. Developmental: age of testicular descent, pubertal age, congenital anomalies of urinary tract or central nervous system
   3. Surgical: orchiopexy, pelvic or retroperitoneal surgery, injury to genitals, spinal cord injury
   4. Medical: venereal disease, mumps, renal disease, diabetes, epididymitis, tuberculosis, or other chronic illnesses
   5. Drugs: many drugs interfere with spermatogenesis, erection, and ejaculation

B. Clinical and Laboratory Features of Germinal Aplasia

	Testis Size		Sperm Count (million/ml)	Hormone Profile				
	Length × Width (cm)	Volume (cc)		FSH (mIU/ml)	LH (mIU/ml)	Testosterone (ng/100 ml)	Testosterone Production Rate (mg/d)	Free Testosterone (ng/100 ml)
Normal men	5.0 × 3.0	16–30	20–100	4–25	4–20	250–1200	7.5	15.3
Germinal aplasia	3.7 × 2.3	8–15	0	25–90	8–25	200–700	3.5	8.6

FSH, follicle-stimulating hormone; LH, luteinizing hormone.

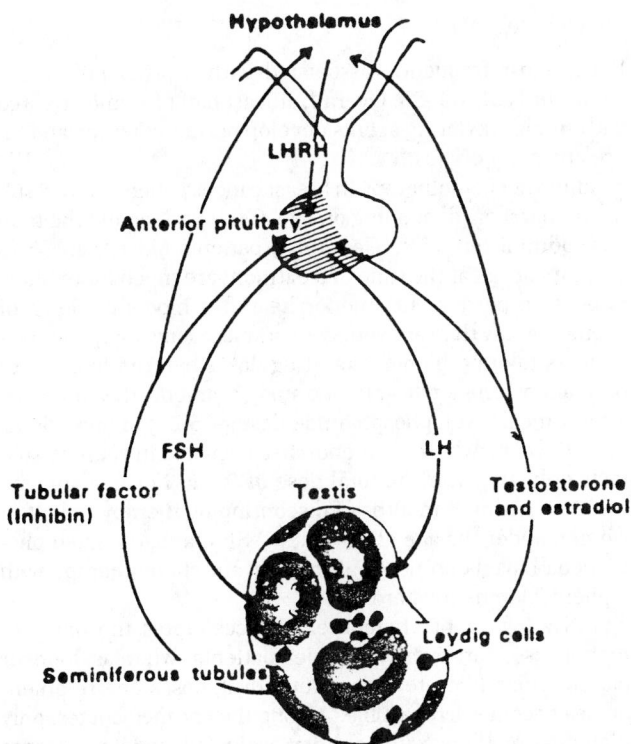

FIGURE 63–9. Hypothalamic-pituitary-testicular interrelations. Notice that leutinizing hormone (LH) acts primarily on Leydig's cells, whereas follicle-stimulating hormone (FSH) primarily affects the seminiferous tubules. LHRH, leutinizing hormone releasing hormone. (Sherins RJ, Winters SJ. Management of disorders of the testis. In: Melmon K, Morelli HP, eds. Clinical pharmacology: Basic principles and therapeutics. 2nd ed. New York: Macmillan, 1978:582)

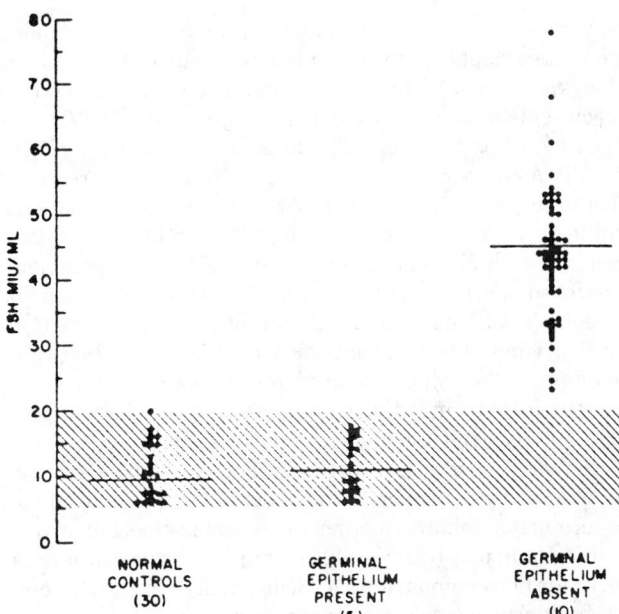

FIGURE 63–10. Serum follicle-stimulating hormone (FSH) levels in normal men and in men with germinal aplasia. (Van Thiel DH, Sherins RJ, Myers GH, et al. Evidence for a specific seminiferous tubular factor affecting follicle-stimulating hormone secretion in man. J Clin Invest 1972;51:1009–1019)

of men receiving single alkylating agents for lymphoma have been a major source of information about drug-related infertility. During alkylating agent therapy, the seminiferous epithelium is depleted in a dose-related fashion. Progressive but reversible oligospermia occurs in men receiving up to 400 mg of chlorambucil, whereas azoospermia and germinal aplasia occur in those patients treated with cumulative doses in excess of 400 mg.[12] Similarly, germinal aplasia is uncommon in patients receiving less than 6 to 10 g of cyclophosphamide.[9–15] Vinblastine, doxorubicin, procarbazine, and cisplatin have all been implicated as being toxic to the germinal epithelium in both animals and humans[13,20–23] although specific dose-toxicity relations have not been established for these drugs. Prospective evaluation of the effects of these and other single agents on testicular function is required to establish reliable data concerning the threshold drug dose above which seminiferous tubular damage becomes irreversible.

COMBINATION CHEMOTHERAPY

Combination drug regimens have a profound impact on spermatogenesis. The effects of nitrogen mustard, vincristine, procarbazine, and prednisone (MOPP) have been most carefully investigated, and it is clear that more than 80% of men receiving this regimen develop testicular atrophy, azoospermia, and elevated serum FSH levels resulting from germinal aplasia.[24–31] Procarbazine leads to particularly long-lasting

testicular damage. Indeed, this drug alone induces germinal aplasia in adult male monkeys.[21]

Whereas the combination of MOPP and cyclophosphamide, vincristine, procarbazine, and prednisone (COPP)[32] produces irreversible germinal aplasia in most patients, this may not be true of other multimodal regimens in use.[33–36] Cyclophosphamide and doxorubicin, when used as adjuvant chemotherapy for soft tissue sarcoma, appear to produce irreversible testicular damage only in men over 40 years of age or in men receiving concomitant irradiation proximal to the gonads. Similar drug doses administered to younger patients produce

TABLE 63–24. Antitumor Agents Associated With Testicular Germ Cell Depletion

Degree of Risk	Drug
Definite	Chlorambucil
	Cyclophosphamide
	Nitrogen mustard
	Busulfan
	Procarbazine
	Nitrosoureas
Probable	Doxorubicin
	Vinblastine
	Cytosine arabinoside
	Cisplatin
Unlikely	Methotrexate
	5-Fluorouracil
	6-Mercaptopurine
	Vincristine
Unknown	Bleomycin

only transient, reversible elevations of serum FSH.[33,36] Among alternative combination chemotherapy regimens for advanced Hodgkin's disease, the combination of doxorubicin (Adriamycin), bleomycin, vinblastine, and dacarbazine (ABVD) has been touted as being equally efficacious and less toxic than MOPP. A comparison of these treatment regimens revealed that azoospermia occurs in 100% of MOPP-treated patients but in only 35% of those receiving ABVD and that spermatogenesis nearly always recovers in the ABVD-treated patients.[37] Improved spermatogenic recovery has also been noted for Hodgkin's patients treated with novantrone, vincristine (Oncovin), vinblastine, and prednisone (NOVP).[38] This information may be important in planning treatment for young men with Hodgkin's disease who are concerned about preservation of fertility during and after treatment.

Similar concerns face patients about to embark on chemotherapy for testicular cancer. Chemotherapy-induced azoospermia that follows treatment with vinblastine, bleomycin, and cisplatin may be reversible within 2 to 3 years after treatment for nonseminomatous testicular cancer.[23,39-44] Evidence suggests that when a standard treatment regimen is used, sperm count and semen quality recover 2 to 3 years after treatment in about half of patients, and these patients are capable of impregnating their partners. Importantly, about 75% of men with nonseminomatous testicular cancer have severely impaired sperm count and semen quality before chemotherapy is instituted[39-44]; and in about 40% of subjects, emission, ejaculation, and sexual function are compromised after retroperitoneal lymph node dissection.[45-47] These observations complicate interpretation of fertility status after therapy. In addition, some men with testicular cancer have been cryptorchid, which predisposes to infertility even when testicular nondescent is unilateral.[7]

CHEMOTHERAPY EFFECTS IN ADULT WOMEN

An assessment of the impact of cancer chemotherapy on ovarian function has been hampered by the relative inaccessibility of the ovary to biopsy and the resultant inability to obtain reliable estimates of the size of the germ cell population. Therefore, one must rely primarily on menstrual and reproductive history and on determinations of serum hormone levels to assess the functional status of the ovary.

CLINICAL PATHOPHYSIOLOGY

Examination of the ovaries of women who have developed chemotherapy-related ovarian failure frequently reveals arrest of follicular maturation or frank destruction of ova and follicles.[48-50] Clinically, these patients become amenorrheic and may complain of menopausal symptoms of estrogen deficiency such as "hot flashes," vaginal dryness, and dyspareunia. Abnormally low circulating estrogen levels result in marked elevation of serum FSH and LH, a manifestation of the loss of feedback inhibition of gonadotropin secretion consequent to drug-induced primary ovarian failure.

SINGLE AGENTS

Drugs most frequently associated with ovarian failure are shown in Table 63–25. Overall, at least half of women treated with single alkylating agents develop permanent ovarian failure and amenorrhea.[48-55]

Adjuvant chemotherapy in breast cancer patients may result in amenorrhea, depending on age of the patient and the total dose administered.[56,57] Generally, patients older than 35 to 40 years of age at the time of treatment are much more likely to develop permanent amenorrhea after moderate doses of chemotherapy than are younger patients. Conversely, younger patients tolerate higher total drug doses before the onset of permanent amenorrhea. In one study,[58] amenorrhea occurred after a mean cyclophosphamide dose of 5.2 g in all patients over 40 years, whereas amenorrhea occurred in younger subjects only after a mean total dose of 9.3 g. Further, menses resumed within 6 months of discontinuing therapy in half of women under the age of 40 years.[58] Similar age-related phenomena have been noted after adjuvant chemotherapy with L-phenylalanine mustard.[59]

Alkylating agent chemotherapy accelerates the onset of menopause, particularly in older patients, whereas younger patients may tolerate higher total drug doses before amenorrhea becomes irreversible. Among the antimetabolites, only high-dose methotrexate has been evaluated, and it appears to have no immediate ovarian toxicity.[60]

COMBINATION CHEMOTHERAPY

Most available information concerning the effects of combination chemotherapy regimens on ovarian function has come from the study of women receiving MOPP for Hodgkin's disease. Unlike the profound effects of this regimen on testicular function, MOPP produces ovarian dysfunction and amenorrhea in only 40% to 50% of treated women.[61-67] The frequency of ovarian injury is related to the age of the patient at the time of treatment, with persistent amenorrhea occurring much more commonly in subjects older than 35 to 40 years of age. Ovarian dysfunction in younger patients appears to be

TABLE 63–25. Antitumor Agents Associated With Ovarian Dysfunction

Degree of Risk	Drug
Definite	Cyclophosphamide
	L-Phenylalanine mustard
	Busulfan
	Nitrogen mustard
Unlikely	Methotrexate
	5-Fluorouracil
	6-Mercaptopurine
Unknown	Doxorubicin
	Bleomycin
	Vinca alkaloids
	Cisplatin
	Nitrosoureas
	Cytosine arabinoside

related to the total chemotherapy dose administered because permanent amenorrhea occurs in women receiving the highest cumulative drug doses. Although it is impossible to predict the effect of MOPP chemotherapy on ovarian function for any individual patient, it appears unlikely that those patients treated under age 25 will experience any significant therapy-related ovarian dysfunction during the initial 5 to 10 years after completion of treatment.[64-67] Continued long-term follow-up of women who maintain normal menses after chemotherapy will be necessary to determine whether these patients are still at risk for the development of premature ovarian failure and early menopause. Clinically, the current view is that changes in number of oocytes have little effect on the age of menopause until significant oocyte destruction is reached, and the rate of oocyte atresia is important.[68,68a]

CHEMOTHERAPY EFFECTS IN CHILDREN

Evaluation of the effects of chemotherapy on gonadal function in children is particularly complex because of the variables introduced by the continuum of sexual development present in this patient population. Knowledge of the pubertal status of the patient at the time of therapy and at the time of evaluation, along with recognition of the need to compare the results of hormonal evaluation with appropriate age-matched normal children, is required before definitive conclusions concerning drug effects can be drawn.

BOYS

Before the onset of puberty, the testicular germinal epithelium appears to be more resistant to moderate doses of alkylating agents than is the adult testis. Cyclophosphamide, in cumulative doses up to 20 g, produces only minor alterations in the testicular histology of prepubertal boys and no abnormalities in serum gonadotropin or testosterone levels.[69-71] At cumulative doses greater than 20 g, however, germinal aplasia has been documented.[72-74] Little information is available concerning the effects of other drugs on the immature testis, although recent data suggest that cytosine arabinoside and nitrosourea may be damaging to the germinal epithelium.[75,76]

Combination chemotherapeutic regimens have variable effects on reproductive function in boys. A commonly used antileukemic regimen, prednisone, 6-mercaptopurine, methotrexate, and vincristine, does not appear to cause damage to the testis in patients at any pubertal stage.[77] By contrast, MOPP administered to male patients during puberty appears to have profound effects on both germ cell production and endocrine function. After MOPP, gynecomastia, accompanied by elevation of both serum FSH and LH levels and by low normal serum testosterone levels, has been noted in many patients.[78,79] Testicular biopsy confirmed the occurrence of germinal aplasia in these patients. In contrast to prepubertal boys, some chemotherapy regimens administered during puberty may result in injury to Leydig's cells and the seminiferous epithelium, with gynecomastia being the clinical manifestation of this endocrine dysfunction. The reasons for the increased sensitivity to cytotoxic chemotherapy during puberty require further study.

GIRLS

Little information is available on the effects of cytotoxic drugs on the prepubertal and pubertal ovary. Postmortem studies of ovarian histology of girls treated with chemotherapy have revealed a spectrum of results ranging from normal histology to arrest of follicular maturation and frank ovarian destruction.[79-81] Most girls display impaired follicular maturation, although the total number of follicles is not reduced.[81] From clinical studies, delay in menarche or interruption of menses in girls treated with single-agent cyclophosphamide is uncommon.[70,74,82,83] Studies of girls with acute lymphocytic leukemia treated with vincristine, methotrexate, and 6-mercaptopurine have revealed normal ovarian function in more than 80% of patients.[84] It appears that the immature ovary is relatively insensitive to cytotoxic chemotherapy; however, follow-up of these patients will be required for many years to determine accurately the long-term effects of this therapy on reproductive potential.

RADIATION THERAPY

Radiation therapy plays a major role in the management of lymphoma, sarcoma, and other malignant diseases. Sometimes it is the only therapy, but varying strategies incorporating chemotherapeutic regimens are common. In considering the potential gonadal toxicity of radiation therapy, one must differentiate the consequences of radiation exposure from those that accrue from the chemotherapeutic agents administered. In contrast to the growing literature describing adverse effects of chemotherapy, there is a paucity of data concerning the effects of irradiation on gonadal function in humans. Furthermore, there are few data about the effects of age, gender, adjunctive chemotherapy, and fractionation of the radiation dose to gonadal toxicity.

MEN

The testis is highly radiosensitive, most likely because of rapid cell division of the germinal epithelium. There is limited discussion in the early literature of the effects of irradiation on testicular function of men receiving radiation therapy.[85,86] Until recently, there were few useful guides to the threshold dose for radiation damage to the human testis.[87-95] Studies of single-dose radiation exposure to normal volunteer men demonstrate a dose-dependent depletion and recovery of the germinal epithelium.[87,88] A marked but transient suppression of sperm production is evident with dosages as low as 15 cGy; transient aspermia is reported with doses of about 50 cGy, and more prolonged periods of aspermia are reported with higher doses. At 200 to 300 cGy, full recovery of sperm production requires 3 years; at 400 to 600 cGy, the interval is about 5 years; and above 600 cGy, sterility appears to be permanent. A recent assessment of the effects of conventionally fractionated irradiation on testicular function of men with Hodgkin's disease indicates that gonadal function is compromised at doses as low as 50 cGy, and that at 200 cGy, cumulative dose testicular dysfunction persists at least to 3 years.[94]

Unfortunately, there are no substantive studies of the effect of low-dose irradiation on testicular function in boys. In the few reports that appear, it is not possible to distinguish between the gonadal toxicity from chemotherapy and that caused by radiation therapy. In several recent studies, however, high doses of radiation (2400 cGy) delivered directly to the testes of boys with gonadal relapse from acute lymphoblastic leukemia produced marked testicular atrophy, with Leydig's cell impairment, androgen deficiency, and clinical hypogonadism.[96-98]

WOMEN

The medical literature is not adequate to counsel women precisely regarding the risks of ovarian dysfunction follow irradiation. There are only broad guidelines regarding the ovarian threshold. In comparison with men, gonadal exposure in women is complicated by the fact that the ovaries lie within the pelvis, often within the direct radiation beam, or considerably closer to major nodal areas where radiation scatter and beam leakage become critical. Although successful pregnancies have been reported after estimated fractionated ovarian doses of about 650 cGy, cessation of ovarian function is progressively more common with gonadal exposure above 150 cGy, and at 500 to 600 cGy, most women remain persistently amenorrheic.[99] Age is a significant factor in that women younger than age 20 have about a 70% chance of retaining regular cyclic menses after total nodal irradiation; whereas by age 30, only 20% of treated women retain normal ovarian function. Older women are virtually all sterile.[100,101] Existing data suggest that chemotherapy plus total nodal irradiation in women with Hodgkin's disease produces additive ovarian toxicity at any age.[100,101]

Further studies of the radiation dose received by the gonads during primary therapy to other sites are needed to determine the contribution to ovarian dysfunction and to define the circumstances under which repositioning or shielding of the ovary is necessary.

TECHNIQUES TO PROTECT FERTILITY

With the recognition that cytotoxic chemotherapy, radiation therapy, and surgery may destroy fertility has come increasing interest to protect the gonads from these adverse effects and to provide methods to store the germ cells for future use.

SUPPRESSION OF PITUITARY GONADOTROPIN

The subject of suppression of germ cell proliferation to prevent gonadal toxicity associated with cancer treatment is well discussed by Redman and Bajorunas.[102] Approaches to the suppression of gonadal function have included administration of testosterone in men,[103] oral contraceptives in women,[104] and hypothalamic gonadotropin-releasing hormone analogs in both men and women.[105] Unfortunately, none of these approaches has been proved effective despite encouraging preliminary results in experimental animals and humans.[106-111] Among the numerous possible factors contributing to these discrepancies is the fact that, in the human, there is usually inadequate time to suppress the germinal epithelium before instituting cancer therapy because of the urgency to treat the tumor as quickly as possible. Interspecies differences in response to pharmacologic manipulations are also well recognized.

TESTICULAR SHIELDING

Techniques to shield the testes from the direct radiation beam are employed during pelvic irradiation when the chance of gonadal injury may be high, but there have been few studies that accurately assess the dose received by the gonad when the treatment beam is directed to anatomically remote sites. Radiation scatter and leakage radiation can be important contributors to gonadal toxicity. For the testes, a threshold as low as 50 cGy, which is less than 1% of a typical treatment dose, means that use of a gonadal shield is required if the distance between the testes and the radiation field edge is less than 30 cm.[112] A simple and practical testicular shield has been developed for use near megavoltage radiation fields. This shield reduces testicular exposure to less than 10% of the patient's prescription dose; this effectively provides a threefold to tenfold reduction in testicular dose, depending on the distance from the field edge to the gonads.[113,114]

OOPHOROPEXY

For women, appropriate gonadal shielding is difficult because of the pelvic position of the ovary. Oophoropexy, a procedure by which the ovaries are surgically placed in the midline behind the uterus, appears to reduce ovarian exposure in about half women receiving pelvic irradiation.[99,115]

SPERM CRYOPRESERVATION

Pretreatment sperm banking is a reasonable approach to preservation of reproductive potential in some men undergoing sterilizing cancer therapy.[116-123] Unlike normal fertile donors whose semen is selected carefully for its subsequent excellent postthaw quality, pretreatment semen from cancer patients often shows both reduced sperm count (less than 20 million/ml) and poor motion characteristics (less than 50% motility). Analysis of semen in men with lymphoma or testicular cancer has shown that about half of patients have suboptimal semen quality before onset of treatment, which precludes cryobanking.[43,119-128]

Contributing factors that can impair semen quality include fever, stress, and the effects of systemic illness on pituitary gonadotropin release. In men with testicular cancer, there is often human chorionic gonadotropin secretion from the tumor, which stimulates increased estrogen production, which can also adversely affect the contralateral testis. Studies of pretreatment testicular function in patients with other malignancies are not yet available to determine if such adverse effects on semen quality are commonly seen with most cancers.

Cryobanking is feasible for men whose pretreatment semen has adequate numbers of reasonably motile cells; generally, more than 20 million/ml with at least 40% progressive motility is required to provide a postthaw specimen of adequate quality for subsequent insemination. For patients with a very low sperm count before cancer therapy, pooling of multiple specimens after freezing is frequently attempted but generally unsuccessful because quality of the postthaw specimen is actually more important than the total number of sperm. Freezing and thawing semen damages sperm and reduces semen quality below that present in the prebanked specimen.[129]

ASSISTED REPRODUCTIVE TECHNIQUES

For men, despite severe oligospermia after cancer treatment, fertility is often preserved and pregnancy achieved by coitus alone; such data are anecdotal. The key issue with return of a low count is retention of high-quality sperm.[130] Physicians can enhance fertility potential by artificial insemination of husband's sperm at the wife's midcycle LH surge. The technique of insemination is important as intrauterine placement of washed sperm appears to give a higher pregnancy rate than intracervical or intravaginal placement.[131] When there are a limited number of frozen specimens or the sperm count is severely reduced, the physician should consider using the sperm specimen for in vitro fertilization (IVF).[132] At IVF, insemination of eggs is usually performed with only 100,000 to 200,000 sperm and can be done with considerably fewer sperm under special conditions. Since multiple eggs are obtained during each IVF cycle, a single cryopreserved sperm specimen has many more eggs to fertilize than would be available if the specimen were used for an intrauterine insemination. In contrast to the egg, embryos can be frozen and subsequently thawed successfully for transfer at a later time.[133,134] IVF offers an important opportunity for both increased egg exposure and cryopreservation of supplemental embryos for a given limited sperm resource.

Assisted reproductive techniques can also be used in cancer patients before treatment is instituted with chemotherapy or radiation therapy. When time permits, IVF can be performed and resulting embryos cryopreserved. If increased estrogen exposure is contraindicated, such as in women undergoing treatment for breast cancer, an attempt can be made to wash out embryos from the uterus during several months of natural coitus and then to cryopreserve the embryos.[135,136] This approach is less efficient, however, because of a high rate of embryo loss in natural conception.[136]

MODIFIED NERVE-SPARING SURGERY

Retroperitoneal lymph node dissection commonly produces severe neurologic dysfunction in men, resulting in failure of emission, retrograde ejaculation, impotence, loss of orgasm, and infertility. Deliberate or inadvertent ligation of the hypogastric arteries may also result in vasculogenic impotence. These factors have stimulated renewed interest in modifying surgical procedures to reduce the adverse reproductive consequences of cancer surgery without diminishing its efficacy. Sexual function can now be preserved in 70% of men undergoing radical prostatectomy for localized prostate cancer[137,138] and in 83% of men undergoing radical cystoprostatectomy for invasive bladder cancer[139] by placing the incision in the lateral pelvic fascia more anteriorly above the neurovascular bundle supplying the penile corpora cavernosa.

Neural injury occurs in most men undergoing standard bilateral retroperitoneal lymph node dissection[45-47] for the staging and treatment of nonseminomatous germ cell tumors

because of injury to the sympathetic innervation of the pelvic viscera. If the area surrounding the aortic bifurcation and sacral prominence is not disturbed, the final common pathways of the sympathetic innervation remain intact, and no neurologic deficit results. A modified bilateral node dissection sparing the final common sympathetic pathway is feasible without missing sites of potential nodal metastases[47] and allows about half of men to preserve ejaculatory function.[46,47] A modified unilateral retroperitoneal lymph node dissection preserves ejaculation in about 70% of men.[140-142]

ELECTROEJACULATION

The technique of electroejaculation, adopted from vast experience in veterinary practice, has been employed successfully to produce semen in neurologically impaired men.[143] From men with paraplegia[143,144] and in those with ejaculatory failure after retroperitoneal lymph node dissection,[145] it has been possible to collect semen of sufficient high quality to obtain pregnancies by insemination or IVF. Advances in sperm cryopreservation enhance the feasibility of using electroejaculation to obtain semen from such patients for subsequent use.

Retrograde ejaculation resulting from retroperitoneal lymph node dissection, however, can occasionally be treated successfully by administering adrenergic or anticholinergic drugs for several days to close the bladder neck.[7] Such treatment before a wife's midcycle ovulation can facilitate pregnancy by coitus. Additionally, sperm can be retrieved from a postejaculatory urine, washed, and then used as an inseminate.[7] If these simple approaches fail, then electroejaculation under anesthesia is a reasonable alternative.

GENETIC CONCERNS

The agents used to treat cancer are specifically designed to interfere with DNA, cellular metabolism, and cell division; hence, there is good reason to suspect that they may cause mutation and genetic disease in humans.[146]

Standard assays in the mouse at the Oak Ridge National Laboratory[147] show a linear dose-response curve for ionizing radiation as a cause of germ cell genetic damage at several loci. The Oak Ridge Laboratory has generated the experimental results used to set guidelines for radiation protection, specifically for germ cell effects in human populations. The data are based on just a few loci in a laboratory species that may not reflect directly the sensitivity of the human organism. For example, species may differ in their capacities to repair damage to germ cell DNA after environmental exposures.

Cancer treatments certainly cause genetic damage to somatic cells in humans. After all, some modern treatments cause cancer themselves and, at the level of the cell, cancer is a genetic disease. Also, cytogenic abnormalities are commonly seen after intensive cancer therapy. Despite considerable information about somatic effects in experimental systems, some data about germ cell effects in experimental animals, and much information about somatic cell mutation in humans, little is known about the sensitivity of the human gonad to mutagens. Dose-dependent abnormalities have been shown in meiotic chromosomes of the human testis after experimental irradiation, but no environmental agent has been causally linked to human germ cell mutation. Yet, in genetic counseling, in the area of mutagenicity of the human gonad, the ultimate measure of concern is human hereditary disease. Does cancer treatment cause hereditary damage in humans? Does it cause actual disease in the offspring, or mutational events without clinical significance? In theory, the effects of mutation may be neutral or even beneficial, as an essential element of biologic evolution.

Atomic bomb survivors in Japan have been extensively studied for possible genetic damage to their offspring.[148,149] The data are limited but are compatible with the interpretation that human germ cells may be much more tolerant of ionizing radiation than the standard laboratory mouse.[95,148-150] A recent evaluation of the same data suggests that the dose required to double the spontaneous mutation rate in humans is five times greater than the dose in the mouse.[148-150]

PREGNANCY OUTCOMES

The actual outcomes of pregnancies in survivors of cancer are published as case reports, small series, and some 14 retrospective case series (Table 63-26).[151-164] These are patients who all had cancer as a child or young adult, mostly finished cancer treatment, and then began a pregnancy. More than 844 cancer patients or survivors, nearly four fifths of them women, initiated a total of 1761 recognized pregnancies. Of 1389 liveborn outcomes, only 53 (about 4%) had a birth defect, a figure that resembles the rate of major malformations in the general population. The range of defects in the 14 studies included common malformations, such as congenital hip dysplasia, that may, in fact, represent deformity or the nongenetic extrinsic molding of fetal features. Only three of the disorders were purely genetic diseases, that is, mendelian traits or cytogenic defects, as were also, perhaps, the two instances of multiple congenital anomalies. Pendred's syndrome (goiter and deafness) is an autosomal recessive disease. Both parents had to have contributed a mutant gene; hence, one cannot be sure that therapy caused the mutation. The other two disorders, the possible trisomy 18 syndrome and Marfan's syndrome, may represent new mutants, but one cannot be sure. Of course, all these studies were hardly comparable and had such relatively small numbers of patients (given the rarity of genetic disease in the general population) that, even in the aggregate, they have low statistical power. With only two instances of possible mutants seen in some 1400 offspring, experience is obviously limited.

A National Cancer Institute study addressed late effects in some 2300 survivors of childhood and adolescent cancer, using siblings as controls. Only 22% had received any chemotherapy, and one third had received radiation therapy. Overall, fertility was slightly depressed in males, to about 85% of the rate in male controls.[165] Fertility was only slightly depressed in women. When fertility was examined as a function of the type of treatment received in the first year after diagnosis, patients (both men and women) who had been treated with alkylating agent chemotherapy and radiation therapy below the diaphragm were most severely affected.

Although fertility rates differed by tumor type and therapy, each case survivor had an average of about one child who had reached a mean age of about 11 years at the time of interview. Seven cancers were reported in the survivors' offspring (5 histologically confirmed), compared with 11 in the offspring of sibling controls (8 histologically confirmed).[166] This represents a slight but not statistically significant excess of cancer in the offspring of case survivors. In the first 5 years of age, the children of cancer survivors had three times the number of cancers expected based on rates from the Connecticut Tumor Registry; children of sibling controls had about half the expected number of cancers. After 5 years of age, there was no statistically significant difference. The excess seemed attributable to some hereditary cancers (retinoblastoma, Sipple's syndrome, and Wilms' tumor) and to some known syndromes of familial cancer.

In short, there does not appear to be an overall excess risk of cancer in offspring.[167-170] What excess risk there was in the offspring appeared to be confined to the first 5 years of life, and could usually be attributable to a known hereditary or familial cancer and not to the cumulative dose of mutagenic agent.[170] There were few person-years of observation in the older adolescent age range, the ages when most of the case survivors were first diagnosed with cancer.

Cancer could be one indication of germ cell mutation. In a preliminary analysis, *genetic disease* was defined as a cytogenic syndrome, a single gene defect, or one of 15 simple malformations tracked for incidence by the Centers for Disease Control, such as neural tube defects, patent ductus arteriosus, and the like.[167] *Potentially mutagenic therapy* was defined as radiation therapy below the diaphragm or above the knee or chemotherapy with an alkylating agent. Finally, *sporadic* indicated that the offspring had no relative with a similar genetic disease; *familial* meant that there was a relative with a similar genetic disease or that the trait in the offspring was a recessive trait. The overall rate of genetic disease was 3.4% and was not different among the offspring of case survivors compared with sibling controls. Some possible differences in the rates of simple defects in the study groups, compared with population rates, probably arose from artifactual differences in defining the defects and differences in the length of follow-up. The case survivors whose offspring had sporadic genetic disease received potentially mutagenic therapies no more often than did those whose offspring were normal.

The study of genetic disease in offspring of cancer survivors had an 87% power for detecting a twofold excess and did not detect this excess, although the power is misleading because it mostly originates from the high background rate of simple birth defects, such as ventricular septal defect or cleft lip. One cannot be sure that such sporadic defects represent new mutations because they also might be due to the polygenic or multifactorial traits that arise from parental genes interacting with environmental factors.

Apart from genetic effects, female survivors may face problems carrying a pregnancy to term. Excess rates of premature delivery and low birth weight have been documented in several studies[158,159,163] but may be confined to women who had abdominal irradiation and were incapable of maintaining a full-term, normal-weight pregnancy, perhaps because of uterine fibrosis or vascular compromise.

TABLE 63–26. Large Series of Pregnancies in and by Survivors of Cancer

Investigations, Years Encompassed	Exposed Parents Total	Females (%)	Completed Pregnancies Total	Fetal Loss*	Elective Abortions	Live Births Normal	With Defect	Types of Defect
Li and Jaffe,[151] ?–1973	45	63	107	15	3	90	2	Hirschsprung's disease, asymptomatic heart murmur‡
Ross,[152] 1956–1973	58†	100	96	18	?	75	3	Pendred's syndrome, tetralogy of Fallot, hemangiomas, eczema and strabismus (1 stillborn with aplasia of the anterior abdominal wall)
Holmes and Holmes,[153] 1944–1975	48	60	93	12	3	77	6	Amblyopia, autism, scleroderma, rectal stenosis, absent fallopian tube and small uterus, slow learner and foot defect
Li et al,[154] ?–1978	146	58	286	45	10	236	8	Possible trisomy 18 syndrome; Marfan's syndrome; deafness, pyloric stenosis; Hirschsprung's disease (same as above); cardiac, brain, and multiple malformations
Blatt et al,[155] ?–1980	30	77	40	12	10	27	1	Congenital hip dysplasia
Horning et al,[156] 1968–1979	20	100	28	5	5	24	0	
Marradi et al,[157] ?–1982	14	57	23	?	?	21	2	Multiple congenital anomalies with mental and growth retardation, panhypopituitarism and cerebral atrophy, gatroschisis
Bundey and Evans,[158] ?–1973	24	83	48	3	0	44	1	Pyloric stenosis
Andrieu et al,[159] 1972–1976	22	100	30	9	4	21	1	Congenital hip dysplasia
Rustin et al,[160] 1958–1980	216†	100	374	90	36	267	8	Spina bifida, tetralogy of Fallot, talipes equinovarus, collapsed lung, umbilical hernia, desquamative fibrosing alveolitis (2 sibs), neonatal tachycardia (plus 2 anencephalic stillbirths and 1 sudden infant death)
Goldstein et al,[161] 1965–1983	?†	100	222	58	6	159	5	Not specified
Mulvihill et al,[162] 1957–1977	66	100	87	22	12	53	6	Neurosensory deafness‡, scoliosis and slow learner‡, hydrocephalus‡, cleft lip and palate‡, tracheomalacia
Li et al,[164] 1931–1979	181	65	246	53	32	190	5	Congenital hip dislocation (2), heart murmur, hypospadias, internal tibial torsion
Total	844	79	1761	373	132	1389	53	(4%)

* Fetal loss is defined as elective abortion, ectopic pregnancy, spontaneous abortion (miscarriage), or stillbirth.
† All gestational trophoblastic neoplasia.
‡ Exposed to cancer treatment during gestation.
(Modified with permission from Mulvihill JJ, Byrne J. Offspring of long-time survivors of childhood cancers. Clin Oncol 1985;4:333–343)

COUNSELING

Infertility must be viewed as an unfortunate complication of cancer chemotherapy and radiation therapy. An additional area of concern is the reproductive dysfunction that can result from cancer and cancer surgery. Not only can tumors directly involve the gonads and the genitalia, but also en bloc dissection of a tumor field may require removal of ovaries or testes. The psychosexual impact of mutilating surgery is not trivial.[171]

Counseling patients facing the high probability of therapy-induced sterility is important.[171-174] Several points should be considered. In cancer patients, there appears to be a high incidence of reduced sexual frequency, low sexual desire, erectile dysfunction, and difficulty reaching orgasm, not to mention infertility.[172-174] There is also the risk of seminal transmission of the mutagenic cancer drugs to the spouse through coitus.[1] Although most of men become infertile after cancer chemotherapy, it is impossible to predict for many drugs if or when spermatogenesis may resume, and standard contraceptive practices should therefore not be abandoned for couples not desiring pregnancy. Factors such as total drug dose administered, duration of time off therapy, and the type of drug or combination administered may be important determinants of reversibility. Recent evidence suggests that the use of procarbazine in combination chemotherapy regimens may be associated with more long-lasting testicular damage than that seen with alkylating agents alone. Certain drug regimens, such as vinblastine, bleomycin, and cisplatin, appear to be associated with a high probability of reversibility. Return of spermatogenesis is uncommon before 1 or 2 years off chemotherapy but may be expected to occur within 4 years off therapy, if at all. Individual patients should be followed carefully, with serial measurements of testicular volume, serum FSH, and sperm count taken as a matter of course.

Pretreatment sperm banking may be valuable to some patients interested in having children after the completion of chemotherapy or radiation therapy. Although the technology of freezing, preserving, and thawing human sperm has advanced considerably, ultimate conception rates using cryopreserved semen remain only 50% to 60% because of loss of semen quality after thawing. Unfortunately, many cancer patients have decreased sperm counts or sperm motility before receiving therapy, which mitigates against successful semen preservation. For example, at least half of patients with Hodgkin's disease and testicular cancer are oligospermic or azoospermic before receiving any therapy. Indeed, it appears that only 10% to 20% of newly diagnosed cancer patients produce semen of sufficient quality to consider cryopreservation. Nevertheless, sperm banking can be offered to patients if they are properly informed of the cost/benefit ratio of the procedure.

Although women older than 40 years of age frequently develop permanent chemotherapy-induced amenorrhea, many younger women maintain normal cyclic menses throughout the treatment period or resume them shortly after therapy is discontinued. Therapeutic guidelines for managing patients with cancer during pregnancy has been well reviewed.[3]

For couples with preserved fertility, genetic counseling should be offered, as outlined in Table 63-27.

REFERENCES

1. Trasler JM, Hales BF, Robaire B. Paternal cyclophosphamide treatment of rats causes fetal loss and malformations without affecting male fertility. Nature 1985;316:144–146.
2. Hales BF, Smith S, Robaire B. Cyclophosphamide in the seminal fluid of treated males: Transmission to females by mating and effect on pregnancy outcome. Toxicol Appl Pharm 1986;84:423–430.
3. Allen HH, Nisker JA. Cancer in pregnancy: Therapeutic guidelines. New York: Futura, 1986.
4. American Cancer Society. Proceedings of the Workshop on Psychosexual and Reproductive Issues Affecting Patients with Cancer— 1987. Chicago: American Cancer Society Publ. No. 87-5M-4515, 1987.
5. Fox BW, Fox M. Biochemical aspects of the actions of drugs on spermatogenesis. Pharmacol Rev 1967;19:21–57.
6. Schilsky RL, Lewis BJ, Sherins RJ, et al. Gonadal dysfunction in patients receiving chemotherapy for cancer. Ann Intern Med 1980;93:109–114.
7. Sherins RJ, Howards SS. Male infertility. In: Harrison JH, ed. Campbell's urology. 4th ed. Philadelphia: WB Saunders, 1978:715–766.
8. Sieber SM, Adamson RH. Toxicity of antineoplastic agents in man: Chromosomal aberrations, antifertility effects, congenital malformations, and carcinogenic potential. Adv Cancer Res 1975;22:57–155.
9. Fairley KF, Berrie JU, Johnson W. Sterility and testicular atrophy related to cyclophosphamide therapy. Lancet 1972;1:568–569.
10. Kumar R, Biggart JD, McEvoy J, et al. Cyclophosphamide and reproductive function. Lancet 1972;1:1212–1213.
11. Miller DG. Alkylating agents and human spermatogenesis. JAMA 1971;217:1662–1665.
12. Richter P, Calamera JC, Morgenfeld MD, et al. Effect of chlorambucil on spermatogenesis in the human with malignant lymphoma. Cancer 1970;25:1026–1030.
13. Meistrich ML, Finch M, da Cunha MF, et al. Damaging effects of fourteen chemotherapeutic drugs on mouse testis cells. Cancer Res 1982;42:122–131.
14. Cheviakoff J, Calamera JC, Morgenfeld M, et al. Recovery of spermatogenesis in patients with lymphoma after treatment with chlorambucil. J Reprod Fertil 1973;33:155–157.
15. Quershi MJA, Goldsmith HJ, Pennington HJ, et al. Cyclophosphamide therapy and sterility. Lancet 1972;2:1290–1291.
16. Van Thiel DH, Sherins RJ, Myers GH, et al. Evidence for a specific seminiferous tubular factor affecting follicle-stimulating hormone secretion in man. J Clin Invest 1972;51:1009–1019.
17. Mecklenberg RS, Sherins RJ. Gonadotropin response to luteinizing hormone releasing hormone in men with germinal aplasia. J Clin Endocrinol Metab 1974;38:1005–1009.
18. Booth JD, Merriam GR, Clark RV, et al. Evidence for Leydig cell dysfunction in infertile men with a selective increase in plasma follicle stimulating hormone. J Clin Endocrinol Metab 1987;64:1194–1198.
19. Sherins RJ, Patterson AP, Brightwell D, et al. Alteration in the plasma testosterone/estradiol ratio: An alternative to the inhibin hypothesis. In: Bardin CW, Sherins RJ, eds. The cell biology of the testis. Ann NY Acad Sci 1982;383:295–306.
20. da Cunha MF, Meistrich ML, Reid HL, et al. Effect of chemotherapy on human sperm production. Proc Am Assoc Cancer Res 1979;20:100.
21. Sieber SM, Correa P, Dalgard DW, et al. Carcinogenic and other adverse effects of procarbazine in nonhuman primates. Cancer Res 1978;38:2125–2134.
22. Vilar O. Effect of cytostatic drugs on human testicular function. In: Mancini RE, Martini L, eds. Male fertility and sterility. New York: Academic Press, 1974:423–440.
23. Drasga RE, Einhorn LH, Williams SD, et al. Fertility after chemotherapy for testicular cancer. J Clin Oncol 1983;1:179–183.
24. Sherins RJ, DeVita VT. Effects of drug treatment of lymphoma on male reproductive capacity. Ann Intern Med 1973;79:216–220.
25. Asbjornsen G, Molne K, Kleep O, et al. Testicular function after combination chemotherapy for Hodgkin's disease. Scand J Haematol 1976;16:66–69.
26. Roeser HP, Stochs AE, Smith AJ. Testicular damage due to cytotoxic drugs and recovery after cessation of therapy. Aust NZ J Med 1978;8:250–254.
27. Chapman R, Sutcliffe SB, Rees L, et al. Prospective study: The effects of Hodgkin's disease and nitrogen mustard, vincristine, procarbazine and prednisolone on male gonadal function. Proc Am Soc Clin Oncol 1979;20:321.
28. Chapman RM, Sutcliffe SB, Rees LH, et al. Cyclical combination chemotherapy and gonadal function. Lancet 1979;1:285–289.
29. Chapman RM, Sutcliffe SB, Malpas JS. Male gonadal dysfunction in Hodgkin's disease. JAMA 1981;245:1323–1328.
30. Waxman JHX, Terry YA, Wrigley PFM, et al. Gonadal function in Hodgkin's disease: Long-term followup of chemotherapy. Br Med J 1982;285:1612–1613.
31. Whitehead E, Shalet SM, Blackledge G, et al. The effects of Hodgkin's disease and

TABLE 63-27. Guidelines for Genetic Counseling of Couples Seeking Pregnancy After Cancer Diagnosis

1. Inquire about family history of cancer.
2. Pregnancy is contraindicated during cancer treatment; birth control should be considered.
3. Discuss risk of infertility after cancer treatment, the option of sperm banking, and the possibility of healthy children if fertility is preserved.
4. Discuss theoretical concerns about mutational damage; data for humans are limited.
5. Pregnancy probably should be monitored with ultrasound; amniocentesis should be offered for usual reasons, not just because of cancer history.
6. Existing data on pregnancy outcome do not indicate an excessive risk of congenital or genetic problems above the 4% risk of any pregnancy resulting in a baby with a major malformation.

combination chemotherapy on gonadal function in the adult male. Cancer 1982;49: 418–422.

32. Kreuser ED, Xiros N, Hetzel WD, et al. Reproductive and endocrine gonadal capacity in patients treated with COPP chemotherapy for Hodgkin's disease. J Cancer Res Clin Oncol 1987;113:260–266.

33. Evenson DP, Arlin Z, Welt S, et al. Male reproductive capacity may recover following drug treatment with the L-10 protocol for acute lymphocytic leukemia. Cancer 1984;53: 30–36.

34. Shamberger RC, Sherins RJ, Rosenberg SA. The effects of post-operative adjuvant chemotherapy and radiotherapy on testicular function in men undergoing treatment for soft tissue sarcoma. Cancer 1981;47:2368–2374.

35. Kreuser ED, Hetzel WD, Heit W, et al. Reproductive and endocrine gonadal functions in adults following multidrug chemotherapy for acute lymphoblastic or undifferentiated leukemia. J Clin Oncol 1988;6:588–595.

36. Meistrich ML, Chawla SP, da Cunha MF, et al. Recovery of sperm production after chemotherapy for osteosarcoma. Cancer, 1989;63:2115–2123.

37. Vivani S, Santoro A, Ragri G, et al. Gonadal toxicity after combination chemotherapy for Hodgkin's disease: Comparative results of MOPP vs ABVD. Eur J Cancer Clin Oncol 1985;21:601–605.

38. Hagemeister FB, Cabanillas FF, Valesquez WS, et al. NOVP: A novel chemotherapeutic regimen with minimal toxicity for treatment of Hodgkin's disease. Semin Oncol 1990;17:34–40.

39. Einhorn LH, Donahue J. Cis-diammine-dichloroplatinum, vinblastine and bleomycin combination chemotherapy in disseminated testicular cancer. Ann Intern Med 1977;87: 293–298.

40. Berthelsen JG, Skakkebaek NE. Gonadal function in men with testicular cancer. Fertil Steril 1983;39:68–73.

41. Berthelsen JG. Andrological aspects of testicular cancer. Int J Androl 1984;7:451–483.

42. Nijman JM, Schraffordt-Koops H, Kremer J, et al. Gonadal function after surgery and chemotherapy in men with stage II and III nonseminomatous testicular tumors. J Clin Oncol 1987;5:651–656.

43. Carroll PR, Whitmore WF Jr, Herr HW, et al. Endocrine and exocrine profiles of men with testicular tumors before orchiectomy. J Urol 1987;137:420–423.

44. Fossa SD, Theodorsen L, Norman N, et al. Recovery of impaired pretreatment spermatogenesis in testicular cancer. Fertil Steril 1990;54:493–496.

45. Kedia KR, Markland C, Fraley EE. Sexual function following retroperitoneal lymphadenectomy. J Urol 1975;114:237–239.

46. Narayan P, Lange PH, Fraley EE. Ejaculation and fertility after extended retroperitoneal lymph node dissection for testicular cancer. J Urol 1982;127:685–688.

47. Lange PH, Narayan P, Fraley EE. Fertility issues following therapy for testicular cancer. Semin Urol II 1984;4:264–274.

48. Belohorsky B, Siracky J, Sandor L, et al. Comments on the development of amenorrhea caused by myleran in cases of chronic myelosis. Neoplasm 1960;4:397–402.

49. Miller JJ, Williams GF, Leissring JC. Multiple late complications of therapy with cyclophosphamide including ovarian destruction. Am J Med 1971;50:530–535.

50. Sobrinio LG, Levine RA, DeConti RC. Amenorrhea in patients with Hodgkin's disease treated with antineoplastic agents. Am J Obstet Gynecol 1971;109:135–139.

51. Louis J, Limarzi LR, Best WR. Treatment of chronic granulocytic leukemia with myleran. Arch Intern Med 1956;97:299–308.

52. Galton DAG, Till M, Wiltshaw E. Busulfan: Summary of clinical results. Ann NY Acad Sci 1958;68:967–973.

53. Fosdick WM, Parsons JL, Hill DF. Long term cyclophosphamide therapy in rheumatoid arthritis. Arthritis Rheum 1968;11:151–161.

54. Uldall PR, Kerr DNS, Tacchi D. Sterility and cyclophosphamide. Lancet 1972;1:693–694.

55. Warne GL, Fairley KF, Hobbs JB, et al. Cyclophosphamide-induced ovarian failure. N Engl J Med 1973;289:1159–1162.

56. Dnistrian AM, Schwartz MK, Fracchia AA, et al. Endocrine consequences of CMF adjuvant therapy in premenopausal and postmenopausal breast cancer patients. Cancer 1983;51:803–807.

57. Samaan NA, DeAsis DN, Buzdar AU, et al. Pituitary-ovarian function in breast cancer patients on adjuvant chemoimmunotherapy. Cancer 1978;41:2084–2087.

58. Koyama H, Wada T, Nishizawa Y, et al. Cyclophosphamide-induced ovarian failure and its therapeutic significance in patients with breast cancer. Cancer 1977;39:1403–1409.

59. Fisher B, Sherman B, Rockette H, et al. L-phenylalanine mustard in the management of premenopausal patients with primary breast cancer. Cancer 1979;44:847–857.

60. Shamberger RC, Rosenberg SA, Seipp CA, et al. Effects of high-dose methotrexate and vincristine on ovarian and testicular function in patients undergoing postoperative adjuvant treatment of osteosarcoma. Cancer Treat Rep 1981;65:739–746.

61. Morgenfeld MC, Goldberg V, Parisier H, et al. Ovarian lesions due to cytostatic agents during the treatment of Hodgkin's disease. Surg Gynecol Obstet 1972;134:826–828.

62. Sherins R, Winokur S, DeVita VT, et al. Surprisingly high risk of functional castration in women receiving chemotherapy for lymphoma. Clin Res 1975;23:343.

63. Chapman RM, Sutcliffe SB, Malpas JS. Cytotoxic-induced ovarian failure in women with Hodgkin's disease: I. Hormone function. JAMA 1979;242:1877–1881.

64. Horning SJ, Hoppe RT, Kaplan HS, et al. Female reproductive potential after treatment for Hodgkin's disease. N Engl J Med 1981;304:1378–1382.

65. Schilsky RL, Sherins RJ, Hubbard SM, et al. Long-term followup of ovarian function in women treated with MOPP chemotherapy for Hodgkin's disease. Am J Med 1981;71: 552–556.

66. Whitehead E, Shalet SM, Blackledge G, et al. The effect of combination chemotherapy on ovarian function in women treated for Hodgkin's disease. Cancer 1983;52:988–993.

67. Specht L, Hansen MM, Geisler C. Ovarian function in young women in long-term remission after treatment for Hodgkin's disease stage II or III. Scand J Haematol 1984;32:265–270.

68. Thomford PJ, Jelovsek FR, Mattison DR. Effect of oocyte number and rate of atresia on the age of menopause. Reprod Toxicol 1987;1:41–51.

68a. Faddy MJ, Gosden RG, Gougeon A, et al. Accelerated disappearance of ovarian follicles in mid-life: Implications for forecasting menopause. Hum Reprod 1992;7:1342–1346.

69. Arneil GC. Cyclophosphamide and the prepubertal testis. Lancet 1972;2:1259–1260.

70. Pennisi AJ, Grushkin CM, Lieberman E. Gonadal function in children with nephrosis treated with cyclophosphamide. Am J Dis Child 1975;129:315–318.

71. Kirkland RT, Bongiovanni AM, Cornfeld D, et al. Gonadotropin responses to luteinizing hormone releasing factor in boys treated with cyclophosphamide for nephrotic syndrome. J Pediatr 1976;89:941–944.

72. Rapola J, Koskimies O, Huttanen NP, et al. Cyclophosphamide and the pubertal testis. Lancet 1973;1:98–99.

73. Etteldorf JN, West CD, Pitcock JA, et al. Gonadal function, testicular histology and meiosis following cyclophosphamide therapy in patients with nephrotic syndrome. J Pediatr 1976;88:206–212.

74. Lentz RD, Bergstein J, Steffes MW, et al. Post-pubertal evaluation of gonadal function following cyclophosphamide therapy before and during puberty. J Pediatr 1977;91: 385–394.

75. Lendon M, Hann IM, Palmer MK, et al. Testicular histology after combination chemotherapy in childhood for acute lymphoblastic leukemia. Lancet 1978;2:439–441.

76. Ahmed SR, Shalet SM, Campbell RHA, et al. Primary gonadal damage following treatment of brain tumors in childhood. J Pediatr 1983;103:562–565.

77. Blatt J, Poplack DG, Sherins RJ. Testicular function in boys after chemotherapy for acute lymphoblastic leukemia. N Engl J Med 1981;304:1121–1124.

78. Sherins RJ, Olweny CLM, Ziegler JL. Gynecomastia and gonadal dysfunction in adolescent boys treated with combination chemotherapy for Hodgkin's disease. N Engl J Med 1978;299:12–16.

79. Whitehead E, Shalet SM, Morris-Jones PH, et al. Gonadal function after combination chemotherapy for Hodgkin's disease in childhood. Arch Dis Child 1981;47:287–291.

80. Himelstein-Braw R, Peters H, Faber M. Morphologic study of the ovaries of leukemic children. Br J Cancer 1978;38:82–87.

81. Nicosia SV, Matus-Ridley M, Meadows AT. Gonadal effects of cancer therapy in girls. Cancer 1985;55:2364–2372.

82. Chiu J, Drummond KN. Long-term followup of cyclophosphamide therapy in frequent relapsing minimal lesion nephrotic syndrome. J Pediatr 1974;84:825–830.

83. DeGroot GW, Faiman C, Winter JSD. Cyclophosphamide and the prepubertal gonad: A negative report. J Pediatr 1974;84:123–125.

84. Siris EJ, Leventhal BG, Vaitukaitis JL. Effects of childhood leukemia and chemotherapy on puberty and reproductive function in girls. N Engl J Med 1976;294:1143–1146.

85. Bateman JL, Bond VP. The effects of radiations of different LET on early response in the mammal. Ann NY Acad Sci 1964;114:32–47.

86. Sanderman RF. The effects of irradiation on male human fertility. Br J Radiol 1966;39: 901–907.

87. Paulsen CA. The study of radiation effects on the human testis: Including histologic, chromosomal and hormonal aspects. Final Progress Report, AEC Contract AT (45-I)-225, Task Agreement 6, RLO–2225–2, 1973.

88. Rowley MJ, Leach DR, Warner GA, et al. Effect of graded doses of ionizing radiation on the human testis. Radiat Res 1974;59:665–677.

89. Ash P. The influence of radiation on fertility in man. Br J Radiol 1980;53:271–278.

90. Hahn EW, Feingold SM, Simpson L, et al. Recovery from aspermia induced by low-dose radiation in seminoma patients. Cancer 1982;50:337–340.

91. Nader S, Schultz PN, Cundiff JH, et al. Endocrine profiles of patients with testicular tumors treated with radiotherapy. Int J Radiat Oncol Biol Phys 1983;9:1723–1726.

92. Tomic R, Bergman B, Damber JE, et al. Effects of external radiation therapy for cancer of the prostate on the serum concentrations of testosterone, follicle stimulating hormone, luteinizing hormone and prolactin. J Urol 1983;130:287–289.

93. Clifton DK, Bremner WJ. The effect of testicular x-irradiation on spermatogenesis in man: A comparison with the mouse. J Androl 1983;4:387–492.

94. Shapiro E, Kinsella TJ, Makoch RW, et al. Effects of fractionated irradiation on endocrine aspects of testicular function. J Clin Oncol 1985;3:1232–1239.

95. Meistrich ML, von Beek MEAB. Radiation sensitivity of the human testis. Adv Radiat Biol 1990;14:227–268.

96. Brauner R, Czernichow P, Cramer P, et al. Leydig cell function in children after direct testicular irradiation for acute lymphoblastic leukemia. N Engl J Med 1983;309: 25–28.

97. Leiper AD, Grant DB, Chessells JM. The effect of testicular irradiation on Leydig cell function in prepubertal boys with acute lymphoblastic leukemia. Arch Dis Child 1983;58:906–910.

98. Blatt J, Sherins RJ, Niebrugge D, et al. Leydig cell function in boys following testicular relapse of acute lymphoblastic leukemia. J Clin Oncol 1985;3:1227–1231.

99. Thomas PRM, Winstantly D, Peckham MJ, et al. Reproductive and endocrine function in patients with Hodgkin's disease: Effects of oophoropexy and irradiation. Br J Cancer 1976;33:226–231.

100. Horning SJ, Hoppe RT, Kaplan HS, et al. Female reproductive potential after treatment for Hodgkin's disease. N Engl J Med 1981;304:1377–1382.

101. Fisher B, Cheung AYC. Delayed effect of radiation therapy with or without chemotherapy on ovarian function in women with Hodgkin's disease. Acta Radiol Oncol 1984;23:43–48.

102. Redman JR, Bajorunas DR. Suppression of germ cell proliferation to prevent gonadal

toxicity associated with cancer treatment. In: Proceedings of the Workshop on Psychosexual and Reproductive Issues Affecting Patients with Cancer. Chicago: American Cancer Society Publ. No. 87-5M-4515, 1987:90–94.

103. Redman J, Davis R, Evenson D, et al. Prospective, randomized trial of testosterone cypionate to prevent sterility in men treated with chemotherapy for Hodgkin's disease: Preliminary results. In: Proceedings of the 14th International Cancer Congress, Budapest. Basel: S Karger, 1986:440.

104. Chapman RM, Sutcliffe SB. Protection of ovarian function by oral contraceptives in women receiving chemotherapy for Hodgkin's disease. Blood 1981;58:849–851.

105. Johnson DH, Linde R, Hainsworth JD, et al. Effect of luteinizing hormone-releasing hormone agonist given during combination chemotherapy on post-therapy fertility in male patients with lymphoma: Preliminary observations. Blood 1985;65:832–836.

106. Glode LM, Robinson J, Gould SF, et al. Protection of spermatogenesis during chemotherapy. Drugs Exp Clin Res 1982;8:367–378.

107. Lewis RN, Dowling KJ, Schally AV. D-Tryptophan-6 analog of luteinizing hormone-releasing hormone as a protective agent against testicular damage caused by cyclophosphamide in baboons. Proc Natl Acad Sci USA 1985;82:2975–2979.

108. Delic JI, Bush C, Peckham MJ. Protection from procarbazine-included damage of spermatogenesis in the rat by androgen. Cancer Res 1986;46:1909–1914.

109. da Cunha MF, Meistrich ML, Nader S. Absence of testicular protection by a gonadotropin-releasing hormone analogue against cyclophosphamide induced testicular cytotoxicity in the mouse. Cancer Res 1987;47:1093–1097.

110. Karashima T, Zalatnai A, Schally AV. Protective effects of analogs of luteinizing hormone releasing hormone agonist chemotherapy induced testicular damage in rats. Proc Natl Acad Sci USA 1988;85:2329–2333.

111. Jegou B, Velez de la Calle JF, Bauche F. Protective effect of medroxyprogesterone acetate plus testosterone against radiation-induced damage to the reproductive function of male rats and their offspring. Proc Natl Acad Sci USA 1991;88:8710–8714.

112. Fraas BA, Kinsella TJ, Harrington FS, et al. Peripheral dose to the testis: The design and use of a practical and effective gonadal shield. Int J Radiat Oncol Biol Phys 1985;11:609–615.

113. Kinsella TJ, Fraas BA, Glatstein E. Late effects of radiation therapy in the treatment of Hodgkin's disease. Cancer Treat Rep 1982;66:991–1001.

114. Pedrick TJ, Hoppe RT. Recovery of spermatogenesis following pelvic irradiation for Hodgkin's disease. Int J Radiat Oncol Biol Phys 1986;12:117–121.

115. Ray GR, Trueblood HW, Enright LP, et al. Oophoropexy: A means of preserving ovarian function following pelvic megavoltage radiotherapy for Hodgkin's disease. Radiology 1970;96:175–180.

116. Sherman JK. Synopsis of the use of frozen human semen since 1964: State-of-the-art of human semen banking. Fertil Steril 1973;24:397–412.

117. Ansbacher R. Artificial insemination with frozen spermatozoa. Fertil Steril 1978;29:375–379.

118. Curie-Cohen M, Luttrell L, Shapiro J. Current practice of artificial insemination by donor in the United States. N Engl J Med 1979;300:585–590.

119. Bracken RB, Smith KD. Is semen cryopreservation helpful in testicular cancer? Urology 1980;15:581–583.

120. Sanger WG, Armitage JO, Schmidt MA. Feasibility of semen cryopreservation in patients with malignant disease. JAMA 1980;244:789–790.

121. Scammell GD, Stedronske J, Edmonds DK, et al. Cryopreservation of semen in men with testicular tumor or Hodgkin's disease: Results of artificial insemination of their partners. Lancet 1985;2:31–32.

122. Rhodes EA, Hoffman DJ, Kaempfer SH. Ten years of experience with semen cryopreservation by cancer patients: Follow-up and clinical considerations. Fertil Steril 1985;44:512–516.

123. Reed E, Sanger WG, Armitage JO. Results of semen cryopresentation in young men with testicular carcinoma and lymphoma. J Clin Oncol 1986;4:537–539.

124. Thacil JV, Jewett MAS, Rider WD. The effects of cancer and cancer therapy on male fertility. J Urol 1981;126:141–145.

125. Chapman RM, Sutcliffe SB, Malpas JS. Male gonadal dysfunction in Hodgkin's disease: A prospective study. JAMA 1981;245:1323–1328.

126. Chlebowski RT, Heber D. Hypogonadism in male patients with metastatic cancer prior to chemotherapy. Cancer Res 1982;42:2495–2498.

127. Vigersky RA, Chapman RM, Berenberg J, et al. Testicular dysfunction in untreated Hodgkin's disease. Am J Med 1982;73:482–486.

128. Marmor D, Elefant E, Dauchez C, et al. Semen analysis in Hodgkin's disease before onset of treatment. Cancer 1986;57:1986–1987.

129. Cross NL, Hanks SE. Effects of cryopreservation on human sperm acrosomes. Hum Reprod 1991;6:1279–1283.

130. Burris AS, Clark RV, Vantman DJ, et al. A low sperm concentration does not preclude fertility in men with isolated hypogonadotropic hypogonadism after gonadotropin therapy. Fertil Steril 1988;50:343–347.

131. Free D, Stutts L, Merryman D, et al. A comparison of donor semen processing techniques for use in intrauterine inseminations and their corresponding pregnancy rates. Abstract #35. Orlando, FL: American Fertility Society, November 1991.

132. Schulman JD, Dorfmann A, Jones S, et al. Outpatient in vitro fertilization using transvaginal oocyte retrieval. N Engl J Med 1985;312:1639.

133. Fugger EF, Bustillo M, Katz LP. Embryonic development and pregnancy from fresh and cryopreserved sibling pronucleate human zygotes. Fertil Steril 1988;50:273–278.

134. Fugger EF, Bustillo M, Dorfmann AD, et al. Human preimplantation embryo cryopreservation: Selected aspects. Hum Reprod 1991;6:131–135.

135. Bustillo, M, Buster JE, Cohen SW, et al. Nonsurgical ovum transfer as a treatment in infertile women: Preliminary experience. JAMA 1984;251:1171–1173.

136. Buster JE, Bustillo M, Rodi IA, et al. Biology and morphology of donated human ova recovered by nonsurgical uterine lavage. Am J Obstet Gynecol 1985;153:211–217.

137. Walsh PC, Lepor H, Eggleson JC. Radical prostatectomy with preservation of sexual function: Anatomical and pathological considerations. Prostate 1983;4:473–485.

138. Quinlan DM, Epstein JI, Carter BS, et al. Sexual function following radical prostatectomy: Influence of preservation of neurovascular bundles. J Urol 1991;145:998–1002.

139. Walsh PC, Mostwin JL. Radical prostatectomy and cystoprostatectomy with preservation of potency: Results using a new nerve sparing technique. Br J Urol 1984;56:694–697.

140. Garnick MB, Richie JP. Toward more rational management for stage I testis cancer: Watch out for "watch and wait." J Clin Oncol 1986;4:1021–1023.

141. Pizzocaro G, Salvioni R, Zononi F. Unilateral lymphadenectomy in intraoperative stage I nonseminomatous germinal testis cancer. J Urol 1985;134:485–489.

142. Jewett MAS, Young-Soo PK, Goldberg SD, et al. Retroperitoneal lymphadenectomy for testis tumor with nerve sparing for ejaculation. J Urol 1988;13:1220–1226.

143. Thomas RJS, McLeisch G. McDonald IA. Electroejaculation of the paraplegic male followed by pregnancy. Med J Aust 1975;2:798.

144. Bennett CJ, Ayers JWT, Randolph JF, et al. Electroejaculation of paraplegic males followed by pregnancies. Fertil Steril 1987;48:1070–1072.

145. Bennett CJ, Seager SWJ, McGuire EJ. Electroejaculation for recovery of semen after retroperitoneal lymph node dissection. J Urol 1987;137:513.

146. Schull WJ. Reproductive problems: Fertility, teratogenesis and mutagenesis. Arch Envir Health 1984;39:207–212.

147. US Congress Office of Technology Assessment. Technologies for detecting heritable mutations in human beings. Washington, DC: US Government Printing Office, 1986.

148. Schull WJ, Otake M, Neel JV. Genetic effects of atomic bombs: A reappraisal. Science 1981;213:1220–1227.

149. Neel JV. Genetic effects of atomic bombs. Science 1981;213:1205.

150. Neel JV, Lewis SE. The comparative radiation genetics of humans and mice. Annu Rev Genet 1990;24:327–62.

151. Li FP, Jaffe H. Progeny of childhood-cancer survivors. Lancet 1974;2:707–709.

152. Ross GT. Congenital anomalies among children born of mothers receiving chemotherapy for gestational trophoblastic neoplasms. Cancer 1976;37:1043–1047.

153. Holmes GE, Holmes FF. Pregnancy outcome of patients treated for Hodgkin's disease: A controlled study. Cancer 1978;41:1317–1322.

154. Li FP, Fine W, Jaffe H, et al. Offspring of patients treated for cancer in childhood. J Natl Cancer Inst 1979;62:1193–1197.

155. Blatt J, Mulvihill JJ, Ziegler JL, et al. Pregnancy outcome following cancer chemotherapy. Am J Med 1980;69:828–832.

156. Horning SJ, Hippe RT, Kaplan HS, et al. Female reproductive potential after treatment for Hodgkin's disease. N Engl J Med 1981;304:1377–1382.

157. Marradi P, Schaison F, Alby N, et al. Les enfants nes de parents leucemiques. Nouv Rev Fr Hematol 1982;24:75–80.

158. Bundey S, Evans K. Survivors of neuroblastoma and ganglioneuroma and their families. J Med Genet 1982;19:16–21.

159. Andrieu JM, Ochoa-Molina ME. Menstrual cycle, pregnancies and offspring before and after MOPP therapy for Hodgkin's disease. Cancer 1983;52:435–438.

160. Rustin GJS, Booth M, Dent J, et al. Pregnancy after cytotoxic chemotherapy for gestational trophoblastic tumors. Br Med J 1984;288:103–106.

161. Goldstein DP, Berkowitz RS, Bernstein MR. Reproductive performance after molar pregnancy and gestational trophoblastic tumors. Clin Obstet Gynecol 1984;27:221–227.

162. Mulvihill JJ, Byrne J. Offspring of long-time survivors of childhood cancer. Clin Oncol 1985;4:333–343.

163. Mulvihill JJ, McKeen EA, Rosner F, et al. Pregnancy outcome in cancer patients: Experience in a large cooperative group. Cancer 1987;60:1143–1150.

164. Li FP, Gimbrere K, Gelber RD, et al. Outcome of pregnancy in survivors of Wilms' tumor. JAMA 1987;257:216–219.

165. Byrne J, Mulvihill JJ, Myers MH, et al. Effects of treatment on fertility in long-term survivors of childhood and adolescent cancer. N Engl J Med 1987;317:1315–1321.

166. Mulvihill JJ, Myers MH, Connelly RR, et al. Cancer in offspring of long-term survivors of childhood and adolescent cancer. Lancet 1987;2:813–817.

167. Mulvihill JJ, Byrne J, Steinhorn SA, et al. Genetic disease in offspring of survivors of cancer in the young. Am J Hum Genet 1986;39:A72.

168. Byrne J, Mulvihill JJ, Myers MH, et al. Reproductive problems and birth defects in survivors of Wilms' tumor and their relatives. Med Pediatr Oncol 1980;16:233–240.

169. Mulvihill JJ, Byrne J. Genetic counseling for the cancer survivor: Germ cell effects of cancer therapy. In: Proceedings of the Workshop on Psychosexual and Reproductive Issues Affecting Patients with Cancer. American Cancer Society Publ. No. #87-5M-4515, 1987:100–104.

170. Green DM, Zevon MA, Lowrie G, et al. Congenital anomalies in children of patients who received chemotherapy for cancer in childhood and adolescence. N Engl J Med 1991;325:141–146.

171. American Cancer Society. Proceedings of the Workshop on Psychosexual and Reproductive Issues Affecting Patients with cancer. American Cancer Society Publ. No. 87-5M-4515, 1987.

172. Schover LR, von Eschenbach AC. Sexual and marital relationships after treatment for nonseminomatous testicular cancer. Urology 1985;25:251–255.

173. Andersen BL. Sexual functioning morbidity among cancer survivors: Current status and future research directions. Cancer 1985;55:1835–1842.

174. Schover LR, Gonzales M, von Eschenbach AC. Sexual and marital relationships after radiotherapy for seminoma. Urology 1986;27:117–123.

SECTION **9**   MARGARET A. TUCKER

Secondary Cancers

As the success of modern cancer therapy has increased the duration of survival and curability of many patients, recognition of long-term complications of therapy also has increased. The successful treatment of first cancers involves radiation therapy and multiagent chemotherapy, each of which is used either as primary therapy or as an adjunct to therapy of the primary tumor, which often includes surgery. The increased use of adjuvant chemotherapy has placed a large number of patients at potential risk for developing a treatment-related malignancy.

In the past, discussion of secondary malignancies emphasized the treatments administered and the potential risk for appearance of a second tumor in relation to a specific agent. Whereas the initial reports considered single cases or small series of patients, there are now large populations of patients, such as those with Hodgkin's disease, pediatric cancers, or breast cancer, from which more accurate assessments of risks can be determined. Proper epidemiologic and statistical methods must be employed to avoid overestimating or underestimating the risks, especially in older populations in whom cancer is a more common occurrence.

More recently, it has become apparent that predisposing factors beyond the treatment itself may have a major impact on the risk for developing a second tumor. Alterations in the retinoblastoma locus, germline mutations in p53, and congenital or acquired immunodeficiency states are examples of some of the host factors that may increase the risk of developing a second tumor.

This chapter covers the important principles related to all these areas, emphasizing data available within the last few years. Some topics, such as the relation between the specific therapeutic agents and secondary cancers, were well reviewed by Li in a previous edition of this book[1] and by others.[2,3] A discussion of late effects and secondary malignancies is possible only if the primary treatment is successful. As more is learned about long-term toxicities, treatments can be altered to decrease these complications without compromising the success of treatments.

METHODS OF STUDYING SECONDARY MALIGNANCIES

Several methods have been used to study secondary cancers. Reports of individual cases or series have been important in establishing the occurrence of secondary cancers but have been of limited use in quantifying risks. The more useful epidemiologic methods for studying secondary cancer risk have included both cohort and case-control studies. In cohort studies, specific groups of patients are identified and observed for a number of years to determine the incidence of specific malignancies. Study groups providing large numbers of patients who may constitute a cohort include population-based tumor registries, multicenter clinical trials, and hospital-based patient groups. The groups to be followed may be defined by a first cancer of interest, such as ovarian cancer or Hodgkin's disease, or by an exposure of interest, such as single-agent cyclophosphamide or interstitial radiation therapy. The person-years of observation are accrued from the start of observation to the date of last follow-up, death, or diagnosis of the second tumor, whichever occurs first.[4] Tumor incidence rates from the general population specific for age, sex, race, and calendar year are multiplied by the accumulated person-years to derive the number of expected tumors. The observed number is then divided by the expected number to estimate the relative risk of a second tumor. When the 95% confidence interval does not include 1.0, the excess risk is statistically significant at the $p < 0.05$ level. This method yields a risk in the cohort that is compared with the general population.

The use of population-based tumor registries has some advantages, including relatively large numbers of patients, which allows the detection of even small risks (*e.g.*, the international cervical cancer study mentioned later[5]). In addition, the actual (observed) and the expected numbers of cancer cases come from the same reference population. Population-based registries have some disadvantages, however, including differential reporting of cancers to the registries by physicians and hospitals, variable follow-up, different autopsy rates, limited treatment data, and different diagnostic criteria for secondary cancers. Many registries record only initial therapy, and patients may be incompletely classified if they receive additional treatment. Finally, comparisons of rates of secondary cancers in cancer patients with rates in the general population are criticized because some types of cancer may have an intrinsically increased risk for specific secondary cancers, such as the retinoblastoma-osteosarcoma association.[6–8] Despite these limitations, these studies are informative and often produce the best data available. They tend, however, to give minimal estimates of risk because of the relatively incomplete follow-up. This source of error is less in the population-based tumor registries that are linked to national health care records.

Clinical trials are valuable sources of information on risks for secondary cancers. In clinical studies, initial evaluation of the patients and follow-up in the comparison arms of the trials are equivalent and usually as complete as possible. Patients within each arm have received comparable treatment, and the risks for secondary tumors may be directly compared between treatment arms. This controls for any intrinsic risk for a secondary cancer associated with the first cancer and also allows the comparison of risks from specific drug therapies or radiation exposure. Complete treatment information, including that administered for relapse, is usually available, so the risk of misclassification of exposure is minimized. The major disadvantage of most of the clinical trials is the relatively small number of study subjects involved. Examples of this type of analysis are the National Surgical Adjuvant Breast Project study of risks of adjuvant chemotherapy for breast cancers,[9] the study of ovarian cancer that combined data from several clinical trials,[10] and the Stanford and Milan Hodgkin's disease studies.[11,12]

Another type of analysis that is useful in the cohort studies is the actuarial or life-table risk.[13] This analysis gives the cumulative risk for a particular event, such as leukemia, expressed in a percentage at a particular time period—for example, 6.2% at 10 years. To calculate this life-table probability, person-years of follow-up, similar to those required for the estimation of relative risk compared with the general population, are necessary. The actuarial risk of a secondary cancer occurring can be compared between treatment arms using methods similar to those employed for the comparison of survival or disease-free survival (Fig. 63–11).[14] The limitation of this method is that it does not account for the baseline tumor rates in the general population. An example is the comparison of acute leukemia by age category in the Stanford population of Hodgkin's disease patients.[15] Within each chemotherapy category, the risk of leukemia is significantly higher among people treated after age 50 years than in those treated at a younger age. When the relative risks are examined, which take into account the higher risk for acute leukemia in the general population over age 50 years, the relative risk for all age groups is essentially the same.[11]

The other major approach is the case-control study, in which exposure to chemotherapy or radiation therapy is compared between patients who develop secondary cancers (cases) and those who do not (controls). The selection of appropriate controls is critical; they should be representative of the entire group from which both the cases and controls are derived. Bias in the selection of the control group can lead to spurious associations or can obscure a true association. Ideally, all therapy given to every person treated in the group from which the cases and controls were selected would be reviewed, and the cases compared with the rest of the subjects. In practice, this is not usually feasible since often hundreds or thousands of patients are involved and few develop secondary cancers. In this circumstance, it is much more cost-effective to collect the information on the cases and controls, the latter being representative of the patients who do not develop secondary cancers. The conclusions from such a study are only as valid as the control group selected.

INDIVIDUAL TREATMENT MODALITIES

RADIATION THERAPY

The carcinogenic effects of ionizing irradiation have been quantified in several groups, including occupational cohorts, people exposed to residential radon, atomic bomb survivors,

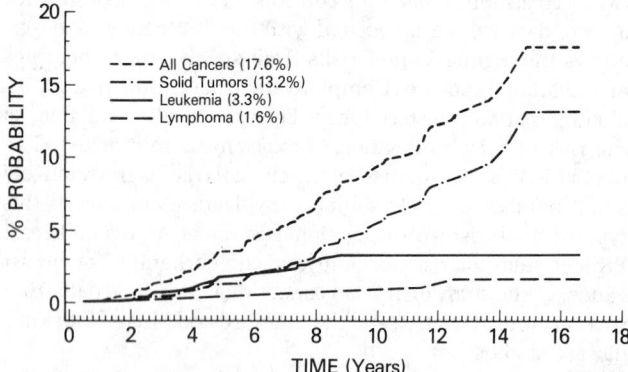

FIGURE 63–11. Actuarial risk of development of secondary malignancy after Hodgkin's disease for 1507 patients treated at Stanford University Medical Center. (Tucker MA, Coleman CN, Cox RS, et al. Risk of second malignancies following Hodgkin's disease after 15 years. N Engl J Med 1988;318:76–81)

and patients who undergo diagnostic and therapeutic procedures. This summary focuses on recent results in atomic bomb survivors and in patients treated with therapeutic irradiation. Many tumor types have been associated, at least in case reports, with irradiation to the tissue in which the malignancy developed; that is, there is no one radiation-induced tumor. With the exception of exposure associated with therapeutic irradiation, the doses have often been low. Extrapolation of radiation effects from low- to high-radiation-dose ranges cannot be done with certainty.[16] In the lower-dose ranges, the risk of a cancer developing increases with dose. Much of the recent effort in radiation epidemiology has focused on the shape (linear versus nonlinear) of the dose-response curves for different tumors. It is thought, however, that at the higher-dose ranges used therapeutically, the risk per centigray decreases, a phenomenon that has been attributed to cell killing at the higher doses.[16] Therapeutic irradiation doses usually fall within a relatively small range, making it difficult to establish a dose-response curve between irradiation doses and risk of a secondary cancer. Therefore, for a patient treated for cancer, the risk per centigray for the development of a secondary tumor cannot necessarily be determined with certainty.[2]

The largest population studies on the carcinogenicity of ionizing irradiation come from survivors of atomic bomb explosions. These people received one whole-body dose that ranged from 0 to 5 Gy. The radiation-related cancers included leukemia, multiple myeloma, and cancers of the lung, female breast, stomach, colon, esophagus, and urinary tract.[17] The relative risk for developing leukemia decreased with time (10.7% per year) after peaking at 5 to 10 years. Although the relative risk for the development of all cancers except leukemia increased with time, the rate of increase was small (4.9% per year).

Recent studies have sought to refine the risk estimates associated with irradiation of these cancers and to evaluate interactions with other known risk factors.[18] Previous evaluations of the cohorts have shown that the risk for breast cancer was greatest in those irradiated as children or adolescents and was lowest in those irradiated when over age 40 years. There was a clear dose response, with risk rising with increased radiation dose to the breast tissue. Parallel analyses of the Life Span Study (LSS) cohort and medically irradiated women in the United States demonstrated that for similar radiation dose levels, ages at exposure, and length of follow-up, similar excess rates of breast cancer were observed. This is remarkable since the age-specific rates of breast cancer are threefold to fivefold higher in the United States than in Japan. To evaluate the potential interaction of radiation with other breast cancer risk factors, Land and colleagues conducted a case-control study.[19,20] Age at first full-term pregnancy (relative risk, 1.08; 95% confidence interval, 1.03–1.13), number of live births (relative risk, 0.81; 95% confidence interval, 0.73–0.90), and cumulative months of lactation (relative risk, 0.98; 95% confidence interval, 0.97–0.99) were strongly associated with both premenopausal and postmenopausal breast cancer risk in the LSS women. Treatment of dysmenorrhea was a risk factor for postmenopausal breast cancer (relative risk, 3.01; $p = 0.07$). The relation between radiation and these risk factors is not simple. The increased risks associated with age at first pregnancy and treatment of dysmenorrhea were even higher in the women who received higher radiation doses, while the protective effects of number of children and cumulative months of lactation were more pronounced in the women who received higher doses. The interaction of radiation with the reproductive factors was not additive but appeared to be more than multiplicative. There was no clear evidence for an additive or multiplicative model for the treatment of dysmenorrhea. Therefore, even in the presence of radiation, the risk may be modulated by other risk factors for a specific tumor.

The risk of lung cancer also rises with increasing irradiation dose to the lungs. In a recent comparison of the histology of lung cancer in the LSS cohort with the lung cancers in uranium miners, 62% of the miners had small cell lung cancer, compared with 13% of the LSS cohort.[21] The percentages of squamous cell cancer were similar (29% in the miners versus 34% in the LSS population) and were related to smoking, but the percentage of adenocarcinomas was different (9% in the miners versus 43% of the LSS population). When the radiation dose was evaluated, there was a tendency for the proportion of small cell lung cancer to increase with radiation dose, while the proportion of adenocarcinomas decreased with increasing dose. The difference in the radiation dose seemed sufficient to explain the differences in the cell types of the lung cancer seen in the two groups.

No one specific type of cancer is seen after therapeutic irradiation. The secondary cancers can occur after any initial cancer when the survival is long enough. Radiation-induced leukemias frequently occur at about 5 years. Solid cancers typically occur more than 10 years after treatment but may occur earlier in particularly susceptible hosts.[9–12] Excess leukemia and cancers of the lung, breast, thyroid, stomach, bone, and connective tissues have been shown after radiation therapy for diverse tumors as described later. When it was evaluated, the risk of secondary solid cancers rose with increasing radiation dose to the site and with increasing time since treatment at least as long as 20 years. Even in the studies in which actual doses to the site were not estimated, the risk was usually highest in the field, lower at the border of the field, and much lower farther away. The excess risk is seen after both external-beam irradiation and interstitial radiation therapy.

The risk for cancer developing after diagnostic irradiation is much lower predominantly because the doses are so much lower. After diagnostic iodine-131 radiation therapy, no increased risk of cancer overall was found, but small increases were noted for endocrine tumors other than thyroid tumors, lymphomas, and leukemias.[22] An increased risk for breast cancer was found after repeated fluoroscopies in tuberculosis patients, particularly those exposed as adolescents[23]; these patients usually received a few gray. In contrast, Linos and associates[24] did not find that the risk of developing leukemia increased after radiation doses of 0 to 3 Gy when these amounts were delivered over long periods of time as part of routine medical care. Evans and colleagues[25] concluded that only about 1% of all cases of leukemia and less than 1% of all cases of breast cancer result from diagnostic radiation therapy.

CHEMOTHERAPY

The predominant secondary cancer associated with chemotherapy is acute nonlymphocytic leukemia (ANLL). Only selected publications of the large number of studies noting this association are mentioned here. Most ANLLs have occurred after treatment with alkylating agents or nitrosoureas for diseases that have prolonged survival. The findings are similar for Hodgkin's disease, pediatric cancers, ovarian cancer, multiple myeloma, polycythemia vera, gastrointestinal cancers, small cell lung cancer, and breast cancer.[9–12,26–33] The risk for leukemia rises with increasing cumulative dose of alkylating agents and nitrosoureas. The relative leukemogenicity of various drugs has not been fully established, but the risk appears to be different with different drugs. Greene and colleagues[10] found that single-agent cyclophosphamide was significantly less leukemogenic than melphalan in women treated for ovarian cancer. All the women who developed leukemia received high cumulative doses of cyclophosphamide or melphalan. This finding was confirmed and extended by Kaldor and colleagues.[34] In a study of 99,113 survivors of ovarian cancer, they found that the risk of leukemia was highest after chlorambucil or melphalan, followed by thiotepa, then cyclophosphamide and Treosulfan. For each drug evaluated, there was clear evidence of increased risk at higher doses. On the basis of small numbers, an elevated risk of leukemia was found after treatment with cisplatin and doxorubicin. In this study, the risk of developing leukemia after combined modality therapy with both radiation therapy and chemotherapy was no higher than the risk after chemotherapy alone.

It has been difficult to disentangle the effects of cumulative dose and duration of treatment, but when these attempts were made, total dose appeared to be more important than duration of treatment.[33–35] The time between cessation of drug treatment and the development of leukemia has also been explored; the risk for leukemia appears to be highest within a few years of completing treatment.[10,33,36] This, too, is difficult to evaluate since treatment of alkylating agents is stopped when people become pancytopenic, which may be a symptom of preleukemia. The observation needs to be evaluated further. The leukemias that occur after alkylating agent or nitrosourea chemotherapy have distinctive characteristics. The cell types are acute myeloblastic, including FAB M6, erythroleukemia. The leukemias typically occur between 2 and 10 years after therapy, with the peak time interval around 5 years. There is usually an antecedent period of pancytopenia, and the leukemia may manifest as part of the spectrum of myelodysplastic syndromes.[37] The leukemias are notoriously refractory to treatment, although there have been some reports of short-term success.[38,39] Clonal alterations in chromosomes 5 and 7 (translocations or deletions) are frequent (occurring in up to about 90% of patients).[40] This has led to the speculation that these chromosomes contain critical genes that are involved in the pathogenesis of the alkylating-agent-induced leukemias. The variance in host susceptibility to develop these leukemias has not been evaluated well but may relate to interindividual variation in drug metabolism.

A few reports were made of ANLL that followed combination chemotherapy including teniposide or etoposide.[41,42] The leukemias differ from those that follow alkylating agents in that they occur sooner (starting at around 15 months after treatment), there is no period of pancytopenia, the leukemias are frequently M4 or M5, and the most frequent chromosomal abnormalities involve chromosome 11q23.[43,44] The specific chromosomal abnormality has been used as corroboration of the importance of the epipodophyllotoxins in the leukemia risk since some in vitro studies indicated that DNA damage induced by these drugs is not random but is particularly frequent in the chromosome 11q regions. Among reported epipodophyllotoxin-related leukemias, however, only 40% to 80% have an abnormality on chromosome 11q.[43] Also, it is not clear that the translocations that have been associated with leukemia occurring after epipodophyllotoxins are due to that exposure since translocations involving chromosome 11q23— specifically, t(4;11)(q21;q23)—are common in acute lymphocytic leukemia (ALL) (the most frequent initial cancer) and since the translocation t(9;11)(p21;q23) is relatively specific for M5 leukemia of any cause. Several potential candidate genes in that region have been identified, including the protooncogene *ETS*1, *THY*1 surface antigen, *CD*3 surface antigen of T lymphocytes, *NCAM*, and a gene for ataxia-telangiectasia.[43]

The higher risks (cumulative risk of 12%) have been reported by Pui and associates[41] in children receiving relatively high doses of teniposide and other drugs, with or without radiation therapy, for ALL. Several of the children developed ANLL during active treatment of ALL. The data are difficult to evaluate because the children also received multiple other drugs, including cyclophosphamide, or radiation therapy. Radiation in much lower doses to equivalent areas in children treated for tinea capitis has caused an excess of leukemia. Potential interactions with radiation therapy and known or suspected leukemogenic drugs were not evaluated. Another unusual aspect of the relation was that the highest risk of leukemia occurred in the arm of the trial in which only 60% of the patients received 90% of the drugs. In the two other arms, with more patients with identical drugs (except for schedule), 84% of the patients received 90% of the drugs, and the risk of subsequent leukemia was much lower. The authors interpret these data as evidence that schedule is more important than dose.[41]

Others reported much lower cumulative risks (about 4% at 5 years) after treatment with etoposide in combination with other drugs.[42] Again, the potential interaction with alkylating or intercalating agents has not been adequately evaluated. Despite the limitations of these data, there is a suggestion that some of the chemotherapy combinations that include epipodophyllotoxins may confer some risk of leukemia. This is an important issue to resolve as soon as possible because of the widespread use of epipodophyllotoxins in curable diseases. Studies are underway to try to quantify the leukemia risk and to start to evaluate interactions with other drugs or radiation therapy.

Few solid tumors have been linked to treatment with chemotherapy. Bladder cancer has been associated with treatment with cyclophosphamide.[45–47] After daily oral cyclophosphamide at 100 mg/m² for 2 to 4 years, the cumulative risk of bladder cancer was 3.5% at 8 years and 10.7% at 12 years. The relative risk of developing bladder cancer was 6.8 (95% confidence interval, 3.2–14.3).[45] Bone sarcomas have also followed treatment with alkylating agents (discussed later).[48] In general, the risk for solid tumors after chemotherapy alone has been difficult to evaluate because the solid tumors occur later than the leukemias and because not enough people survive long enough after treatment by chemotherapy alone to detect substantial risks for solid tumors.

SECONDARY TUMORS IN PEDIATRIC, HODGKIN'S DISEASE, AND BREAST CANCER POPULATIONS

The two patient populations from which most of the secondary malignancy data have been derived are patients treated for pediatric malignancies and those treated for Hodgkin's disease. The spectrum of pediatric malignancies includes a number of diseases that have been correlated with specific genetic abnormalities, such as retinoblastoma,[8,49,50] Wilms' tumor,[51,52] and some soft tissue sarcomas.[53] The Hodgkin's disease populations treated in the modern era have received radiation therapy or chemotherapy or both; this is similar in the major series. Specific aspects of the treatment regimens can be studied for their carcinogenicity. Immunity, however, often is impaired in Hodgkin's disease patients, even long after treatment has been completed.[3] Despite the potential confounding factors, the excellent cure rates among these relatively young patients, coupled with the long-term follow-up of relatively large patient populations, have provided important data on the risk of developing secondary neoplasms. With the widespread use of adjuvant chemotherapy and primary radiation therapy for breast cancer, a third large patient population is available for study of treatment-related malignancy.

PEDIATRIC MALIGNANCIES

After treatment of childhood malignancies, there is a distinctive pattern of secondary cancers that has been well described.[54] The most common secondary cancer is bone sarcomas, followed by soft tissue sarcomas, leukemias, and cancers of the brain, thyroid, and breast. The most frequent initial cancer is retinoblastoma, followed by Hodgkin's disease, soft tissue sarcomas, Wilms' tumor, and brain cancers. This is not the usual distribution of childhood cancers; it reflects both the genetic predisposition to develop multiple tumors of heritable retinoblastoma and soft tissue sarcoma associated with Li-Fraumeni syndrome, the treatment associated with the specific cancers, and perhaps the immune dysfunction associated with Hodgkin's disease. Among 9170 patients treated for childhood cancers by members of the Late Effects Study Group (LESG) who survived 2 or more years, the risk of a secondary bone sarcoma was 133-fold increased (95% confidence interval, 98–176).[48] The relative risks by initial diagnosis were 999 for retinoblastoma, 649 for Ewing's sarcoma, 297 for rhabdomyosarcoma, 127 for Wilms' tumor, and 106 for Hodgkin's disease. The cumulative probability of developing secondary bone sarcoma at 20 years was 2.8% for the whole cohort and 14.1% for patients with retinoblastoma.[48]

To evaluate the relation between radiation dose and the risk of bone sarcoma, individual radiation dosimetry at the site of the development of the bone sarcoma was done for each case and its matched controls. The dosimetry accounted for the absorption characteristics of bone for different types of radiation. When the doses in cases and controls were compared, the risk for bone sarcoma rose dramatically to a 38-fold increase after radiation doses up to 60 Gy.[48] There was concern that the effect was due to an extremely high risk in the retinoblastoma patients, so the retinoblastoma patients were separated from all other patients, and the doses were compared. In each category of dose up to 40 Gy or more, the risks were equivalent in the retinoblastoma patients and all other patients. Although the cumulative risks for developing bone sarcoma are much higher after retinoblastoma than after other cancers, the relative risks, dose for dose, are similar. This is explained by the case-control matching on bilaterality of the retinoblastomas, which controlled for the genetic factors. Patients with heritable retinoblastomas have a higher baseline risk for secondary bone sarcoma, but their response to radiation is similar to patients with other childhood cancers.

In addition to the radiation dose, the exposure to chemotherapy was also evaluated (Table 63–28). There was an independent effect of exposure to alkylating agents in the risk for bone cancer (relative risk, 4.7; 95% confidence interval, 1.0–22).[48] The risk rose with increasing total dose of alkylating agents, suggesting a dose response. The effect of alkylating agents was much smaller than that of the radiation. In the presence of radiation to the site of the bone sarcoma, the alkylating agents added little to the risk. Other drugs did not appear to be associated with the risk of developing bone sarcoma. Although an increased risk for bone sarcoma associated with alkylating agents had not been previously reported, an increased risk for bone sarcoma after cyclophosphamide had been suggested after Ewing's sarcoma by Strong and colleagues[55] and after retinoblastoma by Draper and colleagues.[6] The findings of this study were consistent with previous observations.

Although the smaller number of secondary soft tissue sarcomas in the LESG cohort prohibited as extensive analyses as the bone sarcomas, the patterns of risk were similar. The risk for soft tissue sarcoma also increased with radiation dose to the site of the sarcoma, and there was a suggestion of a small effect of alkylating agent chemotherapy.[55a]

The risk for leukemia was also quantified in this cohort of 9170 survivors of pediatric cancer. Overall, the relative risk of developing leukemia was increased 14-fold (95% confidence interval, 9–22) and was highest (89-fold) after treatment of Hodgkin's disease.[33] The risk was associated with treatment with alkylating-agent chemotherapy, and it increased with the total dose of alkylating agents. Radiation dosimetry was done to estimate the radiation dose to the active bone marrow. In this study, no effect of radiation dose to the bone marrow was found, but the comparison group for the radiation-exposed cases and controls included patients who had received alkylating agents. There was no additional effect of the radiation that could be detected. This group did not include patients who had been treated with epipodophyllotoxins.

Thyroid cancer risk after treatment of childhood cancer is increased 53-fold compared with general population rates.[56] The risk is highest after treatment of neuroblastoma (relative risk, 350); Wilms' tumor (relative risk, 132); non-Hodgkin's lymphoma (relative risk, 81); and Hodgkin's disease (relative risk, 67). Although there have been many quantifications of risk for thyroid cancer after radiation, most of the studies have evaluated much lower doses. This study evaluated therapeutic range radiation doses. Radiation dosimetry was done for the cases and controls to calculate the total dose to the thyroid. Doses to the thyroid of 2 Gy or more were associated with a 13-fold increased risk of thyroid cancer (95% confidence interval, 1.7–104). In this study, the comparison group received less than 2 Gy because all the case patients had received some irradiation to the thyroid. In other studies, patients receiving similar doses have been shown to have about a 10-fold increased risk of thyroid cancer compared with those receiving no radiation therapy. Therefore, the 13-fold increase shown in comparison with patients receiving less than 2 Gy may be about 130-fold increased compared with nonirradiated patients. The risk for thyroid cancer rose with increasing dose ($p < 0.001$), but this was derived almost entirely from the increase from less than 2 Gy to 2 Gy or more. The risk did not decrease, however, at radiation doses as high as 60 Gy related to the total dose of radiation to the thyroid. There was no increased risk of thyroid cancer associated with alkylating-agent chemotherapy. One of the a priori hypotheses to be tested by the study was whether or not dactinomycin protects against radiation-induced solid tumors, as had been previously suggested.[57] There was no diminution of risk associated with dactinomycin in conjunction with radiation therapy.[56]

The Children's Cancer Study Group also evaluated the risk for secondary cancers after ALL and found a sevenfold increased risk of developing a secondary cancer.[58] Most of this risk was due to the 22-fold risk of brain cancer. There was also a fourfold increased risk for lymphoma (n = 8) and leukemia, but the authors did not split the two cases of ANLL from the lymphomas. It is unlikely that the risk for ANLL would have been significantly increased. The brain cancers occurred in patients who were diagnosed before age 5 years and who received cranial or whole-body irradiation.

TABLE 63–28. Risk of Bone Sarcoma by Radiation Dose and Alkylator Score in LESG Study

Radiation Dose	Alkylator Score		
	0	1 or 2	≥3
None			
Relative risk	1.0*	4.8	8.5†
No of cases:controls	6:44	1:4	3:3
<1000 cGy			
Relative risk	1.3	0.4	1.3
No. of cases:controls	5:43	1:13	3:14
≥1000 cGy			
Relative risk	37.4‡	14.2‡	59.2‡
No. of cases:controls	21:45	11:26	13:12

LESG, Late Effects Study Group.
* Referent category.
† Trend in alkylator score in subjects not exposed to radiation; *p* = 0.05.
‡ *p* < 0.05.
(Tucker MA, D'Angio GJ, Boice JD, et al. Bone sarcoma linked to radiotherapy and chemotherapy in children. N Engl J Med 1987;317: 588–593)

HODGKIN'S DISEASE

One of the most widely reported secondary cancers is leukemia after Hodgkin's disease. Virtually every group with an interest in Hodgkin's disease has reported their experience with treatment-related leukemias. These reports, however, are limited by the relatively small number of leukemias reported by any one center. Although the treatment-induced leukemias are a well-recognized phenomenon, several areas

TABLE 63–29. Relative Risk of Acute or Nonlymphocytic Leukemia According to Radiation Dose to Bone Marrow and Dose of Mechlorethamine-Procarbazine Chemotherapy

No. of Cycles	Radiation Dose (Gy)			
	0	<10	10–20	>20
0		1.0	1.6 (0.3–10)	8.2 (1.7–39)
≤6	9.1 (1.6–53)	8.6 (1.9–39)	22 (5.1–99)	9.4 (2–45)
>6	50 (8.1–310)	26 (4.4–150)	63 (9.6–410)	22 (3.7–130)

(Adapted from Kaldor JM, Day NE, Clarke EA, et al. Leukemia following Hodgkin's disease. N Engl J Med 1990;322:7–13)

of controversy persist. It is clear that the leukemias are related to alkylating-agent chemotherapy, but a major area of controversy is whether combined modality therapy confers a higher risk of leukemia than chemotherapy alone. Other areas of discussion are whether splenectomy contributes to risk of leukemia and whether age at treatment is important. One recent study had sufficient numbers of Hodgkin's disease patients and cases of leukemia to address these issues.[35] One hundred and sixty-three leukemias occurred among 29,552 patients with Hodgkin's disease. There was no difference in the relative risk of leukemia after chemotherapy alone (relative risk, 9; 95% confidence interval, 4.1–20) and after combined-modality therapy (relative risk, 7.7; 95% confidence interval, 3.9–15). The highest risk was after mechlorethamine-procarbazine, cyclophosphamide-procarbazine, or chlorambucil. Kaldor was able to evaluate risks associated with radiation and mechlorethamine-procarbazine therapy (Table 63–29).[35] A small risk for leukemia was seen after radiation therapy alone, and this risk rose with increasing radiation dose. The risk did not significantly or consistently vary across radiation doses for either number of chemotherapy cycles, but increased consistently with more cycles of chemotherapy in each radiation dose range. These investigators also found a twofold increased risk

of leukemia in the patients who had undergone splenectomy, even when the dose of chemotherapy was taken into account.[35]

Although many studies have found an increased actuarial risk of leukemia in patients over age 50 years, Tucker and colleagues[11] found equivalent relative risks of acute nonlymphocytic leukemia in those treated over and under age 50 years (116 and 114, respectively). Kaldor and associates[35] reported that the relative risk for leukemia in patients treated under 38 years of age was higher than the relative risk in patients over 38 years old. The apparent discrepancy in the actuarial and relative risks is due to the higher rate of ANLL at older ages in the general population. When the age-specific rates are used, as in the relative risks, the risk for leukemia is equivalent in the different age groups. The risks for solid cancers at 15 years after treatment of Hodgkin's disease have also been quantified (Table 63–30).[11] Significantly elevated risks were found for lung cancer, non-Hodgkin's lymphoma, melanoma, stomach cancer, and bone and connective tissue sarcomas. This pattern of secondary cancers is distinctive and is similar to the distribution of cancers seen in immunosuppressed populations, such as renal transplantation patients or patients with non-Hodgkin's lymphoma. All cancers of the stomach, bone, and connective tissue (as well as a leiomyosarcoma of the small bowel) occurred within areas previously treated with radiation therapy. All those who developed lung cancer received radiation therapy and smoked. The relative risks for solid tumors increased with time, consistent with a radiation effect. The melanomas occurred without association with a specific treatment in patients who had dysplastic nevi.[59] Similar to patients with renal transplantation who develop melanoma, there is minimal lymphocytic host response at the base of the melanomas, which is an important prognostic factor.

Although an excess of thyroid cancer and breast cancer was anticipated at the 15 year follow-up (mean follow-up, 6.2 years), significant excesses were not seen.[11] Hancock and colleagues[60] subsequently found a 16-fold excess of thyroid cancer (mean follow-up, 9.9 years). The actuarial risk of developing thyroid cancer was 1.7% at 20 years. An insignificantly elevated breast cancer risk of 1.7 was seen after 15 years.[11] When the data were examined by age at radiation, because of the findings seen with tuberculosis fluoroscopy pa-

TABLE 63–30. Relative Risk of Second Cancers After Hodgkin's Disease

Site	Observed Cases	Expected Cases	Observed/Expected Cases (95% Confidence Interval)
All cancers	83	15.9	5.2 (4.2–6.5)
Acute nonlymphocytic leukemia	27	0.2	115 (76–167)
Solid tumors	46	14.5	3.2 (2.3–4.3)
Lung	14	1.8	7.7 (4.2–12.9)
Non-Hodgkin's lymphoma	9	0.5	18 (8.1–33.5)
Stomach	4	0.4	10 (2.8–26.4)
Melanoma	4	0.4	8.9 (2.4–22.8)
Bone	2	0.1	31 (3.5–111.8)
Connective tissue	2	0.1	15 (1.6–52.7)
Breast	3	1.8	1.7 (0.3–4.9)

(Adapted from Tucker MA, Coleman CN, Cox RS, et al. Risk of second malignancies following Hodgkin's disease after 15 years. N Engl J Med 1988;318:76–81)

tients and atomic bomb survivors, a 12-fold increased risk was seen in women who were treated before age 30. Hancock and colleagues[61] reevaluated this risk after more prolonged follow-up, and found a significantly elevated (fourfold) risk for breast cancer. Again, the highest risk was in women radiated before age 30.

The actuarial risks for leukemia, non-Hodgkin's lymphoma, and solid tumors at 15 years is demonstrated in Figure 63–11.[11] The risk for any secondary cancer (excluding nonmelanoma skin and simultaneous cancers) was 17.6% (±3.1%) compared with 2.6% (±1%) in the general population. The major component of the risk was due to the solid tumors, which, after a steep rise after 10 years, was 13.2% at 15 years. The risk for leukemia was 3.6%, with no new cases appearing after 9 years; the 1.6% risk for lymphoma rose slowly throughout the study period.[11] The 20-year cumulative risks have not yet been published. The risk for leukemia is unchanged, but the risks for non-Hodgkin's lymphoma and solid tumors have continued to increase, as anticipated.

The same pattern of second solid tumors has been confirmed in many subsequent studies, with some variations. Groups that did not use the spade field of irradiation as commonly did not report an excess of stomach cancer. The largest analysis of combined data sets was done by the International Database on Hodgkin's Disease.[62] The risks for secondary cancers were quantified 1 or more years after start of treatment of the Hodgkin's disease in 12,411 patients who accrued 82,850 person-years. Three hundred and sixty-seven solid secondary cancers, including basal cell carcinomas, occurred. The risk for solid tumors increased with time since treatment. The most common second solid tumor was lung cancer in both men and women. An excess of breast cancer was not seen until 15 to 19 years after treatment. Similar to the Stanford data, the risk for non-Hodgkin's lymphoma continued to increase over time and was not related to any treatment group.

Hodgkin's disease is one of the few tumors that occurs in both children and adults, and it is treated in similar manners in the two age groups. Age-at-treatment effects on the risk for secondary cancers can thus be evaluated (Table 63–31).[11,63] The risks for leukemia were similar. The risks for bone, connective tissue, and thyroid cancers, however, varied by age at treatment. In the Stanford data, the two patients who developed bone cancer were irradiated during their teenage years. Bone sarcomas, therefore, appear to be a consequence of irradiating growing bone rather than adult bone. In a similar manner, the risk for connective tissue sarcoma appears to be somewhat lower in adults. The risk for thyroid cancer also is much greater in those irradiated at an early age, which is consistent with data from atomic bomb survivors and from most groups developing radiation-induced thyroid cancer. The patients treated in the pediatric cohort have not yet attained the age when the "adult" cancers would likely manifest, so that the risks for lung, breast, and stomach cancers and melanoma cannot easily be compared.

In summary, the occurrence of a secondary leukemia after treatment of Hodgkin's disease is related to the cumulative dose of alkylating agents and, to a lesser extent, radiation. The radiation effect is only detectable in the patients who have not received alkylating agents. Secondary solid tumors and lymphomas occur with equal frequency in all treatment schemes, indicating that it is the disease itself or radiation therapy, or both, that is the etiologic agent. Given the increasing risk of the development of solid tumors and lymphomas, careful lifelong surveillance is indicated for Hodgkin's disease patients, with special attention given to new clinical signs or symptoms. Patients must be taught the necessity of not smoking, and for females, the importance of monthly breast self-examination. Mammography should be considered starting at 15 years after treatment. Patients with dysplastic nevi must be taught the necessity of monthly skin self-examinations, avoidance of sunburn, and routine professional skin examinations. With the knowledge of the substantial risks of secondary cancers, clinical trials are seeking to decrease this risk by attempting to decrease the exposure to both radiation therapy and alkylating agents without compromising the excellent therapeutic results.

BREAST CANCER

With the recommendations for the widespread use of adjuvant treatment of even low-stage disease, a large number of women are being exposed to cytotoxic therapy and can be expected to live for a long time.[64] Only relatively limited data are available to address the risk for secondary cancers. The follow-up

TABLE 63–31. Relative Risk of Specific Second Cancers After Treatment for Hodgkin's Disease in Two Age Groups

Site	LESG Study (n = 1036; average follow-up = 5.1 y; average age = 12 y)	Stanford Study (n = 1507; average follow-up = 6.2 y; average age = 29 y)
All cancers	16	7.4
Leukemia	89	66
Bone	106	31
Connective tissue	39	15
Thyroid	68	16*

* Risk of 16 from 1787 patients reported by Hancock and colleagues.[60]
(Adapted from Tucker MA, Coleman CN, Cox RS, et al. Risk of second malignancies following Hodgkin's disease after 15 years. N Engl J Med 1988;318:76–81; and Tucker MA, Meadows AT, Boice JD Jr, et al. Cancer risk following treatment of childhood cancer. In: Radiation carcinogenesis: Epidemiology and biological significance. New York: Raven 1984:211–224)

period in most groups is too short to adequately evaluate solid tumors, but several studies have examined the risk for leukemia associated with treatment of breast cancer.

Fisher and associates[9] reported the risk for leukemia in the National Surgical Adjuvant Breast Project clinical trials. The 10-year cumulative risk for leukemia after surgery alone was 0.06% (±0.05%) and was 1.37% (±0.74%) in the surgery plus locoregional radiation therapy group. Of note, two of the six cases of leukemia that occurred in the surgery plus radiation group were chronic lymphocytic leukemia, which is not a radiation-related cancer. The risk for leukemia plus myelodysplastic syndrome was 1.54% (±0.36%) after surgery plus chemotherapy that included melphalan. This risk was significantly higher than the risk with surgery alone. In contrast, Valagussa and associates[65] found no leukemia in 666 women treated with adjuvant cyclophosphamide, methotrexate, and fluorouracil.[65] These findings were extended by Curtis and associates[66] in a study of 82,700 women treated for breast cancer. The risk for leukemia after regional radiation alone was increased twofold, with an average dose of 7.5 Gy to active bone marrow. The risk associated with treatment with alkylating agents, without radiation, was increased tenfold; and with both radiation and alkylating agents, it was increased 17-fold. These radiation doses and chemotherapy doses are much higher than those used with adjuvant treatment or primary radiation therapy after lumpectomy. Women receiving melphalan were ten times more likely to develop leukemia than those receiving cyclophosphamide (relative risk, 31.4 versus 3.1). All the leukemias that developed after cyclophosphamide occurred in women who had received over 20,000 mg of cyclophosphamide.[66] The difference in the total dose of cyclophosphamide may explain the varying leukemia risks in these populations. Based on the risks found in their study, Curtis and associates[66] estimated that only about 5 in 10,000 patients treated with 6 months of a cyclophosphamide-based adjuvant regimen would be expected to develop a treatment-induced leukemia within about 10 years of breast cancer diagnosis.

Boice and colleagues[67] reported the risk of breast cancer in the contralateral breast of women who received radiation therapy for breast cancer between 1935 and 1982 in Connecticut. There was a small increase in risk associated with an average dose of about 3 Gy to the contralateral breast. Although the treatment varied substantially from recent practices, the total dose was within the range of what is delivered to the contralateral breast with current techniques. Fewer than 3% of all second breast cancers in the study could be attributed to previous radiation treatment. Consistent with the studies discussed previously, the risk was highest in women treated at a young age (under 45 years old). There was no increased risk in the women treated over age 45 years.

In summary, leukemia risk after breast cancer is due to treatment with alkylating agents, particularly melphalan. Risk is related to total dose of drug and is low in the dose range of cyclophosphamide currently used in the adjuvant setting. The risk for leukemia after older techniques of regional radiation therapy (chest wall and nodes) also appears to be minimally increased but is unknown after breast-conserving radiation therapy. The most common solid second primary cancer that occurs after breast cancer is contralateral breast cancer, but fewer than 3% of these tumors could be attributed to radiation. The effect of adjuvant tamoxifen and its increased use[64] on

this radiation consequence is also unknown. Breast cancer patients are an important group to follow over time because, although the risks are much lower than those after treatment of Hodgkin's disease, breast cancer is a common tumor, and even a substantially decreased risk for secondary cancers compared with Hodgkin's disease could translate into a larger number of affected patients.

HOST FACTORS

Although the risks for second tumors after specific drugs and radiation doses are now being quantified, many questions remain. Several host characteristics have been identified that have a substantial effect on the level of risk associated with treatment. One of these is age at exposure. It is clear from multiple populations, including atomic bomb survivors, tuberculosis fluoroscopy patients, Hodgkin's disease patients, and breast cancer patients, that age at irradiation to the breast is a major determinant of risk for breast cancer. Women exposed over age 30 to 45 years, depending on the study, do not appear to be at increased risk for breast cancer, while those exposed at younger ages, particularly in adolescence, have an extremely high risk. From atomic bomb survivors, there is evidence that, in addition to the radiation, other host factors, such as age at first pregnancy, remain important in those who received relatively low doses to the breast. The effects of age and dose have not been fully explored, particularly at the therapeutic ranges, but it appears that in Hodgkin's disease patients, even doses in the therapeutic range confer high risk in young patients.

The risk for radiation-induced thyroid cancer is also modulated by the age at exposure to radiation. From several populations, including atomic bomb survivors, Marshall Islanders, tinea capitis patients, and Hodgkin's disease patients, the risk is higher after early childhood exposure. From the LESG study, the markedly increased risk is also seen not only at the lower doses previously reported, but also after therapeutic range doses up to 60 Gy or more. The data for an age effect in the development of bone sarcomas and perhaps connective tissue sarcomas are less compelling. The much smaller risks of bone, and to a lesser extent connective tissue sarcomas, after treatment of Hodgkin's disease in adults indicates an age effect. The difference in risk for bone sarcoma after treatment of childhood cancer in general versus adult cancers (such as cervical cancer[5]) again suggests that growing bone (and perhaps connective tissue) is more susceptible to treatment-induced sarcomas.

Age does not appear to have the same type of effect in alkylating-agent-induced leukemia. The relative risks by age groups are remarkably similar. The significantly increased actuarial risk of ANLL after Hodgkin's disease that is routinely seen in older patients (over 50 years) in most clinical series is due to the increased rate of ANLL in the general population at that age. The rates in children treated for Hodgkin's disease appear comparable to those in adults.

Immunosuppression also appears to have an effect on the risk for secondary cancers. The similarity in patterns of tumors after Hodgkin's disease, non-Hodgkin's lymphoma,[68] renal transplantation, and congenital or acquired immunodeficiency syndromes suggests that specific tumors are particularly affected by the immune status of the host. Non-Hodgkin's lymphoma, sarcomas, melanoma, and to a lesser extent lung cancer and stomach cancer, appear to be modulated by the immune system.

Probably the most important host factor is the patient's genetic susceptibility to developing cancer. The prototype of this is heritable retinoblastoma, in which patients with germline alterations in the RB locus have an excess of both radiation-induced and spontaneous osteosarcomas, with similar RB changes. As more tumor-suppressor genes, oncogenes, protooncogenes, and other important control genes are discovered and characterized, the individual susceptibility to specific agents may be clarified. The role of interindividual variation in the metabolism of specific drugs is only starting to be explored and may be a potent predictor of patients at risk for alkylating-agent-induced cancers. As the mechanisms of carcinogenesis are clarified, chemotherapy drugs may be able to be chemically modified to reduce risk without sacrificing efficacy.

CONCLUSION

Secondary, treatment-related cancers are seen because the initial treatment is successful. Attempts should be made to reduce this complication. Indeed, most investigators studying pediatric and Hodgkin's disease populations are developing treatment strategies to minimize late complications. Changes in therapy to minimize secondary cancers are best made in the context of a carefully designed study that includes the codification of treatment and follow-up procedures. It is through such careful studies that current treatments can be made less toxic while their efficacy is maintained or improved. Practicing oncologists are encouraged to participate in such studies so that this evolutionary process can proceed as expeditiously as possible.

REFERENCES

1. Li FP. Secondary cancers. In: DeVita VT Jr, Hellman S, Rosenberg SA, eds. Cancer: Principles and practice of oncology. 2nd ed. Philadelphia: JB Lippincott, 1985:2040–2049.
2. Coleman CN. Adverse effects of cancer therapy: Risk of secondary neoplasms. Am J Pediatr Hematol Oncol 1982;4:103–111.
3. Coleman CN. Secondary neoplasms in patients treated for cancer: Etiology and perspective. Radiat Res 1982;92:188–200.
4. Monson RR. Analysis of relative survival and proportional mortality. Comput Biomed Res 1974;7:325–332.
5. Boice JD Jr, Day NE, Anderson A, et al. Second cancer following radiation treatment for cervical cancer: An international collaboration among cancer registries. J Natl Cancer Inst 1985;74:955–975.
6. Draper GJ, Sanders BM, Kingston JE. Second primary neoplasms in patients with retinoblastoma. Br J Cancer 1986;53:661–671.
7. Abramson DH, Ellsworth RM, Kitchi FD, et al. Second nonocular tumors in retinoblastoma survivors: Are they radiation-induced? Ophthalmology 1984;91:1351–1355.
8. Hansen FM, Koufson A, Gallie BL, et al. Osteosarcoma and retinoblastoma: A shared chromosomal mechanism revealing recessive predisposition. Proc Natl Acad Sci USA 1986;82:6216–6220.
9. Fisher B, Rockette H, Fisher ER, et al. Leukemia in breast cancer patients following adjuvant chemotherapy or postoperative radiation: The NSABP experience. J Clin Oncol 1985;3:1640–1658.
10. Greene MH, Harris EL, Gershenson DM, et al. Melphalan may be a more potent leukemogen than cyclophosphamide. Ann Intern Med 1986;105:360–367.
11. Tucker MA, Coleman NC, Cox RS, et al. Risk of secondary malignancies following Hodgkin's disease after 15 years. N Engl J Med 1988;318:76–81.
12. Valagussa P, Santoro A, Bellani-Fossati F, et al. Second acute leukemia and other malignancies following treatment for Hodgkin's disease. J Clin Oncol 1986;4:830–837.
13. Kaplan EL, Meier P. Nonparametric estimation from incomplete observation. J Am Stat Assoc 1958;53:457–481.
14. Gehan EA. A generalized Wilcoxon test for comparing arbitrarily singly censored samples. Biometrika 1965;52:203–223.
15. Coleman CN, Kaplan HS, Cox R, et al. Leukemias, non-Hodgkin's lymphomas and solid tumours in patients treated for Hodgkin's disease. Cancer Surv 1982;1:733–744.
16. National Research Council, Committee on the Biologic Effects of Ionizing Radiations. Health effects of exposure to low levels of ionizing radiation. Washington, DC: National Academy of Science, 1990.
17. Preston DL, Kato H, Kopecky KJ, et al. Studies of the mortality of A-bomb survivors. Radiat Res 1987;111:151–178.
18. Land CE. A nested case-control approach to interactions between radiation dose and other factors as causes of cancer. RERF Commentary and Review Series CR 1-90. Hiroshima: Radiation Effects Research Foundation, 1990.
19. Land CE, Hayakawa N, Machado S, et al. A case-control interview study of breast cancer among Japanese A-bomb survivors. I. Main effects. RERF Technical Report (in press).
20. Land CE, Hayakawa N, Machado S, et al. A case-control interview study of breast cancer among Japanese A-bomb survivors. II. Interactions between epidemiologic factors and radiation dose. RERF Technical Report (in press).
21. Land CE. Histological types of lung cancer in Japanese A-bomb survivors and Colorado plateau uranium miners. Proceedings of the International Conference on Radiation Effects and Protection. Mito, Japan, 1992.
22. Holm LE, Wiklund KE, Lundell GE, et al. Cancer risk in population examined with diagnostic doses of ^{131}I. J Natl Cancer Inst 1989;81:302–306.
23. Hrubec Z, Boice JD Jr, Monson RR, Rosenstein M. Breast cancer after multiple chest fluoroscopies: Second follow-up of Massachusetts women with tuberculosis. Cancer Res 1989;49:229–234.
24. Linos A, Gray JE, Orvis AL, et al. Low-dose radiation and leukemia. N Engl J Med 1980;302:1101–1105.
25. Evans JS, Wennberg JE, McNeil BJ. The influence of diagnostic radiography on the incidence of breast cancer and leukemia. N Engl J Med 1986;315:810–815.
26. Reimer RR, Hoover RN, Fraumeni JF Jr, et al. Acute leukemia after alkylating-agent therapy for ovarian cancer. N Engl J Med 1982;307:1416–1421.
27. Greene MH, Boice JD Jr, Greer BE, et al. Acute nonlymphocytic leukemia after therapy with alkylating agents for ovarian cancer. N Engl J Med 1982;307:1416–1421.
28. Boice JD Jr, Greene MH, Killen JY, et al. Leukemia after chemotherapy with semustine (methyl-CCNU): Evidence of a dose-response effect. N Engl J Med [Letter] 1986;314:119–120.
29. Bergsagel DE, Bailey AJ, Langley GR, et al. The chemotherapy for plasma-cell myeloma and the incidence of acute leukemia. N Engl J Med 1979;301:743–748.
30. Berk PD, Goldberg JD, Silverstein MN, et al. Increased risk of acute leukemia in polycythemia vera associated with chlorambucil therapy. N Engl J Med 1981;304:441–447.
31. Boice JD Jr, Greene MH, Killen, et al. Leukemia and preleukemia after adjuvant treatment of gastrointestinal cancer with semustine (methyl-CCNU). N Engl J Med 1983;309:1079–1084.
32. Chak LY, Sikic BI, Tucker MA, et al. Increased incidence of acute nonlymphocytic leukemia following therapy in patients with small cell carcinoma of the lung. J Clin Oncol 1984;2:385–390.
33. Tucker MA, Meadows AT, Boice JD Jr, et al. Leukemia after therapy with alkylating agents for childhood cancer. J Natl Cancer Inst 1987;78:459–464.
34. Kaldor JM, Day NE, Pettersson F, et al. Leukemia following chemotherapy for ovarian cancer. N Engl J Med 1990;322:1–6.
35. Kaldor JM, Day NE, Clarke A, et al. Leukemia following Hodgkin's disease. N Engl J Med 1990;322:7–13.
36. Cuzik J, Erskine S, Edelman D, et al. A comparison of the incidence of the myelodysplastic syndrome and acute myeloid leukemia following melphalan and cyclophosphamide treatment for myelomatosis. Br J Cancer 1987;55:523–529.
37. Greene MH. Epidemiologic studies of chemotherapy-related acute leukemia. In: Cascinelli A, ed. Epidemiology and quantitation of environmental risk in humans from radiation and other agents. New York: Plenum, 1985:499–514.
38. Preisler HD, Early AP, Raza A, et al. Therapy of secondary nonlymphocytic leukemia with cytarabine. N Engl J Med 1983;308:21–23.
39. Vaughan WP, Karp JE, Burke PJ. Effective chemotherapy of acute myelocytic leukemia occurring after alkylating agent or radiation therapy for prior malignancy. J Clin Oncol 1983;1:204–207.
40. Le Beau MM, Albain KS, Larson RA, et al. Clinical and cytogenetic correlations in 63 patients with therapy-related myelodysplastic syndromes and acute nonlymphocytic leukemia: Further evidence for characteristic abnormalities of chromosomes no. 5 and 7. J Clin Oncol 1986;4:325–345.
41. Pui CH, Ribeiro RC, Hancock ML, et al. Acute myeloid leukemia in children treated with epipodophyllotoxins for acute lymphoblastic leukemia. N Engl J Med 1991;325:1682–1687.
42. Pedersen-Bjergaard J, Daugaard G, Hansen SW, et al. Increased risk of myelodysplasia and leukaemia after etoposide, cisplatin, and bleomycin for germ-cell tumours. Lancet 1991;338:359–363.
43. Whitlock JA, Greer JP, Lukens JN. Epipodophyllotoxin-related leukemia: Identification of a new subset of secondary leukemia. Cancer 1991;68:600–604.
44. Pedersen-Bjergaard J, Philip P, Larsen SO, et al. Chromosome aberrations and prognostic factors in therapy-related myelodysplasia and acute nonlymphocytic leukemia. Blood 1990;76:1083–1091.
45. Pedersen-Bjergaard J, Ersboll J, Hansen VL, et al. Carcinoma of the urinary bladder

after treatment with cyclophosphamide for non-Hodgkin's lymphoma. N Engl J Med 1988;318:1028–1032.

46. Wall RL, Clausen K. Carcinoma of the urinary bladder in patients receiving cyclophosphamide. N Engl J Med 1975;293:271–273.

47. Travis LB, Curtis RE, Boice JD Jr, Fraumeni JF Jr. Bladder cancer after chemotherapy for non-Hodgkin's lymphoma. N Engl J Med 1989;321:544–545.

48. Tucker MA, D'Angio GJ, Boice JD Jr, et al. Bone sarcomas linked to radiotherapy and chemotherapy in children. N Engl J Med 1987;317:588–593.

49. Cavenee WK, Murphee AL, Shull, et al. Prediction of familial predisposition to retinoblastoma. N Engl J Med 1986;314:1201–1207.

50. Lee WH, Bookstein R, Hong F, et al. Human retinoblastoma susceptibility gene: Cloning, identification, and sequence. Science 1987;235:1394–1399.

51. Arthur DC. Genetics and cytogenetics of pediatric cancers. Cancer 1986;58:534–540.

52. Koufos A, Hansen MF, Lampkin BC, et al. Loss of alleles at loci on human chromosome 11 during the genesis of Wllms' tumor. Nature 1984;309:170–172.

53. Malkin D, Li FP, Strong LC, et al. Germ line p53 mutations in a familial syndrome of breast cancer, sarcomas, and other neoplasms. Science 1990;250:1233–1238.

54. Meadows AT. Risk factors for second malignant neoplasms: Report from the Late Effects Study Group. Bull Cancer (Paris) 1988;75:125–130.

55. Strong LC, Herson J, Osborne BM, et al. Risk of radiation-related subsequent malignant tumors in survivors of Ewing's sarcoma. J Natl Cancer Inst 1979;62:1401–1406.

55a. Tucker MA, unpublished data. National Cancer Institute, 1992.

56. Tucker MA, Morris Jones PH, Boice JD Jr, et al. Therapeutic radiation at a young age is linked to secondary thyroid cancer. Cancer Res 1991;51:2885–2888.

57. D'Angio GJ, Meadows AT, Mike V, et al. Decreased risk of radiation-associated second malignant neoplasms in actinomycin-D treated patients. Cancer 1976;37:1177–1185.

58. Neglia JP, Meadows AT, Robison LL, et al. Second neoplasms after acute lymphoblastic leukemia in childhood. N Engl J Med 1991;325:1330–1336.

59. Tucker MA, Misfeldt D, Coleman CN, et al. Cutaneous malignant melanoma after Hodgkin's disease. Ann Intern Med 1985;102:37–41.

60. Hancock SL, Cox RS, McDougall IR. Thyroid diseases after treatment of Hodgkin's disease. N Engl J Med 1991;325:599–605.

61. Hancock SL, Tucker MA, Hoppe RT. Breast cancer after treatment for Hodgkin's disease. J Natl Cancer Inst (in press).

62. Kaldor JM, Lasset C. Second malignancies following Hodgkin's disease. In: Somers R, Henry-Amar M, Meerwaldt JH, et al, eds. Treatment strategy in hodgkin's disease. Colloque INSERM/John Libbey Eurotext 1990;196:139–150.

63. Tucker MA, Meadows AT, Boice JD Jr, et al. Cancer risk following treatment for childhood cancer. In: Boice JD Jr, Fraumeni JF Jr, eds. Radiation carcinogenesis: Epidemiology and biological significance. New York: Raven, 1984:211–224.

64. Early Breast Cancer Trialists' Collaborative Group. Systemic treatment of early breast cancer by hormonal, cytotoxic, or immune therapy. Lancet 1992;339:1–15, 71–85.

65. Valagussa P, Tancini G, Bonadonna G. Second malignancies after CMF for resectable breast cancer. J Clin Oncol 1987;5:1138–1142.

66. Curtis RE, Boice JD Jr, Stovall M, et al. Dose-dependent leukemia risk after drug and radiation treatment for breast cancer. N Engl J Med 1992;326:1745–1751.

67. Boice JD Jr, Harvey EB, Blettner M, et al. Cancer in the contralateral breast after radiotherapy for breast cancer. N Engl J Med 1992;326:781–785.

68. Travis LB, Curtis RE, Boice JD Jr, et al. Second cancers following non-Hodgkin's lymphoma. Cancer 1991;67:2002–2009.

Cancer: Principles & Practice of Oncology, Fourth Edition,
edited by Vincent T. DeVita, Jr., Samuel Hellman, Steven A. Rosenberg.
J.B. Lippincott Co., Philadelphia © 1993.

CHAPTER **64**

Supportive Care and the Quality of Life of the Cancer Patient

SECTION **1**   KATHLEEN M. FOLEY

Management of Cancer Pain

Pain is one of the most common symptoms leading to medical evaluation of the cancer patient. Numerous national and international surveys have demonstrated that 30% to 50% of patients in active therapy and as many as 60% to 90% of patients with advanced disease have pain.[1–6] Several studies that have focused on both patient and physician attitudes toward cancer pain suggest that cancer pain is perceived as the most feared consequence of cancer.[7,8] Sixty-nine percent of patients interviewed reported that they would consider suicide if their cancer pain became intolerable. For the clinician, pain represents a difficult diagnostic and therapeutic medical problem.[9,10]

Advances in the diagnosis and treatment of cancer, coupled with recent advances in our understanding of the anatomy, physiology, pharmacology, and psychology of pain perception, have led to improved care of the patient with pain of malignant origin. Specialized methods of cancer diagnosis and treatment provide the most direct approach to treating cancer pain by treating the cause of the pain. However, before the introduction of successful antitumor therapy, when treatment of the cause of the pain has failed, or when injury to bone, soft tissue, or nerve has occurred as a result of therapy, appropriate pain management is essential. Patients with cancer are managed most effectively by a multidisciplinary approach, using the expertise of a wide range of medical personnel.[2,11,12] The goal of pain therapy for patients receiving active treatment is to provide them with sufficient relief to tolerate the diagnostic and therapeutic approaches required to treat their cancer. For patients with advanced disease, pain control should be sufficient to allow them to function at a level that they choose and to die relatively free of pain. Critical to the management of cancer pain is the establishment of trust between the patient and physician; the physician must respect the pain complaint as serious, assess its nature and severity, and implement pain relief therapy.

BARRIERS TO CANCER PAIN RELIEF

Several barriers interfere with the appropriate management of patients with pain and cancer. Although pain can be controlled in most patients, an analysis of 11 published reports of cancer pain treatment covering nearly 2000 patients in nonhospice settings estimated that 50% to 80% did not have adequate control.[2] Several reports have focused on the observation that cancer pain is often improperly treated.[2,6–8,13–15] Various reasons have been cited for inadequate cancer pain management, including fear of addiction, lack of knowledge of analgesic drug therapy, assignment of low priority to pain management, lack of understanding of the pathophysiology of cancer pain, and overconcern about tolerance to analgesic medications. Patient-physician communication about pain symptoms is reported to be poor, and patients often underreport the amount of pain they experience or fail to report inadequate relief. Patients may also resist taking narcotic analgesics because of the stigma attached, and only take them when their pain is severe. Limited availability and lack of use of alternatives to systemic analgesics (*i.e.*, nerve blocks, palliative neurosurgery, and behavioral treatments) have also been reported to prevent adequate treatment.[4]

Finally, the attitudes of health-care providers toward pain and its impact on the patient influence the priority they and their patients place on pain therapy. Cleeland and colleagues have assessed the factors influencing the pain management practices of clinicians caring for cancer patients.[8] The authors studied clinicians' knowledge and attitudes toward cancer pain and its treatment in 91 physicians who participated in a statewide study. Of the participating physicians, 69% had managed the care of over 100 cancer patients in their current practice setting, and they represented the major medical and surgical subspecialties. Two groups of respondents were identified: one represented younger physicians with more specialized oncology training who had a liberal attitude toward pain management, while the larger group had a more conservative approach, placing a lower priority on pain management.

To further study these issues, Van Roenn and associates assessed physicians' knowledge and attitudes about cancer pain through a survey of the Eastern Cooperative Oncology group.[9] The 1177 oncologists who responded ranked the barriers as detailed in Table 64–1. This study clarified the current status of cancer pain treatment in the United States. Eighty-five percent of the respondents agreed that most patients with pain are undermedicated. Only half reported that pain control in their practice setting was either good or very good. Poor pain assessment was identified as the most important barrier to adequate pain management by 76% of physicians surveyed. In response to a case scenario, adjuvant medications were underused, and physicians failed to include a potent opioid in their most aggressive analgesic regimen 14% of the time. Concern about side effects by 65% of the physicians was cited as the reason for their reluctance to prescribe maximum analgesic therapy.

These data confirm the results of previous studies that have focused on the problems of inadequate pain control and serve

TABLE 64–1.   ECOG Survey of Barriers to Adequate Cancer Pain Management

Characteristic	Percent
Inadequate assessment of pain and pain relief	76
Patient reluctance to report pain	48
Patient reluctance to take opiates	48
Medical staff reluctance to prescribe opiates	46
Lack of equipment skills	39
Nursing staff reluctance to administer opiates	28
Excessive state regulation of prescribing analgesics	12
Lack of psychological support services	8
Lack of available neurodestructive procedures	4
Lack of access to a wide range of analgesics	2
Lack of access to professionals who practice specialized methods	2

This table lists the percentage of 1177 oncologists' responses to a questionnaire survey describing their knowledge and attitudes about cancer pain management.
(Van Roenn JH, Cleeland CS, Gonin R, Hatfield A, Pandya KJ. Physicians' attitudes towards cancer pain management [in press])

as a useful outline for education to improve health-care professionals' and patients' knowledge about cancer pain and its treatment.

EPIDEMIOLOGY

Although large-scale national epidemiologic studies on the incidence and severity of cancer pain are lacking, existing studies suggest that moderate to severe pain is experienced by one third of cancer patients receiving active therapy and by 60% to 90% of patients with advanced cancer. These data have been generated from several surveys of small groups of patients in specific medical-care settings.

Patients with cancer often have multiple causes of pain. In one survey 81% of patients reported two or more distinct pain complaints; 34% reported three pains.[3] More recent studies have focused on the factors that influence the prevalence of cancer pain.[5,10,13–18] Primary tumor type is one factor.[18] Patients with bone tumors and breast and prostate cancer have a much higher incidence of pain (60% to 80%) as compared with patients with lymphoma or leukemia.[1] The stage of disease is also a contributing factor. For example, only 15% of patients with nonmetastatic disease report pain. Certain types of tumors, because of their tendency for bony involvement or their occurrence in sites with proximity to neural structures, have a greater incidence of pain. Moreover, patient variables, such as anxiety and depression, markedly influence the patient's report and experience of pain.[17]

The data are very consistent in cross-cultural studies. Data from India, Thailand, Vietnam, and the Philippines report a similar prevalence of cancer pain in patients in active therapy and advanced disease.[4,20,21]

Studies have also focused not only on the prevalence of pain, but on its intensity, the degree of pain relief, and the impact of pain on quality of life. In one prospective study of pain prevalence and characteristics, 91 ambulatory patients with lung or colon cancer were interviewed.[22] They had reported persistent or frequent pain during the previous 2 weeks. One third of patients had more than one pain. The median pain duration was 4 weeks and the average pain intensity was moderate. Ninety percent experienced pain more than 25% of the time and 50% reported that pain interfered moderately or more with their general activity or work. A similar percentage reported moderate or greater pain interference with sleep, mood, and enjoyment of life. These data support the theory that pain is prevalent among well-functioning ambulatory patients and substantially compromises function in about half the patients who experience it.

In a study of patients with far-advanced disease cared for in a palliative care program, pain was the most common physical symptom associated with patients' perception of not feeling well. This symptom was significantly improved with analgesic therapies, but several other prominent symptoms, including weakness, anxiety, anorexia, nausea and vomiting, and confusion, were less readily treated. Several studies, including this one, have focused on the important observation that pain symptoms often represent only the "tip of the iceberg," and there is an enormous need to evaluate, rank, and treat all symptoms in dying patients to improve their quality of life.[24–27]

DEFINITION AND TYPES OF CANCER PAIN

DEFINITION OF PAIN

The definition of pain proposed by the International Association for the Study of Pain is "an unpleasant sensory and emotional experience associated with actual or potential tissue damage or described in terms of such damage."[28] Because pain is a subjective complaint, there is no definitive way to distinguish pain occurring in the absence of tissue damage from pain resulting from such damage. Pain as a somatic delusion or a masked depression is rare in cancer patients, and the presence of pain usually implies a pathologic process.

ANATOMY AND PHYSIOLOGY OF PAIN

Extensive investigations over the last 25 years have expanded our knowledge of ascending and descending central nervous system pathways that process and modulate nociceptive information. These advances provide a scientific rationale for the use of new and improved methods of cancer pain treatment.[29] A brief review of the neuroanatomy and physiology and pharmacology of pain provides a background for the later discussions of specific drug, anesthetic, and neurosurgical approaches.

Detailed information now supports the theory that activation of peripheral receptors in both superficial and deep structures as well as viscera by mechanical and chemical stimuli excites afferent discharges in two types of nerve fibers: thinly myelinated A-delta fibers and unmyelinated C fibers. These primary sensory afferents have their cell bodies in the dorsal root ganglion, and their axons enter the spinal cord via the dorsal root.

They ascend or descend from one or two segments in Lissauer's tract and synapse in specific lamina in the dorsal horn. There, they give rise to an extensive, highly branched terminal field. The small-diameter afferents that enter the cord in the lateral division of the dorsal root project densely to lamina I and lamina II in the dorsal horn. This projection includes both the unmyelinated and myelinated nociceptors, as well as some afferents that respond to innocuous thermal stimuli. Evidence suggests that myelinated nociceptors project to lamina I and V, unmyelinated nociceptors project to lamina II and possibly lamina I, and nonnociceptive myelinated afferents project to only deep lamina. Anatomic localization of nociceptive pathways within the dorsal horn reflects a very distinct relation between different lamina and their role in pain modulation.

The dorsal horn is an important site for modulating sensory input. Several ascending pathways arise from second-order neurons and decussate in the central gray of the spinal cord to become the neospinothalamic and paleospinothalamic tracts. These tracts project to discrete regions of the thalamus and cortex. The neospinothalamic pathways subserve pain intensity and localization, whereas the phylogenetically older paleospinothalamic pathway subserves the arousal and emotional component of pain. Descending pathways, the most important of which originate from the periaqueductal gray nuclei of the midbrain, synapse in the raphae magnus nucleus of the medulla. From this nucleus, a medial pathway, the dorsal longitudinal fasciculus, projects to the dorsal horn to mod-

ulate pain transmission. This pathway represents an important descending inhibitory pathway. A more laterally placed descending pathway from the locus ceruleus to the dorsal horn also plays a role in pain modulation at the spinal cord level.[30]

Neurotransmitters play a significant role in this modulatory system.[31] At the level of the nociceptive primary afferent, the neurotransmitters that appear to play an important role include substance P and the excitatory neurotransmitters glutamate, aspartate, and adenosine diphosphate. Dopamine, serotonin, norepinephrine, and the endogenous opioids enkephalin, β-endorphin, and dynorphin modulate pain at both the spinal and supraspinal sites. Attempts to enhance and mimic the role of these neurotransmitters in pain modulation have led to a series of clinical analgesic studies of, for example, amitriptyline.[32] Amitriptyline has analgesic properties independent of its antidepressant effects.[33,34] It appears to work by enhancing serotonin activity centrally by presynaptic inhibition of its reuptake and by activation of the descending inhibitory pain system. Recent studies with an NMDA antagonist suggest that pain can be inhibited at the level of the primary afferent by the use of these compounds, which alter the activity of the excitatory amino acid glutamate.[31]

Opiate receptors, stereospecific binding sites on the end of free nerve endings that bind endogenous and exogenous opioids, are localized in the ascending and descending pain pathways.[35] These receptors mediate the multiple pharmacologic effects of the opioid analgesics. Subpopulations of opioid receptors, including high-affinity and low-affinity μ receptors and δ, κ, and σ receptors, are localized to specific areas of the brain and spinal cord.

The identification of these subclasses of receptors that mediate different pharmacologic effects and that are located in specific cerebral and spinal sites offers the possibility of developing new analgesics targeted for specific receptors. For example, mu receptors modulate predominantly supraspinal analgesia, whereas delta receptors are the important receptors in modulating analgesia of the spinal cord level. The periaqueductal gray (PAG) region in the midbrain and the dorsal horn in the spinal cord are rich in these opioid receptors and are the supraspinal and spinal sites that mediate opioid analgesia.[36] These areas were identified as selective sites of analgesia after studies in animals and humans showed that electrical stimulation of the PAG region produces total body analgesia without motor or sensory changes. Administration of opioids directly into the PAG region inhibits pain transmission at the level of the spinal cord by activating this medial descending inhibitory pathway. The use of brain stem stimulation and the administration of the opioid analgesics directly into the cerebrospinal fluid bathing these selective sites in animals and cancer patients with pain are procedures based on this research. Pain transmission at the spinal cord level can be inhibited by the direct application of morphine, and these studies have led to the use of spinal opioid analgesia in clinical pain states.[37,38]

These advances in our understanding of pain modulatory systems and their neuroanatomic and neuropharmacologic correlates have had a major impact on the management of patients with pain. As our understanding of the neurobiology of pain expands, future studies will investigate therapeutic approaches directed at the primary afferent to prevent release of neurotransmitters as well as to modulate neurotransmitters within the central nervous system to enhance inhibitory pain systems.

TYPES OF PAIN

Three types of pain have been described based on the neuroanatomy and the neurophysiology of pain pathways: somatic, visceral, and neuropathic pain.[39] Each type results from either activation and sensitization of nociceptors and mechanoreceptors in the periphery (tumor compression or infiltration) by chemical (epinephrine, serotonin, bradykinin, prostaglandin, histamine) stimuli.

When nociceptors are activated in cutaneous or deep tissues, somatic pain results, typically characterized by a dull or aching but well-localized pain. Metastatic bone pain, postsurgical incisional pain, and myofascial and musculoskeletal pain are common examples of somatic pain.

Visceral pain results from activation of nociceptors from infiltration, compression, extension, or stretching of the thoracic, abdominal, or pelvic viscera. This typically occurs in patients with intraperitoneal metastases and is common with pancreatic cancer. This type of pain is poorly localized, is often described as deep, squeezing, and pressure-like, and when acute is often associated with significant autonomic dysfunction, including nausea, vomiting, and diaphoresis. Visceral pain is often referred to cutaneous sites that may be remote from the site of the lesion (*e.g.,* shoulder pain with diaphragmatic irritation). It may be associated with tenderness in the referred cutaneous site.

Neuropathic pain results from injury to the peripheral or central nervous system as a consequence of tumor compression or infiltration of peripheral nerves or the spinal cord, or from chemical injury to the peripheral nerve or spinal cord caused by surgery, irradiation, or chemotherapy. Examples of neuropathic pain include both metastatic and radiation-induced brachial and lumbosacral plexopathies, chemotherapy-induced peripheral neuropathies, paraneoplastic peripheral neuropathies, and phantom limb pain. Pain from nerve injury is often severe and is described as burning or dysesthetic, with a viselike quality. The pain is typically most common in the site of sensory loss and may be associated with hypersensitivity to nonnoxious and noxious stimuli. Intermittently, patients complain of paroxysms or burning or electric shock-like sensations.

These three types of pain may occur in the same patient, who may have pure somatic or visceral pain, or mixed somatic and neuropathic pain. These different types of pain account for different responses to drug and nondrug approaches. For instance, the nonsteroidal antiinflammatory drugs reduce chemical activation of nociceptors peripherally (*e.g.,* bone pain), whereas anesthetic approaches suppress the pain transmission in peripheral nerves. Management of both somatic and visceral pain suggests that these types of pain respond to a wide variety of approaches. The management of neuropathic pain is more complicated: changes in the peripheral nervous system and the central nervous system make this type of pain less responsive to a wide variety of pharmacologic, anesthetic, and neurosurgical approaches.

Evidence suggests that most cancer patients have both somatic and visceral pain, with neuropathic pain representing 15% to 20% of the significant pain problems in this population.[11,12,24,25] Certain adjuvant drugs appear to be more appropriate in the management of neuropathic pain; these issues are discussed in a later section.

TEMPORAL ASPECTS OF PAIN

Acute pain is characterized by a well-defined temporal pattern of pain onset, generally associated with subjective and objective physical signs and with hyperactivity of the autonomic nervous system. These signs provide the physician with objective evidence that substantiates the patient's complaint of pain. Acute pain is usually self-limited and responds to treatment with analgesic drug therapy and to treatment of its precipitating cause.

Acute pain can be further subdivided into subacute and episodic. Subacute pain comes on over several days, often with increasing intensity, and represents a pattern of progressive pain symptomatology. Episodic or intermittent pain occurs during confined periods of time on a regular or irregular basis. All of the pains in this category of acute pain have associated autonomic hyperactivity.

Chronic pain is the persistence of pain for more than 3 months, with a less well-defined temporal onset. The autonomic nervous system adapts, so chronic pain patients lack the objective signs common to those with acute pain. Chronic pain leads to significant changes in personality, lifestyle, and functional ability. For these patients, the management approach must include both the treatment of the cause of the pain and the treatment of the complications affecting their functional status, social interactions, and personalities.[40] This group of patients is a challenge to physicians in pain management, and this group also colors physicians' attitudes toward the management of acute pain problems. Treatment of chronic pain in the cancer patient is especially challenging because it requires a careful assessment of not only the intensity of the pain but its broad multidimensional aspects. Evidence suggests that the persistence of pain plays a major negative role in the quality of life of patients with pain and cancer.

Recently investigators have identified a series of specific pains in cancer patients with both acute and chronic pain states. Baseline pain is the average pain intensity experienced for 12 or more hours during a 24-hour period. Breakthrough pain is a transient increase in pain to greater than moderate intensity occurring on a baseline pain of moderate intensity or less. In a study of 70 adult inpatient cancer patients, 65% reported breakthrough pain.[41] The median number of reported pains was four, with a wide range. Most pains had a rapid onset and a brief duration. Breakthrough pain has a diversity of characteristics. In some patients, it marks the onset or worsening of pain at the end of the dosing interval or the regularly scheduled analgesic. In other patients, it is caused by an action of the patient, referred to as incident pain; sometimes the incident pain has a nonvolitional precipitant, such as flatulence. Most breakthrough pains are thought to be associated with a known malignant cause from direct tumor infiltration.

INTENSITY OF PAIN

Pain may also be defined on the basis of intensity, but there are limitations to a concept of pain based solely on its intensity.

In a study by Tearnan and associates, 451 cancer patients were asked to describe their pain in their own words.[42] A total of 129 distinct words were used by the patients; each patient used an average of 1.8 words. Ten words accounted for 67% of the total words used. Patients with specific pain etiologies could not be differentiated using word descriptors; in fact, the nature of the word did not define either the nature of the pain syndrome or its affective component.

Specific categorical scales of pain intensity have been used in which patients are asked to describe their pain as mild, moderate, severe, or excruciating.[43] Visual analogue scales have also been used.[19] These are often a 10-cm line anchored on either end by two points—no pain or worst possible pain—and the patient is asked to mark on the line the intensity of the pain. Numerical scales are commonly used, asking patients to rate their pain between "1=no pain" and "10=worst possible pain."

These scales have their limitations, but they are part of a series of validated instruments that include a measure of pain intensity as one of the components of the pain experience to be defined. In a study of physicians' and nurses' understanding of the language to describe pain, there was a close correlation among them of the level of intensity meant by the terms "ache," "hurt," or "pain."[44] Although health-care professionals may understand the common language of pain, there is an enormous discrepancy between their assessment and the patient's report of pain, particularly when the patient reports pain as moderate or severe. Peteet and colleagues interviewed cancer patients and physicians to obtain complete and direct information about pain treatment and the reasons for inadequate pain relief in individual cases.[10] They compared the ratings of pain severity by patients with those by physicians and found that patients tended to rate their pain as more intense than do physicians. In a study by Grossman and associates, the cancer patients' report of pain and the physicians' concurrent observation had a close correlation when patients reported mild pain.[45] However, when patients reported moderate to severe pain, the correlation of the nurse, house officer, and oncology fellow differed significantly from that of the patient: the concordance dropped from 78% for patients with mild pain to 20% for those with moderate to severe pain.

MEASUREMENT OF PAIN

These problems in communication about pain intensity strongly support the argument that multiple dimensions of the pain experience should be used to assess it adequately. Several validated instruments for pain measurement attempt to look at it in a multidimensional nature. The use of such methods can provide rapid evaluation in clinical settings of the major aspects of the pain experienced by cancer patients. Growing evidence suggests that they should be integrated into clinical trials and should be available for use on a routine basis to better define the pain symptomatology and to study the impact on pain by various treatment approaches.

Brief Pain Inventory

The Wisconsin Brief Pain Questionnaire is a self-administered, easily understood, brief method to assess pain.[46] It addresses the relevant aspects of pain (history, intensity, location, and

quality) and the pain's ability to interfere with the patient's activities, and helps to provide an understanding of its cause. The history of pain and its relation to the patient's disease is assessed initially. If the patient admits to pain in the last month, he or she answers questions about current manifestations of pain. If the patient has no pain, he or she skips to the end of the questionnaire to complete demographic information. For patients with pain, a human figure drawing is provided for the patient to shade the area corresponding to the pain. Patients are asked to rate their pain at its worst, usual pain, and pain now. The pain scales consist of numbers from zero to ten; zero is labeled "no pain" and ten is labeled "pain as bad as you can imagine." Patients are asked to report the medications or treatments they receive for pain, the percent relief that these medications or treatment provide, and their belief about the cause of their pain. Finally, they are asked to rate how much the pain interferes with their mood, relations with other people, and functional ability (walking, sleeping, working, enjoying life). All patients, including those without pain, are asked for basic demographic information about marital status, education, occupation, spouse's occupation, and months since diagnosis.

This inventory has been translated into several languages and has been used to assess pain in cancer patients in such diverse settings as Vietnam, Mexico, the Philippines, and the University of Wisconsin Cancer Center.[20,21] Data from these studies suggest that cancer pain patients from widely different cultural and linguistic backgrounds respond in a similar fashion to rating the severity of their cancer-related pain and the interference caused by the pain.

McGill Pain Questionnaire

The McGill Pain Questionnaire (MPQ) is an extensively used pain assessment instrument that produces scores on four empirically derived dimensions, as well as several summary scores.[47] The instrument consists of 78 adjectives that cluster in 20 categories. Within each category, the adjectives are arranged in order of intensity from low to high. The categories are divided into four dimensions: sensory, affective, evaluative, and miscellaneous. The patient is asked to choose one adjective from each applicable category that describes an aspect of his or her current pain, and the score for each dimension is obtained by adding the rank values of the selected adjectives. A total summary score is derived by adding the scores across the four dimensions, and a total word count is also obtained. Finally, a rating of present pain intensity is made on a five-point scale.

Studies with this instrument have demonstrated that the factors derived reflect specific sensory qualities and combined emotional and sensory dimensions. This tool has also been used to assess distinct score profiles according to the nature of pain. For instance, patients with acute pain tend to use more sensory words, but patients with chronic pain tend to use more affective and reaction word subgroups.

Graham and associates obtained detailed findings for both single and multiple administrations of the MPQ with subject samples each composed of 18 cancer outpatients with pain.[47] The results were compared with similar but less extensive data from cancer patients reported by Melzack, and the data were remarkably similar.[48] Patients in both the Melzack and

Graham studies had a high consistency of pain descriptor subclass choice, ranging from 66% to 80% over four administrations.

The MPQ offers a methodologic approach to assess the sensory, affective, and evaluative components of pain, but it may be more difficult and cumbersome for patients to understand and complete and may be limited by its language constraints.

Memorial Pain Assessment Card

The Memorial Pain Assessment Card (MPAC) (Fig. 64–1) was initially developed by the Analgesic Studies Section of Memorial Sloan-Kettering Cancer Center to assess the relative potency of new and standard analgesic drugs. In that context, this method was found repeatedly to be a valid, reliable, efficient, and sensitive measure.[49]

The MPAC consists of three visual analog scales (VAS) that measure pain intensity, pain relief, and mood, and a set of pain severity descriptors adapted from the Tursky rating scale.[50] The card is 8.5″ by 11″ and is folded in the middle so that the four sides can be quickly presented to the patient. Three sides are imprinted with the 100-mm-long VAS scale; the fourth side is the set of Tursky adjectives. The pain intensity VAS is anchored by the terms "least possible pain" and "worst possible pain." The patient is asked to place a mark along the line to indicate his or her subjective judgment of pain intensity. The score on this and the other VAS is obtained by measuring in millimeters the distance between the left end of the line and the patient's mark. The Tursky pain adjective scale is a categorical measure of pain intensity. Eight intensity descriptors, ranging from "no pain" to "excruciat-

ing," are printed in a random arrangement and the patient is asked to circle the adjective that describes his or her subjective experience of pain severity. Side 3 of the MPAC is a pain relief VAS. Patients are asked to indicate with a mark the degree of pain reduction they experience after the most recent intervention, which is usually the administration of an analgesic drug. On side 4 the VAS measures the subjective experience of mood; on this side patients are asked to rate their current feeling, from "worst" to "best." The instructions for administration of these scales are simple and readily understood, and an experienced patient can complete the four ratings in less than 20 seconds.

The MPAC has been compared to the MPQ, the Profile of Mood States Questionnaire (a standardized self-report instrument that measures six dimensions of mood, reflecting degree and type of psychological distress), the Hamilton Rating Scale for Depression (an interviewer-rated scale evaluating the presence and severity of 17 symptoms typical of clinical depression), and the Zung Anxiety Scale (a standardized self-report scale that reports the presence and severity of various symptoms of anxiety).[49,51-53] The MPAC and the MPQ both provide reasonably equivalent assessments of the intensity dimension of pain. However, the evaluative scales of the MPQ did not correlate significantly with any of the measures of the MPAC, suggesting that the cognitive judgmental dimension of pain may be independent of the experiences of intensity, relief, and mood. None of the MPQ subscales correlated significantly with the VAS ratings of mood and pain relief.

These observations have led to the conclusion that the VAS mood scale on the MPAC represents a much more global assessment of general psychological distress rather than a spe-

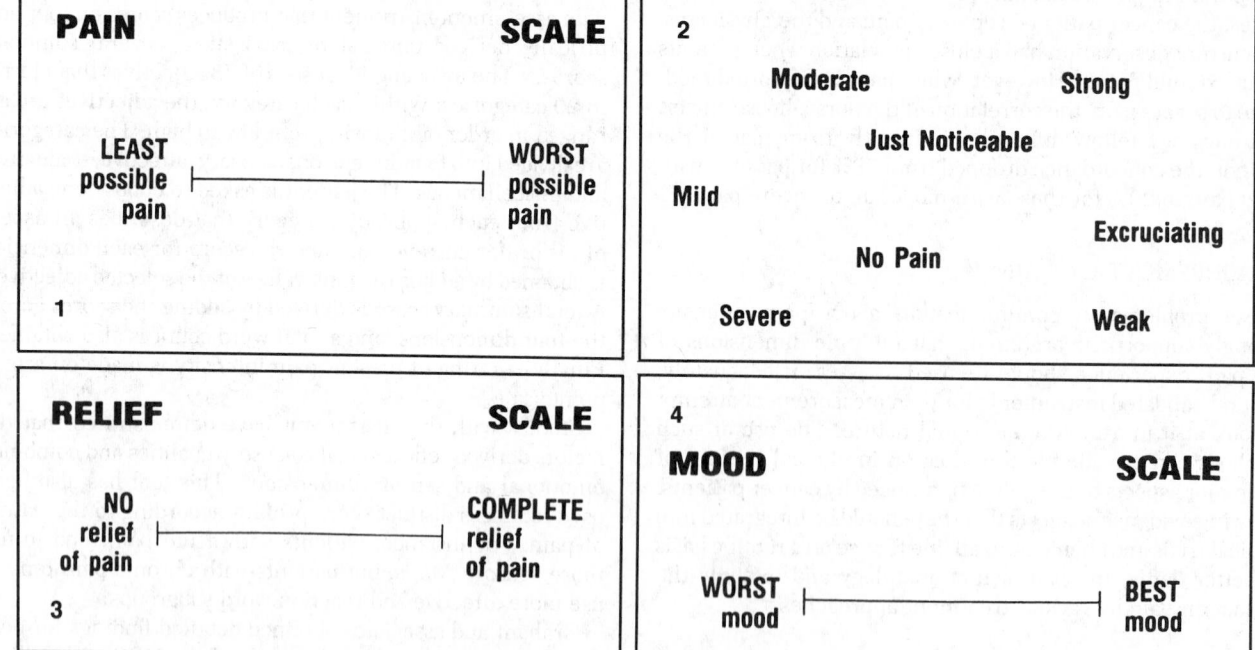

FIGURE 64–1. Memorial Pain Assessment Card, front (**1** and **4**) and back (**2** and **3**) sides. The card is folded along the broken line, and each measure is presented to the patient separately, in the numbered order. (1) Visual Analog Scale (VAS) Pain Intensity. (2) Modified Tursky Pain Descriptors Scale. (3) VAS Pain Relief. (4) VAS Mood. (Fishman B, Pasternak S, Wallenstein SL, Houde R, Holland JC, Foley KM. The Memorial Pain Assessment Card: A valid instrument for the evaluation of cancer pain. Cancer 1987;60:1151)

cific pain-related affect. This would suggest that the MPAC provides a broader assessment of the patient by its use of the mood scale, whereas the MPQ has a more narrow focus of simply representing pain-related emotional distress. What was particularly impressive was that in the use of any of the available scales, patients could differentiate pain and mood when they were explicitly asked. The perceptions of pain intensity and pain relief have different weights as components of psychological distress. The existence of such distinctions has important clinical and theoretical significance. Although the perception of pain intensity was found to contribute significantly to subjective distress, the perception of inadequate pain relief was a more important factor.

The MPAC provides valid, multidimensional information for the evaluation of pain and distress in cancer patients. It can distinguish pain intensity from pain relief and from global suffering, and it can be used to study the subtle interactions of these factors. With repeated administration it has now been demonstrated to be valid, reliable, easy to use, and nondisruptive. The MPAC and the BPI are the tools recommended for use in the clinical evaluation of individual patients and as an outcome measure in clinical trials.

CLASSIFICATION OF PATIENTS WITH CANCER PAIN

Five types of cancer pain patients can be identified, exemplifying the distinctions between acute and chronic pain (Table 64–2).[55] Although these categories are artificial, they serve as a useful preamble for discussion of the specific therapeutic approaches to the management of this group of patients.

Group I: Acute Cancer-Related Pain

Group I, patients with acute cancer-related pain, can be subdivided further according to etiology.

GROUP IA: TUMOR-ASSOCIATED PAIN. For Group IA patients, those with tumor-associated pain, pain is the major symptom prompting medical consultation and the diagnosis of cancer. In addition, pain has a special significance as the harbinger of their illness. Recurrent pain during the course of the illness or after successful therapy has the immediate

TABLE 64–2.   Types of Patients With Pain From Cancer

I. Patients With Acute Cancer-Related Pain
   a. Associated with the diagnosis of cancer
   b. Associated with cancer therapy (surgery, chemotherapy, or radiation)
II. Patients With Chronic Cancer-Related Pain
   a. Associated with cancer progression
   b. Associated with cancer therapy (surgery, chemotherapy, or radiation)
III. Patients With Preexisting Chronic Pain and Cancer-Related Pain
IV. Patients With a History of Drug Addiction and Cancer-Related Pain
   a. Actively involved in illicit drug use
   b. In methadone maintenance program
   c. With a history of drug abuse
V. Dying Patients With Cancer-Related Pain

implication of recurrent disease. Defining the cause of the pain may present a diagnostic problem, but effective treatment of its cause (*e.g.*, radiation therapy to bone metastases) usually is associated with dramatic pain relief in most patients.[56]

GROUP IB: PAIN ASSOCIATED WITH CANCER THERAPY. Group IB patients have postoperative pain, pain secondary to oral ulceration from chemotherapy, or myalgias secondary to steroid withdrawal. The cause of the pain is readily identifiable, and its course is predictable and self-limiting. These patients do not represent difficult diagnostic problems. Pain treatment directed at the cause of the pain is used to manage the transient symptoms. These patients endure significant pain for the promise of a successful outcome.

Group II: Chronic Cancer-Related Pain

Group II patients, those with chronic cancer-related pain, represent difficult diagnostic and therapeutic problems, in contrast to patients with acute cancer-related pain. They can be divided for discussion purposes into two groups: those with chronic pain from tumor progression, and those with chronic pain related to cancer treatment. Both groups share the characteristic of a pain symptom that has persisted for more than 3 months.

GROUP IIA: CHRONIC PAIN FROM TUMOR PROGRESSION. In patients with chronic pain associated with progression of disease (*e.g.*, patients with carcinoma of the pancreas, metastatic melanoma to bone, or Pancoast's syndrome), the pain escalates in intensity secondary to tumor infiltration of adjacent bone, nerve, or soft tissue.[58,59] Combinations of antitumor therapy, analgesic drug therapy, anesthetic blocks, and behavioral approaches to pain control are all applied with varying degrees of success. Psychological factors play a significant role in this group of patients, in whom palliative cancer therapy may be of little value and is physically debilitating.[60] The sense of hopelessness and fear of impending death may further add to and exaggerate the pain complaint; pain then becomes an aspect of the global "suffering" component.[61] Identifying both the pain and the "suffering" component is essential to the development of adequate therapy for these patients. The chronicity of the pain is associated with a series of psychological symptoms and signs, including sleep disturbances, reduced appetite, impaired concentration, or irritability, mimicking a depressive disorder. Management must be directed at controlling the pain, recognizing that antitumor therapy has failed. Analgesic therapy combined with a wide range of alternative approaches is necessary to provide adequate analgesia. Such patients are candidates for palliative care programs that address not only pain symptoms but the broader aspects of symptom management and psychological support.[23–25,62]

GROUP IIB: CHRONIC PAIN ASSOCIATED WITH CANCER THERAPY. Group IIB includes patients with chronic pain associated with cancer therapy, such as patients who develop pain after mastectomy, limb amputation (phantom limb), or thoracotomy. The nature of pain in these patients is secondary to nerve injury with the development of a traumatic neuroma. Treatment of the pain for these patients is limited by the lack of available methods to remove the cause of the pain. Again, treatment is directed at the symptoms, not the cause. These patients closely parallel those in the general population with chronic intractable pain syndromes. Psychological factors play a significant role in how these patients adapt to and function with chronic pain. Defining this group is imperative: identifying the cause of the pain as not directly related to tumor markedly alters the patient's therapy, prognosis, and psychological state. Each of the primary modalities of cancer therapy is associated with a series of specific chronic pain syndromes with characteristic pain patterns and clinical presentations (Table 64–3). Although it is consoling to both the patient and the physician to realize that the pain does not represent recurrent or progressive disease, the persistence of the pain is a constant reminder of the previous diagnosis of cancer.

In these patients, all approaches aimed at maintaining the patient's functional status should be used. Alternative methods of therapy, in contrast to drug therapy, represent the major management approach. This group of patients is increasing in number and accounts for 25% of patients referred to a medical pain clinic.

Group III: Preexisting Chronic Pain and Cancer-Related Pain

Group III includes patients with a history of chronic nonmalignant pain who develop cancer and pain. Psychological factors play a significant role in this group of patients, whose psychological and functional status is already compromised by their chronic nonmalignant pain state.[28] These patients are at high risk of developing further functional incapacity and escalating chronic pain symptoms. However, their history should not be used in a punitive way to minimize or deny their complaints. Identifying this group of patients as a high-risk group helps to improve their psychological assessment and intervention.

TABLE 64–3.   Pain Syndromes in Patients With Cancer

	References		References
Pain Syndromes Associated With Direct Tumor Involvement	1, 67	**Pain Syndromes Associated With Cancer Therapy**	
		Postsurgical Pain Syndromes	
Tumor Infiltration of Bone		Acute	67, 82
Metastases to the cranial vault	68	Postoperative pain	
Metastases to the base of skull	69	Chronic	
Jugular foramen syndrome		Postthoracotomy syndrome	
Clivus metastases		Postmastectomy syndrome	67, 83
Sphenoid sinus metastases		Postradical neck syndrome	67, 84, 85
Vertebral body syndromes	70, 71	Phantom limb syndrome	53
Fracture of the odontoid	72	*Postchemotherapy Pain Syndromes*	
C7–T1 metastases	59	Acute	57, 87
L1 metastases	73	Oral mucositis	
Sacral syndrome	74	Bladder spasms	88
Tumor Infiltration of Nerve		Jaw pain	89
Peripheral nerve	67	Diffuse bone pain	90
Peripheral neuropathy		Headache	90
Intercostal neuropathy	67	Chronic	89
Plexus	75, 76	Peripheral neuropathy	
Brachial plexopathy		Aseptic necrosis fo the femoral head	91
Lumbosacral plexopathy	73, 77	Steroid pseudorheumatism	92
Celiac plexopathy	58	Postherpetic neuralgia	33, 34, 93
Root	70	*Postradiation Pain Syndromes*	26
Radiculopathy		Acute	57
Leptomeningeal metastases	78, 79	Oral mucositis, esophagitis	
Spinal cord	70, 71	Skin burns	26
Epidural spinal cord compression		Chronic	75, 94
Intramedullary metastases	71	Radiation fibrosis of brachial and lumbar plexus	
Brain	68	Radiation myelopathy	95
Intracranial metastases		Radiation-induced second primary tumor	96, 97
Tumor Infiltration of Viscera		Radiation fibrosis of bone	98
Infiltration of pleura	80	*Infection-Induced Pain Syndromes*	
Small and large bowel obstruction	81	Infected fistula in genitourinary and gynecologic cancers	74
Infiltration of pelvis and bladder wall	74	Infected head and neck sites in head and neck cancer	99

Group IV: Patients With a History of Drug Addiction and Pain

Group IV includes patients with a history of drug addiction who have cancer-related pain. Three subgroups can be identified: patients actively involved in illicit drug use and drug-seeking behavior, those receiving methadone in a maintenance program, and those who have not used drugs for several years. Undertreatment with analgesic drugs occurs most commonly in this group of patients. Assessment of reported pain by physicians and nurses is colored by the fact that the pain symptoms are confused with drug-seeking behavior. Attention to the medical and psychological needs of these patients requires individualized assessment and consultation with experts in drug-related problems. The first subgroup represents a major management problem, straining the most tolerant of medical care systems.[63,64] Pain in the other two subgroups is readily managed, with the recognition that the psychological stresses consequent to the pain and cancer may place the patient at a high risk for recidivism.

Group V: Dying Patients With Pain

In dying patients in pain, diagnostic and therapeutic considerations are directed at maintaining the patient's comfort. This group is identified separately from Group II patients because the psychological factors further compound adequate pain management. The issues of hopelessness, death, and dying become more prominent, and the suffering component must be addressed.

Inadequate control of pain in the dying patient exacerbates the suffering component and demoralizes the family and the caregivers, who feel that they have failed in treating the patient's pain at a time when adequate treatment may matter the most. Rapid escalation of analgesic drug therapy, usually by the intravenous route, and attempts to ameliorate psychological symptoms should be used.

The risk-to-benefit ratios in analgesic approaches become less of an issue when the goal of pain therapy is the patient's comfort. In these patients, the physician must understand the temporal setting of pain in assessing the indications for and usefulness of the pain management approaches.

COMMON PAIN SYNDROMES

The common pain syndromes associated with cancer or cancer therapy are listed in Table 64–3. Numerous studies have demonstrated that pain in the cancer patient may have multiple causes. Several investigators have demonstrated that pain associated with direct tumor involvement is the most common cause; 78% of patients in an inpatient cancer pain population and 65% in an outpatient pain clinic were in this category.[11,65,66] Pain in bone is the most common site. Tumor infiltration of nerve and hollow viscus are the second and third most common painful sites.

A second category includes pain syndromes associated with cancer therapy. About 19% of patients in an inpatient population and 25% of those in an outpatient population were in this group.[1,12,66] The group includes patients in whom pain occurred during the course of therapy, during a therapeutic procedure, or as a result of chemotherapy, surgery, or radiation therapy. Each of these primary therapeutic modalities is associated with a series of specific pain syndromes with characteristic pain patterns and clinical presentations that have been well described in the literature.

The third major category of pain syndromes includes those unrelated to the cancer and the cancer therapy. About 3% of inpatients have pain unrelated to their cancer or cancer therapy; this figure increases to 10% in an outpatient cancer population.[1,12,65,66] Common syndromes seen in this population include osteoarthritis, lumbar disc disease, osteoporosis with a collapsed vertebral body, and peripheral neuropathy.

CLINICAL ASSESSMENT OF PAIN

Certain general principles should be followed in evaluating cancer patients who complain of pain. Lack of attention to these general principles is the major cause for misdiagnosis of a specific pain syndrome. As discussed above, multiple barriers exist in the assessment of pain, including the multidimensional nature of the subjective complaint of pain, the lack of a clearly defined language of pain, and poor communication between the patient and physician about pain (*e.g.*, underreporting by the patient and underassessing by the physician or nurse).[8] Sufficient information is now available on the scope of the problem of pain in cancer patients, and there are various assessment tools to refine and define the sensory and affective components of pain in this population; they should be integrated into clinical practice.

Adequate assessment is a critical component for defining the appropriate therapeutic strategy for each patient. The general principles are:

Believe the patient's complaint of pain.
Take a careful history of the patient's pain complaint.
Evaluate the patient's psychological state.
Perform a careful medical and neurologic examination.
Order and personally review the appropriate diagnostic studies.
Treat the pain to facilitate the appropriate workup.
Reassess the patient's response to therapy.
Individualize the diagnostic and therapeutic approaches.
Discuss advance directives with the patient and family.

Believe the Patient's Complaint of Pain

Critical to the management of the patient with cancer pain is the establishment of a trusting relationship with the physician. The complaint of pain is a symptom, not a diagnosis. Pain perception is not simply a function of the amount of physical injury sustained by the patient, but is a complex state determined by multiple factors. The diagnosis of a specific pain syndrome and a complete understanding of the patient's psychological state is not always made during the initial evaluation. In fact, it may take several weeks to define its nature because of the lack of radiologic or pathologic verification. It may take a similar period to fully comprehend each patient's psychological makeup. Numerous examples in the assessment of patients with pain and cancer highlight the limitation of the diagnostic process. It is not uncommon for patients with tumor infiltration of the brachial plexus from either lung or breast cancer to have pain for several weeks or months before the onset of objective radiologic and neurologic findings.[59,67]

A comprehensive evaluation involves taking a careful history, performing a detailed medical, neurologic, and psychological evaluation, developing a series of diagnosis-related hypotheses, and ordering the appropriate diagnostic studies.

Take a Careful History of the Patient's Pain Complaint

This should include the patient's description of:

Site of pain
Quality of pain
Exacerbating and relieving factors
Temporal pattern
Exact onset
Associated symptoms and signs
Interference with activities of daily living
Impact on the patient's psychological state
Response to previous and current analgesic therapies.

Multiple pain complaints are common in patients with advanced disease and must be ranked and classified.[3]

Evaluate the Patient's Psychological State

The patient's current level of anxiety and depression must be clarified and his or her past history of such symptoms must be defined. Knowledge of the patient's previous psychiatric history and need for past hospitalization for psychiatric care helps to clarify the patient's potential psychological risk.[60] Information on how the patient has handled previous painful events may provide insight into whether the patient has demonstrated chronic illness behavior or has a past history of a chronic pain syndrome.[40] It is important to know about a personal or family history of alcohol or drug dependence, to understand why the patient may be fearful or refuse to take opioid drugs.

Because each patient has his or her own understanding of the meaning of pain, it is useful to have the patient elaborate this meaning. Does he or she think it represents recurrent tumor, or is he or she convinced it is simply arthritis? Evidence suggests that when patients have a clear understanding of the meaning of their pain as representing recurrent tumor, they have increased psychological distress.

The importance of defining the psychological makeup of the patient with pain is supported by a variety of studies that have focused on the impact of suffering in patients with pain. Psychological factors play a significant role in accounting for the differences in pain experiences in cancer patients. A series of psychiatric syndromes have been described for cancer patients, with depression occurring in as many as 25% of patients.[60] The depression presents either as an acute stress response or as a major depression. Awareness of the common psychiatric syndromes when evaluating the pain complaint expands the physician's understanding of such a complaint.[60]

Although it is critical to know as much as possible about each patient with pain, some information may not be readily available in the first interview; in some instances it may never be available because of the lack of intellectual competence on the patient's part to define clearly the various components of the pain complaint. It is often necessary to verify the history from a family member who may provide information that the patient is unable or unwilling to provide. The family may be more objective in assessing a disability of a patient who underreports his or her symptoms. Similarly, in a patient who is a poor historian, the family member may be able to provide essential information that may alter the diagnostic approach. All attempts should be made to compile a careful history and define the medical, neurologic, and psychological profile of the pain complaint.

As patients become more active in defining advance directives and as they focus on the quality of life, it is critical to ask patients to define what they would do if the pain were intractable or intolerable. Do they have suicidal thoughts or a pact with a family member?[100] Do they have a family history of suicide? Do they have a family member who died a painful death? From our experience, patients who have had such an experience are particularly fearful of their own death.[16] Does the patient have drugs in reserve or a gun in the house that he or she might use in desperation? Such questions allow patients to discuss openly their fears of death and their need to take matters into their own hands rather than trust the healthcare professional. Such open discussions can allow the physician to better define for the patient the options for care and to reassure the patient of the physician's commitment to care.[16] Because patients rarely offer this information unless requested, it is critical to develop specific questions that can be readily integrated into the initial history taken by the physician.

Perform a Careful Medical and Neurologic Examination

A medical and neurologic examination helps provide the necessary data to substantiate the history. Knowledge of the referral patterns of pain and the common cancer pain syndromes can direct the examination.[101] The characteristics of pain in breast-cancer patients with brachial plexopathy are so specific that they can help define the diagnosis of tumor infiltration of the brachial plexus from radiation fibrosis of the brachial plexus.[67,70] Similarly, the commonly described pain syndromes in cancer patients associated with a postmastectomy pain syndrome can readily be defined as separate from tumor infiltration of the brachial plexus.[71]

The physical and neurologic examination allows the physician to visually inspect and palpate the site of pain and to look for the associated physical and neurologic signs that might help to better define the nature of the pain symptom. Defining the degree of motor or sensory changes can help define the specific site in the nervous system that may be involved. Similarly, in patients with sensory loss, the presence of allodynia and hyperesthesia can further define the nature of the sensory problem. Moreover, the degree of muscle spasm, gait instability, and impaired coordination can only be fully assessed by such an evaluation.

Order and Personally Review the Appropriate Diagnostic Studies

Diagnostic studies confirm the diagnosis and define in patients with metastatic disease the site and extent of tumor infiltration. Computed transaxial tomography and MRI are the most useful diagnostic procedures in evaluating cancer patients with pain. The bone scan is a useful screening device and is more sensitive for demonstrating abnormalities in bone before changes appear on plain radiographs. However, a negative bone scan does not rule out bony metastatic disease, nor does a positive bone scan confirm the diagnosis of metastatic tumor. The physician should review the results personally with the radiologist to correlate any pathologic change with the site of pain.

Evaluation of the extent of metastatic disease may help to discover the relation of the pain complaint to possible recurrent disease. The use of tumor markers such as CEA, CA125, CA153, and PSA can be very useful in a patient in whom recurrent tumor is suspected. In certain pain syndromes the presence of recurrent disease is closely associated with the onset of pain (*e.g.,* in the appearance of late postthoracotomy pain syndrome in a patient after initial resolution of the postoperative pain).[72]

Treat the Pain to Facilitate the Appropriate Workup

No patient should be evaluated inadequately because of a significant pain problem. Early management of the pain while investigating the source will markedly improve the patient's ability to participate in the necessary diagnostic procedures. During the initial evaluation of the pain complaint, early consideration of the use of alternative methods of pain control, including anesthetic and neurosurgical approaches, should be considered (*e.g.,* the temporary use of a local anesthetic via an epidural catheter to manage sacral pain or the use of a percutaneous cordotomy in the patient with unilateral pain below the waist from a lumbosacral plexopathy). These approaches should not be considered for use only when all else fails, but should be an integral part of the assessment of the patient with pain.

Reassess the Patient's Response to Therapy

Continual reassessment of the response of the patient's pain complaint to the prescribed therapy provides the best method to validate the initial diagnosis as correct. If relief is less than predicted or if the pain worsens, reassessment of the treatment approach or a search for a new cause of the pain should be considered. A common example is the patient with epidural cord compression who develops a second block proximal to the one being radiated, with neurologic signs mimicking the original one.

Individualize the Diagnostic and Therapeutic Approach

Evaluation of the patient must be closely linked to the patient's level of function, ability to participate in the diagnostic workup, and willingness to undergo the necessary diagnostic approaches; objective evidence that treatment approaches may be beneficial; and life expectancy. Careful judgment is required to select diagnostic approaches that will have a direct impact on the choice of the therapeutic strategy or will answer a specific question. The random use of diagnostic procedures in these patients, particularly those with advanced cancer and significant pain, is inappropriate because it may have an adverse effect on their quality of life. Open discussion with the

patient about the need for assessment as well as the therapeutic options is critical to allow the patient to be part of the decision-making process. In some patients, diagnostic procedures such as myelography or MRI are inappropriate because they will simply confirm the existence of a disease for which no treatment is available, or for which the treatment would be a major surgical procedure (*e.g.,* vertebral body resection) that would be inappropriate for a dying patient. Patient refusal of evaluation or treatment must be respected when the physician has fully explained the options and is convinced that the patient has an accurate understanding of the implications of no further workup or treatment.[16,103,104]

Discuss Advance Directives With the Patient and Family

When developing approaches for treatment, there must be an open discussion about advance directives so that the physician has a clear understanding of the patient's goal for therapy or his or her ambivalence in developing a therapeutic strategy. The physician must have unconditional positive regard for the patient, placing the control of symptoms of pain and treatment of psychological distress in the highest regard. Knowledge of the patient's decisions about resuscitation, living wills, and symptom management should he or she become incompetent improves the physician's ability to appropriately and humanely care for the dying patient with advanced disease.[73,74]

IMPACT OF A COMPREHENSIVE EXAMINATION ON THE MANAGEMENT OF CANCER PAIN

Although a comprehensive medical and neurologic evaluation is needed in cancer pain treatment, the full impact of such approaches are currently under study. The following information comes from a study of pain service consultations in a retrospective review of 226 consecutive consultations in a total of 190 patients and in 50 consecutive consultations evaluated prospectively in 46 patients.[66] Based on the history, examination, and results of imaging procedures, a pain diagnosis was derived and included the delineation of a somatic, visceral, or neuropathic lesion. Sixty percent of the consultations were requested in patients with known metastatic disease; in 64% of retrospectively studied consult patients and 64% of consultations evaluated prospectively a lesion was newly identified through the pain evaluation performed by the consultant. More than 50% of diagnoses were neurologic; the most common diagnosis was epidural spinal cord compression. The pain service evaluation resulted in a change of treatment and provided an opportunity for primary antineoplastic therapies to be considered. Radiation therapy was offered to 19% of the retrospective group and to 12% of the prospective study patients. Two percent of patients from both studies received chemotherapy, and 1% of retrospective study patients and 4% of prospective study patients were referred to surgery on the basis of the pain evaluation.

The prospective survey also tabulated specific neurologic diagnoses both related and unrelated to the pain complaint. Thirty-four percent (17 patients) had a neurologic diagnosis before evaluation by the pain consultant. Nine of the 17 diagnoses were confirmed, and the consultation led to a new neurologic diagnosis in an additional 18 patients. Thus, neurologic evaluation by the pain consultant confirmed neurologic diagnoses in 54% of patients; the most prevalent of these were epidural spinal cord compression in 9 and lumbosacral plexopathy in 9. Eight more cases of malignant lumbosacral plexopathy were identified by the pain consultant, far more than any other neurologic condition in this group of patients.

This study supports the observation that new pathology is commonly identified through a comprehensive assessment of pain in cancer patients. Equally important, many of these lesions were amenable to primary therapy, which may have direct analgesic consequences. About one fifth of the patients received primary antineoplastic therapy based on the pain evaluation, and another 6% received antibiotics.

Although the high prevalence of neurologic diagnoses may represent a bias in this Memorial study, it is critical to recognize that neurologic lesions make up a substantial portion of painful lesions in the cancer population. In a prospective study of the neurologic symptoms, neurologic diagnoses, and primary tumors in all patients with a history of systemic cancer referred to the Memorial Hospital's Neurology Consultation Service, the three most common symptoms in 851 patients were back pain (18.2%), altered mental status (17.1%), and headache (15.4%).[75] The most common neurologic diagnoses was brain metastases (15.9%), followed by metabolic encephalopathy (10.2%), pain associated with bone metastases only (9.9%), and epidural extension or metastases of tumor (8.4%). Physicians evaluating patients with cancer pain must have sufficient knowledge of these neurologic complications of cancer to appropriately evaluate and treat these patients.

MANAGEMENT OF CANCER PAIN

Recent advances in pain research provide the scientific rationale for using new, improved methods of treatment, including better and more effective use of standard drug therapy (nonnarcotic, narcotic, and adjuvant analgesic drugs), the development of new drugs, the use of novel methods and routes of drug administration, and the use of selective anesthetic and neurosurgical approaches to control pain. A variety of medical and surgical approaches to the management of cancer pain are currently available. The use of such techniques often depends on the clinical expertise in a particular center. Approaches such as drug therapy and some of the behavioral methods should be within the armamentarium of any physician or nurse who cares for patients with pain and cancer. Other approaches, such as specific anesthetic and neurosurgical techniques, require trained medical personnel who have clinical experience in managing cancer pain.

DRUG THERAPY

Analgesic drugs can be divided into three groups: nonnarcotic analgesics, such as aspirin and acetaminophen, and the nonsteroidal antiinflammatory drugs (NSAIDs), which act on the peripheral mechanisms of pain; narcotic agonist and antagonist drugs, which activate opiate receptors in the central and peripheral nervous system and mediate analgesia; and adju-

vant analgesic drugs that produce analgesia in certain pain states (*e.g.*, amitriptyline in postherpetic neuralgia) or potentiate the opioid analgesics (Table 64–4).

Nonopioid Analgesics

Nonopioid analgesics are the drugs of choice for mild to moderate pain. The mechanism of action of their analgesic effect is controversial, but it is thought that they reduce or prevent sensitization of pain receptors to nociceptive stimuli by preventing prostaglandin synthesis through inhibition of cyclooxygenase activity. Their mechanism of action also includes nonprostaglandin inhibitory effects.[106] This class of drugs consists of a heterogenous group of substances that differ in chemical structure and pharmacologic action. Many of these drugs have analgesic, antiinflammatory, and antipyretic properties. All of the drugs in this class have an analgesic potency similar to or greater than that of aspirin. However, the analgesic effects of these drugs have a ceiling; that is, escalating the dose beyond a certain level does not produce additive analgesia. Experimental evidence suggests that these drugs may play a special role in the pain management of patients with bone metastases because of the documented role of prostaglandins in bone resorption in metastatic bone disease. Aspirin has been shown to have an antitumor effect in an animal bone tumor model.[107]

TABLE 64–4. Guidelines for the Rational Use of Analgesics in the Management of Cancer Pain

Start with a specific drug for a specific type of pain
Know the pharmacology of the drug prescribed
    Know the relative potency of the drug
    Know the duration of the analgesic effect
    Know the pharmacokinetics of the drug
    Know the equianalgesic doses for the drug and its route
      of administration
Administer analgesic on a regular basis
Gear the route of administration to the patient's needs

Oral	Sublingual
Buccal	Transmucosal
Rectal	Transdermal
Subcutaneous	Intravenous
Intrathecal	Intraventricular

Use a combination of drugs to provide additive analgesia
    Narcotic plus nonnarcotic (aspirin, acetaminophen, NSAIDs)
    Narcotic plus adjuvants
Anticipate and treat side effects
    Sedation
    Respiratory depression
    Nausea and vomiting
    Constipation
    Multifocal myoclonus and seizures
Management of the tolerant patient
    Use combinations of nonopioid and opioid drugs
    Use combinations of drug therapy, anesthetic and neurosurgical
      procedures
    Switch to an alternative opioid analgesic starting with half the
      equianalgesic dose
    Use epidural local anesthetics
    Reassess the nature of the pain
Prevent and treat acute withdrawal
    Taper drugs slowly
Anticipate complications
    Overdose
    Psychological dependence

In clinical practice, this class of drugs represents the first-line approach to the management of cancer pain with analgesics, but the choice and use of the nonnarcotic must be individualized. Each patient should be given an adequate trial of one nonnarcotic analgesic before switching to an alternative one. Such a trial should include administration of the drug to maximal levels at regular intervals. The gastrointestinal and hematologic side effects often limit their long-term use. There is controversy over the use of prophylactic antiulcer agents in cancer patients receiving these drugs. Histamine H_2 antagonist drugs reduce the incidence of gastroscopically diagnosed NSAID-induced duodenal ulcers.[108] It is unclear whether such an effect is associated with a decreased rate of perforation or bleeding. The duration of treatment with antiulcer agents concurrent with the use of these drugs is also under study. In cancer patients, the concurrent use of steroids should be avoided to limit the gastric effects of these two combinations.

For the patient with moderate pain, adding a narcotic to the nonnarcotic provides additive analgesia. Combinations with codeine, oxycodone, and propoxyphene are available, but these combinations often contain less than the full dose of 650 mg aspirin or acetaminophen. Prescribing each drug separately provides for a better method of individualizing pain control. This is particularly important when the patient requires escalation of the combination to provide analgesia, in which case the additional dosage of the NSAID may become excessive.

Several NSAIDs have been approved by the Food and Drug Administration for use as analgesics for mild to moderate pain and are listed in Table 64–5.

Guidelines for the use of NSAIDs in patients with cancer pain are largely empiric and drawn from clinical experience. If antiinflammatory effects are not essential and analgesia is the only goal, acetaminophen is probably safer than other NSAIDs, although it clearly has the potential for renal toxicity. Appropriate first-line drugs in patients with a bleeding diathesis or peptic ulcer disease should include acetaminophen and two of the salicylates—choline magnesium trisalicylate and salicylate. These are reported to have lower ulcer potential than other NSAIDs and at usual clinical doses do not impair platelet aggregation.

Because there is great variability among patients in their responses to different drugs, patients may require trials with several NSAIDs before finding an effective drug and dose regimen. Some authors have suggested that several weeks are necessary to judge the efficacy of the dose in the treatment of rheumatologic disorders. However, as an analgesic, pain relief should be obtained once steady-state levels are achieved (these depend on the drug's half-life and occur within three to five half-lives). If pain relief is not obtained, an alternative drug trial should be considered.

Opioid Agonists and Antagonists

The opioid analgesics, of which morphine is the prototype, vary in potency, efficacy, and adverse effects. These drugs produce their analgesic effects by binding to discrete opiate receptors in the peripheral and central nervous system. This group also includes a series of heterogenous substances with varying chemical structures. In contrast to the nonopioid analgesics, opioid analgesics do not appear to have a ceiling effect; that is, as the dose is escalated on a log scale, the increment in analgesia is linear to the point of loss of consciousness. Effective use of the opioid analgesics requires the balancing of the most desirable effects of pain relief to the undesirable effects of nausea, vomiting, mental clouding, sedation, constipation, tolerance, and physical dependence. These undesirable effects impose a practical limit on the dose useful for a particular patient.

Much of the difficulty encountered in the clinical use of these drugs arises from individual variation and differences of response of specific patients to the same drug dose. This difficulty is compounded by the lack of pharmacologic and pharmacokinetic data on many of the narcotic analgesics. This lack of information on the clinical pharmacology of these drugs and a series of uncontrolled survey-type studies have led to several controversies in the drug management of cancer pain. These include the type of pain that is responsive to opioid analgesics, the choice of the opioid drug, the appropriate route and method of administration, the extent to which tolerance limits the usefulness of opioid analgesics chronically, and concern about the risk of psychological dependence and substance abuse.[15,110,111] These controversies continue to affect the rational use of opioid analgesics in clinical practice.

Table 64–6 summarizes the most commonly used agents.

Principles of Opioid Drug Therapy

Start With a Specific Drug for a Specific Type of Pain. The WHO Cancer Pain Relief Program has advocated the use of an analgesic ladder (Fig. 64–2).[4] This approach advocates the use of nonopioid, opioid, and adjuvant analgesics alone or in combinations titrated to the needs of each patient.

Nonopioid drugs are the first-line approach for the patient with mild to moderate pain.[112] If pain is not relieved or if the side effects of the nonopioid are intolerable, opioid analgesics should be used.

Codeine, propoxyphene, and oxycodone (5 mg) make up the second step of the WHO analgesic ladder. These drugs have a higher analgesic potential than the nonopioids and are most often used in fixed oradose mixtures, limiting their use in increasing doses.

For moderate to severe pain—the third step of the ladder—morphine-hydromorphone, oxycodone, levorphanol, methadone, and oxymorphone are the drugs most commonly used. Chronic administration of meperidine produces central nervous system irritability and is not recommended for chronic cancer pain management.[113] Heroin is unavailable in the United States but has been demonstrated to be comparable to morphine in its analgesic, mood, and side effects.[114] Heroin does not bind to the opiate receptor and represents a pro-drug that must be metabolized to morphine and 6-acetylmorphine to produce it analgesic effects.[115]

WHO has recommended morphine as the drug of choice for cancer pain by the oral route based on its position on the Essential Drug List and has requested that it be made available worldwide. Alternatives to morphine include hydromorphone and levorphanol, both congeners of morphine. Hydromorphone has poor oral bioavailability with a short half-life. It is highly soluble and available in high-potency form (10 mg/ml). It is a useful alternative to morphine and to levorphanol. Levorphanol has good bioavailability but a long plasma half-life (12 to 16 hours). It must be used cautiously because with

TABLE 64–5. Nonopioid and Adjuvant Analgesic Drugs in the Management of Cancer Pain

Class/Drug	Indications	Starting Oral Dose (mg) and Range/24 h)	Comments
NSAIDs			
Aspirin	Soft-tissue and metastatic bone pain	650 650–1000	Used together with opioids, GI and hematologic effects; avoid combination with steroids
Acetaminophen	Like aspirin	650 650–1000	Fewer GI effects, no effects on platelet function, no significant antiinflammatory effects
Ibuprofen		400 200–800	Higher analgesic potential than aspirin, fewer GI and hematologic effects than aspirin
Choline magnesium trisalicylate	Like aspirin	1500 1000–4000	Antiinflammatory and analgesic effects, similar to aspirin without hematologic effects
Fenoprofen	Like aspirin	200 200–400	Like ibuprofen
Diflunisal	Like aspirin	500 500–1000	Longer duration of action than ibuprofen, higher analgesic potential than aspirin
Naproxen	Like aspirin	250 250–500	Like diflunisal
Anticonvulsants			
Phenytoin	Neuropathic pain acute lancinating type (tic)	100 100–300	Start with low dose, titrate slowly
Carbamazepine	Neuropathic pain acute lancinating type (tic)	100 200–800	Useful in paroxysmal nerve pain
Antidepressants			
Amitriptyline Imipramine	Neuropathic pain (*e.g.*, postherpetic neuralgia)	10 10–150	Start at low dose and titrate slowly; has analgesic properties
Antihistamines			
Hydroxyzine	Somatic and visceral pain	25 25–100	Additive analgesia in combination with opioids; antiemetic, antianxiety properties
Phenothiazines			
Methotrimeprazine	Somatic and visceral pain; useful in opioid-tolerant patients with GI obstruction and pain	5–15 IM	Anxiolytic and antiemetic effects; available only in IM preparation
Steroids			
Prednisone	Somatic and neuropathic pain (*e.g.*, inflammatory bone pain)	5 5–60	Antiinflammatory, antiemetic, analgesic effects
Dexamethasone	Reflex sympathetic dystrophy; brachial, lumbar plexopathy	0.5–16	
Neurostimulants			
Dextroamphetamine	Somatic and visceral pain (*e.g.*, postoperative pain)	2.5 2.5–10	Additive analgesia in combination with opioids; reduces sedative effects
Methylphenidate	Opioid-induced sedation	5 5–15	Additive analgesia in combination with opioids; reduces sedative effects
Caffeine		300 300–600	Additive analgesia in combination with opioids; reduces sedative effects

TABLE 64-6. Opioid Analgesics for Management of Cancer Pain

Drug and Equianalgesic Dose Relative Potency	mg IM/PO	Plasma Half-Life (h)	Starting* Oral Dose (mg)	Available Commercial Preparations
Morphine	10 IM 60 PO	3–4	30–60	Oral: tablet, liquid, slow-release tab Rectal: 5 mg–30 mg Injectable: SC, IM, I.V., epidural, intrathecal
Hydromorphone	1.5 IM 7.5 PO	2–3	2–48	Oral: tablets: 1, 2, 4, mg Injectable: SC, IM, I.V. 2 mg/ml & HP 10 mg/ml
Methadone	10 IM 20 PO	12–24	5–10	Oral: tablets, liquid Injectable: SC, IM, I.V.
Levorphanol	2 IM 4 PO	12–16	2–4	Oral: tablets Injectable: SC, IM, I.V.
Oxymorphone	1	2–3	NA	Rectal: 10 mg Injectable: SC, IM, I.V.
Heroin	5 IM 60 PO	3–4	NA	NA
Meperidine	75 IM 300 PO	3–4 (normeperidine, 12–16)	75	Oral: tablets Injectable: SC, IM, I.V.
Codeine	130 200	3–4	60	Oral: tablets and combination with ASA, acetaminophen, liquid
Oxycodone	15 30	—	5	Oral: tablets, liquid, oral formulation in combination with acetaminophen (tab and liquid) and aspirin (tab)

For these equianalgesic IM doses, the time of peak analgesia in nontolerant patients ranges from 30 minutes to 1 hour and the duration from 4 to 6 hours. The peak analgesic effect is delayed and the duration prolonged after oral administration.
* These doses are recommended starting IM doses from which the optimal dose for each patient is determined by titration and the maximal dose limited by adverse effects.

repeated administration accumulation will occur. Oxymorphone is only available in parenteral and suppository forms, limiting its wide use.

The role of methadone in cancer pain remains the most controversial.[109,116,117] Its bioavailability is 85%, and in single-dose studies its oral-to-parenteral potency ratio is 1:2. Its plasma half-life averages 24 hours but may range from 13 to 50 hours; its duration of analgesia is often only 4 to 8 hours. Repetitive analgesic doses of methadone lead to drug accumulation because of the discrepancy between its plasma half-life and the duration of analgesia. Sedation, confusion, and even death can occur when patients are not carefully monitored. The clinical use of methadone requires greater sophistication, and it should be considered as a second-line drug most useful in the patient with some prior opioid experience and a degree of tolerance. In the opioid-naive patient, initial doses should be titrated carefully.

The roles of the narcotic partial agonists such as buprenorphine and the mixed agonist-antagonists such as pentazocine, butorphanol, and nalbuphine are limited in cancer pain management.[118] Buprenorphine is available in the United States in a parenteral form only but is available worldwide in sublingual form. It is a useful first-line drug before the use of full agonist drugs because its analgesic efficacy is reduced in patients receiving narcotic-agonist drugs. Pentazocine is the only mixed agonist-antagonist available orally, but in the

United States it is available only in combination with naloxone, aspirin, or acetaminophen. Escalation of the dose of pentazocine produces psychotomimetic effects, limiting its usefulness in chronic cancer pain management.

In short, the choice of the opioid analgesic depends on the patient's prior opioid experience and physical and neurologic status. Individualization is the rule.

Know the Equianalgesic Dose of the Drug and Its Route of Administration. Knowing the equianalgesic dose can ensure more appropriate drug use. Lack of attention to these differences in drug dose is the most common cause of undermedication of pain patients.[8] These doses have been derived from assessment of the relative analgesic potency of a drug.[119] Relative potency is the ratio of the doses of two analgesics required to produce the same effect. Estimates of relative potency allow calculation of the equianalgesic dose, which provides the basis for selecting the appropriate dose when switching drugs or the route of administration of the same drug. The values in Table 64–6 are based on studies in which 10 mg morphine was the standard dose. The equianalgesic dose is the recommended starting dose, with the optimal dose for each patient determined by dose adjustment.

Table 64–6 can be useful, but its limitations also need to be understood. One important controversy is the reported difference in relative potency for morphine. On the basis of a

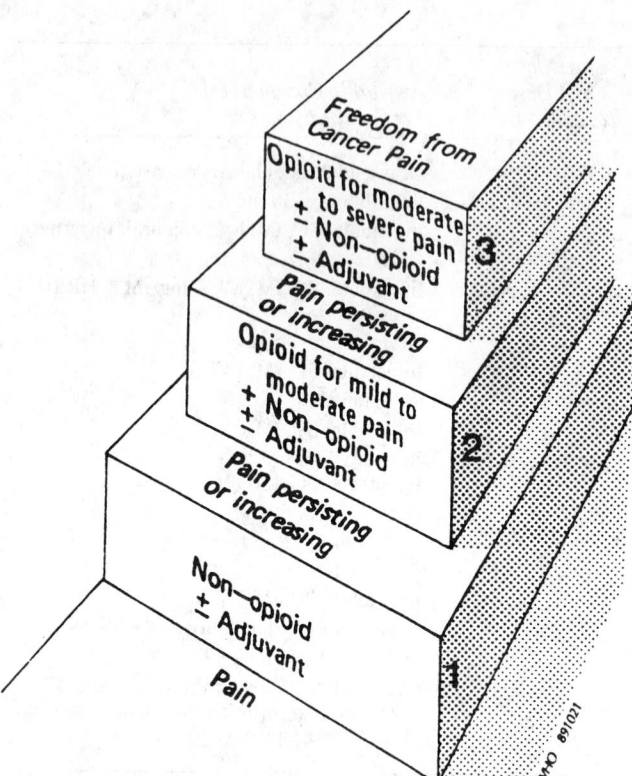

FIGURE 64–2. The World Health Organization's three-step ladder approach to analgesic drug therapy. (World Health Organization. Cancer pain relief. Geneva: World Health Organization, 1986)

series of survey studies, Twycross has suggested that the relative potency of morphine with repeated administration is 1:2 or 1:3.[120] As judged by single-dose studies in patients with both acute and chronic pain, the relative potency of intramuscular to oral morphine is 1:6.[119] The reason for this discrepancy relates to the fact that relative potency may differ in single-dose and repeated-dose studies. In practice, the 1:6 relative analgesic potency ratio should be used for patients with acute pain, the 1:2 or 1:3 ratio in patients treated with repeated doses on a chronic basis. Because of this discrepancy, patients are often undermedicated with morphine during the initial titration when a 1:3 ratio is used. Recent evidence suggests that morphine has an active metabolite, morphine-6-glucuronide, that may account for this difference.[121–123]

Administer Analgesics Regularly After Initial Titration. Medication should be given regularly, even if it means awakening the patient. The pharmacologic rationale of this approach is to maintain the plasma level of the drug above the minimum effective concentration for pain relief. In the initial titration patients should be advised to take their medication as needed to determine their total 24-hour requirements. This is also the timeframe for reaching the steady-state level of drug, which depends on the drug's half-life. For morphine, steady state can be reached in 24 hours; with methadone it may take up to 5 to 7 days to reach steady state. Therefore, full assessment of the analgesic efficacy of a drug regimen may take several days.

In patients on a fixed schedule, rescue medications equivalent to one half-life of the standing dose should be available to patients for breakthrough pain. This allows the physician to start with a safe dose and to use the total dose of rescue medication added to the fixed dose as the dose necessary on a 24-hour basis. Continuous intravenous and subcutaneous opioid infusions to manage both acute and chronic cancer pain are commonly used with a patient-controlled analgesic pump. The pump can be programmed to the patient's needs with a set "lock-out time" to prevent overdosing. This method of drug administration is very useful to manage patients with breakthrough pain. It is a significant advance in facilitating adequate titration of analgesics in chronic cancer patients, allowing discharge to home and hospice settings.[125]

Gear the Route of Administration to the Patient's Needs. Various methods of drug delivery of opioids have been developed in an attempt to maximize pharmacologic effects and minimize side effects. A recent review of the patterns of drug use in cancer pain patients throughout their illness demonstrates that from the onset of pain until death, most patients needed at least two routes of drug administration; 20% needed up to four approaches.[24] These data emphasize the need for these alternative routes and the development of guidelines for chronic drug management.

The oral route is preferable and easy. In general, orally administered drugs have a slower onset of action, delayed peak time, and longer duration of effect; drugs given parenterally have a rapid onset of action but a shorter duration of effect. Sustained-release preparations of morphine allow more convenient dosing of cancer pain patients every 8 to 12 hours. These preparations have found wide acceptance in clinical practice.[127,128]

For cancer therapy by the sublingual route, sublingual buprenorphine is used as part of the second step of the WHO analgesic ladder. The tablet is rapidly absorbed in 3 to 5 minutes with a 55% bioavailability.[118] In contrast, morphine is poorly absorbed by this route but reported anecdotally to be effective, probably secondary to swallowing the drug. Both fentanyl and methadone are well absorbed sublingually, but no commercial preparations exist.[129]

The buccal route has been studied with morphine, and absorption occurs if the tablet remains in contact with the gum for 1 to 2 hours.[130] This approach is impractical.

The transmucosal route has more advantages than the buccal route. Oral transmucosal fentanyl citrate (OTFC) is a new formulation of fentanyl incorporated into a palatable form for dissolution and absorption through the oral mucosa.[131] It produces rapid onset of analgesia, anxiolysis, and sedation in pediatric preoperative patients and in a pilot study in cancer pain has been used to provide rapid onset of analgesia in breakthrough pain.

For the rectal route, oxymorphone, hydromorphone, and morphine are available in suppositories. Oxymorphone suppositories (10 mg) produce analgesia equivalent to 10 mg of parenteral morphine.[132] Morphine pharmacokinetics after rectal absorption are controversial, and there are not enough data to clarify whether this route, like the oral route, undergoes presystemic elimination via the liver. Several studies support the use of sustained-release preparations of morphine that provide comparable analgesia via rectal absorption. The route similarly is practical for patients who require parenteral drug administration.

The transdermal route is a convenient way to deliver a potent, short-acting opioid on a continuous basis.[133] The drug is released through skin patches at a nearly constant amount per unit time with a concentration gradient from patch to skin. Serum fentanyl concentrations increase and steady-state levels are approached at 12 to 24 hours. After patch placement, the drug persists on the skin, with falling blood levels over 24 hours. In calculating the equianalgesic dose, a 1:20 to 1:30 ratio of fentanyl to parenteral morphine is being used in patients not tolerant to opioids.[133]

Parenteral routes include intermittent and continuous subcutaneous, intravenous, epidural, intraventricular, or intrathecal infusions.

The use of intermittent and continuous subcutaneous infusions avoids presystemic clearance by the liver and is most useful in patients who cannot tolerate oral analgesics because of gastrointestinal obstruction or intractable nausea and vomiting. It is the approach of choice for the patient with gastrointestinal obstruction and pain. Numerous series have reported the usefulness of this technique using morphine, heroin, hydromorphone, methadone, and levorphanol.[125,134,135] Pumps designed to infuse continuously but with options for bolus administration are connected to a 27-gauge butterfly needle that the patient can insert into a new subcutaneous site every third to sixth day. Focal erythematous swelling at the site of injection has been reported to occur for both morphine and methadone, appearing several months after the start of therapy.[135] Limited pharmacokinetic studies have demonstrated that systemic absorption of the drug from subcutaneous sites at steady state has a 70% to 100% bioavailability with hydromorphone.[136]

Intermittent and continuous intravenous infusions are used if intravenous access is available and the patient is hospitalized. This route allows for rapid titration of a patient in acute pain. Specific guidelines for the use of continuous infusions in patients with chronic pain have been developed.[137] This approach, as well as continuous subcutaneous infusion, is used to manage the dying cancer pain patient. The goal of therapy must be clearly delineated for patients, families, and staff to alleviate any concern that such an approach is a form of euthanasia. The intent is to provide patients with continuous relief of pain and suffering.[16]

Intermittent and continuous epidural and intrathecal opioid infusions are based on the demonstration of opiate receptors in the dorsal horn of the spinal cord and the ability of opioid drugs to suppress noxious stimuli at the spinal cord level.[35,36] Localized selective analgesia is produced without motor or sensory blockade. This approach has been developed to minimize the distribution of drugs to receptors in the brain stem and cerebral hemispheres, thereby avoiding the problematic side effects of systemic administration of opiates (sedation, drowsiness, and respiratory depression). The use of an intermittent bolus of opioid via an epidural catheter has been compared with continuous opioid administration, and both approaches provide effective analgesia.[138] The pharmacokinetics of epidural opioid administration demonstrate that there is significant systemic uptake after epidural injection, comparable to an intramuscular injection of the same drug and dose.[138] However, distribution of the drug directly into the cerebrospinal fluid is 10 to 100 times greater. Continuous epidural and intrathecal infusions have also been used with implanted pumps. Intrathecal administration has limited systemic uptake, making this theoretically a more useful approach. However, after both epidural and intrathecal administration there is significant rostral redistribution of drug in the cerebrospinal fluid, and rapid development of tolerance has been reported.

The clinical dilemmas are at what point should this approach be considered in the management of cancer patients with pain, and what are the risk-to-benefit ratios in the individual patient. Significant cross-tolerance is induced by systemic opiates, confounding the indications for this approach. Controlled analgesic studies of this approach in the long-term management of cancer patients are needed. Existing studies demonstrate that 10% of cancer patients need this approach to maximize analgesia. It is particularly useful when combined with local anesthetics in patients with neuropathic pain.[37,38,138–140]

For intermittent and continuous intraventricular opioid infusion, the major indication is pain in the cervical and craniofacial region from tumor infiltration. Doses between 1 and 7.5 mg/24 hours have been used, and patients have reported 70% excellent results, 25% good results, and 5% poor results.[141–143] The indications for this procedure, the type of pain, and the prior opioid exposure of the patients have not been fully delineated, making this a rarely used approach.

Use a Combination of Drugs. The use of a combination of drugs enables the physician to increase analgesic effects without escalating the narcotic dose. Combinations that produce additive analgesic effects include a narcotic plus a nonnarcotic (aspirin, acetaminophen, ibuprofen, choline magnesium trisalicylate), a narcotic plus an antihistamine (100 mg intramuscular hydroxyzine), and a narcotic plus an amphetamine (10 mg intramuscular dextroamphetamine).[144,145] Studies demonstrating the efficacy of these combinations were single-dose studies. Hydroxyzine in 25-mg doses has been used regularly, with anecdotal observations that it is an effective combination. Certain combinations do not provide additive analgesia; these include a narcotic plus a benzodiazepine or a narcotic plus a phenothiazine.

Anticipate and Treat Side Effects. The side effects of the narcotic analgesics often limit their effective use. The most common side effects are sedation, respiratory depression, nausea, vomiting, constipation, and multifocal myoclonus and seizures.

Sedation and drowsiness vary with the drug and dose and may occur after both single and repeated administration. They are mediated through activation of opiate receptors in the reticular formation and diffusely throughout the cortex. Management of these effects includes reducing the individual drug dose but prescribing the drug more frequently, or switching to an analgesic with a shorter plasma half-life. Amphetamines, methylphenidate, and caffeine can be used to counteract these sedative effects.[145–147] It is important to discontinue all other drugs that might exacerbate the sedative effects of the narcotic analgesic, including a wide variety of medications such as cimetidine, barbiturates, and other anxiolytic medications.

Respiratory depression is the most serious adverse effect of the opioid drugs. It occurs most commonly after short-term administration of the narcotic and is usually associated with other signs of central nervous system depression, including sedation and drowsiness. The narcotic-agonist drugs act on brain stem respiratory centers to produce, as a function of dose, increasing respiratory depression to the point of apnea. Tolerance to this effect develops rapidly with repeated drug administration, thereby allowing prolonged use without significant risk of respiratory depression.

Respiratory depression can be reversed by giving the short-acting narcotic antagonist naloxone (suggested dose, 0.4 mg/ ml). Repeated administration, including an intravenous drip, may be necessary to prevent respiratory arrest in such patients. In patients receiving narcotics for prolonged periods who develop respiratory depression, diluted doses of naloxone (0.4 mg in 10-ml saline) should be titrated carefully to prevent the precipitation of severe withdrawal symptoms while reversing the respiratory depression. A useful dosing normogram for continuous intravenous infusion of naloxone has been developed in which two thirds of the initial bolus is started on an hourly basis and titrated against the patient's symptoms.[148]

In some patients the use of naloxone to reverse drug-induced respiratory depression can be dangerous. An endotracheal tube should be placed in the comatose patient before giving naloxone to prevent aspiration from excessive salivation and bronchial spasm induced by naloxone administration. In patients receiving meperidine over a longer period, naloxone may precipitate seizures by lowering the seizure threshold and by allowing the convulsant activity of the active metabolite normeperidine to become evident. In this instance, special attention must be given to the potential seizure effect of naloxone. If naloxone is used, diluted doses, slow titration, and appropriate seizure precautions are advised. There is insufficient clinical evidence to make more specific recommendations. If respiratory support can be effected by other means (that is, continuous stimulation to maintain the patient's wakefulness), such an approach may place the patient at less risk and clearly in less discomfort.

The narcotic analgesics produce nausea and vomiting by an action limited to the medullary chemoreceptor trigger zone. The incidence of nausea and vomiting is markedly increased in ambulatory patients. Tolerance develops to these side effects with repeated administration. Nausea with one drug does not mean that all drugs will produce it. Switching to alternative narcotic analgesics or using an antiemetic together with the narcotic analgesics is the way to obviate this effect.

Constipation results from the action of these drugs at multiple sites in the gastrointestinal tract and in the spinal cord to produce a decrease in intestinal secretions and peristalsis, resulting in a dry stool and constipation. When narcotic analgesics are started, a regular bowel regimen, including cathartics and stool softeners, should also be instituted. Several bowel regimens have been suggested because of their specific ability to counteract the effects of the narcotic drugs, but none has been studied in a controlled way.[149] Anecdotal surveys suggest that doses far above those used for routine bowel management are needed, and that careful attention to dietary factors along with the use of a bowel regimen can reduce patient complaints dramatically. Tolerance to this effect develops over time, but relatively slowly.

Multifocal myoclonus may occur with high doses of all of the opioid drugs. Multifocal myoclonus and seizures have been reported in patients receiving multiple doses of meperidine (250 mg or more per day), although signs and symptoms of central nervous system hyperirritability may occur with toxic doses of all the narcotic analgesics. In a series of cancer patients receiving meperidine, accumulation of the active metabolite normeperidine was associated with these neurologic signs and symptoms.[69] However, in a similar group of cancer patients with pain, subtle mood effects were noted after meperidine administration, which suggests a spectrum of central nervous system effects. Management of this hyperirritability includes discontinuing the meperidine, using intravenous diazepam if seizures occur, and substituting morphine to control the persistent pain. Because the half-life of normeperidine is 16 hours, it may take 2 or 3 days for the signs of central nervous system hyperirritability to clear completely. Meperidine is contraindicated in patients with chronic renal disease, but these complications noted in cancer pain occurred in patients with normal renal function.[113] In dying patients with myoclonus, the use of benzodiazepines or barbiturates has been reported anecdotally to suppress this sign, improving the patient's comfort.

Manage Tolerance. The earliest sign of the development of tolerance is the patient's complaint that the duration of effective analgesia has decreased. For reasons not yet understood, the rate of development of tolerance varies greatly among cancer patients.[111] Some demonstrate tolerance within days of initiating narcotic therapy; others remain controlled for many months on the same dose. Studies in an outpatient clinic population, a hospitalized population, and a homecare population revealed three patterns of drug use: those who rapidly increase their opioid requirements, those who stabilize at one dose for several weeks or months, and those who decrease or eliminate opioids.[24,65,137] Increased opioid requirements are most commonly associated with disease progression rather than tolerance alone. With the development of tolerance, increases in the frequency or the dose of the opioid are required to provide continued pain relief. Because the analgesic effect is a logarithmic function of the dose of opioid, a doubling of the dose may be needed to restore full analgesia. There appears to be no limit to the development of tolerance, and with appropriate dose adjustments patients can continue to obtain pain relief. Cross-tolerance among the opioid analgesics is not complete; therefore, it is advantageous to change to an alternate opioid, selecting half the predicted equianalgesic dose as the starting dose.

The use of analgesic combinations can reduce the amount of opioid required. Similarly, the use of bolus or continuous epidural local anesthesia in patients with perineal pain can dramatically reduce the need for systemic opioids and reverse tolerance.

Taper Drugs Slowly. The long-term administration of narcotic analgesics is associated with the development of physical dependence, a state in which the sudden cessation of the narcotic analgesic will produce signs and symptoms of withdrawal: agitation, tremors, insomnia, fear, marked autonomic nervous system hyperexcitability, and exacerbation of pain. Slowly tapering the dose of the narcotic analgesic will prevent such symptoms. The appearance of abstinence symptoms from the time of drug withdrawal is related to the elimination half-life for the particular drug. The type of abstinence syndrome similarly varies with the drug. For example, with morphine, withdrawal symptoms occur within 6 to 12 hours after drug cessation. Reinstituting the drug in doses of about 25% of the previous daily dose suppresses these symptoms.

Anticipate Complications. Overdose with narcotic analgesics occurs either intentionally, when a patient takes an excessive amount of drug in a suicide attempt, or unintentionally, when the recommended dosage accidentally produces excessive sedation and respiratory depression. In both instances, the complication can be treated effectively with naloxone. Intentional overdose in cancer patients occurs rarely, and concern for this is overemphasized. Overdose in patients previously stabilized on a narcotic regimen for cancer pain rarely is caused by drug intake alone. More commonly, it is the medical deterioration of the patient with a superimposed metabolic encephalopathy. Reducing the narcotic drug dosage and carefully assessing the patient's metabolic status usually provide the differential diagnosis. Patients who have taken an unintentional drug overdose should be scrutinized carefully to rule out other causes of excessive sedation, confusion, or respiratory depression. In such cases a reversal of these effects with naloxone is more therapeutic than diagnostic.

Psychological dependence or addiction is characterized by a concomitant behavioral pattern of drug abuse characterized by craving a drug for other than pain relief and overwhelming involvement in the use and procurement of the drug. This is a state distinct from tolerance and physical dependence, which are responses to the pharmacologic effects of long-term narcotic administration. The profound fear of causing psychological dependence plays a major role in a physician's reluctance to prescribe narcotic analgesics, particularly in cancer patients in the early phase of their disease.[8,9] Patients may share this fear, consistently taking less analgesic drug than is effective to control their pain. Increasing evidence suggests that cancer patients with pain can take narcotic analgesics for prolonged periods but can discontinue such drugs when adequate pain relief is achieved from other approaches. In almost all instances, dramatic escalation of drug intake is associated with progression of disease and subsequent death.[24,65,137] Very few patients with cancer and pain become psychologically dependent on the drugs and participate in drug-seeking and illicit drug use. Careful evaluation of patients who might be at risk for this complication is necessary, but such concern should not be punitive to the patient with severe cancer pain.

Adjuvant Analgesic Drugs

These drugs have a unique place in the management of cancer pain, but knowledge about their use is empirical. This group includes several heterogenous substances used to increase the analgesic effects of the opioid analgesics, to counteract their side effects, or to act as analgesics themselves. Any discussion of the use of these adjuvants must be prefaced with caveats:

1. These drugs have been developed and released for clinical indications other than analgesia, including nausea, vomiting, anxiety, mania, depression, and delirium.
2. These drugs are not as effective in relieving pain as are the narcotic analgesics, except for methotrimeprazine (Levoprome).

3. There are no efficacy studies for their co-analgesic properties in cancer patients.
4. The choice of these drugs should be individualized, using the simplest but most potent combination of drugs.

ANTICONVULSANTS. Phenytoin and carbamazepine are anticonvulsant drugs that suppress spontaneous neuronal firing and are the drugs of choice for treating trigeminal neuralgia and other neuropathic pains.[150] In cancer pain, carbamazepine has been useful in managing the acute shocklike neuralgic pain in the cranial and cervical distribution caused by either tumor infiltration or surgical nerve injury. It also has been effective in patients with stump pain secondary to traumatic neuroma and in patients with lumbosacral plexopathy. The starting dose is 100 mg slowly titrated to 400 to 800 mg/day, depending on the patient's needs.

Several studies have reported the use of clonazepam and valproate in patients with acute lancinating pain.[151,152] Clonazepam has been reported to be effective in patients with both trigeminal and posttraumatic neuralgia. Valproate has also been reported to be effective in both trigeminal and postherpetic neuralgia in a series of uncontrolled surveys.

In cancer patients, the use of carbamazepine is limited by the fact that the drug can cause both leukopenia and thrombocytopenia in about 2% of patients. Because cancer patients commonly have a compromised hematologic reserve, this effect may limit the use of carbamazepine. A trial of clonazepam or valproate may be indicated in patients who cannot tolerate carbamazepine.

PHENOTHIAZINES. Of the phenothiazine drugs, methotrimeprazine has definitive analgesic properties. In single-dose studies in patients with postoperative pain and chronic cancer pain, 15 mg intramuscular methotrimeprazine is equivalent to 15 mg intramuscular morphine.[153] This drug is useful in special circumstances. In the patient who is tolerant, it provides a temporary approach to produce analgesia by a non-opiate receptor mechanism. In the patient with bowel obstruction and pain, it avoids the constipating effects of the narcotics. In patients whose respiration is compromised, it avoids the respiratory-depressant effects of the narcotics, although it can produce significant sedative effects. In patients with pain and narcotic-induced nausea and vomiting, it acts as both an analgesic and an antiemetic.

Long-term administration of this drug in patients with cancer pain has not been fully assessed. The usual starting dose is 5 to 10 mg parenterally. Patients should be carefully observed for orthostatic hypotension and sedation.

BUTYROPHENONES. Haloperidol is the first-line drug in the management of the cancer patient with acute psychosis and delirium, but its role in pain management is less clear.[60] In animals it potentiates morphine analgesia. Several authors have reported its clinical usefulness in cancer patients with pain, suggesting that it works as a co-analgesic and thus allows reduction of the narcotic dose.[154] The doses suggested to produce co-analgesic effects are lower than those used to manage psychiatric symptoms; 0.5 to 1 mg orally two to three times daily is the suggested starting dose.

ANTIDEPRESSANTS. The tricyclic antidepressants may be the most useful group of psychotropic drugs used in pain management. Their analgesic effects are mediated by enhancement of serotonin activity. Animal studies demonstrate the direct analgesic effects of amitriptyline as well as its ability to enhance morphine analgesia. Amitriptyline has been reported to be useful in the management of patients with migraine, postherpetic neuralgia, diabetic neuropathy, and a series of chronic pain states.[33,34] No controlled studies in cancer patients with neuropathic pain have been done, but strong anecdotal information suggests a role for these drugs in the management of such patients and in the management of pain-related sleep disturbances.

The doses used for analgesia are far below those needed to produce an antidepressant effect, and the analgesic properties of these drugs appear to occur independently of their mood-altering effects. Patients should be started on low doses of 10 to 25 mg, then titrated up to achieve adequate analgesia in a 2- to 4-week trial. Blood levels should be measured to determine both patient compliance and drug absorption, because there are wide individual variations.

Recent studies suggest that both continuous dysesthesias as well as lancinating pains may respond to the use of these drugs. Most studies support the analgesic efficacy for amitriptyline, imipramine, and doxepin, with less impressive data for nortriptyline and desipramine. Side effects such as cardiotoxicity, sedation, dry mouth, constipation, and urinary retention may occur and affect the choice of drug.

In the management of the cancer patient with pain, these drugs are the first-line therapeutic approach to the management of patients with postherpetic neuralgia, posttraumatic nerve injury, peripheral neuropathy, and central pain states.

STEROIDS. A series of controlled and uncontrolled surveys suggest that the use of chronic steroid therapy improves the quality of life and reduces pain in patients with breast and prostate cancer. In a controlled study of corticosteroid use in patients with far-advanced disease, transient improvement in appetite, analgesia, and mood were noted, but they were not sustained after the initial effect.[155] Corticosteroids have been reported to have both specific and nonspecific benefits in managing acute and chronic pain. Their ability to produce euphoria, increased appetite, and weight gain contributes greatly to the sense of well-being in the cancer patient with pain.[156] Steroids reportedly reduce bone pain of metastatic origin and are used as oncolytic agents with certain types of tumors. Several studies demonstrate prolonged survival time and reduced narcotic doses to control pain in terminal cancer patients receiving steroids.[157] In certain cancer pain syndromes such as epidural cord compression, 85% of patients receiving 100 mg of dexamethasone as part of a radiation therapy protocol reported significant pain relief associated with marked reduction in analgesic requirements.[46] In patients with tumor infiltration of the brachial and lumbosacral plexus, steroids provide additive analgesic effects. In patients with leptomeningeal metastases or headache from increased intracranial pressure from tumor or superior sagittal sinus occlusion, steroids play a major role in controlling head pain or neck and back pain.

ANTIHISTAMINES. Hydroxyzine is the drug most widely studied as an analgesic in the management of patients with pain and cancer. A dose of 100 mg parenterally provides analgesia that is additive to morphine.[93] No data support the analgesic effectiveness of oral doses of 10 or 25 mg of hydroxyzine, although good evidence supports the observation that these doses are associated with anxiolytic and mild antiemetic effects. Hydroxyzine is indicated to provide additive analgesia in a cancer patient requiring additive anxiolysis or an antiemetic effect.

NEUROSTIMULANTS. Evidence supports the analgesic effects of dextroamphetamine, methylphenidate, and caffeine.[145-147] These drugs are most commonly used in patients with excessive sedation from opioids. In a controlled repeated-dose trial of oral methylphenidate in patients with advanced cancer, opioid-induced sedation was reversed and supplemental analgesia was concurrently provided.[146] In a follow-up survey of 50 advanced cancer patients receiving 15 mg of methylphenidate in divided doses, beneficial effects were noted in more than 90% of patients, but evidence suggested the need for escalating doses to maintain a comparable effect in some patients. Because cocaine was commonly used in the Brompton cocktail, it was evaluated for both its analgesic and mood-altering effects. In a well-controlled single-dose analgesic assay, cocaine 10 mg orally influenced mood but had no impact on analgesic efficacy or reversal of sedation.[158]

In clinical practice, dextroamphetamine in doses of 2.5 to 5 mg twice daily, methylphenidate in doses of 15 mg twice daily, and caffeine in doses of 300 mg twice daily are commonly used to reverse opioid-induced sedation. This is particularly useful in patients who are receiving effective analgesia but whose functional status is compromised by drowsiness.

DIPHOSPHONATES. This novel group of drugs, also named biphosphonates, includes four main groups.[159] These drugs act by inhibiting the bone-resorption effects of osteoclasts and have been found particularly useful in conditions characterized by osteoclastic hyperactivity, such as Paget's disease and malignant hypercalcemia.

Osteoclasts have been associated with pain due to bone metastases, and several authors have studied the effects of diphosphonates on cancer bone pain.[159,160] Three small uncontrolled studies in 8, 12, and 17 patients have suggested the presence of diphosphonate-induced analgesia.[161,163]

In a randomized study of 131 patients with metastatic bone cancer, diphosphonate APD 15 mg twice a day orally was studied against a control group.[164] Patients continued to receive antineoplastic therapy, and the authors reported a significant decrease in the incidence of fractures, hypercalcemia, bone pain, and the need for radiation therapy in patients receiving APD as compared with controls. The main limitations of this study were its unblinded nature and the fact that no stratification was made according to the prognostically relevant tumor variables.

In a randomized study of 57 patients with painful bone metastases from prostate cancer, Smith evaluated four protocols: 7.5 mg/kg intravenous etidronate followed by 200 mg of etidronate twice a day orally; 7.5 mg/kg intravenous etidronate plus placebo only; intravenous placebo plus 200 mg twice a day orally; or intravenous placebo plus placebo orally.[165] This randomized double-blind study assessed pain and analgesic consumption for 1 month. Smith reported no significant analgesic effects. The limitation of this study is its limited statistical power: only 14 patients received only drug and 14 patients received only placebo.

Bruera and associates studied 23 consecutive patients with cancer-related bone pain who participated in a double-blind crossover trial of intravenous clodronate 600 mg versus placebo; after 1 week the patients received the alternative therapy.[166] Pain intensity, analgesic consumption, and the investigators' blinded choice favored clodronate. No significant clinical or laboratory side effects were noted.

The utility of these compounds in the management of patients with bone pain remains to be clarified. They may provide interesting mechanisms that might be associated with additive analgesia.

MISCELLANEOUS ADJUVANT DRUGS.   The use of local anesthetics and barbiturates is discussed below in the section on anesthetic approaches.

PSYCHOLOGICAL APPROACHES

Psychological approaches should be an integral part of the care of the cancer patient with pain. New disciplines in psychooncology and psychosocial oncology have developed that focus on the psychological and psychosocial complications of cancer.[60] A series of psychological variables contribute to the cancer pain experience and suffering, such as perception of control, the meaning of pain, fear of death, depressed mood, and hopelessness. The level of psychological distress experienced by each patient varies depending on personality, coping ability, social support, and medical factors. Pain has a profound impact on levels of emotional distress, and psychological factors such as depression and anxiety intensify the pain experience. Measures of emotional disturbance have been reported to be predictors of pain in advancing latter stages of cancer.

Cancer patients with lower levels of neuroticism, anxiety, and depression are less likely to report pain. From a study by the Psychosocial Collaborative Oncology Group, an increased frequency of psychiatric disorders was found in cancer patients with pain, in particular anxiety and depression. Of the patients studied by this group who received a psychiatric diagnosis, 39% had significant pain.[60]

The incidence of pain, depression, and delirium increases with high levels of physical debilitation in advanced disease. About 25% of all cancer patients experience severe depressive symptoms, with the prevalence increasing to 77% in those with advanced illness. Uncontrolled pain is a major factor in cancer suicide.[68] While relatively few cancer patients commit suicide, studies suggest that they are at increased risk.

Various psychological interventions have been advocated for patients with cancer pain. Optimal treatment is multimodal and requires pharmacologic, psychotherapeutic, and cognitive-behavioral approaches. The roles of the psychiatrist, psychologist, and social worker in cancer pain management are well described in the literature.[68,167]

The goals of short-term psychotherapy are to provide emotional support, continuity, and information and to assist patients in adapting to the crisis. Communication skills are of paramount importance for patient and family, particularly about pain and analgesic issues. The needs of the patient and family must be addressed. Psychotherapy in the cancer pain setting is primarily nonanalytic and focuses on current issues and exploration of reactions to cancer, which often provide insight into other life issues. Group interventions may also be helpful.

A specialized approach called cognitive-behavioral therapy has been used to treat pain disorders, including cancer pain.[167] This approach uses short-term therapeutic interventions based on theoretically and empirically derived principles that can be adapted to each patient's problems and needs. It includes a set of systematic mental and behavioral techniques designed to modify specific emotional, behavioral, and social problems as well as the global experiences of pain and distress. Its major goal is to enhance the sense of personal control or self-efficacy. In a multidisciplinary approach to cancer pain, not every patient needs referral for this therapy, but it is useful if all members of the pain team follow a cognitive-behavioral model. Because cognitive-behavioral therapy is a commonsense psychological approach consisting of specific techniques, it can be learned and practiced by any interested clinician, nurse, or social worker who can gain practical training in the use of these techniques and apply them effectively.

Various intervention methods have been developed and are arbitrarily divided into behavioral and cognitive methods for discussion purposes. These approaches must be targeted to each patient's needs.

Behavioral techniques include ways to modify physiologic pain reactions and pain behaviors. Relaxation training can be used by all caregivers who manage patients with pain and cancer. Its mechanism of action includes the reduction of muscle tension and it can provide the patient with a sense of improved self-control and a calming diversion of attention, breaking the associated pain/anxiety/tension cycle. Techniques include simple deep-breathing exercises to more specialized methods of biofeedback and hypnosis. Contingency management is another behavioral approach designed to modify dysfunctional pain behaviors and replace them with "well" behaviors.

Cognitive techniques are designed to modify dysfunctional mental processes or to teach adaptive coping strategies. Cognitive coping and cognitive modification are approaches in which distraction, focusing, and perception and interpretation of the meaning of pain are assessed.

ANESTHETIC AND NEUROSURGICAL APPROACHES

Anesthetic and neurosurgical approaches are most effective in treating patients with well-defined localized pain. Tables 64–7 and 64–8 outline the indications for their use. About 10% to 20% of cancer pain patients need these approaches together with pharmacologic approaches to provide adequate analgesia.

In a prospective study, Ventafridda and colleagues evaluated

TABLE 64–7. Types of Anesthetic Procedures Commonly Used in Cancer Pain

Type of Procedure	Most Common Indications
Inhalation therapy with nitrous oxide	Breakthrough pain, incident pain in patients with diffuse poorly controlled pain
Intravenous barbiturates (sodium pentobarbital)	Diffuse body pain and suffering inadequately controlled by systemic opioids
Local anesthetic by intravenous, subcutaneous, or transdermal application	Neuropathic pain in any site with local application to the area of hyperesthesia or allodynia
Trigger-point injections	Focal muscle pain
Nerve block:	
Peripheral	Pain in discrete dermatomes in chest and abdomen or in distal extremities
Epidural	Unilateral lumbar or sacral pain
	Midline perineal pain
	Bilateral lumbosacral pain
Intrathecal	Mildine perineal pain
	Bilateral lumbosacral pain
Autonomic	
Stellate ganglion	Reflex sympathetic dystrophy
Lumbar sympathetic	Reflex sympathetic dystrophy of the lower extremity
	Lumbosacral plexopathy
	Vascular insufficiency of the lower extremity
Celiac plexus	Midabdominal pain from tumor infiltration
Intermittent or continuous epidural infusion with local anesthetics	Unilateral and bilateral lumbosacral pain
	Midline perineal pain
	Neuropathic pain from the midthoracic region down
Intermittent or continuous epidural or intrathecal with local opioid analgesics	Unilateral and bilateral pain below the midthoracic region; often combined with local anesthetics
Intermittent or continuous intraventrical infusions with opioid analgesics	Head and neck pain and upper chest
Chemical hypophysectomy	Diffuse bone pain

two groups of patients for 3 months who presented with intractable cancer pain not responsive to specific anticancer therapies.[11] One group was treated with sequential pharmacologic approaches using the analgesic ladder. The second group was treated with a multimodal approach of analgesic therapy followed by the use of neurolytic blocks or chronic spinal opioid administration. Patients treated with neurolytic procedures combined with pharmacologic therapy showed a statistically significant degree of greater pain relief than those treated with drugs alone by the third week of therapy. However, by 6 weeks there was no statistical difference between the two groups. Complete pain relief without the need for analgesic drug therapy persisted up to 3 months in 29% of the patients who received spinal opiates, 25% treated with celiac ganglion neurolytic block, 24% with percutaneous cor-

dotomy, 12% with chemical rhizotomy, and 7% with gasserian thermorhizotomy. This study demonstrated that although analgesic therapy is the mainstay of treatment, anesthetic and neurosurgical procedures provide an important but limited contribution to adequate analgesia.

In a study comparing a multimodal pain treatment approach combined with a home-based supportive care program, the same authors noted markedly improved analgesia and quality of life in the patients who were followed in a supportive care program compared with those who received pain therapy alone.[23] Again, these data support the construct that treating cancer pain requires a multidisciplinary approach that includes not only pain therapy but also symptom management and treatment of psychological distress.

Several factors are important in selecting the appropriate procedure for each patient. Because diffuse pain problems are common in cancer patients and most of the procedures are useful for well-defined localized pain, the role of these approaches is limited at best. Further complicating their use is the limited number of professionals who have expertise in these procedures. As patients become more cognizant of their disease and treatment options, they are often hesitant to undergo neurodestructive procedures. Patients often consider their pain to be an important marker for their disease and are frightened of the potential, although unlikely, complications of these procedures. As a result, these procedures are often performed late in the illness, and full evaluation of their effectiveness and duration of action is limited by the patient's overriding medical problems.

These procedures are often not very effective in managing neuropathic pain, except for the use of local anesthetics, and are most helpful in managing most types of somatic and visceral pain. However, cancer patients often have a mixed somatic, visceral, and neuropathic pain syndrome. We advocate early consideration for the use of some of these anesthetic and neurosurgical procedures in patients to improve their quality of life through adequate pain management.

ANESTHETIC APPROACHES

Nitrous Oxide

Nitrous oxide has analgesic properties and has been used in the management of patients with far-advanced disease to provide added analgesia. It is administered with oxygen through a nonrebreathing face mask in concentrations from 25% to 75%. Its use in combination with systemic narcotic analgesics is associated with improvement of symptoms of pain and anxiety and a demonstrable improvement in alertness.[168] Although long-term nitrous oxide use has been associated with the development of pancytopenia, its short-term use is relatively safe. This anesthetic approach should be considered in patients with breakthrough pain or incident pain to provide adequate analgesia to facilitate their care. The method offers a simple means to treat transient pain if excessive side effects occur from increasing opioid doses.

Intravenous Barbiturates

This approach has been advocated to manage dying patients who have inadequate analgesia or uncontrolled symptoms,

TABLE 64–8.   Neuroablative and Neurostimulatory Procedures for Relief of Pain From Cancer

Site	Procedure	Indications
Neuroablative Procedures		
Nerve root	Rhizotomy	Useful in somatic and neuropathic pain from tumor infiltration of the cranial and rarely intercostal nerves
Spinal cord	Dorsal root entry zone lesion (DREZ)	Useful in unilateral neuropathic pain from brachial, intercostal, and lumbosacral plexopathy and postherpetic neuralgia
	Cordotomy	Useful in unilateral pain below the waist. Often combined with local neurolytic blocks in perineal and bilateral lumbosacral plexopathy; may be performed bilaterally
	Myelotomy	Useful in midline pain below the waist but rarely used because it involves extensive surgery
Brain stem	Mesencephalic tractomy	Useful in pain in the nasopharynx and trigeminal region
Thalamus	Thalamotomy	Useful in unilateral neuropathic pain in the chest and lower extremity
Cortex	Cingulotomy	Useful through a stereotactic approach for diffuse pain
Pituitary	Transsphenoidal hypophysectomy	Useful in pain control of bone metastases in endocrine-dependent tumors, breast, and prostate
Neurostimulatory Procedures		
Peripheral nerve	Transcutaneous and percutaneous electrical nerve stimulation	Useful in reducing painful dysesthesias from tumor infiltration of nerve or trauma (*e.g.*, neuroma)
Spinal cord	Dorsal column stimulation	Of limited use in neuropathic pain in the chest, midline, and lower extremities
Thalamus	Thalamic stimulation	Of rare use in neuropathic pain in the chest, midline, or lower extremity

who ask to be maintained in a sedated state. Intravenous thiopental titrated to a level of sedation was the approach advocated in a series of 17 terminally ill patients.[169] The authors suggested that the value of this approach is based on the use of one agent to treat both physical and psychological symptoms. This approach may be seen as a more generalized one to palliative care and should be considered only if the standard approaches with opioid analgesics and adjuvant drugs fail to provide adequate analgesia with minimal side effects. However, because it is the physician's responsibility to manage not only pain but also suffering, this may be a reasonable approach, particularly in the dying patient with profound dyspnea, myoclonus, or agitation. Further studies are needed to clarify the usefulness of this approach. In the published study, 13 of 17 patients developed somnolence and died; the somnolence lasted from 2 hours to 4 days, with an average of 23 hours. Four patients died without being somnolent.

The doses of thiopental varied. A standard solution consisted of 500 mg of thiopental in 250 ml of 5% dextrose and water. The drug was delivered at 20 to 80 mg/hour, titrated to the patient's need for sedation; the average dose was 107 mg/hour. In patients receiving ventilatory assistance the standard dose of thiopental was a 100- to 150-mg bolus followed by a continuous infusion of 150 mg/hour. The doses used in these studies were below those used in patients receiving respiratory assistance.

Several problematic symptoms often arise in the management of the dying patient, including intractable vomiting, profound dyspnea, extreme agitation and anxiety, and uncontrolled pain. Several authors have reported that most cancer patients have crescendo symptoms before death, requiring somnolence.[24,25,170] This approach offers one method to manage these difficult patients. Tachyphylaxis to thiopental has been described, but both the advantages and disadvantages of this approach must be further debated to define its place in the management of patients with advanced disease.

Local Anesthetics

Anecdotal reports and several controlled studies support the use of intravenous, subcutaneous, transdermal, intrapleural, and epidural local anesthetics in the management of patients with somatic, visceral, and neuropathic pain.[171–175]

Intravenous lidocaine should be considered as both a diagnostic and therapeutic approach in patients with neuropathic pain. If such patients obtain an analgesic response, a trial of oral mexiletine or the use of continuous subcutaneous lidocaine should be considered to determine whether prolonged relief may be possible. Although no studies have confirmed that the response to lidocaine predicts a response to mexiletine for pain, a comparable predictive value exists in the cardiac literature, where intravenous lidocaine's effectiveness in controlling ventricular arrhythmias predicts the usefulness of mexiletine for this same disorder.[171]

Cousins and colleagues reported the use of continuous subcutaneous infusions in two patients with cancer-related neuropathic pain, advocating this approach as an alternative one in patients who do not respond to standard opioid and adjuvant treatments as well as anesthetic approaches for neuropathic pain.[172]

The transdermal application of lidocaine using a 2%, 5%, or 10% ointment has been reported to be useful in patients with superficial hyperesthesia, dysesthesias, and significant allodynia. Spreading the ointment on the painful site can often provide transient pain relief. This has been best demonstrated in patients with postherpetic neuralgia. The advantage of such an approach is the limited degree of systemic uptake of the drug and the ability to reduce pain at its peripheral site of origin. This approach has been used in patients with peripheral skin lesions and open draining sores with associated inflammatory changes. Topical ointments used in and around the rectal area or oral solutions can provide pain relief in patients with superficial rectal/anal pain or oral mucositis or esophagitis.

Intrapleural local anesthetics have been used for acute pain in the chest wall and have been adapted for the management of chronic cancer pain.[174] A subcutaneously tunneled intrapleural catheter offered long-term relief of right upper quadrant pain from hepatic metastases in a patient with significant pain from tumor infiltration of the liver. This approach was successful for 6 weeks. The patient used 0.5% preservative-free bupivacaine given every 8 hours. This novel method offers an alternative approach for patients with local regional pain in the pleural and abdominal regions.

Epidural local anesthetics are used to manage patients with localized pain syndromes, usually below the waist. Intermittent and continuous epidural infusions of local anesthetics have been used to manage the difficult chronic pain associated with metastatic disease below the waist, often involving the sacrum and lumbosacral plexus.[140,175,176] This method consists of infusing a local anesthetic into a subcutaneous infusion pump or Ommaya reservoir that is connected to a catheter temporarily or permanently placed in the epidural space. If the amount and concentration of the anesthetic are varied, effective pain relief can be achieved without interrupting significant motor or autonomic function. The risk of infection is minimized because local anesthetics have antimicrobial effects. The use of continuous low-dose infusions of local anesthetics is associated with minimal systemic side effects. Further studies on the use of this technique in comparison with standard therapies are needed to define its place in the management of the cancer patient. Its major advantages are that the resultant analgesia is not cross-tolerant with the analgesic produced by the opioid analgesic, and that temporary use of this technique allows for reduction in the amount of systemic opiate drugs, therefore partially reversing tolerance. This has been a useful preliminary approach in patients for whom the use of spinal opiate analgesia is considered but who have developed tolerance from large doses of systemic opiates. Because tolerance develops to these analgesic effects, this approach is temporary (days to weeks) rather than long term. This approach is most useful in patients who experience an acute pain crisis, such as the patient with a pathologic hip fracture who is not a surgical candidate; this approach would allow the patient to move about in bed.

Peripheral Nerve Blocks

Peripheral nerve blocks are used both diagnostically to localize the nerve distribution and therapeutically to interrupt pain transmission within a determined nerve distribution.[140] This technique is limited to areas of the body in which the interruption of both motor and sensory function will not interfere with the patient's functional status. This approach is most commonly used with patients who have pain in the head, chest, or abdomen. This technique is also limited by the fact that each peripheral nerve subserves sensory function over many levels, and usually several nerves must be blocked to provide adequate analgesia. These techniques are most useful in patients with somatic pain; neuropathic pain is rarely controlled by peripheral nerve blocks alone. Examples of successful blocks include gasserian ganglion block for craniofacial pain, intercostal blocks for chest wall infiltration from tumor, and paravertebral blocks for radicular pain.[140,176]

In patients with somatic pain who respond to a local anesthetic block, neurolytic blockade with either alcohol or phenol may provide more prolonged relief. A block produced by phenol tends to be less profound and of shorter duration than that produced by alcohol. Phenol has local anesthetic as well as neurolytic effects. This is an advantage because it is painless to inject and provides a clear indication of the area affected by neurolysis. Some authors report that phenol has a more marked effect on blood vessels than does alcohol. It was originally believed that phenol's action as a neurolytic agent was based on its differential sparing of large myelinated fibers while destroying the small unmyelinated C fibers. However, this differential effect is not clinically significant, and a wealth of experimental evidence demonstrates these facts.[140]

Whatever the agent used, the most common peripheral neurolytic block is a paravertebral block for localized intercostal pain. From our experience in treating patients with chest wall pain, we advise that this procedure be done under fluoroscopic control or CT localization to accurately interrupt the individual intercostal nerve.

Epidural and intrathecal neurolytic blocks have been used primarily to manage patients with far-advanced disease whose pain is either unilateral in the chest or abdomen or midline in the perineum.[177] These approaches are less useful in managing upper and lower limb pain associated with brachial and lumbosacral plexopathy because of the high risk of motor weakness associated with effective neurolytic blockade by this route. Epidural phenol blocks are useful in chest wall pain over several dermatomes. Such an approach obviates the need for multiple paravertebral injections. Phenol is injected in small increments (1 to 2 ml per segment) over 2 or 3 days by an epidural catheter, and preliminary data demonstrate 80% pain relief in patients with documented somatic pain. Epidural and intrathecal phenol blocks have been used to manage perineal pain, but no studies have delineated the superiority of one approach to the other.

For an intrathecal block, a phenol-glycerine solution, which is viscous and hyperbaric, can be directed to the site by gravity. An 18-gauge spinal needle is used to introduce the phenol intrathecally, and the substance is injected in small increments (0.4 ml) to a total of 1 to 1.5 ml. With the use of alcohol, to produce a precise block of profound intensity and adequate duration, the patient must be carefully positioned so that the maximum concentration of the hypobaric alcohol solution reaches the posterior nerve roots. This means that the patient is placed in a lateral oblique position with the painful side uppermost. For bilateral pain, to produce a saddle or perineal block, the patient must be placed in a prone position with the affected segment uppermost over the break in the operating table. The injected alcohol will then spread over both posterior roots. Alternatively, each side may be blocked on separate occasions, 2 to 3 days apart, when the effect of the initial injection can be assessed before the second procedure is attempted.

A review of a large number of alcohol subarachnoid blocks reports an average of 60% good relief, 21% fair relief, and 18% poor relief.[140,176–178] Because the duration of pain relief has seldom been documented with careful follow-up studies, the overall estimate for relief of pain with both subarachnoid alcohol and phenol blocks suggests a mean duration of pain relief of between 2 weeks and 3 months.

Complications are of two kinds. With intrathecal injection a self-limiting spinal headache may occur. Complications that result from the action of neurolytic substances on nerve fibers include motor paresis, loss of sphincter function, impairment of touch and proprioception, and troublesome dysesthesias. Injection in the thoracic region has a low complication rate. In our experience, many cancer patients already have both motor and autonomic dysfunction before the use of neurolytic blockade; these often remain the same or may worsen. Patients should be informed of the risk of these procedures, with particular attention to the fact that they may develop motor paresis and bladder dysfunction, specifically incontinence, after the blockade.

The selection of patients for management with epidural or intrathecal neurolytic agents should be based on the following criteria: exhaustion of appropriate antitumor approaches; clear clinical and radiologic definition of the pain; poor candidacy for percutaneous cordotomy; failure of nonopioid, opioid, and adjuvant analgesics to produce adequate analgesia without significant side effects; a favorable response to diagnostic or epidural or intrathecal blocks, producing at least 75% pain relief; and myelography done before the procedure to rule out tumor infiltration of the subarachnoid space.

Autonomic Nerve Block

Sympathetic block is effective in conditions with vasomotor or visceromotor hyperactivity. This hyperactivity accompanies many of the cancer-related pain syndromes such as visceral pain or plexopathies. The most commonly used sympathetic block is that of the celiac ganglion for pain due to abdominal malignancy, including cancer of the pancreas, stomach, duodenum, liver, gallbladder, adrenal gland, and colon. Nociceptive fibers of the splanchnic, sympathetic, vagal, phrenic, and somatic nerves converge on the celiac ganglion, which is amenable to a regional block that is successful in from 70% to 85% of patients treated.[138,179,180]

Standardized approaches for the use of this technique have been described using CT monitoring or fluoroscopic control. After placement of the needle, 25 ml of absolute alcohol mixed with local anesthetic and contrast is injected. Bilateral needle placement has been reported to provide the best results, but anecdotal reports suggest that unilateral needle placement on the right provides comparable analgesia. The major side effect of the procedure is transient hypotension, and patients must be well hydrated and monitored carefully during the procedure and for 4 to 6 hours afterward. Significant neurologic complications occur in less than 1% of patients if proper technique is used. Complications include paraparesis, postural hypotension, and urinary difficulties.

Although there has been recent debate about the usefulness of this procedure in patients with pancreatic cancer, it should be considered as one of the approaches, together with pharmacologic approaches, in managing these patients.

Lumbar sympathetic block may provide significant relief of intractable urogenital pain or pain due to carcinomatous invasion of local nerves and plexus in the perineum and lower extremity.[181] This ganglion conveys visceral nociceptive afferents from the pelvic viscera. Pain caused by cancer of the sigmoid colon or rectum may be relieved by bilateral lumbar sympathetic block if the disease is confined to those viscera. Pain caused by cancer of the seminal vesicles or prostate may sometimes be relieved by bilateral lumbar sympathetic block. Similarly, pain caused by uterine cancer may be relieved if the disease is confined to the body of the uterus. In many instances, however, the block must be extended to the T12 ganglion. Good evidence suggests that lumbar sympathetic block alone is not useful in patients with lumbosacral plexopathy; therefore, the role of this procedure is limited to specific anatomic sites of pain.

Stellate ganglion block may sometimes be useful for pain in the face, upper neck, ear, and hemicranium. However, the potential complications of stellate ganglion block limit the use of this technique with neurolytic solution, as there is a high risk of spillage of the neurolytic material into the brachial plexus, with secondary nerve injury and focal pain.

Neuroadenolysis of the Pituitary

Chemical hypophysectomy is a special use of a neurolytic method. Several studies suggest that 35% to 95% of patients undergoing this approach report pain relief, with a median duration of 6 to 7 weeks and a maximum duration of 20 weeks.[182–184] The mechanism by which analgesia is produced may result from alcohol tracking up the pituitary stalk into the hypothalamus, with consequent disruption of the hypothalamic-thalamic endorphinergic pain pathways. Side effects include diabetic insipidus, cranial nerve palsies, cerebrospinal fluid leakage, and rarely meningitis. The lack of detailed clinical data limits critical assessment of these studies. This technique is rarely if ever used in patients with diffuse pain.

Trigger Point Injections

The use of trigger point injections is within the scope of the practicing physician.[185] Patients with significant musculoskeletal pain often describe specific, tender trigger point areas that, when injected with either saline or local anesthetic, are associated with significant pain relief. Effective relief of pain from trigger point injections, however, is not diagnostic of musculoskeletal pain alone, and an evaluation of the cause of the pain is still necessary to rule out the specific etiology.

NEUROSURGICAL APPROACHES

Neurosurgical approaches for cancer pain can be divided into two major categories—antitumor and antinociceptive.[186,187] These approaches are often used alone or in combination by neurosurgeons to provide improved pain relief.

Antitumor Approaches

Antitumor approaches are often more acceptable to patients because they focus on cancer treatment, offering the hope of prolonged survival. The major procedures are listed in Table 64–8 and include tumor removal from the spine, epidural space, or adjacent plexi; stabilization procedures for spinal fracture, instability, and subluxation; and implantation of regional delivery devices for epidural, intrathecal, and intraventricular opioid drugs.

Tumor removal through resection of spinal metastases is associated with dramatic improvement in pain in 70% to 90% of patients.[188,189] With the use of improved methods of internal fixation with methyl methacrylate and improved stabilizing procedures, the use of this approach has increased in patients with intractable continuous or incidental back and neck pain. Patients may also have an associated segmental instability associated with a pathologic fracture of the vertebral body or subluxation, syndromes that place patients at significant risk for neurologic dysfunction. Careful radiologic workup is necessary to define the specific anatomic basis for the spinal pain, but aggressive surgical approaches have improved the quality of life for many patients bedridden by uncontrolled back pain. In patients with epidural cord compression, the indications for surgery include uncontrolled pain in a patient with a pathologic fracture or a solitary relapse in the epidural space or vertebral body from a radioresistant tumor. In patients with radiosensitive tumors who relapse after radiation therapy, spinal surgery should be considered as a reasonable approach and is specifically indicated in the patient with an acute neurologic deterioration during radiation therapy. When percutaneous or open vertebral body biopsy is impossible, surgical resection should be strongly considered to define the primary tumor type in patients with undiagnosed lesions; this serves as both a diagnostic and therapeutic procedure.

In patients with paraspinal tumor or tumor infiltration of the plexus, en bloc resection of tumor has successfully provided pain relief and has served as a debulking antitumor procedure. In patients with Pancoast's syndrome, invasion of the spine or epidural extension is present in 20% at initial presentation and is associated with significant morbidity in up to 50% of patients when local treatment is ineffective. In the good-risk patient with plexopathy and spinal invasion, Sundaresan recommends surgery in which tumor is removed from the lower plexus, C8-T1, and the vertebral body is resected, with brachytherapy to provide further tumor control.[189]

In patients with tumor invasion of the paraspinal area (specifically the psoas and iliacus), radical resection of these tumor masses concurrent with spinal surgery, followed by brachytherapy, combines antitumor and antinociceptive therapies.

When considering the use of these neurosurgical procedures to provide palliative surgery with an antinociceptive component, the patient's extent of disease, performance score, prognosis, and ability to tolerate the surgery must all be weighed.

Antinociceptive Procedures

Antinociceptive procedures include neuroablative, neurostimulatory, and neuropharmacologic approaches.

Neuroablative procedures involve the production of a surgical or radiofrequency lesion along the nociceptive neural pathway. Sectioning of the posterior roots (rhizotomy), lesioning the lateral dorsal horn (dorsal root entry zone lesion), and interrupting the ascending neospinothalamic pathway (cordotomy) or the crossing interneuronal fibers (myelotomy) in the spinal cord are examples of neuroablative procedures performed for pain relief.

Cordotomy, either percutaneous or open, is the most common neuroablative procedure used to manage cancer pain.[187,190–192] It is the neurosurgical procedure of choice for patients with unilateral pain below the waist with a relatively short life expectancy. Cordotomy is usually effective for 1 to 3 years, with dysesthesias substituting for analgesia in patients living longer than 3 years. Pain in the chest wall or upper extremity may be successfully treated initially with cordotomy, but extensive data demonstrate that, with time, the level of analgesia drops, limiting the effectiveness of this approach. Somatic pain appears to be most responsive to cordotomy; visceral and neuropathic pain are less responsive for reasons that are not fully understood.

Percutaneous cordotomy is performed in a supine, awake patient through a lateral C1-2 approach.[187,190] A needle is advanced under fluoroscopic control until cerebrospinal fluid is obtained. A mini-myelogram is done to identify the dentate ligament. A cordotomy electrode is passed through the spinal needle and the spinal cord is punctured with the aid of impedance monitoring. Electrophysiologic stimulation is done to identify the spinothalamic tract and then a radiofrequency lesion is made in the appropriate painful site. Such a lesion interrupts pain and temperature on the contralateral side of the lesioned site. Patients typically report spontaneous relief of pain in this lesioned area.

The anatomic area at the lesion site includes fibers mediating respiration and autonomic function. These fibers are adjacent to the anterior horn and the cervical spinothalamic fibers. Near the lumbar spinothalamic tract are the fibers governing the intercostal muscles. This quadrant of the spinal cord also contains the sacral fibers to and from the bladder, which are closer to the spinothalamic fibers. These anatomic relations explain some of the complications associated with cordotomy: bladder dysfunction, respiratory compromise, and ipsilateral motor weakness.

From the literature that does not provide comparative studies in cancer patients with pain, pain relief can be obtained in 60% to 80% of patients immediately after cordotomy; results at 6 to 12 months are 40% to 50%.[187–190] In a retrospective survey of 40 percutaneous cordotomies in patients with predominant unilateral pain below the waist, 70% of patients obtained complete relief with continued use of some supplemental analgesics, 16% had moderate relief, and 13% did not benefit from the procedure.[186] In another study, Arbit reported that 16% of patients referred for percutaneous cordotomy could not undergo the procedure because of difficulty in positioning or with participating in the procedure, even with the use of increased analgesic drug doses and anesthetic assistance.[187] Careful patient selection is necessary for this procedure.

Open cordotomy is usually done below the cervicothoracic junction through a hemilaminectomy or full laminectomy. Open cordotomy should be reserved for the patient who cannot tolerate a percutaneous approach or for the patient with limited motor or sensory dysfunction from tumor infiltration below the waist in whom bilateral cordotomy is to be done for bilateral or midline pain.

The complications of cordotomy vary with the type of procedure (percutaneous or open) and are also strongly influenced by the patient's premorbid neurologic condition. Many patients have borderline bladder function and mild paresis from tumor infiltration that is transiently or permanently exacerbated by these procedures. In our series at Memorial Sloan-Kettering Cancer Center, 45% of patients had transient or permanent urinary retention.[192] After cordotomy there is often an unmasking of pain ipsilateral to the cordotomy site. This pain was reported in 22% of patients in our series.[187] In some patients it was difficult to clarify if this nerve pain was caused by unidentified tumor and really represented mirror pain, or was caused by the unmasking of tumor-related pain. In 60% of patients in the Arbit series, unmasking of pain on the contralateral side occurred because many patients had bilateral lumbosacral plexopathy. Dysesthesias characterized by burning pain in the area of sensory loss are reported in 1% to 2% of patients after a delay of several months to 2 years after the procedure. Ipsilateral motor weakness results from an inadvertent anterior extension of the lesion to involve the corticospinal tract. In our series, 7% of patients had transient paresis and 22% had permanent paresis. Most series report motor paresis in 10% to 20% of patients.

Respiratory complications occur in patients with a dysfunctional lung contralateral to the site of cordotomy. This is a predictable risk when patients undergo cordotomy on the same side as their only functioning lung: interruption of the reticulospinal fibers controlling the intercostal muscles and of the phrenic nerve may occur because of their proximity to the lateral spinothalamic tract in this spinal cord quadrant.

Several other complications, including headache, fever, and meningismus, are associated with the percutaneous procedure, as well as a Horner's syndrome because of interruption of the sympathetic tract.

In our series, 30% of patients demonstrated a profound depressive syndrome associated with significant pain relief.[192] Patients should be warned about this complication, but the factors contributing to its development have not been fully clarified. Rapid reduction in opioids, realization that with pain relief they must face their terminal illness, and other factors, including exhaustion, depression, and preexisting psychopathology, may all play a role in the appearance of this problematic complication. Psychological intervention and the use of tricyclic antidepressants have been effective in managing these patients.

Dorsal rhizotomy is the next most common neuroablative procedure used for cancer pain. It is performed by sectioning the posterior sensory rootlets, and a specific localized dermatomal pain level can be identified. It can be performed by an operative section of the nerve or as previously discussed by a neurolytic block. In patients with chest wall pain from tumor invasion, improved analgesia in 50% to 80% has been reported with dorsal rhizotomy.[193] Arbit has adapted this procedure to manage patients with significant chest wall pain.[194]

Rhizotomies of the trigeminal nerve, nervus intermedius, glossopharyngeal nerve, and portions of the vagus nerve are effective in controlling pain from head and neck tumors that invade the base of the skull.[195] Bilateral sacral rhizotomy has been reported to treat sacral or perineal pain involving the sacral plexus at the S2 and S3 levels. However, these patients have often had extensive radiation therapy, and wound closure in the irradiated skin over the sacrum may complicate recovery and increase the risk-to-benefit ratio. A neurolytic, epidural, or subarachnoid block is usually considered before surgical sacral rhizotomy.

The use of a dorsal root entry zone lesion is based on the recognition that nociceptive fibers enter lamina I and lamina II at the dorsal horn; interruption of this anterior lateral site has been associated with reduction in neuropathic pain in experimental animals. This approach has been used most commonly in avulsion of the brachial plexus, postherpetic neuralgia, and postradiation plexopathy. Because this approach has not been widely used in cancer pain, its usefulness for brachial and lumbosacral plexopathy is not established, but it is an interesting approach for such patients.[196] The procedure requires a several-level laminectomy to provide an adequate approach to this anatomic site, and this may be too extensive a procedure for the cancer patient with advanced disease. Further studies are necessary to determine its usefulness.

The midline commissural myelotomy approach has been used in patients with midline perineal or coccygeal pain or bilateral pain in the lower extremities. Using a limited midline myelotomy, Gildenberg and Hirschberg reported satisfactory pain relief in 10 of 14 patients with midline pain below the waist from cancer.[197] This procedure is based on the fact that nociceptive fibers cross in the anterior commissure from the dorsal horn to the contralateral spinothalamic pathway. This approach is used rarely if ever in patients with bilateral pain.

Cingulotomy has recently received attention in the treatment of some patients with cancer pain, using a stereotactic procedure with MRI to permit a radiofrequency lesion. Four patients with pain from widely metastatic, diffuse bone disease who were receiving opioid analgesics reported immediate pain relief with bilateral cingulate lesions.[198] The pain relief persisted until death in 2 to 6 weeks. This procedure was previously used to treat psychiatric illness and has a long history of use in severe chronic pain from a variety of neuropathic syndromes. The literature suggests that up to 50% of cancer patients have had moderate, marked, or complete relief for 3 months after the procedure. The extent to which the development of this improved method will alter the use of this technique needs to be clarified.

Neurostimulatory procedures involving the peripheral nerve and spinal cord are generally based on the gate theory of pain.[199] The original theory suggests that there is a neurophysiologic gating mechanism in the spinal cord, probably within the substantia gelatinosa. Noxious sensation is conducted via small-diameter peripheral nerve fibers and nonnoxious sensation via large-diameter fibers, and both send collaterals to the substantia gelatinosa and up the spinal dorsal columns. Stimulation of the small fibers tends to promote pain or "open the gate," whereas stimulation of the large fibers tends to inhibit pain or "close the gate." Because the large nerve fibers ascend in a compact bundle through the dorsal columns, they are accessible to selected electric stimulation. Retrograde firing of the large fibers ensues and pain sensation is inhibited at multiple levels of the spinal cord below that being stimulated.

Based on reports that high-frequency (50 to 100 Hz) percutaneous electrical nerve stimulation relieved chronic neurogenic pain, the use of transcutaneous electrical nerve stimulation (TENS) was reported effective in treating neuropathic pain. Although control studies are lacking, numerous clinical surveys suggest that this approach is useful for nociceptive and neuropathic pain. With the advent of sophisticated electronic devices, various patterns of electric stimulation are currently in use transcutaneously, including pulsed (burst), modulation (ramped), random, and complex wave forms, all designed to improve efficacy. Patients are instructed in proper electrode placement in a dermatomal pattern and are instructed to try both intermittent and continuous stimulation. By trial and error, analgesic effects should be observed either immediately or, in some cases, after the stimulation is discontinued.

TENS is used for a wide variety of pains and serves as a safe, noninvasive approach. Clinical experience suggests its usefulness in some patients with peripheral nerve pain. Several investigators have reported that it is useful in cancer pain for a wide variety of tumor-related and neuropathic pain syndromes.[200,201] Further studies are necessary to define the usefulness of TENS in the cancer patient with pain.

The dorsal column-stimulating technique involves the introduction of an electrode into the epidural or intrathecal space and advancing it to the appropriate level overlying the dorsal columns. This is done under local anesthesia and biplane fluoroscopy. Once in place, the electrode is implanted subcutaneously and an external transmitting electrode is placed over the receiving electrode and connected to a transmitter. A trial is then done to assess the efficacy of the electrode, check its position, and determine the patient's stimulatory parameters (frequency, amplitude, and duration of stimulatory cycles). The electrode that we have found most suitable is the quadripolar lead, a multielectrode lead that permits the physician to choose the pair of electrodes that produces the best response.[202,203]

The main indications for placement of a dorsal column stimulator are intractable dysesthetic or deafferentation pain of the limbs or trunk, such as radiation-induced brachial or lumbosacral plexopathy. This procedure is effective in 43% to 75% of patients and carries a low morbidity rate. The most common complication is failure of the device itself, which occurs in about 10% of patients annually. Other complications include infection, cerebrospinal fluid fistula, allergic or rejection response to the device material, and changes in stimulation over time, which may be related to cellular changes around the electrode or shifts in its position.

Thalamic stimulation involves the placement of electrodes in the medial thalamus and has been reported to be most useful for managing neuropathic pain from lesions in the central and peripheral nervous system. There are a series of reports on the usefulness of this technique in patients with head and neck cancer and prominent cranial neuropathic pain, but the limited use of this technique in these patients makes it difficult to define its specific role.[204]

Acupuncture has been used to treat both acute and chronic pain and is based on a sophisticated, elaborate system of diagnosis. The selected acupuncture points are manually or electrically stimulated with a needle until the patient feels the sensation. A wide variety of acupuncture techniques are available, ranging from a traditional Chinese approach to a Western adaptation. Laser acupuncture with external laser probes has also been used. The studies in cancer patients with pain represent large, uncontrolled, retrospective surveys. Minimal stimulation in manual acupuncture was used in all cases, and three acupuncture treatments represented an adequate trial. Fifty-two percent and 56% of patients reported some pain improvement for at least 7 days; an additional 30% and 22% had pain relief for 2 days or less or reported increased mobility alone.[205] A lack of detailed pain assessment in specific acupuncture techniques or a critical review of the patient population make it difficult to interpret these observations. Based on its current empirical use, this approach is relatively safe and may have some benefit in cancer patients with pain, but further studies are necessary to define its role.

PHYSIATRIC APPROACHES

Rehabilitation medicine plays an important role in the multidisciplinary approach to the patient with cancer pain. Physiatrists are concerned with a patient's physical functioning and provide expertise in assessing how impairment in a patient's physical capacity affects his or her ability to function. A wide variety of interventions are available, including TENS, diathermy (heating pads, ultrasound, hydrotherapy), and cryotherapy (ice and vapo-coolants). Assistive devices and braces, as well as therapeutic exercise and massage, are important. Trigger point injections and acupuncture have also been used. These interventions are commonly used in combination with other pain-therapy approaches, particularly behavioral and pharmacologic approaches.

A large body of data supports the use of rehabilitative interventions in acute and chronic nonmalignant pain, but similar studies have not addressed the rehabilitation needs of the cancer pain patient.[206] From our experience, neurologic dysfunction is one of the common components in patients with cancer pain, and aggressive neurorehabilitation is necessary to ambulate these patients and provide them with functional independence.

ALGORITHM FOR CANCER PAIN MANAGEMENT

An algorithm has been developed that integrates all of these management approaches for cancer pain. It attempts to integrate assessment techniques, drug therapy, behavioral approaches, and anesthetic and neurosurgical approaches and stresses continuity of care. Treatment begins with a diagnostic evaluation that addresses the medical, psychological, and social components of pain. A plan is developed to treat the cancer and the pain. If the anticancer treatment is effective, pain relief usually occurs and the drugs used for analgesia can be discontinued without difficulty. Pain treatment begins with the use of analgesic drugs as described in the analgesic ladder (see Fig. 64–2), starting with nonopioid drugs alone or in combination. If they are successful, no further therapy is necessary. If severe persistent pain does not respond to analgesic drugs or if the side effects of the drugs are not tolerated, the physician should consider switching analgesics (*e.g.*, from oral morphine to methadone), changing the route of administration (*e.g.*, from oral to subcutaneous), or performing a cordotomy for localized pain. A trial of an adjuvant drug together with the opioid and nonopioid drug would also be appropriate. In patients with excessive sedation or confusion, the use of a neurostimulant or haloperidol provides adequate treatment of the side effects of the opioid drugs and maintains the patient's analgesia while markedly reducing concurrent side effects. Alternatively, epidural or intrathecal opioids may be considered if systemic analgesics produce excessive side effects such as confusion or sedation. If the pain is localized (*e.g.*, intercostal pain from tumor infiltration of the chest wall), neurolytic blocks are indicated. If the pain is unilateral and below the waist, cordotomy should be considered. For diffuse pain, nitrous oxide inhalation may be tried. Cognitive-behavioral approaches must be integrated from the onset of treatment and should be used along with the medical and surgical approaches.

Whatever pain management techniques are used, the physician is responsible for providing continuing care, constantly reassessing both the diagnosis and the treatment to achieve optimum relief of pain and suffering for both patient and family.

The care of patients with cancer and chronic pain strains the resources of a single physician, especially after the patient's discharge from the hospital. Various supportive care and continuing care programs have been developed to manage dying patients, both in the hospital and at home. In these patients the focus of treatment shifts to symptom control and palliative comfort care. Palliative care services, home- and hospital-based palliative care teams, home- and hospital-based hospices, and high-technology home care programs are some of the approaches to care for patients with terminal illness.

A model of continuity of care for cancer centers has been developed at Memorial Sloan-Kettering Cancer Center.[207] This program centers on the patient and family and is coordinated by a nurse, using the expertise of the nurse, physician, and social worker. The nurse is responsible for day-to-day management of the patient's pain and works with the patient, family, and community physicians and nurses in symptom control and supportive care. Community health professionals work with the patient at home, and the team is available to the patient, family, and community health workers on a 24-hour-a-day basis.

To achieve continuity of care, the nurse-clinician, together with the social worker and the patient's primary physician, provides the essential link between the primary treating hospital (the cancer center), the patient, and the community. With the use of sophisticated cancer pain management, patients can die at home with adequate pain management.

FUTURE DIRECTIONS

The study of pain in cancer patients offers a unique opportunity to use clinical observations to advance our biologic knowledge. There is a critical need to expand both the research and educational efforts in cancer pain to improve the control of pain in these patients. Information on the basic mechanisms of pain modulation can be culled only from a careful study of these clinical pain problems. These patients can teach us the physiologic and psychological differences between acute and chronic pain problems, the importance of the evolution of psychological factors, the difference between pain and suffering, the clinical pharmacology of analgesic drugs, and the behavioral mechanisms humans use to suppress pain. The use of innovative approaches based on sound scientific principles and advances in research technology offer the opportunity to understand the complex phenomenon of pain.

REFERENCES

1. Foley KM. Pain syndromes in patients with cancer. In: Bonica JJ, Ventafridda V, eds. Advances in pain research and therapy. New York: Raven Press, 1979:59–75.
2. Bonica JJ. Cancer pain. In: Bonica JJ, ed. The management of pain. Philadelphia: Lea & Febiger, 1990:400.
3. Twycross RG, Fairfield S. Pain in far-advanced cancer. Pain 1982;14:303–310.
4. World Health Organization. Cancer pain relief. Geneva: World Health Organization, 1986.
5. Daut RL, Cleeland CS. The prevalence and severity of pain in cancer. Cancer 1982;50: 1913–1918.
6. Levin D, Cleeland CS, Dar R. Public attitudes toward cancer pain. Cancer 1985;56: 2337–2339.
7. Cleeland CS. Pain control: Public and physicians' attitudes. In: Hill CS, Fields WS, eds. Advances in pain research and therapy. New York: Raven Press, 1989:81–89.
8. Cleeland CS, Cleeland LM, Dar R, Rinehardt LC. Factors influencing physician management of cancer pain. Cancer 1986;58:796–800.
9. Van Roenn JH, Cleeland CS, Gonin R, Hatfield A, Pandya KJ. Physicians' attitudes towards cancer pain management: Results of the Eastern Cooperative Oncology Group Survey. Ann Intern Med (in press).
10. Peteet J, Tay V, Cohen G, MacIntyre J. Pain characteristics and treatment in an outpatient cancer population. Cancer 1986;57:1259–1265.
11. Ventafridda V, Tamburini M, DeConno F. Comprehensive treatment of cancer pain. In: Fields HL, Dubner R, Cervero F, eds. Advances in pain research and therapy. New York: Raven Press, 1985:617–628.
12. Moulin DE, Foley KM. A review of a hospital-based pain service. In: Foley KM, Bonica JJ, Ventafridda V, eds. Advances in pain research and therapy. New York: Raven Press, 1990:413–428.
13. Vainio A. Treatment of terminal cancer in Finland: A questionnaire survey. Acta Anesth Scand 1988;32:260–265.
14. Dorrepaal KL, Aaronson NK, van Dam F. Pain experience and pain management among hospital cancer patients. Cancer 1989;63:593–598.
15. Foley KM. The decriminalization of cancer pain. In: Hill CS, Fields WS, eds. Advances in pain research and therapy. New York: Raven Press, 1989:5–18.
16. Foley KM. The relationship of pain and symptom management to patient requests for physician-assisted suicide. J Pain Sympt Manag 1991;6:289–297.
17. Ahles TA, Blanchard EB, Ruckdeschel JC. The multidimensional nature of cancer-related pain. Pain 1983;17:277–289.
18. Ahles TA, Ruckdeschel JC, Blanchard EB. Cancer-related pain I. Prevalence in an outpatient setting as a function of stage of disease and type of cancer. J Psychosom Res 1984;28:115–119.
19. Ahles TA, Ruckdeschel JC, Blanchard EB. Cancer-related pain II. Assessment with visual analogue scales. J Psychosom Res 1984;28:121–124.
20. Cleeland CS, Ladinsky JL, Serlin RC, Thuy NC. Multidimensional measurement of cancer pain: Comparisons of US and Vietnamese patients. J Pain Symptom Manag 1988;3:23–27.
21. Cleeland CS. Assessment of pain in cancer: Measurement issues. In: Foley KM, Bonica JJ, Ventafridda V, eds. Advances in pain research and therapy. New York: Raven Press, 1990:47–56.
22. Portenoy RK, Miransky J, Thaler HT, et al. Pain in ambulatory patients with lung or colon cancer: Prevalence, characteristics and impact. Cancer 1992;70:1616–1624.
23. Ventafridda V, DeConno F, Ripamonti C, Gamba A, Tamburini M. Quality-of-life assessment during a palliative care programme. Ann Oncol 1990;1:415–420.
24. Coyle N, Adelhardt J, Foley KM, Portenoy RK. Character of terminal illness in the advanced cancer patient: Pain and other symptoms during the last 4 weeks of life. J Pain Sympt Manag 1990;5:83–93.
25. Ventafridda V, Ripamonti C, DeConno F, Tamburini M. Symptom prevalence and control during cancer patients' last days of life. J Palliat Care 1990;6:7–11.
26. Twycross R, Lack SA. Symptom control in far-advanced cancer. In: Pain Relief. London: Pitman Books, 1984.
27. Walsh TD, West TS. Controlling symptoms in advanced cancer. Br Med J 1988;296: 477–481.
28. IASP Subcommittee on Taxonomy. Pain terms: A list with definitions and notes on usage. Pain 1980;8:249–252.
29. Payne R. Pathophysiology of cancer pain. In: Foley KM, Bonica JJ, Ventafridda V, eds. Advances in pain research and therapy. New York: Raven Press, 1990:13–16.

30. Basbaum AI, Fields HL. Endogenous pain control mechanisms: Review and hypothesis. Ann Neurol 1978;451–462.

31. Wilcox GL. Excitatory neurotransmitters and pain. In: Bond MR, Charlton JE, Woolf CJ, eds. Pain research and clinical management. New York: Elsevier, 1991:97–118.

32. Spiegel K, Kalb R, Pasternak GW. Analgesic activity of tricyclic antidepressants. Ann Neurol 1983;13:462–465.

33. Watson CP, Evan RJ, Reed K, et al. Amitriptyline versus placebo in post-herpetic neuralgia. Neurology 1982;32:671–673.

34. Max MB, Culnane M, Shafer SC, et al. Amitriptyline relieves diabetic neuropathy pain in patients with normal or depressed mood. Neurology 1987;37:589–593.

35. Pasternak GW. Multiple opiate receptors. JAMA 1988;2599:1362–1367.

36. Yaksh TL. Spinal opiate analgesia: Characteristics and principles of action. Pain 1981;11:293–346.

37. Max MB, Inturrisi CE, Kaiko RF, Grabinski PY, Li CH, Foley KM. Epidural and intrathecal opiates: Distribution in CSF and plasma and analgesic effects in patients with cancer. Clin Pharm Ther 1985;38:631–641.

38. Onofrio BM, Yaksh TL. Long-term pain relief: Intrathecal morphine infusion in 53 patients. J Neurosurg 1990;72:200–209.

39. Besson JM, Chrouch A. Peripheral and spinal mechanisms of nociception. Physiol Rev 1987;67:67–186.

40. Sternbach RA. Pain patients: Traits and treatment. New York: Academic Press, 1974.

41. Portenoy RK, Hagen N. Management of breakthrough pain. Prim Care Cancer 1991;11:24–27.

42. Tearnan J, Blake H, Cleeland CS. Unaided use of pain descriptors by patients with cancer pain. J Pain Sympt Manag 1990;5:228–232.

43. Wallenstein SL. Measurement of pain and analgesia in cancer patients. Cancer 1984;53:2217–2234.

44. McGrath PJ, Beyer J, Cleeland CS, Eland J, McGrath PA, Portenoy RK. Report of a subcommittee on assessment and methodologic issues in the management of childhood cancer. Pediatrics 1990;86:813–834.

45. Grossman SA, Sheidler VR, Swedeen K, Mucenski J, Pianladosi S. Correlation of patient and caregiver ratings of cancer pain. J Pain Sympt Manag 1991;6:53–57.

46. Daut RL, Cleeland CS, Flanery RC. The development of the Wisconsin Brief Pain Questionnaire to assess pain in cancer and other diseases. Pain 1983;17:197–210.

47. Graham C, Bond SS, Gertrovitch MM, Cook MR. Use of the McGill Pain Questionnaire in the management of cancer pain—replicability and consistency. Pain 1980;8:377–387.

48. Dubuison D, Melzack R. Classification of clinical pain descriptions by multiple group discriminant analysis. Exp Neurol 1976;51:480–487.

49. Fishman B, Pasternak S, Wallerstein SL, et al. The Memorial Pain Assessment Card: A valid instrument for the assessment of cancer pain. Cancer 1986;60:1151–1157.

50. Tursky B. The development of a pain perception profile: A psychophysical approach. In: Weisenberg M, Tursky B, eds. Pain: New perspectives in therapy and research. New York: Plenum Press, 1976:171–194.

51. Pollack V, Cho D, Reker D, Volavka J. Profile of mood states. The factors and their psychological correlates. J Nerv Ment Dis 1979;167:612–614.

52. Hamilton M. A rating scale for depression. J Neurol Neurosurg Psychiatry 1960;23:56–62.

53. Zung W. The measurement of affects: Depression and anxiety. Mod Probl Pharmacopsych 1974;7:170–188.

54. Fishman B, Pasternak S, Wallenstein SL, et al. The Memorial Pain Assessment Card: A valid instrument for the assessment of cancer pain. Cancer 1986;60:1151–1157.

55. Foley KM. The treatment of cancer pain. N Engl J Med 1985;313:84–95.

56. Hellman S. The role of radiation therapy in the management of cancer. In: Foley KM, Bonica JJ, Ventafridda V, eds. Advances in pain research and therapy. New York: Raven Press, 1990:41–46.

57. Chapman CR, Hill HF. Prolonged morphine self-administration and addiction liability: Evaluation of two theories in a bone marrow transplant unit. Cancer 1989;63:1636–1655.

58. Saltzburg D, Foley KM. The management of pancreatic cancer pain. In: Reber H, ed. Surgical clinics of North America. Philadelphia: WB Saunders, 1989:629–650.

59. Kanner RM, Martini N, Foley KM. Incidence of pain and other clinical manifestations of superior pulmonary sulcus tumor (Pancoast's tumors). In: Bonica JJ, Ventafridda V, eds. Advances in pain research and therapy. New York: Raven Press, 1982:27–38.

60. Holland J, Rowland JH, eds. Handbook of psycho-oncology: Psychological care of the patient with cancer. New York: Oxford Press, 1989:369–382.

61. Cassell EJ. The nature of suffering and the goals of medicine. N Engl J Med 1982;306:639–45.

62. Bruera E, Brenneis C, Michaud M, MacDonald RN. Influence of the pain and symptom control team on the patterns of treatment of pain and other symptoms in a cancer center. J Pain Sympt Manag 1989;4:112–116.

63. Macaluso C, Weinberg D, Foley KM. Opioid abuse and misuse in a cancer pain population. J Pain Sympt Manag 1988;3:S54.

64. Portenoy RK, Payne R. Acute and chronic pain. In: Lowinson JH, Ruiz P, Millman RB, eds. Comprehensive textbook of substance abuse. Baltimore: Williams & Wilkins, 1992.

65. Kanner RM, Foley KM. Patterns of narcotic drug use in a cancer pain clinic. Ann NY Acad Sci 1981;362:161–172.

66. Gonzales GR, Elliott KJ, Portenoy RK, Foley KM. Impact of a comprehensive evaluation in the management of cancer pain. Pain 1991;47:141–144.

67. Elliott K, Foley KM. Neurologic pain syndromes in patients with cancer. Neurol Clin North Am 1989;7:333–360.

68. Patchell R, Posner JB. Neurologic complications of systemic cancer. Neurol Clin North Am 1985;3:729–750.

69. Greenberg HS, Deck MD, Vikram B, et al. Metastasis to the base of the skull: Clinical findings in 43 patients. Neurology 1981;31:530–537.

70. Portenoy RK, Lipton RB, Foley KM. Back pain in the cancer patient: An algorithm for evaluation and management. Neurology 1986;37:134–138.

71. Posner JB. Back pain and epidural spinal cord compression. Med Clin North Am 1987;71:185–205.

72. Sundaresan N, Galicich JH, Lane J. Treatment of odontoid fractures in cancer patients. J Neurosurg 1981;54:468–472.

73. Jaeckle KA, Young DF, Foley KM. The natural history of lumbosacral plexopathy in cancer. Neurology 1985;35:8–15.

74. Stillman M. Perineal pain: Diagnosis and management, with particular attention to perineal pain of cancer. In: Foley KM, Bonica JJ, Ventafridda V, eds. Advances in pain research and therapy. New York: Raven Press, 1990:359–378.

75. Kori S, Foley KM, Posner JB. Brachial plexus lesions in patients with cancer: Clinical findings in 100 cases. Neurology 1981;31:45–50.

76. Foley KM. Brachial plexopathy in patients with breast cancer. In: Harris JR, Hellman S, Henderson IC, Kinne D, eds. Breast diseases. Philadelphia: JB Lippincott, 1991:722–729.

77. Evans RJ, Watson CPN. Lumbosacral plexopathy in cancer patients. Neurology 1985;35:1392–1393.

78. Glass PJ, Foley KM. Carcinomatous meningitis. In: Harris JR, Hellman S, Henderson IC, Kinne D (eds). Breast diseases. Philadelphia: JB Lippincott, 1991:700–719.

79. Wasserstrom WR, Glass JP, Posner JB. Diagnosis and treatment of leptomeningeal metastases for solid tumors. Experience with 90 patients. Cancer 1982;49:759–768.

80. Macaluso C, Foley KM. Managing pain in patients with lung cancer. J Resp Dis 1988;9:59–80.

81. Baines M, Oliver DJ, Carter RL. Medical management of intestinal obstruction in patients with advanced malignant disease: A clinical and pathological study. Lancet 1985;2:990–993.

82. Kanner RM, Martini N, Foley KM. Nature and incidence of post-thoracotomy pain. Proc ASCO 1982;1:152.

83. Granek I, Ashikari R, Foley KM. Postmastectomy pain syndrome: Clinical and anatomical correlates. Proc ASCO 1983;3:122.

84. Swift TR, Nichols FT. The droopy shoulder syndrome. Neurology 1984;34:212–215.

85. MacDonald DR, Strong E, Nielson S, et al. Syncope from head and neck cancer. J Neuro-oncol 1983;1:257–267.

86. Sherman RA, Sherman CJ, Parker L. Chronic phantom and stump pain among American veterans. Pain 1984;18:83–95.

87. Aker SN. Oral findings in the cancer patient. Cancer 1979;43:2103–2107.

88. Fair WR. Urologic emergencies. In: DeVita VT, Hellman S, Rosenberg SA, eds. Principles & Practice of Oncology. Philadelphia: JB Lippincott, 1985:1894–1906.

89. Lequesne PM. Neuropathy due to drugs. In: Dyck PJ, Thomas PK, Lambert EH, et al., eds. Peripheral neuropathy. 2d ed. Philadelphia: WB Saunders, 1983:2126–2179.

90. Huang ME, Ye YC, Chen SR, et al. Use of transretinoic acid in the treatment of acute promyelocytic leukemia. Blood 1988;72:567–572.

91. Ihde DC, DeVita VT. Osteonecrosis of the femoral head in patients with lymphoma treated with intermittent combination chemotherapy (including corticosteroids). Cancer 1975;36:1585–1588.

92. Rotstein J, Good RA. Steroid pseudorheumatism. Arch Intern Med 1957;99:545–555.

93. Portenoy RK, Duma C, Foley KM. Acute herpetic and postherpetic neuralgia: Review of clinical features and current therapy. Ann Neurol 1987;20:651–664.

94. Thomas JE, Cascino TE, Earle JD. Differential diagnosis between radiation and tumor plexopathy of the pelvis. Neurology 1985;35:1–7.

95. Jellinger K, Sturm KW. Delayed radiation myelopathy in man. J Neurol Sci 1971;14:389–408.

96. Foley KM, Woodruff JM, Ellis F, et al. Radiation-induced malignant and atypical peripheral nerve sheath tumors. Ann Neurol 1980;7:311–318.

97. Payne R, Foley KM. Exploration of the brachial plexus in patients with cancer. Neurology 1986;36:329.

98. Harrington KD. Orthopaedic management of metastatic bone disease. Washington: CV Mosby, 1988.

99. Bruera E, MacDonald N. Intractable pain in patients with advanced head and neck tumors: A possible role for infection. Cancer Treat Rep 1986;70:691–692.

100. Breitbart WS, Holland J. Psychiatric aspects of cancer pain. In: Foley KM, Bonica JJ, Ventafridda V, eds. Advances in pain research and therapy. New York: Raven Press, 1990:73–88.

101. Kellgren JH. On the distribution of pain arising from deep somatic structures with charts of segmental pain areas. Clin Sci 1939–1942;4:35–46.

102. Journal of Pain and Symptom Management, Special Issue on Medical Ethics: Physician-Assisted Suicide and Euthanasia, 1991.

103. Emanuel LL, Emanuel EJ. The medical directive: A new comprehensive advance care document. JAMA 1989;261:3288–3293.

104. Annas G. The health care proxy and the living will. N Engl J Med 1991;324:1210–1213.

105. Clouston P, DeAngelis L, Posner JB. The spectrum of neurologic disease in patients with systemic cancer. Ann Neurol 1992;31:268–273.

106. Brooks PM, Day RO. Drug therapy: Nonsteroidal antiinflammatory drugs. N Engl J Med 1991;324:1718–1725.

107. Galasko CSB. Mechanisms of bone destruction in the development of skeletal metastases. Nature 1976;263:507–510.

108. Langman MJS. Treating ulcers in patients receiving anti-arthritic drugs. Q J Med 1989;73:1089–1091.

109. Foley KM. Controversies in cancer pain—medical perspective. Cancer 1989;63:2257–2266.

110. Portenoy RK, Foley KM, Inturrisi CE. The nature of opioid responsiveness and its implications for neuropathic pain: New hypotheses derived from studies of opioid infusions. Pain 1990;43:273–286.

111. Foley KM. Clinical tolerance to opioids. In: Basbaum AI, Besson JM, eds. Towards a new pharmacotherapy of pain. Chichester: John Wiley & Sons, 1991:181–204.

112. Ventafridda V, DeConno F, Panerai AE, Maresca V, Monza GC, Ripamonti C. Nonsteroidal antiinflammatory drugs as the first step in cancer pain therapy: Double-blind, within-patient study comparing nine drugs. J Intl Med Res 1990;18:21–29.

113. Kaiko RF, Foley KM, Grabinski PY, et al. Central nervous system excitatory effects of meperidine in cancer patients. Ann Neurol 1983;13:180–185.

114. Kaiko RF, Wallenstein SL, Rogers AG, et al. Analgesic and mood effects of heroin and morphine in cancer patients with postoperative pain. N Engl J Med 1981;304:1501–1505.

115. Inturrisi CE, Max M, Foley KM, Chen J, Schultz M, Houde R. The pharmacokinetics of heroin in patients with chronic pain. N Engl J Med 1984;310:1213–1217.

116. Ventafridda V, Ripamonti C, Bianchi M, Sbanotto A, DeConno E. A randomized study on oral administration of morphine and methadone in the treatment of cancer pain. J Pain Sympt Manag 1986;1:203–207.

117. Sawe J, Hansen J, Ginsman C, et al. Patient-controlled dose regimen for methadone for chronic cancer pain. Br Med J 1981;282:771–773.

118. Ventafridda V, DeConno F, Guarise G, et al. Chronic analgesic study on buprenorphine action in cancer pain—comparison with pentazocine. Drug Res 1983;33:587–590.

119. Houde RW. Methods for measuring clinical pain in humans. Acta Anaesthesiol Scand (Suppl) 1982;74:25–29.

120. Twycross RG. Clinical experience with diamorphine in advanced malignant disease. Int J Clin Pharmacol Therap Toxicol 1974;9:184–198.

121. Paul D, Standifier KM, Inturrisi CE, Pasternak GW. Pharmacological characterization of morphine-6-glucuronide, a very potent morphine metabolite. J Pharmacol Exp Ther 1989;251:477–483.

122. Portenoy RK, Thaler HT, Inturrisi CE, Friedlander-Klar H, Foley KM. The metabolite, morphine-6-glucuronide, contributes to the analgesia produced by morphine infusion in pain patients with normal renal function. Clin Pharmacol Therap 1992;51:422–431.

123. Portenoy RK, Foley KM, Stulman J, et al. Plasma morphine and morphine-6-glucuronide during chronic morphine therapy for cancer pain: Plasma profiles, steady-state concentrations and the consequences of renal failure. Pain 1991;47:13–19.

124. Hagen N, Foley KM, Cebrone DJ, Portenoy RK, Inturrisi CE. Chronic nausea and morphine-6-glucuronide. J Pain Sympt Manag 1991;6:125–128.

125. Citron ML, Johnston-Early A, Boyer M, Brasnow SH, Hood M, Cohne MH. Patient-controlled analgesia for severe cancer pain. Arch Int Med 1986;146:734–736.

126. Coyle N, Adelhardt J, Foley KM, Portenoy RK. character of terminal illness in the advanced cancer patient: Pain and other symptoms during the last 4 weeks of life. J Pain Sympt Manag 1990;5:83–93.

127. Kaiko RF. Controlled-release oral morphine for cancer-related pain: The European and North American experiences. In: Foley KM, Bonica JJ, Ventafridda V, eds. Advances in pain research and therapy. New York: Raven Press, 1990:171–190.

128. Shepard K. Review of controlled-release morphine preparation Roxanol SR. In: Foley KM, Bonica JJ, Ventafridda V, eds. Advances in pain research and therapy. New York: Raven Press, 1990:191–202.

129. Weinberg DS, Inturrisi CE, Reidenberg B, et al. Sublingual absorption of selected opioid analgesics. Clin Pharm Therap 1988;44:335–342.

130. Bell MDD, Mishra P, Weldon P, et al. Buccal morphine—a new route of analgesia. Lancet 1985;1:71–73.

131. Fine PG, Marcus M, DeBaer AJ, Van der Oord B. An open-label study of oral transmucosal fentanyl titrate for the treatment of breakthrough cancer pain. Pain 1991;45:149–155.

132. Beaver WT, Feise GA. A comparison of the analgesic effects of oxymorphones by rectal suppository and intramuscular injection in patients with postoperative pain. J Clin Pharmacol 1977;17:276–291.

133. Portenoy RK, Southam MA, Gupta SK, et al. Transdermal fentanyl for cancer pain: Repeated dose pharmacokinetics. Anesthesiology 1992 (in press).

134. Coyle N, Mauskop A, Maggard J, et al. Continuous subcutaneous infusions of opiates in cancer patients with pain. Oncol Nurs Forum 1986;13:53–57.

135. Bruera E, Fainsinger R, Moore M, Thibault R, Spoldi E, Ventafridda V. Local toxicity with subcutaneous methadone. Pain 1991;45:141–145.

136. Moulin DE, Kreeft JH, Murray-Parsons N, Bouquillon AI. Comparison of continuous subcutaneous and intravenous hydromorphone infusions for management of cancer pain. Lancet 1991;337:465–468.

137. Portenoy RK, Moulin DE, Rogers A, Inturrisi CE, Foley KM. Intravenous infusion of opioids in cancer pain: Clinical review and guidelines for use. Cancer Treat Rep 1985;70:575–581.

138. Gourlay GK, Plummer JL, Cherry DA, et al. Comparison of intermittent bolus with continuous infusions of epidural morphine in the treatment of severe cancer pain. Pain 1991;47:135–140.

139. Vainio A, Tigerstedt I. Opioid treatment for radiating cancer pain: Oral administration versus epidural techniques. Acta Anaesthesiol Scand 1988;32:179–185.

140. Cousins MJ, Bridenbaugh PO, eds. Neural blockade in clinical anesthesia and management of pain. 2d ed. Philadelphia: JB Lippincott, 1988.

141. Leavens ME, Hill CS, Cech DA, et al. Intrathecal and intraventricular morphine for pain in cancer patients: Initial study. J Neurosurg 1982;56:241–243.

142. Lobato RD, Madrid JL, Fatela LV, et al. Intraventricular morphine for control of pain in terminal cancer patients. J Neurosurg 1983;59:627–633.

143. Dennis CG, DeWitty RL. Long-term intraventricular infusion of morphine for intractable pain in cancer of the head and neck. Neurosurgery 1990;26:404–408.

144. Beaver WT. Comparison of analgesic effects of morphine sulfate, hydroxyzine and other combination in patients with postoperative pain. In: Bonica JJ, Ventafridda V, eds. Advances in pain research and therapy. New York: Raven Press, 1976:553–557.

145. Forrest WH, Brown B, Brown C, et al. Dextroamphetamine with morphine for the treatment of postoperative pain. N Engl J Med 1977;296:712–715.

146. Bruera E, Chadwich S, Brenneis C, et al. Methylphenidate associated with narcotics for the treatment of cancer pain. Cancer Treat Rep 1987;71:67–71.

147. Laska EM, Sunshine A, Mueller F, et al. Caffeine as an analgesic adjuvant. JAMA 1984;251:1711–1714.

148. Goldfrank L, Weisman RS, Errick JK, Lo MW. A normogram for continuous intravenous naloxone. Ann Emerg Med 1986;15:566–570.

149. Portenoy RK. Constipation in the cancer patient: Causes and management. In: Payne R, Foley KM, eds. Medical Clinics of North America: Cancer pain. New York: Raven Press, 1987:303–310.

150. Swerdlow M. Anticonvulsant drugs and chronic pain. Clin Neuropharmacol 1984;7:51–82.

151. Caccia MR. Clonazepam in facial neuralgia and cluster headache: Clinical and electrophysiological study. Eur Neurol 1975;13:560–566.

152. Peris JB, Perera GLS, Devendra SV, et al. Sodium valproate in trigeminal neuralgia. Med J Aust 1980;2:278–281.

153. Beaver WT, Wallenstein SL, Houde RW, Rogers AG. A comparison of the analgesic effect of methotrimeprazine and morphine in patients with cancer. Clin Pharmacol Ther 1983;7:436–446.

154. Brevik H, Rennemo F. Clinical evaluation of combined treatment with methadone and psychotropic drugs in cancer patients. Acta Anesthesiol Scand (Suppl) 1982;74:135–140.

155. Bruera E, Roca E, Cedaro L, Carraro S, Chacon R. Action of oral methylprednisolone in terminal cancer patients: A prospective randomized double-blind study. Cancer Treat Rep 1985;69:751–756.

156. Weissman DE. Glucocorticoid treatment for brain metastases and epidural spinal cord compression—a review. J Clin Oncol 1988;6:543–551.

157. Tannock I, Gospodarowicz M, Meakin W, Panzarella T, Stewart L, Rider W. Treatment of metastatic prostate cancer with low-dose prednisone—evaluation of pain and quality of life as prognostic indices of response. J Clin Oncol 1989;7:590.

158. Kaiko RF, Kanner R, Foley KM, et al. Cocaine and morphine in cancer patients with chronic pain. Pain (Suppl 2) 1984;S203.

159. Fleisch H. Bisphosphonate: Mechanism of action. In: Burckhardt P, ed. Disodium pamidronate in the treatment of malignancy-related disorders. Bern: Hans Huber, 1989:21–35.

160. Bisvoet OLM. Pamidronate in cancer therapy—the pharmacological background. In: The management of bone metastases and hypercalcemia by osteoclast inhibition. Switzerland: Hogrefe & Huber, 1990:9–11.

161. Schnur V. Etidronate for the relief of metastatic bone pain. J Urol 1984;131:404–407.

162. Hayward ML, Howell DA, O'Donnell JF, et al. Hypercalcemia complicating small-cell carcinoma. Cancer 1981;48:1643–1646.

163. Adami S, Salvago G, Guarrera G, et al. Dichloromethylene-diphosphonate in patients with prostatic carcinoma metastatic to the skeleton. J Urol 1985;134:1152–1154.

164. Van Holten A, Bijvoet ALM, Cleton FJ. Reduced morbidity from skeletal metastases in breast cancer patients during long-term biphosphonate treatment. Lancet 1987;2:983–985.

165. Smith JA. Palliation of painful bone metastases from prostate cancer using sodium etidronate: Results of a randomized prospective, double-blind, placebo-controlled study. J Urol 1989;141:85–87.

166. Ernst DS, MacDonald RN, Paterson AHG, Jasen J, Bruera E. A double-blind, crossover trial of I.V. clodronate in metastatic bone pain. J Pain Sympt Manag 1992;7:4–11.

167. Loscalzo M, Amendola J. Psychosocial and behavioral management of cancer pain: The social work contribution. In: Foley KM, Bonica JJ, Ventafridda V, eds. Advances in pain research and therapy. New York: Raven Press, 1990:429–442.

168. Fosburg MT, Crone RK. Nitrous oxide analgesia for refractory pain in the terminally ill. JAMA 1983;250:511–513.

169. Green WR, David WH. Titrated intravenous barbiturates in the control of symptoms in patients with terminal cancer. South Med J 1991;84:332–337.

170. Roy D. Need they sleep before they die. J Palliat Care 1990;6:3–4.

171. Edwards WT, Habib F, Burney RG, Begin G. Intravenous lidocaine in the management of various chronic pain states. Reg Anesth 1985;10:1–6.

172. Brose WG, Cousins MJ. Subcutaneous lidocaine for treatment of neuropathic cancer pain. Pain 1991;45:141–148.

173. Rowbotham MC, Fields HL. Post-herpetic neuralgia: The relation of pain complaint, sensory disturbance, and skin temperature. Pain 1989;39:129–144.

174. Waldman SD, Cronen MC. Thoracic epidural morphine in the palliation of chest wall pain secondary to relapsing polychondritis. J Pain Sympt Manag 1989;4:38–40.

175. Jacobsen L, Chabal C, Brody MC, Mariano AJ, Chaney EF. A comparison of the effects of intrathecal fentanyl and lidocaine on established post-amputation stump pain. Pain 1990;40:137–142.

176. Ferrer-Brechner T. Anesthetic management of cancer pain. Semin Oncol 1985;12:431–437.

177. Kuzucu EY, Derrick WS, Wilber SA. Control of intractable pain with subarachnoid alcohol block. JAMA 1966;195:541–548.

178. Swerdlow M. Complications of neurolytic blockade. In: Cousins MJ, Bridenbaugh PO, eds. Neural blockade in clinical anesthesia and management of pain. Philadelphia: JB Lippincott, 1980.

179. Ischia S, Luzzani A, Ischia A, et al. A new approach to the neurolytic block of the caeliac plexus: The transaortic technique. Pain 1983;16:333–341.

180. Brown DL, Bulley CK, Quiel EL. Neurolytic caelic plexus block for pancreatic cancer pain. Anesth Analg 1987;66:869–873.

181. Lofstrom B, Cousins MJ. Sympathetic neural blockade. In: Cousins MJ, Bridenbaugh PO, eds. Neural blockade in clinical anesthesia and management of pain. Philadelphia: JB Lippincott, 1980.

182. Gianasi G. Neuroadenolysis of the pituitary: An overview of development, mechanisms, technique and results. In: Benedetti C, Chapman CR, Moricca G, et al., eds. Advances in pain research and therapy. New York: Raven Press, 1984:647–678.

183. Katz J, Levin AB. Treatment of diffuse metastatic cancer pain by installation of alcohol into the sella turcica. Anesthesiology 1977;46:115.

184. Moricca G. Pituitary neuroadenolysis in the treatment of intractable pain from cancer. In: Lipton S, ed. Persistent pain: Modern methods of treatment. New York: Grune & Stratton, 1977.

185. Travell JG, Simons DG. Myofascial pain and dysfunction: The trigger-point manual. Baltimore: Williams & Wilkins, 1983.

186. Sundaresan N, DiGiacinto GV, Hughes EO. Neurosurgery in the treatment of cancer pain. Cancer 1989;63:2365–2377.

187. Arbit E. Neurosurgical management of cancer pain. In: Foley KM, Bonica JJ, Ventafridda V, eds. Advances in pain research and therapy. New York: Raven Press, 1990:289–300.

188. Sundaresan N, Galicich JH, Lane JM, Scher H. Stabilization of the spine involved by cancer. In: Dunsker DB, Schmidek HH, eds. The unstable spine. Orlando: Grune & Stratton, 1986:249–274.

189. Sundaresan N, Hilaris BS, Martini N. The combined neurosurgical-thoracic management of superior sulcus tumors. J Clin Oncol 1987;5:1739–1745.

190. Lahuerta T, Lipton SA, Wells JD. Percutaneous cervical cordotomy: Results and complications in a recent series of 100 patients. Ann Royal Col Surg Exp 1985;67:41–47.

191. Ischia S, Luzzani A, Ischia A, et al. Subarachnoid neurolytic block (L5, S1) and unilateral percutaneous cervical cordotomy for the treatment of neoplastic vertebral pain. Pain 1984;19:123.

192. Macaluso C, Arbit E, Foley KM. Cordotomy for lumbosacral, pelvic, and lower extremity pain of malignant origin: Safety and efficacy. Neurology 1988;38:110.

193. Barrash JM, Milan EL. Dorsal rhizotomy for the relief of pain of malignant tumor origin. J Neurosurg 1973;38:755–757.

194. Arbit E, Galicich JH, Burt M, et al. Modified open thoracic rhizotomy for treatment of intractable chest wall pain of malignant etiology. Ann Thoracic Surg 1989;48:820–823.

195. Giorgi C, Broggi G. Surgical treatment of glossopharyngeal neuralgia and pain from cancer of the nasopharynx. J Neurosurg 1984;61:952–955.

196. Nashold BS, Ostdahl RH. Dorsal root entry zone lesions for pain relief. J Neurosurg 1979;51:59–69.

197. Gildenberg PL, Hirschberg RM. Limited myelotomy for the treatment of intractable cancer pain. J Neurol Neurosurg Psychiatry 1984;47:94–96.

198. Hassenbusch SJ, Pillay PK, Barnett GH. Radiofrequency cingulotomy for intractable cancer pain using stereotaxis guided by magnetic resonance imaging. Neurosurgery 1990;27:220–223.

199. Melzack R, Wall PD. Pain mechanisms: A new theory. Science 1965;150:971–979.

200. Ventafridda V. Transcutaneous nerve stimulation in cancer pain. In: Bonica JJ, Ventafridda V, eds. Advances in pain research and therapy. New York: Raven Press, 1979: 509–515.

201. Thompson JW, Filshie J. Transcutaneous electrical nerve stimulation and acupuncture in palliative care medicine. In: Doyle D, Hanks G, MacDonald N, eds. Oxford University Press, 1992 (in press).

202. Hosobuchi Y. Subcortical electrical stimulation for control of intractable pain: Report of 122 cases. J Neurosurg 1986;64:543–553.

203. Levy RM, Lamb S, Adams JE. Treatment of chronic pain by deep brain stimulation: Long-term followup and review of the literature. Neurosurgery 1987;21:885–893.

204. Young RF, Brechner T. Electrical stimulation of the brain for relief of intractable pain due to cancer. Cancer 1986;57:1266–1272.

205. Filshie J. Acupuncture and malignant pain problems. Acupuncture in Medicine 1990;8: 38–39.

206. King JC, Kellcher MJ. The chronic pain syndrome: The interdisciplinary rehabilitative behavioral modification approach. Physical Medicine: State of the Art Reviews 1991;5: 165–186.

207. Coyle N, Monzillo E, Loscalzo M, et al. A model of continuity of care for cancer patients with pain and neuro-oncologic complications. Cancer Nurs 1985;8:111–119.

SECTION **2**

MARGUERITE S. LEDERBERG
MARY JANE MASSIE

Psychosocial and Ethical Issues in the Care of Cancer Patients

PSYCHOSOCIAL ISSUES: HISTORICAL BACKGROUND

The word cancer refers to a group of diseases that has struck fear in people's hearts for centuries. In the past, its fatal outcome, absence of known cause or cure, and association with pain and disfigurement made it particularly frightening. Physicians regarded the diagnosis as too painful to reveal to the patient and conspired, often unsuccessfully, with the family to create the illusion of a lesser illness. The same fear prevented the word from appearing in the press; patients and their families kept the diagnosis a secret from all but the closest acquaintances. A person who even suspected that he or she had cancer would often refuse to go to the doctor out of fatalistic resignation. Cancer was widely used as a metaphor for an insidious, destructive force in society. Fear, secrecy, and mythologic elaboration compounded the emotional burden and social stigma borne by patients and families.

In 1913, the American Cancer Society was founded to counter the public's fears and teach that early diagnosis and surgical treatment could be curative. However, negative attitudes have persisted. Only in the past 4 decades has a real, albeit still incomplete, change occurred in attitudes toward cancer in the United States. There is greater openness in public discussion and more candor in revealing the diagnosis to patients. Except for Scandinavia, few other countries have moved as far as the United States, but similar trends are under way throughout Western Europe.[1]

Several factors contributed to the change in attitudes in the United States:

1. Physicians and patients became more optimistic as radiation therapy and chemotherapy began to cure several common neoplasms of children and young adults.

2. Clinicians who spoke more openly with their patients found that such candor was unexpectedly well tolerated. A better understanding of the rationale for treatment helped patients handle side effects better, and truthful communication enhanced trust in the physician. During the 1950s, psychological studies showed that patients given accurate information adapted better to radical surgery.

3. Terminal care practices were reexamined. Following the lead of the European hospice movement and the pioneering work of Elizabeth Kubler-Ross, it became more widely understood that terminally ill patients benefited from an opportunity to discuss not only their illness but also their feelings and fears about death.

4. In the 1970s, advocacy of patients' rights became increasingly vocal. Physicians were required to discuss all diagnostic and treatment options to enable patients to participate in decisions. Informed consent for research patients became mandated by federal guidelines. In routine clinical care, the patient autonomy issue overlapped with and reinforced a growing demand for greater attention to quality of life during treatment. This problem was particularly acute in oncology, where the often severe side effects of treatment made special demands on patient trust. As physicians came to depend more on laboratory data and spent less time at the bedside, patients complained increasingly about the diminished

closeness to their new, more technology-oriented doctors.

Another impetus to exploring psychosocial issues in cancer was the recognition that psychological factors and their resulting behaviors are critical to the prevention and early detection of cancer. Much of the research effort in cancer prevention today, particularly that of smoking cessation, depends on the social sciences to develop ways of understanding and altering behavior.[2,3] Most recently, studies of the possible role of personality factors in altering not only risk but also survival, through neuroendocrine and neuroimmune mechanisms, has generated enormous public interest, far beyond what the scientific evidence can currently support. It has also stimulated extensive research that will, we hope, resolve the controversies during the next decades.[4,5] This issue is discussed later in this chapter.

The subspecialty of psychooncology developed in the wake of these developments. Since the mid-1970s, it has established a large body of information based on systematic clinical observations and scientific investigations, addressing two broad areas[6]:

1. The impact of cancer and its treatment on the psychological and social functioning of patients, their families, and the treating staff
2. The role of psychosocial factors and behaviors in cancer risk and survival.

PSYCHOLOGICAL IMPACT OF CANCER

Acute psychological distress is to be expected as a patient confronts the implications of cancer: possible death, pain, dependence on others, disability, disfiguring changes in the body, and loss of function, all of which endanger his or her relationships to others. The initial crisis is just the first of many, each requiring resiliency and rapid adaptation. Most patients cope adequately, keeping distress in a manageable range; some do not. To treat and prevent pathologic reactions, it is important to understand their causes, which are of three kinds: societal, biomedical, and patient-related (personal and interpersonal).

SOCIETAL FACTORS

Social factors play an immediate and important role in a patient's psychological adaptation to cancer but are seldom obvious to the patient.

In the past, patients came to the physician with a sense of doom at the mention of cancer, along with a deep sense of shame and the associated desire for secrecy. At the same time, they were more ready to trust their physician and accept his or her recommendations without question. Today—paradoxically in the face of far better outcomes—patients may come with less simple hope, more fear of treatment, and more mistrust of the doctor and the medical establishment.

The financial side of medical care is affecting physicians and patients more and more acutely. The issue of national health insurance is thought to have caused a major upset in the 1991 Pennsylvania senatorial election, making it clear how deeply the public fears medical pauperization. Patients and families may become easily angered when they perceive their physician as careless about this aspect of care. The same physician is also under enormous pressure to contain costs from both public and private sectors and may have to restrict length of stay or certain procedures in ways that also draw patient and family resentment. These sources of friction between physician and patient are less acute in countries with socialized medicine.

In the United States there is a large uninsured population whose health-care problems are well known. But even among the initially insured, identified cancer patients often become uninsurable. The policyholder becomes locked into a given job so as not to lose insurance benefits, causing a downward social drift that has yet to be fully documented.

Recent studies have shown a major effect of social class on cancer incidence and outcomes (see further discussion later in the chapter).[7,8] While this is mediated through many routes, psychological factors figure prominently among them. Socially disadvantaged patients are often more fatalistic and hopeless in their outlook and hence delay and seek less treatment. They also have many of the psychological risk factors outlined below.

Social rejection and job discrimination remain problems for cancer patients, although there has been a marked change in the handling of cancer in the media, and many famous personalities have come forward to speak about their own experience in ways that can be very meaningful to patients.

Alternative cancer therapies enjoy enduring popularity.[9] But there are now many naturalistic therapies that, while not scientifically proven, may increase a patient's sense of control and well-being and thus improve quality of life, as long as they are not used instead of proven treatments. They are becoming increasingly visible and popular, in direct proportion to the disillusionment with or mistrust of traditional medicine. (The possible scientific basis for claims of improved survival are discussed later in this chapter.)

These trends are affecting the practice of oncology in many ways. The growth of bioethics and the patients' rights movement have resulted in many changes of law and custom, including:

1. Many states require that a woman with stage I or II breast cancer be given the choice between breast-conserving treatment and mastectomy.
2. New York State gives the patient or family the ultimate authority in demanding resuscitation.
3. The Federal Patient Self-Determination Act requires all hospitals and nursing homes to advise patients at the time of admission of their right to refuse treatment.

The most dramatic intrusion of social policy into the practice of medicine is the debate over the legalization of euthanasia, which is discussed in the section below on ethical issues.

While these developments have brought difficult transition periods, the overall movement toward enabling patients to participate as fully and as early as possible in planning for their own care is a welcome one. One of the very positive outcomes of increased consumerism has been the emphasis on quality-of-life issues in evaluating cancer treatment. Today, an increasing number of treatment protocols that aim for prolonged survival rather than cure are factoring quality-of-life measures into the final outcomes.[10,11]

MEDICAL FACTORS

Once a patient receives a diagnosis of cancer, the vicissitudes of the disease and the treatment assume a central role in the patient's existence and emotional state.

Transition Points

Adaptational needs and distress are greatest at certain crises or transition points such as diagnosis, the start of primary treatment, the end of primary treatment (when concerns about possible recurrence increase), a change in treatment modalities, relapse, the transition from curative to supportive treatment, and during advanced and terminal disease.[12] The oncologist must be especially attuned to psychological distress at these points. For example, patients terminating an intensive course of treatment should be given an early follow-up appointment, reassured of the physician's ongoing availability, and warned that they may go through an unexpected period of increased anxiety.

Fear of Treatment

Today's patient is often very aware of the paradoxical toxicity of most cancer treatments and of the many unpleasant side effects they may have observed in friends or family members. Patient compliance and psychological adaptation improve if the oncologist is aware of these anxieties and allows the patient to discuss them.

Symbolically Meaningful Symptoms and Losses

Each patient brings his or her own history to bear on the illness. Construction workers value their stamina, computer operators their manual dexterity. Each will react with special intensity to a loss in their area of special functioning and may need special support.

Two related areas are of special significance to almost all patients: altered physical appearance and altered sexual functioning.[13-16] The first is easier to address; the second is often ignored out of patient and doctor embarrassment. Patients are deeply relieved and grateful when the doctor broaches these sensitive topics in an open, matter-of-fact manner.

Communication Problems

Physicians are often baffled when patients claim ignorance about matters they have clearly been told. Because anxiety interferes with information-processing, it is predictable that patients will need repeated statements to absorb complex and unwelcome news. This is particularly problematic when patients use an unusual amount of denial and systematically screen out the "bad" parts of the news. It becomes the oncologist's difficult task to gently confront denial when it interferes with important decision-making or necessary life adaptations.

Denial is a ubiquitous psychological defense mechanism that can range from very adaptive to very destructive. *Instrumental denial* prevents the patient from being active on his or her own behalf and must be confronted. *Affective denial* allows the patient to maintain an upbeat, hopeful stance even while making decisions that flow from a realistic assessment of his or her situation. This form of denial can be encouraged and is associated with better compliance and better quality of life.

Terminal Illness

In the past, terminal patients were often kept in the dark about their condition because protective families and physicians felt this was the most humane thing to do. This approach has been made obsolete by society's attention to patient's rights to participate in decisions about instituting and foregoing life-sustaining measures, especially cardiopulmonary resuscitation. The 1991 Federal Patient Self-Determination Act requires that all patients be asked on admission about their wishes concerning resuscitation. While both physicians and families may wish to avoid frank discussions with the fatally ill patient, almost all patients, even disturbed ones, are better off having frank discussions. Concern for how the patient may react, guilt for having failed the patient, and self-consciousness about how to present the issue cause many physicians to delay and avoid the discussion. This improves with encouragement, role-modeling, and practice. (The ethical problems associated with the terminal care period are discussed below.)

PATIENT-RELATED FACTORS

The patient's contribution to adaptation to illness is derived from several sources. Patients with a stable personality, no current psychiatric disorder, and no history of significant prior psychological problems can be expected to adapt well to cancer. These patients confront the facts, seek available information, and actively pursue treatment. They respond to the disease as a challenge, while poorer copers often try to avoid the implications of the illness and delay the decisions required for optimal care. The best predictor of good patient adjustment is good adaptation to prior life crises. However, some prior crises can make the diagnosis of cancer much more upsetting even in psychologically healthy patients. These include cancer in a close relative or friend, especially when it involves the same site as the patient's disease, and the coincidence of cancer with other crises such as grief, divorce, job loss, or another illness. Without the support of close, caring people, many patients unravel under the stress of cancer. Social supports have even been found to influence mortality rates and measures of immune function.[17,18]

Normal Psychological Responses to Cancer

The expected range of psychological responses to cancer must be defined to recognize when a patient requires further evaluation and support. The observed response to a diagnosis of cancer is similar to that of other life-threatening illnesses or major life changes. Initially, the person is often disbelieving. "I feel numb," "as if I am watching someone else," are common expressions used by patients at this time. This is a constructive attempt at keeping awareness within tolerable levels. The next stage is one of mixed anxious and depressed feelings, preoccupation with the implications of the illness, foreboding thoughts about the future, and a sense of helplessness. Attention and concentration are impaired; sleeping and eating patterns are disrupted. These acute symptoms dissipate over a few weeks as a treatment plan is agreed on and undertaken. During this critical time, the psychological distress and associated physiologic arousal make it difficult for the patient to fully absorb the diagnosis and treatment recommendations. Therefore, the physician should plan to repeat information several times and should not be surprised when patients appear to have poor comprehension and even poorer recall.

Although the acute response is limited to a few weeks, the overall adaptation lasts much longer. Weisman and Worden described the first 100 days after diagnosis as one of continuing "existential plight," and of course some level of concern remains indefinitely.[19] Psychologically healthy patients use ways of coping that have worked well in the past, obtaining and processing information about the treatment as well as help and advice from experienced others.

Psychosocial and Medical Factors Associated With Poor Adjustment

The vulnerability factors that identify patients at increased risk of poor adjustment and psychiatric problems fall into three major categories: psychological, social, and medical factors (Table 64–9). Prior psychiatric problems, alcohol or drug abuse, depression, and chronic anxiety are strong predictors for poor adjustment and for exacerbation of previous psychiatric difficulties. Evidence of unusually high initial distress that persists usually long with high levels of anxiety and depression, especially when coupled with behavioral evidence of poor coping, is also reason for concern. A negative attitude toward physicians and treatment and low expectations for the future do not bode well. Medical factors suggesting high vulnerability are advanced disease and poorly controlled symptoms, particularly pain and insomnia.[20] Several social factors are associated with poor adjustment: low socioeconomic status, chronic marital or family problems, perceived or actual poor support from others, and absence of affiliation with a meaningful social group, especially a religious one.

Abnormal Psychological Responses to Cancer

It is important for the oncologist to recognize when a patient's response is normal and self-limited and when it has become pathologic. The diagnosis of psychiatric disorders in cancer patients has been clouded by assumptions that severe depression is "normal" in cancer patients. In fact, when the level and severity of physical illness are controlled for, cancer patients have the same frequency of depression as other medically ill patients.[21]

TABLE 64–9. Psychological Problems of Cancer Survivors

Fears of termination of treatment
Preoccupation with minor physical problems
Adjustment to physical losses and handicaps
Difficulty with reentry into normal life (the Lazarus syndrome)
Perceived loss of job mobility
Awareness of insurance discrimination
Persistent sense of vulnerability to illness and death (the Damocles syndrome)
Persistent guilt (the survivor syndrome)

The incidence of psychiatric disorders in cancer patients has been determined by assessing ambulatory and hospitalized patients in three cancer centers using standard diagnostic criteria (Fig. 64–3).[22] Fifty-three percent of patients interviewed, although showing signs of stress, were coping adequately. The remaining 47% had a diagnosable psychiatric disorder. The most common by far was adjustment disorder with anxious and depressive symptoms, seen in two thirds of those with psychiatric disorders and one third of all patients interviewed. Depression was next, seen in 13% of those with a psychiatric diagnosis. Central nervous system complications resulting in organic mental disorders were present in 4%; prior psychiatric problems accounted for only 4% of cases.

Among hospitalized and more seriously ill patients, the frequency of major depression rises to 20%.[21] Organic mental disorders, primarily delirium, increase with worsening illness to a frequency of 20% in hospitalized cancer patients and 80% in the terminally ill.[20,23]

Six psychiatric disorders occur frequently enough in cancer patients to warrant a description of their clinical picture. Three represent a direct reaction to the illness: adjustment disorders (reactive anxiety and depression), major depression, and delirium. The others (primary anxiety disorders, personality disorders, and major mental illness) are preexisting conditions often exacerbated by illness.

ADJUSTMENT DISORDER WITH DEPRESSED, ANXIOUS, OR MIXED FEATURES (REACTIVE ANXIETY AND DEPRESSION). These common disorders are an exaggeration of the mixed anxiety and depression seen in self-limited stress responses. The key features are unusual persistence and undue interference with functioning.

Interventions are aimed at helping the patient resume successful coping by use of several modalities. Individual psychotherapy focuses on clarifying the medical situation and the meaning of illness and on reinforcing the patient's positive coping strategies. It is often desirable to include a spouse or family member to enhance support at home. Group therapy, with a focus on illness, is often helpful, as are behavioral methods such as relaxation and hypnosis. Couple and family therapy may be helpful when interpersonal issues are prominent. The decision to prescribe a psychotropic drug requires a high level of distress and the inability to carry out daily activities. Low doses of alprazolam, lorazepam, or oxazepam control symptoms and need not cause undue daytime sedation or risk withdrawal or dependence in these psychologically healthy patients. Alprazolam, because of its rapid onset and combined anxiolytic and antidepressant action, is particularly effective starting at doses of 0.25 mg one to three times per day. Bedtime sedation with a benzodiazepine (triazolam or temazepam) or a sedating antidepressant (amitriptyline) is effective and may improve daytime symptoms as well.

MAJOR DEPRESSION. All depression in cancer has a strong reactive component. However, major depressive episodes also occur and are responsive to treatment. Unfortunately, because it is often assumed that the patient is "appropriately" depressed, major depression is often undiagnosed and untreated.

Because of the associated medical illness, diagnosis cannot depend on vegetative signs such as fatigue, insomnia, weight

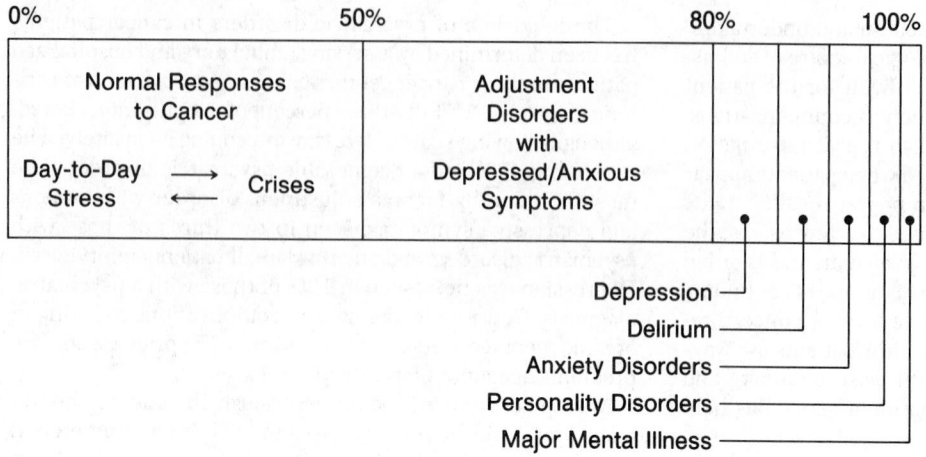

FIGURE 64–3. Incidence of psychiatric disorders in cancer patients. (Derogatis LB, Morrow GR, Fetting J, et al. The prevalence of psychiatric disorders among cancer patients. JAMA 1983;249:751)

loss, and anorexia, but rests on a constellation of psychological symptoms: dysphoric or sad mood, feelings of helplessness and hopelessness, loss of self-esteem and feelings of worthlessness or guilt, and a wish to die. Patients at high risk for major depression are those with a history of prior depression, inadequately controlled pain, an advanced stage of illness, and disease at certain sites such as the pancreas.[24] Some of the endocrine and ectopic hormone-secreting tumors also produce depression. Several drugs can produce severe depression as part of their central nervous system toxicity, both singly and additively; among chemotherapy agents, these include interferon, steroids, BCNU, vincristine, tamoxifen, and L-asparaginase.[25] Other commonly used drugs are antihypertensives, benzodiazepines, antiparkinsonian agents, and beta-blockers.

The presence of suicidal ideation requires careful assessment to determine if it reflects depressive illness or expresses a wish to have ultimate control over intolerable symptoms. Thoughtful clinical judgment is required to make this differentiation, especially in the patient with advanced disease. Breitbart has outlined factors that place a cancer patient at a high risk for suicide: poor prognosis and advanced illness, depression and hopelessness, uncontrolled pain, delirium, prior psychiatric history, history of previous suicide attempts or family history of suicide, history of recent death of friends or spouse, history of alcohol abuse, and few social supports.[26] At Memorial Sloan-Kettering Cancer Center, patients who have attempted suicide have been characterized by poorly controlled pain, mild encephalopathy, disinhibition secondary to medications, and hopelessness combined with distress about being unable to communicate discomfort to caregivers. If a patient is suicidal, a 24-hour companion is provided to establish constant observation, monitor the suicidal risk, and reassure the patient.

Depressed patients are usually treated with a combination of supportive psychotherapy and antidepressants. There are several reports of the efficacy of antidepressants in depressed patients with cancer.[27–30] The antidepressant agents that can be considered for use in cancer patients are the tricyclic antidepressants (TCAs), heterocyclic antidepressants, atypical antidepressants, monoamine oxidase inhibitors (MAOIs), psychostimulants, lithium carbonate, and benzodiazepines.[31]

Table 64–10 shows the starting dose and range of therapeutic daily doses for drugs in these classes.

The antidepressants best documented in the oncology setting are the tricyclic antidepressants. They are started at a low dose (10 to 25 mg at bedtime), especially in debilitated patients, and the dose is increased by 25 mg every 1 to 2 days until a beneficial effect is achieved. For reasons that are unclear, depressed cancer patients often show a therapeutic response to a TCA at much lower doses (75 to 125 mg daily) than are usually required in physically healthy, depressed patients (150 to 300 mg daily). Patients are usually maintained on a TCA for 4 to 6 months after symptoms improve, after which time the dose is gradually lowered and discontinued.

The choice of TCA depends on the nature of the depressive symptoms, medical problems present, and side effects of the TCA. The depressed patient who is agitated and has insomnia will benefit from the use of a TCA with sedating effects, such as amitriptyline or doxepin. Patients with psychomotor slowing will benefit from use of the compounds with the least sedating effects, such as protriptyline or desipramine. The patient who has stomatitis secondary to chemotherapy or radiation therapy or who has slow intestinal motility or urinary retention should receive a TCA with the least anticholinergic effects, such as desipramine or nortriptyline.

Patients who cannot swallow pills may be able to take an antidepressant in an elixir (amitriptyline, nortriptyline, or doxepin) or in an intramuscular form (amitriptyline or imipramine). Intramuscular administration causes discomfort because of the volume of the vehicle; hence, 50 mg is usually the maximum dosage that can be delivered per intramuscular injection. Although TCAs have not yet been approved for intravenous use in the United States, several studies from Europe indicate their efficacy and safety by this route.[31] Hospital pharmacies can prepare some TCAs in rectal suppository form, but absorption by this route has not been studied in cancer patients.

Imipramine, doxepin, amitriptyline, desipramine, and nortriptyline are often used in the management of neuropathic pain in cancer patients. Dosing is similar to the treatment of depression, and analgesic efficacy, if it occurs, is usually observed at a dose of 50 to 150 mg daily; higher doses are needed occasionally. While the initial assumption

TABLE 64–10. Antidepressant Medications Used in Cancer Patients

Drug Name	Starting Daily Dosage mg (PO)	Therapeutic Daily Dosage mg (PO)
Tricyclic Antidepressants		
Amitriptyline	25	75–100
Doxepin	25	75–100
Imipramine	25	75–100
Desipramine	25	75–100
Nortriptyline	25	50–100
Heterocyclic Antidepressants		
Maprotiline	25	50–75
Amoxapine	25	100–150
Atypical Antidepressants		
Buproprion	15	200–450
Fluoxetine	20	20–60
Trazodone	50	150–200
Monoamine Oxidase Inhibitors		
Isocarboxazid	10	20–40
Phenelzine	15	30–60
Tranylcypromine	10	20–40
Lithium Carbonate	300	600–1200
Psychostimulants		
Dextroamphetamine	2.5 at 8 A.M. and noon	5–30
Methylphenidate	2.5 at 8 A.M. and noon	5–30
Pemoline	18.75 in A.M. and noon	37.5–150
Benzodiazepines		
Alprazolam	0.25–1.00	0.75–6.00

(Massie MJ, Holland JC. The cancer patient with pain: Psychological complications and their management. J Symptom Pain Manage [in press])

was that the analgesic effect resulted indirectly from the effect on depression, it is now clear that these tricyclics have a separate, specific analgesic action, probably mediated through several neurotransmitters, most prominently norepinephrine and serotonin.[32]

If a patient does not respond therapeutically to adequate blood levels of a TCA or cannot tolerate its side effects, a heterocyclic (maprotiline or amoxapine) or a second-generation (bupropion, trazodone, fluoxetine, sertraline) antidepressant can be used. The heterocyclic antidepressants have side-effect profiles similar to the TCAs. Maprotiline should be avoided in patients who are at high risk for seizures, because the incidence of seizures can be increased with this medication. Amoxapine has strong dopamine-blocking activity, so patients taking other dopamine blockers (*e.g.*, antiemetics) have an increased risk of developing extrapyramidal symptoms and dyskinesias.

The atypical antidepressants are generally considered to be less cardiotoxic than the TCAs and are increasingly being used. Bupropion is a relatively new drug in the United States, and there is little experience with its use in the medically ill. At present, it is not the first drug of choice for depressed patients with cancer, but it should be considered if a patient has a poor response to other antidepressants. Bupropion may be somewhat activating in medically ill patients. Because of its seizure potential it should be avoided in patients with seizure disorders and brain tumors and those who are malnourished.

Trazodone is strongly sedating and in low doses (50–100 mg at bedtime) is helpful in the treatment of the depressed cancer patient with insomnia. Effective antidepressant doses are often greater than 300 mg per day. Trazodone has been associated with priapism and should therefore be used with caution in male patients.

Fluoxetine, a selective inhibitor of neuronal serotonin uptake, has fewer sedative and autonomic effects than the TCAs. The most common side effects are mild nausea and a brief period of increased anxiety; hyponatremia is an uncommon adverse effect.[33] Fluoxetine can cause appetite suppression, which usually lasts for several weeks. Some cancer patients experience transient weight loss, but weight usually returns to baseline level and the anorectic properties of this drug have not been a limiting factor in this population. Fluoxetine may be particularly useful in depressed cancer patients who are additionally distressed from weight gain resulting from chemotherapy. Overall, the side-effect profile of fluoxetine suggests that it may be a relatively favorable treatment for depressed cancer patients; a multicenter study of its efficacy is currently under way. Sertraline, a recently approved serotonergic agent, has a shorter duration of action than fluoxetine, and possibly a more benign side effect profile. It is increasingly being used, starting with 25 mg per day, in the medically ill.

Patients who were taking lithium carbonate before cancer should be maintained on it throughout cancer treatment, although close monitoring is necessary when the intake of fluids and electrolytes is restricted, such as during preoperative and postoperative periods. The maintenance dose of lithium may need to be reduced in seriously ill patients. Lithium should be prescribed with caution in patients receiving cisplatin due to the potential nephrotoxicity of both drugs. Although several authors have reported that the leukocytosis produced by lithium could be beneficial in neutropenic cancer patients, the functional capabilities of these leukocytes have not been determined.[34] The bone-marrow stimulation appears to be transient; no mood changes have been noted in these patients.

If a patient has responded well to an MAOI for depression before treatment for cancer, its continued use is warranted. However, most psychiatrists are reluctant to start depressed cancer patients on MAOIs because the need for dietary restriction is poorly received by patients who already have dietary limitations and nutritional deficiencies secondary to cancer illness and treatment.

In cancer patients, low doses of the psychostimulants (dextroamphetamine, methylphenidate, and pemoline) promote a sense of well-being, decrease fatigue, and stimulate appetite.[35,36] An advantage of these drugs is their rapid onset of antidepressant action, compared with that of the TCAs. Psychostimulants can potentiate the analgesic effects of narcotic analgesics and are commonly used to counteract opioid-induced sedation. Occasionally they can produce nightmares, insomnia, and even psychosis.

Treatment with dextroamphetamine and methylphenidate is usually started at a dose of 2.5 mg at 8 A.M. and noon. Typically patients are maintained for 1 to 2 months, after which time about two thirds can be withdrawn without a recurrence of depressive symptoms. Those who develop recurrence of depressive symptoms can be maintained for up to 1 year. Tolerance may develop, and adjustment of the dose may be necessary.

Pemoline, a less potent and longer-acting psychostimulant, comes in a chewable tablet so patients who have difficulty swallowing can absorb the drug through the buccal mucosa.[36] We have begun to use pemoline frequently in a population of cancer patients with depressive symptoms, and it appears to be as effective as methylphenidate or dextroamphetamine. Pemoline should be used with caution in patients with renal impairment; liver function tests should be monitored periodically with long-term treatment.

The triazolobenzodiazepine alprazolam has been shown to be an effective antidepressant as well as an anxiolytic.[37] Alprazolam is particularly useful in cancer patients who have mixed symptoms of anxiety and depression.[38] Treatment is initiated with doses of 0.25 mg three or four times a day and titrated up to effective antidepressant doses, usually 4 to 6 mg per day.

Benzodiazepines are usually readily discontinued by cancer patients when the symptoms of anxiety abate. Concerns about addiction should not interfere with their use in the cancer setting. In fact, cancer patients often must be encouraged to take enough medication to provide relief from anxiety. Benzodiazepines should be tapered to avoid withdrawal.

DELIRIUM FROM CNS COMPLICATIONS. Delirium, the second most common psychiatric diagnosis among cancer patients, is due both to the direct effects of cancer on the CNS and the indirect CNS complications of the disease and treatment. Posner reported that 15% to 20% of hospitalized cancer patients have abnormalities of cognitive function that are not related to structural disease.[39] About one fifth of all consultation requests made to a psychooncology service were requests for assistance in the management of symptoms of delirium. Early symptoms are often unrecognized or misdiagnosed by medical and nursing staff as symptoms of depression or "poor coping." Early recognition is important: the underlying cause may be a treatable complication of cancer.

Any patient who shows the acute onset of agitation, impaired cognitive function, altered attention span, or a fluctuating level of consciousness should be suspected of having delirium. It is usually due to one or more of these causes: medications, electrolyte imbalance, failure of a vital organ or system, nutritional state, infections, vascular complications, or hormone-producing tumors. In a study of terminally ill cancer patients, over three fourths developed delirium with a multifactorial etiology.[23]

Many drugs can cause acute confusional states. Confusion is a common adverse effect of opioids. Among the more than 280 chemotherapeutic agents now available for cancer, delirium has been associated with methotrexate (with intrathecal or intravenous administration), 5-fluorouracil (5-FU), vin-

cristine, vinblastine, bleomycin, BCNU, cisplatin, asparaginase, procarbazine, cytosine arabinoside, ifosfamide, and corticosteroids.[40,41] Other medications commonly prescribed to cancer patients that can cause confusional states are interleukin-2, amphotericin, and acyclovir.

All steroid compounds can cause symptoms ranging from minor mood disturbance to frank psychosis.[42] Disturbances may include affective changes (emotional lability, euphoria, depressed mood, anxiety), fears, paranoid interpretation of events and suspiciousness of others, with illusions, delusions, and hallucinations. Symptoms often develop 4 to 5 days after high-dose steroids are begun or when the dose is rapidly tapered, but they can also develop while patients are on maintenance dosages. It may be necessary to continue steroids despite psychiatric symptoms, in which case neuroleptics such as haloperidol can be used for symptom control. A steroid psychosis during one course of treatment does not necessarily predict recurrence with subsequent courses of steroids. No relation has been shown between the development of steroid psychosis and premorbid personality or psychiatric history.

Whole-brain irradiation, especially when combined with intrathecal chemotherapy, strongly predisposes patients to the development of later cognitive deficits. These are more severe in the very young and the very old, and result in IQ drops of as much as 20 to 25 points. Learning disabilities have been found even in the absence of documented IQ losses. Thus, despite some controversy, the preponderance of studies shows some residual deficits, leading to a search for new regimens to minimize them.[43,44]

Haloperidol is the most effective drug for prompt control of delirium and agitated or disruptive behavior. Intramuscular or intravenous injection of 0.5 to 2.0 mg reduces agitation without causing sedation or hypotension. It can be given intravenously at 1 mg/minute, if necessary, and repeated at 60-minute intervals, titrated against behavior. The patient should be changed to an oral dose of three-fourths the parenteral dose as soon as possible. For milder symptoms, 1 to 2 mg of trifluoperazine or 10 to 25 mg of thioridazine may be given orally twice a day.

ANXIETY DISORDERS: PREEXISTING PHOBIAS, PANIC ATTACKS, AND GENERALIZED ANXIETY. Persistent and incapacitating anxiety symptoms in cancer patients usually represent worsening of preexisting problems. Phobias, the most common form of abnormal fears, often revolve around physical illness, death, pain, needles, claustrophobia, or fear of solitude. Panic attacks may be precipitated, and chronic generalized anxiety syndromes are severely exacerbated. Long scanning procedures are intolerable to many patients, who require special handling and medication.[45] Agoraphobic patients may be unable to tolerate the night before surgery alone in the hospital and require relaxation of rules to allow the presence of a relative. They also need longer and higher levels of preoperative sedation, with coordination between the psychiatrist and the anesthesiologist. Specific fears of needles, pain, or the sight of blood require acknowledgment and individualized management, including medication, distraction, and desensitization.[46] Given this special care, patients are generally cooperative, grateful, and able to proceed with treatment.

Benzodiazepines are the drugs of choice for both acute and

chronic anxiety states. The most common side effects—sedation and confusion—occur more frequently in older patients and in those with impaired liver function. Short-acting benzodiazepines such as alprazolam, lorazepam, and oxazepam are often prescribed. Oxazepam and lorazepam are metabolized by conjugation and excreted by the kidney; hence, they are better tolerated by patients with impaired hepatic function and by those taking other medications with sedative effects (*e.g.,* analgesics). Lorazepam reduces vomiting in cancer patients receiving emetogenic cancer chemotherapies.

Clonazepam has been found useful in patients with organic mental disorders or seizure disorders who develop symptoms of depersonalization or anxiety. This longer-acting benzodiazepine is particularly useful for patients who have end-of-dose failure with recurrence of anxiety symptoms. It is effective in patients with organic mood disorders with symptoms of mania and as an adjuvant analgesic in patients with neuropathic pain.

PERSONALITY DISORDERS. Patients or families with "difficult" personalities frustrate and anger those who treat them. The stress of cancer exaggerates their normally maladaptive coping strategies and they become even more difficult than usual. The disorders can be recognized by the exaggeration of common characteristics: the paranoid person who is suspicious and constantly threatens litigation; the obsessive person whose excessive attention to details of care is accompanied by repeated criticism; the dependent person who demands care far beyond objective needs and who may be dependent on alcohol or drugs; the patient with borderline disorder who cannot conform to rules and who manipulates, divides, and may disturb other patients as well as staff; and the histrionic person who overdramatizes symptoms and distress.

Because personality disorders are not seen by patients as a problem, management usually depends on helping staff to understand the pattern and to contain their behavior. Many of these patients benefit from consistent limit-setting, applied in a quiet, kindly manner.

MAJOR MENTAL ILLNESS. Schizophrenia and bipolar (manic-depressive) illness are rare in the general population and hence uncommon in cancer patients. Careful management is needed to ensure the patient's cooperation with treatment and to prevent escalation of symptoms under stress. Previously prescribed neuroleptics should be continued, and management must be coordinated with the anesthesiologist when surgery is required because of potential paradoxical blood pressure reactions. Lithium should also be continued but may need to be stopped briefly during periods of fluid loss or restriction.

Indications for Psychiatric Evaluation

Many mild to moderately severe psychiatric disorders are managed successfully by the oncologist and a sensitive staff. However, as the above discussion makes clear, cancer patients experience several psychiatric disorders requiring accurate diagnosis for precise, effective treatment. Once treatment is outlined, management may often be done by the physician with help of social workers or other mental-health profes-

sionals. The more severe psychiatric problems require close collaboration between the oncologist and psychiatrist.

Table 64–11 outlines the indications for psychiatric consultation. Disorders directly related to illness, preexisting psychiatric disorders exacerbated by illness, and major mental disorders have been described, but four additional indications warrant discussion.

CAPACITY TO CONSENT TO OR REFUSE TREATMENT. A psychiatric consultation may be needed when a patient refuses a procedure critical to survival or when the capacity to give informed consent is in question. Rarely is legal advice or a judge's decision necessary for emergency treatment. However, when elective treatment is planned for a mentally impaired patient with no family, court direction may be needed. An increasingly common concern is the patient who refuses a clearly life-sustaining treatment, such as dialysis, as part of a decision to forego all further treatment. Physicians and nurses often are uncertain whether the patient is truly capable of assessing all the options. The presence of acute depression, which dulls mental processes and strongly biases decisions, poses a difficult and sometimes urgent reason for psychiatric consultation.

LEAVING AGAINST MEDICAL ADVICE. Requests to leave the hospital against advice are most commonly due to the presence of a confusional state secondary to illness or medication and as such often represent an acute danger to self, allowing for brief restraint and treatment after psychiatric evaluation. An acutely psychotic state or an exacerbated prior psychiatric disorder may also result in poor judgment. The cause of the behavior must be determined and a decision made as to whether the patient can be managed safely at home or whether he or she must remain in the hospital with a relative or companion. Often the severity of the patient's illness prevents safe transfer to a medical-psychiatric unit, but improvement occurs rapidly under the care of familiar medical staff, with one-to-one observation and low doses of a neuroleptic drug such as haloperidol.

SEXUAL DYSFUNCTION. Infertility and sexual dysfunction are often unavoidable consequences of irradiation, surgery, and chemotherapy. In men, the opportunity for sperm banking before treatment can both arouse and assuage con-

TABLE 64–11. Indications for Psychiatric Evaluation

Disorders directly related to illness
　Adjustment disorders (reactive anxiety and depression)
　Major depression and suicidal risk
　Delirium from CNS complications
Preexisting disorders exacerbated by illness
　Anxiety disorders
　Personality disorders
Major mental disorders
　Schizophrenia
　Unipolar and bipolar mood disorder
Capacity to consent or to refuse treatment
Leaving against medical advice
Sexual dysfunction
Significant distress from conflict with family or staff

---

cerns about infertility. In women, psychological preparation for the premature menopause and sterility associated with chemotherapy or the altered sexual function that results from gynecologic surgery is very useful in diminishing the inevitable adverse reactions. Soon after completion of treatment, patients are reluctant to bring up sexual problems, and physicians and staff are equally reluctant to ask about them. In later follow-up visits, the burden is on the oncologist to inquire into the sexual problems common with several tumor sites: breast, testicular, and gynecologic neoplasms; prostate, bladder, and head and neck tumors; and Hodgkin's disease. An increasingly sophisticated literature on diagnosis and treatment is developing in this area.[15,16]

SIGNIFICANT DISTRESS FROM CONFLICT WITH FAMILY OR STAFF. Sometimes a case becomes imbued with persistent conflict. This may stem from the patient's personality but often involves the family's problems or, more rarely, the staff's inadvertent mishandling. A psychiatric consultation can provide an objective assessment that identifies and confronts the sources of the problematic behavior. Family meetings, possibly with the patient and selected staff members present, often help to ease family distress; similarly, staff conferences encourage a more concerted and effective approach to the family and patient.

Therapeutic Interventions in Cancer

The problems outlined above are amenable to three main types of therapeutic intervention: psychopharmacologic, psychological, and behavioral. Psychopharmacologic treatment has been described. The primary indications for all three modalities are reviewed in Table 64–12. An aggressive and eclectic approach combining several modalities is most useful.

The cornerstone is psychological support, which can take many forms, some carried out by many nonpsychiatric staff. Individual sessions for both patients and families offer counseling, advice, and information about illness, treatment, and expectation of side effects. Spiritual counseling is meaningful for many patients as they turn to their religion during the existential crisis created by cancer. The chaplain can offer not only spiritual solace but also the concrete support and services of others of the same faith. Psychotherapy usually consists of brief, crisis-oriented sessions to help patients regroup their defenses and cope successfully with the problems of illness. The one-to-one visit of a veteran patient who has successfully negotiated the same experience is often very helpful.

Group interventions have also proved to be useful for cancer patients in several ways. The first is an educational function: orientation and learning what is needed to adapt to a treatment or its consequences (*e.g.*, radiation, laryngectomy, ostomy). Second, groups encourage emotional learning and relieve anxiety by allowing patients to see how others are coping with the same problems and by encouraging the expression of feelings without fear of being ridiculed. Third, the advocacy provided by cancer groups often becomes a voice for more social awareness and change, while at the same time giving participants a valuable sense of strength and empowerment. These consumer groups can be effective whether led by a professional or self-directed, such as CanSurmount and I Can Cope. A recent and provocative use of groups is suggested by two

TABLE 64–12. Primary Indications for Each Therapeutic Approach

Intervention	Treatment Modality
Psychological	
Professional crisis intervention at points of maximal stress	
At time of diagnosis	Individual and group counseling
Before a new treatment	
At relapse	Crisis intervention
At treatment failure	Psychotherapy
Ongoing psychotherapy for patients with preexisting psychiatric disorders	Counseling by clergy
Nonprofessional (self-help)	
Provision of "practical" advice at times of crisis	Veteran and fellow patient counseling
Ongoing support	Self-help groups
Empowerment during chronic and survival phases	
Psychopharmacologic	
Some adjustment disorders	Antianxiety agents
Anxiety disorders	Antidepressants
Major depression	Analgesics
Delirium/dementia	Antipsychotics
Schizophrenia	
Manic-depressive illness	
Pain	
Nausea and vomiting	
Insomnia	
Behaviorial Interventions	
Anxiety and discomfort with procedures (bone-marrow aspiration, lumbar puncture)	Relaxation
	Biofeedback
Pain (adjunct to analgesics)	Systematic desensitization
Nausea and vomiting (anticipatory treatment-related)	Suggestion/imagery/hypnosis
Eating disorders	Distraction
Some anxiety disorders	

studies in which immune function was improved and survival time increased by a group intervention; see below for further discussion.[47,48]

Behavioral interventions such as relaxation, posthypnotic suggestion, autohypnosis, desensitization, and distraction are the newest additions to patient management and are particularly useful for the acute anxiety surrounding painful procedures or feared surgery, and for the conditioned nausea, vomiting, food aversions, and possible immune suppression found in patients receiving chemotherapy.[49–53]

An important role for the oncologist is to ensure that the patient and family have optimal access to the full range of financial, social, religious, psychological, and community resources available to them. In a large center social workers are trained to perform this function, but in more decentralized settings the oncologist should become familiar with a few key local resources and should use them systematically. The resulting improvements in coping benefit the patient and ease case management.

LONG-TERM SURVIVORS

Advances in cancer treatment have resulted in a rapidly growing population of over 5 million long-term survivors, many of them children and young adults. Early psychological studies using crude measures such as marriage and level of education showed few psychological effects, but recent investigators, using more refined measures, have shown more symptoms.[54-56] Figure 64–4 illustrates the magnitude of the effect in male leukemia survivors, who are about one standard deviation above the mean in their level of distress. The results for female survivors are comparable.

Much attention has been paid to the late medical effects of cancer. The ones with the most far-ranging psychological consequences include cognitive dysfunction secondary to brain radiation, which is most marked in the very young and very old; growth retardation in children; problems with sexual response and fertility (these are often submerged at the time of treatment but reemerge acutely later); chronic organ failure at all ages; and most poignantly the occurrence of a second malignancy.

The psychological issues outlined in Table 64–9 occur at many levels. There is a documented but paradoxical increase in distress when treatment is successfully terminated, because of the loss of the emotionally protective effect of the ongoing treatment. Psychiatric intervention is useful at this time. Memorial Sloan-Kettering Cancer Center has established a posttreatment resource program to address this and other issues important to survivors. Survivors forever remain aware of their vulnerability to disease, and remain more frightened of minor physical discomforts. Some manifest the guilt of the survivor syndrome, others rejoice in a sense of special worthiness and good fortune. Reentry into normal life can be very difficult for a patient with strong dependency traits or a patient whose family is very much out of tune with the patient's needs and capabilities. At work, survivors must cope with altered co-worker attitudes and with pervasive insurance discrimination, which in turn may lead to a loss of a career mobility; the dimensions of this need to be fully explored. Yearly checkups with the oncologist remain a recurrent frightening experience even after years pass. However, they are also an excellent opportunity for the physician to assess the survivor's overall adjustment and to institute appropriate supportive measures in psychological as well as physical areas.

Peer support has been found especially valuable for survivors, who provide each other with unique understanding and advocacy. Many patients can be referred to the National Coalition of Cancer Survivorship, and the American Cancer Society can direct patients to many other special survivor organizations, such as those for laryngectomy, ostomy, and mastectomy patients.

THE "WORRIED WELL": PSYCHOLOGICAL PROBLEMS IN HIGH-RISK GROUPS

The current explosion of information about the genetic contribution to the development of cancer has produced a new population: people whose family history is such that they are clearly at high risk for certain cancers. Table 64–13 lists cancers already known to be occasionally associated with recessive chromosomal abnormalities. With new DNA technologies, these numbers are increasing rapidly, creating psychological, social, legal, and ethical problems.

Psychologically, it is useful to differentiate between people who are afraid they *might* be at risk and people who are afraid because they know they *are* at risk. The first group can benefit from careful education about their increased risk, if any. Some will remain excessively anxious even in the absence of objective reason and may be said to suffer from cancerophobia; they benefit from psychological support and regular checkups with a trusted oncologist to prevent them from squandering

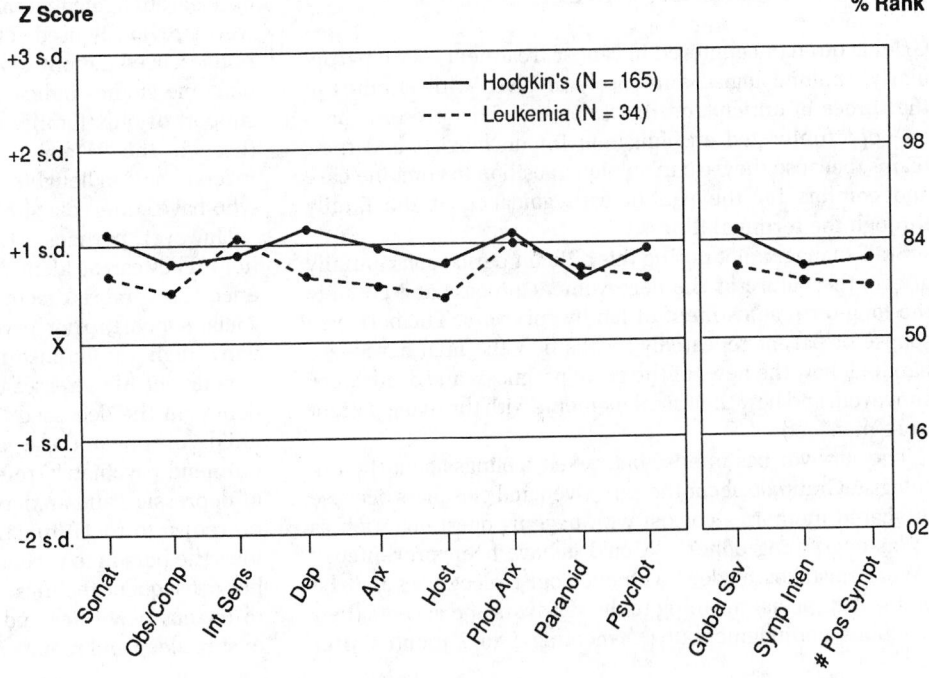

FIGURE 64–4. Comparison of psychological distress of male Hodgkin's disease and leukemia survivors in relation to normals: brief symptom inventory. (Lesko LM, Ostroff J, Smith K. Life after cancer: Survival and beyond. In: Current concepts in psycho-oncology. Memorial Sloan-Kettering Cancer Center, 1991, and Korn-blith AB, et al. Quality of life assessment of Hodgkin's disease survivors: A model for cooperative clinical trials. Oncology 1990; 4:93)

TABLE 64–13. Human Cancers Associated With Recessive Chromosomal Abnormalities

Cancer	Chromosome or Region
Bilaterial acoustic neuroma	22q
Bladder cancer	11p
Breast cancer	13q, 17p, 17q
Colorectal cancer	5q, 17p, 18, 22
Familial renal cell carcinoma	3p
Gastric carcinoma	13q
Multiple endocrine neoplasia (type 2A)	10
Neuroblastoma	1p32
Ovarian cancer	6q
Small cell lung cancer	3q13-p24, 13q, 17p
Uveal melanoma	2
Wilms' tumor	11p13

(Bodmer WF. Cancer genetics and the human genome. Hosp Prac 1991;29:73–85)

time and resources on numerous physicians.[58] The second group benefits from the same education but may need detailed genetic and psychological counseling to help them make difficult decisions regarding marriage, child-bearing, prenatal testing, and further personal testing or medical interventions such as prophylactic mastectomy.

Breast cancer is the most common cancer known to have a possible genetic component (in up to 30% of cases), and high-risk surveillance programs have been developed that have medical, surgical, educational, and psychological components.[59,60] Support groups have proven very helpful and have enabled many women who were too frightened to practice breast self-examination to begin to do it regularly.[60]

MANAGEMENT OF GRIEF

Grief is often encountered in cancer treatment. More particularly, the oncologist is intensely involved with families in the throes of anticipatory bereavement. This presents both an opportunity and an obligation for oncologists and their teams, because they are in a unique position to combine care and comfort for the patient with guidance of the family through the terminal illness.

Staff management during this difficult period substantially affects the nature of the bereavement process and possibly the long-term adjustment of family survivors. The bereaved spouse or parent repeatedly recalls how the final days were handled, how the news of the grave prognosis and death were conveyed, and how their final moments with the dying patient were managed.

The survivor has intense but mixed feelings about the oncologist. Gratitude about the care given and closeness because of shared memories coexist with nagging questions such as "Was everything done?" "Could it have been prevented?" "Were mistakes made?" The oncologist recognizes that he or she has special meaning to the survivors and accepts their reactions nonjudgmentally. A meeting 1 to 2 months after the death serves as an important setting in which troubling questions can be discussed. Autopsy findings, if available, provide a good opportunity to clarify concerns and relieve guilt. The meeting can also be used to monitor the course of grieving. The hallmarks of normal and abnormal grief are outlined below.[61,62]

Even when a death is clearly anticipated, the reaction of a relative to the actual event is often one of temporary disbelief. Despite visible deterioration in a dying spouse, the surviving partner may be unable to tolerate any real emotional awareness of the death and of what life will be like without the person. Available information suggests, however, that grief is tolerated better when the loss is expected and there has been some psychological preparation.

Once death has occurred, grieving has acute and chronic components. Acute waves of an overwhelming sense of loss, associated with crying and agitation, and usually precipitated by a reminder of the deceased, are superimposed on a chronic background of social withdrawal, preoccupation with the deceased, diminished concentration and attention, restlessness, depressed mood, anxiety, insomnia, and anorexia. The intense distress of the first few months looks like depression and may be clinically indistinguishable from it.

Over several months, the acute symptoms diminish in intensity and frequency. Reorganization of activities with resurgence of interest is seen. Preoccupation with the deceased is replaced by recall of memories associated with both pleasure and sadness. Satisfactory resolution of grief is marked by the readiness to invest deeply in new relationships and is assumed to be usually achieved by 1 year. However, the duration of normal grieving is quite variable and often extends well beyond a year. Parents, for example, are never the same again after the death of a child, and some never really recover. Older spouses from a long union often grieve acutely for 2 to 4 years, and some much longer.

The morbidity and mortality related to grief have been actively explored in the past decade. The symptoms were described above. Bereaved people often become more dependent on cigarettes, alcohol, and drugs to reduce distress, if these were previously used. They visit physicians more often than nonbereaved patients, with various physical complaints. Yet outcome studies indicate that most people recover with the support of only family, friends, and clergy. Peer counseling through the Widow-to-Widow programs, Compassionate Friends, or Candlelighters offers excellent support from others who have suffered a similar loss.

However, perhaps 20% of family survivors require special help. They can be identified early in bereavement by the presence of several risk factors, including perceived or actual poor social support, prior psychiatric history (especially alcoholism), high and intense initial distress, unanticipated death, concurrent life stresses or losses, prior high level of dependency on the deceased for primary support, and death of a child. Any one of these risk factors is sufficient reason to recommend psychiatric referral, particularly when high levels of depression and anxiety are sustained and there is little or no return to social functioning. Bereavement counseling allows the person to recount the details of the death and his or her subsequent feelings, to explore new ways of coping, and to try out new roles and experiences. An antidepressant to ensure sleep and reduce high levels of distress permits better daily functioning and often facilitates the exploration of painful feelings.

STRESSES ON ONCOLOGISTS

While recent studies have painted an increasingly clear picture of the emotional reaction of patients and their relatives, few studies have addressed the stresses on oncologists and their staffs, and the effect of these stresses on their personal and professional life.[63-65] These issues are important both for the well-being of medical professionals and for their impact on patient care. Studies consistently show that despite recurrent criticism that medicine has become uncaring and commercial, patients accept arduous treatment regimens largely because of their personal trust in their physician, and still expect to obtain their primary psychological support from him or her.[66] The harried, stressed oncologist cannot give sufficient attention to this aspect of medicine.

Physicians generally tolerate work stresses well. They have a strong intellectual and emotional commitment to their work and a well-tested capacity for hard work and discipline. However, they also have characteristics that predispose them to chronic stress. Many work long hours and seek little recreation, straining marital relations and upsetting children. Socializing becomes minimal except with colleagues. Strains in marriage and family life compound stresses at work. Conflicts with close colleagues endanger job performance and satisfaction and are especially difficult because resolution may be impossible. The need to care for patients while pursuing research and teaching activities adds special strains in the academic setting. Physical illness and frequent sleep loss are transient additional stressors; chronic fatigue is more insidious.

The practice of oncology brings special strains: the uncertainty inherent in treatment decisions; the unique toxicity inherent in treatments, especially those known to predispose to life-threatening complications such as bone-marrow transplants; and the repeated impact of patient deaths, especially patients to whom the oncologist has become attached. Some personal distress is inherent in confronting decisions about withholding or stopping life-sustaining measures and in discussing these decisions with the patient and family. The impact of patients' unrealistic expectations and the strain associated with the care of "problem" patients are additional sources of stress.[65] Caring for a colleague with cancer, while a compliment, is a double burden when treatments fail, and the loss is felt as a personal and a medical failure. Malpractice threats and suits increase, as do paperwork and outside intrusions on the ability to give the desired quality of care. Finally, it is poignantly clear that conscientious medical staff are not immune to irrational guilt, much less to ordinary sorrow. The wonder is not that symptoms of stress are observed, but rather how well physicians continue to cope.

The actual incidence of serious psychiatric problems in physicians is probably underreported. Depression, suicide, and alcohol and drug abuse are the most common psychiatric disorders seen. The rate of suicide among physicians is 100 physicians per year, or the equivalent of one medical-school class. When combined with the significant number who become dependent on drugs or alcohol, the reasons for concern become apparent; alcoholism is estimated to occur in 7% to 10% and drug abuse in 2% to 3% of physicians.

While neither of these have been examined in oncologists per se, the constant and continuing care of cancer patients, when combined with personality traits or personal problems, may provide a matrix for depression and psychological burnout. At the extreme it may lead to the need for peer review of professional competence. New legislation places increasing attention on physician competence and encourages doctors to identify their dysfunctional colleagues at an earlier and more treatable stage. Depressed physicians who continue to work cannot provide solid emotional support and therefore deprive their patients of a vital source of empathy.

What are the symptoms of emotional fatigue and burnout? The physician notices less zest and enthusiasm for work, with a sense of having to "drag in" to work. This may be coupled with feeling chronically tense, easily frustrated, and easily angered; depressed "down" moods frequently ensue. The need for a "few drinks after work" or experimentation with psychotropic drugs to "relax" are ominous signs, because the habits usually escalate. Insomnia is common, with either difficulty falling asleep, frequent awakening, or early-morning awakening. Appetite change may lead to weight gain or loss. Feeling exhausted or "tired all the time," headaches, and aches and pains are other indicators of distress.

Physicians tend to ignore these symptoms. At this point, the physician may "tune out" and feel detached from patients and unable to empathize. This is an early sign of stress in house staff, who say they feel less able to care and are cynical and pessimistic about the meaning of their work. They may begin working longer hours with a sense that "nobody can do it right but me" and "nobody works around here but me," when in fact they are less effective and efficient.

Physicians often delay seeking help for physical symptoms; unfortunately, they delay even longer in admitting to psychiatric problems and seeking help for them. To avoid becoming identified as a psychiatric patient, physicians hide their symptoms from family and colleagues, fearing the impact on their job and practice if it should become known. The warning signs of depression, the taking of secret drinks, and surreptitious use of pills are ignored. Family, colleagues, and even patients often collude in pretending nothing is wrong. The result is a paradoxical delay in identification and treatment of the physician.

Monitoring oneself for symptoms of emotional fatigue and acknowledging one's stress is very important in oncology. Survival tactics include recognizing one's limitations, not taking oneself too seriously, accepting the inadequacies of medicine, using gallows humor to lighten the meaning of painful events, working a "normal" work day for a few weeks, stopping when others do, taking a long weekend at recurrent intervals, maintaining a regular exercise program, and bringing to these measures the same care and consistency given to other responsibilities. When symptoms do not remit, psychiatric consultation should be sought.

Some training programs in oncology encourage awareness of personal reactions and provide regular meetings in which difficult patients and management of personal stresses are reviewed. They have proven useful and have been well described with oncology fellows.[65] Hospitals with liaison psychiatrists also have a built-in mechanism for attending to staff problems, especially among nurses and house staff. However, few resources exist for practicing oncologists after leaving training, and it is at this time when stresses may be greatest and the physician the most vulnerable. Actively seeking a supportive peer group is important.

More willingness to confront colleagues and to encourage them to seek treatment is necessary when significant symptoms are noted, especially because the professional arena is usually the *last* to be impaired, after personal and family functioning is already damaged. The motivation for intervention is human concern for a friend, together with the demands of optimal patient care, which require physicians to be strong enough to provide support and understanding to their patients. The severely distressed physician cannot meet this important requirement and endures much unnecessary personal suffering at the same time.

With the increasing complexity of therapeutic regimens, oncologists are working more and more as leaders or coleaders of treatment teams. Such leaders play a critical role in maintaining group morale, thereby diminishing staff stress and improving patient care. The main principles of good leadership are:

1. Modeling and expecting the delivery of high-quality patient care while also acknowledging realistic human limitations
2. Exercising authority clearly and consistently where appropriate, while supporting teamwork where appropriate
3. Encouraging and respecting in others the self-monitoring described above
4. Educating oneself about sources of help for one's staff, making them known, and using them.

Staff support groups are reportedly very effective in decreasing staff stress.[65,67] Oncologists may participate directly in such groups, but even if they choose not to, their well-publicized and genuine support for such groups is a key element of success.

PSYCHOSOCIAL AND BEHAVIORAL FACTORS IN CANCER RISK AND SURVIVAL

Psychosocial and behavioral factors affect both the risk of developing cancer and the length of survival once cancer has developed. Patients ask many questions about these issues as they attempt to understand why they got cancer and how they can positively affect the treatment outcome. Oncologists must be familiar with the present state of research to respond accurately and usefully.

Holland has reviewed the psychosocial and behavioral factors that may alter cancer risk and survival and has divided them into five areas: lifestyle and behaviors, social environments, personality and coping style, life events and emotional states, and behavioral and lifestyle interventions.[4,5]

LIFESTYLE AND BEHAVIORS

The effect of individual behaviors on altering exposure to carcinogens and the incidence of many cancers is well known. Cancer-prevention programs depend heavily on insights and techniques derived from psychology, psychiatry, and the social sciences for help in reducing smoking and alcohol intake and altering dietary practices and sexual behavior.[2,3] In addition, much of the improvement in survival for common cancers, such as breast and colon cancer, depends on early detection; psychiatry and the social sciences are needed to understand the complex factors that make people delay seeking consultation long after they have suspicious symptoms.

SOCIAL ENVIRONMENT

Socioeconomic status has been shown to be a key variable in the incidence and survival rates for many cancers, even under standardized treatment conditions.[6-8,68] This includes factors such as premorbid state of health and access to care, and also the other psychosocial factors described in this section. The absence of social ties also has been shown to prejudice cancer incidence and mortality, and in one study had an impact on natural killer-cell activity in women with breast cancer.[18]

PERSONALITY AND COPING STYLE

Although this area is of great interest to patients and to the lay press, data still do not strongly support the theory that a particular personality style predisposes to cancer. Early studies on type C personality have not been replicated.[69] Type A personality was shown to have at a most a 1.5 risk.[70] Greer's early work on the protective effect of the "fighting spirit" has been contradicted by three later studies.[71-74]

LIFE EVENTS AND EMOTIONAL STATES

The contribution of grief and depression to mortality from cancer does not appear to be as great as was previously assumed. Early studies showing some effects have been contradicted by later, better-designed ones.[75-79] While immune functions are perturbed after bereavement and in some other stressed states, the effects are probably too small to have clinical significance.[80]

BEHAVIORAL AND LIFESTYLE INTERVENTIONS

The impact of "mind on body" has been given impetus by two small but well-designed studies of group interventions that showed a positive effect on survival of breast-cancer patients and a positive effect on immune function in stage I and II melanoma patients.[47,48] However, three studies have shown no effects on mortality of intensive holistic supportive behavioral programs.[81-83] Follow-up and duplication attempts of the positive studies are currently under way.

Despite the sobering research trends described above, the wish, often translated into a magical belief, that one can cure the body with the power of the mind remains compelling. Its implied promises have spawned a growth industry of clinics and healers who encourage patients to use their mental powers to fight their cancer, with or without the help of traditional treatments. The accompanying emphasis on a healthy lifestyle and careful attention to nutrition is commendable. However, confusion is rampant between risk and survival factors. The well-known and powerful risk factors are conflated with ambiguous and weak survival factors, while the role of personality factors is inflated far beyond the existing evidence. The intense, cultlike aspect of many alternative programs encourages extreme hopes and beliefs and leads to equally extreme disappointments.

By placing the locus of power over cancer in the patient's mind, "healers" play into patients' (and families') universal tendency to feel they are to blame for their illness. It is only too common to see a nauseated, anorectic patient being badgered to eat by family members who demand that he or she demonstrate a "positive attitude." Worst of all, healers let patients bear personal responsibility for failure, or blame it on their having sought traditional treatment. The hapless patient has no choice but to join the universal chorus by blaming himself or "the cancer establishment."

Yet some of these programs have a core of constructiveness. Patients who feel energized and empowered to act on their own behalf, who maintain a healthful lifestyle, and who have a better subjective sense of hope and well-being will pursue and tolerate treatment more effectively and will have a better ongoing quality of life. If survival is improved, so much the better. The best traditional medical treatment has aimed for these results, but not often and not vigorously enough, as the demands of technology have elbowed aside the time- and labor-intensive demands of psychosocial interventions. It is to be hoped that the future will see a reconciliation between traditional cancer care and the more constructive aspects of alternative care.

COMMON ETHICAL DILEMMAS CONFRONTING THE CAREGIVER IN CANCER

The practice of medicine has been greatly affected by the development of the discipline of applied bioethics. Clinicians can no longer follow only their personal sense of what is right; they must now answer to a more informed and demanding public, as well as ethics committees and legal precedents. Oncology is at the heart of many controversial areas. Today's oncologists must have an understanding of the basic issues and the basic arguments.[84,85] We will present a brief review of the contemporary code of medical ethics and a description of the main areas likely to affect clinical oncologists.

MEDICAL CODE OF ETHICS

The medical code of ethics goes back to the Hippocratic oath and was restated by the American Medical Association in 1980. In the past two decades it has come under searching criticism and redefinition by bioethicists, who have criticized the profession as too paternalistic and monopolistic.

Beauchamp and Childress reviewed four basic principles that should guide the contemporary physician[85]:

1. *Respect for the patient's autonomy* implies honoring the patient's right to self-governance, privacy, and individual choice.
2. *Nonmaleficence* implies the obligation to do no harm.
3. *Beneficence* implies the obligation to help others to further their own best interests.
4. *Justice* is the hardest to define without many qualifiers,

but in the context of clinical practice can be said to imply the duty to apply the first three principles to one's patients fairly and consistently.

From these principles are derived four sets of rules of conduct that should characterize the physician-patient relationship:

1. *Rules of veracity* bear directly on truth-telling and informed consent.
2. *Rules of privacy* stipulate that the physician must honor conditions of limited access to the patient. These two sets of rules have figured prominently in past statements of the profession.
3. *Rules of confidentiality* have long figured in medical codes of ethics, but are in fact profoundly eroded by economic, political, and legal developments, as well as purely technologic ones.
4. *Rules of fidelity* address the contractual nature of the physician-patient relationship in the legal arena, but also a broader concept of "promise-keeping" in the moral arena.

TRUTH-TELLING

A diagnosis of cancer can immediately present caregivers with an ethical dilemma, depending on the area in which they practice. In countries where the principle of autonomy is valued above all others, the physician is expected to tell the patient the diagnosis without any evasion. However, in many more countries, the principle of autonomy is much less valued than the principle of beneficence, or more exactly the principle of nonmaleficence. Thus, physicians are expected to shield the patient and to enter into a conspiracy with the patient's family. Practitioners who do not follow the locally accepted mode are surrounded by controversy.

INFORMED CONSENT FOR TREATMENT

Patients cannot give informed consent for treatment if they have not been given adequate information about their condition. Because there is an increasing pressure to require informed consent before treatment, truth-telling will probably become more widespread, especially because many cancer treatments are toxic. Public awareness of the toxicity of cancer treatment has risen steadily and has caused fear and anxiety. Improvements in outcomes in the last decade have been measured more by small but steady increments than by any major breakthroughs. Statistical analyses that point toward improved outcomes have been criticized.[86] Hence, the general public is even less likely to trust caregivers blindly.

Bone-marrow transplantation is an exception to the incremental improvement model because it offers a chance of cure to patients who would otherwise die. Unfortunately, the mortality rate from the procedure has remained around 15% to 20%, and the best results are obtained by selecting the healthiest patients, preferably those in remission. In a democratic society, it would appear difficult, or at the very least inconsistent, to justify putting a patient into such a high-risk/high-gain situation without obtaining consent from a fully informed patient. Nevertheless, this is still accepted practice in some countries. For the practice to be acceptable in these countries, the moral and professional caliber of the caregivers must be very high, and societal approval of the practice must run very deep.

INVESTIGATIONAL TREATMENTS

The special issues that surround investigational treatment are not unique to cancer. Being a clinical investigator puts the physician into a possibly irreducible conflict between concerns for research and his or her duty to the individual patient. Major abuses in previous decades have led to the development of mandatory institutional review boards (or ethics committees, as they are more often called in Western Europe).[87] A well-constituted, well-functioning institutional review board is the first and most important safeguard of the individual patient's welfare in a protocol (and the physician's, as well). But how can patients be protected from a caregiver's earnest zeal to accrue subjects who might not wish to participate in a given protocol? The best safeguard is a well-informed patient, aware of his or her right to refuse and able to give fully informed consent.

A second major controversy arises at the very core of the investigational process: Are randomized trials, by their very nature, unethical? This question was most recently highlighted by two articles in the May 30, 1991, issue of the *New England Journal of Medicine*. Hellman and Hellman invoked several arguments against the ethical validity of clinical trials[88]:

1. There is an irreducible conflict between the physician's duty to his or her patient and the researcher's responsibility to randomize.
2. Although patients may waive their rights to individual treatment, it is inconsistent with the physician's role to ask that they do so.
3. Terminally ill patients, said to have least to lose and most to gain, may also be least able to give informed consent that is truly voluntary.

The authors made a plea for pursuing research methods that avoid randomization.

In rebuttal, Passamani described the conditions for an ethical clinical trial[89]:

1. A fully informed patient
2. A condition of clinical equipoise where no treatment branch is clearly preferable to any other
3. A trial designed as a critical test of the alternatives
4. A data-monitoring committee prepared to stop the trial if that state of equipoise no longer exists.

He pointed out that many randomized trials have answered questions with counterintuitive results that might not have been established any other way.

TERMINAL CARE ISSUES

Although good medical care has resulted in the curing of many patients and has changed cancer from a rapidly fatal to a chronic disease, terminal care issues continue to present themselves regularly.

Truth-telling often recurs as an issue because many caregivers find it difficult to bring the patient or family to confront the grim reality. Sometimes the family will demand that the patient not be told, and may even remove the patient from a given physician's care when they fear he or she would be too frank. The ethics of surrogate decision-making are particularly important when family members must make decisions for newly incompetent patients. Currently, ethical and legal expectations are that the family, knowing the patient best, will act in a way that most closely approximates what the patient's wishes would have been. In reality, however, families often follow their own wishes. Furthermore, there are no guidelines to establish the competence of family surrogates. Many terminal care situations become quite chaotic when a very disturbed spouse or parent becomes the main decision-maker.

Medical technology has also brought about the need to make decisions for which our social, political, legal, ethical, and spiritual history has not prepared us: namely, decisions regarding the maintenance of life. These can be roughly divided into three categories: stopping the fight against death and winding down from active treatment to palliative care; accepting the arrival of death (namely, overcoming the magical expectations of cardiopulmonary resuscitation and allowing the dead to stay dead); and hastening the coming of death, which includes forms of passive and active euthanasia and assisted suicide.

In the United States these three areas have been the focus of intense public debate and changing policy. The first occurred during the 1970s, when increasing consumer disillusionment with the outcome of "high-tech" medicine led to more readiness on the part of physicians and patients to forego aggressive treatments. The second phase evolved during the 1980s, when there was a confrontation between the increasingly automatic practice of resuscitation and consumers' growing dread of "prolonged dying." This resulted in the development of "do not resuscitate" (DNR) regulations and the use of living wills and advance directives, by which patients can make their own wishes known while they are still competent. The last phase has only begun and is being discussed on many political and social fronts. It addresses the growing demand for the legalization of physician-assisted suicide and possibly euthanasia. Medical and legal organizations and many professional ethicists have opposed these measures, but grassroots support runs deep. A legal initiative to allow physician-assisted suicide was narrowly defeated in the state of Washington in November 1991, but further initiatives are expected in several western states.

THE PREGNANT CANCER PATIENT

The pregnant cancer patient is thrust into the furious crossfire of the right-to-life versus pro-choice debate, and such a patient almost always creates acute management controversies. Most recently, the Stoner case created a possible precedent. Mrs. Stoner had been forced to undergo a cesarean section against her will in a desperate effort to save her 23-week fetus while she was dying of advanced cancer. When both mother and infant died within a few days, the Stoner family sued the hospital. The case was settled out of court and the hospital published a set of guidelines designed to prevent future violation of the rights of pregnant patients. This is a welcome development in an era in which Curran has noted a rise in involuntary cesarean sections.[90] Nevertheless, the often competing interests of the mother and fetus make all treatment decisions momentous and conflict-ridden.

THE RIGHTS OF TRANSPLANT DONORS

The rights of transplant donors have also been a subject of controversy as increasingly bold recipients or their family members pursue potential donors. One patient sued his hospital to release the name of matched but unrelated and unwilling donors, and lost on the grounds of protecting the donor's right to privacy. This begged the issue of how much pressure could be brought to bear on a known donor. This was most recently addressed by the case of two half-siblings whose absent father sued to force their mother to permit them to provide a bone-marrow transplant for his older son from another union. The courts upheld the mother's refusal in a thoughtful opinion that, although it will not generalize automatically to other cases, will provide a useful guide to help caregivers analyze similar troubling situations.[90]

THE RIGHTS OF MINORS AS DECISION-MAKERS

Considering the rights of children and adolescents as decision-makers can profoundly complicate the practice of pediatric oncology due to potential conflicts between parents and children, especially adolescents. For every overt conflict, there are probably many that never become apparent to the caregivers. In keeping with the current trend toward empowering the recipient of medical care, King and Cross[91] and Leikin[92] offered guidelines for assessing and enhancing children's decision-making potential and for dealing with issues of death and dying.

THE RIGHTS OF GENETICALLY AT-RISK PATIENTS

As the ability to identify genetic markers for cancer has improved, the potential problems this may create for identified patients have become clearer. Lack of confidentiality leading to job discrimination, loss of insurability, and even loss of procreative freedom have already been reported. These and other related problems are being addressed by the Committee on Ethical, Legal, and Social Issues of the Human Genome Project and have been the focus of an Office of Technology Assessment Task Force.[93,94] Their publication on genetic monitoring in the workplace contains a current review of the legal and regulatory situation.[95]

REFERENCES

1. Holland JC, Marchini A, Tross S. An international survey of physician attitudes and practice in regard to revealing the diagnosis of cancer. Cancer Invest 1987;5:151–154.
2. Lerman C, Rimer BK, Engstrom PF. Reducing avoidable cancer mortality through prevention and early detection. Cancer Res 1989;49:4955–4962.
3. Ockene JK, Lindsay E, Berger L, Hymowitz N. Health-care providers as key change agents in the Community Intervention Trial for Smoking Cessation (COMMIT). Int Q Commun Health Educ 1990-1991;11:223–237.
4. Holland JC. Psychosocial variables: Are they factors in cancer risk or survival? In: Holland JC, Rowland J, Massie MJ, eds. Current concepts in psycho-oncology. New York: Memorial Sloan-Kettering Cancer Center, 1991.
5. Levenson JC, Bemis C. The role of psychological factors in cancer onset and progression. Psychosomatics 1991;32:125–132.
6. Holland JC, Rowland J, eds. Handbook of psycho-oncology: Psychological care of the patient with cancer. New York: Oxford University Press, 1989.
7. Baquet CR, Horm JW, Gibbs T, Greenwald P. Socioeconomic factors and cancer incidence among blacks and whites. JNCI 1991;83:551–557.
8. Freeman H. Race, poverty and cancer. JNCI 1991;83:526–527, 1991.
9. Cassileth BR, Lusk EJ, Strouse TB, Bodenheimer BJ. Contemporary unorthodox treatments in cancer medicine: A study of patients, treatments and practitioners. Ann Intern Med 1984;101:105–12.
10. Aaronson NK. Methodologic issues in assessing the quality of life of cancer patients. Cancer 1991;67:844–850.
11. Hillner BE, Smith TJ. Efficacy and cost effectiveness of adjuvant chemotherapy in women with node-negative breast cancer. N Engl J Med 1991;324:160–168.
12. Holland JC. Clinical course of cancer. In: Holland JC, Rowland JC, eds. Handbook of psycho-oncology. New York: Oxford University Press, 1989:134–145.
13. Bronheim H, Strain JJ, Biller JH. Four aspects of head and neck surgery, Part I: New surgical techniques and psychiatric consequences. Gen Hosp Psychiatry 1991;13:165–176.
14. Bronheim H, Strain JJ, Biller JH. Four aspects of head and neck surgery, Part II: Body image and interventions. Gen Hosp Psychiatry 1991;13:225–232.
15. Auchincloss S. Sexual problems in cancer patients; evaluation and management issues. In: Holland JC, Rowland JH, eds. Psycho-oncology: The psychological care of the patient with cancer. New York: Oxford University Press, 1989:383–413.
16. Schover LR, Jensen SB. Sexuality and chronic illness: A comprehensive approach. New York: Guilford Press, 1988.
17. House JS, Landis KR, Umberson D. Social relationship and health. Science 1988;240:540–545.
18. Levy SM, Herberman RB, Whiteside T, et al. Perceived social support and tumor estrogen/progesterone receptor status as predictors of natural killer cell activity in breast cancer patients. Psychosom Med 1990;52:73–85.
19. Weisman AD, Worden JW. The existential plight in cancer: Significance of the first 100 days. Int J Psychiatry Med 1976;7:1–17.
20. Massie MJ, Holland JC. The cancer patient with pain: Psychiatric complications and their management. J Sympt Pain Manage 1992;7:99–109.
21. Bukberg J, Penman D, Holland JC. Depression in hospitalized cancer patients. Psychosom Med 1984;46:199–212.
22. Derogatis LB, Morrow GR, Fetting J, et al. The prevalence of psychiatric disorders among cancer patients. JAMA 1983;249:751–757.
23. Massie MJ, Holland JC, Glass E. Delirium in terminally ill cancer patients. Am J Psychiatry 1983;140:1048–1050.
24. Holland JC, Korzun AH, Tross S, et al. Comparative psychological disturbance in patients with pancreatic and gastric cancer. Am J Psychiatry 1986;143:982–986.
25. Lederberg MS, Holland JC. Psycho-oncology. In: Kaplan HI, Sadock BJ, eds. Comprehensive textbook of psychiatry. Baltimore: Williams & Wilkins, 1989:1249–1264.
26. Breitbart W. Suicide in cancer patients. In: Holland JC, Rowland JH, eds. Handbook of psycho-oncology: Psychological care of the patient with cancer. New York: Oxford University Press, 1989:291–299.
27. Rifkin A, Reardon G, Siris S, et al. Trimipramine in physical illness with depression. J Clin Psychiatry 1985;46:4–8.
28. Popkin MK, Callies AI, MacKenzie TB. The outcome of antidepressant use in the medically ill. Arch Gen Psychiatry 1985;42:1160–1163.
29. Costa D, Mogos I, Toma T. Efficacy and safety of mianserin in the treatment of depression of women with cancer. Acta Psychiatr Scand 1985;72(suppl 320):85–92.
30. Massie MJ, Lesko L. Psychopharmacological management. In: Holland JC, Rowland JH, eds. Handbook of psycho-oncology: Psychological care of the patient with cancer. New York: Oxford University Press, 1989:470–491.
31. Mucha H, Lange E, Bonitz G. Amitriptyline in der psychiatrischen therapie. Psychiatr Neurol Med Psychol [Leipz] 1970;22:116–120.
32. France RD. The future for antidepressants: Treatment of pain. Psychopathology 1987;20:99–113.
33. Vishwanath BM, Navalgund AA, Cusano W, Navalgund KA. Fluoxetine as a cause of SIADH. Am J Psychiatry 1991;148:542–543.
34. Lyman GH, Williams CC, Preston D. The use of lithium carbonate to reduce infection and leukopenia during systemic chemotherapy. N Engl J Med 1980;302:257–260.
35. Fernandez F, Adams F, Holmes VF, et al. Methylphenidate for depressive disorders in cancer patients. Psychosomatics 1987;28:455–461.
36. Chiarello RJ, Cole JO. The use of psychostimulants in general psychiatry: A reconsideration. Arch Gen Psychiatry 1987;44:286–295.
37. Rickels K, Feighner JP, Smith WT. Alprazolam, amitriptyline, doxepin, and placebo in the treatment of depression. Arch Gen Psychiatry 1985;42:134–141.
38. Holland JC, Morrow GR, Schmale A, et al. A randomized clinical trial of alprazolam versus progressive muscle relaxation in cancer patients with anxiety and depressive symptoms. J Clin Oncol 1991;9:1004–1011.
39. Posner JB. Neurologic complications of systemic cancer. 1978;2:7–60.
40. Young DF. Neurological complications of cancer chemotherapy. In: Silverstein A, ed. Neurological complications of therapy: Selected topics. New York: Futura. 1982:47–113.
41. Drugs of choice for cancer chemotherapy. Medical Letter 1991;33:21–28.
42. Stiefel FC, Breitbart WS, Holland JC. Corticosteroids in cancer: Neuropsychiatric complications. Cancer Invest 1989;7:479–491.
43. Fletcher JM, Copeland DR. Neurobehavioral effects of central nervous system prophylactic treatment of cancer in children. J Clin Exp Neurol 1988;10:495–538.
44. Cousens P, Waters B, Said J, Stevens M. Cognitive effects of cranial irradiation in leukemia: A survey and meta-analysis. J Child Psychol Pyschiatr 1988;29:839–852.
45. Brennan SC, Redd WH, Jacobsen PB, et al. Anxiety and panic during magnetic resonance scans. Lancet 1988;2:512.
46. Jacobsen PB. Treating a man with needle phobia who requires daily injections of medication. Hosp Comm Psychiatry 1991;42:877–878.
47. Spiegel D, Bloom J Kraemer HC, et al. Effects of psychosocial treatment on survival of patients with metastatic breast cancer. Lancet 1989;2:888–891.
48. Fawzy FI, Kemeny ME, Fawzy NW, et al. A structured psychiatric intervention for cancer patients: II. Changes over time in immunologic measures. Arch Gen Psych 1990;47:729–735.
49. Loscalzo M, Jacobsen PB. Practical behavioral approaches to the effective management of pain and distress. J Psychosocial Oncol 1991;8:139–169.

50. Jacobsen PB, Redd WH. The development and management of chemotherapy-related anticipatory nausea and vomiting. Cancer Invest 1988;6:329–336.
51. Andrykowski MA, Otis JL. Development of learned food aversions in humans: Investigation in a natural laboratory of cancer chemotherapy. Appetite 1990;14:145–158.
52. Bovbjerg DH, Redd WH, Maier LA, et al. Anticipatory immune suppression and nausea in women receiving cyclic chemotherapy for ovarian cancer. J Consult Clin Psych 1990;58:153–157.
53. Manne SL, Redd WH, Jacobsen PB, Gorfinkle K, Schorr O, Rapkin S. Behavioral intervention to reduce child and parent distress during venipuncture. J Consult Clin Psych 1990;58:565–572.
54. Welch-McCaffrey D, Hoffman B, Leigh LA, et al. Surviving adult cancers, Part 2: Psychosocial implications. Ann Intern Med 1989;111:517–524.
55. Smith K, Ostroff J, Tan C, Lesko LM. Alterations in self-perceptions among adolescent cancer survivors. Cancer Invest 1991;9:581–588.
56. Mumma GH, Mashberg D, Lesko LM. Long-term psychosexual impact of marrow transplantation versus conventional chemotherapy. Gen Hosp Psychiatry 1992;14:43–55.
57. Loescher L, Welch-McCaffrey D, Leigh SA, et al. Surviving adult cancers, Part 1: Physiological effects. Ann Intern Med 1989;111:411–432.
58. Holland JC. Fears and abnormal reactions to cancer in physically healthy individuals. In: Holland J, Rowland JR, eds. Handbook of psycho-oncology: Psychological care of the patient with cancer. New York: Oxford University Press, 1989:13–21.
59. Scalfani L. Management of the high-risk patient. Sem Sup Oncol 1991;7:261–266.
60. Kash KM, Holland JC, Halper MS, Miller DG. Psychological distress and surveillance behaviors of women with a family history of breast cancer. JNCI 1992;84:24–30.
61. Osterweis M, Solomon F, Green M, eds. Bereavement: Reactions, consequences and care. Washington DC: National Academy Press, 1984.
62. Chochinov H, Holland JC. Bereavement: A special issue in oncology. In: Holland J, Rowland JR, eds. Handbook of psycho-oncology: Psychological care of the patient with cancer. New York: Oxford University Press, 1989:612–627.
63. Mount BM. Dealing with our losses. J Clin Oncol 1986;4:1127–1134.
64. Kash K, Holland JC. Special problems of physicians and house staff. In: Holland J, Rowland JR, eds. Handbook of psycho-oncology: Psychological care of the patient with cancer. New York: Oxford University Press, 1989.
65. Lederberg MS. Psychological problems of staff and their management. In: Holland J, Rowland JR, eds. Handbook of psycho-oncology: Psychological care of the patient with cancer. New York: Oxford University Press, 1989.
66. Penman D, Holland Jc, Bahna G, et al. Informed consent for investigational chemotherapy: Patients' and physicians' perceptions. J Clin Oncol 1984;2:849–855.
67. Lederberg MS. Group support for medical staff in high-stress settings. In: Alonzo A, Swiller HI, eds. Group psychotherapy in clinical practice. APA Press, 1992.
68. Cella DF, Orav J, Kornblith AB, Holland JC, et al. Socioeconomic status and cancer survival. J Clin Oncology 1991;9:1500–1509.
69. Temoshok L, Heller BW, Sageviel RW, et al. The relationship of psychological factors of prognostic indicators in cutaneous malignant melanoma J Psychosom Res 1985;29:139–153.
70. Fox BH, Ragland DR, Brand RJ, Rosenman RH. Type A behavior and cancer mortality. Ann NY Acad Sci 1987;496:620–627.

71. Greer S, Morris T, Pettingale KW. Psychological response to breast cancer: Effect on outcome. Lancet 1979;2:785–787.
72. Cassileth BR, Lusk EJ, Miller DJ, et al. Psychological correlates of survival in advanced malignant disease? N Engl J Med 1985;312:1551–1555.
73. Holland JC, Korzun AH, Tross S, Cella DF, et al. Psychosocial factors and disease-free survival in Stage II breast cancer. Proc Am Soc Clin Oncol [Abstract] 1986;5:237.
74. Jamison RN, Burish TG, Wallston KA. Psychogenic factors in predicting survival of breast cancer patients. J Clin Oncol 1987;5:768–772.
75. Helsing KJ, Szklo M. Mortality after bereavement. Am J Epidemiol 1981;1124:41–52.
76. Bieliauskas LA, Garron DC. Psychological depression and cancer. Gen Hosp Psychiatry 1982;4:187–195.
77. Hahn RC, Petitti DB. Minnesota Multiphasic Personality Inventory-rated depression and the incidence of breast cancer. Cancer 1988;61:845–848.
78. Kaplan GA, Reynolds P. Depression and cancer mortality and morbidity: Prospective evidence from the Alameda County study. J Behav Med 1988;11:1–13.
79. Zonderman AB, Costa PT, Jr, McCrae RR. Depression as a risk for cancer morbidity and mortality in a nationally representative sample. JAMA 1989;262:1191–1195.
80. Stein M, Miller AH, Trestman RL. Depression of the immune system and health and illness. Arch Gen Psych 1991;48:171–177.
81. Bagenal FS, Easton DF, Harris E, et al. Survival of patients with breast cancer attending Bristol Cancer Help Centre. Lancet 1990;336:606–610.
82. Cassileth BR, Lusk EJ, Guerry D, et al. Survival and quality of life among patients receiving unproven as compared with conventional cancer therapy. N Engl J Med 1991;324:1180–1185.
83. Morganstein H, Gellert GH, Walter SD, et al. The impact of a psychosocial support program on survival with breast cancer; the importance of selection bias in program evaluation. J Chron Dis 1984;37:273–282.
84. Jonsen AR, Siegler M, Winslade WJ. Clinical ethics: A practical approach to ethical decisions in clinical medicine. New York: Macmillan, 1982.
85. Beauchamp TL, Childress JF. Principles of biomedical ethics. New York: Oxford University Press, 1989.
86. Bailar JC, Smith, EM. Progress against cancer? N Engl J Med 1986;314:1226–1232.
87. Beecher HK. Ethics and clinical research. N Engl J Med 1966;274:1354–1360.
88. Hellman S, Hellman DS. Of mice but not men: Problems of the randomized clinical trial. N Engl J Med 1991;324:1585–1589.
89. Passamani E. Clinical trials: Are they ethical? N Engl J Med 1991;324:1589–1592.
90. Curran WJ. Beyond the best interests of a child: Bone marrow transplantation among half-siblings. N Engl J Med 1991;324:1818–1819.
91. King NMP, Cross AW. Children as decision makers: Guidelines for pediatricians. J Pediatr 1989;115:10–16.
92. Leikin S. A proposal concerning decisions to forgo life-sustaining treatment for young people. J Pediatr 1989;115:17–22.
93. Wexler NS. Genetic jeopardy and the new clairvoyance. Prog Med Genet 1985;6:1.
94. Nelkin D, Tancredi L. Dangerous diagnostics: The social power of biological information. New York: Basic Books, 1989.

LESLIE R. SCHOVER
DROGO K. MONTAGUE
WENDY S. SCHAIN

SECTION 3

Sexual Problems

Sexual rehabilitation is an important aspect of restoring the quality of life to men and women who survive cancer treatment. Despite the attention to sexuality in our society, most cancer patients remain poorly informed about the impact of their disease and its treatment on sexual function, and about options available to them to overcome sexual problems related to cancer therapy. In the last 20 years we have seen important advances in our knowledge of the mechanisms of sexual function and how it may be impaired by cancer treatment. We also have evaluated treatment strategies in both the medical and psychological realms. However, this broader research base has had only a minimal impact on the counseling of cancer patients in clinical settings. The challenge of the 1990s is to implement sexual rehabilitation programs that are practical, economical, and effective.

The concept of sexual rehabilitation used in this chapter is not restricted to restoring firmer erections or overcoming dyspareunia, although these are common goals of treatment after cancer therapy. We also define sexual rehabilitation as remediation of the emotional impact of cancer diagnosis and treatment on body image, relationship satisfaction, and reproductive capacity.

Cancer treatments may damage one or more phases of the sexual response by affecting attitudes and emotions, central or peripheral components of the nervous system, the pelvic vascular system, and the hypothalamic-pituitary-gonadal axis. Sexual dysfunctions can be classified according to the phases of the sexual response cycle: desire, arousal, and orgasm.[1] It is very rarely a malignancy itself that interferes with sexual function, but rather the therapy needed to eradicate cancer that is the culprit. Not only does each treatment have its own peculiar impact on the various substrates of sexual function, but given that most types of cancer occur more often with age, many patients have a previous history of medical factors that could interfere with arousal or orgasm.

Clinicians need a clear idea of the types of problems to expect after specific cancer therapies. It is of limited value to study or make generalizations about groups of patients with the same diagnosis but different treatments (*i.e.,* gynecologic cancer survivors, or men with prostate cancer).[2] Thus, we will review the known impact of a variety of cancer treatments on sexual function.

PSYCHOLOGICAL IMPACT OF CANCER ON SEXUAL FUNCTION

In examining the impact of cancer treatment on sexual function, one must be aware of the general psychological effect of receiving a diagnosis of cancer as well as the more specific physiologic impairments related to certain types of cancer therapy. The diagnosis of cancer has traditionally been a source of terror and stigmatization. Cancer patients were viewed as unclean and marked for death. Although a very large change in these attitudes has occurred in the United States in this century, some men and women still regard cancer as a disease that renders them untouchable. Occasionally the spouse is the one who has these beliefs. A cessation of sexual activity because of a phobia about venereal contagion of cancer is seen more often in patients who are less educated and come from a rural or traditional ethnic background. Another common belief is that because sex is sinful and unclean, staying sexually active would interfere with cancer treatment. Some patients believe that the cancer is a punishment for some past sex-related behavior, such as having had an affair, sex with a prostitute, or an abortion. Obviously those who feel a high degree of sexual guilt are more likely to become celibate after a cancer diagnosis.

Cancer can also change a person's concept of his or her sexual attractiveness. Sometimes a very visible change results from treatment, such as loss of a nose or facial scarring from basal cell carcinoma. Other changes, such as a mastectomy or urostomy, are invisible to a casual observer but will be seen by the sexual partner. This creates dilemmas not only for married couples about whether to be open about nudity or try to conceal the change, but for single people about when to disclose the history of cancer treatment to a potential mate.[3] During chemotherapy, alopecia, pallor, skin changes, and weight changes are visible. Afterwards the patient may regain a physical appearance almost identical to that before the cancer treatment, but the experience of stigmatization lingers and can interfere with feeling sexually attractive. For example, about a quarter of long-term survivors of testicular cancer in one survey felt less attractive than before their illness.[4]

Affective disorders are increased in prevalence in cancer patients, although the prevalence depends on the type of assessment used.[5-7] In a study of sexual rehabilitation cases in a cancer center, low sexual desire was more common in men and women who were depressed and coping poorly with their cancer.[8] Several studies suggest that younger men and women who go through cancer treatment are more apt to be psychologically distressed, probably because they suffer more disruption of daily life goals, such as establishing a committed relationship, child-bearing, parenting, and advancing in their careers.[7,8] Clinical experience suggests that younger patients are also more apt to express distress over sexual dysfunction related to cancer treatment.

Cancer treatment does not result in an increased rate of divorce for adult patients.[9] Several studies suggest that the diagnosis does not produce marital distress in happy couples but may exacerbate conflict in couples already having problems. Sexual dysfunction and marital unhappiness tend to occur in tandem.[10-13] Some problems are related to disruption of traditional gender roles. For example, expression of nonsexual affection decreases more in couples in which the woman is the cancer patient.[8] This may be viewed as a result of the roles that society assigns to men and women. Women are socialized to be nurturant, and thus may feel quite competent to deal with an ill spouse. Men often feel helpless when faced with the disease, however, because there is little they can do to alleviate the wife's physical pain or fear, and they are often not skilled in providing emotional support. For both men and women, having a spouse go through cancer surgery produces significant psychological distress.[8,14] When a man has cancer, loss of sexual function and earning power are two events he often sees as a symbolic loss of masculinity.[15]

For younger, childless men, infertility after chemotherapy or radiation therapy also can cause long-term distress.[16] Unfortunately, many of these men do not take advantage of opportunities for sperm banking because they refuse to believe that their cancer treatment can really damage their fertility.[17] In young women survivors, not only is infertility a problem, but many fear that pregnancy could promote a cancer recurrence, especially those who had a hormone-sensitive breast cancer.[18] Current evidence suggests, however, that pregnancy at diagnosis of early-stage breast cancer or after successful local treatment does not affect disease-free survival in node-negative women.[19-21]

A problem that has both psychological and physiologic elements is loss of sexual desire during the debilitation of cancer treatment. Often chronic fatigue, nausea, or specific pain interfere with well-being. For most men and women, the energy level improves and pain decreases after cancer therapy is over. It is often at that time that they request help for a sexual problem that has become more salient as other areas of life are brought under control.

PHYSIOLOGIC IMPACT OF SYSTEMIC THERAPIES

Little research has been done on the impact of various systemic cancer therapies on sexual function. This section reviews what is known about sexual side effects of hormonal, chemotherapeutic, and biologic response modifiers.

HORMONAL THERAPY IN MEN

Men with metastatic prostate cancer typically receive hormonal regimens designed to reduce their amount of circulating serum testosterone. With the advent of luteinizing hormone-releasing hormone (LHRH) agonists such as buserelin or goserelin, the use of estrogenic compounds has decreased. The LHRH-agonist drugs do not have the estrogenic side effects of gynecomastia or cardiovascular toxicity.[22] Some men still prefer surgical orchiectomy, however, to avoid the expense or inconvenience of taking medication.[23] Although one might hypothesize that bilateral orchiectomy would impair sexual function because of a poor body image, one small case series found no difference in sexual function in men treated with surgery versus medication.[24] No evidence exists to suggest the superiority of one particular hormonal modality in preserving sexual function. All have the effect of reducing serum testosterone to prepubertal levels.

The typical dysfunctions related to hormonal therapy include a severe reduction in spontaneous desire for sex, difficulty getting subjectively aroused, difficulty achieving and maintaining rigid erections, and difficulty achieving orgasm. Men who can reach orgasm typically note reduced semen volume and sometimes decreased intensity of orgasmic pleasure.[25] It is also clear, however, that perhaps 15% to 20% of men can function quite normally after hormonal therapy has reduced serum testosterone levels to near zero.[22] This is true even in men treated with either orchiectomy or an LHRH-agonist plus the anti-androgen flutamide.[24] From clinical experience, men who maintain good sexual function are almost always under age 65. Some men cannot achieve good erections but have sufficient desire and arousability that they wish to have treatment to promote erectile rigidity.

The physician should avoid the word *castration* in educating patients about hormonal therapy, and should encourage positive expectations about maintaining sexual activity if desired.

HORMONAL THERAPY IN WOMEN

Women with breast cancer, and to a lesser extent those with endometrial cancer, face two issues related to hormonal therapy. The first is that they have traditionally been told not to risk using estrogens for postmenopausal hormonal replacement. The second is that many women with estrogen-receptor-positive disease are offered antiestrogen therapy, usually with tamoxifen.

Data increasingly demonstrate that women who take postmenopausal estrogen replacement live longer.[26,27] One factor is reduced risk of cardiovascular disease because of the beneficial effect of estrogen on lipid levels. Women who take estrogens also are less likely to have osteoporosis, with its increased risk of fatalities from complications of hip fractures. Without estrogen replacement, postmenopausal women may develop dyspareunia related to vaginal atrophy. Changes include decreased vaginal blood supply, less elasticity of the vaginal walls, decreased lubrication, and thinning of the mucosa. Although there have been conflicting epidemiologic studies, a recent review suggests that conjugated estrogens taken in a daily dose of 0.625 mg or less do not increase a woman's relative risk of breast cancer.[27] In another recent, large prospective study, women who used estrogen replacement therapy actually had reduced mortality from breast cancer compared with women who took no hormones.[26] Because of the known benefits of postmenopausal estrogen replacement, the American College of Obstetricians and Gynecologists recently stated that some clinicians may consider postmenopausal estrogen replacement for breast-cancer survivors who appear free of disease. The decision must be made on the basis of individual risks and benefits, the woman's informed consent must be elicited, and her oncologist must be informed.[28]

Tamoxifen has both estrogenic and antiestrogenic effects on different tissues.[29,30] While it can inhibit the growth of estrogen-receptor-positive breast-cancer cells, tamoxifen may actually produce estrogenic changes in the vaginal mucosa of postmenopausal women.[29,30] The impact of tamoxifen in exacerbating or alleviating symptomatic vaginal atrophy is unknown. Some women report increased hot flashes while on the drug.[30] Tamoxifen seems to prevent bone loss and lowers total serum cholesterol in women, making it a possible alternative to estrogens in breast-cancer survivors for long-term prevention of cardiovascular disease and osteoporosis.

CHEMOTHERAPY IN MEN

Although the toxic effects of chemotherapy on spermatogenesis are well known, recent evidence suggests that many men also develop dysfunction in the testicular Leydig's cells that produce testosterone.[31] Elevations in luteinizing hormone (LH) and decreases in total and free serum testosterone, as well as excessive rises in LH after LHRH stimulation, have been observed. It is unclear how often this translates into sexual dysfunction, but hypogonadal states are not uncommon in young men who survive treatment with combination chemotherapy.[31-33] In men with testicular cancer, low testosterone levels may also reflect congenital abnormalities in the remaining testicle.[34] Treatment with long-acting injectable forms of replacement testosterone can often alleviate loss of sexual desire or erectile dysfunction in these patients. In a pilot study of 46 men who had survived bone-marrow transplants for hematologic malignancies, both endocrine and autonomic nervous system abnormalities were predictive of sexual dysfunction.[33] Patients' psychological adjustment and the presence of graft versus host disease were also related to sexual variables.

Some chemotherapy drugs cause autonomic or sensory neuropathies, another possible mechanism for sexual dysfunction. No data are available on the association of autonomic neuropathy with erectile dysfunction after chemotherapy, but failure of the initial, emission phase of the male orgasm after chemotherapy has been observed.[34,35] Emission is mediated by short adrenergic neurons and involves contractions of the prostate and seminal vesicles, with simultaneous closure of the bladder neck. These men have dry orgasms, with pleasurable sensation and the striated muscle contractions of ejaculation, the second phase of orgasm, but no semen.

It is difficult to find case series detailing the sexual function of men treated with chemotherapy alone. The data available include men who also received radiation therapy or in some cases surgery. Nevertheless, it is helpful to look at the prevalence of sexual problems in men surviving treatment for hematologic, lymphatic, or testicular malignancies. In 60 men treated for Hodgkin's disease, sexual function was significantly worse than in a group of matched, healthy controls.[36] Eighteen percent of men reported a distinct worsening of sexual function after cancer therapy. In a group of men who had bone-marrow transplants, reports of sexual problems increased from 22% of the sample to 48% after cancer treatment.[33] The most common dysfunctions were low sexual desire, erectile dysfunction, and dry orgasm. In men treated for testicular cancer, including both studies of men with seminoma and nonseminomatous tumors, rates of low sexual desire ranged from 4% to 12%, erectile dysfunction from 9% to 15%, and difficulty reaching orgasm from 6% to 10%. About 20% of men reported engaging in sexual activity very infrequently or not at all. Diminished pleasure with orgasm is also a common complaint. Across studies, sexual dysfunction has been associated with more emotional distress and marital unhappiness, although causal relations could not be addressed in cross-sectional designs.[4,11-13,35]

Information is sparse on sexual function in patients given biologic response modifiers. There is one report that men treated with interferon-α for hairy cell leukemia had no unusual sexual problems.[37]

CHEMOTHERAPY IN WOMEN

Even less is known about the prevalence of sexual dysfunction in women after chemotherapy. Clinicians are increasingly concerned about measuring quality-of-life issues, hoping to determine the cost-benefit ratio for giving adjuvant chemotherapy, for example, in node-negative women with breast cancer.[38] As in men, alkylating agents seem to be the most damaging to the female gonads.[31] In premenopausal women receiving combination chemotherapy, those who are over age 30 are more apt to cease menstruating and less apt to resume menses after treatment. Even in younger women who recover menstrual cycles, permanent menopause tends to occur prematurely.[31,39,40] Because androgens are the hormones that promote sexual desire in women, it would be helpful to know what happens to ovarian androgen production after chemotherapy.[41,42] This issue has not been addressed. Loss of sexual desire is quite common clinically during extended chemotherapy treatment and afterwards.[26-28] It is unknown whether this represents psychological distress, impaired body image, or actual hormonal changes.

In addition to the typical symptoms of premature menopause, including severe vaginal dryness and loss of elasticity and vulnerability to urinary tract infections, women receiving drugs that cause stomatitis often report periodic vaginal irritation during courses of chemotherapy.[39,40] This exacerbates problems of dyspareunia. Monilial infections are also common, perhaps because of changes in vaginal pH related to premature menopause. Women who have viral sexually transmitted diseases, such as genital herpes or human papillomavirus, may have florid recurrences because of being immunosuppressed.

PHYSIOLOGIC IMPACT OF LOCAL THERAPIES

RADIATION THERAPY IN MEN

Radiation therapy can impair sexual function if treatment fields include the pelvis, or when gonadal or genital tissue receives radiation scatter from an adjacent field. In rare cases, the testes may receive enough radiation to damage Leydig's cell function, for example when testicular relapse of acute lymphocytic leukemia in pubertal boys was treated with a 2400-rad dose directly to the testes.[31] Circulating testosterone values have also been observed to decline temporarily after external-beam irradiation for prostate cancer, with full recovery to normal levels by 6-month follow-up.[43] During this period, men may experience a loss of sexual desire or have difficulty achieving erection, but such problems should be transient.

More controversy exists about the prevalence of permanent loss of erectile capacity after definitive external-beam irradiation to the pelvis for prostate cancer. Reported rates of erectile dysfunction have varied from 22% to 84%.[44] Unfortunately, most case series have been studied retrospectively. Because men with prostate cancer are typically elderly and have complex medical histories, many already have erectile dysfunction unrelated to their cancer diagnosis.[45,46] Goldstein has theorized that the fibrotic process taking place after radiation therapy accelerates existing pelvic arteriosclerosis or causes new stenoses in the arterial system necessary for erection.[44] In a retrospective case series, he and his colleagues found evidence of reduced arterial flow to the penis after pelvic irradiation for prostate cancer. One small prospective case series has not confirmed their findings, however.[47] Furthermore, the measure they used of vascular integrity has since been largely discredited.[48] One repeated finding is that men with excellent health and sexual function have a low rate of new erectile dysfunction after radiation therapy for prostate cancer, whereas those with barely adequate sexual function and risk factors for cardiovascular disease are more likely to develop severe impairments.[44,45] In one prospective study of 85 men, at 8 to 12 months after radiation therapy only 27% of those with unequivocally normal pretreatment sexual function had developed erection problems, versus 54% of the men who reported only "borderline" erectile rigidity and coital frequency before prostate cancer.[49] It would be helpful to have longer-term follow-up, however, because the vascular effects of posttreatment fibrosis may manifest themselves gradually, beginning at 6 to 12 months after treatment.

Other elements of sexual function may also be affected by external-beam irradiation for prostate cancer. Toward the end of the course of treatment, men often experience dysuria and gastrointestinal complications. Not only do these problems temporarily interfere with sexual desire, but urethral irritation can cause pain at ejaculation. These are usually transient symptoms, but the destruction of the prostate and seminal vesicles also leads to a permanent decline in semen volume at ejaculation. Many men notice only a few drops of semen or have completely dry orgasms.

Similar side effects on sexual function may be seen after radiation therapy for testicular cancer, but are less prevalent. The dose of radiation to the pelvic area is lower, but three retrospective surveys of testicular cancer patients suggest that men who received radiation therapy to the pelvis and retroperitoneum had increased rates of erectile dysfunction.[12,13,35] Men whose only cancer treatment was radiation therapy for seminoma also often reported decreases in semen volume.[13]

In the case of noninvasive penile cancer, interstitial irradiation can sometimes be used as definitive treatment, with preservation of the penis. The incidence of long-term side effects, such as radiation ulcers or fibrosis, that could interfere with functional erections is unknown.[50]

RADIATION THERAPY IN WOMEN

Pelvic irradiation in women produces sexual dysfunction through two mechanisms. One is the destruction of ovarian function, producing premature menopause in younger women. The prevalence of amenorrhea increases with doses over 150 rad. Although attempts have been made to shield the ovaries in women with Hodgkin's disease by moving them to the pelvic midline behind the uterus, results have been mixed.[31] As with chemotherapy, women under age 30 have more chance of regaining menses or perhaps having a successful pregnancy than do women over 30 treated with pelvic radiation therapy. In young adult women, a dose of 600 to 1000 rad to the ovaries will permanently destroy their function.[40] As with chemotherapy, researchers have not addressed the question of whether ovaries damaged by irradiation still produce androgens.

In addition to the effects of estrogen deprivation on the vagina and vulva, irradiation permanently damages the basal layer of vaginal epithelium, the endothelium of small vessels in the genital area, and the fibroblasts of the connective tissues in the subepithelium.[51] The net result is a gradual process of fibrosis that may continue for several years after treatment. After definitive external-beam plus intracavitary irradiation for cervical cancer, most women have some stenosis of the upper vagina.[51] In some women, fibrosis of the vaginal walls is severe enough to cause dyspareunia. Other common changes include pallor and thinning of the vaginal mucosa. Less lubrication is produced and intercourse may cause small lacerations, experienced as postcoital bleeding and irritation. A few women develop vaginal ulcers that can take months to heal. For the first several months after radiation therapy, the irritated vagina is in danger of agglutination or of developing tight, fibrous bands of scar tissue unless the woman continues to have sexual activity or uses a vaginal dilator to stretch the tissue several times a week.[52] Although estrogen replacement therapy has less effect on the irradiated vagina, it can relieve dyspareunia in some women.[53]

Few case series are available of women treated with irradiation alone.[51] Most gynecologic cancer patients studied have had a combination of surgery and irradiation, making it difficult to isolate the impact of one specific treatment on sexual function.[2,52] One study of women with early-stage cervical cancer randomized subjects to receive either definitive irradiation or radical hysterectomy.[54] Comparable and mild levels of sexual dysfunction were found in both groups at 6-month follow-up. A more recent case series compared 26 women treated with radical hysterectomy alone to 23 who underwent radiation therapy.[10] Sexual function in the two groups was equivalent when they were interviewed before treatment and at 6 months posttreatment. By 1-year follow-up however, women who had undergone radiation therapy had decreased sexual desire (27% versus 22% for the hysterectomy group), more arousal phase problems (29% versus 6%), and more dyspareunia (22% versus 0%). Their reports of painful intercourse correlated with gynecologists' ratings of the vaginal mucosa, vaginal size, and pain during pelvic examination. Despite conventional wisdom that women need a vaginal lubricant to have comfortable intercourse after pelvic irradiation, only about a quarter of the women reported a need for a lubricant by the 1-year mark. Compliance in using vaginal dilators was quite poor, despite sexual counseling given to each woman.

RADICAL PELVIC SURGERY IN MEN

Men have dreaded the possibility of radical pelvic cancer surgery because of the high rate of resultant erectile dysfunction.

In recent years the work of Walsh and colleagues has elucidated the mechanism of erectile failure. The autonomic nerves of the prostatic plexus had been damaged by the removal of organs centrally located in the pelvis (the prostate, seminal vesicles, bladder, or rectum).[55] A method of sparing the prostatic nerve plexus was devised and applied to radical prostatectomy, radical cystectomy, and abdominoperineal resection.

When radical prostatectomy (removal of the prostate and seminal vesicles) was performed in the traditional manner, only about 10% of men recovered erections with normal rigidity. Using nerve-sparing procedures, Walsh reported a recovery rate of 74% when both neurovascular bundles are preserved and 69% with higher-stage tumors when only one bundle is left intact.[55] Recovery of erectile rigidity is gradual, taking a year or more for many men. The most recent and extensive case series from Johns Hopkins confirms earlier findings that men under age 50, those in whom both neurovascular bundles can be spared, and those with lower-stage tumors are more likely to recover functional erections.[56] Controversy remains, however. Other surgeons have not reported these success rates, although nerve-sparing certainly represents an advantage over conventional techniques.[57] Although two large case series suggested that nerve-sparing did not compromise surgical margins, a recent report questioned the efficacy of nerve-sparing prostatectomy either in preserving erectile capacity or in achieving good surgical margins in men with bulky clinical stage B2 tumors.[55,57,58] In a sample of 77 men, only 32% had clear margins and preserved potency.

Another troublesome issue is the definition used of potency. All of these studies use the criterion that the erection is firm enough to allow vaginal penetration and orgasm. Unfortunately, most men who ask for help for erectile dysfunction fit this definition. Most men do have partial erections after radical cancer surgery, and these can be sufficient for penetration with some difficulty and thrusting to the point of orgasm.[56,59] Nevertheless, the erection may not be fully rigid, so the ability to use different coital positions and produce pleasure for the woman are still unsatisfactory. When Walsh and colleagues assessed the quality of erections in finer detail in a group of men with preservation of only one neurovascular bundle, 69% met their usual criteria for potency, but only 32% described erections of normal rigidity.[60] This point is important, because men with nonrigid erections may wish further sexual rehabilitation, ending up in very much the same category as men with partial erections after traditional radical prostatectomy.

The surgeon often focuses exclusively on erectile function in discussing sexuality with a patient undergoing radical prostatectomy. It is important to inform men that desire for sex should not be impaired by surgery, because hormonal production is not altered. Sensation on the genital skin also remains normal, because the sensory nerves that innervate the genitals course along the pelvic sidewalls, where they are protected by fascia and are not in the surgical field. Because these same nerves control the striated muscle contractions of ejaculation and afferent impulses to the brain during orgasm, men can reach orgasm after radical prostatectomy, although without any ejaculation of semen, given the absence of the prostate and seminal vesicles. Many men have no idea that orgasm is possible without a firm erection and without semen. Thus, they make no attempt to resume sexual activity after radical prostatectomy, even though pleasure and orgasm from manual or oral stimulation are still options.

A few men (6% in one recent series) also suffer urinary incontinence after radical prostatectomy.[61] Seepage of urine during sexual activity may be embarrassing, although use of a condom can help.

Radical cystectomy includes not only removal of the prostate and seminal vesicles, but also the urinary bladder. In most cases only the prostatic urethra is removed, but complete urethrectomy is done if there is a risk of tumor extension to the urethral mucosa. As with radical prostatectomy, a pelvic lymphadenectomy is also part of the standard procedure. Urinary diversion may be done with an ileal conduit or more recently with alternate procedures to create a continent urinary reservoir.[62,63] Quality of life, including resumption of sexual activity, has been reported to be superior with a continent urinary diversion.[62] It is difficult to compare patient groups, however, because those who choose the longer surgery and risk of complications to have a continent diversion are often younger and more active than those who choose an ileal conduit.

Before the advent of the nerve-sparing procedure, 73 consecutive men were assessed before and at least 6 months after radical cystectomy with ileal conduit diversion.[59] Before surgery, 20% of the men were sexually inactive and 35% had at least mild erection problems. After surgery these rates increased to 50% and 91%, respectively. Men were more likely to have achieved orgasm after surgery if they had tried sexual activity more often and had recovered fuller erections. About half of the men who were orgasmic reported a reduction in the intensity of their pleasure. Treatment with preoperative pelvic irradiation or with complete urethrectomy did not have measurable additional impact on sexual function. Some reports suggest, however, that complete urethrectomy may further damage the autonomic nerves that control blood flow to the penis.[64] Two European studies also found some evidence that penile blood flow may be reduced after radical cystectomy because of intraoperative arterial ligation.[65,66]

Walsh and colleagues reported an 83% recovery of erections in men who had nerve-sparing radical cystectomy, dropping to 40% in men who had a subsequent complete urethrectomy.[55] Subsequently they reported a 71% rate of potency after cystectomy with ileocolic bladder reconstruction. They noted, however, that their patients were younger than most men undergoing radical cystectomy.[63] Although Walsh's group found that nerve-sparing did not compromise surgical margins, others warn that a nerve-sparing cystectomy may leave behind lymph nodes that are often the first site of metastatic disease in bladder cancer, compromising the completeness of surgery.[63,67]

Walsh has also suggested that nerve-sparing techniques should be applied to abdominoperineal resection.[55] He suggests that injury to nerves may be avoided with better recognition of the anatomy, not only of the prostatic plexus, but of the sacral nerve roots, the pelvic plexus, the neurovascular bundles in the perineum, and the hypogastric nerves in the retroperitoneum that mediate the emission phase of male orgasm. Sparing the prostatic nerve plexus may be most applicable to smaller, lower-stage tumors, however.[68]

After standard abdominoperineal resection, rates of erectile dysfunction have been reported from 15% to 80% in various case series.[68–76] Tumor stage does not predict recovery of erections, but as with other radical pelvic operations, younger men are more likely to recover fully.[68,70,72,73] Poor specification of the severity of erection problems in these studies makes it difficult to compare findings from different centers. Patients who underwent low anterior resection had a lower incidence of postoperative erectile dysfunction than those who had abdominoperineal resection.[69,71,77] For example, La Monica and colleagues reported a 55% rate of erection problems after abdominoperineal resection, compared with 20% after low anterior resection.[71] In another case series the respective rates were 67% and 30%.[74] Procedures that merely preserve the anal sphincter are not as successful in preventing erectile dysfunction, perhaps because the prostatic nerve plexus is often injured during surgery at that level.[72] Very low anterior resection may also damage the prostatic plexus.[68]

Impaired emission is also common after abdominoperineal resection because of dissection in the presacral area or between the seminal vesicles and rectum.[68,75] The prevalence of dry orgasm after surgery is unclear, because most published case series confuse failure of emission with inability to reach orgasm at all, or omit assessment of orgasm phase dysfunctions completely, focusing only on erectile capacity. Sympathetic nerve plexi involved in emission also are damaged during node dissections for tumors of the sigmoid colon. The incidence of dry orgasm increases with the extent of the dissection.[78] Although men who have dry orgasm still experience intense pleasure and have ejaculatory contractions of the bulbocavernosus muscles, they will need infertility treatment to have any hope of fathering a child.[79,80] Men in their reproductive years should consider sperm-banking before surgery.

Another surgical procedure that impairs the neurologic control of emission is retroperitoneal lymphadenectomy (RLND), performed to diagnose metastases from nonseminomatous testicular tumors. The standard bilateral node dissection usually damages sympathetic ganglia that send input to the short adrenergic neurons stimulating contractions of the prostate and seminal vesicles during emission.[12,81] This adrenergic system also mediates closure of the bladder neck at emission, so that dry orgasm after RLND sometimes is caused by simple retrograde ejaculation related to failure of the internal sphincter, and sometimes represents a more profound failure of the smooth muscle contractions of emission. The simplest way to differentiate the two patterns is to test for fructose and spermatozoa in urine voided after orgasm.[82]

Only two case series report detailed information on sexual function in a large sample of survivors of RLND who did not have additional chemotherapy or radiation therapy.[12,82] In one group of 47 men, only 38% consistently had dry orgasm.[12] In the other sample of 63 men, 85% had dry orgasm.[82] This discrepancy may represent different surgical technique, a shorter follow-up time in the second case series, or a different way of asking about the problem. RLND does not increase the prevalence of erectile dysfunction (seen in 6% of one and 2% of the other sample). Difficulty reaching orgasm was also rare (2% of men), but 24% of the men reported that their orgasms were less intense than before RLND.[12]

To preserve fertility and avoid dry orgasm, RLND has been

modified to spare some of the crucial sympathetic ganglia.[81,83] A recent review of nerve-sparing RLND in 75 patients found all were free of disease at 2 years postdiagnosis and none had dry orgasm.[81] The advent of highly successful combination chemotherapy for nonseminomatous testicular cancer has also led to surveillance programs for men with stage I tumors, avoiding RLND altogether.[84,85] These programs work best with highly motivated men who can travel to a regional center regularly for diagnostic tests, however, and relapse rates remain controversial.[81] Men who undergo RLND and have impaired emission can be treated by sympathomimetic agents to induce antegrade ejaculation of semen.[82,86] Another treatment that has value for some men is electrical stimulation of ejaculation.[87]

Only anecdotal accounts are available of sexual function after less common radical operations, including total pelvic exenteration, partial penectomy, and total penectomy.[25] Total pelvic exenteration is performed occasionally in men with large, localized tumors (for example, prostatic sarcomas). Given the extent of surgery, sparing the prostatic plexus is rarely possible. As with other radical pelvic procedures, however, sexual desire, penile sensation, and the ability to reach orgasm with striated muscle contractions are not impaired. Because most patients are relatively young, they often are interested in options to restore erectile function.

Penectomy is necessary when invasive, localized malignancies are found in the urethra or penis. Most are squamous cell carcinomas. There is growing evidence that cancer of the penis, like squamous cell carcinomas of the cervix, vulva, and anus, is promoted by the human papillomavirus.[88] Partners of men with penile cancer should be screened for evidence of human papillomavirus infection, although the efficacy of treatment of either partner in preventing cervical dysplasia is debatable.[89] Partial penectomy is usually chosen when the penile stump is long enough to allow a man to direct his urinary stream away from his body. After partial penectomy, most men have sufficient penile length and rigidity with erection to penetrate for intercourse. With thrusting, men report reaching a satisfying orgasm, even without the sensitive glans penis. For more proximal tumors, total penectomy is performed, including the creation of a perineal urethrostomy behind the scrotum. Because the internal sphincter is intact, men can control urination. Some men learn to reach orgasm after total penectomy, either through erotic dreams or fantasies, or from caressing the remaining erotically responsive areas.[25,90] Ejaculation of semen occurs through the perineal urethrostomy.

RADICAL PELVIC SURGERY IN WOMEN

As with men, there are several common misconceptions about the destructive impact of radical pelvic cancer surgery on a woman's sexual function. It is also difficult to find case series that assess sexual function in women who have had surgery alone, rather than combined treatment programs including chemotherapy or pelvic irradiation. Enough information exists to give a fairly complete picture, however.

Even having an abnormal Pap smear or experiencing the early symptoms of gynecologic cancer can disrupt sexual function.[91,92] Thus, estimates of changes in sexual function after cancer treatment should be based on recall of sexual function before gynecologic symptoms began to interfere.

Radical hysterectomy is a standard treatment for invasive early-stage cancer of the cervix. It includes removal of the uterus and surrounding ligaments, a pelvic node dissection, and resection of the cervix and upper one third to one half of the vagina. In women under age 40, at least one ovary is usually spared to avoid premature menopause. Some sex researchers have theorized that the cervix and uterus are essential for a woman's ability to have satisfying orgasms during intercourse, although empiric evidence from physiologic studies does not support this view.[93-95] If this were true, women after radical hysterectomy should experience a reduction in the frequency of coital orgasm and the intensity of orgasmic pleasure. One prospective study of women who had cervical conization found no impairment of sexual desire, frequency of activity, or ability to reach orgasm.[96] The percentage of women experiencing impaired sexual function after radical hysterectomy has ranged in several case series from 6% to 42%.[10]

To make sense of these variable results, one needs a large sample of women, studied prospectively and at adequate follow-up intervals using assessment techniques that examine sexual dysfunction in detail.[2,10] Only one case series meets these criteria and reports data for women treated with surgery alone.[10] Twenty-six women were interviewed and filled out questionnaires before radical hysterectomy and at 6 months and 1 year after surgery. No significant changes were observed in women's ability to reach orgasm from masturbation, partner noncoital stimulation, or intercourse. Only one woman felt that her orgasms had become less intense. Women also reported that sexual desire, arousal, and overall satisfaction were maintained at pre-illness levels. Dyspareunia occurred only 10% of the time for women evaluated at 1 year follow-up.

Vaginal sensory thresholds were studied in 26 women treated for cervical cancer.[51] There was some sensory loss at 6 and 12 months after surgery, compared with initial levels or with healthy control women. A good deal of recovery was seen by 2 years, however. Half of the women had also received radiation therapy, so that the impact of surgery alone cannot be assessed.

Only two studies of women treated for endometrial cancer are available, and both include women who had a combination of abdominal hysterectomy and pelvic radiation therapy.[97,98] Women experienced high rates of dyspareunia and decreased vaginal lubrication, as well as impairment in sexual frequency and satisfaction.

In women with invasive bladder cancer, radical cystectomy includes not only removal of the bladder and urethra, but also the uterus, adjacent ligaments, cervix, ovaries, and most of the anterior vaginal wall. The vagina is reconstructed, using the posterior wall to form either a shallower or narrowed vaginal barrel, depending on the approach taken.

Women with bladder cancer tend to be an elderly group, and many are no longer sexually active. Out of 39 consecutive women having radical cystectomy at one institution, only 9 were sexually active at the time of cancer diagnosis.[99] Interviews before and after surgery revealed that all women had severe dyspareunia on first attempting to resume coitus. By at least 6-month follow-up, however, 6 women were having regular sexual intercourse with at most mild pain. All of these women had been orgasmic with intercourse at least 50% of the time before the bladder cancer diagnosis, and continued to be orgasmic at least as often after surgery. No changes occurred in the type of stimulation needed to reach orgasm, and indeed 2 women became more easily orgasmic than in the past. Although 6 women also had pelvic radiation therapy, no additional impact of this treatment was evident in this very small sample.

The use of continent urinary diversions and modifications in surgical technique to spare more of the anterior vaginal wall are current trends that should improve women's sexual recovery after radical cystectomy.

Abdominoperineal resection for rectal cancer sometimes also includes removal of the uterus, cervix, uterine ligaments, ovaries, and posterior vaginal wall. The extent of surgery depends on tumor size and location, as well as the surgeon's preference. Little information has been published on women's sexual function after abdominoperineal resection. In one recent series of 18 women who were all sexually functional by self-report before cancer diagnosis, 78% had loss of sexual desire after surgery, 44% reported decreased overall satisfaction with sex, 34% had dyspareunia, and 6% (1 woman) could no longer achieve coital orgasm.[76] These rates of sexual dysfunction are about as expected. The loss of cushioning of the posterior vagina, as well as pelvic adhesions after surgery are common causes of dyspareunia. As with other pelvic cancer operations, loss of orgasmic capacity would not be expected. The colostomy may also affect a woman's body image and sexual desire.

Total pelvic exenteration is the most radical surgery performed for gynecologic cancer, most commonly locally recurrent cervical cancer. The uterus, tubes, ovaries, cervix, vagina, urethra, bladder, and rectum are excised. Both urinary and bowel diversions are needed. The vulva is usually left intact. The most common method currently of vaginal reconstruction is to use myocutaneous gracilis flaps from the thighs.[100] Although creating a neovagina extends the duration of surgery, it fills the defect created, helping the healing process. A neovagina created with myocutaneous flaps has the advantage of creating cushioned walls, but the vaginal lining consists of normal skin, rather than a mucosa that becomes self-lubricating as occurs with a split-thickness skin graft.[101] Women need to douche regularly to prevent odor from the neovagina, and also need a water-based lubricant for comfortable intercourse. It is unknown how many women learn to experience the sensation of thrusting during intercourse as erotic, but a few have complained that they perceive stimulation of the vaginal walls as coming from the inner thighs instead. When the clitoris is still present, many women continue to have orgasms from noncoital stimulation after total pelvic exenteration.[102,103] Many women do not resume sexual activity after exenteration, even if a vaginal reconstruction is performed.[104–106]

Radical vulvectomy not only removes the most erotically sensitive tissue of a woman's genital area, but often leads to dyspareunia because the vaginal introitus is narrowed by scar tissue and the exposed urethra is vulnerable to irritation. The pelvic lymph node dissection usually done as part of the procedure also usually produces severe lymphedema in the legs, which is both unsightly and uncomfortable. In women with in situ disease, use of wide local excision is superior to radical vulvectomy in preserving sexual function.[107,108] After radical vulvectomy, many women discontinue sexual activity, especially if they are older, or if the woman and her partner receive no sexual counseling.[109,110] Common sexual problems include loss of desire, loss of pleasurable genital sensations, dyspareunia, and difficulty reaching orgasm.[109,111]

The loss of the clitoris is not the major determining factor in whether women continue to be orgasmic after various surgical procedures to treat vulvar cancer, however.[112] A careful prospective study of 10 women undergoing radical vulvar surgery revealed that 50% regained the ability to reach orgasm, although there were elevations in genital sensory thresholds and increases in unpleasant sensations during sex that endured up to 2 years after treatment.[111] The most striking observation was that women's sexual satisfaction and level of activity recovered to pretreatment levels and seemed to depend more on the psychological intimacy of the marital relationship than on physiologic sexual function.

LOCAL TREATMENT FOR BREAST CANCER

A recent finding from two large studies is that women with early-stage breast cancer do not differ from healthy women of similar demographic background in terms of psychiatric disorders, sexual problems, or marital happiness.[113,114] This contradicts the conventional wisdom that the diagnosis of breast cancer and treatment by mastectomy is a permanent disruption of most women's sexual and marital relationships.

With the advent of breast-conservation surgery plus radiation therapy as an effective alternative to mastectomy for stage I or II disease, researchers have compared psychological and sexual adjustment after the two procedures. A recent review of 12 such studies, including four with randomized patient assignment to cancer treatment, reveals that the only consistent difference between treatment groups is a better body image for women with breast conservation.[9] This seemed to be true no matter how body image was measured, whether by standardized scales or by questions about feeling attractive sexually or feeling comfortable with nudity. Breast conservation has no clear advantage in terms of marital satisfaction, frequency of sex, sexual dysfunction, or sexual practices. Studies of breast reconstruction had similar results. One caveat, however, is that most researchers have not assessed the more subtle aspects of sexuality that might differ in women with a conserved or reconstructed breast compared to mastectomized women. These include duration of foreplay, use of breast caressing, erotic pleasure from breast caressing, and partner sexual satisfaction.

TREATMENT FOR PEDIATRIC CANCER

Little information is available about the impact of treatment for pediatric cancer on adult sexual function. Two large series of young adult survivors of childhood cancer reveal that rates of marriage are lower than in the general population.[115,116] In a study of over 2000 cancer survivors and sibling controls, there was no excess divorce rate among the cancer survivors.[116]

Only one research group has studied sexual issues. Twenty-eight young men who survived treatment for leukemia were compared to 25 men who survived other childhood cancers.[117] Overall, the men lagged behind developmental norms in terms of sexual attitudes, interest, and experience. The leukemia survivors were the most impaired, however. Only 32% of the leukemia group, compared with 64% of other survivors, were age-appropriate in their psychosexual development. Eighty-four percent of the mixed survivor group but only 57% of the leukemia group had experienced adolescent masturbation.

As more patients survive to adulthood, we need much better knowledge about the impact of pediatric cancer on sexual function.

ASSESSING SEXUAL FUNCTION IN CANCER PATIENTS

As this chapter illustrates, we now have a good knowledge of the impact of cancer on sexual function. In our work as clinicians and educators, however, it is painfully obvious to us that most men and women treated for cancer are never asked about sexual issues by their medical team. The most common reason clinicians give for not assessing sexuality is time pressure. Not only physicians but medical social workers and oncology nurses often are overwhelmed by the demands of a busy clinic. Complaints about time often mask other common concerns, however. Clinicians fear that discussing sexuality will be awkward or that they will not have remedies to offer for the patient's sexual problems.

We hope that this chapter helps clinicians feel more informed about sexual function and rehabilitation after cancer treatment, and more aware of the importance of these issues to patients. We urge the health-care professional to include one generic question about sex in an initial history or follow-up visit. The question can be prefaced by a statement emphasizing the normalcy of providing sexual health care: "I always ask patients about sexuality as part of a history," or "One aspect of every person's health is sexual health." The actual question should be open-ended, to elicit maximal information. For example, "What impact has your cancer diagnosis had on your sex life?" or "How concerned are you about the sexual side effects of your cancer treatment?" or "How well are you functioning now in your sex life?"

When cancer treatment is likely to cause sexual problems, options for rehabilitation should be mentioned at least briefly at the time of treatment disposition. Many clinicians think that this would be disruptive, and that discussing sex should wait until a follow-up visit. In our experience, however, knowing what to expect and what can be done to treat iatrogenic dysfunctions reduces the patient's anxiety.

It may be practical in a multispecialty setting to designate one trained physician, nurse, psychologist, or social worker as the sexual rehabilitation expert. If the primary physician is willing to invest a few minutes of extra time, however, we estimate that 80% to 90% of patients can benefit from brief sexual advice and information without a specialty consult.

A few patients need more intensive help. The patients at high risk to have significant sexual concerns are often younger and unmarried and may not have finished having children. Other common risk factors are being in a newer relationship

or in a marriage that is troubled, with poor communication. Men who have many extramarital affairs often seek help for sexual problems after cancer treatment. The clinician should also be alert for the patient who has a history before the cancer diagnosis of poor psychological coping, sexual or physical abuse as a child, chemical dependency, or sexual dysfunction. High-risk patients should be identified and offered more intensive assessment and counseling.

ASSESSMENT BY INTERVIEW

The interview is the heart of a sexual assessment.[95] In a hospital setting it is important that interviews take place in a private setting, and that the patient can be assured that details of sexual behavior will not be documented in the medical chart. If the patient has a committed relationship, whether heterosexual, homosexual, marital, or cohabiting, we prefer to include both partners in the session. Not only do both partners have a chance to express their perspectives and hear information given by the clinician, but their behavior during the session provides insight into their relationship. If time permits, a few minutes alone with each partner can be added to assess sensitive issues such as masturbation or affairs. The clinician must hold such information in confidence, however.

Assessing General Issues

It is helpful to gain rapport by beginning the interview reviewing nonsexual issues, including the patient's demographic background, reaction to the cancer diagnosis and treatment plan, symptoms of major depression or anxiety, use of alcohol and street drugs, compliance with medical instructions, the quality of the patient's social support, shared leisure activities for the couple, expressions of caring and anger in the relationship, and communication of emotions each partner has about the cancer.

Some useful questions include the following:

1. "How has the illness affected your private time with your partner?" Especially for young couples with children, cancer treatment disrupts the family schedule so that spouses have no time just to sit together and talk, let alone have sex.
2. "Has there been a change in the amount of physical affection you show to each other?" A decrease in sexual activity is often paralleled by declining expressions of love and caring, especially in couples with marital conflict or when the wife is the cancer patient.[8] Even for the terminally ill, touching and intimacy continue to be important.[118]
3. "Every couple disagrees sometimes. If the two of you get angry with each other, how do you each express it?" The stress of cancer can accentuate marital conflict.
4. "Has the cancer diagnosis caused disagreements in the extended family?"
5. "Are you under serious financial stress?" Financial problems related to the illness can contribute to marital and sexual conflict.

Discussion of these issues leads naturally into an assessment of sexuality, as one more facet of the relationship.

Assessing Sexual Function

Questions about sexual function should be detailed and specific. The clinician's comfort in discussing sex will help ease the patient's embarrassment. It is helpful to begin with more general topics, such as:

1. How often does lovemaking occur?
2. Who is the initiator?
3. Does activity include manual or oral genital caresses? Can each partner reach orgasm through noncoital caressing, or only during intercourse? Patients who have tried having orgasms from manual or oral stimulation are more likely to resume sex if cancer treatment impairs erections.[59]
4. Do the partners communicate preferences for touch either verbally or nonverbally during sex? Cancer treatment can interfere with a long-term sexual routine, necessitating more sexual communication and negotiation than usual.
5. How has sex changed since the cancer diagnosis in terms of frequency, variety, and function?

The interviewer can ask about each phase of the response cycle:

1. How often does the patient feel a desire for sex?
2. Can a man get and keep firm erections? If he loses erections, at what point in the lovemaking does this occur?
3. Can a woman produce enough vaginal lubrication for comfort during sexual caressing?
4. Is there pain during sex? Describe the location and quality of the pain.
5. What kinds of stimulation help each partner to reach orgasm?
6. Has the quality of orgasmic pleasure changed?
7. Does the male partner have premature ejaculation?

When a dysfunction is identified, further questions should be asked about whether the onset was sudden or gradual and about the timing of onset in relation to cancer diagnosis and treatment. Other life stresses or medical problems that could have led to sexual dysfunction should not be overlooked. Does the problem occur with all types of sexual stimulation? With all partners? On every occasion? What about response to erotic materials? Does alcohol or drug use (including prescription medications) have an impact on the problem?

Some cancer patients are seropositive for the human immunodeficiency virus (HIV) and thus are at risk for transmitting it to a sexual partner. Others may be of unknown serologic status but have engaged in high-risk behaviors. Currently, any adult who is not in a monogamous relationship with a person known to be seronegative or at very low risk for HIV should be counseled about safer sex practices.[119]

ASSESSMENT BY QUESTIONNAIRE

Asking patients to fill out questionnaires can save valuable clinician time, especially in screening large numbers of patients to identify those with high levels of psychological, marital, or sexual distress. Such patients can then be targeted for more detailed interview assessment. If a screening program is set up, the inventories should be presented to the patient by a member of the health-care team with a rationale, a discussion of confidentiality, and an opportunity for the patient to ask questions or refuse to participate. Table 64–14 lists some questionnaires that we have found particularly useful.

The Sexual History Form is a multiple-choice inventory designed to be used on an item-by-item basis to arrive at a diagnosis of sexual dysfunction.[95] Some researchers who are comparing treatment groups or diagnostic groups prefer inventories with items that cluster into a numeric scale. Such questionnaires have been devised to study sexual function in female cancer patients and in male patients.[2,46]

MEDICAL ASSESSMENT OF MALE DYSFUNCTIONS

Medical assessment of men's sexual problems has focused on identifying the causes of erectile dysfunction. Several specialized examinations are available to evaluate the complex hormonal, vascular, and neurologic impacts of cancer treatment.

History

The evaluation begins with a clear definition of the sexual problem, as discussed above. The interviewer obtains a complete review of systems; past and current medication; surgeries; major injuries; radiation therapy, chemotherapy, angioplasty, or other medical treatments; illicit drug use; and a quantitative estimate of alcohol and tobacco consumption.

Physical Examination

The examiner notes the presence or absence of secondary sex characteristics and gynecomastia. After an abdominal examination, the femoral pulses are palpated. The external genitalia are carefully examined, including palpating the penis to identify plaques or fibrosis. During a rectal examination, anal sphincter tone, bulbocavernosus reflex, and the prostate are checked. The patient's gait is observed. Motor strength, sensation, and deep tendon reflexes in the lower extremities are also assessed.

Laboratory Studies

A complete blood count and screening profile check for occult systemic disorders such as hepatic or renal disease are done.

TABLE 64–14. Questionnaires for Cancer Patients With Sexual Problems

Area of Assessment	Questionnaire
Sexual function	Sexual History Form[95]
Marital satisfaction	Dyadic Adjustment Inventory[120]
Psychological distress	Brief Symptom Inventory[121]
Illness-related distress	Psychosocial Adjustment to Illness Scale[122]
Adjustment to cancer	Cancer Rehabilitation Evaluation System[123]

Serum testosterone and prolactin levels are also determined.[124] Some groups of cancer patients are at risk for hormonal abnormalities.[32-34] Because diabetes mellitus is a common cause of male erectile and ejaculatory disorders, a glucose tolerance test should be ordered when there is no other obvious cause for the sexual dysfunction.[125] Thyroid function can be assessed by determining serum thyroxine and thyroid stimulating hormone levels.

Nocturnal Penile Tumescence

Men normally have several erections each night during rapid-eye-movement sleep. When these erections are normal in number, duration, and rigidity, significant vascular, neurologic, or hormonal impairment is rarely a cause for erectile dysfunction during waking sexual activity. If nocturnal erections are impaired, an organic cause of the dysfunction is likely.[126,127] A cost-effective and accurate way to monitor erections during sleep is a Rigiscan home monitor.[128] This is one of the most helpful tests in planning treatment, because a normal study suggests that sexual counseling can be of benefit and obviates the need for further expensive, specialized examinations. An abnormal study, however, is not as definitive, because nocturnal erections can be impaired by sleep disorders, depression, low sexual desire, or the impact of normal aging in men who are still sexually functional.[127,129,130] Indeed, lower norms for rigidity should be used in men over age 60.

Vascular Assessment

Erection is initiated with neurotransmitter changes within the spongy tissue of the corpora cavernosa. Usually, the sinusoidal spaces within the corpora are small because of contraction of cavernosal smooth muscle, mediated by tonic α-adrenergic activation.[131] As an erection begins, neurotransmitter release, mediated by parasympathetic nerves, results in cavernosal smooth muscle relaxation. The sinusoidal spaces enlarge and blood flow into the corpora increases greatly. At the same time, small veins that normally drain the corpora are compressed between the expanding soft tissue and the tunica albuginea, resulting in decreased outflow of blood. At first the penis grows in length and circumference, but as the pressure continues to build within the corpora, the shaft becomes rigid.

Assessment of the arterial and venous hemodynamics of erection has been revolutionized by the discovery that erections can be induced by the injection of vasoactive substances directly into the corpora cavernosa.[48,132] A test penile injection of drugs such as papaverine, phentolamine, prostaglandin E_1, or combinations thereof will produce a firm erection in many men who do not have disease processes in the arterial or venous systems. However, anxiety can override the drugs, producing a false-positive test result in men with psychogenic erectile dysfunction.[133,134]

A further refinement of injection testing is dynamic infusion cavernosometry, in which a test injection is given while a needle with a pressure transducer is placed in the opposite corpus cavernosum. If full erection does not result after 10 to 20 minutes, saline is pumped into the penis briefly to attempt to obtain rigidity. Both the rate of infusion needed to maintain full erection and the intracavernous pressure 30 seconds after the infusion pump is stopped are noted. This evaluation attempts to measure the adequacy of the mechanism of venous occlusion during erection.[134,135] Although using Doppler technology to obtain penile blood pressures in the flaccid penis is no longer considered an adequate diagnostic test, pressures in the cavernosal arteries can be assessed successfully during these dynamic studies. When the cavernosometry is abnormal, the study can be repeated using contrast medium so that venous outflow can be radiographically assessed. Unfortunately, the dynamic cavernosometry procedure is also subject to interference by anxiety. Healthy young men who describe situational erection problems and have very normal Rigiscan studies may appear to have severe venous occlusive dysfunction on cavernosometry.[134]

Another important diagnostic study performed first before and then after intracavernous injection is the duplex ultrasound scan.[48] Changes in arterial circumference and rate of blood flow are an index of the adequacy of arterial supply to the penis.

The utility of these vascular evaluations may be limited in cancer patients. A simple test injection can help determine whether a man is a good candidate for using penile injections at home to obtain erections for sexual activity, although results in the office are often not as good as those in a sexual situation at home. Infusion cavernosometry and duplex ultrasound provide valuable information if vascular surgery is a treatment option, but that is rare in posttreatment cancer patients.

Neurologic Assessment

Unfortunately we still do not have a direct means to assess autonomic nervous system dysfunction that contributes to erectile problems.[136] Tests such as sacral evoked response or dorsal nerve somatosensory evoked potential testing assess only somatic nerve function and are rarely helpful with routine problems. Such tests could perhaps be useful in evaluating sexual function after treatment for tumors of the brain or spinal cord, especially in research studies. Penile sensory thresholds can be measured through either vibratory or electric stimulation tests.[137] Such testing can help assess complaints of loss of erotic penile sensation after cancer treatment.

MEDICAL ASSESSMENT OF FEMALE SEXUAL DYSFUNCTIONS

Methods available to the clinician who wants to determine the cause of a woman's sexual problem are far less sophisticated than the array of tests available for male dysfunctions. The pelvic examination continues to be the mainstay of the evaluation for female sexual problems. In women who are experiencing ovarian failure, indices of vaginal atrophy such as skin elasticity, thickness of pubic hair, fullness of the labia, caliber of the vaginal introitus, color and rugation of the vaginal mucosa, and vaginal depth are important.[138] The physician can use a speculum or fingers to attempt to reproduce pelvic pain that a patient experiences during intercourse.[139] The cause of the pain then becomes more evident.

Clinicians who examine women during systemic chemotherapy should look for an irritated vaginal mucosa. Immunosuppression also leaves a woman vulnerable to florid recurrences of genital herpes or human papillomavirus. The effects of pelvic and vaginal irradiation can include reduced vascularization of the mucosa, vaginal ulcers or stenosis, or more diffuse fibrous changes in the vaginal walls or adnexae.[52] A recently described syndrome of superficial pain and dyspareunia at the vaginal introitus, vulvar vestibulitis, can easily be missed during a routine pelvic examination.[140] Erythematous lesions in the vestibule produce exquisite pain when a cotton swab is touched to the local area. Ulcerations can often be seen on colposcopy. In our experience, vulvar vestibulitis is often triggered after gynecologic procedures such as topical chemotherapy or laser treatment for human papillomavirus.[141]

Researchers have attempted to measure vaginal blood flow, analogous to noninvasive examinations of penile vascular integrity. Unfortunately, such measurements in women must occur during sexual arousal and involve placing an instrument in the vagina. Many women are uncomfortable undergoing erotic stimulation under laboratory conditions. The instruments used also have limited reliability.[94] Neurologic measures of genital reflex arcs in women have also proven unreliable and have no clear correlation with sexual symptoms.[142,143] Sensory thresholds in women can be measured with electric stimulation, however, providing useful information on changes in sensitivity after cancer treatment.[51] Radioimmunoassays to measure serum levels of estradiol, prolactin, thyroid hormones, and follicle-stimulating hormone during amenorrhea or in the first 5 days of a menstrual cycle can help in deciding whether to prescribe replacement hormones for women showing signs of premature menopause after chemotherapy for cancers that are not hormone-sensitive (*e.g.*, leukemia or Hodgkin's disease).[40]

TREATING SEXUAL PROBLEMS IN CANCER PATIENTS

Our biggest challenge is to ensure that cancer patients benefit from the techniques of sexual rehabilitation now available. There is a dearth of outcome research on the effectiveness of such programs. Even in major cancer centers, it is rare to have a specialist in sexual health care on staff. When such a program does exist, our experience is that few physicians refer patients consistently to get help. The first step is to make sexual assessment routine in the clinic and hospital. A clinician within the primary treatment setting should be available to provide brief sexual counseling. The most effective way to present sexual rehabilitation to patients is as part of a more comprehensive program of psychosocial support. Sexuality is just one of the emotional issues facing men and women treated for cancer. It is increasingly obvious that psychological adjustment and supportive relationships are more important determinants of sexual satisfaction than is physiologic functioning.[51,95]

BRIEF SEXUAL COUNSELING

Brief counseling, the backbone of sexual rehabilitation, involves at least a few minutes and more often takes an hour or two. Of patients referred for sexual consultation in a cancer center, 73% were seen once or twice; 16% had three to five sessions.[8] Only a few of the patients who have brief counseling will need medical consultation by a urologist, gynecologist, or specialist in sexual medicine. Such experts should be linked in a referral network, however. Because sexual problems after cancer treatment are usually complex, a combined program of both counseling and medical or surgical intervention is often optimal. Thus, the clinician doing sexual counseling must have good communication and collaboration with the other specialists. They, in turn, should be well versed in treating sexual problems and in the iatrogenic effects of cancer treatment.

Table 64–15 lists the components of brief sexual counseling for cancer patients. Brief counseling has been described in more detail in a previous publication.[95] The American Cancer Society has developed guidebooks for men and women on sexuality and cancer.[144,145] They include diagrams, explanations of the sexual side effects of cancer treatments, and advice on sexual rehabilitation.

INTENSIVE SEX THERAPY

Perhaps 10% to 20% of cancer patients have severe sexual dysfunctions that call for the specialty skills of a trained sex therapist.[95] Indicators for referral to sex therapy include a sexual problem that preceded the cancer and remains a source of distress, sexual issues related to severe marital conflict, a dysfunction that has not responded to brief sexual counseling, or a sexual problem that is just one feature of poor psychological coping. Some patients endure cancer treatments that are so mutilating, such as total pelvic exenteration, total penectomy, radical vulvectomy, or facial disfigurement, that consultation with a mental-health professional trained in sex therapy should be routine during recovery, unless the patient declines.

Formal sex therapy is a short-term, symptom-focused treatment that ideally includes both partners.[146] Patients are assigned tasks between sessions that include sensate focus exercises and learning other sexual techniques found effective in reversing specific dysfunctions. Work on marital communication and individual psychological well-being are often part of treatment. Sex therapy can also enhance the results of medical or surgical rehabilitation, such as breast reconstruction or treatment of organic erectile dysfunction.

TREATING ORGANIC ERECTILE DYSFUNCTION

Most men with erectile dysfunction related to cancer treatment are candidates for one of three treatments: intracavernous injection therapy, a vacuum erection device, or a penile prosthesis. Surgery to improve arterial flow to the penis or to ligate penile veins is rarely appropriate in these patients.[147]

Intracavernous injection of vasoactive drugs to obtain an erection has become a popular method of treatment in recent years.[148] Men are taught how to inject themselves safely with a proper dose of medication just before beginning sexual activity at home. Men with neurologic damage from radical pelvic surgery often can obtain erections with quite low doses of medication.[149] Those with mild to moderate vascular impairment of erection may need larger doses or may be unable to use injections successfully. To be a good candidate for this treatment, a man should have the cognitive ability to learn the injection technique and the manual dexterity to perform the procedure. A committed spouse can also learn to give the injection. The patient should be compliant enough to follow

TABLE 64–15.   Elements of Brief Sexual Counseling

Education

Illustrate genital and pelvic anatomy using models or pictures

Explain the normal sexual response cycle

Explain the impact of specific treatments on sexual function

Give advice on options for sexual rehabilitation:

    Sex therapy

    Vaginal dilators

    Hormone replacement

    Water-based lubricants

    Vacuum erection device

    Home penile injections

    Penile prostheses

    Changes in medication

Minimizing Physical Handicaps

Time sex to avoid pain and fatigue

Learn to cope with ostomy appliance, limb prosthesis, laryngectomy, and so forth

Find comfortable positions

Female dyspareunia can benefit from lubricants and dilators

Erectile dysfunction can be treated appropriately

Use open sexual communication, verbal and nonverbal

Attitude Change

Debunk myths on cancer and sex:

    Venereal contagion of cancer

    Cancer as punishment for sins

    Resuming sex is unhealthy

Accept noncoital sex when coitus not possible

Sex cannot always be spontaneous

Sex is not just for the young and healthy

Advice on Resuming Sex

Either partner can initiate sex

Increase expression of nonsexual affection

Start slowly using sensate focus format[146]

Discuss how to deal with physical attractiveness (mastectomy, ostomy, and so forth): desensitize to reality vs camouflage

Resolving Couple Conflict

Make private time for each other

Discuss fears and sadness

Negotiate illness-related changes in marital roles (wage-earner, childcare, budgeting, and so forth)

Act as team in dealing with conflict in extended family

---

instructions precisely and to come in for reversal if priapism occurs.

Although priapism is rare at recommended doses, penile fibrosis becomes progressively more frequent with prolonged use of papaverine and phentolamine, the most popular drug combination.[150] In severe cases, fibrosis can cause pain and curvature of erection. Although prostaglandin E_1 has been recommended as a superior drug, a significant minority of men experience prolonged penile pain after using it.[151] In our program, a smaller but still significant rate of fibrosis is also seen with long-term use of prostaglandin E_1.[152] Thus, periodic follow-up examinations are crucial in treating men on intracavernous injection programs. This form of treatment is not ideal for a young man with a long life expectancy, but is often a good alternative to a penile prosthesis in an older patient who does not wish to have elective surgery.

The vacuum erection device (VED), shown in Figure 64–5, has also gained increasing popularity.[153,154] The VED works on a negative pressure principle. Either before starting sexual activity or preferably after obtaining some partial tumescence with foreplay, the man places the VED over his penis and uses a hand pump to create a vacuum around his penis. The vacuum leads to congestion of the spongy tissue of the corpora cavernosa and increased arterial inflow.[154] A constriction band is then transferred from the base of the pump to encircle the base of the erect penis, and the cylindrical pump is removed.

The resulting erection may be larger in circumference than a natural one, but unfortunately is often not firm proximal to the constriction band, so that the penis pivots. This can in-terfere with thrusting during intercourse. The band is also tight enough to constrict the urethra, resulting in retention of semen and occasional discomfort at orgasm for at least half the men who use the device. Most men can obtain usable erections, however. Over the first few months of use, drop-out rates have been reported to be only about 20%.[153,154]

Complications of the VED are minimal. Some men experience bruising or discomfort with the device. It should be used with caution in men with low platelet counts or those on

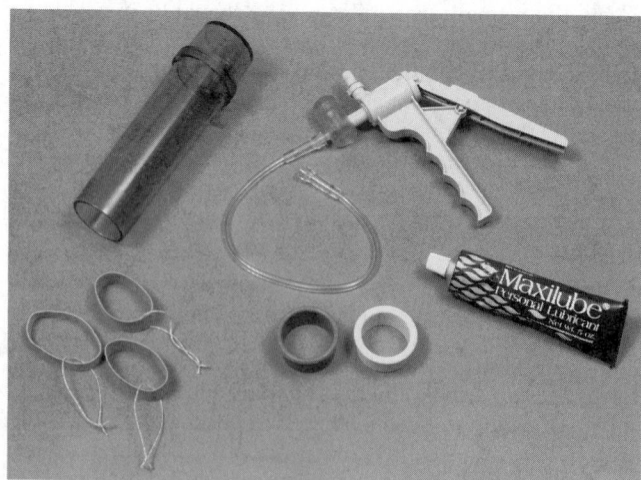

FIGURE 64–5.   Vacuum erection device.

anticoagulants. The constriction band should not be used for more than 30 minutes, because penile ischemia can occur with the device.[155] Skin necrosis has been reported in one man with genital hypesthesia.[156] Men who obtain partial tumescence with sexual stimulation tend to have better erections with a VED than do men who no longer have any erectile changes at all.

Implantation of a penile prosthesis has the disadvantage of being potentially irreversible. If the prosthesis malfunctions or is removed, the capacity to have a normal erection may not return. On the other hand, with the improved reliability of prosthetic devices, surgery represents a permanent solution to erectile dysfunction for the vast majority of men who choose it.[157] A penile prosthesis may be the optimal treatment for irreversible erectile dysfunction in a patient with a long life expectancy.

Penile prosthesis surgery is successful in over 95% of cases. Infection around the prosthesis occurs in about 2% to 5% of cases and invariably requires removal of the prosthesis.[158] Later complications are usually mechanical device failures that require surgical revision. Late hematogenous infections of penile prostheses are rare.[159] No data are available on prosthetic complications related to the immunosuppression of cancer treatment, but the experience with organ transplant recipients suggests that the prosthesis is a safe treatment option.[160]

Although prosthesis implantation at the time of pelvic cancer surgery has been advocated, this practice has not gained widespread acceptance.[161] Surgeons are reluctant to prolong the cancer operation or to incur a risk of periprosthetic infection. Because many patients also recover erectile rigidity gradually after nerve-sparing surgery, an optimal time for prosthesis implantation appears to be at least 6 months after cancer surgery.

Prosthesis implantation is often done through a single 2- to 4-cm incision, without removing tissue and with minimal blood loss. Transfusions are rarely necessary. Some surgeons implant prostheses under local anesthesia on an outpatient basis, but more commonly the procedure is done under general or spinal anesthesia with a 1- to 2-day hospital stay.[162]

Three major types of penile prosthesis are most commonly used today: the rod prosthesis, the single-component hydraulic, and the multicomponent inflatable. Device failures are least likely to occur with simple rod prostheses but increase in frequency with increasing device complexity. A malleable prosthesis is one of the most simple, but even when the penis is bent for concealment, it does not look or feel flaccid. The erection obtained is shorter and narrower than a full, natural erection. The single-component hydraulic prosthesis (Fig. 64–6) also produces an erection similar to that with a malleable model, but the flaccid penis appears more natural for concealment.[163] In cancer patients who have had either pelvic irradiation or pelvic surgery, a malleable or single-component hydraulic prosthesis may be optimal, because no abdominal reservoir needs to be placed. The hydraulic type may be superior when repeated cystoscopies will be necessary.

Some men, however, desire the full penile girth and complete concealment of a multicomponent inflatable prosthesis (Fig. 64–7). The newest inflatable prosthesis also allows some elongation of the corpora cavernosa, so that the erect penis is more normal in length.[164] The fluid reservoir of a multi-

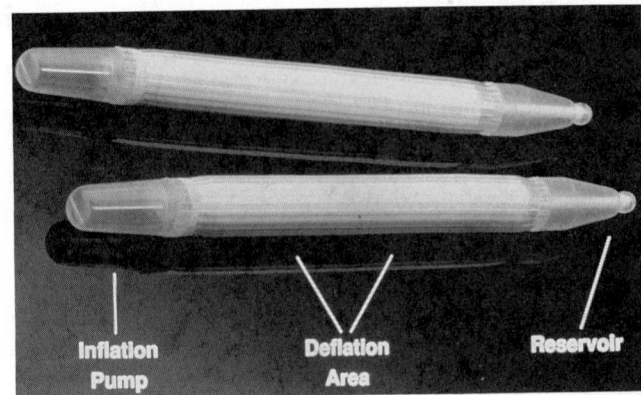

FIGURE 64–6. Single-component hydraulic penile prosthesis.

component prosthesis is usually implanted in the retropubic space via the penoscrotal incision, using special insertion tools. If the patient has had pelvic surgery or irradiation, however, the surgeon can avoid the risk of bowel injury by placing the reservoir extraperitoneally behind a rectus muscle.[165] A multicomponent inflatable prosthesis can also compensate for some of the loss of penile girth after urethrectomy.

None of these treatments for erectile dysfunction can directly improve sexual desire, penile sensation, or the ability to reach orgasm, but often the renewed ability to have erections has a positive impact on a man's self-esteem and interest in initiating sex. If intercourse was a man's preferred aspect of sexual activity, the ability to engage in coitus again can improve sexual pleasure and facilitate reaching orgasm. None of these treatments is a cure for premature ejaculation, but that is the one sexual problem that does not increase in prevalence with cancer treatment.[8]

MEDICAL OR SURGICAL INTERVENTIONS FOR WOMEN

In contrast to the specific treatments for men's sexual problems, interventions for women are more closely linked to specific cancer therapies. Breast reconstruction can be considered a type of sexual rehabilitation, although enhancing sexual pleasure is not the primary motivation of most women who choose this surgery. Vaginal reconstructive surgery more

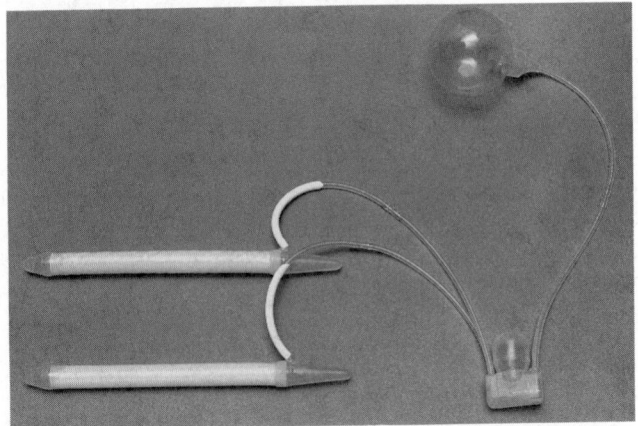

FIGURE 64–7. Multicomponent inflatable penile prosthesis.

closely parallels the penile prosthesis in that it restores the functional capacity for intercourse. After radical vulvectomy, some women need split-thickness skin grafts to repair stenosis of the vaginal introitus. Myocutaneous flap technology has also been used to perform reconstruction of the labia, both for cosmetic appearance and to provide cushioning for the urethra and vaginal entrance.[166]

Women who undergo premature menopause after cancer treatment need medical intervention. Those who do not have hormone-sensitive tumors should definitely be considered for hormonal replacement, given the benefits in preventing cardiovascular disease and osteoporosis, as well as the favorable impact on vaginal lubrication and elasticity.[26] As discussed above, even some women who are long-term survivors of node-negative breast cancer may decide that the benefits of estrogen replacement outweigh the risks.[28]

Women who have dyspareunia after cancer treatment can often benefit from learning exercises to relax the muscles that surround the vaginal entrance.[139] When a woman feels she can contract or relax these muscles at will, she may want to use a series of vaginal dilators of graduated size (Fig. 64–8). The goal of dilation is not usually to stretch the vagina physically, but to give the woman a sense that she can relax the vaginal entrance and accommodate penile penetration without pain. Steps in dilation include inserting the dilator and removing it, inserting it and holding it in the vagina for a few minutes, and being able to move the dilator without pain. Dilator size varies from about the length and thickness of a finger to that of an erect penis. When the woman can use the largest dilator without pain, she can approach penile penetration by gradually tolerating first one and then two fingers in her vagina during lovemaking, and then slowly guiding her partner's penis into her vagina while she stays relaxed in the female-superior position.

Water-based nonprescription lubricants are very helpful, not only in preventing pain with the use of dilators, but also in sexual activity for the woman with chronic vaginal dryness. Gel lubricants include Astroglide and Today Personal Lubricant. Suppositories can be used before sexual activity (Lubrin or Condommate). A vaginal moisturizer, Replens, can be used three times a week to provide more consistent hydration of the vaginal mucosa. Women with persistent superficial dyspareunia should be examined for vulvar vestibulitis, because combined surgery and counseling can often alleviate the pain.[141]

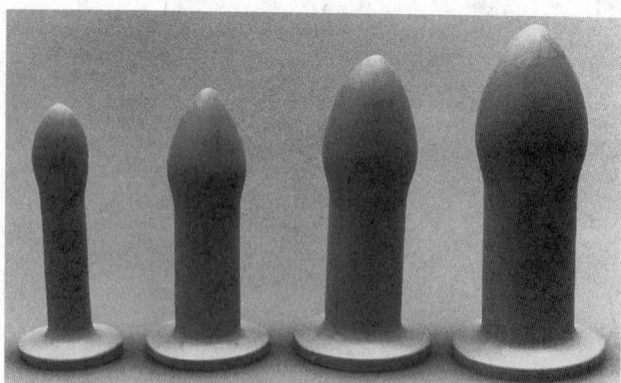

FIGURE 64–8. Graduated sizes of vaginal dilators.

REFERENCES

1. Schover LR, Friedman J, Weiler S, et al. The multiaxial problem-oriented system for sexual dysfunctions. Arch Gen Psychiatry 1982;39:614–619.
2. Andersen BL, Anderson B, deProsse C. Controlled prospective longitudinal study of women with cancer: I. Sexual functioning outcomes. J Consult Clin Psychol 1989;57:683–691.
3. Dackman L. Up front: Sex and the post-mastectomy woman. New York: Penguin Books, 1990.
4. Gritz ER, Wellisch DK, Wang H, et al. Long-term effects of testicular cancer on sexual functioning in married couples. Cancer 1989; 64:1560–1567.
5. Derogatis LR, Morrow GR, Fetting J, et al. The prevalence of psychiatric disorders among cancer patients. JAMA 1983;249:751–757.
6. Bukberg J, Penman D, Holland JC. Depression in hospitalized cancer patients. Psychosom Med 1984;46:199–212.
7. Kathol RG, Mutgi A, Williams J, Clamon G, Noyes R. Diagnosis of major depression in cancer patients according to four sets of criteria. Am J Psychiatry 1990;147:1021–1024.
8. Schover LR, Evans RB, von Eschenbach AC. Sexual rehabilitation in a cancer center: Diagnosis and outcome in 384 consultations. Arch Sex Behav 1987;16:445–461.
9. Schover, LR. The impact of breast cancer on sexuality, body image, and intimate relationships. CA 1991;41:112–120.
10. Schover LR, Fife M, Gershenson DM. Sexual dysfunction and treatment for early stage cervical cancer. Cancer 1989;63:204–212.
11. Rieker PP, Edbril SD, Garnick MB. Curative testis cancer therapy: Psychosocial sequelae. J Clin Oncol 1985;3:1117–1126.
12. Schover LR, von Eschenbach AC. Sexual and marital relationships after treatment for nonseminomatous testicular cancer. Urology 1985;25:251–255.
13. Schover LR, Gonzales M, von Eschenbach AC. Sexual and marital relationships after radiotherapy for seminoma. Urology 1986;27:117–123.
14. Keitel MA, Zevon MA, Rounds JB, Petrelli NJ, Karakousis C. Spouse adjustment to cancer surgery: Distress and coping responses. J Surg Oncol 1990;43:148–153.
15. Liss-Levinson WS. Clinical observations on the emotional responses of males to cancer. Psychother Theory Res Pract 1982;19:325–330.
16. Rieker PP, Fitzgerald EM, Kalish LA. Adaptive behavioral responses to potential infertility among survivors of testis cancer. J Clin Oncol 1990;8:347–355.
17. Cella DF, Najavits L. Letter to the editor: Denial of infertility in patients with Hodgkin's disease. Psychosomatics 1986;27:71.
18. Nugent P, O'Connell TX. Breast cancer and pregnancy. Arch Surg 1985;120:122–124.
19. Knob P. Physical and psychological distress associated with adjuvant chemotherapy in women with breast cancer. J Clin Oncol 1986;4:678–684.
20. Querleu D, Laurent JC, Verhaeghe M. Pregnancy following surgery for cancer of the breast. J Gynecol Obstet Biol Reprod 1986;15:633–639.
21. Riberio G, Jones DA, Jones M. Carcinoma of the breast associated with pregnancy. Br J Surg 1986;73:607–609.
22. Peeling WB. Phase III studies to compare goserelin (Zoladex) with orchiectomy and with diethylstilbestrol in treatment of prostatic carcinoma. Urology (Suppl) 1989;33:45–52.
23. Cassileth BR, Soloway MS, Vogelzang NJ, et al. Patients' choice of treatment in stage D prostate cancer. Urology (Suppl) 1989;33:57–62.
24. Rousseau L, Dupont A, Labrie F, Couture M. Sexuality changes in prostate cancer patients receiving antihormonal therapy combining the antiandrogen flutamide with medical (LHRH agonist) or surgical castration. Arch Sex Beh 1988;17:87–98.
25. Schover LR. Sexuality and fertility in urologic cancer patients. Cancer 1987;60(Suppl):553–558.
26. Henderson BE, Paganini-Hill A, Ross RK. Decreased mortality in users of estrogen replacement therapy. Arch Intern Med 1991;151:75–78.
27. Dupont WD, Page DL. Menopausal estrogen replacement therapy and breast cancer. Arch Intern Med 1991;151:67–72.
28. American College of Obstetricians and Gynecologists. Technical Bulletin 158: Carcinoma of the breast. Washington DC, 1991.
29. Jordan VC. Long-term adjuvant tamoxifen therapy for breast cancer: The prelude to prevention. Cancer Treatment Rev 1990;17:15–36.
30. Love RR. Antiestrogen chemoprevention of breast cancer: Critical issues and research. Prev Med 1991;20:64–78.
31. Gradishar WJ, Schilsky RL. Effects of cancer treatment on the reproductive system. Crit Rev Oncol Hematol 1988;8:153–171.
32. Vigersky RA, Chapman RM, Berenberg J, et al. Testicular dysfunction in untreated Hodgkin's disease. Am J Med 1982;73:482–486.
33. Baruch J, Benjamin S, Treleaven J, et al. Male sexual function following bone marrow transplantation for haematological cancer. Tenth World Congress for Sexology, Amsterdam, 1991.
34. Fossa SD, Klepp O, Molne K, et al. Testicular function after unilateral orchiectomy for cancer and before further treatment. Int J Androl 1982;5:179–184.
35. Nijman JM. Some aspects of sexual and gonadal function in patients with nonseminomatous germ-cell tumor of the testis (dissertation). Groningen, The Netherlands: Drukkerij Van Denderen BV, 1987.
36. Cella DF, Tross S. Psychological adjustment to survival from Hodgkin's disease. J Consult Clin Psychol 1986;54:616–622.
37. Schilsky RL, Davidson HS, Magid D, et al. Gonadal and sexual function in male patients with hairy cell leukemia: Lack of adverse effects of recombinant alpha-2-interferon. Cancer Treat Rep 1987;71:179–181.

38. Gelber RD, Goldhirsch A, Cavalli F, et al. Quality-of-life-adjusted evaluation of adjuvant therapies for operable breast cancer. Ann Int Med 1991;114:621–628.

39. Suttcliffe SB. Clinical problems and their management: Clinical problems in females with lymphoma. In: Proceedings of Workshop on Psychosexual and Reproductive Issues of Cancer Patients. Chicago: American Cancer Society, 1987.

40. Chapman RM. Effect of cytotoxic therapy on sexuality and gonadal function. Semin Oncol 1982;9:84–94.

41. Davidson JM, Myers LS. Endocrine factors in sexual psychophysiology. In: Rosen RC, Beck JG, eds. Patterns of sexual arousal: Psychophysiological processes and clinical applications. New York: Guilford Press, 1988:189–211.

42. Sherwin BB. A comparative analysis of the role of androgen in human male and female sexual behavior: Behavioral specificity, critical thresholds, and sensitivity. Psychobiology 1988;16:416–425.

43. Tomic R, Bergman B, Damber JE, Littbrand B, Lofroth PO. Effects of external radiation therapy for cancer of the prostate on the serum concentrations of testosterone, follicle-stimulating hormone, luteinizing hormone and prolactin. J Urol 1983;130:287–289.

44. Goldstein I, Feldman MI, Deckers PJ, et al. Radiation-associated impotence: A clinical study of its mechanism. JAMA 1984;251:903–910.

45. van Heeringen C, De Schryver A, Verbeek E. Sexual function disorders after local radiotherapy for carcinoma of the prostate. Radiother Oncol 1988;13:47–52.

46. Zinreich ES, Derogatis LR, Herpst J, et al. Pre- and posttreatment evaluation of sexual function in patients with adenocarcinoma of the prostate. Int J Radiat Oncol Biol Phys 1990;19:729–732.

47. Mittal B. A study of penile circulation before and after radiation in patients with prostate cancer and its effect on impotence. Int J Radiat Oncol Biol Phys 1985;11:1121–1125.

48. Lue TF, Abber JC. Penodynamics: Diagnostic studies of vasculogenic impotence. In: Montague DK, ed. Disorders of male sexual function. Chicago: Year Book Medical Publishers, 1988:95–104.

49. Banker FL. The preservation of potency after external beam irradiation for prostate cancer. Int J Radiat Oncol Biol Phys 1988;15:219–220.

50. Schover LR, von Eschenbach AC. Letter to the editor: Sexual rehabilitation of urologic cancer patients. CA 1985;35:319–320

51. Weijmar Schultz WCM, van de Weil HBM. Sexual functioning after gynaecological cancer treatment (dissertation). Groningen, The Netherlands: Drukkerij Van Denderen BV, 1991.

52. Abitbol MM, Davenport JH. The irradiated vagina. Obstet Gynecol 1974;44:249–256.

53. Pitkin RM, van Voorhis LW. Postirradiation vaginitis: An evaluation of prophylaxis with topical estrogen. Ther Radiol 1971;99:417–421.

54. Vincent CE, Vincent B, Griess FC, et al. Some marital-sexual concomitants of carcinoma of the cervix. South Med J 1975;68:552–558.

55. Walsh PC, Schlegel PN. Radical pelvic surgery with preservation of sexual function. Ann Surg 1988;208:391–400.

56. Quinlan DM, Epstein JI, Carter BS, Walsh PC. Sexual function following radical prostatectomy: Influence of preservation of neurovascular bundle. J Urol 1991;145:998–1002.

57. Catalona WJ, Dresner SM. Nerve-sparing radical prostatectomy: Extraprostatic tumor extension and preservation of erectile function. J Urol 1985;134:1149–1151.

58. Bigg SW, Kavoussi LR, Catalona WJ. Role of nerve-sparing radical prostatectomy for clinical stage B2 prostate cancer. J Urol 1990;144:1420–1424.

59. Schover LR, Evans RB, von Eschenbach AC. Sexual rehabilitation and male radical cystectomy. J Urol 1986;136:1015–1017.

60. Walsh PC, Epstein JI, Lowe FC. Potency following radical prostatectomy with wide unilateral excision of the neurovascular bundle. J Urol 1987;138:823–827.

61. Middleton RG, Smith JA, Melzer RB, et al. Patient survival and local recurrence rate following radical prostatectomy for prostatic carcinoma. J Urol 1986;136:422–424.

62. Boyd SD, Feinberg SM, Skinner DG, et al. Quality of life survey of urinary diversion patients: Comparison of ileal conduits versus continent Kock ileal reservoirs. J Urol 1987;138:1386–1389.

63. Marshall FF, Mostwin JL, Radebaugh LC, Walsh PC, Brendler CB. Ileocolic neobladder post-cystectomy: Continence and potency. J Urol 1991;145:502–504.

64. Kitamura T, Moriyama N, Shibamoto K, et al. Urethrectomy is harmful for preserving potency after radical cystectomy. J Urol 1987;42:375–379.

65. Bergman B, Sivertsson S, Suurkala M. Penile blood pressure in erectile impotence following cystectomy. Scand J Urol Nephrol 1982;16:81–84.

66. Tizzani A, Casetta G, Carone R, et al. Defective erection in patients subjected to radical cystectomy: Diagnosis by Doppler test and stimulated sacral reflex. Minerva Urol Nephrol 1985;37:335–339.

67. Pritchett TR, Schiff WM, Klatt E, Lieskovsky G, Skinner DG. The potency-sparing radical cystectomy: Does it compromise the completeness of the cancer resection? J Urol 1987;140:1400–1403.

68. Santangelo ML, Romano G, Sassaroli C. Sexual function after resection for rectal cancer. Am J Surg 1987;154:502–504.

69. Balslev I, Harling H. Sexual dysfunction following operation of carcinoma of the rectum. Dis Colon Rectum 1983;26:785–788.

70. Danzi M, Ferulano GP, Abate S, et al. Male sexual function after abdominoperineal resection for rectal cancer. Dis Colon Rectum 1983;26:665–668.

71. La Monica G, Audisio RA, Tamburini M, et al. Incidence of sexual dysfunction in male patients treated surgically for rectal malignancy. Dis Colon Rectum 1985;28:937–940.

72. Neal D. The effects on pelvic visceral function of anal-sphincter-ablating and anal-sphincter-preserving operations for cancer of the lower part of the rectum and for benign colorectal disease. Ann R Coll Surg Engl 1984;66:7–13.

73. Kinn C, Ohman V. Bladder and sexual function after surgery for rectal cancer. Dis Colon Rectum 1986;29:43–48.

74. Williams NS, Johnston D. The quality of life after rectal excision for low rectal cancer. Br J Surg 1983;70:460–462.

75. Yeager ES, Van Heerden JA. Sexual dysfunction following proctocolectomy and abdominoperineal resection. Ann Surg 1980;191:169–170.

76. Cirino E, Pepe G, Pepe F, et al. Sexual complications after abdominoperineal resection. Ital J Surg Sci 1987;17:315–318.

77. Hjortrup A, Kirkegaard P, Friis J, et al. Sexual dysfunction after low anterior resection for midrectal cancer. Acta Chir Scand 1984;150:687–688.

78. Tomoda H, Furosawa M. Sexual and urinary dysfunction following surgery for sigmoid colon cancer. Jpn J Surg 1985;15:355–360.

79. Bergman B, Nilsson S, Petersen I. The effect on erection and orgasm of cystectomy, prostatectomy and vesiculectomy for cancer of the bladder: A clinical and electromyographic study. Brit J Urol 1982;51:114–120.

80. Biester RJ, Howards SS. Failure of seminal emission and retrograde ejaculation. In: Tanagho EA, Lue TF, McClure RD, eds. Contemporary management of impotence and infertility. Baltimore: Williams & Wilkins, 1988:285–290.

81. Donohue JP, Foster RS, Rowland RG, et al. Nerve-sparing retroperitoneal lymphadenectomy with preservation of ejaculation. J Urol 1990;144:287–292.

82. Nijman JM. Some aspects of sexual and gonadal function in patients with nonseminomatous germ-cell tumor of the testis (dissertation). Groningen, The Netherlands: Drukkerij Van Denderen BV, 1987.

83. Jewett MAS, Kong YP, Goldberg SD, et al. Retroperitoneal lymphadenectomy for testis tumor with nerve sparing for ejaculation. J Urol 1988;139:1220–1224.

84. Freedman LS, Parkinson MC, Jones WG, et al. Histopathology in the prediction of relapse of patients with stage I testicular teratoma treated by orchidectomy alone. Lancet 1987;2:294–298.

85. Herr HW, Whitmore WF, Sogani PC. Selection of testicular tumor patients for omission of retroperitoneal lymph node dissection. J Urol 1986;135:500–503.

86. Lange PH, Narayan P, Fraley EE. Fertility issues following therapy for testicular cancer. Semin Urol 1984;11:264–274.

87. Ohl DA, Denil J, Bennett CJ, et al. Electroejaculation following retroperitoneal lymphadenectomy. J Urol 1991;145:980–983.

88. Barrasso R, De Brux J, Croissant O, Orth G. High prevalence of papillomavirus-associated penile intraepithelial neoplasia in sexual partners of women with cervical intraepithelial neoplasia. N Engl J Med 1987;317:916–923.

89. Krebs HB, Helmkamp BF. Does the treatment of genital condylomata in men decrease the treatment failure rate of cervical dysplasia in the female sexual partner? Obstet Gynecol 1990;76:660–663.

90. Witkin MH, Kaplan HS. Sex therapy and penectomy. J Sex Marital Ther 1982;8:209–221.

91. Andersen BL, Lachenbruch PA, Anderson B, DeProsse C. Sexual dysfunction and signs of gynecologic cancer. Cancer 1986;57:1880–1886.

92. Campion MJ, Brown JR, McCance DJ, et al. Psychosexual trauma of an abnormal cervical smear. Br J Obstet Gynaecol 1988;95:175–181.

93. Ladas AK, Whipple B, Perry JD. The G spot. New York: Holt, Rinehart & Winston, 1982.

94. Rosen RC, Beck JG. Patterns of sexual arousal: Psychophysiological processes and clinical applications. New York: Guilford Press, 1988.

95. Schover LR, Jensen SB. Sexuality and chronic illness: A comprehensive approach. New York: Guilford Press, 1988.

96. Kilkku P, Gronroos M, Punnonen R. Sexual function after conization of the uterine cervix. Gynecol Oncol 1982;14:209–212.

97. Cochran SD, Hacker NF, Wellisch DK, Berek JS. Sexual functioning after treatment for endometrial cancer. J Psychosoc Oncol 1987;5:57–63.

98. Jenkins B. Patients' reports of sexual changes after treatment for gynecological cancer. Oncol Nursing Forum 1988;15:349–354.

99. Schover LR, von Eschenbach AC. Sexual function and female radical cystectomy: A case series. J Urol 1985;134:465–468.

100. Edwards CL, Loeffler M, Rutledge FN. Vaginal reconstruction. In: von Eschenbach AC, Rodriguez DB, eds. Sexual rehabilitation of the urologic cancer patient. Boston: GK Hall, 1981:251–264.

101. Masters WJ, Johnson VE. Human sexual response. Boston: Little, Brown, 1966.

102. Lamont JA, De Petrillo AD, Sargeant EJ. Psychosexual rehabilitation and exenterative surgery. Gynecol Oncol 1978;6:236–242.

103. Dempsey GM, Buchsbaum HJ, Morrison J. Psychosocial adjustment to pelvic exenteration. Gynecol Oncol 1975;3:325–334.

104. Morley GW, Lindenauer SM, Youngs D. Vaginal reconstruction following pelvic exenteration: Surgical and psychological considerations. Am J Obstet Gynecol 1973;116:996–1002.

105. Vera MI. Quality of life following pelvic exenteration. Gynecol Oncol 1981;12:355–366.

106. Andersen BL, Hacker NF. Psychosexual adjustment following pelvic exenteration. Obstet Gynecol 1983;61:331–338.

107. Disaia PJ, Creasman WT, Rich WM. An alternative approach to early cancer of the vulva. Am J Obstet Gynecol 1979;133:825–832.

108. Andersen BL, Turnquist D, LaPolla J, Turner D. Sexual functioning after treatment of in situ vulvar cancer: Preliminary report. Obstet Gynecol 1988;71:15–19.

109. Andreasson B, Moth J, Jensen SB, Bock JE. Sexual function and somatopsychic reactions in vulvectomy-operated women and their partners. Acta Obstet Gynecol Scand 1986;65:7–10.

110. Stellman RE, Goodwin JM, Robinson J, Dansak D, Hilgers RD. Psychological effects of vulvectomy. Psychosomatics 1984;25:779–783.

111. Weijmar Schultz WCM, van de Wiel HBM, Bouma J, Janssens J, Littlewood J. Psy-

chosexual functioning after the treatment of cancer of the vulva. Cancer 1990;66:402–407.

112. Andersen BL, Hacker NF. Psychosexual adjustment after vulvar surgery. Obstet Gynecol 1983;62:457–462.

113. Psychological Aspects of Breast Cancer Study Group. Psychological response to mastectomy: A prospective comparison study. Cancer 1987;59:189–196.

114. Vinokur AD, Threatt BA, Caplan RD, Zimmerman BL. Physical and psychosocial functioning and adjustment to breast cancer: Long-term follow-up of a screening population. Cancer 1989;63:394–405.

115. Green DM, Zevon MA, Hall B. Achievement of life goals by adult survivors of modern treatment for childhood cancer. Cancer 1991;67:206–213.

116. Byrne J, Fears TR, Steinhorn SC, et al. Marriage and divorce after childhood and adolescent cancer. JAMA 1989;262:2693–2699.

117. Ropponen P, Aalberg V, Rautonen J, Kalmari H, Siimes MA. Psychosexual development of adolescent males after malignancies in childhood. Act Psychiatr Scand 1990;82:213–218.

118. Lieber L, Plumb MM, Gerstenzang ML, et al. The communication of affection between cancer patients and their spouses. Psychosom Med 1976;38:379–389.

119. Goedert JJ. What is safe sex? Suggested standards linked to testing for human immunodeficiency virus. N Engl J Med 1987;316:1339–1341.

120. Spanier GB. Measuring dyadic adjustment: New scales for assessing the quality of marriage and similar dyads. J Marriage Fam 1976;38:15–28.

121. Derogatis LR, Melisaratos N. The Brief Symptom Inventory: An introductory report. Psychol Med 1983;13:595–605.

122. Derogatis LR. Psychosocial Adjustment to Illness Scale (PAIS and PAIS-SR): Scoring procedures and administration manual. Baltimore: Clinical Psychometric Research, 1983.

123. Ganz PA, Schag CAC, Cheng HL. Assessing the quality of life: A study in newly diagnosed breast cancer patients. J Clin Epidemiol 1990;43:75–86.

124. Maatman TJ, Montague DK, Martin LM. Cost-effective evaluation of impotence. Urology 1986;27:132–135.

125. Maatman TJ, Montague DK, Martin LM. Erectile dysfunction in men with diabetes mellitus. Urology 1987;29:589–592.

126. Meisler AW, Carey MP. A critical reevaluation of nocturnal penile tumescence monitoring in the diagnosis of erectile dysfunction. J Nerv Mental Dis 1990;178:78–89.

127. Schiavi RC. Nocturnal penile tumescence in the evaluation of erectile disorders: A critical review. J Sex Mar Ther 1988;14:83–97.

128. Kaneko S, Bradley WE. Evaluation of erectile dysfunction with continuous monitoring of rigidity. J Urol 1986;136:1026–1029.

129. Thase ME, Reynolds CF, Jennings JR, et al. Diagnostic performance of nocturnal penile tumescence studies in healthy, dysfunctional (impotent), and depressed men. Psychiatry Res 1988;26:79–87.

130. Schiavi RC, Schreiner-Engel P. Nocturnal penile tumescence in healthy aging men. J Geront 1988;43:146–150.

131. Lue TF, Tanagho EA. Functional anatomy and mechanism of penile erection. In: Tanagho EA, Lue TF, McClure RD, eds. Contemporary management of impotence and infertility. Baltimore: Williams & Wilkins, 1988:39–50.

132. Abber JC, Lue TF, Orvis BR, et al. Diagnostic tests for impotence: A comparison of papaverine injection with the penile-brachial index and nocturnal penile tumescence monitoring. J Urol 1986;135:923–925.

133. Buvat J, Buvat-Herbaut M, Dehaene JL, et al. Is intravascular injection of papaverine a reliable screening test for vascular impotence? J Urol 1986;135:476–478.

134. Montague DK, Lakin MM, Medendorp SV, Tesar LJ. Infusion pharmacocavernosometry and nocturnal penile tumescence findings in men with erectile dysfunction. J Urol 1991;145:768–771.

135. Lue TF. Functional study of penile veins. In: Tanagho EA, Lue TF, McClure RD, eds. Contemporary management of impotence and infertility. Baltimore, Williams & Wilkins, 1988:65–69.

136. Padma-Nathan H, Goldstein I. Neurologic assessment of the impotent patient. In: Montague DK, ed. Disorders of male sexual function. Chicago: Year Book Publishers, 1988:86–94.

137. Rowland DL, Greenleaf W, Mas M, Myers L, Davidson JM. Penile and finger sensory thresholds in young, aging, and diabetic males. Arch Sex Beh 1989;18:1–12.

138. Leiblum SR, Bachmann G, Kemmann E, et al. Vaginal atrophy in the postmenopausal woman: The importance of sexual activity and hormones. JAMA 1983;249:2195–2198.

139. Fordney DS. Dyspareunia and vaginismus. Clin Obstet Gynecol 1978;21:205–221.

140. Friedrich EG. Vulvar vestibulitis syndrome. J Reprod Med 1987;32:110–114.

141. Schover LR, Youngs DD, Cannata R. Psychosexual aspects of the evaluation and management of vulvar vestibulitis. Am J Obstet Gynecol 1992;167:630–636.

142. Blaivas JG, Zayed AAH, Labib KB. The bulbocavernosus reflex in urology: A prospective study of 299 patients. J Urol 1981;126:197–199.

143. Haldeman S, Bradley WE, Bhatia WN, et al. Pudendal evoked responses. Arch Neurol 1982;39:280–283.

144. Schover LR, Randers-Pehrson M. Sexuality and cancer: For the woman who has cancer, and her partner. Atlanta: American Cancer Society, 1991.

145. Schover LR, Randers-Pehrson M. Sexuality and cancer: For the man who has cancer, and his partner. Atlanta: American Cancer Society, 1991.

146. Wincze JP, Carey MP. Sexual dysfunction: A guide for assessment and treatment. New York: Guilford Press, 1991.

147. Lue TF, Carroll PR, Moore C. Treatment of impotence in cancer patients. Import Adv Oncol 1989;1:193–203.

148. Virag R, Shoukry K, Floresco J, Nollet F, Greco E. Intracavernous self-injection of vasoactive drugs in the treatment of impotence: 8-year experience with 615 cases. J Urol 1991;145:287–293.

149. Dennis RL, McDougal WS. Pharmacological treatment of erectile dysfunction after radical prostatectomy. J Urol 1988;139:775–776.

150. Lakin MM, Montague DK, Medendorp SV, Tesar L, Schover LR. Intracavernous injection therapy: Analysis of results and complications. J Urol 1990;143:1138–1141.

151. Stackl W, Hasun R, Marberger M. Intracavernous injection of prostaglandin E1 in impotent men. J Urol 1988;140:66–68.

152. Lakin MM, Montague DK, Schover LR, Chen RN, Ignaut CA. Fibrosis with intracavernous injection therapy utilizing prostaglandin E1 (PGE-1). [Abstract] Presented at the Annual Meeting of the American Urological Association, Washington, DC, May 1992.

153. Sidi AA, Becher EF, Zhang G, Lewis JH. Patient acceptance of and satisfaction with an external negative pressure device for impotence. J Urol 1990;144:1154–1156.

154. Turner LA, Althof SE, Levine SB, et al. Treating erectile dysfunction with external vacuum devices: Impact upon sexual, psychological and marital functioning. J Urol 1990;144:79–82.

155. Katz PG, Haden HT, Mulligan T, Zasler ND. The effect of vacuum devices on penile hemodynamics. J Urol 1990;143:55–56.

156. Meinhardt W, Kropman RF, Lycklama AAB, Nijeholt A, Zwartendijk J. Skin necrosis caused by use of negative pressure device for erectile impotence. J Urol 1990;144:983.

157. Montague DK. Penile prostheses: An overview. Urol Clin N Amer 1989;16:7–12.

158. Montague DK. Periprosthetic infections. J Urol 1987;138:68–69.

159. Carson CC, Robertson CN. Late hematogenous infection of penile prostheses. J Urol 1988;139:50–52.

160. Kabalin JN, Kessler R. Successful implantation of penile prostheses in organ transplant patients. Urology 1989;33:282–284.

161. Bennett AH. Placement of penile prosthesis during surgery for malignancies. Urology 1987;20:276–277.

162. Kaufman JJ. Penile prosthetic surgery under local anesthesia. J Urol 1982;128:1190–1191.

163. Mulcahy JJ. The Hydroflex penile prosthesis. Urol Clin N Amer 1989;16:33–38.

164. Montague DK, Lakin MM. Early experience with the controlled girth- and length-expanding cylinder of the AMS Ultrex penile prosthesis. J Urol 1992;148:1444–1446.

165. Scott FB, Light JK, Fishman IJ. Treatment of impotency caused by cancer therapy: The inflatable penile prosthesis. Cancer Bull 1982;34:33–39.

166. Spauwen PHM, Bouma J, Burger MPM. Vulval reconstruction after cancer excision. Tenth World Congress of Sexology, Amsterdam, 1991.

JOHN M. DALY
MICHAEL H. TOROSIAN

SECTION 4

Nutritional Support

Proper preparation of cancer patients for major surgery, chemotherapy, and radiation treatment requires both physiologic and psychological intervention and support. The goal of therapy during the perioperative period in surgical patients is to prepare the patient to withstand the stress of major surgery and to minimize postoperative complications. The appropriate duration of the preoperative support period depends on the relative urgency of the surgical procedure compared with the operative risk and the natural history of the disease. A multitude of factors such as the patient's chronologic and physiologic age, the degree of metabolic derangements and nutritional deficits, the presence of organ dysfunction, the extent of obesity, and the stage of the primary disease should be considered relative to the timing and magnitude of the surgical procedure.

Protein-calorie malnutrition is a common problem in hospitalized medical and surgical cancer patients and occurs in most patients undergoing major upper-abdominal surgery. Among hospitalized patients, those with cancer have the highest incidence of protein-calorie malnutrition. Thus, evaluation of nutritional deficits is critical to determining operative risk and can influence the timing and extent of surgery.

Protein-calorie malnutrition results from decreased oral intake, increased enteral losses secondary to malabsorption or intestinal fistula, various forms of antineoplastic therapy, and tumor-induced alterations in host metabolism. In the absence of adequate exogenous nutrients, the body uses endogenous substrates to satisfy the ongoing requirements of both the host and the tumor for energy and protein. In patients with malignant obstruction of the gastrointestinal tract, the tumor itself may cause diminished nutrient intake. Multimodal therapy for malignant disease including surgery, chemotherapy, and radiation therapy exacerbates these metabolic derangements, further increasing the risk of significant postoperative morbidity and mortality.

Malnutrition associated with malignancy has major prognostic significance, and the association between weight loss and increased mortality in cancer patients has been known for several decades. The use of enteral and total parenteral nutrition allows clinicians to have an impact on the malnutrition associated with cancer. However, controversy remains as to whether nutritional intervention benefits the host and the tumor, and to what extent nutritional intervention affects clinical endpoints such as morbidity, mortality, and response to therapy.

CANCER CACHEXIA

Cancer cachexia is a group of symptoms and signs that includes inanition, anorexia, weakness, tissue wasting, and organ dysfunction. Common in patients with advanced metastatic disease, cachexia also occurs in patients with localized disease (Table 64–16). DeWys and associates noted substantial weight loss in some patients with breast cancer and most patients with gastric or pancreatic carcinoma.[1] The relation of cachexia to tumor burden, stage of disease, and tumor histology is in-

TABLE 64–16. Potential Etiologies of Cancer Cachexia

Tumor	*Antineoplastic Therapy*
Dysphagia	Reduced intake in preparation for diagnostic and therapeutic intervention
Early satiety	
Bowel obstruction	
Malabsorption	Ileus
Competition for substrate	Malabsorption
Alteration of host metabolism	Increased energy requirements
Anorexia	Anorexia
Alteration of taste	Anosmia
	Nausea and vomiting
	GI mucosal damage
	Mastication and swallowing dysfunction
	Xerostomia
	Oropharyngeal ulcerations/infections

consistent, and no single theory satisfactorily explains the cachectic state. Recent results suggest that cytokines and peptides secreted by the host in response to the tumor play a major role in the development of cachexia (Fig. 64–9). These mediators, such as cachectin/tumor necrosis factor and interferon-γ, exert profound effects on the host's intermediary metabolism. In the short term, these effects promote an acute-phase response by rerouting nutrients from the periphery to the liver. However, over the long term, these cytokines result in anorexia and abnormalities in carbohydrate, protein, and lipid metabolism.

DIMINISHED NUTRIENT INTAKE

Anorexia accompanies most neoplasms to some extent and is a major contributing factor to the development of the cachectic state. Often, loss of appetite is an important symptom of an underlying tumor. Several physiologic derangements have been cited as possible reasons for anorexia. Abnormalities in taste perception, such as reduced thresholds for sweet, sour, and salty flavors, have been shown. DeWys and Walters noted that a reduced taste sensitivity for sucrose and urea is associated with reduced caloric intake; reduced oral threshold for urea correlates with an aversion for red meat.[2] Deficiencies in zinc and other trace elements may contribute to altered taste sensation. Patients with hepatic metastases accompanied by hepatic insufficiency may develop anorexia and nausea from reduced clearance of lactate produced by anaerobic tumor metabolism of glucose.

The specific metabolic processes that affect nutrient intake in cancer patients are unclear. Lucke and colleagues noted the presence of a humoral factor that reproduces the metabolic characteristics of the tumor-bearing state in non-tumor-bearing animals.[3] DeWys and coworkers suggested that tumor peptides acting through neuroendocrine cells and neuroreceptors alter metabolic pathways.[1] Nakahara described a "toxohormone" capable of mimicking the cachectic state when injected into normal animals.[4] Antibodies to interferon-γ partially reversed the cachexia in animals with end-stage tumors.[5] Endogenously produced tumor necrosis factor/cachectin may also be a mediator in the development of cachexia in the tumor-bearing host. Krause and associates noted that abnormalities in the central nervous system metabolism of serotonin may be responsible for the anorexia associated with the tumor-bearing state.[6]

The local effect of the tumor may also lead to reduced food intake, particularly when the tumor obstructs the upper alimentary tract. Patients with cancer of the oral cavity, pharynx, or esophagus may have reduced nutrient intake because of dysphagia or odynophagia due to partial or complete obstruction. Patients with gastric cancer often have reduced gastric capacity or partial gastric outlet obstruction, leading to nausea, vomiting, and early satiety. Intestinal tumors and abdominal carcinomatosis can cause partial obstruction or blind-loop syndrome to interfere with nutrient absorption. Pancreatic carcinomas often cause exocrine enzyme deficiencies and malabsorption syndromes. Finally, psychological factors such as depression, grief, or anxiety resulting from the disease or its treatment may lead to poor appetite, abnormal eating behavior, and learned food aversions and thus to a diminished or unbalanced dietary intake.

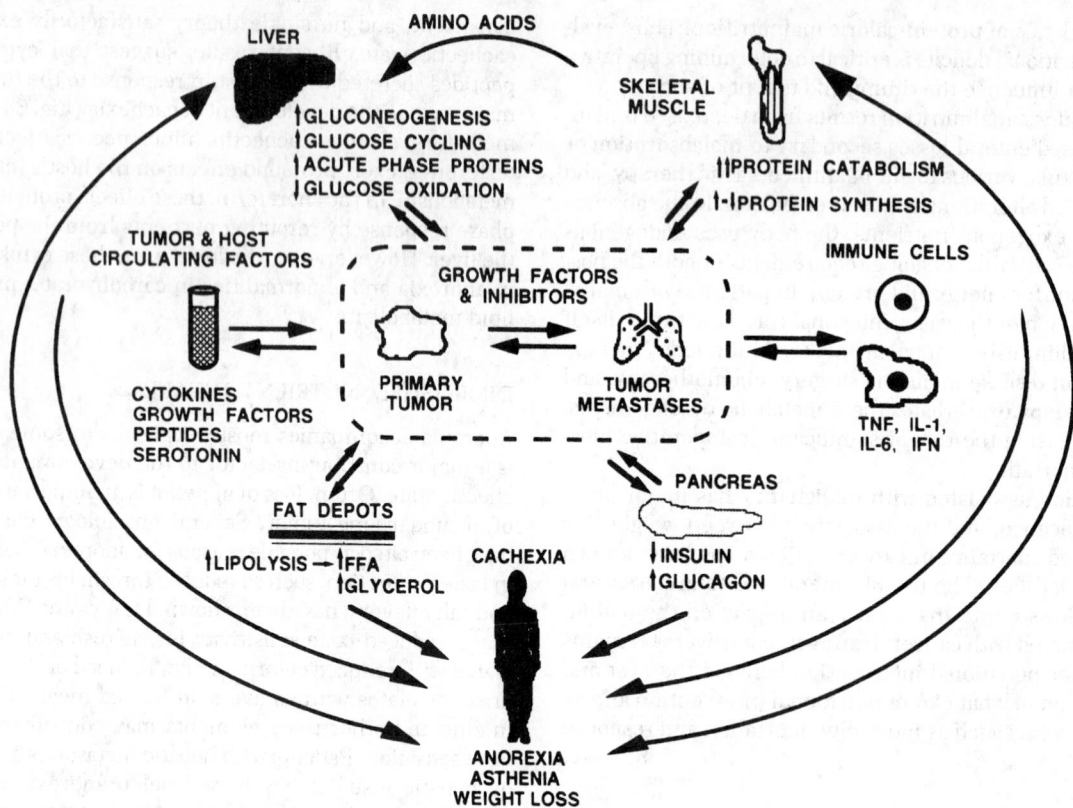

FIGURE 64–9.   Mechanisms of metabolic abnormalities in tumor-bearing hosts.

ABNORMALITIES OF SUBSTRATE METABOLISM

Extensive changes in energy, carbohydrate, lipid, and protein metabolism have been demonstrated in patients with malignant disease.[7–9] Increased energy expenditure and inefficient energy use are frequently cited causes of malnutrition in tumor-bearing hosts.[10] The normal response to diminished food intake is a reduction in the basal metabolic rate (BMR); the BMR or resting energy expenditure consists of all the energy-requiring processes of vegetative function and accounts for 75% of total energy expenditure in normal people. The lack of a decreased response of BMR to semistarvation likens cancer cachexia to the septic state.

Energy requirements of cancer patients have been studied prospectively. Young could not conclude that resting metabolism was consistently elevated in cancer patients, although increased resting energy expenditure was found in leukemia and lymphoma patients.[10] Increases in resting metabolic rate paralleled advancing disease and reduced nutrient intake. Other investigators have shown an elevation in resting energy expenditure in patients with lymphomas, lung cancer, and head and neck cancers.[11] Shike and colleagues demonstrated in a group of patients with small cell lung carcinoma that basal energy expenditure was elevated compared with controls.[12] Responders to chemotherapy had a significant decrease in basal energy expenditure, while nonresponders exhibited no change. In 1983 Knox and coworkers measured energy expenditure in 200 malnourished cancer patients by indirect calorimetry.[13] Only 41% had a normal resting energy expenditure, while decreased and increased resting energy expen-

diture was observed in 33% and 26%, respectively. Similarly, Heber and associates found no clear evidence of hypermetabolism in noncachectic lung-cancer patients.[14] They argued that because malnourished patients normally have a decreased BMR as an adaptation to starvation, even predicted metabolic rates are inappropriately elevated in malnourished cancer patients.

Shaw and colleagues concluded that the alteration in metabolic rate depends on the type of tumor.[15] They demonstrated an elevated rate of energy expenditure in sarcoma-bearing patients associated with increased Cori cycle activity and glucose turnover, reduced glucose oxidation, and increased protein catabolism. Buzby and colleagues noted a reduction in metabolic rate associated with pancreatic cancer.[16] Patients with lower gastrointestinal neoplasms tended to be metabolically similar to normal volunteers, but patients with upper gastrointestinal tumors had an elevated metabolic rate.

Inefficient energy use by the tumor-bearing host was studied by Holroyde and Reichard, who reported increased Cori cycle activity in patients with malignancy.[9] This futile cycle, in which glucose is converted to lactic acid and subsequently reconverted to glucose by hepatocytes, wastes energy. The highest level of Cori cycle activity was seen in patients with the greatest energy expenditure and weight loss. Young suggested that increased rates of protein turnover also result in significant energy losses due to the failure of normal adaptation to starvation.[10] During the first 2 days of fasting, endogenous glycogen stores of muscle and the liver are depleted. Glucose use by the brain, leukocytes, and other tissues continues, resulting in the breakdown of protein for gluconeogenesis. In noncancer patients, muscle protein breakdown is gradually replaced by fat fuel metabolism, in which fatty acids are converted to ketone bodies. These are used for energy by peripheral tissues and eventually for up to 95% of energy use by the brain; this results in decreased glucose use, with sparing of muscle protein. In cancer patients, these adaptive mechanisms occur less commonly, resulting in increased glucose production and protein catabolism.

Although cancer patients have normal levels of circulating insulin and glucose, they have impaired insulin sensitivity (Table 64–17). Glucose intolerance is documented by hyperglycemia and delayed clearance of blood glucose in cancer patients after oral or intravenous glucose administration.[9,14,17] Glucose intolerance is due in part to decreased peripheral tissue sensitivity to insulin, but may also involve an attenuated islet cell secretory response to glucose.[17] Cancer patients also exhibit increased hepatic gluconeogenesis from alanine and lactate. Using carbon 14-labeled alanine, Waterhouse and coworkers found that the apparent increase in gluconeogenesis from alanine reflected a very rapid glucose turnover.[18] Feedback control of glucose production may be impaired because gluconeogenesis and Cori cycle activity are not inhibited by glucose administration in the cancer patient. Moley and associates[19] and Peacock and Norton[20] studied sarcoma-bearing rats and found that supplemental insulin administration preserves host lean body mass and even influences the duration of survival.

Shaw and Wolfe recently noted that patients with gastrointestinal tumors had elevated rates of basal hepatic glucose production.[21] They found a direct relation between tumor burden and the increased rate of gluconeogenesis. Furthermore, patients with the largest tumor burdens failed to suppress their own endogenous glucose production during glucose infusions.

Alterations in lipid metabolism in cancer patients include decreased fat stores and increased lipid mobilization.[22,23] Decreases in total body fat are common in these patients and

TABLE 64–17. Metabolic Changes in the Cancer Patient

Carbohydrate Metabolism
Insulin resistance
Glucose intolerance
Increased gluconeogenesis
Increased Cori cycle activity
Increased glucose turnover
Increased serum lactate

Fat Metabolism
Increased fatty acid mobilization
Increased fatty acid turnover
Increased glycerol turnover
Hyperlipidemia
Decreased lipoprotein lipase

Protein Metabolism
Increased whole body protein turnover
Increased skeletal muscle catabolism
Decreased skeletal muscle anabolism
Impaired keto-adaptation

are most likely related to insulin resistance. Increased oxidation of fatty acids also occurs. Glycerol and fatty acids, the byproducts of lipolysis, serve as substrates for gluconeogenesis and energy production, respectively, during periods of nutrient deprivation. Waterhouse found that fatty acids are the major substrates used in patients with progressive malignant disease.[24] Increased plasma clearance of endogenous fat stores and exogenously administered fat emulsions occurs in cancer patients in both fasting and fed states. Patients with malignancy fail to suppress lipolysis after glucose administration and continue to oxidize fatty acids.[25]

Because loss of body fat occurs often in patients with cancer cachexia, Wilson and colleagues measured changes in intravenous fat clearance and the effects on such clearance by operation and total parenteral nutrition (TPN) in patients with colorectal cancer.[26] Fifteen out of 21 patients had increased rates of fat clearance. Fat clearance rates were reduced to nearly normal in the 14 patients who were retested 12 weeks after curative resection. In 7 malnourished patients who received intravenous nutrition, fat clearance was also reduced.

Several abnormalities of protein metabolism occur in cancer patients, including nitrogen depletion, decreased muscle protein synthesis, and abnormal plasma aminograms.[8] Nitrogen balance is negative in most patients with progressive malignancy. Amino acid trapping by tumor cells has been demonstrated clinically and experimentally. Norton and coworkers found that sarcoma-bearing limbs released less than 50% of the amount of amino acids released from tumor-free limbs.[27] Evidence obtained with whole-body protein studies using nitrogen 15-labeled glycine indicates that cancer patients have increased whole-body protein turnover, which contributes to increased energy expenditure.[27]

Muscle wasting and decreases in serum protein levels are common in patients with malignant disease. Eventually, severe wasting of host muscle mass occurs along with depletion of visceral and circulating proteins, due primarily to increased protein breakdown. Kien and Carmitta noted a close association of accelerated rates of whole-body protein turnover and energy expenditure in children with acute lymphocytic leukemia.[28] Fearon and associates demonstrated no correlation between increased turnover and increased resting energy expenditure in adults.[29]

While tumor-induced increases in muscle and visceral protein breakdown contribute to host cachexia, evidence is emerging that tumor tissues may regulate their own protein degradation. Recent work by Tayek and colleagues compared the rate of host muscle protein synthesis and tumor protein synthesis and degradation in rats bearing either syngeneic sarcoma or hepatoma.[30] Eighteen days after tumor implantation, synthesis of rat muscle protein was decreased, but liver protein synthesis increased, with a net decrease in total protein synthesis. The metabolic cost to the host of increased protein flux may be substantial and may contribute to the development of cachexia.

Changes in body composition occur in cachexia, such as increased extracellular fluid and total body sodium and decreased intracellular fluid and total body potassium. Cohn and coworkers, using prompt γ-neutron activation to evaluate total body nitrogen and a whole-body counter to measure potassium 40, found that total body potassium was diminished out of proportion to total body nitrogen.[31] On the basis of this finding, they concluded that endogenous nutrient losses in cancer patients were predominantly in the skeletal muscle compartment, because muscle makes up 45% of total body nitrogen and 85% of total body potassium. In normal volunteers, body cell mass (BCM) tended to decrease with increasing age as an absolute value and as a percentage of total body weight. In anorexia nervosa patients, there was a significant depletion of BCM but relative sparing of the BCM when expressed as a percentage of body weight. This reflects the normal adaptation to starvation, where fat use predominates and endogenous protein is spared. In cancer patients, there was a significant degree of weight loss accompanied by a proportional decline in BCM, indicating that protein is depleted to the same extent as fat stores.

A variety of micronutrient abnormalities (vitamin and trace metals) may occur in cancer patients. Because vitamin A plays a role in the histology of certain types of epithelia, it has been suggested that cancer patients may have abnormally low total carotenoid levels. However, no difference in total carotenoids and pro-vitamin A precursors have been noted between well-nourished normal volunteers and cancer patients.

ETIOLOGY OF CANCER CACHEXIA

The etiology of cancer cachexia remains controversial but is undoubtedly multifactoral. Cachexia is not simply a local effect of the tumor but is caused by systemic factors induced by the tumor (*i.e.*, a type of paraneoplastic syndrome). Most current theories hypothesize that tumors do not directly produce the mediators of cachexia but induce host tissues to secrete circulating factors that cause cachexia. Two classes of cachexia mediators believed to be important in the development of cancer cachexia are cytokines and regulatory hormones (Table 64–18).

Cytokines are soluble proteins secreted by host tissues in response to various stimuli, including cancer, sepsis, inflammation, starvation, and other pathophysiologic insults. Cytokines exert their effects on host tissues by autocrine, paracrine, or circulating/systemic mechanisms. Tumor necrosis factor/cachectin, interleukin-1, and interleukin-6 are specific cyto-

kines implicated in the development of cancer cachexia by recent experimental evidence.

Tumor necrosis factor (TNF) or cachectin is a 17-kilodalton molecular weight protein secreted by macrophages in response to endotoxin or malignancy. When given to animals, TNF can reproduce many, but not all, of the changes seen in cancer cachexia. Anorexia, weight loss, depletion of fat stores, loss of protein mass, hypoproteinemia, and increased total body water have been documented in TNF-treated animals. Some of these effects can be prevented by inducing tolerance to TNF or can be reversed with anti-TNF antibodies. Thus, TNF may cause some of the adverse host effects of cancer cachexia, but it is certainly not the sole mediator. Furthermore, it has been difficult to detect circulating levels of TNF in cancer patients even with severe degrees of cachexia.

Interleukin-1 (IL-1) is a cytokine secreted by macrophages in response to endotoxin. This inflammatory cytokine causes anorexia, pyrexia, hypotension, decreased systemic vascular resistance, and increased cardiac output. Gene amplification of the IL-1 locus has been found in one cachectic, tumor-bearing animal model, and both IL-1 and TNF produce alterations in hepatic protein synthesis similar to the tumor-bearing state.

Interleukin-6 (IL-6) is secreted by macrophages stimulated by endotoxin and by fibroblasts in response to TNF or IL-1. This cytokine, also called β_2-interferon, hepatocyte-stimulating factor, and hybridoma growth factor, has many activities similar to TNF and IL-1. Elevated levels of IL-6 have been found in tumor-bearing animals and correlate with the hepatic acute-phase response to cancer.

Abnormalities in anabolic regulatory hormones may also play an important role in the development of cancer cachexia. Cancer is associated with numerous aberrations of intermediary metabolism, including glucose intolerance, increased glucose cycling, impaired glucose oxidation, and increased lipolysis. Hormonal changes may be integral to these metabolic alterations, and cachexia from cancer and other catabolic states has been associated with decreased insulin and increased glucagon levels. The resulting insulin:glucagon ratio, an anabolic hormone index, is significantly reduced and is asso-

TABLE 64–18.   Circulating Host Factors That May Cause Cancer Cachexia

Factor	Food Intake	Body Weight	Lipid Mass	Protein Mass	Measured in Circulation	Antibody Studies
Cachectin/tumor necrosis factor	Decrease	Decrease	Decrease	Decrease	Animal studies correlate with cachexia (with stimulation). Human did not correlate with cachexia.	AB to TNF reversed anorexia and body composition changes in tumor-bearing mice
Interleukin-1	Decrease	Decrease	NA	NA	Undetectable levels in cancer cachexia	NA
Interleukin-6	NA	NA	NA	NA	Levels increased with increasing tumor burden	NA
Interferon-γ	Decrease	Decrease	NA	NA	NA	AB reversed cachexia and prolonged survival of tumor-bearing rat

NA, data not available; AB, antibody; TNF, tumor necrosis factor.
(Langstein H, Norton JA. Mechanisms of cancer cachexia. Hematol Oncol Clin North Am [February] 1991)

ciated with weight loss and continued catabolism. Although insulin alone is inadequate to reverse these metabolic abnormalities, the combined administration of the anabolic hormones insulin, growth hormone, and somatostatin can effectively treat some of the adverse host changes seen in cancer cachexia.[32]

Additional clinical and basic research is required to further elucidate the role of cytokines, hormones, and other circulating factors in the development of cancer cachexia and to devise effective therapeutic strategies to treat the cancer patient.

EFFECTS OF ANTITUMOR THERAPY ON NUTRITION

Antineoplastic therapy invariably affects the host, either by mechanical or physiologic alterations due to surgery, or at the cellular level with chemotherapy or radiation therapy.[33] The effects of therapy may add to the cachexia of malignancy and exacerbate the severe nutritional deficiency of cancer patients.

Surgery is the primary treatment modality of most solid cancers, particularly those of the gastrointestinal tract. The immediate metabolic response to major surgery in patients with cancer is similar to that of patients who have surgery for benign disease: increased nitrogen losses and energy requirements.[34] However, because cancer patients may have significant weight loss before surgery, their ability to cope with stress is impaired, resulting in increased morbidity and mortality. The physical insult, the associated pain, and the emotional and physiologic response to surgery cause an integrated endocrine and metabolic reaction designed to maintain homeostasis. There is an increased output of catecholamines, glucagon, and cortisol that results in hypermetabolism, weight loss, negative nitrogen balance, and retention of sodium and water. In addition to this general response to injury, operations on the oropharynx and gastrointestinal tract have specific nutritional sequelae, depending on the site of surgery.

Cancer chemotherapy may profoundly alter the host's nutritional state. The effects may be direct (by interfering with host cell metabolism or DNA synthesis and cellular replication) or indirect (by producing nausea, vomiting, changes in taste sensation, and learned food aversions). Most agents have the ability to stimulate the chemoreceptor trigger zone, resulting in nausea and vomiting. The rapid cell turnover in the alimentary tract mucosa makes it especially vulnerable to chemotherapy, resulting in stomatitis, ulceration, and decreased absorptive capacity. These effects result, in turn, in decreased intake and absorption of nutrients and further predispose the cancer patient to malnutrition. The bone marrow is another organ with a high cell turnover; toxicity is manifested by anemia, leukopenia, and thrombocytopenia. Neutropenia is, in turn, associated with an increased risk of sepsis.

Radiation therapy may also affect the host's nutritional state by its effects on the gastrointestinal tract. The severity of radiation injury is related to the dose of radiation and the volume of tissue treated. The adverse effects of radiation therapy are classified as early or late. Early effects are transient and are manifested by diarrhea, xerostomia, alterations in taste, and food aversions. Late radiation effects include intestinal strictures, fistulae, and malabsorption.

CONSEQUENCES OF MALNUTRITION IN THE CANCER PATIENT

The clinical relevance of severe malnutrition has been demonstrated by increased morbidity and mortality and poor treatment tolerance in malnourished tumor-bearing patients.[35,36] In 1932 Warren noted that malnutrition was a major factor contributing to mortality in cancer patients.[37] The protein-calorie malnutrition produced by the cancer-bearing state leads not only to obvious weight loss, but also to visceral and somatic protein depletion that compromises enzymatic, structural, and mechanical body functions. Impaired immunocompetence and increased susceptibility to infection often result, and these changes may be exacerbated by chemotherapy. Moreover, poor wound healing, increased wound infections, prolonged postoperative ileus, and longer hospital stays have all been linked to poor nutritional status in cancer patients. In patients undergoing colorectal cancer operations, the return to adequate oral food intake was significantly delayed in those patients classified as malnourished based on preoperative assessment.[38] Morbidity and mortality in malnourished patients was 52% and 12% respectively, compared with 31% and 6% in well-nourished patients.

In animal studies, severe protein restriction depressed both humoral and cellular immune responses. Daly and colleagues demonstrated that only 30% of tumor-bearing rats had a delayed hypersensitivity response to intradermal purified protein derivative after 2 weeks on an oral protein-free diet.[39] Protein repletion with 7 days of TPN or oral ad libitum feeding restored the response in 91% and 78% of rats, respectively. Only 17% of animals who remained on protein-free diets for 7 or more days showed a delayed hypersensitivity response. Law and associates found reduced titers of antibodies, reduced IgM-producing cells, reduced lymphocyte response to mitogens, and decreased delayed hypersensitivity in rats after 6 weeks on protein-free nutrition.[40]

In human studies, there is evidence for increased morbidity and mortality with depressed immunocompetence. In addition, it has been documented that nutritional therapy reverses anergy. Harvey and coworkers reported on 161 cancer patients undergoing nutritional support.[41] Of these, 32 were anergic before therapy. In 27 of these patients anergy was reversed, and three of this group died. Of the 5 patients who remained anergic, all died. Daly and associates documented that 51% of anergic patients undergoing cancer treatment had restoration of skin-test reactivity in response to TPN.[42]

The effect of malnutrition on host immune function is to depress host immune competence, particularly cell-mediated immunity. McEntee and coworkers further delineated the effects of malnutrition and nutrient administration in malnourished patients undergoing major surgery.[43] Acutely malnourished patients had significant reductions in absolute lymphocyte counts but no significant alterations in the proportion of T cells or T-cell helper and suppressor subsets. There was a marked impairment of the delayed cutaneous hypersensitivity response: 20 of 29 patients failed to respond to any of the seven antigens. Twenty patients responded positively to nutritional support with significant improvement in serum protein levels, absolute lymphocyte count, and delayed cutaneous hypersensitivity response, with a mean duration of 15 days of nutritional support. Other factors such as sepsis, trauma, steroids, and medications influence host immune function, but nutritional support is an important therapeutic intervention that can improve immunocompetence.

NUTRITIONAL ASSESSMENT

General indications of the need for nutritional assessment and therapeutic intervention with enteral or parenteral nutritional support include the patient's inability to eat or unwillingness to eat enough, and specific nutritional requirements due to cardiac, hepatic, or renal dysfunction. Using data from the patient's history, physical examination, and laboratory tests, together with knowledge of the anticipated method of treatment, the degree and duration of nutritional disability can be estimated and a nutritional management plan formulated.

The ability to ingest adequate quantities of nutrients orally is evaluated by dietary history and the extent of recent weight loss. A history of a recent (within 3 months) loss of 10% or more of body weight signifies substantial protein-calorie malnutrition. In our society, this determination is more important than measurement of the percentage of ideal body weight, because obesity is prevalent and the rapidity of weight loss indicates the severity of illness. Patient history includes questions regarding usual body weight; recent weight changes; special diets; problems with taste, chewing, or swallowing; food allergies and medications; alcohol ingestion; and bowel habits related to dietary intake. Physical examination may reveal evidence of undernutrition such as dry, scaly, and atrophic skin; muscle wasting; pitting, presacral, or pretibial edema; loss of muscle strength; and depletion of fat stores.

A thorough history and physical examination by an experienced physician is the simplest and one of the best methods of nutritional assessment. An excellent correlation has been demonstrated between the clinical diagnosis of malnutrition and nutritional status as determined by a battery of anthropometric and laboratory tests as well as analyses of total body potassium and total body nitrogen (Table 64–19). Thus, although laboratory tests and research tools such as total body potassium and nitrogen measurements allow quantification of nutritional status for comparative purposes, the diagnosis of malnutrition can be made by experienced medical personnel.

Several sophisticated tests have been devised to detect milder forms of malnutrition and to objectively quantify the patient's response to nutritional therapy. Anthropometric measurements quantify body habitus and body compartments and relate them to measurements of an age- and sex-matched normal population. The creatinine-height index, defined as the patient's 24-hour creatinine excretion divided by the expected 24-hour excretion of creatinine by a normal adult of the same height, provides another estimate of skeletal muscle mass in a patient with normal renal function. Substantial protein-calorie malnutrition is a level 75% or less of standard. A method for estimating body cell mass has also been developed by determining the ratio of exchangeable sodium to exchangeable potassium using isotope dilution techniques. This ratio increases with chronic malnutrition to a value greater than 1.22. Use of a whole-body counter allows determination of ^{40}K, a naturally occurring radioisotope, within the skeletal muscle mass. From this measurement total body potassium can be calculated, allowing an estimate of lean body mass. Measurement of total body nitrogen by γ-neutron activation is the gold standard for determining total body protein. These last three tests are not available for routine use in hospital centers, but they have been useful research tools in the assessment of body composition changes.

The degree of visceral protein depletion can be estimated by determining concentrations of serum proteins such as retinal-binding protein, prealbumin, transferrin, and albumin. The correlation of serum protein levels with protein-calorie malnutrition is directly related to the metabolic half-life of the individual serum proteins and the patient's hydrational state. Prealbumin and retinal-binding protein have the shortest half-lives and are depressed first, followed by serum transferrin and albumin levels. The half-lives of these proteins are 0.5, 2, 8, and 20 days, respectively. Thus, changes in prealbumin and retinal-binding protein reflect recent dietary changes, whereas transferrin and albumin are more closely related to nutritional status. A decrease in the serum concentration of these proteins may also be related to changes in the patient's salt and water balance. For example, serum albumin concentrations commonly decline after starting a malnourished patient on TPN. This depression in serum albumin concentration results from hydrational effects and does not reflect a worsening malnourished state (Fig. 64–10). With effective nutritional support, significant increases in serum transferrin

TABLE 64–19. Nutritional Assessment Using Clinical Evaluation and Objective Tests

Clinical Assessment	Normal	Malnutrition	
		Mild	Severe
% Ideal body weight	112 ± 3	105 ± 5	81 ± 3
Albumin (g/dl)	39 ± 0.1	3.6 ± 0.3	3.1 ± 0.1
Transferrin (mg/dl)	208 ± 16	175 ± 27	147 ± 16
Total body nitrogen	1.80 ± 0.10	1.77 ± 0.20	1.40 ± 0.11
Total body potassium	0.108 ± 0.007	0.121 ± 0.011	0.077 ± 0.006
% Positive skin test	80	53	50

Mean ± SEM.
(Adapted from Baker JP, et al. N Engl J Med 1982;306:969–972)

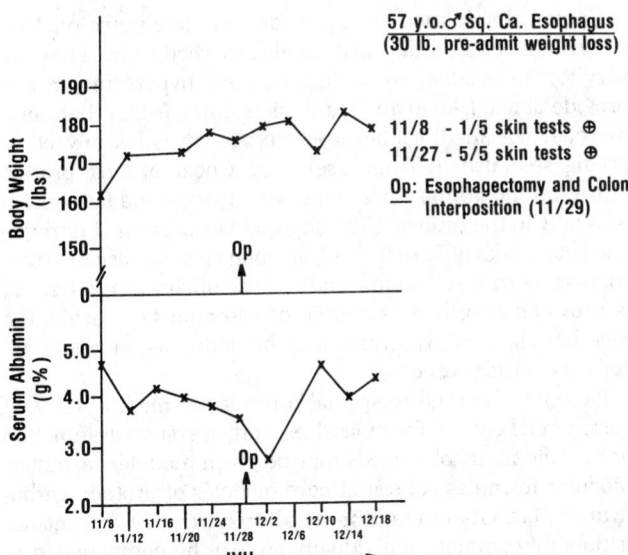

FIGURE 64–10. Body weight increases while serum albumin levels decrease during parenteral nutrition (IVH) before and after operation for a 57-year-old man with esophageal carcinoma.

and albumin levels typically occur after 7 to 10 days and 4 weeks of therapy, respectively.

The degree of visceral protein depletion has also been evaluated by determining the status of cell-mediated immunity as manifested by recall antigen skin testing and by the total blood lymphocyte count. Loss of immunocompetence is *not* a sensitive indicator of visceral protein depletion because weight loss usually exceeds 10% of the body weight before anergy develops secondary to malnutrition. Therefore, anergy associated with malnutrition signifies a significant deficiency of visceral protein and portends increased morbidity and mortality in hospitalized patients. Several factors result in anergy to recall skin testing, including age, presence of malignant disease, immunosuppression due to exogenous medications such as steroids, radiation therapy, stress, or sepsis. In the absence of these factors, nutritional repletion of the malnourished patient can result in reversal of skin-test anergy, and this reversal is associated with improved treatment outcome. Usually, however, improvement in other measurements of nutritional status such as body weight occur much in advance of improvement in delayed cutaneous hypersensitivity.

Complete nutritional assessment provides an estimate of body composition (fat, skeletal muscle protein, and visceral protein) to help identify and quantify the magnitude of clinical or subclinical malnutrition. A nutritional status scale can be used for classifying patients into nutritional categories of normal status, mild malnutrition, or severe malnutrition. The nutritional assessment should help to determine whether the goal of anabolic nutritional therapy should be repletion of nutritional deficits or maintenance of existing status. All of these measurements have proved accurate in population surveys, but they have varying sensitivity and lack specificity in individual patients. Thus, their major value lies in supporting the clinical diagnosis of malnutrition made by an experienced observer. Finally, blood analysis documents specific deficiencies that require correction.

Objective data can thus define the nebulous term nutritional status and allow both initial assessment of the patient and repeated evaluation of the efficacy of nutritional therapy. A prognostic nutritional index (PNI) to quantify the extent of malnutrition can be calculated as follows:

$$PNI (\%) = 158 - 16.6 (Alb) - 0.78 (TSF)$$
$$- 0.20 (TPN) - 5.8 (DH)$$

where Alb is albumin in g/dl, TSF is triceps skin fold in mm, TFN is transferrin in mg/dl, and DH is delayed hypersensitivity (0=negative, 1=less than 5 mm reactivity, and 2=5 or more mm reactivity).[16] In a large retrospective series of surgical patients, a PNI of below 30 (low risk) was associated with an 11.7% complication rate and 2% mortality. A PNI of 60 or above (high risk) was associated with an 81% complication rate and 59% mortality.

Studies such as these have helped to establish the relative importance of nutritional indices as predictive factors for postoperative morbidity and mortality in surgical patients. Almost all nutritional support teams have devised nutritional status scoring systems that allow repeated estimates of nutritional status during diagnostic and therapeutic management of the patient. A simple, practical definition of malnutrition that can be readily applied clinically includes an unintentional or unexplained loss of 10% or more of body weight, a serum transferrin level less than 150 mg/dl, and a serum albumin level less than 3.4 g/dl. Any two of these three criteria is an indication for nutritional support or therapy.

PREOPERATIVE NUTRITIONAL SUPPORT

After the need for preoperative nutritional support has been established, the most appropriate feeding regimen and the duration of nutritional support are determined (Fig. 64–11). The optimum duration of preoperative nutritional support varies with each patient. Generally, patients with severe malnutrition should receive at least 7 days of nutritional therapy during their workup and preparation for a major elective procedure. They should continue to receive postoperative nutritional support until oral intake is adequate. Obviously, the urgency of the operation determines the length of time available to correct existing nutritional deficiencies.

NASOENTERAL TUBE FEEDING

Nasoenteral tube feeding is the preferred method for providing short-term nutrition when the gastrointestinal tract is intact and sufficiently functional to tolerate and absorb adequate nutrients. When an elective operation is delayed and allows for longer preoperative preparation, nasointestinal or a surgical, endoscopic, or laparoscopic-placed tube feeding is preferred. Examples include patients with head and neck, esophageal, and gastric malignancies who are receiving preoperative chemotherapy or radiation therapy.

Solutions

The solution used should be nutritionally adequate, well tolerated, easy to prepare, and economical. Four types of enteral

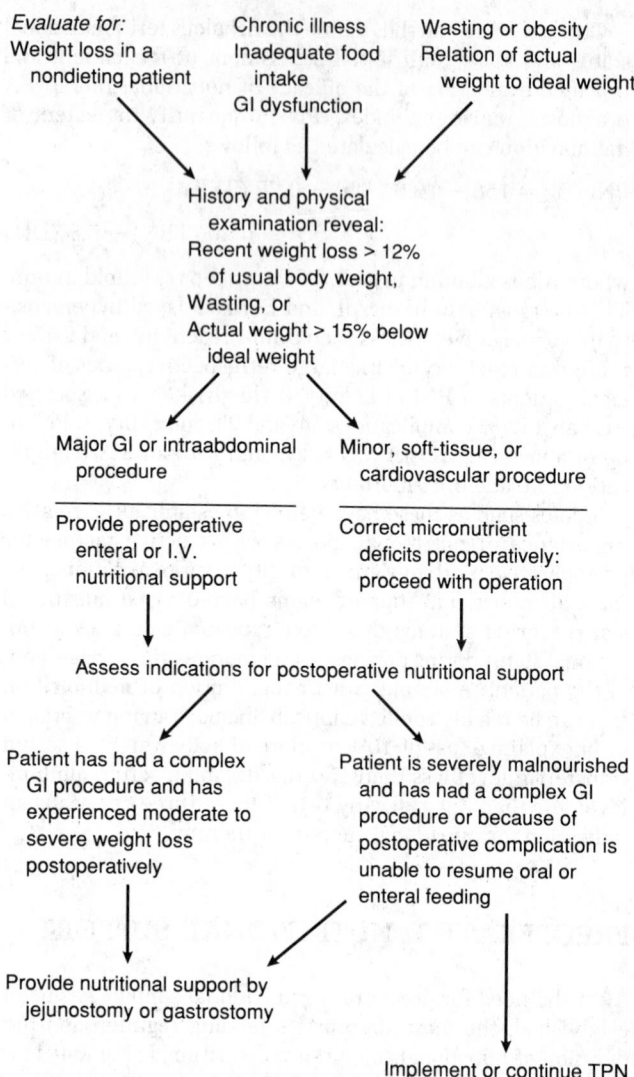

FIGURE 64–11. Nutritional management schema for cancer patients undergoing surgery.

formulas are available: blenderized tube-feeding formulas, nutritionally complete commercial formulas, chemically defined liquid diets, and modular formulas.

Blenderized tube feedings may be composed of any food that can be blenderized such as meat, whole or skim milk, vegetables, fruit, and cereal. Soy, safflower, sunflower, and corn oil are often used to increase caloric density and to supply a source of essential fatty acids. Other additives such as corn syrup or modular formulas can also be used to increase caloric density. Additional protein can be provided using dry milk powder, strained meats, or egg. Caloric concentrations of these formulas vary from 0.6 to 1.3 kcal/ml. These feedings are the least expensive but require both a larger-bore tube (14 Fr) and longer preparation time.

Nutritionally complete commercial formulas vary in protein, carbohydrate, and fat composition and are low to moderate in residue content. Most are lactose-free and contain about 1 to 1.5 kcal/ml. These formulas are the regimens of choice because they are relatively inexpensive and easily prepared and provide adequate nutrients.

Chemically defined diets provide complete nutritional requirements in a predigested, easily absorbed form. They are very low in residue, are lactose free and hyperosmolar, and provide about 1 kcal/ml. These diets differ from other commercial tube feedings because the protein is hydrolyzed or predigested, usually from casein, soy, wheat, or meat protein or crystalline amino acids. The carbohydrate and fat content is usually in the ratio of 150 nonprotein kcal/gram of nitrogen and represents 60% to 90% of the total calories, usually from sucrose, corn syrup solids, and glucose oligosaccharides. Fat is provided mainly as a source of essential fatty acids, but medium-chain triglycerides may be added as an easily absorbed caloric source.

Patients who require special formulas or modifications of commercial enteral formulas due to organ system dysfunction or specific metabolic needs may be given modular formulas. Modular formulas consist of core modules of protein, carbohydrate, fat, vitamin, and mineral mixtures that are not nutritionally complete individually but can be compounded to provide a complete diet specific to a patient's needs.

Tube Selection and Placement

Small-bore (8 to 10 Fr) flexible nasoenteral tubes of polyurethane and silicone elastomer have reduced major patient discomfort caused by large-bore rubber tubes. Nasogastric feeding uses a 91-cm-long tube, while the 109-cm tube with tungsten weight is used for spontaneous or directed passage of the tip through the pylorus into the distal duodenum or upper jejunum. Longer nasojejunal tubes should be used to reduce the risk of pulmonary aspiration. Placement of the weighted tube tip through the pylorus is facilitated by fluoroscopy and an inner stylet that stiffens the catheter. The exact position of the catheter tip must be documented by fluoroscopy or x-rays before starting feeding.

The bore size of the tube is determined by the viscosity and osmolality of the formula to be used. Isotonic formula flows well through a #8 French tube, while a high calorie-density (2 kcal/ml) formula requires at least a #10 French tube for proper infusion. As a general rule, the smallest bore tube that allows the formula to flow without clogging should be used for greater patient acceptance.

If preoperative enteral nutritional support is indicated for more than 6 weeks, the nutrient solution may be infused through a gastrostomy or jejunostomy tube. A gastrostomy tube has the advantage of being easy to care for because it is readily available and visible to the patient. Gastrostomy feedings are well tolerated because of the stomach's storage and dilutional functions, but the risk of aspiration is higher than with jejunostomy feedings. The tube may be placed using a percutaneous endoscopic technique, laparoscopic technique, or a minor surgical procedure under local, regional, or general anesthesia. Percutaneous endoscopic and laparoscopic gastrostomy have become quite popular as cost-effective and less morbid methods of permanent gastric intubation.

Tube feedings should be administered by continuous gravity drip or with pump infusion. Bolus feedings have been used in patients with nasogastric tubes, but this method is unsuitable for use with chemically defined hyperosmolar diets because of gastrointestinal complications. Clinical tolerance of the enteral nutrient solution is determined by the osmolality of the solution as well as the rate of infusion. The most common method is to begin infusion with a full-strength solution at 30 ml/hour and increase the rate every 12 to 24 hours over 2 to 4 days in increments of 10 ml/hour. Preoperative enteral feeding can be supplemented with peripheral parenteral nutrition to provide adequate caloric intake more quickly and safely. Nutritional/metabolic patient monitoring is performed as in patients receiving TPN. In addition, gastrointestinal complications such as nausea, vomiting, bloating, cramping, and diarrhea are common, and thus close monitoring is indicated (Table 64–20).

TOTAL PARENTERAL NUTRITION

Patients with severe malnutrition (weight loss greater than 12% of their usual body weight, serum albumin 2.5 g/dl or less, and serum transferrin 150 mg/dl or less) usually require intravenous nutritional support in the preoperative period. TPN is also indicated when nausea, vomiting, gastrointestinal tract obstruction, fistulae, or malabsorption make the gastrointestinal tract unavailable for nutrient administration and when rapid nutritional repletion becomes necessary to maximize the safety of operative intervention.

The hypertonic nutrient solution most commonly used for TPN consists of 15% to 25% dextrose, 4% to 5% crystalline amino acids, 10% fat emulsion, electrolytes, and vitamins. Each unit of base solution provides about 5.25 to 6.0 g nitrogen and 900 to 1000 calories in 1000 to 1100 ml of water. Specific water, electrolyte, calorie, and nitrogen requirements are individualized to avoid metabolic complications. Fluid requirements for normal maintenance can be estimated from either body weight (30 ml/kg) or body surface area (1400 ml/m^2) and adjusted for existing deficits and ongoing excessive losses. In febrile patients, insensible water losses can be appreciable. Knowledge of fluid and electrolyte losses occurring from the gastrointestinal tract are critical to proper intravenous replacement.

In patients who are at or above ideal body weight and have lost less than 12% of their usual body weight, protein is provided at 1.0 to 1.5 g per kg of current body weight for maintenance of body protein status (Table 64–21). If these patients exhibit a serum albumin level less than 3 g/dl or a serum transferrin concentration less than 150 mg/dl or if weight loss has exceeded 12%, then 1.5 to 2.0 g of protein per kg of current body weight is provided. In obese patients whose current body weight exceeds 120% ideal body weight, 1.0 to 1.5 g of protein per kg *ideal* body weight is given.

Daily caloric requirements for each patient are most precisely defined by measuring resting energy expenditure using indirect calorimetry. However, the costs involved prohibit the routine use of this approach outside the research setting. Caloric requirements can also be calculated on the basis of the Harris-Benedict formula:

Male: Basal Energy Expenditure (kcal) = 66 + 13.7

$$\times \text{ weight (kg)} + 5 \times \text{height (cm)} - 6.8 \text{ age (y)}$$

Female: Basal Energy Expenditure (kcal) = 655 + 9.6

$$\times \text{ weight (g)} + 1.7 \times \text{height (cm)} - 4.7 \times \text{age (y)}$$

Daily caloric requirements are met by providing 1000 kcal above the patient's basal energy expenditure or by giving 150% of the calculated or measured resting energy expenditure. An alternate method for determining caloric requirements is to calculate 35 kcal/kg/day for maintenance and 45 kcal/kg/day for anabolism. Dietary nitrogen requirements per day should be provided in a ratio of 1 g nitrogen to 125 to 150 calories. In obese patients whose body weight exceeds 120% ideal body weight, a caloric goal of 90% to 100% resting energy expenditure should be given to allow the use of excess endogenous fat tissue for calories.

The maximal rate of glucose oxidation in the adult is 7 g/kg/day. Patients with extremely high caloric requirements or severe glucose intolerance should have calories in excess of this amount supplied by lipid. Insulin should be given as needed to maintain serum glucose levels between 130 and 250 mg/dl. In intensive care unit patients who have fluctuating needs, insulin can be given as a separate intravenous infusion using a pump under close supervision. Glucose that is not oxidized is stored as either glycogen or lipids. Fatty infiltration of the liver and increased carbon dioxide production are clinical complications of excess glucose administration.

Lipid as a 10% solution is isotonic and can therefore be administered via either central or peripheral vein. This allows administration of more calories in the form of free fatty acids, which are a major source of energy for most peripheral tissues. Most patients can tolerate up to 2 g fat/kg/day, limiting the caloric supply of fat to 18 kcal/kg/day, or 1260 kcal/day for a 70-kg person. The daily dosage should not exceed 4 g fat/kg/day. Fat emulsions, supplied as either 10% or 20% solutions, can be infused over 6 to 8 hours. The more common practice is to have all nutrients (fat, glucose, and amino acids) admixed in a 3-L bag for administration. Serum triglyceride levels should be monitored to ensure that the patient can metabolize this amount of lipid. Energy requirements are best met by using a mixed fuel system supplying 30% of the nonprotein calories as lipids. If a predominantly glucose-based system is used, at least 1000 ml of a 10% lipid emulsion per week or 4% of calories per day should be given to prevent essential fatty acid deficiency.

In addition to calories and protein, electrolytes, vitamins, and trace elements are required nutrients. Daily requirements of electrolytes are as follows: sodium, 60 to 120 mEq; potassium, 60 to 100 mEq; chloride, 60 to 120 mEq; magnesium, 8 to 10 mEq; calcium, 200 to 400 mg; and phosphorus, 300 to 400 mg. These electrolyte maintenance requirements must be met daily. In selecting the proper nutrient formula, preexisting deficits, ongoing urine and gastrointestinal losses, and organ dysfunction (cardiac, hepatic, and renal) must be considered. Vitamin and trace metal preparations are commercially available to provide daily parenteral requirements. The latter formulation contains zinc, copper, chromium, and manganese. In some centers, 1000 units of heparin are added to each liter to reduce the risk of central venous catheter occlusion and subclavian vein thrombosis.

Administration of TPN and Patient Monitoring

The safest and most effective infusion route for administering hypertonic TPN solutions in adults has been the infraclavicular, percutaneous subclavian venous catheters. Tunneling of the catheters subcutaneously and use of the Seldinger method may reduce catheter-related infections. Double- and triple-

TABLE 64–20.   Potential Complications of Enteral Nutritional Support

Problem	Diagnosis	Therapy	Prevention
Gastrointestinal Complications			
Offensive smell/taste	c/o smell, nausea, vomiting	Add flavorings	Use polymeric formulas
Gastric retention	Gastric residual >100 ml 4 h after a bolus, or >115% of vol/h, nausea and vomiting	Dilute formula, reduce bolus volume	Dilute formula and gradually increase toxicity and volume
Rapid infusion	Nausea and vomiting	Decrease rate, advance 25 ml/h q 12–24 h	Start gastr. feedings at 40–50 ml/h, jej. & duo feedings at 20–25 ml/h, advance 25 ml/h q 12–24 h
Lactose intolerance	Review of history, diarrhea, nausea, vomiting, lactose intolerance test	Switch to nonlactose formula	Use formulas with low lactose content
Excessive fat in diet	Review of history, nausea, vomiting	Switch to low-fat diet	Provide <30–40% of calories by fat
Fat malabsorption	Review of history, 72-h fecal fat assessment	Pancreatic enzyme supplements	Use low-fat formulas
Hyperosmolar solution	Osmolality > 300 mOsm, diarrhea, increased stool water content	Dilute to isotonicity, stop for 12 h, resume at slow rate, use Kaopectate, Lomotil	Use isotonic solutions, start at slow rate (40–50 ml/h), increase in 12–24 h increments
Cold feedings	Tubing cold to touch, diarrhea	Discontinue feedings until formula is warm	Start recently refrigerated formulas at 40 ml/h
Protein malnutrition	Albumin < 3 g/dl, diarrhea	Dilute solutions to isotonicity, use antidiarrheal	Start at slow rate (20–25 ml/h), increase in 12–24 h increments
Malabsorption	Diarrhea	Decrease flow rate to 25–50 ml/h or discontinue, use parenteral feeding	Start at slow rate (20–25 ml/h), increase gradually
Dehydration	Orthostatic hypotension, dry mucous membranes, constipation	Supplemental fluids	Monitor intake and output
Impaction	Rectal examination, constipation	Digital disimpaction	Monitor intake and output
Obstruction	Nausea, vomiting, constipation, obstructive series	Surgery	
Mechanical Complications			
Nasopharyngeal discomfort	Mouth breathing, sore throat, hoarseness	Sugarless gum, gargling with warm water and mouthwash, anesthetic lozenges, viscous or spray topical anesthetics	Use soft small-bore tubes or surgically inserted tubes for long-term nutrition
Nasal erosions	Erosions of nasal ala	Tape tube without pressure on nasal ala	Use soft small-bore tubes
Abscess of nasal septum	Pain, fever, chills	Remove tube, drainage, antibiotics	Use soft small-bore tubes, proper taping
Acute sinusitis	Pain, nasal congestion, fever, malodorous breath	Remove tube, hot compresses, analgesics	Use soft small-bore tubes
Acute otitis media	Severe throbbing ear pain, fever, chills, dizziness	Change tube to other nostril, antibiotics	
Rupture of esophageal varices	Hematemesis, melena, radiographic studies	Sedation, rest of esophagus	Use soft small-bore tube
Esophagitis	Heartburn, substernal & epigastric burning	Remove tube	Keep head of bed at 45°, keep gastric pH > 7 with H_2-blockers or antacids
Esophageal ulceration	Dysphagia, radiologic studies	Remove tube, esophagoscopy, and dilation	Use soft small-bore tube; with persistent vomiting, consider a jej. tube
TE fistula	Fistula present	Symptomatic	Use soft small-bore tube, gastric or jej. tube
Knotting of tube	Unable to remove tube	Cut tube and allow to pass per rectum; use McGill forceps to bring tube out mouth to cut tube	None

(continued)

TABLE 64–20.   *(Continued)*

Problem	Causes	Therapy	Prevention
Metabolic Complications			
Hypokalemia	Insulin administration, diarrhea, severe malnutrition	K$^+$ supplements	Check electrolytes
Hypophosphatemia	Insulin administration, severe malnutrition	Phosphate supplements	
Hyponatremia	Over hydration	Water restriction	
Hypomagnesemia	Decreased carrier protein, inadequate delivery	Magnesium supplements	
Elevated transaminase	Activation of hepatic enzymes, excess caloric load	Reduce carbohydrates	
Vitamin K deficiency	Inadequate delivery	Vitamin K replacement	
Essential fatty acid deficiency	Low linoleic acid	Parenteral fat, 5 ml safflower oil qd	

lumen catheters are often used, with one port for TPN and other ports for blood-drawing, antibiotic administration, or chemotherapy administration. These functions must be carefully performed and monitored to preserve catheter sterility.

Meticulous care and maintenance of the catheter are critical to ensure long-term success with TPN. At any sign of unexplained fever or sepsis, the catheter should be changed over a guidewire using aseptic technique. Blood should be removed from the catheter for culture and the catheter tip cultured after its removal over the guidewire. A new catheter can be inserted using the Seldinger guidewire technique to reduce catheter-insertion complications until catheter sterility can be determined. If catheter infection is confirmed, a new catheter should be inserted at a distant site.

Parenteral nutrition is usually initiated by administering 1000 ml of the hypertonic solution at a constant rate using a pump over 24 hours. Once the patient can metabolize dextrose and amino acids in 1000 ml of the hypertonic solution during the 24-hour period, the flow rate can be increased to 2000 ml every 24 hours. Within 2 to 3 days of nutritional repletion, average adults should be able to tolerate their caloric and protein requirements intravenously. Close monitoring and the use of a nutrition support team can dramatically reduce the incidence of TPN-associated complications (Table 64–22).

TABLE 64–21.   Solutions Used for Parenteral Nutrition

Solution	Unit Volume (ml)	Amino Acids (g)	Dextrose (g)	Total Calories (kcal)
Standard	1000	50	250	850
High-calorie	1000	50	350	1200
Low nitrogen	750	25	250	850
Low nitrogen/ high-calorie	750	25	350	1250
Peripheral	1000	29	50	170
Fat emulsion 10%	500	—	—	550
Fat emulsion 20%	500	—	—	1100

NUTRITION IN THE PERIOPERATIVE PERIOD

Planning for the operative procedure should take into account all aspects of treatment and monitoring and should meld nutritional support into the operative approach and postoperative management. Patients undergoing complex upper-gastrointestinal procedures such as esophagogastrectomy, total gastrectomy, and pancreaticoduodenectomy who have experienced moderate to severe weight loss preoperatively should have a feeding jejunostomy placed for postoperative nutritional support. Standard methods use a #8, #10, or #12 French catheter placed into the proximal jejunum using a Witzel technique and suturing the bowel to the anterolateral abdominal wall. A needle-catheter jejunostomy can also be used by inserting a small-diameter catheter for 15 cm into the proximal jejunum. Because small-bowel function returns within 6 hours of the operation, D$_5$W can be infused at a constant rate of 25 ml/hour in the recovery room. On the first postoperative day, a full-strength feeding formula is begun at a rate of 25 ml/hour. Usually the rate of infusion is increased in increments of 10 ml/hour every 12 to 24 hours until adequate caloric and protein goals are achieved. It is important to clinically assess the patient *frequently* to ensure that the infusion rate can be increased safely. Early postoperative enteral feeding may also be indicated in cancer patients requiring adjuvant chemotherapy or radiation therapy shortly after surgery.

In the malnourished patient undergoing a major, complex intraabdominal procedure, TPN is indicated when enteral feeding cannot be accomplished by jejunostomy. Use of TPN is also indicated in the patient who develops a major postoperative complication that does not allow resumption of adequate enteral or oral feeding. However, the metabolic profile of the malnourished preoperative patient differs from that of the stressed, complicated postoperative patient. In the absence of sepsis, resting energy expenditure postoperatively may be similar or slightly increased over preoperative levels. However, the altered hormonal milieu in the septic postoperative patient results in increased protein catabolism, gluconeogenesis, and glucose intolerance. Protein should be given at 1.5

TABLE 64–22.   Potential Complications Associated With Total Parenteral Nutrition

Complications	Diagnosis	Treatment	Prevention
Mechanical			
Pneumothorax	Dyspnea, CXR	Tube thoracostomy, observation	Avoid emergency procedures, use Trendelenburg
Hemothorax	Dyspnea, CXR	Remove catheter, observation	
Venous thrombosis	Inability to cannulate	Remove catheter, heparin therapy	Use silicone catheters; add heparin to solution
Air embolism	Dyspnea, cyanosis, hypotension, tachycardia, precordial murmur	Trendelenburg; left lateral decubitus; attempt aspiration through line	Trendelenburg, Valsalva maneuver; tape intravenous connections
Catheter embolism	Sheared catheter	Fluoroscopic retrieval	Never withdraw catheter through needle
Arrhythmias	Catheter tip in right atrium	Withdraw catheter to SVC	Fluoroscopy, CXR
Subclavian artery injury	Pulsatile red blood	Remove needle, apply pressure, CXR	Review anatomy
Catheter tip misplacement	CXR	Redirect with a guidewire	Direct bevel of needle caudally
Metabolic			
Hyperglycemic, hyperosmolar, nonketotic coma	Dehydration with osmotic diuresis, disorientation, lethargy, stupor, convulsions, coma, glu 1000 mg/dl, osm 350 mOsm/L	Discontinue TPN, D1/2NS at 250 ml/h, insulin 10–20 u/h, bicarbonate, monitor glu, K, pH	Monitor glucose
Hypoglycemia	Headache, sweating, thirst, convulsion, disorientation, paresthesias	$D_{50}W$ I.V.	Taper TPN by 1/2 for 12 h then 12 h of $D_{50}W$ at 100 ml/h
CO_2 retention	Ventilator dependence, high RQ	Reduce glucose load	Provide 30–40% of calories with fat
Azotemia	Dehydration, elevated BUN	Reduce protein load, increase nonprotein calories, increase fluid	Monitor fluid balance
Hyperammonemia	Lethargy, malaise, coma, seizures	Discontinue amino acid infusions, infuse arginine	Avoid casein or fibrin hydrolysate
Essential fatty acid deficiency	Xerosis, hepatomegaly, impaired healing, bone changes	Fat administration	Provide 25–500 mg/kg/day of essential fatty acids
Hypophosphatemia	Lethargy, anorexia, weakness, arrhythmias	Supplemental phosphate	Treat causative factors: alkalosis, gram neg, sepsis, vomiting, malabsorption, provide 20 mEq/ 1000 cal
Abnormal liver function tests	Fatty infiltrate	Rule out other etiologies (*e.g.,* sepsis)	Provide balanced TPN solution
Hypomagnesemia	Weakness, nausea, vomiting, tremors, depression, hyporeflexia	Infuse 10% $MgSO_4$	Supply 0.35–0.45 mEq/kg/day
Hypermagnesemia	Drowsiness, nausea, vomiting, coma, arrhythmia	Dialysis, infuse calcium gluconate	Monitor serum levels

CXR, chest x-ray; RQ, respiratory quotient; BUN, blood urea nitrogen; SVC, superior vena cava; TPN, total parenteral nutrition.

g/kg/day. Lipid emulsions are used to provide at least 30% to 40% of calculated resting energy expenditure caloric requirements to reduce the occurrence of hyperglycemia, glycosuria, and abnormal fluid and electrolyte losses.

NUTRITION AND HOST METABOLISM

Despite the demonstration of metabolic abnormalities in cancer patients, it is unclear how efficacious enteral or parenteral nutrient administration can be in reversing derangements of substrate use. Jeevanandam and colleagues evaluated changes in whole-body protein kinetics before and after administration of TPN in malnourished cancer patients using a primed-continuous infusion of ^{15}N glycine.[44] After 10 days of TPN, whole-body protein breakdown decreased by 50% and 59% in cancer and noncancer patients respectively, whereas protein synthesis decreased by 21% and 33%. The mechanism of improved nitrogen balance during intravenous repletion is probably due to a significant reduction in protein breakdown. During oral or enteral nutritional repletion, improvement in nitrogen balance may be due to stimulation of protein synthesis.

To further define the alteration in protein kinetics that occur in patients with malignancy, Shaw and Wolfe performed a series of studies to determine rates of whole-body protein synthesis and metabolism in normal volunteers and in patients with either early or advanced gastrointestinal cancer.[45] This study demonstrated that gastrointestinal cancer patients and normal volunteers had similar basal rates of whole-body protein catabolism, but cancer patients had an increased rate of net protein loss. In patients with advanced disease and marked weight loss, a state of net protein synthesis could not be achieved, although whole-body protein synthesis became nearly equivalent to whole-body protein catabolism.

The effects of nutritional support in cancer patients are often complicated by the adverse effects of antineoplastic therapy. Drott and coworkers randomized 23 patients with metastatic testicular carcinoma to receive either TPN or spontaneous oral intake during their hospital stay coincident with multidrug chemotherapy.[46] Energy and nitrogen intakes were profoundly decreased in the spontaneous oral intake group, whereas intake decreased in the TPN group only at home while patients relied on oral intake alone. Despite the cytotoxic drugs, the TPN group remained in nitrogen balance when undergoing TPN. However, they lost substantial body weight and nitrogen over 10 weeks, which was a result of the prolonged anorexia all patients had after termination of chemotherapy. Thus, intermittent periods of adequate intravenous nutrition had only a marginal long-term impact. The clinical significance of improved nitrogen balance during chemotherapy administration remains controversial.

Several animal models have suggested that dietary nutritional depletion decreases tumor growth but results in marked wasting of the host (Fig. 64–12). Controversy exists as to whether nutritional repletion stimulates tumor growth out of proportion to enhancement of host nutritional status (Table 64–23). Numerous studies have demonstrated accelerated tumor growth in animals receiving nutrition support. Torosian and associates reported significant increases in the S, or DNA synthetic, phase of tumor cell cycle kinetics with potentiation of chemotherapy efficacy during parenteral nutrient administration.[47] Karpeh and colleagues reported that nutritional repletion resulted in significantly smaller tumors in the moderately immunogenic C1300 neuroblastoma and larger tumors in the nonimmunogenic TBJ neuroblastoma.[48] These results suggest that the influence of nutritional repletion on the tumor-bearing host varies specifically with the presence of an antitumor immune response.

Other studies in tumor-bearing animal models have demonstrated effects of specific nutrient alterations on tumor growth. Skeef and coworkers noted that zinc deficiency had a stimulatory effect on cAMP synthesis that was selective for hepatoma cells in an animal tumor model.[49] Both zinc deficiency and zinc excess resulted in a tendency toward decreased tumor growth in their hepatoma model. The effect of a protein-free diet or restricted intake and subsequent host repletion with TPN was examined by Grossie and associates.[50] Host body weight was significantly reduced both by the administration of a protein-free diet and restriction of standard diets

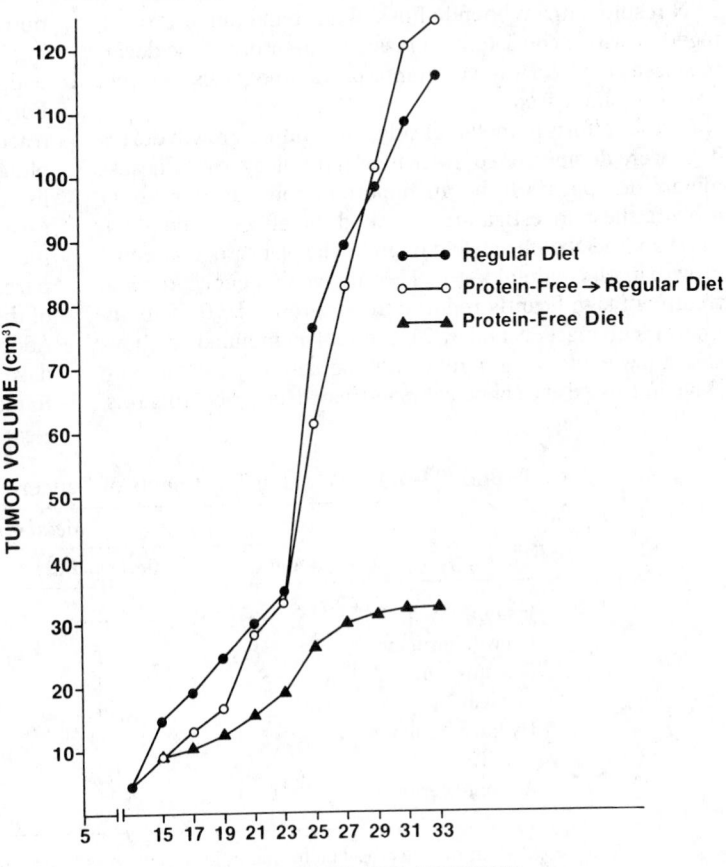

FIGURE 64–12. Tumor volume plateaus in animals on a protein-free diet. Animals switched from a protein-free to a regular diet on day 15 show a rapid increase in tumor volume to become similar to the regular diet group.

TABLE 64–23. Effects of Nutrition Supplementation on Tumor Growth

Animal/Tumor System	Nutrition	Results
W rats/AC-33	I.V. AA ± dextrose	↑ Tumor growth, no change tumor/host weight
	I.V. AA or TPN	↑ Tumor protein synthesis
	TPN	↑ Tumor weight, no change tumor/host weight
	TPN	↑ % S-phase tumor cells
F344/rats/MCA sarcoma	TPN	↑ Tumor weight proportional to TPN infused; tumor/host weight
SD rats/W256	Oral prot/carb diet	↑ Tumor volume
	Oral prot/carb diet or TPN	↑ Tumor volume, no change tumor/host weight
	TPN	↑ Tumor growth
		↑ Tumor mitotic acitivty
		↑ Tumor/host weight
Buff rats/Morris hepatoma	TPN	↑ H³-thymidine labeling index of tumors
W rats/W-256	TPN	No significant ↑ tumor weight
ACI-N rats/Morris hepatoma	TPN	No change in tumor weight, protein content, or DNA synthesis

TPN, total parenteral nutrition; AA, amino acids; MCA, methylcholanthrene; SD, Sprague-Dawley; W, Walker.
(Adapted from Torosian M, Daly JM. Nutritional support in the cancer-bearing host. Cancer 1986;58: 1915–1929)

with diminished tumor growth. Subsequent host repletion with TPN resulted in a rebound of host weight and tumor growth, together with a consistent increase in tumor ornithine decarboxylase activity. However, tumor polyamine levels were not uniformly increased.

Further efforts to metabolically affect tumor growth during TPN were demonstrated by Chance and colleagues.[51] Because glutamine appears to be an important substrate for tumor growth, these investigators evaluated the effect of the glutamine antimetabolite acivicin on methylcholanthrene sarcoma growth in rats maintained on TPN or given rat chow. Acivicin treatment significantly reduced tumor growth by 67% in animals receiving TPN and by 71% in rats maintained on chow. Carcass weights were significantly increased by TPN in both acivicin-treated and saline-solution-treated tumor-bearing rats.

Thus, interest continues in methods to manipulate specific nutrients to selectively promote host anabolism while "starving" the tumor (Table 64–24). Unfortunately, this desired endpoint may be complicated by host metabolic requirements. For example, glutamine is an energy substrate of the intestinal tract. Recently, Grant and Snyder evaluated the use of L-glutamine in TPN in an animal model.[52] They noted that adding either 1% or 2% L-glutamine to TPN solutions did not result in any toxic clinical effects. Glutamine preserved the intestinal nitrogen content of the stomach and the colon compared with standard TPN and increased the nitrogen content of the small bowel greater than that seen in chow-fed animals. Adding 1% and 2% glutamine increased mucosal disaccharidase activity and protected the liver from fatty infiltration found with administration of standard TPN. Use of glutamine-

TABLE 64–24. Potential Treatments of Cancer Cachexia

Therapy	Metabolic Abnormalities				
	Anorexia	Carbohydrate	Protein	Fat	Host Weight
Insulin	+	++	+	+	+
Growth hormone	+	+	++		+
Somatostatin	+	+	+		
Acivicin		+	+		+
Hydrazine sulfate	+	++	+		+
Anti-TNF	+			+++	+
Anti-interferon-γ	++	+		+++	+

TNF, tumor necrosis factor. +, mild improvement; ++, moderate improvement; +++, marked improvement.

supplemented TPN may substantially reduce the adverse side effects of chemotherapy such as mucositis and enterocolitis.

Enterocolitis induced by radiation therapy and chemotherapy is a significant problem and often is the sole limiting side effect from the administration of antineoplastic therapy. Previous work in our laboratory noted that administration of an elemental diet to rats given methotrexate resulted in 100% mortality from severe enterocolitis (Fig. 64–13). Enteral feeding with polypeptides protected completely (100% survival) against methotrexate-induced enterocolitis.[53] Administration of glutamine with the elemental diet also resulted in increased survival (30%).[54] Thus, administration of a peptide-based diet or an elemental diet supplemented with glutamine, either enterally or parenterally, can protect against intestinal injury when either liquid elemental diets or TPN are used. Further studies in humans are clearly indicated to confirm these experimental results.

NUTRITION AND IMMUNITY

Immunosuppression is a common finding in the cancer patient. Malignancy, malnutrition, surgery, anesthesia, blood transfusions, chemotherapy, and radiation treatment have all been found to depress the immune system. Patients with cancer show depression of both cellular and humoral immune functions. Classically, T-cell proliferative responses to both mitogen and alloantigen are reduced with increasing tumor

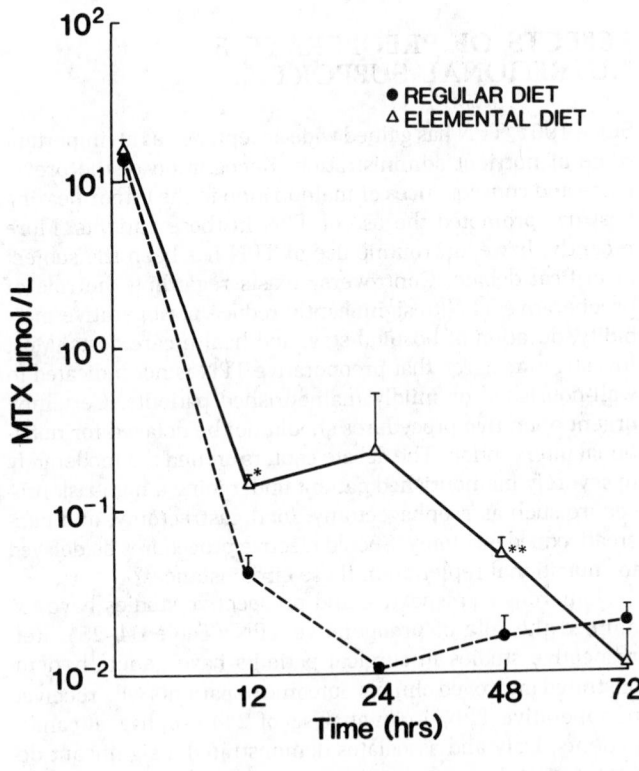

FIGURE 64–13. Plasma clearance of methotrexate (MTX) was significantly slower in animals given an elemental diet compared with a regular diet. Significantly greater toxicity (enterocolitis) was noted in the former group after receiving 20 mg/kg MTX.

burden. Patients with advanced disease often lack a delayed-type hypersensitivity reaction to skin-recall antigens (anergy). Anergy is clearly predictive of increased sepsis and mortality in patients undergoing major surgery.[55]

In analyzing anergy, defects in T-cell activation have been found to be the primary abnormality in the delayed hypersensitivity response.[56] When removed from the "anergic environment" and cultured in vitro with recall antigen, however, T cells proliferate normally. These activated T cells then can elicit the delayed-type hypersensitivity response when reinjected into the patient. Cytotoxic T lymphocytes isolated from patients with breast, lung, and colon carcinomas as well as from sarcomas demonstrate decreased cytotoxicity to autologous tumor.[57] Natural killer cells, the body's putative first line against cancer, are also less active when isolated from tumor-bearing animals and patients.

In addition to the immunosuppression that occurs in the presence of malignancy, operative therapy intended to eradicate tumor may promote metastatic tumor growth. Patients undergoing diverting colostomy followed by colectomy for cancer have been shown to do less well than those treated by one operation.[58] Controlled experiments in animal models corroborate enhancement of tumor growth, but mechanisms remain obscure.[59] Functionally, T cells show depressed responses to mitogen or alloantigen. Although blood transfusions are often unavoidable in oncologic surgery, they may adversely affect outcome in the cancer patient. Perioperative blood transfusion has been associated with significantly poorer prognosis in patients with breast carcinoma, colon cancer, non-small cell lung cancer, and sarcoma.[60–63] The mechanisms involved are complex and multifactoral, but multiple blood transfusions depress the immune response manifested in vitro by poor T-cell proliferative indices and decreased effector-cell response to various lymphokines.

Certain nutrient substrates may have a major role in the nutritional support of the cancer patient. Specific amino acids, RNA, ω-3 fatty acids, and trace metals such as zinc have all been shown to affect host immune function.

Arginine is a semi-essential dibasic amino acid that is a component of the urea cycle (Fig. 64–14). It is converted by the enzyme arginase into ornithine and urea. Arginine has potent secretagogue effects on several endocrine and neuroendocrine glands.[64,65] Administration of arginine induces the secretion of growth hormone, prolactin, insulin, glucagon, insulin-like growth factor-1, pancreatic polypeptide, somatostatin, and catecholamines. In laboratory studies, arginine supplementation has thymotropic properties and enhances the responsiveness of thymic lymphocytes to mitogens in normal and traumatized animals.[66,67] Arginine enhances cellular immunity, as evidenced by improved skin allograft rejection in normal mice and improved delayed-type hypersensitivity responses and improved bacterial containment and survival in animal burn models. Arginine has also been demonstrated to have antitumor effects in both chemically and virally induced and transplanted solid tumor models. Studies from our laboratory have demonstrated beneficial effects of supplemental arginine in the tumor-bearing host by noting increased concanavalin A (con-A) mitogenic responses and IL-2 production by host splenocytes and increased host reactivity against tumor antigens in the tumor-bearing group.[68] Supplemental arginine significantly retarded the growth of C1300 neuroblastoma in protein-depleted mice and prolonged

ARGININE METABOLISM

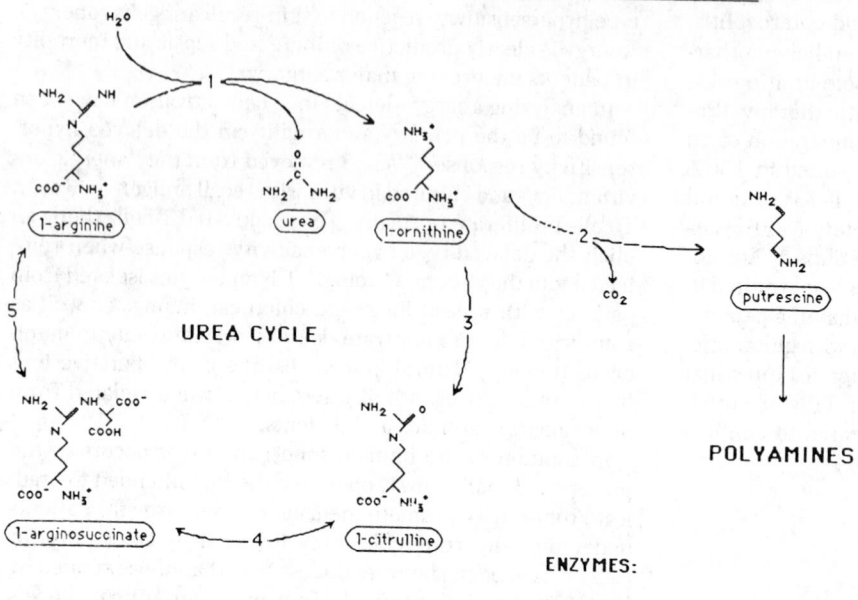

FIGURE 64–14. Arginine is a semi-essential amino acid within the urea cycle.

median host survival.[69] These effects were dependent on tumor antigenicity.

Few clinical studies have examined the role of oral or intravenous supplemental arginine in humans. In healthy volunteers, supplemental dietary arginine increased peripheral blood lymphocyte mitogenic response to con-A and phytohemagglutinin (PHA).[70] Our group investigated the effects of supplemental arginine in cancer patients undergoing major surgery.[71] Thirty patients were randomized to receive either supplemental arginine (25 g/day) or isonitrogenous L-glycine (43 g/day) as part of the graduated enteral diet for 7 days after surgery (Fig. 64–15). Supplemental arginine significantly increased mean mitogenic responses to con-A and PHA on postoperative days four and seven compared to postoperative day one (Fig. 64–16). No differences were found in the glycine-treated group. Mean CD4 phenotype levels on postoperative day seven were also significantly increased compared to the glycine group. Mean plasma levels of somatomedin-C were also significantly increased on day seven in the arginine group compared with the glycine group.

RNA has been demonstrated to be essential for the continued maturation of T cells in animal models. Absence of RNA from the diet results in depressed cell-mediated immune function, decreased survival after *Staphylococcus aureus* injection, and diminished rejection of allografts.[72] Fatty acids in the diet affect levels of arachidonic and eicosapentaenoic acid, resulting in changes in prostaglandin synthesis. Increased intake of ω-3 fatty acids has been reported to improve immunologic function by decreasing prostaglandin E_2 production after major injury. Animal studies by Alexander and coworkers have demonstrated improved response to infectious challenges in animals supplemented with ω-3 fatty acids.[73] Recent studies in cancer patients undergoing major upper gastrointestinal surgery demonstrated a significant reduction in postoperative infections, wound complications, and hospital length of stay in patients receiving arginine, RNA, and ω-3 fatty acids compared with patients receiving a standard diet (Fig. 64–17).[74]

EFFECTS OF PREOPERATIVE NUTRITIONAL SUPPORT

Since 1967, TPN has gained wide acceptance as an important route of nutrient administration. Recognition of the prevalence and consequences of malnutrition in the tumor-bearing host has promoted the use of TPN in these patients. More recently, however, routine use of TPN has been the subject of critical debate. Controversy exists regarding the role of preoperative TPN to significantly reduce perioperative morbidity, duration of hospital stay, and health-care costs. Most investigators agree that preoperative TPN is not indicated in well-nourished or mildly malnourished patients. Certainly, urgent operative procedures should not be delayed for nutritional intervention. The debate centers around the moderately to severely malnourished patient undergoing a high-risk procedure such as esophagectomy, total gastrectomy, and pancreaticoduodenectomy. Should elective procedures be delayed for nutritional repletion in these circumstances?

Numerous retrospective and prospective studies have examined the role of preoperative TPN (Table 64–25). Retrospective studies in surgical patients have generally demonstrated improved clinical outcome in patients who received perioperative TPN. In an analysis of 244 esophageal cancer patients, Daly and associates demonstrated a significant decrease in major complications in patients who received 5 or more days of TPN preoperatively compared with both concurrent and historical controls who did not receive TPN.[75] In other studies, preoperative TPN significantly reduced com-

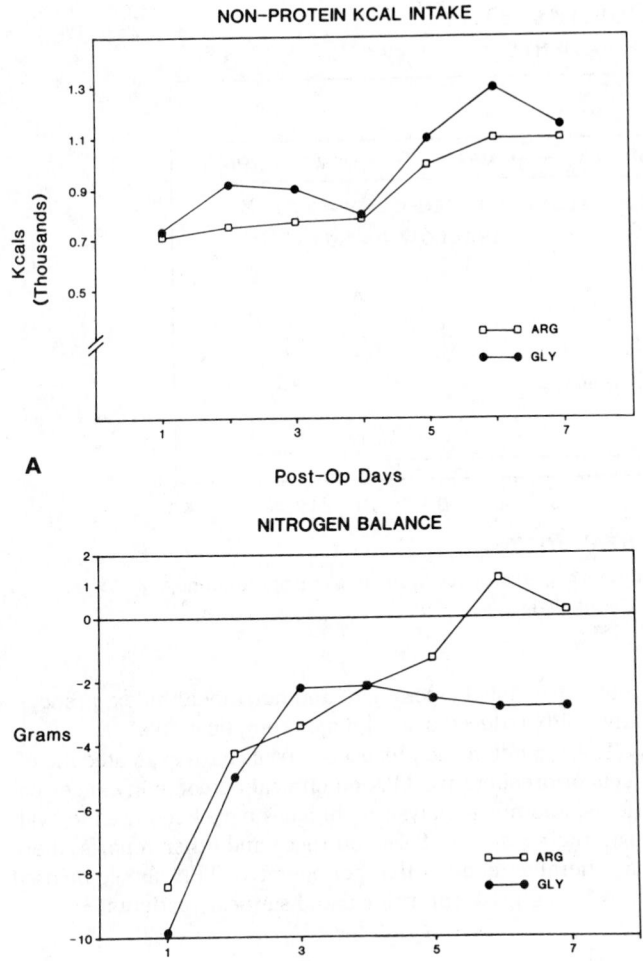

NON-PROTEIN KCAL INTAKE

A

Post-Op Days

NITROGEN BALANCE

B

Post-Op Days

FIGURE 64–15. Postoperative patients were randomized to receive arginine (25 g/day) or glycine (43 g/day) in addition to standard enteral feeding by jejunostomy. Although caloric intake was similar, nitrogen balance was slightly improved in the arginine group.

lated to the patient and the planned operation. It also allows use of postoperative enteral feeding, which may be significantly more cost-effective.

In 1979 Heatley and associates studied 74 gastric cancer patients who either received preoperative TPN for 7 to 10 days or served as controls.[76] TPN patients had fewer wound infections and lost less body weight perioperatively than corresponding control patients. Muller and colleagues studied 125 patients with gastrointestinal cancer who were randomized to receive 10 days of preoperative TPN or standard diet.[77] Postoperative major morbidity and mortality were significantly lower in the TPN group. Muller and coworkers reported an extension of their work that included three groups: control, TPN (amino acids/glucose), and TPN-L (amino acids/glucose/lipid emulsion) patients.[78] Significant differences were seen in body-weight change, protein and immune parameters, and major complications and mortality comparing the TPN (amino acid/glucose) and control groups. The trial was changed before completion by stopping the TPN-L (amino acids/glucose/lipid emulsion) group due to greater complications in this group.

Studies by Starker[79] and Bellantone[80] and their colleagues included patients with benign and malignant disease. In the former study, 59 malnourished patients were divided into three groups based on initial response to TPN. Patients received TPN for 5 days to 6 weeks. The authors noted a high morbidity and mortality in patients who remained hypoalbuminemic after 1 week of TPN, suggesting the importance of administering preoperative TPN until nutritional deficits have been corrected.

Foschi and coworkers studied 64 patients who underwent preoperative transhepatic catheter biliary diversion for obstructive jaundice with or without preoperative TPN.[81] The nutritionally repleted group had significantly fewer major complications (18% versus 47%) and mortality (3.5% versus 12.5%) compared with control patients.

A multiinstitutional prospective randomized trial evaluated

plications in patients deemed to be at high risk by their prognostic nutritional index.

Thus, clinical trials of perioperative TPN have demonstrated improved nutritional status as reflected by gain in body weight, improvement in serum protein levels, restoration of immune function, and improved nitrogen balance. Effects on clinical outcome remain less well defined. Preoperative TPN probably results in a significant reduction in postoperative complications and reduced mortality in the *severely malnourished, high-risk* group when given for an *adequate* length of time. Failure to demonstrate improved outcome with TPN in other trials may accurately reflect the limited value of TPN in well-nourished or moderately malnourished patients or in patients undergoing low-risk procedures. It is also possible that in these patients, the complications associated with TPN and the increased risk of nosocomial infections due to prolonged hospitalization negate any benefit and may result in net harm.

A useful approach to the nutritional management of elective surgical patients is shown in Figure 64–10. This approach uses a clinical assessment of nutritional and medical risk re-

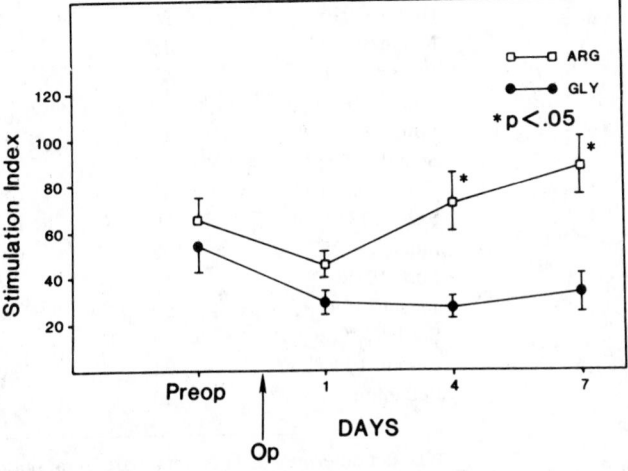

T LYMPHOCYTE ACTIVATION
Conconavalin A (7 ugs/ml)

FIGURE 64–16. Peripheral blood T lymphocyte activation to ConA was significantly improved on postoperative days 4 and 7 in the arginine group compared with the glycine group.

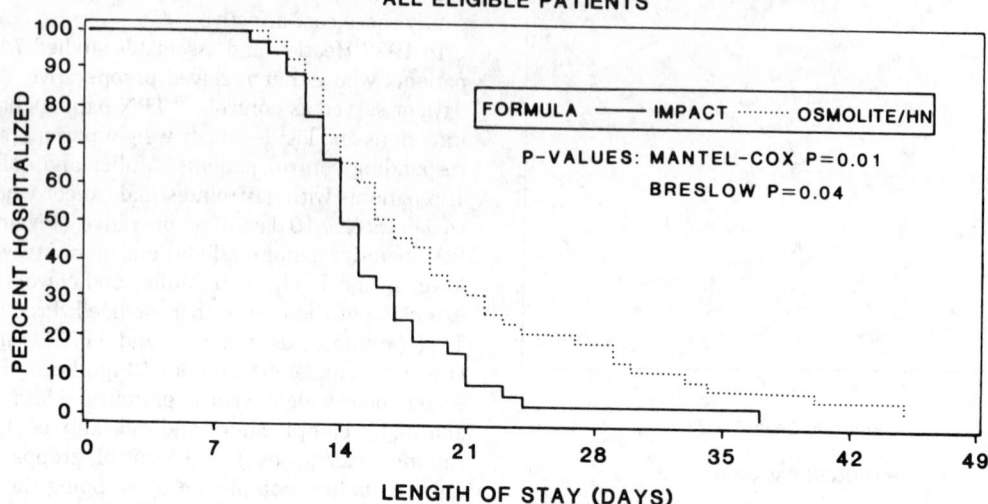

FIGURE 64–17.   Length of hospital stay was significantly less in the group receiving supplemental arginine, RNA, and omega-3 fatty acids compared with a standard enteral diet.

TPN in surgical patients.[82] Two hundred and thirty-one TPN and 228 control patients were studied at ten Veterans Administration Medical Centers across the United States. Mortality rates and major postoperative complications were similar for both groups. A higher incidence of infectious complications was noted in the TPN group, while a higher noninfectious complication rate occurred in controls. In the subgroup of patients with severe malnutrition, measured by subjective global assessment and nutritional index, preoperative TPN reduced overall major complications.

These randomized prospective trials have evaluated the effects of preoperative TPN on clinical outcome in cancer patients, and meta-analysis techniques have been used to evaluate their results.[83] Based on these and other reports, there is general agreement that perioperative TPN should be used only in high-risk (nutritional and surgical) patients.

TABLE 64–25.   Prospective Randomized Trials of Preoperative TPN in Surgical Patients

Investigations	No. of Patients	Preoperative TPN Duration (days)	Complication Rate (%) TPN vs Control	Mortality Rate (%) TPN vs Control
Holter, 1977	56	3	13 vs 19	7 vs 8
Heatley, 1979[76]	74	7–10	28 vs 25	15 vs 22
Holter, 1976	26	2	16 vs 18	ND
Moghissi, 1977	15	5–7	30 vs 50	ND
Preshaw, 1979	47	1	33 vs 17	ND
Simms, 1980	40	7–10	ND	0 vs 10
Lim, 1981	19	21–28	30 vs 50	10 vs 20
Schildt, 1981	15	14	38 vs 57	0 vs 0
Thompson, 1981	41	5–14	17 vs 11 vs 10	0 vs 0 vs 0
Sako, 1981	69	8–32	50 vs 56	50 vs 25
Mueller, 1982	125	10	11 vs 19	3 vs 11
Burt, 1982	18	14	ND	ND
Jenson, 1982	20	2	Sig in TPN group	ND
Starker, 1986[79]	59	5–42	12.5 vs 45	0 vs 10
Foschi, 1986[81]	64	20	18 vs 47	3.5 vs 12.5
Bellantone, 1988[80]	100	7	5.3 vs 22	5.3 vs 6.6

ND, not determined; TPN, total parenteral nutrition.
(Modified from Redmond HP, Daly JM. Preoperative nutritional therapy in cancer patients is beneficial. In: Simmons R, ed. Debates in clinical surgery. Chicago: Mosby-Year Book, 1991)

NUTRITIONAL SUPPORT WITH CHEMOTHERAPY AND RADIATION THERAPY

The use of nutritional support in the cancer patient receiving chemotherapy and radiation therapy remains controversial because of the lack of appropriate prospective randomized clinical trials to evaluate the effect of nutritional support on host survival and morbidity in these patients. Major flaws exist in most published clinical studies, including inadequate numbers of patients, inadequate duration/amount of nutritional support, heterogenous patient populations, and inappropriate study populations. Many clinical trials do not even stratify patients into malnourished versus well-nourished groups.

Numerous clinical reviews have correlated malnutrition with decreased survival in patients with advanced cancer receiving chemotherapy. Despite retrospective studies suggesting improved tolerance to chemotherapy in patients receiving nutritional support, prospective randomized trials have provided limited support for this concept. The primary toxicities evaluated in these trials include gastrointestinal (nausea, vomiting, stomatitis, and diarrhea), hematologic (leukopenia, anemia, and thrombocytopenia), and septic complications. The results are summarized in Table 64–26. In six trials that studied gastrointestinal toxicity, reduced toxicity was demonstrated in only one study and increased toxicity (stomatitis) was found in two studies; no difference in toxicity was found comparing TPN and control groups in three studies. Only two of eleven trials documented less hematologic toxicity in patients receiving TPN; in one trial of patients with advanced colorectal cancer, increased hematologic toxicity was observed. Finally, two of five clinical trials observed an increased incidence of septic complications in patients receiving TPN compared with the control group. A review of tumor response and length of survival in these clinical trials demonstrated similar outcome between patients receiving parenteral nutrition and control groups.

Weisdorf and associates in 1987 performed a prospective study of 137 bone-marrow transplant patients. In this large clinical trial, patients receiving TPN demonstrated improved overall survival, improved disease-free survival, and decreased incidence of relapse compared with control patients. This large prospective study demonstrates the possibility of using TPN to support patients through extremely aggressive chemotherapy treatment regimens.

Radiation therapy increases the potential for the development of severe nutritional deficits, and toxicity is related to degree of preexisting malnutrition, radiation site, and dose of radiation given. Published clinical trials of the efficacy of nutritional support in patients receiving radiation therapy suffer from the same defects as studies in chemotherapy patients. Most clinical radiation therapy studies have been conducted in patients with head and neck, esophageal, and abdominal/pelvic cancer (Table 64–27). An almost universal finding in studies of patients with advanced malignancy receiving radiation therapy is that TPN significantly increases weight gain. The significance of this weight gain is limited, however, as reduced toxicity and improved survival are difficult to demonstrate. Improved survival was found in one prospective study of 40 cancer patients receiving abdominal/pelvic radiation therapy, and fewer interruptions in radiation therapy treatments were seen in a similar patient population. However, insufficient numbers of patients have been evaluated to establish or refute the efficacy of nutritional support in patients receiving radiation therapy.

In summary, the efficacy of nutritional support in patients receiving adjuvant chemotherapy and radiation therapy remains to be determined. Few conclusions can be made from the limited information provided by existing prospective randomized trials. Nutritional support may play a more important role as adjuvant therapy regimens become more intense, such as bone-marrow transplantation. Furthermore, specific nutrients such as glutamine, arginine, and ω-3 fatty acids may play either a nutritive or pharmacologic role to prevent organ-

TABLE 64–26. Effect of Parenteral Nutrition on Chemotherapy Toxicity

Tumor Type	No. of Patients	Gastrointestinal	Hematologic	Infections
Lymphoma	41	—	ND	—
Colorectal	45	ND	↓	—
Testicular	30	ND	↑	↓
Metastatic sarcoma	27	—	ND	ND
Childhood metastatic	19	—	—	↓
Acute leukemia	23	—	ND	—
Lung, small cell	39	ND	ND	—
Lung, small cell	39	↓	ND	ND
Lung, small cell	31	—	ND	—
Lung, adenocarcinoma	43	↓	ND	ND
Lung, non-small cell	27	—	ND	—
Lung, squamous cell		↑	↑	—

↑, TPN group had reduced toxicity vs control group; ↓, TPN group had increased toxicity vs control group; —, information not provided; ND, no difference.
(Adapted from Koretz RL. J Clin Oncol 1984;2:535)

TABLE 64–27. TPN and Radiation Therapy

Cancer	No. of Patients	Weight	Toxicity	% XRT Given		Survival	
				TPN	Control		
Pelvic	32	↑TPN	ND	—	—	—	—
Abdominal/pelvic	20	↑TPN	ND	92	100	—	ND
Abdominal/pelvic	40	↑TPN	—	—	—	↑	—
Ovarian	81	—	—	—	—	ND	—
Abdominal/pelvic	25	—	ND	100	100	—	ND
Abdominal/pelvic	29	↑TPN	ND	91	82	ND	—

TPN, total parenteral nutrition; ND, no difference; XRT, radiation therapy.

specific toxicity. Once the mechanism of cancer cachexia and cellular mechanisms of adjuvant therapy toxicity have been elucidated, more specific nutrient regimens may be designed to prevent the development of cancer cachexia and reduce host toxicity associated with antineoplastic therapy.

REFERENCES

1. DeWys WE, Begg C, Lavin PT, et al. Prognostic effect of weight loss prior to chemotherapy in cancer patients. Am J Med 1980;69:491–497.
2. DeWys WD, Walters K. Abnormalities of taste sensation in cancer patients. Cancer 1975;36:1888–1896.
3. Lucke B, Borwick M, Zeckwer I. Liver catalase activity in parabiotic rats with one partner tumor bearing. J Natl Cancer Inst 1952;13:681–686.
4. Nakahara W. A chemical basis for tumor host relations. J Natl Cancer Inst 1960;24:77–86.
5. Langstein H, Fraker D, Norton JA. Reversal of cancer cachexia by antibodies to interferon-gamma but not cachectin/tumor necrosis factor. Surg Forum 1989;40:408–410.
6. Krause R, Humphreys C, von Meyenfeldt M. A central mechanism for anorexia in cancer: A hypothesis. Cancer Treat Rep 1981;65(suppl):15–21.
7. Brennan MF. Uncomplicated starvation versus cancer cachexia. Cancer Res 1977;37:2359–2364.
8. Brennan MF, Burt ME. Nitrogen metabolism in cancer patients. Cancer Treat Rep 1981;65(suppl):67–78.
9. Holroyde CP, Reichard A. Carbohydrate metabolism in cancer cachexia. Cancer Treat Rep 1981;65(suppl):55–59.
10. Young VR. Energy metabolism and requirements in the cancer patient. Cancer Res 1977;37:2336–2347.
11. Warnold I, Lundholm K, Schersten T. Energy balance and body composition in cancer. Cancer Res 1978;38:1801–1807.
12. Shike M, Russell D, Detsky A, et al. Changes in body composition in patients with small cell lung cancer: The effect of TPN as an adjunct to chemotherapy. Ann Intern Med 1984;101:303–309.
13. Knox LS, Crosby LO, Feurer ID, et al. Energy expenditure in malnourished cancer patients. Ann Surg 1983;197:152–162.
14. Heber D, Chlebowski RT, Ishibashi DE, et al. Abnormalities in glucose and protein metabolism in non-cachectic lung cancer patients. Cancer Res 1982;42:4815–4819.
15. Shaw JM, Humberstone DM, Wolfe RR. Energy and protein metabolism in sarcoma patients. Ann Surg 1988;207:283–289.
16. Buzby GP, Mullen JL, Matthews DC, et al. Prognostic nutritional index in gastrointestinal surgery. Am J Surg 1980;139:160–167.
17. Schein PS, Kesner D, Haller D, et al. Cachexia of malignancy: Potential role of insulin in nutritional management. Cancer 1979;43:2070–2076.
18. Waterhouse C, Jeanpretre N, Keilson J. Gluconeogenesis from alanine in patients with progressive malignant disease. Cancer Res 1979;39:1968–1972.
19. Moley JF, Morrison SD, Gornschboty DM, Norton JA. Body composition changes in rats with experimental cancer cachexia: Improvement with exogenous insulin. Cancer Res 1988;48:2784–2787.
20. Peacock JL, Norton JA. Impact of insulin on survival of cachectic tumor-bearing rats. J Parenter Enteral Nutr 1988;12:260–264.
21. Shaw JHF, Wolfe RR. Whole-body protein kinetics in patients with early and advanced gastrointestinal cancer—the response to glucose infusion and total parenteral nutrition. Surgery 1977;103:148–155.
22. Lundholm K, Edstron S, Edman L, et al. Metabolism in peripheral tissues in cancer patients. Cancer Treat Rep 1981;65(suppl):79–83.
23. Brennan MF. Cancer cachexia and rate of whole-body lipolysis. Metabolism 1986;35:304–310.
24. Waterhouse C. Nutritional disorders in neoplastic diseases. J Chron Dis 1963;16:637–644.
25. Waterhouse C, Kemperman JH. Carbohydrate metabolism in subjects with cancer. Cancer Res 1971;31:1273–1278.
26. Wilson AW, Kirk CJC, Goode AW. The effect of weight loss, operation and parenteral nutrition on fat clearance in patients with colorectal cancer. Clin Sci 1987;73:489–495.
27. Norton JA, Stein TP, Brennan MF. Whole-body protein synthesis and turnover in normal and malnourished patients with and without known cancer. Ann Surg 1981;194:123–128.
28. Kien CL, Carmitta BN. Close association of accelerated rats of whole-body protein turnover (synthesis and breakdown) and energy expenditure in children with newly diagnosed acute lymphocytic leukemia. J Parenter Enteral Nutr 1987;11:129–134.
29. Fearon KCH, Hansell DT, Preston T, et al. Influence of whole-body protein turnover rate on resting energy expenditure in patients with cancer. Cancer Res 1988;48:2590–2595.
30. Tayek JA, Blackburn GL, Bistrian BR. Alterations in whole-body, muscle, liver and tumor tissue protein synthesis and degradation in Novikoff hepatoma and Yoshida sarcoma tumor growth studied in vivo. Cancer Res 1988;48:1554–1558.
31. Cohn SH, Gartenhaus W, Sawitsky A, et al. Compartmental body composition of cancer patients by measurement of total body nitrogen, potassium, and water. Metabolism 1981;30:222–229.
32. Bartlett DL, Torosian MH. Specific metabolic therapy of cancer cachexia. Arch Surg (in press).
33. McAnena OJ, Daly JM. Impact of antitumor therapy on nutrition. Surg Clin N Am 1986;66:1213–1228.
34. Stein JP, Buzby GP. Protein metabolism in surgical patients. Surg Clin N Am 1981;61:519–527.
35. Copeland EM, Daly JM, Dudrick SJ. Nutrition as an adjunct to cancer treatment in the adult. Cancer Res 1977;37:2451–2456.
36. Nixon DW, Heymsfield SB, Cohen AE. Protein-calorie malnutrition in hospitalized cancer patients. Am J Med 1980;68:683–690.
37. Warren S. The immediate cause of death in cancer. Am J Med Sci 1932;184:610–615.
38. Meguid M, Mughal MM, Debonis D, et al. Influence of nutritional status on the resumption of adequate food intake in patients recovering from colorectal cancer operations. Surg Clin N Am 1986;66:1167–1176.
39. Daly JM, Copeland EM, Dudrick SJ. Effect of intravenous nutrition on tumor growth and host immunocompetence in malnourished animals. Surgery 1978;84:655–658.
40. Law DK, Dudrick SJ, Abdou NI. The effects of protein-calorie malnutrition on immunocompetence of the surgical patient. Surg Gynecol Obstet 1974;139:257–266.
41. Harvey KB, Bath A, Jr, Blackburn GL. Nutritional assessment and patient outcome during oncological therapy. Cancer 1979;43(suppl):2065–2069.
42. Daly JM, Dudrick SJ, Copeland EM. Intravenous hyperalimentation: Effect on delayed cutaneous hypersensitivity in cancer patients. Ann Surg 1980;192:587–592.
43. McEntee GP, Forster S, Duignan JP, O'Malley E. The effect of parenteral nutritional support on cell-mediated immunity. Int Ther Clin Monit 1988;8:138–143.
44. Jeevanandam M, Legaspi A, Lowry SF, Horowitz GD, Brennan MF. Effect of total parenteral nutrition on whole-body protein kinetics in cachectic patients with benign or malignant disease. J Parenter Enteral Nutr 1988;12:229–236.
45. Shaw JHF, Wolfe RR. Whole-body protein kinetics in patients with early and advanced gastrointestinal cancer—the response to glucose infusion and total parenteral nutrition. Surgery 1977;103:148–155.
46. Drott C, Unsgaard B, Schersten T, Lundholm K. Total parenteral nutrition as an adjuvant to patients undergoing chemotherapy for testicular carcinoma: Protection of body composition—a randomized, prospective study. Surgery 1977;103:499–506.
47. Torosian MH, Tsou KC, Daly JM, et al. Alteration of tumor cell kinetics by total parenteral nutrition: Potential therapeutic implications. Cancer 1984;53:1409–1415.
48. Karpeh MS, Kehne JA, Choi SH, et al. Tumor immunogenicity, nutritional repletion and cancer. Surgery 1987;102:283–290.
49. Skeef NS, Duncan Jr. A possible relation between dietary zinc and cAMP in the regulation of tumor cell proliferation in the rat. Br J Nutr 1988;59:437–442.
50. Grossie VB Jr, Ota DM, Ajani JA, Chang THE, Pateniz D, Nishioka K. Influence of total parenteral nutrition on tumor growth and polyamine biosynthesis of fibrosarcoma-bearing rats after induced-cachexia. J Parenter Enteral Nutr 1988;12:441–444.

51. Chance WT, Cao L, Nelson JL, Foley-Nelson T, Fischer JE. Acivicin reduces tumor growth during total parenteral nutrition. Surgery 1987;102:386–394.

52. Grant JP, Snyder PJ. Use of L-glutamine in total parenteral nutrition. J Surg Res 1988;33:506–513.

53. McAnena OJ, Harvey LP, Bonau RA, Daly JM. Alteration of methotrexate toxicity in rats by manipulation of dietary components. Gastroenterology 1987;92:354–360.

54. Fox AD, Kripke SA, DePaula J, Berman JM, Settle RG, Rombeau JL. Effect of a glutamine-supplemented enteral diet on methotrexate-induced enterocolitis. J Parenter Enteral Nutr 1988;12:325–331.

55. Meakins JL. Pietsch JB, Bubenik O, et al. Delayed hypersensitivity indicator of acquired failure of host defenses in sepsis and trauma. Ann Surg 1977;186:241–246.

56. Rode HN, Christou NV, Bubenik O, et al. Lymphocyte function in anergic patients. Clin Exp Immunol 1982;47:156–161.

57. Tartter PI, Martinelli G, Steinberg B, et al. Changes in peripheral T-cell subsets and natural killer cytotoxicity in relation to colorectal cancer surgery. Cancer Detect Prev 1987;9:359–364.

58. Lundy J, Lovett EJ, Hamilton S, et al. Immune impairment and metastatic tumor growth. Cancer 1979;43:945–951.

59. Weese JL, Ottery FD, Emoto SE. Does operation facilitate tumor growth? An experimental model in rats. Surgery 1986;100:273–277.

60. Tartter PI, Burrows L, Papatesta AE, et al. Perioperative blood transfusion has prognostic significance for breast cancer. Surgery 1985;97:225–230.

61. Burrows L, Tartter P. Effects of blood transfusions on colonic malignancy recurrence rate. Lancet 1982;2:662–664.

62. Blumberg N. Agarwal MM, Chuang C. Relation between recurrence of cancer of the colon and blood transfusion. Br Med J 1985;290:1037–1039.

63. Rosenberg SA, Siepp CA, White DE, et al. Perioperative blood transfusions are associated with increased rates of recurrence and decreased survival in patients with high-grade soft-tissue sarcoma of the extremities. J Clin Oncol 1985;3:698–709.

64. Merimee TJ, Lillicrap DA, Rabinowitz D. Effect of arginine on serum levels of human growth hormone. Lancet 1965;2:668–670.

65. Rakoff JS, Siver TM, Sinha YM, et al. Prolactin and growth hormone release in response to sequential stimulation by arginine and TRF. J Clin Endocrin Metab 1973;37:641–644.

66. Barbul A, Wasserkrug HL, Sisto DA, et al. Thymic and immune stimulatory actions of arginine. J Parenter Enteral Nutr 1980;4:446–449.

67. Barbul A, Wasserkrug HL, Seifter E, et al. Immunostimulatory effects of arginine in normal and injured rats. J Surg Res 1980;29:228–235.

68. Reynolds JV, Zhang SM, Thom AK, et al. Arginine as an immunomodulator. Surg Forum 1988;38:415.

69. Reynolds JV, Thom AK, Ziegler M, et al. Arginine, protein calorie malnutrition and cancer. J Surg Res 1987;45:513.

70. Barbul A, Sisto DA, Wasserkrug HL, et al. Arginine stimulates lymphocyte immune response in healthy humans. Surgery 1981;90:244.

71. Daly JM, Reynolds JV, Thom AK, et al. Immune and metabolic effects of arginine in surgical patients. Ann Surg 1988;208:512.

72. Rudolph RF, Kulkami AD, Schandle VB, et al. Involvement of dietary nucleotides in T-lymphocyte function. Adv Exp Med 1984;165:175–178.

73. Alexander JW, Saito H, Oglle C, Trocki O. The importance of lipid type in the diet after burn injury. Ann Surgery 1986;204:1–8.

74. Daly JM, Lieberman MD, Goldfine J, et al. Enteral nutrition with supplemental arginine, RNA and omega-3 fatty acids in postoperative patients: Immunologic, metabolic and clinical outcome. Surgery 1992;112:56–67.

75. Daly JM, Massar E. Giacco G, et al. Parenteral nutrition in esophageal cancer patients. Ann Surg 1982;196:203–208.

76. Heatley RV, Williams RHP, Lewis MH. Preoperative intravenous feeding: A controlled trial. Postgrad Med J 1979;35:541–45.

77. Muller JM, Dienst C, Brenner U, Pichlmaier H. Preoperative parenteral feeding in patients with gastrointestinal carcinoma. Lancet 1982;1:68–71.

78. Muller JM, Keller HW, Brenner U, Walter M. Holzmuller W. Indications and effects of preoperative parenteral nutrition. World J Surg 1986;10:53–63.

79. Starker PM, LaSala PA, Askanazi J, et al. The influence of preoperative total parenteral nutrition upon morbidity and mortality. Surg Gyn Obstet 1986;162:569–574.

80. Bellantone R. Doglietto G, Bossola M, et al. Preoperative parenteral nutrition of mal-nourished surgical patients. Acta Chir Scand 1988;22:249–251.

81. Foschi D, Cavagna G, Callioni F, et al. Hyperalimentation of jaundiced patients on percutaneous transhepatic biliary drainage. Br J Surg 1986;73:716–719.

82. Buzby GP, The Veterans Affairs TPN Cooperative Study Group. Perioperative TPN in surgical patients. N Engl J Med 1991;325:525–543.

83. Klein S, Simes J, Blackburn G. Total parenteral nutrition and cancer clinical trials. Cancer 1986;58:1378–1386.

SECTION 5

FRANK J. BRESCIA

Specialized Care of the Terminally Ill

The modern concepts of palliative medicine were firmly established because of frustration with physicians and the health-care system to deliver effective, compassionate treatment to the dying.[1–3] In the roots of our past agricultural society, death at home was expected and familiar. However, by 1950, nearly half of the population in the United States died in the hospital. Today, at least 75% of Americans die in institutions.[4] Because medicine's primary objective became focused on curative intervention, the basic needs of terminally ill patients were often neglected. Unfortunately, prolonged and extensive diagnostic investigation was considered necessary by some physicians before the bothersome symptoms of dying patients were relieved. Often no treatment of symptoms was offered because the patient was considered terminal, or misdirected therapy was given to patients for every complaint without searching for an appropriate cause and remedy.

In 1974 America's first hospice opened in New Haven, Connecticut, starting with a home-care program and progressing to a 44-bed inpatient facility. Nearly 2000 American hospice programs and over 200 Canadian hospices flourished within 15 years. Of the patients they served, 92% had advanced malignancy.

In 1978 a hospice task force was started by the Department of Health, Education, and Welfare to examine the federal government's role in the care of the terminally ill.[5] Two years later, the Health Care Finance Administration funded 26 demonstration hospice programs to study the quality and utilization of hospice care by these organizations.

The terminally ill were reported to use 22% of all Medicare reimbursement expenses.[6] Because of an expected cost savings to the Medicare system of $30 million to $150 million, there was momentum to pass reimbursement legislation, which also had enormous political appeal.[7] Therefore, effective November 1, 1983, hospice services became part of the Medicare benefits program, featuring the following major components:

1. Physician-certified patient prognosis of 6 months or less
2. Annual reimbursement cap per patient to any individual hospice (initially this cap was $6,500)
3. Maximum of 210 days of hospice reimbursement
4. To encourage home-care usage, a 20% reimbursement cap on inpatient hospice days
5. Mandated home care and inpatient care, and spiritual, bereavement, and volunteer services.

PHILOSOPHY OF CARE

Despite the enormous advances in understanding and treating malignant illness, half of patients diagnosed will die of their disease.[8] The success in managing diverse, multiple, and difficult symptoms, which is important for all patients at all stages of disease, becomes the overriding imperative for those facing incurable cancer. The oncology literature began to aggressively examine measures to relieve pain and other symptoms in advanced disease as well as the unacceptable side effects of beneficial anticancer therapies.[9] With the initial promise of possible cure, the magnitude of side effects in cancer therapy seem unimportant to many patients.[10,11] However, when the reality of tumor recurrence and incurability must be faced, the patient is exceptionally wounded and vulnerable, sometimes more so than at the initial diagnosis.

Principles of good palliative medicine are no different from those of other medical care: clinical competency, experienced technical skills, and a compassionate bedside manner. However, at some point in the overall management of failing cancer therapy, the health-care team must recognize that the dying process has started. It is not death, but the indignity of the dying process, that terrifies most terminal patients.[12]

It has always been difficult to define the point that signals the beginning of the dying process. The decision that no further treatment should be directed against the tumor may create conflict between the patient and family. If the physician demands a trial of more conventional or experimental treatment in a patient who accepts his or her dying, this can create confusion, tension, and anger. The timing and acceptance among those involved with care decisions are crucial for preparing for the patient's imminent death.

Who are the known dying, the terminal (Table 64–28)? All patients known to be dying of advanced cancer are time-bound, but the terminal phase may be quite immediate, long-term, or indeterminate. Lynn considers the use of categorical terms such as terminal to be cumbersome, inadequate, and pejorative.[13] Unfortunately, these terms are used commonly for hospice admission criteria, court decisions, insurance claims, and public policy decisions.

The ability to effectively relieve the wide spectrum of difficult clinical problems begins with an understanding of tumor behavior and malignant pathophysiology. Ideally, if the tumor burden is diminished, the patient will experience subjective improvement of symptoms. A knowledge of both the natural history and tempo of progression for a specific malignancy allows the clinician to anticipate and therefore manage the changing signs and symptoms. The primary origin of the neoplasm, histology, grade, extent of disease (stage), and metastatic behavior must be evaluated early in the course of disease when the initial plan of care is formulated. The tumor's tempo of progression may vary among patients, even among those having the same primary site, histology, and stage. The patient's age, disease-free interval, tumor markers, hormone

receptors, performance status, and previous response to adequate clinical trials all help to clarify the potential outcome.

The following are important considerations and questions when deciding the clinical options for patients with extensive disease:

1. Establish with certainty that the disease is beyond curative intervention.
2. What are the etiology, severity, and relation of the patient's tumor to the patient's present symptoms?
3. Are the symptoms compatible with the natural history of the specific cancer under treatment?
4. What potential limitations of function do the disease, diagnostic intervention, or treatment impose?
5. Where is the patient on the disease trajectory?
6. What issues need to be communicated with members of the treatment team, family, and patient?
7. What is a realistic therapeutic goal? Should the patient be treated at all?
8. Should systemic treatment be initiated for the overall illness, or should local therapy (*e.g.*, radiation therapy) be given for the specific complaint (*e.g.*, bone pain)?
9. Is the patient a reasonable candidate for experimental therapy?
10. Are there any other possible options, if the patient refuses the clinician's recommendations?[14,15]

The appropriateness of antineoplastic treatment in the asymptomatic patient with widespread disease may be questionable, because complete remissions are seldom noted and survival is not prolonged in most common advanced solid tumors.[16-18] Good clinical trials should be initiated if there is any degree of uncertainty for any possible useful outcome. Most importantly, patients with treatable cancer should never be referred to hospice settings.[19] Physicians, supported by their knowledge, training, and experience, must base their decisions not on what they would like to happen for their patients, but on the clinical reality, and must accept what most likely will occur. Decisions may be different when factors such as the patient's age, functional status, mental status, and concurrent illness are considered. Finally, the clinician's goal for the dying patient is quite simple: to relieve only by reducing the intensity of the distressful symptoms, canceling certain forms of treatment without avoiding the person as a patient. This is the ultimate meaning of patient nonabandonment.

SYMPTOM CONTROL

Traditionally, patients with end-stage cancer have not been the focus of major research interest. Yet these incurable patients may spend weeks to years suffering the poorly understood symptoms that normally accompany progressive malignancy. The emotional, social, and spiritual influences on a person's perception of any symptom, including pain, are personal and complex and become especially evident when the disease process is progressive, the tumor is advanced, the patient's lifestyle is limited, and the patient is expected to die.

For patients, persistent, unattended, and unrelieved pain may be linked to disturbing questions of suffering, abandonment, and perhaps for some even spiritual atonement. Furthermore, stressed and overwhelmed families may feel guilty

---

TABLE 64–28.   Terminal Illness Syndrome

- Causal illness with a progressive evolution
- Survival defined in days to weeks
- Karnofsky score < 40%
- Single or multiple organ failure
- Failure of conventional or proven treatment measures
- Absence of any other potential proven or experimental therapy
- Irreversible progressive complications

(Apilanez RV, Gonzalez de Langarica LR, Arribas EG. Terminal illness syndrome. Fourth European Conference on Clinical Oncology and Cancer Nursing. Madrid: Federation of European Cancer Societies, 1987:193)

and helpless, as well as angry at the caregivers for allowing unrelieved symptoms to continue until death.

The great variability of pain intensity and opioid usage as patients approach death underscores the need for careful ongoing assessment of distressing symptoms throughout the disease process.[20,21] A pain-free state may be an unrealistic goal in patients with advanced cancer.

The ability to control and manage physical complaints other than pain is extraordinarily difficult in patients who exhibit complicated multisystem signs and symptoms.[22-25] The clinician's dilemma is worsened by the patient's inability to undergo extensive or definitive diagnostic studies. Many distressing complaints may themselves be related to ongoing symptom-control therapy (*e.g.*, opioid-induced nausea, constipation, sedation; steroid-induced myopathy, insomnia, confusion).[26-38] Some symptoms are more easily corrected than others as the patient approaches death; others may be perceived as difficult or unacceptable by the family but are unnoticed by the patient (*e.g.*, moaning, grimacing, death rattles). Although the pathophysiology and treatment of cancer pain have been widely reviewed, there are no clear recommendations to manage every complex malignant symptom as patients approach death. (The reader is referred to a more comprehensive discussion of cancer pain by Dr. Kathleen Foley earlier in this chapter.) Common symptoms of advanced cancer are summarized in Table 64–29.

Unrelieved intolerable symptoms that accompany progressive malignancy are influenced by a variety of factors.[10,11] Similar tumor pathology will produce variable symptoms in different patients. Cancer patients may note distress of normal bodily sensations or minor symptoms may become exaggerated if recurrence of the cancer is feared. Thoughtful discussions of the true nature of a patient's complaints may help palliate the intensity of these somatic symptoms.

The difficulty of witnessing distressing symptoms in the dying patient may lead family members to seek hospitalization. Comfort measures directed toward these symptoms become the most important aspect of care once the patient enters the dying process. The clinician should have less concern about the potential negative consequences of the chosen symptom-control therapy (*e.g.*, steroid-induced bleeding, immunosuppression, narcotic masking pain).[39] In the last few days it may be appropriate and less distressing to eliminate much of the patient's medication for nonproblematic concurrent diseases (*e.g.*, hypertension, diabetes, thyroid).

TERMINAL EVENTS

There is little change in the quality of life of patients until 4 to 6 months before death, but the last weeks of life are especially dramatic, with increased dependency, weakness, confusion, and inability to manage simple functional and personal tasks such as bathing, walking, and continence. Coyle reviewed the prevalence and change of symptoms volunteered by 90 patients during the last 4 weeks of their terminal disease (Table 64–30).[32] Nearly 75% had three or more separate complaints near death, while some had as many as nine distinct symptoms. Less than 5% of these dying patients reported hallucinations, diarrhea, nightmares, hiccups, itch, or panic attacks.

The final phase of the dying process can be frightening for both patient and family, and sometimes is managed by clinicians with confusion, inadequacy, negligence, and apathy. Escalating symptoms during the last 48 to 72 hours usually foreshadow death. A prospective study of 120 terminal patients demonstrated that 63 had uncontrollable symptoms that appeared an average of 48 hours before death. Dyspnea appeared to be the most common uncontrollable problem, especially as death approached.[40] National Hospice Study data indicated that dyspnea occurred in 70.2% of dying patients during the last 6 weeks of life, and was usually associated with lung or pleural disease.[41] Other studies had a much lower incidence of this symptom.[35,42] It is rare, however, for symptoms to be

TABLE 64–29. Relation of Cancer Diagnosis and Symptoms Present at Time of Admission (n = 1103)

	Symptoms					
	Severe Pain (%)	Confusion (%)	Anorexia (%)	Dyspnea (%)	Dysphagia (%)	Nausea (%)
Total Patients	38	33	31	27	22	19
Primary Diagnosis						
Lung	31	43	35	51	21	16
Breast	39	38	30	30	22	13
Colon	36	25	34	17	12	30
Rectum and sigmoid	49	32	28	17	15	15
Prostate	57	32	18	28	22	8
Pancreas	44	21	54	21	13	35
Head and neck	42	11	22	11	62	2
Cervix	68	27	27	21	22	39
Ovary	32	38	35	21	17	56
Stomach	23	17	40	10	15	47

(Brescia FJ, Adler D, Gray G, et al. Hospitalized advanced cancer patients: A profile. J Pain Symptom Manage 1990;5:221–227)

TABLE 64–30.   Prevalence of Symptoms 4 Weeks and 1 Week Before Death

Symptom	4 Weeks Before Death (%)	1 Week Before Death (%)
Fatigue	58	52
Pain	54	34
Generalized weakness	43	49
Mental haziness/confusion	24	28
Anxiety	21	18
Cough	6	7

(Modified from Coyle N, Adelhardt J, Foley KM, et al. Character of terminal illness in the advanced cancer patient: Pain and other symptoms during the last 4 weeks of life. J Pain Symptom Manage 1990;5: 83–93)

TABLE 64–31.   Diagnoses and Survival (Diagnosis to Death) (n = 1107)

	Duration of Illness (%)			
	6 Mo or Less	7–12 Mo	1–2 Y	2 Y or More
Total Patients	24	18	21	37
Leading Diagnoses				
Lung	39	26	21	15
Breast	5	5	18	72
Colon	15	12	24	49
Rectum and sigmoid	16	16	24	45
Prostate	4	6	20	71
Pancreas	54	30	9	6
Head and neck	17	29	31	24
Cervix	8	11	38	43
Ovary	19	16	16	48
Stomach	50	28	11	11

(Calvary Hospital Clinical Database, 1989 [unpublished data])

so unmanageable near death that total sedation is required to ease the patient's suffering.

PREDICTING SURVIVAL

The ability to predict the life expectancy of an advanced cancer patient has been poor, even among experienced clinicians.[43–45] The life expectancy of 108 hospice patients was overly optimistic by an average of 3.4 weeks.[46] The patient's functional status (Karnofsky score) appears to be the most important variable in estimating survival. One study showed that half the patients whose Karnofsky scores were 10% to 20% died within 53 days if no symptoms were present, compared with 50% within 16 days if dry mouth, dyspnea, anorexia, dysphagia, and weight loss were present.[47]

Terminal cancer patients, despite the setting (home, hospital, or nursing home), appear to share a common three-step decline in the last weeks of life (15 weeks, 2 months, and 2 weeks before death), with the greatest functional dependency, obviously, close to death.[48,49] The interval from the initial cancer diagnosis to death was examined in 1107 patients admitted to a palliative care setting (Table 64–31). Of these patients, 63% were diagnosed with cancer and subsequently died within 2 years. Survival was inversely related to age: patients under 74 years were more likely to survive longer than older patients.[50] These data are important because they show that physicians have difficulty with the Medicare requirement to certify a 6-month prognosis and eligibility for hospice benefits.

CHALLENGES AND QUESTIONS

Numerous challenges face palliative medicine, and there are many barriers to appropriate terminal care, such as inadequate physician education regarding symptom control; government regulations hindering the prescribing of narcotics; retail pharmacy restrictions; reimbursement limits because of Medicare hospital regulations (*e.g.*, 6-month prognosis); and the fear of opioid addiction or tolerance by the physician,

nurses, family, and patient.[19,51–53] Some important issues that must be further explored in the care of the dying are discussed below.

SITE OF DEATH

Despite the difficulties in keeping patients at home, most patients prefer to die at home.[54–57] The ability to allow patients to die at home in home-care hospice programs (55% to 72% of patients) may reflect the attitudes of staff and communication of the hospice philosophy rather than specific patient characteristics.[58] Wilkes found that only 3% of relatives of patients who died at home would have preferred the hospital setting.[59] The site of death was the consistent issue on which hospice-treated families demonstrated greater satisfaction over those families who received conventional care. However, in urban environments, dying at home may be difficult if not impossible, for example in the case of an elderly patient who lives alone, a patient with severe agitation, a patient who cannot get narcotics in pharmacies, or if such services are not covered by insurance.

A retrospective analysis of a home-care hospice program showed that pain was the single most important symptom that made hospitalization necessary, but this study could not determine whether the patients, despite the pain, could have remained at home.[60] The National Hospice Study reported that patients followed in hospital-based hospice programs were less likely to report having persistent pain, but this finding needs further analysis because a randomized trial of hospice care found no difference in pain-control outcomes between hospice and conventional care.[61] Another hospice program affiliated with a university hospital had 47% of their patients die at home, while 38% of patients had their care managed entirely without hospitalization.[62] In this study 71% of hospitalized patients received an average daily morphine dose of 75 mg; 53% of patients in the home had an average daily dose of 25 mg.

Dying at home is not always superior to the hospital setting. Families who strongly advocate death at home may not appreciate the enormous burden of 24-hour care of the sickest of patients and may eventually feel abandoned by their physicians and the health-care system. Unfortunately, many communities do not have the resources and trained professionals to meet the complex needs of terminal patients. The specific features of the patient, family, physician, program, or disease that impel hospitalization remain poorly defined.

LEGAL AND ETHICAL QUESTIONS IN HOSPICE CARE

There is always a rational place for therapy that comforts. In recent years, a medical consensus has emerged that patients have the right to refuse a treatment that no longer can remedy illness but only extends the agony of the dying process.[63-71] On whose authority are decisions of care finally made? Patients as people have the right to decide their own destiny; this premise is grounded in both common and constitutional law in the United States.[13,72] Thus, when competency exists, the patient's moral and legal right defines the soundness of the clinical action. However, situations may become quite complex for the physician. The patient may be competent and may understand the clinical issue at hand and the potential consequences of therapy, but because of his or her advanced state of illness, the symptoms endured, or the intensity, duration, and type of toxicity to past treatments, the patient's decisions may differ from those the physician anticipated.[73] The clinician may have moral conflicts if the patient talks of despair, harm to himself or herself, or avoidance of some treatment thought to be beneficial.[74,75]

Family members have the right to speak for their incompetent loved ones, but they often assume decision-making power for patients who are dying and frail but still competent. When patients lose the capacity to make decisions for themselves, family members usually render a substitute judgment of the patient's past wishes, not their own.

In some clinical situations there is an obligation *not* to provide some form of medical intervention to a dying patient. For example, both hunger and thirst are rarely recognized as problems in terminal patients by experienced clinicians.[76] Forcing fluid and food to patients is not warranted and is perhaps harmful with the onset of pulmonary congestion and edema and the need for a urinary catheter to manage increased urine output. Dehydration may result in some benefit to the dying person by enhancing sedation if hemoconcentration, hyperosmolality, azotemia, and hypercalcemia occur.

Trials of therapy should always be given when there is a clinical uncertainty of the outcome, but bad outcomes do not always mean the medical decisions of care were incorrect. For example, it is wrong to believe that therapy once begun cannot be stopped, because clinicians may omit clinical trials to patients who may benefit. Withdrawing treatment often appears to be more damaging and serious to the caregivers than if nothing had been initiated in the first place. What is indicated should be tried, and what is a failure should be stopped. Due to this misunderstood distinction and the fear of liability among good physicians, patients have suffered because clinicians have failed to give an adequate therapeutic trial or have kept patients on some form of futile intervention for long, exhausting, and costly periods of time.[77]

Major issues of conflict for clinicians in palliative settings include the futility of resuscitation, and inappropriate demands for resuscitation by the patient or family; the withholding of treatments such as chemotherapy, blood products, or antibiotics; and the withdrawal of some form of intervention, such as total parenteral nutrition, food, or hydration.[75,78-80] Physician-assisted suicide and active euthanasia are dilemmas that will soon confront physicians as attempts are made in our society to morally justify these actions as part of medical practice.[81-86]

Physicians must not have ill-conceived plans of medical care based on what they believe the patient's quality of life should be.[87] The urgency and challenge to promote adequate, acceptable patient comfort escalate as the patient enters the final days and hours. The anguish of any difficult manner of dying must be diminished, even if death is hastened—if not directly caused—by such therapy. These therapeutic decisions should be made with the patient's comfort as the objective, but should not be based on any public policy to seek death. The experience of most physicians who care for the dying is that there are few "unmanageable" patients, too few to change traditional medical practices and promote euthanasia and risk all the possible future abuses. However, as cost-containment controls are enacted, the criteria for limiting some treatments for certain patients must be publicly discussed and closely monitored.[88]

PERSONNEL ISSUES

Personnel remains the largest expenditure in hospice care and has the biggest impact on quality. It is difficult to attract and keep emotionally mature, competent, compassionate physicians to care for the dying.[89,90] Those involved in this work know both the gratification and the stress of dealing with the incurably ill. Witnessing dying and communicating tragic news to patients and their families produces an enormous strain on physicians.[91] The clinician is responsible for the timing and manner of discussing worsening clinical states. Attempting to offer realistic hope as well as helping the patient and family face the awful reality is no easy task, especially if the physician has previously avoided communication or is uncertain about treatment and outcome options. Other physicians, as well as family members, may feel that symptoms during the terminal phase are caused by the toxicity of some cancer treatment, and not by the obvious progressive cancer, and may blame the oncologist.

RESOURCE MANAGEMENT

Should those expected to die soon, despite therapy, use the scarce resources of well-trained clinicians and institutions?[92] Should oncologic treatment against the tumor continue because of demands by the patient or family, despite cost concerns? Because palliative care demands the skills of different disciplines, it remains costly.[93] Filling empty beds or meeting reimbursement needs should not be reasons for institutions to consider caring for the dying. Studies document that home-care hospice programs may save 10% to 20% of the total health care costs in the last year of life over inpatient medical care.[6,94-96] Savings of hospice care are more dramatic during the last 1 or 2 months of a patient's life, when diagnostic intervention and high-tech procedures are usually performed. Hospice care at home before the last 2 months of life appears more costly because of the need for expensive home services not usually seen in the conventional setting.[97] On average, conventional care of the cancer patient is more costly during the last year of a patient's life. There is an estimated annual savings of $4,000 if the patient is in a home-care hospice program and $1,300 if in a hospital-based hospice. If the patient remains in the hospice longer than 4 months, however, the costs are higher than conventional care.[98]

A study from western Australia found that the costs of providing 24-hour comprehensive medical and nursing care at home were comparable to those in acute hospitals during the last 3 months of life.[99] Vinciguerra reported a cost benefit of $256 per day for terminal patients receiving comprehensive multidisciplinary services for home treatment versus hospital care.[100] Despite the cost differences during the last 2 months of life, no negative effects were found in the National Hospice Study of patients who received hospice care.[95]

QUALITY ASSURANCE

How do we monitor the quality of medicine when the morbidity and mortality of advanced cancer is anticipated?[101] The problem is compounded because real alternatives of therapy and viable clinical options are severely limited in this population. Quality studies of patient care mandate the use of defined indicators of clinical care.[102–104] Mechanisms to monitor palliative care objectives, documentation of treatment outcomes, and evaluation of staff performance all must be included in these ongoing reviews of quality assurance.[19,75,105–112] Because these patients are so close to death, the review process must identify any inappropriate treatment or intervention. For example, an examination of the use of blood products in the terminally ill revealed that patients in conventional medical settings were five times more likely to get blood than in a hospital-based hospice and ten times more likely than those patients in home-care hospices.[113] Because satisfaction and comfort outcome measures appear similar in all three groups, this specific issue would suggest monitoring the use of blood products in this population.

Because the experience of terminal disease is interwoven with issues involving quality of life, psychosocial status, and suffering, as well as the devastating physical problems, outcome measurements can be cumbersome, complex, and almost impossible to interpret. The National Hospice Study examined 1754 patients to determine whether hospice care (home- or hospital-based) improved physical and overall quality of life outcomes compared to conventional medical care.[58] Home-care hospice patients did no worse than those in conventional care, with considerably lower cost. In general, studies showed that hospice care may offer equal or more satisfaction to patients and their families than conventional settings.[114]

RESEARCH

Although clinical studies are important in all medicine, advanced cancer patients are vulnerable and must be protected. Some clinical protocols may be inappropriate for this population. Therefore, the value and safety of the research project must be established beyond doubt. Symptom-control studies

are ideal, if patients understand what is required and if possible adverse effects for patients are minimal.[19]

SUFFERING

Physicians should reflect on the concept of suffering in their daily work, especially if they are treating the dying. The objectives of medical care must emphasize patients' general well-being.[115] For example, patients may have distress beyond the severity of their pain, encompassing their psychosocial, spiritual, and cultural existence. Cassell addressed the need for medicine to recognize the patient as a person and to omit the traditional assignment of the body to medicine, and of the person to the category only of the mind.[116,117] If we accept this dichotomy, we depersonalize the patient and become the source of further suffering. This is especially evident as we examine the technological imperative of present-day medicine: doing something for patients because we *can* do it before asking whether we *ought* to do it.

Dying patients may reflect on and sometimes come to know the reasons for their own suffering because they have anguish that no other person can truly understand.[118] Suffering attacks a person's integrity and wholeness and dominates the patient's consciousness, causing sustained interior agony.[119] The diseased body becomes objectified, bound to time, place, and physical insult, and feels pain. When this perception of pain or physical insult can no longer be tolerated, the person assumes the role of a patient and seeks the advice of a physician.

It is the personal quest of the human spirit to search for meaning that enhances human dignity. The search for purpose is important and necessary because only the patient can give meaning to his or her life. Rosenthal, in an account of his own impending death, repeats that it is not death people are afraid of, but the incompleteness of their lives.[120] Indeed, each life and death have their own tempo and character. Somehow, the patient must touch the moment of discontinuity between life and death and at the same time discover that it was meaningful and worth something to have lived.

CONCLUSION

Uniting the humanity of the physician and those needing care requires an appreciation of our human drama.[121] The social ethic of medicine requires shared goals that allow patients a safe, comforting passage to a compassionate end. It is the unique ability of good clinicians to be concerned yet detached that allows a clear, logical awareness of what needs to be done for the sickest of human beings. Physicians must share the distress yet keep some distance, or they will become wounded and vulnerable themselves. These difficult cases call for attention to details that weaken the destructiveness of illness and aim to comfort.

Death is the only true democratic event. Although we must all die alone, our dependence on one another makes each death intensely shared. Illness radically tears apart the normal harmony of this interconnection of human lives, and the experience of patients dying with advanced cancer raises powerful, emotional, and sometimes conflicting issues for the physician. It is the compassionate and competent manner in which care is delivered at the end of life that helps these sickest of humans to transcend their suffering.

REFERENCES

1. Stoddard S. The hospice movement. Briarcliff Manor: Stein & Day, 1978.
2. Feifel H, ed. The meaning of death. New York: McGraw-Hill, 1959.
3. Kubler-Ross E. On death and dying. New York: Macmillan, 1969.
4. President's Commission for the Study of Ethical Problems in Medicine & Biomedical & Behavioral Research. Deciding to forego life-sustaining treatment. Washington DC, 1983:17.
5. Evolution of hospice. In: Mor V, ed. Hospice care systems. New York: Springer, 1987: 2.
6. Wachtel TJ, Mor V. Physicians' use of health resources for terminal cancer patients: Clinical setting versus physician specialty. South Med J 1987;80:1120–1124.
7. Bayer R, Feldman E. Hospice under the Medicare wing. Hastings Cent Rep 1982;12: 5–6.
8. Boring CC, Squires TS, Tong T. Cancer statistics, 1991. CA 1991;41:19–36.
9. Symposium on clinical pharmacology of symptom control. Med Clin North Am 1982;66.
10. Barsky AJ. Palliation and symptomatic relief. Arch Intern Med 1986;146:905–909.
11. Kane RL, Klein SJ, Bernstein L, et al. Hospice role in alleviating the emotional stress of terminal patients and their families. Med Care 1985;23:189–197.
12. Brescia FJ. An overview of pain and symptom management in advanced cancer. J Pain Symptom Manage 1987;2(Suppl):S7–S11.
13. Lynn J. Legal and ethical issues in palliative health care. Semin Oncol 1985;12:476–481.
14. Richter MP, Coia LR. Palliative radiation therapy. Semin Oncol 1985;12:375–383.
15. Abrams RA, Hansen RM. Radiotherapy, chemotherapy and hormonal therapy in the management of cancer pain. In: Abram SE, ed. Cancer pain: Current management of pain. Boston: Kluwer Academic, 1989:49–66.
16. Stoll BA. Quality of life as an objective in cancer treatment. In: Stoll BA, ed. Cancer treatment: Endpoint evaluation. New horizons in oncology. New York: John Wiley, 1983:113–138.
17. Braverman AS. Medical oncology in the 1990s. Lancet 1991;337:901–902.
18. Cellerino R, Tummarello D, Guidi F, et al. A randomized trial of alternating chemotherapy versus best supportive care in advanced non-small cell lung cancer. J Clin Oncol 1991;9:1453–1461.
19. Potter JF. A challenge for the hospice movement. N Engl J Med 1980;302:53–55.
20. Portenoy RK, Coyle N. Controversies in the long-term management of analgesic therapy in patients with advanced cancer. J Pain Symptom Manage 1990;5:307–319.
21. Brescia FJ, Portenoy RK, Ryan M, et al. Pain, opioid use and survival in hospitalized patients with advanced cancer. J Clin Oncol 1992;10:149–155.
22. Levy MH, Catalano RB. Control of common physical symptoms other than pain in patients with terminal disease. Semin Oncol 1985;12:411–429.
23. DeWys W. Management of cancer cachexia. Semin Oncol 1985;12:452–460.
24. Twycross RG, Lack SA. Symptom control in far-advanced cancer. London: Pitman Books, 1983.
25. Osoba D, ed. Effect of cancer on quality of life. Boston: CRC Press, 1991.
26. Kris MG, Gralla RJ. Management of vomiting caused by anticancer drugs. In: Foley KM, Bonica JJ, Ventafridda V, eds. Second International Congress on Cancer Pain: Advances in pain research and therapy, Vol. 16. New York: Raven Press, 1990:337–344.
27. Twycross RG. Management of constipation in the cancer patient with pain. In: Foley KM, Bonica JJ, Ventafridda V, eds. Second International Congress on Cancer Pain: Advances in pain research and therapy, Vol. 16. New York: Raven Press, 1990:317–326.
28. Baines MJ. Management of malignant intestinal obstruction in patients with advanced cancer. In: Foley KM, Bonica JJ, Ventafridda V, eds. Second International Congress on Cancer Pain: Advances in pain research and therapy, Vol. 16. New York: Raven Press, 1990:327–335.
29. Baines M. Nausea and vomiting in the patient with advanced cancer. J Pain Symptom Manage 1988;3:81–85.
30. Bruera E, MacDonald RN. Asthenia in patients with advanced cancer. J Pain Symptom Manage 1988;3:9–14.
31. Cowcher K, Hanks GW. Long-term management of respiratory symptoms in advanced cancer. J Pain Symptom Manage 1990;5:320–330.
32. Coyle N, Adelhardt J, Foley KM, et al. Character of terminal illness in the advanced cancer patient: Pain and other symptoms during the last 4 weeks of life. J Pain Symptom Manage 1990;5:83–93.
33. DeConno F, Ventafridda V, Saita L. Skin problems in advanced and terminal cancer patients. J Pain Symptom Manage 1991;6:247–256.
34. Hagen NA. An approach to cough in cancer patients. J Pain Symptom Manage 1991;6: 257–262.
35. Higginson I, McCarthy M. Measuring symptoms in terminal cancer: Are pain and dyspnoea controlled? J Royal Soc Med 1989;82:264–267.
36. Kolodzik PW, Eilers MA. Hiccups (singultus): Review and approach to management. Ann Emerg Med 1991;20:565–573.
37. Madden EJ. Itch. J Pain Symptom Manage 1986;1:97–99.
38. Collaud T, Rapin CH. Dehydration in dying patients: Study with physicians in French-speaking Switzerland. J Pain Symptom Manage 1991;6:230–240.
39. Levy MH. Integration of pain management into comprehensive cancer care. Cancer 1989;63:2328–2335.
40. Ventafridda V, Ripamonti C, DeConno F, et al. Symptom prevalence and control during cancer patients' last days of life. J Palliat Care 1990;6:7–11.
41. Reuben DB, Mor V. Dyspnea in terminally ill cancer patients. Chest 1986;89:234–236.
42. Fishbein D, Kearon C, Killian KJ. An approach to dyspnea in cancer patients. J Pain Symptom Manage 1989;4:76–81.
43. Pearlman RA. Inaccurate predictions of life expectancy: Dilemmas and opportunities. Arch Intern Med 1988;148:2537–2538.
44. Addington-Hall JM, MacDonald LD, Anderson HR. Can the Spitzer Quality of Life Index help to reduce prognostic uncertainty in terminal care? Br J Cancer 1990;62: 695–699.
45. Schonwetter RS, Teasdale TA, Storey P, et al. Estimation of survival time in terminal cancer patients: An impedance to hospice admissions? Hosp J 1991;6:65–79.
46. Forster LE, Lynn J. Predicting life span for applicants to inpatient hospice. Arch Intern Med 1988;148:2540–2543.
47. Reuben DB, Mor V, Hiris J. Clinical symptoms and length of survival in patients with terminal cancer. Arch Intern Med 1988;148:1586–1591.
48. Morris JN, Sherwood S. Quality of life of cancer patients at different stages in the disease trajectory. J Chronic Dis 1987;40:545–553.
49. Morris JN, Suissa S, Sherwood S, et al. Last days: A study of the quality of life of terminally ill cancer patients. J Chronic Dis 1986;39:47–62.
50. Brescia FJ, Adler D, Gray G, et al. Hospitalized advanced cancer patients: A profile. J Pain Symptom Manage 1990;5:221–227.
51. Adams AB. Dilemmas of hospice: A critical look at its problems. CA 1984;34:183–190.
52. Hyman RB, Bulkin W. Physician-reported incentives and disincentives for referring patients to hospice. Hosp J 1991;6:39–64.
53. Problems in the care of the dying patient. In Zimmerman JM, ed. Hospice: Complete care for the terminally ill. Baltimore: Urban & Schwarzenberg, 1981:1–12.
54. Parkes CM. Terminal care: Home, hospital, or hospice? Lancet 1985;1:155–157.
55. Ventafridda V, DeConno F, Vigano A, et al. Comparison of home and hospital care of advanced cancer patients. Tumori 1989;75:619–625.
56. Townsend J, Frank AO, Fermont D, et al. Terminal cancer care and patients' preference for place of death: A prospective study. Br Med J 1990;301:415–417.
57. McCusker J. The use of home care in terminal cancer. Am J Prev Med 1985;1:42–52.
58. Quality of life outcomes. In: Mor V, ed. Hospice care systems. New York: Springer, 1987:125–176.
59. Wilkes E. Dying now. Lancet 1984;1:950–952.
60. Brescia FJ, Sadof M, Barstow J. Retrospective analysis of a home care hospice program. Omega 1984;15:37–44.
61. Kane RL, Bernstein L, Wales J, et al. Hospice effectiveness in controlling pain. JAMA 1985;253:2683–2686.
62. Vinciguerra V, Degnan TJ, Sciortino A, et al. A comparative assessment of home versus hospital comprehensive treatment for advanced cancer patients. J Clin Oncol 1986;4: 1521–1528.
63. Smith DH, Granbois JA. The American way of hospice. Hastings Cent Rep 1982;12: 8–10.
64. Scham M, Scham A. Hospices: Medical and legal considerations. Leg Med 1985;297–322.
65. Veatch RM. Cross-cultural perspectives in medical ethics. Boston: Jones & Bartlett, 1989.
66. Wanzer SH, Federman DD, Adelstein SJ, et al. The physician's responsibility toward hopelessly ill patients: A second look. N Engl J Med 1989;320:844–849.
67. Tobias JS, Tattersall MH. Doing the best for the cancer patient. Lancet 1985;1:35–37.
68. Lo B, Jonsen AR. Ethical decisions in the care of a patient terminally ill with metastatic cancer. Ann Intern Med 1980;92:107–111.
69. Novack DH, Plumer R, Smith RL, et al. Changes in physicians' attitudes toward telling the cancer patient. JAMA 1979;241:897–900.
70. Roy DJ. Ethical issues in the treatment of cancer patients. J Palliat Care 1989;5:56–60.
71. Goetzler RM, Moskowitz MA. Changes in physician attitudes toward limiting care of critically ill patients. Arch Intern Med 1991;151:1537–1540.
72. Meisel A. Legal myths about terminating life support. Arch Intern Med 1991;151: 1497–1502.
73. Brock DW, Wartman SA. When competent patients make irrational choices. N Engl J Med 1990;322:1595–1599.
74. Brescia FJ. A philosophy of care: Notes of a death watcher. J Pain Symptom Manage 1988;3:212–214.
75. Brescia FJ. The goals and challenges of palliative care: Thoughts of a death watcher. J Pain Symptom Manage 1990;5:382–384.
76. Lynn J, ed. By no extraordinary means. Bloomington: Indiana University Press, 1986.
77. Brescia FJ. Killing the known dying: Notes of a death watcher. J Pain Symptom Manage 1991;6:337–339.
78. Cimino JE. Medical ethics and the decision to feed or not to feed: A physician speaks. Top Clin Nutr 1991;6:72–75.
79. Tomlinson T, Brody H. Futility and the ethics of resuscitation. JAMA 1990;264:1276–1280.
80. Emanuel EJ. A review of the ethical and legal aspects of terminating medical care. Am J Med 1988;84:291–301.
81. Battin MP. Euthanasia: The way we do it, the way they do it. J Pain Symptom Manage 1991;6:298–305.
82. Clouser KD. The challenge for future debate on euthanasia. J Pain Symptom Manage 1991;6:306–311.
83. Klagsbrun SC. Physician-assisted suicide: A double dilemma. J Pain Symptom Manage 1991;6:325–328.
84. Lachs J. Active euthanasia. J Clin Ethics 1990;1:113–115.
85. Goodwin JS. Mercy killing: Mercy for whom? JAMA 1991;265:326.
86. Singer PA, Siegler M. Euthanasia—a critique. N Engl J Med 1990;322:1881–1883.

87. Magno JB. The role of the physician when cure is no longer possible. Linacre Q 1991;58: 79–88.
88. Bayer R, Callahan D, Fletcher J, et al. The care of the terminally ill: Morality and economics. N Engl J Med 1983;309:1490–1494.
89. Cimino JE. Global trends of hospice care (unpublished data).
90. Ajemian I, Mount BM, eds. The R.V.H. manual on palliative/hospice care. Salem, N.H.: Ayer, 1980.
91. Whippen DA, Canellos GP. Burnout syndrome in the practice of oncology: Results of a random survey of 1000 oncologists. J Clin Oncol 1991;9:1916–1920.
92. Mor V, Kidder D. Cost savings in hospice: Final results of the National Hospice Study. Health Serv Res 1985;20:407–422.
93. Brody H, Lynn J. The physician's responsibility under the new Medicare reimbursement for hospice care. N Engl J Med 1984;310:920–922.
94. Hazzard WR. Geriatric medicine: Life in the crucible of the struggle to contain health-care costs. In: McCue JD, ed. The medical cost-containment crisis. Ann Arbor: Health Administration Press, 1989:266.
95. The cost of hospice. In: Mor V, ed. Hospice care systems. New York: Springer, 1987: 177–212.
96. Warren BH, Bell PL, Isikoff S, et al. Cost-containment and quality of life: An experiment in compassion for physicians. Arch Intern Med 1991;151:741–744.
97. Kidder D. The impact of hospices on the health-care costs of terminal cancer patients. In: Mor V, Greer DS, Kastenbaum R, eds. The hospice experiment. Baltimore: Johns Hopkins University Press, 1988:48–68.
98. Kidder D. Hospice services and cost savings in the last weeks of life. In: Mor V, Greer DS, Kastenbaum R, eds. The hospice experiment. Baltimore: Johns Hopkins University Press, 1988:69–87.
99. Gray D, MacAdam D, Boldy D. A comparative cost analysis of terminal cancer care in home hospice patients and controls. J Chronic Dis 1987;40:801–810.
100. Vinciguerra V, Degnan TJ, Budman DR, et al. Comparative cost analysis of home and hospital treatment. In: Mortensen LE, Engstrom PF, Anderson PN, eds. Advances in cancer control: Health care financing and research. New York: Alan R. Liss, 1986: 155–164.
101. Bulkin W, Lukashok H. Rx for dying: The case for hospice. N Engl J Med 1988;318: 376–378.

102. Donovan K, Sanson-Fisher RW, Redman S. Measuring quality of life in cancer patients. J Clin Oncol 1989;7:959–968.
103. Zweibel NR. Measuring quality of life near the end of life. JAMA 1988;260:839–840.
104. Latimer E. Auditing the hospital care of dying patients. J Palliat Care 1991;7:12–17.
105. Mor V, Masterson-Allen S. A comparison of hospice versus conventional care of the terminally ill cancer patient. Oncology 1990;4:85–91.
106. Rhymes J. Hospice care in America. JAMA 1990;264:369–372.
107. Krakoff IH. The case for active treatment in patients with advanced cancer: Not everyone needs a hospice. CA 1991;29:108–111.
108. McCann BA, Enck RE. Standards for hospice care: A JCAH hospice project overview. In: Engstrom PF, Anderson PN, Mortensen LE, eds. Advances in cancer control: Epidemiology and research. New York: Alan R. Liss, 1984:431–440.
109. Rees WD. Role of the hospice in the care of the dying. Br Med J 1982;285:1766–1768.
110. Powers JS, Burger MC. Terminal care preferences: Hospice placement and severity of disease. Public Health Rep 1987;102:444–449.
111. Wallston KA, Burger C, Smith RA, et al. Comparing the quality of death for hospice and nonhospice cancer patients. Med Care 1988;26:177–182.
112. Cimino JE. Concerns for hospice. N Y Med Q 1980;2:46.
113. Wachtel TJ, Mor V. The use of transfusions in terminal cancer patients: Hospice versus conventional care setting. Transfusion 1985;25:278–279.
114. Mor V, Greer DS, Kastenbaum R, eds. The hospice experiment. Baltimore: Johns Hopkins University Press, 1988.
115. Portenoy RK. Pain and quality of life: Theoretical aspects. In: Osoba D, ed. Effect of cancer on quality of life. Boston: CRC Press, 1991:279–292.
116. Cassell EJ. Recognizing suffering. Hastings Cent Rep 1991;21:24–31.
117. Cassell EJ. The nature of suffering and the goals of medicine. New York: Oxford University Press, 1991.
118. Frankl VE. Man's search for meaning. New York: Pocket Books, 1984.
119. Gunderman RB. Medicine and the question of suffering. Second Opin 1990;14:15–25.
120. Rosenthal T. How could I not be among you? New York: George Braziller, 1973.
121. Bennahum DA. Intimations of mortality reconsidered: Terminal care. Am J Med 1980;69: 488–490.

SECTION **6**

DONNA SAMMARINO

Dealing With the Dying Patient

Despite all our advances in health care, life can only be prolonged; death cannot be eradicated. As such, we must find ways of providing optimal care to people at all stages in their lives. This seemingly fundamental notion has become a complicated challenge in our increasingly technologic arena of health care. This chapter is intended to:

1. Identify and help one understand institutional obstacles that impede the provision of optimal care to the dying in hospitals
2. Provide insight into the issues and personal difficulties that arise for caregivers when dealing with the dying
3. Identify some of the specific care needs of the terminally ill
4. Formulate practical suggestions to maximize our effectiveness when dealing with the dying.

INSTITUTIONAL OBSTACLES

Acute-care hospitals remain the most common setting for death in our society due to the large concentration of caregivers and resources within these institutions.[1] Throughout life, until the dying process begins, a person's understanding of a hospital's mission to treat health-care needs is aligned with the hospital's ability to do so. However, the care of the dying is not necessarily within the hospital's repertoire of subspecialties.

Dealing with the dying can be a positive challenge and a rewarding experience, depending largely on what caregivers bring to the situation. We must gain a clearer understanding of the needs of the dying and also must appreciate the obstacles within our health-care system that can impede even the most well-intentioned of us from providing quality care to the dying.

Balfour Mount elucidated the differences between the needs of the terminally ill and the goals of an acute-care hospital.[2] He saw the mission of a general hospital to be fourfold: "to investigate, to diagnose, to cure, and to prolong life." For the terminally ill, the only appropriate goal is improvement of the quality of life through palliative care. The problem arises when we introduce into the acute-care environment patients who challenge the expertise of the health-care team. In the management of the dying, the skills of investigating and diagnosing are important, but with a view toward palliation and symptom management rather than cure and prolongation of life. What results is a misalignment between what the patient needs and what the staff can offer. The perception exists in this acute-care setting that "nothing can be done" for the dying patient. Therefore, the health-care team may feel frustrated and incompetent and may become angry or apathetic. What may appear on the surface as indifference may actually be a manifestation of guilt, anxiety, and insecurity. Often the staff distance themselves from patients and families, aggravating the problem.

Mount's study of attitudes toward the dying at the Royal Victoria Hospital in Montreal confirmed that there were deficiencies in the care of the dying. The medical, emotional, and spiritual needs of these patients and their families were often neglected. The staff felt inadequately prepared to meet their needs. Nurses did not welcome being assigned to dying patients. Physician visits decreased in frequency as the patients' length of stay increased. Nursing care decreased as death approached, despite the fact that patients' needs increased. For example, it took longer to answer the call bells of dying patients than those of patients with a better prognosis. Lack of communication and deficiencies in care led to patient isolation and to feelings of suspicion and mistrust among patients, family members, nurses, and physicians. Physicians and nurses felt poorly prepared to communicate openly and honestly with patients and families and as a result spent less time with the dying. Moreover, the staff felt that the efficient execution of their regular routines was disrupted by the dying patients.[2]

Hospital routines are designed to promote efficiency and to satisfy the needs of the staff in acute-care units.[2] Such routines can serve as obstacles as death approaches and the total emphasis is on diminution of suffering. Similarly, the physical environment of an acute-care hospital is not optimal for dying patients. Often, even if staff have the skills to render palliative care, the constraints of an acute-care environment can impede the implementation of such interventions. Visiting hours and policies are restrictive. Private rooms are reserved for isolation cases, not for the terminally ill. There is little room or time to deal with families. There is little training for staff to communicate appropriately with families, let alone include them as a unit of care.[3]

Terminally ill patients should always have the option of having loved ones present and available to them throughout this final phase of their illness. Most acute-care hospitals will make this provision only when the patient is deemed to be at the point of death. Even when loved ones are permitted, there is limited space; the room is crowded with sophisticated equipment of little value in the care of the terminally ill, and it is often difficult to remove. Acute-care hospitals also must comply with building codes, governmental regulations, and accreditation standards that make the creation of a more homelike environment for the terminally ill very difficult.[1]

There are real concerns about where to put the dying in an acute-care hospital. The impact of the death on the living, both bereaved family members and other patients, must be considered. Postmortem care and the transport of the body to the morgue are visible on the unit, despite institutional efforts to conceal them. Grieving families are entitled to time with the newly dead as part of the bereavement process. This is often impractical in an acute-care hospital: either another patient is waiting for the bed of the deceased, or the roommate needs treatment and support.

In their study of the hospitalized dying, Glaser and Strauss pointed out that as these patients are trying to exert some control over their remaining lives, they must expend a large amount of energy trying to learn how to be acceptable patients while in the hospital.[4] This type of energy expenditure is inappropriate and unfair: these patients are already struggling to enhance the quality of their remaining lives. Continued and inevitable loss of physical control is demoralizing, and the terminally ill have the ever-present awareness that they will soon cease to have any influence over anything.

PERSONAL OBSTACLES

It is not uncommon for dying patients to be perceived as socially dead even before their physical death occurs. The irony is that this occurs at the time of a person's greatest need.[5]

Dying patients thus become victims of our inability to deal with them. Such distancing thwarts the patients' and families' attempts to process and integrate all that is happening. Rather, patients are left to analyze the reason for our abandonment and remain with a sense of shame for being terminal. There is a pervasive tendency to equate the inability to cure the incurable with failure. Dying patients are very sensitive to this notion, as it is often communicated to them by physicians.

Caring for and dealing with dying patients can be unsettling for caregivers, as it forces each of us to confront our mortality and arouses our preconceptions about dying. Ultimately we must gain some understanding, both as humans and collectively as a profession, of what it is that makes us uncomfortable around dying patients.[6] Only by acknowledging our personal limitations, as well as those of our health-care system in a death-denying society, can we even begin to help those at the most vulnerable, frightening part of their lives.

Part of understanding the plight of the dying is to question why we have been allowed to be remiss in this area of health care for so long, and why the deficiencies in terminal care are not more widely recognized. Mount offered two explanations.[2] First, health-care providers prefer to see themselves as sensitive and responsive to the needs of others. Second, patients are loath to criticize their physicians. Mount found that staff members were more likely to identify inadequacies in care on the parts of their colleagues than they were to acknowledge their own deficiencies. The staff attributed to their colleagues greater avoidance of discussions with patients about dying than they recognized in themselves.

A final possible explanation is that both the bereaved and the caregiver are likely to repress recollections of the dying experience of a loved one or patient. This decreases the chance that the caregiver's wisdom and expertise in this area will grow. It also makes it less likely that caregivers will be motivated—from without or within—to improve their delivery of terminal care.

THE DYING PROCESS

As with any other stage of life, there are tasks and needs unique to those living through the final stage. As with all developmental phases of life, there is pain and change, which ideally results in adaption. But how does one adapt to dying? There is a vast difference between having the cognitive awareness that death is universal and we each will someday die, and being the person confronted with the terminal illness. The crisis of dying calls into question our previous coping mechanisms of denial and repression of death.

People who are dying must reorient themselves by adjusting to all present and impending losses. The dying person experiences loss and death on various levels. There is social death, in which the dying person must learn to separate from the living. The phenomenon of losing our status and who we are is known as phenomenologic death. Psychological death involves the loss of the personality, the essence of a person. Psychological death occurs as the patient acknowledges that he or she will no longer exist. Simultaneously, a biologic death is occurring, and physical deterioration is an ever-present reminder that at the end of this experience, all that will be left are a person's remains.[7]

Our goal as caregivers is to make this overwhelming process

of dying more manageable for patients, families, and ourselves.

MEDICAL AND NURSING NEEDS OF THE TERMINALLY ILL

The care of the dying is both a science and an art. We must help patients cope with the high-tech medical environment that commonly surrounds them at the point of death. The concept of a "good death" should mean more than simply withholding aggressive measures. It also demands that we create an environment that allows for a peaceful, comfortable death. Doing so requires familiarity with the unique care needs of the terminally ill.

Inadequate or inappropriate management of pain and other symptoms is a major source of distress for dying patients. The pain of a terminal illness is not just physical pain. By the time a person has reached the terminal stage of disease, he or she suffers from many other types of pain, including mental, financial, interpersonal, and spiritual. Caregivers must pay attention to the whole person if they expect to affect this type of pain. However, a common error is to focus solely on the psychological and emotional needs of the dying; physical comfort comes first. Counseling a dying patient who is lying in a wet bed is ineffective.

Although the basic goals of pain management are somewhat similar in both cure-oriented and palliative contexts, the distinctive aspects of the situation of dying patients demand distinctive responses.

Acute pain can be significant but is usually of short duration. It can be classified as mild, moderate, or severe in intensity. Acute pain is associated with resolvable or reversible problems. For acute pain, treatment on a prn or as-needed basis is usually adequate. The patient's expectation is that the pain will be of finite duration, which is correct.

Unlike acute pain, chronic pain cannot be easily classified according to severity. Chronic pain can be seen as a "circular continuum of aching to agony."[8] The difference between tolerable chronic aching and intolerable chronic agony sometimes depends on the nature of the physical cause (*e.g.*, tumor involvement in bone or nerve plexus). However, equally important are the psychoemotional and social factors that inevitably exacerbate the pain. Unlike acute pain, chronic pain is not associated with recovery. It does not resolve rapidly, which in and of itself generates more anxiety and depression, which then lead to feelings of isolation and hostility.[8] Acute pain warns of a malfunction; chronic pain often dominates the patient's life to the exclusion of all else.

The terminally ill patient must receive whatever is necessary to control pain. Despite the recent advances in care of the dying, many practitioners still struggle with this concept. They continue to fear the legal repercussions of liberal narcotic use, which may depress respirations and blood pressure. They are also in a dilemma about the implications of assisted suicide or euthanasia. These fears are certainly well founded in an age of defensive medicine. The outcome, however, is a pervasive fear among patients, families, and the public at large that inadequate pain control will result in needless suffering. Fear of dying in pain is a common concern expressed by patients and families, and these fears are often valid.

A recent article in the *New England Journal of Medicine*

took a strong stand on minimizing pain and suffering in a patient whose dying process is irreversible, even if this means potentially hastening death.[9] Wanzer and associates wrote that it is morally correct to use whatever narcotics are needed, in whatever doses and by whatever routes, even if this may decrease blood pressure or respirations or cause a loss of consciousness. Fears of addiction have no place in terminal care, and physicians, patients, and families alike must be reminded of this. Reassurance from the physician to patients and families that pain will be controlled should begin at the outset, when a fatal disease is diagnosed.

Other common physical symptoms experienced by the terminally ill that require skilled management are anorexia, nausea and vomiting, dry mouth, dyspnea, cough, hiccups, anxiety, confusion, depression, insomnia, constipation, incontinence, diarrhea, itch, and mental distress.[10] Narcotic and nonnarcotic medications are needed for the management of these and other symptoms. Benzodiazepines, metaclopramide, antihistamines, tricyclic antidepressants, phenothiazines, and other major and minor tranquilizers are used frequently.

The care needs of the terminally ill usually increase as death approaches. The patient becomes increasingly debilitated and dependent on staff for performing activities of daily living. Things that are usually taken for granted, such as mobility and personal hygiene, must now be performed by one human for another. Controlling all the symptoms requires tremendous time, patience, and compassion on the part of the caregivers. As Wanzer and associates wrote, "Dying patients may require palliative care of an intensity that challenges even that of curative efforts. . . [P]rofessionals . . . are still called upon to use intensive measures—extreme responsibility, extraordinary sensitivity and heroic compassion."[9]

PSYCHOEMOTIONAL NEEDS OF THE TERMINALLY ILL

The implications of a cancer diagnosis are vast. The emotional responses range from the expectation of cure, to hope for chronicity, to expectation of a terminal illness. For cancer patients, it is often difficult to determine when the dying process begins. Kastenbaum wrote that dying usually begins as a psychosocial event.[11] The optimal course of events is initiated by the physician's recognition that effective treatment options are no longer available. This should then be communicated to the patient. Ideally, the patient accepts the fact that nothing more can be done medically to preserve life. Once an acutely ill cancer patient becomes terminally ill, a grief response begins for all present, past, and future losses.

Merely contemplating one's own mortality causes some degree of anxiety. For terminally ill people, forced to confront their own imminent death, immense anxiety composed of specific fears is a major emotional response. There are fears of the unknown, loneliness, loss of self-control, loss of all loved ones, and loss of bodily functions. There are fears of pain and suffering, sorrow, regression, mutilation, decomposition, and premature burial.[7] Caregivers and family must help the dying to break down their anxiety into its components to make it manageable.

Depression, anger, guilt, and shame are common responses of the dying. Acceptance, withdrawal, detachment, and hope are also central issues. The nature and quality of hope change as the patient progresses through the stages of terminal illness. It is no longer hope of cure, but hope for a certain quality of remaining life. It is a day-to-day hope that enables the person to keep some control, dignity, and sense of worth.[7]

Caregivers also have an emotional response to cancer and to death and dying. With acute-care patients, although the prognosis is uncertain, caregivers can rely on experience to predict the direction things will take. In terminal care, the prognosis is known but what lies beyond is unknown to all.

To enable the dying to perform the last tasks of their lives with some degree of dignity and self-determination, caregivers must create a maximally supportive environment for those with limited energy. To do this, we are asked to put aside our professional and personal egos for a time and become active listeners. This requires a role reversal of sorts, which is often uncomfortable for physicians and nurses to perform. It means allowing the dying patients and their families to be our teachers and to communicate to us their real needs and concerns. This is not only the beginning, but the essence of what it takes to deal with dying patients.

WHAT CAN BE DONE?

Those who work closely with the terminally ill would like to maximize their effectiveness, despite institutional obstacles and individual limitations. A recent survey at a comprehensive cancer center revealed the following notable trends among the medical attending and nursing staff at the study institution.[12] The staff confirmed the existence of a patient population identified as terminally ill who required a significant amount of time and resources. They recognized the unique care needs of the terminally ill and acknowledged that certain institutional obstacles led to deficiencies in the care of this group in deference to the more acutely ill. For example, the staff recognized a tendency to respond first to the acutely ill patient if both types of patients required attention at the same time; they also admitted to some discomfort with this choice. They perceived that the continuity of care was inadequate in the present system, and the staff strongly preferred to follow their primary patients from the point of diagnosis through their final stages of life. They expressed an interest in finding solutions to more effectively deal with dying patients, and there was overwhelming support for the development of a formal program devoted to this end.

Irrespective of the setting of death, certain ways of relating to the dying person are essential. Thanatologic conversation is a unique type of communication between caregiver and patient. It is not ordinary conversation that occurs among friends, it is not the hierarchical conversation typical of the physician-patient relationship, and it is not the professional conversation of psychotherapy. It is an interaction between two humans, both acknowledging their common fate. It is a flexible communication that takes place in the present, with the awareness of the inevitable downhill course to follow. It requires a tremendous amount of empathy on the caregiver's part, with no place for sympathy or pity. It acknowledges the entire ambience of the dying process and thereby extends to family members and friends as well. The goals of such an interaction are to support and comfort patients and to help them find value in their remaining days.

For any interaction with the dying person to be effective,

the caregiver must not fear the patient. A certain amount of death anxiety is normal when seeing a human who is dying or dead. However, caregivers must distinguish this general anxiety from more specific fears of the particular dying patient to whom they are attending. Caregivers commonly express fears that, although irrational, are important to recognize and deal with. Death and the process of dying are not contagious. Avoiding the dying patient does not confer immortality. Practitioners should not view their patients who become terminally ill as failures. This perception is self-serving and egocentric and creates additional anxiety for caregivers and patients. No patient wants to be seen as a failure, and it is equally uncomfortable for a practitioner to cast himself or herself as a failure.

Death has been viewed as the great equalizer among us, and this notion can help allay our fears of being with a dying patient. As Ajeman and Mount wrote, "The doctor, being himself a mortal man, should be diligent and tender in relieving his suffering patients inasmuch as he himself must one day be a like sufferer."[13]

Our efforts will be continually thwarted if we try to have every patient die a peaceful death with total acceptance and freedom from denial. This is rarely the case. We do ourselves and our patients an injustice by setting unrealistic goals. It is a myth to think we can help a person accept death. We cannot make the unknown familiar and eradicate all associated fears. We cannot render good and pretty that which is often bad and ugly. We as caregivers should repress this societally enforced tendency of avoiding unpleasantness when dealing with the dying.

To varying degrees throughout our lives, we all use the defense mechanism of denial with regard to death. Death is something we hold in abeyance somewhere out there in the distant future. Therefore, it is unrealistic for us as caregivers to believe that we can completely break down this protective mechanism, which has been nurtured for a lifetime. It is also unfair to our patients. At best, what usually occurs is that patients acknowledge the inevitable outcome: they will cease to be. As caregivers, we should strive to help the patients cope with the ramifications of this recognition.

It is equally important to acknowledge other limitations as clinical practitioners. Sometimes it is impossible to effectively manage all the symptoms of dying patients. This is particularly true when patients, along with other physically distressing problems, present with an altered mental state or mental distress of questionable etiology. These symptoms are often resistant to treatment, and we tend to throw up our hands in dismay due to our frustration and feelings of helplessness.

In these extraordinarily difficult cases, the desirable patient outcome of a peaceful, comfortable death will not be achieved. This can raise doubts for even the most caring and tenacious oncology practitioners as to our purpose: if we cannot even help a person die comfortably, what is the point? The main goal in this situation is not to turn away from the patient and family. Honest disclosure of the difficulty in controlling such symptoms can allay anxieties and offer reassurance that the symptom is not being ignored. We should also avoid focusing on the refractory symptoms to the exclusion of others. One is not seen as an inadequate physician or nurse because of the inability to manage *all* the distressing symptoms of the dying.

We caregivers must direct our energy toward what we can do for the dying. In many ways, it is the simplest offering of all. Yet perhaps because of its fundamental nature, we fail to recognize its importance and instead focus on our feelings of inadequacy or impotence. The most important thing we can offer our patients is our presence. We can easily relieve patients' fears that we will abandon and reject them because they are dying. We bring our skills and expertise in management and control of the symptoms of dying, but to be most effective we need to do more, and in this case, the more is less. We must learn to just be there: to listen, look, and try to understand what is happening for the particular person at this point in time. This concept is foreign to us and represents the total antithesis of our medical training. We need to relinquish control and take our cues from the patient. We should refrain from our tendency to stereotype and assume we know the needs of the dying. They will tell us if we just give them the time to do so.

From clinical experience, the willingness and ability to *listen* is the single most important characteristic a caregiver can bring to a dying patient. I have seen a sincerely concerned housekeeper, having daily contact and conversation with a dying patient, be more effective than the physician who was rushing in and out of the patient's room each morning reciting the plan for the day. In such circumstances, the greatest effectiveness comes from eliciting information from the patient about what he or she considers important and valuable. Not all dying patients want their hands held or their families maintaining a vigil at the bedside. We may assume this is how it should be because it makes us feel better, but we should not write the scripts for the dying.

The only way to overcome our trained tendency "to do" is to occupy our time by being with the patient and listening. This need not take endless hours that health-care professionals seldom have to spare. Rather, it is our sincerity and the quality of the time we give the person when we are present that is important. Certainly it is the dying patient who is most acutely aware of the passage of time.

Asking questions of the patient is encouraged. Certain questions may facilitate conversation, such as are you comfortable, do you feel like talking, what's on your mind, are you frightened. Then wait for the answer. Do not start something you cannot finish; if you are pressed for time, say so. Reassuring patients of your routine and thereby explaining your absences goes a long way toward allaying their fears of abandonment. Often is is us, not our dying patients, who impose unrealistic expectations on caregivers.

The dying often are acutely aware of and gain a sense of peace from the notion that life goes on. This brings a certain sense of familiarity and comfort in knowing that although life will cease to be for them, it goes on for others. This is why it is common for those of us who routinely talk with the dying to find ourselves discussing a multitude of topics totally unrelated to death. This, too, can be therapeutic and consoling; it should not be viewed as wasted time.

Entering into a relationship with a dying person involves some of the same dynamics as any other human interaction. Trust must be built through mutual understanding. The difference is that time is of the essence, so it behooves us to get it right the first time for the sake of the patient. Maintaining reasonable expectations of ourselves and our dying patients will allow a mutually fulfilling experience to occur. Caregivers need not underestimate the contribution their presence and genuine expressions of concern bring to a dying person. One of the few tangible guarantees we can give our patients is that we will not abandon or reject them, however threatened we are by their dying.

We must view the dying person from several different perspectives: in relation to the illness and the physical symptoms, in light of his or her psychological response to impending death, and in relation to others. There may come a time of pulling back on the patient's part. Usually this state of self-involvement comes after a period of enhanced emotional connection with and affirmation of feelings for those around him or her, both family and caregivers. At this time, it is helpful for us to shift our focus to the family and reassure them that their efforts have not been in vain. We should remember this advice for ourselves too at this time. This again requires our unselfish understanding, to step back and give the dying patient space and permission to begin to disconnect from all that he or she will soon lose totally.

There are few rules in thanatologic communication, but some pointers can enrich the experience. Throughout the dying process, honest communication must be maintained. To lie to or withhold information from the dying is cruel. Depriving them of such information could deny them crucial control over their remaining time. However, such disclosures should be handled sensitively, with the patient guiding the pace. Let the patient's level of comfort and understanding determine the pace, not your own. Ask questions and wait for answers. Of course, the ultimate question of "why" is completely unanswerable. As we discussed above, through all of this, hope is never totally taken away, but its nature changes. It is no longer hope for cure, but a hope to get through the next day with a sense of purpose and worth.

In being with people who are dying, try not to be afraid of them. Touch them, look at them, maintain eye contact, be aware of your body language. Pull up a chair so you are looking at them equally and not standing up and looking down at them in their beds. Listen and accept what you hear. Elicit their fears and concerns. Take action where you can and accept things over which you have no control. You cannot prevent death, but you can do your best to ensure that the dying guide their course to the extent possible.

It is really quite simple. Running away and leaving the matters of the dying to the clergy alone does not yield immortality or even professional fulfillment. The plight of the dying cannot be reversed, but it can be made easier if all members of the health-care team remember that the dying are still among the living; they are not yet dead. They should be treated with respect and sensitivity.

Greater effectiveness in dealing with the dying can really only be taught from doing so and being there. It is hoped that this chapter might make each of us more willing and able to learn.

REFERENCES

1. Grinslades S, Reko R. Hospital-based inpatient hospice units: Planning considerations. In: Corr CA, Corr DM, eds. Hospice care—principles and practice. New York: Springer, 1983:294–307.
2. Mount BM. The problem of caring for the dying in a general hospital: The palliative care unit as a possible solution. Can Med Assoc J 1976;115:119–121.
3. McNulty EB, Holdershy RA. Hospice, a caring challenge. Chicago: Charles L. Thomas, 1983.

4. Glaser BG, Strauss AL. Time for dying. Chicago: Aldine, 1968.

5. Cox JJ. Caring for the dying: Reflections of a medical student. Can Med Assoc J 1987;136: 577–579.

6. Bulkin W, Lukashok H. Rx for dying: The case for hospice. N Engl J Med 1988;318: 376–378.

7. Rando T. Grief, dying and death. Chicago: Research Press, 1984.

8. Lipman AG. Drug therapy of chronic pain. In: Corr CA, Corr DM, eds. Hospice care—principles and practice. New York: Springer, 1983:73–87.

9. Wanzer SH, Federman DD, Adelstein SJ, et al. The physician's responsibility toward hopelessly ill patients. N Engl J Med 1989;320:844–849.

10. Barnes M. Drug control of common symptoms. In: Corr CA, Corr DM, eds. Hospice care—principles and practice. New York: Springer, 1983:89–97.

11. Kastenbaum RJ. Death, society and human experience. St. Louis: CV Mosby, 1981.

12. Sammarino D. Caring for the terminally ill cancer patient within an acute-care cancer center: Analysis and alternatives. Unpublished master's thesis, Department of Health and Nutrition Science, Brooklyn College, 1990.

13. Ajeman I, Mount BM, eds. The R.V.H. manual on palliative hospice care. Salem, NH: Ayer, 1982.

GRACE H. CHRIST
ROSEMARY T. MOYNIHAN
MATTHEW LOSCALZO
LOIS L. WEINSTEIN

SECTION 7

Providing Community Resources for Cancer Patients

A patient diagnosed with cancer may require a range of services over the course of the illness. As a consequence of the disease, treatment, and rehabilitation, the patient may need concrete services such as personal care, household assistance, medical equipment, child care, financial assistance, transportation, and information and counseling. These needs also may arise as a result of the demands of the health-care system, bureaucratic complications, financial limitations, and the emotional problems that patients and families often experience during a major illness. If these needs are unmet, patients may be unable to comply with intensive treatment regimens, may experience low morale that affects treatment-related decisions, may fail to resume active functioning after acute episodes of illness, and may experience an overall reduction in functioning and quality of life.

Resources to meet patients' concrete and emotional needs have never been more essential to treatment and recovery than in the contemporary medical climate. In recent years, the trend in the United States toward "dehospitalization" has affected oncology as well as other fields. Extended outpatient care, ambulatory surgical and radiation treatment centers, day treatment hospitals, and home administration of complex chemotherapies and associated treatments testify to the move away from the hospital as the locus of care. At the same time, cancer has become a chronic rather than an acute illness for increasing numbers of patients. The net effect of these trends is that greater demands are placed on informal and formal support systems in the family and community.

Demands for practical assistance in the home arise from patients' inability to meet daily living and treatment-related tasks. These tasks increase as the disease progresses and are complicated by the toxic side effects of treatment. Many of these needs, formerly handled in the hospital, must now be met by family members and other informal caregivers. Studies have documented, however, that this assistance often is inadequate.[1–3] In response to these changed conditions, studies on the prevalence of such needs identified barriers to service delivery and led to the development of new methods of delivery, new models of provision of care, different types of community services, and more comprehensive systems of care.

The services that cancer patients need can be divided into six categories:

1. *Cancer information, education, and counseling:* Individual or family counseling, support groups, veteran patient programs, marital counseling, sexual counseling, and spiritual counseling[4]
2. *Home care:* Personal care, including injections, care of catheters, stoma management, nasogastric tube feeding, pain management, occupational therapy, and so on; household assistance such as housecleaning, meal preparation, laundry, and shopping[5–7]
3. *Alternatives to home care:* Nursing homes, hospices, and so forth
4. *Equipment:* Wheelchairs, walkers, bath benches, hospital beds, intravenous poles and pumps, stoma bags, and the like[6,7]
5. *Financial assistance:* Income maintenance and help with the cost of treatment
6. *Transportation:* Ambulances, ambulettes, taxis, car services, and so on.[8]

This chapter presents the findings of recent research on the prevalence of these needs, defines the range of community resources available to meet them, describes new intervention models, and identifies evolving problems in the provision of community services. It also presents the range of resources available, reviews the indicators of need for such services, and describes ways of finding services in the community.

PREVALENCE OF NEEDS

Several recent studies have attempted to estimate the prevalence of cancer patients' needs for concrete assistance. Although earlier studies documented the importance of these needs and the fact that needs increased with progression of the disease and with age, their use of different definitions and measures of need and heterogenous samples of patients made it difficult to compare results.[3,9,10] In the more recent studies, careful definition of needs, better methods of data collection, and use of specific populations of patients at different stages of disease and treatment allowed comparisons of results.

In a randomized survey of 629 cancer patients selected from the Pennsylvania Cancer Registry and 397 support persons, Houts and colleagues found that 59% of the patients had at least one unmet psychosocial need during the first year after diagnosis.[2] The unmet need cited most often was for emotional support (25% of the patients cited this need). In a second study conducted with a stratified random sample of 433 significant others of patients who had recently died, Houts and colleagues found that 72% of the patients had had at least one unmet need during their final month of life.[11] The unmet needs reported most often were help with activities of daily living (42%), emotional support (21%), physical assistance (21%), communication problems with medical staff (20%), insurance (19%), and financial support (15%).

Mor and associates surveyed the unmet needs for concrete services of 217 patients with advanced cancer and family members who were already receiving agency services in New York City and found that age, duration of disease, education, income, gender, marital status, living arrangements, and pain were related to the degree of need.[3] More than half of the patients (51%) reported at least one unmet need, and most indicated unmet instrumental needs such as meal preparation, housekeeping, shopping, and home health care.

In a subsequent study, Guadagnoli and Mor interviewed 412 patients, 70% of whom received care in a private oncology practice in Rhode Island.[12] Ninety percent of these patients needed help with an activity of daily living. The unmet needs cited most often were help with heavy housework, shopping, and completing forms and other paperwork. Fewer than a third (26.7%) received help with at least one activity of daily living from a formal source. The vast majority (84%) received help with at least one daily living activity from informal sources (usually a family member). The level of unmet need (26%) in the second study was lower than expected, possibly because the patients lived in rural areas and fewer than two thirds of them (62%) had advanced disease.

The differences in these results were attributable to the fact that Houts assessed the need for emotional support, which accounted for 25% of the prevalence rate, but Mor did not. In the latter studies, the level of unmet need varied as a function of the level of confidence in the ability of others to provide help and the number of helpers available, as well as physical functioning and age.

Siegel and colleagues conducted in-depth interviews with 200 outpatients with advanced disease who were receiving chemotherapy at Memorial Sloan-Kettering Cancer Center and found that 62% reported at least one unmet need within the previous month; 39% reported two or more.[13,14] The mean number of unmet needs was about 1.7. Furthermore, the patients exhibited a marked lack of knowledge about the services available in their community. The estimation of prevalence of needs was based on a cross-sectional design and included patients who had been in treatment for different periods of time. If the sample had been followed longitudinally, the proportion of patients with one or more unmet needs at any point in the course of treatment would have been significantly greater.

Finally, in a survey of caregiver burden and unmet patient needs among 483 patients and their informal caregivers that did not include an assessment of the need for psychological counseling, only 18.9% of the patients reported an unmet need.[15] Because a more restricted definition of unmet need was used in this study, the prevalence rate was lower. In addition, patients with early- and late-stage cancer were included. Significant predictors of unmet needs were:

1. The patient's illness and treatment resulted in restricted ability to perform tasks of daily life.
2. The patient's financial resources were so limited that he or she was forced to apply for Medicaid or welfare.
3. The spouse was not the patient's caregiver.
4. The care provided was associated with a high level of burden.

Table 64–32 summarizes the results of these studies. The varying percentages of unmet needs were the result of dif-

TABLE 64–32. Recent Studies on the Prevalence of Cancer Patients' Unmet Psychosocial Needs

Source	Study Population	Prevalence
Included the Need for Emotional Counseling		
Houts et al[2]	Randomized survey of 629 patients and 397 support persons	59% reported at least one unmet need; 25% needed emotional support
Houts et al[11]	Randomized survey of 433 significant others of patients who had died	72% reported at least one unmet need during the final month of life
Did Not Include the Need for Emotional Counseling		
Mor et al[3]	217 patients and family members already receiving help from a cancer service agency	51% reported at least one unmet service need; the longer the duration of the disease, the higher the prevalence rate
Christ and Siegel[14]	200 outpatients with advanced disease	62% reported at least one unmet need; 39% reported two or more.
Used a Restricted Definition of Concrete Needs and Did Not Include the Need for Emotional Counseling		
Guadagnoli and Mor[12]	410 outpatients with early and late-stage disease	25% reported at least one unmet need
Siegel et al[24]	483 patients with early and late-stage disease and their informal caregivers	19% reported at least one unmet need

ferent stages of disease, inclusion or exclusion of the need for emotional support, and varying definitions of unmet need.

BARRIERS TO THE USE OF COMMUNITY RESOURCES

Several recent studies suggest that the primary reasons that patients have unmet needs is their lack of awareness that services exist and their inability to negotiate complex bureaucracies to obtain them in a timely manner.[6,8,13,16,17] In Siegel's study, for instance, in response to the question, "If the areas we have been talking about became a problem for you, would you know where to go to obtain help from an agency or a service?," 68% of the patients answered no. In addition to finding that patients and families were unaware of community resources, Parsons found that many lacked the mobility or strength to search for them, cope with the arduous process of establishing eligibility, and follow through on an application.[7]

Many authors have stressed the importance of informing patients and their families about available resources and providing guidance on how to use them to maximize comfort and functioning at home and to avoid unnecessary hospitalization. Dwyer and Held, who focused on the chronic phase of cancer and periodic changes in needs, wrote that patients and families should be told in advance about home-care services so they will know where to turn when they need help.[18] Lurie suggested a case advocacy approach that would ensure that programs are accessible to appropriate patients.[19]

Bennet pointed out that because of anxiety, physically ill patients have difficulty comprehending and integrating information.[20] After distributing written material on concrete services to 80 patients, she found, during a follow-up interview, that only 12 patients had read the material and that none of the patients believed it would be helpful. Thus, she concluded that written material should be distributed to patients in conjunction with individualized contact.

Grobe and associates recommended the use of a glossary of available services in the context of an extensive educational program that would enhance patients' awareness of potential needs and available resources.[7] Edstrom and Miller used a three-session course on home care to teach patients about aspects of physical care and how to find community resources to meet concrete needs.[16]

All of these studies, together with clinical experience, reveal several attitudinal and psychological barriers that prevent patients from learning about and using community resources. First, because they want to be independent, they would rather not ask for help and therefore usually do so only in a medical emergency. They are especially reticent about reporting nonmedical needs; however, if asked, they can specify which nonmedical needs are not being met and often want to know about the services available. Furthermore, asking patients if they need certain kinds of help implies that other patients have the same needs, which makes it easier for them to acknowledge their unmet needs. For these reasons, a system of universal outreach is essential.

Second, because patients are understandably focused primarily on their illness and treatment, they have difficulty assimilating information about services that are not relevant to their current needs. Some patients are threatened by information that forces them to acknowledge a probable deterioration in their functional status. Therefore, the timing of information should be individualized and patient-specific. Guadagnoli and coworkers postulated that intervention strategies are more effective when they are matched to a patient's readiness—that is, patients should be classified according to the following stages[21]:

1. The *precontemplation* stage, in which the patient needs help with a daily living activity but would not consider using formal services
2. The *contemplation* stage, in which the patient reports a need and is willing to receive help from a formal service, but has not yet received it
3. The *action* stage, in which the patient is trying to obtain formal services
4. The *maintenance* stage, in which the patient has used formal services in the past and would be willing to do so again.

Third, because their needs change over time, patients may need to be followed up. However, the growing number of patients treated on an outpatient basis and the limited staff available to serve them means that social work, nursing, or discharge planning staff cannot regularly follow up all outpatients. Hence, patients often are left to recognize their own unmet needs and to make those needs known.

NEW INTERVENTIONS

Using the findings from these prevalence studies, new interventions have been proposed and developed to address the problems that typically arise in obtaining community resources and to monitor patients' care:

1. A case-management training program for patients and families
2. A case-management patient and family monitoring program
3. A computer-automated telephone outreach system
4. New community resource manuals for patients and families and information hotlines
5. A training program for health professionals to heighten their awareness of the psychosocial needs of cancer patients and available resources.

All these programs aim to be cost-effective and focus primarily on outpatient care. Except for the case-management training program for patients and families, they focus on intervention over a longer period of time than earlier rehabilitation programs, which tended to focus on inpatients, were expensive, and covered a relatively brief period.

CASE-MANAGEMENT TRAINING PROGRAM

On the basis of Mor's survey,[3] Wool and colleagues[22] developed a 12-week training program for high-risk patients and their families to improve their problem-solving skills. The program combined an educational and counseling approach in which the case manager assessed patients' needs, provided information about existing resources, and guided patients in gaining access to these resources. The goal was to increase the family's autonomy and mastery, reduce their unmet needs, and counteract the common feeling of helplessness associated with serious illness. Thus, training patients to recognize problems as they arose was an important aspect of the program. To accomplish these goals, the case manager had regular meetings, both in person and on the telephone, with patients and caregivers to teach them problem-solving skills and impart information about current and anticipated needs. The case manager acted as a direct intermediary only when necessary. This training model is currently being tested in a randomized trial.

CASE-MANAGEMENT MONITORING PROGRAM

Polinsky and associates developed a 12-month case-management program for patients with stage I or stage II breast cancer that began 3 to 5 weeks after surgery and extended for 1 year.[23] This intervention included an initial assessment followed by periodic reassessments conducted primarily by telephone as well as in person if indicated, at least once every 6 weeks. During the initial in-depth assessment, patients received information about a broad range of resources. Throughout the 12 months that followed, the case manager provided new information about support-group meetings, presentations, and recent research findings, either by telephone or mail.

Although the program was not designed to include direct provision of counseling, case managers often provided counseling in the form of reassurance. Over the year, their time was accounted for by reassurance (58%), information (38%), and referrals (4%). They also served as advocates when a patient's efforts seemed ineffective (*e.g.,* correcting hospital billing errors). The average time of each case-management contact was 15.3 minutes. One case manager spent 374 hours during the year on the program with 69 newly diagnosed patients. The average case-management time spent on each patient per year was 5.4 hours. The efficacy of this program in improving patients' functional status, mood, and quality of life is now being studied in a randomized trial.

TELEPHONE OUTREACH

In the second phase of their study, Siegel and associates attempted to reduce the prevalence of unmet needs by developing an intervention that would permit cost-effective, universal assessment of outpatients' needs as well as periodic reassessments to identify changing or emerging needs in a timely manner.[24] A computerized system telephoned patients periodically to conduct a brief needs assessment. This fully automated outreach system consisted of a specifically configured computer and custom-designed software that accepted a virtually unlimited number of patients and did not require a human operator.

In their earlier cross-sectional study, Christ and Siegel extracted a set of only 12 questions that allowed them to identify about 93% of the patients who reported one or more unmet concrete needs in response to the extensive list of concrete services covered during personal interviews with patients (see Appendix).[14] These 12 questions (Table 64–33) were then adapted for use in the telephone survey with the expectation

TABLE 64–33. Survey Questions Used in the Automated Telephone Outreach System to Assess Patients' Concrete Needs

Now, here is the first question, which is about the cost of your transportation to the hospital, including the cost of public transportation, other fares, parking, tolls, and gas. During the past month, when you came to the hospital, could you have used any help with these costs?

The second question is about the kind of transportation you usually take to the hospital. During the past month, would another kind of transportation have made the trip to the hospital easier?

The third question is about your medical prescriptions. During the past month, could you have used any help either paying for your prescriptions or getting them filled?

The fourth question is about the time you spend alone at home. During the past month, was there any time when you were alone in the house and felt too sick or weak to be alone?

The fifth question is about how you are managing bathing. During the past month, was there any time when you needed more help than you had when you were showering or bathing?

The sixth question is about how you are managing food shopping. During the past month, was there any time when you needed more help than you had to shop for food?

The seventh question is about how you are managing meal preparation. During the past month, was there any time when you needed more help than you had to prepare a meal?

The eighth question is about how you are managing light housekeeping like dusting, washing dishes, or making beds. During the past month, was there any time when you needed more help than you had to do light housework?

The ninth question is about how you are managing heavy housekeeping like mopping, vacuuming, doing the laundry, or cleaning the bathroom. During the past month, was there any time when you needed more help than you had to do heavy housework?

The tenth question is about how you are managing medical bills. Do you currently need help either understanding or paying your medical bills?

The eleventh question is about how you are managing to get medical information. Do you currently need help getting more information about your illness and its treatment?

Is there any other problem connected with your illness which you would like to discuss with a social worker?

that they would capture a similarly high proportion of patients who had one or more unmet needs. The questions specifically addressed needs related to the cost and mode of transportation to and from the hospital, medical prescriptions, supervision at home, personal care, food shopping, meal preparation, light and heavy housekeeping, medical bills, and medical information. If a patient said yes to any of the questions, a social worker called the patient within a week to discuss ways of solving the problem. In this way, the intervention coupled computer automation with professional service delivery.

The ability of the intervention to reduce the prevalence of unmet needs was then evaluated in an experimental trial. Patients were preassigned to the experimental or control group before accrual. The experimental group was entered onto the computer system to begin a series of three automated telephone surveys scheduled about 6 weeks apart. The results showed that the prevalence of unmet needs in the control group was higher than in the experimental group for 15 of the 21 specific needs; for eight of these needs, the difference exceeded 10%. Furthermore, in every domain of need, the proportion of patients who reported unmet needs for assistance with any task was lower among the patients in the experimental group than in the control group. Significant findings and trends in the data supported the conclusion that patients in the experimental group were less likely to experience unmet needs than were patients in the control group.

This automated outreach system appeared to be an especially cost-effective way of addressing the changing needs of the large number of patients who move in and out of outpatient care. It did not incur the considerable expense associated with other strategies used to screen patients needs. The expensive professional time was used for problem-solving in the return call. Because the problem was already identified, social workers found that the average length of a call was only 18 minutes.

In summary, the automated telephone screening survey holds promise as an effective strategy for early identification of patients with unmet needs. These patients can then be contacted by professionals who can further explore the nature and severity of their needs and their receptivity to and eligibility for available services in a timely way. The vast majority of patients with unmet needs may not otherwise come to professional attention, given the shortage of staff. In Siegel's cross-sectional study, only 11% of the patients had contact with a social worker in the 6 months before the intervention.

NEW RESOURCE AND EDUCATIONAL MATERIALS

Several new resource manuals and materials have been developed to inform patients about the community services available to them. Of particular note is the book *Facing Forward*, developed by the National Cancer Institute. This useful resource manual for cancer survivors can be obtained along with other materials by calling the Cancer Information Service (1-800-4-CANCER).

Another excellent resource manual for cancer patients and families is *Helping People Cope: A Guide for Families Facing Cancer*, which was developed by the Cancer Control Plan of the Pennsylvania Department of Health. This manual not only provides information about a broad range of community resource needs but also contains clear directions about how to obtain these services. It can be obtained by calling 1-800-537-4063.

These two sources of information take into account the changing health-care environment and data from recent studies of patients' needs, and are more comprehensive and practical than previous publications on the subject. Additional written materials for patients can be obtained from agencies listed in the appendix.

TRAINING PROGRAM FOR PROFESSIONALS

In response to Houts' survey, Barg and colleagues conducted a statewide 3-day continuing education program for health professionals in oncology in Pennsylvania.[25] The goals of the program were to:

1. Enhance the participants' knowledge regarding psychosocial support services
2. Develop consumer guides to community resources to improve and expand the use of existing support services

3. Increase the participants' knowledge about pain and symptom control to meet patients' physical and psychological needs
4. Increase the effectiveness of communication among patients, families, and caregivers.

When the program ended, the 409 participants were assessed to determine whether their attitudes and beliefs had changed as a result of the program. Later, the participants were assessed again to determine whether the program had led to new psychosocial initiatives within their institutions. The changes in both domains were significant and subsequently led to the development of a network for health providers who were interested in the psychosocial aspects of cancer. One recommendation from the program was to computerize regional resources for patients as a more timely, accurate, and cost-effective way to organize this information than the development of multiple directories. This led to a toll-free number that patients could call to obtain information about any cancer-related resource in the state. The information is updated every 6 months.

SERVICES FOR EVOLVING NEEDS

The fact that cancer has become a chronic illness in many instances has resulted in growing numbers of survivors who need rehabilitation. At the same time, the constant search for ways to reduce health-care costs is affecting the kinds of services available and how those services are delivered. Patients with prolonged chronic illness must deal with gradual debilitation, progression of disease, and fear of losing control over the disease. These stresses are heightened by the cost of medical care and surveillance, which can exhaust medical insurance and the family's resources.

Finally, chronically ill patients, although their numbers are increasing, have few positive models to emulate. Society's models tend to be either cured patients who can fill their roles in the community with no apparent impediments, or those who die heroically. Thus, cancer patients, as well as other chronically ill people, need new role models who illustrate the courage it takes to live day by day in this society with a chronic, sometimes terminal illness.

Cured patients must reenter a culture that values people who emerge unscathed from a crisis, yet they need ongoing social and psychological rehabilitation. They may have lost their hair or a breast, limb, or other organ; they may have gained or lost weight or suffered other effects of the disease or treatment, including infertility. They must live with the fear that the cancer will recur or that a new cancer will develop, possibly because of the treatment for the original cancer. Finally, they may confront discrimination from employers and medical insurance carriers.

Although most survivors adjust well to their illness, they are frustrated by the common notion that they can pick up where they left off. To most patients whose treatment has been successful, the illness represents a major discontinuity that brings about lasting changes in how they perceive themselves and their future. New resources are now being developed in the community to help survivors deal with these obstacles to developing meaningful and productive lives.[26]

Reducing the cost of health care is the dominant issue in

health-care policy for the 1990s. All purchasers of health care—governments, businesses, and people—experience the burden of mushrooming costs of medical care and the efforts to control them. These financial pressures are affecting patients in the following ways:

1. Their insurance premiums have increased but fewer costs are covered.
2. The number who lack insurance or have only limited coverage has increased dramatically.[27]
3. The kinds of treatment covered for a given diagnosis, the places where treatment can be provided, and coverage for outpatient care are increasingly restricted. The result is high turnover among staff of community agencies and changes in the way services are delivered and who is billed for them.

All these conditions have created an atmosphere in which patients are uncertain whether they will be able to obtain or afford the treatments that will prolong their lives. In other words, the cost of a particular treatment is becoming a major factor in a patient's decision about which course of treatment to pursue. Patients can no longer assume, as they have in the past, that the insurance company, the government, or the hospital will make it possible for them to receive recommended treatments. Furthermore, because of regulatory changes, a patient's financial liability may change during the course of treatment. For example, a new Medicare regulation asserts that hospitals must refer patients to selected outside vendors for equipment, absorb the cost of billing, and pay the vendors themselves if such services are not covered by Medicare. In the past, to avoid unfair restriction of trade, hospitals often avoided referring patients to specific vendors; this gave patients more choices of service providers.

Because less money is available for community resources at a time when those resources are increasingly necessary, it is even more urgent that professionals find cost-effective ways of facilitating patients' timely access to resources and thus reduce the risk of costly, uncomfortable medical crises that occur at home.

LIMITATIONS OF DISCHARGE-PLANNING SERVICES

In recent years, the emphasis on discharge planning has heightened the awareness of health professionals about the importance of careful coordination of posthospital care for cancer patients. Such coordination is crucial to ensure an uninterrupted flow of health services that will maximize patients' chances of recovering their normal functional status to the degree possible and will minimize the cost of care.[28] When the prospective payment system began to be phased into the health-care system in 1983, the length of stay for inpatients began to decline and the demand for outpatient services increased proportionately. Clearly, helping patients return home and remain there have become national priorities, and identifying supportive resources in the community and developing new services are necessary to achieve this end.

Until recently, most of the literature on the community resources available for cancer patients focused either on planning for the discharge of patients after an acute episode of illness or on patient care (at home or in a hospice) during the terminal phase of illness.[8,29–35] Little was written about

patients' needs in the chronic phase, when progression of the disease and intensified treatment make the patient more and more debilitated but not yet in need of hospitalization or hospice care.[6,16,18]

Chronically ill patients may experience not only symptoms of the disease but also the sequelae of chemotherapy and radiation therapy, such as nausea and vomiting, anorexia, weight loss, aplastic anemia, and weakness.[16] As a result of improved methods of medical management, patients have greater tolerance for highly cytotoxic chemotherapeutic agents and can be treated on an outpatient basis.[18] However, because of variations in the course of the disease and the unpredictability of the side effects of treatment, medical crises may develop abruptly and cause concomitant changes in the types of home care a patient needs.[18] Discharge plans that appear to be satisfactory immediately after hospitalization cannot always anticipate a patient's future needs as the disease progresses. Thus, when further deterioration occurs months later, the patient is an outpatient and thus not as easily identified as requiring services because fewer screening mechanisms are available to determine his or her needs.[36]

NEED FOR A COMMUNITY RESOURCES NETWORK

To direct patients in a timely manner to the broad range of services available, practitioners must be aware of agencies and community services that address patients' needs. By so doing, they will be able to match individual patients with the appropriate community resources.[37] Most hospitals, clinics, and private physicians have developed resource manuals or computerized lists of cancer-specific resources available in their area. Ideally these manuals and lists are developed after needs assessments are conducted based on the diagnoses, treatments, and other characteristics of the patients treated and after the cost, quality, and appropriateness of the services provided by agencies have been reviewed.[37]

Private practitioners may have to give one person the responsibility for making referrals, maintaining relationships with vendors, reviewing the quality and performance of vendors periodically, and updating the list of resources. Auditing, surveying, or interviewing patients who have been referred to such services is necessary to evaluate the service providers. Generally, the most practical way to monitor the quality of the service is through ongoing communication with the vendors of these services. Establishing ongoing relationships with vendors and institutions ensures that the needs of all are presented and that changes are effectively made and maintained.

NEED FOR FINANCIAL ASSISTANCE

Medical Insurance

Medical insurance coverage is usually obtained through an employer or the federally and state-funded programs of Medicaid and Medicare. Because an employer may discontinue an employee's health insurance if the employee goes on leave without pay for an extended period and because individual policies are expensive and difficult to obtain, patients should make every effort to pay for their work-related group policy rather than allow it to lapse. Unfortunately, even people who have been free of disease for many years may have difficulty obtaining new or additional coverage. The state insurance representative and religious, fraternal, or advocacy organizations such as the American Association of Retired Persons and the National Coalition of Cancer Survivors may be helpful in finding individual policies for patients who have lost their insurance coverage.

Those who cannot obtain group insurance through an employer may be able to purchase direct-payment insurance. For example, Blue Cross/Blue Shield offers open enrollment in 12 states and high-risk pools have been set up in 22 states. To find out about Blue Cross/Blue Shield enrollment, call the organization's Washington office (202-626-4827). In states that do not have open enrollment, information about high-risk insurance can be obtained by calling (612) 854-9005 in Minneapolis.

Medicaid is funded by both federal and state governments and pays the medical expenses of people receiving welfare and those who fall within the Social Security Administration's definition of disability. In most states, people who are disabled but whose income exceeds the financial eligibility standards for Supplemental Security Income (SSI) are still eligible for Medicaid benefits, especially if they owe large medical bills not covered by other insurance. In some hospitals, applications for Medicaid can be made through the hospital billing department; otherwise, the patient must apply at a local welfare or social services office.

Medicare is a federal health-insurance program for people 65 or older. Medicare insurance is also extended to people who have received Social Security disability benefits for 2 years. Patients with disabilities such as kidney failure are eligible for Medicare without a 2-year wait. Specific instructions for obtaining these benefits can be obtained from the local Social Security office or by calling 1-800-234-5772.

Because Medicare does not cover medical bills completely, recipients may want to buy a Medicare supplementary insurance policy (Medigap). If the patient is older than 65, the American Association of Retired Persons and Blue Cross/Blue Shield have several policies for people diagnosed with cancer. People younger than 65 should call their state insurance department and ask for the names of the companies that sell Medicare supplementary policies to people under 65 on Medicare.

The American Cancer Society (ACS), the Leukemia Society of America, and other local religious and philanthropic agencies provide financial assistance for equipment, home care, transportation, certain pharmacy costs, and prostheses. The Crippled Children's Fund, managed by state health departments and funded by the federal government, also pays for some costs such as hospitalization, surgery, and appliances for patients younger than 21. (For sources of medical insurance, see the Appendix.)

Income Support

Because an ongoing source of income is a major concern for patients once paid-leave benefits from an employer are exhausted, Social Security disability benefits should be applied for early, because processing of claims can be time-consuming. Patients are eligible if they have accumulated sufficient quarters of Social Security coverage in the recent past. Children also are eligible for Social Security insurance on the basis of diagnosis and family income. The telephone number for children is 1-800-342-3009. Although the availability of other assets is not considered in the determination of eligibility for this benefit, the disease must have existed for 6 months and must be expected to last for at least 1 year. Also, the patient must be unable to work. (The requirement that the disease has existed for 6 months is often met while the application is being processed.) Application forms and detailed information can be obtained from the local Social Security office.

Patients can apply for SSI at the same time they apply for Social Security disability benefits. SSI provides income to elderly and disabled patients with extremely limited income and few assets and thus involves a means test. The amount of income or assets allowable varies from state to state. The SSI program may provide patients with income while they wait for disability benefits, then may be terminated once disability benefits are obtained and their income exceeds the limit. Children who have cancer may be eligible for this benefit if their parents' income meets the eligibility requirement.

State-administered public assistance programs provide financial assistance of various kinds, but the assistance varies greatly from state to state and within different jurisdictions. Generally, however, a patient's income must be extremely limited to qualify for these programs (*i.e.*, the patient must be receiving Aid to Dependent Children, food stamps, or general emergency relief funds). Additional pension funds and income support may be available from the Veterans Administration and from religious and fraternal organizations with which the patient is affiliated.

NEED FOR HOME HEALTH-CARE SERVICES

Home care for cancer patients consists of a wide range of health and personal services and equipment to support optimum recovery, restore functioning, and enhance patients' and families' quality of life throughout the course of care. The basic components of home care include personal care, medical care, skilled nursing, supportive counseling, case management, physical therapy, occupational therapy, nutritional counseling, and homemaking services.

Because of the variety of personnel who provide home care to patients and the fact that the titles used to denote these personnel vary according to geographic region, professionals and patients alike are often confused about the functions performed by home health-care personnel. In general, home-care personnel can be categorized as nonprofessionals or professionals according to their level of skill and training. Nonprofessional home-care personnel will be categorized here as companions, housekeepers, homemakers, and home health aides. Professional personnel include registered nurses, licensed practical nurses, social workers, physical therapists, and occupational therapists.

A companion may have little or no specific training and may stay with a patient to either supervise or ensure the patient's safety because he or she is confused or demented, weak, or extremely anxious. A housekeeper is responsible only for maintaining the household by performing such tasks as grocery shopping, cooking, and cleaning. A homemaker usually takes care of children in addition to maintaining the household. A home health aide has some training in the essentials of patient care and helps patients with bathing, dressing, toileting, and mobility; reminds them to take medications; gets their prescriptions filled; accompanies them to medical appointments; and performs light, minimal housekeeping tasks directly related to patient care (*e.g.*, changes the bed).

Registered nurses and practical nurses are responsible for monitoring the patient, making ongoing assessments of the patient's medical status, communicating this information to the physician, giving medications, supervising nonprofessional home health-care personnel, and teaching the patient and family how to manage special medical equipment or devices such as oxygen tanks and Broviac catheters and how to care for wounds or stomas. The social worker visits the patient and family at home and provides psychosocial counseling about adjusting to cancer, the stress of caring for the patient, and the family's fears or anticipation of the patient's death. In addition, the worker often assists with case management of entitlements and home-care services provided or funded by various agencies with the care rendered by the referring physician or hospital; more than one agency is often involved.

Medical Indicators of Need

The medical indicators of the type and intensity of home health-care services that a patient needs vary considerably and should be determined by evaluating several factors simultaneously:

1. The symptoms of the disease as defined by type, site, and stage of cancer
2. The type of treatment required (surgery, radiation therapy, chemotherapy)
3. Whether the treatment will be given on an inpatient or outpatient basis
4. The patient's insurance and personal and family resources.

Differences in need can be assessed most clearly at the time of the initial treatment, during treatment for recurrent or metastatic disease, and during palliative treatment for terminal illness.

Recently diagnosed patients tend to be less symptomatic and more functional and therefore usually require short-term (if any) home health care focused on their recovery from the initial treatment. Because surgery and radiation therapy, unlike chemotherapy, are discrete and time-limited, the patients' functioning is either compromised to a limited degree or affected significantly only for the immediate period of recuperation. Thus, there is a realistic expectation of increased functioning as each day passes. However, although the physical functioning of these patients usually improves quickly, the psychological impact of permanent or altered body functioning can create major impediments to adjustment at most stages of illness. Counseling to help the patient cope with bodily changes such as sexual functioning, the ability to communicate, appearance, and ambulation can significantly facilitate adjustment at home. Furthermore, any procedure that is done in the hospital reduces the need for home care because the patient receives complete care in the hospital and thus recuperates to a great extent before returning home. As a result, home care consists of teaching the patient to care for a surgical wound or ostomy or to manage a prosthesis, helping

maintain the household while the patient regains strength and stamina, and providing physical or occupational therapy or special equipment during the recuperation period.

Because patients with recurrent or metastatic disease are often more symptomatic, their treatment is often long-term or chronic rather than acute. Consequently, many of these patients need some form of home care, usually for an indefinite period. Patients receiving systemic chemotherapy, which can be debilitating, are especially in need of this type of care. Furthermore, chemotherapy is often given on an outpatient basis, which taxes the patient's already limited energy by requiring frequent trips to the hospital or oncologist's office and increased interactions with a complex medical system. These patients (and those who receive similarly fatiguing radiation therapy on an outpatient basis, especially if it requires many daily treatments) usually need home health care to manage the side effects of treatment and the activities of daily living.

For patients with metastatic disease who are in the terminal stage of disease and require palliative treatment, home health care is a primary issue. Can the patient be managed at home rather than in an inpatient setting, given the nearly total care he or she requires? Because arranging appropriate home care for terminally ill patients involves acknowledging and preparing for their death both practically and psychologically, it is emotionally stressful. At this stage of the illness, most patients require home care from outside agencies because of their poor functional status and the exhaustion of family members who have cared for them during earlier stages of disease.

The home health-care team for terminally ill patients usually includes—in addition to traditional professional and nonprofessional home health-care personnel—clergy, volunteers, and a physician or a specially trained nurse or nurse practitioner who makes house calls. Hospice programs, which often help families to maintain their dying members safely and comfortably at home, attempt to provide such comprehensive services. For these reasons, the planning of appropriate home care for terminally ill patients is a complex process in which the patient's and family's medical, practical, and psychosocial needs must be addressed.

Social and Behavioral Indicators of Need

Several social and behavioral characteristics can be important indicators of the need for home health care. One indicator is the family's or friends' commitment and ability to care for the patient. The home-care needs of most patients are met by family members; patients who live alone are more likely to require help from outside agencies. Even if a patient lives with his or her family or has relatives nearby, however, the degree of the relatives' involvement can vary greatly. The family members' availability and willingness to help usually is demonstrated by their presence or absence at medical visits and the degree to which they take an active role in discussing treatment, the symptoms and progress of the disease, medications, and the general care of the patient. A family's ability to provide care also depends on its economic status, especially on the type of employment, work schedules, and other family illnesses and responsibilities.

A second behavioral indicator is the patient's Karnofsky status and general appearance at medical appointments.[38]

Does the patient appear relatively well-groomed? Does the patient's personal hygiene seem adequate? Are wounds or special medical devices being properly cared for? Are there any signs of decubitus ulcers or other symptoms that indicate the patient may not be well cared for? Is the patient's nutritional status adequate? Because of emotional stress, a patient may not recognize the degree of need and thus may not mention a need for home-care services until the situation becomes severe. Thus, problems observed by the physician may be an earlier indication of need for such services.

A third, often subtle, indicator is a noticeable change in the patient's or family's communication with the treatment team. For example, an increased number of telephone calls about the patient's condition—especially if they occur after normal office hours—from a patient or family member who typically calls infrequently and during office hours is often a sign that the patient requires more help at home than is available. Similarly, reduced contact with the medical system, manifest by missed or canceled medical appointments, also may indicate that the patient feels too ill to make the visits without additional help or that family members can no longer help as much as before. Finally, patients who make an increased number of emergency visits, either at the hospital emergency room or in unscheduled office visits, may well be signaling that they are uncomfortable with the existing home-care plan. In this situation, the family members also may be indicating that they feel overwhelmed by the responsibility of managing the patient's medical and emotional needs at home. These changes can alert the physician to the possibility that the patient or family is indirectly requesting additional help.

Resources

Patients receiving in- or outpatient care from a hospital can ask the hospital's social work or discharge planning department for information about home-care services and referrals. These hospital-based professionals have special expertise in assessing and enhancing the problem-solving abilities of patients and families concerning the medical plan and can link patients and families with entitlements and health resources in the community that will provide the needed services.

Patients who are not being treated by a hospital system can turn to a community agency, a local unit of the ACS, the departments of social work or discharge planning at a local hospital, or the local Visiting Nurse Association office. The type of care that patients need and their ability to pay for it are two major factors in exploring home-care resources. Three basic types of agencies provide home-care services: nonprofit (voluntary) home-care agencies, proprietary (for-profit) home-care agencies, and government-based services.

The services of nonprofit agencies are reimbursed by Medicare, Medicaid, and insurance carriers. These agencies, which include the Visiting Nurse Association, often have a sliding scale of fees based on the patient's ability to pay. These agencies regulate their own eligibility criteria and referral procedures. For example, a patient referred to the Visiting Nurse Association must demonstrate the need for skilled nursing to activate other services such as a home health aide. Because these agencies differ geographically in the hours of service per week they will provide, a patient who needs a great deal of care may require a plan that coordinates the services of several different agencies, including a visiting nurse for skilled nursing care, Meals on Wheels for nutrition, and a home health aide for general care. Other services can be coordinated through hospital-based home-care agencies or a community-based hospice in many areas.

Proprietary home-care agencies are privately owned businesses that recruit, train, and supervise a full range of home health-care workers who are assigned to clients under their supervision. Some are local; others have a nationwide network of offices. These agencies are listed in the Yellow Pages under "Home Health Agencies." Although the agencies provide comprehensive services and equipment at home 24 hours a day, 7 days a week, they are expensive and thus accessible only to patients who have strong financial support or excellent insurance coverage for home care for chronic diseases. Only proprietary agencies that are certified by Medicare will be reimbursed (80%) by Medicare. To be eligible for this type of home care under Medicare, patients must meet the following criteria:

1. A physician must certify the need for services and develop a specified plan of treatment.
2. The patient needs skilled care from a nurse or other therapist (skilled nursing services are strictly defined and interpreted by governmental and insurance company guidelines).
3. The patient cannot leave the house without help from another person, special transportation, or the aid of equipment such as a cane or wheelchair.

NEED FOR ALTERNATIVES TO HOME CARE

Patients who need care in an extended-stay facility after acute care in the hospital usually have preterminal or terminal disease. The most common social reasons for long-term institutional care are the lack of available family members or the need for home services 24 hours a day but an inability to pay. The usual medical indications for extended care are the progressive nature of the disease, coupled with a regimen of care that the family cannot manage at home. The decision to use this form of care must be made jointly by the patient, the family, and the treatment team to ensure that family relationships and the integrity of the family unit are maintained.

Many communities have institutions that provide extended care for patients with chronic illnesses; in some instances, a floor or wing of a building may be designated for patients who need long-term care. Most extended-care institutions accept cancer patients, and a few are devoted exclusively to them. The institutions can be nonprofit, proprietary, or under public auspices. Proprietary nursing homes accommodate the largest number of patients in extended-care institutions. Institutions that seek reimbursement from Medicare must meet Social Security Administration standards.

Terminal or preterminal cancer patients, in particular, tend to exceed Medicare's limit of 100 days of extended care. If a patient's stay is likely to exceed 100 days, the family must be prepared to assume the continuing financial responsibility. To avoid interrupting a patient's care, many institutions, including some proprietary ones, make financial arrangements with families of limited means, such as helping them file an application for Medicaid.

NEED FOR TRANSPORTATION SERVICES

In areas where services are accessible, transportation is available to patients with certain degrees of need and the financial resources to pay for it. Because the first step in obtaining such services is an awareness of their existence and the ability to apply for them, a social worker or discharge planner should arrange for transportation. Researchers have found that disadvantaged patients are more likely to keep medical appointments if transportation is arranged for them.[39] Because transportation services vary greatly in quality, they must be monitored constantly to protect patients. Certainly, patients should be surveyed concerning the quality of services; however, the most effective way to provide safe, reliable, and comfortable transportation is through ongoing communication with vendors to sensitize them to cancer patients' specific needs and concerns.

Ambulances

An ambulance is indicated when the patient's physical or mental condition is so serious that transport is impossible by any other means; in other words, if patients cannot sit, if they experience intense pain when they move, or if they have other conditions that require rapid transport to a hospital in optimal comfort in a vehicle containing life-saving equipment such as intravenous poles and tubes, oxygen tanks, cardiac monitors, and suction devices.

Transport by ambulance is expensive and seldom is completely covered by insurance. Medicare usually pays up to 80% of the customary charges of a one-way trip. The cost of transferring patients to their home, a nursing home, or another hospital (if that hospital provides treatment that is unavailable at the first hospital) also is reimbursed. In all these cases, however, a hospital or physician must provide documentation of the need for the service. Medicaid usually pays the entire cost of transport by ambulance for situations similar to those partially covered by Medicare. Because the reimbursement policies of private and commercial insurance carriers vary greatly, reviewing the specific policy is essential. Social workers and discharge planners often can negotiate with the ambulance and insurance companies to arrange the best accommodations for all involved.

Social work departments in medical centers maintain lists of ambulance services and the names of people to contact to arrange them. Although the Yellow Pages also lists ambulances, determining the quality and reliability of these services is impossible. In an emergency, a local police emergency unit can be called; in New York City, the police transport emergency cases to the emergency room of the nearest municipal hospital free of charge.

Ambulettes

An ambulette is the transportation of choice for patients who cannot walk or climb stairs without assistance but who can sit in a wheelchair and do not require acute care while in transit. The most common medical and physical reasons for using an ambulette are physical or mental senility, orthopedic impairments, neuromuscular disorders, severe cardiac disease, and acute side effects from treatments.

Ambulette service usually costs about 25% less than an ambulance. Medicare does not cover this service. In most states, Medicaid does cover it, but the hospital or physician must document the need. Private and commercial carriers sometimes pay for this service. Although insurance carriers initially may refuse to pay for the service, social workers often can negotiate with them by pointing out the higher cost of an ambulance.

Van, Car, and Taxi Services

Van, car, and taxi services are indicated for patients who are visually, physically, or cognitively impaired; weakened by illness or treatment; or otherwise unable to use public transportation. These services tend to be much less expensive than ambulances and ambulettes, and they are more convenient than mass transportation because they provide door-to-door service. Medicare and private and commercial insurance carries do not pay for these services; Medicaid usually does. Because vans usually pick up several patients during the same trip, patients often are forced to wait and may become uncomfortable.

These services can be obtained through social work departments in medical centers, which maintain lists and sometimes have special relationships with vendors to ensure quality and provide reduced rates to patients who need financial help.

Rail Services

Some wheelchair-bound patients who must travel long distances prefer to go by train. Carriers must be notified 48 hours in advance to make appropriate arrangements. (A slide board is useful for transferring the patient easily to a regular seat.) The patient should have a reservation, which should be confirmed before the patient arrives at the station. Trains lack facilities for stretcher patients.

The cost of transporting a wheelchair-bound patient by train is the same as for ordinary passengers. Medicare and private and commercial insurance carriers usually do not pay for train travel; however, some Medicaid programs do under certain circumstances. Travel arrangements are usually made simply by calling the railroad's reservation desk.

Airlines

For wheelchair-bound, stretcher-bound, or acutely ill patients who must travel long distances, air travel is often the best solution. Although each airline has different regulations, most require a letter from a physician describing the patient's condition and stating that the patient can tolerate the trip. If the patient must spend the entire trip on a stretcher, most airlines must be notified 48 hours in advance.

Medicare and private and commercial insurance companies usually do not pay for air travel. In many states, however, Medicaid does if the circumstances are unusual. A wheelchair-bound patient who can be moved to a regular seat pays the same fare as any other passenger. Stretcher-bound patients, on the other hand, must pay for a first-class seat (which must be physically removed) plus a second- or third-class seat if they are accompanied by a nurse or by equipment such as an intravenous pole and pump.

To make appropriate arrangements, notify the airline in advance. In addition, contact the airline before the flight to ensure that the flight will leave at the scheduled time and that the airline has all the necessary information about the patient. The necessary documentation should remain with the patient at all times, and a member of the health-care team should be available by telephone until the plane actually departs.

Volunteer Services

Volunteer transportation services are often underused because people do not know how to find them. Ground transportation is obtained most easily, but its availability, degree of comfort, predictability, and reliability vary greatly, depending on the volunteers' resources and commitment. Free air travel also is available under certain circumstances.

To locate services, contacting the local chapter of the ACS is a good first step. Other sources of information include the Red Cross, volunteer police and fire departments, religious groups, local men's and women's groups, visiting or public health nurses, and hospital social work departments. In addition, many commercial vendors who serve hospitals will provide free services for specific patients when asked. Obtaining free services is often limited only by one's imagination and by gaining access to the people who control the services. To save time when seeking free service, always try to contact the person at the top of the system.

The Corporate Angel Network (914-328-1313) offers free air travel by corporate jets, primarily for cancer patients who can sit up and do not need life-sustaining equipment. The network also will transport as many as three additional people (*e.g.*, a family member, a bone-marrow donor, and so on), depending on the size of the aircraft. The patient's physician must provide clearance for the patient in writing. Similar service is offered by an air transportation network in Toronto and Missouri, in cooperation with the Canadian Cancer Society (416-924-9333). Patients, family members, or social workers can contact these services directly. Using them requires advance notice and flexibility.

NEED FOR COUNSELING SERVICES

Counseling can be provided by self-help groups and by professional counselors, either individually or in groups. Counseling can range in duration from a single session to long-term traditional psychotherapy.

Many patients are reluctant to request professional counseling or even a self-help group, despite overwhelming reactions to a cancer diagnosis. Some are psychologically immobilized and cannot exert the emotional energy needed to get help. Others view a request for support as reflecting an inability to cope, a loss of autonomy, or a sign of mental illness. Many are unaware that counseling can help assuage the existential terror evoked by a cancer diagnosis or can alleviate grief over the loss of body function or appearance. Ironically, these same patients may later resent not having received enough emotional support. Such patients are more likely to use counseling services if those services are presented as an acceptable adjunct to the medical treatment plan, are universally prescribed, and are easily available.[40]

Because of increased coverage in the lay press, however, counseling has become more acceptable to patients. Consequently, increasing numbers of them are requesting professional counseling or self-help groups to solve the psychological, social, and practical problems created by their disease and treatment. Spiegel and colleagues suggested that group support that enhances mental health also may slow progression of the disease.[41]

Self-Help Groups

The number of self-help groups for people with a chronic illness such as cancer has grown astronomically. A self-help group now exists for every major disease listed by the World Health Organization.[42] All these groups share the philosophy that people who have experienced a crisis can make a unique contribution to others who are undergoing the same experience.

Several mechanisms have been suggested to explain the appeal of self-help groups. First, because they have been through the same crisis (*i.e.*, they have "experiential knowledge"), "veterans" can provide new members with insight and understanding.[43] As Katz and associates said, sharing a central problem is what defines members of a self-help group.[44]

A second mechanism through which group members experience benefits is the destigmatization and normalization of conditions and problems. A third mechanism is the helper-therapy principle, which suggests that "helpers" may benefit more than recipients of help because their role as adviser increases their sense of interpersonal competence, they learn from those they help, they receive social approval for helping others, and their own success in coping is reinforced.[45] Because members of self-help groups are both givers and receivers of care, all can benefit. Another benefit of self-help groups is the modeling of successful recovery—a role that veteran patients, such as Reach to Recovery volunteers, consciously adopt to encourage members' successful adaptation.

Contacts with veteran patients are reported to be helpful to almost all patients in highlighting the normal and universal nature of their reactions and reducing their sense of isolation. Patients learn from other patients about different coping strategies that can be used to deal with the myriad stresses associated with the disease and its treatment.

Some groups are organized and run by mental-health professionals; others are organized and controlled by patients. Some sponsor intense, short-term sessions for several months and then disband. Others have ongoing programs that involve the same members and are closed to newcomers. Still others are always open to new members. In all cases, the underlying group mechanisms are the same: members help one another by sharing their problems, being role models of successful recovery, and destigmatizing the illness.

Self-help groups in a specific geographic area can be found by contacting the local office of the ACS or the Cancer Information Service (1-800-4-CANCER), the National Self-Help Clearinghouse (1-800-422-6237), the social work or nursing department at the local hospital, or community organizations such as family service agencies or private counseling groups.

Professional Counseling

Although patients rarely report adverse reactions to self-help groups, they may feel that such groups are insufficient to meet their need for emotional support. Therefore, when patients are emotionally overwhelmed by their disease and treatment, are in an acute psychological crisis, have specific individual problems, or need to deal with preexisting personal and interpersonal problems that have been exacerbated by disease, professional counseling is recommended.

In addition to the traditional individual and group counseling, some medical centers now offer specialized counseling for patients and families. Specialized counseling has been developed in response to research findings that have documented the prevalence of particular concerns among cancer patients:

1. Marital counseling for couples whose relationship has been damaged by the stresses of diagnosis and treatment
2. Sexual counseling, especially for people with tumors directly related to areas of the body associated with sexuality
3. Drug or alcohol abuse counseling for patients or family members who have problems with substance abuse that either existed before the cancer diagnosis or have been exacerbated by the diagnosis and treatment.

Patients who need professional counseling represent a continuum ranging from those who are seriously mentally ill to those who are psychosocially vulnerable to those who, although resilient and well supported, can benefit from some counseling. Indeed, some *must* receive counseling to maintain their functioning and prevent their social and emotional breakdown.

Cancer patients with a history of mental illness or psychiatric treatment generally have an ongoing relationship with several supportive services in the community that may need information about their medical condition. Such patients should be urged to contact their therapists or mental health counselors about their medical condition or to ask a social worker or other mental health professional to transmit information about their medical status and arrange for continued psychological treatment and care. Because a cancer diagnosis can exacerbate mental illness or seriously affect day-to-day functioning, early psychosocial intervention may prevent a breakdown of functioning that would have lasting negative effects on the quality of a mentally ill patient's life, such as loss of a job or alienation of friends and relatives. Therefore, a referral for counseling is essential for these patients.

A much larger group of patients are not mentally ill but have social and psychological characteristics that place them at risk of emotional and social breakdown when confronted with a cancer diagnosis. Such reactions may interfere with their daily functioning and compliance with treatment. These patients are likely to have one or more of the following characteristics:

1. They live alone and have few friends or relatives to help them.
2. They are older than 75.
3. They have dependent children.
4. They are financially stressed (lack medical insurance or have only limited insurance).
5. They are undergoing multiple stresses or have experienced severe stress in the past.
6. They are experiencing other life crises such as loss of a job or a divorce.
7. Their family has a history of violence or sexual abuse or drug and alcohol abuse.
8. They have multiple cancers or other diseases.
9. They have another family member who also is ill.
10. They have a history of cancer in the family.

Although such patients may be more difficult to identify, they will benefit by obtaining emotional support services.

Finally, patients who are resilient and psychologically strong and have numerous personal, social, practical, and financial resources tend to express their needs specifically and are grateful when help is provided. Unfortunately, however, professionals often overlook their psychological and support needs and view them as coping well. These patients usually make rapid and highly effective use of emotional support services to better meet their high standards for functioning and often resent not having access to counseling services. As one patient said, "I knew I could cope well with a cancer diagnosis and I did, but I might have coped better with some help and would have liked to have known about counseling that could have been available to me."

In hospitals, counseling services are typically provided by social workers, nurses, psychiatrists, psychologists, and chaplains. Some hospitals refer patients directly for counseling; others offer counseling as part of routine psychosocial assessments. Mental health professionals in private practice provide these therapies, as do many special agencies for cancer patients, such as some local chapters of the ACS, religious organizations, and other mental health and family service agencies. Counseling services also can be found by contacting the social work or psychiatric department in the local hospital or cancer center or by calling the local ACS office or another cancer or community agency.

Resources and Services

FINANCIAL ASSISTANCE FOR INCOME SUPPORT

Social Security Administration. Social Security Disability Insurance (SSDI) makes monthly payments to patients who cannot work because of disease or treatment. Eligibility does not depend on assets or income. Supplemental Security Income (SSI) makes monthly payments to disabled people with extremely limited income and assets.

State Departments of Social Services. Aid for Dependent Children provides monthly support for children of disabled parents. General Relief provides cash assistance in short-term emergencies. Food Stamps provides coupons to purchase food.

Veterans Administration. The State Disability Benefits Office provides payments through employers.

FINANCIAL ASSISTANCE FOR TREATMENT

Insurance. State departments of insurance can provide information about private insurance carriers. Medicaid pays the expenses of disabled patients. Eligibility requirements include limited assets and income. Medicare pays the medical expenses of patients older than 64 and those who have received SSDI for 2 years. Coverage for outpatient treatment and care is limited.

Philanthropic Agencies. The ACS pays some of the costs of transportation, treatment, home care, and dressings. The Crippled Children's Program pays for approved hospitalizations, operations, and appliances. The Leukemia Society of America pays some of the costs for leukemia patients such as transportation, drugs, and radiation therapy in specific instances.

HOME HEALTH CARE

Hospital-based home-care programs provide home-care personnel, and hospital departments of social work and discharge planning provide information about local home-care resources.

The Visiting Nurse Association and public health nurses provide home-care personnel and information about local proprietary agencies and other resources. Their services are covered by most insurance carriers.

Private home-care agencies provide personnel and usually require private pay or major medical insurance to cover the services of registered nurses only. These agencies are listed in the Yellow Pages or are recommended by hospital departments of social work and discharge planning or local visiting nurse services.

The ACS pays some home health-care fees, and the Leukemia Society of America selectively provides home-care services.

Hospices provide coordinated home care for terminally ill patients by using visiting nurse services and volunteers. Insurance coverage for these services varies.

Meals on Wheels, which delivers meals to patients' homes, is administered by a range of local social service and religious agencies.

EQUIPMENT

Hospital-based home-care programs, surgical supply companies, and pharmacies provide medical equipment for the home.

ALTERNATIVES TO HOME CARE

Terminal care and cancer-specific chronic care facilities provide inpatient care for terminally ill patients. Nursing homes provide chronic and terminal care of patients who cannot be cared for at home. Veterans Administration hospitals provide residential placement for veterans.

TRANSPORTATION

Private transportation companies provide ambulance, ambulette, taxi, van, or car transportation. See listings in the Yellow Pages.

The ACS provides transportation or money for transportation to the treatment center.

The American Red Cross provides free transportation to and from treatment centers when volunteers are available.

The Corporate Angel Network provides free air transport on corporate aircraft from home to the treatment center when flights are available. These flights are for ambulatory patients only.

Hospital transportation services arrange transportation to and from the hospital and, in some situations, provide funding for transportation.

The Leukemia Society of America provides some money for transportation to the treatment center.

Local religious organizations provide a range of vans and car services for members of their religious community.

Local volunteer ambulance and fire departments often provide free transportation to and from treatment centers when volunteers are available.

EMOTIONAL SUPPORT AND PLANNING SERVICES

The ACS sponsors the following self-help groups:

Candlelighters: emotional support and information for parents of children with cancer

CanSurmount: emotional support and information for patients with various cancer diagnoses

International Association of Laryngectomees: emotional support and information to patients having their larynx removed

Reach to Recovery: emotional support, exercises, and temporary prostheses for women undergoing mastectomy

United Ostomy Association: emotional support, information, and advice to ostomy patients

Family service agencies provide information, practical help, emotional support, and psychological and behavioral therapies.

Hospital social work, psychiatric, nursing, and pastoral staff provide information, emotional support, and psychological and behavioral therapies.

Make Today Count provides group and individual emotional support and problem-solving for cancer patients with all diagnoses.

The National Coalition of Cancer Survivors is a clearinghouse for publications, self-help organizations of cancer survivors, and a resource for political advocacy.

The National Self-Help Clearinghouse provides information about self-help groups throughout the country.

Pastoral care and religious agencies provide emotional support and spiritual guidance.

Private practitioners provide emotional support and psychological and behavioral therapies.

EDUCATION AND INFORMATION

The ACS is a source of information about prevention, treatment, services, and rehabilitation.

The Breast Cancer Advisory Center provides medical advice to newly diagnosed breast cancer patients, makes referrals, and disseminates information.

The National Cancer Institute sponsors two services: the Cancer Information Service, a free nationwide telephone information service, and the National Cancer Information Clearinghouse, a source of indexes, abstracts, information, and free searches of resources.

AGENCIES AND ORGANIZATIONS

American Cancer Society. A voluntary organization that offers programs of cancer research and education and patient services and rehabilitation. Address: National Headquarters, 3340 Peachtree Road NE, Atlanta, GA 30326; (404) 329-7625

American Red Cross. Provides free transportation when volunteers are available. Address: National Headquarters, Washington, DC 20006; (202) 737-8300

Breast Cancer Advisory Center. Provides medical advice to breast cancer patients, makes referrals, disseminates information, gives lectures, and maintains a library of materials on breast cancer. Address: 11426 Rockville Pike, Suite 406, Rockville, MD 20859; (301) 984-1020

Cancer Information Service. A free, confidential, nationwide telephone information service sponsored by the National Cancer Institute that provides current, reliable information on research about cancer, local sources of cancer care, and free publications on a variety of subjects. The toll-free number 1-800-4-CANCER automatically connects callers to the Cancer Information Service serving their area. New York business number for professionals: (212) 794-7984

Candlelighters. An international organization that provides emotional support to parents of children with cancer. Address: National Headquarters, 2025 I (Eye) Street NW, Suite 1011, Washington, DC 20006; (202) 659-5136

Compassionate Friends, Inc. A self-help group that offers friendship and understanding to bereaved parents. Its primary goals are to aid parents in the positive resolution of grief experienced after a child's death and to foster the physical and emotional health of bereaved parents and siblings. Address: P.O. Box 1347, Oak Brook, IL 60521; (312) 323-5010

Concern for Dying. A nonprofit educational council dedicated to the belief in each person's right to participate in treatment decisions made during terminal illness. It offers counseling and information on death, dying, and burial, and provides copies of the living will. Address: 250 West 57th Street, New York, NY 10019; (212) 246-6962

Corporate Angels Network. Provides free air transportation on corporate planes *from* home *to* the treatment center when flights are available. Address: Westchester County Airport Building, White Plains, NY 10604; (914) 328-1313

Crippled Children's Program. Listed under Bureau of Handicapped Children in the telephone directory.

Hodgkin's Disease and Lymphoma Organization. Provides information and emotional support for patients with Hodgkin's disease and their families. Address: 518 Wingate Drive, East Meadow, NY 11154; (516) 999-6813

International Association for Enterostomal Therapy. Organizes enterostomal therapy nurses to promote education of patients, nurses, physicians, and other allied health professionals for rehabilitation of patients with abdominal stomas, fistulas, draining wounds, incontinence, and pressure sores. Address: 505 A Tustan Avenue, Suite 282, Santa Ana, CA 92705; (714) 972-1725

International Association of Laryngectomees. A voluntary organization of 286 member clubs that coordinates the activities of local laryngectomee clubs, which provide mutual support and encourage total rehabilitation. Address: 777 Third Avenue, New York, NY 10017; (212) 371-2900

Leukemia Society of America, Inc. A national voluntary health agency, supported primarily by donations from the public, that seeks to control and eradicate leukemia, Hodgkin's disease, and lymphomas. It supports a three-pronged program of research, patient aid, and public and professional education. Address: National Headquarters, 800 Second Avenue, New York, NY 10017; (212) 573-8584

Make-a-Wish Foundation of America. Grants the special wishes of seriously or terminally ill children, and consists of a network of 50 chapters. Located in Phoenix, AZ; (602) 234-0960

National Cancer Information Clearinghouse. Facilitates the exchange of information on public and patient educational materials; indexes, abstracts, and stores information received from people and organizations; and provides free searches of resources. Address: Office of Cancer Communication, National Cancer Institute, 9000 Rockville Pike, Bethesda, MD 20205; (800) 422-6237

National Home Caring Council. Provides a quick reference to all homemaker/home health aide services across the United States, including those it accredits. Address: 235 Park Avenue South, New York, NY 10003; (202) 547-6586

National Hospice Organization. A nonprofit, privately funded association of health professionals that promotes better, more appropriate care for terminally ill patients and ensures hospice care at the highest level. Publishes a quarterly newsletter, locator directory, and several reports. Address: 1909 North Fort Myer Drive, Suite 307, Arlington, VA 22209; (703) 243-5900

National League for Nursing. Provides a list of visiting nurse organizations in local areas. Address: American Public Health Association, 10 Columbus Circle, New York, NY 10019; (212) 582-1022

National Self-Help Clearinghouse. Provides information about self-help groups in specific communities and places patients in contact with one of 27 regional clearinghouses, which may be available to provide help in organizing self-help groups. Address: Graduate School and University Center, City University of New York, 33 West 43 Street, New York, NY 10036

Starlight Foundation. Grants the special wishes of terminally, chronically, and critically ill children. Address: 9021 Melrose Avenue, Suite 204, Los Angeles, CA 90069; (213) 205-0631

United Ostomy Association, Inc. A nonprofit service agency organized and run by ostomates that helps ostomy patients return to normal living through mutual aid and moral support by educating patients and the public about ostomy, contributing to improvement of ostomy equipment and supplies, and publishing the *Ostomy Quarterly* and educational literature for patients, the public, and professionals. At present, more than 500 local chapters exist through the United States and Canada. Address: 2001 W. Beverly Blvd., Los Angeles, CA 90057; (213) 481-2811

REFERENCES

1. Grobe ME, Ahmann DL, Ilstrup DM, et al. Assessment of the needs of cancer patients undergoing active anticancer therapy and the needs of their family members. Am Soc Clin Oncol 1983;2:61.
2. Houts PS, Yasko JM, Kahn B, et al. Unmet psychological, social and economic needs of persons with cancer in Pennsylvania. Cancer 1986;58:2355-2361.
3. Mor V, Guadagnoli E, Wool M. An examination of the concrete service needs of advanced cancer patients. J Psychosoc Oncol 1987;5:1-17.
4. Hermann, JF, Wojkowiak SL, Houts PS, Kahn SB. Helping people cope: A guide for families facing cancer. Harrisburg: Pennsylvania Department of Health, 1988.
5. Googe MC, Varriccio CG. A pilot investigation of home health-care needs of cancer patients and their families. Oncol Nurs Forum 1981;8:24-28.
6. Parsons J. A descriptive study of intermediate stage terminally ill cancer patients at home. Nurs Dig 1977;5:1-26.
7. Grobe ME, Ahmann DL, Alstrup DM. Needs assessment for cancer patients and their families. Oncol Nurs Forum 1982;9:26-30.
8. Putnam ST, McDonald MM, Miller MM, et al. Home as a place to die. Am J Nurs 1980;80:1451-1453.
9. Gold M. Life support: Families speak about hospital, hospice, and home care for the fatally ill. Mount Vernon, NY: Consumers Union Foundation, Institute for Consumer Policy Research, 1983.
10. Greer DS, Mor V, Morris JN, et al. An alternative in terminal care: Results of the National Hospice Study. J Chron Dis 1985;39:9-26.
11. Houts PS, Yasko JM, Harvey HA, et al. Unmet needs of persons with cancer in Pennsylvania during the period of terminal care. Cancer 1988;62:627-634.
12. Guadagnoli E, Mor V. Daily living needs of cancer outpatients. J Commun Health 1991;16:37-47.
13. Siegel K. Continuing care of cancer patients—concrete needs: Progress report. New York: Memorial Sloan-Kettering Cancer Center, 1987.
14. Christ GH, Siegel K. Monitoring the quality-of-life needs of cancer patients. Cancer 1990;65:760-765.
15. Siegel K, Raveis VH, Houts P, et al. Caregiver burden and unmet patient needs. Cancer 1991;68:1131-1140.
16. Edstrom S, Miller MW. Preparing the family to care for the cancer patient at home: A home-care course. Cancer Nurs 1981;4:53.
17. Rose MA. Problems families face in home care. Am J Nurs 1976;76:416-418.
18. Dwyer JE, Held DM. Home management of the adult patient with leukemia. Nurs Clin North Am 1982;17:666-675.
19. Lurie A. The social work advocacy role in discharge planning. Soc Work Health Care 1982;8:75-85.
20. Bennet C. Testing the value of written information from patients and families in discharge planning. Soc Work Health Care 1984;9:95-100.
21. Guadagnoli E, Rice C, Mor V. Cancer patients' knowledge of and willingness to use agency-based services: Toward application of a model of behavioral change. J Psychosoc Oncol 1991;9(3):1-21.
22. Wool MS, Guadagnoli E, Thomas M, et al. Negotiating concrete needs: Short-term training for high-risk cancer patients. Health Soc Work 1989;14:184-195.
23. Polinsky ML, Fred C, Ganz PA. Quantitative and qualitative assessment of a case management program for cancer patients. Health Soc Work 1991;16:176-183.
24. Siegel K, Mesagno FP, Karus DG, et al. Reducing the prevalence of unmet needs for concrete services of patients with cancer. Cancer 1992;69:1813-1883.
25. Barg FK, McCorkle R, Jepson R, et al. A statewide plan to address unmet psychosocial needs of patients with cancer. J Psychosoc Oncol 1991;10(3).
26. Siegel K, Christ GH. Psychosocial consequences of long-term survivorship. In: Redman J, Lacher M, eds. Hodgkin's disease: Consequences of survival. Philadelphia: Lea & Febiger, 1989.
27. Vincenzino JV. Trends in medical care costs. Statistical Bulletin 1990;28-35.
28. Jessee WF, Doyle BJ. Discharge planning: Using audit to identify areas that need improvement. Quality Rev Bull 1979;5:25-29.
29. Hunter G, Johnson SH. Physical support systems for the homebound oncology patient. Oncol Nurs Forum 1980;7:21-23.
30. Shragen J, Halman M, Myers D, et al. Impediments to the cause and effectiveness of discharge planning. Soc Work Health Care 1978;4:65-80.
31. Wellisch DK, Fawzy FI, Landsverk J, et al. Evaluation of psychosocial problems of the homebound cancer patient: The relationship of disease and the sociodemographic variables of patients to family problems. J Psychosoc Oncol 1983;1(3):1-15.

32. Amado A, Cronk BA, Mileo R. Cost of terminal care: Home hospice versus hospital. Nurs Outlook 1979;27:522–526.

33. Cassileth BR, Donovan JA. History and implications of the new legislation. J Psychosoc Oncol 1983;1(1):59–69.

34. Marker WM, Simon VG. The hospice concept. Cancer 1978;28:225–237.

35. Rosenbaum EH, Rosenbaum DR. Principles of home care for the patient with advanced cancer. JAMA 1980;244:1484–1489.

36. Lindenberg RE, Coulton C. Planning for post-hospital care: A follow-up study. Health Soc Work 1980;5:45–50.

37. Polinsky ML, Ganz PA, Rofessart-O'Berry J, et al. Developing a comprehensive network of rehabilitation resources for referral of cancer patients. J Psychosoc Oncol 1987;5:1–10.

38. Mor V, Laliberte L, Morris JN, et al. The Karnofsky Performance Status Scale: An examination of its reliability and validity in a research setting. Cancer 1984;53:2002–2007.

39. Bryan JL, Greger HA, Miller ME, et al. An evaluation of the transportation needs of disadvantaged cancer patients. J Psychosoc Oncol 1991;9(3):23–36.

40. Christ GH, Bowles ME, Kleban R, et al. Educational and support programs for breast-cancer patients and their families. In: Harris JR, Hellman S, Henderson C, eds. Breast diseases, 2d ed. Philadelphia: JB Lippincott, 1991:866–871.

41. Spiegel D, Kramer H, Bloom JR, et al. Effect of psychosocial treatment on survival of patients with metastatic breast cancer. Lancet 1989;2:888–891.

42. Gussow Z, Tracey GS. The role of self-help clubs in adaptation to chronic illness and disability. Soc Sci Med 1978;10:407.

43. Borkman T. A cross-national comparison of stutterers' self-help organizations. Speech Ther J 1974;29:6.

44. Katz S, Hedrick S, Henderson N. The measurement of long-term needs and impact. Health Med Care Serv Rev 1979;2:2–21.

45. Riessman F. The helper therapy principle. Soc Work 1965;10:27.

Cancer: Principles & Practice of Oncology, Fourth Edition,
edited by Vincent T. DeVita, Jr., Samuel Hellman, Steven A. Rosenberg.
J.B. Lippincott Co., Philadelphia © 1993.

John J. Mulvihill

CHAPTER **65**

Genetic Counseling of the Cancer Patient

Genetic counseling is a communication process that deals with the human problems associated with the occurrence or the risk of occurrence of a genetic disorder in a family. This process involves an attempt by one or more appropriately trained persons to help the individual or family: (1) comprehend the medical facts, including the diagnosis, the probable course of the disorder, and the available management; (2) appreciate the way heredity contributes to the disorder and the risk of recurrence in specified relatives; (3) understand the options for dealing with the risk of recurrence; (4) choose the course of action that seems appropriate to them in view of their risk and their family goals and act in accordance with that decision; and, (5) make the best possible adjustment to the disorder in an affected family member or to the risk of recurrence of that disorder.[1]

At the level of the cell, cancer is a genetic disorder, and it is appropriate that the total care of every patient with cancer includes attention to all five elements of genetic counseling. The definition emphasizes that genetic counseling is not a one-time event but rather an ongoing process of communication with the patient and his or her family. Such communication is a task for all clinicians and not exclusively for geneticists. One practical result of genetic counseling is addressing an inevitable question that most patients have but that some clinicians may not have time to consider in the midst of making a diagnosis and devising optimal therapy: "Why me?" This point was made in the ground-breaking book by cancer patient and advocate, Rose Kushner.[2] The answer is often unknown, but sometimes a patient's erroneous notions can be corrected with current evidence. In any case, it seems useful to offer the patient and relatives an opportunity to explore the known or perceived causes of his or her cancer; sometimes they are conspicuously genetic.

In practice, the need for formal genetic counseling of cancer patients may arise in three settings: at the time of diagnosis, to address questions of etiology; at the time of therapy, to address issues of reproduction and possible teratogenicity; and after survival has been achieved, to address the possibility of recurrence, risk in family members, and reproductive issues.

COUNSELING ABOUT GENETIC CAUSES OF CANCER

Genetics plays a role in the development of most human cancers. Four questions about the cancer patient may be posed to screen for the likelihood of genetic origins of the cancer:

1. Did the patient have a prior cancer, tumor, or growth?
2. Are there birth defects, dysmorphic features, or precursor lesions found on examination or by history?
3. Is there any clue in the pathology or description of the primary tumor that may suggest genetic origins?
4. Does any family member have cancer or a preneoplastic syndrome?

There are many features that suggest a person has a cancer of genetic origins and should be considered for more formal genetic counseling than usual (Table 65–1).[3–5] Some factors are suggested only by case series, and some are rigorously proved by analytic epidemiologic and prospective studies.

The criteria may identify persons or relatives at high risk for cancer because of genetic, congenital, or familial factors. The explanation may lie in a cytogenetic defect, a mendelian

2529

TABLE 65–1. Identifying Patients and Families for Possible Genetic Counseling

Criterion	Example
Patients With a Cancer That Has One of These Features	
Bilateral, as separate primary neoplasms	Both kidneys, both breasts
Multifocal, within one organ	Multicentric colorectal cancers
An additional primary malignancy	Endometrial after colon cancer
At an atypical age	Breast cancer before 40 years
At an atypical site	Osteosarcoma of the mid-humerus
In the sex not usually affected	Breast cancer in a male
Associated with birth defects	Wilms' tumor with aniridia
Associated with a mendelian trait	Sarcoma in neurofibromatosis 1
Associated with a precursor lesion	Melanoma in dysplastic nevus syndrome
Associated with a rare disease	Lymphoma in immunodeficiency
A rare or unusual tumor type	Pheochromocytoma, sarcoma
Families With	
One first-degree relative* with a cancer with any of the above features	Siblings and children of a person with pheochromocytoma or melanoma arising in a dysplastic nevus.
Two first-degree relatives* with *any* cancer	Parents and siblings of a boy with sarcoma and his sister with brain tumor

* Brother, sister, parent, or child.
(Parry DM, Berg K, Mulvihill JJ, et al. Strategies for controlling cancer through genetics: Report of a workshop. Am J Hum Genet 1987;41:63–69; Parry DM, Mulvihill JJ, Miller RW, et al. Strategies for controlling cancer through genetics. Cancer Res 1987;47:1814–1817; Mulvihill JJ. Prospects for cancer control and prevention through genetics. Clin Genet 1989;36:313–319)

single-gene trait, in multifactorial inheritance or familial clustering, or even in environmental catalysts.

CHROMOSOMES AND SINGLE-GENE TRAITS

Every cancer probably has abnormal chromosomes, but they are usually acquired and doe not occur in every body cell.

Cancer can be a complication of a recognized syndrome of multiple malformations that has underlying constitutional chromosomal defects.[6] Such cytogenetic syndromes include Down's syndrome (trisomy 21) with various acute leukemias and perhaps testicular cancer; Klinefelter's syndrome (47,XXY) with nongonadal germ cell tumors and breast cancer; gonadal dysgenesis, including the full Turner's syndrome (if some Y chromosome material is present), with gonadoblastoma; trisomy 8 with preleukemia; the Miller syndrome of aniridia with Wilms' tumor and a deletion of 11q13; retinoblastoma with or without birth defects and a deletion of 13q14; and the fragile X syndrome with unusual cancers, including testicular cancer.[7]

Rare familial aggregations of specific cancers have been explained by constitutional translocations: t(3;8) in one family with renal cell carcinoma, an insertion of 11p13 into chromosome 2q32 with familial Wilms' tumor, an insertion of 13q14 into 3p12 with familial retinoblastoma, and a t(14;22) with familial meningioma.[8–11] Recognition of these rare families provides excellent opportunities for clinicians to make presymptomatic or prenatal diagnoses by vigorous identification and screening of persons at high risk. These families also present research opportunities for cancer biologists.

The ninth edition of *Mendelian Inheritance in Man* enumerates 2636 definite single-gene traits and 2281 others with suggestive but inconclusive evidence of mendelian inheritance behavior.[12] Of the 4917 traits, 338 conditions (in addition to 56 protooncogenes) have neoplasia as the sole feature, a frequent concomitant, or a rare complication.[13] The inference can be drawn that some 9% of known human genes influence the expression or suppression of neoplasia. Because these disorders have known or likely patterns of mendelian inheritance (*i.e.*, autosomal dominant, autosomal recessive, or X-linked inheritance), it is a simple matter to quote recurrence risks and offer counseling to a patient with a cancer that arose because of one of these mutant genes.

FAMILIAL AGGREGATION

As suggested in Table 65–1, no firm definition of a cancer family is available, and only empiric guidelines can be offered. Because 1 of every 4 Americans develops cancer, most persons have some relatives with cancer, and some, by chance, have many. In two clinical surveys, 6% of persons with cancer said they had three or more first-degree relatives with cancer.[14,15] Half of the cancer patients said they had no first-degree relative with cancer, about 30% said one, and 12% said two. The accuracy of a patient's report of cancer among relatives has been independently validated with medical records. The primary site of cancer was correct in 83% of first-degree, 67% of second-degree, and 60% of third-degree relatives.[16]

A working definition of familial cancer depends on the type and site of cancer, the age at diagnosis, the sex, the number of tumors, and the absolute numbers of affected relatives. It may be chance when 2 of 8 elderly sisters have breast cancer.

It would be unusual if both sisters were premenopausal or had bilateral disease. If brothers of any age had breast cancer, intuition recognizes a significant familial aggregation.

There are many reports of familial recurrences of exactly the same cancer, such as cancer of the breast, colorectum, ovary, or lung. Occasionally, closely related tumor types aggregate in relatives, such as squamous carcinomas of the lung and larynx or adenocarcinomas of the breast and ovary. The same pair of tumor types that cluster to excess in families also tend to occur as multiple primary neoplasms in one person. Of course, family members share many environmental factors, and there are clear instances of familial cancer due to environmental exposures, such as familial lung cancer and mesothelioma due to exposure to asbestos brought into the home on work clothes.[17]

At least two distinct patterns occur repeatedly enough to have gained the label of "cancer family syndrome." Many other patterns of familial cancer probably await delineation. One is the *cancer family syndrome of Lynch,* which is characterized by two or more generations with cancer of the colon and endometrium (and sometimes ovaries and breast) with diagnosis at an early age and with an excess of persons with multiple primary cancers.[18] Alternate names for the disorder are Lynch syndrome 2 or hereditary nonpolypotic colonic cancer, type 2; Lynch syndrome 1 is the term reserved for familial aggregation of colon cancers without polyposis or other cancers (*i.e.,* site-specific familial colon cancer). It is not clear that either Lynch syndrome is inherited as a simple single-gene trait.

The second distinct pattern is the *Li-Fraumeni cancer family syndrome* or *SBLA syndrome,* an acronym for the tumor types seen to excess: *s*arcomas; *b*reast, *b*one, and *b*rain tumors; *l*ung cancer, *l*aryngeal cancer, and *l*eukemia; and *a*drenal cortical neoplasia.[19] Constitutional mutations of the gene *p53* on chromosome 17p have been documented, and the predisposition to the syndrome is clearly a mendelian dominant trait with high penetrance.[20]

CLINICAL RECOMMENDATIONS

Identifying persons at high risk of cancer because of cytogenetic, mendelian, or familial determinants can lead to effective cancer screening and prevention through proper genetic counseling (see Table 65–1).[3–5] It is a persistent misperception that nothing can be done to manage genetic disease; in fact, the routes to prevention are numerous. Those at high risk for cancer may be enrolled in screening programs. Prenatal diagnosis can be offered for certain cytogenetic and mendelian predispositions to cancers. Patients with one cancer can be specifically screened for possible additional neoplasms. Prophylactic surgery may remove the target organ and prevent an inevitable cancer.[21] For example, prophylactic colectomy is done for patients with a polyposis syndrome or those at risk for familial colon cancer; gonadectomy is performed for cryptorchism, familial ovarian cancer, or gonadal dysgenesis; mastectomy is performed for familial breast cancer; and thyroidectomy is done for persons with the multiple mucosal neuroma syndrome. Interrupting gene-environmental interactions may prevent cancer by limiting environmental exposures in especially susceptible persons (*e.g.,* use of sun-

screen, sun avoidance, chemoprevention in patients with xeroderma pigmentosum or albinism).

To offer genetic counseling to a person with or at high risk of developing cancer, the physician or counselor must first collect and interpret the family and personal medical histories, recognize any preneoplastic syndromes, assess the risk, begin counseling, and follow through with medical surveillance and perhaps prophylactic surgery.

Strategies for cancer prevention or for cancer genetics clinics, modeled after the practice of clinical genetics, have been advanced.[3–5,22–29] Disease-specific registries have expedited research and advanced preventive management (*e.g.,* syndromes of colorectal polyposis reported to the Immunodeficiency–Cancer Registry, NCI's research efforts on the Li-Fraumeni cancer family and dysplastic nevus syndromes).[19,30–33] Population-based registries of cancer families are underway in Iceland, Israel, and Utah, but only the latter seems to provide active prevention, probably because so many clinical studies are being conducted.[34–36] An innovative approach to identifying potential cancer families has been demonstrated in Utah and Texas.[37] In required health education classes, high school students complete a systematic medical family history. From 1980 through 1986, 24,332 family trees were collected at an estimated direct cost of $8.30 each; 1.7% were considered cancer-prone families.

The published experience indicates that the cancer prevention clinic serves mostly self-referred women who are concerned about a family history of breast cancer. Intake is done by a nurse or genetic counselor and usually includes family and medical histories for the consultant to complete. Medical records are sought to confirm reported diagnoses. In the University of Wisconsin model, a 3-hour clinic session is held in three parts: preview and general cancer prevention counseling (including a 16-minute videotape) by a social worker; instruction on disease-specific prevention and early detection by a health educator; and a review of family history and other risk factors leading to a specific age-adjusted risk assessment.[24] The Creighton University model (Fig. 65–1) emphasizes the research opportunities and the need for long-term follow-up with families.[23]

In the ideal situation, the genetic counseling of a person with an unusual personal or family history of cancer should include the following:

1. Review of the patient's family history for evidence of a preneoplastic syndrome or constellation of cancers that is considered to have a genetic etiology;
2. Review of the patient's environmental history for evidence of any unusual occupational, demographic, or medical exposures that may lead to cancer in a genetically susceptible person;
3. Review of the patient's medical history for evidence of a genetic condition predisposing to malignancy;
4. Clinical examination searching for dysmorphic features, congenital anomalies, abnormal cutaneous manifestations, or other abnormal findings that could form the basis for a syndromic diagnosis; and
5. Studies (*e.g.,* radiographs, peripheral blood karyotype) to confirm or rule out specific diagnoses.

If a single-gene disorder or chromosomal syndrome predisposing to cancer is diagnosed, the clinician can provide

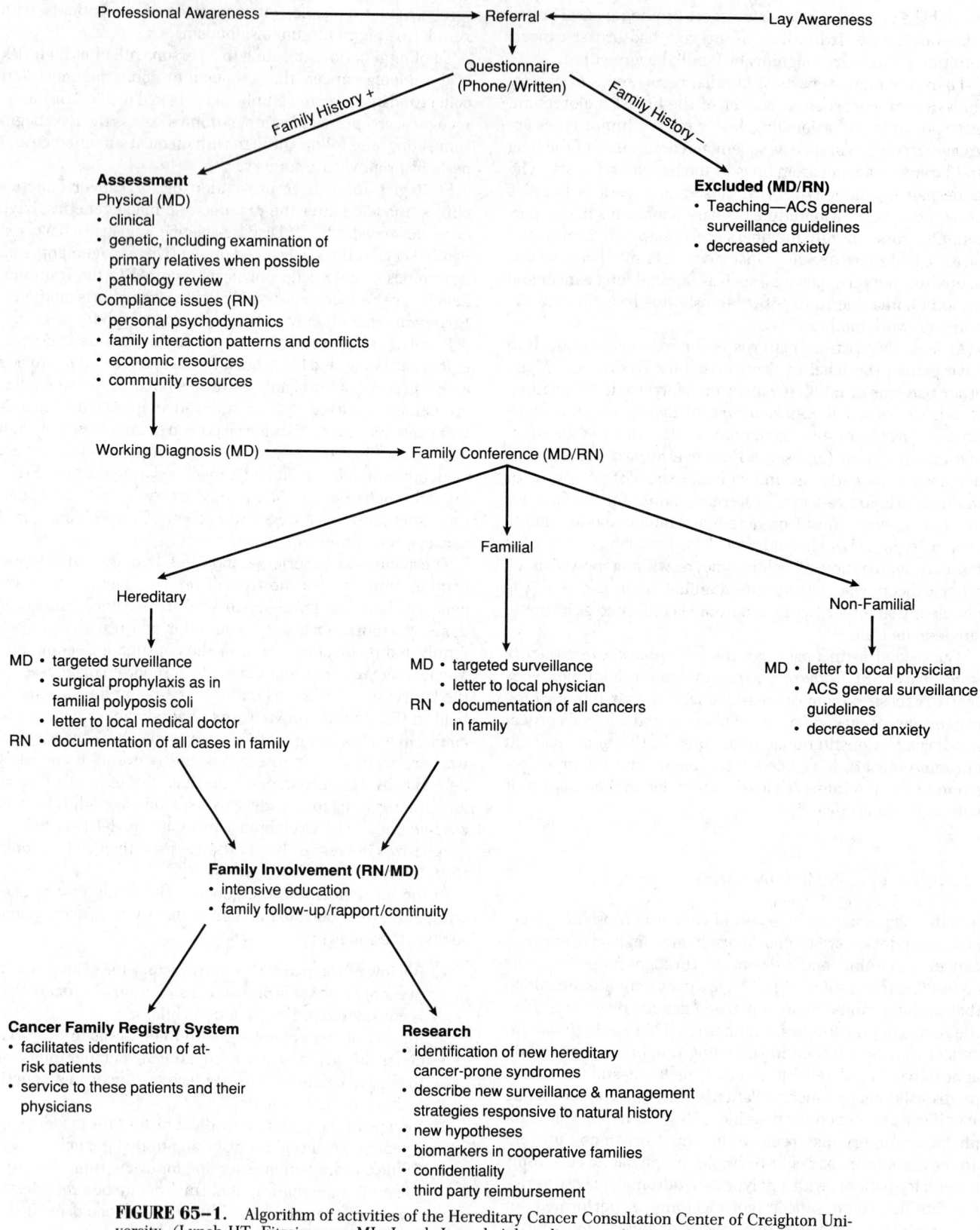

FIGURE 65–1. Algorithm of activities of the Hereditary Cancer Consultation Center of Creighton University. (Lynch HT, Fitzsimmons ML, Lynch J, et al. A hereditary cancer consultation clinic. Nebraska Med J 1989;74:351–359)

information on prognosis, offer appropriate genetic counseling, and recommend medical surveillance for the patient and at-risk family members with the intention of detecting early any further complications of the underlying condition, including cancer. For an increasing number of genetic disorders with neoplastic manifestations, it is becoming possible to identify affected fetuses or asymptomatic gene carriers in the family through the use of DNA tests (*e.g.*, for retinoblastoma, neurofibromatosis 1, Fanconi's anemia).

EMPIRIC RISK COUNSELING

For most patients, it is not possible to diagnose a specific cytogenetic or mendelian disorder. A counselor experienced in evaluating cancer families can sometimes offer empiric-risk estimates for future disease. In general, if a person develops a cancer, first-degree relatives (*i.e.*, parents, children, brothers, sisters) have a threefold risk of developing the same type of cancer. Until specific genes are found for common adult cancers, efforts are beginning to refine gross risk estimates by modifying them with information on other risk factors, calculating individual probabilities of disease, and discussing management options.

Breast Cancer Risk Counseling

One attempt to combine information on risk factors for breast cancer used age at menarche, age at first full-term livebirth, number of previous biopsies, and number of first-degree relatives with breast cancer.[38] A model of relative risks for various combinations of these factors was developed from case-control data from the Breast Cancer Detection Demonstration Project (Table 65-2). The baseline age-specific hazard rate (*i.e.*, rate for a patient without identified risk factors) was computed as the product of the observed age-specific composite hazard rate times the quantity 1 minus the attributable risk. The individualized breast cancer probabilities were calculated from information on relative risks and the baseline hazard rate. The resulting percentages, best applied to women undergoing regular mammography, are point estimates of the absolute probability of a woman's developing breast cancer in 10, 20, or 30 years after counseling (Table 65-3). This approach to individualizing the probability of developing breast cancer is used in the clinical research trial of tamoxifen as a way to prevent new clinical breast cancers.[39]

Another strategy for individualizing breast cancer risks assumes a genetic model of breast cancer predisposition that involves a rare dominant gene.[26,40] The counselor can offer calculated probabilities based on that model and on the specific pattern of affected relatives and their ages at diagnosis. This strategy has the disadvantage of ignoring other individual risk factors and assuming a genetic model for every familial case. (Familial does not always mean genetic.) Regardless of the method used to estimate risk, it is hoped that hearing a quantitative estimate of risk in a clinical setting may motivate women at high risk to undertake scrupulous surveillance. Some women have undergone prophylactic mastectomy, a controversial procedure that may be indicated for some women especially fearful of developing breast cancer.[41] If considered at all, proper counseling should precede a decision to operate.[42-44]

TABLE 65-2. Relative Risks for Selected Risk Factors

Risk Factor		Relative Risk
Age at menarche (y)		
≥14		1.00
12–13		1.10
<12		1.21
Number of breast biopsies		
Age <50 y		
0		1.00
1		1.70
≥2		2.88
Age ≥ 50 y		
0		1.00
1		1.27
≥2		1.62
Age at first term livebirth (y)	Number of first-degree relatives with breast cancer	
<20	0	1.00
	1	2.61
	≥2	6.80
20–24	0	1.24
	1	2.68
	≥2	5.78
25–29 or nulliparous	0	1.55
	1	2.76
	≥2	4.91
≥30	0	1.93
	1	2.83
	≥2	4.17

(Gail MH, Brinton LA, Byar DP, et al. Projecting individualized probabilities of developing breast cancer for white females who are being examined annually. JNCI 1989;81:1879–1886)

Follow-up studies of women counseled about their high risk of cancer revealed a low percentage who complied with the complete recommendation for surveillance.[41,45] One study showed only 40% performed monthly breast self-examination, and 69% went for clinic examinations; a surprising 94% had regular mammography.[45] The behavior seemed to reflect psychological distress from high anxiety. A small study found participation in a cancer prevention clinic correlated with prior involvement in cancer prevention activities, interest in cancer-specific information, and perceived risk level.[46]

Other Cancers

Table 65-4 summarizes familial recurrence risk estimates for several common sites of cancers. These common cancers are infrequently due to a single-gene trait inherited as a dominant or recessive trait, but more often, they have a low risk of recurrence. For the many people with no identifiable genetic determinants, the genetic counselor may reassure the patient that, based on current knowledge, the development of cancer was most likely a chance event, and that the risk of developing additional cancers in the patient or relatives is

TABLE 65–3. Projected Probability of Developing Breast Cancer Within 30 Years of Follow-up

Initial Age (y)	Later Relative Risk*	Initial Relative Risk (%)*					
		1	2	5	10	20	30
20		1.7	3.4	8.3	15.9	29.3	40.5
30	1	3.2	4.8	9.5	16.9	29.9	40.8
	2	4.7	6.3	10.9	18.2	30.9	41.7
	5	8.9	10.4	14.9	21.8	34.0	44.3
	10	15.6	17.1	21.2	27.6	38.8	48.3
	20	27.6	28.8	32.3	37.8	47.4	55.5
	30	37.7	38.7	41.8	46.4	54.7	61.7
40	1	4.4	5.6	9.1	14.6	24.6	33.5
	2	7.4	8.6	11.9	17.3	27.0	35.6
	5	15.9	17.0	20.0	24.9	33.7	41.5
	10	28.3	29.2	31.8	35.9	43.4	50.0
	20	47.5	48.1	50.0	53.1	58.5	63.4
	30	61.2	61.6	63.1	65.3	69.3	72.8
50		4.4	8.5	19.9	35.5	57.8	71.7

* The initial relative risk corresponds to the initial age at consultation. If the age is under 50 and the 30-year projection exceeds 50, a later relative risk at age 50 should be specified, because risk due to the number of biopsies varies with age (see Table 65–2).
(Gail MH, Brinton LA, Byar DP, et al. Projecting individualized probabilities of developing breast cancer for white females who are being examined annually. JNCI 1989;81:1879–1886)

TABLE 65–4. Empiric Familial Recurrence Risks for Selected Common Cancers

Cancer	Mendelian Risk	Empiric Recurrence Risk*
Skin (Basal cell or squamous cell)		
General		1% (Depending on skin exposure)
Nevoid basal cell carcinoma syndrome	AD	
Xeroderma pigmentosum	AR	
Lung		
General		Relative risk of 3.0
Interstitial pulmonary fibrosis	AD	
P450-susceptible	AD	
Colorectal		
General		3–5%
Many polyposis syndromes	AD	
Turcot polyposis syndrome	AR	
Adenoma-carcinoma syndrome	AD	
Pancreas		
General		<1%
Hereditary pancreatitis	AD	
Breast		
General		See Tables 65–2 and 65–3
Cowden's disease	AD	
Certain families, especially with ovarian, linked to chromosome 17q	AD	
Ovarian carcinoma		
General		3–5%
Certain rare families	AD	
Prostate		
General		3%
Rare families	AD	

AD, autosomal dominant; AR, autosomal recessive.
* For first-degree relative (brother, sister, parent, child) with the same cancer.
(Mulvihill JJ. McKusick's mendelian inheritance in man: Oncology. Baltimore: Johns Hopkins University Press, 1993)

no greater than that of the population at large. The caveat should be added that future developments in the patient's or family's medical history may alter the patient's risk and that such developments should be brought to the counselor's attention.

GENETIC COUNSELING AT THE BEGINNING OF THERAPY

RISKS TO THE PATIENT

It is important to counsel the new cancer patient about the potential for decreased fertility caused by the cancer and its treatment. Cancer may affect the reproductive organs directly, or cancer surgery may impair reproduction. More likely, the use of alkylating agents, especially combined with radiotherapy below the diaphragm, predictably diminish reproductive potential. Alternate regimens that maintain excellent survival rates but decrease reproductive toxicity may be considered. Women have been offered oophoropexy to position ovaries outside radiotherapy fields to try to preserve fertility. Men may consider sperm banking before the therapy starts if they are interested in improving their potential for having natural children after the completion of cancer treatment, although the systemic effects of the cancer may have already impaired or reduced sperm production to below levels that can be effectively cryopreserved.

TERATOGENICITY

A rare but extremely unfortunate situation is the simultaneous diagnosis of cancer and pregnancy.[47] Pregnancy is contraindicated during cancer therapy because most cancer therapies are teratogens that are toxic to the fetus. Part of the advice at the onset of cancer therapy of a woman of reproductive age is to recommend birth control or at least to alert the woman of the potential for teratogenicity.

In human beings, largely based on experience of pregnant women exposed to the atomic bombs in Japan, as few as 10 cGy to the developing fetus between 8 and 15 weeks of gestational age is thought to result in some loss on IQ performance.[48,49] Microcephaly and short stature are the results of fetal exposure to higher doses of ionizing radiation. Each 100 cGy of fetal dose is calculated to lower IQ by 30 points. The older fetus is quite radioresistant. We documented normal findings in a 52-year-old man who, as a 30-week fetus, had been exposed to 180 to 300 cGy of radiation to the brain, given in the course of treating his mother's cervical cancer.[50]

If therapy has been inadvertently given to a woman with cancer who is later recognized to be pregnant or if life-saving therapy for a pregnant woman with cancer must begin, it may be possible to modify therapy to agents that are less likely to be teratogenic than others. For this purpose of genetic counseling, a registry of pregnancies exposed to cancer therapy was established at the NCI and is maintained at the University of Pittsburgh.[51] Because cancer treatment during pregnancy is a rare and sometimes accidental event, the exact teratogenicity of various chemotherapeutic agents will never be the subject of rigorous analytic epidemiologic study. It seems best to register the rare human experience as it accrues. The registry is available to answer immediate questions, for example, about the published and unpublished experience of vincristine given to women who are 5- to 6-weeks pregnant. Contrary to expectations, even substantial chemotherapy in the first trimester is not inevitably teratogenic. If a pregnancy exposed to cancer treatment is much wanted, there is some room for reassurance that gross malformations are not inevitable. However, given the experience with other human teratogens (*e.g.*, fetal alcohol syndrome), the least apparent manifestation of toxicity to the developing fetus is often a loss of higher brain function (*i.e.*, behavioral traits, IQ). It is better to expose no embryo or fetus to chemotherapy or radiotherapy.

GENETIC COUNSELING AFTER THERAPY ENDS

Former cancer patients should be told that there are major theoretical concerns about possible somatic and germ cell mutations. Cancer treatments are specifically designed to interfere with DNA, cellular metabolism, and cell division. There is good reason to suspect a priori that cancer treatments can cause mutation and genetic disease in human beings. They do so in mice and in somatic cells of human beings (*e.g.*, sustained chromosomal breakage or second cancers after cancer treatment). However, no environmental agent has been causally linked to human germ cell mutation, contrary to expectations. Despite intensive study of various parameters, genetic damage has not been seen in the offspring of the survivors of the atomic bombs in Japan.[52] Indicators of possible genetic damage have been birth defects, newborn survival, chromosomal abnormalities, a change in protein structure or function, and growth or development of malignancies.

In several large retrospective case series (Table 65–5), there was some room for reassurance that, despite expectations, no excess of birth defects or genetic diseases has been seen in the offspring of cancer survivors who maintain fertility enough to bear or father children. In 3687 liveborns from 15 cases series in the literature, the summary rate of birth defects and genetic disease is 4%, a rate comparable to that in the general population. The studies were not all directly comparable in how cancer survivors were identified and pregnancy outcomes were defined. In the single largest study, the NCI Five Center Study, family controls and population expected numbers were used, and no excess of genetic disease was seen.[66] That study alone had a 94% power to detect a 50% increase and did not find it.

Based on just two offspring with interventricular septal defects of the heart, the question was raised of possible adverse effects on pregnancies of women who had received dactinomycin.[67] Special analysis of the Five Center Study data could not confirm the association.[68]

Among 4256 offspring of survivors of childhood and adolescent cancer followed for over 32,000 person-years, 33 offspring had cancer; 25 of them had retinoblastoma, as did a parent of each.[69,70] Except for known hereditary or familial cancer syndromes, the offspring of survivors of cancer seem to have no excess of cancer.

TABLE 65–5. Large Series of Pregnancies Among Survivors of Cancer

	Exposed Parents		Completed Pregnancies			Liveborns		
Investigations	Total	Females (%)	Total	Fetal Loss*	Elective Abortions	Total	With Defects	Type of Defects
Li and Jaffe, ?–1973[53]	45	63	107	15	3	90	2	Hirschsprung's disease, asymptomatic heart murmur‡
Ross, 1956–1973[54]	58†	100	96	18	?	75	3	Penred's syndrome, tetralogy of Fallot, hemangiomata, eczema and strabismus (1 stillborn with aplasia of the anterior abdominal wall)
Holmes and Holmes[55]	48	60	93	12	3	77	6	Amblyopia, autism, scleroderma, rectal stenosis, absent fallopian tube and small uterus, slow learner and foot defect
Li et al[56]	146	58	286	45	10	236	8	Possible trisomy 18 syndrome, Marfan's syndrome, deafness, pyloric stenosis, Hirschsprung's disease (same as above), cardiac, brain, and multiple malformations
Blatt et al, ?–1980[57]	30	77	40	12	10	27	1	Congenital hip dysplasia
Horning et al, 1968–1979[58]	29	100	28	5	5	24	0	
Marradi et al, ?–1982[59]	14	57	23	?	?	21	2	Multiple congenital anomalies with mental and growth retardation, panhypopituitarism and cerebral atrophy, gastroschisis
Bundey and Evans, ?–1973[60]	24	83	48	3	0	44	1	Pyloric stenosis
Andrieu and Ochoa-Molina, 1972–1976[61]	22	100	30	9	4	21	1	Congenital hip dysplasia
Rustin et al, 1958–1980[62]	216†	100	374	90	36	267	8	Spina bifida, tetralogy of Fallot, talipes eqinovares, collapsed lung, umbilical hernia, desquamative fibrosing alveolitis (2 sibs), neonatal tachycardia (plus 2 anencephalic stillbirths and 1 sudden infant death)
Goldstein et al, 1965–1983[63]	?†	100	222	58	6	159	5	Not specified
Mulvihill et al, 1959–1977[64]	66	100	87	22	12	53	6	Neurosensory deafness‡, scoliosis and slow learner‡, hydrocephalus‡, cleft lip and palate‡, hydrocephalus, tracheomalacia
Li et al, 1931–1979[65]	181	65	246	53	32	190	5	Congenital hip dislocation (2), heart murmur, hypospadias, internal tibial torsion
Mulvihill et al, 1945–1975[66]	2308	~50	?	?	?	2198	75	(Rate no different than control)
Green et al, 1960–1984[67]	60	58	?	?	?	100	8	Ventricular septal defect, tetralogy of Fallot, hydrocele, birth marks (2), skin tags, epidermal nevus
Total	3212	58	>4059	>373	132	3687	136	

* Fetal loss is defined as elective abortion, ectopic pregnancy, spontaneous abortion (miscarriage), or stillbirth; ?, uncertain.
† All gestational trophoblastic neoplasia.
‡ Exposed to cancer treatment during gestation.
(Modified from Mulvihill JJ, Byrne J. Offspring of long-time survivors of childhood cancers. Clin Oncol 1985;4:333–343)

CONCLUSION

Many questions remain about the proper care and counseling of survivors of cancer. Because no center and few nations will in the near future have much experience with pregnancies in or by cancer patients, it is hoped that collaborative international studies will prove feasible and gain wide support from clinicians. Currently, the ideal situation is that genetic and reproductive counseling should take place as soon as cancer is diagnosed (before therapy starts) and again when pregnancy is contemplated.

REFERENCES

1. Fraser FC. Genetic counseling. Am J Hum Genet 1974;26:636–659.
2. Kushner R. Why me? New York: Holt, Rinehart, and Winston, 1982.
3. Parry DM, Berg K, Mulvihill JJ, et al. Strategies for controlling cancer through genetics: Report of a workshop. Am J Hum Genet 1987;41:63–69.
4. Parry DM, Mulvihill JJ, Miller RW, et al. Strategies for controlling cancer through genetics. Cancer Res 1987;47:6814–1817.
5. Mulvihill JJ. Prospects for cancer control and prevention through genetics. Clin Genet 1989;36:313–319.
6. Mulvihill JJ. Childhood cancer, the environment, and heredity. In: Pizzo PA, Poplack DG, eds. Principles and practice of pediatric oncology, 2nd ed. Philadelphia: JB Lippincott, 1993.
7. Phelan MC, Stevenson RE, Collins JL, et al. Fragile X syndrome and neoplasia. Am J Med Genet 1988;30:77–82.
8. Cohen AJ, Li FP, Berg S, et al. Hereditary renal cell carcinoma associated with a chromosomal translocation. N Engl J Med 1979;301:592–595.
9. Yunis JJ, Ramsay NKC. Familial occurrence of the aniridia-Wilms' tumor syndrome with deletion 11p13–14.1. J Pediatr 1980;96:1027–1030.
10. Strong LC, Riccardi VM, Ferrell RE, et al. Familial retinoblastoma and chromosome 13 deletion transmitted via an insertional translocation. Science 1981;213:1501–1503.
11. Bolger GB, Stamberg J, Kirsch IR, et al. Chromosome translocation t(14;22) and oncogene (c-*sis*) variant in a pedigree with familial meningioma. N Engl J Med 1985;312:564–567.
12. McKusick VA. Mendelian inheritance in man. 9th ed. Baltimore: Johns Hopkins, 1990.
13. Mulvihill JJ. McKusick's mendelian inheritance in man: Oncology. Baltimore: Johns Hopkins University Press, 1993.
14. Müller HJ. Familial cancer in Basel: Some aspects. In: Müller HJ, Weber W, eds. Familial cancer. Basel: Karger, 1985:1–5.
15. Albano WA, Lynch HT, Recabaren JA, et al. Family cancer in an oncology clinic. Cancer 1981;47:2113–2118.
16. Love RR, Evans AM, Josten DM. The accuracy of patient reports of a family history of cancer. J Chron Dis 1985;38:289–293.
17. Li FP, Lokich J, Lapey J, Neptune WB, Wilkins EW Jr: Familial mesothelioma after intense asbestos exposure at home. JAMA 1978;240:467.
18. Lynch HT, Lynch JF, Cristofaro G. Genetic epidemiology of colon cancer. In: Lynch HT, Hirayama T, eds. Genetic epidemiology of cancer. Boca Raton: CRC Press, 1989:251–277.
19. Li FP, Fraumeni JF Jr, Mulvihill JJ, et al. A cancer family syndrome in twenty-four kindreds. Cancer Res 1988;48:5358–5362.
20. Malkin D, Li FP, Strong LC, Fraumeni JF Jr, et al. Germ line *p53* mutations in a familial syndrome of breast cancer, sarcomas, and other neoplasms. Science 1990;250:1233–1238.
21. Weber W, Dürig M, eds. Hereditary cancer and preventive surgery. Basel: Karger, 1990:118.
22. Blattner WA. The interdisciplinary approach to cancer families. In: Mulvihill JJ, Miller RN, Fraumeni JF Jr, eds. Genetics of human cancer. New York: Raven Press, 1972.
23. Lynch HT, Fitzsimmons ML, Lynch J, et al. A hereditary cancer consultation clinic. Nebraska Med J 1989;74:351–359.
24. Josten DM, Evans AM, Love RR. The cancer prevention clinic: A service program for cancer-prone families. J Psychosoc Oncol 1986;3:5–20.
25. Ponder BAJ. Familial cancer: Opportunities for clinical practice and research. Eur J Surg Oncol 1987;13:463–473.
26. Kelly PT. Risk counseling for relatives of cancer patients: New information, new approaches. J Psychosoc Oncol 1987;5:65–79.
27. LeMarec B, LeGail E, Journel H, et al. Le conseil génétique en cancérologie. Presse Med 1986;15:1369–1371.
28. Williams CJ. Managing families genetically predisposed to cancer: The "cancer-family syndrome" as a model. In: Chaganti RSK, German J, eds. Genetics in clinical oncology. New York: Oxford University Press, 1985:222–240.
29. Philippe P. Les familles à cancer. Paris: Éditions Maloine, 1985:181–191.
30. Bussey HJF. Familial polyposis coli. Baltimore: Johns Hopkins, 1975:104.
31. Burt RW, Bishop DT, Lynch HT, et al. Risk and surveillance of individuals with heritable factors for colorectal cancer. Bull World Health Org 1990;68:655–665.
32. Kersey JH, Shapiro RS, Filipovich AH. Relationship of immunodeficiency to lymphoid malignancy. Pediatr Infect Dis J 1988;7:S10–S12.
33. Goldstein AM, Dracopoli NC, Ho EC, et al. Further evidence for a locus for cutaneous malignant melanoma-dysplastic nevus (CMM/DN) on chromosome 1p and evidence for genetic heterogeneity. Am J Hum Genet (in press).
34. Tulinius H. Familial cancer registration in Iceland. In: Müller HJ, Weber W, eds. Familial cancer. Basel: Karger, 1985:263–267.
35. Steinitz R, Costin C, Ben-Hur M, et al. Clusters of families in a population-based cancer registry: Methodological problems. In: Müller HJ, Weber W, eds. Familial cancer. Basel: Karger, 1985:272–274.
36. Skolnick M. The Utah genealogical data base: A resource for genetic epidemiology. In: Cairns J, Lyon JL, Skolnick M, eds. Banbury report 4. Cold Spring Harbor, NY: Cold Spring Harbor Laboratory, 1980:285–297.
37. Williams RR, Hunt SC, Barlow GK, et al. Health family trees: A tool for finding and helping young family members of coronary and cancer prone pedigrees in Texas and Utah. Am J Public Health 1988;78:1283–1286.
38. Gail MH, Brinton LA, Byar DP, et al. Projecting individualized probabilities of developing breast cancer for white females who are being examined annually. JNCI 1989;81:1879–1886.
39. Fisher B, Redmond C. New perspective on cancer of the contralateral breast: A marker for assessing tamoxifen as a preventive agent. JNCI 1991;464:1278–1280.
40. Claus EB, Risch N, Thompson WD. Autosomal dominant inheritance of early onset breast cancer: Implications for risk prediction. Cancer (in press).
41. Mulvihill JJ, Safyer AW, Bening JK. Prevention in familial breast cancer: Counseling and prophylactic mastectomy. Prev Med 1982;11:500–511.
42. Lynch HT, Lynch JF, Fusaro RM. Clinical importance of familial cancer. In: Müller HJ, Weber W, eds. Familial cancer. Basel: Karger, 1985:6–12.
43. Lerman C, Rimer B, Engstrom P. Cancer risk notification: Psychosocial and ethical implications. J Clin Oncol 1991;9:1275–1282.
44. Wapnir IL, Rabinowitz B, Greco R. A reappraisal of prophylactic mastectomy. Surg 1990;171:171–184.
45. Kash KM, Holland JC, Helper MS, Miller DG. Psychological distress and surveillance behaviors of women with a family history of breast cancer. JNCI 1992;84:24–30.
46. Evans AM, Love RR, Meyerowitz BE, et al. Factors associated with active participation in a cancer prevention clinic. Prev Med 1985;14:358–371.
47. Allen HH, Nisker JA, eds. Cancer in pregnancy: Therapeutic guidelines. Mt. Kisco, NY: Futura Publishing, 1986.
48. United Nations Environment Programme. Radiation: Doses, effects, risks. Oxford, Blackwell, 1991:89.
49. Miller RW, Mulvihill JJ. Small head size after atomic irradiation. Teratology 1976;14:355–357.
50. Mulvihill JJ, Harvey EB, Boice JD Jr, et al. Normal findings 52 years after in utero radiation exposure. Lancet 1991;338:1202–1203.
51. Mulvihill JJ, Stewart KR. A registry of pregnancies exposed to chemotherapeutic agents. Teratology 1986;33:80C.
52. Neel JV, Satoh C, Goriki K, et al. Search for mutations altering protein charge and/or function in children of atomic bomb survivors: Final report. Am J Hum Genet 1988;42:663–676.
53. Li FP, Jaffe H. Progeny of childhood-cancer survivors. Lancet 1974;2:707–709.
54. Ross GT. Congenital anomalies among children born of mothers receiving chemotherapy for gestational trophoblastic neoplasms. Cancer 1976;37:1043–1047.
55. Holmes GE, Holmes FF. Pregnancy outcome of patients treated for Hodgkin's disease: A controlled study. Cancer 1978;41:1317–1322.
56. Li FP, Fine W, Jaffe H, et al. Offspring of patients treated for cancer in childhood. JNCI 1979;62:1193–1197.
57. Blatt J, Mulvihill JJ, Ziegler JL, et al. Pregnancy outcome following cancer chemotherapy. Am J Med 1980;69:828–832.
58. Horning SJ, Hippe RT, Kaplan HS, et al. Female reproductive potential after treatment for Hodgkin's disease. N Engl J Med 1981;304:1377–1382.
59. Marradi P, Schaison F, Alby N, et al. Les enfants nés de parents leucémiques. Nouv Rev Fr Hematol 1982;24:75–80.
60. Bundey S, Evans K. Survivors of neuroblastoma and ganglioneuroma and their families. J Med Genet 1982;19:16–21.
61. Andrieu JM, Ochoa-Molina ME. Menstrual cycle, pregnancies and offspring before and after MOPP therapy for Hodgkin's disease. Cancer 1983;52:435–438.
62. Rustin GJS, Booth M, Dent J, et al. Pregnancy after cytotoxic chemotherapy for gestational trophoblastic tumours. Br Med J 1984;288:103–106.
63. Goldstein DP, Berkowitz RS, Bernstein MR. Reproductive performance after molar pregnancy and gestational trophoblastic tumors. Clin Obstet Gynecol 1983;27:221–227.
64. Mulvihill JJ, McKeen EA, Rosner F, et al. Pregnancy outcome in cancer patients: Experience in a large cooperative group. Cancer 1987;60:1143–1150.
65. Li FP, Gimbrere K, Gelber RD, et al. Outcome of pregnancy in survivors of Wilms' tumor. JAMA 1987;257:216–219.
66. Mulvihill JJ, Byrne J, Steinhorn SA, et al. Genetic disease in offspring of survivors of cancer in the young. Am J Hum Genet 1986;39:A72.
67. Green DM, Zevon MA, Lowrie G, et al. Congenital anomalies in children of patients who received chemotherapy for cancer in childhood and adolescence. N Engl J Med 1991;325:141–146.
68. Byrne J, Nicholson HS, Mulvihill JJ. Absence of birth defects in offspring of women treated with dactinomycin. N Engl J Med 1992;326:137.
69. Mulvihill JJ, Myers MH, Connelly RR, et al. Cancer in offspring of long-term survivors of childhood and adolescent cancer. Lancet 1987;2:813–817.
70. Hawkins MM, Draper GJ, Smith RA. Cancer among 1,348 offspring of survivors of childhood cancer. Int J Cancer 1989;43:975–978.

Cancer: Principles & Practice of Oncology, Fourth Edition,
edited by Vincent T. DeVita, Jr., Samuel Hellman, Steven A. Rosenberg.
J.B. Lippincott Co., Philadelphia © 1993.

Lynn H. Gerber   Patrice Gallelli

Stephen Levinson   Jessie Whitehurst

Jeanne E. Hicks   Donna Scheib

Barbara C. Sonies

CHAPTER **66**

Evaluation and Management of Disability: Rehabilitation Aspects of Cancer

The oncologist or oncologic surgeon may be most concerned with the ablation of tumor and with the ultimate survival of the patient, and the patient may be just as concerned with issues of function, quality of life, and with independence in life routines. Factors predicting whether a patient will have a good functional outcome after cancer treatment include the site, stage, type, and rate of growth of tumor, but other factors may be as influential. These typically include coexisting medical conditions, concomitant use of medications, age or life stage, and psychosocial variables such as motivation, depression, or optimism. The impact of cancer treatments on function, much of which is not appreciated until well after primary treatment has been completed, is often significant. Key examples of this are the long-term effects of irradiation on the brachial plexus or the central nervous system (CNS).

Often, as a result of the underlying disease process or of its treatment, patients are forced to accept a degree of physical dependence on others. Long-term disability, however, is a treatable and often preventable complication of cancer and cancer therapy. Early intervention by the cancer rehabilitation team can significantly reduce the morbidity associated with malignant disorders.

Disability in a significant portion of patients undergoing treatment for cancer has been well documented.[1] The causes of disability are varied and often difficult to predict from the tumor type alone. Most obvious are the direct effects of primary and metastatic lesions. Invasion of soft tissues can cause pain and, if skeletal structures are involved, loss of bony in-

tegrity.[2] Invasion of the digestive tract or liver can lead to generalized wasting, and invasion of the lungs or pleura can lead to respiratory compromise.

CNS involvement can result in cognitive impairment, or if the spinal column is involved, in quadriplegia or paraplegia. This can affect mobility and gross physical function, and it may interfere with essential body functions such as respiration and waste elimination. Bulbar involvement may impede autonomic or motor control, and it may lead to dysfunctional speech and swallowing. Peripheral nerves may be compromised by the direct effects of a tumor or its metastases, resulting in the loss of critical sensory or motor functions.

Venous compression may result in edema or in deep venous thrombosis that can lead to life-threatening pulmonary embolus. Edema can result from lymphatic obstruction. Left untreated, the swollen extremity can become a major burden to the patient, impeding mobility, causing pain and discomfort, and leading to the development of permanent changes in skin consistency. The edematous extremity can become infected or necrotic, with tissue breakdown leading to severe morbidity and mortality.

A tumor may result in disability through its systemic effects. Paraneoplastic syndromes resulting in myopathy, neuropathy, and cerebellar dysfunction are well documented.[3,4] Perhaps the most significant causes of disability are related to cancer treatment. Chemotherapy-related neuropathies are commonly related to agents such as vincristine, cisplatin, DDC, and DDI. Radiation treatment often results in neuropathies, plexopathies, and myelopathies in lymphedema and in tissue fibrosis. Irradiation effects are often not evident until months or years after the completion of all treatment. Surgery can lead to the loss of a limb or of important functional elements. Prolonged bed rest can lead to severe deconditioning and significant psychological morbidity.

New treatment strategies may be associated with disability and with new challenges to the rehabilitation specialist. Limb-salvage procedures may preserve anatomy and body image, although occasionally at the expense of function. Early involvement of the cancer rehabilitation team can help to predict the degree of disability and to help the patient make an informed decision about a variety of treatment options. Strategies to help adapt to the loss of critical musculoskeletal elements can often be devised before treatment actually begins.

The patient undergoing immunotherapy with agents such as interleukin-2 (IL-2) presents another set of challenges, including phenomenal fluid shifts.[5] Intraoperative irradiation can result in a more concentrated delivery of radiation to the tumor bed, but it has been our experience that severe delayed peripheral neuropathy and pain are frequent sequelae. Rehabilitation can play a role in the evaluation, treatment and prevention of disability.

THE ROLE OF REHABILITATION

Rehabilitation is a phased process, which should begin soon after diagnosis if a disability is anticipated. It should continue until the patient has reached maximal functional benefit.

THE PRETREATMENT EVALUATION

A complete functional assessment should be made at the time of staging, with particular attention to the home environment, the patient's occupation, and his or her valued roles. This assessment focuses attention on strategies that can preserve the aspects of function that are most important to the patient. Potential problem areas can be identified and possible solutions explored.

If multiple treatment options exist, discussion should center on the functional impact of each potential treatment program and the rehabilitation strategies that are required to maintain or restore full function. When surgery is planned, the rehabilitation team can make preparations in advance, such as the provision of adaptive equipment and gait aids to promote independence. Prosthetic and orthotic devices can be planned before surgery, and initial prosthetic fitting can even take place in the operating room. When radiation therapy is planned, the patient can be trained in an exercise program designed to minimize the effects of radiation fibrosis.

REHABILITATION DURING THE TREATMENT PHASE

Treatment should begin with mobility to prevent the complications of prolonged bed rest. Pain management using heat, cold transcutaneous electrical nerve stimulation (TENS) can help prevent a patient becoming a chronic pain patient. Gait and functional retraining can the proceed even as the patient receives chemotherapy or radiation therapy. Other problems such as peripheral neuropathies, myopathies, myelopathies,

and pathologic fractures can be addressed as rapidly as they arise.

REHABILITATION OF THE CANCER SURVIVOR

After treatment has been completed, the cancer patient may need continued treatment to maintain strength and range of motion (ROM), control pain, and return to normal activity. There may be residual effects of the disease or its treatment, and the patient may suffer from nutritional deficits and from a loss of physical capacity. Psychosocial issues may be a critical factor.[6] The survivor often has an impaired body image, and patients always perceive themselves as being different from the rest of the world. The fear of recurrence is a real one, but cancer survivors often deny obvious signs of recurrent tumor.[7]

Vocational counseling and retraining are important aspects of returning the cancer patient to the community. Adaptive strategies are often needed to facilitate the return to work. Job discrimination is a real problem that may interfere with the rehabilitative process and that must be overcome.[8,9] The clinical oncology and cancer rehabilitation teams often must serve in an advocacy role.

Sexual rehabilitation is an important aspect of cancer survivorship that is often ignored.[10,11] Pain during intercourse is a common problem that can often be overcome using modified sexual practices. Infertility may be a secondary issue during the acute phase of cancer treatment, only to emerge as a primary concern in the survivor.[12] Teratogenesis and the complications of pregnancy may be concerns.[13]

The child with cancer presents a special set of circumstances.[14-16] The rehabilitation team often must treat the entire family. Siblings may feel particularly vulnerable, or they may feel resentment about the attention received by the patient. Parents may feel guilt that they may have inadvertently caused the illness, and parents may sometimes place blame on each other. Classmates may have difficulty understanding what the patient has been through, and they may, out of their own fear, treat the patient as if cancer were a communicable disease. Growth and development are frequently impaired. Although the survivor of childhood cancer usually regains much of the development that was lost or delayed after treatment has been completed, residual short stature, uneven growth, and cognitive impairment are frequent long-term sequelae of treatment.[17-20]

Late neurologic complications of cancer include plexopathies, peripheral neuropathies, and myelopathies, all of which can be the result of late radiation effects or of tumor recurrence. Abnormal brain development or cognitive impairment can result from intrathecal chemotherapy or from brain irradiation, although late deterioration should always lead to the suspicion of recurrent metastatic disease. Paraneoplastic syndromes, including cerebellar degeneration, encephalomyelitis, subacute necrotizing myelopathy, peripheral neuropathies, myopathies, and myasthenic syndrome, are uncommon but documented late complications that may not resolve with resolution of the malignancy.[3,21] Chronic pain related to radiation fibrosis, radiation neuritis, or tumor recurrence may result in the need for late rehabilitative interventions.

A swollen extremity in the cancer survivor always warrants further investigation. Swelling may be the result of deep venous thrombosis, lymphatic tumor invasion, or venous obstruction by tumor. Lymphedema, often related to radiation fibrosis or previous surgery, should be a diagnosis of exclusion. Rehabilitation management may require the use of compressive garments or pumps, exercise, and the use of moisturizing creams. The use of a compression pump in the face of recurrent lymphatic involvement may increase the likelihood of further tumor spread. Radiation fibrosis may require the use of exercise, splinting, orthotic appliances, moisturizing creams, or surgery.

REHABILITATION OF THE TERMINAL PATIENT

Even in the patient in whom there is no chance of survival, rehabilitation can play a critical role in the prevention of unnecessary morbidity. Pain control is of utmost importance. Prevention of skin ulcers, contractures, and generalized wasting can improve the quality of life. Maintaining mobility through the use of exercises and adaptive devices can maximize patient independence and minimize the burden to others.

THE CANCER REHABILITATION TEAM

Rehabilitation is a complex discipline that involves the interaction of numerous treatment providers, each with a particular area of training. The rehabilitation team is usually composed of physiatrists, occupational and physical therapists, speech and language pathologists, vocational counsellors, and a variety of other professionals as determined by the particular needs of the individual patient.

Although any rehabilitation specialist can serve as the team leader, we feel that, if possible, the rehabilitation team should be led by a medical rehabilitation specialist. A *physiatrist* is a physician who has specialty training in the field of physical medicine and rehabilitation. This training includes a core of information about the causes and effects of functional disability, the basic biomechanics of human motion, methods of functional assessment, and adaptive strategies. This physician is usually well equipped to prescribe and train patients in the use of orthotics, prosthetics, and adaptive equipment.

The *physical therapist* is an allied health specialist well informed in the basic mechanics of human motion and exercise. Physical therapists often institute and supervise an exercise program to improve mobility, strength, and stamina. If involved early in the course of treatment, they can instruct the patient and the family in a basic exercise program to prevent muscle atrophy or contractures and maintain fitness. Typically, physical therapists provide assessments of ROM, manual muscle testing, and gait. They use orthotics and other adaptive devices to correct specific neuromuscular impairments, such as a foot drop, and they may treat edema using exercise, compressive pumps, and elastic stockings. They are particularly adept at the use of superficial and deep heating modalities, traction, hydrotherapy, and electrical stimulation in the management of open wounds, contractures, and pain. Working with occupational therapists, they may address issues such as bed mobility and the use of wheel chairs or custom seating.

Occupational therapists are specialists who evaluate and treat dysfunction in daily living activities, including self-care, work, and leisure-related activities, placing emphasis on those roles and activities that the patient most values. They often help to develop alternative strategies for performing basic self-care activities and other valued roles, making use of adaptive equipment where indicated. Bathroom safety is an issue of particular importance to the cancer patient, and occupational therapists frequently recommend or provide devices such as a raised toilet seat or bedside commode, a tub or shower transfer bench or chair, a hand-held shower hose, and grab bars.

Occupational therapists are often involved with the evaluation of wheelchairs and custom seating for assisted mobility. They play a major role in the assessment and management of hand dysfunction and often make use of therapeutic hand exercises, splints, and braces to restore function. Vocational issues are often the responsibility of the occupational therapist, although in some institutions, a separate *vocational counselor* is a part of the rehabilitation team. In some cases, the occupational therapist performs a home visit to evaluate the home environment and physical changes that are needed for the patient to be safe and independent.

The *social worker* provides important input into the rehabilitation process for the cancer patient, evaluating the complete home environment and determining the availability, willingness, and strengths of family members who can assist with care and support of the patient. The social worker may help the family evaluate its financial resources and provide information on available support services.

Speech pathologists evaluate communication skills and the mechanics of speech and swallowing. In many institutions, they perform cognitive assessments and training in basic memory skills. They may provide vocal retraining and instruction in alaryngeal speech, and they may provide equipment for alternative methods of communication such as with an alphabet board or a computer. They assess functional integrity and compensatory ability of structures and mechanisms needed to achieve adequate communication, deglutition, nutrition, hydration, and cognition. They are often involved with the evaluation and treatment of dysphagia and work with *maxillofacial prosthetists* in the restoration of facial appearance and oral function.

Audiologists assess the integrity of the peripheral and central auditory mechanism in relation to presurgical and postsurgical, intraoperative, and ototoxic effects on hearing. They provide advice for preserving or restoring hearing using augmentative devices.

A *psychologist* can play a crucial role as a member of the cancer rehabilitation team. Virtually all cancer patients must address issues of death and dying and many need the support of someone trained in this area. Patients may have difficulty dealing with changes in their body image, particularly with the loss of a limb. *Clinical neuropsychologists* may be involved with the evaluation of cognitive impairment.

The *rehabilitation nurse* is a nurse who has specialty training in rehabilitative aspects of nursing care. Particular emphasis is placed on bowel and bladder management in the patient with neurogenic disorders of waste elimination and on wound management. The rehabilitation nurse may be involved with ostomy care and with the training of the patient or family in the management of catheters, ostomy equipment, and surgical dressings.

The *prosthetist-orthotist* is involved with the fitting and fabrication of braces and artificial limbs. In oncology, the prosthetists often provide valuable input about appropriate prosthetic or orthotic components that may be used. In cases of limb-sparing procedures, the orthotist often needs to fabricate devices that substitute for weak muscle groups or unstable joints.

A variety of other practitioners may be involved as part of the rehabilitation team. These may include the chaplains, recreational therapists, nutritional services, psychiatrists, and pain management specialists. By assembling an optimal mix of specialists, it is possible to minimize the disability that results from malignancy and its treatment.

FUNCTIONAL EVALUATION

It is necessary for rehabilitation specialists to evaluate the impact of cancer diagnoses on complex behaviors and activities and its impact on anatomic structures and physiologic processes. These evaluations, often called global or functional assessments, are multidimensional and combine objective measures and subjective reports.

Typically, the evaluations include joint ROM data, strength measures and measurements of stamina and often measures of pain intensity. Some evaluations include measures of the psychological impact of cancer on patients and their adjustment to it.[22] Most functional assessments include indices that reflect independence in self-care, mobility, bowel or bladder functioning, and cognitive performance if indicated.

These measurement tools are useful as long as they are reliable, sensitive to the magnitude of change expected, easy to use, and standardized for the cancer population.[23]

COMMON FUNCTIONAL IMPAIRMENTS IN ONCOLOGY

The common functional impairments caused by cancer therapy are summarized in Table 66–1.

IMMOBILITY AND ITS IMPACT

Bed rest in cancer patients is associated with numerous metabolic and physiologic changes that may impair the patient's medical and functional recovery.[24] Bone loss is well documented and, in extreme cases, may lead to hypercalcemia.[25-27] In patients who are already osteoporotic or who have metastatic involvement of the skeletal system, this may predispose to pathologic fractures and further disability. The use of agents to minimize bone loss is somewhat controversial.[28,29] Muscle atrophy can be quite rapid, often leading to an inability to walk in as short a time as a week. Changes in muscle physiology and fiber type have been documented as well.[30,31] As muscle mass becomes reduced, the amount of soft tissue covering bony prominences can become marginal, predisposing to the development of pressure ulcers (decubiti). Prolonged pressure over the nerves and particularly over the peroneal nerve as it crosses the fibular head may lead to a mononeuropathy and foot drop. Lack of motion about the joints may result in contractures and changes in muscle and joint physiology.[32,33] Lack of mobility can lead to the development of deep venous thrombosis and pulmonary embolus.[34] All of these factors can significantly reduce mobility and independence.

Generalized Deconditioning

As a rule of thumb, each week of immobility requires as much as a month of rehabilitation to regain functional mobility.

TABLE 66–1. Functional Impairments Caused by Cancer Therapy

Musculoskeletal Problem	Primary Cancer Therapy			
	Surgery	Chemotherapy	Irradiation	Immunotherapy
Atrophy/weakness	X	X	X	X
Contracture	X		X	
Decubiti/wound complications	X	X	X	X
Edema	X	X	X	X
Gait deficits	X	X	X	
Joint instability	X		X	
Neuropathy (sensory and motor)	X	X	X	
Pain	X		X	
Generalized deconditioning (cardiotoxicity)		X	X	X
CNS involvement (UMN/LMN)	X	X	X	
Cosmetic deficits	X		X	

UMN/LMN, upper motor neuron/lower motor neuron.
(Modified from Gerber LH, McGarvey CL. Musculoskeletal deficits and rehabilitation intervention in the cancer patient. In: Wittes RE, ed. Manual of oncologic therapeutics. Philadelphia: JB Lippincott, 1991:417)

Complications such as pathologic fractures and pressure ulcers can further prolong the hospital stay. Although it is sometimes impossible to fully mobilize a patient receiving chemotherapy or major surgery, some degree of mobilization under a physical therapist's supervision may significantly reduce morbidity. For the patient who is mildly restricted by disease or treatment, active ambulation at least once or twice daily should be strongly encouraged. If this is not possible, an exercise program in bed may be started, using resistance against gravity or against an elastic band. A tilt table may be used to maintain or restore cardiovascular conditioning in the patient who is unable to stand. This helps to minimize heel cord contractures. In patients with severe dependent edema, compressive garments may help to maintain the vascular volume and to reduce the degree of the edema while facilitating ambulation. Exercises, by increasing muscular tone and facilitating venous compression, can help to maintain cardiovascular volume.

Skin Care

Prevention of skin breakdown should be of utmost importance in the bed-bound patient. Above all else, the patient must not be allowed to remain in a single position for more than 2 hours. If the patient is unable to position himself or herself in bed, repositioning should be done with pillows or cushions, taking care not to encourage the development of contractures by, for example, persistently flexing the neck, hips, or knees. Air-cushioned beds can help to reduce the incidence of pressure injuries, but they do not substitute for proper nursing care. Sequential air chamber mattresses seem to be as effective as older designs, provided that an intervening cushion such as an egg-crate or sheepskin mattress is not used. Shear forces and direct pressure may be important in the development of decubiti. Care should therefore be taken to avoid leaving the patient slouched in a chair or in bed with the head elevated, because these positions can predispose to ischial and sacral pressure wounds, respectively.

If skin becomes dry, aqueous remoisturizing creams should be applied. Greasy agents can predispose to maceration and breakdown. Irradiated skin is of particular concern, due to the loss of normal resilience and healing capacity. Moisturizing agents may be required for the remainder of the patient's lifetime. Careful attention to hygiene is important with irradiated skin, and all open cuts and abrasions should receive scrutiny, because these can easily become infected.

When complications arise, they should be treated promptly. Areas of skin redness that do not blanch should be considered to be early pressure ulcers (stage I) and treated by removing pressure over the affected area. Most tissue damage in pressure ulcers occurs in the deep layers of the dermis and underlying tissues, such that the visible portion of the ulcer may represent only a fraction of the total extent. If actual skin breakdown occurs, care should be taken to keep the wound clean and to avoid the accumulation of purulent exudates. Packing should be used to prevent loculation of fluid, and frequent dressing changes should be used to keep the wound clean. All necrotic tissue should be debrided daily, if necessary. In many instances, hydrotherapy (whirlpool) can aid in the process of debridement and cleansing.

Packing the wound with an antiseptic solution such as Dakin's or povidone-iodine should be done only if the wound is known to be clinically infected, because such solutions can actually retard the healing process. In the case of noninfected small lesions, absorptive hydrocolloid occlusive dressings can be effective in promoting healing, provided they are used in accordance with the manufacturer's recommendations. The use of occlusive dressings with larger wounds is controversial. Although we have seen many cases of complete resolution with the use of absorptive granules and occlusive dressings in deeper wounds, the potential exists for developing a superinfection. Occlusive dressings cannot be used as a substitute for adequate nursing care.

With proper management, virtually any pressure ulcer can heal in a healthy well-nourished patient. Unfortunately, most cancer patients do not have the luxury of a healthy intact immune system with which to lay down new connective tissue. For this reason, it is often necessary to maintain care to an open pressure or surgical wound until well after all chemotherapy has been completed. In any case, good nutrition should never be ignored as a factor in would healing. Dietary supplementation with ascorbic acid, B complex vitamins, and minerals, particularly zinc, should always be considered in cases of delayed wound healing. In some cases, it may be necessary to use a skin graft or myocutaneous transfer (flap) procedure to close a wound. This is particularly true over irradiated tissues, in which the capacity for healing may be permanently impaired.

Contractures

In cases of prolonged disuse, collagen fibers within muscles, tendons, and ligaments shorten, resulting in a loss of joint motion and the development of a contracture. This problem is particularly evident at the shoulder, where the joint capsule is fairly redundant, but also occurs in all major joints of the body. Heel cords are prone to severe shortening, with hamstring and hip flexor contractures contributing to impaired mobility.

ROM exercises should be done actively by the debilitated patient or passively by nursing or by the family at least two to three times each day, moving all major joints through their full ROM in all directions. In the case of the shoulder, this includes external and internal rotation full abduction, and flexion. If flexion and abduction need to be limited (*e.g.*, in the patient after mastectomy or axillary lymph node dissection), internal and external rotation should be done to stretch the joint capsule.[35] Splinting may be used to maintain functional hand and foot position. An example of each is presented in Figures 66–1 and 66–2.

Radiation fibrosis may potentiate the development of contractures, and its continuing long-term effects may make recovery of ROM especially difficult. The rehabilitation team should instruct the patient in a home stretching program at the earliest possible time, impressing the need to continue this faithfully. A long-term stretching program may be required because of the tendency for irradiated tissues to develop persistent fibrosis. Compliance with the exercise recommendations is essential.

If contractures do occur, they may require months of therapy to regain full motion. Stretching exercises should be done at least once or twice daily under the guidance of a physical therapist. This may be supplemented by the use of superficial

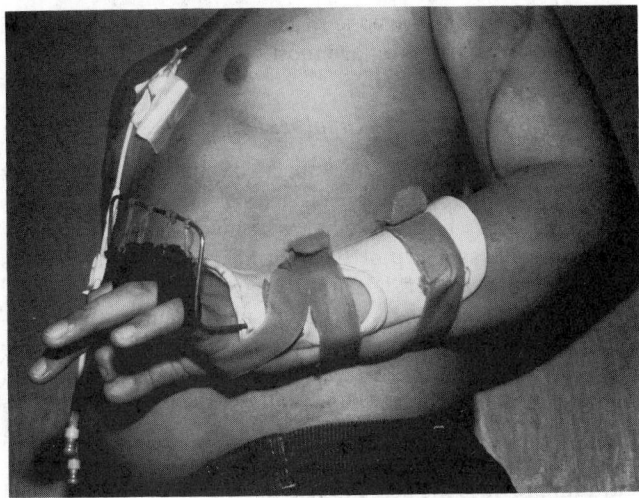

FIGURE 66–1. Functional, dynamic hand splint used to compensate for weak extensors.

or deep heating modalities, particularly ultrasound, which can help to increase the pliability of collagen, facilitating stretching. However, ultrasound may increase the tendency for metastasis, and caution should be used if it is thought that malignant cells may be present in the insonofied area.[36] This problem is of minimal concern in systemic malignancies. In extreme conditions, surgical release or manipulation under anesthesia may be considered.

METABOLIC PROBLEMS

Metabolic problems can result from tumor involving the endocrine organs, metastasis to these organs, the secretion of ectopic hormones by tumors, or cancer treatments.[37,38]

Rehabilitation professionals should be aware of the metabolic changes produced by malignancy and cancer treatments. The chemical alterations, symptoms, and physical findings produced by these entities can influence rehabilitation goal and treatment planning for patients. The metabolic changes often include electrolyte disturbances as hyponatremia, hy-

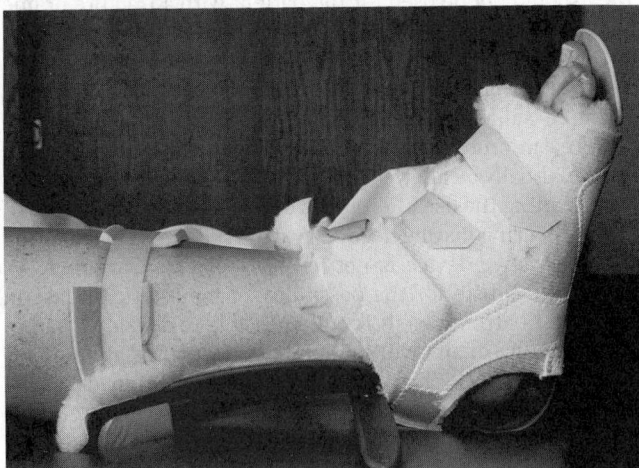

FIGURE 66–2. Multipodus splint to maintain foot and ankle in functional (neutral) position.

percalcemia, hypoglycemia, hyperuricemia, hyperkalemia; lactic acidosis; and hormonal overactivity syndromes such as hypercortisolism, hyperthyroidism, and hyperparathyroidism. Signs and symptoms related to these metabolic disturbances include anorexia, nausea, vomiting, myalgias, altered mental states, seizures, psychosis, cardiac arrhythmias, muscle weakness, lethargy, fatigue, and hyperpnea. These problems limit the delivery of rehabilitation programs.

Exercise may produce lactic acidosis and hypoglycemia, and it should be avoided in these patients. Patients with hyperkalemia or hypokalemia may be more susceptible to arrhythmia. Patients have problems following directions and have poor carryover with altered mental states due to metabolic problems. In this instance, rehabilitation programs may have to be put on hold.

When symptoms or findings that may suggest metabolic problems are observed, staff should notify the primary care physician. In treating patients with cancer, it is good to review the patient chart before each treatment session to see if any new metabolic problems that may alter the rehabilitation program have occurred.

MYOPATHY

Tumor-associated myopathy may result in mobility and activities-of-daily-living (ADL) deficits. The myopathy may be a result of direct tumor invasion of muscle and other soft tissues, paraneoplastic syndrome, carcinomatous myopathy, steroid myopathy, or carcinomatous neuromyopathy.

Direct Tumor Invasion

Tumors that invade muscle include soft tissue sarcomas, rhabdomyosarcoma, lymphoma, osteogenic sarcoma, and metastatic tumor. The invasion of muscle by tumor is usually nonreversible and the resultant myopathy remains. Rhabdomyosarcoma and lymphoma may respond to chemotherapy and irradiation with shrinkage of the tumor and improvement in muscle strength. Soft tissue tumors are often excised with surrounding muscle and other soft tissue. Metastatic tumors may be irradiated or removed. After tumor and muscle resection, exercise to increase or preserve joint motion and to strengthen remaining muscles is essential to ensure optimal functioning of the limb. Re-education of surgically transposed muscles may need to be done. Radiation causes soft tissue changes that may produce muscle shortening and joint contracture. A stretching program should be prescribed and supervised for the duration of the radiation course.

Paraneoplastic Syndrome

Nonmetastatic paraneoplastic syndromes of malignancy have been recognized with polymyositis and dermatomyositis. Malignancy primarily occurs in association with dermatomyositis rather than with polymyositis.[39] The incidence is thought to be higher in men over 50 years of age.[40] The literature between 1975 and 1983 reports an incidence of malignancy of 7% to 8%.[41] A study by Lakhanpal mentions a 25% incidence of malignancy in a polymyositis and dermatomyositis group and a 17% incidence in the control group.[42] The most commonly associated malignancies with polymyositis and dermatomyositis are breast (18%) and lung (16%).[43]

Patients with this syndrome have decreased endurance, muscle weakness, pain, decreased joint motion, and problems with ambulation, self-care, sexual performance, and work related activity. Treatment to increase joint motion with stretching exercise, to increase muscle strength with isometric exercise, to improve mobility with gait aides and bracing, and to improve ADL with assistive devices are all appropriate. The patient should be instructed in energy conservation, joint protection, and sexual and vocational counseling.[44,45]

Carcinomatous Myopathy

Carcinomatous myopathy may be seen with metastatic malignant disease. Histologically, there is widespread muscle necrosis and minimal or no inflammatory response. Clinically, there is proximal muscle weakness in this type of myopathy.[46]

Because of the necrosis of muscle, it is thought that these patients would probably not respond well to an exercise program, but function should be maintained if possible. They should be given appropriate pain relieving modalities and assistive and mobility devices to help with ADL and safe ambulation. The environment should be altered to help ensure safety and easy access.

Carcinomatous Neuropathy and Myopathy

This entity occurs with metastatic disease and affects peripheral nerve and muscle due to toxic or immunopathologic effects of the tumor. Diminished reflexes and sensation occur.[46]

The rehabilitation treatment is similar to that recommended in the management of carcinomatous myopathy. However, distal weakness occurs in addition to the proximal weakness, and appropriate bracing to improve ankle dorsiflexion may be needed. If weakness is severe, an electric scooter may be needed. Several assistive devices to help with hand function are useful.

Steroid Myopathy

Steroid muscle weakness is really a selective atrophy of type II fibers in proximal muscles. It tends not to affect neck flexor muscles. It may be superimposed on the weakness of carcinomatous myopathy or polymyositis and dermatomyositis associated myopathy and exacerbate it. It is caused by catabolic and anabolic effects of steroid on muscle. Amino acids leak into the circulation, and there is decreased incorporation of protein into muscle. The condition may be diminished by providing exercise to enhance protein metabolism by muscle.[47] Isometric exercise can be used to accomplish this goal. It may take up to 1 year after cessation of steroids for steroid-induced muscle weakness to return to normal.[48]

BONE DESTRUCTION

For several types of cancer, many patients develop metastases to bone during the course of the disease.[28,49,50] Most metastatic lesions result from carcinoma of the breast, lung, kidney, and colon, and prostate, bladder, ovaries, and uterus are frequent sites of primary lesions.[51] Leukemias, lymphomas, and my-

elomas may invade the bone marrow. The axial skeleton and the proximal extremities are most often affected.

Evaluation of Skeletal Involvement

The most frequent symptom associated with bony involvement is pain, usually localized, dull, aching, and more severe at night. Patients with multiple sites of involvement frequently describe pain as sharp or burning in nature. If this pain is brought on by weight bearing it may indicate a pathologic fracture. Bone involvement may result in neuropathic or radicular pain through entrapment or compression of nerves or nerve roots. Any cancer patient with new localized pain symptoms or cancer survivor with atypical pain should be evaluated for skeletal metastases. A bone scan provides the simplest means of screening for bony lesions. The plain x-ray film provides the best method for characterizing the local extent of lesions. A computed tomography (CT) scan may be needed to further evaluate the extent of cortical involvement. Magnetic resonance imaging (MRI) does not provide good visualization of bone and is not suitable for this purpose.

Prevention and Management of Pathologic Fractures

Pathologic fractures can limit mobility in a marginally functioning patient and, in some cases, lead to significant morbidity and mortality. Hip fractures are particularly debilitating and often difficult to stabilize, and they may lead to a significant hemorrhage. Prevention of pathologic fracture is important. Fracture should be considered imminent if the size of a lytic lesion exceeds 60% of the total bone width, if cortical involvement exceeds 50%, or if the axial extent of cortical destruction exceeds 13 mm in the femoral neck and 30 mm elsewhere.[52] Pain with weight bearing suggests a need to reduce load on the affected structure.

A cane used in the hand opposite the affected extremity can theoretically remove about 50% of body weight from that extremity. Attachments, such as a quadruped base (quad-cane) or a forearm support (forearm or Lofstrand crutch), may help to stabilize the cane, but they cannot overcome the simple physics of gravitation loading. Canes or single crutches can be used for the patient who has pain with weight bearing, but they should not be used for the patient with a fracture or one that is imminent.

Bilateral support is essential for the patient in whom no weight bearing is required. For the more debilitated patient, a simple walker suffices. For the more active patient, axillary or forearm crutches may be used. Toe touch of the affected leg can usually be allowed, but in the patient who has difficulty coordinating the use of crutches or walker, total avoidance of weight bearing may be needed to avoid sudden weight bearing if the assistive device is not properly placed. Care must be taken to evaluate for the possibility of metastatic disease in the upper extremities. It is quite possible to develop a pathologic fracture of an involved humerus if it is used as a weight-bearing structure. The patient should be cautioned against torquing the affected extremity, because this can often lead to fracture, even without weight bearing.

After an affected extremity has been unweighted, options for stabilization can be considered. Radiation often can be used to treat lesions of the long bones. Irradiation does not directly repair damaged bone, and irradiated bone heals much more slowly than normal bone. For small lesions, irradiation with the use of a cane may be all that is required. For larger lesions, surgical stabilization should be considered if possible. Intramedullary rods or methylmethacrylate can be used to increase strength of the invaded bone or, if used prophylactically, to stabilize a painful lesion and prevent fractures.[53] This gives the patient a more functional limb and allows increased mobility.

Destruction of the femoral head or acetabulum may be treated with hip joint arthroplasty, making ambulation a possibility while providing excellent palliation of pain. Fractures of the ischium may be painful during sitting and should be treated with cushions to reduce weight bearing over the fracture. Fractures of a single portion of the pelvic ring are generally not a problem. Multiple fractures, however, can interfere with ambulation and should be addressed appropriately. Fractures of the iliac wing may be painful during active hip flexion and abduction, due to the attachments of the iliacus and gluteal abductors, respectively. Assistive devices used to avoid activation of these muscles during ambulation can provide significant relief of pain.

Ribs are a common site of bony involvement and fracture. Generally, only a rib belt is required. Pathologic fractures of nonweight-bearing bones can be managed with splinting or sling immobilization while irradiation is delivered. ROM or isometric exercises may be appropriate to maintain function. If a dominant upper extremity is involved, assistive devices and training in one-handed strategies by an occupational therapist can significantly improve function. Devices such as reachers and dressing aids can help the patient to avoid torquing the spine or hips if the risk of fracture is high.

SPINAL COLUMN INVOLVEMENT

The emergency management of tumor-related spinal cord compression is discussed elsewhere. The rehabilitation team can assist in the prediction, prevention, and rehabilitation of vertebral column and spinal cord dysfunction resulting from malignant invasion or as a side effect of treatment. Prevention of disabling vertebral collapse requires a high index of suspicion for any patient with known or suspected malignancy, past or present, that frequently metastasizes to bone, such as tumors of breast, lung, and prostate.

Evaluation of Suspected Spine Involvement

One of the earliest indicators of spine involvement is pain.[54] The diagnosis of mechanical back pain should be one of exclusion in this population. Particular features that should alert the clinician are pain that is unrelated to activities or position, pain that is worse at night or when lying down, and pain associated with neurologic symptoms such as sciatica, muscle weakness, sensory loss, and particularly loss of bowel or bladder control. Hyperreflexia may be masked by peripheral neuropathy or plexopathy related to chemotherapy or irradiation, and patients with extensive metastatic involvement of the vertebral column may have little or no pain.

In the patient who presents with neurologic deficits, the physician must always rule out spinal cord compression by tumor. Other causes of paraparesis in the cancer patient include peripheral neuropathy, lumbosacral plexitis, radiation myelitis, and pseudotumor, often from radiation fibrosis. Radiation-related paraparesis may not occur for some time after the completion of all treatment. We have seen patients with radiation myelitis presenting as long as 7 years after having been declared free of disease.

Screening of suspected spinal involvement with a bone scan can be helpful, although this technique may not image epidural or intramedullary tumors. Myelography, previously the method of choice for detection of epidural involvement in cases of neurologic symptoms, has largely been supplanted by the use of magnetic resonance imaging (MRI).[55–58] Intramedullary tumors are particularly difficult to detect by any imaging modality, and they may mimic radiation myelitis.[59] Suspicion is often based on clinical grounds alone.

Issues of Stability

The prevention of serious spinal cord injury should be the primary initial goal of the cancer rehabilitation team in treating the patient with known vertebral destruction by primary or metastatic disease. Although radiation treatment may be used to control tumor growth and to relieve spinal cord compression, this does not address the issue of spinal stability.

Although no good models of vertebral collapse from tumor exist, it has been assumed that spinal stability in the cancer patient can be addressed in much the same way that it is in the patient with a traumatic injury of the spine.[60] The most widely accepted method of stability evaluation involves the concept of three columns.[61,62] This method considers the spine to be made up of three supporting columns, consisting of the anterior, middle, and posterior structures of the vertebrae, roughly divided into equal thirds. Any two of these supporting columns must be intact for the spine to be stable. For example, complete destruction of a vertebral body is usually unstable, because the posterior structures (facet joints) can easily sublux. A simple compression fracture, however, is usually stable because the posterior and middle columns are relatively intact. Of particular concern are lesions at the atlantoaxial and thoracolumbar junctions, due to the significant bending and torquing moments generated at these interfaces.

Whenever possible, an unstable lesion of the bony spine should be stabilized surgically, because virtually no brace can be completely effective in preventing subluxation. Irradiated bone heals slowly and often incompletely, and continued malignant destruction may sometimes occur. It is desirable from the rehabilitation standpoint to mobilize the patient as quickly as possible to prevent the complications associated with immobility. Even if there is extensive vertebral destruction, surgical stabilization can usually be accomplished by means of rods, strut grafts, and cement.[63,64] Occasionally, extensive multilevel involvement may make it impossible to find adequate healthy bone to which stabilizing hardware can be attached, or the patient's health may preclude any surgical option. In such cases, bracing may provide the only means of protecting the spinal canal.

Although a variety of spinal orthotics is available, some commonly used neck and back braces have no place in the management of the unstable spine. The soft cervical collar, for example, may provide comfort to the patient with neck pain, but it provides virtually no significant limitation in cervical motion. Beyond a doubt, the only cervical orthotic that provides virtually complete immobilization of all but the lowest cervical segments is the halo brace.[65] This device is attached directly to the skull using bone pins and to the chest using a plastic vest or plaster cast. Unfortunately, many cancer patients cannot tolerate the degree of chest immobilization resulting from this type of brace.

If it becomes necessary to use a more "practical" cervical stabilization orthotic, selection should be based on the level of potential instability and the directions of motion that might lead to instability.[66] The Philadelphia collar, consisting of a foam collar with rigid supports, provides moderately successful stabilization of higher segments in flexion and extension but inadequate stabilization at lower levels and inadequate stabilization for side bending and rotation, and it is of limited usefulness as a spinal stabilization brace.

Two alternatives that provide excellent stabilization of lower segments in flexion and extension are the two-poster and sternal occipital mandibular immobilization (SOMI) braces. The SOMI is particularly useful in managing debilitated patients, due to its open design and the ease with which it can be applied, because all components are attached from the front. It can be used with a light-weight chest piece as supplied, or it can be bolted onto a lower spinal orthotic, as shown in Figure 66–3, making it useful in cases of multilevel instability. An alternative cervical thoracic orthosis is the Yale brace, which essentially consists of a Philadelphia collar attached to a thoracic extension. With any of these orthotics, the patient must be informed that the brace is a compromise solution, and that care is indicated, particularly with motions not well supported by the particular brace.

Stabilization of the thoracolumbar regions is generally done using two basic types of bracing. Metal braces such as the Jewitt or the Taylor-Knight orthoses can be fit to the patient rapidly, providing optimal limitation of flexion and extension (Fig. 66–4). The custom-molded plastic thoracolumbosacral orthotic, or body jacket, additionally provides limitation in rotation as well. Body jackets can be padded to enhance comfort, and they can be perforated to reduce heat build-up, which is a frequent problem. They can be fabricated using a one-piece anterior opening design that can be applied independently by the patient, although a two-piece "clam shell" design is preferred in the unstable spine, because it can be donned and doffed with assistance by "log-rolling" the patient to apply first the back half and then the front half. Unfortunately, these braces are frequently poorly tolerated in the debilitated patient with atrophic skin. Elastic back braces and corsets, often used in the management of mechanical low back pain, do not provide adequate limitations in motion to be used for spinal stabilization, although rigid corsets may be worthy of consideration in the patient who absolutely cannot tolerate anything else.

High thoracic lesions and cases of extensive vertebral involvement may require the use of a combination orthotic. A cervical extension or SOMI brace can, for example, be attached to a body jacket, providing restricted mobility of the entire spine, as shown in Figure 66–5. These braces should be worn whenever the patient is upright or travels in a motor vehicle. When the patient lies in bed without the brace, the head of the bed should not be elevated by more than 30°. Patients should be cautioned against twisting or torquing their backs, because this may potentiate the injury. Cervical orthoses should be worn even when the patient is recumbent and removed only in a supervised setting.

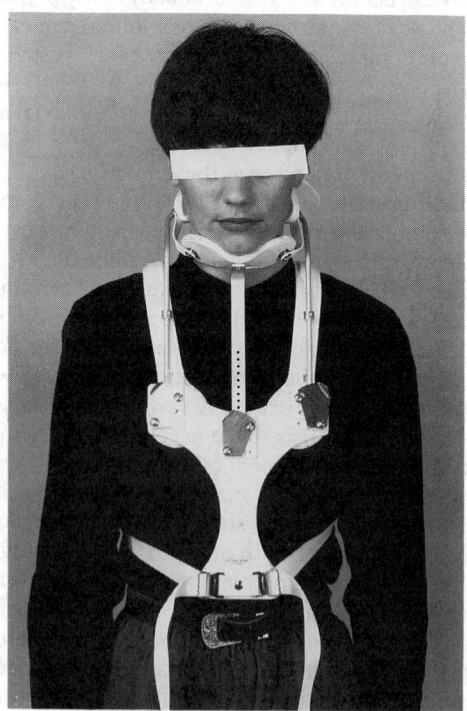

FIGURE 66–3.   Sternal occipital mandibular immobilization brace (SOMI).

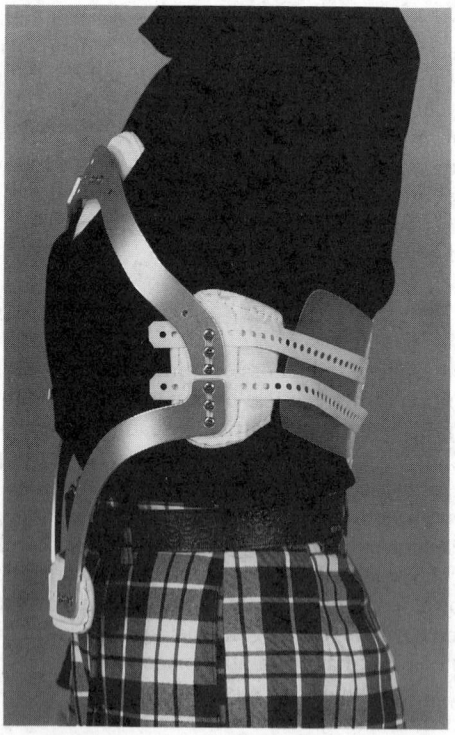

FIGURE 66–4.   Taylor-Knight orthosis.

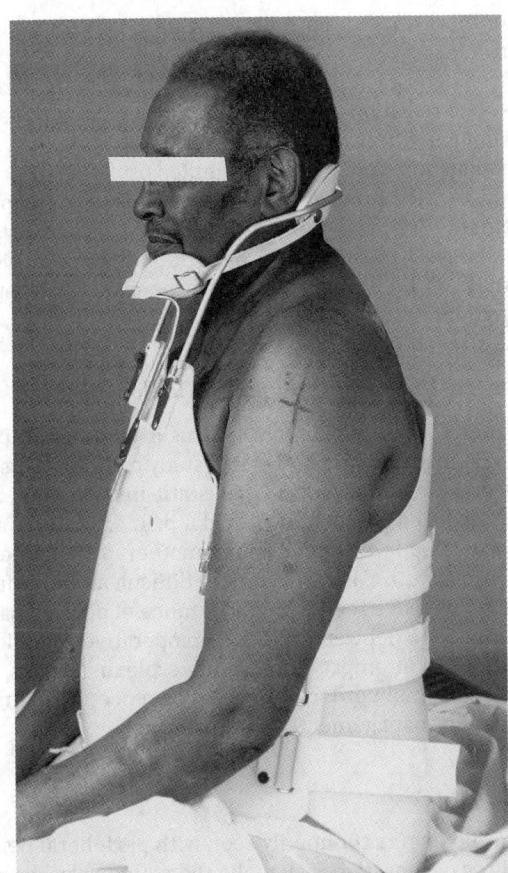

FIGURE 66–5. SOMI brace attached to a body jacket.

Spinal Cord Injury Syndromes

Spinal cord disorders in cancer patients may result from malignant invasion, bony compression or trauma, syrinx or hematoma formation, radiation myelitis, or vascular events. Radiation myelitis is directly related to radiation dose and often does not develop until years after the completion of therapy.[67] Spinal cord dysfunction has been associated with high-dose intrathecal chemotherapy.[68,69]

The degree of functional impairment in a spinal cord disorder is related to the level of the lesion and to its degree of completeness. The level of a lesion is by American convention the last fully functional spinal root level. For example, a C5 (cervical root 5) quadriplegic has intact function of the biceps brachii (innervated primarily by C5 and C6), with intact sensation over the shoulders and lateral aspects of the arms. A C5 quadriplegic is able to bring the hand to the mouth but requires assistance for most self-care. A level of C4 is required for unassisted breathing. C6 quadriplegics have intact wrist extension, allowing some light grasp through the tenodesis effect. C7 quadriplegics are able to extend the elbows, making it possible for them to lift themselves, performing their own weight shifts. C8 and T1 are required for intact hand function.

The remaining thoracic segments are of significance primarily in the motor control of trunk stability. In the lower spine, the degree of functional use of the legs is more vague due to the extensive overlap of motor segments. Generally, hip and knee extensor strength of sufficient magnitude to overcome gravity (3/5) are essential for safe ambulation. Although long leg braces can be used for paraplegic ambulation, the level of energy required is usually beyond the capability of many healthy persons, let alone the patient debilitated by cancer. Short leg braces or ankle-foot orthoses (AFOs) can be used effectively to compensate for the loss of ankle dorsiflexors and plantarflexors. In selected patients with intact hip musculature, AFOs that limit dorsiflexion can be used to create an extension moment at the knee, substituting for quadriceps function during the stance phase of gait.

Damage of the central portion of the spinal cord may occur with the outer portions being spared. This may occur with intramedullary tumors, with syrinx formation, or in certain vascular events. The central cord syndrome is characterized by loss of upper extremity function, with relative sparing of function in the legs. If only one side of the spinal cord is involved, the Brown-Sequard syndrome results, in which motor function is affected on the ipsilateral side while most sensory function is affected on the contralateral side.

Rehabilitation in Spinal Cord Impairment

Because of the complexities involved with spinal cord dysfunction, rehabilitation should be provided by those familiar with management of spinal cord injury. Assisted mobility using manual or motorized wheel chairs or crutches or canes with braces are usually required. Adaptive equipment and strategies for self-care may be needed in the cancer patient with spinal cord involvement.

Bowel and bladder dysfunction in this patient population is virtually universal, requiring particular attention. Even in the patient with apparent normal voiding, silent bladder, and sphincter spasticity may lead to infection, bladder reflux, and significant morbidity. We have seen cases of hydronephrosis with almost complete destruction of the kidneys in asymptomatic persons. Foley catheters may be used for short-term management if there are other medical indications. Otherwise, intermittent catheterization done frequently enough to keep the bladder volume less than 500 ml is the method of choice during the acute phase. A urologist should be consulted after the patient has stabilized. Regular use of laxatives as part of a bowel training program are frequently required.

Autonomic dysreflexia or hyperreflexia is a true emergency in the spinal cord impaired patient. When the spinal cord level is T6 or above, uncontrolled vasoconstriction and severe hypertension may result. Paradoxically, the heart rate is often slowed due to the intact vagus nerve. The first objective should be to lower the blood pressure as quickly as possible. Sitting the patient upright helps to reduce intracerebral pressure. A fast-acting agent such as sublingual nifedipine may be used initially, followed by a longer-acting agent such as nitroprusside, if needed. After the blood pressure has been stabilized, the cause, usually a noxious stimulus, should be isolated and corrected. The most common cause is an overdistended bladder, and distended bowel and skin trauma are other possible explanations.

NEUROPATHIES AND PLEXOPATHIES

Peripheral nerve involvement is a common diagnostic dilemma in the cancer patient. Dysfunction of peripheral nerves usually results from the use of cisplatin or vincristine and irradiation.[20,70–74] Peripheral neuropathies and plexopathies can be the result of direct tumor invasion or a paraneoplastic syndrome.

Chemotherapy-Induced Neuropathies

Generally chemotherapy-related neuropathies tend to be distal and symmetric. Occasionally, initial symptoms are unilateral, mimicking a mononeuritis or invasive lesion. Vincristine and cisplatin are documented causes of autonomic neuropathies.[75,76] In some instances, this has been severe enough to mimic spinal cord involvement.[77] Cytarabine (ara-C) has caused brachial plexus neuropathy.[78] Suramin, largely an experimental drug, has caused a profound polyneuropathy mimicking Guillain-Barré syndrome. Agents that are lipid soluble or that have metabolites with a prolonged half-life may lead to a progressive neuropathy, even after discontinuance of the drug.[79]

Vincristine seems to induce distal axonal degeneration similar to that of other toxic neuropathies.[20] Because of this, the duration of the neuropathy tends to be prolonged because of the time needed for nerve fiber regeneration. Many patients receiving this agent develop sensory complaints of numbness and paresthesias. Some patients develop severe neuropathic pain. Often the degree of motor neuropathy is significant, sometimes resulting in a virtual quadriparesis. Although it may take months after cessation of chemotherapy to recover function, recovery is usually complete. Neurotoxicity is one of the most common reasons for limiting the dosage of vincristine chemotherapy.

Neuropathies due to cisplatin generally tend to be less frequent and often milder. Unfortunately, we have treated several patients who have developed a severe permanent neuropathy from the use of cisplatin. There does not seem to be any common factor that can be used to predict the development of lasting neuropathy. Rarely is an adjustment in cisplatin dosage indicated.[70]

Brachial Plexopathies

Radiation-induced brachial plexopathy is an uncommon problem in the conservative management of breast cancer if supraclavicular and axillary lymph nodes are irradiated. It may be seen as a late effect of mantle irradiation for Hodgkin's disease. Onset of symptoms is usually delayed. In one study, onset of symptoms occurred with a median time of 4.5 months after the cessation of radiation treatment, and full recovery was usually observed.[74] In another study, symptoms began more than 1 year after therapy, and the overall prognosis for recovery was poor.[72]

Differentiation of radiation from neoplastic plexitis is essential. Severe pain has been documented in 80% of patients with infiltrating tumor, but only 19% of patients with radiation injury described this finding.[80] Horner's syndrome is more common in cases of tumor involvement, and lymphedema is a much more common concomitant finding in radiation injury. The distribution of involvement of the brachial plexus is an important diagnostic criterion, with 72% of patients with invasive tumor having involvement of the lower trunk and 78%

of patients with radiation injury having involvement of the upper trunk.

Electrodiagnostically, myokymic discharges are virtually diagnostic of radiation plexitis, occurring in 63% of patients.[81] Other abnormalities are common in both types of injury, with nerve conduction studies being of limited usefulness.[82] Tumor detection by MRI provides definitive evidence of neoplastic involvement. Even without visible tumor during surgery, neoplastic disease has sometimes been found microscopically, and it may not be possible to rule out neoplastic plexopathy for many months after the onset of symptoms.[73,83]

Lumbosacral Plexopathy and Radiculopathy

Involvement of the lumbosacral plexus is common in pelvic tumors due to direct invasion.[84] In a study of 11 patients with lumbosacral plexopathy, 6 had metastatic involvement, 2 had radiation-induced plexopathy, 1 had a primary tumor, and 2 had neuritis due to intraarterial chemotherapy.[85] Direct imaging of tumor with CT or MRI may be difficult after irradiation or surgery. We have seen a preponderance of delayed painful plexopathy in patients receiving intraoperative radiation. It is important to attempt to differentiate plexus lesions from those of the spinal cord, due to the difference in treatment, rehabilitation management, and prognosis.

Management

Neuropathic pain is commonly seen with peripheral neuropathies. Loss of sensation may make the patient susceptible to skin injury. The patient with insensate skin should be cautioned about the avoidance of potential injuries from burns and sharp objects and about the need for daily skin inspection to avoid the development of infection. Loss of proprioceptive feedback, particularly in the patient with impaired vision, may interfere with simple fine motor tasks and with ambulation. A cane can provide proprioceptive feedback to the upper extremities in the patient with impaired proprioception in the lower extremities. Motor impairment is treated similarly to other neurologic disorders, with bracing and adaptive devices as needed.

REHABILITATION ASPECTS OF PAIN CONTROL

In addition to the use of narcotic agents, which has become the mainstay of palliative treatment in the cancer patient, the physical modalities of pain control may significantly help to alleviate suffering. More aggressive approaches, including nerve blocks and rhizotomies, have been used with limited success. Sympathetic nerve blocks and sympathectomies may be effective in patients with the reflex sympathetic dystrophy syndrome. Trigger point injections are sometimes helpful in musculoskeletal pain disorders.

The use of physical modalities can be particularly effective adjunct in the management of pain in the cancer patient. Heat modalities, including superficial heat, shortwave diathermy and ultrasound may provide relief in musculoskeletal pain syndromes, but ultrasound may help to spread lymphatic disease. Other heat modalities increase circulation to the affected area, questionably increasing the potential for metastatic spread. Therapeutic cold can sometimes help to reduce pain.

Electrical stimulation has met with increasing criticism in the literature, but we have found electrical stimulation to be effective in reducing narcotics usage in a variety of cancer patients with a variety of pain syndromes. It seems to be particularly effective in the management of phantom limb pain and in treating radiculopathy and incisional pain. If effective, the patient can be provided with a pocket-sized TENS unit, which can be used as needed. Electrodes should be placed at the site of maximum pain or, in the case of referred pain, at the site of the lesion. A conventional high-frequency setting is usually most effective. Many TENS units are available at modest cost.

LYMPHEDEMA AND DEEP VENOUS THROMBOSIS

The swollen extremity is often a diagnostic dilemma in the patient with a history of cancer. Because of the possibility of malignant compression or invasion of lymphatics or venous drainage, and because of the possibility of deep venous thrombosis, a swollen extremity should always be fully evaluated in the cancer patient or cancer survivor. Idiopathic lymphedema, rather than edema secondarily caused by infection or tumor, should be a diagnosis of exclusion. Tumor can usually be excluded by imaging studies such as CT, MRI, or bone scan, or in extreme instances, by lymphangiogram.

Deep venous thrombosis can usually be ruled out using impedance plethysmography or ultrasound.[86,87] If certainty is required, a venogram can be done. Suspected pulmonary embolism can be evaluated with a ventilation-perfusion scan or more definitively by pulmonary angiography. The greatest risk of embolization is from proximal thromboses.[88]

Lymphedema in the cancer patient is frequent with lymph node involvement or after lymph node dissection. Late edema is usually related to radiation therapy and the gradual development of fibrous tissue. Edema in a nonirradiated extremity should always be thoroughly evaluated, and remediable causes, such as infection or cardiovascular causes, should be treated.

The simplest means of minimizing edema is to keep the affected extremity elevated as often as possible. Legs should be placed on an elevated foot support, preferably keeping the feet above the level of the heart. Arms should be rested on a high table surface. A sling may be of short-term benefit. Isometric exercises, by increasing muscle tone, may help to minimize edema.

The mainstay of lymphedema management is the compressive garment. Compressive stockings in the legs and elastic sleeves in the arms can significantly reduce swelling. These are designed with a pressure gradient such that the pressure exerted by the garment distally is greater than that proximally. This is to ensure fluid flow in a proximal direction. Compressive garments should always be used over the entire extent of the edema. A stocking that only reaches the knee tends to develop tightness and occlude lymphatic and venous return if there is significant edema in the thigh. Ready-made garments are available in a variety of sizes. These should not be confused with the thin elastic support hose frequently used on hospital wards that are ineffective in edema management. Patients with long-standing lymphedema should usually be fitted for custom-made compressive garments, which provide an optimized pressure gradient. Care should be taken with the use of compressive garments in insensate patients and in those with open wounds due to the potential for impaired circulation and local ischemia. The one major drawback of elastic garments is that they are extremely difficult to don and doff. A newer nonelastic compressive orthotic, which consists of a series of adjustable straps, is much easier to apply, but it is rather unsightly.[89]

In some patients, the use of compressive garments alone is not sufficient to manage severe lymphedema. For these patients, compressive pumps may provide the answer. These pumps consist of an inflatable garment that is cyclically filled with air, pressing fluid out of the affected extremity. There are two types of pumps: single-chamber devices and sequential multichamber devices. Single-chamber pumps are relatively inexpensive and can easily be used by the patient at home. Sequential devices can be extremely effective, although at a higher cost.[90] Sequential pumping can be so effective as to put the patient with cardiovascular compromise into cardiovascular overload. It is often preferable to start use of this device in an inpatient setting. In some cases, it may be necessary to use the sequential pump at home on a nightly basis, wearing compressive stockings during the day. Caution when using compressive pumps and other techniques should be taken if there is a potential for residual tumor to be mobilized into venous or lymphatic channels.

BOWEL AND BLADDER DISORDERS

Oncologic patients develop bowel and bladder difficulties for a variety of reasons. Bowel obstruction or urethral or ureteral compromise is usually the result of malignant invasion or compression. Constipation and urinary hesitancy are frequently related to the use of medication, particularly narcotics and drugs with anticholinergic properties. Input from the rehabilitation team is most often needed if there is neurologic dysfunction or in ostomy care.

Management of Bowel Dysfunction

Disorders of fecal elimination are frequently the most significant complaint of the cancer patient. Constipation is extremely common and is best treated using dietary modifications and medication. Often, a high-fiber diet with copious fluid intake is all that is required to ensure regularity. If fiber supplements are used, the patient should be cautioned about the absolute need for fluid intake, because bulk in the absence of fluid can lead to impaction. If necessary, stool softeners such as docusate (*e.g.*, docusate sodium, 50–200 mg/day) can be added to reduce straining. A stimulant medication such as metoclopramide (metoclopramide hydrochloride, 10 mg 30 minutes before meals and at bedtime) can be used for delayed gastric emptying.

When spontaneous defecation does not occur, a stimulant agent may be required. A mild preparation with a well-controlled transit time, such as an over-the-counter senna preparation, is preferred. A standard dose of senna (*e.g.*, Senokot, 2 tablets) at bedtime usually results in controlled defecation in the morning. Stronger agents such as bisacodyl (5–15 mg) or magnesium hydroxide (milk of magnesia, 30 ml) may be used in more recalcitrant cases, although it should be kept in mind that magnesium is mildly nephrotoxic. Cathartics such as magnesium citrate should be used as a last resort and only if there is no suspicion of obstruction or impaction.

In the patient with neurogenic bowel dysfunction, stimulation from below may be required. Digital stimulation, or if needed, use of a glycerin or bisacodyl (10 mg) suppository, should usually be sufficient to initiate evacuation. Rarely, an enema may be required. By instituting a regular bowel training program in which full evacuation is achieved on a daily or every-other-day basis through the use of medications and rectal stimulation, it is usually possible to achieve continence.

Diarrhea in the cancer patient is usually the result of chemotherapy. Standard antidiarrheal preparations, narcotics, and anticholinergics may be used. If occurring in the face of antibiotics, pseudomembranous colitis resulting from infection with *Clostridium difficile* should always be ruled out. Other bacterial or parasitic diarrheas should be treated with appropriate antibiotics, as determined by stool culture or smear. Narcotic antidiarrheals should be avoided in this case due to the potential for developing toxic megacolon. Viral diarrhea should be allowed to run its course.

Management of the Neurogenic Bladder

Proper evaluation and management of bladder dysfunction in cancer patients with neurologic abnormalities is essential to the prevention of significant morbidity. Although bladder dysfunction is often arbitrarily divided into disorders of incontinence or reduced bladder capacity and disorders of retention, this model is overly simplistic. Patients with spinal cord or brain stem involvement should always undergo formal evaluation of bladder function.

There may be various combinations of a spastic or flaccid bladder and a spastic or flaccid urinary sphincter.[91] The combination of a spastic bladder and sphincter is the most dangerous, because this can lead to reflux, causing hydronephrosis or upper tract infection, or to autonomic hyperreflexia. Medications such as oxybutynin (oxybutynin chloride, 5 mg 2–4 times daily) can be used to reduce bladder spasticity, but mechanical means of drainage may be needed.[92] Urinary tract infections are frequent in the patient with neurogenic bladder, and proper evaluation and treatment is mandatory.

In the acute phase of management, an indwelling catheter is usually sufficient if there are appropriate medical indications. Catheters should be removed as soon as the patient is stable, so as to minimize the risk of infection. In the patient who appears to be voiding normally, evaluation for possible retention should still be done. Postvoid residual urine volumes as determined by catheterization or by ultrasound should be less than 50 ml. If the patient does exhibit retention, intermittent catheterization should be instituted, taking care to catheterize frequently enough to keep bladder volumes less than 500 ml. In the incontinent patient without retention, condom (Texas) catheters may be used for men. Collection devices for women are often less than satisfactory.

Management of the Ostomy Patient

Cancer patients may have ostomies for a variety of reasons. Ureteral stints are often used in patients with ureteral obstruction, occasionally in combination with a temporary ostomy for kidney drainage. Patients with bladder carcinoma may have a ureteral diversion to an ileal loop, which is drained through an ostomy. Patients with bowel carcinoma or other types of bowel obstruction may need a temporary or permanent ostomy for fecal elimination. This may be required at any level of the small bowel or colon. Ileostomies, involving diversion of the terminal small bowel, are sometimes problematic because of the volume of fluid present in the fecal contents before entry into the colon. An ileal pouch is sometimes created surgically as a reservoir for urine or ileal fluid as a means of providing continence.

In cases of neck tumors or if there is impaired swallowing, a gastrostomy may be required for supplemental nutrition. This can often be placed by percutaneous endoscopic gastrostomy (PEG), eliminating the need for major surgery. Tracheostomies are often used in cases of head or neck tumors or if there is a need for prolonged access to the airway, as in the patient with severe cognitive impairment and uncontrolled tracheal secretions. Gastrostomies and tracheostomies are discussed in more detail in the section on head and neck cancer.

Ostomy training should be a regular part of the cancer patient's rehabilitation process.[93] Proper clean technique avoids the likelihood of infection. Proper attention to skin care should avoid maceration and breakdown. Occasionally, a bowel training program can be instituted for colostomy patients, regularizing emptying and sometimes eliminating the need for an ostomy bag. A variety of ostomy collections systems are available, including one-piece collection bags that are applied directly to the skin using an adhesive and two-piece collection bags involving an occlusive seal that is applied to the skin and a separate detachable bag.[94] Collection bags may be closed and disposed of with each use or open, allowing for drainage and reuse. One- and two-piece barriers may be used to help patients maintain continence. Support groups for ostomy patients are available in most areas, and a variety of patient information materials are available.[95–100]

PSYCHOSOCIAL ASPECTS OF CANCER REHABILITATION

The rehabilitation team has an opportunity to help plan, supervise, and reinforce behaviors that may ameliorate symptoms of distress. These should be directed toward reducing stress and anxiety, improving fitness and performance, enhancing coping, and maintaining optimism.

Management of Stress

Cancer staging and treatment planning often require patients to go through multiple steps, during or after which choices have to be made. This is a particularly stressful time for patients and their families. Relaxation training using relaxation tapes and a low-level aerobic program is effective in reducing anxiety and depression. The rehabilitation process requires a commitment to participate in therapies on the part of the patient. This therapeutic alliance, oriented toward patient valued outcomes often addresses some aspects of the uncertainty that lies ahead and permits patients to be proactive in their own care.

Management of Depression

Cancer patients are psychologically vulnerable for several reasons. Often these include facing a serious illness with concerns about life expectancy and disability. Some cancer patients worry that the treatments and their results may cause family and friends to spurn them. The rehabilitation team can provide support and can suggest exercise at an appropriate level that may confer a sense of mastery, control, and offer the antidepressant benefits associated with exercise.

REHABILITATION AND MANAGEMENT OF SPECIFIC TUMORS

BREAST CARCINOMA

Rehabilitation interventions for patients undergoing modified or radical mastectomy, lumpectomy, and axillary dissection have usually included treatment for painful or immobile shoulders or swollen upper extremities or to restore functional activity. Because treatments for control of breast cancer vary widely, the rehabilitation interventions must be customized. Clinical experience has taught that a three-level axillary dissection is associated with more lymphedema than a less complete dissection. The patient with the more extensive surgery needs closer monitoring of upper extremity edema. The patient receiving chest irradiation is likely to experience chest wall tenderness and possible rib fractures and should be informed and monitored for the occurrence of these problems.

The prognosis of breast cancer is good and because its expression may occur in any decade of life after the first, early rehabilitation may play an important role in preserving function and returning the patient to her previous level of activity. A direct relation between physical therapy and good shoulder motion is established.[101] The converse has been demonstrated. Delaying physical therapy as little as 7 to 10 days postoperatively results in moderately severe limitation of shoulder abduction.[102] Some caution must be exercised in introducing shoulder motion immediately postoperatively, because this may result in increased axillary drainage and delayed wound healing.[35,102]

Most of the studies cited were performed in women receiving radical or modified radical mastectomy. However, one prospective study compared radical mastectomy with lumpectomy patients with respect to arm motion and found the latter group had better motion at 3 months.[103] None of the women received axillary dissection. Another study demonstrated no difference between a group receiving modified radical mastectomy or lumpectomy and axillary dissection at 1 or 2 years after definitive therapy.[104]

Typically, arm mobilization begins on postoperative day 1 or 2, with joint rotation to tolerance but restricted abduction and flexion to 40°. By day 4, flexion is gradually advanced to 45° and increased by 10° to 15° per day if tolerated. Abduction is held at 45° until the drains are removed and then advanced to tolerance.[35]

The incidence of lymphedema is not precisely known. This is in part a result of lack of uniform measurement techniques to assess it and few prospective, long-term studies to evaluate it. There are several types of upper extremity lymphedema, each of which may be characterized by its time of onset after treatment and associated clinical findings. The first is acute, transient, and mild, occurring within a few days of surgery, and is a result of cutting of lymphatic channels. It usually responds within a week of onset after arm elevation and hand pumping (*i.e.*, making a fist and releasing it). The second is acute, painful, and occurs 4 to 6 weeks postoperatively as a result of acute lymphangitis or phlebitis. This type can successfully be treated with arm elevation and use of antiinflammatory medication. The third type is an acute erysipeloid form, often occurring after an insect bite or minor injury or burn. It may be superimposed on a chronic edematous limb. This form of edema often requires arm elevation and antibiotics. Compression pumping or wrapping is contraindicated if there is infection. The fourth and most common form of lymphedema is usually insidious and painless and not associated with erythema. This form is most frequently apparent 18 to 24 months after surgery. If it develops much later than that, the physician should suspect recurrent tumor in the axilla or chest wall. This form of edema is thought to be due to lymphatic ablation and resultant increased interstitial pressure causing impedance of lymph flow. Successful treatment of this form of edema usually requires the use of compression pumps, single channel or multichannel systems, plus a compression garment. Careful attention to arm positioning so that gravity is eliminated and protection from sun, insect bites, and trauma are important therapeutic interventions.

Although arm motion and lymphedema are two of the most common findings seen in the breast cancer patient, a variety of other sequelae are common to this population (Table 66–2).

The patient undergoing mastectomy is usually provided with a temporary prosthesis that is Dacron filled. This may be used

TABLE 66–2. Clinical Problems After Mastectomy or Axillary Dissection Often Requiring Rehabilitation

Problem	When Likely to Occur
Pain	
Incisional	0–2 wk
Dysesthesiae	0–2 wk
Muscle spasm	0–2 wk
Chest wall	3 mo–2 y (usually with radiation)
Edema	
Transient (arm)	0–2 mo
Persistent (arm)	>1 y
Breast	0–2 mo
Weakness	
Serratus anterior	0–3 mo
Loss of motion	
Shoulder	0–3 mo

even if the patient is not comfortable wearing a bra and is simply pinned to an undergarment. After the incision is well healed, a definitive breast prosthesis can be fitted. This is usually done at 3 to 6 weeks postoperatively. There are a variety of types available.[105] Patients who elect breast reconstruction often have a tissue expander placed initially in anticipation of a definitive reconstruction. These patients may benefit from a temporary prosthesis until they are reconstructed.

HEAD AND NECK CANCER

There are approximately 42,000 new cases of oral, pharyngeal, and laryngeal cancers every year.[106] Despite constituting only about 5% of all malignancies, they present with profound deficits and cosmetic deformities. Because these cancers involve body parts that are highly visible, structurally complex, and crucial to survival, optimal interactions between medical treatment and rehabilitative care are necessary to assure adequate physiologic function, socially acceptable cosmesis, and quality psychosocial status.

Approximately 50% of these patients are expected to be disease free after a 5-year period.[106] Survivorship presents major challenges to patients, their families, and their acquaintances. To maintain medical and therapeutic compliance and disease-free status, long-standing habits of tobacco and alcohol abuse must be addressed. Vocational adaptations or changes may be required if return to work is necessary. Alternations of self-concept and body image may lead to seclusion and avoidance of activities such as eating in restaurants or attendance at social and religious activities. Due to isolation and pain, many patients become depressed and fail to thrive. We cannot measure survival in this population just by looking at morbidity or mortality statistics.

The goals of the rehabilitation team in the management of head and neck cancer are to provide counseling and therapeutic intervention aimed at maximizing functional capabilities, compensating for lost function, and preventing secondary complications that may result from disuse and cancer treatment. If we view head and neck cancer as a chronic disease, we must address these goals throughout the course of the disease and provide timely and appropriate interventions in the pretreatment, treatment, posttreatment (survivorship), and terminal stages of the illness.

The functional deficits (items 1 through 7) and needs (items 8 and 9) common to head and neck patients are as follows:

1. Psychosocial deficits
2. Communication or speech deficits
3. Mastication, deglutition, and nutrition deficits
4. Sensory deficits of taste, smell, or vision
5. Auditory and vestibular dysfunction
6. Neck and shoulder dysfunction
7. Disfigurement
8. Tracheostomy management
9. Oral hygiene management

The patient undergoing partial glossectomy or removal of small tumors of the tonsil or palate may experience mild deficits in speech and swallowing that can easily be addressed by therapeutic exercises and prosthetic management. A partial laryngectomy could result in severe swallowing difficulties,

including aspiration, but only mild problems with speech and voice. A total laryngectomy requires extensive speech therapy training to use augmentative communication systems or to learn new voice production techniques. In some cases, secondary surgical procedures such as tracheoesophageal fistula (TEF) or tracheoesophageal puncture (TEP) for voice restoration are suggested. The patient undergoing total glossectomy and laryngectomy may require alternative communication systems, or synthetic speech devices, and text telephone (TT) for the communicatively impaired (formerly called telecommunication devices for the deaf [TDD]) and computers for communication.

Tumors of the Aerodigestive System

Tumor sites are from the nose and nasopharynx to the lower border of the cricoid cartilage, including the accessory sinuses and glands. Primary locations of head and neck cancers include:

> Oral cavity: tongue, floor of mouth, buccal mucosa, retromolar region, gingivae, lips, roof of mouth, cheeks
> Oropharynx: tongue base, pharyngeal walls, soft palate, tonsils, faucial pillars
> Nasopharynx
> Hypopharynx: pyriform sinuses, postcricoid
> Larynx: glottic, supraglottic, subglottic
> Salivary glands: parotid, submandibular glands
> Cervical nodes

A summary of assessment and treatment components for head and neck cancer patients is given in Table 66–3.

Pretreatment Evaluation

Most head and neck cancers are squamous cell carcinomas arising from the epithelial lining of the aerodigestive tract.[107] Most grow and present as malignant ulcerations of the surface mucosa, sores that do not heal, or areas of leukoplakia and erythema. The most common sites for head and neck cancers are in the oral cavity (including the lips), pharynx, larynx, and salivary glands.[107] Signs and symptoms depend on the tumor location and may include dysphagia, vocal changes, sensory and motor deficits, or pain. In-depth medical evaluation to asses the extent of the tumor begins with diagnostic staging procedures, including a biopsy.

Thorough dental and maxillofacial prosthetic evaluations are needed to examine the structure and function of the oral cavity before medical intervention. Evaluation includes radiographs, impressions and casts, and recording of baseline data. The prosthetist consults with the oncologist and surgeon about the therapy plan, design, and fabrications of the initial surgical prosthesis, implants, and obturators (Fig. 66–6). For patients receiving irradiation and chemotherapy, a plan is developed for dental and oral care before or early in the medical intervention program to control oral infections, stomatitis, and conditions that may lead to later problems. Some patients require dental extractions before irradiation.[108]

Pretreatment evaluation by the clinical social worker, vocational rehabilitation counselor, and an occupational therapist can help to alleviate emotional distress by anticipating

TABLE 66–3. Assessment and Treatment Components for Head and Neck Cancer Patients

Components	Pretreatment	Treatment	Survivorship
Oral sensorimotor examination	×	×	
Clinical examination of oropharyngeal swallow	×	×	
Hearing and balance assessment	×	×	
Speech and voice assessment	×	×	
Dental examination and treatment	×	×	×
Nutrition assessment	×	×	
Instrumental swallowing assessment		×	
Speech and voice therapy		×	
Augmentative/alternative communication		×	×
Dysphagia therapy		×	×
Prosthetic management		×	×
Feeding and dietary management		×	×
Physical therapy		×	
Medical/surgical management	×	×	×
Nursing education	×	×	
Intubation, tracheostomy, stoma management		×	×
Cognitive and memory assessment	×	×	
Communication, language, reading, writing, assessment	×	×	
Lifestyle counseling	×	×	×
Family counseling	×	×	×
Vocational rehabilitation		×	
Community support groups		×	×

changes in vocational and family roles and financial resources.[109]

Before surgery, chemotherapy, or irradiation, a series of baseline diagnostic procedures should be performed to assess premorbid levels of speech and swallowing function that can be used after treatment for assessment of progress. It is important to establish whether any changes are due to treatment or were preexisting. The sensory motor function of the oropharynx, including the tongue, jaw, velum, teeth, oral mucosa, face, and neck areas must be assessed clinically. This examination should include an oral motor examination of the sensation and motion of the structures innervated by cranial nerves V, VII, VIII, IX, X, and XII, which are essential to speech, swallowing, hearing, oral sensation, taste, smell, and saliva-

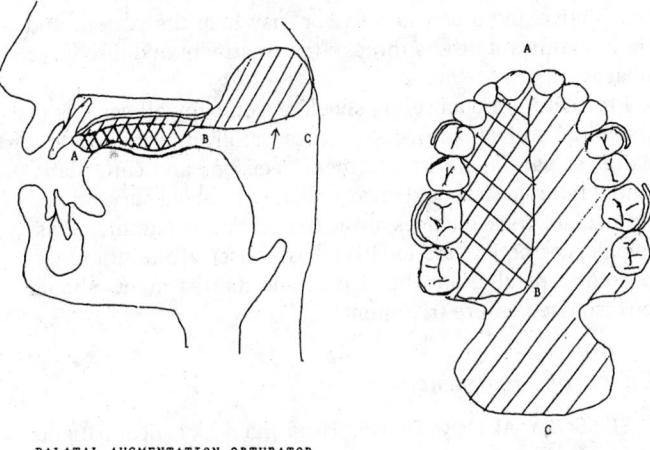

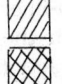 PALATAL AUGMENTATION OBTURATOR

A-B PALATAL AUGMENTATION SECTION
(COMPENSATE FOR HEMIGLOSSECTOMY- PALATAL CONTACT)

B-C OBTURATOR IN NASOPHARYNGEAL SECTION
(OBTURATION OF SOFT PALATE RESECTION)

FIGURE 66–6. Palatal augmentation obturator: Speech prosthesis for a hemiglossectomy with soft palate resection. (Courtesy of Jack Light, DDS)

tion.[110] In a complete workup of preoperative function the aerodigestive system should be examined radiographically for masses, lesions, and structural deviations. Speech should be assessed and recorded to determine whether articulation, vocal quality, pitch, resonance, frequency, or prosody has changed subsequent to disease progression. Long-standing patterns of deviant speech or misarticulations should be described, because old errors can contribute to the success of speech therapy.

Because many tumors and medications can affect the VIII (auditory) nerve and its pathway to the cortex and cause hearing impairment, hearing levels, emission, balance, and vestibular functioning should be assessed by an audiologist or an otolaryngologist before surgery.[111] Impaired auditory acuity can reduce ability of the patient to monitor his or her speech production, and the patient may not demonstrate maximal progress during speech rehabilitation.

Before starting cancer treatment, it is important to evaluate the nutritional status and food preferences of each patient.[112,113] A pretreatment screening assessment should examine mastication, jaw alignment, dental status and deviations, oral hygiene, periodontal condition, and salivary flow. The examiner should question whether there are any complaints of difficulty swallowing pills, painful swallowing, choking, reflux or heartburn, or avoidance of certain food textures or prolonged duration of eating. Patients at risk of aspiration should be advised that they may require a temporary or permanent feeding tube.

Screening for existence of cognitive dysfunction (*e.g.*, memory, reasoning, problem-solving ability) and personality or affective disorders is important to determine potential areas of noncompliance. Language usage and comprehension, reading, written expressions, and fine motor coordination should be assessed informally or through interviews, especially for patients who have CNS involvement.

Pretreatment Counseling

Rehabilitation begins at the time of diagnosis and often requires a support team of medical and lay specialists, including the oncologist, dentist, prosthodontist, surgeon, nurse, social worker, and speech-language pathologist.[114] A religious representative and a cancer survivor may help the patient and their significant others through the treatment and discharge phases.

Pretreatment counseling should accompany all aspects of the initial evaluation process, because a fully informed patient can best participate in treatment decisions and care plans. Initial interviews should uncover concerns about survival and immediate consequences of the treatments. Anatomic, physiologic, cosmetic, functional, and psychosocial alterations expected to result from the disease and its treatments should be discussed before treatment.

Effects of Treatment

SENSORY ALTERATIONS. Head and neck cancer patients may experience temporary or permanent auditory or vestibular deficits related to ototoxic medications. Surgical or radiation treatments may affect the functions of the ear or eustachian tubes and diminish auditory acuity. Before treatment,

auditory and vestibular testing procedures should be explained, and the need for follow-up monitoring should be mentioned during early counseling sessions. Because these patients are likely to experience alterations in taste and smell as a consequence of the disease and its treatments, counseling should increase awareness of hazards from smoke, spoiled foods, and oral hygiene and include the compensatory use of other senses.[115–117]

SWALLOWING AND NUTRITION. Nutritional status before and during cancer treatment influences recovery.[118] Previous lifestyles and food preferences, combined with the effects of the disease, may cause compromised nutritional status and weight loss. Swallowing abilities may be impaired due to muscular, structural, and sensory changes. Patients need to be informed that they can experience added structural and functional changes from irradiation, chemotherapy, or surgery that can further alter eating and swallowing.[119,120] They should know that there are therapeutic interventions that can restore those functions and reduce the risk of aspiration. Occasionally, swallowing techniques and compensations may be taught and practiced during these pretreatment sessions. The major reason for pretreatment counseling about potential difficulties in swallowing is to prepare the patient for the possibility of therapy and to facilitate compliance and success.

COMMUNICATION ISSUES AND ALTERNATIVES. Because alterations of speech and voice occur after treatment for head and neck cancer, discussion of possible communication changes is important. Counseling allows for exploration of current communication abilities, styles, and needs and the introduction to alternative and augmentative communication methods. It is imperative that the patient be provided with options for communication of basic needs immediately after surgery.[121] A variety of alternatives should be offered, such as use of a buzzer or a bell for general alerting, writing (*i.e.*, pad and pencil, magic slate), or an alphanumeric and picture board communication system. Several types of electrolarynx (*e.g.*, neck and intraoral instruments) should be demonstrated before medical or surgical treatment. Voice and telephone amplifiers can enhance whispered or dysphonic speech. Patients should be assured that a variety of communication options and voice restoration procedures are available later in their course of treatment. This can be accomplished with visits from cancer survivors who have undergone successful speech rehabilitation or with films and literature from the American Cancer Society.

DENTAL PROSTHETIC AND ORAL HYGIENE ISSUES. Counseling, education, and dental evaluation should begin in the pretreatment phase of the disease to effect positive treatment outcomes. Consultation from a maxillofacial prosthetist should be sought for patients who undergo ablative surgery.[122,123] Dental damage and infections may be prevented if patients are seen before or early in their treatment. Regular oral hygiene, attention to dental health, and prophylactic use of fluorides and other soft tissue treatment may be necessary for the remainder of the patient's life.[124] Prophylactic extraction of viable teeth within the field of radiation exposure is often recommended to prevent subsequent jaw necrosis secondary to dental decay.[108]

LIFESTYLE ISSUES. The association between tobacco and oral cancer has been well established, and multiple studies confirm an independent and synergistic relation between head and neck cancer and consumption of alcohol and tobacco.[125] Successful rehabilitation and subsequent survival can be greatly compromised if habits are not changed. Counseling efforts, strategies, and support groups must be introduced early to facilitate modifications in lifestyles that allow the best recovery and prevent mortality from intercurrent and recurrent disease.

Presurgical nursing, self-care counseling, and education may be needed to educate the patient and family to manage tracheostomy or laryngectomy tubes, stoma and secretions, tube feedings, and associated equipment and supplies and to introduce suctioning, oral hygiene, and irrigation techniques.

PAIN. Because pain occurs in most head and neck cancers, pain control issues, including pharmacologic intervention, should be discussed early and throughout the course of care. Tolerances, past experiences, and coping styles need exploration. Whenever possible, objective scales and subjective descriptions of pain should be used.[126,127]

Rehabilitation Issues

CANCER TREATMENT INVENTIONS. Rehabilitation that includes preservation of function and acceptable appearance is a prime consideration for surgical planning. Many surgical reconstructive approaches for voice and cosmetic rehabilitation have been developed during the last 40 years; some are performed as part of the primary surgery, and others are secondary procedures.[128] The surgeon and maxillofacial prosthodontist must evaluate and consult preoperatively, sharing information about the dynamics and limitations of various prosthetics in relation to surgical reconstruction and clinical conditions. If voice restoration surgery (*i.e.*, TEF) is considered as a primary procedure, consultation with and evaluation by a trained speech-language pathologist can provide information that is critical to successful vocal rehabilitation.[129,130]

Neurophysiologic intraoperative monitoring by trained audiologists neurologists, anesthetists, and other physicians is becoming an accepted standard of care in many hospital settings.[131,132] The application of evoked potential measurements and techniques to surgical monitoring may help to avoid or reduce the risk of injury to the auditory and facial nerve pathways.[133]

POSTOPERATIVE SWALLOWING, SPEECH, AND COMMUNICATION EVALUATIONS. On referral of the physician, depending on patient tolerance, the speech-language pathologist reassesses the structure and function of the orolaryngopharyngeal mechanisms for speech and swallowing capabilities postoperatively. In most instances, postsurgical nutrition is provided nonorally (*e.g.*, PEG, nasogastric tube, Keo feed tube). Before resumption of oral intake, the speech-language pathologist conducts a clinical evaluation of oropharyngeal swallow (bedside swallowing evaluation). Careful clinical evaluation of the anatomy and physiology, including range, rate, and coordination of movement, tone and reflexes during a variety of tasks that may include manipulation of

material in the mouth, and sensory and speech observations, can reveal much about the oral stages of swallowing, including mastication, bolus preparation and transport.[110,134] However, only instrumental approaches, such as the modified barium swallow, provide objective information about the neuromuscular events of the pharyngeal phase to reveal dangers such as pooling, reflux, reduced peristalsis and aspiration.[134–137] Endoscopy, ultrasound, and scintigraphy provide critical objective information about pharyngeal and laryngeal events, tongue and hyoid movements, and the presence and amount of aspiration.[138] After clinicians gain a thorough understanding of the swallow, they can introduce and objectively judge the efficacy of a variety of management techniques during the radiographic studies.

Dynamic radiographic evaluation by videofluoroscopy and ultrasound can provide useful feedback in evaluation of speech.[139] Some medical centers assess vocal and resonance parameters with instrumentation such as videostroboscopy, nasometry, acoustic spectrographic analysis, palatometers, and glossometers.[140] The severity of speech disorders in this population is a direct result of site and size of the tumor and the variety of reconstructive surgical procedures and prosthetic applications. Reduction of speech intelligibility is due to deviations in articulation, oral and nasal resonance patterns, voice production and quality characteristics, changes of speaking rate and prosody, and preexisting speech impairment. Tests of articulation in a variety of contexts, voice and resonance ratings, measures of diadochokinesis, speaking rate, speech and breathing efficiency, and judgments of overall intelligibility are administered postoperatively. Video and audio tape recordings are useful for patient feedback and documenting progress. A clinical tool called Performance Status Scales assesses the specific areas of dysfunction unique to this population, which is understandability of speech, normalcy of diet, and eating in public.[141] This scale can be administered by untrained professionals, is reliable, and can discriminate across the broad range of head and neck cancers. The scale can be a useful tool to screen patients who deviate from the expected course of recovery and who are in need of further rehabilitation.

As soon as the patient is medically or surgically stable, oral-motor exercises should be initiated to aid maximal return of the sensorimotor functions requisite for speech and swallowing. These exercises are designed to facilitate, maintain, and increase the ROM, strength, speed, flexibility, and sensation of the oral muscles and structures. Exercises are especially important to reduce mandibular fixation and increase range of jaw motion in patients who have had jaw reconstruction.[142] Lingual, labial, and velar exercises are important in retraining speech articulation and often involve teaching compensatory movement patterns or using sensory and reflex stimulation to enhance perception and execution of motion.[143–145] Fibrosis or contractions of facial and neck muscles can often be prevented by early and ongoing application of sensory stimulation and massage coupled with specific exercises to increase ROM.[146]

Irradiation and chemotherapy cause a variety of symptoms, including significant diminution of salivary flow and oral dryness (xerostomia); thick, sticky oral secretions; mucositis of the oropharyngeal mucosa; esophagitis; oral pain; dental caries; and taste changes, appetite loss, and nausea.[147–149] Use of various tastes, spices, textures, or olfactory input may be used to stimulate salivary flow in postirradiation patients and for swallowing treatment. Artificial saliva and spray have limited or temporary benefits.[149] Pilocarpine appears to have some potential for increasing salivary flow in selected patients.[149] Careful continual dietary planning and modification are necessary to ensure proper nutrition and to encourage eating when it is so unpleasant. Foods may need to be modified to make them taste better or to be less spicy. The addition of sauces, gravy, margarine, or butter may compensate for oral dryness. Moist, soft, or smooth foods such as buttered noodles, puddings, yogurt, ices, hot or cold soups, juice, purees, liquids, and dietary supplements (*e.g.*, Ensure or Sustacal) are moist and are easier to swallow if there is mouth pain or dryness. Papain dissolves thick oral secretions and can be swabbed in the mouth before eating.[150,151] If pain is more severe, topical anesthetics can be applied orally before a meal.[124] The use of fluoride trays can help to manage dental caries.[152] Dental monitoring and good oral hygiene are essential throughout treatment.

Because most head and neck patients have excisions of the structures needed for swallowing and bolus transport, swallowing retraining is an essential component of rehabilitation.[150,151,153–156] Although some patients may benefit from prosthetic swallowing devices or obturators, most can be retrained to swallow by therapeutic techniques. Modification of head, trunk, or body position may be crucial in swallowing retraining to improve bolus flow and reduce pooling in the hypopharynx that may lead to aspiration after swallowing. For many patients, a safe swallow procedure combines airway protection and head positioning to reduce the threat of aspiration or bolus penetration into the laryngeal vestibule.[155] This technique is especially important because aspiration is a major complication of head and neck cancer and a major cause of respiratory complications.[157]

Swallowing treatment is done by the speech-language pathologist or swallowing therapist and involves indirect and direct strategies for feeding and deglutition.[155] Indirect swallowing treatment does not involve the use of food, but direct treatment strategies involve modifications of temperature, bolus size, and texture of the food and in feeding positions. Indirect treatment strategies to retrain patterns needed for bolus manipulation and transport can be used while the patient is taking nothing orally and intubated. Because many head and neck cancer patients can not handle thin liquids or tough, sinuous foods after surgery, thickeners are often added to foods. Many patients benefit from preparing all foods to pureed consistency. A variety of special spoons, syringes, and adapted eating devices may be necessary to transport food from the oral cavity to the pharynx in patients who have had glossectomies or other oral surgical procedures.[119,158] Because the effects of irradiation or chemotherapy treatment are not immediately apparent, the patient may have progressive changes in dental status, smell, taste, and salivary flow that should be monitored. If the patient is found to have hoarseness or a gurgling voice that persists after eating, aspiration into the laryngeal area may occur. Elevated temperature can indicate aspiration pneumonia that should be monitored by periodic chest radiographs.

TRACHEOSTOMY CARE AND PRECAUTIONS. Head and neck surgery often involves creation of a temporary or permanent tracheostomy. The nursing staff can teach self-care and hygiene techniques and stress the importance of keeping the airway open and free of foreign substances. Patients should be encouraged to cough deeply to aerate the lungs and bring secretions to the tube opening. In the early postsurgical period, suctioning may be needed to remove thick secretions from the airway. Patients usually require continuous humidity in the inspired air just after surgery and may continue to need humidification to reduce mucosal crusting from dried secretions. The stoma must be protected from dust, aerosol sprays, powders, and other foreign substances by wearing a crocheted bib or other coverings. A protective stoma cover must be worn during showering to prevent water from entering the airway. Special stoma equipment (Keith-White tracheostomy Snorkel, Gauthier Medical Inc., Rochester, MN or Larkel Snorkel, Seidel Medicine, West Germany) is available for those who wish to resume swimming and water sports. Neck breathers should be instructed to wear medical alert bracelets (American Cancer Society), carry medical data cards, and place emergency instructions in their cars and homes so that special procedures such as mouth-to-neck breathing are clearly visible when needed.

EARLY COMMUNICATION OPTIONS. After head and neck surgery, especially if the laryngopharyngeal area has been changed, verbal communication may be sufficiently altered or compromised so that written communication becomes the primary mode of expression. Premorbid spelling, grammar, legibility, condition of the hands, and composition abilities dictate the ease of using writing to substitute for speaking. In most cases, the written conversational interchanges should be short phrase-length units, rather than long narratives. The patients and their families often need instruction on how to use key ideas and telegraphic writing to facilitate written interactions.

In the early stages of treatment and recovery, an artificial speaking device is widely recommended by head and neck surgeons and speech-language pathologists. These instruments are relatively inexpensive ($200–$600) and are reimbursable through most insurance policies. They are easy to operate and often can be used successfully after a few training sessions. The most commonly used instruments are the neck and intraoral electrolarynx devices. They are battery powered tone generators that convey sound through tissue of the neck or directly into the mouth by catheter to be articulated into speech. However, inability to obtain a good neck seal with the instrument or soreness and pain due to surgery or irradiation may preclude the early use of this type of speech aid. Despite adjustment for loudness and pitch levels, these instruments produce a monotonous, robot-like sound. The third type of electrolarynx, the Pneumatic External Reed larynx, diverts air from the tracheostomy site past a vibrating membrane into the mouth by rubber tubing and is not commonly used in this country.

Speech synthesizers and other communication aids with digital displays and paper printouts are available. One inexpensive device allows the user to request basic needs, spell words, generate simple questions and statements, and to phone the police, fire department or medical help in an emergency (Vocaid, Texas Instruments). A variety of more sophisticated synthetic speech systems have been developed for the severely speech and motor handicapped person. These devices can be eed successfully by the laryngectomized glossectomy patient

tomized glossectomy patient

used successfully by the laryngectomized glossectomy patient who is unable to use an electrolarynx. The use of the TT and fax machines may be helpful for electronic communication needs in the work setting.

REHABILITATION OF IMPAIRED SPEECH PRODUCTION. Speech production requires precise coordination of respiration, phonation, resonation, articulation, and cognition. If these are impaired by head and neck cancer, speech therapy can restore function and is essential for rehabilitation.

For laryngectomized patients, speech rehabilitation may consist of several techniques; esophageal speech, voice restoration through TEP or TEF, and voice prosthesis.[159-161] The electrolarynx was discussed in the previous section.

Esophageal Speech. To produce esophageal speech, air is injected or inhaled and trapped in an esophageal reservoir and then released with volitional control through the pharyngoesophageal (PE) segment and articulated in a normal manner. The PE segment is formed by the inferior pharyngeal constrictor, cricopharyngeal, and upper esophageal sphincter muscles. These serve as the substitute vibratory source for the production of voice.[160,161] Attainment of esophageal speech is successful in only 26% to 46% of patients because of several limiting factors. Among these are scarring of the tissues, nerve damage, poor relaxation or tension of the sphincter, impaired intellectual ability, hearing loss, and unavailability of trained instructors.[162-166] The combination of pharyngectomy and esophagectomy along with laryngectomy make learning esophageal speech impossible. Partial glossectomy or base of the tongue resection also compromises ability to learn esophageal speech.

TEP and TEF Prostheses. Singer and Blom described a procedure for voice restoration that creates a fistula or puncture between the tracheal stoma and the esophagus.[167] The puncture is stented with a catheter, and after maturation of the fistula (approximately 2–10 days), a one-way valved silicone voice prosthesis is sized and inserted into the fistula (Figs. 66–7 and 66–8).[130,168] The TEP prosthesis protects the airway during swallowing. If the tracheostomy is occluded with a finger or a tracheostomy valve, the prosthesis opens to shunt air from the lungs into the area of the PE segment.[159]

Speech restoration treatment for TEP requires collaboration of the speech-language pathologist and the surgeon. Patients are selected preoperatively using results of the air insufflation test, radiographic studies, and pharyngeal plexus blockade to rule out pharyngeal spasm.[164,169,170] The procedure may be unsuccessful if the patient has pharyngoesophageal spasm, myopharyngeal strictures, or hypotonia of the PE segment.[171] To alleviate failure, several procedures can be used: presurgical selective myotomy of the pharyngeal constrictor muscles, lysis of scar tissue that prevents vibration of the PE segment, constriction bands or digital pressure to increase tension of the PE segment, or dilation of the esophageal sphincter.[168,171] TEP surgery has been found to be successful for patients with reconstruction flaps and gastric pull-up procedures, advanced tumors and those who have had large doses of radiation.[171]

The speech-language pathologist and otolaryngologist fit the patient with the appropriate speaking valve after the surgery. Patients are then trained on insertion, care, and management of the TEP and valve. Patients must learn to coordinate the timing of the occlusion of the stoma with exhalation to achieve

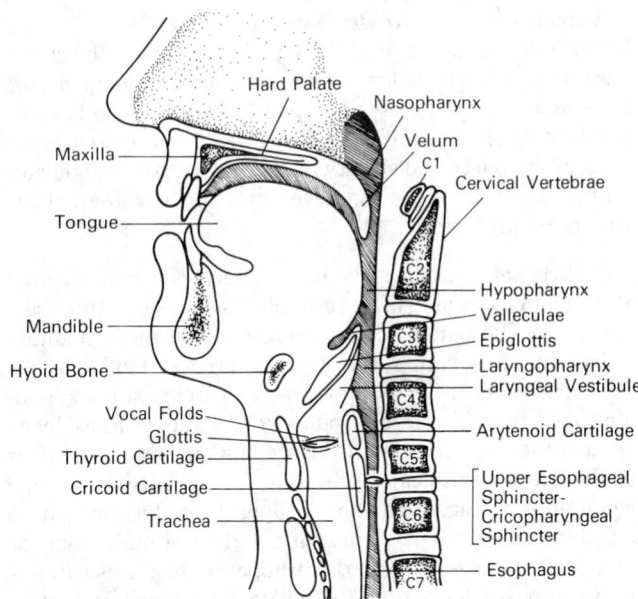

FIGURE 66–7. Sagittal view of oropharyngeal structures.

optimal speech production. A tape on voice reconstruction after total laryngectomy is available to train patients and professionals (Blom, Singer, Cine-med, Woodbury, CT). Functional communication is often achieved after a few therapy sessions. Perceptual and acoustic studies and subjective speech rating suggest near-normal speech characteristics and excellent intelligibility.[162,167,172] Self sufficiency in care and self-insertion may take longer in patients with impaired visual acuity, manual dexterity or cognitive capacity.

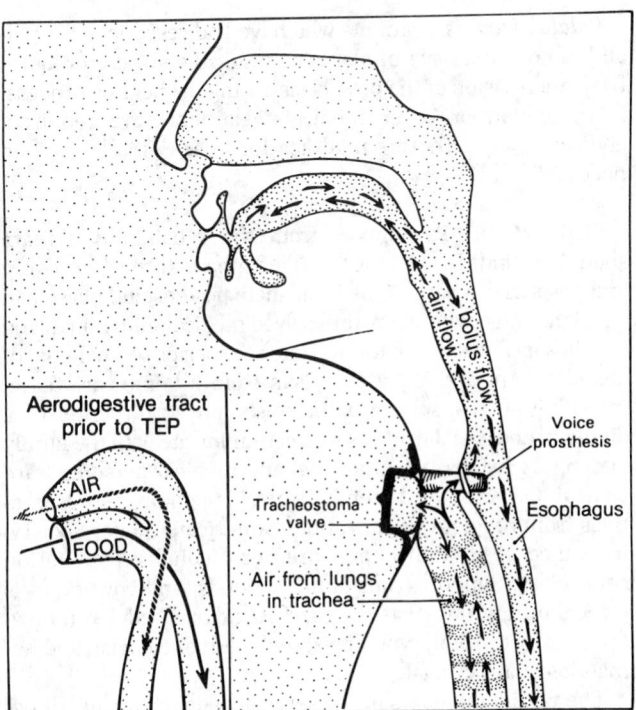

FIGURE 66–8. Sagittal view of oropharyngeal structures after tracheoesophageal puncture, with voice prosthesis and breathing valve in place.

A tracheostomy valve developed by Baxter, Mueller, and Bivona eliminates the need for digital occlusion of the stoma during speech. An airflow sensitive diaphragm opens during quiet breathing and closes for speech. Patients who have irregularities of the configuration of the stoma or excessive mucous discharge and secretions may not be good candidates for the valve. The stoma and valve can be modified for patients with these problems.[173-175]

Glossectomy. Patients who have undergone partial or total glossectomies usually achieve intelligible speech after therapy.[143-145] The patient can be taught to use the remaining tongue stump and other articulators to produce modifications of normal articulatory patterns that are perceptually indistinguishable from the target sound.[144,176] Patients must learn compensatory gestures of the lips, velum, mandible, and floor of the mouth muscles to substitute for the missing tongue when approximating phonemes. Speech production can be aided in these patients by use of a variety of oral, velar, or lingual prostheses. A properly fitting oral prosthesis can improve appearance and can simulate tongue-palate contact needed to produce speech sounds and achieve correct oral resonance.[177,178] Fitting prosthetic appliances and dentures in some irradiated patients may have to wait for several years after treatment.[108] Speech therapy may continue to be needed for 3 to 12 months beyond the surgical treatments, depending on the extent and type of tumor and treatments, cognitive factors, and the complexity of new speech, voice, and communication systems.

Composite Resections. Patients who have had composite resections that involve the tongue, jaw, and neck usually experience the greatest difficulty with speech and swallowing rehabilitation. Major problems after surgery can be caused by surgical ankyloglossia and absence of buccal gingival sulci.

Palatal Tumors. Patients who have had resections for palatal tumors and have implants or surgical obturators require frequent revision of the prosthesis during the healing process. If irradiation or other medical treatments are required, additional prosthetic modifications are likely to be needed.[108,123,179,180]

SURVIVORSHIP. Support from the rehabilitation team should continue beyond the treatment phase, through recovery and hospital discharge. The immediate posthospital phase can be frightening, with many unresolved medical, functional, and psychosocial issues. Patients often experience feelings of abandonment and isolation. Visits from a home-care team, including nurses, speech pathologists, physical therapists, a dietitian, and social workers who communicate with the family and act as liaisons with hospital and medical personnel are critical. Other helpful members of the team are representatives from religious organizations, American Cancer Society, insurance or disability, and drug or alcohol rehabilitation counselors. Support from family, friends, and coworkers is critical during this phase of care. Regular scheduled followup visits by the otolaryngologist, radiation oncologist, and hematologist are crucial.

The family members of the seriously and terminally ill patient need counseling about their feelings and fears. Social workers, psychologists, hospice workers, and clergy are best prepared to deal with the issues of death and feelings of anxiety. The speech pathologist, although not specifically trained, is often involved in assisting the patient to develop methods for expression of feelings and may be the person who initiates referral for counseling.[163]

SUPPORT GROUPS. The interactions and support of the various community and lay groups for cancer patients under the auspices of the American Cancer Society can be a crucial factor in adjustment to the disease and in maintenance of a healthy life style. These groups can provide educational materials, counseling, recreational activities, equipment, transportation, and financial and vocational assistance for cancer survivors. The International Association of Laryngectomies is one group that provides cancer patients with specific activities for speech and swallowing retraining, purchase of an electrolarynx, and hospital visitation and provides family members with counseling and other assistance. Groups to reduce smoking and alcohol abuse can often provide a positive milieu and enhance the quality of life of these patients.

TUMORS OF THE CENTRAL NERVOUS SYSTEM

CNS tumors may be primary or metastatic. In the case of metastatic lesions, the prognosis is related to the particular type of primary malignancy, but the neurologic deficits observed are related to the location of the metastatic lesions.[181] Chemotherapy and irradiation may cause CNS deficits in the absence of an intracranial lesion.[182] Primary malignant neoplasms of the CNS are most commonly gliomas, most frequently glioblastoma multiforme.[183,184] Lymphomas, relatively rare among CNS neoplasms, are relatively common in patients with the acquired immunodeficiency syndrome (AIDS).[185-187] Additional CNS neoplasms are angiosarcoma and germinomas.[188-191]

Although the long-term prognosis of glioblastomas is poor, many patients live for several years, during which time rehabilitation can play a significant role in minimizing disability and improving the quality of life. In children, advances have resulted in significant improvements in survival.[192,193] Long-term sequelae in survivors of childhood cancer may result in residual cognitive deficits that may require ongoing measures.[17,194]

The type, location, and depth of the CNS tumor dictate the severity and form of deficits in speech, language, cognition, memory, and personality. Different symptoms result from lesions of the right or left hemisphere, from frontal, temporal, parietal, and occipital tumors, and from surface versus deep tumors. Primary tumors can cause a wide variety of deficits in the areas of cognition, language, memory, perception, reading, writing, behavior, and affect. Whenever possible, it is important to have some premorbid, pretreatment assessment or estimate of these functions for comparison and for use in later family counseling sessions.

Changes in cognitive function may resemble those usually associated with patients who have had strokes if the lesions are specific to a specific lobe or hemisphere. If the lesions are spotty throughout the CNS, cognitive behavior may resemble that of the dementias. Subcortical lesions, especially to the left ventral tract of the thalamus, most often mimic cortical lesions to the language areas. Sensory and motor deficits are related to the area of involvement, with unilateral cortical lesions often presenting a picture virtually identical to that of stroke.

Rehabilitation treatments should include intellectual and communicative assessment as soon as possible after diagnosis of a tumor. The speech-language pathologist or neuropsychologist uses standardized test batteries of the various modalities, including speech, language, writing, auditory and visual perception, attention, reading, memory, gesture, comprehension, and verbal and nonverbal problem solving in their assessment of patient status. The results of these tests are used to formulate an individualized treatment plan and to evaluate progress of disease or progress in treatment. For some patients with severe disability, a variety of augmentative and alternative communication systems may be used to substitute for verbalization. Specialized switches and adaptations to other equipment and environmental control systems, assistive technology, and computer use may be useful avenues for rehabilitation.

Because swallowing abnormalities are common in CNS tumors, a high index of suspicion is necessary. The swallowing evaluation should include an oral motor examination and a modified barium swallow using video fluoroscopy. Swallowing and dietary modifications or tube feedings may be needed by some patients.

Difficulties with mobility and self-care should be handled similarly to that of other neurologic impairment syndromes. Orthotics and assistive devices may be used to substitute for lost motor function. In some cases, a wheel chair may be needed. Particular attention should be given to the avoidance of shoulder, hand and heel cord contractures in the hemiplegic patient, using splinting and ROM exercises as appropriate. Additional adaptive equipment, such as reachers, dressing aids, and bathroom equipment, may be used as needed. Treatment should involve counseling about the modification of expectations of work ability, life style, and roles. The spouse and family should be included in counseling before, during, and after treatment.

SARCOMAS OF THE EXTREMITIES

The three most commonly seen extremity sarcomas requiring rehabilitation are soft tissue sarcomas, osteosarcoma, and Ewing's sarcoma. Management of these usually is surgical, often amputation. Early detection and treatment has made limb-sparing surgeries possible without compromising outcome.[195-197] Sixty percent of all soft tissue sarcomas occur in the extremities with a 3:1 ratio of lower extremity (45%) to upper extremity (15%) involvement.[197] Approximately 75% of lower extremity sarcomas originate at or above the knee. Osteosarcomas are the most common primary bone malignancy of children and adolescents.[198] This type of tumor is most frequently located in the metaphyseal ends of long bones. Seventy-five percent of all osteosarcomas occur in the extremities, with most occurring in the femur (40%).[199] The axial skeleton, clavicle, and scapula are rarely involved.[198] Ewing's sarcoma is second only to osteosarcoma as the most common malignant bone tumor of children and adolescents.[200] As with soft tissue sarcomas and osteosarcomas, Ewing's most frequently affects the extremities. Approximately 60% of these sarcomas originate in the extremities (*i.e.*, femur, 21%; tibia or fibula, 23%; foot, 2%; humerus, 11%; hand or forearm, 2%), and approximately 40% appear in the flat bones (*e.g.*, pelvis, vertebral body, scapula).[200,201]

Pretreatment Phase

During the pretreatment phase, the rehabilitation staff should be familiar with the medical history, perform a thorough musculoskeletal evaluation and a functional assessment, and educate the patient and family about the expected course of treatment. An effort should be made to ascertain the patient's prognosis and his or her understanding of the disease and treatment options available. Knowledge of the patient's support system, vocational and avocational interests is useful in planning the optimal treatment program.

After the history is obtained, a complete musculoskeletal evaluation should be performed. This should include a general observation of the patient and close inspection of the affected area. Particular attention should be paid to the overall ROM, strength, sensation, pain intensity, edema, deep tendon reflexes, pulses, and joint alignment. The functional assessment to determine the patient's level of independence for bed mobility, transfers, ambulation, and self-care should be added at this time. The team must evaluate endurance levels for basic activities, such as walking on level surfaces, inclines and stairs, and use of gait assistance.

A crucial aspect of the pretreatment evaluation is the education of the patient and family. Patients who have a good understanding of what they may face and with whom they may need to interact postoperatively often progress faster, are more satisfied with their levels of progress, and cooperate more with their specialists than those who are unaware of their treatment. Patients need information about what their functional capabilities will be after surgery. For example, a patient who is to receive an above-knee amputation should be shown a prosthesis that would be appropriate for him or her or be introduced to another above-knee amputee of similar age, size, and medical history. A patient receiving a forearm excision may be shown a splint or brace appropriate for this type of surgery or view photographs of patients who have received a similar procedure. The pretreatment phase is an ideal time to instruct patients on the use of assistive devices such as crutches, cane, or walker that may be necessary for use after surgery. It is an appropriate time for demonstrating exercises that may be beneficial after surgery.

Surgery Phase

Before the early 1970s, amputation was the standard treatment for soft tissue sarcomas and osteosarcomas of the extremities. Despite this radical surgical approach, the 5-year survival rate for these patients was less than 50%.[202,203] However, advances in diagnosis and treatment have dramatically improved 5-year survival rates for patients with extremity soft tissue sarcomas to 70% to 80% and for osteosarcoma to 50% to 60%, and they have improved functional use of the extremity.[204] Surgical advances in limb-salvage procedures and the use of neoadjuvant and adjuvant chemotherapy and radiation therapy have promoted limb-sparing procedures as an alternative to more ablative procedures such as amputation.[205]

These procedures seem to preserve function, although they may prolong rehabilitation postoperatively.

AMPUTATIONS. Despite advances in treatment, there are cases in which amputation is indicated as the primary surgical option. Figure 66–9 shows various amputation levels. If the tumor is located in such a position that its removal would not ensure resection of all gross disease or if resection would sacrifice major nerves, blood vessels, or muscle, resulting in a poorly functioning limb, amputation is the treatment of choice. Other considerations that may favor amputation are pathologic fracture and skeletal immaturity. However, advances in endoprosthetic replacement have resulted in the increased ability to perform limb-salvage surgeries despite these factors and are discussed elsewhere in this chapter.[206] This chapter does not discuss basic amputee management because there are many other resources for this topic.[207] It is more important to discuss the problems unique to the oncologic amputee. The rehabilitation of patients with high-level amputations, including shoulder disarticulation, forequarter amputation, hip disarticulation, and hemipelvectomy, is the primary focus of this section.

Amputation of a limb, for any reason, has many psycholog-

ical, social, and physical impacts. Amputations due to trauma, although devastating in their abrupt nature, are usually not life threatening. In contrast, the oncologic amputee often confronts a life-threatening diagnosis in which anxiety about the extent of involvement and choices about how to treat it are anxiety inducing. Treatments and their side effects (*e.g.,* alopecia, nausea, vomiting, fatigue) may produce fear, pain, altered body image, and change in customary roles. All these factors must be addressed for successful rehabilitation of this patient population, who tends to be younger and may have more significant problems with acceptance of their loss than vascular patients. The oncologic amputee often has greater rehabilitation potential.

Oncologic amputations are usually at higher levels than those due to other medical problems. The use of prosthetic devices in such cases requires higher energy expenditure and may result in the patient having limited physical capacity.[208] In the extreme case, some older patients may not be able to use a prosthetic limb because of the amount of energy required. Prostheses for above the knee amputees with very short residual limbs, hip disarticulations, or hemipelvectomy (and prostheses for the shoulder disarticulation or forequarter amputee) are difficult to fit, because there is less area to anchor

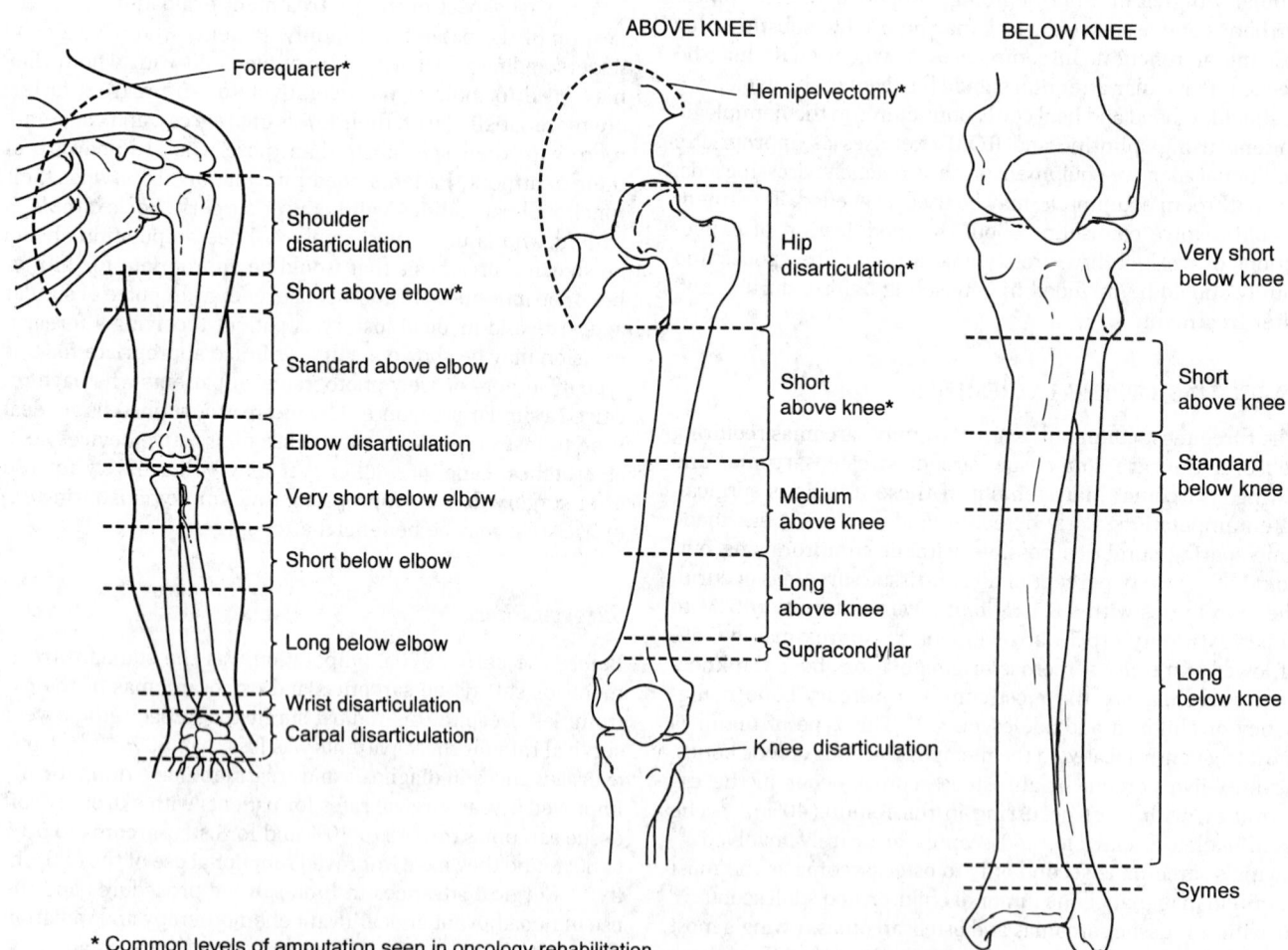

* Common levels of amputation seen in oncology rehabilitation.

FIGURE 66–9. Schematic drawing of upper- and lower-extremity amputation levels.

or suspend the prosthesis. The weight of the prosthesis is often considerable, and the problem of adequately distributing pressure to minimize discomfort becomes a major aspect of prosthetic fitting. Interim inspections are essential so that modifications can be made to alleviate high-pressure areas before fabrication of the final prosthesis.

The oncologic amputee may undergo additional treatments, such as chemotherapy and radiation therapy, that may delay healing of the incision or produce stump volume fluctuations secondary to chemotherapy side effects. A rigid dressing applied in the operating room may aid in reducing edema and promoting healing. After a prosthetic socket is fabricated, maintaining a proper fit is always challenging in this patient population. Volume changes and muscle atrophy occur, and weight maintenance is difficult due to the chemotherapy-induced nausea, vomiting, and loss of appetite. If the period of chemotherapy lasts for only a few months, prosthetic fitting should be delayed until completion of chemotherapy and weight stabilization. However, the obvious psychological and physical disadvantages of delaying prosthetic fitting must be kept in mind and considered in the rehabilitation team's decisions. In general, it is advisable to obtain a prosthesis as soon as the incision is healed. Socket fit can be adapted by changing stump sock thickness, using a temporary flexible socket with adjustable closures, using a series of flexible sockets in a rigid frame, or modifying a permanent socket by filling it entirely or by padding specific areas.[199]

During this treatment time, prosthetic training may be hampered by decreased stamina, fatigue, and anemia. Daily fluctuations may require alterations in rehabilitation treatments. Occasionally, an amputated limb may receive irradiation that may interfere with prosthetic fitting by causing pain and skin breakdown in the irradiated area. Extra padding and vigorous stump management can aid in coping with the resulting problems.

Shoulder Disarticulation or Forequarter Amputation. The rehabilitation of high-level upper extremity amputations should concentrate on training the patient in one-handed activities, training the uninvolved hand in fine motor activities such as writing skills if the amputated limb was the dominant one, strengthening of the remaining extremity, and addressing postural and cosmetic issues (Figs. 66–10 and 66–11). The patient may tend to lean toward the affected side due to the weight imbalance, resulting in neck and back problems. This can be avoided with ROM exercises of the neck and trunk and postural training exercises using a mirror for visual feedback. A functional prosthesis is rarely recommended and is often rejected by patients because of its weight, lack of coordinated multiarticular movement, psychological unacceptability, and ready adaptation to one-handed activities.[209] The patient who desires a functional prosthesis is usually the exception and requires extensive training to coordinate shoulder and elbow movement with hook opening and closing. Despite the ineffectiveness of a functional prosthesis for most patients, all patients should be fitted with a cosmetic shoulder cap to provide symmetry and a shelf for clothing. A purely cosmetic, light-weight full arm and hand may be used to assist with psychological adjustment.[209] Rehabilitation team members can provide ideas for clothing modification and instruction in the use of assistive devices, as needed.

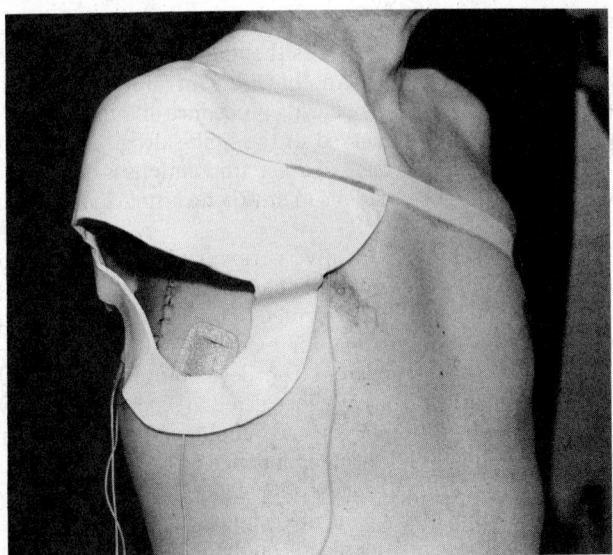

FIGURE 66–10. Custom-molded plastic shoulder cap for a forequarter amputee.

Hip Disarticulation and Hemipelvectomy. Malignant, bony lesions of the middle and distal femur and soft tissue tumors of the middle and lower thigh that are not amenable to limb salvage usually require hip disarticulation. This surgical procedure involves disarticulation of the hip joint, with complete removal of the femur and most muscles of the lower extremity. Hemipelvectomy, removal of the entire lower extremity and hemipelvis with disarticulation of the sacroiliac joint and pubic symphysis, is most often used for lesions of the proximal thigh

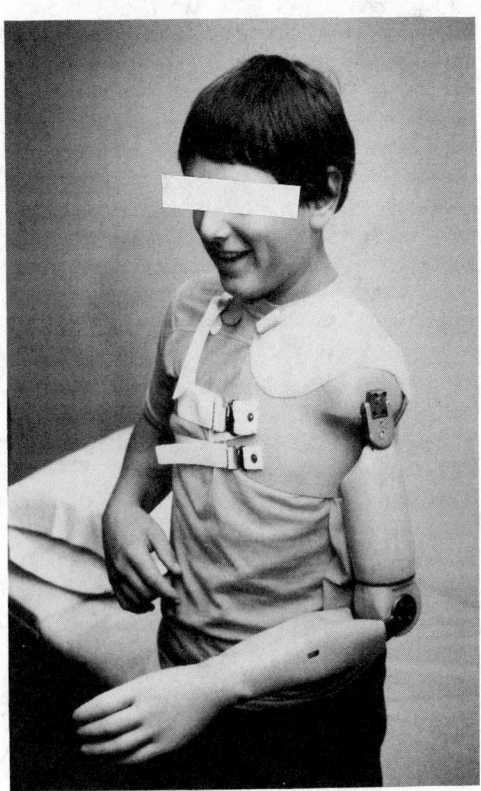

FIGURE 66–11. Forequarter prosthesis.

and buttocks. Similar to the standard hemipelvectomy is a modified version that preserves the iliac wing and improves patient rehabilitation.[210] Another version of the standard hemipelvectomy is a limb-sparing procedure of internal hemipelvectomy that is discussed in the limb-salvage section of this chapter. Rehabilitation of these amputations is quite similar, with only slight variations in prosthetic fitting and training (Fig. 66–12).

The immediate postoperative period is usually one of bed rest for 3 to 5 days. During this period, exercises on the uninvolved limb should be performed to maintain strength and promote circulation. Special air mattresses are usually provided to prevent pressure areas from developing in the surgical site, and the patient is usually instructed to lie predominantly on the uninvolved side. A trapeze bar should be placed over the patient's bed to allow independence in bed mobility and for upper extremity strengthening. Pain and phantom sensation are managed by pain medications, but TENS can be used if TENS pads are not placed on the flap area. Placement of pads to the translumbar area has given some relief of phantom pain. Compression wrapping with elastic bandages or the use of a commercial girdle with the involved side sewn closed aids in reducing pain and controlling postoperative edema.

After the period of bed rest, increased mobility should be encouraged. Initially, the patient may start on the tilt table to accommodate to the upright position. However, sitting on or at the bedside for several short periods may aid in adjusting

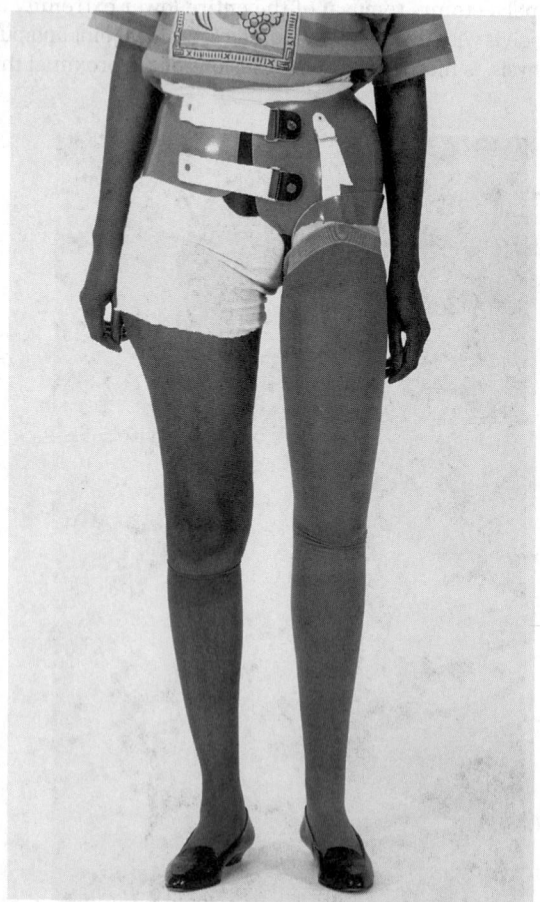

FIGURE 66–12. Hemipelvectomy prosthesis.

to this position. Re-educating the patient to become ambulatory involves a series of steps. Parallel bars are used initially, with the patient advancing to a walker and finally crutches as he or she develops increased strength, balance, and coordination. Activities that promote improved sitting and standing balance include sitting at the edge of a mat and reaching, catching, or kicking a foam or rubber ball with and without upper extremity support. Catching and throwing activities within the parallel bars challenge and improve standing balance. During sitting activities, a wedge or air (*e.g.*, Roho) cushion should be provided to enable equal weight distribution. This is particularly important for the hemipelvectomy patient who lacks a bony weight-bearing surface on the amputated side. After good balance and independent ambulation on level surfaces have been achieved, the patient may be advanced to more difficult activities such as stair climbing, getting up and down from the floor, opening doors, and riding on escalators.

Fitting for a prosthesis should occur after the suture line is well healed, surgical swelling has subsided, and the residual limb appears firm and nontender. Before obtaining a prosthesis, all patients should be informed of the potential benefits and the limitations of prosthetic use at this level. After such discussion with the rehabilitation team, the patient should be fitted if he or she so desires and prosthetic wearing is thought appropriate. The prosthetic socket is usually a plastic laminate that contours the remaining pelvis or abdomen and extends around the intact pelvis for additional pressure distribution. An endoskeletal unit with a foam covering is usually prescribed because it weighs less than a wooden exoskeletal type, but the exoskeletal type may be prescribed for the very active child or adult. The knee unit most often prescribed is a constant friction single axis knee, but occasionally, a safety knee may be prescribed. The safety knee allows increased stability in stance phase from a weight activated breaking system. A SACH (single axis, cushioned heel) foot is adequate at this level, but some patients are fitted with energy-storing feet, such as the Seattle foot or the Carbon Copy II, that simulate more natural foot mechanics.

Interim examinations are essential in this population. Modifications can be made to the socket, length, and alignment. The stability of the prosthesis depends on proper alignment of the hip, knee, and ankle joints and is crucial for successful ambulation. The prosthesis should be 1 to 2 cm shorter than the sound limb to aid in foot clearance. Other specific items to be checked are well documented elsewhere.[207]

After completion of the prosthesis, prosthetic training should begin. Instruction in an exaggerated pelvic tilt is necessary for bending of the prosthetic knee. This movement is more easily accomplished by those patients who have had hip disarticulations or modified hemipelvectomy because they have retained their entire pelvis or their iliac crest on the amputated side. Other gait deviations include vaulting and hip hiking to aid in advancement of the prosthetic limb. Vaulting is done to clear the prosthetic foot and to use up time needed for the prosthesis to take a step. It is sometimes impossible to eliminate vaulting, particularly in the younger amputee who needs and wants to walk fast. Vaulting is contraindicated only if there are leg or foot problems on the sound side.[207]

Patients with hip disarticulation may ambulate without any assistive devices, but most require at least a cane. Almost all patients with hemipelvectomy require a cane or pair of crutches for ambulation. Because these levels require increased energy expenditure for prosthetic use, some patients abandon the prosthesis and use crutches. It has been the experience of these authors that patients older than 50 and those younger than 18 prefer to use crutches, despite adequate prosthetic training. Few patients require the use of wheelchairs. Back pain and scoliosis should be monitored, especially in the growing child. If prosthetic use is impractical or not desired, a custom-made sitting jacket may be prescribed to stabilize the remaining pelvis and equalize the sitting surface.

Patients undergoing lower extremity amputation should be referred to occupational therapy to assess their safety in bathroom activity, need for adaptive devices for dressing and to review vocational and avocational interests. Adaptation of the environment may be useful to this population in preserving independence and conserving energy.

LIMB SALVAGE. Limb-sparing surgery implies removal of a soft tissue or bone sarcoma while preserving the extremity with a satisfactory functional and cosmetic result. Reconstruction should provide limb function that is equal or superior to the function of a prosthetic device. Sarcomas may arise in any part of the extremity. The functional outcome is determined in most part by the extent of soft tissue and bony structures resected. Knowledge of the anatomy and function of the musculoskeletal and nervous systems is fundamental in the treatment of these patients. With this knowledge, the rehabilitation team can better predict the outcome of the intended treatments and plan for the appropriate rehabilitation interventions.

Buttockectomy is an en bloc resection of the gluteus maximus muscle. Hip ROM and stretching exercises are recommended postoperatively. Gait deviations are usually absent, except for minor difficulty in stair climbing. A prosthetic buttock contour can be fabricated out of thermoplastic material or cloth covered foam and attached to the patient's underwear to provide a cosmetic appearance.

Internal hemipelvectomy is a procedure in which a portion of the hemipelvis and proximal femur are resected while leaving the extremity intact. A prolonged period of bed rest with skeletal traction is required postoperatively to allow fusion of the femur with the remaining pelvis. Strengthening and ROM exercises of the uninvolved extremities would be appropriate during this time. After the period of bed rest, a hip spica cast is most often indicated until further stabilization occurs, but ambulation with partial weight bearing can be performed while in the cast. Leg-length discrepancies are common and should be corrected with shoe lifts. Partial weight-bearing restrictions are usually maintained until total union occurs.[199] Most patients are independent ambulators with bilateral Lofstrand crutches, but depending on the extent of surgical resection, some may only require a cane. Common gait deviations include Trendelenburg and lateral trunk bending due to hip weakness and leg-length discrepancies. Rehabilitation efforts should be directed at minimizing these deficits.

Adductor group excisions typically result in significant postoperative drainage. Bed rest is recommended until drainage has decreased or drainage tubes are removed. Lower extremity edema and mild tightness are common after this procedure. Leg elevation, compression garments, active ROM exercises, and stretching are recommended to manage these problems. Gait deviations are rare, as is the need for assistive devices after this procedure.

Rehabilitation after quadriceps excision requires a period of bed rest with the extremity in a knee immobilizer for proper positioning and healing of the surgical site. Exercises on the uninvolved extremity should be encouraged and ankle exercises and hip isometrics on the operated limb. After drainage has decreased, ambulation may begin with partial weight bearing. An AFO should initially be prescribed that blocks dorsiflexion and allows 5° of plantarflexion. This creates an extension moment at the knee to provide knee stability during stance phase. With training, it has been shown through biomechanical analysis that some patients can learn to substitute hip extensors and plantarflexors adequately to control the knee joint. In such cases, ambulation can occur without an orthosis.

Management of patients after hamstring group excisions should include strengthening exercises for the quadriceps, knee ROM program, and stretching exercises to prevent knee flexion contractures. Little functional loss is attributed to this surgery if the sciatic nerve is not sacrificed. If the nerve is resected, motor and sensory loss below the knee occurs. The patient should be placed in an ankle splint in the neutral position postoperatively to prevent ankle contractures. Instruction in proper foot care including shoe wear is necessary to prevent skin ulcerations. A dorsiflexion-assist AFO is needed to provide foot clearance.[199]

Gastrocnemius muscle excision interferes with the patient's ability to properly push off at the end of stance phase. A rocker bottom on the sole of the patient's shoe aids in this motion. Active heel cord stretching should be performed to prevent heel cord tightening.[199]

Tumors involving the distal femur or proximal tibia can, in selected patients, be treated by limb-salvage surgery. Surgical treatment options include en bloc resection of the involved bone and soft tissue with autogenous grafting or allografting and arthrodesis of the knee, replacement with an endoskeletal prosthesis, or rotationplasty.[206,211] An expandable endoprosthesis has been developed that allows this procedure to be performed on a growing child.[206]

Rehabilitation after arthrodesis or arthroplasty is generally prolonged. Postoperative bed rest is recommended for 1 to 2 weeks with the leg elevated and immobilized in a posterior knee splint. If no wound healing problems are encountered, active exercises may begin after the period of bed rest. Quadriceps setting, gluteal setting, ankle pumps, and assisted straight-leg raising are encouraged. Weight-bearing limitations are determined on an individual basis, but most patients are progressed initially from no weight bearing to partial weight bearing to full weight bearing. Active ROM of the knee for those receiving arthroplasty usually begins 3 weeks postoperatively.[212]

Arthrodesis has the advantage of providing a stable limb that can withstand greater physical demands than arthroplasty, but the functional and cosmetic deficit of a fused knee must be considered. Successful arthroplasty has its advantages over arthrodesis in that it provides improved mobility of the reconstructed limb. However, complications of the endoprosthesis are common and can interfere with full functional restoration.[211]

Rotationplasty is a procedure that is performed instead of above-knee amputation. In this procedure, the distal femur is resected, and the distal portion of the limb is rotated 180°. The ankle is in a reversed position, and acts as the knee joint. The plantarflexors of the ankle act to extend the knee, and the dorsiflexors act to flex the knee. The functional result is that of a below-knee amputation and is superior to the function of an above-knee amputation. Vigorous rehabilitation should be instituted to achieve 90° of plantar flexion and to restore strength in the ankle musculature for the ankle to adequately perform as a knee joint. Prosthetic fitting includes weight-bearing surfaces to be distributed to the ischium and heel pad and has been described elsewhere.[206,213]

Soft tissue sarcomas adjacent to the scapula may require partial or total scapulectomy. A partial scapulectomy removes any extent of the scapula while preserving the glenohumeral joint, but the glenohumeral joint is sacrificed in a total scapulectomy. Near-total shoulder function with mild limitations in ROM can be expected after partial scapulectomy. However, after total scapulectomy, active motion at the shoulder is severely limited, and strength at the shoulder girdle is lost.[214] Preservation of function at the elbow and hand make this procedure superior to forequarter amputation.

Sarcomas deep to the scapula or involving the proximal humerus that do not involve the brachial plexus or axillary vessels can be treated with a Tikhoff-Lindberg resection. This procedure involves resection of the distal clavicle, upper humerus, and part or all of the scapula.[210] Partial shoulder and elbow function is maintained by muscle transfers and skeletal reconstruction. A custom prosthesis is used to maintain the length of the humerus. All patients should be fitted with a cosmetic shoulder mold similar to that for the forequarter amputee. If the cosmetic deficit is not as great, an off-the-shelf shoulder pad can be used instead of the shoulder mold.

Postoperatively, the arm should be maintained in an arm sling to restrict abduction and prevent distal traction on the reconstructed shoulder. Arm edema should be controlled with elastic stockinet. Active hand exercises aid in preventing and controlling edema. After drain removal and incisional healing, active exercises at the elbow can begin within the sling. At approximately 3 weeks postoperatively, passive ROM at the shoulder and forearm can begin. Progressive ROM and strengthening exercises should be encouraged after the arm is out of the sling. Excesses of 9 kg (20 lb) should not be lifted with the reconstructed arm.[199] Although shoulder function is limited, elbow, wrist, and hand function is usually preserved, making the functional outcome of this procedure more desirable than the alternative of forequarter amputation.

Other surgical resections in the upper extremity, including deltoid and triceps excisions, result in the obvious limitations. Due to the proximity of the major neurovascular structures in the upper extremity, many resections involve the median, radial, or ulnar nerves. After such resections, static and dynamic splinting must be employed to preserve functional use of the involved areas.

This information about rehabilitation progression constitutes general guidelines. Each surgical procedure must be individualized. Most limb-sparing surgeries are combined with other modalities, such as chemotherapy and radiation therapy. The effects of these treatments on the functional outcomes of the surgical procedures must be considered and are discussed in subsequent sections.

Effects of Chemotherapy

Extremity sarcoma patients receiving chemotherapy may experience complications that warrant rehabilitation intervention. Common musculoskeletal sequelae associated with chemotherapy that may affect mobility include nausea, vomiting, edema, peripheral neuropathy, cardiopulmonary toxicity, CNS dysfunction, immunosuppression, and delayed wound healing. Early rehabilitation intervention can lessen the degree of functional deficits that may result from the above sequelae. The rehabilitation varies in accordance with the medical status changes of the patient during or proceeding the chemotherapy course. Bouts of nausea and vomiting require careful monitoring and adjustment of treatment goals.

Fluctuations in fluid volume of the involved extremity should be treated using compression garments, active exercise, and, if appropriate, compression pumping or manual lymph drainage. Heat, cold, vibration, or compression can decrease the tingling or sharp pain associated with chemotherapy-induced neuropathies. If partial or complete loss of muscle function has occurred (*e.g.*, foot drop), ROM exercises and stretching of the affected joint can prevent contractures. Similarly, if muscle function has been disrupted, appropriate bracing can improve ambulation or basic daily living skills.

Cardiopulmonary toxicity can limit a patient's stamina and overall activity level. A carefully prescribed, closely monitored walking program is an excellent choice of exercise for increasing endurance in a patient with a compromised cardiovascular system. The goal of this form of endurance training is to progress the patient from a level of low exercise tolerance to a functionally and physiologically improved level.

CNS dysfunction resulting from chemotherapy treatment can manifest itself in motor and sensory losses. Motor dysfunction can range from subjective weakness with no objective findings to objective weakness with impaired function or even paralysis. Sensory loss can vary from mild paresthesia to severe objective sensory loss that significantly limits function. Rehabilitation can intervene by providing appropriate exercise and functional training, adaptive devices for assistance with impaired daily living activities, and assistive devices to aid in gait abnormalities resulting from weakness or sensory loss.

Immunosuppression may limit a patient's activity level, possibly confining them to bed rest. An exercise program that may be performed at bedside can be designed to decrease the unwanted effects of bed rest. Exercises can include active-assistive ROM, active ROM, isometrics, or resistive exercises. An immunosuppressed patient's blood counts should be closely monitored, and progression on therapy should follow medical status improvement (see Table 66–1).[215] Chemotherapy treatment can often delay wound healing. Delayed or inadequate wound healing should be treated immediately and can be managed by whirlpool or protection of the involved extremity by splinting or bracing.

Effects of Irradiation

Extremity sarcoma patients frequently receive radiation therapy preoperatively to reduce size and deep fixation of a tumor or postoperatively to eliminate or reduce residual tumor.[216] Radiation may produce pain, edema, delayed wound healing, leg-length discrepancy, or significant tissue fibrosis with possible contracture of the affected joint, any of which may occur early or remote from treatment. The goal of rehabilitation is to lessen the degree of functional deficit that may subsequently occur.

Pain control is often achieved with a TENS unit used on a high-frequency conventional setting. Modalities such as heat and cold can be used after the course of irradiation but should be avoided during treatment due to skin sensitivity or radioenhancement. Edema resulting from fibrosis of lymphatic channels can often be controlled with proper extremity positioning, compression garments or, if necessary, intermittent compression pumping. The use of whirlpool, debridement, or splinting or bracing of the involved area may be indicated for facilitation of wound healing.

Irradiation of growing bones, as in the case of adjuvant treatment of Ewing's sarcoma, may result in epiphyseal closure and leg-length discrepancy. Rehabilitation can supply shoe lifts, reducing future risk of scoliosis or muscle or joint imbalances. Fibrosis of joint tissues secondary to radiation treatment is a challenging problem for the rehabilitation specialist. Tissue fibrosis may continue 6 to 12 months after treatment. Patients must be encouraged to stretch and perform ROM exercises during and for 1 year after radiation treatment.

LUNG CANCER

Lung cancer may be one of four types: squamous cell, large cell, small cell, and adenocarcinoma. These four types are further classified as non-small cell lung cancer (NSCLC) and small cell lung cancer (SCLC). SCLC often has extensive local disease when diagnosed and is associated with early widespread metastasis. It carries the worst prognosis and has the lowest long-term 5-year survival rate. All types of lung cancer can metastasize to brain, liver, and bone.[217]

The treatment for lung cancer depends on the type and stage of the disease. Surgery is indicated for primary resectable lesions without distant metastasis. The primary tumor may be resected with a solitary brain metastasis, in which case, there is a 25% 5-year survival rate.[218] Surgical resection varies in extent and may include a pneumonectomy, lobectomy, or wedge segmental resection. At times, resection of the chest wall with reconstruction and insertion of plastic mesh may be needed.

Radiotherapy may be used as a preoperative adjunctive treatment to shrink the tumor, allowing surgery to be done. In this instance, it is associated with increased survival.[219] Radiotherapy as a primary treatment for unresectable tumor has a 5% 5-year survival rate.[220] Radiotherapy may be used in low doses for palliative treatment of superior vena cava syndrome secondary to tumor compression. High-dose radiation therapy is associated with lung tissue radiation effects.

Rehabilitation of the patient with lung cancer is generally divided into a preoperative or pretreatment phase and a postoperative phase. The pretreatment phase consists of a medical review of the chart to ascertain the stage and type of the tumor and whether metastasis is present. The physician should review the planned medical treatment. In addition to assessment of current medical status in regard to cardiopulmonary function, tests should be done for hemoglobin, hematocrit, and electrolytes. The current vocational status and family support situation should be assessed. A preoperative physical examination with particular attention to chest wall expansion, mus-

culoskeletal status, and cardiopulmonary status is requisite. The patient is generally educated in proper coughing and breathing techniques (*i.e.*, diaphragmatic, segmental). It should be explained to the patient that these exercises help air to enter the lungs better, increase the efficiency of the respiratory muscles, increase chest mobility, and decrease risk of pneumonia.[221] Lower extremity exercises after surgery to prevent thrombophlebitis are explained.

During the postoperative stage, the patient's pulmonary function and chest excursion are again assessed.[221] Specific breathing exercises are started after the patient is extubated. Posture and lower extremity exercises are addressed. Chest wall pain is often relieved by use of a TENS unit. After pain is controlled and the patient is allowed to ambulate, some assessment of endurance should be made. Endurance exercises should be gradually introduced into the rehabilitation program.

In patients with metastatic disease of the brain, speech and language deficits should be included in a cognitive, language, and swallowing evaluation. Depending on the location of the metastasis, there may be focal motor and sensory deficits. Ambulatory aids, bracing or splinting, and occupational therapy intervention for assistive devices and safety equipment may be needed. Bone metastasis may need unweighting with crutches or a walker and spinal bracing and pain management.

Depending on the prognosis of the patient, there should be discussions with him or her and the family about adjustment to whatever disabilities there may be. Careful assessment of whether the person can continue working should be made.

HEMATOPOIETIC TUMORS

Leukemias

Leukemia is the uncontrolled proliferation and incomplete maturation of leukocyte and lymphocyte precursors appearing in bone marrow and peripheral blood. The type of leukemia depends on the cell line affected—myeloid, monocyte, or lymphocyte. Leukemia may occur in acute or chronic forms.

The acute leukemias include acute myelogenous leukemia (AML) and acute lymphoblastic leukemia (ALL). They are more common in childhood. Both leukemias are associated with anemia, fatigue, fever, bleeding gums, gastrointestinal tract or urinary tract symptoms, easy bruising, and pallor. Headache, mental changes, and cranial nerve palsy are common in ALL with CNS involvement. Joint pain is often seen with ALL but rarely in AML. The prognosis for AML even with treatment is poor.[222] ALL responds much better to treatment, and complete remissions are often seen. Treatment of AML consists of cytosine ara-C, daunorubicin, and m-amsacrine. The mainstay treatment in ALL consists of vincristine and prednisone.

Chronic myelogenous leukemia (CML) is not usually seen before 20 years of age, and chronic lymphocytic leukemia (CLL) is generally seen after 50 years of age. Both present with abdominal discomfort, organ enlargement, malaise, and fatigue. Anemia, low platelet count, bruising, and cutaneous bleeding are seen with CML. Chemotherapeutic agents may suppress the disease, but only bone marrow transplantation is curative.[223]

The rehabilitation team must address the effects of the leukemia itself and the side effects of medications and irradiation.

A leukemia that doesn't respond completely to treatment has a course of remissions and exacerbations that seriously affects the ability to attend school or continue working. Long periods of rest may be needed during treatment or during times of low platelets. Generalized deconditioning and decreased muscle strength occur. Steroids contribute to decreased strength when they cause a myopathy. They may be associated with osteoporosis, compression fractures, and painful aseptic necrosis of bone. CNS leukemia is associated with altered cognition, cranial nerve abnormalities, and other neurologic deficits. Vincristine causes peripheral neuropathy. Hair loss occurs with some chemotherapeutic agents. Bone marrow transplantation requires a 6-week hospital stay, usually with confinement in a bone marrow hospital unit because of the necessary immunosuppression (*e.g.*, leukocyte count <1000/mm^3).

Management of muscle weakness, decreased endurance, focal neurologic deficits, joint pain, cosmesis, and psychosocial and vocational problems are a challenge to rehabilitation specialists in this group of patients. The type and intensity of exercises allowable depends mainly on the platelet count and hemoglobin level. Exercise should be nonresistive when the platelet count is less than 50,000/mm^3. No exercise is performed with counts below 20,000/mm^3.[224] Aerobic or endurance exercise is limited when hemoglobin is less than 8 to 10 g/dl.[225] Whenever exercise and activity is possible, it should be encouraged. Patients undergoing bone marrow transplantation are always placed on an exercise program to increase strength and endurance. They are on high-dose steroid therapy and particularly susceptible to steroid myopathy, osteoporosis, and aseptic necrosis. Their exercise program includes weight-bearing activities, upper extremity ROM, an isometric program, and back extension exercises. An aerobic program is introduced when platelet and hemoglobin levels permit.[224,225]

Bracing and splinting are needed for neurologic deficits. Assessment of activity of daily living and issuance of safety equipment and assistive devices may be needed. Energy-conservation education is important. Assisting the patient and family with coping with acute and chronic problems is essential. A wig should be available during hair loss due to chemotherapy. Children should be tutored while they are unable to attend school.

Lymphomas

Lymphomas represent a malignant group of tumors that arise principally from lymph node cellular structures, other reticuloendothelial organs, and bone marrow. These tumors are classified as Hodgkin's disease and non-Hodgkin's lymphomas. The type of cells and their growth pattern help to differentiate the types of lymphomas. Knowledge of the stage of the disease is important because medical and rehabilitation treatment regimens are oriented to the stage-specific problems and prognosis.

Hodgkin's disease arises in lymph nodes and commonly involves bone marrow, liver, lung, and bone. There is a bimodal distribution of incidence, with peaks between 15 and 35 years of age and above age 50. Significant progress has been made in the medical management of this disease, and 75% of patients are cured.[226] Stage IV disease carries a less favorable prognosis, as does disease occurring after age 50. Relapses may occur anytime during the life of the patient.

Treatment consists of combination chemotherapy and radiation therapy. Many multidrug regimens exist. Choice of an appropriate drug regimen depends on the stage of the disease. Most of the regimens include prednisone, and side effects of osteoporosis, compression fracture, myopathy, and aseptic necrosis may be seen in 10%.[227] Other drugs with potential side effects that need to be addressed by rehabilitation include doxorubicin (Adriamycin), which produces decreased cardiac ejection fraction, and vincristine, which causes peripheral neuropathy. Combination regimens may result in hair loss, aspermia, and early menopause. Prolonged bed rest results in muscle weakness and decreased endurance. Treatment with radiotherapy can result in skin tightness, restricted joint motion, and aspermia.

The disease itself can be asymptomatic subtype (A) or symptomatic subtype (B). Systemic symptoms of fever, night sweats, weight loss, and decreased endurance are present with stage I through IVB disease.

Non-Hodgkin's lymphoma (NHL) is three times as common as Hodgkin's disease. The peak incidence occurs between the ages of 50 and 59.[228] These lymphomas are tumors of B and T cells and can originate in any lymphatic organ. Staging is similar to Hodgkin's disease (stage I–IVA or B). An international classification of NHL is based on the grade of the tumor (*i.e.*, low, intermediate, high). For purposes of prognosis, NHL can be classified according to its biologic behavior into indolent (favorable) lymphomas and aggressive (unfavorable) lymphomas. Indolent lymphomas are low grade and progress over many years. They are not currently curable by medical treatment. The aggressive lymphomas are fatal in a short time if not treated. Long-term disease-free survival occurs for 50% of patients. Aggressive high-grade lymphomas, such as Burkitt's, have a high propensity for metastasis to the CNS (*i.e.*, meningeal carcinomatosis), causing symptoms of headache, diplopia, cranial nerve palsy, and weakness. Spinal cord compression can occur if lymphoma involves the epidural space. CNS and spinal cord involvement can occur with NHL and Hodgkin's disease.

Other problems that arise with lymphomas include increased susceptibility to infection, pleural and pericardial effusion, and superior vena cava syndrome due to compression of the superior vena cava by enlarged lymph nodes.

Chemotherapy and irradiation regimens for NHL are chosen according to the grade and type of tumor. Vincristine, prednisone, and cyclophosphamide are commonly used in these regimens. Side effects are similar to those described under Hodgkin's disease.

As for patients with any type of cancer, it is important to know the type and stage of lymphoma, the treatment indicated, side effects, and the general prognosis when planning a rehabilitation regimen. In general, patients have to cope with disease-related problems and the effects of complex chemotherapeutic and radiotherapy regimens. Some patients may have an early complete cure and be left with no residual problems. Others may have had more advanced or more malignant disease with incomplete remissions or recurrences and disease- and treatment-related morbidity. In this latter group, vocational and school status should be assessed. All members of the rehabilitation team are involved in the management of these patients.

Neurologic involvement may require bracing, mobility aides, assistive devices, and speech and language evaluation.

Unweighting lower extremity joints involved with aseptic necrosis is appropriate. Muscle weakness and deconditioning should be addressed with appropriate strengthening and endurance exercises. The same precautions about platelet and hemoglobin levels hold true for lymphomas and leukemias.

Particular attention should be paid to unweighting bony lower extremity lesions if there is more than 50% cortical involvement. Appropriate spinal bracing for vertebral involvement should be addressed. Unstable lesions should be evaluated surgically. If the patient has advanced disease and surgery cannot be done, choice of a body jacket for thoracic and lumbar lesions and a four-poster brace for cervical lesions may need to be used to help prevent spinal cord compression. When treating patients in rehabilitation, any early signs of spinal cord compression such as new weakness, sensory deficits, or reflex changes should be reported to the primary physician, because radiation therapy may be effective in reducing the size of spinal metastasis and relieving spinal compression. Likewise, any signs of superior vena cava syndrome such as increased dyspnea, facial edema, and dilated chest wall veins should be reported, because irradiation may palliate these symptoms.

REFERENCES

1. Lehmann JF, DeLisa JA, Warren CG, deLateur BJ, Bryant PLS, Nicholson CG. Cancer rehabilitation: Assessment of need, development and evaluation of a model of care. Arch Phys Med Rehabil 1976;59:410.
2. Habermann ET, Lopez RA. Metastatic disease of bone and treatment of pathological fractures. Orthop Clin North Am 989;20:469.
3. Palma G. Paraneoplastic syndromes of the nervous system. West J Med 1985;142: 787.
4. Bateman DE, Weller RO, Kennedy P. Stiffman syndrome: A rare paraneoplastic disorder? J Neurol Neurosurg Psychiatry 1990;53:659–696.
5. Van Healst-Pisani CM, Pisani RJ, Kovach JS. Cancer immunotherapy: Current status of treatment with interleukin 2 and lymphokine-activated killer cells. Mayo Clin Proc 1989;64:451.
6. Welch-McCaffrey D, Hoffman B, Leigh SA, Loescher LJ. Surviving adult cancers. Part 2: Psychosocial implications. Ann Intern Med 1989;111:517.
7. Hoffman B. Current issues of cancer survivorship. Oncology 1989;3:85.
8. Hoffman B. Cancer survivors at work: Job problems and illegal discrimination. Oncol Nurs Forum 1989;16:39.
9. Tebbi CK, Bromberg C, Piedmonte M. Long-term vocational adjustment of cancer patients diagnosed during adolescence. Cancer 1989;63:213.
10. Schover LR, Schain WS, Montague DK. Sexual problems of patients with cancer. In: De Vita VT Jr, Hellman S, Rosenberg SA, eds. Cancer: Principles and practice of oncology. Philadelphia: JB Lippincott, 1989:2206.
11. Smith DB. Sexual rehabilitation of the cancer patient. Cancer Nurs 1989;12:10.
12. Levy MJ, Stillman RJ. Reproductive potential in survivors of childhood malignancy. Pediatrics 1991;18:61.
13. Green DM, Zevon MA, Lowrie G, Seigelstein N, Hall B. Congenital anolmalies in children of patients who received chemotherapy for cancer in childhood and adolescence. N Engl J Med 1991;325:141.
14. Kazak AE. Psychological issues in childhood cancer survivors. J Assoc Pediatr Oncol Nurses 1989;6:15.
15. Chang PN. Psychosocial needs of long-term childhood cancer survivors: A review of literature. Pediatrician 1991;18:20.
16. List MA, Ritter-Sterr C, Lansky SB. Cancer during adolescence. Pediatrician 1991;18: 32.
17. Glauser TA, Packer RJ. Cognitive deficits in long-term survivors of childhood brain tumors. Childs Nerv Syst 1991;7:2.
18. Goldwein JW. Effects of radiation therapy on skeletal growth in childhood. Clin Orthop Rel Res 1991;262:101.
19. Maguire A, Murray JJ, Craft AW, Kernahan J, Welbury RR. Radiological features of the long-term effects from treatment of malignant disease in childhood. Br Dental J 1987;162:99.
20. Ryan JR, Emami A. Vincristine neurotoxicity with residual equinocavus deformity in children with acute leukemia. Cancer 1983;51:423.
21. Hammack JE, Kimmel DW, O Neill BP, Lennon VA. Paraneoplastic cerebellar degeneration: A clinical comparison of patients with and without Purkinje cell cytoplasmic antibodies. Mayo Clin Proc 1990;65:1423.
22. Derogatis L, Abeloff M, Melisaratos N. Psychological coping mechanisms and survival time in metastatic breast cancer. JAMA 1979;242:1504.
23. Bergner M, Bobbitt R, Carter W, Gilson B. The sickness impact Profile: Development and final revision of a health status measure. Med Care 1981;19:787.
24. Wilmore DW. Catabolic illness: Strategies for enhancing recovery. N Engl J Med 1991;325:695.
25. Gross M, Roberts JG, Foster J, Shankardass K. Calcaneal bone density reduction in patients with restricted mobility. Arch Phys Med Rehabil 1987;68:158.
26. Stewart AF, Adler M, Byers CM, Segre GV, Broadus AE. Calcium homeostasis in immobilization: An example of resorptive hypercalcemia. N Engl J Med 1982;306:1136.
27. Claus-Walker J, Halstead LS, Rodrigues GP, Henry YK. Spinal cord injury hypercalcemia: Therapeutic profile. Arch Phys Med Rehabil 1982;63:108.
28. Scher HI, Yagoda A. Bone metastases: Pathogenesis, treatment, and rationale for use of resorption inhibitors. Am J Med 1987;82:6.
29. Vico L, Chappard D, Alexandre C, et al. Effects of a 120 day period of bedrest on bone mass and bone cell activities in man: Attempts at countermeasure. Bone Miner 1987;2: 383.
30. Booth FW. Physiologic and biochemical effects of immobilization on muscle. Clin Orthop Rel Res 1987;219:15.
31. Häggmark T, Eriksson E, Jansson E. Muscle fiber type changes in human skeletal muscle after injuries and immobilization. Orthopedics 1986;9:181.
32. Akeson WH, Amiel D, Abel MF, Garfin SR, Woo SL-Y. Effects of immobilization on joints. Clin Orthop Rel Res 1987;219:28.
33. Woo SL-Y, Gomez MA, Sites TJ, Newton PO, Orlando CA, Akeson WH. The biomechanical and morphological changes in the medial collateral ligament of the rabbit after immobilization and remobilization. J Bone Joint Surg 1987;69-A:1200.
34. Mohr DN, Ryu JH, Litin SC, III ECR. Recent advances in the management of venous thromboembolism. Mayo Clin Proc 1988;63:281.
35. Lotze MT, Duncan MA, Gerber LH, Woltering EA, Rosenberg SA. Early versus delayed shoulder motion following axillary dissection. Ann Surg 1981;193:288.
36. Lehmann JF, De Lateur BJ. Diathermy and superficial heat, laser and cold therapy. In: Kottke FJ, Lehmann JF, eds. Krusen's handbook of physical medicine and rehabilitation. Philadelphia: WB Saunders, 1990:283.
37. Glover D. Metabolic emergencies. New York: JB Lippincott, 1991:7.
38. Glover D. Paraneoplastic syndrome: Endocrine effects. Philadelphia: JB Lippincott, 1991.
39. Dalakas M. Polymyositis dermatomyositis, and inclusion body myositis. N Engl J Med 1991;325:1487.
40. Cairncross GJ. Effects of cancer on the nervous system. In: Wiites R, ed. Manual of oncological therapeutics. New York: JB Lippincott, 1991.
41. Manchul LA, Jina-Prichard KI, Tenenbaum J, et al. The frequency of malignant neoplasms in patients with polymyositis-dematomyositis. Arch Intern Med 1985;145:1835.
42. Lakhanpal S, Bunch TW, Strup IL, et al. Polymyositis-dermatomyositis and malignant lesions: Does an association exist? Mayo Clin Proc 1986;61:645.
43. Bohm A. Clinical presentation and diagnosis of polymyositis and dermatomyositis. In: Dalakas M, ed. Polymyositis and dermatomyositis. London: Butterworths, 1987:28.
44. Hicks JE. Comprehensive rehabilitation management of patients with polymyositis and dermatomyositis. In: Dalakas M, ed. Polymyositis and dermatomyositis. London: Butterworths, 1987:293.
45. Hicks JE, Miller F, Plotz P, et al. Strength improvement without CPK elevation in a polymyositis patient on isometric exercise program. Arthritis Rheum 1988;31:559.
46. Rosenberg N, Carry M, Rengel S. Association of inflammatory myopathies with other connective tissue disorders and malignancies. In: Dalakas M, ed. Polymyositis and dermatomyositis. London: Butterworths, 1987.
47. Dalakas M. Treatment of polymyositis and dermatomyositis with corticosteroids. In: Dalakas M, ed. Polymyositis and dermatomyositis. London: Butterworths, 1987.
48. David DS, Greico H, Cushman P. Adrenal glucocorticoids after twenty years: A review of their clinically relevant consequences. J Chron Dis 1970;22:637.
49. Paterson AHG. Bone metastases in breast cancer, prostate cancer and myeloma. Bone 1987;1(suppl 1):S17.
50. Nielsen OS, Munro AJ, Tannock IF. Bone mestastases: Pathophysiology and management policy. J Clin Oncol 1991;9:509.
51. Bocchi L, Lazzeroni L, Maggi M. The Surgical treatment of metastases in long bones. Ital J Orthop Traumatol 1988;14:167.
52. Menck H, Schulze S, Larsen E. Metastasis size in pathologic femoral fractures. Acta Orthop Scand 1988;59:151.
53. Galasko CSB. Skeletal metastases. Clin Orthop Rel Res 1986;210:18.
54. Rodichok LD, Harper GR, Ruckdeschel JC, et al. Early diagnosis of spinal epidural metastases. Am J Med 1981;70:1181.
55. Rodichok LD, Ruckdeschel JC, Harper GR, et al. Early detection and treatment of spinal epidural metastases: The role of myelography. Ann Neurol 1986;20:696.
56. Beltran J, Noto AM, Chakeres DW, Christofordis AJ. Tumors of the osseous spine: Staging with MR imaging versus CT. Radiology 1987;162:565.
57. Godersky JC, Smoker WRK, Knutzon R. Use of magnetic resonance imaging in the evaluation of metastatic spinal Disease. Neurosurgery 1987;21:676.
58. Smoker WRK, Godersky JC, Knutzon RK, Keyes WD, Normal D, Bergman W. The role of MR imaging in evaluating metastatic spinal disease. Am J Neuroradiol 1987;8: 901.
59. Winkelman MD, Adelstein DJ, Karlins NL. Intramedullary spinal cord metastasis. Arch Neurol 1987;44:526.
60. Errico TJ, Kostuik JP. Diagnosis and treatment of metastatic disease of the spinal column: A review. Contemp Orthop 1986;13:15.
61. Denis F. Spinal Instability as defined by the three-column spine concept in acute spinal trauma. Clin Orthop Rel Res 1984;189:65.
62. Pal GP, Sherk HH. The vertical stability of the cervical spine. Spine 1988;13:447.
63. Onimus M, Schraub S, Bertin D, Bosset JF, Guidet M. Surgical treatment of vertebral metastasis. Spine 1986;11:883.
64. Galasko CSB. Spinal instability secondary to metastatic cancer. J Bone Joint Surg [Br] 1991;73:104.

65. Cooper PR, Marvilla DR, Sklar FH, Moody SF, Clark K. Halo immobilization of cervical spine Fractures. Indications and results. J Neurosurg 1979;50:603.

66. Johnson RM, Owen JR, Hart DL, Callahan RA. Cervical orthoses. A guide to their selection and use. Clin Orthop Rel Res 1981;154:34.

67. Sutherland IA, Myers SJ. Radiation myelopathy. Arch Phys Med Rehabil 1976;57:81.

68. Hahn AF, Feasby TE, Gilbert JJ. Paraparesis following intrathecal chemotherapy. Neurology 1983;33:1032.

69. Werner RA. Paraplegia and quadriplegia after intrathecal chemotherapy. Arch Phys Med Rehabil 1988;69:1054.

70. Loehrer PJ, Einhorn LH. Drugs five years later. Cisplatin. Ann Intern Med 1984;100:704.

71. Reinstein L, Ostrow SS, Wiernik PH. Peripheral neuropathy after cis-platinum (II) (DDP) therapy. Arch Phys Med Rehabil 1980;61:280.

72. Basso-Ricci S, della Costa C, Viganotti G, Ventafridda V. Report on 42 cases of post-irradiation lesions of the brachial plexus and their treatment. Tumori 1980;66:117.

73. Barr LC, Kissin MW. Radiation-induced brachial plexus neuropathy following breast conservation and radical radiotherapy. Br J Surg 1987;74:855.

74. Salner AL, Botnick LE, Herzog AG, et al. Reversible brachial plexopathy following primary radiation therapy for breast cancer. Cancer Treat Rep 1981;65:797.

75. Wheeler JS Jr, Siroky MB, Bell R, Babayan RK. Vincristine-induced bladder neuropathy. J Urol 1982;130:342.

76. Rosenfeld CS, Broder LE. Cisplatin-induced autonomic neuropathy. Cancer Treat Rep 1984;68:659.

77. Raphaelson MI, Stevens JC, Newman RP. Vincristine neuropathy with bowel and bladder atony. Mimicking spinal cord compression. Cancer Treat Rep [Letter] 1983;67:604.

78. Scherokman B, Filing-Katz MR, Tell D. Brachial plexus neuropathy following high-dose cytarabine in acute monoblastic leukemia. Cancer Treat Rep 1985;69:1005.

79. La Rocca RV, Meer J, Gilliatt RW, et al. Suramin-induced polyneuropathy. Neurology 1990;40:954.

80. Kori SH, Foley KM, Posner JB. Brachial plexus lesions in patients with cancer: 100 cases. Neurology 1981;31:45.

81. Harper CM Jr, Thomas JE, Cascino TL, Litchy WJ. Distinction between neoplastic and radiation-induced brachial plexopathy, with emphasis on the role of EMG. Neurology 1989;39:502.

82. Mondrup K, Olsen NK, Pfeiffer P, Rose C. Clinical and electrodiagnostic findings in breast cancer patients with radiation-induced brachial plexus neuropathy. Acta Neurol Scand 1990;81:153.

83. Hoang P, Ford DJ, Burke FD. Post-mastectomy pain after brachial plexus palsey: Metastases or radiation neuritis. J Hand Surg 1986;11B:441.

84. Jaeckle KA, Young DF, Foley KM. The natural history of lumbosacral plexopathy in cancer. Neurology 1985;35:8.

85. Pettigrew LC, Glass JP, Maor M, Zornoza J. Diagnosis and treatment of lumbosacral plexopathies in patients with cancer. Arch Neurol 1984;41:1282.

86. Ricci MA. Deep venous thrombosis in orthopedic patients. Current techniques in precise diagnosis. Orthop Rev 1984;13:185.

87. Dauzat MM, Laroche J-P, Charras C, et al. Real-time B-mode ultrasonography for better specificity in the noninvasive diagnosis of deep venous thrombosis. J Ultrasound Med 1986;5:625.

88. Moser KM, LeMoine JR. Is embolic risk conditioned by location of deep venous thrombosis. Ann Intern Med 1981;94:439.

89. Vernick SH, Shapiro D, Shaw FD. Legging orthosis of venous and lymphatic insufficiency. Arch Phys Med Rehabil 1987;68:459.

90. Klein MJ, Alexander MA, Wright JM, Redmond CK, LeGasse AA. Treatment of adult lower extremity lymphedema with the Wright linear pump: Statistical analysis of a clinical trial. Arch Phys Med Rehabil 1988;69:202.

91. Madersbacher H. The various types of neurogenic bladder dysfunction: An update of current therapeutic concepts. Paraplegia 1990;28:217.

92. Wyndaele JJ. Pharmacotherapy for urinary bladder dysfunction in spinal cord injury patients. Paraplegia 1990;28:146.

93. Broadwell DC, Jackson BS. Principles of ostomy care. St. Louis: CV Mosby, 1982.

94. ConvaTec. A professionals guide for counseling ostomy patients. Princeton, NJ: Squibb and Sons, 1989.

95. Broadwell DC, Sorrells SL. Ileostomy care. Plainfield, NJ: Patient Education Press, 1988:21.

96. Broadwell DC, Broadhurst BB. Colostomy care. Plainfield, NJ: Patient Education Press, 1989:26.

97. Broadwell DC, Broadhurst BB. Urinary diversion. Plainfield, NJ: Patient Education Press, 1989:24.

98. ConvaTec. An ostomy is for living. Princeton, NJ: Squibb & Sons, 1983.

99. ConvaTec. For a better way of living with a colostomy . . . everyday. Princeton, NJ: Squibb & Sons, 1985.

100. ConvaTec. For a better way of living with an ileostomy . . . everyday. Princeton, NJ: Squibb & Sons, 1985.

101. Pollard K, Callum K, Altman D. Shoulder movement following mastectomy. Clin Oncol 1976;2:343.

102. Flew TJ. Wound drainage following radical mastectomy: The effect of restriction of shoulder movement. Br J Surg 1966;66:302.

103. Atkins H, Hayward JL, Klugman DJ. Treatment of early breast cancer: A report after 10 years of a clinical trial. Br Med J 1972;2:423.

104. Gerber L, Lampert M, Wood C. Comparison of pain, motion and edema after modified radical mastectomy or local excision with axillary dissection and radiation. Breast Cancer Res Treat 1992;21:139.

105. After mastectomy: Finding the right prosthesis. Consumer Reports 1975;105:652.

106. Mathog RH. Rehabilitation of head and neck cancer patients: Consensus on recommendations from the International Conference on Rehabilitation of the Head and Neck Cancer Patient. Head Neck 1991;Jan/Feb:1–2.

107. Zagar G, Norante J. Head and neck tumors. 6th ed. Atlanta: American Cancer Society, 1983.

108. Silverman S. Radiation effects. 3rd ed. Atlanta: American Cancer Society, 1990:9.

109. Dudgeon B, DeLisa L, Miller R. Head and neck cancer: A rehabilitation approach. Am J Occup Ther 1980;34:243.

110. Sonies BC, Weiffenbach J, Atkinson J, Brahim J, Macynski A, Fox P. Clinical examination of motor and sensory function of the adult oral cavity. 1987;1:178.

111. Blakley BW, Black O, Meyers SF, Rintelmann WF, Schweitzer V, Schwan SA. Ototoxicity. Head Neck 1991;Jan/Feb:2–3.

112. Aker S, Tilmont G, Harrison V. A guide to good nutrition during and after chemotherapy and radiation. Health Sciences Learning Research Center. Fred Hutchinson Cancer Research Center, 1976.

113. Bradford K. A practical application of nutrition for the patient with head and neck cancer. Cancer Bull 1977;29:35.

114. Argerakis GP. Psychosocial considerations of head and neck cancer patients. Dent Clin North Am 1990;34:285.

115. DeWys WD, Walters K. Abnormalities of taste sensation in cancer patients. CA 1975;36:1888.

116. Kelly D. Speech rehabilitation of the laryngectomized patient. Cancer Bull 1977;29:39.

117. Marunick MT, Kapur K, Beumer J, McGregor IA, Urken M. Mastication. Head Neck 1991;Jan/Feb:6–7.

118. Donaldson S. Nutrititional consequences of radiotherapy. Cancer Res 1977;37:2407.

119. Fleming S, Hamlet S, Nelson R, Muz J. Deglutition. Head Neck 1991;Jan/Feb:4–5.

120. Hamlet S, Jones L, Patterson R, Michou G, Cislo C. Swallowing recovery following anterior tongue and floor of mouth surgery. Head Neck 1991;13:334.

121. McKenna JP, Fornataro-Clerici LM, Menamin PGM, Leonard RJ. Laryngeal cancer: diagnosis, treatment and speech rehabilitation. Am Fam Physician 1991;44:123.

122. Urken ML, Buchbinder D, Weinberg H, et al. Functional evaluation following microvascular oromandibular reconstruction of the oral cancer patient: A comparative study of reconstructed and nonreconstructed patients. Laryngoscope 1991;101:935.

123. Burgess EM. Surgery as related to prosthetics and orthotics. Bull Prosthet Res 1974;Fall:15–21.

124. Wright WE, Haller JM, Harlow SA, Pizzo PA. An oral disease prevention program for patients receiving radiation and chemotherapy. J Am Dent Assoc 1985;110:43.

125. Silverman S, Shillitoe E. Etiology and predisposing factors. 3rd ed. Atlanta: American Cancer Society, 1990:32.

126. Ingall JRF, Saper JR, Kish J, Kuch K, Evans R. Pain. Head Neck 1991;Jan/Feb:9–10.

127. McCaffery M, Beebe A. Pain: Clinical manual for nursing practice. St Louis: CV Mosby, 1989.

128. Siddoway JR, Gursel E, Sullivan W, Hayden R. Cosmetic rehabilitation of the head and neck cancer patient. Head Neck 1991;Jan/Feb:3.

129. Hamaker RC, Singer MI, Blom ED. Primary voice restoration of laryngectomy. Arch Otolaryngol 1985;111:182.

130. Singer MI. Tracheoesophageal speech: Vocal rehabilitation after total laryngectomy. Laryngoscope 1983;93:1454.

131. Instrumental guidelines for diagnosis of dysphagia. American Speech and Hearing Association, 1992;34(Suppl):7.

132. Miller A, Miller B. Does intraoperative monitoring of auditory evoked potentials reduce incidence of hearing loss as a complication of microvascular decompression of the cranial nerves? Neurosurgery 1989;Feb.

133. Hammerschlag PE, Cohen NL. Introperative monitoring of facial nerve function in cerebellopontine angle surgery. Otolaryngol Head Neck Surg 1990;Nov.

134. Logemann JA. Manuel for the videofluorographic study of swallowing. San Diego: College-Hill Press, 1986.

135. Staple TW, Ogura JH. Cineradiography of the swallowing mechanism following supraglottic subtotal laryngectomy. Radiology 1966;87:226.

136. Muz J, Mathog RH, Hamlet SL, Kling LPDA. Objective assessment of swallowing function in head and neck cancer patients. Head Neck 1991;13:33.

137. Litton WB, Leonard JR. Aspiration after partial laryngectomy: Cineradiographic studies. Laryngoscope 1969;79:887.

138. Sonies BC. Instrumental procedures for dysphagia diagnosis. New York: Thieme Medical Publishers, 1991:13.

139. Sonies BC. Ultrasound imaging and swallowing. New York: Springer-Verlag, 1991:10.

140. Fletcher SG, Jacobs RF, Kelly D. Speech Production. Head Neck 1991;Jan/Feb:8–9.

141. List MA, Ritter-Sterr C, Lansky SB. A performance status scale for head and neck cancer patients. CA 1990;66:564.

142. Beumer J, Zlotolow I, Curtis T. Rehabilitation. 3rd ed. Atlanta: American Cancer Society, 1990:21.

143. Skelly M, Spector DJ, Donaldson RC. Compensatory physiologic phonetics for the glossectomee. J Speech Hear Disord 1971;36:101.

144. Skelly M, Donaldson RC, Fust RS. Changes in phonatory aspects of glossectomee intelligibility through vocal parameter manipulation. J Speech Hear Disord 1972;37:379.

145. Skelly M, Donaldson R, Schinsky I. Substitution consistency as a factor in glossectomy intelligibility. J Missouri Hear Assoc 1972;5:21.

146. Stockmeyer S. An interpretation of the approach of Rood to the treatment of neuromuscular dysfunction. Am J Phys Med 1967;46:1.

147. Mendenhall WM, Parsons JT, Stringer SP. The role of radiation therapy in laryngeal cancer. CA 1990;40:3.

148. Moore GK, Getchell T, Mistretta C, Mozell M, Kern R. Taste/smell. Head Neck 1991;Jan/Feb:7–8.

149. Nelson R, Fox P, Marks J. Salivation. Head Neck 1991;Jan/Feb.

150. Larsen G. Guidelines for head and neck rehabilitation. Fred Hutchinson Cancer Research Center, 1979.

151. Larsen G. Rehabilitating dysphagia mechanica, paralytica, pseudobulbar. J Neurosurg Nurs 1976;8:14.

152. Keyes HM, McCasland JP. Techniques and results of a comprehensive dental care program in head and neck cancer patients. Int J Radiat Oncol Biol Phys 1976;1:859.

153. Doberneck RC, Antoine JE. Deglutition after resection of oral, laryngeal, and pharyngeal cancers. Surgery 1974;75:87.

154. Trible WM. The rehabilitation of deglutition following head and neck surgery. Laryngoscope 1967;77:518.

155. Logemann JA. Swallowing and communication rehabilitation. Semin Oncol Nurs 1989;5:205.

156. Desjardins RP, Laney WR. Prosthetics rehabilitation after cancer resection in the head and neck. Surg Clin North Am 1977;57:809.

157. Fine R, Krell W, Ranella K, Sessions D, Williams M. Respiratory problems and rehabilitation in the head and neck cancer patient. Head Neck 1991;Jan/Feb.

158. Fleming S. Treatment of mechanical swallowing disorders. Boston: Butterworths, 1984:157.

159. Westmore SJ, Johns ME, Baker SR. The Singer-Blom voice restoration procedure. Arch Otolaryngol 1981;107:674.

160. Schaefer SD, Johns DF. Attaining functional esophageal speech. Arch Otolaryngol 1982;108:647.

161. Miller S. The role of the speech-language pathologist in voice restoration after total laryngectomy. CA 1990;40(3).

162. Robbins J, Fisher HB, Blom EC, Singer MI. A comparative acoustic study of normal esophageal and tracheoesophageal speech production. J Speech Hear Disord 1984;49:202.

163. Keith RL, Darley FL. Laryngectomee rehabilitation. Houston: College-Hill Press, 1979.

164. Singer MI, Blom ED. Medical techniques for voice restoration after total laryngectomy. CA 1990;40(3).

165. Jacobs JR, Pearson BW, Singer M, Hamaker R, Blom E, Tucker H. Rehabilitation of the patient following total laryngectomy. Biol Assoc Med 1989;8(11):455–457.

166. Lehmann W, Krebs H. Interdisciplinary rehabilitation of the laryngectomees. Recent Results Cancer Res 1991;121:442.

167. Singer MI, Blom ED. An endoscopic technique for restoration of voice after laryngectomy. Ann Otol Rhinol Laryngol 1980;89:529.

168. Singer MI, Blom ED, Hamaker RC. Further experience with voice restoration after total laryngectomy. Ann Otol Rhinol Laryngol 1981;90:498.

169. Blom ED, Singer MI, Hamaker RC. An improved esophageal insufflation test. Arch Otolaryngol 1985;111:211.

170. Juarbe C. Overview of results with trachea esophageal puncture after total laryngectomy. Bol Assoc Med Puerto Rico 1989;8:455.

171. Baugh RF, Lewin JS, Baker SR. Vocal rehabilitation of tracheoesophageal speech failures. Head Neck 1990;Jan/Feb:69–73.

172. Baggs T, Pine S. Acoustic characteristics: Tracheo-esophageal speech. J. Commun Disord 1983;16:299.

173. Doyle P, Grantmyre A, Myers C. Clinical modification of the tracheostoma breathing valve for voice restoration. J Speech Hear Disord 1989;54:189.

174. Cantu E, Shagets FW, Fifer RC. Customized valve housing. Laryngoscope 1986;96:1065.

175. Barton D, DeSanto L, Pearson BW, Keith R. Anendostomal tracheostomy tube for leakproof retention of the Blom-Singer stomal valve. Otolaryngol Head Neck Surg 1988;999:38.

176. Heller KS, Levy J, Sciubba JJ. Speech patterns following partial glossectomy for small tumors of the tongue. Head Neck 1991;13:340.

177. Aramy MA, Down JA, Berry QC. Prosthodontic rehabilitation for glossectomy patients. J. Prosthet Dent 1982;48:78.

178. Davis JW, Lazarus C, Hurst PS. Effects of a maxillary glossectomy prosthesis on articulation and swallowing. J Prosthet Dent 1987;57:715.

179. Drane J. Role of maxillofacial prosthetics. Cancer Bull 1977;29:41.

180. Panje WR. Mandibular reconstruction with the trapezius osteomusculocutaneous flap. Arch Otolaryngol 1985;111:223.

181. Zochodne DW, Cairncross JG. Metastasis to the central nervous system. Cancer Growth Prog 1989;8:32.

182. Pluss JL, DiBella NJ. Reversible central nervous system dysfunction due to tamoxifen in a patient with breast cancer. Ann Intern Med 1984;101:652.

183. Paoletti P, Spanu G. Surgical therapy of malignant gliomas. J Neurosurg Sci 1990;34:289.

184. Brandes A, Soesan M, Fiorentino MV. Medical treatment of high grade malignant gliomas in adults: An overview. Anticancer Res 1991;11:719.

185. O Neill BP, Illig JJ. Primary central nervous system lymphoma. Mayo Clin Proc 1989;64:1005.

186. Grote TH, Grosh WW, List AF, Wiley R, Cousar JB, Johnson DH. Primary lymphoma of the central nervous system. A report of 20 cases and a review of the literature. Am J Clin Oncol 1989;12:93.

187. Remick SC, Diamond C, Migliozzi JA, et al. Primary central nervous system lymphoma in patients with and without the acquired immune deficiency syndrome. A retrospective analysis and review of the literature. Medicine (Baltimore) 1990;69:345.

188. Mena H, Ribas JL, Enzinger FM, Parisi JE. Primary Angiosarcoma of the central nervous system. Study of eight cases and review of the literature. J Neurosurg 1991;75:73.

189. Horowitz MB, Hall WA. Central nervous system germinomas. A review. Arch Neurol 1991;48:652.

190. Black PM. Brain tumors. (II.) N Engl J Med 1991;324:1555.

191. Black PM. Brain tumors. (I.) N Engl J Med 1991;324:1471.

192. Friedman HS, Horowitz M, Oakes WJ. Tumors of the central nervous system. Improvement in outcome through a multimodality approach. Pediatr Clin North Am 1991;38:381.

193. Harwood-Nash DC. Primary neoplasms of the central nervous system in children. Cancer 1991;67(suppl 4):1223.

194. Gamis AS, Nesbit ME. Neuropsychologic (cognitive) disabilities in long-term survivors of childhood cancer. Pediatrician 1991;18:11.

195. Eilber R, Huth J, Mina J. Progress in the recognition and treatment of soft tissue sarcomas. Cancer 1990;65:660.

196. Quill G, Gitelis S, Morton T. Complications associated with limb salvage for extremity sarcomas and their management. Clin Orthop Rel Res 1990;260:242.

197. Sondak V, Economow J, Eilber F. Soft tissue sarcoma of the extremity and retroperitoneum: Advances in management. Adv Surg 1991;24:333.

198. Meyer W, Malawer M. Osteosarcoma. Ped Clin North Am 1991;38:317.

199. Lampert M, Gahagen C. Rehabilitation of the sarcoma patient. In: McGarvey CL, ed. Physical therapy for the cancer patient. New York: Churchill-Livingstone, 1990:123.

200. Horowitz M. Ewing's sarcoma: Current status of diagnosis and treatment. Oncology 1989;3:101.

201. Delephine N, Delephine G, Desbois J. Present trends in the treatment of Ewing's sarcoma. Biomed Pharmacother 1990;44:249.

202. Kraybill W, Emani B, Lyss A. Management of soft tissue sarcomas of the extremities. 1991;109:333.

203. Eilber F, Eckhardt J, Morton D. Advances in the treatment of sarcomas of the extremity: Current status of limb salvage. 1984;54:2695.

204. Yang JC, Rosenberg SA. Surgery for patients with soft tissue sarcomas. Semin Oncol 1989;16(4):289–296.

205. Elias AE. Advances in the diagnosis and management of sarcomas. 1990;2:474.

206. Finn HA, Simon MA. Limb salvage surgery in the treatment of osteosarcoma in skeletally immature individuals. 1991;262:108.

207. Lower limb prosthetics. New York: New York University Medical Center, 1987.

208. Nowroozi F, Salvanelli M, Gerber L. Energy expenditure in hip disarticulation and hemipelvectomy amputees. Arch Phys Med Rehabil 1983;64:300.

209. Griffith E. Rehabilitation of children with bone and soft tissue sarcomas: A physiatrist's viewpoint. NCI Monogr 1981;56:137.

210. Sugarbaker P, Nicholson T. Atlas of extremity sarcoma surgery. Philadelphia: JB Lipincott, 1984.

211. Harris I, Leff A, Gitelis S. Function after amputation, arthrodesis or arthroplasty for tumors about the knee. 1990;72A:1477.

212. Rao B, Champion J, Gore D. Limb salvage procedures for children with osteosarcoma: An alternative to amputation. 1983;18:901.

213. Murray M, Jacobs P, Gore D. Functional performance after tibial rotationplasty. 1985;67A:392.

214. Ward B, McGarvey C, M. L. Excellent shoulder function is obtainable after partial or total scapulectomy. Arch Surg 1990;125:537.

215. Pfalzer C. Aerobic exercise for patients with disseminated cancer. Clin Management 1988;8:28.

216. Shiu M, Hadju S. Management of soft tissue sarcoma of the extremity. Semin Oncol 1981;8:172.

217. Shank B, Sher H. Controversies of treatment of small cell carcinoma of the lung. Cancer Invest 1985;3:367.

218. Magilligan DJ. Surgical approach to lung cancer with solitary cerebral metastasis: Twenty five years' experience. Ann Thorac Surg 1986;42:360.

219. Warren J. Preoperative irradiation of cancer of the lung: Final report of a therapeutic trial: A collaborative study. Cancer 1975;36:914.

220. Perez CA, Stanley K, Grundy G, et al. Impact of irradiation technique and tumor extent in tumor control and survival of patients with un resectable oal cell carcinoma of the lung. Report by the Radiation Therapy Oncology Group. Cancer 1982;50:1091.

221. Shea B, Vlad G. Rehabilitation of the lung cancer patient. In: McGarvey CL, ed. Clinics in physical therapy: Physical therapy for the cancer patient. New York: Churchill-Livingstone, 1990:29.

222. Robinson J, Nesbit ME. Treatment of acute leukemia in childhood. In: Wierner PH, ed. Contemporary issues in clinical oncology: Leukemia and lymphomas. New York: Churchill-Livingstone, 1985:1.

223. Marmont AM. Allogenic bone marrow transplantation for chronic granulocytic leukemia: Progress and controversies. Acta Haematol (Basel) 1987;78(suppl 1):181.

224. Holtzman L, Chesney K. Rehabilitation of the leukemia/lymphoma patient. New York: Churchill-Livingstone, 1990:85.

225. Hicks JE. Exercise for cancer patients. In: Basmajian JV, Wolf S, eds. Therapeutic exercise. Baltimore: Williams & Wilkins, 1990:351.

226. Fisher RI. Hodgkins disease. New York: JB Lippincott, 1991:268.

227. Proswitz LR, Lawson JP, Firedlander GE, et al. Avascular necrosis of bone in Hodgkin's disease patients treated with combined modality therapy. Cancer 1981;47:2793.

228. Fisher RI. Non-Hodgkin's lymphoma. New York: JB Lippincott, 1991.

Cancer: Principles & Practice of Oncology, Fourth Edition,
edited by Vincent T. DeVita, Jr., Samuel Hellman, Steven A. Rosenberg.
J.B. Lippincott Co., Philadelphia © 1993.

Ellen J. Gallina

CHAPTER **67**

Practical Guide to Chemotherapy Administration for Physicians and Oncology Nurses

Chemotherapy administration in an office, hospital, or home should be performed only by specially trained personnel. Physicians and oncology nurses must be knowledgeable about cytotoxic agents, proficient in drug administration, skilled in venipuncture, and familiar with recommendations for safe handling and disposal of chemotherapeutic agents to provide safe treatment, protect themselves, and conserve the environment.

Although certain aspects of all drug administration, such as verification of correct drug, dose, and route of administration, are similar, chemotherapeutic agents differ because their lethal potential is greater if errors in dosing or administration occur. It is essential to patient safety that the persons preparing and administering these drugs have in-depth knowledge about each cytotoxic agent, its classification, mechanism of action, routes of administration, coinciding normal dosage ranges, common side effects and toxicities, special precautions, and management of symptoms.[3-6,8-10,17,24]

Before initiating treatment, a baseline assessment of the patient, including current height and weight, should be obtained and recorded. Throughout the course of treatment, monitoring for toxicity and adverse side effects should continue.[1,4,5,15]

This data provides the basis for decisions about the current treatment. The importance of asking the patient specific questions cannot be overemphasized. Patients often respond by saying that things are "okay," but when queried about specific points, they provide details that may alter the treatment plan. For instance, a patient being treated with vincristine may not advise the clinician about having difficulty buttoning shirts or opening pill containers, because the patient may be unaware of the association between the symptom and the drug.

At the beginning of each cycle of therapy, weight should be rechecked. For patients who have excess weight from ascites, edema, or overeating, consideration should be given to adjusting dosing for "ideal" body weight. Patients should be weighed without prostheses.

Chemotherapy is generally ordered in units of mg/m². Because errors in calculating body surface areas (BSA) can easily occur, it is prudent to recalculate the BSA and dosage before preparing the drug.[5,20] Doses should be compared against standard practice or against a protocol, if appropriate, and with dispensed drug before actual drug administration. Accuracy in dosing is crucial to patient safety.

Pertinent laboratory data and clinical assessment should be monitored before each treatment. Education of the patient and family regarding the treatment regimen, side effects of each agent, and how to manage them and a discussion about the risks associated with treatment must be initiated before the first treatment and reviewed periodically. Patients must understand what measures they can take to alleviate symptoms and which symptoms and problems require prompt reporting. Instructions should include appropriate phone numbers to call.[1,8-11,15,20] The information should be given verbally and in writing for later reference. Having information in writing allows the patient to refresh his or her memory and provide a family member with pertinent information. Educational information designed for patients about chemotherapy in general, specific drugs, clinical trials, and eating hints are available through the National Cancer Institute (NCI) and other agencies. Many institutions have preprinted materials for patient education that can be purchased.

DRUG ADMINISTRATION

After reverifying the drug, dose, and route of administration and checking the labels on the dispensed drug, confirm the patient's identification. This is particularly important in busy outpatient settings where patients do not wear identification bands. Verify before treatment that informed consent has been obtained from patients participating in clinical trials. Additional questions about the protocol and research trial should be addressed at this time.

When you choose an intravenous site for drug administration, begin by carefully inspecting both arms for the best vein.[1,4,5,9,20] Choose a distal site first, feeling and palpating for soft, pliable veins, large enough to handle the needle. Avoid veins that are hard, sclerosed, or fragile. Using arms with compromised or impaired circulation, such those on the side of a mastectomy, lymph node dissection, invading neoplasm, or with active phlebitis or extravasation, is not recommended. Upper extremities should not be used in patients with superior vena cava syndrome. Lower extremities should be generally avoided and never be used to administer vesicant agents. (Specific information regarding vesicant administration is discussed later in the chapter.) The distal veins of the hand and arms should be used first. Avoid areas over wrists and antecubital fossae if possible. Measures such as using warm packs or holding the patient's arm under warm water may assist in obtaining access.

In choosing a catheter for venipuncture, clinicians should use the one with which they are most comfortable. Needle gauge and size are determined by the size of the vein, the chemotherapy, and the fluid needed for drug administration.[5,6,17,20] Choose the smallest-gauge needle to meet these criteria. For patients with difficult access, seek assistance of a colleague if more than two venipunctures are attempted.

If access continues to be problematic, alternate means of vascular access should be discussed with the patient. The clinician should consider several questions when recommending alternate access devices for the patient. Will more than one intravenous line frequently be needed for blood, blood products, and therapy? Will continuous infusions of vesicants be part of the long-term treatment plan? In these situations, external Silastic catheters are more appropriate for patient care and safety. If an implantable venous port is planned, placement should be on the side of the nondominant arm whenever possible. This decreases the chances of needle dislodgement or coring of the port septum during continuous infusions resulting from increased movement of the dominant arm.

After a suitable line is placed, it should be secured, allowing visualization of the insertion site, particularly if irritants or vesicants are to be administered. Never use the chemotherapeutic agent to test the line. Venous integrity can be assessed using a running line of normal saline or dextrose and water. Observe the site for swelling or pain. Assess blood return by gently drawing back with a syringe, being careful not to exert undue pressure, particularly if vesicants are to be administered. Gently palpate the tip of the needle as fluid runs through for a "buzz" or "bruit" sensation. Observe the flow rate of the intravenous fluid. Consideration should be given to securing the venous line with an arm board if increased mobility could disrupt the line integrity. These steps to monitor venous patency should be taken throughout the treatment.

The control of chemotherapy-induced nausea and vomiting is integral to quality patient care, fostering patient compliance, and maximizing quality of life.[1-10] Antiemetics should be administered before chemotherapy and prophylactically at predetermined intervals based on the emetogenic characteristics of the drugs, the patients's age and gender, and the patients's response to prior antiemetics. In the outpatient setting, caution should be used with agents that have a sedative effect especially if patients are traveling alone or driving.

Chemotherapy should be administered sequentially, as ordered, especially if the patient is being treated on a clinical trial. If multiple drugs are being administered, flush the line with 5 to 10 ml of a compatible solution between agents and again at the end of the infusion to prevent the drug from leaking as the line is discontinued.

Monitor the patient throughout treatment for adverse or allergic reactions. Be prepared to intervene promptly. For patients who are at increased risk for sensitivity or anaphylactic reactions to chemotherapy, attempts to block the histamine receptors before retreatment have been successful in some circumstances. One regimen used at Memorial Sloan-Kettering Cancer Center includes diphenhydramine (50 mg every 6 hours), around-the-clock (ATC) with cimetidine (300 mg every 6 hours), ATC or ranitidine (150 mg every 6 hours), and ATC beginning the evening before chemotherapy. Dexamethasone (20 mg) is administered intravenously immediately before initiating the therapy.

For patients on continuous infusions of chemotherapy, inspection and assessment of the intravenous site for signs and symptoms of infiltration should be performed every 4 hours. Patients should be advised of the signs and symptoms to report. Care should be taken to ensure compatibility of chemotherapy with maintenance intravenous fluids, additives, and antiemetics to prevent precipitation or other adverse drug interactions. Flush the line before and after any drug of unknown compatibility is administered. If compatibility of a concomitant infusion cannot be ascertained, use separate intravenous lines. Instruct all staff involved in caring for these patients to follow these principles. Continuous infusions of chemotherapy should be placed on a rate controller device to avoid inadvertent bolus of the drug and to maintain consistent blood levels.

Administration of chemotherapy through central access lines has become increasingly common, particularly in patients with difficult venous access and those who require intensive or long-term therapy. Verify the location of the catheter tip before the line is used. If treatment may be given in a variety of settings or by various persons, a standardized policy outlining specific procedures should be in place to verify the purpose, location, and patency of the device. Implantable ports used for purposes other than venous access may be surgically placed in locations on the body where venous ports are usually placed. Ports used for epidural drug administration may be found in the upper chest area; venous ports may be placed below the nipple line, where a peritoneal port or a hepatic artery port may be located. Even the most experienced clinician would have difficulty making a determination based on physical assessment in these cases. Making an assumption about the purpose of these devices is risky.

As alternate uses for implantable ports increase, it becomes the challenge and the responsibility of the care givers to maintain detailed records of placement, removal, type, and anatomic locations of these devices.[14] Although the burden of this should not be on the patient, educating the patient about the specific purpose of the port can help to decrease problems. Advising patients to alert or remind health care personnel about the device in place and what it is or is not to be used for can help, especially if the patient may require care outside of the usual setting. Written documentation about the device, carried by the patient, minimizes the risk of inappropriate port use. Telling a patient that the port is for "chemotherapy" is inadequate and could lead to delivery of medications or intravenous fluids into an inappropriate region such as the peritoneal cavity or epidural space. This clearly opens a new area in risk management.

Before administering therapy through an intravenous implantable port, assess catheter integrity for presence of blood return and for signs and symptoms of infection, prior infiltration, or port erosion through the skin.[13,14] Use only a noncoring, nonsiliconized needle long enough to pass through the skin and touch the back of the port without being easily dislodged. Ports located deeply in tissue or ones placed in overweight patients require the longest needles. Needle gauge depends on type and volume of the fluid and drug to be administered. Larger-gauge needles are better suited for administration of high volumes of fluids and blood products, and smaller-gauge needles are better for continuous infusions.

Access the port after it is cleansed with a bactericidal agent. Spread the skin taut over the port using the thumb and forefinger to anchor it while the already fluid-primed needle is inserted with the other hand at a 90° angle directly into the center of the port. The back of the port can be felt by gently pressing on the needle at the bend of the angle or at the hub if a straight noncoring needle is used. Patients can be taught easily to reconfirm needle placement using this technique. The angled needle can be supported with a 2-in × 2-in gauze before covering it with a clear occlusive dressing. For patients who experience pain during port access, the skin over the port can be numbed with an ice pack before needle insertion. It is not uncommon for a patient to be admitted to have a port placed and to have treatment initiated immediately after. Ask the surgical team to access the device and leave the noncoring needle in place at the completion of the surgical procedure. The postoperative pain and swelling over the port insertion site are severe enough in many cases that accessing the port after the patient has returned from surgery becomes impossible. Postoperative swelling makes it more difficult to ascertain if fluid is infiltrating around the needle exit site.

Venous access ports may not have a blood return after just a few uses. This can result from a positional line, a fibrin sheath at the end of the catheter, an intraluminal clot, or venous thrombosis.[2,5] Assessment is necessary to ascertain the cause of any lack of blood return. Verify that the needle is in the port septum by pressing on the needle until it comes in contact with the base of the port. Attempt to withdraw

blood again. If there is still no blood return, reaccess the port, making sure that the needle is directly in the center of the septum, and retest for blood return. Sometimes this simple measure corrects the problem. In other cases, the catheter tip may have temporarily adhered to the vein wall resulting in lack of blood return. Use a 3- to 5-ml syringe to flush, and gently pull back on the line. Have the patient change position from side to side, raise hands above his or her head, sit forward and cough, or bear down with a Valsalva maneuver while opening his or her mouth. Attempt to withdraw blood again.

If none of these measures is effective, a fibrin sheath may cover the tip of the catheter. Initiate an infusion of normal saline or 5% dextrose and water, and run the line wide open. Observe the intravenous flow rate. Inspect the port site for symmetry and signs of swelling or leakage around the needle entry site. Have the patient slowly turn his or her head from side to side, and observe for changes in the fluid flow. If none of these symptoms exist, it is probably safe to use the port without a blood return. However, if swelling occurs or if the intravenous flow rate changes as the patient changes position, the catheter may be kinked or partially occluded. Reconfirmation of the location and of overall catheter integrity using a contrast agent is recommended before proceeding with chemotherapy, especially if vesicants are to be administered. Communicate the specific problem to the radiology department or service personnel so that they may thoroughly evaluate the problem. The catheter may be kinking when the patient turns his or her head, causing back pressure in the line. The radiologic examination should include such an assessment.

After line placement and catheter integrity are radiologically confirmed, consider using an antiembolic agent, such as urokinase, to attempt to dissolve an intraluminal clot. Catheter occlusion may also be the result of venous thrombosis. Clinicians should be mindful of the signs and symptoms associated with thrombosis when assessing for these complications.

REGIONAL DRUG ADMINISTRATION

Chemotherapy can be administered directly into a particular cavity or region. These regions may have temporary or semipermanent lines in place through which drugs are delivered. The physician or oncology nurse must understand the general principles of chemotherapy and its administration and the unique aspects of regional therapy.

Therapy can be delivered into the peritoneal cavity by a percutaneous catheter or an implantable port. Before initiating treatment, fluid distribution within the cavity is assessed radiologically using contrast material. This provides information about cavity perfusion and patient tolerance to the amount of fluid administered during the flow study, which can be useful in predicting treatment problems.

Further assessment of the patient includes inspection of the abdominal area for symmetry, infection, and existing ascites. Ascites may need to be drained before treatment for comfort and to allow adequate drug distribution. Access the catheter to assess patency and to determine if drainage is possible. These catheters frequently have a one-way valve effect that interferes with fluid drainage. Drug delivery fluid volume may need to be altered or therapy may need to be postponed until the peritoneal cavity can be drained. Perform these assessments before drug preparation to avoid drug waste and increased cost.[2,18]

Patients should have information about the rationale for intraperitoneal therapy and about the specific agents so that they may fully participate in the treatment and report problems promptly.[17] Therapy should begin after the patient has emptied his or her bladder to facilitate comfort. Although the goal is to deliver the treatment in approximately 20 minutes, factors such as pain, bloating, increased pressure on the diaphragm, and restricted fluid flow frequently alter delivery time. Narcotic analgesia may be required during treatment particularly with vesicant drugs. Close supervision of the patient and needle entry site is necessary to avoid extravasation of a vesicant. Patients should remain in bed, with the head of the bed slightly elevated for comfort. After the treatment, instruct the patient to change position (*e.g.*, side to side, flat and upright) to enhance fluid distribution throughout the peritoneal cavity. Because approximately 1 L of fluid is absorbed in 24 hours, patients should understand that some of the uncomfortable side effects, like bloating, will decrease over 24 hours but not subside until after the last dose of the cycle. Some patients find it painful to have their ports accessed; using ice to chill the skin covering the port sometimes decreases the discomfort associated with needle insertion. For patients receiving treatment every 12 hours, consider leaving the noncoring needle in place. Flush the catheter with normal saline, and cover the site with a dry sterile dressing. Reconfirm needle placement in the septum before initiating each treatment.

Implantable pumps and ports can be placed into the hepatic artery. Implantable pumps deliver drugs as a continuous infusion over a maximum of 14 days, followed by a 2-week rest period.[2,17,19] The pump is emptied of remaining drugs and refilled with 10,000 U of heparin and enough saline to make a 50-ml solution. Fifty milliliters of 50% glycerol may be used in the main chamber to maintain pump function after treatment. The glycerol lasts 5 to 6 weeks. Boluses of a drug may be delivered through the side port of the pump. Depending on the patient's anatomy, there may be one or two side ports.

For patients with two side ports, the total dose of the drug is divided and delivered into each port. As with other implanted devices, an initial flow study using radiopaque dye is performed to assess the degree of perfusion. The study is repeated periodically for therapeutic assessment and to evaluate mechanical problems. Experience and technical expertise are particularly important because the septa of the pump and side ports are smaller than other venous access devices. Familiarity with normal pressure and resistance when using this device is essential for early identification of problems and intervention. Assess pump and catheter integrity promptly whenever a question arises. Assessment, recording, and monitoring of the amount of residual fluid remaining in the pump is important to determine pump functioning and therapeutic management.

Education is integral for this population of patients. Patients should not fly in airplanes or have significant changes in altitude without notifying their physician or oncology nurse. Changes in altitude can alter the pump's rate of flow, as can changes in body temperature from fever or hot baths, possibly increasing the toxicity from accelerated drug infusion. Premature emptying of the pump could result in the pump's clotting off. Patient education literature about the pump is available from the manufacturer of the device.

The drugs most frequently administered through the pump are FUDR with or without leucovorin and Decadron. Mitomycin or BCNU are most frequently administered through the side ports. Drug infusion through the side port requires a pump to deliver the drug against the arterial pressure.

Implantable access devices placed into the hepatic artery are used in patients who are not candidates for the implantable pump but who would benefit from drug delivery directly into the region. Assessment of catheter integrity, tip location, and degrees of pressure and resistance when the line is flushed are essential for ports placed in the hepatic artery. The port is accessed as is any other vascular access device; however, do not attempt to aspirate for blood return to minimize the risk of clotting. The line is flushed with normal saline after the port is accessed with a fluid-primed noncoring, nonsiliconized needle to evaluate patency. In some patients, a pulsing of the saline in the line can be observed. The catheter patency is maintained on a weekly basis and after discontinuance of treatment with 300 to 1000 U of heparin, depending on physician preference.

Patients must be instructed to keep the area around the catheter clean, because the port is often located in the upper pubic region. Frequent inspection for signs and symptoms of infections must be emphasized in practice and in patient education. Bolus therapy or continuous infusions are administered through the port. Carefully selected patients can manage effectively at home with an ambulatory infusion pump connected to the port. Flushing the port at home by the patient or family member is frequently taught.

Chemotherapy can be administered intrapleurally though chest tubes immediately postoperatively for therapeutic management or after chest tube placement for the management of pleural effusions. Experience in determining air leaks and the side effects of agents is essential. Patients require narcotic analgesics when drugs such as mitomycin are infused, despite incomplete recovery from anesthesia. Resealable chest tubing is required to prevent leakage of the chemotherapy from the tubing and prevent exposure to these agents by the staff caring for the patient. Chest drainage is treated as chemotherapy waste.

Drug administration though the Ommaya reservoir requires extreme caution, meticulous technique, and verification of the drug dose, volume, and route of administration.[6] Drug errors can be fatal in this situation.

CUTANEOUS REACTIONS ASSOCIATED WITH CHEMOTHERAPY ADMINISTRATION

Chemotherapy agents are described as irritants, nonirritants, and vesicants. Irritants are capable of producing venous pain at the injection site or along the vein, with or without an inflammatory reaction.[12,20] The symptoms do not usually last for long periods and present themselves as complaints of local discomfort and burning. The symptoms can be reduced by decreasing the flow rate of the chemotherapy and increasing the simultaneous intravenous hydration. Other measures to minimize the venous discomfort include applying ice to numb the area or heat, which is thought to dilate the veins and decrease discomfort.[1] The application of topical hydrocortisone cream (1%) has been effective in some patients. Drugs more commonly associated with irritation include dacarbazine, carmustine, and plicamycin. Doxorubicin, a potent vesicant, can be irritating without causing underlying tissue damage. The clinician must respond promptly to any patient complaint of pain or burning. Differentiating the irritating effects of these agents from the signs and symptoms of extravasation is crucial and a challenge even for the most experienced clinician. Continuous monitoring of venous patency throughout treatment with attention to any changes is essential for determining the situation. If either problem occurs, promptly stop administration of the drug and allow the maintenance intravenous line to flow freely. Patients usually feel relief from the irritant effects within 10 to 15 minutes. If there are no signs of infiltration of the drug and the discomfort has been altered by stopping the drug, slowly restart it. The rate of the drug should be adjusted in accordance with the patient's tolerance.

VESICANT DRUG ADMINISTRATION

A vesicant is an agent capable of producing severe tissue damage and necrosis if the drug is extravasated into the surrounding tissue.[12] Drugs capable of causing extravasation include dactinomycin, daunorubicin, doxorubicin, idarubicin, mitomycin, mechlorethamine, vinblastine, and vincristine.

The best management of a vesicant extravasation continues to be prevention. It cannot be emphasized enough that the person administering a vesicant must be highly skilled in techniques of intravenous line placement and well versed in the risks, signs, symptoms, and interventions of extravasation. He or she must be sensitive to subtle changes in venous patency during drug delivery and attentive to all patient complaints and comments during treatment.

Good lighting, a relaxed approach, and application of heat to the arm facilitate selection of a site for vesicant administration. The clinician must critically assess the veins of both upper extremities, with attention to overall venous integrity, visibility, evidence of compromised circulation, location, and time of previous venipunctures above the site of potential access. Veins above a recent site of access or attempted access should not be used for 24 or more hours. Veins chosen should be resilient and large; however, smaller veins may be used if the needle can be easily threaded. Veins over joints, wrists, and the antecubital area should be avoided. Lower extremities should never be used for vesicants, because extravasation in these areas can result in greater injury and have a more negative effect on quality of life. The forearm often offers the best choices of veins because there is more soft tissue and fewer nerves and tendons. Distal veins of the forearm should be chosen first. The overall guiding principle should be to choose a vein that, if the drug did infiltrate, would have the least debilitating effects on the extremity.

It is recommended that the physician or oncology nurse responsible for the vesicant administration should be the person to place the line. This allows the care giver to understand the type of vein being used and the amount of trauma associated with needle insertion. Clinicians must be willing to recommend a short delay in treatment if choices of access are impaired by recent venipunctures or if access is poor enough to recommend an alternate means of access. In the hospital setting, it is a good idea to coordinate routine blood sampling with the phlebotomy team to avoid delays in treatment resulting from limited venous choice because of phlebotomy in the antecubital area.

For patients receiving mechlorethamine, which can cause immediate vomiting, or for those who may have difficulty keeping the extremity still, an arm board or some other method of gentle restraint should be used to minimize the risk of needle dislodgement and infiltration from the sudden movement. Patients are usually amenable to this precaution if they comprehend the risks associated with the administration of vesicants.

After suitable access is obtained using a needle or catheter, the line should be gently secured with tape, leaving the insertion site exposed. Using the degree of ease of needle or catheter insertion as a baseline, the physician or oncology nurse can begin to monitor the site for any signs or symptoms of impaired venous integrity by running a maintenance intravenous line with normal saline. Initial baseline assessment also includes evaluation for swelling or inflammation around the insertion site, changes in rate of flow of the maintenance intravenous solution, a blood return, a "buzz" or "bruit" when the needle or catheter tip is gently palpated with the forefinger, and complaints of pain or burning by the patient.

These criteria must be continuously assessed throughout treatment. Before injecting the vesicant, gently flush the line using a syringe with 5 to 10 ml of saline. Never test venous integrity with the vesicant. Inject the vesicant at a rate of 1 to 2 ml at a time, pausing to allow additional maintenance fluid to infuse. Continue to recheck patency and to ask the patient for feedback.

Respond to complaints promptly by stopping the drug immediately and assessing the situation to determine if this is an extravasation, an irritation, or an flare reaction, which is described later. There may not be a disruption in blood return if there is a tiny leak or if an underlying part of the vein was punctured. Apply a tourniquet above the intravenous site; if the vein is intact, the intravenous flow rate should slow down. If there is any doubt, discontinue the infusion and administer the therapy in an alternate site. With vesicants, it is better to err on the side of safety. After vesicant administration, allow additional maintenance intravenous fluid to infuse. The severity of the extravasation depends on the drug, its concentration, and the amount of drug infiltrated, and the use of additional intravenous fluid further dilutes the drug.

Continuous infusions of vesicants used in the treatment of leukemias, lymphomas, and sarcomas present additional challenges. Vesicants prescribed for this route of administration should only be initiated though a central venous line resting in the superior vena cava. The intensive monitoring required for these infusions precludes peripheral administration. Extreme caution must be exercised with these infusions because of the risk of vesicant infiltration into the chest or neck area. Before initiating therapy, catheter tip location and catheter integrity must be confirmed. Questionable lines should be verified radiologically using contrast medium. Standardized orders for monitoring infusions and specific interventions for suspected infiltrations should be initiated at the time of therapy and reviewed with the personnel who will be caring for the patient (Fig. 67–1). This is particularly important if the drug is being infused through an implanted venous port. Needle dislodgement can occur at any time but especially when the patient is asleep or sedated. Because of this increased risk, the use of venous access ports for home infusions of vesicants is strongly discouraged.

In rare instances, such as the patient with superior vena cava syndrome, a catheter may be placed in the inferior vena cava for the delivery of a vesicant. To minimize the risk of extravasation and avert the significant damage resulting from such an extravasation, the line should be placed immediately before the initiation of therapy. The patient must remain on bed rest. Interventions to reduce chances of catheter kinking or breakage from increased flexion of the leg must be taken. The patient needs to understand thoroughly the risks associated with the use of ports and inferior vena cava catheters for this drug therapy. Documentation of the patient's consent and understanding should be placed in the medical record.

EXTRAVASATIONS

The management of extravasations resulting from chemotherapy continues to be controversial. Studies in humans are limited because of incidence and ethical issues. Many studies in animals have been inconclusive.[12,17,20]

Despite the best efforts, extravasations do occur and can present in a delayed fashion, because they are undetected at the time of drug administration. After extravasation is suspected, prompt intervention is essential. Stop the drug immediately. Attempt to withdraw any remaining drug from the line. Administer an antidote in accordance with institutional guidelines and policies through the infiltrated line or subcutaneously around the site of infiltration. Apply heat or cold as indicated.[12] Table 67–1 lists antidotes recommended by the Oncology Nursing Society. In many institutions, a plastic surgery consultation is immediately initiated, especially if the clinician is sure that the drug did infiltrate.

A standardized plan for systematic follow-up of the patient should be in place and initiated with each suspected or actual extravasation. It should include the following data: patient demographics, name of the vesicant infiltrated, dose, amount suspected to have infiltrated, specific location of infiltration, presenting signs and symptoms (*e.g.*, redness, swelling, pain, blisters, necrosis), and range of motion at time of presentation. Management of extravasation, interventions, and plans for follow-up must be included. Patients should receive written information about the home care of the infiltration and be advised of the appropriate persons to contact with questions or problems. Because a delay in intervention can adversely affect the outcome and because patients can be reluctant to call if they are uncertain if it is appropriate, the care giver should follow-up at specified intervals by phone or office visit (Fig. 67–2). For monitoring purposes, baseline and periodic photographs are recommended. These serve as a visual record of the efficacy of treatments and interventions and as an educational tool for colleagues.

FLARE REACTION

A flare reaction can occur with the administration of anthracyclines, particularly doxorubicin. This reaction occurs within minutes of initiating treatment and is evidenced by erythematous streaking around the injection site and along the vein. Pruritus, urticaria, and patchy erythema may be present. Pain and burning at the site occur infrequently and aid in differentiating a flare reaction from an infiltration. The reaction is transient, often subsiding within 30 to 45 minutes of onset. It may recur with future doses of doxorubicin.

Prompt intervention is essential to determine whether the reaction is a flare phenomenon or an infiltration. Stop the drug immediately and allow the intravenous solution to infuse freely. Reassess catheter patency and assess for signs and symptoms of extravasation. After extravasation has been ruled out, hydrocortisone cream (1%) may be applied to the areas of inflammation. Restart the drug administration at a slower rate. These measures may alleviate the symptoms.

The occurrence of a flare reaction does not preclude future

(*text continues on page* 2579)

PHYSICIAN'S ORDERS

Chemotherapy: Continuous Infusion of a Vesicant

DATE AND TIME OF ORDER: _____

START DATE: _____ STOP DATE: _____

_____ is receiving a continuous infusion of a
   (patient name)

vesicant, _____ for _____ days.
     (name of drug(s))

1. Infuse chemotherapy via **CENTRAL ACCESS ONLY**. Do not administer the vesicant peripherally.
2. Check the catheter insertion site and needle entry site every 2 hours for signs and symptoms of infiltration.

   If there are signs of redness, swelling or leakage at the needle or catheter insertion site OR if there is any question regarding the integrity of the infusion, take the following steps:

   A. STOP the chemotherapy infusion **IMMEDIATELY.**

   B. STOP other fluids infusing through the line.

   C. Flush the line with normal saline and the appropriate amount of heparin, specific to the device.

   D. Notify the following persons **IMMEDIATELY:**

     Attending Physician: _____ M.D.

     Medical Oncology Fellow: _____ M.D.

        BEEPER #: _____

     House Officer

     Plastic Surgery Service

     Chemotherapy Nursing/Pharmacy

   E. After medical consultation, discontinue all IV's infusing through the affected site.

   F. Save chemotherapy and tubing in a plastic bag for chemotherapy to pick up.

   G. Apply _____ compresses for 24 hours.

   H. Medications to be administered IN THE EVENT OF A VESICANT INFILTRATION: (VERIFY orders with attending physician/fellow prior to administration.)

   _____

   _____

Physician Name: _____ Date: _____

Physician Signature: _____ M.D.

FIGURE 67–1. Physician's orders for chemotherapy.

TABLE 67–1. Antidotes for Vesicant or Irritant Drugs

Drug Classification	Specific Agent	Local Antidote	Positive Effect		Antidote Preparation	Method of Administration	Comments
			Animal Studies	Clinical Case Reports			
Alkylating agents	Mechlorethamine (nitrogen mustard)	Isotonic sodium thiosulfate 1 g/10 ml (manufacturer's recommendations)	None	Yes[1]	Mix 4 ml of 10% Na thiosulfate with 6 ml sterile water for injection (1/6 molar solution results)	1. Inject 5–6 ml (0.2–0.24 g) I.V. through the existing line and SQ into the extravasated site with multiple injections. 2. Repeat dosing SQ over the next several hours. 3. Apply cold compresses. 4. No total dose established.	1. ACTION: chemical neutralization 2. Initiate treatment immediately and liberally.
	Mitomycin C (Mutamycin)	Topical DMSO (RIMSO)	Yes[2]	None	1–2 ml of 1 mmol DMSO 50–100%	1. Apply topically one time to the site.	1. Probably not effective for distal or delayed ulcers 2. Initiate treatment immediately. 3. ACTION: carrier solvent or oxygen radical scavenger
Plant alkaloids	Vinblastine (Velban) Vincristine (Oncovin)	Hyaluronidase (Wydase) 150 U/ml (manufacturer's recommendations)	Yes[3]	None	Add 1 ml USP sodium chloride (150 U/ml results)	1. Inject 1–6 ml (150–900 U) SQ into the extravasated site with multiple injections. 2. Repeat dosing SQ over the next several hours. 3. Apply warm compresses. 4. No total dose established.	1. ACTION: enhances absorption and dispersion of the extravasated drug 2. Corticosteroids and topical cooling appear to worsen toxicity 3. Warm compresses increase systemic absorption of the drug.
	Vindesine (Eldisine)	Hyaluromidase (Wydase)	Yes[4]	None			

Drug		Antidote	Availability	Dose	Application	Comments
Teniposide (VM-26)	150 U/ML					
Etoposide (VP-16-213 VePesid)						
Anthracycline antibiotics						
Doxorubicin (Adriamycin) Daunomycin (Cerubidine)		Topical DMSO	Yes[5-9] Yes[10-11]	1–2 ml of 1 mmol DMSO 50–100%	1. Apply topically one time to the site. 2. Apply cold compresses.	1. Probably best to initiate treatment immediately 2. ACTION: carrier solvent or oxygen free radical 3. Cold compresses block cytotoxicity of doxorubicin.
Bisanirene		Sodium bicarbonate 1 mEq/1 ml (premixed)	Yes[12] Yes[12]	Mix equal parts of 1 mEq/ml sodium bicarbonate with sterile normal saline (1:1 solution). Resulting solution is 0.5 mEq/ml	1. Inject 2–6 ml (1.0–3.0 mEq) I.V. through the existing line and SQ into the extravasated site with multiple injections. 2. Appy cold compresses. 3. Total dose not to exceed 10 ml of 0.5 mEq/ml solution (5.0 mEq).	1. ACTION: chemical activation 2. Dilute bicarbonate chemically degrades the drug.

1. Owen O, Dellatorre DL, Scott EJ, Cohen MR. Accidental intramuscular injection of mechlorethamine. Cancer 1980;45:2225–2226.
2. Dorr R, Soble MJ, Liddil JD. Keller JH. Mitomycin C skin toxicity studies in mice: Reduced ulceration and altered pharmokinetics with topical dimethyl sulfoxide. J Clin Oncol 1986;4:1399–1404.
3. Dorr RT, Alberta DS, Woods MW. Vinca alkaloid ulceration: Experimental mouse model and effects of local antidotes. Proc Am Assoc Cancer Res 1982;23:109.
4. Dorr RT, Alberts DS. Skin ulceration potential without therapeutic anticancer activity for epipodophyllotoxin commercial diluents. Invest New Drugs 1983;1:151–159.
5. Desai MH, Teres D. Prevention of doxorubicin-induced skin ulcers in the rat and pig with dimethyl sulfoxide (DMSO). Cancer Treat Rep 1982;66:1371–1374.
6. Svingen BA, Powis G, Appel PL, Scott M. Protection against Adriamycin-induced skin necrosis in the rat with dimethyl sulfoxide and alpha tocopherol. Cancer 1981;41:3395–3399.
7. Dorr RT, Alberta DS. Failure of DMSO and vitamin E to prevent doxorubicin skin ulceration in the mouse. Cancer Treat Rep 1983;67:499–501.
8. Nobbs P, Barr RD. Soft tissue injury caused by antineoplastic drugs is inhibited by topical dimethyl sulphoxide and alpha tocopherol. Br J Cancer 1983;48:873–876.
9. Soble M, Dorr R, Plezia P, Breckenridge S. Dose dependent skin ulcers in mice treated with DNA binding antitumor antibiotics. Cancer Chemother Pharmacol 1987.
10. Olver IN. Use of dimethyl sulfoxide in limiting tissue damage caused by extravasation of doxorubicin. Cancer Treat Rep 1983;67:407–408.
11. Lawrence HJ, Goodnight SH. Dimethyl sulfoxide and extravasation of anthracycline agents. [Letter] Ann Intern Med 1983;98:1025.
12. Dorr RT, Peng YM, Alberts DS. Bisantrene solubility and skin toxicity studies: Efficacy of sodium bicarbonate as a local antidote. Invest New Drug 1984;2:351–357. (With permission from the ONS Cancer Chemotherapy Guidelines—Module V. Recommendations for the management of extravasations and anaphylaxis. Oncology Nursing Society, 1988:8–9)

CHEMOTHERAPY NURSING

Extravasation Flow Sheet

Pt. Name _____   M.R. # _____

Date _____   Date Extravasation Occurred _____

Name and Volume of Drug Extravasated _____

Attending Physician _____   Physician Notified _____

Patient Telephone # _____   Preferred Calling Time _____

Appearance of Extravasation Site
Exact Location (*describe and doc. on diagram*)

_____

_____

Dimensions _____

Appearance of Skin at Site _____

_____

_____

Nursing Interventions (* *indicates requires M.D. order*)

_____ Antidote Administered* _____   _____ Hydrocortisone cream applied

_____ Cold Compresses   _____ Warm Compresses

_____ Dermatology Consult*   _____ Plastic Surgery Consult*

_____ Initiated Wound Care (*describe*) _____

_____ Patient Education Card Reviewed   _____ Plan for Follow-up Reviewed

_____ Baseline Photograph Obtained

Follow Up Flow Sheet

	Day 1	Day 3	Day 5	Day 7	Day 14	Day 21	Day 28	Day 35**	Day 42**
Pain									
Edema									
Skin Changes									
Change Mobility									
Color of area									
Fever									
Date									
R.N. Initial									
Tel. Call. Visit									

** may omit if patient without positive signs of extravasation

FIGURE 67–2. Flow sheet for managing extravasations.

treatment. The flare may recur at the next treatment, but it is usually milder than the first reaction. The literature suggests pretreatment with antihistamines or corticosteroids. Documentation of the event should be included in the medical record.

HANDLING AND DISPOSAL OF CHEMOTHERAPY

Because chemotherapy is currently administered in many settings, health care personnel and support personnel (*e.g.*, maintenance, sanitation) continue to be at increased risk of exposure to antineoplastic drugs. Many are rightfully concerned. Because the risks from prolonged exposure are unknown and no safe level of exposure has been identified, meticulous attention must be given to handling and disposal of these agents.[1,3–11,33]

The goal must be to protect health care personnel, support persons, and the environment from the potential hazards of these agents. The Office of Safety and Health Administration has issued guidelines for safe handling and disposal, which focus on minimizing exposure through absorption and inhalation.[28]

All personnel having contact with cytotoxic agents must become aware of the possible risks and how to effectively minimize them before they handle the chemotherapy drugs.[29–32] Antineoplastic drug preparation requires specific training and attention to manufacturer guidelines.[36–38]

All drugs should be prepared aseptically in a class II biologic safety cabinet, which is cleaned, serviced, and maintained at specified intervals. The environment should be clean and free of interruptions; no food, drinks, or cosmetics should be present.

Personnel preparing chemotherapy should wear disposable surgical gowns, which tie in the back and have cuffs. Unpowdered latex gloves should be worn at all times when preparing chemotherapy.[28,36,37] Gloves should be changed hourly or more frequently if needed. A thermoplastic face shield or goggles and an air purifying respirator should be worn when drugs are prepared outside of a biologic safety cabinet. Measures to avoid exposure to drug leakage or aerosolization should be taken, no matter where the drug is prepared. Care should be taken to ensure that intravenous tubing is secured in the infusion container and all lines are clamped and capped to avoid inadvertent drug spills. Drugs should be transported to the patient in a sealed, zip-closed plastic bag.

Proper administration techniques provide optimal protection from exposure. Physicians and nurses must be well versed in proper handling and disposal of chemotherapy.[30–32] Many clinicians wear lab coats as a barrier, rather than gowns, but drug can be readily absorbed into a lab coat, and it does not provide maximal protection. If the coat is to have any barrier benefit, it should be worn closed, with the sleeves down, and changed frequently.

To reduce further potential exposure, intravenous tubing should be primed in the biologic safety cabinet. If this is not feasible, the clinician can back-prime the secondary tubing that is connected to the chemotherapy by piggybacking it into the side arm of a compatible intravenous solution. This technique maintains a closed system. An alternative method is to wrap a sterile gauze around the tip of the needle and slowly prime the chemotherapy tubing into a zip-closed bag. Care must be taken to protect the sterility of the infusion line. Syringes containing chemotherapy can be primed in a similar fashion. After chemotherapy is discontinued, gauze should be held at the disconnection site to catch any droplets of the drug. All waste should be disposed of in the zip-closed bag and discarded as hazardous waste.

All chemotherapy should be disposed of in accordance with applicable state, local, and federal regulations for handling hazardous waste. Written guidelines should be placed in all areas where chemotherapy is dispensed, administered, or handled.[34,35,38]

All waste associated with chemotherapy—gloves, gowns, gauze, tubings, and syringes—should be treated as hazardous waste. Drugs containing solutions to be wasted should first be transferred to resealable containers. Needles and syringes should be disposed of intact into a leak-proof, puncture-proof container to avoid aerosolization leaks or spills. Gloves should be worn by all persons handling bodily waste of a patient who has received chemotherapy within the last 48 hours.

Patients receiving therapy at home must also be educated in proper handling and disposal of chemotherapy waste.[38] The Environmental Protection Agency has made available patient fact cards, entitled "Disposal Tips For Home Health Care," which explain how to handle needles and syringes. Patients should be urged to contact their state or community environmental programs or local sanitation departments for specific details in their areas.

In cases of accidental exposure to the drug, contaminated clothing should be removed promptly and the affected skin washed thoroughly with soap and water. If the eye is involved, immediately flood the eye for 5 minutes with water or isotonic eye wash. Prompt medical follow-up is recommended after all exposures. Document exposure of personnel according to institutional policy.[28,34–38]

A spill kit should be maintained in all dispensing and treatment areas in the event of an accidental drug spill. These kits can be purchased or assembled. They should contain two pairs of disposable gloves, disposable protective garments including shoe covers, safety goggles, respirator, absorbent plastic-backed pads, disposable towels, two resealable hazardous waste bags, a scoop for picking up glass, and a container for disposal of glass fragments.

Spills should be cleaned promptly. Traffic through the area should be restricted until clean-up is completed. Windows and doors should remain closed to minimize aerosolization. After the waste is cleaned and disposed of, the area should be washed three times with detergent and then flushed with water.

Smaller spills of less than 5 ml of unconcentrated drug should be promptly cleaned using absorbent toweling. Wash the affected area three times with soap and water. Reusable items can be washed by specially trained personnel wearing a double pair of unpowdered latex gloves.

Physicians and oncology nurses have a responsibility to protect themselves and the environment from the potential hazards of chemotherapeutic agents through safe practice techniques. An ongoing review of the current literature regarding practice issues and changes should be basic to all clinical practice settings using this treatment modality.

CONCLUSION

Successful treatment and management of chemotherapy requires in-depth knowledge and skill by the physician and oncology nurse. Clinicians must maintain competency and clinical expertise to deliver continued quality of care in a complex, changing climate.

REFERENCES

1. Perry MC. The chemotherapy source book. Baltimore: Williams & Wilkins, 1992:780–882.
2. Lokich JJ. Cancer chemotherapy by infusion. Chicago: Precept Press, 1987:3–113, 502–524.
3. Carter S, Bakowski M, Hellman K. Chemotherapy of cancer. 3rd ed. New York: Wiley Medical, 1987:325–340.
4. Baird SB, McCorkle R, Grant M. Cancer nursing. Philadelphia: WB Saunders, 1991: 291–321.
5. Otto SE. Oncology nursing. St. Louis: Mosby, 1991:253–317.
6. Chabner BA, Collins JM. Cancer chemotherapy principles and practice. Philadelphia: Lippincott, 1990:449–464.
7. Groenwald SL, Frogge MH, Goodman M, Yarbro CH. Cancer nursing principles and practice. Boston: Jones and Bartlett, 1990:230–284.
8. Cancer chemotherapy guidelines. Recommendations for cancer chemotherapy. Pittsburgh: Oncology Nursing Society, 1988.
9. Cancer chemotherapy guidelines. Recommendations for nursing practice in the acute care setting. Pittsburgh: Oncology Nursing Society, 1988.
10. Cancer chemotherapy guidelines. Recommendations for nursing practice in the outpatient setting. Pittsburgh: Oncology Nursing Society, 1988.
11. Cancer chemotherapy guidelines. Recommendations for nursing practice in the home care setting. Pittsburgh: Oncology Nursing Society, 1988.
12. Cancer chemotherapy guidelines. Recommendations for the management of extravasation and anaphylaxis. Pittsburgh: Oncology Nursing Society, 1988.
13. Access device guidelines. Recommendations for nursing education and practice. Modules 1–3. Pittsburgh: Oncology Nursing Society, 1989.
14. Wickman R. Advances in venous access devices and nursing management strategies. Nurs Clin North Am 1990;25:345–364, 1990.
15. Brown MH, Kiss ME, Outlaw E, Viamontes C. Standards for oncology nursing practice. Somerset, NJ: Wiley and Sons, 1986:59–101, 595–610.
16. Brager BL, Yasko JM. Care of the client receiving chemotherapy. Reston, VA: Reston Publishing, 1984:53–89.
17. DeVita VT, Hellman S, Rosenberg SA. Cancer: Principles and practice of oncology. 3rd ed. Philadelphia: Lippincott, 1989:2369–2402.
18. Swenson KK, Erikkson JH. Nursing management of intraperitoneal chemotherapy. Oncol Nurs Forum 1986;13:33–39.
19. Roemeling R, MacDonald M, Langevin T, et al. Chemotherapy via implanted infusion pump: New perspectives for delivery of long-term continuous treatment. Oncol Nurs Forum 1986;13:17–24.
20. Fischer DS, Tish Knobf M. The cancer chemotherapy handbook. 3rd ed. Chicago: Year Book Medical, 1989:199–233, 557–558.
21. Ziegfeld CR. Core curriculum for oncology nursing. Philadelphia: WB Saunders, 1987: 225–234.
22. Ashwanden P, Belcher A, Hubbard Mattson EA, et al. Oncology nursing advances, treatments and trends into the twenty-first century. Rockville, MD: Aspen, 1990:53–57, 303–309.
23. Lynch M, Yanes L. Flowsheet documentation of chemotherapy administration. Oncol Nurs Forum 1991;18:777–782.
24. Dorr RT, Fritz WL. Cancer chemotherapy handbook. New York: Elsevier, 1980:75–93, 101–137.
25. Alberts DS, Dorr RT. Case report: Topical DMSO for mitomycin-C-induced skin ulcerations. Oncol Nurs Forum 1991;18: 693–695.
26. Rudolf R, Larson DL. Etiology and treatment of chemotherapeutic agent injuries: A review. J Clin Oncol 1987;5:1116–1126.
27. Reed WP, Newman KA, Applefeld MM, Sutton FJ. Drug extravasation as a complication of venous access ports. Ann Intern Med 1985;102:788–790.
28. U.S. Department of Labor, Office of Occupational Medicine, Occupational Safety and Health Administration. Work practice guidelines for personnel dealing with cytotoxic (antineoplastic) drugs, No 8-1.1, Washington, DC: U.S. Government Printing Office, 1986.
29. Venitt S, Crofton-Sleigh C, Hunt J, et al. Monitoring exposure of nursing and pharmacy personnel to cytotoxic drugs: Urinary mutation assays and urinary platinum as markers of absorption. Lancet 1984;1:74–76.
30. Miller S. Issues in cytotoxic drug handling safety. Semin Oncol Nurs 1987;3:133–141.
31. Valanes M, Shortridge L. Self-protective practices of nurses handling antineoplastic drugs. Oncol Nurs Forum 1987;14:23–27.
32. Cloak M, Connor T, Stevens K, et al. Occupational exposure of nursing personnel to antineoplastic agents. Oncol Nurs Forum 1985;12:33–39.
33. Stellman JM, Zoloth R. Cancer chemotherapeutic agents as occupational hazards: A literature review. Cancer Invest 1986;4:127–135.
34. Gullo SM. Safe handling of antineoplastic drugs: Translating the recommendations into practice. Oncol Nurs Forum 1988;15:595–601.
35. Barhammand BA. Difficulties encountered in implementing guidelines for handling antineoplastics in the physician's office. Cancer Nurs 1986;9:138–143.
36. Power LA, Anderson RW, Cortopassi R, Gera JR, Lewis RM. Update on safe handling of hazardous drugs: The advice of experts. Am J Hosp Pharm 1990;47:1050–1060.
37. ASHP technical assistance bulletin on handling cytotoxic and hazardous drugs. Am J Hosp Pharm 1990;48:1033–1049.
38. Stevens KR. Safe handling of cytotoxic drugs in home chemotherapy. Semin Oncol Nurs 1989;5:15–20.

Cancer: Principles & Practice of Oncology, Fourth Edition,
edited by Vincent T. DeVita, Jr., Samuel Hellman, Steven A. Rosenberg.
J.B. Lippincott Co., Philadelphia © 1993.

CHAPTER **68**

Information Systems in Oncology

SECTION **1**   SUSAN MOLLOY HUBBARD

Information Retrieval Systems

Ready access to current information on effective and promising new investigational therapies is crucial if patients with cancer are to receive state-of-the-art treatment. This is particularly important given the explosive growth of knowledge and the pace of research advances in the field of medicine. Results of a survey of 432 primary care practitioners and 88 of their opinion leaders indicated that two of three physicians claimed that the volume of medical literature was unmanageable.[1] More than 78% reported that they had problems sorting out irrelevant material when examining the medical literature. Fifty-four percent were unaware of recently proven clinical advances regarding the use of digitalis preparations in the elderly, and knowledge deficiencies were documented for five other medical advances that were used as marker studies. Survey data indicated that these physicians felt that critical, "validated" reviews were the most useful means of meeting their information needs. Experts in continuing medical education and information science have been attempting to develop innovative systems that assist physicians to manage what promises to be an ongoing information explosion.[2-10]

Automated systems for improving access to medical knowledge and accelerating the pace of technology transfer have been developed by the National Cancer Institute (NCI). These computerized resources provide ready access to bibliographic citations of the published cancer research literature (*i.e.*, CANCERLIT database) and validated, peer-reviewed syntheses of current information on the prognosis and treatment of all major cancers (*i.e.*, PDQ database). Both of these com-

puterized information systems are designed to facilitate research and patient care by assisting health professionals to maximize use of current medical knowledge. This chapter summarizes the information systems that are currently available from the NCI, existing mechanisms for distributing these resources, enhancements that are under development, and ongoing efforts to electronically link patient records, clinical and laboratory information, and decision support to our automated information systems.

HISTORICAL PERSPECTIVE

Index Medicus, inaugurated in 1879, was the first systematic classification of the medical literature. The first year's volume contained 17,000 citations from 700 periodicals. In 1992, a single month of *Index Medicus* averaged more than 31,000 citations and annual coverage exceeded 373,000 articles.[11,12] The rapid growth of the medical literature manual preparation of *Index Medicus* a logistic nightmare by the early 1950s, prompting the staff of the National Library of Medicine (NLM) to develop a computer-based medical literature analysis and retrieval system (MEDLARS). MEDLARS automated the process of organizing, indexing, publishing, and searching *Index Medicus.* This pioneering use of early computing technology led to the introduction of MEDLINE in 1971, an online version of the *Cumulated Index Medicus.* Rapid acceptance of MEDLINE by the medical and scientific community stimulated the growth of nationwide access systems by commercial telecommunication networks and the development of a variety of additional scientific and medical databases for distribution over the MEDLARS system. By the end of 1991, MEDLINE alone contained over 7 million medical references.

In 1971, the National Cancer Act mandated the creation of an international databank to foster rapid and effective exchange of cancer data throughout the world.[13] Faced with responsibility for organizing, updating, and disseminating a rapidly growing collection of knowledge, staff at the NCI decided to establish a computerized information program to complement its peer-reviewed scientific journals. NCI staff immediately began to develop cancer databases for distribution on MEDLARS and a series of database-derived publications designed to meet the information needs of those who without access to on-line systems.[14]

The first on-line information system to be made available was a bibliographic database called CANCERLIT, created in 1974.[5,6] Each literature citation was formatted in a unit record structure similar to the records in MEDLINE to enable NCI to distribute CANCERLIT on the NLM's computer system. Because NCI staff anticipated that users would want access to summary data from each article, abstracts were created and included in each citation. CANCERLIT is a comprehensive resource of the published cancer literature containing over 900,000 citations screened, indexed, abstracted, and keyed from over 3000 biomedical journals, books, monographs, government-sponsored reports, and proceedings.

Other than presenting abstracts of ongoing research from conference proceedings, the CANCERLIT database does not provide information on clinical research in progress. To fill this need, in 1974, NCI staff developed CLINPROT, a computerized database that summarized the investigational treatment protocols sponsored by the Institute. Each protocol record was created using the full clinical research protocol as the source document and indexed with special terms that allowed users to retrieve protocols by tumor type and treatment. As with CANCERLIT, each unit record was formatted to allow distribution and on-line searching on the NLM computer system. However, the CLINPROT database did not provide information on state-of-the-art treatment. Moreover, summaries were not indexed by stage, histologic type, participating investigators, or institutions. This made it difficult for physicians to identify clinical trials appropriate for cancer patients that were being conducted in a particular location. CLINPROT did not lend itself to use in clinical care or decision making, but it instead served as an on-line catalog of clinical research that provided physicians designing treatment protocols with information on research performed by others. Moreover, as with all MEDLARS databases, effective information retrieval required knowledge of the NLM's specialized searching language. A trained search intermediary, usually a medical librarian, was required to search the cancer databases effectively.

The growing power of personal computers in the 1980s and the introduction of powerful operating systems permitted greater speed and flexibility in telecommunications among computers and an enormous increase in the capacity to store and manipulate large quantities of data. New software technologies quickly emerged to support the development and distribution of large factual databases. Recognizing the power of this computer technology, the director of the NCI conceived PDQ, an on-line database containing up-to-date information on state-of-the-art cancer treatment to speed the diffusion of information about advances in cancer treatment and to facil-

itate the integration of new medical knowledge and research advances into clinical practice.[15]

THE PDQ SYSTEM

The PDQ information system is a computerized resource that provides three general types of information: up-to-date guidelines cancer treatment that are synthesized, peer reviewed, and continually updated by cancer experts; summaries of clinical trials that are open to patient accrual; and a directory of physicians and organizations that provide cancer care. The information in PDQ enables users to identify the full range of treatment alternatives that are state-of-the-art therapy for all major cancers; locate clinical trials for patients who are candidates for treatment research; and identify physicians and treatment facilities for consultation and referral. The PDQ information retrieval system that is distributed on NLM's MEDLARS system is designed with a user-friendly, menu-driven interface that internally links diverse types of information and allows users to search and display information without learning a specialized search language (Fig. 68–1).[16]

PDQ's cancer information file contains treatment recommendations that summarize current state-of-the-art therapy for all major cancers. Treatment information is presented in two formats: a peer-reviewed file of "state-of-the-art statements" that are written to meet the information needs of clinicians and a corresponding file of overviews written in simpler language for patients, their families, and the general public. The state-of-the-art statements provide current information that can assist clinicians in deciding whether a standard or investigational therapy is appropriate for their cancer patient. Each state-of-the-art statement provides up-to-date data on prognosis, relevant staging and histologic classifications, therapies that constitute current standards of cancer care, and references to seminal literature. Abstracts have been incorporated into the system, allowing users to retrieve them for review if so desired. Each patient information summary contains references to patient education materials that are readily available through NCI and other sources.

PDQ's cancer information file is being enhanced with information on the cause and management of untoward sequelae of cancer or its treatment. PDQ contains 20 "supportive care" summaries on the management of patient care issues, such as pain, nutrition, sleep disorders, radiation enteritis, nausea, vomiting, and oral complications. The file is being expanded to peer-reviewed information on innovative approaches to cancer prevention and promising investigational drugs. Prognostic and treatment information for rare tumors is also under development.

The cancer information file contains a *news file* that contains items of interest, including summaries of the most recent changes to the state-of-the-art statements; NCI's clinical alerts; NIH Consensus Development Conferences dealing with cancer; information on NCI's group C drugs and its treatment referral center; current database vendors, including foreign MEDLARS centers; and NCI's high-priority clinical trials.

The prognostic and treatment information in the cancer information file was developed and is maintained by an Editorial Board of cancer specialists with input from experts

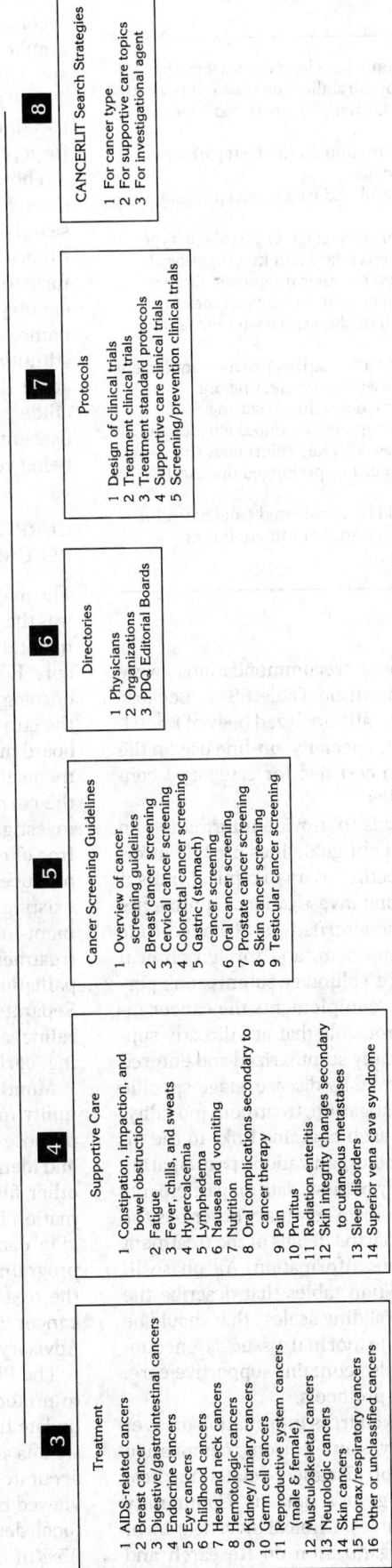

FIGURE 68–1. The PDQ file structure. This diagram from the PDQ User Guide depicts the menu hierarchy from the "main PDQ menu," shown at the top of the diagram. PDQ's user interface uses menu selections to prompt users to select the information desired. Each item of the main PDQ menu has a series of submenus that are arranged in hierarchical order. User commands provide shortcuts for moving through the hierarchy of menus.

PDQ Menu

The following information is available in PDQ.

1 Information about PDQ   5 Screening
2 PDQ News   6 Directories
3 Treatment   7 Protocols
4 Supportive Care   8 CANCERLIT
      Search Strategies

9 Exit PDQ

3 Treatment

1 AIDS-related cancers
2 Breast cancer
3 Digestive/gastrointestinal cancers
4 Endocrine cancers
5 Eye cancers
6 Childhood cancers
7 Head and neck cancers
8 Hematologic cancers
9 Kidney/urinary cancers
10 Germ cell cancers
11 Reproductive system cancers
    (male & female)
12 Musculoskeletal cancers
13 Neurologic cancers
14 Skin cancers
15 Thorax/respiratory cancers
16 Other or unclassified cancers

4 Supportive Care

1 Constipation, impaction, and
    bowel obstruction
2 Fatigue
3 Fever, chills, and sweats
4 Hypercalcemia
5 Lymphedema
6 Nausea and vomiting
7 Nutrition
8 Oral complications secondary to
    cancer therapy
9 Pain
10 Pruritus
11 Radiation enteritis
12 Skin integrity changes secondary
    to cutaneous metastases
13 Sleep disorders
14 Superior vena cava syndrome

5 Cancer Screening Guidelines

1 Overview of cancer
    screening guidelines
2 Breast cancer screening
3 Cervical cancer screening
4 Colorectal cancer screening
5 Gastric (stomach)
    cancer screening
6 Oral cancer screening
7 Prostate cancer screening
8 Skin cancer screening
9 Testicular cancer screening

6 Directories

1 Physicians
2 Organizations
3 PDQ Editorial Boards

7 Protocols

1 Design of clinical trials
2 Treatment clinical trials
3 Treatment standard protocols
4 Supportive care clinical trials
5 Screening/prevention clinical trials

8 CANCERLIT Search Strategies

1 For cancer type
2 For supportive care topics
3 For investigational agent

TABLE 68–1. Guidelines for the Development of Treatment Statements

1. Open with a prognostic statement that clearly describes the success of treatment in terms of curability (or treatability) with current modalities and states whether prognostic variables influence treatment outcome.
2. Provide clinically relevant information on the histopathologic classification of the malignant cells.
3. Describe the most clinically useful and widely accepted staging classification.
4. Provide current survival data for each stage or histologic type.
5. Provide treatment information (standard and investigational) options by stage of dissemination or other prognostic factors such as histology (*e.g.*, lung cancer), sites of involvement (*e.g.*, rhabdomyosarcoma), or location of the primary tumor (*e.g.*, brain neoplasms).
6. Indicate whether the therapeutic alternatives produce equivalent results and whether there are reasons for selecting one treatment over another in a particular clinical setting.
7. List only therapies with superior and documented efficacy as potential therapeutic alternatives with key references that document treatment efficacy if cure or prolonged disease-free survival is achievable.
8. Clearly state that patients should be considered candidates for investigational therapies currently under evaluation if no effective treatment exists.

around the country. Treatment recommendations were drafted using the guidelines shown on Table 68–1. Because PDQ provides a current and critically analyzed body of knowledge that encompasses an entire specialty, on-line use on the NLM implementation has been certified for category I continuing medical education credits.

Because a major goal of PDQ is to provide information on therapeutic research, the treatment guidelines provide information on ongoing studies, directing users to clinical trials if effective therapies do not exist and investigational approaches represent important therapeutic alternatives. A *protocol file* containing over 1500 active American and foreign clinical trials, 30% to 35% of which are voluntary submissions performed without federal support, complements the cancer information file. All treatment protocols that are directly supported by the NCI are automatically summarized and entered into PDQ. Each protocol is indexed by disease, stage-specific eligibility criteria, phase of investigation, treatment modality, drugs, and drug regimens, and each contains links to the directory records of physicians and organizations participating in the trial so that users can easily retrieve data on participants by geographic location. Each protocol summary describes the study objectives, eligibility criteria, the details of the treatment program, and dose and schedule information. All phase III protocols contain dose-modification tables that describe the dose and schedule adjustments (sliding scales) that should be used when significant toxicity to normal tissue is encountered.[17] The PDQ protocol file also contains supportive care, early detection, and prevention protocols.

A *physician directory* contains address information on over 19,000 physicians. This directory is an electronic compilation of the membership directories of 17 cancer-related medical societies, NCI's clinical trials groups, and its Community Clinical Oncology Program grantees. Clinical investigators of the NCI and the European Organization on Research and

Treatment of Cancer (EORTC) are also listed. Each person's record includes the physician's full name, address, telephone number, medical specialties, information on oncologic subspecialty board certification, and organizational affiliations. The PDQ implementation that distributed on the NLM system uses interfile linkages to automatically retrieve all protocols for a physician if requested by the user.

The *organization directory* includes information on more than 2500 organizations at which NCI supports clinical research and hospitals with cancer programs certified by the American College of Surgeons' Commission on Cancer. Information on organizations is retrievable by name, city, state, country, or postal code. Each organization record includes the name, address, and telephone number of a person at the institution who has agreed to answer questions from PDQ users about the organization's cancer treatment programs and facilities. As in the physician directory, PDQ on the NLM system uses interfile linkages to automatically retrieve all protocols being conducted at an organization if requested by the user.

CURRENCY OF THE TREATMENT RECOMMENDATIONS

The major rationale for developing PDQ as an on-line database was the ability to use computer technology to rapidly and easily maintain the currency of the information. A multidisciplinary core Editorial Board of 30 cancer specialists (including an oncology nurse) and an 80-member Advisory Board maintains the currency of the treatment information. Each month, core board members receive a printout of the state-of-the-art statements that fall within their purview and relevant articles from the current literature that report cure with an established or investigational treatment program; improvement in disease-free or overall survival that is equivalent to or better than that produced by regimens cited as "standard" treatment in the existing statement; significantly less acute or long-term treatment-induced toxicity with equivalent results to standard treatments cited in the existing statement; and significant palliation for cancers for which no effective therapies exist. Separate Editorial Boards have been established to develop, refine, and update the state-of-the-art information on screening, early detection, cancer prevention, and supportive care.

Monthly meetings of the Board afford members the opportunity to discuss data from the current treatment literature, propose modifications and refinements to PDQ statements, and identify the need for new state-of-the-art statements and other file enhancements. Modifications to the cancer information file are based on Board discussions. Articles that provide data suggesting improved results with investigational programs are also reviewed and highlighted or referenced in the text if the data merit. On average, 20% to 25% of the cancer information statements are modified each month. The Advisory Board provides input and peer review by mail.

The PDQ protocol file is maintained by a monthly mailing to protocol coordinators at medical centers nationwide who update the status and update the matrix of participating physicians and organizations to ensure that the protocols remain accurate. Twice each year, the protocol summaries are reviewed by the principal investigators to ensure that the protocol details remain accurate. Each month, approximately 35% of the active protocols in PDQ undergo a change of description, status, or investigators. On average, 60 new protocols are abstracted, indexed, and entered into PDQ each month and about 50 are closed and transferred to the closed protocol file.

Each physician and organization in PDQ is sent a printout of the directory record annually and must validate the accuracy of the listing by return mail. Update requests are mailed to one twelfth of the PDQ directory each month. Physicians and organizations are encouraged to submit changes whenever they occur. More than 93% of the directory records have been revalidated or corrected by return mail every year, making the file one of the most accurate directories in existence.

In September of 1992, the PDQ Screening and Prevention file was introduced on-line. It includes *Guidelines* for screening for cancers of the breast, cervix, colon and rectum, stomach, oral cavity, prostate, skin, and testes. For each site, in addition to the actual screening *Guideline*, there is background information describing studies of the efficacy of screening as a means of accomplishing the early detection of cancer in asymptomatic individuals and reducing mortality.

The Screening and Prevention Editorial Board reviews the published literature and discusses the clinical data at a bimonthly meeting. The data are analyzed with regard to whether the specific technique detects cancers earlier and whether there is evidence that earlier detection results in improved treatment outcome. The editorial board determines whether the narrative should be changed to accommodate the new literature and whether new evidence is sufficient to change actual guidelines. Board members discuss the quality of the data and the gaps in knowledge as the basis for their decisions about establishing or revising screening guidelines. Critical parameters considered for a specific technique include sensitivity, specificity, and predictive value. Four measures of improved outcome are considered: (1) a decrease in cause-specific mortality; (2) a reduction in the incidence of advanced stage cancers; (3) an increase in survival; and (4) a shift in stage distribution. Evidence of improved outcome is categorized into five levels in decreasing order of strength:

1. Evidence obtained from at least one properly randomized well-designed and well-conducted trial
2. Evidence obtained from well-designed and well-conducted trials without randomization

3. Evidence obtained from well-designed cohort or case-control analytic studies, preferably from more than one center or research group
4. Evidence obtained from multiple time series with or without the intervention
5. Opinions of respected authorities based on clinical experience, descriptive studies, or reports of expert committees

The levels of evidence supporting improved outcome are specified in the narrative and taken into account by the editorial board in arriving at screening guidelines. Statements are sent yearly to an external advisory board for review and comment.

SYSTEM IMPLEMENTATION

As implemented on the NLM's MEDLARS system, PDQ is completely menu driven. The main menu (see Fig. 68–1) prompts users to select a number to select information about PDQ (*i.e.*, a description of the database and instructions on database searching); a list of the members of the various PDQ Editorial Boards; the news file; cancer information; directories of physicians and organizations; protocols, or information on preformulated CANCERLIT searches. Throughout a PDQ search, users may return to previous menus and change files by entering a simple command, restart from the main menu, or exit from PDQ at any time during a search.

Prognostic and treatment information contained in the cancer information file are selectable options from a menu that is dynamically generated when the user selects a cancer diagnosis. Treatment information for each cancer diagnosis is provided in two formats: state-of-the-art information and information for patients (Fig. 68–2). Because, for many users, the cancer information file is the entry point into the PDQ files, each description of stage-specific treatment options on the NLM implementation indicates the number of clinical trials that may be found in the protocol file for that subset of patients. PDQ also offers users the opportunity to review the abstracts of any of the literature that is cited in the state-of-the-art statements. A series of preformulated search statements that enable the user to search the CANCERLIT database

FIGURE 68–2. The cancer treatment information menu. Once a specific clinical diagnosis is selected this menu is displayed for that diagnosis. By making *selections 1 → 3*, the user can display information written for patients based on the state-of-the-art recommendations made for physicians. These summaries are written in lay language with references to printed materials written for cancer patients. By making *selections 4 → 7*, the user can display the state-of-the-art statements that are written to meet the technical information needs of clinicians caring for cancer patients. Key references from the medical literature, abstracts, and the number of active trials for each type and stage are available for review. *Selection 8* allows the user to display all of the information. *Selection 9* contains the continuation options that are available for the selected diagnosis. If the user has selected treatment information about a particular stage, the diagnosis and stage are used for continuing searches.

CANCER INFORMATION MENU

Breast Cancer

Information for Patients

1 Description
2 Stage Explanations
3 General Treatment Options

State-of-the-Art Information

4 Prognosis
5 Cellular Classification
6 Stage Information
7 Treatment by Cell Type/Stage

8 Display all information
9 Continuation options for citation abstracts, **CANCERLIT** searches and protocols.

* Enter desired number and press CR

for additional literature on treatment questions are available as a menu selection (see Figs. 68–1 and 68–2).

Users may select protocols for a particular cancer diagnosis and stage by choosing the continuation option on the cancer information menu (see Fig. 68–2). This option automatically retrieves all trials that are open to the last type or stage of cancer defined by the user from the protocol file without re-formulation of the search criteria. Users may also select protocols as the primary retrieval option from the main menu or by typing a simple command (*i.e.*, prot) at most prompts. Users can retrieve protocols from PDQ by diagnosis, stage, therapeutic agent, treatment modality, phase of clinical investigation, title word, patient age, geographic region, cancer center, cooperative group, ID number, and any combination of these parameters (see lower part of Fig. 68–1). In 1992, PDQ began to provide users with the capability of narrowing their protocol retrievals by patient-related criteria, such as menopausal status, and protocol-specific eligibility criteria, such as prior chemotherapy. Dose and schedule modifications for normal tissue toxicity are provided for all phase III and standard therapy protocols and most adjuvant trials. Detailed summaries describing the administration of treatment regimens considered to be state-of-the-art (*e.g.*, CMF, MOPP, ABVD) are provided as *standard therapy protocols*.

After a protocol set is defined, PDQ informs the user how many protocols met the search criteria. At this point, the user may redefine the criteria or decide to display or print information in a range of formats by selecting one of PDQ's print options. A customized print format can be created from a menu containing all protocol data elements. Users can select and order the items as desired and can maintain the customized format for the entire session or redefine it any time. In 1991, NCI incorporated a large portion of its CLINPROT database into PDQ. Users who wish to retrieve information on over 7000 closed and completed protocols may now do so.

Users can retrieve information about physicians by entering a name, medical specialty, a particular geographic location, or a combination of these parameters. After a data set is defined, PDQ offers a variety of print and display options that enable the user to review physician profiles in varying degrees of detail. Protocols for which a physician is a principal investigator or those that are being conducted at an organization can also be displayed using interfile linkages. The directory of organizations can be searched in a similar fashion.

AVAILABILITY

More than 35,000 domestic and 4000 foreign centers have access to the cancer databases on the MEDLARS system. Over 3500 student codes are also in effect. There are currently 16 principal foreign MEDLARS centers that offer database access to foreign medical institutions and physicians. Sixteen, including the Pan American Health Organization, offer access to CANCERLIT, and 12 offer access to PDQ. An on-line service, called EuroCODE, operated by the EORTC makes PDQ available to its participating organizations.[18] Once logged into the EORTC's EuroCODE computer system, physicians can register, randomize, and enter patients on EROTC clinical trials, search PDQ, or exchange electronic mail with colleagues.[19] NCI staff plan to make PDQ and CANCERLIT widely available to Latin American and Caribbean countries

on the academic network, BITNIS, with an easy to use front end that will permit users to formulate their search query before logging onto the on-line system. Any hardware that can emulate an 80-character ASCII terminal can be used to search PDQ by a 300, 1200, or 2400 baud modem. Transmission of PDQ data over commercial telecommunication networks allows users to access PDQ without incurring long-distance charges. PDQ is also licensed to commercial vendors and academic and nonprofit health care organizations with computerized medical information systems.

A wide range of implementations exist for access by PDQ users. Some have been developed by the NCI and others by private vendors. Implementations fall into two general categories: on-line time-sharing systems with dial-up access and "local" implementations that reside on a single computer or a local area network for use by groups of individuals. Local access to PDQ is currently available from NCI as MUMPS or C language versions. PDQ is also offered as a local system on CD-ROM by two commercial sources. Subscriptions to the CD-ROM products are sold on an annual basis. They can be purchased to run on a DOS-based personal computer or a local area network. PDQ is provided alone on CD-ROM and as a component of products that also contain oncologic textbooks and other bibliographic databases. At least one vendor plans to release a CD-ROM product for the Macintosh computer family. The availability of NCI databases on CD-ROM should serve to markedly increase the awareness and usage of PDQ and CANCERLIT throughout the world, particularly in regions where access to on-line systems is difficult and cost is a consideration.

As part of an initiative to increase information dissemination to underserved populations, NCI is providing subscriptions to a commercial CD-ROM product containing PDQ and CANCERLIT to over 40 demonstration sites in selected domestic and foreign underserved areas for a 3-year demonstration period. These sites will serve as cancer information distribution centers, enabling the NCI to disseminate up-to-date information on cancer research findings and current standards of patient care to new and hitherto largely unreachable audiences.

NCI's Cancer Information Service (CIS) network uses CD-ROM technology to handle PDQ inquiries from the public. NCI plans to augment the CIS system with a new 800 number that will handle inquiries from physicians and other health professionals. The new service will be introduced in early 1993 and provide rapid and easy access to PDQ to those who do not have ready access to PDQ in other ways, especially disadvantaged and underserved health care professionals.

USER DOCUMENTATION AND PDQ ACCESS

Enhancements are continually being incorporated into PDQ to increase its clinical and educational value and ease of use. User documentation consists of a User Guide for the version that is distributed over the NLM system, which provides an overview of the system, explicit instructions for the inexperienced user on how to search each file, and advanced searching techniques for the expert searcher.[20] The guide is sold through the National Technical Information Service and subscribers automatically receive updates as they are printed. There is also a Quick Reference Guide that summarizes frequently used system functions and commands and a publication on the terminology in PDQ that explains how PDQ is indexed, the associations among indexed terms, and an index of drug synonyms. These resources are available free of charge through the NCI.

PDQ ACCESS is a telecommunications program that totally automates the dial up and log-on procedures to the NLM's MEDLARS system. The PDQ ACCESS software is provided free of charge to everyone who subscribers to the PDQ User Guide. Two versions of the PDQ ACCESS program are available: one for IBM-compatible computers and the other for the Macintosh family of computers.[21]

The PDQ ACCESS program automatically captures each search session to disk, enabling users to print the search after the on-line session is over. The PDQ ACCESS program also automates a link from PDQ to CANCERLIT. After a preformulated literature search in PDQ is selected, the PDQ AC-CESS program connects the user to CANCERLIT and automatically executes the search and captures the results to a disk file. When the CANCERLIT search is complete, the PDQ ACCESS program returns the user to the PDQ search session. NLM's telecommunications package, GRATEFUL MED, also provides access to CANCERLIT, PDQ, and all of the preformulated CANCERLIT searches in PDQ.

CANCERFAX

Recent advances in technology allow facsimile (fax) boards to be placed inside personal computers so that the computer can act as a fax machine, sending and receiving documents simultaneously. When coupled with digital voice technology and software that interprets user selections from a touch-tone telephone, information from a database like PDQ can be delivered to a caller without human intervention. In 1991, NCI staff began distributing the treatment guidelines from PDQ using fax technology.[22] The service, CancerFax, allows users to dial into one of NCI's computers (301-402-5874) from the handset on their fax machine and retrieve a faxed image of any of PDQ's state-of-the-art, patient information statements or news articles. The service is available 24 hours each day, and there is no cost to the user other than the telephone call. In addition to the prognostic and treatment information contained in PDQ's cancer information file, CancerFax provides the current information on databases vendors, NCI's scientific journals, its database-derived publications, and its patient education materials. At the end of 1992, the CancerFax service had handled over 29,000 calls approximately 2400 queries per month.

Advances in computer technology have led to the development of natural language processing systems that have programs for speech recognition, language understanding, and language generation.[23] A text processing translation system has been used to facilitate the translation of text from PDQ's cancer information file into Spanish for distribution on CancerFax. The machine translator processes the source language text, producing a literal translation. This draft is reviewed, edited, and finalized by Spanish-speaking health professionals and oncologists and distributed on CancerFax.

In July 1992, NCI also introduced CancerNet, an electronic service that enables computer users to obtain free access to the treatment guidelines in PDQ 24 hours a day, 7 days a week on INTERNET's electronic bulletin board. INTERNET, a web of computer networks that reaches all over the world, trades information over high-speed datalines. This new service is another example of the NCI's efforts to make effective and efficient use of technology to facilitate its information dissemination initiatives. In the first 6 months, CancerNet was accessed over 8000 times (1400 times/month); one third of the users were from foreign countries. The technology is expected to play an increasingly important role in the dissemination of ICIC services and products as high-speed networks become more widely used.

NEW INITIATIVES

As part of its challenge to develop novel communication technologies, NCI is identifying emerging communication technologies that can facilitate the dissemination of information on cancer through the federal government's small business innovation research (SBIR) program. Areas of research include improving telecommunication access; optimizing the user interface; the ongoing refinement of touch-tone interfaces to facsimile (CancerFax); the development of other advanced personal computing technologies such as portable digital storage devices; and voice-recognition interfaces for information dissemination applications.[24]

Future plans include the development of links in PDQ that will make it easy for users to move between protocol summaries and published abstracts or articles on the trial that are cited in the CANCERLIT database. A drug file that would provide information on indication, does, mechanism of action, pharmacology and phase of development of investigational agents listed in the PDQ protocol file is under development. This enhancement will enable users to move easily between a protocol summary or state-of-the-art statement in the cancer information file to a relevant summary in the drug file or citations in the CANCERLIT database. Advances in fiberoptic communication technology offer the potential for future integration of images into PDQ as new developments in computer and communication technologies make it feasible.

CLINICAL INFORMATION SYSTEMS FOR DECISION SUPPORT

Hospital-based information systems have been developed to automate the collection, retrieval, and analysis of information for rapid and flexible access in clinical settings. Most systems process clinical, laboratory, and administrative data to support inpatient care, clinical research, and hospital operations. Some also use computer-based logic to support clinical decision making without additional data entry requirements.[25,26] The logic incorporated in these systems generates medical alerts that provide physicians with interpretations of physiologic data and medical advice (*e.g.*, drug interaction warnings, recommendations for additional tests) and guide them in the efficient management of patients in light of their past medical history and current problem list. Information systems also have been designed to deal specifically with diagnostic problems.[5,6,10,27,28]

Protocol-derived clinical algorithms have been developed to specify data-collection requirements (*e.g.*, frequency of radiologic studies, laboratory tests), to flag abnormal values, and to help oncologists to administer treatments as prescribed in a written protocol. Many of the oncology systems developed during the last decade also provided clinical databanks for statistical analysis, often with special displays or prompts to help remind physicians about protocol details.[29-32] Advice provided through algorithms implemented on a computer have been shown by investigators to improve oncology protocol compliance significantly for the cooperative group with which they worked.[33] However, this system was unable to analyze complex, ambiguous, or unusual clinical situations, involved data entry and program management centrally at the university rather than at the cooperating oncologist's office, and required considerable central effort to prepare the appropriate algorithm for each clinic visit. These limitations precluded the system's use in routine practice.

There is ongoing interest in the development of decision-support systems that formulate advice by following lines of reasoning similar to those used by human experts. Systems such as these capture and analyze patient data, apply medical knowledge, and interact with the physician to provide patient-specific recommendations on a course of action.[6,9,10] ONCOCIN is a decision-support system that integrates a clinical data management environment with an expert system provides customized treatment advice for cancer patients and clinical trial data management.[34] It presents, on a picture-quality display screen, a flow sheet that duplicates the traditional paper version. The graphic flow sheet is divided into sections, similar to those that separate classes of data on the paper flow sheet, and the physician can open sections for review or data entry by selecting them with a mouse device. ONCOCIN has several features that facilitate clinical trials data management:

1. *Registers and menus for data entry.* When physicians wish to enter data such as the current white blood cell count, they select the corresponding box on the flow sheet. An appropriate register containing values appears on the screen. They can use a mouse to indicate the proper value, which appears in the appropriate box on the flow sheet.

2. *Graphic data entry.* A paper flow sheet traditionally includes drawings of the human torso and chest x-ray views on which a physician is able to indicate areas of disease involvement. ONCOCIN also permits data to be entered and retrieved with a mouse.

3. *Guidance during data entry.* ONCOCIN uses current and past data on the patient to guide its assessment of the appropriate protocol-directed treatment for the current visit. The program indicates what information is needed to make an informed recommendation by displaying question marks in the appropriate boxes on the flow sheet. As clinical data are entered on the graphic flow sheet, they are passed to a "reasoner" that uses them plus knowledge about the protocol or treatment program to consider whether therapy should be administered and, if so, whether dosage adjustments are indicated. This decision-support program then displays its recommendations in the appropriate column on the flow sheet. If physicians wish to administer different dosages or to delay therapy, they indicate their changes in treatment by entering the new doses.

In addition to knowing the rules for chemotherapy administration in specific clinical trials, ONCOCIN keeps track of the data required by the protocol and provides reminders to the physician when laboratory studies or radiologic examinations are indicated. ONCOCIN can generate order forms, which can be printed and used to arrange tests on subsequent appointments. At the end of each clinic visit, ONCOCIN produces a hard copy of the flow sheets that can be placed in the patient's chart for backup and review. Although it has been documented that the data management and clinical consultation provided by this system can exert a significant influence on physician behavior, the overall impact of this and other systems on medical practice has been limited to selected settings.[35] However, there is increasing interest in using computer technology to meet the practicing physician's need for up-to-date medical information and expert medical advice.[6,10,11,36,37] Interest is due in part to the availability of increasingly powerful and sophisticated microcomputers, greatly improved graphical interfaces, and affordable, easily used, software tools, coupled with the growing concern about the increase in medical knowledge, medicolegal accountability, and cost-effective practice.[38,39] A key requirement for physician acceptance of automated information and decision support systems appears to be the smooth integration of the computer programs into the routine patient-care environment. Narrowly defined systems that serve a single purpose and require users to make special or duplicate efforts to access them have met with limited success, even though the information they provide has been shown in some cases to be accurate and valuable for patient care.[40,41]

Several recent developments may accelerate the pace at which the logistic problems are addressed. In an initiative to address technologic solutions to the current health care crisis, the Institute of Medicine (IOM) commissioned an 18-month study to examine the status of patient records and computer-based approaches to their management.[42] The study recommended the development of information systems to address the deficiencies in the paper-based medical record and help physicians to access and manage clinical information effectively.[43] Acknowledging that such systems must provide a critical mass of capabilities to achieve widespread and routine use, the IOM has recommended the establishment of a public and private computer-based patient record institute to develop and implement standards to ensure intersystem compatibility and data sharing.

Research in medical informatics is focusing on intersystem compatibility. Physician workstations are being designed with an "open systems architecture" that allows new applications to be added easily.[44] This permits the development of cost-effective systems that can integrate innovations in user interface and database technology as well as data from computer-based hospital information systems and decision support tools.[45] Designers of such systems have begun to systematically study the work patterns of physicians and analyze clinical practices to identify information needs in the context of patient care.[46] Future systems should help physicians find pertinent information and provide innovative ways to assist them in determining how the data apply to a specific clinical question.[47]

Several academic centers have developed and successfully implemented strategically placed computer workstations developed under grants from the NLM. These networked workstations are designed to instill query habits in the daily clinical activities of young physicians in training.[48-50] They facilitate one-stop, integrated information shopping.

One of these systems allows users to maintain patient records, check findings with two diagnostic decision support systems (*i.e.*, RECONSIDER and DXplain), look up drugs on various databases, and search PDQ by a licensed, local implementation and search the medical literature.[48]

In radiation therapy, two groups have reported their experiences with the development and use of workstation-based expert systems designed to serve as consulting resources to the practicing radiotherapist and as a teaching aid to residents in training.[51,52] Both groups reported satisfaction with the power, capability, and utility of the workstations and expressed enthusiasm about the development and integration of anatomic atlases, treatment planning guides, dosimetric calculations, tutorials, and decision-support tools like ONCOCIN for protocol management.

DEVELOPMENT OF AN INTEGRATED ONCOLOGY WORKSTATION

NCI is currently supporting efforts to enhance computerized support for clinical decision-making through the development of an *integrated oncology workstation* (IOW). This workstation integrates an electronic patient record; automated clinical and laboratory systems; access to information resources such as PDQ, CANCERLIT, the full text of this and other oncologic textbooks (through OncoDisc); and access to decision-support software such as ONCOCIN, which is currently undergoing refinement. A prototype for this workstation has been designed as an advanced, yet affordable, desk-top personal computer or technical workstation. Extensive integration of this data-management function with laboratory, financial, and office-management systems is under development to enhance the utility of the IOW.

Users on networked workstations will be able to retrieve and manipulate patient records, integrate laboratory and diagnostic test results into the medical record and the flow sheet, obtain decision support, manage clinical trials data, and easily obtain context-specific (*i.e.*, patient- or problem-specific) information from integrated electronic databases and textbooks. Commercial development of the workstation is being conducted as a collaborative project with the medical informatics group at Stanford University and private industry under the auspices of the Federal Technology Transfer Act (FTTA).[53] The FTTA authorizes the NCI to enter into a Cooperative Research and Development Agreement (CRADA). The CRADA is a mechanism for facilitating commercial development that permits private sector partners to obtain exclusive license rights in exchange for participation in product development and marketing.

Another development that may hasten the integration of computer technology into medical practice is the introduction of a fully electronic medical journal, the *Online Journal of Clinical Trials*.[54,55] Subscribers must have a personal computer with a 286 or higher-level processor, two megabytes of memory, a VGA monitor, a modem, and Microsoft's Windows software. Subscribers will be notified of new articles by fax and can have instant access to them, complete with tables and figures, on their video terminals. The software also allows readers to browse through previously published articles. The concept is innovative but not without its critics. Concern has been expressed about the fate of traditional customs of review, authorship, and attribution. However, the introduction of an online journal reflects a growing recognition that the current process by which clinical research is reviewed, edited, and published requires substantial streamlining to expedite the rapid dissemination of important clinical advances—the principal goal of PDQ, CancerFax, CancerNet, and NCI's clinical alert mechanism.[56-58]

As the biologic revolution continues, it has become clear that computer and communication technology has a major role to play in information management and decision support. Future systems should assist physicians not only to find pertinent information but also to determine how the data apply to specific clinical situations. An improved understanding of the nature of medical knowledge, the way it should be used for optimal decision-making, and the logistical issues that serve as barriers to widespread use, pose continued challenges for system developers.

REFERENCES

1. Williamson JW, German PS, Weiss R, Skinner EA, Bowes F. Health science information management and continuing education of physicians. A survey of U.S. primary care practitioners and their opinion leaders. Ann Intern Med 1989;110:151–160.
2. Association of Medical Colleges. Physicians of the twenty-first century: Report of the panel on the general education of the physician and college preparation for medicine. J Med Educ 1984;59:1–208.
3. Covell DG, Uman GC, Manning PR. Information needs in office practice: Are they being met? Ann Intern Med 1985;103:596–599.
4. Medical education in the information age. Proceedings of the Symposium on Medical informatics. Washington, DC: Association of Medical Colleges, 1986.
5. Bankowitz RA, Mc Neill MA, Challinor SM, Parker RC, Kapoor WN, Miller RA. A computer-assisted medical diagnostic consultation service. Ann Intern Med 1989;110:824–832.
6. Greenes RA, Shortliffe EH. Medical informatics: An emerging academic discipline and institutional priority. JAMA 1990;263:1114–1120.
7. Connelly DP, Rich EC, Curley SP, Kelly JT. Knowledge resource preferences of family physicians. J Fam Pract 1990;3:353–359.
8. Osheroff JA, Forsythe DE, Buchanan BG, Bankowitz RA, Blumenfeld BH, Miller RA. Physicians' information needs: Analysis of questions posed during clinical teaching. Ann of Intern Med 1991;114:576–581.
9. Wyatt J. Uses and sources of medical knowledge. Lancet 1991;338:1368–1373.
10. Wyatt J. Computer-based knowledge systems. Lancet 1991;338:1431–1436.
11. Lindberg DAB, Schoolman HM. The National Library of Medicine and medical informatics. West J Med 1986;145:786–790.
12. Lindberg DAB. Information systems to support medical practice and scientific discovery. Method Inform Med 1989;28:202–206.
13. 92nd Congress. National Cancer Act of 1971. Public Law 92–218, Sec. 1828, Dec. 23, 1971.
14. Masys DR, Hubbard SM. Technical information progress of the National Cancer Institute. J Am Soc Info Sci 1987;38:60–64.
15. Hubbard SM, Henney JE, DeVita VT. A computer database for information on cancer treatment. N Engl J Med 1987;316:315–318.
16. Hubbard SM, DeVita VT. PDQ: An innovation in information dissemination linking cancer research and clinical practice. In: DeVita VT, Hellman S, Rosenberg SA, eds. Important advances in oncology: 1987. Philadelphia: JB Lippincott, 1987:263–277.
17. Perry, DJ, Hubbard, SM, Masys, DR, Tingley, DE. Dose modification for PDQ. In: Stead WW, ed. Symposium on Computer Applications in Medical Care. 11th ed. Los Angeles: Computer Society Press, 1987:739–742.
18. Perry DJ, Hubbard SM, Young RC. PDQ: A new source of information on cancer therapy. Eur J Cancer Clin Oncol 1989;25:1907–1908.
19. EuroCODE. A new approach to collaborative research in clinical oncology. Eur J Cancer Clin Oncol 1989;25:1905–1906.
20. Van Camp AJ. PDQ search aids. Database Searcher 1990;6:24–28.
21. Perry DJ, Sloane EM, Hubbard SM, Tingley DE, DeVita VT. Keeping up with the cancer literature—PDQ and CANCERLIT. J Clin Oncol 1988;6:1649–1652.
22. Hubbard SM. Getting the "fax" on cancer treatments. Oncology Times [Editorial] 1991;13:2.
23. Joshi AK. Natural language processing. Science 1991;254:1242–1249.
24. Gomez E, Demetriades JE, Babcock D, Peterson J. The Department of Veteran's Affairs optical patient card workstation. In: Clayton PD, ed. Assessing the value of medical informatics. New York: McGraw Hill, 1992:378–380.

25. Warner HR. Computer-assisted medical decision-making. New York: Academic Press, 1979.

26. McDonald CJ, Hui SL, Smith DM, et al. Reminders to physicians from an introspective computer medical record. Ann Intern Med 1984;100:130–138.

27. Barnett GO, Cimino JJ, Hupp JA, et al. DXplain: An evolving diagnostic decision-support system. JAMA 1987;258:67–74.

28. Miller RA, Pople HE, Myers JD. Internist-1: An experimental computer-based diagnostic consultant for general internal medicine. N Engl J Med 1982;307:468–476.

29. Friedman RH, Frank AD. Use of a conditional rule structure to automate clinical decision support: A comparison of artificial intelligence and deterministic programming techniques. Comput Biomed Res 16:378–394.

30. Friedman RB, Entine SM, Carbone PP. Experience with an automated cancer protocol surveillance system. Am J Clin Oncol 1983;6:583–592.

31. Wirtschafter DD, Scalise M, Henke C, et al. Do information systems improve the quality of clinical research? Results of a randomized trial in a cooperative multi-institutional cancer group. Comput Biomed Res 1981;14:78–90.

32. Lenhard RE, Blum BI, Sunderland JM. The Johns Hopkins oncology clinical information system. J Med Syst 1983;7:147–174.

33. Wirtschafter DD, Carpenter JT, Mesel E. A consultant-extender system for breast cancer adjuvant chemotherapy. Comput Biomed Res 1979;90:396–401.

34. Hickam DH, Shortliffe EH, Bischoff MB, et al. The treatment advice of a computer-based chemotherapy protocol advisor. Ann Intern Med 1985;103:928–936.

35. Kent DL, Shortliffe EH, Carlson RW, et al. Improvements in data collection through physician use of a computer-based chemotherapy treatment consultant. J Clin Oncol 1985;3:409–417.

36. Schwartz WB, Patil RS, Szolovits P. Artificial intelligence in medicine: Where do we stand? N Engl J Med 1987;316:685–688.

37. Perry CA. Knowledge bases in medicine: A review. Bull Med Libr Assoc 1990;78:271–282.

38. Shortliffe EH. Computer programs to support clinical decision making. JAMA 1987;258:67–74.

39. Shortliffe EH, Wulfman CE, Rindfleisch TC, Carlson RW. An integrated oncology workstation. Bethesda: National Cancer Institute, 1990.

40. Kent DL, Shortliffe EH, Carlson RW, et al. Improvements in data collection through physician use of a computer-based chemotherapy treatment consultant. J Clin Oncol 1985;3:409–417.

41. Hickam DH, Shortliffe EH, Bischoff MB, et al. The treatment advice of a computer-based chemotherapy protocol advisor. Ann Intern Med 1985;103:928–936.

42. Institute of Medicine. Committee on Improving the Patient Record. The computer-based patient record: An essential technology for health care. Washington, DC: National Academy Press, 1991.

43. Shortliffe EH, Tang PC, Detmer DE. Patient records and computers. Ann Intern Med 1991;115:979–981.

44. Young CY, Tang PC, Annevelink J. An open systems architecture for development of a physicians workstation. In: Clayton PD, ed. Assessing the value of medical informatics. New York: McGraw Hill, 1992:491–495.

45. Annevelink J, Young CY, Tang, PC. Heterogenous database integration in a physician's workstation. In: Clayton PD, ed. Assessing the value of medical informatics. New York: McGraw Hill, 1992:368–372.

46. Fafchamps D, Young CY, Tang PC. Modelling work practices: Input to the design of a physician's workstation. In: Clayton PD, ed. Assessing the value of medical informatics. New York: McGraw Hill, 1992:788–792.

47. Rennels GD, Shortliffe EH, Miller PM, et al. A computational model of reasoning from the clinical literature. Comput Method Prog Biomed 1987;24:139–149.

48. Broering N. The MAClinical workstation project at Georgetown University. Bull Med Libr Assoc 1991;79:276–281.

49. Clayton PD, Anderson RK, Hill C, McCormack M. An initial assessment of the cost and utilization of the integrated academic information system (IAIMS) at Columbia Presbyterian Medical Center. In: Clayton PD, ed. Assessing the value of medical informatics. New York: McGraw Hill, 1992:109–113.

50. Clark AS, Shea S. Free text database in an integrated academic information system (IAIMS) at Columbia Presbyterian Medical Center. In: In: Clayton PD, ed. Assessing the value of medical informatics. New York: McGraw Hill, 1992:333–337.

51. Laramore GE, Altschular MD, Banks G, et al. Applications of databases and AI/expert systems in radiation therapy. Am J Clin Oncol 1988;11:387–393.

52. Zusag TW, McDonald S, Miller BA, Purdy JA, Rubin P. Radiation oncology resident's computer workstations. Int J Radiat Oncol Biol Phys 1991;22:147–157.

53. Esterhay R, Hubbard S. The integrated oncology workstation (IOW): A collaborative project under the Federal Technology Transfer Act (FTTA). Proc ASCO (in press).

54. Palca J. New journal will publish without paper. Science 1991;253:1480, 1991

55. Kassirer JP. Journals in bits and bytes. N Engl J Med 1992;326:195–196.

56. DeVita VT, Hubbard SM. NCI's breast cancer clinical alert: Rationale and results. Resident Staff Physician 1989;35:49–55.

57. Huth EJ. Prepublication release of scientific data and the right of the public to know: Adapting to our times. J Infect Dis 1989;159:407–411.

58. Steinbrook R. Informing physicians about promising new treatments for severe illness. JAMA 1990;263:2078–2082.

SECTION 2

COLIN B. BEGG

Research Data Management

Every prospective clinical research study is constructed with the goal of addressing specific scientific objectives, and each is completed, if successful, with an interpretive analysis of the results. However, to progress from the initial idea to the results, the researcher must have a system for conducting the study and collecting the data. Research data management is the discipline devoted to the collection, storage, retrieval, and quality control of the data required for evaluating the scientific objectives of the study. It plays a crucial role in determining the success or failure of the study. This role is especially important in cancer studies because of the relative complexity of the clinical interventions in this field and the fact that the endpoints are frequently multifaceted, subjectively interpreted, and involve follow-up over a significant period.

There are two motivating factors for paying careful attention to data management in the development phase of a research study. The first is that medical records are rarely maintained with the kind of detail that is necessary to answer the scientific objectives of research studies, and any data assembled retrospectively from the medical record is likely to be incomplete and of poor quality. Second, the data collection methods should be uniform for all patients and should be developed in close conformity with the methodologic principles of good study

design. This can only be ensured with careful attention to these principles during the design and development of the study. If not, there is the possibility that unforeseen biases may compromise a study that appears to be methodologically sound. For example, in a randomized trial involving long-term follow-up, it is important that the schedules for evaluating patients over time are similar for the treatments under comparison, or reporting biases may influence one of the treatment groups disproportionately. In studies with multiple endpoints, such as phase I and II studies of new agents in which a variety of adverse reactions are possible, absence of careful data collection tools may lead to underreporting of toxicities.

There are four key components to research data management: protocol development, data collection, computing, and quality control. The protocol should contain, in addition to the scientific background and the goals of the study, detailed information on all important logistical aspects of the study, including the data collection forms and a schedule for their completion. After the protocol is open to patient accrual, it is important that there is a system for checking patient eligibility and for prospective registration and randomization of all patients entered in the study. Collection and abstraction of the data is often complex because the medical intervention is often delivered over a period of weeks or months, may have to be adjusted over time in the individual patient due to adverse reactions, and may be multimodal. The outcomes, such as graded toxicities, may have to be derived from secondary data collected over time (*e.g.*, blood counts) or subjectively interpreted. Because of the volume of data collected and the requirements of the statistical analysis, computerization of the data is invariably required. A system of quality control is necessary to protect the integrity of the database, because errors can occur in a variety of ways and are especially likely in complex studies.

In addition to being crucial to the success of the study, the process of data management spans a number of disciplines. Forms development and data abstraction can be performed by data managers, people who have knowledge of biology, medical terminology, and the medical record. This role is often played by nurses, who can also apply their expertise in protocol development to check that details of the intervention under study are factually correct, consistent, and feasible. However, the active involvement of the principal investigator and a statistician is also extremely important to ensure that the appropriate data are being targeted, that the data are being coded in a manner amenable to statistical analysis, and that the logistics of data collection are structured in such a way as to validate the scientific principles embedded in the study design. A team approach of this nature is essential for a successful study with high-quality data.

PRINCIPLES OF STUDY DESIGN

There are many methodologic principles and related techniques that are relevant to the design of clinical research studies, far too many to discuss in a comprehensive way in this chapter. This section instead addresses a few general principles and the relevance of data management planning to ensuring their observance. These principles are concerned with the composition of the source population of patients, the integrity of the sampling procedure (*e.g.*, the patients selected for the trial), the degree to which the intervention under study is prescribed, and the accuracy and completeness of the endpoints. In practice, the role of the statistician or epidemiologist is to make sure that the appropriate design is selected to address the targeted hypotheses of the study.

Typically, the composition of the source population is defined by a set of eligibility criteria in the study protocol. The study may target a broad or a focussed group of patients, depending on the extensiveness of these criteria, and there has been considerable debate on the relative merits of broad or strict criteria.[3] In any event, the results of the trial will be interpreted in the context of the population under study, and the clear characterization of the source population is important from a reporting standpoint. From the data management perspective, the primary goal is to ensure that the patients recruited to the study belong to the source population by fulfilling the eligibility criteria.

In reporting the results of therapeutic trials, the principle of "intent to treat" is frequently invoked, especially in randomized trials.[41] The data analyst includes all patients randomized in the analysis, even though some patients may never have received the allocated treatment for one reason or another. In this way, any bias that may be caused by conscious or inadvertent exclusion of patients with an unrepresentative prognostic profile is avoided, at the cost of reporting aggregate results for groups of patients, not all of whom received the intervention under study. This principle is equally important in uncontrolled or nonrandomized studies. To ensure that the analyst has at least the opportunity to assess the outcome of the study in the total sample of patients selected for inclusion in the study, it is essential to have a system for prospective registration of patients, with the registration taking place after completion of the informed consent but before initiation of the intervention. A registration system of this nature, using an independent office, is in place in all of the cooperative groups and many of the cancer centers. In the absence of a formal system of registration, it is important that all patients recruited to the study be cataloged, so that there is full information on all the patients for whom there was intent to treat.

If the study is randomized, the legitimacy of the process of randomization is crucial to the integrity of the study. The treating physician must play no role in or be able to predict the selection of treatment. Many organizations have an independent office to control the randomization process, but if the study is conducted locally, the logistics of the randomization process must be constructed to ensure the blinding of the allocation procedure.[2] Organizational issues are crucial in studies in which the treatment selection remains unknown to the physician and the patient during the study (*i.e.*, double-blind studies).

A clinical research study invariably involves one or more prescribed interventions on the patients. These could be medical, surgical, radiotherapeutic, diagnostic, or a combination of modalities. The prescribed nature of the intervention distinguishes the experimental nature of a clinical trial from an observational study, in which the extent of the intervention is determined on a patient by patient basis by the physician. This distinction is extremely important with regard to the credibility of the study in that, in an observational study, it is likely that the aggressiveness of the intervention is influenced by the prognosis of the patient, with the result that any apparent treatment difference observed may be spurious (*i.e.*, due to systematic differences in the prognostic composition of the groups of patients being compared, rather than due to the intervention).[4] Because the major methodologic advantage of a study is the fact that the intervention strategies are prescribed rather than elective, it is important that the interventions actually be delivered as prescribed. Such protocol compliance is necessary to validate the results of the research, and monitoring its success is an important data management objective.

The quality of the study depends on the accuracy and completeness of the data. Of paramount importance are the primary endpoints, which must be carefully defined to ensure that the necessary supportive data are collected. For example, if reduction in tumor volume (*i.e.*, tumor response) is the endpoint, measurements at predefined times are required; if survival is the endpoint, regular follow-up of surviving patients is necessary to validate the statistical analysis; and graded toxicities require regular monitoring of the patient and scheduling of laboratory tests. If the outcomes must be assessed subjectively, carefully defined assessment scales are essential to reduce interobserver and intraobserver variability, and the logistical circumstances of the assessment must be constructed to minimize observer biases. For example, in studies of diagnostic technologies, it is sometimes necessary to "blind" test raters from information from other tests conducted on the patient. Care in developing study forms, coding conventions, documentation of codes, and precise data collection schedules is necessary to ensure that the special methodologic requirements of the study are protected.

In structuring the data management system to satisfy important methodologic goals, the data collected must conform to the specific objectives of the study. The required data and the tools for their collection are different from those that are necessary for regular clinical support. The research database is different from a clinical database, even though there may be a lot of overlap in practice. For example, in diagnostic imaging studies, information on the suspected presence of disease usually are carefully coded by site in a manner that permits precise anatomic correlations between the tests and the surgical and pathologic evaluations to a far greater level of precision than is necessary in everyday clinical care. An important conceptual error that is frequently made is the belief that clinical databases, if complete, are adequate resources for clinical research. In fact, only by constructing research databases prospectively, in a manner designed to address the preceding methodologic concerns, can an appropriate resource for clinical research be developed.[5]

RESEARCH DATA MANAGEMENT METHODOLOGY

In the following sections, the major components of a system for research data management are discussed. In each case, the most important tasks are identified and cataloged, tools for facilitating the tasks are described, and the expertise necessary at each stage of the process is discussed. Most of the concepts are sufficiently general that they apply to all kinds of clinical research studies, even though the examples presented are primarily derived from medical oncology trials.

PROTOCOL DEVELOPMENT

The research protocol is the guiding document for the study, and it should specify in detail all important logistical components of the plans for data collection and analysis. Although the format of protocols may vary considerably across modalities, every protocol should address a number of key issues, as indicated in Table 68–2. Care in protocol development is vital to a successful study, and a major data management role is to ensure that the study plan as embodied in the protocol is feasible, consistent, and unambiguous and that the necessary tools for conducting the protocol are in place before the study commences.

TABLE 68–2. Skeleton of Protocol

Study objectives
Definition of the patient population
Registration and randomization of patients
Description of the interventions
Definitions of endpoints
Data collection
Biostatistics
Informed consent procedures

The study population is usually defined in terms of a list of eligibility criteria. Ideally, this list is short, and the exclusion factors are designed only to exclude patients inappropriate to the hypothesis under study, those for whom the intervention is inappropriate on medical grounds, or those for whom evaluation of the endpoints is likely to be compromised. Experienced data managers and nurses can play a useful role in ensuring that the appropriate tests for determining eligibility are planned and that the relevant data are recorded on the data collection forms.

The prospective registration of all patients entered on the study is important for ensuring the scientific integrity of the results. This process is usually accomplished together with randomization if the study is randomized. At a minimum, the protocol must contain enough information about the registration and randomization procedures to enable study participants to enter patients into the trial in an efficient manner and to convince scientific reviewers of the validity of the treatment assignment processes and treatment blinding procedures, if appropriate.

The interventions under study should be entirely prescribed. In practice, the treatment of cancer patients is sufficiently complex and dynamic that modifications are frequently necessary during the progress of the study. Guidelines for protocol modifications should be specified in the protocol to the maximal extent possible to minimize the likelihood of elective treatment modifications and to preserve the experimental nature of the study.

Careful, objective definitions of the primary endpoints are essential. Their absence can introduce "noise" into the results and inhibit the meaningful comparison of the results with those of similar studies. Wherever possible, accepted reporting standards should be used, such as the National Cancer Institute's (NCI) common toxicity criteria.[6] It is important that the endpoints correspond to the written study objectives in the protocol and that, if there are multiple objectives, precisely quantified endpoints be defined for each of them.

The protocol should contain a summary of the data collection schedules and a list of data collection forms to ensure that all personnel contributing to the conduct of the study are familiar with the plans. It is wise to have these materials in place before the study is activated, because it is often impossible to retrieve data retrospectively.

There are several biostatistical issues that are essential to successful protocol development. The design of the study must be justified in logical and quantitative statistical terms, and the latter must address a projected sample size. This usually involves calculations specifying the power of the study to detect statistically significant effects or the precision to which the targeted endpoints can be estimated. Formal calculations of this nature are neither relevant nor meaningful for small exploratory (*i.e.*, pilot) studies. The feasibility of the study should be addressed by projecting the accrual rate and the time required to complete the study.

Protocol development should be a team effort, with all relevant parties contributing to and understanding all aspects of the protocol. From the biostatistical and data management perspective, the major task is to ensure that the study design is capable of addressing the stated scientific hypotheses and that the logistical plans for managing the conduct of the study and collecting the data can produce a database that contains high-quality, complete data that are free from methodologic biases.

DATA COLLECTION

The process of data collection is greatly facilitated if attention is given to the creation of protocol-specific data management tools. These tools include data collection forms and various checklists to guide the study participant in the conduct of the study.

The design of the data collection forms is central to the conduct of the study, and this task requires the active involvement of the principal investigators in addition to the data manager. The forms embody the database for the study; it is in their design that the investigators come to grips with the nuts and bolts of how the scientific objectives are going to be reflected in the data with regard to the coding of endpoints and the demarcation of subsets of patients.

It is advisable to create forms that are self-coding to the maximal extent possible; text responses are minimized and as many items as possible are translated into single or multiple digit codes. This facilitates the eventual computer data entry and retrieval, and it ensures that the appropriate data summarization takes place at the optimal time with regard to access to secondary data, minimizing the risk of interpretive errors in data abstraction.[7] Another important consideration is the layout of the paper forms. They should be designed so that data items collected at approximately the same time are contiguous. The values to be entered on the computer should be positioned to maximize efficiency and ease of data entry (*e.g.*, all codes on the left-hand margin of the form, with explanatory text to the right of the code). Using boxes to collect the codes can help to enforce proper form completion, because the boxes dictate maximal field length.

Another ideal attribute of data forms is that they should be parsimonious. Investigators are inclined to want to record every datum imaginable to prevent items from being missed that eventually turn out to be important. However, the volume of data collected is inversely associated with quality.[8] The scientific credibility of any observed association is qualitatively greater if the hypothesis is targeted in the design of the study, and the collection of excessive data is likely to lead to unscientific data dredging. For all of these reasons, a tightly-organized, defined, parsimonious dataset is ideal.

If a variety of studies are being conducted on an ongoing basis, the form design and the coding conventions should reflect the continuity of the research effort. Coding conventions for outcomes, pathology, staging, and other relevant variables should be consistent across studies if feasible. This reduces the risk of transcription errors because data managers and other persons are less likely to be confused by conflicting conventions, and it facilitates the aggregation of data across studies for general statistical analyses. Consistency of coding also simplifies the task of computer database management.

Timing of data collection is usually important in cancer studies, and the precise schedule for completing the forms deserves attention. In medical oncology studies, flow sheets are often used in the clinic to record supplementary data and as a primary source for toxicity data. The flow sheets are unusual in that they represent an amalgamation of the goals of collecting data for research and providing data for clinical support.

Data collection can take place in a variety of settings, depending on the type of study. If the study investigators or nurses complete the data forms, the role of the data manager may be focussed on entering data into the computer and retrieving data for reports of the study results. In studies in which the data collection is performed by data managers and abstraction of results from the medical record or from flow sheets is involved, the data managers generally require significant knowledge of medical terminology, anatomy, and biology and expertise in specific aspects of the protocol, such as formulas for evaluating the correctness of drug dosages and similar technical issues.

It can be helpful for the data manager to create additional tools to assist in the conduct of the study and to improve protocol compliance. An eligibility checklist is useful to guard against the registration of ineligible patients. If the study is in any way complex, a patient calendar can be a useful resource to remind the physicians and nurses of the required tests and treatments throughout the course of the study. Table 68–3 displays part of such a calendar from a study of E-MVAC chemotherapy and recombinant human granulocyte colony-stimulating factor in the treatment of urothelial tract tumors. The calendar serves as a daily reminder and is designed to maximize protocol compliance. It can be amended if unscheduled delays in protocol treatment occur.

COMPUTING

Computing has become an essential feature of research data management for all but the smallest studies. A computer database allows easy and flexible access to the data for quality control and reporting purposes. Statistical analyses invariably involve the use of a computer, and many modern statistical methods are impossible to use without a computer.

What are the attributes of a good computer system for storing a clinical research study? First, it must be structured in such a way that retrieval and analysis of the data are relatively simple. An important ingredient of this is the user friendliness of the software; fortunately, the computer industry has made enormous strides in this respect in recent years. Second, the system should be designed to minimize the number of errors in the data. Many coding errors can be detected at data entry if built-in checks ensure that coded values are in the admissible range for the data item. Other logical checks can be built into any system to ensure that logically related items are consistent with each other. For example, a date of relapse should not occur later than a date of remission. Double entry of data is a technique that can virtually eliminate coding errors, at the expense of doubling the time required to enter the data. However, the quality of the computer support is only of limited usefulness without a carefully organized data management system, as outlined in the preceding sections.

The creation of a research database to encompass multiple studies presents a far greater database management challenge. It is necessary to consider the overlapping features of the individual studies, and in addition to the preceding attributes, there are many other desirable characteristics. The first concerns the consistency of a number of database features across studies. Data items that are common to different studies should

TABLE 68–3. Patient Calendar for Study of Urothelial Tumors

Day 0	Methotrexate (34 mg/m²)	Day 8	rh-G-CSF (5 µg/kg/day SQ)
Day 1	PE & KPS	Day 9	rh-G-CSF (5 µg/kg/day SQ)
	CBC & Differential counts	Day 10	CBC & differential counts
	LAP		Bone marrow (selected patients)
	SMA-12		rh-G-CSF (5 µg/kg/day SQ)
	Creatinine	Day 11	rh-G-CSF (5 µg/kg/day SQ)
	Vinblastine (3.4 mg/m²)	Day 12	rh-G-CSF (5 µg/kg/day SQ)
	Adriamycin (45 mg/m²)	Day 14	PE & KPS
	Cisplatin (70 mg/m²)		CBC & differential counts
Day 2	Differential count		LAP
Day 3	PE		SMA-12
	Differential count		Creatinine
	Creatinine		Bone marrow (selected patients)
Day 4	rh-G-CSF (5 µg/kg/day SQ)		Methotrexate (34 mg/m²)
Day 5	rh-G-CSF (5 µg/kg/day SQ)		Vinblastine (3.4 mg/m²)
Day 6	rh-G-CSF (5 µg/kg/day SQ)	(Note: Dose modification schedules should be	
Day 7	PE & KPS	examined)	
	CBC & differential count	Day 15	rh-G-CSF (5 µg/kg/day SQ)
	LAP	Day 16	rh-G-CSF (5 µg/kg/day SQ)
	SMA-12	Day 17	rh-G-CSF (5 µg/kg/day SQ)
	Creatinine	Day 18	rh-G-CSF (5 µg/kg/day SQ)
	rh-G-CSF (5 µg/kg/day SQ)	Day 19	rh-G-CSF (5 µg/kg/day SQ)
		Day 21	Methotrexate (34 mg/m²)

PE, physical examination; KPS, Karnovsky performance status; CBC, complete blood counts; LAP, leukocyte alkaline phosphatase; SMA-12, standard chemistry screen; rh-G-CSF, recombinant granulocyte colony-stimulating factor; SQ, subcutaneous.

be coded in a consistent manner, if feasible. Important common variables include stage, pathologic classifications, and tumor response criteria. Most items collected in cancer studies are applicable to a variety of sites and types of studies. Consistency of this nature facilitates aggregate analyses of multiple studies, in addition to expediting data transfer, education of new personnel, and the maintenance of quality control. A second type of consistency involves the naming of data items, and this has benefits similar to consistent coding. A third area concerns the user interface for data entry and retrieval. For example, if data entry screens are constructed with a consistent layout, data entry efficiency is improved when data entry operators or data managers are involved in a variety of studies.

A second general goal that becomes increasingly important as the number of studies and data items increase is the performance of the system. Most modern database management systems are relational, and the performance (*i.e.*, speed of operation) is determined by the manner in which the database architecture is constructed and maintained in an on-going manner by performance tuning.[9] These activities require the input of an experienced database administrator. The integration of multiple studies and investigators necessitates an effective and flexible security system to ensure that access to individual studies is limited to designated persons. As a general rule, it is advisable that data entry privileges for an individual study be severely restricted, ideally to a single person, but that access for retrieval of data be more broadly available.

There are many commercial software packages to aid in the construction of the database. Typically, database man-

agement packages provide a convenient structure and a language of commands to achieve this goal. For all but the simplest databases, it is necessary to use the package to construct the database system in the required format, and the extent of the developmental effort increases with the complexity of the database. Because the market is changing rapidly and there are many products available, it is not worthwhile to discuss the merits of individual products. However, there are two general characteristics of a product that have an important bearing on its usefulness, depending to some extent on the size and complexity of the database. The first issue is hardware independence. Many products available are designed specifically for the host computer and its operating system. However, there are nonproprietary packages that have been designed to work on a variety of hardware platforms. This capability increases the opportunity to develop a distributed database, in which parts of the database can reside on different computers, and it increases the options for changing the hardware in the future with minimal disruption. Therefore, hardware independence is an insurance against future unforeseen changes in hardware requirements. Second, many packages can now communicate with each other. This greatly facilitates data transfer. Of special importance is the link between the database and the statistical packages that are to be employed. For some products, direct links of this nature are available, permitting interactive statistical analysis and data retrieval without the user having to log in and log out of each product.

Computing is an essential component of research data

management. Modern technology offers the potential for efficient storage, retrieval, and analysis of the data, in addition to providing a valuable tool for enhancing quality control of the data. However, the construction of the database is a complex task for all but the simplest studies and requires significant expertise in computer science.

QUALITY CONTROL

There are several areas in which the quality and reliability of a research study can be compromised. We can group these into three broad categories, each of which requires an entirely different approach to quality control: accuracy of the computer record, compliance with the protocol, and accurate reporting of the results of the study.

Accuracy of the Computer Record

In transcribing results from their source (*e.g.*, point of collection, medical records, data forms) to the computer, it is desirable to minimize the number of random errors. This is an objective issue, and quality control can be influenced in an algorithmic manner. Because most computer errors are due to transcription errors by the data manager on abstracting the data (*e.g.*, from the chart) or typing errors during data entry, some of the errors are potentially identifiable by computer logical checks. For example, if a keyed value of a coded item is outside the admissible range, it can be flagged at data entry. More complex checking is also possible. For example, stage can be logically mapped to disease extent, such that inconsistencies can be identified when either item is keyed. These logical associations can apply to key dates, such as date of registration and date of response or date of death. There are many potential logical inconsistencies in a typical research database that can be used to advantage in flagging errors.

An alternative approach that can dramatically reduce typing errors is to enter all data twice, to allow the computer to match each item with itself. This technique is guaranteed to virtually eliminate all simple typing errors, at the cost of doubling the time for data entry. Although it may be advisable in some situations, it is not always necessary or practical to implement double data entry. For example, if an experienced data entry operator is keying the data, the error rate may be so low that double data entry is not cost effective. In a busy clinic environment where a nurse or data manager is keying the data, it may be unrealistic to consider this technique.

Protocol Compliance

A good research protocol clarifies in detail all aspects of the research study. Of particular importance are the definition of the source population of patients, the description of the prescribed interventions, and the definitions and schedules for evaluating endpoints. To ensure that the results of a study are reliable, it is important that the study be conducted in compliance with these protocol guidelines. Quality control in this context involves techniques for monitoring and enhancing protocol compliance.

One way to promote protocol compliance for an individual study is to carefully prepare data management tools to facilitate the conduct of the study, as outlined previously. Realistically, long-term success in this area also requires on-going evaluations of individual investigators with regard to patient management and endpoint assessment and feed-back of the results to improve performance. A useful approach is to perform random, retrospective audits for individual patients. Typically, this is not a simple thing to do because it can involve a detailed examination of the medical record for information regarding eligibility, work-up, protocol modifications, and endpoint evaluation. Medical judgments are an important ingredient of this process, and audits of this nature usually involve a team of data managers, clinicians, and possibly nurses, depending on the nature of the study. Routine audits have become a standard requirement for most of the cooperative group cancer trials in recent years.[10] Audits can be beneficial in identifying problems with the accuracy of the data recorded on forms. By comparing the study forms with the medical record, it may be possible to identify relevant events that were not reported on the forms, such as laboratory values missing from a flow sheet.

Accurate Reporting of Results

An institutional or global concern is the accuracy of the study results that are eventually disseminated through journals, conference presentations, and other media. It is vital for the process of science that the published findings be an accurate reflection of the results of the study as conducted, or the study will not be reproducible and may be misleading. For example, if the study involves 50 patients, but the investigators report the results as if only 40 had been studied without at least documenting the number of exclusions and reasons for exclusion and if the chosen 40 are selected (even unconsciously) on the basis of favorable outcomes, the implications of the reported results will be misleading and overoptimistic. It is important that the results of clinical research studies be reported factually and completely.

Quality control of research reporting is not an issue that is commonly addressed, although it is an extremely important aspect of the research process. The induced biases are probably more profound in this area than in the areas discussed in the previous sections.[11] Moreover, recent incidents of false reporting of scientific research have led to tremendously adverse publicity for the host institutions and for the field of research in general. Practical problems in setting up a system of review include the fact that individual protocols may spawn many publications, perhaps only involving subgroups of patients, but other publications may involve aggregation of data from many protocols. The sampling frame for selecting studies for auditing purposes is not obvious. This is an issue that requires development in the future.

MULTIINSTITUTIONAL STUDIES

A considerable proportion of clinical research studies undertaken are multiinstitutional studies. The multiinstitutional approach was developed in response to the need for studies with relatively large numbers of patients, especially large randomized clinical trials and studies of rare diseases. Although individual multiinstitutional studies are occasionally organized to tackle a specific high-priority objective, most of the multiinstitutional studies in cancer are conducted by one of the numerous cooperative groups of institutions, each of which conducts many studies in an ongoing basis.

The conduct of multiinstitutional studies compared with single-institution studies, presents a special organizational challenge to data management. The challenge is to ensure protocol compliance, standardization of data, and timely data collection from a large group of contributing investigators scattered geographically. The role of the coordinating center is crucial to the development and conduct of these studies. The coordinating center orchestrates all logistical aspects of the study, including registration and randomization of patients, protocol development, forms development, creation of the computer database, quality control of submitted data, and statistical analysis.

The coordinating center is responsible for consistently conducting the study at each of the contributing institutions, and it must ensure that the data are submitted in a timely fashion. To accomplish this as effectively as possible, a system of reminders is necessary to trigger the submission of relevant data forms at each stage of the protocol. Special data management tools are necessary over and above those described earlier for local studies. The coordinating center is also responsible for quality control, and much of its data processing function is geared toward monitoring the quality of the data submitted to identify inconsistencies and missing data. This can be accomplished by computer logical checks and by manual examination of the submitted data by experienced data managers. To evaluate protocol compliance, eligibility and accuracy of the data occasional audits of individual institutions are useful. This is now mandated by the NCI for the cooperative groups.[12]

Recent advances in computer technology have offered the opportunity for many of the manual aspects of this process to be bypassed by allowing remote data entry at the participating institutions, including on-line registration and randomization. In this setting, the task of the coordinating center is to create a computing environment that preserves the quality control capabilities of a central office and database, while allowing the local institutions to take advantage of the new technology. The challenge is to create a software environment that allows, for example, registration and randomization on a local workstation in a manner that preserves the scientific integrity of the registration process.

Another role of the coordinating center is the sequential monitoring of the data. The statistical monitoring of the primary endpoints may or may not involve a formal plan for terminating the study, and in this respect, the monitoring is similar to a single-institution study.[13] An additional data management role is to detect the occurrence of unforeseen adverse side effects while the trial is in progress, because individual reactions may not cause concern locally.

The general principles of data management outlined earlier are applicable to multiinstitutional studies. The multiinstitutional setting merely creates some additional logistical complexities. Multiinstitutional studies are necessary for the conduct of many types of trials due to sample size limitations at individual institutions.

CONCLUSIONS

Planning the data management of a clinical research study is a task that is crucial to its success. Failure to determine the precise data requirements for achieving the scientific objectives of the study and a suitable schedule for the data collection can seriously compromise the validity of the study, because use of medical records to obtain outcome data retrospectively is frequently problematic. Data management plans should be initiated in the earliest stages of planning the study and should address all aspects of the study, encompassing protocol development, forms development, patient registration, data collection procedures, computing, and quality control. This resource-intensive approach to data management is only worthwhile if the study objectives are of sufficient scientific importance. As Medawar pointed out, "An experiment not worth doing is not worth doing well."[14]

The conduct of the study is enhanced by the development and use of specially developed data management tools. These include carefully prepared data collection forms, eligibility checklists, patient-specific calendars to prompt scheduled interventions and tests, and other reminders and supportive documentation. The precise coding of the data and the schedule for their collection are especially important for standardizing the results.

The conclusions of the study are limited in their validity by the quality of the data, and quality control is therefore an important aspect of the process. It should involve methods to limit the number of transcription errors in abstracting and keying the data and efforts to evaluate protocol compliance, patient eligibility, and the correctness of outcomes involving judgment, such as the determination of tumor response. A frequently ignored aspect of quality control concerns the veracity of the results eventually reported in publications. Of particular concern is the completeness of the census of patients registered in the study, because the selective reporting of subgroups of patients has an important bearing on the credibility of the results.

Computing plays an increasingly important role in the conduct of clinical research. The computer is essential for data storage and statistical analysis, but it can also be used to provide tools for enhancing the conduct of the study and for improving quality control. The construction of a computer research database is not a simple task when many different kinds of studies are involved, and this aspect of clinical research is assuming an increasing share of the budget for conducting studies. For example, the conversion of the Southwest Oncology Group from a hierarchical to a relational system took 5 programmers 4 years to complete.[15] Other groups have had similar experiences.

The successful implementation of a data management system for supporting clinical research requires the input of several disciplines. The active involvement of the principal investigator and a statistician is essential to ensure that the appropriate data are recorded in a manner capable of addressing the scientific objectives of the study but free from analytic biases. Computer science personnel are usually necessary to develop and maintain an efficient database management system, except for relatively simple, individual studies. A team approach is essential for the successful conduct of clinical research.

REFERENCES

1. Peto R, Pike MC, Armitage P, et al. Design and analysis of randomized clinical trials requiring prolonged observation of each patient: I. Introduction and design. Br J Cancer 1976;34:585–612.
2. Zelen M. The randomization and stratification of patients to clinical trials. J Chron Dis 1974;27:365–375.
3. Begg CB. Selection of patients for clinical trials. Semin Oncol 1988;15:434–440.
4. Silverman WA. Human experimentation: A guided step into the unknown. New York: Oxford University Press, 1985.
5. Byar DP. The use of data bases and historical controls in treatment comparisons. Recent Results Cancer Res 1988;111:95–98.
6. Wittes RE. Manual of oncologic therapeutics. Philadelphia: JB Lippincott, 1989:627–632.
7. Van der Patten E, van der Valden JW, Siers A, Hamersma EAM. A pilot study on the quality of data management in a cancer clinical trial. Controlled Clin Trials 1987;8:96–100.
8. Knatterud GL. Methods of quality control and of continuous audit procedures for controlled clinical trials. Controlled Clin Trials 1981;1:327–332.
9. Sandberg G. A primer on relational data base concepts. IBM Syst J 1981;20:23–40.
10. Wolter JM. Quality assurance in a cooperative group. Cancer Treat Rep 1985;69:1189–1193.
11. Begg CB: Publication bias and the dissemination of clinical research. JNCI 1989;81:107–115.
12. Mauer JK, Hoth DF, Macfarlane DK, et al. Site visit monitoring program of the clinical cooperative groups: Results of the first 3 years. Cancer Treat Rep 1985;69:1177–1187.
13. O'Brien PC, Fleming TR. A multiple testing procedure for clinical trials. Biometrics 1979;35:549–556.
14. Medawar PW. The threat and the glory. New York: Harper Collins, 1990.
15. Blumenstein BA. The relational database model and multiple multicenter clinical trials. Controlled Clin Trials 1989;10:386–406.

Cancer: Principles & Practice of Oncology, Fourth Edition,
edited by Vincent T. DeVita, Jr., Samuel Hellman, Steven A. Rosenberg.
J.B. Lippincott Co., Philadelphia © 1993.

CHAPTER **69**

Newer Approaches to Cancer Treatment

SECTION **1**

STEVEN A. ROSENBERG

Gene Therapy of Cancer

Gene therapy can be defined as a therapeutic technique in which a functioning gene is inserted into the cells of a patient to correct an inborn genetic error or to provide a new function to the cell. Increased understanding of gene regulation in eukaryotic cells and the development of improved techniques for inserting and expressing foreign genes into mammalian cells have opened new possibilities for cancer therapy based on these gene transfer techniques. In May 1989, the first successful transfer of foreign genes into a human was performed in a patient with advanced melanoma.[1] This early trial using a bacterial "marker" gene led to the first gene therapy approaches with advanced cancer that began in January 1991. This chapter reviews the current status and potential future applications of gene therapy in the treatment of patients with cancer.

INTRODUCTION OF FOREIGN GENES INTO MAMMALIAN CELLS

A variety of techniques are available for the introduction of DNA into eukaryotic cells (Table 69–1), including coprecipitation with calcium phosphate, the use of polycations or lipids complexed with DNA, encapsulation of DNA in lipid vesicles or erythrocyte ghosts, or the exposure of cells to rapid pulses of high voltage electric current (*i.e.*, electroporation).[2] DNA has also been introduced into cells by direct microinjection or by the use of high-velocity tungsten microprojectiles. These techniques are capable of integrating multiple copies of DNA into the genome although the efficiency of the integration varies widely with the technique, different genes, and different cell types. The efficiency of most of these physical transfection techniques is less than 1 in 10,000 and can be lower than 1 in 1 million.

Recently techniques have been developed using viral vectors to introduce DNA into mammalian cells.[2–12] These techniques have the potential for infecting all cells exposed to the virus. In developing techniques for the use of viral vectors, it was necessary to develop vectors that stably incorporated into the target cell without damaging it. Early work used transforming DNA viruses such as papovaviruses, simian virus 40, polyomavirus, or adenoviruses. More recently, murine and avian retroviruses have been used for DNA transduction and have proven practical and safe. These retroviral vectors can infect multiple cell types, although cell replication is necessary for integration into the genome using this approach.

Retroviruses are viruses in which the viral genes are encoded in RNA rather than DNA. After infection of the cell the viral RNA is converted to DNA by the action of reverse transcriptase. The DNA then enters the nucleus and integrates randomly into the genome. This integrated provirus is indistinguishable from other cellular genes and replicates with the cell during mitosis. The integration of the provirus into the cell genome and the subsequent formation of progeny virus may have no effect on the viability of the infected cell.

Because practical applications of gene therapy involve in-

TABLE 69–1. Methods for Inserting Genes Into Mammalian Cells

Coprecipitation with calcium phosphate
Polycations complexed with DNA
Lipids complexed with DNA
Encapsulation of DNA in lipid vesicles
Exposure of cells to pulses of high-voltage electric current
 (electroporation)
Microinjection
High-velocity tungsten microprojectiles
Retroviruses
DNA viruses (*e.g.*, adenoviruses, vaccinia, herpes simplex)

---

troduction of the foreign gene by the retrovirus without actual replication of new retroviral particles in the host, special techniques using packaging cell lines have been developed.[2–12] Retroviral vectors can be produced with the deletion of the viral protein coding sequences and introduction of the exogenous gene. These modified retroviruses retain the encapsulation sequences required for production of RNA transcripts into virions and the necessary sequences for integration and expression of the vector in the host cell genome.

To obtain these replication defective vector preparations, special "packaging cell lines" were produced that contain the helper virus genome but lack the encapsulation or psi sequence. The packaging cell line cannot produce active virions that contain viral RNA. Introduction of the retroviral vector provides the necessary encapsulation sequence that in conjunction with the viral coding sequences in the packaging cell line produces virions containing the vector RNA. The most popular packaging cell lines have been derived from NIH 3T3 cells.[2–12] The possibility exists however that replication competent virus may be produced by recombination of the vector encapsulation sequences with the viral coding sequences present in the packaging cell line. A variety of workers, have engineered modifications of the packaging cell lines and the retroviral vectors to minimize the possibility of helper virus generation including deletions if specific sequences in the 5' and 3' long terminal repeats (LTR), thereby requiring at least two recombinations to produce replication competent virus. The particular retroviral vector that we have used, designated LNL6 derived from the N2 vector, was engineered to contain a stop codon at the site of the *GAG* start codon, further reducing the possibility that any competent virus would be produced.[6,7]

The development of improved retroviral vectors for introduction of genes into eukaryotic cells is an active area of current investigation. The need exists for the consistent production of high-titer virus capable of efficient transduction into a broad array of target cell lines. The need for cell replication and DNA synthesis required for provirus integration limits the usefulness of these retroviruses to the introduction of DNA into rapidly dividing cells. Although integration of the retroviral genome is often stable, in some cases, there is substantial instability of the inserted genes, and loss of inserted genetic material with cell replication can occur. The random integration of the retrovirally derived DNA into the cell genome can lead to insertional mutagenesis through disruption of es-

sential cellular genes or by activating otherwise quiescent cellular genes. A major area of current interest involves the development of retroviral vectors with appropriate internal promoters that can express multiple genes in the same retroviral construct. In retroviral vectors in which one gene is promoted by the retroviral LTR and another from internal promoters the interactions between these promoters can lead to marked inhibition of expression of one of the inserted genes.

Despite these problems, retroviral vectors represent the most efficient means of stably integrating DNA into large numbers of target cells by coincubation of the packaging cell line or the retroviral vector preparation with the target cell. Future developments are aimed at the development of retroviral vectors that can be introduced systemically into an intact animal and targeted specifically to selected cells. Although techniques for accomplishing this are not currently feasible, this represents an area of active investigation.

Viruses other than the murine and avian retroviruses are being explored for possible use as expression vectors (reviewed elsewhere[13]). Human adeno-associated viruses can be achieved in high concentrations and appear to be nonpathogenic, however difficulties in producing these preparations in the absence of contaminating helper viruses and concern about the long-term consequences of integration of these adenoviruses into cells have limited their usefulness. Vaccinia viruses, herpesviruses, bovine viruses, and papillomaviruses and others are being explored for their usefulness in gene transduction into human cells.

CANCER THERAPY USING GENE-MODIFIED TUMOR-INFILTRATING LYMPHOCYTES

STUDIES OF TUMOR-INFILTRATING LYMPHOCYTES

Tumor-infiltrating lymphocytes (TIL) are lymphocytes that infiltrate into growing tumors and can be grown by culturing single-cell suspensions obtained from tumors in interleukin-2 (IL-2).[14–21] TIL cultures can be readily established from most murine and human tumors. To prepare TIL, a single-cell suspension is made from a freshly resected tumor, generally by enzymatic digestion, and is incubated in complete medium containing IL-2. Although lymphocytes comprise a minor subpopulation of the enzymatic digest, some lymphocytes contain IL-2 receptors, presumably because of their interaction with antigens in the tumor cell surface. These lymphocytes begin to grow under the influence of IL-2 in the culture medium. Although tumor cells also grow, the lymphocytes outgrow the tumor cultures, and when these lymphocytes have specific lytic activity or lymphokine-activated killer (LAK) activity, tumor cells are destroyed. By 2 to 3 weeks after initiating the culture, pure populations of lymphocytes without contaminating tumor cells can be obtained.

Extensive studies of murine TIL have been conducted in vitro and in vivo. In vitro, murine TIL are CD8[+] and often have specific cytolytic function directed against the tumor from which they were derived.[22] TIL can specifically secrete cytokines when cocultured with their specific tumor.[23,24] Extensive in vivo studies have demonstrated the effective therapeutic impact of the administration of TIL into mice with established cancer.[14,15,23,25]

The administration of TIL plus IL-2 is from 50 to 100 times more effective than LAK cells and IL-2 in treating established 3-day lung micrometastases.[14,15] Although TIL can be specifically lytic, it appears that specific secretion of cytokines such as interferon-γ and tumor necrosis factor (TNF) are the best correlates of the in vivo antitumor effectiveness of TIL.[23] Although most specifically lytic TIL are therapeutically effective in vivo, nonlytic TIL that specifically secrete interferon-γ can also effectively eliminate established lung micrometastases. These studies of transplantable mouse tumors led to the study and application of TIL derived from human cancers.

TIL can be grown from approximately 80% of human cancers of various histologies, including melanoma, renal cell cancer, colon cancer, breast cancer, and bladder cancer.[16–21] From approximately 33% of patients with melanoma, TIL can be derived that have specific cytolytic activity for fresh cancer cells and not normal cells from the same patient, including lymphocytes, fibroblasts, or Epstein-Barr virus (EBV)-transformed B cells.[16,17,21] It is difficult, however, to generate specifically cytolytic TIL from tumors other than melanoma, and we have been unsuccessful in finding TIL with specific lysis with patients with colon cancer and breast cancer. Rare cultures from patients with renal cancer can exhibit specific cytolytic activity.[26] TIL derived from human tumors are mainly CD3$^+$ and can be CD8$^+$ or CD4$^+$ or mixtures of both. Some cultures contain CD56$^+$ non-MHC-restricted killer cells.

The specific lysis of autologous tumor by TIL is MHC restricted. Specific lysis of TIL can be inhibited by antibodies to CD3 or MHC class I molecules.[21] When specific TIL are tested against a panel of HLA-typed allogeneic melanomas, the cross-reactivity of lysis follows a pattern of HLA specificities.[27] HLA-A2 appears to be a common restriction element for the recognition of melanoma antigens on allogeneic melanomas. We transfected the gene for HLA-A2 into allogeneic non HLA-A2 melanomas and showed that HLA-A2-restricted TIL could lyse allogeneic melanomas expressing the transfected HLA-A2 gene in 6 of 6 patients.

The recognition of specific antigens by TIL has led to studies attempting to define the nature of these antigens. By repeated immunoselection using TIL with specific lysis tumor lines can be isolated that are resistant to lysis by autologous TIL.[28] These immunoselected tumors can then be used to identify multiple tumor antigens present on a single tumor.

In seeking other assays for detecting tumor specific antigens, we determined that specific cytokine release by TIL cocultured with the autologous human tumor is an indicator of specific immune recognition of tumor antigens.[24] The specific secretion of cytokines, such as granulocyte-macrophage colony-stimulating factor (GM-CSF), TNF, and interferon-γ after incubation with autologous tumor have shown patterns similar to that seen with the use of lytic TIL. Using this cytokine release assay, specific reactivity has been identified in TIL from patients with breast cancer and melanoma. We are currently exploring the use of this assay to identify tumor-specific antigens in other tumors.

In pilot trials, the treatment of patients with advanced melanoma using TIL plus IL-2 has resulted in objective responses in 38% of 50 patients.[29] This is approximately twice the level of response seen with IL-2 alone or LAK cells plus IL-2. Prior nonresponsiveness to therapy with IL-2-based regimens does not compromise the ability to respond to TIL plus IL-2 therapy. In vitro lysis of autologous tumor by TIL has a weak but significant correlation with clinical response, and we are currently testing whether specific cytokine release correlates with clinical response.[30]

Studies have been conducted in patients with metastatic melanoma treated with TIL labeled with indium 111 to test whether administered TIL localized to tumor deposits.[31–32] Clear tumor localizations of TIL were seen on 13 of 18 nuclear scan series. Similarly, paired biopsies of tumor and normal skin showed a substantial concentration of ^{111}In-labeled TIL in tumor compared with normal skin. It appears that TIL can concentrate in tumor deposits. Approximately 0.015% of the injectate accumulates per gram of tumor. The accumulation of TIL in tumor has played an important role in the development of gene therapies using TIL transduced with cytokine genes.

GENE TRANSFERS INTO HUMANS USING TUMOR-INFILTRATING LYMPHOCYTES

Attempts to follow the in vivo distribution and survival of human TIL after systemic administration to humans were limited by the problems associated with using radioactive ^{111}In as a label for the cells. ^{111}In has a half-life of 2.8 days, and the combination of the natural decay of the isotope and the spontaneous release of ^{111}In from the cell limited the time we could use these cells for study to 1 to 2 weeks. The autoirradiation of the TIL by the ^{111}In led to potential damage of the TIL, which could alter their function. Information was needed about how long infused TIL persisted in vivo, where they were located in the body, and whether the in vivo accumulation of TIL at the tumor site, draining lymph nodes, or in the circulation correlated with clinical antitumor effect. The opportunity to reisolate administered TIL from the tumor site would also provide information about the functional characteristics of TIL that traffic to tumor sites and whether any of these properties correlated with in vivo antitumor effects.

The introduction of new genes into TIL provided a possibility for genetically marking the cell to answer many of these questions. An introduced gene has many potential advantages as a cell marker that no other exogenous label can provide. The label becomes part of the permanent genome of the cell and does not leach away from the original cell, as would a radioactive label. The label is not diluted as the cells proliferate, and every daughter cell is labeled. The label is lost as soon as the cell dies and does not become sequestered or reused in other cells. The vital function of the cells is not changed by the marker label. A new functional property, such as the use of a selectable marker gene, can be introduced into the cell that would permit the specific recovery of the marked cells. Depending on the gene inserted, sensitive detection methods are available, such as the polymerase chain reaction (PCR), which enable the identification of as few as one marked cell in one million unmarked cells.

A clinical protocol was conducted using retroviral mediated gene transfer to introduce the gene coding for neomycin phosphotransferase, a bacterial protein capable of rendering the cell resistant to G418, a neomycin analog otherwise lethal to all eukaryotic cells.[1] Because gene transfer studies had never been approved in humans, the potential risks and benefits of this proposed technology were carefully analyzed by a variety of review groups, including the Clinical Research Committees of the National Cancer Institute; the National Heart, Lung and Blood Institute; the National Institutes of Health (NIH) Biosafety Committee; the Gene Therapy Subcommittee of the Recombinant DNA Advisory Committee (RAC), the full RAC, and the Food and Drug Administration. Final approval was required from the Director of the NIH, who gave his approval to proceed in January 1989. A variety of factors were considered by these review groups. It was necessary to demonstrate that marker genes could insert and express in human TIL, that the marked TIL were not significantly altered, that the marked cells could be detected in animal models, and that there was low risk to the patient and no risk to the public in using this new technology.

In initial studies, TIL obtained from cancer patients were grown in culture and transduced with the retroviral vector N2 from the PA317 packaging cell line.[6] N2 was a derivative of the Moloney murine leukemia virus in which the *GAG*, *POL*, and *ENV* genes were removed or truncated and the bacterial NeoR gene inserted. To further decrease the development of replication, competent virus the LNL6 vector was derived from the N2 vector.[7] This vector contained a stop codon at the site of the gag start codon. Substitution of the 5′

Moloney leukemia virus sequences with those of the Moloney sarcoma virus sequences minimized the homology between the vector and helper virus genome, which decreased the potential frequency of recombination. The PA317/LNL6-C8 cell line was used to produce the transduction vector used in these clinical studies and provided high-titer retroviral vector without helper virus contamination.

A variety of preclinical studies preceded the clinical administration of gene transduced TIL into humans.[33-34] These studies were conducted with the N2 and the LNL6 vectors.

The gene coding for neomycin phosphotransferase could be readily introduced into human TIL using these vectors.[1,33,34] An example of the growth of the nontransduced and transduced TIL in IL-2 is shown in Figures 69–1 and 69–2. Examples of the ability of the transduced cells to resist exposure to the neomycin analog G418 are also shown in these figures. Only the transduced and not the nontransduced cells could grow in G418 concentrations of 0.4 mg/ml or higher.

The proviral sequences in transduced TIL populations were demonstrated on Southern blots by hybridization of *Sac*1-digested DNA with ^{32}P-labeled NeoR probes (Fig. 69–3). A single copy of the expected 3.2-kb NeoR-hybridizing fragment was present without rearrangement or deletion in the transduced TIL populations but was not detectable in nontransduced cells. The integration and expression of the transduced TIL

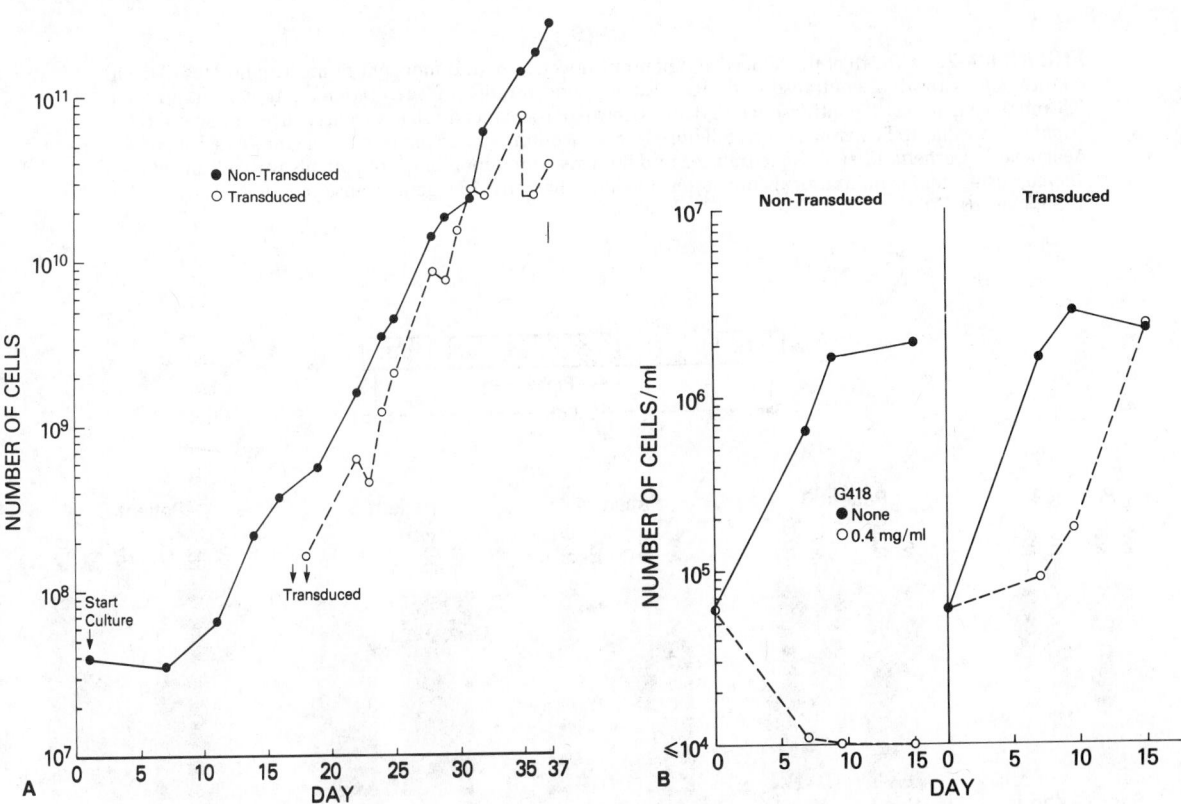

FIGURE 69–1. Growth of nontransduced and transduced human tumor-infiltrating lymphocytes (TIL) in culture. When TIL reach approximately 3×10^8 cells, an aliquot is transduced, and the transduced and nontransduced cells are grown in parallel. **(A)** Growth rates for the two populations appear to be similar. **(B)** The effect of 0.4 mg/ml of G418 on nontransduced and transduced TIL. The nontransduced TIL die in the presence of G418. The transduced TIL show a short lag after exposure to G418 and then begin to grow at a rate equivalent to that of the nontransduced cells. (Kasid A, Morecki S, Aebersold P, et al. Human gene transfer: Characterization of human tumor-infiltrating lymphocytes as vehicles for retroviral-mediated gene transfer in man. Proc Natl Acad Sci USA 1990;87:473–477)

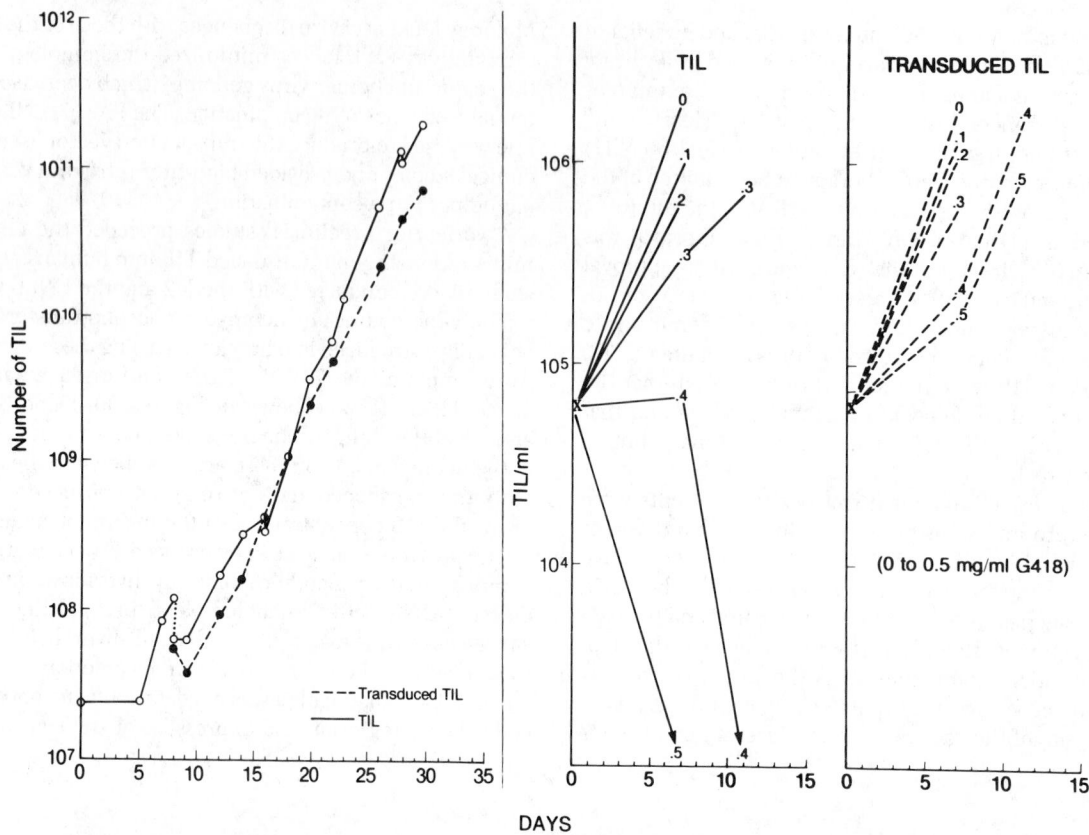

FIGURE 69–2. Growth of transduced and nontransduced human tumor-infiltrating lymphocytes (TIL) in culture (*left*). Growth of nontransduced TIL in varying concentration of G418 (*middle*). At concentrations of 0.4 and 0.5 mg/ml G418, nontransduced TIL die. Growth of transduced TIL in various concentrations of G418 (*right*). Transduced TIL grow successfully in G418 concentrations as high as 0.5 mg/ml. (Rosenberg SA, Aebersold P, Cornetta K, et al. Gene transfer into humans—Immunotherapy of patients with advanced melanoma, using tumor-infiltrating lymphocytes modified by retroviral gene transduction. N Engl J Med 1990;323:570–578)

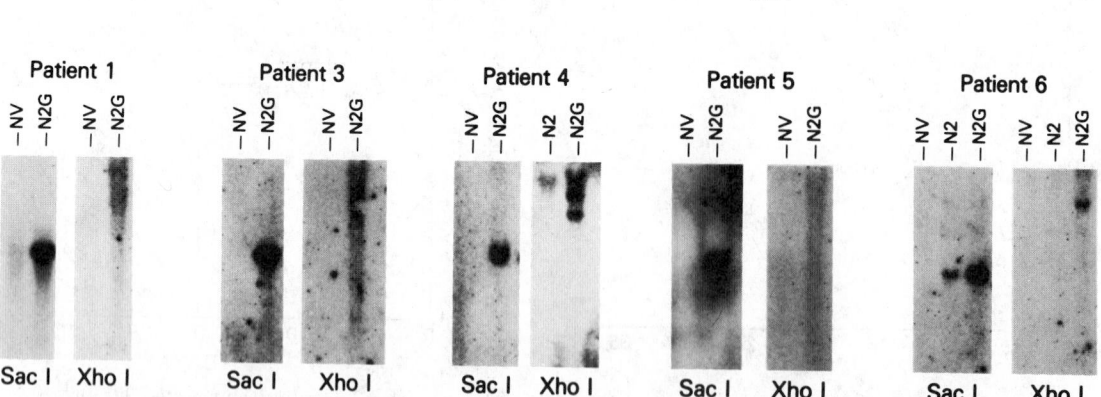

FIGURE 69–3. Detection and integration of vector DNA in human tumor infiltrating lymphocytes (TIL) transduced with the *NeoR* gene. The *Sca*1-digested DNA shows the expected 3.2 kilobase *NeoR* hybridizing fragment in the transduced but not in the nontransduced cells. The *Sca*1-digested DNA revealed multiple clones of transduced TIL containing proviral DNA integrated into different sites of the host chromosome. (Kasid A, Morecki S, Aebersold P, et al. Human gene transfer: Characterization of human tumor-infiltrating lymphocytes as vehicles for retroviral-mediated gene transfer in man. Proc Natl Acad Sci USA 1990;87:473–477)

appeared stable during extended cell cultures even in the absence of G418. Restriction digest with *Sca*, which did not cut within the provirus, revealed multiple clones of transduced TILs containing proviral DNA integrated into different sites of the chromosome. Neomycin phosphotransferase activity could also be demonstrated in the transduced cells.

Extensive tests were performed on the transduced and nontransduced populations to test whether the transduction procedure altered the phenotypic and functional characteristics of the TIL.[1,33] Because the antigenic specificity of the TIL depended on the presence of T-cell receptors, we used human genomic and cDNA probes specific for β and γ T-cell receptors to study the pattern of gene rearrangement in the TIL.[33] As illustrated in Figure 69–4, T-cell receptor-β gene rearrangements appeared similar in the nontransduced and transduced selected populations. The study of Northern blots for cytokine mRNA expression revealed similar patterns between the transduced and the nontransduced TIL; TIL expressed mRNA for TNF-α and TNF-β but not for IL-6, GM-CSF, IL-1β or interferon-γ.[33] Similarly, studies of the phenotype and cytotoxicity of transduced and nontransduced cells appeared to reveal substantial similarity unaffected by cell transduction. It appeared from these studies that the gene for *NeoR* could be inserted and expressed in human TIL and that the marked TIL were not significantly altered.

Before initiating clinical trials, studies were performed to see if marked cells could be detected in animals.[34] Despite extensive efforts, it has not been possible to introduce genes into short-term murine lymphocyte cultures by any available technique. Extensive efforts have been made using retroviral vectors, calcium phosphate precipitation, and electroporation to stably insert genes into short-term murine cultures without

success. It has, however, been possible to insert genes into selected long-term mouse lymphocyte lines, and these long-term cultures were used to test the detection and recovery of marked cells in animal models. Culver and coworkers inserted the *NeoR* gene into long-term cultures of sperm whale myoglobin specific murine helper T cells (clone 14.1), which were maintained by repeated cycles of stimulation in vitro with myoglobin in the presence of antigen presenting cells.[34] These murine helper T cells were transduced with the N2 vector and the retroviral SAX vector, which expressed *NeoR* and human adenosine deaminase genes. After selection of these cells in G418, they were injected into nude mice to test the persistence of the cells in vivo. In these studies, G418-resistant cells were readily recovered from the spleens of recipient animals several months after injection. These cells could be grown in vitro and shown to express neomycin phosphotransferase activity. Animal experiments suggested that marked cells could survive and could be recovered in animal models, although it should be emphasized that these studies were not performed with murine TIL.

Safety considerations were paramount in our preclinical evaluation of the use of retroviral vectors for transduction of human cells.[1,35] Sterility tests and tests for replication competent virus capable of detecting one viral particle per milliliter of solution were performed on the viral supernatants and on the gene modified cells after expansion in culture. In no case did we ever find evidence of replication competent viruses in cells administered to patients.

After presentation of much of this information to the appropriate regulatory committees, permission was received to treat as many as 10 patients with advanced melanoma having life expectancies of 90 days or less. In these trials patients

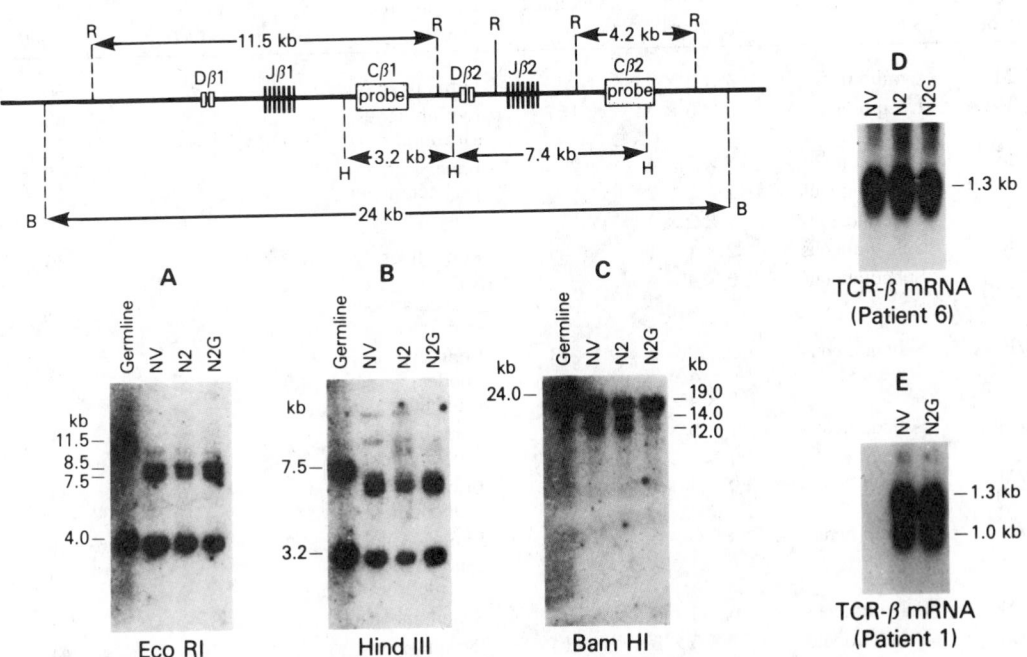

FIGURE 69–4. T-cell receptor-β gene rearrangements in nontransduced and transduced tumor-infiltrating lymphocytes. Similar patterns of gene rearrangements were seen in the transduced and nontransduced populations. (Kasid A, Morecki S, Aebersold P, et al. Human gene transfer: Characterization of human tumor-infiltrating lymphocytes as vehicles for retroviral-mediated gene transfer in man. Proc Natl Acad Sci USA 1990;87:473–477)

received an aliquot of gene modified cells with nonmodified cells as part of their standard TIL treatment for advanced melanoma.[1,29] Ten patients with advanced melanoma were treated using *NeoR* gene-modified cells. The results in the first 5 patients have been published.[1] The characteristics of the 10 patients are presented in Table 69–2. They vary in age from 26 to 52, and all had extensive melanoma with multiple lesions, including lesions in brain, lung, liver, subcutaneous tissue, adrenal gland, and other sites. Characteristics of the infused gene transduced and nontransduced TIL administered to the first 5 patients are also presented in Table 69–3.

Lymphocytes grew to a maximum of 63,400-fold over a 65-day period. Estimates of the percent of transduced cells by semiquantitative PCR analysis revealed that from 1% to 11% of the cells were transduced. Semiquantitative Southern blot analysis estimated that 4% to 18% of cells were transduced. In each patient, evidence for the insertion of the *NeoR* gene was demonstrated using Southern blots. Expression of the neomycin phosphotransferase was detected in all of the transduced cell populations and none of the nontransduced cells. The expression of the *NeoR* gene was demonstrated by successfully culturing TIL from 4 of the 5 initial patients in the neomycin analog G418.

A primary goal of our studies was the detection of these gene-marked cells in blood and tumor samples. Samples of peripheral blood and tumor samples were taken from all pa-tients before and at various times after the infusion. Because of the pattern of tumor spread, multiple tumor biopsies could not be obtained from all patients. PCR analyses were performed in a blinded fashion by at least two investigators, and the results on all positive samples were confirmed in a second independent assay. The results of these assays on the first 5 patients is presented in Figure 69–5. Circulating peripheral blood mononuclear cells containing the *NeoR* gene were consistently present in the first 19 to 22 days after cell infusion. Cells were detected in the peripheral blood on day 51 in 1 patient and on day 60 on another patient. One of the patients underwent resection of a lesion 64 days after the infusion of gene modified cells. TIL in this specimen contained the *NeoR* gene, and TIL were reinfused on day 94. In this patient, gene-modified cells were detected in the circulation on day 121 and day 189 after the initial infusion.

An attempt was made to estimate the number of gene-modified cells in the circulation using semiquantitative PCR analysis.[1] In patient 1 the incidence of transduced TIL in peripheral blood was approximately 1 in 5000 mononuclear cells on day 1, 1 in 8000 on day 2, and 1 in 16,000 on day 4 after cell infusion. Another patient had 1 transduced cell in 300 on day 3, 1 in 1500 on day 6, 1 in 3000 on day 14, and 1 in 10,000 on day 19. TIL grown from the tumor in one of the patients grew successfully in G418, indicating that the *NeoR* gene was present and was expressed in these cells. Multiple

TABLE 69–2. Characteristics of Patients Receiving Tumor-Infiltrating Lymphocytes Transduced With the NeoR Gene

Patient	Age/Sex	Site	Size (cm)	Total No. of Cells Obtained ($\times 10^{-7}$)	Sites of Evaluable Disease	Day of Transduction	Total Days of Growth	Fold Expansion*
1	52/M	Lymph node	4 × 4 × 2	33	Lung, liver spleen	13	60	16,100
2	46/F	Lymph node	5 × 5 × 3	157	Lymph nodes, intramuscular	19	65	5,000
3	42/M	Lymph node	6 × 5 × 4	205	Lung, subcutaneous	12	48	35,100
		Subcutaneous	2 × 2 × 2					
		Subcutaneous	2 × 2 × 2					
4	41/M	Subcutaneous	2 × 1 × 1	41	Lung, liver, lymph nodes, subcutaneous brain	16	36	9,500
		Subcutaneous	5 × 4 × 4					
5	26/F	Subcutaneous (6 sites)	2 × 2 × 2 to 5 × 4 × 2	71	Lung, lymph nodes, subcutaneous	8	30	5,300
6	38/M	Subcutaneous	17 × 9 × 6	150	Lymph nodes, subcutaneous	21	36	12,818,000
7	43/M	Lymph node	5 × 4 × 3	100	Brain, subcutaneous	21	71	4,000
8	53/M	Lymph node	4 × 3 × 3	22	Lung, subcutaneous, retroperitoneum,	20	36	79,400
9	30/M	Subcutaneous	6 × 4 × 3	100	Subcutaneous	31	41	2,300
10	30/M	Subcutaneous	5 × 5 × 3	14	Lymph nodes, intraperitoneal	20	41	10,000

* Calculated fold expansion of cells administered. Not all cultured cells were given; some cells were diverted for experimental studies or lost to contamination.

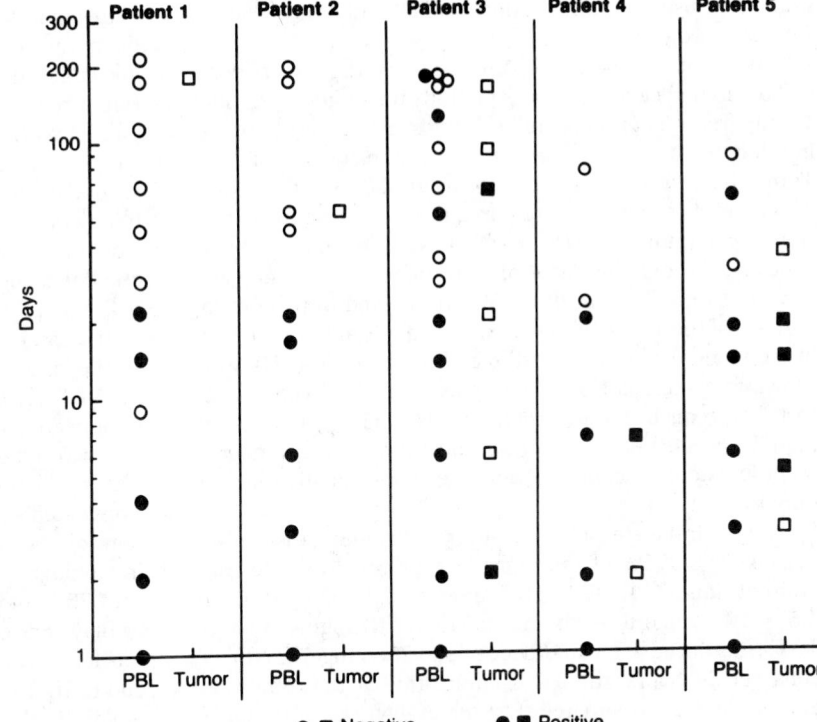

FIGURE 69–5. Results of polymerase chain reaction assays on peripheral blood mononuclear cells and tumor biopsy of 5 patients receiving *NeoR* gene-modified tumor-infiltrating lymphocytes (TIL). Gene-modified cells were consistently seen in the circulation for approximately 21 days after infusion. *NeoR* gene-modified TIL were found in tumor biopsies up to 64 days after TIL infusion. (Rosenberg SA, Aebersold P, Cornetta K, et al. Gene transfer into humans—Immunotherapy of patients with advanced melanoma, using tumor-infiltrating lymphocytes modified by retroviral gene transduction. N Engl J Med 1990;323:570–578)

specimens taken at autopsy performed on 3 patients who received gene-modified cells about 6 months earlier revealed no PCR-positive cells, with the exception of one specimen in a single renal cortex biopsy that was thought to be a false positive; the opposite renal cortex was negative.

Two of the 10 patients had an objective regression of cancer, including 1 patient who had complete regression of multiple lung lesions, subcutaneous deposits, and oral mucosal deposits, which has persisted for more than 2 years. The antitumor effects were due to the TIL and IL-2 treatment and not to any direct function of the modified gene.

All of the safety studies in the patients have been negative. All viral supernatants used for gene transduction and all infused TIL were sterile for bacteria, fungi, and mycoplasma and negative on S⁺L⁻ assays for ecotropic, xenotropic, and amphotropic infectious viruses and on NIH 3T3 amplification tests. PCR analysis for the presence of the amphotropic helper virus 4070A envelope genes and reverse transcriptase assays of all TIL were negative. All infused TIL stopped growing shortly after IL-2 was withdrawn from the culture medium. Western Blot assays of the patient's serum to antibodies to 4070A viral P30 GAG protein and S⁺L⁻ assays for virus performed at various times up to 180 days after cell infusion were negative.[1]

These studies demonstrated that it was possible to use retroviral mediated gene transfer to introduce foreign genes into cells that could be readministered safely to humans.[1] These studies also showed that small numbers of lymphocytes could persist for long periods in the circulation and at tissue sites and suggested that TIL might be suitable vehicles for the introduction of other genes that might improve the therapeutic efficacy of these cells or be suitable for the introduction of genes to correct inherited genetic defects, such as severe combined immunodeficiency disease based on adenosine deaminase deficiency.

THERAPY USING TUMOR-INFILTRATING LYMPHOCYTES TRANSDUCED WITH THE GENE FOR TUMOR NECROSIS FACTOR

Initial studies using TIL transduced with the *NeoR* gene provided the basis for attempts of the gene therapy of cancer using TIL transduced with genes that would increase their therapeutic efficacy. The first gene selected for these studies was the gene coding for production and secretion of the cytokine TNF.

A variety of considerations led to the hypothesis that TIL secreting large amounts of TNF would increase the therapeutic efficacy of the TIL. Extensive animal research in the Surgery Branch, NCI, and in many other groups demonstrated that the injection of recombinant TNF could mediate the necrosis and regression of a variety of established experimental murine cancers.[36–38] The combined administration of TNF and IL-2 mediated far greater antitumor effects against subcutaneous and liver tumors than either cytokine alone.[39] The exact mechanisms of the antitumor effects of TNF are not clearly understood, although it appears that TNF has a significant effect on the vascular supply of tumors.[38] Membrane-bound TNF may be involved in direct tumor lysis as well.[40]

The animal experiments led to extensive tests of recombinant human TNF administered to humans with advanced cancer.[41–45] In the Surgery Branch, NCI, 38 patients with advanced cancer were treated using escalating doses of recombinant TNF administered in conjunction with IL-2.[41] No antitumor effects of TNF administration were seen in these studies nor were antitumor responses seen after bolus or continuous infusion administration of TNF in multiple other studies as well.

The reason for the discrepancy between the effectiveness of TNF in mice and humans is not fully understood, although an important factor appears to be the substantial differences in tolerance of mice and man to the administration of TNF. Tumor-bearing mice can tolerate from 400 to 500 μg/kg of TNF, and these doses are required to mediate tumor regression; the administration of less TNF is far less effective.[38] In contrast, the maximal dose of TNF tolerated by humans is approximately 8 μg/kg/day.[41] When injected intravenously, only 2% of the TNF dose required to mediate antitumor effects in the mouse can be administered to man. Because TIL were shown to accumulate at tumor deposits, it was hypothesized that TIL producing large amounts of TNF might generate very high TNF concentrations in the local tumor microenvironment and achieve concentrations capable of mediating antitumor effects.

Using ^{111}In-labeled TIL, measurements in humans showed that about 0.015% of the injected cells can traffic to each gram of tumor.[31,32] Of 3×10^{11} injected TIL, approximately 4.5×10^7 traffic to each gram of tumor. If highly selected TNF-transduced TIL can produce up to 2500 mg of TNF/10^6 cells per 24 hours, the TIL accumulating at the tumor site can produce approximately 112 mg of TNF/kg of tumor. If we estimate that only a small percentage of the tumor is the interstitial fluid volume, the equivalent TNF concentration in the interstitial fluid should exceed the 400 ug/kg that murine models predict is necessary to mediate tumor destruction. These concentrations at the tumor site are approximately 100 times the concentration that can be achieved at the tumor in humans by the intravenous injection of TNF.

An indirect estimate of the impact of high local concentrations of TNF at the tumor site may be achieved by introducing the gene for TNF into murine tumors and studying the effects of this TNF secretion on the growth of these tumor cells when injected in vivo. These studies using cytokine genes transduced into tumors are considered in more detail in a subsequent section of this chapter. Transduction of tumors with the TNF gene can result in the production of from 10 to 12 ng of TNF/10^6 cells/24 hours.[46] Nontransduced tumor cells do not produce TNF. When the murine tumors producing TNF are injected into syngeneic mice, they grow to about 5 mm and then often spontaneously regress, leading to the cure of mice. Nontransduced tumors or tumors transduced with *NeoR* gene alone grow and kill the mice.

In similar studies, the TNF gene was introduced into human melanoma cells and injected into nude mice. These tumor cells grow and then often regress while nontransduced human tumors grow and kill the nude mice. Local production of TNF by human tumors can also lead to their destruction. We have not detected TNF in the serum of animals bearing TNF-transduced tumors. When transduced tumors have been removed from animals and placed back into culture, assays of culture supernatants have shown that these cells are continuing to make TNF.

These studies have shown that high local concentrations of TNF in the tumor microenvironment can lead to tumor regression and hold promise that TIL accumulating at tumor sites producing large amounts of TNF might lead to tumor regression in humans.

In support of this hypothesis are studies in which TNF has been injected directly into tumor nodules in humans. Bartsch and colleagues injected TNF directly into tumors and observed tumor regression in 1 of 3 melanoma patients.[47] An additional patient with a squamous cell cancer of the oral pharynx and a patient with malignant histiocytoma also showed significant shrinkage after TNF was injected into the tumor. A double blind, randomized, placebo-controlled study of the intralesional injection of recombinant TNF was reported by Kahn and colleagues.[48] One Kaposi's sarcoma lesion was injected with recombinant TNF and another Kaposi's sarcoma lesion in the same patient was injected with the same volume of sterile saline. The TNF reduced the cross-sectional area of 12 (92%) of 13 of the injected lesions and caused a complete disappearance of two lesions. The placebo response rate was 7%, with no complete response observed ($p < 0.01$). There was no observed disease progression in any TNF treated lesion. These studies suggested that achieving high local concentrations of TNF at the tumor site could lead to tumor regression in humans.

In 25 patients with metastatic renal cell cancer reported by Blay and colleagues using LAK cells and IL-2, a correlation was found between serum levels of TNF at 48 hours after the end of IL-2 infusion and response to this immunotherapy.[49] Studies in the Surgery Branch using TIL in animals also suggested that those TIL that specifically secreted cytokines, including TNF, were the TIL with the most potent antitumor activities, and this cytokine secretion correlated far better than direct tumor lysis with the antitumor efficacy of TIL against established metastases.[23] These studies suggested that secretion of TNF by lymphocytes might play a role in the response to immunotherapy and increased production of TNF might increase therapeutic effects. Clinical trials were begun with humans using the systemic administration of TIL transduced with the gene for TNF.

The TNF retroviral vector used in these studies was generated by inserting the native full-length human TNF-cDNA gene containing the native signal peptide sequence into the retroviral vector LXSN developed by Miller and colleagues.[10–12] A schematic representation of the TNF retroviral vector is shown in Figure 69–6. The human TNF gene is promoted by the retroviral LTR and the *NeoR* gene by the SV40 early promoter. Both the promoters are placed in the same orientation. To prevent synthesis of viral proteins from the vector, alterations have been made in the basic vector backbone, including insertion of a stop codon in place of the *GAG* start codon. Similarly, part of the vector has been replaced with the homologous region from the Moloney murine sarcoma virus which is very similar to the Moloney murine leukemia virus but does not make a glycosylated protein. The TNF vector producing cell lines were generated by transfection of the PA317 packaging cell line as discussed earlier in this review.

Although this retroviral vector readily transduced murine and human tumor cells with *TNF* and *NeoR* genes, it was more difficult to get consistent transduction and expression of the *TNF* gene in human TIL. Despite multiple attempts to optimize the transduction procedure, transduction efficiencies in the range of 0.1% to 10% have been common. Some patients' TIL appear to be more readily transduced than others, and the reasons underlying this difference are unclear. Using se-

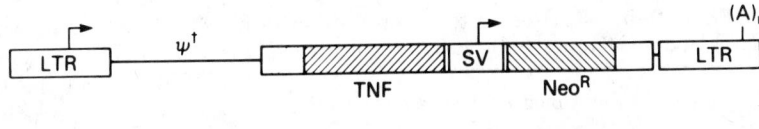

FIGURE 69–6. Schematic diagram of the tumor necrosis factor (TNF) *NeoR* retroviral construct. The TNF gene is promoted by the retroviral long terminal repeat (LTR) and the *NeoR* gene promoted by the SV40 early promoter.

lection in G418, it was possible in one study to increase the percent of transduced cells from $3.2 \pm 1.0\%$ to $57.8 \pm 7.5\%$ (Table 69–3). The increased secretion of TNF was stable over time (Table 69–4). It has been possible to achieve TNF production by transduced TIL in selected patients in excess of 100 pg/10^6 cells/24 hours, and in selected cells, TNF levels in excess of 500 pg/10^6 cells/24 hours have been achieved in some patients. TIL producing TNF grow well in culture and retain their growth dependence on IL-2.

After extensive review, the protocol for the use of these TNF gene-modified TIL was approved and treatment of patients with TNF-modified TIL begun on January 29, 1991. A schema of the approved protocol is shown in Table 69–5. In this protocol, escalating numbers of TNF transduced TIL are administered to patients in the absence of IL-2 administration. This cautious escalation of the use of TNF-transduced TIL was instituted because of the potential toxic side effects that could be induced in patients due to the TNF secretion. As of April, 1992, 6 patients have been entered into this protocol, and it is too early to determine whether TIL producing TNF will be more effective than unmodified TIL (Table 69–6). These studies represent a prototype for the use of TIL potentially modified by other genes for use in the gene therapy of cancer.

OTHER POTENTIAL MODIFICATIONS OF TUMOR-INFILTRATING LYMPHOCYTES FOR CANCER THERAPY

In addition to the introduction of the *TNF* gene into TIL, several other genetic modifications of TIL may improve their therapeutic efficacy. A list of some of these possibilities is shown in Table 69–7.

TABLE 69–3. Transduction of Human Tumor-Infiltrating Lymphocytes With the Genes for Tumor Necrosis Factor and Neomycin Phosphotransferase

Concentration of G418 Used for Selection (mg/ml)	No. of Patients	Percentage of Transduced Cells (Mean ± SEM)*
0	10	3.2 ± 1.0
0.1	4	9.0 ± 2.0
0.3	12	40.9 ± 6.5
0.5	9	57.8 ± 7.5

* Estimated on semiquantitative Southern blots after 5 days of selection in G418.
(Hwu, et al. J Immunol [in press])

The increased local secretion of interferon-α or interferon-γ by TIL may have antitumor effects for several reasons. Interferon-α has a direct antiproliferative effect against some tumor cell types, and high local concentrations at the tumor site may impede tumor growth. In addition, interferon-α and interferon-γ can upregulate major histocompatibility antigens and other molecules on the cell surface, such as tumor antigens or adhesion molecules and increase the immunogenicity of these tumor cells. The introduction of other cytokine genes that may be involved in antitumor activity such those for as IL-6, IL-1α, IL-7, and RANTES, may also have antitumor effects because of their ability to modulate the immune response at the tumor site.

Modifications of tumor cells that do not affect secretory functions but could alter a different functional aspect of the cell might be useful. TIL do not bear Fc receptors and therefore cannot mediate antibody-dependent cellular cytotoxicity. However, because TIL target to tumor sites and have cytolytic capacity, the transduction of TIL with the gene for Fc receptors may induce the ability to mediate antibody-dependent cellular cytotoxicity and be a potent therapeutic tool in conjunction with the administration of monoclonal antibodies.

TIL depend on IL-2 for their continued survival, and the high doses of IL-2 required to cause TIL proliferation in vivo can be associated with substantial toxicity when administered to patients. Transduction of the gene for IL-2 receptors into TIL may increase the sensitivity of TIL to administered IL-2 and lessen the need for the high doses currently required.

TABLE 69–4. Tumor Necrosis Factor Production in Transduced Tumor-Infiltrating Lymphocytes

Patient Number	Days After Transduction	TNF (pg/ml/10^6 cells/ 24 h) No Vector	Transduced*
1142.9†	34	5	380
	45	10	119
	52	8	554
1143.A†	24	55	245
	31	62	216
	49	53	228
888 MEL‡	18	0	28,280
	97	0	31,170

* Transduced TIL selected in 0.3–0.5 mg/ml G418 for 5 days. Transduced tumor (888 MEL) selected continuously in 0.6 mg/ml G418. The increased secretion of TNF was stable over time.
† Representative patient TIL cultures.
‡ Melanoma cell line.

TABLE 69–5. Revised Protocol for Administering *TNF*-Modified Tumor-Infiltrating Lymphocytes

1. Escalate *TNF*-modified TIL *twice weekly;* no IL-2.
$$10^8 \text{ cells}$$
$$3 \times 10^8$$
$$10^9$$
$$3 \times 10^9$$
$$10^{10}$$
$$3 \times 10^{10}$$
$$10^{11}$$
$$3 \times 10^{11}$$
2. Reduce cell dose to *one tenth* of maximal tolerated dose. Escalate as in (1) every *3 weeks* with 180,000 IU of IL-2 per 1 kg body weight.
3. After treating 3 patients, discuss with the FDA (possibly start at a higher cell dose with IL-2).

Eshhar and his coworkers provided an intriguing possibility for extending the use of TIL to tumors for which reactive monoclonal antibodies exist.[50] These workers made chimeric T-cell receptors by combining the genes coding for the constant region of the T-cell receptor with the variable region of monoclonal antibodies. When these genes are transfected into hybridoma cells, they confer the reactivity of the monoclonal antibody to the hybridoma. These chimeric T-cell receptors can result in triggering lysis or cytokine release from the appropriate hybridoma line. An example of this phenomenon is shown in Table 69–8. We are currently attempting to produce chimeric T-cell receptors by using the constant region of the human T-cell receptor with the variable region of monoclonal antibodies that recognize human gastrointestinal or ovarian tumors. The transduction of these chimeric T-cell receptor genes into TIL may induce the TIL to exhibit the non MHC restricted reactivity of the monoclonal antibody.

GENE THERAPY OF CANCER USING TUMOR TRANSDUCED WITH CYTOKINE GENES TO INCREASE IMMUNOGENICITY

The introduction of genes coding for cytokines into tumor cells can increase the immunogenicity of tumor cells and decrease tumor growth.[46,51-58] The potential use of these gene-modified tumor cells for active immunization against cancer or for the generation of lymphocytes to be used in adoptive immunotherapy represents an attractive approach to the gene therapy of cancer. The introduction of cytokine genes into tumor cells can also provide a sensitive assay for identifying cytokines with antitumor activity and elucidate the types of tumor cells susceptible to this type of cytokine gene therapy. A summary of studies introducing cytokine genes into murine tumors is shown in Table 69–9.

Tepper and colleagues introduced the gene for interleukin-4 (IL-4) into the J558L BALB/c plasmacytoma and the K485

TABLE 69–6. Gene Therapy With Tumor-Infiltrating Lymphocytes Transduced With the Gene for Tumor Necrosis Factor

Patient Number	Age	Sex	Sites of Metastatic Disease	Cell Doses Administered
1	30	F	Brain, subcutaneous, adrenal	1.1×10^8
				3.0×10^8
				1.0×10^9
				3.0×10^9
				5.4×10^9
2	44	M	Lymph nodes, subcutaneous, intramuscular	1.0×10^8
				3.1×10^8
				1.1×10^9
				3.0×10^9
3	53	F	Liver, subcutaneous, retroperitoneum	1.0×10^8
				3.0×10^8
				9.6×10^8
				3.0×10^9
				1.0×10^{10}
				2.4×10^{10}
				1.0×10^{11}
				$1.0 \times 10^{10} + \text{IL-2}$
				$2.8 \times 10^{10} + \text{IL-2}$
				$9.0 \times 10^{10} + \text{IL-2}$
4	25	M	Brain, lung, subcutaneous, mediastinum	1.0×10^9
				1.0×10^{10}
				4.2×10^{10}
5	30	M	Lymph nodes, subcutaneous	$8.5 \times 10^9 + \text{IL-2}$
				$1.1 \times 10^{11} + \text{IL-2}$
6	48	M	Lung, lymph nodes	$3.0 \times 10^{10} + \text{IL-2}$
				$4.9 \times 10^{10} + \text{IL-2}$

TABLE 69–7. Genetic Modification of Tumor-Infiltrating Lymphocytes for Use in the Gene Therapy of Cancer

Gene Insertion	Rationale
Tumor necrosis factor	Interfere with the blood supply of tumors
Interferon-α or -γ	Upregulate major histocompatibility antigens on tumors and increase susceptibility to T-cell killing
Cytokines, (e.g., IL-1 α, IL-6, IL-7, RANTES)	Modulate immune response to tumors
Fc receptor	Enable TIL to mediate antibody dependent cellular cytotoxicity
Chimeric T-cell receptor (constant region of T-cell receptor and variable region of monoclonal antibody)	Broaden the specificity of TIL recognition of tumors
IL-2 receptor	Increase the sensitivity of TIL to administered IL-2

mammary cancer.[51] IL-4 was studied because of its ability to activate MHC-restricted and MHC-unrestricted cytotoxic lymphocytes and macrophages. Tumor cells expressing the IL-4 gene showed reduced tumor growth that was related to the secretion of IL-4. The mixture of nontransfected with transfected tumor cells resulted in growth inhibition, indicating that the local production of IL-4 could lead to antitumor effects against parental tumor cells at the same site although no effect was seen on tumor cells at distant sites. The rejection of the IL-4-producing tumors was associated with a dense macrophage and eosinophil infiltrate at the tumor site.

Many workers, including Fearon and coworkers,[52] Gansbacher and colleagues,[53] and Ley and associates,[54] introduced the *IL2* gene into tumor cells using calcium phosphate transfection or retroviral mediated gene transduction. These workers used different tumors including colon cancer, melanoma, sarcomas, and mastocytomas, and all showed that introduction and expression of the *IL2* gene could lead to inhibition of growth of the tumor. This activity could be blocked by anti-CD8 or anti-MHC class I antibodies. CD8$^+$ cells were required in vivo to mediate these effects. Fearon and colleagues hypothesized that the failure of the immune response to the parental tumor was due in part to the failure of T-cell help that could be overcome by the local production of cytokines such as IL-2.[52]

Asher and coworkers conducted extensive studies of the retroviral mediated transduction of the *TNF* gene into mouse sarcomas, and these studies are used here as an example of the results obtained by other workers using the *TNF* gene and genes coding for other cytokines.[46] The introduction of *TNF* genes into a murine sarcoma and subsequent cloning of the tumor cells revealed that different clonal tumor populations had widely varying but stable expression of TNF secretion. An example of the variation of TNF secretion in clonal tumor lines is shown in Figure 69–7. TNF can exist in a secreted or membrane-bound form and both types of TNF were found in these tumor cells.

Cells secreting high levels of TNF would grow to a size of several millimeters and then often spontaneously regressed. In contrast, cells producing low or no levels of TNF grew progressively and killed the animals (Fig. 69–8). The growth inhibition could be inhibited by the administration of anti-TNF antibodies, as shown in Figure 69–9. The mechanism of tumor rejection was related to an immune effect in the host; lymphocyte depletion in the mouse using antibodies to CD4$^+$ or CD8$^+$ T-cell subpopulations could result in abrogation of tumor inhibition. It appeared that both cell subpopulations were necessary to mediate antitumor effects. As was shown by other investigators using other cytokine genes, the mixture of cytokine-producing cells and noncytokine-producing parental cells resulted in the inhibition of the mixture. Studies by Blankenstein and associates[55] and Teng and colleagues[56] using a BALB/c plasmacytoma and a UV-induced skin tumor, respectively, showed tumor growth inhibition that could be blocked by anti-TNF antibody and *TNF* gene-modified tumor cells.

Other cytokines are being studied for their potential to reduce tumor growth when introduced into tumor cells. No effect

TABLE 69–8. Transfecting Chimeric T-Cell Receptor Genes That Alter the Specificity of MD.45 Hybridoma Line

Transfected Chimeric Genes*	Stimulator Cells					
	EL-4†	A20‡	TNP A20	TNP Mouse Spleen	TNP Human Lymphocyte	TNP KLH
	(IL-2 production, U/ml)					
	17	0	0	0	0	0
$V_L C_\beta$	50	0	0	1	1	0
$V_H C_\beta$	15	0	23	5	2	6
$V_H C_\beta + V_L C_\alpha$	72	0	108	10	20	150

* Variable region from anti-TNP antibody plus constant region of T cell receptor
† MD.45: Murine hybridoma that lyses H-2^b target cells (EL-4)
‡ A20: B cell lymphoma from BALB/c mice (H-2^d)
(Gross G, Waks T, Eshhar Z. Expression of immunoglobulin T-cell receptor chimeric molecules as functional receptors with antibody-type specificity. Proc Natl Acad Sci USA 1989;86:10024–10028)

TABLE 69–9. Introduction of Cytokine Genes Into Murine Tumors

Gene Inserted	Investigations	Tumor	Method	Comments
IL-4	Tepper et al[51]	J558L BALB/c plasmacytoma K485 mammary cancer	Electroporation or calcium phosphate	Tumor growth reduced or eliminated; related to IL-4 secretion; nontransfected cells at same site inhibited; dense macrophage and eosinophil infiltrate
IL-2	Fearon et al[52]	CT26 BALB/c colon cancer B16 C57BL/6 melanoma	Calcium phosphate	Mediated generation of CTL; activity blocked by anti-CD8 and anti-MHC class I antibodies; tumor growth inhibited; CD8+ cells required in vivo
	Gansbacher et al[53]	CMS-5 BALB/c sarcoma	Retroviral transduction	Tumor growth inhibited; correlated with IL-2 secretion; CTL activity induced; nontransduced cells at same site
	Ley et al[54]	P815 DBA/2 mastocytoma	Not stated	Growth inhibited
TNF	Asher et al[46]	MCA-205 C57BL/6 sarcoma	Retroviral transduction	Tumor growth inhibited; correlated with TNF secretion; blocked by anti-TNF antibody; membrane-associated TNF detected; nontransduced cells at same site inhibited
	Blankenstein et al[55]	J558L BALB/c plasmacytoma	Retroviral transduction	Tumor growth inhibited; blocked by anti-TNF antibody and anti-TNF antibody and anti-CR3 antibody; dense macrophage infiltrate (IL-6 transfected tumor showed no growth inhibition)
	Teng et al[56]	1591 UV induced skin tumor	Liopfection or calcium phosphate	Tumor growth inhibited; mediated generation of CTL; increased membrane class I expression
Interferon-γ	Gansbacher et al[57]	CMS-5 BALB/c sarcoma	Retroviral transduction	Tumor growth inhibited; mediated generation of CTL; increased membrane class I expression
G-CSF	Colombo et al[58]	C-26 BALB/c colon cancer	Retroviral transduction	Tumor growth inhibited; blocked by anti-G-CSF antibody; tumor growth inhibited in nude mice

IL, interleukin; TNF, tumor necrosis factor; G-CSF, granulocyte colony-stimulating factor.

was seen by Blankenstein and coworkers after introducing the *IL6* gene into tumors.[55] Gansbacher and associates saw tumor growth inhibition after introducing the gene for interferon-γ into the CMS-5 BALB/c sarcoma.[57] This growth inhibition was associated with an increased expression of membrane class I antigens. Colombo and colleagues introduced the gene for granulocyte colony stimulating factor (G-CSF) into the C26 BALB/c colon cancer and showed growth inhibition that could be blocked by anti-G-CSF antibody.[58]

Golumbek and colleagues demonstrated that active immunization with *IL4* gene-modified tumor cells could reduce the growth of established tumor deposits at distant sites in mice.[59] It is possible that the use of other cytokines or cytokines in combination may provide a more potent immune stimulus sufficient to reduce growth or cause regression of distant tumors.

Alternatively, the use of gene-modified tumor cells could be used to generate immune lymphocytes for use in the adoptive immunotherapy of cancer. Fearon and coworkers[52] and

Gansbacher and colleagues[53] showed that IL-2-modified tumor cells could induce the generation of specific cytotoxic T lymphocytes that could not be raised to the original parental tumor. Experiments are underway to use these cytolytic cells for the adoptive therapy of established tumor deposits.

Based on these considerations, a clinical protocol has been developed to use tumor cells modified by transduction with the *IL2* and *TNF* genes for the treatment of patients with advanced cancer. A schema of the protocol is shown in Table 69–10.

OTHER APPROACHES TO GENE THERAPY

Many innovative techniques are being proposed to apply the technology of gene manipulation to cancer treatment. Several of these current approaches are summarized in Table 69–11.

In contrast to gene modification of lymphocytes and tumor cells ex vivo as discussed previously, several groups have ex-

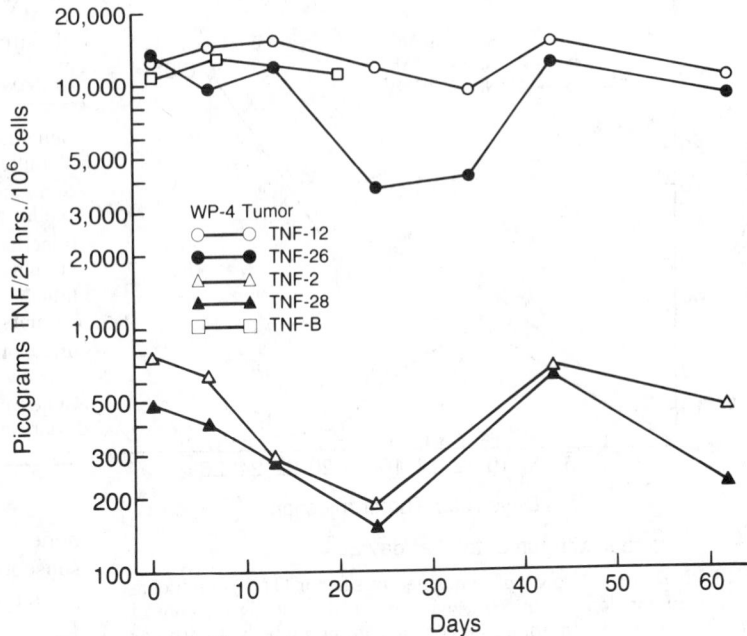

FIGURE 69–7. Secretion of tumor necrosis factor (TNF) by transduced murine tumor cell lines. Some clones produced higher levels of TNF than other clones and this production was consistent over 2 months of growth in culture. (Asher AL, Mulé JJ, Reichert CM, et al. Studies of the anti-tumor efficacy of systemically administered recombinant tumor necrosis factor against several murine tumors in vivo. J Immunol 1987;138:963–974)

plored approaches to the direct injection of genes into tumors in situ. Nabel and colleagues have proposed using DNA in liposomes for direct injection of the gene coding for the HLA-B7 alloantigen into tumors.[60] Murine studies have suggested that these liposomes are taken up by cancer cells and the DNA is incorporated into the cell genome. The expressed foreign alloantigen is then designed to trigger an immune response that stimulates immune reactions against bystander nonmodified tumor cells. Roth and colleagues have proposed injecting, directly into tumors, antisense genes intended to block the effects of the K-RAS gene that is involved in cell proliferation.[61,62] Alternate approaches to inject P53 suppressor genes directly into cancers in an attempt to suppress cell growth are also being explored.

Several groups are attempting to use "suicide" genes in cancer treatment. Culver and colleagues have developed an approach to the treatment of experimental brain tumors using the direct injection into brain cancers of a cell line producing retroviral particles carrying the herpes thymidine kinase (TK) gene.[63] The incorporation of the TK gene into tumor cells will make them sensitive to the drug gancyclovir. In this approach it is hoped that the death of cells containing the TK gene will cause a "bystander effect," which will result in the death of adjacent cancer cells as well. Attempts to use this approach in patients with brain cancer have begun at the National Institutes of Health. Freeman and colleagues have proposed using the TK gene inserted into ovarian cancer cells that will then be injected into the tumor-bearing host. Treatment with

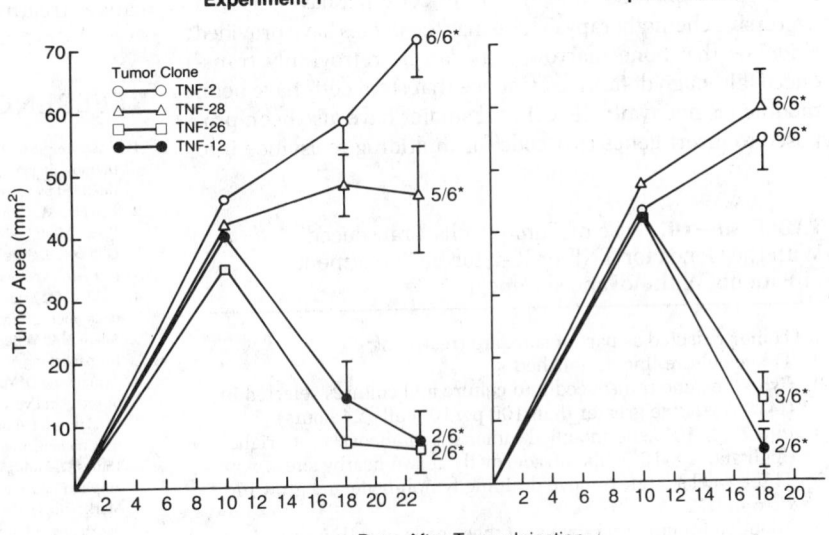

FIGURE 69–8. Growth of tumor necrosis factor (TNF)-producing murine tumor clones after injection into mice. High-producing TNF clones grew for about 10 days and then regressed, but low-producing clones grew progressively and resulted in death of the mice. (Asher AL, Mulé JJ, Reichert CM, et al. Studies of the anti-tumor efficacy of systemically administered recombinant tumor necrosis factor against several murine tumors in vivo. J Immunol 1987;138:963–974)

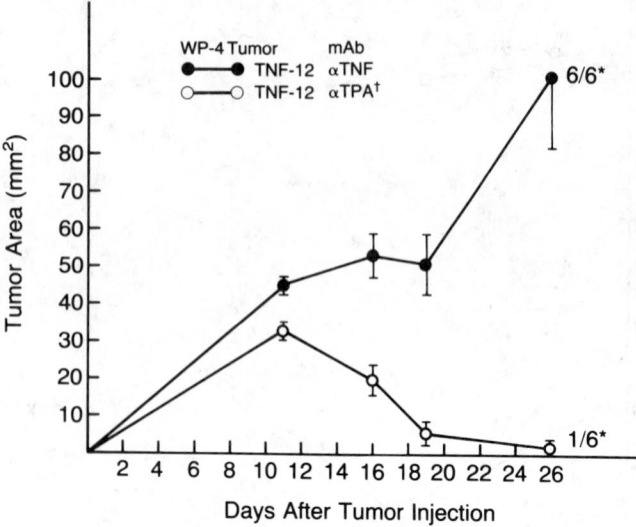

*Number with tumor/total at day 28

FIGURE 69–9. Growth of tumor necrosis factor (TNF)-producing murine tumor clones in mice receiving anti-TNF antibody or a control anti-TPA antibody. In animals receiving control antibody, the tumor grew for approximately 11 days and then regressed. Progressive tumor growth was seen after anti-TNF antibody was administered, indicating that TNF production is involved in the regression of these TNF gene-modified tumors. (Asher AL, Mulé JJ, Reichert CM, et al. Studies of the anti-tumor efficacy of systemically administered recombinant tumor necrosis factor against several murine tumors in vivo. J Immunol 1987;138:963–974)

gancyclovir results in the destruction of these cells and possible lysis of adjacent tumor cells as well. This approach is being directed toward the treatment of patients with diffuse intraperitoneal ovarian cancer.

Approaches to introduce foreign genes into bone marrow cells have also been proposed in patients with cancer. Brenner and colleagues at St. Jude Children's Research Hospital have inserted marker genes into the bone marrow cells of children with acute myeloid leukemia or neuroblastoma. These studies are designed to determine whether recurrence after autologous bone marrow transplantation is caused by cancer cells in the retransplanted bone marrow or cells that have survived aggressive chemotherapy. These marker studies have provided evidence that bone marrow cells can be retrovirally transduced, although definitive evidence that stem cells have been modified is not available. Clinical studies have also been proposed to insert genes that code for multidrug resistance into

TABLE 69–10. Use of Tumor Cells Transduced With the Genes for TNF or IL-2 for the Treatment of Patients With Advanced Cancer

1. Tumor resected as part of standard treatment
2. Tissue culture line established
3. Cytokine gene transduced into culture and cultures selected in G418 (cytokine greater than 100 pg/10^6 cells/24 hours)
4. Inject 2×10^8 gene-modified tumor subcutaneously into right thigh and 2×10^7 cells intradermally at two nearby sites.
5. Three weeks later, remove draining lymph node and grow in vitro in IL-2.
6. Adoptive immunotherapy using these cells plus IL-2

TABLE 69–11. Current Approaches to the Gene Therapy of Cancer in Humans

Approach	Aim
Gene modification of lymphocytes	Increase antitumor activity
Gene modification of tumor cells	Increase tumor immunogenicity
Injection of class I genes into tumors	Increase tumor immunogenicity
Injection of antisense genes into tumors	Block expression of oncogenes
Injection of retroviral producer lines into tumors	Introduce "suicide" genes into cancer cells
Gene modification of bone marrow cells	Increase resistance to chemotherapeutic drugs

bone marrow cells to attempt to protect the marrow against subsequent aggressive chemotherapy treatment. This approach may allow larger doses of chemotherapy to be used.

CONCLUSIONS

Ongoing studies are using gene transfer technology for the development of new approaches to cancer treatment. Initial studies using TIL modified by transduction with the *NeoR* gene showed that retroviral mediated gene transfer can be safely and practically used for the introduction of genes into humans. Attempts are underway to use this technology to introduce the genes for TNF into TIL to attempt to improve the therapeutic efficacy of these cells. Other approaches to the gene therapy of cancer involve attempts to modify tumor cells to increase their immunogenicity for use in active immunization against cancer or to raise immune lymphocytes for use in adoptive transfer. Some researchers are attempting to clone the gene that codes for tumor antigens in animal and human systems. The identification of these genes could potentially result in their incorporation into viruses for use in active immunization against cancer that may have applications for cancer treatment and prevention.

REFERENCES

1. Rosenberg SA, Aebersold P, Cornetta K, et al. Gene transfer into humans—Immunotherapy of patients with advanced melanoma, using tumor-infiltrating lymphocytes modified by retroviral gene transduction. N Engl J Med 1990;323:570–578.
2. Kriegler M. Gene transfer and expression. A laboratory manual. New York: Stockton Press, 1990:1–242.
3. Gilboa E, Eglitis MA, Kantoff PW, et al. Transfer and expression of cloned genes using retroviral vectors. Biotechniques 1986;4:504–512.
4. Eglitis MA, Anderson WF. Retroviral vectors for introduction of genes into mammalian cells. Biotechniques 1988;6:608–614.
5. Adam MA, Miller AD. Identification of a signal in a murine retrovirus that is sufficient for packaging of nonretroviral RNA into virions. J Virol 1988;62:3802–3806.
6. Armentano D, Yu SF, Kantoff PW, et al. Effect of internal viral sequences on the utility of retroviral vectors. J Virol 1987;61:1647–1650.
7. Bender MA, Palmer TD, Gelinas RE, et al. Evidence that the packaging signal of Moloney murine leukemia virus extends into the *gag* region. J Virol 1987;61:1639–1646.
8. Danos O, Mulligan RC. Safe and efficient generation of recombinant retroviruses with amphotropic and ecotropic host ranges. Proc Natl Acad Sci USA 1988;85:6460–6464.
9. Markowitz D, Goff S, Bank A. Construction and use of a safe and efficient amphotropic packaging cell line. Virol 1989;167:400–406.
10. Miller AD, Buttimore C. Redesign of retrovirus packaging cell lines to avoid recombination leading to helper virus production. Mol Cell Biol 1986;6:2895–2902.

11. Miller AD, Trauber DR, Buttimore C. Factors involved in the production of helper virus-free retrovirus vectors. Somatic Cell Mol Genet 1986;12:175–183.

12. Miller AD, Rosman GJ. Improved retroviral vectors for gene transfer and expression. Biotechniques 1989;7:980–986.

13. Friedmann T. Progress toward human gene therapy. Science 1989;244:1275–1281.

14. Rosenberg SA, Spiess P, Lafreniere R. A new approach to the adoptive immunotherapy of cancer with tumor-infiltrating lymphocytes. Science 1986;223:1318–1321.

15. Spiess PJ, Yang JC, Rosenberg SA. In vivo antitumor activity of tumor-infiltrating lymphocytes expanded in recombinant interleukin-2. JNCI 1987;79:1067–1075.

16. Muul LM, Spiess PJ, Director EP, et al. Identification of specific cytolytic immune responses against autologous tumor in humans bearing malignant melanoma. J Immunol 1986;138:989–995.

17. Itoh K, Tilden AB, Balch CM. Interleukin 2 activation of cytotoxic T-lymphocytes infiltrating into human metastatic melanomas. Cancer Res 1986;46:3011–3017.

18. Kurnick JT, Kradin RL, Blumberg R, et al. Functional characterization of T lymphocytes propagated from human lung carcinomas. Clin Immunol Immunopathol 1986;38:367–380.

19. Rabinowich H, Cohen R, Bruderman I. Functional analysis of mononuclear cells infiltrating into tumors: Lysis of autologous human tumor cells by cultured infiltrating lymphocytes. Cancer Res 1987;47:173–177.

20. Miescher S, Whiteside TL, Moretta L, et al. Clonal and frequency analyses of tumor-infiltrating T lymphocytes from human solid tumors. J Immunol 1987;138:4004–4011.

21. Topalian SL, Solomon D, Rosenberg SA. Tumor-specific cytolysis by lymphocytes infiltrating human melanomas. J Immunol 1989;142:3714–3725.

22. Barth RJ, Bock SN, Mulé JJ, et al. Unique murine tumor-associated antigens identified by tumor infiltrating lymphocytes. J Immunol 1990;144:1531–1537.

23. Barth RJ, Mulé JJ, Spiess PJ. Interferon gamma and tumor necrosis factor have a role in tumor regressions mediated by murine CD8⁺ tumor-infiltrating lymphocytes. J Exp Med 1991;173:647–658.

24. Schwartzentruber DJ, Topalian SL, Mancini M, et al. Specific release of granulocyte-macrophage colony-stimulating factor, tumor necrosis factor-α, and IFN-γ by human tumor-infiltrating lymphocytes after autologous tumor stimulation. J Immunol 1991;146:3674–3681.

25. Yang JC, Perry-Lalley D, Rosenberg SA. An improved method for growing murine TIL with in vivo antitumor activity. J Biol Response Modif 1990;9:149–159.

26. Belldegrun A, Muul LM, Rosenberg SA. Interleukin 2 expanded tumor-infiltrating lymphocytes in human renal cell cancer: Isolation, characterization, and antitumor activity. Cancer Res 1988;48:206–214.

27. Hom SS, Topalian SL, Simoni ST, et al. Common expression of melanoma tumor-associated antigens recognized by human tumor-infiltrating lymphocytes: Analysis by HLA restriction. J Immunother 1991;10:153–164.

28. Topalian SL, Kasid AL, Rosenberg SA. Immunoselection of a human melanoma resistant to specific lysis by autologous tumor infiltrating lymphocytes: Possible mechanism for immunotherapeutic failures. J Immunol 1990;144:4487–4495.

29. Rosenberg SA, Packard BS, Aebersold PM, et al. Use of tumor-infiltrating lymphocytes and interleukin-2 in the immunotherapy of patients with metastatic melanoma. A preliminary report. N Engl J Med 1988;319:1676–1680.

30. Aebersold P, Hyatt C, Johnson S, et al. Lysis of autologous melanoma cells by tumor infiltrating lymphocytes: Association with clinical response. JNCI 1991;83:932–937.

31. Fisher B, Packard BS, Read EJ, et al. Tumor localization of adoptively transferred indium-111 labeled tumor infiltrating lymphocytes in patients with metastatic melanoma. J Clin Oncol 1989;7:250–261.

32. Griffith KD, Read EJ, Carrasquillo JA, et al. In vivo distribution of adoptively transferred indium-111 labeled tumor infiltrating lymphocytes and peripheral blood lymphocytes in patients with metastatic melanoma. JNCI 1989;81:1709–1717.

33. Kasid A, Morecki S, Aebersold P, et al. Human gene transfer: Characterization of human tumor-infiltrating lymphocytes as vehicles for retroviral-mediated gene transfer in man. Proc Natl Acad Sci USA 1990;87:473–477.

34. Culver K, Cornetta K, Morgan R, et al. Lymphocytes as cellular vehicles for gene therapy in mouse and man. Proc Natl Acad Sci USA 1991;88:3155–3159.

35. Cornetta K, Morgan RA, Anderson WF. Safety issues related to retroviral-mediated gene transfer in humans. Human Gene Ther 1991;2:5–14.

36. Carswell EA, Old LJ, Kassel RC, et al. An endotoxin-induced serum factor that causes necrosis of tumors. Proc Natl Acad Sci USA 1975;72:3666–3670.

37. Wang AM, Creasy AA, Ladner MB, et al. Molecular cloning of the complementary DNA for human tumor necrosis factor. Science 228:149–154.

38. Asher AL, Mulé JJ, Reichert CM, et al. Studies of the anti-tumor efficacy of systemically administered recombinant tumor necrosis factor against several murine tumors in vivo. J Immunol 1987;138:963–974.

39. McIntosh JE, Mulé JJ, Merino MJ, et al. Synergistic antitumor effects of immunotherapy with recombinant interleukin-2 and recombinant tumor necrosis factor-alpha. Cancer Res 1988;48:4011–4017.

40. Kriegler M, Perez C, DeFay K, et al. A novel form of TNF/cachectin is a cell surface cytotoxic transmembrane protein: Ramifications for the complex physiology of TNF. Cell 1988;53:45–53.

41. Rosenberg SA, Lotze MT, Yang JC, et al. Experience with the use of high-dose interleukin-2 in the treatment of 652 cancer patients. Ann Surg 1989;210:474–485.

42. Spriggs Dr, Sherman ML, Michie H, et al. Recombinant human tumor necrosis factor administered as a 24-hour intravenous infusion. A phase I and pharmacologic study. JNCI 1988;80:1039–1044.

43. Sherman ML, Spriggs DR, Arthur KA, et al. Recombinant human tumor necrosis factor administered as a five-day continuous infusion in cancer patients: Phase I toxicity and effects on lipid metabolism. J Clin Oncol 1988;6:344–350.

44. Feinberg B, Kurzrock R, Talpaz M, et al. A phase I trial of intravenously-administered recombinant tumor necrosis factor-alpha in cancer patients. J Clin Oncol 1988;6:1328–1334.

45. Moritz T, Niederle N, Baumann J, et al. Phase I study of recombinant human tumor necrosis factor alpha in advanced malignant disease. Cancer Immunol Immunother 1989;29:144–150.

46. Asher AL, Mulé JJ, Kasid A, et al. Murine tumor cells transduced with the gene for tumor necrosis factor-α. Evidence for paracrine immune effects of tumor necrosis factor against tumors. J Immunol 1991;146:3227–3234.

47. Bartsch HH, Pfizemaier K, Schroeder M, et al. Intralesional application of recombinant human TNF factor alpha induces local tumor regression in patients with advanced malignancies. Eur J Cancer Clin Oncol 1989;25:285–291.

48. Kahn J, Kaplan J, Zeigler P, et al. Phase II trial of intralesional recombinant tumor necrosis factor alpha (rTNF) for aids associated Kaposi's sarcoma (KS). Proc Am Soc Clin Oncol 1989;8:4.

49. Blay JY, Favrot MC, Negrier S, et al. Correlation between clinical response to interleukin-2 therapy and sustained production of tumor necrosis factor. Cancer Res 1990;50:2371–2374.

50. Gross G, Waks T, Eshhar Z. Expression of immunoglobulin T-cell receptor chimeric molecules as functional receptors with antibody-tupe specificity. Proc Natl Acad Sci USA 1989;86:10024–10028.

51. Tepper RI, Pattengale PK, Leder P. Murine interleukin-4 displays potent anti-tumor activity in vivo. Cell 1989;57:503–512.

52. Fearon ER, Pardoll DM, Itaya T, et al. Interleukin-2 production by tumor cells bypasses T helper function in the generation of an antitumor response. Cell 1990;60:397–403.

53. Gansbacher B, Zier K, Daniels B, et al. Interleukin 2 gene transfer into tumor cells abrogates tumorigenicity and induces protective immunity. J Exp Med 1990;172:1217–1224.

54. Ley V, Roth C, Langlade-Demoyen P, et al. A novel approach to the induction of specific cytolytic T cells in vivo. Res Immunol 1990;141:855–863.

55. Blankenstein T, Qin Z, Uberla K, et al. Tumor suppression after tumor cell-targeted tumor necrosis factor α gene transfer. J Exp Med 1991;173:1047–1052.

56. Teng MN, Park BH, Koeppen HKW, et al. Long-term inhibition of tumor growth by tumor necrosis factor in the absence of cachexia or T-cell immunity. Proc Natl Acad Sci USA 1991;88:3535–3539.

57. Gansbacher B, Bannerji R, Daniels B, et al. Retroviral vector-mediated γ-interferon gene transfer into tumor cells generates potent and long lasting antitumor immunity. Cancer Res 1990;50:7820–7825.

58. Colombo MP, Gerrari G, Stoppacciaro A, et al. Granulocyte colony-stimulating factor gene transfer suppresses tumorigenicity of a murine adenocarcinoma in vivo. J Exp Med 1991;173:889–897.

59. Golumbek PT, Lazen by AJ, Levitsky, HI, et al. Treatment of established renal cancer by tumor cells engineered to secrete interleukin-4. Science 1991;254:713–716.

60. Stewart MJ, Plautz GE, Del Buono L, et al. Gene transfer in vivo with DNA-liposome complexes: Safety and acute toxicity in mice. Hum Gene Ther 1992;3:267–275.

61. Roth JA, Mukhopadhyay T, Tainsky MA, et al. Molecular approaches to prevention and therapy of aerodigestive tract cancers. Review article. Monogr Natl Cancer Inst 1992;13:15–21.

62. Mukhopadhyay T, Tainsky M, Cavender AC, Roth JA. Specific inhibition of K-ras expression and tumorigenicity of lung cancer cells by antisense RNA. Cancer Res 1991;51:1744–1748.

63. Culver KW, Ram Z, Wallbridge S, et al. In vivo gene transfer with retroviral vector-producer cells for treatment of experimental brain tumors (see comments). Cellular Immunology Section, National Cancer Institute, National Institutes of Health, Bethesda, MD. Science 1992;256:1550–1552.

SECTION **2**

ZVI Y. FUKS
SAMUEL HELLMAN

Three-Dimensional Conformal Radiotherapy

Three-dimensional conformal radiation therapy (3D-CRT) is a mode of high precision radiotherapy. It is based on treatment designs which shape the isosurface of a given radiation dose to accurately conform the anatomic boundaries of the tumor in its entire three-dimensional configuration. Dynamic modes or multiple static coplanar and noncoplanar field arrangements are used to build the tumor dose while concomitantly minimizing the dose to the surrounding normal tissues. This approach permits increased tumor doses beyond those feasible with current conventional two-dimensional (2D) radiotherapy without increasing the risk of normal tissue complications. The improved tumor coverage and the increased tumor dose are likely to improve tumor control, although the benefit from 3D-CRT still must be demonstrated. 3D-CRT has been implemented using photon beams, protons, or heavy charged particles. In this chapter, we limit the discussion to 3D conformal photon-beam radiotherapy only.

Until several years ago, photon-beam 3D therapy was not considered practical, because its planning and implementation require the use of powerful computers not readily available at the time. The emergence of new computer technologies in the last decade enabled an accelerated development of several of the systems essential for full-scale 3D-CRT programs. New 3D treatment planning systems, powerful workstations capable of fast computations of elaborate mathematical functions, specialized computer-driven radiation producing machines, multileaf collimators, and on-line imaging devices that monitor automated treatments and assure their quality, have recently been introduced for patient use in several centers. The current clinical experience, although based on only a few hundred patients treated so far, indicates that this approach has an enormous potential and should become available for routine clinical use in the foreseeable future.

BIOLOGIC BASIS OF THREE-DIMENSIONAL CONFORMAL RADIOTHERAPY

The specific goal of 3D conformal radiotherapy is to improve the likelihood of local tumor control. Efforts to develop 3D-CRT in this context can be justified only if improved local control can be shown to have a significant impact on the overall therapeutic outcome. Because of the inability to define the boundaries between tumor and normal tissues, radiation target volumes have classically included a "safety" margin of surrounding normal tissue. Treatments have been frequently constrained by normal tissue tolerance rather than by specific tumor parameters. When attempts were made to increase tumor doses, reductions in the normal tissue safety margins were required, frequently leading to inadvertent tumor misses and subsequent marginal recurrences.[1-4] Although the intro-

duction of computed tomography (CT)-assisted treatment planning has significantly improved the ability to define tumor target volumes for radiation beams, the problem of geographic misses has not been completely eliminated because of the limited use of CT information in conventional 2D treatment planning.[5,6] Only one or a few CT slices are used, mostly at the level of the central axis, and treatment planning at off-center levels is not based on detailed CT anatomic information.

The new techniques of 3D treatment planning provide complete anatomic and dose information for the entire tumor volume, and recent studies using 3D systems have indeed documented significant improvements in target coverage as compared with CT-assisted 2D treatment planning.[7,8] However, improved tumor coverage in itself is apparently not sufficient to produce maximal local tumor control. Local failure after radiotherapy is related to the degree of inherent radioresistance of the tumor clonogenic stem cells and to a variety of epigenetic and microenvironmental factors.[9-13] Because some of these parameters vary significantly even within the same tumor, it leads to clonal heterogeneity in terms of the sensitivity to the effects of radiation.[14] This apparently contributes to the observed phenomenon that in many human tumors the relation of tumor control probability to dose is substantially shallower than would be expected from the Poisson distribution that describes the randomness of cell killing by ionizing radiation.[15] There have been concerns that in many human tumors a significant dose escalation will be required before an effect on local control is detected.[15] However, underdosed regions within the tumor or marginal misses may contribute to "flattening" of dose-response curves. Besides causing local failures, such geometric and dosimetric inaccuracies would flatten the population average of dose-response curves and obscure the beneficial effects of dose increases in achieving improved local control. The use of 3D-CRT is likely to eliminate or minimize these sources of uncertainty and should maximize the likelihood of observing dose effects on the probability of local control.

Another major concern has been that efforts to improve survival by enhancement of local control alone may be offset by the subsequent appearance of metastatic disease, arising from micrometastases already present at the time of initial diagnosis.[16,17] However, clinical and experimental studies on patterns of failure after curative locoregional therapy (*i.e.,* surgery, radiotherapy) show that the incidence of metastatic disease significantly increases when initial treatment fails to control the primary tumor.[1,4,18] A recent study of 679 surgically staged B-C/NO prostatic cancer patients treated at Memorial Sloan-Kettering Cancer Center with interstitial ^{125}I source implantations showed that the actuarial 15-year distant metastasis-free survival for 351 locally controlled patients was 77%, compared with 24% in 328 patients who relapsed locally ($p > 0.001$).[18] The association of the local failure and the development of metastatic disease was uniformly observed across the spectrum of biologic variants, from the less aggressive stage B1N0–grade I to the highly malignant stage CN0–grade III tumors.[18] Similar associations between local failure and metastatic disease have been reported in carcinoma of the breast, lung, rectum, prostate, uterine cervix, endometrium and vagina, tumors of the head and neck, and in soft tissue sarcoma (Table 69–12).[18-37] These data suggest that

TABLE 69–12. Impact of Local Control on the Incidence of Distant Metastases in Human Tumors

Investigations	Site	Stage	No. of Patients	Distant Metastases (%)	
				LC	LF
Chauvet[20]	Breast	T1–2/N0–1	202	9	20
Perez[51]	Lung	III	365	46	58
Chung[52]	Lung	T1–2/N0–2	118	39	89
		N0	51	24	90
		N1–2	67	52	59
Merino[49]	Head and neck	I–IV	5019	8	17
Leibel[48]	Head and neck	I–IV	2860	17	40
Lee[50]	Nasopharynx	I	196	3	20
Fuks[47]	Prostate	B–C/N0	679	24	77
Perez[58]	Prostate	B–C	317	22	58
Kuban[59]	Prostate	A2–C	286	18	61
Paunier[53]	Cervix	I–IV	1705	6	30
Anderson[54]	Cervix	IIB–IV	122	30	90
Perez[55]	Cervix	I–IV	1054	18	66
Stokes[56]	Endometrium	I	304	4	50
Perez[57]	Vagina	I–IV	149	20	54
Schild[60]	Rectum	B2–C3	139	28	90
Vigliotti[61]	Rectosigmoid	B1–C3	103	32	93
Markhede[62]	Soft tissue sarcoma	All	97	41	71
Suit[63]	Soft tissue sarcoma	All	204	25	61
Gustafson[36]	Soft tissue sarcoma	All	375	25	56

LC, local control; LF, local failure.

local failure exerts a dominant effect on the probability of spread to remote sites even in tumors with an inherent propensity for early and frequent metastatic dissemination (*e.g.*, breast, lung).

The association of local relapse and metastatic spread has led to the postulate that improving the local control can decrease the incidence of metastatic failure.[1,4,18] This hypothesis is consistent with recent investigations on the mutagenic origin of metastatic tumor cells. There is compelling evidence that cancer arises by a pleiotropic and multistage process. Mutagenic alterations in positive and negative regulatory genes seem equally prevalent among human cancers, because genetic instability and growth requirements grant selective advantages to to specific tumor clonogens.[37–40] The acquisition of metastatogenic properties seems to represent the ultimate outcome of tumor progression in this selective process.[37–42] It has been postulated that multiple mutational events in several recessive suppressor and dominant regulatory genes are involved in the transformation of nonmetastatic clonogens into cells with metastatic potential.[1,4,37–43] Mutagenic deactivation of recessive suppressor genes, such as *RB1*, *NM23*, and *p53* were shown to be associated with the metastatic conversion, and the function of several normal genes has been shown to be suppressed, ectopically expressed, or upregulated in metastatic tumor cells.[41–46] Suppressed expression of the major histocompatibility complex (MHC), increased expression of several oncogene and regulatory protooncogene products,

and ectopic expression of enzymes involved in the metastatic cascade (collagenase type IV, heparanase, and cathepsin proteases) were found to be upregulated in metastatic versus nonmetastatic cells, and their demonstration has been considered evidence for the metastatic phenotypes.[43,46–50]

The realization that this multistep mutational process exists may elucidate the mechanism by which local failure enhances the rate of metastatic disease. It is likely that tumor cell clonogens remaining in residual tumors after failure to eradicate the primary lesion are primed with at least some of the initial events required for completion of the metastatic conversion. The enhanced mitotic activity that is typical for the early phases of the regrowth of locally failing primary residual lesions provides an opportunity for a rapid progression of the mutations required for completion of the metastatic conversion, facilitating subsequent events of metastatic spread and the increase in metastatic disease (Fig. 69–10).[51–53]

If a reasonably similar growth rate is assumed for the locally relapsing tumor and for the distant metastases in a given patient, the hypothesis previously described suggests that the relapsing tumor would become clinically detectable first and the distant metastases only later on. Clinical studies on the temporal relation between local relapse and distant metastases in prostatic cancer patients are consistent with this assumption.[18] Figure 69–11 shows that the median for local relapse-free survival after ^{125}I implantation in patients with stage B-C/N0 prostate cancer was 51 months, compared with 71

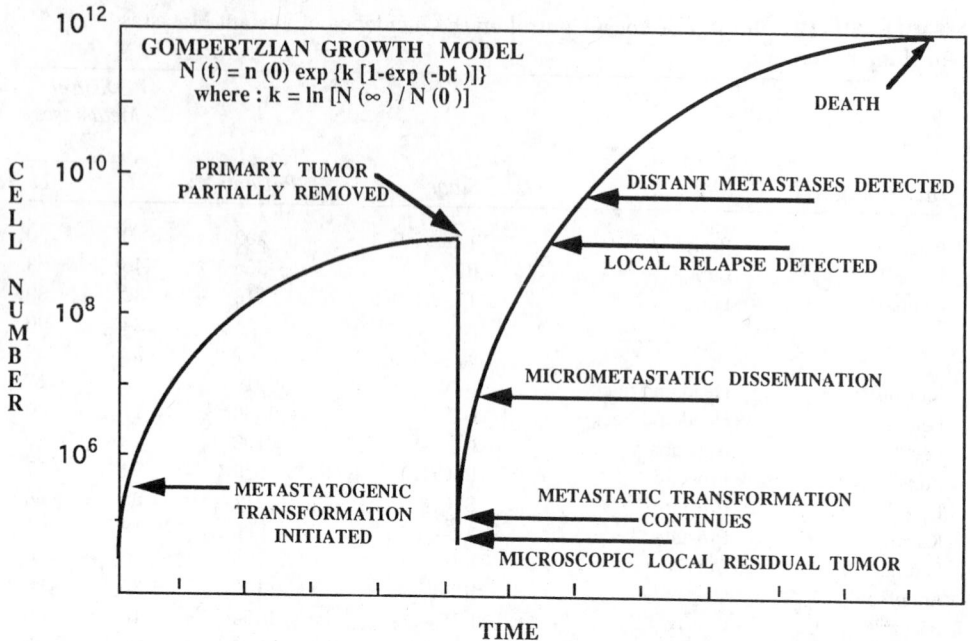

FIGURE 69–10. A hypothetical model that describes the effect of local failure on the development of metastatic disease. The growth pattern of the tumor is modeled according to Gompertzian growth kinetics. In this case, an assumption is made that the multistep process of mutations responsible for the metastatic conversion is initiated in stem cell clonogens of the primary lesion early in its subclinical growth phase, when the mitotic frequency is high. Another hypothetical assumption made is that the metastatic conversion is not completed when the primary lesion is clinically detected and only partially removed. The growth kinetic of the residual microscopic primary lesion is significantly accelerated according to the Gompertzian model. This provides an opportunity for an accelerated completion of the mutational metastatic transformation within residual tumor stem cell clonogens. According to this model, the clinical detection of the primary tumor lesion should precede the detection of metastatic disease.

months for the distant metastases-free survival in the same group of patients ($p < 0.001$). The same line of logic suggests that distant metastases in patients with local control, apparently already existing as micrometastases before treatment, would be detected earlier than metastases resulting from local relapse. Figure 69–12 shows that the median time to distant

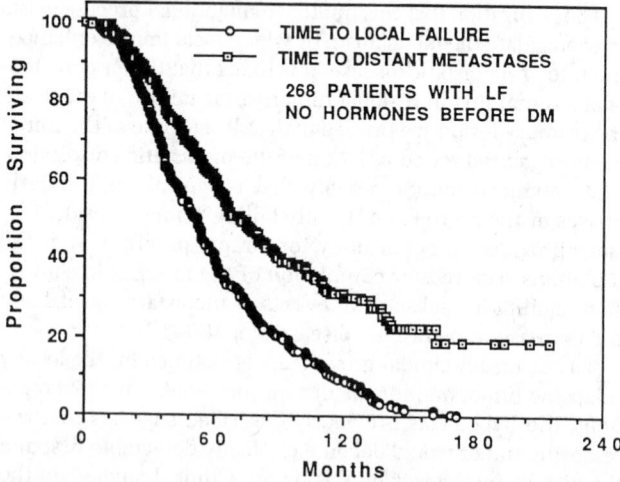

FIGURE 69–11. Kaplan-Meier time-adjusted analysis comparing local relapse-free survival (LRFS) and distant metastases-free survival (DMFS) in 268 patients with stage B-C/N0 carcinoma of the prostate who developed local failures after retropubic ^{125}I implantations. The criteria for inclusion in this analysis required that patients did not receive hormonal therapy before distant metastases were detected.

metastases in patients with stage B-C/N0 carcinoma of the prostate in local control after ^{125}I implantation was 36 months, compared with 54 months in patients with local relapse ($p > 0.001$). The hypothetical impact of local failure on the metastatic outcome highlights the need for a complete eradication of the primary tumor lesion during the initial attempt at curative therapy, and the concept serves as a basis for recent protocols designed to test the effect of improved local control by 3D-CRT on the metastatic outcome.[1,4]

THREE-DIMENSIONAL SIMULATION PROCEDURES

Essentially all imaging methods are suitable sources for acquisition of the detailed anatomic information required for 3D treatment planning, but dose calculation formalisms require that the anatomic information be presented in terms of electron density ratios, which can be obtained only from CT images.[54] Although magnetic resonance imaging (MRI), PET scanning, ultrasound, and monoclonal imaging are useful in providing complementary anatomic information on the target volume and the adjacent normal organs, the simulation process for 3D treatment planning is essentially based on CT. Conventional simulators are still used in 3D treatment planning, mainly to determine the positioning of the patient, fit the patient immobilization devices (*e.g.*, facial or body thermoplastic masks, alpha cradle body molds, head and feet rests), define the isocenter, and produce localization marks

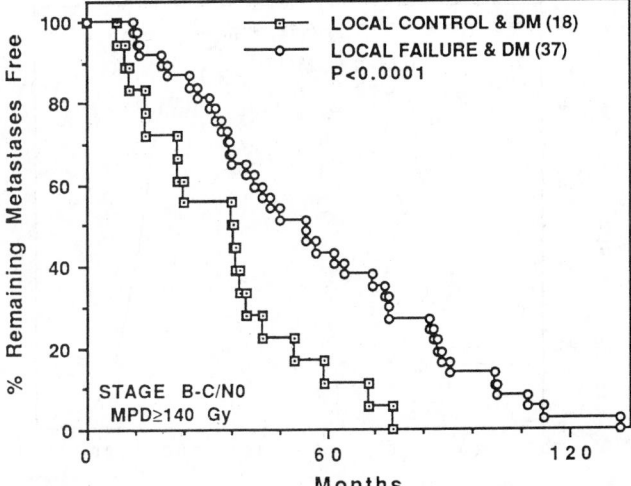

FIGURE 69–12. Time-dependent probability of remaining distant metastases free for 37 patients who developed local and distant relapses and for 18 locally controlled patients who developed distant metastases. Times to distant failure were calculated from ^{125}I implantation. Inclusion in this analysis required that patients received a mean peripheral implant dose (MPD) to the prostate of 140 Gy or more (to decrease the likelihood of occult local relapse), developed distant metastases regardless of whether they developed local recurrences, and did not receive hormonal therapy before distant metastases were detected.

on the patient's skin. The patient is then scanned on a flat table top in the treatment position, with opaque catheters placed over the predetermined simulation skin marks, so that the isocenter location can be visualized on the CT scans. The number of CT slices obtained and the spacing between slices depends on the size, shape, and location of the region of interest and the treatment technique. To produce the best 3D reconstruction, the interslice spacing should be 3 to 5 mm, and the slice thickness should be chosen to avoid overlaps or gaps between images.

BIOLOGIC TARGET VOLUME AND CRITICAL ORGANS

The biologic target volume (BTV) for treatment is defined as the volume of tissue that includes the tumor and the regions considered to be at risk for microscopic tumor extensions.[55] Usually, 5- to 10-mm margins are added to the BTV as visualized on CT to compensate for treatment set-up errors and other uncertainties. The contours of the BTV and the surrounding normal tissues are delineated manually on every CT slice with the aid of a track ball, digitizer pad, or light pen. The degree of effort required for manual extraction of anatomic features from the large number of CT slices and the lack of accuracy associated with the extraction of low contrast structures represent two of the challenging problems of current 3D treatment planning systems. Artificial intelligence and new image processing technologies are being explored for their potential to facilitate the anatomic extraction process.

A 3D structural reconstruction of the BTV and its surrounding normal organs is then performed using the beam's eye view (BEV) technique, in which the anatomic structures are

displayed as if the viewer is positioned at the beam's source, observing the structures that are in the path of the beam from every spatial angle possible around the isocenter.[56,57] This mode of display facilitates the selection of beam shapes and directions that minimize radiation to the normal tissues while simultaneously conforming to the accurate shape of the tumor. Real time display of solid surfaces has recently been introduced to enhance the imaging involved in this process.[58]

SELECTION OF BEAMS AND CALCULATION OF DOSE DISTRIBUTIONS

Most current 3D-CRT plans are based on a multidirectional coplanar and noncoplanar static field arrangements. After beam directions and shapes are defined with the BEV technique, dose calculations are performed and dose distributions are displayed to evaluate the adequacy of the treatment plan. Dose computations are performed for the entire 3D space, and because of their enormous complexity, they require the use of powerful computers. Modern methods of 3D dose calculations are based on parameters of radiation transport through the entire geometry of the tissues and its pleiotropic interactions with absorbing media and account for variations in tissue composition and density.[59]

The techniques most commonly used are the radiologic path length method, the scatter integration technique, and the more advanced delta-volume method, differential pencil beam dosimetry, and the Fourier convolution methods.[59–65] The pencil beam method, for example, divides the beams into many narrow beams (*i.e.*, pencils), and the dose is computed by summation of the contributions from the individual pencil beams. The method accounts for the transport of radiation in the full three dimensions to include contributions from the primary photons, scattered photons, and secondary electrons, and it improves the accuracy of the computed dose distributions for curved patient surfaces and inhomogenous internal structures.[66]

After the field arrangement and dose calculations are completed, the selected beam shapes are used to produce treatment blocks. The digital information of the computer-stored images can be used to produce reconstructed beam films that serve as templates for block fabrication.[66] The digital data can be used for automated block fabrication by numerically controlled milling machines or to guide individual leaf positioning in computer controlled multileaf collimators.[66]

QUANTITATIVE EVALUATION OF TREATMENT PLANS

The traditional method for evaluation of dose distributions, in which isodose curves are superimposed onto 2D CT displays of body sections, is inadequate for 3D treatment plan evaluation. New methods for graphic presentation of spatial 3D dose distributions superimposed or covering 3D anatomic configurations of the tumor and normal organ structures have been described.[67,68] To differentiate anatomy from dose information, different surface rendering techniques must be used. For example, the anatomy may be shown as a stack of contours and the dose as a mesh of points or as a solid transparent surface. Volumetric displays of the 3D CT data with dose can be implemented, in which the entire volume of CT pixel data can be shown in a semitransparent manner, much like a radiograph from arbitrary angles. Graphic presentations of spatial dose distributions are highly useful for rapid qualitative evaluations of treatment plans and for the identification of "hot" or "cold" spots within a given plan. However, such methods are by themselves insufficient for the final selection of the most appropriate plan, and complementary information must be obtained from quantitative numeric evaluation methods.

Integral dose-volume histograms (DVH) represent the current most useful numeric evaluation method.[69,70] In this approach, the volume (or the percentage of the total organ volume) receiving at least the dose D is presented as a function of D (Fig. 69–13). DVHs are convenient condensations of the dose distribution data. One DVH is generated for the tumor and one for each organ involved in the treatment plan. The compilation of the curves is used for evaluating or comparing treatment plans in a convenient and rapid manner. However, there are limitations to the use of DVHs. If the dose-volume histograms do not cross one another, the curve that is found furthest to the left in the case of normal organ DVHs or furthest to the right in the case of tumor DVHs (see Fig. 69–13A) is regarded as the best plan. Frequently, the ranking of the DVHs in rival plans is more ambiguous, because the histograms often cross one another (see Fig. 69–13B), and it is not evident which plan is better. If there are several rival plans and many organs, DVH comparisons can become quite complex and demanding. DVHs do not provide spatial information, and the positions of hot or cold regions cannot be obtained directly from the DVH; spatial dose distributions must be used. DVHs do not incorporate the complex trade-offs between tumor control and normal tissue toxicities. Although dose-volume histograms represent an advancement over spatial dose distribution displays, numeric scoring functions that correlate with biologic endpoints have been suggested to improve the selection process of the best plan.

The most popular numeric scoring functions are the normal tissue complications probabilities (NTCP) and tumor control probabilities (TCP), which employ a further condensation of dose distribution data to yield a single number for each structure.[71–74] Normal tissue tolerance doses required for NTCP calculations are derived from clinical data and are fit to a function that has a sigmoid shape. Complication probability data for normal tissues, even for uniform whole organ irradiation, are scarce, and the accuracy of the available data is unknown. A recent compilation of organ tolerance doses has been developed by Emami and coworkers.[71] The aim was to obtain tolerance doses for 5% and 50% complication probabilities for uniform whole organ and for two-thirds and one-third partial organ irradiation. Whenever possible, the data were obtained from the literature, and otherwise, the dose was based on the best judgment of the participating investigators, but the consistency and accuracy of the input data were not adequately tested. Although the absolute value of the calculations based on these data may have large uncertainties, their relative values may still prove useful in evaluating rival plans (Fig. 69–14), because certain systematic errors are likely to cancel out in ranking treatment plans.

The model currently used to calculate TCP is based on the

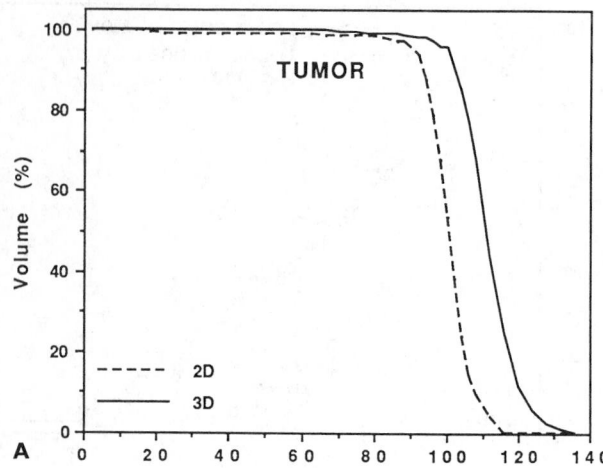

A

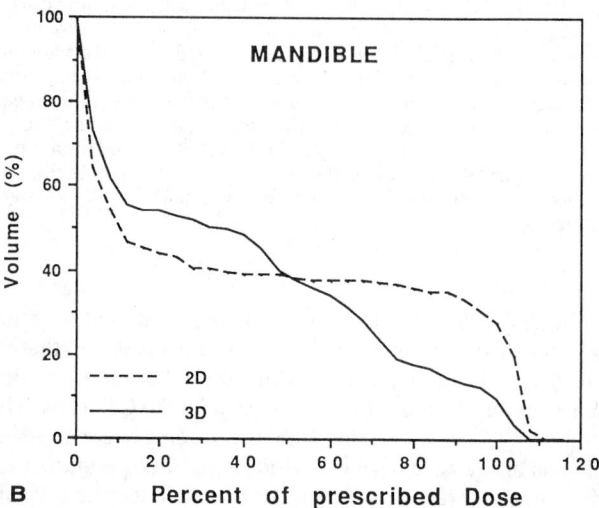

B

FIGURE 69–13. Dose-volume histograms (DVH) derived from a conventional 2D and a conformal 3D treatment plan for a patient with carcinoma of the nasopharynx. The doses were normalized to the prescribed minimum tumor dose, and the volumes are presented as the percentage of the total target volume. **(A)** This graph demonstrates the tumor DVH. Both plans cover the total target volume with at least 80% of the prescribed dose, but the 2D treatment plan shows a steep fall-off beginning at approximately 80% of the prescribed dose, and the 3D plan carries the total tumor volume to 100%, with portions of the tumor receiving up to 120% of the prescribed dose. **(B)** DVHs for the mandible in the same patient. At the low dose levels, the 2D plan seems to offer less mandibular dose. However, the two DVHs cross each other at approximately 50% of the prescribed dose, and 40% of the mandible is carried to significantly higher doses with the 2D plan than the 3D plan.

work of Goitein.[75] TCP is given by the product of the TCPs for small subvolumes of the tumor in which the dose is uniform. The tumor control for each subvolume is obtained from the estimated control for the whole tumor using binomial statistics. This model, although similar to one developed by Brahme, includes the effect of population heterogeneity on TCP.[76] The input data for these calculations are the target dose-volume histogram, TCP at the prescribed dose, and the normalized slope of the dose-response function at the 50% tumor control level. Because of microscopic disease there can be a nonzero TCP at zero dose, and an additional parameter, the probability of no tumor, is included.

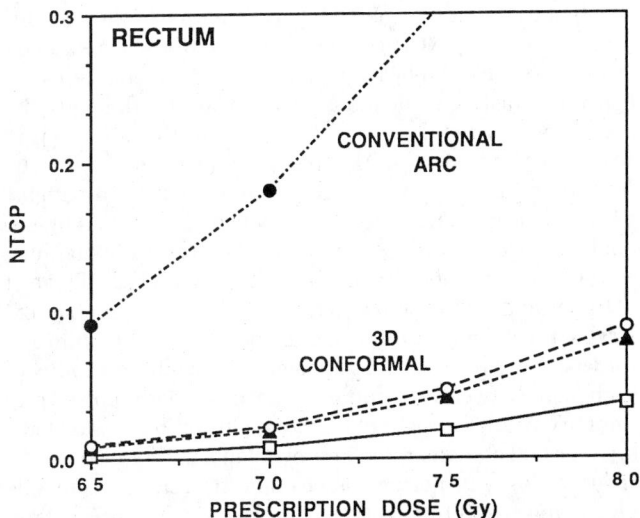

FIGURE 69–14. Calculated rectal normal tissue complication probabilities (NTCP) as a function of dose in a patient with carcinoma of the prostate. Treatment was planned with a conventional 2D, bilateral, 120° arc approach (●) or with three different 3D conformal plans involving four fields (□), six fields (▲), or eight fields (○). Rectal NTCP for each plan was calculated for a range of prescribed doses of between 65 and 80 Gy. Calculations were made assuming a strong volume effect for rectal NTCP. A potential for tumor dose escalation is demonstrated with the 3D plans because the calculated risks of toxicity to the rectum remained at acceptably low levels with all 3D planned doses.

The primary utility from calculating NTCP and TCP is that they can be used to rank treatment plans. Even though the absolute value of the calculations may be uncertain, it is their relative values that are needed for numeric evaluations. Together with DVHs and spatial dose distributions, these parameters yield a fairly complete representation of a treatment plan as required for its evaluation.

COMPUTER-AIDED OPTIMIZATION OF TREATMENT PLANNING

The process of 3D treatment planning described so far indicates that the amounts of data that need to be managed and analyzed in each plan is so voluminous that decisions regarding the selection of the most adequate plan may become an intellectually demanding task. Because there are no restrictions for the use of coplanar and noncoplanar field combinations, the number of evaluations and decision making processes involved in the planning of a single case may easily exceed practical constraints in terms of manpower and time factors involved.

There has been great interest in the development of expert systems for computer-aided optimization of 3D treatment planning.[6,74,77] Because there is virtually an infinite number of combinations possible, the specifications for this approach in terms of input of beam arrangements, weights, intensity, distributions, NTCP, TCP, and machine parameters to yield the highest possible therapeutic ratio need to be restricted to make computer-aided optimization a practical tool. However, the probability of finding a better solution increases as the domain of search for the optimal solution increases. Because

a larger number of beams can improve the ratio of tumor dose to normal tissue dose, optimized 3D conformal plans, in general, contain a larger number of beams than a conventional 3D plan. The maximal benefit from computer-aided optimization is associated with the availability of new treatment machines that are capable of rapidly delivering large numbers of arbitrarily shaped fields under automated computer control.

THREE-DIMENSIONAL CONFORMAL THERAPY DELIVERY SYSTEMS

The application of 3D-CRT requires new performance standards of treatment delivery systems and the formulation of new specifications for their function. Most commercial linear accelerators have been reconfigured to allow automated computer controlled movements of the gantry and the treatment couch, as required for the delivery of successive multisegment or dynamic treatments within a reasonable treatment time. Another major development has been the introduction of new beam shaping devices. Three-dimensional plans frequently entail 10 or more fields, with all fields delivered every day. The introduction of multileaf collimators (MLC) provides an ideal solution for this need. The multileaf collimator is a secondary collimator system, which consists of independently movable high-Z material rods or leaves. Each leaf is operated by an individual motor, and the function of all motors is coordinated under computer control. The leaves on both sides can be automatically positioned to shape the treatment beam according to a preprogrammed plan. Successive multisegment therapy can be employed, in which each segment's aperture conforms to the specific shape of the tumor from that angle. A photograph of a recently developed MLC is shown in Figure 69–15. This MLC can be retrofitted onto existing linear accelerators, and other types of MLCs are currently designed as built-in components. The spatial resolution with currently available MLCs is approximately the projected leaf width in the patient plane (usually 1 cm), although narrower leaf widths may be available in the future for treatment of small target volumes. Integration of automated collimator beam shaping with other automated motions of the machine is being developed to produce the full range of static and dynamic conformal therapy.

Other modes of beam modulation within the aperture or the open part of the field are frequently needed. This has been classically accomplished by custom-made compensators manually attached to the head of the treatment machine. For multifield conformal therapy, however, automated systems are preferred, and such capabilities have been provided by techniques of beam scanning within the radiation field. For example, the Scanditronix MM50 racetrack microtron is capable of scanning photon and electron beams under computer control. The elementary electron fields used in this scanning process can be as narrow as 1.4 cm for 50-MeV electrons. Although the elementary field widths for scanning photon beams are considerably larger, they can still be used to obtain field shaping where less resolution is acceptable, or they can be used in conjunction with MLC if finer resolution is required.

Another useful system recently introduced is the on-line treatment imaging system that permits fluoroscopy-like reviews of the actual treatment fields as given daily to the patient. Although the component structure of these devices differs

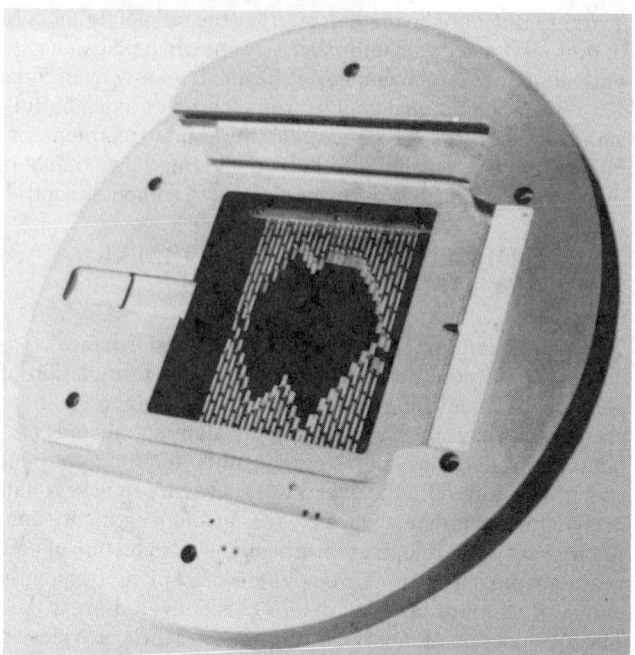

FIGURE 69–15. A computer-controlled multileaf collimator for photon beam shaping. This particular multileaf collimator features 52 leaves, each driven by a dedicated motor, and the function of all motors is coordinated by a computer. The resolution of each leaf is 10 mm at the 100-cm isocenter. The leaves can be driven under the computer control to shape the beam according to preplanned specifications. (Courtesy of Varian Associates)

between manufacturers, they all have in common an imaging detector attached to the machine gantry, methods of digitizing and analyzing image data with a computer, and a video display system. The images can be contrast enhanced or modified in other ways to highlight and enhance details that are difficult to observe with conventional screen film systems. The major potential of these systems for conformal therapy is the speed with which each field can be verified. It should be possible in the near future to use these systems in a feedback mode to compensate for set-up errors or patient movements. For example, before daily treatment begins, two orthogonal images can be obtained, the output can be compared with a preplanned configuration by the computer, and deviations that exceed tolerance limits can be adjusted automatically by computer controlled movements of the gantry, couch, and the MLC setting positions. On-line imaging devices will play a crucial role in the verification of conformal 3D treatments and probably contribute to improving the accuracy of all radiation treatments.

PRELIMINARY CLINICAL EXPERIENCE

The clinical application of 3D conformal radiotherapy is still in its developmental phase. Because 3D treatment planning systems are only beginning to emerge and treatment delivery systems are still in a testing mode, the number of published reports on clinical experiences with 3D conformal therapy is small. A major development has been the completion of a

collaborative multiinstitutional study organized by the National Cancer Institute (NCI) on the evaluation of treatment planning for 3D photon-beam radiotherapy.[78] The study established the basic specifications and standard for this modality and demonstrated the potential benefit of this approach in several disease entities. Although patients were not actually treated by 3D-CRT in this study, anatomic data on patients with various malignancies were provided and planned in parallel in several institutions on 2D and 3D treatment planning systems. The results demonstrated the potential advantage of 3D planning and treatment in tumors of the nasopharynx, larynx, breast, lung, uterine cervix, prostate, and rectum and for Hodgkin's disease and the potential for reproducibility of such plans between institutions.[78] Other studies reported preliminary results in patients treated with prototype 3D-CRT systems and demonstrated improvements in target coverage, reduced doses to normal tissues, and decreased acute side effects in several tumors types.

NASOPHARYNX

Leibel and colleagues studied at Memorial Sloan-Kettering Cancer Center (MSKCC) the advantages of 3D-CRT in patients with carcinoma of the nasopharynx.[8] The study entailed 10 previously untreated patients and 5 patients treated for locally recurrent disease. The previously untreated patients received initially 5040 cGy with conventional two lateral opposed fields to the primary tumor and the cervical lymph nodes, and the 3D-CRT component was limited to a boost of 1980 cGy given to the region of the primary tumor. The patients with locally recurrent disease received the entire treatment (1620–2160 cGy; median, 1960 cGy) by 3D-CRT. All patients were planned independently by two teams. One team performed a conventional 2D plan employing bilateral opposed fields, and the other performed a 3D plan using the BEV technique to select the most optimal field configurations and BEV-derived tumor-conforming blocks for delivery of treatment. Comparisons of dose distributions, DVHs, TCPs, and NTCPs for the 2D and 3D plans were performed for the target volume and for each normal organ in each patient. Overall, the 3D plans consistently showed improved tumor coverage and reduced underdosed tumor volumes. Despite the fact that there was no intentional effort to increase the dose beyond prescription dose, the mean dose with the 3D plan was found to be higher in all cases tested (Fig. 69–16), resulting in an overall mean increase of 13%. This was achieved mainly from the improved ability to avoid tumor underdosage. The 3D plans also resulted in a significant reduction of normal tissue doses, with the traditional 2D plans involving almost twice as much normal tissue volumes carried to high-dose levels as compared with the 3D plans. An analysis of the uncomplicated tumor control probability demonstrated that with the 3D approach there was with an overall mean increase of 15% in the predicted uncomplicated control (Fig. 69–17). This translates roughly to an expected advantage from an increment of approximately 1000 cGy in effective tumor dose. Whether further escalation of the tumor volume dose is possible without exceeding normal tissue tolerance in this disease is currently being investigated in a phase I dose escalation study.

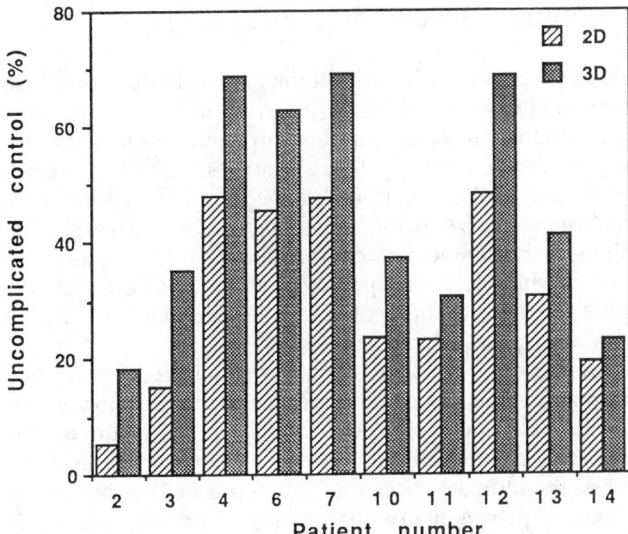

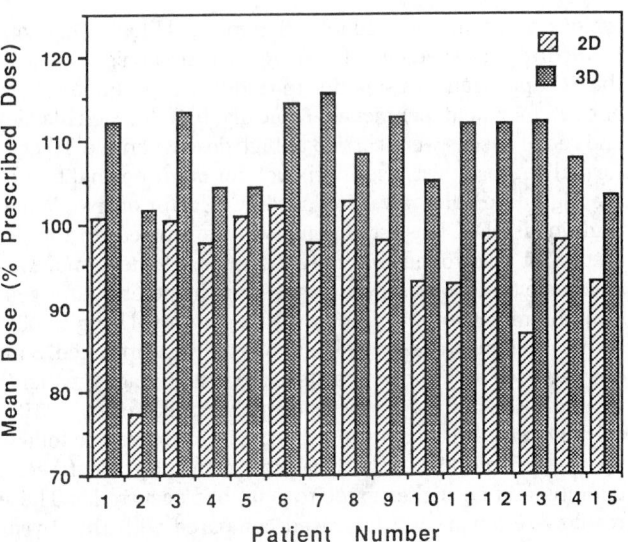

FIGURE 69–16. The probability of uncomplicated control in patients with carcinoma of the nasopharynx. The treatment was prescribed to deliver 50 Gy through conventional two lateral opposed fields to the nasopharynx and the cervical lymph node-bearing areas. Subsequently, a 19.6-Gy boost dose was planned by traditional 2D or a 3D conformal approach. The score in each case was calculated from the normal tissue complication probabilities and tumor control probabilities for the entire prescribed course of 70 Gy. Because the complication probability for the parotid gland is near unity, this organ was excluded from the calculations.

FIGURE 69–17. Comparison of the mean tumor dose in patients with carcinoma of the nasopharynx planned with a conventional 2D or a conformal 3D treatment plan. The mean dose is expressed in terms of the percentage of the prescribed minimum tumor dose.

BRAIN

The University of Michigan conducted a series of studies on 3D-CRT of brain tumors.[79-81] To demonstrate that 3D planning is practical and applicable to the treatment of high-grade astrocytomas, 50 patients were treated with cerebral irradiation delivered in a focussed, nonaxial techniques employing from two to five beams.[79] Patients were immobilized with a mask-marker immobilization system, using a commercially available thermoplastic mesh indexed and mounted to a rigid frame attached to the therapy couch. Studies employing weekly simulation indicate that patient treatment position movement can be restricted by this immobilization system to 2 mm over the course of treatment.[80] The tumor plus a 3.0-cm margin was treated to 4500 cGy and the tumor plus a 1.5-cm margin were then boosted to 5940 cGy using beam orientations that maximally spared normal parenchyma. DVH curves demonstrate dosimetric advantages to nonaxial techniques over conventional parallel-opposed orientations. Assessment of the nonaxial techniques in selected cases indicated that uniform target volume coverage could be maintained with a typical reduction of 30% in the total amount of brain tissue treated to the 95% isodose line.[79] DVH analysis demonstrated an approximation of brachytherapy dose confinement through the use of multiple nonaxial noncoplanar beam orientations. Of 12 patients with recurrent astrocytoma treated with this technique to a dose of 3060 cGy, 7 showed improvement in Karnofsky status or decrease in steroid dependence and the average survival exceeded 9 months, demonstrating the potential of this approach.[81]

LUNG

Armstrong and colleagues compared 3D conformal treatment planning with the traditional 2D approach for 10 patients with non-small cell lung cancer.[82] Patients were simulated in custom Alpha-cradle molds and scanned with CT using 1.0-cm slice thicknesses from below the larynx to the upper abdomen and 0.5-cm thickness through the levels containing visible nodal and primary disease. The objective was to deliver 5040 cGy to elective nodal volumes and 7020 cGy to all visible disease. Significant underdosing occurred in 2% of the gross target volume with the 3D approach, compared with 15% with 2D. Three-dimensional treatment reduced significantly the dose to normal tissues outside of the target volume. In some patients, as much as 30% of the uninvolved lung received 2000 cGy or more with the 2D plan, although no portion of the contralateral lung received over 2000 cGy with the 3D plan. Esophageal NTCPs were reduced from 33% with 2D to 22% with 3D. Using the doses generally delivered to normal tissues with traditional 2D planning methods as constraints, the data suggest that with the 3D approach the dose to the primary tumor can be escalated by at least 20% to 30% in appropriate cases.

PROSTATE

The University of Michigan carried out several studies on 3D-CRT for prostate cancer. Ten Haken and colleagues compared 3D treatment plans with conventional 2D plans in 17 patients with stage C carcinoma of the prostate.[7] CT scans and BEV displays were used to generate a six-field 3D treatment plan consisting of a two parallel lateral opposed fields and two sets of oblique fields directed at ±45° with respect to the lateral fields. For each field, an interactive BEV display was produced showing the target in its correct 3D perspective, and an autoblock program was used to design focused blocks that conformed to that specific volume. Normal tissue sparing with the 3D approach was superior to traditional 2D bilateral arc or open four-field techniques. Typically, half as much bladder and rectal tissues were carried to high dose when the 3D conformal approach was used, although for other normal tissues the high-dose volume was reduced by a factor of five. When traditional 2D CT-assisted plans were evaluated on the 3D system, it was found that only 72 ± 7% of the tumor was covered by the 95% isodose, suggesting the potential for geographic misses in 20% to 35% of the patients. Using the 3D six-field technique, a dose escalation study was initiated. Sandler reported preliminary results in the first 15 stage C patients treated with 4500 cGy to the whole pelvis, followed by a 3100-cGy 3D-guided boost to the prostate. Within an average follow-up of 16.5 months, only 2 patients showed grade I rectal toxicity, and no higher grade toxicity had occurred.[83] These results are apparently improved compared with the 2-year 60% moderate to severe rectal complications reported in a recent study of patients treated with conventional techniques to 7500 cGy or higher, but longer follow-up is required to confirm this observation.[84]

Soffen and colleagues from the Fox Chase Institute in Philadelphia compared a four-field 3D conformal static technique with conventional 2D techniques to determine the advantages of the 3D approach in treating patients with B1 (Gleason Score 2–5) disease.[85,86] A DVH analysis demonstrated that an average of 14% of the bladder, and the rectal dose was eliminated using the 3D approach. Grade 2 or higher acute toxicity occurred in 60% of the 2D treated patients, compared with 31% in the 3D treated patients ($p > 0.05$). The researchers emphasized the need for careful patient immobilization so that the margins of normal tissue surrounding the prostate in the high-dose radiation volume can be reduced without compromising the precision of treatment.

At MSKCC, Leibel and colleagues treated 73 patients with stages A2 through C disease in a phase I dose escalation study to explore the highest feasible tumor doses and their effect on the outcome.[87] The entire prostate, seminal vesicles, and the pelvic organs were reconstructed in their full 3D configuration from consecutive 5 to 10 mm CT slices obtained throughout the pelvis. The BEV planning technique was used to select the most optimal field configurations for the individual patient, and BEV-derived tumor-conforming blocks were used for individualized treatment in each case. Thirty-six patients received 6480 cGy, 25 received 7020 cGy, and 12 received 7560 cGy. Complete tumor regressions in all patients were confirmed by digital rectal examinations. Sixty-seven patients have been followed for more than 6 months (median, 12 months, with 36 followed for at least 1 year and 10 for >2 years), regarded as sufficient to analyze acute toxicity and response to treatment. Serum PSA normalized within a median of 3 months after treatment (range, 1–9 months) in 80% of the patients. Eleven of the 14 patients with abnormal posttreatment PSA have developed bone metastases, although the prostates remained normal to rectal digital examination. Acute toxicities were mild. Grade 1 or acute gastrointestinal toxicity developed in 49% and grade 1 or 2 acute genitourinary toxicity in 76% of the patients, but severe acute toxicities were not observed. There have been no late complications within a median follow-up of 12 months (range, 6–36).

PROSPECTS FOR THE FUTURE

The experience with early prototypes of 3D planning and treatment systems, although based on only a few hundred patients treated so far, indicates an enormous potential for this approach, but the full exploitation of 3D-CRT requires significant additional effort. It is necessary to develop more sophisticated 3D treatment planning tools and to test and implement the new automated treatment delivery systems. The rate at which technical progress can be made critically depends on the availability of new and faster computers and on new approaches to software design.

An important development is the anticipated introduction of treatment planning optimization, which is essential if conformal 3D radiotherapy is to become practical for routine clinical use at the community level. But beyond technical progress, the ultimate success of this approach depends on the ability to deliver high radiation doses to a large variety of tumors without significantly increasing the toxicity to transited normal tissues. If higher radiation doses are indeed feasible without adverse effects on the surrounding normal tissues, the ultimate limitation to 3D-CRT could be due to dose directly applied to the tumor bed. As with all irradiated tissue, the maximal tolerable dose within the tumor bed is a function of volume. Large volumes are expected to have a lower tolerance than smaller volumes, for which primary integrity may rely on migration of important stromal elements from adjacent less irradiated normal tissues. More should be done to understand the limitations on dose due to the target volume, rather than the transited normal tissues. Current 3D-CRT systems are adequate to support phase I or II dose escalation and toxicity studies, and several institutions have already initiated such studies.

The efficacy of the treatment depends on the tumor being reasonably well defined by the imaging procedures, so that a relatively small margin can be added with the expectation that a target volume has been appropriately identified and covered. If this is not the case and tumor extends beyond the target volume, conformal therapy offers no better opportunity for control; in fact, it may offers less likelihood of tumor control, because simpler techniques would more likely include unidentified tumor. There are no imaging techniques that can provide information about the existence of microscopic deposits of tumor cells. The current resolutions of magnetic resonance and radiolabeled monoclonal antibody imaging are not sufficient to provide such information, although there is potential for such developments in the future, especially with magnetic resonance spectroscopy. Anther exciting prospect of magnetic resonance spectroscopy is its potential to add biologic information to 3D conformal radiotherapy, such as the state of tumor oxygenation, cell cycle parameters, and other biologic variables that can be used to determine appropriate time-dose relations. As chemotherapy becomes more effective in controlling occult micrometastatic disease, as evidenced by the current success of adjuvant treatment, combined-modality approaches for improving local control increase in their importance. Three-dimensional conformal radiotherapy will afford opportunities for improved local control, and it will reduce the dose to transited normal tissues and decrease toxicities associated with combinations of radiation and chemotherapy.

The extraordinary increase in the complexity of treatment that results from the application of conformal radiotherapy should be recognized. This invites possibilities for errors and requires extraordinary attention to assurances that the treatment is being given in accordance with the treatment plan. With conventional radiotherapy, quality control depends on static portal images made at periodic intervals through treatment. For 3D-CRT to be regarded as safe, much more sophisticated on-line verifications are required, which should allow feedback and control loops to provide automated mechanisms for error corrections during treatment. All of this suggests that treatment will be quite expensive and extremely time consuming, raising issues of cost-benefit evaluations and cost containment. The true clinical advantages of 3D conformal therapy and the justification for its high cost will not be known until future phase III studies are conducted to test whether improved local control can be achieved and whether it affects the outcome in several human cancers.

REFERENCES

1. Fuks Z, Leibel SA, Kutcher GE, Mohan R, Ling CC. Three dimensional conformal treatment: A new frontier in radiation therapy. In: DeVita VT Jr, Hellman S, Rosenberg SA, eds. Important advances in oncology. Philadelphia: JB Lippincott, 1991:151–172.
2. Suit H, Urie M. Proton beams in radiation therapy. JNCI 1992;84:155–164.
3. Castro JR, Chen GT, Blakley EA. Current considerations in heavy charged particle radiotherapy. Radiat Res 1985;8:227S–234S.
4. Leibel SA, Ling CC, Kutcher GJ, Mohan R, Cordon-Cardo C, Fuks Z. The biological basis of conformal three-dimensional radiation therapy. Int J Radiat Oncol Biol Phys 1991;21:805–811.
5. Munzenrider JE, Pilepich M, Rene-Ferrero JB, Tchakarova I, Carter BL. Use of body scanner in radiotherapy treatment planning. Cancer 1979;40:170–179.
6. Goitein M. The utility of computed tomography in radiation therapy: An estimate of outcome. Int J Radiat Oncol Biol Phys 1979;5:1799–1807.
7. Ten Haken RK, Perez-Tamayo C, Tesser RJ, McShan DL, Fraass BA, Lichter AS. Boost treatment of the prostate using shaped fixed beams. Int J Radiat Oncol Biol Phys 1989;16:193–200.
8. Leibel SA, Kutcher GJ, Harrison LB, et al. Improved dose distributions for 3D conformal boost treatments in carcinoma of the nasopharynx. Int J Radiat Oncol Biol Phys 1991;20:823–833.
9. Deacon JM, Peckham MJ, Steel GG. The radioresponsiveness of human tumours and the initial slope of the cell survival curve. Radiat Oncol 1984;2:317–323.
10. Fertil B, Malaise EP. Intrinsic radiosensitivity of human cell lines is correlated with radioresponsiveness of human tumors: Analysis of 101 published survival curves. Int J Radiat Oncol Biol Phys 1985;11:1699–1707.
11. Steel GG, McMillan TJ, Peacock JH. The picture has changed in the 1980s. Int J Radiat Biol 1989;56:525–537.
12. Suit HD, Baumann M, Skates S, Convery K. Clinical interest in determinations of cellular radiation sensitivity. Int J Radiat Biol 1989;56:725–737.
13. Weichselbaum RR, Rotmensch J, Swan SA, Beckett MA. Radiobiological characterization of 53 human tumor cell lines. Int J Radiat Biol 1989;56:553–560.
14. Peters LJ, Withers HR, Thames HD, Fletcher GH. Keynote address. The problem: Tumor radioresistance in clinical radiotherapy. Int J Radiat Oncol Biol Phys 1981;8:101–108.
15. Thames HD, Schulthheiss TE, Hendy JH, Tucker SL, Dubry BM, Brock WA. Can modest escalations of dose be detected as increased tumor control? Int J Radiat Oncol Biol Phys 1991;22:241–246.
16. DeVita VT, Lippman M, Hubbard SA, Idhe DC, Rosenberg SA. The effect of combined modality therapy on local control and survival. Int J Radiat Oncol Biol Phys 1986;12:487–501.
17. Suit HD. Potential for improving survival rates for the cancer patient by increasing the efficacy of treatment of the primary lesion. Cancer 1982;50:1227–1234.
18. Fuks Z, Leibel SA, Wallner KE, et al. The effect of local control on metastatic dissemination in carcinoma of the prostate: Long term results in patients treated with ^{125}I implantation. Int J Radiat Oncol Biol Phys 1991;21:549–566.
19. Fisher B, Anderson S, Fisher ER, et al. Significance of ipsilateral breast tumour recurrence after lumpectomy. Lancet 1991;338:327–331.
20. Chauvet B, Reynaud-Bougnoux A, Calais G, et al. Prognostic significance of breast relapse after conservative treatment in node-negative early breast cancer. Int J Radiat Oncol Biol Phys 1990;9:1125–1230.
21. Perez CA, Pajak TF, Rubin P, et al. Long term observations of the pattern of failure in patients with unresectable non-oat cell carcinoma of the lung treated with definitive radiotherapy. Report by the Radiation Therapy Oncology Group. Cancer 1987;59:1874–1881.
22. Chung CK, Stryker JA, O'Neill M, DeMuth WE. Evaluation of adjuvant postoperative radiotherapy for lung cancer. Int J Radiat Oncol Biol Phys 1982;8:1877–1880.
23. Merino OR, Lindberg RD, Fletcher GH. An analysis of distant metastases from squamous cell carcinoma of the upper respiratory and digestive tracts. Cancer 1977;40:145–151.
24. Leibel SA, Kutcher GJ, Harrison LB, et al. Improved dose distributions for 3D conformal boost treatments in carcinoma of the nasopharynx. Int J Radiat Oncol Biol Phys 1991;20:823–833.
25. Lee AW, Sham JS, Poon YF, Ho JH. Treatment of stage I nasopharyngeal carcinoma: Analysis of the patterns of relapse and the results of withholding elective neck irradiation. Int J Radiat Oncol Biol Phys 1989;17:1183–1190.
26. Kuban DH, El-Mahdi AM, Schellhammer PF. Effect of local tumor control on distant metastasis and survival in prostatic adenocarcinoma. Urology 1987;30:420–426.
27. Perez CA, Pilepich MV, Zivnuska F. Tumor control in definitive irradiation of localized carcinoma of the prostate. Int J Radiat Oncol Biol Phys 1986;12:523–531.
28. Paunier JP, Delclos L, Fletcher GH. Cause, time of death, and sites of failure in squamous cell carcinoma of the uterine cervix on intact uterus. Radiology 1967;88:552–562.
29. Anderson P, Dische S. Local tumor control and subsequent incidence of distant metastatic disease. Int J Radiat Oncol Biol Phys 1981;7:1645–1648.
30. Perez CA, Kuske RR, Camel HM, et al. Analysis of pelvic tumor control and impact on survival in carcinoma of the uterine cervix treated with radiation therapy alone. Int J Radiat Oncol Biol Phys 1988;14:613–621.
31. Stokes S, Bedwinek J, Kao MS, Camel HM, Perez CA. Treatment of stage I adenocarcinoma of the endometrium by hysterectomy and adjuvant irradiation: A retrospective analysis of 304 patients. Int J Radiat Oncol Biol Phys 1986;12:339–344.
32. Perez CA, Camel HM, Galakatos AE, et al. Definitive irradiation in carcinoma of the vagina: Long-term evaluation of results. Int J Radiat Oncol Biol Phys 1988;15:1283–1290.
33. Schild SE, Martenson JA Jr, Gunderson LL, et al. Postoperative adjuvant therapy of rectal cancer: An analysis of disease control, survival and prognostic factors. Int J Radiat Oncol Biol Phys 1989;17:55–62.
34. Vigliotti A, Rich TA, Romsdahl MM, Withers HR, Oswald MJ. Postoperative adjuvant radiotherapy for adenocarcinoma of the rectum and rectosigmoid. Int J Radiat Oncol Biol Phys 1987;13:999–1006.
35. Markhede G, Angervall L, Stener B. A multivariate analysis of the prognosis after surgical treatment of soft tissue tumors. Cancer 1982;49:1721–1733.
35a. Suit HD, Mankin HJ, Wood WC, et al. Treatment of the patient with stage MO soft tissue sarcoma. J Clin Oncol 1988;6:854–862.
36. Gustafson P, Rooser B, Rydholm A. Is local recurrence of minor importance for metastases in soft tissue sarcoma? Cancer 1991;67:2083–2086.
37. Vogelstein B, Fearon ER, Kern SE, et al. Allelotype of colorectal carcinomas. Science 1989;244:207–211.
38. Fearon ER, Vogelstein B. A genetic model for colorectal tumorigenesis. Cell 1990;61:759–767.
39. Hollstein M, Sidransky D, Vogelstein B, Harris CC. Mutations in human cancers. Science 1991;253:49–53.
40. Bishop M. Molecular themes in oncogenesis. Cell 1991;64:235–249.
41. Kerbel RS. Towards an understanding of the molecular basis of the metastatic phenotype. Invasion Metastasis 1989;9:329–337.
42. Sobel ME. Metastasis suppressor genes. JNCI 1990;82:267–276.
43. Liotta LA, Steeg PS, Stettler-Stevenson WG. Cancer metastasis and angiogenesis: An imbalance of positive and negative regulation. Cell 1991;64:327–336.
44. Steeg PS, Bevilacqua G, Kopper L, et al. Evidence for a novel gene associated with low tumor metastatic potential. JNCI 1988;89:200–203.
45. Cance WG, Brennan MF, Dudas ME, Cordon-Cardo C. Altered expression of the retinoblastoma gene product in human sarcomas. N Engl J Med 1990;323:1457–1462.
46. Cordon-Cardo C, Fuks Z, Eisenbach L, Feldman M. Expression of HLA-A,B,C antigens on primary and metastatic tumor cell populations of human carcinomas. Cancer Res 1991;51:6327–6380.
47. Greenberg AH, Egan SE, Wright JA. Oncogenes and metastatic progression. Invasion Metastasis 1989;9:360–378.
48. Muschel R, Liotta RA. Role of oncogenes in metastasis. Carcinogenesis 1988;9:705–710.
49. Vlodavsky I, Michaeli RI, Bar-Ner M, et al. Involvement of heparanase in tumor metastasis and angiogenesis. Isr J Med Sci 1988;24:464–470.
50. Sloane BF, Dunn TR, Honn KV. Lysosomal cathepsin B. Correlation with metastatic potential. Science 1981;212:1151–1153.
51. Steel GG, McMillan TJ, Peacock JH. The picture has changed in the 1980s. Int J Radiat Biol 1989;56:525–537.
52. Tubiana M. Repopulation in human tumors. Acta Oncol 1988;27:83–88.
53. Withers HR, Taylor JMG, Maciejewski B. The hazards of accelerated tumor clonogens repopulation during radiotherapy. Acta Oncol 1988;27:131–146.
54. Mohan R. Three-dimensional radiation treatment planning. Aust Phys Eng Sci Med 1989;12:73–91.
55. Urie MM, Goitein M, Doppke K, et al. The role of uncertainty analysis in treatment planning. Int J Radiat Oncol Biol Phys 1991;21:91–107.
56. McShan DL, Silverman A, Lanza DM, Reinstein LE, Glicksman AS. A computerized three-dimensional treatment planning system utilizing interactive colour graphics. Br J Radiol 1979;52:478–481.
57. Goitein M, Abrams M, Rowell D, Pollari H, Wiles J. Multi-dimensional treatment planning: II. Beam's eye-view, back projection, and projection through CT sections. Int J Rad Oncol Biol Phys 1983;9:789–797.
58. Three-dimensional displays in planning radiation therapy: A clinical perspective. Photon

Treatment Planning Collaborative Working Group. Int J Radiat Oncol Biol Phys 1991;21: 79–89.

59. Three-dimensional dose calculations for radiation treatment planning. Photon Treatment Planning Collaborative Working Group. Int J Radiat Oncol Biol Phys 1991;21:25–36.
60. Cunningham JR. Scatter-air Ratios. Phys Med Biol 1972;17:42–51.
61. Larson KB, Prasad SC. Absorbed-dose computations for inhomogeneous media in radiation treatment planning using differential scatter-air ratios IEEE. Proceedings of the Second Annual Symposium on Computer Application in Medical Care, 1978:93–99.
62. Wong JW, Slessinger ED, Hermes RE, Offutt CJ, Roy T, Vannier MW. Portal dose images. I. Quantitative treatment plan verification. Int J Radiat Oncol Biol Phys 1990;18: 1455–1463.
63. Chui CS, Mohan RM. Extraction of pencil beam kernels by the deconvolution method. Med Phys 1988;15:138–144.
64. Mohan R, Chui CS. Use of Fourier transforms in calculating dose distributions for irregularly shaped fields for three dimensional treatment planning. Med Phys 1987;14: 70–77.
65. Boyer AL, Mok EC. Fourier convolution incorporating inhomogeneities. Med Phys 1985;12:507.
66. Mohan R, Chui C, Lidofsky L. Differential pencil beam dose computation model for photons. Med Phys 1986;13:64–73.
67. Photon Treatment Planning Collaborative Working Group. State of the art of external photon beam radiation treatment planning. Int J Radiat Oncol Biol Phys 1991;21:9–23.
68. Photon Treatment Planning Collaborative Working Group. Three-dimensional displays in planning radiation therapy: A clinical perspective. Int J Radiat Oncol Biol Phys 1991;21:79–89.
69. Shipley WU, Tepper JE, Prout GR, et al. Proton radiation as boost therapy for localized prostatic carcinoma. JAMA 1979;241:1912–1915.
70. Drzymala RE, Mohan R, Brewster L, et al. Dose-volume histograms. Int J Radiat Oncol Biol Phys 1991;21:71–78.
71. Emami B, Lyman J, Brown A, et al. Tolerance of normal tissue to therapeutic irradiation. Int J Radiat Oncol Biol Phys 1991;21:109–122.
72. Burman C, Kutcher GJ, Emami B, Goitein M. Fitting of normal tissue tolerance data to an analytic function. Int J Radiat Oncol Biol Phys 1991;21:123–135.
73. Kutcher GJ, Burman C, Brewster L, Goitein M, Mohan R. Histogram reduction method for calculating complication probabilities for three-dimensional treatment planning evaluations. Int J Radiat Oncol Biol Phys 1991;21:137–146.
74. Munzenrider JE, Brown AP, Chu JC, et al. Numerical scoring of treatment plans. Int J Radiat Oncol Biol Phys 1991;21:147–163.

75. Goitein M. The probability of controlling an inhomogeneously irradiated tumor. In: Evaluation of treatment planning for particle beam radiotherapy. Bethesda: National Cancer Institute, 1987:5.8.1–5.8.17.
76. Brahme A. Dosimetric precision requirements in radiation therapy. Acta Radiol Oncol 1984;23:379–391.
77. Mohan R, Mageras GS, Baldwin MS, et al. Clinically relevant optimization of 3D conformal treatments. Med Phys 1992;19:933–943.
78. Three-dimensional photon treatment planning: Report of the Collaborative Working Group on the evaluation of treatment planning for external beam radiotherapy. Int J Radiat Oncol Biol Phys 1991;21:1–206.
79. Thornton AF, Hegarty TJ, Ten-Haken RK, et al. Three-dimensional treatment planning of astrocytomas: A dosimetric study of cerebral irradiation. Int J Radiat Oncol Biol Phys 1991;20, 1309–1315.
80. Thornton AF, Ten-Haken RK, Gerhardsson A, Correll M. Three-dimensional motion analysis of an improved head immobilization system for simulation, CT, MRI, and PET imaging. Radiother Oncol 1991;20:224–228.
81. Thornton AF, Sandler HM Jr, Ten-Haken RK, Greenberg HS. Retreatment of recurrent high grade astrocytoma using three-dimensional external beam treatment planning. [Abstract] Proceedings of the 9th Annual Meeting of the European Society for Therapeutic Radiology and Oncology (ESTRO), Notectini, Italy, 1990:274.
82. Armstrong JG, Burman C, Leibel SA, et al. Conformal three dimensional treatment planning may improve the therapeutic ratio of high dose radiation therapy for lung cancer. Int J Radiat Oncol Biol Phys 1991;21(suppl 1):146.
83. Sandler HM Jr, Perez-Tamayo C, Licter A. Dose escalation in the treatment of stage C (T3) prostate cancer: Report on the rectal toxicity observed in a prospective series using a conformational external beam technique. [Abstract] Proceedings of the 9th Annual Meeting of the Europeen Society for Therapeutic Radiology and Oncology (ESTRO), Notectini, Italy, 1990:329.
84. Smit WGJM, Helle PA, van Putten WLJ, Wijnmaalen AJ, Seldenrath JJ, van der Werf-Messing BHP. Late radiation damage in prostate cancer patients treated by high dose external radiotherapy in relation to rectal dose. Int J Radiat Oncol Biol Phys 1990;18: 23–29.
85. Soffen EM, Hanks GE, Hwang CC, Chu JHC. Conformal static field therapy for low volume low grade prostate cancer with rigid immobilization. Int J Radiat Oncol Biol Phys 1991;20:141–146.
86. Soffen EM, Epstein BE, Hunt MA, Hanks GE. Decreased acure morbidity with conformal static field radiation therapy treatment of early prostate cancer as compared to nonconformal techniques. Int J Radiat Oncol Biol Phys 1991;21(suppl 1):152.
87. Leibel S. Personal communication.

ELLEN S. VITETTA
JONATHAN W. UHR
PHILIP E. THORPE

SECTION **3**

Immunotoxin Therapy

GENERAL PRINCIPLES

Chemotherapy and radiotherapy have been used successfully to treat a variety of malignancies. They act by killing rapidly dividing or metabolizing cells whether malignant or normal. For this reason, there have been increasing efforts to develop new approaches that offer better selectivity for malignant cells. One emerging modality is immunotoxin therapy.

The concept of immunotoxin therapy is appealing. An antibody or other cell-binding ligand with specificity for tumor cells is biochemically or genetically linked to a potent toxin. When injected into a patient with cancer, the ligand carries the toxin to the tumor cells. Once bound to the cells, the toxin is internalized and kills the cell. Even though monoclonal antibodies and other ligands are rarely tumor specific, they often react with a limited array of normal tissues that are not life sustaining.

Despite its conceptual simplicity, the development of immunotoxins for clinical use has been challenging. Immunotoxins are large, complex molecules in which each component,

including the cell-binding moiety, the crosslinker, and the toxin, plays a critical role in the effectiveness of the agent.

COMPONENTS OF AN IMMUNOTOXIN

LIGAND PORTION

Antibodies and Antibody Fragments

Monoclonal antibodies directed against molecules on tumor cells have been most frequently used as the ligand portion of immunotoxins. Such antibodies are seldom tumor specific and often recognize differentiation antigens present on the nonneoplastic cell at the time it became malignant. Immunotoxins directed against tumor-associated antigens often kill the tumor cells and certain nonneoplastic cells of the same lineage. Antibodies can crossreact with molecules on normal cells in a spurious and unpredictable fashion. When the nonmalignant cells are not life sustaining, this damage may be acceptable. In contrast, cross-reactions with life-sustaining tissue, even if minor, may be life threatening when these reagents are administered in vivo.[1] These cross-reactions are often difficult to detect by screening monoclonal antibodies on cell lines and normal tissues. For example, if the density of the cross-reacting antigen is low, it may not be possible to visualize cross-reactions by standard techniques of immunofluorescence or immunoperoxidase. Thus, even antigens of low density may be effective targets for immunotoxins.[2,3] Nonhuman primates can be useful for determining toxicities for the rare instances where a monoclonal antibody crossreacts with epitopes expressed on the cells.

A second consideration in the use of monoclonal antibodies as targeting agents is their immunogenicity. Because most monoclonal antibodies are of murine origin, they induce antibody responses in patients, unless they are immunosuppressed because of their disease or prior therapy. The development of chimeric antibodies having human constant (C_H and C_L) domains and murine variable (V_H and V_L) domains and of humanized murine antibodies having mouse hypervariable regions grafted onto human framework regions have reduced the immunogenicity of murine monoclonal antibodies.[4-7] However, even if this approach is successful in reducing the immunogenicity of the antibody portion of an immunotoxin, the toxin will probably induce an immune response. This has led to the practical consideration of treating persons who are immunosuppressed because of their disease or using various immunosuppressive regimens in conjunction with immunotoxin therapy.[8-10] However, the use of immunosuppressive agents may not be desirable if an intact immune system is needed to suppress regrowth of tumors.

Antibodies can be used as intact IgG molecules or as their F(ab')$_2$, Fab', or Fab fragments.[11,12] Fv fragments have also been used to generate fusion proteins.[13,14] IgG and F(ab')$_2$ molecules are divalent and bind to target cells more avidly than Fab or Fab' fragments. They generally have superior cytotoxic activity as immunotoxins.[15] Although F(ab')$_2$ molecules are less immunogenic and do not bind to Fc receptors, they are often partially inactivated by coupling to toxins.[12] Because they lack an Fc portion, they have a shorter half-life in vivo.[16] Univalent fragments have little antigenicity but often have lower potencies as immunotoxins and rapid clearance in vivo both of which reduce their antitumor activity relative to their IgG and F(ab')$_2$ counterparts.[12,15-18]

Although not often appreciated, only 5% to 25% of specific monoclonal antibodies make potent immunotoxins. For an immunotoxin to be effective, it must bind avidly to cells, be rapidly internalized, and be routed to intracellular compartments where toxins can translocate into the cytosol.[19-22] Many antibodies must be screened to select the ones which make effective immunotoxins.[23] Screening involves an indirect immunotoxin assay in which appropriate target cells are first treated with the test antibody and then with a Fab' immunotoxin directed against the immunoglobulin portion of the immunotoxin.[23,24] If effective killing is obtained, the test antibody invariably makes a potent immunotoxin when directly conjugated to the same toxin or ribosome-inactivating protein (RIP).

Even when an effective immunotoxin is used, the heterogeneity of tumor cells undoubtedly leads to the escape of antigen-negative mutants, necessitating the use of combinations (*i.e.,* "cocktails") of effective immunotoxins directed against different target cell antigens.[25,26]

Growth Factors

Growth factors can sometimes be used as carriers for toxins, and these constructs are called oncotoxins. Although growth factors bind to normal cells, tumor cells frequently express elevated levels of growth factor receptors.[27-30] If the normal cells are not life sustaining, it may be possible to devise dose-regimens that provide an acceptable therapeutic index. Fibroblast growth factor (FGF), melanocyte-stimulating hormone-α (MSH-α), epidermal growth factor (EGF), transforming growth factor-α (TGF-α), insulin-like growth factor (IGF), and interleukin-2, -4, and -6 have been coupled to toxins to create oncotoxins (Table 69–13). Advantages of using growth factors as ligands include their lack of immunogenicity, generally high affinity for their receptors, and the availability of cloned genes for generating growth factor-toxin fusion proteins.[31-38] However, many growth factors are rapidly cleared in vivo and may require continuous administration for long periods.[39] Another potential problem is that growth of some tumor cells may be stimulated by a few molecules of bound oncotoxins, insufficient to kill the cells.[40,41] Circulating levels of these ligands or their soluble receptors can be elevated in animals and patients with malignant disease resulting in competition for the oncotoxin and inhibition of its target cell cytotoxicity.[42,43] Despite these considerations, the use of oncotoxins has enormous potential and is currently being explored in animal studies and in phase I clinical trials.

TOXIN PORTION

The toxins that have been used to form immunotoxins are derived from bacteria and plants and are inhibitors of protein synthesis.[44] They are the most powerful cell poisons known, and when effectively targeted, fewer than 10 molecules in the cytosol of the target cell can be lethal.[45,46] Because toxins inhibit protein synthesis, they kill resting cells and, hence,

TABLE 69–13. Growth Factor–Toxin Fusion Proteins

Growth Factor	Toxin	Type of Cancer	References
IL-2	PE40	T-cell leukemia	14
	DAB486	Hodgkin's lymphoma	63, 137
		non-Hodgkin's lymphoma, T-cell leukemia	138
IL-4	DAB389	Non-Hodgkin's lymphoma	139
	PE40	Sarcoma, colon adenocarcinoma	140
IL-6	PE40	Myeloma, hepatoma	141
			142
TGF-α	PE40	Epidermoid carcinoma, prostate carcinoma, ovarian carcinoma, liver carcinoma, breast carcinoma	143 144
EGF	PE40	Epidermoid carcinoma	144
IGF	PE40	Breast carcinoma, hepatoma	145
FGF	Saporin		146
	PE40	Hepatoma, colon carcinoma, ovarian carcinoma, breast carcinoma	147
MSH-α	DT	Melanoma	148

IL, interleukin; TGF, tumor growth factor; EGF, epidermal growth factor; IGF, insulin-like growth factor; MSH, melanocyte-stimulating hormone.

have the potential of killing tumor cells that are not in cycle at the time of the treatment and that are spared by conventional chemotherapy. Toxins that have been used for the construction of immunotoxins are described in Table 69–14.[47] They share several features. All are synthesized as single chain peptides and are processed posttranslationally or in the target cell to which they are delivered into two-chain molecules with interchain disulfide bonds.[44,48,49] All have subunits or domains devoted to binding to cells, to translocation across membranes, and to the destruction of the protein synthetic machinery of the cell.[36]

The most frequently used plant toxins are ricin and abrin, both of which are synthesized as single chain polypeptides and then processed posttranslationally into mature toxins consisting of disulfide bonded A and B subunits.[44] The B-chain is a galactose-specific lectin that binds to glycoproteins and glycolipids on the surface of all cell types in higher animals and the A-chain is an N-glycosidase that translocates across the membrane of an intracellular vesicle and inhibits protein synthesis by removing an adenine residue from the 28S RNA (60S ribosomal subunit) that is needed for the binding of elongation factor-2 (EF-2).[44,50,51] The B-chain, and probably the A-chain, contain translocation domains that enable the A-chain to traverse cell membranes and enter the cytosol.[52]

RIPs analogous to the A-subunit of ricin (RTA) or abrin have been found in many plants and several of these have been used to form immunotoxins, such as bryodin, momordin, saporin, gelonin, trichosanthin, and pokeweed antiviral protein (PAP).[53–61] These single-chain RIPs are evolutionarily related to RTA and inactivate ribosomes in an identical fashion. However, because they lack the equivalent of the B-chain, they can only enter cells after being targeted by an appropriate ligand. Their main advantage over the toxin A-chains is that rigorous purification to eliminate B-chain or toxin is not required.

The bacterial toxins, like the plant toxins, are also synthesized as single polypeptide chains and have domains devoted to binding, translocation, and inhibition of protein synthesis.[36] The most frequently used bacterial toxins are *Pseudomonas* exotoxin A (PE) and diphtheria toxin (DT). DT is processed by the bacterium into the mature form consisting of two disulfide bonded chains analogous to the A- and B-chains of ricin and abrin.[48,49] PE is processed in the target cell to which it is delivered into a disulfide-bonded two-chain molecule.[36] The enzymatic domain of these toxins kills cells by catalyzing a modification of EF-2 that prevents its participation in protein synthesis.[62] The bacterial toxins have been successfully cloned, expressed and truncated into versions containing the active A-chain and the translocation domain without the nonspecific cell-binding domain.[63,64] These have been coupled to a variety of ligands (see Table 69–13) and the resulting oncotoxins are highly potent to target cells.

CROSSLINKER

For their use in in vivo therapy, the ligand and the toxin portions of the immunotoxins must be coupled in such a way as to remain stable in the blood and tissues and yet be labile within the target cell so the toxin subunit can enter the cytosol. A variety of crosslinkers that generate linkages that meet these requirements have been developed. The choice of a cross-

linker depends on whether an intact toxin, A-chain, or RIP is used.

Holotoxin Immunotoxins

Linkers used to couple holotoxins usually introduce a free thiol group into the antibody or ligand and an alkylating function into the toxin.[65,66] The two derivatized proteins are then reacted to produce a conjugate containing a thioether linkage. This linkage is stable to reduction and precludes dissociation of the toxin from the antibody. Holotoxin-immunotoxins retain the natural disulfide bond between the A- and B-chain that is necessary for the release of the A-chain inside the cell. For in vivo use, the lectin site on the B-chain must be blocked to prevent the immunotoxin from binding to and killing cells nonspecifically. The blockade can be accomplished sterically by attaching the ligand by a short crosslinker to the toxin or by using galactose-based affinity labels that bind covalently to the lectin site of the toxin.[67–70]

A-Chain Immunotoxins

Unlike holotoxin-containing immunotoxins, those containing toxin A-chains must have a disulfide bond introduced between the ligand and the A-chain, because bonds that cannot be reduced (*e.g.*, thioethers) generate ineffective immunotoxins.[15] The linker used to couple the A-chain to the ligand is usually a heterobifunctional crosslinker that introduces an activated thiol group into the ligand. The derivatized ligand is then mixed with reduced A-chain and the free thiol group in the A-chain displaces the leaving group from the activated thiol group of the ligand to form a disulfide linkage. The resulting immunotoxin is then purified to remove free A-chain and free antibody. These constructs retain full antigen-binding activity but the disulfide bond is usually not as stable as that generated with a thioether linkage.[17,71,72] A-chain can be released in vivo in the circulation or in the tissues. This is probably due to reduction by glutathione, albumin or other thiol-containing molecules. Immunotoxins prepared with hindered crosslinkers (*e.g.* SMPT) are much more stable and may have fewer side effects probably because less A chain is released in vivo.[72]

Fab and Fab' fragments of antibodies are coupled to A-chain by forming a disulfide bridge between the free cysteine residue near the hinge region and the free cysteine residue of the A-chain.[73] The thiol group in the antibody fragment is generally activated with Ellman's reagent and the derivative is mixed with reduced A-chain. Coupling then occurs by a thiol-disulfide exchange reaction. Because the thiol group of the antibody fragment is distant from the antigen combining site, the A chain does not interfere with the antigen-binding activity of the Fab'/Fab fragment.[73]

Ribosome-Inactivating Protein Immunotoxins

Immunotoxins containing RIPs are formed by linking the antibody and the RIP by a disulfide bond. However, unlike toxin A-chains, RIPs do not contain a free thiol group, and one must be introduced by treating the RIP with a thiolylating reagent.[47,74,75] The coupling reaction between the thiolylated RIP and the antibody is then performed in the same manner as for the A-chain immunotoxins.

TABLE 69–14. Structure and Function of Toxins and Ribosome-Inactivating Proteins Used for Immunotoxin Therapy

Toxin	Structure of Mature Form	Receptor	A-Chain Action
DT		Heparin-binding EGF-like growth factor precursor[149]	ADP-ribosylation of EF-2
DT(CRM-45)		None	ADP-ribosylation of EF-2
PE		α_2-macroglobulin receptor-LDL receptor-related protein[150]	ADP-ribosylation of EF-2
PE40		None	ADP-ribosylation of EF-2
Ricin, abrin		Galactose-containing oligosaccharide	N-glycosidase for 28S ribosomal RNA
Blocked ricin, abrin		None	N-glycosidase for 28S ribosomal RNA
RTA		None	N-glycosidase for 28S ribosomal RNA
RIP (gelonin, saporin)		None	N-glycosidase for 28S ribosomal RNA

▨, translocation domain; A, cytotoxic domain; B, binding domain; DT, diphtheria toxin; PE, *Pseudomonas* endotoxin A; EF-2, elongation, factor-2.

Recombinant Immunotoxins

Recombinant oncotoxins have been prepared with truncated PE or DT (see Table 69–13). This has been accomplished by cloning the genes for the toxins and mutagenizing them to delete segments encoding the cell-binding domain. The truncated forms of PE are PE40 and PE40lys, and the truncated forms of DT are CRM45, DAB486, and DAB389. The genes for the modified toxins are spliced to the gene encoding the ligand, and the entire oncotoxin is synthesized as a fusion protein in *E. coli*. Oncotoxins retain the activities of the ligand and the toxin, and they are highly stable in vivo because they contain a nonreducible peptide bond.[76]

PRECLINICAL EVALUATION

CYTOTOXIC POTENCY

The potency of an immunotoxin depends on the affinity of the antibody, the cell surface molecule that the antibody recognizes, and the capacity of that cell surface molecule to enter an intracellular compartment that is effective for A-chain translocation.[12,20,77,78] In the case of DT-containing immunotoxins, A-chain translocation occurs in an acidic compartment, such as late endosomes.[79,80] In the case of ricin and RIP immunotoxins, translocation occurs in a nonacidic compartment, possibly the trans-Golgi network.[81] The epitope on the surface molecule that the antibody recognizes may also play a critical role in intracellular routing and subsequent potency of the immunotoxin.[20,22,82] Those epitopes lying closer to the membrane appear to provide better targets possibly because they position the toxin closer to the lipid bilayer through which the toxin must ultimately pass to kill the cell.[82]

Immunotoxins containing blocked holotoxin or genetically engineered bacterial toxins are usually more potent that those containing A-chains or RIPs, although there are exceptions.[37,69,78,83,84] In the case of blocked abrin and ricin immunotoxins, their superior potency is probably attributable to the fact that the immunotoxin is partially degraded inside the target cell, and the unblocked toxin or toxin fragments that are released then kill the cell.[85] In the case of the oncotoxins, translocation domains in the toxin may form pores in the membrane that enable the A-chain-like domain to enter the cytosol and kill the cell. Immunotoxins prepared with A-chains and RIPs often have greatly enhanced toxicity in the presence of lysosomotropic amines and carboxylic ionophores.[86–88] These agents work by slowing the fusion of endosomes with lysosomes (where A-chains are enzymatically destroyed), or by delaying the transit of the immunotoxin through a compartment favorable for A-chain translocation (such as the trans-Golgi). B chains and B-chain immunotoxins also enhance the toxicity of some A-chain immunotoxins presumably by facilitating intracellular events involved in translocation.[89–91] Carboxylic ionophores have also been used successfully to potentiate the activity of immunotoxins in vivo by administering them in emulsions or coupled to albumin.[92,93]

HEPATOTOXICITY AND LIVER CLEARANCE

Immunotoxins prepared with blocked ricin, RTA, abrin A-chain, DT, PE, and certain RIPs (*e.g.* saporin) cause hepato-

toxicity in rodents of a severity that varies from moderate to dose limiting.[64,94–99] However, the mechanisms by which these immunotoxins cause liver damage are not the same. In the case of RTA, mannose and fucose-containing oligosaccharides are recognized by avid receptors on parenchymal and non-parenchymal cells of the liver and by other cells of the RES.[100,101] This results in rapid clearance, modest hepatic damage, and reduction in antitumor activity.[25,72,94,99] This problem has been circumvented by using chemically or enzymatically deglycosylated RTA or by using recombinant RTA expressed in a nonglycosylating cell.[102,103] In the case of blocked ricin-immunotoxins, the natural oligosaccharides on the A- and B-chains and those used to block the B-chain's lectin sites result in liver homing and marked liver damage.[100–102,104] Deglycosylation of the B-chain reduces its ability to potentiate the toxicity of A-chain immunotoxins and is therefore predicted to reduce their potency.[105] In the case of immunotoxins containing DT, PE, saporin, or abrin A-chain, the mechanisms underlying hepatotoxicity have not been elucidated. However, hepatotoxicity is not mediated through recognition of oligosaccharides on the toxin because none of these toxins is glycosylated. Conceivably, liver cells express a receptor for some portion of the toxin molecule. Alternatively, these toxins, like RTA, may bind to serum proteins for which liver cells have avid receptors.[106]

ANTITUMOR EFFECTS

A variety of animal tumor models have been used to evaluate immunotoxin therapy. In these models, immunotoxins are usually administered shortly after animals are injected with tumor cells to ascertain their effectiveness in treating minimal disease. In other studies, they have been administered to animals with large, established tumors. Although immunotoxins are generally more efficacious in the setting of minimal disease, some immunotoxins have had major antitumor effects on established tumors.[3,18,25,61,107–112] Chemotherapy or radiotherapy given in conjunction with immunotoxin therapy markedly improves their antitumor effects, as do β-adrenergic blockers and emulsified monensin.[92,113–118]

Cocktails of immunotoxins directed against different determinants on tumor cells have antitumor activity that is superior to that of single immunotoxins because the cocktail diminishes the probability that antigen-deficient variants or mutants will escape killing.[25,26] Taken together, these results indicate that immunotoxins will have their greatest impact in the clinic when used as a cocktail in conjunction with other debulking therapies. The ideal scenario is probably to administer an immunotoxin cocktail at a time when patients have minimal residual disease. It is encouraging that combined modalities have in certain experimental tumors reduced the tumor burden to a level where the immune system of the host can suppress the growth of remaining tumor cells.[3,115] If the immune system is functional, it may not be necessary to kill every tumor cell to induce a prolonged remission.

IMMUNOTOXIN-RESISTANT MUTANTS

Subpopulations of tumor cells that are resistant to immunotoxins pose the same problem for immunotoxin therapy as it does for chemotherapy. In several rodent tumor models, the inability of immunotoxin therapy to cure the animals is due to the survival and subsequent outgrowth of immunotoxin-resistant tumor cells.[25,26] Various types of mutants have been identified. The most common are antigen-loss mutants that lack the target antigen entirely or express it at levels too low for immunotoxin-mediated killing.[25,26] This type of mutant can be eradicated with cocktails of two or more immunotoxins recognizing different target antigens. Rarely, the mutants express the target antigen but have some deficiency in their intracellular transport system.[25,26] This type of mutant should also succumb to an immunotoxin cocktail provided that the deficiency in entry is not common to both antigen-entry pathways. Mutants having toxin-resistant ribosomes have not been observed despite deliberate attempts to raise them. Mutations in ribosomes that confer A-chain resistance may be lethal. Alternatively, there may be multiple copies of genes encoding ribosomal components that make simultaneous mutations in all copies highly improbable.

CLINICAL TRIALS

SOLID TUMORS

The first clinical trials with RTA and PE-based immunotoxins were carried out in patients with solid tumors, including melanoma, breast cancer, and colon cancer. For several reasons, these tumors are among the least likely to respond to immunotoxin therapy. Tumor cells in solid epithelial tumors are not very accessible to immunotoxins. Compression of draining lymphatics and elevation of interstitial pressure within the tumor reduce the amount of an antibody that enters the tumor to approximately 0.001% of the injected dose per gram of tumor.[120,121] The immunotoxin that enters the tumor is absorbed by tumor cells adjacent to the vasculature and often fails to reach tumor cells deeper in the tumor mass.[122] Patients with solid tumors are usually not intrinsically immunosuppressed and frequently develop neutralizing antibodies against the immunotoxin that preclude further courses of immunotoxin therapy.[123,124] Antibodies raised against antigens on solid epithelial tumors frequently crossreact with life-sustaining normal tissues.[1,125]

Few phase I–II clinical trials involving systemic therapy with immunotoxins in solid tumors are ongoing. The results of several trials are presented in the next sections, and their major features are summarized in Table 69–15.

Melanoma

The first phase I immunotoxin trial was carried out in patients with metastatic melanoma.[126] The antibody portion of the immunotoxin was directed against a high molecular weight antigen on melanoma cells and the toxin was native RTA. The two components were linked by a disulfide bond generated with the SPDP-crosslinker. Twenty-two patients were treated in the phase I trial. Toxicities included hypoalbuminemia in 20 patients, weight gain and edema in 6 patients, and low voltage electrocardiograms in 16 patients. These toxicities are characteristic of vascular leak syndrome (VLS). The maximal tolerated dose (MTD) was greater than 3 mg/kg, and 17 of the patients made antibody against the immunotoxin. One

patient had a complete remission, and 9 had mixed responses or stabilized disease. Pharmacokinetic data are not available, but immunoperoxidase staining indicated the presence of RTA and mouse immunoglobulin in the metastatic lesions of 5 patients after 24 hours of therapy. In the ensuing phase II trial, 43 patients were treated, and 3 had partial responses, 1 had a mixed response, and 9 had stabilization of their disease.[127] Toxicities were similar to those described in the phase I trial. In another phase II trial, the immunotoxin was administered in conjunction with cyclophosphamide to decrease the antibody response against the immunotoxin.[123] In this trial, 1 patient developed seizures, neutropenia, and anemia, but this may have been attributable to cyclophosphamide rather than the immunotoxin. Four of the 20 patients treated had partial responses. Thirteen patients evaluated for an immune response made antibodies against the immunotoxin. Cyclophosphamide did not reduce the immunogenicity of the immunotoxin, and it is unclear if it contributed to the clinical responses.

Colon Carcinoma

A phase I study of an immunotoxin containing native RTA and a monoclonal antibody that recognizes glycoprotein, gp72, on the surface of colon carcinoma cells was conducted in 17 patients with metastatic colorectal carcinoma.[124] Toxicities included fever, hypoalbuminemia, flu-like symptoms, proteinuria, and mental status changes (*e.g.,* fatigue, slurred speech, irritability, expressive aphasia), all of which reversed when treatment was discontinued. The MTD was greater than 1 mg/kg. Five of the 16 patients had mixed tumor regressions, including 2 with a reduction of hepatic metastases, 3 with a reduction in subcuticular metastases, and 1 with a decrease in pulmonary metastases. Virtually all patients made antibodies against the RTA (HARA) and the mouse Ig (HAMA) of the IgM and IgG classes.

Breast Carcinoma

Nine patients with metastatic breast carcinoma were treated with recombinant RTA coupled to an antibody (260F9) that reacts with an antigen expressed on approximately 50% of breast cancer cells. The immunotoxin was administered by bolus injection (4 patients) or continuous infusion (5 patients).[1,128] The patients receiving the bolus infusion developed symptoms of VLS, even at the lower doses. Continuous infusion of the immunotoxin in 5 patients resulted in less severe VLS, but severe neurologic toxicity occurred in 3 patients, commencing with plexopathies at the site of previous chest wall irradiation and progressing to sensor motor neuropathies in all extremities. Neuropathies worsened over a period of 2 to 3 months. During the following 6 months, the patients recovered motor function but had persistent paresthesias. A nerve biopsy of 1 patient at the time of maximal symptoms revealed axonal loss and segmental demyelination consistent with toxic injury to the Schwann cells. It was found that the 260F9 antibody intensely stained the nerve sheath, suggesting that the antibody recognized an epitope present on Schwann cells or myelin.

The major dose-limiting toxicity of this immunotoxin was due to targeting of the RTA to normal neural tissue, rather

TABLE 69–15. Summary of Clinical Trials

Disease	Phase	Immunotoxin	Maximal Tolerated Dose (Total)	Toxicity	Antibody Response	$T_{1/2}$ (h)	Clinical Response	Reference
Metastatic melanoma	I	Xomazyme-Mel	>3 mg/kg	VLS, myalgia	17/21 (81%)	ND	1/22 CR 9/22 mixed or stabilized	126
	II	Xomazyme-Mel		VLS	ND	ND	3/43 PR 1/43 MR' 9/43 stabilization	127
	II	Xomazyme-Mel plus cyclophosphamide		VLS	13/13 (100%)	ND	4/20 PR	123
Colorectal carcinoma	I	Anti-gp72-RTA	>1 mg/kg	VLS, aphasia	15/16 HARA (94%) 16/17 HAMA (94%)	ND	5/16 mixed tumor regressions	124
Metastatic breast carcinoma	I	260F9-rRTA (bolus)	>50 µg/kg	VLS, myalgia paresthesia	4/4 (100%)	8.3	1/4 resolution of lung nodules	128
	I	260F9-rRTA (continuous infusion)	0.4 mg/kg	VLS, myalgia, neuropathies	4/5 HARA (80%) 3/5 HAMA (60%)	4–6	0/5	1
Ovarian carcinoma	I	Anti-OVB3-PE		SGOT/SGPT elevations, abdominal pain, encephalopathy		ND	0/23	125
Non-Hodgkin's lymphoma	I/II	Anti-CD19-blocked ricin (bolus)	0.25 mg/kg	SGOT/SGPT elevations thrombocytopenia	12/15 (78%)	ND	1/25 CR 2/25 PR 10/25 mixed or transient	129
	I	Anti-CD19-blocked ricin (continuous infusion)	0.35 mg/kg	SGOT, SGPT elevations thrombocytopenia edema	26/43 (60%)	ND	2/43 CR 5/43 PR 11/43 transient	130
	I	Fab' anti-CD22-dgA	75 mg/m² (1.8 mg/kg)	VLS, myalgia, pulmonary edema rhabdomyolysis	4/14 HARA (29%) 1/14 HAMA (7%)	1.4	5/13 PR	131
	I	IgG anti-CD22-dgA	30 mg/m² (0.7 mg/kg)	VLS, myalgia, pulmonary edema, rhabdomyolysis	8/24 HARA (33%) 7/24 HAMA (29%)	7.8	6/24 PR 1/24 CR	Amlot et al (submitted)
B-cell chronic leukemia	I	Anti-CD5 (T101)-RTA	ND	Fever	1/4 HARA (25%) 0/4 HARA	ND	4/5 transient rapid fall in circulating leukemic cells	132
T-cell lymphoma	I	Anti-CD5 (H65)-RTA	3.3 mg/kg	VLS, dyspnea	10/12 (86%)	1.2–2.9	4/14 PR	133
NHL, Hodgkin's disease	I	IL-2-DAB486		Hepatic transaminase elevations, hypoalbuminemia, hypersensitivity, creatine elevations, thrombocytopenias	(60%)	0.08	3/47 CR	134 (J. Nichols, personal communication)
Steroid-resistant GVHD	II	Anti-CD5 (H65)-RTA		VLS, myalgia; hematuria, tremors	6/23 HAMA (26%) 6/23 HARA (26%)	1.5–3.9	9/32 CR 7/32 PR 6/32 MR	135

ND, not determined; VLS, vascular leak syndrome; CR, complete response; PR, partial response.

than nonspecific effects common to all RTA-immunotoxins. In the bolus infusion protocol, the MTD was approximately 50 μg/kg, and in the continuous infusion protocol, the MTD was 400 μg/kg. After bolus administration, the peak serum concentrations of immunotoxin were between 200 and 850 μg/ml, the $T_{1/2}$ was 1.8 hours, and the $T_{1/2}\beta$ was 8.3 hours. Using the continuous infusion protocol the $T_{1/2}$ was 4-6 hours. One of 4 patients who received bolus administration showed resolution of a lung nodule, which was the sole site of disease. All 4 patients made antibody against the immunotoxin. None of 5 patients who received the continuous infusion of immunotoxin showed clinical responses, and 4 patients made HARA and 3 made HAMA. Because of the cross-reactivity of this immunotoxin with normal neural tissue, trials with this immunotoxin were discontinued.

Ovarian Carcinoma

OVB3 antibody linked to PE was administered intraperitoneally to 23 patients with advanced ovarian carcinoma.[125] Therapeutic levels of immunotoxin were achieved in peritoneal fluid at all doses of the immunotoxin. At higher doses, therapeutic levels were also achieved in the serum. Side effects included transient elevations of liver enzymes, fever and abdominal pain that was sufficiently severe to require treatment. The dose-limiting toxicity was neurologic. Two patients developed encephalopathy (*e.g.,* confusion and aphasia) after two doses of the immunotoxin and took several months to recover. A third patient developed severe encephalopathy after three doses resulting in seizures, coma, and ultimately death. It was found that the OVB3 antibody was weakly reactive with cells in the cerebellum. No objective responses were achieved.

HEMATOLOGIC MALIGNANCIES

Several clinical trials have been conducted in which immunotoxins have been used to treat lymphomas and leukemias. Hematologic tumors are particularly likely to respond to immunotoxin therapy for several reasons. It is possible to treat such diseases with immunotoxins directed against normal lymphocyte and myeloid cell markers, because the normal cells that are killed with the tumor cells are rapidly replenished from progenitor cells in the marrow. Many antibodies that react with tumor cells but not with life-sustaining tissues are available. The tumor cells in large solid lymphomas may be more accessible than those in epithelial tumors, which frequently contain dense connective tissue. Patients with lymphoid malignancies are often immunosuppressed by their disease and by prior therapy. Not all patients make antiimmunotoxin antibodies so that immunotoxin therapy can be given in multiple courses.

Four types of immunotoxin constructs have been used to treat lymphomas and leukemias, as described in the next few sections.

Blocked-Ricin Immunotoxins

In two phase I trials, an anti-CD19-blocked ricin immunotoxin was administered to patients with refractory lymphomas and leukemias.[129,130] This immunotoxin was highly potent and specific in vitro. CD19 is present on virtually all B-cells and tumor cells from non-Hodgkin's lymphoma (NHL), chronic lymphocytic leukemia (CLL), and some types of non-T-cell acute lymphocytic leukemia (ALL). In the first phase I trial, daily bolus injections of the immunotoxin were administered to 23 patients with NHL, 1 with non-T-ALL, and 1 with CLL. All patients had relapsed after prior chemotherapy or bone marrow transplantation. Toxicities included transient elevation of hepatic transaminase, transient thrombocytopenia, low-grade fevers, and hypoalbuminemia without edema. Of the 25 patients treated, 1 had a complete response after 3 courses of therapy, 2 had partial responses, and 10 had transient or mixed responses. The two partial responses occurred in patients where bone marrow was the only site of tumor. The MTD was 250 μg/kg. Twelve of the 15 patients made antibodies against the immunotoxin. Blood levels of the immunotoxin were approximately 200 nM but were maintained only transiently. In a subsequent trial, anti-CD19-blocked ricin immunotoxin was administered by a 7-day continuous infusion protocol. Forty-three patients were treated, including 33 with NHL, 5 with CLL, and 5 with non-T-ALL. Toxicities that defined MTD included elevations of SGOT and SGPT that lasted from 1 to 2 weeks and thrombocytopenia. In addition, 23 patients developed transient hypoalbuminemia, 11 developed peripheral edema, and 30 developed fever. Twenty-six of the 43 patients made HAMA or HARA. Of the 43 patients treated, there were 2 complete responses, 5 partial responses, and 11 transient responses. Almost 50% of the patients with low- and intermediate-grade NHL or CLL had significant responses; less frequent responses were seen in patients with high-grade NHL and non-T-ALL.

Deglycosylated-RTA Immunotoxins

Two phase I trials have been carried out with immunotoxins consisting of anti-CD22 antibody coupled to chemically deglycosylated RTA.[131] The patient population was similar to that treated with the CD19-blocked ricin immunotoxin. CD22 is a normal B-lymphocyte antigen that is expressed on cells from 60% to 70% of patients with B-cell lymphomas. A total of 41 patients with CD22$^+$ tumor cells were entered into the two trials. An average of 50% of the tumor cells in the patients expressed CD22. The remaining tumor cells lacked the antigen or expressed it at levels too low to be detected by indirect immunofluorescence analyses. One immunotoxin consisted of an intact IgG antibody (RFB4) coupled by a stable crosslinker (SMPT) to chemically deglycosylated ricin A-chain. The other immunotoxin was an Fab' fragment of the same antibody coupled by a cystine bond to deglycosylated ricin A-chain. The RTA was deglycosylated to prevent the immunotoxins from homing to and damaging cells in the liver and RES that have receptors for the mannose and fucose residues on native RTA. The IgG immunotoxin had an IC$_{50}$ on Daudi cells in vitro of 10^{-12} M, and the Fab' immunotoxin had an IC$_{50}$ of 10^{-11} M. Both constructs were more than 100,000 times more toxic to cells expressing CD22 than they were to cells lacking CD22. Fifteen patients were treated with the Fab' immunotoxin and 26 with the IgG immunotoxin.

In both cases, dose-related toxicities included VLS and myalgia, and dose-limiting toxicities included aphasia, pulmonary edema, and rhabdomyolysis. In the earlier phases of the trial, the presence of pulmonary parenchymal lymphoma predisposed patients to rapidly appearing and severe pulmonary edema during treatment; therefore, patients with pulmonary lymphoma were later excluded from entry.

The MTD for the Fab' immunotoxin was 75 mg/m^2 (1.8 mg/kg) and the MTD for the IgG immunotoxin was 30 mg/m^2 (0.7 mg/kg). The $T_{1/2}$ of the Fab' immunotoxin averaged 1.3 hours, but that of the IgG immunotoxin averaged 7.8 hours. Only a single phase of clearance was visible in the recipients of the Fab' immunotoxin, but in 9 patients receiving IgG-IgA, distinct α and β phases of clearance were observed, with a $T_{1/2}\beta$ that ranged from 6 to 17 hours. The highest serum levels obtained were 15.8 μg/ml for the Fab' immunotoxin and 11.3 μg/ml for the IgG immunotoxin. In 2 patients treated with the IgG immunotoxin, serum was taken 24 hours after administration of the IgG immunotoxin and the concentration and cytotoxic activity of this circulating immunotoxin were determined. The immunotoxin was fully active, indicating that it was highly stable in vivo. Overall, 28% of the patients treated with the Fab' immunotoxin and 37% treated with the IgG immunotoxin made antibodies against the RTA, the mouse immunoglobulin, or both, but the Fab' portion of the immunotoxin was less immunogenic than the IgG portion. After one course of treatment, the clinical responses for the Fab' and the IgG immunotoxin were very similar. At 1 month, 6 of 24 evaluable patients who had received the IgG immunotoxin had partial responses, and an additional patient had a complete response. Five of 12 patients who received the Fab' immunotoxin had partial responses. In all cases, responses were transient and lasted between 1 and 4 months.

It can be concluded that the Fab' construct was less immunogenic than the IgG construct. The Fab' construct was shorter lived but similar in efficacy. VLS and myalgias were observed in patients treated with both constructs. Because these side effects were the same as those observed in patients treated with immunotoxins containing other antibodies and recombinant or native RTA, they cannot be attributed to the specificity of the antibody, the Fc portion of the antibody, or the carbohydrate portion of the A-chain.

Native RTA Immunotoxins

Five patients with refractory CLL were treated with 24 mg/m^2 of anti-CD5-RTA prepared with the T101 antibody.[132] Toxicities included VLS and fever. No objective responses were achieved although 4 of 5 patients had a rapid and transient decreases in circulating leukemic cells. One of the 4 patients made HARA, and none made HAMA. The lack of efficacy may be due to the fact that CLL cells internalize the immunotoxins poorly.

In another trial, an anti-CD5-RTA prepared with the H65 antibody was administered to 14 patients with cutaneous T-cell lymphoma in a dose escalation protocol.[133] VLS was observed in virtually all patients and the dose-limiting toxicity was dyspnea. The MTD was 3.3 mg/kg and the $T_{1/2}$ ranged from 1.2 to 2.9 hours. Ten of 12 patients evaluated made HAMA/HARA, and in 7 of 11 cases, this antibody blocked immunotoxin-mediated killing. All patients but 1 had a decrease in circulating CD3$^+$/CD5$^+$ lymphocytes, and 4 of 14 patients had partial responses lasting from 3-5 months. Palliation of disease was observed in all patients.

Diphtheria Toxin Oncotoxins

Human IL-2 fused to DT-AB486 has been used to treat a variety of malignancies of lymphoid, epidermoid, or sarcomatoid types.[134] The fusion protein was administered to 72 patients with IL-2R$^+$ malignancies, and 47 were evaluable for a response. Side effects at MTD included transient hepatic transaminase elevations, hypoalbuminemia, hypersensitivity-like syndromes, and occasional transient creatine elevations and thrombocytopenias. Antibodies against DT were present in approximately 30% of the patients before treatment and in 60% after one or two courses of therapy. Preliminary studies indicated that the response rates in patients with circulating antibodies were similar to those without antibodies. However, the $T_{1/2}$ of this oncotoxin was so short (5–10 minutes) that the presence of antibodies may have been irrelevant. Of 47 patients treated with different dose schedules ranging from bolus injection to 6-hour infusions, complete responses were seen in 3 patients and these responses lasted from 9 to 24 months. Although the IL-2 oncotoxin is directed against the tumor cells, it also has the potential of killing activated IL-2R$^+$ T cells in these patients. Elimination of T cells may be directly or indirectly involved in tumor regressions. This possibility remains to be explored.

GRAFT-VERSUS-HOST DISEASE

Although not a malignant disease, we include a description of the efficacy of an immunotoxin in treating GVHD, because it makes the important point that immunotoxins are extremely effective therapeutic agents in settings where the target cells are readily accessible to the blood and where it is not necessary to kill all the target cells for benefit to be obtained.

Thirty-two patients were treated with anti-CD5(H65)-RTA.[135] The CD5 antigen is expressed on most T cells and a minority of B cells. Most of the patients had visceral and skin involvement. The immunotoxin was administered in 7 to 14 doses, and the $T_{1/2}$ ranged from 1.5 to 3.9 hours. Toxicities included VLS, hematuria, and tremors. Nine of the 32 patients had a complete response, 7 had a partial response, and 6 had mixed responses. In 26 patients with evaluable skin disease, 11 had complete resolution of their disease, and 8 showed improvement. Resolution of disease was seen in 6 of the 22 patients with gastrointestinal involvement, and 3 of 22 patients with liver involvement. The success of these trials demonstrates that clinical responses could be induced at safe doses of the immunotoxin and that the side effects were tolerable. There was marked reduction in mononuclear cells staining with anti-CD5 and anti-CD3 antibodies in all 7 patients studied, demonstrating that the target cells were eliminated. It is not clear whether the responses are attributable to elimination of the CD5$^+$ T cells, the CD5$^+$ B cells, or both.

CONCLUSIONS

Several important lessons have been learned from the phase I–II clinical trials. The side effects of immunotoxin therapy are different from those of conventional chemotherapy. In particular, the damage to rapidly regenerating normal tissues observed with conventional chemotherapy is absent with immunotoxin therapy, with the exception of anti-CD19-blocked ricin immunotoxins and IL2-DAB486 that, for obscure reasons, cause thrombocytopenia. Liver toxicity is a consistent side effect in recipients of DT- and PE-containing immunotoxins. Blocked ricin immunotoxins cause liver toxicity, VLS, and myalgias. Immunotoxins containing native RTA cause VLS and myalgias but little liver toxicity, and those containing recombinant or deglycosylated RTA cause VLS and myalgias but no liver toxicity.

Because the side effects of immunotoxin therapy and chemotherapy differ, it is important to test these modalities in combination. In vitro and animal studies indicate that these two forms of therapy are markedly synergistic.

VLS observed with immunotoxins containing ricin or RTA rapidly reverses after treatment is discontinued or corticosteroids are given. The mechanism underlying VLS is not known. Possibilities include a direct effect of the RTA on vascular endothelium (for which we have some preliminary experimental evidence) or RTA-induced release of cytokines (*e.g.* TNF, IFN-, IL-2) that cause increased vascular permeability. Myalgias and muscle weakness may be caused by VLS-induced extravasation of immunotoxins into skeletal muscle. A generalized reduction in cardiac voltage, as determined by electrocardiogram, is usually observed after administration of RTA immunotoxins. The cause is unknown, but it could be a result of fluid accumulation in the chest wall. Electrocardiographic changes have not been associated with any other abnormalities, including abnormalities in echocardiograms, elevations in cardiac enzymes in sera, or clinical evidence of cardiac dysfunction.

There are circumstances in which VLS or myalgia become dose limiting, including rhabdomyolysis, pulmonary edema (particularly if there is a concomitant pulmonary neoplasia or infection), and psychoneurologic alterations. The latter are usually manifested by mental confusion and aphasia and are transient. The mechanisms involved in neurologic changes are not known, but they could be related to VLS. No permanent sequelae have resulted.

The severe neurotoxicity observed in two trials for breast and ovarian carcinoma emphasizes the importance of carefully screening antibodies for unexpected cross-reactivities with life-sustaining tissues and, if possible, for selecting antibodies that are cross-reactive with their homologs in nonhuman primates.

Optimal regimens for administration of the immunotoxins have not yet been devised so that the $T_{1/2}$s are generally shorter than would be predicted to induce an optimal therapeutic response. The short $T_{1/2}$s are due to a combination of factors. Immunotoxins prepared from antibodies that lack an Fc portion are not resorbed into the blood after filtration in the glomerulus, and they have inherently short serum half-lives. Immunotoxins prepared from glycosylated toxins (*e.g.* ricin) are cleared by cells with carbohydrate receptors in the liver and the RES. The crosslinkers used to form the immunotoxins that were used in some of the first clinical trials were unstable, and this instability has been shown in animal tumor models to diminish antitumor activity. Because of the short $T_{1/2}$, it is probably advisable to consider continuous infusion protocols. It should be noted, however, that sustaining the blood levels of immunotoxins over days or weeks could lead to additional toxicities from cross-reactions with cells in less accessible tissues.

Antibody responses against the antibody portion and the toxin portion of the immunotoxins have been observed. It is not known to what extent these antibodies can prevent repeated courses of therapy. A high and sustained level of serum antibody will probably inhibit further therapy by increasing the rate of clearance from the blood or neutralizing the toxin. However, little is known about the persistence of these antibody responses, the generation of memory cells, and what proportion of the antibodies are neutralizing. HAMA can probably be partially overcome by humanizing the antibodies, but it is unlikely that humanization will significantly reduce antibody responses against the toxins. The latter will probably require the prior or simultaneous administration of immunosuppressive agents or the derivatization of immunotoxins with agents that render them nonimmunogenic. In patients who are immunosuppressed because of their disease, immune responses are less frequent, but even in these patients, immune responsiveness depends on the immunogenicity of the construct. Blocked ricin-immunotoxins are considerably more immunogenic than RTA-immunotoxins in a similar population of patients.

Clinical responses in phase I and II patients are encouraging considering that most patients had bulky disease and that the targeted antigen may not have been expressed on all tumor cells. This is particularly true in lymphoma and leukemia. In one trial, as few as 15% of the tumor cells in some patients were positive for the targeted antigen.[131] This situation may also be true for some of the other targeted antigens, although it has not been reported. In future trials, it will be important to determine the phenotype of residual tumor cells to establish whether their escape is due to deficiency of the target antigen, to other resistance mechanisms, or to inaccessibility to the immunotoxin. If the first possibility is true, survival of the residual cells might be prevented by the use of immunotoxin cocktails directed against two or more target antigens. It will also be important to correlate response rates in phase II trials with the percentage of antigen-positive cells in tumor samples and with the size, location, and grade of the tumors. The response rate may also correlate with the incidence of VLS, because a moderate degree of VLS may promote access of the immunotoxin to the tumor. If clinical responses were not achieved in phase I trials but unacceptable toxicities were absent, it is possible that clinical responses may be achieved in the setting of minimal disease.

Although not specifically addressed in the clinical trials carried out to date, a general problem in targeting immunotoxins is the identification and phenotype of the malignant progenitor cell. In the case of NHL, it appears that the renewal cell bears surface immunoglobulin and has the phenotype of a mature B cell. This can be deduced from the complete remissions induced by treatment with antibody to the tumor immunoglobulin idiotype in some patients with NHL.[136] In contrast, the bulk of tumor cells in CLL are mature, nondividing lymphocytes, and the phenotype of their progenitor cell has not yet been determined. It is important to develop in vitro assays for progenitor cells to verify that candidate immunotoxins have cytotoxic activity against the malignant stem cells in the neoplastic disease to be treated.

The immunotoxin field has undergone an impressive evolution since its inception one decade ago. Although drug development is a lengthy and complex process (and no less so for the immunotoxins), it is extremely encouraging that one immunotoxin (*i.e.*, anti-CD5-A-RTA) has received approval to be marketed for the treatment of GVHD. The speed with which this occurred is due in no small part to the impact of immunology, pharmacology, and molecular and cell biology on the rational design of these reagents. Optimization of immunotoxins for cancer therapy will be more complex, but there is every reason to believe that success for treating some tumors will be achieved.

REFERENCES

1. Gould BJ, Borowitz MJ, Groves ES, et al. Phase I study of an anti-breast cancer immunotoxin by continuous infusion: Report of a targeted toxic effect not predicted by animal studies. JNCI 1989;81:775–781.
2. Fulton RJ, Uhr JW, Vitetta ES. In vivo therapy of the BCL1 tumor: Effect of immunotoxin valency and deglycosylation of the ricin A chain. Cancer Res 1988;48:2626–2631.
3. Krolick KA, Uhr JW, Slavin S, Vitetta ES. In vivo therapy of a murine B cell tumor (BCL1) using antibody-ricin A chain immunotoxins. J Exp Med 1982;155:1797–1809.
4. Morrison SL, Johnson MJ, Herzenberg LA, Oi VT. Chimeric human antibody molecules: Mouse antigen-binding domains with human constant region domains. Proc Natl Acad Sci USA 1984;81:6851–6855.
5. Shaw DR, Khazaeli MB, Lobuglio AF. Biological activity of mouse/human chimeric antibodies of the four human IgG subclasses with specificity for a tumor-associated antigen. Proc Am Assoc Cancer Res 1988;29:421.
6. Jones PT, Dear PH, Foote J, Neuberger MS, Winter G. Replacing the complementarity-determining regions in a human antibody with those from a mouse. Nature 1986;321:522–525.
7. Shaw DR, Khazaeli MB, Sun LK, et al. Characterization of a mouse/human chimeric monoclonal antibody (17-1A) to a colon cancer tumor-associated antigen. J Immunol 1987;138:4534–4538.
8. Lederman JA, Begent RHJ, Bagshawe KD, et al. Repeated anti-tumor antibody therapy in man with suppression of the host response by cyclosporin A. Br J Cancer 1988;58:654–657.
9. Lobuglio AF, Khazaeli MB, Lee J, et al. Pharmacokinetics and immune response to Xomazyme-Mel in melanoma patients. In: Antibody Immunoconj Radiopharm 1988;1:305–310.
10. Pai LH, FitzGerald DJ, Tepper M, Schacter B, Spitalny G, Pastan I. Inhibition of antibody response to *Pseudomonas* exotoxin and an immunotoxin containing *Pseudomonas* exotoxin by 15-deoxyspergualin in mice. Cancer Res 1990;50:7750–7753.
11. Raso V, Griffin T. Specific cytotoxicity of a human immunoglobulin directed Fab'-ricin A conjugate. J Immunol 1980;125:2610–2616.
12. Ghetie M-A, May RD, Till M, et al. Evaluation of ricin A chain-containing immunotoxins directed against CD19 and CD22 antigens on normal and malignant human B-cells as potential reagents for in vivo therapy. Cancer Res 1988;48:2610–2617.
13. Batra JK, FitzGerald DJ, Chaudhary VK, Pastan I. Single-chain immunotoxins directed at human transferrin receptor containing *Pseudomonas* exotoxin A or diphtheria toxin: Anti-TFR (Fv)-PE40 and DT388-anti-TFR (Fv). Mol Cell Biol 1991;11:2200–2205.
14. Chaudhary VK, Gallo MG, FitzGerald DJ, Pastan I. A recombinant single-chain immunotoxin composed of anti-tac variable regions and a truncated diphtheria toxin. Proc Natl Acad Sci USA 1990;87:9491–9494.
15. Masuho Y, Kishida K, Saito M, Umeto N, Hara T. Importance of the antigen-binding valency and the nature of cross-linking bond in ricin A chain conjugates with antibody. J Biochem 1982;91:1583–1591.
16. Holton OD, III, Black CDV, Parker RJ, et al. Biodistribution of monoclonal IgG1, F(ab')2 and Fab' in mice after intravenous injection. Comparison between anti-B cell (anti-LyB8. 2) and irrelevant (MOPC21) antibodies. J Immunol 1987;139:3041.
17. Fulton RJ, Tucker TF, Vitetta ES, Uhr JW. Pharmacokinetics of tumor-reactive immunotoxins in tumor-bearing mice: Effect of antibody valency and deglycosylation of the ricin A chain on clearance and tumor localization. Cancer Res 1988;48:2618–2625.
18. Engert A, Martin G, Pfreundschuh M, et al. Anti-tumor effects of ricin A chain immunotoxins prepared from intact antibodies and Fab' fragments on solid human Hodgkin's disease tumors in mice. Cancer Res 1990;50:2929–2935.
19. Bjorn MJ, Ring D, Frankel A. Evaluation of monoclonal antibodies for the development of breast cancer immunotoxins. Cancer Res 1985;45:1214–1221.
20. Engert A, Burrows F, Jung WE, et al. Evaluation of ricin A chain-containing immunotoxins directed against CD30 as potential reagents for the treatment of Hodgkin's disease. Cancer Res 1989;50:84–88.
21. Goldmacher VS, Scott CF, Lambert JM, et al. Cytotoxicity of gelonin and its conjugates with antibodies is determined by the extent of their endocytosis. J Cell Physiol 1989;141:222–234.
22. Press OW, Martin P, Thorpe PE, Vitetta ES. Ricin A-chain containing immunotoxins directed against different epitopes on the CD2 molecule differ in their ability to kill normal and malignant T cells. J Immunol 1988;141:4410–4417.
23. Till M, May RD, Uhr JW, Thorpe PE, Vitetta ES. An assay that predicts the ability of monoclonal antibodies to form potent ricin A chain-containing immunotoxins. Cancer Res 1988;48:1119–1123.
24. Weltman JK, Pedroso P, Johnson S-A, Davignon D, Fast LD, Leone LA. Rapid screening with indirect immunotoxin for monoclonal antibodies against human small cell lung cancer. Cancer Res 1987;47:5552–5556.
25. Thorpe PE, Wallace PM, Knowles PP, et al. Improved anti-tumor effects of immunotoxins prepared with deglycosylated ricin A chain and hindered disulfide linkages. Cancer Res 1988;48:6396–6403.
26. Thorpe PE, Blakey DC, Brown AN, et al. Comparison of two anti-Thy 1.1-abrin A-chain immunotoxins prepared with different cross-linking agents: Antitumor effects, in vivo fate, and tumor cell mutants. JNCI 1987;79:1101–1112.
27. Libermann TA, Nusbaum HR, Razon N, Kris R, Lax I, Soreq H. Amplification, enhanced expression and possible rearrangement of EGF receptor gene in primary brain tumors of glial origin. Nature 1985;313:144–147.
28. Leonard WJ, Depper JM, Robb RJ, Waldmann TA, Greene WC. Characterization of the human receptor for T cell growth factor. Proc Natl Acad Sci USA 1983;80:6957–6961.
29. Hendler FJ, Ozanne BW. Human squamous cell lung cancers express increased epidermal growth factor receptors. J Clin Invest 1984;74:647–651.
30. Kronke M, Depper JM, Leonard WJ, Vitetta ES, Waldmann TA, Greene WC. Adult T cell leukemia: A potential target for ricin A chain immunotoxins. Blood 1985;65:1416–1421.
31. FitzGerald D, Pastan I. Targeted toxin therapy for the treatment of cancer. JNCI [Review] 1989;81:1455–1463.
32. FitzGerald D, Pastan I. Redirecting *Pseudomonas* exotoxin. Semin Cell Biol 1991;2:31–38.
33. Greenfield L, Bjorn MJ, Horn G, et al. Nucleotide sequence of the structural gene for diphtheria toxin carried by corynebacteriophage beta. Proc Natl Acad Sci USA 1983;80:6853–6857.
34. Gray GL, Smith DH, Baldridge JS, et al. Cloning, nucleotide sequence, and expression in Escherichia coli of the exotoxin A structural gene of *Pseudomonas aeruginosa*. Proc Natl Acad Sci USA 1984;81:2645–2649.
35. Leong D, Coleman KD, Murphy JR. Cloned fragment A of diphtheria toxin is expressed and secreted into the periplasmic space of *Escherichia coli* K12. Science 1983;220:515–517.
36. Ogata M, Chaudhary VK, Pastan I, FitzGerald DJ. Processing of *Pseudomonas* exotoxin by a cellular protease results in the generation of a 37,000 Da toxin fragment that is translocated to the cytosol. J Biol Chem 1990;256:20678–20685.
37. Kondo T, FitzGerald D, Chaudhary VK, Adhya S, Pastan I. Activity of immunotoxins constructed with modified *Pseudomonas* exotoxin A lacking the cell recognition domain. J Biol Chem 1988;263:9470–9475.
38. Johnson VG, Wilson D, Greenfield L, Youle RJ. The role of the diphtheria toxin receptor in cytosol translocation. J Biol Chem 1988;263:1295–1300.
39. Bacha P, Forte S, Kassam N, et al. Pharmacokinetics of the recombinant fusion protein DAB486IL-2 in animal models. Cancer Chemother Pharmacol 1990;26:409–414.
40. Walz G, Zanker B, Murphy JR, Strom TB. A kinetic analysis of the effects of interleukin-2 diphtheria toxin fusion protein upon activated T cells. Transplantation 1990;49:198–201.
41. Walz G, Zanker B, Brand K, Waters C, Genbauffe F, Zeldis JB, Murphy JR, Strom TB. Sequential effects of interleukin-2/diphtheria toxin fusion protein of T-cell activation. Proc Natl Acad Sci USA 1989;86:9485–9488.
42. Balkwill F, Osborne R, Burke F, Naylor S, Talbot D, Durbin H, Tavernier J, Fiers W. Evidence for tumor necrosis factor/cachectin production in cancer. Lancet 1987;2:1229–1232.
43. Kay NE, Burton J, Wagner D, Nelson DL. The malignant B-cells from B-chronic lymphocytic leukemia patients release TAC-soluble interleukin-2 receptors. Blood 1988;72:447–450.
44. Olsnes S, Pihl A. Toxic lectins and related proteins. In: Cohen P, van Heyningen S, eds. Molecular action of toxins and viruses. New York: Elsevier, 1982:51–105.
45. Eiklid K, Olsnes S, Pihl A. Entry of lethal doses of abrin, ricin and modeccin into the cytosol of HeLa cells. Exp Cell Res 1980;126:321–326.
46. Yamaizumi M, Mekada E, Uchida T, Okada Y. One molecule of diphtheria toxin fragment A introduced into a cell can kill the cell. Cell 1978;15:245–250.
47. Thorpe PE, Ross WC. The preparation and cytotoxic properties of antibody-toxin conjugates. Immunol Rev 1982;62:119–158.
48. Gill DM, Dinius LL. Observations on the structure of diphtheria toxin. J Biol Chem 1971;246:1485–1491.
49. Collier RJ. Diphtheria toxin: Mode of action and structure. Bacteriol Rev 1975;39:54–85.
50. Endo Y, Tsurugi K. RNA N-glycosidase activity of ricin A-chain. Mechanism of action of the toxic lectin ricin on eukaryotic ribosomes. J Biol Chem 1987;262:8128–8130.
51. Endo Y, Mitsui K, Motizuki M, Tsurugi K. The mechanism of action of ricin and related toxic lectins on eukaryotic ribosomes. The site and the characteristics of the modification in 28S ribosomal RNA caused by the toxins. J Biol Chem 1987;262:5908–5912.
52. Neville DM Jr, Hudson TH. Transmembrane transport of diphtheria toxin, related toxins, and colicins. Annu Rev Biochem 1986;55:195–224.
53. Casellas P, Dussossoy D, Falasca AI, et al. Trichokirin, a ribosome-inactivating protein from the seeds of *Trichosanthes kirilowii* Maximowicz. Purification, partial characterization and use for preparation of immunotoxins. Eur J Biochem 1988;176:581–588.
54. Stirpe F, Wawrzynczak EJ, Brown ANF, et al. Selective cytotoxic activity of immunotoxins composed of a monoclonal anti-Thy 1.1 antibody and the ribosome-inactivating proteins, bryodin and momordin. Br J Cancer 1988;58:558–561.

55. Wang QC, Ying WB, Xie H, Zhang Z, Yang Z, Ling L. Trichosanthin-monoclonal antibody conjugate specifically cytotoxic to human hepatoma cells in vitro. Cancer Res 1991;51:3353–3355.

56. Ramakrishnan S, Houston LL. Prevention of growth of leukemia cells in mice by monoclonal antibodies directed against Thy 1.1 antigen disulfide linked to two ribosomal inhibitors: Pokeweed antiviral protein or ricin A chain. Cancer Res 1984;44:1398–1404.

57. Uckun FM, Ramakrishnan S, Houston LL. Increased efficiency in selective elimination of leukemia cells by a combination of a stable derivative of cyclophosphamide and a human B-cell-specific immunotoxin containing pokeweed antiviral protein. Cancer Res 1985;45:69–75.

58. Stirpe F, Barbieri L. Ribosome-inactivating proteins up to date. FEBS Lett 1986;195:1–8.

59. Thorpe PE, Brown AN, Ross WC, et al. Cytotoxicity acquired by conjugation of an anti-Thy1.1 monoclonal antibody and the ribosome-inactivating protein, gelonin. Eur J Biochem 1981;116:447–454.

60. Stirpe F, Gasperi-Campani A, Barbieri L, Falasca A, Abbondanza A, Stevens WA. Ribosome-inactivating proteins from the seeds of Saponaria officinalis L. (soapwort), of Agrostemma githago L. (corn cockle) and of Asparagus officinalis L. (asparagus), and from the latex of Hura crepitans L. (sandbox tree). Biochem J 1983;216:617–625.

61. Thorpe PE, Brown AN, Bremner JA Jr, Foxwell BM, Stirpe F. An immunotoxin composed of monoclonal anti-Thy 1.1 antibody and a ribosome-inactivating protein from Saponaria officinalis: Potent antitumor effects in vitro and in vivo. JNCI 1985;75:151–159.

62. Vasil ML, Kabat D, Iglewski BH. Structure-activity relationships of an exotoxin of Pseudomonas aeruginosa. Infect Immunol 1977;16:353–361.

63. Williams DP, Parker K, Bacha P, et al. Diphtheria toxin binding domain substitution with interleukin-2: Genetic construction and properties of a diphtheria toxin-related interleukin-2 fusion protein. Protein Eng 1987;1:493–498.

64. Jinno Y, Chaudhary VK, Kondo T, Adhya S, FitzGerald DJ, Pastan I. Mutational analysis of domain I of Pseudomonas exotoxin. Mutations in domain I of Pseudomonas exotoxin which reduce cell binding and animal toxicity. J Biol Chem 1988;263:13203–13207.

65. Houston LL, Nowinski RC. Cell-specific cytotoxicity expressed by a conjugate of ricin and murine monoclonal antibody directed against thy 1.1 antigen. Cancer Res 1981;41:3913–3917.

66. Youle RJ, Neville DM Jr. Anti-Thy 1.2 monoclonal antibody linked to ricin is a potent cell-type-specific toxin. Proc Natl Acad Sci USA 1980;77:5483–5486.

67. Thorpe PE, Ross WC, Brown AN, et al. Blockade of the galactose-binding sites of ricin by its linkage to antibody. Specific cytotoxic effects of the conjugates. Eur J Biochem 1984;140:63–71.

68. Houston LL. Inactivation of ricin using 4-azidophenyl-β-D-galactopyranoside and 4-diazophenyl-β-D-galactopyranoside. J Biol Chem 1983;258:7208–7212.

69. Breitmeyer J, Nadler L, Coral F, Eliseo L, Blattler WA, Schlossman S. Blocked ricin immunotoxin therapy of malignant lymphoma. Proceedings of Monoclonal Antibody Immunoconjugates in Cancer Therapy, Chicago, September, 1989:28–29.

70. Moroney SE, Dalarcao LJ, Goldmacher VS, Lambert JM, Blattler WA. Modification of the binding site(s) of lectins by an affinity column carrying an activated galactose-terminated ligand. Biochemistry 1987;26:8390–8398.

71. Blakey DC, Watson GJ, Knowles PP, Thorpe PE. Effect of chemical deglycosylation of ricin A chain on the in vivo fate and cytotoxic activity of an immunotoxin composed of ricin A chain and anti-Thy 1.1 antibody. Cancer Res 1987;47:947–952.

72. Thorpe PE, Wallace PM, Knowles PP, et al. New coupling agents for the synthesis of immunotoxins containing a hindered disulfide bond with improved stability in vivo. Cancer Res 1987;47:5924–5931.

73. Stanworth DR, Turner MW. Immunochemical analysis of immunoglobulins and their sub-units. In: Weir DM, ed. Handbook of experimental immunology. Oxford: Blackwell Scientific Publications, 1978:1–102.

74. Wawrzynczak EJ, Thorpe PE. Methods for preparing immunotoxins: Effects of the linkage on activity and stability. In: Vogel CW, ed. Immunoconjugates: Antibody conjugates in radioimaging and therapy of cancer. New York: Oxford University Press, 1987:28–55.

75. Lambert JM, Senter PD, Yau-Young A, Blattler WA, Goldmacher VS. Purified immunotoxins that are reactive with human lymphoid cells. J Biol Chem 1985;260:12035–12041.

76. Murphy JR, Bisha W, Williams D, et al. Genetic assembly and selective toxicity of diphtheria-toxin-related polypeptide hormone fusion proteins. Biochem Soc Symp 1987;53:9–23.

77. Ramakrishnan S, Houston LL. Comparison of the selective cytotoxic effects of immunotoxins containing ricin A chain or pokeweed antiviral protein and anti-Thy 1.1 monoclonal antibodies. Cancer Res 1984;44:201–208.

78. Shen G-L, Li J-L, Ghetie M-A, et al. Evaluation of four CD22 antibodies as ricin A chain-containing immunotoxins for the in vivo therapy of human B-cell leukemias and lymphomas. Int J Cancer 1988;42:792–797.

79. Guillemot JC, Sundan A, Olsnes S, Sandvig K. Entry of diphtheria toxin linked to concanavalin A into primate and murine cells. J Cell Physiol 1985;122:193–199.

80. Bacha P, Williams DP, Waters C, Williams JM, Murphy JR, Strom TB. Interleukin 2 receptor-targeted cytotoxicity. Interleukin 2 receptor-mediated action of a diphtheria toxin-related interleukin 2 fusion protein. J Exp Med 1988;167:612–622.

81. Van Deurs B, Tønnessen TI, Petersen OW, Sandvig K, Olsnes S. Routing of internalized ricin and ricin conjugates to the Golgi complex. J Cell Biol 1986;102:37–47.

82. Press OW, Vitetta ES, Farr AG, Hansen JA, Martin PJ. Evaluation of ricin A-chain immunotoxins directed against human T cells. Cell Immunol 1986;102:10–20.

83. Thorpe PE, Mason DW, Brown AN, et al. Selective killing of malignant cells in a leukaemic rat bone marrow using an antibody-ricin conjugate. Nature 1982;297:594–596.

84. Bacha P, Murphy JR, Reichlin S. Thyrotropin-releasing hormone-diphtheria toxin-related polypeptide conjugates. J Biol Chem 1983;258:1565.

85. Wawrzynczak EJ, Watson GJ, Cumber AJ, et al. Blocked and non-blocked ricin immunotoxins against the CD4 antigen exhibit higher cytotoxic potency than a ricin A-chain immunotoxin potentiated with ricin B-chain or with a ricin B-chain immunotoxin. Cancer Immunol Immunother 1991;32:289–295.

86. Casellas P, Bourrie BJP, Gros P, Jansen F. Kinetics of cytotoxicity induced by immunotoxins. Enhancement by lysosomotropic amines and carboxylic ionophores. J Biol Chem 1984;259:9359–9364.

87. Ramakrishnan S, Houston LL. Inhibition of human acute lymphoblastic leukemia cells by immunotoxins: Potentiation by chloroquine. Science 1984;223:58–61.

88. Raso V, Lawrence J. Carboxylic ionophores enhance the cytotoxic potency of ligand- and antibody-delivered ricin A chain. J Exp Med 1984;160:1234–1240.

89. McIntosh DP, Edwards DC, Cumber AJ, et al. Ricin B chain converts a non-cytotoxic antibody-ricin A chain conjugate into a potent and specific cytotoxic agent. FEBS Lett 1983;164:17–20.

90. Vitetta ES, Cushley W, Uhr JW. Synergy of ricin A chain-containing immunotoxins and ricin B chain-containing immunotoxins in in vitro killing of neoplastic human B cells. Proc Natl Acad Sci USA 1983;80:6332–6335.

91. Vitetta ES, Fulton RJ, Uhr JW. Cytotoxicity of a cell-reactive immunotoxin containing ricin A chain is potentiated by an anti-immunotoxin containing ricin B chain. J Exp Med 1984;160:341–346.

92. Ramakrishnan S, Bjorn MJ, Houston LL. Recombinant ricin A chain conjugated to monoclonal antibodies: Improved tumor cell inhibition in the presence of lysosomotropic compounds. Cancer Res 1989;49:613–617.

93. Casellas P, Jansen FK. Immunotoxin enhancers. In: Frankel AE, ed. Immunotoxins. Norwell, MA: Kluwer Academic Publishers, 1988;351–371.

94. Harkonen S, Stoudemire J, Mischak R, Spitler LE, Lopez H, Scannon P. Toxicity and immunogenicity of monoclonal anti-melanoma antibody-ricin A chain immunotoxin in rats. Cancer Res 1987;47:1377–1382.

95. Stirpe F, Derenzini M, Barbieri L, et al. Hepatotoxicity of immunotoxins made from saporin, a ribosome-inactivating protein from Saponaria officinalis. Virchows Arch [B] 1987;53:259–271.

96. Blakey DC, Skilleter DN, Price RJ, et al. Comparison of the pharmacokinetics and hepatotoxic effects of saporin and ricin A-chain immunotoxins on murine liver parenchymal cells. Cancer Res 1988;48:7072–7078.

97. Kanellos J, MacKenzie IF, Pietersz GA. In vivo studies of whole ricin monoclonal antibody immunoconjugates for the treatment of murine tumours. Immunol Cell Biol 1988;66:403–415.

98. Zaleberg JR, Pietersz G, Toohey B, Zimet A, Hennessy O, McKenzie IFC. Phase I–II study of a ricin monoclonal antibody conjugate in colon cancer. In: Monoclonal antibody immunoconjugates for cancer. San Diego, CA: Abstract from 4th International Conference, 1989.

99. Jansen FK, Blythman HE, Carriere D, et al. Immunotoxins: Hybrid molecules combining high specificity and potent cytotoxicity. Immunol Rev 1982;62:185–216.

100. Blakey DC, Skilleter DN, Price RJ, Thorpe PE. Uptake of native and deglycosylated ricin A-chain immunotoxins by mouse liver parenchymal and non-parenchymal cells in vitro and in vivo. Biochim Biophys Acta 1988;968:172–178.

101. Skilleter DN, Paine AJ, Stirpe F. A comparison of the accumulation of ricin by hepatic parenchymal and non-parenchymal cells and its inhibition of protein synthesis. Biochim Biophys Acta 1981;677:495–500.

102. Thorpe PE, Detre SI, Foxwell BMJ, et al. Modification of the carbohydrate in ricin with metaperiodate-cyanoborohydride mixtures. Effects on toxicity and in vivo distribution. Eur J Biochem 1985;147:197–206.

103. O'Hare M, Roberts LM, Thorpe PE, Watson GJ, Prior B, Lord JM. Expression of ricin A chain in Escherichia coli. FEBS Lett 1987;216:73–78.

104. Skilleter DN, Price RJ, Thorpe PE. Modification of the carbohydrate in ricin with metaperiodate and cyanoborohydride mixtures: Effect on binding, uptake and toxicity to parenchymal and non-parenchymal cells of rat liver. Biochim Biophys Acta 1985;842:12–21.

105. Vitetta ES, Thorpe PE. Immunotoxins containing ricin A or B chains with modified carbohydrate residues act synergistically in killing neoplastic B cells in vitro. Cancer Drug Deliv 1985;2:191–198.

106. Ghetie MA, Uhr JW, Vitetta ES. Covalent binding of human 2-macroglobulin to deglycosylated ricin A chain and its immunotoxins. Cancer Res 1991;51:1482–1487.

107. Jansen FK, Blythman HE, Carriere D, et al. High specific cytotoxicity of antibody-toxin hybrid molecules (immunotoxins) for target cells. Immunol Lett 1980;2:97–102.

108. FitzGerald DJ, Willingham MC, Pastan I. Antitumor effects of an immunotoxin made with Pseudomonas exotoxin in a nude mouse model of human ovarian cancer. Proc Natl Acad Sci USA 1986;83:6627–6630.

109. Manske JM, Buchsbaum DJ, Hanna DE, Vallera DA. Cytotoxic effects of anti-CD5 radioimmunotoxins on human tumors in vitro and in a nude mouse model. Cancer Res 1988;48:7107–7114.

110. Hara H, Luo Y, Haruta Y, Seon BK. Efficient transplantation of human non-T-leukemia cells into nude mice and induction of complete regression of the transplanted distinct tumors by ricin A-chain conjugates of monoclonal antibodies SN5 and SN6. Cancer Res 1988;48:4673–4680.

111. Bernhard MI, Foon KA, Oeltmann TN, et al. Guinea pig line 10 hepatocarcinoma model: Characterization of monoclonal antibody and in vivo effect of unconjugated antibody and antibody conjugated to diphtheria toxin A chain. Cancer Res 1983;43:4420–4428.

112. Hwang KM, Foon KA, Cheung PH, Pearson JW, Oldham RK. Selective antitumor effect on L10 hepatocarcinoma cells of a potent immunoconjugate composed of the A chain of abrin and a monoclonal antibody to a hepatoma-associated antigen. Cancer Res 1984;44:4578–4586.

113. Weil-Hillman G, Uckun FM, Manske JM, Vallera DA. Combined immunochemotherapy of human solid tumors in nude mice. Cancer Res 1987;47:579–585.

114. Pearson JW, Sivam G, Manger R, Wiltrout RH, Morgan AC Jr, Longo DL. Enhanced therapeutic efficacy of an immunotoxin in combination with chemotherapy against an intraperitoneal human tumor xenograft in athymic mice. Cancer Res 1989;49:4990–4995.

115. Sironi M, Canegrati MA, Romano M, Vecchi A, Spreafico F. Chemotherapy-increased antineoplastic effects of antibody-toxin conjugates. Cancer Treat Rep 1984;68:643–645.

116. Pirker R, FitzGerald DJP, Raschack M, Frank Z, Willingham MC, Pastan I. Enhancement of the activity of immunotoxins by analogues of verapamil. Cancer Res 1989;49:4791–4795.

117. Yokota S, Hara H, Luo Y, Seon BK. Synergistic potentiation of in vivo anti-tumor activity of anti-human T-leukemia immunotoxins by recombinant interferon and daunorubicin. Cancer Res 1990;50:32–37.

118. Pearson JW, FitzGerald DJP, Willingham MC, Wiltrout RH, Pastan I, Longo DL. Chemoimmunotoxin therapy against a human colon tumor (HT-29) xenografted into nude mice. Cancer Res 1989;49:3562–3567.

119. Smyth MJ, Pietersz GA, McKenzie IF. Use of vasoactive agents to increase tumor perfusion and the antitumor efficacy of drug-monoclonal antibody conjugates. JNCI 1987;79:1367–1373.

120. Jain RK, Baxter LT. Mechanisms of heterogeneous distribution of monoclonal antibodies and other macromolecules in tumors: Significance of elevated interstitial pressure. Cancer Res 1988;48:7022–7032.

121. Sands H. Radioimmunoconjugates: An overview of problems and promises. Antibody Immunoconjugates Radiopharm 1988;1:213–226.

122. Osdol WV, Fujimori K, Weinstein JN. An analysis of monoclonal antibody distribution in microscopic tumor nodules: Consequences of a "binding site barrier." Cancer Res 1991;51:4776–4784.

123. Oratz R, Speyer JL, Wernz JC, et al. Anti-melanoma monoclonal antibody-ricin A chain immunoconjugate (XMMME-001-RTA) plus cyclophosphamide in the treatment of metastatic malignant melanoma: Results of a phase II trial. J Biol Response Modif 1990;9:345–354.

124. Byers VS, Rodvien R, Grant K, et al. Phase I study of monoclonal antibody-ricin A chain immunotoxin XomaZyme-791 in patients with metastatic colon cancer. Cancer Res 1989;49:6153–6160.

125. Pai LH, Bookman MA, Ozols RJ, et al. Clinical evaluation of intraperitoneal *Pseudomonas* exotoxin immunoconjugate OVBB-PE in patients with ovarian cancer. J Clin Oncol 1991;9(12):2095–2103.

126. Spitler LE, del Rio M, Khentigan A, et al. Therapy of patients with malignant melanoma using a monoclonal anti-melanoma antibody-ricin A chain immunotoxin. Cancer Res 1987;47:1717–1723.

127. Spitler LE. Clinical studies: Solid tumors. In: Frankel AE, ed. Immunotoxins. Norwell, MA: Kluwer Academic Publishers, 1988;493–515.

128. Weiner LM, O'Dwyer J, Kitson J, et al. Phase I evaluation of an anti-breast carcinoma monoclonal antibody 260F9-recombinant ricin A chain immunoconjugate. Cancer Res 1989;49:4062–4067.

129. Grossbard ML, Freedman AS, Kinsella JM, Epstein CL, Blattler WA, Nadler LM. Immunotherapy with anti-B4-blocked ricin (Anti-B4–BR): Phase 1 trials of continuous infusion in patients with B-cell neoplasms. Am Soc Hematol [Abstract] 1991;.

130. Grossbard ML, Freedman AS, Ritz J, et al. Serotherapy of B-cell neoplasms with anti-B4-blocked ricin: A phase 1 trial of daily bolus infusion. Blood 1992;79:576–585.

131. Vitetta ES, Stone M, Amlot P, et al. A phase I immunotoxin trial in patients with B cell lymphoma. Cancer Res 1991;15:4052–4058.

132. Hertler AA, Schlossman DM, Borowitz MJ, Blythman HE, Casellas P, Frankel AE. An anti-CD5 immunotoxin for chronic lymphocytic leukemia: Enhancement of cytotoxicity with human serum albumin-monensin. Int J Cancer 1989;43:215–219.

133. Le Maistre CF, Rosen S, Frankel A, et al. Phase I trial of H65-RTA immunoconjugate in patients with cutaneous T-cell lymphoma. Blood 1991;78:1173–1182.

134. Le Maistre F, Rosenblum M, Reuben J, et al. Phase I study of genetically engineered DAB486IL-2 in IL-2-receptor expressing malignancies. Blood 1990;76:360a.

135. Byers VS, Henslee PJ, Kernan NA, et al. Use of an anti-pan T-lymphocyte ricin A chain immunotoxin in steroid-resistant acute graft-versus-host disease. Blood 1990;75:1426–1432.

136. Miller RA, Maloney DG, Warnke R, Levy R. Treatment of B-cell lymphoma with monoclonal anti-idiotypic antibody. N Engl J Med 1982;306:516–522.

137. Waters CA, Schimke PA, Snider CE, et al. Interleukin 2 receptor-targeted cytotoxicity. Receptor binding requirements for entry of a diphtheria toxin-related interleukin 2 fusion protein into cells. Eur J Immunol 1990;20:785–792.

138. Kiyokawa T, Shirono K, Hattori T, et al. Cytotoxicity of interleukin 2-toxin toward lymphocytes from patients with adult T cell leukemia. Cancer Res 1989;49:4042–4046.

139. Lakkis F, Steele A, Pacheco-Silva A, Rubin-Kelly V, Strom TB, Murphy JR. Interleukin 4 receptor targeted cytotoxicity: Genetic construction and in vivo immunosuppressive activity of a diphtheria toxin-related murine interleukin 4 fusion protein. Eur J Immunol [Abstract] 1991;21:2253–2258.

140. Puri RK, Ogata M, Leland P, Feldman GM, FitzGerald D, Pastan I. Expression of high-affinity interleukin 4 receptors on murine sarcoma cells and receptor-mediated cytotoxicity of tumor cells to chimeric protein between interleukin 4 and *Pseudomonas* exotoxin. Cancer Res 1991;51:3011–3017.

141. Siegall CB, Chaudhary VK, FitzGerald DJ, Pastan I. Cytotoxicity of an interleukin 6–*Pseudomonas* exotoxin fusion protein on human myeloma cells. Proc Natl Acad Sci USA 1988;85:9738–9742.

142. Siegall CB, Kreitman RJ, FitzGerald DJ, Pastan I. Antitumor effects of interleukin 6–*Pseudomonas* exotoxin chimeric molecules against the human hepatocellular carcinoma, PLC/PCF/5 in mice. Cancer Res 1991;51:2831–2836.

143. Pai LH, Gallo MG, FitzGerald DJ, Pastan I. Antitumor activity of a transforming growth factor a-*Pseudomonas* exotoxin fusion protein (TGF-a-PE40). Cancer Res 1991;51:2808–2812.

144. Siegall CB, FitzGerald DJ, Pastan I. Selective killing of tumor cells using EGF or TGFa-*Pseudomonas* exotoxin chimeric molecules. Cancer Biology 1990;1:345–350.

145. Prior TI, Helman LJ, FitzGerald DJ, Pastan I. Cytotoxic activity of a recombinant fusion protein between insulin-like growth factor I and *Pseudomonas* exotoxin. Cancer Res 1991;51:174–180.

146. Lappi DA, Maher PA, Martineau D, Baird A. The basic fibroblast growth factor-saporin mitotoxin acts through the basic fibroblast growth factor receptor. J Cell Physiol 1991;147:17–26.

147. Siegall CB, Epstein S, Spein E, et al. Cytotoxic activity of chimeric proteins composed of acidic fibroblast growth factor and *Pseudomonas* exotoxins on a variety of cell types. FASEB J 1991;5:2843–2849.

148. Murphy JR, Bishai W, Borowski M, Miyanohara A, Boyd J, Nagle S. Genetic construction, expression, and melanoma-selective cytotoxicity of a diphtheria toxin-related melanocyte-stimulating hormone fusion protein. Proc Natl Acad Sci USA 1986;83:8258–8262.

149. Naglich JG, Methereal JE, Russel DW, Erdels L. Expression cloning of a diphtheria toxin receptor: Identity with a heparin-binding EGF-like growth factor precursor. Cell 69:1051–1061.

150. Kounnas MZ, Morris RE, Thompson MR, FitzGerald DJ, Strickland DK, Saelinger CB. The α_2-macroglobulin receptor/low density lipoprotein receptor-related protein binds and internalizes *Pseudomonas* exotoxin A*. J Biol Chem 1992;267:12420–12423.

SECTION 4

CHARLES W. YOUNG
RAYMOND P. WARRELL, JR

Differentiating Agents

Cancer can be perceived as an inappropriate accumulation of cells that are capable of varying degrees of differentiation. This concept is inherent in the familiar diagnostic adjectives, which range from "well differentiated" through "poorly differentiated" to "anaplastic." In the usual course of disease progression, there is an inverse relation between the degree of cytologic differentiation and the clinical aggressiveness of the neoplastic condition. It is now clear that the neoplastic change is not immutable; some cancer cells can be induced to undergo phenotypic changes, characterized by morphologic maturation along the expected pattern for the tissue of origin and by the loss of replicative capacity. This process is referred to as "terminal" differentiation, and drugs that predictably induce these changes are considered to be differentiating agents.

For several decades it had been recognized that a residual mass comprised solely of differentiated cells may be observed after aggressive therapy of certain tumors, particularly neuroblastoma and germ cell neoplasms. Whether this phenomenon resulted from treatment-induced cytodifferentiation or selective destruction of less differentiated tumor cell population was not established. In the past 2 decades, interest in differentiation therapy of cancer as a planned therapeutic approach was aroused by reports that cytodifferentiation of cancer cell lines could be produced in vitro by treatment with a wide variety of physiologic and xenobiotic molecules.[1-4] Although the theoretic interest of these cell culture observations has been widely accepted, their clinical relevance was considered to be questionable. However, clinical applications of this approach have been convincingly established in at least one disorder, acute promyelocytic leukemia.[5-9]

Cancer is associated with genetic abnormalities that range in extent from translocations, such as t(9;22) in chronic myelogenous leukemia (CML) and t(15;17) in acute promyelocytic leukemia, to the extensive multichromosomal defects that characterize colorectal cancer and breast cancer.[10-14] In colorectal cancer, anatomic and physiologic correlations exist between the progressive loss of genetic integrity and sequential changes from an apparently normal mucosa to one that shows hyperproliferation and then dysplasia, adenoma, locally invasive carcinoma, and eventually metastatic carcinoma. Similarly, in CML progression from the chronic to the accelerated and blastic phases is accompanied by further chromosomal loss, particularly at the p53 locus.[15-17] Simplistically, the genetic abnormalities in cancer cells result in a physiologic block at a stage of differentiation that retains proliferative capacity; moreover, the neoplastic cells no longer respond to controls that normally govern growth and differentiation. Differentiation therapy reasserts certain critical aspects of normal control that eventually leads to loss of proliferative capacity. Because these controls are presumably physiologic, differentiation therapy should be considerably less toxic than conventional cytotoxic therapies.

A wide variety of drugs or physical conditions induce cytodifferentiation (Table 69–16). Not all cancer cells or cancer cell lines are responsive to inducing agents in vitro; frequently, those that do respond differentiate under the influence of several different agents. These observations suggest that, although responding cells may have a rather "localized" block to dif-

ferentiation, they retain sufficient intact genetic information to fully respond after the localized block has been circumvented. Conceivably, nonresponding lines have undergone more extensive genetic injury or may have multiple blocks that not relieved by a single agent. Extending this concept, dysplastic or precancerous cells that have undergone minimal genetic change may have only a partial block to differentiation and be quite responsive to induced maturation. Accordingly, the early stages of preneoplastic transition may also be an appropriate place for the use of differentiating agents. This idea is supported by the considerable overlap between agents that produce differentiation and those that have chemopreventive activity in model systems.

This chapter summarizes relevant clinical and laboratory information related to differentiation agents currently undergoing extensive clinical testing. Because mechanisms of drug-induced differentiation are largely unknown, clinical trials have usually been empirically based on activity observed for a given drug in model systems. Hematologic disorders, largely leukemia and myelodysplastic syndromes, have received particular attention because phenotypic stages of normal differentiation in blood cells are well characterized. Furthermore, because the neoplastic cell population in these patients can be conveniently and repeatedly sampled during the course of treatment, there is an opportunity to delineate whether cytotoxicity or cytodifferentiation is occurring in responding patients.

RETINOIDS

BACKGROUND

The term retinoids includes the naturally occurring and synthetic analogues of vitamin A (retinol) a fat-soluble dietary substance essential for growth, normal embryologic development, and vision.[18,19] The physiologic morphogen, all-*trans*-retinoic acid (tretinoin) is synthesized in vivo from retinol; when supplied exogenously, tretinoin can replace retinol in all biologic functions except that of supporting vision. Retinoids produce biologic effects by interaction with a series of nuclear receptors that are analogous to the receptors of steroids and thyroid hormone.[20-23] At least three RA-receptor (RAR) subtypes—α, β, and γ—have been identified, along with a second receptor family, termed RXR.[23] Tretinoin and its naturally occurring isomer 13-*cis*-retinoic acid (isotretinoin) induce cytodifferentiation of a wide variety of tissues and cells in culture.[2,3,24,25] RARA is expressed in hematopoietic cells and has been shown to mediate RA-induced differentiation in certain myeloid cells.[26]

TABLE 69–16. Cytodifferentiation Agents in Cell Culture

Class	Example
Retinoids	All-*trans*-retinoic acid
	13-*cis*-retinoic acid
Vitamins	1,25-Dihydroxyvitamin D_3
Fatty acids	Butyrate
Interferons	
Phorbol esters	
Planar/polar compounds	Dimethyl sulfoxide (DMSO)
	Hexamethylene bisacetamide (HMBA)
	Dimethylformamide (DMF)
Cytotoxics	Cytosine arabinoside (ara-C)
	Tiazofurin
	5-Bromodeoxyuridine
	Antifolates
	Aclacinomycin
Cyclic-AMP Modulators	Cholera toxin
	Forskolin
	Isobutylmethylxanthine
Analogs	8-Cl/Br-cyclic-AMP
	Dibutyryl-cyclic AMP

ALL-*TRANS*-RETINOIC ACID IN ACUTE PROMYELOCYTIC LEUKEMIA

Clinical evaluation of tretinoin (all-*trans*-retinoic acid; RA) in acute promyelocytic leukemia (APL) was undertaken because of numerous reports that documented retinoic acid-induced differentiation of APL cells in vitro.[3,24,27] Studies of normal human bone marrow progenitor cells treated with RA in vitro suggest that normal granulopoiesis is stimulated, possibly by increasing responsiveness to cytokines and growth factors.[28] Leukemic blasts freshly obtained from patients with acute myeloid leukemia (AML) show variable responsiveness to RA exhibiting stimulation and inhibition of colony formation.[29]

REMISSION INCIDENCE

Since the original report by Huang and colleagues in 1988, studies from China, France, and the United States have conclusively documented the activity of all-*trans*-RA in (APL).[5] Table 69–17 summarizes the clinical activity of the drug in APL from reported studies in 207 of these cases.[5–9,30] The treatment groups are not homogenous because previously treated and newly diagnosed patients were included in these series. Moreover, with the recent advances using molecular genetic techniques for the diagnosis of APL, a number of patients were included in these series who had a morphologic diagnosis of APL but who did not have the disease as it can now be molecularly defined. These issues notwithstanding, the initial response to all-*trans*-RA in a patient with APL documented by cytogenetics or molecular studies is very high (95–100% if patients who died before being fully evaluated are excluded).

REMISSION DURATION

The actual number of patients maintained solely on all-*trans*-RA in continuous complete remission (CR) is quite small; nonetheless, it is clear that CRs induced by all-*trans*-RA tend to be brief. The median duration of CR in the New York series was 4 months, ranging from 1 to 10 months for 13 patients.[8] CR durations in other series are similar although a few patients in China are reported to have had CR durations exceeding 1 year.[5,6,9] Three groups have indicated that induction treatment with all-*trans*-RA, followed by "consolidation" or "maintenance" with standard chemotherapy, yields a CR duration that seems to be at least equivalent to results achieved with conventional chemotherapy, albeit with considerably shorter follow-up.[7–9] There appears to be no benefit (and there may be some disadvantage) to continuous treatment with all-*trans*-RA during complete remission.

RETINOID RESISTANCE

Patients who relapse while taking all-*trans*-RA usually cannot be reinduced into CR by further treatment with all-*trans*-RA, although there seems to be no increased resistance to reinduction with conventional chemotherapy.[5–9] One report from China suggested that occasional patients who were induced with RA and then taken off could be successfully retreated at relapse.[9] In the New York series, CR could not be recaptured in any patient who relapsed during all-*trans*-RA treatment despite a twofold escalation of the daily drug dosage.[8,31] The reasons for relapse and acquired resistance to retinoid therapy are subjects of intense research interest. Potential mechanisms include accelerated drug clearance from plasma, further acquired mutations in retinoid receptors, or sequestration by cellular retinoic acid binding proteins in normal tissues.

CLINICAL PHARMACOLOGY

Retinoic acid is normally found in the body and circulates in plasma at concentrations of approximately 1 to 2 ng/ml. Physiologic amounts of RA are likely derived by oxidation of vitamin A (retinol) that has been absorbed from the gastrointestinal tract.[18,19] An isomerase reaction may convert some of the material to 13-*cis*-RA. Pharmacologic amounts of all-*trans*-RA are highly protein bound, probably nonspecifically to albumin.[32] A membrane transport mechanism has not been identified and the drug appears to enter cells by simple diffusion where it is bound to several cellular retinoic acid-binding proteins (CRABP). RA bound to CRABP is transferred to the cell nucleus and then binds to various retinoic acid receptors. Signaling events after receptor binding of RA are poorly characterized, although a number of RA-responsive genes have been identified.

After a single oral all-*trans*-RA dose of 45 mg/m^2, peak plasma drug concentrations of approximately 300 ng/ml (10^{-6} M) are achieved within 1 to 2 hours.[31,32] The drug rapidly disappears from plasma with a half-life of approximately 40 minutes. The plasma half-life of 13-*cis*-RA is 12–14 hours.[33] Only trace amounts of RA metabolites (<1% of the administered dose) are excreted in urine. The drug does not penetrate the cerebrospinal fluid and thus the agent is not effective treatment for CNS leukemia.[32]

Continuous daily treatment with all-*trans*-RA is associated with a marked decrease in plasma drug concentrations,[31,32] an effect not observed with other retinoids.[34,35] The reduction in plasma levels has been correlated with clinical relapse in patients with APL.[31] Conceivably, relapse from remissions induced by all-*trans*-RA may be due to an inability to sustain effective "cytodifferentiating" concentrations in vivo during prolonged administration.

TABLE 69–17. Clinical Trials Using All-*trans*-Retinoic Acid as Remission Induction Treatment for Acute Promyelocytic Leukemia

Site	No. of Patients	No. in Complete Remission	Complete Responses (%)	References
Shanghai	100	85	85	5, 6
Suzhou	50	47	94	9
Paris	22	14	64	8
New York	35	27	77	8*

* And R. P. Warrell, Jr, unpublished data.

PREDICTING RESPONSE TO RETINOIC ACID WITH CELL CULTURE, CYTOGENETIC, AND MOLECULAR STUDIES

Short-term (7-day) cultures of freshly aspirated blasts from patients with APL can be cultured in the presence of RA at various concentrations (usually 10^{-6} or 10^{-7} M). The Chinese and French groups have reported that the in vitro response to all-*trans*-RA predicts for clinical effectiveness.[5,7,9] However, the interpretation of differentiation in vitro is somewhat more qualitative than quantitative, and clinical exigencies often dictate the choice of treatment before obtaining such results. Relapsing patients may retain in vitro sensitivity to the drug yet remain clinically resistant.[31]

APL is associated with a specific cytogenetic abnormality, t(15;17), that results in the fusion of the *RARA* gene on chromosome 17 with a previously unknown gene, initially named *MYL*, and now renamed *PML* (for promyelocytic leukemia).[36–38]

It appears that the initial clinical response to all-*trans*-RA is most closely correlated with presence of the t(15;17) translocation as assessed by conventional cytogenetics or by molecular detection of the rearranged RARA receptor.[39,40] Molecular testing is usually performed using probes for *RARA* and Northern blot analysis or by reverse transcriptase-polymerase chain reaction (RT/PCR) using specific primers.[41] Each of these tests varies in its sensitivity and specificity, and proper interpretation of the laboratory result is critical. A cytogenetic result that indicates the presence of the t(15;17) is pathognomonic for APL, is associated with molecular rearrangement of the RARA receptor, and is positively correlated with clinical response to all-*trans*-RA. A "negative" result—indicating a normal karyotype or technical failure—is problematic. Some patients with typical or equivocal evidence of APL by light microscopy and with reportedly normal karyotypes have shown the typical rearrangement of RAR-α by molecular testing, and each of these patients subsequently responded to all-*trans*-RA. All patients tested who have had a negative RT/PCR test for the *RARA* mutation also failed to exhibit t(15;17) by cytogenetic analysis, and none of these patients responded clinically.[41] This result is not surprising, because relatively few metaphases are evaluated by cytogenetics, but only minute amounts of rearranged *RARA*-encoded mRNA are necessary to detect the mutation.

ADVERSE CLINICAL EFFECTS

Compared with most anticancer drugs used in oncologic practice, all-*trans*-RA must be considered highly safe with few serious adverse reactions. The drug shares adverse reactions common to other retinoids and its principal side effects are listed in Table 69–18.

Headache occurring several hours after drug ingestion is the most common side effect of all-*trans*-RA. Mild analgesics generally suffice for control and the patient usually develops a tolerance to the effect. Pseudotumor cerebri, a known consequence of vitamin A toxicity, has been documented in several patients. These persons have required serial lumbar punctures, high-dose corticosteroids, and narcotic analgesics. Children have proven markedly more sensitive than adults to the CNS effects of all-*trans*-RA, and this effect is dose limiting in children.

TABLE 69–18. Adverse Effects of All-*Trans*-Retinoic Acid

Skin or Mucous Membranes
Skin dryness, itching, peeling
Genital excoriations
Angular cheilitis, lip cracking

Central Nervous System
Headache
Intracranial hypertension ("pseudotumor cerebri")

Metabolic Effects
Hypertriglyceridemia
Hypercholesterolemia

Hematologic Effects
Marked leukocytosis

Gastrointestinal Effects
Hepatic toxicity (increased SGOT, alkaline phosphatase, bilirubin)

Cardiovascular Effects
Congestive heart failure
Fluid overload
Lower extremity edema
Episodic hypotension
Decreased left ventricular ejection fraction
Pericardial effusion

Pulmonary Effects
Respiratory distress
Pleural effusion
Radiographic infiltrates

Dry skin, itching, flaking, nasal stuffiness, xerostomia, and cheilitis are relatively common although these reactions rarely disabling. Skin and mucous membrane effects can be managed with topical lubricants. Occasional scrotal and penile ulcerations have been observed. Bone pain occurs in 10% to 20% of patients. This effect tends to occur early during remission induction and usually remits despite continued therapy. The pain may transiently become quite intense and narcotics can be required for adequate analgesia.

Hypertriglyceridemia, a known side effect of other retinoids, has been observed with all-*trans*-RA. Hypercholesterolemia occurs to a less striking degree. Adverse consequences specifically related to hyperlipidemia have not been described. Retinoids are fat soluble and restrictions on dietary fat may decrease bioavailability of the drug. Hepatic toxicity is a well-known side effect of retinoids. Transient increases in serum transaminases, alkaline phosphatase, and bilirubin have been observed during RA treatment, and these effects may persist for several weeks after the drug is stopped. Permanent liver damage (even in posttransplant patients) has not been reported. As a group, the retinoids are exceptionally potent teratogens. All-*trans*-RA should not be administered to women who are pregnant, and a pregnancy test should be performed before therapeutic use in women of child-bearing age.

Leukocytosis (increase in peripheral leukocytes to $\geq$20,000 cells/mm^3) may occur in as many as 40% of APL patients treated with all-*trans*-RA. Although the development of leukocytosis was originally equated with an unfavorable outcome, additional experience suggests that an elevated leukocyte count, unaccompanied by the "retinoic acid syndrome," actually represents a positive biologic response to the drug and requires no specific treatment in the absence of other signs of leukostasis.[7] The peripheral blood leukocytes comprise a spectrum of myeloid cells including myeloblasts, promyelocytes, "intermediate cells", and granulocytes. Disseminated intravascular coagulopathy is usually not exacerbated by the leukocytosis.

Approximately 10% to 20% of patients with APL treated with all-*trans*-RA have experienced a syndrome characterized by high fever, respiratory distress, radiographic pulmonary infiltrates, and pleural or pericardial effusions.[42] This syndrome has occasionally been accompanied by impaired myocardial contractility and episodic hypotension. Although originally attributed to pneumonia or congestive heart failure, this reaction is now seen as a characteristic feature of all-*trans*-RA treatment in APL and represents by far the most serious reaction encountered with the use of this agent. Autopsy has revealed extensive infiltration of myeloid cells into lungs, skin, kidney, liver, and lymph nodes. Although leukocytosis is frequently observed with this syndrome, onset of the reaction may occur with a relatively normal leukocyte count in up to one third of cases.[42]

After reports of benefit in the "capillary leak syndrome" associated with interleukin-2 treatment, short courses of corticosteroids (*e.g.*, dexamethasone, 10 mg intravenously every 12 hours for 3 or more days) have been used and clinical symptoms have reversed in some patients.[42,43] Early recognition of the syndrome (especially unexplained fever and dyspnea) is critical, and the appearance of these signs should prompt immediate steroid treatment.

RETINOIC ACID-INDUCED DIFFERENTIATION

Although differentiation as a practical method of cancer treatment has been difficult to document conclusively, several lines of suggest that differentiation is a principal effect of all-*trans*-RA. This evidence includes changes in morphology, increased proliferative activity demonstrated by RNA/DNA flow cytometry, emergence of mature antigens on the surface of leukemic cells by immunophenotype studies, and persistence of the 15;17 translocation in morphologically mature cells documented by fluorescence in situ hybridization. One of the most distinctive aspects of all-*trans*-RA treatment is the appearance of cells derived from the leukemic clone visibly undergoing maturation. This process is obvious in the bone marrow and in the peripheral blood where cells can be found that are intermediate in maturation between promyelocytes and neutrophils.[8] Typically, these cells form indented vacuolated nuclei and lose their hypergranular appearance. Occasionally, one or more Auer rods can be found in the peripheral blood in cells that otherwise appear as mature polymorphonuclear neutrophils.

Using DNA/RNA flow cytometry, the S-phase component generally remains unchanged or increases during treatment with all-*trans*-RA.[44,45] This effect is clearly distinct from cytotoxic therapy (including low-dose cytosine arabinoside) wherein the proportion of cells in S-phase decreases markedly.

Consistent with the phenomenon of leukocytosis described above, this effect probably indicates that cells treated with all-*trans*-RA in vivo undergo one or more cycles of mitosis before maturing to a cell incapable of further division. In studies of APL patients, cell surface immunophenotyping of the neoplastic cells showed progression from a pattern of immature marker expression at presentation toward the appearance of mature granulocytic markers during remission; however, midway during remission induction, morphologically maturing cells were observed in the peripheral blood that simultaneously expressed mature and immature markers on the same cell (Fig. 69–18).[8] Using fluorescence in situ hybridization (FISH), the karyotypes of maturing cells in peripheral blood have been examined for the presence of clonal abnormalities by using a molecular probe for chromosome 17.[46] The PCC/FISH studies showed that approximately one third of these mature cells contained the chromosome 17 translocation while patients were undergoing induction treatment. After achieving complete remission, however, no mature cells containing the chromosome 17 translocation could be found.

Although this evidence is important, none of these data conclusively document that differentiation is the only mechanism whereby all-*trans*-RA exerts a therapeutic effect. To the extent that leukemic cells suppress normal hematopoiesis, all-*trans*-RA may cause a modest antiproliferative effect on the leukemic clone that could still be sufficient to eventually permit regrowth of normal cells. There is also no evidence that an abundance of mature cells derived from the leukemic

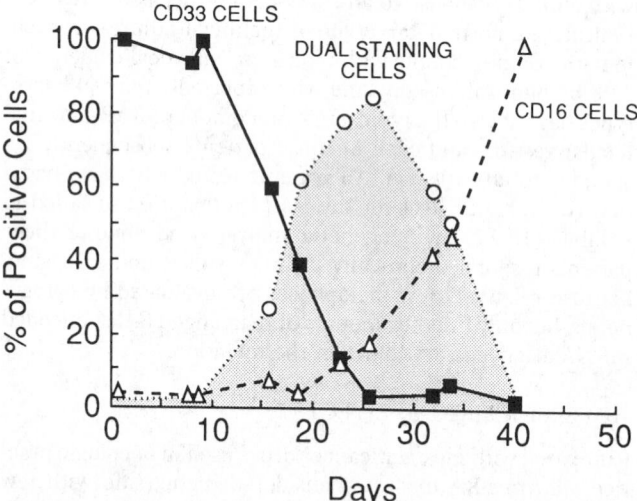

FIGURE 69–18. Cell immunophenotyping studies of peripheral blood leukocytes taken from a patient with acute promyelocytic leukemia undergoing treatment with all-*trans*-retinoic acid. Surface marker studies were performed to show the presence of cells that expressed only immature (CD33; *closed squares, solid line*) or mature (CD16; *open diamonds, dashed line*) myeloid surace antigens. A unique population of "intermediate" cells transiently appeared between days 15 and 33 of treatment (*open circles, dotted line*) that simultaneously disappeared as the patient entered complete remission (day 40), when only mature cell surface antigens were expressed. (Data provided by D. A. Scheinberg and reprinted with permission from Warrell RP Jr, Frankel SR, Miller WH Jr, et al. Differentiation therapy of acute promyelocytic leukemia with tretinoin [all-*trans*-retinoic acid]. N Engl J Med 1991;324:1385–1393)

clone persist during complete remission. However, the tests used to evaluate ongoing differentiation during remission (*e.g.*, immunophenotyping, PCC/FISH) are relatively insensitive. Studies using detection of restriction fragment length polymorphisms are clearly desirable to further explore this proposed mechanism.[47]

13-*CIS*-RETINOIC ACID

Due to its widespread availability, 13-*cis*-retinoic acid (isotretinoin) has been broadly evaluated as a method of cancer treatment and cancer prevention; the field has been extensively reviewed.[48,49] Because of the established relation between retinoic acid and the physiologic maturation of squamous epithelium, particular emphasis has been placed on the study of isotretinoin in preneoplastic and fully cancerous lesions of that tissue.

Effects in Squamous Neoplasms

Hong and colleagues demonstrated isotretinoin to be effective in reversing oral leukoplakia, a known precursor to squamous cancer.[50] The principal toxic effects of cheilitis, facial erythema, and dryness and peeling of the skin were acceptable in most patients. They were able to maintain remission of leukoplakia by a low-dose regimen of isotretinoin.[51] In a follow-up study, Hong and colleagues demonstrated that 12 months of therapy with high oral doses of isotretinoin significantly reduced the incidence of second primary cancers in patients who were free of disease from a previously treated squamous cell carcinoma of the head and neck.[52] The isotretinoin therapy had no evident effect on the rate or timing of recurrence of the original primary cancer. The isotretinoin dosage used in the study produced significant side effects; one third of the isotretinoin patients did not complete the planned 12-month course because of toxicity or noncompliance. Less toxic regimens are being sought.

Meyskens and Lippman observed objective antitumor effects of isotretinoin in advanced squamous cell carcinoma of the skin; however, the major response rates with the drug as a single agent were low.[53,54] Lippman and coworkers subsequently evaluated the combination of isotretinoin and interferon-α-2a in patients with advanced squamous cell cancer of the skin or cervix.[55,56] The preclinical basis for this combination was that interferon, a known differentiating agent, was synergistic with retinoic acid in differentiation induction of HL-60 and neuroblastoma and in growth inhibition in four additional human cell lines.[4,57-59] The drug dosages were identical in the skin and cervix cancer trials (isotretinoin, 1 mg/kg/day orally; interferon α-2a, 3 million units daily by subcutaneous injection).

In 32 patients with advanced cutaneous squamous cell carcinoma of the skin, 19 of 28 evaluable patients had a major response; the response was complete in 7 patients (25%).[55] Major response was observed in 13 of 14 patients with advanced local disease, 4 of 6 with regional disease, and 2 of 8 with distant metastases. The median duration of response was greater than 5 months. In the trial in patients with squamous cervix cancer, the isotretinoin plus interferon combination produced a major response in 13 of 26 patients; at the time

of assessment, 9 of the 13 "nonresponders" had stable disease, and only 4 patients demonstrated frank progression.[56] Although it cannot be stated that these antitumor responses are the result of drug-induced differentiation rather than immune modulation or some other mechanism, the two drugs produce synergistic differentiating effects in at least two cell model systems. Moreover, cytotoxic side effects in normal organ systems were limited to granulocytopenia in a small proportion of the treatment population.

Effects in Hematopoietic Neoplasms and Embryonal Tumors

Because of the differentiation induction of retinoic acid in leukemic and embryonal tumor models isotretinoin has also been evaluated in myeloproliferative disorders and germ cell neoplasms. It is not clear whether 13-*cis*-retinoic acid has significant activity APL. There are scattered reports of responses and failures in this disorder; however, a detailed assessment has not been undertaken.[27,60-63]

Isotretinoin has produced transient responses in patients with mycosis fungoides, but it did not produce useful effects in an extended evaluation in patients with myelodysplastic syndromes.[64,65,66-68] It was also inactive in a phase II assessment in patients with nonseminomatous germ cell tumors.[69]

1,25-DIHYDROXYVITAMIN D₃

$1\alpha,25$-dihydroxyvitamin D₃ ($1,25(OH)_2D_3$), the active form of the hormone, contributes to physiologic differentiation in a variety of cell types.[70] The biologic effects of $1,25(OH)_2D_3$ are mediated through interaction with nuclear receptors analogous to thyroid, steroid, and retinoic acid receptors.[71] These receptors have been identified in a variety of cells, including normal and neoplastic cells of hematopoietic, colonic, and breast epithelial lineages.[72-74] Epidemiologic data suggest that an adequate dietary vitamin D intake reduces the incidence of colorectal cancer, and calcium or vitamin D supplementation protects against induction of colon cancer in some rodent models.[75-77] $1,25(OH)_2D_3$ is growth inhibitory to breast, colonic, and melanoma cancer cell lines, but does not induce differentiation;[78-81] However, it greatly enhances butyrate-induced differentiation in colon cancer cell lines.[79,80]

$1,25(OH)_2D_3$ induces differentiation of HL-60 cells along the monocyte-macrophage pathway.[82-84] Koeffler and colleagues demonstrated that a high concentration of $1,25(OH)_2D_3$ (10^{-6} M) induced in vitro differentiation of blast cells from patients with acute myeloblastic leukemia as assessed by morphology, phagocytosis, and superoxide production.[85] At a lower concentration (10^{-9} M), there was no effect. Based on these results, this group treated 18 patients with myelodysplastic syndrome with 2 μg/day of $1,25(OH)_2D_3$; 8 patients had partial or minor peripheral blood responses during the period of drug administration. However, no patient showed significant improvement of peripheral blood or bone marrow findings, and 9 patients developed hypercalcemia that precluded further study.[85] New analogs of vitamin D₃ have been synthesized that retain the differentiating activity while minimizing effects on calcium mobilization.[86-88] Several of these agents have been proposed for clinical investigation.

LOW-DOSE CYTOSINE ARABINOSIDE

In low concentrations, cytosine arabinoside (ara-C) induces terminal cytodifferentiation in HL-60 and K562 leukemia cells.[89-92] At higher concentrations, ara-C produces cytotoxic effects by inhibition of DNA synthesis and by incorporation into DNA and RNA. The mechanism by which ara-C and other inhibitors of DNA synthesis produce cellular differentiation in culture is not established. In HL-60 and K562 cells it is postulated that a low but predictable rate of terminal differentiation occurs in the absence of added inducers. At "subcytotoxic" concentrations, ara-C may slow the rate of DNA synthesis and prolong the S phase, causing a shift in the cellular balance from proliferation toward differentiation.

Low-dose ara-C has been extensively evaluated in patients with myelodysplastic syndromes and in elderly persons with AML.[93-97] A variety of dosages and schedules have been examined. Although complete remissions have been induced in some patients, it remains unclear whether low-dose ara-C merits an established place in the management of these diseases. It is also uncertain to what extent these regimens produce their effects by cytodifferentiation, rather than by cytotoxicity.

In a review of the published results on 751 patients treated with low-dose ara-C up to 1986, Cheson and coworkers projected the following CR rates for the 507 evaluable patients: 32% for patients with primary AML; 16% for AML secondary to prior chemotherapy; and 16% for patients with myelodysplastic syndromes (MDS).[98] The median survival of these three groupings was 9 months, 3 months, and 15 months, respectively.[98] The status of low-dose ara-C has also been reviewed for MDS.[99,100] In a randomized prospective comparison study of low-dose ara-C versus supportive therapy, the CR rate from low-dose ara-C was only 8%.[101] Despite a longer progression-free survival in ara-C treated patients, total survival was similar in the two groups (8.7 versus 6.9 months with ara-C and supportive care). Although response rates may be higher in some subgroups of the myelodysplastic syndromes, low-dose ara-C does not have an established role in management of MDS.

Although some contribution of differentiation induction to the therapeutic effects produced by low-dose ara-C can not be excluded, the available data suggest that the principal mechanism was cytotoxicity. Myelosuppression was evident in 88% of patients.[98] In patients for whom bone marrow hypoplasia was not observed, concerns have been raised about the frequency of observation. Although examples of mature cells with the malignant genotype have been reported in patients undergoing low-dose ara-C therapy, the heterogeneity of the entities under treatment and the paucity of observations do not permit definitive conclusions.

TIAZOFURIN

Tiazofurin is one of a numerous inhibitors of purine synthesis developed as candidate anticancer agents. Their synthesis was stimulated by observations that cancer cells commonly have upregulated the guanylate biosynthetic pathway by increased expression of inosine 5'-monophosphate (IMP) dehydrogenase, the rate-limiting step in guanylate biosynthesis.[102] Recent studies demonstrate that two isoenzymes of IMP dehydrogenase exist in human cells.[103] Neoplastic cells display a selective increase in mRNA for the type II isoenzyme, while the rate of expression of type I IMP dehydrogenase mRNA remains relatively constant.[103-105]

Tiazofurin (2-β-D-ribofuranosylthiazole-4-carboxamide), is metabolized to tiazofurin adenine dinucleotide, a highly selective inhibitor of IMP dehydrogenase.[106,107] The drug has displayed cytotoxic and cytodifferentiating effects in cell culture systems, with a clear correlation between these effects and a decrease in cellular levels of GTP.[108-111] Consistent with this proposed relation, tiazofurin-induced differentiation in cell culture can be reproduced by mycophenolic acid, another inhibitor of IMP dehydrogenase, and abrogated by the addition of guanosine to the culture medium.[107-111]

Tricot and colleagues have treated patients with refractory acute myeloblastic leukemia and blast crisis of chronic myelocytic leukemia with a protocol combining tiazofurin and allopurinol.[112,113] The concept of the protocol is to lower cellular GTP pools by the combined effects of inhibition of IMP dehydrogenase (through tiazofurin) and inhibition of guanine salvage (guanine plus hypoxanthine/guanine phosphoribosyl transferase plus PRPP with or without guanylate plus ribose-1-phosphate) by elevating plasma hypoxanthine levels through the use of allopurinol. Hypoxanthine and guanine are competitive substrates for the purine salvage pathway but hypoxanthine would enter the guanylate pools only through the action of IMP dehydrogenase.

The regimen appears to have produced the greatest therapeutic effect in patients with blast crisis of CML; 9 of 11 patients returned to the chronic phase of the disorder.[113] One patient with AML in first relapse achieved a complete remission of 10 months duration.[112] Although the response in AML was considered to be due to the drug's cytotoxic effects, the absence of marrow hypoplasia and the consistent presence of chromosomal abnormalities in the responding CML patients suggested differentiation induction as a contributing mechanism.[112] Although of considerable theoretic interest, this program is not readily extended to wide usage as it required frequent specialized biochemical observations and tiazofurin dose adjustments. Adverse effects included drowsiness, nausea, vomiting, pleuropericarditis, headache, skin rash, myalgia and hypertension.

PLANAR-POLAR INDUCERS

Hexamethylene bisacetamide (HMBA) entered clinical trials largely because of its capacity to induce terminal differentiation in murine erythroleukemia cells (MELC). The studies with HMBA extended the original observations of Friend and colleagues with dimethyl sulfoxide (DMSO).[114] HMBA and related planar-polar compounds induce differentiation in numerous other neoplastic cell lines.[115] This field has been the subject of several recent reviews.[1,116,117] Numerous biochemical events have been associated with HMBA-induced differentiation; recent data indicate that the drug produces an activation of the β isozyme of protein kinase C.[118,119] The effects of HMBA mimic those of transforming growth factor-β (TGF-β) in a number of systems. The two agents are synergistic in MELC.[120] However, in the HT29 colon cancer cell line, the effects of HMBA appear to result from its capacity to induce the synthesis of TGF-β1.[121,122]

The initial clinical evaluations of HMBA have been based on drug concentrations and durations of exposure derived from the extensive studies in the MELC system. In all cell culture models, prolonged exposure to HMBA has been required to induce cellular commitment to differentiation. In MELC, 1 mM was the minimal effective concentration in 5-day cultures; 5 mM was optimal, producing erythroid differentiation in over 95% of cells, and 10 mM was cytotoxic. Most clinical studies of HMBA have employed continuous intravenous infusions given for 5 or 10 days. The 5-day regimens used steady-state HMBA levels between 1 and 2 mM.[123,124] In the 10-day regimens, the [HMBA]$_{ss}$ has been 1 mM.[125] Renal and central nervous system toxicity precluded the use of steady state concentrations $\geq$2 mM.[123,124] The limiting side effect of prolonged infusions has been thrombocytopenia. Because HMBA is rapidly cleared from plasma, and the drug is only moderately soluble, intravenous treatment programs have required administration of large fluid volumes.[123-126] Although extended studies of the intravenous drug have been limited, these impediments may be obviated by the development of an oral formulation and the documentation that oral HMBA is fully bioavailable.[127]

There have been no major clinical responses to HMBA given by the 5-day schedule in the phase I studies or in a subsequent phase II assessment in patients with myelodysplastic syndromes (MDS).[123,124,128] With the 10-day schedule, one sustained complete response has been observed in a patient with lung cancer.[125] Although 5-day courses of HMBA produced no apparent remissions in MDS, Andreeff and coworkers observed 2 CRs and 6 PRs in 22 evaluable patients with MDS or acute myeloid leukemia treated on a 10-day schedule.[128,129] In 1 patient with monosomy 7 who entered CR, HMBA administration produced an increase in granulocytes with the monosomy 7 marker, as demonstrated by direct FISH.

The extensive excretion of HMBA and active metabolites in the urine, coupled with the availability of an oral formulation of HMBA, make it a potentially useful chemotherapeutic or chemopreventive agent in patients with recurrent superficial bladder tumors.[126,130,131] Russo and colleagues have demonstrated that HMBA has growth-inhibitory effects on bladder cancer cells in studies with short-term culture of shed cells and with an established cell line.[132]

Future studies of planar-polar compounds may also involve assessment of newer analogs, several of which are approximately 100-fold more active than HMBA in differentiation induction in the MELC system.[133] One of these compounds demonstrates a 33-fold increase in growth-inhibitory potency against the HT-29 human colon cancer line.

CYCLIC AMP MODULATION

Increase cytodifferentiation is observed in a broad range of cell culture systems with the combined use of "triggering agents" (*e.g.*, retinoic acid, HMBA, interferons) and substances that increase intracellular levels of 3',5'-cyclic adenosine monophosphate (cAMP) by inducing an increase in its synthesis (*e.g.*, cholera toxin, PGE$_1$, forskolin, isoproterenol) or a decrease in its degradation by phosphodiesterase

(*e.g.*, isobutylmethylxanthine).[134-137] Analogs of cAMP (*e.g.*, dibutyryl-cAMP, 8-Br-cAMP) are also effective for this purpose.[138,139] cAMP modulation is only a weak inducer of cytodifferentiation in the absence of the triggering agents. Although widely examined in the preclinical systems, differentiation regimens including a cAMP modulatory component have not yet received a meaningful clinical assessment.

CONCLUSIONS

With the striking exception of the major therapeutic activity of all-*trans*-retinoic acid in treating APL, the use of single agents to induce differentiation and eventual regression of advanced cancer has been clinically disappointing. Success of differentiation therapy may be increased by the use of combination regimens. Except for the combination of isotretinoin and interferon-α, combination regimens have not received extended clinical evaluation. Nevertheless combination regimens of differentiating agents themselves are possible and justified by preclinical data. Many of the triggering agents (*e.g.*, retinoic acid, DMSO, HMBA, 1,25(OH)$_2$D$_3$, interferons) have nonoverlapping toxicities but produce enhanced differentiation effects in combination.[140] It is reasonable to explore the combined use of inducers with pharmacologic modulators needed to maintain adequate plasma concentrations of the active agent, or inducers with enhancing agents (*e.g.*, cAMP-elevating regimens).

Differentiation therapy was initially conceived as altering the phenotypic behavior of neoplastic cells, rather than eliminating that population. Theoretically, this could result in a pseudochimeric state in which a morphologically normal mixture of genetically normal and abnormal cells would be present on a continuing basis. In APL patients in complete remission after therapy with all-*trans*-retinoic acid, the *RARA/PML* gene fusion is frequently detectable by PCR techniques; however, the numbers of genetically abnormal cells are dramatically decreased, implying a therapy-induced adjustment of the proliferative balance between the normal and neoplastic cell populations.

What is the proper dosage schedule and duration for new candidate differentiation regimens? In the successful treatment of APL and the encouraging regimens for squamous cancers of skin and cervix the drugs are given daily for weeks or months. Because drug-induced differentiation does not kill cells acutely, even differentiated cells may survive for prolonged periods, and some tumor cells may resume proliferation when therapy is interrupted. Chronic therapy of some weeks' duration may be more likely to show a clinical effect than a more intense course that can only be given a few days each month.

It is reasonable to explore possible interface between cytotoxic and differentiation regimens. Currently, differentiation therapy appears to work best when the target cells have a low number of genetic mutations. When this concept is extended to precancerous lesions, differentiation therapy merges with chemoprevention. The use of isotretinoin in delaying the development of new primary head and neck cancer provides a paradigm for differentiation therapy after initial ablative therapy of cancer. In ongoing APL studies, the sequence is reversed. Tretinoin is used to induce remission with good patient tolerance; however, because resistance to continuous retinoid therapy is expected in most patients, responding patients are shifted to cytotoxic regimens while still in remission; the utility of this approach will be assessable over the next several years.

REFERENCES

1. Reuben RC, Khanna PL, Gazitt Y, et al. Inducers of erythroleukemic differentiation. Relationship of structure to activity among planar-polar compounds. J Biol Chem 1978;253:4214–4218.
2. Strickland S, Mahdavi V. The induction of differentiation in teratocarcinoma stem cells by retinoic acid. Cell 1978;15:393–403.
3. Breitman TR, Selonick SE, Collins SJ. Induction of differentiation of the human promyelocytic leukemia cell line (HL-60) by retinoic acid. Proc Natl Acad Sci USA 1980;77:2936–2940.
4. Rossi GB. Interferons and cell differentiation. In: Gresser I, ed. Interferon. London: Academic Press, 1985:31–68.
5. Huang ME, Ye YC, Chen JR, et al. Use of all-*trans* retinoic acid in the treatment of acute promyelocytic leukemia. Blood 1988;72:567–572.
6. Wang ZY, Sun GL, Lu JX, et al. Treatment of acute promyelocytic leukemia with all-*trans* retinoic acid in China. Nouv Rev Fr Hematol 1990;32:34–36.
7. Castaigne S, Chomienne C, Daniel MT, et al. All-*trans* retinoic acid as a differentiation therapy for acute promyelocytic leukemia: I. Clinical results. Blood 1990;76:1704–1709.
8. Warrell RP Jr, Frankel SR, Miller WH Jr, et al. Differentiation therapy of acute promyelocytic leukemia with tretinoin (all-*trans*-retinoic acid). N Engl J Med 1991;324:1385–1393.
9. Zi-Xing C, Yong-Quan X, Ri Z, et al. A clinical and experimental study of all-*trans* retinoic acid-treated acute promyelocytic leukemia patients. Blood 1991;78:1413–1419.
10. Vogelstein B, Fearon ER, Hamilton SR, et al. Genetic alterations during colorectal-tumor development. N Engl J Med 1988;319:525–532.
11. Fearon ER, Cho KR, Nigro JM, et al. Identification of a chromosome 18q gene that is altered in colorectal cancers. Science 1990;247:49–56.
12. Baker SJ, Preisinger AC, Jessup JM, et al. *P53* gene mutations occur in combination with 17p allelic deletions as late events in colorectal tumorigenesis. Cancer Res 1990;50:7712–7722.
13. Miyaki M, Seki M, Okamoto M, et al. Genetic changes and histopathological types in colorectal tumors from patients with familial adenomatous polyposis. Cancer Res 1990;50:7166–7173.
14. Sato T, Akiyama F, Sakamoto G, et al. Accumulation of genetic alterations and progression of primary breast cancer. Cancer Res 1991;51:5794–5799.
15. Kelman Z, Prokocimer M, Peller S, et al. Rearrangements in the p53 gene in Philadelphia chromosome positive chronic myelogenous leukemia. Blood 1989;74:2318–2324.
16. Mashal R, Shtalrid M, Talpaz, et al. Rearrangement and expression of p53 in the chronic phase and blast crisis of chronic myelogenous leukemia. Blood 1991;75:180–189.
17. Feinstein E, Cimino G, Gale RP, et al. *P53* in chronic myelogenous leukemia in acute phase. Proc Natl Acad Sci USA 1991;88:6293–6297.
18. Blomhoff R, Green MH, Green JB, et al. Vitamin A metabolism: New perspectives on absorption, transport, and storage. Physiol Rev 1991;71:951–990.
19. De Luca LM. Retinoids and their receptors in differentiation, embryogenesis, and neoplasia. FASEB J 1991;5:2924–2933.
20. Evans RM. The steroid and thyroid hormone superfamily. Science 1992;240:889–895.
21. Petkovich M, Brand NJ, Krust A, et al. A human retinoic acid receptor which belongs to the family of nuclear receptors. Nature 1987;330:444–450.
22. Giguere V, Ong ES, Segui P, et al. Identification of a receptor for the morphogen retinoic acid. Nature 1987;330:624–629.
23. Mangelsdorf DJ, Ong ES, Dyck JA, et al. Nuclear receptor that identifies a novel retinoic acid response pathway. Nature 1990;345:224–229.
24. Breitman TR, Collins SJ, Keene BR. Terminal differentiation of human promyelocytic leukemic cells in primary culture in response to retinoic acid. Blood 1981;57:1000–1004.
25. Sidell N, Altman A, Haussler M, et al. Effects of retinoic acid on the growth and phenotypic expression of several human neuroblastoma cell lines. Exp Cell Res 1983;148:21–30.
26. Collins SJ, Robertson KA, Mueller LM. Retinoic acid-induced granulocytic differentiation of HL-60 myeloid leukemia cells is mediated directly through the retinoic acid receptor (RAR-alpha). Mol Cell Biol 1990;10:2154–2163.
27. Flynn PJ, Miller WJ, Weisdorf DJ, et al. Retinoic acid treatment of acute promyelocytic leukemia: In vitro and in vivo observations. Blood 1983;62:1211–1217.
28. Douer D, Koeffler PH. Retinoic acid enhances colony stimulating factor induced growth of normal human myeloid progenitor cells in vitro. Exp Cell Res 1982;138:193–198.
29. Lawrence HJ, Conner K, Kelly MA, et al. *Cis*-retinoic acid stimulates the clonal growth of some myeloid leukemia cells in vitro. Blood 1987;69:302–307.
30. Chen Z, Sun G-L, Chen S-S, et al. All-*trans*-retinoic acid and acute promyelocytic leukemia in China: From clinic to molecular biology. Conference Proceedings for Retinoids: New Trends in Research and Clinical Application, Palermo, 1991:102.
31. Muindi J, Frankel SR, Miller WH Jr, et al. Continuous treatment with all-*trans* retinoic acid causes a progressive reduction in plasma drug concentrations: Implications for

32. Muindi J, Frankel SR, Huselton, C, et al. Clinical pharmacology of oral all-*trans* retinoic acid in patients with acute promyelocytic leukemia. Cancer Res 1992;52:2138–2142.
33. Goodman GE, Einspahr JG, Alberts DS, et al. Pharmacokinetics of 13-*cis*-retinoic acid in patients with advanced cancer. Cancer Res 1982;42:2087–2091.
34. Brazzell RK, Colburn WA. Pharmacokinetics of the retinoids isotretinoin and etretinate: A comparative review. J Am Acad Dermatol 1982;6:643–651.
35. Brazell RK, Vane FM, Ehmann CW, et al. Pharmacology of isotretinoin during repetitive dosing to patients. Eur J Clin Pharmacol 1983;24:695–702.
36. Larson RA, Kondo K, Vardiman JW, et al. Evidence for a 15;17 translocation in every patient with acute promyelocytic leukemia. Am J Med 1984;76:827–841.
37. de The H, Chomienne C, Lanotte M, et al. The t(15;17) translocation of acute promyelocytic leukaemia fuses the retinoic acid receptor gene to a novel transcribed locus. Nature 1990;347:558–561.
38. Kakizuka A, Miller WH Jr, Umesono K, et al. Chromosomal translocation t(15;17) in human acute promyelocytic leukemia fuses the RAR-alpha receptor with a novel putative transcription factor PML. Cell 1991;66:663–674.
39. Biondi A, Rambaldi A, Alcalay M, et al. *RAR-α* gene rearrangements as a genetic marker for diagnosis and monitoring in acute promyelocytic leukemia. Blood 1991;77:1418–1422.
40. Miller WH Jr, Warrell RP Jr, Frankel S, et al. Novel retinoic acid receptor-α transcripts in acute promyelocytic leukemia responsive to all-*trans*-retinoic acid. JNCI 1990;82:1932–1933.
41. Miller WH, Kakizuka A, Frankel SR, et al. Reverse transcriptase/polymerase chain reaction amplification for *PML/RAR-alpha* clarifies diagnosis and detects minimal residual disease in acute promyelocytic leukemia. Proc Natl Acad Sci USA 1992;89:2694–2698.
42. Frankel SR, Weiss M, Warrell RP. A "retinoic acid syndrome" in acute promyelocytic leukemia: Reversal by corticosteroids. Blood 1991;78:380a.
43. Vetto JT, Papa MZ, Lotze MT, et al. Reduction of toxicity of Interleukin-2 and lymphokine-activated killer cells in humans by the administration of corticosteroids. J Clin Oncol 1987;5:496–503.
44. Andreeff M, Darzynkiewicz, Sharpless TK, et al. Discrimination of human leukemia subtypes by flow cytometric analysis of cellular DNA and RNA. Blood 1980;55:282–293.
45. Frankel SR, Scheinberg DA, Miller WH Jr, et al. Differentiation therapy of acute promyelocytic leukemia with all-trans retinoic acid. Proc Am Soc Clin Oncol 1991;10, 225.
46. Pinkel D, Strauma T, Gray JW. Cytogenetic analysis using quantitative, high sensitivity, fluorescence hybridization. Proc Natl Acad Sci USA 1986;83:2934–2938.
47. Fearon ER, Burke PJ, Schiffer CA, et al. Differentiation of leukemia cells to polymorphonuclear leukocytes in patients with acute nonlymphoblastic leukemia. N Engl J Med 1986;315:15–24.
48. Lippman SM, Kessler JF, Meyskens FL Jr. Retinoids as preventive and therapeutic anticancer agents (Part I). Cancer Treat Rep 1987;71:391–405.
49. Lippman SM, Kessler JF, Meyskens FL Jr. Retinoids as preventive and therapeutic anticancer agents (Part II). Cancer Treat Rep 1987;71:493–515.
50. Hong WK, Endicott J, Itri LM, et al. 13-*Cis*-retinoic acid in the treatment of oral leukoplakia. N Engl J Med 1986;315:1501–1505.
51. Lippman SM, Toth BB, Batsakis JG, et al. Low-dose 13-cis-retinoic acid maintains remission in oral premalignancy: More effective than β-carotene in randomized trial. Proc Am Soc Clin Oncol 1990;9:59.
52. Hong WK, Lippman SM, Itri LM, et al. Prevention of second primary tumors with isotretinoin in squamous cell carcinoma of the head and neck. N Engl J Med 1990;323:795–801.
53. Meyskens FL Jr, Gilmartin E, Alberts DS, et al. Activity of isotretinoin against squamous cell cancers and preneoplastic lesions. Cancer Treat Rep 1982;66:1315–1319.
54. Lippman SM, Meyskens FL Jr. Treatment of advanced squamous cell carcinoma of the skin with isotretinoin. Ann Intern Med 1987;107:499–501.
55. Lippman SM, Parkinson DR, Itri LM, et al. 13-*Cis*-retinoic acid and interferon α-2a: Effective combination therapy for advanced squamous cell carcinoma of the skin. JNCI 1992;84:235–241.
56. Lippman SM, Kavanagh JJ, Paredes-Espinoza M, et al. 13-*Cis*-retinoic acid plus interferon α-2a: Highly active systemic therapy for squamous cell carcinoma of the cervix. JNCI 1992;84:241–245.
57. Hemmi H, Breitman TR. Combinations of recombinant human interferons and retinoic acid synergistically induce differentiation of the human promyelocytic leukemia cell line HL-60. Blood 1987;69:501–507.
58. Higuchi T, Hannigan GE, Malkin D, et al. Enhancement by retinoic acid and dibutyryl cyclic adenosine 3',5'-monophosphate of the differentiation and gene expression of human neuroblastoma cells induced by interferon. Cancer Res 1991;51:3958–3964.
59. Frey JR, Peck R, Bollag W. Antiproliferative activity of retinoids, interferon α and their combination in five human transformed cell lines. Cancer Lett 1991;57:223–227.
60. Nilsson B. Probable in vivo induction of differentiation by retinoic acid of promyelocytes in acute promyelocytic leukemia. Br J Haematol 1984;57:365–371.
61. Daenen S, Vellenga E, van Dobbenburgh OA, et al. Retinoic acid as antileukemic therapy in a patient with acute promyelocytic leukemia and *Aspergillus* pneumonia. Blood 1986;67:559–561.
62. Fontana JA, Rogers JS, Durham JP. The role of 13 cis-retinoic acid in the remission induction of a patient with acute promyelocytic leukemia. Cancer 1989;57:209–217.
63. Wijermans PW, Rebel VI, Ossenkoppele GJ, et al. Combined procoagulant activity

and proteolytic activity of acute promyelocytic leukemic cells: Reversal of the bleeding disorder by cell differentiation. Blood 1989;73:800–805.

64. Kessler JF, Meyskens FL Jr, Levine N, et al. Treatment of cutaneous T-cell lymphoma (mycosis fungoides) with 13-cis-retinoic acid. Lancet 1983;1:1345–1347.

65. Warrell RP Jr, Coonley CJ, Kempin SJ, et al. Isotretinoin in cutaneous T-cell lymphoma. Lancet 1983;1:629.

66. Greenberg BR, Durie BGM, Barnett TC, et al. Phase I–II study of 13-cis-retinoic acid in myelodysplastic syndrome. Cancer Treat Rep 1985;69:1369–1374.

67. Picozzi VJ, Swanson GF, Morgan R, et al. 13-Cis retinoic acid treatment for myelo-dysplastic syndromes. J Clin Oncol 1986;4:589–595.

68. Koeffler HP, Heitjan D, Mertelsmann R, et al. Randomized study of 13-cis retinoic acid vs placebo in the myelodysplastic disorders. Blood 1988;71:703–708.

69. Gold EJ, Bosl GJ, Itri LM. Phase II trial of 13-cis retinoic acid in patients with advanced nonseminomatous germ cell tumors. Cancer Treat Rep 1984;68:1287–1288.

70. Suda T, Shinki T, Takahashi N. The role of vitamin D in bone and intestinal cell differentiation. Annu Rev Nutr 1990;10:195–211.

71. Fuller PJ. The steroid receptor superfamily: Mechanisms of diversity. FASEB J 1991;5: 3092–3099.

72. Kizaki M, Norman AW, Bishop JE, et al. 1,25-dihydroxyvitamin D_3 receptor RNA. Expression in hematopoietic cells. Blood 1991;77:1238–1247.

73. Meggouh F, Lointier P, Saez S. Sex steroid and 1,25-dihydroxyvitamin D_3 receptors in human colorectal adenocarcinoma and normal mucosa. Cancer Res 1991;51:1227–1233.

74. Eisman JA, Suva LJ, Sher E, et al. Frequency of 1,25-dihydroxyvitamin D_3 receptor in human breast cancer. Cancer Res 1981;41:5121–5124.

75. Garland C, Shekelle RB, Barrett-Connor E, et al. Dietary vitamin D and calcium and risk of colorectal cancer: A 19 year prospective study in men. Lancet 1985;1:307–309.

76. Pence BC, Buddingh F. Inhibition of dietary fat-promoted colon carcinogenesis in rats by supplemental calcium or vitamin D. Carcinogenesis 1988;9:187–190.

77. Sitrin MD, Halline AG, Abrahams C, et al. Dietary calcium and vitamin D modulate 1,2-dimethylhydrazine-induced colonic carcinogenesis in the rat. Cancer Res 1991;51: 5608–5613.

78. Frampton RJ, Omond SA, Eisman JA. Inhibition of human cancer cell growth by 1,25-dihydroxyvitamin D_3 metabolites. Cancer Res 1983;43:4443–4447.

79. Tanaka Y, Bush KK, Klauck TM, et al. Enhancement of butyrate-induced differentiation of HT-29 human colon carcinoma cells by 1,25-dihydroxyvitamin D_3. Biochem Pharmacol 1989;38:3859–3865.

80. Tanaka Y, Bush KK, Eguchi T, et al. Effects of 1,25-dihydroxyvitamin D_3 and its analogs on butyrate-induced differentiation of HT-29 human colonic carcinoma cells and on the reversal of the differentiated phenotype. Arch Biochem Biophys 1990;276:415–423.

81. Colston K, Colston MJ, Feldman D. 1,25-Dihydroxyvitamin D_3 and malignant melanoma: The presence of receptors and inhibition of cell growth in culture. Endocrinology 1981;108:1083–1086.

82. McCarthy DM, San Miguel JF, Freake HC, et al. 1,25-Dihydroxyvitamin D_3 inhibits proliferation of human promyelocytic leukemia (HL60) cells and induces monocyte-macrophage differentiation in HL60 and normal human bone marrow cells. Leuk Res 1983;7:51–55.

83. Tanaka H, Abe E, Miyaura C, et al. 1,25-Dihydroxyvitamin D_3 induces differentiation of human promyelocytic leukemia cells (HL-60) into monocyte-macrophages, but not into granulocytes. Biochem Biophys Res Comm 1983;117:86–92.

84. Manglesdorf DJ, Koeffler HP, Donaldson CA, et al. 1,25-Dihydroxyvitamin-D_3-induced differentiation in a human promyelocytic leukemia cell (HL-60): Receptor-mediated maturation to macrophage-like cells. J Cell Biol 1984;98:391–398.

85. Koeffler HP, Hirji K, Itri L, et al. 1,25-Dihydroxyvitamin D_3: In vivo and in vitro effects on human preleukemic and leukemic cells. Cancer Treat Rep 1985;69:1399–1407.

86. Zhou J-Y, Norman AW, Lubbert ED, et al. Novel vitamin D analogues that modulate leukemic cell growth and differentiation with little effect on either intestinal calcium absorption or bone calcium mobilization. Blood 1989;74:82–93.

87. Perlman K, Kutner A, Prahl J, et al. 24-Homologated 1,25-dihydroxyvitamin D_3 compounds: Separation of calcium and cell differentiation activities. Biochemistry 1990;29: 190–196.

88. Norman AW, Jhou JY, Henry HL, et al. Structure-function studies on analogues of 1α,25-dihydroxyvitamin D_3: Differential effects on leukemic cell growth, differentiation, and intestinal calcium absorption. Cancer Res 1990;50:6857–6864.

89. Lotem J, Sachs L. Different blocks in the differentiation of myeloid leukemic cells. Proc Natl Acad Sci USA 1974;71:3507–3511.

90. Sachs L. The differentiation of myeloid leukaemic cells: New possibilities for therapy. Br J Haematol 1978;40:509–517.

91. Griffin J, Munroe D, Major P, et al. Induction of differentiation of human myeloid leukemia cells by inhibitors of DNA synthesis. Exp Hematol 1982;10:774–781.

92. Luisi-DeLuca C, Mitchell T, Spriggs D, et al. Induction of terminal differentiation in human K562 erythroleukemia cells by arabinofuranosylcytosine. J Clin Invest 1984;74: 821–827.

93. Baccarani M, Tura S. Differentiation of myeloid leukemia cells: New possibilities for therapy. Br J Haematol 1979;42:485–487.

94. Castaigne S, Daniel MT, Tilly H, et al. Does treatment with ara-C in low dosage cause differentiation of leukemic cells? Blood 1983;62:85–86.

95. Wisch JS, Griffin JD, Kufe DW. Response of preleukemic syndromes to continuous infusion of low-dose cytarabine. N Engl J Med 1983;309:1599–1602.

96. Ishikura H, Sawada H, Okazaki T, et al. The effect of low dose ARA-C in acute non-lymphoblastic leukaemias and atypical leukaemia. Br J Haematol 1984;58:9–18.

97. Degos L, Castaigne S, Tilly H, et al. Treatment of leukemia with low-dose ara-C. A study of 160 cases. Semin Oncol 1985;12(suppl 3):196–199.

98. Cheson BD, Jasperse DM, Simon R, et al. A critical appraisal of low-dose cytosine arabinoside in patients with acute non-lymphocytic leukemia and myelodysplastic syndromes. J Clin Oncol 1986;4:1857–1864.

99. Cheson BD. The myelodysplastic syndromes: Current approaches to therapy. Ann Intern Med 1990;112:932–941.

100. List AF, Garewal HS, Sandberg AA. The myelodysplastic syndromes: Biology and implications for management. J Clin Oncol 1990;8:1424–1441.

101. Miller KB, Kim K, Morrison FS, et al. Evaluation of low dose ara-C versus supportive care in the treatment of myelodysplastic syndromes: An intergroup study by the Eastern Cooperative Oncology Group and the Southwest Oncology Group. Blood 72(suppl 1): 215A.

102. Weber G. Biochemical strategy of cancer cells and the design of chemotherapy: G.H.A. Clowes Memorial Lecture. Cancer Res 1983;43:3466–3492.

103. Natsumeda Y, Ohno S, Kawasaki H, et al. Two distinctive cDNAs for human IMP dehydrogenase. J Biol Chem 1990;265:5292–5295.

104. Konno Y, Natsumeda Y, Nagai M, et al. Expression of human IMP dehydrogenase types I and II in Escherichia coli and distribution in human normal lymphocytes and leukemic cell lines. J Biol Chem 1991;266:506–509.

105. Nagai M, Natsumeda Y, Konno Y, et al. Selective up-regulation of type II inosine 5′-monophosphate dehydrogenase messenger RNA expression in human leukemias. Cancer Res 1991;51:3886–3890.

106. Cooney DA, Jayaram HN, Gebeyehu G, et al. The conversion of 2-β-D-ribofuranosyl-thiazole-4-carboxamide to an analogue of NAD with potent IMP dehydrogenase inhibitory properties. Biochem Pharmacol 1982;31:2133–2136.

107. Jayaram HN, Dion RL, Glazer RI, et al. Initial studies on the mechanism of action of a new oncolytic thiazole nucleoside, 2-β-D-ribofuranosylthiozole-4-carboxamide (NSC 286193). Biochem Pharmacol 1982;31:2371–2380.

108. Olah E, Natsumeda Y, Ikegami T, et al. Induction of erythroid differentiation and modulation of gene expression by tiazofurin in K562 leukemic cells. Proc Natl Acad Sci USA 1988;85:6533–6537.

109. Kharbanda SM, Sherman ML, Spriggs DR, et al. Effects of tiazofurin on protooncogene expression during HL-60 cell differentiation. Cancer Res 1988;48:5965–5968.

110. Yamaji Y, Natsumeda Y, Yamada S, et al. Synergistic action of tiazofurin and retinoic acid on differentiation and colony formation of HL-60 leukemia cells. Life Sci 1990;46: 435–442.

111. Kiguchi K, Collart FR, Henning-Chubb C, et al. Induction of cell differentiation in melanoma cells by inhibitors of IMP dehydrogenase: Altered patterns of IMP dehydrogenase expression and activity. Cell Growth Diff 1990;1:259–270.

112. Tricot GJ, Jayaram HN, Lapis E, et al. Biochemically directed therapy of leukemia with tiazofurin, a selective blocker of inosine 5′-phosphate dehydrogenase activity. Cancer Res 1989;49:3696–3701.

113. Tricot G, Jayaram HN, Zhen W, et al. Biochemically directed therapy with tiazofurin of refractory leukemia and myeloid blast crisis of chronic granulocytic leukemia. Proc Am Assoc Cancer Res 1991;32:184.

114. Friend C, Scher W, Holland JG, et al. Hemoglobin synthesis in murine erythroleukemia cells in vitro: Stimulation of erythroid differentiation by dimethylsulfoxide. Proc Natl Acad Sci USA 1971;68:378–382.

115. Sekiya S, Kimura H, Yamazawa K, et al. Induction of human embryonal carcinoma cell differentiation using N,N′-hexamethylene bisacetamide in vitro. Gynecol Oncol 1990;36:69–78.

116. Reuben RC, Rifkind RA, Marks PA. Chemically induced murine erythroleukemic differentiation. Biochim Biophys Acta 1980;605:325–346.

117. Marks PA, Sheffery M, Rifkind RA. Induction of transformed cells to terminal differentiation and the modulation of gene expression. Cancer Res 1987;47:659–666.

118. Melloni E, Pontremoli S, Michetti M, et al. Protein kinase C activity and hexamethy-lenebisacetamide-induced erythroleukemia cell differentiation. Proc Natl Acad Sci USA 1987;84:5282–5286.

119. Melloni E, Pontremoli S, Sparatore B, et al. Introduction of the β-isoenzyme of protein kinase C accelerates induced differentiation of murine erythroleukemia cells. Proc Natl Acad Sci USA 1990;87:4417–4420.

120. Yamashita T, Eto Y, Shibai H, et al. Synergistic action of activin A and hexamethylene bisacetamide in differentiation of murine erythroleukemia cells. Cancer Res 1990;50: 3182–3185.

121. Schroy P, Rifkin J, Coffey RJ, et al. Role of transforming growth factor β_1 in induction of colon carcinoma differentiation by hexamethylene bisacetamide. Cancer Res 1990;50: 261–265.

122. Hafez MM, Infante D, Winawer S, et al. Transforming growth factor β_1 acts as an autocrine-negative growth regulator in colon enterocytic differentiation but not in goblet cell maturation. Cell Growth Different 1990;1:617–626.

123. Egorin MJ, Sigman LM, Van Echo DA, et al. Phase I clinical and pharmacokinetic study of hexamethylene bisacetamide (NSC 95580) administered as a five-day continuous infusion. Cancer Res 1987;47:617–523.

124. Rowinsky EK, Ettinger DS, Grochow LB, et al. Phase I and pharmacologic study of hexamethylene bisacetamide in patients with advanced cancer. J Clin Oncol 1986;4: 1835–1844.

125. Young CW, Fanucchi MP, Walsh TD, et al. Phase I trial and clinical pharmacological evaluation of hexamethylene bisacetamide administration by ten-day continuous intravenous infusion at twenty-eight-day intervals. Cancer Res 1988;48:7304–7309.

126. Egorin MJ, Zuhowski EG, Cohen AS, et al. Plasma pharmacokinetics and urinary excretion of hexamethylene bisacetamide metabolites. Cancer Res 1987;47:6142–6146.

127. Ward FT, Kelley JA, Roth JS, et al. A phase I bioavailability and pharmacokinetic

study of hexamethylene bisacetamide (NSC 95580) administered via nasogastric tube. Cancer Res 1991;51:1803–1810.

128. Rowinsky EK, Conley BA, Jones RJ, et al. Efficacy of hexamethylene bisacetamide in myelodysplastic syndromes: 5-Day exposure to maximal levels. Proc Am Assoc Cancer Res 1990;31:190.

129. Andreeff M, Stone R, Young C, et al. Treatment of myelodysplastic syndromes and acute myeloid leukemia with hexamethylene bisacetamide. Blood 1990;76(suppl 1): 251a.

130. Snyder SW, Egorin MJ, Geelhaar LA, et al. Induction of differentiation of human promyelocytic leukemia cells (HL60) by metabolites of hexamethylene bisacetamide. Cancer Res 1988;48:3613–3616.

131. Subramanyam B, Callery PS, Egorin MJ, et al. An active, aldehydic metabolite of the cell-differentiating agent hexamethylene bisacetamide. Drug Metab Dis 1989;17:398–401.

132. Russo P, Sheinfeld J, Cordon-Cardo C, et al. Changes in phenotype and growth induced by hexamethylene bisacetamide and *cis*-retinoic acid in human urothelial carcinoma cells obtained from bladder washings. Surg Forum 1990;38:685–688.

133. Breslow R, Jursic B, Yan ZF, et al. Potent cytodifferentiating agents related to hexamethylenebisacetamide. Proc Natl Acad Sci USA 1991;88:5542–5546.

134. Olsson IL, Breitman TR. Induction of differentiation of the human histiocytic lymphoma cell line U-937 by retinoic acid and cyclic adenosine 3',5'-monophosphate-inducing agents. Cancer Res 1982;42:3924–3927.

135. Fontana J, Munoz M, Durham J. Potentiation between intracellular cyclic-AMP-elevating agents and inducers of leukemic cell differentiation. Leuk Res 1985;9:1127–1132.

136. Strickland S, Smith KK, Marotti KR. Hormonal induction of differentiation in teratocarcinoma stem cells: Generation of parietal endoderm by retinoic acid and dibutyryl cAMP. Cell 1980;21:347–355.

137. Lando M, Abemayor E, Verity MA, et al. Modulation of intracellular cyclic adenosine monophosphate levels and the differentiation response of human neuroblastoma cells. Cancer Res 1990;50:722–727.

138. Cho-Chung YS. Role of cyclic AMP receptor proteins in growth, differentiation, and suppression of malignancy: New approaches to therapy. Cancer Res 1990;50:7093–7100.

139. Tagliaferri P, Katsaros D, Clair T, et al. Synergistic inhibition of growth of breast and colon human cancer cell lines by site-selective cyclic AMP analogues. Cancer Res 1988;48:1642–1650.

140. Breitman TR, He R. Combinations of retinoic acid with either sodium butyrate, dimethyl sulfoxide, or hexamethylene bisacetamide synergistically induce differentiation of the human myeloid leukemia cell line HL60. Cancer Res 1990;50:6268–6273.

SECTION **5**

C.A. STEIN

Antisense Inhibition of Gene Expression

HISTORICAL BACKGROUND

Antisense oligodeoxynucleotides are short fragments of DNA, usually 15 nucleotide bases or longer. The term "antisense" refers to the fact that these molecules are complementary to the "sense" strand of mRNA. Due to Watson-Crick base pairing, antisense oligodeoxynucleotides form DNA-mRNA duplexes in an antiparallel fashion. In theory, this process can inhibit the function of the mRNA, which normally is translated into protein in the cytoplasm by the ribosome. If the protein in question is vital for cellular or viral growth and reproduction, inhibition of its synthesis by antisense oligodeoxynucleotides could lead to a diminution in cellular or viral viability. The use of oligodeoxynucleotides as antisense inhibitors of gene expression holds forth the promise of a specific, genetically based therapeutic approach.

There are two other antisense approaches to inhibition of gene expression that are being actively investigated. The first is antisense RNA. For example, a plasmid expressing the *MYC* gene cloned in the antisense orientation produces *MYC*-encoded mRNA, also with the antisense orientation.[1] The RNA-RNA hybrids formed may result by several different mechanisms in inhibition of *MYC* mRNA translation into protein. However, because this method is not currently at a stage of therapeutic consideration, it is not covered in this chapter. An additional antisense approach is provided by the ribozyme, an oligoribonucleotide that catalyzes the specific scission of a complementary mRNA strand.[2–4] Their development as therapeutic agents, while of potentially great interest, is behind that of oligodeoxynucleotides.

Since the commercialization of the oligomer synthetic process in the mid-1980s, the relative ease of availability of these materials has led to wide variety of antisense experiments in various test systems, many successful, others not. There are also many reviews on the subject.[5–18]

CLASSES OF OLIGODEOXYNUCLEOTIDES

In the quest for nuclease-resistant oligomers, many modifications to the structure of normal or phosphodiester (PO) DNA (Fig. 69-19) have been made. Some of these are briefly described in the following sections.

METHYLPHOSPHONATE OLIGOMERS

The biochemistry and biologic effects of these materials have been reviewed by Miller and colleagues.[19] As shown in Figure 69–19, they possess four different substituents at each phosphorus atom, a property known as chirality; lack ionizable groups; and are uncharged. This can lead to solubility problems at long chain length that may be overcome by including, for example, a single PO residue at the 5' end. Methylphosphonate oligomers have significant antiviral activity, especially against

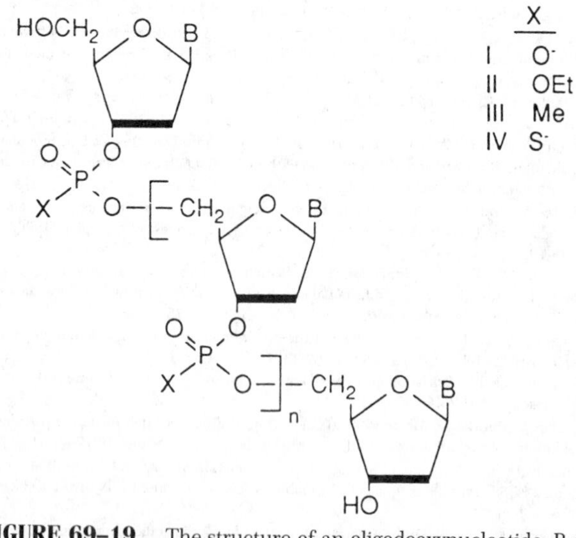

FIGURE 69–19. The structure of an oligodeoxynucleotide. B represents the nucleotide bases adenine, cytosine, guanine, or thymine. When X = O, the structure is that of a phosphodiester (PO) or normal oligodeoxynucleotide. When X = methyl (Me), methylphosphonate; X = S, phosphorothioate (PS) oligodeoxynucleotide. (Stein CA, Cohen J. Oligodeoxynucleotides as inhibitors of gene expression: A review. Cancer Res 1988;48:2659–2668)

vesicular stomatitis virus and human immunodeficiency virus-1 (HIV-1), but they do not elicit RNase H activity.[20,21]

PHOSPHOROTHIOATE OLIGOMERS

The subject of phosphorothioate oligomers has been reviewed elsewhere.[22,23] The compounds (see Fig. 69–19) were first synthesized by Stec and coworkers.[24] The charge and solubility are retained, but hybridizability with complementary mRNA is poorer than that of the PO oligomers. Phosphorothioate (PS) oligomers are nuclease resistant and have been shown to be sequence-specific inhibitors of HIV-1 and herpes simplex virus (HSV) replication.[25–28] However, they also have several nonsequence specific effects on HIV-1 replication, including competitive inhibition of the viral reverse transcriptase with respect to template primer binding and binding to cell surface CD4 and interference with the binding of the HIV-1 envelope glycoprotein gp120, a ligand for CD4.[29,30] These compounds are also chiral.

INTERACTIONS OF OLIGONUCLEOTIDES WITH CELLS

Many classes of oligonucleotides are polyanions. Because of their charge, it had been supposed that they could not readily pass through cell membranes. However, the existence of cell-surface DNA has been recognized for several years. Bennett and associates discovered a 30-kd protein on the surface of peripheral blood lymphocytes that binds double stranded DNA.[31] Lymphocytes that bear this membrane protein can cap the bound DNA over a period of 30 to 45 minutes, with internalization occurring within 2 hours.[31,32] The DNA receptor protein, however, does not seem to bind oligodeoxynucleotides. Loke and colleagues demonstrated that cellular association of oligomer could be inhibited by other phosphodiester homopolymers and phosphorothioate oligomers, but not by heparin, ribose-5-phosphate, or uncharged thymidine methylphosphonate oligomers.[33] They isolated an 80-kd cell-surface protein that appeared to be responsible for specific oligomer binding to HL60 cells. Yakubov and coworkers found two cell-surface oligomer binding proteins (79 kd and 90 kd).[34] Gasparro and associates identified three high-affinity double-stranded DNA-binding proteins on the surface of human peripheral blood lymphocytes.[35] These included a 28-kd species, a 79-kd species, and a protein of approximately 59 kd. The researchers did not comment on the role that any of these proteins might have with respect to internalization of cell-surface DNA.

Stein and colleagues demonstrated by flow cytometric analysis in HL60 cells that the Michaelis Constant (K_m) of a 5'-fluorescein (F)-labeled phosphodiester 15-mer homopolymer of thymidine from the cell surface is 22 nM.[36] It has also been shown in HL60 cells that there is only one unique site on the cell surface that binds oligonucleotides. A phosphorothioate 28-mer homopolymer of cytidine, known as SdC28, is a competitor of oligomer binding, and has a $K_c \sim 3$ nM. Cell membrane-bound fluorescence can be seen to cluster on the cell surface and the specific binding of oligomers to HL60 cells is calcium dependent. Cell surface-bound oligonucleotide appears to be nuclease resistant.[37] However, most oligomer in-

ternalization appears to be consequent to pinocytosis or fluid-phase endocytosis. This is a process in which the cell entraps and internalizes external liquid that contains dissolved solute (*e.g.*, oligonucleotide). It is mechanically similar to the process of receptor mediated endocytosis, although no specific receptors are present. It is likely that a smaller percentage of oligomer internalization may be accounted for by adsorptive endocytosis. In HL60 cells, we have shown that the pinocytosis rate is under the control of protein kinase C, a major signal transduction protein.

Several strategies, mostly relying on 5' modification, have been employed to increase the cellular internalization of oligonucleotides. Investigators have linked poly-L-lysine (which is internalized by pinocytosis) to the 5' terminus of an oligomer complementary to vesicular stomatitis virus or HIV mRNA sequences. Enhanced antiviral activity was observed.[38–41] Oligomers modified with a 5' cholesteryl or lipid residue increase intracellular internalization, and the cholesteryl modification renders homopolymeric PS oligomers more potent HIV inhibitors than the unmodified parent. These effects may relate to the ability of 5'-cholesteryl oligomers to bind to low-density lipoprotein (LDL) and to be at least partially internalized by the LDL receptor.[42–46] However, the detergent properties of these molecules may contribute to nonspecific cellular cytotoxicity. A phosphorothioate oligomer complementary to an *MYC*-encoded mRNA sequence has been liposome encapsulated and shown to reduce levels of MYC protein in HL60 cells after fusion.[47]

After a phosphodiester oligonucleotide is internalized in a cell, it is vulnerable to nuclease digestion by cellular DNAses. For example, in microinjected *Xenopus* oocytes, an unmodified 17-mer was degraded with a half-life of only about 10 minutes.[48] In *Xenopus* embryos and in human plasma ($T_{\frac{1}{2}}$ = 7.7 minutes), this process occurred primarily because of 3' exonuclease activity, and is vitiated by heat inactivation.[49–51] Some label originating from intracellularly digested oligomer (as nucleotide 5' triphosphate) may be incorporated into the de novo synthesis of genomic DNA, but relatively long oligomers may be expelled from the cell by the process of exocytosis.[52] On the other hand, oligonucleotides that have been microinjected into cells seem to be quickly translocated to the nucleus.[53,54] This is unlike the behavior observed when fluorescent oligomers are allowed to "passively diffuse" into cells. In this case, a perinuclear pattern of fluorescence with nuclear sparing has been observed.[36] Little is known about the intracellular organellar distribution of oligonucleotides.

PHARMACOLOGY OF OLIGODEOXYNUCLEOTIDES

Relatively little information exists about the pharmacology of oligodeoxynucleotides because of the difficulties and cost involved in large-scale oligonucleotide synthesis. Preliminary studies with a methylphosphonate oligomer (8-mer) targeted to the splice acceptor junction of the HSV-1 immediate early mRNA 4 and 5 have shown efficacy in preventing the development of herpetic lesions when applied to the ear skin of a mouse.[9] The oligomer was distributed to all tissues except the brain, although other investigators, using ^{14}C-labeled methylphosphonates complementary to rat insulin mRNA, found accumulation preferentially in the brain, followed by kidney, lung, heart, and muscle.[55] Organ accumulation was sequence independent. As much as 99% of a 12-mer methylphosphonate oligomer may be eliminated in the urine within one hour.[56]

Iverson and coworkers studied the pharmacokinetics of a single injection of phosphorothioates of different lengths in rats.[57] Included was a 27-mer complementary to the HIV-1 rev sequence used by Matsukura and associates.[27,28] The plasma concentration of oligomer versus time could be fitted to a two-compartment model. Peak plasma levels were achieved in 10 to 20 minutes after intravenous injection and at 90 minutes after intraperitoneal injection. Little of the compound was associated with formed blood elements. The initial distribution half-time, representing distribution out of the plasma ($t_{1/2}\alpha$, intravenous administration) was 23 ± 3 minutes, and the actual half-time, representing total body elimination ($t_{1/2}\beta$) was 33.9 hours. Similar values were determined for an intraperitoneal injection approach. The plasma clearance of oligomer was not affected by length (*e.g.*, 21-, 27-, and 40-mer) or base composition. The researchers suggest that the long elimination half-time can lead to infrequent repetitive dosing to maintain therapeutically effective tissue concentrations.

Oligomer, within 3 hours, was found to appear in liver, fat, and muscle. Within 12 hours, the liver contained over 40% of the administered dose. About 5% of the dose accumulated in the kidney. After 12 hours, less than 1% of the injected dose remained circulating in the plasma, compared with the 58% that was tissue associated. Approximately one third of a 100 μg-dose of oligomer was recovered in the urine within 24 hours of injection and virtually all of it, as the parent compound, within 3 days. Fecal excretion was minimal. Toxicity included a twofold to sixfold rise in lactate dehydrogenase, peaking at 24 hours and normalizing within 3 days. Smaller increases in serum glutamic oxalacetic transaminase (SGOT) and serum glutamic pyruvic transaminase (SGPT) were seen.

MECHANISM OF THE ANTISENSE EFFECT

After internalization, and presumably after liberation from an endosomal compartment, sequence-specific oligomers can bind to their complement, forming an RNA-DNA hybrid. RNAse H is a virtually ubiquitous cytoplasmic enzyme that cleaves the RNA strand of an RNA-DNA duplex, and it is this activity, rather than translation inhibition, that may account for most antisense effects.[58] RNAse H activity can be elicited when the DNA strand is phosphodiester. This activity is also present when the DNA strand is phosphorothioate, but it is absent with methylphosphonate oligomers.[25,59] If a sample of the cell-free reticulocyte lysate translation system, which is poor in RNAse H activity, is doped with exogenously added RNAse H, translation into protein of an added mRNA proceeds poorly in the presence of a complementary 17-mer oligomer.[60] Antisense activity is also diminished in reticulocyte lysate if a competitive inhibitor of RNAse H activity (poly(rA)-oligo dT) is added.[61] Because the cleavage of mRNA by RNAse H is irreversible and should lead to dissociation of the oligomer from its target, the process of RNase H cleavage of mRNA is catalytic with respect to oligomer. After enzymatic cleavage, the mRNA appears to be rapidly degraded and usually cannot

support translation. In one report of a cell-free translation system, incubation of rabbit globin mRNA with oligomers complementary to β-globin led to loss of the intact message and the appearance of RNA fragments.[62,63] The size of these mRNA pieces corresponded to cleavage occurring at binding sites complementary to the oligomer. However, in intact cell systems, mRNA fragments are rarely observed. Successful sequence specific antisense experiments have been performed with nuclease-resistant methylphosphonate oligomers, which are not substrates for RNAse H activity. Translation arrest in this case must occur through another, yet unknown mechanism.

The location of the best targets for antisense oligonucleotides has been discussed by several researchers.[14,64] In a cell free translation system, the best inhibition results from targeting of the 5' cap or the initiation codon (AUG) regions of the globin message molecule. In contrast, in HL60 cells, the 5' cap region of the *MYC* message, which is thought to occur as a stem and bulge region, was a significantly better target than the initiation codon region.[65] The first splice junction site was about as effective a target as the initiation codon region. Effectiveness was dependent on oligomer length, with an 18-mer complementary to the initiation codon region being twice as effective as a 15-mer and a 12-mer only 25% as effective. Daaka and colleagues targeted the 5' cap region of the *HRAS* message, as expressed in NIH3T3 fibroblasts.[37] Other regions targeted included a region upstream of the initiation codon, and the initiation codon region. Cells were treated with 25 or 50 μM oligomer, and dose-dependent decreases in the amount of p21 HRAS protein were observed. All three oligomers were effective, but the most effective oligomer was the one targeted to the 5' cap region. Other workers constructed PO oligomers complementary to regions on the HIV-1 mRNA.[66] Greatest efficacy, as assessed by ability to inhibit HIV-1 induced syncytia formation and to diminish viral p24 GAG protein production, was found for an oligomer complementary to the polyadenylation signal region (*i.e.*, 5' to the mRNA poly A tail). This was followed by oligomers targeted to the 5' cap and untranslated regions. The internal *TAT* splice acceptor site and the splice acceptor site upstream of the *ENV* initiator were also good targets. On the basis of currently available information, it is clear that there is no general rule about the preferred target site.

SEQUENCE-SPECIFIC ANTISENSE INHIBITION OF GENETIC EXPRESSION

HEMATOPOIETIC CELL LINES

MYC

The initial work with antisense *MYC* constructs was performed in peripheral blood lymphocytes by Heikkila and coworkers.[67] The oligomer was a 15-mer complementary to the first five codons of the human *MYC*-encoded mRNA and included the initiation codon. A single addition of the oligomer (30 μM) blocked the increase in MYC protein production after mitogen (*e.g.*, phytohemagglutinin) stimulation. The effect persisted for 24 hours, and treatment with noncomplementary oligomers was ineffective. The treatment with antisense oligomer and concomitant decrease in MYC protein levels led to cell cycle blockade at the G_1/S interface, but did not block cell cycle traversal from G_0 to G_1. Treatment was associated with a dramatic decrease in the mitotic index. Similar results, including blockade of entry into S phase, were found in human T lymphocytes, in which an anti-MYC phosphodiester oligomer blocked the proliferative response to interleukin-2 (IL-2).[68] The identical 15-mer was used by Wickstrom and associates in HL60 cells to inhibit MYC translation.[69] In this cell line, the *MYC* gene is amplified as much as 30-fold and is expressed in large quantities. A significant reduction in MYC protein levels at a concentration of 10 μM was observed. The antisense oligomer decreased proliferation by 50% at 4 μM.

Holt and colleagues, using HL60 cells, employed oligomers complementary to the 5' initiation codon region, but the sequences were different than those cited previously.[70] Evidence was found for the formation of an RNA-DNA duplex that was S1 nuclease resistant, and the antisense oligomer could inhibit MYC translation by 50% to 90% at 4 μM. The growth rate of the cells was decreased by 50% over the 5-day experiment, and some of the cells underwent myeloid differentiation. No accumulation of cells in any one phase of the cell cycle was observed.

Other experiments with HL60 cells have produced very different results. Loke and coworkers found that a 50 μM concentration of antisense oligomer was required to decrease intracellular MYC protein to 30% of control; this decrease took place over a 24-hour period.[47] An identical phosphorothioate oligomer was ineffective at reducing intracellular MYC protein levels. However, the PO and PS antisense, but not sense oligomers, when encapsulated in liposomes, could inhibit MYC protein expression within several hours after fusion, but the effect was transient. Other experiments using HL60 cells revealed little inhibition after incubation with an antisense MYC oligomer, even if it was dosed daily.[71] There was, however, a decrease in ability to form colonies in soft agar, and an increase in nitroblue tetrazolium and sudan black staining, indicating at least partial, intermediate granulocytic differentiation.

When the 15-mer anti MYC oligomer was linked to poly-L-lysine and complexed with heparin, 50% inhibition of the growth of L929 cells was achieved at 1 μM.[72] This was associated with a decrease in MYC protein expression and in MYC mRNA levels, although no degraded RNA products could be detected. A 21-mer oligomer, targeted to the aberrantly transcribed first intron of *MYC*, inhibited growth of several Burkitt's lymphoma cell lines in culture.[73] Such transcripts are not found in normal cells nor in the Burkitt's cell line KK124, in which the oligomer had no effect. Levels of MYC protein were decreased after 48 hours. Experiments of this type demonstrate the attractive therapeutic potential of oligodeoxynucleotides, because, theoretically, translation of the normal MYC transcripts were unaffected.

In an in vitro system, transcription of *MYC* could be suppressed by a 27-mer targeting 115 base pairs upstream from

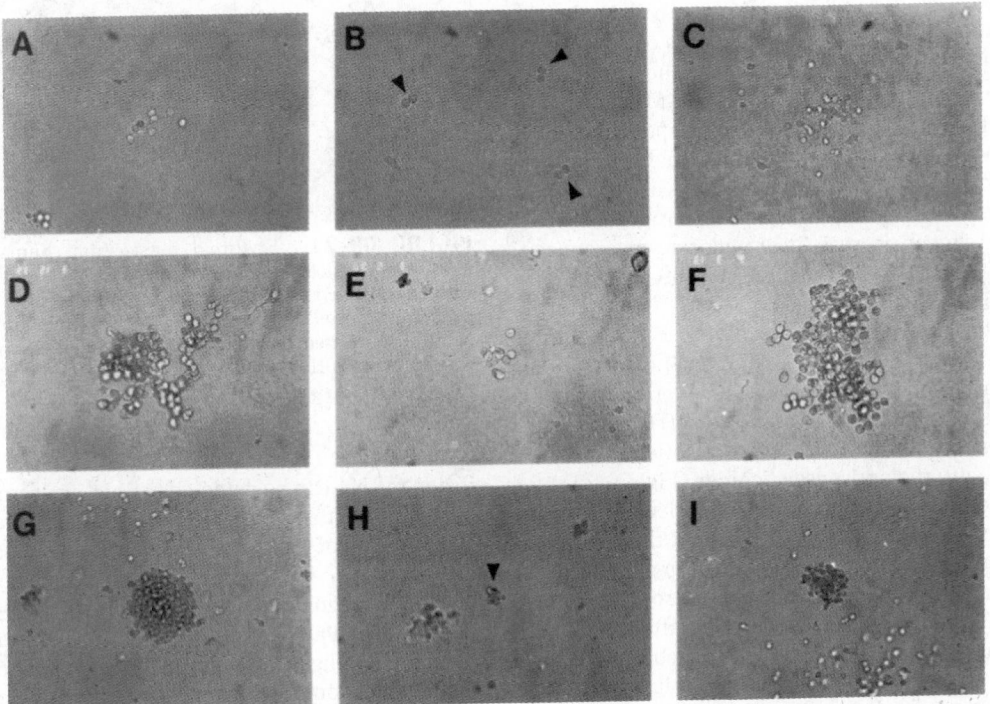

FIGURE 69–20.   Development of human hematopoietic colonies cloned in plasma clot culture from normal bone marrow cells in the presence of oligonucleotides. **(A–F)** CFU-GM-derived colonies; **(G–I)** CFU-E-derived colonies. GM colony development after 4 days of exposure to c-*MYB* sense, C-*MYB* antisense, or myeloperoxidase antisense PO oligonucleotides is depicted in **A, B,** and **C,** respectively. Arrows in **B** point to cell doublets. GM colony development after 12 days of exposure to c-*MYB* sense, c-*MYB* antisense, or myeloperoxidase antisense PO oligomers is shown in **D, E,** and **F,** respectively. Erythroid colony development after 7 days of exposure to c-*MYB* sense, c-*MYB* antisense, or coagulation factor V antisense PO oligomers is shown in **G, H** (*arrow*), and **I,** respectively. (Gewirtz A, Calabretta B. A c-*myb* antisense oligodeoxynucleotide inhibits normal human hematopoiesis in vitro. Science 1988;242:1303–1306)

the transcription origination site.[74] This is presumably due to the formation of a DNA triple helix. The oligomer can insert itself into the major groove of a Watson-Crick double helix. Binding of the oligomer to the double helix is a consequence of so-called Hoogsteen base pairing and is stable, in the presence of divalent cations, for CG . . . C and TA . . . T triplets. It is unclear to what extent triple helix formation is a process that can occur in vivo.

MYB

The protein product of this protooncogene appears to play a role in the maintenance of the dedifferentiated phenotype in hematopoietic cells. The 18-mer PO oligomers targeted to the 5′ regions of the *MYB*-encoded mRNA were effective at suppressing the growth of HL60 cells after 5 days in culture.[75] An oligomer with a two-base mismatch was only slightly effective. Measurement of DNA content revealed that most cells were in the G_1 phase of the cell cycle. This finding is similar to that after antisense inhibition of *MYC*. However, no phenotypic differentiation was observed after treatment. In peripheral blood T lymphocytes, incubation with the 18-mer led to decreased proliferation after phytohemagglutinin stimulation.[76] Intranuclear expression of MYB protein decreased with the 18 mer PO oligomer, and with a 15-mer and the 18-mer, cells were also blocked at the G_1/S interface.[77] *MYB*-encoded mRNA detected by the polymerase chain reaction (PCR) was markedly diminished after 12 hours of treatment with antisense oligomer.[78] Antisense inhibition of *MYB* translation was also accompanied by decreases in cellular levels of DNA polymerase-α and PCNA mRNAs, both of whose protein products play a role in de novo DNA synthesis.[79]

One problem with the eventual use of an anti-MYB oligomer in clinical practice in, for example, the extracorporeal purging of autologous bone marrow, is that the normal function of *MYB* is compromised. For example, in cultures of normal human bone marrow, incubation with the 18-mer antisense PO oligomer caused a mean decrease in granulocyte-macrophage colony-forming units (CFU-GM) of 68% (Fig. 69-20), in CFU-E of 67% (Fig. 69-21), and in CFU-Meg of 76%.[80] The number of cells per colony was also dramatically reduced. CFU-CM colonies, even in the presence of GM-CSF or IL-3, and CFU-G colonies, even in the presence of G-CSF, were reduced in number of cells per colony after antisense *MYB* treatment. Levels of *MYB*-encoded mRNA were also dramatically reduced after treatment with the antisense oligomer (Fig. 69-22).

It has been demonstrated that normal and leukemic cells exhibit differential sensitivity to the effects of the antisense oligomer.[81] In mixed cultures of blast cells from patients with acute myelogenous leukemia and normal marrow elements, only the normal elements could be detected after antisense treatment. If this treatment is generally applicable to the leukemic marrow, and can be shown to effect a high cell kill, it may become therapeutically attractive.

BCL2

The *BCL2* gene plays a role in the survival and growth of normal lymphoid cells. It is also implicated in the t(14:18) translocation that is found in most cases of follicular lymphoma, in which high levels of *BCL2*-encoded mRNA is found. In 65% to 75% of these cases, a novel BCL2/immunoglobulin

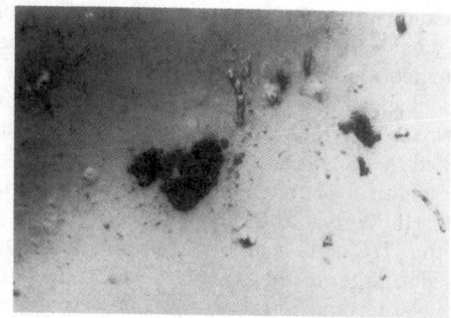
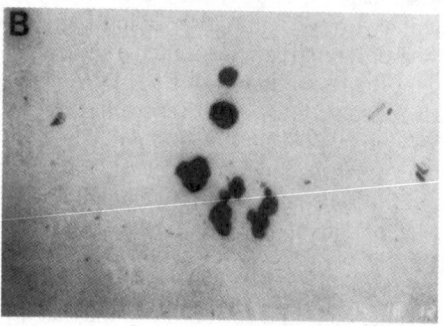
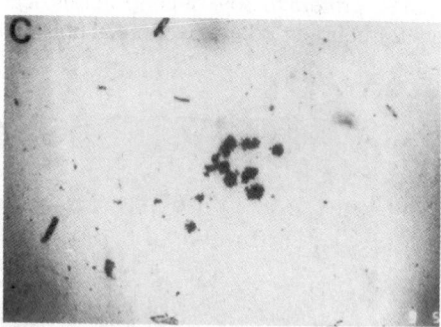

FIGURE 69–21. Erythroid bursts from human bone marrow MY10⁺ mononuclear cells. **(A)** Control. **(B)** Colonies after treatment with a c-*MYB* sense PO oligomer. **(C)** Colonies after treatment with a c-*MYB* antisense PO oligomer. (Caracciolo D, Venturelli D, Valtieri M, et al. Stage-related proliferative activity determines c-*myb* functional requirements during normal hematopoiesis. J Clin Invest 1990;85:55–61)

fusion mRNA can be detected.[82] Reed and associates used 20-mer PO and PS oligomers complementary to the initiation codon region of the human BCL2 mRNA.[83] Both inhibited the growth of 697 leukemia cells in a dose dependent fashion, but the PS oligomer was more potent (Fig. 69-23). However, although the PO oligomer inhibited proliferation after 2 to 3 days, the PS oligomer required 3 to 6 days for maximal effect. A concentration-dependent decrease in BCL2 protein expression (Fig. 69-24) was also observed (75–95%, PO oligo, 150 μM, 4 days: 70% PS oligomer, 25 μM). Cellular viabilities rapidly declined after 3 days of treatment (PO and PS oligomers), which was attributed to the role of *BCL2* in promoting lymphoid survival. These results highlight some of the similarities and differences between PO and PS oligomers with respect to their biologic interactions. However, the *BCL2* gene appears to be an excellent target for the purging of autologous bone marrow in patients with follicular lymphoma.

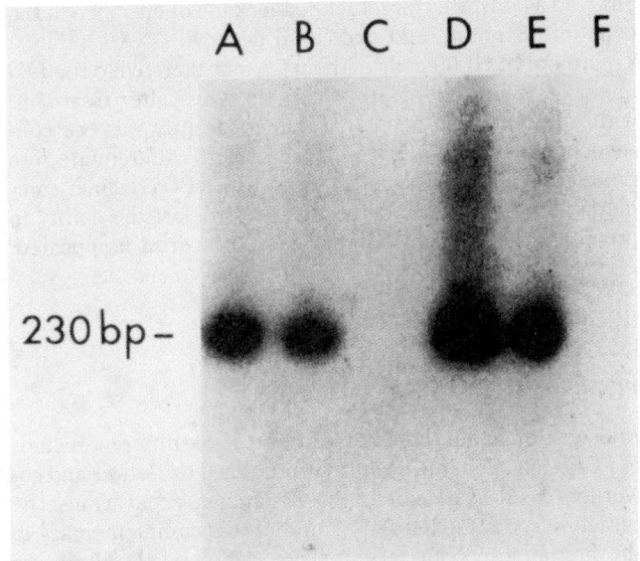

FIGURE 69–22. Expression of c-*MYB* mRNA in bone marrow progenitors cultured in the presence of c-myb oligomers. MY10⁺ mononuclear cells are shown in lanes A–C. Mononuclear cells depleted of adherent phagocytic cells and T lymphocytes are shown in lanes D–F. Control lanes (no oligomer) are A and D. mRNA from cells incubated with c-*MYB* sense is in lanes B and E. mRNA from cells incubated with c-*MYB* antisense is in lanes C and F. C-*MYB* mRNA was amplified by the polymerase chain reaction and detected by a radiolabeled 50-mer spanning the nucleotide region 2351 to 2400. (Caracciolo D, Venturelli D, Valtieri M, et al. Stage-related proliferative activity determines c-*myb* functional requirements during normal hematopoiesis. J Clin Invest 1990;85:55–61)

CSF1R and CSF1

Differentiation of HL60 cells into macrophages, induced by phorbol esters or 1,25-dihydroxy vitamin D₃, is associated with increased transcription of the *CSF1R* (formerly called FMS) message, which codes for the CSF1 receptor.[84,85] Treatment with an antisense PO oligomer complementary to the *CSF1R*-encoded mRNA inhibited macrophage formation induced by phorbol ester, but not by 1,25-dihydroxy vitamin D₃. Granulocytic differentiation induced by DMSO was not affected. Similar results were obtained using oligomers targeted against the mRNA of CSF1. Synergistic inhibition of macrophage formation was suggested by combination of the two oligomers. In a murine cell line, a 15-mer PO oligomer targeted to the initiation codon region of the CSF1 mRNA (5 μM) reduced cell proliferation by 63% at 24 hours, and decreased membrane levels of CSF1 protein over a 3-hour period.[86] Inhibition of proliferation could be increased to 95% if an anti-CSF1 monoclonal antibody was added to the cell cultures.

Myeloblastin

This is a serine protease, initially described by Bories and colleagues in HL60 cells.[87] It is down regulated during differentiation of myeloblasts with DMSO or 1,25-dihydroxy vitamin D₃. Specific diminution of myeloblastin mRNA translation was accomplished by an 18-mer PO oligomer complementary to a sequence beginning at position 95 downstream of the initiation codon. Oligomer was added to the growing cells every 8 hours, and by 7 days, cells began to assume a differentiated phenotype. After 10 days, myeloblastin protein had also markedly decreased. By day 12, 80% of the cells exhibited the typical morphologic characteristics of monocytic differentiation, and few cells remained in S phase. The changes are virtually identical to what was seen after treatment of HL60 cells with phorbol esters, which are known to induce monocytic differentiation. Use of the antisense oligomer, in this case, has allowed the function of the myeloblastin protein to be ascertained, a task that otherwise would have been possible only with difficulty.

BCR-ABL

This fusion gene results from the translocation of the *ABL* protooncogene from chromosome 9 to the *BCR* (breakpoint cluster region) of chromosome 22.[88] Transcripts of this hybrid gene are found only in patients with hematologic neoplasms, predominately chronic myelogenous leukemia. After determination of the base sequence of the *BCR-ABL* junction region, a complementary 18-mer PO oligomer was constructed and added to cells derived from a patient with CML.[88] The number of colonies formed in soft agar in 10 days declined from 60% to 90%. An oligomer with a two-base mismatch was ineffective. The antisense oligomer did not affect clonogenic growth

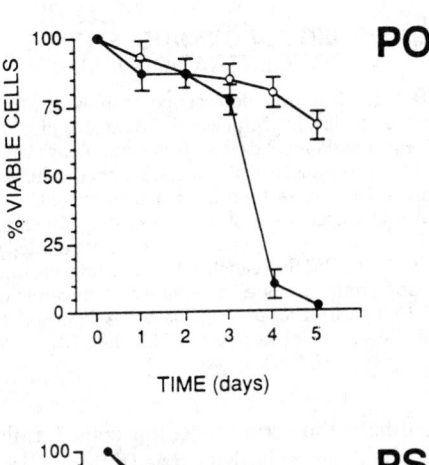

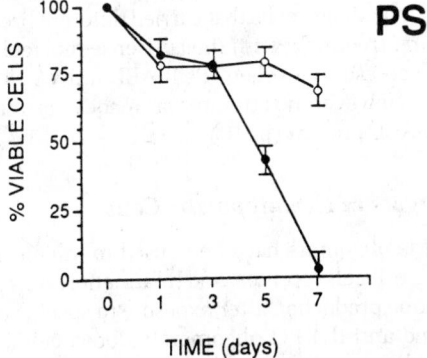

FIGURE 69–23. Influence of *BCL2* antisense oligonucleotides on the viability of 697 leukemia cells. The leukemia cells were cultured with PO and PS oligomers. The percentage of viable cells was determined by trypan blue dye exclusion. Open circles indicate sense oligomers, and closed circles indicate antisense oligomers. (Reed JC, Stein CA, Subasinghe C, et al. Antisense-mediated inhibition of BCL2 protooncogene expression and leukemic cell growth and survival: Comparisons of phosphodiester and phosphothioate oligodeoxynucleotides. Cancer Res 1990;50:6565–6570)

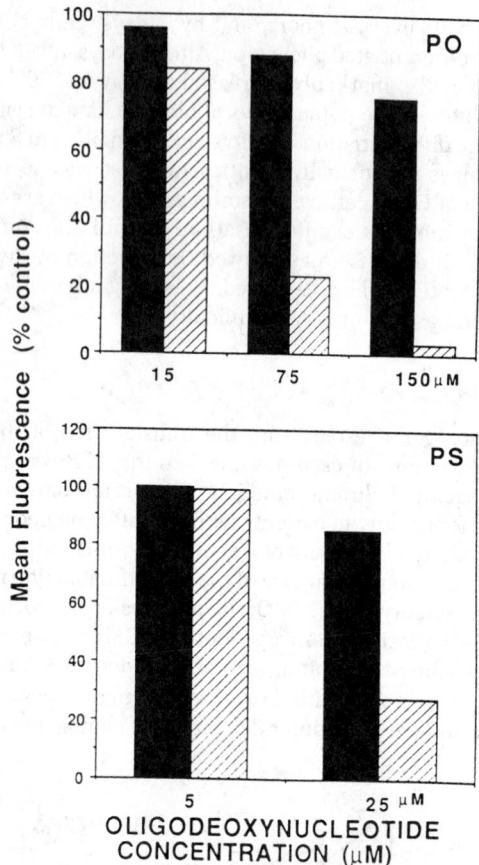

FIGURE 69–24. Immunofluorescence analysis of *BCL2*-encoded protein levels after oligodeoxynucleotide treatment of 697 leukemia cells. Cells were treated for 2 days with PO and 4 days with PS oligomers. Black columns are sense oligomers, hatched columns are antisense oligomers. Cells were then labeled with anti-*BCL2* antiserum and analyzed by fluorescence-activated cell sorting. Data are expressed as percent of mean fluorescence relative to cells not treated with oligomer. (Reed JC, Stein CA, Subasinghe C, et al. Antisense-mediated inhibition of *BCL2* protooncogene expression and leukemic cell growth and survival: Comparisons of phosphodiester and phosphothioate oligodeoxynucleotides. Cancer Res 1990;50:6565–6570)

from normal hematopoietic progenitor cells. Similar results were found in patients' cells that carried different breakpoints. Furthermore, treatment with the antisense molecule led to a dramatic decrease in levels of BCR-ABL mRNA as detected by RT-PCR. However, no attempt was made to quantitate levels of BCR-ABL protein (p210).

Other Targets in Hematopoietic Cells

PO antisense oligomers have been used to inhibit the α and β genes of the T-cell receptor, and treatment results in failure of lymphokine production after exposure to specific antigen.[89] Anti-IL2 and anti-IL4 PO oligomers reduced cellular proliferation and levels of lymphokine message in two different T-cell lines, and a PO oligomer targeted to the growth hormone mRNA reduced secreted immunoreactive growth hormone levels and the cellular proliferation of rat lymphocytes.[90,91] The gene *CDC2*, which codes for a p34 serine-threonine protein kinase, increases in expression as cells traverse the cell cycle after G_1.[92] Treatment of T cells with a PO oligomer

directed against this target led to blockade of entrance of the cells into S phase, and decreased de novo DNA synthesis. Treatment of HL60 cells with an 18-mer targeted to the *FES* message caused cell death within 24 hours after treatment with differentiating agents.[77] This apparently was the consequence of the inability of these cells to differentiate into granulocytes. Myeloma cells treated with a PO oligomer complementary to the prothymosin-α mRNA lost the ability to proliferate for 24 hours.[93] By day 2, the effect had disappeared.

GROWTH REGULATORY TARGETS IN NONHEMATOPOIETIC CELLS

FGFB

Antisense oligomers complementary to three different regions of *FGFB*-encoded mRNA were synthesized by Becker and co-workers.[56] These included a PO oligomer directed against the initiation codon region (#1); another was complementary to the first splice donor-acceptor site (#2), and the third was complementary to the second splice donor-acceptor site at codons 94–95 (#3). WM75 cells, derived from a human melanoma in the vertical growth phase, when treated with a single dose (50 μM) of oligomer #2, were growth inhibited by 60% at day 8. When the metastatic melanoma line WM 983-B was treated with oligomer #3, similar growth inhibition was observed. The sense and five-base mismatched oligomers had no effect on proliferation. Competition experiments performed with sense oligomer in the presence of antisense oligomer revealed that the inhibition of growth was reversible within 48 hours. Treatment with the antisense oligomers reduced the ability of the melanoma cells to clone in soft agar.

Another source of FGFB is in neural tissue, particularly the brain. It has been suggested that this fibroblast growth factor may directly promote glial cell tumor growth directly or indirectly secondary to stimulation of angiogenesis.[94] PO 15-mer oligomers were synthesized and targeted, as previously described, to the initiation codon (#1) and first splice donor-acceptor regions (#2) of the FGFB mRNA. Incubation with oligomer #2 markedly reduced the growth rate of SNB-19 human glioma cells (25 μM). The effect was dose dependent and plateaued at higher concentrations. The sense strand had no effect on growth, and the antiproliferative effect was vitiated by addition of exogenous FGFB. Similar results were obtained after incubation with oligomer #1. This correlated with a 67% reduction in FGFB protein content and a 55% reduction in cell number, implying that the diminution in cell number was directly related to the inhibitory effects on FGFB mRNA translation by the oligomer. The proliferation of nontransformed astrocytes, prepared from temporal lobe biopsies, was not inhibited by either antisense oligomer. These results suggest the possibility of a local therapeutic strategy for high-grade human glioma, a uniformly fatal disease.

HRAS

The protein product of the *HRAS* gene is involved in signal transduction across cell membranes, and p21, the protein product of the *HRAS* oncogene, binds guanosine nucleotide phosphates, and possesses GTPase activity. Yu found that the most common pathway of *RAS* activation in human cancer involves a point mutation in the 12th or 61st amino acid codon of *HRAS*.[95] This mutation is found in a variety of radiation-induced and chemically induced tumors.

Brown and associates inserted the murine RAS p21 coding region into an RNA expression vector.[96] A methylphosphonate oligonucleotide was targeted to the first 11 nucleotides of the initiation codon region. When the in vitro run off mRNA transcripts were translated in cell-free systems in the presence of the antisense oligomer, a 59% inhibition of translation was observed at 25 μM. The effect was dose dependent and was maximal (virtually 100%) above 100 μM. Lower levels of inhibition were observed for oligomers with one- and two-base mismatches. Because methylphosphonate oligomers do not elicit RNAse H activity, it was proposed that the mechanism of the antisense effect depended on blocking the ribosome from interacting with the translation initiation site.[97] At no point was the morphology of the cells affected.

Yu and colleagues targeted methylphosphonate oligomers (8-mers) to the twelfth amino acid codon of a wild type and a mutant *HRAS*-encoded mRNA transcript.[95] The oligomers effectively inhibited translation in cell-free systems, and the translation inhibition was diminished in the presence of oligomers with one- or two-base mismatches. The exquisite sequence specificity was further demonstrated when the mutant HRAS transcript was used in the cell-free translation system. There was a single nucleotide change, from guanine to thymine, in the twelfth amino acid codon. At 200 μM, inhibition was most pronounced (84%) with the oligomer containing the single-base mismatch and somewhat less so (65%) with the oligomer complementary to the wild type gene. At 50 μM, only the exact complement of the mutated HRAS message produced any inhibition whatsoever in the cell-free translation system. Experiments of this type suggest an important role for antisense oligomers in which the transcripts from normal and mutant alleles must be discriminated and highlights novel potential therapies if these results can be applied in cellular or tissue systems.

MYCN

The 15-mer PO oligomers were synthesized as targets to the initiation codon of the *MYCN*-encoded mRNA in the CHP 100 neuroepithelial cell line.[98] CHP 100 cells contain only one copy of the *MYCN* gene. Diminished cellular staining for MYCN protein was observed after 16 hours of exposure to 100 μM oligomer. The sense oligomer was ineffective at reducing cellular MYCN protein levels, and no effects on *MYC* expression were seen. Cellular proliferation and DNA synthesis were also reduced by the antisense oligomer. Morphologically, there was a decrease in cellular heterogeneity, with an increase in the number of flat, epithelial-like cells (*i.e.*, S cells), which are contact inhibited, do not clone in soft agar, and are not tumorigenic in nude mice. The researchers suggested using implantable microinfusion pumps to study the effects of antisense oligomers when infused at a constant rate into nude mice.

Other Targets In Nonhematopoietic Cells

Cope and coworkers treated the malignant keratinocyte line SCC-25 with 15-mer PO oligomers complementary to the cellular retinol-binding protein 1 (cRBP) and to the human nuclear retinoic acid receptor-α (hnRARA).[99] At a concentration of 30 μM antisense cRBP, a 90% loss of retinol binding in the cytoplasm was observed over 16 hours. This oligomer had no effect on the binding of retinoic acid to hnRAR. When the cells were treated with the antisense hnRARA construct, nuclear binding of retinoic acid was blocked to a similar extent. These decreases in binding were shown to directly correlate with decreases in levels of the respective retinoid binding proteins. In cells treated with either oligomer, the typical retinol-dependent induction of alkaline phosphatase activity did not occur. Cells treated with the cRBP antisense construct rounded up, lost cell-cell attachments, and exhibited decreased adherence to the substratum. Sense oligomers had few if any biologic effects.

The colonic adenocarcinoma line, LoVo, and its doxorubicin-resistant subline, LoVo/Dx, overexpress the *MYB* oncogene.[100] The researchers treated the cells with 18-mer PO oligomers complementary to codons 2–7 of the MYB mRNA. The proliferative rate was markedly decreased, as was *MYB* expression.

Proliferating cell nuclear antigen (PCNA) is a nuclear protein that is a cofactor of DNA polymerase-δ. Jaskulski and colleagues prepared 18 mer PO oligomers extending from nucleotides 4–21 and 22–39 of the mouse PCNA mRNA.[101] The mitotic index of the cells treated with the antisense oligomer was decreased, and by 16 hours, no cells undergoing mitosis could be detected. These effects were even more striking when the oligomers were used individually and could be correlated with a decrease in levels of PCNA protein. After determination of the amount of DNA per cell, it was concluded that the cell cycle block must have occurred at the G_1/S boundary or early in the S phase.

The use of antisense oligomer to reverse the pleiotropic drug-resistant phenotype has been considered. Rivoltini and coworkers, using the LoVo cell line and its resistant sublines LoVo/H and LoVo/Dx, treated these cells with 15-mer PO oligomers complementary to the initiation codon region of the p170 mRNA (160 μM on day 1 and 80 μM on day 2).[102] After 3 days, cell-surface p170 was down-modulated, and in the LoVo/Dx cells, the MDR phenotype was reverted, with the cells becoming almost as sensitive to doxorubicin as after treatment with verapamil. Studies further investigating these intriguing observations should appear shortly.

Although the potential of specific genetic therapy is huge and theoretically within reach, in reality, daunting problems remain. Technically, foremost among these are the problems of scale and cost. Although it is soon likely that several grams of an antisense oligomer can be relatively easily synthesized, it is not clear that technology exists to cost effectively synthesize the at least 1 kg of material required for adequate phase I testing in humans. This problem is reflected in the relative paucity of pharmacokinetic and pharmacodynamic data referable to oligonucleotides. Nevertheless, the breathtaking progress in this field over a very short span of years and the ever increasing number of targets known to be susceptible to antisense inhibition of gene expression must be taken as an excellent harbinger of the eventual development of a novel, specific, antineoplastic therapy, which is in its earliest stages.

REFERENCES

1. Griep A, Westphal H. Antisense myc sequences induce differentiation of F9 cells. Proc Natl Acad Sci USA 1988;85:6806–6810
2. Cech T, Bass B. Biological catalysis of RNA. Ann Rev Biochem 1986;55:599–629.
3. Haseloff J, Gerlach W. Simple RNA enzymes with new and highly specific endoribonuclease activities. Nature 1988;334:585–591.
4. Sarver N, Cantin E, Chang P, et al. Ribozymes as potential anti-HIV-1 therapeutic agents. Science 1990;247:1222–1225.
5. Stein CA, Cohen J. Oligodeoxynucleotides as inhibitors of gene expression: A review. Cancer Res 1988;48:2659–2668.
6. Zon G. Oligonucleotide analogues as potential chemotherapeutic agents. Pharm Res 1988;5:539–549.
7. van der Krol AR, Mol JN, Stuije AR. Modulation of eukaryotic gene expression by complementary RNA or DNA sequences. Biotechniques 1988;6:958–976.
8. Marcus-Sekura C. Techniques for using antisense oligodeoxyribonucleotides to study gene expression. Analyt Biochem 1988;172:289–295.
9. Miller PS, Ts'o POP. A new approach to chemotherapy based on molecular biology and nucleic acid chemistry: Matagen (masking tape for gene expression). Anticancer Drug Des 1987;2:117–128.
10. Paoletti C. Anti-sense oligonucleotides as potential antitumour agents: Prospective views and preliminary results. Anticancer Drug Des 1988;2:325–331.
11. Goodchild J. Conjugates of oligonucleotides and modified oligonucleotides: A review of their synthesis and properties. Bioconjugate Chem 1990;1:165–183.
12. Tidd D. A potential role for antisense oligonucleotide analogues in the development of oncogene targeted cancer chemotherapy. Anticancer Res 1990;10:1169–1182.
13. Dolnick B. Antisense agents in pharmacology. Biochem Pharmacol 1990;40:671–675.
14. Helene C, Toulme JJ. Specific regulation of gene expression by antisense, sense and antigene nucleic acids. Biochim Biophys Acta 1990;1049:99–125.
15. Knorre D, Vlassov V. Antisense oligonucleotide derivatives as gene-targeted drugs. Biomed Sci (USSR) 1990;1:334–343.
16. Uhlmann E, Peyman A. Antisense oligonucleotides: A new therapeutic principle. Chem Rev 1990;90:543–584.
17. Calabretta B. Inhibition of protooncogene expression by antisense oligodeoxynucleotides: Biological and therapeutic implications. Cancer Res 1991;51:4505–4510.
18. Cohen J, ed. Oligodeoxynucleotides: Antisense inhibitors of gene expression. London: Macmillan, 1989.
19. Miller P. Non-ionic antisense oligonucleotides. In Cohen J, ed. Oligodeoxynucleotides: Antisense inhibitors of gene expression. London: Macmillan, 1989:79–95.
20. Agris C, Blake D, Miller P, et al. Inhibition of vesicular stomatitis virus protein synthesis and infection by sequence-specific oligodeoxyribonucleoside methylphosphonates. Biochemistry 1986;25:6268–6275.
21. Sarin P, Agrawal S, Civeira M, et al. Inhibition of acquired immunodeficiency syndrome virus by oligodeoxynucleoside methylphosphonates. Proc Natl Acad Sci USA 1988;85:7448–7451.
22. Stein C, Cohen J. Phosphorothioate oligodeoxynucleotide analogues. In Cohen J, ed. Oligodeoxynucleotides: Antisense inhibitors of gene expression. London: Macmillan, 1989:97–117.
23. Stein C, Tonkinson J, Yakubov, L. Phosphorothioate oligodeoxynucleotides. Pharmacol Ther 1991;52:365–384.
24. Stec W, Zon G, Egan T. Automated solid-phase synthesis, separation and stereochemistry of phosphorothioate analoges of oligodeoxyribonucleotides. J Am Chem Soc 1984;106:6077–6079.
25. Stein C, Subasinghe C, Morgan N, et al. Physicochemical properties of phosphorothioate oligodeoxynucleotides. Nucleic Acids Res 1988;16:3209–3221.
26. Matsukura M, Zon G, Shinozuka K, et al. Phosphorothioate oligodeoxynucleotides as inhibitors of the replication of HIV. Gene 1988;72:343–347.
27. Matsukura M, Zon G, Shinozuka K, et al. Regulation of viral expression of HIV in vitro by an antisense phosphorothioate oligodeoxynucleotide against rev in chronically infected cells. Proc Natl Acad Sci USA 1989;86:4244–4248.
28. Gao W, Hanes R, Vazquez-Padua M, et al. Inhibition of herpesvirus type 2 growth by phosphorothioate oligodeoxynucleotides. Antimicrob Agents Chemother 1990;34:808–821.
29. Majumdar C, Stein C, Cohen J, et al. HIV reverse transcriptase stepwise mechanism: Phosphorothioate oligodeoxynucleotide as primer. Biochemistry 1989;28:1340–1346.
30. Stein C, Pal R, Hoke G, et al. Phosphorothioate oligodeoxynucleotide interferes with binding of CD4 to gp 120. J Acquir Immune Defic Syndr 1991;4:686–693.
31. Bennett R, Gabor GT, Merritt M. DNA binding to human leukocytes: Evidence for a receptor-mediated association, internalization, and degradation of DNA. J Clin Invest 1985;76:2182–2190.
32. Rogers J, Kerstiens J. Capping of DNA on phytohemagglutinin-stimulated human lymphoblasts. J Immunol 1981;126:703–705.
33. Loke SL, Stein, CA, Zhang XH, et al. Characterization of oligonucleotide transport into living cells. Proc Natl Acad Sci USA 1989;86:3474–3478.
34. Yakubov LA, Deeva EA, Zarytova VF, et al. Mechanism of oligonucleotide uptake by cells: Involvement of specific receptors? Proc Natl Acad Sci USA 1989;86:6454–6458.
35. Gasparro FP, Dall'Amico R, O'Malley M, et al. Cell membrane DNA. A new target for psoralen photoadduct formation. Photochem Photobiol 1990;52:315–321.
36. Stein CA, Tonkinson J, Zhang LM, et al. Unpublished observations.
37. Daaka Y, Wickstrom E. Target dependence of antisense oligodeoxynucleotide inhibition of c-Ha-ras p21 expression and focus formation in T24–transformed NIH3T3 cells. Oncogene Res 1990;5:267–275.
38. Leonetti JP, Degols G, LeBleu B. Biological activity of oligonucleotide-poly(L-lysine) conjugates: Mechanism of cell uptake. Bioconjugate Chem 1990;1:149–153.
39. Lemaitre M, Bayard B, Lebleu B. Specific antiviral activity of a poly(L-lysine)-conjugated oligodeoxyribonucleotide sequence complementary to vesaicular stomatitis virus N protein mRNA initiation site. Proc Natl Acad Sci USA 1989;84:648–652.
40. LeMaitre M, Bayard B, Lebleu B. Specific antiviral activity of a poly(L-lysine)-conjugated oligodeoxyribonucleotide sequence complementary to vesicular stomatitis virus N protein mRNA initiation site. Proc Natl Acad Sci USA 1987;84:648–682.
41. Stevenson M, Iversen P. Inhibition of human immunodeficiency virus type 1-mediated cytopathic effects of poly(L-lysine)-conjugated synthetic antisense oligodeoxyribonucleotides. J Gen Virol 1989;70:2673–2682.
42. Boutourin A, Gus'kova E, Ivanova E, et al. Synthesis of alkylating oligonucleotide derivatives containing cholesterol or phenazinium residues at their 3' terminus and their interaction with DNA within mammalian cells. FEBS Lett 1989;254:129–132.
43. Shea R, Marsters J, Bischofberger N. Synthesis hybridization properties and antiviral activity of lipid-oligodeoxynuycleotide conjugates. Nucleic Acids Res 1990;18:3777–3783.
44. Letsinger R, Zhang G, Sun D, et al. Cholesteryl-conjugated oligonucleotides: Synthesis, properties, and activity as inhibitors of replication of human immunodeficiency virus in cell culture. Proc Natl Acad Sci USA 1989;86:6553–6556.
45. Stein CA, Pal R, DeVico A, et al. Mode of action of 5'-linked cholesteryl phosphorothioate oligodeoxynucleotides in inhibiting syncytia formation and infection by HIV-1 and HIV-2 in vitro. Biochemistry 1991;30:2439–2444.
46. Stein CA, Tonkinson J, Yakubov L, et al. unpublished observations
47. Loke SL, Stein CA, Zhang XH, et al. Delivery of c-myc antisense phosphorothioate oligodeoxynucleotides to hematopoietic cells in culture by liposome fusion: Specific reduction in c-myc protein expression correlates with inhibition of cell growth and DNA synthesis. Curr Top Microbiol Immunol 1988;141:282–289.
48. Cazenave C, Chevrier M, Thuong N, et al. Rate of degradation of [α]- and [β]-oligodeoxynucleotides in Xenopus oocytes. Implications for anti-messenger strategies. Nucleic Acids Res 1987;15:10507–10521.
49. Dagle J, Walder J, Weeks D. Targeted degradation of mRNA in Xenopus oocytes and embryos directed by modified oligonucleotides: Studies of An2 and cyclin in embryogenesis. Nucleic Acids Res 1990;18:4751–4757.
50. Dagle J, Weeks D, Walder J. Pathwasys of degradation and mechanism of action of antisense oligonucleotides in Xenopus laevis embryos. Antisense Res Devel 1991;1:11–20.
51. Eder P, DeVine R, Dagle J, Walder J. Substrate specificity and kinetics of degradation of antisense oligonucleotides by a 3'-exonuclease in plasma. Antisense Res Devel 1991;1:141–151.
52. Zon G. Pharmaceutical considerations. In Cohen J, ed. Oligodeoxynucleotides: Antisense inhibitors of gene expression. London: Macmillan, 1989:243–248.
53. Chin DJ, Green GA, Zon G, et al. Rapid nuclear accumulation of injected oligodeoxyribonucleotides. New Biologist 1990;12:1091–1100.
54. Leonetti JP, Mechti N, Degols G, et al. Intracellular distribution of microinjected antisense oligonucleotides. Proc Natl Acad Sci USA 1991;88:2702–2706.
55. Maguire DK, Han H. Synthesis and metabolism of oligonucleoside methylphosphonates. Proc Austral Biochem Soc 1988;20:26.
56. Becker D, Meier C, Herlyn M. Proliferation of human malignant melanomas is inhibited by antisense oligodeoxynucleotides targeted against basic fibroblast growth factor. EMBO J 1989;8:3685–3691.
57. Iverson P, Mata J, Zon G. The single injection pharmacokinetics of an antisense phosphorothioate oligodeoxynucleotide against rev (art/trs) for the human immunodeficiency virus (HIV) in the adult male rat. Personal communication.
58. Wintersberger U. Ribonucleases H of retroviral and cellular origin. Pharmacol Ther 1990;48:259–280.
59. Cazenave C, Stein CA, Loreau N, et al. Comparative inhibition of rabbit globin mRNA translation by modified antisense oligodeoxynucleotides. Nucleic Acids Res 1989;17:4255–4273.
60. Minshull J, Hunt T. The use of single-stranded DNA and RNase H to promote quantitive hybrid arrest of translation of mRNA/DNA hybrids in reticulocyte lysate cell-free translation. Nucleic Acids Res 1986;14:6433–6451.
61. Walder R, Walder J. Role of RNase H in hybrid-arrested translation by antisense oligonucleotides. Proc Natl Acad Sci USA 1988;85:5011–5015.
62. Dash P, Lotan I, Knapp, M, et al. Selective elimination of mRNAs in vivo: Complementary oligodeoxynucleotides promote RNA degradation by an RNase H-like activity. Proc Natl Acad Sci USA 1987;84:7896–7900.
63. Cazenave C, Loreau N, Thuong N, et al. Enzymatic amplification of translation inhibition of rabbit β-globin mRNA mediated by anti-messgnger oligodeoxynucleotides covalently linked to intercalating agents. Nucleic Acids Res 1987;15:4717–4736.
64. Goodchild J. Inhibition of gene expression by oligonucleotides. In Cohen J, ed. Oligodeoxynucleotides, antisense inhibitors of gene expression. London: Macmillan, 1989:53–77.
65. Bacon T, Wickstrom E. Walking along human c-myc mRNA with antisense oligodeoxynucleotides: Maximum efficacy at the 5' cap region. Oncogene Res 1991;6:13–19.
66. Goodchild J, Agrawal S, Civeira M, et al. Inhibition of human immunodeficiency virus replication by antisense oligodeoxynucleotides. Proc Natl Acad Sci USA 1988;85:5507–5511.
67. Heikkila R, Schwab G, Wickstrom E, et al. A c-myc antisense oligodeoxynucleotide inhibits entry into S phase but not progress from G$_0$ to G$_1$. Nature 1987;328:445–449.
68. Harel-Bellan A, Ferris D, Vinocour M, et al. Specific inhibition of c-myc protein biosynthesis using an antisense synthetic deoxyolignucleotide in human T lymphocytes. J Immunol 1988;140:2431–2435.
69. Wickstrom EL, Bacon T, Gonzalez A, et al. Human promyelocytic leukemia HL-60 cell proliferation and c-myc protein expression are inhibited by an antisense penta-

decadeoxynucleotide targeted against c-myc mRNA. Proc Natal Acad Sci USA 1988;85: 1028–1032.

70. Holt J, Redner R, Nienhuis A. An oligomer complementary to c-myc mRNA inhibits proliferation of HL-60 promyelocytic cells and induces differentiation. Mol Cell Biol 1988;8:963–973.

71. Bacon T, Wickstrom E. Daily addition of an anti-c-*myc* DNA oligomer induces granulocytic differentiation of human promyelocytic leukemia HL-60 cells in both serum-containing and serum-free media. Oncogene Res 1991;6:21–32.

72. Degols G, Lenoetti JP, Mechti N, et al. Antiproliferative effects of antisense oligonucleotides directed to the RNA of c-*myc* oncogene. Nucleic Acids Res 1991;19:945–948.

73. McManaway ME, Neckers LM, Loke SL, et al. Tumour-specific inhibition of lymphoma growth by an antisense oligodeoxynucleotide. Lancet 1990;335:808–811.

74. Cooney M, Czernuszewicz G, Postel E, et al. Site-specific oligonucleotide binding represses transcription of the human c-*myc* gene in vitro. Science 1988;241:456–459.

75. Anfossi G, Gewirtz A, Calabretta B. An oligomer complementary to c-*myb*-encoded mRNA inhibits proliferation of human myeloid leukemia cell lines. Proc Natl Acad Sci USA 1989;86:3379–3383.

76. Gewirtz A, Anfossi G, Venturelli D, et al. G_1/S transition in normal human T-lymphocytes requires the nuclear protein encoded by c-*myb*. Science 1989;245:180–183.

77. Ferrari S, Donelli A, Manfredini R, et al. Differential effects of c-*myb* and c-*fes* antisense oligodeoxynucleotides on granulocytic differentiation of human myeloid leukemia HL60 cells. Cell Growth Differ 1990;1:543–548.

78. Churilla A, Braciale T, Braciale V. Regulation of T lymphocyte proliferation: Interleukin 2-mediated induction of c-*myb* gene expression is dependent of T lymphocyte activation state. J Exp Med 1989;170:105–121.

79. Venturelli D, Travale S, Calabretta B. Inhibition of T-cell proliferation by a MYB antisense oligomer is accompanied by selective down-regulation of DNA polymerase α expression. Proc Natl Acad Sci USA 1990;87:5963–5967.

80. Gewirtz A, Calabretta B. A c-*myb* antisense oligodeoxynucleotide inhibits normal human hematopoiesis in vitro. Science 1988;242:1303–1306.

81. Calabretta B, Sims R, Valtieri M, et al. Normal and leukemic hematopoietic cells manifest differential sensitivity to inhibitory effects of c-*myb* antisense oligodeoxynucleotides: An in vitro study relevant to bone marrow purging. Proc Natl Acad Sci USA 1991;88:2351–2355.

82. Weiss L, Warnke R, Sklar J, et al. Molecular analysis of the t(14;18) chromosomal translocation in malignant lymphoma. N Engl J Med 1987;317:1185–1189.

83. Reed JC, Stein CA, Subasinghe C, et al. Antisense-mediated inhibition of BCL2 protooncogene expression and leukemic cell growth and survival: Comparisons of phosphodiester and phosphothioate oligodeoxynucleotides. Cancer Res 1990;50:6565–6570.

84. Wu J, Zhu JQ, Han KK, et al. The role of the c-*fms* oncogene in the regulation of HL-60 cell differentiation. Oncogene 1990;5:873–877.

85. Sherr C, Rettenmier C, Sacca R, et al. The c-*fms* proto-oncogene product is related to the receptor for the mononuclear phagocyte growth factor, CSF-1. Cell 1985;41:665–676.

86. Birchenall-Roberts M, Ferrer C, Ferris D, et al. Inhibition of murine monocyte proliferation by a colony-stimulating factor-1 antisense oligodeoxynucleotide. J Immunol 1990;145:3290–3296.

87. Bories D, Raynal MC, Solomon DH, et al. Down-regulation of a serine protease, myeloblastin, causes growth arrest and differentiation of promyelocytic leukemia cells. Cell 1989;59:959–968.

88. Szczylik C, Skorski T, Nicolaides N, et al. Selective inhibition of leukemia cell proliferation by BCR-ABL antisense oligodeoxynucleotides. Science 1991;253:562–565.

89. Zheng H, Sahai B, Kilgannon P, et al. Specific inhibition of cell-surface T-cell receptor expression by antisense oligodeoxynucleotides and its effect on the production of an antigen-specific regulatory T-cell factor. Proc Natl Acad Sci USA 1989;86:3758–3762.

90. Harel-Bellan A, Durum S, Muegge K, et al. Specific inhibition of lymphokine biosynthesis and autocrine growth using antisense oligonucleotides in Th1 and Th2 helper T cell clones. J Exp Med 1988;168:2309–2318.

91. Weigent D, Blalock J, LeBoeuf R. An antisense oligodeoxynucleotide to growth hormone messenger ribonucleic acid inhibits lymphocyte proliferation. Endocrinology 1991;128:2053–2057.

92. Furukawa Y, Piwnica-Worms H, Ernst T, et al. CDC2 gene expression at the G_1 to S transition in human T lymphocytes. Science 1990;250:805–808.

93. Sburlati A, Manrow R, Berger S. Prothymosin α antisense oligomers inhibit myeloma cell division. Proc Natl Acad Sci USA 1991;88:253–257.

94. Morrison R. Suppression of basic fibroblast growth factor expression by antisense oligodeoxynucleotides inhibits the growth of transformed human astrocytes. J Biol Chem 1991;266:728–734.

95. Yu A, Chen D, Black R, et al. Sequence specific inhibition of in vitro translation of mutated or normal *ras* p21. J Exp Pathol 1989;4:97–108.

96. Brown D, Yu A, Miller P, et al. Modulation of *ras* expression by anti-sense, nonionic deoxyoligonucleotide analogs. Oncogene Res 1989;4:243–254.

97. Miller P, McParland K, Jayaraman K, et al. Biochemical and biological effects of nonionic nucleic acid methylphosphonates Biochemistry 1981;20:1874–1880.

98. Rosolen A, Whitesell L, Ikegaki N, et al. Antisense inhibition of single copy N-*myc* expression results in decreased cell growth without reduction of c-*myc* protein in a neuroepithelioma cell line. Cancer Res 1990;50:6316–6322.

99. Cope F, Wille J. Retinoid receptor antisense DNAs inhibit alkaline phosphatase induction and clonogenicity in malignant keratinocytes. Proc Natl Acad Sci USA 1989;86:5590–5594.

100. Melani E, Rivoltini L, Parmiani G, et al. Inhibition of proliferation by c-*myb* antisense oligodeoxynucleotides in colon adenocarcinoma cell lines that express c-*myb*. Cancer Res 1991;51:2897–2901.

101. Jaslkulski D, DeRiel J, Mercer W, et al. Inhibition of cellular proliferation by antisense oligodeoxynucleotides to PCNA cyclin. Science 1988;240:1544–1546.

102. Rivoltini L, Colombo M, Supino R, et al. Modulation of multidrug resistance by verapamil or *mdr1* anti-sense oligodeoxynucleotide does not change the high susceptibility to lymphokine-activated killers in *mdr*-resistant human carcinoma (LoVo) line. Int J Cancer 1990;46:727–732.

103. Caracciolo D, Venturelli D, Valtieri M, et al. Stage-related proliferative activity determines c-*myb* functional requirements during normal hematopoiesis. J Clin Invest 1990;85:55–61.

SECTION **6**

WILLIAM S. DALTON

Overcoming the Multidrug-Resistant Phenotype

The problem of clinical drug resistance is well known to those involved in the care of cancer patients. Despite improvements in the treatment of many cancers, including hematologic and solid tumors, most patients will relapse and die of their disease. Modern chemotherapeutic regimens are capable of inducing remissions in many newly diagnosed patients, but treatment of relapsed disease is usually less rewarding. The drug resistance that eventually develops in the patients with recurrent disease is one of "acquired" resistance. Drugs that were initially effective in reducing tumor burden become ineffective by selecting for drug-resistant cells over time. Hematologic tumors such as acute leukemia and malignant lymphoma are good examples of diseases that manifest acquired resistance. Unlike acquired drug resistance, tumors that are relatively insensitive to chemotherapeutic drugs from the onset of disease, such as non-small cell lung cancer and colon cancer, are described as having "intrinsic" drug resistance.

Failure of chemotherapy to induce a response may be due to several different factors. These factors may be considered at the level of the entire organism or at the level of individual cells. At the level of the entire organism, physiologic factors play a major role in the successful outcome of therapy. The physiologic disposition of drugs considers absorption, distribution, metabolism, and elimination as key principles in successful cancer chemotherapy. These factors determine whether the drug actually reaches the tumor and can be manipulated by changing route of administration, drug dosage, and scheduling. Because these factors may be more readily addressed they have been given the term "temporary resistance."[1]

A more permanent form of drug resistance occurs at the genetic level. Compared with normal cells, malignant cells are genetically more unstable.[2] Genetic changes such as mutations, deletions, translocations, and gene amplification can lead to an inheritable form of drug resistance that is passed from one generation of cells to another. These genetic changes can lead to altered protein products that may be directly involved in the development of drug resistance. Chemotherapy becomes a selection factor, eradicating drug-sensitive cells and leaving behind a smaller population of drug-resistant cells. The resistant cells eventually proliferate, resulting in recurrent disease that is drug resistant.

Individual mechanisms of cellular drug resistance vary according to tumor type and the family of drugs used in the treatment of disease. One form of cellular drug resistance is the overexpression of an integral plasma membrane protein given the name P-glycoprotein or P-170.[3,4] This resistance may be acquired or intrinsic and is usually associated with natural product drugs such as the anthracyclines and vinca alkaloids. P-glycoprotein acts as a drug efflux pump that actively extrudes drugs from tumor cells, preventing a cytotoxic drug from reaching the cellular site of action. Although there are other important mechanisms of cellular drug resistance, this section focuses on multidrug resistance due to the overproduction of P-glycoprotein. Overcoming or preventing this form of drug resistance may represent a new approach to cancer treatment and improve treatment outcomes.

Multidrug resistance (MDR) is a term that describes the phenomenon by which a cancer becomes resistant to multiple drugs that have little similarity in their chemical structure and mechanism of action.[3,4] The drugs involved in MDR are primarily natural products and include antibiotics such as doxorubicin and mitomycin C and plant products, including the vinca alkaloids and podophyllotoxins. However, even certain antimetabolites such as trimetrexate and synthetic compounds such as mitoxantrone may be involved in the MDR mechanism.[5,6] Table 69–19 lists some of the drugs that have been associated with MDR.

STRUCTURE AND FUNCTION OF P-GLYCOPROTEIN

P-glycoprotein (P-gp) consists of 1280 amino acids that are arranged in such a way that the protein appears to have two similar halves.[4] The amino acid sequence predicts that each half consists of six separate segments that span the entire width of the cell membrane. The sequence information also reveals two segments of the protein that are likely to bind the energy-containing molecule ATP. Only a small portion of the protein extends to the outside of the cell, and it is this portion of the protein that is glycosylated. Most of the protein resides inside the cell and consists of two homologous domains that bear the ATP-binding sites. These ATP-binding sites on the P-gp molecule suggest that the protein is involved in an energy-requiring function, such as the transport of molecules from inside the cell to the outside.

The structural similarities between P-gp and other known membrane transport proteins support the contention that P-

gp is involved in drug transport.[7,8] Presumably, chemotherapeutic drugs enter the cell and, before they reach their critical target, are bound to P-gp and actively pumped out of the cell, reducing the overall intracellular accumulation of drug (Fig. 69–25). How drugs actually bind to the P-gp and are extruded from the cell is unknown. An alternative explanation likens the mammalian P-gp to the bacterial transport protein, hemolysin-B, which transports the toxin α-hemolysin.[9] In this setting, drugs bind a carrier protein and the drug protein complex is actively transported from the cell (Fig. 69–26). No candidate for a carrier protein has been identified. In either case, P-gp must be in high concentrations in the plasma membrane if it is involved in the transport of drugs out of the cell.

Although P-gp is involved in the transport of drugs out of neoplastic cells, its normal function is unknown. Analyzing for the presence of P-gp in normal tissue may give us clues to the normal function of this molecule. Fojo and colleagues were the first to report on a large survey of *MDR1* expression in normal human tissues.[10] Using a technique to detect MDR1 mRNA, they found a high degree of expression in normal adrenal gland and kidney. Intermediate levels were detected in the lung, liver, and colon. Tumors derived from those tissues that express a higher intermediate level of MDR1 RNA (*e.g.*, renal cell carcinoma) may explain the intrinsic drug resistance observed in these tumors.

Using flow cytometry, Chaudhary and Roninson examined *MDR1* expression in human bone marrow.[11] These investigators found that early hematopoietic precursor cells, defined as high expressors of CD34 antigen and capable of self-renewal in tissue culture, produce high levels of P-gp. Functional analysis demonstrated that these cells could exclude the dye rhodamine 123 (a substrate for P-gp) and that this exclusion could be attenuated by inhibitors of P-gp (*e.g.*, verapamil). Using the polymerase chain reaction (PCR), it was shown that the lymphoid region of the bone marrow—where most of early progenitor cells are thought to reside—express MDR1 RNA. P-gp expression has been associated with the

TABLE 69–19. Chemotherapeutic Drugs Exhibiting Cross-Resistance in Multidrug Resistance

Doxorubicin	Taxol
Daunorubicin	Trimetrexate
Vincristine	Mitomycin C
Vinblastine	Dactinomycin
Etoposide	Mitoxantrone

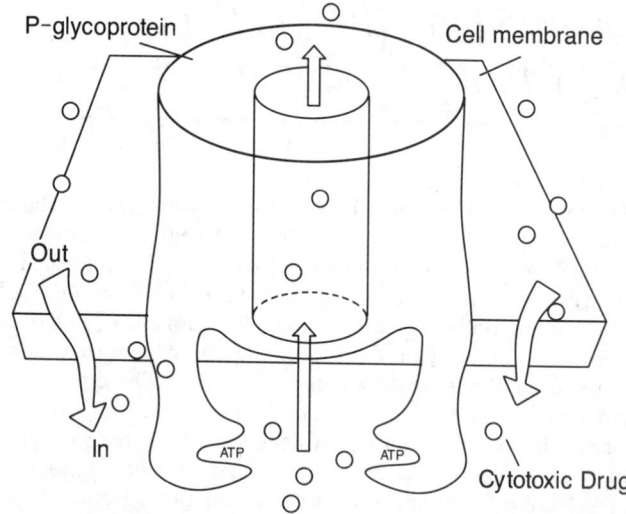

FIGURE 69–25. Model of P-glycoprotein as an energy-dependent drug efflux pump. In this model, cytotoxic drugs bind directly to P-glycoprotein and are transported from the intracellular to the extracellular space.

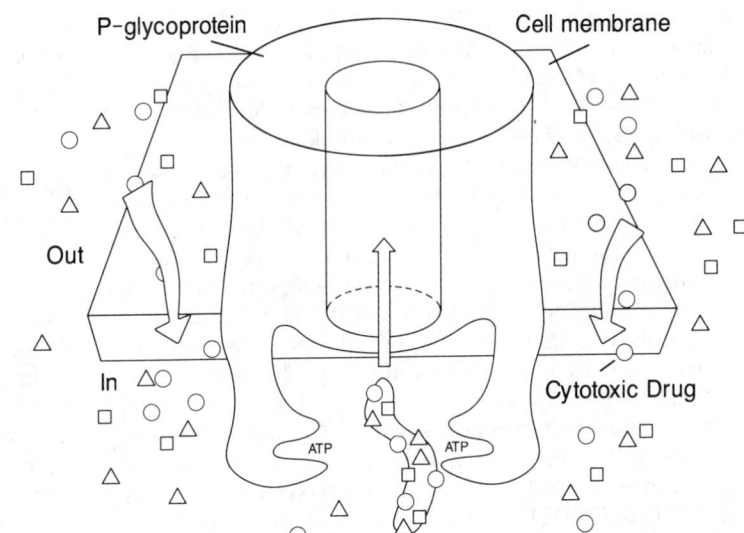

FIGURE 69–26. In this model, P-glycoprotein transports an intracellular protein that serves as a carrier for cytotoxic drugs. This model is analogous to other transport molecules known to transport proteins to the extracellular space.

CD34 phenotype in myelodysplastic syndrome and acute myeloid leukemia.[12] These hematopoietic stem cell malignancies are notoriously resistant to drugs.

With the development of monoclonal antibodies against P-gp, the cellular location of P-gp can be determined. Using the monoclonal antibody MRK-16, Thiebaut and coworkers found that P-gp was distributed in a highly site-specific fashion.[13] Immunohistochemical staining with the MRK-16 antibody demonstrated that P-gp was distributed along the apical surface of epithelial cells of the proximal tubules of the kidney, superficial columnar epithelial cells of the colon in jejunum, and limited to hepatocytes lining the biliary canaliculi of the liver. These results suggested that P-gp served a function in the normal excretion of compounds and possibly drugs into the urine, gastrointestinal tract, and bile. Immunohistochemical studies using monoclonal antibodies HYB-241 and HYB-612 have shown that endothelial cells of human capillary blood vessels in the brain and testes express high levels of P-gp.[14] This finding suggests a physiologic role for P-gp in reducing the amount of drugs in critical anatomic sites that have been known to be sanctuaries for malignant cells.

METHODS OF DETECTION OF MULTIDRUG RESISTANCE

General methods of detecting MDR in tissues are shown in Table 69–20. These approaches include assessing DNA amplification, measuring messenger mRNA, and quantitating the amount of protein. Although the amplification of the *MDR1* gene has been observed in tumor cell lines, gene amplification is an uncommon event in the clinical setting, and overexpression of the *MDR1* gene is usually not associated with gene amplification.[15] Most investigators have turned to measuring the *MDR1* message or actual detection of the gene product, P-gp. To evaluate the role of P-gp in clinical drug resistance, it is important to develop assays that are specific for the *MDR1* gene but sensitive enough to detect minute concentrations that may be present in small tissue specimens.[16] An added confounding factor in the clinical setting is the fact that P-gp

is expressed in certain normal tissues. Assays must be specific and sensitive and be able to discriminate between normal and neoplastic tissue.

Initial studies analyzing the role of *MDR1* in human tumor specimens used biochemical analyses of bulk tumor tissue. Bell and colleagues first reported the presence of P-gp in ovarian cancer by detecting the protein in bulk tumor specimens using an immunoblot analysis.[17] Gerlach and associates, using a similar immunoblot technique, detected P-gp in a series of sarcoma patients.[18] Fojo and colleagues[10] and later Goldstein and colleagues[19] were successful in measuring MDR1 RNA in various human tumors by extracting total RNA from bulk tissue and detecting the *MDR1* message with gene-specific probes. Although these initial analyses were considered to be specific for *MDR1*, they were relatively insensitive and did not differentiate between normal and neoplastic tissue.

Methods to differentiate expression of *MDR* in normal and tumor cells have been developed. In situ hybridization with nucleic acid probes on tissue sections allows the detection of MDR mRNA in tumor cells.[20] This technique, however, is very laborious and can be difficult to interpret. Because of the difficulties in performing mRNA in situ hybridization, attention has been directed to the use of monoclonal antibodies in immunohistochemical detection.

Several antibodies are available for detection of P-gp. The

TABLE 69–20. Methods of Detecting Multidrug Resistance

1. DNA analysis for amplification (Southern blot)
2. Analysis of RNA
   Northern blot
   Slot-blot
   RNase protection assay
   In situ hybridization
   Polymerase chain reaction analysis
3. Analysis for protein
   Western blot
   Immunohistochemistry
   Flow cytometry

monoclonal antibody C219, developed by Victor Ling and associates, was among the first antibodies to be developed.[21] This antibody is used in immunoblot analysis and immunohistochemical detection of P-gp. The epitopes for C219 have been mapped to conserve cytoplasmic domains, which requires that cells be fixed so that the antibody may gain entrance into the cell. There is also a problem of specificity in using C219, because it recognizes *MDR1* and *MDR3* isoforms of P-gp.[22] Cross-reactivities of C219 have been observed in striated musculature.[23] Several monoclonal antibodies in addition to C219 react with different epitopes of the MDR1 P-gp. The C494 antibody is MDR1 specific and does not cross-react with the non-MDR-related *MDR3* gene of P-gp.[22] This antibody also recognizes an epitope in the cytoplasm and requires fixation before immunohistochemical staining. A third monoclonal antibody, JSB-1, recognizes a highly conserved epitope in the cytoplasm, which is different from the epitope recognized by C219.[24] Like C494, JSB-1 is specific for MDR1 P-gp.[25]

Tsuruo and colleagues developed a monoclonal antibody, MRK-16, that has a high affinity for MDR1.[26] Unlike the antibodies mentioned previously, MRK-16 recognizes an external epitope on the outer surface of the plasma membrane of living cells. The use of MRK-16 does not require prior fixation to detect P-gp. This particular characteristic allows the use of flow cytometry in detecting P-gp in living cells. Two new monoclonal antibodies, HYB-241 and HYB-612, have been developed by Hybritech (San Diego, CA) in collaboration with Biedler and associates at Memorial Sloan-Kettering Cancer Center in New York.[14] These two antibodies recognize external epitopes of MDR1 but recognition is restricted to a 180-kd P-gp, and they do not recognize the 170-kd form of P-gp. Whether this limits the usefulness of these antibodies in P-gp detection in clinical samples is unknown.

Immunohistochemical detection of P-gp in clinical samples holds particular promise, because it is a practical, readily performed procedure.[16,27] The primary advantages of immunohistochemistry in the clinical setting include the ability to detect P-gp a single cell, allowing for small sample size, and the ability to discriminate P-gp expression in normal cells from that found in tumor cells. This latter feature is especially important considering the heterogenous nature of clinical specimens. The sensitivity and specificity of immunohistochemical detection of P-gp have been improved, and this method holds considerable promise for practical application in the clinical setting.[23-30]

The advent of the PCR provided probably the most sensitive and reliable means of detecting MDR1 RNA. Using this approach, it is possible to analyze the most minute of clinical specimens.[31] PCR is so sensitive, however, that it raises the question of what threshold level of *MDR1* expression is necessary to confer multidrug resistance. Levels detected below a theoretical threshold level may actually cause a tumor to be called drug resistant although it is still sensitive to drugs. This problem illustrates the need for proper controls, usually in the form of drug-sensitive and drug-resistant cell lines for a particular tumor type, when performing assays for MDR detection. Several PCR methods have been developed to quantitate MDR1 RNA in tumor specimens.[32-34]

The multitude of assays and techniques used in clinical studies may produce various results for a given tumor type, and investigators must be aware of the strengths and weaknesses of each assay. In the clinical situation, a combination of complementary assays such as immunohistochemistry and PCR may provide the best information about the presence of MDR in human tumors.

MULTIDRUG RESISTANCE IN HEMATOLOGIC TUMORS

When first diagnosed, hematologic tumors are sensitive to most chemotherapeutic agents used. However, after relapse, the response rate is less and usually of shorter duration. The anthracyclines, vinca alkaloids, and epipodophyllotoxins are integral components of treatment regimens used in the treatment of leukemias, malignant lymphomas, and multiple myeloma. Complete remissions are common with initial induction therapy, but if relapse occurs, patients usually acquire drug resistance and frequently die of their disease.

ACUTE LYMPHOCYTIC LEUKEMIA

Complete hematologic remissions are achieved in 70% to 90% of patients with newly diagnosed adult or childhood acute lymphoblastic leukemia (ALL).[35] Sustained remissions are more common in childhood than adult ALL. Expression of P-gp in ALL blast cells is detected infrequently at initial diagnosis (Table 69-21). Goldstein and coworkers[19] and Rothenberg and colleagues[36] found overexpression of the *MDR1* gene in fewer than 15% of patients with childhood ALL at presentation or at relapse. Acquisition of the MDR phenotype, however, may be more frequent in adult ALL. As shown in Table 69-21, Musto and associates[37] and others[38-40] have found expression of the MDR phenotype in 50% or more of cases of re-

TABLE 69-21. Multidrug Resistance in Acute Leukemias

Malignancy/ Investigations	Pretreatment		Relapsed	
	No. of Patients	MDR+ (%)	No. of Patients	MDR+ (%)
Acute Lymphocytic Leukemia (ALL)				
Childhood ALL				
Goldstein et al[19]	9	1 (11)	20	3 (15)
Rothenberg et al[36]	9	1 (11)	19	3 (16)
Adult ALL				
Goldstein et al[19]	15	2 (13)		
Musto et al[37]	20	2 (10)	12	7 (58)
Herweijer et al[38]	8	4 (50)	1	1
Adult T-cell Leukemia-Lymphoma (ATL)				
Kuwazuru et al[41]	20	8 (40)	6	6 (100)
Acute Non-Lymphocytic Leukemia (ANLL)				
Goldstein et al[19]	24	3 (13)	5	4 (80)
Herweijer et al[38]	7	1 (14)	10	8 (80)
Holmes et al[45]	8	2 (25)	8	5 (62)
Ito et al[46]	10	1 (10)	14	2 (15)
Musto et al[37]	12	1 (8)	8	6 (75)
Nooter et al[47]	6	1 (17)	10	6 (60)
Sato et al[44]	36	9 (25)	17	9 (53)

lapsing adult ALL. These observations are consistent with the lower rate of successful reinduction in relapsed adult ALL.

Patients with adult T-cell leukemia-lymphoma (ATL) syndrome appear to have a high prevalence of P-gp overexpression. Remissions are usually of short duration and are associated with the emergence of acquired drug resistance despite the use of intensive chemotherapy induction regimens. In a study by Kuwazuru and colleagues, 25 patients with the ATL syndrome were studied for the presence of P-gp using immunoblot analyses.[41] At initial presentation, 8 of 20 patients were positive for P-gp. Of 6 patients who had relapsed and were refractory to chemotherapy, all were positive for P-gp. Similarly, Herweijer and coworkers found a higher frequency of *MDR1* expression in T-cell-lineage ALL, implying that lymphoblast lineage may relate to *MDR* overexpression.[38]

ACUTE NONLYMPHOCYTIC LEUKEMIA

Like ALL, patients with acute nonlymphocytic leukemia (ANLL) have a high probability of going into a complete remission; however, if relapse occurs, they are unlikely to be cured due to the emergence of drug resistance.[42] The anthracycline daunorubicin is one of the most active agents used in the treatment of ANLL. Studies have shown that the intracellular concentration of daunorubicin in leukemic cells is an important determinant of response to therapy.[43] The presence of P-gp on cells could lower the intracellular concentration of daunorubicin, thereby decreasing efficacy.

Table 69-21 shows the incidence of P-gp in newly diagnosed and relapsed ANLL patients from several studies using different methods of detection for *MDR1*. Between 10% and 20% of cases of newly diagnosed ANLL appear to express the *MDR1* message or its P-gp product. Although few patients have been studied serially, P-gp or its message occurs in more than 50% of patients with relapsed ANLL. In a study by Sato and colleagues, 88% of patients who had P-gp-negative disease obtained a complete remission, compared with 58% of patients whose leukemic cells contained moderate of high levels of *MDR1* message.[44] The number of patients requiring two courses of induction therapy to obtain a complete remission was substantially higher among patients with high *MDR* expression. Moreover, the median duration of response for patients with low levels of *MDR* expression was twice as long as that observed for patients with high levels of *MDR* expression, indicating that *MDR* expression affects overall outcome in patients receiving conventional cytarabine-daunorubicin induction and consolidation treatment.

The prevalence of P-gp in myelodysplastic syndromes has been investigated. Holmes and associates found elevated levels of MDR1 RNA in 7 of 19 cases of myelodysplastic syndrome (MDS).[45] List and colleagues, using immunocytochemical staining and flow cytometry to detect P-gp, found increased expression in 7 of 32 patients (22%).[12] P-gp detection was limited to blast cells and leukemic monocytes and was otherwise absent from terminally differentiated blood cells. Among patients who developed ANLL that was preceded by a myelodysplastic syndrome, the incidence of P-gp increased to 75%. Among patients with secondary leukemia related to prior treatment for hematologic disorders including Hodgkin's disease, 9 (82%) of 11 patients had overexpression of P-gp on their leukemic cells.

Patients with acute leukemias preceded by myelodysplastic syndrome or patients with secondary leukemias related to treatment of other hematologic disorders usually have a poor response to conventional induction therapy. The high incidence of *MDR1* expression in these patient populations may explain the poor treatment outcome.

CHRONIC LEUKEMIAS

The expression of P-gp has also been examined in chronic lymphocytic and chronic myelocytic leukemias. Chronic lymphocytic leukemia (CLL) is characterized by the progressive increase in malignant lymphocytes in the peripheral blood, bone marrow, and lymphoid tissues. Chemotherapy is able to control proliferation of these abnormal lymphocytes; however, cure is generally not possible. In a study by Holmes and coworkers measuring *MDR1* expression, moderate levels of MDR1 RNA were found in 4 of 7 untreated CLL patients and 14 of 27 previously treated patients.[48] In a study by Herweijer and colleagues using a sensitive RNAse protection assay, 17 of 17 patients expressed at least some MDR1 mRNA in their cells.[38] These same investigators found detectable message for the *MDR3* gene in all CLL patients. No correlation was observed between *MDR1* expression and prior treatment. However, the *MDR3* expression was generally higher in treated patients than in untreated patients. The investigators speculated that a particular splice variant of *MDR3* may be functional in conferring drug resistance in CLL.

The importance of the type of method used in detecting MDR in CLL was reported by Cumber and colleagues.[49] These investigators used the monoclonal antibody MRK-16, which recognizes an external epitope of P-gp on the external surface of cells. Initial studies using this antibody showed only 12% of the lymphocyte samples from CLL patients had increased P-gp on their cells. Treatment of the leukemic cells with neuraminidase to remove sialic acid residues increased the proportion of patients expressing P-gp on their cells from 12% to 52%. The investigators think that abnormal sialalation patterns on the surface of cells masked the epitope recognized by MRK-16, creating false-negative results.

In chronic myelocytic leukemia, *MDR1* expression generally has been limited to blast cells seen in the terminal phase of the disease. Goldstein and associates analyzed the RNA of 9 patients with chronic myelogenous leukemia.[19] Three patients were in the chronic phase of their CML, and 6 patients were in the blast phase. All 3 patients who were in chronic phase showed no *MDR1* expression in their leukemic cells. In contrast, 5 of 6 patients in the blast phase of their disease showed overexpression of *MDR1*. Similarly, two different studies using immunocytochemistry or RNA analysis found that 50% of patients in the blast phase of their CML expressed *MDR1*.[50,51] This increased expression may partially explain the poor results of treatment for the blast phase of CML.

LYMPHOMA

The clinical course of patients with malignant lymphoma closely parallels the laboratory animal models of acquired drug resistance. Most patients with newly diagnosed non-Hodgkin's lymphomas and advanced Hodgkin's disease respond to initial chemotherapy. Responses to treatment are observed with a wide variety of single agents or combinations of drugs. However, most patients relapse and eventually develop drug-resistant disease.

The parallel to animal models of multidrug resistance is even more striking when the frequency of P-gp expression is considered. Newly diagnosed and untreated patients rarely express the P-gp in detectable amounts, but patients with recurrent and drug-refractory disease frequently have detectable levels of P-gp. In a consecutive series of 42 patients with newly diagnosed malignant lymphomas, Miller and colleagues using immunocytochemistry found detectable levels of P-gp in only 1 patient.[52] Goldstein and coworkers, using RNA slot blot methods, found P-gp in 4 of 18 previously untreated patients.[19] These findings contrast with the high frequency of P-gp expressed in previously treated patients with recurrent and clinically drug-resistant disease. Miller and colleagues[52] found P-gp in 7 (64%) of 11 patients, and Goldstein and associates[19] found it in 3 (60%) of 5 patients. These studies suggest that incidence of detectable levels of P-gp closely parallels the clinical response to chemotherapy.

MULTIPLE MYELOMA

Multiple myeloma is a malignancy of the plasma cell, the most mature cell in the B-cell series. Advances in the treatment of multiple myeloma have been made over the last 3 decades and are manifest both in prolongation of survival from less than 1 year to almost 3 years and in a better quality of life.[53,54] These improvements are attributed to the development of more effective chemotherapy, which includes the natural products vincristine and doxorubicin. Despite initial responses seen in most patients, all patients develop drug resistance and eventually die of their disease.

At the University of Arizona, over 100 patients with multiple myeloma have been studied for the expression of P-gp.[55] In newly diagnosed patients, fewer than 5% of patients have P-gp on their cells. When treated with alkylating agents alone (*e.g.,* melphalan), the incidence of P-gp remains basically unchanged. As patients receive more treatment, including vincristine and doxorubicin, the incidence of P-gp increases. When patients become refractory to vincristine and doxorubicin (Adriamycin), as used in the VAD regimen of continuous infusion of vincristine and doxorubicin given over 4 days, more than 75% of patients express P-gp on their tumor cells. Epstein and colleagues, using the C219 monoclonal antibody and flow cytometry, found that most patients who failed VAD treatment had P-gp-positive myeloma cells.[56] In multiple myeloma, the development of MDR appears to be acquired and related to the type of chemotherapy received.

MULTIDRUG RESISTANCE IN SOLID TUMORS

The incidence of MDR in human tumors was first shown in a series of five ovarian cancer patients who had undergone chemotherapy before surgery. In the study, Bell and coworkers found two tumors exhibiting overproduction of P-gp as revealed by Western blot analysis using the monoclonal antibody C219.[17] Since this first paper appeared in 1985, several studies have been performed using various methods of detection to determine the incidence of MDR in solid tumors. The largest study performed was reported by Goldstein and colleagues.[19] These investigators studied over 400 human cancers and were able to group tumors into four groups based on their level of expression of MDR1 RNA (Table 69–22). Not surprisingly, tumors that had a high level of *MDR1* message tended to originate from normal cells that were also known to express high levels. These tumors included most untreated colon cancers, renal carcinomas, hepatoma, adrenal cortical carcinoma, pheochromocytoma, islet cell tumors of the pancreas, and carcinoid tumors. Tumors that occasionally expressed *MDR1* were neuroblastoma, breast cancer, and bladder cancer. Those untreated cancers that rarely if ever expressed *MDR1* were esophageal carcinoma, gastric carcinoma, head and neck cancer, Wilms' tumor, and ovarian cancer. The investigators found that posttreatment relapsed breast cancers, pheochromocytoma, and neuroblastoma had increased levels of *MDR1* expression.

Perhaps the most impressive studies demonstrating the value of P-gp as a prognostic factor comes from the retrospective studies of Chan and associates.[57] These investigators studied 30 cases of rhabdomyosarcoma and undifferentiated sarcoma from children. P-gp was detected in 9 patients, 4 at diagnosis and 5 at subsequent biopsy. All 9 patients who had P-gp-positive tumors relapsed after chemotherapy. Of the 20 patients who had P-gp-negative tumors and responded to chemotherapy, only 1 relapsed. The overall probability of survival was significantly different in these two groups of patients with childhood soft tissue sarcoma.

TABLE 69–22. Expression of *MDR1* in Untreated Solid Tumors

Tumor	No. of Samples	Percent Positive
Tumors With Moderate to High Expression		
Colon	41	85
Renal	50	80
Hepatoma	12	100
Adrenocortical	9	77
Pheochromocytoma	20	75
Islet cell	4	50
Carcinoid	9	77
Tumors With Low Expression		
Breast	57	15
Bladder	6	16
Esophageal	14	0
Gastric	2	0
Head and Neck	14	0
Melanoma	3	0
Ovarian	16	0
Prostate	3	0
Thyroid	4	0
Wilms' Tumor	20	0

(Modified from Goldstein LJ, Galski H, Fojo A, et al. Expression of a multidrug resistance gene in human cancers. JNCI 1989;81:116–124)

Similar results have been reported in children with neuroblastoma.[58] Tumors positive for P-gp as detected by immunocytochemistry predicted for poor response to chemotherapy compared with P-gp negative tumors. Relapse-free survival and overall survival were also worse in patients whose tumors were positive for P-gp. Although these studies were retrospective, they provide strong preliminary evidence that P-gp is an important prognostic factor in these childhood solid tumors.

Studies to detect P-gp in breast cancer have produced interesting results regarding level of expression and stage of disease. Several studies using various methods, including immunodetection or measurement of RNA, have shown that the level of expression in breast cancer is relatively low.[59,60] However, two studies, both involving locally advanced breast cancer, have shown that most patients express P-gp on their tumors. Using the C219 monoclonal antibody, Ro and colleagues observed frequent expression of P-gp in tumors after preoperative chemotherapy.[61] This expression was significantly associated with a poor response to chemotherapy. In a second study by Verrelle and coworkers,[62] the expression of P-gp in locally advanced breast cancer was analyzed using immunohistochemical staining with the monoclonal antibody C494, which is considered specific for the MDR1 protein.[22] This study of 20 previously untreated patients found a surprisingly high incidence of P-gp expression in tumor cells from patients with primary, locally advanced breast cancer. Eighty-five percent of the patients expressed P-gp in at least some of their tumor cells. Seven patients who had a high degree of staining in most tumor cells had a worse prognosis, with fewer patients responding to therapy and with shorter durations of response.

These studies demonstrate that, as a tumor grows, there may be a higher likelihood of expressing P-gp. The numbers of patients in these studies were small, and confirmatory studies are necessary.

Cordon-Cardo and colleagues studied 22 patients with non-small cell lung cancers using an immunohistochemical stain.[63] Only two of the 22 lung cancers showed any positive staining cells in the tumor. A similar study by Lai and associates found very low levels of MDR1 RNA in small cell and non-small cell lung cancers.[64] It would appear that MDR1 expression plays an insignificant role in drug resistance in lung cancer.

REVERSING MULTIDRUG RESISTANCE

Efforts to overcome drug resistance that can be attributed to overexpression of MDR1 include several possibilities: the use of high-dose chemotherapy to increase intracellular concentrations; the use of noncross-resistant regimens as proposed by the Goldie-Coldman hypothesis; targeting P-gp-positive cells with monoclonal antibodies or conjugates; and the use of chemosensitizing agents or agents that are able to inhibit the function of P-gp. This last approach has received much attention in the laboratory and in the clinic. Tsuruo and colleagues observed that the calcium channel blocker verapamil was able to overcome resistance in vivo and in vitro to vincristine and doxorubicin.[65] Since the initial observation of Tsuruo and coworkers, a great deal of effort has been devoted to identifying other chemosensitizing agents capable of reversing MDR.[66,67]

All of these agents have been identified empirically, and several them are listed in Table 69–23. These agents share the property of inhibiting anticancer drug binding to P-gp, blocking enhanced drug efflux and allowing increased intracellular concentrations of the anticancer drug (Fig. 69–27).[7,8,9] Exactly how these chemosensitizing agents inhibit P-gp function is unknown, but it has been shown that the chemosensitizers themselves bind to P-gp.[68,69] What is not clear is the nature of the P-gp binding sites. It is unknown whether the chemosensitizers share binding sites with anticancer drugs or whether these agents inhibit P-gp function through allosteric changes. Because some of these agents can modulate calcium metabolism (e.g., verapamil, trifluoperazine), it is possible that the MDR reversal effect is mediated by indirect means, through modulation of calcium-dependent P-gp phosphorylation.[70]

The effect of chemosensitizers such as verapamil and cyclosporine on cytotoxic drug accumulation has been investigated in tumor cells from patients with drug-resistant disease.[36,71,72] In these studies of patients with hematologic neoplasms, verapamil increased the accumulation of vincristine or daunorubicin. In studies of patients with myeloma or acute lymphocytic leukemia, verapamil increased drug accumulation in cells shown to express P-gp.[36,71] In a study by Nooter and colleagues, cyclosporin A was more effective than verapamil in increasing daunorubicin intracellular accumulation in leukemic cells from patients with acute nonlymphocytic leukemia.[72] The degree of cyclosporin-A-induced increase in daunorubicin accumulation correlated with the levels of overexpression of the MDR1 gene in these leukemic cells. This in vitro analysis of human leukemic cells obtained from patients with drug-resistant, P-gp-positive disease demonstrated that drug accumulation can be increased by chemosensitizers such as verapamil and cyclosporin A. What remains to be demonstrated, however, is an increase in cellular drug accumulation when chemosensitizers are given in the clinical situation.

With the evidence that P-gp overexpression occurs in patients with drug-resistant diseases, pilot studies have been conducted to determine if verapamil is capable of overcoming

TABLE 69–23. Chemosensitizers Known to Modulate P-glycoprotein Function

Chemical Class	Example
Calcium channel blockers	Verapamil
Calmodulin inhibitors	Trifluoperazine
Indole alkaloids	Reserpine
Quinolines	Quinine
Lysosomotropic agents	Chloroquine
Steroids	Progesterone
Triparanol analogs	Tamoxifen
Detergents	Cremophor EL
Cyclic peptide antibiotics	Cyclosporines

(Citations for individual agents can be found in Beck WT. Modulators of P-glycoprotein associated multidrug resistance. In: Ozols RF, ed. Drug resistance, vol. II. Norwell, MA: Kluwer Academic Publishers, 1991)

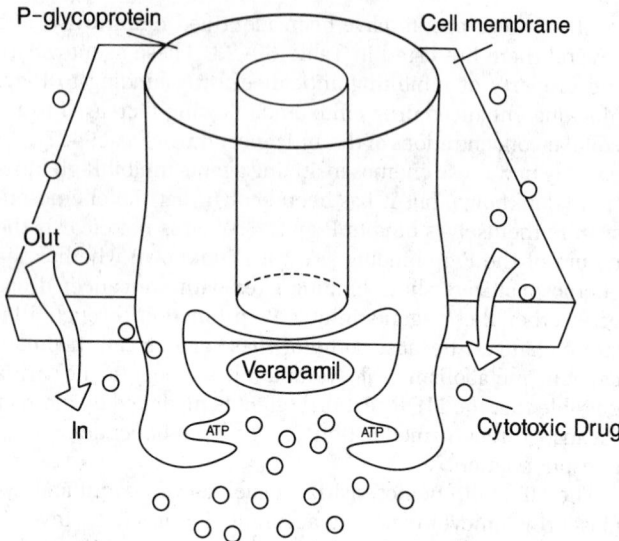

FIGURE 69–27.   Chemosensitizers, such as verapamil, may block the enhanced efflux of cytotoxic drugs by directly binding to P-glycoprotein and inhibiting its function.

clinical drug resistance.[71,73–78] Benson and associates reported preliminary findings of a phase I study investigating the combination of vinblastine and verapamil in 17 patients with solid tumors.[73] Both verapamil and vinblastine were given as continuous infusion for 5 days. Cardiac toxicity was dose limiting, and there was no augmentation of vinblastine toxicity. In a similar study, Ozols and colleagues examined the combination of intravenous verapamil with doxorubicin in 8 patients who had drug-resistant ovarian cancer.[75] No patients benefitted from this treatment, and cardiac toxicity was dose limiting.

In a study of multiple myeloma patients with drug-resistant disease by Dalton and coworkers, 5 of 7 patients overexpressed P-gp on their tumor cells as determined by immunohistochemical staining and RNA analysis.[71] All patients had developed progressive disease while receiving a regimen containing vincristine and daunorubicin (VAD). At the time of progressive disease, continuous infusion verapamil was added to the VAD regimen. Two of the 7 patients who were refractory to VAD alone responded after verapamil was added to the regimen. Both patients who responded had P-gp-positive tumors. In two patients whose tumors overexpressed P-gp, verapamil increased the intracellular accumulation of vincristine or doxorubicin in vitro. This study has been expanded to 22 patients, with 5 patients showing a partial response.[76] Durations of response have been short, with a median response duration of 5.4 months. Two other studies using verapamil as a chemosensitizing agent have been reported in preliminary form in patients with drug-resistant myeloma.[77,78]

In a report by Gore and colleagues, 7 patients who were resistant to 4-day continuous infusion vincristine and doxorubicin were administered a low dose of verapamil by continuous infusion.[77] Four of 7 patients had a further reduction in paraprotein levels of greater than 25%. Two patients had a greater than 50% response with the addition of verapamil to the chemotherapeutic regimen. A second preliminary report by Trumper and associates studied 10 patients who had developed drug-resistant myeloma.[78] Only 1 of 10 patients re-

sponded after verapamil was added to the VAD regimen. Based on these pilot studies, prospective, randomized, controlled studies are indicated. A prospective randomized study is being conducted by the Southwest Oncology Group to determine the value of adding verapamil to the VAD chemotherapy regimen.

A similar pilot study was conducted in patients with drug-resistant non-Hodgkin's lymphoma.[52] Verapamil was administered as a continuous 5-day infusion at escalating doses until dose-limiting cardiotoxicity intervened. The verapamil was combined with cyclophosphamide and a 4-day infusion of vincristine and doxorubicin and oral dexamethasone. Patients were carefully selected for drug resistance based on disease progression while receiving combination chemotherapy or a relapse within 3 months of receiving doxorubicin and vincristine-containing chemotherapy regimen. Clinical drug resistance was confirmed by a high incidence of *MDR1* expression. Five complete remissions (28%) and eight partial remissions (44%) were observed among 18 patients studied. Cardiovascular side effects observed most frequently included first-degree heart block, hypotension, sinus bradycardia, and junctional rhythms.[79] Effects on mean arterial pressure, heart rate, and PR interval were time- and dose-related. Severe, symptomatic congestive heart failure was rarely observed. The most common noncardiovascular side effects were constipation, peripheral edema, and weight gain.

From these studies it can be concluded that the cardiovascular side effects associated with continuous, high-dose intravenous verapamil therapy are significant and dose limiting. Further research is clearly needed to develop less toxic and more efficacious chemosensitizers to be used clinically.

Clinical studies using other chemosensitizers listed in Table 69–23 have been reported. Miller and colleagues reported that the calmodulin inhibitor, trifluoperazine, was capable of causing a second response to doxorubicin in patients who had received this drug in prior regimens.[80] Drug-limiting toxicity was due to extrapyramidal site effects commonly seen with trifluoperazine. Trump and coworkers reported a phase I clinical trial of high-dose oral tamoxifen administered in conjunction with 5-day continuous infusion vinblastine.[81] Neurotoxicity was dose limiting and resolved rapidly when tamoxifen was discontinued. There was no indication that tamoxifen enhanced the expected toxicity of vinblastine. Like verapamil, the dose-limiting toxicities of these potential chemosensitizers have been attributed to the inherent toxicity of the chemosensitizer and not due to enhanced chemotherapy toxicity.

Theoretically, chemosensitizers may alter or enhance the toxicity of chemotherapeutic drugs by inhibiting the function of P-gp in normal tissues, including the kidney, liver, colon, and capillary endothelial cells of the brain. Preliminary studies using high doses of cyclosporin A as a chemosensitizer found hyperbilirubinemia as a side effect.[82–84] This toxic effect may be related to cyclosporin A inhibiting the normal function of P-gp in hepatic biliary canaliculi.[23] A phase II study of epidoxorubicin plus cyclosporin A in patients with colorectal cancer observed a greater than expected frequency of severe neutropenia.[85] P-gp occurs in normal hematopoietic (CD34 positive) precursor cells.[11] High doses of cyclosporin A may have increased intracellular concentrations of epidoxorubicin in this hematopoietic compartment, resulting in severe neutropenia. A second explanation for this enhanced toxicity may be changes in clearance of the cytotoxic drug by cyclosporin A. Studies of cyclosporin A plus etoposide have reported a prolonged clearance of etoposide when cyclosporin A was added.[82] These studies illustrate the importance of measuring pharmacokinetics of chemosensitizers and cytotoxic drugs in clinical trials so that therapeutic and toxicity results may be interpreted correctly.

Strategies for developing new chemosensitizing agents are outlined in Table 69–24. Currently, compounds are screened for activity on an empiric basis using in vitro cytotoxicity assays. Promising agents are then evaluated in in vivo models to determine the therapeutic index and efficacy. Studies of structure-activity relations of chemosensitizers performed by Beck and colleagues have demonstrated that modulators of P-gp are usually lipid soluble at physiologic pH and possess a basic nitrogen atom and at least one planar aromatic ring.[86,87] Notable exceptions to these generalities exist (*e.g.*, cyclosporin A). Rationale drug design by molecular modeling as proposed by Beck and colleagues should ultimately provide more effective and less toxic chemosensitizers, but more basic information about P-gp binding sites and exactly how P-gp exports anticancer drugs is needed.[86]

One approach to reducing toxicity is to develop stereoisomers of effective chemosensitizers that have fewer side effects. Both the R and S optical isomers of verapamil are equally effective in reversing MDR, but the R isomer is 10 times less cardiotoxic than the S isomer.[88] Clinical studies are using R-verapamil as a chemosensitizer. The optical isomers quinine and quinidine also appear to have equal activity in reversing resistance. Quinine is less toxic than quinidine, and the therapeutic index for quinine may be superior in the clinical setting.[89]

A transgenic mouse was developed for testing agents as potential chemosensitizers in reversing drug resistance. In this model developed by Mickisch and associates, transgenic mice express the multidrug resistance gene in their bone marrow cells and are resistant to leukopenia induced by natural products such as anthracyclines.[90] This drug resistance can be circumvented in a dose-dependent manner by simultaneous administration of agents such as verapamil and quinine. This *MDR1*-transgenic mouse model may serve as a reliable system for evaluating the bioactivity of potential chemosensitizing agents.

TABLE 69–24. Strategies for Developing Chemosensitizers to Overcome Multidrug Resistance

1. Drug screening of candidate drugs
   A. Evaluate efficacy using in vitro cytotoxicity assays with drug-resistant cell lines and short-term cultures of fresh tumor specimens
   B. Determine therapeutic index by analyzing in vivo activity in murine tumors, xenografts, or transgenic mouse models
2. Develop analogs of known chemosensitizers for
   A. Molecular modeling
   B. Structural activity relations
3. Identify P-glycoprotein binding sites by
   A. Biochemical methods—competitive photoaffinity labeling experiments
   B. Molecular methods—effect of P-glycoprotein site-directed metagenesis on drug binding

TABLE 69–25. Clinical Evaluation of Chemosensitizing Agents to Overcome Multidrug Resistance

1. Select promising agents from preclinical screening (see Table 69-23)
2. Phase I trials of chemosensitizing (CS) agent plus chemotherapy
   A. Determine maximal tolerated dose of CS for phase II trials
   B. Evaluate pharmacokinetics of CS (serum levels of CS agent should approximate levels known to be active in vitro)
3. Phase II trials of CS agent plus chemotherapy
   A. Choose tumor types known to be associated with MDR
   B. Monitor P-glycoprotein before and after therapy
   C. Monitor pharmacokinetic levels of both CS and chemotherapy
4. Phase III trials of CS agent plus chemotherapy in MDR-positive tumors
   A. Patients randomized to chemotherapy alone versus chemotherapy plus CS. Consider cross-over design for patients receiving chemotherapy alone to chemotherapy plus CS at time of progressive disease
   B. Monitor P-glycoprotein levels before and after therapy

After a promising potential chemosensitizing agent has been identified by a preclinical means, it is important to design clinical trials so that meaningful data may be obtained regarding potential activity of chemosensitizing agents (Table 69–25). In phase I trials, it is important to perform pharmacokinetic analyses of the chemosensitizers to ensure that levels required for activity in vitro can be obtained clinically. If toxicity of the chemosensitizer plus chemotherapy is acceptable and adequate concentrations of the chemosensitizer are obtained, phase II testing may be performed. Cancers known to be associated with MDR and P-gp should be treated in phase II trials, and analysis for P-gp in individual patients enrolled in study should be attempted. Pharmacokinetic analysis of anticancer drugs would be helpful in determining if chemosensitizers alter the physiologic disposition of anticancer drugs. Ultimately, phase III testing of the chemosensitizer and chemotherapy will be required to determine if treatment outcome is improved in specific diseases by the use of chemosensitizers.

Tumors that are considered drug-sensitive at diagnosis but acquire an MDR phenotype at relapse pose an interesting problem for protocol design. It is unclear how these initially drug-sensitive tumors become P-gp positive at relapse, but tumor heterogeneity and cell selection by cytotoxic drugs presumably play a role. At diagnosis, only a minority of tumor cells may express P-gp and treatment with chemotherapy provides a selection advantage for the few cells that are P-gp positive early in the course of disease. An alternative explanation is that natural-product-derived chemotherapy actually induces the expression of *MDR1*, leading to P-pg-positive tumors at relapse. A possible therapeutic approach to tumors that acquire MDR is outlined in Table 69–26. Using chemosensitizers early in the course of disease may prevent the emergence of MDR by eliminating the few cells that are P-gp positive at the beginning. In vitro studies have shown that selection of drug-resistant cells by combining verapamil and doxorubicin does prevent the emergence of P-gp, but that an alternative drug resistance mechanism develops, which is secondary to altered topoisomerase II function.[91]

Reasons for possible failure of chemosensitizers to reverse

TABLE 69–26. Possible Approaches to Overcoming Clinical Multidrug Resistance in Tumors With Acquired Drug Resistance

1. Use chemosensitizers plus natural product agents (*e.g.,* anthracyclines, vinca alkaloids) as initial treatment to prevent *MDR* overexpression.
2. Follow with noncross-resistant drugs, such as antimetabolites and alkylating agents.
3. Consider high-dose chemotherapy as a form of consolidation therapy.
4. Use biologics or differentiating agents as maintenance therapy.

clinical MDR as shown in Table 69–27. Other mechanisms of natural product resistance may emerge after treatment with cytotoxic drugs and chemosensitizers. One such non-P-gp mechanism is due to altered topoisomerase II function that may confer resistance to anthracycline and epipodophyllotoxins.[92] A second mechanism of MDR that involved enhanced drug efflux but is non-P-gp mediated has also been described.[93,94] This mechanism of drug resistance due to enhanced drug efflux is unaffected by verapamil or other commonly known chemosensitizers. The clinical relevance of these alternative drug resistance mechanisms remains to be determined.

CONCLUSIONS

There are many ways by which a cancer may develop drug resistance at the cellular level. Clinical studies suggest that a common form of multidrug resistance in human cancers results from the expression of the *MDR1* gene that encodes for P-gp. This glycoprotein functions as a plasma membrane, energy-dependent, multidrug efflux pump that reduces the intracellular concentration of cytotoxic drugs. This mechanism of resistance may account for de novo resistance in common tumors, such as colon cancer and renal cancer, and for acquired resistance, as observed in common hematologic tumors such as acute nonlymphocytic leukemia and malignant lymphomas. Although this type of drug resistance may be common, it is by no means the only mechanism by which cells become drug resistant.

With the understanding that P-gp is a common mechanism of drug resistance in certain tumors, it is reasonable to try to prevent or circumvent this form of resistance. Pilot studies

TABLE 69–27. Possible Reasons for Failure of Chemosensitizers to Reverse Clinical Multidrug Resistance

1. Levels of the chemosensitizing agents are inadequate at the tumor site.
2. Levels of P-glycoprotein increase as the tumor progresses.
3. The *MDR1* gene mutates, resulting in decreased binding of the chemosensitizing agent to P-glycoprotein.
4. Alternative non-P-glycoprotein mechanisms of resistance emerge during treatment that are unaffected by chemosensitizers.

using chemosensitizers indicate that these agents may reverse resistance in a subset of patients. These same preliminary studies also indicate that drug resistance is multifactoral, because not all drug-resistant patients have P-gp-positive tumor cells and only a few patients appear to benefit from the use of chemosensitizers. The development of more efficacious and less toxic agents may improve the therapeutic outcome when they are added to cytotoxic drugs.

To define the role of chemosensitizers in reversing multidrug resistance in the clinic, it will be important to perform randomized, prospective, controlled clinical trials. Factors that should be considered in designing these trials include the type of tumor studied, which should have a high expression of P-gp, de novo or acquired; the presence or absence of P-gp on patients' tumor cells at the time of administering chemosensitizers; and the type and dose of chemosensitizer used. Only after demonstrating efficacy in well-designed clinical trials can the use of chemosensitizers be integrated into the everyday practice of clinical oncology.

REFERENCES

1. DeVita VT. The problem of resistance. PPO Updates 1990;4:11.
2. Goldie JH, Coldman AJ. Genetic instability in the development of drug resistance. JNCI 1989;81:116–124.
3. Pastan I, Gottesman M. Multiple-drug resistance in human cancer. N Engl J Med 1987;316:1388–1393.
4. Bradley G, Guranka PF, Ling V. Mechanisms of multidrug resistance. Biochem Biophys Acta 1988;948:87–128.
5. Assaraf YG, Molina A, Schimke RT. Sequential amplification of dihydrofolate reductase and multidrug resistance genes in Chinese hamster ovary cells selected for stepwise resistance to the lipid-soluble antifolate trimetrexate. J Biol Chem 1989;264:18324–18326.
6. Dalton WS, Durie BGM, Alberts DS, Gerlach JH, Cress AE. Characterization of a new drug resistant human myeloma cell line which expresses P-glycoprotein. Cancer Res 1986;46:5125–5130.
7. Higgins CF, Hiles ID, Salmond PC, et al. A family of related ATP-binding submits coupled to many distinct biological processes in bacteria. Nature 1986;323:448–450.
8. Gros P, Croop J, Housman D. Mammalian multidrug resistance gene: Complete cDNA sequence indicates strong homology to bacterial transport proteins. Cell 1986;47:371–380.
9. Gerlach JH, Endicott JA, Juranka PF, et al. Homology between P-glycoprotein and a bacterial hemolysin transport protein suggests a model for multidrug resistance. Nature 1986;316:820.
10. Fojo AT, Ueda K, Slamon DJ, et al. Expression of a multidrug resistance gene in human tumors and tissues. Proc Natl Acad Sci USA 1987;84:265–269.
11. Chaudhary PM, Roninson IB. Expression and activity of P-glycoprotein, a multidrug efflux pump, in human hematopoietic stem cells. Cell 1991;66:85–94.
12. List AF, Spier CM, Cline A, et al. Expression of the multidrug resistance gene product (P-glycoprotein) in myelodysplasia is associated with a stem cell phenotype. Br J Haematol 1991;78:28–34.
13. Thiebaut F, Tsuruo T, Hamada H, et al. Cellular localization of the multidrug-resistance gene product P-glycoprotein in normal human tissues. Proc Natl Acad Sci USA 1987;84:7735–7738.
14. Cordon-Cardo C, O'Brien JP, Casals D, et al. Multidrug-resistance gene (P-glycoprotein) is expressed by endothelial cells at blood-brain barrier sites. Proc Natl Acad Sci 1989;86:695–698.
15. Fuqua SAW, Moretti-Rojas IM, Schneider SL, et al. P-glycoprotein expression in human breast cancer cells. Cancer Res 1987;47:2103–2106.
16. Dalton WS, Grogan TM. Does P-glycoprotein predict response to chemotherapy, and if so, is there a reliable way to detect it? JNCI 1991;83:80–81.
17. Bell DR, Gerlach JH, Kartner N, et al. P-glycoprotein expression in ovarian cancer: Evidence for multidrug resistance. J Clin Oncol 1985;3:311–315.
18. Gerlach JH, Bell DR, Karakousis C, et al. P-glycoprotein in human sarcoma: Evidence for multidrug resistance. J Clin Oncol 1987;5:1452–1460.
19. Goldstein LJ, Galski H, Fojo A, et al. Expression of a multidrug resistance gene in human cancers. JNCI 1989;81:116–124.
20. Chabner BA, Fojo A. Multidrug resistance: P-glycoprotein and its allies—the elusive foes. JNCI 1989;81:910–913.
21. Kartner N, Evernden-Porelle D, Bradley G, et al. Detection of P-glycoprotein in multidrug-resistant cell lines by monoclonal antibodies. Nature 1985;316:820–823.
22. Georges E, Bradley G, Gariepy J, et al. Detection of P-glycoprotein isoforms by gene-specific monoclonal antibodies. Proc Natl Acad Sci USA 1990;87:152–156.
23. Thiebaut F, Tsuruo T, Hamada H, et al. Immunohistochemical localization in normal

tissues of different epitopes in a multidrug transport protein P170: Evidence for localization in brain capillaries and crossreactivity of one antibody with a muscle protein. J Histochem Cytochem 1989;37:159–164.

24. Scheper RJ, Bulte JWM, Brakke JGP, et al. Monoclonal antibody JSB-1 detects a highly conserved epitope on the P-glycorptoein associated with multi-drug-resistance. Int J Cancer 1988;42:389–394.

25. Schinkel AH, Roelofs MEM, Borst P. Characterization of the human MDR3 P-glycoprotein and its recognition by PGP-specific monoclonal antibodies. Cancer Res 1991;51:2628–2635.

26. Hamada H, Tsuruo T. Functional role for the 170- to 180-kDa glycoprotein specific to drug-resistant tumor cells revealed by monoclonal antibodies. Proc Natl Acad Sci USA 1986;83:7785–7789.

27. Weinstein RS, Kuszak JR, Kluskens LF, Coon JS. P-glycoproteins in pathology: The multidrug resistance gene family in humans. Human Pathol 1990;21:34–48.

28. Chan HSL, Bradley G, Thorner P, et al. A sensitive method for immunocytochemical detection of P-glycoprotein in multidrug-resistant human ovarian carcinoma cell lines. Lab Invest 1988;59:870–875.

29. Dalton WS, Grogan TM, Rybski JA, et al. Immunohistochemical detection and quantitation of P-glycoprotein in multiple drug-resistant human myeloma cells: Association with level of drug resistance and drug accumulation. Blood 1989;73:747–752.

30. Grogan TN, Dalton WS, Rybski J, et al. Optimization of immunocytochemical P-glycoprotein assessment in multidrug resistant plasma cell myeloma using 3 antibodies. Lab Invest 1991;63:815–824.

31. Saiki RK, Scharf S, Faloona F, et al. Enzymatic amplification of β-globin genomic sequences and restriction site analysis for diagnosis of sickle cell anemia. Science 1985;230:1350–1354.

32. Noonan KE, Beck C, Holzmayer TA, et al. Quantitative analysis of MDR1 (multidrug resistance) gene expression in human tumors by polymerase chain reaction. Proc Natl Acad Sci USA 1990;87:7160–7164.

33. Murphy LD, Herzog CE, Rudick JB, Tito Fojo A, Bates SE. Use of the polymerase chain reaction in the quantitation of the *mdr1* gene expression. Biochemistry 1990;29:10351–10356.

34. Futscher BW, Blake LL, Grogan TM, Dalton WS. Quantitative PCR analysis of *mdr1* expression in clinical specimens. Anal Biochem 1993 (in press).

35. Champlin R, Gale RP. Acute lymphoblastic leukemia in recent advances in biology and therapy. Blood 1989;73:2051–2066.

36. Rothenberg ML, Mickley LA, Cole DE, et al. Expression of the *mdr1*/P-170 gene in patients with acute lymphoblastic leukemia. Blood 1989;74:1388–1395.

37. Musto P, Melillo L, Lombardi G, Matera R, Di Giorgio G, Carotenuto M. High risk of early resistant relapse for leukemic patients with presence of multidrug resistance associated P-glycoprotein positive cells in complete remission. Br J Haematol 1991;77:50–53.

38. Herweijer H, Sonneveld P, Baas F, Nooter K. Expression of mdr1 and mdr3 multidrug-resistance genes in human acute and chronic leukemias and association with stimulation of drug accumulation by cyclosporine. JNCI 1990;82:1133–1140.

39. Kato S, Ideguchi H, Muta K, Nishimura J, Nawata H. Mechanisms involved in the development of Adriamycin resistance in human leukemias. Leuk Res 1990;14:567–573.

40. Mattern J, Efferth T, Back M, Ho AD, Volm M. Detection of P-glycoprotein in human leukemias using monoclonal antibodies. Blut 1989;58:215–217.

41. Kuwazuru Y, Hanada S, Furukawa T, et al. Expression of P-glycoprotein in adult T-cell leukemia cells. Blood 1990;76:2065–2071.

42. Champlin R, Gale RP. Acute myelogenous leukemia: Recent advances in therapy. Blood 1987;69:1551–1562.

43. Kokenberg E, Sonneveld P, Delwel R, Sizoo W, Hagenbeek A, Lowenberg B. In vivo uptake of daunorubicin by acute myeloid leukemia (AML) cells measured by flow cytometry. Leukemia 1988;2:511–517.

44. Sato H, Preisler H, Day R, et al. Mdr1 transcript levels as an indication of resistant disease in acute myelogenous leukemia. Br J Haematol 1990;75:340–345.

45. Holmes J, Jacobs A, Carter G, Janowska-Wieczorek A, Padua RA. Multidrug resistance in haemapoietic cell lines, myelodysplastic syndromes and acute myeloblastic leukemia. Br J Haematol 1989;72:40–44.

46. Ito Y, Tanimoto M, Kumazawa T, et al. Increased P-glycoprotein expression and multidrug-resistant gene (mdr1) amplification are infrequently found in fresh acute leukemia cells: Sequential analysis of 15 cases at initial presentation in relapse stage. Cancer 1989;63:1534–1538.

47. Nooter K, Sonneveld P, Oostrum R, Herweijer H, Hagenbeek T, Valerio D. Overexpression of the mdr1 gene in blast cells from patients with acute myelocytic leuekmia is associated with decreased anthracycline accumulation that can be restored by cyclosporine. Int J Cancer 1990;45:263–268.

48. Holmes JA, Jacobs A, Carter G, et al. Is the *mdr1* gene relevant in chronic lymphocytic leukemia? Leukemia 1990;4:216–218.

49. Cumber PM, Jacobs A, Hay T, Fisher J, Whittaker JA, Tsuruo T. Expression of the MDR gene (*mdr1*) and epitope masking in chronic lymphatic leukemia. Br J Haematol 1990;76:226–230.

50. Tsuruo T, Sugimoto Y, Hamada H, et al. Detection of multidrug resistance markers, P-glycoprotein and *mdr1* mRNA, in human leukemia cells. Jpn J Cancer Res 1987;78:1415–1419.

51. Carulli G, Petrini M, Marini A, et al. P-glycorptoein in acute nonlymphoblastic leukemia and in the blastic crisis of myeloid leukemia. N Engl J Med 1988;319:797–798.

52. Miller TP, Grogan TM, Dalton WS, Spier CM, Scheper RJ, Salmon SE. P-glycoprotein expression in malignant lymphoma and reversal of clinical drug resistance with chemotherapy plus high dose verapamil. J Clin Oncol 1991;9:17–24.

53. Kyle RA. Diagnosis and management of multiple myeloma and related disorders. Prog Hematol 1986;14:257–282.

54. Buzaid AC, Durie BGM. Management of refractory myeloma: A review. J Clin Oncol 1988;6:889–905.

55. Grogan TM, Spier CM, Salmon SE, et al. P-glycoprotein expression in human plasma cell myeloma: An acquired trait related to prior chemotherapy. Blood 1993 (in press).

56. Epstein J, Xiao H, Oba BK. P-glycoprotein expression in plasma-cell myeloma is associated with resistance to VAD. Blood 1989;74:913–917.

57. Chan HSL, Thorner PS, Haddad G, Ling V. Immunohistochemical detection of P-glycoprotein: Prognostic correlation is soft tissue sarcoma of childhood. J Clin Oncol 1990;8:689–704.

58. Chan HSL, Haddad G, Thorner PS, et al. P-glycoprotein expression as a predictor of the outcome of therapy for neuroblastoma. N Engl J Med 1991;325:1608–1614.

59. Merkel DE, Fuqua SAW, Tandon AK, et al. Electrophoretic analysis of 248 clinical breast cancer specimens for P-glycoprotein overexpression or gene amplification. J Clin Oncol 1989;7:1129–1136.

60. Schneider J, Bak M, Efferth TH, et al. P-glycoprotein expression in treated and untreated human breast cancer. Br J Cancer 1989;60:815–818.

61. Ro J, Sahin A, Ro JY, et al. Immunohistochemical analysis of P-glycoprotein expression correlated with chemotherapy resistance in locally advanced breast cancer. Hum Pathol 1990;21:787–791.

62. Verrelle P, Meissonnier F, Fonck Y, et al. Clinical relevance of immunohistochemical detection of multidrug resistance P-glycoprotein in breast carcinoma. JNCI 1991;83:111–116.

63. Cordon-Cardo C, O'Brien JP, Boccia J, Casals D, Bertino JR, Melamed MR. Expression of the multidrug resistance gene product (P-glycoprotein) in human normal and tumor tissues. J Histochem Cytochem 1990;38:1277–1287.

64. Lai S-L, Goldstein LJ, Gottesman MM, et al. *MDR1* gene expression in lung cancer. JNCI 1989;81:1144–1150.

65. Tsuruo T, Iida H, Tsukagoshi S, et al. Overcoming of vincristine resistance in P388 leukemia in vivo and in vitro through enhanced cytotoxicity of vincristine and vinblastine by verapamil. Cancer Res 1981;41:1967–1972.

66. Kessel D, Wilberding C. Anthracycline resistance in P388 murine leukemia and its circumvention by calcium antagonists. Cancer Res 1985;45:1687–1691.

67. Ramu A, Spanier R, Rahaminoff H, et al. Restoration of doxorubicin responsiveness in doxorubicin-resistant P388 murine leukemia cells. Br J Cancer 1984;50:501–507.

68. Yang CPH, Mellado W, Horwitz SB. Azidopine labeling of multidrug resistance-associated glycoproteins. Biochem Pharmacol 1988;37:1417–1421.

69. Safa AR. Photoaffinity labeling of the multidrug resistance-related P-glycoprotein with photoactive analogs of verapamil. Proc Natl Acad Sci USA 1988;85:7187–7191.

70. Hamada H, Hagiwara KI, Nakajima T, et al. Phosphorylation of the 170,000 to 180,000 glycoprotein specific to multidrug-resistant tumor cells: Effects of verapamil, trifluoperazine, and phorbol esters. Cancer Res 1987;47:2860–2865.

71. Dalton WS, Grogan TM, Meltzer PS, et al. Drug-resistance in multiple myeloma and non-Hodgkin's lymphoma: Detection of P-glycoprotein and potential circumvention by addition of verapamil to chemotherapy. J Clin Oncol 1989;7:415–424.

72. Nooter K, Sonneveld P, Oostrum R, Herweijer H, Hagenbeek T, Valerio D. Overexpression of the *mdr1* gene in blast cells from patients with acute myelocytic leukemia is associated with decreased anthracycline accumulation that can be restored by cyclosporin-A. Int J Cancer 1990;45:263–268.

73. Benson AB, Trump DL, Koeller JM, et al. Phase I study of vinblastine and verapamil given by concurrent IV infusion. Cancer Treat Rep 1985;69:795–799.

74. Presant CA, Kennedy PS, Wiseman C, et al. Verapamil reversal of clinical doxorubicin resistance in human cancer. Am J Clin Oncol 1986;9:355–357.

75. Ozols RF, Cunnion RE, Klecker RW, et al. Verapamil and Adriamycin in the treatment of drug-resistant ovarian cancer patients. J Clin Oncol 1987;5:641–647.

76. Salmon SE, Dalton WS, Grogan TM, et al. Multidrug-resistant myeloma: Laboratory and clinical effects of chemosensitizers. Blood 1991;78:44–50.

77. Gore ME, Selby PJ, Millar B, et al. The use of verapamil to overcome drug resistance in myeloma. Proc Am Soc Clin Oncol 1988;7:228.

78. Trumper LH, Ho AD, Wulf G, et al. Addition of verapamil to overcome drug resistance in multiple myeloma. Preliminary clinical observations in 10 patients. J Clin Oncol 1989;7:1578–1579.

79. Pennock GD, Dalton WS, Roeske WR, et al. Systemic toxic effects associated with high dose verapamil infusion and chemotherapy administration. JNCI 1991;83:105–110.

80. Miller RL, Bukowski RM, Budd GT, et al. Clinical modulation of doxorubicin resistance by the calmodulin inhibitor trifluoperazine: A phase I trial. J Clin Oncol 1988;6:880–888.

81. Trump D, Rogers M, Fine R, et al. Phase I trial of high dose Tamoxifen and 5 day infusion of vinblastine as an approach to reverse multidrug resistance. Proc Am Assoc Cancer Res [Abstract] 1990;31:205.

82. Yahanda AM, Adler KM, Hardy R, Brophy NA, Halsey J, Sikic B. A phase I trial of etoposide with cyclosporine as a modulator of multidrug resistance. Proc Am Soc Clin Oncol [Abstract] 1991;10:102.

83. Samuels B, Ratain M, Mick R, et al. Phase I trial of multidrug resistance modulation with cyclosporin-A. Proc Am Assoc Cancer Res [Abstract] 1991;32:195.

84. List AF, Spier C, Greer J, Azar C, Hutter J, Wolff S, Salmon S, Futscher B, Dalton W. Biochemical modulation of anthracycline resistance (MDR) in acute leukemia with cyclosporin-A [Abstract]. Proc Am Soc Clin Oncol [Abstract] 1992;11:264.

85. Verweij J, Herweijer H, Oosterom R, et al. A phase II study of epidoxorubicin in colorectal cancer and the use of cyclosporin-A in an attempt to reverse multidrug resistance. Br J Cancer 1991;64:361–364.

86. Beck WT. Modulators of P-glycoprotein associated multidrug resistance. In: Ozols RF, ed. Drug resistance, vol II. Norwell, MA: Kluwer Academic Publishers, 1991.

87. Zamora JM, Pearce HL, Beck WT. Physical-chemical properties shared by compounds that modulate multidrug resistance in human leukemia cells. Mol Pharmacol 1988;33:454–462.

88. Keilhauer C, Emling F, Raschack M, et al. The use of R-verapamil (R-VPM) is superior to racemic VPM in breaking multidrug resistance (MDR) of malignant cells. Proc Am Assoc Cancer Res 1989;30:503.

89. Lehnert M, Dalton WS, Roe D, Emerson S, Salmon SE. Synergistic inhibition by verapamil and quinine of P-glycoprotein-mediated multidrug resistance in a human myeloma cell line model. Blood 1991;77:348–354.

90. Mickisch GH, Merlino GT, Galski H, Gottesman MM, Pastan I. Transgenic mice that express the human multidrug-resistance gene in bone marrow enable a rapid identification of agents that reverse drug resistance. Proc Natl Acad Sci USA 1991;88:547–551.

91. Dalton WS. Reversing multidrug resistance in the laboratory and clinic. Proc Am Assoc Cancer Res 1990;31:520.

92. Danks MK, Yalowich JC, Beck WT. Atypical multiple drug resistance in a human leukemic cell line selected for resistance to teniposide (VM-26). Cancer Res 1987;47:1297.

93. Dalton WS, Cress AE, Alberts DS, Trent JM. Cytogenetic and phenotypic analysis of a human colon carcinoma cell line resistant to mitoxantrone. Cancer Res 1988;48:1882.

94. Taylor CW, Dalton WS, Parrish PR, et al. Different mechanisms of decreased drug accumulation in doxorubicin and mitoxantrone resistance variants of the MCF7 human breast cancer cell line. Br J Cancer 1991;63:923–929.

SECTION **7**

WILLIAM J.M. HRUSHESKY
GEORG A. BJARNASON

The Application of Circadian Chronobiology to Cancer Chemotherapy

Most clinicians give little thought to the time of day at which a drug is given. In general, patients receive drugs at times that are convenient for the staff administering them. A growing body of data suggests that therapeutic effect may be maximized and toxicity may be minimized if drugs are administered at carefully selected times of the day.[1] This potential for a marked improvement in therapeutic index is especially critical for therapies with narrow ratios of efficacy to toxicity, like most anticancer treatment regimens.[2]

The toxicities of at least 20 chemotherapeutic agents depend on the time of day in murine systems. The anticancer efficacy of many of these agents, given singly or in combinations, depends on circadian factors.[3] Clinical data show that the dosing time of 5-fluorouracil (5-FU), floxuridine, 4'-O-tetrahydropyranyl-doxorubicin, and oxaliplatin markedly affect their toxicities, safely achievable dose intensity, and perhaps their therapeutic efficacy.[4–9] The toxicity and therapeutic efficacy of combination chemotherapy with cisplatin and doxorubicin were found to depend on the time of day that they were administered.[10–12]

This reproducible temporal variability in antitumor effect and normal tissue toxicity can be explained in part by two important observations. First, experimental and clinical studies have documented that the pharmacokinetics of many anticancer drugs (and most other drugs studied) show consistent and reproducible circadian temporal variation, depending on the time of their administration.[1,13–16] Second, most normal tissues are reproducibly rhythmically more or less sensitive to the effects of drugs at specific times of day.[17] Some tumors also exhibit similar rhythmic susceptibility patterns during the circadian cycle.[18,19] These circadian rhythmic variations in drug pharmacokinetics and tissue susceptibility may be exploited to select a time for treatment that results in an increased tumor cell killing and reduced toxicity.

The availability of portable infusion pumps capable of delivering a single or multiple drugs, each with their optimal circadian scheduling, has made the clinical application and testing of these principles possible.

CHRONOBIOLOGY

Chronobiology is the quantitative study of the temporal relations of biologic phenomena. Even the most superficial quantitative study of biodynamics demonstrates that biophysical and biochemical processes vary with respect to time in a regular and predictable periodic manner across several rhythmic frequencies.[20,21] De Mairan's early 18th century observations that the leaves of the mimosa plant open during the day and close at night and that this pattern continues faithfully in constant darkness constitutes an important partial proof of the endogenicity of circadian time structure.[22] Richter further generalized these findings to mammals, documenting the persistence of diurnal activity rhythms in rats housed in constant darkness.[23] In a landmark study, Johnson found that the activity rhythm of animals under constant darkness fit a period different from 24 hours and postulated an internal physiologic rhythm that was not directly dependent on the daily fluctuations of environmental conditions.[24]

Endogenous biologic rhythms have been demonstrated at all biologic levels, from yeasts and nucleated unicells to man, and at all levels of biologic organization, including the entire organism, organ system, organ tissue, cell, and subcellular unit.[20,21,25] Each patient's hospital record demonstrates tight coordination of all vital signs. Figure 69–28 demonstrates the circadian rhythms of activity, pulse, temperature, and systolic, diastolic, and mean blood pressure in a typical person.

The existence of a molecular time-keeping mechanism, "clock-gene," was first inferred for *Drosophila melanogaster* by Konopka and Benzer.[26] Subsequently, molecular biologists used several mutant strains to identify an important "clock gene" that has been named *per* (for period). In several other species (*e.g., Neurospora, Chlamydomonas*), single-gene mutations have been shown to alter such basic clock properties as period length, light entrainability, and temperature compensation.[27,28] A mammalian clock gene mutation was found that dramatically alters the period of the circadian locomotor rhythm of golden hamsters.[29]

There is considerable evidence to suggest that the suprachiasmatic nucleus (SCN) of the hypothalamus is a site of critically important circadian pacemaker cells in mammals. Meijer and Rietveld reviewed this subject.[30] The most definitive experimental evidence for primacy of the SCN in circadian organismic time keeping demonstrates that circadian rhythmicity can be restored to SCN-lesioned arrhythmic hamsters by implantation of fetal brain tissue containing SCN cells.[31–34] Ralph and colleagues demonstrated that small neural grafts from the SCN of normal hamsters and τ-mutant ham-

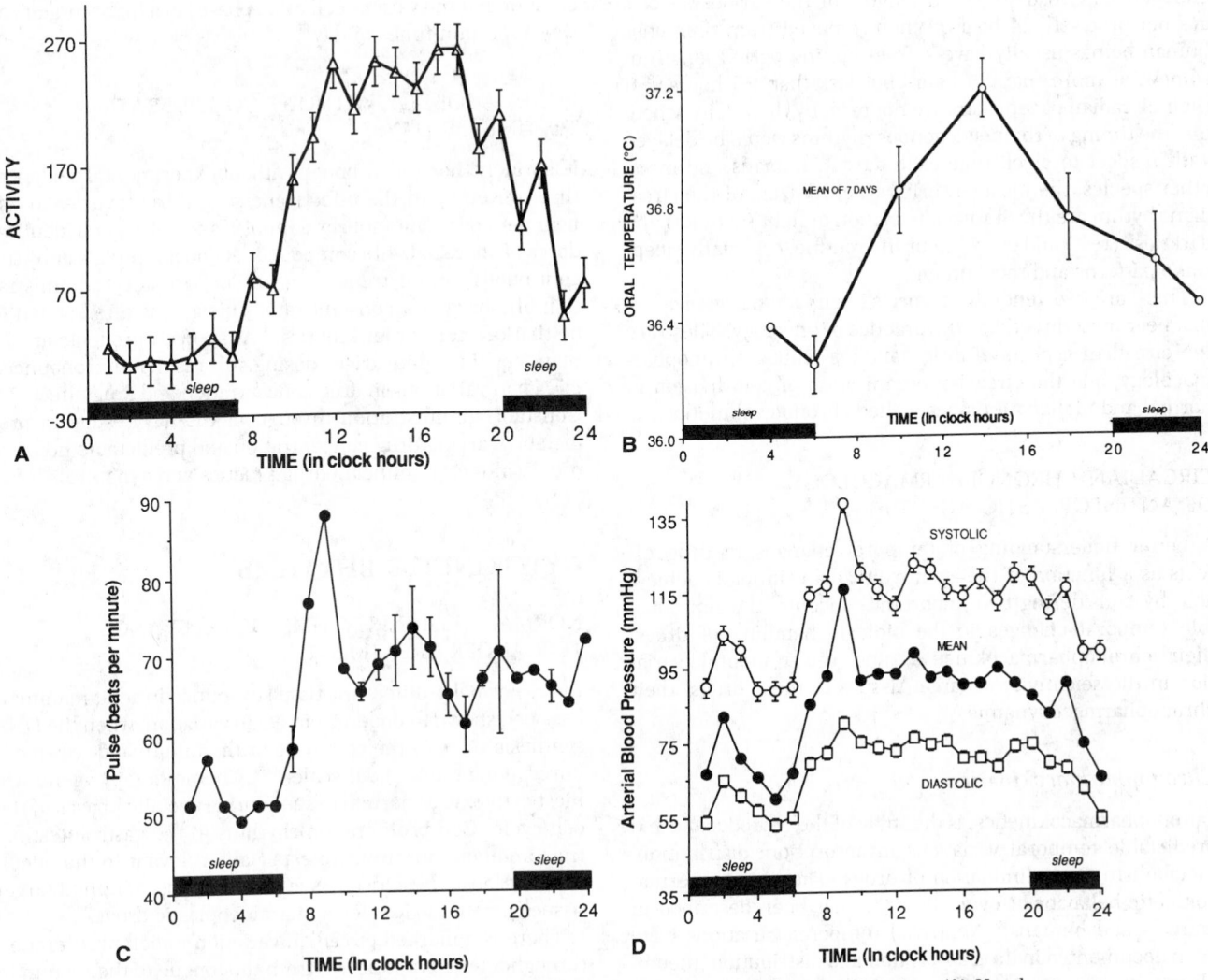

FIGURE 69–28.   All physiologic functions are temporally organized within circadian time. **(A)** Hourly averages of continuously monitored activity. **(B)** Intermittent oral temperature obtained every 4 hours for 7 consecutive days. **(C)** Hourly averages of continuously monitored pulse. **(D)** Hourly averages of continuously monitored systolic, diastolic, and mean arterial blood pressure. The activity pattern documents the sleep onset, wakefulness onset, and amount of activity throughout the day. The temperature pattern documents the daily rise of temperature, which anticipates daily arising, peaks in the afternoon, and falls throughout each night. Pulse and blood pressure behave similarly throughout the day, dropping substantially during sleep and rising sharply after morning arousal. This rapid morning rise in circadian hemodynamic variables has been prominently associated with a high frequency of heart attacks and strokes at this time of day.

sters restored circadian rhythms to arrhythmic animals whose own nucleus had been ablated.[35] The restored rhythms always exhibited the period of the donor genotype.

Genetic time-keeping mechanisms most likely evolved in response to regular variations in physical demands of the environment. The two motive forces for this temporal evolution would be biologic economy and systematic stability. It could be thermodynamically wasteful if not lethal for cellular and organismic tasks to be unordered in time or too easily affected by environmental cycles. The multifrequency resonance structure of living organisms helps to keep the life processes within acceptable homeostatic limits by reinforcing temporal order. Biologic processes are sequential, ordered, and depend on the completion of one event to initiate the next.

At least three major biologic rhythms have been defined

that correspond to obvious periodic changes in the environment: the circadian rhythm (20–28 hours, the solar day); the circatrigintan rhythm (30 ± 7 days, the lunar month); and the circannual rhythm (12 ± 2 months, the year). These three rhythms weave the temporal fabric from which each earth-born organism is tailored, and they have left an indelible imprint on every biologic process. Of each of the biofrequency domains, the circadian rhythm has been most thoroughly investigated. Moore-Ede and coworkers reviewed its potential importance in health and disease.[36,37] The basic properties of biologic rhythms are similar in plants and animals; they are endogenous and genetic in origin, persist without time cues, and are regularly influenced by cyclic variations of certain environmental factors called synchronizers.[20]

When precisely measured under constant conditions, the

endogenous circadian period lengths of the various species are not precisely 24 hours. When removed from time cues human beings usually have a free-running period length of somewhat more than 24 hours but less than 25 hours.[38] If their circadian pacemakers are not reset by their daily schedule, the timing of their endogenous rhythms would be delayed with respect to clock time each day. In humans and many other species, the most powerful synchronizers of the circadian rhythm are the diurnal alternation of light (activity) and darkness (rest) and our 24-hour life routine, especially sleep-wake patterns and meal timing.

There are two general categories of circadian organization that bear most directly on the practice of oncology. These are the circadian aspects of drug handling, called chronopharmacology, and the circadian organization of cell division in normal and malignant tissues, called chronocytokinetics.

CIRCADIAN CHRONOPHARMACOLOGY OF ANTINEOPLASTIC AGENTS

A better understanding of temporal changes in drug effects as a function of the agents circadian timing is achievable by considering two important concepts: the reproducible temporal changes in the biologic handling of drugs, their chronopharmacokinetics, and the temporal variation in the sensitivity of target tissues to these drugs, their chronopharmacodynamics.

Chronopharmacokinetics

Chronopharmacokinetics, is the study of the reproducible and predictable temporal variations in absorption, distribution, metabolism, and elimination of drugs. The chronopharmacokinetic behavior of over 100 drugs has been described in animals and humans.[1] Nontrivial temporal variations have been documented in drug absorption and distribution, metabolism, and excretion.[39–42] This has been well documented in vivo for many drugs metabolized through the P-450 system. This may be due to temporal variation in the microsomal concentration of the various P-450 isoenzymes. Reproducible circadian variation has been documented in the activity of at least 13 major hepatic drug metabolizing enzyme systems, including those responsible for hepatic glucuronidation and sulfation and for glutathione conjugation.[43,44]

Chronopharmacodynamics

Rhythmic changes in the susceptibility of a biosystem is well documented for many cytotoxic agents, in vivo and in vitro, for cells removed at specific circadian phases. Sometimes the susceptibility can be explained and quantified in terms of bioperiodic changes in the concentration of receptors of a given system for a given drug. Circadian rhythms in cellular defense mechanisms such as oxygen free radical defense mechanisms, such as glutathione and the concentration of other nonprotein-bound sulfhydryl compounds can also be responsible for time-of-day dependence of drug effect.[45–51]

For cytotoxic anticancer drugs, rhythmic changes in specific normal tissue functions, such as cell division, can also help explain the temporal variation in sensitivity of rapidly proliferating tissues. The cells of every tissue appropriately studied

enter or exit the various cell cycle phases in a highly organized way at certain times of day.[52]

PHARMACOLOGY WITHOUT CONSIDERATION TO TIME OF DAY

It is widely thought, although without experimental evidence, that constancy in the effectiveness of a drug over each 24-hour period is achievable by administration of several identical doses of short-half-life compounds at equal intervals or by the continuous enteral, transcutaneous, or parenteral administration of a drug at a constant rate. This goal is often stated to be that of "zero-order kinetics." As shown in rodents and in man, equal time-invariant dosing still results in pronounced circadian variations in drug concentration and drug effect.[25,53] Constant administration throughout the day results in predictably varying drug concentration and predictable nonzero order (in fact, nonlinear) drug kinetics and dynamics.[14,54]

CYTOKINETIC RHYTHMS

NORMAL TISSUE RHYTHMS OF RELEVANCE TO CANCER TREATMENT

Every normal proliferating tissue examined in adult mammals has been shown to undergo circadian variation, when the DNA synthesis stage of the cell cycle or the mitotic index is monitored along the 24-hour scale.[55,56] Chemotherapy agents are most cytotoxic to normal tissues during specific phases of the cell cycle. Cell proliferation rhythms in the gastrointestinal tract and bone marrow are especially relevant to the oncologist, because these two tissues are the most common target tissues for the toxic effects of antineoplastic drugs.

There is a marked circadian variation in cell proliferation throughout the gut mucosa, from the tongue to the rectum in mice and rats.[52,57] There are major variations seen in the amplitude of the rhythms in the various regions, but the phasing in the different regions of the gut is remarkably similar. Similar rhythms have been thoroughly documented in the gastrointestinal tract in humans, with the highest DNA synthetic activity each day between 5 to 9 A.M. each morning (Fig. 69–29A).[58]

The bone marrow is the most common tissue to limit dose intensity of common anticancer treatment. The production of all types of blood cells undergoes strong regular temporal variations, and circadian and seasonal rhythms in blood cell production have been described.[59] The relative number of bone marrow stem cells and progenitor cells, such as CFU-S, CFU-GM and CFU-E, have significant, predictable circadian variation in rodents. These findings have been confirmed in normal humans.[60–64] The marrow activity rhythms are reflected by circadian rhythms in the cellular components of the peripheral blood.[65,66] The studies of Smaaland of a group of 16 normal controls unequivocally confirmed the earlier findings of Mauer and Killman.[62–64] The percentage of cells in DNA synthesis measured by flow cytometry demonstrated a large variation along the circadian time scale for each 24-hour profile, with a range of variation from 29% to 339% from the lowest to highest value. The mean value of the lowest DNA synthesis for each 24-hour period was 8.7% ± 0.6% (8

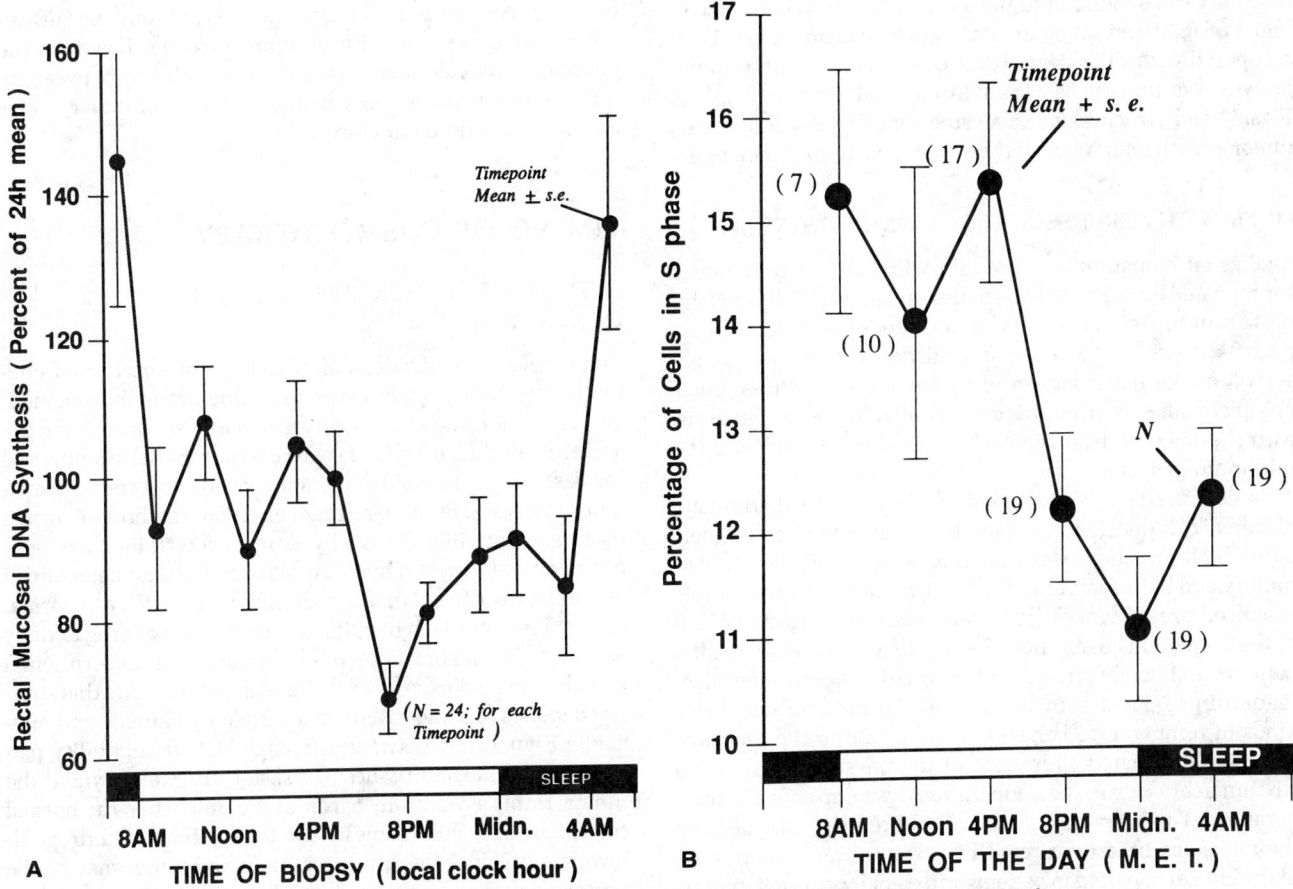

FIGURE 69–29. **(A)** The pattern of tritiated thymidine uptake by samples of human colorectal mucosa as a function of the time of day the samples were obtained. The data are presented as averages for 24 persons, each expressed relative to that person's 24-hour mean DNA synthetic capacity. Flexible colonoscopy was performed every 2 hours, round the clock, in each of 24 normal persons. Three mucosal tissue samples were obtained at each time of day from each subject, and one of these samples was immediately incubated with labeled thymidine. After appropriate washing and processing, the amount of radioactively labeled thymidine incorporated into DNA was measured. This histogram demonstrates that DNA synthetic capacity is highest in the early morning, before usual daily awakening (4 A.M. and 6 A.M. samples). DNA synthetic capacity is lowest in the evening hours, before daily sleep onset (8 P.M. and 10 P.M. samples). This tight circadian organization ($p < 0.001$) is similar in phasing and amplitude in fed and fasted states (data not shown). (Buchi KN, Moore JG, Hrushesky WJM, Sothern RB, Rubin NH. Circadian rhythm of cellular proliferation in the human rectal mucosa. Gastroenterology 1991;101:410–415). **(B)** The cytofluorometrically determined average percentage of cells in S phase actively synthesizing DNA. Bone marrow punctures were performed on as many as 19 healthy persons at up to six times of day. Samples were stained appropriately and then evaluated by flow cytometry. Samples obtained between 6 A.M. and 2 P.M. had the greatest average proportion of cells undergoing DNA synthesis. Samples obtained around midnight averaged much lower DNA synthesis activity ($p < 0.001$). (Smaaland R, Laerum OD, Lote K, Sletvold O, Sothern RB, Bjerknes R. DNA synthesis in human bone marrow is circadian stage dependent. Blood 1991;77:2603–2611). Concurrent inspection of these two panels reveals that the morning hours are associated with the greatest DNA synthetic activity for both chemotherapy-sensitive tissues. The evening hours are associated with far less DNA synthetic capacity in the bone marrow and the gut.

P.M. to 4 A.M.), and the mean value of the highest was 17.6% ± 0.6% (8 A.M. to 4 P.M.), which was a twofold difference, with the highest DNA synthetic activity between 7 A.M. and 4 P.M. (see Fig. 69–29B). This has now been confirmed in cancer patients.[66a]

MURINE TUMOR TISSUE CYTOKINETIC RHYTHMS

Another focus of interest has been the investigation of whether tumor cells proliferate rhythmically within the circadian reference frame and how their circadian pattern of cell division

relates to those of nonmalignant host target tissues. Earlier-stage better-differentiated hepatomas seem more tightly tied to host circadian time structure than are later-stage more-undifferentiated malignancies.[18] Similar circadian variations in DNA synthesis have been demonstrated in Lewis lung carcinoma cells after implantation into mice.[19,67]

In an attempt to determine whether tumor tissue communicates with circadian control mechanisms, Waldorp investigated whether the length of the daily photoperiod altered tumor growth rate in a mouse colon adenocarcinoma cell line.[68] Significantly greater tumor size, weight, and group mortality were found in tumor-bearing mice exposed to a 12 hours of light and 12 hours of darkness schedule (12L:12D) compared with 6L:18D or 18L:6D. In this model the tumor growth was influenced by environmental circadian milieu. Blask[69] and Hrushesky[70] suggested that this day length and tumor growth interaction may be mediated through melatonin.

HUMAN TUMOR TISSUE CYTOKINETIC RHYTHMS

Studies on human tumors are more difficult due to the need for repeated biopsies. In two studies of patients with skin nodules from breast cancer, the mitotic index was determined over 24 hours.[71,72] A large interindividual variation was observed in the daily pattern of tumor mitotic indices, but a group circadian rhythm was documented by cosinor analysis, with the maximum in the early afternoon (3 P.M.) and the minimum near 3 A.M.[73]

Some investigators have tried to correlate the rhythmicity of tumor cell division with measured tumor surface temperature. Stoll investigated the relation between uptake of ^{32}P in tumors and skin temperature in 19 women with inoperable advanced breast cancer.[74] He demonstrated periodicity in 9 of the 19 patients examined. The cycle was circadian in all 9 patients and demonstrated a close relation to circadian fluctuation in adjacent skin temperature. Gautherie found two kinds of temperature behavior, attributable to the presence of cancer associated alterations of the physiologic circadian rhythm in breast surface temperature, by comparing the temperature of the healthy contralateral breast to that bearing the untreated breast cancer.[75] First, there was a shortening of the circadian period in patients with rapidly growing tumors. These cancers subsequently proved to be poorly differentiated. Second, he found the persistence of a normal 24-hour rhythm in the slow-growing tumors, but with a decreased amplitude and a 6-hour phase advance, compared with the temperature pattern of the contralateral normal breast. The maximal mitotic index and maximal surface temperature coincided in circadian time.

Klevecz looked at cell proliferation in the ascites fluid from 30 patients with ovarian cancer.[76] A highly significant circadian rhythm in tumor cell DNA synthesis was found. Its peak (*i.e.*, mid to late morning) was found to be almost 12 hours out of phase with the proliferation in benign mesothelial cells from the same patients.

Smaaland has documented coordinated circadian patterns of DNA synthesis in the malignant lymph nodes of 24 patients with non-Hodgkin's lymphoma. Fine-needle aspirates were obtained from each patient every 4 hours for at least 24 hours. Flow cytometry was used to determine the proportion of cells in each sample that were actively synthesizing DNA (S-phase). DNA synthesis of these lymphomas was coordinated within the day, peaking during early sleep, out of phase with normal bone marrow, which peaks in the first half or middle of each day.[77] Both raw data and best fitting cosine curves can be used to demonstrate this phase relation of DNA synthesis in normal bone marrow and malignant lymph node tissue involved with non-Hodgkin's lymphoma. S-phase active bone marrow toxins may therefore be less toxic and more effective in the treatment of malignant lymphoma.

In summary, there is some evidence to suggest that human tumors preserve circadian cytokinetic synchrony. Because of clear host synchrony with different phasing, however, the possibility of exploiting a cytokinetic asynchrony between tumor and host tissue is real, whether an individual tumor retains any circadian time structure.

TIMING OF CHEMOTHERAPY

OPTIMIZING THE CIRCADIAN TIMING OF CHEMOTHERAPY

The clinical investigations of circadian optimization of chemotherapy have been based on prior findings in murine models. These murine studies consider the best time(s) for the anticancer effect on one or several tumor model systems and the best time(s) to avoid or to minimize one or several normal-tissue toxicities. Because relevant circadian rhythms of normal tissue susceptibility are usually easier to determine than those of tumor cells, most clinical studies have to date been aimed at finding the time of delivery causing least toxicity to normal tissue. This approach has allowed a reduction of drug toxicity and the safe maximization of dose intensity in experimental and clinical studies.[3,6,8,10,78,81] Clinical benefit using this strategy depends to some extent on a certain cytokinetic and metabolic asynchrony between the circadian susceptibility patterns of the normal tissues at risk for drug toxicity and the tumor. If this asynchrony exists, at the time when the normal tissues are less vulnerable to the toxic effects of a drug, allowing more dose intensive treatment, the tumor may not be protected to the same extent, providing for an improved therapeutic index.

Some researchers have given chemotherapy treatment to tumor-bearing animals at a time when a high percentage of the malignant cell population in the tumor is occupying a more drug-sensitive cell-cycle phase. In mice bearing methylcholanthrene-induced sarcoma, cyclophosphamide was given during the time of day associated with the highest G_2-phase distribution of sampled tumor cells. This strategy achieved 44% growth inhibition and 13% tumor cures.[79] Based on the finding that cyclophosphamide could synchronize tumor cells in M phase, tumor cure rate was improved to 53%, if vinblastine was given 12 hours after cyclophosphamide during the M phase of synchronized tumor cells.[80] Similar results have been reported for cyclophosphamide treatment in Lewis lung carcinoma-bearing mice.[67]

In a clinical trial based on these murine findings, 63 cancer patients with various tumors were randomized to receive the same 40-hour sequential chemotherapy regimen (*i.e.*, methotrexate or 5-FU, followed by vinblastine and cyclophosphamide). In the group receiving the treatment, at times taking into account the circadian rhythm of tumor proliferation, the antitumor effectiveness appeared better with respect to response rate (85% versus 58%), duration of response, and survival.[82] Braly and Klevecs are currently conducting a clinical trial in ovarian cancer patients in which intraperitoneal tumor cell samples are obtained every 1 to 4 hours for as long as 72 hours before treatment. Treatment timing is assigned to that time of day at which the predictably highest tumor cell S-phase fraction occurs.

METHODOLOGY FOR DETERMINING OPTIMAL CIRCADIAN DRUG TIMING

The clinical study design that ensures discovery of the optimal time of day for a given anticancer agent requires at least six arms; randomization to treatment at one of six equispaced times of day. This is unfortunately difficult because of the number of patients required. Therefore, surrogate information, such as DNA synthesis rhythms in target tissues and circadian pharmacokinetic changes, is combined with information obtained in large groups of mice or rats treated at each of six equispaced circadian stages. Preclinical experiments are usually performed in rats or mice of the same strain, sex, and age with free access to food and water. Like human beings with cancer who are living on a regular schedule of nocturnal sleep and diurnal activity, these animals have been synchronized for 2 weeks or longer in a lighting regimen usually consisting of 12 hours of light and 12 hours of darkness (LD 12: 12) or an other specified LD-time regimen. As a time reference in these studies, the hours after light onset (HALO) in the animal cage is universally accepted. This circadian reference point corresponds approximately to the time humans go to sleep, and it has proven helpful in extrapolating rhythm data from nocturnally active rodents to humans.[83] Sleep or rest onset is a particularly stable reference point, because many endocrinologic rhythms are fixed and reinforced by light regimen and sleep onset secondarily.[83]

Data Analysis

Biodynamics are described by time series analyses that resolve rhythmic patterns and trends in biologic variability. Time series record the values of the variable(s) in question over at least one full period, for circadian rhythms at least 24 hours, and depict these values as a function of sampling time. Several excellent specialized methods are available to analyze rhythmic time series data objectively.[84,85] A method commonly used to complement Chi squared standard ANOVA and life table analysis is the cosinor method. This method was originally described by Halberg and colleagues.[86] This method is a simple regression technique that uses the least squares fit of the raw data or data as percentage of daily mean to the best fitting cosine function.

Marker Rhythms for Cancer Chronochemotherapy

In assigning a time of day to administer chemotherapeutic agents, certain assumptions about interindividual circadian synchrony are made. This can easily be checked by establishing internal timing markers, which can be used as reference points independently of and complementary to clock hour.[87] Hrushesky and associates studied this in patients with small and large tumor burdens.[88] Biologic measurements were done every 2 hours during wakefulness and once during midsleep over three circadian cycles. At this sampling frequency and duration, oral temperature, heart rate, and blood pressure were poor choices as reference rhythms. Urinary volume and sodium excretion rhythms were affected by tumor burden. The rhythm characteristics of urinary potassium excretion were not different in patients with large or small tumor burden.

The daily time peak of potassium excretion was near its usual afternoon timing. Urinary cortisol excretion was highly rhythmic in all patients studied. The daily peak was quite normal in patients with good performance status and moderate tumor burden. In bedridden patients with large tumor burdens, the peak occurred somewhat later in the day, with a higher circadian amplitude and mean cortisol excretion, indicating that circadian treatment studies should be limited to persons with good performance status. When markers of circadian time structure are obtained densely over several cycles (5–7 days), it has been discovered that circadian coordination with the environment is maintained up until very shortly before death from widespread cancer. Ultimately, marker rhythms may be used to tailor the timing of chemotherapy to each patient. Currently, we may realistically aim to give chemotherapy in the correct sixth to quarter of the day (*i.e.*, the best predicted timing ±2–3 hours).

CHRONOBIOLOGIC DATA FOR CHEMOTHERAPY AGENTS

Preclinical chronotoxicologic studies have investigated whether mice or rats tolerate the same dose of an anticancer agent differently depending on when in their circadian cycle it is given.[89] Table 69–28 summarizes data for 20 antineoplastic agents given to normal mice or rats by bolus or continuous infusion, intravenously, or intraperitoneally, evaluating a range of toxicities from lethal toxicity to organ specific toxicities. Table 69–29 summarizes 10 studies involving seven antineoplastic agents in seven different transplantable tumor systems in mice and rats. In these experimental systems, giving chemotherapy at the optimal time with regard to reduced toxicity improved the effectiveness of the treatment. In these nocturnally active animals, hours after light onset (HALO) correspond to hours after humans go to sleep.

FLUOROPYRIMIDINES

FUDR Animal Data

Animal studies have shown FUDR bolus and continuous infusion to be highly circadian stage dependent with regard to toxicity and antitumor activity.[90,130] Single boluses of FUDR in doses from 1000 mg/kg to 2000 mg/kg were given at one of six equally distributed circadian stages to more than 300 CD_2F_1 mice. Survival varied reproducibly by more than 50%, depending on the circadian stage of injection, with the best drug tolerance in the daily late activity span (18–20 HALO). The animals died with severe gut and bone marrow damage.[90]

Because of its short half-life, FUDR is usually given by prolonged infusion. Therefore, circadian patterned infusion studies were performed. FUDR (1000 mg/kg) was given by continuous intravenous infusion over 48 hours to female 344 Fisher rats. Drug was delivered by constant rate infusion or by variable rate infusion, with peak drug delivery during one of six different times of day. FUDR lethal toxicity, which was secondary to gut damage, was lowest 4 to 6 hours later (22–04 HALO) than the best time for bolus FUDR. This was also the best time with regard to tumor response in animals with

TABLE 69-28. Chronotoxicity of Anticancer Agents in Murine Models

Agent and Route	Least Toxic Time in Rodents, HALO* (no. of tested times)†	Least Toxic Time for Humans‡ Resting 22-06	Measure of Toxicity§
Antimetabolites			
FUDR I.V. bolus[90]	18–20 (6)	16–18	Lethal toxicity
FUDR I.V. infusion[91]	22–04 (6)	20–02	Lethal toxicity
FUDR IP[92]	02 (6)	24	Lethal toxicity
5-FU IP[93]	19 (11)	17	Gastrointestinal
5-FU IP[94]	02 > 12 (2)	24 > 10	Marrow
5-FU I.V.[95]	20 > 14 (2)	18 > 12	Marrow
5-FU IP[96]	05–07 (6)	03–05	Lethal toxicity
5-FU IP[97]	05 > 17 (2)	03 > 15	Lethal toxicity
5-FU IP[92]	10 (6)	08	Lethal toxicity
Methotrexate I.V.[98,99]	17.5 (4)	15.5	Lethal, marrow, renal, liver
Methotrexate IP[100]	14 (4)	12	Weight loss
Ara-C IP[101]	03–12 (8)	01–10	Lethal toxicity
Antitumor Antibiotics			
Doxorubicin IP[102,103]	08–10 (6)	06–08	Lethal—early, marrow
Doxorubicin I.V.[102,103]	15 (6)	13	Lethal—late, cardiac
Daunorubicin IP[104]	10 (6)	8	Lethal toxicity
Epirubicine IP[105]	02–06 (6)	24–04	Lethal toxicity
THP-doxorubicin I.V.[106]	07–10 (6)	05–08	Lethal, marrow
Mitoxantrone IP[107]	16 (4)	14	Lethal toxicity
Platinum Analogs			
Cisplatin IP, I.V.[108,109]	17–19 (6)	16–18¶	Lethal, renal, marrow
Oxaliplatin I.V.[110]	16 (6)	14	Lethal, marrow, jejunal
Caboplatin I.V.[111]	16 (6)	14	Lethal, marrow, jejunal
Vinca Alkaloids			
Vinblastine I.V.[112]	18–19 (6)	16–17	Lethal
Vincristine IP[113]	13 (6)	11	Lethal
Etoposide I.V.[114,115] ‖	07–11 (6)	05–09	Lethal
Alkylating Agents			
Cyclophosphamide IP[116]	07, 19 (6)	05, 17	Bladder
Cyclophosphamide IP[117,118]	12–13 (6, 5)	10–11	Lethal
Ifosfamide IP[119]	22–23 (6)	20–21	Lethal
Peptichemio I.V.[120]	15 (6)	13	Lethal, marrow, intestinal
Mitomycin C I.V.[121,122]	17–20 (6)	15–18	Lethal
Melphalan IP[123]	10 (6)	08	Marrow

* HALO, Hours after light on in animal cage; least toxic time refers to the time when treatment results produce least toxicity to the target tissue or the whole animal. Toxicity was not always tested at the same times for the same agents.

† Number of circadian times tested in the given experiment. If only a few times tested, 2 > 15 indicates that treatment was less toxic if given at 2 than if given at 15 HALO.

‡ Extrapolated from animal data for humans sleeping from 10 P.M. to 6 A.M. Human time = (HALO + 22) − 24.

§ Usually lethal toxicity. If autopsy was performed to determine tissue sustaining most toxcity, this is mentioned.

‖ The vehicle is more toxic to moce than VP-16 plus the vehicle; therefore, these data may reflect vehicle toxicity and are suspect.

¶ L:D–8:16 schedule used. May transfer later.

TABLE 69–29. Effectiveness of Anticancer Agents in Murine Tumor Systems When Each Agent is Given at Its Least Toxic Circadian Time

Agent	Tumor	HALO*	Index†	Control‡	Circadian Timed
				Effectiveness (%)	
CY (+ Ara-C)	L1210 leukemia	8	Cure rate	44	94[124]
Doxorub (+CY)	L1210 leukemia	13	Cure rate	0–8	56–68[125]
Ara-C	L1210 leukemia	8	Cure rate	11	23[126]
L-PAM + D	Breast-adeno ca	10	PR	12.5	50[127]
Cisplatin (+D)	Immunocytoma	18	CR	24	60[128]
FUDR infusion	Breast-adeno ca	22–04	PR	0	25[91]
5-FU	Colon-adeno ca	2	PR	§[94]	
CY	T9 + T10 sarcoma	2	Cure rate	14% improvement[79]	
CY	L1210 leukemia	12	Cure rate	27% improvement[118]	
CY	Ehrlich's ascites	4	Cure rate	13% improvement[129]	

CY, cyclophosphamide; D, doxorubicin.
* If more than one agent was given, HALO (hours after light onset) refers to the timing of the agent outside the brackets.
† Index of effectiveness as measured by cure rate; PR, partial response; CR, complete response.
‡ Effectiveness of treatment if not given at the best circadian time.
§ Tumor growth delay was significantly better with treatment at 2 HALO than at 12 HALO.

a transplanted 13762-adenocarcinoma given 700 mg/kg of FUDR as a 48-hour intravenous infusion. Because some of the circadian shaped infusions studied were toxicologically and therapeutically inferior to constant rate infusion, the circadian pattern and not the quasi-intermittency of circadian FUDR administration was primarily responsible for these circadian pharmacodynamic differences.[90,91]

FUDR Clinical Data

In a series of clinical studies, von Roemeling and Hrushesky used a 14-day continuous infusion of FUDR. To achieve a variable rate infusion pattern, the daily drug dose was divided into four portions of 68%, 15%, 2%, and 15%. Each portion was infused over a 6-hour span. This type of infusion with its peak drug delivery between 3 P.M. and 9 P.M. was found to give substantially less toxicity than a constant infusion of the same dose.[6] In a crossover study and a second randomized study, patients with metastatic malignancies treated with equal dose intensities experienced less frequent and less severe diarrhea, nausea, and vomiting after the variable-rate infusion described previously compared with a flat-rate infusion. In a third study, the dose intensity of variable rate infusion was escalated stepwise to determine the maximal tolerated dose. Patients receiving the time-modified FUDR infusion tolerated an average of 1.45-fold more drug per unit time while experiencing minimal toxicity. Valvassori confirmed in 111 cancer patients that FUDR is well tolerated when given by this circadian schedule.[131]

This FUDR schedule was found to be active in 63 consecutive evaluable patients with metastatic renal cell cancer, with five complete responses and ten partial responses to give a 24 ± 5.1% (95% confidence limits) objective response rate.[5] Other researchers have confirmed this. Huben similarly treated a group of good performance status patients without prior therapy and found a 60% objective response rate.[132] Damaschelli also found the regimen to be active.[133] More re-

cently, Venook treated 29 patients and also found a 21% objective response rate. Dexeus and colleagues, using a somewhat different circadian schedule of FUDR in 42 patients with metastatic renal cell cancer, reported a partial response in 4 patients (10%; 95% confidence limits 3–24%). Another 4 patients (10%) had partial responses at metastatic sites but no response in the primary kidney tumor.[134] Hrushesky and colleagues are conducting a prospective randomized multicenter trial comparing a 14 day circadian infusion of FUDR with a 14 day flat FUDR infusion in patients with metastatic renal cell cancer.

Continuous FUDR intravenous infusion for 14 out of 21 to 28 days is the most consistently active and useful chemotherapy for metastatic RCC. FUDR toxicity and safely achievable dose intensity are each favorably modified by circadian infusion, giving most of each day's dose in the evening hours. An NCI-sponsored multicenter international study is currently determining the effect of circadian optimization on response frequency and quality and patient survival.

In 50 patients with liver metastases from colorectal cancer receiving FUDR as intrahepatic infusion, toxicity in the form of cholestasis and jaundice was several-fold less frequent, less severe, and occurred later when circadian infusion was employed compared with a flat infusion. Patients receiving the circadian modified infusion tolerated a 70% higher average dose intensity. Response rates in the two groups were similar.[7]

Focan and colleagues have reported preliminary data from a randomized study of intravenous 5-FU and intrahepatic FUDR in 38 previously untreated patients with liver metastases from colorectal cancer.[133a] Patients in arm A received a flat infusion, and patients in arm B received a circadian infusion with peaks for 5-FU at 4 A.M. and for FUDR at 4 P.M. Stomatitis was dose limiting. No hepatic toxicity was noted. After the third course, toxicity (alopecia, neutropenia, and skin) became lower in arm B despite a higher dose intensity. More courses could be delivered in arm B. The response rate was similar in both arms (50–60%). The median survival was superior in arm B (40+ months versus 19.6 months in arm A).

More recent animal studies indicate that the optimal systemic FUDR infusion should most likely peak 4 to 6 hours later than was originally extrapolated from the bolus studies.[91] Even more benefit may be expected in future clinical studies using FUDR infusion if this is taken into account.

5-Fluorouracil Animal Data

Popovic found that the best tolerance to 5-FU, with 30% mortality, was in middle to late rest phase (5–7 HALO), but 100% mortality was observed in animals treated in the late activity phase (20–22 HALO).[96] Burns randomized mice to receive 5-FU treatment at 5 or 17 HALO. The single intraperitoneal bolus dose of 5-FU killing 50% of the animals (LD_{50}) was significantly higher in early rest (5 HALO) than in midactivity (17 HALO) phase.[97] Gonzales and coworkers concurrently tested the lethal toxicity of a single intraperitoneal 5-FU and FUDR bolus injections at one of six different time points in Balb/c mice.[92] 5-FU was least toxic in late rest (10 HALO), and FUDR was least toxic in early rest (2 HALO). Gardner found that the impairment of water absorption by small intestine in vitro and the incidence of diarrhea in vivo differed as a function of treatment time when 5-FU was given to rats.[93] The intestinal toxicity was minimal after treatment in late activity (19 HALO) when the maximum of small intestine mucosa cells were in the postmitotic resting phase (G_1) and less susceptible to the effects from 5-FU. Peters and colleagues tested the antitumor and bone marrow toxicity of 5-FU in transplantable mouse colon cancer-bearing mice. Better antitumor activity and less marrow toxicity was found in the early rest phase compared with treatment given in the early activity phase.[94] Minshull has confirmed these data with regard to bone marrow toxicity in Wistar rats.[95] Overall, these preclinical data indicate that this drug, like FUDR, is probably best given in the first half of the daily sleep span.

5-Fluorouracil Clinical Data

Murine data from investigating 5-FU-induced lethal toxicity and human pharmacology data for 5-FU were the basis for subsequent clinical trials, giving the highest dose of 5-FU centered in the second half of the daily sleep span at 4 A.M.[14,96,97] Lévi and associates used a 5-day circadian continuous infusion of 5-FU every 3 weeks in 30 patients with metastatic colorectal cancer. The delivery rate varied in a circadian manner and was highest at 4 A.M. and null from 6 to 10 P.M. An intrapatient dose escalation by 1 g/m²/course was planned from 5 g/m²/course (usual schedule) to 9 g/m²/course according to toxicity criteria. The mean highest tolerated dose was 7.5 g/m²/course, considerably higher than that recommended for a constant infusion of 5-FU.[4,9]

The clinical data available indicate that the combination of 5-FU and leucovorin (LV) is more effective in shrinking tumors than 5-FU alone in patients with metastatic colorectal cancer.[135] In a phase II trial using patients with metastatic colorectal cancer, 5-FU, LV, and oxaliplatin were infused continuously for 5 days every 3 weeks.[9] Oxaliplatin (25 mg/m²/day) was infused for 12 hours, with peak delivery at 4 P.M., and 5-FU (700 mg/m²/day) and LV (300 mg/m²/day)

were infused concurrently for 12 hours with peak delivery at 4 A.M. Fifty-four of the 93 patients had an objective response (58%; 95% confidence limits, 48% to 68%) regardless of previous chemotherapy. In a subsequent phase II study, this circadian schedule was used in 37 patients with fluoropyrimidine-resistant colorectal cancer. After a mean number of eight courses, a partial response rate was achieved in 16 of 37 patients (43%).[135a] The timing of oxaliplatin was based on previous experimental and clinical studies.[78,110] These findings await confirmation in a ongoing randomized study comparing a flat infusion of these agents with the schedule described here.

A phase I trial was conducted to identify the optimal dose rate of delivery for admixtures of 5-FU and LV given for 14 days as a flat continuous infusions.[136] The optimal dose rate for 5-FU and LV was found to be 200 mg/m²/day and 5 mg/m²/day, respectively. In a phase I study of a 14-day circadian infusion of 5-FU and LV, with the infusion peaking at 4 A.M., Bjarnason and colleagues determined the maximum tolerated dose (MTD) for 5-FU and LV, given as a continuous circadian infusion over 14 days, with 64% of the daily dose given over 7 hours around 3 to 4 A.M.[137] LV was first escalated by 5 mg/m²/day to 20 mg/m²/day, followed by escalation of 5-FU by 50 mg/m²/day. Patients who developed ≥grade II toxicity had the peak of the infusion shifted from 3 to 4 A.M. to 9 to 10 P.M., to determine if this reduced toxicity. This timing corresponds to the time of least toxicity from 5-FU in more recent murine studies, testing nonlethal doses.[93–95] Recent clinical studies of 5-FU pharmacokinetics, 5-FU metabolism, and gut cytokinetics also suggest that an evening infusion peak may be less toxic than an infusion peaking at 3 to 4 A.M.[54,58,146] The MTD for an infusion peaking at 3 to 4 A.M. was reached at dose level 5 (5-FU 250 mg/m²/day-LV 20 mg/m²/day). In 6 patients developing ≥grade II toxicity, the peak of the infusion was shifted to 9 to 10 P.M. Toxicity was reduced in all 6 patients and further dose escalation was possible in 3 patients. The MTD for an infusion peaking at 9–10 P.M. was reached at dose level 6 (5-FU 300 mg/m²/day-LV 20 mg/m²/day). Stomatitis and hand-foot syndrome was dose limiting. There was no bone marrow toxicity. The recommended dose for phase II studies using this schedule is 5-FU 250 mg/m²/day and LV 20 mg/m²/day with the infusion peak at 9 to 10 P.M. This is a 300% and 25% higher dose for LV and 5-FU, respectively, than was suggested to be safe for a flat infusion. A phase II study is ongoing in metastatic colorectal cancer. The addition of leucovorin may alter the circadian time-dependent toxicity of 5-FU by diverting its mechanism of action more toward the inhibition of thymidylate synthetase and away from incorporation into RNA. Preliminary animal studies of 5-FU and LV pharmacodynamics indicate that the addition of LV may change the circadian optimum for 5-FU from the second half toward the first half of the daily sleep span.[138]

Mechanisms of Fluropyrimidine Circadian Pharmacodynamics

Several studies have shown that plasma drug levels vary significantly during continuous infusion of 5-FU.[139–141] Two studies demonstrated a circadian rhythm in the plasma concentration of 5-FU in patients receiving this drug as a continuous venous infusion at a constant rate for 5 to 14 days.[14,54]

Harris found the peak value for plasma 5-FU at 11 A.M. and the trough value at 11 P.M. The ratio of the maximal concentration of 5-FU to the minimal concentration observed was almost fivefold higher.[54] Petit found the peak value for plasma 5-FU at 1 A.M. and the trough value at 1 P.M., 10 hours earlier than Harris.[14] The difference may be related to the fact that the patients in the second study received cisplatin at a fixed time of day before each 5-day 5-FU infusion (450–966 mg/m²/day), but the patients in the first study received only 5-FU in a lower dose (300 mg/m²/day) and for a longer time span. Pharmacokinetic interactions between cisplatin and 5-FU have been documented, with a single dose of cisplatin increasing subsequent plasma levels of 5-FU given by continuous infusion.[142]

More than 80% of an administered dose of 5-FU is rapidly catabolized in the liver and extrahepatic sites.[143] Catabolism largely determines the availability of 5-FU for anabolism to its active nucleotide analogs. The activity of dihydropyrimidine dehydrogenase (DPD), the rate-limiting enzyme for fluoropyrimidine catabolism, is highly circadian stage dependent ($p < 0.0001$) in the rat liver, with a peak in late rest (10 HALO).[144] Harris showed that this leads to a circadian variation of 5-FU catabolism in the isolated perfused rat liver with the peak and trough elimination rates of 5-FU in late activity (19 HALO) and midrest (7 HALO) respectively. There was a reciprocal relation between the elimination rates of 5-FU and 5-FU catabolites.[145]

Tuchman[146] and Harris[54] independently demonstrated a circadian variation of DPD activity in human mononuclear cells with peak values occurring at 10 P.M. to 2 A.M. and at 1 A.M., respectively (*i.e.*, early rest period). A inverse relation between DPD activity in peripheral blood mononuclear cells and plasma 5-FU concentration was demonstrated by Harris in his study of cancer patients receiving a protracted continuous infusion if 5-FU.[54] The timing of peak values for DPD activity in humans (*i.e.*, early rest) differs somewhat from the time of peak values of DPD activity determined in rats (*i.e.*, late rest). The reason for this discrepancy is not clear, but it emphasizes the variability that may exist between species. The activity of the initial enzyme in fluoropyrimidine anabolism, thymidine kinase, recently has been shown to be rhythmic in the rat spleen, with a pattern opposite to that of DPD.[146a]

The activities of other enzymes of importance in fluoropyrimidine activation; dihydrouracil dehydrogenase, uridine phosphorylase, and thymidine phosphorylase have each been shown to be circadian rhythmic in the mouse liver.[147] Daher did not find a circadian variation in the activity of thymidine phosphorylase in the rat liver.[148] Thymidine phosphorylase is the major enzyme responsible for the phosphorolysis of FUDR to 5-FU.

Reproducible circadian patterns in the activities of catabolic and anabolic enzymes relevant to the biochemical pharmacology of fluoropyrimidines are responsible, at least in part, for the marked circadian pharmacodynamics of 5-FU and FUDR.

ANTHRACYCLINES

Animal Toxicity Studies

Early chronotoxicity studies of intraperitoneal doxorubicin in hybrid mice and F344 rats demonstrated its profound circa-

dian pharmacodynamics.[149] When doxorubicin was given in early activity (14 HALO), it was much better tolerated than when given in early rest (2 HALO). These results were confirmed by Sothern in a more detailed study, in which the toxicity of doxorubicin given intravenously and intraperitoneally was investigated.[103] The timing of best tolerance for doxorubicin was found to be to some extent dependent on the route of administration.[102,103] Early mortality (*i.e.*, day 5–20) from doxorubicin was only seen after intraperitoneal administration, with late rest (8 HALO) being the time of least toxicity. Late mortality, starting on day 40, was found to be similar for intraperitoneal and intravenous administration, with early activity (15 HALO) the time of least toxicity for both routes. Sothern has demonstrated that circadian stage, not time of day, characterizes doxorubicin susceptibility rhythms of mice in continuous light.[83] The time of least toxicity coincided with the low point of the rectal temperature rhythm in animals in constant light and in animals on a schedule of alternating light and darkness. Intraperitoneal daunorubicin, compared with doxorubicin, had an earlier time of least toxicity (10 HALO versus 14 HALO).[104] Experimental data are also available for the time of epirubicin and 4′-O-tetrahydropyranyl doxorubicin.[105,106]

Mitoxantrone was tested at four circadian times in $B_6D_2F_1$ mice, and found to be most toxic in early rest (3–7 HALO). Pharmacokinetic monitoring showed that this coincided with the time for the longest half-life and the largest area under the curve (AUC) for mitoxantrone compared with treatment at the three other time points.[107] The least toxic time was at 16 HALO, about 8 hours later than for doxorubicin.

The time of day associated with lowest doxorubicin toxicity to bone marrow, gut, and heart tissue, as well as its best antitumor activity occurs just before usual daily awakening, when normal tissue oxidative defense systems are most robust.

Animal Tumor Response Studies

In LOU rats bearing an immunocytoma, a single injection of doxorubicin induced a faster tumor regression, but a faster regrowth of tumor, when doxorubicin was given near the time of best tolerance, just before daily awakening (06 HALO).[150]

Several studies have used doxorubicin in combination with other chemotherapy agents. Halberg and coworkers gave sequential chemotherapy with doxorubicin and melphalan to female Fisher rats that were previously inoculated with 13762 mammary adenocarcinoma.[127] The best responses to treatment, as measured by tumor size, complete remissions, and duration of remission, were observed when the drugs were given just before usual awakening (10 HALO), near the time of best normal tissue tolerance in rodents.

Studies of intraperitoneal doxorubicin and cisplatin in immunocytoma-bearing LOU rats documented a striking circadian stage dependence of tumor response and toxicity. The maximal tumor response and least toxicity was observed when cisplatin was administered in the middle to latter part of the daily activity span, and doxorubicin was administered near the end of the daily resting span.[128]

Scheving studied the response rate to intraperitoneal doxorubicin and cyclophosphamide in mice bearing advanced L1210 leukemia.[125] The variation in cure rate ranged from 8% to 68% in male animals and 0% to 56% in female animals, depending on the time of treatment. The maximal cure rate was recorded when the two drugs were administered 3 hours apart during the early activity cycle, corresponding to the time of best tolerance for doxorubicin.

Clinical Studies

Several clinical studies have used the combination of doxorubicin and cisplatin. In the first randomized-crossover study, which accrued 23 patients between 1979 and 1982, patients with metastatic ovarian cancer (11) and bladder cancer (12) alternated between treatments with doxorubicin (60 mg/m²) at 0600 or 1800 with cisplatin (60 mg/m²) given 12 hours later.[151] Nadir blood counts were moderate, and recovery was complete within 21 days, using morning doxorubicin and evening cisplatin. Evening doxorubicin and morning cisplatin produced statistically significantly lower nadirs with less than full recovery by day 28. Nephrotoxicity from the first course of treatment was entirely avoided by the use of the favorable circadian schedule, but treatment with morning cisplatin and evening doxorubicin resulted in an average creatinine clearance fall of 30 ml/minute after the first course of treatment. Cisplatin urinary pharmacokinetics were concurrently studied and contrasted in patients receiving morning or evening cisplatin. These studies were performed in a general clinical research center, where vigorous comparability of all oral and intravenous fluid and calorie delivery were maintained. It was found that peak urinary cisplatin concentration and the AUC of cisplatin concentration were each much higher for the patients receiving cisplatin in the morning. There was a good correlation between the peak urinary concentration and degree of subsequent permanent kidney damage.[13,151] These data are consistent with the animal data described previously.[128]

In a study conducted between 1982 and 1986, 37 patients with ovarian cancer were accrued and randomized to receive doxorubicin (60 mg/m²) at 0600 (schedule A) or 1800 (schedule B), with cisplatin (60 mg/m²) given 12 hours later, monthly for 9 months.[10,151] Evaluation of bone marrow toxicity in patients who received at least 8 of 9 planned treatments revealed more cumulative marrow toxicity in patients treated on schedule B. Most patients on this schedule had to have greater than 33% doxorubicin dose reductions and some treatment delays because of marrow toxicity. Patients on schedule A had fewer dose reductions, treatment delays, and fewer episodes of infection, bleeding, and transfusions (Fig. 69–30). This study confirmed all the preliminary toxicity results uncovered in the initial crossover study. Average achievable dose intensity, expressed in mg/kg/week or as percentage of planned dose intensity, was lower for schedule B than schedule A. This prospectively randomized study hinted at a survival advantage for patients treated on schedule A. At 5 years, 44% of patients treated on schedule A were alive, but 11% of those treated using schedule B survived 5 years.

The same two-drug combination of doxorubicin and cisplatin was given to 43 patients with advanced transitional cell carcinoma of the bladder. Patients were randomized to receive schedule A or schedule B. Overall, 57% had an objective response, and 23% had a complete response (35 evaluable patients). The numbers of patients per treatment group did not allow interpretation of schedule-dependent differences in response, but toxicity evaluation confirmed that schedule A was superior, with lower toxicity despite higher dose intensity.[12]

Similar schedule dependency with regard to toxicity was observed by Lévi using 4′tetrahydropyranyl doxorubicin (THP) and cisplatin in patients with advanced ovarian cancer.[8] Thirty-one patients were randomized to chemotherapy according to one of two schedules (*i.e.*, schedule A or schedule B). Patients on schedule A received their chemotherapy at times predicted to be least toxic by animal experiments: THP (50 mg/m²) by intravenous bolus at 6 A.M. and cisplatin (100 mg/m²) by a 4-hour infusion from 4 to 8 P.M. Patients on schedule B received THP at 6 P.M. and cisplatin infusion from 4 to 8 A.M. The overall response rate was 64%, 73% on schedule A and 57% on schedule B. Schedule A was associated with two to three times less hematologic and renal toxicity than schedule B ($p < 0.01$). Three of 4 patients withdrawn from this protocol because of severe toxicity were on schedule B. Full planned doses of these drugs could be given for three or more courses to fourfold as many patients on schedule A compared with schedule B. A randomized trial is ongoing.

The Gynecology Oncology Group has reported a phase II study of patients with advanced or recurrent endometrial cancer.[152] Doxorubicin (60 mg/m²) was given over 30 minutes at 6 A.M., followed by cisplatin (60 mg/m²) given over 30 minutes at 6 P.M. every 28 days. The number of treatment courses ranged from two to eight, with a median of six. A preliminary review of 25 evaluable patients shows 4 (16%) of 25 complete responses, 9 (36%) of 25 partial responses, and 8 (32%) of 25 with stable disease. This 52% objective response rate was three times the predicted response rate and is currently being followed-up with additional clinical trials.

Lévi is studying chronotherapy with doxorubicin in patients with metastatic breast cancer, comparing a flat infusion with a sinusoid infusion, giving the highest dose of doxorubicin from 3 to 7 A.M.[153] Stomatitis was the main dose limiting factor on both schedules, but hematologic toxicity was more pronounced on the flat infusion schedule. In another study Lévi found better hematologic tolerance to 4′-O-tetrahydropyranyl doxorubicin if this agent was given at 0600 compared with 1800 in patients with metastatic cancer.[154]

Each of several circadian clinical trials of doxorubicin or its analogs with cisplatin or its analogs demonstrate substantial advantage to timing the anthracycline early at, or just before, usual awakening and platinum compounds late in the afternoon or in the early evening.

Mechanism

Circadian variation of plasma concentration of doxorubicin was noticed in mice.[155] In humans receiving bolus or infusional therapy with doxorubicin, similar circadian changes in doxorubicin pharmacokinetics were found with higher levels late in the day.[156]

Some of the bone marrow toxicity and all of the cardiac toxicity of doxorubicin may be related to the NADPH-dependent doxorubicin semiquinone-mediated generation of free radicals, such as hydroxyl and superoxide anions, that can be detoxified by several pathways, primarily the glutathione cycle.[157] A circadian rhythm in the level of total glutathione and reduced glutathione (GSH) in cardiac tissue has been documented in mice and rats, with highest levels in the early activity span, corresponding to the time of lowest lethal toxicity of intravenous doxorubicin in these animals.[50,158] He-

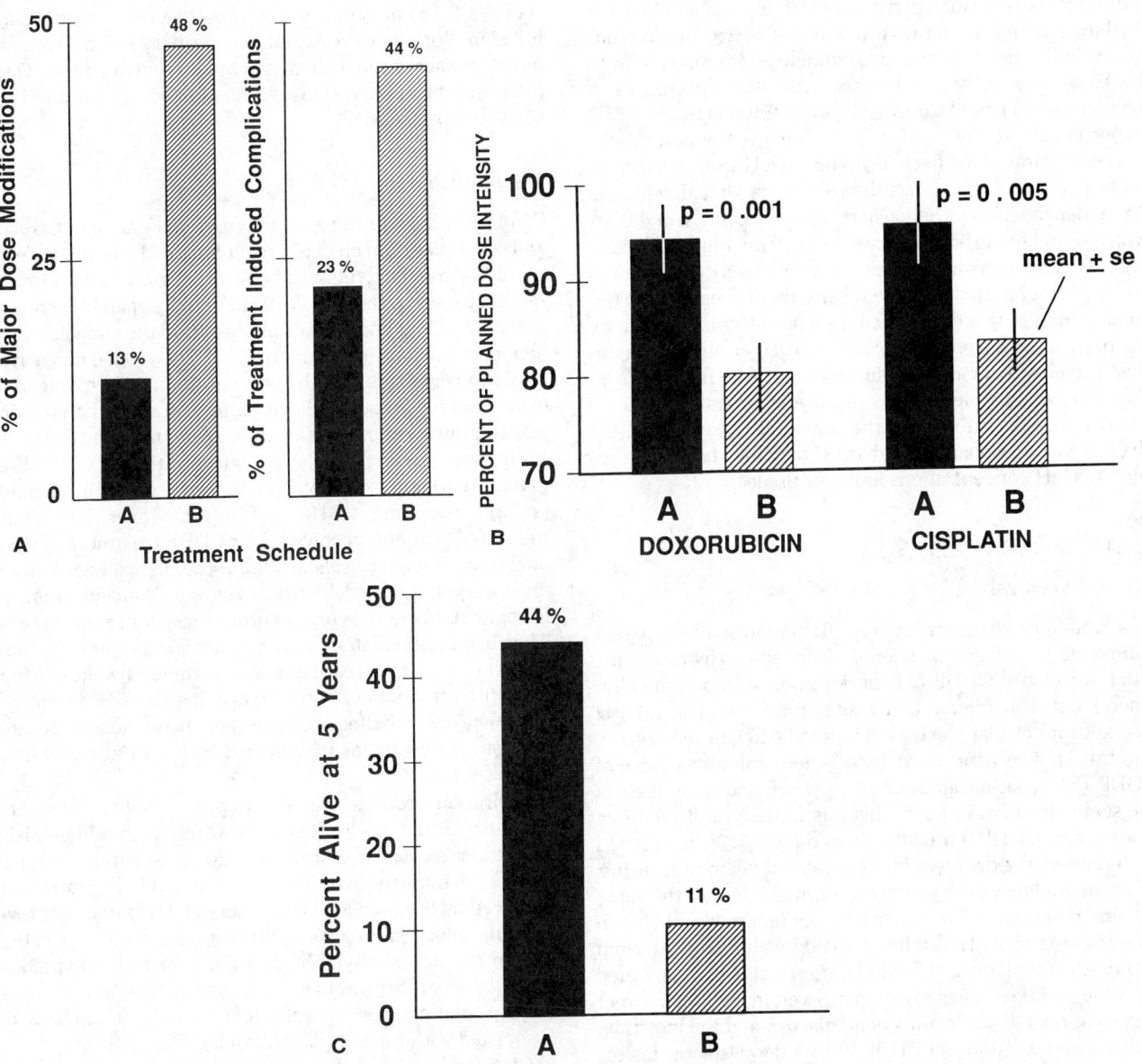

FIGURE 69–30. **(A)** The frequency of dose modifications and treatment delays forced by therapy on each circadian schedule and the frequency of treatment-associated complications. Each of 37 patients were randomized to receive monthly treatment courses of doxorubicin and cisplatin at one of two times of the day. Patients randomized to receive morning doxorubicin and evening cisplatin (A, *solid bars*) had to have only about 1 in 10 of their treatment courses modified (13%), but treatment with doxorubicin in the evening and cisplatin in the morning (B, *hatched bars*) forced major dose or schedule modifications in almost one of every two treatment courses (48%) ($p < 0.001$). On the right of the first panel, it can be seen that patients treated on schedule A had serious complications in almost one of every five treatment courses (23%); patients treated on schedule B had complications in more than three of every five courses (44%) ($p < 0.001$), even though this group of patients received less drug less frequently. **(B)** The average achievable dose intensity of each drug for patients treated on schedule A (*solid*) or schedule B (*hatched*) for doxorubicin and cisplatin. Toxicity forced reduction of doxorubicin dose if schedule A (*solid bars*) was used to 95% of the planned dose. When schedule B (*hatched bars*) was employed, only 80% of planned dose could safely be given ($p < 0.001$). Moreover, 96% of scheduled cisplatin could be given if schedule A (*solid bars*) was employed, but only 83% of the planned dose could be administered if schedule B (*hatched bars*) was used ($p < 0.005$). **(C)** This panel contrasts the relative probability that patients treated with schedule A (*solid bar*) are alive 5 years after study entry (44%) with the relative probability of survival for patients treated on schedule B (*hatched bar*), which was 11%.

patic GSH concentration in rodents exhibits a similar circadian rhythmicity, and similar rhythmicity in GSH occurs in other tissues in the rat, differing in amplitude and frequency from the hepatic cycle.[159,160] Substantial circadian differences in the nonprotein-bound sulfhydryl concentration (>90% GSH) in nucleated cells of human bone marrow has been documented.[49] More than fivefold higher levels were present at 8 A.M. than at 8 P.M. in 5 healthy volunteers. Smaaland found a time-dependent covariation between GSH content and DNA synthesis in human bone marrow from 10 healthy volunteers, when 70 bone marrow samples were collected every 4 hours over a 24-hour period.[51] These results are in keeping with the human findings that doxorubicin produced less myelotoxicity when given in the morning. The toxicity of other antineoplastic agents that cause the formation of free radicals (*e.g.,* alkylating agents, bleomycin, mitomycin C, antitumor antibiotics) could be affected by the temporal variation in GSH levels. Cyclophosphamide and ara-C toxicities have been related to GSH concentrations in target tissues.[48]

PLATINUM ANALOGS

Animal Studies

Cis-diamminedichloroplatinum (CDDP) represents the parent compound in this group. There is a circadian rhythm in the lethal toxicity of CDDP (11 mg/kg given intraperitoneally) when studied in female 344 Fisher rats.[108,161] The highest tolerance for cisplatin occurred in middle to late activity 17–19 HALO). The nephrotoxicity of a lower nontoxic dose of CDDP (5 mg/kg intraperitoneally) was found to be least at the same circadian time.[162] This was further confirmed in a study giving CDDP intravenously to male $B_6D_2F_1$ mice.[163] In both species, the drug was best tolerated if given near or just after the middle of the activity span, regardless of the route of administration. CDDP induced renal failure was the main cause of drug-related mortality. Two nonnephrotoxic platinum analogs, carboplatin and oxaliplatin, are also best tolerated near the middle of the activity span, even though their target organs of toxicity are mainly bone marrow and the intestine, rather than the kidney for CDDP.[110,111] A new cisplatin analog, B-85-0040, is likewise best tolerated near the middle activity span.[164]

Cisplatin and each of its analogs, which have been studied, are least toxic and most effective when given in the second half of the daily activity span.

Clinical Studies

Modern cancer treatment is polypharmaceutical, and most clinical studies with CDDP have been done with combination chemotherapy. Combinations with doxorubicin have been discussed previously and have confirmed the time of least toxicity in humans to be in the evening.

Caussanel has reported a randomized phase I trial of a 5-day flat continuous venous infusion of oxaliplatin compared with a circadian-modulated infusion with its peak at 1600.[78] Toxicity was assessed for 94 courses in 23 patients. There was far less neutropenia ($p < 0.05$) and less frequent and less severe distal paresthesias ($p < 0.001$) and a trend to less eme-

sis ($p = 0.15$) in patients receiving the circadian-modulated infusion. With dose escalation, the mean dose was 33% higher in the circadian-modulated arm by the fourth course. Oxaliplatin has been studied in combination with 5-FU and LV as discussed previously.[9]

Mechanism

Cisplatin's dose-limiting toxicity is renal damage. Cisplatin and other platinum analogs are eliminated from the body primarily by renal excretion. The fact that glomerular filtration rate increases in the middle of the activity span in laboratory rodents and in humans could play a part in the circadian stage-dependent toxicity of platinum.[165,166] The renal damage from cisplatin correlates with the concentration of free drug in the urine, and the greatest tubular damage occurs when the drug is given during the phase of the circadian cycle that results in highest urinary cisplatin concentration.[108,162,167] Free-platinum urinary excretion kinetics were studied in 11 cancer patients receiving CDDP (60 mg/m²) over 30 minutes monthly.[13] Patients received their CDDP treatment at 6 A.M. or at 6 P.M. Evening cisplatin administration resulted in greater urine output, lower peak urinary platinum concentration, and lower areas under the curve of urinary cisplatin concentration. The normal circadian rhythm, characteristic of urine volume, 1 month after the treatment was disrupted by the morning CDDP treatment but not by the evening CDDP treatment.[168] Plasma protein binding of cisplatin has been found to be circadian stage dependent in humans, with its daily maximum around 4 P.M.[169]

Hydration reduces cisplatin nephrotoxicity.[170] An intraperitoneal saline load was given or withheld in female Fisher rats concurrently with cisplatin at six separate circadian times.[109] A marked rhythm in the amount of kidney protection achieved by the fluid load was observed. Hydration improved outcome most when given with platinum at its optimal circadian timing. Diethyldithiocarbamate or tetraethylthiocarbamate, which act through nucleophile excretion, protected from cisplatin induced nephrotoxicity only at times of day associated with high cisplatin toxicity.[171]

Cisplatin and its analogs are not cell cycle specific, but circadian rhythms have been well documented for renal cytokinetics.[172,173] Other cellular defenses of importance may be tied to cell cycle; for example, the urinary activity of many metabolically important renal tubular enzymes has a circadian rhythm in animals and healthy human volunteers.[162,174–176] A specific index of proximal tubular damage is an increase in the urinary excretion of (β-N-acetylglucosaminidase (β-NAG), a lysosomal enzyme released into the urine by normal proximal tubular cells.[177] Lévi documented in rats that β-NAG was released into the urine in proportion to the degree of histologically confirmed renal dysfunction induced by cisplatin.[162] This enzyme was present in the urine of normal animals, and its base line concentration was found to display a high-amplitude circadian rhythm. When cisplatin was given at its most toxic time, the circadian rhythm of urinary β-NAG was maintained, but the mean and peak levels increased fivefold in direct proportion to the subsequent rise in BUN. When cisplatin was given at a favorable circadian stage, these groups demonstrated a smaller β-NAG rise and had little histologic renal damage with only a small rise in BUN. Other thiol-rich proteins or amino acids such as GSH may play a role in the mechanism of circadian renal toxicity from platinum.[178]

Boughattas has looked at tissue concentration of cisplatin and carboplatin in spleen, kidney, and colon of mice given eight weekly courses of these drugs at one of three dosing times.[179] There was half the tissue accumulation of platinum when these drugs were given at their least toxic circadian times.

ALKYLATING AGENTS

Melphalan, peptichemio, cyclophosphamide, ifosfamide, and threosulfan toxicities are all characterized by circadian rhythms in murine tolerance.[117–120,123,180,181] These drugs have different times for best tolerance (see Table 69–28), perhaps because some of them must be metabolized to become active by different metabolic processes.

Three studies looked at the time-dependent anticancer activity of alkylating agents. Badran gave a single intraperitoneal dose of cyclophosphamide to female mice bearing transplantable mammary carcinoma at one of six circadian stages. Animals treated in the resting span (2, 6, and 10 HALO) developed significantly smaller tumors.[182] Focan treated sarcoma bearing mice with cyclophosphamide. Best antitumor effect was found if the drug was given early rest (02 HALO), coinciding with the G_2 phase of the sarcoma cells.[79] Cardoso observed maximal cure rate and least toxicity in leukemic mice when cyclophosphamide was given at the end of the rest period (12 HALO).[118] Anticancer activity was usually superior when the cytoxan was given in the second half of the daily sleep span, or just before or just after usual daily awakening.

Bladder toxicity from cyclophosphamide in male CD1-mice was minimal after dosing in midrest (7 HALO) or midactivity (19 HALO).[116] Most mucosal damage was induced with dosing in late rest (11 HALO) or late activity (23 HALO). These results suggest a 12-hour cycle in the sensitivity of the bladder to cyclophosphamide.

Mitomycin C can produce prolonged myelosuppression among other toxicities.[121,122] This drug was least toxic when given to mice in mid to late activity (17–20 HALO). Histologic evaluation of all target organs revealed that the lethal toxicity so profoundly modified by drug timing may well be related to the vexing clinical problem of mitomycin C induced microangiopathic disease.[122] No clinical work has been done to investigate this possibility.

Although the circadian timing of each alkylating agent studied markedly affects its toxicity, their optimal times are quite different. Clinical trials are needed to follow-up on the murine data.

CYTOSINE ARABINOSIDE

A single fixed dose of cytosine arabinoside (ara-C) administered daily for 6 days to mice was found to be least toxic when given in the rest span (2,5–7 HALO). The same dose of ara-C killed 15% of the animals if given in the rest span compared with 75% if given in the activity span.[183,184] Haus applied this finding to the treatment of leukemic mice.[126] Each animal received eight intraperitoneal injections of ara-C at 3-hour intervals over 24 hours. This was given on days 1, 6, 10, and 14. In one group of animals, the doses at the various injection times varied in amount according to a sinusoidal pattern, ranging from 7.5 mg/kg given at the predicted time of lowest resistance to 67.5 mg/kg given at the predicted time of highest resistance. Another group of animals received the same total doses in eight equal doses over each 24-hour period. A doubling of survival was observed in the sinusoidally treated group (23%) compared with the group given constant doses (11%).

In an attempt to unequivocally demonstrate rhythmic variation in tolerance to ara-C, studies were carried out by two different laboratories using the same experimental design as described previously, but on nontumor-bearing mice.[101] Eight differently timed circadian-shaped treatment schedules and one constant-dose schedule were used. The most favorable survival was achieved in the sinusoidal treatment arms in which the highest dose was given in the rest period (from 3.5–12.5 HALO). The homeostatic treatment achieved only 12.5% survival; 25% to 38% of the animals given treatment on "unfavorable" sinusoidal schedules survived, and the "favorable" sinusoidal treatments produced survival rates of 73% to 80%.

Hromas used flow cytometry to look at the effect of ara-C on the chronobiology of the bone marrow DNA synthesis in mice.[185] At all times, ara-C flattened the rhythm of bone marrow DNA synthesis; however, it had it's greatest effect if given when there were relatively more cells moving into S phase (18 HALO) or in S phase (0 HALO) than if few cells were in S phase (12 HALO) or cells were leaving S phase (6 HALO).

Scheving treated L1210 leukemic mice with a combination of intraperitoneal ara-C and cyclophosphamide at one of six circadian stages.[124] Best results with regard to cure rate and survival were observed when cyclophosphamide was given in late rest (8 HALO) and ara-C given by the sinusoidally shaped schedule found to be optimal in previous studies. In the animals receiving ara-C in the optimal fashion, the cure rate ranged from 44% to 94%, depending on the timing of the cyclophosphamide dose. Only 1.4% of these animals died from drug toxicity. When another group of animals was treated with the same drugs without chronobiologic consideration, 30% died from acute drug toxicity.

When vincristine was added to the best schedule of ara-C and cyclophosphamide described previously, best results (52% cure rate) were achieved when vincristine was given in late activity (23 HALO). When methylprednisolone was added to this three-drug scheme, best results were obtained when prednisolone was given in early activity (11 HALO or 14 HALO).[186] Attempts were made to improve the response rate further by adding cisplatin to this schedule.[187] The least toxic time for cisplatin was in late activity (20 HALO). With reduced drug dosage to decrease toxicity from this combination chemotherapy regimen, a 88% cure rate was obtained in these L1210 leukemic animals.

Rose confirmed the circadian variation in toxicity for ara-C and cyclophosphamide given as single agents.[188] The optimal therapeutic responses of leukemic mice treated in the least toxic way by ara-C or cyclophosphamide at maximal tolerated dose levels were no better than those achieved in leukemic mice receiving equitoxic, but results were achieved lower doses of these drugs by the conventional method and at other circadian stages. The design and analysis of this study have been criticized.[189]

Cytosine arabinoside alone or in combination with other cytotoxic agents was much more effective and much less toxic when given during the usual daily sleep span.

METHOTREXATE

Intravenous methotrexate was found to be most toxic in rats in late activity (23.5 HALO), with least toxicity in terms of marrow, renal, and liver toxicity in midactivity (17.5 HALO).[98] The pharmacokinetics of methotrexate were found to be circadian stage dependent, with the longest half-life after treatment at the most toxic time. The time of day of maximal toxicity coincided with the nadir for plasma corticosterone concentration. In subsequent studies by the same researchers, high plasma levels of exogenously administered corticosterone protected against methotrexate toxicity, but suppressed levels markedly increased toxicity unrelated to time.[99] Giving oral melatonin daily for 6 weeks before methotrexate treatment increased its toxicity at all time points.[190]

Labat found intraperitoneal methotrexate to be most toxic to male Swiss mice when given in early rest (2 HALO), as estimated by the relative weight loss after therapy.[100] The highest AUC values in this study were found after treatment in early rest. This observation is consistent with the work of English and with his earlier data, showing that the inhibition by methotrexate of the activity of renal dihydrofolate reductase (DHFR), the target enzyme for methotrexate, is maximal in the early rest period.[191] These results indicate clearly that methotrexate is least toxic when given in the middle of the daily activity span.

In a very limited two times of day study, Robinson did not find circadian variation in the pharmacokinetics for methotrexate in six lymphoma patients receiving the drug as a part of the CHOP chemotherapy.[16] Methotrexate was given as a 30 minute continuous infusion starting at 0600 or 1800, with each patient serving as his own control. The timing of oral methotrexate may be important in children on maintenance therapy for acute lymphoblastic leukemia.[192]

Methotrexate is metabolized only to a minor extent in rodents and is excreted largely unchanged in roughly equal amounts in the urine and in the bile, but in humans, the major route is renal excretion.[193] Variation in plasma clearance rate in rodents may be caused by variations in renal filtration rate or biliary output.

6-MERCAPTOPURINE

The course of 118 children with ALL, who had achieved complete remission with a standard induction protocol and had received meningeal prophylaxis with intrathecal methotrexate and cranial irradiation, was reviewed.[192] Maintenance therapy consisted of daily 6-mercaptopurine (6-MP), weekly methotrexate (MTX), and monthly vincristine and prednisone. For compliance reasons, 82 children took their 6-MP and MTX in the morning, and 36 children took these medications in the evening. Regression analysis showed that, for those children surviving free of disease for longer than 78 weeks, the

risk of relapsing was 4.6 times greater for the morning schedule than for the evening schedule ($p = 0.006$).

Studies of orally administered 6-MP and MTX have shown a poor correlation between the given dose and peak serum levels.[194] Absorption of MTX and 6-MP is better if the drugs are taken in a fasting state.[195,196] The bioavailability of 6-MP can be very low and unpredictable, and in some patients, the drug is undetectable in blood.[197] Evans and colleagues have shown that relapsing children have significantly faster clearance rates of MTX and therefore are exposed to substantially lower serum concentrations of the drug.[198] Peeters and associates reported that relapsing patients receive significantly less methotrexate during the first and second years of therapy.[199]

Balis and colleagues could not demonstrate any difference in the pharmacokinetics of MTX and 6-MP between morning and evening dosing in 17 children with ALL.[200] Koren and colleagues have studied the pharmacokinetics of intravenous MTX at 10 A.M. and 9 P.M. in 6 children with ALL.[200a] There was a significant fall in MTX plasma clearance at night ($p < 0.05$). Langevin and coworkers studied the pharmacokinetics of 6-MP in 6 children on this treatment for ALL.[201] After evening dosing, the AUC was significantly larger, and 6-MP had a longer half-life compared with morning dosing. Koren and colleagues compared the disposition pharmacokinetics of 6-MP administered in the morning or in the evening in 13 children with ALL.[202] The elimination half-life was longer, and the AUC, especially the AUC of the postdistributive phase, was significantly larger after evening dosing of the drug. In the same study, 12 children receiving the 6-MP in the morning were switched to an evening dose. Within 2 weeks there was a sharp fall in peripheral leukocyte counts in all patients. The leukocyte count during maintenance therapy was found to be significantly related to risk of relapse, giving patients with higher cell counts the poorer outcome.[203] The antileukemic effect of 6-MP is related to the incorporation of 6-MP derived neucleotides (6-TGN) into DNA. The erythrocyte concentration of 6-TGN achieved after a standard dose of 6-MP varied widely and was not correlated with the dose of 6-MP but was predictive of outcome in children on maintenance therapy (6-MP given in the morning after overnight fasting) for ALL.[204] Giving a constant dose of MTX and 6-MP, without modification with regard to achieved serum concentrations or induced toxicity, may expose these children to very different amounts of drugs over time and can affect their ultimate prognosis.

The anticancer pharmacodynamics of these antimetabolites, as reflected by the survival of children with ALL, is superior if the drugs are given in the evening. The time of day also affects the pharmacokinetics of each of these agents.

PLANT ALKALOIDS

The time for least toxicity in mice varies considerably for plant alkaloids. Vincristine is least toxic in early activity (13 HALO), and vinblastine is least toxic in midactivity (18 HALO).[112,113] Etoposide is best tolerated in late rest (7–11 HALO).[115] The solvent for VP-16 was more toxic to rodents than the combination of solvent and VP-16, and therefore these data may not truly reflect the circadian pharmacodynamics of VP-16.[114] The toxic response to the VP-16 plus solvent and solvent alone were time dependent, and the lethality patterns were about 180° out of phase with one another.

Focan demonstrated a circadian variation in vindesine serum concentration in 9 patients receiving this drug as a 48-hour continuous constant-rate infusion, with peak at about midday.[15] In a study of 34 patients receiving cisplatin (given at 6 P.M. daily for 3 days) and etoposide (given at 7 A.M. or 7 P.M., daily for 3 days), less hematologic toxicity was found in the group receiving etoposide at 7 A.M.[205] Focan reported a randomized trial using 124 patients with previously untreated advanced lung cancer.[206] Etoposide (100 mg/m^2) was given on days 1, 2, and 3 at 6 A.M. (group A) or at 6 P.M. (group B). Cisplatin (100 mg/m^2) was given on day 4 at 6 P.M. Animal studies have predicted that the 6 A.M. etoposide dose (group A) would be less toxic. Interim analysis of 76 patients and 126 courses confirmed lesser hematologic toxicity in group A, but cisplatin was better tolerated in group B. No differences could be established in the overall dose intensities of drugs or in the frequency of tumor response. The most commonly used plant alkaloids, vincristine and vinblastine, may be less toxic if given during the first half of the daily activity span.

ADRENAL CORTICOSTEROIDS

Adrenal corticosteroids are widely used as antiemetic agents in patients receiving chemotherapy and as an integral part of the chemotherapy protocol in some hematologic malignancies. The activity of several hepatic drug-metabolizing enzymes are influenced by corticosterone in mice.[44] It is not surprising that these agents can modulate the efficacy and toxicity of some chemotherapy agents. English and colleagues documented that the time of maximal toxicity for methotrexate is in the late activity period.[98] This coincides with the time of the lowest level of serum corticosterone. In another study, these researchers gave dexamethasone or corticosterone to the animals for 10 days before a dose of methotrexate.[99] The dexamethasone suppressed the corticosterone level and abolished its normal circadian rhythm, but the corticosterone resulted in high corticosterone plasma levels throughout the day. The dexamethasone-treated animals all died from the methotrexate treatment within 5 days, regardless of the time of administration. Less toxicity was observed in the animals receiving the corticosterone than in those receiving either dexamethasone or placebo steroids before treatment. In the control group, the late activity span was again found to be the time of worst methotrexate toxicity. In vitro work with L1210 murine leukemia cells has indicated that cortisol and methylprednisolone can inhibit uptake of methotrexate by these lymphoblastoid cells.[207] Prednisolone has improved the therapeutic index of several alkylating agents in nonsteroid-responsive cancer cell lines, but exogenous corticosteroids decreased the antitumor effect of cyclophosphamide in Erlich ascites carcinoma-bearing female mice.[129,208] Giving ACTH 24 hours before doxorubicin raised GSH levels to their circadian maxima in a variety of murine tissues and protected against toxicity from intravenous doxorubicin in mice.[102] Children with ALL had better survival rates when maintenance chemotherapy consisting of daily 6 mercaptopurine and weekly methotrexate was given in the evening rather than in

the morning.[192] This time coincides with the lowest level of plasma cortisol.

ACTH, corticosteroids, and melatonin are agents that demonstrate the potential for manipulating some circadian toxicity patterns.[190] Giving oral melatonin daily for 6 weeks before methotrexate treatment increased the toxicity at all time points in rats, but especially at time points for which melatonin was artificially high.[190] Extending the period during which melatonin is high is theoretically equal to extending the dark phase in photoperiodic species.[209] This chronobiotic approach to making each time of day predictably the optimal time requires much more preclinical and clinical work to make it practical. There is every reason to believe, for example, that the optimal chronobiotic for one cytotoxic agent may differ from that for another. The effective use of a chronobiotic depends intimately on when it is given—when in circadian terms and when relative to the drugs whose toxic to therapeutic ratios are to be modulated.

BIOLOGIC RESPONSE MODIFIERS AND GROWTH FACTORS

Biologic response modifiers are a new important class of weapon in the armamentarium against cancer. We are at a very early stage in our understanding of these agents and their potential therapeutic applications. Early data indicate that these agents may be even more circadian stage dependent with regard to toxicity and therapeutic efficacy than the traditional chemotherapeutics. This is logical because the xenobiotics, reactive chemicals, and antimetabolites that have served as the mainstay for systemic cancer therapy usually have multiple metabolites and many subcellular targets, unlike the receptor-mediated and highly specific activity of peptides.

In humans, erythropoietin, which stimulates bone marrow erythroid precursors to produce new erythrocytes, peaks at around 8 P.M., and reticulocyte numbers peak some 5 hours later.[210,211] Wood gave recombinant human erythropoietin (rhEPO) to female CD$_2$F$_1$ mice at one of six circadian stages. The reticulocyte response to rhEPO varied almost sevenfold as a function of its circadian timing, with the greatest response occurring when rhEPO was given before usual awakening compared with later in the day.[212] Vysula and colleagues have looked at the time-dependent activity of G-CSF in rodents.[216a] In two separate studies, 89 female C3HeB/FeJ mice were given either G-CSF or sterile normal saline. In the first study, G-CSF was given in a dose of 5 µg/kg for 5 consecutive days at one of six equispaced times of day. Leukocytes were measured at baseline and daily for 13 days after G-CSF administration. In the second study, mammary adenocarcinoma was inoculated and a single 25 µg/kg dose of G-CSF was given 7 days later when tumor was palpable. Tumor volume was measured daily for 9 days after the G-CSF administration. The rise in leukocytes after G-CSF was found to be circadian-stage dependent, with the maximum rise in total leukocyte count after dosing in the mid-activity phase. Unexpectedly, G-CSF was found to have antitumor activity, with the maximum tumor reduction at the time of best leukocyte count response.

Interleukin-2 (IL-2) has profound circadian-dependent effects on DNA synthesis in many organs of CD2F1 mice.[213,214] Feuers studied the circadian-dependent effect of IL-2 on enzymes of lipid, amino acid, and carbohydrate metabolism in male CD2F1 mice.[215] IL-2 had no significant effect if given during the light span. When treatment was given in the dark span, IL-2 produced statistically significant increases in enzymes of glycolysis and lipid synthesis, but amino acid metabolism was decreased. Von Roemeling gave recombinant IL-2 to mice at one of six circadian stages.[216] Significant circadian rhythmicity (>50% of daily mean) affected spleen weight of control mice, as well as the proportion of suppressor T cells in spleen and bone marrow, and Lyt-5.2$^+$ cells in bone marrow. IL-2 increased the number of spleen cells by 16% overall, but up to threefold more when it was given during the activity span of the animals ($p < 0.02$). Toxicity as gauged by wet-dry lung weight was minimal but clearly circadian stage dependent. Daily administration of IL-2 to mice bearing Meth A sarcoma had opposite effects on the balance between host and cancer, depending on the time of administration. IL-2 given just before usual daily awakening halved tumor growth compared with diluent-treated mice. IL-2 given in the middle of daily activity more than doubled tumor growth rate compared with concurrent diluent treatment or to IL-2 treatment just before awakening.[70]

The toxicity of tumor necrosis factor (TNF) in mice is highly circadian stage dependent, with 90% mortality in late rest (10 HALO) and only 10% mortality in midactivity (18 HALO) after a 750 to 1000 μg/kg dose was given intravenously.[217]

Clinical experience with toxicity and some physiologic observations indicate that the best time to give interferon may be in the evening.[218-220] Under physiologic conditions, interferon plasma levels are negligible in the morning, but they tend to increase in the late afternoon.[221] There is a circadian variation of several lymphocyte subsets, including monocytes, with the lowest level in the morning and highest levels at night.[211] These are one type of the effector cells for interferon. Interferon causes a marked but transient rise in the plasma 11-hydroxycorticosteroids, with a peak about 8 hours after injection. Evening administration did not interfere with the normal rhythm of corticosteroids, with a peak in the morning.[220] However, a peak in plasma steroids in the evening, induced by morning interferon, may hinder the normal rise in circulating lymphocytes in the evening. Gatti looked at circadian changes in the enhancement of the natural killer (NK) cell activity after exposure to interferon-γ of peripheral blood mononuclear cells obtained from 7 healthy volunteers over 24 hours.[222] Maximal enhancement of NK activity was attained in blood removed in the second part of the night or in the early morning, in phase with the peak of the spontaneous NK activity in these volunteers. A phase I clinical trial of a 21-day circadian infusion of interferon-α has been reported.[223] The investigators gave interferon-α2 as a continuous circadian modulated infusion to 10 patients with metastatic melanoma or renal cell cancer for 21 days with a treatment-free interval of 10 days between courses. The largest proportion of the 24-hour dose was given from 6 P.M. to 10 P.M. The starting dose was 15 MU/m²/day. Doses were escalated as high as 20 MU/m²/day. Dose-limiting toxicity was fatigue in 9 of the 10 patients. All patients experienced a grade I flu-like syndrome limited to the first 4 to 5 days of each treatment course. A mild dose-dependent somnolence was noted in 2 patients. Grade III–IV neutropenia was observed in 25% of all courses in 5 patients.

PRACTICAL IMPLICATIONS OF CIRCADIAN EFFECTS

Each cytotoxic or biologic agent that has been tested at different circadian stages in rodents shows a significant circadian stage dependency for toxicity. In most cases of tumor-bearing animals given chemotherapy, the time of least toxicity has coincided with or was close to the time of best antitumor activity. There are compelling experimental data suggesting that the therapeutic index of commonly applied anticancer agents can be improved by the optimal circadian timing of treatment. Clinical trials have confirmed the decreased toxicity and demonstrated that maximal safe dose intensity is dependent on the time of drug therapy. Additional prospective, randomized studies are required to demonstrate if a better response rate or survival can be achieved in patients given chemotherapy based on these principles.

These data have significant implications for new anticancer drug discovery and development. Usually, drugs leave murine toxicology, done at the beginning to middle of the daily rest span in the mice and rats, and are immediately tested in humans at a similar clock hour, in the first half or middle of the patient's daily activity span (*i.e.*, the opposite circadian time). It is not common practice to optimize or fix the circadian stage of drug administration in phase I–II trials. This process of anticancer drug selection introduces a clear selection bias for agents that are safe and active in the rest span and may explain in part why many drugs reaching phase I–II studies are ultimately abandoned because of toxicity or lack of activity at achievable doses. Phase III studies, comparing a "standard treatment" to a new treatment, may be comparing apples and oranges if all agents in all arms are not given at their optimal times. These concepts apply even more urgently to research using the various new biologic response modifiers and growth factors. Early data indicate that these agents are even more profoundly circadian stage dependent with regard to response and toxicity than the classic cytotoxic agents.

Toxicity is an important endpoint in itself in patients receiving chemotherapy. Chemotherapy-induced toxicity affects the quality of life for these patients and increases costs of health care. Even if we observe similar response rates but less toxicity by using chronochemotherapy, something important has been gained. Toxicity becomes an important issue with regard to adjuvant treatment. A large proportion of patients receiving adjuvant treatment are not destined to have recurrence of their cancer, but receive adjuvant chemotherapy as an insurance policy against future relapse. It is important to be able to offer patients in this situation safe and effective chemotherapy.

Evidence from studies with chronochemotherapy in animals and humans confirm that this scheduling method reduces bone marrow toxicity but also reduces other types of toxicity such as gastrointestinal and renal toxicity. This scheduling method therefore offers the possibility of giving more dose-intensive chemotherapy without more toxicity and could work well in conjunction with other strategies for high-dose chemotherapy. Dose intensity is in itself a time-dependent variable, because the pharmacokinetics and pharmacodynamics of the major anticancer agents depend on the time of delivery. This fact complicates even further the practice of dose-intensity calculation.

We are still at an early stage in understanding the mechanisms responsible for the circadian dependency of toxicity and efficacy. Interindividual variation in the best timing for certain drugs is a potential problem. Ideally, the best treatment time should be determined for each person according to measurable internal marker rhythms.[88] More work is needed in this area to optimize the benefits of chronochemotherapy for each patient. Clinical trials have, however, documented that we can gain substantially by delivering many drugs at or near the optimal time of day for that drug.

REFERENCES

1. Reinberg A, Smolensky MH. Circadian changes of drug disposition in man. Clin Pharmacokinet 1982;7:401–420.
2. Hrushesky WJ. Chemotherapy timing: An important variable in toxicity and response. In: Perry MC, Yarbro JM, eds. Toxicity of chemotherapy. Orlando: Grune & Stratton, 1984:449–477.
3. Lévi F, Boughattas NA, Blazsek I. Comparative murine chronotoxicity of anticancer agents and related mechanisms. In: Reinberg A, Smolensky M, Labrecque G, eds. Annual review of chronopharmacology, vol 4. Oxford: Pergamon Press, 1987:283–331.
4. Lévi F, Soussan A, Adam R, Caussanel J, Metzger G, Misset JL. Programmable-in time pumps for chronotherapy of patients with colorectal cancer with 5-day circadian-modulated venous infusion of 5-fluorouracil. Proc Am Soc Clin Oncol [Abstract] 1989;8:A429.
5. Hrushesky WJM, von Roemeling R, Lanning RM, Rabatin JT. Circadian-shaped infusion of floxuridine for progressive metastatic renal cell carcinoma. J Clin Oncol 1990;8:1504–1513.
6. von Roemeling R, Hrushesky WJM. Circadian patterning of continuous floxuridine infusion reduces toxicity and allows higher dose intensity in patients with widespread cancer. J Clin Oncol 1989;7:1710–1719.
7. Wesen C, Hrushesky WJM, Roemeling R, Lanning R, Rabatin J, Grage T. Circadian modification of intra-arterial 5-fluoro-2'-deoxyuridine infusion rate reduces its toxicity and permits higher dose intensity. J Infus Chemother 1992;2(2):69–75.
8. Lévi F, Benavides M, Chevelle C, et al. Chemotherapy of advanced ovarian cancer with 4'-O-tetrahydropyranyl doxorubicin and cisplatin: A randomized phase II trial with an evaluation of circadian timing and dose-intensity. J Clin Oncol 1990;8:705–714.
9. Lévi F, Misset JL, Brienza S, et al. A chronopharmacologic phase-II clinical trial with 5-fluorouracil, folinic acid, and oxaliplatin using an ambulatory multichannel programmable pump. Cancer 1992;69:893–900.
10. Hrushesky WJM. Circadian timing of cancer chemotherapy. Science 1985;228:73–75.
11. Hrushesky JM. Circadian scheduling of chemotherapy increases ovarian patient survival and cancer responses significantly. Proc Annu Meet Am Soc Clin Oncol [Abstract] 1987;6:A473.
12. Hrushesky WJM, Roemeling RV, Wood PA, Langevin TR, Lange P, Farley E. High-dose intensity systemic therapy of metastatic bladder cancer. J Clin Oncol 1987;5:450–455.
13. Hrushesky WJM, Borch R, Levi F. Circadian time dependence of cisplatin urinary kinetics. Clin Pharmacol Ther 1982;32:330–339.
14. Petit E, Milano G, Levi F, Thyss A, Bailleul F, Schneider M. Circadian rhythm-varying plasma concentration of 5-fluorouracil during a five day continuous infusion at a constant rate in cancer patients. Cancer Res 1988;48:1676–1679.
15. Focan C, Mazy JM, Zhou J, Rahmani R, Cano JP. Circadian variation of vindesine serum concentrations during continuous infusion. In: Reinberg A, Smolensky M, Labreque G, eds. Annual review of chronopharmacology, vol 5. Oxford: ergamon Press, 1988:411–414.
16. Robinson BA, Begg EJ, Colls BM, Jefferey GM, Sharman JR. Circadian pharmacokinetics of methotrexate. Cancer Chemother Pharmacol 1989;24:397–399.
17. Scheving LE. Chronobiology of cell proliferation in mammals: Implications for basic research and cancer chemotherapy. In: Edmunds LN, ed. Cell cycle clocks. New York: Marcel Dekker, 1984:455–499.
18. Nash RE, Echave Llanos JM. Circadian variation in DNA synthesis of fast-growing and slow-growing hepatoma: DNA synthesis rhythm in hepatoma. JNCI 1971;47:1007–1012.
19. Burns ER, Scheving LE, Tsai TH. Circadian rhythms in DNA synthesis and mitosis in normal mice and in mice bearing the Lewis lung carcinoma. Eur J Cancer 1979;15:233–242.
20. Aschoff J. Comparative physiologyurnal rhythms. Ann Rev Physiol 1963;25:581.
21. Bünning E. Die physiologische Uhr. Berlin: Springer Verlag, 1963.
22. De Mairan J. Observation botanique. Hist Acad R Sci Paris 1729;:35–36.
23. Richter CPA. A behavioristic study of the activity of the rat. Comp Physiol Monogr 1922;1.
24. Johnson MS. Activity and distribution of certain wild mice in relation to biotic communities. J Mammal 1926;7:245–277.
25. Reinberg A. Clinical chronopharmacology, an experimental basis for chronotherapy. Drug Res 1978;28:1861.
26. Konopka RJ, Benzer S. Clock mutants of drosophila melanogaster. Proc Nat Acad Sci USA 1971;68:2112–2116.
27. Hall JC, Rosbash M. Mutations and molecules influencing biological rhythms. Ann Rev Neurosci 1988;11:373–393.
28. Dunlap JC. Closely watched clocks: Molecular analysis of circadian rhythms in Neurospora and Drosophila. Trends Genet 1990;6(5).
29. Ralph MR, Menaker M. A mutation of the circadian system in golden hamsters. Science 1988;241:1225–1227.
30. Meijer JH, Reitveld WJ. Neurophysiology of the suprachiasmatic circadian pacemaker in rodents. Physiol Rev 1989;69:671–707.
31. Sawaki Y, Nihonmatsu I, Kawamura H. Transplantation of the neonatal suprachiasmatic nuclei into rats with complete bilateral suprachiasmatic lesions. Neurosci Res 1984;1:67–72.
32. Drucker-Colin R, Aguilar-Roblero F, Garcia-Hernandez F, Fernandez-Cancinoa F, Rattoni FB. Fetal suprachiasmatic nucleus transplants: Diurnal rhythm recovery of lesioned rats. Brain Res 1984;311:353–357.
33. DeCoursey PJ, Buggy J. Restoration of locomotor rhythmicity in SCN-lesioned golden hamsters by transplantation of fetal SCN. Neurosci Abstr 1986;12:210.
34. Lehman MN, Silver R, Gladstone WR, Kahn RM, Gibson M, Bittman EL. Circadian rhythmicity restored by neural transplant. Immunocytochemical characterization of the graft and its integration with the host brain. J Neurosci 1987;7:1626–1638.
35. Ralph MR, Foster RG, Davis FC, Menaker M. Transplanted suprachiasmatic nucleus determines circadian period. Science 1990;247:975–978.
36. Moore-Ede MC, Czeisler CA, Richardson GS. Circadian timekeeping in health and disease. Part 1. Basic properties of circadian pacemakers. N Engl J Med 1983;309:469–476.
37. Moore-Ede MC, Czeisler CA, Richardson GS. Circadian timekeeping in health and disease. Part 2. Clinical implications of circadian rhythmicity. N Engl J Med 1983;309:530–536.
38. Aschoff J. On the perception of time during prolonged temporal isolation. Hum Neurobiol 1985;4:41–52.
39. Bruguerolle B. Temporal aspects of drug absorption and drug distribution. In: Lemmer B, ed. Chronopharmacology: Cellular and biochemical interactions. New York: Markel Dekker, 1989:3–13.
40. Belanger MP, Labreque G. Temporal aspects of drug metabolism. In: Lemmer B, ed. Chronopharmacology: Cellular and biochemical interactions. New York: Markel Dekker, 1989:15–34.
41. Waterhouse JM, Minors DS. Temporal aspects of renal drug elimination. In: Lemmer B, ed. Chronopharmacology: Cellular and biochemical interactions. New York: Markel Dekker, 1989:35–50.
42. Koopman MG, Krediet RT, Arisz L. Circadian rhythms and the kidney. Neth J Med 1985;28:416–423.
43. North C, Feuers RJ, Scheving LE, Pauli JE, Tsai TH, Casciano DA. Circadian organization of thirteen liver and six brain enzymes of the mouse. Am J Anat 1981;162:184–199.
44. Radzialowski FM, Bousquet WF. Daily rhythmic variation in hepatic drug metabolism in rat and mouse. J Pharmacol Exp Ther 1968;163:229–238.
45. Hughes A, Jacabon HI, Wagner RK, Jungblut PW. Ovarian independent fluctuations of estradiol receptor levels in mammalian tissues. Mol Cell Endocrinol 1976;5:379–388.
46. Wirz-Justice A. Neuropsychopharmacology and biological rhythms. In: Mendlewics J, ed. Biological rhythms and behavior. Basel: Karger, 1982.
47. Wirz-Justice A, Wehr TA, Goodwin FK, et al. Antidepressant drugs slow circadian rhythm in behaviour and brain neurotransmitter receptors. Psychopharmacol Bull 1980;16:45.
48. Adams J, Carmichael J, Wolf CR. Altered mouse bone marrow glutathione transferase levels in response to cytotoxins. Cancer Res 1985;45:1669–1673.
49. Bellamy WT, Alberts DS, Dorr RT. Daily variation in non-protein sulfhydryl levels of human bone marrow. Eur J Cancer Clin Oncol 1988;24:1759–62.
50. Hrushesky WJM, Dell I, Eaton J, Halberg F. Circadian-stage-dependent effect of doxorubicin upon reduced glutathione in the murine heart. Proc Annu Meet Am Assoc Cancer Res [Abstract] 1982;23:12.
51. Smaaland R, Svardal AM, Lote K, Ueland PM, Laerum OD. Glutathione content in human bone marrow and circadian stage relation to DNA synthesis. JNCI 1991;83:1092–1098.
52. Scheving LE, Tsai TS, Feuers RJ, Scheving LA. Cellular mechanisms involved in the action of anticancer drugs. In: Lemmer B, ed. Chronopharmacology: Cellular and biochemical interactions. New York and Basel: Markel Dekker, 1989:317–369.
53. Haus E, Halberg F, Kuhl JFW, Lakatua DJ. Chronopharmacology in animals. Chronobiologia 1974;1(suppl 1):122.
54. Harris BE, Song R, Soong SJ, Diasio RB. Relationship between dihydropyrimidine dehydrogenase activity and plasma 5-fluorouracil levels with evidence for circadian variation of enzyme activity and plasma drug levels in cancer patients receiving 5-fluorouracil by protracted continuous infusion. Cancer Res 1990;50:197–201.
55. Scheving LE. Circadian rhythms in cell proliferation: Their importance when investigating the basic mechanism of normal versus abnormal growth. In: von Mayersbach H, Scheving LE, Pauli JE, eds. 11th International Congress of Anatomy, part C: Biological rhythms in structure and function. New York: Alan R Liss, 1981:39–79.
56. Hrushesky WJM, Merdink J, Abdel-Monem M. Circadian rhythmicity characterizes monoacetyl polyamine urinary excretion. Cancer Res 1983;43:3944–3947.
57. Scheving LE, Burns ER, Pauli JE, Tsai TH. Circadian variation and cell division of

the mouse alimentary tract, bone marrow and corneal epithelium. Anat Rec 1978;191:479–486.

58. Buchi KN, Moore JG, Hrushesky WJM, Sothern RB, Rubin NH. Circadian rhythm of cellular proliferation in the human rectal mucosa. Gastroenterology 1991;101:410–15.

59. Sletvold O, Smaaland R, Laerum OD. Cytometry and time-dependent variations in peripheral blood and bone marrow cells: A literature review and relevance to the chronotherapy of cancer. Chronobiol Int 1991;8:235–250.

60. Stoney PJ, Halberg F, Simpson HW. Circadian variation in colony-forming ability of presumable intact murine bone marrow cells. Chronobiologia 1975;2:319–324.

61. Bartlett P, Haus E, Tuason T, Sacket-Lundeen L, Lakatua D. Circadian rhythm in number of erythroid and granulocytic colony forming units in culture (ECFU-C and GCFU-C) in bone marrow of BDF1 male mice. In: Haus E, Kabat HF, eds. Proceeding of the 15th International Conference on Chronobiology. Basel: S Krager, 1984:160–164.

62. Killman SA, Cronkite EP, Fliedner TM, Bond VP. Mitotic indices of human bone marrow cells. I. Number and cytologic distribution of mitosis. Blood 1962;19:743–750.

63. Mauer AM. Diurnal variation of proliferative activity in the human bone marrow. Blood 1965;26:1–7.

64. Smaaland R, Laerum OD, Lote K, Sletvold O, Sothern RB, Bjerknes R. DNA synthesis in human bone marrow is circadian stage dependent. Blood 1991;77:2603–2611.

65. Morley AA. A neutrophil cycle in healthy individuals. Lancet 1966;ii:1220.

66. Ponassi A, Morran L, Bonanni F, et al. Normal range of blood colony forming cells (CFU-C) in humans. Blut 1979;39:257.

66a. Smaaland R, Abrahamsen JF, Svardal AM, Lote K, Ueland PM. DNA cell cycle distribution and glutathione (GSH) content according to circadian stage in bone marrow of cancer patients. Br J Cancer 1992;66:39–45.

67. Flentje M, Akokan G, Reinecke D, Klein HO. Diurnal variations of tumor growth and its influence on cytostatic treatment. Blut 1981;43:85–88.

68. Waldrop RD, Saydjari R, Rubin NH, Rayford PL, Townsend CM, Thompson JC. Photoperiod influences the growth of colon cancer in mice. Life Sci 1989;45:737–744.

69. Blask DE, Pelletier DB, Hill SM, et al. Pineal melatonin inhibition of tumor promotion in the N-nitroso-N-methylurea model of mammary carcinogenesis: Potential involvement of antiestrogenic mechanisms in vivo. J Cancer Res Clin Oncol 1991;117:1–7.

70. Hrushesky WJM, Sánchez P, Wood PA, et al. Heterogeneity of interleukin-2 therapeutic activity. Proc Am Assoc Cancer Res [Abstract] 1992;33:A1791.

71. Voutilainen A. Über die 24-stunden-rhythmik der mitozfrequenz in malignen tumoren. Acta Pathol Microb Scan 1953;99(Suppl):1–104.

72. Tähti E. Studies of the effect of x-irradiation on 24 hour variations in the mitotic activity in human malignant tumours. Acta Pathol Microbiol Scand 1956;117:1–61.

73. Garcia-Sainz M, Halberg F. Mitotic rhythms in human cancer reevaluated by electronic computer programs. Evidence for chronopathology. JNCI 1966;37:279–292.

74. Stoll BA, Burch WM. Surface detection of circadian rhythm in ^{32}P content of cancer of the breast. Cancer 1968;21:193–196.

75. Gautherie M, Gros C. Circadian rhythm alteration of skin temperature in breast cancer. Chronobiologia 1974;4:1–17.

76. Klevecz RR, Shymko RM, Blumenfeld D, Braly PS. Circadian gating of S phase human ovarian cancer. Cancer Res 1987;47:6267–6271.

77. Smaaland R, Lote K, Sothern RB, Laerum OD. Circadian and circannual variation in DNA synthesis in non-Hodgkin's lymphoma. Biological rhythms and medications: The Fifth International Conference of Chronopharmacology, Amelia Island, FL [Abstract] 1992;:AIV-12.

78. Caussanel JP, Lévi F, Brienza S, et al. Phase I trial of 5-day continuous venous infusion of oxaliplatin at circadian rhythm-modulated rate compared with constant rate. JNCI 1990;82:1046–1050.

79. Focan C, Barbason H, Betz EH. Influence du rythme nycthéméral des division cellulaires sur l'efficacité de la cyclophosphamide contre des sarcomes induits par le méthylcholanthréne. C R Acad Sci (Paris) 1973;276:136–137.

80. Focan C, Schyns-Mosen J, Barbason H, Betz EH. Kinetically scheduled sequential chemotherapy with cyclophosphamide and vinblastine in methylcholanthrene-induced sarcoma of mice. In: Reinberg A, Smolensky M, Labrecque G, eds. Annual review of chronopharmacology, vol 3. Oxford: Pergamon Press, 1986:191–194.

81. Bjarnason GA, Hrushesky WJM. Circadian cancer chemotherapy: Clinical trials. J Infus Chemother 1992;2(2):79–88.

82. Focan C. Sequential chemotherapy and circadian rhythm in human solid tumors. Cancer Chemother Pharmacol 1979;3:197–202.

83. Sothern RB, Halberg F, Hrushesky WJM. Circadian stage not time of day characterizes doxorubicin susceptibility rhythm of mice in continuous light. In: Reinberg A, Smolensky M, Labrecque G, eds. Annual review of chronopharmacology, vol 5. Oxford: Pergamon Press, 1988:385–388.

84. Scheving LE. Chronobiology, a new perspective for chronobiology in medicine. In: Saletu B, ed. Proceedings of the 11th International Neuro-psycho-pharmacologium Congress. Oxford: Pergamon Press, 1978:629–646.

85. Benton LA, Berry SJ, Yates FE. Ultradian rhythmic models of blood pressure variation in normal human daily life. Chronobiologia 1990;17:95–116.

86. Halberg F, Johnson EA, Nelson W, Runge W, Sothern E. Autorhythmometry procedures for physiological self measurement and their analysis. Physiol Tech 1972;1:1–11.

87. Haus E, Nicolau GY, Lakatua D, Sackett-Lundeen L. Reference values for Chronopharmacology. In: Reinberg A, Smolensky M, Labrecque G, eds. Annual review of chronopharmacology, vol 4. Oxford: Pergamon Press, 1987:333–424.

88. Hrushesky WJM, Haus E, Lakatua DJ, Halberg F, Langevin T, Kennedy BJ. Marker rhythms for cancer chrono-chemotherapy. In: Haus E, Kabat HF, eds. Chronobiology 1982–1983. New York: Krager, 1985:493–499.

89. Mormont C, Boughattas N, Lévi F. Mechanisms of circadian rhythms in the toxicity and efficacy of anticancer drugs: Relevance for the development of new analogs. In: Lemmer B, ed. Chronopharmacology: Cellular and biochemical interactions. New York and Basel: Markel Dekker, 1989:395–437.

90. Roemeling Rv, Hrushesky WJM. Circadian pattern of continuous FUDR infusion reduces toxicity. In: Pauli JE, Scheving LE, eds. Advances in chronobiology, Part B. New York: Alan R Liss, 1987:357–373.

91. von Roemeling R, Hrushesky WJM. Determination of the therapeutic index of floxuridine by its circadian infusion pattern. JNCI 1990;82:386–393.

92. Gonzalez RB, Sothern RB, Thatcher G, Nguyen N, Hrushesky WJM. Substantial difference in timing of murine circadian susceptibility to 5-fluorouracil and FUDR. Proc Annu Meet Am Assoc Cancer Res [Abstract] 1989;30:A2452.

93. Gardner MLG, Plumb JA. Diurnal variation in the intestinal toxicity of 5-fluorouracil in the rat. Clin Sci 1981;61:717–722.

94. Peters GJ, Van Dijk J, Nadal JC, Van Groeningen CJ, Lankelman J, Pinedo HM. Diurnal variation in the therapeutic efficacy of 5-fluorouracil against murine colon cancer. In Vivo 1987;1:113–118.

95. Minshull M, Gardner MLG. The effect of time of administration of 5-fluorouracil on leukopenia in the rat. Eur J Cancer Clin Oncol 1984;20:857–858.

96. Popovic P, Popovic V, Baughman J. Circadian rhythm and 5-fluorouracil toxicity in C₃H mice. Biomed Thermol 1982;25:185–187.

97. Burns RE, Beland SS. Effect of biological time on the determination of the LD₅₀ of 5-fluorouracil in mice. Pharmacology 1984;28:296–300.

98. English J, Aherne GW, Marks V. The effect of timing of a single injection on the toxicity of methotrexate in the rat. Cancer Chemother Pharmacol 1982;9:114–117.

99. English J, Aherne GW, Marks V. The effect of abolition of the endogenous corticosteroid rhythm on the circadian variation in methotrexate toxicity in the rat. Cancer Chemother Pharmacol 1987;19:287–290.

100. Labat C, Mansour K, Malmary MF, Terrissol M, Oustrin J. Chronotoxicity of methotrexate in mice after intraperitoneal administration. Chronobiologia 1987;14:267–75.

101. Scheving LE, Haus E, Kuhl JFW, Pauly JE, Halberg F, Cardoso SS. Different laboratories closely reproduce characteristics of circadian rhythm in tolerance of mice for arabinofuranosylcytosine. Cancer Res. 1976;36:113–1137.

102. Lévi F, Halberg F, Haus E, et al. Synthetic adrenocorticotropin for optimizing murine circadian chronotolerance for Adriamycin. Chronobiologia 1980;7:227–244.

103. Sothern RB, Nelson WL, Halberg F. A circadian rhythm in susceptibility of mice to the anti-tumor drug Adriamycin. In: Proceedings of the 12th International Conference of the International Society for Chronobiology. Milano: Il Ponte, 1977:433–438.

104. Sothern RB, Halberg F, Good R, Simpson H, Grage T. Differing characteristics of circadian rhythms in murine tolerance to chemically related antibiotics: Adriamycin and daunomycin. In: Walker CA, Soliman K, Winget C, eds. Chronopharmacology. Gainesville, FL: University Presses of Florida, 1981.

105. Mormont MC, Roemeling RV, Sothern RB, et al. Circadian and seasonal dependence in the toxicological response of mice to epirubicin. Invest New Drugs 1988;6:273–284.

106. Lévi F, Mechkouri M, Roulon A, et al. Circadian rhythm in tolerance of mice for the new anthracycline analog 4'-tetrahydropyranyl Adriamycin (THP). Eur J Cancer Clin Oncol 1985;121:1245–1251.

107. Metzger G, Bizi E, Mechkouri M, Halleck M, Lévi F. A pharmacokinetic mechanism for the circadian rhythm in mitoxantrone toxicity in mice. Proc Am Ass Cancer Res [Abstract] 1990;31:A2375.

108. Hrushesky WJM, Lévi F, Halberg F, Kennedy BJ. Circadian stage dependence of cisdiamminedichloroplatinum lethal toxicity in rats. Cancer Res 1982;42:945–949.

109. Lévi F, Hrushesky WJM, Halberg F, Langevin TR, Haus E, Kennedy BJ. Lethal nephrotoxicity and hematologic toxicity of cis-diamminedichloroplatinum ameliorated by optimal circadian timing and hydration. Eur J Cancer Clin Oncol 1982;18:471–477.

110. Boughattas N, Lévi F, Fournier C, et al. Circadian rhythm in toxicities and tissue uptake of 1,2-diamminocyclohexane (trans-1)oxalatoplatinum(II) in mice. Cancer Res 1989;49:3362–3368.

111. Boughattas N, Lévi F, Hecquet B, et al. Circadian time dependence of murine tolerance for carboplatin. Toxicol Appl Pharmacol 1988;96:233–247.

112. Mormont MC, Berestka J, Mushiya T, et al. Circadian dependence of vinblastine toxicity. In: Reinberg A, Smolensky M, Labrecque G, eds. Annual review of chronopharmacology, vol 3. Oxford: Pergamon Press, 1986:187–190.

113. Halberg F, Gupta B, Haus E, et al. Steps toward a chronopolychemotherapy. Proceedings of the 14th International Congress of Therapeutics. Paris: L'Expansion Scientifique Francaise, 1977:151–196.

114. Tsai TH, Scheving LE. Murine circadian variation in susceptibility to epipodophillotoxin (VP16) as well as to the solvent alone in which it was suspended. In: Reinberg A, Smolensky M, Labrecque G, eds. Annual review of chronopharmacology, vol 3. Oxford: Pergamon Press, 1984:389–392.

115. Lévi F, Mechkouri M, Roulon A, et al. Circadian rhythm in tolerance of mice for etoposide. Cancer Treat Rep 1985;69:1443–1445.

116. Hacker MP, Ershler WB, Newman RA, Fagan MA. Chronobiologic fluctuation of cyclophosphamide induced urinary bladder damage. Chronobiologia 1983;10:301–306.

117. Haus E, Fernandes G, Kuhl JFW, Yunis EJ, Lee JP, Halberg F. Murine circadian susceptibility rhythm to cyclophosphamide. Chronobiologia 1974;1:270–277.

118. Cardoso SS, Avery T, Venditti JM, Goldin A. Circadian dependence of host and tumor response to cyclophosphamide in mice. Eur J Cancer 1978;14:949–954.

119. Snyder NK, Smolensky M, Hsi BP. Circadian variation in the susceptibility of male Balb/c mice to iphosphamide. Chronobiologia 1981;8:33–44.

120. Lévi F, Horvath C, Mechkouri M, et al. Circadian-time dependence of murine tolerance for the alkylating agent peptichemio. Eur J Cancer Clin Oncol 1987;23:487–497.

121. Klein F, Danober L, Roulon A, Lemaigre G, Mechouri M, Lévi F. Circadian rhythm in murine tolerance for the anticancer agent mitomycin C. In: Reinberg A, Smolensky M, Labrecque G, eds. Annual review of chronopharmacology, vol 5. Oxford: Pergamon Press, 1988:367–370.

122. Sothern RB, Haus R, Langevin TR, et al. Profound circadian stage dependence of mitomycin-C toxicity. In: Reinberg A, Smolensky M, Labrecque G, eds. Annual review of chronopharmacology, vol 5. Oxford: Pergamon Press, 1988:389–392.

123. Simpson HW, Stoney PJ. Circadian variation of melphalan (L-phenylalanine nitrogen mustard) toxicity to murine bone marrow: Relevance to cancer treatment protocols. Br J Haematol 1977;35:459–464.

124. Scheving LE, Burns R, Pauly JE, Halberg F, Haus E. Survival and cure of leukemic mice after circadian optimization of treatment with cyclophosphamide and 1-β-D-arabinofuranosylcytosine. Cancer Res 1977;37:3648–3655.

125. Scheving LE, Burns ER, Pauly JE, Halberg F. Circadian bioperiodic response of mice bearing advanced L1210 leukemia to combination therapy with Adriamycin and cyclophosphamide. Cancer Res 1980;40:1511–1515.

126. Haus E, Halberg F, Scheving L, et al. Increased tolerance of mice to arabinosylcytosine given on schedule adjusted to circadian system. Science 1972;177:80–82.

127. Halberg F, Nelson W, Lévi F, Culley D, Bogden A, Taylor DJ. Chronotherapy of mammary cancer in rats. Int J Chronobiol 1980;7:85–99.

128. Sothern RB, Levi F, Haus E, Halberg F, Hrushesky WJ. Control of a murine plasmacytoma with doxorubicin-cisplatin: Dependence on circadian stage of treatment. JNCI 1989;81:135–145.

129. Kodama M, Kodama T. Influence of corticosteroid hormones on the therapeutic efficacy of cyclophosphamide. Gann 1982;73:661–666.

130. Roemeling R, Mormont MC, Walker K, Olshefski R. Cancer control depends upon the circadian shape of continuous FUDR infusion. Proc Annu Meet Am Assoc Cancer Res [Abstract] 1987;28:A1293.

131. Valvassori L, Bellegotti L, Marchiano A, et al. Continuous circadian-shaped infusion FUDR effectively reduces toxicity. Proc Am Soc Clin Oncol [Abstract] 1989;8:A427.

132. Huben RP, Dragone N, Perrapato SD. Continuous infusion FUDR chemotherapy in the treatment of metastatic renal cell carcinoma. Am Urol Assoc [Abstract] 1990;:A413.

133. Damascelli B, Marchiano A, Spreafico C, et al. Circadian continuous chemotherapy of renal cell carcinoma with an implantable, programmable infusion pump. Cancer 1990;66:237–241.

133a. Focan C, Lévi F, Couturier SL, et al. Chronotherapy of hepatic metastases from colorectal cancer by local and general infusion. Proc Annu Meet Am Soc Clin Oncol [Abstract] 1992;11:A542.

134. Drexus FH, Logothetis CJ, Sella A, et al. Circadian infusion of floxuridine in patients with metastatic renal cell carcinoma. J Urol 1991;146:709–713.

135. Arbuck SG. Overview of clinical trials using 5-fluorouracil and leucovorin for the treatment of colorectal cancer. Cancer 1989;63(suppl 6):1036–1044.

135a. Lévi F, Brienza JL, Misset R, et al. Circumvention of clinical resistance of metastatic colorectal cancer to 5-fluorouracil (5-FU) with circadian rhythm modulated chemotherapy. Proc Am Soc Clin Oncol [Abstract] 1992;11:A500.

136. Anderson N, Lokich J, Bern M, Wallach S, Moore C, Williams D. A phase I clinical trial of combined fluoropyrimidines with leucovorin in a 14-day infusion. Demonstration of biochemical modulation. Cancer 1989;63:233–237.

137. Bjarnason GA, Kerr I, Doyle N, MacDonald M, Sone M. Phase I study of 5-fluorouracil (5-FU) and leucovorin (LV) by 14 day continuous infusion chronotherapy in patients with metastatic adenocarcinoma. Eur J Cancer [Abstract] 1991;2:A528.

138. Markiewicz M, Martynowicz M, Sanchez S, Wood P, Hrushesky WJM. Reversal of circadian 5-fluorouracil lethality pattern by leucovorin in mouse. 20th international conference on chronobiology. Israel [Abstract] 1991;.

139. Erlichman C, Fine S, Elhakim T. Plasma pharmacokinetics of 5-FU given by continuous infusion with allopurinol. Cancer Treat Rep 1986;70:903–904.

140. Poplin E, Chabot G, Rutkowski K, Baker L. Continuous infusion (CI), low-dose 5-fluorouracil (FUra): Plasma concentrations. Proc Am Assoc Cancer Res [Abstract] 1988;29:A753.

141. Gudauskas G, Goldie JH. The pharmacokinetics of high-dose continuous 5-fluorouracil infusion. Proc Am Assoc Cancer Res and Am Soc Clin Oncol [Abstract] 1978;18:C-230.

142. Bastian G, Demarcq C, Leteutre F, et al. Pharmacokinetics of 5 fluorouracil: Effect of association with cisplatinum during long term infusion. Proc Am Soc Clin Oncol [Abstract] 1986;5:A213.

143. Mayers CE. The pharmacology of fluoropyrimidines. Pharmacol Rev 1981;33:1–15.

144. Harris BE, Song R, HE Y, Diasio RB. Circadian rhythm of rat liver dihydropyrimidine dehydrogenase. Biochem Pharmacol 1988;37:4759–4762.

145. Harris BE, Song R, Soong S, Diasio RB. Circadian variation of 5-fluorouracil catabolism in isolated perfused rat liver. Cancer Res 1989;49:6610–6614.

146. Tuchman M, Roemeling R, Lanning R. Source of variability of dehydropyrimidine dehydrogenase (DPD) activity in human blood mononuclear cells. In: Reinberg A, Smolensky M, Labrecque G, eds. Annual review of chronopharmacology, vol 5. Oxford: Pergamon, 1988:399–402.

146a. Zhang R, Liu T, Soong SJ, Diasio RB. Circadian rhythm of rat spleen cytoplasmic thymidine kinase: Possible relevance to 5-fluorodeoxyuridine chemotherapy. Biological rhythms and medications: The Fifth International Conference of Chronopharmacology, Amelia Island, FL [Abstract] 1992;:AIV-12.

147. el Kouni MH, Naguib FMN, Cha S. Circadian rhythm of dihydrouracil dehydrogenase (DHUDase), uridine phosphorylase (UrdPase), and thymidine phosphorylase (dThdase) in mouse liver. FASEB J 1989;3:A397.

148. Daher G, Zhang R, Soong SJ, Diasio RB. Circadian variation of fluoropyrimidine catabolic enzymes in rat liver: Possible relevance to 5-fluorodeoxyuridine chemotherapy. Drug Metab Dispos 1991;19:285–287.

149. Kuhl JFW, Grage F, Halberg F, Rosene G, Scheving LE, Haus E. Ellen-effect: Tolerance of Adriamycin by mice and rats depend on circadian timing of injection. Int J Chronobiol 1973;1:335–336.

150. Good RA, Sothern RB, Stoney PJ, Simpson E, Halberg E, Halberg F. Circadian stage dependence of Adriamycin-induced tumor regression and recurrence rates in immunocytoma bearing LOU rats. Chronobiologia 1974;4:177–183.

151. Hrushesky WJM, von Roemeling R, Sothern B. Circadian chronotherapy: From animal experiments to human cancer chemotherapy. In: Lemmer B, ed. Chronopharmacology: Cellular and biochemical interactions. New York: Marcel Dekker, 1989:439–473.

152. Barrett R, Blessing J, Webster K, Twiggs L. Circadian-timed combination doxorubicin-cisplatin chemotherapy for advanced endometrial carcinoma. Gynecol Oncol 1990;36:285–297.

153. Bailleul F, Lévi F, Metzger G, Regensberg C, Reinberg A, Mathé G. Chronotherapy of advanced breast cancer with continuous doxorubicin infusion via an implantable programmable device. Proc Annu Meet Am Assoc Cancer Res [Abstract] 1987;28:A771.

154. Lévi F, Bailleul F, Misset JL, et al. Clinical chronopharmacologic optimization of hematologic tolerance for the anticancer agent 4'-O-tetrahydropyranyl Adriamycin. Preliminary results. In: Reinberg A, Smolensky M, Labrecque G, eds. Annual review of chronopharmacology, vol 3. Oxford: Pergamon Press, 1986:199–202.

155. Sqalli A. Chronopharmacociétique clinique et expérimentale de la doxorubicine. Thésis Doctorat Es-Sciences. Toulouse, France: Université Paul Sabatier, 1988.

156. Sqalli A, Oustrin J, Houin G, Bugat R, Carton M. Clinical chronopharmacokinetics of doxorubicin. In: Reinberg A, Smolensky M, Labreque G, eds. Annual review of chronopharmacology, vol 5. Oxford: Pergamon Press, 1988:393–396.

157. Bachur NR, Gordon SL, Gee MW. A general mechanism for microsomal activation of quinone anticancer agents to free radicals. Cancer Res 1978;38:1745–1750.

158. Boor PJ. Cardiac glutathione: Diurnal rhythm and variation in drug-induced cardiomyopathy. Res Commun Chem Pathol Pharmacol 1979;24:27–36.

159. Jakoby WB, Habig WH. Glutathione transferases. In: Enzymatic basis of detoxification, vol 2. New York: Academic Press, 1980.

160. Farooqui MYH, Ahmed AE. Circadian periodicity in tissue glutathione and its relationship with lipid peroxidation in rats. Life Sci 1984;34:2413–2418.

161. Halberg E, Halberg F, Venner KJ, et al. Twenty-four hour synchronized chronotolerance of cisdiamminedichloroplatinum (II) by rats on 8-h and 12-h photofraction gauged by acrophase and paraphase of rectal temperature. In: Reinberg A, Halberg F, eds. Chronopharmacology. New York: Pergamon Press, 1979:377.

162. Lévi FA, Hrushesky WJM, Blomquist CH, et al. Reduction of cis-diamminedichloroplatinum nephrotoxicity in rats by optimal circadian drug timing. Cancer Res 1982;42:950–955.

163. Boughattas AN, Levi F, Roulon A, et al. Similar circadian rhythm in murine host tolerance for two platinum analogs: Carboplatin (cbdca) and oxaliplatin (i-ohp). Proc Annu Meet Am Assoc Cancer Res [Abstract] 1987;28:451.

164. von Roemeling R, Portuese E, Salzer M, et al. Improved therapeutic index of cisplatin analogue: B-85-0040 by circadian timing. Prog Clin Biol Res 1990;341B:11–20.

165. Cal JC, Dorian C, Cambar J. Circadian and circannual changes in nephrotoxic effects of heavy metals and antibiotics. In: Reinberg A, Smolensky M, Labrecque G, eds. Annual review of chronopharmacology, vol 3. Oxford: Pergamon Press, 1986:143–176.

166. Wesson LG. Diurnal circadian rhythms of renal function and electrolytes excretion in heart failure. Int J Chronobiol 1979;6:109–117.

167. Guarino AM, Moller DS, Arnold ST, et al. Platinate toxicity: Past, present, and prospects. Cancer Treat Rep 1979;63:1475–1483.

168. Kanabrocki EL, Scheving LE, Halberg F, Brewer RL, Bird TJ. Circadian variations in presumably healthy men under conditions of peace time army reserve unit training. Space Life Sci 1973;4:258–270.

169. Hecquet B, Maynadier J, Bonneterre J, Adenis L, Demaille A. Time dependency in plasmatic protein binding of cisplatin. Cancer Treat Rep 1985;69:79–83.

170. Ozols RF, Corden BF, Jacob J. High-dose cisplatin in hypertonic saline. Ann Intern Med 1984;100:19–24.

171. Roemeling RV, Olshefski R, Langevin T, et al. Cisplatin Chronotherapy and disulfiram rescue reduce toxicity without interfering with anticancer activity: Animal findings and preliminary clinical experiences. Chronobiol Intern 1986;3:55–64.

172. Ivanova LN. Diurnal rhythm of the mitotic activity of the various regions of the mouse nephron. Bull Exp Biol Med 1967;64:88–89.

173. Farutina LM, Bogatova RI. Circadian rhythm of mitotic division of kidney cells in rats of different sexes. Bull Exp Biol Med 1969;67:78–80.

174. Lindahl PE, Surowiak J. The circadian fluctuation of the amount of free phosphate and the activity of acid phosphatase in the kidneys of mice and the effect of UV radiation upon this rhythm. Acta Physiol Scand 1970;80:254–268.

175. Margolis R. The effect of continuous illumination (LL) and continuous darkness (DD) on the daily rhythms of membrane-bound and microsomal enzymes in the adrenal gland and kidney of the rat. Am J Anat 1977;149:469–476.

176. Maruhn D, Stozyk K, Gielow L, Bock KD. Diurnal variations of urinary enzyme excretion. Clin Chim Acta 1977;75:427–433.

177. Robinson D, Price RG, Dance N. Rat urine glycosidases and kidney damage. Biochem J 1967;102:533–538.

178. Nakano S, Gemba M. Potentiation of cisplatin-induced lipid peroxidation in kidney cortical slices by glutathione depletion. Jpn J Pharmacol 1989;50:87–92.

179. Boughattas NA, Lévi F, Fournier C, et al. Stable circadian mechanism of toxicity of two platinum analogs (cisplatin and carboplatin) despite repeated dosage in mice. J Pharmacol Exp Ther 1990;256:672–679.

180. Sothern RB, Rosene G, Nelson W, Jovonovich JA, Wurcher T, Halberg F. Circadian rhythm in tolerance of melphalan by mice. In: Proceedings of the 12th International Conference of the International Society for Chronobiology. Milano: Il Ponte, 1977: 443–450.

181. Anagnou J, Mayer D, von Mayersbach H. Circadian toxicity of cytostatic drugs. Chronobiologia 1979;6:73.

182. Badran AF, Echave-Llanos JM. Persistence of mitotic circadian rhythm of a transplantable mammary carcinoma after 35 generations: Its bearing on the success of treatment with endoxan. JNCI 1965;35:285–290.

183. Cardoso SS, Scheving LE, Halberg F. Mortality of mice as influenced by the hour of the day of drug (ara-C) administration. Pharmacologist 1970;12:302.

184. Scheving LE, Cardoso SS, Pauly JE, Halberg F, Haus E. Variation in susceptibility of mice to the carcinostatic agent arabinosylcytosine. In: Scheving LE, Pauly JE, eds. Chronobiology. Tokyo: Igaku-Shoin, 1974:213–217.

185. Hromas RA, Hutchinson JT, Markel DE, Scholes VE. Flow cytometric analysis of the effect of ara-C on the chronobiology of bone marrow DNA synthesis. Chronobiologia 1981;8:369–373.

186. Burns ER, Scheving LE. Circadian optimization of the treatment of L 1210 leukemia with 1-β-D-arabinofuranasylcytosine, cyclophosphamide, vincristine and methylprednisolone. Chronobiologia 1980;7:41–51.

187. Scheving LE, Burns ER, Halberg F, Pauly JE. Combined chronotherapy of L1210 leukemic mice using 1-β-D-arabinofuranasylcytosine, cyclophosphamide, vincristine, methylprednisolone and cisdiamminedichloroplatinum. Chronobiologia 1980;7:33–40.

188. Rose WC, Trader MW, Laster WR, Schabel FM. Chronochemotherapy of 11210 leukemic mice with cytosine arabinoside or cyclophosphamide. Cancer Treat Rep 1978;62:1337–1349.

189. Halberg F, Haus E, Scheving LE, Good RA. On methods for testing and achieving cancer chronotherapy. Cancer Treat Rep 1979;63:1428–1430.

190. English J, Aherne GW, Arend J. Effect of corticosteroids and melatonin on the circadian rhythm of methotrexate toxicity in the rat. In: Reinberg A, Smolensky M, Labrecque G, eds. Annual review of chronopharmacology, vol 1. Oxford: Pergamon Press, 1984: 145–148.

191. Malmary-Nebot MF, Labat C, Casanovas AM, Oustrin J. Aspect chronobiologique de l'action du méthotrexate sur la dihydrofolate réductase. Ann Pharm Fr 1985;43:337–343.

192. Rivard GE, Infante-Rivard C, Hoyoux C, Champagne J. Maintenance chemotherapy for childhood acute lymphoblastic leukemia: Better in the evening. Lancet 1985;2:1264–1266.

193. Henderson ES, Adamson RH, Denham C, Oliverio VT. The metabolic fate of tritiated methotrexate. 1. Absorption, excretion and distribution in mice, rats, dogs and monkeys. Cancer Res 1965;25:1008.

194. Poplack DG, Balis FM, Zimm S. The pharmacology of orally administered chemotherapy. A reappraisal. Cancer 1986;58(suppl 2):473–480.

195. Pinkerton CR, Welshman SG, Glasgow JFT, Bridges JM. Can food influence the absorption of methotrexate in children with acute lymphoblastic leukemia? Lancet 1980;2:944–945.

196. Riccardo R, Balis FM, Ferrara P, Lasorella A, Poplack DG, Mastrangelo R. Influence of food intake on bioavailability of oral 6-mercaptopurine in children with acute lymphoblastic leukemia. Pediatr Hematol Oncol 1986;3:319–324.

197. Zimm S, Collins J, Roccardi R, et al. Variable bioavailability of oral mercaptopurine: Is maintenance chemotherapy in acute lymphoblastic leukemia being optimally delivered? N Engl J Med 1983;308:1005–1009.

198. Evans WE, Crom WR, Abromowitch M, et al. Clinical pharmacodynamics of high dose methotrexate in acute lymphocytic leukemia: Identification of a relation between concentration and effect. N Engl J Med 1986;314:471–477.

199. Peeters M, Koren G, Jakubovicz D, Zipursky A. Physician compliance and relapse rates of acute lymphoblastic leukemia in children. Clin Pharmacol Ther 1988;43:228–232.

200. Balis FM, Jeffries SL, Lange B, et al. Chronopharmacokinetics of oral methotrexate and 6-mercaptopurine: Is there diurnal variation in the disposition of antileukemic therapy? Am J Pediatr Hematol Oncol 1989;11:324–326.

200a. Koren G, Ferrazzini G, Sohl H, Robieux I, Johnson D, Giesbrecht E. Chronopharmacology of methotrexate pharmacokinetics in childhood leukemia. Chronobiol Intern 1992;9(6):424–438.

201. Langevin AM, Koren G, Soldin S, Greenberg M. Pharmacokinetic case for giving 6-mercaptopurine maintenance doses at night. Lancet [Letter] 1987;2:505–506.

202. Koren G, Langevin AM, Olivieri N, Giesbrecht E, Zipursky A, Greenberg M. Diurnal variation in the pharmacokinetics and myelotoxicity of mercaptopurine in children with acute lymphocytic leukemia. Am J Dis Child 1990;144:1135–1137.

203. Schmiegelow K, Pulczynska MK, Seip M. White cell count during maintenance chemotherapy for standard-risk childhood acute lymphoblastic leukemia: Relation to relapse rate. Pediatr Hematol Oncol 1988;5:259–267.

204. Lennard L, Lilleyman JS. Variable mercaptopurine metabolism and treatment outcome in childhood lymphoblastic leukemia. J Clin Oncol 1989;7(12):1876–1823.

205. Krakowski I, Levi F, Mechkouri M, et al. Dose intensity of etoposide (VP16)-cisplatin (CDDP) depends upon dosing time. Proc Annu Meet Am Assoc Cancer Res [Abstract] 1988;29:A776.

206. Focan C. Chronotherapy in lung and ovarian cancer. J Cancer Res Clin Oncol [Abstract] 1990;116:16.20.04.

207. Zagar RF, Frisby SA, Oliverio VT. Cellular transport and antitumor activity of methotrexate in combination with clinically useful drugs. Proc Am Assoc Cancer Res [Abstract] 1972;13:33.

208. Shepherd R, Harrap KR. Modulation of the toxicity and antitumor activity of alkylating drugs by steroids. Br J Cancer 1982;45:413.

209. Carter DS, Goldman BD. Antigonadal effects of timed melatonin infusion in pinealectomised male Djungarian hamsters (*Phodopus sungorus sungorus*): Duration is the critical parameter. Endocrinology 1983;113:1267–1267.

210. Wide L, Bengtsson C, Birgegard G. Circadian rhythm of erythropoetin in human serum. Br J Haematol 1989;72:85–90.

211. Haus E, Lakatua DJ, Swoyer J, Sackett LL. Chronobiology in hematology and immunology. Am J Anat 1983;168:467–517.

212. Wood PA, Sanchez de la Peña S, Hrushesky WJM. Evidence for circadian dependency of recombinant human erythropoietin (rhEPO) response in the mouse. In: Reinberg A, Smolensky M, Labreque G, eds. Annual review of chronopharmacology. Oxford: Pergamon Press, 1990;7:173–176.

213. Scheving LA, Tsai TH, Feuers RJ, Smolensky MH, Young JD, Scheving LE. Differential effect of interleukin-2 on [³H]TdR incorporation into DNA in the thymus, spleen and bone marrow of CD2F1 male mice. In: Reinberg A, Smolensky M, Labrecque G, ed. Annual review of chronopharmacology, vol 5. Oxford: Pergamon Press, 1988;381–382.

214. Tsai TH, Scheving LA, Feuers RJ, Young JD, Scheving LE. Circadian influence of IL-2 in stimulating DNA synthesis in the lung, liver and pancreas of CD2F1 male mice. In: Reinberg A, Smolensky M, Labreque G, eds. Annual review of chronopharmacology, vol 5. Oxford: Pergamon Press, 1988;397–398.

215. Feuers RJ, Scheving LA, Tsai TH, Young JD, Scheving LE. A preliminary report of circadian effects of interleukin-2 (IL-2) on the activity of enzymes of intermediary metabolism of mice. Prog Clin Biol Res 1990;341B:473–482.

216. von Roemeling R, DeMaria L, Salzer M, et al. Circadian stage dependent response to IL-2 in mouse spleen and bone marrow. In: Reinberg A, Smolensky M, Labreque G, eds. Annual review of chronopharmacology. Oxford: Pergamon Press, 1990;7:211–214.

216a. Vyzula R, Whighton T, Traynor K, et al. Comparative circadian organization of the myelopoetic and unexpected oncomodulary effects of granulocyte colony stimulating factor. Third Meeting of the Society for Research on Biological Rhythms, Amelia Island, FL [Abstract] 1992;:A139.

217. Langevin T, Young J, Walker K, Roemeling R, Nygaard S, Hrushesky WJM. The toxicity of tumor necrosis factor (TNF) is reproducibly different at specific times of the day. Proc Annu Meet Am Assoc Cancer Res [Abstract] 1987;28:A1580.

218. Bocci V. Administration of interferon at night may increase its therapeutic index. Cancer Drug Deliv 1985;2:313–318.

219. Abrams PG, McClamrock E, Foon KA. Evening administration of alpha interferon. N Engl J Med [Letter] 1985;312:443–4445.

220. Morgano A, Puppo F, Criscuolo D, Lotti G, Indiveri F. Evening administration of alpha interferon: Relationship with the circadian rhythm of cortisol. Med Sci Res 1987;15:615–616.

221. Bocci V. The physiological interferon response. Immunol today 1985;6:7–9.

222. Gatti G, Masera R, Cavallo R, et al. Circadian variation of interferon-induced enhancement of human natural killer (NK) cell activity. Cancer Detect Prevent 1988;12:431–438.

223. Deprés-Brummer P, Lévi F, DiPalma M, et al. A phase I trial of 21-day continuous venous infusion of α-interferon at circadian rhythm modulated rate in cancer patients. J Immunol 1991;10:440–447.

HARVEY I. PASS
THOMAS F. DELANEY

SECTION **8**

Photodynamic Therapy

It is only recently that photodynamic therapy (PDT) has been investigated on a large scale, although the concept of a light-activated sensitizer resulting in specific or nonspecific cell death is not new. PDT was first used in 1900, when acridine and light were combined to kill paramecia, and the first oncologic use of PDT was in 1903, when eosin and light were employed in the treatment of skin cancer.[1,2] In the following years, many chemicals were used to promote photochemically induced cytotoxicity.[3]

Since Hauseman's initial experiments in 1911 with hematoporphyrin (HP), there has been a continued interest in porphyrin-based photosensitizers.[3] During the late 1940s, a key development was made. HP (probably a fairly impure preparation) was found to selectively concentrate or to be preferentially retained in malignant tissues.[4,5] Lipson improved the tumor-localizing properties of HP by synthesizing a complex porphyrin mixture called hematoporphyrin derivative (HPD).[6–9] Gregorie extended Lipson's observations by demonstrating that HPD is retained in a large percentage of squamous and adenocarcinomas.[10] Lipson's work on tumor detection resulted in a single attempt to manage a large, recurrent breast cancer by multiple injections of HPD and light treatments. The tumorous lesion was not cured, but there was objective evidence of photodynamically induced cytotoxic effect.[11] Several years later, Kelly reported results with intravenous HPD followed by light delivered through a fiberoptic device to treat a patient with recurrent bladder cancer. Shortly afterward, Dougherty described his first of a sustained series of studies throughout the 1970s and 1980s exploring the mechanism and applications of HPD-based PDT for the treatment of diverse human malignancies.[12–17] It was through Dougherty's continued efforts that PDT evolved to the level it is practiced today.

MECHANISM OF PHOTODYNAMIC THERAPY

Photodynamic therapy requires three simultaneously present components for cytotoxicity: a sensitizer, light, and oxygen. PDT is an oxygen-dependent photochemical oxidative process that should not be confused with laser techniques, including carbon dioxide or neodymium-yttrium-aluminum-garnet lasers. The laser techniques, used at much longer wavelengths (10,600 and 1064 nm, respectively), are associated with heat production to produce a desiccating-cutting action. Moreover, the wavelength of the sensitizers used dictates the proper light spectrum and the depth of treatment effect with photodynamic therapy. PDT may have more promise as a primary cancer modality than the laser techniques, primarily because PDT offers some tumor selectivity due to selective sensitizer retention compared with sensitizer concentrations in normal tissue. This differential cytotoxicity separates PDT from other chemically based forms of cancer treatment.

COMPONENTS OF PHOTODYNAMIC THERAPY

PHOTOSENSITIZERS

The most widely used sensitizers in clinical studies have been hematoporphyrin derivative (HPD; Photofrin I) or a further purified mixture of HPD known as dihematoporphyrin ether (DHE; Photofrin II). HPD localizes in tumors and has photodynamic properties that, when activated by 630-nm light, lead to cytotoxicity. The absorption at longer wavelengths, although small in comparison with its major absorptive peak, allows greater tissue penetration and obviates the problems associated with light absorbance by naturally present biologic chromophores such as hemoglobin.[18] The relative impurity of HPD has been improved by the availability of Photofrin II (PII) that, although more homogenous, also contains hematoporphyrin, hydroxyethylvinyl deuteroporphyrin, and protoporphyrin.

The distribution of different porphyrins is determined by the individual chemical properties, including lipophilicity or hydrophilicity, polarity, pH, anionic or cationic change, and aggregate size.[19] HPD is predominantly associated with the lipoproteins LDL and VLDL, and the components not associated with tumor localization (*i.e.*, HP, HVD, protoporphyrin) are associated with albumin.[20] LDL is the main early carrier, but it later becomes almost exclusively associated with HDL. PII accumulates in and is retained by vascular endothelium by endocytosis, but its selectivity to tumor as a result of abnormal tumor vascular endothelium remains to be elucidated.[21–23] Intracellular accumulation of the drug is most certainly affected by the concentration of soluble and structural protein such as collagen and may be influenced by diminished local lymphatic drainage in tumors. Although the serum half-life is relatively short in humans (20–30 hours for a 5-mg bolus), the photosensitizing component remains in the skin or at least at low levels (2–5%) in the serum for at least 4 to 6 weeks.[18]

SELECTIVE TUMOR RETENTION

One of the attributes of porphyrin-based photodynamic therapy is the ability of tumor tissue to retain substantial levels of sensitizer for a longer period than normal tissue. Why DHE is retained to a greater extent in tumors than in normal tissues is unknown. In vitro studies to determine if tumor cells are more photosensitive or selectively retain HPD fail to show a difference between normal and cancerous cells. NIH3T3 cells transformed by the *RAS* oncogene have identical PDT survival curves compared with the parent NIH3T3 line, and Perry found no differences in sensitivity to PDT or in vitro survival curves of thoracic oncologic lines compared with a normal lung fibroblast.[24,25] Differences in in vivo retention of sensitizer between tumor and normal tissues have been demonstrated by numerous methods, including using fluorescent and radioactively labeled sensitizer. In examining and kinetics of PII delivery in flank tumors of animals in vivo, sensitizer levels fall significantly in tumor only after 48 hours and are significantly greater than those seen in the muscle and the skin.[24] Route of delivery and the type of tumor play a role in the kinetics of delivery. Maximal tumor to tissue ratios shortly after HPD administration were demonstrated by Tochner after intraperitoneal injection of HPD in an ovarian cancer ascites model.[26] Because the drug was directly injected into the ascites fluid containing the tumor cells, drug availability was greater because there was no dependence on vascular delivery.

The difference between in vivo tumor and normal cell sensitizer uptake and retention probably depends on several environmental factors. Leaky tumor neovascular effects, retention within the tumor vascular endothelial cells with subsequent disruption of tumor oxygen and nutrient delivery, poorly developed tumor lymphatics, lower tumor pH, binding to lipoproteins, and subsequent receptor mediated endocytosis may all contribute to the selective retention. The trapping of porphyrin aggregates by macrophages may be favored in tumor-associated monocytes, which could contribute to a host of immunologic circumstances.

LIGHT

Any source of light having the appropriate spectral characteristics can be used for photodynamic therapy. Lasers, specifically argon pump-dye lasers, are used, exciting Kiton red or rhodamine B to produce up to 5 watts of red light, which corresponds to one of the minor spectral peaks of Photofrin II. The laser can be coupled to one or more fiberoptic cables to propagate the light with minimal energy loss to the tip, cleaved (for forward light projection), bulbous (for isotropic spherical distribution), or coated with cylindrical scattering material to yield light perpendicular to the midpoint of the fiber axis. The amount of energy delivered depends on the dose rate of light from the fiber and the duration of light delivery. The light distribution can be calibrated with a power meter at the tip before treatment, and the rate of light delivery is always gauged to prevent hyperthermic effects.

OXYGEN

PDT cytotoxicity probably occurs through photooxidative reactions. When oxygen is absent from the system or present at levels less than 2%, cells are resistant to photodynamic therapy cytotoxicity.[27,28] The light-excited sensitizer loses or accepts an electron with oxygenation of secondary radicals or transfer of energy to oxygen to yield singlet oxygen with resultant hydroperoxyl products.[29] Such products, although short lived, lead to cell death at various targets.

The most striking and immediate cellular response observed after PDT is damage to membranes, particularly the plasma membrane.[30,31] Shortly after light treatment, cells withstand trypsin removal from plastic surfaces. Such early changes imply that membrane proteins have cross-linked with residual double bonds of the plastic. Within hours of treatment, visible damage is seen by cessation of normal cellular movement and the formation of multiple membrane blebs.[32] The blebs, which are often as large as the cell itself, develop as balloon-like structures protruding from the cell membrane and indicate severe membrane damage.[33,34] After cell blebbing, there is no longer cell division, and cell lysis follows. Other experimental indications of membrane distortion after PDT are constituent leakage from intact cells or isotope from red blood cell ghosts.[35,36] Other cellular membranes may be at risk, including the nucleus, mitochondria, lysosome, Golgi apparatus,

and endoplasmic reticulum. Membranes, by virtue of the HPD or DHE water-lipid partition coefficient, are good targets for PDT damage. Mitochondrial damage after PDT has been demonstrated by specific inhibition of oxidative phosphorylation and electron transport enzymes and reduction in cellular ATP levels.[37,38]

Although production of DNA strand breaks has been observed after PDT, such lesions may not be responsible for cellular death.[39,40] Incorporation of bromodeoxyuridine into cellular DNA has been shown to sensitize cells to ionizing radiation and chemotherapy drugs but not to PDT.[41,42] PDT is not mutagenic in in vitro systems.[43,44] These last two facts indicate that DNA is not a primary target for PDT-induced cytotoxicity. The HPD or DHE uptake studies clearly define initial binding within the plasma membrane followed, in time, by migration to internal cellular regions.[45]

MECHANISMS OF PHOTODYNAMIC THERAPY

SENSITIZER DOSE

Cells exposed to increasing amounts of sensitizer exhibit an increase in light-induced cytotoxicity, and drug uptake depends on drug concentration, length of incubation (i.e., the longer the incubation with PII, the greater the PDT cytotoxicity), and protein concentration of the media environment (i.e., the higher the protein concentrations, the less the PDT cytotoxicity).[46] As the volume of cells increase, there is a linear increase in HPD uptake, and larger cells may have greater susceptibility to PDT than smaller cells treated under identical conditions.[47]

DOSE RATE EFFECTS

The degree of PDT cytotoxicity depends on the rate at which the dose of energy is given. The greater the dose rate delivery to the tumor cells at a given energy, the greater the PDT cytotoxicity.[48] The ability of the cells to escape PDT cytotoxicity at low dose rates, but equal energies, may be related to their ability to repair sublethal damage or remove toxic oxidative products. These potential repair capabilities may have significant clinical implications, because light dose delivery to the tumor falls off exponentially as a function of the distance from the light point of entry. With low levels of light at low dose rates, tumor tissue may escape treatment and may locally recur.

INHERENT PHOTODYNAMIC THERAPY SENSITIVITY OF CELL LINES

Despite various histologies of malignancies at a given anatomic site, no real differences in the parameters that influence survival after similar doses of PDT has been elucidated. Corrections of sensitizer uptake with regard to total cellular protein, volume, and cell size make no difference, and the survival characteristics in vitro of adenocarcinoma, squamous cell carcinoma, large cell carcinoma, small cell carcinoma, and mesothelioma are quite similar.[25] The modest difference in cell survival after PDT may be partially explained by the cells inherent ability to form colonies (i.e., its plating efficiency).

IMMUNE MECHANISMS
AND PHOTODYNAMIC THERAPY

One of the more interesting aspects of PDT that is being pursued is the relation between immune mechanisms and PDT. An immunosuppressive element of PDT was recognized in the 1980s. Elmets and Bauer reported a 50% suppression of contact hypersensitivity after PDT treatment, and this was a sustained phenomenon for a period of at least 2 weeks.[49] Moreover, the immunosuppressive characteristics could be adoptively transferred. A direct effect on effector cells and evidence that PDT could cause release of vasoactive peptides, priming factors, or substances that influence immune status as a secondary messenger has been demonstrated. Ortner illuminated murine peritoneal mast cells previously incubated with protoporphyrin and documented progressive inhibition of histamine secretion at low fluences, while histamine was released at high dose rates.[50] Henderson and Donovan have reported release of proctoglandins from peritoneal murine macrophages after PII-based PDT.[51] This release was associated with cellular membrane disruption. Lynch was able to demonstrate that the macrophage was the cell that mediates the adoptively transferred suppression of contact hypersensitivity after PDT.[52]

Tumor necrosis factor is released in a dose-dependent fashion from PDT stimulated peritoneal murine macrophages, and it is possible to potentiate this TNF release with pretreatment with interferon.[53] Such an effect could have implications for indirect mechanism of tumor killing by PDT though cytokine stimulation or effect of the cytokine on tumor vascular to cause hemorrhagic necrosis due to endothelial cell destruction.

A great interest in the use of immune mechanisms for increasing specificity of PDT has developed. Levy conjugated hematoporphyrin to monoclonal antibody and selectively eliminated a suppressor subset of T lymphocytes.[54] Elimination resulted in tumor regression by the HP-monoclonal antibody becoming an immunotoxin that selectively destroys the suppressor T cell alone so other cytotoxic T lymphocytes can destroy the cancer. A more direct use of monoclonal antibody-sensitizer conjugates has been reported by Pogrebniak; greater specificity, less normal tissue destruction, and greater long-term cures were described for a in vivo murine model.[55]

Whether these immune mechanisms are truly active in vivo in humans requires further verification. Nevertheless, Shumaker[56] described an increase in T-cell lymphocytes and plasma cells in bladders of patients undergoing bladder PDT, and Nseyo[57] documented cytokine production in the urine of patients receiving bladder PDT. Clinically, psoralen photosensitization has been used as a light-activated therapy with extracoporeal photophoresis to treat cutaneous T-cell lymphoma.[58] Patients who respond have a selective destruction of the malignant T-cell clone.

TISSUE EFFECTS IN VIVO

The response to PDT in vivo is rapid, with no palpable tumor present within 1 to 2 days after treatment. Where there is regrowth of tumor, it usually occurs after 1 to 2 weeks at the edges of the wound.[18] The original injury to the tumor is a marked coagulation necrosis, and regrowth could be due to inherent tumor cell resistance, hypoxia, inadequate drug uptake, or inadequate drug-light dose concentration. Vascular damage is probably one of the primary targets of in vivo PDT, and tumor blood flow studies confirm a marked decrease in blood flow with PDT. Such vascular damage results in tumor hypoxia and cytotoxicity. This PDT induced vascular damage can be amplified with use of hypoxic cell sensitizers just before or within 30 minutes of the PDT treatment. Misonidazole selectivity binds hypoxic cells and once within the tumor helps amplify the PDT effect.[59]

PHOTODYNAMIC THERAPY
FOR MALIGNANCIES

CLINICAL STUDIES

Initial efforts with HPD photodynamic therapy were in patients with cutaneous and subcutaneous malignancies. Since that time, several thousand patients have been treated with PDT for a wide variety of malignancies involving various organ systems. For most patients, conventional treatment had failed or it had been refused. The first trials were designed to develop techniques to treat particular anatomic sites and to gather dose, toxicity, and response information. As additional experience with this modality has accumulated, there has been increasing emphasis on the development of controlled clinical studies to help define the role of modality in the current management of patients with cancer.

CUTANEOUS AND SUBCUTANEOUS TUMORS

Malignancies involving the skin that have been treated with PDT include basal and squamous cell carcinomas, malignant melanomas, mycosis fungoides, recurrent metastatic breast carcinoma, and Kaposi's sarcomas (Table 69–30).[60] Patients received sensitizer by intravenous injection and were treated with red light 72 to 96 hours after injection of HPD. Both external surface illumination and interstitial implantation have been used for some larger lesions. Most patients in the early reports had disease that had not been controlled by prior surgery, chemotherapy, and ionizing radiation. Although investigators used different criteria to judge response, it is clear that responses have been obtained even after extensive prior treatment, and differential responses are seen between tumor and adjacent normal tissue within the light field.

Treatment is effective to a depth of 5 to 10 mm, depending on the drug and light doses and the mode of light delivery. The discovery of photobleaching (photodestruction) of porphyrins during illumination has been an important development in the treatment of skin lesions.[61] By reducing the injected dose of photosensitizer, the drug concentration in the normal skin surrounding tumors may be low enough that any residual drug is photobleached and destroyed during light delivery. This permits large increases in light delivery to the tumors (which still contain active photosensitizer) with much less risk of injury of normal skin. For primary lesions involving skin, investigators report high complete response rates that are often durable. Complete responses have been achieved, lasting up to 4 years.[60]

Bandieramonte and coworkers treated 43 basal cell carcinomas and 18 metastatic breast cancer lesions. Using light

TABLE 69–30. Results of Photodynamic Therapy for Cutaneous or Subcutaneous Tumors

Investigations	Tumor Type	Patients/Sites	Light Dose (J/cm²)	Response Rate (%) CR	PR	NR	Comments
Kennedy[65]	Basal cell	3/38	90	100	0	0	None recur at 35 mo
Bandieramonte[62]	Basal/breast	7/61	60–100	50	31	19	Follow-up 4–16 mo
Waldow[64]	Basal/SCCa	6/9	8–60	100	0	0	Follow-up 8–24 mo
Pennington[66]	Basal/SCCa	6/53	30	68	NA	NA	Most recur at 6 mo
Wilson[67]	Basal/SCCa	37/151	56–216	88	12	0	61% PR retreated to CR
Santoro[63]	Basal cell	50/292	120–150	93.5	6.5	0	Topical porphyrin
Schuh[73]	Breast	14/NA	26–288	15	69	15	Palliative, longest CR was 6 mo

J, joules; CR, complete response, eradication of tumor; PR, partial response, greater than 50% reduction in tumor size; NR, no response; SCCa, squamous cell carcinoma; NA, not available.

doses of 60 to 120 J/cm², clinically complete responses were seen in 26 (43%) of 61, and 16 (26%) of 61 had partial responses.[62] Side effects included cutaneous photosensitivity and discomfort during and after treatment. Pain appeared to be related to tumor necrosis and was more severe with larger and more deeply infiltrating lesions. This group reported using a topically applied porphyrin, tetraphenylporphinesulfonate, for the treatment of 50 patients with 292 basal cell carcinomas less than 2 mm thick.[63] Complete responses were seen with 273 lesions (93.5%). Recurrences were observed in 29 (10.6%). The advantage of the topically applied photosensitizer is that the patient is spared cutaneous photosensitivity. Because of limited depth of penetration by the topical photosensitizer preparation, this approach is only suitable for patients with superficial lesions (<2 mm thick).

Waldow and associates reported treatment of six basal cell lesions and three cases of Bowen's disease or squamous cell carcinomas.[64] All lesions had clinically complete responses, with follow-up times of 8 to 24 months. Kennedy reported durable, complete responses for 38 primary basal cell carcinomas in 3 patients.[65] Pennington and coworkers, however, reported a less favorable experience for 53 primary basal cell or squamous cell skin tumors.[66] Using HPD 5 mg/kg and 30 J/cm², complete responses were achieved in 52% of the basal cell lesions and 81% of the squamous cell lesions. However, over half of the squamous lesions and most of the basal cell lesions recurred at the time of the 6 month follow-up visit. No attempts were made to determine whether alterations of the drug or light dose would affect the response duration.

The group at Roswell Park reported 133 complete and 18 partial responses in 151 basal cell lesions in 37 patients with acceptable normal tissue response and excellent cosmesis.[67] They delivered light doses of 180 to 133 J/cm² 48 to 72 hours after injection of 1 mg/kg of DHE. With 12 months minimum follow-up, recurrences were seen in 13 of 133 complete responders. Most patients who had recurrences had morpheoform basal cell epitheliomas, which the researchers suggested might be more effectively treated with higher light doses or intralesional fiber optic implantation. Eleven of the 18 partial responders were given a repeat course of photoradiation therapy. All had complete responses and remained free of disease at 1 year after treatment.

Excellent treatment results have been reported for managing multiple basal cell carcinomas in patients with nevoid basal cell carcinoma syndrome, with an 82.5% pathologic complete response rate.[68] A higher complete response rate was seen for power densities above 40 mW/cm² and total light doses greater than 70 J/cm². Multiple lesions of Bowen's disease have been treated with excellent response, although complete eradication of tumors required more than one course of treatment.[69]

Of particular interest is the finding by Kennedy that ALA (5-aminolevulinic acid), a precursor of protoporphyrin IX in the biosynthetic pathway for heme, can be applied *topically* to photosensitize skin tumors.[70] Because ALA in aqueous solution passes readily through abnormal keratin but not through normal keratin, topical application induces photosensitization that is restricted primarily to abnormal epithelium. This permits photodynamic therapy to these lesions without causing systemic photosensitivity. The response rate for basal cell carcinomas after a single treatment has been 90% complete response and 7.5% partial response for the first 80 lesions treated.

Dose-seeking studies to determine the optimal treatment schedule for skin lesions are in progress. Gilson and colleagues found more complete responses with 1.5 or 2.0 mg/kg of DHE than with 1.0 mg/kg, although this was accompanied by higher frequency of skin necrosis (which healed in all cases). The relation between the drug and light dose necessary to control tumor is complex and nonlinear.[71] Lower drug doses (*e.g.*, 1.0 mg/kg of DHE) offer the advantage of greater normal tissue sparing and superior depth of treatment effect because of photobleaching of photosensitizer. However, drug dose reductions are accompanied by dramatic increases in the light dose necessary to control tumor, which may be a practical problem for large lesions.

Pigmented melanomas are almost completely unresponsive to PDT because of extremely efficient light absorption by melanin. Nonpigmented lesions, however, can be effectively controlled by PDT. Control of Kaposi's sarcomas as large as 3 cm in diameter has been reported.[60]

Photoradiation has been evaluated for treatment of recurrent breast cancer on the chest wall. Such patients have disease that is difficult to control on the chest wall despite multiple local therapies. Chest wall recurrence of breast cancer is frequently associated with the development of distant metastases. Although focal tumor nodules on the chest wall can be controlled with PDT, new lesions often appear outside of the treatment field. Attempts at treatment of the entire ipsilateral chest wall in patients with diffuse or multifocal involvement have only produced transient responses.[72–74]

HEAD AND NECK TUMORS

Photodynamic therapy should prove to be a useful addition to head and neck oncology because of the accessibility of this area to endoscopy and laser light and because these patients tend to develop multiple primary malignancies. Photodynamic therapy can be repeated when necessary and can be used in sites that have been previously irradiated. Treatment appears to be more effective in early-stage lesions, but relative indications for its use with respect to radiation or surgery need to be defined. Although PDT was initially attempted for patients with lesions that had not been controlled with surgery or irradiation, it appears to be most effective in patients with *early* tumors of the head and neck.[75,76] These patients often have curative surgical or irradiation options; PDT must establish itself as highly reliable and effective before it can be deemed "standard treatment" for such patients. It may have an important role in patients with field cancerization with large areas of superficial premalignant and malignant change for which PDT may be able to produce complete responses with normal tissue preservation.[76]

Wile and coworkers reported on 21 patients with head and neck tumors recurrent in the primary site who were treated with HPD and red light (Table 69–31).[77] Most had squamous cell carcinomas refractory to conventional therapy. Complete responses were seen in 6 patients (29%), and partial responses were seen in 11 patients (52%). The complete responses were durable in 4 of the 6 patients at follow-up times from 8 to 18 months. These occurred in patients with tongue, soft palate, and nasopharyngeal lesions. In 10 patients with regional head and neck cancer recurrences in soft tissues, results were less favorable: 2 complete responses and 3 partial responses. In these patients, tumor rapidly recurred at the margins of the treated field, and the overall disease process did not appear substantially altered by treatment.

Schuller and colleagues documented short response durations in patients with recurrent or metastatic tumors in the head and neck region.[78] Takata found significant necrosis of tumors of the larynx, oropharynx, and tongue by PDT, but pathologic examination of biopsy and surgical specimens revealed nests of viable tumor below the mucosa, suggesting inadequate light delivery and dose inhomogeneity.[79] Grossweiner described 10 patients with early-stage squamous cell carcinoma of the head and neck region who had refused or could not tolerate conventional therapy or with advanced or recurrent disease after conventional therapy who were treated with photodynamic therapy by superficial or interstitial illumination. With follow-up of 6 to 18 months, eight complete responses and one partial response were seen. One patient failed to respond to treatment.[80] Gluckman found encouraging results with photodynamic therapy for earlier-stage squamous carcinomas of the oropharynx and larynx, with control of tumor of up to 2 years.[76] Twenty-five of 41 patients with superficial, less advanced tumors were treated (13 with oral cavity and oropharynx, 6 with recurrent laryngeal lesions after radiation therapy, 6 with tumors at miscellaneous sites). Eleven of the 13 with oropharyngeal lesions obtained complete responses, but less success was seen with the laryngeal and miscellaneous lesions.

Durable control of carcinoma in situ with PDT was reported by Schweitzer.[81] Freche and De Corbiere reported treatment of 32 patients with severe dysplasia, carcinoma in situ, or microinvasive carcinoma of the true vocal cord without anterior commissure involvement.[82] Twenty five patients (72%) had eradication of their disease, with follow-up times as long as 4.5 years. Seven patients had tumors that failed to respond to treatment, probably due to inadequate light delivery. All patients developed a local laryngeal reaction of a laryngitis type with edema and petechiae. Dysphonia persisted for 1 to 2 months, but normal voice returned in all cases.

Photodynamic therapy has been effective in eradicating papillomas caused by papillomavirus in animals and is being evaluated clinically for the eradication of laryngeal papillomatosis.[83]

TABLE 69–31.   Results of Photodynamic Therapy for Head and Neck Tumors

Investigations	Tumor Type	No. of Patients	Light Dose (J/cm²)	Response Rate (%) CR	PR	NR	Comments
Takata[79]	Squamous	6	34–390	0	100	0	Primary site
Wile[77]	Squamous	21	17–91	29	52	19	Primary site
Wile[77]	Squamous	10	17–91	20	30	50	Regional soft tissue
Grossweiner[80]	Squamous	10	60–100	80	10	10	9 of 10 have early cancer
Freche[82]	Squamous	23	~270 J	72	0	28	Early cancer
Gluckman[76]	Squamous	25	50–100	56	24	20	Early cancer
Gluckman[76]	Squamous	8	50–100	87.5	12.5	0	Carcinoma in situ
Gluckman[76]	Squamous	8	50–100	0	0	100	Advanced cancers

J, joules; CR, complete response, eradication of tumor; PR, partial response, greater than 50% reduction in tumor size; NR, no response; NA, not available.

CENTRAL NERVOUS SYSTEM MALIGNANCIES

Because of the grim prognosis with high-grade gliomas, there has been interest in PDT for these tumors (Table 69–32). Diamond and coworkers reported the inactivation of glioma cells in tissue culture with hematoporphyrin and light and significant destruction of gliomas transplanted subcutaneously and intracranially in rats.[84–87]

Perria and associates first reported the use of PDT as part of a treatment program for malignant brain tumors, with intraoperative PDT using a low power helium-neon laser to a modest dose of 9 J/cm² to the tumor bed after resection.[88] Survival ranged from 6 to 44 weeks, and no significant complications of treatment were seen.

Laws and coworkers from the Mayo Clinic reported a phase I feasibility study with PDT for the treatment of malignant brain tumors.[89] All patients were thought to be surgically incurable and had gross recurrent tumor after conventional therapy at the time of treatment. Two of the patients showed a transient decrease in the size of the mass or resultant mass effect on computed tomography (CT) scans after the procedure. In a subsequent report, Laws described a total of 23 patients with brain tumors treated with PDT, most of whom were treated after tumor resection.[90] Two patients developed transient worsening of neurologic function, and 2 had wound infections after PDT. The longest survivor in this series lived 37 months after PDT.

McCulloch described the use of intraoperative PDT delivered by external illumination to the resection cavity in patients with primary gliomas or recurrent metastatic lesions.[91] The patients with glioblastoma all underwent radical resection with PDT and received radiation therapy. Three patients were alive 17 to 42 months after treatment. Energy densities of 100 to 150 J/cm² and total energies of 2000 to 2500 J were employed. In their experience, cerebral edema was encountered after PDT but was manageable with steroids and osmotic agents.

Kostron reported intraoperative intratumoral injection and intraarterial injection of hematoporphyrin derivative in a modification of the usual intravenous photosensitization for PDT. Their approach was well tolerated, although the intratumoral injection required a second operation 3 days later for light delivery. Histologic examination immediately after intravenous and intraarterial injection demonstrated a predominantly vascular effect, but the direct injection resulted in a direct cellular effect with few vascular changes.[92]

Two series by Kaye[93] and Muller[94] demonstrated that high-dose adjuvant photoradiation therapy can be delivered at the time of resection of cerebral gliomas with an acceptable level of risk, although increased intracranial pressure and cerebral edema may be seen in some patients. Higher light doses appear to be more effective than lower light doses. Investigators in this area are exploring the use of a light diffusing lipid solution or a lipid-filled balloon to homogenously illuminate the resection cavity to high dose. However, the limited depth of photodynamic effects, ranging from 0.5 to 1.0 cm, which has been seen after illumination of the resection cavity highlights the need for the development of photosensitizers and techniques to adequately treat deep-seated tumors and infiltrating gliomas cells beyond the limits of grossly evident tumor, possibly using multiple interstitial fibers.

LUNG NEOPLASMS

The primary use of PDT in patients with lung cancer or endobronchial metastases has been to palliate endobronchial obstruction in patients with intrinsic lesions of the bronchus causing partial or complete obstruction. The patient receives 2 mg/kg of PII intravenously 48 to 72 hours before endobronchial illumination and is then removed from direct contact with sunlight but may be exposed to incandescent or fluorescent lighting for up to 12 hours each day. After the elapsed time, the patient is then exposed to 630-nm light usually from an argon pump-dye laser. Two methods are used to accomplish tumor illumination, both of which require quartz fibers linked to the laser for light transmission. The tumor can be directly implanted with the fiber for a length 0.5 to 2.0 cm, which shields the normal bronchus to the greatest extent and results in more uniform tumor illumination. For this interstitial treatment, a cylindrical fiber illuminator provides uniform illumination in all planes perpendicular to the fiber. Alternatively, an "end-cleaved" fiber can be used for surface illumination of the tumor. In both techniques, the light dose can be calibrated before treatment using a light power meter. The length of time that the tumor is exposed to the light dictates the total amount of energy (J) that constitutes the treatment. The amount of energy used for endobronchial tumor illumination has been loosely standardized but depends on the site and method of treatment and ranges from 5 to 900 J/cm².

TABLE 69–32. Results of Photodynamic Therapy for Brain Tumors

Investigations	Tumor Type	No. of Patients	Light Dose (J/cm²)	Response Rate (%)			Comments
				CR	PR	NR	
Laws[89]	Glioma/Met	5	810 J	NA	NA	NA	No toxicity; phase I
McCulloch[91]	Glioma/Met	16	1260–2520 J	NA	NA	NA	Cerebral edema after PDT
Kaye[93]	Glioma/Met	23	70–230	NA	NA	NA	No toxicity; phase I–II
Kostron[92]	Glioma	14	15/120	NA	NA	NA	Well tolerated
Muller[94]	Glioma	32	8–68	19	13	68	25% cerebral edema
Perria[88]	Glioma	8	720–2400 J	NA	NA	NA	PDT after resection

J, joules; CR, complete response, eradication of tumor; PR, partial response, greater than 50% reduction in tumor size; NR, no response; Met, tumors metastatic to the brain; PDT, photodynamic therapy.

PDT has no immediate effect on hemostasis; after the patient is treated with light, no attempt is made to remove the obstruction until 72 hours later at a "clean-up" bronchoscopy. During this second bronchoscopy, multiple biopsies are performed without hemorrhage, which enables to bronchus to be opened to the bronchial wall. After hemorrhage is encountered, the endoscopist is beyond the phototherapy effect, and the session is terminated after ensuring airway hemostasis.

The relative advantages of PDT for endobronchial obstruction relief include its nonthermal nature and selective retentive properties that make it more akin to a specific cytotoxic modality. There is no real chance for airway ignition due to high inspired oxygen tensions, and the treatment takes relatively little time to perform (*i.e.*, 10–12 minutes to deliver 250 J/cm^2). The superficial nature of the treatment is a mixed blessing because, unlike Nd:YAG laser, there is no chance for extra-airway perforation of vessels. The delay in relieving the airway obstruction to allow the avascular necrosis to occur and a second bronchoscopy are obvious disadvantages of this technique, along with the inability to have an impact on acute hemostasis that can be performed with the Nd:YAG laser. Because PII is the only sensitizer approved in the United States for human use, and even that use is confined to experimental investigations, the obligatory 4 to 6 week avoidance of sunlight can severely limit the patient's independence. An ongoing prospective, randomized trial is attempting to define efficacy and toxicity comparisons between endobronchial PDT and Nd:YAG therapy for bronchial obstruction. Until definitive advantages are illustrated, it is the endoscopist's choice as to which method of airway relief is used, depending on training and equipment constraints.

The ability to compare results of PDT for management of malignant endobronchial lesions has been limited by the lack of standardization of protocols regarding the timing of laser treatment after sensitizer injection, sensitizer dose, treatment energy, and method of treatment (*i.e.*, tumor insertion or surface treatment). Moreover, the definition of a response has not been uniform, with some investigators defining a complete response as an anatomical improvement in the endobronchial component, while others call no evidence of tumor histologically, cytologically, or endoscopically a complete response. In a series of 10 patients treated uniformly with regard to dose rate (400 mW/cm^2, and energy (200–250 J/cm^2 with 2 mg/kg of sensitizer 72 hours before light), 80% of the patients were objectively improved, and there was a 20% histologically complete response rate. A summary of the published results is given in Table 69–33.[95-107]

The complications of endobronchial PDT can be immediate or late, depending on previous treatments, technique, or patient compliance. Hemorrhage can occur in previously irradiated patients. Pneumothorax after PDT and reversible pulmonary infiltrates may represent sensitized lung with injury.[95] Skin sensitization is the most common complication and can be minimized by limiting patient sun exposure for at least 4 weeks.

Photodynamic techniques have been investigated in the diagnosis of early lung cancer in an attempt to detect the small carcinoma (in situ lesions) or superficial lung tumors that cover a large endobronchial area. The method involves intravenous injection of hematoporphyrin D (HpD) or PII.[98-101] All of the current systems function by using the selective retention properties of malignant tissue in a temporal fashion after the sensitizer is delivered to the patients. With the use of an imaging intensifying, wavelength detecting device, wavelengths of approximately 405 nm (blue-violet) are used to selectively produce characteristic reddish fluorescence from tissue containing significant amounts of the sensitizer. As described by Lam, due to the preferential retention of the PII by the tumor, tumor fluorescence is higher than surrounding normal tissues.[108] The endoscopist can image the areas of red fluorescence distinct from the green autofluorescence, or a ratio for different areas of red to green fluorescence can be calculated, with the areas of highest ratios indicating the likely sites of tumor.

The most striking disadvantage of this technique is the requirement that patients receiving the sensitizer avoid sunlight for 4 to 6 weeks to avoid severe skin burn. Lam reported the use of low dose (0.25 mg/kg) PII instead of the usual 2 to 3 mg/kg dose in conjunction with a ratioing fluorometer probe.[108] The red-green ratios of known normal areas was 0.9

TABLE 69–33. Results of Photodynamic Therapy for Bronchial Obstruction

Investigations	No. of Patients	Response Rates (%)		
		Complete	Partial	Minimal
Kato et al[96]	13	77	22	0
Kato et al[97]	60	0	48	52
Edell and Cortese[98]	30	70	30	0
Doiron and Balchum[99]	38	34	66	0
Balchum et al[100]	22	91	9	0
Balchum et al[100]	236	100	0	0
Vincent et al[101]	21	12	83	5
Forbes et al[103]	17	22	30	48
Lam et al[104]	7	89	11	0
Hugh-Jones and Gardner[105]	15	80	20	0
Pass et al[95]	10	20	60	20
Li and Zhao[106]	74	14	78	8
Benov et al[107]	25		76	24

to 1.8, and the red-green ratio in biopsy-proven tumor areas was 4.8 (3.0–9.5). Increasing the dose of PII by 700% (to 2 mg/kg) increased the ratio in the tumor area by only 64% (to 7.9). Moreover, skin photosensitivity testing after the 0.25 mg/km PII but before the additional 1.75 mg/g revealed no skin reaction to as high a dose as 30 J/cm², a light dose commonly used to eradicate recurrent skin malignancies (after giving the patient the usual 2 mg/kg dose of sensitizer).

Success in detecting these occult neoplasms has been reported from all centers involved in their development. Nevertheless, the systems still lack specificity because areas of cellular atypia or moderate or marked digress concentrate sensitizer and have low levels of fluorescence. Moreover, false positives have been reported with metaplasia. Ongoing efforts must concentrate on the miniaturization of the system, simultaneous digital computerized video imaging of the airway, fluorescence ratios, and methods to decrease the chance for nonspecific skin toxicity that may involve alternate routes of sensitizer delivery or use of differences in autofluoresence between normal and tumor tissue without sensitizer use.

It would seem logical that, if these areas of early or occult lung cancer could be localized by standard bronchoscopic methods or by the fluorescence activation principles as covered above, these superficial lesions would be most amenable to possible complete eradication by endobronchial photodynamic therapy. The Japanese were among the first to recognize this potential route of treatment and reported a series of 8 patients who had "early-stage central type" lung cancer (*i.e.*, x-ray and endoscopic findings suggesting the absence of lymph node involvement, and disease confined to the bronchial wall) who did not undergo resection due to patient refusal or medical contraindication, who were treated with photodynamic therapy.[109] Complete tumor remission as defined by no evidence of endoscopic, cytologic, or histologic tumor was obtained in all cases. Variable sensitizer doses, from 2.5 to 5 mg/kg were used, with a wide range of energies (90–600 J/cm²).[104] Of these 8 patients, 1 was described in a follow-up report as the first 5-year disease-free survivor treated only by photodynamic therapy.[110] This pioneering group has subsequently updated their results in early-stage lung cancer in 40 cytology-positive only patients, of which 26 were treated without surgical resection. An impressive 100% initial complete remission rate has been reported, with 3 (12%) late recurrences, although autopsy confirmation in 10 deaths supposedly unrelated to cancer was not 100%.[111] The 16 surviving patients are free of disease 21 to 112 months post PDT at the time of the report (July 1990). More sobering results were recorded for 14 patients who, due to uncertainty of the PDT effect, had surgical resection of 15 PDT-treated lesions, of which 67% showed residual carcinoma.

In smaller but similar series of 13 patients with 14 carcinomas who had a complete endobronchial response to PDT, 11 of 13 had no local recurrence 3 to 53 months after treatment.[98] Most of these squamous carcinomas were less than 1 cm² in surface area. This surface area corresponds to the most recent recommendations from Hayatas group for best PDT results in early lung cancer.

The concept of endobronchial PDT for occult or early-stage lung cancer will be the subject of numerous reports in the future; currently, the best therapy for the patient with no medical contraindication to resection is surgical removal of the cancer. Moreover, thoracic surgeons and pulmonary physicians must keep in mind that if an "early" lung cancer is visible endoscopically, there is a 25% chance that the regional lymph nodes are involved with metastatic cancer. With the current sensitizers, the nodal basins will not be affected by endobronchial PDT. Moreover, the major problem with early-stage or occult lung cancers is the development of a second primary malignancy, often in the airway. Unless this disease is thought to be occult multicentric disease and all visible airways are illuminated, this late cause of death will be unaffected.

The number of patients for whom this therapy would be relevant must be mentioned. Because only 1% of patients on initial screening were found to have early lung cancer (which raises doubts about the cost effectiveness of such screening), few patients will then fall into the favorable cytologically positive, roentgenographically and endoscopically negative group with lesions smaller than 1 cm². Perhaps more patients can be defined in the future as high-risk patients on the basis of more sophisticated sputum analysis with monoclonal antibody markers and be followed for the development of in situ cancer amenable to PDT.

We need to refine the sensitizers to circumvent the 6-week avoidance of light. Newer sensitizers, conjugation of sensitizers to monoclonal antibody, or perhaps aerosol delivery of sensitizer topically to the airway will affect these problems.

The use of PDT for treatment of large pleural surfaces contaminated by malignancy, such as stage IIIB lung cancer, isolated pleural metastases, or mesothelioma, has been addressed at the National Cancer Institute, with the groundwork beginning in 1986. A series of in vitro, in vivo, small and large animal, and phantom modeling experiments were designed as a prelude to human investigations. A feasibility and phase I trial of intrapleural PDT for the treatment of pleural malignancies, including stage IIIB lung cancer isolated pleural metastases to the hemithorax, and mesothelioma has been ongoing since November of 1989 to define the maximal tolerated dose of photodynamic therapy that can be delivered to the chest cavity after maximal cytoreductive surgery. Light delivery to the thorax is accomplished after pleurectomy or modified extrapleural pneumonectomy to debulk the disease to 5 mm thickness maximum using dilute intralipid for light dispersion.[112] Seven photodiodes are strategically placed in the chest to record ongoing cumulative and real time light dose. After the maximal tolerated dose of PDT has been defined, a phase II trial of efficacy in the treatment of uniform histologic types (*e.g.*, mesothelioma) is planned. In such patients, whose curative options are close to zero with standard treatment, the advent of an intraoperative adjuvant that may obtain at least local control could be the first step toward improving survival.

OCULAR TUMORS

PDT has been attempted for control of choroidal malignant melanoma, a tumor managed traditionally by enucleation, but in recent years, there has been interest in local or external particle beam irradiation in addition to laser photocoagulation or transscleral diathermy (Table 69–34).[113–115] Complete responses have been seen in patients with small or medium lesions, with the final appearance of the tumor that of a large

TABLE 69–34. Results of Photodynamic Therapy for Ocular Tumors

Investigations	Tumor Type	Patients/Eyes	Light Dose (J/cm²)	Response Rate (%) CR	PR	NR	Comments
Murphree[116]	Melanoma	9/9	50–400	22	66	12	CRs nonpigmented
Bruce[113]	Melanoma	24/24	300–3000	41	6	53	CRs in small tumors
Murphree[116]	Retinoblastoma	6/9	50–400	11	78	11	All recur later

J, joules; CR, complete response, eradication of tumor; PR, partial response, greater than 50% reduction in tumor size; NR, no response.

chorioretinal scar. Posttreatment complications include transient chemosis, iritis, and lid swelling in all patients, managed with cycloplegics and corticosteroid drops. Exudative retinal detachment worsened or developed in most patients.

Most investigators have used high energy densities for treatment, and there are no comments about the pigmentation in the lesions treated. Melanin is an efficient absorber of red light, and high energy densities must be used if sufficient light is to reach the deepest portions of pigmented lesions. Thermal effects may have been present at the power densities (dose rates) employed and increased the risk of damage to uninvolved normal tissue. Murphree and Gomer achieved no complete responses in patients with pigmented choroidal melanomas.[116]

Photodynamic destruction of retinoblastoma cells in vitro has been reported, but generally the response to PDT in humans has been disappointing.[117]

ESOPHAGEAL MALIGNANCIES

PDT has been attempted for cure and palliation of esophageal malignancies (Table 69–35). In the United States, where patients most often present with bulky tumor and adjacent nodal involvement indicative of advanced-stage disease, investigators have reported palliation of esophageal obstruction using PDT. In Japan and China, where mass screening clinics have been able to detect early esophageal carcinomas, PDT has been attempted with curative intent.

McCaughan and coworkers reported the treatment of 40 patients with esophageal tumors (19 adenocarcinomas, 19 squamous carcinomas, and 2 melanomas) in whom conventional treatments were unsuccessful.[118] Patients received HpD or DHE, followed by the delivery of red light by an optical fiber passed through a flexible endoscope. Four patients with stage I tumors had a complete response. One with squamous cancer subsequently died of recurrent disease at 18 months, but 2 with adenocarcinoma were alive and free of disease at 11 and 23 months after treatment. A third patient with melanoma died of another cancer 31 months after treatment. Of the 35 patients who could be evaluated 1 month after PDT, the average improvement in food intake was from a liquid to a soft diet. Of the 28 patients assessable one month after PDT, the average minimal esophageal diameter opening increased from 6 to 9 mm. Nine patients with complete obstruction were treated; of the 7 survivors at 1 month, all were able to tolerate oral intake of food. Side effects of treatment included six pleural effusions, of which five resolved without treatment; six strictures requiring dilation, and three tracheoesophageal fistulas (one in a patient with tracheal invasion and one in a patient who had had prior laryngeal surgery). Because of the advanced nature of most of their cases, overall survival was poor, averaging 7.7 months for patients with adenocarcinoma and 5.8 months for patients with squamous carcinomas.

Thomas and colleagues treated 14 patients with locally advanced esophageal cancer using high-dose photodynamic

TABLE 69–35. Results of Photodynamic Therapy for Esophageal and Gastric Tumors

Investigations	Tumor Type	No. of Patients	Light Dose (J/cm²)	Response Rate (%) CR	PR	NR	Comments
McCaughan[118]	Esophagus	40	300–600 J/c	10	NA	NA	Most improve swallowing
Thomas[119]	Esophagus	14	60–337	14	86	0	All improve swallowing
Aida[120]	Esophagus	4	270–360	50	50	0	Early stage; CR's NED at 1, 2 y
Aida[120]	Esophagus	5	270–360	0	100	0	Advanced stage
Hayata[121]	Gastric	4	34–960	100	0	0	3/4 recur by 27 mo.
Hayata[121]	Gastric	12	34–960				Resected after PDT; 5 of 12 had no tumor in specimen

J, joules; J/c: joules per centimeter; CR, complete response, eradication of tumor; PR, partial response, greater than 50% reduction in tumor size; NR, no response; NED, no evidence of disease.

therapy.[119] All patients achieved a measurable improvement in the severity of dysphagia persisting from 1 to 28 weeks. Two patients had complete eradication of tumor proven by histologic examination of the subsequently resected esophagus. The complication rate was 16% and included mediastinitis and bronchoesophageal fistula.

Aida and Hirashima treated 4 patients with superficial carcinomas of the esophagus.[120] Two had endoscopically complete responses and remained disease-free at one and two years after treatment. The other two patients went on to surgical resection and were found to have residual tumor cells in portions of the tumor thought to have been inadequately illuminated. Their advanced cases showed partial responses.

UPPER GASTROINTESTINAL MALIGNANCIES

PDT may have some applicability in early-stage gastric cancer for patients who cannot undergo curative surgery. The shape of the stomach and deep rugae complicate the delivery of light. The technical aspects of light delivery must be addressed if adequate PDT is to be given. Because of the difficulty in diagnosing early-stage cases and the propensity of gastric carcinomas to metastasize to adjacent lymph nodes, PDT for most gastric cancers in the United States will probably be limited to palliation of medically inoperable cases.

The practice of screening for gastric cancers in Japan has detected some early gastric cancers that have been treated by PDT in patients who refused or were not eligible for surgery. Hayata and coworkers in Japan treated 16 patients with early-stage gastric carcinoma (see Table 69–35).[121] Four were treated by PDT alone because of medical inoperability or refusal of surgery, while the other 12 patients had resection after PDT. Complete disappearance by endoscopic visualization was obtained in all 4 patients treated with PDT alone. One patient remained disease free at 30 months, 1 had a recurrence at 27 months and was retreated, and 2 patients died with recurrent disease at 5 and 13 months. Of the 12 patients who had resection after PDT, there was no evidence of tumor

in the operative specimen in 5. Okuda reported endoscopic PDT treatment of 5 patients with early and 1 patient with advanced gastric cancer.[122]

LOWER GASTROINTESTINAL MALIGNANCIES

Fluorescence assays of human and murine colorectal cancers that had received intravenous HpD demonstrate preferential localization of HpD in adenocarcinomas and tubular adenomas, with the mean HpD concentration twofold to sixfold higher in tumor compared with surrounding normal mucosa.[123–125] It has been possible to destroy experimental colon cancers without producing any damage to adjacent normal colon exposed to similar light doses.[126] For experimental tumors undergoing necrosis caused by PDT slough, the defect heals by regeneration of the normal colon, and photosensitization does not reduce the mechanical strength of the colonic wall.[127] Barr treated 10 patients with colorectal cancers unsuitable for operation because of metastatic disease or underlying medical debility.[128] Light was delivered with an optical fiber passed through the colonoscope and into from 1 to 4 points within the lesion. Intraluminal ultrasound measurements showed a reduction in mean tumor depth from 18.8 to 12.6 mm with four patients reporting some degree of symptomatic improvement. PDT was suitable for treatment of small tumors or for small areas of persistent tumor where the bulk of tumor could be removed by alternative techniques.

GENITOURINARY MALIGNANCIES

The first reported human use of PDT was for a patient with transitional cell carcinoma of the bladder. Kelly and Snell observed destruction of tumor in the subsequent cystectomy specimen only in sites that had been illuminated.[12] This has been one of the most active areas of interest in PDT (Table 69–36). Emphasis has been on treatment of superficial transitional cell cancers not involving the muscularis of the bladder (*e.g.*, Tis, Ta, T1 tumors).

TABLE 69–36. Results of Photodynamic Therapy for Urinary Bladder Tumors

Investigations	Tumor Type	Patients/Sites	Light Dose (J/cm²)	Response Rate (%)			Comments
				CR	PR	NR	
Hisazumi[133]	TCCa	9/36	F 50–300	50	19	31	Ta, T1 tumors; all CR ≤2 cm
Tsuchiya[132]	TCCa	8/NA	F 120–360	100	0	0	Ta-T2; two recur at 6–18 mo
Benson[134]	TCCa	4/NA	F 150	100	0	0	CIS; recur elsewhere in bladder
Benson[136]	TCCa	10/NA	WB 25–45	60	20	20	CIS or CIS and T2 tumors
Prout[135]	TCCa	19/50	F 100–200	24	50	26	Ta, T1, CIS tumors
Nseyo[138]	TCCa	19/NA	WB 5–60	37	53	10	Ta, T1, CIS tumors
Harty[140]	TCCa	7/NA	WB 25+F	78	0	22	4/7 develop contracted bladder
Dugan[143]	TCCa	12/NA	WB 15				PDT prophylaxis reduces recurrences, 33% vs 83%

J, joules; CR, complete response, eradication of tumor; PR, partial response, greater than 50% reduction in tumor size; NR, no response; TCCa, transitional cell carcinoma; F, focal; WB, whole bladder; CIS, carcinoma in situ; Ta, papillary tumor confined to mucosa; T1, tumor invading lamina propria; T2, tumor invading muscle superficially; PDT, photodynamic therapy.

Sensitizer is selectively retained by murine bladder tumors and tumor destruction can be achieved with the appropriated combination of photosensitizer and light.[129,130] Benson demonstrated localization of sensitizer in transitional cell carcinoma in situ and severely dysplastic epithelium in the urinary bladder after intravenous administration and subsequent illumination of the bladder with violet light.[131] Their observations were confirmed at histologic examination of the bladders after cystectomy with the only false-positive findings at sites of regenerative mucosal activity around healing biopsy areas. Other groups have found preferential fluorescence in tumors compared with normal bladder mucosa.[132,133]

Light dose and light delivery technique have been important for tumor control and complications of treatment. High-dose (100–200 J/cm²) focal light treatment has been used to control papillary lesions. However, much lower doses (~15 J/cm²) have been used for the whole-bladder treatment, which has been used to control carcinoma in situ or microscopic disease after resection of papillary lesions. The Mayo Clinic group initially reported biopsy-proven complete tumor responses in 4 patients with recurrent, previously treated transitional cell carcinomas of the bladder that were focally illuminated using optical fibers introduced through the cystoscope after intravenous HpD injection.[134] A collaborative group of American and Chinese urologists treated 50 papillary tumors and three areas of carcinoma in situ in 20 patients with focal PDT to the involved sites.[135] The carcinomas in situ were all eliminated, and 74% of the papillary lesions had complete responses to treatment. The complete response rate was only 33% for lesions larger than 1.5 cm. Two groups from Japan reported that the highest complete remission rate was seen for lesions smaller than 1 cm.[132,133]

Because of the tendency of tumors to later recur at other sites in the bladder that had not been illuminated and because of the interest in treating diffuse, multifocal carcinoma in situ, several groups switched to using a modified optical fiber with a spherical diffusing bulb to illuminate the entire bladder.[136,137] In 10 patients with carcinoma in situ alone, biopsy and urinary cytology at follow-up examination 3 months after treatment showed complete disappearance of tumor.[136] Two patients with both carcinoma in situ and papillary, noninvasive lesions were found to have disappearance of the former but persistence of the latter. Of these 12 patients, 3 subsequently developed focal recurrent disease at 6 to 9 months after treatment. Hisazumi treated 2 other patients with carcinoma in situ, both of whom had a complete response to treatment. Both developed acute posttreatment inflammatory symptoms for 2 to 3 weeks and a transient reduction in bladder capacity that resolved by 3 months.[137]

Nseyo and colleagues treated 19 patients with resistant superficial transitional cell carcinoma of the bladder.[138,139] Seven patients (37%) had complete responses to treatment, and 10 (53%) had partial responses. All patients had irritative urinary tract symptoms after treatment; 4 patients developed bladder shrinkage that did not resolve. Among 4 patients treated with muscle invading disease (≥T2), control of gross hematuria was the only benefit seen. Harty and associates described the development of a contracted bladder with hydroureteronephrosis and vesicoureteral reflux in 4 of 7 patients treated with 25 J/cm² to the whole bladder, with or without additional focal treatment.[140] Deep bladder biopsies showed replacement of smooth muscle by fibrous tissue. Careful attention to light

dose and treatment technique and photosensitizer localization in tumor compared with normal bladder is important if this is to be a safe and effective treatment for superficial bladder cancer.[141,142]

In a controlled trial, the toxicity of the therapy appears acceptable. Dugan and associates reported the preliminary results of a randomized trial of observation versus PDT after transurethral resection for patients with high-grade or recurrent low-grade papillary superficial bladder cancer.[143] PDT patients received 2 mg/kg of DHE followed 40 to 50 hours later by 15 J/cm² with 630-nm red light to the whole bladder. With median follow-up of 1 year, there were 10 recurrences (83%) of 12 in the observation group, compared with 4 (33%) of 12 in the PDT group ($p = 0.0014$); 91% of the PDT patients experienced acute irritative symptoms after treatment, but these were self-limited. Bladder capacity over time was equivalent in both groups. The final report from this trial will be an important factor in determining the efficacy and safety of bladder PDT. In another ongoing trial, patients with refractory or recurrent superficial transitional cell carcinoma in situ in the bladder are being treated with PDT as an alternative to cystectomy.

GYNECOLOGIC MALIGNANCIES AND INTRAABDOMINAL PHOTODYNAMIC THERAPY

An early report on the use of PDT for gynecologic malignancies described treatment of 5 patients with recurrent tumors involving the vaginal vault.[144] Two complete responses were seen, one in a patient with recurrent ovarian cancer and the other in a patient with melanoma. These were durable at 10 and 12 months. The only toxicity observed was cutaneous phototoxicity.

Multiple other reports subsequently appeared, primarily describing cases of gynecologic cancer recurring in the vagina or skin after conventional treatment (Table 69–37).[145-150]

PDT is being investigated as an adjuvant therapy to be delivered to patients with ovarian cancer at the time of second-look laparotomy. Tochner and coworkers were able to control an experimental murine ovarian ascites tumor in 17 of 20 animals using intraperitoneally administered HpD and four intraperitoneal light treatments.[26] On the basis of these experimental findings, a phase I study was initiated in which PDT was administered to the peritoneal surface of patients with minimal thickness intraperitoneal tumor at the time of surgical resection.[152-154] The study was completed with the determination of a maximal tolerated dose of photodynamic therapy that could be delivered to the peritoneal cavity after major cytoreductive surgery. Of the 54 patients with refractory ovarian cancer, sarcoma, colon cancer, or mucinous adenocarcinoma diffusely involving the peritoneal cavity, 39 were able to undergo adequate surgical cytoreduction to receive intraoperative photodynamic therapy. With median follow-up of 22 months, 9 of 39 patients remained free of disease. Phase II studies at the maximal tolerated dose are planned.

CONCLUSIONS

PDT represents another modality for the treatment of human malignancy. Light-activated photosensitizers have definite antitumor activity in in vitro and in vivo experimental systems.

TABLE 69–37. Results of Photodynamic Therapy for Gynecologic Tumors

Investigations	Tumor Type	Patients/Sites	Light Dose (J/cm²)	Response Rate (%) CR	PR	NR	Comments
Ward[144]	Vagina	5/5	NA	40	60	0	CRs durable at 10, 12 mo
Soma[145]	Vagina	1/NA	NA	100	0	0	NED at 1 y
Dahlman[146]	Vulva	2/2	NA	50	0	50	CR in carcinoma in situ
Rettenmaier[147]	Vagina/perineum	6/9	20–40	22	45	33	Treatment well tolerated
McCaughan[148]	Vulva/vagina	5/5	Variable	80	20	0	Follow-up 5–15 mo
Lobraico[151]	Vulva/vagina	7/45	Variable	76	18	6	Edema, erythema after PDT
Corti[149]	Vagina	15/15	60–240	53	40	7	Duration of CR 2.5–25 mo
Lele[150]	Skin	7/NA	Variable	100	0	0	PDT with palliative intent
Lele[150]	Vagina/cervix	11/NA	Variable	18	18	64	CRs durable at 28, 36 mo

J, joules; CR, complete response, eradication of tumor; PR, partial response, greater than 50% reduction in tumor size; NR, no response; NED, no evidence of disease; PDT, photodynamic therapy; NA, not available.

Much of the early clinical work involved treatment of patients with advanced, recurrent disease who had not responded to conventional therapy. Because good responses with acceptable toxicity have been obtained in these patients, active investigation continues and is aimed at defining the most appropriate sites and applications for the technique. Because of the limited depth of light penetration in tissue, the most promising sites may be those where there is limited thickness of tumor, such as in superficial skin lesions or early-stage carcinomas involving the aerodigestive tract, bronchial tree, or the genitourinary tract. Other potential uses include those where PDT could be combined with surgical or chemotherapeutic debulking, such as pleural mesothelioma or advanced stage ovarian cancer. Whether PDT can be of benefit in surgical cases for which the margins of resection are close is an interesting question.

The hematoporphyrin derivative, dihematoporphyrin ethers, and benzoporphyrin monoacid ring A are currently only approved for use as investigational compounds in clinical studies. If ongoing trials of PDT in superficial bladder cancer, obstructing esophageal cancer, and non-small cell lung cancer show encouraging results, application to the Food and Drug Administration for approval of DHE as a photosensitizer for general clinical use for these indications is planned. Laboratory work to better understand mechanism of photosensitizer localization and cytotoxicity continues, as do investigations into alternative photosensitizers with improved tumor localization, less cutaneous photosensitivity, and absorption peaks at deeper penetrating wavelengths of light. Attempts at measurement of singlet oxygen, if successful, will permit the development of more meaningful dosimetry to correlate response with actual tissue levels of the purported cytotoxic agent. Hopefully, these and other developments in the field of PDT will improve the treatment for patients with cancer.

REFERENCES

1. Raab O. Uber die Wirkung Fluoreszierenden Stoffen. Infusoria Z Biol 1900;39:524.
2. Jesionek A, Tappeiner VH. Zur Behandlung der hautcarcinomit mit fluorescierenden stoffen. Muench Med Wochenshr 1903;47:2042.
3. Hausman W. Die sensibilisierende Wirkung des hematoporphyrins. Biochem Z 1911;30:276.
4. Auber H. Banger G. Unter suchungen uber die rolle der porphyrine bei geschwulstkranken menschen und tieren. Z Krebsforsch 1942;53:65.
5. Figge FHJ, Weiland GS, Manganiello LOJ. Cancer detection and therapy. Affinity of neoplastic embryonic and traumatized tissue for porphyrins and metalloporphyrins. Proc Soc Exp Biol Med 1948;68:640.
6. Lipson RL, Baldes EJ. The photodynamic properties of a particular hematoporphyrin derivative. Arch Dermatol 1960;82:508.
7. Lipson RL, Blades EJ. The use of a derivative of hematoporphyrin in tumor detection. JNCI 1961;26:1.
8. Lipson RL, Baldes EJ. Hematoporphyrin derivative: A new aid for endoscopic detection of malignant disease. J Thorac Cardiovasc Surg 1961;42:623.
9. Grey M, Lipson RL, Mack JVS, et al. Use of hematoporphyrin derivative in detection and management of cervical cancer. Am J Obstet Gynecol 1967;9:766.
10. Gregorie HG, Horger EO, Ward JL, et al. Hematoporphyrin derivative for detection and management of cancer. Ann Surg 1968;167:82.
11. Lipson RL, Gray MJ, Baldes EJ. Hematoporphyrin derivative for detection and management of cancer. Proceedings of the 9th International Cancer Congress, Tokyo, 1966:393.
12. Kelly JF, Snell NE, Berenbaum MC. Photodynamic destruction of human bladder carcinoma. J Urol 1976;115:150.
13. Dougherty RJ. Activated dyes vs anti-tumor agents. JNCI 1974;51:1333.
14. Dougherty TJ, Crindley GE, Fiel R, et al. Photoradiation therapy II. Cure of animal tumors with hematoporphyrin and light. JNCI 1975;55:115.
15. Dougherty TJ, Kaufman JE, Goldfarb A, et al. Photoradiation therapy for the treatment of malignant tumors. Cancer Res 1978;38:2628.
16. Dougherty TJ. Photoradiation therapy. Urology 1984;23:61.
17. Dougherty TJ. Photosensitizers: Therapy and detection of malignant tumors. Photochem Photobiol 1987;45:874.
18. Pass HI Photodynamic therapy for lung cancer. Chest Surg Clin North Am 1991;1:135–151.
19. Lin C-W. Selective localization of photosensitizers in tumors: A review of the phenomenon and possible mechanisms. In: Kessel D, ed. Photodynamic therapy of neoplastic disease. Boston: CRC Press, 1990:79–101.
20. Barel A, Jori G, Perin A, Romandini P, Pagnan A, Biffanti S. Role of high-, low-, and very low-density lipoproteins in the transport and tumor-delivery of hematoporphyrin, in vivo. Cancer Lett 1986;32:145.
21. Bugelski PJ, Porter CW, Dougherty TJ. Autoradiographic distribution of hematoporphyrin derivative in normal and tumor tissue of the mouse. Cancer Res 1981;41:4606.
22. Selman SH, Kreimer-Birnbaum M, Klaunig JE, Goldblatt PJ, Keck RW, Britton SL. Blood flow in transplantable bladder tumors treated with hematoporphyrin derivative and light. Cancer Res 1984;44:1924.
23. Star WM, Marijnissen HPA, van den Berg-Blok AE, Versteeg JAC, Franken KA, Reinhold HS. Destruction of rat mammary tumor and normal tissue microcirculation by hematoporphyrin derivative photoradiation observed in vivo in sandwich observation chambers. Cancer Res 1986;46:2532.
24. Pass HI, Evans S, Matthews WA, et al. Photodynamic therapy of oncogene-transformed cells. J Thorac Cardiovasc Surg 1991;101:795–799.
25. Perry RR, Matthews W, Pass HI, et al. Sensitivity of different human lung cancer histologies to photodynamic therapy. Cancer Res 1990;50:4272–4276.
26. Tochner Z, Mitchell JB, Smith P, et al. Photodynamic therapy of ascites tumours within the peritoneal cavity. Br J Cancer 1986;53:733.
27. Mitchell JB McPherson S, DeGraff W, et al. Oxygen dependence of hematoporphyrin derivative-induced photoinactivation of Chinese hamster cells. Cancer Res 1985;45:2008.
28. Lee See K, Forbes IJ, Betts WH. Oxygen dependency of phototoxicity with maematoporphyrin derivative. Photochem Photobiol 1984;39:631.

29. Foote CS. Mechanisms of photooxygenation. In: Doiron DR, Gomer CJ, eds. Porphyrin localization and treatment of tumors. New York: Alan R Liss, 1984:3.

30. Christensen T, Moan J, Smedshammer L, et al. Influence of hematoporphyrin derivative (HPD) and light on the attachment of cells to the substratum. Photochem Photobiophys 1985;10:53.

31. Denstaman SC, Dillehay LE, Williams JR. Enhanced susceptibility of HPD-sensitized phototoxicity and correlated resistance to trypsin detachment in SV40 transformed IMR-90 cell. Photochem Photobiophys 1985;10:53.

32. Volden G, Christensen T, Moan J. Photodynamic membrane damage of hematoporphyrin derivative-treated NHIK 3025 cells in vitro. Photochem Photobiophys 1981;3:105.

33. Jewell SA, Bellomo G, Thor H, et al. Bleb formation in hepatocytes during drug metabolism is caused by disturbances in thiol and calcium ion homeostatis. Science 217:1257.

34. Borrelli MJ, Wong RSL, Dewey WC. A direct correlation between hyperthermia-induced blebbing and survival in synchronous G_1 CHO cells. J Cell Physiol 1986;126:181.

35. Tom M, Dubhelman AR, Prinsze C, et al. Photodynamic therapy membrane and enzyme photobiology. In: Henderson B, Dougherty T, eds. Photodynamic therapy. New York: Marcel Dekker, 1992.

36. Sonoda M, Murali-Krishna C, Riesz P. The role of singlet oxygen in the photochemolysis of red blood cells sensitized by phthalocyanine sulfonates. Photochem Photobiol 1987;46:635.

37. Hilf R, Murant RS, Narayanan U, Gibson SL. Hematoporphyrin derivative-induced photosensitivity of mitochondrial succinate dehydrogenase and selected cytosolic enzymes of R3230AC mammary adenocarcinomas of rats. Cancer Res 1984;44:1483.

38. Hilf R, Murant RS, Narayanan U, Gibson SL. Relationship of mitochondrial function and cellular adenosine triphosphate levels to hematoporphyrin derivative-induced photosensitization in R3230AC mammary tumors. Cancer Res 1986;46:211.

39. Gomer CJ. DNA damage and repair in CHO cells following hematoporphyrin photoradiation. Cancer Lett 1980;11:161.

40. Moan J, Waksvik H, Christensen T. DNA single-stand breaks and sister chromatid exchanges induced by treatment with hematoporphyrin and light or by x-rays in human NHIK 3025 cells. Cancer Res 1980;40:2915.

41. Mitchell JB Russo A, Kinsella TJ, Glatstein E. The use of non-hypoxic cell sensitizers in radiobiology and radiotherapy. Int J Radiat Oncol Biol Phys 1986;12:1513.

42. Russo A, DeGraff W, Kinsella TJ, et al. Potentiation of chemotherapy cytotoxicity following iododeoxyuridine incorporation in Chinese hamster cells. Int J Radiat Oncol Biol Phys 1986;12:1418.

43. Gomer CJ, Rucker N, Banerjee A, Benedict WF. Comparison of mutagenicity and induction of sister chromatid exchange in Chinese hamster cells exposed to hematoporphyrin derivative, ionizing radiation, or ultraviolet radiation. Cancer Res 1983;43:2662.

44. Ben-Hur E, Fujihara T, Suzuki F, Elkind MM. Genetic toxicology of the photosensitization of Chinese hamster cells by phthalocyanines. Photochem Photobiol 1987;45:227.

45. Kessel D. Sites of photosensitization by derivatives of hematoporphyrin. Photochem Photobiol 1986;44:489.

46. Rizzoni WE, Matthews W, Pass HI, et al. In vitro photodynamic therapy of human lung cancer. Influence of dose rate, hematoporphryn concentration and incubation, and cellular targets. Surg Forum 1987;38:452–455.

47. Bohmer RM, Morstyn G. Uptake of hematoporphyrin derivative by normal and malignant cells: Effect of serum, pH, temperature, and cell size. Cancer Res 1985;45:5328–5334.

48. Matthews W, Cook J, Pass HI. In vitro photodynamic therapy of human lung cancer: Investigation of dose-rate effects. Cancer Res 1989;49:1718–1721.

49. Elmets CA, Bowen KD. Immunological suppression in mice treated with hematoporphyrin derivative photoradiation. Cancer Res 1986;46:1608–1611.

50. Ortner MJ, Abhold RH, Chignell CF. The effect of protoporphyrin on histamine secretion by rat peritoneal mast cells: A dual phototoxic reaction. Photochem Photobiol 1981;33:355–360.

51. Henderson BW, Donovan JM. Cellular prostaglandin E release after photodynamic therapy. Lasers Med Sci 1988;3:103.

52. Lynch DH, Haddad S, King VJ, Ott MJ, Straight RC, Jolles CJ. Systemic immunosuppression induced by photodynamic therapy (PDT) is adoptively transferred by macrophages. Photochem Photobiol 1989;49:453–458.

53. Evans S, Matthews W, Perry R, Fraker D, Norton J, Pass HI. Effect of photodynamic therapy on tumor necrosis factor production by murine macrophages. JNCI 1990;82:34–39.

54. Jiang FN, Liu D.J Neyndorff H, et al. Photodynamic killing of human squamous cell carcinoma cells using a monoclonal antibody-photosensitizer conjugate. JNCI 1991;83:1218–1225.

55. Pogrebniak HW, Matthews W, Black C, et al. Targeted phototherapy with sensitizer-monoclonal antibody and light. Surg Forum 1991;42.447–449.

56. Shumaker BP, Hetzel FW. Clinical laser photodynamic therapy in the treatment of bladder carcinoma. Photochem Photobiol 1987;46:899–901.

57. Nseyo UO, Whalen RK, Duncan MR, Berman B, Lundahl SL. Urinary cytokines following photodynamic therapy for bladder cancer. Urology 1990;36:167–171.

58. Heald PW, Perez MI, McKiernan G, Christensen I, Edelson RL. Extracorporeal photochemotherapy for CTCL. Prog Clin Biol Res 1990;337:443–447.

59. Gonzalez S, Arnfield MR, Meeker BE, et al. Treatment of Dunning R3327-AT rat prostate tumors with photodynamic therapy in combination with misonidazole. Cancer Res 1986;46:2858–2862.

60. Dougherty TJ. Photosensitization of malignant tumors. Semin Surg Oncol 1986;2:24.

61. Mang TS, Dougherty TJ, Potter WR, et al. Photobleaching of porphyrins used in photodynamic therapy and implications for therapy. Photochem Photobiol 1987;45:501.

62. Bandieramonte C, Marchesini R, Melloni E, et al. Laser phototherapy following HpD administration in superficial neoplastic lesions. Tumori 1984;70:327.

63. Santoro O, Bandieramonte G, Melloni E, et al. Photodynamic therapy by topical mesotetraphenylporphinesulfonate tetrasodium salt administration in superficial basal cell carcinoma. Cancer Res 1990;50:4501.

64. Waldow SM, Lobraico RV, Kohler IK, et al. Photodynamic therapy for treatment of malignant cutaneous lesions. Lasers Surg Med 1987;7:451.

65. Kennedy J. Photoradiation therapy for cancer at Kingston and Hamilton. In: Kessel D, Dougherty TJ, eds. Pophyrin photosensitization. New York: Plenum Press, 1983:53.

66. Pennington DG, Waner M, Knox A. Photodynamic therapy for multiple skin cancers. Plast Reconst Surg 1987;82:1067.

67. Wilson BW, Mang TS, Cooper MC, et al. Use of photodynamic therapy for the treatment of extensive basal cell carcinomas. Facial Plastic Surgery 1990;6:185.

68. Tse DT, Kerstein RC, Anderson RL. Hematoporphyrin derivative photoradiation therapy in managing nevoid basal-cell carcinoma syndrome: A preliminary report. Arch Opthalmol 1984;102:990.

69. Robinson PJ, Carruth JAS, Fiarris GM. Photodynamic therapy: A better treatment for widespread Bowen's disease. Br J Dermatol 1988;119:59.

70. Kennedy JC, Pottier RH, Pross DC. Photodynamic therapy with endogenous protoporphyrin IX. Basic principles and present clinical experience. J Photochem Photobiol B 1990;6:143.

71. Potter WR, Mang TS, Dougherty TJ. The theory of photodynamic therapy dosimetry: Consequences of photodestruction of sensitizers. Photochem Photobiol 1987;46:97.

72. Aberizk WJ, Silver B, Henderson IC, et al. The use of radiotherapy for treatment of isolated locoregional recurrence of breast carcinoma after mastectomy. Cancer 1986;58:1214.

73. Schuh M, Nseyo UO, Potter WR, et al. Photodynamic therapy for palliation of locally recurrent breast carcinoma. J Clin Oncol 1987;5:1766.

74. Sperduto PW, DeLaney TF, Thomas G, et al. Photodynamic therapy for chest wall recurrence in breast cancer. Int J Radiat Oncol Biol Phys 1991;21:441.

75. Gluckman JL, Waner M, Shumrick K, et al. Photodynamic therapy. A viable alternative to conventional therapy for early lesions of the upper aerodigestive tract. Arch Otolaryngol Head Neck Surg 1986;112:949.

76. Gluckman JL. Hematoporphyrin photodynamic therapy. Is there truly a future in head and neck oncology? Laryngoscope 1991;191:36.

77. Wile AG, Novotny J, Mason GR, et al. Photoradiation therapy of head and neck cancer. Am J Clin Oncol 1984;6:39.

78. Schuller DE, McCaughan JS Jr, Rock RP. Photodynamic therapy in head and neck cancer. Arch Otolargyngol 1985;111:351.

79. Takata C, Imakiire M. Cancer of the ear, nose, and throat. In: Hayata Y, Dougherty TJ, eds. Lasers and hematoporphyrin derivative in cancer. New York: Igaku-Shoin, 1983:70.

80. Grossweiner LI, Hill JH, Lobraico RV. Photodynamic therapy of head and neck squamous cell carcinoma: Optical dosimetry and clinical trial. Photochem Photobiol 1987;46:911.

81. Schweitzer VG. Photodynamic therapy for treatment of head and neck cancer. Otolarygol Head Neck Surg 1990;102:225.

82. Freche C, De Corbiere S. Use of photodynamic therapy in the treatment of vocal cord carcinoma. J Photochem Photobiol 1990;B6:291.

83. Shikowitz MJ, Steinberg BM, Abramson A.L. Hematoporphyrin derivative therapy of papillomas: Experimental study. Arch Otolaryngol Head Neck Surg 1986;112:42.

84. Diamond I, Granelli SG, McDonough AF, et al. Photodynamic therapy of malignant tumours. Lancet 1972;2:1175.

85. Boggan JE, Walter R, Edwards MSB, et al. Distribution of hematoporphyrin derivative in the rat 9L gliosarcoma brain tumour analyzed by digital videofluorescence microscopy. J Neurosurg 1984;61:1113.

86. Little FM, Gomer CJ, Hyman S, et al. Observations in studies of quantitative kinetics of tritium labelled hematoporphyrin derivatives (HpDI and HpDII) in the normal and neoplastic rat brain model. J Neurooncol 1984;2:361.

87. Berenbaum MC, Hall GW, Hoyes AD. Cerebral photosensitization by hematoporphyrin derivative. Evidence for an endothelial site of action. Br J Cancer 1986;53:81.

88. Perria C, Carai M, Balzoi A, et al. Photodynamic therapy of malignant brain tumors: Clinical results of difficulties, with questions about and future prospects for the neurosurgical applications. Neurosurgery 1988;23:557.

89. Laws ER Jr, Cortese DA, Kinsey JH, et al. Photoradiation therapy in the treatment of malignant brain tumors: A phase I (feasibility) study. Neurosurgery 1981;9:672.

90. Laws ER Jr, Wharen RE, Anderson RE. Photoradiation therapy of malignant gliomas. In: Wilkens RH, Rengachary SS, eds. Neurosurgery Update, 1990:260.

91. McCulloch GAJ, Forbes IJ, See KL, et al. Phototherapy in malignant brain tumors. In: Doiron DR, Gomer CJ, eds. Porphyrin localization and treatment of tumors. New York: Alan R Liss, 1984:709.

92. Kostron H, Weiser G, Fritsch E, et al. Photodynamic therapy of malignant brain tumors: Clinical and neuropathological results. Photochem Photobiol 1987;46:937.

93. Kaye AH, Morstyn G, Brownbill D. Adjuvant high-dose photoradiation therapy in the treatment of cerebral glioma: A phase 1–2 study. J Neurosurg 1987;67:500.

94. Muller PJ, Wilson BC. Photodynamic therapy of malignant primary brain tumors: Clinical effects, post-operative ICP, and light penetration of the brain. Photochem Photobiol 1987;46:929.

95. Pass HI, Delaney T, Smith PD, et al. Bronchoscopic phototherapy at comparable dose rates: Early results. Ann Thorac Surg 1989;47:693–699.

96. Kato H. Lung cancer. In: Hayata Y, Dougherty TJ, eds. Lasers and hematoporphyrin derivative in cancer. Tokyo: Kgaka-Shion, 1983:39.

97. Kato H, Aizawa K, Ono J, et al. Clinical measurement of tumor fluorescence using a

new diagnostic system with hematoporphyrin derivative, laser photoradiation, in a spectroscope. Lasers Surg Med 1984;4:49–58.

98. Edell ES, Cortese DA. Detection and phototherapy of lung cancer. In: Morstyn G, Kaye A, eds. Phototherapy of cancer. London: Harwood Academic Publishers, 1990:185.

99. Doiron DR, Balchum OJ. Hematoporphyrin derivative photoradiation therapy of endobronchial lung cancer. In: Andreoni A, Bucedda R, eds. Porphyrin in tumor phototherapy. New York: Plenum Press, 1984:195.

100. Balchum OJ, Doiron DR, Huth GC. Photodynamic therapy of obstructing lung cancer. In: Doiron DR, Gomer CJ, eds. Porphyrin localization and treatment of tumors. New York: Alan R Liss, 1984:721.

101. Balchum OJ. Photodynamic therapy of endobronchial lung tumors. [Abstract] Clayton Foundation Conference, 1987.

102. Vincent RG, Dougherty TJ, Rao U. Photoradiation therapy in the treatment of advanced carcinoma of the trachea and bronchus. In: Doiron DR, Gomer CJ, eds. Porphyrin localization and treatment of tumors. New York: Alan R Liss, 1984:759.

103. Forbes IJ, Ward AD, Jacka FJ, et al. Multidisciplinary approach to phototherapy in tumors. In: Doiron DR, Gomer CJ, eds. Porphyrin localization and treatment of tumors. New York: Alan R. Liss, 1984:693.

104. Lam S, Kostashuk EC, Coy P, et al. A randomized comparative study of the safety and efficacy of photodynamic therapy using Photofrin II combined with palliative radiotherapy alone in patients with inoperable non-small cell bronchogenic carcinoma: A preliminary redport. Photochem Photobiol 1987;5:893–898.

105. Hugh-Jones P, Gardner WN. Laser photodynamic therapy for inoperable bronchogenic carcinoma. J Med 1987;243:565–581.

106. Li JH, Zhao HZ. Photodynamic therapy of bronchogenic carcinoma. Proceedings of the Third Biennial Meeting of the International Photodynamic Association [Abstract] 1990:8:5–10.

107. Benov E, Kostadinov D, Vlasov V. Photoradiation therapy of bronchial cancer. Proceedings of the Third Biennial Meeting of the International Photodynamic Association [Abstract] 1990:8:3–31.

108. Lam S, Palcic B, McLean D, et al. Detection of early lung cancer using low dose Photofrin II. Chest [Abstract] 1990;97:333–337.

109. Hayata Y, Kato H, Konaka C, et al. Photoradiation therapy with hematoporphrin derivative in early and stage 1 lung cancer. Chest 1984;86:169–177.

110. Kato H, Konaka C, Kawate N, et al. Five-year disease-free survival of a lung cancer patient treated only by photodynamic therapy. Chest 1986;90:768–770.

111. Kato H, Konaka C, Yamamoto H, et al. Photodynamic therapy in early stage lung cancer. Proceedings of the Third Biennial Meeting of the International Photodynamic Association [Abstract] 1990;8:4–31.

112. Pass HI, Tochner Z, Delaney T, et al. Intraoperative photodynamic therapy for malignant mesothelioma. [Abstract] Ann Thorac Surg 1990;50:687–688.

113. Bruce RA Jr, McCaughan JS. Lasers in uveal melanoma. Ophthamol Clin North Am 1989;2:597.

114. Tse DT, Dutton JJ, Weingeist TA, et al. Hematoporphyrin photoradiation therapy for intraocular and orbital malignant melanoma. Arch Opthalmol 1984;102:833.

115. Sery TW, Shield JA, Augsburger JJ, et al. Photodynamic therapy of human ocular cancer. Ophthal Surg 1987;18:413.

116. Murphree AL, Cote M, Gomer CJ. The evolution of photodynamic therapy techniques in the treatment of intraocular tumors. Photochem Photobiol 1987;46:919.

117. Sery TW. Photodynamic killing of retinoblastoma cells with hematoporphyrin and light. Cancer Res 1979;39:96.

118. McCaughan JS Jr, Nims TA, Guy JT, et al. Photodynamic therapy for esophageal tumors. Arch Surg 1989;124:74.

119. Thomas RJ, Abbott M, Bhathal PS, et al. High-dose photoradiation of esophageal cancer. Ann Surg 1987;206:193.

120. Aida M, Hirashima T. Cancer of the esophagus. In: Hayata Y, Dougherty TJ, eds. Lasers and hematoporphyrin derivative in cancer. New York: Igaku-Shoin, 1983:57.

121. Hayata T, Kato H, Okitsu H, et al. Photodynamic therapy with hematoporphyrin derivative in cancer of the upper gastrointestinal tract. Semin Surg Oncol 1985;1:1.

122. Okuda S, Mimura S, Otani T, et al. Experimental and clinical studies on HpD-photoradiation therapy for upper gastrointestinal cancer. In: Andreoni A, Cubeddu R, eds. Porphyrins in tumor phototherapy. New York: Plenum Press, 1984:413.

123. Agrez MV, Wharen RE, Anderson RE, et al. Hematoporphyrin derivative: Quantitative derivative: Quantitative uptake in demethylhydrazine-induced murine colorectal carcinoma. J Surg Oncol 1983;24:173.

124. Wooten RS, Ahlquist DA, Anderson RE, et al. Localization of hematoporphyrin derivative to human colrectal cancer. Cancer 1989;64:1569–1576.

125. Dal Fanter M, Bottiroli G, Spinelli P. Behavior of hematoporphyrin derivative in adenomas and adenocarcinomas of the colon: A microfluorometric study. Lasers Med Sci 1988;3:165.

126. Barr H, Tralau CJ, Lewin M, et al. Selective destruction of experimental colon cancer using photodynamic therapy. Br J Surg 1988;75:611.

127. Barr H, Tralau CJ, MacRobert AJ. Photodynamic therapy in the normal rat colon with phthalocyanine sensitisation. Br J Cancer 1987;56:111.

128. Barr H, Krasner N, Boulos PB. et al. Photodynamic therapy for colorectal cancer: A quantitative pilot study. Br J Surg 1990;77:93.

129. Shulok JR, Klaunig JE, Selman SH, et al. Cellular effects of hematoporphyrin derivative photodynamic therapy on normal and neoplastic rat bladder cells. Am J Pathol 1986;122:277.

130. Jocham D, Staehler G, Chaussy C, et al. Laserbehandlung von blasentumoren nach photosensibilisierung mit hämatoporphyrin-derivat. Urologe 1981;20:340.

131. Benson RC Jr, Farrow GM, Kinwey JH, et al. Detection and localization of in situ carcinoma of the bladder with hematoporphyrin derivative. Mayo Clin Proc 1982;57:548.

132. Tsuchiya A, Obara N, Miwa M, et al. Hematoporphyrin derivative and laser photoradiation in the diagnosis and treatment of bladder cancer. J Urol 1983;130:79.

133. Hisazumi H, Misaki T, Miyoshi N. Photoradiation therapy of bladder tumors. J Urology 1983;130:685.

134. Benson RC Jr. Laser photodynamic therapy for bladder cancer. Mayo Clin Proc 1986;61:859.

135. Prout GR Jr, Lin C, Benson R Jr, et al. Photodynamic therapy with hematoporphyrin derivative in the treatment of superficial transitional-cell carcinoma of the bladder. N Engl J Med 1987;317:1251.

136. Benson RC Jr. Treatment of diffuse transitional cell carcinoma in situ by whole bladder hematoporphyrin derivative photodynamic therapy. J Urology 1985;134:675.

137. Hisazumi H, Miyoshi N, Naito K, et al. Whole bladder wall photoradiation therapy for carcinoma in situ of the bladder: A preliminary report. J Urology 1984;131:884.

138. Nseyo UO, Dougherty TH, Sullivan L. Photodynamic therapy in the management of resistant lower urinary tract carcinoma. Cancer 1987;60:3113.

139. Nseyo UO, Whalen TK, Duncan MR, et al. Urinary cytokines following photodynamic therapy for bladder cancer: A preliminary report. Urology 1990;36:167.

140. Harty JI, Amin M, Wieman TJ, et al. Complications of whole bladder dihematoporphyrin ether photodynamic therapy. J Urol 1989;141:1341.

141. Nseyo UO, Dougherty TJ, Boyle DG, et al. Study of factors mediating effect of photodynamic therapy of bladder in canine bladder model. Urology 1988;32:41.

142. Star W, Marijnissen HPA, Jansen H, et al. Light dosimetry for photodynamic therapy by whole bladder wall irradiation. Photochem Photobiol 1987;46:619.

143. Dugan M, Crawford E, Nseyo U, et al. A randomized trial of observation (obs) vs photodynamic therapy after transurethral resection (TUR) or superficial papillary bladder carcinoma. Proc Am Soc Clin Oncol [Abstract] 1991;10:173.

144. Ward BG, Forbes IJ, Cowled PA, et al. The treatment of vaginal recurrences of gynecologic malignancy with phototherapy following hematoporphyrin derivative pretreatment. Am J Obstet Gynecol 1982;142:356.

145. Soma H, Akiya K, Nutahara S, et al. Treatment of vaginal carcinoma with laser photoirradiation following administration of haematoporphyrin derivative. Ann Chir Gynaecol 1982;71:133.

146. Dahlman A, Wile AG, Burns RG, et al. Laser photoradiation therapy of cancer. Cancer Res 1983;43:430.

147. Rettenmaier MA, Berman ML, Disaia PJ, et al. Gynecologic uses of photoradiation therapy. In: Doiron DT, Gomer CJ, eds. Porphyrin localization and treatment of tumors. New York: Alan R Liss, 1984:767.

148. McCaughan JS Jr, Schellhas HF, Lomano J, et al. Photodynamic therapy of gynecologic neoplasms after presensitization with hematoporphyrin derivative. Lasers Surg Med 1985;5:491.

149. Corti L, Tomio L, Maluta S, et al. Photodynamic therapy in gynecological cancer. Lasers Med Sci 1989;4:155.

150. Lele SB, Piver MS, Mang TS, et al. Photodynamic therapy in gynecologic malignancies. Gynecol Oncol 1990;34:350.

151. Lobraico RV, Waldow SM, Harris DM, et al. Photodynamic therapy for cancer of the lower female genital tract. Colops Gynecol Laser Surg 1986;2:185.

152. DeLaney TF, Sindelar W, Smith P, et al. Initial experience with photodynamic therapy for intraperitoneal carcinomatosis. In: Sharp F, Mason WP, Leake RE, eds. Ovarian cancer: Biological and therapeutic challenges. London: Chapman and Hall Medical, 1990:371.

153. Sindelar WF, DeLaney TF, Tochner Z, et al. Technique of photodynamic therapy for disseminated intraperitoneal malignancies: Phase I study. Arch Surg 1991;126:318.

154. DeLaney TF, Sindelar WG, Tochner Z, et al. Phase 1 study of debulking surgery and photodynamic therapy for disseminated intraperitoneal tumors. Int J Radiat Oncol Biol Phys [Abstract] 1991;21:183.

CLAIR J. BEARD
C. NORMAN COLEMAN
TIMOTHY J. KINSELLA

SECTION **9**

Radiation Sensitizers

The cause of the failure of irradiation to locally control solid tumors is multifactorial but may be divided into three broad categories: an excessive number of clonogenic cells, intrinsic cellular characteristics, and environmental factors. Intrinsic cellular characteristics include cell kinetics of a tumor and the capacity to repair radiation damage.[1,2] Intratumoral cellular and environmental heterogeneity makes it likely that multiple factors are operative.[3-7]

A cell that might be sensitive to irradiation under normal physiologic conditions may become resistant due to its microenvironment within the tumor.[8] The nutritional status, pH, and degree of oxygenation contribute to treatment resistance.[9-11] Although each factor is likely to be important, clinical and laboratory research has focused on tumor hypoxia as a potentially important factor limiting local control after treatment with radiation therapy.[12-16] This chapter emphasizes two major areas of radiation sensitization under investigation: the hypoxic cell sensitizers and the halopyrimidines. Although a substantial effort in the development of radiation sensitizers has focused on the oxygen effect and the halopyrimidines, there are numerous potential factors causing radiation failure, and even an effective hypoxic cell or halopyrimidine sensitizer is not a panacea for local tumor persistence.[9,17-20]

THERAPEUTIC STRATEGIES FOR HYPOXIC CELLS

Hypoxic cell sensitizers fall within the broader category of chemical modifiers of cancer treatment.[8,9,21-23] Chemical modifiers are usually not cytotoxic by themselves but modify or enhance the tissue response to standard radiation therapy. The ultimate utility of a radiotherapy or chemotherapy modifier depends on its ability to alter the therapeutic index, which is the ratio of toxicity to efficacy. For a modifier to be beneficial, it must enhance curability more than toxicity; tumor cells must be more affected than normal tissues. Conceptual knowledge of the mechanism of radiation cell killing, the competition model, and the physiology of hypoxia are briefly reviewed to facilitate the understanding of the current therapeutic approaches.

MECHANISMS OF RADIATION CELL KILLING AND THE COMPETITION MODEL

Radiation causes cell death by damaging a critical target within the cell. Evidence for chromosomal DNA as the principle target is circumstantial but overwhelming; nuclear membrane damage may also be important.[24] Ionizing radiation interacts with molecules inside the cell to produce free radicals directly within the DNA (direct effect) or in molecules able to diffuse to and damage the DNA (indirect effect). Cell death probably occurs after a sufficient number of double-stranded DNA breaks are produced by ionization of the DNA or during the enzymatic repair process.[25]

Although the precise mechanism of radiation damage is not fully understood, the competition model is useful for visualizing the potential roles of hypoxic sensitizers and protectors. Figure 69–31 illustrates the competition model. DNA· represents ionized (damaged) DNA; its fate is determined by two competing processes, protection and sensitization.

In theory, an oxygen mimetic hypoxic cell sensitizer can replace oxygen leading to the stable lesion, DNA-sensitizer; the precise chemistry of this interaction is unknown.[26] The processes in which DNA radicals are stabilized by oxygen or an oxygen-mimetic sensitizer is called sensitization. Two of the primary clinical approaches to irradiation and chemotherapy modification are hypoxic-cell sensitization and thiol modulation. Before reviewing the currently available literature, it may be helpful to review the physiology and clinical importance of tumor hypoxia.

THE OXYGEN EFFECT

Awareness of the importance of oxygen in tissue response to irradiation can be traced back to 1921, when Holthusen found

THE COMPETITION MODEL

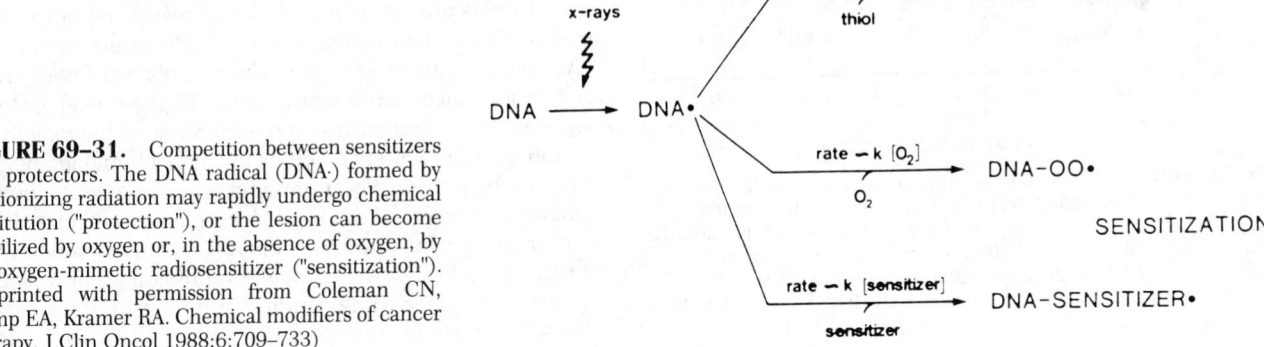

FIGURE 69–31. Competition between sensitizers and protectors. The DNA radical (DNA·) formed by the ionizing radiation may rapidly undergo chemical restitution ("protection"), or the lesion can become stabilized by oxygen or, in the absence of oxygen, by an oxygen-mimetic radiosensitizer ("sensitization"). (Reprinted with permission from Coleman CN, Bump EA, Kramer RA. Chemical modifiers of cancer therapy. J Clin Oncol 1988;6:709–733)

that larger doses of radiation were needed to inactivate sea urchin eggs rendered hypoxic by liquid nitrogen.[15] Since that time, it has been repetitively demonstrated in vitro that to achieve the same proportion of cell killing, about three times the radiation dose is required for hypoxic cells compared with that for well oxygenated cells.[27] The ratio of dose required for a given level of cell killing under hypoxic conditions compared with the dose needed in air is called the oxygen enhancement ratio (OER) (Fig. 69–32).[24] It is estimated that even a 2% or 3% proportion of hypoxic cells within a tumor may double the radiation dose needed for permanent local control.[14,27] For relatively large single doses of radiation, the OER is in the range of 3, and for clinically relevant smaller doses of radiation (200 cGy per fraction) the OER is approximately 2.[28,29] Oxygen has the ability to sensitize cells to ionizing radiation even at clinically relevant radiation doses.

Hypoxic cells are relatively radioresistant, but how important is hypoxia in clinical radiotherapy? Although the answer to this question remains unknown, this is an area of intense laboratory and clinical research and much information suggests that hypoxia may be important in certain situations.

TYPES OF HYPOXIA

The classic model of chronic hypoxia was developed by Thomlinson and Gray who found the pathologic appearance in lung cancer specimens of small necrotic volumes at set distances from capillaries.[30] They calculated that hypoxic but viable cells could be present at a radial distance of up to 130 to 150 μm from the nearest capillary, because oxygen is metabolized and consumed by the cells closest to the vessel. In this model, it is assumed that the nutrient vessel remains patent and that the hypoxic cells are confined to the area surrounding the necrosis (Fig. 69–33). These chronically hypoxic cells have diffusion limited hypoxia.

A second kind of hypoxia can be demonstrated in animal tumors. Due to the dysfunctional opening and closing of tumor vessels, transient or intermittent hypoxia occurs.[31,32] In the intermittent hypoxia model, cells irradiated when blood flow is present behave radiobiologically as oxygenated cells. When blood flow transiently stops, existing oxygen and other nutrients are rapidly exhausted, leaving cells that were perfused by that vessel in a temporarily ischemic state. If irradiation is given when these cells are not perfused, these cells will behave radiobiologically as hypoxic cells. These intermittently hypoxic cells can be conceived as having perfusion-limited hypoxia. Experiments in murine systems indicate that, in general, the percentage of hypoxic cells within a tumor remains relatively stable during a course of fractionated irradiation rather than increasing, as might be expected with the selective killing of aerobic cells.[16,33,34] A process called reoxygenation occurs between radiation fractions and may explain the success of fractionated radiotherapy in curing relatively large size tumors.[33] The mechanism of reoxygenation is unknown, and the degree to which it occurs during radiation therapy in the clinic awaits the further development of methods to identify and quantitate hypoxic cells.

Although the dominant form of tissue hypoxia in human tumors is unknown, the potential existence of two types of hypoxia has important implications for attempts to overcome hypoxic radioresistance. A radiosensitizer that diffuses well through tissue without being rapidly metabolized should reach the inner core of chronically hypoxic cells as well as the well-perfused intermittently hypoxic cells.

IDENTIFYING HYPOXIC CELLS

Clinical assays able to identify and quantitate hypoxic cells in a simple and reproducible manner would have great utility in the evaluation of tumor hypoxia. Ideally, these assays would identify areas of chronic and intermittent hypoxia. Although indirect evidence of tumor hypoxia exists, attention has recently been turned to direct measurement of hypoxia in tumors. Oxygen electrodes can be introduced directly into tumors with visual or under computed tomography (CT) guidance.[35–38] Although these techniques are complicated and most tumors are not accessible for implantation of the electrodes, Vaupel and colleagues were able to measure the in vivo oxygen partial pressure values of normal breast tissue and breast cancer, as demonstrated by Figure 69–34. Gatenby and colleagues demonstrated the presence of hypoxia in the lymph nodes of patients with head and neck malignancies.[38] Despite the presence of intratumoral heterogeneity, the preradiation oxygen content in the lymph nodes correlated well with treatment outcome. For tumors of 4 cm in diameter, the mean tumor PO_2 in the complete remission group was 20.6 mm Hg, compared with 8.8 mm Hg for the partial responders and 4.7 mm Hg for the nonresponders.

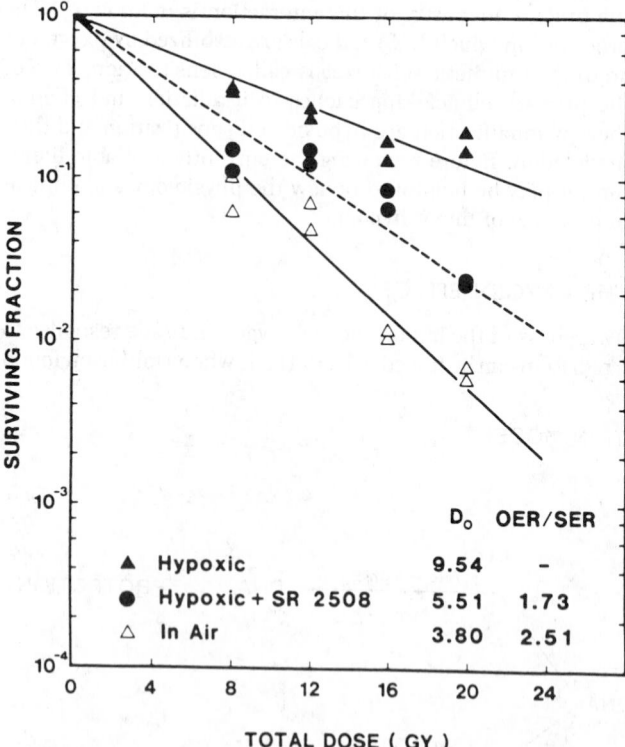

	D_0	OER/SER
▲ Hypoxic	9.54	–
● Hypoxic + SR 2508	5.51	1.73
△ In Air	3.80	2.51

FIGURE 69–32.   Radiation survival curves demonstrating the oxygen enhancement ratio (OER) and sensitizer enhancement ratio (SER) at clinically relevant doses. Oxygen or sensitizer increase the hypoxic cell killing by irradiation. (Reprinted with permission from Brown JM, Yu NY. Radiosensitization of hypoxic cells in vivo by SR 2508 at low radiation doses. Int J Radiat Oncol Biol Phys 1984;10:1207–1212)

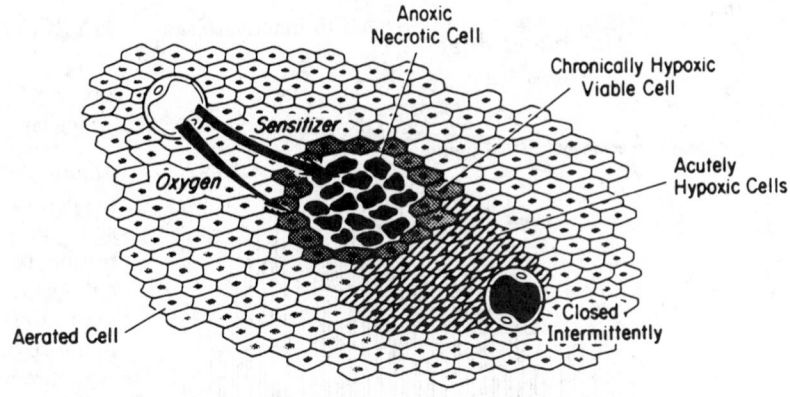

Anoxic
Necrotic Cell

Chronically Hypoxic
Viable Cell

Acutely
Hypoxic Cells

Sensitizer

Oxygen

Closed
Intermittently

Aerated Cell

FIGURE 69–33. Chronic and intermittent hypoxia. Chronically hypoxic cells (*left side*) are diffusion limited. Intermittently hypoxic cells (*right side*) are perfusion limited in that they are hypoxic only if blood flow stops in their nutrient vessel. Possible methods of overcoming acute and chronic hypoxia are suggested. (Reprinted with permission from Coleman CN. Chemical modification of radiation and chemotherapy. In: Cancer: Principles and practice of oncology. Philadelphia: JB Lippincott, 1989:2435–2449)

Approaches to Chronic Hypoxia

- Increase Oxygen Delivery
  Transfusion
  Hyperbaric Oxygen
  Perfluorochemical
  Altered Hgb Affinity for O_2
- Hypoxic Cell Sensitizers
  ± Thiol modification
- Bioreductive Agents
  Mitomycin-C
  Nitroimidazoles
- ? Hyperthermia

Approaches to Acute Hypoxia

- Altered Oxygen Delivery
  Likely to have minimal impact
- Hypoxic Cell Sensitizers
  ± Thiol modification
- Bioreductive Agents
  Would need rapid action
  under hypoxia
- ? Hyperthermia
- ? Chemotherapy

^{31}P magnetic resonance spectroscopy (MRS) can be used to examine intact tissue and has the advantage of being non-invasive and easily repeated. ^{31}P techniques measure intratumoral phosphorus metabolites and assess tumor metabolism. Metabolism is affected by several physiologic factors including blood flow and oxygen tension. Several investigators have attempted to correlate MRS readings with hypoxia but the heterogeneity of MRS spectral parameters, interfering signals from surrounding tissues, and the presence of hypoxic but metabolically active tumor cells have limited its usefulness.[36,39–42] A similar technique that may be useful is positron emission tomography (PET) scanning for measuring anaerobic glycolysis (indirectly representing hypoxia).[43]

Hypoxic cells preferentially reduce and bind misonidazole at a rate that is three times faster that oxygenated cells.[44] Radiolabeled misonidazole can then be used to indicate the presence of tumor hypoxia.[45–48] Tumor selective retention of fluorinated nitroimidazoles has been demonstrated in vivo by Maxwell and coworkers using magnetic resonance spectroscopy.[49] ^{3}H-misonidazole has been used to identify hypoxic cells in solid animal tumors, multicellular spheroids, and human tumors labeled in vivo.[50–57] Unfortunately, the large doses of ^{3}H required limit the use of this technique in the clinic.

A histologic technique allowing direct visualization of chronic and intermittently hypoxic cells in mice involves sequential intravenous injection of two fluorescent stains, Hoechst 33342, a DNA-binding dye, and DiOC7, a carbocyanine dye.[3,58] Each dye defines cells near blood vessels that were open for the few minutes after administration of the stains. The presence of cells containing one dye and not the other indicates that their perfusion was intermittent.[59]

Ideally, it should be possible to assess the hypoxic state of the cell using intrinsic markers of properties of the cells.

Chronic or severe hypoxia can induce metabolic and phenotypic changes in the tumor. Sutherland and colleagues have observed the increased production of a group of proteins, oxygen regulated proteins (ORPs), and reduction of intracellular glutathione content. The induction of ORPs is a general phenomenon that has been observed in a variety of human and rodent cell lines.[60] Although the kinetics vary for the different ORPs, in general synthesis peaks by about 12 hours into hypoxic incubation and declines to aerobic levels after 12 hours of reoxygenation.[61] Whether or not it will be possible to detect stress protein levels or other intrinsic markers in tumors remains to be determined.

A model being used to evaluate cellular phenotypic changes induced by ischemia and reperfusion described by Hlatky and coworkers has demonstrated metabolic (reductive enzyme induction) and phenotypic changes (differentiation) caused by the cellular environment.[62] Although the ideal technique to assess tissue hypoxia remains to be established, methods such as those described will be critical for the understanding of the cellular biology and may be ultimately useful for the tailoring of a treatment plan based on the pretreatment characteristics of the particular tumor.

APPROACHES TO HYPOXIA IN THE CLINIC

Clinicians have attempted to increase oxygen delivery to hypoxic tumors with the use of hyperbaric oxygen, erythrocyte transfusions, and perfluorocarbons.[63–70] The use of the hyperbaric oxygen chamber was the first widely explored approach. A total of nine prospective randomized trials were performed, but only three gave statistically significant positive results for the use of hyperbaric oxygen.[71] Because of the difficulty in hyperbaric oxygen administration, radiation therapy

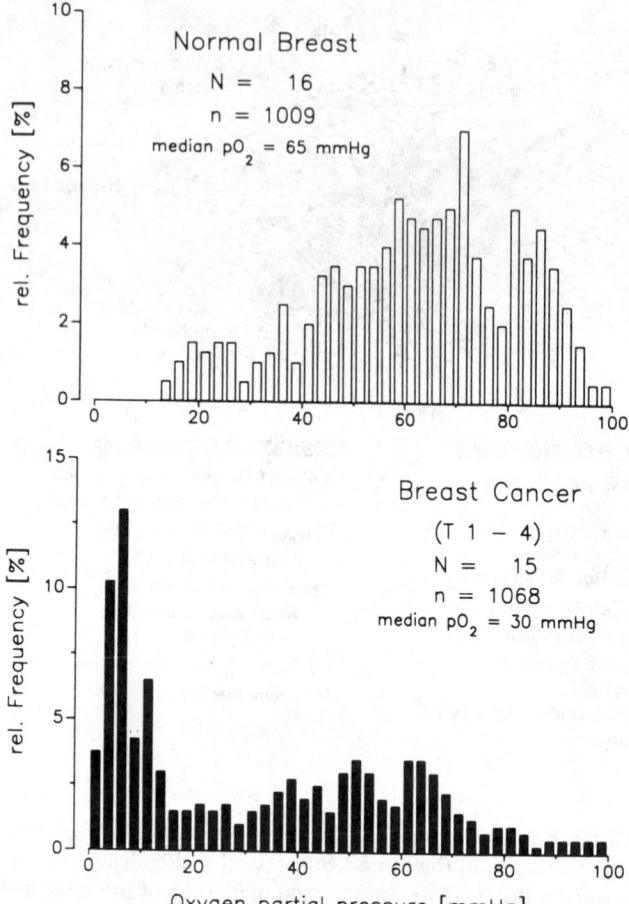

FIGURE 69–34. Frequency distributions of measured oxygen partial pressures (pO$_2$ histograms) for normal breast tissue (*top*) and for breast cancers (pooled data for pathologic stages T1–T4, *bottom*). (Reprinted with permission from Vaupel P, Schlenger K, Knoop C, Hockel M. Oxygenation of human tumors: Evaluation of tissue oxygen distribution in breast cancers by computerized O$_2$ tension measurements. Cancer Res 1991;51:3316–3332)

was often administered in few high-dose fractions that did not take full advantage of reoxygenation and that might have led to increased normal tissue injury.[69,71] Nevertheless, the results were of biologic interest.

A second approach toward increased oxygen delivery involved the use of erythrocyte transfusions. Retrospective studies looking at the effect of low initial hemoglobin on local tumor control or overall survival yielded indirect evidence that radiotherapy is less effective in the presence of anemia.[67–70] These findings should be interpreted with caution, because it can be difficult to correct for other important prognosticators such as stage and size of tumors in a retrospective setting.[72] However, a prospective, randomized trial using erythrocyte transfusion did improve the results of treatment of cervical cancer.[68] A phase I–II study of the perfluorochemical oxygen-carrying emulsion Fluosol-DA and 100% O$_2$ as adjunct to radiotherapy in the treatment of advanced malignancies of the head and neck was sufficiently promising to proceed to a phase III trial (now in progress).[72–74] Although these data are not conclusive, they are sufficiently encouraging to lead to efforts to develop other methods of overcoming hypoxia.

HYPOXIC CELL SENSITIZERS

METRONIDAZOLE, MISONIDAZOLE, AND DESMETHYMISONIDAZOLE

Adams and colleagues described the properties that would be needed for a hypoxic cell sensitizer.[75] The compound should selectively sensitize hypoxic cells at a clinically safe concentration, be chemically stable with slow metabolic breakdown, be capable of diffusing a considerable distance through a tumor mass, and be effective at clinically relevant radiation doses.[33] In the 1970s, researchers began to study drugs with a chemical structure associated with increased electron affinity. The nitroimidazole compounds have been the most interesting and most tested class of drugs meeting these criteria.

The effectiveness of a sensitizer is generally expressed as the sensitizer enhancement ratio (SER). The SER (like the OER) is the dose of radiation required to produce a defined level of killing without sensitizer divided by the dose of radiation required for the same level of cell killing with the sensitizer. Because oxygen is the best "oxygen-like" sensitizer, the SER should, at best, equal the OER, unless the sensitizer has inherent cytotoxic properties or provides sensitization by mechanisms beyond the oxygen effect.[76]

The first compound tested was the 5-nitroimidazole, metronidazole. Marketed as Flagyl and already approved for use in humans as an antitrichimonal agent, metronidazole had an SER of 1.3 to 1.6, depending on the dose of drug used.[27] In the classic randomized trial by Urtasun and colleagues, patients with glioblastoma multiforme were treated with 330 cGy three times a week for 3 weeks with metronidazole plus irradiation or irradiation alone.[77] The median survival of the sensitizer group, 7 months, was superior to the 3 month median survival of the controls ($p = 0.02$). However, almost all the patients died by 1 year, and the results of the sensitizer group were not superior to historical controls given standard radiation therapy. This study indicated that an oxygen-mimetic sensitizer could demonstrate clinical activity, but that it should be added to the most effective irradiation schema.

Misonidazole was the first in a series of 2-nitroimidazole compounds to be used in the clinic. Because the 2-nitroimidazole compounds are more electron affinic than metronidazole, they are more efficient as hypoxic cell sensitizers (*i.e.,* they produce a greater amount of sensitization for a given dose). Oral misonidazole was evaluated in clinical trials for a wide range of tumor sites. Unfortunately, the maximal tolerated single dose that could be administered was limited by nausea and vomiting and the total dose that could be administered was limited by neuropathy.[78,79] Because of the toxicities associated with misonidazole, it was necessary to use a modest drug dose with only a few radiation fractions, yielding a low SER and leaving most of the radiation fractions unsensitized. In retrospect, it would have been surprising if misonidazole produced a major therapeutic benefit in the clinic.[8]

When Dische reviewed the results of 33 clinical trials with misonidazole, only five showed some possible benefit to the use of this drug.[80] Four of these five positive trials were from twelve head and neck cancer studies. A large randomized trial in Denmark (1979–1985) suggested that misonidazole was of benefit for male patients with pharyngeal cancer, with an overall disease-free survival rate of 46% for the misonidazole group, compared with 26% for controls. The misonidazole group had a superior 3-year survival rate, 59% compared with 39% for controls (*p* value not stated).[81] This finding was not confirmed in a retrospective analysis of the RTOG trial, in which patients with stage III and IV head and neck malignancies experienced no benefit with the addition of misonidazole to standard radiotherapy in terms of local or regional control, disease-free survival, or overall survival.[82]

ETANIDAZOLE

Using pharmacokinetic principles, Brown, Lee, Workman, and coworkers developed a series of misonidazole analogs designed to be as potent as misonidazole but less toxic.[83–88] These drugs were designed to be less lipid soluble to decrease their ability to permeate nervous system tissue and to facilitate metabolic clearance. Because the critical element in oxygen mimetic sensitization is the concentration of drug only at the time of irradiation, rapid elimination is desirable because drug remaining after irradiation would produce toxicity without benefit. The two compounds judged to be of greatest interest were etanidazole (SR 2508) and pimonidazole (Ro-03- 8799).[83–89]

Etanidazole produces significantly less neurotoxicity than misonidazole and doses of up to 36 to 40 g/m^2 can be given over 4 to 6 weeks.[90,91] In the RTOG phase I trial, 30% of patients experienced a peripheral neuropathy when receiving a total of 34 to 36 g/m^2.[90,91] A retrospective evaluation of the phase I data indicated that the risk of neuropathy in any given patient could be predicted from their individual pharmacokinetic profile (Fig. 69–35).[91] A series of plasma levels obtained at several specific time points after administration of etanidazole are used to generate the area under the concentration versus time curves (AUC) that remains constant throughout a course of treatment.[91,92] For a single dose of 2 g/m^2, a typical single-dose AUC is approximately 2.2 mM.hour but can be more than 5 mM.hour. Multiplying the single dose AUC by the number of drug administrations yields the total AUC, a measure of drug exposure. The risk of neurotoxicity increases with increasing AUC with slightly more drug being tolerated as the overall treatment course lengthened.

As part of a phase II trial for patients with locally advanced adenocarcinoma of the prostate, this model was tested prospectively. The ability to predict, and subsequently prevent, peripheral neuropathy was investigated.[93] Single-dose and total-dose AUCs were calculated for all patients (Fig. 69–36). Group I patients received "standard" etanidazole, 2 g/m^2, three times per week for a total of 17 doses or 34 g/m^2 without schedule modification. Group II patients underwent a schedule modification for an individual AUC more than 2.2 mM.hour (predicted cumulative AUC 36 mM.hour). Group III patients were scheduled to receive 1.8 g/m^2 for 19 doses, but their individual dose size was adjusted to limit their cumulative AUC to approximately 40 mM.hour. The baseline incidence of neurotoxicity in the group I patients was decreased from 65% to 55% with simple dose or schedule modification (group II). However, using pharmacokinetically derived dose individualization, group III patients received 19 treatments as scheduled, but the incidence of neuropathy was decreased to 1 in 19 patients (see Fig. 69–36). By eliminating the high single-dose AUC, the patients in schedule III actually received a higher total dose of drug. Future trials will incorporate the

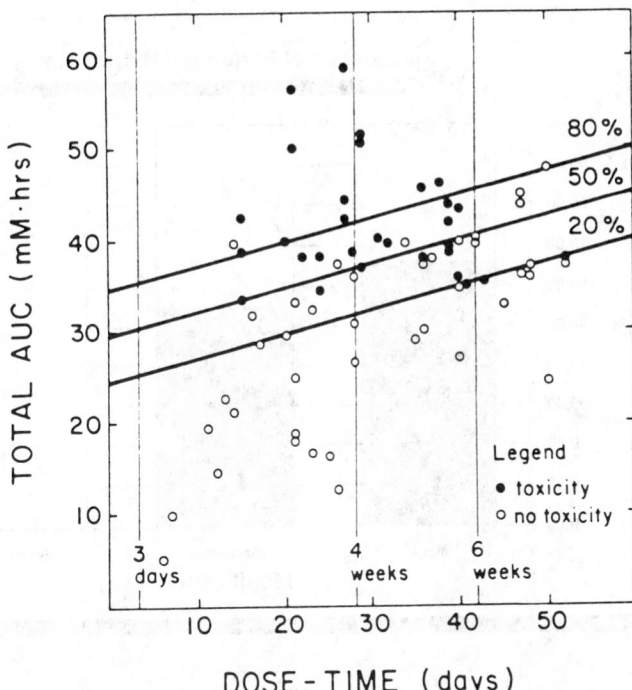

FIGURE 69–35.   Risk of developing peripheral neuropathy by drug exposure and duration of treatment course. The total area under the curve (AUC) (mM·h) is derived from the single-dose AUC times the number of doses given. Circles indicate patients without neuropathy (*open circle*) and those with neuropathy (*closed circle*). The three curves indicate the 20%, 50%, and 80% risk of developing peripheral neuropathy. (Reprinted with permission from Coleman CN, Halsey J, Cox RS, et al. Prediction of the neurotoxicity of the hypoxic cell radiosensitizer SR 2508 from the pharmacokinetic profile. Cancer Res 1987;47:319–322)

principle of pharmacokinetic monitoring and dose individualization in an attempt to minimize the incidence of peripheral neuropathy and optimize the total amount of sensitizer administered.

Efficacy data for etanidazole are not yet available. Randomized clinical trials for head and neck cancer are ongoing under the auspices of the RTOG and in a multicenter European trial.[94,95] Because etanidazole is excreted in the urine, high concentrations have been found in bladder tumors.[96,97] This has generated interest in the use of etanidazole in bladder and prostate cancer. For esophageal tumors, combined-modality treatment with cisplatin, 5-fluorouracil and irradiation plus etanidazole (on the nonchemotherapy weeks) is being evaluated. Because of the relatively high likelihood of distant disease for many of these patients with esophageal cancer, a major improvement in local control rate, possibly with the avoidance of surgery, would affect the quality of life more than survival. The data using combined-modality therapy for esophageal cancer is encouraging in this regard.[98]

Although etanidazole does not appear to penetrate the normal blood-brain barrier (BBB), the BBB integrity may be lost in the presence of a brain tumor.[99–101] As part of a phase I continuous infusion etanidazole plus brachytherapy protocol, the ability of etanidazole to penetrate into malignant gliomas was investigated.[102] In this study, all of the 22 brain tumor patients studied had various concentrations of etanidazole in their brain tumor tissue, confirming the results of Newman

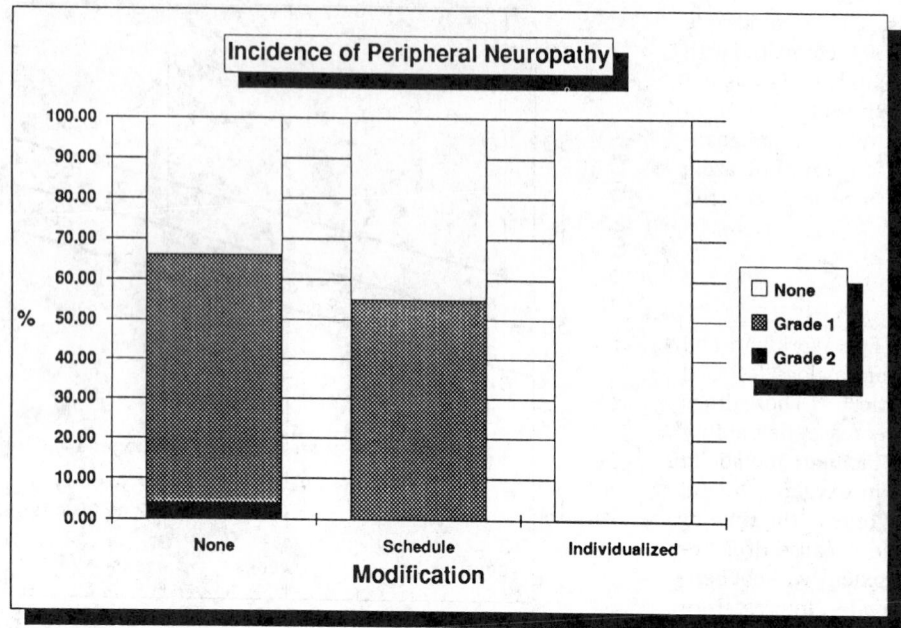

FIGURE 69–36. Risk of developing peripheral neuropathy by modification of etanidazole exposure during treatment using single and total AUC measurements. (Reprinted with permission from Coleman NC, Buswell L, Noll L, et al. The efficacy of pharmacokinetic monitoring and dose modification of etanidazole in the incidence of neurotoxicity: Results from a phase II trial in locally advanced prostate cancer. Radiother Oncol 1991)

and coworkers[103] Etanidazole is currently being evaluated as part of a phase I study of accelerated fraction external-beam irradiation with or without a sensitized implant for patients with newly diagnosed high-grade glioma.

Etanidazole has been evaluated as a continuous infusion accompanying brachytherapy based on laboratory data indicating that a continuous exposure of etanidazole may produce an SER that could exceed the OER.[27,76,104] The precise mechanism of this additional enhancement is unknown but involves metabolic reduction of the drug under hypoxic conditions. Seventy-seven patients were treated on a phase I protocol using continuous infusion etanidazole of 48 or 96 hours' duration while undergoing brachytherapy for locally advanced tumors.[105] A previously unreported toxicity called the cramping arthralgia syndrome limited dose escalation to 20 to 21 g/m² over 48 hours and 23 to 24 g/m² for patients receiving 96-hour infusions. The cramping arthralgia syndrome consists of relatively severe muscle and joint aches that disappear within hours or days after discontinuing the etanidazole.[93,106] The more classic peripheral neuropathy was only seen in 2 patients. Phase II trials are now ongoing.

Pimonidazole is a basic, lipophilic drug that is concentrated in the acidic environment within tumors.[107,108] It is a more efficient hypoxic cell sensitizer than etanidazole on a molar basis due to its higher electron affinity.[109] A phase I trail using pimonidazole plus etanidazole was conducted in an attempt to increase hypoxic cell sensitization by combining two drugs with different dose-limiting toxicities.[110] For the 48 patients who received both drugs, there was some evidence for toxicity interaction with 40% of the patients not receiving the planned cumulative dose secondary to toxicity.[111] Similar results were reported by Newman and colleagues in their phase I trial and phase I–II trial in brain tumor patients.[112,113] In a recently completed phase III trial of external-beam irradiation (5000 cGy in 5 weeks) with or without pimonidazole, followed by intracavitary treatment, cervical cancer patients who were randomized to receive pimonidazole actually had a lower in-

cidence of clinical complete regression, and statistically significantly lower local control, freedom from distant metastases, disease-free survival, and overall survival.[114] Known prognosticators seemed to be balanced between the two arms of the trial, and the reason for the poor outcome of the sensitizer patients is currently being investigated, although there is speculation that the pimonidazole may have decreased tumor perfusion. No additional clinical trials with pimonidazole are planned.

NIMORAZOLE

The Danish Head and Neck Cancer Group (DAHANCA) is evaluating a 5-nitroimidazole, nimorazole, in a randomized trial of 421 patients with squamous cell cancer of the larynx and pharynx.[115] Patients were randomized to nimorazole (1.2 g/m²) or placebo with each of the 30 fractions of radiotherapy. Results to date demonstrate a statistically significant improvement in locoregional control (52% versus 33% at 4 years, $p = 0.013$). The dose-limiting toxicity of nimorazole was nausea and vomiting. Although not as electron affinic as the 2-nitroimidazole compounds, an advantage of nimorazole may be the ability to administer it with each radiation treatment. The final results of this study will be of great interest.

DUAL-FUNCTION HYPOXIC CELL SENSITIZERS

This group of compounds is preferentially activated to their toxic species in the presence of hypoxia. This series of 2-nitroimidazole compounds under development additionally has a dual action: oxygen-mimetic sensitization (from the 2-nitroimidazole ring) and an alkylating function (from the aziridine side chain). The prototype for this group is RSU-1069, a 2-nitroimidazole containing a monofunctional, alkylating aziridine ring. RSU-1069 induced a dose-dependent loss of up to 50% of the clonogenic KHT cells in the absence of radiation and greater hypoxic cell sensitization activity than misonidazole in experimental systems.[116–120] Phase I testing revealed severe nausea, limiting its use in the clinic at the present time.[121] However, less toxic analogs, such as RB 6145, are under preclinical development.[122]

BENZOTRIAZINE DIOXIDE

SR 4233 (3-amino-1,2,4-benzotriazine-1,4-dioxide) is a newly developed bioreductive agent developed by Zeman, Brown, and coworkers.[123] It is particularly cytotoxic to hypoxic cells in vitro with 25 to 100 times more drug required to produce a given level of cell killing in aerobic conditions compared with anaerobic ones.[123–125] The mechanism of action remains to be fully defined, but the drug appears to induce DNA strand scission resulting from an oxidative damage to pyrimidines.[126] The free radical 1-electron reduction product, formed rapidly under hypoxic conditions, is thought to be the toxic species.[124,127,128] Analysis of DNA and chromosomal breaks after hypoxic exposure to SR 4233 suggest that DNA double-strand breaks are the primary lesion causing cell death.[129]

Due at least in part to its hypoxic cell cytotoxicity, SR 4233 has been shown to markedly enhance radiation-induced tumor killing in vitro.[124,128,130] This enhancement is seen when SR 4233 is given before or after irradiation.[131] The theoretical benefit to the use of an effective bioreductive agent is indicated in Figure 69–37, which shows the surviving fraction of cells after radiation doses with sensitizers of different properties.[132] Brown mathematically simulated cell survival curves under hypothetical and varied scenarios of irradiation and tumor properties, demonstrating the theoretical benefit to the use of a hypoxic cell toxin.[132,133] In Figure 69–37, it is assumed that a tumor has 20% hypoxic cells and that complete reox-

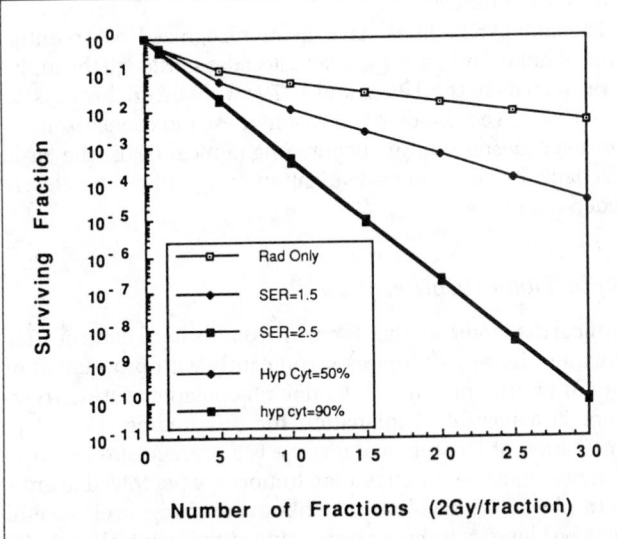

FIGURE 69–37. Surviving fraction of cells of a tumor with 20% hypoxic cells as a function of the number of 2-Gy fractions, assuming no reoxygenation between fractions and no tumor cell repopulation. The lines for SER = 1.5 or 2.5 and Hyp Cyt = 50% or 90% show the projected effect of adding to each radiation dose a hypoxic cell radiosensitizer or a hypoxic cell cytotoxin, each with two efficacies. The lines for SER = 2.5 and Hyp Cyt = 50% and 90% are superimposed. (Reprinted with permission from Brown JM. Therapeutic advantage of hypoxic cells in tumors: A theoretical study. JNCI 1991;83:1778–1784)

ygenation occurs between 200-cGy fractions. Each time a treatment is given, the tumor has 20% hypoxic cells. The curves for SER 1.5 and 2.5 indicate the impact of a hypoxic cell radiosensitizer (*e.g.,* etanidazole) of various potentcies. Similarly, Hyp Cyt indicates the impact of a hypoxic cytotoxic agent that is given with each treatment of irradiation and that kills 50% or 90% of the hypoxic cells. A hypoxic cell sensitizer is less effective than a hypoxic cell cytotoxin if a sufficient number of doses of the hypoxic cell cytotoxin can be administered. Such laboratory and theoretical modeling results are intriguing, and SR 4233 is now in phase I clinical trials.

TREATMENT WITH RADIATION SENSITIZERS

ALTERATION OF BLOOD FLOW

As a consequence of the introduction of bioreductive agents, attention has been turned to agents that modify blood flow within the tumor and actually induce hypoxia so that the hypoxic cells may then be targeted with bioreductive-cytotoxic radiation sensitizers or hyperthermia.[134] The microcirculation of tumors has been studied extensively and is characterized by low pressure, intermittent stasis, spontaneous hemorrhage, bidirectional flow, and regions of hypoxia.[36,135–137] Tumor vessels are generally thin walled and fragile, lacking the muscular and neuronal components necessary for normal dilation and constriction in response to vasoactive stimuli.[138] Because tumors already have compromised blood flow, a minor change in blood pressure may increase their proportion of hypoxic cells. There is a major interest in the use of systemically administered agents, such as hydralazine, nicotinamide, or flunarazine to alter tumor blood flow and secondarily modulate hypoxia.

Studies have centered on hydralazine, primarily because of its use as an antihypertensive agent. In transplanted rodent and dog tumors, intravenously administered hydralazine has resulted in rather dramatic reductions in tumor blood flow as measured by flow cytometry, MRS, and laser Doppler flowmetry.[139–142] The reduced blood flow and resulting hypoxia seem to potentiate the activity of bioreductive drugs used alone or with irradiation or irradiation with hyperthermia.[128,139,140,143] Unfortunately, the dramatic decrease in blood flow seen in animal tumors has been difficult to recreate in transplanted human tumors xenografted into mice.[144,145] Additionally, Horsman and coworkers demonstrated that a 10% decrease in blood pressure actually resulted in a blood flow increase of approximately 30%.[146]

Another factor that may limit the use of blood flow reduction in the clinic includes the possibility that high doses of agents such as hydralazine could produce focal areas of hypoxia in critical normal tissues and increase the normal tissue toxicity of the bioreductive agents.[139,140] A second potential problem is the heterogeneity of blood vessels within a single tumor mass. Studies have shown that tumor vessels in different parts of the same tumor may respond differently to hydralazine with induction of complete vascular stasis in some areas with relatively normal perfusion in others. The reason for this is unclear but more work will be needed before it is known if this overall approach of blood flow modification is effective or safe in the clinic.

GLUTATHIONE MODIFICATION

Glutathione (GSH), a ubiquitous tripeptide thiol, has important functions in a wide range of cellular functions including metabolism, transport, and protection. GSH is involved in the free radical scavenging of radiation-induced lesions such as hydroxyl radicals, peroxy radicals, and organic radicals, and is a substrate for enzymatic reduction and detoxification of electrophiles such as alkylating agents by means of glutathione-S-transferase. It is the protective functions that are of interest in cancer therapy (see Fig. 69–33).[8] The discovery by Griffith and Meister that GSH synthesis could be manipulated by BSO (D,L-buthionine-S,R-sulfoximine) has generated great interest in glutathione manipulation as a method of sensitizing cells to the effects of irradiation.[147,148]

L-BSO

Glutathione is a tripeptide, gammaglutamyl-cysteinyl-glycine. The enzyme γ-glutamylcysteine synthetase acts to combine glutamate with cysteine to produce gammaglutamylcysteine. Glutathione synthetase then acts on this product plus glycine to produce glutathione. L-BSO inhibits the enzyme gammaglutamylcysteine synthetase and prevents the de novo synthesis of GSH. The kinetics of GSH depletion depend on the pharmacokinetics of L-BSO and on the rate of depletion and resynthesis of GSH. Although data from human studies are not yet available, Kramer and colleagues demonstrated that after a single-dose of L-BSO to mice, the time course for depletion and recovery of GSH concentration varies from tissue to tissue with liver, stomach, and lung recovering faster than kidney and heart.[149]

To understand and optimally use L-BSO, it is critical to be able to monitor GSH concentration within tumor and normal tissue. O'Dwyer and coworkers are measuring GSH concentration in circulating monocytes to monitor GSH depletion, but it is not clear that this correlates with thiol content of tumor or critical normal tissues.[150] Ongoing work with MRS to measure the cellular thiol reduction-oxidative state is encouraging but the technique has not yet been applied to solid tumors.[151] BSO is currently under investigation in the phase I setting as a chemomodifier of alkylating agents, and no toxicity has been demonstrated with doses of 1000 to 4800 mg/m²/dose in the twenty patients entered.[150,152]

GSH Depletion and Radiation Therapy

The clinical utility of GSH depletion to decrease protection, as illustrated in Figure 69–33, depends greatly on the therapeutic ratio (*i.e.*, extent of depletion, loss of protection) in the target tissue compared with the effect of GSH depletion (*i.e.*, loss of protection and other functions) in normal tissues. Some researchers have found that GSH depletion alone sensitizes hypoxic cells to radiation without affecting the sensitivity of aerobic cells.[153–156] Under these circumstances, GSH depletion would produce a therapeutic advantage. Other investigators found various degrees of aerobic sensitization after GSH depletion, a discrepancy due to the much greater degree of GSH depletion in the latter experiments.[157–161] In any case, GSH depletion by itself is not likely to be a useful strategy to enhance the radiation effect.

Hodgkiss and colleagues demonstrated that GSH depletion can greatly enhance the efficacy of a single dose of misonidazole.[162] Similar results have been obtained with BSO and other hypoxic cell sensitizers such as etanidazole and pimonidazole.[162–167] The work by Kramer and coworkers revealed that BSO significantly enhanced the SER of etanidazole with fractionated radiotherapy in vitro from 1.2 to 1.4 in the relatively aerobic RIF tumor model and from 1.4 to 1.8 in the relatively hypoxic MCA tumor model.[149] Etanidazole toxicity, measured as the LD_{50} dose, was doubled in animals receiving BSO but only at doses of etanidazole that exceeded the optimal therapeutic dose.

The enhancement of hypoxic sensitization by L-BSO may be most important in cells that have a high endogenous concentration of GSH, a phenomena seen in several human tumor cell lines.[168–170] This hypothesis was tested by Degraff and coworkers who analyzed five nitroimidazole hypoxic cell sensitizers in A549 cells (high in GSH) and V79 cells (low in GSH).[184] They were able to demonstrate enhanced sensitization in the A549 cells after pretreatment with BSO, particularly with the sensitizer pimonidazole but also with etanidazole. Although the available data are limited, these results are interesting and it may be that L-BSO can be used to enhance the cytotoxicity and sensitizing effects of clinically available hypoxic cell sensitizers like etanidazole.

HALOPYRIMIDINE RADIOSENSITIZERS

Another strategy to improve the efficacy of radiation therapy is the use of the halogenated pyrimidine analogs (*e.g.*, IUDR, BUDR, FUDR, 5-FU). These drugs are taken up and metabolized only by cells actively synthesizing DNA.[194,195] Drug uptake by adjacent or dose-limiting normal tissues could limit the therapeutic gain for radiosensitization of tumor compared with normal tissues.

The halopyrimidines have been recognized as potential clinical radiosensitizers for over 3 decades. Although the initial clinical trials in the 1960s and 1970s were inconclusive, several trials have rekindled interest in these radiosensitizers.[196] However, despite these encouraging clinical trials, the basic mechanisms of radiosensitization are still not clearly understood.

Rapid Tumor Proliferation

Clinical data indicate that for some tumors local control after radiation therapy decreases significantly with protraction of overall treatment time.[171] Tumor repopulation during treatment is a possible explanation for this finding. Complete eradication of locoregional disease is a prerequisite for cure. Although most common human tumors are perceived to grow quite slowly with volume doubling occurring over several weeks or longer, it must be recognized that clinical or radiographic volume changes reflect a combination of tumor cell proliferation and tumor cell loss. Cell loss factors in human tumors have been estimated to be as high as 80% to 99%.[197] Tumor volume doublings over many weeks can disguise clonogenic doubling times that can be as rapid as 1 week or less. In a typical conventional fractionated radiotherapy course lasting 6 to 7 weeks, such potentially rapid tumor cell proliferation could significantly reduce tumor cell killing by up to 3 to 4 logs and result in a treatment failure.

With the use of in vivo BrdUrd/IdUrd labeling of S-phase DNA in human tumors followed by analysis with flow cytometry, there is limited but confirmatory data supporting the argument that a sizable proportion of human tumors are proliferating rapidly as measured by the potential doubling time (T_{pot}) as seen in Table 69–38.[171,184] T_{pot} is equal to the cell cycle time divided by the growth fraction (multiplied by log 2). T_{pot} measurements before treatment are thought to be of importance because they may be a reliable indicator of a human tumor's ability to proliferate during therapy.[198] The clinical relevance of pretreatment T_{pot} measurements in at least one common human tumor (head and neck) was highlighted recently.[172]

Metabolic Studies

IUDR, BUDR, and FUDR are a family of deoxyuridine analogs in which the halogen atom is substituted for the methyl group at the 5 position on the pyrimidine ring. FUDR is the deoxyribonucleoside derivative of 5-fluorouracil (5-FU). Structurally, IUDR and BUDR are analogs of thymidine (TDR) and are recognized by the same cellular enzymes that process thymidine to its triphosphate form (dTTF). Thymidine kinase (TK) is the rate-limiting enzyme in this salvage pathway. DNA polymerase then uses IdUTP or BUTP as a substrate for synthesis of DNA. The radiosensitizing effect of IUDR and BUDR are closely associated with DNA incorporation (*i.e.*, radiosensitization parallels the percentage of TDR replacement).[173,174]

The molecular mechanism of radiosensitization by IUDR and BUDR is thought to be induction of highly reactive free radicals (*e.g.*, uracilyl radical) within DNA.[196] Radiation damage as measured by clonogenic survival and induction of single- and double-strand DNA breaks may be increased twofold to threefold with prior incorporation of these analogs.[199,200] This effect on irradiation is most noticeable in the clinically relevant range of radiation dose as measured by changes in the shoulder, alpha component of the LQ formula, or survival at 200 cGy.[174–177]

Although the fluoropyrimidines (FUDR, 5-FU) share similar metabolic pathways as the TDR analogs, the mechanism of radiosensitization is less well understood and presumably does not involve DNA incorporation. Both FUDR and 5-FU inhibit

TABLE 69–38. Summary of Potential Doubling Times in Some Common Human Tumors After S-phase Radiosensitizers Have Been Used

Tumor Site (*no. of tumors*)	T_{pot} (*median*)	T_{pot} (*range*)
Colorectal (100)	5.9 d	2–23 d
Esophageal and gastric (22)	9.8 d	6.8–14 d
Head and neck (102)	5.5 d	1.8–30 d
Malignant glioma (10)	8.4 d	2–13.5 d

(Modified from Miller EM, Kinsella TJ. Radiosensitization by fluorodeoxyuridine: Effects of thymidylate synthase inhibition and cell synchronization. Cancer Res 1992 [in press])

thymidylate synthase (TS) after conversion to FdUMP using TK. This inhibition is believed to be the principle mechanism of cytotoxicity and possibly radiosensitization mediated through imbalances in the triphosphate pool and subsequent altered DNA damage repair.[178] Because 5-FU affects processing of nuclear RNA to ribosomal RNA, these RNA effects might be related to radiosensitization.

Although the interaction of fluoropyrimidines and irradiation has been recognized for over 30 years, there are surprisingly few in vitro data despite the renewed clinical interest.[179] In vitro radiosensitization by 5-FU appears to be schedule dependent, with maximal sensitization occurring only if cytotoxic doses of 5-FU are administered after irradiation.[180,181] In vivo, the combination of 5-FU and irradiation has proved to be slightly greater than additive in cell killing, but the schedule dependency was weak.[182,183] Another laboratory has been evaluating the in vitro interaction of FUDR and irradiation in human colon cancer cells to further relate TS inhibition and radiosensitization.[184] FUDR was selected instead of 5-FU because FUDR is a more specific inhibitor of TS and has no RNA effects. These results suggest that FUDR radiosensitization occurs with preincubation and does not require extended drug exposure. It appears more related to the effect of extended TS inhibition on cell kinetic changes than to the actual time course of inhibition. Several questions persist regarding the in vitro and in vivo mechanisms of fluoropyrimidine radiosensitization that need further study.

Clinical Results and Future Trial Design

Over the last decade, there has been a resurgence in clinical investigation of halogenated pyrimidines as radiosensitizers for several different tumor sites. As a result, there appears to be an improvement in locoregional tumor control and survival with acceptable normal tissue toxicities.[185–187,189–193] A better understanding of halogenated pyrimidine metabolism opens the possibility of using biochemical modulators of key enzymes (*e.g.*, leucovorin, 5-aminothymidine) to further improve clinical radiosensitization.

Most clinical trials with the TDR analogs (*e.g.*, BUDR, IUDR) have been phase I and II studies involving continuous prolonged (several days or longer) infusions in patients with poorly radioresponsive tumors such as high-grade gliomas and sarcomas, colorectal liver metastases.[185–187] Phase III trials are ongoing for these tumor types and others at the NCI and within RTOG. The optimal clinical approach for BUDR or IUDR has not been clearly defined. Theoretically, the clinical approach should result in adequate DNA replacement (probably only 3% to 10%) in all tumor cells.[188] Based on tumor cell kinetic and radiobiologic data, this most likely will require prolonged continuous relatively low-dose infusion.[188] The use of nontoxic modulators might improve the therapeutic gain, and clinical protocols are being designed to address this approach.

Clinical trial results with the fluoropyrimidine (principally 5-FU) are even more impressive. Several phase III studies have documented an improvement in local control and survival in cancers of the rectum, anus, esophagus, pancreas, and larynx.[189–193] In some trials, study design did not allow a direct comparison to irradiation alone.[192] 5-FU has been administered by bolus or continuous infusion alone or with other drugs (*e.g.*, mitomycin C, cisplatin) that cloud the issue of additive cytotoxicity compared with true sensitization of irradiation.[191,193]

Many ongoing trials have assumed that continuous infusion 5-FU (±leucovorin modulation) is superior as a radiosensitizer, although the preclinical data are confusing.[184,201] It is hoped that further experimental studies will help shape the next generation of clinical trials in fluoropyrimidine radiosensitization.

CONCLUSIONS

This chapter has only addressed two general approaches to radiosensitization. The lack of success to date has been due in part to the toxicities of these compounds at therapeutic doses (*e.g.*, misonidazole) and lack of knowledge of optimal drug timing and scheduling in conjunction with the radiotherapy. Nevertheless, these early efforts have yielded much important information, including identification and quantification of hypoxia in human tumors, newer aspects of assessing tumor cell kinetics, a better understanding of drug pharmacokinetics and toxicities, and interesting results in some of the clinical hypoxic radiosensitizer and halopyrimidine trials. Other radiation-modification approaches are being developed and include the use of altered irradiation schedules based on cell survival parameters or on tumor cell kinetics, and combinations of irradiation and systemic therapies such as chemotherapy, hormonal therapy, biologics, and radioprotectors. Entirely novel approaches, such as GSH depletion and hypoxic cytotoxic therapies, are undergoing evaluation in early clinical trials. Through incremental advances in cancer biology and drug development, there has been steady progress in the radiation modifier field. Combined with improved systemic therapies and surgical approaches, these have the possibility to improve local control, survival, and quality of life.

REFERENCES

1. Barker JL, Montague ED, Peters LJ. Clinical experience with irradiation of inflammatory carcinoma of the breast with and without elective chemotherapy. Cancer 1980;45:625–629.
2. Norin T, Onyango J. Radiotherapy in Burkitt's lymphoma: Conventional or superfractionated regimen. Int J Radiat Oncol Biol Phys 1977;2:399–406.
3. Fertil B, Malaise EP. Intrinsic radiosensitivity of human cell lines is correlated with radioresponsiveness of human tumors: Analysis of 101 published survival curves. Int J Radiat Oncol Biol Phys 1985;11:1699–1707.
4. Courtenay VD. Radioresistant mutants of L5178Y cells. Radiat Res 1969;38:186–203.
5. Peters LJ, Withers HR, Thames HD, Fletcher GH. Keynote address: The problem: Tumor radioresistance in clinical radiotherapy. Int J Radiat Oncol Biol Phys 1982;8:101–108.
6. Weichselbaum RR, Nove J, Little JB. Radiation Response of human tumor cells in vitro. In: Radiation biology in cancer research. New York: Raven Press, 1980:345–352.
7. Carmichael J, Hickson ID. Keynote address: Mechanisms of cellular resistance to cytotoxic drugs and x-irradiation. Int J Radiat Oncol Biol Phys 1991;20:197–202.
8. Coleman CN, Bump EA, Kramer RA. Chemical modifiers of cancer therapy. J Clin Oncol 1988;6:709–733.
9. Coleman CN. Hypoxia in tumors: A paradigm for the approach to biochemical and physiological heterogeneity. JNCI 1988;80:310–317.
10. Koch CJ, Meneses JJ, Harris JW. The effect of extreme hypoxia and glucose on the repair of potentially lethal and sublethal radiation damage by mammalian cells. Radiat Res 1977;70:542–551.
11. Varnes ME, Dethlefsen LA, Biaglow JA. The effect of Ph on potentially lethal damage recovery in A549 cells. Radiat Res 1986;108:80–90.
12. Dische S. Review of hypoxic cell sensitizers. Int J Radiat Oncol Biol Phys 1991;20:147–152.
13. Gray LH, Conger AO, Ebert M, et al. The concentration of oxygen dissolved in tissues at the time of irradiation as a factor in radiotherapy. Br J Radiol 1953;26:638–648.
14. Hall EJ. Welcome and overview. Int J Radiat Oncol Biol Phys 1982;8:323–325.
15. Holthusen H. Beitrage zur biologie der Strahlenwirkung; untersuch ungen an ascarideneiern. Arch Ges Physiol 1921;187:1–24.
16. Howes AE. An estimation of the changes in the proportions and absolute numbers of hypoxic-cells after irradiation of transplanted C3H mouse mammary tumors. Br J Radiol 1969;42:441–447.
17. Adams GE. Hypoxia-mediated drugs for radiation and chemotherapy. Cancer 1980;48:696–709.
18. Brown JM. Keynote address: Hypoxic cell radiosensitizers: Where next? Int J Radiat Oncol Biol Phys 1989;16:987–993.
19. Fowler JF. Chemical Modifiers of radiosensitivity-theory and reality: A review. Int J Radiat Oncol Biol Phys 1985;11:665–674.
20. Gonzalez DG. Hypoxia and local tumor control. Part I. Radiother Oncol 1991;20:5–7.
21. Coleman CN, Glover DJ, Turrisi AT. Radiation and chemotherapy sensitizers and protectors. Cancer chemotherapy: Principles and practice. Philadelphia: WB Saunders, 1989:225–252.
22. Coleman CN. Modification of radiotherapy by radiosensitizers and cancer chemotherapy agents. I. Radiosensitizers. Semin Oncol 1989;16:169–175.
23. Coleman CN. Hypoxic cell radiosensitizers: Expectations and progress in drug development. Int J Radiat Oncol Biol Phys 1985;11:323–329.
24. Hall EJ. Cell survival curves. In: Radiobiology for the radiologist. 3rd ed. Philadelphia: JB Lippincott, 1988:1–16.
25. Ward JF. Mechanisms of DNA repair and their potential modification for radiotherapy. Int J Radiat Oncol Biol Phys 1986;12:1027–1032.
26. Finklestein E, Glatstein E. Seduced by oxygen. Int J Radiat Oncol Biol Phys 1988;14:205.
27. Hall EJ, Astor MA, Biaglow J, et al. The enhanced sensitivity of mammalian cells to killing by x-rays after prolonged exposure to several nitroimidazoles. Int J Radiat Oncol Biol Phys 1982;8:447–451.
28. Brown JM, Yu NY. Radiosensitization of hypoxic cells in vivo by SR 2508 at low radiation doses. Int J Radiat Oncol Biol Phys 1984;10:1207–1212.
29. Skarsgard LD, Harrison I, Durand RE, et al. Radiosensitization of hypoxic cells at low doses. Int J Radiat Oncol Biol Phys 1986;12:1075–1078.
30. Thomlinson RH, Gray LH. The histological structure of some human lung cancers and the possible implications for radiotherapy. Br J Cancer 1955;9:539–549.
31. Chaplin DJ, Durand RE, Olive PL. Acute hypoxia in tumors: Implications for modifiers of radiation effects. Int J Radiat Oncol Biol Phys 1986;12:1279–1282.
32. Chaplin DJ, Olive PL, Durand RE. Intermittent blood flow in a murine tumor: Radiobiological effects. Cancer Res 1987;47:597–601.
33. Hall EJ. The oxygen effect and reoxygenation. In: Radiobiology for the radiologist. 3rd ed. Philadelphia: JB Lippincott, 1988:137–160.
34. van Putten LM. Tumor reoxygenation during fractionated radiotherapy: Studies with a transplantable osteosarcoma. JNCI 1968;40:441–451.
35. Carter DB, Silver IA. Quantitative measurements of oxygenation in normal tissues and in the tumors of patients before and after radiotherapy. Acta Radiol 1960;53:233–256.
36. Vaupel P, Frinak S, O'Hara M. Direct measurement of reoxygenation in malignant mammary tumors after a single large dose of irradiation. Adv Expt Med Biol 1984;180:773–782.
37. Vaupel P, Schlenger K, Knoop C, Hockel M. Oxygenation of human tumors: Evaluation of tissue oxygen distribution in breast cancers by computerized O_2 tension measurements. Cancer Res 1991;51:3316–3322.
38. Gatenby RA, Kessler HB, Rosenblum JS, et al. Oxygen distribution in squamous cell carcinoma metastases and its relationship to outcome of radiation therapy. Int J Radiat Oncol Biol Phys 1988;14:831–838.
39. Fu KK, Wendland MF, Iyer SB, et al. Correlations between in vivo 31P NMR spectroscopy measurements, tumor size, hypoxic fraction and cell survival after radiotherapy. Int J Radiat Oncol Biol Phys 1990;18:1341–1350.
40. Okunieff P, Kallinowski F, Vaupel R, Neuringer LJ. Effects of hydralazine-induced vasodilation on the energy metabolism of murine tumors studied by in vivo 31P-nuclear magnetic resonance spectroscopy. JNCI 1988;80:745–750.
41. Okunieff P, Ramsay J, Tokuhiro T, et al. Estimation of tumor oxygenation and metabolic rate using 31P MRS. correlation of longitudinal relaxation with tumor growth rate and DNA synthesis. Int J Radiat Oncol Biol Phys 1988;14:1185–1195.
42. Rofstad EK, DeMuth P, Fenton BM, et al. 31P NMR spectroscopy and HbO_2 cryospectrophotometry in prediction of tumor radioresistance caused by hypoxia. Int J Radiat Oncol Biol Phys 1989;16:919–924.
43. Frank JA, Alger JR, Bizzi A, et al. In vivo proton magnetic resonance spectroscopy (1HMRS) of human gliomas. Annual Meeting of the American Society for Clinical Oncology, Bethesda, 1990:349.
44. Chapman JD, Franko AJ, Sharplin JA. A marker for hypoxic cells in tumors with potential clinical applicability. Br J Cancer 1981;43:546–550.
45. Biaglow JE. Cellular electron transfer and radical mechanisms for drug metabolism. Radiat Res 1981;86:212–242.
46. Ling L, Streffer C, Sutherland R. Decreased hypoxic toxicity and binding of misonidazole by low glucose concentration. Int J Radiat Oncol Biol Phys 1986;12:1231–1234.
47. Biaglow JE, Varnes ME, Roizin-Towle L, et al. Biochemistry of reduction of nitroheterocycles. Biochem Pharm 1986;35:77–90.
48. Raleigh JA, Franko AJ, Treiber EO, et al. Covalent binding of a fluorinated 2-nitroimidazole to EMT-6 tumors in Balb/C mice: Detection by F-19 nuclear magnetic resonance at 2.35 T. Int J Radiat Oncol Biol Phys 1988;12:1243–1246.
49. Maxwell RJ, Workman R, Griffiths JR. Demonstration of tumor-selective retention of

fluorinated nitroimidazole probes by ^{19}F magnetic resonance spectroscopy in vivo. Int J Radiat Oncol Biol Phys 1989;16:925–930.

50. Chapman JD. The detection and measurement of hypoxic cells in solid tumors. Cancer 1984;54:2441–2449.

51. Horowitz M, Blasberg R, Molnar P, et al. (^{14}C) Misonidazole binding to EMT-6 and V-79 spheroids. Cancer Res 1983;43:3800–3807.

52. Rasey JS, Koh W, Grierson JR, Grunbaum Z, Krohn KA. Radiolabeled fluoromisonidazole as an imaging agent for tumor hypoxia. Int J Radiat Oncol Biol Phys 1989;17:985–991.

53. Franko AJ, Chapman JD, Koch CJ. Binding of misonidazole to EMT-6 and V-79 spheroids. Int J Radiat Oncol Biol Phys 1982;8:737–739.

54. Hlatky L, Hong C, Sachs R. Patterns of misonidazole binding as observed in the sandwich system. Int J Radiat Oncol Biol Phys 1989;16:943–948.

55. Hlatky L, Ring CS, Sachs RK. Detection of an intrinsic marker in hypoxic cells. Cancer Res 1989;49:5162–5166.

56. Sutherland RM, Sordat B, Bamat J, et al. Oxygenation and differentiation in multicellular speroids of human colon carcinoma. Cancer Res 1986;46:5320–5329.

57. Urtasun RC, Chapman JD, Raleigh JA, et al. Binding of ^{3}H-misonidazole to solid human tumors as a measure of tumor hypoxia. Int J Radiat Oncol Biol Phys 1986;12:1263–1267.

58. Olive PL, Chaplin DJ, Durand RE. Pharmacokinetics, binding and distribution of Hoechst 33342 in spheroids and murine tumours. Br J Cancer 1985;52:739–746.

59. Trotter MJ, Chaplin DJ, Durand RE, Olive PL. The use of fluorescent probes to identify regions of transient perfusion in murine tumors. Int J Radiat Oncol Biol Phys 1989;16:931–934.

60. Heacock CS, Sutherland RM. Induction characteristics of oxygen regulated proteins. Int J Radiat Oncol Biol Phys 1986;12:1287–1290.

61. Kwok TT, Sutherland RM. The relationship between radiation response of human squamous carcinoma cells and specific metabolic changes induced by chronic hypoxia. Int J Radiat Oncol Biol Phys 1989;16:1301–1305.

62. Hlatky L, Coleman CN. Modification of cell phenotype by ischemia/reperfusion. Seventh International Conference on Chemical Modifiers of Cancer Treatment. Clearwater, FL, 1991:27–28.

63. Brady LW, Plenk HP, Hanley JA, et al. Hyperbaric oxygen therapy for carcinoma of the cervix—stages IIb, IIIA, IIIB, and IVA. Results of a randomized study by the Radiation Therapy Oncology Group. Int J Radiat Oncol Biol Phys 1981;7:991–998.

64. Churchill-Davidson I, Sanger C. High pressure oxygen and radiotherapy. Lancet 1955;10:1091–1095.

65. Dische S. Hyperbaric oxygen. The Medical Research Council's trials and their clinical significance. Br J Radiol 1978;51:888–894.

66. Rubin P, Hanley J, Keys HM, et al. Carbogen breathing during radiation therapy. The Radiation Therapy Oncology Group study. Int J Radiat Oncol Biol Phys 1979;5:1963–1970.

67. Bush RS. The significance of anemia in clinical radiation therapy. Int J Radiat Oncol Biol Phys 1986;12:2047–2050.

68. Dische S, Saunders MI, Wharburton MF. Hemoglobin, radiation, morbidity, and survival. Int J Radiat Oncol Biol Phys 1986;12:1335–1337.

69. Henk JM. Does hyperbaric oxygen have a future in radiation therapy? Int J Radiat Oncol Biol Phys 1981;7:1125–1131.

70. Hong A, Rojas A, Dische S. Normobaric oxygen as a radiosensitizer of hypoxic tumor cells. Int J Radiat Oncol Biol Phys 1989;16:1097–1100.

71. Dische S. Hypoxia and local tumor control. Part 2. Radiother Oncol 1991;20:9–11.

72. Dische S. Radiotherapy and anaemia: The clinical experience. Radiother Oncol 1991;20:35–40.

73. Rose C, Lustig R, McIntosh N, et al. A clinical trial of Fluosol-DA 20% in advanced squamous cell carcinoma of the head and neck. Int J Radiat Oncol Biol Phys 1988;12:1325–1327.

74. Lustig R, McIntosh LN, Rose C, et al. Phase I/II study of Fluosol DA and 100% oxygen as an adjuvant to radiation in the treatment of advanced tumors of the head and neck. Int J Radiat Oncol Biol Phys 1989;16:1587–1593.

75. Adams GE, Dische SE, Fowler JF, Thomlinson RH. Hypoxic cell sensitizers in radiotherapy. Lancet 1976;1:186–188.

76. Taylor YC, Brown JM. Radiosensitization in multifraction schedules, II. Greater sensitization by 2-nitroimidazoles than by oxygen. Radiat Res 1987;112:134–145.

77. Urtasun RC, Bond P, Chapman JD, et al. Radiation and high-dose metronidazole in supratentorial glioblastomas. N Engl J Med 1976;294:1364–1367.

78. Dische S, Saunders MI, Flockhart IR, et al. Misonidazole—A drug for trial in radiotherapy and oncology. Int J Radiat Oncol Biol Phys 1979;5:851–860.

79. Wasserman TH, Phillips TL, Johnson RJ, et al. Initial United States clinical and pharmacologic evaluation of misonidazole (Ro-07-0582), an hypoxic cell radiosensitizer. Int J Radiat Oncol Biol Phys 1979;5:775–786.

80. Dische SE. Chemical sensitizers for hypoxic cells: A decade of experience in clinical radiotherapy. Radiother Oncol 1985;3:97–115.

81. Overgaard J, Hansen HS, Anderson AP. Misonidazole combined with split course radiotherapy in the treatment of invasive carcinoma of the larynx and pharynx. Int J Radiat Oncol Biol Phys 1989;16:1065–1068.

82. Fazekas J, Pajak TF, Wasserman T, et al. Failure of misonidazole-sensitized radiotherapy to impact upon outcome among stage III–IV squamous cancers of the head and neck. Int J Radiat Oncol Biol Phys 1987;13:1155–1160.

83. Brown JM, Lee WW. Pharmacokinetic considerations in radiosensitizer development. In: Radiation sensitizers, their use in the clinical management of cancer. New York: Masson Publishing, 1980:2–13.

84. Brown JM, Yu NY. The optimum time for irradiation relative to tumor concentration of hypoxic cell sensitizers. Fr J Radiol 1980;53:915.

85. Brown JM, Yu NY, Brown DM, et al. SR-2508: A 2-nitroimidazole amide which should be superior to misonidazole as a radiosensitizer for clinical use. Int J Radiat Oncol Biol Phys 1981;7:695–701.

86. Brown JM. Clinical perspectives for the use of new hypoxic cell sensitizers. Int J Radiat Oncol Biol Phys 1982;8:1491–1497.

87. Dische S, Bennett MH, Orchard R, et al. The uptake of the radiosensitizing compound Ro 03-8799 (pimonidazole) in human tumors. Int J Radiat Oncol Biol Phys 1989;16:1089–1092.

88. Hall EJ, Biaglow J. Ro-07-0582 as a radiosensitizer and cytotoxic agent. Int J Radiat Oncol Biol Phys 1977;7:521–530.

89. Maughan TS, Newman HFV, Bleehan NM, et al. Abnormal clinical pharmacokinetics of the developmental radiosensitizers pimonidazole (Ro 03-8799) and etanidazole (Sr 2508). Int J Radiat Oncol Biol Phys 1990;18:1151–1156.

90. Coleman CN, Wasserman TH, Urtasun RC, et al. Phase I trial of the hypoxic cell radiosensitizer SR-2508: The results of the five to six week drug schedule. Int J Radiat Oncol Biol Phys 1986;12:1105–1108.

91. Coleman CN, Halsey J, Cox RS, et al. Prediction of the neurotoxicity of the hypoxic cell radiosensitizer SR 2508 from the pharmacokinetic profile. Cancer Res 1987;47:319–322.

92. Workman P, Ward R, Maughan TS, et al. Estimation of plasma area under the curve for etanidazole (SR 2508) in toxicity prediction and dose adjustment. Int J Radiat Oncol Biol Phys 1989;17:177–181.

93. Coleman CN, Buswell L, Noll L. The efficacy of pharmacokinetic monitoring and dose modification of etanidazole on the incidence of neurotoxicity: Results from a phase II trial in locally advanced prostate cancer. Int J Radiat Oncol Biol Phys1992;22(3):565–568.

94. Wasserman TH, Lee DJ, Cosmatos D, et al. Clinical trials with etanidazole (SR-2508) by the Radiation Therapy Oncology Group (RTOG). Radiother Oncol 1991;20:129–135.

95. Chassagne D, Sancho-Garnier H, Charreau I, et al. Progress report of a phase II and III trial with etanidazole (SR-2508): A multicentre European study. Radiother Oncol 1991;20:121–127.

96. Awwad HK, El Merzabani MM, El Badawy S, et al. Misonidazole in the preoperative and radical radiotherapy of bladder cancer. In: Radiation sensitizers, their use in the clinical management of cancer. New York: Masson Publishing, 1980:381–386.

97. Awwad H, el Badawy S, Zagloul M, et al. Pharmacokinetics of etanidazole (SR-2508) in bladder and cervical cancer: Evidence of diffusion from urine. Proceedings of the Chemical Modifiers of Cancer Treatment, Paris, 1988:3–13.

98. Whittington R, Coia LR, Haller DG, et al. Adenocarcinoma of the esophagus and esophago-gastric junction: The effects of single and combined modalities on the survival and patterns of failure following treatment. Int J Radiat Oncol Biol Phys 1990;19:813–815.

99. Eifel PJ, Brown JM. Pharmacokinetics and toxicology of continuously infused nitroimidazoles. Int J Radiat Oncol Biol Phys 1983;10:1311–1314.

100. Pardridge WM. Recent advances in blood-brain barrier transport. Ann Rev Pharmacol Toxicol 1988;28:25–39.

101. Workman P. Controversy in drug delivery to tumors in the brain. In: Drug delivery in cancer treatment. European School of Oncology Monograph. Berlin: Springer Verlag, 1990:1–50.

102. Hurwitz SJ, Coleman CN, Riese N, et al. Distribution of etanidazole into human brain tumors: Implications for treating high grade gliomas. Int J Radiat Oncol Biol Phys 1992;22(3):573–576.

103. Newman HFV, Bleehan NM, Ward R, Workman P. Hypoxic cell radiosensitizers in the treatment of high grade gliomas: A new direction using combined Ro 03-8799 (pimonidazole) and SR 2508 (etanidazole). Int J Radiat Oncol Biol Phys 1988;15:677–684.

104. Fu K, Hurst A, Brown JM. The effects of misonidazole and continuous low dose irradiation. In: Radiation sensitizers, their use in the clinical management of cancer. New York: Masson Publishing, 1980:167–175.

105. Coleman CN, Noll L, Howes AE, et al. Initial results of a phase I trial of continuous infusion SR 2508 (etanidazole): A Radiation Therapy Oncology Group study. Int J Radiat Oncol Biol Phys 1989;16:1085–1088.

106. Coleman CN, Noll L, Riese N, et al. Final report of the phase I trial of continuous infusion etanidazole (SR 2508): A Radiation Therapy Oncology Group study. Int J Radiat Oncol Biol Phys 1992;22(3):577–580.

107. Cobb LM, Nolan J, Butler SA. Distribution of pimonidazole and RSU 1069 in tumour and normal tissues. Br J Cancer 1990;62:314–318.

108. Lespinasse F, Thomas C, Bonnay M, et al. Ro 03-8799: Preferential relative uptake in human tumor xenografts compared to a murine tumor: Comparison with SR-2508. Int J Radiat Oncol Biol Phys 1989;16:1105–1109.

109. Bleehan NM, Maughan TS, Workman P, et al. The combination of multiple doses of etanidazole and pimonidazole in 48 patients: A toxicity and pharmacokinetic study. Radiother Oncol 1991;20:137–142.

110. Honess DJ, Wasserman TH, Workman P, et al. Additivity of radiosensitization by the combination of SR 2508 (etanidazole) and Ro 03-8799 (pimonidazole) in a murine tumor system. Int J Radiat Oncol Biol Phys 1988;15:671–675.

111. Bleehan NM, Newman HFV, Maughan TS, Workman P. A multiple dose study of the combined radiosensitizers Ro 03-8799 (pimonidazole) and SR 2508 (etanidazole). Int J Radiat Oncol Biol Phys 1989;16:1093–1096.

112. Newman H, Bleehan NM, Workman P. A phase I study of the combination of two hypoxic cell radiosensitizers, Ro-03-8799 and SR 2508: Toxicity and pharmacokinetics. Int J Radiat Oncol Biol Phys 1986;12:1113–1116.

113. Newman HFV, Ward R, Workman P, Bleehan NM. The multi-dose clinical tolerance

and pharmacokinetics of the combined radiosensitizers, Ro 03-8799 (pimonidazole) and SR 2508 (etanidazole). Int J Radiat Oncol Biol Phys 1988;15:1073–1084.

114. Dische S, Chassagne D, Machin D. Randomized controlled trial of the use of pimonidazole (Ro 03-8799) in the treatment of advanced carcinoma of the cervix. Seventh International Conference on Chemical Modifiers of Cancer Treatment. Clearwater, FL, 1991;7:172–173.

115. Overgaard J, Hansen HS, Lindelov B, et al. Nimorazole as a hypoxic radiosensitizer in the treatment of supraglottic larynx and pharynx carcinoma. First report from the Danish Head and Neck Cancer Study (DAHANCA) protocol 5-85. Radiother Oncol 1991;20:143–149.

116. Adams GE, Ahmed I, PWS, Stratford IJ. Radiation sensitization and chemopotentiation with RSU 1069, a compound more effective than misonidazole in vitro and in vivo. Br J Cancer 1984;49:571–578.

117. Ahmed I, Jenkins TC, Walling JM. Analogues of RSU-069: Radiosensitization and toxicity in vitro and in vivo. Int J Radiat Oncol Biol Phys 1986;12:1079–1081.

118. Chaplin DJ, Durand RE, Stratford IJ. The radiosensitizing and toxic effects of RSU-1069 on hypoxic cells in a murine tumor. Int J Radiat Oncol Biol Phys 1986;12:1091–1095.

119. Deacon JM, Holliday SB, Ahmed I, et al. Experimental pharmacokinetics of RSU-1069 and its analogs: High tumor/plasma ratios. Int J Radiat Oncol Biol Phys 1986;12:1087–1090.

120. Stratford IJ, O'Neill P, Sheldon PW, et al. RSU 1069, a nitroimidazole containing a aziridine group. Biochem Pharm 1986;35:105–109.

121. Horwich A, Holliday SB, Deacon JM, Peckham MJ. A toxicity and pharmacokinetic study in man of the hypoxic cell radiosensitizer RSU1069. Br J Radiol 1986;59:1238–1240.

122. Sebolt-Leopold JS, Vincent PW, Beningo KA, et al. Pharmacologic/pharmacokinetic evaluation of emesis induced by RSU 1069 and its control by antiemetic agents. Seventh International Conference on Chemical Modifiers of Cancer Treatment. Clearwater, FL, 1991:152–153.

123. Zeman EM, Brown JM, Lemmon MJ, et al. SR-4233: A new bioreductive agent with high selective toxicity for hypoxic mammalian cells. Int J Radiat Oncol Biol Phys 1986;12:1239–1242.

124. Zeman EM, Hirst VK, Lemmon MJ, et al. Enhancement of radiation-induced tumor cell killing by the hypoxic cell toxin SR 4233. Radiother Oncol 1988;12:209–218.

125. Baker MA, Zeman EM, Hirst VK, Brown JM. Metabolism of SR 4233 by Chinese hamster ovary cells: Basis of selective hypoxic cytotoxicity. Cancer Res 1988;48:5947–5953.

126. Edwards DI, Virk NS. Repair of DNA damage induced by SR 4233. Seventh International Conference on Chemical Modifiers of Cancer Treatment. Clearwater, FL, 1991:229–230.

127. Laderoute KR, Eryavec E, McClelland RA, et al. The production of strand breaks in DNA in the presence of the hydroxylamine of SR-2508 (1-[N-(2- hydroxyl-ethyl)acetamido]-2-nitroimidazole at neutral pH. Int J Radiat Oncol Biol Phys 1986;12:1215–1218.

128. Brown JM, Lemmon MJ. Potentiation by the hypoxic cytotoxin SR 4233 of cell killing produced by fractionated irradiation of mouse tumors. Cancer Res 1990;50:7745–7749.

129. Biedermann KA, Wang J, Giaccia AI, et al. DNA and chromosomal damage and repair after hypoxic treatment of cells with SR 4233. Seventh International Conference on Chemical Modifiers of Cancer Treatment. Clearwater, FL, 1991:227–228.

130. Brown JM, Lemmon MJ. SR 4233: A tumor specific radiosensitizer active in fractionated radiation regimens. Radiother Oncol 1991;20:151–156.

131. Zeman EM, Brown JM. Pre- and post-irradiation radiosensitization by SR 4233. Int J Radiat Oncol Biol Phys 1989;16:967–971.

132. Brown JM. Therapeutic advantage of hypoxic cells in tumors: A theoretical study. JNCI 1991;83:178–184.

133. Brown J, Koong A, Lemmon MJ. A comparison of the relative efficacies of combining either a hypoxic cell radiosensitizer, increased tumor oxygenation or a hypoxic cytotoxin, with fractionated irradiation. Seventh International Conference on Chemical Modifiers of Cancer Treatment. Clearwater, FL, 1991:272–273.

134. Chaplin DJ, Horsman MR, Peters CE, et al. Tumour blood flow and its modulation: Implications for bioreductive drug activity in vivo. In: Selective activation of drugs by redox processes. New York: Plenum, (in press).

135. Warren BA. The vascular morphology of tumors. In: Tumor blood circulation. Boca Raton: CRC Press, 1978:1–47.

136. Eddy HA, Cassarett GW. Development of the vascular system in hampster malignant neurilemmoma. Microvasc Res 1973;6:63–82.

137. Dewhirst MW, Oliver R, Tso CY, et al. Heterogeneity in tumor microvasculature response to radiation. Int J Radiat Oncol Biol Phys 1990;18:559–568.

138. Denekamp J, Hill S. Angiogenic attack as a therapeutic strategy for cancer. Radiother Oncol 1991;20:103–112.

139. Chaplin DJ, Horsman MR. Changes in tumour blood flow induced by chemical modifiers of radiation response. Seventh International Conference on Chemical Modifiers of Cancer Treatment. Clearwater, FL, 1991:56–57.

140. Chaplin DJ, Peters CE, Horsman MR, Trotter M. Drug induced perturbations in tumor blood flow:therapeutic potential and possible limitations. Radiother Oncol 1991;20:93–101.

141. Horsman MR, Chaplin DJ, Brown JM. Radiosensitization by nicotinamide in vivo: A greater enhancement of tumor damage compared to that of normal tissue. Radiat Res 1987;109:479–489.

142. Okunieff P, Walsh CS, Vaupel P, et al. Effects of hydralazine on in vivo tumor energy metabolism, hematopoietic radiation sensitivity, and cardiovascular parameters. Int J Radiat Oncol Biol Phys 1989;16:1145–1148.

143. Horsman MR, Overgaard J, Chaplin DJ. The interaction between RSU 1069, hydralazine,

and hyperthermia in a C3H mammary carcinoma as assessed by tumor growth delay. Acta Oncol 1988;27:861–862.

144. Cole S, Robbins L. Manipulation of oxygenation in a human tumor xenograft with BW12C or hydralazine: Effect of misonidazole or RSU 1069. Radiother Oncol 1989;16:235–243.

145. Guichard M, Lespinasse F, Trotter M, Chaplin D. The effect of hydralazine on blood flow and misonidazole toxicity in human tumor xenografts. Radiother Oncol 1991;20:117–123.

146. Horsman MR, Christensen KL, Overgaard J. Relationship between the hydralazine-induced changes in murine tumor blood supply and mouse blood pressure. Seventh International Conference of Chemical Modification of Cancer Treatment. Clearwater, FL, 1991:54–55.

147. Griffith OW, Meister A. Potent and specific inhibition of glutathione synthesis by bu-thionine sulfoximine (S-n-butylhomocysteine sulfoximine). J Biol Chem 1979;254:7558–7560.

148. Griffith OW. Mechanism of action, metabolism, and toxicity of buthionine sulfoximine and its higher homologs, potent inhibitors of glutathione synthesis. J Biol Chem 1982;254:13704–13712.

149. Kramer RA, Soble M, Howes AE, Montoya VP. The effect of glutathione (GSH) depletion in vivo by buthionine sulfoximine (BSO) in the radiosensitization of SR 2508. Int J Radiat Oncol Biol Phys 1989;16:1325–1329.

150. O'Dweyer PJ, Hamilton TC, Young RC, et al. Depletion of glutathione in normal and malignant tumor cells in vivo by buthionine sulfoximine: Clinical and biochemical results. Seventh International Conference of Chemical Modifiers of Cancer Treatment. Clearwater, FL, 1991:313–315.

151. Livesey JC, Golden RN, Shankland Z, et al. Magnetic resonance spectroscopic measurement of cellular thiol reduction-oxidation state. Seventh International Conference on Chemical Modifiers of Cancer Treatment. Clearwater, FL, 1991:307–308.

152. Bailey H, Spriggs D, Tutsch K, et al. Phase I trial of intravenous L-buthionine sulfoximine and melphalan: An attempt at modulation of glutathione chemoprotection. Seventh International Conference of Chemical Modifiers of Cancer Treatment. Clearwater, FL, 1991:319–320.

153. Brown JM. The mechanisms of cytotoxicity and chemosensitization by misonidazole and other nitroimidazoles. Int J Radiat Oncol Biol Phys 1982;8:675–682.

154. Bump EA, Yu NY, Brown JM. Radiosensitization of hypoxic tumor cells by depletion of intracellular glutathione. Science 1982;127:544–545.

155. Clark EP, Epp ER, Biaglow JE, Morse-Gaudio E. Glutathione depletion, radiosensitization, and misonidazole potentiation in hypoxic Chinese hamster ovary cells by buthionine sulfoximine. Radiat Res 1984;98:370–380.

156. Louie KG, Behrens BC, Kinsella TJ, et al. Radiation survival parameters of antineoplastic drug-sensitive and -resistant human ovarian cancer cell lines and their modification by buthionine sulfoximine. Cancer Res 1985;45:2110–2115.

157. Mitchell JB, Cook JA, DeGraff W, et al. Keynote address: Glutathione modulation in cancer treatment: Will it work? Int J Radiat Oncol Biol Phys 1989;16:1289–1295.

158. Biaglow JE, Varnes ME, Tuttle SW, et al. The effect of L-buthionine sulfoximine on the aerobic radiation response of A549 human lung carcinoma cells. Int J Radiat Oncol Biol Phys 1986;12:1139–1142.

159. Rice GC, Bump EA, Shrieve DC, et al. Quantitative analysis of cellular glutathione by flow cytometry utilizing monochlorobimane: Some applications to radiation and drug resistance in vitro and in vivo. Cancer Res 1986;46:6105–6110.

160. Russo A, Mitchell JB, Finkelstein E, et al. The effects of cellular glutathione elevation on the oxygen enhancement ratio. Radiat Res 1985;103:232–239.

161. Van der Schans GP, Vos O, Roos-Verheij WSD, et al. The influence of oxygen on the induction of radiation damage in DNA in mammalian cell after sensitization by intracellular glutathione depletion. Int J Radiat Biol 1986;50:453–465.

162. Hodgkiss RJ, Middleton RW. Enhancement of misonidazole radiosensitization by an inhibitor of glutathione biosynthesis. Int J Radiat Biol 1983;43:179–183.

163. Lespinasse F, Biscay P, Malaise EP, Guichard M. SR-2508 plus buthionine sulfoximine or SR-2508 alone: Effects on the response and the glutathione content of a human tumor xenograft. Radiat Res 1987;110:149–154.

164. Ling CG, Wong RSL, Basas RD. Glutathione depletion and cytotoxicity of buthionine sulphoximine and SR2508 in rodent and human cells. Int J Radiat Oncol Biol Phys 1990;16:325–330.

165. McNally NJ, Soranson JA. Radiosensitization by misonidazole during recovery of cellular thiols following depletion by BSO or DEM. Int J Radiat Oncol Biol Phys 1989;16:1331–1334.

166. Phillips TL, Mitchell JB, DeGraff WG, et al. Modification in SR 2508 sensitization in hypoxic V79 cells by manipulation of glutathione (GSH) levels. Int J Radiat Oncol Biol Phys 1989;16:1335–1340.

167. Yu NY, Brown JM. Depletion of glutathione in vivo as a method of improving the therapeutic ratio of misonidazole and SR 2508. Int J Radiat Oncol Biol Phys 1984;10:1265–1269.

168. DeGraff WG, Russo A, Gamson J, Mitchell JB. Evaluation of nitroimidazole hypoxic cell radiosensitizers in a human tumor cell line high in intracellular glutathione. Int J Radiat Oncol Biol Phys 1989;16:1021–1024.

169. Phillips TL, Mitchell JB, DeGraff W, et al. Variation in sensitizing efficiency for SR 2508 in human cells dependent on glutathione content. Int J Radiat Oncol Biol Phys 1986;12:1627–1635.

170. Stratford IJ, Hickson ID, Robson CN, Stephens M. Radiosensitizing and cytotoxic effects of nitroimidazoles in CHO cells expressing elevated levels of glutathione-s-transferase. Int J Radiat Oncol Biol Phys 1989;16:1307–1310.

171. Fowler JF, Lindstrom MJ. Loss of local control with prolongation of radiotherapy. Int J Radiat Oncol Biol Phys 1992;22(2):457–467.

172. Begg AC, Hofland I, Moonen L, et al. The predictive value of cell kinetic measurements in a European trial of accelerated fractionation in advanced head and neck tumors: An interim report. Int J Radiat Oncol Biol Phys 1990;19:1449–1453.

173. Kinsella TJ, Mitchell JB, Russo A, et al. The use of halogenated thymidine analogs as clinical radiosensitizers: Rationale, current status, and future prospects: Monhypoxic sensitizers. Int J Radiat Oncol Biol Phys 1984;10:1399–1406.

174. Kinsella TJ, Dobson PP, Mitchell JB, et al. Enhancement of x-ray induced DNA damage by pretreatment with halogenated pyrimidine analogs. Int J Radiat Oncol Biol Phys 1987;13:733–739.

175. Iliakis G, Kurtzman S, Pantelias G, et al. Mechanism of radiosensitization by halogenated pyrimidines: Effect of BrdU in radiation induction of DNA and chromosome damage and its correlation with cell killing. Radiat Res 1989;119:286–304.

176. Fornace AJ, Dobson PP, Pantelias G, et al. Enhancement of radiation damage of cellular DNA following unifilar substitution with iododeoxyuridine. Int J Radiat Oncol Biol Phys 1990;18:873–878.

177. Lawrence TS, Davis MA, Maybaum J, et al. The effect of single versus double stranded substitution on halogenated pyrimidine-induced radiosensitization and DNA strand breakage in human tumor cells. Radiat Res 1990;123:192–198.

178. Berger SH, Berger FG. Thymidylate synthase as a determinant of 5-fluoro-2'-deoxyuridine response in human colonic tumor cell lines. Mol Pharmacol 1988;34:474–479.

179. Heidelberger C, Griesbach L, Montag BJ, et al. Studies on fluorinated pyrimidines II. Effects on transplanted tumors. Cancer Res 1958;18:305–317.

180. Byfield JE, Calabro-Jones P, Klisak I, et al. Pharmacologic requirements for obtaining sensitization of human tumor cells in vitro to combined 5-fluorouracil and x-rays. Int J Radiat Oncol Biol Phys 1982;8:1923–1933.

181. Ishikawa T, Tanaka Y, Ishituska H, et al. Comparative antitumor activity of 5-fluorouracil and 5-deoxy-5-fluorouridine in combination with radiation therapy in mice bearing colon 26 adenocarcinoma. Jap J Cancer Res 1989;80:583–591.

182. Nakajima M, Miyamoto M, Tamabe T, et al. Enhancement of mammalian cell killing by 5-fluorouracil in combination with x-rays. Cancer Res 1979;39:3763–3767.

183. Weinberg MJ, Rauth AM. 5-Fluorouracil infusion and fractionated doses of radiation: Studies with a murine squamous cell carcinoma. Int J Radiat Oncol Biol Phys 1987;13:1691–1699.

184. Miller EM, Kinsella TJ. Radiosensitization by fluorodeoxyuridine: Effects of thymidylate synthase inhibition and cell synchronization. Cancer Res 1992;52(7):1627–1684.

185. Tochner Z, Kinsella TJ, Rowland J, et al. Treatment of unresectable sarcomas of adults with hyperfractionated irradiation and iododeoxyuridine. Br J Radiol 1989;19:107–111.

186. Rodriguez R, Kinsella TJ. Halogenated pyrimidines as radiosensitizers for high grade glioma. Int J Radiat Oncol Biol Phys 1991;21:859–862.

187. Chang AE, Kinsella TJ, Rowland J, et al. A phase I study of intra-arterial iododeoxyuridine in patients with colorectal liver metastases. J Clin Oncol 1989;7:662–668.

188. Rodriquez R, Miller E, Fowler JF, et al. Continuous infusion of halogenated pyrimidines. Int J Radiat Oncol Biol Phys 1991;20:1380–1381.

189. Gastrointestinal Tumor Study Group. Prolongation of the disease-free interval in surgically treated rectal carcinoma. N Engl J Med 1985;312:1465–1472.

190. Gastrointestinal Tumor Study Group. Further evidence of effective adjuvant combined radiation and chemotherapy following curative resection of pancreatic cancer. Cancer 1987;59:2006–2010.

191. Krook JE, Moertel CG, Gunderson LL, et al. Effective surgical adjuvant therapy for high risk rectal carcinoma. N Engl J Med 1991;423:709–715.

192. The Department of Veterans Affairs Laryngeal Cancer Study Group. Induction chemotherapy plus radiation compared with surgery plus radiation in patients with advanced laryngeal cancer. N Engl J Med 1991;324:1685–1690.

193. Sischy B, Doggett RLS, Krall JM. Definitive irradiation and chemotherapy for radiosensitization in management of anal carcinoma: Interim report in Radiation Therapy Oncology Group No. 8314. JNCI 1989;81:850–856.

194. Goz B. The effects of incorporation of 5-halogenated deoxyuridines into the DNA of eukaryotic cells. Pharmacol Rev 1978;29:249–272.

195. Myers CE. The pharmacology of the fluoropyrimidines. Pharmacol Rev 1981;33:1–13.

196. Kinsella TJ, Mitchell JB, Russo A, et al. The use of halogenated thymidine analogs as clinical radiosensitizers: Rationale, current status, and future prospects: Nonhypoxic sensitizers. Int J Radiat Oncol Biol Phys 1984;10:1399–1406.

197. Steel G. Growth kinetics of tumors. Oxford: Clarendon Press, 1977.

198. Fornace AJ, Dobson PP, Pantelias G, et al. Enhancement of radiation damage of cellular DNA following unifilar substitution with iododeoxyuridine. Int J Radiat Oncol Biol Phys 1990;18:873–878.

199. Kinsella TJ, Dobson PP, Mitchell JB, et al. Enhancement of x-ray induced DNA damage by pretreatment with halogenated pyrimidine analogs. Int J Radiat Oncol Biol Phys 1987;13:733–739.

200. Fowler JF. Potential for increasing the differential response between tumors and normal tissues: Can proliferation rate be used? Int J Radiat Oncol Biol Phys 1986;12:641–645.

201. Lawrence TS. The effects of leucovorin and dipyridamole on fluoropyrimidine-induced radiosensitization. Int J Radiat Oncol Biol Phys 1991;20:377–381.

SECTION **10**

THOMAS W. GRIFFIN
MARY AUSTIN-SEYMOUR

Heavy Particle Beam Radiation Therapy

Advances in the field of radiation oncology have substantially improved the outlook for significant numbers of cancer patients, but failure to control locoregional disease is still a major problem. Heavy particle radiation therapy can address at least a part of this problem by offering a therapeutic gain over conventional photon and electron radiation therapy in several clinical situations.

Heavy particle beams in clinical use include fast neutrons, protons, helium ions, heavy ions (*e.g.* carbon, neon, argon), and negative pions.[1–3] Fast neutrons are used for their radiobiologic properties that potentially are superior to those of conventional photons and electrons. Protons and helium ions are used for their ability to achieve dose distributions that are potentially superior to those obtainable with conventional radiations. Heavy ions and pions have potential biologic and dose distribution advantages.

BIOLOGIC EFFECTS OF HEAVY PARTICLE BEAMS

The biologic effects of a radiation beam depend on the spatial distribution of the ionizing events produced in tissue. The rate at which charged particles deposit energy per unit distance is known as the linear energy transfer (LET), expressed in keV/μm. Protons, helium ions, electrons, and photons are sparsely ionizing, characterized by a low LET. Conversely, fast neutrons, heavy ions, and pions are densely ionizing and are referred to as high-LET radiations. Review of the possible causes of cancer treatment failure with conventional radiation therapy suggests that there are major areas in which neutrons and other high-LET radiations may offer a biologic advantage.

TUMOR CELL HYPOXIA

The oxygen enhancement ratio (OER) is defined as the ratio of the dose of radiation required to produce a specified biologic effect under anoxic conditions to the dose required to produce the same effect under well-oxygenated conditions. With photons, the oxygen enhancement ratio for most mammalian cells is 2.5 to 3.0. With neutrons, heavy charged particles, or pions, the oxygen enhancement ratio is significantly smaller (1.4 to 1.7), and the protection conferred on tumor cells by hypoxia is diminished. In practice, the clinical advantage of high-LET radiations may be less than suggested by the differences in oxygen enhancement ratios. Not all tumor cells are severely hypoxic, and reoxygenation may occur during intervals between dose fractions, diminishing the influence of hypoxic cells on tumor recurrence.[4]

RELATIVE BIOLOGIC EFFECTIVENESS

The relative biologic effectiveness (RBE) of an ionizing radiation is the ratio of the dose of that radiation compared with the dose of a reference radiation required to produce a specific endpoint in a specific tissue. A potential area of therapeutic gain from high-LET radiations exists if tumor cells are relatively radioresistant because of their increased capacity to accumulate sublethal radiation injury. This situation is reflected in a wide shoulder for the tumor-cell-survival curve. With neutrons and other high-LET radiations, most cell killing results from single lethal events, producing cell-survival curves that are almost exponential in the range of clinical relevance. Tumors characterized by a large capacity to accumulate and repair sublethal radiation injury should have a higher value of relative biologic effectiveness for high-LET radiations than for normal tissues.[5] However, Howlett and others have shown that RBE values of neutrons for different experimental tumors vary considerably, and no general statement about which types of tumors are best treated with high-LET radiations can be made.[6]

TUMOR CELL KINETICS

The cell-cycle-dependent variation of radiosensitivity is similar for neutrons and γ-rays, but the magnitude of the difference is smaller for neutrons and other high-LET particle beams.[7] Whether this properly constitutes a therapeutic advantage for high-LET radiations cannot always be predicted. Tumors in which cells are slowly cycling, tumors in which cells redistribute poorly between phases of their cell cycles, and tumors in which the cell cycle spectrum is dominated by cells in resistant phases are more effectively treated with high-LET radiations.

REPAIR OF POTENTIALLY LETHAL DAMAGE

Repair of potentially lethal damage occurs after low-LET irradiation, but it is observed less frequently after high-LET irradiation.[8] If, as has been suggested by Hall and Kraljevic, potentially lethal damage repair after low-LET irradiation occurs in nutritionally deprived tumor cells but not in normal tissue cells, the use of high-LET radiation beams would be therapeutically advantageous in tumors with these types of cell populations.[9]

PHYSICAL EFFECTS OF PARTICLE BEAMS

Fast neutron beams can be generated for radiation therapy by bombarding a target containing tritium (T) with accelerated deuterium (d) ions in a dT generator or by bombarding a suitable target, such as beryllium (Be) with protons (p) or deuterons (d) accelerated in a cyclotron or linear accelerator. The dT generator produces a monoenergetic 14-MeV neutron beam, and the proton-on-beryllium (p-Be) reactions produce neutron beams with a spectrum of energies. High-energy particle accelerators are required to produce medically useful beams of heavy charged particles.

Neutrons have no dose distribution advantages over photons, but protons, helium ions, heavy ions, and negative pions have significant dose distribution advantages over conventional photons and electrons. These charged particles preferentially deposit energy and more effectively destroy tumor cells near the end of their path. By appropriate determination of range (or path length) in tissue and by spreading the peak area, the

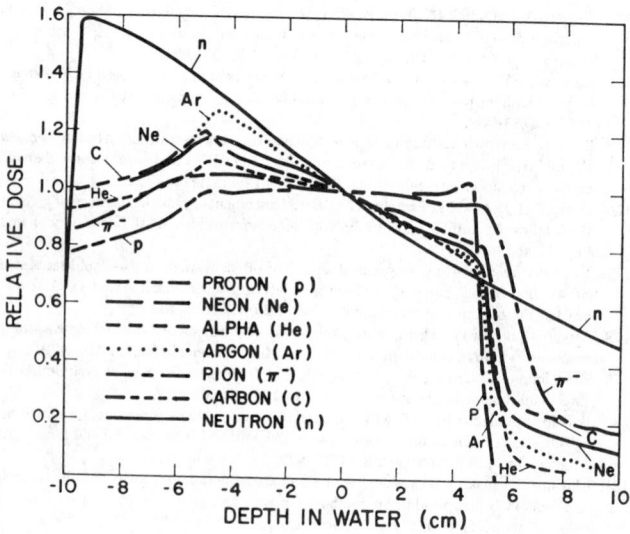

FIGURE 69–38. Comparison of depth dose (spread peak curves) for various charged particles of clinical interest.

high-effect region (*i.e.* the spread Bragg peak) can be made to correspond to the target volume.

The complex effects of heavy particles in tissues are a function of the energy, weight, velocity, and tract structure of the accelerated particle and the technique of beam delivery. Figure 69–38 compares the physical parameters of the clinically useful heavy particles. Table 69–39 illustrates the biologic and physical characteristics of these particles.

FAST NEUTRON CLINICAL STUDIES

Fast neutron radiation therapy was first used as a cancer treatment tool by Robert Stone at the Lawrence Berkeley Laboratory in 1938.[10] Using the Berkeley cyclotron, Dr. Stone treated a series of patients with advanced malignancies in various locations to high doses. Almost all of the long-term survivors from that clinical trial had severe radiation sequelae in their normal tissues. This result was initially thought to be due to an increased RBE of neutrons for late effects, and it deterred further clinical investigation of fast neutrons for approximately 20 years. Later experiments, however, showed that the daily treatment doses used in Stone's clinical work corresponded to a much higher equivalent photon dose than Stone had assumed.[11] An exhaustive review of Stone's work revealed that the early and late normal tissue effects observed in his patients could be accounted for by the equivalent photon doses received.[12] The influence of his fractionation scheme on tissue response, and the change of RBE with fraction size, caused his patients to be inadvertently treated to extremely high radiation doses.

Dr. Catterall reintroduced fast neutrons as a cancer treatment in the late 1960s on the basis of the new knowledge gained from the early neutron therapy experience. After several hundred patients were treated on the Hammersmith Hospital cyclotron, she concluded that fast neutron radiation therapy, using appropriate fractionation, was well tolerated

TABLE 69–39. Comparison of Relative Physical and Biologic Parameters of Particles in Clinical Use

High LET Advantage	Protons	Helium	Pions	Neutrons	Heavy Ions			
					C	Ne	Si	Ar
Physical depth dose	+++	+++	+++	No	+++	+++	++	+
RBE	No	+	+	++	++	++	+++	+++
OER	No	+	+	+++	+	++	+++	+++

+, slight advantage; ++, moderate advantage; +++, very significant advantage.

and that many advanced tumors responded amazingly well.[13] Based on her encouraging results, 38 cancer treatment centers in North America, Europe, Asia, and Africa began clinical treatments with fast neutron beams of various energies. Initially, clinical trials were confined to converted physics-laboratory-based particle accelerators that were poorly suited for patient treatment. In the mid-1980s, hospital-based neutron generators became available with treatment delivery systems comparable to those of modern, conventional linear accelerators. Approximately 15,000 patients have been treated with neutrons, resulting in a fairly extensive worldwide database.

SALIVARY GLAND CANCERS

The case for high-LET radiation therapy is strong for salivary gland tumors. Tumors with low growth fractions and long doubling times are predicted to be more sensitive to high-LET than to low-LET radiations. Reduced variation in radiosensitivity throughout the cell cycle predicts that slowly growing tumors with slowly cycling cells, such as salivary gland cancers, would be advantageously treated with high-LET radiations. Batterman and colleagues published pioneering work clinically defining the RBE of fast neutrons for various human malignancies.[14] One of the highest RBEs of neutrons was found in adenoid cystic carcinomas (8.0 with fractionated neutron therapy), which indicates an inherent radiosensitivity of this tumor to high-LET radiation. The RBE for adenoid cystic carcinomas is substantially higher than that for normal mesenchymal tissues. Treating an adenoid cystic carcinoma with 2000 neutron cGy would be approximately equivalent to 16,000 photon cGy in its tumor effect, but equivalent to only 6000 to 6600 photon cGy in its effect on normal tissues. This differential effect gives rise to a therapeutic gain factor of approximately 2.5 and is thought to be the underlying reason for the success of high-LET radiations in salivary gland malignancies. Clinical trials have confirmed these predictions.

In excess of 300 patients have been treated for locally advanced, unresectable salivary gland tumors with fast neutrons.[15] Patients have been treated with neutrons alone and mixed beam irradiation over short (4 weeks) and long (8 weeks) overall treatment times. The results are remarkably consistent and demonstrate long-term locoregional tumor control rates of approximately 67% compared with average long-term locoregional tumor control rates of approximately 26% for low-LET radiations (Tables 69–40 and 69–41).[15-37] The normal tissue complication rates have been marginally

higher with low-energy, fixed-beam neutron generators, but they have been equivalent to megavoltage photons when high-energy or isocentric hospital-based neutron generators were employed.[24,30,31] Subsequently, the National Cancer Institute (NCI) and the Medical Research Council (MRC) of Great Britain jointly sponsored a prospective, randomized phase III clinical trial directly comparing fast neutron to megavoltage photon and electron radiation therapy for patients with locally advanced, unresectable salivary gland tumors using laboratory-based and hospital-based neutron generators.[24] This study demonstrated a long-term locoregional tumor control rate of 67% for neutrons compared with 17% for photons ($p < 0.005$) in this group of patients with advanced tumors (up to 16 cm. in maximum dimension) (Table 69–42). The normal tissue toxicities were not statistically significantly different between the two groups.

An analysis of patients treated on the national neutron registry in a phase IV fashion at the University of Washington was recently accomplished.[37] Grouping patients according to

TABLE 69–40. Local Control Rates for Malignant Salivary Gland Tumors Treated With Low LET Radiotherapy

Investigations*	Local Control (patients)	Local Control Rate (%)
Borthne[16]	8/35	23
Fitzpatrick[17]	6/50	12
Fu[18]	6/19	32
Shidnia[19]	6/16	38
Elkon[20]	2/19	11
Rossman[21]	6/11	54
Rafla[22]	9/25	36
Dobrowsky[23]	7/17	41
Griffin[24]	2/12	17
Vikram[25]	5/49	10
Stewart[26]	9/19	47
Guillamondegui[27]	9/15	60
Ravasz[28]	3/12	25
Total	79/299	26

* Patients were treated with photon or electron-beam irradiation with or without radioactive implants. Patients treated de novo and for gross disease after a postsurgical recurrence are included but not patients who were treated postoperatively for microscopic residual disease.

TABLE 69–41. Local Control Rates for Malignant Salivary Gland Tumors Treated With Neutron Radiotherapy

Investigations*	Local Control (patients)	Local Control Rate (%)
Saroja[29]	71/113	63
Catterall[30]	50/65	77
Duncan[31]	12/22	55
Ornitz[32]	3/8	38
Batterman[33]	21/32	66
Maor[34]	6/9	67
Eichhorn[35]	3/5	60
Skolyszewski[36]	2/3	67
Buchholz[37]	40/52	77
Total	208/309	67

* Patients treated de novo and for gross disease after a postsurgical recurrence are included but not patients who were treated postoperatively for microscopic residual disease.

treatment status, actuarial 5-year locoregional tumor control rates were 92% for patients treated definitively with fast neutrons (without a prior surgical procedure), 63% for patients treated postoperatively for gross (measurable by computed tomography) residual disease, and 51% for patients treated for recurrent disease after a surgical procedure. (Fig. 69–39) The p values associated with these differences were 0.12 and 0.01, respectively (two-sided log rank test). There were no cases of radiation-induced facial nerve damage. Figure 69–40 illustrates patient survival as a function of presentation. The difference between patients treated primarily and those treated for recurrent disease is significant at the $p = 0.03$ level. These results have been confirmed by other series.[30]

PROSTATE CANCER

Fast neutron radiation therapy has been predicted to be advantageous in this tumor system for many of the same reasons as it was for salivary gland tumors. Based on these same biologic considerations, an RTOG-sponsored phase III study was designed and conducted between 1977 and 1983 randomizing patients between photons and a mixture of neutrons and photons using physics-laboratory-based machines. The 10-year results are now available from this study. These results confirm the radiobiology-based predictions, and they demonstrate statistically significant advantages for neutrons in terms of

locoregional tumor control, survival, and disease-specific survival.[38] Ten-year locoregional control rates on this study were 70% for mixed beams compared with 58% for photons ($p = 0.03$); 10-year survival rates were 46% for mixed beams compared with 29% for photons ($p = 0.04$); and 10-year disease-specific survival rates were 58% for mixed beams compared with 43% for photons ($p = 0.05$). No significant differences were found in complication rates. Although statistically significant advantages were seen with neutron therapy for all relevant endpoints at 10 years, this study has been criticized on the basis of photon locoregional tumor control and survival rates that appear to be inferior to other photon retrospective series published in the medical literature. Although these differences are probably due to patient selection factors, a confirmatory study was designed using state-of-the-art, hospital-based cyclotrons.

One hundred seventy-eight patients were randomized on this follow-up study comparing 2040 neutron cGy delivered in 12 fractions over 4 weeks against 7000 photon cGy delivered in 35 fractions over 7 weeks. The depth-dose properties and isocentric delivery capabilities of the hospital-based, high-energy neutron beams allowed treatment with neutrons alone to this deep-seated tumor, whereas the prior study using lower energy physics-laboratory-based equipment was limited to mixtures of photons and neutrons in the experimental treatment arm. After stratification for stage, Gleason grade, and the presence or absence of surgical nodal staging, 89 patients were randomized to each treatment arm. Patients with high grade, stage B2, stage C, or stage D1 tumors were eligible for the study. The two treatment arms were balanced for all known prognostic factors.

A preliminary analysis of this study is presented in Figures 69–41 and 69–42. The median follow-up time at the time of this analysis is only two years. Currently, locoregional tumor control rates favor neutrons with a 94% control rate for neutron-treated patients compared with an 86% control rate for photon-treated patients ($p = 0.04$). It is too early (with this slow growing tumor system) to expect any significant differences to show up in survival rates, and no significant differences have been seen. Survival rates are 85% for neutron-treated patients compared with 80% for photon-treated patients ($p = $ not significant). Only two deaths can be attributed to prostate cancer (both on the photon treatment arm); the rest have been due to intercurrent disease or homicide. The preliminary results from this second generation randomized study confirm the results of the prior study showing an increased effectiveness for fast neutron beam irradiation over standard photon radiation therapy in the radiation field.

TABLE 69–42. Salivary Gland RTOG-MRC Randomized Study Results

Endpoint	Treatment	Total Evaluable	One-Year Survival	Two-Year Survival
Locoregional tumor control	Photons	12	17% (±11)	17% (±11)
	Neutrons	13	67% (±14)	67% (±14)
Survival	Photons	12	67% (±12)	25% (±14)
	Neutrons	13	77% (±12)	62% (±14)

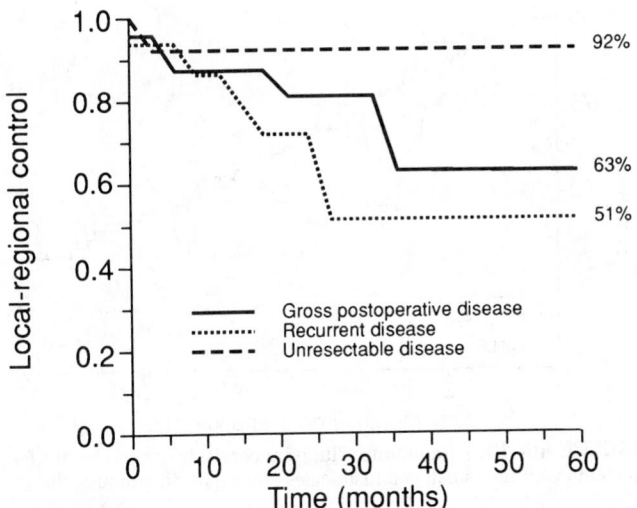

FIGURE 69–39.   Actuarial locoregional control of salivary gland tumors for patients stratified according to their disease status at presentation. Curves are shown as a function of time from the start of neutron irradiation. The patients with unresectable disease are shown by the dashed curve, the patients with gross postoperative disease are shown by the solid curve, and patients with recurrent disease are shown by the dotted curve.

NON-SMALL CELL LUNG CANCER

Fast neutron radiation therapy was first systematically investigated for lung cancer by Einhorn and colleagues using a Russian cyclotron generating a neutron beam of 6.2 MeV mean energy.[39] Although no improvements were seen in survival rates, combinations of neutrons and photons demonstrated at autopsy an increased tumor sterilization with increasing neutron dose. The disease sterilization rates in the chest at autopsy were 33% (149 of 429) for photon-treated patients, 48% (45 of 93) for patients receiving 20% of their

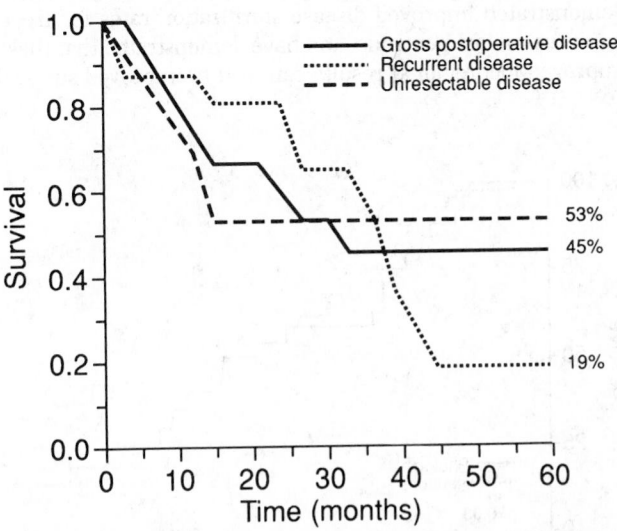

FIGURE 69–40.   Actuarial survival for patients with salivary gland tumors stratified according to their disease status at presentation. Curves are shown as a function of time from the start of the neutron irradiation. The patients with unresectable disease are shown by the dashed curve, the patients with gross postoperative disease are shown by the solid curve, and patients with recurrent disease are shown by the dotted curve.

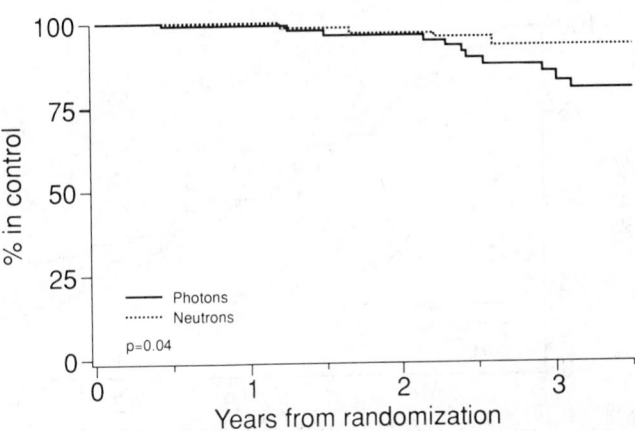

FIGURE 69–41.   Locoregional tumor control rates from a randomized prostate cancer study comparing 20.4 neutron Gy with 70 photon Gy. The results are significant at the $p = 0.04$ level.

total dose with neutrons, and 57% (49 of 65) for patients receiving 37% of their total dose with neutrons. The University of Washington reported a 70% local control rate using high-energy neutrons, and M.D. Anderson reported a 91% high-energy neutron local control rate for patients with superior sulcus tumors.[40,41] Sawada, using the NIRS facility in Chiba, Japan, demonstrated improved survival rates for neutron radiation therapy over photon radiation therapy for patients in this same situation.[42] An RTOG-sponsored randomized trial comparing photons to neutrons to mixtures of photons and neutrons using low-energy equipment failed to demonstrate significant differences in median survival or local control, although local tumor control was difficult to evaluate due to obscuring pneumonitis in the low-energy neutron and mixed beam treatment fields. Early treatment failures tended to be dominated by distant metastases, and longer-term (3-year) survival rates favored the neutron-treated and mixed beam-treated patient groups over the photon-treated group (37% versus 25% versus 12%). The normal tissue severe complication rate was significantly higher in patients treated with low-energy neutrons than it was for patients treated with mixed beam or photons (30.9% versus 14.5% versus 5.4%).[43]

A definitive phase III clinical trial using hospital-based, state-of-the-art neutron equipment was subsequently designed for

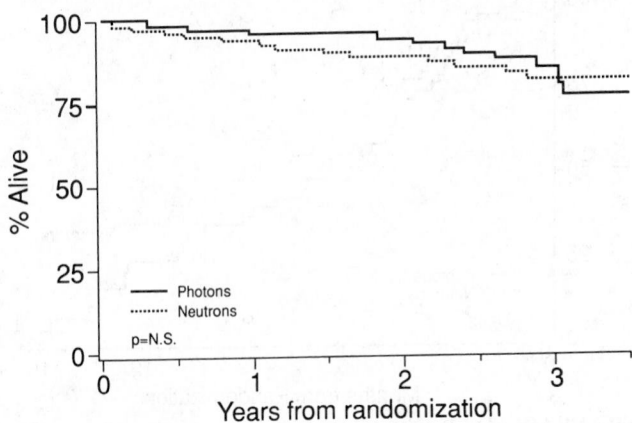

FIGURE 69–42.   Survival rates from a randomized prostate cancer study comparing 20.4 neutron Gy with 70 photon Gy.

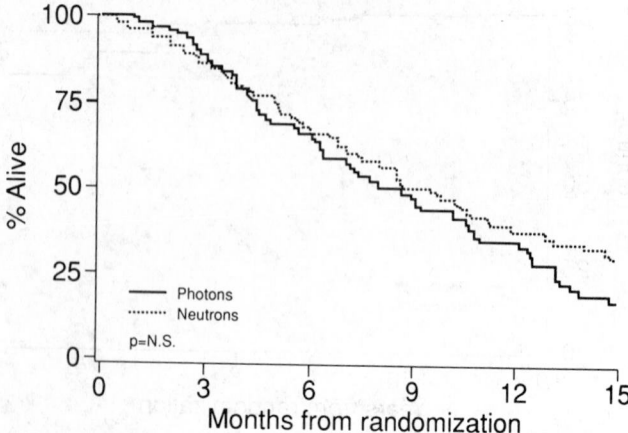

FIGURE 69–43. Results of overall survival from a randomized study comparing fast neutrons with photons for locally advanced non-small cell lung cancer. The differences in the survival curves fail to reach statistical significance.

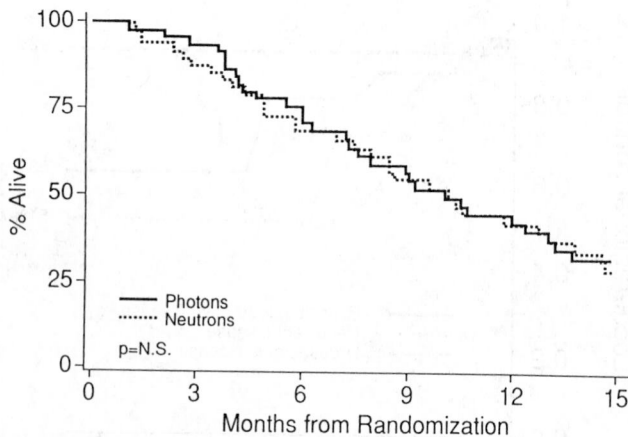

FIGURE 69–45. Randomized lung cancer study survival results for patients with non-small cell histologies other than squamous cell.

patients with inoperable non-small cell carcinomas of the lung. After stratification by prognostic factors and treating institution, patients were randomized to receive 6600 photon cGy delivered in 33 fractions over 7 weeks or 2040 neutron cGy delivered in 12 fractions over 4 weeks. Two hundred patients were entered on this study; 99 patients were randomized to photons, and 101 patients were randomized to neutrons. Tumors confined to the ipsilateral hemithorax and draining regional lymph nodes in patients with a Karnofsky performance score of 70 or better were eligible. The two treatment arms were balanced for all known prognostic factors.

Local tumor control was difficult to evaluate, as it is on all lung cancer studies, due to obscuring radiation pneumonitis in the treatment fields. Actuarial survival curves are depicted for the entire group, patients with squamous cell histologies, patients with non-squamous cell histologies, and patients with favorable prognostic factors in Figures 69–43 through 69–46. There is a trend favoring neutrons in the entire study population that is statistically significant in patients with

squamous cell carcinomas ($p = 0.02$; Fig. 69–44). No differences are observed in patients with non-squamous cell histologies. The advantage for neutrons in the patient population with favorable prognostic factors (patients without pleural effusions, without weight loss greater than 5% of body weight, without T4 or N3 tumors) is significant at the $p = 0.03$ level (see Fig. 69–46). There were only four major treatment-related complications (grades 4 or 5) in this study population, with two complications observed in each treatment arm (p = not significant).

Locoregional treatments of non-small cell lung cancer can only show survival benefits in patients who do not have a high probability of harboring occult distant metastases at the time their disease presents itself. Patients with squamous cell cancers, superior sulcus tumors, and patients with favorable prognostic indicators fall into this category. Prior studies have demonstrated improved disease sterilization rates for treatments using fast neutrons, and have demonstrated that these improved locoregional results can lead to improved survival

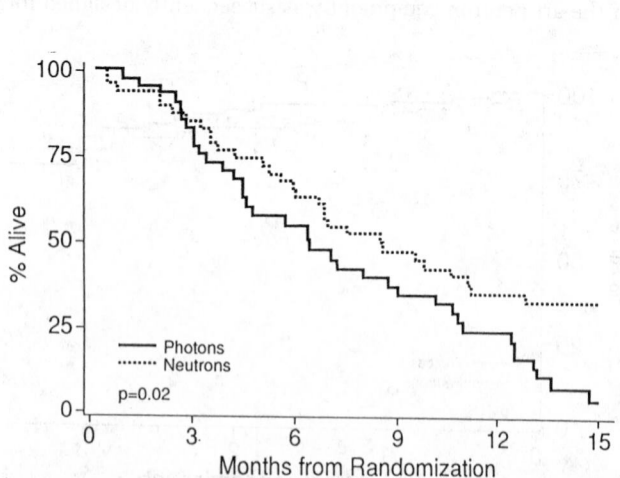

FIGURE 69–44. Randomized lung cancer study survival results for patients with squamous cell histologies. The differences are significant at the $p = 0.02$ level.

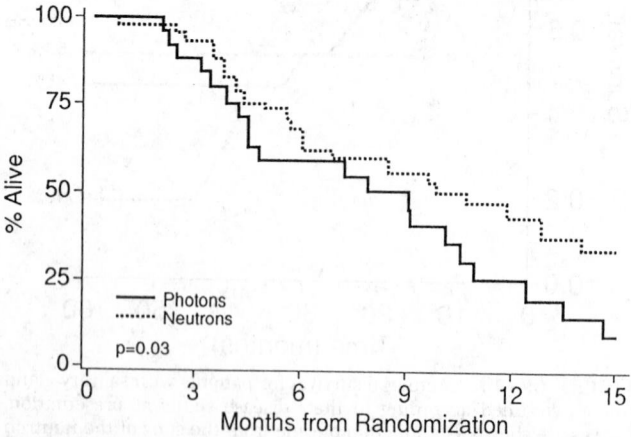

FIGURE 69–46. Randomized lung cancer study results for patients with non-small cell histologies and in good prognostic categories (excludes patients with T4, N3, pleural effusions, weight loss >5% of body weight). The difference is significant at the $p = 0.03$ level.

rates in patients where the risk of distant metastases is not overwhelming. The results of this study thus far appear to confirm these findings.

SQUAMOUS CELL HEAD AND NECK CANCERS

More patients have been treated for squamous cell carcinomas of the head and neck with neutrons than have been treated with neutrons for any other tumor system. Seven phase III randomized studies have been completed; six using low-energy or laboratory-based neutron generators of marginal capability, and a seventh using state-of-the-art equipment. Results from the six low-energy, laboratory-based studies were equivocal. Some reported dramatic improvement in complete response rates and locoregional tumor control with neutrons, and others reported no significant differences.[44-49] Direct comparisons of these trials are made difficult due to the diversity of treatment techniques and equipment, total radiation doses, and patient populations. A seventh prospective, randomized, phase III study using hospital-based cyclotrons was designed to definitively answer questions concerning the role of fast neutrons in treatment of squamous cell carcinomas of the head and neck.

One hundred and seventy-eight patients were entered on this study directly comparing state-of-the-art fast neutron radiation therapy with state-of-the-art photon and electron radiation therapy; 89 patients were randomized to each treatment arm. Patients with T3 or T4 tumors, or T2N+ tumors originating in the oral cavity, oropharynx, hypopharynx, supraglottic larynx, and glottic larynx received 7000 photon cGy in 35 fractions over 7 weeks or 2040 neutron cGy in 12 fractions over 4 weeks. The complete response rate in the neutron-treated group of patients is 70%, compared with 50% in the low-LET-treated group of patients ($p = 0.003$); with relatively short follow-up, this increased complete response rate has resulted in an improvement in locoregional tumor control (53% for neutrons compared with 35% for low-LET radiations). The survival rates are illustrated in Figure 69–47. There are no significant differences in major complication rates between the two groups.

Although fast neutron radiation therapy may ultimately

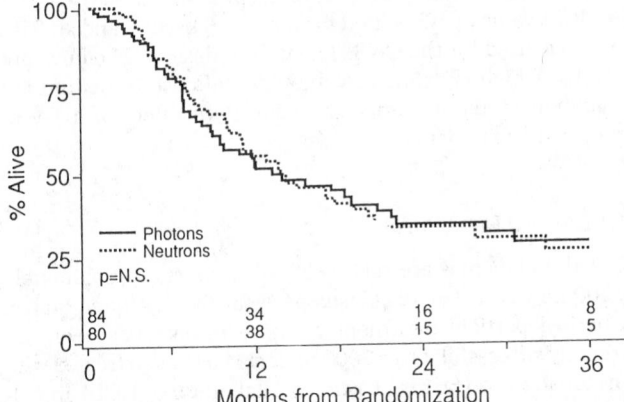

FIGURE 69–47. Survival results from a randomized study comparing 20.4 neutron Gy with 70 photon Gy for squamous cell carcinomas of the head and neck.

TABLE 69–43. Local Control Rates for Soft Tissue Sarcomas Treated Definitively With Radiotherapy

Investigations*	Local Control (patients)	Local Control Rate (%)
Neutrons		
Hammersmith[49]	26/50	52
NIRS[50]	7/12	58
Fermi Laboratory[51]	13/26	50
MANTA[32]	4/10	40
TAMVEC[52]	18/29	62
Edinburgh[53]	5/12	42
Hamburg/Eppendorf[54]	27/45	60
Heidelberg/Essen[55]	31/60	52
Louvain[56]	4/19	21
Amsterdam[57]	8/13	61
Seattle[58]	15/21	71
Total	158/297	53
Photons or Electrons		
McNeer[59]	14/25	56
Windeyer[60]	13/22	59
Duncan[63]	5/25	20
Tepper[61]	17/51	33
Leibel[62]	0/5	0
Total	49/128	38

* Patients treated de novo or for gross disease after surgery are included but not patients treated postoperatively for microscopic residual disease or for limited macroscopic residual disease.

demonstrate a statistically significant improvement in locoregional tumor control in this tumor system, it is unlikely, based on the shapes of the survival curves, that this improvement will result in an associated improvement in survival.

SARCOMAS

Although no phase III randomized studies have been completed investigating the role of fast neutrons in treatment of sarcomas of soft tissue, bone, or cartilage, a considerable experience has been amassed in non-randomized settings. Tables 69–43 through 69–45 compare neutron results with historical photon results reported in the literature for soft tissue sarcomas, osteogenic sarcomas, and chondrosarcomas, respectively.[49-69] The summed locoregional tumor control rates for inoperable, locally advanced soft tissue sarcomas are 53% for neutrons compared with 38% for low-LET photons and electrons. The locoregional results for locally advanced osteogenic sarcomas are 55% for neutrons compared with 21% for photons and electrons, and the results for locally advanced chondrosarcomas are 49% for neutrons compared with 33% for low-LET radiations. The results of fast neutron radiation therapy for these sarcomas are remarkably consistent and appear to demonstrate an improvement in locoregional tumor control rates over historical results. These results cannot be considered definitive until randomized studies are completed.

TABLE 69–44. Local Control Rates for Osteogenic Sarcomas Treated Definitively With Radiotherapy

Investigations*	Local Control (patients)	Local Control Rate (%)
Neutrons		
MANTA[32]	1/1	100
TAMVEC[52]	0/1	0
Fermi Laboratory[51]	2/9	22
Amsterdam[57]	0/3	0†
Edinburgh[63]	1/5	20
NIRS[64]	33/41	80
Seattle[58]	3/13	23
Total	40/73	55
Photons		
DeMoor[65]	9/43	33
Beck[66]	1/21	5
Tudway[67]	5/9	56
Total	15/73	21

* Patients treated postoperatively for microscopic residual disease or for limited macroscopic residual disease are not included.
† Persistent mass and calcification treated as failure, and local control rates may be underestimated.

TABLE 69–45. Local Control Rates for Chondrosarcomas Treated Definitively With Radiotherapy

Investigations*	Local Control (patients)	Local Control Rate (%)
Neutrons		
MANTA[32]	7/9	78
TAMVEC[52]	4/4	100
Fermi Laboratory[51]	9/16	56
Amsterdam[57]	0/6	0†
Edinburgh[63]	0/5	0†
NIRS[64]	1/2	50
Seattle[58]	4/9	44
Total	25/51	49
Photons		
McNanny[68]	3/10	30
Harwood[69]	7/20	35
Total	10/30	33

* Patients treated postoperatively for microscopic residual disease or for limited macroscopic residual disease are not included.
† Persistent mass and calcification treated as failure, and local control rates may be underestimated.

CHARGED PARTICLE CLINICAL STUDIES

As with neutrons (uncharged particles), charged particle radiation therapy was first suggested by physicists. However, despite 2 decades of small volume treatment for pituitary diseases, the investigation of large field charged particle cancer treatment did not begin until the mid 1970s. The first clinical cancer trials in the United States used protons (hydrogen nuclei) at the Harvard Cyclotron Laboratory (HCL), helium ions (α particles) at the University of California Lawrence Berkeley Laboratory (LBL), and pi mesons (subatomic particles) at the Los Alamos Meson Physics Facility. Heavier nuclei (*e.g.*, neon, carbon, silicon) were introduced at LBL later in that decade.

The initial accrual of clinical data to heavy charged particle studies was slow because of limitations on beam availability and the need to develop pioneering treatment techniques. In the United States almost 3600 cancer patients have been treated with protons and helium ions.[70] In other parts of the world, smaller numbers of patients have been treated at several proton facilities including the USSR, Switzerland, and Japan. Almost 230 patients were treated with pi mesons in the United States before that project was closed.[71] Subsequently over 700 patients have been treated with pi mesons in Switzerland and Canada. Heavy charged particle therapy has been used in over 400 patients. Virtually all patients receiving treatment with charged particles have been treated in laboratory-based treatment facilities located at some distance from their affiliated medical centers.

PROTONS AND HELIUM IONS

Protons and helium ions are charged particles that have a finite penetration in tissue. This unique characteristic results in dose distributions that are superior in many clinical situations to those obtainable with photons or electrons. The finite range and well-defined lateral edge allows smaller treatment volumes and lower doses to adjacent critical organs when compared with photons or electrons. Figure 69–48 shows a helium ion treatment plan for a chordoma at C2; in this plan the distal edge of the posterior field (with a cord block) is matched exactly to the lateral penumbra of the lateral fields.

Although the primary distinguishing characteristic of protons and helium ions compared with photons is their finite range in tissue, protons and helium ions differ slightly in relative biologic effectiveness (RBE) compared with megavoltage photons. The RBE for protons is 1.1.[72,73] Dose is expressed in the units of cobalt Gray equivalent (CGE) where CGE equals proton Gy × 1.1. The RBE for helium ions depends on fraction size, position in the spread out Bragg peak and tissue type.[74,75] An RBE value of 1.3 is used for non-CNS tissues, and an RBE of 1.6 is used for the CNS. The unit of dose is Gy-equivalent (GyE), which is defined as the physical dose of helium ion radiation required to give the equivalent effect of 1 Gy of megavoltage radiation.

UVEAL MELANOMAS

Uveal melanomas are relatively rare tumors; approximately 1200 new cases are diagnosed per year in the United States. Charged particle treatment of these tumors has been extremely successful. Over 2000 patients have been treated with protons at the Harvard Cyclotron Laboratory (HCL) in collaboration with Massachusetts General Hospital and Massachusetts Eye and Ear Infirmary or with helium ions at the Lawrence Berkeley Laboratory (LBL) in collaboration with the University of California-San Francisco.[70]

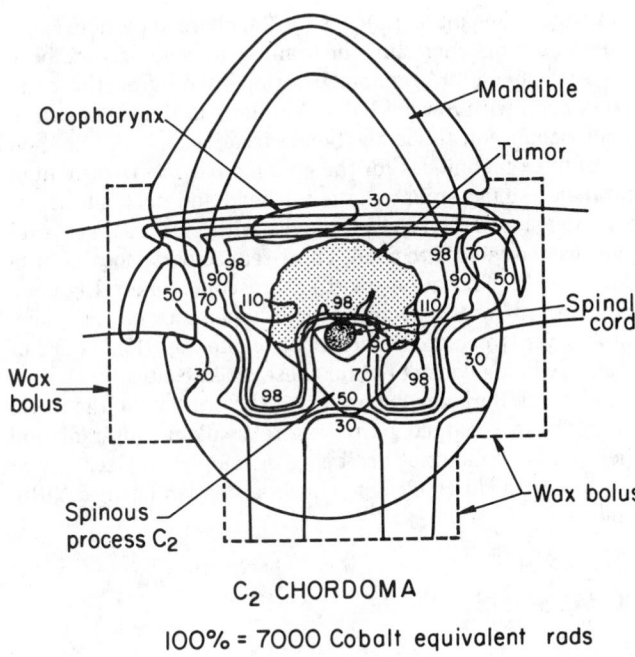

FIGURE 69-48. Composite treatment plan for precision high-dose helium irradiation of a chordoma of the upper cervical spine.

Charged particle treatment of uveal melanoma has employed high doses of radiation. Most patients have received the equivalent of 7000 cGy in five fractions over 8 to 9 days.[76,77] The treatment volume is small because the charged particles have minimal scatter and there is no radiation distal to the end of the particle range. Precise planning and delivery methods have been used for these treatments.[78]

The goal of charged particle treatment is to eradicate the melanoma while preserving a cosmetically intact eye and visual function. Local control rates after charged particle treatment have been very high (Table 69-46): the actuarial 5-year local control rate is 96.3% for the HCL patients and 96.8% for the LBL patients.[79,80] All but a small number of patients have maintained a cosmetically intact eye. In the HCL experience the 5-year actuarial eye retention rate is 89%, and in the LBL experience, the rate is 83%.[81,80] Vision of 20/200 or better has been maintained in 65% to 70% of the HCL patients.[82,83] At 5 years, 80% of the HCL patients and 76% of the LBL patients are without evidence of metastatic disease.[84] Survival rates for patients treated with protons have been compared using known prognostic factors with survival rates for patients undergoing enucleation.[80,85] The results show no differences in survival after the two different treatments.

SARCOMAS

The next largest group of cancer patients receiving proton or helium ion treatment are patients with sarcomas of the skull base and cervical spine. Charged particle radiation in the postoperative setting has achieved a significant clinical gain for patients with these uncommon tumors. Despite the rarity of these tumors, 320 patients with chordomas or chondrosarcomas in the skull base or cervical spine have been treated with protons or helium ions.[85,215] These tumors are locally

TABLE 69-46. Results of Charged Particle Treatment for Uveal Melanoma

Results	Protons*	Helium Ions*
Local control	96.3%	96.8%
Eye retention	89%	83%
Survival without metastases	80%	76%

* Five-year actuarial rates.

aggressive and are located immediately adjacent to critical structures such as the brain stem, spinal cord, temporal lobes, and optic nerves and chiasm. Surgical resection is usually incomplete. Postoperative photon radiation achieves local control in approximately 35% to 40% of patients.[86] Proton and helium ion radiation can deliver a substantially higher dose than photons to the residual tumor. The 5-year actuarial local control rates are 60% to 77% for patients treated with helium ions or protons after surgery.[87,88] Survival rates at 5 years are 62% to 88%.

In the HCL proton experience, patients received a median dose of 68.5 CGE (range, 56.8–77.4 CGE) using 1.8 CGE fractions. Patients with chondrosarcomas have a better prognosis than patients with chordomas. The 5-year actuarial local control rate is 91% for chondrosarcomas (85 patients) and 65% for chordomas (130 patients).[70] Tumor volume is another prognostic factor with small volumes having higher local control rates.[89] Patients treated with helium ions at LBL have received a mean dose of 67 GyE (range, 36–80 GyE). The usual fractionation was 2.0 to 2.5 GyE four days per week. Patients with tumor volume less than 20 ml had a 5-year actuarial local control rate of 80% while patients with larger tumor volumes had a 33% local control rate.[87] Patients with recurrent disease had a poorer outcome than previously untreated patients.[90] A small number of patients with sacral chordomas have received helium ion treatment.[91]

The achievements of proton therapy discussed in this section have been accomplished using physics laboratory facilities with fixed, horizontal beams. The next generation of proton facilities in the United States will be hospital based machines with isocentric gantries. Such a facility has been built at Loma Linda University and plans for several other facilities are being developed.

HEAVY CHARGED PARTICLES

Heavy charged particle radiotherapy has been investigated at the University of California Lawrence Berkeley Laboratory in collaboration with the University of California-San Francisco Department of Radiation Oncology. Heavy charged particles have high-LET properties and improved dose localization properties compared with x-rays because of a defined depth of penetration in tissue. Most of the clinical work with heavy charged particles has been done with neon. A small number of patients have been treated with silicon and carbon.

Between 1979 and 1988, a total of 239 patients had received neon treatment with a neon dose of 1000 cGy or greater.[92] Neon doses were gradually escalated while acute and late toxicities were monitored until toxicity limits were reached. The preclinical in vitro and in vivo measurements of neon RBE relative to megavoltage x-rays were 2.0 to 3.5, depending on fraction size, beam energy, size of the extended Bragg peak, type of tissue irradiated and biologic endpoint chosen.[93-98] The clinical RBE for acute normal tissue reactions was consistent with the experimental data in the range of 2.0 to 3.5 (average 2.5). The RBE for the CNS is higher and the dose to the brain and spinal cord is limited to 1000 cGy whenever possible.[4,5] The neon dose is expressed as equivalent dose using the units of GyE (GyE=neon physical Gy × RBE).

Neon treatment of many different tumor sites has been explored and include prostate cancer, soft tissue and bone sarcomas, paranasal sinus cancers, salivary gland tumors, advanced head and neck cancer, malignant gliomas, lung cancer, esophageal cancer, gastric cancer, pancreatic cancer, biliary tract cancer, and melanoma. Promising results were seen in advanced prostate cancer, macroscopic soft tissue and bone sarcomas, paranasal sinus cancers, macroscopic salivary gland cancers, and biliary tract cancers (Table 69–47). Further studies including randomized trials are in progress or are being initiated for these disease sites.

Twenty-one patients with locally advanced prostate cancer received a neon boost after megavoltage treatment to the pelvis. The median total dose was 7500 cGy, and the median neon dose was 11 Gy. The 5-year actuarial local control rate is 89%, and the disease-specific survival (DSS) is 61%.[100] Disease-specific survival analysis reflects the events of death from disease or treatment complications. A phase III trial is in progress for patients with stage C and D1 disease; this trial compares neon and photon boosts to the prostate.

Twelve patients with soft tissue sarcomas were treated with a median total dose of 60 GyE and a median neon dose of 14 Gy. Nineteen patients with bone sarcomas were treated. The median total dose used in this group of patients was 69.6 GyE and the median neon dose was 16.8 Gy. The actuarial 5-year local control rate is 56% for patients with macroscopic soft tissue sarcoma and 59% for patients with macroscopic bone sarcoma.[92] The excellent dose localization properties of neon allow treatment in challenging tumor locations where high doses of x-rays or neutrons cannot be delivered safely. These tumor locations include soft tissue sarcomas of the retroperitoneum and trunk and bone sarcomas arising in the spine

TABLE 69–47. Results of Neon Treatment for Malignant Disease

Tumor	No. of Patients	5-Year Local Control (%)	5-Year Disease-Specific Survival (%)*
Prostate	21	89	61
Soft tissue sarcoma	12	56	56
Bone sarcoma	19	59	45
Paranasal sinuses	12	69	69
Salivary gland	18	61	59
Biliary tract	8	44	29

* Disease-specific survival scores death from disease and treatment complications as events.

and clivus. Elegant techniques for the charged particle treatment of tumors encircling the brain stem or spinal cord have been developed.[100] A randomized trial is in progress that compares neon with lower-LET helium ions in the treatment of macroscopic soft tissue and bone sarcomas.

Complex techniques for the charged particle treatment of paranasal sinus tumors and other head and neck sites have been developed.[101] Twelve patients with paranasal sinus tumors were treated with neon. The 5-year actuarial local control rate was 69% for patients with macroscopic tumor. Eighteen patients with locally advanced major and minor salivary gland tumors were treated. The local control rate was 61%.[92] Further trials are being considered for these disease sites.

Lawrence Berkeley Laboratory is the only site in the world where heavy charged particles are available for radiation therapy. New facilities are being developed in Germany at G.S.I. Darmstadt-Heidelberg University and in Japan at NIRS, Chiba.

PI MESONS

Pi mesons (pions) were first investigated clinically at the Los Alamos Meson Physics Facility (LAMPF) between 1974 and 1981. Patient treatment with pions were later started at the TRI University Meson Facility (TRIUMF) in Vancouver, Canada, and the Paul Scherrer Institute (PSI) in Villigen, Switzerland. Clinical investigations are continuing at these facilities. Pions have improved depth dose characteristics and increased RBE compared with photons. The interaction of pions with tissue is characterized by the pion star that is formed as pions are captured by nuclei. Preclinical in vivo measurements of RBE indicated a pion RBE of 1.5 in the range of 2 to 3 Gy per fraction.[102-104] Phase I–II clinical experience at LAMPF is consistent with an RBE in the range of 1.4 to 1.6 for acute normal tissue reactions and late sequelae.[71] Phase III studies are planned for gliomas, sarcomas, and prostate. Encouraging phase I–II results for the treatment of unresectable soft tissue sarcomas have been reported.[105]

BORON NEUTRON-CAPTURE THERAPY

An isotope of boron, boron 10 has the capacity to capture neutrons and concentrate their cell killing effects in a small volume. When the nucleus of a boron atom captures a neutron, it undergoes a fission reaction producing lithium and helium nuclei that deposit approximately 2.35 million electron volts in energy over short distances comparable to cellular dimensions. If boron atoms are selectively concentrated in tumor cells, by attaching them to tumor-specific antibodies or through other means, this energy could be removed from an external neutron beam and concentrated in malignant cells. If a sufficient concentration differential of boron atoms is achieved between tumor and normal tissues, then the destruction of target tumor cells will be selectively enhanced relative to surrounding normal tissue structures, and the effectiveness of neutron radiotherapy would be greatly increased.

Shortly after the neutron was discovered by Chadwick in 1932, Locher proposed the use of boron neutron capture therapy (BNCT) as a possible treatment for human malignancies.[106] A few years later, Kruger[107] and Zahl[108] demonstrated the biologic effectiveness of the fission fragments produced by the interaction of slow neutrons with ^{10}B. The first clinical trials for human malignancies were carried out for malignant gliomas of the brain using a reactor beam at the Brookhaven National Laboratories with borax used as the ^{10}B carrier agent.[109,110] These and other subsequent trials carried out in the 1960s showed no therapeutic benefit for this form of treatment and moreover, showed considerable damage to the endothelial linings of the blood vessels. This was attributed to the high concentration of ^{10}B in the blood at the time of treatment and to the poorly penetrating characteristics of the collimated reactor beams used for treatment. The development of new ^{10}B-carrier agents has led to a resurgence of interest in BNCT on the part of the medical community.

Although most BNCT work has used thermal and epithermal nuclear reactor generated slow neutron beams, it is possible to enhance accelerator-produced fast neutron beams by BNCT. When a fast neutron beam penetrates tissue, a small "thermalized" neutron flux develops naturally due to neutron-nuclear interactions, and it is possible to use this thermalized component to specifically enhance the microdosimetric radiation dose to tumor cells via BNCT techniques.[111] The use of fast neutrons for BNCT avoids the problems of poor depth dose, poor skin sparing, poor collimation, and the radiation safety considerations associated with slow neutron beams generated from nuclear reactors. Typical fast neutron doses used in a course of radiotherapy are in the range of 18 to 20 neutron Gy.

Because only low-energy neutrons can be captured by boron atoms, the effective low-energy component of fast neutron beams has been measured by activation of Sodium in a $NaNO_3$ solution, and model calculations have been performed based on Monte Carlo simulations for cell survival. This model predicts that over a standard course of fast neutron radiotherapy, 30 $\mu g/g$ concentrations of boron in the tumor cells would result in a tenfold to 100-fold increase in tumor cell kill. Using a Poisson model for tumor control, a tenfold improvement in cell kill would increase a tumor control rate from 20% to 85%. Concentration differentials (tumor to normal tissue) of 30 to 50 $\mu g/g$ have been achieved with modern boron carrier technology. These newer carriers include: sodium borocaptate, tumor specific antibodies, chlorpromazine, misonidazole, thiouracil, porphyrins, amino acids, nucleosides, and steroids.

Radiobiologic measurements made in vitro verify these model calculations (Fig. 69–49), and the size of these measured effects agree with the models.[112]

Boron neutron capture therapy, in a theory described by Lochner in 1936, should result in a dramatic improvement in the results of treatment for tumors that can concentrate quantities of boron in excess of 30 $\mu g/g$ of tumor above surrounding normal tissue. With the development of new carrier agents for boron and with studies that now demonstrate that cyclotron-generated fast neutron beams can be enhanced by boron capture, BNCT has the potential to become a practical clinical reality.

REFERENCES

1. Griffin TW, Wambersie A, Laramore GE, et al. High LET heavy particle trials. Int J Radiat Oncol Biol Phys 1988;14:583.
2. Suit HD, Griffin TW, Castro JR, et al. Particle radiation therapy research plan. Am J Clin Oncol 1988;11:330.
3. Von Essen CF, Blattman H, Crawford JF, et al. The piotron: Initial experience, preparation and experience with pion therapy. Int J Radiat Oncol Biol Phys 1982;8:1499.
4. Gray LH, Conger AE, Ebert M, et al. Concentration of oxygen dissolved in tissues at time of irradiation as a factor in radiotherapy. Br J Radiol 1950;26:638.
5. Tenforde TJ, Azal SM, Parr, SS, et al. Cell survival in rat rhabdomyosarcoma tumors irradiated in vivo with extended peak silicon ions. Radiat Res 1982;92:208.
6. Howlett JF, Thomlinson RH, Alper T. A marked dependence on the conformative effective causes of neutrons on tumor line and its implications for clinical trials. Br J Radiol 1975;48:40.
7. Gragg RL, Humphrey RM, Thomas HT, et al. The response of Chinese hamster ovary cells to fast neutron radiotherapy beams. I. Variations in relative biologic effectiveness with position in the cell cycle. Radiat Res 1978;76:283.
8. Gragg RL, Humphrey RM, Meyn RE. The response of Chinese hamster ovary cells to fast neutron radiotherapy beams. II. Sublethal and potentially lethal damage recovery capabilities. Radiat Res 1977;71:461.
9. Hall EJ, Kraljevic J. Repair of potentially lethal radiation damage: Comparison of neutron and x-ray RBE and implications for radiation therapy. Radiology 1976;121:731.
10. Stone RS, Larkin JC. Treatment of cancer with fast neutrons. Radiology 1942;39:608.
11. Fowler JF, Morgan RL. Pre-therapeutic experiments with fast neutron beam from Medical Research Council's cyclotron. VIII: General review. Br J Radiol 1963;36:115.
12. Sheline GE, Phillips TL, Field SB, et al. Effects of fast neutrons on human skin. AJR 1971;111:31.
13. Catterall M. The treatment of advanced cancer by fast neutrons from the Medical Research Council's cyclotron at Hammersmith Hospital, London. Eur J Cancer 1974;10:343.
14. Batterman JJ, Breur K, Hart GAM, et al. Observations on pulmonary metastases in patients after single doses and multiple fractions of fast neutrons and cobalt-60 gamma rays. Eur J Cancer 1981;17:539.
15. Koh W, Laramore GE, Griffin TW, et al. Fast neutron radiation for inoperable and recurrent salivary gland cancers. Am J Clin Oncol 1989;12:316.
16. Borthne A, Kjellevold K, Kaalhus O, et al. Salivary gland malignant neoplasms: Treatment and prognosis. Int J Radiat Oncol Biol Phys 1986;12:747.
17. Fitzpatrick PJ, Theriault C. Malignant salivary gland tumors. Int J Radiat Oncol Biol Phys 1986;12:1743.
18. Fu KK, Leibel S, Levine M, et al. Carcinoma of the major and minor salivary glands: Analysis of treatment results and sites and causes of failures. Cancer 1977;40:2882.
19. Shidnia H, Hornback N, Hamaker R, et al. Carcinoma of major salivary glands. Cancer 1980;45:693.
20. Elkon D, Colman M, Hendrickson F. Radiation therapy in the treatment of malignant salivary gland tumors. Cancer 1978;41:502.
21. Rossman K. The role of radiation therapy in the treatment of parotid carcinomas. AJR 1975;123:492.
22. Rafla S. Malignant parotid tumors: Natural history and treatment. Cancer 1977;40:136.
23. Dobrowsky W, Schlappack O, Karcher KH, et al. Electron-beam therapy in treatment of parotid neoplasm. Radiother Oncol 1986;6:293.
24. Griffin TW, Pajak TF, Laramore GE, et al. Neutron vs. photon irradiation of inoperable salivary gland tumors: Results of an RTOG-MRC cooperative study. Int J Radiat Oncol Biol Phys 1988;15:1085.

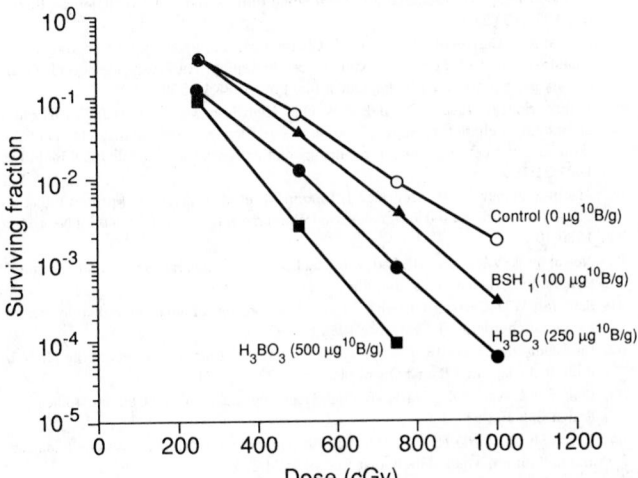

FIGURE 69–49. Survival of Chinese hamster ovary cells after fast-neutron-beam irradiation. Cells incubated with boron-containing compounds before irradiation show enhanced cell killing.

25. Vikram B, Strong EW, Shah JP, et al. Radiation therapy in adenoid-cystic carcinomas. Int J Radiat Oncol Biol Phys 1984;10:221.

26. Stewart JG, Jackson A, Chew M. The role of radiation therapy in the management of malignant tumors of the salivary glands. AJR 1968;102:100.

27. Guillamondegui OM, Byers RM, Luna MA, et al. Aggressive surgery in the treatment for parotid cancer: The role of adjunctive postoperative radiotherapy. AJR 1975;123:49.

28. Ravasz LA, Terhhard CHJ, Hordijk GJ. Radiotherapy in epithelial tumors of the parotid gland: Case presentation and literature review. Int J Radiat Oncol Biol Phys 1990;19:55.

29. Saroja KR, Mansell J, Hendrickson R, et al. An update on malignant salivary gland tumors treated with neutrons at Fermilab. Int J Radiat Oncol Biol Phys 1987;13:1319.

30. Catterall M, Errington RD. The implications of improved treatment of malignant salivary gland tumors by fast neutron radiotherapy. Int J Radiat Oncol Biol Phys 1987;13:1313.

31. Duncan W, Orr JA, Arnott SJ, et al. Neutron therapy for malignant tumors of the salivary glands: A report of the Edinburgh experience. Radiother Oncol 1987;8:97.

32. Ornitz R, Herskovic A, Bradley E, et al. Clinical observations of early and late normal tissue injury and tumor control in patients receiving fast neutron irradiation. In: High LET radiations in clinical radiotherapy. Elmsford, NY: Pergamon Press, 1979.

33. Battermann JJ, Mijnheer BJ. The Amsterdam fast neutron therapy project: A final report. Int J Radiat Oncol Biol Phys 1986;12:2093.

34. Maor M, Hussey D, Fletcher GH, et al. Fast neutron radiotherapy for locally advanced head and neck tumors. Int J Radiat Oncol Biol Phys 1981;7:155.

35. Eichhorn HJ. Pilot study on the applicability of neutron radiotherapy. Radiobiol Radiother 1981;3:262.

36. Skolyszewski J, Byrski E, Chrzanowska A, et al. A preliminary report on the clinical application of fast neutrons in Krakow. Int J Radiat Oncol Biol Phys 1982;8:1781.

37. Buchholz TA, Laramore GE, Griffin BR, et al. The role of fast neutron radiotherapy in the management of advanced salivary gland malignancies. Cancer 1992:2779–2788.

38. Laramore GE, Krall JM, Thomas FJ, et al. Fast neutron radiotherapy for locally advanced prostate cancer: Final report of an RTOG randomized clinical trial. Am J Clin Oncol (in press).

39. Eichhorn HJ. Results of a pilot study on neutron therapy with 600 patients. Int J Radiat Oncol Biol Phys 1982;8:1561.

40. Livingston RB, Griffin BR, Higano C, et al. Combined treatment with chemotherapy and neutron irradiation for limited non-small cell lung cancer: A SWOG study. J Clin Oncol 1987;5:1756.

41. Komaki R, Mountain C, Holbert J, et al. Superior sulcus tumors: Treatment selection and results for 85 patients without metastases at presentation. Int J Radiat Oncol Biol Phys 1990;19:31.

42. Sawada K, Fukuma S, Seki Y, et al. Clinical experience in patients with Pancoast tumor treated by fast neutron radiotherapy. Gan No Rinsho 1983;A7:111.

43. Laramore GE, Bauer M, Griffin TW, et al. Fast neutron and mixed beam radiotherapy for inoperable non-small cell carcinoma of the lung. Am J Clin Oncol 1986;9:233.

44. Catterall M, Bewley D, Sutherland I. Second report on a randomized clinical trial of fast neutrons compared with x or gamma rays in treatment of advanced cancers of the head and neck. Br J Med 1977;1:1942.

45. Maor M, Schoenfeld DA, Hendrickson FR, et al. Evaluation of a neutron boost in head and neck cancer: Results of the randomized RTOG trial 78-08. Am J Clin Oncol 1986;9:61.

46. Duncan W, Orr JA, Arnott SJ, et al. Fast neutron therapy for squamous cell carcinoma in the head and neck region: Results of a randomized trial. Int J Radiat Oncol Biol Phys 1987;13:171.

47. Griffin TW, Davis R, Hendrickson F, et al. Fast neutron radiation therapy for unresectable squamous cell carcinomas of the head and neck: The results of a randomized RTOG study. Int J Radiat Oncol Biol Phys 1984;10:2217.

48. Griffin TW, Pajak T, Maor M, et al. Mixed neutron/photon irradiation of unresectable squamous cell carcinomas of the head and neck: The final report of a randomized trial. Int J Radiat Oncol Biol Phys 1989;17:959.

49. Catterall M. The treatment of advanced cancer by fast neutrons from the Medical Research Council's cyclotron at Hammersmith Hospital, London. Eur J Cancer 1974;10:343.

50. Tsunemoto H, Morita S, Arai T, et al. Results of clinical trial with 30 MeV d-Be neutrons at NIRS. In: Treatment of radioresistant cancers. Amsterdam, Elsevier-North Holland, 1974.

51. Cohen L, Hendrickson F, Mansell J, et al. Response of sarcomas of bone and soft tissue to neutron beam therapy. Int J Radiat Oncol Biol Phys 1984;10:821.

52. Salinas R, Hussey DH, Fletcher GH. Experience with fast neutron therapy for locally advanced sarcomas. Int J Radiat Oncol Biol Phys 1980;6:267.

53. Duncan W, Dewar JA. A retrospective study of the role of radiotherapy in the treatment of soft tissue sarcoma. Clin Radiol 1985;36:629.

54. Franke HD, Hess A, Brassow F, et al. Clinical results after irradiation of intracranial tumors, soft tissue sarcomas, and thyroid cancers with fast neutrons at Hamburg-Eppendorf. In: Progress in Radio-Oncology II. New York: Raven Press, 1982.

55. Schmitt G, Schnabel K, Sauerwein W, et al. Neutron and neutron-boost irradiation of soft tissue sarcomas: A 4.5 year analysis of 139 patients. Radiother Oncol 1983;1:23.

56. Wambersie A. The European experience in neutron therapy at the end of 1981. Int J Radiat Oncol Biol Phys 1982;8:2145.

57. Battermann JJ, Breur K. Fast neutron therapy for locally advanced sarcomas. Int J Radiat Oncol Biol Phys 1981;7:1051.

58. Laramore GE, Griffeth JT, Boespflug M, et al. Fast neutron radiotherapy for sarcomas of soft tissue, bone, and cartilage. Am J Clin Oncol 1989;12:320.

59. McNeer GP, Cantin J, Chu F, et al. Effectiveness of radiation therapy in the management of sarcoma of the soft somatic tissues. Cancer 1968;22:391.

60. Windeyer W, Dische S, Mansfield CF. The place of radiotherapy in the management of fibrosarcoma of the soft tissues. Clin Radiol 1966;17:32.

61. Tepper JE, Suit HD. Radiation therapy alone for sarcoma of soft tissue. Cancer 1985;56:474.

62. Leibel SA, Tranbaugh RF, Wara WF, et al. Soft tissue sarcomas of the extremities: Survival and patterns of failure with conservative surgery with postoperative irradiation compared to surgery alone. Cancer 1985;56:475.

63. Duncan W, Arnott SJ, Jack WJL. The Edinburgh experience of treating sarcomas of soft tissue and bone with neutron irradiation. Clin Radiol 1986;37:317.

64. Hokada E, Maruyama K, Takada N, et al. Multimodality treatment, including fast neutron radiotherapy, for osteosarcoma. Cancer Bull 1979;31:216.

65. deMoor NG. Osteosarcoma: A review of 72 cases treated by megavoltage radiation therapy with or without surgery. S Afr J Surg 1975;13:137.

66. Beck JC, Wara WM, Bovill EG, et al. The role of radiation therapy in the treatment of osteosarcoma. Radiology 1976;120:163.

67. Tudway RC. Radiotherapy for osteogenic sarcoma. J Bone Joint Surg 1961;43:61.

68. McNaney D, Lindberg RD, Ayala AG, et al. Fifteen year radiotherapy experience with chondrosarcoma of bone. Int J Radiat Oncol Biol Phys 1982;8:187.

69. Harwood AR, Krajbich JI, Fornasier VL. Radiotherapy of chondrosarcoma of bone. Cancer 1980;45:2769.

70. Suit H, Urie M. Clinical gains to be realized from proton beams in radiation therapy (in press).

71. Schmitt G, von Essen CF, Greiner R, et al. Review of the SIN and Los Alamos pion trials. Radiat Res 1985;104:272.

72. Urano M, Goitein M, Verhey L, et al. Relative biological effectiveness of a high energy modulated proton beam using a spontaneous murine tumor in vivo. Int J Radiat Oncol Biol Phys 1980;6:1187.

73. Urano M, Verhey LJ, Goitein M, et al. Relative biological effectiveness of modulated proton beams in various murine tissues. Int J Radiat Oncol Biol Phys 1983;10:509.

74. Phillips TL, Fu KK, Curtis SB. Tumor biology of helium and heavy ions. Int J Radiat Oncol Biol Phys 1977;3:109.

75. Lyman JT. Computer modeling of heavy charged-particle beams. In: Pion and heavy ion radiodtherapy pre-clinical and clinical studies. New York: Elsevier Biomedical, 1979.

76. Gragoudas ES, Goitein M, Koehler A, et al. Proton irradiation of choroidal melanomas. Arch Ophthalmol 1978;96:1583.

77. Saunders WM, Char DH, Quivey JM, et al. Precision high dose radiotherapy: Helium ion treatment of uveal melanoma. Int J Radiat Oncol Biol Phys 1985;11:227.

78. Goitein M, Miller T. Planning proton therapy of the eye. Med Phys 1983;10:275.

79. Munzenrider JE, Verhey L, Gradoudas ES, et al. Conservative treatment of uveal melanoma: Local recurrence after proton beam therapy. Int J Radiat Oncol Biol Phys 1989;17:493.

80. Linstadt D, Castro J, Char D, et al. Long-term results of helium ion irradiation of uveal melanoma. Int J Radiat Oncol Biol Phys 1990;19:613.

81. Munzenrider JE, Gragoudas ES, Seddon JM, et al. Conservative treatment of uveal melanoma: Probability of eye retention after proton treatment. Int J Radiat Oncol Biol Phys 1988;15:553.

82. Seddon JM, Gragoudas ES, Polivogianis L, et al. Visual outcome after proton beam irradiation of uveal melanoma. Ophthalmology 1986;93:666.

83. Gragoudas ES, Seddon JM, Egan K, et al. Long-term results of proton beam irradiated uveal melanomas. Ophthalmology 1987;94:349.

84. Gragoudas ES, Seddon JM, Egan K, et al. Metastasis from uveal melanoma after proton beam irradiation. Ophthalmology 1988;95:992.

85. Seddon JM, Gragoudas ES, Egan KM, et al. Relative survival rates after alternative therapies for uveal melanoma. Ophthalmology 1990;97:769.

86. Austin-Seymour M, Munzenrider JE, Goitein M, et al. Progress in low-LET heavy particle therapy: Intracranial and paracranial tumors and uveal melanomas. Radiat Res 1985;104:219.

87. Berson AM, Castro JR, Petti P, et al. Charged particle irradiation of chordoma and chondrosarcoma of the base of skull and cervical spine: The Lawrence Berkeley Laboratory experience. Int J Radiat Oncol Biol Phys 1988;15:559.

88. Munzenrider JE, Liebsch NJ, deBois W, et al. High dose fractionated combined proton and photon radiation therapy of chordomas and low-grade chondrosarcomas of the skull base and cervical spine. I. results in adult patients. Int J Radiat Oncol Biol Phys 1991;21:166.

89. Austin-Seymour M, Munzenrider J, Goitein M, et al. Fractionated proton radiation therapy of chordoma and low-grade chondrosarcoma of the base of the skull. J Neurosurg 1989;70:13.

90. Nowakowski VA, Castro JR, Petti PL, et al. Charged particle radiotherapy of paraspinal tumors. Int J Radiat Oncol Biol Phys 1991;22:1.

91. Saunders WM, Castro JR, Chen GTY, et al. Early results of ion beam radiation therapy for sacral chordoma. J Neurosurg 1986;64:243.

92. Lindstadt DE, Castro JR, Phillips TL. Neon ion radiotherapy: Results of the phase I/II clinical trial. Int J Radiat Oncol Biol Phys 1991;20:761.

93. Blakely EA, Ngo FQH, Curtis SB, et al. Heavy-ion radiobiology: Cellular studies. Adv Radiat Biol 1984;11:295.

94. Curtis SB, Tenforde TS, Parks D, et al. Response of a rat rhabdomyosarcoma to neon- and helium-ion irradiation. Radiat Res 1978;74:274.

95. Curtis SB, Schilling WA, Tenforde TS, et al. Survival of oxygenated and hypoxic tumor cells in the extended-peak regions of heavy charged-particle beams. Radiat Res 1982;90:292.

96. Leith JT, Woodruff KH, Howard J, et al. Early and late effects of accelerated charged particles on normal tissues. Int J Radiat Oncol Biol Phys 1977;3:103.

97. Leith JT, Smith P, Ross-Riveros P, et al. Cellular response of a rat brain tumor to a therapeutic neon ion beam. Int J Radiat Biol 1977;32:401.
98. Tobias CA, Blakely EA, Alpen EL, et al. Molecular and cellular radiobiology of heavy ions. Int J Radiat Oncol Biol Phys 1982;8:2109.
99. Castro J. Personal communication.
100. Castro JR, Collier M, Petti PL, et al. Charged particle radiotherapy for lesions encircling the brain stem of spinal cord. Int J Radiat Oncol Biol Phys 1989;17:477.
101. Castro JR, Reimers MM. Charged particle radiotherapy of selected tumors in the head and neck. Int J Radiat Oncol Biol Phys 1988;14:711.
102. Raju MR, Carpenter S, Tokita N, et al. Effects of fractionated pions on normal tissues. I. Mouse skin. Int J Radiat Oncol Biol Phys 1980;6:2663.
103. Peters LJ, Withers HR, Mason KA, et al. Effects of fractionated pions on normal tissues. II. Mouse jejunum. Int J Radiat Oncol Biol Phys 1980;6:1667.
104. Chaplin DJ, Douglas BG, Saito T, et al. Preclincal evaluation of pions in vivo: Experience at TRIUMF. Radiother Oncol 1990;17:7.
105. Greiner RH, Blattmann JH, Thum P, et al. Dynamic pion irradiation of unresectable soft tissue sarcoma. Int J Radiat Oncol Biol Phys 1989;17:1077.

106. Locher GL. Biological effects and therapeutic possibilities of neutrons. Am J Roentgenol Radium Ther 1936;36:1.
107. Kruger PG. Some biological effects of nuclear disintegration products on neoplastic tissue. Proc Natl Acad Sci 1940;26:181.
108. Zahl PA, Cooper FS, Dunning JR. Some in vivo effects of localized nuclear disintegration products on a transplantable mouse sarcoma. Proc Natl Acad Sci 1940;26:589.
109. Farr LE, Sweet WH, Robertson JS, et al. Neutron capture therapy with boron in the treatment of glioblastoma multiforme. AJR 1954;71:279.
110. Godwin JT, Farr LE, Sweet WH, et al. Pathological study of eight patients with glioblastoma multiforme treated by neutron capture therapy using boron-10. Cancer 1955;8:601.
111. Waterman FM, Kuchnir FT, Skaggs LS, et al. The use of ¹⁰B to enhance the tumour dose in fast-neutron therapy. Phys Med Biol 1978;23:592.
112. Laramore GE, Livesey J, Wootton P, et al. Boron neutron capture therapy: A means of increasing the effectiveness of fast neutron radiotherapy. In: Proceedings of the 9th International Congress of Radiation Research. Academic Press, San Diego (in press).

SECTION 11

JAMES R. OLESON

Hyperthermia

Temperature elevation to 42°C to 45°C for 10 to 60 minutes can lethally damage bacterial and mammalian cells. This fact, first observed in ancient times, was rediscovered in the 19th century when patients with malignant tumors who had fevers related to bacterial infections occasionally had regressions in tumor size. Coley deliberately induced fevers in cancer patients using pyrogenic bacterial toxins and observed some partial responses.[1]

The development of radiofrequency generators in the early 1900s and their application in diathermy allowed the testing of effects due to temperature rise localized to a tumor, rather than whole-body hyperthermia.[2,3] Although investigation of combined hyperthermia and irradiation soon followed, a series of reports by Crile in the 1960s probably stimulated the modern quantitative study of effects of hyperthermia on cancer.[4-6] Crile demonstrated thermal enhancement of radiation effect and cure of melanomas implanted on the feet of mice with water bath heating; no normal tissue damage was observed from exposures to 44°C for 30 minutes. Since the early 1960s, systematic laboratory investigation of hyperthermia has expanded, and these investigations continue to support use of hyperthermia in cancer therapy. Several reviews provide further information.[7-10]

BIOLOGIC BACKGROUND

EFFECTS OF HYPERTHERMIA ALONE

When the logarithm of the surviving fraction of cells is plotted as a function of time of exposure to given temperatures above 41°C, the resulting cell survival curve is similar to that resulting from radiation exposure (Fig. 69–50). An initial shoulder region for short exposure times is followed by a linear portion representing cell killing that is an exponential function of time.[11] At temperatures below 42.5°C, the rate of cell killing diminishes with exposure times longer than about 200 minutes, providing evidence of the development of thermotolerance, a fundamentally important and universal phenome-

non.[12] For a given effect, such as the percentage of cell killing, the exposure time must be reduced by one half for each 1°C increase in temperature. For temperatures below 42.5°C in thermotolerant cells, the heating time must be reduced by about one half for each 0.5°C increase in temperature for an isoeffect.

Thermal sensitivity varies during the cell cycle. Chinese hamster ovary (CHO) cells exhibit the greatest thermal sensitivity during M and S phases, and mild thermal exposure of CHO causes a cell cycle delay in G₂ of about 6 hours.[13,13a,14] Relative thermal sensitivity varies with different cell lines and is not correlated with radiation sensitivity.[15] Earlier reports suggested erroneously that malignant cells were intrinsically more thermally sensitive than normal cells, but the

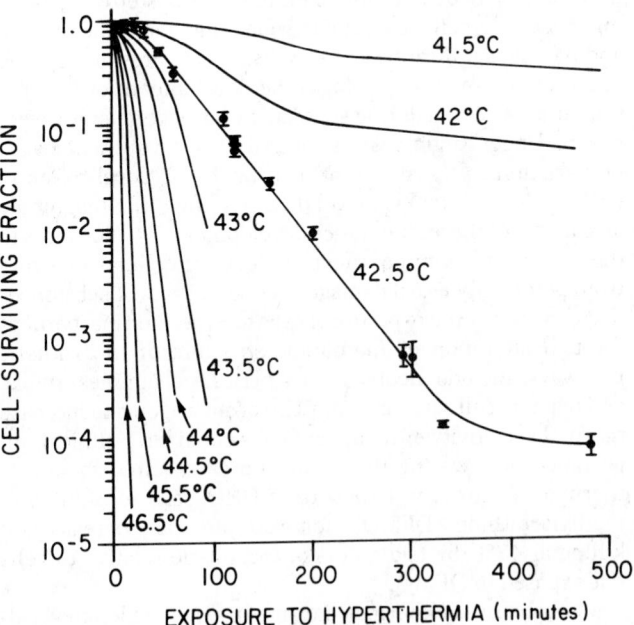

FIGURE 69–50. Survival curves for Chinese hamster ovary cells in vitro exposed to various temperatures for different periods. Similar to radiation survival curves, there is a shoulder and an exponential portion. Prolonged exposure to 42.5°C and below leads to flattening of the curves with minimal further cell killing, corresponding to thermotolerance induction. (Modified from Dewey W, Hopwood L, Sapareto S, et al. Cellular responses to combinations of hyperthermia and radiation. Radiology 1977;123:463–474)

altered physiologic milieu of malignant cells in vivo may lead to thermal sensitization relative to normal cells.[16,17] The shoulder of the survival curve of preheated cells is reproduced with a second exposure, implying recovery from sublethal damage produced with the first exposure. Part of this recovery is separate from thermotolerance induction.[18]

The ratio of slopes of survival curves for preheated and single heated cells, respectively, gives a thermotolerance ratio (TTR) that varies as a function of the fractionation interval. Exposure to temperatures above 42.5°C for more than 30 minutes induces a maximal TTR at 6 to 16 hours, after the first or priming exposure. This effect requires at least 24 hours for complete decay in L1A2 cells.[19] The magnitude and kinetics of thermotolerance vary with cell lines and may vary within subclonogenic lines.[20,21]

Acidic pH inhibits the magnitude and rate of expression of thermotolerance, although the pH effects in cells adapted to low pH are less marked.[22-24] Intracellular, not extracellular, pH determines the thermosensitivity of cells.[24a] Induction of thermotolerance is associated temporally with synthesis of proteins with molecular masses in the range of 20 to 100 kd, particularly 70 kd, which are called heat shock proteins (HSP).[25-27] If these proteins are induced by agents other than heat, cells can become thermotolerant. Whether the HSP are enzymes or structural proteins is unknown. HSP are highly conserved in prokaryotic and eukaryotic cells, suggesting an important role of the HSP in the cellular stress response.[27a] A possible function is that HSP may participate in "rescuing" denatured proteins.[28]

Other agents and conditions can modify the cellular effects of hyperthermia from those illustrated in Figure 69–50. Incubation of cells at temperatures from 40°C to 43°C after an initial exposure of 45°C for 20 minutes (*i.e.,* "step down heating") leads to cell survival curves lacking a shoulder region and having significantly increased slopes.[29] Presumably, the initial exposure at 45°C blocks the development of thermotolerance observed during subsequent lower temperature exposure. Under conditions controlled for pH and nutrient levels, no variation in thermal sensitivity with PO_2 level exists in CHO cells, and the PO_2 level does not affect the magnitude or kinetics of thermotolerance development.[30,31] Nutrients in the culture medium do affect the level of cellular recovery from potentially lethal damage.[32] Other classes of substances that can modify the exposure of cells to hyperthermia, perhaps through alteration of membrane structure or biosynthetic pathways, include alcohols, anesthetics, polyamines, thiols, and hypoxic cell sensitizers.[7,33] Use of such agents to increase thermal sensitivity of malignant cells could have clinical importance by lowering the temperatures required for direct thermal cytotoxicity. Exposure of CHO cells to α-difluoromethylornithine (DFMO), for example, can increase cell killing at 43°C by two orders of magnitude relative to cells not exposed to DFMO.[34]

Mechanisms of thermal damage are not understood, although effects on the cell membrane and nucleus are associated with heat exposure.[35-37a] An Arrhenius plot analysis gives the energy of activation of the assumed chemical reaction that is rate limiting for thermal cell killing to be about 140 to 150 kilocalories per mole, similar to that required for protein denaturation.[14] This implies that heat-induced aggregation of cellular proteins is involved in cell killing.

A rapid mode of interphase cell death can occur. At lower levels of heat, stressed cells become morphologically abnormal with multinucleation; these are nonclonogenic.[37b,37c] Thermotolerant cells have fewer heat-induced morphologic changes immediately after a second heat challenge, suggesting a protective role of thermotolerance in stabilizing cell structures. Other observations indicate that recovery from heat-induced changes is stimulated in the thermotolerant cell, suggesting induction or activation of repair enzymes by HSP.

EFFECTS OF COMBINED HYPERTHERMIA AND IRRADIATION

In 1963, Belli and Bonti demonstrated temperature dependence of the radiation response of mammalian cells in tissue culture, suggesting thermal lability of enzymes involved in repair of radiation damage.[38] Ben-Hur and colleagues showed that temperature elevation above 41°C increases the slope of the exponential portion of the radiation survival curve of CHO cells, confirming enhancement of lethal damage expression.[39] The effects of incubation at temperatures below 40.5°C after irradiation are principally on the shoulder of the survival curve, indicating a reduced capacity for sublethal damage repair. At 41°C, the shoulder of the survival curve is absent. Survival of CHO cells depends on the sequence of hyperthermia and irradiation, with sixfold lower survival resulting from simultaneous exposure to 42.5°C and irradiation compared with heat preceding or after the irradiation by more than 5 minutes.[40] Thermal radiosensitization is greater for S-phase cells than G_1 cells, complementary to the cell cycle dependence of survival from irradiation alone.[13] Survival also is lower for the very low dose rates typical of brachytherapy than for those used in teletherapy.[41,42] Cell survival with hyperthermia and irradiation depends on intracellular pH; this is of particular significance in vivo, because acid pH also reduces the rate of thermotolerance development at 42°C to 42.5°C.[24,43-46] The effect of thermotolerance on thermal cytotoxicity, radiosensitivity, and thermal radiosensitization is complex, but in general terms, thermotolerance does not modify radiation sensitivity of cells but does decrease direct thermal cytotoxicity and thermal radiosensitization.[47-51]

EFFECTS OF HYPERTHERMIA COMBINED WITH CHEMOTHERAPEUTIC AGENTS

Many chemotherapeutic agents (*e.g.,* doxorubicin, bleomycin, cisplatin, mitomycin C, nitrosoureas) have increased cytotoxicity in vivo with an increase in temperature.[7] When thermotolerance is induced, an associated tolerance for the effects of drugs occurs in some cases.[52,53] Wallner and Li illustrated the importance of the duration of exposure of cells to a drug and heat-drug sequencing.[54] Maximal potentiation with simultaneous exposure also occurs with cyclophosphamide and mitomycin. Although an increased number of DNA crosslinks in CHO cells exposed to cisplatin at 43°C compared with 37°C exists, the precise mechanisms of thermal potentiation of drug effects are not known. In vivo, pH, PO_2, and drug pharmacokinetics can lead to more complex sequencing effects.[54-55d]

Acquired resistance to some chemotherapeutic agents can be partially overcome by hyperthermia, suggesting a role for hyperthermia in treating drug-resistant disease.[55e] Hyperthermia can increase uptake and retention of monoclonal antibodies in solid tumors.[55f]

IN VIVO EFFECTS OF HYPERTHERMIA

Effects of hyperthermia alone or in combination with other agents in vivo have been studied in rodents, large animals, and humans. Many variables can influence the effects of hyperthermia in vivo.[56] Most importantly, blood circulation is a mechanism for transporting heat, affecting the temperatures produced in tissues with heating by any means.[57,58] The amount of blood flow and temperature dependence of flow itself influence the delivery of nutrients to the cells and the metabolic status and pH.[59] Tumor vessels resemble leaky capillaries and venous sinusoids without the vascular smooth muscle that allows normal vasoactivity, such as thermally induced vasodilation.[58] Stasis of blood flow and vascular destruction can occur in tumor microcirculation under conditions that produce only reversible reactive change in normal tissues, creating one of the most important rationales for advantageous differential effects of hyperthermia between tumors and normal tissues. Areas of low blood perfusion in tumors can reach preferentially higher temperatures than normal tissue, further enhancing the differential effects of heat.

Measurements of extracellular pH in animal and human tumors confirm that acidic pH conditions occur in some tumors, presumably from low PO_2 and nutrient levels producing anaerobic glycolysis and high lactic acid levels.[45] The pH shift does not correlate consistently with tumor size, histology, or other characteristics. Glucose infusions to lower tumor pH during hyperthermia may take advantage of increased thermal cytotoxicity, reduced thermotolerance, and reduced recovery from sublethal hyperthermic damage.[60,61]

Thermotolerance occurs in vivo.[62] A priming treatment of 43.5°C for 30 minutes in C3H mammary carcinoma tumors, for example, leads to maximal thermotolerance 16 hours later and a complete decay time of 120 hours.[63] Thermotolerance can also be induced in the tumor vessels.[59a] The implications of thermotolerance development for fractionation of hyperthermia and irradiation in treatment regimens are complex and significant.

The kinetics of repair of sublethal damage and thermotolerance induction and decay in vivo may vary between tumor and normal tissue. Simultaneous irradiation and heat results in equal sensitization of tumor and normal tissue under uniform temperature conditions, producing no therapeutic gain.[64,65] When an interval of at least 2 hours separates radiation and heat, with radiation administered before heat, there is consistently a ratio of enhancement of radiation effect in tumor compared with normal tissue (*i.e.*, therapeutic gain) of 1.2 to 1.5.

The expression of direct thermal injury in normal tissues follows that expected from interphase death of cells rather than postmitotic death as in the case of radiation injury.[37b] Studies involving scoring of development of rodent leg contracture, for instance, show peak damage between 2 and 15 days after hyperthermia, and radiation damage peaks at 20 to 25 days and then progresses for as long as 365 days.[66] This pattern of difference is found in intestinal crypts, testis, and kidney. In normal feline brain, the histologic appearance and

time course of repair of thermal injury are similar to the acute necrosis produced by vascular infarction.[67] In murine jejunal tissue, hyperthermia accelerates the expression and increases the magnitude of late radiation fibrosis.[68]

The threshold for normal tissue injury is sharply marked as a function of time and temperature of exposure. A 20% increase in time of exposure or a 0.5°C increase in temperature in the range of 42.0°C to 45.5°C increases the likelihood of necrosis from 0% to 100% in rodent tissue.[69] Few clinical studies report severe normal tissue thermal injury or potentiation of radiation effects in superficial tissues if there has been careful monitoring of the temperatures achieved and the patients' perceptions. Normal tissue temperatures rarely exceed safe limits of 42°C to 43°C and usually reach highest levels corresponding to locations predictably receiving the greatest power deposition. Hyperthermia techniques causing temperature elevation in deep visceral sites infrequently cause serious injury; however, the potential location and magnitude of temperature elevation is more difficult to predict and is less well perceived by the patient. Little information exists on the toxic or therapeutic in vivo effects of combined hyperthermia and chemotherapeutic agents, although hyperthermia can alter drug pharmacology.[69a–72]

Relating the tissue effects of hyperthermia to a thermal dose is a desirable but elusive goal. From Arrhenius associations, formulas for combinations of time and temperature can be derived that give isoeffects in cultured cells and in animal tissues.[73] The formulas may be useful for comparing clinical treatments, but they do not predict absolute levels of effects, are difficult to apply to nonuniform temperature distributions, do not express effects of fractionated therapy, and may not express correctly the variation of thermal radiosensitization with pH.[74] The use of a thermal isoeffective dose is still investigational.

The prospective, randomized phase III study of Dewhirst and collaborators was one of the most important therapeutic trials in animals.[75] Treatment with combined hyperthermia and radiotherapy produced a statistically significant improvement in freedom from disease progression compared with radiotherapy or hyperthermia alone. The complete response rate and duration were inversely correlated with the tumor volume, but the relative improvement in response was greater for large tumors than small tumors. The average site-nonspecific minimal temperature was the thermal measure best correlating with response; the equivalent of 41.3°C for 30 minutes, plus radiation, nearly doubled the complete response rate from 35% to 65% compared with radiotherapy alone.

TECHNICAL ASPECTS

THERMOMETRY

Typical temperature distributions in tumors are nonuniform. Methods for measuring temperatures are limited in practice to invasive placement of probes at only a few sites, introducing the problem of inferring the overall temperature distribution from spatially limited samples.[76,77] Methods of calculating temperature distributions are being developed but cannot be applied routinely because the principal determinants of temperature rise, absorbed power density, and blood perfusion rate are not accurately known.[78] Proper choice, use, and calibration of thermometers to limit errors of measurement require many different considerations for each hyperthermia technique.[79] Standard practice includes the use of single sensors, multiple sensors, or periodically translated sensors within catheters placed into tumor sites.[80] The selection of the number of sensors and sites of measurement bears directly on the likelihood of sampling prognostically important temperatures or defining prospectively what temperature distributions are required for efficacious treatment. Adherence to quality assurance guidelines can help to systematize treatments.[81]

METHODS OF HEATING

Available heating methods include ultrasound or electromagnetic applicators. The principle of heat production is that energy is absorbed in tissue in doing work against the molecular viscosity or electrical resistance of tissue constituents.[82,83] These dissipative processes causing heat production do not involve ionization, unlike absorption mechanisms for diagnostic and therapeutic radiation. Local heat production results in a temperature rise that depends on the specific heat of the tissue and the heat transport processes of conduction and convection (*i.e.*, blood flow); chemical or metabolic heat production levels are themselves temperature dependent and may contribute to the local temperature rise.[57] Heating methods consist of noninvasive and invasive techniques of depositing power in localized volumes, regional vascular perfusion techniques, and whole-body hyperthermia techniques. Heating superficial tumors in a water bath is common for laboratory study of small rodent tumors, but this technique is inappropriate for bulky human tumors. Special techniques are required for achieving temperature uniformity even in small rodent tumors.[84] Many of these methods have been evaluated in a multiinstitutional effort.[84a]

NONINVASIVE TECHNIQUES

Ultrasound applicators with focused or unfocused stationary beams and with focused scanning beams are available for the frequency range of 0.5 to 10 MHz, for which the penetration depth in tissue varies from about 10 to 0.5 cm, respectively. Lack of ultrasound propagation across air spaces, marked absorption in bone, and reflections from tissue interfaces constitute fundamental problems with ultrasound. The depths of penetration and ability to focus, however, are advantages over electromagnetic techniques, especially for deep-seated tumors.[85,85a]

Electric currents in the frequency range of 0.2 to 13 MHz can be capacitively coupled into tissue to result in resistive heating by using two or more surface electrodes or plates.[82] The currents flow in divergent paths between the plates, and large plates must be used for significant power absorption in deep sites relative to superficial sites near the plates. The power absorption is not focused or localized in tumor, and excessive superficial fat heating is a problem for fat layers thicker than about 1.5 cm. At frequencies of 10 to 30 MHz, current carrying coils external to the body can create an intense magnetic field that in turn induces eddy current flow within the body.[86] The resulting power deposition generally

diminishes with increasing depth, so these techniques are best suited for tumors at superficial and intermediate depths. Radiated electromagnetic fields in the frequency range of 60 to 2450 MHz penetrate to depths of about 15 to 1.5 cm, respectively. Single microwave applicators commonly are limited to heating superficial lesions, and multiapplicator arrays can achieve heating at depth in the body without excessive superficial normal tissue heating.[87]

Sharp focusing of the power is not possible with these techniques, and as with the other electromagnetic approaches, it is necessary to rely on blood perfusion in tumor lower than normal tissue for preferential temperature elevation in tumor.

INVASIVE TECHNIQUES

Interstitial Hyperthermia

Greater localization and control of power deposition within a tumor volume is possible using interstitial techniques that can be combined with conventional interstitial irradiation treatments.[88] Electric current at 0.5 MHz flowing between implanted metallic needles results in resistive heating of intervening tumor.[89] Alternatively, nonmetallic catheters can accommodate miniature microwave antennas operating at 433 to 2450 MHz that radiate power into surrounding tumor.[90] Interstitial ferromagnetic seeds can be heated inductively to produce conductive or "hot source" heating of the implanted tumor.[91]

Regional Vascular Perfusion

Isolation of the major artery and vein of an extremity from the systemic circulation and connection of these vessels to an extracorporeal heated perfusion circuit results in temperature elevation of an entire limb.[92] This approach has been used for treating extremity melanoma and sarcoma with chemotherapy-containing heated perfusates.

Whole-Body Hyperthermia Techniques

Currently used methods of inducing systemic temperature rise depend on limiting the heat loss from the body while inducing heat absorption through conduction across the skin surface from heated water or infrared power absorption.[93-95]

CLINICAL RESULTS

EFFICACY OF COMBINED HYPERTHERMIA AND RADIOTHERAPY

Several studies reported treatment to small superficial metastatic nodules by hyperthermia alone, radiotherapy alone, or combined radiotherapy and hyperthermia. A variety of heating techniques and radiation fractionation schemes was used, and temperature distributions were not always characterized. Despite these problems, there is surprising consistency in results as summarized by Overgaard and as updated in Table 69–48.[98] Complete response rates with hyperthermia alone are about 15%, about 35% with radiotherapy, and about 70% with combined radiotherapy and hyperthermia. The rate of toxicity, principally thermal burns and blisters, is usually about 10%

TABLE 69–48. Complete Response of Superficial Tumors to Treatment

Investigations	Lesions	Total No. of Tumors	Radiotherapy Alone†	Radiotherapy and Hyperthermia†	Significance (p)
Valdagni et al[132] *	Neck nodes	43	36.8%	82.3%	0.015
Arcangeli et al[99,133]	Neck nodes; melanoma mets.	81	42%	79%	<0.05
			14% (24 mo)	58% (24 mo)	<0.05
Steeves et al[134]	Superficial tumors	90	31%	65%	
Lindholm et al[120]	Superficial tumors, superficial matched pairs only	85	25%	46%	
		56	25%	57%	0.0027
Van der Zee et al[121]	Breast cancer recurrences	113	55%	90%	<0.001
Kim et al[122,126]	Melanoma recurrences	97	45%	66%	
Li et al[123]	Superficial tumors	124	29%	53.8%	
	Superficial matched pairs only	62	29%	68%	
Scott et al[131]	Superficial tumors, matched pairs only	62	39%	87%	<0.01
Corry et al[125]	Superficial tumors	21	30%	62%	
Perez et al[101a]	Superficial tumors	218	28%	32%	
	Subset ≤3 cm dia. CR ≥12 mo	48	15%	80%	

* Prospective, randomized trials; *p* values shown when reported.
† Complete response rates.

to 15%. No evidence exists of enhanced late effects of radiotherapy in these studies. These trials have established safety and efficacy for combined treatment in superficial lesions, particularly if prior radiotherapy limits additional doses to suboptimal levels.

Other trials, summarized in Table 69–49, confirm that tumor volume, radiation dose, and measures of minimal tumor temperature are prognostic factors for response to hyperthermia and radiotherapy. Arcangeli and coworkers found a highly significant correlation of complete response rate with minimal thermal isoeffective dose.[99] Dunlop and colleagues found improvement in response rates from 35% to 86% with at least two hyperthermia treatments in which a tumor minimal isoeffective dose of 20 minutes at the equivalent of 43°C (Eq 43) was achieved.[100] Kapp and coworkers randomized prospectively treatment to small superficial lesions with radiotherapy plus two or six weekly fractions of hyperthermia and observed no differences in complete response rate or duration of response.[101] Perez and colleagues found no overall difference in complete response rates of tumors treated with radiotherapy or radiotherapy plus hyperthermia treatment and argued that poorly defined criteria for matching microwave applicators to tumor size resulted in inadequate treatment of tumors larger than 3 cm in diameter.[101a] These researchers proposed that quality assurance and control for hyperthermia treatments would be essential for obtaining good results.

For superficial tumors treated with radiotherapy plus one or two hyperthermia treatments per week, the complete response rate depended greatly on the cumulative time for which 90% of intratumoral temperatures exceeded 40.5°C.[101b]

These results imply that the number of hyperthermia treatments is less important for complete response than the cumulative duration and extent of temperature elevation.[101b–d] Radiation dose is important, and in specific diseases, many other prognostic factors may be important.[101e,101f] The use of frequency distribution of temperature parameters (*e.g.*, temperature exceeded by 10% or 50% of tumor temperatures) and cumulative time may provide the basis for a hyperthermia treatment dosimetry.[102]

TABLE 69–49. Prognostic Variables for Complete Response to Hyperthermia and Radiotherapy

Investigations	Prognostic Variables
Kim et al[122,126]	Volume, radiation dose/fx, T_{min}
Dewhirst and Sim[75]	Volume, T_{min} (not site specific)
Oleson et al[105]	Volume, radiation dose, T_{min} averaged over all treatments, HT technique
Sim et al[127]	Volume, radiation dose, HT technique, number of intratumoral sites ≥ 42.5°C
Arcangeli et al[99,133]	Volume, minimum equivalent time at 42.5°C
Luk et al[128]	Total radiation dose, recurrence status, minimum daily average temperature, volume
Van der Zee et al[130]	Mean minimum tumor temperature
Dunlop et al[100]	Number of HT treatments for which T_{min} ≥ 20 min equals 43
Scott et al[124,131]	T_{ave} ≥ 43°C, greatest tumor diameter, site and histology
Kapp et al[101,101e]	Histology, radiation dose, volume; mean T_{min} (borderline significance); no dependence on 2 vs 6 HT treatments
Leopold et al[101b]	Cumulative min for T_{90} ≥ 40.5°C, radiation dose, tumor depth

HT, hyperthermia treatment.

EVALUATION OF HYPERTHERMIA FOR DEEP TUMORS

The reported trials on superficial tumors define important biologic aspects of treatment with hyperthermia and radiotherapy. Control of bulky deep locoregional disease, however, limits the curability of many common human tumors.[103] Development and phase I equipment evaluation for inducing hyperthermia in deep sites, especially interstitial techniques, magnetic induction coils, and capacitively coupled plates, annular microwave phased arrays, and focused ultrasound, is the subject of extensive current investigation.[104] If deep sites can be implanted, interstitial hyperthermia techniques can provide higher average temperatures than noninvasive techniques.[105] Toxicity is similar to irradiation alone, except that in pelvic sites, tumor necrosis and slough can occur acutely, precipitating development of fistulas.

Trials using a commercially available magnetic induction coil (Magnetrode) that included extensive temperature measurements revealed that most intratumoral sites do not exceed 42°C to 43°C with this device, although marked temperature elevation in core regions of bulky tumors is possible, presumably because of low blood perfusion.[107,108] Japanese investigators reported clinical testing of capacitively coupled radiofrequency devices (13.6 MHz and 8 MHz), and a report of multipoint measurements in 60 deep-seated tumors revealed a maximal tumor center temperature of more than 43°C in 38% of tumors, a lowest intratumoral temperature of more than 42°C in 11%, and temperature variation greater than 2°C in 81%.[109,109a,110] Localized pain was the major power-limiting factor.[111] The capacitively coupled radiofrequency device can produce significant temperature rise in deep tumors at a variety of anatomic locations with limited toxicity and with significant nonuniformity of the temperature distribution.

Investigators at the University of Utah have extensively evaluated an annular microwave array (AA) for heating intraabdominal and pelvic malignancies.[108,112,112a] Measurement of temperature distributions across at least one tumor diameter was typical. In pelvic tumors, pain during the hyperthermia treatments occurred in most of 43 patients, and there were 8 patients with serious late complications. In 73% of 175 treatments for 43 patients, temperatures over 42°C were achieved. Applied electromagnetic power levels were limited by patient discomfort and safety considerations. Serious toxicity with these techniques has been infrequent. In deep sites, most of the tumor volume may not reach temperatures and durations of temperature elevation sufficient to result in direct thermal cytotoxicity, and enhancement of radiation effect by hyperthermia may be more limited than is evident in superficial tumors.[112b,112c] Determining the extent and distribution of temperature elevation and number of treatments needed for significant improvement in local control compared with radiation alone will require prospective studies.

Study of focused ultrasound for treatments of deep tumors has been limited. Lele used scanned focused ultrasound transducers to treat tumors at depths of 12 cm with volumes up to about $10 \times 10 \times 10$ cm.[85] The incidence of pain from bone or periosteum heating and other toxic effects was negligible, and the desired temperature of 43°C were achieved in 43 of 44 tumors in 30 patients. Similar success has been demonstrated by others.[113]

Few reports exist using electromagnetically produced locoregional hyperthermia with chemotherapy. A trial of ifosfamide plus etoposide combined with hyperthermia for soft tissue sarcoma and bone sarcoma did show activity (complete responses in 6 of 38 patients) and temperature parameters such as T_{20mean}, T_{90mean}, and T_{50mean} (*i.e.*, mean temperature exceeded by 20%, 90%, 50% of monitored sites) correlated with outcome.[69b,69c]

Most reports of whole-body hyperthermia have been phase I trials that showed considerable toxicity. However, a radiant heating device has allowed routine heating of mildly sedated patients to 41.8°C for 2 hours with minimal toxicity.[94] This device promises to facilitate more systematic study of whole-body hyperthermia with chemotherapy and localized radiotherapy. Selection of a chemotherapeutic agent for which there is clear evidence of therapeutic gain with whole-body hyperthermia is difficult. Carboplatin with whole-body hyperthermia improved therapeutic gain in rat tumors.[69a] Altered pharmacokinetics of systemic agents, acid pH in tumors, and thermal modulation of macrophage activity are factors that can be exploited for therapeutic gain.[114,115]

TRENDS IN HYPERTHERMIA

There has been considerable progress in analyzing mechanisms of action of hyperthermia alone and in combination of chemotherapy and irradiation. Significant potentiation of some chemotherapeutic agents and radiation is possible, and efficacy of thermoradiotherapy has been demonstrated in small superficial tumors. Research supports a strong rationale for hyperthermia in cancer therapy.

It is pertinent to question why clinical testing of hyperthermia treatment has not led to more demonstrations of efficacy over the last 10 to 15 years and why most clinical trials of hyperthermia treatment are still phase I feasibility and toxicity studies. To demonstrate dose-effect relations (phase II), it is necessary to establish a dosimetry system. This has been difficult for temperature distributions that are typically highly nonuniform. Even the sophisticated technology for measuring temperatures at multiple intratumoral sites has been developed only with difficulty in recent years; in early trials, the temperature at only one site in a tumor may have been monitored, and this approach gives no indication whatsoever of spatial nonuniformity of tumor temperature. After a dosimetry system is established, there must be heating devices available that are capable of producing and controlling the desired temperature distribution. In general, electromagnetic heating systems do not produce highly focused power deposition in tumors, and applied power levels are limited by excessive normal tissue temperatures rather than tumor temperatures. The marked limitations of heating devices have been recognized slowly and in retrospect. Concepts of thermal dosimetry are being developed that may provide a basis for treatment prescription.[102]

Many of these problems can be addressed through adequate quality assurance programs, and the importance of such programs was recognized in a series of articles.[81,116–119] Lack of quality assurance guidelines in the past has contributed to the difficulty of performing meaningful single or multiple institutional trials.

There is little justification for phase III trials of hyperthermia until a dose-response relation has been demonstrated for the tumor studied and until there is demonstration that the desired thermal dose can be delivered routinely to the tumor site being studied.

REFERENCES

1. Coley-Nauts H, Swife W, Coley B. The treatment of malignant tumors by bacterial toxins as developed by the late William B. Coley, M.D., reviewed in light of modern research. Cancer Res 1946;6:205–216.
2. Susskind C. The "story" of nonionizing radiation research. Bull N Y Acad Med 1979;55: 1152–1163.
3. Westermark N. The effect of heat upon rat-tumors. Skandin Arch F Physiol 1927;52: 257–322.
4. Rohdenburg GL, Prime F. The effect of combined radiation and heat on neoplasms. Arch Surg 1921;2:116–129.
5. Selawry OS, Carlson JC, Moore GE. Tumor response to ionizing rays at elevated temperatures. AJR 1958;80:833–839.
6. Crile G Jr. The effects of heat and radiation on cancers implanted on the feet of mice. Cancer Res 1963;23:372–380.
7. Hahn GM. Hyperthermia in cancer. New York: Plenum Press, 1982.
8. Urano M, Double EB, eds. Hyperthermia and oncology, vols 1 and 2. Zeist, Netherlands: VSP, 1988.
9. Hand JW, James JR, eds. Physical techniques in clinical hyperthermia. Letchworth, England: Research Studies Press, 1986.
10. Oleson JR, Calderwood SR, Coughlin CT, et al. Biological and clinical aspects of hyperthermia in cancer therapy. Am J Clin Oncol 1988;11:368–380.
11. Dewey WC, Hopwood LE, Sapareto SA, et al. Cellular responses to combinations of hyperthermia and radiation. Radiology 1977;123:463–474.
12. Gerner E, Schneider M. Induced thermal resistance in HeLa cells. Nature 1976;256: 500–502.
13. Westra A, Dewey WC. Variation in sensitivity to heat shock during the cell-cycle of Chinese hamster cells in vitro. Int J Radiat Biol 1971;19:467–477.
13a. Dewey WC, XiLian L, Wong RSL. Cell killing, chromosomal aberrations, and division delay as thermal sensitivity is modified during the cell cycle. Radiat Res 1990;122: 268–274.
14. Sapareto SA, Hopwood LE, Dewey WC, et al. Effects of hyperthermia on survival and progression of chinese hamster ovary cells. Cancer Res 1978;38:393–400.
15. Gerweck LE, Burlett P. The lack of correlation between heat and radiation sensitivity in mammalian cells. Int J Radiat Oncol Biol Phys 1978;4:283–285.
16. Giovanella BC, Stehlin JS Jr, Morgan AC. Selective lethal effect of supranormal temperatures on human neoplastic cells. Cancer Res 1976;36:3944–3950.
17. Overgaard J, Nielsen OS. The role of tissue environmental factors on the kinetics and morphology of tumor cells exposed to hyperthermia. Ann N Y Acad Sci 1980;335: 254–278.
18. Nielsen OS, Overgaard J. Effect of extracellular pH on thermotolerance and recovery of hyperthermic damage in vitro. Cancer Res 1979;39:2772–2778.
19. Nielsen OS, Overgaard J. Influence of time and temperature on the kinetics of thermotolerance in L1A2 cells in vitro. Cancer Res 1982;42:4190–4196.
20. Rofstad EK, Midthjell H, Brustad T. Heat sensitivity and thermotolerance in cells from five human melanoma xenografts. Cancer Res 1984;44:4347–4354.
21. Leith JT, Bliven SF, Glicksman AS. Similarity of thermotolerance characteristics in heterogeneous human colon tumor subpopulations after exposure to fractionated heat doses (44°C). Radiat Res 1985;104:128–139.
22. Gerweck LE. Modification of cell lethality at elevated temperatures: The pH effect. Radiat Res 1977;70:224–235.
23. Holahan PK, Dewey WC. Effect of pH and cell cycle progression on development and decay of thermotolerance. Radiat Res 1986;106:111–121.
24. Hahn GM, Shiu EC. Adaptation to low pH modifies thermal and thermochemical responses of mammalian cells. Int J Hyperthermia 1986;2:379–387.
24a. Chu GL, Wang Z, Hyun WC, et al. The role of intracellular pH and its variance in low pH sensitization of killing by hyperthermia. Radiat Res 1990;122:288–293.
25. Hahn GM, Li GC. Thermotolerance and heat shock proteins in mammalian cells. Radiat Res 1982;92:452–457.
26. Li GC. Elevated levels of 70,000 Dalton heat shock protein in transiently thermotolerant chinese hamster fibroblasts and in their stable heat resistant variants. Int J Radiat Oncol Biol Phys 1985;11:165–177.
27. Lindquist SL. The heat shock response. Ann Rev Biochem 1986;55:535–572.
27a. Carper SW, Duffy JJ, Gerner EW. Heat shock proteins in thermotolerance and other cellular processes. Cancer Res 1987;47:5249–5255.
28. Pelham HRB. Speculations on the function of the major heat shock proteins. Cell 1986;46:959–961.
29. Henle KJ. Sensitization to hyperthermia below 43°C induced in Chinese hamster ovary cells by step-down heating. JNCI 1980;64:1479–1483.
30. Gerweck LE, Richards B, Jennings M. The influence of variable oxygen concentration on the response of cells to heat or x-irradiation. Radiat Res 1981;85:314–320.
31. Gerweck LE, Bascomb F. Influence of hypoxia on the development of thermotolerance. Radiat Res 1982;90:356–361.
32. Li GC, Shiu EC, Hahn GM. Recovery of cells from heat-induced potentially lethal damage: Effects of pH and nutrient environment. Int J Radiat Oncol Biol Phys 1980;6: 577–582.
33. Stone HB, Dewey WC. Biologic basis and clinical potential of local-regional hyperthermia. In: Phillips T, Wara W, eds. Radiation oncology, vol 2. New York: Raven Press, 1987:1–41.
34. Fuller DJM, Gerner EW. Sensitization of chinese hamster ovary cells to heat shock by alpha-difluoromethylornithine. Cancer Res 1987;47:816–820.
35. Lepcock JR. Involvement of membranes in cellular responses to hyperthermia. Radiat Res 1982;92:433–438.
36. Konings AWT, Ruifrok ACC. Role of membrane lipids and membrane fluidity in thermosensitivity and thermotolerance of mammalian cells. Radiat Res 1985;102: 86–98.
37. Roti Roti JL, Uygur N, Higashikubo R. Nuclear protein following heat shock: Protein removal kinetics and cell cycle rearrangements. Radiat Res 1986;107:250–261.
37a. Dewey WC. Failla Memorial Lecture: The search for criticial cellular targets damaged by heat. Radiat Res 1989;120:191–204.
37b. Vidair CA, Dewey WC. Two distinct modes of hyperthermic cell death. Radiat Res 1988;116:157–171.
37c. Borrelli MJ, Thompson LL, Cain CA, Dewey WC. Time-temperature analysis of cell killing of BHK cells heated at temperatures in the range of 43.5°C to 57.0°C. Int J Radiat Oncol Biol Phys 1990;19:389–399.
38. Belli JA, Bonte FJ. Influence of temperature on the radiation response of mammalian cells in tissue culture. Radiat Res 1963;18:272–276.
39. Ben-Hur E, Elkind MM, Bronk BV. Thermally enhanced radioresponse of cultured chinese hamster cells: Inhibition of repair of sublethal damage and enhancement of lethal damage. Radiat Res 1974;58:38–51.
40. Sapareto S, Raaphorst G, Dewey WC. Cell killing and the sequencing of hyperthermia and radiation. Int J Radiat Oncol Biol Phys 1979;5:343–347.
41. Spiro IJ, McPherson S, Cook JA, et al. Sensitization of low-dose rate irradiation by nonlethal hyperthermia. Radiat Res 1991;127:111–114.
42. Jones EL, Lyons BE, Double EB, Dain BJ. Thermal enhancement of low dose rate irradiation in a murine tumour system. Int J Hyperthermia 1989;5:509–523.
43. Gillette EL, Ensley BS. Effect of heat, radiation, and pH on mouse mammary tumor cells. Int J Radiat Oncol Biol Phys 1983;9:1521–1525.
44. Wike-Hooley JL, Haveman J, Reinhold HS. The relevance of tumour pH to the treatment of malignant disease. Radiother Oncol 1984;2:343–366.
45. Thistlethwaite AJ, Leeper DB, Moylan DJ III, et al. pH distribution in human tumors. Int J Radiat Oncol Biol Phys 1985;11:1647–1652.
46. Chu GL, Wang Z, Hyun WC, et al. The role of intracellular pH and its variance in low pH sensitization of killing by hyperthermia. Radiat Res 1990;122:288–293.
47. Haveman J. Influence of pH and thermotolerance on the enhancement of x-ray induced inactivation of cultured mammalian cells by hyperthermia. Int J Radiat Biol 1983;43: 281–289.
48. Holahan EV, Highfield DP, Holahan PK, et al. Hyperthermic killing and hyperthermic radiosensitization in Chinese hamster ovary cells: Effects of pH and thermal tolerance. Radiat Res 1984;97:108–131.
49. Holahan PK, Dewey WC. Effect of pH and cell cycle progression on development and decay of thermotolerance. Radiat Res 1986;106:111–121.
50. Haveman J, Luinenburg M, Wondergem J, et al. Effects of hyperthermia on the linear and quadratic parameters of the radiation survival curve of mammalian cells: Influence of thermotolerance. Int J Radiat Biol 1987;51:561–565.
51. Wynstra JH, Wright WD, Roti JL. Repair of radiation-induced DNA damage in thermotolernce and nonthermotolerant LeLa cells. Radiat Res 1990;124:85–89.
52. Morgan JE, Honess DJ, Bleehen NM. The interaction of thermal tolerance with drug cytotoxicity in vitro. Br J Cancer 1979;39:422–428.
53. Herman TS, Sweets CC, White DM, et al. Effect of heating on lethality due to hyperthermia and selected chemotherapeutic drugs. JNCI 1982;68:487–491.
54. Wallner KE, Li GC. Effect of drug exposure duration and sequencing on hyperthermic potentiation of mitomycin-C and cisplatin. Cancer Res 1987;47:493–495.
55. Meyn RE, Corry PM, Fletcher SE, et al. Thermal enhancement of DNA damage in mammalian cells treated with cis-diaminadichloroplatinum(II). Cancer Res 1980;40: 1136–1139.
55a. Double EB, Jones EL, Kellogg KC, Van Buren T. Treatment sequence effects of combined cisplatin and hyperthermia in a murine tumor system. Hyperthermic oncology, 1988, vol 1, summary papers. London: Taylor & Francis, 1989:221–222.
55b. Herman TS, Teicher BA, Holden SA. Trimodality therapy (drug/hyperthermia/radiation) with BCNU or Mitomycin C. Int J Radiat Oncol Biol Phys 1990;18:375–382.
55c. Raaphorst GP, Feeley MM, Martin L. Enhancement of sensitivity to hyperthermia by lonidamine in human cancer cells. Int J Hypethermia 1991;7:763–772.
55d. Herman TS, Teicher BA, Collins LS. Effect of hypoxia and acidosis on the cytotoxicity of four platinum complexes at normal and hyperthemric temperatures. Cancer Res 1988;48:2342–2347.
55e. Laskowitz DT, Elion GB, Dewhirst MW, et al. Hyperthermia-induced ehancement of melphalan activity against a melphalan-resistant human rhabdomyosarcoma xenograft. Radiat Res 1992;129:218–223.
55f. Cope DA, Dewhirst MW, Friedman HS, et al. Enhanced delivery of a monoclonal antibody (Fab′) 2 fragment to subcutaneous human glioma xenografts using local hyperthermia. Cancer Res 1990;50:1803–1809.
56. Urano M, Gerweck LE, Epstein R, et al. Response of a spontaneous murine tumor to hyperthermia: Factors which modify the thermal response in vivo. Radiat Res 1980;83:312–322.
57. Jain RK, Ward-Hartley K. Tumor blood flow—Characterization, modifications, and role in hyperthermia. IEEE Trans Sonics Ultrasonics 1984;SU-31:504–526.

58. Reinhold HS, Endrich B. Tumor microcirculation as a target for hyperthermia. Int J Hyperthermia 1986;2:111–137.

59. Streffer C. Metabolic changes during and after hyperthermia. Int J Hyperthermia 1985;1:305–319.

59a. Song CW, Chelstrom LM, Sung JH. Effects of a second heating on blood flow in tumors. Radiat Res 1990;122:66–71.

60. Ward-Hartley KA, Jain RK. Effect of glucose and galactose on microcirculatory flow in normal and neoplastic tissues in rabbits. Cancer Res 1987;47:371–377.

61. Thistlethwaite AJ, Alexander GA, Moylan DJ III, et al. Modification of human tumor pH by elevation of blood glucose. Int J Radiat Oncol Biol Phys 1987;13:603–610.

62. Urano M. Kinetics of thermotolerance in normal and tumor tissues: A review. Cancer Res 1986;46:474–482.

63. Nielsen OS, Overgaard J, Kamura T. Influence of thermotolerance on the interaction between hyperthermia and radiation in a solid tumor in vivo. Br J Radiol 1983;56:267–273.

64. Dewey WC, Freeman ML, Raaphorst GP, et al. Cell biology of hyperthermia and radiation. In: Meyn RE, Withers HR, eds. Radiation biology in cancer research. New York: Raven Press, 1980:589–621.

65. Overgaard J. Simultaneous and sequential hyperthermia and radiation treatment of an experimental tumor and its surrounding normal tissue in vivo. Int J Radiat Oncol Biol Phys 1980;6:1507–1517.

66. Stone HB, Harding RP. Reversible injury after mild hyperthermia. Int J Radiat Oncol Biol Phys 1986;12:823–827.

67. Lyons BE, Obona WG, Borcich JK, et al. Chronic histological effects of ultrasonic hyperthermia on normal feline brain tissue. Radiat Res 1986;106:234–251.

68. Peck JW, Gibbs FA Jr. Assay of premorbid murine jejunal fibrosis based on mechanical changes after x-irradiation and hyperthermia. Radiat Res 1987;112:525–543.

69. Morris CC, Meyers R, Field SB. The response of the rat tail to hyperthermia. Br J Radiol 1977;50:576–580.

69a. Ohno S, Siddik ZH, Baba H, et al. Effect of carboplatin combined with whole body hyperthermia on normal tissue and tumor in rats. Cancer Res 1991;51:2994–3000.

69b. Issels RD, Wadepohl M, Tiling K, et al. Regional hyperthermia combined with systemic chemotherapy in advanced abdominal and pelvic tumors: First results of a pilot study employing an annular phased array applicator. Rec Res Cancer Res 1988;107:236–243.

69c. Issels RD, Prenninger SW, Nagele A, et al. Ifosfamide plus etoposide combined with regional hyperthermia in patients with loclly advanced sarcomas: A phase II study. J Clin Oncol 1990;8:1818–1829.

70. Marmor JB. Interactions of hyperthermia and chemotherapy in animals. Cancer Res 1979;39:2269–2276.

71. Zakris EL, Dewhirst MW, Riviere JE, et al. Pharmacokinetics and toxicity of intraperitoneal cisplatin combined with regional hyperthermia. J Clin Oncol 1987;5:1613–1620.

72. Page RL, Thrall DE, George SL, et al. Quantitative estimation of the thermal dose-modifying factor for cis-diamminedichloroplatinum (CDDP) in tumor-bearing dogs. Int J Hyperthermia 1992;8:761–769.

73. Field SB. Studies relevant to a means of quantifying the effects of hyperthermia. Int J Hyperthermia 1987;3:291–296.

74. Overgaard J. Some problems related to the clinical use of thermal isoeffect doses. Int J Hyperthermia 1987;3:329–336.

75. Dewhirst MW, Sim DA. The utility of thermal dose as a predictor of tumor and normal tissue responses to combined radiation and hyperthermia. Cancer Res 1984;44:4772s–4780s.

76. Fessenden P, Lee ER, Samulski TV. Direct temperature measurement. Cancer Res 1984;44:4799s–4804s.

77. Divrik AM, Roemer RB, Cetas TC. Inference of complete temperature fields from a few measured temperatures: An unconstrained optimization method. IEEE Trans Biomed Eng 1984;31:150–160.

78. Strohbehn JW, Roemer RB. A survey of computer simulations of hyperthermia treatments. IEEE Trans Biomed Eng 1984;31:136–149.

79. Cetas TC. Thermometry. In: Lehmann JR, ed. Therapeutic heat and cold. 3rd ed. Baltimore: Williams & Wilkins, 1982:35–69.

80. Gibbs FA Jr. Thermal mapping in experimental cancer treatment with hyperthermia: Description and use of a semiautomatic system. Int J Radiat Oncol Biol Phys 1983;9:1057–1063.

81. Dewhist MW, Phillips TL, Samulski TV, et al. RTOG quality assurance guidelines for clinical trials using hyperthermia. Int J Radiat Oncol Biol Phys 1990;18:1249–1259.

82. Guy AW. Biophysics of high frequency currents and electromagnetic radiation. In: Lehmann JF, ed. Therapeutic heat and cold. 3rd ed. Baltimore: Williams & Wilkins, 1982:199–277.

83. Frizzell LA, Dunn F. Biophysics of Ultrasound. In: Lehmann JF, ed. Therapeutic heat and cold. 3rd ed. Baltimore: Williams & Wilkins, 1982:353–385.

84. Gibbs FA Jr, Peck JW, Dethlefsen LA. The importance of temperature uniformity in the study of radiosensitizing effects of hyperthermia in vivo. Radiat Res 1981;87:187–197.

84a. Final report on the NCI hyperthermia equipment evaluation contractors group, part 1. London: Taylor & Francis, In: J Hyperthermia [Special issue] 1988;4:1–132.

85. Lele PP. Physical aspects and clinical studies with ultrasonic hyperthermia. In: Storm FK, ed. Hyperthermia in cancer therapy. Boston: GK Hall Medical, 1983:333–365.

85a. Ebbini ES, Cain CA. A spherical-section ultrasound phased array applicator for deep localized hyperthermia. IEEE Trans Biomed Eng 1991;38:634–643.

86. Oleson JR. A review of magnetic induction methods for hyperthermia treatment of cancer. IEEE Trans Biomed Eng 1984;31:91–97.

87. Bach Andersen J. Regional electromagnetic heating. In: Hand JW, James JR, eds. Physical techniques in clinical hyperthermia. Letchworth, England: Research Studies Press, 1986:65–97.

88. Oleson JR. Interstitial hyperthermia. In: Withers HR, Peters LJ, eds. Innovations in Radiation Oncology Research. Berlin: Springer-Verlag, 1987:303–312.

89. Joseph C, Astrahan M, Lipsett J, et al. Interstitial hyperthermia and interstitial iridium-192 implantation: A technique and preliminary results. Int J Radiat Oncol Biol Phys 1981;7:827–833.

90. Lyons BE, Britt RH, Strohbehn JW. Localized hyperthermia in the treatment of malignant brain tumors using an interstitial microwave antenna array. IEEE Trans Biomed Eng 1984;31:53–62.

91. Stea B, Cetas TC, Cassady JR. Interstitial thermoradiotherapy of brain tumors: Preliminary results of a phase I clinical trial. Int J Radiat Oncol Biol Phys 1990;19:1463–1471.

92. Cavaliere R, Mondovi B, Moricca G, et al. Regional perfusion hyperthermia. In: Storm FK, ed. Hyperthermia in cancer therapy. Boston: GK Hall Medical, 1983:369–399.

93. Bull J, Lees D, Schuette W, et al. Whole body hyperthermia: A phase I trial of a potential adjuvant to chemotherapy. Ann Intern Med 1979;90:317–323.

94. Robins HI, Dennis WH, Neville AJ, et al. A nontoxic system for 41.8°C whole body hyperthermia: Results of a phase I study using a radiant heat device. Cancer Res 1985;45:3937–3944.

95. Parks L, Minaberry C, Smith D, et al. Treatment of far advanced bronchogenic carcinoma by extracorporeally induced systemic hyperthermia. J Thorac Cardiovasc Surg 1979;78:883–892.

98. Overgaard J. Rationale and problems in the design of clinical studies. In: Overgaard J, ed. Hyperthermic oncology 1984, vol 2. London: Taylor & Francis, 1985:325–338.

99. Arcangeli G, Benassi M, Cividalli A, et al. Radiotherapy and hyperthermia. Analysis of clinical results and identification of prognostic variables. Cancer 1987;60:950–956.

100. Dunlop PRC, Hand JW, Dickinson RJ, et al. An assessment of local hyperthermia in clinical practice. Int J Hyperthermia 1986;2:39–50.

101. Kapp DS, Petersen IVA, Cox RS. Two or six hyperthermia treatments as an adjunct to radiation therapy yield similar tumor responses: Results of a randomized trial. Int J Radiat Oncol Biol Phys 1990;19:1481–1495.

101a. Perez CA, Gillespie B, Pajak T, et al. Quality assurance problems in clinical hyperthermia and their impact on therapeutic outcome: A report by the Radiation Therapy Oncology Group. Int J Radiat Oncol Biol Phys 1989;16:551–558.

101b. Leopold KL, Dewhirst MW, Samulski TV, et al. Cumulative minutes with T_{90} greater than Temp index is predictive of response to hyperthermia and radiation. Int J Radiat Oncol Biol Phys 1993 (in press).

101c. Oleson JR, Dewhirst MW, Harrelson JM, et al. Tumor temperature distributions predict hypethermia effect. Int J Radiat Oncol Biol Phys 1989;16:559–570.

101d. Leopold KA, Dewhirst M, Samulski T, et al. Relationship among tumor temperature, treatment time, and histopathological outcome using preoperative hyperthermia with radiation in soft tissue sarcoma. Int J Radiat Oncol Biol Phys 1992;27:989–998.

101e. Kapp DS, Barnett TA, Cox RS. Hyperthermia and radiation therapy of local-regional recurrent breast cancer: Prognostic factors for response and local control of diffuse or nodular tumors. Int J Radiat Oncol Biol Phys 1991;20:1147–1164.

101f. Valdagni R, Liu F-F, Kapp DS. Important prognostic factors influencing outcome of combined radiation and hyperthermia. Int J Radiat Oncol Biol Phys 1988;15:959–972.

102. Oleson JR, Samulski TV, Leopold KA, et al. Sensitivity of hyperthermia trial outcomes to temperature and time: Implications for thermal goals of treatment. Int J Radiat Oncol Biol Phys 1993 (in press).

103. Kapp DS. Site and disease selection for hyperthermia clinical trials. Int J Hyperthermia 1986;2:139–156.

104. Gibbs FA Jr. Regional hyperthermia: A clinical appraisal of noninvasive deep-heating methods. Cancer Res 1984;44:4765s–4770s.

105. Oleson JR, Sim DA, Manning MR. Analysis of prognostic variables in hyperthermia treatment of 161 patients. Int J Radiat Oncol Biol Phys 1984;10:2231–2239.

107. Oleson JR, Manning MR, Heusinkveld RS. Hyperthermia by magnetic induction: II. Clinical experience with concentric electrodes. Int J Radiat Oncol Biol Phys 1984;10:2231–2239.

108. Sapozink MD, Gibbs FA Jr, Thomson JW, et al. A comparison of deep regional hyperthermia from an annular phased array and a concentric coil in the same patients. Int J Radiat Oncol Biol Phys 1985;11:179–190.

109. Abe M, Hiraoka M, Takahashi M, et al. Multi-institutional studies on hyperthermia using an 8-MHz radiofrequency capacitive heating device (Thermotron RF-8) in combination with radiation for cancer therapy. Cancer 1986;58:1589–1595.

109a. Kakehi M, Ueda K, Mukojima T, et al. Multi-institutional clinical studies on hyperthermia combined with radiotherapy or chemotherapy in advanced cancer of deep-seated organs. Int J Hyperthermia 1990;6:719–740.

110. Hiraoka M, Shiken J, Alzuta K, et al. Radiofrequency capacitive hyperthermia for deep-seated tumors. I. Studies on thermometry. Cancer 1987;60:121–127.

111. Hiraoka M, Shiken J, Akuta K, et al. Radiofrequency capacitive hyperthermia for deep-seated tumors. II. Effects of thermoradiotherapy. Cancer 1987;60:128–135.

112. Sapozink MD, Gibbs FA Jr, Egger MJ, et al. Regional hyperthermia for clinically advanced deep-seated pelvic malignancy. J Clin Oncol 1986;9:162–169.

112a. Sapozink MD, Joszef G, Astrahan MA, et al. Adjuvant pelvic hyperthermia in advanced cervical carcinoma. I. Feasibility, thermometry and device comparison. Int J Hyperthermia 1990;6:985–996.

112b. Feldman HJ, Molls M, Adler S, et al. Hyperthermia in eccentrically located pelvic tumors: Excessive heating of the perineal fat and normal tissue temperatures. Int J Radiat Oncol Biol Phys 1991;20:1017–1022.

112c. Petrovich Z, Langholz B, Gibbs FA. Regional hyperthermia for advanced tumors: A clinical study of 353 patients. Int J Radiat Oncol Biol Phys 1989;16:601–607.

113. Hynynen K, Shimm D, Anhalt D, et al. Temperature distributions during clinical scanned, focused ultrasound hypethermia treatments. Int J Hyperthermia 1990;6:891–908.

114. Riviere JE, Page RL, Dewhirst MW, et al. Effect of hyperthermia on cisplatin pharmacokinetics in normal dogs. Int J Hyperthermia 1986;2:351–358.

115. Klostergaard J, Barta M, Tomasovic SP. Hyperthermic modulation of tumor necrosis factor-dependent monocyte/macrophage tumor cytotoxicity in vitro. J Biol Response Modif 1989;8:262–277.

116. Shrivastava P, Luk K, Oleson J, et al. Hyperthermia quality assurance guidelines. Int J Radiat Oncol Biol Phys 1989;16:559–587.

117. Waterman FM, Dewhirst MW, Fessenden P, et al. RTOG quality assurance guidelines for clinical trials using hyperthermia administered by ultrasound. Int J Radiat Oncol Biol Phys 1991;20:1099–1107.

118. Sapozink MD, Corry PM, Kapp DS, et al. RTOG quality assurance guidelines for clinical trials using hyperthermia for deep-seated malignancy. Int J Radiat Oncol Biol Phys 1991;20:1109–1115.

119. Emami B, Stauffer P, Dewhirst MW. RTOG quality assurance guidelines for interstitial hyperthermia. Int J Radiat Oncol Biol Phys 1991;20:1117–1124.

120. Lindholm CE, Kjellen E, Nilsson P, et al. Microwave-induced hyperthermia and radiotherapy in human superficial tumors: Clinical results with a comparative study of combined treatment versus radiotherapy alone. Int J Hyperthermia 1987;3:393–411.

121. van der Zee J, van Rhoon GC, Wike-Hooley, et al. Thermal enhancement of radiotherapy in breast carcinoma. In: Overgaard J, ed. Hyperthermic oncology 1984, vol 1. London: Taylor & Francis, 1985:345–348.

122. Kim JH, Hahn EW, Ahmed SA, et al. Clinical study of the sequence of combined hyperthermia and radiation therapy of malignant melanoma. In: Overgaard J, ed. Hyperthermic oncology 1984, vol 1. London: Taylor & Francis, 1985:387–390.

123. Li R-Y, Zhang T-Z, Lin S-Y, et al. Effects of hyperthermia combined with radiation in the treatment of superficial malignant lesions in 90 patients. In: Overgaard J, ed. Hyperthermic oncology 1984, vol 1. London: Taylor & Francis, 1985:395–397.

124. Scott RS, Johnson RJR, Story KV, et al. Local hyperthermia in combination with definitive radiotherapy: Increased tumor clearance, reduced recurrence rate in extended follow-up. Int J Radiat Oncol Biol Phys 1984;10:2119–2123.

125. Corry PM, Spanos WJ, Tilchen EJ, et al. Combined ultrasound and radiation therapy treatment of human superficial tumors. Radiology 1982;145:165–169.

126. Kim JH, Hahn EW, Antich P. Radiofrequency hyperthermia for clinical cancer therapy. NCI Monogr 1982;61:339–342.

127. Sim DA, Oleson JR, Grochowski KJ. An update of the University of Arizona human clinical hyperthermia experience including estimates of therapeutic advantage. In: Overgaard J, ed. Hyperthermic oncology 1984, vol 1. London: Taylor & Francis, 1985:367–370.

128. Luk KH, Pajak TF, Perez CA, et al. Prognostic factors for tumor response after hyperthermia and radiation. In: Overgaard J, ed. Hyperthermic oncology 1984, vol 1. London: Taylor & Francis, 1985:353–358.

130. van der Zee J, van Putten WLJ, van den Berg AP, et al. Retrospective analysis of the response of tumors in patients treated with a combination of radiotherapy and hyperthermia. Int J Hyperthermia 1986;2:337–349.

131. Scott R, Gillespie B, Perez CA, et al. Hyperthermia in combination with definitive radiation therapy: Results of a phase I/II RTOG study. Int J Radiat Oncol Biol Phys 1988;15:711–716.

132. Valdagni R, Armichetti M, Pani G. Radical radiation alone versus radical radiation plus microwave hyperthermia for N3 (TNM-UICC) neck nodes: A prospective clinical trial. Int J Radiat Oncol Biol Phys 1988;115:13–24.

133. Arcangeli G, Arcangeli GC, Guerra A, et al. Tumor response to heat and radiation: Prognostic variables in the treatment of neck node metastases from head and neck cancer. Int J Hyperthermia 1985;1:207–217.

134. Steeves RA, Severson SB, Paliwal BR, et al. Matched-pair analysis of response to local hyperthermia and megavoltage electron therapy for superficial human tumors. Endocurietherapy/Hyperthermia Oncol 1986;2:163–170.

Cancer: Principles & Practice of Oncology, Fourth Edition,
edited by Vincent T. DeVita, Jr., Samuel Hellman, Steven A. Rosenberg.
J.B. Lippincott Co., Philadelphia © 1993.

Gregory A. Curt

CHAPTER **70**

Unsound Methods of Cancer Treatment

Things are seldom what they seem, skim milk masquerades as cream.

—Gilbert and Sullivan, "HMS Pinafore"

DEFINITION AND MAGNITUDE OF THE PROBLEM

In earlier editions of this text, this chapter was called "Unproven Methods of Cancer Treatment." However, the term *unproven* is nonjudgmental and at best is a euphemism for the unsound therapies described in this chapter. After all, many of the newer methods of cancer treatment described elsewhere in this edition are, in some sense, "unproven" in that their precise role in clinical treatment remains uncertain. The two distinguishing characteristics of *unsound* methods of cancer treatment (whether we want to label them unproven, unorthodox, nontraditional, complementary, or alternative therapies) are promotion without sufficient preclinical data to justify use in patients, and unmethodical treatment of patients that cannot detect either meaningful responses or therapy-related side effects.

A recent and somewhat surprising development has been the beginning of scientific and impartial evaluation of alternative cancer treatments. This healthy trend has been seen with the Bristol Cancer Help Centre (holistic care), the Livingston Wheeler Clinic (autogenous vaccines and diet), and the Burzynski Research Institute (antineoplaston therapy). These are discussed later in this chapter.

Not surprisingly, purveyors of unsound methods generally offer "nontoxic" or "natural" approaches to cancer treatment.

These unorthodox practitioners are largely physicians who escape regulatory control by the Food and Drug Administration (FDA) and offer their particular treatment approach to well-educated patients with early-stage disease. At a time when 50% of the serious cancers diagnosed in the United States are curable with existing therapies, and access to scientifically sound experimental trials has been considerably simplified with the National Cancer Institute's Physician Data Query computerized information system, it seems inconsistent that unsound methods of cancer treatment should continue to be a significant public health problem. However, the problem remains enormous.

Until recently, it was difficult to accurately estimate the magnitude of the use of unsound cancer remedies. In 1984 the Subcommittee on Health and Long-Term Care of the U.S. House of Representatives concluded that Americans spent $10 billion on unsound and unscientific remedies, with some $4 billion to $5 billion being spent annually on useless cancer treatments.[1] The cost in human terms is impossible to estimate.

One survey found that 13% of inpatients treated at a large urban cancer center had used or were using an unorthodox treatment regimen in addition to therapy prescribed by their oncologists.[2] Although this represents a highly selected inpatient population at a university referral center, this estimate of the frequency of use of unsound treatments is supported by a more recent Harris telephone survey of over 6000 American households. The study, undertaken for the Division of Consumer Affairs of the Food and Drug Administration in 1986, reports that 15% of all cancer patients had used one or more questionable cancer treatments.[3] This sample estimate, applied to the 6 million Americans who are alive today with a previous diagnosis of cancer, would project that about one million Americans have used one or more unsound cancer treatments.

What factors contribute to the continuing appeal of "alternative" cancer treatments? An interesting and perhaps predictable component to cancer quackery has always been an element of faddism. Indeed, the popularity of different methods of unsound cancer treatment has often paralleled advances in orthodox clinical cancer medicine. In the 1940s and 1950s, when radiation therapy was beginning to improve control of locoregional disease, cancer quackery became device-oriented: cancer patients were treated with the oscilloclast (a device that supposedly "retuned" disharmonic electrons and restored health) and the orgone energy accumulator (purportedly capable of concentrating a visible and ubiquitous cosmic energy into depleted erythrocytes). During the 1960s and 1970s, when chemotherapy was beginning to become accepted as an effective treatment for patients with advanced cancer, useless drugs were offered by nonscientific practitioners. This era saw the use of krebiozen and laetrile in thousands of cancer patients, and "freedom of choice" became the banner under which cancer patients demanded access to organized quackery.

There have been two recent fundamental shifts in the practice of unsound cancer treatment. The first, and most predictable, is a new focus on treatments that might be called "biologic." Since the beginning of the 1980s, thousands of cancer patients have paid millions of dollars for treatment with antineoplastons (proteins derived from urine that are said to be capable of differentiating tumors) or with Dr. Lawrence Burton's immunoaugmentative therapy (falsely represented as being able to boost immune response). Differentiating agents and immunotherapy are among the most promising leads in mainstream cancer treatment, and the biologic trend in unsound cancer therapy in the 1980s continues the device orientation of the 1940s and 1950s and the drug orientation of the 1960s and 1970s. In each case, the unsound practitioners echo the most promising theories of the day in offering their own peculiar brand of optimism. This optimism is derived from the promise that, in addition to being scientifically avant-garde, the alternative therapy is safer, more natural, less toxic, yet uniquely effective.

The second recent shift in alternative medicine involves the perception of cancer and other diseases as symptoms of metabolic imbalance rather than illnesses in and of themselves. The lifestyle approach to cancer holds that the disease can be effectively prevented and treated by changes in diet, supplements of enzymes and vitamins, or avoidance of stress, pollutants, and impurities. This is the world of "metabolic therapy," where laetrile is no longer a drug, but instead is reborn as "vitamin B_{17}." In addition, because metabolic therapy holds that the cancer is merely a symptom of more fundamental underlying processes, tumor progression does not necessarily indicate treatment failure. Instead, the effectiveness of treatment can be monitored by subjective feelings, by blood assays available only to the practitioner, or through other irrelevant observations, such as iridology (anatomic diagnosis by examination of the iris).

The result of all of these unsound approaches is the same: patients spend time and money on useless therapies. The potential for greater harm is obvious. Cancer patients who seek and obtain unsound therapy may not receive treatments of proven efficacy or appropriate experimental treatment approaches based on sound science. In addition, some of the most popular unsound treatments are potentially harmful in themselves.

A list of unsound therapies is given in Table 70–1, and detailed statements on each approach are available from the American Cancer Society.

TREATMENT REGULATION

It is useful, from an historical perspective, to understand how quackery affected drug regulation in the United States before reviewing the evolution of past and present unsound cancer treatments. The FDA is responsible for regulating the avail-

TABLE 70–1. Unsound Methods of Cancer Treatment

Alivizatos therapy (Greek cancer cure)	Dimethyl sulfoxide (DMSO)	Koch antitoxins
Antineoplastons	Dotto electronic reactor	Krebiozen
Bamfolin	Ferguson plant products	Laetrile (amygdalin, vitamin B_{17})
Beard method	Fonti method	Low's method
Bonifacia anticancer goat serum	Francis diet	Macrobiotic diet
Cancer-lipid concentrate	Fresh cell therapy	Makari intradermal cancer test
Carcin and neo-carcin	Frost method	Metabolic therapy
Carzodelin	Gerson method	Mucorhicin
C.N.T.	Glover serum	Multiple enzyme therapy
CH-23	Grape diet	Orgone energy devices
Chase dietary method	Hill Hadley vaccine	Polonine
Collodaurim and bichloracetic acid	Hemacytology index	Psychic surgery
Chaparral tea	Hett cancer serum	Revici method
Clam extracts (mercenene)	Hoxsey method	Spears hygenic system
Contreras method	Immunoaugmentative therapy (IAT)	Ultraviolet blood irradiation
Cresson method	Iscador	
Crofton immunization	Issel's combination therapy	
Cytec lung cancer screening	KC-555	
Diamond carbon compound	Kanfer handwriting test	
	Kelly malignancy index	

ability of drugs, biologicals, and medical devices in the United States and has the ultimate authority to approve or disapprove new treatments in cancer and other diseases. Much of the FDA's current regulatory authority came from an obvious hoax in cancer therapy at the turn of the century—the so-called "golden age of quackery."[4]

The case involved Dr. O.A. Johnson of Kansas City, Missouri, and his "Mild Combination Treatment" for cancer. As shown in Figure 70–1, prospective patients were invited to send for Dr. Johnson's books, *Cancer and Its Cure* and *My 125-Page Testimonial Book*—titles that have a contemporary ring in today's world of unsound cancer treatments. Those who could not visit the doctor were asked to fill out a symptom sheet so that cures could be "effected at home." Recognizing that the Mild Combination Treatment was fraudulent, the Bureau of Chemistry (the forerunner of today's FDA) prosecuted Dr. Johnson under the Food and Drug Act of 1906. The case eventually reached the Supreme Court and was decided in favor of Dr. Johnson. Justice Oliver Wendell Holmes, writing the majority opinion, interpreted existing laws to pertain only to drug labeling and not therapeutic claims. As long as the treatment materials were properly labeled, Dr. Johnson could not be prosecuted for "mistaken praise" of the Mild Combination Treatment.[4]

President Taft and Congress responded by amending the Food and Drug Act, making "false and fraudulent" therapeutic claims a criminal offense. However, legal proof of fraudulence was often difficult in practice, and in 1938 Congress passed a new Food and Drug Act that required proof of safety before a drug could be marketed. The new law strengthened the FDA's ability to cope with fraudulent cancer therapists, and the subsequent years saw a series of successful criminal prosecutions. During this era the Koch therapy, Hoxsey's herbal tonic, and krebiozen became subjects of highly visible public trials that also resulted in seizures of drug supplies and in-

junctions against further drug distribution. By 1960, FDA Commissioner George Larrick could state, "The Food and Drug Administration has had considerable success in combatting quackery in the courts. There have been some heavy fines and some prison sentences. Such actions have had a strong deterrent effect."[5]

In 1962, however, the FDA's responsibilities and priorities changed with the passage of the Kefauver-Harris amendments to the 1938 Food and Drug Act. These amendments required evidence of drug efficacy and safety before marketing. As a result, the FDA increasingly turned its attention to the control of the pharmaceutical industry. Between 1962 and 1987, over 7000 previously available prescription drugs were removed from the U.S. market. During the same interval, the FDA's commitment to combatting quackery decreased proportionately; less than 0.001% of the FDA budget is currently committed to combatting health fraud.

THE ERA OF UNSOUND DEVICES

The period between 1940 and 1950 saw the use of several fraudulent devices in the treatment of cancer. One of the more interesting therapists was Dr. Wilhelm Reich, a Viennese colleague of Sigmund Freud. Reich's studies of character analysis and sexuality during the 1930s were considered seminal to the new discipline of psychoanalysis.

Between 1936 and 1939, Reich's research took him to Norway, where he claimed discovery of orgone, a visible and ubiquitous cosmic energy that he described as "the most powerful force in the universe." In 1940, Reich emigrated to the United States, where he purchased a 300-acre estate in Rangeley, Maine, which he named, appropriately enough, Organon. The estate eventually housed the Orgone Energy Ob-

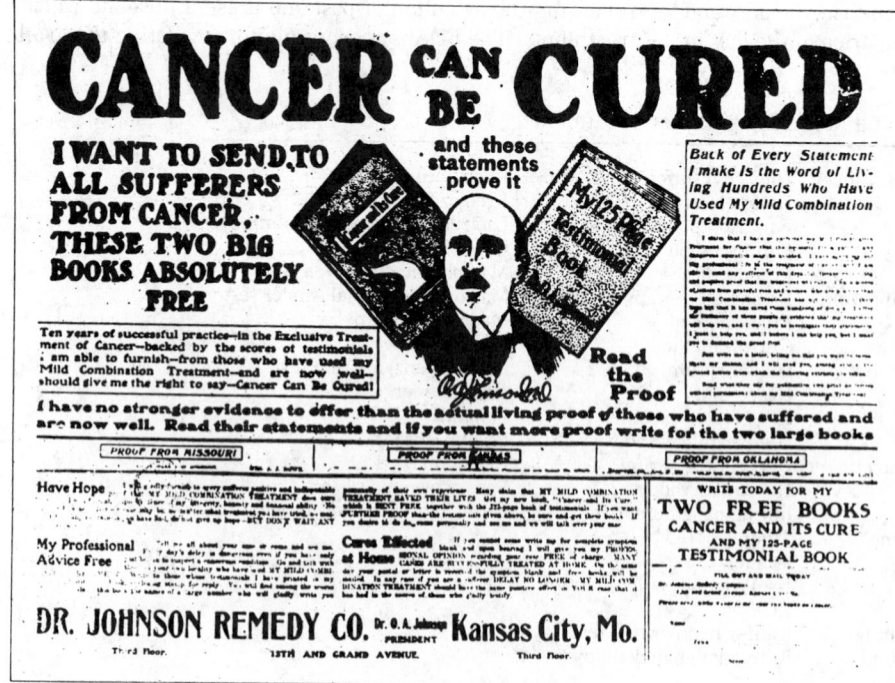

FIGURE 70–1. A 1908 advertisement of Dr. Johnson's Mild Combination Cancer Treatment. Litigation involving this reached the Supreme Court and resulted in important changes in U.S. drug regulation. (Courtesy of the U.S. Food and Drug Administration History Office)

servatory, the Wilhelm Reich Foundation, laboratories, and its own printing facilities.[6]

In Rangeley Reich designed and built "orgone energy accumulators," treatment devices resembling telephone booths constructed of metal, wood, and asbestos board. Specialized cone-shaped instruments were also designed to treat the head. Hundreds of these devices were leased throughout the United States at the then-remarkable cost of $250 per month. Treatment response was judged by blood tests performed in Reich's laboratories. Volume I of the 1942 edition of *The International Journal of Sexual Economy and Orgone Research* has a strangely contemporary tone in describing the four blood tests for cancer: a culture test, a biologic resistance test, a disintegration test, and a blue margin test. This battery of studies was purported to be capable of distinguishing between healthy and "cancerous" blood and was even purported to be able to detect cancer *before* the development of a tumor.

Reich had developed not only his own theories of cancer etiology (orgone depletion in erythrocytes) but also a completely self-contained system for diagnosis, treatment, and prevention of cancer.[7,8] It was an unimpeachable and self-fulfilling system that anticipated many common characteristics of unsound cancer therapies today.

However, this was an era of organized opposition to cancer quackery. The FDA consulted a group of independent clinicians and physicists who examined several orgone accumulators and concluded that orgone energy could be neither accumulated nor measured, and that Reich's principles had no scientific merit or clinical utility. In 1954 a federal injunction was issued against Reich and his foundation, demanding a recall of orgone accumulators and banning interstate advertisements in Reich's pamphlets and magazines.

Proponents of the orgone energy theories charged that the FDA investigation interfered with freedom of the press and was part of an organized government effort to prevent effective and nontoxic cancer treatments from being widely distributed.[9] Reich was held in criminal contempt of the FDA injunction when he continued to lease and distribute orgone accumulators, claiming that courts and juries had no jurisdiction in matters of "natural law."[4] Despite an appeal to the Supreme Court, Reich was sentenced to 2 years in prison, where he died in 1957.

Although orgone energy devices are not part of the contemporary scene of cancer quackery, several common themes remain all too familiar: a charismatic "scientist" with an appealing—albeit unsupportable—theory of cancer and its treatment; unverifiable measures of success; and faithful proponents who believe that orthodox medicine wants to suppress innovation.

At the same time on the west coast of the United States, Dr. Albert Abrams was pioneering other devices—equally unsound in principle and profitable in practice—for the diagnosis and treatment of cancer. Abrams' diagnostic technique involved analyzing patient blood specimens in a "radioscope"— a tuning apparatus capable of detecting radiofrequencies associated with disease. After a blood specimen was dried on filter paper and inserted into the machine, the patient had to hold metal plates connected to the radioscope while the operator completed an examination with a plastic wand. This examination was described as sufficiently sensitive to "inform the doctor whether or not the patient has cancer, or a tendency

towards cancer, long before there has been any visible disturbance of tissue."[10] To treat what the radioscope diagnosed, Abrams developed the oscilloclast, a device said to be capable of restoring electronic vibrations in diseased tissue.

Eventually the fraud blossomed into a mail-order business sponsored by the Electronic Medical Foundation. Radioscopes were "perfected" to diagnose blood specimens mailed in on postcards by practitioners who rented an oscilloclast directly from Abrams. A diagnosis was promptly returned with recommended oscilloclast treatment settings. At the height of its popularity in 1950, oscilloclasts were rented to more than 3000 practitioners for a $250 deposit and $5 per month. As a result, Abrams was able to endow his Electronic Medical Foundation with some $3 million.[11]

However, a comprehensive investigation by the FDA demonstrated that the radioscope could not distinguish colored water from blood. The radioscope diagnosis of a specimen from an 11-week-old rooster was sinus infection and bad teeth.[12] In 1958, after a series of appeals, the Electronic Medical Foundation was prohibited from interstate shipment of the devices. In 1962 the Foundation was dissolved.

The story has an ironic twist: the officers of the Electronic Medical Foundation subsequently founded the National Health Federation, an organization established to represent, protect, and promote alternative medicine in the United States. During the ensuing years, the National Health Federation would become increasingly organized supporters of the Hoxsey therapy, krebiozen, and laetrile.

THE ERA OF UNSOUND DRUGS

The 1950s saw the first successful use of cancer chemotherapy but also was an era in which fraudulent drugs were promoted.

THE HOXSEY TREATMENT

One of the most popular health scams of the 1950s was the Hoxsey method of cancer treatment. In his 1956 book *You Don't Have to Die*, Harry Hoxsey described his approach as "essentially chemotherapy" for "the systemic treatment of cancer."[13] The Hoxsey method involved two medicines: the "pink medicine" (potassium iodide and pepsin) and the "black medicine" (cascara in an extract of licorice, red clover, burdock root, stillingia root, berberis root, poke root, and the bark of the buckthorn and prickly ash).[14] This complex of plant products was attributed to Hoxsey's great-grandfather, who observed that his horse was cured of cancer after grazing on these plants.

Hoxsey initially peddled his therapy from state to state and was convicted of practicing medicine without a license in Illinois and Iowa. He finally established clinics in Texas and Pennsylvania, where patients were examined, uniformly diagnosed as having cancer, and routinely offered treatment at a cost of $400. At the height of its popularity in the late 1950s, more than 10,000 "cancer" patients were receiving Hoxsey's medicines.[4]

Because of the treatment's popularity, there were many contemporary attempts to validate antitumor activity by independent review. In 1957, a site visit by the University of British Columbia to Hoxsey's Texas clinic concluded, "The medications are of no value in the treatment of cancer. We have found that the methods of diagnosis are inadequate, that treatments do not affect the progress of disease, that no serious attempt is made to evaluate results and that no significant research has been done."[15]

This was followed by a detailed FDA examination of 400 cases of cancer "cured" by Hoxsey's regimen. Patients were found to fall into one of three categories: those who never had a diagnosis of cancer, those who had been previously cured of cancer by conventional therapy, or those (the majority) who had cancer that had not responded to the regimen.[16] In short, no cures could be documented and no evidence of antitumor activity was found.

These reviews led to a series of highly public trials during which Hoxsey proponents countered the prosecution by lobbying Congress with a prayer campaign against the FDA. After ten years of litigation, the Hoxsey cancer treatment was finally banned from U.S. sales, although by that time over $50 million had been spent on the drugs.[17] This approach is still available in Mexico.

KREBIOZEN

The growing popularity of krebiozen in the late 1950s and early 1960s, after the invalidation of Hoxsey's herbal medicines, began a new era in unsound cancer treatments. Unlike Hoxsey's folksy midwestern tonics, krebiozen and subsequent popular unsound remedies had a pseudoscientific ring of authenticity and were increasingly promoted by more convincing, scientifically trained proponents with the support of an organized constituency.

Krebiozen was initially manufactured as an antihypertensive by Dr. Stevan Durovic, a Yugoslavian physician who claimed to produce the drug by extracting the serum of horses injected with sterile extracts of *Actinomyces bovis,* a pathogenic fungus that causes lumpy jaw disease in animals. The original 2 grams of krebiozen (an estimated 200,000 doses) were purportedly produced from 2000 horses in Argentina and brought into the United States in Durovic's suitcase in 1949.

In the United States, Durovic met Dr. Andrew Ivy, a professor emeritus at the University of Illinois. Ivy became convinced that krebiozen had antitumor activity after an experiment in which Durovic demonstrated disease "improvement" in seven of twelve animals treated with the drug.[18] These results were never reproduced. Instead, Ivy, a respected scientist, began treating a series of patients after deciding that the drug was nontoxic by administering it to himself.

In 1951, the results of krebiozen treatment in 22 cancer patients were announced at a press conference at the Drake Hotel in Chicago. The results of the trial were never submitted for publication; instead, pamphlets published by the newly organized Krebiozen Research Foundation were distributed to the press, claiming improvement in most patients treated. Although 8 patients had died during the course of the trial, death was said not to be due to progressive cancer, and the fact was omitted that 2 additional patients had died in the interval between publication of the pamphlet and the press conference.

After Ivy's announcement, small quantities of krebiozen were provided to several medical centers to allow them to reproduce the results of the initial clinical trial. During the subsequent 12 years, independent investigators could not confirm that krebiozen had any antitumor activity. However, this did not stop the Krebiozen Research Foundation from issuing reports and independently publishing monographs claiming impressive treatment responses in individual patients.

Between 1951 and 1963, krebiozen was distributed by the Krebiozen Research Foundation to thousands of general practitioners throughout the United States. Physicians could receive an injectable ampule of krebiozen for a "research donation" of $9 and use it in any way they saw fit. Business was brisk. The initial 200,000 doses were rapidly depleted, and in 1960 Durovic manufactured an additional 100,000 ampules from horse serum and horse meat. It was claimed that, like the original batch of krebiozen, the treatment material contained lipopolysaccharides consisting of galacturonic acid, glucosamine, arabinose, and xylose, combined with glycerol.

In 1962 the Kefauver-Harris amendments to the Food and Drug Act required sponsors of investigational drugs to submit plans for the rational clinical development of new agents. Although Durovic submitted such a plan for krebiozen to the FDA in June 1963, he withdrew the package without review a month afterward, making interstate shipment of krebiozen illegal. Several concurrent observations led to subsequent criminal proceedings. In 1963 FDA chemists analyzed samples of krebiozen submitted by Ivy and Durovic. The white power was found to be creatine, a simple organic acid widely distributed in muscle tissues and inactive as an antitumor agent. Analysis of pre-1960 ampules of krebiozen revealed nothing but mineral oil, while those vials manufactured after 1960 contained mineral oil and trace quantities of methylhydantoin, a soluble form of creatine.

Independent analysis of the clinical results of krebiozen treatment was equally revealing. In 1962 the Krebiozen Research Foundation selected its 504 best responses (from over 4000 patients on whom records were available) and sent them to the National Cancer Institute (NCI) for independent review and analysis. Because these cases were inadequately documented for careful review, FDA officials spent considerable effort confirming diagnoses and reconstructing treatment duration, dose, and response. This information was submitted to an independent 24-member panel of experts appointed by the NCI. In 1963 that committee reported that review of all 504 cases established that krebiozen had no antitumor activity. From the NCI's perspective, the case was closed and there was no justification to pursue clinical trials.[19]

The FDA undertook its own independent analysis of an additional 4307 cases submitted by the Krebiozen Research Foundation. Again, no convincing evidence for antitumor activity could be demonstrated.

In short, krebiozen had been promoted for the treatment of thousands of cancer patients at a cost of millions of dollars. The treatment materials were falsely labeled. Moreover, although indiscriminate prescription made retrospective review of the thousands of available records particularly time-consuming and expensive, there was no evidence of reproducible antitumor activity in any malignancy.

In 1964 Ivy, Durovic, and the Krebiozen Research Foundation were indicted on 49 counts of violation of the Food, Drug and Cosmetic Act, including mail fraud, mislabeling of drugs, and conspiracy to defraud the public. Although the defendants were found innocent after a highly public 9-month trial, the interstate distribution of krebiozen was stopped.[20]

This decision was followed by a series of demonstrations by krebiozen supporters, who argued that the government, industry, and organized medicine had worked in concert to deny the public an effective and nontoxic cancer treatment. Proponents blocked the FDA Commissioner's office and lobbied Congress to reverse the FDA decision. Eventually, 11 senators demanded an impartial trial of krebiozen. Durovic offered to sell the NCI bulk krebiozen for such a study for $170,000 per gram; the same quantity of pure creatine from chemical suppliers was available for 30 cents.

However, interest in krebiozen evaporated when Durovic unexpectedly left the United States for Switzerland after withdrawing substantial amounts of cash from Foundation bank accounts. At the time, he was under investigation by the Internal Revenue Service for nonpayment of taxes on $904,907 of unreported income. Ivy renamed krebiozen "carcalon"—Greek for a natural substance that slows down a cancerous process—and continued to prescribe the drug from his Chicago office.[21] At the request of the Illinois State Medical Society, the governor appointed the Illinois Krebiozen Committee to oversee continued "controlled scientific testing of krebiozen" by Ivy. The committee never gave a report, and at the time of Ivy's death in 1977 there was still no evidence that krebiozen was useful in the treatment of cancer.

LAETRILE

Laetrile is a generic term for a group of cyanogenic glucosides that can be isolated from several natural sources, including the pits of edible fruits such as apricots, cherries, pears, apples, and peaches.[22,23] The term was coined by E.T. Krebs, "because this apricot-kernel preparation was *lae*vorotary to polarized light and because amygdalin was chemically a malo*nitrile*."[24] The principal constituent of laetrile is amygdalin, a compound first isolated in 1830 and chemically synthesized in 1924.[25,26] As early as 1935 it was found that the β-glycoside linkage in amygdalin could be hydrolyzed by emulsin (an enzyme found in almonds) or specific β-glucosidases to release one molecule of hydrogen cyanide and benzaldehyde and two molecules of glucose.

In the 1920s, Ernest Krebs Sr. was the first to use oral amygdalin in the treatment of cancer. The preparation proved toxic, however, and it was not until 1952 that Krebs' son, E.T. Krebs, reported the development of a "safe" parenteral formulation.

Laetrile's purported mechanism of action is shown below. It was hypothesized that β-glucosidases would activate amygdalin to glucose, benzaldehyde, and toxic hydrogen cyanide. Hydrogen cyanide could be itself detoxified by rhodanese (thiosulfurtransferase), which would convert the hydrogen cyanide to inactive thiocyanate.[27]

$$\text{Amygdalin} \xrightarrow{\text{glycosidases}} \begin{array}{c} \text{HCN} \\ \text{benzaldehyde} \\ \text{glucose} \end{array} \xrightarrow{\text{rhodanese}} \text{thiocyanate}$$

To explain amygdalin's specific antitumor effects and lack of toxicity, proponents further postulated that cancer cells have high intracellular levels of β-glucosidase and low levels of rhodanese, while the opposite is true in normal tissues.

There are several critical flaws in this theory. First, normal and malignant tissues appear to have comparable levels of rhodanese, and tumor tissues lack β-glucosidase activity.[28,29] Indeed, there appears to be little detectable in vivo β-glucosidase activity, so that virtually all of a parenteral amygdalin dose is excreted intact in the urine.[23] Moreover, laetrile itself is inactive in vitro and in vivo against murine and human tumors in several preclinical assays, even when β-glycosidase is administered concurrently.[30-34] Indeed, control animals in comparative studies showed improved survival, suggesting that amygdalin is toxic without being active against disease.

Because β-glycosidase is not found in mammalian tissues, up to 10 grams of amygdalin can be administered intravenously without toxicity. However, gut bacteria have glycosidase and can release cyanide from amygdalin. Cyanide toxicity can occur after the administration of oral laetrile, and death from cyanide poisoning has been reported after such treatment.[35] Moreover, although cyanide is proposed as the active component to laetrile, cyanide itself has been tested as a potential antitumor agent and appears to be more toxic to normal than malignant tissues.[36-38]

Thus, there is no evidence for selective activation of amygdalin by malignant tissues, preferential inactivation of hydrogen cyanide by normal tissues, or usefulness of hydrogen cyanide as a chemotherapeutic agent. The drug has proved inactive in every in vivo and in vitro system in which it was tested. So why did laetrile become the most popular and celebrated unsound cancer therapy of contemporary medicine?

As Wallace Jansen has noted, by the mid-1950s the laetrile business was controlled by Andrew McNaughton, an international entrepreneur with a flair for manipulating the press.[4] In 1961 McNaughton founded Bioenzymes International, Ltd., and began to manufacture laetrile in Mexico and Canada. In 1963 a strongly pro-laetrile paperback book, *Laetrile—Control for Cancer, The Authorized Story*, was published with an introduction by McNaughton.[39] Several of the chapters were reprinted in newspapers and magazines, and so began an intense public interest in and demand for the drug. However, with neither preclinical nor clinical evidence that laetrile was useful in the treatment of cancer, the FDA began a series of actions against Krebs and the McNaughton Foundation. The Canadian FDA followed by prohibiting distribution of laetrile in Canada. Manufacture and distribution continued in Mexico, where apricot pits were largely imported from the California fruit-packing industry.

In 1970 the McNaughton Foundation of Canada submitted an investigational new drug application (INDA) to the U.S. FDA. The INDA was granted, but the FDA withdrew its approval a month later. Dr. Charles Edwards, then FDA commissioner, cited "serious preclinical and clinical deficiencies" in the application.[40] For example, while chemical analysis of Canadian laetrile in the 1960s found amygdalin contents between 87% and 98%, Mexican production suffered from problems in quality control.[41] FDA analysis of laetrile from Mexican laboratories indicated that a 500-mg tablet might contain anywhere from 42 to 450 mg of amygdalin, while the parenteral product was 14% to 87% pure. Indeed, vials of injectable laetrile were found to be contaminated with bacteria, fungus, and isopropyl alcohol.[42]

However, the FDA's reversal only strengthened the public's conviction that the "establishment" was intent on keeping a useful product away from patients. An article in the *Harvard Political Review* ignored available evidence and concluded that "vested interests have prevented the use of an inexpensive and effective cancer cure."[43] At the same time, the legal prosecution of the ultraconservative physician Dr. John Richardson under a California law that made prescription of laetrile a felony galvanized the John Birch Society. Laetrile proponents established the International Association for Cancer Victims and Friends in 1963, and in 1972 Robert Bradford, a John Bircher, founded the Committee for Freedom of Choice in Cancer Therapy. Together with the National Health Foundation, these organizations mounted an effective campaign to "legalize" laetrile on the premise that the patient and physician should have ultimate authority in choosing treatment and that the government should not regulate medical practice. As Lerner notes in assessing the laetrile phenomenon, this was a time when antiestablishment groups and ultraconservatives united in the name of "freedom of choice."[44]

Their efforts at the state level were highly successful. In a 1977 *New England Journal of Medicine* editorial entitled "Laetrilomania," Dr. F.J. Ingelfinger summarized contemporary developments: "In Alaska, Laetrile may be prescribed by doctors, and an Oklahoma judge legalized importation of drug from Mexico. Indiana, if the physician-governor signs the bill passed by his legislature, would become the first state to approve the manufacture and sale of the substance as well as its use. Bills that prohibit interference with the sale or use of laetrile are well on their way in Arizona, Florida, Massachusetts, and Minnesota."[45]

During the next year, additional legislation to approve laetrile at the state level followed the celebrated case of Rutherford versus the United States. In this 1978 case, Glenn Rutherford enjoined the FDA from interfering with his constitutional right to obtain nontoxic therapy (laetrile) for his terminal malignancy. Both the U.S. District Court in Oklahoma and the Court of Appeals ignored the fact that Rutherford's "terminal" rectal polyp had been surgically cured. Instead, they ruled that safety and efficacy have no meaning in the treatment of terminally ill patients and that the designation of terminal illness could be made by any licensed physician. The FDA was directed to provide regulations for the distribution of laetrile to any terminal cancer patient who desired it.[46] Although this decision was eventually overturned by the Supreme Court, laetrile gained additional political credibility and 23 states moved to legalize laetrile therapy.

Despite widespread laetrile use, evidence that the drug was effective remained unconvincing. By 1978 it was estimated that more than 70,000 Americans had been treated with laetrile.[47] A small retrospective analysis of laetrile treatment response was undertaken by the California Cancer Commission in 1953; no antitumor activity was found in 44 patients with a variety of tumors.[48] By far the largest retrospective analysis of laetrile efficacy was undertaken by the NCI in 1978.[47] Case reports of patients who might have benefited from laetrile were solicited from 385,000 physicians, 70,000 health professionals, and pro-laetrile groups. Only 93 cases were submitted, of which 67 could be evaluated. Of these, 6 patients were felt to have had an objective treatment response (2 lymphoma, 2 adenocarcinoma, 1 carcinoid, 1 squamous cell lung cancer). The authors admitted that the design of the study made it impossible to rule out intentional or unintentional submission of inaccurate information, but concluded that if laetrile has antitumor activity, it must be vanishingly small. The proper denominator for the six responses is not the 67 cases selected for best response but the 70,000 patients known to have been treated with the drug.

The issue of laetrile's usefulness in cancer treatment remained unsettled. Some prominent physicians urged legalization as a way to "make forbidden fruit less tempting," while others urged prospective clinical trials.[45,49] In 1978 the NCI submitted its own INDA for a clinical trial of amygdalin to the FDA. The NCI ensured quality control in the production of the drug as well as prospective, well-designed, and well-implemented clinical trials. In a small phase I study, a single patient developed cyanide toxicity after eating almonds during laetrile treatment; almonds not only contain small quantities of amygdalin but also have β-glycosidase activity.[50] In the larger phase II trial, no responses were seen in 178 patients with a variety of cancers.[51] The resolution of laetrile's activity as an anticancer drug came 30 years and 70,000 patients too late.

UNSOUND CANCER TREATMENTS POPULAR TODAY

As discussed at the beginning of this chapter, there have been two fundamental developments in the contemporary practice of unsound cancer medicine. The first is a predictable shift towards treatments that might be considered biologic, while the second is the development of the concept that cancer is a symptom of underlying metabolic disturbances and can be prevented and treated by diet, vitamins, and avoiding stress.

IMMUNOAUGMENTATIVE THERAPY

Immunoaugmentative therapy (IAT) is a scientifically unsupportable treatment dispensed by the Immunology Researching Center in Freeport, Bahamas. The center was established in 1977 by Lawrence Burton, a PhD zoologist, after he failed to receive approval for clinical studies of IAT in the U.S. from the FDA.[52] The treatment is based on the theory that cancer develops because of "immunoincompetence," which Burton can measure and restore using a series of protein fractions derived from the blood of patients and healthy donors.

Patients receiving IAT first undergo a series of immunocompetence blood tests that are computer-analyzed to select each patient's treatment regimen. The treatment itself consists of four "immune serum protein fractions" called blocking protein, tumor antibody, tumor complement, and deblocking protein. Based on the computer analysis of the patient's immune profile, some or all of these fractions may be prescribed as daily subcutaneous injections. Stabilization of the immune system usually requires several weeks on the island, after which patients leave with a cache of sera and computer projections for further treatment.[53] The initial treatment costs about $10,000, and patients are required to make follow-up visits for immune system "tune-ups."[53] The clinic also provides patients with assistance in filing claims for third-party reimbursement.

In 1978, a year after the clinic was established, the Bahamian government requested a review of IAT by a committee of physician-scientists from the Pan-American Health Organization. This panel found neither a scientific rationale for IAT nor clinical evidence for its efficacy, and unanimously recommended that the center be closed.[54] Despite these findings, the clinic remained open (for the treatment of non-Bahamians only) and over 3000 patients, most of them Americans with cancer, have received IAT for cancer treatment or prevention.

Because of political pressure at the state level, IAT was approved for the treatment of cancer in Florida and Oklahoma in 1981.[55,56] In addition, there have been unsuccessful congressional proposals to exempt IAT from FDA control.[57] As with laetrile in the previous decade, an unsound cancer treatment was essentially legalized by individual states without regard to either therapeutic effectiveness or potential toxicity.

However, subsequent independent analysis of IAT treatment materials has shown them to be devoid of purported content or biologic activity. In each case, analysis of the IAT treatment reagents revealed diluted blood proteins, the major component of which was albumin.[58] Specific immunoglobulins, macroglobulins, and complement activity said to be essential to the activity of the regimen were undetectable. Treatment materials were found to be uniformly contaminated with bacteria and hepatitis, and an epidemic of nocardia abscess formation was reported at IAT injection sites.[59,60] Even more worrisome was Burton's use of IAT in the treatment of acquired immunodeficiency syndrome (AIDS), a disease that he ascribes to the immunodepressant effects of sexual lubricants.[61] Since the IAT laboratories pool blood specimens before processing them into treatment reagents, contamination of reagents with the human immunodeficiency virus (HIV) is possible. Indeed, of 72 vials of IAT treatment materials available to the NCI for analysis, 37 (51%) were positive for antibodies to HIV, and the Centers for Disease Control were subsequently reproducibly able to culture viable AIDS virus from Burton's treatment materials.[58,62]

Therefore, IAT is without scientific rationale or documented clinical activity; rather, patients are treated with a series of inert blood products capable of transmitting bacterial infection, hepatitis, and AIDS. Because of these findings, in July 1985 the Bahamian clinic was closed as a hazard to its laboratory workers. After 6 months of demonstrations in Freeport and Washington, the clinic reopened. By then, Burton had already moved to establish clinics in Mexico.

IAT is an unsound and potentially harmful approach to the treatment of cancer and AIDS. Unfortunately, as reported by the Congressional Office of Technology Assessment, which devoted considerable attention to IAT in its report on alternative cancer treatments, attempts to evaluate this approach impartially have not met with Burton's cooperation.[63]

ANTINEOPLASTONS

Antineoplaston treatment is an alternative biologic therapy offered by Dr. Stanislaw Burzynski at the Burzynski Research Institute in Houston. The treatment is based on the theory that medium-sized peptides normally present in urine are capable of controlling tumor growth and differentiating cancer cells in vivo. In the early 1970s Burzynski, then a faculty member at the Baylor College of Medicine, used gel filtration techniques to isolate peptides from normal urine that inhibited in vitro growth of several human cell lines.[64]

In 1977 Burzynski left Baylor to establish the Burzynski Research Institute. There, the initial peptide fraction, called antineoplaston A, was subfractionated into antineoplaston A_1, A_2, A_3, A_4, A_5, A_{10}, and AS2-1.[65] Each fraction is said to be composed of low-molecular-weight peptides in the 2000 to 5000 dalton range. The active component in each of these peptides has recently been identified as 3-[N-phenylacetyl-aminopiperidine]-2,5-dione, a substance that is not known to occur in urine.[65] In treating cancer patients, the dosage of each antineoplaston fraction is determined individually by first measuring pretreatment levels of antineoplastons in serum and urine. Burzynski claims that this ambient antineoplaston profile is a valuable aid in cancer diagnosis and also uses the assay to monitor response to antineoplaston therapy.[66]

The period of full-dose antineoplaston treatment may require from 6 weeks to more than a year.[67] Therapy is administered via Hickman catheter, although newly available capsules for oral administration "appear to produce better results in some forms of cancers."[67] The cost of each treatment (exclusive of monitoring and laboratory testing) is $45, regardless of dose, and the therapy is claimed to be nontoxic. The clinic accepts responsibility for billing third-party insurers, although a cash deposit of $5000 has been requested from patients at the beginning of therapy.[68]

In small phase I studies, clinical activity, including complete responses, is claimed in carcinoma of the lung, prostate, stomach, colon, breast, and bladder.[69–72] Independent confirmation of these results, however, has not yet occurred. A site visit to the Burzynski Research Institute by the Canadian Ministry of Health in 1982 found no evidence of therapeutic efficacy, and medical claims for antineoplaston treatments were subsequently disallowed in Canada.[73] In 1985 a follow-up of 36 antineoplaston-treated patients followed by 25 Canadian physicians found no evidence of partial or complete responses. Indeed, 34 of the 36 patients had died, and the only two survivors had had prior curative therapy.[74]

The NCI has always had a policy of investigating potential new treatments from alternative practitioners, so long as the methods could be evaluated and prioritized using the science criteria for development of other agents; that is, these unorthodox approaches should play on a level field with orthodox medicine. As part of an effort to uncover new leads from alternative medicine, NCI investigators from the Cancer Therapy Evaluation Program examined a series of best-case responses submitted by the Burzynski clinic.[75] Seven patients with primary brain tumors on no other therapy showed disease response on antineoplaston therapy. Based entirely on this clinical evidence, the NCI will sponsor a phase II trial of antineoplastons in high-grade glioma, low-grade glioma, anaplastic glioma, and pediatric brain tumors in 1993. The drug will be supplied by Burzynski, but the trials will be performed by NCI-supported investigators. We hope that well-implemented and impartial studies will determine, 15 years after broad clinical use, whether this approach has any merit.

METABOLIC THERAPIES

Current metabolic approaches to the treatment of cancer represent a wide spectrum of alternative interventions, including enzyme therapy, cellular therapy, dietary manipulation, vitamin treatment (including vitamin B_{17} [laetrile] and megavitamins), and detoxification with enzymes or hydrogen peroxide. In each case, cancer is viewed as a symptom of a more basic and underlying metabolic imbalance. Therefore, the metabolic therapist believes that cancer can be prevented and treated with metabolic interventions.

The idea is not new. In the early 1900s, Dr. William Koch prescribed a regimen of cancer treatment that was based on the theory that malignancies were nothing more than a protective response to toxic compounds generated within the body.[76] Cancer could be treated by oxidizing these toxic compounds with Koch's "antitoxin" preparation in combination with diet and enema therapy. Although Koch's antitoxin was, in essence, distilled water (Koch actually labeled the drug one part glyoxylide to one trillion parts water), the treatment was enormously popular and remains available today.[4]

There has been a renaissance of interest in the metabolic and holistic therapy of cancer. Treatments offered at these centers vary widely, depending on the philosophy of the program. For example, the International Health Institute was established by dentist William Kelley, who believes that cancer is caused by pancreatic enzyme deficiency. He developed the Kelley enzyme test or the "self-test for cancer." For a "donation" of $50, patients receive a nutritional lifestyle program and the procedure for the enzyme test. Patients are instructed to take six to eight pancreatic tablets after each meal for 4 weeks. The analysis then runs as follows:

> If at the end of this time:
> You feel worse, have a loss of appetite, nausea, headache, goopy, sick, toxic or in general listless: you can be assured there is a cancerous condition present in your body.
> You feel better, have more energy and a brighter, happier outlook: you can be assured there is a precancerous condition in your body.
> You feel no different: you can be reasonably assured there is not a cancerous condition present in your body.[77]

Overall, not very reassuring, although the institute's nutritional program explains "how to avoid cancer or how to proceed if you're a victim." The program might include a low-protein diet (buttermilk allowed), mineral supplements (for example, blackstrap molasses), yogurt enemas, and induced sweating.

Some of the clinics offer more "traditional" alternative treatments. For example, the Biomedical Center in Tijuana still uses herbal tonics based on Hoxsey's original methods. Most of the clinics have evolved with the times, however. Diet, an important component of many metabolic therapies, is especially emphasized by the East West Center for Macrobiotics and the Kushi Foundation. The emphasis here is on the traditional Oriental philosophy of yin and yang: cancers of "yin" organs (colon, stomach, bladder) are treated with "yang" foods (cooked vegetables, fruit, fish), and cancer of "yang" organs (lung, liver) are treated with "yin" food (raw vegetables, no fruit, no fish).[78–80] Kushi recommends that patients avoid meat, dairy products, sweets, processed foods, hot spices, and "toxic and unnatural" conventional cancer treatments.[81] Because the macrobiotic diet is deficient in calories, vitamins D and C, and iron, nutritional deficiencies have been reported in children and adults, and there is no evidence that this approach is useful as a cancer treatment.[82–88]

Others, most notably Dr. Linus Pauling, have espoused nutritional supplements as primary cancer treatment. Ewan

Cameron, in the mid-1960s, hypothesized that vitamin C might inhibit tumor cell invasion and metastasis. The theory, also called the orthomolecular treatment of cancer, is predicated on the notion that vitamin C augments collagen production or stabilization and decreases tumor cell production of enzymes, such as hyaluridase, required for basement membrane invasion.[89,90] An initial clinical trial of high-dose vitamin C (10 g/day) appeared to improve survival, at least when compared with historical controls.[91] However, because of the problems inherent in this kind of retrospective analysis, the NCI supported two successive trials at the Mayo Clinic. The first, a standard phase II study, used vitamin C therapy in patients who had disease refractory to standard therapy; no evidence of tumor regression or subjective benefit was observed.[92] The second study was a randomized, double-blind, placebo-controlled trial of high-dose vitamin C in patients who had had no prior therapy; again, no evidence of tumor regression was observed.[93]

Interestingly, vitamin C can prevent development of carcinogen-induced malignancies in some animal models, and the NCI is supporting chemoprevention studies using vitamin C. However, available evidence now indicates that ascorbic acid has no role in primary cancer treatment.[94]

However, nutritional and megavitamin therapy for the treatment of cancer and other diseases has developed into a profitable health-fraud industry in the United States.[87,95] Here, practitioners can obtain degrees in "nutrition" by mail: $1000 for a bachelor's degree, $2000 for both bachelor's and master's degrees, and $4000 for bachelor's, master's, and PhD degrees.[96,97] Some diploma mills even provide a computer program that will prescribe specious nutritional supplements based on the patient's dietary history. In addition to high-dose vitamin C, these "health and wellness" clinics might prescribe:

Megadose vitamin A (3000 to 300,000 units/day) for "immune stimulation" and "epithelial integrity."[86] These doses of vitamin A are not known to have such effects and may, in fact, be associated with significant toxicity. Indeed, the ingestion of 5000 to 10,000 units of vitamin A for 30 days can cause increased intracranial pressure, fetal abnormalities, and hepatic and renal toxicity.[98,99]

Megadose vitamin E (up to 3200/IU/day) as an "antioxidant."[100] Vitamin E has no known use in cancer treatment. Although doses of 300 IU or less a day are considered nontoxic, increased triglycerides are seen at 600 IU/day, depression and fatigue at 900 IU/day, and nausea, diarrhea, headache, and blurred vision at 3200 IU/day.[101–103] Double-blind studies have shown no effect of vitamin E on work performance or libido, and high doses in experimental animals can cause teratogenesis, depressed bone calcification, and testicular atrophy.[101,104]

Vitamin B_{15} (also known as pangamic acid, 15, or pangamate). Vitamin B_{15} is not known to be a vitamin at all. Prescribed as a dietary supplement in health stores, analysis reveals that preparations consist of dimethylglycine hydrochloride (DMG) or diisopropylamine dichloroacetate (DIPA).[105] Both compounds are, indeed, known carcinogens of no nutritional value.[106,107] Although pangamic acid is illegal in the United States as either a drug or a vitamin, it remains freely available in health stores because the FDA cannot trace the thousands of vitamin B_{15} retailers.[88,108]

Most metabolic clinics offer a combined program of diet, vitamin therapy (sometimes including laetrile), and detoxification with wheatgrass therapy or coffee enemas. Again, the underlying principle for these approaches is the theory that reversing the metabolic imbalances that "actually caused" the malignancy will control or cure the disease. For example, the portal delivery of caffeine to the liver by a coffee enema is thought to increase bile production, alkalinize the intestine, and detoxify impurities.[109,110] Yet there are internal inconsistencies to the theory; for example, drinking coffee is prohibited during treatment.

The Centro Medico Del Mar in Mexico, established by Dr. Ernesto Contreras, also offers orthodox treatment in addition to its metabolic program of laetrile, cell therapy, interferon, and enzyme enemas. However, laboratory tests, chemotherapy, and surgery are not included in the cost of Contreras' 3-week program. Other practitioners, such as Hans Nieper of Germany, routinely include standard anticancer chemotherapy as part of a metabolic program that includes tumor vaccines, vitamin A, anavit (enzymes extracted from pineapple), squalene (shark-liver extract), carnivora (Venus flytrap extract), laetrile, and selenium and zinc (minerals that supposedly promote tissue healing). Should the tumor respond to effective drugs, practitioner and patient can ascribe the regression to the chemotherapy or any other aspect of the program.

IRIDOLOGY

Metabolic therapists may offer not only an unsound cancer treatment but also may compound the problem with unsound methods of cancer diagnosis. One such technique is iridology, the science of reading the iris to diagnose disease.[111,112] As shown in Figure 70–2, the iridologist studies a homunculus superimposed within the iris, and from the physiologic black stripes therein can make organ-specific diagnoses. Because the technique is purported to be more sensitive than standard diagnostic imaging techniques, the iridologist claims to be able to detect preclinical or subclinical disease. Of course, this can then be conveniently "cured" (*i.e.*, reversal of iris changes) with a medically useless intervention. Double-blind studies in which ophthalmologists and iridologists have examined photographs from patients and healthy controls have shown the technique to be without merit.[113,114] Still, iridology is a common technique for diagnosing disease and following therapeutic response in homeopathic and metabolic clinics.

INVESTIGATING ALTERNATIVE THERAPIES

There have been two recent attempts to investigate the clinical efficacy of alternative therapies. These studies are important because they were conducted with the approval of the unorthodox clinic by impartial investigators trained in science. Cassileth and coworkers studied 158 matched cohorts of patients with metastatic or recurrent colon cancer treated at either the Livingston-Wheeler Clinic in San Diego (autogenous immune-enhancing vaccine, bacillus Calmette-Guérin, vegetarian diet, and coffee enemas) or the University of Pennsylvania.[115] Although there was no difference in survival between these two groups, the quality of life was significantly and uniformly better in those patients receiving only conventional care. This study, then, does not support the assumption

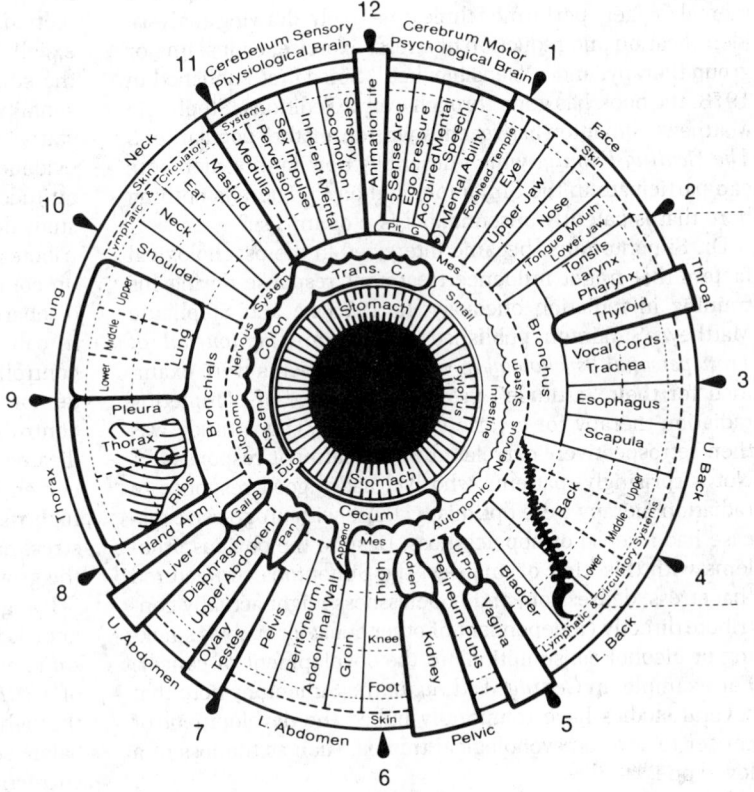

FIGURE 70–2. The iridology homunculus. Metabolic and holistic practitioners commonly use changes in the iris to diagnose organ-specific cancer and follow "disease response." Although inexpensive and noninvasive, iridology is also useless. (Adapted from Worrall RS. Iridology: Diagnosis or delusion. In: Stalker D, Glymour C, eds. Examining holistic medicine. Buffalo: Prometheus, 1985)

that alternative therapies (with emphasis on self-help and absence of the toxicity of conventional treatments) lead to a better quality of life.

The Bristol Cancer Help Centre (BCHC) was established in Great Britain in 1979 to offer a more holistic approach to cancer treatment, including a vegetarian diet, counseling, healing, and development of a more positive attitude. Patients also may continue conventional treatment. Bagenal and associates studied 334 women with breast cancer followed for 3 years at BCHC, comparing them with 461 consecutive breast-cancer patients seen at a single cancer center or two general hospitals over the same time period.[116] Overall, women seen at BCHC were about twice as likely to die from their disease and three times more likely to develop metastases as women receiving conventional care. These results must be interpreted with caution, however, since the BCHC cohort was significantly younger than the more general population. However, for the first time, alternative approaches are being evaluated scientifically, and preliminary evidence does not suggest any clinical advantage.

THE SIMONTON METHOD: AN UNPROVEN ADJUNCT TO CANCER TREATMENT

There is one unproven (as opposed to unsound) method that deserves mention in this chapter, if only because of its current popularity. The Simonton method of relaxation and imagery is basically a self-help program designed to be used in conjunction with standard medical treatment.[117] The program is described in detail in Dr. O. Simonton's best-selling book *Getting Well Again*.[118] The techniques, which are simple and largely easily self-taught, include a program of relaxation and mental imagery performed three times daily, drawing analysis, identification and reduction of stress, exercise, counseling or group therapy, and a "sensible diet." Since first published in 1978, the book has gone through over 20 editions. Stephanie Matthews-Simonton has recently written another popular text, *The Healing Family*, which describes now family members can participate in the Simonton method.[119] There is nothing here that is patently unsound, but is it of any use?

Dr. Simonton first became interested in the psychological factors that might influence treatment response during his training in radiation oncology. In 1975 he and Stephanie Matthews-Simonton published a study in *The Journal of Transpersonal Psychology* in which 152 patients were examined for their "attitude" profile at the time of completing radiation therapy for a variety of cancers. This attitude was then retrospectively correlated with treatment responses.[120] Not surprisingly, patients who had had a good response to radiation therapy were optimistic; those with progressive disease had a sense of hopelessness. Despite the obvious problems with this kind of analysis, the Simontons conjectured that stress, depression, and hopelessness might actually contribute directly (independent of other behavior such as smoking or alcohol consumption) to the development of cancer. For example, in *Getting Well Again* the Simontons note that several studies have temporally linked the development of cancer to severe psychological trauma, such as the loss of a loved one.[121-124]

In a leap of faith, the Simontons hypothesized that positive thinking and stress reduction might be useful as therapy and established the Cancer Counseling and Research Center (recently renamed the Simonton Cancer Center) in Fort Worth, Texas, to teach and administer their program. The center conducts regular counseling and training workshops for patients and professionals. A 10-day "phase I" program of group therapy, training in relaxation and imagery, and counseling, intended primarily for patients, is offered at the Simonton's Southern California clinic. In addition, more extensive "phase II" workshops are conducted to instruct professionals in the Simonton techniques; more than 4000 such counselors have been trained.[125] Finally, the Simontons have produced a series of audiotape cassettes describing the program that can be purchased by mail.[126]

In today's climate of "self-help" or "how-to" literature, the Simonton techniques have become enormously popular, and there are certain appealing facets to the program. It is relatively inexpensive and recommended only as an adjunct to proven therapy. An American Cancer Society review notes other potentially positive aspects to the method: it gives the patient a sense of control, promotes relaxation and well-being, and has no known deleterious effects.[127] R.M. Mack, a physician with metastatic lung cancer, detailed the usefulness of the Simonton techniques in a deeply personal note in *The New England Journal of Medicine,* and equal praise has appeared in other journals as well.[128-132]

However, the literature on mindset and cancer is much more confused than the Simontons would have us believe. For example, *Getting Well Again* limits its discussion to studies in which development of cancer has followed bereavement and asks the reader to accept that depression and carcinogenesis are causally linked. Alternative explanations are not discussed. For example, a patient under stress may be more likely to visit a doctor—behavior that might lead to early detection.[133] Moreover, as Wellisch and Yager discuss in their excellent review, "Is There a Cancer-Prone Personality?," the studies that link depression and disease use faulty personality measurements, have inherent selection bias, and are statistically imprecise.[134] Indeed, there is an equal body of evidence to suggest that no relationship between psychological attitude and cancer exists.[135-137] For example, a controlled study demonstrated no correlation between psychological attributes and development of breast cancer.[136] A 24-year follow-up comparison of a large number of World War II veterans discharged because of "psychoneurosis" showed no increase in cancer incidence compared with controls.[138] A carefully controlled 22-year study of 191 chronically depressed patients demonstrated an incidence of cancer equal to age-matched controls.[139] A recent, well-controlled, prospective study indicated that attitude appears to have no effect on time to recurrence or survival of patients with stage II breast cancer or high-risk melanoma.[140] Indeed, animal studies suggest that stress has a protective effect in carcinogenesis and can inhibit the growth of implanted experimental tumors.[141]

By ignoring this information, the Simontons fail to acknowledge that this is an area of controversy; indeed, although some of these studies have appeared since the first printing of *Getting Well Again*, the book has remained unrevised through more than 20 printings.[142] Friedlander has written a balanced review of the Simonton hypothesis and concludes, correctly, that the method is unproven.[143] Only well-designed negative studies can show if it is unsound.

PATIENT CHARACTERISTICS AND THE ROLE OF HEALTH PROVIDERS

Logic might suggest that patients who adopt unsound methods of cancer treatment might be unsophisticated consumers with diseases for which there is no effective standard therapy. However, analysis in this area once again defies logic. In one important review of the contemporary popularity of unsound cancer treatments, Cassileth and coworkers compared 304 cancer inpatients at the University of Pennsylvania Cancer Center with 356 cancer patients under the care of 138 alternative practitioners at 19 clinics.[2] In decreasing order of popularity, unsound or unproven cancer treatments included metabolic therapy (161 patients), diet (134 patients), megavitamins (92 patients), imagery (89 patients), spiritual healing (71 patients), and immunotherapy (57 patients). Practitioners of unsound therapies were likely to be physicians (60%) and 18% had subspecialty boards. Insurance covered some costs of treatment in a third of the patients being treated.

When compared with patients being treated with standard therapy, those adopting unsound or unproven (imagery) approaches were more likely to be white ($p > 0.00001$) and better educated ($p > 0.00001$). Of these, patients who selected imagery were the most educated, with 79% having some college education. This finding is also supported by the recent FDA telephone survey of 6000 American households in which higher levels of education were the single best predictor of likelihood to adopt an unsound treatment approach.[3]

Another surprising finding of the Cassileth study is that patients who opted for unsound therapy were more likely to be asymptomatic and have earlier (and perhaps more conventionally curable) stages of disease. Of the 325 patients concomitantly receiving both standard and unsound treatments, 40% discontinued standard therapy in favor of the unorthodox approach. One expected finding was that patients who opted for nontraditional care distrusted the medical establishment.

There are some important lessons for health professionals in this analysis. Patients who seek alternative or unsound cancer therapies are intelligent and inquisitive and unlikely to be persuaded that an approach is useless simply because the proponent lacks scientific credentials or has not published in peer-reviewed journals. Moreover, those who offer these useless approaches are generally convinced that they can help the patient. The clinician needs to understand and be able to discuss the seemingly attractive although useless treatments patients hear about through the media or from well-intentioned friends.

There are various sources of updated information on unsound remedies. The American Cancer Society and the American Society of Clinical Oncology maintain committees that critically review and publish the facts on questionable treatments. Other organizations, such as the National Council Against Health Fraud (Box 1276, Loma Linda, CA 92354), the Center for Medical Consumers and Health Care Information (237 Thompson Street, New York, NY 10012), the Consumer Product Safety Commission (Food & Drug Administration, Rockville, MD 20892), and the National Consumer League (1028 Connecticut Avenue, NW, Washington, DC 20036), have additional consumer-oriented information.

However, the most important protection against health fraud is the practitioner's willingness to discuss the disease and available treatments in an open and supportive fashion.[144,145] The NCI's Physician Data Query computer database on current state-of-the-art (phase III) and scientifically sound experimental (phase I and II) therapies is a useful resource in guiding patients to the best available care. In addition, a recent NCI booklet, *What Are Clinical Trials All About?*, is a helpful educational tool that explains how bona-fide clinical studies are performed and gives patients the information they need to know to learn if a trial is logical and well-run.[146] In today's world of alternative treatments, education has replaced legislation as the first defense against unsound cancer therapy.

REFERENCES

1. Quackery: A $10 billion scandal. Subcommittee on Health and Long-Term Care, of the Select Committee on Aging, House of Representatives, 98th Congress, 2d session, 1984 (Committee publication 98-435).
2. Cassileth BR, Lusk EJ, Strouse TB, Badenheimer BA. Contemporary unorthodox treatments in cancer medicine: A study of patients, treatments and practitioners. Ann Intern Med 1984;101:105–112.
3. Louis Harris Survey on the Use of Questionable Cancer Products. Food and Drug Administration, Division of Consumer Affairs, 1987.
4. Jansen WF. Cancer quackery, the past in the present. Semin Oncol 1976;6:526–536.
5. Why the FDA doesn't crack down. Consumer Reports, May 1985:282–284.
6. Reich W. The Orgone Energy Accumulator: Its scientific and medical use. Rangeley, Maine: Orgone Institute Press, 1951.
7. Reich W. Selected writings, an introduction to orgonomy. New York: Farrar, Strauss & Cudahy, 1960.
8. Reich W. Cosmic superimposition: Man's orgonotic roots in nature. Rangeley, Maine: Wilhelm Reich Foundation, 1951.
9. Orgone energy devices. In: Unproven methods of cancer management. New York: American Cancer Society, 1975:176.
10. Hart FJ, ed. Electronic Medical Digest. San Francisco: Electronic Medical Foundation, 1952.
11. Young J. The medical messiahs: A social history of health quackery in 20th-century America. Princeton, NJ: Princeton University Press, 1987.
12. Milstead JL, Davis JB, Dubiele M. Quackery in the medical device field. Proceedings of the Second National Congress on Medical Quackery, 1963:30–35.
13. Hoxsey HM. You don't have to die—The amazing story of the Hoxsey cancer treatment. New York: Milestone Books, 1956.
14. Food and Drug Administration. Report on the background of Harry M. Hoxsey and the Hoxsey Cancer Center, 1952.
15. Mather JM, et al. Report of a committee of faculty members of the University of British Columbia concerning the Hoxsey treatment for cancer. December 19, 1957.
16. FDA Notices of Judgment DD 5654, 5212 and 5202.
17. Press Release HEW-020, U.S. Department of Health, Education & Welfare, Food & Drug Administration, September 21, 1960.
18. Durovic S. Cancer and krebiozen: A new concept in cancer. Today Japan Orient West 1961;6:51–55.
19. Report of the Director, National Cancer Institute, to the Secretary, Department of Health, Education and Welfare, concerning decision of the Institute not to undertake clinical testing of krebiozen. Released October 16, 1963.
20. FDA Notices of Judgment No. 121, FDA Papers, June 1968, p. 43.
21. Hartwell W. Dr. Ivy: Life begins anew at 74. Chicago's American, April 2, 1967.
22. Vierhover A, Mach H. Biochemistry of amygdalin. Am J Pharm 1935;197:392–450.
23. Greenberg DM. The vitamin fraud in cancer quackery. West J Med 1975;122:345–348.
24. Beard HH. A new approach to the conquest of cancer, rheumatic and heart disease. New York: Pageant Press, 1958.
25. Robiquet B. Les amande ameres et l'iele volafle qu'elles focurscent. Ann Chim Phys 1830;14:352–382.
26. Van Meter CT, Gennaro AR. Natural products. In Remington's pharmaceutical sciences, 14th ed. Easton, Pa.: Merck, 1915:474–475.
27. Dorr RT, Paxinos J. The current status of laetrile. Ann Int Med 1978;89:389–397.
28. Gal EM, Fung FH, Greenberg DM. Studies on the biological action of malonitriles. II. Distribution of rhodanese (transulfurase) in tumor-bearing animals, and the effect of malonitriles thereon. Cancer Res 1952;12:574–579.
29. Conchie J, Findley J, Levvy GA. Mammalian glycosidases: Distribution in the body. Biochemistry 1959;71:318–325.
30. Koeffler PH, Lowe L, Golde DL. Amygdalin (laetrile): Effect of clonogenic cell from human myeloid leukemia cells and normal human marrow. Cancer Treat Rep 1980;64:105–110.
31. Stock CC, Martin DS, Suiguira K, et al. Antitumor tests of amygdalin in animal tumor system. Surg Oncol 1978;10:81–88.
32. Wodinsky I, Swiniarski J. Antitumor activity of amygdalin set on a spectrum of transplantable rodent tumors. Cancer Chemo Rep 1975;59:939–950.
33. Laster WR, Schabel FM. Experimental studies of the antitumor activity of amygdalin MF (NSC 15780) above and in combination with beta-glucosidase (NSC 128056). Cancer Chemo Rep 1975;59:957–965.
34. Toxicity of laetrile. FDA Drug Bull 1977;7:25.

35. Laetrile, not so harmless. Emerg Med 1978;10:155–156.
36. Bickis IJ, Quastel JH. Effects of metabolic inhibitors on energy metabolism of Ehrlich ascites carcinoma cells. Nature 1965;205:44–46.
37. Browne WE, Wood CD, Smith AW. Sodium cyanide as a cancer chemotherapeutic agent: Laboratory and clinical studies. Am J Obstet Gynecol 1960;80:907–915.
38. Perry IH. The effect of prolonged cyanide treatment on body and tumor growth in rats. Am J Cancer 1935;25:592–598.
39. Kittler GD. Laetrile: Control for cancer, the authorized story. New York: Paperback Library, 1963.
40. Edwards CC. Statement before the Subcommittee on Intergovernmental Relations of the Committee on Government Operations. June 9, 1970:21–22.
41. Levi L, French WW, Bickis IJ, Henderson WB. Laetrile: A study of its physiochemical and biochemical properties. Can Med Assoc J 1965;92:1057–1061.
42. Davignon P, Trissel LA, Kleinman LM. Pharmaceutical assessment of amygdalin (laetrile products). Cancer Treat Rep 1978;62:99–104.
43. Diamond GEB. Cancer research: Who profits? Harvard Political Review 1977;5(3):17–21.
44. Lerner IJ. The whys of cancer quackery. Cancer 1984;53:815–819.
45. Ingelfinger FJ. Laetrilomania. N Engl J Med 1977;296:1167–1168.
46. Rutherford vs. United States, 524F 2d 1137 (10th Cir 1976).
47. Ellison NM, Byar DP, Newell GR. Results of the National Cancer Institute's retrospective laetrile analysis. N Engl J Med 1978;299:549–557.
48. California Medical Association, Cancer Commission: The treatment of cancer with "laetrile." Calif Med 1953;78:320–326.
49. Moertel CG. A trial of laetrile now. N Engl J Med 1977;298:218–219.
50. Moertel CG, Ames MM, Kovach JS, et al. A pharmacologic and toxicological study of amygdalin. JAMA 1978;255:591–594.
51. Moertel CG, Fleming TR, Rubins J, et al. A phase II trial of amygdalin (laetrile) in human cancer. N Engl J Med 1982;306:201–206.
52. Immunoaugmentative therapy. Food and Drug Administration publication T82-14. Rockville, MD: U.S. Department of Health and Human Services, 1982.
53. Immunoaugmentative therapy: Cancer research and treatment (IAT Information Center patient brochure). Freeport, Bahamas: Immunology Researching Center, 1984.
54. Report to the Ministry of Health of Bahamas on the site visit to the Immunology Researching Center, Ltd., Freeport, Grand Bahamas Island, Bahamas. Washington DC: Pan-American Health Organization, Regional Office of the World Health Organization, 1978:29–31.
55. The cancer therapeutic research act. Fla. Stat. 402.36, 1982.
56. The immunoaugmentative therapy act, Oklahoma House Bill 1633, 1982.
57. Page H. Easy "cures" for cancer still support. JAMA 1981;246:714–715.
58. Curt GA, Katterhagen G, Mahaney FX. Immunoaugmentative therapy: A primer on the perils of unproven treatment. JAMA 1986;255:505–507.
59. Curt GA. Warning on immunoaugmentative therapy. N Engl J Med 1984;311:859.
60. Cutaneous nocardiosis in cancer patients receiving immunotherapy—Bahamas. MMWR 1984;33:471–477.
61. Burton L. Immunoaugmentative therapy. Read before the Fourth Annual "Health by Choice" Conference, Atlanta, May 1983.
62. Isolation of human T-lymphotropic virus type III/lymphoadenopathy-associated virus from serum proteins of cancer patients—Bahamas. MMWR 1985;34:489–490.
63. Congressional Office of Technology Assessment Report. U.S. Congress, Office of Technology Assessment, Unconventional Cancer Treatments, OTA-H-405. Washington, DC: U.S. Government Printing Office, September 1990.
64. Burzynski SR, Georgiades J. Effect of urinary peptides on DNA, RNA and protein synthesis in normal and neoplastic cells. Fed Proc 1973;32:766.
65. Burzynski SR. Antineoplastons: History of research. Drugs Exper Clin Res 1986;12:1–9.
66. Liau MC, Szopa M, Burzynski B, Burzynski SR. Quantitative assay of plasma and urinary peptides as an aid for the evaluation of cancer patients undergoing antineoplaston therapy. Drugs Exper Clin Res 1986(Suppl 2);13:61–70.
67. Burzynski Research Institute, Houston, TX. Patient information brochure, undated.
68. Antineoplastons. CA 1983;33:57–59.
69. Burzynski SR, Kubove E. Toxicology studies on antineoplaston A$_{10}$ injections in cancer patients. Drug Exper Clin Res 1987(Suppl 1);12:1–12.
70. Burzynski SR, Kubove E. Initial clinical study with antineoplaston A$_2$ injections in cancer patients with 5 years follow-up. Drug Exper Clin Res 1987(Suppl 1);12:1–12.
71. Burzynski SR, Kubove E, Burzynski B. Phase I clinical studies of antineoplaston A$_3$ injections. Drug Exper Clin Res 1987(Suppl 1);13:37–43.
72. Burzynski SR, Kubove E, Burzynski B. Phase I clinical studies of antineoplaston A$_5$ injections. Drug Exper Clin Res 1987(Suppl 1);13:37–43.
73. Blackstein and Sagal. The treatment of cancer patients with antineoplastons at the Burzynski Clinic in Houston, Tex. Report to the Ministry of Health, Province of Ontario, 1982.
74. Antineoplastons A2, AS2-1, A$_3$, A$_5$ and A$_{10}$. Memorandum from JD Sproul, Bureau of Prescription Drugs, to Dr. Ian Henderson, Director, Toronto, Ontario, Canada, March 15, 1985.
75. Mead JAR. Developmental Therapeutics Program, NCI: Letter to JD Sproul. Preclinical evaluation of antineoplastons by Southern Research Institute, December 1, 1983.
76. Koch WF. A new and successful treatment and diagnosis of cancer. Detroit Medical Journal, July 1979.
77. Kelley WD. One answer to cancer—An ecological approach to the successful management of malignancy. Grapevine, TX: The Kelley Research Foundation, 1969.
78. Kohler JC, Kohler MA. Healing miracles from macrobiotics: A diet for all diseases. New York: Parker, 1979.
79. Esko E. The cancer prevention diet. Brookline, MA: East West Foundation, 1981.
80. Enloe CH. Yin Yang and Mao. Nutrition Today 1974;9:24.
81. Kushi M. A dietary approach to cancer. In: Diet and Cancer. Brookline, MA: East West Foundation, 1981.
82. Sherlock P, Rothchild EO. Scurvy produced by a Zen macrobiotic diet. JAMA 1987;199:794–798.
83. Roberts IF, West RJ, Ogilvie D, et al. Malnutrition in Infants receiving cult diets: A form of child abuse. Br Med J 1979;1:296–298.
84. Robson JRK, Konlande JE, Larkin FA, et al. Zen macrobiotic dieting problems in infancy. Pediatrics 1974;53:326–329.
85. Bowman BB, Kushner RF, Dawson SC, Levin B. Macrobiotic diets for cancer treatment and prevention. J Clin Oncol 1984;2:702–711.
86. Herbert V. Unproven (questionable) dietary and nutritional methods in cancer prevention and treatment. Cancer 1986;58:1930–1941.
87. Herbert V. Faddism and quackery in cancer nutrition. Nutr Cancer 1984;6:196–206.
88. Shils ME, Hermann MG. Unproved dietary claims in the treatment of patients with cancer. Bull NY Acad Med 1982;58:323–340.
89. Cameron E, Campbell A. The orthomolecular treatment of cancer. Clinical trial of high-dose ascorbic acid supplements in advanced human cancer. Chem Biol Interact 1974;9:285–315.
90. Cameron E. Hyaluronidase and cancer. New York: Pergamon Press, 1966.
91. Cameron E, Pauling L. Supplemental ascorbate in the supportive treatment of cancer: Prolongation of survival times in terminal human cancer. Proc Natl Acad Sci USA 1976;73:3685–3689.
92. Greagen ET, Moertel CG, O'Fallon JR, et al. Failure of high-dose vitamin C (ascorbic acid) therapy to benefit patients with advanced cancer. N Engl J Med 1979;301:687–690.
93. Moertel CG, Fleming TR, Creagen ET, et al. High-dose vitamin C versus placebo in the treatment of patients with advanced cancer who have had no prior therapy: A randomized double-blind comparison. N Engl J Med 1985;312:137–141.
94. Abdel-Galil AM. Preventive effect of vitamin C (L-ascorbic acid) on methylcholanthrene-induced soft tissue sarcomas in mice. Oncology 1986;43:335–337.
95. Herbert V, Barnet S. Vitamins and "health" foods: The great American hustle. Philadelphia: George F. Stickley, 1981.
96. Herbert V, Jarvis WT, Monaco GP. Commentary: Obstacles to nutrition education. Health Values 1983;7:38–41.
97. Herbert V. Will questionable nutrition overwhelm nutrition? Sci Am J Clin Nutr 1981;34:2848–2853.
98. Yaffe SF, Filer LJ Jr. Use and abuse of vitamin A. In ADA Handbook of Clinical Dietetics. New Haven: Yale University Press, 1981:81–83.
99. Dubiele MA, Rucker RB. Dietary supplements and health foods. A critical evaluation—vitamins and minerals. J Nutr Ed 1983;2:47–53.
100. Jukes TH. Megavitamins and food fads. In: Hodes RE, ed. Human nutrition, Vol. 4. New York: Plenum Press, 1979:257–292.
101. Tsai AC, Kelley JJ, Peng B, Cook N. Study on the effect of megavitamin E supplementation in man. Am J Clin Nutr 1978;31:831–837.
102. DiPalma JR, Richie DM. Vitamin toxicity. Am Rev Pharm Toxicol 1977;17:133–148.
103. Anderson TW. Vitamin E in angina pectoris. Can Med Assoc J 1974;110:401–406.
104. Roberts HJ. Perspective on vitamin E as therapy. JAMA 1981;246:129–131.
105. Herbert V. Pangamic acid (vitamin B$_{15}$). Am J Clin Nutr 1979;32:1534–1540.
106. Colman N, Herbert V, Bardner A, Gelernt M. Mutagenicity of dimethylglycine when mixed with nitrite: Possible significance in human use of pangamates. Proc Soc Exp Biol Med 1980;164:9–12.
107. Gelernt MD, Herbert V. Mutagenicity of diisopropylamine dichloroacetate, the "active constituent" of vitamin B$_{15}$ (pangamic acid). Nutr Cancer 1982;3:129–133.
108. McPherrin EW, Herbert V, Herbert R. Vitamin B$_{15}$: Anatomy of a health fraud. New York: American Council of Science and Health, 1981.
109. Manner HW, DiSanti SJ, Michalsen TL. The death of cancer. Chicago: Advanced Century Publishing Corporation, 1978.
110. Eisele JWS, Reay DT. Deaths related to coffee enemas. JAMA 1980;244:1608–1609.
111. Banner D. Applied iridology and herbology. Orem, UT: Bioworld Publishers, 1982.
112. Worrall RS. Iridology: Diagnosis or delusion? In: Stalker D, Glymour C, eds. Examining holistic medicine. Buffalo: Prometheus Books, 1985:167–179.
113. Simon A, Worthen DM, Mites JA. An evaluation of iridology. JAMA 1979;242:1385–1387.
114. Worrall RS. Pseudoscience—A critical look at iridology. J Am Optom Assoc 1984;55:735–739.
115. Cassileth BR, Lusk EJ, Guerry D, et al. Survival and quality of life among patients receiving unproven compared with conventional cancer therapy. N Engl J Med 1991;324:1180–1185.
116. Bagenal FS, Eastor DF, Harris E, et al. Survival of patients with breast cancer attending Bristol Cancer Help Centre. Lancet 1990;336:606–610.
117. Simonton Cancer Counseling and Research Center brochure, undated.
118. Simonton OC, Matthews-Simonton S, Creighton JL. Getting well again. New York: Bantam, 1980.
119. Matthews-Simonton S. The healing family. New York: Bantam, 1984.
120. Simonton OC, Matthews-Simonton S. Belief systems and management of the emotional aspects of malignancy. J Transpersonal Psychology 1975;7:29–47.
121. Greene WA, Young LE, Swisher SW. Psychological factors and reticuloendothelial disease: Observations on a group of women with lymphomas and leukemias. Psychosom Med 1956;18:1252–303.
122. Greene WA. The psychosocial setting of the development of lymphoma and leukemia. Ann NY Acad Sci 1966;164:394–406.
123. Schamle AH, Iker HP. The effect of hopelessness in the development of cancer in women with atypical cytology. Psychosom Med 1964;26:634–635.
124. LeShan L, Worthington RE. Some recurrent life history patterns observed in patients with malignant disease. J Ment Dis 1954;124:460–465.

125. Kolata G. Texas counselors use psychology in cancer therapy. Smithsonian 1980:49–56.

126. Publications CCRC brochure, undated.

127. Simonton OC. Unproven methods of cancer management. CA 1982;32:58–61.

128. Mack RM. Lessons from living with cancer. N Engl J Med 1984;311:1640–1644.

129. Kennedy AM. Coping with cancer: New ways to deal with its physic devastation. Medical World News, Oct. 15, 1979:36–46.

130. Scarf M. Images that heal: A doubtful idea whose time has come. Psychology Today 1986;14:32–46.

131. Kirsch ML. The Simonton method of visualization: Nursing implications and a patient's perspective. Cancer Nursing 1980;3:295–300.

132. Wright ME. Book review of Getting Well Again. Contemporary Psychology 1979;24:1019–1020.

133. Hanley CA. Illness behavior and psychosocial correlates of cancer. Soc Sci Med 1977;11:223–225.

134. Wellisch DK, Yager J. Is there a cancer-prone personality? CA 1983;33:145–153.

135. Graham S, Snell LM, Graham JB, et al. Social trauma in the epidemiology of cancer of the cervix. J Chronic Dis 1971;24:711–725.

136. Green S, Maris T. Psychological attributes of women who develop breast cancer: A controlled study. J Psychosom Res 1975;19:147–153.

137. Muslin HL, Gyarfas K, Pieper WJ. Separation experience and cancer of the breast. Ann NY Acad Sci 1966;125:802–806.

138. Keehn RJ, Goldberg ID, Beebe GW. 24-Year follow-up of any veteran with disability separations for psychoneurosis in 1944. Psychosom Med 1978;26:27–46.

139. Niani T, Jasskleainen J. Cancer morbidity in depression persons. J Psychosom Res 1978;22:117–120.

140. Cassileth B, Lusk EJ, Miller DS, Brown LL, Miller C. Psychosocial correlates of survival in advanced malignant disease. N Engl J Med 1984;312:1551–1555.

141. Fox BH. Current theory of psychogenic effects on cancer incidence and prognosis. J Psychosoc Oncol 1983;1:17–31.

142. Fox BH. Premorbid psychological factors as related to cancer. J Behavioral Med 1978;1:45–133.

143. Friedlander ER. Dream your cancer away: The Simontons. In: Stalker D, Glymour C, eds. Examining holistic medicine. Buffalo: Prometheus Books, 1985:273–285.

144. Monaco GP. The primary care physician: The first line of defense in the battle against health fraud. Medical Times 1986;114:43–48.

145. Jarvis W. Helping your patients deal with questionable cancer treatments. CA 1986;36:293–301.

146. Nealon E. What are clinical trials all about? NIH Publication No. 86-2706, 1986.

Index

Page numbers followed by *f* indicate figures; those followed by *t* indicate tabular material; **CF** indicates color figures.

ISBN 0-397-51214-7